HEMATOLOGY

BASIC PRINCIPLES AND PRACTICE

HEMATOLOGY

BASIC PRINCIPLES AND PRACTICE

FIFTH EDITION

Ronald Hoffman MD

Albert A. and Vera G. List Professor of Medicine; Hematology/Oncology Section; Mount Sinai Cancer Institute, Department of Medicine, Cell and Gene Medicine, Mount Sinai School of Medicine New York, New York

Edward J. Benz, Jr. MD

Richard and Susan Smith Professor of Medicine, Professor of Pediatrics, and Professor of Pathology, Harvard Medical School; President and CEO, Dana-Farber Cancer Institute; Director, Dana-Farber/Harvard Cancer Center, Boston, Massachusetts

Sanford J. Shattil MD

Professor of Medicine and Chief, Hematology-Oncology Division, University of California San Diego; Adjunct Professor of Molecular and Experimental Medicine, The Scripps Research Institute, La Jolla, California

Bruce Furie MD

Professor of Medicine, Harvard Medical School; Chief, Division of Hemostasis and Thrombosis, Beth Israel Deaconess Medical Center, Boston, Massachusetts

Leslie E. Silberstein MD

Professor of Pathology, Harvard Medical School; Director, Joint Program in Transfusion Medicine, Children's Hospital Boston, Brigham and Women's Hospital, and Dana-Farber Cancer Institute; and Director, Center for Human Cell Therapy, Immune Disease Institute, Boston, Massachusetts

Philip McGlave MD

C.J. Watson Land Grant Chair in Medicine; Director, Division of Hematology, Oncology and Transplantation; Deputy Director, Masonic Cancer Center, University of Minnesota, Academic Health Center, Minneapolis, Minnesota

Helen E. Heslop MD

Professor of Medicine and Pediatrics, Dan L Duncan Chair, Center for Cell and Gene Therapy, Baylor College of Medicine, The Methodist Hospital and Texas Children's Hospital, Houston, Texas

Hematology Image Consultant

John Anastasi MD

Associate Professor of Pathology, Assistant Director, Hematopathology, University of Chicago, Pritzker School of Medicine, Chicago, Illinois

CHURCHILL LIVINGSTONE

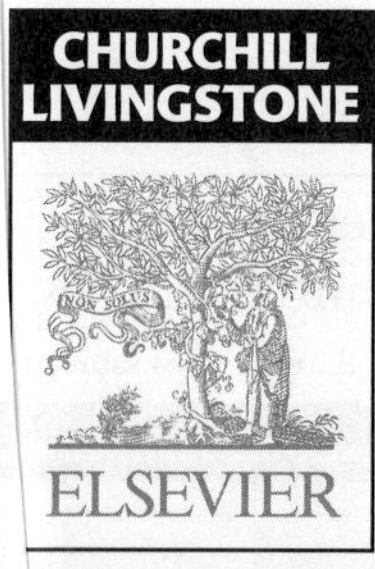

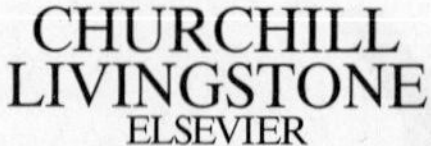

1600 John F. Kennedy Blvd.
Ste 1800
Philadelphia, PA 19103-2899

HEMATOLOGY: Basic Principles and Practice

ISBN: 978-0-443-06715-0 (Expert Consult)
978-0-443-06713-6 (Expert Consult Premium Ed.)

Notice

Knowledge and best practice in this field are constantly changing. As new research and experience broaden our knowledge, changes in practice, treatment and drug therapy may become necessary or appropriate. Readers are advised to check the most current information provided (i) on procedures featured or (ii) by the manufacturer of each product to be administered, to verify the recommended dose or formula, the method and duration of administration, and contraindications. It is the responsibility of the practitioner, relying on their own experience and knowledge of the patient, to make diagnoses, to determine dosages and the best treatment for each individual patient, and to take all appropriate safety precautions. To the fullest extent of the law, neither the Publisher nor the Editors assumes any liability for any injury and/or damage to persons or property arising out of or related to any use of the material contained in this book.

The Publisher

Cover images by Vesna Najfeld, Ph.D., Professor of Pathology and Medicine, Tumor Cytogenetics Laboratory of the Mount Sinai Medical Center, New York, New York

Library of Congress Cataloging-in-Publication Data
Hematology : basic principles and practice / editors, Ronald Hoffman . . . [et al.] ; photomicrograph editor, John Anastasi.—5th ed.
p. ; cm.
Includes bibliographical references and index.
ISBN 978-0-443-06715-0
1. Hematology. 2. Blood–Diseases. I. Hoffman, Ronald, 1945–
[DNLM: 1. Hematologic Diseases–diagnosis. 2. Blood Physiology. 3. Hematologic Diseases–therapy. WH 120 H487 2008]
RC633.H434 2008
616.1′5–dc22
2008020092

Acquisitions Editor: Dolores Meloni
Developmental Editor: Lucia Gunzel
Publishing Services Manager: Frank Polizzano
Senior Project Manager: Peter Faber
Design Direction: Lou Forgione

Printed in China

Last digit is the print number: 9 8 7 6 5 4 3 2 1

To my wife Nan and my children Michael and Judith who have been so supportive of my efforts during the numerous editions of the book. To the staff at Elsevier, especially Dolores Meloni and Lucia Gunzel who have made this fifth edition especially enjoyable and have permitted us to move this edition forward as an outstanding contribution to the field of hematology. I remain indebted to each of the contributors to this volume who have continued to provide incredibly wonderful contributions; this monumental task could never have been completed on time without your collective efforts. I finally would like to acknowledge the monumental efforts of each of my co-editors; it remains a pleasure and an honor to purse this project with each of you.

Ronald Hoffman, MD

To my wife, Peggy, for your support, inspiration, and partnership; to our children, Tim, Jenny, Julie, and Rob, for your understanding; to my mentors, for your support and guidance; and to Janet Cameron, Sharon Olsen and Rebecca Velasquez, for your incredible skill, patience, and good humor throughout this project.

Edward J. Benz, Jr. MD

To my wife Gloria, my son Jason, my sister Sherry, and my late parents Helen and Arthur. I would like to thank my mentors at the Harvard Medical Unit of the Boston City Hospital, Drs. Richard Cooper, Neil Abramson and the late James H. Jandl and late William B. Castle who instilled in me a profound respect for the importance of basic research in blood diseases and a deep appreciation for the privilege of contributing to this endeavor.

Sanford J. Shattil, MD

To my wife Barbara and my sons Eric and Gregg. To my late parents, Bernice Wolfe Furie and J. Leon Furie. And to my trainees who have made this all worthwhile. And to my colleagues in the field of hematology who have become lasting friends.

Bruce Furie, MD

To my friends and family for their love and support. To my mentors Eugene M. Berkman and Robert S. Schwartz, who have provided me with invaluable guidance. To my colleagues at the University of Pennsylvania and Harvard, who have helped me develop academic transfusion medicine programs; and to the trainees, who make this endeavor enjoyable and worthwhile.

Leslie E. Silberstein, MD

To my wife, Anne, and my children, Alice, Pavel, and Claire, for their love and support. To my colleagues past and present at the University of Minnesota, for their help, guidance, and, most of all, friendship.

Philip McGlave, MD

To my family, friends and to all my present and past colleagues and trainees for their support and encouragement. To all my mentors in hematology who have provided guidance in particular Michael Beard and Malcolm Brenner.

Helen Heslop, MD

CONTRIBUTORS

Janis L. Abkowitz MD
Professor of Medicine, Director, Hematology Clinic, Seattle Cancer Care Alliance; Head, Division of Hematology, University of Washington, Seattle, Washington

Janet L. Abrahm MD
Associate Professor, Department of Medicine and Anesthesia, Harvard Medical School; Director, Pain and Palliative Care Program, Department of Medical Oncology, Dana-Farber Cancer Institute; Director, Palliative Care Program, Department of Medicine, Brigham and Women's Hospital, Boston, Massachusetts

Charles S. Abrams MD
Associate Professor, Department of Medicine, Division of Hematology-Oncology, University of Pennsylvania School of Medicine; Attending Physician, Division of Hematology-Oncology, Department of Medicine, Hospital of the University of Pennsylvania, Philadelphia, Pennsylvania

Steven J. Ackerman PhD
Professor of Medicine (Hematology-Oncology), Biochemistry and Molecular Genetics, Department of Biochemistry and Molecular Genetics, University of Illinois at Chicago College of Medicine, Chicago, Illinois

Sharon Adams MT CHS
HLA Laboratory Supervisor, National Institute of Health, Warren G. Magnuson Clinical Center, Bethesda, Maryland

Adeboye H. Adewoye MD
Assistant Professor of Medicine, Boston University School of Medicine; Attending Physician, Boston Medical Center, Boston, Massachusetts

Claudio Agostinelli MD
Researcher, Bologna University School of Medicine, Bologna, Italy

Amin Alousi MD
Assistant Professor of Medicine, Department of Stem Cell Transplant and Cellular Therapy, University of Texas, M.D. Anderson Cancer Center, Houston, Texas

Claudio Anasetti MD
Professor, Department of Interdisciplinary Oncology, University of South Florida School of Medicine; Leader, Blood and Marrow Transplant Program, H. Lee Moffitt Cancer Center and Research Institute, Tampa, Florida

John Anastasi, MD
Associate Professor of Pathology, University of Chicago, Pritzker School of Medicine, Chicago, Illinois

Nancy C. Andrews MD, PhD
Dean and Vice Chancellor, Duke University School of Medicine, Durham, North Carolina

Aśok C. Antony MD
Professor, Department of Medicine, Division of Hematology-Oncology, Indiana University School of Medicine; Attending Physician and Consultant, Indiana University Hospitals; Roudebush Veterans Affairs Medical Center, Indianapolis, Indiana

Robert J. Arceci MD, PhD
King Fahd Professor of Pediatric Oncology; Professor of Pediatrics, Oncology and Cellular and Molecular Medicine, Kimmel Comprehensive Cancer Center at Johns Hopkins, Bunting-Blaustein Cancer Research Building, Baltimore, Maryland

Scott A. Armstrong MD, PhD
Assistant Professor of Pediatrics, Harvard Medical School; Attending Physician, Department of Hematology/Oncology, Children's Hospital/ Dana-Farber Cancer Institute, Boston, Massachusetts

Irit Avivi MD
Senior Lecturer, Bruce Rappaport Faculty of Medicine, Technion, Israel Institute of Technology; Senior Attending Hematologist, Department of Hematology and Bone Marrow Transplantation, Rambam Medical Center, Haifa, Israel

Farrukh T. Awan MD, MS
Clinical Instructor, Clinical Fellow-Hematology Oncology, James Cancer Center, The Ohio State University, Columbus, Ohio

Aleksandar Babic PhD, MD
Instructor in Pathology, Harvard Medical School; Associate Medical Director, Adult Transfusion Service, Brigham and Women's Hospital, Boston, Massachusetts

Tiziano Barbui MD
Professor of Hematology, Scientific Director, Research Foundation, Ospedali Riuniti di Bergamo, Bergamo Italy

Giovanni Barosi MD
Director, Unit of Clinical Epidemiology and Center for the Study of Myelofibrosis, IRCCS Policlirico S. Matteo Foundation, Pavia, Italy

Robert A. Barrington MD
Postdoctoral Fellow, Department of Pathology, Harvard University Medical School and CBR Institute for Biomedical Research, Boston, Massachusetts

Kenneth A. Bauer MD
Professor of Medicine, Harvard Medical School, Boston; Chief, Hematology Section, VA Boston Healthcare System, West Roxbury; Director, Thrombosis Clinical Research, Division of Hemostasis and Thrombosis, Beth Israel Deaconess Medical Center, Boston, Massachusetts

Linda G. Baum MD
Professor, Department of Pathology and Laboratory Medicine, David Geffen School of Medicine at UCLA, Los Angeles, California

Johanna Bendell MD
Instructor, Department of Medicine, Harvard Medical School, Assistant, Department of Medicine, Massachusetts General Hospital Cancer Center, Boston, Massachusetts

Joel S. Bennett MD
Professor of Medicine and Pharmacology, University of Pennsylvania School of Medicine; Attending Physician, Hospital of the University of Pennsylvania, Philadelphia, Pennsylvania

Don M. Benson, Jr. MD, PhD
Assistant Professor of Medicine, The Ohio State University; Attending Physician, Comprehensive Cancer Center, The Ohio State University Columbus, Ohio

Edward J. Benz, Jr. MD
Richard and Susan Smith Professor of Medicine, Professor of Pediatrics, and Professor of Pathology, Harvard Medical School; President and CEO, Dana-Farber Cancer Institute; Director, Dana-Farber/Harvard Cancer Center, Boston, Massachusetts

Stacey L. Berg MD
Professor of Pediatrics, Section of Hematology/Oncology, Baylor College of Medicine Houston, Texas

Nancy Berliner MD
Professor of Medicine, Brigham and Women's Hospital, Harvard Medicine School, Boston, Massachusetts

Kapil N. Bhalla MD
Director, Medical College of Georgia Cancer Center; Professor, School of Medicine, Medical College of Georgia; Vice-Dean for Cancer Research and Services, Medical College of Georgia; Chief, Clinical Cancer Services, MCG Health System, Augusta, Georgia

Nina Bhardwaj MD, PhD
Professor of Medicine, Pathology and Dermatology, New York University School of Medicine; Director, Tumor Vaccine Program, New York University Cancer Institute, New York, New York

Ravi Bhatia MD
Professor, Division of Hematology and Hematopoietic Cell Transplantation, Director, Division of Hematopoietic Stem Cell and Leukemia Research, City of Hope National Medical Center, Duarte, California

Smita Bhatia MD, MPH
Professor and Chair, Division of Population Sciences, City of Hope National Medical Center, Duarte, California

Craig D. Blinderman MD, MA
Instructor, Harvard Medical School; Co-Director, MGH Cancer Pain Clinic; Attending Physician, Palliative Care Service, Massachusetts General Hospital, Boston, Massachusetts

Catherine M. Bollard MBChB, FRACP, FRCPA
Associate Professor, Department of Pediatrics, Baylor College of Medicine; Department of Pediatric Hematology/Oncology, Texas Children's Hospital, Houston, Texas

Douglas E. Brandoff MD
Instructor in Medicine, Harvard Medical School; Attending Physician and Co-Director of Outpatient Services, Pain and Palliative Care Program, Dana-Farber Cancer Institute/Brigham and Women's Hospital, Boston, Massachusetts

Lawrence F. Brass MD, PhD
Professor of Medicine and Pharmacology, University of Pennsylvania School of Medicine, Philadelphia, Pennsylvania

Malcolm K. Brenner MD, PhD
Professor of Medicine and Pediatrics, Director, Center for Cell and Gene Therapy; Fayez Sarofim Chair, Baylor College of Medicine; Director, Center for Cell and Gene Therapy, The Methodist Hospital, Texas Children's Hospital, Houston, Texas

Gary M. Brittenham MD
James A. Wolff Professor of Pediatrics and Medicine, Columbia University College of Physicians and Surgeons; Attending Pediatrician, Children's Hospital of New York–Presbyterian, Hospital New York, New York

Robert A. Brodsky MD
Director, Division of Hematology, Johns Hopkins University School of Medicine, Johns Hopkins University, Baltimore, Maryland

Hal E. Broxmeyer PhD
Chairman and Mary Margaret Walther Professor of Microbiology and Immunology; Professor of Medicine; Indiana University School of Medicine; Scientific Director, Walther Oncology Center, Indianapolis, Indiana

Claudio G. Brunstein MD, PhD
Assistant Professor, Division of Hematology, Oncology, and Transplantation Department of Medicine, University of Minnesota, Medical School; Attending Physician, Medical Director of Unrelated Donor Transplant, University of Minnesota Medical Center, Minneapolis, Minnesota

Michael P. Busch MD, PhD
Professor of Laboratory Medicine, University of California, San Francisco, School of Medicine; Vice President, Blood Systems Research Institute, San Francisco, California

James B. Bussel MD
Professor of Pediatrics and Professor of Pediatrics in Obstetrics and Gynecology and in Medicine, Weill Medical College of Cornell University; Director, Platelet Research and Treatment Program, and Attending, Department of Pediatric Hematology Oncology, New York Hospital; Attending Pediatrician, New York Presbyterian Hospital, New York, New York

Joseph H. Butterfield MD
Professor of Medicine, Mayo Medical School, Mayo Clinic, Rochester, Minnesota

John C. Byrd MD
Professor of Medicine and Medical Chemistry, D Warner Brown Professor of Leukemia Research, The Ohio State University, Columbus, Ohio

Michael A. Caligiuri MD
Professor, The Ohio State University; Director/Chief Executive Officer, Comprehensive Cancer Center, Arthur James Cancer Hospital and Richard Solove Research Institute, Columbus, Ohio

Alan B. Cantor MD, PhD
Assistant Professor of Pediatrics, Harvard Medical School; Assistant in Medicine, Children's Hospital Boston, Dana-Farber Cancer Institute, Boston, Massachusetts

Christopher L. Carpenter MD, PhD
Assistant Professor, Department of Medicine, Harvard Medical School; Department of Medicine, Beth Israel Deaconess Medical Center, Boston, Massachusetts

Michael C. Carroll PhD
Professor of Pediatrics and Pathology, Harvard Medical School; Senior Investigator, CBR Institute for Biomedical Research, Boston, Massachusetts

Paula M. Charuhas MS, RD, FADA, CD, CNSD
Nutrition Education Coordinator, Nutrition Program Seattle Cancer Care Alliance, Seattle, Washington

David H.K. Chui MD
Professor of Medicine, Boston University School of Medicine, Boston, Massachusetts

Douglas Cines MD
Professor, Department of Pathology and Laboratory Medicine, University of Pennsylvania School of Medicine; Director, Coagulation Laboratory, Hospital of the University of Pennsylvania, Philadelphia, Pennsylvania

David B. Clark PhD
President, Platte Canyon Consulting, Inc., Shawnee, Coloràdo

Thomas D. Coates MD
Professor of Pediatrics and Pathology, University of Southern California Keck School of Medicine; Section Head of Hematology, Children's Center for Cancer and Blood Disease, Children's Hospital Los Angeles, Los Angeles, California

Aileen C, Cohen MD PhD
Instructor of Pediatrics, Division of Hematology/Oncology, Department of Pediatrics, Stanford University School of Medicine; Attending Physician at Lucile Packard Children's Hospital, Lucile Packard Children's Hospital, Stanford, California

Désiré Collen MD, PhD
Professor Center for Molecular and Vascular Biology, University of Leuven Faculty of Medicine, Leuven, Belgium

Barry S. Coller MD
David Rockefeller Professor of Medicine, Rockefeller University School of Medicine; Head, Laboratory of Blood and Vascular Biology and Physician-in-Chief, Rockefeller University Hospital; Clinical Professor of Medicine, Mount Sinai School of Medicine, New York, New York

Elizabeth Diana Cooke RN MN ANP AOCN
School of Medicine, Hamilton, Ontario, Canada

Richard J. Creger PHARM D
Associate Professor of Medicine, Case Western Reserve University; Ireland Cancer Center, University Hospitals Case Medical Center, Cleveland, Ohio

Mark A. Crowther MD, MSc, FRCPC
Professor of Medicine (Hematology and Thromboembolism), McMaster University; Senior Research Specialist and Nurse Practitioner, Department of Nursing, Beckman Research Institute at the City of Hope, Duarte, California

Melissa M. Cushing MD
Assistant Professor, Department of Pathology and Laboratory Medicine, Weill Cornell Medical College; Assistant Director, Transfusion Medicine and Cellular Therapy, New York—Presbyterian Hospital-Weill Cornell Medical Center, New York, New York

Gary V. Dahl MD
Professor of Pediatrics, Department of Pediatric Hematology/Oncology, Lucile Packard Children's Hospital, Stanford University School of Medicine, Palo Alto, California

Richard Dahl PhD
Research Assistant Professor, University of New Mexico Health Sciences Center, Albuquerque, New Mexico

Björn Dahlbäck MD, PhD
Professor of Blood Coagulation Research, Department of Laboratory Medicine, Section of Clinical Chemistry University Hospital, Lund University, Malmő, Sweden

Alan D. D' Andrea MD
Fuller-American Cancer Society Professor, Department of Radiation Oncology, Harvard Medical School; Dana-Farber Cancer Institute, Boston, Massachusetts

Chi Van Dang MD, PhD
Professor of Medicine, Oncology, Pathology and Cell Biology, Johns Hopkins University School of Medicine; Attending Physician, Johns Hopkins Hospital, Baltimore, Maryland

Ayelet Dar PhD
Weizmann Institute of Science, Rehovot, Israel

Stella M. Davies MBBS, PhD, MRCP
Professor of Pediatrics, University of Cincinnati; Director, Blood and Marrow Transplantation Program, Division of Hematology/Oncology, Cincinnati Children's Hospital Medical Center, Cincinnati, Ohio

Marcos De Lima MD
Associate Professor of Medicine, Department of Stern Cell Transplantation and Cell Therapy, University of Texas M.D. Anderson Cancer Center, Houston, Texas

Daniel J. De Angelo MD, PhD
Assistant Professor of Medicine, Harvard Medical School; Attending Physician, Dana-Farber Cancer Institute, Boston, Massachusetts

H. Joachim Deeg MD
Professor of Medicine, Division of Oncology, University of Washington; Member, Fred Hutchinson Cancer Research Center, Clinical Research Division, HCRC, Seattle, Washington

David De Remer PHARM D, BCOP
Clinical Assistant Professor, University of Georgia; Clinical Hematology/Oncology Pharmacy Specialist, Medical College of Georgia, Augusta, Georgia

Bimalangshu R. Dey MD, PhD
Assistant Professor of Medicine, Harvard Medical School, Massachusetts General Hospital, Bone Marrow Transplantation Program, Boston, Massachusetts

Volker Diehl MD
Professor, Department of Medicine, University of Cologne Faculty of Medicine, Cologne, Germany

Mary C. Dinauer MD, PhD
Nora Letzter Professor of Pediatrics (Hematology/Oncology) and Professor of Microbiology/Immunology and of Medical and Molecular Genetics, Department of Pediatrics, Indiana University School of Medicine; Professor of Pediatrics, Riley Hospital for Children, Indianapolis, Indiana

Angela Dispenzieri MD
Consultant, Division of Hematology, Mayo Clinic, Associate Professor of Medicine, Mayo Clinic College of Medicine; Mayo Clinic, Rochester, Minnesota

Michele L. Donato MD
Core Faculty, Touro University College of Medicine; Collection Facility Medical Director, Blood and Marrow Transplantation Program, Hackensack University Medical Center, Hackensack, New Jersey

Kenneth Dorshkind PhD
Professor, Department of Pathology and Laboratory Medicine, David Geffen School of Medicine at UCLA, Los Angeles, California

William N. Drohan PhD (Deceased)
Professor, Graduate Program in Genetics, George Washington University, Washington, District of Columbia; Vice President, STB, Ltd., Gaithersburg, Maryland, deceased-contact David B, Clark, co-author

Kieron Dunleavy MD
Metabolism Branch, National Cancer Institute, Bethesda, Maryland

Benjamin L. Ebert MD, PhD
Clinical Fellow, Department of Adult Oncology, Dana-Farber Cancer Institute and Harvard Medical School, Boston; Research Fellow, Broad Institute of Harvard and MIT, Cambridge, Massachusetts

William E. Evans PHARMD
St. Jude Endowed Chair and Professor of Pediatrics, College of Medicine, University of Tennessee; Director and CEO, St. Jude Children's Research Hospital, Memphis, Tennessee

Brunangelo Falini MD
Professor of Haematology, Director of Haematopathology, Perugia University School of Medicine; Perugia, Italy Director of Haematopathology, Monteluce Hospital, Perugia, Italy

Donald I. Feinstein MD, MACP
Professor of Medicine (Emeritus), Keck School of Medicine, University of Southern California, Attending Physician, USC/Norris Comprehensive Cancer Center, USC—University Hospital, LAC/USC Medical Center, Los Angeles, California

Adolfo A. Ferrando MD, PhD
Assistant Professor of Pediatrics and Pathology, Institute for Cancer Genetics, Columbia University, New York, New York

James L. M. Ferrara MD
Professor of Internal Medicine and Pediatrics, University of Michigan Medical School; Doris Duke Distinguished Clinical Scientist and Director, Blood and Marrow Transplantation Program, University of Michigan Cancer Center, Ann Arbor, Michigan

Eberhard W. Fiebig MD
Associate Professor of Clinical Laboratory Medicine, University of California, San Francisco, School of Medicine; Chief, Transfusion Services and Hematology, Laboratory Division, Clinical Laboratory, San Francisco General Hospital, San Francisco, California

Guido Finazzi MD
Teaching Position Professor of Hematology; Universita Milano Bicocea, Milan, Italy; Director, Transfusion Medicine Service Institution, dspedali Riuniti di Bergamo, Bergamo, Italy

Bernard G. Forget MD
Professor, Department of Internal Medicine and Genetics, Yale University School of Medicine; Attending Physician, Department of Internal Medicine, Yale-New Haven Hospital, New Haven, Connecticut

Stephen J. Forman MD
Director, Hematologic Neoplasia Program, City of Hope Comprehensive Cancer Center, Duarte, California

Bridget Fowler PHARMD
Clinical Assistant Professor, Northeastern University; Clinical Pharmacy Specialist, Pain and Palliative Case Program, Dana-Farber Cancer Institute, Boston, Massachusetts

Melvin H. Freedman MD, FRCPC, FAAP
Professor (Emeritus), Department of Pediatrics, University of Toronto Faculty of Medicine; Toronto, Ontario, Canada Honorary Consultant, Division of Hematology/Oncology, Hospital for Sick Children, Toronto, Ontario, Canada

Barbara C. Furie PhD
Professor of Medicine, Harvard Medical School; Chief, Division of Hemostasis and Thrombosis, Beth Israel Deaconess Medical Center, Boston, Massachusetts

Bruce Furie MD
Professor of Medicine, Harvard Medical School; Chief, Division of Hemostasis and Thrombosis, Beth Israel Deaconess Medical Center, Boston, Massachusetts

David Gailani MD
Associate Professor of Pathology and Medicine, Vanderbilt University; Medical Director, Clinical Coagulation Laboratory, Vanderbilt University Medical Center Nashville, Tennessee

Lawrence B. Gardner MD
Assistant Professor of Medicine and Pharmacology, Division of Hematology, Department of Medicine, New York University School of Medicine New York, New York

Sharon M. Geaghan MD
Associate Professor, Department of Pathology and Pediatrics, Stanford University School of Medicine; Chief, Pathology, Department of Pathology, Pediatrics, Lucile Salter Packard Children's Hospital, Palo Alto, California

Adrian P. Gee PhD
Professor of Medicine and Pediatrics, Baylor College of Medicine; Technical Director, GMP Laboratories, Center for Cell and Gene Therapy, Texas Children's Hospital and the Methodist Hospital, Houston, Texas

Stanton L. Gerson MD
Professor of Medicine, Director, Case Comprehensive Cancer Center; Director, Center for Stem Cell and Regenerative Medicine, Case Western Reserve University; Director, Ireland Cancer Center, University Hospitals Case Medical Center, Cleveland, Ohio

Morie A. Gertz MD
Consultant, Division of Hematology, Mayo Clinic; Professor of Medicine, Mayo Clinic College of Medicine, Mayo Clinic, Rochester, Minnesota

Alan M. Gewirtz MD
C. Winnard Robinson Professor, Division of Hematology/Oncology, Department of Medicine, University of Pennsylvania School of Medicine; Attending Physician, Hospital of the University of Pennsylvania, Philadelphia, Pennsylvania

Patricia J. Giardina MD
Professor of Clinical Pediatrics, Weill Medical College of Cornell University; Attending Pediatrician, New York Presbyterian Hospital, New York, New York

D. Gary Gilliland MD, PhD
Professor of Medicine, Harvard Medicine School; Investigator, Howard Hughes Medical Institute; Senior Physician, Brigham and Women's Hospital, Boston, Massachusetts

David Ginsburg MD
James V. Neel Distinguished University Professor of Internal Medicine and Human Genetics, Howard Hughes Medical Institute, University of Michigan Ann Arbor, Michigan

Jeffrey S. Ginsberg MD, FRCPC
Professor, Department of Medicine; McMaster University Faculty of Medicine; Head, Thromboembolism Unit, Hamilton Health Sciences, McMaster Site, Hamilton, Ontario, Canada

Sergio Giralt MD
Professor of Medicine, Department of Stem Cell Transplantation and Cell Therapy, University of Texas M. D. Anderson Cancer Center, Houston, Texas

Bertil Glader MD, PhD
Professor, Department of Pediatrics, Stanford University School of Medicine, Stanford; Attending Physician, Department of Hematology/Oncology, Lucile Salter Packard Children's Hospital, Palo Alto; Attending Physician, Department of Pediatrics, Stanford University Hospital, Stanford, California

Nicola Gökbuget MD
Medical Clinic III, University Hospital of J.W. Goethe University, Frankfurt, Germany

Alfred L. Goldberg PhD
Professor of Cell Biology, Harvard Medical School; Boston, Massachusetts

Todd R. Golub MD
Associate Professor of Pediatrics, Harvard Medical School; Charles A. Dana Investigator, Associate Investigator HHMI, Department of Pediatric Oncology, Dana-Farber Cancer Institute, Boston; Director, Cancer Program, Broad Institute of Harvard and MIT, Cambridge, Massachusetts

Stephen Gottschalk MD
Associate Professor, Departments of Pediatrics and Immunology, Center for Cell and Gene Therapy, Texas Children's Cancer Center, Baylor College of Medicine, Houston, Texas

Gregory A. Grabowski MD
Professor of Pediatrics, University of Cincinnati College of Medicine; Director, Division of Human Genetics, Cincinnati Children's Hospital Medical Center, Cincinnati, Ohio

Steven Grant MD
Professor of Medicine, Biochemistry and Pharmacology, Virginia Commonwealth University, Associate Director for Translational Research; Massey Cancer Center, VCU Health Systems Richmond, Virginia

Xylina T. Gregg MD
Utah Cancer Specialists, Salt Lake City, Utah

Timothy C. Greiner MS, MD
Associate Professor, Department of Pathology and Microbiology, University of Nebraska College of Medicine; Medical Director, Molecular Diagnostic Laboratory, The Nebraska Medical Center, Omaha, Nebraska

John G. Gribben MD, DSc
Professor of Experiment Cancer Medicine, Barts and the London School of Medicine, Institute of Cancer; Consultant, Medical Oncology, St. Bartholomew's Hospital, London, United Kingdom

Thomas G. Gross MD, PhD
Associate Professor, Department of Pediatrics, School of Medicine, The Ohio State University; Chief, Division of Hematology/Oncology/BMT, Nationwide Children's Hospital, Columbus, Ohio

Joan Guitart MD
Associate Professor of Dermatology, Department of Dermatology, Northwestern University Medical School; Northwestern Memorial Hospital, Chicago, Illinois

Alejandro Gutierrez MD
Instructor of Pediatrics, Hematology/Oncology Department, Harvard Medical School; Dana-Farber Cancer Institute and Children's Hospital, Boston, Massachusetts

Parameswaran Nair Hari MD, MS, MRCP
Division of Neoplastic Diseases, Assistant Professor of Medicine, Medical College of Wisconsin; Assistant Scientific Director, Center for International Blood and Marrow Transplant Research, Milwaukee, Wisconsin

John Harlan MD
Professor of Medicine, University of Washington; Chief, Section of Hematology–Oncology, Harborview Medical Center, Seattle, Washington

John H. Hartwig PhD
Professor of Medicine, Harvard Medical School; Senior Biologist, Brigham and Women's Hospital, Boston, Massachusetts

Evdoxia Hatjiharissi MD
Department of Hematology, Theagenio Cancer Institute, Thessaloniki, Greece

Suzanne R. Hayman MD
Consultant, Division of Hematology, Mayo Clinic; Assistant Professor of Medicine, Mayo Clinic College of Medicine, Mayo Clinic, Rochester, Minnesota

Robert P. Hebbel MD
Regents Professor, George Clark Professor, Department of Medicine, Director, Vascular Biology Center, University of Minnesota Medical School, Minneapolis, Minnesota

Helen E. Heslop MD
Professor of Medicine and Pediatrics, Dan L Duncan Chair, Center for Cell and Gene Therapy, Baylor College of Medicine, The Methodist Hospital and Texas Children's Hospital, Houston, Texas

Katherine A. High MD
William Bennett Professor of Pediatrics, University of Pennsylvania School of Medicine, Investigator, Howard Hughes Medical Institute, Children's Hospital of Philadelphia, Attending Physician, Director, Center for Cellular and Molecular Therapeutics, Children's Hospital of Philadelphia, Philadelphia, Pennsylvania

Christopher D. Hillyer MD
Professor, Emory University School of Medicine, Department of Pathology and Laboratory Medicine; Director, Center for Transfusion and Cellular Therapies, Medical Director, Transfusion Services, Emory University Hospital Atlanta, Georgia

David M. Hockenberry PhD
Adjunct Associate Professor, Department of Immunology, and Associate Professor, Department of Medicine, University of Washington School of Medicine; Associate Member, Clinical Research and Human Biology, Fred Hutchinson Cancer Research Center, Seattle, Washington

Dieter Hoelzer MD
Professor of Internal Medicine, Johan Wolfgang Goethe University School of Medicine; Chief, Department of Hematology, Zentrum der Inneren Medizin, Medizinische Klinik III, Frankfurt, Germany

Ronald Hoffman MD
Albert A. and Vera G. List Professor of Medicine; Hematology/Oncology Section; Mount Sinai Cancer Institute, Department of Medicine, Cell and Gene Medicine, Mount Sinai School of Medicine New York, New York

Mary M. Horowitz MD, MS
Chief Scientific Director, Center of International Blood and Marrow Transplant Research—CIBMTR®, Department of Medicine, Medical College of Wisconsin, Milwaukee, Wisconsin

Robert Hromas MD
Professor, Chief, Hematology/Oncology, University of New Mexico Health Sciences Center, Albuquerque, New Mexico

Joseph E. Italiano, Jr. PhD
Assistant Professor of Medicine, Harvard School of Medicine; Assistant Professor of Medicine, Brigham and Women's Hospital, Boston, Massachusetts

Elaine S. Jaffe MD
Chief, Hematopathology Section, Laboratory of Pathology Center for Cancer Research, National Cancer Institute, Bethesda, Maryland; Staff Pathologist, Clinical Center, National Institutes of Health, Bethesda, Maryland

Petr Jarolim MD, PhD
Assistant Professor of Pathology, Harvard Medical School; Staff Pathologist, Brigham and Women's Hospital, Boston, Massachusetts

Sima Jeha MD
Professor of Pediatrics, University of Tennessee Health Science Center, Member, Department of Oncology, St. Jude Children's Research Hospital, Memphis, Tennessee

Cassandra Josephson MD
Associate Professor, Pathology Laboratory Medicine and Pediatrics, Emory University School of Medicine, Associate Direction, Children's Healthcare of Atlanta, Blood Tissue Services, Department of Pathology, Atlanta, Georgia

Sarita A. Joshi MB BS, MD
Staff Physician, Blood and Marrow Transplantation Program, Cincinnati Children's Hospital Medical Center, Division of Hematology/Oncology, Cincinnati, Ohio

Leo Kager MD
Associate Professor of Pediatrics, Medical University Vienna; Associate Professor of Pediatrics, St. Anna Children's Hospital, Vienna, Austria

Aly Karsan MD
Professor, Pathology and Laboratory Medicine, University of British Columbia; Hematopathologist/Senior Scientist, British Columbia Cancer Agency, Vancouver, BC, Canada

Randal J. Kaufman PhD
Investigator, Howard Hughes Medical Institute, Chevy Chase, Maryland; Professor, University of Michigan, Ann Arbor, Michigan

Richard M. Kaufman MD
Assistant Professor of Pathology, Harvard Medical School; Medical Director, Adult Transfusion Service, Brigham and Women's Hospital, Boston, Massachusetts

Frank G. Keller MD
Associate Professor, Department of Pediatrics, Emory University School of Medicine; Children's Healthcare of Atlanta, Atlanta, Georgia

Geoffrey Kemball-Cook PhD
Divisional Posteraduate Administrator, Senior Scientist, MRC Clinical Sciences Center, London, United Kingdom

Craig M. Kessler MD
Professor of Medicine, Department of Medicine; Georgetown University School of Medicine; Chief, Division of Hematology, Department of Medicine, Hematology-Oncology, Georgetown University Hospital, Washington, District of Columbia

Nigel S. Key MB, ChB, FRCP
Harold R. Roberts Distinguished Professor, Chief Section of Hematology, Division of Hematology-Oncology, University of North Carolina School of Medicine; Director, Harold R. Roberts Comprehensive Diagnostic and Treatment Center, UNC Memorial Hospital, Chapel Hill, North Carolina

Arati Khanna-Gupta PhD
Lecturer, Brigham and Women's Hospital, Department of Hematology; Harvard Medical School, Boston, Massachusetts

Harvey G. Klein MD
Chief, Department of Transfusion Medicine, Warren G. Magnuson Clinical Center, National Institutes of Health, Bethesda, Maryland

Beate Klimm MD
Department of Internal Medicine I, University Hospital of Cologne, Cologne, Germany

Orit Kollet PhD
Weizmann Institute of Science, Rehovot, Israel

Barbara A. Konkle MD
Professor of Medicine, Pathology, and Laboratory Medicine, University of Pennsylvania, Director, Penn Comprehensive Hemophilia and Thrombosis Program, Philadelphia, Pennsylvania

Stanley J. Korsmeyer MD (Deceased)
Sidney Farber Professor of Pathology and Professor of Medicine, Harvard Medical School; Director, Program in Molecular Oncology, Department of Cancer Immunology and AIDS, Dana-Farber Cancer Institute, Boston, Massachusetts; Investigator, Howard Hughes Medical Institute, Chevy Chase, Maryland

Elizabeth F. Krakow MD, CM, FRCPC
Hematology Fellow, McMaster University; Clinical Scholar, Department of Medicine, Hamilton Health Sciences, Hamilton, Ontario, Canada

Amrita Krishnan MD, FACP
City of Hope, Duarte, California

Magdalena Kucia PhD
University of Louisville, School of Medicine, Developmental Biology Research Program, Louisville, Kentucky

Thomas J. Kunicki PhD
Associate Professor Tenure, The Scripps Research Institute, La Jolla, California, Canada

Timothy M. Kuzel MD, RACP
Professor of Medicine, Division of Hematology/Oncology, Department of Medicine, Northwestern University Feinberg School of Medicine, Chicago, Illinois

Martha Q. Lacy MD
Consultant, Division of Hematology, Mayo Clinic, Associate Professor of Medicine, Mayo Clinic College of Medicine, Mayo Clinic, Rochester, Minnesota

Viswanathan Lakshmanan PhD
Research Associate, Lewis Sigler Institute for Integrative Genomics, Princeton University, Princeton, New Jersey

Wendy Landier RN, MSN, CPNP
Assistant Clinical Professor, School of Nursing, University of California at Los Angeles, Los Angeles; Clinical Director Center for Cancer Survivorship, City of Hope National Medical Center, Duarte, California

Tsvee Lapidot PhD
Professor, Weizmann Institute of Science, Rehovot, Israel

Peter J. Larson MD
Director, Global Clinical Strategy, Bayer Healthcare, Biological Products, Research Triangle Park, North Carolina

Jacob Laubach MD
Instructor of Medicine, Harvard Medical School, Dana-Farber Cancer Institute, Department of Medical Oncology, Boston, Massachusetts

Ellen F. Lazarus MD, FCAP
Visiting Scientist, Department of Transfusion Medicine, Warren G. Magnuson Clinical Center, National Institutes of Health, Bethesda; Division of Human Tissue, FDA Center for Biologics Evaluation and Research, Rockville, Maryland

Stewart H. Lecker MD, PhD
Assistant Professor of Medicine, Harvard Medical School; Attending Physician, Renal Unit, Beth Israel Deaconess Medical Center, Boston, Massachusetts

William M.F. Lee MD
Associate Professor of Medicine, University of Pennsylvania School of Medicine, Philadelphia, Pennsylvania

Xavier Leleu MD
Hematology, CHRU-Lille, Maladies du Sang, Rue Michel Polonovski, Lille, France

Michael J. Lenardo MD
Adjunct Professor of Pathology, University of Pennsylvania School of Medicine, Philadelphia; Section Chief and Senior Investigator, Molecular Development Section, National Institute of Allergy and Infections Disease, Bethesda, Maryland

Polly Lenssen MS, RD, CD, FADA
Director, Clinical Nutrition, Children's Hospital and Regional Medical Center, Seattle, Washington

Georg Lenz MD
Center for Cancer Research, National Cancer Institute, NIH, Bethesda, Maryland

Nancy D. Leslie MD
Professor of Pediatrics, University of Cincinnati College of Medicine, Director, Metabolic Lab, Director, Clinical Operations, Cincinnati Children's Hospital Medical Center, Cincinnati, Ohio

Alexandra M. Levine MD
Distinguished Professor of Medicine, (Emeritus), Keck School of Medicine, University of Southern California, Los Angelcs; Chief Medical Officer, City of Hope National Medical Center, Duarte, California

David B. Lewis MD
Professor of Pediatrics and Member of the Program in Immunology, Division of Immunology and Transplantation Biology, Department of Pediatric, Stanford University School of Medicine, Attending Physician at Lucile Packard Children's Hospital, Stanford, California

Howard A. Liebman MD
Associate Professor of Medicine and Pathology, Jane Anne Nohl Division of Hematology, Keck USC School of Medicine; Attending Physician, Norris Comprehension Cancer Center Keck USC School of Medicine, Los Angeles, California

Henri Roger Lijnen PhD
Fenta Por Molecular and Vascular Biology, University of Leuven, Faculty of Medicine, Leuven, Belgium

Wendy Lim MD, MSc
Assistant Professor, Department of Medicine, McMaster University, Hamilton, Ontario, Canada

Thomas S. Lin MD, PhD
Associate Professor of Medicine, The Ohio State University, Columbus, Ohio

Michael P. Link MD
Lydia J. Lee Professor of Pediatrics, and Chief, Division of Hematology/Oncology, Department of Pediatrics, Stanford University School of Medicine, Stanford; Director, Center for Cancer and Blood Disease, Lucile Salter Packard Children's Hospital at Stanford, Palo Alto, California

Evelyn Lockhart MD
American Red Cross, Carolina Region, Charlotte, North Carolina

Mignon Loh MD
Associate Professor of Pediatrics, University of California, San Francisco, California

A. Thomas Look MD
Professor, Department of Pediatrics, Harvard Medical School; Vice Chair for Research, Pediatric Oncology Department, Dana-Farber Cancer Institute, Boston, Massachusetts

José A. López MD
Executive Vice President of Research, Puget Sound Blood Center, Puget Sound, Washington

Jaroslaw P. Maciejewski MD, PhD
Chief, Experimental Hematology and Hematopoiesis Section, Taussig Cancer Center; Staff Physician, Department of Hematologic Malignancies and Blood Disorders, Taussig Cancer Center Professor of Medicine, Cleveland Clinic Lerner College of Medicine, Case Western Reserve University, Cleveland, Ohio

Navneet Majhail MD, MS
Assistant Professor, Division of Hematology, Oncology and Transplantation, University of Minnesota, Minneapolis, Minnesota

Olivier Manches PhD
Research Assistant, New York University Cancer Institute, New York, New York

Robert Mandle PhD
Investigator, Center for Blood Research, Boston, Massachusetts

Catherine S. Manno MD
Professor, Department of Pediatrics, University of Pennsylvania School of Medicine; Associate Chair for Clinical Activities, The Children's Hospital of Philadelphia, Philadelphia, Pennsylvania

Simon Mantha MD
Hematologist, Laney Clinic Medical Center, Burlington, Massachusetts

Francesco M. Marincola MD
Director, Immunogenetics Program, Department of Transfusion Medicine, Warren G. Magnuson Clinical Center, National Institutes of Health, Bethesda, Maryland

Peter W. Marks MD, PhD
Associate Professor of Medicine, Yale University School of Medicine; Attending Physician, Yale-New Haven Hospital, New Haven, Connecticut

Steffen Massberg MD, PhD
Deutsches Herzzentrum Muenchen, Technische Universitaet Muenchen, Munich, Germany

Peter M. Mauch MD
Professor, Department of Radiation Oncology, Harvard Medical School; Senior Physician, Department of Radiation Oncology, Brigham and Women's Hospital, Boston, Massachusetts

Ruth McCorkle PhD, RN, FAAN
Florence S. Wald Professor of Nursing; Director, Center for Excellence in Chronic Illness Care; Chair, Doctoral Program, Department of Nursing, Yale University; Program Leader, Cancer Control, Yale Comprehensive Cancer Center, New Haven, Connecticut

Keith R. McCrae MD
Associate Professor of Medicine, Case Western Reserve University School of Medicine; University Hospitals of Cleveland, Cleveland, Ohio

Rodger P. McEver MD
Member and Chair, Cardiovascular Biology Program, Oklahoma Medical Research Foundation, Oklahoma City, Oklahoma

Philip McGlave MD
C.J. Watson Land Grant Chair in Medicine; Director, Division of Hematology, Oncology and Transplantation; Deputy Director, Masonic Cancer Center, University of Minnesota, Academic Health Center, Minneapolis, Minnesota

John H. McVey BSc, HONS, PhD
Weston Professor of Molecular Medicine, Thrombosis Research Institute, London, United Kingdom

Jay E. Menitove MD
Clinical Professor of Medicine, University of Missouri–Kansas City School of Medicine; Clinical Professor of Medicine, Kansas University School of Medicine; Executive Director and Medical Director, Administration, Community Blood Center of Greater Kansas City, Kansas City, Missouri

Giampaolo Merlini MD
Biotechnology Research laboratories, IRCCS Policlinico San Matteo Hospital, Department of Biochemistry, University of Pavia, Pavia, Italy

Ara Metjian MD
Hematology Fellow, Duke University School of Medicine, Durham, North Carolina

Anna Rita Migliaccio PhD
Professor of Medicine, Hematology Oncology Section, Mount Sinai School of Medicine, New York, New York

Jeffrey S. Miller MD
Professor of Medicine, Division of Hematology, Oncology and Transplantation, University of Minnesota Medical School, Minneapolis, Minnesota

Kenneth B. Miller MD
Director of Clinical Hematology, Bone Marrow Transplantation and Hematological Malignancy Unit, Beth Israel Deaconess Medical Center, Boston, Massachusetts

John G. Monroe PhD
Professor and Vice-Chair, Department of Pathology and Laboratory Medicine, University of Pennsylvania School of Medicine, Philadelphia, Pennsylvania

Michael R. Moore BSc, PhD, DSc
Professor of Medicine and Director, National Research Centre for Environmental Toxicology, University of Queensland Faculty of Medicine; Director, Queensland Health Scientific Services, Queensland Health, Brisbane, Queensland, Australia

Kari C. Nadeau MD, PhD
Assistant Professor of Pediatrics, Center of Excellence in Pulmonary Biology, Department of Pediatrics, Stanford University School of Medicine; Attending Physician, Lucile Packard Children's Hospital, Stanford, California

Vesna Najfeld PhD
Professor of Pathology and Medicine Director, Tumor Cytogenetics, The Mount Sinai School of Medicine, New York, New York

Kavita Natarajan MBBS
Assistant Professor of Medicine, Section of Hematology/Oncology, Medical College of Georgia, Augusta, Georgia

Benjamin G. Neel MD, PhD
Senior Scientist, Division of Stem Cell and Development Biology; Director, Ontario Cancer Institute, Toronto, Ontario, Canada

Anne T. Neff MD
Vanderbilt University Medical Center, Division of Hematology/Stem Cell Transplant, Vanderbilt University; Medical Director, Vanderbilt Hemostasis and Thrombosis Clinic, Medical Director, Blood Cell Collection Center, Vanderbilt University Medical Center, Nashville, Tennessee

Robert S. Negrin MD
Associate Professor of Medicine, Department of Medicine, Stanford University School of Medicine, Stanford, California

Paul M. Ness MD
Professor, Department of Pathology and Medicine, Johns Hopkins University School of Medicine; Director, Department of Transfusion Medicine, Johns Hopkins Hospital, Baltimore, Maryland

Ellis J. Neufeld MD, PhD
Associate Professor of Pediatrics, Harvard Medical School, Associate Chief, Hematology, Children's Hospital, Boston, Massachusetts

Andrea K. Ng MD, MPH
Associate Professor in Radiation Oncology, Harvard Medical School; Brigham and Women's Hospital, Dana-Farber Cancer Institute, Boston, Massachusetts

Diane J. Nugent MD
Director, Hemostasis Thrombosis Research and Proteomic Core, Children's Hospital of Orange County, Orange, California

Sarah H. O'Brien MD, MSc
Assistant Professor of Pediatrics, The Ohio State University College of Medicine; Assistant Professor of Pediatrics, Pediatric Hematology/Oncology, Nationwide Children's Hospital, Columbus, Ohio

Thalia Papayannopoulou MD
Professor, Department of Medicine, Division of Hematology, University of Washington School of Medicine, Seattle, Washington

Animesh D. Pardanani MBBS, PhD
Assistant Professor, Mayo Medical School, Consultant in Hematology, Mayo Clinic, Rochester, Minnesota

Effie W. Petersdorf MD
Professor of Medicine, Department of Medicine, Division of Oncology, University of Washington School of Medicine; Attending Physician, Seattle Cancer Care Alliance; Member, Division of Clinical Research, Fred Hutchinson Cancer Research Center, Seattle, Washington

LoAnn C. Peterson MD
Professor, Department of Pathology, Northwestern University Feinberg School of Medicine, Chicago, Illinois

German A. Pihan MD
Assistant Professor, Department of Pathology, Harvard Medical School; Director, Hematopathology, Beth Israel Deaconess Medical Center, Boston, Massachusetts

Stefano A. Pileri MD
Professor of Pathology, Director of the Haematopathology Unit and of the Doctorate Research Project in Clinical and Experimental Haematology anal Haemetopathology, Bologna University School of Medicine; Director of the Haematopathology Unit, ST Orsota-Malpighi Hospital, Bologna, Italy

Stefania Pittaluga MD, PhD
Staff Clinician, Hematopathology Section, Laboratory of Pathology, Center for Cancer Research; Staff Pathologist, National Institutes of Health, Bethesda, Maryland

Edward F. Plow PhD
Chair, Department of Molecular Cardiology, Cleveland Clinic Foundation/Lerner Research Institute, Cleveland, Ohio

David G. Poplack MD
Professor of Pediatrics, Section of Hematology/Oncology, Department of Pediatrics, Baylor College of Medicine, Texas Children's Cancer Center Houston, Texas

Laura Popolo PhD
Associate Professor, Universita' Degli Studi di Milano, Milano, Italy

Leland D. Powell MD, PhD
Associate Clinical Professor of Medicine, Department of Medicine, David Geffen School of Medicine at UCLA, Los Angeles; Olive View–UCLA Medical Center, Sylmar, California

Amy Pocoers MD
Instructor in Pathology, Harvard Medical School; Medical Director, Aphenesis and Infusion Services, Beth Israel Deaconess Medical Center, Boston, Massachusetts

Josef T. Prchal MD
Professor of Medicine, Department of Pathology and Genetics, University of Utah School of Medicine, Salt Lake City, Utah

Elizabeth A. Price MD
Instructor in Medicine Hematology, Division of Hematology, Department of Medicine, Stanford University School of Medicine, Stanford, California

Felipe Prosper MD, PhD
Professor, School of Medicine, University of Navarra; Co-Director, Department of Hematology and Director of Cell Therapy Area, Clinica Universîtaria De Navarra, Panflowa, Spain

Ching-Hon Pui MD
Professor of Pediatrics, University of Tenneisee Health Suenie Center; Chair, Department of Oncology, American Cancer Society Professor, St. Jude Children's Research Hospital, Memphis, Tennessee

Karen R. Rabin MD
Assistant Professor of Pediatrics, Section of Hematology/Oncology, Baylor College of Medicine, Houston, Texas

Jerald P. Radich MD
Professor, Fred Hutchinson Cancer Research Center, University of Washington School of Medicine, Seattle, Washington

Margaret V. Ragni MD, MPH
Professor of Medicine, Department of Medicine, Division of Hematology/Oncology, University of Pittsburgh School of Medicine; Director, Hemophilia Center of Western Pennsylvania, Pittsburgh, Pennsylvania

Janina Ratajczak MD, PhD
University of Louisville School of Medicine, Developmental Biology Research Program, Louisville, Kentucky

Marius Z. Ratajczak MD, PhD
Professor of Medicine, Stem Cell Institute at James Graham Brown Cancer Center, University of Louisville, Louisville, Kentucky

David J. Rawlings MD
Professor, Division of Pediatric Immunology, University of Washington, Section Head, Immunology, Seattle Children's Hospital Research Institute, Seattle, Washington

Daniel Re MD
Internal Medicine, Hematology and Medical Oncology, Centre Hospitalier Antibes Juan-les-Pins, Antibes Cédex, France

Pavan Reddy MD
Assistant Professor of Medicine, Department of Internal Medicine, University of Michigan Medical School; University of Michigan Comprehensive Cancer Center, Ann Arbor, Michigan

Mark T. Reding MD
Assistant Professor of Medicine, Division of Hematology, Oncology, and Transplantation, Department of Medicine, University of Minnesdta Medical School; Director, Center for Bleeding and Clotting Disorders, University of Minnesota Medical Center–Fairview, Minneapolis, Minnesota

Marion E. Reid PhD
Director, Immochemistry Laboratory, New York Blood Center, New York, New York

Alan C. Rigby PhD
Assistant Professor of Medicine, Harvard Medical School, Division of Molecular and Vascular Medicine, Both Israel Deaconess Medical Center, Boston, Massachusetts

A. Kim Ritchey MD
Professor Department of Pediatrics, University of Pittsburgh School of Medicine; Chief, Pediatric Hematology/Oncology, Children's Hospital of Pittsburgh, Pittsburgh, Pennsylvania

Jerome Ritz MD
Professor of Medicine, Harvard Medical School; Medical Director, The Connell and O'Reilly Families Cell Manipulation Core Facility, Dana-Farber Cancer Institute, Boston, Massachusetts

David J. Roberts MD, PhD
Professor of Haematology, Naffield Department of Clinical Laboratory Science, University of Oxford, Consuntant Haematologist, National Health Service Blood and Transplant Oxford, United Kingdom

Aldo Roccaro MD
Dana-Farber Cancer Institute, Boston, Massachusetts

Cliona M. Rooney PhD
Professor, Department of Pediatrics and Department of Molecular Virology and Microbiology, Baylor College of Medicine; Center for Cell and Gene Therapy, Texas Children's Cancer Center, Texas Children's Hospital, Houston, Texas

Steven T. Rosen MD
Professor of Medicine, Northwestern University Feinberg School of Medicine; Director, Robert H. Lurie Comprehensive Cancer Center, Northwestern Memorial Hospital, Chicago, Illinois

David S. Rosenthal MD
Professor of Medicine, Harvard Medical School; Attending Physician, Brigham and Women's Hospital, Dana-Farber Cancer Institute, Boston, Massachusetts

Rachel Rosovsky MD
Instructor in Medicine, Harvard Medical School; Attending Physician, Massachusetts General Hospital, Boston, Massachusetts

David A. Roth MD
Assistant Vice President, Clinical Research and Development, Therapeutic Area Director, Hematology, Wyeth Research, Cambridge, Massachusetts

Jacob M. Rowe MD
Dresner Professor of Hemato-Oncology, Bruce Rappaport Faculty of Medicine, Technion, Israel; Institute of Technology; Director, Department of Hematology and Bone Marrow Transplantation, Rambam Medical Center, Haifa, Israel

Scott D. Rowley MD, FACP
Clinical Associate Professor, UMDNJ-School of Medicine, Newark, New Jersey; Chief, Adult Blood and Marrow Transplantation Program, Hackensack University Medical Center, Hackensack, New Jersey

J. Evan Sadler MD, PhD
Professor of Medicine, Professor of Biochemistry and Molecular Biophysics, Washington University School of Medicine, St. Louis, Missouri

John T. Sandlund, Jr. MD
Professor of Pediatrics, University of Tennessee College of Medicine; Member, Department of Hematology/Oncology, St. Jude Children's Research Hospital, Memphis, Tennessee

Tomo Saric MD, PhD
University of Cologne, Medical School, Group Leader, Institute for Neurophysiology, Cologne, Germany

Yogen Saunthararajah MB, BCh
Associate Professor, Cleveland Clinic Foundation, Cleveland, Ohio

David T. Scadden MD
Associate Professor, Harvard Medical School; Co-Director, Harvard Stem Cell Institute, Massachusetts General Hospital, Boston, Massachusetts

Alvin H. Schmaier MD
Chief, Hematology and Oncology, Robert W. Kellermeyer Professor of Hematology and Oncology, Case Western Reserve University, School of Medicine; University Hospitals Case Medical Center, Cleveland, Ohio

Paul I. Schneiderman MD
Clinical Professor, Department of Dermatology, Columbia University College of Physicians and Surgeons; Department of Dermatology, Columbia Presbyterian Medical Center, New York, New York

Hélène Schoemans MD
Fellow in Hematology, PhD Student, Katholieke Universiteit Leuven, Leuven, Belgium

Jeffrey R. Schriber MD, FRCP
Banner Good Samaritan Medical School, Phoenix, Arizona

Stanley L. Schrier MD
Professor of Medicine (Hematology) Active Emeritus, Department of Medicine, Division of Hematology, Stanford University School of Medicine; Stanford University Medical Center, Stanford, California

Bart L. Scott MD, MS
Assistant Professor, University of Washington, Assistant Member, Fred Hutchinson Cancer Research Center, Seattle, Washington

Montaser Shaheen MD
Adjunct Clinical Assistant Professor, Indiana University; Physician, Providence Medical Group, Terre Haute, Indiana

Sanford J. Shattil MD
Professor of Medicine and Chief, Hematology-Oncology Division, University of California San Diego; Adjunct Professor of Molecular and Experimental Medicine, The Scripps Research Institute, La Jolla, California

Mark J. Shlomchik MD, PhD
Professor, Department of Laboratory Medicine and Immunobiology, Yale University School of Medicine; Associate Director, Transfusion Service, Yale New Haven Hospital, New Haven, Connecticut

Susan B. Shurin MD
Deputy Director, National Heart, Lung and Blood Institute NIH, Bethesda, Maryland

Leslie E. Silberstein MD
Professor of Pathology; Director, Joint Program in Transfusion Medicine and Director, Center for Human Cell Therapy, Harvard Medical School, Boston, Massachusetts

Franklin O. Smith MD
Professor of Pediatrics, University of Cincinnati College of Medicine; Marjory J. Johnson Endowed Chair, Director, Division of Hematology/Oncology, Cincinnati Children's Hospital Medical Center, Cincinnati, Ohio

Edward L. Snyder MD
Professor of Laboratory Medicine, Yale University School of Medicine; Director, Transfusion/Apheresis/Cell Processing/Tissue Bank, Yale New Haven Hospital, New Haven, Connecticut

Thomas R. Spitzer MD
Professor of Medicine, Harvard Medical School; Director, Bone Marrow Transplant Program, Massachusetts General Hospital, Boston, Massachusetts

Louis M. Staudt MD, PhD
Deputy Chief and Chief of Lymphoid Malignancies Section, Center for Cancer Research, National Cancer Institute, Bethesda, Maryland

Harald Stein MD
Professor of Pathology; Charite-University Medicine Berlin, Campus Benjamin Franklin; Director of the Pathology Department, Benjamin Franklin Clinic, Berlin, Germany

Martin H. Steinberg MD
Professor of Medicine, Pediatrics, Pathology and Laboratory Medicine, Department of Medicine, Boston University School of Medicine; Director, Center of Excellence in Sickle Cell Disease, Boston Medical Center, Boston, Massachusetts

Johan Stenflo MD, PhD
Professor of Clinical Chemistry, Department of Laboratory Medicine, Section of Clinical Chemistry, University Hospital, Malmo, Sweden

C. Philip Steuber MD
Professor of Pediatrics, Section of Hematology/Oncology, Baylor College of Medicine; Texas Children's Cancer Center, Houston, Texas

Richard M. Stone MD
Associate Professor of Medicine, Harvard Medical School; Boston, MA Director of Clinical Research, Adult Leukemia Program, Dana-Farber Cancer Institute, Boston, Massachusetts

Ronald G. Strauss MD
Professor of Pathology and Pediatrics, University of Iowa College of Medicine; Medical Director, U.I. DeGowin Blood Center, University of Iowa Hospitals and Clinics, Iowa City, Iowa

David F. Stroncek MD
Chief, Laboratory Services Section, Department of Transfusion Medicine, Warren G. Magnuson Clinical Center, National Institutes of Health, Bethesda, Maryland

Zbigniew M. Szczepiorkowski MD, PhD
Director, Transfusion Medicine Service and Cellular Therapy Center, Darmouth-Hitchcock Medical Center, Lebanon, New Hampshire

Martin S. Tallman MD
Professor, Division of Hematology/Oncology, Northwestern University Feinberg School of Medicine, Chicago, Illinois

Ayalew Tefferi MD
Professor of Medicine and Hematology, Mayo College of Medicine, Mayo Clinic, Rochester, Minnesota

Ramon V. Tiu MD
Cleveland Clinic Taussig Cancer Center, Research Scholar in Bone Marrow Failure, Cleveland, Ohio

Cameron C. Trenor III MD
Instructor in Pediatrics, Harvard Medical School; Staff Physician, Division of Pediatric Hematology/Oncology, Children's Hospital Boston, Dana-Farber Cancer Institute, Boston, Massachusetts

Steven P. Treon MD, PhD
Bing Program for Waldenström's Macroglobulinemia, Division of Hematologic Oncology; Associate Professor, Harvard Medical School Dana-Farber Cancer Institute, Boston, Massachusetts

Guido Tricot MD, PhD
Professor, Department of Medicine; Director, Utah Blood and Marrow Transplant and Myeloma Program, University of Utah School of Medicine, Salt Lake City, Utah

Edward G. Tuddenham MD
Professor of Haemophilia, University College, Director, Royal Free Hospital Haemophilia Centre, Royal Free Hospital Trust, London, United Kingdom

Catherine Verfaillie MD
Professor of Medicine, Director, Stem Cell Institute, Katholieue Universiteit Leuven, Leuven, Belgium

Elliott P. Vichinsky MD
Adjunct Professor of Pediatrics, University of California, San Francisco, School of Medicine, San Francisco; Director, Department of Hematology/Oncology, Children's Hospital and Research Center at Oakland, Oakland, California

Ulrich H. von Andrian MD, PhD
Mallinckrodt Professor of Immunopathology, Harvard Medical School, Senior Investigator Immune Disease Institute; Boston, Massachusetts

Andrew J. Wagner MD, PhD
Instruction of Medicine, Harvard Medical School; Staff Oncologist, Center for Sarcoma and Bone Oncology, Dana-Farber Cancer Institute, Boston, Massachusetts

Denisa D. Wagner PhD
Professor, Department of Pathology, Harvard Medical School; Senior Investigator, CBR Institute for Biomedical Research, Boston, Massachusetts

John E. Wagner Jr. MD
Professor and Director, Division of Hematology/Oncology and Transplantation, Department of Pediatrics, University of Minnesota, Medical School; Attending Physician, Co-Director of the Blood and Marrow Transplant Program, University of Minnesota Medical Center and Children is Hospital, Minneapolis, Minnesota

Ena Wang MD
Staff Scientist, Department of Transfusion Medicine, National Institutes of Health, Bethesda, Maryland

Theodore E. Warkentin MD
Professor, Department of Pathology and Molecular Medicine, and Department of Medicine, Michael G. DeGroote School of Medicine, McMaster University, Regional Director, Transfusion Medicine, Hamilton Regional Laboratory Medicine Program, Hamilton Health Sciences, Hamilton General Hospital Site, Hamilton, Ontraio, Canada

Michael C. Wei MD, PhD
Instructor, Division of Pediatric Hematology/Oncology, Stanford University School of Medicine; Lucile Packard Children's Hospital, Palo Alto California

Howard J. Weinstein MD
Alan R. Ezekowitz Professor of Pediatrics, Harvard Medical School; Chief, Pediatric Hematology and Oncology, Massachusetts General Hospital for Children, Boston, Massachusetts

Daniel J. Weisdorf MD
Professor, Department of Medicine, University of Minnesota Medical School; Director, Adult Blood and Marrow Transplant Program, University of Minnesota Hospitals, Minneapolis, Minnesota

Jeffrey I. Weitz MD, FRCPC, FACP
Professor of Medicine and Biochemistry, Canada, Research Chair (Tier I) in Thrombosis, Heart and Stroke Foundation of Ontario/J.F. Mustard, Chair in Cardiovascular Research, McMaster University; Director, Henderson Research Centre, Hamilton Health Sciences-Henderson Site, Hamilton, Ontario, Canada

Ilene Ceil Weitz MD
Assistant Clinical Professor of Medicine, Jane Anne Nohl Division of Hematology, Keck-USC School of Medicine; Norris Comprehensive Cancer Center, Keck-USC School of Medicine, Los Angeles, California

Gerlinde Wernig MD
Harvard Medical School; Brigham and Women's Hospital, Boston, Massachusetts

Connie M. Westhoff PhD
Adjunct Professor, Division of Transfusion Medicine, Department of Pathology and Laboratory Medicine, University of Pennsylvania; Scientific Director, American Red Cross, Philadelphia, Pennsylvania

Gilbert C. White, II MD
Professor of Medicine, Biochemistry, Pharmacology and Toxicology Associate Dean for Research, Medical College of Wisconsin; Executive Vice President for Research, Director, Blood Research Institute, Richard H. and Sara E. Aster Chair for Medical Research, Blood Center of Wisconsin, Milwaukee, Wisconsin

James S. Wiley MD, FRACP, FRCPA
Professor, Department of Medicine, Nepean Clinical School, University of Sydney; Head, Department of Haematology, Nepean Hospital, Penrith, New South Wales, Australia

Wyndham H. Wilson MD, PhD
Senior Investigator, Metabolism Branch, National Cancer Institute, National Institutes of Health, Bethesda, Maryland

Thomas E. Witzig MD
Professor of Medicine, Mayo Clinic College of Medicine; Consultant, Mayo Clinic, Rochester, Minnesota

Joanne Wolfe MD, MPH
Assistant Professor of Pediatrics, Harvard Medical School, Harvard University; Director, Pediatric Palliative Care, Dana-Farber Cancer Institute and Children's Hospital of Boston, Boston, Massachusetts

Yan Yun Wu MD, PhD
Assistant Professor of Laboratory Medicine, Yale University School of Medicine; Assistant Director, Blood Bank/Apheresis/Transfusion Cellular Therapy, Yale New Haven Hospital, New Haven, Connecticut

Kai W. Wucherpfennig MD, PhD
Professor, Harvard Medical School, Professor, Dana-Farber Cancer Institute, Boston, Massachusetts

Ming Jiang Xu MD, PhD
Assistant Professor, Hematology/Oncology Section, Mount Sinai Cancer Institute, Mount Sinai School of Medicine, New York, New York

Donald C. Yee MD
Assistant Professor, Department of Pediatrics, Hematology/Oncology Section, Department of Medicine, Thrombosis Research Section, Baylor College of Medicine, Texas Children's Cancer Center and Hematology Service, Houston, Texas

Mervin C. Yoder MD
Richard and Pauline Klingler Professor of Pediatrics, Professor of Biochemistry and Molecular Biology and of Cellular and Integrative Physiology, Indiana University School of Medicine; Attending Physician, James Whitcomb Riley Hospital for Children, Indianapolis, Indiana

Jo-Anne Hertha Young MD
Associate Professor, Department of Medicine; Director, Transplant Infectious Diseases, University of Minnesota, Minneapolis, Minnesota

Neal Stuart Young MD
Chief, Hematology Branch, National Heart, Lung and Blood Institute, National Institutes of Health, Bethesda, Maryland

Anaadriana Zakarija MD
Clinical Instructor, Division of Hematology/Oncology, Northwestern University Feinberg School of Medicine, Chicago, Illinois

PREFACE TO THE FIFTH EDITION

This volume represents the fifth edition of *Hematology: Basic Principles and Practice*. The initial concept for this textbook was formulated over two decades ago, and each edition of the book has evolved in response to the dramatic advances that have occurred in hematology. This evolution is a testimony to the continued energy of the editors, contributors, and readers of the book. The editorial board has incorporated scientific and diagnostic and therapeutic advances in hematology into each edition so that that the practicing hematologist, laboratory researcher, clinical researcher, student, or healthcare professional might more easily keep pace with this field and more effectively practice their craft. This text is intended to make modern hematology an exciting discipline that can be easily accessed by its diverse readership.

There have been several changes in the leadership of the book that have resulted in this fifth volume moving in new and exciting directions. Six of the editors of the previous edition, Ronald Hoffman, Edward J. Benz Jr., Sanford J. Shattil, Bruce Furie, Leslie E. Silberstein and Philip McGlave, have enthusiastically participated in the fifth edition. Remarkably, Drs. Hoffman, Benz, Shattil, and Furie have been with the book from its conception. Dr. Harvey J. Cohen, who was one of the editors of each of the previous four editions, unfortunately was not able to participate in this edition due to other responsibilities. Dr. Cohen made numerous important contributions to each of the previous editions and was an important ingredient to the success of this textbook. Each of the editors would like to express their sincere appreciation for his efforts. Dr. Cohen has been replaced by Dr. Helen Heslop from the Baylor College of Medicine in Houston, Texas. Dr. Heslop is an outstanding, internationally renowned scientist, pediatrician, and hematologist. Her participation has led to further improvements and expansion of chapters dealing with clinical immunology, pediatric hematology, pediatric stem cell transplantation, and gene therapy—additions that have substantially improved this edition.

The editorial board recognizes the pivotal role that hematopathology plays in the practice of modern hematology. This requires a close interaction between the clinician and the hematopathologist, each using their various clinical tools to serve patients with hematologic disorders. To improve the number and quality of hematopatology images in the fifth edition, we have invited Dr. John Anastasi, a well-respected hematopathologist from the University of Chicago, Pritzker School of Medicine, to join our editorial board as Hematopathology Image Consultant. Dr. Anastasi has reviewed each chapter and added or replaced photomicrographs with more illustrative images. One just has to thumb through this volume to gain a sense of the contribution that Dr. Anastasi has made to the fifth edition.

Another modification that is being implemented in this edition deals with references in each chapter. In previous editions, a significant proportion of the pages of many chapters were devoted to long lists of references. Such referencing of the literature is critical to the maintenance of the book as an academic enterprise. In order to retain this feature, a complete reference list of each chapter is provided on the Expert Consult Website that accompanies this volume. This strategy has allowed us to expand the actual number of pages devoted to useful text and to provide a short list of 20–30 general references at the end of each chapter. This modification has allowed us to maintain this textbook as a single volume. We hope that this compromise will be received in a favorable manner by our readership and that the website containing the full reference list will be accessible and useful.

Hematology: Basic Principles and Practice has become a leader among other textbooks dealing with the same subject matter. The close interaction between the members of the editorial board has, in the creation of each edition, led to novel concepts that have subsequently been incorporated into a number of other medical textbooks. As we finish this fifth edition of our book, it is important for the readership to be aware that this unique group of editors and authors will shortly begin to plan the sixth edition. These efforts and responsibilities are truly labors of love, which have provided us with enormous satisfaction. We all hope that this edition of *Hematology: Basic Principles and Practice* will not only find its way onto your bookshelf or your computer, but be your constant companion as you navigate the field of modern hematology.

Ronald Hoffman, MD
Edward J. Benz Jr., MD
Sanford Shattil, MD
Bruce Furie, MD
Leslie E. Silberstein, MD
Philip McGlave, MD
Helen Heslop, MD
John Anastasi, MD

CONTENTS

PART I

Molecular and Cellular Basis of Hematology

CHAPTER 1

ANATOMY AND PHYSIOLOGY OF THE GENE

Andrew J. Wagner, Nancy Berliner, and Edward J. Benz, Jr

Normal blood cells have limited life spans; they must be replenished in precise numbers by a continuously renewing population of progenitor cells. Homeostasis of the blood requires that proliferation of these cells be efficient yet strictly constrained. Many distinctive types of mature blood cells must arise from these progenitors by a controlled process of commitment to, and execution of, complex programs of differentiation. Thus, developing red blood cells must produce large quantities of hemoglobin, but not the myeloperoxidase characteristic of granulocytes, the immunoglobulins characteristic of lymphocytes, or the fibrinogen receptors characteristic of platelets. Similarly, the maintenance of normal amounts of coagulant and anticoagulant proteins in the circulation requires exquisitely regulated production, destruction, and interaction of the components. Understanding the basic biologic principles underlying cell growth, differentiation, and protein biosynthesis requires a thorough knowledge of the structure and regulated expression of genes, because the gene is now known to be the fundamental unit by which biologic information is stored, transmitted, and expressed in a regulated fashion.

Genes were originally characterized as mathematical units of inheritance. They are now known to consist of molecules of deoxyribonucleic acid (DNA). By virtue of their ability to store information in the form of nucleotide sequences, to transmit it by means of semiconservative replication to daughter cells during mitosis and meiosis, and to express it by directing the incorporation of amino acids into proteins, DNA molecules are the chemical transducers of genetic information flow. Efforts to understand the biochemical means by which this transduction is accomplished have given rise to the discipline of molecular genetics.

THE GENETIC VIEW OF THE BIOSPHERE: THE CENTRAL DOGMA OF MOLECULAR BIOLOGY

The fundamental premise of the molecular biologist is that the magnificent diversity encountered in nature is ultimately governed by genes. The capacity of genes to exert this control is in turn determined by relatively simple stereochemical rules, first appreciated by Watson and Crick in the 1950s. These rules constrain the types of interactions that can occur between two molecules of DNA or ribonucleic acid (RNA).

DNA and RNA are linear polymers consisting of four types of nucleotide subunits. Proteins are linear unbranched polymers consisting of 21 types of amino acid subunits. Each amino acid is distinguished from the others by the chemical nature of its side chain, the moiety not involved in forming the peptide bond links of the chain. The properties of cells, tissues, and organisms depend largely on the aggregate structures and properties of their proteins. The central dogma of molecular biology states that genes control these properties by controlling the structures of proteins, the timing and amount of their production, and the coordination of their synthesis with that of other proteins. The information needed to achieve these ends is transmitted by a class of nucleic acid molecules called RNA. Genetic information thus flows in the direction DNA → RNA → protein. This central dogma provides, in principle, a universal approach for investigating the biologic properties and behavior of any given cell, tissue, or organism by study of the controlling genes. Methods permitting direct manipulation of DNA sequences should then be universally applicable to the study of all living entities. Indeed, the power of the molecular genetic approach lies in the universality of its utility.

One exception to the central dogma of molecular biology that is especially relevant to hematologists is the storage of genetic information in RNA molecules in certain viruses, notably the retroviruses associated with T-cell leukemia/lymphoma and the human immunodeficiency virus. When retroviruses enter the cell, the RNA genome is copied into a DNA replica by an enzyme called *reverse transcriptase*. This DNA representation of the viral genome is then expressed according to the rules of the central dogma. Retroviruses thus represent a variation on the theme, rather than a true exception to or violation of the rules.

ANATOMY AND PHYSIOLOGY OF GENES

DNA Structure

DNA molecules are extremely long, unbranched polymers of nucleotide subunits. Each nucleotide contains a sugar moiety called deoxyribose, a phosphate group attached to the 5′ carbon position, and a purine or pyrimidine base attached to the 1′ position (Fig. 1–1). The linkages in the chain are formed by phosphodiester bonds between the 5′ position of each sugar residue and the 3′ position of the adjacent residue in the chain (Fig. 1–1). The sugar phosphate links form the backbone of the polymer, from which the purine or pyrimidine bases project perpendicularly.

The haploid human genome consists of 23 long, double-stranded DNA molecules tightly complexed with histones and other nuclear proteins to form compact linear structures called *chromosomes*. The genome contains 3 billion nucleotides; each chromosome is thus 50 to 200 million bases in length. The individual genes are aligned along each chromosome. The human genome contains about 30,000 genes. Blood cells, like most somatic cells, are diploid. That is, each chromosome is present in two copies, so that there are 46 chromosomes consisting of approximately 6 billion base pairs (bp) of DNA.

The four nucleotide bases in DNA are the purines (adenosine and guanosine) and the pyrimidines (thymine and cytosine). The basic chemical configuration of the other nucleic acid found in cells, RNA, is quite similar, except that the sugar is ribose (having a hydroxyl group attached to the 2′ carbon, rather than the hydrogen found in deoxyribose) and the pyrimidine base uracil is used in place of thymine. The bases are commonly referred to by a shorthand notation: the letters A, C, T, G, and U are used to refer to adenosine, cytosine, thymine, guanosine, and uracil, respectively.

The ends of DNA and RNA strands are chemically distinct, because of the 3′ → 5′ phosphodiester bond linkage that ties adjacent bases together (see Fig. 1–1). One end of the strand (the 3′ end) has an unlinked (free at the 3′ carbon) sugar position, and the other (the 5′ end) a free 5′ position. There is thus a polarity to the sequence of bases in a DNA strand: the same sequence of bases read in a 3′ → 5′ direction carries a different meaning than if read in a 5′ → 3′ direction. Cellular enzymes can thus distinguish one end of a nucleic

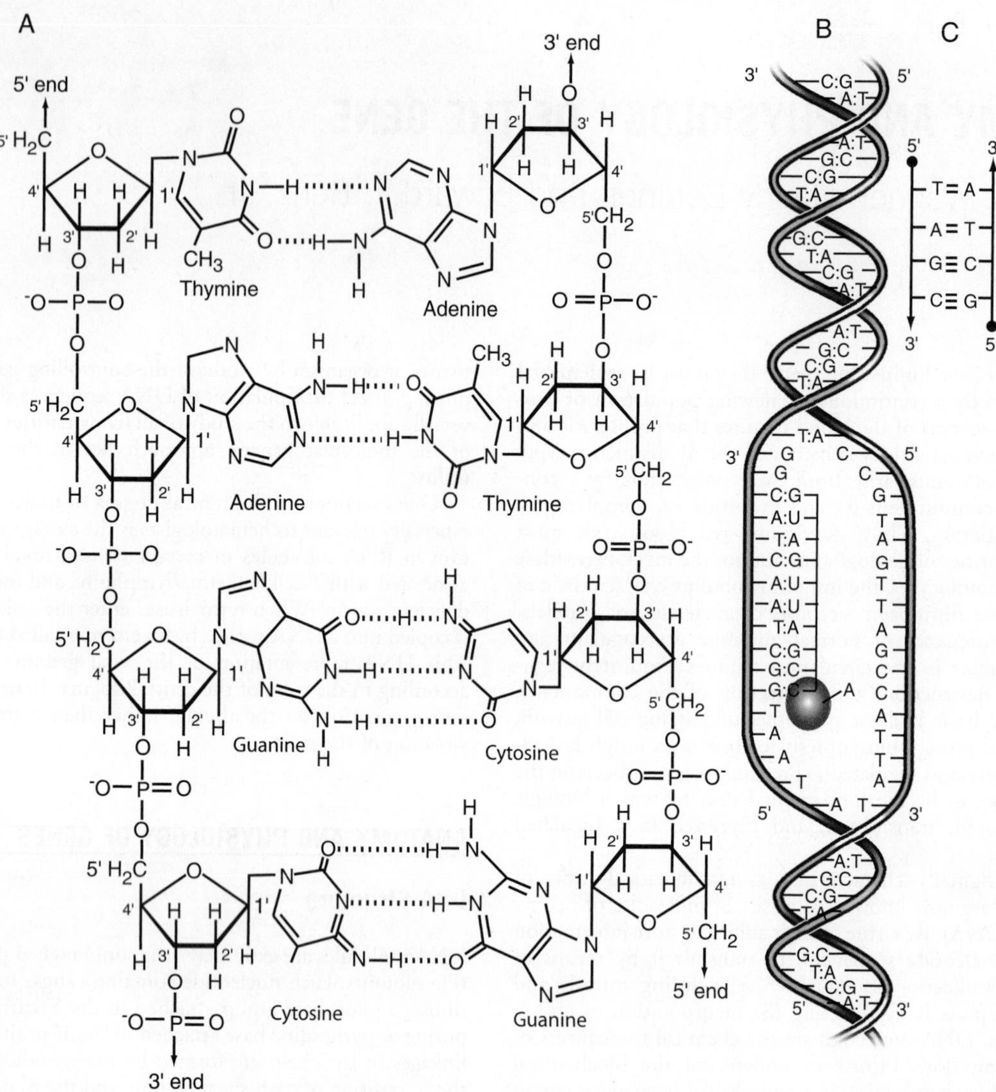

Figure 1–1 STRUCTURE, BASE PAIRING, POLARITY, AND TEMPLATE PROPERTIES OF DNA. **A,** Structures of the four nitrogenous bases projecting from sugar phosphate backbones. The hydrogen bonds between them form base pairs holding complementary strands of DNA together. Note that A–T and T–A base pairs have only two hydrogen bonds, whereas C–G and G–C pairs have three. **B,** The double helical structure of DNA results from base pairing of strands to form a double-stranded molecule with the backbones on the outside and the hydrogen-bonded bases stacked in the middle. Also shown schematically is the separation (unwinding) of a region of the helix by mRNA polymerase, which is shown using one of the strands as a template for the synthesis of an mRNA precursor molecule. Note that new bases added to the growing RNA strand obey the rules of Watson-Crick base pairing (see text). Uracil (U) in RNA replaces T in DNA and, like T, forms base pairs with A. **C,** Diagram of the antiparallel nature of the strands, based on the stereochemical $3' \rightarrow 5'$ polarity of the strands. The chemical differences between reading along the backbone in the $5' \rightarrow 3'$ and $3' \rightarrow 5'$ directions can be appreciated by reference to part **A.** A, adenosine; T, thymine; C, cytosine; G, guanosine.

acid from the other; most enzymes that "read" the DNA sequence tend to do so only in one direction ($3' \rightarrow 5'$ or $5' \rightarrow 3'$, but not both). Most nucleic acid-synthesizing enzymes, for instance, add new bases to the strand in a $5' \rightarrow 3'$ direction.

The ability of DNA molecules to store information resides in the sequence of nucleotide bases arrayed along the polymer chain. Under the physiologic conditions in living cells, DNA is thermodynamically most stable when two strands coil around each other to form a double-stranded helix. The strands are aligned in an "antiparallel" direction, having opposite $3' \rightarrow 5'$ polarity (see Fig. 1–1). The DNA strands are held together by hydrogen bonds between the bases on one strand and the bases on the opposite (complementary) strand. The stereochemistry of these interactions allows bonds to form between the two strands only when adenine on one strand pairs with thymine at the same position of the opposite strand, or guanine with cytosine; the Watson-Crick rules of base pairing. Two strands joined together in compliance with these rules are said to have "complementary" base sequences.

These thermodynamic rules imply that the sequence of bases along one DNA strand immediately dictates the sequence of bases that must be present along the complementary strand in the double helix. For example, whenever an A occurs along one strand, a T must be present at that exact position on the opposite strand; a G must always be paired with a C, a T with an A, and a C with a G. In RNA–RNA or RNA–DNA double-stranded molecules, U–A base pairs replace T–A pairs.

STORAGE AND TRANSMISSION OF GENETIC INFORMATION

The rules of Watson-Crick base pairing apply to DNA–RNA, RNA–RNA, and DNA–DNA double-stranded molecules. Enzymes that replicate or polymerize DNA and RNA molecules obey the base-pairing rules. By using an existing strand of DNA or RNA as the template, a new (daughter) strand is copied (transcribed) by reading

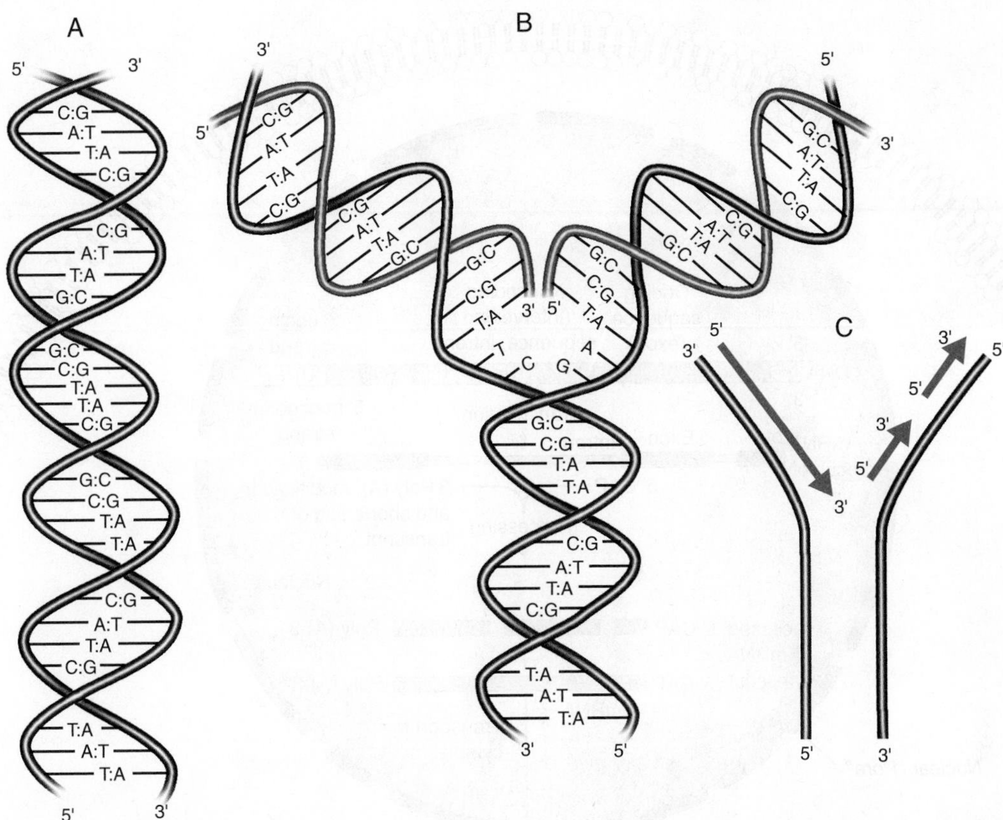

Figure 1–2 SEMICONSERVATIVE REPLICATION OF DNA. **A,** The process by which the DNA molecule on the left is replicated into two daughter molecules, as occurs during cell division. Replication occurs by separation of the parent molecule into the single-stranded form at one end, reading of each of the daughter strands in the 3′ → 5′ direction by DNA polymerase, and addition of new bases to growing daughter strands in the 5′ → 3′ direction. **B,** The replicated portions of the daughter molecules are identical to each other (*red*). Each carries one of the two strands of the parent molecule, accounting for the term *semiconservative replication.* Note the presence of the replication fork, the point at which the parent DNA is being unwound. **C,** The antiparallel nature of the DNA strands demands that replication proceed toward the fork in one direction and away from the fork in the other (*red*). This means that replication is actually accomplished by reading of short stretches of DNA, followed by ligation of the short daughter strand regions to form an intact daughter strand.

processively along the base sequence of the template strand, adding to the growing strand at each position only that base that is complementary to the corresponding base in the template according to the Watson-Crick rules. Thus, a DNA strand having the base sequence 5′-GCTATG-3′ could be copied by DNA polymerase only into a daughter strand having the sequence 3′-CGATAC-5′. Note that the sequence of the template strand provides all the information needed to predict the nucleotide sequence of the complementary daughter strand. Genetic information is thus stored in the form of base-paired nucleotide sequences.

If a double-stranded DNA molecule is separated into its two component strands, and each strand is then used as a template to synthesize a new daughter strand, the product will be two double-stranded daughter DNA molecules, each identical to the original parent molecule. This semiconservative replication process is exactly what occurs during mitosis and meiosis as cell division proceeds (Fig. 1–2). The rules of Watson-Crick base pairing thus provide for the faithful transmission of exact copies of the cellular genome to subsequent generations.

EXPRESSION OF GENETIC INFORMATION THROUGH THE GENETIC CODE AND PROTEIN SYNTHESIS

The information stored in the DNA base sequence achieves its impact on the structure, function, and behavior of organisms by governing the structures, timing, and amounts of protein synthesized in the cells. The primary structure (ie, the amino acid sequence) of each protein determines its three-dimensional conformation and therefore properties (eg, shape, enzymatic activity, ability to interact with other molecules, stability). In the aggregate, these proteins control cell structure and metabolism. The process by which DNA achieves its control of cells through protein synthesis is called *gene expression.*

An outline of the basic pathway of gene expression in eukaryotic cells is shown in Fig. 1–3. The DNA base sequence is first copied into an RNA molecule, called *premessenger RNA,* by messenger RNA (mRNA) polymerase. Premessenger RNA has a base sequence identical to the DNA coding strand. Genes in eukaryotic species consist of tandem arrays of sequences encoding mRNA (exons); these sequences alternate with sequences (introns) present in the initial mRNA transcript (premessenger RNA) but absent from the mature mRNA. The entire gene is transcribed into the large precursor, which is then further processed (spliced) in the nucleus. The introns are excised from the final mature mRNA molecule, which is then exported to the cytoplasm to be decoded (translated) into the amino acid sequence of the protein, by association with a biochemically complex group of ribonucleoprotein structures called *ribosomes.* Ribosomes contain two subunits: the 60S subunit contains a single, large (28S) ribosomal RNA molecule complexed with multiple proteins, whereas the RNA component of the 40S subunit is a smaller (18S) ribosomal RNA molecule.

Ribosomes read mRNA sequence in a ticker tape fashion three bases at a time, inserting the appropriate amino acid encoded by each three-base code word or codon into the appropriate position of the growing protein chain. This process is called *mRNA translation.* The glossary used by cells to know which amino acids are encoded by each DNA codon is called the *genetic code* (Table 1–1). Each amino acid is encoded by a sequence of three successive bases. Because there

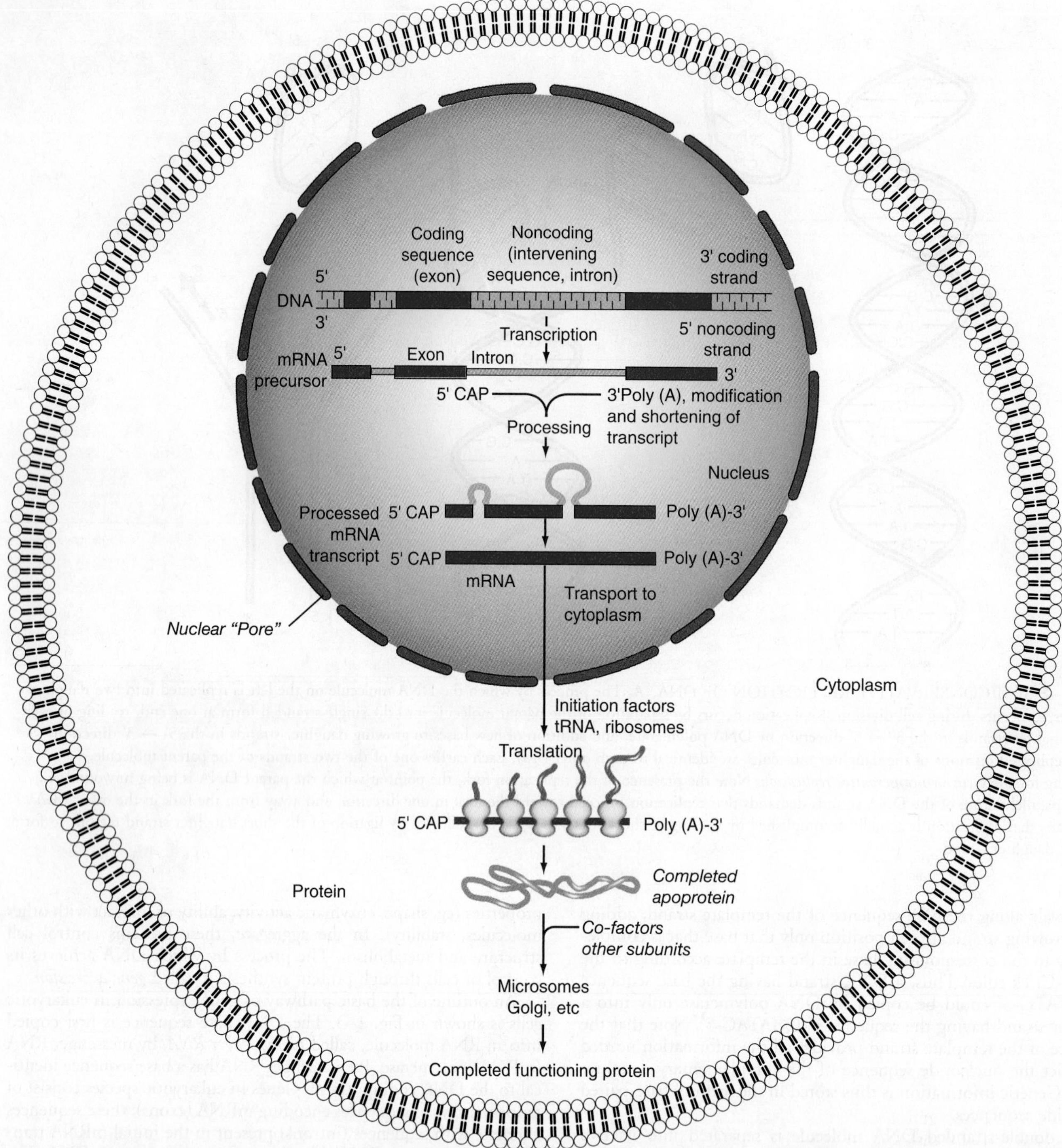

Figure 1–3 SYNTHESIS OF MRNA AND PROTEIN—THE PATHWAY OF GENE EXPRESSION. The diagram of the DNA gene shows the alternating array of exons (*red*) and introns (*shaded color*) typical of most eukaryotic genes. Transcription of the mRNA precursor, addition of the 5′-CAP and 3′-poly (A) tail, splicing and excision of introns, transport to the cytoplasm through the nuclear pores, translation into the amino acid sequence of the apoprotein, and posttranslational processing of the protein are described in the text. Translation proceeds from the initiator methionine codon near the 5′ end of the mRNA, with incorporation of the amino terminal end of the protein. As the mRNA is read in a 5′ → 3′ direction, the nascent polypeptide is assembled in an amino → carboxyl terminal direction.

are four code letters (A, C, G, and U), and because sequences read in the 5′ → 3′ direction have a different biologic meaning than sequences read in the 3′ → 5′ direction, there are 4^3, or 64, possible codons consisting of three bases.

There are 21 naturally occurring amino acids found in proteins. Thus, more codons are available than amino acids to be encoded. As noted in Table 1–1, a consequence of this redundancy is that some amino acids are encoded by more than one codon. For example, six distinct codons can specify incorporation of arginine into a growing amino acid chain, four codons can specify valine, two can specify glutamic acid, and only one each methionine or tryptophan. In no case does a single codon encode more than one amino acid. Codons thus predict unambiguously the amino acid sequence they encode. However, one cannot easily read backward from the amino acid sequence to decipher the *exact* encoding DNA sequence. These facts are summarized by saying that the code is degenerate but not ambiguous.

Some specialized codons serve as punctuation points during translation. The methionine codon (AUG), when surrounded by a consensus sequence (the Kozak box) near the beginning (5′ end) of the mRNA, serves as the initiator codon signaling the first amino acid to

Table 1–1 The Genetic Code* Messenger RNA Codons for the Amino Acids

Alanine	Arginine	Asparagine	Aspartic Acid	Cysteine
5′-GCU-3′	CGU	AAU	GAU	UGU
GCC	CGC	AAC	GAC	UGC
GCA	CGA			
GCG	AGA			
	AGG			

Glutamic Acid	Glutamine	Glycine	Histidine	Isoleucine
GAA	CAA	GGU	CAU	AUU
GAG	CAG	GGC	CAC	AUC
		GGA		AUA
		GGG		

Leucine	Lysine	Methionine	Phenylalanine	Proline‡
UUA	AAA	AUG†	UUU	CCU
UUG	AAG		UUC	CCC
CUU				CCA
CUC				CCG
CUA				
CUG				

Serine	Threonine	Tryptophan	Tyrosine	Valine
UCU	ACU	UGG	UAU	GUU
UCC	ACC		UAC	GUC
UCA	ACA			GUA
UCG	ACG			GUG
AGU				
AGC				

Chain Termination§
UAA
UAG
UGA

*Note that most of the degeneracy in the code is in the third base position (eg, lysine, AA[G or C]; asparagine, AA[C or U]; valine GUN [where N is any base]).
†AUG is also used as the chain-initiation codon when surrounded by the Kozak consensus sequence.
‡Hydroxyproline, the 21st amino acid, is generated by posttranslational modification of proline. It is almost exclusively confined to collagen subunits.
§The codons that signal the end of translation, also called nonsense or termination codons, are described by their nicknames *amber* (UAG), *ochre* (UAA), and *opal* (UGA).

be incorporated. All proteins thus begin with a methionine residue, but this is often removed later in the translational process. Three codons, UAG, UAA, and UGA, serve as translation terminators, signaling the end of translation.

The adaptor molecules mediating individual decoding events during mRNA translation are small (40 bases long) RNA molecules called *transfer RNAs* (tRNAs). When bound into a ribosome, each tRNA exposes a three-base segment within its sequence called the *anticodon*. These three bases attempt to pair with the three-base codon exposed on the mRNA. If the anticodon is complementary in sequence to the codon, a stable interaction among the mRNA, the ribosome, and the tRNA molecule results. Each tRNA also contains a separate region that is adapted for covalent binding to an amino acid. The enzymes that catalyze the binding of each amino acid are constrained in such a way that each tRNA species can bind only to a single amino acid. For example, tRNA molecules containing the anticodon 3′-AAA-5′, which is complementary to a 5′-UUU-3′ (phenylalanine) codon in mRNA, can only be bound to or charged with phenylalanine; tRNA containing the anticodon 3′-UAG-5′ can only be charged with isoleucine, and so forth.

Transfer RNAs and their amino acyl tRNA synthetases provide for the coupling of nucleic acid information to protein information needed to convert the genetic code to an amino acid sequence. Ribosomes provide the structural matrix on which tRNA anticodons and mRNA codons become properly exposed and aligned in an orderly, linear, and sequential fashion. As each new codon is exposed, the appropriate charged tRNA species is bound. A peptide bond is then formed between the amino acid carried by this tRNA and the C-terminal residue on the existing nascent protein chain. The growing chain is transferred to the new tRNA in the process, so that it is held in place as the next tRNA is brought in. This cycle is repeated until completion of translation. The completed polypeptide chain is then transferred to other organelles for further processing (eg, to the endoplasmic reticulum and the Golgi apparatus) or released into cytosol for association of the newly completed chain with other subunits to form complex multimeric proteins (eg, hemoglobin), and so forth, as discussed in Chapter 2.

mRNA METABOLISM

In eukaryotic cells, mRNA is initially synthesized in the nucleus (Figs. 1–3 and 1–4). Before the initial transcript becomes suitable for translation in the cytoplasm, mRNA processing and transport occur by a complex series of events including excision of the portions of the mRNA corresponding to the introns of the gene (mRNA splicing), modification of the 5′ and 3′ ends of the mRNA to render them more stable and translatable, and transport to the cytoplasm. Moreover, the amount of any particular mRNA moiety in both prokaryotic and eukaryotic cells is governed not only by the composite rate of mRNA synthesis (transcription, processing, and transport) but also by its degradation by cytoplasmic ribonucleases (RNA degradation). Many mRNA species of special importance in hematology (eg, mRNAs for growth factors and their receptors, protooncogene mRNAs, acute-phase reactants) are exquisitely regulated by control of their stability (half-life) in the cytoplasm.

Posttranscriptional mRNA metabolism is complex. Only a few relevant details are considered in this section.

mRNA Splicing

The initial transcript of eukaryotic genes contains several subregions (see Fig. 1–4). Most striking is the tandem alignment of exons and introns. Precise excision of intron sequences and ligation of exons is critical for production of mature mRNA. This process is called *mRNA splicing*, and it occurs on complexes of small nuclear RNAs and proteins called snRNPs; the term *spliceosome* is also used to describe the intranuclear organelle that mediates mRNA splicing reactions. The biochemical mechanism for splicing is complex. A consensus sequence, which includes the dinucleotide GU, is recognized as the donor site at the 5′ end of the intron (5′ end refers to the polarity of the mRNA strand coding for protein); a second consensus sequence ending in the dinucleotide AG is recognized as the acceptor site, which marks the distal end of the intron (Figs. 1–4 and 1–5). The spliceosome recognizes the donor and acceptor and forms an intermediate lariat structure that provides for both excision of the intron and proper alignment of the cut ends of the two exons for ligation in precise register.

Messenger RNA splicing has proved to be an important mechanism for greatly increasing the versatility and diversity of expression of a single gene. For example, some genes contain an array of more exons than are actually found in any mature mRNA species encoded by that gene. Several different mRNA and protein products can arise from a single gene by selective inclusion or exclusion of individual exons from the mature mRNA products. This phenomenon is called *alternative mRNA splicing*. It permits a single gene to code for multiple mRNA and protein products with related but distinct structures and functions. The mechanisms by which individual exons are selected or rejected remain obscure. For present purposes, it is sufficient to note that important physiologic changes in cells can be regulated by altering the patterns of mRNA splicing products arising from single genes.

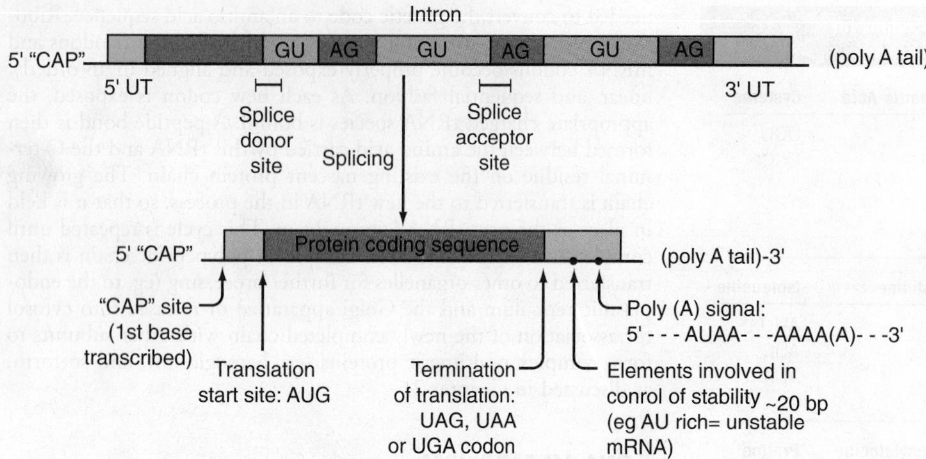

Figure 1–4 ANATOMY OF THE PRODUCTS OF THE STRUCTURAL GENE (MRNA PRECURSOR AND MRNA). This schematic shows the configuration of the critical anatomic elements of an mRNA precursor, which represents the primary copy of the structural portion of the gene. The sequences GU and AG indicate, respectively, the invariant dinucleotides present in the donor and acceptor sites at which introns are spliced out of the precursor. Not shown are the less stringently conserved consensus sequences that must precede and succeed each of these sites for a short distance.

Many inherited hematologic diseases arise from mutations that derange mRNA splicing. For example, some of the most common forms of the thalassemia syndromes and hemophilia arise by mutations that alter normal splicing signals or create splicing signals where they normally do not exist (activation of cryptic splice sites).

Modification of the Ends of the mRNA Molecule

Most eukaryotic mRNA species are polyadenylated at their 3′ ends. mRNA precursors are initially synthesized as large molecules that extend further downstream from the 3′ end of the mature mRNA molecule. Polyadenylation results in the addition of stretches of 100 to 150 A residues at the 3′ end. Such an addition is often called the poly-A tail and is of variable length. Polyadenylation facilitates rapid early cleavage of the unwanted 3′ sequences from the transcript and is also important for stability or transport of the mRNA out of the nucleus. Signals near the 3′ extremity of the mature mRNA mark positions at which polyadenylation occurs. The consensus signal is AUAAA (see Fig. 1–4). Mutations in the poly-A signal sequence have been shown to cause thalassemia.

At the 5′ end of the mRNA, a complex oligonucleotide having unusual phosphodiester bonds is added. This structure contains the nucleotide 7-methyl-guanosine and is called CAP (see Fig. 1–4). The 5′-CAP enhances both mRNA stability and the ability of the mRNA to interact with protein translation factors and ribosomes.

5′ and 3′ Untranslated Sequences

The 5′ and 3′ extremities of mRNA extend beyond the initiator and terminator codons that mark the beginning and the end of the sequences actually translated into proteins (see Figs. 1–4 and 1–5). These so-called 5′ and 3′ untranslated regions (5′ UTR and 3′ UTR) are involved in determining mRNA stability and the efficiency with which mRNA species can be translated. For example, if the 3′ UTR of a very stable mRNA (eg, globin mRNA) is swapped with the 3′ UTR of a highly unstable mRNA (eg, the c-*myc* protooncogene), the c-*myc* mRNA becomes more stable. Conversely, attachment of the 3′ UTR of c-*myc* to a globin molecule renders it unstable. Instability is often associated with repeated sequences rich in A and U in the 3′ UTR (see Fig. 1–4). Similarly, the UTRs in mRNAs coding for proteins involved in iron metabolism mediate altered mRNA stability or translatability by binding iron-laden proteins.

Transport of mRNA From Nucleus to Cytoplasm: mRNP Particles

An additional potential step for regulation or disruption of mRNA metabolism occurs during the transport from nucleus to cytoplasm. mRNA transport is an active, energy-consuming process. Moreover, at least some mRNAs appear to enter the cytoplasm in the form of complexes bound to proteins (mRNPs). mRNPs may regulate stability of the mRNAs and their access to translational apparatus. There is some evidence that certain mRNPs are present in the cytoplasm but are not translated (masked message) until proper physiologic signals are received.

GENE REGULATION

Virtually all cells of an organism receive a complete copy of the DNA genome inherited at the time of conception. The panoply of distinct

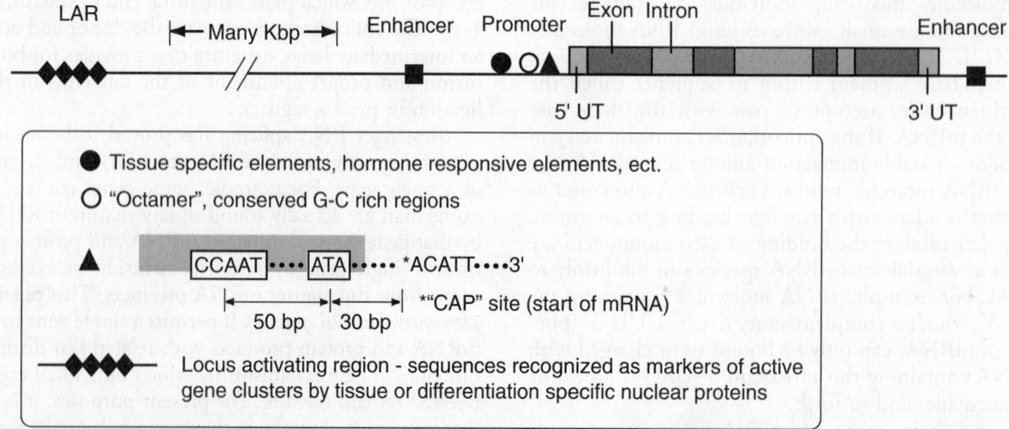

Figure 1–5 Regulatory elements flanking the structural gene.

cell types and tissues found in any complex organism is possible only because different portions of the genome are selectively expressed or repressed in each cell type. Each cell must "know" which genes to express, how actively to express them, and when to express them. This biologic necessity has come to be known as *gene regulation* or *regulated gene expression*. Understanding gene regulation provides insight into how pluripotent stem cells determine that they will express the proper sets of genes in daughter progenitor cells that differentiate along each lineage. Major hematologic disorders (such as the leukemias and lymphomas), immunodeficiency states, and myeloproliferative syndromes result from derangements in the system of gene regulation. An understanding of the ways that genes are selected for expression thus remains one of the major frontiers of biology and medicine.

EPIGENETIC REGULATION OF GENE EXPRESSION

Most of the DNA in living cells is inactivated by formation of a nucleoprotein complex called *chromatin*. The histone and nonhistone proteins in chromatin effectively sequester genes from enzymes needed for expression. The most tightly compacted chromatin regions are called *euchromatin*. Heterochromatin, less tightly packed, contains actively transcribed genes. Activation of a gene for expression (ie, transcription) requires that it become less compacted and more accessible to the transcription apparatus. These processes involve both *cis*-acting and *trans*-acting factors. *Cis*-acting elements are regulatory DNA sequences, within or flanking the genes. They are recognized by *trans*-acting factors, which are nuclear DNA-binding proteins needed for transcriptional regulation.

DNA sequence regions flanking genes are called *cis*-acting because they influence expression of nearby genes only on the same chromosome. These sequences do not usually encode mRNA or protein molecules. They alter the conformation of the gene within chromatin in such a way as to facilitate or inhibit access to the factors that modulate transcription. These interactions may twist or kink the DNA in such a way as to control exposure to other molecules. When exogenous nucleases are added in small amounts to nuclei, these exposed sequence regions become especially sensitive to the DNA-cutting action of the nucleases. Thus, nuclease-hypersensitive sites in DNA have come to be appreciated as markers for regions in or near genes that are interacting with regulatory nuclear proteins.

Methylation is another structural feature that can be used to recognize differences between actively transcribed and inactive genes. Most eukaryotic DNA is heavily methylated, that is, the DNA is modified by the addition of a methyl group to the 5 position of the cytosine pyrimidine ring (5-methyl-C). In general, heavily methylated genes are inactive, whereas active genes are relatively hypomethylated, especially in the 5′ flanking regions containing the promoter and other regulatory elements (see "Enhancers, Promoters, and Silencers"). These flanking regions frequently include DNA sequences with a high content of Cs and Gs (CpG islands). Hypomethylated CpG islands (detectable by methylation-sensitive restriction endonucleases) serve as markers of actively transcribed genes. For example, a search for undermethylated CpG islands on chromosome 7 facilitated the search for the gene for cystic fibrosis.

DNA methylation is facilitated by DNA methyltransferases. DNA replication incorporates unmethylated nucleotides into each nascent strand, thus leading to demethylated DNA. For cytosines to become methylated, the methyltransferases must act after each round of replication. After an initial wave of demethylation early in embryonic development, regulatory areas are methylated during various stages of development and differentiation. Aberrant DNA methylation also occurs as an early step during tumorigenesis, leading to silencing of tumor suppressor genes and of genes related to differentiation. This finding has led to induction of DNA demethylation as a target in cancer therapy. Indeed, 5-azacytidine, a cytidine analog unable to be methylated, and the related compound decitabine, are approved by the United States Food and Drug Administration for use in myelodysplastic syndromes, and their use in cases of other malignancies is being investigated.

Although it is poorly understood how particular regions of DNA are targeted for methylation, it is becoming increasingly apparent that this modification targets further alterations in chromatin proteins that in turn influence gene expression. Histone acetylation, phosphorylation, and methylation of the *N*-terminal tail are currently the focus of intense study. Acetylation of lysine residues (catalyzed by histone acetyltransferases), for example, is associated with transcriptional activation. Conversely, histone deacetylation (catalyzed by histone deacetylase) leads to gene silencing. Histone deacetylases are recruited to areas of DNA methylation by DNA methyltransferases and by methyl–DNA-binding proteins, thus linking DNA methylation to histone deacetylation. Drugs inhibiting these enzymes are being studied as anticancer agents.

The regulation of histone acetylation/deacetylation appears to be linked to gene expression, but the roles of histone phosphorylation and methylation are less well understood. Current research suggests that in addition to gene regulation, histone modifications contribute to the "epigenetic code" and are thus a means by which information regarding chromatin structure is passed to daughter cells after DNA replication occurs.

ENHANCERS, PROMOTERS, AND SILENCERS

Several types of *cis*-active DNA sequence elements have been defined according to the presumed consequences of their interaction with nuclear proteins (see Fig. 1–5). *Promoters* are found just upstream (to the 5′ side) of the start of mRNA transcription (the CAP). mRNA polymerases appear to bind first to the promoter region and thereby gain access to the structural gene sequences downstream. Promoters thus serve a dual function of being binding sites for mRNA polymerase and marking for the polymerase the downstream point at which transcription should start.

Enhancers are more complicated DNA sequence elements. Enhancers can lie on either side of a gene, or even within the gene. Enhancers bind transcription factors and thereby stimulate expression of genes nearby. The domain of influence of enhancers (ie, the number of genes to either side whose expression is stimulated) varies. Some enhancers influence only the adjacent gene; others seem to mark the boundaries of large multigene clusters (gene domains) whose coordinated expression is appropriate to a particular tissue type or a particular time. For example, the very high levels of globin gene expression in erythroid cells depend on the function of an enhancer that seems to activate the entire gene cluster and is thus called a locus-activating region (see Fig. 1–5). The nuclear factors interacting with enhancers are probably induced into synthesis or activation as part of the process of differentiation.

Silencer sequences serve a function that is the obverse of enhancers. When bound by the appropriate nuclear proteins, silencer sequences cause repression of gene expression. There is some evidence that the same sequence elements can act as enhancers or silencers under different conditions, presumably by being bound by different sets of proteins having opposite effects on transcription. *Insulators* are sequence domains that mark the "boundaries" of multigene clusters, thereby preventing activation of one set of genes from "leaking" into nearby genes.

TRANSCRIPTION FACTORS

Transcription factors are nuclear proteins that exhibit gene-specific DNA binding. Considerable information is now available about these nuclear proteins and their biochemical properties, but their physiologic behavior remains incompletely understood. Common structural features have become apparent. Most transcription factors have DNA-binding domains sharing homologous structural motifs (cytosine-rich regions called zinc fingers, leucine-rich regions called leucine zippers, etc), but other regions appear to be unique. Many factors implicated in the regulation of growth, differentiation, and development (eg, homeobox genes, protooncogenes, antioncogenes) appear to be DNA-binding proteins and may be involved in the steps needed for activation of a gene within chromatin. Others bind to or modify DNA-binding proteins. These factors are discussed in more detail in several other chapters.

REGULATION OF MRNA SPLICING, STABILITY, AND TRANSLATION (POSTTRANSCRIPTIONAL REGULATION)

It has become increasingly apparent that posttranscriptional and translational mechanisms are important strategies used by cells to govern the amounts of mRNA and protein accumulating when a particular gene is expressed. The major modes of posttranscriptional regulation at the mRNA level are regulated alternative mRNA splicing, control of mRNA stability, and control of translational efficiency. As discussed elsewhere (see Chapter 2), additional regulation at the protein level occurs by mechanisms modulating localization, stability, activation, or export of the protein.

A cell can regulate the relative amounts of different protein isoforms arising from a given gene by altering the relative amounts of an mRNA precursor that are spliced along one pathway or another (alternative mRNA splicing). Many striking examples of this type of regulation are known—for example, the ability of B lymphocytes to make both IgM and IgD at the same developmental stage, changes in the particular isoforms of cytoskeletal proteins produced during red blood cell differentiation, and a switch from one isoform of the *c-myb* protooncogene product to another during red blood cell differentiation. The effect of controlling the pathway of mRNA processing used in a cell is to include or exclude portions of the mRNA sequence. These portions encode peptide sequences that influence the ultimate physiologic behavior of the protein, or the RNA sequences that alter stability or translatability.

The importance of the control of mRNA stability for gene regulation is being increasingly appreciated. The steady-state level of any given mRNA species ultimately depends on the balance between the rate of its production (transcription and mRNA processing) and its destruction. One means by which stability is regulated is the inherent structure of the mRNA sequence, especially the 3′ and 5′ UTRs. As already noted, these sequences appear to affect mRNA secondary structure or recognition by nucleases, or both. Different mRNAs thus have inherently longer or shorter half-lives, almost regardless of the cell type in which they are expressed. Some mRNAs tend to be highly unstable. In response to appropriate physiologic needs, they can thus be produced quickly and removed from the cell quickly when a need for them no longer exists. Globin mRNA, on the other hand, is inherently quite stable, with a half-life measured in the range of 15–50 hours. This is appropriate for the need of reticulocytes to continue to synthesize globin for 24 to 48 hours after the ability to synthesize new mRNA has been lost by the terminally mature erythroblasts.

The stability of mRNA can also be altered in response to changes in the intracellular milieu. This phenomenon usually involves nucleases capable of destroying one or more broad classes of mRNA defined on the basis of their 3′ or 5′ UTR sequences. Thus, for example, histone mRNAs are destabilized after the S phase of the cell cycle is complete. Presumably this occurs because histone synthesis is no longer needed. Induction of cell activation, mitogenesis, or terminal differentiation events often results in the induction of nucleases that destabilize specific subsets of mRNAs. Selective stabilization of mRNAs probably also occurs, but specific examples are less well documented.

The amount of a given protein accumulating in a cell depends on the amount of the mRNA present, the rate at which it is translated into the protein, and the stability of the protein. Translational efficiency depends on a number of variables, including polyadenylation and presence of the 5′ cap. The amounts and state of activation of protein factors needed for translation are also crucial. The secondary structure of the mRNA, particularly in the 5′ UTR, greatly influences the intrinsic translatability of an mRNA molecule by constraining the access of translation factors and ribosomes to the translation initiation signal in the mRNA. Secondary structures along the coding sequence of the mRNA may also have some impact on the rate of elongation of the peptide.

Changes in capping, polyadenylation, and translation factor efficiency affect the overall rate of protein synthesis within each cell. These effects tend to be global, rather than specific to a particular gene product. However, these effects influence the relative amounts of different proteins made. mRNAs whose structures inherently lend themselves to more efficient translation tend to compete better for rate-limiting components of the translational apparatus, whereas those mRNAs that are inherently less translatable tend to be translated less efficiently in the face of limited access to other translational components. For example, the translation factor eIF-4 tends to be produced in higher amounts when cells encounter transforming or mitogenic events. This causes an increase in overall rates of protein synthesis but also leads to a selective increase in the synthesis of some proteins that were underproduced before mitogenesis.

Translational regulation of individual mRNA species is critical for some events important to blood cell homeostasis. For example, as discussed in Chapter 31, the amount of iron entering a cell is an exquisite regulator of the rate of ferritin mRNA translation. An mRNA sequence called the *iron response element* is recognized by a specific mRNA-binding protein, but only when the protein lacks iron. mRNA bound to the protein is translationally inactive. As iron accumulates in the cell, the protein becomes iron bound and loses its affinity for the mRNA, resulting in translation into apoferritin molecules that bind the iron.

Tubulin synthesis involves coordinated regulation of translation and mRNA stability. Tubulin regulates the stability of its own mRNA by a feedback loop. As tubulin concentrations rise in the cell, it interacts with its own mRNA through the intermediary of an mRNA-binding protein. This results in the formation of an mRNA–protein complex and nucleolytic cleavage of the mRNA. The mRNA is destroyed and further tubulin production is halted.

These few examples of posttranscriptional regulation emphasize that cells tend to use every step in the complex pathway of gene expression as points at which exquisite control over the amounts of a particular protein can be regulated. In other chapters, additional levels of regulation are described (eg, regulation of the stability, activity, localization, and access to other cellular components of the proteins that are present in a cell).

SMALL INTERFERING RNA AND MICRO RNA

Recently, posttranscriptional mechanisms of gene silencing involving small RNAs were discovered. One process is carried out by *small interfering RNAs* (siRNAs): short, double-stranded fragments of RNA containing 21 to 23 bp (Fig. 1–6). The process is triggered by perfectly complementary double-stranded RNA, which is cleaved by Dicer, a member of the RNase III family, into siRNA fragments. These small fragments of double-stranded RNA are unwound by a helicase in the RNA-induced silencing complex. The antisense strand anneals to mRNA transcripts in a sequence-specific manner, and in doing so brings the endonuclease activity within the RNA-induced silencing complex to the targeted transcript. An RNA-dependent RNA polymerase in the RNA-induced silencing complex may then create new siRNAs to processively degrade the mRNA, ultimately leading to complete degradation of the mRNA transcript and abrogation of protein expression.

Although this endogenous process likely evolved to destroy invading viral RNA, the use of siRNA has become a commonly used tool for evaluation of gene function. Sequence-specific synthetic siRNA may be directly introduced into cells or introduced via gene transfer methods and targeted to an mRNA of a gene of interest. The siRNA will lead to degradation of the mRNA transcript, and accordingly prevent new protein translation. This technique is a relatively simple, efficient, and inexpensive means to investigate cellular phenotypes after directed elimination of expression of a single gene. The

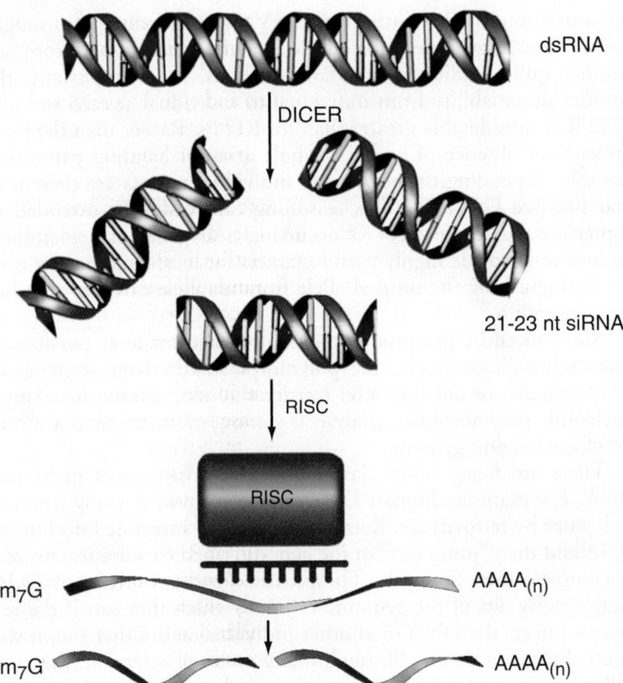

Figure 1–6 mRNA DEGRADATION BY siRNA. Double-stranded RNA is digested into 21- to 23-bp siRNAs by the Dicer RNase. These RNA fragments are unwound by RISC and bring the endonucleolytic activity of RISC to mRNA transcripts in a sequence-specific manner, leading to degradation of the mRNA. mRNA, messenger RNA; RISC, RNA-induced silencing complex; siRNA, small interfering RNA.

2006 Nobel Prize in Physiology or Medicine was awarded to two discoverers of RNA interference, Andrew Fire and Craig Mello.

Micro RNAs (miRNAs) are 22 nt small RNAs encoded by the cellular genome that alter mRNA stability and protein translation. These genes are transcribed by RNA polymerase II, and capped and polyadenylated like other RNA polymerase II transcripts. The precursor transcript of approximately 70 nucleotides is cleaved into mature miRNA by the enzymes Drosha and Dicer. One strand of the resulting duplex forms a complex with the RNA-induced silencing complex that together binds the target mRNA with imperfect complementarity. Through mechanisms that are still incompletely understood, miRNA suppresses gene expression, likely either through inhibition of protein translation or through destabilization of mRNA. miRNAs appear to have essential roles in development and differentiation, and may be aberrantly regulated in cancer cells. The identification of miRNA sequences, their regulation, and their target genes are areas of intense study.

ADDITIONAL STRUCTURAL FEATURES OF GENOMIC DNA

Most DNA does not code for RNA or protein molecules. The vast majority of nucleotides present in the human genome reside outside structural genes. Structural genes are separated from one another by as few as 1 to 5 kilobases, or as many as several thousand kilobases of DNA. Almost nothing is known about the reason for the erratic clustering and spacing of genes along chromosomes. It is clear that intergenic DNA contains a variegated landscape of structural features that provide useful tools to localize genes, identify individual human beings as unique from every other human being (DNA fingerprinting), and diagnose human diseases by linkage. A more detailed discussion of these techniques is included in Chapter 2. Only a brief introduction is provided here.

The rate of mutation in DNA under normal circumstances is approximately $1/10^6$. In other words, 1 of 1 million bases of DNA will be mutated during each round of DNA replication. A set of enzymes called *DNA proofreading enzymes* corrects many but not all of these mutations. When these enzymes are themselves altered by mutation, the rate of mutation (and therefore the odds of neoplastic transformation) increases considerably. If these mutations occur in bases critical to the structure or function of a protein or gene, altered function, disease, or a lethal condition can result. Most pathologic mutations tend not to be preserved throughout many generations because of their unfavorable phenotypes. Exceptions, such as the hemoglobinopathies, occur when the heterozygous state for these mutations confers selective advantage in the face of unusual environmental conditions, such as malaria epidemics. These "adaptive" mutations drive the dynamic change in the genome with time (evolution).

Most of the mutations that accumulate in the DNA of *Homo sapiens* occur in either intergenic DNA or the "silent" bases of DNA, such as the degenerate third bases of codons. They do not pathologically alter the function of the gene or its products. These clinically harmless mutations are called *DNA polymorphisms.* DNA polymorphisms can be regarded in exactly the same way as other types of polymorphisms that have been widely recognized for years (eg, eye and hair color, blood groups). They are variations in the population that occur without apparent clinical impact. Each of us differs from other humans in the precise number and type of DNA polymorphisms that we possess.

Like other types of polymorphisms, DNA polymorphisms breed true. In other words, if an individual's DNA contains a G 1200 bases upstream from the α-globin gene, instead of the C most commonly found in the population, that G will be transmitted to that individual's offspring. Note that if one had a means for distinguishing the G at that position from a C, one would have a linked marker for that individual's α-globin gene.

Occasionally, a DNA polymorphism falls within a restriction endonuclease site. (Restriction enzymes cut DNA molecules into smaller pieces, but only at limited sites, defined by short base sequences recognized by each enzyme.) The change could abolish the site or create a site where one did not exist before. These polymorphisms change the array of fragments generated when the genome is digested by that restriction endonuclease. This permits detection of the polymorphism by use of the appropriate restriction enzyme. This specific class of polymorphisms is thus called *restriction fragment length polymorphisms* (RFLPs).

Restriction fragment length polymorphisms are useful because the length of a restriction endonuclease fragment on which a gene of interest resides provides a linked marker for that gene. The exploitation of this fact for diagnosis of genetic diseases and detection of specific genes is discussed in Chapter 2; Fig. 1–7 shows a simple example.

Restriction fragment length polymorphisms have proved to be extraordinarily useful for the diagnosis of genetic diseases, especially when the precise mutation is not known. Recall that DNA polymorphisms breed true in the population. For example, as discussed in Chapter 116, a mutation that causes hemophilia will, when it occurs on the X chromosome, be transmitted to subsequent generations attached to the pattern (often called a framework or haplotype) of RFLPs that was present on that same X chromosome. If the pattern of RFLPs in the parents is known, the presence of the abnormal chromosome can be detected in the offspring.

An important feature of the DNA landscape is the high degree of repeated DNA sequence. A DNA sequence is said to be repeated if it or a sequence very similar (homologous) to it occurs more than once in a genome. Some multicopy genes, such as the histone genes and the ribosomal RNA genes, are repeated DNA sequences. Most repeated DNA occurs outside genes, or within introns. Indeed, 30% to 45% of the human genome appears to consist of repeated DNA sequences.

The function of repeated sequences remains unknown, but their presence has inspired useful strategies for detecting and characterizing individual genomes. For example, a pattern of short repeated DNA sequences, characterized by the presence of flanking sites recognized by the restriction endonuclease Alu-1 (called Alu-repeats), occurs approximately 300,000 times in a human genome. These sequences

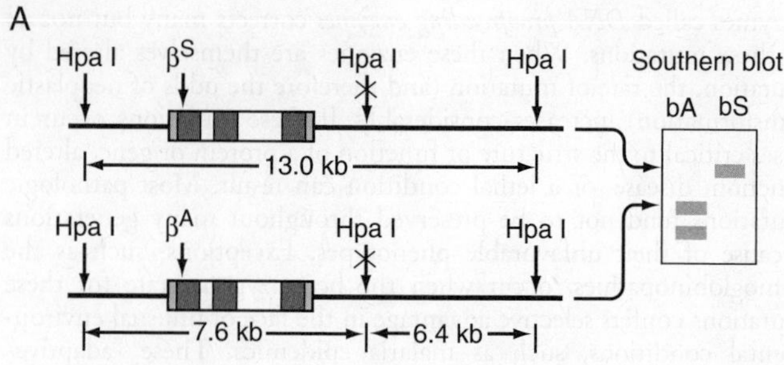

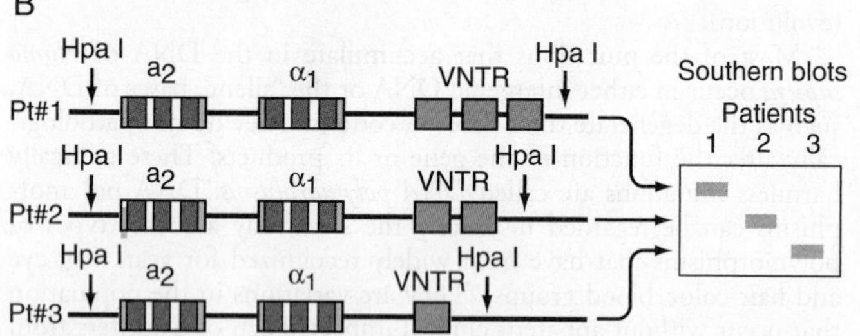

Figure 1–7 TWO USEFUL FORMS OF SEQUENCE VARIATION AMONG THE GENOMES OF NORMAL INDIVIDUALS. **A,** Presence of a DNA sequence polymorphism that falls within a restriction endonuclease site, thus altering the pattern of restriction endonuclease digests obtained from this region of DNA on Southern blot analysis. (Readers not familiar with Southern blot analysis should return to examine this figure after reading later sections of this chapter.) **B,** A variable-number tandem repeat (VNTR) region (defined and discussed in the text). Note that individuals can vary from one to another in many ways according to how many repeated units of the VNTR are located on their genomes, whereas restriction fragment length polymorphism differences are in effect all-or-none differences, allowing for only two variables (restriction site presence or absence).

are not present in the mouse genome. If one wishes to infect mouse cells with human DNA and then identify the human DNA sequences in the infected mouse cells, one simply probes for the presence of Alu-repeats. The Alu-repeat thus serves as a signature of human DNA.

Classes of highly repeated DNA sequences (tandem repeats) have proved to be useful for distinguishing genomes of each human individual. These short DNA sequences, usually less than a few hundred bases long, tend to occur in clusters, with the number of repeats varying between individuals (see Fig. 1–6). Alleles of a given gene can therefore be associated with a variable number of tandem repeats (VNTR) in different individuals or populations. For example, there is a VNTR near the insulin gene. In some individuals or populations, it is present in only a few tandem copies, whereas in others it is present in many more. When the population as a whole is examined, there is a wide degree of variability from individual to individual as to the number of these repeats residing near the insulin gene. It can readily be imagined that if probes were available to detect a dozen or so distinct VNTR regions, each human individual would differ from virtually all others with respect to the aggregate pattern of these VNTRs. Indeed, it can be shown mathematically that the probability of any two human beings' sharing exactly the same pattern of VNTRs is exceedingly small if approximately 10 to 12 different VNTR elements are mapped for each person. A technique called DNA fingerprinting that is based on VNTR analysis has become widely publicized because of its forensic applications.

Variable-number tandem repeats can be regarded as normal sequence variations in DNA that are similar to, but far more useful than, single-base-change RFLP polymorphisms. Note that the odds of a single base change altering a convenient restriction endonuclease site are relatively small, so that RFLPs occur relatively infrequently in a useful region of the genome. Moreover, there is only one state or variable that can be examined—that is, the presence or absence of the restriction site. By contrast, many VNTRs are scattered throughout the human genome. Most of these can be distinguished from one another quite readily by standard methods. Most important, the amount of variability from individual to individual at each site of a VNTR is considerably greater than for RFLPs. Rather than the mere presence or absence of a site, a whole array of banding patterns is possible, depending on how many individual repeats are present at that site (see Fig. 1–6). This reasoning can readily be extended to appreciate that those VNTRs occurring near genes of hematologic interest can provide highly useful markers for localizing that gene, or for distinguishing the normal allele from an allele carrying a pathologic mutation.

More recently, genomic technologies have made it possible to characterize single nucleotide polymorphisms in large stretches of DNA whether or not they alter restriction endonuclease sites. Single nucleotide polymorphism analysis is gaining momentum as a means for characterizing genomes.

There are many other classes of repeated sequences in human DNA. For example, human DNA has been invaded many times in its history by retroviruses. Retroviruses tend to integrate into human DNA and then "jump out" of the genome when they are reactivated, to complete their life cycle. The proviral genomes often carry with them nearby bits of the genomic DNA in which they sat. If the retrovirus infects the DNA of another individual at another site, it will insert this genomic bit. Through many cycles of infection, the virus will act as a transposon, scattering its attached sequence throughout the genome. These types of sequences are called *long interspersed elements.* They represent footprints of ancient viral infections.

KEY METHODS FOR GENE ANALYSIS

The foundation for the molecular understanding of gene structure and expression is based on fundamental molecular biologic techniques that were developed in the 1970s and 1980s. These techniques allow for the reduction of the multibillion nucleotide genome into smaller fragments that are more easily analyzed. Several key methods are outlined here.

Restriction Endonucleases

Naturally occurring bacterial enzymes called *restriction endonucleases* catalyze sequence-specific hydrolysis of phosphodiester bonds in the DNA backbone. For example, *Eco*RI, a restriction endonuclease isolated from *Escherichia coli,* cleaves DNA only at the sequence 5′-GAATTC-3′. Thus, each DNA sample will be reproducibly reduced to an array of fragments whose size ranges depend on the distribution with which that sequence exists within the DNA. A specific six-nucleotide sequence would be statistically expected to appear once every 4^6 (or 4096) nucleotides, but in reality the distance between specific sequences varies greatly. Using combinations of restriction endonucleases, DNA several hundred million base pairs in length can be reproducibly reduced to fragments ranging from a few dozen to tens of thousands of base pairs long. These smaller products of enzymatic digestion are much more manageable experimentally. Genetic "fingerprinting," or restriction enzyme maps of genomes, can be constructed by analyzing the DNA fragments resulting from digestion. Many enzymes cleave DNA so as to leave short, single-stranded overhanging regions that can be enzymatically linked to other similar fragments, generating artificially recombined, or *recombinant,* DNA molecules. These ligated gene fragments can then be inserted into bacteria to produce more copies of the recombinant molecules or to express the cloned genes.

DNA, RNA, and Protein Blotting

There are many ways that a cloned DNA sequence can be exploited to characterize the behavior of normal or pathologic genes. Blotting

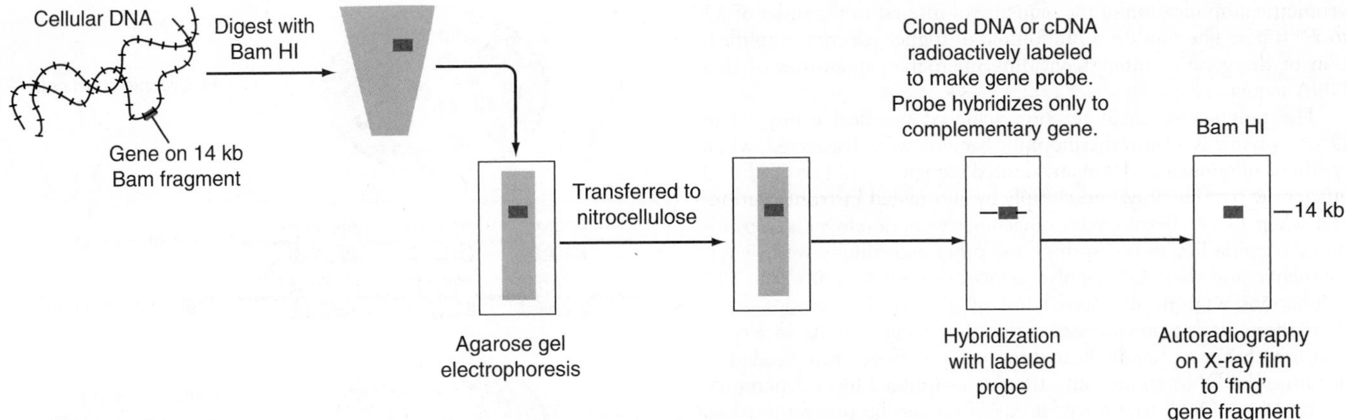

Figure 1–8 SOUTHERN GENE BLOTTING. Detection of a genomic gene (*red*) that resides on a 14-kilobase Bam HI fragment. To identify the presence of a gene in the genome and the size of the restriction fragment on which it resides, genomic DNA is digested with a restriction enzyme, and the fragments are separated by agarose gel electrophoresis. Human genomes contain from several hundred thousand to 1 million sites for any particular restriction enzyme, which results in a vast array of fragments and creates a blur or streak on the gel; one fragment cannot be distinguished from another readily. If the DNA in the gel is transferred to nitrocellulose by capillary blotting, however, it can be further analyzed by molecular hybridization to a radioactive cDNA probe for the gene. Only the band containing the gene yields a positive autoradiography signal, as shown. If a disease state were to result in loss of the gene, alteration of its structure, or mutation (altering recognition sites for one or more restriction enzymes), the banding pattern would be changed.

methods deserve special mention because of their widespread use in clinical and experimental hematology. A cloned DNA fragment can be easily purified and tagged with a radioactive or nonradioactive label. The fragment provides a pure and highly specific molecular hybridization probe for the detection of complementary DNA or RNA molecules in any specimen of DNA or RNA. One set of assays that has proved particularly useful involves Southern blotting, named after Dr E. Southern, who invented the method (Fig. 1–8). Southern blotting allows detection of a specific gene, or region in or near a gene, in a DNA preparation. The DNA is isolated and digested with one or more restriction endonucleases, and the resulting fragments are denatured and separated according to their molecular size by electrophoresis through agarose gels. By means of capillary action in a high salt buffer, the DNA fragments are passively transferred to a nitrocellulose or nylon membrane. Single-stranded DNA and RNA molecules attach noncovalently but tightly to the membrane. In this fashion, the membrane becomes a replica, or blot, of the gel. After the blotting procedure is complete, the membrane is incubated in a hybridization buffer containing the radioactively labeled probe. The probe hybridizes only to the gene of interest and renders radioactive only one or a few bands containing complementary sequences. After appropriate washing and drying, the bands can be visualized by autoradiography.

Digestion of a DNA preparation with several different restriction enzymes allows a restriction endonuclease map of a gene in the human genome to be constructed. Southern blotting has thus become a standard way of characterizing the configuration of genes in the genome.

Northern blotting represents an analogous blotting procedure used to detect RNA. RNA cannot be digested with restriction enzymes (which cut only DNA); rather, the intact RNA molecules can be separated according to molecular size by electrophoresis through the gel (mRNAs are 0.5–12 kilobases in length), transferred onto membranes, and probed with a DNA probe. In this fashion, the presence, absence, molecular size, and number of individual species of a particular mRNA species can be detected.

Western blotting is a similar method that can be used to examine protein expression. Cellular lysates (or another source of proteins) can be electrophoresed through a polyacrylamide gel so as to separate proteins on the basis of their apparent molecular sizes. The resolved proteins can then be electrically transferred to nitrocellulose membranes and probed with specific antibodies directed against the protein of interest. As with RNA analysis, the relative expression levels and molecular sizes of proteins can be assessed with this method.

Polymerase Chain Reaction

The development of the polymerase chain reaction was a major breakthrough that has revolutionized the utility of a DNA-based strategy for diagnosis and treatment. It permits the detection, synthesis, and isolation of specific genes and allows differentiation of alleles of a gene differing by as little as one base. It does not require sophisticated equipment or unusual technical skills. A clinical specimen consisting of only minute amounts of tissue will suffice; in most circumstances, no special preparation of the tissue is necessary. Polymerase chain reaction thus makes recombinant DNA techniques accessible to clinical laboratories. This single advance has produced a quantum increase in the use of direct gene analysis for diagnosis of human diseases.

The polymerase chain reaction is based on the prerequisites for copying an existing DNA strand by DNA polymerase: an existing denatured strand of DNA to be used as the template, and a primer. Primers are short oligonucleotides, 12 to 100 bases in length, having a base sequence complementary to the desired region of the existing DNA strand. The enzyme requires the primer to "know" where to begin copying. If the base sequence of the DNA of the gene under study is known, two synthetic oligonucleotides complementary to sequences flanking the region of interest can be prepared. If these are the only oligonucleotides present in the reaction mixture, then the DNA polymerase can only copy daughter strands of DNA downstream from those oligonucleotides. Recall that DNA is double stranded, that the strands are held together by the rules of Watson-Crick base pairing, and that they are aligned in antiparallel fashion. This implies that the effect of incorporation of both oligonucleotides into the reaction mix will be to synthesize two daughter strands of DNA, one originating upstream of the gene and the other originating downstream. The net effect is synthesis of only the DNA between the two primers, thus doubling only the DNA containing the region of interest. If the DNA is now heat denatured, allowing hybridization of the daughter strands to the primers, and the polymerization is repeated, then the region of DNA through the gene of interest is doubled again. Thus, two cycles of denaturation, annealing, and elongation result in a selective quadrupling of the gene of interest. The cycle can be repeated 30 to 50 times, resulting in a selective and geometric amplification of the sequence of interest to the order of 2^{30} to 2^{50} times. The result is a millionfold or higher selective amplification of the gene of interest, yielding microgram quantities of that DNA sequence.

The polymerase chain reaction achieved practical utility when DNA polymerases from thermophilic bacteria were discovered, when synthetic oligonucleotides of any desired sequence could be produced efficiently, reproducibly, and cheaply by automated instrumentation, and when DNA thermocycling machines were developed. Thermophilic bacteria live in hot springs and other exceedingly warm environments, and their DNA polymerases can tolerate 100°C (212°F) incubations without substantial loss of activity. The advantage of these thermostable polymerases is that they retain activity in a reaction mix that is repeatedly heated to the high temperature needed to denature the DNA strands into the single-stranded form. Microprocessor-driven DNA thermocycler machines can be programmed to increase temperatures to 95°C to 100°C (203°F to 212°F) (denaturation), to cool the mix to 50°C (101°F) rapidly (a temperature that favors oligonucleotide annealing), and then to raise the temperature to 70°C to 75°C (141.4°F to 151.5°F) (the temperature for optimal activity of the thermophilic DNA polymerases). In a reaction containing the test specimen, the thermophilic polymerase, the primers, and the chemical components (eg, nucleotide subunits), the thermocycler can conduct many cycles of denaturation, annealing, and polymerization in a completely automated fashion. The gene of interest can thus be amplified more than a millionfold in a matter of a few hours. The DNA product is readily identified and isolated by routine agarose gel electrophoresis. The DNA can then be analyzed by restriction endonuclease, digestion, hybridization to specific probes, sequencing, further amplification by cloning, and so forth.

USE OF TRANSGENIC AND KNOCKOUT MICE TO DEFINE GENE FUNCTION

Recombinant DNA technology has resulted in the identification of many disease-related genes. To advance the understanding of the disease related to a previously unknown gene, the function of the protein encoded by that gene must be verified or identified, and the way changes in the gene's expression influence the disease phenotype must be characterized. Analysis of the role of these genes and their encoded proteins has been made possible by the development of recombinant DNA technology that allows the production of mice that are genetically altered at the cloned locus. Mice can be produced that express an exogenous gene and thereby provide an in vivo model of its function. Linearized DNA is injected into a fertilized mouse oocyte pronucleus and reimplanted in a pseudopregnant mouse. The resultant *transgenic mice* can then be analyzed for the phenotype induced by the injected transgene. Placing the gene under the control of a strong promoter that stimulates expression of the exogenous gene in all tissues allows the assessment of the effect of widespread overexpression of the gene. Alternatively, placing the gene under the control of a promoter that can function only in certain tissues (a tissue-specific promoter) elucidates the function of that gene in a particular tissue or cell type. A third approach is to study control elements of the gene by testing their capacity to drive expression of a "marker" gene that can be detected by chemical, immunologic, or functional means. For example, the promoter region of a gene of interest can be joined to the cDNA encoding green jellyfish protein, and activity of the gene assessed in various tissues of the resultant transgenic mouse by fluorescence microscopy. Use of such a reporter gene demonstrates the normal distribution and timing of expression of the gene from which the promoter elements are derived. Transgenic mice contain exogenous genes that insert randomly into the genome of the recipient. Expression can thus depend as much on the location of the insertion as it does on the properties of the injected DNA.

In contrast, any defined genetic locus can be specifically altered by targeted recombination between the locus and a plasmid carrying an altered version of that gene (Fig. 1–9). If a plasmid contains that altered gene with enough flanking DNA identical to that of the normal gene locus, homologous recombination can occur, and the altered gene in the plasmid will replace the gene in the recipient cell. Using a mutation that inactivates the gene allows the production of a null mutation, in which the function of that gene is completely lost. To induce such a mutation, the plasmid is introduced into an embryonic stem cell, and the rare cells that undergo homologous recombination are selected. The "knockout" embryonic stem cell is then introduced into the blastocyst of a developing embryo. The resultant animals are chimeric; only a fraction of the cells in the animal contain the targeted gene. If the new gene is introduced into some of the germline cells of the chimeric mouse, then some of the offspring of that mouse will carry the mutation as a gene in all of their cells. These heterozygous mice can be further bred to produce mice homozygous for the null allele. Such knockout mice reveal the function of the targeted gene by the phenotype induced by its absence. Genetically altered mice have been essential for discerning the biologic and pathologic roles of large numbers of genes implicated in the pathogenesis of human disease.

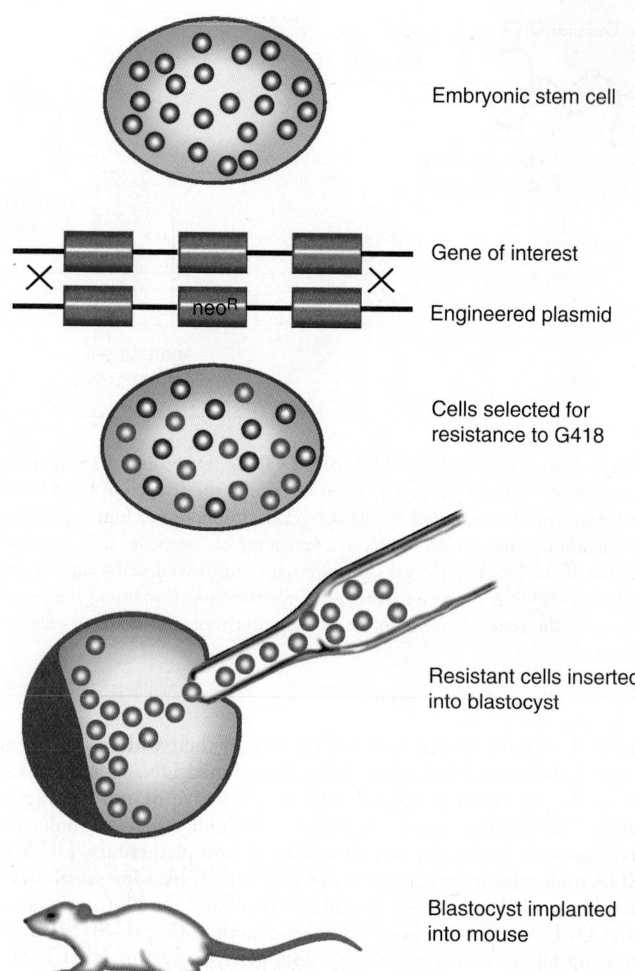

Figure 1–9 GENE "KNOCKOUT" BY HOMOLOGOUS RECOMBINATION. A plasmid containing genomic DNA homologous to the gene of interest is engineered to contain a selectable marker positioned so as to disrupt expression of the native gene. The DNA is introduced into embryonic stem cells, and cells resistant to the selectable marker are isolated and injected into a mouse blastocyst, which is then implanted into a mouse. Offspring mice that contain the knockout construct in their germ cells are then propagated, yielding mice with heterozygous or homozygous inactivation of the gene of interest.

DNA-BASED THERAPIES

Gene Therapy

The application of gene therapy to genetic hematologic disorders is an appealing idea. In most cases, this would involve isolating hematopoietic stem cells from patients with diseases with defined genetic lesions, inserting normal genes into those cells, and reintroducing the genetically engineered stem cells back into the patient. A few candidate diseases for such therapy include sickle cell disease, thalassemia, hemophilia, and adenosine deaminase-deficient severe combined immunodeficiency. The technology for separating hematopoietic stem cells and for performing gene transfer into those cells has advanced rapidly, and clinical trials have begun to test the applicability of these techniques. However, despite the fact that gene therapy has progressed to the enrollment of patients in clinical protocols, major technical problems still need to be solved, and there are no proven therapeutic successes from gene therapy. However, progress in this field continues rapidly. The scientific basis for gene therapy and the clinical issues surrounding this approach are discussed in Chapter 102.

Antisense Therapy

The recognition that abnormal expression of oncogenes plays a role in malignancy has stimulated attempts to suppress oncogene expression to reverse the neoplastic phenotype. One way of blocking mRNA expression is with antisense oligonucleotides. These are single-stranded DNA sequences, 17 to 20 bases long, having a sequence complementary to the transcription or translation start of the mRNA. These relatively small molecules freely enter the cell and complex to the mRNA by their complementary DNA sequence. This often results in a decrease in gene expression. The binding of the oligonucleotide may directly block translation and clearly enhances the rate of mRNA degradation. This technique has been shown to be promising in suppressing expression of *bcr-abl* and to suppress cell growth in chronic myelogenous leukemia. The technique is being tried as a therapeutic modality for the purging of tumor cells before autologous transplantation in patients with chronic myelogenous leukemia.

SUMMARY

The elegance of recombinant DNA technology resides in the capacity it confers on investigators to examine each gene as a discrete physical entity that can be purified, reduced to its basic building blocks for decoding of its primary structure, analyzed for its patterns of expression, and perturbed by alterations in sequence or molecular environment so that the effects of changes in each region of the gene can be assessed. Purified genes can be deliberately modified or mutated to create novel genes not available in nature. These provide the potential to generate useful new biologic entities, such as modified live virus or purified peptide vaccines, modified proteins customized for specific therapeutic purposes, and altered combinations of regulatory and structural genes that allow for the assumption of new functions by specific gene systems.

Purified genes facilitate the study of gene regulation in many ways. First, a cloned gene provides characterized DNA probes for molecular hybridization assays. Second, cloned genes provide the homogeneous DNA moieties needed to determine the exact nucleotide sequence. Sequencing techniques have become so reliable and efficient that it is often easier to clone the gene encoding a protein of interest and determine its DNA sequence than it is to purify the protein and determine its amino acid sequence. The DNA sequence predicts exactly the amino acid sequence of its protein product. By comparing normal sequences with the sequences of alleles cloned from patients known to be abnormal, such as the globin genes in the thalassemia or sickle cell syndromes, the normal and pathologic anatomy of genes critical to major hematologic diseases can be established. In this manner, it has been possible to identify many mutations responsible for various forms of thalassemia, hemophilia, thrombasthenia, red blood cell enzymopathies, porphyrias, and so forth. Similarly, single base changes have been shown to be the difference between many normally functioning protooncogenes and their cancer-promoting oncogene derivatives.

Third, cloned genes can be manipulated for studies of gene expression. Many vectors allowing efficient transfer of genes into eukaryotic cells have been perfected. Gene transfer technologies allow the gene to be placed into the desired cellular environment and the expression of that gene or the behavior of its products to be analyzed. These surrogate or reverse genetics systems allow analysis of the normal physiology of expression of a particular gene, as well as the pathophysiology of abnormal gene expression resulting from mutations.

Fourth, cloned genes enhance study of their protein products. By expressing fragments of the gene in microorganisms or eukaryotic cells, customized regions of a protein can be produced for use as an immunogen, thereby allowing preparation of a variety of useful and powerful antibody probes. Alternatively, synthetic peptides deduced from the DNA sequence can be prepared as the immunogen. Controlled production of large amounts of the protein also allows direct analysis of specific functions attributable to regions in that protein.

Finally, all of the aforementioned techniques can be extended by mutating the gene and examining the effects of those mutations on the expression of or the properties of the encoded mRNAs and proteins. By combining portions of one gene with another (chimeric genes), or abutting structural regions of one gene with regulatory sequences of another, the researcher can investigate in previously inconceivable ways the complexities of gene regulation. These activist approaches to modifying gene structure or expression create the opportunity to generate new RNA and protein products whose applications are limited only by the collective imagination of the investigators.

The most important impact of the genetic approach to the analysis of biologic phenomena is the most indirect. Diligent and repeated application of the methods outlined in this chapter to the study of many genes from diverse groups of organisms is beginning to reveal the basic strategies used by nature for the regulation of cell and tissue behavior. As our knowledge of these rules of regulation grows, our ability to understand, detect, and correct pathologic phenomena will increase substantially.

SUGGESTED READINGS

Bentley D: The mRNA assembly line: Transcription and processing machines in the same factory. Curr Opin Cell Biol 14:336, 2002.

Dykxhoorn DM, Novina CD, Sharp PA: Killing the messenger: Short RNAs that silence gene expression. Nat Rev Mol Cell Biol 4:457, 2003.

Fischle W, Wang Y, Allis CD: Histone and chromatin cross-talk. Curr Opin Cell Biol 15:172, 2003.

Grewal SI, Moazed D: Heterochromatin and epigenetic control of gene expression. Science 301:798, 2003.

Kloosterman WP, Plasterk RHA: The diverse functions of microRNAs in animal development and disease. Dev Cell 11:441, 2006.

Klose RJ, Bird AP: Genomic DNA methylation: The mark and its mediators. Trends Biochem Sci 31:89, 2006.

Lee TI, Young RA: Transcription of eukaryotic protein-coding genes. Annu Rev Genet 34:77, 2000.

Tefferi A, Wieben ED, Dewald GW, et al: Primer on medical genomics, part II: Background principles and methods in molecular genetics. Mayo Clinic Proc 77:785, 2002.

Wilusz CJ, Wormington M, Peltz SW: The cap-to-tail guide to mRNA turnover. Nat Rev Mol Cell Biol 2:237, 2001.

CHAPTER 2

GENOMIC APPROACHES TO THE STUDY OF HEMATOLOGIC SCIENCE

Benjamin L. Ebert, Todd R. Golub, and Scott A. Armstrong

The publication of the initial sequence of the human genome heralded the beginning of a period in biomedical research that will be heavily influenced by the field of genomics.[1] Just as molecular biology changed the face of biomedical research in the 1970s and 1980s, genomics promises a novel perspective into biological questions and human disease. Broadly defined, genomics is the study of biological processes in a manner that takes advantage of the information that has come from the sequencing of the genomes of humans and other organisms. The new technologies that have been developed allow quantitative and parallel assessment of thousands of variables in a single experiment, including mRNA expression, microRNA expression, DNA copy number, single nucleotide polymorphisms, and epigenetic modifications.

This new comprehensive approach to biology has already provided an improved understanding of a number of biological processes and disease states including hematologic malignancies. As has often been the case, the study of hematologic malignancies has proven to be an attractive training ground for the application of new technologies. Genomic analysis has progressed more rapidly in hematologic malignancies than in other diseases such as solid tumors a result of extensive knowledge about the lineage specific gene expression programs present in developing blood cells and the ability to obtain relatively pure populations of cells. Combined with the detailed characterization of recurrent chromosomal abnormalities in leukemia and lymphoma, this provides a foundation of knowledge that has aided in the interpretation of complex datasets. Finally, the development of sophisticated model systems that faithfully recapitulate human diseases represent valuable tools necessary for validation of the hypotheses that come from genomic experiments.

The massive increase in the size of datasets has subsequently led to an expansion of the field of bioinformatics, which has become a critical part of genomic experiments. The datasets generated by genomic technologies are large and potentially contaminated by experimental or biological noise. Since genomic datasets typically involve the assessment of thousands of variables in a relatively modest number of samples, analyses are prone to overinterpretation. "Traditional" clinical trials, in contrast, generally have few variables and are assessed in larger numbers of samples or patients. Genomic experiments require careful assessment of statistical significance, and validation by independent datasets or experimental systems. When carefully performed, such global genomic views provide different types of insight into disease than do narrow but deeper traditional views. In this chapter, we will outline the current technologies available for genomic analysis, describe some of the bioinformatic tools that are available, and highlight some of the applications of this technology to the study of hematologic diseases.

TECHNOLOGY PLATFORMS

Comparative Gene Expression Analysis

The most well developed and widely used genomic technology is genome-wide expression profiling. Gene expression profiling allows one to quantitatively assess the RNA expression level for thousands of genes simultaneously. The most commonly used platforms on which to perform such an analysis are DNA microarrays. A DNA microarray generally consists of a glass slide or silica wafer to which either complementary DNA (cDNA) or oligonucleotide probes are attached. The probes can be chosen based on knowledge of genes expressed in a particular cell type (eg, the "lymphochip")[2] or they can be chosen from genomic databases, which do not require previous knowledge about gene expression in a given cell type. Current microarray technology allows a density of over one million oligonucleotide probes per array. Since current estimates suggest the human genome consists of approximately 26,000 genes, we now have the capability to assess the expression of almost all genes in a given sample in a single experiment.

Oligonucleotide arrays can be generated by depositing oligonucleotides onto glass slides or directly synthesizing oligonucleotides between 25 and 60 nucleotides long on a solid support.[3–5] The most widely used oligonucleotide arrays are commercially available from Affymetrix (Santa Clara, CA). These arrays are produced by photolithographically synthesizing oligonucleotides onto a silica support. For experiments with this type of array, one labels the RNA sample of interest by first producing double stranded DNA, and then performing an in vitro transcription reaction that incorporates biotinylated nucleotides into the resulting chromosomal RNA (cRNA) (Fig. 2–1A). The labeled cRNA is then hybridized to the array, and the amount of hybridized cRNA is quantitated by a streptavidin-phycoerythrin conjugate. The major limitation of this technology is the high cost of the arrays, but their ease of use has made this technology the dominant platform for global gene expression profiling.

Alternative technologies for gene expression profiling include cDNA arrays and sequencing strategies. cDNA arrays are produced by robotic-spotting of thousands of polymerase chain reaction (PCR)-amplified cDNA clones onto glass slides.[6–8] The RNA sample of interest is then reverse-transcribed to produce cDNA labeled with a fluorescent dye (generally either Cy3 or Cy5). This labeled cDNA is then hybridized to the array in conjunction with a reference cDNA sample that is labeled with the second die (Fig. 2–1B). The relative abundance of a given RNA species in the experimental sample is then determined by comparing the intensity of the fluorescent signals from each of the dies for a given probe. The major advantage of such array technology is that once one has an appropriate cDNA library and the spotting device, they theoretically should be able to produce many arrays at a relatively low cost. In practice though, it has proven more difficult to produce high quality cDNA arrays than expected unless the center has significant expertise in such techniques.

Another method to assess genome-wide gene expression is serial analysis of gene expression (SAGE).[9] The first step in performing SAGE is to perform PCR with oligonucleotides that allow for amplification of all cDNA species within a sample. After this has been performed, high throughput sequencing is performed on many thousands of PCR amplicons and the number of unique sequences determined. This allows one to determine the number of RNA transcripts that were present in the initial sample. Therefore, SAGE is a method that counts the number of transcripts, whereas microarrays only allow one to look at the relative abundance of a given gene across two samples. The ability to compare the number of transcripts within a given sample is one of the major advantages of this technology; microarray analysis cannot do this because of the different hybridization efficiencies of different probes. The sequencing of large numbers of transcripts is expensive, so SAGE is not currently a commonly used approach to gene expression profiling. The development of single

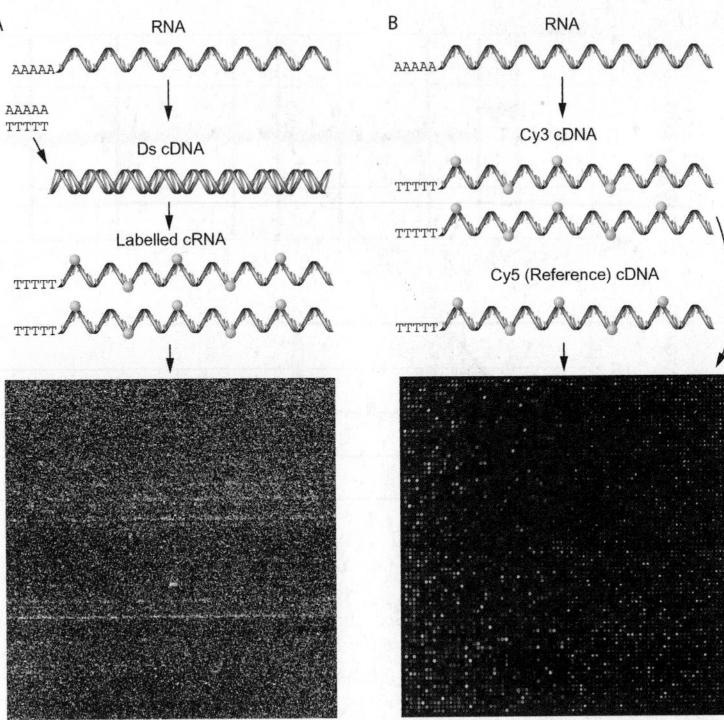

Figure 2–1 GENE EXPRESSION PROFILING USING DNA MICROARRAYS. Images from an Affymetrix oligonucleotide array (**A**) and a complementary DNA (cDNA) array (**B**). RNA labeling techniques are shown. **A,** For an Affymetrix oligonucleotide array experiment, double-stranded cDNA is first produced, and then an in vitro transcription reaction is performed with biotinylated nucleotides, to give labeled cRNA. This RNA sample is then hybridized to the array without the addition of a control sample. **B,** For hybridization to a cDNA array, Cy3- or Cy5-labeled cDNA is produced from experimental and control RNA samples. Hybridization experiments performed on cDNA arrays compare the relative amounts of a given RNA species in the labeled experimental and control samples that are hybridized to the array simultaneously.

molecule sequencing technologies, discussed below, may make a sequencing-based, high-throughput sequencing technologies may make SAGE a more attractive platform.

Analysis of MicroRNA Expression

MicroRNAs (miRNAs) are small (approximately 22 nucleotides) RNAs that do not encode for proteins, but bind to mRNA transcripts to regulate translation and mRNA stability. In *Caenorhabditis elegans*, zebrafish, and other model organisms, miRNAs play a critical role in development through regulation of translation of key proteins. In mammalian cells, a role for miRNAs has been recognized in the regulation of cellular differentiation. Not only are many miRNAs differentially expressed across hematopoietic lineages, but several miRNAs have been demonstrated to play key functional roles in hematopoietic lineage specification and differentiation.[10] Moreover, the expression or function of several miRNAs is altered by chromosomal translocations, deletions, or mutations in leukemia.[10]

Several methodologies have been developed for the detection of miRNAs. As with mRNA, individual miRNAs can be assayed by Northern blots or quantitative reverse-transcription PCR. Global miRNA profiles can be detected using microarrays or bead-based technologies using platforms that are highly analogous to the mRNA gene expression profiles.[11,12] Global miRNA profiles are sufficient to distinguish different differentiation states and can be used for the classification of cancers.[12] The expression of miRNAs is a key aspect of the complete genomic characterization of cellular states and, in some cases, may provide critical insights into the biology of the malignant transformation of hematopoietic cells.

Analysis of Changes in Gene Copy Number

Gains (amplifications) or losses (deletions) of genetic material at specific loci are recognized as playing an important role in the pathophysiology of disease. Dramatic examples of this association come from the study of inherited cancer predisposition syndromes. The most prominent example emanated from the study of families demonstrating a predisposition for development of retinoblastoma. In a landmark set of studies, it was shown that tumors from patients who inherit a mutant copy of the retinoblastoma tumor suppressor gene often contain deletions of the remaining allele.[13–16] This process has been termed *loss of heterozygosity*, and the search for genetic loci showing loss of heterozygosity in tumor samples has identified a number of genes that are involved in critical cellular processes and are important for cancer progression. Similarly, amplification of genomic loci can play an important role in oncogenesis and cancer biology. For example, amplification of the HER2/Neu oncogene in human breast cancer is associated with a poor prognosis, and HER2/Neu has been shown to be an important therapeutic target in this disease.[17,18]

The search for gains and losses of genetic material can be done using a number of techniques that require various levels of expertise, and allow assessment of genomic integrity at various resolutions. The first method developed to assess genomic integrity, *cytogenetic analysis*, is still used today, but it allows identification only of abnormalities that encompass large regions of DNA. Nevertheless, cytogenetic analysis has provided tremendous insight into the pathophysiology of disease, particularly for leukemogenesis.[19] Cytogenetic analysis remains a key part of the diagnostic workup for new cases of leukemia.

Another, more recently developed technology is that of *comparative genomic hybridization* (CGH).[20] To perform CGH analysis, tumor DNA and normal genomic DNA are labeled with different fluorescent dyes and are hybridized to a metaphase spread that is prepared in a fashion similar to that used in routine cytogenetic analysis. Gains and losses are determined on the basis of the relative fluorescence at any given location along the chromosome. Although this technique allows assessment of genomic integrity at a greater resolution than is possible with cytogenetic analysis, the resolution is still only in the 10- to 20-megabase (Mb) range. Also, CGH requires that the sample of interest has been characterized by cytogenetic analysis.

A recently developed method that has improved genomic resolution to less than 1 Mb and has all but replaced standard CGH is array CGH (aCGH).[21–23] Although this method still requires significant expertise to produce custom arrays, it allows high resolution and does not require any previous characterization such as cytogenetic analysis. Analogous to the design of gene expression microarrays, aCGH probes can be derived from oligonucleotides, cDNAs, or larger DNA fragments produced from bacterial artificial chromosomes (BACs).

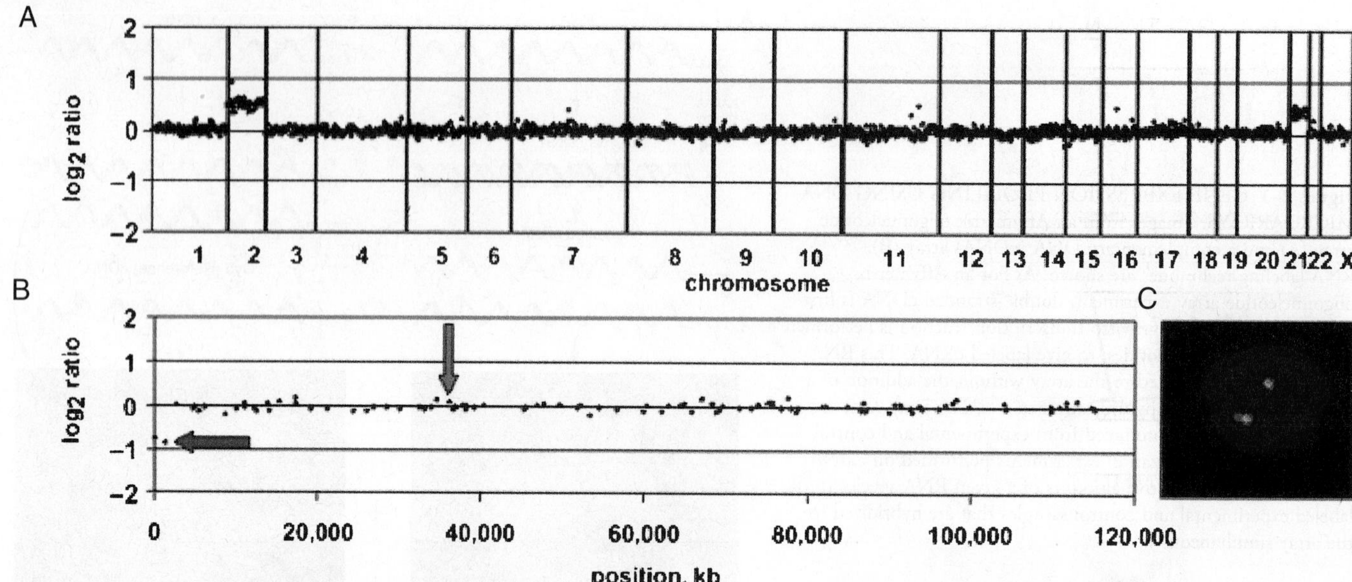

Figure 2–2 **A,** An example of array-based comparative genomic hybridization (CGH) performed on a cell line known to be trisomic for chromosomes 2 and 21. This technique entails comparison of fluorescence intensities of triplicate spots for each given BAC clone, represented graphically by individual spots. The data are presented for chromosomes 1p to Xq (oriented from *left* to *right*), and *bars* separate clones on different chromosomes. It is evident from the array CGH data that there are extra copies of chromosomes 2 and 21, as determined originally by FISH analysis. **B,** Array CGH data from a cell line on BACs from chromosome 9. The $\log_2$ ratio of −1 for two of the clones *(red arrow)* indicates a single-copy deletion in this region on chromosome 9. Colored arrows indicate the clones that were labeled and used to perform FISH analysis to verify the array CGH data. **C,** FISH analysis of the cell line analyzed in B using the BAC probes identified by the *colored arrows*. Note only one signal from the BAC, corresponding to the *red arrow*. BAC, bacterial artificial chromosome; FISH, fluorescence in situ hybridization. *(From Snijders AM, Nowak N, Segraves R, et al: Assembly of microarrays for genome-wide measurement of DNA copy number. Nat Genet 29:263, 2001.)*

Probes that correspond to a known location within the human genome are spotted onto glass microarrays, and the experimental genomic DNA and normal genomic DNA are labeled with either Cy3 or Cy5, as in glass slide-based microarray analysis. Relative gains or losses of genomic material are then determined on the basis of the relative Cy3 or Cy5 fluorescence at any given spot (Fig. 2–2).

Oligonucleotide microarrays designed for the detection of single nucleotide polymorphisms (SNPs) are also being widely utilized for the analysis of copy number change in tumor samples. In addition to the detection of gains and losses of chromosomal material, SNP arrays can be used to detect loss of heterozygosity in a chromosomal region that has not had a change in copy number. Unlike aCGH, in which tumor and control samples are labeled with different fluors and hybridized to the same array, a single sample is hybridized to a SNP array. SNP arrays have been utilized to identify novel genes contribute to the pathogenesis of acute leukemia.[24]

Single-Nucleotide Polymorphisms

Since the initial proposal to look for association of certain inherited diseases with common genetic polymorphisms found in the human genome,[25] linkage analysis has been a particularly successful method for identification of disease-associated genes, such as those responsible for chronic granulomatous disease and cystic fibrosis.[26,27] This method is limited, however, by the number of individuals in a family with the disease, and by the number of polymorphisms present in the region of the genome where the disease gene resides. The latter of these two problems is becoming less of an issue as the number of recognized SNPs increases. SNPs represent single nucleotides within the human genome that are polymorphic and thus constitute potential signposts in the search for linkage to a gene responsible for a given disease. Current estimates suggest that 400,000 SNPs will be required to tag each of the common haplotype blocks in the human genome. Genome-wide scans are just beginning to be performed with the approximately 2×10^6 SNPs that have been identified.[28] SNPs identified within the coding region of genes may be of particular importance, as these changes may have functional consequences and predispose carriers of these variants to the development of conditions such as thrombosis. The importance of coding-region SNPs is discussed later in the section highlighting the use of this technology. SNP analysis can be performed in a number of ways, but the most commonly used methodologies are PCR-based approaches and SNP arrays. The PCR-based approaches are the least expensive and require the least expertise, but the array-based approaches are capable of assessing thousands of SNPs simultaneously.

DIRECT SEQUENCING OF CANDIDATE GENES

The Human Genome Project helped accelerate the development of high throughput sequencing strategies. Now, high-throughput sequencing efforts are increasingly being directed towards the sequencing of cancer genomes to identify somatic mutations. Such an approach is being taken to characterize kinase mutations in cancers.[29,30] Based on the fact that kinases are frequently activated by mutation in cancer cells and that small molecule therapeutics are particularly effective against these proteins,[31] a number of groups have undertaken an effort to sequence all kinases in particular cancers. The first major discovery from such an effort was the identification of activating mutations in the serine/threonine kinase BRAF in melanoma (Fig. 2–3).[29] JAK2 mutations in polycythemia vera and other hematologic malignancies were identified by high-throughput sequencing as well as other genetic approaches. Small molecule inhibitors of BRAF and JAK2 are currently in clinical development.

Several new sequencing technologies are under development; these promise to lower the costs of sequencing by one or more orders of magnitude. Single molecule sequencing technologies either sequence a single DNA strand directly or amplify a single DNA molecule prior to sequencing.[32] By sequencing a single DNA molecule, mutations can be identified that are present in a rare subpopulation of cells. Novel sequencing technologies promise to enable the

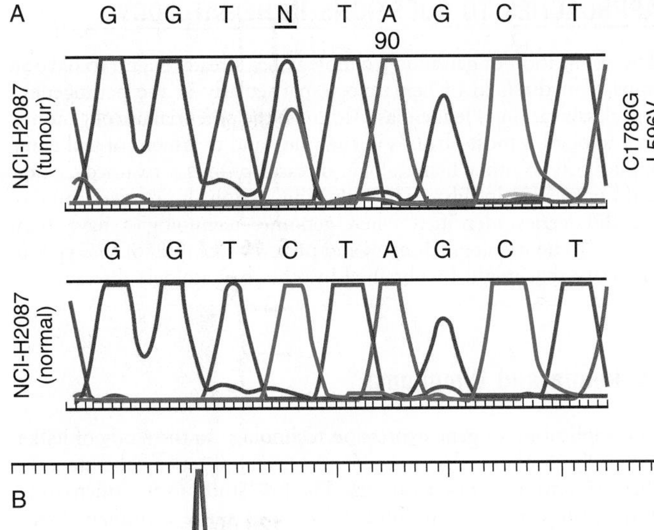

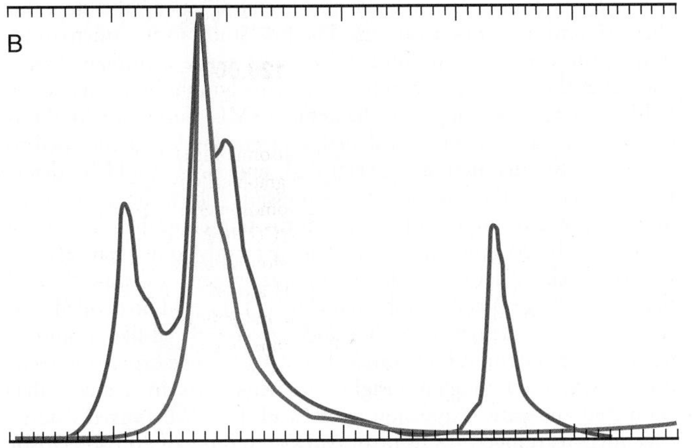

Figure 2–3 Activating mutations of *BRAF* were identified in melanoma using high-throughput DNA sequencing and heteroduplex analysis. The DNA sequencing traces are from a melanoma sample (*upper panel* in **A**) and from a normal sample (*lower panel* in **A**) for a region of the *BRAF* gene. A capillary-based heteroduplex analysis performed on normal (*green*) and cancer (*red*) DNAs from the same person is shown in (**B**). The melanoma sample has acquired a mutation that results in constitutive activation of *BRAF*. *(From Davies H, Bignell GR, Cox C, et al: Mutations of the BRAF gene in human cancer. Nature 417:949, 2002.)*

sequencing of entire genomes from biopsy specimens, allowing scientists and clinicians to catalog all of the somatic mutations present in a given sample and to correlate these mutations with phenotype and response to therapy. Moreover, the identification of novel somatic mutations may reveal important new therapeutic targets for the treatment of cancer.

SAMPLE ACQUISITION AND PREPARATION

Acquisition of the appropriate samples for a genomic experiment is arguably the most crucial step for the production of a dataset that will be rich with biological information. This is particularly true for gene expression analysis, in which a number of processes may affect the data. Since gene expression is a dynamic process that can be affected by any type of cellular manipulation, RNA abundance measurements are potentially complicated by changes that occur between the time that the biopsy is taken and the time that the RNA is isolated from the specimen. In general, the highest quality RNA is obtained if, as soon as possible after harvesting a sample, cells are dissolved in a solution such as TRIzol (Invitrogen) that inactivates RNase enzymes, and the sample is stored at −80°C (−112°F) until RNA can be extracted. Paraffin-embedded samples represent an even more difficult situation for extraction of RNA of sufficient quality for microarray analysis. Most microarray experiments require approximately 5 μg of total RNA (a few million cells) for labeling and hybridization, and thus small biopsies or rare cell populations may not produce enough RNA for standard analysis. A number of amplification procedures have been described, including those that utilize two rounds of in vitro transcription and those that take advantage of the PCR.[33]

Another extremely important, but complicated issue is the complexity of the mixture of cells present in the sample. If the goal is to assess genomic changes that represent somatic rather than germline differences, the sample needs to be enriched (often to >75%) in the cell of interest. This may not be an issue for bone marrow samples from patients with newly diagnosed leukemia, in which the number of blasts often approaches 90% or greater. But, it may become an issue if the goal is to analyze leukemia at the time of relapse. In this scenario, the relapse is often detected long before the bone marrow is completely replaced with leukemia, and thus the blasts may represent fewer than 50% of the mononuclear cells. Multiple methods are available for enrichment and selection of cells of interest from a biopsy sample including flow-cytometry, immunomagnetic bead sorting, and laser-capture microdissection.[34] All have the benefit of enrichment of the cell of interest but also increase the amount of processing time and sample manipulation. Alternatively, "contaminating" nonmalignant cells may be included in gene expression signatures as these cells may reflect the tumor environment and may therefore carry important information.[35] This is most obvious for solid tumors where the tumor stroma and infiltrating inflammatory cells likely influence the neoplastic cells, but all diseased cells exist in a complex environment and are thus no doubt influenced by their interactions. Thus, dismissing these cells as contamination must be done with caution.

BIOINFORMATICS

As the technologies described previously have become increasingly easy to use and more accessible to investigators, the rate-limiting step for turning the data thus acquired into important discoveries has become data analysis. As a result, the field of bioinformatics has become an integral part of genomic analysis. The single most difficult question that arises when genomic experiments are performed is whether the differences identified are important or are just results of measuring too many variables in too few samples and thus represent chance associations. This difficulty is further complicated because it can be difficult to separate signal from noise in genomic experiments. The issues regarding data analysis are the subjects of entire textbooks; here, we outline in broad terms two different analytic approaches: unsupervised and supervised learning.

Unsupervised Learning Approaches

Unsupervised learning approaches (often referred to as clustering) have become an important part of the discovery process in genomic analysis. This type of analysis involves grouping or separating samples based solely on the data obtained without regard to any previous knowledge that one might have had about the samples or the disease. Thus, one can obtain the predominant "structure" of the dataset without imposing any prior bias. For example, unsupervised learning approaches have been used to cluster leukemia or lymphoma samples based on their gene expression profiles with the goal of uncovering the most robust classification schemes.[36–39] Clustering algorithms can also cluster genes that have a similar expression profile in a gene expression data set. There are a number of methods for clustering genes and samples, all of which have computational strengths and weaknesses. Comparing the clustering methods is beyond the scope of this chapter, but all will identify major associations within a given data set if the signature is robust. Great care must be taken in the interpretation of clustering results because clusters with distinct gene expression profiles may be caused not only by biologically important distinctions, but also by artifacts of sample processing. Unsupervised learning methods that have been used include hierarchical clustering[40] (freely available at http://rana.lbl.gov/), self-organizing maps (SOM)[41] (freely available at http://www.broad.mit.edu/cancer/) principal component analysis (PCA),[42] nonnegative matrix factorization (NMF),[43] and k-means clustering.[44]

Supervised Learning Approaches

Supervised learning approaches are best suited for comparing data between two or more classes of samples that can be distinguished by some known property (or class distinction) such as biologic subtype or clinical outcome. For example, to determine the gene expression differences between two leukemia subtypes with distinct genetic abnormalities, one would employ a supervised approach. The same genes might be clustered together based on the unsupervised approaches described above, but they might also be obscured by a more dominant gene expression signature that had nothing to do with the distinction of interest; if there was another major signature within the data (ie, a stage of differentiation signature) the differences that the investigator was searching for might be lost. There are a number of metrics that can be used to identify genes that are differentially expressed between two groups of samples, all of which are best suited to identify genes that are uniformly highly expressed in one group.[37,39,41] Although the different metrics may generate slightly different lists of gene expression differences, all should give comparable results if the gene expression difference is robust.

No matter which metric is used for comparison of two classes of samples, one must determine if the association is greater than what would be found by chance alone. This is particularly important when analyzing genomic datasets because one is most often assessing many more variables (>10,000) than one has samples (<500). When such an analysis is performed there will always be differential gene expression. Most methods that address this question rely on some type of permutation analysis. To determine if observed differences in gene expression are greater than random associations, the class labels that define the two groups are randomly assigned to samples and the gene expression differences of the two classes is determined. This random assignment is performed multiple times (usually 1000 or greater), and the greatest differences in gene expression identified in the randomly permuted set are compared to the differences found in the initial experiment. Given the large number of comparisons, a critical step in statistical analysis is correction for multiple hypotheses, for example by calculation of the False Discover Rate. Thus, one can determine how likely it is that the observed correlation is not a chance association.

Another common goal is the creation of a gene expression-based classifier. Most studies use a supervised approach to determine which genes discriminate the classes of interest, and then build an expression-based prediction model using these genes. Validation of classifiers can be performed using a leave-one-out cross validation scheme or, preferably, by testing the classifier in an independent dataset. Many such classifiers have been developed using machine learning algorithms such as weighted voting, k-nearest neighbors, artificial neural networks, support vector machines, nearest centroid algorithms, and decision trees.[37,41,42,45–47] While each algorithm has strengths and weaknesses, in most cases, similar results should be obtained if the gene expression differences are significant.

The statistical methods for analyzing complex genomic datasets continue to evolve, but most of the currently available methods will uncover similar structure within a dataset. But, one should keep in mind that the predominant structure within a dataset may not be the most biologically important, and identifying the more subtle structures may be obscured by other gene expression signatures. A continuing challenge is how to infer the biological importance of any such structure. Since determining the biological importance of the observed differences is a highly subjective exercise, many refer to such experiments as "hypothesis generating" experiments that require validation in model systems.

APPROACHES TO QUESTIONS IN HEMATOLOGY

The application of genomic technology has already begun to have an impact on the field of hematology, particularly in the pathogenesis and classification of leukemias. Although the potential use of genomic technologies is most obvious in the study and treatment of leukemia, application to other hematologic diseases promises to uncover new and unexpected insights. The following section summarizes some of the discoveries identified when genomic technologies have been applied to hematologic diseases and presents examples of the types of discovery that might be obtained in other hematologic diseases.

Leukemia and Lymphoma

The application of gene expression technology to the study of leukemia and lymphoma has opened new avenues, setting the stage for characterization of other cancers. The first study to use microarray-based gene expression technology to characterize a human disease compared the gene expression between acute lymphoblastic leukemia (ALL) and acute myelogenous leukemia (AML) samples.[41] Methods of supervised and unsupervised analyses were developed and used to show that the distinction between ALL and AML could be determined solely on the basis of gene expression. Thus, the study demonstrated that an important clinical distinction could be made using microarray-based gene expression. The first study to use gene expression-based classification to identify unique subsets of disease showed that diffuse large B-cell lymphomas (DLBCLs) could be divided into two subsets—germinal center-like and activated B cell-like tumors—having different clinical outcomes (Fig. 2–4).[37] Gene expression technology was used to gain insight into leukemias in a study that compared the gene expression profiles of 17 *MLL* (*m*ixed *l*ineage *l*eukemia)-rearranged B-precursor ALLs with those of 20 B-precursor ALLs without this rearrangement.[36] With these tumors, the presence of an *MLL* translocation is most often found in infant ALL and generally carries a poor prognosis.[48] On the basis of the significant differences in gene expression, it was hypothesized that *MLL* rearrangements specify a unique disease with features that probably contribute to the poor prognosis for this leukemia. Support for the idea that chromosome translocations specify unique subsets of ALL comes from a large gene expression study showing that all chromosome translocations found in ALL are associated with unique gene expression profiles.[39]

The presence of cytogenetic abnormalities in T-cell acute lymphoblastic leukemias (T-ALLs) is not as clearly associated with differences in outcome as it is in B-precursor ALLs; therefore, classification based on gene expression could provide needed insight. In the first study addressing this question,[49] 39 T-ALL samples were grouped with respect to high-level expression of the oncogenes LYL1, *HOX11*, and *TAL/SCL1*—genes known to be important in the pathogenesis of T-ALL.[50] Only one of the oncogenic transcription factors was highly expressed in most of the leukemia samples. Analysis of gene expression using oligonucleotide arrays suggested that LYL1-, *HOX11*-, and *TAL/SCL1*-expressing samples were arrested at the double-negative, early cortical, and late cortical stages of thymocyte development, respectively. The type of classification system also may have prognostic importance because the patients with high-level *HOX11* expression appeared to have better prognoses than those in the other groups.

Gene expression analysis of leukemias also might be used to predict response to therapy and identify important new therapeutic avenues for targeted therapies. A number of studies of hematologic malignancies have reported that gene expression-based prediction models can improve on current clinical stratification schemes.[2,38,39] If these findings can be validated prospectively and confirmed by other studies, such models will be of great clinical usefulness. Large studies are needed to determine the clinical usefulness of such analyses, and to determine if prospective gene expression-based disease stratification is feasible.

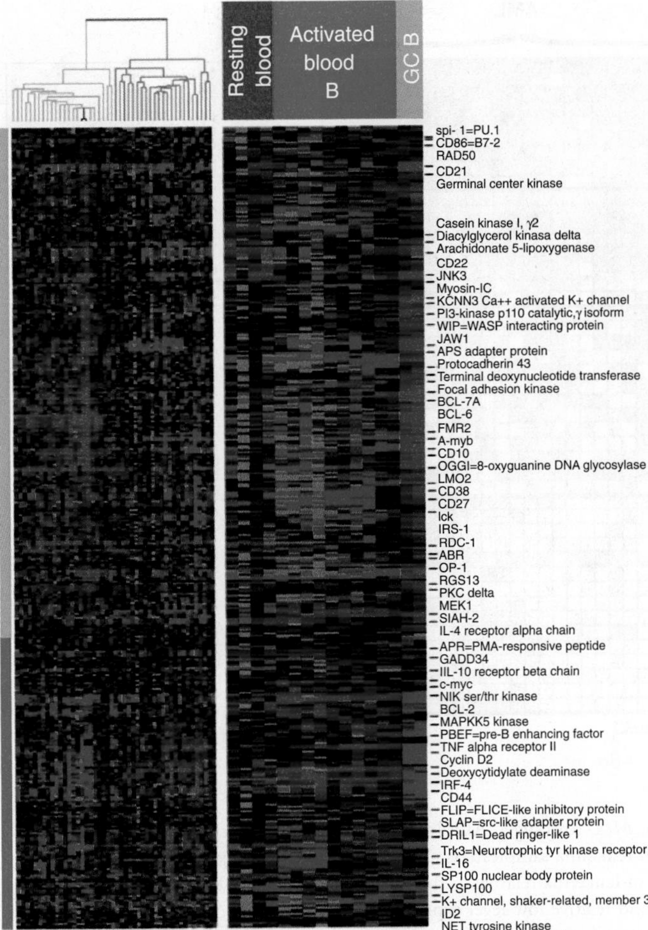

Figure 2–4 Diffuse large B-cell lymphomas (DLBCLs) classified by hierarchical clustering of genes. Gene expression in DLBCL samples was analyzed by the complementary DNA (cDNA) arrays containing approximately 17,000 genes, and the samples were clustered according to inherent differences in gene expression by hierarchical clustering. Patients with DLBCLs that had a gene germinal center-like gene expression pattern (*orange*) had a higher likelihood of survival than those with DLBCLs with an activated B cell-like expression pattern (*blue*). Each column represents a patient sample, and each row a gene. *Red* represents relative high-level expression and relative low-level expression. *(From Alizadeh AA, Eisen MB, Davis RE, et al: Distinct types of diffuse large B-cell lymphoma identified by gene expression profiling. Nature 403:503, 2000.)*

One of the most exciting potential uses of gene expression and other genomic technologies is the identification of unexpected new therapeutic avenues. In particular, gene expression analysis has the potential to identify oncogenes that are expressed to a higher level in one disease than another. High-level expression of a gene, however, does not necessarily mean anything about the function of the encoded protein. Despite this caveat, it does appear that gene expression-based comparisons can uncover important therapeutic targets in a given subset of disease. For example, when the gene expression profile of *BCR-ABL*-rearranged ALL is compared with those of other ALLs, the *ABL* gene is identified as one of the most highly expressed genes in this disease.[39] Similarly, α-*KIT* is highly expressed in gastrointestinal stromal tumors relative to other spindle cell tumors.[51] The importance of targeting *Abl* and *Kit* with the small-molecule inhibitor imatinib mesylate (Gleevec) is now well documented.[31,52] Thus, even if these molecules were not previously known to be important in these diseases, gene expression analysis probably would have identified them as such.

Along these lines, and as a result of gene expression studies (Fig. 2–5), the receptor tyrosine kinase Flt3 (*F*MS-*l*ike *t*yrosine kinase-3) has been validated as a potential therapeutic target in *MLL*-rearranged ALLs.[53] Because small-molecule Flt3 inhibitors were already being developed for the therapy of Flt3-mutated AML, the discovery of Flt3 in *MLL*-rearranged ALL prompted the initiation of clinical trials testing small-molecule Flt3 inhibitors in this disease.

Another approach that can be employed to identify potential therapeutic avenues in a given disease is to search for evidence of activation of a particular signaling pathway in the disease. This might be done by looking for high-level expression of multiple members of a pathway or by searching for a gene expression profile that is associated with activation of a particular pathway. Although analytic tools that can do this type of search in an automated fashion are still in development, activation of the nuclear factor-κB (NF-κB) pathway in activated B cell-like DLBCL was identified in this manner.[54]

Analysis of chromosome abnormalities has a long and rich history in the study of leukemogenesis. Although leukemia genomes have been studied extensively, the introduction of aCGH and SNP analysis will allow an even more thorough assessment of recurrent abnormalities in leukemia. A particularly powerful approach will be the combination of methods such as gene expression analysis and chromosome analysis by methods such as aCGH and SNP. This increase in "dimensionality" of genomic data should give an unprecedented view of the workings of a neoplastic cell. Indeed a recent study used SNP analysis to identify new recurrent genetic abnormalities in childhood leukemia that appear to be contributing to the neoplastic phenotype.[24]

Although such analyses are still in their infancy, important insights into leukemia classification and pathogenesis are beginning to be realized. Most of the discoveries await further validation in model systems, but it is clear that the addition of whole-genome expression analysis and detailed characterization of changes in DNA structure/sequence to our previous base of knowledge will provide further understanding. Finally, the development of more specific therapeutic regimens and new targeted therapeutic molecules is likely to arise from these studies. The integration of refined molecular classification and targeted therapies based on our understanding of leukemogenesis should lead to an improvement in the care of patients with leukemia.

Sickle Cell Disease

Although significant effort already has been put toward genomic analyses of diseases such as cancer, other hematologic diseases stand to benefit from such analyses. With the explosion of genomic information and the ever-increasing number of SNPs, we may now be able to begin to identify genes that modify the severity of human disease. For example, although most children with sickle cell anemia have similar genetic defects, the severity of the disease varies from individual to individual. Some patients have a predilection for the development of acute chest syndrome, stroke, or other devastating manifestations of the disease; others have a relatively benign course. Some of the genetic factors for such disease variability are known. An example is increased levels of hemoglobin F. The reason for most of the variability in disease expression, however, remains obscure. Although the cause of this variability will be multifactorial, disease modifier genes are likely to play an important role. Questions such as this can now be addressed using high-throughput SNP analysis to assess for polymorphisms that are either linked to or reside in sickle cell modifier genes. An example of an SNP that may provide information about disease severity in sickle cell disease lies within the gene encoding vascular cell adhesion molecule-1 (VCAM-1), which is associated with an increased risk of stroke.[55] Although such findings must be validated in larger studies and in models of the disease, experiments to investigate questions such as this one can be performed relatively easily and quickly. Of course, large, well-designed studies will need to be performed to take full advantage of the technology, but many centers have the clinical infrastructure to perform such studies.

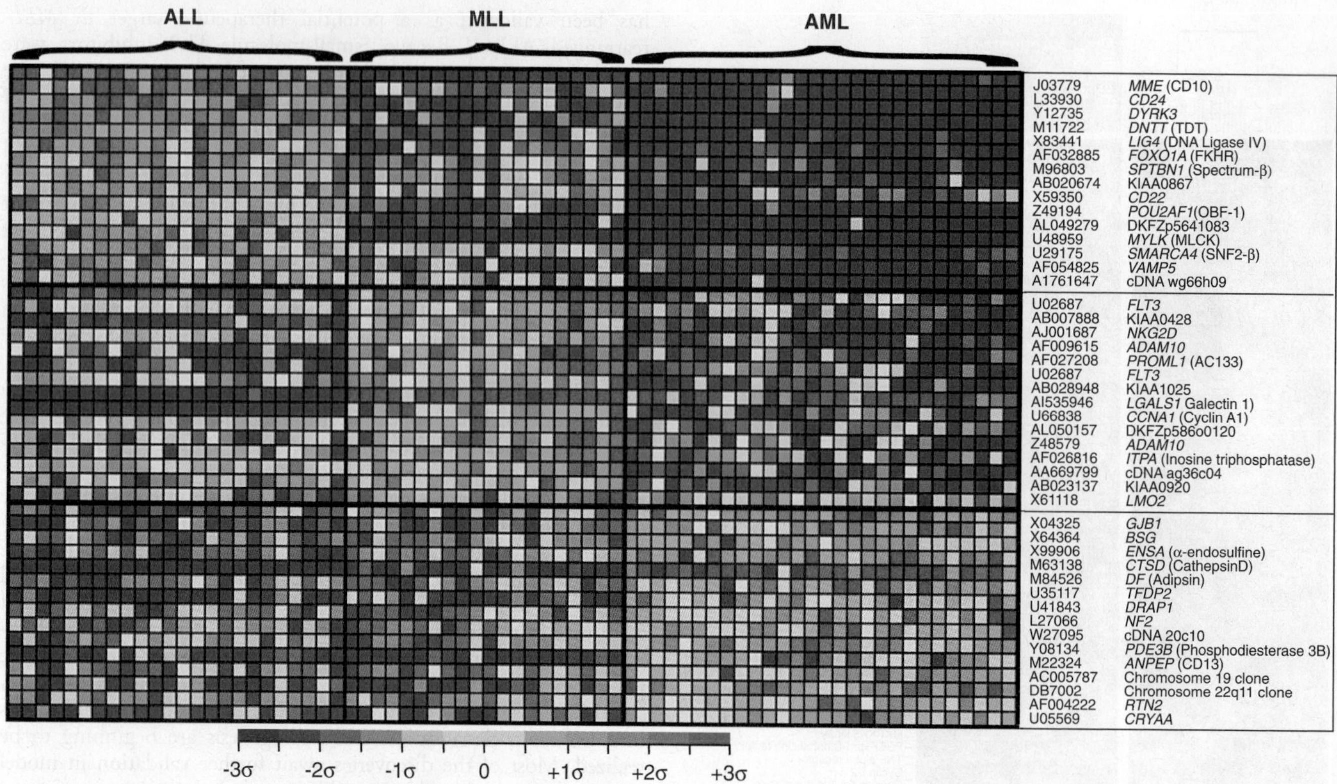

Figure 2–5 Comparison of gene expression in acute lymphocytic leukemia (ALL), *MLL*-rearranged ALL (designated MLL), and acute myelogenous leukemia (AML) samples using a supervised learning approach. Gene expression in leukemia samples was analyzed using Affymetrix microarrays (U95AV2) containing 12,600 unique probe sets. Genes that are highly expressed in one type of leukemia relative to the other two are shown. Each column represents a patient sample, and each row a gene. *Red* represents relative high-level expression and relative low-level expression. *(From Armstrong SA, Staunton JE, Silverman LB, et al: MLL translocations specify a distinct gene expression profile that distinguishes a unique leukemia. Nat Genet 30:41, 2002.)*

Thrombosis

The importance of SNPs in inherited predisposition to thrombotic episodes is well documented. The factor V Leiden and the prothrombin 20210A mutations associated with prothrombotic risk both are coding-region SNPs that predispose affected persons to venous thrombotic episodes.[56,57] Although these mutations were identified before large-scale SNP analysis, they provide evidence that further SNP analysis in persons who have experienced thrombotic episodes is likely to be of benefit. Identification of such mutations should be less time consuming because of the high-throughput nature of SNP analysis. Also, such analysis may provide insights into the mechanisms of predisposition to arterial thrombosis, stroke, and myocardial infarction in the general population.

In one such analysis, three SNPs surrounding the lymphotoxin-α gene were found to segregate with predisposition to myocardial infarction.[58] Of interest, one of the SNPs was shown to lead to increased lymphotoxin-α expression, which subsequently increased the expression of VCAM-1. A VCAM-1 polymorphism is also associated with stroke in sickle cell anemia, so this may be a particularly important association. Large follow-up studies and functional analyses are needed to validate these associations, but it appears evident that SNP analysis will provide new insights into the predisposition to thrombotic episodes.

PHARMACOGENETICS

A field that will benefit from the high-throughput technologies of genomics is that of pharmacogenetics. Pharmacogenetics encompasses the attempt to understand the clinical variability in toxicity and efficacy of particular therapeutics. The field historically has focused largely on the characterization of polymorphic variants of enzymes involved in drug metabolism. One of the earliest examples noted that an inherited deficiency in red blood cell glucose-6-phosphate dehydrogenase (G6PD deficiency) led to red cell hemolysis when affected patients were given antimalarial therapy. Since this early discovery, a number of genetic polymorphisms have been shown to modify the way a particular person responds to a given therapy. Because most drug-metabolizing enzymes are polymorphic, it is possible that a significant amount of variability in toxicity can be attributed to these polymorphisms. Drug toxicity probably represents an interplay among the multiple proteins involved in drug metabolism, proteins involved in drug clearance, and proteins that are the drug targets responsible for the toxicity; therefore, more comprehensive assessment will be required if we are to develop an understanding that can be used to predict clinical responses.[59]

Because of the complexities described earlier, the field of *pharmacogenomics* (the study of the relationship between drug effects and genome-wide variations among different people) stands to affect the manner in which we treat our patients. Studies are now under way to perform genome-wide assessment of SNPs and gene expression with a goal of correlating these changes with either toxicity or efficacy. One example of such an analysis was the correlation of gene expression with the development of secondary leukemia in patients with ALL who were given the topoisomerase II inhibitor etoposide.[39] In this study, the investigators were able to show a gene expression profile, present in lymphoblasts before treatment with etoposide, which was robust enough to predict the occurrence of the secondary leukemia. Because this study looked only at the gene expression profile of the leukemic blasts, it is not known whether this profile is the result of germline polymorphisms in some critical genes or whether it is acquired in the lymphoblasts. Despite the need for further study, this example highlights the potential power of this type of genome-wide analysis.

Another approach is to directly assess the polymorphisms responsible for toxicity or efficacy by genome-wide SNP analysis. Such an analysis would assess the greater than 2×10^6 currently known SNPs and look for association either with response to a given drug or with toxicity. For an SNP within the coding or upstream regulatory region of a gene, the effect of this polymorphism on the gene of interest could be directly assessed.

As the technology for high-throughput genome-wide analysis continues to improve, and the types of analyses described here are performed on a large scale within the setting of carefully designed clinical trials, we should see an improvement in our ability to predict not only which drugs will be efficacious in which disease but also to identify patients who have an increased risk for severe toxicity.

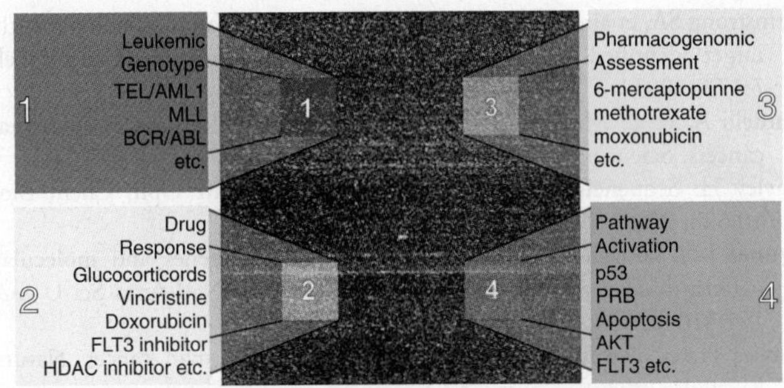

Figure 2–6 GENOMIC ANALYSIS OF LEUKEMIA IN THE FUTURE? A DNA microarray could be produced that would be able to identify molecular genetic information within the leukemia. This array could determine oncogenic mechanisms, drug resistance profiles, and the likelihood of drug toxicity. This information could then be used to develop a personalized treatment plan that would be most efficacious and least toxic for the particular type of leukemia and an individual patient.

CLINICAL IMPLEMENTATION

Although tremendous interest exists in how genomic views of hematologic diseases will be used clinically, most of the techniques described here are not routinely used for patient care decisions. The major reason for this limitation is the need for prospective validation of genomic studies performed to date. Furthermore, it remains uncertain whether techniques such as genome-wide gene expression analyses are feasible in the setting of routine clinical care, in view of the intricacies of sample acquisition, RNA handling, and informatic analysis described previously. Most studies performed to date have been done with rigorous controls designed to manage such variables.

The genomic discoveries that are most easily translated into clinical tests that can be used widely are those that involve assessing for polymorphisms. The best example of such translatability is the speed with which the assessment for resistance to activated protein C (factor V Leiden) began to be used clinically. Similarly, many centers can routinely test for the prothrombin 20210A mutation when assessing for predisposition to thrombosis. It is predicted that the ongoing large SNP studies will find similar polymorphism associations that can be quickly developed into useful tests.

Gene expression-based classifiers of leukemia and lymphoma represent a more difficult genomic discovery in terms of how to use this information clinically. For example, new gene expression-based classifiers of DLBCLs appear to be robust and add important information to current classification schemes. A gene expression classifier could be implemented as a multigene quantitative PCR assay, as a custom microarray that only detects the expression of key genes, or a genome-wide microarray. Clinical trials utilizing a quantitative PCR-base approach are currently underway. Whatever technology is ultimately used, most investigators believe that the information obtained by genomic studies will be incorporated into routine clinical practice in the not-too-distant future, whether or not the clinical tests are performed on the platforms used during the discovery process.

FUTURE DIRECTIONS

Genomic analysis promises to give an unprecedented view into the molecular composition of a diseased cell. These new discoveries are likely to be of both biologic and clinical importance and therefore require intense collaboration between clinical and basic scientists, so that the information gathered can be used to its full potential. Numerous studies have shown that such large-scale analysis can produce important information about disease, but an ongoing challenge is validation of hypotheses from such studies. Another current challenge is the integration of data obtained using different platforms across multiple institutions. The ability to compare genomic data sets produced by different investigators will be of great value and should help in the refinement of hypotheses. Similarly, genomic studies aimed at predicting outcome are being assessed in large prospective studies, which should provide information regarding the validity of the gene expression classifiers already developed. Finally, major effort is being put forth to develop high-throughput methods to allow rapid validation of biologic hypotheses. These studies will provide crucial tools for the future.

As the ability to use genomic technologies has become more widely available, integration of multiple types of analysis has become possible. Such multicomponent analysis should lead to an ever-increasing precision and ability to focus on biologically important information. For example, analysis of a leukemia sample by gene expression, aCGH, SNP, and direct sequencing of kinases may yield clinically useful prognostic information and uncover new therapeutic avenues that might go unrecognized if any of the strategies were used alone. An important goal will be to integrate genomic information to get a complete molecular description of cancer cells: the mutations, chromosomal abnormalities, gene expression, miRNA expression, and epigenetic state of the cells that determine the clinical phenotype and response to therapy.

We can now begin to imagine a time in the near future when we will truly be able to develop personalized medicine. For example, when a patient presents to the hospital or clinic with a new diagnosis of leukemia, a sample of the leukemic cells might be taken and assessed for gene expression and SNP analysis (Fig. 2–6). From these data, the physician might learn that the patient's leukemia cells have a particular chromosome translocation, a mutant tyrosine kinase, and a gene expression profile that predicts response to certain chemotherapeutics in combination with a specific tyrosine kinase inhibitor. Also, SNP analysis might predict that the patient would have severe toxicity to one of the chemotherapeutic agents commonly used in this disease. On the basis of these data, the physician would decide to manage the patient with a combination of drugs that has the greatest likelihood of efficacy with the least toxicity.

Although this type of personalized medicine is now on the horizon, its implementation will require an intense collaboration among clinical scientists, laboratory scientists, and pharmaceutical companies. Because all of this constitutes new territory for clinicians and scientists alike, it will not be an efficient process. Also, implementation of truly personalized medicine will have to be performed in a manner that does not compromise the current standards of care. Although this may make the pace of change in clinical medicine uncertain, there is great motivation for such a change.

SUGGESTED READING LIST

Armstrong SA, Staunton JE, Silverman LB, et al: MLL translocations specify a distinct gene expression profile that distinguishes a unique leukemia. Nat Genet 30:41, 2002.

Armstrong SA, et al: Inhibition of FLT3 in MLL: Validation of a therapeutic target identified by gene expression based classification. Cancer Cell 3:173, 2003.

Bardelli A, et al: Mutational analysis of the tyrosine kinome in colorectal cancers. Science 300:949, 2003.

Bayley H: Sequencing single molecules of DNA: Curr Opin Chem Biol 10:628, 2006.

Brunet J-P, Tamayo P, Golub TR, Mesirov J: Metagenes and molecular pattern discovery using matrix factorization. Proc Natl Acad Sci U S A 101:4164, 2004.

Davies H, et al: Mutations of the BRAF gene in human cancer. Nature 417:949, 2002.

Demetri GD, et al: Efficacy and safety of imatinib mesylate in advanced gastrointestinal stromal tumors. N Engl J Med 347:472, 2002.

Efron B, Tibshirani R: Empirical Bayes methods and false discovery rates for microarrays. Genet Epidemiol 23:70, 2002.

Ferrando AA, et al: Gene expression signatures define novel oncogenic pathways in T cell acute lymphoblastic leukemia. Cancer Cell 1:75, 2002.

Liu CG, et al: An oligonucleotide microchip for genome-wide microRNA profiling in human and mouse tissues. Proc Natl Acad Sci U S A 101:9740, 2004.

Lu J, et al: MicroRNA expression profiles classify human cancers. Nature 435:834, 2005.

Mullighan CG, et al: Genome-wide analysis of genetic alterations in acute lymphoblastic leukaemia. Nature 446:758, 2007.

Ozaki K, et al: Functional SNPs in the lymphotoxin-alpha gene that are associated with susceptibility to myocardial infarction. Nat Genet 32:650, 2002.

Pomeroy S, et al: Gene expression-based classification and outcome prediction of embryonal tumors of the CNS: Nature 415:436, 2002.

Shipp MA et al: Diffuse large B-cell lymphoma outcome prediction by gene-expression profiling and supervised machine learning. Nat Med 8:68, 2002.

Shivdasani RA: MicroRNAs: regulators of gene expression and cell differentiation. Blood 108:3646, 2006.

Taylor JG, et al: Variants in the VCAM1 gene and risk for symptomatic stroke in sickle cell disease. Blood 100:4303, 2002.

Yeoh EJ, et al: Classification, subtype discovery, and prediction of outcome in pediatric acute lymphoblastic leukemia by gene expression profiling. Cancer Cell 1:133, 2002.

REFERENCES

For complete list of references log onto www.expertconsult.com

CHAPTER 3

PROTEIN SYNTHESIS, PROCESSING, AND TRAFFICKING

Randal J. Kaufman and Laura Popolo

Proteins are the final executers of the genetic program of a cell and are responsible for the remarkable diversity in cell specialization that is typical of metazoan organisms. To perform this role, after synthesis, proteins need to be properly folded, assembled into oligomeric complexes, and transported to their final destinations. In many cases, protein folding and processing are coupled with protein trafficking so that the targeting process is unidirectional and irreversible. Eukaryotic cells contain membrane-bound compartments, termed *organelles*, such as the mitochondria, the endoplasmic reticulum (ER), the peroxisomes, and the nucleus. Each organelle serves a particular purpose. The capacity of any organelle to fulfill its role in intracellular physiology depends on a characteristic set of protein components. This chapter briefly describes how proteins are synthesized and then focuses on their processing and delivery to appropriate destinations within the cell. An understanding of the mechanisms that catalyze protein folding, assembly, and targeting is necessary for the study of hematology and can help explain how malfunctions in these processes can cause blood disorders.

PROTEIN SYNTHESIS

Among all the biosyntheses of macromolecules occurring in a cell, protein synthesis is the most important in quantitative terms. It is a highly energy-consuming process and proceeds through a mechanism that has been conserved during evolution. Proteins are synthesized by the joining of amino acids, through peptide bonds, each of which has characteristic physical–chemical properties (see Table 3–1 for single-letter designations). Peptide bonds are created by the condensation of the carboxyl group (COOH) of one amino acid with the amino group (NH_2) of the next. The free NH_2 and COOH groups of the terminal amino acids define the amino- or N-terminal end and the carboxyl- or C-terminal end, respectively, of the resulting polypeptide chain. In many cases, multiple polypeptide chains assemble into a functional protein. For example, hemoglobin is formed by four polypeptide chains, two α-globin chains and two β-globin chains that assemble with heme, an iron-containing prosthetic group, to yield the functional protein designed to deliver molecular oxygen to all cells and tissues.

The whole process of protein synthesis is orchestrated by a large ribonucleoprotein complex, called the *ribosome*, which is composed of a large subunit of 60S and a small one of 40S (S stands for Svedberg unit, and refers to the rate of sedimentation). Eukaryotic mRNA molecules typically contain a 5′-untranslated region (5′-UTR), a protein coding sequence that begins with an AUG and ends with one of three stop codons (UAA, UAG, UGA), and a 3′-untranslated region (3′-UTR). The 5′ end carries a 7-methylguanosine forming a structure called a "cap" (m^7GpppN mRNA), whereas the 3′ end is polyadenylated. These modifications are required to protect the mRNA from degradation, for export out of the nucleus and for efficient recruitment of ribosomes for translation. Once in the cytoplasm, the 40S ribosomal subunit binds to the cap and then scans the mRNA toward the 3′ end until the translation start codon is encountered (usually the first AUG). At that time, the 60S subunit assembles with the 40S to produce an 80S ribosome. A special tRNA specific for methionine, called the initiator ($tRNA_i^{Met}$), is required for the initiation of protein synthesis at the start codon. Other charged tRNA molecules ferry amino acids to the ribosome, where they are joined together in sequence as the ribosome moves toward the 3′ end of the mRNA. The codons in the mRNA interact by base-pairing with the anticodon of the tRNAs so that amino acids are incorporated into the nascent polypeptide chain in the right order. Translation is terminated on encountering a stop codon, when the polypeptide is released. Typically, multiple ribosomes are engaged in the translation of a single mRNA molecule in a complex termed a *polyribosome* or *polysome*.

Protein synthesis is divided into three phases: initiation, elongation, and termination. Each phase requires a set of soluble proteins called initiation, elongation, and termination or release factors that are termed eIFs, eEFs, and eRFs, respectively, where the prefix *e* indicates their eukaryotic origin.

REGULATION OF mRNA TRANSLATION

There are two major general regulatory steps in mRNA translation that are mediated by the initiation factors eIF2 and eIF4. All cells regulate the rate of protein synthesis through reversible covalent modification of eIF2, a soluble factor required for the binding and recruitment of the Met-$tRNA_i^{Met}$ to the 40S subunit. eIF2 is a heterotrimeric G-protein (guanine nucleotide-binding protein) that can exist in an inactive form bound to guanosine diphosphate (GDP) or in an active form bound to guanosine triphosphate (GTP). The eIF2–GTP–Met-$tRNA_i^{Met}$ ternary complex binds to the 40S ribosomal subunit. Joining of the 60S subunit triggers hydrolysis of GTP to GDP and thus converts eIF2 to the inactive form, whereas the opposite reaction is catalyzed by a guanine nucleotide exchange factor (GEF) called eIF2B. In reticulocytes, which synthesize hemoglobin almost as a sole protein, heme starvation blocks the synthesis of α- and β-globins by activating a protein kinase, called hemin-regulated inhibitor (HRI), that specifically phosphorylates the eIF2α subunit of eIF2. The phosphorylated form of eIF2 binds more tightly than usual to eIF2B, so that eIF2B is sequestered and not available for the exchange reaction. Thus, eIF2 molecules remain in the GDP-bound form and translation of globin mRNA comes to a halt. This mechanism of translational inhibition is of more general significance because eIF2 is a target of phosphorylation by additional protein kinases that cause translational arrest in response to different conditions of cell stress, such as amino acid starvation, glucose starvation, and viral infection.

A second major control point of general protein synthesis is mediated by the eIF4 protein complex that binds the cap and uses an ATP-dependent RNA helicase activity to unwind the structural elements in the 5′ end of mRNA to make it accessible for 40S ribosome binding. The subunit that binds the cap, eIF4E, is the least abundant factor regulating translation in mammalian cells. Increased levels of eIF4E stimulate protein synthesis and can contribute to oncogenesis. The cap-binding activity of eIF4E is inhibited by the eIF4E-binding protein (eIF4EBP), which is regulated by phosphorylation by the protein kinases AKT and TOR. Because phosphorylated eIF4BP cannot bind eIF4E, eIF4EBP phosphorylation stimulates translation initiation.

The efficiency of translation can also be modulated by cellular factors that bind mRNA in a sequence-specific manner. An example of this mode of regulation is the control of iron metabolism in animal cells. Key players of this system are (a) the iron-responsive element

Table 3–1 Examples of Targeting Signals

Organelle	Signal Location*	Example
Posttranslational Uptake		
Nucleus	Internal	PKKKRKV (import; SV40 large T antigen)
		LQLPPLERLTLD (export; HIV-1 Rev)
Mitochondrion	N-terminal	MLGIRSSVKTCFKPMSLTSKRL (iron–sulfur protein of complex III)
Peroxisomes	C-terminal	KANL (PTS1, human catalase)
	N-terminal	RLQVVLGHL (PTS2, human 3-ketoacyl-CoA thiolase)
Cotranslational Uptake		
ER	N-terminal	MMSFVSLLLVGILFWATEAEQLTKCEVFQ (ovine lactalbumin)

ER, endoplasmic reticulum; HIV, human immunodeficiency virus; PTS1, peroxisomal targeting signal-type 1; PTS2, peroxisomal targeting signal-type 2, SV40, simian virus 40.

*Acidic residues (negatively charged) are in *italic* type; basic residues (positively charged) are in bold type. Amino acids: A, alanine; C, cysteine; *D*, aspartic acid; *E*, glutamic acid; F, phenylalanine; G, glycine; **H**, histidine; I, isoleucine; **K**, lysine; L, leucine; M, methionine; N, asparagine; P, proline; Q, glutamine; **R**, arginine; S, serine; T, threonine; V, valine; W, tryptophan; Y, tyrosine.

(IRE), a hairpin structure that is formed in the untranslated regions of the mRNAs, and (b) iron regulatory proteins (IRPs) that bind IRE. In the transferrin receptor (Tfr) mRNA and ferritin mRNA, IREs are located in the 3′-UTR and 5′-UTR, respectively. In iron-starved cells, the binding of IRPs to IREs results in the stabilization of Tfr mRNA and inhibition of translation initiation of ferritin mRNA. Conversely, when iron is abundant, IRPs have a lower affinity to IREs and as a result Tfr mRNA is degraded whereas ferritin mRNA translation is stimulated. In this manner, cells can coordinately regulate iron uptake and iron sequestration in response to the changes in iron availability.

PROTEIN SORTING

The transport of newly synthesized polypeptides to their destination requires navigation through several sorting branch points (Fig. 3–1). These sorting events are governed by sorting signals (ie, short linear sequences or three-dimensional patches of particular amino acids) and by their cognate receptors. The first sorting decision occurs after approximately 30 amino acids of the nascent polypeptide have been extruded from the ribosome. If the nascent polypeptide lacks a "signal sequence," most often found near the amino-terminal end, the translation of the polypeptide is completed in the cytosol. Then the protein can either stay in the cytosol or be posttranslationally incorporated into one of the indicated organelles (Fig. 3–1, pathways 7, 8, and 9). If the protein does contain an amino–terminal signal sequence is imported cotranslationally into the ER, from where it can be targeted to the other compartments of the secretory pathway (Fig. 3–1, pathway 1).

PROTEIN FOLDING

Proteins are not functional in the extended linear conformation in which they emerge from the ribosome. The polypeptide chain must fold into a conformation that is basically dictated by the primary structure. Although some proteins can acquire their mature three-dimensional conformation in a test tube by a self-assembly process, most polypeptides require assistance to fold. Molecular chaperones either directly assist protein folding or act to prevent aberrant interactions, such as aggregation, that can occur in a highly crowded environment, similar to the cytosol of eukaryotic cells (protein concentrations of 200–300 mg/mL). Most molecular chaperones are members of the heat-shock protein (hsp) family. Chaperones bind to short-sequence protein motifs, in many cases containing hydrophobic amino acids. By undergoing cycles of binding and release (linked to ATP hydrolysis), chaperones help the nascent polypeptide to find its native conformation, one aspect of which is hiding hydrophobic sequence motifs in the protein interior so that they no longer contact the hydrophilic environment of the cytosol. Some properly folded protein monomers are assembled with other proteins to form multi-subunit complexes. The population of chaperones that assist folding and assembly in the cytosol is distinct from those that operate within the ER or mitochondria.

PROTEIN DEGRADATION

Proteins can contain mutations that prevent them from folding properly. Such misfolded proteins are marked for destruction and are degraded. In addition to carrying out the disposal of damaged and misfolded proteins, the cellular protein degradation machinery is responsible for regulating a wide array of cellular processes, including cellular differentiation, tissue development, induction of inflammatory responses, antigen presentation, and cell cycle progression through the controlled destruction of key regulatory proteins. Degradation of these molecules is achieved in two major phases. First, the molecules are tagged with a polypeptide moiety termed *ubiquitin.* Second, the tagged molecules are ferried to an ATP-dependent protease complex called the proteasome for destruction. Chapter 4 provides an overview of the ubiquitin-mediated protein degradation pathway.

SORTING FROM THE CYTOSOL INTO OTHER COMPARTMENTS

Most of the proteins synthesized on free polysomes remain in the cytosol as cytosolic or soluble proteins. These include enzymes involved in metabolic and signal transduction pathways or proteins required for the assembly of the cytoskeleton. Other proteins are imported into the organelles, including the nucleus, the mitochondrion, and the peroxisome (see Fig. 3–1).

In general, there are two types of protein trafficking. In one type, the protein crosses a lipid bilayer. The polypeptide crosses the membrane in an unfolded state through an aqueous channel composed of proteins. In the second type, the protein does not traffic across a lipid bilayer and is exemplified by trafficking into the nucleus or from the ER to the Golgi compartment. In these cases, proteins and protein complexes are transported in their folded/assembled state.

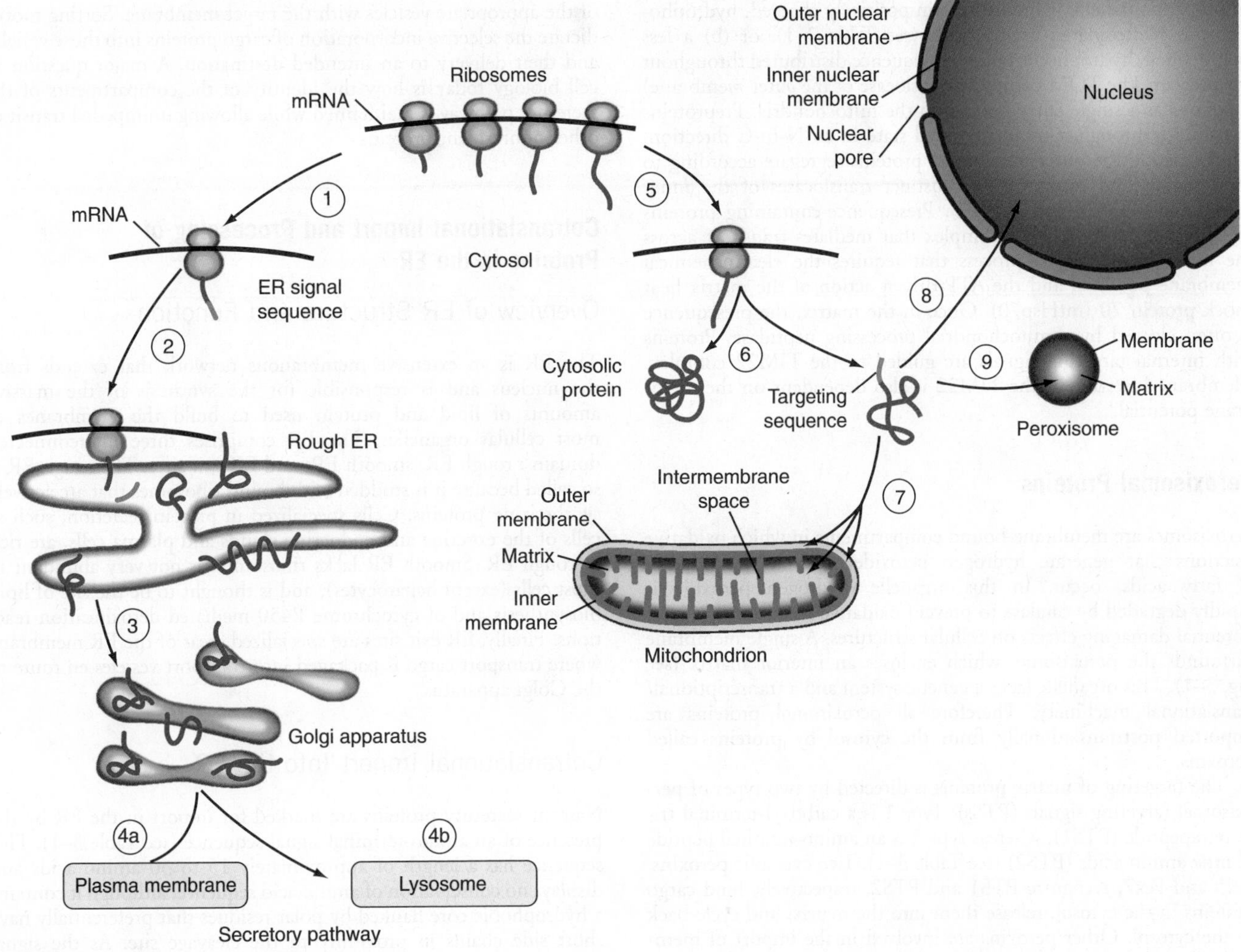

Figure 3–1 Intracellular protein trafficking.

Nuclear Proteins

The nucleus contains the genome of a cell and is bounded by a double membrane that forms the nuclear envelope (see Fig. 3–1). The outer membrane is continuous with the ER and has a polypeptide composition distinct from that of the inner membrane. Approximately 3000 nuclear pore complexes (NPCs) perforate the nuclear envelope in animal cells. NPCs are approximately 120 nm in diameter and comprise approximately 50 different proteins (nucleoporins). Although NPCs allow unrestricted, bidirectional movement of molecules smaller than 40,000 to 50,000 daltons, traversal of NPCs by larger molecules is tightly regulated.

NPCs are capable of importing and exporting molecules or complexes, provided that the molecules have an exposed nuclear localization signal or nuclear export signal (see Table 3–1). Candidates for nuclear import (ie, transcription factors, DNA repair enzymes, ribosomal proteins, mRNA processing factors, etc) or export (ribosomal subunits, mRNA-containing particles, tRNAs, etc) are transported through the NPC in association with carrier proteins, called importins, that bind their cargo on one side of the NPC and release it on the other. In contrast, other proteins called exportins bind the cargo in the nucleus and release it in the cytoplasm. A monomeric G-protein called Ran controls both the docking of carrier proteins with their cargo and the directionality of transport through cycles of GTP binding and hydrolysis. The movement of carrier proteins across the NPC requires their interaction with nucleoporins that bear phenylalanine–glycine (F–G) repeats.

The lack of a nuclear localization or nuclear export signal removal during transport through the NPC enables multiple cycles of nuclear entry and exit, which is a particularly important mechanism for regulating the activity of proteins involved in DNA and RNA metabolism.

Mitochondrial Proteins

The mitochondrion is an essential cellular compartment in eukaryotes. Although it contains a genome organized in a circular DNA molecule and an independent transcriptional/translational machinery, 98% of the approximately 1000 proteins that constitute mitochondria are encoded by nuclear DNA and are imported from the cytosol after their synthesis. A small number of proteins is encoded by mitochondrial DNA and is synthesized by ribosomes within the mitochondria.

Like nuclei, mitochondria have two membranes: an outer one that contacts the cytosol and an inner one in which reside the enzymes that synthesize ATP through reactions of the electron transport chain and oxidative phosphorylation. Where the outer membrane is permeable to small molecules and ions, the inner membrane is highly impermeable, a property essential for creating an electrochemical gradient necessary to drive the synthesis of ATP. The space enclosed by the two membranes is the intermembrane space and the space enclosed in the inner membrane is the *matrix* (see Fig. 3–1).

Translocation and sorting of nuclear-encoded proteins into the various mitochondrial subcompartments are achieved by the concerted action of translocases. Precursor proteins usually have one of two targeting signals: (a) an amino-terminal presequence that is generally between 10 and 80 amino acid residues long and forms an amphipathic α-helix, which is rich in positively charged, hydrophobic, and hydroxylated amino acids (see Table 3–1), or (b) a less well-defined, hydrophobic targeting sequence distributed throughout the protein. The TOM complex (*t*ranslocase of the *o*uter *m*embrane) functions as a single entry point into the mitochondria. Preproteins translocate through it in an unfolded state in an N-to-C direction. After crossing the outer membrane, proteins segregate according to their signals and recognize two distinct *t*ranslocases of the *i*nner *m*embrane (TIM23 and TIM22). Presequence-containing proteins are directed to the TIM23 complex that mediates transport across the inner membrane, a process that requires the electrochemical membrane potential and the ATP-driven action of the matrix heat shock protein 70 (mtHsp70). Once in the matrix, the presequence is often cleaved by a mitochondrial processing peptidase. Proteins with internal targeting signals are guided to the TIM22 complex. Membrane insertion at the TIM22 is also dependent on the membrane potential.

Peroxisomal Proteins

Peroxisomes are membrane-bound compartments in which oxidative reactions that generate hydrogen peroxide, such as β-oxidation of fatty acids, occur. In this organelle, hydrogen peroxide is rapidly degraded by catalase to prevent oxidative reactions that have potential damaging effects on cellular structures. A single membrane surrounds the peroxisome, which encloses an interior matrix (see Fig. 3–1). This organelle lacks a genetic system and a transcriptional/translational machinery. Therefore all peroxisomal proteins are imported posttranslationally from the cytosol by proteins called peroxins.

The targeting of matrix proteins is directed by two types of peroxisomal targeting signals (PTSs). Type 1 is a carboxyl-terminal tri- or tetrapeptide (PTS1), whereas type 2 is an amino-terminal peptide of nine amino acids (PTS2) (see Table 3–1). Two cytosolic peroxins, Pex5 and Pex7, recognize PTS1 and PTS2, respectively, bind cargo proteins in the cytosol, release them into the matrix, and cycle back to the cytosol. Other peroxins are involved in the import of membrane proteins. Although the mechanism of translocation is not known, cargo proteins appear to cross the membrane in a folded state, or even as oligomers. In this regard, the process is more similar to protein import into the nucleus, although a structure similar to the nuclear pore has not been identified to date.

One consequence of the existence of two different mechanisms for protein import is that when the import of matrix proteins is defective, membrane ghosts of peroxisomes persist in the cells. In contrast, when the import of membrane proteins is impaired, neither normal peroxisomes nor membrane ghosts are present. Defects in *PEX3* underlie Zellweger syndrome, which is characterized by the presence of empty peroxisomes and abnormalities of the brain, liver, and kidney that cause death shortly after birth.

PROTEIN TRAFFICKING WITHIN THE SECRETORY PATHWAY

Proteins that enter the ER are transported toward the plasma membrane through a route that is called the secretory pathway (Fig. 3–2). Specific signals cause proteins to be retained in the ER, Golgi, or plasma membrane. Proteins may also be targeted from the Golgi compartment to lysosomes or from the plasma membrane to endosomes (Fig. 3–2, pathways 8 and 9). Initially the study of this complex protein trafficking took advantage of mutants in this pathway isolated in the lower eukaryote *Saccharomyces cerevisiae*. Many genes encoding products involved in secretion were found to be conserved from yeast to mammals, indicating the importance of this pathway for the life of a eukaryotic cell.

Transport through the secretory pathway is mediated by vesicles. Different sets of structural and regulatory proteins control the fusion of the appropriate vesicles with the target membrane. Sorting motifs dictate the selective incorporation of cargo proteins into those vesicles and their delivery to an intended destination. A major question in cell biology today is how the identity of the compartments of the secretory pathway is maintained while allowing unimpeded transit of other nonresident proteins.

Cotranslational Import and Processing of Proteins in the ER

Overview of ER Structure and Function

The ER is an extensive membranous network that extends from the nucleus and is responsible for the synthesis of the massive amounts of lipid and protein used to build the membranes of most cellular organelles. The ER comprises three interconnected domains: rough ER, smooth ER, and ER exit sites. The rough ER is so called because it is studded with bound ribosomes that are actively synthesizing proteins. Cells specialized in protein secretion, such as cells of the exocrine and endocrine glands and plasma cells, are rich in rough ER. Smooth ER lacks ribosomes, is not very abundant in most cells (except hepatocytes), and is thought to be the site of lipid biosynthesis and of cytochrome P450-mediated detoxification reactions. Finally, ER exit sites are specialized areas of the ER membrane where transport cargo is packaged into transport vesicles en route to the Golgi apparatus.

Cotranslational Import Into the ER

Nascent secretory proteins are marked for import in the ER by the presence of an amino-terminal signal sequence (see Table 3–1). This sequence has a length of approximately 15 to 30 amino acids and displays no conservation of amino acid sequence, although it contains a hydrophobic core flanked by polar residues that preferentially have short side chains in proximity to the cleavage site. As the signal sequence emerges from the ribosome, it is recognized by the signal recognition particle (SRP), a ribonucleoprotein, and this binding induces a temporary arrest in translational elongation (Fig. 3–3). The docking of ribosomes to the ER occurs by interaction of the SRP with the SRP receptor. Upon binding of GTP to both the SRP and its receptor, the ribosome and the nascent chain are transferred to the Sec61 complex, allowing translation to resume. Preproteins translocate through the Sec61 complex in an N-to-C direction. As the nascent polypeptide emerges from the luminal side of the translocon, its signal sequence is cleaved by a signal peptidase.

In the absence of specific targeting sequences, proteins that completely translocate into the ER lumen traffic through bulk flow to the cell surface. In contrast, proteins that have specific targeting signals may be localized to the lumen of the ER, the Golgi compartment, or lysosomes. Other proteins that reside in membranes of the cell contain topological sequences called transmembrane domains that consist of approximately 20 largely apolar amino acids. When a transmembrane domain enters the translocon, the polypeptide is released laterally from the Sec61 channel into the lipid bilayer.

Protein Folding in the Lumen of the ER

Protein chaperones facilitate protein folding in the ER, but amino acid posttranslational modifications such as asparagine(N)-linked-glycosylation and disulfide bond formation are also involved. Proteins start to fold cotranslationally by interaction with a host of chaperones, including the hsp70 family member BiP. In addition, there are folding catalysts that increase the rate of protein folding. For example, the proper pairing and formation of disulfide bonds is catalyzed by oxidoreductases, such as protein disulfide isomerase (PDI). In

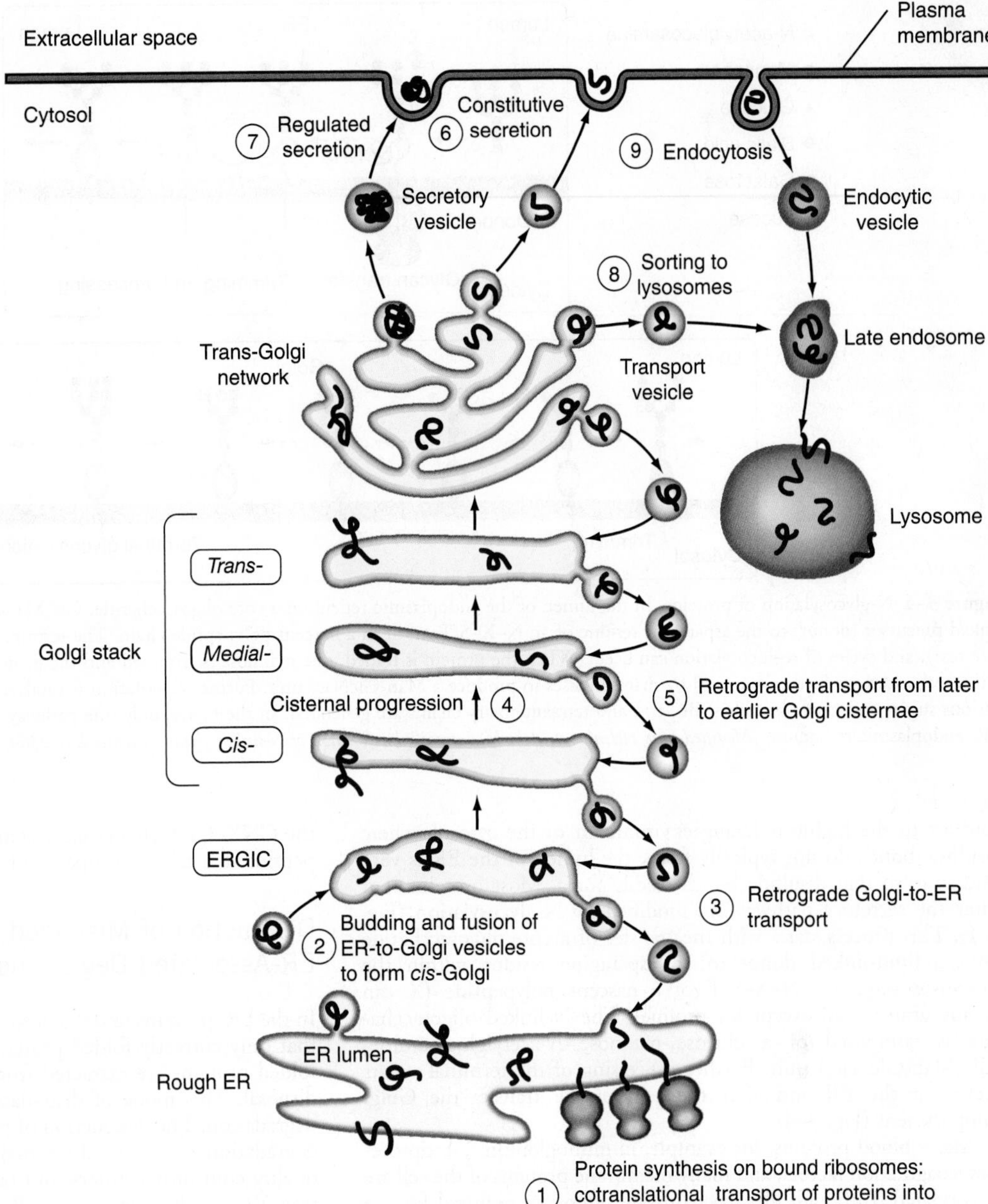

Figure 3–2 Protein trafficking through the secretory pathway. For details, see the text.

Figure 3–3 Protein translocation into the endoplasmic reticulum.

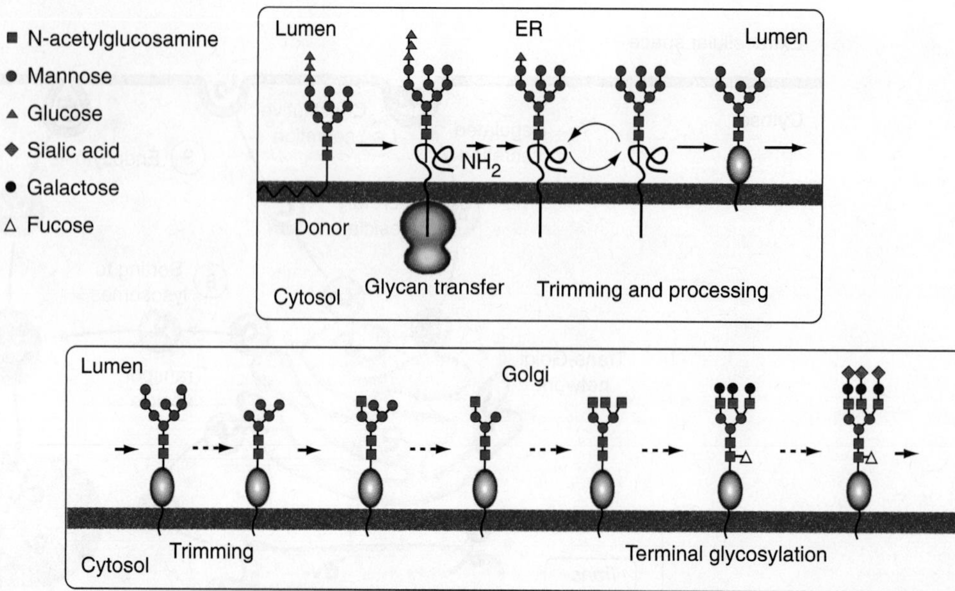

Figure 3–4 N-glycosylation of proteins. In the lumen of the endoplasmic reticulum a core oligosaccharide, $Glc_3Man_9GlcNac_2$, is transferred from a lipid-linked precursor (donor) to the asparagine residue of an N–X–S/T motif in a nascent polypeptide chain. The terminal glucoses are removed by GI and GII (see text), and cycles of reglucosylation can occur. When the protein is folded, one mannose is trimmed and the protein is transported to the Golgi. Core oligosaccharides are further trimmed by mannosidases to produce a $Man_5GlcNac_2$ unit. Further elaboration is catalyzed by glycosyltransferases, which add various sugars and create branches. Bi-, tri-, and tetraantennary chains are generated. In the figure, only one pathway of terminal glycosylation is shown. ER, endoplasmic reticulum. *(Modified from Helenius A, Aebi M: Intracellular function of N-linked glycans. Science 291:2364, 2001.)*

contrast to the highly reducing environment of the cytosol, where disulfide bonds do not typically form, the lumen of the ER is very oxidizing, so that disulfide bonds readily form. Most proteins that enter the secretory pathway are modified by N-glycosylation (Fig. 3–4). This process starts with the transfer of a core oligosaccharide from a lipid-linked donor to an asparagine residue within the consensus sequence N–X–S/T of a nascent polypeptide (X can be any amino acid except for proline). The N-linked oligosaccharide is composed of a glucose$_3$-mannose$_9$-*N*-acetylglucosamine$_2$ ($Glc_3Man_9GlcNac_2$) unit. Further processing of the terminal sugars occurs in the ER and after the polypeptide transits the Golgi compartment (Fig. 3–4).

Many blood proteins, for example, immunoglobulins, antiproteases, coagulation factors, and many membrane proteins of the cell are glycosylated. Although glycan chains are often not required for the enzymatic activity of glycoproteins, they are important for the physical properties they confer and for many physiological functions. Glycans protect proteins from protease digestion and heat denaturation, confer hydrophilicity and adhesive properties to the proteins, and mediate interaction with other proteins or receptors. A remarkable example is the hormone erythropoietin that requires a particular complex type of *N*-glycan chains for its biological function to stimulate erythropoiesis.

In recent years, several studies have revealed the importance of protein N-glycosylation in promoting folding. The addition of glycan chains may prevent aggregation or provide steric influences that affect polypeptide folding and disulfide bond formation and also mediate interaction with specific chaperones. In mammalian cells, N-linked oligosaccharides are also used as signal for monitoring protein folding. They are substrates for a complex chaperone system composed of the lectin chaperones calnexin (CNX) and calreticulin (CRT), Erp57 (an oxidoreductase), two glucosidases (GI and GII), and one folding sensor (UGT1) endowed with reglucosylation activity (UDP-glucose: glycoprotein glucosyltransferase). GI and GII remove the two terminal glucose residues to form a monoglucosylated N-linked chain (see Fig. 3–4) that is a ligand for CNX and CRT. Then another glucose residue is removed. UGT1 recognizes and reglucosylates N-linked oligosaccharides on proteins that have not completed the folding process. The addition of glucose residues allows reassociation with the CNX–CRT chaperone system for another attempt for the polypeptide to attain its proper conformation.

Destruction of Misfolded or Misassembled Proteins: ER-Associated Degradation

In the ER, proteins undergo a so-called quality control which ensures that only correctly folded proteins exit the ER. Consequently, misfolded proteins are extracted from the ER folding environment for disposal. This mode of degradation is referred to as ER-associated degradation. The destruction of proteins that undergo ER-associated degradation occurs in three major steps: (a) detection by the ER quality control machinery and targeting for ER-associated degradation, (b) transport across the ER membrane into the cytosol, and (c) ubiquitination and release in the cytosol for degradation by the proteasome. One model for misfolded protein recognition is that hydrophobic patches or sugar moieties, which remain exposed on the protein for an extended period of time, are recognized by chaperone proteins like PDI or by the CNX–CRT chaperone system. In a number of cases retrotranslocation appears to require reduction of disulfide bridges by PDI. Similarly, BiP association with substrates (eg, unassembled immunoglobulin light chains) can direct them to ER-associated degradation. If a protein remains in its unfolded state for an extended period of time, trimming of the $Man_8GlcNac_2$ occurs. The ER-resident lectin EDEM/Htm1p binds to the remaining mannose residues and assists the retrotranslocation. Proteins retrotranslocate to the cytosol through a protein-conducting channel, possibly formed by derlin and/or the Sec61 complex. On their emergence at the cytosolic face of the ER membrane, substrates targeted for degradation start undergoing ubiquitination. Tagged peptides are released into the cytosol in an ATP-dependent fashion, where they are degraded by the 26S proteasome.

The Unfolded Protein Response

The ER monitors the amount of unfolded protein in its lumen. When that number exceeds a certain threshold, ER sensors activate a signal transduction pathway. The set of responses activated by this pathway is called the unfolded protein response (UPR). A number of cellular insults disrupt protein folding and cause unfolded protein accumulation in the ER lumen. The UPR is an adaptive response signaled through three ER-localized transmembrane proteins, PERK, IRE1, and ATF6, to limit the accumulation of unfolded protein by reducing protein synthesis, increasing the degradation of unfolded protein, and increasing the ER protein folding capacity. IRE1 is conserved in all eukaryotic cells and has protein kinase and endoribonuclease activities that, upon activation, mediate unconventional splicing of a 26-base intron from the XBP1 mRNA to produce a potent transcription factor. ATF6 is a basic leucine zipper-containing transcription factor that, upon accumulation of unfolded protein in the ER lumen, transits to the Golgi compartment, where it is cleaved to yield a cytosolic fragment that migrates to the nucleus to activate gene transcription. Finally, PERK-mediated phosphorylation of eIF2α attenuates general mRNA translation, however, paradoxically increasing translation of the transcription factor ATF4 mRNA to also induce transcription of UPR genes. If the UPR adaptive response is not sufficient to correct the protein folding defect, the cells enter apoptotic death. Activation of the UPR and defects in UPR are now known to be important factors that contribute to many disease processes ranging from metabolic disease, neurologic disease, infectious disease, and cancer.

Control of Exit From the ER

On achieving transport competence, proteins are granted access to higher-ordered membrane domains termed ER exit sites. At ER exit sites, membrane-bound and membrane-soluble proteins are concentrated into transport vesicles for trafficking to a network of smooth membranes called the ER–Golgi intermediate compartment (ERGIC; see Fig. 3–2). COPII complex, composed of *co*at *p*roteins, concentrate and package the protein cargo into vesicles. COPII binds to cargo molecules either directly, if they span the membrane, or through intermediate cargo receptors and then provides some of the force that causes vesicle budding, thereby linking cargo acquisition to vesiculation. Overall, the mechanisms involved in cargo recognition are poorly defined.

ER resident proteins are selectively sequestered in the ER both for the absence of export signals and for the presence of ER retention signals. Soluble luminal ER resident proteins are retained through a C-terminal ER tetrapeptide retention motif KDEL. Frequently, transmembrane proteins have either a C-terminal dilysine motif KKXX or an N-terminal diarginine motif XXRR, or variants thereof. However, it is more accurate to indicate ER localization signals as "retrieval motifs" because proteins bearing these signals can transiently escape from the ER into the ERGIC, from which they are returned to the ER through the retrograde vesicular transport (see Fig. 3–2).

For the KDEL motif of luminal ER proteins, a specific retrieval receptor has been identified, first in yeast and then in mammals. The KKXX motif has been shown to interact directly with the COPI-coated protein complex that is involved in retrograde transport from the ER to the Golgi. Retrograde transport also serves to replenish the vesicle components lost as a result of anterograde (forward) transport. In conclusion, selective protein exit from the ER is achieved by monitoring and regulating (a) transport competence of nascent proteins, (b) capture of cargo in transport vesicles, and (c) protein retention/retrieval for ER-localized proteins.

Receptor-Mediated Protein Transport in the Secretory Pathway

The LMAN1–MCFD2 complex is the only well-defined cargo receptor in mammalian cells. LMAN1, *L*ectin *man*nose-binding protein 1 (also referred to as ERGIC-53), is a transmembrane protein with a C-terminal cytoplasmic tail containing an endoplasmic reticulum (ER)-exit motif (two phenylalanine residues, FF). This motif allows the interaction of LMAN1 with the COPII-coat proteins. The luminal domain of LMAN1 recognizes mannose residues and binds MCFD2, a luminal protein, in a Ca^{2+}-dependent manner. Both LMAN1 and MFDC2 are required in a complex for the recruitment of coagulation factors V and VIII into specific cargo vesicles. Of interest, loss-of-function mutations in either *LMAN1* or *MCDF2* cause a bleeding disorder as a result of the combined deficiency of factors V and VIII. It has been shown that mutant forms of both LMAN1 and MFCD2 fail to recruit factor VIII into the vesicles. Thus, the deficiency of coagulation factors is caused by a block in their export from the ER. Interestingly, the LMAN1–MCFD2 complex appears to only be required for the secretion of factors V and VIII, as there are no significant reductions in any other plasma proteins.

Intra-Golgi Transport and Protein Processing

Organization of the Golgi Apparatus

The Golgi complex comprises a stack of flattened, membrane-bound cisternae that are highly dependent on microtubules for structural integrity. The stack of cisternae can be subdivided into three parts, referred to as *cis*, *medial*, and *trans*, with the *cis* and *trans* sides facing the ER and the plasma membrane, respectively (see Fig. 3–2). Both the *cis* and *trans* faces are associated with tubulovesicular bundles of membranes. The ERGIC comprises the bundle on the *cis* side of the Golgi stack and is the site where incoming proteins from the ER are sorted into those directed for anterograde or for retrograde transport. The tubulovesicular bundle at the *trans* side is the *trans*-Golgi network (TGN; see Fig. 3–2).

A major feature of the Golgi is polarity. The processing events are temporally and spatially ordered because the processing enzymes have a characteristic distribution across the Golgi stack. In the Golgi, other types of modifications also take place, for example, protein O-glycosylation, phosphorylation of oligosaccharides, and sulfation of tyrosines.

Retention of Resident Golgi Proteins

Extensive analysis has failed to reveal a clear retention motif enabling subdomain-specific retention of resident Golgi proteins. Two possible models have been proposed. One model is *retention by preferential interaction with membranes of optimal thickness.* It is based on the finding that the transmembrane domains of Golgi proteins are shorter than the transmembrane domains of plasma membrane proteins. These differences should allow a preferential interaction with the Golgi membrane lipid bilayer that is thinner than that of plasma membrane. The other model is *kin-recognition/oligomerization.* It postulates that proteins of a given subdomain of the Golgi membrane can aggregate into large detergent-insoluble oligomers as a way of minimizing lipid–protein contact. This would prevent the entry of proteins into the vesicles and thus their traffic to more distal cisternae. There is evidence in support of both models.

Protein Trafficking To and Through the Golgi Apparatus

Cargo proteins exit the ER in COPII-coated vesicles that enter the ERGIC and are ultimately delivered to the *cis*-Golgi either in vesicles or along extended tubules. However, the means whereby cargo proteins move across the Golgi complex from *cis* to *trans* remain controversial. Two models have been proposed. The vesicular transport model contends that anterograde transport occurs in vesicles or tubules. The second suggests that there is a cisternal maturation. This alternative model proposes that Golgi cisternae are not fixed structures but move forward from the *cis* side to the *trans* side, generating an anterograde movement. As cisternae mature, resident Golgi proteins that belong to more *cis*-like cisternae must be selectively pinched off in vesicles and trafficked back to the *cis* side of the Golgi stack. This would occur by COPI-mediated retrograde vesicular transport (see Fig. 3–2). Although which of these models is correct is currently unclear, a majority of the experimental data supports the cisternal maturation model.

Sorting Events at the *Trans*-Golgi Network

Overview

The TGN is an important site of intracellular sorting, where proteins bound for lysosomes or regulated secretory vesicles are separated from those entering the constitutive pathway leading to the plasma membrane (see Fig. 3–2, pathways 6, 7, and 8). The secretion process is called exocytosis. The molecular basis for diversion of proteins into lysosomes and regulated secretory granules are described below.

Sorting Into Lysosomes

Lysosomes are acidic (pH of ~5.0–5.5), membrane-bound organelles containing numerous hydrolytic enzymes designed to degrade proteins, carbohydrates, and lipids. Soluble hydrolases are selectively marked for sorting into lysosomes by phosphorylation of their N-linked saccharides, which creates the mannose-6-phosphate (M6P) sorting signal. On arrival at the TGN, the modified hydrolase is bound by a cargo receptor, the M6P receptor (M6P-R), which delivers it first to a "late endosomal compartment," where the low pH releases the hydrolase from the M6P-R. Subsequently, the hydrolase is delivered to the lysosome, and the M6P-R is recycled to the TGN.

The motif responsible for targeting M6P-R to lysosomes is YSKV and is recognized by all three distinct adaptor protein (AP) complexes (AP-l, -2, and -3) that contribute to the delivery of cargo to lysosomes by linking cargo acquisition to vesiculation. Cargo recruitment occurs in a manner similar to that described for the COPI- and COPII-dependent vesicles, except that the cytosolic coat complex is clathrin. In addition to luminal hydrolases, lysosomes also contain a wide array of membrane proteins that are targeted to lysosomes via one of two consensus motifs: (a) YXXe, where X is any amino acid and e is any amino acid with a bulky hydrophobic side chain, and (b) a leucine-based motif (LL or LI). Trafficking of these membrane-bound proteins to lysosomes is indirect, proceeding first to late endosomes or the plasma membrane prior to their retrieval to lysosomes. Failure to accurately target lysosomal hydrolases underlies Hurler syndrome and I-cell disease.

Sorting Into Regulated Secretory Granules

In regulated secretion, proteins are condensed into stored secretory granules that are released to the plasma membrane after the cell has received an appropriate stimulus (see Fig. 3–2, pathway 7). After budding from TGN, the granule proteins are concentrated (up to 200-fold in some cases) by selective removal of extraneous contents from clathrin-coated vesicles. Mature secretory granules are thought to be stored in association with microtubules until the stimulation of a surface receptor triggers their exocytosis. One example of stimulus-induced exocytosis is the binding of a ligand to the T-cell antigen receptor complex on a cytotoxic T lymphocyte. Conjugation of a cytotoxic T cell with its target causes its microtubules and associated secretory granules to reorient toward the target cell. Subsequently, the granules are delivered along microtubules until they fuse with the plasma membrane, releasing their contents for lysis of the target cell. Following release of the granule contents, the granule membrane components are internalized and transported back to the TGN, where the granule can be refilled with cargo proteins.

Endocytic Traffic

Overview

Substances are imported from the cell exterior by a process termed *endocytosis* (see Fig. 3–2, pathway 9). Endocytosis also serves to recover the plasma membrane lipids and proteins that are lost by ongoing secretory activity. There are three types of endocytosis: (a) phagocytosis (cell eating), (b) pinocytosis (cell drinking), and (c) receptor-mediated endocytosis. Defects in endocytosis can underlie human diseases. For example, patients with familial hypercholesterolemia have elevated serum cholesterol because of mutations in the low-density lipoprotein receptor that prevents the endocytic uptake of low-density lipoprotein and its catabolism in lysosomes.

Phagocytosis

During *phagocytosis*, cells are able to ingest large particles (greater than 0.5 μm in diameter). Phagocytosis serves not only to engulf and destroy invading bacteria and fungi but also to clear cellular debris at wound sites and to dispose of aged erythrocytes. Primarily, specialized cells such as macrophages, neutrophils, and dendritic cells execute phagocytosis. Phagocytosis is triggered when specific receptors contact structural triggers on the particle, including bound antibodies, complement components as well as certain oligosaccharides. Then the polymerization of actin is stimulated, driving the extension of pseudopods, which surround the particle and engulf it in a vacuole called phagosome. The engulfed material is destroyed when the phagosome fuses with a lysosome, exposing the content to hydrolytic enzymes. In addition, phagocytosis is a means of "presenting" the pathogen's components to lymphocytes, thus eliciting an immune response.

Pinocytosis

Pinocytosis refers to the constitutive ingestion of fluid in small pinocytotic (endocytotic) vesicles (0.2 μm in diameter) and occurs in all cells. Following invagination and budding, the vesicle becomes part of the endosome system that is described below. The plasma membrane portion that is ingested returns later through exocytosis. In some cells, pinocytosis can result in turnover of the entire plasma membrane in less than 1 hour.

Receptor-Mediated Endocytosis

This is a means to import macromolecules from the extracellular fluid. More than 20 different receptors are internalized through this pathway. Some receptors are internalized continuously whereas others remain on the surface until a ligand is bound. In either case, the receptors slide laterally into coated pits that are indented regions of the plasma membrane surrounded by clathrin and pinch off to form clathrin-coated vesicles. The immediate destination of these vesicles is the endosome.

The endosome is part of a complex network of interrelated membranous vesicles and tubules termed the *endolysosomal system.* The endolysosomal system comprises four types of membrane-bound structures: early endosomes, late endosomes, recycling vesicles, and lysosomes. It is still a matter of debate whether these structures rep-

Influence of MHC-I and MHC-II Biosynthesis on Type of Antigen Presented

Peptide antigens are presented to T lymphocytes in association with either class I or class II major histocompatibility complexes (MHCs). Peptides presented by class I derive from endogenously synthesized proteins (or viruses), whereas those presented by class II derive from proteins found in the extracellular space. This results from differences in the intracellular trafficking of class I and class II MHC. Class I MHC molecules are held in the endoplasmic reticulum (ER) in association with molecular chaperones until they acquire a cytosolic peptide that is transported into the ER. In contrast, class II molecules are prevented from acquiring a peptide in the ER by an associated protein called invariant chain, which plugs the class II binding pocket. Moreover, invariant chain possesses sorting signals that divert class II molecules into the endosome–lysosome pathway, where proteolytic removal of invariant chain allows acquisition of peptides that were derived from degradation of material internalized by endocytosis. Thus, the respective roles of class I and class II molecules in presenting antigens to the immune system are dramatically influenced by their biosynthesis.

resent independent stable compartments or one structure matures into the next. The interior of the endosomes is acidic (pH ~6). Endocytosed material is ultimately delivered to the lysosome, presumably by fusion with late endosomes. Lysosomes are also used for digestion of obsolete parts of the cell in a process called autophagy.

During the formation of clathrin-coated vesicles, clathrin molecules do not recognize cargo receptors directly but rather through the adaptor proteins, which form an inner coat. The AP-2 components bind both clathrin and sorting signals present in the cytoplasmic tails of cargo receptors close to the plasma membrane. These internalization motifs are YXXϕ (where ϕ is a hydrophobic amino acid), as a most common motif, and the NPXY signal, which was first identified in the low-density lipoprotein receptor. For receptors that are internalized in response to ligand binding, the internalization signal may also be generated by a conformational change induced by the binding of the ligand. Through the specificity of the AP-2 complex, the capture of a unique set of cargo receptors is linked to vesiculation, resulting in concentration of the cargo. The coated pit pinches off from the plasma membrane by the action of a GTP-binding protein, dynamin, which forms a ring around the neck of each bud and contributes to vesicle formation. After release and shedding of the clathrin coat, the vesicle fuses with the early endosome compartment.

SPECIFICITY OF VESICULAR TARGETING

As described above, COPI- and COPII-coated vesicles transport material early in the secretory pathway whereas clathrin-coated vesicles transport material from the plasma membrane and Golgi. Coating proteins assemble at specific areas of the membrane in a process controlled by the coat-recruitment GTPases: Arf1 is responsible for the assembly of COPI coats and clathrin coats at Golgi membranes whereas Sar1p is responsible for COPII coat assembly at the ER membrane. Clathrin-coat assembly at the plasma membrane is also thought to involve a GTPase but its identity is unknown. These regulatory proteins also ensure that membrane traffic to and from an organelle are balanced.

After budding, vesicles are transported to their final destination by diffusion or motor-mediated transport along the cytoskeletal network (microtubules or actin). The molecular motors kinesin, dynein, and myosin have been implicated in this process. The vesicles undergo an uncoating process before fusion with the correct target membrane. Both transport vesicles and target membranes display surface markers that selectively recognize each other.

Three classes of proteins guide the selectivity of transport vesicle docking and fusion: (a) complementary sets of *v*esicles SNAREs, v-SNAREs (*s*oluble *N*SF *A*ssociation Protein *Re*ceptor), and *t*arget membrane SNAREs (t-SNAREs) that are crucial for the fusion; (b) a class of GTPases, called Rabs; and (c) protein complexes called tethers that, together with Rabs, facilitate the initial docking of the vesicles to the target membrane.

CONCLUSIONS

The mechanisms regulating protein synthesis, processing, degradation, and transport are under intense evaluation. Protein motifs and their cognate receptors have been identified for many intracellular sorting and processing reactions. Investigations are now directed to elucidate these processes at a molecular level by resolution of the three-dimensional structures of the proteins involved in protein processing and trafficking. The future challenge will be to find ways of exploiting this knowledge to intervene in the numerous disease states that result from errors in these processes.

SUGGESTED READINGS

Baines AC, Zhang B: Receptor-mediated protein transport in the early secretory pathway. TIBS 32:381, 2007.

Beraud-Dufour S, Balch W: A journey through the exocytic pathway. J Cell Sci 115:1779, 2002.

Cal H, Reinisch K, Ferro-Novick S: Coats, tethers, Rabs and SNAREs work together to mediate the intracellular destination of a transport vesicle. Dev Cell 12:671, 2007.

Gingras AC, Raught B, Sonenberg N: Regulation of translation initiation by FRAP/mTOR. Genes Dev 15:807, 2001.

Heiland I, Erdmann R: Biogenesis of peroxisomes. FEBS J 272:2362, 2005.

Helenius A, Aebi M: Intracellular functions of N-linked glycans. Science 291:2364, 2001.

Kaufman RJ: Orchestrating the unfolded protein response in health and disease. J Clin Invest 110:1389, 2002.

Moremen K, Molinari M: *N*-linked glycan recognition and processing: The molecular basis of endoplasmic reticulum control. Curr Opin Struct Biol 16:592, 2006.

Rehling P, Brandner K, Pfanner N: Mitochondrial import and the twin-pore translocase. Nat Rev Mol Cell Biol 5:519, 2004.

Ron D, Walter P: Signal integration in the endoplasmic reticulum unfolded protein response. Nat Rev Mol Cell Biol 8:519, 2007.

Rouault TA: The role of iron regulatory proteins in mammalian homeostasis and disease. Nat Chem Biol 2:406, 2006.

Schroder M, Kaufman RJ: The mammalian unfolded protein response. Annu Rev Biochem 74:739, 2005.

Sitia R, Braakman I: Quality control in the endoplasmic reticulum factory. Nature 426:891, 2003.

Stewart M, Baker RP, Bayliss R, et al: Molecular mechanism of translocation through nuclear pore complexes during nuclear protein import. FEBS Lett 498:145, 2001.

Wickner W, Sheckman R: Protein translocation across biological membranes. Science 310:1452, 2005.

CHAPTER 4

PROTEIN DEGRADATION IN CELLS

Stewart H. Lecker, Tomo Saric, and Alfred L. Goldberg

Nearly all proteins within cells and most in the extracellular space are in a state of continuous turnover, being synthesized from amino acids and then broken back down. Individual proteins in the nucleus and cytosol, as well as in the endoplasmic reticulum (ER) and mitochondria, are degraded at widely differing rates that vary from minutes for some regulatory enzymes or mutated polypeptides, to days or weeks for long-lived proteins, such as actin and myosin in skeletal muscle, and to months for hemoglobin in the red cell.

In eukaryotic cells, there are two principal systems for the complete degradation of proteins: the lysosomal system, where proteolysis occurs within membrane-enclosed vesicles, and the highly selective ubiquitin–proteasome pathway, which functions both in the cytosol and nucleus. These pathways involve very different enzymes and serve different functions in the cell. Proteolytic systems are also present in mitochondria for the degradation of organelles or proteins. One critical feature of these intracellular degradative systems is that they require metabolic energy, unlike the typical proteases that function in the extracellular space. These energy-dependent steps help ensure exquisite selectivity and allow precise regulation of the proteolytic enzymes. Other proteolytic enzymes also exist in the cytosol. A set of Ca^{2+}-activated cysteine proteases termed *calpains* appear to be activated when cell membranes are injured and cytosolic Ca^{2+} rises (eg, in muscular dystrophy). They play an important role in tissue injury, necrosis, and autolysis. Another important family of cytosolic proteases is the caspases that cleave proteins following aspartic acid residues. These enzymes, which are also cysteine proteases, are critical in the destruction of cell constituents during apoptosis. It remains unclear exactly what role the calpains or caspases play, if any, in the continuous degradation of proteins in normal cells.

WHY ARE PROTEINS CONTINUALLY TURNING OVER?

Because cells must use significant amounts of energy for new RNA and protein synthesis and protein folding (see Chapter 3), the continual destruction of cell proteins might appear to be highly wasteful. However, this process serves multiple functions that are essential for life:

1. The degradation of intracellular proteins is a highly selective and tightly regulated process. The rapid removal of many regulatory proteins (transcription factors, oncogenes, tumor suppressors) and many key rate-limiting enzymes is essential for maintaining cellular homeostasis (Table 4–1). Unlike most regulatory mechanisms, peptide bond cleavage is an irreversible process, and proteases therefore act as unidirectional biological switches. The only way that nondividing or slowly dividing cells can rapidly reduce the level of a particular protein is by proteolytic degradation, because decreases in the synthesis of a protein will not lead to a decreased protein content unless the protein itself turns over rapidly. Thus, continual protein degradation permits cells to adapt to changes in the cellular environment. For example, adaptation of the liver to fasting involves net degradation of enzymes for glycogen production, whereas synthesis of enzymes for gluconeogenesis rises.
2. Also of enormous importance in cellular regulation is that protein half-lives can vary dramatically under different conditions. Probably the most important example is the regulation of the cell cycle. Each transition between phases of the cell cycle involves programmed destruction of one of the cyclins, whose presence controls the activity of critical kinases, or of key kinase inhibitory proteins, CKIs, which prevent progression through the mitotic or meiotic cycles.

   In many cases, these degradative processes are triggered by phosphorylation of key residues, which marks them for selective degradation. Another medically important example of such regulation is in the activation of the inflammatory response. In response to the inflammatory mediators TNFα or lipopolysaccharide, the inhibitor of NFκB, IκB, is phosphorylated, leading to its rapid destruction by the ubiquitin–proteasome pathway, which allows NFκB to enter the nucleus and trigger the inflammatory response.

   In these cases, cellular responses are triggered by the conversion of a long-lived protein to one with a short half-life. In addition, several important regulatory responses proceed through stabilization of a normally short-lived protein. For example, in response to hypoxia, the very rapidly degraded transcription factor, HIF-1α, becomes stable and transcribes genes for erythropoietin, VEGF, and glycolytic enzymes. As these various examples suggest, degradation of key proteins by the ubiquitin–proteasome pathway probably regulates most cellular pathways.
3. Protein breakdown also functions as a quality control mechanism that selectively removes abnormal misfolded proteins. Such proteins may arise through mutations, biosynthetic errors (eg, premature terminations), postsynthetic damage (eg, by oxygen radicals), failure to form multienzyme complexes or to bind key cofactors, or failure of normal folding and assembly (which may be a common event in the cytosol or ER) (see Chapter 3 by Kaufman). Some of the clearest examples of protein misfolding leading to disease are the hemoglobinopathies. Some "unstable hemoglobins" demonstrate reduced heme binding and result in lower (or no) oxygen-carrying capacity. This failure of the mutant globins to fold generally leads to intracellular denaturation and rapid destruction often within minutes of synthesis. In thalassemia, mutations that reduce the levels or association of globin-α and globin-β chains lead to rapid degradation of the unassociated chains tend to be degraded in reticulocytes. Their selective degradation is noteworthy because normal hemoglobin is among the most stable intracellular proteins, lasting the life span of the red cell (in humans, ~90 days).

   The failure to degrade misfolded proteins in the cytosol and nucleus seems to account for the accumulation of intracellular inclusions in various neurodegenerative diseases (eg, Lewy bodies in Parkinson disease, τ inclusions in Alzheimer disease). Of particular medical interest in several diseases is the quality control system (termed ERAD) that catalyzes the extraction of misfolded and mutant proteins from the ER for degradation in the cytosol (see Endoplasmie Reticulum-Associated Degradation).
4. Proteins in cells also constitute a reservoir of amino acids that can be mobilized under poor nutritional conditions for generation of new proteins or for energy metabolism. When deprived of essential amino acids, all cells show a general acceleration of protein degradation, but in mammals, skeletal muscle comprises the primary mobilization pool of amino acids, and the net degradation of muscle proteins in fasting or disease provides amino acids that can be used for hepatic gluconeogenesis, direct oxidation, synthesis of acute-phase proteins, or wound repair (Muscle Protein Breakdown and Cachexia).

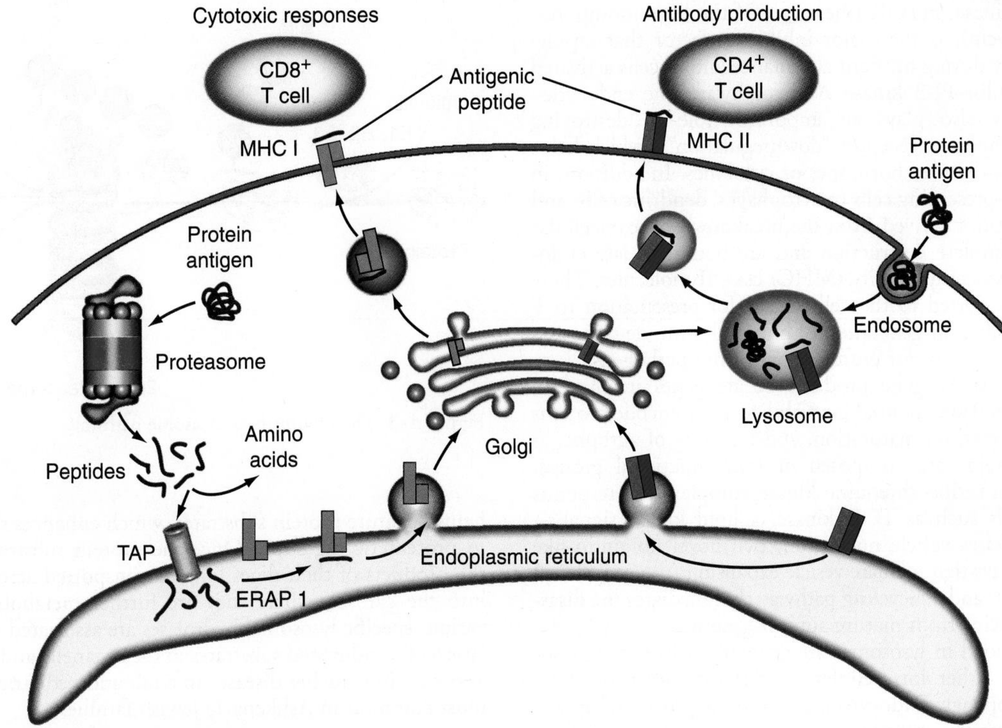

Figure 4–1 Protein degradation and the immune response.

Table 4–1 Important Growth-Regulatory Proteins Rapidly Degraded by the Ubiquitin–Proteasome Pathway

Oncogene Products and Tumor Suppressors
p53 and MDM2 (degrades p53)
c-fos, c-jun, c-Mos
E2A proteins
Cell Cycle Regulators
CDK inhibitors (p27, p21, . . .)
Cyclins (mitotic cyclins, G1 cyclins, . . .)
Transcriptional Regulators
IκB and NF-κB—controls inflammation
HIF1—controls response to hypoxia (VEGF, erythropoietin)
STAT proteins—control response to interferon
β-Catenins—critical in many cancers

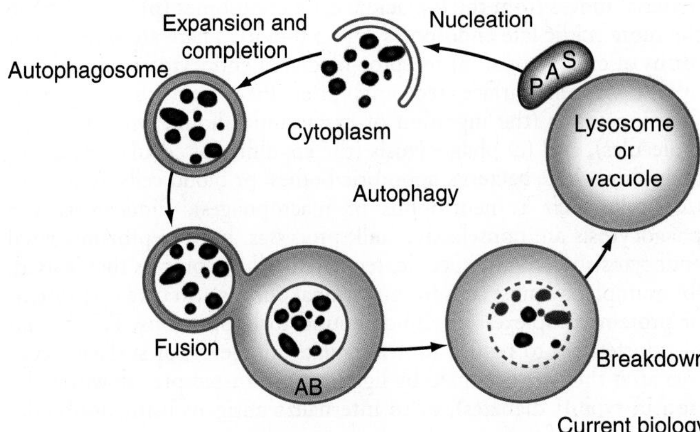

Figure 4–2 Formation of autophagic vacuoles.

5. The continuous degradation of cellular constituents is also critical for recognition of foreign proteins by the immune system. Immune surveillance against intracellular pathogens (eg, viruses and certain bacteria) or pathogens and toxins in the extracellular space (eg, bacteria) is dependent on the continual production of peptide fragments generated from cell proteins by the ubiquitin–proteasome pathway. These antigenic peptides are displayed on surface major histocompatibility complex (MHC) class I molecules, and the appearance of nonnative peptide (eg, of viral origins) triggers cytolytic T-cell responses (see below), whereas the breakdown of bacteria or viruses in lysosomes leads to the fragments' being displayed on surface MHC class II molecules, where they elicit antibody responses (Fig. 4–1).

ENDOCYTIC–LYSOSOMAL PATHWAY

Lysosomes are single membrane-bound organelles found in the cytoplasm. They were discovered by Christian de Duve and coworkers in the mid-1950s and are found in all eukaryotic cells except mature red blood cells. Most extracellular proteins (eg, plasma proteins or cytokines) taken up by receptor-mediated endocytosis are degraded in lysosomes, as are phagocytosed cells (eg, bacteria or red cells in macrophages), and most membrane proteins in all cells. In addition, lysosomes are the sites of degradation of cellular organelles, for example, mitochondria, and cytoplasmic proteins in the process of autophagy that occurs at a low rate in all eukaryotic cells but is of increased importance upon nutrient deprivation (Fig. 4–2). In this process, bits of the cytosol become surrounded by a limiting membrane to form an autophagosome or autophagic vacuole. The outer membrane of this autophagosome then fuses with the lysosome to deliver the inner vesicle to the lysosomal lumen. This process involves a highly conserved set of proteins that covalently modify membranes to promote vacuole formation. Degradation of the sequestered organelles and cytosolic material generates nucleotides, amino acids, and free fatty acids that are reutilized in macromolecular synthesis or are oxidized for energy. Autophagy is rapidly induced in cells lacking nutrients or growth factors (eg, during fasting or low-insulin states) and allows cells to rid themselves of damaged organelles or viruses (eg, during oxidative stress, infection, and accumulation of protein aggregates). The kinase, mTOR (the target of the immunosuppression drug, rapamycin), is the major inhibitory factor that rapidly turns off autophagy during nutrient abundance and in cells activated by the IGF-1–insulin–PI-3 kinase–AKT pathway. The endocytic–lysosomal pathway also plays an important role in destroying receptor–ligase complexes (receptor "downregulation"), which helps reduce cellular sensitivity to hormones or cytokines. In addition, in specialized antigen-presenting cells (macrophages, dendritic cells, and B cells), some peptides derived from the breakdown of extracellular proteins escape complete destruction and are bound in late endosomes by major histocompatibility (MHC) class II molecules. These complexes are transported to the cell surface for presentation to T helper cells responsible for generation of humoral immune responses against nonnative proteins, for example, ones from pathogens.

There are at least 17 gene products or atg genes involved in autophagy and several are essential for viability. They encode proteins needed for the generation, maturation, and recycling of autophagosomes. These proteins are composed of four functional groups, including a protein serine–threonine kinase complex that responds to upstream signals such as TOR kinase, a lipid kinase signaling complex that mediates vesicle nucleation, two novel ubiquitin-like conjugation pathways that mediate vesicle expansion (the Atg8/LC-3 and Atg12 systems), and a recycling pathway that mediates the disassembly of Atg proteins from mature autophagosomes.

Substrates degraded in lysosomes are generally delivered by lysosomal fusion with other intracellular vesicles that are formed by endocytosis or autophagy. Endocytosis refers to the process of uptake of extracellular material or membrane proteins by invagination of the cell membrane, followed by formation of vesicles inside the cell. Before these vesicles reach the lysosomes (pH 4.5–5.0), ingested material moves from the less acidic early endosomes (pH 6.0–6.5) to the more acidic late endosomes (pH 5.0–6.0). There are three major forms of endocytosis: (a) receptor-mediated endocytosis (the specific uptake of cell surface receptors after they bind their ligands), (b) pinocytosis (the ingestion of extracellular liquid with its solute molecules), and (c) phagocytosis (the engulfing of cellular materials, including whole bacteria, apoptotic bodies, or blood cells by specialized cells such as neutrophils or macrophages). Pinocytosis and phagocytosis are nonselective bulk processes, but receptor-mediated endocytosis is a highly specific, regulated cellular process that is used, for example, by most cells for nutritional purposes to take up proteins or protein complexes (eg, lipids bound to lipoproteins, Fe^{2+} bound to transferrin), to reduce (downregulate) the levels of surface receptors after they are occupied by ligands (insulin-receptor downregulation in type II diabetes), or to internalize antigens using antibodies on the cell surface as receptors.

LYSOSOMAL PROTEOLYSIS

Lysosomes contain at least 50 different hydrolytic enzymes, which catalyze the breakdown of proteins, nucleic acids, carbohydrates, and lipids into their components. It is important that lysosomal hydrolases normally do not escape into the cytoplasm, and their isolation in this vesicular compartment is essential for protecting cells from nonspecific degradation of key cell constituents. However, during necrotic cell death, lysosomes release their contents, which helps destroy cellular constituents. Release of lysosomal enzymes outside of cells contributes to severe inflammation and the symptoms of some diseases (eg, gout) and may facilitate tumor metastases and invasiveness. Most lysosomal enzymes are optimally active at an acidic pH of 4 to 6, and the pH within this organelle is maintained acidic by a membrane hydrogen ion pump (a proton-ATPase). Thus upon release or breakage of lysosomes, these enzymes are not as destructive as within the lysosomes. Lysosomal proteases are traditionally called cathepsins, and most belong to the cysteine protease family. The most abundant lysosomal proteases are cathepsins D and L (endopeptidases) and cathepsins B and H (exopeptidases), but there are well over a dozen distinct cathepsins. The acidic milieu in lysosomes not only keeps lysosomal enzymes at their most active state, but it also helps denature protein substrates, which enhances their susceptibility to proteolytic digestion. Once the protein substrates are degraded, the products of their digestion are transported across the membrane into the cytosol, where they are further metabolized. The lack of various specific lysosomal hydrolases are associated with the accumulation of nondigested substrates in the organelle and cell enlargement, as occurs in Gaucher disease, an adult and pediatric inherited disease most common in Ashkenazic Jewish families.

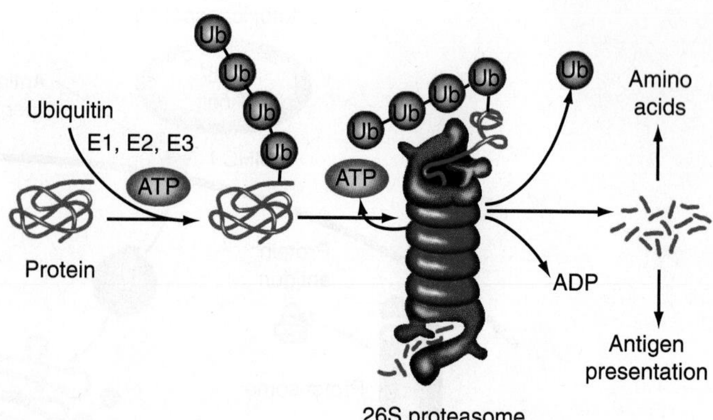

Figure 4–3 The ubiquitin–proteasome pathway.

THE UBIQUITIN–PROTEASOME PATHWAY

Most cytosolic and nuclear proteins are degraded by the highly selective ubiquitin–proteasome pathway (Fig. 4–3). This system catalyzes the breakdown of short-lived proteins that regulate a wide variety of essential cellular processes, ranging from cell cycle progression to signal transduction and gene transcription, as well as most normal long-lived proteins, which comprise the bulk of proteins in cells. In addition, it catalyzes the rapid elimination of misfolded or denatured proteins, which are continuously produced as a result of mutations, biosynthetic errors, failure of successful folding, and postsynthetic damage. The discovery of the ubiquitin–proteasome pathway resulted from the finding that the rapid breakdown of such misfolded proteins was nonlysosomal and was an ATP-dependent process, which was surprising because peptide bond cleavage per se should not require energy. Biochemical dissection of this pathway in the 1980s revealed that it consists of two ATP-dependent processes: the covalent conjugation of a small protein ubiquitin to proteins to mark them for degradation, and the hydrolysis of ubiquitinated proteins by the very large ATP-dependent proteolytic machine, the 26S proteasome (S refers to the rate of sedimentation in the ultracentrifuge in Svedberg units). The ubiquitination step provides exquisite specificity to the degradation process and regulates cellular responses. For their discovery of ubiquitin and the biochemistry of its conjugation to substrate proteins, Avram Hershko, Aaron Ciechanover, and Irwin Rose were awarded the Nobel Prize in Chemistry in 2004.

UBIQUITIN CONJUGATION

Formation of Polyubiquitin Chains

To be degraded by 26S proteasomes, most intracellular proteins must be first covalently linked to a chain of ubiquitin molecules. Ubiquitin is a 76-residue globular protein, and unlike typical peptide bonds formed on the ribosome, ubiquitin is linked to proteins via isopeptide linkages, where the C-terminal carboxyl group of ubiquitin forms an amide bond with the ε-amino group of lysine residues. Formation of a ubiquitin chain ensures that only selected substrates are degraded in a regulated manner and prevents the uncontrolled degradation of

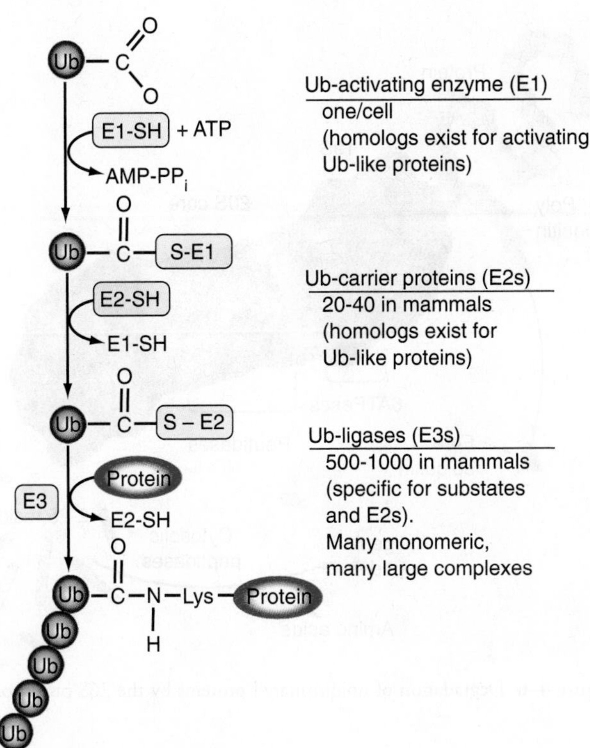

Figure 4–4 Ubiquitin conjugation to protein substrates.

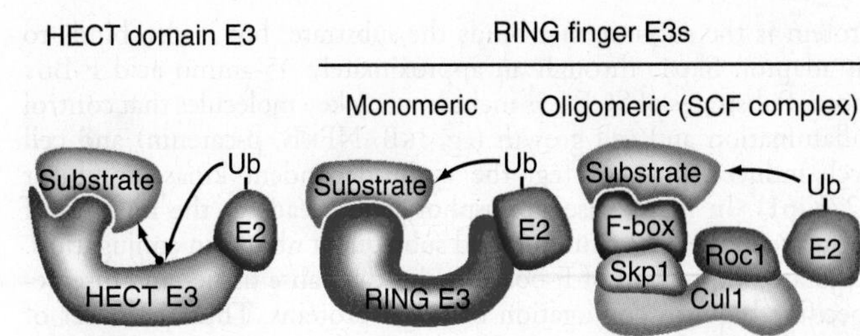

Figure 4–5 Ubiquitin protein ligases or E3s. HECT, homologous to E6-AP carboxy terminus.

other cellular proteins. Ubiquitin can also be conjugated to proteins as a monomer (rather than as a typical ubiquitin chain). This type of tagging can trigger cell surface protein internalization and targeting to the lysosome and can regulate transcription, as with the monoubiquitination of histones. Ubiquitin conjugation to proteins and the formation of polyubiquitin chains is mediated by the sequential action of three types of enzymes (Fig. 4–4). In this ATP-dependent process, the ubiquitin-activating enzyme (E1) initially forms a highly reactive thiolester linkage between the C terminus of ubiquitin and the thiol group in the active site of the E1. The activated ubiquitin is then transferred to a sulfhydryl group on one of the cell's 30 to 40 ubiquitin-conjugating enzymes (ubiquitin-carrier proteins or E2s).

The exquisite specificity of protein degradation is due to the large variety of the ubiquitin-protein ligases or E3 enzymes. The human genome contains between 500 and 1000 different E3s, most of which act on a small number of substrates, thus providing enormous specificity to the ubiquitination process. E3s catalyze the transfer of the activated ubiquitin from a specific E2 initially to a lysine on the target protein and subsequently to lysines present in the preceding ubiquitin, yielding a substrate-anchored chain of ubiquitin molecules. A single E2 may function with multiple E3s and a single E3 with multiple E2s to provide further specificity in a combinatorial fashion. Generally, E3s fall into two broad structural classes based on their enzymatic mechanism; some contain HECT (homologous to E6-AP carboxy terminus) domains but most catalyze ubiquitination through their RING finger domains (Fig. 4–5). Although many RING finger E3s are small monomeric proteins, many are large multisubunit complexes.

HECT domain proteins are large monomeric E3s that consist of two functionally distinct domains. The C-terminal HECT domain accepts the activated ubiquitin from the E2, by forming a thiolester linkage with ubiquitin, enabling it to be transferred to the substrate. HECT-domain E3s directly bind activated ubiquitin and are actual components of the enzymatic conjugation cascade. The prototypical member of this family is the E6-associated protein (E6AP). Lack of this enzyme causes Angelman syndrome, an inherited neurologic disorder, but E6AP is also utilized by oncogenic strains of human papilloma virus for the destruction of host p53 tumor suppressor protein.

The vast majority of E3s contain RING finger domains, which are 40- to 60-residue zinc-binding motifs that are rich in cysteine and histidine residues and facilitate transfer of the activated ubiquitin to the substrate. These E3s serve as scaffolds that bring the substrate and the E2 into close proximity but, unlike the HECT E3s, do not covalently bind the activated ubiquitin. Monomeric RING finger E3s include the oncoprotein Mdm2, a physiological regulator of p53 stability in normal cells, and c-Cbl, which catalyzes ubiquitination of certain cell surface receptors and tyrosine, and cIAP and XIAP inhibitors of apoptosis that function as oncogenes. Two E3s that are important in the processes of muscle atrophy and cachexia, Muscle Ring Finger-1 (MuRF-1) and E3α, belong to this group; E3α was the first of the E3s to be biochemically identified and recognizes protein substrates on the basis of their N-terminal amino acid. Proteins beginning with large basic or hydrophobic residues are targeted for degradation by E3α. This "N-end rule" pathway seems to be important in the destruction of protein fragments, for example, cohesins during the cell cycle, certain signaling molecules, and the enhanced protein degradation in atrophying muscle.

Another group of enzymes with ubiquitin ligase activity are small monomeric proteins that contain anomalous RING finger motifs termed *U boxes*. One important U-box-domain protein is CHIP, which catalyzes the removal of abnormally folded proteins, for example, misfolded CFTR in cystic fibrosis, mutated tau protein, and polyglutamine repeat proteins present in several neurodegenerative diseases (eg, Huntington disease). Degradation of these abnormal proteins begins when they are bound by specific molecular chaperones, Hsp70 (or its homolog, Hsc70) and Hsp90, which associate with misfolded protein domains triggering selective ubiquitination. This binding of molecular chaperones to the unfolded domains helps prevent irreversible aggregation and promotes refolding. However, if refolding is impossible (as occurs with many mutant proteins), binding to the Hsp70 or Hsp90 recruits CHIP, leading to the ubiquitination and degradation of the potentially toxic polypeptides. Interestingly, in conditions where cells accumulate large amounts of misfolded or damaged proteins (eg, during heat shock or oxidative stress), they adapt by expressing large amounts of these heat-shock proteins, ubiquitin, and certain ubiquitination enzymes. This transcriptional response (termed the *heat-shock response*) protects cells against many toxic insults and disease processes.

Other RING finger E3s contain many subunits that serve as scaffolds to bring together the substrate and an E2 conjugated to the activated ubiquitin. The largest (1.5 MDa), most complex E3 is the anaphase-promoting complex, which is essential for the ubiquitination of mitotic cyclins and other proteins involved in progression of the cell cycle. A very large group of E3s is the cullin–RING ubiquitin ligase family. The basic core of these E3s is the elongated, rigid cullin subunit. At one end of these subunits is the RING component (typically Rbx1/Roc1), which binds the E2, whereas at the other end, the substrate-interacting protein is bound, generally through an additional adaptor protein. Because of the large number of cullins and substrate-binding subunits, the same multisubunit organization can recognize and ubiquitinate a large number of diverse proteins.

The best-understood group of cullin–RING ligases are the medically important Skp1–Cul1–F-box (SCF) complexes. The F-box protein is the subunit that binds the substrate, but it also binds to an adaptor, Skp1, through an approximately 45-amino acid F-Box motif. Substrates of SCF E3s include many key molecules that control inflammation and cell growth (eg, IκB, NFκB, β-catenin) and cell cycle-induced proteins (eg, the cyclin-dependent kinase inhibitor p27Kip1). In many cases, phosphorylation leads to the binding of substrate to the F-box subunit and subsequent ubiquitin conjugation. Regulated expression of F-box proteins can cause tissue- and disease-specific ubiquitin conjugation of target proteins. Thus the onset of the inflammatory and most immune responses involve the phosphorylation of the NFκB inhibitor, IκB, which leads to its rapid ubiquitination by the SCF family member β-TRCP and destruction in the proteasome. This step then allows NFκB to enter the nucleus and transcribe key inflammatory mediators (IL-1, Il-6, TNFα, iNOS, etc).

Other types of protein modifications can also stimulate ubiquitination. For example, under normal oxygen tension in cells, the key transcription factor, HIF-1α, which triggers expression of angiogenic genes (VEGF), erythropoietin, and glycolytic enzymes, is very short-lived. Under these conditions, a proline in HIF-1α is hydroxylated by molecular oxygen, and this single change to a hydroxyproline is recognized by the VBC–ubiquitin ligase, leading to its ubiquitination and its proteasomal destruction. The subunit in this E3 that recognizes the oxygen-modified HIF-1α is the von Hippel–Lindau (VHL) protein, and VHL mutations are associated with highly vascular tumors in the kidney, presumably due at least in part to the presence of stable, active HIF-1α. When intracellular oxygen tension falls, the HIF-1α is not modified, not recognized by VHL, and is not degraded. This response is quite important in many human cancers as it promotes angiogenesis and expression of glycolytic enzymes (a hallmark of most cancers). The VBC complex is another cullin–RING ligase, made up of Cul2 and a substrate-interacting domain made up of the VHL protein and the adaptors elonginB and elonginC. Other protein modifications that have been shown to recruit E3s include glycosylation, nitrosylation, and deacetylation. Thus, substrate modification adds another layer of regulation to the ubiquitin–proteasome pathway by integrating cell signaling and cell metabolism with the ubiquitin-conjugation degradation machinery.

DEUBIQUITINATION

Ubiquitin conjugation to cellular proteins can be reversed by deubiquitinating enzymes, which are all cysteine proteases that catalyze the disassembly of ubiquitin conjugates. Several such isopeptidases are found in the 26S proteasome, and during degradation of ubiquitin-conjugated proteins they play important roles in recycling monomeric ubiquitin. There are also many cytosolic deubiquitinating enzymes. Certain deubiquitinating enzymes also probably serve as proofreading systems, which ensures that no erroneous or inappropriate ubiquitination of substrates takes place. However, there is growing evidence that specific isopeptidases function to regulate key enzymes and to prevent their degradation (eg, isopeptidases' control of p53 longevity in the cell) by the opposing actions of E3s. In fact, mutations in certain deubiquitinating enzymes can cause neuronal degeneration and may contribute to the occurrence of cancer.

PROTEIN DEGRADATION

The 26S Proteasome

The rapid degradation of ubiquitinated proteins is catalyzed by the 26S proteasome (Fig. 4–6). This structure is found in the nucleus and the cytosol of all cells and constitutes approximately 1% to 2% of a cell's mass. The 26S particle is composed of approximately 50 subunits and is thus approximately 50 to 100 times larger than the typical proteases that function in the extracellular environment (eg, in digestion or blood clotting). Unlike such enzymes, the proteasome

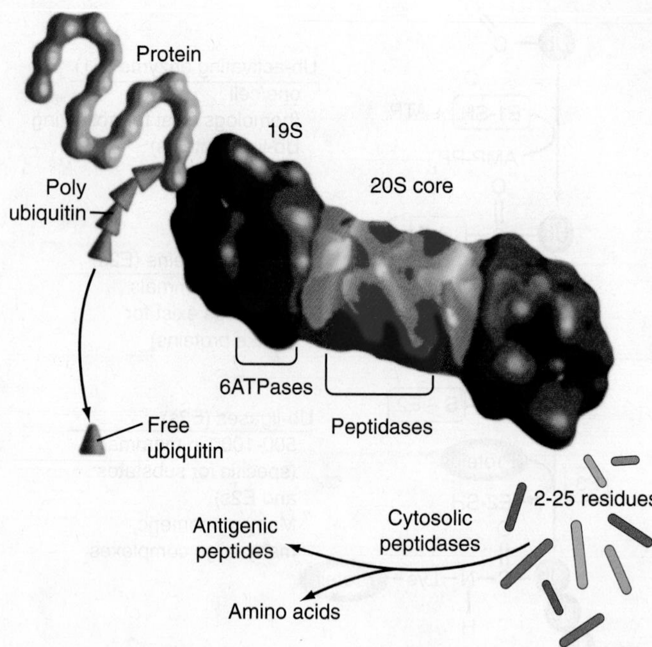

Figure 4–6 Degradation of ubiquitinated proteins by the 26S proteasome.

is a very complex proteolytic machine in which protein degradation is linked to ATP hydrolysis and substrate deubiquitination. The 26S complex is composed of the hollow cylindrical 20S proteasome, within which proteins are cleaved to small fragments, plus a 19S regulatory particle at either or both of its ends. Substrate entry is a complex ATP-dependent process catalyzed by the 19S particle. This architecture evolved to isolate proteolysis within a nano-sized compartment and thus to prevent the nonspecific destruction of cell proteins. One can view protein ubiquitination and the functioning of the 19S particle as mechanisms to ensure that proteolysis is exquisitely selective and that only certain particles and degraded molecules get translocated into the 20S.

The 20S Core Particle: The 20S proteasome is composed of four stacked rings, each containing seven homologous subunits. There are two identical outer α rings and two identical inner β rings. Three of the subunits in each inner β ring contain proteolytic active sites. The outer α rings surround the narrow openings into the 20S particle at either end, through which substrates can enter into the inner proteolytic chamber. These openings are tightly gated, and gate opening and substrate entry occur upon the association of α rings with the 19S regulatory particle. The proteasomal active sites in the β rings are confined to the interior of the cylinder where proteins are cleaved to small peptides 2 to 24 residues long. Each of the three active subunits has a different substrate preference: the "chymotrypsin-like" site cleaves preferentially after large hydrophobic residues, the "trypsin-like" site after basic amino acids, and the "caspase-like" site after acidic residues. The active-site nucleophile of these sites is the threonine hydroxyl group at the amino terminus of the β subunits.

19S Regulatory Particle: The 19S particle consists of at least 18 different subunits and associates with α rings on one or both ends of the 20S proteasome. Two functionally different substructures of this complex have been distinguished: the base and the lid. The base, which touches the α rings of the 20S core particle, contains eight polypeptides, including six ATPases in a ring-like configuration. These ATPases bind substrates and use the energy of the ATP to unfold globular protein substrates. In the ATP-bound state, these ATPases open the gate in α rings and promote rapid translocation of the unfolded substrates into the 20S core particle. The lid contains eight non-ATPase subunits, including a ubiquitin-binding subunit and two deubiquitinating enzymes. Although the lid is required for degradation of ubiquitinated proteins, much remains to be learned about the mechanisms by which these different subunits function in recognition, binding, and disassembly of the ubiquitin chain.

Mechanism of Protein Degradation

Upon binding of the polyubiquitinated substrate to the proteasome, the substrate is unfolded in an energy-dependent manner by the action of ATPases localized in the base of the 19S particle. Conformational changes induced by ATP binding trigger opening of the gate in α rings followed by translocation of the unfolded substrate into the inner chamber of the proteasome. Successful translocation of the substrate requires removal and disassembly of the attached polyubiquitin chain by deubiquitinating enzymes attached to the 19S particle. Translocation of the substrate can occur from either its amino or carboxyl terminus, or even internally by the process in which a polypeptide loop enters the axial channel to permit initial endoproteolytic cleavage. Unlike traditional proteases, the proteasome does not simply cleave a protein and release the partially digested fragments; on the contrary, a protein substrate, once bound by the proteasome, is cut repeatedly by the six active sites until small peptides 3 to 25 residues in length are generated. This behavior ensures that partially digested proteins do not accumulate within cells. However, in several instances, the 26S proteasome degrades substrates only partially, yielding biologically active proteins, as in the generation of the p50 subunit of the transcription factor NFκB from the larger 105-kD precursor, and in the processing of some membrane-bound transcription factors. The complete process of degradation of one substrate molecule requires several hundred molecules of ATP and is completed generally in seconds (<1 min), depending on the size of the substrate. Although generally substrates must be ubiquitinated in order to be rapidly degraded, 26S proteasomes can degrade certain polypeptides in a ubiquitin-independent manner, though the physiological importance of this ubiquitin-independent degradation remains uncertain.

PROTEASOME INHIBITORS AND CANCER THERAPY

Because the proteasome's proteolytic mechanism is novel, highly specific inhibitors of its active sites have been synthesized or are found as microbial products. These inhibitors (eg, MG132, lactacystin, epoxymycin) have been widely used as research tools that have enabled investigators to discover many of the key functions of the ubiquitin–proteasome pathway. Proteasome inhibitors were initially synthesized in an attempt to develop agents that could block the excessive breakdown of muscle proteins in various cachectic states, but it was discovered that they could also block the activation of NFκB, the critical transcription factor that mediates production of many inflammatory cytokines. NFκB also has important antiapoptotic roles, which could block the death of cancer cells. Subsequently, inhibition of the proteasome was found to induce apoptosis, especially in neoplastic cells. One synthetic inhibitor, bortezomib (Velcade, PS-341), has now emerged as an important new treatment for hematologic malignancies. Bortezomib is a peptide boronate inhibitor widely used for the treatment of multiple myeloma and for mantle cell lymphoma. This agent is a potent inhibitor of the 20S proteasome's chymotrypsin-like active sites and, at therapeutic doses, it spares the other two types of active sites, thus allowing significant proteasomal protein degradation, but at a reduced rate.

Surprisingly, Bortezomib induces apoptosis in myeloma cells, even when protein degradation by the proteasome in these cells is only partially compromised. Although NFκB is antiapoptotic in all cells, myeloma cells are particularly dependent upon NFκB for production of essential autocrine growth factors (especially IL-6). In addition, plasma cells and myeloma cells require high expression of the ER chaperone system, termed the *unfolded protein response* (see Chapter by Kaufman) because they synthesize large quantities of immunoglobins. Exposure of the myeloma cells to proteasome inhibitors augments this stress response by blocking the degradation of abnormal immunoglobins by the ERAD pathway (Endoplasmic Reticulum-Associated Degradation), which activates JNK kinase and causes apoptosis. Bortezomib in combination with other chemotherapeutic agents are being currently tested against a broad range of other malignancies. Surprisingly, proteasome inhibitors also have benefits in animal models of stroke and various inflammatory disease models. The compounds appear to reduce postischemia adhesion of macrophages to ischemic endothelia and reperfusion injury. Again, the mechanism of the inhibitors seems to largely involve inhibiting the activation of NFκB.

THE PROTEASOME AND ANTIGENIC PRESENTATION

In addition to its essential roles in regulating cell growth and metabolism and in the elimination of misfolded proteins, in higher vertebrates the ubiquitin–proteasome pathway and the lysosomal–endosomal system also serve critical roles as information-gathering mechanisms for the immune system (see Fig. 4–1). The continual breakdown of intracellular proteins including foreign proteins that arise during viral or bacterial infection or with cancer, allows the immune system to screen for nonnative proteins within cells. Although the great majority of peptides generated by the proteasome during breakdown of intracellular proteins are digested within seconds to free amino acids, some escape this fate and are transported into the ER. Here, they bind to nascent MHC class I molecules and are delivered to the cell surface for presentation to cytotoxic $CD8^+$ lymphocytes. If nonnative epitopes (eg, ones derived from viruses or intracellular parasites) are presented on the cell surface, the presenting cells are quickly killed by cytotoxic ($CD8^+$) T cells. Whereas the presence of abnormal polypeptides within cells elicits cytolytic responses, foreign proteins in the extracellular space elicit antibody production. The degradation of such proteins by the endosomal–lysosomal system generates the antigenic peptides that are displayed on surface MHC class II molecules, are recognized by circulating $CD4^+$ lymphocytes, and trigger production of specific antibodies. Thus, both arms of the immune system respond to peptide fragments generated by the cell's two main proteolytic systems and are presented on surface MHC molecules.

To bind to most MHC class I molecules, antigenic peptides need to be 8 to 9 residues long; however, at least 70% to 80% of proteasome products are shorter than that length. Proteasome products longer than 8 to 9 residues (ie, with additional amino acids on their amino termini) can also be presented on MHC class I molecules after trimming in the ER. Peptides are taken up into the ER by a specific ATP-dependent peptide transporter, called TAP. Although some peptides arrive in the ER at the optimal length to bind directly to the MHC class I molecules, most contain additional N-terminal residues that are clipped off by the ER aminopeptidase 1 (ERAP1). This enzyme has the unusual ability to trim extra amino acids off the longer precursors, stopping at 8 to 9 residues, the precise length for binding to MHC molecules.

Several proteasome adaptations that enhance the efficiency of antigen presentation are evident in cells of the immune system (splenocytes, dendritic cells, or thymocytes), and in most other cells in inflammatory states. In response to the immune modifier, γ-interferon, cells express novel types of proteasomes, termed *immunoproteasomes*, that play a major role in modulating MHC class I antigen presentation. The immunoproteasomes differ because they contain three novel β subunits with peptidase activity that replace the normal β subunits containing the active sites. These specialized subunits exhibit different specificities that enable them to cleave proteins in distinct factions, so that more of the products have the correct features (eg, hydrophobic C-terminal residues) for binding to MHC class I molecules. In addition, interferon-γ induces a special proteasome-activating complex, PA28, that binds to one end of the 20S proteasome and forms a hybrid 26S particle that has a 19S complex at the other end. These hybrid particles degrade ubiquitinated proteins at normal rates, but cleave them differently, generating an even higher fraction of peptides capable of serving as antigenic precursors.

At the same time, interferon-γ can cause cells to express higher amounts of TAP (transporter associated with antigen processing), ERAP1, and MHC molecules. Presumably, antigen processing by these systems normally function well below maximal levels until activation of host's defenses is necessary. On the other hand, a number of viruses (eg, herpesviruses) have evolved sophisticated mechanisms to escape immune detection by inhibiting the uptake of proteasome products into the ER by the TAP or by promoting the degradation of MHC class I molecules from the cell surface. Interferon-γ also stimulates the lysosomal generation of antigenic peptides presented on MHC class II molecules. Thus, these two arms of the immune system increase the efficiency of immune surveillance by adaptation of the cells' two proteolytic systems.

ENDOPLASMIC RETICULUM-ASSOCIATED DEGRADATION

Newly synthesized proteins destined for secretions are translocated into the lumen of the ER and if destined to serve as components of the surface membrane, they are incorporated directly into the ER membrane. The ER contains a large set of molecular chaperones and enzymes that assist newly synthesized proteins and glycoproteins in attaining their final conformations (see Chapter 3), but sometimes, this maturation process fails, or mutations prevent proper folding. Such misfolded proteins are efficiently removed from the ER so as not to form potentially toxic aggregates by a disposal process, often called ER-associated degradation (ERAD). In this process, the misfolded proteins are retrotranslocated from the ER back into the cytosol, where they are ubiquitinated, by ER-associated ubiquitin ligases and degraded by 26S proteasomes. This export is necessary because the ER does not contain proteolytic enzymes for protein degradation. In a variety of human diseases, including cystic fibrosis and α-antitrypsin deficiency, the mutant proteins are rapidly digested by this process. ERAD is also used by some viruses (eg, cytomegalovirus) to downregulate MHC class I molecules in the ER as a means to block antigen presentation and escape the detection by the immune system. In addition, the ERAD pathway functions in the regulated degradation of critical ER-associated proteins, such as the key enzyme for cholesterol biosynthesis, HMG-CoA reductase, which is rapidly degraded when cholesterol levels are high. Also in the liver, the nascent β-lipoproteins that deliver triglycerides to peripheral tissues are rapidly degraded in the ER under conditions when lipid levels are low.

PROTEOLYSIS IN MITOCHONDRIA

As in the cytosol and nucleus, proteins in mitochondria also have widely different half-lives, and mitochondria can selectively degrade misfolded proteins, or ones damaged by free radicals. Although mitochondria as a whole can be degraded in lysosomes by autophagy, this process is nonselective and cannot account for different turnover rates of regulatory mitochondrial proteins. The matrix and the inner membrane of mitochondria contain their own autonomous proteolytic systems, which consist of several ATP-dependent proteases that belong to the AAA superfamily of ATPases (like the six 26S proteasomal ATPases). These proteasomes function independently of ubiquitin and can mediate the complete degradation of nonassembled or misfolded proteins. The matrix of mammalian mitochondria contains two kinds of soluble ATP-dependent proteases that are homologous to bacterial proteases (Lon, ClpXP) and responsible for degradation of matrix proteins. The mitochondrial inner membrane also contains two complex multimeric proteases whose catalytic sites extend into the matrix or intermembrane space. Their ATPases catalyze protein unfolding and facilitate subsequent degradation by the proteolytic sites. Substrates of these proteases are proteins located in the inner membrane, and their activity is essential for the maintenance of oxidative phosphorylation. Impaired function of

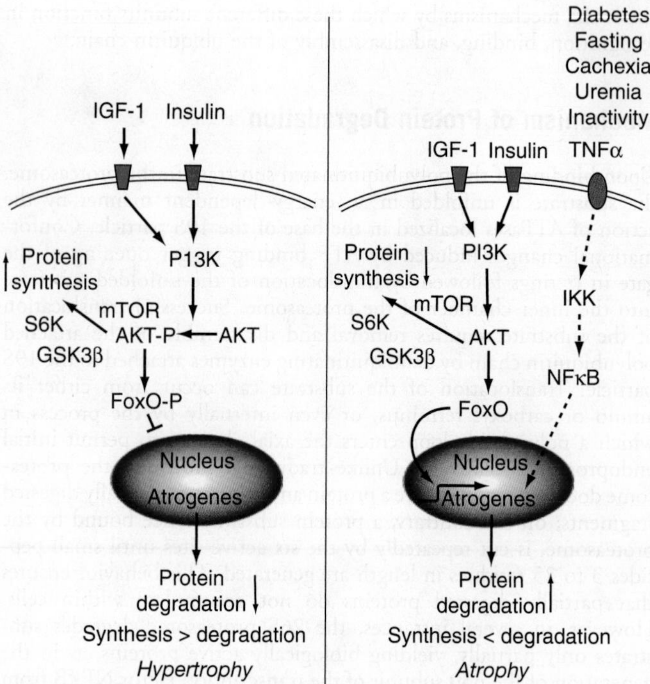

Figure 4–7 Mechanisms leading to enhanced protein breakdown, second reduced protein synthesis in atrophying muscle.

these proteases has been associated with rare neurodegenerative diseases.

MUSCLE PROTEIN BREAKDOWN AND CACHEXIA

Muscle proteins serve as a primary protein reservoir that can be rapidly mobilized through enhanced protein breakdown to provide amino acids for hepatic gluconeogenesis and energy production. This catabolic response is marked and can be highly debilitating in many disease states, especially cancer, sepsis, untreated diabetes, and chronic renal failure. Cachexia occurs in the majority of cancer patients and may contribute to death in as many as 20% of cases, especially when the wasting process affects respiratory muscles. A similar atrophy of muscles is seen with inactivity, which in hospitalized patients is a major cause of loss of body protein stores and weaknesses. In these diverse situations, a similar series of adaptations have been found in the atrophying muscles (but not in other tissues), indicating a common cellular program that involves excessive breakdown of proteins through the ubiquitin–proteasome pathway, as well as autophagy. Microarray analyses of muscles atrophying in response to diverse diseases have identified a set of approximately 100 coordinately regulated genes, or atrogenes. These transcriptional changes include induction of ubiquitin, two atrophy-specific ubiquitin–protein ligases, proteasome subunits, and autophagy-related genes. Recent studies have established that in fasting, and in insulin-deficient (eg, diabetes) or insulin-resistant states (eg, sepsis or cancer cachexia), the general rise in proteolysis is due to decreased signaling by the PI3 kinase/AKT pathway, which in normal states is activated by insulin or IGF-1 (Fig. 4–7). When the activity of PI3 kinase is reduced, there is decreased phosphorylation and activity of the serine/threonine kinase, AKT. Activated AKT is a major stimulus of growth-related processes and, when overproduced, AKT causes muscle hypertrophy via enhanced protein synthesis and decreased protein degradation generally. The reduction in signaling by the IGF-1–PI3K–AKT pathway leads to reduced translation and protein synthesis. One of the targets of activated AKT is the forkhead family of the transcription factors (FoxO1, 3, 4); when these are not phosphorylated, they migrate into the nucleus and catalyze the transcription of certain atrogenes, leading to excessive protein breakdown and muscle atrophy. By itself, FoxO3 can cause profound muscle wasting. There also is evidence that like FoxO factors, NFκB, if overproduced, can cause muscle atrophy specifically following muscle disuse or in cancer cachexia. These advances raise the possibility for development of rationale therapies to reduce this excessive proteolysis in these catabolic states.

OUTLOOK

This chapter hopes to make two points clear: (a) that protein degradation is an exquisitely selective, tightly regulated process that is essential in the normal control of cell division, cell metabolism, as well as immune responses, and (b) that proteolysis by the ubiquitin–proteasome pathway also is critical in the pathogenesis of multiple human diseases, especially many cancers. The recent emergence of the proteasome inhibitor, bortezomib, as a very useful treatment for multiple myeloma and mantle cell lymphoma illustrates the importance and promise of this area for pharmacologic intervention. It is likely that selective inhibitors of the activity or expression of specific ubiquitin ligases will emerge in coming years and will offer new possibilities for the treatment of specific cancers as well as cachexia.

Acknowledgments

We are grateful to Mary Dethavong, Alice Callard, and Joan Goldberg for assistance and advice in preparing this chapter and to the NIH for support of our work (grants R01 GM46147 and R01 GM51923 to A. L.G. and R01 DK62307 to S.H.L.).

SUGGESTED READINGS

Ciechanover A: Proteolysis: From the lysosome to ubiquitin and the proteasome. Nat Rev Mol Cell Biol 6:79, 2005.

Cuervo AM: Autophagy: In sickness and in health. Trends Cell Biol 14:70, 2004.

Glickman MH, Ciechanover A: The ubiquitin-proteasome proteolytic pathway: Destruction for the sake of construction. Physiol Rev 82:373, 2002.

Goldberg AL: Protein degradation and protection against misfolded or damaged proteins. Nature 426:895, 2003.

Goldberg AL: Nobel committee tags ubiquitin for distinction. Neuron 45:339, 2005.

Goldberg AL: Functions of the proteasome: From protein degradation and immune surveillance to cancer therapy. Biochem Soc Trans 35:12, 2007.

Kaelin WG Jr: How oxygen makes its presence felt. Genes Dev 16:1441, 2002.

Kisselev AF, Goldberg AL: Proteasome inhibitors: From research tools to drug candidates. Chem Biol 8:739, 2001.

Lecker S, Goldberg AL, Mitch W: Protein degradation by the ubiquitin-proteasome pathway in normal and disease states. J Am Soc Nephrol 17:1807, 2006.

Levine B, Yuan J: Autophagy in cell death: An innocent convict? J Clin Invest 115:2679, 2005.

Meusser B, Hirsch C, Jarosch E, Sommer T: ERAD: The long road to destruction. Nat Cell Biol 7:766, 2005.

Petroski MD, Deshaies RJ: Function and regulation of cullin-RING ubiquitin ligases. Nat Rev Mol Cell Biol 6:9, 2005.

Rock KL, York IA, Saric T, Goldberg AL: Protein degradation and the generation of MHC class I-presented peptides. Adv Immunol 80:1, 2002.

Salvesen GS, Dixit VM: Caspases: Intracellular signaling by proteolysis. Cell 91:443, 1997.

Sandri M, Sandri C, Gilbert A, et al: Foxo transcription factors induce the atrophy-related ubiquitin ligase atrogin-1 and cause skeletal muscle atrophy. Cell 117:399, 2004.

Smith D, Benaroudj N, Goldberg AL: Proteasomes and their associated ATPases: A destructive combination. J Struct Biol 156:72, 2006.

Voges D, Zwickl P, Baumeister W: The 26S proteasome: A molecular machine designed for controlled proteolysis. Annu Rev Biochem 68:1015, 2000.

CHAPTER 5

PROTEIN ARCHITECTURE: RELATIONSHIP OF FORM AND FUNCTION

Alan C. Rigby, Bruce Furie, and Barbara C. Furie

Previous chapters described how the information stored in the gene is transcribed into messenger RNA (mRNA), how the mRNA template is translated to synthesize proteins, and how newly synthesized proteins are transported to their appropriate site of function. Proteins are linear polymers made up of amino acids linked together by peptide bonds. Twenty different amino acids are incorporated into these polymers when protein is synthesized from mRNA. The features distinguishing one protein from another are determined not by the polypeptide backbone but by the different side chains of the amino acids incorporated into the protein and the sequence in which they occur. Proteins fold to form compact structures with a specific three-dimensional architecture that is determined by their unique amino acid sequences. Folded proteins have the capacity to accomplish many different tasks: formation of larger structures (as in the assembly of fibrin monomers into polymers), transport of ligands (as in the binding of oxygen by hemoglobin), catalysis of chemical reactions (as in proteolytic zymogen activation during the propagation of blood coagulation), and modulation of biologic processes (as in regulation of DNA function by DNA-binding proteins). A mutation that alters the sequence of a protein can result in failure to function either because a critical functional residue has been lost or because alterations in amino acid sequence prevent the protein from achieving its proper three-dimensional structure.

AMINO ACIDS: THE BUILDING BLOCKS OF PROTEINS

In an amino acid, the central or α-carbon atom bears four substituents: an amino group, a carboxyl group, a group of variable chemical structure (R, usually referred to as the side chain), and a hydrogen atom. The side chains of the amino acids provide each one with its distinct chemical character. The amino acids can be divided into three general classes on the basis of the properties of their side chains. *Hydrophobic* amino acids include alanine, valine, leucine, isoleucine, proline, tryptophan, phenylalanine, and methionine. The side chains of aspartic acid, glutamic acid, lysine, and arginine are charged at physiologic pH. The side chains of serine, threonine, tyrosine, histidine, cysteine, asparagine, and glutamine are considered *polar*. Additional amino acids can be found in proteins. These amino acids, for example, hydroxyproline, γ-carboxyglutamic acid, and phosphotyrosine, are formed posttranslationally by modification of one of the amino acids incorporated into a protein during translation of mRNA. Hydrogen bonds may be formed between these polar side chains and water molecules, making them adaptable to the aqueous milieu. Hydrogen bonds also may form between two polar side chains (Fig. 5–1). Glycine has as its side chain a second hydrogen atom. Histidine is unique in that it is the only amino acid whose side chain may be protonated or unprotonated, and therefore charged or uncharged, at physiologic pH. This property of the histidine side chain is functionally significant. For example, the catalytic mechanism of serine proteases, such as the enzymes in the blood coagulation cascade or the complement pathways, is dependent on the ability of a histidine residue in the active site of the enzyme to act as a general base, accepting and then releasing a proton in sequential steps of the enzymatic reaction.

NATURE OF THE PEPTIDE BOND

An amino acid becomes incorporated into a protein when the carboxyl group of one amino acid condenses with the amino group of a second, forming a peptide bond, eliminating water, and establishing the covalent link between these amino acids. The peptide bond is formed between the carbonyl carbon of one amino acid and the nitrogen of the next amino acid in the protein sequence. This process is repeated as the polypeptide chain elongates. The amino group of the first amino acid in the chain and the carboxyl group of the last are not usually modified: a protein's polypeptide chain, the main chain or backbone, is described as running from its N terminus to its C terminus. The peptide backbone is composed of the repeating unit NH—C_α—C′=O. (The carbonyl carbon of the protein backbone is referred to as C′ for ease of identification.)

The fundamental properties of the peptide bond dictate the conformation of the main chain of a protein. The chemical nature of the peptide bond (partial double bond) requires that each segment of the polypeptide chain between one C_α and the next one in the main chain be planar (Fig. 5–2). The conformation of the polypeptide backbone is thus dictated by the angles between these planar segments. The angle of rotation or torsion about the N—C_α bond (Φ, phi angle) and the angle of rotation about the C_α—C′ bond (Ψ, psi angle) are restricted because some angles of rotation would result in steric interference between the main chain and amino acid side chains. The only exceptions to these restrictions are the angles of rotation permissible for glycine residues.

DISULFIDE BRIDGES

In addition to the peptide bond, one other covalent bond between amino acid residues frequently occurs in proteins. The sulfhydryl groups on cysteine residues can be oxidized to form cystine, which contains a disulfide bond (Fig. 5–3). This reaction requires an oxidizing environment. Because the intracellular space is a reducing environment, disulfide bonds are not usually found in intracellular proteins. The disulfide bonds found in extracellular soluble and integral membrane proteins are formed in the lumen of the endoplasmic reticulum (ER), the initial compartment of the secretory pathway. Disulfide bonds form between cysteines that are members of the same polypeptide chain, probably stabilizing an already-folded polypeptide backbone. Disulfide bonds may also serve to covalently join two different polypeptide chains, for example, the heavy and light chains of immunoglobulins.

ELEMENTS OF SECONDARY STRUCTURE

The amino acid sequence of a protein is termed its *primary structure*. This structure is coded in the gene. When a number of consecutive amino acid residues have similar angles of rotation about N—C_α and C_α—C′, the main chain of the protein will assume a regular structure. Two regular protein structures, termed *secondary structures*,

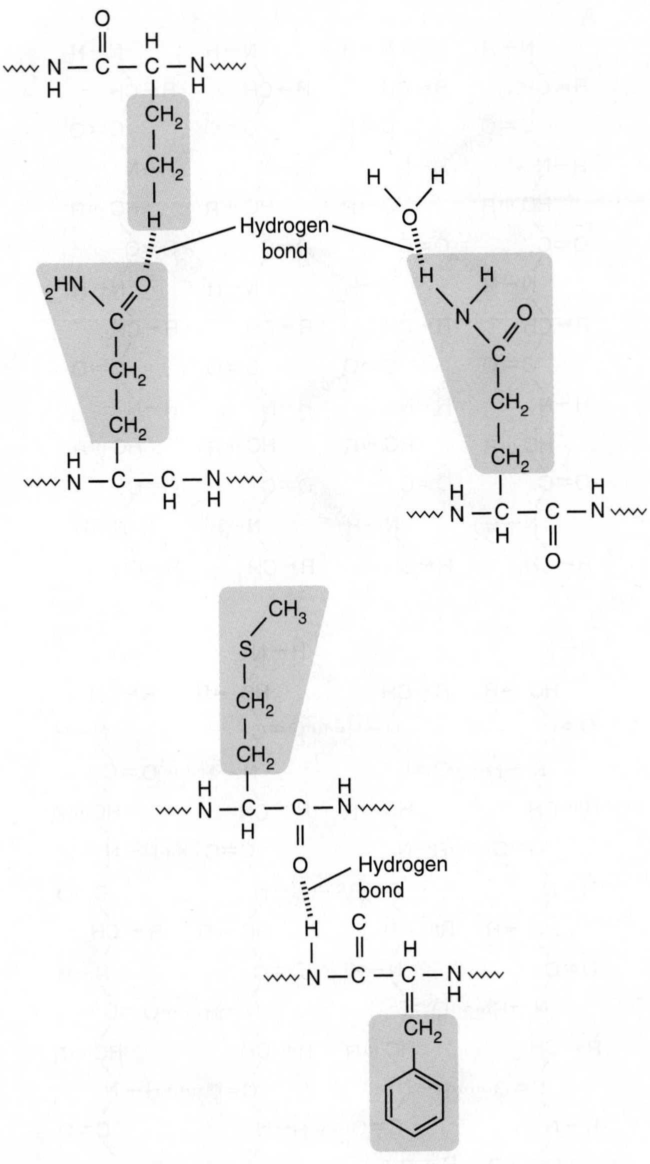

Figure 5–1 In a hydrogen bond, two electronegative atoms share a single proton. The proton is located at the normal covalent distance from the atom to which it is formally bound and at a somewhat shorter distance than the normal van der Waals contact from the other. Hydrogen bonds form in proteins between electronegative atoms in two polar side chains (shown between serine and glutamine side chains), between water and a polar amino acid side chain (shown between water and the glutamine side chain), between carbonyl oxygen atoms and amide nitrogen atoms of the protein backbone (shown between the carbonyl oxygen of a methionine residue and the amide nitrogen of a phenylalanine residue), and between polar side chains and the polypeptide backbone (not shown). Amino acid side chains are shaded.

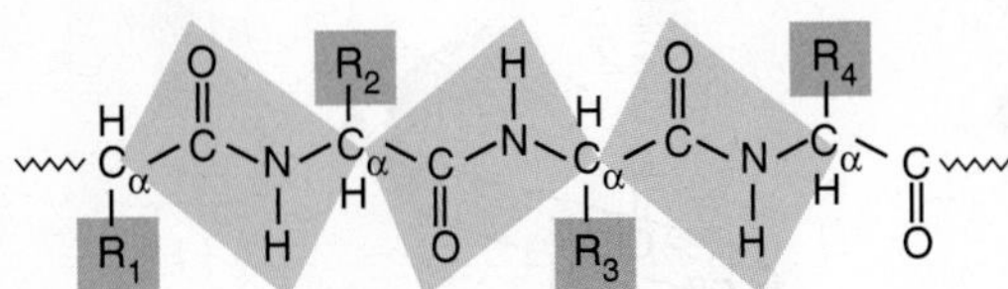

Figure 5–2 In a peptide bond, the amide nitrogen shares its lone pair of electrons with the carbonyl oxygen, lending a considerable double-bond character to the C′—N bond. As a consequence, the main chain of a protein is planar from one C_α to the next C_α. Each planar unit has two degrees of freedom; it can rotate about the N—C_α bond and about the C_α—C′ bond. The peptide bonds of the polypeptide depicted are in the trans configuration; adjacent C_α carbons and the side chains they bear are on opposite sides of the planar C′—N bond. This is the preferred configuration for most amino acids, as it minimizes steric hindrance. For proline, the trans configuration is not favored as much as for other amino acids, and the cis configuration occurs with significant frequency. The planar units of the polypeptide backbone are enclosed in gray boxes. The amino acid side chains are highlighted.

are *α helices* and *β sheets.* A third important element of secondary structure is a *β turn.*

Formation of these secondary structures resolves a dilemma posed by the folding of a polypeptide chain by permitting formation of hydrogen bonds between the NH groups and the C′=O groups of the protein main chain. The major driving force for folding proteins in the aqueous environment is to remove nonpolar amino acid side chains from water by sequestering them in the hydrophobic core of the protein. To bring the nonpolar side chains into the hydrophobic interior of the protein, the main chain must follow. The main chain of a protein with its NH and C′=O groups is highly polar. The hydrophilic nature of the main chain is neutralized in regions of secondary structure by the formation of hydrogen bonds between its polar elements, as illustrated in Figs. 5–4 and 5–5.

α HELIX

α Helices ranging in length from 4 or 5 to 40 residues are found in compact globular proteins such as hemoglobin, whereas long rodlike proteins like the tail of the cytoskeletal protein myosin are made up of long helices twisted around each other to form coiled coils. The membrane-spanning regions of integral membrane proteins, for example, glycophorin and the α_2-adrenergic (epinephrine) receptor, are α helices of approximately 20 amino acids. An α helix is formed from a continuous sequence of amino acid residues in a protein. One turn of an α helix contains 3.6 amino acid residues, with hydrogen bonds between the carbonyl oxygen of residue *n* and the amide hydrogen of residue $n + 4$ (see Fig. 5–4). The distance between one turn of an α helix and the next, its pitch, is 5.4 Å. With 3.6 residues per turn, the rise per residue along the vertical axis of the helix is 1.5 Å. Theoretically, an α helix can be either right-handed or left-handed with regard to direction of "screw." In proteins, left-handed helices are rarely seen, as the side chains of L-amino acids approach

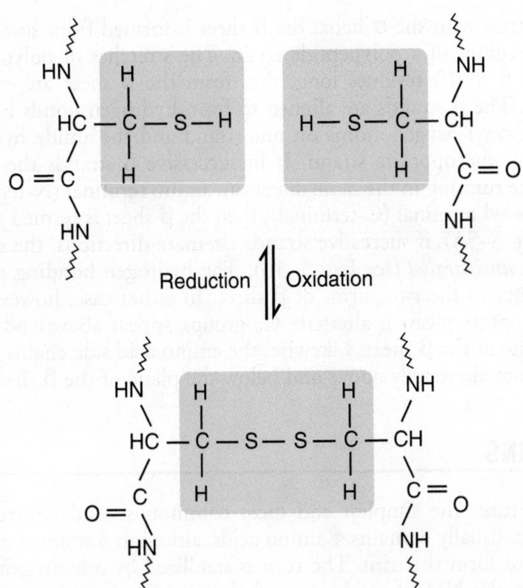

Figure 5–3 Disulfide bonds are formed between neighboring cysteine residues in an oxidizing environment. The side chains of cysteine and cystine are shaded.

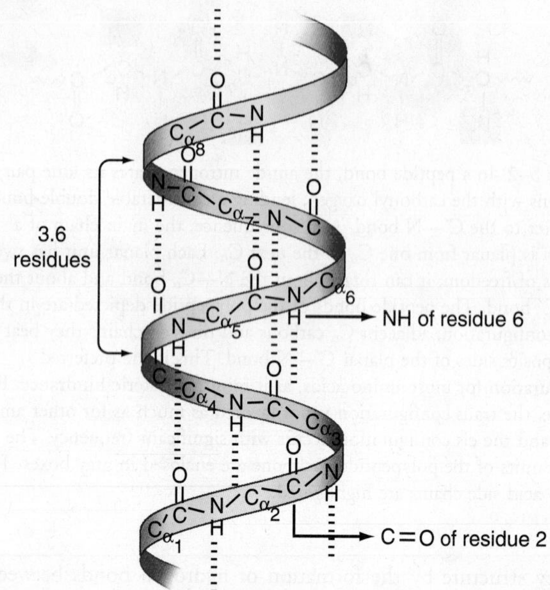

Figure 5–4 The α helix is formed from a continuous sequence of amino acids. A right-handed α helix is illustrated. The hydrogen bonds between residue *n* and residue *n* + 4, which stabilize the helix, are depicted as lines composed of stacked dashes.

the C′=O group too closely. Collagen is a notable exception: it assumes a left-handed helical conformation.

With the exception of proline, there are no strong predictors of whether or not a particular amino acid side chain is likely to be incorporated into an α helix. The last atom of the proline side chain is bonded to the main-chain nitrogen atom, preventing the nitrogen atom from participating in hydrogen bond formation. In addition, the proline side chain sterically hinders the α-helical conformation, producing a bend in the helix if it appears after the first turn.

β SHEETS

In contrast with the α helix, the β sheet is formed from several different regions of a polypeptide chain. The stretches of polypeptide, usually 5 to 10 residues long, that form the β sheet are called *β strands*. The β strands are aligned to form hydrogen bonds between the carbonyl oxygen atoms on one strand and the amide hydrogen atom on the opposite strand. If in successive β strands the amino acids are running in the same direction, amino terminal (N-terminal) to carboxyl terminal (C-terminal), then the β sheet is termed *parallel* (see Fig. 5–5A); if successive strands alternate directions, the sheet is termed *antiparallel* (see Fig. 5–3B). The hydrogen bonding pattern is distinct in the two forms of β sheet. In either case, however, the sheet appears pleated; alternate C_α groups appear above and below the plane of the β sheet. Likewise, the amino acid side chains on a β strand are alternately above and below the plane of the β sheet.

β TURNS

The β turn, the simplest and most common secondary structural element, usually contains 4 amino acids, although 3 residues are sufficient to form the turn. The turn is stabilized by a hydrogen bond between the NH of residue *n* and the C=O of residue *n* + 3. β Turns typically link successive α helices and/or β strands and generally are found on the surface of proteins exposed to the aqueous environment (Fig. 5–6).

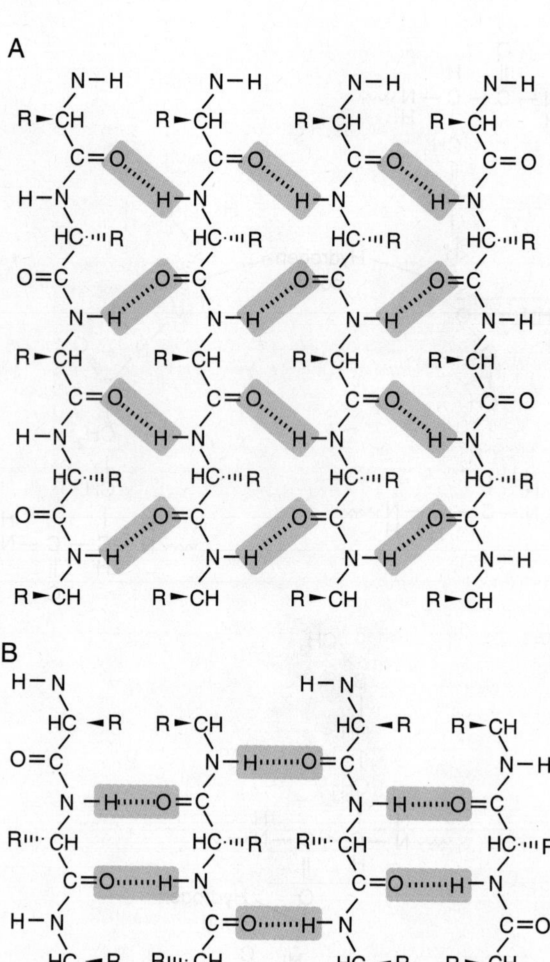

Figure 5–5 β Sheets are formed from several regions of a polypeptide chain. The strands of polypeptide assembled in a β sheet may be parallel, that is, aligned in the same direction from amino to carboxyl (N to C) terminus, or the strands may be antiparallel, that is, aligned in alternating direction from N to C terminus. **A,** Schematic drawing of a parallel β sheet. **B,** Schematic drawing of an antiparallel β sheet. The hydrogen bonds that stabilize these structures are *highlighted.*

PROTEIN TERTIARY STRUCTURE: ASSEMBLY OF SECONDARY STRUCTURES

Most proteins are made up of combinations of α helices and β sheets connected by regions of less regular structure usually termed *loops.* The α helices and β sheets pack together to form the hydrophobic core of a protein, whereas the loop regions tend to appear on the surface of the protein. Loops are stabilized by side chain-to-main chain hydrogen bonds or are extended structures that do not contain stabilizing hydrogen bonds. Comparison of homologous proteins among species suggests greater mutability of loop regions than of regions of regular secondary structure. The structures of the folded cores of the proteins are preserved during evolution, although insertions or deletions of several amino acids occur primarily in loop regions. Protein surface loops are important determinants of a protein's functional specificity, for example, substrate recognition by enzymes or ligand recognition by adhesion molecules.

The arrangement of secondary structures within a polypeptide defines its tertiary structure. The packing of secondary structural elements into a compact, folded form brings distant parts of the polypeptide chain into close proximity. Most proteins may be assigned to one of four classes depending on the content and arrangement of secondary structure within the core of the protein. Proteins of the α class are made up primarily of α helices with connecting loop structures. Similarly, β proteins are made up of β sheets connected by loop regions. In αβ proteins, the two elements of secondary structure alternate, again connected by loops. A fourth class of proteins, α + β, incorporates both α helices and β sheets, but these elements are not arranged in an easily identifiable pattern.

Figure 5–6 shows examples of α, β, and αβ proteins.. The vesicular transport protein α-SNAP (soluble NSF attachment protein from yeast) is an α protein composed of an N-terminal twisted sheet of α-helical hairpins and a C-terminal α-helical bundle (Fig. 5–6A). It is structurally related to several other α/α proteins that are known to mediate protein–protein interactions. Homologous proteins mediate membrane fusion events in platelets and other mammalian cells. A β structure, the seven-bladed β-propeller domain, is found in integrins, adhesion proteins that mediate cell–cell interactions and intracellular signaling. This domain is illustrated in Fig. 5–6B by two seven-bladed β-propeller domains of the *Caenorhabditis elegans* homolog of the Actin interacting protein 1 (Aip1) found in yeast. Figure 5–6C shows an example of an αβ protein, a monomer of the hexameric D2 domain of *N*-ethylmaleimide-sensitive fusion protein, Nsf-D2, a cytosolic ATPase required for intracellular vesicle fusion reactions. The monomer is made up of two domains. The first contains a central five-stranded parallel β sheet flanked by α helices (an αβ domain). The second domain consists of four α helices topped by two short antiparallel β strands.

With the explosion of information on protein sequence and structure in recent years, large databases classifying proteins on the basis of structural characteristics are now available (see Databases and Related Literature at the end of this chapter).

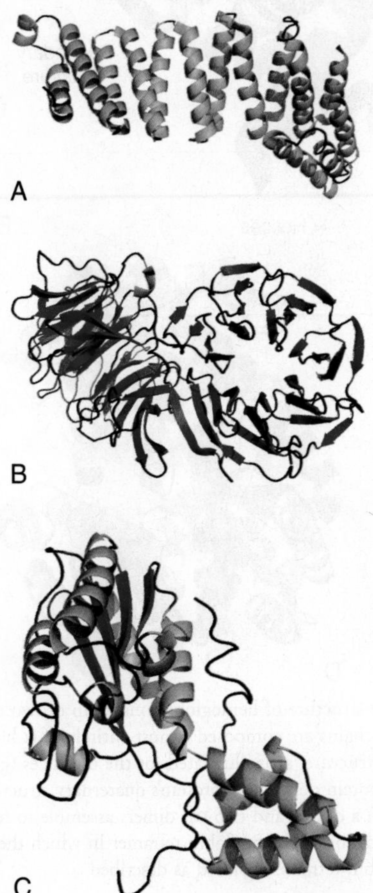

Figure 5–6 Models illustrating the three-dimensional structures of proteins composed almost exclusively of secondary structural elements. The protein backbones are illustrated using ribbon traces that make it easy to discern the elements of secondary structure. α Helices are shown as blue ribbon traces and β sheets are shown as purple ribbon traces, with arrows indicating the direction of the β strand from the N-terminal to the C-terminal. Connecting loops are indicated in black. **A,** α-SNAP (from yeast) composed of an amino (N)-terminal twisted sheet of α-helical hairpins and a carboxyl (C)-terminal α-helical bundle. **B,** Two seven-bladed β-propeller domains of the *Caenorhabditis elegans* homolog of the actin-interacting protein 1 (Aip1) found in yeast. The two β propellers are at 90° to one another. **C,** A monomer of the hexameric D2 domain of *N*-ethylmaleimide-sensitive fusion protein, Nsf-D2, is composed of two domains: a central five-stranded parallel β sheet flanked by α helices (an αβ domain) and the second four α helices topped by two short antiparallel β strands (not shown as ribbons).

PROTEIN DOMAINS

Many proteins are made up of domains. A protein domain, frequently encoded in a single exon, is a region of a polypeptide chain that can fold autonomously into a stable tertiary structure. The packing of secondary structural units into a globular or folded unit yields the tertiary structure of a domain or protein. The spatial relationship of independent domains within a protein is part of the description of its tertiary structure. The relationship between the secondary and the tertiary structure is illustrated for hemoglobin in Fig. 5–7.

During evolution, a limited number of protein domains have been used repeatedly. Related domains from different proteins share enough sequence homology to preserve the polypeptide fold but may have markedly different amino acid sequences and functions. Such domains appear to be associated with exon shuffling and duplication. Examples of proteins whose tertiary structures are built from such conserved domains abound in plasma and as components of cells within the vasculature. A demonstration of the assembly of discrete proteins from such domains is given in Chapter 118 for the proteins involved in hemostasis and fibrinolysis. These proteins incorporate, among others, epidermal growth factor (EGF)-like domains, kringle domains, and type I and type II fibronectin domains, all of which are widely distributed in mammalian proteins. The domains within a given class share a stable core structure with discrete functions determined by the nonconserved amino acids expressed on the module's surface.

Several common domain structures are illustrated in Fig. 5–8. The Src family tyrosine kinases are found in many cell types and are essential components of many signal transduction pathways. The Src homology 2 (SH2) domain is a regulatory domain that binds phosphorylated tyrosine residues in a sequence-specific manner and is found in phosphatases as well as kinases. Src-like kinases contain a second ligand-binding regulatory domain, the SH3 domain. EGF domains are common to many different classes of proteins, including blood coagulation proteins, Factors VII, IX, and X (see Chapter 118). Some of these domains contain calcium ion-binding sites. C2 domains are common to a number of phospholipid-binding proteins, including the coagulation proteins factor V and factor VIII.

Protein motifs are common arrangements of secondary structure that are incorporated into many protein domains. Motifs are characterized by highly conserved amino acid sequences and by conserved function. Examples of protein motifs are shown in Fig. 5–9. Zinc finger-containing proteins are one of the most abundant families of proteins within the eukaryotic genomes. The EF-hand is the most common calcium-binding motif. The basic leucine zipper (bZIP) motif binds to DNA. The β barrel of OmpT, an integral

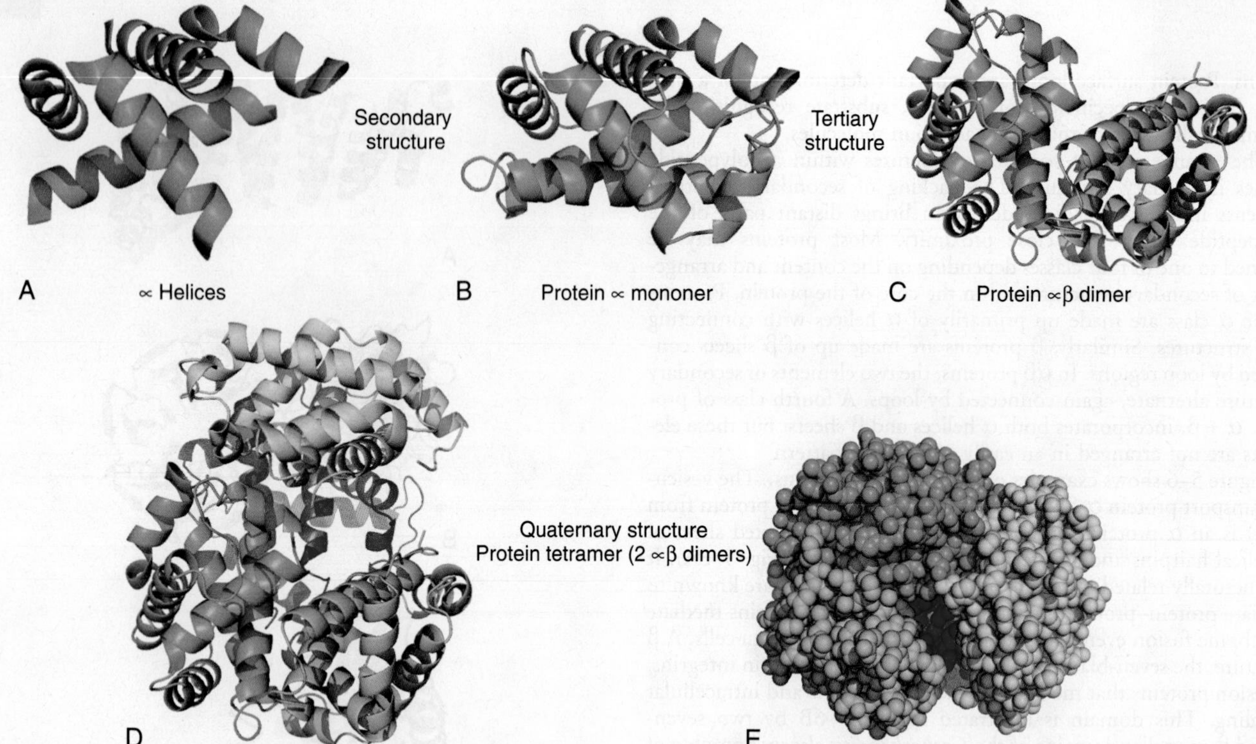

Figure 5–7 The structure of hemoglobin, made up of two α-globin chains and two β-globin chains, is used to illustrate the hierarchical nature of protein folding. Globin chains are composed almost entirely of α helices. The organization of secondary structural elements within a domain or protein defines the fold or tertiary structure, as is illustrated for the α helices (green ribbon) of an α-globin chain of deoxyhemoglobin. The spatial relationship of subunits in the assembled protein defines the protein's quaternary structure. To form a hemoglobin molecule, an α- and a β-globin chain (green and blue, respectively) assemble to form a dimer, and two αβ dimers assemble to form the hemoglobin tetramer (α chains, green and magenta; β chains, blue and yellow). A space-filling model of the hemoglobin tetramer in which the atoms are represented by spheres with radii proportional to their van der Waals radii is shown for the hemoglobin tetramer, colored as described.

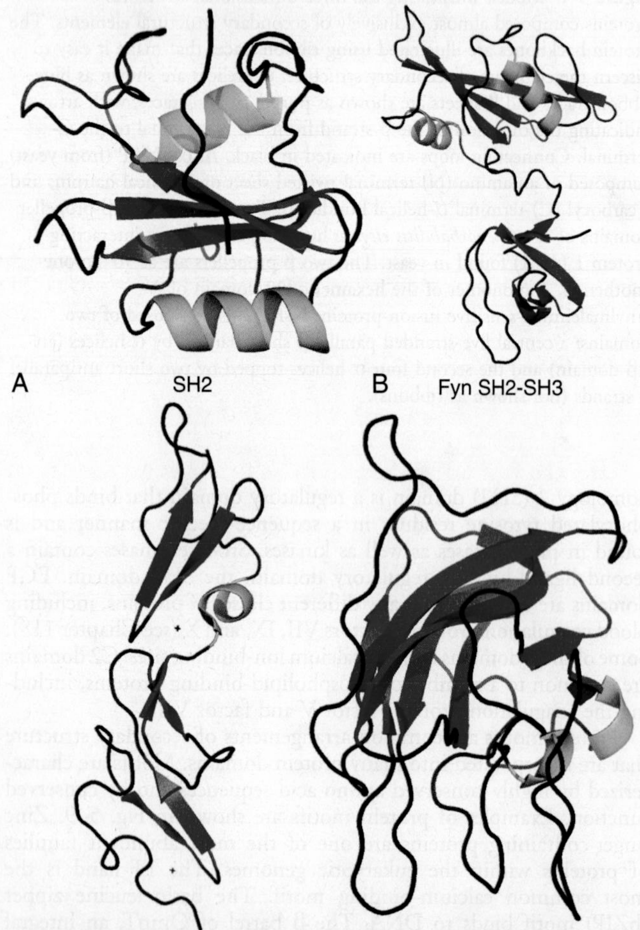

Figure 5–8 The amino-terminal SH2 domain of the tyrosine phosphatase Syp demonstrates the highly conserved central core of SH2 domains. The Src family kinases are composed of a catalytic tyrosine kinase domain preceded by two ligand-binding regulatory domains, SH3 and SH2. The backbone trace of the SH3-SH2 regulatory pair from the Src nonreceptor tyrosine kinase Fyn is illustrated with the SH2 domain oriented toward the top of the figure. Comparison of the SH2 domain of Fyn with the SH2 domain of Syp indicates differences outside the conserved SH2 core, including an additional β strand in the Fyn SH2 domain and more extensive loops in the Syp SH2 domain. These differences demonstrate that the surface topography of SH2 domains can be altered, resulting in changes in binding specificity. Fibrillin-1, a major component of connective tissue fibrils associated with Marfan syndrome, is a mosaic protein composed of 43 calcium-binding epidermal growth factor (cbEGF)-like domains. The backbone trace of calcium-bound cbEGF11–12 exhibits the linear arrangement of these domains with a single interdomain linker region. The carboxyl-terminal C2 domain of the procoagulant cofactor, factor VIII, contains critical determinants that are essential for binding to anionic phospholipids and von Willebrand factor. This structure is a β-sandwich core that possesses two solvent-exposed β turns that include the hydrophobic and positively charged residues that interact with membranes.

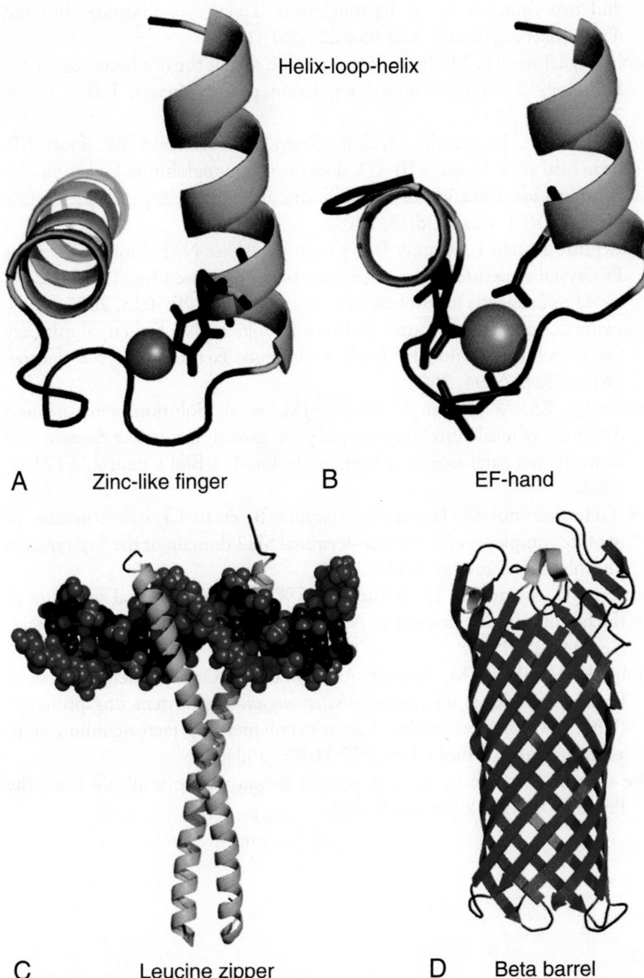

Figure 5–9 The transcriptional adaptor protein CBP contains two copies of a zinc finger motif called the *TAZ finger* that are implicated in binding to transcription factors and viral oncoproteins. The structure of the TAZ1 domain is shown. One of three bound zinc atoms is shown bound by His362, Cys366, Cys379, and Cys384. His362 is shown in black; the zinc ion is red. The most common calcium-binding motif in proteins is the EF-hand motif, which is illustrated for the calcium-bound B-chain of human psoriasin. This protein is abundant in many cell types and is upregulated in keratinocytes in psoriasis. The calcium-chelating residues of this canonical acidic helix-loop-helix motif, Asp62, Asn64, Asp66, Lys68, and Glu73, are shown in black. The calcium ion is red. The basic leucine zipper (bZIP) DNA-binding motif of GCN4 is a parallel-coiled coil. The coiled coil is oriented perpendicular to the DNA double helix, which forms numerous contacts between its major groove and the amino-terminal amino acids of GCN4. The GCN4 coiled coil is in blue. The carbons atoms of one strand of the DNA helix are black and the other purple. The 10-stranded antiparallel β barrel of OmpT of *Escherichia coli* is illustrated as a purple ribbon. The structure of OmpT is depicted with the extracellular portion of the protease that is involved in lipopolysaccharide binding oriented up.

outer-membrane protease found in *Escherichia coli,* binds to lipopolysaccharide.

QUATERNARY STRUCTURE: ASSEMBLY OF POLYPEPTIDE CHAINS

For some proteins, the functional unit is made up of more than one independently synthesized polypeptide chain. The orientation of the polypeptide chains to one another within the functional unit is termed the *quaternary structure* of a multimeric protein. A multimeric protein may be made up of identical subunits or polypeptide chains, as in glucosephosphate isomerase, a dimer of two identical polypeptide chains, or different subunits, as in hemoglobin, in which the functional protein contains two α and two β subunits. The relationship between the tertiary and the quaternary structure for hemoglobin is illustrated in Fig. 5–7. The interaction between the subunits of a multimeric protein may be stabilized by disulfide bonds between the polypeptide chains. The light and heavy chains of immunoglobulin molecules and the Aα chains, Bβ chains, and γ chains of fibrinogen are examples of such proteins.

The subunits of a multimeric protein may influence one another, as in the binding of oxygen to hemoglobin, in which the occupancy of one heme group with oxygen influences the affinity of the heme groups of the remaining three subunits for oxygen (see Chapter 33). Alternatively, the subunits of the assembled multimeric protein may provide a unique function, as in the formation of the antigen-binding site of an immunoglobulin, the complementarity-determining site being formed by the variable regions of both the heavy and light chains of the immunoglobulin molecule. Finally, there are multisubunit proteins in which each subunit has a distinct function; RNA polymerase is an example of such a protein.

Ribbon diagrams that trace the α-carbon backbone of a protein identify the fold of the protein, but they provide a misleading impression that a large amount of empty space exists within proteins. This is not the case, as most folded, globular proteins possess a hydrophobic core that is enclosed by the secondary structural elements that make up the tertiary fold. The core of globular proteins is actually densely packed with atoms contributed by both the backbone carbonyls and amine hydrogen atoms and by the atoms of the amino acid side chains, as is demonstrated by a space-filling model of the hemoglobin tetramer in which the atoms are represented by spheres with radii proportional to their van der Waals radii (see Fig. 5–7). Very little empty space remains within the core of proteins when they are in their active conformation. The cavity at the center of the assembled tetramer is filled by the four heme prosthetic groups.

SUGGESTED READINGS

Alberts B, Bray D, Lewis J, et al: Molecular Biology of the Cell, 4th ed. New York, Garland Press, 2002.

Branden C, Tooze J: Introduction to Protein Structure, 2nd ed. New York, Garland Press, 1998.

Creighton TE: Proteins: Structures and Molecular Properties, 2nd ed. New York, WH Freeman, 1993.

Janin J, Chothia C: Domains in proteins: Definitions, location and structural principles. Methods Enzymol 115:420, 1985.

Richardson JS: The anatomy and taxonomy of protein structure. Adv Protein Chem 34:167, 1981.

Richardson JS: Describing patterns of protein tertiary structure. Methods Enzymol 115:349, 1985.

Richardson JS, Richardson DC: Principles and patterns of protein conformation. In Fasman GD (ed.): Prediction of Protein Structure and the Principles of Protein Conformation. New York, Plenum Press, 1989, p 1.

Richardson DC: The origami of proteins. In Gierasch LM, King J (eds.): Protein Folding: Deciphering the Second Half of the Genetic Code. Washington, DC, American Association for the Advancement of Science, 1990, p 5.

Databases and Related Literature

Class, Architecture, Topology and Homologous (CATH) superfamily database (http://www.biochem.ucl.ac.uk/bsm/cath/): Employs a rigorous hierarchical classification of protein domain structure using both sequence and structural properties. The organization of protein structure has been more thoroughly characterized using this database.

Orengo CA, Michie AD, Jones S, et al: CATH-a hierarchic classification of protein domain structures. Structure 5:1093, 1997.

Pearl FMG, Lee D, Bray JE, et al: Assigning genomic sequences to CATH. Nucleic Acids Res 28:277, 2000.

SCOP (structural classification of proteins) database (http://scop.mrc-lmb.cam.ac.uk/scop/): A comparative pairwise analysis of individual structures that has the potential to identify subtle relationships often not detected in an automated process.

Lo Conte L, Brenner SE, Hubbard TJP, Chothia C, Murzin A: SCOP database in 2002: Refinements accommodate structural genomics. Nucleic Acids Res 30:264, 2002.

Pfam (protein families) database (http://www.sanger.ac.uk/Software/Pfam/index.shtml): A large collection of multiple sequence alignments and hidden Markov models covering many common protein domains and families. For each family in Pfam, the database user can look at multiple alignments, view protein domain architectures, examine species distribution, and view known protein structures.

Bateman A, Birney E, Cerruti L, et al: The Pfam protein families database. Nucleic Acids Res 30:276, 2002.

Protein Structures

Ellenberger TE, Brandl CJ, Struhl K, Harrison SC: The GCN4 basic region leucine zipper binds DNA as a dimer of uninterrupted alpha helices: crystal structure of the protein-DNA complex. Cell 71:1223, 1992.

Brodersen DE, Nyborg J, Kjeldgaard M: Zinc-binding site of an S100 protein revealed. Two crystal structures of Ca^{2+}-bound human psoriasin (S100A7) in the Zn^{2+}-loaded and Zn^{2+}-free states. Biochemistry 38:1695, 1999.

De Guzman RN, Wojciak JM, Martinez-Yamout MA, Dyson HJ, Wright PE: CBP/p300 TAZ1 domain forms a structured scaffold for ligand binding Biochemistry 44:490, 2005.

Liddington R, Derewenda Z, Dodson E, Hubbard R, Dodson G: High resolution crystal structures and comparisons of T-state deoxyhaemoglobin and two liganded T-state haemoglobins: T(alpha-oxy)haemoglobin and T(met)haemoglobin. J Mol Biol 228:551, 1992.

Arold ST, Ulmer TS, Mulhern TD, et al: The role of the Src homology 3-Src homology 2 interface in the regulation of Src kinases. J Biol Chem 276:17199, 2001.

Spiegel PC, Jr, Jacquemin M, Saint-Remy JM, Stoddard BL, Pratt KP: Structure of a factor VIII C2 domain-immunoglobulin G4kappa Fab complex: identification of an inhibitory antibody epitope on the surface of factor VIII. Blood 98:13, 2001.

Vandeputte-Rutten L, Kramer RA, Kroon J, Dekker N, Egmond MR, Gros P: Crystal structure of the outer membrane protease OmpT from *Escherichia coli* suggests a novel catalytic site. EMBO J 20:5033, 2001.

Hamiaux C, van Eerde A, Parsot C, Broos J, Dijkstra BW: Structural mimicry for vinculin activation by IpaA, a virulence factor of *Shigella flexneri*. EMBO Rep 7:794, 2006.

Smallridge RS, Whiteman P, Werner JM, et al: Solution structure and dynamics of a calcium binding epidermal growth factor-like domain pair from the neonatal region of human fibrillin-1. J Biol Chem 278:12199, 2003.

Lee CH, Kominos D, Jacques S, Margolis B, et al: Crystal structures of peptide complexes of the amino-terminal SH2 domain of the Syp tyrosine phosphatase. Structure 2:423, 1994.

Lenzen CU, Steinmann D, Whiteheart SW, Weis WI: Crystal structure of the hexamerization domain of *N*-ethylmaleimide-sensitive fusion protein. Cell 94:525, 1998.

Mohri K, Vorobiev SM, Fedorov AA, Almo SC, Ono S: Identification of functional residues on *Caenorhabditis elegans* actin-interacting protein 1 (UNC-78) for disassembly of actin depolymerizing factor/cofilin-bound actin filaments. J Biol Chem 279:31697, 2004.

The coordinates of most known protein structures are available from the Protein Data Bank (www.pdb.org).

CHAPTER 6

REGULATION OF CELLULAR RESPONSE

Benjamin G. Neel and Christopher L. Carpenter

INTRODUCTION AND OVERVIEW

Hematopoiesis is a dynamic process in which a small number of self-renewing stem cells generate large numbers of terminally differentiated cells, which carry out multiple essential functions. For the hematopoietic system to maintain homeostasis, cell proliferation, differentiation, adhesion, migration, and death must be carefully controlled. Small changes in this balance can lead to marked alterations in blood cell number and function, resulting in marrow failure (eg, aplastic anemia), abnormal proliferation (eg, leukemia), or defective effector cell function (eg, lymphocyte defects in autoimmunity or immunodeficiency). Understanding the regulatory systems controlling normal hematopoietic cells and delineating how these mechanisms are deranged in disease should facilitate the rational development of novel and improved diagnostic and therapeutic modalities.

Hematopoietic cells can respond to a wide range of stimuli or signals. These include *extrinsic* signals (eg, hormones, growth factors, and cytokines) and *intrinsic* (intracellular) signals that indicate exposure to toxic stimuli (eg, ionizing radiation or toxic drugs) and/or cell damage. Some hematopoietic cell signals are similar, even identical to, those acting on other cell types. For example, insulin-like growth factors (IGFs) act on hematopoietic and nonhematopoietic cells, and all cells share most elements of the DNA damage response pathway. Other signals, such as antigens and immune complexes, complement, and certain bacterial products, are more specific to hematopoietic cells. Indeed, with the possible exception of neurons, hematopoietic cells respond a greater variety of signals than any other cell type.

To react appropriately to such a diverse array of signals, cells must solve six fundamental problems: (a) most signals must be transmitted across the cell membrane; (b) detection must be sufficiently sensitive and (c) specific; (d) multiple signals must be interpreted and integrated; (e) analog signals must be converted to digital outputs; and (f) the signaling response must be terminated. The extracellular and intracellular milieus are aqueous environments separated by a hydrophobic cell membrane. Cells must have a mechanism to transmit extracellular signals across this diffusion barrier. The second problem is more general, and arises because most signals are present at very low levels. Hormones and cytokines typically act at low nanomolar or even picomolar concentrations. Likewise, white blood cells must detect and respond to extremely low numbers of invading microbes, lest the host be rapidly overcome. Cells also must recognize very low levels of DNA damage, as even one double-stranded DNA break can have disastrous consequences. Therefore, cells must be able to respond to signals with adequate *sensitivity*. A third, equally important challenge is the *specificity* of the cellular response. Hematopoietic progenitors must be able to discern a signal to proliferate from one to differentiate. Lymphocytes must distinguish foreign antigens from self, when that difference may be as small as a single amino acid in a short peptide sequence. Again, failure to achieve adequate specificity can result in serious disease. Under physiological conditions, cells are simultaneously barraged by multiple signals; hence, *signal integration* is a fourth key problem in cellular regulation. Ultimately, the cellular response consists of regulating protein expression and function. Integration of the ambient and extrinsic signals can result in fine-tuning of the cellular set point to maintain the basal state. However, when the appropriate signals are present, a change in cellular state ensues. For example, a quiescent cell is stimulated to enter the cell cycle and proliferate, or an activated lymphocyte is triggered to undergo cell death. Cellular response systems therefore must have both analog (ie, the ability to generate continuous levels of signals) and digital (ie, on–off) characteristics, and the ability to switch between these two signaling modes. Accordingly, cells must effect *analog–digital conversions*. Finally, once initiated, signals must be terminated appropriately (*signal termination*).

Cells solve these fundamental problems by means of signal transduction pathways. A typical signal transduction pathway consists of a ligand (or sometimes more than one ligand), a receptor, and a set of downstream signaling molecules (Fig. 6–1). Downstream signals converge on the nucleus to regulate transcription, RNA processing, and/or nuclear import/export, on the protein synthetic machinery to control translation, and/or on the mitochondria or various metabolic enzymes to affect cellular energetics and cell survival. Signal transduction pathways may also regulate cytoskeleton-dependent functions, such as motility or phagocytosis. Transmembrane receptors allow the cell to solve the diffusion barrier problem, and specific receptors for discrete ligands help contribute to response specificity. Downstream signaling cascades involve the formation of multiprotein complexes, phosphorylation/dephosphorylation or proteolytic cascades, and/or second messenger generation, facilitating amplification of the initial signal. Such *signal amplification* enhances the response sensitivity. Downstream signaling molecules often contain one or more small domains or *modules* (eg, SH2, SH3, PTB, PH; see below) that recognize specific *motifs* on other signaling molecules. Multiprotein complexes are assembled through these interactions. Like a molecular bar code, the combinatorial use of signaling modules and motifs contributes to specificity, amplification and efficiency of signal transmission. Signaling is terminated via several mechanisms, including degradation or posttranslational modification of the ligand, its receptor, and/or critical downstream signaling components. Many signal termination mechanisms are activated by downstream signaling pathways, thereby coupling initial pathway stimulation to its eventual inactivation. Analog-digital conversions are accomplished by signaling circuits in which pathway-stimulating and -inactivating mechanisms are regulated coordinately in opposing directions, leading to the generation of positive feedback loops.

In this chapter, we survey the types of signaling molecules found in hematopoietic cells and review the general features of their receptors and signal transduction pathways. Our goal is to emphasize the general principles that these pathways illustrate, rather than to provide a comprehensive accounting of each pathway. For details about any of the individual systems discussed, the reader is urged to consult the more detailed reviews cited at the end of the chapter.

SIGNAL DETECTION: LIGANDS AND RECEPTORS

Signals

Hematopoietic cells respond to an enormous variety of extrinsic and intracellular stimuli and generate an impressive number of signals (Table 6–1). *Extrinsic signals* important for hematopoietic cell function include proteins and peptides (eg, growth factors, hormones, cytokines, most chemokines), lipids (eg, LPA, PAF, eicosanoids),

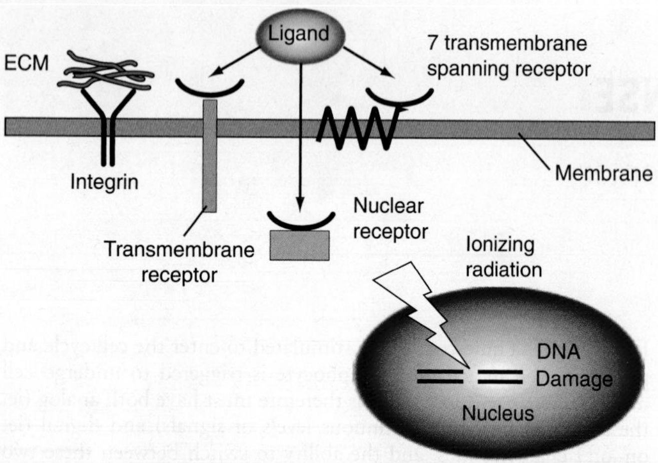

Figure 6–1 Examples of ligands and receptors. Signals can originate from fixed ligands like extracellular matrix (ECM). Soluble ligands that are not membrane permeable bind to extracellular regions of transmembrane receptors. Membrane permeable ligands bind to intracellular receptors, such as the nuclear receptor family. Signals can also originate from within the cell, such as DNA damage caused by ionizing radiation.

Table 6–1 Signals in the Hematopoietic System

Types of Ligands	Examples
Peptide/protein	
Soluble	Growth factors/cytokine
ECM	Fibronectin, collagen
Cell surface-bound	ICAM, Kit ligand
Small Organics	Thyroid hormone
Nucleotides	
Soluble	ADP
DNA	Double-strand breaks
Lipids	Eicosanoids, LPA
Gases	H_2O_2, Nitric oxide*

*Indicates function in hematopoietic system not well-defined

nucleotides (eg, ADP), and gases (eg, nitric oxide, hydrogen peroxide, and possibly superoxide). These signals can be grouped into two general classes based on their activation of two fundamentally distinct types of receptors. Signals such as steroid hormones (androgens, estrogens, glucocorticoids) and gases diffuse into the cell (*transcellular signals*) where they encounter their cognate receptors or targets. The vast majority of signals are lipid-insoluble (*extracellular signals*), however, and thus cannot transit the plasma membrane. These ligands bind to specific cell surface receptors, which transduce the signal through the membrane to the cell interior.

Extracellular signals can be further grouped into subclasses (Table 6–1). *Soluble signals* include most growth factors, hormones, chemokines, and nucleotides; as their name implies, these signals diffuse freely in the extracellular space. Often, soluble signals are further characterized based on the distance over which they act. *Endocrine* signals (classical hormones) typically act over fairly long distances. For example, IGFs are produced in the liver in response to growth hormone that, in turn, is secreted by the pituitary. *Paracrine* signals are produced by one cell and act on an adjacent one. For example, T helper lymphocytes produce cytokines that stimulate antibody production by adjacent B lymphocytes. Although the distinction is not absolute, paracrine signals are generally viewed as acting over smaller distances than endocrine signals. *Autocrine* signals are produced by, and act on, the same cell. For example, interleukin-2 is produced in response to T cell-antigen receptor activation, and stimulates further cell cycle progression of T lymphocytes. Although terms like endocrine, paracrine, and autocrine are useful, they only describe the function of a particular signal in a given physiological setting; they are not fundamental properties of a specific signal. Indeed, the same signal can act in an endocrine fashion in some contexts and as a paracrine or autocrine factor in others.

Contrasting with soluble signals are solid-state signals. Many extracellular matrix (ECM) molecules (eg, collagen and fibronectin), in addition to mediating cell–matrix adhesion, have signaling roles. Other ECM components, such as heparin sulfate proteoglycans, bind soluble growth factors. Such interactions can either concentrate or sequester the growth factor, facilitating or acting as a mechanism to localize or terminate cell signaling, respectively. Cell–cell adhesion molecules also have signaling functions. Cadherins and PECAM (platelet–endothelial cell adhesion molecule; aka CD31), among others, participate in *homotypic* interactions, in which a molecule on one cell acts as both ligand and receptor for the cognate molecule on an apposing cell. Other interactions (eg, P-selectin/PSGL-1) are *heterophilic*. Still other solid-state signals have no apparent cell adhesion function, acting only as signaling molecules. Examples include the Serrate family of ligands for Notch signal transducers. Interestingly, in the case of ephrins and Eph receptors, both heterophilic partners transduce signals into their respective cell (as well as transmitting signals to the adjacent cell), thereby muddying the distinction between "ligand" and "receptor."

Some ligands have a complex nature and/or a complicated life history. The ligands for T cell-antigen receptors (TCRs) are complexes comprising a short peptide bound to major histocompatibility complex (MHC) proteins. Epidermal growth factor family members are synthesized as transmembrane precursors, with the mature growth factor released only upon appropriate proteolytic cleavage. Although the transmembrane forms of these ligands may signal in some contexts, in others, the soluble growth factor is essential. Stem cell factor (SCF, also known as Kit Ligand), which plays an essential role in hematopoietic progenitors and mast cells, also exists in both transmembrane and soluble forms, but its transmembrane form is required for function. Wnts are secreted proteins, yet they effectively function as solid-state signal transducers because they are so tightly associated with the ECM. Still other signals, most notably TGF beta superfamily members, are secreted in a latent form that must be activated by specific proteolysis. Perhaps the most baroque example is provided by the thrombin receptor (and its relatives); here, the receptor (a G-protein coupled receptor; see below) and its cryptic ligand are contained within a single polypeptide chain. Exposure to thrombin (a protease activated during coagulation) results in cleavage of the receptor and exposure of the ligand, which then binds intramolecularly to the receptor, resulting in its activation.

Cell signals also differ in temporal quality. Most soluble signals are released only under specific conditions to enable cell–cell communication. In contrast, ECM-derived signals typically transmit continuous information about cell attachment and/or cell–cell interactions. However, solid-state signals can also be inducible. Examples include the ICAM/LFA-1 interactions that follow TCR activation and the increase in affinity of GP IIB/IIIA for its ligand fibrinogen that occurs upon platelet activation. Continuous and intermittent signaling modes probably have different cellular effects, although this issue remains poorly understood.

Finally, important signals arise from within cells. (Some investigators have termed these signals *intracrine*, but because this terminology is not in general usage, we prefer the more general *intrinsic* to refer to this type of signals.) Important examples include checkpoint pathways, which ensure orderly progression of the cell cycle, sense and repair damaged DNA, and detect and respond to cellular stresses, such as nutrient and/or energy deprivation or unfolded proteins. When activated, these pathways lead to cell-cycle arrest, which allows time for the damage to be repaired and/or cellular stress to be alleviated, or to cell death.

TABLE 6–2 Receptors in the Hematopoietic System

Types of Receptors	Examples	Types of Ligands
RTK	Insulin, Kit, Fms	Kit ligand, M-CSF
RSK	TGF-β Receptors	Activin, BMPs, TGF-β
GPCR	Thrombin receptor, CXC, CC receptors	Thrombin Chemokines
PTK-associated MIRR	Cytokine receptors BCR/TCR/FcR	Epo, Interleukins, IFN Peptide/MHC, Fc domains
TNF family	Fas, TNFR, CD40	Fas, TNF, CD40L
Notch	Notch	Delta-Serrate-LAG-2
Frizzled family	Wnt receptors	Wnts
Toll receptors	TLR1-10	Bacterial DNA, LPS
RPTP	CD45	Unknown
Nuclear receptors	AR, RAR	Testosterone, retinoids
Adhesion receptors	Integrins	Fibronectin, Collagen

AR, androgen receptor; BCR, B-cell antigen receptor; BMPs, Bone morphogenetic proteins; CC, CXC, types of chemokine receptors; CD40L, Ligand for CD40; Epo, erythropoietin; FcR, receptors for Fc portion of antibodies; GPCR, G protein-coupled receptor; M-CSF, macrophage colony stimulating factor; MIRR, multichain immune recognition receptor; RAR, retinoic acid receptor; RPTP, receptor protein-tyrosine phosphatase; RSK, receptor serine kinase; RTK, receptor tyrosine kinase; TCR, T-cell antigen receptor; TGF-β, transforming growth factor-β; TNF, tumor necrosis factor.

Receptors

Nearly all extrinsic signaling pathways begin with a ligand binding to its receptor. Signaling gases, which directly modify intracellular protein targets by nitrosylation (nitric oxide) or oxidation (peroxide, superoxide), are the exception to this general rule. Below, we briefly describe the major families of signaling receptors in hematopoietic cells (Table 6–2).

Intracellular Receptors

Intracellular receptors include those that sense DNA damage and cell cycle checkpoints, guanylate cyclase and the nuclear receptors. The checkpoint receptors are, in general, not well understood, and guanylate cyclase has little known role in hematopoietic cells, so we focus on the nuclear receptors.

The Nuclear Receptor Superfamily

The best understood intracellular receptors are members of a large superfamily of molecules that transduce signals by ligands as diverse as amino acid derivatives (eg, thyroid hormone), steroids (eg, glucocorticoids, estrogens, progesterone, androgens), vitamins (eg, retinoids, Vitamin D), xenobiotics, and fatty acids and/or their derivatives (eg, prostaglandins). Initially termed *steroid–thyroid hormone* receptors, they are now referred to as "nuclear receptors" in recognition of the wide range of signals they transduce. Unfortunately, this nomenclature also is a bit of a misnomer; some family members (eg, the progesterone receptor) bind ligand in the cytoplasm and only then move to the nucleus.

Nuclear receptors share a modular structure, consisting of domains A through E (some family members have a C-terminal extension that is termed F or E/F), which allows them to function as ligand-dependent transcription factors. Domain C is a double-stranded DNA-binding domain that binds to specific palindromic target sequences in the genome. Accordingly, nuclear receptors bind DNA as dimers, with some (eg, glucocorticoid, steroid hormone receptors) acting as homodimers, but most binding as heterodimers with a group of nuclear receptors termed RXRs (eg, thyroid hormone signals through thyroid hormone receptor/RXR heterodimers; retinoids employ retinoic acid receptor (RAR)/RXR pairs). The E (or E/F) domain functions both in ligand binding and transcriptional activation (transactivation). These two functions are coupled in a remarkable example of "induced fit." In the absence of ligand, the critical residues for transactivation are inaccessible, only to be exposed on the surface when ligand binds. The A/B domain also has a transactivation function, although this is ligand-independent. The D domain serves mainly as a hinge to join the C and E/F domains, although it also plays an important role in binding certain coregulatory molecules.

In addition to their structural similarity, nuclear receptors share the ability to bind ligand and then directly alter cellular transcription. Some data suggest that these receptors also have extranuclear functions. For example, the estrogen receptor binds to and affects the activity of the cell cycle regulatory protein cyclin D, as well as the signal transducers Src, Erk, and PI-3 kinase (see Signal Propagation: The Intermediaries). These alternative functions of nuclear receptors remain controversial and an area of active study. The ability of nuclear receptors to regulate transcription is also modified by other signal transduction pathways. For example, phosphorylation of some nuclear receptors can enhance their transactivation potential or even render them ligand-independent. Like other transcription factors, nuclear receptors transmit activation signals by means of coactivators that are associated with histone acetylase activity; phosphorylation of coactivators also can modify nuclear receptor signaling. Although ligands are known for a large number of nuclear receptors, others, known as "orphan receptors" have no known ligands. Identifying ligands remains an active area of investigation, but some nuclear receptors may not have ligands. Such molecules, of course, are not functional "receptors" (because they lack ligand-binding ability). By competing with ligand-binding family members for the same response elements, orphan receptors act as repressors and/or ligand-independent transcription factors.

Extracellular Receptors

Extracellular receptors have adopted several strategies to solve the diffusion barrier problem. *Enzyme-linked* receptors directly couple extracellular ligand binding to intracellular enzyme activation. The enzymatic activity may be intrinsic to the receptor (eg, receptor tyrosine kinases, receptor serine kinases, receptor protein-tyrosine phosphatases) or enzymes can associate noncovalently with one or more ligand-binding subunits (eg, integrins, cytokine receptors, multichain immune recognition receptors). G protein-coupled receptors (GPCRs) couple ligand binding to the activation of heterotrimeric GTP-binding proteins (G proteins). Upon activation, TNF and Toll-like receptors generate protein surfaces for the assembly of multimolecular complexes, whereas activation of members of the Notch family results in cleavage of their intracellular domain and release of a signaling fragment that translocates to the nucleus to modulate transcription. The structure of these receptor families and the initial events in receptor activation are discussed briefly below.

Enzyme-Linked Receptors

Receptor Tyrosine Kinases

Receptor tyrosine kinases (RTKs) consist of an extracellular ligand-binding domain, a transmembrane domain, and an intracellular protein-tyrosine kinase (PTK) domain. RTKs can be further grouped into subfamilies based on structural motifs found in their extracellular (ectodomains) and intracellular domains, with members of the same RTK subfamily often binding structurally related ligands. The ligands for RTKs typically are soluble proteins or peptides; examples include epidermal growth factor (EGF), platelet-derived growth factors (PDGFs), the fibroblast growth factors (FGFs) and insulin and the insulin-like growth factors (IGFs). However, as mentioned above, some RTK ligands (eg, SCF) are cell surface proteins or have cell surface-associated forms. Indeed, the largest subfamily of RTKs, Eph receptors, respond to a number of glycerophosphoinositide (GPI)-linked or transmembrane ligands known as Ephrins. One RTK (DDR) is activated by specific subtypes of collagen, and recent data suggest that ROR is activated by certain Wnts (see below). The ligands for some RTKs (eg, ROS) remain unknown.

In the absence of ligand, most RTKs are monomers, but this is not an absolute rule. The hepatocyte growth factor (HGF) receptor (also termed Met) and its relatives, including RON, which plays an important role in the hematopoietic system, are cleaved posttranslationally to generate heterodimers. Members of the insulin receptor subfamily are heterotetramers in which the subunits are linked by disulfide bonds.

Ligands activate RTKs by promoting receptor oligomerization. Juxtaposition and activation of their (intracellular) kinase domains results, followed by cross (trans)-phosphorylation. Although for historical reasons, this process often is termed *autophosphorylation*, "trans-phosphorylation" is a more accurate description. Ligands can stimulate receptor oligomerization in a variety of ways. Some, such as PDGF, are dimeric, so that one ligand molecule binds two receptors simultaneously. Others, such as EGF, are monomers but have two receptor-binding sites that facilitate receptor dimerization. FGFs also are monomers, but they have only a single receptor-binding site. However, FGFs bind to heparin sulfate proteoglycans, which effectively oligomerize the ligand. Cell surface-bound ligands (eg, Ephrins) presumably promote RTK activation on opposing cells by clustering in localized regions of the plasma membrane.

The insulin and IGF-1 receptors are exceptions to this general scheme. These RTKs act as heterotetramers in the absence of ligand. Although their activation mechanism remains incompletely understood, most likely, ligand binding induces higher-order oligomerization and/or a conformational change that alters the orientation of the intracellular domain and leads to kinase activation. In addition, a hydrophobic residue in the juxtamembrane region of the receptor inhibits the basal activity of the IR and many other RTKs (eg, PDGFRs, Eph RTKs). Ligand binding may disrupt this autoinhibitory interaction, resulting in kinase activation.

RTK transphosphorylation occurs on multiple sites. Phosphorylation within the RTK "activation loop" locks the kinase into a high-activity conformation, and may also render it less accessible to inactivating phosphatases. Other tyrosines phosphorylated on RTKs become docking sites for *signal relay* molecules that contain SH2 (Src Homology domain-2) or PTB (phosphotyrosine-binding) domains, which are short (approximately 100 amino acid) modules that recognize phosphotyrosine (pY) within specific sequence contexts. For example, the motif pY-X-N-X (X—any amino acid), binds the SH2 domain of the signal relay molecule Grb2, whereas pY-X-X-M specifies interaction with the SH2 domains of regulatory subunit (p85) of an enzyme known as phosphoinositide-3 kinase (PI3K). Multiple proteins containing SH2 or PTB domains can assemble on an activated RTK, resulting in the formation of signaling complexes. The sequence motifs surrounding tyrosyl phosphorylation (pTyr) sites differ among RTKs. Consequently, RTKs recruit distinct combinations of signal relay molecules, providing an initial layer of specificity to RTK signaling. Although SH2 domains only bind pTyr-containing peptide sequences, some PTB domains can recognize specific motifs (NPXY) containing an unphosphorylated tyrosine.

SH2/PTB domain-containing proteins fall into two general classes: enzymes and adapters. Examples of the former include the tyrosine phosphatase Shp-2, phospholipase Cγ (PLCγ) and Ras GTPase-activating protein (RasGap). Although not enzymes per se, the SH2 domain-containing transcription factors known as Stats (Signal transducers for activating transcription) should probably be grouped within this class. Adapters lack intrinsic catalytic activity and instead serve as regulatory and/or targeting subunits for enzymes. For example, Grb2 binds the Ras guanine nucleotide exchange factor Sos, whereas PI3K p110 catalytic subunits are bound to SH2 domain-containing p85 regulatory subunits. Binding of an SH2/PTB domain-containing protein to an activated RTK can relocate an enzyme to the vicinity of its substrate (eg, PLCγ, Sos, RasGap) and/or activate the enzyme. Enzyme activation can result from binding of the SH2/PTB domain protein to its cognate pTyr motif (eg, Shp2, PI-3K). Alternatively (or in addition), many signal relay molecules are substrates for the activated RTK, and tyrosyl phosphorylation can result in enzyme activation (eg, PLCγ, Stats, and possibly Shp2).

Although this simplified paradigm applies to signaling by all RTKs, complexity abounds. For example, the EGF receptor (ERBB) family alone comprises four receptors (ERBB1–4) that respond to a large number of ligands. A single growth factor can stimulate receptor homodimerization as well as heterodimerization with other family members. ERBB3 retains the overall structure of an RTK and can bind to neuregulins (themselves, a large family of ligands). But the ERBB3 kinase domain is inactive, so that it signals *only* upon heterodimerization with an active family member (typically, ERBB2 or ERBB4). An important consequence of all of this complexity is that a single ligand can activate different signaling pathways, with distinct downstream effects, depending on which ErbB family members are expressed. For example, heparin-binding EGF-like growth factor (HB-EGF) stimulates mitogenesis but not chemotaxis when it activates the EGF receptor, but is both mitogenic and chemotactic when it activates ERBB4. Conversely, the same receptor, when stimulated by different ligands, can transduce distinct signals. Ligands may induce specific conformational changes that lead to the phosphorylation of different sets of tyrosine residues on the receptor, and consequently, phosphorylation of distinct sets of substrates. Alternatively (or in addition), the affinity of a given EGFR ligand for its receptor may influence signaling, by determining the length of time that it remains bound and thus signal duration. Finally, recent data indicate that at least some RTKs can translocate to the nucleus and have direct effects on transcription. In some cases (eg, EGFR, ERBB2, the entire receptor appears to enter the nucleus by as an yet unresolved pathway. For others (eg, ERBB4), the C-terminal tail is cleaved from the rest of the RTK and enters the nucleus in a manner somewhat analogous to that used by Notch family members (see Notch Receptors).

Receptor Protein-Tyrosine Phosphatases

Tyrosyl phosphorylation is exquisitely regulated not only by PTKs, but also by a large superfamily of protein-tyrosine phosphatases (PTPs). Like the PTKs, PTPs exist as transmembrane, receptor-like molecules and nontransmembrane (often misleadingly termed *cytosolic*) family members. Similar to the RTKs, receptor PTPs (RPTPs) have an extracellular domain(s), a single transmembrane-spanning domain, and cytoplasmic catalytic domains. The extracellular domains of many RPTPs contain fibronectin and immunoglobulin repeats, suggesting that at least some of them may recognize adhesion molecules as ligands. Several RPTPs are capable of homotypic interaction, but the ligands for most RPTPs remain either unknown or controversial. Interestingly, most RPTPs have two catalytic (PTP) domains. Although both are active in some RPTPs, in nearly all, the more the N-terminal of the two PTP domains (D1) has substantially greater activity and appears to play the major role in substrate dephosphorylation, the more the C-terminal domain (D2) is evolutionarily conserved (however, often to a greater extent than the N-terminal PTP domain), indicating that it must have an important function. Some possibilities that have been suggested for the function of D2 include substrate binding, regulation of oxidation of the D1 domain, and/or binding to certain lipids. Although at first glance, one might think that RPTPs (and other PTP superfamily members) would act to attenuate signaling initiated by PTKs, the situation is far more complicated. For example, CD45 plays both positive and negative roles in MIRR signaling (see Receptors Asscoiated with Protein-Tyrosine Kinases), keeping receptor-associated kinases inactive prior to activation but also required for activation on ligand binding.

Serine-Threonine Kinase Receptors

The transforming growth factor-β (TGF-β) receptor family, which includes receptors for TGFβ, bone morphogenetic proteins (BMPs) and activins, comprises transmembrane proteins with intrinsic serine-threonine kinase activity. Each active receptor consists of two subunits, termed Type I and Type II receptors, respectively. Signaling occurs as a result of ligand-dependent oligomerization of these receptor subunits. Type II receptors are constitutively active but do not normally phosphorylate substrates, whereas the type I receptors are normally inactive. Ligand-induced dimerization results in phosphorylation of the Type I receptor subunit by the Type II receptor, which converts the former into an active kinase. Signal propagation is dependent on the kinase activity of the Type I receptor and phosphorylation of its downstream substrates, the most important of which are the Smad family transcription factors.

Receptors Associated with Protein-Tyrosine Kinases

Three distinct families of receptors lack intrinsic enzymatic activity, but signal via associated PTKs. These include cytokine receptors, multichain immune recognition receptors (MIRRs) and integrins.

Cytokine receptors exist in several configurations, all of which associate with and signal via Janus family protein tyrosine kinases (Jaks). Some receptors, such as those for erythropoietin, prolactin, and growth hormone, combine ligand binding and signaling functions in a single transmembrane protein. Others (eg, IL3, GM-CSF, IL-5) have separate high-affinity ligand-binding and signaling subunits. Still others (eg, IL2 receptor) have a high-affinity ligand-binding subunit, and two signaling subunits, one of which also has a low affinity for ligand. The same signaling subunit can be shared by different ligand-binding subunits; for example, the IL3, GM-CSF and IL-5 receptors have different ligand binding α chains, but share a β-common (βc) chain.

The signaling subunits of cytokine receptors have two general functions: they direct association with specific Jaks and become tyrosyl phosphorylated in response to receptor stimulation. As with RTKs, ligand binding evokes Jak activation. Jaks are unusual in that besides an active kinase domain, they have an additional kinase-like domain (known as a Jak homology-2, or JH2, domain). This domain is important for regulating kinase activity, as illustrated by the association of V617F mutations (which lie in the JH2 domain) in Jak2 with nearly all cases of polycythemia vera and a significant fraction of essential thrombocythemia and myeloid metaplasia. Once activated, Jaks phosphorylate the cytokine receptor signaling subunit(s), although other PTKs also may contribute. The signaling subunits of cytokine receptors, together with their associated Jak, are the functional equivalents of RTK cytoplasmic domains. This allows analogous pTyr-dependent recruitment of signal relay molecules to the receptor. Stat family transcription factors are particularly important in cytokine receptor signaling. In addition to their DNA-binding and transcriptional-activation domains, Stat proteins contain an SH2 domain that has two functions. First, it recruits Stat monomers to the cytokine receptor, where they become tyrosyl phosphorylated. The SH2 domain on one Stat monomer then interacts with the pTyr residue on another, resulting in Stat dimers. These then translocate to the nucleus and activate specific gene expression. Cytokine receptors also activate other downstream pathways (eg, RAS/ERK P13K/AKT) in a manner similar to RTKs.

Multichain immune recognition receptors (MIRRs) include the antigen receptors on B and T lymphocytes, activating receptors on NK cells, and Fc receptors. As their name implies, these receptors tend to have several subunits (at least 2 and as many as 10 or more). At least one subunit is responsible for ligand binding and at least one other serves as the signaling subunit. Other subunits function either in receptor assembly, cell surface transport or as additional signaling subunits. MIRR signaling subunits are characterized by the presence of one or more specialized pTyr-based motifs called ITAMs (immune tyrosine-based activation motifs), which consist of two pTyr-X-X-L sequences separated by 10 amino acids.

Unlike cytokine receptors, signaling by MIRRs involves the sequential activation of Src (SFK), Syk, and Tec family PTKs. Ligand binding results in activation of one or more receptor-associated SFKs. How this occurs remains unknown. Conceivably, receptor clustering may have an effect analogous to dimerization/oligomerization by RTKs and cytokine receptors. However, some evidence, particularly for the T cell-antigen receptor (TCR) suggests that receptor-associated SFKs (eg, Lck for the TCR) are maintained in an inactive state by the adjacent receptor protein-tyrosine phosphatase, CD45. On ligand engagement, CD45 is excluded from the receptor complex, leading to SFK activation and phosphorylation of the ITAMs in the associated signaling subunits. Phosphorylated ITAMs then bind and activate Syk family PTKs (Syk or ZAP-70). The unique features of ITAMs are designed to fit optimally into the two SH2 domains of these PTKs. Activated Syk/ZAP70, in turn, phosphorylate coreceptors (eg, CD28 in T cells, CD19 in B cells) as well as adapters (eg, LAT in T cells and BLNK in B cells). Phosphorylation sites on these proteins bind signal relay molecules and activate downstream signaling. Tec family kinases (eg, Btk, Itk, Rlk) also are recruited by specific downstream adapters, activated by receptor-associated SFKs and, in turn, phosphorylate key enzymes, such as PLCγ. Thus, in MIRR signaling, three functions normally encoded on a single RTK molecule (ligand binding, kinase activation, docking site generation) are fragmented into separate receptor subunits and accessory signaling chains. Nevertheless, the same general signaling strategy applies.

Integrins, which are composed of heterodimers of α and β subunits, comprise the third group of receptors associated with PTKs. There are 18 α and 8 β subunits, allowing the generation of a large number of different heterodimers. Integrins act as both adhesion receptors and signaling molecules. Binding to an integrin requires the presence of one of two motifs, either arginine–glycine–aspartate (RGD) or leucine–aspartate–valine (LDV). These motifs typically are found in ECM molecules; hence, most integrins mediate cell–matrix adhesion and signaling. Some important integrin ligands, such as ICAM-1, are cell surface proteins. ICAM-1 is expressed on antigen-presenting cells and, by binding the integrin LFA-1, mediates cell–cell adhesion.

Activation of integrin signaling involves both ligand binding and clustering of integrins. Inactive integrins adopt a conformation in which the extracellular domains of α and β are bent, blocking ligand binding. The intracellular regions of α and β are bound to each other, preventing binding of downstream effectors. Binding of ligand to the extracellular domain separates the cytoplasmic portions of α and β, allowing them to interact with the cytoskeleton and transmit signals (outside-in signaling). Intracellular signals, such as phosphorylation, also can cause separation of the cytoplasmic domains of α and β; this can propagate in the reverse direction to open the head group and enhance ligand binding (inside-out signaling or affinity modulation). The conformational change that occurs on activation can facilitate transmembrane domain interaction, leading to cluster formation. Integrin clustering, in turn, results in increased avidity for ligand (avidity modulation).

Integrins also signal via PTKs. Integrin engagement stimulates SFKs, focal adhesion kinase (Fak), and in some cell types, the Fak relative Pyk. How this occurs is poorly understood. The so-called PBD domain of talin binds to a conserved NPXY motif in the β-integrin tail. Talin can recruit paxillin, which in turn binds Fak. Partial Fak activation and autophosphorylation appears to create a binding site for SFKs, which may phosphorylate and further activate Fak/Pyk2. However, the precise order and mechanism of activation of SFKs and Fak/Pyks during integrin signaling remains an area of controversy and active research.

G Protein-Coupled Receptors

G protein-coupled receptors (GPCRs) are by far the most numerous receptors. The human GPCR family contains nearly 700 members, making it the second most common protein family after protein kinases. GPCRs are characterized by seven membrane-spanning domains, resulting in four extracellular and four cytoplasmic regions. GPCRs bind a large variety of ligands, including proteins and peptides, lipids, amino acids, and nucleotides. Not surprisingly, the ligand-binding regions of GPCRs are quite diverse. In the hematopoietic system, chemokine receptors probably comprise the most important group of GPCRs.

GPCRs are so named because of their associated signaling subunits, the heterotrimeric GTP-binding proteins (G proteins). Most GPCR ligands bind to the receptor extracellular domain, but others bind to the transmembrane domain or to both the transmembrane and extracellular domains. In the absence of ligand, GPCRs exist in an inactive conformation resulting from intramolecular bonds between residues in the transmembrane or juxtamembrane regions. Heterotrimeric G proteins are bound to the inactive receptor. Following ligand binding, the receptor undergoes a conformational change that stimulates an intrinsic guanine nucleotide exchange activity for the associated G protein. This catalyzes dissociation of the associated G protein into α and βγ subunits (see below), either of which can then bind to and activate different downstream signaling molecules. For example, $G\alpha_s$ subunits activate adenylate cyclase, resulting in cAMP generation, whereas some Gβγ subunits stimulate phosphoinositide phospholipases. Many GPCRs also activate PTKs via a complex trans-activation pathway. Although the details remain controversial, this pathway appears to involve initial GPCR-activated signals that result in stimulating the cleavage and releasing the transmembrane-bound form of HB-EGF, which in turn stimulates the EGFR in an autocrine or paracrine manner.

Wnt Receptors

Wnts are a family of secreted proteins that are palmitoylated and thus relatively insoluble. They bind to extracellular matrix and can be transported by cellular extensions or lipid particles. Consequently, Wnts have properties of both solid-state and soluble signals. In the hematopoietic system, specific Wnts appear to play critical roles in stem cell homeostasis.

Wnts activate several downstream pathways by means of different receptor complexes. The canonical pathway culminates in the activation of β catenin, and is mediated by a regulatory complex comprising the Apc (adenomatous polyposis coli) tumor suppressor gene, axin, glycogen synthase kinase beta (GSK-3b), and casein kinase-1 (CK-1). In the absence of a Wnt signal, GSK-3β phosphorylates β-catenin (which is bound to the complex), promoting its degradation by the ubiquitin ligase β-TRCP. Wnts bind to primary receptors known as Frizzled proteins (relatives of *Drosophila frizzled*) which, like GPCRs, span the membrane seven times. In addition to the 10 human Frizzled family members, canonical pathway activation requires Wnt binding to the coreceptors LRP5 or LRP6, which have single membrane spanning regions and belong to the low-density-lipoprotein-related protein family. Binding results in inhibition of GSK-3β activity within the complex, a process mediated by the PDZ domain-containing adapter protein Dishelved (Dsh), and axin destabilization, which involves recruitment of axin to the LRP subunit and its phosphorylation and degradation.

Wnts also can activate noncanonical pathways. One is termed the "planar cell polarity (PCP) pathway," reflecting its key role in regulating this process during development. The PCP pathway is less well defined, but appears to involve binding to Frizzled family members (but not LRPs), Dsh phosphorylation, recruitment of Rho family small G proteins, and activation of the serine kinase JNK and downstream transcription. Wnts can also increase intracellular calcium via a second noncanonical pathway that appears to involve heterotrimeric G protein activation and phospholipase C activation. Remarkably, one Wnt family member (Wnt 5a) can bind to the receptor tyrosine kinase ROR-2, which can activate the PCP-pathway. Even more complexity is conferred by a variety of soluble receptors that modulate Wnt activity.

Notch Receptors

Notch signaling plays a critical role in cell fate determination within multiple hematopoietic lineages. Notch family receptors have a large extracellular domain, a single transmembrane domain, and a cytoplasmic domain. Their ligands (Jagged and Delta) are also transmembrane proteins expressed on the surface of adjacent cells. Activation of a Notch receptor results in a unique signal transduction mechanism. The extracellular domain of Notch is cleaved, probably by a member of the ADAM protease family, leaving the transmembrane and cytoplasmic domains intact. Following endocytosis, Notch undergoes a second proteolytic cleavage, which requires presenilin, releasing a soluble form of the receptor. This intracellular domain (ICD) fragment translocates to the nucleus and binds to a transcriptional repressor, CBF1 (the ortholog of Suppressor of Hairless in Drosophila). Binding to CBF1 relieves its inhibitory function, leading to transcriptional activation. Activation of Notch-responsive genes also requires ICD interaction with members of the Mastermind family of transcriptional coactivators. The importance of this novel signaling pathway has been vividly illustrated by mutations in Notch that result in constitutive cleavage and transcriptional activation; such mutations are found in a high percentage of T-cell acute lymphoblastic leukemia patients.

The Tumor Necrosis Factor Receptor Family

Tumor necrosis factor (TNF) family receptors (TNFRs) are single membrane-spanning proteins with a cysteine-rich extracellular ligand-binding region and a cytoplasmic tail that often contains a "death" domain. Ligand binding leads to receptor oligomerization, which is necessary to activate downstream signaling. A protein-binding surface is generated by the oligomerized receptor, leading to the recruitment of cytoplasmic proteins that form a large multiprotein complex. TNFR family members generate a least three types of downstream signals. Proapoptotic signaling is mediated via activation of a cytoplasmic protease, caspase 8, that initiates the extrinsic pathway of programmed cell death. TNFRs also can activate multiple members of the MAP kinase family of serine/threonine kinases. Some of these, in particular Jnk and possibly p38, also can have proapoptotic effects. Most TNFRs are also capable of generating survival signals. These signals depend on receptor-binding proteins known as TRAFs (TNF-associated factors) to mediate activation of the NF-κB family of transcription factors.

Whether pro- or antiapoptotic TNFR signals dominate depends on the particular cellular context as well as other signals. Some family members (eg, TRAIL) are professional death-inducers, whereas others (eg, CD30, CD40), lack a death domain and primarily generate survival signals. An additional feature of the TNFR system is the existence of so-called decoy receptors. Such receptors lack all or part of the cytoplasmic tail and thus cannot transmit a signal, but they bind and sequester ligand. Decoy receptors provide a unique mechanism for inhibiting and further regulating signaling. The pharmaceutical industry has utilized this strategy in the production of Enbrel, a recombinant soluble TNFR, which acts as a decoy receptor for TNF signals, and thus is a potent antiinflammatory agent.

Toll-Like Receptors

Toll-like receptors (TLRs), which get their name from the founding member of the family, a *Drosophila* ortholog, are expressed at particularly high levels on granulocytes and monocyte/macrophages and play critical roles in the innate immune response. Ten human TLRs have been identified. Each has a single transmembrane domain and a conserved cytoplasmic region known as the Toll/IL-1 receptor (TIR) domain. Two classes of TLRs can be defined on the basis of their extracellular domains: those with leucine-rich repeats and those with immunoglobulin domains. The most extensively studied mammalian

TLRs function to sense and respond to infection by acting as receptors for the products of microorganisms, such as lipopolysaccharide (TLR2 and TLR4) and the CpG DNA (TLR9) found in bacteria.

As for TNFRs, TLR signaling also appears to involve the formation of multimeric receptor complexes. Once activated, different TLRs recruit one or more adapters such as MyD88 and TRIM, sometimes by means of bridging adapters such as Mal (for MyD88) or TRAM (for TRIF). MyD88 recruits IRAK (interleukin-1 receptor-associated kinase) family members, which bind TRAF6 and in turn result in activation of various MAPK family members. TRIF-containing complexes promote activation of the NFκB pathway. The result is release of inflammatory cytokines, which help to activate the adaptive immune system, although some TLRs can also activate proapoptotic or prosurvival signaling pathways.

SIGNAL PROPAGATION: THE INTERMEDIARIES

Activation of a receptor usually results in transmission of signals to the cell interior. In some cases (eg, Notch or hormone receptors) receptor activation leads directly to transcriptional regulation. In other cases, receptors stimulate downstream signaling cascades that regulate many aspects of cell function. Still other receptors (eg, some RTKs, cytokine receptors, TGFβ family receptors) directly activate transcription factors (Stats, Smads) and secondary signaling cascades. Many downstream signaling pathways are shared by multiple receptors, and include protein kinases and phosphatases, small GTP-binding proteins, lipid kinases, and small molecules. This section provides an overview of these signal relay components.

Protein Kinases

Protein kinases (PKs) are divided into three classes according to the residues they phosphorylate: PTKs (some of which have been discussed above), protein serine-threonine kinases, and dual-specificity kinases, which phosphorylate serine, threonine, and tyrosine residues. Important issues in understanding the role and regulation of protein phosphorylation are how kinases phosphorylate specific substrates and sites and how phosphorylation alters protein function.

All protein kinases share the same overall three-dimensional structure, and most, if not all, shuttle between inactive and activated states. Phosphorylation of the so-called T loop serves as a general activation mechanism. The T loop forms a lip within the catalytic pocket and can occlude the active site, preventing binding of the protein substrate and/or ATP. Upon phosphorylation, the T loop undergoes a conformational change, moving out of the active site and permitting substrate access. T loop phosphorylation can be catalyzed by an upstream kinase or by kinase dimerization (eg, as in RTKs; see above).

Once activated, PKs phosphorylate specific substrates on particular sites. Specificity relies on two properties: colocalization of the kinase with the substrate and the presence of sequences in the substrate that can be phosphorylated by the kinase. Substrate motifs have been identified that in some cases, absolutely govern whether a protein will be a substrate. For example MAP kinases and cyclin-dependent kinases can only phosphorylate serines or threonines that are followed by a prolyl residue. Other kinases are slightly more promiscuous, but they too favor particular motifs as phosphorylation sites, probably because these motifs fit best into their catalytic clefts. Sequences distant from the site of phosphorylation can also mediate low-affinity association of a kinase with a substrate, which enhances both catalytic specificity and efficiency. This theme of "combinatorial control of specificity" is common to many signaling molecules and pathways.

Phosphorylation of a substrate can have two general effects: it can lead to a conformational change, thereby altering the activity of the protein, or it can create binding sites for specific domains. Examples of such binding modules are SH2 and PTB domains, which bind pTyr-containing peptides, as well as FHA domains, polo box domains, and 14–3-3 proteins, which bind phosphoserine and phosphothreonine motifs. Interaction of modules with their cognate motifs can result in the assembly of multiprotein signaling complexes.

Regulation can involve both of the above strategies. Tyrosine phosphorylation of different sites within SFKs can stimulate or inhibit their activity. Phosphorylation of a C-terminal tyrosine residue results in an intramolecular interaction between this phosphotyrosine and the SH2 domain of the SFK. This association contorts the catalytic domain, preventing substrate binding. In contrast, phosphorylation of a tyrosine in the T loop of the catalytic domain stimulates kinase activity by stabilizing the catalytic pocket in an active conformation. Once activated, SFKs can bind other phosphotyrosyl proteins via their SH2 domains; many of these proteins then serve as substrates for the SFK.

Mammalian serine-threonine kinases have been subdivided into 11 subfamilies on the basis of primary sequence homology. Kinases having significant homology often have related functions. Like tyrosine kinases, serine-threonine kinases are activated by phosphorylation of the T loop. Serine-threonine kinases also are regulated by other mechanisms. Small-molecule "second messengers" stimulate some serine-threonine kinases. Examples include cAMP and protein kinase A, calcium and diacylglycerol, and members of the protein kinase C family, and calcium and calmodulin for the calcium/calmodulin-dependent protein kinases (CAM kinases). Akt and PDK1, among others, contain Pleckstrin homology (PH) domains, which bind phosphoinositides. The Akt and PDK1 PH domains are specific for the phosphatidylinositol phosphate products of phosphoinositide 3-kinases (PI3K). Binding to PI3 lipids colocalizes PDK1 and Akt at the plasma membrane, which allows PDK1 to phosphorylate the T loop on Akt, resulting in the Akt activation. Protein–protein interactions, such as the association of cyclins with cyclin-dependent kinases, also can regulate kinase activity.

Many kinases participate in "kinase cascades." For example, activation of Raf results in phosphorylation and activation of Mek1, which in turn leads to activation of the Erk MAP kinases and, subsequently, pp90Rsk and Mnk. Kinase cascades allow cells to regulate pathway activity at multiple levels, thereby promoting signal integration. Equally important, cascades allow for remarkable levels of signal amplification, such that nanomolar or even picomolar levels of cytokines and growth factors can affect intracellular components at micromolar concentrations.

Protein Phosphatases

Protein phosphatases can activate or inactivate signaling pathways, depending on the specific sites that they dephosphorylate. Like the kinases, protein phosphatases can be classified on the basis of their substrate preference as tyrosine-, serine-threonine-, or dual-specificity phosphatases (DSPs). However, unlike kinases, which share the same general domain structure, protein phosphatases have several distinct structurally and mechanistically distinct superfamilies, which makes for a more informative classification scheme.

The PTP superfamily includes most known tyrosine-specific and dual-specificity phosphatases. PTPs are characterized by a conserved signature motif that centers on an essential cysteine residue. Catalysis by these enzymes involves the production of a cysteinyl-phosphate intermediate by this conserved residue. Although all PTP superfamily members contain a signature motif, classic PTPs, which are specific for phosphotyrosine, also contain a number of other conserved residues within a 240- to 250-amino acid PTP domain. Classic PTPs, in turn, can be subdivided into RPTPs (see above) and nontransmembrane families. All known DSPs lack a transmembrane domain, and their catalytic domains are smaller and more similar to each other than to those of the classic PTPs. In addition, some DSPs, although they can dephosphorylate artificial phosphopeptide substrates in vitro, actually target specific phosphoinositides. These include several enzymes that, when mutated, play important roles in the pathogenesis of hematopoietic and other types of disease. The best known of these is the tumor suppressor gene PTEN, which specifically targets

PI3,4P2 and PI3,4,5P43. Other examples include myotubularin and its relatives, which target PI-3P. When mutated, these enzymes can cause several types of neuromuscular disease.

Structural and enzymological studies have provided several insights into how PTPs are regulated. As indicated above, at least some RPTPs (CD45, PTPα) may be inactivated by dimerization. The nontransmembrane family members Shp1 and Shp2 (Shps) have, in addition to their PTP domains, two N-terminal SH2 domains and C-terminal tyrosyl phosphorylation sites. In the basal, inactive state, the catalytic cleft of the Shps is blocked by their respective N-terminal SH2 (N-SH2) domain. Binding of a pTyr peptide to the N-SH2 induces a conformational change that allows substrate access to the catalytic domain. This regulatory mechanism is altered by mutations in the autosomal dominant genetic disorder Noonan syndrome, about 50% of which is caused by germline mutations in various residues that comprise the N-SH2–PTP domain interface. Similar mutations occur sporadically in juvenile myelomyelogenous leukemia and CALLA+ B-cell acute lymphoblastic leukemia. In addition, tyrosyl phosphorylation of the Shp2 C-terminus has been shown to enhance Shp2 biological activity by an as yet uncertain mechanism. A more recently appreciated, potentially general, mechanism of PTP regulation capitalizes on the high reactivity of the catalytic cysteine residue in PTPs. This allows it to undergo reversible oxidation by reactive oxygen species such as hydrogen peroxide, which have recently been shown to act as second messengers in RTK and cytokine receptor signaling pathways.

PTPs act both to attenuate signals that require tyrosine phosphorylation and to activate pathways inhibited by tyrosine phosphorylation. The two Shps provide examples of each of these types of regulatory function. Shp1 functions primarily as a negative regulator of RTK, cytokine, and immune receptor signaling. Despite its strong sequence (>50% identity) and structural similarity, Shp2 acts mainly as a positive signal transducer, although it also may downregulate signaling in some contexts. As discussed above, CD45 also has both positive and negative effects on MIRR signaling.

The protein-serine/threonine phosphatases (PSPs) also comprise a large superfamily of enzymes that differ from the PTPs in catalytic mechanism, structure, and regulation. PSP catalysis utilizes an essential bound metal ion to activate water and promote dephosphorylation. Whereas PTPs typically have catalytic and regulatory functions encoded within the same polypeptide chain, most PSPs have distinct catalytic and regulatory subunits. The regulatory subunits have two general functions: they target specific PSPs to different intracellular locales and they regulate catalytic activity. Both types of subunits also can be inducibly modified by phosphorylation and/or other post-translational modifications (eg, methylation), resulting in changes in activity and/or localization.

PSPs are subdivided into families based on shared biochemical and structural features. Protein Phosphatase 1 (PP1) enzymes contain a catalytic subunit and one regulatory (targeting) subunit. With four different catalytic and approximately 50 regulatory subunits, a large number of different PP1 holoenzymes can be generated. PP2A enzymes are heterotrimers of scaffolding A, regulatory B, and catalytic C subunits. There also are a large number of possible A-B-C subunit combinations; thus, PP2A and PP1 do not each represent a single activity but rather, more than a hundred different enzymes. PP2B, better known as calcineurin, is a multimeric enzyme that, in addition, binds to calmodulin and is regulated by calcium. Calcineurin is a particularly important enzyme for immune cells, where it acts as a positive transducer of antigen receptor signals by dephosphorylating and activating NFAT (*N*uclear *F*actor of *A*ctivated *T* cells) transcription factors, and is the target of the immunosuppressant drugs cyclosporin and FK506. PP2C family members represent the final group of PSP activities. Unlike other PSPs, these enzymes tend to have a single subunit, and their regulatory mechanisms and functions are less well known.

Recently, selected members of the haloacid dehalogenase (HAD) family have been found to act as protein phosphatases. The best described of these are the Eyes absent (Eya) transcription factors, which play critical roles in developmental pathways. There is disagreement over whether Eya proteins dephosphorylate phosphotyrosine selectively or have dual-specificity phosphatase activity, and more importantly, their physiological targets remain undefined. Whether these or other HAD family members have roles in the hematopoietic system also remains to be determined.

Guanosine Triphosphate-Binding Proteins

GTP-binding proteins (G proteins) are activated by many receptors, and transmit their signals by binding to and altering the activity and/or localization of downstream effector proteins. G proteins come in two varieties: heterotrimeric and Ras-like (small). Both types use a similar signaling strategy that involves shuttling between GDP- and GTP-bound states. When bound to GDP, G proteins cannot bind effectors and are thus inactive. GTP binding leads to a conformational change that exposes an effector-binding site (often termed the *effector domain* of the G protein). Transit of G proteins from the inactive to the active state is catalyzed by guanine nucleotide-exchange proteins (GEFs). G protein inactivation is catalyzed by GTPase-activating proteins (GAPs), which stimulate their intrinsic GTPase activity (see below). The extent to which any given G protein, heterotrimeric or small, is active at any given time depends on the relative activity of its GEFs and GAPs. Most G proteins also have lipid modifications, such as farnesylation or geranylgeranylation, that promote membrane association and are required for biological activity.

Although all G proteins share this general regulatory mechanism, there are important differences between them. Heterodimeric G proteins consist of α, β, and γ subunits. Although these proteins are synthesized as individual polypeptide chains, β and γ are bound to each other extremely tightly and never dissociate within the cell; hence, they are usually referred to as βγ subunits. Mammals have 20 α subunits, 6 β subunits, and 12 γ subunits, resulting in the generation of a large number of active heterotrimers. In the GDP-bound state, the heterotrimers are stable and associate with a GPCR, which acts as a ligand-activated GEF (see above). Following activation, GTP binds the α subunit, resulting in dissociation of βγ. Both types of subunit transduces signals by binding to different types of effectors. Examples include adenylate cyclase, which is stimulated by some Gα subunits and inhibited by others, phospholipases, protein kinases, and ion channels. "Regulators of G protein Signaling" (RGS) domains have GAP activity and attenuate signaling by the α subunit. Many, if not all, RGS proteins are Gα effectors, thereby coupling signal transmission and termination in a single protein.

In contrast, Ras-like G proteins function as monomers. There are five families of Ras-like GTP-binding proteins: the Ras, Rho, Rab, Arf, and Ran proteins. The Ras and Rho families regulate cell growth, transcription, and the actin cytoskeleton; the Arfs regulate phospholipase D and vesicle trafficking; Rabs regulate vesicle trafficking; and the Ran family regulates nuclear import. Receptors do not act directly as GEFs for exchange for Ras-like G proteins. Instead, a large number of specific GEFs catalyze activation of Ras-like G proteins in response to specific cellular events. There also are multiple and specific GAPs to direct inactivation of these proteins. Ras-like G proteins have a number of downstream effectors, including protein and lipid kinases, protein phosphatases and lipases.

Phosphoinositide Kinases

Phosphoinositides (phosphorylated isoforms of phosphatidylinositol) recruit signaling molecules to intracellular membranes and some act as substrates for specific phospholipases. The regulation of the synthesis of PI-4-P and PI-4,5-P_2, the two most abundant phosphoinositides, is not well understood. PI 4-kinases synthesize PI-4-P from PI. Type I phosphatidylinositol phosphate kinases (PIPKs) phosphorylate PI-4-P at the 5 position to make PI-4,5-P_2. A related group of enzymes, the class II PIPKs, phosphorylate PI-5-P at the 4 position to make PI-4,5-P_2. PI 3-kinases phosphorylate PI, PI-4-P, and PI-4,5-P_2 at the 3-position of the inositol ring, generating PI-3-P, PI-3,4-P_2, and PI-3,4,5-P_3, respectively. Phosphoinositide levels also are regulated by phosphatases. As indicated above, the tumor suppressor protein PTEN dephosphorylates the 3′P on PI-3,4P2 and PI-3,4,5P_3. Distinct enzymes, SHIP in hematopoietic cells and SHIP2 in other cell types, remove the phosphate from the 5 position of PtdIns-3,4–5-P_3.

Phospholipases

Three distinct types of phospholipases play important roles in cellular signaling. Phospholipases A (PLA) cleave the acyl groups from phospholipids, producing a lysophospholipid and a free fatty acid. PLA2, for example, catalyzes the first step in the production of eicosinoids by generating free arachidonic acid. Phospholipases C (PLC) cleave PI-4,5-P_2 to produce diacylglycerol and inositol trisphosphate (IP_3), both of which are second messengers (see below). Phospholipases D (PLD) hydrolyze phosphatidylcholine to produce phosphatidic acid and choline. Phosphatidic acid (PA) also can be made by diacylglycerol kinases. The function of PA is poorly understood, although it too is believed to act as a second messenger.

Small-Molecule Second Messengers

Small molecules that regulate cell signaling are generated in response to many "first messengers" that activate cell surface receptors, such as growth factors or hormones. Second messengers generally bind noncovalently to protein targets, affecting their function. The best known small-molecule signal is cAMP, the first second messenger discovered. Adenylate cyclase, activated by heterotrimeric G proteins, catalyzes the synthesis of cAMP from ATP. The primary target of cAMP is protein kinase A (PKA), which in its inactive form is a tetramer of two catalytic and two regulatory subunits. The regulatory subunits contain two cAMP-binding sites. Binding of cAMP to the first site causes a conformational change that exposes the second site; binding of cAMP to the second site dissociates the regulatory and catalytic subunits. The free catalytic subunits are active kinases that phosphorylate a variety of important intracellular targets. Although for many years PKA was thought to be the only target of cAMP in mammalian cells, other targets, including a cAMP-dependent GEF, are now known to exist.

Many activated receptors also stimulate PLCs. PLC action results in the generation of two second messengers, inositol trisphosphate (IP_3) and diacylglycerol (DAG). DAG binds to the C1 domains of members of the protein kinase C (PKC) family of serine/threonine kinases, thereby localizing this enzyme to the plasma membrane and contributing to their activation. IP3 binds to specific receptors in the endoplasmic reticulum (ER), which leads to the release of calcium from intracellular stores. Depletion of intracellular calcium stores leads to an influx of extracellular calcium via capacitative calcium channels at the plasma membrane. In unstimulated cells, cytosolic calcium is quite low (100 nM), so opening channels in the endoplasmic reticulum or plasma membrane allows calcium to flow into the cytoplasm, temporarily raising the cytoplasmic calcium to micromolar levels. Calcium returns to basal levels as a result of closing the channels and stimulation of calcium pumps. The latter include molecules that pump calcium back into the ER (SERCA), and plasma membrane-bound calcium ATPases (PMCA). Recent evidence indicates that PMCAs also can be regulated, and may be an important target of inhibitory signaling in immune cells. Calcium has many cellular effects, including directly regulating enzymatic activities, ion channels, and transcription. Specific calcium-binding domains are known, including the C2 domain and EF hands, and are found in several cell signaling molecules. In addition, calmodulin serves as a professional calcium-binding protein that regulates a number of key intracellular signaling enzymes, including CAM-kinases and calcineurin.

Eicosanoids are ubiquitous lipid signaling molecules that bind to some GPCRs and nuclear receptors. Synthesized in response to multiple stimuli, eicosanoids, unlike most second messengers, can be produced in one cell, and then both stimulate that cell and diffuse freely into nearby cells to transmit signals. Eicosanoids are produced from arachidonic acid (AA), which in turn is produced by the action of diglyceride lipases and phospholipases A on DAG and phospholipids, respectively. PLA2s cleaves the sn-2 acyl group of phospholipids to produce free AA and a lysophospholipid. The calcium-regulated form of PLA2 shows a preference for substrates containing arachidonic acid. Further metabolism of arachidonic acid results in the synthesis of prostaglandins and leukotrienes, which function as ligands for receptors. These molecules have a large array of important physiological functions, including major roles in controlling the interaction between platelets and endothelial cells. For this reason, enzymes regulating these pathways are important targets for drugs to control hemostasis and thrombosis.

EFFICIENCY AND SPECIFICITY: MULTIPROTEIN SIGNALING COMPLEXES

Effective signal transduction requires that signaling molecules find their targets rapidly and specifically. The likelihood of any two proteins coming into contact is proportional to their concentrations. Hence, diffusion is the bane of signal transmission. Even in pure aqueous solutions, diffusion rates are slow compared to the molecular dimensions of the cell and its biomolecules, and diffusion also is nonspecific and dilutes the signal. Furthermore, the intracellular milieu is closer to a proteinaceous gel than a bag of water, making diffusion-limited processes even less efficient.

To overcome this problem, most signaling occurs in complexes, more like a solid-state rather than an aqueous process. Restricting a signaling protein to a specific compartment or complex increases the local concentration of that protein and the probability that it will interact with other proteins or small molecules in the same compartment or complex. Colocalization of proteins in a signaling pathway is achieved by recruitment to the same membrane surface or organelle (eg, plasma membrane versus ER) and ultimately by protein–protein and/or protein–lipid interactions. Conversely, separating proteins or second messengers (or both) into distinct compartments can be used to turn off signaling pathways and/or to prevent gratuitous interactions.

Protein complexes can assemble on membranes by binding to specific lipids. Creating such an environment is an important function of the products of phosphoinositide kinases. For example, PI-3,4-P_2 and PI-3,4,5-P_3 colocalize the kinases Akt and PDK1, resulting in Akt activation. Other signaling molecules bind to PI4,5P2 specifically. Higher-order membrane structures, such as lipid rafts, also may direct the formation of localized signaling complexes.

Signaling molecules also can be concentrated in organelles. Nuclear localization of the NFAT transcription factors illustrates this concept. In response to antigen receptor activation, intracellular calcium rises and activates calcineurin, which dephosphorylates NFAT. Dephosphorylated NFAT binds to importins, and NFAT, along with calcineurin, is transported through nuclear pores into the nucleus. NFAT also contains a nuclear export signal (NES). Phosphorylation of NFAT leads to binding to exportin, resulting in transport to the cytoplasm and signal attenuation.

Compartmentalization also occurs on a smaller scale. Proteins involved in a sequential pathway can exist in a preformed, but inactive, complex that is activated in response to upstream signals. This strategy was first appreciated by studies of a yeast MAP kinase module composed of the Ste11, Ste7, and MAP kinases bound to the scaffolding protein Ste5. A signal activates the first kinase in the cascade, Ste20 kinase, which initiates the relay. Ste20 phosphorylates and activates Ste11, which activates the kinase cascade on Ste5. Activation of the Jnk kinase pathway in mammalian cells uses an analogous preformed complex bound to a scaffolding protein. JIP-1 (Jnk inhibitory protein) binds to MLK1, MKK7, and JNK and facilitates the activation of JNK, through colocalization with the upstream kinases. Analogous scaffolding complexes exist for, and regulate, other MAP kinase cascades. "A Kinase-Anchoring Proteins" (AKAPs) perform a related function by binding to the regulatory subunit of PKA and targeting it to a variety of locations, including ion channels, endosomes, and mitochondria. Most AKAPs also bind other signaling molecules in addition to PKA, including phosphatases that act to terminate PKA signaling.

A common theme utilized by such signaling complexes is that of reinforcing negative feedback loops. For example, a given kinase may be colocalized with the phosphatase that inactivates its signals, and the system "wired" such that the kinase inactivates the phosphatase (eg, by directly phosphorylating it or a regulatory molecule), whereas the phosphatase dephosphorylates and inactivates the kinase. The upstream signal is designed to simultaneously activate the kinase and inactivate the phosphatase. Mathematical modeling as well as kinetic analysis indicates that such a configuration leads to switch-like behavior of the module, so that the system can oscillate between what is essentially an "off" and "on" state. Other types of pathway "wiring" can lead to more analog types of signaling.

Protein–Protein Binding Domains

The formation of multiprotein signaling complexes often involves regulated protein–protein binding (Fig. 6–2). These interactions are typically mediated by modular domains that recognize particular peptide sequences and modifications or small molecules (Table 6–3).

SH2 domains and most PTB domains bind to motifs containing pTyr residues (some PTB domains can bind to nonphosphorylated peptide motifs). All SH2 domains share a similar structure, as do PTB domains, but in an example of convergent evolution, SH2 and PTB domains have no structural similarity. PTKs and PTPs regulate the formation of SH2- and PTB-domain-containing complexes by determining the state of tyrosine phosphorylation on specific proteins. The specificity of these interactions derives from both phosphorylation of particular tyrosine residues and recognition of a motif surrounding the phosphorylated tyrosine by the SH2 or PTB domain. An example of this type of protein–protein interaction is the binding of PI3K, SHP2, and p120 RASGAP to specific phosphorylated tyrosines on the PDGFR. In addition to mediating protein–protein interactions, binding of SH2 domains to pTyr residues stimulates the enzymatic activities of such proteins as PI3K, SHP2, and SFKs. The crystal structures of many SH2 domains have been determined, revealing a pocket that binds the phosphotyrosine and a groove that determines binding specificity based on the fit of the residue's C-terminal (or, in a few cases, N-terminal) to the phosphotyrosine.

Recognition of motifs containing a phosphorylated serine provides also an important means of protein–protein interaction. Fork-head-associated domains, 14–3-3 proteins, polo boxes, and some WD40 and WW domains bind to regions of proteins containing phosphoserine. WD40 domains in F-box proteins mediate phosphorylation-dependent ubiquitination and subsequent proteolysis of some proteins, such as the inhibitor of κB (IκB).

TABLE 6–3 Protein–Protein Interaction Domains and Motifs

Motif	Binding Domain	Examples of Proteins Containing this Domain
pTyr	SH2	SFK, PI3K, Shp2, PLCγ
	PTB	Ship, Shc
pSer	WD40	Apaf, PP2A-alpha subunit
	14-3-3	14–3-3 proteins
	WW	Pin1*
	FHA	Rad 53
	Polo Box	Plk
Proline-rich	SH3	SFK, Grb2, PI3K, PLCγ
	WW	YAP
	EVH1	VASP, ENA, WASp
C-terminal sequences	PDZ	Disheveled, ZO-1

PI3K, phosphatidylinositol 3-kinase; pSer, phosphoserine peptides; pTyr, phosphotyrosyl peptides; SFK, Src family kinases; YAP, yes-associated protein.
*Note that Pin1 is the only known case of a pSer-specific WW domain.

Other domains (Src homology 3 [SH3], WW, and Ena-Vasp homology [Eva] domains) mediate protein–protein interactions by binding to proline-rich sequences. Like SH2 and PTB domains, these domains are structurally quite different. Many proteins that contain SH3 domains have proline-rich regions themselves that mediate intramolecular binding. A conformational change in such a protein could disrupt intramolecular binding and allow the SH3 domain to interact *in trans* with other proteins. Similarly, the accessibility of proline-rich regions to SH3 domains may be regulated by conformational changes that expose the proline-rich region or disrupt an intramolecular interaction. Protein phosphorylation or binding of a small G protein to its effector domain can alter such interactions, resulting in a biological response. For example, binding of the SH3 domain containing protein Nck or the small G protein Rac to WASP, the protein mutated in Wiskott–Aldrich syndrome, can disrupt an intramolecular inhibitory interaction and promote new actin polymerization.

PDZ domains recognize specific motifs in the C-termini of proteins. These domains are found in cytoplasmic proteins, and many proteins contain multiple PDZ domains. PDZ domain-containing proteins can function to aggregate transmembrane proteins, such as the ion channels. Alternatively, they can act to assemble intracellular signaling complexes. Binding of PDZ domains to their motifs can be disrupted by phosphorylation of an amino acid in or near the binding site, thereby allowing regulation of the signaling complex assembly.

Protein/Lipid-Binding Domains

Localization of proteins to membrane surfaces reduces their diffusion, increasing the probability of enzyme–substrate contact. A number of protein modules have evolved to mediate binding to specific lipids (Table 6–4). The C1 domains present in PKCs and other signaling molecules bind to DAG. Membrane recruitment of PKC is also aided by the C2 domains, which binds to anionic phospholipids in the presence of calcium. The lipid phosphatase PTEN is also targeted to

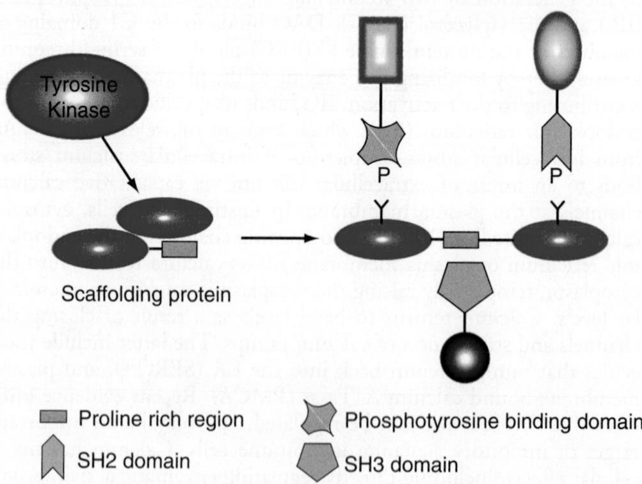

Figure 6–2 Formation of signaling complexes. Many signals are transmitted by complexes of signaling molecules that form in response to receptor activation. Scaffolding proteins are sites of complex formation. They can be activated by tyrosine phosphorylation, which allows proteins containing phosphotyrosine recognition domains (PBD and SH2 domains) to bind. Proteins that contain SH3 domains bind to proline-rich sequences, whose accessibility can be regulated. Signaling complexes solve the problem of diffusion and result in efficient transmission of signals to nearby proteins.

TABLE 6–4 Lipid-Binding Domains in Signaling Proteins

Lipid	Binding Domain
DAG	C1
PA	PX
PI-4-P	PH
PI-3-P	PX, PH, FYVE
PI-3,4-P_2	PH
PI-3,5-P_2	PH
PI-4,5-P_2	PH, Tubby, FERM, Sprouty, ENTH, ANTH
PI-3,4,5-P_3	PH

DAG, diacylglycerol; PA, phosphatidic acid.

membranes by means of a C2 domain. Several structurally unrelated domains bind to phosphoinositides. PH domains bind specifically to PI-3,4-P2, PI-3,4,5-P3, or PI-4,5P-2. PX and FYVE domains bind specifically to PI-3-P, whereas FERM domains bind PI-4,5-P_2. The physiological importance of such interactions is demonstrated by the fact that mutation of a single residue within the PH domain of the Tec family kinase BTK eliminates its ability to bind to PI3,4,5P3 and causes the disease X-linked agammaglobulinemia.

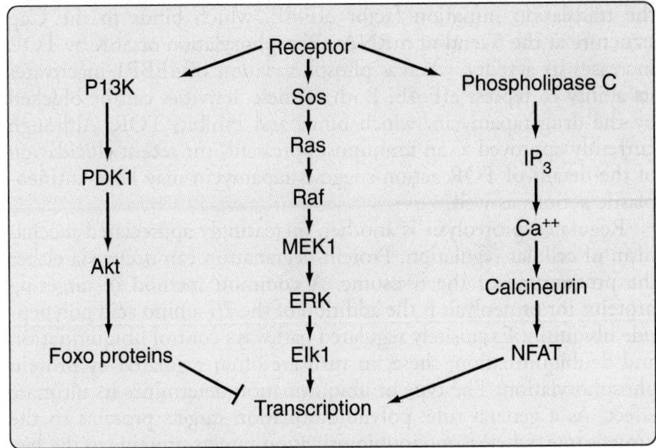

Figure 6–3 Examples of signaling pathways that regulate transcription. Transcriptional regulation is a common target of many signaling pathways and receptors often stimulate multiple pathways that can regulate common and distinct transcription factors. In the examples shown here, production of PtdIns-3,4,5-P_3 by phosphoinositide 3-kinase (PI3K) leads to the activation of the serine/threonine kinase Akt. Akt phosphorylates Foxo transcription factors, leading to their cytoplasmic sequestration and inactivation. Ras is activated by the guanine nucleotide exchange factor son of sevenless (Sos). Ras activation initiates a cascade of serine/threonine kinase activity: Ras activates Raf, Raf phosphorylates and activates Mek1, and Mek1 phosphorylates and activates Erk. Phosphorylation of the transcription factor Elk1 by Erk stimulates its activity. Increased intracellular calcium is also a common signaling event. Activation of phospholipase C leads to hydrolysis of PtdIns-4,5-P_2 and production of IP_3. IP_3 binds to its receptor, leading to intracellular calcium release and then extracellular calcium influx. Calcium activates the serine phosphatase calcineurin, which dephosphorylates NFAT proteins, allowing them to enter the nucleus and stimulate transcription.

SIGNALING OUTPUTS

Signal transduction pathways regulate most aspects of cellular and organismic function. Decisions about cell division, differentiation, and death are the result of inputs from multiple signaling pathways. Similarly, metabolism, cell motility, and cell-specific functions such as antibody production are regulated by specific signaling events. Most of these outputs require changes in protein expression, which is mediated by altering transcription, translation, and protein stability.

Regulation of gene transcription is the primary outcome of many signaling pathways. Microarray studies attest to the magnitude of this effect. Addition of a single growth factor to a cell can alter the transcription of hundreds of genes. The ability to transcribe a gene is regulated at many levels, including the structure of chromatin in the region of the gene, modifications of the promoter regions, and the activity of specific transcription factors and coactivators. Signal transduction pathways affect all of these steps.

Transcription factors are stimulated by many different mechanisms (Fig. 6–3). In the simplest case, binding of ligands to the nuclear receptor family of transcription factors results in a change in conformation of the ligand-binding domain, which simultaneously results in corepressor dissociation and creates a surface for binding to coactivators. Also, as discussed above, phosphorylation of STAT family transcription factors in response to stimulation of cytokine receptors or RTKs allows them to dimerize through their SH2 domains, enter the nucleus to bind DNA, and activate transcription. TGFβ family receptors activate transcription by phosphorylating SMAD proteins on seryl residues. This promotes heterodimerization with SMAD4 and exposes the DNA-binding domain. Activated SMADs translocate to the nucleus, complex with a protein called FAST1, and bind DNA to regulate transcription.

Other transcription factors are activated by more complicated signal transduction pathways. Antigen receptor signaling leads to PLCγ activation, which, in turn, leads to an increase in intracellular calcium release and activation of calcineurin. Calcineurin dephosphorylates and activates NFAT family members, which translocate into the nucleus and activate transcription. Several immediate early genes (genes whose transcription is induced without the need for new protein synthesis) are activated by growth factors, hormones, and cytokines. A major mechanism of regulation of such genes is via Ets family transcription factors such as ELK-1, which is under the control of a canonical MAP kinase cascade. Stimulation of the transcriptional activity of ELK-1 by EGF requires activation of a RAS-GEF, which leads to GTP binding and activation of RAS. RAS stimulates the kinase RAF, which in turn phosphorylates and activates MEK1. MEK1 phosphorylates and activates ERK, which translocates to the nucleus and phosphorylates and stimulates ELK-1. An analogous pathway, involving another family of MAP kinases, serves to activate the transcription factor c-JUN. In this case, receptor activation leads to activation of the MAP kinase JNK (again, via activation of the upstream kinases MEK4/7 and MEKK1, respectively), which phosphorylates c-JUN on a specific site to enhance its transcriptional activation activity. In addition to directly activating transcription factors, phosphorylation cascades can also affect the activity of coactivators and corepressors.

Messenger RNA export from the nucleus and translation also are controlled at multiple levels by cellular signaling pathways. A particularly important means of regulating translation involves the action of several protooncogene and tumor suppressor gene products. Activation of many receptors results in the activation of PI3K, which in turn activates AKT (both protooncogenes). AKT has several downstream targets, but among them is TSC2 (Tuberin), one of two tumor suppressor genes mutated in tuberous sclerosis patients. TSC2 forms a complex with the other tuberous sclerosis-associated gene, TSC1 (Hamartin); together, this protein complex inhibits the protein kinase TOR. TOR exists as part of two large protein complexes, which function to direct it to specific substrates and probably to regulate its activity. Two important targets of TOR complex 1 are p70S6 kinase (S6K) and 4EBP1. Both of these targets regulate transcription: S6K phosphorylates the ribosomal protein S6 and the RNA-binding protein SKAR, which may enhance the translation or export of specific mRNAs, respectively. 4EBP1 acts as a repressor for the translation initiation factor eIF-4E, which binds to the Cap structure at the 5′ end of mRNAs. Phosphorylation of S6K by TOR increases its activity, whereas phosphorylation of 4EBP1 inactivates its ability to repress eIF-4E. Both of these activities can be blocked by the drug rapamycin, which binds and inhibits TOR. Although currently approved as an immunosuppressant, the recent elucidation of the details of TOR action suggests rapamycin may have antineoplastic actions as well.

Regulated proteolysis is another, increasingly appreciated mechanism of cellular regulation. Protein degradation can occur via either the proteosome or the lysosome. A common method of targeting proteins for proteolysis is the addition of the 76-amino acid polypeptide ubiquitin. Exquisitely regulated pathways control ubiquitination and deubiquitination; these, in turn are often regulated by protein phosphorylation. The type of ubiquitination determines its ultimate effect. As a general rule, polyubiquitination targets proteins to the proteosome, whereas monoubiquitination targets proteins to the lysosome. In some cases, however, monoubiquitination does not lead to lysosomal targeting, but instead alters protein function.

The NF-κB family of transcription factors provides a classic example of the interplay between phosphorylation and ubiquitination. NF-κB is sequestered in the cytoplasm by IκB proteins. A variety of receptor-mediated signaling pathways lead to the activation of a large protein complex with IκB kinase (IKK) activity. Phosphorylation of IκB causes its dissociation from NF-κB, which allows NF-κB to enter the nucleus and bind DNA. Phosphorylation of IκB also makes it a substrate for a specific ubiquitin ligase that catalyzes its polyubiquitination and degradation by the proteosome. One of the many NF-kB targets is the IκB gene, which leads to restoration of IκB levels, and resets the system.

The second major pathway of protein degradation is the lysosomal pathway, which also plays a key role in signal transduction. An early response to the stimulation of receptors is their internalization into endosomes; some evidence suggests that signaling persists at this location after endocytosis. In the case of RTKs, ligand-dependent PTK activity is necessary for endocytosis, mediated by clathrin-coated pits. After endocytosis, either receptors may either recycle to the plasma membrane or the endosomes may fuse with lysosomes, leading to degradation of the receptor. A key control of this pathway is effected by a group of monoubiquitin ligases, the Cbl proteins.

SUMMARY AND PERSPECTIVE

This brief introduction has illustrated the complexity of cellular regulation and some examples of how this regulation, when perturbed, can result in diseases of lymphohematopoietic tissues. With the completion of the Human Genome Project, most of the critical participants in cell regulation are now known, and much of the core signaling circuitry has been elucidated. The challenge for the future is to understand how these pathways are integrated to control hematopoiesis and to utilize this knowledge to develop more effective treatments for disease.

SUGGESTED READINGS

Aggarwal BB: Signalling pathways of the TNF superfamily: A double-edged sword. Nat Rev Immunol 3:745, 2003.

Akira S: TLR signaling. Curr Top Microbiol Immunol 311:1, 2006.

Arnaout MA, Mahalingam B, Xiong JP: Integrin structure, allostery, and bidirectional signaling. Annu Rev Cell Dev Biol 21:381, 2005.

Bray SJ: Notch signalling: A simple pathway becomes complex. Nat Rev Mol Cell Biol 7:678, 2006.

Cho W, Stahelin RV: Membrane-protein interactions in cell signaling and membrane trafficking. Annu Rev Biophys Biomol Struct 34:119, 2005.

Clevers H: Wnt/beta-catenin signaling in development and disease. Cell 127:469, 2006.

Cole CN, Scarcelli JJ: Transport of messenger RNA from the nucleus to the cytoplasm. Curr Opin Cell Biol 18:299, 2006.

Engelman JA, Luo J, Cantley LC: The evolution of phosphatidylinositol 3-kinases as regulators of growth and metabolism. Nat Rev Genet 7:606, 2006.

Ferrell JE Jr: Self-perpetuating states in signal transduction: Positive feedback, double-negative feedback and bistability. Curr Opin Cell Biol 14:140, 2002.

Freedman BD: Mechanisms of calcium signaling and function in lymphocytes. Crit Rev Immunol 26:97, 2006.

Gilmore TD: Introduction to NF-kappaB: Players, pathways, perspectives. Oncogene 25:6680, 2006.

Hogan PG, Chen L, Nardone J, Rao A: Transcriptional regulation by calcium, calcineurin, and NFAT. Genes Dev 17:2205, 2003.

Jaffe AB, Hall A: Rho GTPases: Biochemistry and biology. Annu Rev Cell Dev Biol 21:247, 2005.

Kerscher O, Felberbaum R, Hochstrasser M: Modification of proteins by ubiquitin and ubiquitin-like proteins. Annu Rev Cell Dev Biol 22:159, 2006.

Kolch W: Coordinating ERK/MAPK signalling through scaffolds and inhibitors. Nat Rev Mol Cell Biol 6:827, 2005.

Levy DE, Darnell JE Jr: Stats: Transcriptional control and biological impact. Nat Rev Mol Cell Biol 3:651, 2002.

Mitin N, Rossman KL, Der CJ: Signaling interplay in Ras superfamily function. *Curr Biol* 15:R563, 2005.

Mor A, Philips MR: Compartmentalized Ras/MAPK signaling. Annu Rev Immunol 24:771, 2006.

Ninfa AJ, Mayo AE: Hysteresis vs. graded responses: The connections make all the difference. Sci STKE 2004:pe20, 2004.

Nourry C, Grant SG, Borg JP: PDZ domain proteins: Plug and play! Sci STKE 2003:RE7, 2003.

Novac N, Heinzel T: Nuclear receptors: Overview and classification. Curr Drug Targets Inflamm Allergy 3:335, 2004.

Osterlund T, Kogerman P: Hedgehog signalling: How to get from Smo to Ci and Gli. Trends Cell Biol 16:176, 2006.

Pasquale EB: Eph receptor signalling casts a wide net on cell behaviour. Nat Rev Mol Cell Biol 6:462, 2005.

Pemberton LF, Paschal BM: Mechanisms of receptor-mediated nuclear import and nuclear export. Traffic 6:187, 2005.

Pierce KL, Premont RT, Lefkowitz RJ: Seven-transmembrane receptors. Nat Rev Mol Cell Biol 3:639, 2002.

Sancar A, Lindsey-Boltz LA, Unsal-Kacmaz K, Linn S: Molecular mechanisms of mammalian DNA repair and the DNA damage checkpoints. Annu Rev Biochem 73:39, 2004.

Schlessinger J: Cell signaling by receptor tyrosine kinases. *Cell* 103:211, 2000.

Schlessinger J, Lemmon MA: SH2 and PTB domains in tyrosine kinase signaling. Sci STKE 2003:RE12, 2003.

Schreck R, Rapp UR: Raf kinases: Oncogenesis and drug discovery. Int J Cancer 119:2261, 2006.

Shaw AS: Lipid rafts: Now you see them, now you don't. Nat Immunol 7:1139, 2006.

Tonks NK: Protein tyrosine phosphatases: From genes, to function, to disease. Nat Rev Mol Cell Biol 7:833, 2006.

Tsygankov AY: Non-receptor protein tyrosine kinases. Front Biosci 8:s595, 2003.

Waters C, Pyne S, Pyne NJ: The role of G-protein coupled receptors and associated proteins in receptor tyrosine kinase signal transduction. Semin Cell Dev Biol 15:309, 2004.

Wettschureck N, Offermanns S: Mammalian G proteins and their cell type specific functions. Physiol Rev 85:1159, 2005.

Willars GB: Mammalian RGS proteins: Multifunctional regulators of cellular signalling. Semin Cell Dev Biol 17:363, 2006.

Wormald S, Hilton DJ: Inhibitors of cytokine signal transduction. J Biol Chem 279:821, 2004.

REFERENCES

For complete list of references log onto www.expertconsult.com

CHAPTER 7

CONTROL OF CELL DIVISION

William M. F. Lee and Chi V. Dang

Somatic cells undergo one of three general fates: They proliferate by mitotic cell division, differentiate and acquire specialized functions, or die and are eliminated. Cell proliferation is necessary for growth of the organism and ensures repletion of cells lost to terminal differentiation, cell death, or cell shedding. In the case of lymphocytes, it serves the additional function of amplifying immune responses to specific antigens. Differentiation provides the organism with a supply of cells to execute specific and specialized functions. In some cell types, such as muscle and nerve cells, differentiation and proliferation are mutually exclusive fates, and cells undergo "terminal differentiation." In other cell types, such as those of the hematopoietic lineage, proliferation may continue after cells acquire differentiated characteristics. For example, erythroblasts, myeloblasts, and megakaryoblasts are committed to particular differentiation pathways and possess lineage-specific markers yet continue to proliferate. T and B lymphocytes are fully differentiated and express antigen-specific receptors but can be induced to proliferate when appropriately stimulated. Cell death is an active process when it is initiated by the cell itself in the process known as *apoptosis* and can be as important as cell proliferation and differentiation for maintaining the integrity of the organism. It allows tissue renewal and changes in cellular composition without undesirable cell accumulation.

When the regulation of any of these three cellular processes—proliferation, death, and differentiation—goes awry and their balance becomes abnormal, the consequences to the organism are usually dire and result in either functional insufficiency or neoplasia. The relevance of these events to normal tissue function and neoplasia has led to investigations of their mechanisms and regulation at a molecular level. This chapter focuses on cell proliferation and its regulation. Cell death is discussed in Chapter 8, and differentiation of specific hematopoietic cell types is discussed in chapters focused on these cell types.

SIGNAL TRANSDUCTION AND CELL PROLIFERATION

Cells normally proliferate and differentiate and sometimes die in response to signals from their environment. Of these, cell proliferation or mitogenic signals and signaling mechanisms are the best studied and provide a paradigm for how cells respond to environmental signals in general. Cell proliferation normally is stimulated by extracellular growth factors interacting with specific receptors located at the cell surface. Signal transduction is the process by which information about growth factors at the cell surface is transmitted to the nucleus, where ultimate control of most cellular events resides. Signal transduction pathways leading to cell differentiation operate on similar principles and use similar mechanisms but produce different outcomes. A brief overview of some of the biochemical events involved in mitogenic signal transduction is provided as introduction and context for the following discussion of cell cycle regulation. A detailed discussion of signal transduction is found in Chapter 5.

Much of what is known about signal transduction is based on studies of the cellular biochemical response to mitogens such as platelet-derived growth factor (PDGF) and epidermal growth factor (EGF).[1,2] When these ligands bind to their cognate cell-surface receptors (PDGF-R and EGF-R, respectively), the receptors dimerize, activate their intrinsic tyrosine kinase activity, and catalyze the transfer of phosphate groups from adenosine triphosphate (ATP) to tyrosine residues of specific cellular proteins, including the receptors themselves (Fig. 7–1).[3] Some other types of receptors, such as the T-cell antigen receptor and CD4 and CD8 co-receptors, are not tyrosine kinases, and the tyrosine phosphorylation that they induce on ligand binding is mediated by associated nonreceptor tyrosine kinases-ZAP-70 in the case of T-cell antigen receptors and Lck in the case of CD4 and CD8.[4]

The presence of phosphotyrosines in target proteins enables them to form noncovalent complexes with proteins containing SH2 domains (Src homology region 2; defined by homology to a region in the Src retroviral oncoprotein), which are peptide domains that bind phosphotyrosine-containing peptides.[5] Thus, phosphorylation of the EGF-R and PDGF-R enables them to interact with SH2-containing proteins near or at the plasma membrane, which initiates downstream signaling events. Certain enzymes with SH2 domains, such as the γ1 isoform of phospholipase C (PLCγ1), directly associate with phosphorylated EGF-R and PDGF-R and become tyrosine phosphorylated by them, which, in the case of PLCγ1, results in enhancement of enzymatic activity. Activation of PLCγ1 catalyzes the hydrolysis of phosphatidylinositol (PIP_3) into diacylglycerol (DAG) and inositol 1,4,5-triphosphate (IP_3), both of which act as "second messengers" that launch additional actions inside cells: DAG activates protein kinase C (PKC), a kinase that phosphorylates serine/threonine residues in substrate proteins, and IP_3 induces Ca^{2+} release from intracellular stores, which in turn activates Ca^{2+}/calmodulin-dependent serine/threonine protein kinases and other Ca^{2+}-dependent events.[6]

Another signaling pathway activated when mitogen receptors bind ligand and become phosphorylated stems from activation of Ras proteins. These are low-molecular-weight guanosine triphosphate (GTP)-binding proteins that are active in their GTP-bound state but inactive in their guanosine diphosphate (GDP)-bound state. The intrinsic GTPase activity of Ras, enhanced by the presence of GTPase-activating proteins (GAPs), hydrolyzes bound GTP to GDP and maintains Ras in its inactive state.[7,8] Following EGF binding by EGF-R, two cytoplasmic proteins, Grb2 and SOS, that exist as heterodimers in unstimulated cells physically link EGF-R with Ras in a quaternary complex through binding of phosphorylated EGF-R with the SH2 domain of Grb2 and the binding of SOS to Ras. Formation of this complex activates the function of SOS as a guanine nucleotide exchange factor (GEF), resulting in the conversion of Ras-GDP to Ras-GTP and Ras activation. Activation of Ras initiates a cascade of serine/threonine kinase activation involving a trio of kinases.[9] Beginning with the association of GTP-Ras with Raf-1 (a mitogen-activated protein kinase [MAPK]), which activates the latter's serine/threonine kinase function, Raf-1 phosphorylates and activates MEK (MAPK kinase). MEK is a kinase that phosphorylates and activates MAPK, which is also known as ERK (*e*xtracellular signal-*r*egulated *k*inase). Modules composed of three sequentially activated serine/threonine kinases are a recurring motif in signaling from the plasma membrane, where Ras and Ras-like molecules reside, to the nucleus, which phosphorylated MAPK or ERK can enter.

Serine/threonine kinases activated following mitogen exposure phosphorylate diverse cellular proteins and modulate their activities.[10] Prominent among these targets are transcription factors.[11] Phosphorylation may directly alter the ability of these factors to bind DNA or

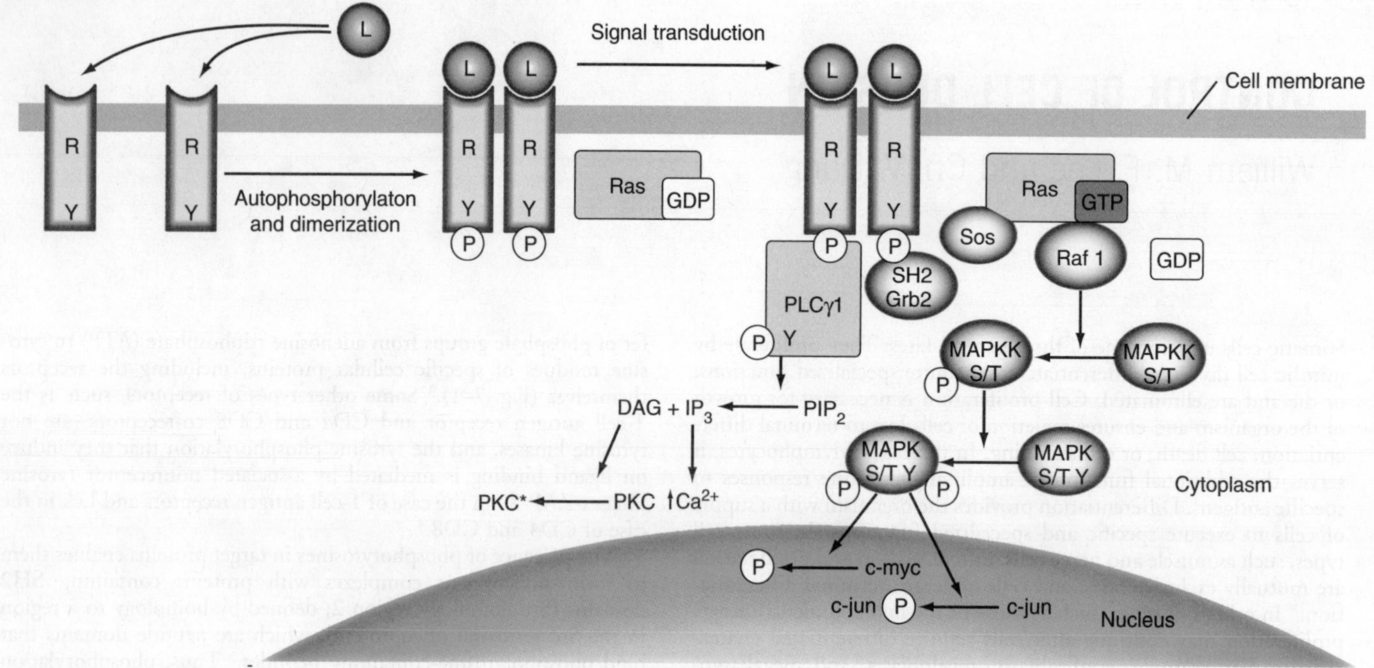

Figure 7–1 MITOGENIC SIGNAL TRANSDUCTION. Shown are signal transduction pathways activated by the binding of mitogenic ligands (L), to their cognate receptors (R) at the cell surface. Binding results in dimerization and autophosphorylation (P) of the receptors on tyrosine residues (Y). This enables them to associate with and activate specific SH2 domain-containing downstream components of the signaling pathway. In the case of phospholipase Cγ1 (PLCγ1), association leads to tyrosine phosphorylation by the receptor kinase and an enhanced ability to hydrolyze phosphoinositol bisphosphate (PIP_2) to diacylglycerol (DAG) and inositol trisphosphate (IP_3); in turn, DAG activates protein kinase C (PKC) and IP_3 mobilizes Ca^{2+} from intracellular stores. In the case of Grb2-SOS, association with phosphorylated receptors stimulates its ability to facilitate Ras GTP-GDP exchange; GTP-Ras activates the MAP kinase (MAPK) cascade, which eventually induces serine (S)/threonine (T) phosphorylation of nuclear proteins that modulate gene transcription. Note that MAPK is activated by serine/threonine and tyrosine phosphorylation and that both result from the activity of a single dual-function kinase, MAPK kinase. EGF, epidermal growth factor; MAP, mitogen-activated protein; PDGF, platelet-derived growth factor.

activate transcription. Alternatively, phosphorylation may indirectly activate transcription factors by inactivating an antagonist of these factors. Mitogen stimulation may result in activation of protein phosphatases that dephosphorylate specific phosphorylated residues in certain transcription factors to alter function.[12] The end result of these rapid posttranslational protein modifications is the first wave of change in cell transcription, which can occur independent of new protein synthesis. "Immediate early" is the description collectively applied to genes whose messenger RNA (mRNA) is rapidly induced by growth factor stimulation in the absence of de novo protein synthesis. Included in their number are genes encoding transcription factors. These initial changes lead to changes in expression of other transcription factor genes (which do require de novo protein synthesis) and culminate in the transcriptional reprogramming of the cell that eventually enables them to undergo DNA synthesis and cell cycling. It should not be surprising that many of the components of the mitogenic signaling pathway are oncogenic when they are inappropriately activated.[1]

Ligands other than EGF and PDGF may use different schemes for signal transduction. Neuroactive and vasoactive peptides (eg, epinephrine and thrombin) activate responsive cells through specific receptors that have seven membrane-spanning domains. These receptors are typically coupled to heterotrimeric G proteins that resemble Ras in being regulated by GTP and GDP.[7,13] These receptor-coupled G proteins are linked to effector enzymes (eg, adenylyl cyclases) that generate molecular signaling intermediates (eg, cyclic adenine monophosphate [cAMP]) on ligand binding. Steroid and thyroid hormones and retinoids can enter cells by virtue of their lipophilic nature. Their receptors are intracellularly located and able to bind sequence-specific DNA and directly modulate the transcription of responsive genes. Thus, the receptors are transcription factors whose activities are influenced by binding of the cognate hormone.[14]

Interferon signaling uses a different signal transduction paradigm. Tyrosine kinases of the Janus kinase (Jak) family associate with interferon receptor subunits. On ligand binding, association of the receptor subunits allows these Jaks to phosphorylate and activate each other and to phosphorylate the associated receptors. Specific members of the STAT (signal transducers and activators of transcription) family of latent cytoplasmic transcription factors, which have SH2 domains, dock to the receptor phosphotyrosines and become phosphorylated by Jak. Tyrosine phosphorylation allows STATs to dimerize and translocate to the nucleus, where they bind sequence-specific DNA and modulate transcription of interferon-responsive genes.[15] Signal transduction using Jak-STAT protein is used by many peptide ligands and cytokines of hematologic interest (eg, erythropoietin; interleukins IL-2, IL-3, IL-4, IL-6, and IL-12).

The signal transduction schemes outlined permit a single event, ligand-receptor interaction, to have several downstream consequences. Its multiplex, frequently cascading nature allows signal amplification and diversification but also permits their modulation and fine regulation. Signaling pathways can intersect and interact at different levels, allowing one ligand to modify the signals generated by another ligand. For example, STATs can be phosphorylated by receptor tyrosine kinases, such as PDGF-R and EGF-R, as well as by Jak, and can undergo serine/threonine phosphorylation, which modulates their transcriptional activity.[15] This allows PDGF and EGF to initiate some events usually initiated by cytokines and interferons, and the phenotypic changes brought about by cytokines and interferons may be altered in the presence of PDGF and EGF.

Transcription factors are final participants in afferent signal transduction pathways and initiators of cellular responses to these signals.[11] In general, they are sequence-specific DNA-binding proteins that modulate the expression of genes to which they bind. When these factors bind their cognate DNA sequence, they interact with the basal transcription machinery either directly or via intermediary proteins ("coactivators" and "corepressors") to initiate, enhance, or inhibit transcription. Transcription factors have peptide domains with characteristic secondary structures that are responsible for their ability to bind DNA. Many bind DNA only as dimers, making the peptide domain responsible for dimerization essential for DNA binding.

Transcription factors use one of a number of peptide motifs to dimerize and bind DNA, among them the zinc finger, the basic region-leucine zipper (bZip), the basic region-helix-loop-helix (bHLH), and the helix-turn-helix motifs.[16] Factors that activate gene transcription generally do so because they have a distinct transcriptional activation domain that is frequently acidic in nature, glutamine rich or proline rich. Transcriptional gene regulation is highly complex, not only because of the multitude of transcription factors present in cells but also because of the ability of many factors to heterodimerize and form combinatorial pairs that have DNA-binding, transactivation, and/or regulatory properties that differ from those of the parental homodimers. A striking example is provided by heterodimers containing the Id protein, which is an HLH protein that can dimerize with selected bHLH proteins, such as the myogenic transcription factor MyoD, but that does not possess a DNA-binding basic region. Id-containing heterodimers are incapable of binding DNA, making Id a negative transcriptional regulator that inhibits the function of positive factors.

Negative gene regulation also occurs by active repression of transcription, and certain transcriptional repressors have been shown to recruit factors that bind histone deacetylases. Histones are a family of nuclear proteins that interact with DNA and organize it into higher-order structures consisting of DNA wrapped around a histone core (nucleosomes). Acetylation of histones masks their basic residues, destabilizes their interaction with DNA, "loosens" nucleosome DNA, and facilitates transcription. Deacetylation of histones, in contrast, stabilizes their interaction with DNA, which "tightens" nucleosome DNA and inhibits transcription. Reversible, regional histone acetylation, through recruitment of co-activators with acetyltransferase activity or recruitment of co-repressors with deacetylase activity, is a general mechanism by which transcription factors facilitate or repress expression of specific genes.[17]

THE CELL DIVISION CYCLE

A cell stimulated to divide passes through a series of states, defined by biochemical and morphologic criteria, collectively termed the *cell cycle* (Fig. 7–2). Passage through the cell cycle provides an ordered sequence to the complex series of events necessary for the production of two identical progeny cells. The normal cell cycle is divided into discrete and sequential phases: S, G_2, M, and G_1.

S Phase

S phase is the period of wholesale DNA synthesis during which the cell replicates its genetic content; a normal diploid somatic cell with a 2N complement of DNA at the beginning of S phase acquires a 4N complement of DNA at its end. (Recall that N = 1 copy of each chromosome per cell [haploid]; 2N = 2 copies [diploid].) The duration of S phase may vary from only a few minutes in rapidly dividing, early embryo cells to a few hours in most somatic cells. Early embryo cells generally "live off" the accumulated stores of maternal RNA and proteins present in the egg and are transcriptionally silent, whereas cells in later development and mature organisms must actively transcribe subsets of their genes to survive and maintain specialized functions. The longer time required for the latter to complete S phase probably allows these cells to coordinate DNA replication with transcription and to preserve higher-order gene and chromatin structural information that influences gene expression for transmission to progeny cells.

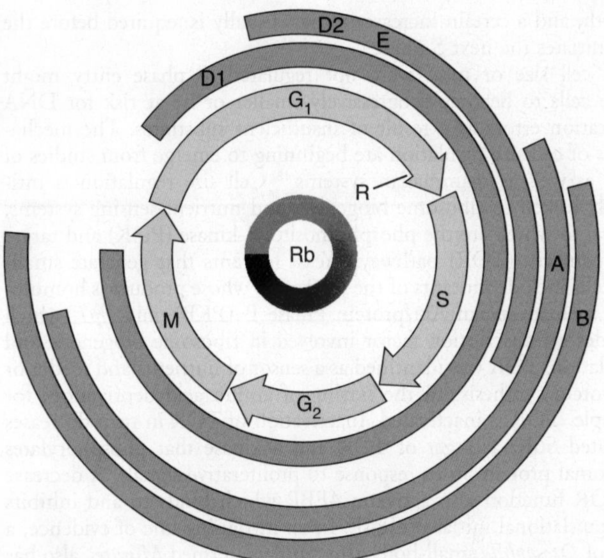

Figure 7–2 THE CELL CYCLE. The somatic cell cycle is divided into phases of DNA replication (S), mitosis (M), and the "gaps" in between (G_1 between M and S; G_2 between S and M). G_0 is not shown for the sake of simplicity but would be a side loop exiting and entering G_1. The point in late G_1 at which cells become committed to DNA replication is called the restriction point (R). The *inner circle* shows the pattern of Rb phosphorylation through the cell cycle, with the density of stippling indicating the degree of Rb phosphorylation. Places in the cell cycle where individual cyclins (A, B, D1, D2, E) appear are shown by the outer arcs.

M Phase

Mitosis, or M phase, is the period of actual nuclear and cell division during which the duplicated chromosomes are divided equally between two progeny cells. It is obvious microscopically as the period of chromosome condensation and segregation, nuclear division (karyokinesis), and physical separation of the two daughter cells (cytokinesis). A cell entering M phase has a 4N DNA content and finishes as two cells, each with an identical 2N complement of DNA. The complex sequence of changes that take place allows M to be subdivided into prophase, prometaphase, metaphase, anaphase, and telophase. *Prophase* is the period of chromatin/chromosome condensation, centrosome separation/migration to opposite poles, and nuclear membrane breakdown. The centrosomes are microtubule organization centers that eventually give rise to the bipole mitotic spindle apparatus that will separate the sister chromatids of each duplicated chromosome. During *prometaphase*, chromosomes attach to microtubules of the mitotic spindle, so that sister chromatids become attached to opposite poles. In *metaphase*, the condensed chromosomes align at the equatorial plate. The cohesive "bond" between sister chromatids of duplicated chromosomes is dissolved, allowing *anaphase*, the period of sister chromatid separation, to proceed. On reaching their poles, nuclear membranes form to envelop each of the two separated sets of chromosomes, which also begin to decondense, marking *telophase* and karyokinesis. This is soon followed by cytokinesis and exit from M.

G_1 and G_2 Phases

G_1 and G_2 phases were originally conceived of as "gaps" between the distinctive M and S phases of the cell cycle. G_1, which occupies the period or gap between M and S, is the interval between the completion of one round of cell division and initiation of the next. Its duration is the most variable, can be prolonged depending on the cell type, and is subject to regulation by environmental factors such as the availability of growth factors and nutrients. It is the period of cell growth, and a certain increase in mass usually is required before the cell initiates the next S phase.

If cell size or mass were not regulated, S phase entry might cause cells to become progressively smaller or be at risk for DNA replication errors as a result of insufficient substrates. The mechanisms of cell size regulation are beginning to emerge from studies of yeast as well as mammalian systems.[18] Cell size regulation is intimately linked to ribosome biogenesis and nutrient-sensing systems, central to which are the phosphoinositol 3-kinase (PI3K) and target of rapamycin (TOR) pathways. Yeast mutants that generate small-size cells include mutants of the *sch9* gene, whose product is homologous to mammalian Akt/protein kinase B (PKB), and *sfp1*, which encodes a transcription factor involved in ribosome biogenesis and translation. TOR was identified as a sensor of nutrients and mediator of protein synthesis. In the setting of amino acid deprivation, for example, TOR is inactivated. Inactivation of TOR in turn decreases activated S6K, a target of TOR and a kinase that phosphorylates ribosomal protein S6 in response to proliferative signals. A decrease in TOR function also activates 4EBP, which binds to and inhibits the translational initiator eIF4E. In an intriguing line of evidence, a class of *Drosophila* small-body-size mutants, termed *Minutes,* also has been shown to be defective in ribosomal protein genes as well as in signal transduction pathways. Specifically, mutations in the *Drosophila* insulin receptor, PI3K, TOR, S6K and Akt/PKB result in the *Minute* phenotype, whereas mutation of *Pten* (phosphatase and tensin homolog deleted on chromosome 10), which negatively regulates the PI3K and Akt/PKB pathways, produces large flies with large cells.

Remarkably, mutations in the *Drosophila Myc* gene also resulted in fewer, smaller cells and small body size, suggesting that protooncogenic *Myc* regulates size as well as cell proliferation. Because Myc pleiotropically affects gene expression, it has emerged as an integrator of cell size regulation and cell proliferation. In particular, mammalian c-Myc regulates both cyclins and *CDK* genes as well as ribosomal protein genes and genes involved in translation. Overexpression of c-Myc in lymphocytes results in both cell size increase and a detectable increase in cell proliferation. However, germline mutation of *myc* in the mouse results in small mice that have fewer but normal-sized cells. An interpretation of these observations is that mammalian cells may be less tolerant of cell size depletion than lower metazoans. In aggregate, studies from a variety of organisms indicate that cell size regulation is linked to cell proliferation, except in specialized cells that undergo endoreplication (see Specialized Cell Cycle).

As a first approximation, the amount of time a cell spends in G_1 is inversely related to its rate of proliferation. When conditions are unsuitable for proliferation (eg, because of insufficient nutrients or absence of mitogens), cells arrest in G_1, and those that are already in S, G_2, or M usually complete the round to which they have been committed and arrest only when they reach G_1 again. On the other hand, when rapid cell proliferation is mandated, as in embryos shortly after fertilization, G_1 is virtually undetectable, and there is no cell enlargement. As a result, the original mass of egg cytoplasm is partitioned among thousands of cells within a few hours without a noticeable increase in size. G_1 has been subdivided into segments and regulatory points based largely on the study of the proliferative response of cells to sequential application of different growth factors, nutrients, and metabolic inhibitors. From the standpoint of cell cycle regulation, a particularly important point in G_1 is the restriction point, or R, which occurs near the G_1-S boundary. This is the point at which cells become committed to entering S phase, regardless of subsequent availability of growth factors or essential nutrients, and is analogous to the commitment point in the yeast cell cycle called Start.

G_2 is the period or gap between S and M when cells have finished replicating their DNA, are preparing to divide, and have a 4N DNA content. For most cells entering S phase, passage through G_2 is "automatic," and the duration of G_2 is fixed except under unusual circumstances. For example, G_2 duration can be extremely short and is essentially undetectable in rapidly proliferating, early embryonic cells.

G_0 Phase

G_0 is a nonproliferative phase in which viable cells may remain for prolonged periods. Cells in G_0 have 2N DNA content and have exited the cell cycle. They may be difficult to distinguish morphologically from cells in a prolonged G_1 phase but in some cases can be distinguished biochemically, as they differ in protein and RNA metabolism. Terminally differentiated cells, such as neutrophilic granulocytes, muscle cells, and neurons, have irreversibly exited the cell cycle during the process of differentiation and are examples of cells that have irreversibly entered G_0. Other cells reversibly enter G_0 and may be induced to return to G_1 and begin cycling with appropriate stimuli. For example, hepatocytes usually are in G_0, unless partial hepatectomy induces them to proliferate to reconstitute the functional mass of the liver. Resting, antigen-specific lymphocytes are in G_0 until antigen and cytokine stimulation induces them to proliferate.

The enforced sequence G_1–S–G_2–M during normal progression through the cell cycle means that a cell must duplicate its DNA before dividing and that it must divide before duplicating its DNA again. This sequence ensures euploidy, and its enforcement maintains genetic stability. The dependence of later events in the cell cycle on successful completion of earlier events is ensured by checkpoint control mechanisms that prevent a cell that has not successfully completed one phase of the cycle from entering the next.[19,20] Certain cell types, such as megakaryocytes, become polyploid as part of their normal development and differentiation. In these cases, the normal cell division cycle script obviously is not followed: M fails to follow S, and DNA replication is allowed to repeat despite this lack of follow-through.

RB AND TRANSCRIPTIONAL REGULATION OF THE CELL DIVISION CYCLE

Progression through the different phases of the cell cycle requires successful execution of a complex series of events. Although each of these is indispensable for a cell to give rise to two identical progeny, the pivotal event during cell proliferation is the replication of its genes. Not surprisingly, therefore, entry into S phase and initiation of DNA replication constitute a highly regulated decision. Without trivializing the other processes involved in cell cycling, those preceding DNA synthesis may be viewed as ensuring that conditions warrant genome replication and preparing for it, whereas those following genome replication may be viewed as making sure that the products are apportioned correctly to progeny cells. The actual process of DNA replication requires the coordinate presence and activity of substrates for DNA synthesis (deoxynucleotide triphosphates), DNA-synthetic enzymes, mechanisms for copying template DNA, mechanisms for checking the integrity of the results and correcting defects if present, and mechanisms for deconstructing and reconstructing chromatin composition and chromosome structure. The task of replicating cellular DNA is complex, as are the enzymatic and regulatory mechanisms that carry them out. Cells entering S phase must possess the proteins and substrates necessary for DNA synthesis (acquiring substrates essentially means acquiring the relevant biosynthetic enzymes), so S phase entry can happen only in cells that have activated expression of genes encoding the needed proteins.

Studies of the Rb protein have revealed fundamental principles underlying transcriptional regulation of cell entry into S phase and DNA replication.[21] Rb is the product of the *Rb* gene, which when defective is responsible for childhood susceptibility to retinoblastoma tumors.[22] Only one functional copy of *Rb* is present in the germline of patients with familial susceptibility to retinoblastomas. Retinoblasts become transformed and proliferate uncontrollably when there is no functional Rb after the remaining good copy of *Rb* is lost or rendered nonfunctional in retinoblastoma tumor cells from these patients. This mechanism is supported by the observation that introduction of wild-type but not mutant Rb into cells without Rb causes

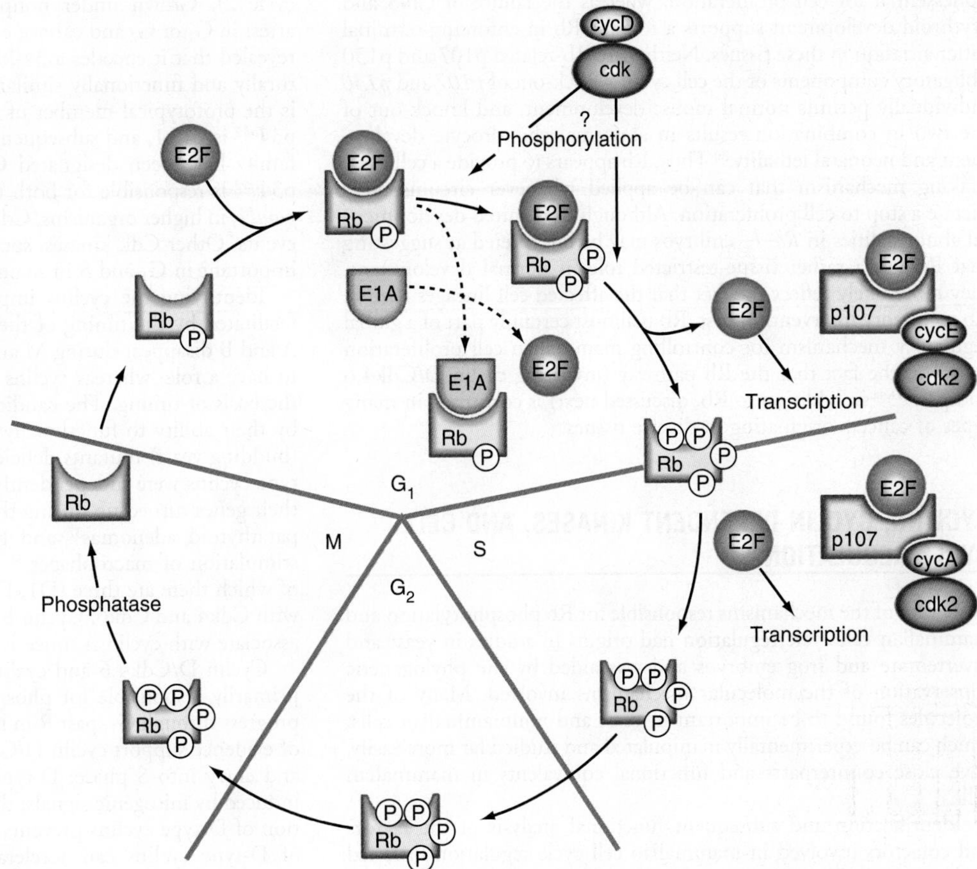

Figure 7–3 REGULATION OF THE RETINOBLASTOMA SUSCEPTIBILITY GENE PRODUCT (RB) THROUGH THE CELL CYCLE. Rb is regulated by serine/threonine phosphorylation (P) through the cell cycle. Non- or hypophosphorylated Rb present in early and mid-G_1 can bind transcription factor E2F and thereby alter or sequester its activity. In late G_1, Rb becomes hyperphosphorylated (perhaps caused by Cdk/cyclin D kinase activity), releasing E2F for transcriptional duties or formation of other complexes. Removal of phosphate groups in M restores Rb to its hypophosphorylated form. In cells transformed by adenovirus E1A, SV40 large T, or HPV E7, these oncoproteins can bind hypophosphorylated RB and displace E2F (*dashed lines*). The Rb-like p107 protein also binds E2F and is found in quaternary complexes with cyclin E/Cdk2 in G_1 or with cyclin A/Cdk2 in S phase.

them to arrest in G_1.[23] Thus, Rb can prevent cell entry into S phase, and retinoblastomas arise when retinoblast proliferation is no longer restrained by Rb.

Rb is widely expressed in normal cells and present at similar levels throughout the cell cycle, indicating that cell proliferation is not regulated primarily by levels of Rb protein. On the other hand, Rb phosphorylation changes markedly in different phases of the cell cycle. It is hypophosphorylated in early G_1, becomes progressively more phosphorylated on serine and threonine residues as cells progress through G_1 and approach S, and maintains this hyperphosphorylated state until M, at which time it is dephosphorylated and returned to its hypophosphorylated, early G_1 state.[24–26]

How Rb phosphorylation controls cell proliferation is understood in terms of Rb binding to transcription factors of the E2F family (Fig. 7–3).[27,28] Originally described as a cellular factor necessary for adenovirus E2 gene transcription, E2F proteins heterodimerize with members of the DP family of proteins to activate gene transcription. E2F-responsive genes include many that encode proteins necessary for DNA synthesis, such as dihydrofolate reductase, thymidine kinase, and others. Hypophosphorylated Rb binds E2F, rendering it transcriptionally inactive or an active repressor of E2F-mediated transcription.[29] Phosphorylation of serine/threonine residues in Rb near or at the site of E2F binding abrogates this interaction and Rb inhibition of E2F transcriptional activity. Thus, E2F activation of gene expression needed for S phase is inhibited by hypophosphorylated Rb in early G_1 and is reinstated as Rb becomes increasingly phosphorylated as cells progress through G_1. The importance of E2F activity for S phase transition is shown by the fact that its gratuitous expression can induce cells to enter S phase. In addition to p105 Rb (molecular mass of 105 kD), two related cellular proteins, p107 and p130, possess similar functional properties, such as the ability to bind E2F.[30] These two Rb-related proteins undoubtedly participate in cell cycle regulation, but their precise roles are still being defined.

The importance of hypophosphorylated Rb in control of cell cycling is underscored by the mechanisms tumorigenic DNA viruses use to deregulate proliferation of infected cells.[31] These viruses possess oncogenes that encode proteins responsible for transforming the infected cells. The E1A oncoprotein of adenovirus, E7 oncoprotein of human papillomavirus, and large T antigen of SV40 virus preferentially bind Rb in its hypophosphorylated state. These oncoproteins interact with Rb in the same molecular pocket as that of E2F, preventing Rb from binding E2F and permitting E2F to carry out its function unimpeded. Thus, transformation by these DNA tumor viruses is associated with cell cycle deregulation caused by viral oncoprotein inactivation of hypophosphorylated Rb function.

In the widely accepted model just described, the key to cell proliferation is release of E2F and other proteins important for S phase from Rb inhibition. This is solved in retinoblastoma and some other tumor cell types by inactivating both copies of the *Rb* gene and in cells transformed by DNA tumor viruses by viral oncoproteins that inactivate hypophosphorylated Rb. Solutions that cause total, irreversible disruption of normal cell cycle regulation present no problems for tumors and help explain their growth deregulation. Normal cells needing to proliferate, however, must use a solution that can be reversed when the need has been satisfied. Their solution is use of kinases that phosphorylate Rb, which results in the progressive phosphorylation of Rb seen during passage of normal cells through G_1.

The model of Rb activity derived from study of tumors and tumor cells implies that Rb is a regulatory protein dispensable for cell cycling. The phenotype of *Rb* knock-out mice[32] suggests that this view also may apply in physiologic situations and during development. $Rb^{-/-}$ embryos arise in expected numbers up to day 14 of gestation but fail to develop beyond that, with evidence of abnormal central nervous system (CNS) development and defective erythropoiesis. Their development more than halfway through gestation and grossly normal appearance up to that time indicate that Rb is nonessential for cell proliferation, whereas the failure of CNS and erythroid development supports a role for Rb in enforcing terminal differentiation in these tissues. Neither are Rb-related p107 and p130 obligatory components of the cell cycle: Knock-out of *p107* and *p130* individually permits normal mouse development, and knock-out of the two in combination results in abnormal chondrocyte development and neonatal lethality.[30] Thus, Rb appears to provide a cell cycle braking mechanism that can be applied whenever circumstances dictate a stop to cell proliferation. Although the limited developmental abnormalities in *Rb–/–* embryos may be interpreted as suggesting that Rb has a rather tissue-restricted role in normal development, they more likely reflect the fact that the affected cell lineages require Rb regulatory intervention first. Rb is almost certainly part of a global regulatory mechanism for controlling mammalian cell proliferation based on the fact that the Rb pathway (involving cyclin D/Cdk4,6 and $p16^{INK4a}$ in addition to Rb, discussed next) is corrupted in many types of cancers originating in diverse tissues.

CYCLINS, CYCLIN-DEPENDENT KINASES, AND CELL CYCLE REGULATION

Discovery of the mechanisms responsible for Rb phosphorylation and mammalian cell cycle regulation had origins in studies in yeast and invertebrate and frog embryos and was aided by the phylogenetic conservation of the molecular mechanisms involved. Many of the molecules found to be important in yeast and nonmammalian cells, which can be experimentally manipulated and studied far more easily, have close counterparts and functional equivalents in mammalian cells.

Identification and subsequent functional analysis of the factors and cofactors involved in mammalian cell cycle regulation have led to the current view that progression through the cell division cycle is driven and regulated by the activity of serine/threonine kinases of the Cdk (*c*yclin-*d*ependent *k*inase) family. As their name implies, the activity of these kinases is under the stringent control of associated regulatory proteins called *cyclins*. These were so named because levels of the first to be described, cyclins A and B, were seen to fluctuate periodically with the cell cycle. Binding to cyclins alters Cdk structure and activates their catalytic function.[33] Numerous Cdk kinases and cyclins exist in the cell, forming combinatorial pairs with distinct activities.

Control of cyclin/Cdk activity occurs at many levels. First is the appearance and disappearance of different cyclins at specific phases of the cell cycle, which dictates the cyclin/Cdk complexes that can form in each phase. Regulation at this level is a result of highly regulated synthesis and degradation of cyclin mRNA and protein at different points in the cell cycle. A second level of regulation is afforded by posttranslational modification of Cdk kinases, which is often necessary to activate their function. A third level of regulation is provided by proteins that inhibit the activity of Cdk kinases or cyclin/Cdk complexes. The importance of regulation by Cdk inhibitors is shown by the fact that cell differentiation signals often act through them to inhibit cell proliferation and by the fact that inhibitor loss allows deregulated proliferation and promotes neoplastic transformation of some cell types. Once active, Cdk kinases phosphorylate other proteins involved in cell cycling, modulating their activity and behavior. Among their important functions is control of cell entry into S and M phases of the cell cycle.

ENTRY INTO S PHASE

The importance of decisions made in G_1 leading into S and their relevance to neoplastic cell behavior have made identification of regulatory factors involved in G_1 and the G_1–S transition a prime objective.[34] The molecular mechanisms regulating cell entry into S phase were first revealed by studies of a conditional cell cycle mutant of *Schizosaccharomyces pombe* (fission yeast) called *cdc2* (cell division cycle 2). Grown under nonpermissive conditions, these mutants arrest in G_1 or G_2 and cannot enter S or M. Cloning of the *cdc2* gene revealed that it encodes a 34-kD serine/threonine kinase. The structurally and functionally similar protein in mammalian cells, $p34^{cdc2}$, is the prototypical member of a family of Cdk kinases. The protein $p34^{cdc2}$ is Cdk1, and subsequently discovered members of this kinase family have been designated Cdk2, Cdk3, and so forth. Whereas $p34^{cdc2}$ is responsible for both the G_1–S and G_2–M transitions in *S. pombe*, in higher organisms, Cdk1 is involved only in G_2 and M phase events. Other Cdk kinases, such as Cdk2 and Cdk4, are the kinases important in G_1 and S in mammalian cells.

Identifying the cyclins important for G_1-S transition has been facilitated by the timing of their appearance (see Fig. 7–2). Cyclins A and B disappear during M and only reappear in S and are unlikely to have a role, whereas cyclins D and E are excellent candidates on the basis of timing. The candidacy of cyclins D and E is supported by their ability to functionally complement *Saccharomyces cerevisiae* (budding yeast) mutants deficient in G_1 cyclin genes (*CLN*).[35,36] D-type cyclins were independently suspected as being important when their genes turned up during the search for an oncogene involved in parathyroid adenomas[37] and for genes induced during mitogenic stimulation of macrophages.[38] Studies indicate that D-type cyclins, of which there are three (D1, D2, and D3), associate predominantly with Cdk4 and Cdk6. Cyclin E associates with Cdk2, which also can associate with cyclin A, once it appears in S phase.

Cyclin D/Cdk4,6 and cyclin E/Cdk2 are considered the kinases primarily responsible for phosphorylating Rb and allowing cells to progress through G_1, past R in late G_1, and into S phase. Several lines of evidence support cyclin D/Cdk4,6 as regulators of G_1 progression and entry into S phase: D-type cyclins appear in early G_1 and are induced by mitogenic signals; they can phosphorylate Rb; neutralization of D-type cyclins prevents cell entry into S; and overexpression of D-type cyclins can accelerate entry into S.[39,40] D-type cyclins appear to be mitogen sensors for the cell cycle, with many steps in their accumulation being sensitive to the presence of extrinsic growth factors and mitogenic signaling. The generally accepted view is that cyclin D/Cdk4,6 complexes initiate Rb phosphorylation in mid-G_1, which leads up to the subsequent complete inactivation of Rb that is needed for the G_1-S transition. Other studies, however, have raised questions about the absolute requirement for cyclin D/Cdk4,6 in the G_1-S transition.[41,42] In mitogen-stimulated cells, cyclin E appears later in G_1, peaks near the G_1/S boundary, and declines in S (see Fig. 7–2). Cyclin E/Cdk2 associates with Rb in G_1 and can phosphorylate Rb, and inhibition of Cdk2 activity blocks cell entry into S. If all of these observations are taken into account, Cyclin E/Cdk2 is probably responsible for phosphorylating Rb at additional sites in late G_1, producing a hyperphosphorylated Rb that can no longer bind E2F.

Cyclin E associates primarily with Cdk2, and the two can be found in complex with transcription factor E2F and members of the Rb family of proteins in cells in G_1. Of interest, this complex disappears as cells enter S, just as a similar complex containing cyclin A instead of E makes its appearance. Thus, cyclin A/Cdk complexes may maintain Rb in its hyperphosphorylated state past this point in the cell cycle. Cyclin A first appears at the beginning of S and declines in G_2 and M and has an expression pattern that parallels but precedes that of cyclin B (see Fig. 7–2). These data and the results of cyclin A inhibition and addition experiments[43] have led to the view that cyclin A/Cdk2 plays a major role in driving events once cells enter S phase. Later in S and G_2, cyclin A in complex with $p32^{cdc2}$ may help trigger the G_2-M transition by phosphorylating Cdc25 and initiating activation of cyclin B/$p32^{cdc2}$.

ENTRY INTO M PHASE

Studies initiated in *S. pombe cdc2* mutants, which arrest in G_1 or G_2 and do not enter S or M, led to the cloning of the evolutionarily conserved $p34^{cdc2}$ (Cdk1) serine/threonine kinase.[44] An independent line of study examining the effect of cytoplasmic extracts from mature

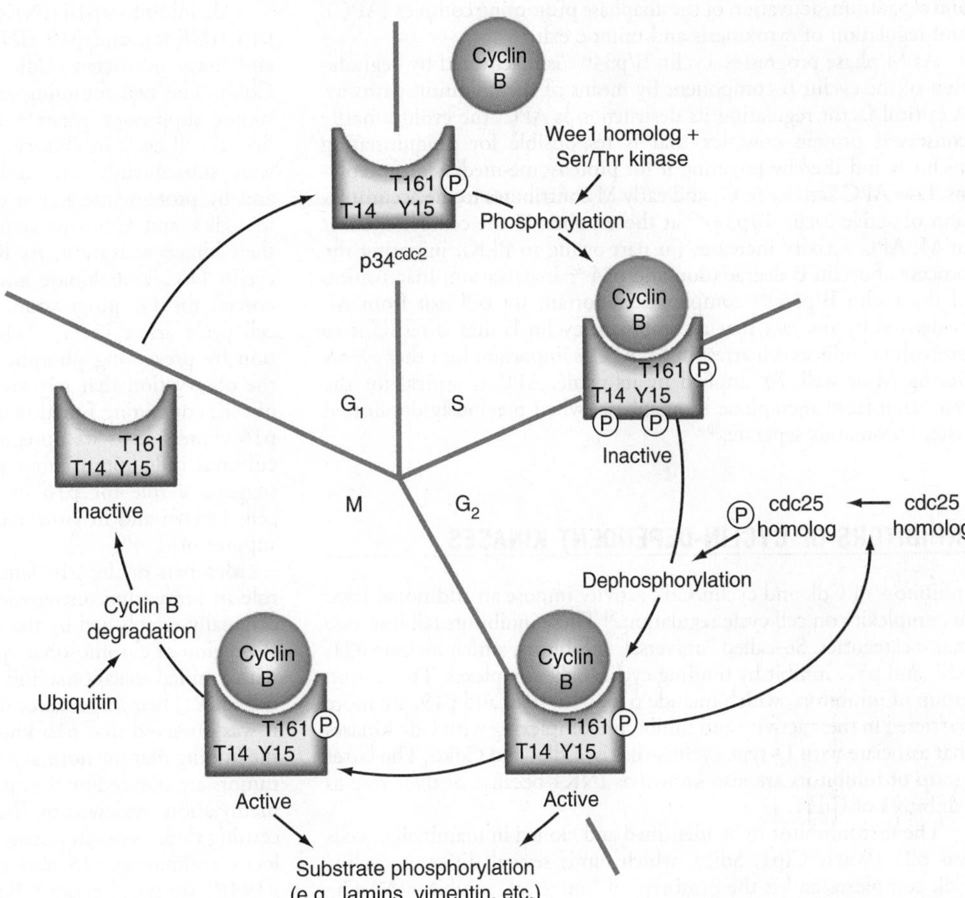

Figure 7–4 Regulation of cell entry into M by cyclin B/p34*cdc2* or Cdk1 (maturation-promoting factor [MPF]). p34*cdc2* kinase activity controls cell entry into M and is regulated during the cell cycle. Association with cyclin B, which first appears during S phase, is necessary for its kinase activity, and formation of the cyclin B/p34*cdc2* or Cdk1 complex (MPF) is stabilized by phosphorylation of Thr(T)161. Accumulating MPF is maintained in an inactive state by phosphorylation of Thr14 and Tyr(Y)15, which is catalyzed by the homolog of the *Schizosaccharomyces pombe wee1* gene product and another kinase. At the G_2/M transition, MPF is activated by dephosphorylation of Thr14 and Tyr15 by the homolog of the *S. pombe cdc25* gene product. This may be a self-amplifying reaction because activated MPF can phosphorylate and activate more Cdc25. Activated MPF phosphorylates cellular substrates and brings about the biochemical changes needed for M phase. During progression through M, degradation of cyclin B generates inactive p34*cdc2* and permits cell exit from M.

Xenopus frog eggs microinjected into immature frog oocytes showed that these extracts contain a material that induces oocytes to mature and undergo M phase changes such as nuclear membrane breakdown. After purification, the maturation-promoting factor (MPF) in these extracts was found to contain two proteins: One is p34*cdc2*, and the other is a B-type cyclin. Cyclin B has a regulatory role in the MPF complex, shown by the fact that p34*cdc2* exhibits kinase/MPF activity only in association with cyclin B.

Cyclin B levels increase during S and G_2 (see Fig. 7–2), and levels of cyclin B/p34*cdc2* complex sufficient for the G_2-M transition are reached well before the onset of M. Mitosis is not prematurely triggered because the complex accumulates in an inactive form (Fig. 7–4). During S and G_2, the p34*cdc2* complexed with cyclin B accumulates as a multiply phosphorylated protein. In mammalian cells, phosphorylation of p34*cdc2* threonine (Thr) 161 stabilizes its association with cyclin B and is essential for activity. The kinase responsible for Thr 161 phosphorylation, CAK (*C*dk-*a*ctivating *k*inase), is itself a Cdk (designated Cdk7) that associates with a novel cyclin, cyclin H. On the other hand, phosphorylation of p34*cdc2* Thr 14 and tyrosine (Tyr) 15 suppresses its kinase activity and keeps the cyclin B/p34*cdc2* complex inactive. The kinase responsible for Tyr 15 phosphorylation is the homolog of the product of the *S. pombe wee1* gene.[45]

Activation of the cyclin B/p34*cdc2* complex is the key to cell entry into M and occurs just prior to M through the action of the dual-specificity phosphatase, Cdc25, causing dephosphorylation of both Thr 14 and Tyr 15. The activities of *wee1* kinase and Cdc25 phosphatase are themselves regulated with phosphorylation, inhibiting *wee1* kinase function and enhancing Cdc25 phosphatase function. Once a little cyclin B/p34*cdc2* is activated, it can phosphorylate Cdc25 and create a self-amplifying feedback loop that generates more active cyclin B/p34*cdc2* from the large preexisting stock of inactive complex.

What starts this sequence of events by initially phosphorylating and activating Cdc25 is unclear. Cyclin A/Cdk complexes have been suggested as candidates because they are active before cyclin B/p34*cdc2* activation and have MPF activity, and because inhibition of cyclin A during S prevents entry into M. However, it is unclear how cyclin A/Cdk complexes, which are abundant and active throughout S, would suddenly initiate the cascade of cyclin B/p34*cdc2* activation that marks cell entry into M phase. Polo-like kinases (PLKs), named after polo kinase, the prototypical member of this evolutionarily conserved serine/threonine kinase family, are[46] reasonable candidates, because they too can phosphorylate and activate Cdc25 and because amplification of cyclin B/p34*cdc2* activity does not occur until PLK becomes activated. Additionally, PLK phosphorylation of cyclin B and Cdc25 promotes nuclear localization of these proteins, enhancing nuclear accumulation of active cyclin B/p34*cdc2* complex.[47]

Cyclin B/p34*cdc2* can phosphorylate serine/threonine residues in many cellular proteins. Discerning its direct physiologic substrates is not simple, however, because many other kinases and cyclin/Cdk kinases are concurrently active. Candidate substrates include the lamins and vimentin, which are, respectively, nuclear and cytoplasmic proteins important for the structural organization of their compartments. These proteins undergo M phase phosphorylation and are cyclin B/p34*cdc2* substrates in vitro. Phosphorylation of lamins is important for nuclear lamina disassembly and envelope breakdown, and phosphorylation of vimentin may cause depolymerization of vimentin intermediate filaments. If these are physiologic substrates, p34*cdc2*/cyclin B kinase activity may initiate the structural reorganization that is essential for mitosis. PLKs, which may be phosphorylated and activated by cyclin B/p34*cdc2*, are found at important structures and sites during M and facilitate many crucial M phase events. For example, in prophase, PLK phosphorylates cohesin and is responsible for removing most of this protein, which holds sister chromatids together following DNA replication.[48] Removal of cohesin is required for subsequent sister chromatid separation during the metaphase to anaphase transition. PLK is also needed for centrosome maturation and separation, activation of the anaphase promoting complex (APC), and regulation of cytokinesis and mitotic exit.[49]

As M phase progresses, cyclin B/p34^{cdc2} is inactivated by degradation of the cyclin B component by means of the ubiquitin pathway. A critical factor regulating its destruction is APC, the evolutionarily conserved protein complex that is responsible for ubiquitinating cyclin B and thereby targeting it for proteosome-mediated proteolysis. Low APC activity in G_2 and early M contributes to the accumulation of active cyclin B/p34^{cdc2} at those points in the cell cycle. Later in M, APC activity increases (in part owing to PLK), initiating the process of cyclin B degradation and p34^{cdc2} inactivation. Inactivation of the cyclin B/p34^{cdc2} complex is important for cell exit from M, evidenced by the fact that recombinant cyclin B that is resistant to proteolysis induces cell arrest in M. APC is important for other events during M as well. As implied by its name, APC is critical for the transition from metaphase to anaphase, when previously duplicated sister chromatids separate.[50]

INHIBITORS OF CYCLIN-DEPENDENT KINASES

Inhibitors of Cdk and cyclin/Cdk activity impose an additional layer of complexity on cell cycle regulation.[51] These inhibitors fall into two major categories. So-called "universal" inhibitors, which include p21, p27, and p57, inhibit by binding cyclin/Cdk complexes. The second group of inhibitors, which include p16, p15, p18, and p19, are more restricted in their activity and inhibit by complexing with Cdk kinases that associate with D-type cyclins-that is, Cdk4 and Cdk6. The latter group of inhibitors are also known as INK4 because of their role as *in*hibitors of Cd*k4*.

The first inhibitor to be identified and cloned in mammalian cells was p21 (Waf1, Cip1, Sdi1), which binds several different cyclin/Cdk complexes and is the prototypical "universal" inhibitor.[52,53] The proteins p27 (Kip1) and p57 (Kip2) were subsequently identified as Cdk inhibitors with structural and functional similarities to those of p21.[54-56] The regulation of p21 expression sheds light on its function. Expression is transcriptionally induced by p53, the tumor suppressor protein activated by DNA damage (see following), and induction of p21 expression provides a mechanism for halting cell proliferation after DNA damage to allow time for damage assessment and repair.[57] The p21 protein also can be expressed in cells lacking functional p53, indicating that p53-independent pathways of expression exist. These other pathways may account for increased p21 expression in other circumstances associated with cell cycle arrest, such as senescence and terminal differentiation.

The p27 protein was originally cloned as the Cdk inhibitor associated with G_1 arrest in cells treated with transforming growth factor-β (TGF-β) or experiencing contact inhibition of growth,[54] but levels also increase in cells induced to differentiate.[58] These observations indicate that p27 often mediates the cell cycle arrest induced by extrinsic inhibitors of cell proliferation. In marked contrast with the transcriptional regulation of p21, regulation of p27 occurs post-transcriptionally, such that mRNA levels remain constant while levels of the protein change. In accordance with the ability of p21 and p27 to inhibit cyclin/Cdk activity and cell cycling, *p21* and *p27* are candidate tumor suppressor genes, but silencing or loss of these genes is very uncommon in cancers. However, decreased levels of p27 are seen in many carcinomas and often correlate with aggressive tumor histology and poor prognosis.[58] In some cancers, p27 levels are normal, but the protein is found in the cytoplasm rather than in the nucleus and thus unable to inhibit nuclear cyclin/Cdk complexes. Recent studies in breast cancer cells (reviewed by Blain and Massague[59]) showed that p27 is banished from the nucleus because of its phosphorylation by AKT, which is frequently constitutively active in these cells. Thus, although the *p27* gene is not genetically inactivated during oncogenesis and therefore cannot be formally counted as a tumor suppressor gene, p27 inhibition of cyclin/Cdk activity seems to be a major obstacle that cells may have to circumvent on their way to malignancy.

Cdk inhibitors p16 (INK4a, MTS1, Cdk4), p15 (INK4b, MTS2), p18 (INK4c), and p19 (INK4d) differ structurally from p21/p27 and have restricted Cdk specificity, binding only Cdk4 and Cdk6. The two founding members, p16 and p15, were cloned as tumor suppressor genes,[60] but both had previously been identified as cell cycle inhibitory proteins.[61,62] The p18 and p19 proteins were subsequently cloned based on homology to p16 and p15 and by protein interaction cloning.[63,64] Binding of these inhibitors to Cdk4 and Cdk6 prevents their association with cyclin D and their kinase activation. As Rb family proteins are prime targets of cyclin D/Cdk4,6 kinase and phosphorylation of these proteins is crucial for G_1 progression, inhibitors of the p16 family induce cell cycle arrest in G_1. Evidence that p16 inhibits cell proliferation by preventing phosphorylation of Rb proteins is provided by the observation that p16 overexpression inhibits proliferation only of cells containing functional Rb proteins.[65] An interesting aspect of p16 expression is its upregulation in tissues of aging mice and in cultured cells approaching proliferative senescence.[66] This finding suggests a role for p16 in limiting the proliferative potential of cells in vivo and in vitro and may reflect on its activity as a tumor suppressor.

Members of the p16 family of inhibitors unquestionably have a role in preventing oncogenic transformation in vivo. This role was originally established by the cloning of the *p16* and *p15* genes from the region of chromosome 9p21 mutated in the germline of patients with familial melanoma and in the genome of many human tumor cell lines. Their importance during oncogenesis was reinforced when it was observed that p16 knock-out mice are cancer prone[67] and by the finding that the normal *p16* and *p15* genes found in many human tumors are silenced by the epigenetic mechanism of promoter hypermethylation (reviewed by Ruas and Peters[68]). A lingering issue concerning these genes in oncogenesis stems from the fact that the 9p21 locus containing *p16* also contains the *p14ARF* (in humans) or *p19ARF* (in mice) genes.[69] Because these genes overlap, *p14/p19ARF* mRNA shares sequence with *p16* mRNA but produces a totally different protein because of translation in an *a*lternative *r*eading *f*rame (ie, ARF). This overlap also means that many inactivating mutations of *p16* (including engineered mutations in mice) also inactivate *p14/p19ARF*. Because p14/p19ARF is a positive regulator of p53 expression and a tumor suppressor protein in its own right, attribution of tumor suppressor effect to each of these two genes is difficult. The more recent results of individual knock-out of each these two genes in mice indicate that loss of either *p14/p19ARF* or *p16INK4a* predisposes mice to tumors and results in abnormal regulation of cell proliferation.[70,71]

The idea that Cdk inhibitors act simply as negative regulators of kinase activity and cell cycling and that p16/p15INK4 arrests cell cycling solely through inhibition of Cdk4,6 activity has been revised (reviewed in 1999 by Sherr and Roberts[51]). It was observed that complexes such as cyclin E/Cdk2 bound to p21/p27 were inactive but that cyclin D/Cdk4,6 complexes containing these inhibitors remained active. This suggested that the latter might sequester inhibitors while maintaining activity and prevent inactivation of Cdk2-containing complexes. Keeping cyclin E/Cdk2 active by preventing its inhibition by p21/p27 is a noncatalytic function of cyclin D/Cdk4,6 that complements and augments its catalytic function of promoting Rb hyperphosphorylation and cell cycling. In addition, p21/p27 was found to promote assembly and nuclear accumulation of active cyclin D/Cdk complexes, suggesting that the presence of these inhibitors in cyclin D/Cdk complexes may actually be facilitatory or obligatory rather than merely optional. If cyclin D/Cdk complexes are positively regulated by p21/p27 and prevent p21/p27 from inactivating cyclin E/Cdk2, the effect of p16/p15 extends beyond inhibition of Cdk4,6 complexes. In binding Cdk4,6 and preventing assembly of cyclin D/Cdk complexes, p16/p15 causes redistribution of p21/p27 onto cyclin E/Cdk2 complexes, resulting in their inactivation and an inability to hyperphosphorylate Rb. Thus, G_1 cell cycle arrest induced by p16/p15INK4 may require and be mediated by p21/p27 proteins.

CELL CYCLE CHECKPOINTS

The welfare of an organism depends on production, by its constituent cells, of normal copies of themselves during mitotic replication. If errors arise, one or both of the progeny cells develop defects in their genome that will be transmitted to successive cell generations in subsequent rounds of mitotic proliferation. Perpetuation and amplification of genetic flaws are fundamentally detrimental, and cell cycle checkpoints, which are control mechanisms that monitor and enforce proper execution of the cell division cycle, defend against development of genomic error and instability.[19]

Cell cycle checkpoints are positioned before entry into S (G_1 checkpoint), in S (S phase checkpoint), and before entry into M (G_2 checkpoint). They enforce the orderly progression of cell cycle events, such that cells must fully duplicate their DNA before they divide and divide before they duplicate their DNA again. They also check for damage sustained by genomic DNA. When problems are detected, checkpoint mechanisms interrupt cell cycling to allow correction of the problem or elimination of the defective cell. Where the mechanisms are known, cell cycling is stopped through inhibition of the cyclins and Cdk kinases that drive normal cell cycle progression. Checkpoints also exist within M, but mitotic checkpoints may exist mostly to prevent chromosome missegregation by enforcing the sequence of M phase events that distribute duplicated genetic material equally between progeny cells. The operation of checkpoints and the consequences of their failure are illustrated by yeast mutants defective in the *RAD9* gene. Although yeasts normally cannot enter M phase until their DNA is fully replicated, defects in the *RAD9* gene allow yeasts to enter M phase even if they are prevented from completing DNA replication. Affected yeasts die more rapidly, as progeny inherit incomplete or damaged genetic material.

The activity of checkpoints in mammalian cells usually is observable after they have been exposed to DNA-damaging agents, such as ionizing radiation, ultraviolet light, or certain chemotherapy agents. Checkpoint activation by these genotoxic insults results in cell division cycle arrest in G_1, S, or G_2 phase, allowing cells time to repair the fault before resuming the cycle or, if the damage is irreparable, to execute a program of programmed cell death or apoptosis. Mechanisms that detect and signal the presence of damaged cellular DNA are incompletely understood, but the ATM and ATR protein kinases are clearly important components (Fig. 7–5). ATM (*a*taxia-*t*elangiectasia *m*utated) kinase is activated by ionizing radiation and the double-strand DNA breaks it causes.[72] Defects in ATM result in cell sensitivity to ionizing radiation, defects in all DNA damage-induced cell cycle checkpoints and susceptibility of patients with ataxia-telangiectasia (AT) to cancer. The ATR (*AT* and *R*AD3-related) kinase responds to UV-induced DNA damage, to stalled intermediates of DNA replication, and to damage from ionizing radiation.

ATM and ATR, both of which bind DNA, plus other proteins with homology to proteins involved in DNA replication, are responsible for sensing damaged DNA or failed DNA replication and initiating checkpoint signaling. As ATM and ATR kinase function is activated in the process, they also transduce the signals by phosphorylating downstream effectors of the checkpoint response (reviewed by Abraham[73]). Among the recipients of ATM/ATR signaling are Chk1 and Chk2. These two structurally distinct serine/threonine kinases are phosphorylated and activated by ATM/ATR. Chk1 is regulated primarily by ATR,[74] whereas Chk 2 is regulated primarily by ATM,[75] but other factors, such as BRCA1, clearly influence their activation in response to DNA damage.[76] Once active, Chk1/Chk2 join ATM/ATR to phosphorylate and activate effectors of the checkpoint response.

Prominent among the effectors activated by these kinases is p53, the tumor suppressor protein missing or inactivated in over 50% of human cancers and an essential component of the G_1 DNA damage checkpoint. ATM/ATR directly phosphorylate p53 and indirectly promote its phosphorylation through Chk1/Chk2 phosphorylation of p53 at additional sites. The effect of this p53 phosphorylation is protein stabilization, a result that is augmented by ATM phosphorylation of the Mdm2 protein and inhibition of its ability to direct rapid p53 turnover.[77] Through this combination of mechanisms, p53 is rapidly induced following DNA damage. A transcription factor, p53 engenders cell cycle arrest by activating transcription of *p21(Waf1/Cip1/Sdi1)* and inhibiting cyclin/Cdk2 activity. The pathway leading from ATM/ATR to Cdk2 inhibition activates the G_1 DNA damage checkpoint by preventing Rb hyperphosphorylation.

Enforcement of the G_2 DNA-damage checkpoint involves Chk1 and Chk2 phosphorylation of Cdc25C, allowing this phosphatase to bind the 14–3-3σ protein and be sequestered in the cytoplasm. Excluded from the nucleus, Cdc25C cannot dephosphorylate Cdc2 and activate the cyclin B/Cdc2 complex needed for M phase entry.[78] Although signaling from ATM/ATR to Chk1/Chk2 to Cdc25C is one G_2 checkpoint mechanism, p53 also plays a role. The p53 protein induces p21 and represses cyclin B and Cdc2 gene expression, reducing levels and activity of cyclin B/Cdc2 complex.[79,80] These effects, plus effects on expression of other genes, result in p53-dependent G_2 arrest following DNA damage. As p53 induction stems from ATM/ATR activation, this pathway complements Cdc25C sequestration to provide multiple ways by which ATM/ATR activation can enact G_2 arrest.

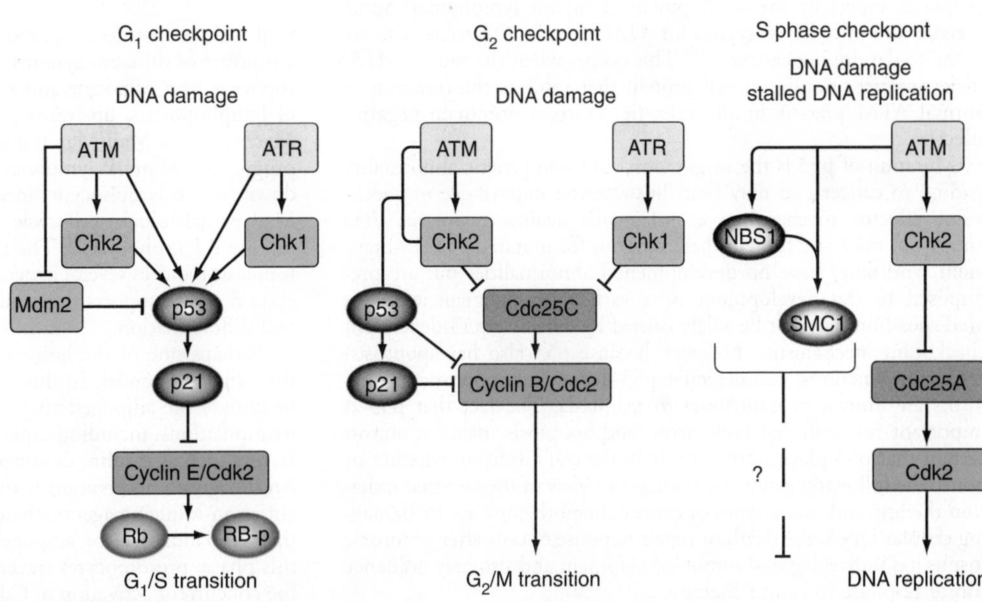

Figure 7–5 CELL CYCLE CHECKPOINTS. Pathways for activating G_1, G_2, and S phase checkpoints are shown. Arrows (Ø) designate activating interactions, and (→) designate inhibitory or inactivating interactions.

The S phase checkpoint arrests cells that experience problems after beginning DNA replication, ie, cells that are in S phase. It does not depend on p53 and is distinct from the G_1 checkpoint, which affects cells that have not yet entered S. When ionizing radiation fails to activate this checkpoint, it results in the phenomenon of radioresistant DNA synthesis (RDS), whereby cells inappropriately continue to initiate new origins of DNA replication and replicate DNA despite DNA damage. ATM plays an important role in this pathway, evidenced by the fact that AT cells display RDS. ATM activates S phase arrest via Chk2, which phosphorylates Cdc25A and accelerates its degradation. Cdc25A normally dephosphorylates Cdk2, activating this kinase and allowing it to promote assembly of replication initiation complexes at replication origins. The inability of ATM-deficient cells to downregulate Cdc25A results in their inability to curb Cdk2 activity and DNA replication in response to ionizing radiation.[81]

More recently, Chk1 also has been shown to participate in Cdc25A regulation and prevention of RDS,[82] but the mechanism of Chk1 activation in this situation remains to be clarified. In a parallel pathway of S phase checkpoint activation, ATM phosphorylates NBS1, the product of the gene mutated in Nijmegen breakage syndrome (NBS). NBS and AT resemble each other in the predisposition of patients to cancer and of their cells to chromosome instability, radiation sensitivity, and RDS. NBS1 is part of a protein complex that binds to and helps repair double-strand DNA breaks,[83,84] and its phosphorylation by ATM is important for inducing S phase arrest following DNA damage and preventing RDS. Recently, the SMC1 (*s*tructure *m*aintenance of *c*hromosomes-1) protein, which has a role in chromosome structure and DNA repair, was found to be phosphorylated by ATM following ionizing radiation exposure. Phosphorylation depended on NBS1 and was important for S phase checkpoint activation.[85,86] Although many details are still unclear, ATM/NBS1/SMC1 and ATM/Chk2/Cdc25A appear to provide parallel and cooperative pathways for S phase checkpoint activation.[87]

The importance of checkpoint mechanisms is shown by the fact that mutant yeasts defective in checkpoint genes and proteins exhibit difficulties with mitotic replication, genomic instability, and death. In mammals, the consequences of failed checkpoint mechanisms can be just as devastating. *ATR* knock-out in mice is lethal at a very early stage (7.5 days) of embryonic development, with cells cultured from the embryos exhibiting loss of genomic integrity and widespread death by apoptosis.[88] Defective checkpoint mechanisms compatible with survival beyond birth, such as loss of *ATM* or *NBS1*, must have less catastrophic consequences but nevertheless produce growth retardation and developmental abnormalities.[89–91] Because organisms deficient in ATM or NBS1 survive, the impact of these proteins on neoplasia can be seen. Deficient mice and humans are predisposed to neoplasia, especially the development of thymic lymphomas. Some humans and mice heterozygous for *ATM* mutations (carriers) also are prone to developing cancers.[92,93] This occurs when the mutant *ATM* allele produces nonfunctional protein that inhibits the function of normal ATM present in the cells (ie, exerts a dominant-negative effect).

Mutation of p53 is the single most common genetic abnormality leading to cancer and may best illustrate the importance of checkpoint effector mechanisms as safeguards against neoplasia. *P53* knock-out mice and humans heterozygous for mutated *p53* (Li-Fraumeni syndrome) have no developmental abnormalities but are predisposed to the development of a variety of malignancies. This predisposition may not be solely caused by defective p53-dependent checkpoint mechanisms, however, because p53 also has apoptosis-activating functions, and defective p53-dependent apoptotic mechanisms are known to contribute to neoplasia. The fact that p53 is important for both cell cycle arrest and apoptosis makes it almost certain that p53 plays a critical role in the cell's decision whether or not to die following genotoxic damage. In view of the fact that radiation therapy and many types of cancer chemotherapy act by damaging cellular DNA, the death or repair response of cells after genotoxic insults has impact beyond tumor development and also may influence tumor response to cancer therapy.

CELL CYCLE ALTERATIONS WITH DIFFERENTIATION

The cell cycle machinery regulates the normal proliferation of cells for both maintenance and replacement purposes. For example, blood cells, skin cells, and the gut epithelia undergo rapid turnover and require constant maintenance of the differentiated cell pools that provide specific differentiated functions. In contrast, liver, muscle, and fat cells may be replaced or expand in response to the metabolic status of the organism or to injury. Either maintenance or replacement of the differentiated cell compartment requires an orchestrated interplay between cell cycle regulation and the cell differentiation program. Although previously thought to be mutually exclusive, cell cycle progression and cell differentiation are tightly linked in the differentiation of specific cell types.

WITHDRAWAL FROM AND ENTRY INTO THE CELL CYCLE AND CELL DIFFERENTIATION

The previous paradigm for cell differentiation suggested, on the basis of studies performed with cell lines, that cell cycle progression and cell differentiation are mutually exclusive. It has become more evident, however, that cell cycle progression is inherently necessary for the differentiation of specific cell types. For example, the hematopoietic stem cell compartment is quiescent until these cells are called on by certain stresses to activate the hematopoietic differentiation program. The cell cycle inhibitors p21 and p27 participate in the regulation of hematopoietic stem cell cycle. Using mice null for either p21 or p27, transplantation experiments have revealed distinct roles for these two cell cycle inhibitors. Hematopoietic stem cells depleted of p21 proliferated, and the absolute number of stem cells doubled.[94] This unrestricted proliferation caused diminished self-renewal potential, resulting in hematopoietic failure in animals that received serially transplanted p21-null bone marrow. In contrast with the findings for p21, depletion of p27 does not affect stem cell numbers, but its absence increases progenitor cell proliferation and pool size.[95] The absence of p27, however, does not affect self-renewal potential. These findings indicate that hematopoietic stem cells differentiate through an orderly progression through the cell cycle for the generation of progenitor cells and the ensuing more differentiated lineage-specific cells.

COUPLING OF MANDATORY CELL CYCLE PROGRESSION AND CELL DIFFERENTIATION

Cell cycle progression required for cell differentiation is illustrated by a number of different systems including lymphopoiesis, myeloerythropoiesis, and adipocyte and keratinocyte differentiation. In the case of lymphopoiesis, upstream regulators of the cell cycle such as the Myc/Max and Mad/Max transcriptional regulators permit cell cycle progression of pre-B lymphocytes for their sequential differentiation down the B-lymphocyte lineage. For example, overexpression of Mad, which blocks cell cycle progression, results in the paucity of mature B lymphocytes.[96] The fact that myeloid and erythroid hematopoiesis requires several generations of differentiating cells to proliferate further supports the requirement of concurrent cell expansion and differentiation.

Perhaps one of the best-studied models of cell differentiation is the adipocyte model. In this model, specific fibroblasts are triggered to initiate the adipogenesis program through a series of cell culture manipulations, including exposure of confluent fibroblasts to specific factors such as insulin, dexamethasone, and methylisobutylxanthine. An intriguing observation is that following exposure to these differentiation-inducing agents, there is a "mitotic clonal expansion" phase that is mandatory for adipogenesis of 3T3L1 fibroblasts.[97] During this phase, preadipocytes traverse through the G_1/S checkpoint with the concurrent activation of Cdk2 activity and turnover of p27. After several rounds of synchronous cell divisions, these cells cease to proliferate and start to express markers of adipocytes.

SPECIALIZED CELL CYCLE: ENDOREPLICATION AND DIFFERENTIATION

A special type of cell cycle progression is featured in the differentiation of cells that have high metabolic profiles required for synthesis of specific proteins, such as plasma proteins produced by hepatocytes, or for the production of platelets by megakaryocytes. Both cell types display endoreplication, or the repeated phases of DNA replication without cell division, resulting in cells that are gigantic and could have large nuclei with DNA content well over 128N.[98] Endoreplication also features prominently in specific plant and insect tissues, indicating that this mechanism is well utilized through evolution.

It stands to reason that endoreplicating cells permit G_1/S transition but have mechanisms to prevent entry into or completion of mitosis. Studies of many types of endoreplicating cells in fact support this notion. In particular, megakaryocytes endoreplicate in response to thrombopoietin with upregulation of cyclin D3. Overexpression of cyclin D3 results in increased megakaryocyte ploidy.[99] As is suspected, megakaryocyte endoreplication occurs at levels of the mitotic cyclin B/Cdk1 significantly below levels in cells that undergo cytokinesis. Similarly, mammalian trophoblasts, which also undergo endoreplication, display increased cyclins D1, E, and A, but the levels of cyclin B are diminished. These observations indicate that depending on the specific cell types, cell cycle progression may be critically required for differentiation of specialized cells.

SUGGESTED READING LIST

Blain SW, Massague J: Breast cancer banishes p27 from nucleus. Nat Med 8:1076, 2002.

Falck J, Petrini JH, Williams BR, et al: The DNA damage-dependent intra-S phase checkpoint is regulated by parallel pathways. Nat Genet 30:290, 2002.

Helt AM, Galloway DA: Mechanisms by which DNA tumor virus oncoproteins target the Rb family of pocket proteins. Carcinogenesis 24:159, 2003.

Iritani BM, Delrow J, Grandori C, et al: Modulation of T-lymphocyte development, growth and cell size by the Myc antagonist and transcriptional repressor Mad1. EMBO J 21:4820, 2002.

Kang J, Bronson RT, Xu Y: Targeted disruption of NBS1 reveals its roles in mouse development and DNA repair. EMBO J 21:1447, 2002.

Kim ST, Xu B, Kastan MB: Involvement of the cohesin protein, Smc1, in Atm-dependent and independent responses to DNA damage. Genes Dev 16:560, 2002.

Narlikar GJ, Fan HY, Kingston RE: Cooperation between complexes that regulate chromatin structure to transcription. Cell 108:475, 2002.

Saucedo LJ, Edgar BA: Why size matters: Altering cell size. Curr Opin Genet Dev 12:565, 2002.

Shiloh Y: ATM and related protein kinases: Safeguarding genome integrity. Nat Rev Cancer 3:155, 2003.

Sorensen CS, Syljuasen RG, Falck J, et al: Chk1 regulates the S phase checkpoint by coupling the physiological turnover and ionizing radiation-induced accelerated proteolysis of Cdc25A. Cancer Cell 3:247, 2003.

Spring K, Ahangari F, Scott SP, et al: Mice heterozygous for mutation in *Atm*, the gene involved in ataxia-telangiectasia, have heightened susceptibility to cancer. Nat Genet 32:185, 2002.

Sumara I, Vorlaufer E, Stukenberg PT, et al: The dissociation of cohesin from chromosomes in prophase is regulated by Polo-like kinase. Mol Cell 9:515, 2002.

Tang QQ, Otto TC, Lane MD: Mitotic clonal expansion: A synchronous process required for adipogenesis. Proc Natl Acad Sci U S A 100:44, 2003.

Toyoshima-Morimoto F, Taniguchi E, Nishida E: Plk1 promotes nuclear translocation of human Cdc25C during prophase. EMBO Rep 3:341, 2002.

Yarden RI, Pardo-Reoyo S, Sgagias M, et al: *BRCA1* regulates the G2/M checkpoint by activating Chk1 kinase upon DNA damage. Nat Genet 30:285, 2002.

Yazdi PT, Wang Y, Zhao S, et al: SMC1 is a downstream effector in the ATM/NBS1 branch of the human S-phase checkpoint. Genes Dev 16:571, 2002.

REFERENCES

For complete list of references log onto www.expertconsult.com

CHAPTER 8

CELL DEATH*

David M. Hockenbery and Stanley J. Korsmeyer

Cell death is a highly organized fundamental activity that is as equivalently complex as cell division and differentiation. In the physiologic contexts of embryonic development and tissue renewal, or as pathologic responses to cell injury and infectious pathogens, cell deaths are orchestrated for multiple purposes that benefit the organism. These include maintenance of epithelial barrier function,[1] destruction of microbes,[2] immune response,[3] recycling of cellular material,[4] intercellular signaling,[5] and preservation of genomic integrity.[6] The majority of mammalian cell deaths have morphologic and biochemical features of apoptosis (Table 8–1), a self-inflicted death program encoded in the genetic material of all cells. Necrosis, an alternative mechanism of cell death, occurs in the aftermath of extreme cellular insults and could be viewed as a failure of cellular homeostasis. Although cells contain their own death apparatus, cell death in multicellular organisms is exquisitely subject to the advice and consent of neighboring cells. As might be expected, the internal cell death machinery is tightly interwoven with other essential cell pathways. Investigations of cell death have also informed our understanding of living cells, for example, the recognition that cellular remodeling shares some machinery with apoptotic cell death.[7]

PHYSIOLOGIC CELL TURNOVER

An adult human loses approximately 1011 cells/day, with skin, intestinal, and hematopoietic tissues accounting for the majority. Physiologic cell death in the adult occurs in the context of continuously (skin and intestine) or cyclically (endometrium and breast) renewing tissues. In most instances, homeostasis balances generation of new cells with loss of terminally differentiated cells. In the intestinal epithelium, for example, one stem cell per epithelial crypt asymmetrically divides to produce a daughter cell that rapidly divides, terminally differentiates (coinciding with exit from cell cycle), migrates onto the epithelium surface, and undergoes a specialized form of apoptosis that leaves behind cytoplasmic bridges that preserve epithelial barrier function, all within 2 to 3 days.

Neutrophils recruited to sites of inflammation undergo apoptosis concurrent with removal of the inflammatory stimulus.[8] Apoptotic neutrophils are unable to degranulate and are silently phagocytosed by macrophages, without stimulating an inflammatory response.[9] This clearance mechanism is specialized to apoptotic neutrophils, as necrotic neutrophils and opsonized cells trigger macrophages to secrete inflammatory cytokines. Apoptotic neutrophils also secrete anti-inflammatory cytokines, such as IL-10 and TGF-β.

Although a hallmark of apoptosis is a characteristic compaction of nuclear chromatin, enucleated cells are also subject to apoptotic processes. Biochemical evidence indicates that red blood cells (RBCs) and platelet life spans can be shortened by apoptosis. A general feature of apoptotic cells is the loss of normal asymmetry of phospholipid distribution in the plasma membrane, with accumulation of phosphatidylserine in the outer leaflet. Loss of erythrocyte and platelet viability during in vitro aging is accompanied by phosphatidylserine exposure and activation of apoptotic proteases, known as caspases. Increased phosphatidylserine exposure in erythrocyte membranes is also found in diseases characterized by shortened RBC life spans, such as sickle cell anemia.

Physiologic cell death is also a mechanism to generate a reserve production capacity for functionally mature cells. The glycoprotein hormone erythropoietin (Epo) is produced by kidney mesangial cells and stimulates excess RBC production in proportion to the demand for blood oxygen-carrying capacity. The erythropoietin receptor is expressed on committed erythrocyte precursors (CFU-E and proerythroblasts). Growth factors, in general, also generate survival signals. The primary in vivo effect of Epo is to rescue erythroid precursors from death. The Epo-responsive erythroid compartment in the bone marrow is maintained at a constant size and rate of cell proliferation under various demands (hypoxia and hypertransfusion), despite widely differing production rates of mature erythroid cells. The rationale appears to be to overproduce CFU-Es and proerythroblasts at low altitudes, with excess cells removed prior to the erythroblast stage; this scheme provides a rapidly accessible reserve under conditions of higher demand. Similar arrangements of excessive production with apoptosis of maturing cells are found in small-intestinal crypts and in spermatogenesis.

A final physiologic form for apoptosis is a mechanism for selection of specific cell phenotypes. A well-known example occurs in the immune system following clonal diversification of T- and B-lymphocyte antigen receptors by gene recombination and error-prone DNA replication. Positive and negative clonal selection to match T-cell receptors to cognate class I and class II histocompatibility antigens on accessory cells, and to eliminate receptors reacting with self-antigens, takes place in the thymus. Affinity maturation of immunoglobulin-bearing B cells takes place in germinal centers of lymphoid organs. In each case, cells run a gauntlet of near-death experiences, with death and survival signals directly linked to the binding properties of the antigen receptor on individual cells.

EMBRYOGENESIS AND SCULPTING

During development, apoptosis is extensively used to sculpt the final shape of the embryo. Regression of vestigial tails, interdigital webs, and the pro- and mesonephros are accomplished by an autophagic type of cell death with biochemical hallmarks of classic apoptosis. Certain anatomic structures, such as hollow viscus organs, are formed by apoptotic excavation of interior cell masses; the final form of other structures, such as the forebrain, is shaped by patterns of apoptotic death within neural precursor cells. A more refined example is matching the number of projecting neurons to the size of a target field, accomplished by apoptosis of surplus neurons. Excess or misdirected neurons fail to find the trophic factors produced by their designated targets.

RESPONSE TO CELL DAMAGE

One striking observation is the similarity between physiologic and pathologic cell deaths, since confirmed using biochemical and genetic approaches. Diverse forms of cellular damage trigger apoptotic death.

*This updated chapter is dedicated to the memory of Stanley J. Korsmeyer, MD, who coauthored the original version.

Table 8–1 Characteristic Features of Mammalian Cell Deaths

Apoptosis	Necrosis
Cell shrinkage and fragmentation	Cell swelling and lysis
Nuclear condensation	Karyolysis
Internucleosomal DNA fragmentation	Random DNA breaks
Loss of asymmetry of phospholipids in plasma membrane bilayer	Loss of plasma membrane integrity
Detachment and engulfment by phagocytes	Recruitment of inflammatory cells

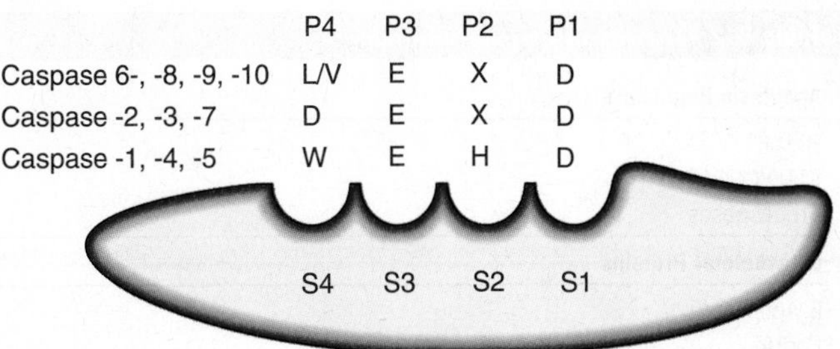

Figure 8–1 Substrate specificity of caspases is determined by the geometry of specificity-binding pockets S4 to S1, recognizing peptide side chains numbered P1 to P4 on the acyl side of the scissile peptide bond. All caspases require Asp in S1 pocket.

DNA damage due to free radicals, alkylating agents, ultraviolet radiation, as well as errors of replication (eg, deficiency of nucleotide pools, topoisomerase inhibition, and mismatch errors) trigger apoptosis via the operation of cellular checkpoints. Apoptotic cell death has been associated with numerous chemical toxins and idiosyncratic drug reactions, often attacking cells prone to physiologic apoptosis.

Recently, attention has been drawn to the role of intracellular protein aggregates and misfolded proteins as a stimulus for apoptosis. Experimental expression of aggregation-prone proteins has been shown to inhibit the ubiquitin–proteasome system, leading to accumulation of multiple proteasomal substrates. Ineffective erythropoiesis in β-thalassemia major is caused by intramedullary apoptotic death of erythroblasts with aggregations of α-globin chains and the erythrocyte membrane proteins spectrin and band 4.1.

GOVERNOR OF CELL BEHAVIOR

Apoptosis also serves a tumor suppressor function to eliminate both excess and damaged cells, including those with genetic instability or DNA mutations. Cells also sense supranormal activation of dominant protooncogenes, such as myc and ras, as apoptotic signals. The list of triggers for apoptotic death seems endless. It appears that many physiologic pathways are closely monitored, with virtually any deviation from normal culled by apoptosis. For epithelia and other cell types attached to extracellular matrix and basement membranes, detachment triggers an apoptotic response, designated as anoikis. Cellular differentiation also appears to have a fail-safe apoptotic response in many lineages, such that cells that do not successfully execute a differentiation program are eliminated.

EXECUTIONERS OF APOPTOSIS

Caspases

The central effectors of apoptosis are a novel family of cysteine proteases, designated as caspases (cysteinyl aspartate-specific protease).[10,11] All caspases are aspartases with a four-residue recognition sequence P4–P1 (Fig. 8–1). Granzyme B is a serine protease involved in cytolytic T-cell killing that also recognizes aspartic acid motifs. Caspase cleavage sites often present as a single site per protein and are found in a variety of cellular proteins, leading to limited digestion of substrate proteins. Approximately 280 substrates have been identified to date.[12] These can be grouped in several categories (Table 8–2).

Although no single caspase substrate has been identified that is obligate for cell death, progress has been made in attributing the biochemical and morphologic features of apoptotic death to proteolysis of specific substrates.[13] Cleavage of structural elements of nuclear scaffolds (lamins) and cytoskeleton (actin, fodrin, and gelsolin) likely actuate membrane blebbing and packaging of chromatin and cytoplasmic material in apoptotic bodies. DNA fragmentation is mediated by an endonuclease, CAD/DFF40, activated following caspase-mediated degradation of an inhibitory binding partner, ICAD/DFF45. Detachment of apoptotic cells from adhesion surfaces accompanies cleavage of proteins in focal adhesion complexes (FAKs).

Caspases also target proteins that participate in energy-consuming cell processes. A classic example is polyADP ribose polymerase (PARP), a nuclear enzyme involved in DNA repair. PARP, activated by DNA damage, consumes nicotinamide adenine dinucleotide (NAD) and ultimately adenosine triphosphate (ATP), as the source of adenosine diphosphate (ADP) ribose. Other caspase substrates are involved in DNA repair (DNA-PKcs, Rad51, MCM3, DNA, RFC140), ribosomal assembly (U1–70KsnRNP), and cell-cycle regulation (p21, p27). One rationale for this category of caspase substrates in apoptosis may be a requirement for energy in the form of ATP. Reducing cellular ATP has been reported to convert apoptosis into necrotic death, with accompanying inflammation.

In the intracellular battle between survival and proapoptotic factors, caspases can swing the advantage toward death by altering the balance of forces. The mitochondrial survival proteins, BCL-2 and BCL-XL, are subject to N-terminal cleavage by caspases. Not only does truncation eliminate their survival functions, but the shortened versions behave as proapoptotic factors experimentally. Activation of a BCL-2-family proapoptotic member, BID, also requires caspase-mediated processing to a truncated factor, tBID, that facilitates translocation to its mitochondrial site of action.

ACTIVATION OF PROCASPASES

Caspases are expressed in healthy cells as zymogens with low to absent protease activity. Strong activation happens upon proteolytic processing into large and small subunits and tetrameric assembly (dimers of heterodimers) (Fig. 8–2). Processing of procaspases occurs adjacent to aspartate residues within caspase recognition motifs.[14] Subsite specificities are distributed among caspases so that most caspase zymogens must be processed in trans by a different caspase, creating a hierarchy of proteolytic activation.[15] The remainder of the caspases have autocatalytic activity at high concentrations (induced proximity model) and are, instead, activated by the regulated assembly of self-activating complexes. Designated as initiator caspases, these zymogens are distinguished by the presence of a long prodomain that serves as a docking site for recruitment into the catalytic complex.[16] Protein associations within these complexes are built around homomeric interactions between three binding cassettes, death (DD), death effector (DED), and CARD domains.

DEATH-INDUCING SIGNALING COMPLEXES AND APOPTOSOMES

Two distinct caspase-activating assemblies are known, although additional structures are expected to be discovered (Fig. 8–3). Caspase-8 is engaged by a family of cell surface receptors known as "death receptors." These include TNF, Fas, and TRAIL (see later). Ligand binding

Table 8–2 Diversity of Caspase Substrates

Category	Substrates
Apoptosis Regulators	Bid*; ICAD/DFF45; Procaspases
Cytoskeletal Proteins	β-Actin; Fodrin; Gelsolin; Keratins 14, 17, 18, and 19
Cell Adhesion	APC; β-Catenin; Focal adhesion kinase
Nuclear Organization	Lamins A, B1; Scaffold attachment factor-A
Cell Cycle	Cdc6; DNA replication factor C; $p21^{waf1/cip1}$; $p27^{Kip1}$; Rb
DNA Repair	DNA-dependent protein kinase catalytic subunit; PolyADP ribose polymerase-1; RAD51
Transcription	GATA-1; NF-κB p65; TAF(II)80δ
RNA Splicing	Acinus; Heterogeneous nuclear ribonucleoproteins; U1–70-kDa small nuclear ribonucleoprotein
Translation	Eukaryotic translation initiation factor 4GI; Death-associated protein 5
Cytokines	Pro-IL-1β; Pro-IL-16; Pro-IL-18; Endothelial monocyte-activating polypeptide-II*
Transmembrane Receptors	Deleted in colorectal cancer; RET
Protein Kinases	AKT; MEK kinase-1; Mammalian STE20-related kinase-1; PKC-δ,ε, η, μ, θ, ζ; PKR; p21-activated kinase 2; Receptor-interacting kinase-1; Rho-associated kinase-1
Protein Degradation	Calpastatin
G-Protein Signaling	D4-GDI; Ras-Gap
Calcium Ion Transport	Inositol 1,4,5-triphosphate receptor-1/2
Neurodegenerative Disorders	β-amyloid precursor protein; Huntington disease; Presenilin-1 and -2
Protein and Membrane Trafficking	BAP31; Golgin-160; p115; Rabaptin-5

induces trimerization of the death receptor. The cytoplasmic tail of the liganded death receptor binds to an adapter protein, FADD/MORT1, by dimerization of homologous death domains from each molecule. A second interaction domain in FADD/MORT1, a death effector domain, binds to a similar DED in the prodomain of caspase-8, leading to localized autocatalysis. The death receptor, FADD, and caspase-8 complex is known as the death-inducing signaling complex (DISC).[17]

The second assembly, the apoptosome, is specialized for activating caspase-9, which has a CARD-type prodomain. Formation of the cytoplasmic apoptosome is initiated by release of the soluble electron carrier, cytochrome c, from mitochondria. Cytochrome c binds to an adapter protein, APAF-1, which exposes its own CARD domain in an ATP/dATP-dependent process. Docking of caspase-9 initiates its autocatalytic processing. Because the prodomains of caspase-8 and caspase-9 are severed from the catalytic enzyme during processing, these initiator caspases are no longer sequestered in the complex and are dispersed to cellular substrates. Both pathways converge with proteolytic activation of caspase-3 by either caspase-8 or -9.

POSTTRANSCRIPTIONAL REGULATION

Because of their active-site cysteines, caspases are also subject to regulation by the thiol status of the cell.[18] These residues appear to be particularly susceptible to stable S-nitrosylation by nitric oxide, in the presence of reactive oxygen species (ROS) and transition metals. This is a physiologically important mechanism in the maintenance of endothelial cell survival by shear-induced stress and prolonged survival of activated neutrophils during a respiratory burst (NADPH-oxidase).[19]

NONAPOPTOTIC ROLES FOR CASPASES

Although justifiably known for their apoptotic functions, there is accumulating evidence that caspases also have roles in healthy cells.[20] Caspase-1 was originally identified as the processing enzyme for IL-1β and recently, another proinflammatory cytokine, IL-18. Caspases are also involved in negative feedback control of erythroblast differentiation by mature erythroblasts through degradation of GATA-1.[21] Finally, several dramatic structural alterations associated with cell differentiation also apparently require transient caspase activation. Cleavage of a limited number of caspase substrates precede nuclear and chromatin changes during terminal erythroid differentiation. Caspase inhibitors also block proplatelet formation from megakaryocytes.[22] The limited caspase activation in these instances may involve some type of compartmentalization.

INHIBITOR OF APOPTOSIS PROTEINS

The only known endogenous caspase inhibitors are members of the inhibitor of apoptosis proteins (IAP) family. IAPs were originally described in insect viruses as viral proteins produced during cellular infection to block host cell apoptosis.[23] In addition to other cellular functions, certain IAPs bind to the active sites of specific caspases (3, 6, 7, and 9) to block catalytic activity or maturation of procaspases.[24] IAP proteins contain one to three BIR (baculovirus IAP repeat) domains that coordinate zinc, and one or more additional protein-interaction domains. Individual IAP proteins use different domains to occlude the substrate grooves of specific caspases. Similar proteins have been identified in yeast, flies, and worms.

Inhibitors of apoptosis proteins also function as ubiquitin E3 ligases, labeling proteins for degradation by the 26S proteasome.[25] The cIAP-1 and cIAP-2 proteins also bind to Traf-1, an adapter protein in TNF receptor signaling to NF-κB and Jun-N kinase pathways. An apoptotic response is reinforced by cIAP-mediated Traf-1 degradation, triggered when TNF binds to the TNF-RII receptor.

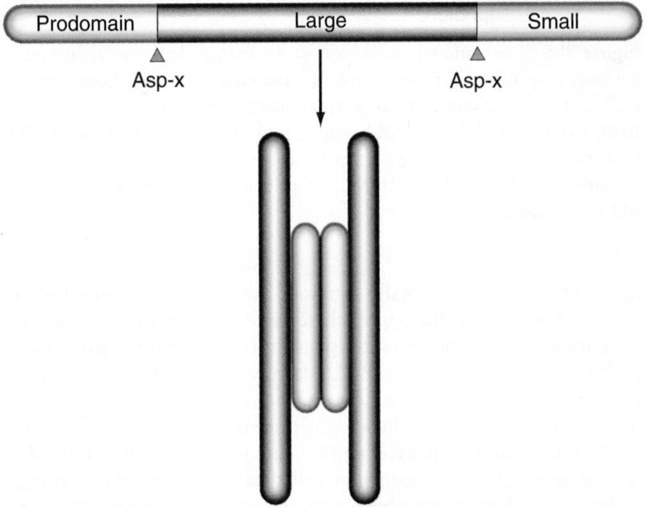

Figure 8–2 Mature caspases are formed by proteolytic processing of procaspases to divide large and small subunits and remove N-terminal peptides. Caspase substrate motifs at cleavage sites enable sequential caspase activation or, in the case of initiator caspases, autoactivation. Caspase dimers are assembled from two large and two small subunits.

SMAC/DIABLO AND OMI/HTRA2

Two proteins normally localized in the mitochondrial intermembrane space, SMAC/Diablo and Omi/HtrA2, can bind IAPs via a conserved NH_2-terminal sequence and competitively displace bound caspases.[26,27] The NH_2 terminus of active SMAC/Diablo is generated by removal of a presequence during mitochondrial import, whereas Omi/HtrA2 is a stress-activated serine protease that is cleaved by autoprocessing. Cytoplasmic translocation of SMAC/Diablo and Omi/HtrA2 during apoptosis provides an additional mechanism for caspase activation. The reaper, grim, hid, and sickle proteins in Drosophila function similarly on fly IAPs and have NH_2-terminal homology to SMAC/Diablo and HtrA2.

Inhibitors of apoptosis proteins can direct self-ubiquitination or ubiquitin ligation to caspases and reaper family proteins, suggesting that IAP complexes can flag a variety of proteins for destruction. This mechanism appears well designed for detecting differences in protein conformation and aggregation state. Although many IAPs inhibit apoptosis, only a subset is known to bind caspases. It is likely that regulation of protein stability has multiple inputs to apoptotic pathways, as found for cell-cycle control.

REGULATORS OF APOPTOSIS

The founding member of this family, BCL2, was discovered as the defining oncogene in follicular lymphomas, located at one reciprocal

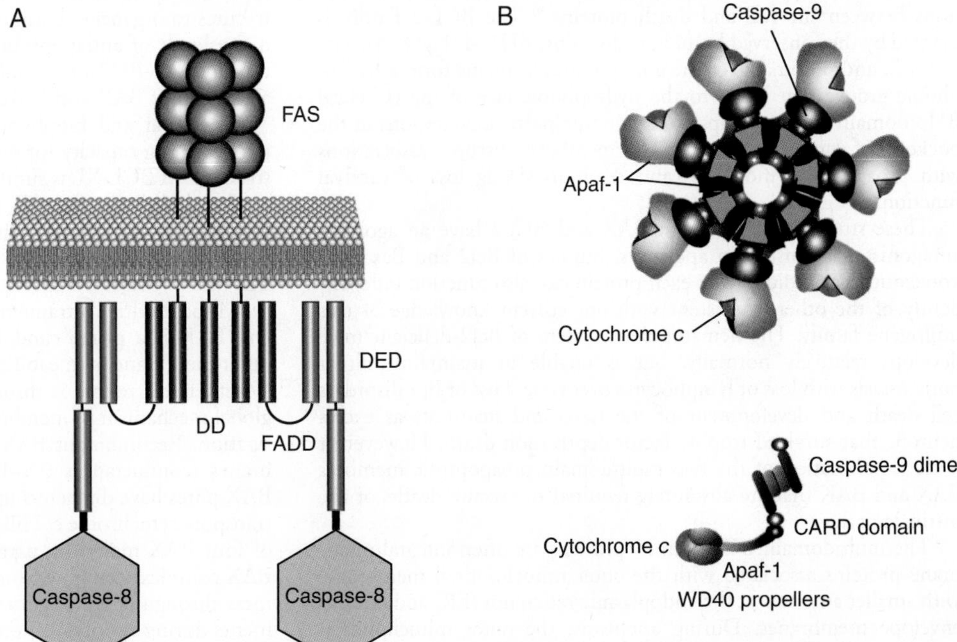

Figure 8–3 Multiprotein complexes govern activation of initiator caspases. **A**, DISC is assembled after binding of ligand (FAS) to death receptor (CD95) at cell surface. Protein interaction domains (DD and DED) mediate associations between the death receptor, initiator caspase (caspase-8), and adapter protein (FADD). **B**, Apoptosome (viewed from above) resembles seven-spoked disk, with procaspase-9 molecules bound at the hub extending above one surface, and Apaf-1 adapters aligned as spokes, presenting CARD interaction domains at the hub and WD40 propellers bound to cytochrome c at the rim. **C**, Side view of unitary cytochrome c–Apaf-1–caspase-9 association.

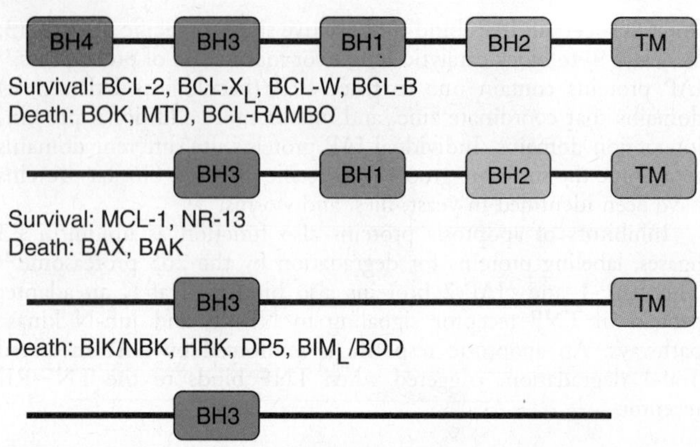

Figure 8–4 Classification of the Bcl2 family according to conserved domains. BH1–3 domains form a surface hydrophobic groove capable of binding BH3 domains of other family members. C-terminal hydrophobic sequences function to target or anchor Bcl2 family proteins to intracellular lipid membranes.

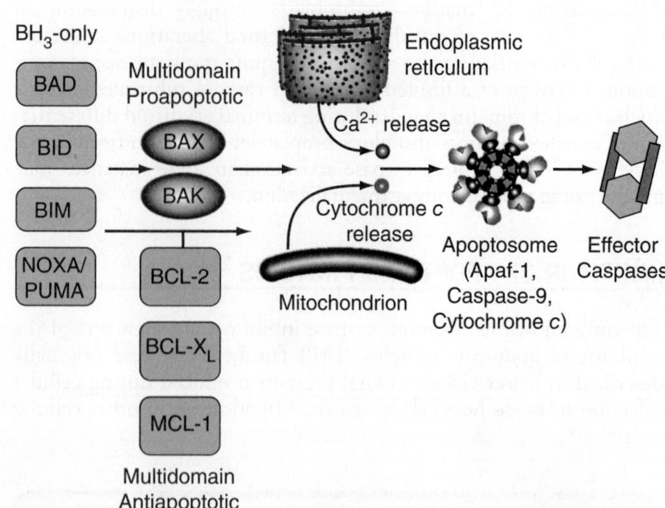

Figure 8–5 Schematic representation of the mammalian core apoptotic pathway in which a BH3-only molecule interacts with a multidomain BCL-2 member upstream of an adapter and a caspase. BH3-only BID, BIM, BAD, and NOXA/PUMA require multidomain proapoptotic BAX/BAK to initiate a cytochrome c, Apaf-1-driven caspase activation. Antiapoptotic BCL-2/BCL-XL/MCL-1 principally inhibits the activated BH3-only molecules.

breakpoint of the t(14;18) (q32;q21) chromosome translocation.[28] Cells transduced with BCL2 remained viable for extended periods in the absence of growth factors. Transgenic mice bearing a BCL2-Ig mini-gene recapitulating the t(14:18) displayed B-cell follicular hyperplasia and progressed over time to diffuse large B-cell lymphomas. The first proapoptotic BCL2 homologous protein to be identified, BAX, coimmunoprecipitated in stoichiometric amounts with BCL2. BAX-transfected cells died rapidly in the absence of growth factor and BAX was subsequently shown to be capable of directly triggering apoptosis. Since the discovery of BCL2 and BAX, the BCL2 family in mammals has expanded to 18 members, with 6 acting principally as survival factors and 12 hastening cell death in various experimental systems.[29] Homologs of BCL2 proteins exist in all metazoans studied to date and several animal DNA viruses.

BCL2 FAMILY PROTEINS

Early experiments showed that relative steady-state levels of antiapoptotic and proapoptotic BCL-2 members correlated with cellular sensitivity to death stimuli, such as growth factor withdrawal. This "rheostat" for apoptosis is manifest, in part, by differential associations between survival and death proteins.[30] The BCL-2 family is marked by the conserved homology domains, BH1–4 (Fig. 8–4). The BH1, 2, and 3 domains of the antiapoptotic proteins form a hydrophobic groove that binds to the hydrophobic face of the α-helical BH3 domain from a proapoptotic binding partner. Mutations in the pockets of antiapoptotic BCL2 members disrupt associations with proapoptotic molecules and result in strong loss of survival function.

These studies indicated that BAX and BCL2 have an agonist–antagonist relationship in apoptosis. Studies of Bcl2 and Bax gene knockout mice indicate that each protein can also function independently of the other, consistent with our current knowledge of this multigene family. The hematopoietic system of Bcl2-deficient mice develops relatively normally, but is unable to maintain cellular homeostasis with loss of lymphocytes over time. Loss of Bax disorders cell death and development of the testis and manifests as excess neurons that survived trophic factor-deprivation death. However, it is the combination of the two multidomain proapoptotic members BAX and BAK that are absolutely required to execute deaths of the intrinsic pathway.

The multidomain BCL2 family proteins are often integral membrane proteins associated with the outer mitochondrial membrane, with smaller amounts at the endoplasmic reticulum (ER) and nuclear envelope membranes. During apoptosis, the outer mitochondrial membrane becomes permeable, with release into the cytoplasm of multiple proteins normally retained within the intermembrane space.[31] One insightful approach to investigating the antiapoptotic functions of BCL2 has been to focus on its role in the mitochondrial pathway of apoptosis. The BCL2 family of pro- and antiapoptotic proteins constitutes a critical control point for apoptosis proximal to irreversible damage to cellular constituents.

A combination of genetic and biochemical studies has ordered the components of the mammalian cell death pathway. The upstream "BH3-only" family members respond to select death signals and subsequently trigger the activation of the multidomain death effectors BAX and BAK.[32–34] Multidomain, proapoptotic BAX and BAK constitute an essential gateway to the intrinsic death pathway operating both at the level of mitochondria and ER Ca^{2+} dynamics.[32,35] Activated, homo-oligomerized BAX or BAK results in the permeabilization of the mitochondrial outer membrane and the release of proteins, especially cytochrome c, which initiates a caspase cascade and contributes to organelle dysfunction. Conversely, cells protected by adequate levels of antiapoptotic BCL2 or BCL-XL bind and sequester translocated BH3-only molecules in stable complexes, preventing activation of BAX and BAK (Fig. 8–5).[33]

Structural and biophysical studies have indicated the intrinsic pore-forming capacity for several BCL2 family proteins. The tertiary structure of BCL-XL is similar to model pore-forming proteins, such as the diphtheria toxin T domain and bacterial colicins.[36] Pore-forming activities have been identified with the antiapoptotic proteins BCL-XL and BCL2, and proapoptotic BAX, BCL-XS, and BID.

Mitochondrial intramembranous homo-oligomerization of BAX and BAK is a prime candidate for a mechanism of mitochondrial outer membrane permeabilization that would release cytochrome c.[37] Whether this release is through a distinct BAX pore or some more global mechanism of membrane permeabilization is still under investigation. Recombinant BAX forms megachannels in artificial membranes (conductances 0.5–1.5 ns). Sizing approaches indicate that BAX pores have diameters up to 22 to 30 Å, and are large enough to transport cytochrome c. Hill plot kinetics indicate that a molecularity of four BAX molecules participates in the release of cytochrome c. BAX complexes ranging from 41 to 260 kd, consistent with homodimers through larger oligomers, are observed in cross-linking experiments during apoptosis. Recently, a novel high-conductance channel in the mitochondrial outer membrane has also been described

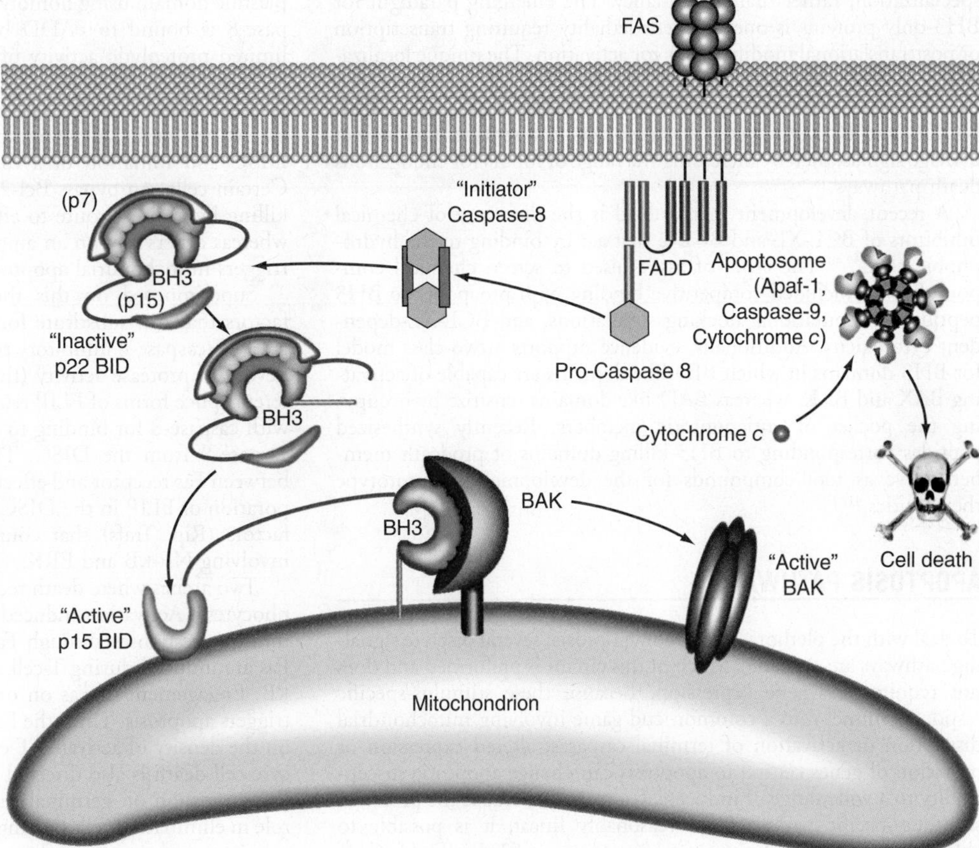

Figure 8–6 Schematic model of proapoptotic activation cascade. Proapoptotic BID to BAK integrates the apoptotic pathway from death receptors to mitochondrial release of cytochrome c.

(mitochondrial apoptosis-induced channel or MAC), coinciding with mitochondrial translocation of BAX.

Alternatively, BAX has been reported to decrease the stability of planar lipid bilayers by decreasing linear tension within the membrane, resulting in hydrophilic pores within the lipid membrane itself. The three-dimensional structure of inactive BAX revealed that its COOH-terminal tail is folded back into the BAX hydrophobic cleft formed by the BH1, 2, and 3 domains. Soon after stimulation of apoptosis, cytoplasmic BAX undergoes a conformational change, exposing an NH_2-terminal epitope, forms homodimers/oligomers, and becomes an integral mitochondrial-membrane protein (Fig. 8–6).[31]

BH3-ONLY PROAPOPTOTIC MEMBERS

The BH3-only molecules constitute the third subset of the BCL2 family and include BID, NOXA, PUMA, BIK, BIM, and BAD. These proteins share sequence homology only in the amphipathic α-helical BH3 region, which mutation analysis indicated is required in proapoptotic members for their death activity. Moreover, the BH3-only proteins require this domain to demonstrate binding to multidomain BCL2 family members. Multiple binding assays indicate that individual BH3-only molecules display some selectivity for multidomain BCL2 members. The BID protein binds proapoptotic BAX and BAK, as well as antiapoptotic BCL2 and BCL-XL. In contrast, BAD and NOXA display preferential binding as intact molecules to antiapoptotic members. However, expression of all of these members, BID, BAD, BIM, and NOXA, results in the activation of BAX and BAK. Their expression in Bax–Bak doubly deficient cells indicates that BAX and BAK are absolutely required for their induction of cell death. Comparison of wild-type with mutant BCL2, BCL-XL indicated that antiapoptotic members sequester all these BH3-only molecules in stable mitochondrial complexes, preventing the activation of BAX and BAK.

BID, the initial BH3-only protein described, is a cytosolic protein that lacks a membrane targeting sequence. Caspase-8 cleaves BID in an unstructured loop, exposing an N-terminal glycine that undergoes posttranslational (rather than classic cotranslational) N-myristoylation. Consistent with its three-dimensional structure, myristoylation enhances the translocation of a p7/myr-p15 BID complex to mitochondria, where the inhibitory p7 fragment is released exposing the BH3 domain. This lipid modification serves as a molecular switch that markedly augments the capacity of activated tBID to release cytochrome c (see Fig. 8–6).

Thus, activation of BH3-only proteins is often directed by specific apoptotic signaling pathways. Proapoptotic activity is associated with exposure of the hydrophobic face of the BH3 helix, enabling it to interact with the hydrophobic groove of multidomain dimerization partners. The specific activation mechanism for BID, a latent proapoptotic protein subject to caspase-mediated cleavage, exposes the BH3 domain.

The BAD BH3-only protein has two consensus binding sites for 14-3-3 scaffold proteins. Phosphorylation at serines 112 and 136 within the 14-3-3 binding site results in binding to 14-3-3 and cytoplasmic sequestration of BAD. Phosphorylation of BAD occurs downstream of growth factor signals and has been attributed to several kinases: protein kinase B/Akt and p70S6 kinase (Ser 136), and mitochondrial-anchored protein kinase A (Ser112). Other BH3 proteins interact with distinct extramitochondrial targets. BIM is localized to the microtubule dynein motor complex by binding to the dynein light chain, DLC1, and BMF associates with dynein light chain 2 (DLC2) in the myosin V actin motor complex.

It is interesting to consider the reasons for having multiple pro- and antiapoptotic BH proteins. In the case of the proapoptotic proteins, the large number of BH3-only members is indicative of specialization, rather than redundancy. The emerging paradigm for BH3-only proteins is one of latent lethality requiring transcription or posttranslational modifications for activation. The unique localizations, protein associations, and mechanisms of activation for the individual proapoptotic BH3-only members BAD, BID, BIM, NOXA, and PUMA suggest that each acts as a sentinel for distinct damage signals, thereby increasing the range of inputs for endogenous death pathways.[38]

A recent development in this field is the discovery of chemical inhibitors of BCL-XL and BCL-2 that act by binding to the hydrophobic cleft.[39,40] The types of assays used to screen chemical compounds have included competitive binding with proapoptotic BH3 peptides, computational docking simulations, and BCL-XL-dependent cytotoxicity. Additionally, evidence supports a two-class model for BH3 domains in which BID-like domains are capable of activating BAX and BAK, whereas BAD-like domains sensitize by occupying the pocket of antiapoptotic members. Recently synthesized peptides corresponding to BH3-killing domains of prodeath members serve as tool compounds for the development of prototype therapeutics.[41]

APOPTOSIS PATHWAYS

To deal with the plethora of cues for apoptosis, several discrete signaling pathways are available. Much of this circuit is preformed and does not require new gene expression. Because these stimulus-specific responses funnel into a common end game involving mitochondrial disruption or activation of terminal caspases, altered expression or mutation of genes central to apoptosis can change apoptotic susceptibility to a wide range of inducers. Conversely, because the proximal stimulus-specific pathways are reasonably linear, it is possible to ablate a stimulus-specific response (eg, mutant p53, Fas/FasL). Core pathways have nonlinear, feed-forward features as well as high levels of redundancy such that complete resistance to apoptosis has not been observed.

DEATH RECEPTOR SIGNALING

Death receptors are expressed on many cell types, especially the immune system, where they function as a restraint on cell viability. The intracellular responses to death receptors appear to be more limited than for growth factors, and the cytoplasmic sequences of members of the death receptor superfamily all contain the death domain (DD 80 aa) protein-interaction motif.[42] Once clustered by receptor–ligand interaction, the DD serves to nucleate formation of an activation "machine" for initiator caspases (caspases 8, 10) with distinct protein interaction motifs in their long prodomains. This multiprotein complex has been designated as a DISC. Death receptors and proximal caspases do not bind each other directly, but through adapter connectors with docking sites for each motif. Like scaffolds in other signal transduction pathways, adapter proteins act to amplify the initial receptor signal and approximate key factors, as well as provide opportunities for flexibility and regulation of signaling circuits.

There are eight mammalian death receptors (TNF-R1, Fas, TRAMP, DR4, DR5, DR6, NGF-R, and EDA-R). The extracellular domains contain several cysteine-rich domains, forming an extended structure stabilized by disulfide bonds. Death receptor ligands share a TNF homology domain and bind as trimers to cysteine-rich domains of the corresponding receptors. All known ligands are expressed as type II transmembrane proteins and are subject to limited proteolysis, generating soluble forms. In most cases, soluble ligands are inferior to membrane-bound forms for receptor activation. Thus, cell-to-cell contacts are necessary for death-receptor signaling, justifying the characterization of subsequent apoptotic deaths as "fratricides."

In the simplest example, binding of the Fas ligand to CD95/Fas receptor triggers allosteric conformational activation of an apparently trimeric receptor. An adapter protein, FADD, binds at the Fas cytoplasmic domain using homotypic DD associations. Similarly, procaspase-8 is bound to FADD by homotypic DED interactions. The limited proteolytic activity of procaspase-8 appears to be sufficient for autoprocessing in trans of neighboring procaspase molecules. An NH_2-proximal cleavage separates the caspase-8 prodomain from the catalytic subunits, allowing untethering of active caspase-8 from the DISC and initiation of a cascade of processing effector caspases. Certain cells can bypass Bcl-2 interdiction at the mitochondria and killing by a direct route to effector caspase activation (type I cells), whereas others rely on an amplification loop in which BID cleavage triggers mitochondrial apoptosis (type II cells).[43]

Superimposed on this three-component model are additional factors that can substitute for one of the core components.[44] FLIP (FLICE/caspase-8 inhibitory protein) is homologous to caspase-8 but devoid of protease activity (the active-site cysteine is replaced). Different splice forms of FLIP retain the DED motif and either compete with caspase-8 for binding to FADD or prevent release of processed caspase-8 from the DISC. Thus, FLIP interrupts communication between Fas receptor and effector caspases, blocking apoptosis. Incorporation of FLIP in the DISC leads to the recruitment of additional factors (Rip, Trafs) that connect to signal transduction pathways involving NF-κB and ERK.

Two arenas where death receptors act physiologically involve lymphocytes. Activation-induced cell death curtails T lymphocyte immune responses through Fas receptor signaling.[45] Fas ligand and Fas are induced during T-cell activation downstream of lck and NF-κB. Engagement of Fas on one cell by Fas ligand on a second cell triggers apoptosis. Thus, the Fas–FasL system provides an upper limit on the density of activated T cells at sites of inflammation. Lymphocyte cell death is also directed by FasL expression on dissimilar cells. Fas expression on germinal center B lymphocytes appears to play a role in eliminating cells bearing self-reactive surface immunoglobulin, as mice expressing Fas only on T lymphocytes acquire high levels of autoantibodies. In this case, FasL expression on T cells delivers the fatal blow. T lymphocytes can also be eliminated by FasL expressed on nonlymphoid cell types.

Immune-privileged zones, such as the eyes and testes, can be transplanted with allogenic tissue owing to the lack of immune surveillance at these sites, enabling corneal transplants from unrelated donors without need for immunosuppression. Gld mice deficient in FasL expression do not manifest site-specific restrictions to immune responses with vigorous inflammatory responses to viral infections and allogenic cells. In place of a physical barrier to lymphocyte trafficking to immune-privileged sites, constitutive expression of FasL by interstitial and support cells in these locations effectively deletes trespassing cells.[46]

Fas expression is constitutively expressed in nonlymphoid tissues (hepatocytes, cardiac muscle, kidney epithelium); in others, it is induced during acute stress responses (UV- and gamma-radiation). FasL–Fas interactions take place during cytotoxic T lymphocyte killing, and in some circumstances, Fas has proved necessary for target cell killing.

Targeted deletions of components of the Fas signaling pathway indicate the importance of this pathway in development. Mouse knockouts for caspase-8, FADD, and FLIP die during embryogenesis with severe cardiac malformations. Although lack of normal developmental death can lead to abnormal morphogenesis, the ability of death receptors to communicate with other signal transduction pathways may have important physiologic consequences. Fas signaling in resting lymphocytes has comitogenic effects, indicating that entry to alternative signaling pathways is dependent on cell activation state and receptor density.

DNA DAMAGE

Among other types of cellular damage, alterations in DNA structure as a result of oxidation, alkylation, single- or double-strand breaks (including stalled replication forks) are notorious for triggering apoptotic pathways. Apoptosis is recognized as part of a larger DNA damage response involving cell cycle checkpoint (control mechanisms ensuring dependency in the cell cycle) and repair pathways.[6]

The transition from repair to dismantling the cell is usually believed to involve some quantitative aspect of DNA damage, perhaps the ability to repair DNA below a certain threshold before apoptotic mechanisms kick in. Some insight into the biochemical mechanism has come from the understanding of p53 protein degradation pathways. In healthy cells, p53 has a half-life of 5 to 20 minutes, its ubiquitin-mediated degradation governed by its interactions with Mdm2. Mdm2 acts as a ubiquitin E3 ligase for p53. p53 functions as a tetrameric, sequence-specific transcription factor; thus, p53 activity is dependent on nuclear levels of p53. At early times following p53 activation, negative feedback control results from transcription of Mdm2, resulting in increased p53 degradation. However, continued stabilization of p53 inactivates another p53 target gene, the lipid phosphatase PTEN.[47] PTEN inactivates the second messenger PI(3,4,5)P3, ultimately resulting in nuclear exclusion of Mdm2 and stabilization of p53.

Several types of changes to the DNA template trigger activation of chromatin-associated kinases over long distances, probably through changes in higher-order chromatin structure. In response to DNA strand breaks, the PI(3)K-related kinase ATM phosphorylates multiple substrates, including p53, Mdm2, and the checkpoint kinase Chk2 (Cds1). Posttranslational modification of p53 at several sites leads to inhibition of Mdm2 association and transcriptional activation. Transcriptional targets of p53 include several proapoptotic BCL2 members (Bax, Noxa, Puma), death receptors (Fas, DR5), oxidation-reduction enzymes (PIG3), and APAF-1.[48] There may also be examples of p53 contributions to apoptosis that are independent of transcriptional activity, including associations of p53 with mitochondria[49] and a cytosolic E3 ligase (Parkin).

UNFOLDED PROTEIN RESPONSE

Protein stress responses are a recent addition to apoptotic pathways. These highly conserved mechanisms provide feedback fidelity control of protein folding, glycosylation, and secretory pathways in the ER. Multiple inputs (amino acid deficiency, glucose deprivation, calcium dysregulation, and proteasomal activity) trigger this pathway through their effects on ER protein folding.

In yeast models, a unique ER transmembrane protein with both serine/threonine kinase and endoribonuclease activities, IRE1, functions as a sensor for misfolded or unfolded ER proteins.[50] IRE1 kinase activity is normally suppressed by binding to the ER chaperone protein GRP78/BiP. Unfolded proteins accumulating within the ER lumen recruit GRP78/Bip away from IRE1, allowing oligomerization and autophosphorylation of IRE1. Phosphorylation stimulates IRE1 endoribonuclease activity for a specific target, the mRNA for a basic leucine zipper transcription factor, HAC1. The HAC1 transcript is constitutively expressed, but contains a nonclassic intron that inhibits translation. IRE1 removes this intron by two site-specific cleavages, and a third factor, Rlg1p, splices the remaining exons. With efficient translation of the spliced mRNA, HAC1 activates transcription of several ER chaperones.

The mammalian version of the UPR incorporates two additional features: general suppression of translation and a connection to apoptotic pathways. Inhibition of translation is accomplished using an ER transmembrane kinase, PERK, related to the dsRNA-dependent kinase PKR. PERK phosphorylates the eukaryotic initiation factor EIF2-α, inhibiting assembly of preinitiation complexes at ribosomes. The precise downstream apoptotic pathway is uncertain, but an ER-localized caspase, caspase-12, has been reported[51] to process IRE1 in response to ER stress.

ONCOGENE-INDUCED APOPTOSIS

Hyperactivity of mitogenic oncogenes, such as Myc, adenovirus E1A, and Ras triggers a common pathway of p53 accumulation via induction of the ARF tumor-suppressor gene.[52] P14ARF (or P19ARF in mice) is encoded by an alternative reading frame in the p16INK4a locus. ARF inhibits Mdm2, the p53 E3 ubiquitin ligase, and transports Mdm2 to the nucleolus, where additional ARF functions are evident. Processing of precursor rRNAs to 28S, 18S, and 5.8S rRNAs is prevented by ARF, independent of p53 or Mdm2. The proximal signals for oncogene-dependent induction of ARF are under exploration.

SURVIVAL SIGNALING PATHWAYS

Cell death has been postulated to serve as a default pathway for single cells, with a need for signals from neighboring cells for survival. The prototypical example of intercellular survival signaling is the insulin-like growth factor-1 (IGF-1)–PI(3)kinase–Akt kinase pathway.[53] Note that survival signal transduction pathways are engaged downstream of most, if not all, growth factors.

The IGF-1 receptor tyrosine kinase is autophosphorylated in trans following ligand binding. An adapter protein (insulin receptor substrate [IRS]) binds to the cytoplasmic domain of the receptor through a phosphotyrosine-binding domain. The IRS adapter is phosphorylated on tyrosines in turn, enabling the p85 regulatory subunit of PI(3) kinase to bind, and relieving inhibition of the catalytic PI(3) kinase. Phosphorylation of phosphatidylinositol in the plasma membrane yields PI3, PI4, 5P3, 4P2, and PI3P; these lipid-signaling molecules function by recruiting signaling proteins containing pleckstrin homology domains to the plasma membrane.[54] One of these, the serine/threonine kinase PDK1, activates downstream kinases, including Akt/PKB, by phosphorylating its active loop.

Several substrates for Akt/PKB and Akt-like serine/threonine kinase are implicated in cell survival. Bad and procaspase-9 are inhibited by phosphorylation. Another set of factors with proapoptotic effects inhibited by Akt/PKB-mediated serine/threonine phosphorylation are the forkhead transcription factors.[55] Phosphorylated forkhead transcription factors bind to 14–3-3 proteins and are exported from the nucleus and degraded in the cytosol. Transcriptional targets of forkhead transcription factors relevant to apoptosis include FasL and Bim. A broader role for forkhead transcription factors includes adaptation to stress and aging (mutants of the homologous DAF-16 in *Caenorhabditis elegans* have shortened life spans).

SUMMARY

Apoptosis is an evolutionarily conserved, highly regulated mechanism for maintaining homeostasis in multicellular organisms. Numerous signals are capable of modulating cell death. After a death stimulus, the signal is propagated and amplified through the activation of caspases, culminating in the ordered disassembly of the cell. The process may transpire through an intrinsic, mitochondria-dependent pathway or an extrinsic pathway—depending on the death signal and the cell type involved. The BCL2 family of proteins is situated upstream of irreversible cell damage in the apoptotic pathway, providing a pivotal checkpoint in the fate of a cell after a death stimulus. The proapoptotic molecules BAX and BAK undergo an allosteric conformational activation to permeabilize mitochondria on receipt of a death stimulus. BH3-only members connect distinct upstream signal transduction pathways with the common, core apoptotic pathway. The distribution and responsiveness of the BH3-only members suggest that they function as sentinels for recognizing cellular damage. For example, BID amplifies minimal caspase-8 activation and BAD patrols for metabolic stress after loss of critical survival factors or glucose. This model would explain how seemingly diverse cellular injuries converge on a final common pathway of cell death.

SUGGESTED READINGS

Aggarwal BB: Signalling pathways of the TNF superfamily: a double-edged sword. Nat Rev Immunol 3:745–756, 2003.

Algeciras-Schimnich A, Barnhart BC, et al: Apoptosis-independent functions of killer caspases. Curr Opin Cell Biol 14:721–726, 2002.

Cantley LC: The phosphoinositide 3-kinase pathway. Science 296:1655–1657, 2002.

Chai J, Du C, Wu JW, et al: Structural and biochemical basis of apoptotic activation by Smac/DIABLO. Nature 406:855–862, 2000.

Cheng EH, Wei MC, Weiler S, et al: BCL-2, BCL-X(L) sequester BH3 domain-only molecules preventing BAX- and BAK-mediated mitochondrial apoptosis. Mol Cell 8:705–711, 2001.

Denault JB, Salvesen GS: Caspases: keys in the ignition of cell death. Chem Rev 102:4489–4500, 2002.

Levine B, Yuan J: Autophagy in cell death: an innocent convict? J Clin Invest 115:2679–2688, 2005.

Li P, Nijhawan D, Budihardjo I, et al: Cytochrome c and dATP-dependent formation of Apaf-1/caspase-9 complex initiates an apoptotic protease cascade. Cell 91:479–489, 1997.

Manion MK, Fry J, Schwartz PS, et al: Small molecule inhibitors of BCL-2. Curr Opin Invest Drugs 2006; in pess.

Savill J, Fadok V: Corpse clearance defines the meaning of cell death. Nature 407:784–788, 2000.

Strasser A, Bouillet P: The control of apoptosis in lymphocyte selection. Immunol Rev 193:82–92, 2003.

Thome M, Tschopp J: Regulation of lymphocyte proliferation and death by FLIP. Nat Rev Immunol 1:50–58, 2001.

Toledo F, Wahl GM: Regulating the p53 pathway: in vitro hypotheses, in vivo veritas. Nat Rev Cancer 6:909–923, 2006.

Vander Heiden MG, Plas DR, Rathmell JC, et al: Growth factors can influence cell growth and survival through effects on glucose metabolism. Mol Cell Biol 21:5899–5912, 2001.

Wei MC, Zong WX, Cheng EH, et al: Proapoptotic BAX and BAK: a requisite gateway to mitochondrial dysfunction and death. Science 292:727–730, 2001.

Yang Y, Fang S, Jensen JP, et al: Ubiquitin protein ligase activity of IAPs and their degradation in proteasomes in response to apoptotic stimuli. Science 288:874–877, 2000.

REFERENCES

For complete list of references log onto www.expertconsult.com

CHAPTER 9

PHARMACOGENOMICS AND HEMATOLOGIC DISEASES

Leo Kager and William E. Evans

The fundamental hypothesis pursued in genetics is that heritable genetic variation (ie, genotypes or haplotypes) translates into inherited phenotypes (eg, disease risk, drug response). On the basis of this hypothesis, the aim of medical genetics and pharmacogenomics is to understand the myriad associations between individual genotypes and specific phenotypes of *disease* or *drug response*, with the ultimate goal of better defining the risk for, or outcome of, diseases and the response to specific medications. Many seminal discoveries in medical genetics were made in the course of investigating hematologic disorders, as exemplified by the fact that the most prevalent monogenic disorders, the hemoglobinopathies, affect approximately 7% of the world's population.[1] Pharmacogenomics also has a long tradition in hematology; one of the first documented clinical observations of inherited differences in drug effects was the relationship between hemolysis after antimalarial therapy and the inherited glucose-6-phosphate dehydrogenase activity in erythrocytes.[2]

In the pregenomic era, efforts concentrated on mapping highly penetrant monogenic (mendelian) loci, for both specific diseases and drug-metabolizing pathways that influence the effects of medications.[3] Since the completion of the first draft of the human genome sequence, genome-wide approaches are being increasingly used to define markers for polygenic loci in complex diseases, identify genetic factors that modify the phenotype of a monogenic disease, and elucidate the interplay of genes encoding proteins involved in multiple pathways of drug metabolism, disposition, and effects.[3,4]

This chapter is not meant to be an exhaustive review; rather, it provides an overview of pharmacogenomics, using selected examples to illustrate its impact on the treatment of hematologic diseases. Recent reviews of the importance and potential of pharmacogenomics are available for readers seeking broader coverage of this burgeoning field.[3,5–7]

HUMAN SEQUENCE VARIATION

The genome-wide systematic identification and functional analysis of genes, their sequence variants, and related products (ie, proteins) are revolutionizing the study of disease, the development of new medications, and the optimization of drug therapy. Genetics increasingly enable clinicians to make reliable assessments of a person's risk of acquiring a particular disease, to identify drug targets, and to explain interindividual differences in the effectiveness and toxicity of medications.[3,6]

For practical purposes, the term *sequence variation* is mainly used herein.[8] *Polymorphisms* are defined as common variations in the DNA sequence. The Human Genome Project has unveiled many types of sequence variations that constitute allelic variants within the 3.2 billion base pairs of the human genetic code. Common variations include single-nucleotide polymorphisms (SNPs), insertions and deletions of nucleotides or entire genes, and variation in the number of repeats of a specific motif (mini- and microsatellites).[9,10]

SINGLE-NUCLEOTIDE POLYMORPHISMS

The most common and important inherited sequence variations are SNPs, positions in the genome where individuals have inherited a different nucleotide.[11] In diploid species such as humans, SNPs are usually biallelic. More than 1.2 million SNPs were identified in the initial sequencing of the human genome, and it is now estimated that several million SNPs exist in humans.[12] Many efforts are currently under way to catalog these variants, because a comprehensive SNP catalog would offer the possibility to pinpoint important variants in which nucleotide changes alter the function or expression of a gene that influences diseases or response to pharmacologic treatment. The main public database is dbSNP (http://www.ncbi.nlm.nih.gov/SNP/), and a rapid increase in the number of SNPs in dbSNP is driven by the HapMap project (http://www.hapmap.org/).[13]

SINGLE-NUCLEOTIDE POLYMORPHISMS AND PHENOTYPES

SNPs are present in exons, introns, promoters, enhancers, and intergenic regions. To elucidate the relationship between SNPs and phenotypes of interest, efforts have concentrated mainly on SNPs that are likely to alter the function or expression of a gene.

Only a small portion of the identified SNPs lie within coding regions, and only approximately half of those SNPs cause amino acid changes in expressed proteins. SNPs that cause amino acid changes are referred to as nonsynonymous SNPs (nsSNPs).[14] nsSNPs are the main sequence variants underlying most of the highly penetrant inherited monogenic diseases currently known, such as hemoglobinopathies. The likelihood that an nsSNP will result in disease or functional change in drug metabolism depends on the localization and nature of the amino acid change within the encoded protein. Although it is intuitively obvious that amino acid substitutions have the potential to change the function of a protein, gene expression also can be affected by SNPs positioned in regulatory sequences or intronic regions. For example, the cytosine-to-thymine nucleotide substitution in the promoter region (−159C>T) of the gene encoding CD14, an important molecule in the innate immune response, has been associated with decreased levels of soluble CD14 and increased total serum immunoglobulin E, resulting in a more severe allergic phenotype.[15] This finding demonstrates that discrete changes in genotype can amplify or damp complex biologic pathways, if those changes affect the regulation of functionally important genes.

HAPLOTYPE AND LINKAGE DISEQUILIBRIUM

The vast majority of SNPs are located in noncoding regions of the genome, which constitute a predominant amount of the human genome sequence. Most SNPs have no obvious effect on gene expression, protein function, or phenotype; however, a growing number of intronic SNPs are being linked to inherited phenotypes. Combinations of SNPs are commonly inherited together in the same region of DNA, forming haplotypes. Genome-wide haplotypes can be constructed by linkage disequilibrium (LD) analysis.[16] LD analysis is a statistical measure of the extent to which particular alleles or SNPs at two loci are associated with each other in the population, and LD occurs when haplotype combinations of alleles or SNPs at different loci occur more frequently than would be expected from random association. SNPs and alleles of interest are presumably inherited together if they are physically close to each other (usually <50 kilobases [kb]), producing strong LD. Therefore, SNPs that are in LD with a disease phenotype or response-to-drug phenotype can *mark* the position on the chromosome where a susceptibility gene is located, even though the SNP itself may not be the cause of the phenotype. Of interest, recent investigations have demonstrated that common SNPs are also in LD with other common variants in the human genome, such as deletions.[17] In addition, studies have suggested that the human genome is organized in blocks of haplotypes with high LD that are separated by regions of low LD.[18]

Considerable debate has arisen over the best strategies for SNP-based association studies to elucidate complex diseases and drug responses.[19] Various methods (eg, polymerase chain reaction [PCR] assay, matrix-assisted laser desorption/ionization [MALDI] mass spectrometry) and study designs (eg, association studies and linkage analysis) promoting access to genetic variation have been developed, and new techniques are still emerging.[20–22]

The great majority of SNPs or haplotypes currently used as molecular diagnostics in hematology are variations that were discovered on account of their direct involvement in altering the function of encoded proteins, as opposed to anonymous SNPs, which have been identified in association studies on the basis of their LD with causative SNPs. For example, hematologists have embraced testing for informative SNPs in factor V Leiden variant as one of several parameters used to determine the appropriate duration of anticoagulant therapy after documented venous thrombosis.[23] Likewise, it is increasingly common to search for three SNPs in the human *TPMT* gene that predispose a patient to thiopurine hematopoietic toxicity upon receiving drugs such as azathioprine (AZA) or mercaptopurine (MP).[24]

GENETIC VARIATIONS INFLUENCING DRUG RESPONSE: PHARMACOGENETICS–PHARMACOGENOMICS

Until relatively recently, genetics has played little or no role in finding the right drug and the optimal dosage for individual patients. Mostly empirical approaches are used to select drug therapy, despite the fact that there is great heterogeneity in the way people respond to medications, in terms of both host toxicity and treatment efficacy. Unfortunately, for almost all medications, interindividual differences are the rule, not the exception, and these differences result from the interplay of many variables, including genetics and environment. Variables influencing drug response include pathogenesis and severity of the underlying disease being treated; drug interactions; the patient's age (ie, *developmental pharmacology*), gender, nutritional status, and renal and liver function; presence of concomitant illnesses; and other medications. In addition to these clinical variables, increasing evidence points to a substantial inherited component of interindividual differences in drug response.[3,6,25]

Clinical observations of inherited differences in drug effects were first documented in the 1950s, and the concept of *pharmacogenetics* was defined initially in 1959 by Friedrich Vogel as "the study of the role of genetics in drug response."[26] The number of recognized clinically important pharmacogenetic traits grew steadily in the 1970s; the elucidation of the molecular genetics underlying these traits began in the late 1980s and 1990s, and their translation to molecular diagnostics is well under way in the 2000s.[6] Of interest, during the last decade, the field of pharmacogenetics was *rediscovered* by the pharmaceutical industry and by a broader spectrum of researchers in academia. This rediscovery has been driven in large part by the Human Genome Project, and by the recognition that inheritance can play a major role in determining drug effects.

The study of pharmacogenetics began with the analysis of genetic variations in drug-metabolizing enzymes and how those variations translate into inherited differences in drug effects. More recently, the field has extended to genome-wide approaches to identify networks of genes that govern the clinical response to drug therapy (ie, pharmacogenomics).[5,6] The terms *pharmacogenetics* and *pharmacogenomics*, however, are synonymous for all practical purposes.[6] Overall, pharmacogenomics can be viewed as a broad strategy to establish pharmacological models by integrating information from functional genomics, high-throughput molecular analyses, and pharmacodynamics. Approaches to establish pharmacogenomic models include candidate gene analyses (which focus on the analysis of single genes or sets of functionally related genes in pathways) and genome-wide analyses. Pharmacogenomic models can be used to both maximize efficacy and reduce toxicity of existing medications, or to identify novel therapeutic targets.[27] The general field of pharmacogenomics is the subject of several recent reviews[3,5–7,27–32] and is not comprehensively addressed here. Rather, clinically relevant examples are provided to illustrate how pharmacogenomics can be used to improve current drug therapy for hematologic disorders, to prevent hematologic toxicity, and to identify novel targets for developing new therapeutic approaches.

OPTIMIZATION OF DRUG THERAPY

Most drug effects are determined by the interplay of several gene products that influence the pharmacokinetics and pharmacodynamics of medications. *Pharmacokinetics* is the study of the absorption, distribution, metabolism, and excretion (ADME) of drugs. *Pharmacodynamics* is the relationship between the pharmacokinetic properties of drugs and their pharmacologic effects, either desired or adverse. The ultimate goal of pharmacogenomics in this context is to elucidate the inherited determinants for drug disposition and response to select medications and dosages on the basis of each patient's inherited ability to metabolize, eliminate, and respond to specific drugs.[3] A model of how polygenic variables can determine drug response is illustrated in Fig. 9–1.

GENETIC VARIATIONS THAT INFLUENCE DRUG DISPOSITION

Drug Metabolism

Metabolism often includes reactions that make lipophilic drugs more water soluble and thus more easily excreted. Pathways of drug metabolism are classified as either phase I reactions, which catalyze changes of functional moieties by oxidation, reduction, or hydrolysis, or phase II conjugation reactions, which conjugate functional moieties by acetylation, glucuronidation, sulfation, or methylation. The names employed to categorize these pathways are purely historical and used for convenience.[30]

The process of metabolic reactions that inactivate drugs or prodrugs is referred to as *catabolism*; for example, cytochrome P450 enzymes catalyze the *N*-dechlorethylation of the cytostatic prodrug cyclophosphamide. However, drug metabolism also includes reactions that convert prodrugs into therapeutically active compounds; these processes are referred to as *anabolism*. Additionally, metabolic reactions can form toxic metabolites. For example, cytochrome P450 catalyzes the 4-hydroxylation of cyclophosphamide into the cytotoxic compound phosphoramide mustard, and when cyclophosphamide is activated, the urotoxic compound acrolein is formed.

Essentially all genes encoding drug-metabolizing enzymes (there are more than 30 families of enzymes in humans) exhibit genetic variations, many of which translate into functional changes in the proteins encoded.[6] Inheritance of genes containing sequence variations that alter the function of enzymes encoded can influence drug disposition and ultimately determine drug effects (either desired or adverse), if those enzymes are involved in crucial pathways of elimination or activation of the administered medication. Numerous variant enzymes have been characterized within the last decade, as reviewed elsewhere[3,30,33]; here we focus on only three relevant examples:

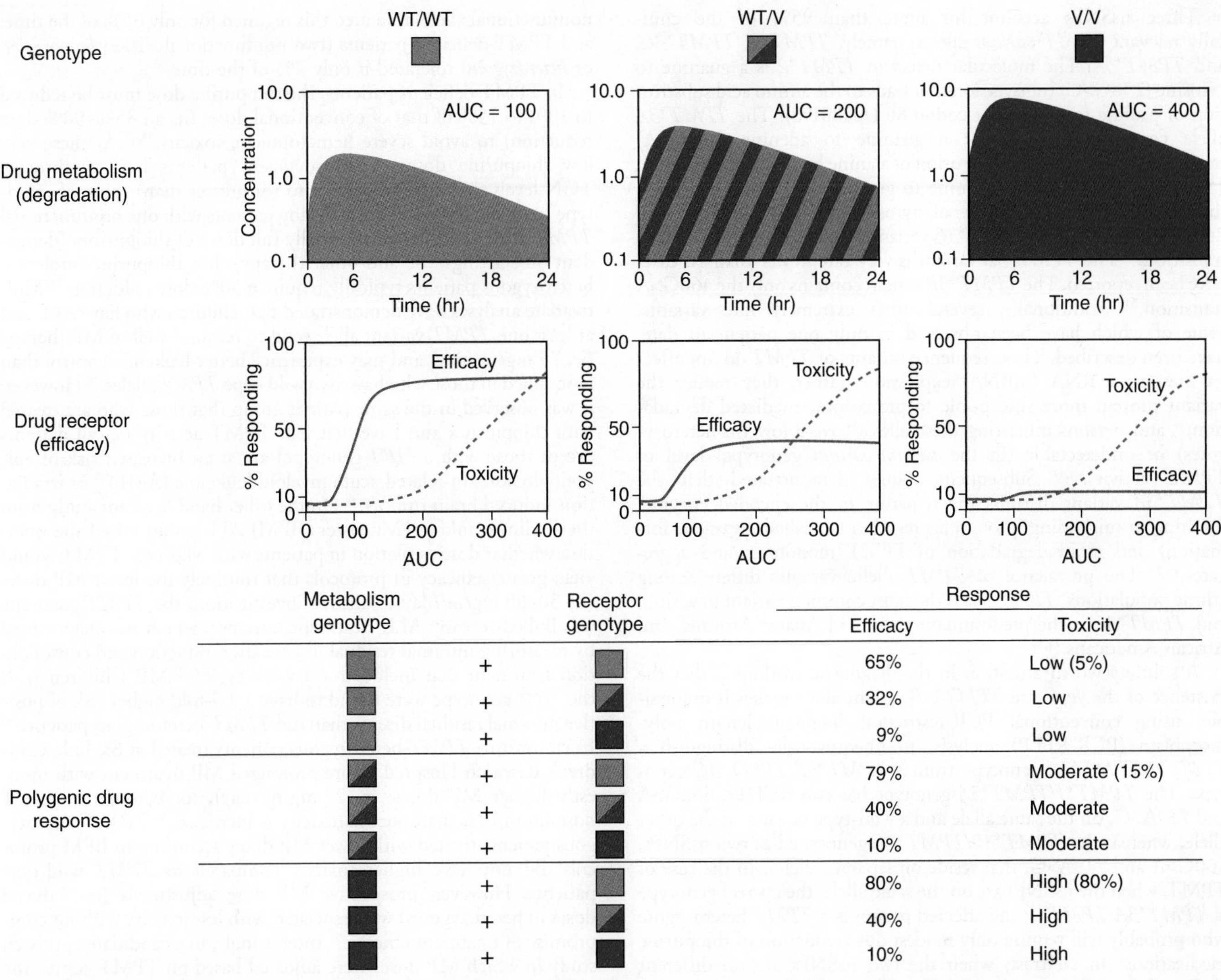

Figure 9–1 Polygenic determinants of drug response. The potential effects of two genetic variants are illustrated. One genetic variant involves a drug-metabolizing enzyme (*top*), and the second involves a drug receptor (*middle*). Differences in drug clearance (or the area under the plasma concentration–time curve [AUC]) and receptor sensitivity are depicted in patients who are either homozygous for the wild-type allele (*WT/WT*) or heterozygous for one wild-type and one variant (*V*) allele (*WT/V*), or have two variant alleles (*V/V*) for the two genetic variants. At the *bottom* are shown the nine potential combinations of drug metabolism, drug-receptor genotypes, and the corresponding drug-response phenotypes, which were calculated with data from the top. The therapeutic indexes (efficacy-to-toxicity ratios) ranged from 13 (65%:5%) to 0.125 (10%:80%).[6] *(Adapted with permission from Evans WE, McLeod HL: Pharmacogenomics—drug disposition, drug targets, and side effects. N Engl J Med 348:538, 2003. Copyright © 2003 Massachusetts Medical Society. All rights reserved.)*

thiopurine *S*-methyltransferase (TPMT), glutathione *S*-transferases (GSTs), and cytochrome P4502C9 (CYP2C9).

Thiopurine *S*-Methyltransferase

The genetic sequence variation of *TPMT* provides one of the best and most thoroughly studied examples of a clinically important pharmacogenetic trait. During the last two decades, studies have established that variations within the *TPMT* gene locus are a major determinant of the effects of thiopurines, which are widely prescribed structural analogs of purines.[24]

The prodrugs MP and thioguanine are among the agents that constitute the backbone of treatment for childhood acute lymphoblastic leukemia (ALL). The MP prodrug AZA is used primarily as an immunosuppressant to treat autoimmune disorders and to prevent rejection reaction after solid organ transplantation.

The hydrophilic thiopurines are transported into target cells, where they undergo extensive metabolism. Metabolic reactions include anabolism to form active cytotoxic thioguanine nucleotides (TGNs) and catabolism including phase I (oxidation via xanthine oxidase) and phase II (*S*-methylation via TPMT) reactions. In hematopoietic cells such as leukemic blasts, xanthine oxidase is low or absent[34]; therefore, degradation via TPMT is the only path by which thiopurines can be inactivated. TPMT activity determines how much of these intracellular prodrugs is inactivated to methylated metabolites and how much remains available for activation to TGNs. TGNs are responsible for the efficacy in leukemic blasts and toxicity in normal hematopoietic tissues.[35,36]

TPMT activity is inherited as an autosomal codominant trait. Approximately 90% to 95% of the population are homozygous for the wild-type allele (*TPMT*1*) and have normal enzyme activity; approximately 5% to 10% are heterozygous for the polymorphism and have intermediate levels of enzyme activity; 1 in 300 persons carries two variant *TPMT* alleles that cause TPMT deficiency.[37,38] TPMT activity typically is measured in erythrocytes, because this measure correlates with the activity in other normal[39] and neoplastic tissues.[40]

Three nsSNPs account for more than 95% of the clinically relevant *TPMT variant* alleles, namely, *TPMT*2, TPMT*3C,* and *TPMT*3A*. The molecular defect in *TPMT*2* is a guanine to cytosine (238G>C) transversion that leads to the amino acid substitution of proline for alanine at codon 80 (Ala80Pro). The *TPMT*3A* allele contains two nsSNPs: a guanine to adenine (460G>A) transition that leads to a substitution of alanine by threonine at codon 154 (Ala154Thr) and an adenine to guanine (719A>G) transition that leads to a substitution of tyrosine by cysteine at codon 240 (Tyr240Cys). The *TPMT*3C* variant contains only the 719A>G transition.[34] The *TPMT*3B* variant is very rare; fewer than 10 cases have been reported. The *TPMT*3B* variant contains only the 460G>A transition.[24] Additionally, several other extremely rare variants, some of which have been observed in only one patient to date, have been described. These sequence variants of *TPMT* do not affect its messenger RNA (mRNA) expression; rather, they render the variant protein more susceptible to proteosome-mediated degradation,[41] and persons inheriting these alleles have a low (in heterozygotes) or undetectable (in the *variant/variant* genotype) level of TPMT activity.[41,42] Subsequent studies demonstrated that the *TPMT*3A* variant disrupts the structure of the encoded enzyme, resulting in misfolding, protein aggregation (so called *aggresome* formation) and rapid degradation of TPMT monomers and aggregates.[43,44] The prevalence of *TPMT* allelic variants differs among ethnic populations. *TPMT*3A* is the most common variant in whites, and *TPMT*3C* is the predominant variant in Asians, Africans, and African Americans.[24,44]

A subtlety worth attention in the diagnostic workup is that the existence of the very rare *TPMT*3B* variant allele makes it impossible, using conventional PCR-restriction fragment length polymorphism (PCR-RFLP) analysis, to unequivocally distinguish a *TPMT*1/TPMT*3A* genotype from a *TPMT*3B/TPMT*3C* genotype. The *TPMT*1/TPMT*3A* genotype has two nsSNPs, 460G>A and 719A>G, on the same allele and a wild-type variant on the other allele, whereas the *TPMT*3B/TPMT*3C* genotype has two nsSNPs, 460G>A and 719A>G, that reside on separate alleles. In the case of TPMT, when the nsSNPs are on the same allele, the correct genotype is *TPMT*3A/TPMT*1*; the affected person is a *TPMT* heterozygote who probably will require only modest dose reduction of thiopurine medications. In contrast, when the two nsSNPs are on different alleles, the correct genotype is *TPMT*3B/TPMT*3C*. This is an important distinction, because both the *TPMT*3B* and the *TPMT*3C* alleles, like *TPMT*3A*, encode proteins that undergo rapid degradation. Therefore, patients with a *TPMT*3B/TPMT*3C* genotype are completely TPMT deficient, which necessitates an 85% to 90% dose reduction. Because *TPMT*3B* is extremely rare and LD is so strong between the nsSNPS 460G>A and 719A>G, the assumption that such patients have a *TPMT*3A/TPMT*1* genotype, necessitating only a modest dose reduction, usually is correct.[45]

Definitive ways are available to determine the correct haplotype structure and thus genotype. However, most of these methods require either family studies, cloning and sequencing, conversion of diploid to haploid cells, or technology that is not widely available (eg, nanotubes). Recently, a relatively simple method was developed to determine molecular haplotype structure for genes like *TPMT*, in which two or more SNPs lie within approximately 30 kb in genomic DNA.[46]

Childhood ALL studies have shown that essentially all homozygous TPMT-deficient patients experience dose-limiting hematotoxicity, and some experience life-threatening hematotoxicity if given conventional doses of thiopurines. Patients with only one nonfunctional *TPMT* allele have intermediate tolerance to thioguanine therapy. Although many patients with only one nonfunctional *TPMT* allele can tolerate thiopurine therapy at essentially full doses, they are at higher risk of dose-limiting hematotoxicity than are those patients who have a wild-type *TPMT* genotype (eg, 35% cumulative risk vs. 7% cumulative risk in a study of ALL patients).[32] Furthermore, patients with no documented *TPMT* mutations *1/*1 and normal enzyme activity tolerated full-dose MP during 84% of the time of scheduled therapy; patients who were *TPMT* heterozygotes (one nonfunctional allele) tolerated this regimen for only 65% of the time; and TPMT-deficient patients (two nonfunctional alleles: *homozygous* or *heterozygous*) tolerated it only 7% of the time.[36]

In TPMT-deficient patients, the thiopurine dose must be reduced to 10% to 15% of that of conventional doses (ie, an 85%–90% dose reduction) to avoid severe hematopoietic toxicity.[34,47] At these very low thiopurine doses, TPMT-deficient patients have erythrocyte TGN levels that are comparable to (or greater than) those of "wild-type" patients given full doses. Many patients with one nonfunctional *TPMT* allele can tolerate essentially full doses of thiopurines (dependent on starting dose and other therapy), but thiopurine-intolerant heterozygous patients typically require a 50% dose reduction.[34] Multivariate analyses have demonstrated that children who have ALL and at least one *TPMT*-variant allele tend to respond well to MP therapy (ie, 75 mg/m^2/day) and may experience better leukemia control than is obtained in those who have two wild-type *TPMT* alleles.[36] However, it was observed in the same patient group that those who are treated with thiopurines and have deficient TPMT activity (ie, all patients except those with a **1/*1* genotype) are at an increased risk of epipodophyllotoxin-related acute myeloid leukemia (AML)[48] or irradiation-induced brain tumors.[49] On the other hand, a recent study from the Berlin–Frankfurt–Muenster (BFM) ALL group raised the question whether dose escalation in patients with wild-type TPMT would yield greater efficacy in protocols that routinely use lower MP doses (ie, 50–60 mg/m^2/day).[50] In this investigation, the *TPMT* genotype was linked to early ALL treatment response, which was determined by measuring minimal residual disease after induction and consolidation treatment that included a 4-week cycle of MP. Children with the **1/*1* genotype were found to have a 2.9-fold higher risk of positive minimal residual disease than did *TPMT*-heterozygous patients.[50] In contrast to *TPMT*-heterozygous patients treated at St. Jude Children's Research Hospital (more prolonged MP treatment with modestly higher MP doses; ie, 75 mg/m^2/day), for whom the risk of dose-limiting hematopoeitic toxicity is increased,[36] *TPMT*-heterozygous patients treated with lower MP doses according to BFM protocols did not have higher toxicity compared to *TPMT* wild-type patients. However, prospective MP dose adjustment (ie, reduced doses in heterozygotes) was associated with less toxicity without compromise in treatment efficacy.[51] Interestingly, in a candidate approach study in which MP doses were adjusted based on TPMT status, the efficacy of childhood ALL therapy was influenced by glutathione *S*-transferase M1 (*GSTM1*) and thymidylate synthetase (*TS*) genotypes.[52]

More than 98% concordance exists between *TPMT* genotype and phenotype, and genotyping is very reliable (90% sensitivity, 99% specificity) in identifying patients who have inherited one or two nonfunctional alleles.[53] Therefore, using the *TPMT* genotype to individualize thiopurine therapy, clinicians can now diagnose inherited differences in drug response to prevent serious toxicities (see box on Mercaptopurine Dosage Adjustment and Fig. 9–2).

Glutathione S-Transferase Polymorphisms

GSTs are ubiquitous in human organs and provide an important line of cellular defense against electrophilic genotoxic compounds. GSTs neutralize these compounds, which arise from both endogenous sources and xenobiotics (eg, anthracyclines, cisplatin), mainly by conjugating them to glutathione. In addition to their catalytic activity, certain GST isoenzymes can regulate mitogen-activated protein kinases by acting as ligand-binding proteins, or can facilitate the addition of glutathione to cysteine residues in target proteins (S-glutathionylation). The GST proteins are divided into three major families: cytosolic, mitochondrial, and microsomal GSTs.[54,55] In humans, there are currently seven subclasses of soluble cytosolic GSTs, with four major classes: GST α, GST μ, GST π, and GST θ. Three of these classes, GST μ, GST θ, and GST π, have been studied extensively in the context of pharmacogenomics and hematology/oncology.[55] Gene clusters of GST μ (*GSTM1, M2, M3, M4,* and *M5*) and GST θ (*GSTT1* and *GSTT2*) are located on chromosomes 1 and 22,

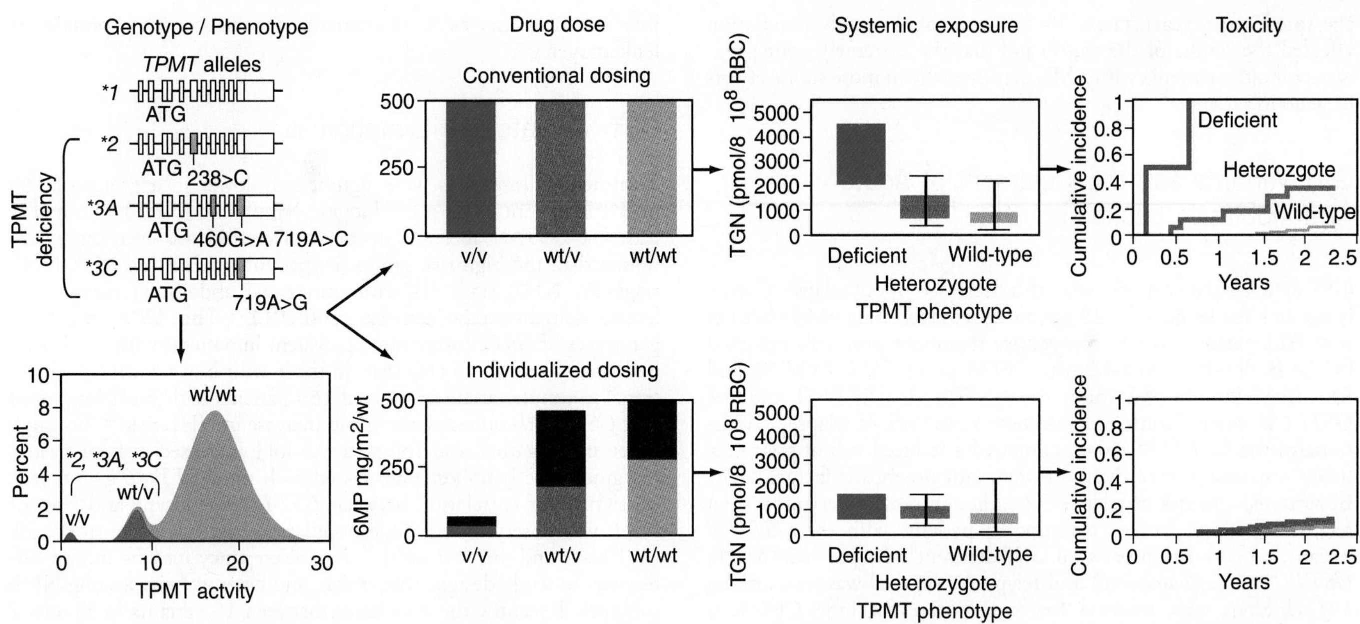

Figure 9–2 Genetic polymorphism of thiopurine methyltransferase (TMPT) and its role in determining toxicity to thiopurine medications. Under "Genotype/Phenotype" (*far left*) are depicted the predominant *TPMT* mutant alleles that cause autosomal codominant inheritance of TPMT activity in humans. As shown in the graphs under "Drug Dose," "Systemic Exposure," and "Toxicity," when uniform (conventional) dosages of thiopurine medications (eg, azathioprine, mercaptopurine [6MP], thioguanine) are administered to all patients, TPMT-deficient patients accumulate markedly higher (10-fold) cellular concentrations of the active thioguanine nucleotides (TGN), and *TPMT*-heterozygous patients accumulate approximately twofold higher TGN concentrations, which translate into a significantly higher frequency of toxicity (*far right*). As depicted in the bottom row of graphs, when genotype-specific dosages of thiopurines are administered, comparable cellular TGN concentrations are achieved, and all three TPMT phenotypes can be treated without acute toxicity. In the two graphs under "Drug Dose," the *solid* or *striped* portion of each bar depicts the mean 6MP doses that were tolerated in patients who presented with hematopoietic toxicity; the *stippled* portion depicts the mean dosage tolerated by all patients in each genotype group, not just those patients presenting with toxicity. (v, variant; wt, wild-type.) *(Reproduced with permission from Evans WE: Thiopurine S-methyltransferase: A genetic polymorphism that affects a small number of drugs in a big way. Pharmacogenetics 12:421, 2002.)*

respectively. GST π is encoded by a single locus (*GSTP1*) on chromosome 11.[56]

Some glutathione *S*-transferases (GSTs) are highly polymorphic. In most populations, approximately 50% of persons have a homozygous deletion of the gene encoding GSTM1, and approximately 25% have a homozygous deletion of the gene encoding GSTT1. These patients have the so-called *null* alleles *GSTM1*0* and *GSTT1*0*, both of which lead to absence of enzyme activity.[57] *GSTP1* also displays genetic variations within its coding region: the nsSNP 1578A>G causes an isoleucine to valine substitution at codon 105 (Ile105Val), and the 2293C>T gives rise to the replacement of alanine by valine at the amino acid position 114 (Ala114Val).[58] The enzymes encoded by the resulting variants, *GSTP1*2* (only the Ile105Val substitution) and *GSTP1*3* (both Ile105Val and Ala114Val), alter catalytic activity and thermal stability.[56] Population frequency distributions of these variants differ widely among geographic regions and ethnic groups; for example, the *GSTM1*0* type occurs more commonly in whites (50%) than in African Americans (35%).[59]

In general, it is hypothesized that patients with the *null* genotype, especially those with the *double-null* genotype (ie, *null* genotype for *GSTM1* and *GSTT1*), exhibit impaired detoxification of environmental toxins and chemotherapy. Therefore, these patients have a higher risk of primary and secondary cancers and treatment-related complications but might have a better response to chemotherapy.[60,61] Indeed, GST deficiency has been associated with increased toxicity of some anticancer drugs, and increased expression of GST has been associated with drug resistance in cell lines.[55] However, some of these results and the underlying hypothesis are challenged by results that appear contradictory.[62,63]

GST Variants and the Treatment of Acute Myeloid Leukemia

In patients receiving intensive treatment for acute myeloid leukemia (AML), the *GSTT1*0* genotype has been associated with greater toxicity and death after chemotherapy.[64,65] Because of GST's putative role in the metabolism of several cytotoxic drugs, such as anthracyclines, which are among the most important drugs used in remission induction therapy for AML, the GST deficiency caused by *null* genotypes might be expected to result in greater response to chemotherapy and higher toxicity. Consequently, a dose reduction would be indicated. However, the situation is probably more complex.

In a multivariate analysis of 106 adults with AML, persons with *GSTM1*0*, *GSTT1*0*, or *double-null* variants were found to have enhanced resistance to induction chemotherapy and a shorter survival rate. In this study, 42% of patients presented with the *GSTM1*0*, 28% with the *GSTT1*1*, and 18% with the *double-null* variant.[62] These results might be explained by the hypothesis that the deficiency of GST enzymes gives rise to higher intracellular levels of glutathione (GSH): GSH is consumed in GST-catalyzed reactions, and patients with *GST-null* genotypes have less (or no) GST to catalyze this reaction; therefore, intracellular GSH levels are higher in these patients. In addition to its role in detoxification, GSH, in high concentration, stimulates cell proliferation and inhibits apoptosis.[66,67] Accordingly, an increased level of GSH in blast cells has been associated with an increased risk of relapse in childhood ALL.[68] In a recent study on 200 adults with AML, Southwest Oncology Group investigators were unable to find associations between *GSTM1*, *GSTT1*, and *GSTA1* genotypes and treatment outcome. It was speculated that the increased age (median 68 years, range 56–88 years) of the study population affected the results of the study; and that the extremely poor prognosis for older patients with AML may overwhelm more subtle effects of genetic variants.[69]

GST Variants and the Treatment of Acute Lymphoblastic Leukemia

GST deficiency was associated with a decreased risk of relapse of acute lymphoblastic leukemia (ALL) in a case–control study of 64 children with ALL treated on two consecutive treatment protocols designed by the Berlin–Frankfurt–Munster (BFM group (ALL-BFM 86 and ALL-BFM 90). In this study, the *GSTM1*0*, *GSTT1*0*, and the *GSTP1*B* variants conferred a decrease in the risk of relapse.[61] Additionally, the *GSTT1*0* variant conferred a reduced risk of poor cortisone response (one of the most important prognostic factors in the BFM trials) and risk of relapse.[70,71] Although central nervous system relapse tended to be less common in patients with the *GSTM*0* variant, no correlation between GST-deficient subtypes (*GSTM1*0*, *GSTT1*0*, and *double-null*) and relapse or survival was seen among 197 children who received five consecutive St. Jude Children's Research Hospital (SJCRH) protocols (Total X, XI, XII, XIIIA, and XIIIB).[59] Additionally, two studies of 710 children with ALL treated by the Children's Cancer Group and 320 children with ALL who received LAL (leucémies aiguës lymphoblastiques) protocols and the protocols developed by the Dana-Farber Cancer Institute (DFCI 87–01, 91–01, and 95–01) found no association between GST genotype (*GSTM1*0*, *GSTT1*0*, and *double-null*) and treatment outcome in childhood ALL.[63,72] Some of the observed discrepancies may be attributed to differences in study designs, number of patients, and treatment protocols. Recently, 246 children with ALL treated on the SJCRH Total XIIIB protocol were screened for 16 genetic germline sequence variants in 13 candidate genes.[52] The *GSTM1* non-null genotype (which is associated with a higher *GSTM1* expression) was significantly associated with an increased relapse rate in children with higher-risk ALL, and the risk was further increased in children carrying the thymidylate synthetase (*TS*) 3/3 genotype (which is associated with higher *TS* expression). Of interest, no genotypes were predictive for outcome in children with lower-risk ALL, which might be due to the small number of treatment failures in this cohort or that other genes are important for the lower-risk treatment protocols.[52] Overall, these data provide evidence that the identified *prognostic genotypes/phenotypes* have to be considered treatment-dependent. If confirmed, however, then dosage modifications of antileukemic medications may overcome these drug resistance genotypes in children who are treated on similar treatment protocols.

GST Variants and the Risk of Leukemia and Myelodysplastic Syndrome

GST variants have been implicated in the development of de novo ALL,[73–76] de novo AML, therapy-related AML (t-AML), and myelodysplastic syndrome (MDS) in children and adults.[56,77–80] It can be argued that the development of these diseases may be due to the limited ability of the GST variants to effectively detoxify carcinogens from the environment or cancer therapy. Results from several studies appear to be contradictory, however. For example, one multicenter study did not reveal an association of *GSTM1*0* or *GSTT1*0* variants with t-AML in the context of epipodophyllotoxin treatment[81]; another study could not find an association between *GSTT1*0* and the risk of AML[82]; and another could not find a relationship between *GSTM1*0*, *GSTT1*0*, and *double-null* variants and the risk of ALL.[64] Overall, as summarized in a recent systematic review and meta-analysis of 30 published case–control studies, it is conceivable that different *GST* genotypes may play a role in leukemogenesis.[83] However, carefully designed further studies are warranted to fully address the possible contributions of GST variants in the complex process of leukemogenesis.

GST Variants and Lymphomas

Treatment failure rates were significantly lower in a group of 169 pediatric patients with non-Hodgkin lymphoma (NHL) who had at least one *GSTM1* allele.[84] This protective effect was even more pronounced in the high-risk group (ie, patients with B-cell ALL, NHL stage IV, NHL stage III with unresected abdominal tumor, and lactate dehydrogenase activity ≥500 U/L).[84] The **2/*2* and **1/*2* genotypes of *GSTP1* were more prevalent in patients with NHL who had small tumors (<5 cm) than in those with larger tumors.[85] Additionally, a multivariate analysis of 169 patients with NHL suggested that *GSTT1*0* conferred a fourfold increase in NHL risk.[86] Although other investigators also found a 9.5-fold increased risk of gastric marginal zone lymphoma associated with the *GSTT1*0* genotype,[87] no significant correlation between *GSTT1*0* genotype and risk for NHL was observed in a large population-based case–control study (351 cases and 467 controls).[88] The discrepancy may be due to differences in study design, cohort size, and heterogeneity among NHL subtypes. Recently, the association between 15 variants in 11 metabolic genes (including *GSTP1* and *GSTM3*) and the risk of NHL was investigated in 1172 cases and 982 controls. Subjects who were heterozygous or homozygous for the cytochrome P450 gene variant *CYP1B1* V432L G allele were found to be at slightly greater risk for NHL; there was no overall association with NHL for the other gene variants examined.[89]

GST variants appear to be of interest in patients with Hodgkin disease (HD), because survivors of HD who receive combination chemotherapy and radiotherapy have an increased risk of treatment-related complications, especially second malignant neoplasms.[90] The GSTT1-null genotype was reported to be associated with a increased risk for HD,[91] and more importantly the *GSTP1*2/*2* variant (which is associated with a lower GSTP1 activity) was shown to be associated with a poor outcome in patients with advanced stage HD (IIB-IV).[92]

In conclusion, GST enzyme variants appear to be important in intracellular metabolism of drugs commonly used to treat hematologic malignancies and in the process of leukemogenesis. However, compared with the highly penetrant *TPMT* variants, *GST* variants appear to have a more complex role. Interestingly, GST variants which result in a higher expression of the genes encoded, seem to be associated with a poorer outcome in patients who receive more intense treatment; for example, for higher-risk ALL and advanced-stage HD.[52,92] Further studies are warranted to establish the importance of GST polymorphisms in determining response to treatment and the risk of leukemogenesis.

Cytochrome P4502C9

Cytochrome P4502C9 (CYP2C9) belongs to the cytochrome P450 (CYP) superfamily, a system of phase I enzymes involved in the metabolism of endogenous substances (eg, steroids, arachidonic acid, vitamin D_3) and exogenous compounds (eg, drugs, environmental chemicals, pollutants).[93] In humans, the CYP enzymes (http://drnelson.utmem.edu/CytochromeP450.html) are encoded by more than 57 genes, and the majority of genes are polymorphic.[94] Updated information regarding the nomenclature and properties of the variant alleles with links to the dbSNP database (http://www.ncbi.nlm.nih.gov/SNP/) is available at the human CYP allele home page (http://www.imm.ki.se/cypalleles/). On the basis of the composition of CYP variant alleles, individuals have been categorized into four major phenotypes: poor metabolizers (having two nonfunctional alleles), intermediate metabolizers (being deficient in one allele), extensive metabolizers (having two copies of functional alleles), and ultrarapid metabolizers (having three or more active gene copies).[94] The *CYP2* gene family, which is the largest subfamily, is encoded by more than

16 genes.[93] CYP2C9 is the principal CYP2C isoenzyme in the human liver, and it is involved in the oxidative metabolism of several clinically important drugs, including oral anticoagulants, phenytoin, and various nonsteroidal anti-inflammatory drugs. To date, numerous polymorphic alleles (*CYP2C9*1* to **30*) have been identified for the known *CYP2C9* gene, at least half of which are associated with diminished enzyme activity in vitro.[94]

The two most common *CYP2C9* variants are *CYP2C9*2* and *CYP2C9*3*. *CYP2C9*2* has a cytosine to thymine transversion at nucleotide 430 (430C>T) that encodes cysteine instead of arginine at amino acid residue 144 (Arg144Cys); *CYP2C9*3* has an adenine to cytosine transversion at nucleotide 1075 (1075A>C) that leads to the substitution of isoleucine by leucine at amino acid residue 359 (Ile359Leu).[95,96] Approximately 35% of whites have one or two of these variant alleles; the overall allelic frequency of *CYP2C9*2* is approximately 10%, and that of *CYP2C9*3* is 8%.[95,96] The **2* and **3* variants are virtually nonexistent in African Americans and Asians; 95% of these persons express the wild-type genotype (ie, extensive metabolizers).[96] Both *CYP2C9*2* and *CYP2C9*3* are important in the metabolism of the oral anticoagulants (vitamin K antagonists) warfarin, acenocoumarol, and phenprocoumon.[95,97–100]

In the United States, warfarin is widely used to prevent thromboembolic events in patients with chronic conditions such as atrial fibrillation, and the drug is prescribed to more than 1 million persons annually. A narrow therapeutic index with a risk of serious hemorrhage (1.3–2.7 per 100 patient-years[101]) and interindividual variability in response to warfarin necessitate individualization of treatment, which is based primarily on monitoring prothrombin time. Several studies have demonstrated that *CYP2C9* genotype influences warfarin anticoagulant dose requirements[95,101–105] and bleeding risks.[105] The required dose of warfarin is lowest if *CYP2C9*3* is present, as predicted by in vitro studies that compared the functional effects of the two variant alleles.[95] In addition, heterozygosity for *CYP2C9*2* significantly affects overall CYP2C9 activity.[95] Recently, a clear association between metabolic clearance of *S*-warfarin and the *CYP2C9* genotype has been demonstrated.[106]

Warfarin is a racemic mixture of *R*- and *S*-enantiomers that differ in their patterns of metabolism and in their potency of pharmacodynamic effect.[95] Although *S*-warfarin exhibits a three- to fivefold higher inhibitory effect on the target enzyme vitamin K epoxide reductase, differences in metabolism result in an approximately twofold higher plasma concentration of *R*-warfarin. It has therefore been suggested that *S*-warfarin accounts for 60% to 70% of the overall anticoagulation response and *R*-warfarin accounts for 30% to 40%.[107] A number of CYP isoforms contribute to warfarin metabolism[95]; however, 6- and 7-hydroxylation by CYP2C9 is the most important inactivation pathway of *S*-warfarin. Compared with the amount of *S*-warfarin metabolized by wild-type enzyme (encoded by the *CYP2C9*1* allele), that metabolized by the enzyme encoded by the *CYP2C9*2* variant is reduced by approximately 30% to 50%, and the amount metabolized by the enzyme encoded by the *CYP2C9*3* variant is reduced by 90%.[95] The substantial reduction in turnover seen with the *CYP2C9*3* variant may be caused by the amino acid substitution Ile359Leu within the substrate-binding site of the enzyme.[95]

It is well established that *CYP2C9* genotype is correlated with warfarin, acenocoumarol, and phenprocoumon metabolism and dose requirement, and genotyping for the more common *CYP2C9* alleles before initiation of anticoagulation therapy may help clinicians choose the appropriate initial anticoagulant treatment and determine the extent of clinical monitoring needed.[95,108] However, because interindividual variability in the dose requirement occurs within the various *CYP2C9* groups, genotyping for additional polymorphic genes that encode clotting factors, transporters, and warfarin targets could possibly further improve anticoagulation therapy. Indeed, a novel pharmacodynamic mechanism underlying warfarin resistance has been elucidated with the recent discovery of sequence variants in the warfarin target gene *VKORC1*, which encodes the vitamin K epoxide reductase complex 1.[109,110] This complex regenerates reduced vitamin K for another cycle of catalysis, which is essential for the posttranslational gamma-carboxylation of vitamin K-dependent clotting factors II (prothrombin), VII, IX, and X (Fig. 9–3). The identification of common variants in *VKORC1* has emerged as one of the most important genetic factors determining coumarin dose requirements.[111–114] Main *VKORC* haplotypes include the putative *ancestral* haplotype *VKORC1*1*, the *low-dose coumarin* haplotype *VKORC1*2*, and the *high-dose coumarin* haplotypes *VKORC1*3* and **4*. There are major differences in the distribution of *VKOCR1* haplotypes among ethnic groups, and this may explain interethnic differences in coumarin requirement. For example, the significantly higher average warfarin requirement in Africans is in line with significantly lower occurrence of the *low-dose coumarin VKORC1*2* haplotype in Africans.[112] Overall, the hereditary pharmacodynamic factor *VKORC1* explains approximately 25% of the variance in coumarin dose requirement, compared with 5% to 10% for the hereditary pharmacokinetic factor *CYP2C9* alone.[112] More recently 201 Caucasians were genotyped for sequence variants in 29 candidate genes involved in the warfarin interactive pathways, and these results combined with several nongenetic factors were tested for the association with warfarin dose requirement. By means of this systematic investigation, 62% of the variance in warfarin dose requirements in Swedish patients could be explained.[115] Clearly, prospective studies that incorporate genetic (eg, *CYP2C9* and *VKORC1*) and nongenetic factors (eg, variable intake of vitamin K) in coumarin dose calculation will be required to demonstrate the safety, cost-effectiveness, and feasibility of individualized dosing regimens.[116]

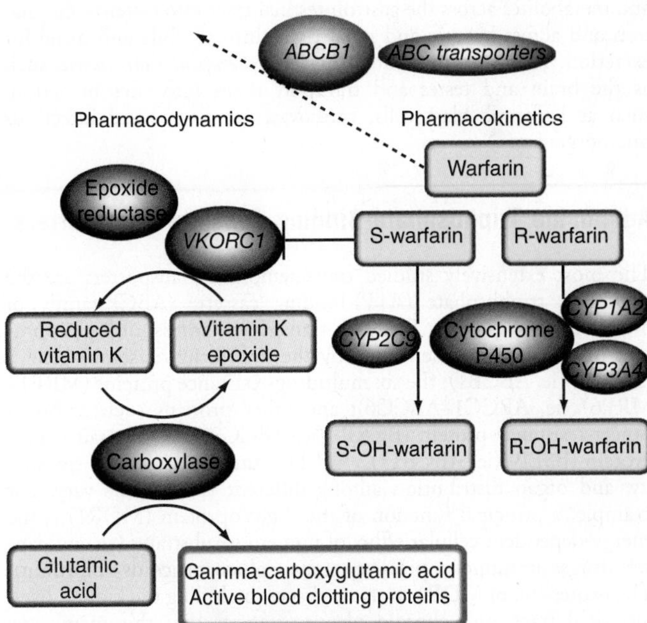

Figure 9–3 The cytochrome P450 isoenzymes *CYP2C9* (to a much lesser extent *CYP3A4* and *CYP1A2*) and vitamin K epoxide reductase complex 1 *VKORC1* genotypes influence warfarin dose requirement. The racemic mixture of *R*- and *S*-warfarin (threefold higher pharmacodynamic effect of *R*-warfarin) inhibits the reductase in the vitamin K cycle, impairing the synthesis of active vitamin K-dependent clotting factors in liver cells and causes bleeding. *R*- and *S*-warfarin are metabolized via hepatic CYP isoenzymes and there is evidence that warfarin is transported out of the liver into the bile via the ATP-dependent transporter (ABC transporter) ABCB1 (or P-glycoprotein).

DRUG TRANSPORTERS

Although passive diffusion accounts for tissue distribution of some drugs and metabolites, for more lipophilic substances and at higher drug concentrations, an increased emphasis is being placed on the role of membrane transporters. Membrane transporters move drugs and metabolites across the gastrointestinal tract into systemic circulation and across hepatic and renal tissue into the bile and urine for excretion. They also distribute drugs into *therapeutic sanctuaries* such as the brain and testes and transport them into sites of action, such as leukemic blast cells, cardiovascular tissue, and infectious microorganisms.[5]

Adenosine Triphosphate-Binding Cassette Transporters

The most extensively studied transmembrane transporters are the adenosine triphosphate (ATP)-binding cassette (ABC) family of membrane transporters. The ABC transporters consist of P-glycoprotein MDR1, which is encoded by the multidrug-resistance gene 1 (*MDR1*) (ie, ABCB1); the six multidrug-resistance proteins (MRP1–MRP6) (ie, ABCC1–ABCC6); and other proteins such as breast cancer-resistance protein (BCRP) (ie, ABCG2) and bile salt export protein (BSEP) (ie, ABCB11).[117,118] The function, substrate specificity, and organ distribution among different transporters vary. For example, a principal function of the P-glycoprotein (MDR1) is the energy-dependent cellular efflux of numerous substrates (eg, anticancer drugs, immunosuppressive agents, glucocorticoids, bilirubin). The expression of MDR1 in many tissues, including the kidney, liver, intestinal tract, and choroid plexus, suggests that this membrane transporter plays an important role in the distribution of xenobiotics; MDR1 excretes xenobiotics and their metabolites into urine, bile, and the intestinal lumen and transports substances across the blood–brain barrier.[6] The genetic polymorphisms of the ABC transporters have been summarized,[119] and their clinical relevance in the field of hematology is being increasingly investigated.[120–122]

Although transporters like MDR1 transport various substrates and thus have rather low substrate specificity, other transporters such as the reduced folate carrier (RFC) transport only a few specific molecules and their analogs, and thus have much higher substrate specificity. Functionally important polymorphisms in transporters with high substrate specificity might be of even greater interest in pharmacogenomics than those with low specificity, because the former can affect the distribution of specific drugs.

Reduced Folate Carrier

At physiologic extracellular folate concentrations or concentrations of antifolates achieved after conventional dosages, folates and their structural analogs (eg, antifolates) enter cells mainly via the reduced folate carrier (RFC or SLC19A1), which is encoded by the *SLC19A1* gene. The antifolate drug methotrexate (MTX) is a key component in the treatment of childhood ALL. Given that passive diffusion of MTX is not of importance (ie, extracellular MTX concentrations are less than 20 μM), SLC19A1 expression and impaired SLC19A1 function appear to influence intracellular MTX accumulation and might confer cellular MTX resistance.[123,124] Gene alterations affecting the transport properties of SLC19A1 have been found in cell lines and in patient lymphoblasts.[124,125] Recently, an nsSNP (80G>A) that replaces histidine with arginine at position 27 (His27Arg) of the SLC19A1 protein has been identified.[126] The *G/G* variant correlated with lower plasma folate and higher homocysteine (Hcy) levels in healthy persons.[126]

Folate and Hcy homeostasis are affected by MTX,[127] and the nsSNP 80G>A in the *SLC19A1* gene may modulate MTX disposition and MTX effects in leukemic blast cells. This question was addressed in a study that assessed the association among the 80G>A genetic variation in *SLC19A1*, MTX plasma levels, and childhood ALL treatment outcome.[128] In this analysis, children with the *80A* variant had worse outcome after receiving MTX-containing combination chemotherapy than that noted in patients with the homozygous *80G* genotype. Additionally, patients homozygous for *80A* had higher MTX plasma concentrations than patients with other *SLC19A1* variants.[128] However, plasma concentrations of MTX are highly variable and influenced by numerous factors (eg, renal function); therefore, plasma MTX level is not a reliable indicator of SLC19A1 function. Currently, it remains unknown whether the 80G>A nsSNP confers a change in SLC19A1 function in human leukemic lymphoblasts.

The *SLC19A1*–MTX example illustrates a common problem in association studies; until causality is established through mechanistic studies, it is not possible to definitely establish the clinical importance of a given genetic variant. One can hypothesize that the association of this *SLC19A1* nsSNP and treatment outcome is caused by decreased MTX uptake into leukemic cells; however, unless it is shown that the *SLC19A1* variant causes altered transmembrane transport of MTX and/or folates, causality remains uncertain. In this regard, the amino acid change (strong to weak basic amino acid) in the first transmembrane domain (TMD1), which is caused by the 80G>A SNP, probably influences SLC19A1 transport properties; in cell lines, several alterations within the TMD1 region were shown to change the ratio of SLC19A1 affinity for MTX relative to that for other folate substrates.[129,130] Likewise, the *80A* variant transporter might have lower affinity for MTX and higher affinity for other folate substrates. However, studies in human erythroleukemia K562 cell lines showed no difference in MTX transport between the *80G* and the *80A SLC19A1* variants.[131] Therefore, additional studies are needed to elucidate the underlying mechanisms linking *SLC19A1* polymorphisms, MTX/folate transport into cells, and ALL outcomes, and these clinical findings also must be independently replicated.

The *SLC19A1* gene is located on chromosome 21, and high expression of *SLC19A1* has been correlated with higher cellular accumulation of MTX and its active polyglutamylated metabolites (MTXPG). Indeed, hyperdiploid ALL cells (ie, ALL blast cells with >50 chromosomes) almost always have extra copies of chromosome 21, and therefore have high *SLC19A1* expression and high MTXPG accumulation after MTX treatment in vivo.[124,132] Moreover, individuals with Down syndrome have germline trisomy 21, and this is associated with overexpression of a number of genes on this chromosome. However, the hypothesis that a constitutive overexpression of the *SLC19A1* gene in cells of patients with Down syndrome may explain why these individuals are more susceptible to MTX toxicity remains to be established.[124] Of interest, ALL cells carrying the *E2A-PBX1* fusion gene, which results from a t(1;19)(q23;p13.3) chromosomal translocation, have low *SLC19A1* expression and correspondingly accumulate low MTXPG levels in vivo.[132] The putative impaired MTX transport into *E2A-PBX1* ALL cells is the first chemotherapy resistance mechanism identified in this ALL subtype; and impaired MTX influx might be overcome by high-dose MTX. Notably, the clinical trials with the best treatment results for *E2A-PBX1* ALL, the St. Jude Total Therapy XIII protocol and the Berlin–Frankfurt–Muenster (ALL-BFM 90) protocol, with 5-year event-free survival rates of 89.5% ± 7.3% and 93% ± 6%, respectively, featured high-dose MTX consolidation therapy.[133,134]

Clearly, further investigations are needed to define the nature of *SLC19A1* function and MTX uptake in hematological malignancies such as acute lymphoblastic leukemia and lymphomas.

GENETIC VARIATIONS INFLUENCING DRUG TARGETS

To exert their pharmacologic effects, most drugs interact with specific target proteins such as receptors, enzymes, or proteins involved in signal transduction, cell cycle control, or other cellular events. Molecular studies have revealed that many of the genes encoding these drug targets exhibit genetic variations, which can alter the sensitivity of these targets to specific medications.[3,5,6,109] Here we focus on three that are potentially relevant in hematology.

Glycoprotein IIIa Subunit of the Glycoprotein IIb/IIIa Receptor

Platelets play a crucial role in thrombosis and the development of acute ischemic coronary artery syndromes (eg, a platelet-rich thrombus forms at the site of the ruptured atherosclerotic plaque). Inhibition of platelet function is an effective strategy in the treatment and prevention of thrombosis of arteriosclerotic origin. Three main classes of antiplatelet agents are available for clinical use: aspirin, the thienopyridines, and intravenous GPIIb/IIIa antagonists.

The glycoprotein (GP) complex GPIIb/IIIa is the most abundant platelet membrane GP; each platelet contains approximately 80,000 copies of this GP. The GPIIb/IIIa complex is believed to be the final common pathway in platelet aggregation, which is mediated by the binding of fibrinogen or von Willebrand factor. The importance of GPIIb/IIIa for thrombus formation is convincingly evidenced by clinical trials, which have successfully used intravenously administered GPIIb/IIIa antagonists to block platelet aggregation and thrombus formation.[135] In addition, aspirin inhibits epinephrine-induced platelet aggregation by inhibiting GPIIb/IIIa activation through interference with intracellular signaling events[136] and acetylation of GPIIb/IIIa molecules.[137]

Theoretically, polymorphisms that change the function of the GPIIb/IIIa receptor might influence the outcome of antiplatelet therapy and contribute to differences in drug effects. A common polymorphism of GPIIIa, *HPA-1* (*Pl(A)*), involving a thymidine to cytosine transition at nucleotide 1565 (1565T>C) results in leucine to proline substitution at position 33 (Leu33Pro) and defines the *Pl(A1)* (*HPA-1a*, Leu33) and *Pl(A2)* (*HPA-1b*, 33Pro) alleles, respectively.[138] The *Pl(A2)* allele is present in 20% to 30% of Caucasians[139] and confers a *hyperreactive* thrombocyte status in vitro (ie, these platelets have a lower threshold for activation, granule release, GPIIb/IIIa activation, and fibrinogen binding).[140] Therefore *Pl(A2)* allele carriers seem to have a higher risk for thrombotic events, for example, ischemic coronary syndromes[141,142] and restenosis after coronary stent placement.[143] Whereas there is consensus on the prothrombotic phenotype of the *Pl(A2)* sequence variant, in part disconcordant results are reported on the sensitivity of platelets to aspirin, thienopyridines, and GPIIb/IIIa antagonists as a function of the *Pl(A)* variant alleles.[140,144–148] Clearly, further studies are needed to elucidate whether the *Pl(A)* variant alters GPIIb/IIIa function and response to aspirin, thienopyridines, or intravenous GPIIb/IIIa antagonists.

IgG Fc Receptor (Subtype FcγRIIIa, CD16)

Rituximab is a chimeric anti-CD20 immunoglobulin G1 (IgG1) monoclonal antibody (mAb) directed against the CD20 antigen present on B lymphocytes. Rituximab was successfully introduced for the treatment of B-lymphoproliferative malignancies, including non-Hodgkin lymphomas (NHL, eg, diffuse large B-cell lymphoma, follicular lymphoma), Waldenstrom macroglobulinemia, and chronic lymphocytic leukemia.[149–153] This drug is associated with severe B-cell depletion from peripheral blood and lymphoid tissue, which makes it useful in autoimmune diseases such as immune thrombocytopenia, by interfering with the production of pathologic antibodies.[154] However, 30% to 50% of patients with NHL, for example, exhibit no clinical response to rituximab therapy, and the actual cause of this treatment failure is largely unknown.[149]

Besides other mechanisms, like mAb-induced apoptotic signaling via CD20[155] and complement-dependent cytotoxicity,[156] antibody-dependent cell-mediated cytotoxicity (ADCC) appears to be an important mechanism in the eradication of $CD20^+$ blast cells by rituximab, and failure in this pathway might confer drug resistance.[157] The initiation of the ADCC program requires leukocyte receptors for the Fc portion of IgG (FcγR). FcγRs link the IgG-sensitized antigens to FcγR-bearing cytotoxic cells and trigger the cell activation mechanisms.[149] Three classes of IgG Fc receptors (ie, FcγRs)—FcγRI, FcγRII, and FcγRIII—have been found in humans, and several genetic variations that influence the IgG-binding properties of these receptors have been described.[157,158]

In the FcγRIIIa (CD16) receptor, a guanine to thymine transition at position 559 of the *FCGR3A* gene (559G>T) leads to substitution of phenylalanine by valine at codon 158 (Phe158Val).[158] Of interest, this genetic variation has the same distribution in various ethnic populations.[149,158] Of the receptor molecule, the affected residue is located at the F-G loop that serves as a binding interface and is surrounded by both chains of the Fc fragments of IgG1.[159] Because the side chain of phenylalanine is hydrophobic and larger than that of valine, the genetic variation can affect the major conformation or the hydrophobicity of the surface of the binding interface; therefore, it may influence the receptor's binding properties.[159] Indeed, human IgG1 binds more strongly to natural killer (NK) cells bearing homozygous FcγRIIIa-158V receptors than to NK cells bearing homozygous FcγRIIIa-158F receptors or NK cells bearing heterozygous FcγRIIIa receptors; this difference might have a profound influence on ADCC.[157,158] Patients with follicular lymphoma,[149,150] diffuse large B-cell lymphoma,[151] and Waldenstrom macroglobulinemia,[152] whose NK cells carry the homozygous FcγRIIIa-158V receptor and who receive rituximab have a greater probability of clinical and molecular response than those patients who carry the FcγRIIIa-158F receptor, a finding that suggests that the ADCC mechanism of rituximab is more effective in the patients with homozygous FcγRIIIa-158V receptors.[149,157] However, FcγRIIIa polymorphisms were not predictive for response to rituximab in patients with chronic lymphocytic leukemia, which suggests that unlike the case with NHL, mechanisms of tumor cell clearance other than ADCC may be more important in chronic lymphocytic leukemia.[153] Interestingly, results from a recent investigation provide evidence that CD20 mAb-induced blood B cell clearance may not necessarily correlate with tissue B cell clearance.[160]

Because FcγRIIIa polymorphism is strongly associated with response to rituximab in NHL, these findings need to be considered in the development of new drugs targeting the CD20 antigen.

5,10-Methylenetetrahydrofolate Reductase

The flavin adenine dinucleotide-dependent enzyme 5,10-methylenetetrahydrofolate reductase (MTHFR) plays a key role in folate and Hcy metabolism. MTHFR resides at a metabolic branch point directing the folate pool toward Hcy remethylation and DNA methylation, at the expense of DNA and RNA biosynthesis, by catalyzing the irreversible conversion of 5,10-methylenetetrahydrofolate to 5-methyltetrahydrofolate.[161] The latter provides methyl groups for methionine synthesis from Hcy and *S*-adenosyl methionine, a common methyl donor for purine and pyrimidine biosynthesis, which is crucial for DNA methylation. Alternatively, the one-carbon unit of 5,10-methylenetetrahydrofolate is used for DNA and RNA synthesis (Fig. 9–4). Because MTHFR affects folate distribution, Hcy metabolism, and DNA methylation, genetic defects that change the activity of MTHFR have the potential to modulate disease risk and effects of medications.

Two common variations in the *MTHFR* gene, a cytosine to thymine transition (677C>T) leading to the amino acid substitution Ala222Val and an adenine to cytosine transition (1298A>C) leading to the amino acid change Glu429Ala, result in diminished enzyme activity owing to enhanced thermolability.[162] The frequencies of the 677C>T and 1298A>C alleles are similarly distributed among many ethnic groups.[162] The most extensively studied MTHFR variant contains the 677C>T nsSNP. The MTHFR enzymatic activity in persons with the homozygous *677TT* genotype (approximately 10% to 16% in white and Asian populations) is approximately 30% that of persons with the wild-type variant (*677CC*). Thus, the *TT* genotype leads to an elevated plasma concentration of Hcy, particularly in persons with low folate status.[162,163] The *TT* variant has been associated with numerous consequences, increased risk of disease (eg, cardiovascular disease, renal failure), congenital abnormalities, pregnancy complications, cancer risk, and altered drug effects (eg, MTX).[161,162] Whereas a meta-analysis published in 2002 suggested that persons with the *TT* genotype and inadequate folate status have a significantly higher risk of coronary heart disease, which is probably due to elevated Hcy levels,[164] a meta-analysis published in 2005 was unable to confirm this previous finding.[165] Nevertheless, Hcy levels can be markedly decreased in persons with the *TT* genotype by daily supplementation of folic acid (0.5 to 2.0 mg).[161] During the past decade, conflicting data have been reported on the impact of variations in the *MTHFR* gene and the risk of thromboembolic disease.[166–171] In most case–

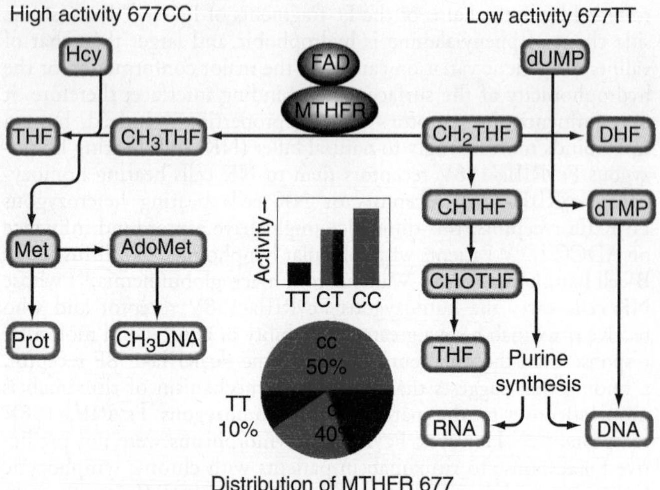

Figure 9–4 The 677C>T methylenetetrahydrofolate reductase (MTHFR) polymorphism affects the distribution between folate species used for DNA and RNA syntheses and the 5-methyltetrahydrofolate form required for homocysteine remethylation and thus protein synthesis. The pie chart in the *center* indicates the genotype prevalence often found in white populations and the associated *vertical boxes*, the relation between genotype and MTHFR activity. AdoMet, *S*-adenosylmethionine; CH_3DNA, DNA methylation; CHOTHF, formyltetrahydrofolate; CHTHF, methenyltetrahydrofolate; CH_2THF, 5,10-methylenetetrahydrofolate; CH_3THF, 5-methyltetrahydrofolate; DHF, dihydrofolate; dTMP, thymidine 5′-monophosphate; dUMP, uracil 5′-monophosphate; FAD, flavin adenine dinucleotide cofactor; Hcy, homocysteine; Met, methionine; Prot, protein; THF, tetrahydrofolate. *(Modified from Ueland PM, Refsum H, Beresford SAA, Vollset SE: The controversy over homocysteine and cardiovascular risk. Am J Clin Nutr 72:324, 2000. With permission from the American Journal of Clinical Nutrition. © Am J Clin Nutr. American Society for Clinical Nutrition.)*

control studies of the risk for venous thromboembolic disease, a leading cause of morbidity and death, no significant associations with *MTHFR* variations were observed[169–171]; therefore, it is unlikely that 677C>T and 1298A>C variants are significant risk factors for venous thromboembolic disease.

Additional examples of consequences of variations in the *MTHFR* gene are potentially relevant in hematology, namely, risk for and outcome of leukemia and MTX toxicity. Low-function *MTHFR* variants conserve intracellular folate in a cyclic pathway by shunting one-carbon groups toward thymidine and purine synthesis.[161] These variants also confer decreased *S*-adenosinemethionine synthesis, which is associated with a lower rate of DNA methylation.[172] Numerous case–control studies have evaluated the association between *MTHFR* variants and the risk of acute leukemia in both adults and children. However, in a recent meta-analysis that included the results of 13 studies, no association between the 1298A>C polymorphism and susceptibility to childhood or adult ALL was disclosed.[173] The 677C>T polymorphism in the *MTHFR* gene might contribute to risk of ALL in adults,[173] but this variant does not seem to play a major role in risk modulation in children with ALL, at least for populations with adequate folate intake.[174,175] These provocative findings require further study to fully elucidate whether a combination of unfavorable folate pathway genotypes, diet, and vitamin B status may be a key factor in susceptibility to ALL.

The response of medications that target folate metabolism (e.g., MTX) could theoretically be modulated by genetic variants of *MTHFR*. Increased toxicity (oral mucositis) was observed in patients with the 677TT genotype (decreased MTHFR activity) who received low-dose MTX as graft-versus-host disease prophylaxis after stem cell transplantation for chronic myelogenous leukemia.[176] It is hypothesized that MTX induces a more extensive folate depletion in patients who have low MTHFR activity and leads to a greater decrease in DNA synthesis and less ability to repair DNA, which results in greater damage and delayed healing.[176] Three other studies in small patient groups confirmed the potentially higher toxicity after low-dose MTX treatment in patients with the *TT* genotype, treated for ovarian cancer,[177] breast cancer,[178] and adult ALL.[179] For example, patients with the *TT* genotype had a 40-fold higher relative risk for severe (G3/G4) toxicity during low-dose MTX treatment (2.5 mg daily for 21 days) for ovarian cancer.[177] Of importance, this finding does not apply to patients receiving high-dose MTX treatment with leucovorin rescue, probably because leucovorin directly bypasses MTX-induced folate depletion to prevent MTX toxicity.[180]

Recently, the effect of the deactivating *MTHFR* allele on treatment outcome of children with ALL was assessed in the Children's Cancer Study Group ALL study CCG-1891, and it was shown that patients who carried the *MTHFR* 677C>T variant allele had significantly higher risk of relapse.[181] If these preliminary data can be confirmed, MTX dose adjustments based on *MTHFR* genotypes may help improve MTX therapy in childhood ALL.

ADVERSE DRUG EFFECTS PRESENTING AS HEMATOLOGIC DISORDERS

Adverse drug reactions (ADRs) constitute a major clinical problem, and strong evidence indicates that ADRs account for approximately 5% of all hospital admissions and increase the length of hospitalization by 2 days.[182] Although the factors that determine susceptibility to ADRs are unclear in most cases, there is increasing interest in the role of genetics[183]; therefore, the availability of a genetic test that identifies patients at risk for rare but serious adverse effects has particular appeal. Several medications whose adverse effects have been associated with variability in candidate genes and manifest predominantly as hematologic abnormalities are listed in Table 9–1. By using genome-wide analyses, gene signatures were recently identified in leukemia cells of children treated for ALL, that were associated with the development of treatment-induced AML[184] and secondary brain tumors.[185] Further investigations are necessary to confirm these data, which suggest that germline-driven gene expression across different tissues may relate to the risk of secondary malignancy following antileukemic treatment.

DRUG DEVELOPMENT

Optimizing the selection and dosage of medications is a principal goal of pharmacogenomics. Another important application is in drug development, which is evolving in parallel with improved insights into the mechanisms by which medications exert their pharmacologic effects. Such improved insights into the mechanism(s) of drug action in target cells will help elucidate mechanisms that confer drug resistance, and they will facilitate the development of strategies to further enhance efficacy. This knowledge can be used as a basis to engineer drugs that amplify treatment effects or bypass resistance mechanisms, or both. For example, identification of the mechanism underlying rituximab resistance, a genetically determined functional change in the Fc receptor domain, enables the design of more specific antibodies for patients bearing the FcγRIIIa-158F variant.[149] Indeed, in contrast to rituximab, anti-CD20 mAb with enhanced affinity for FcγRIIIa has been demonstrated to activate NK cells and ADCC effectively irrespective of FcγRIIIa polymorphism.[186]

One of the most powerful tools to study mechanisms of drug action is genome-wide analysis of gene expression profiles by means of high-density microarrays. In addition, this approach offers the opportunity to identify previously unknown drug targets. The feasibility of this method has been recently demonstrated in studies of several hematologic diseases.[187–195] For example, recent pharmacogenomic studies shed light on the biological basis of treatment failure in childhood ALL, by investigating gene expression signatures that

Table 9–1 Selected Pharmacogenetic Defects That Lead to Adverse Drug Reactions Manifesting as Hematologic Disorders

Adverse Effect	Causative Drug(s)	Altered Protein	Important Genetic Variant(s)*	Hypotheses on Pathophysiology	References
Myelosuppression	6-Mercaptopurine 6-Thioguanine azathioprine	Thiopurine-6-methyltransferase (TPMT)	TPMT*2: 238G>C; TPMT*3A: 460G>A; 719A>G; and TPMT*3C: 719A>G	In hematopoietic cells, TPMT inactivates cytotoxic thioguanine nucleotides (TGNs) by methylation. Accumulation of TGNs as a result of the functionally defective TPMT variants causes severe hematotoxicity.	See text
Myelosuppression (diarrhea)	Irinotecan (CPT-11) Active metabolite: 7-ethyl-10-hydroxycamptothecine (SN-38)	UDP-Glucuronosyltransferase (UGT) isoenzyme 1A1 (UGT1A1)	UGT1A1*28: promotor polymorphism; dinucleotide insertion in the TATA box [wild-type: (TA)6TAA] resulting in (TA)7TAA	The cytotoxic metabolite of CPT-11, SN-38, is mainly inactivated by UGT1A1. Accumulation of cytotoxic SN-38 in hematopoietic and intestinal cells is due to decreased inactivation (glucuronidation) by the variant enzyme.	References 206–208
Myelosuppression (mucositis, neurotoxicity)	5-Fluorouracil (5-FU)	Dihydropyrimidine dehydrogenase (DPD)	DPYD*2A: G to A mutation in the invariant GT splice donor site flanking exon 14 (IVS14+1G>A); leading to skipping of exon 14 during splicing	DPD is the rate-limiting enzyme in 5-FU catabolism. Skipping exon 14 during splicing renders the enzyme inactive and can, therefore, be one cause of severe 5-FU toxicity as a result of prolonged 5-FU exposure.	References 209 and 210
Venous thrombosis	Oral contraceptives	Prothrombin (FII, F2)	Factor II 20210G>A; SNP in the 3 untranslated regions (UTR) at position 20210	Factor II 20210G>A causes elevated prothrombin level, which is a risk factor for thrombosis. Oral contraceptives are an additional independent risk factor, and both (FVL) raise the risk of thrombosis	References 212–215
Venous thrombosis	Oral contraceptives	Factor V (FV, F5)	FVL: 1691G>A (in exon 10 of the FV gene) leads to Arg506Gln change lies within the activated protein C cleavage site	FVL causes activated protein C resistance, which is a thrombotic risk factor. Oral contraceptives are an additional independent risk factor, and both (+ factor II 20210G>A) raise the risk of thrombosis	References 212–215
Bleeding risk	Warfarin and other coumarin derivatives	Cytochrome P450 isoenzyme 2C9 (CYP2C9)	CYP2C9*2: 430C>T in exon 3 leads to an Arg144Cys change. CYP2C9*3: 1075A>C in exon 7 leads to an Ile359Leu change.	CYP2C9 is the most important enzyme in the catabolism of *S*-warfarin. The CYP2C9*3 allele leads to an amino acid change in the substrate-binding site, a decrease in enzyme activity (additionally seen in CYP2C9*2 allele), and an accumulation of S-warfarin, which enhances the risk of bleeding.	See text

*Nucleotide bases: A, adenine; C, cytosine; G, guanine; T, thymine.
Ig, immunoglobuline; SNP, single-nucleotide polymorphism; UDP, uridine diphosphate.

were associated with in vitro sensitivity of diagnostic ALL cells to prednisolone, vincristine, L-asparaginase, and daunorubicin. Importantly, only few of the identified intrinsic drug resistance genes have been previously linked to drug resistance, and the identified gene expression signatures discriminated patients who were at higher risk for relapse.[193,194] Moreover, using genome-wide gene expression analyses, the FMS-like tyrosine kinase 3 (*FLT3*) gene was identified as being overexpressed in *MLL*-rearranged and hyperdiploid ALL.[189] FLT3 inhibitors have been shown to inhibit growth in cells that overexpress FLT3.[196,197] Thus, the inclusion of FLT3 inhibitors seems

Relevance to Clinical Hematology

Mercaptopurine Dosage Adjustment Based on TPMT Genotypes in Acute Lymphoblastic Leukemia

Mercaptopurine (MP) is a mainstay of treatment of childhood acute lymphoblastic leukemia (ALL). However, conventional doses of this prodrug can induce severe hematotoxicity in patients who have impaired thiopurine metabolism in hematopoietic tissues owing to less-stable thiopurine *S*-methyltransferase (TPMT) enzyme variants. The three major variant alleles (*TPMT*2, TPMT*3C,* and *TPMT*3A*) encoding the variant proteins can quickly be determined by commercially available Clinical Laboratories Improvement Act-certified molecular diagnostics or in special laboratories (eg, Prometheus Labs, San Diego, CA) using samples obtained from peripheral blood before MP therapy. In patients with two nonfunctional alleles (1 out of 300), MP dosage must be reduced to 10% to 15% of conventional dosages. Patients with one variant allele (5%–10% of the population) can tolerate MP at full dosage; however, in intolerant patients, a dose reduction of 50% often is required.

worthy of being investigated in the therapy of the poor prognostic ALL subtype with *MLL* rearrangements, and perhaps hyperdiploid ALL that also overexpress FLT3.[188] Most recently, a new approach was used to computationally connect disease-associated gene expression signatures (eg, ALL blast cells that are intrinsically sensitive or resistant to glucocorticoid (GC)-induced apoptosis in vitro) to drug-associated gene expression profiles (ie, the so called Connectivity Map; http://www.broad.mit.edu/cmap/)[198] in order to identify molecules that reverse a drug resistance signature.[199] This strategy builds on prior findings that small molecules can induce treatment-specific changes in gene expression in leukemia cells in vivo.[195] Indeed, the profile induced by the mTOR inhibitor rapamycin was found to match the signature of GC sensitivity in ALL cells. Moreover, it was shown that rapamycin sensitized a resistant leukemia cell line to GC-induced apoptosis via a modulation of antiapoptotic protein MCL-1.[199] This is consistent with earlier work revealing MCL-1 overexpression in steroid-resistant ALL.[193] This work suggests that GC in combination with rapamycin could be an effective approach to overcome intrinsic GC resistance in ALL, and provides evidence that such a chemical genomic approach based on gene expression might be useful to identify molecules with the potential to overcome intrinsic drug resistance in leukemia.

CHALLENGES FOR THE FUTURE

Pharmacogenomics has already been proved to be an important approach to improve drug therapy. For example, the FDA has recently approved a label for irinotecan to prevent severe hematotoxicity based on the assessment of sequence variants in the uridine diphosphate glucuronosyltransferase (UGT) 1A1 gene; ie, a reduction in the starting dose is recommended for patients homozygous for *UGT1A1*28* allele. In most occasions, however, testing for a single allele of a single gene is unlikely to provide sufficient information to establish precise pharmacogenomic models that help explain all differences in drug effects among individuals. Clearly, further progress depends on the development and refinement of strategies and methods to elucidate the inherited determinants of drug effects. For the development of strategies, a number of crucial issues must be considered; a major one is that the inherited component of drug response often is polygenic (see Fig. 9–1). Approaches to elucidate polygenic determinants of drug response include, for example, the use of anonymous SNP maps to perform genome-wide searches for genetic variants that are associated with the effects of certain drugs and the *candidate-gene strategy*. The latter is based on existing knowledge of a medication's mechanisms of action and pathways of metabolism and disposition. These approaches and their potential value and limitations have been the subjects of recent reviews.[31,200] The candidate-gene strategy offers the advantage of focusing on a manageable number of genes, and variations within, that are likely to be of importance in the pharmacokinetic and pharmacodynamic pathways of certain drugs. However, lack of knowledge of these pathways is an inherent limitation of this approach. Gene expression profiling, proteomic studies,[201] and metabonomic investigations[202] are additional evolving strategies for identifying genes and the mechanisms by which their products may contribute to drug response.

Epigenetic changes, mainly methylation, have recently been demonstrated to be implicated in the regulation of drug-metabolizing enzyme activity.[203,204] This indicates that genetic and epigenetic mechanisms may act separately or in concert to influence pharmacological effects. In addition, in hematologic malignancies like leukemias, allele-specific copy number differences exist between host cells (ie, germline genotype) and malignant cells (which often contain cytogenetic aberrations including trisomies and gene amplification). As recently documented, these differences can cause disconcordance between germline genotypes and leukemia cell phenotypes.[205] Therefore, qualitative and quantitative genomic investigations and the analysis of epigenetic factors may be necessary to establish precise pharmacogenomic models in hematologic malignancies.

In order to define valid pharmacogenetic traits, rigorous correlations between genotype and phenotype have to be established and validated. This implicates the need for well-characterized patient groups who have been uniformly treated and systematically evaluated to make it possible to estimate drug response more objectively. To this end, investigators should try to obtain genomic DNA for pharmacogenetic studies from all patients enrolled in clinical drug trials, with appropriate informed consent. Racial and ethnic differences in the frequency and nature of genetic variants also must be recognized in attempting to extrapolate research from one population to another. For example, approximately 35% of whites have variant alleles in the *CYP2C9* gene, but these variants are virtually nonexistent in African Americans and Asians. Therefore, pharmacogenomic relations must be validated for each therapeutic indication in different racial and ethnic groups, as well as in different treatment and disease contexts. Remaining cognizant of these caveats will help ensure accurate elucidation of genetic determinants of drug response and facilitate the translation of pharmacogenomics into the field of hematology.[6]

SUGGESTED READINGS

Cheok MH, Evans WE: Acute lymphoblastic leukaemia: A model for the pharmacogenomics of cancer therapy. Nat Rev Cancer 6:117, 2006.

Eichelbaum M, Ingelman-Sundberg M, Evans WE: Pharmacogenomics and individualized drug therapy. Annu Rev Med 57:119, 2006.

Evans WE, Relling MV: Moving towards individualized drug therapy with pharmacogenomics. Nature 429:464, 2004.

Evans WE, McLeod HL: Pharmacogenomics—drug disposition, drug targets, and side effects. N Engl J Med 348:538, 2003.

Kamali F. Genetic influences on the response to warfarin. Curr Opin Hematol 13:357, 2006.

Need AC, Motulsky AG, Goldstein DB: Priorities and standards in pharmacogenetic research. Nat Genet 37:671, 2005.

Rocha JC, Cheng C, Liu W, et al: Pharmacogenetics of outcome in children with acute lymphoblastic leukemia. Blood 105:4752, 2005.

Szakacs G, Paterson JK, Ludwig JA, et al: Targeting multidrug resistance in cancer. Nat Rev Cancer 5:219, 2006.

Wang L, Weinshilboum R: Thiopurine *S*-methyltransferase pharmacogenetics: Insights, challenges and future directions. Oncogene 25:1629, 2006.

Wilkinson GR: Drug metabolism and variability among patients in drug response. N Engl J Med 352:2211, 2005.

REFERENCES

For complete list of references log onto www.expertconsult.com

PART

II

IMMUNOLOGIC BASIS OF HEMATOLOGY

CHAPTER 10

OVERVIEW AND COMPARTMENTALIZATION OF THE IMMUNE SYSTEM

Leland D. Powell and Linda G. Baum

The human immune system is assigned the seemingly impossible role of keeping at bay the universe of pathogens seeking to invade and take advantage of the permissive conditions found in mammals for growth. It also plays a less celebrated but equally important role in the clearance of dead cells and tissues, promoting wound healing, and recognition of transformed cells. It is a complex, multilayered system that has evolved over millions of years, and early vestiges of our current immune system can be found in simple invertebrate species. The tasks assigned to it are to recognize and rapidly neutralize invading pathogens and their toxins, with minimal damage to host tissues in the process; to recognize new pathogens, including those with a high degree of likeness to the host; to discriminate between trace amounts of virulent organisms or toxins and more abundant amounts of foreign yet benign dietary or environmental structures; and to distinguish between healthy viable cells and apoptotic or necrotic cells. Disorders that are the consequence of immune underreactivity or overreactivity are found in all medical specialties. Methods of manipulating the immune system in the areas of infectious disease, transplantation biology, and tumor immunology are active frontiers of medical research.

Conceptually, the immune response may be divided into innate and adaptive systems (Table 10–1). The innate system is evolutionarily the oldest, with many components found in invertebrate species. It is a system of cells and constitutively expressed membrane-bound or soluble receptors on those cells that recognize specific pathogens without the requirement of prior exposure. Pathogen–receptor binding results in the immediate activation of specific protective humoral and cellular responses. In contrast, cells of the adaptive system do not mount an effective response on first encounter with a pathogen because of the limited numbers of antigen-specific T and B cells present in a naive host. However, recurrent infections or infections by pathogens that escape the innate immune system result in the expansion of populations of pathogen-specific lymphocytes (ie, formation of immunologic memory).

The innate and adaptive immune systems have been characterized in depth at the cellular and molecular levels. The principal goal of these systems is defense against pathogens seeking entry through one of four anatomic sites: the respiratory, gastrointestinal, and genitourinary tracts and the skin. Consequently, immune function can be fully understood only by examining the anatomy of these four entry points and their relation to lymphatics, blood vessels, and lymphoid organs. This chapter provides an introduction to the molecular and cellular components of innate and adaptive immunity with an overview of their anatomic relationships.

THE INNATE IMMUNE SYSTEM

Pathogen Recognition Receptors and Pathogen-Associated Molecular Patterns

Pathogen recognition receptors (PRRs) are proteins that recognize and bind to pathogen-associated molecular patterns (PAMPs); they are the cornerstones of the innate immune response.[1,2] PAMPs are molecular motifs common to bacteria, fungi, and some viruses but not viable mammalian cells. They frequently are characterized by a repeating pattern of hydrophobic or charged molecules. Common PAMPS include lipopolysaccharide (LPS or endotoxin of gram-negative bacteria), peptidoglycans and teichoic acids (gram-positive and negative bacteria), mannans (fungi), single or double-stranded RNA (viruses), or dsDNA (viruses or necrotic/apoptotic cells). An important feature of PAMPs is that they are derived from structures essential for the viability of the particular pathogen. Consequently, selective evolutionary pressure has not yielded organisms lacking them, which is reflected in the evolutionary endurance and invariance of the innate immune system. As such, they are ideal targets for immune recognition by a host organism, which is accomplished by the PRRs (Table 10–2). PRRs are germ-line encoded and constitutively expressed, key features that distinguish them from the adaptive immune system. PRRs may be soluble proteins found in the serum, lymphatic fluid, or cell cytosol or as type I transmembrane proteins expressed on the surface of marrow-derived effector cells. They are also found on the surface of or secreted by epithelial cells in the gut,[3] bronchial airways,[4] renal tubules,[5] uterus,[6] skin,[7] and endothelial cells in the liver.[8] As such, they are poised at the four major portals of pathogen entry.

PRRs encompass several different structural families (Table 10–2). Two PRR families—peptidoglycan receptor proteins (PGRPs) and the Toll-like receptors (TLRs)—were first identified in *Drosophila* and only later demonstrated in vertebrate organisms.[9] In flies, PGRPs help defend against gram-negative bacteria, and four PGRP homologs have been identified in the human genome.[10] In humans, 10 TLRs have been identified; their ligands include bacterial lipopeptides (TLR1, TLR2, TLR6), peptidoglycans (TLR2), LPS (TLR2, TLR4), fungal saccharides (TLR2, TLR6), ds and ssRNA (TLR3, TLR7, TLR8), flagellin (TLR5), and dsDNA and CpG DNA fragments (TLR9).[1,2,11] Although the TLRs may be the most characterized family of PRRs, other receptor families include the C-type lectins (including the mannose-binding lectin [MBL] and pulmonary surfactant proteins),[12,13] dectin-1,[14] macrophage scavenger receptors,[15,16] peptidoglycan recognition proteins,[10] NOD-like receptors (NLRs),[17] and RNA helicases.[18,19] Many of these receptors are transmembrane proteins and function as cellular receptors and activation molecules, whereas others are soluble serum proteins and function by neutralizing or inducing the opsonization of pathogens. Other PRRs are found as soluble proteins within the cytoplasm of cells, where they recognize intracellular bacterial components resulting from lysosomal degradation or the products of replicating viruses (NLRs and RNA helicases).

Consequences of PRR–PAMP Ligation: Phagocytosis, the Cytokine Response, and Priming the Adaptive Immune Response

PRR–PAMP ligation triggers immune and inflammatory responses in three stages. In the first, ligation induces clearance of pathogens or foreign molecules by monocytes, macrophages, and neutrophils. This process is initiated by pathogen binding directly to PRRs on the surfaces of these cells or the opsonization of pathogens bound by a soluble PRR. Internalized pathogens are destroyed by a combination of hydrolytic and oxidation reactions within vacuoles inside the phagocytic cells. Phagocytosis also triggers degranulation and the

Table 10–1 Human Innate Versus Adaptive Immune System

Feature	Innate	Adaptive
Response time	Hours to days	>5 Days
Expression	Constitutive	Induced by pathogen exposure
Shaped by pathogen exposure	No	Yes
Approximate number of gene products involved in direct pathogen recognition	10^2 to 10^3	10^{10} to 10^{14}
Clonal response	No	Yes
Found in invertebrate species	Yes	No

release into tissues of bactericidal or bacteriostatic molecules such as lysozyme, lactoferrin, myeloperoxidase, antimicrobial peptides, nitrous oxide, and superoxide radicals. These products are toxic to pathogens and induce a local inflammatory response that can lead to tissue injury. Other molecules released, including elastase and collagenase, participate in tissue injury and wound healing.[12,20–24]

The second stage is cytokine production. Despite the diversity of the PRRs, intracellularly they share common pathways, leading to the synthesis and secretion of proinflammatory cytokines, chemokines, and type I interferons, molecules that are essential for the initiation, amplification, and maintenance of innate and adaptive immune responses.[25] Many PRRs function by activating NF-κB, whereas others signal through the caspases, IRF3/5/7, MyD88, and other kinase cascade pathways. Cytokines may be categorized according to similarities in cell source, receptor structure, or biologic consequences.[26] In general, interleukins are produced by monocytes/macrophages, lymphocytes, or specialized or inflamed epithelial cells. They act on these and other cells to amplify the innate and initiate the adaptive immune responses. The interferons are produced by virtually all cells. Acting on T and natural killer (NK) cells, they propagate antiviral and antitumor responses. Chemokines are produced primarily by cells of the innate immune system and function dually as chemoattractants (ie, recruiting cells) and cytokines (ie, activating cells). Members of the tissue necrosis factor family mediate the sepsis response and cell death and they participate in the development of lymphoid organs. A simplified organization of some of the better-characterized cytokines by biologic effects is presented in Table 10–3, and a more detailed discussion of some cytokines can be found in Chapter 6.

The final stage is activation of the adaptive immune response. Both by the production of cytokines, which activate lymphocytes, and by the processing, transport, and presentation of antigens directly to T cells (primarily done by dendritic cells), PRRs and cells of the innate immune system are essential for the development of adaptive immune responses. The biology of T cells, B cells, and dendritic cells is discussed in detail in Chapters 11 to 14.

IMMUNE DEFICIENCY CONDITIONS DUE TO MUTATIONS IN THE INNATE IMMUNE SYSTEM

Studies in mice and in tissue culture cell lines have been instrumental in characterizing the roles of many PRRs listed in Table 10–2. Their significance to humans is established by diseases linked to naturally occurring mutations in either the PRRs or their intracellular signaling molecules.

In humans, 10 different MBL haplotypes have been identified, and serum levels may vary 1000-fold. Low MBL levels may contribute to more severe infections with encapsulated organisms in normal hosts and are associated with more significant infectious complications in immunocompromised individuals (such as patients with cystic fibrosis or chemotherapy-induced neutropenia).[27,28] Differences in MBL haplotype may contribute to responses to viral infections as well, including hepatitis B.

Within the TLR system, two classes of mutations have been identified: polymorphisms in the TLRs themselves and defects in the common intracellular signaling pathway used by the different TLRs. Two forms of ectodermal dysplasia with immunodeficiency (EDA-ID) are characterized multiple developmental abnormalities and with recurrent pyogenic infections.[29] These two disorders are due to mutations in IKKγ and IκBα—intracellular proteins essential for linking PRR–PAMP ligation to cell activation. The intracellular kinase IRAK4 is essential for the function of all of the 10 TLRs, and IRAK4 deficiency too has been identified in a small number of individuals. As with those affected by EDA-ID, these individuals are also affected by recurrent infections by gram-positive organisms. However, affected individuals become less susceptible with adulthood, likely owing to the development of the adaptive immune system.[30] Although these immunodeficiency disorders are rare, a larger number of individuals have been identified with specific polymorphisms within the TLRs. Studies using case–control methodologies have attempted to link these polymorphisms to susceptibility to specific infections (eg, invasive pyogenic infections, pulmonary tuberculosis, Legionnaire disease, or septic shock). Although some of these studies have suggested that specific TLR polymorphisms increase an individual's risk of these infections, not all studies have been in agreement.[31]

Mutations in NLRs have also been linked to specific diseases. The transcriptional activation CIITA is suggested to be an NLR on the basis of its similarity to established NLRs and TLRs, and CIITA mutations result in the bare lymphocyte syndrome, which is characterized by vulnerability to fungal, bacterial, and viral infections.[32] The NLR NOD2 functions intracellularly by binding to bacterial peptidoglycan and activating mitogen-activated protein kinases and NF-κB, and NOD2 mutations have been directly linked to both Crohn disease and Blau syndrome.[33] Polymorphisms in the TLRs and CD14 may be related to the development of asthma and other atopic disorders.[34] Single-nucleotide polymorphisms in *NOD2* correlate with complications (GVHD and transplant survival) after allogeneic bone marrow transplant.[35]

INNATE IMMUNITY AND TISSUE HOMEOSTASIS

Although PRRs and cells of the innate immune system are essential for microbial defense, they also function in normal tissue homeostasis. Specific PRRs are involved in the clearance of serum clotting factors, hormones, lysosomal hydrolases, senescent cells, and proteins and in wound healing.[34–37] The class A scavenger receptor on macrophages is involved in the internalization of oxidized low-density lipoprotein, the development of atherosclerosis, and the clearance of apoptotic T cells in the thymus.[15] Another aspect of tissue homeostasis is the surveillance against transformed or malignant cells, which involves interferon-γ (IFN-γ), γδ T cells, NK cells, and cytotoxic T lymphocytes (CTLs).

ADAPTIVE IMMUNE RESPONSE

The adaptive immune response deals primarily with the generation of T-cell receptor (TCR) and B-cell receptor ([BCR] or immunoglobulin [Ig]) diversity. The adaptive system achieves two goals not met by the innate system: generation of a receptor repertoire far more diverse than that represented by PRRs and the amplification of specific populations of pathogen-specific cells as a consequence of pathogen exposure (ie, generation of specific immunologic memory). Whereas innate immune function depends on germline-encoded molecules, the adaptive immune response arises from somatic mutations in TCR and BCR/Ig genes that occur during T- and B-cell development. This process results in a remarkable diversification and amplification of the repertoire of pathogen-specific recognition molecules (see Table 10–1).

Table 10–2 Human Pathogen Recognition Receptors

Receptor	Location	Ligands or PAMPS	Features
Toll-like receptors (TLRs) Leucine-rich protein)	Leukocytes and some epithelial cells in bronchial airways, urogenital tract, and gut	Cell wall components of gram-positive and gram-negative bacteria (peptidoglycans and lipopeptides), viral dsDNAs, ds- and ssRNAs, bacterial flagellin, and other pathogen-derived molecules	A family of 10 different proteins (TLR1–TLR10) found as transmembrane proteins on the surface of cells or internal endosomes, or as free cytosolic proteins; trigger cell activation and cytokine response
CD14 (Leucine-rich protein)	Soluble and membrane-bound forms found on monocytes, macrophages, and endothelial cells	LPS from gram-negative bacteria	Binding of LPS on the cell surface forms a complex including TLR4 that results in cytokine production and the sepsis response
Serum mannose-binding lectin (MBL) (C-type lectin)	Soluble protein found in serum and lymphatic fluid	Pathogen-derived carbohydrate structures containing mannose, fucose, or *N*-acetylglucosamine	Secreted by hepatocytes; binding to pathogen triggers complement activation and assembly of the membrane attack complex
Pulmonary surfactant proteins (C-type lectin)	Soluble proteins found extracellularly on pulmonary mucosal surfaces	Carbohydrate structures or lipid motifs on viral, bacterial, or fungal pathogens, and inhaled irritants including pollens	Secreted by alveolar type II cells and nonciliated bronchiolar epithelial cells; binding to pathogen induces opsonization and leukocyte activation (including alveolar macrophages)
Macrophage mannose receptor (C-type lectin)	Surface of monocytes and macrophages	Pathogen-derived carbohydrate structures similar to MBP	Ligand binding results in phagocytosis and monocytes/macrophage activation
NKG2 (C-type lectin)	Surface of NK cells	Carbohydrates on HLA molecules or other host molecules	Involved in recognition and destruction of virally infected or transformed host cells
Dectin-1 (C-type lectin)	Surface of macrophages, neutrophils, and dendritic cells	β-Glucan structures on fungi and plants	Binding results in cell activation, cytokine production, and internalization of pathogen
Class A scavenger receptors (SR-A I/II/III) (Scavenger receptor family)	Monocytes, macrophages, and epithelial cells	Modified low-density lipoprotein, cell wall components of gram-positive and gram-negative organisms	Phagocytosis of nonopsonized particles and macromolecules triggers macrophage activation and cytokine release; plays a role in the generation of atherosclerotic plaques and diabetic nephropathy
MACRO (Scavenger receptor family)	More restricted macrophage populations than SR-A, including alveolar, peritoneal, and thymic macrophage populations	Similar to SR-A, including silica particles	Phagocytosis of nonopsonized particles and macromolecules triggers macrophage activation and cytokine release
RNA helicases (RIG-I, Mda-5)	Cell cytoplasm	dsRNA	Bind to dsRNA produced during intracellular replication of certain classes of viruses
C-reactive proteins and Serum Amyloid P (Pentraxins)	Serum proteins	Bind to and affect clearance or activation of host proteins (C1q and DNA fragments) as well as constituents of some pathogenic organisms	Secreted by the liver during early acute phase response and influence clearance and complement activation of recognized macromolecules
Peptidoglycan recognition proteins	Soluble proteins found intracellularly in leukocyte granules or synthesized by the liver and secreted into the serum	Peptidoglycan structures	Direct bactericidal or bacteriostatic activity by interfering with bacterial peptidoglycan wall biosynthesis
NOD-LRR receptor family (NLR) (includes NOD, NALP, CIITA, IPAF, and NAIP proteins)	Soluble intracellular proteins	NOD1 and NOD2 bind bacterial peptidoglycan; PAMPs for other proteins not identified	Survey intracellular compartment for intracellular pathogens, binding to bacterial wall fragments produced either during bacteria proliferation or lysosomal degradation; ligand binding triggers activation of NF-κB inflammation pathway
$\alpha_v\beta_3$ (Integrin)	Epithelial cells	*Trypanosome cruzi*	Binding induces opsonization and cell activation
CD11b/ CD18 (also CR3) (Integrin)	Monocytes, macrophages, and epithelial cells	LPS, constituents of *Mycobacterium tuberculosis*, yeast saccharides (including zymosan)	Binding induces opsonization and cell activation
Sialic acid-binding immunoglobulin-like lectins (Siglecs)	Surface receptors on onocytes, macrophages, NK cells, and myeloid cells	Sialylated complex carbohydrates (found on endogenous proteins and some pathogenic organisms)	Role for binding and phagocytosis of pathogenic organisms proposed

Table 10–3 The Cytokines

Cytokines and Cellular Targets	Examples	Biologic Consequences
Interleukins		
Monocyte/macrophages, endothelial cells	IL-1, IL-2, IL-6, IL-10, IL-13, IL-16, TNF-α	Local inflammation, cell recruitment, hepatic acute phase reaction, sepsis response
B cells	IL-2, IL-4, IL-6, IL-7, IL-9, IL-14	Recruitment, activation, differentiation of B cells
T cells (type 1 cytokines)	IL-2, IL-12, IL-15, IFN-α/β/γ	Type 1 helper T cell (T_H1) response
T cells (type 2 cytokines)	IL-4, IL-5, IL-6, IL-10, IL-13	Type 2 helper T cell (T_H2) response
Interferons		
T cells and NK cells	IFN-α, IFN-β, IFN-γ	Upregulates activity of T cells and NK cells against virally infected cells and malignant cells
Tissue Necrosis Factors		
All cells except erythrocytes	TNF-α, TNF-β	Pyrexia, tissue hyperemia, capillary leak, sepsis/shock syndrome, enhancement of target cell effector functions, expansion of lymphoid compartments
Chemokines		
Monocytes/macrophages, granulocytes, dendritic cells, lymphocytes	MCPs, eotaxin, TARC, MDC, MIPs, RANTES, PF-4	Recruit and activate cells of innate and adaptive immune system to specific sites of pathogen exposure, inflammation, and/or tissue damage
Hematopoietic Growth Factors		
Hematopoietic cells in marrow and peripheral compartments	G-CSF, GM-CSF, M-CSF, SCF	Maintenance, growth, and differentiation of hematopoietic cells

G-CSF, granulocyte colony-stimulating factor; GM-CSF, granulocyte–macrophage colony-stimulating factor; IFN, interferon; IL, interleukin; MCP, macrophage/monocyte chemotactic protein; M-CSF, macrophage colony-stimulating factor; MDC, macrophage-derived chemokine; MIPs, macrophage inflammatory proteins; PF-4, platelet factor-4; RANTES, regulated on activation, normally T cell expressed and segregated chemokine; SCF, stem cell factor; TARC, thymus and activation-regulated chemokine; TNF, tumor necrosis factor.

The complex steps involved in TCR and BCR/Ig generation requires a close interplay between the innate and adaptive immune systems. A particular pathogen gaining entry through a specific anatomic site first encounters the innate defenses. The initial response, which depends on PRRs, triggers the production of cytokines that activate resident dendritic cells (DCs). DCs phagocytose and process the antigens by cleaving them into small peptides. These peptides are then presented on the DCs' surfaces bound to MHC molecules. T and B cells that recognize the processed antigens become activated and begin to divide. This antigen presentation step may occur at the site of pathogen exposure, or it may require the migration of antigen-containing DC from the point of pathogen entry through lymphatic channels to lymphoid tissues. Other consequences of the inflammatory response induced by the innate response include changes in vascular permeability, chemotaxis, and lymphocyte adhesion. These steps result in local inflammation and the recruitment of additional lymphocytes to the site of pathogen entry. DCs, B cells, and T cells are discussed in depth in Chapters 11 to 13.

CELLS OF THE INNATE AND ADAPTIVE IMMUNE SYSTEMS

Lymphocytes

The major lymphocyte subsets are B and T cells; NK cells are a specialized lymphoid population. Lymphocytes initially arise in the bone marrow and subsequently undergo maturation in peripheral lymphoid organs (ie, thymus for T cells and lymph nodes, spleen, or other lymphoid tissues for B cells). Different populations of T and B cells can be identified by unique surface phenotypes, a characteristic that has been useful in understanding normal biology and in the diagnosis of inflammatory or malignant conditions.

Mature B cells are characteristically identified by CD19 and CD20 expression. Most B cells, called B2 cells, have a $CD5^-$ phenotype and require T-cell cooperation for function. A minority population of B cells, called B1 cells, expresses CD5, does not require T-cell help, and appears to function in pleural and peritoneal immunity. Given their $CD20^+CD5^+$ phenotype, B1 lymphocytes may be the population from which chronic lymphocytic leukemia arises. B cells represent approximately 10% of the lymphocytes in the marrow or circulation but account for up to 50% of the population in spleen and lymph nodes.

After emerging from the bone marrow compartment, T cells develop further into αβ T-cell or γδ T-cell populations. The αβ T cells are the most abundant subset and include $CD3^+CD8^+$ and $CD3^+CD4^+$ T-cell populations. $CD3^+CD8^+$ T cells, which develop into CTLs, are involved in defense against virally infected or transformed cells. $CD3^+CD4^+$ T cells can be further subdivided into T_H1 cells (stimulate development of CTLs), T_H2 cells (stimulate isotype switching and antibody production in B cells), T_H17 cells (induce or enhance tissue damage secondary to autoimmune or infectious processes), or T_{reg} cells (control or limit autoimmune responses).[36–38] The γδ T cells are $CD3^+CD4^-CD8^-$ T cells that can develop in the thymus and the gut.[39] As the γδ antigen receptor on this T-cell subset is rearranged embryonically before antigen exposure, these cells may function in innate immunity. The γδ T cells represent only 1% to 5% of circulating T cells but up to 50% of the T cells in certain epithelial sites (eg, skin, intestinal tract), where their activity is influenced by local inflammation. Stimulatory and suppressive roles of γδ T cells' response to bacterial and viral infections and possibly malignant transformation have been demonstrated in experimental systems.

NK cells are a distinct lymphocyte subset and comprise approximately 10% of the circulating lymphocyte population. NK cells are identifiable by their $CD3^{-}CD56^{+}$ phenotype. They function in defense against virally infected cells and transformed cells through the generation of cytotoxic cytokines, direct cytolytic activity, and antibody-dependent cellular cytotoxicity. Pathogen recognition is accomplished through three classes of receptors, including killer-cell immunoglobulin receptors (KIRs), C-type lectins (CD94/NKG2s), and natural cytotoxicity receptors (NCRs).[40,41]

Monocytes, Macrophages, and Dendritic Cells

Monocytes develop in the bone marrow and then circulate through the blood and lymphatics with an average half-life of 1 to 3 days before migrating into tissues and maturing into macrophages.[42,43] Macrophages can be found in all tissues, particularly at points of entry for pathogens such as the skin, respiratory tract, gastrointestinal tract, and genitourinary tract. Tissue-specific macrophage populations include Kupffer cells (liver), alveolar macrophages (lung), osteoclasts (bone), microglia (central nervous system), and type A lining cells (synovia), which can be identified morphologically and by surface immunophenotype.

DCs are specialized antigen-presenting cells. Like macrophages, DCs are found at points of pathogen entry, including skin and mucosal surfaces, and locations of lymphocyte proliferation, such as germinal centers. DC biology is described further in Chapter 14.

Granulocytes

Granulocytes can be further subclassified into neutrophils, basophils, and eosinophils by the types of cytoplasmic granules that they contain. Neutrophils mature in the marrow, where 80% to 90% of the body's store of mature neutrophils resides. The recruitment of neutrophils from the marrow into the circulation and inflamed tissues can occur within hours of exposure to bacterial endotoxin. Neutrophil effector functions include phagocytosis and cytokine production, both of which are activated through PRR-, FcR-, or CR3-dependent triggering.

The basophilic leukocytes—mast cells and basophils—have several structural and functional similarities. Functionally, they are key mediators of immediate allergic and inflammatory responses, with mast cells being more predominant in tissues and basophils in circulation. Both cell types express $Fc\varepsilon R$, which induces rapid degranulation when triggered by aggregated IgE. Both cell types have granules containing histamine, platelet-activating factor, and bioactive proteoglycans. Degranulation can be rapid, producing anaphylaxis, or sustained, inducing a more sustained inflammatory response. Degranulation is also associated with leukotriene production. Differences between basophils and mast cells include the expression of receptors on basophils for IgG, C3a, and C5a and receptors on mast cells for stem cell factor, interleukin-2 (IL-2), and IL-3, and in the spectrum of cytokines produced by each cell type. Basophils and diseases related to basophils are discussed in Chapter 73.

Eosinophils are found predominantly in tissues, with a smaller fraction found in circulation. The eosinophilic granules of this subset contain hydrolytic enzymes that may be damaging to invading pathogens and host tissues. Eosinophil activation also triggers leukotriene production and the release of an array of cytokines. A role in allergic responses and defense against helminth pathogens has long been presumed according to the eosinophilia characteristic of these conditions; however, the true physiologic necessity of eosinophils has yet to be demonstrated. Eosinophils may be viewed as effector cells of the adaptive immune system, because they are acutely triggered by a B-cell product (IgE) and their development in part depends on T cells. Disorders of eosinophils are discussed in Chapter 72.

Non–Marrow-Derived Cells Involved in Immune Function

Populations of non–marrow-derived cells function in innate immunity. Renal tubular cells and epithelial cells in the gut, bronchial airways, reproductive organs, and dermis express different PRRs. In these cells, the receptors function in pathogen clearance or by triggering pathogen-dependent inflammatory responses. Bronchial airway cells secrete pulmonary surfactants and antimicrobial peptides, creating a very localized antimicrobial barrier. Liver endothelial cells use several PRRs, including the $Fc\gamma$, scavenger, and mannose receptors, to clear senescent serum proteins and pathogens. The functions of these cells dovetail with those of the leukocytes in pathogen defense and tissue homeostasis.

ANATOMY OF THE IMMUNE SYSTEM

An array of soluble mediators and a repertoire of immune cells mediate the host response to microbial pathogens, to tumors, to self-antigens in autoimmunity, and to foreign antigens in graft rejections. Where do these cells and mediators come from, and where do these interactions take place?

Immune Cell Development: Primary and Secondary Lymphoid Organs

Most immune cells or their precursors arise in the bone marrow. Bone marrow anatomy and hematopoiesis are discussed in detail in Part III of this textbook. The cellular components of the innate immune response—the neutrophils, eosinophils, basophils, and monocytes—leave the marrow as mature, functional cells. In contrast, the cellular components of the adaptive immune response leave the marrow as immature precursors (in the case of T cells) or as naive cells (in the case of B cells).

T-Cell Maturation

T-cell precursors mature into functional T cells in the thymus.[36,44,45] Thymic architecture is shown in Fig. 10–1. The thymus is composed of lymphocytes, DCs, epithelial cells, and stromal components. The thymic stroma arises primarily from the third and fourth pharyngeal pouches during fetal development, and the stroma is then populated with lymphocyte precursors emigrating from the bone marrow. The stromal meshwork of the thymus, including various types of epithelial cells, is essential for thymic development. The requirement for thymic stroma in T-cell development is demonstrated in patients with DiGeorge syndrome, otherwise known as 22q11 deletion (del22q11) syndrome. These patients have deletions of one or more genes critical for fetal development, resulting in failure of involution of the third and fourth pharyngeal pouches, and consequent absence of thymic stroma. Although DiGeorge patients have T-cell precursors in the bone marrow, they have no thymus organ and have markedly reduced numbers of mature T cells in the peripheral circulation and in tissues. As discussed in "Secondary Lymphoid Tissue", the observation that most DiGeorge patients do have small numbers of circulating mature T cells suggests that extra-thymic sites in these patients may partially substitute for the thymus in promoting T-cell maturation.

The thymus is divided histologically into two general zones, the cortex and the medulla, although these zones have microdomains where the maturing T cells, or thymocytes, are phenotypically and functionally distinct.[45–47] Thymic precursors leave the bone marrow, circulate in the blood, and selectively home to the thymus, entering the organ to populate the subcapsular cortex. At this site, TCR rearrangement begins, and maturing thymocytes move to the cortex, where continued proliferation occurs. During this phase of TCR

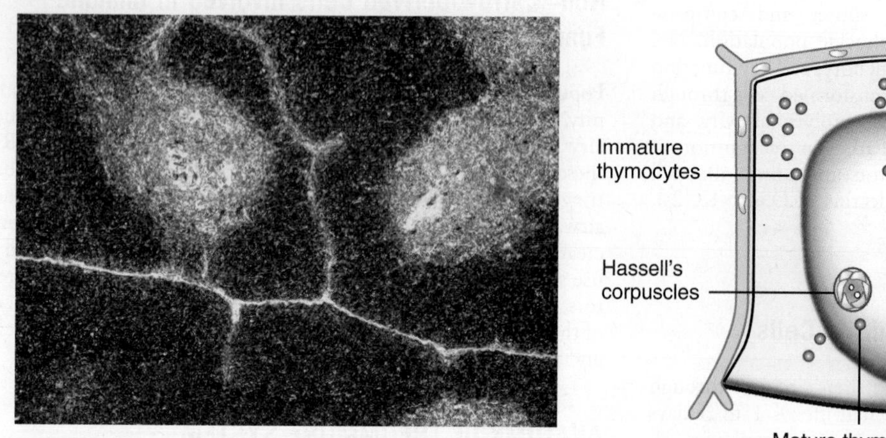

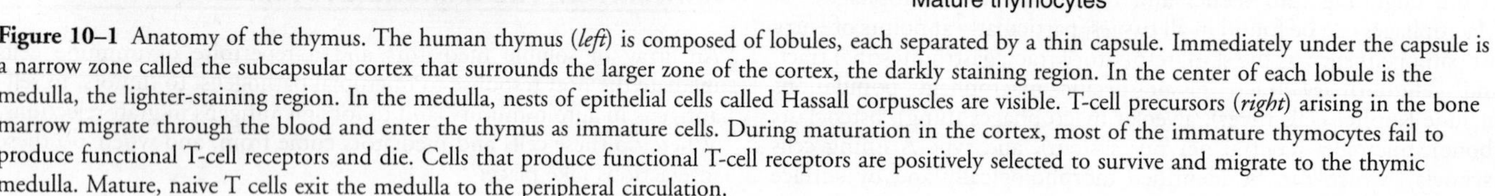
Figure 10–1 Anatomy of the thymus. The human thymus (*left*) is composed of lobules, each separated by a thin capsule. Immediately under the capsule is a narrow zone called the subcapsular cortex that surrounds the larger zone of the cortex, the darkly staining region. In the center of each lobule is the medulla, the lighter-staining region. In the medulla, nests of epithelial cells called Hassall corpuscles are visible. T-cell precursors (*right*) arising in the bone marrow migrate through the blood and enter the thymus as immature cells. During maturation in the cortex, most of the immature thymocytes fail to produce functional T-cell receptors and die. Cells that produce functional T-cell receptors are positively selected to survive and migrate to the thymic medulla. Mature, naive T cells exit the medulla to the peripheral circulation.

rearrangement and proliferation, more than 90% of the cells die in a process called *selection.* A large fraction of thymocytes fail to express a functional TCR, and these cells could never recognize antigens; these cells die of *nonselection* (ie, programmed cell death) because the cells do not receive a survival signal through a functional TCR. Of the thymocytes that do express a functional TCR, many recognize self-antigens and die through a process called *negative selection.* Negative selection is not completely understood, but involves recognition of abundant or high-affinity self-antigens that trigger robust TCR signaling, so that elimination of these developing T cells by negative selection is proposed to reduce self-reactivity and autoimmune disease. A genetic defect in presentation of self-antigens by thymic epithelial cells results in the autoimmune syndrome APECED (autoimmune endocrinopathy–candidiasis–ectodermal dystrophy).[48] Apoptotic T cells that are killed by nonselection or by negative selection are phagocytized and degraded by macrophages in the thymus. The remaining few surviving thymocytes express a functional TCR that does not appear to be autoreactive; these cells survive via a process termed *positive selection.* Positively selected thymocytes migrate to the thymic medulla, where they commit to a particular T-cell lineage (CD4 or CD8) and finally leave the thymus as functional but naive T cells.

B-Cell Maturation

In the adult, naive B cells leave the marrow and traffic to secondary lymphoid tissues, including the spleen, the lymph nodes, and the mucosa- or epithelium-associated lymphoid tissue such as Peyer patches in the small intestine. Although these tissues are critical for proper B-cell development, they are called *secondary lymphoid tissues* because these sites are also where the mature cells of the adaptive immune system encounter non-self-antigens and become activated.

B-cell maturation is described in detail in Chapter 11. Briefly, naive cells enter primary follicles in the cortex of the secondary lymphoid tissue, such as the lymph node shown in Fig. 10–2.[49] As B cells in primary follicles encounter antigens that are recognized by BCR/Ig on the cell surface, the cells begin to proliferate, and also undergo somatic hypermutation of immunoglobulin genes that results in positive selection of cells with increasing BCR affinity for antigen. Once B-cell proliferation begins, the primary follicle becomes a secondary follicle.[50] The secondary follicle has two general regions, a germinal center filled with the proliferating B cells, some T cells, macrophages, and DCs, surrounded by a mantle zone of nonproliferating B cells that have not encountered an antigen they recognize. The germinal center can be further divided into dark and light zones, depending on the stage of proliferation, as discussed below in "Systemwide Surveillance."

ENCOUNTERS WITH ANTIGEN

A primary function of the immune system is to provide protection against microbial pathogens. The most common sites for microbes to breach the protective barriers of epithelium are the skin and the respiratory, gastrointestinal, and genitourinary tracts. These tissues directly encounter the outside world, and they have evolved complex, multifaceted mechanisms for dealing with antigens.[51,52]

The local defense system is immediately activated when pathogens disrupt the epithelial barriers in these sites. These tissues are rich in components of the innate immune system, including macrophages and DCs, which perform a surveillance function in tissues. Some tissues have specialized or unique populations of macrophages and DCs (see Chapter 14), although these cells have many common features in different tissues. Macrophages provide a critical first line of defense against pathogens by directly phagocytosing microorganisms. Macrophages also send the first signals that recruit granulocytes from the circulation into the tissues (Fig. 10–3). These signals include cytokines, nitrous oxide, and leukotrienes that cause vasodilatation, endothelial cell activation, leukocyte adhesion to endothelial cells at the inflammatory site, and diapedesis of leukocytes into the tissues (see Chapter 17). The resulting exudate fluid at the site of vasodilatation is also rich in plasma proteins that participate in innate immunity, such as complement and soluble PRRs. The soluble mediators may be directly toxic to microbes or may opsonize microbes to facilitate phagocytosis and killing by granulocytes. The soluble and cellular components of the innate immune system provide the first line of defense at the tissues where pathogens invade.

These tissues contain resident lymphocytes and plasma cells. The lymphoid cells can also respond to cytokines secreted by resident macrophages, such as IL-2 that stimulates T-cell proliferation. The ability of macrophages to secrete mediators that cause vasodilatation and recruit granulocytes, as well as initiate T-cell activation, illustrates the interplay between innate and adaptive immunity in the tissues where antigens are encountered and underscores the point that the

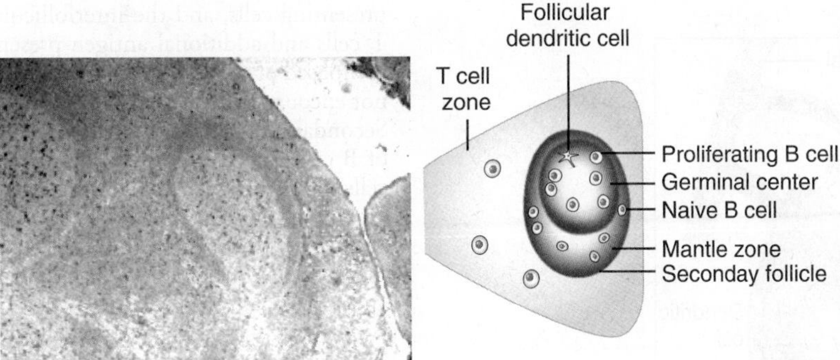

Figure 10–2 B-cell proliferation in lymph nodes. B cells primarily populate the lymphoid follicles. A section of tonsil (*left*) demonstrates a secondary follicle with a pale germinal center filled with proliferating B cells, scattered T cells, and specialized antigen-presenting cells called follicular dendritic cells (*dark staining*). The germinal center is surrounded by a darker mantle zone, populated by nonproliferating B cells. Adjacent to the follicle is the T cell-rich zone of the cortex. The schematic of a section of lymph node (*right*) demonstrates a secondary follicle with a germinal center and a mantle zone. The T cells reside primarily adjacent to the follicles. However, scattered T cells can be found in the germinal center and are typically helper T cells stimulating B-cell proliferation.

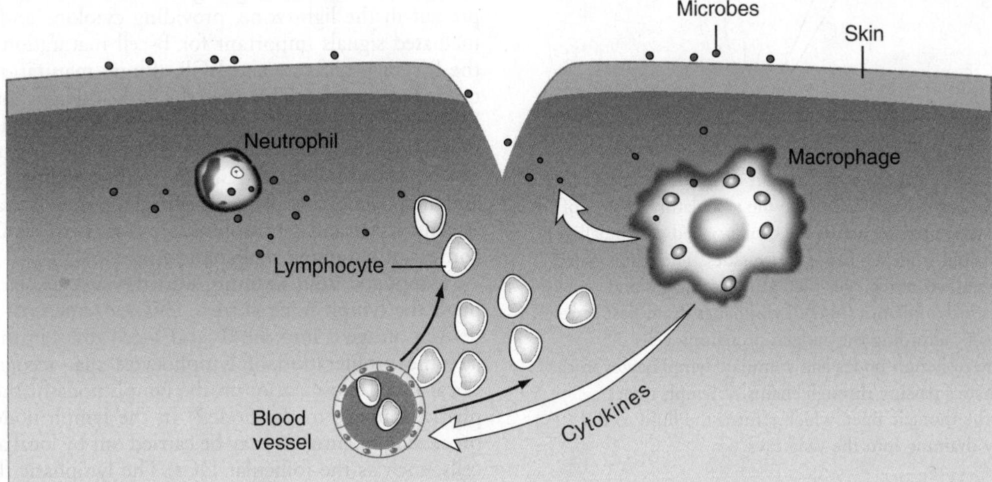

Figure 10–3 Encounters with antigen. The immune system evolved primarily to protect against invading microorganisms that penetrate the epithelial coverings of the body. In this schematic, microbes entering through a break in the skin epithelium are phagocytosed by resident macrophages as the first line of defense in innate immunity. The macrophages can secrete products that are directly microbicidal (*hatched arrow*), as well as cytokines and other mediators (*open arrow*) that cause vasodilatation and endothelial cell separation to allow influx of soluble mediators and inflammatory cells such as neutrophils and lymphocytes into the skin. Neutrophils, as a component of innate immunity, can also directly kill microorganisms, typically by releasing granular contents. Lymphocytes responding to microbial antigens proliferate and contribute to the adaptive immune response against microbes.

innate and adaptive immune systems work in concert in host defense. Resident T cells and plasma cells in the tissue can respond to antigen, with local activation of antigen-specific effector T cells and increased antibody secretion, respectively, so that the adaptive immune response is stimulated locally after pathogens are sensed by the innate immune system.

SYSTEMWIDE SURVEILLANCE: THE ROLE OF LYMPHATIC CIRCULATION

During the local inflammatory response in tissues, the exuded fluid, along with antigen-loaded DCs, T cells, and cytokines, drains from the tissues back through the lymphatic channels. Lymphatics are an essential component of the vascular system (Fig. 10–4). Even in the absence of inflammation, a fraction of the fluid component of blood leaves the capillary bed continually during circulation, because of the pressure drop between the arterial and venous sides of the vasculature. This fluid bathes the tissues, picking up antigens and cells, and drains into lymphatic channels that interdigitate in every capillary bed. At sites of inflammation, the amount of fluid and cells that drain into local lymphatics increases in response to effects on vascular tone and permeability by chemokines, lipid mediators, and oxygen radicals produced locally by activated macrophages and neutrophils. Lymphatic fluid eventually returns to the circulation by draining through the thoracic duct into the vena cava. However, before returning to the venous circulation, the lymphatic fluid travels through the secondary lymphoid tissue such as lymph nodes and spleen, which serve as sites of systemic surveillance. Signals from cells within the lymph nodes can also expand the lymphatic network, again resulting in increased drainage of DCs and antigens into the nodes.[53] The movement of lymphatic fluid through secondary lymphoid tissue is an essential component of the adaptive immune system.

Lymph node anatomy is shown schematically in Fig. 10–5; the anatomy of lymph nodes and the spleen is also discussed in Chapter 11. Fluid and cells enter the lymphatics in the tissues and travel through the lymphatics to the lymph nodes. The fluid and cells enter the lymph nodes on the convex surface through the afferent lymphatics that drain into the subcapsular sinus. Under the subcapsular sinus is the cortex of the lymph node. The cortex is composed of follicles that contain primarily B cells, along with some T cells and antigen-

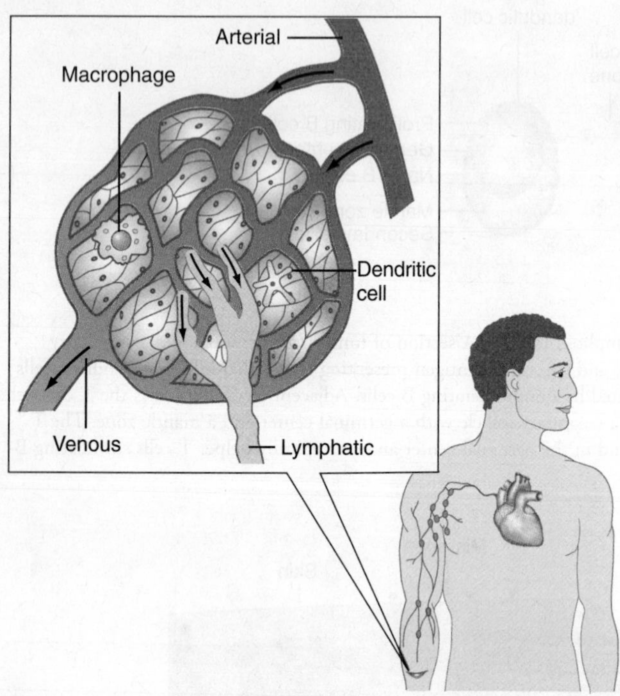

Figure 10–4 Lymphatic drainage is a critical part of immune surveillance. As shown in Figure 10–3, fluid and cells leave the vasculature at sites of inflammation. Hydrostatic pressure across the capillary bed continually drives transudation of fluid from the blood into tissues. The extravasated fluid, along with antigen-presenting cells such as macrophages and dendritic cells, collects in lymphatics (*inset*). Lymphatics drain past series of lymph nodes (*dark ovals*), affording the antigen-presenting cells the opportunity to migrate to lymph nodes and stimulate lymphocytes in the nodes. Fluid in lymphatics passing through chains of lymph nodes eventually collects in the thoracic duct, which returns the fluid to the vascular circulation by draining into the vena cava.

presenting cells, and the interfollicular zones that contain primarily T cells and additional antigen-presenting cells. Primary follicles are composed of naive B cells that are not proliferating because they have not encountered antigen recognized by BCR/Ig on the B-cell surface. Secondary follicles have a germinal center that is composed primarily of B cells that are proliferating in response to antigens presented by cells in the germinal center, and a surrounding mantle zone containing primarily quiescent naive B cells that have not encountered an antigen they recognize. The central part of the lymph node, the medulla, contains additional antigen-presenting cells, some T cells, and numerous plasma cells. Plasma cells differentiate from follicular B cells and migrate to the medulla, where most plasma cells leave the lymph node to traffic to peripheral tissues.

The germinal center can be further divided into a light zone and a dark zone.[54,55] The dark zone consists primarily of rapidly dividing immature B cells called centroblasts. In the light zone, nondividing B cells called centrocytes undergo positive selection, similar to the process described for T cells in the thymus, to select for B cells that express functional BCR/Ig. In the light zone, centrocytes interact with a unique population of DCs, called *follicular DCs*, that present antigens to B cells undergoing selection. $CD4^+$ helper T cells are also present in the light zone, providing cytokine and cell–cell contact-mediated signals important for B-cell maturation and selection. As the B cells proliferate and BCR affinity maturation occurs, the cells traffic back and forth between the dark and light zones, to continually encounter DCs and T cells that provide essential signals for B cell maturation and survival. B cells that fail this selection process (ie, do not express a functional BCR) die in the germinal center by apoptosis and are phagocytized by macrophages. Some of these cell types, such as centrocytes and centroblasts, are discussed (see Chapter 75) in the context of lymphoid malignancies.

Lymphatic fluid draining into the subcapsular sinus travels through the lymph node cortex. This movement of antigen-rich fluid delivers antigens into the B- and T-cell zones in the cortex to stimulate the proliferation of lymphocytes that recognize the antigens. Local B-cell proliferation in the lymph node further stimulates lymphatic drainage to the node.[53] In the lymph node follicles, further processing of antigens may be carried out by local antigen-presenting cells, such as the follicular DCs. The lymphatic fluid draining into the node collects through the trabecular sinuses that run through the cortex between follicles, perpendicular to the capsule, into the

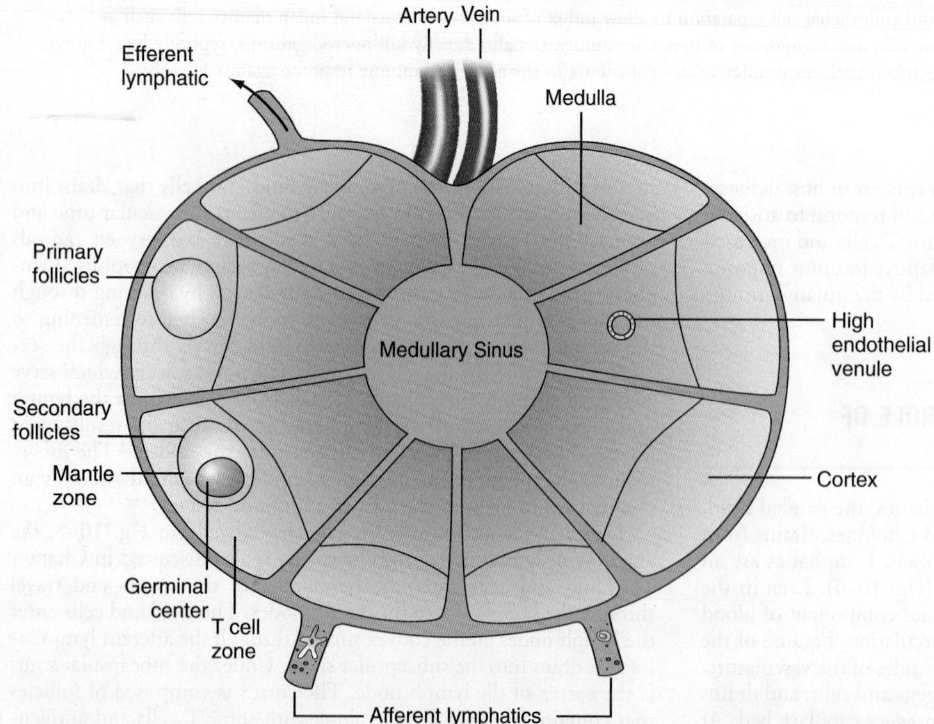

Figure 10–5 Lymph node anatomy. The lymph node is surrounded by a capsule. Afferent lymphatics draining tissues enter the node on the convex side into the capsule. Fluid and cells drain through the node and collect in the medullary sinus, where the fluid leaves the node through efferent lymphatics to rejoin the lymphatic circulation. The outer rim of the node is called the cortex and contains primary follicles composed of naive, nonproliferating B cells that have not encountered antigens and secondary follicles with proliferating B cells in the germinal center. The germinal center can be subdivided into dark and light zones. Each lymph node is supplied with blood by the arterial circulation. Arterioles expand into a meshwork of capillaries within each follicle, and venous blood drains back out of the node. Naive T cells in the peripheral circulation can exit the blood and enter the lymph node through the high endothelial venules.

medullary sinus. From the medullary sinus, the lymphatic fluid leaves the node by efferent lymphatics exiting the hilum of the node to travel through additional lymph nodes on the way to the thoracic duct. Thus, antigens and cells draining from sites of inflammation travel through chains of lymph nodes. Trace amounts of microbial proteins or toxins, together with activated monocytes/macrophages, DCs, lymphocytes, and the cytokines produced (the direct consequence of PAMP–PRR ligation), are kept in anatomic proximity, providing numerous opportunities for the antigens to encounter antigen-specific lymphocytes and stimulate the adaptive immune system.

In addition to lymphatic fluid, blood must also travel through lymph nodes, to provide oxygen and nutrients to the tissue and also to deliver new B and T cells to the tissue. Although lymphatic fluid contains lymphocytes from tissues that have already encountered antigens, lymphocytes in blood are predominantly naive T cells that have emigrated from the thymus but not yet encountered an antigen they can recognize. Arterial blood enters the lymph node at the hilum, where arterioles branch off toward each follicle. Naive T cells leave the blood to enter lymph nodes through specialized vessels called *postcapillary venules*, which arise from follicular capillary beds, and travel through the T cell-rich interfollicular zones. Naive T cells exit from postcapillary venules into the T-cell zone, and if the naive T cells encounter antigens they recognize, the cells remain in the node and proliferate. If the naive T cells do not encounter antigens they recognize, the cells drain by means of lymphatic fluid back to the blood and continue the circular route from the blood through lymph nodes to lymphatics and back to blood.

Egress of lymphocytes from lymph nodes, and from the thymus, is regulated by a specialized lipid, sphingosine-1-phosphate (S1P), that is produced in lymphoid tissues. Lymphocytes express S1P receptors that are important for facilitating lymphocyte egress from tissues into blood. Novel immunosuppressive therapeutics are being developed that are S1P antagonists; these S1P antagonists reduce release of lymphocytes from lymphoid tissues into blood.[56]

SECONDARY LYMPHOID TISSUE: COMMON AND UNIQUE ANATOMY AND FUNCTIONS

The spleen is an important site for B-cell development and for antigen presentation and stimulation of the adaptive immune system. Key differences between splenic and lymphoid anatomy are worth noting.[57] Antigens enter lymph nodes primarily by afferent lymphatics. Because the spleen has no afferent lymphatic drainage, blood enters through the splenic artery. Unlike other organs that have a closed vascular circulation in which blood travels from arterial to venous circulation through capillary beds, branches of the splenic artery penetrate into the lymphoid area of the spleen, the white pulp, and then open into marginal sinuses. From the marginal sinuses, blood filters through the parenchyma of the spleen. As lymphocytes in lymph nodes monitor lymphatic fluid for antigens, lymphocytes in the spleen monitor blood for antigens. As seen in the lymph node cortex, B cells in the splenic white pulp also form follicles, primary follicles containing naive B cells and secondary follicles with germinal centers. Surrounding the follicles are marginal zones that are populated by specialized subsets of B cells and macrophages. In the splenic white pulp, as in lymph nodes, the B- and T-cell zones are separate but contiguous.[58,59] In the splenic white pulp, the T-cell zone is found primarily surrounding a central artery, and this region is called the *periarterial lymphatic sheath* (PALS). The spleen does have efferent lymphatics, and fluid and cells that do not exit through the splenic vein collect by means of lymphatics that originate in the white pulp and drain into the lymphatic circulation.

Beyond the white pulp, the splenic artery sends additional branches into the red pulp. The red pulp contains numerous myeloid cells, including many macrophages that phagocytose unwanted components such as opsonized microbes and damaged red blood cells. The splenic red pulp is also the site of extramedullary hematopoiesis early in fetal life; extramedullary hematopoiesis in the spleen may also occur postnatally in patients with diseases in which the bone marrow is not competent to support hematopoietic cell development.

In addition to lymph nodes and the spleen, there are numerous other sites of secondary lymphoid tissue.[60] A critical part of the secondary lymphoid system is the mucosa-associated lymphatic tissue (MALT). As the name implies, the MALT is in physical proximity with the mucosa (ie, the epithelium and associated connective tissue that line the surfaces of the body). MALT is found at sites where antigens most commonly breach these epithelial barriers: the gastrointestinal, respiratory, and genitourinary tracts. In some tissues, the MALT forms relatively large structures that can be clearly distinguished histologically, such as the Peyer patches in the ileum and in the lymphoid tissue under the epithelium of the appendix. In these sites, perhaps because of the constant stimulation by microbial pathogens in the intestine, the MALT resembles lymphatic tissue in the spleen and lymph nodes, with well-demarcated primary and secondary follicles that contain primarily B cells and intervening T cell-rich zones. In other tissues, such as the genitourinary tract and the salivary glands, the microscopic anatomy of the MALT may not be as well defined as that seen in Peyer patches, but the stromal tissue underlying the epithelium contains numerous lymphocytes and antigen-presenting cells. These sites provide an additional compartment of secondary lymphoid tissue where antigens can be accumulated, processed, and presented to lymphocytes to stimulate an adaptive immune response. In addition to serving as part of the secondary lymphoid tissue, the MALT may also provide an alternative site of primary lymphoid tissue for T-cell development.[61] In support of this theory, it has been observed that children with DiGeorge syndrome, in which the thymus does not develop, do have some circulating mature T cells, although the number of T cells is greatly reduced. This suggests that the T-cell precursors emigrating from the bone marrow can mature in other sites, such as the intestine, if the thymus is absent.

Whereas the MALT constitutes a lymphoid population beneath the surface epithelium, a separate population of lymphocytes, primarily T cells, traffics directly through the epithelium in certain tissues, such as the gastrointestinal tract, on surveillance for pathogens. These intraepithelial lymphocytes (IELs) include $\alpha\beta$ T cells and $\gamma\delta$ T cells, and comprise 1 in every 5 to 10 cells in the intestinal epithelium. As the lining of the intestine is the largest organ surface area of the body, IELs are one of the largest T cell populations. These IEL T cells are comprised of different subpopulations, some of which are conventional T cells that recognize foreign antigens and some are regulatory T cells that limit the extent of an immune response and maintain immune homeostasis, a critical function in the antigen-rich milieu of the gut.[52,62]

SUGGESTED READINGS

Akira S, Uematsu S, Takeuchi O: Pathogen recognition and innate immunity. Cell 124:783, 2006.

Belardelli F, Ferrantini M: Cytokines as a link between innate and adaptive antitumor immunity. Trends Immunol 23:201, 2002.

Cheroutre H: IELs: enforcing law and order in the court of the intestinal epithelium. Immunol Rev 206:114, 2005.

Crocker PR, Paulson JC, Varki A: Siglecs and their roles in the immune system. Nat Rev Immunol 7:255, 2007.

Cyster JG, Ansel KM, Reif K, et al: Follicular stromal cells and lymphocyte homing to follicles. Immunol Rev 176:181, 2000.

Guan R, Mariuzza RA: Peptidoglycan recognition proteins of the innate immune system. Trends Microbiol 15:127, 2007.

Iwasaki A, Medzhitov R: Toll-like receptor control of the adaptive immune responses. Nat Immunol 5:987, 2004.

Kawai T, Akira S: Innate immune recognition of viral infection. Nat Immunol 7:131, 2006.

Medzhitov R, Janeway CA Jr: Decoding the patterns of self and nonself by the innate immune system. Science 296:298, 2002.

Meylan E, Tschopp J, Karin M: Intracellular pattern recognition receptors in the host response. Nature 442:39, 2006.

Steinman L: A brief history of T(H)17, the first major revision in the T(H)1/T(H)2 hypothesis of T cell-mediated tissue damage. Nat Med 13:139, 2007.

Takahashi K, Ip WE, Michelow IC, et al: The mannose-binding lectin: A prototypic pattern recognition molecule. Curr Opin Immunol 18:16, 2006.

Trinchieri G, Sher A: Cooperation of Toll-like receptor signals in innate immune defence. Nat Rev Immunol 7:179, 2007.

Turvey SE, Hawn TR: Towards subtlety: Understanding the role of Toll-like receptor signaling in susceptibility to human infections. Clin Immunol 120:1, 2006.

Villasenor J, Benoist C, Mathis D: AIRE and APECED: Molecular insights into an autoimmune disease. Immunol Rev 204:156, 2005.

REFERENCES

For complete list of references log onto www.expertconsult.com

CHAPTER 11

B-CELL DEVELOPMENT

Kenneth Dorshkind and David J. Rawlings

B cells are the subset of lymphocytes specialized to synthesize and secrete immunoglobulin (Ig). Their name derives from the finding, made in the mid-1950s, that removal of the avian bursa of Fabricius severely compromises antibody production.[1] In mammals, B-cell differentiation initiates during fetal life in various tissues, including the liver. However, during postnatal life the bone marrow is the site of B-cell production.[2–4]

The bone marrow is a primary lymphoid organ, and the generation of B cells in that tissue is referred to as *primary* B-cell production. B lymphopoiesis is dependent on the commitment of immature, multipotential hematopoietic precursors to the B-cell lineage. Subsequently, these B lineage precursors proliferate and progress through a highly regulated maturation process that culminates in the production of immature, surface Ig-expressing B lymphocytes. These newly produced, immature B lymphocytes then migrate into *secondary* lymphoid organs such as the spleen, where they undergo further maturation. These cells subsequently recirculate through the bloodstream and enter peripheral lymph nodes and spleen and are poised to respond to antigens encountered in those organs.

The aim of this chapter is to summarize B-cell development in primary and secondary lymphoid tissues. The discussion focuses initially on B-cell development during fetal and adult life and the regulation of that process by local and systemic signals. The final sections of the chapter outline B-cell development in secondary lymphoid tissues. The information presented provides a basis for understanding abnormalities of B-cell development, such as leukemia, lymphoma, and immunodeficiency states that are discussed in other chapters. Because this is a clinical textbook, the discussion preferentially focuses on human B-cell development. However, murine studies have contributed much to what is known about B-cell development, so references to the extensive literature in that species are frequent.

THE HEMATOPOIETIC HIERARCHY AND B-LINEAGE COMMITMENT

B lymphocytes, like all hematopoietic cells, are derived from hematopoietic stem cells (HSC).[5] HSC, by definition, can sustain long-term, multilineage blood cell production for the lifetime of the organism. They are able to function in this capacity because upon division they can self-renew, thereby producing additional HSC as well as more committed progenitors that ultimately give rise to myeloid and lymphoid cells.[6,7] Advances in the development of monoclonal antibodies to leukocyte cell surface antigens and achievements in flow cytometric analysis have led to isolation of these committed lymphoid and myeloid progenitors in both mouse and man (Fig. 11–1).

The *common myeloid progenitor* is an immature cell population whose downstream progeny include megakaryocyte–erythroid and granulocyte–macrophage progenitors.[8] The identification of the most immature HSC proximal lymphoid precursor is an area of active investigation. Most recent schemes of murine hematopoiesis place a cell termed the *common lymphoid progenitor*, defined in mice by its c-kit^{low} Sca-1^{low} interleukin-7 (IL-7) receptor positive (IL-7R$^+$) lineage-negative (Lin$^-$) phenotype, as the precursor from which all T and B cells arise.[9] Lin$^-$ indicates that the cells lack expression of determinants present on mature myeloid, erythroid, and lymphoid lineage cells. However, an emerging view is that CLP so defined are primarily destined to generate B lineage cells and that they are downstream progeny of an earlier lymphoid-specified precursor that does not yet express IL-7R.[10]

The definition of stages of human B-cell development has recently been reviewed in depth.[3] There is general agreement that the most immature human lymphoid progenitors are included in a Lin$^-$CD34$^+$ subpopulation of hematopoietic cells.[11,12] Galy and colleagues described a Lin$^-$CD34$^+$CD38$^+$CD10$^+$ bone marrow cell that could generate B and T cells but whose myeloid potential was attenuated.[13] Expression of the CXCR4 chemokine receptor on Lin$^-$CD34$^+$ cells also has been used to define human lymphoid precursor populations.[14] However, single cells were not manipulated in these studies, which is a prerequisite for drawing conclusions regarding a population's lineage potential.[15] Accordingly, a later study of cord blood CD34$^+$CD38$^-$CD7$^+$IL-7R$^-$ cell population is of interest. Clonal analysis has demonstrated that these cells are devoid of myeloid and erythroid potential but can generate B and T cells with high efficiency.[16]

As a result of these types of studies, increasingly detailed models of hematopoiesis, as shown in Fig. 11–1, have been formulated. These schemes imply that lineage branch-points occur at precise cellular stages of development. However, the reported existence of distinct cellular intermediates that do not fit easily into these hierarchical schemes, such as those with B, T, granulocytic, and macrophage but not megakaryocytic and erythroid developmental potential, suggests that this may not be the case.[17] In addition, Fig. 11–1 indicates that commitment to a particular developmental pathway occurs as an all-or-none phenomenon, but this almost certainly does not occur. Instead, emerging evidence suggests that lineage commitment is a gradual progression. This process has been described as occurring in two phases. In the first, termed *specification*, developmental potential becomes narrowed but cells still retain multilineage potential. On the other hand, lineage *commitment* implies an inability to generate cells other than those in a specific lineage.[18]

That specification and commitment occur gradually reflects the fact that the process of activating selected genes while suppressing the expression of others takes place in a stepwise manner. In this regard, it is increasingly accepted that these evolving patterns of gene expression ultimately resulting in lineage commitment reflect the sum total effect of transcription factors expressed and the epigenetic changes that follow in developing precursors.[19,20] Genetic studies in mice in which genes controlling expression of specific transcription factors have been disrupted have made it possible to identify where within the hierarchical model of hematopoiesis expression of a particular transcription factor is critical (see Fig. 11–1).

For example, early blood cell development is dependent on *PU.1*, an Ets family member. Mice in which this gene is not expressed can produce erythroid and megakaryocytic but not monocytic, granulocytic, and lymphoid cells. As a result of this severe defect, *PU.1* knock-out mice die during embryonic development.[19–21] The developmental potential of hematopoietic cells is further narrowed toward a lymphoid fate by products of the *Ikaros* gene. Ikaros is an interesting transcription factor because rather than activating gene expression, it acts as a repressor by associating with transcriptionally silent genes in foci containing heterochromatin.[22]

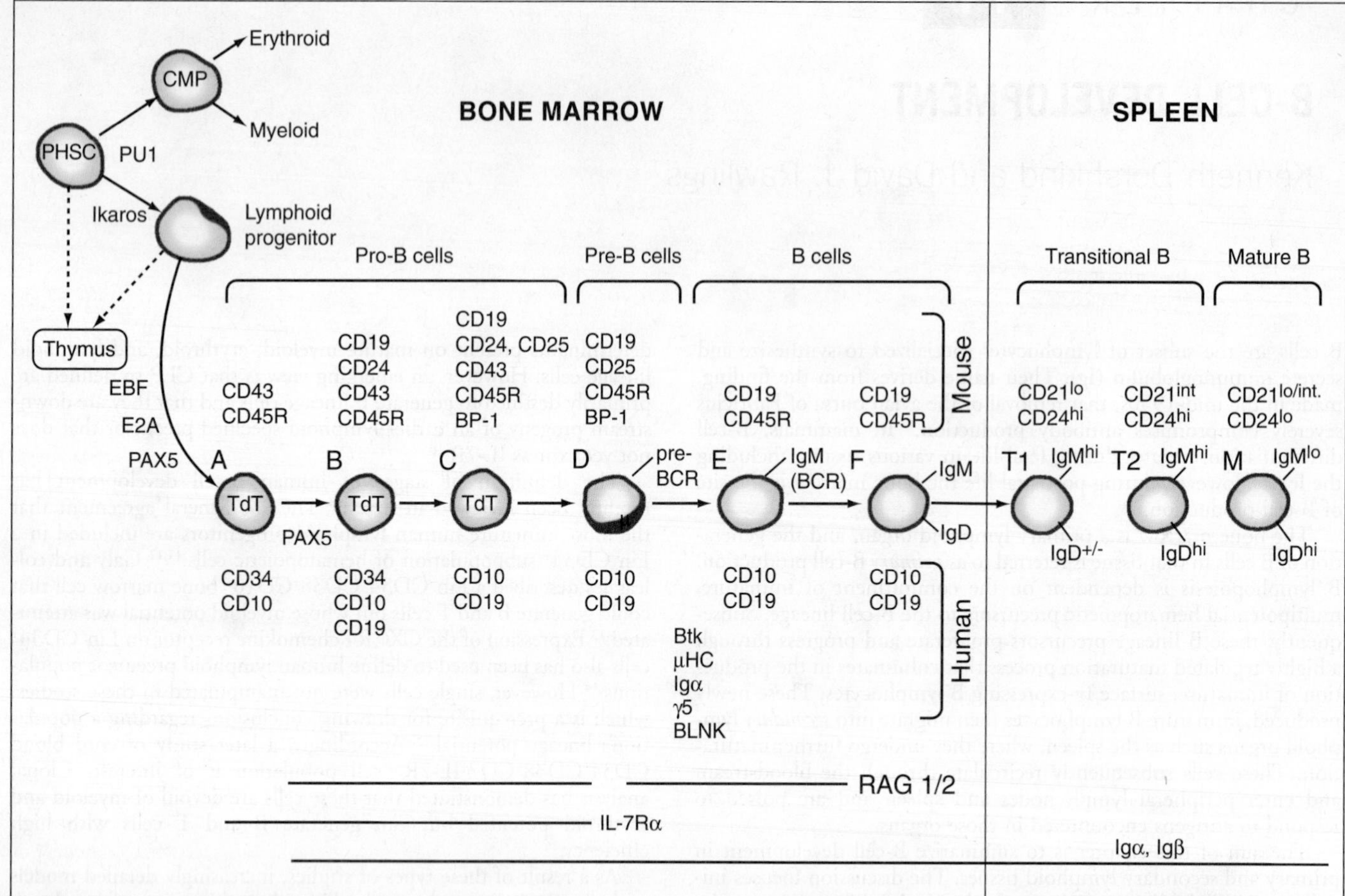

Figure 11–1 Hematopoiesis with an emphasis on B-cell development. Stages of human and murine B-cell development, and the cell surface, cytoplasmic, and nuclear determinants expressed on those cells are indicated. When comparing this scheme to others, it is important to appreciate that a uniform terminology for stages of development has not been adopted. Placement of lineage markers at various stages of development is an approximation. T1, transitional 1B cells; T2, transitional 2B cells; M, mature, naive B cells. The precise characteristics of the earliest lymphoid specified progenitor are unresolved.

T-cell, but not B-cell, progenitors can be detected in *Ikaros*-null mice, indicating that specification toward the B lineage is *Ikaros* dependent.[23] Further specification toward the B-cell lineage is dependent on expression of additional transcription factors that include early B-cell factor (EBF) and the *E2A*-encoded splice variants E12 and E47.[24–28] Each of these DNA-binding proteins regulates the expression of a variety of B-lineage target genes and induces expression of additional transcription factors that play a role in B-cell development. That EBF and E2A expression plays a critical role in B lymphopoiesis has been demonstrated by the fact that mice in which these gene products are no longer expressed exhibit an almost complete block in B-cell development at the pro-B-cell stage.

EBF- and E2A-expressing progenitors can still exhibit some myeloid potential, indicating that the expression of these DNA-binding proteins does not result in absolute commitment of cells to the B lineage. Instead, this is dependent on subsequent expression of the Pax5 transcription factor. Phenotypically identifiable B-cell precursors are present in *Pax5* knock-out mice, and when placed under appropriate conditions, they can differentiate into myeloid, T, and natural killer (NK) cells. However, if the gene encoding Pax5 is introduced into these Pax5-deficient precursors, this developmental promiscuity is no longer observed. Thus, a critical function of Pax5 is to suppress non-B lineage potential.[29,30] One way in which this is accomplished is by extinguishing expression of myeloid growth factor receptors, such as those for macrophage colony-stimulating factor. Pax5 also may inhibit the T-cell potential of lymphoid-restricted progenitors by antagonizing expression of Notch1, a cell-surface receptor whose stimulation activates signaling pathways required for commitment to the T-cell lineage.[31] Thus, Pax5-deficient pro-B cells constitute a good example of cells that have undergone specification without full commitment to the B lineage. In addition to regulating commitment to the B-cell lineage, continued Pax5 expression is necessary to maintain lineage fidelity even in relatively mature B cells.[32]

STAGES OF ADULT B-CELL DEVELOPMENT

As indicated previously, the precise characteristics of the cellular intermediates between the HSC and the most immature, B-lineage-committed progenitors are still being refined. On the other hand, there is greater certainty about the properties of B cell-committed progenitors and their downstream progeny. As a result, detailed schemes of B-cell development in mouse and human have been formulated.[2–4,33] The earliest B-lineage progenitor is termed the *pro-B cell* in both species. Ig heavy-chain gene rearrangement is under way in these cells, and if the rearrangement is successful, an Ig heavy chain of μ class is expressed in the cytoplasm. At this stage, the cells are defined as *pre-B cells*. Finally, once light-chain gene rearrangements have occurred and light-chain protein is expressed, pre-B cells mature into newly produced B lymphocytes that express the assembled Ig molecule on their surface. The designation of a cell as a B lymphocyte should be restricted to cells that express surface Ig.

Detailed phenotypic analyses of cells at various stages of pro-, pre- and B-cell development have been made, and subpopulations of cells within each compartment have been described. For example, the pro-B-cell compartment is subdivided into pre-pro-B and pro-B stages, and protocols have been described in which up to 11 different antibody combinations are used to resolve stages within the murine B-cell developmental pathway.[34] The terminology used in this chapter is that defined originally by Hardy and colleagues[35] and is based on the differential expression of CD19, CD45R (B220), CD24 (heat-stable antigen), CD43, BP-1 IgM, and IgD (see Fig. 11–1). The ability to isolate cells on the basis of the expression of one or more of these determinants has contributed much to what is known about their molecular characteristics and how they respond to various microenvironmental and systemic signals.

Figure 11–1 shows the comparable stages of human B-cell development. The most immature B-lineage-committed pro-B cells coexpress CD10, CD34, and CD19.[36] Cells at this stage of development have initiated Ig heavy-chain gene rearrangements. CD19 can be considered to be a B-lineage-specific determinant. Once an Ig heavy-chain gene has undergone productive rearrangement and is expressed, μ heavy-chain protein is detected in the cytoplasm of pre-B cells. CD10 and CD19 are present on the pre-B-cell surface, but CD34 expression is extinguished.[37,38] Finally, productive rearrangement and expression of an Ig light-chain gene result in maturation to the surface IgM-expressing B-cell stage of development. A number of additional cell-surface determinants are expressed on developing and mature B-lineage cells and include CD20, CD21, CD22, CD24, and CD40.[39] Many of these determinants are linked to critical intracellular signaling pathways (see Chapter 14). Antibodies against the CD20 determinant (rituximab) are in widespread clinical use for the treatment of lymphoma and, increasingly, autoimmune diseases.[40]

As cells mature from pro-B cells into B lymphocytes, they pass through two critical checkpoints. The first occurs at the pro-B to pre-B-cell transition and is dependent on expression of Ig heavy-chain protein. The second occurs at the pre-B to B-cell transition, where signaling through the pre-B-cell receptor (pre-BCR) leads to expression of light-chain protein and surface expression of the mature B-cell antigen receptor (BCR).

THE PRO-B TO PRE-B-CELL TRANSITION

The expression of Ig heavy-chain protein is dependent on the functional rearrangement of an Ig heavy-chain gene. If this occurs successfully, Ig heavy-chain protein of the μ class is expressed in the cytoplasm of pre-B cells.

Organization of Immunoglobulin Heavy-Chain Genes

The genes that encode Ig heavy-chain protein are located on human chromosome 14 (Fig. 11–2).[41] The heavy-chain gene consists of distinct variable (V), diversity (D), joining (J), and constant (C) regions. The V region genes are located at the 5′ end of the Ig heavy-chain gene, and each consists of approximately 300 base pairs. These genes, which are separated by short intron sequences, are organized into seven families based on sequence homology. There are approximately 25 human D region genes located 3′ to the V region. These also are grouped into families, and at least 10 have been described in humans. Downstream of the D region are six human J region genes. Finally, 10 C region genes representing alternative Ig isotypes are arranged in tandem.[42,43]

STERILE TRANSCRIPTS

Ig heavy-chain gene rearrangement is preceded by transcription at the unrearranged heavy-chain locus. This results in the production of developmentally regulated transcripts of unrearranged Ig genes, referred to as germline transcripts, or *sterile transcripts*. Multiple species of sterile transcripts have been described, and some could conceivably encode proteins. A mechanistic link between transcription and Ig gene rearrangement has been hypothesized. For example, transcription might make unrearranged Ig genes accessible to both RNA polymerase and V(D)J recombinase, the germline transcripts could function in the rearrangement reaction, or transcription could alter structural characteristics of DNA, making the recombination signal sequences (see later) better targets for recombination.[44–46]

IMMUNOGLOBULIN HEAVY-CHAIN (H) GENE REARRANGEMENT

Subsequent to the appearance of sterile transcripts, Ig heavy-chain gene rearrangements occur. Because the coding regions of the V, D, and J region segments are separated from one another, their juxtaposition with deletion of the intervening intron must occur. The initial event during heavy-chain gene rearrangement juxtaposes a D region segment to a J_H segment. Although in theory any D region gene can join with equal frequency to any one J_H region gene, there may be preferential utilization of selected D and J_H region genes at various stages of development. Following successful D–J_H recombination, a V_H region gene rearranges to the D–J_H complex. Evidence suggests that biased usage of J_H proximal V_H genes occurs in the newly generated repertoire of neonatal mice and humans.[47] The heavy-chain C region remains separated from the rearranged V_HDJ_H complex by an intron, and this entire sequence is transcribed. RNA processing subsequently leads to deletion of the intron between the V_HDJ_H complex and the most proximal C region genes. Following translation, μ heavy-chain protein is expressed in the cytoplasm of pre-B cells.[44]

The process just described is dependent on an enzymatic machinery that deletes intronic sequences and joins coding segments of DNA.[48–50] The enzymes that mediate these functions act through recognition of recombination signal sequences that are located 3′ of each heavy-chain V region exon, 5′ of each heavy-chain J segment, and 5′ and 3′ of each heavy-chain D region gene. Figure 11–2 shows the association of these recognition sequences with the various heavy-chain exons. Each recombination signal sequence consists of conserved heptamer and nonamer sequences, separated by nonconserved DNA segments of 12 or 23 base pairs. During Ig gene recombination, these recognition sequences form loops of DNA, which in turn bring the coding exons in apposition to one another. These noncoding loops are subsequently deleted and degraded.

The expression of two highly conserved proteins, referred to as RAG-1 and RAG-2, is required for heavy- and light-chain gene recombination.[51,52] Mice[53,54] and humans[55] in whom these recombinase-activating genes (*RAGs*) are not expressed do not generate B or T cells. Results from cell-free systems that measure V(D)J recombination indicate that RAG proteins are involved in cleavage of DNA at recombination signal sequences. The RAG proteins also are needed for subsequent efficient joining of coding sequences to one another.[50] In addition to the RAG proteins, general DNA repair enzymes, and those encoded by the Ku complex of genes in particular, also play a critical role in Ig heavy-chain gene recombination.[56,57]

ALLELIC EXCLUSION

Each pro-B cell has two Ig heavy-chain genes, but only one of these encodes μ protein in any given cell. This phenomenon is known as *allelic exclusion*.[51] One theory for how this occurs is that functional Ig rearrangements are rare, so the chance that two functional rearrangements will occur in an individual cell is extremely low.[58] An increasingly accepted second model of allelic exclusion is that the expression of μ protein from a successfully rearranged allele inhibits rearrangements at the other heavy-chain allele.[59] As discussed subsequently, these signals may be mediated through the pre-BCR complex.[60] However, if rearrangements are unsuccessful at one heavy-chain locus during B-cell development, recombination will initiate at the second one. If productive, these cells will then mature into pre-B

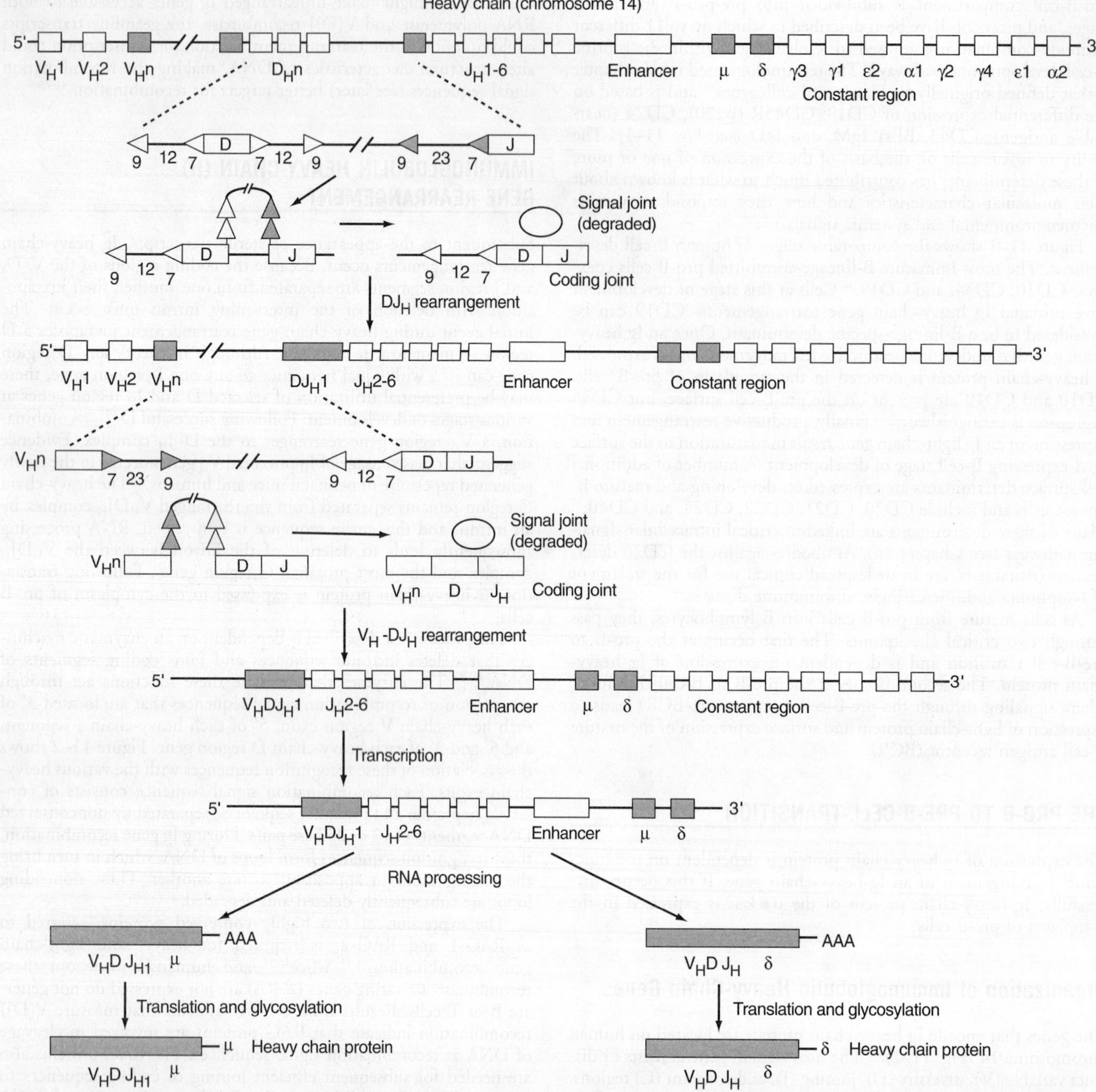

Figure 11–2 Rearrangement and expression of the human immunoglobulin heavy-chain gene. The figure shows the Ig heavy-chain gene and the signal sequences 3′ of each V region locus, 5′ and 3′ of each D region locus, and 5′ of each J region locus. These consist of heptamer and nonamer sequences separated by either 12 or 23 base pairs. During Ig recombination, a signal sequence of 12 base pairs can only join to another of 23 base pairs (the so-called 12–23 rule). As shown in the figure, initial heavy-chain gene rearrangements form coding joints between D and J regions as well as signal joints that are ultimately degraded. Subsequently, the joining of the V region gene to the DJ complex occurs. Following a successful rearrangement, the VDJ complex, the μ intron, and portions of the constant regions are transcribed. RNA processing and differential splicing results in formation of an mRNA molecule that is then translated. In the example shown, the rearranged VDJ complex and the constant region, with the μ and δ C region genes, is transcribed. Following RNA processing and translation, a particular B cell could then express μ and/or δ protein.

cells. If this rearrangement is also defective, cells will undergo apoptosis.

IMMUNOGLOBULIN HEAVY-CHAIN GENE EXPRESSION

Following the productive rearrangement of at least one heavy-chain gene, transcription of the rearranged locus occurs. Transcription is dependent on the binding of various transcription factors to specific promoter sequences located 5′ of each heavy-chain V region and one or more heavy-chain enhancer regions located 3′ of the J region genes and downstream from the C_H region genes (see Fig. 11–2).[44–46]

Many of the transcription factors that bind within these sites have been identified. These include the previously described E12 and E47 proteins encoded by the *E2A* gene. Before Ig gene rearrangement, E12 and E47 proteins may be in an inactive state owing to their heterodimeric association with another protein known as Id. In this configuration, DNA binding by E12 and E47 does not occur.[61] Thus, successful transition from the pro-B to pre-B-cell stage is dependent

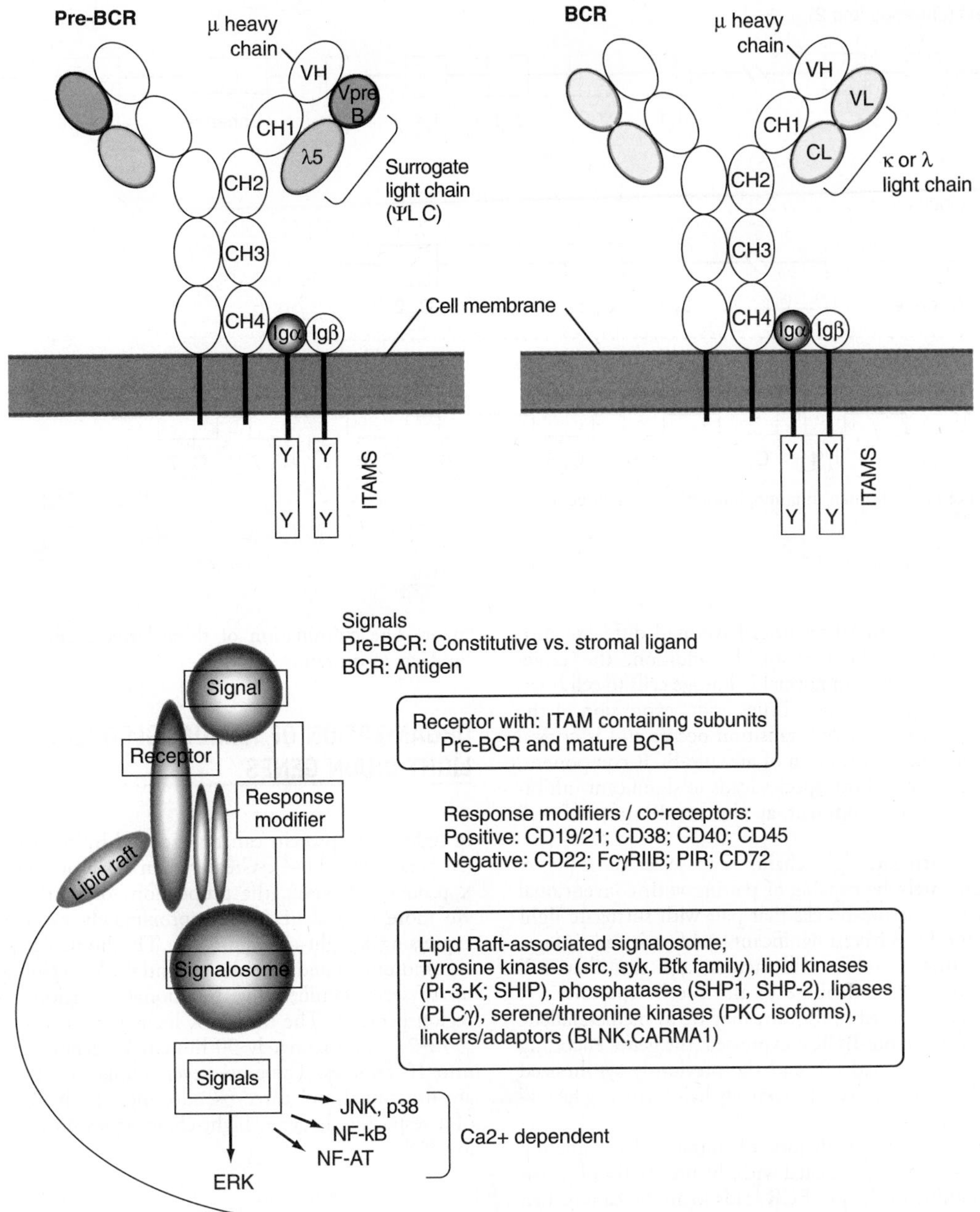

Figure 11–3 The pre-B-cell receptor (pre-BCR) and B-cell receptor (BCR) and associated signaling intermediates. **Top,** μ heavy-chain protein in pre-B cells is associated with the surrogate light chains v-pre-B and λ5 (*left*). In newly produced B lymphocytes, μ heavy chain is associated with conventional light chain (*right*). Associated with heavy chain in both pre-B and B cells are two additional transmembrane proteins, Ig-α and Ig-β, that contain immunoreceptor tyrosine activation motifs (ITAMs) critical to the signaling function. **Bottom,** Expression of the pre-BCR (or possibly its binding to a stromal ligand) or binding of antigen to the mature BCR, respectively, initiates the assembly of a lipid raft, BCR-associated "signalosome" composed of multiple signaling molecules, ultimately leading to transcriptional events that promote cell proliferation, survival, and differentiation.

on cessation of Id expression. This conclusion is consistent with the fact that mice expressing an Id transgene have a complete block in B-cell differentiation.[62]

THE PRE-B-CELL RECEPTOR

When μ heavy-chain protein is first synthesized, it associates with a chaperone protein known as Bip.[63] However, it subsequently associates on the cell surface with two additional proteins that together function in a manner analogous to that identified for conventional light chains. These proteins, referred to as Vpre-B and λ5, are non-covalently linked to one another, forming the surrogate light chain.[64,65] These proteins are encoded by genes located on chromosome 16 in mice[66] and on chromosome 22 in humans.[67] λ5 is covalently linked to the C_H1 domain of the μ heavy chain via a carboxyl-terminal (C-terminal) cysteine.[64] This μ heavy chain-surrogate light-chain complex is associated with two additional transmembrane proteins, Igα and Igβ, that together form the pre-BCR.[68] The intracellular tails of both Igα and Igβ contain immunoreceptor tyrosine activation motifs critical to the signaling function of both the pre-BCR and the BCR (Fig. 11–3, upper panel).

There has been considerable confusion regarding the stage of development at which the pre-BCR is expressed on human B-lineage cells.[33] For example, evidence has been presented that surrogate light chains are detected on pro-B cells before the expression of μ heavy-chain protein,[69] whereas other reports indicate that it is restricted to a late stage of pre-B-cell differentiation.[70] One reason for these diver-

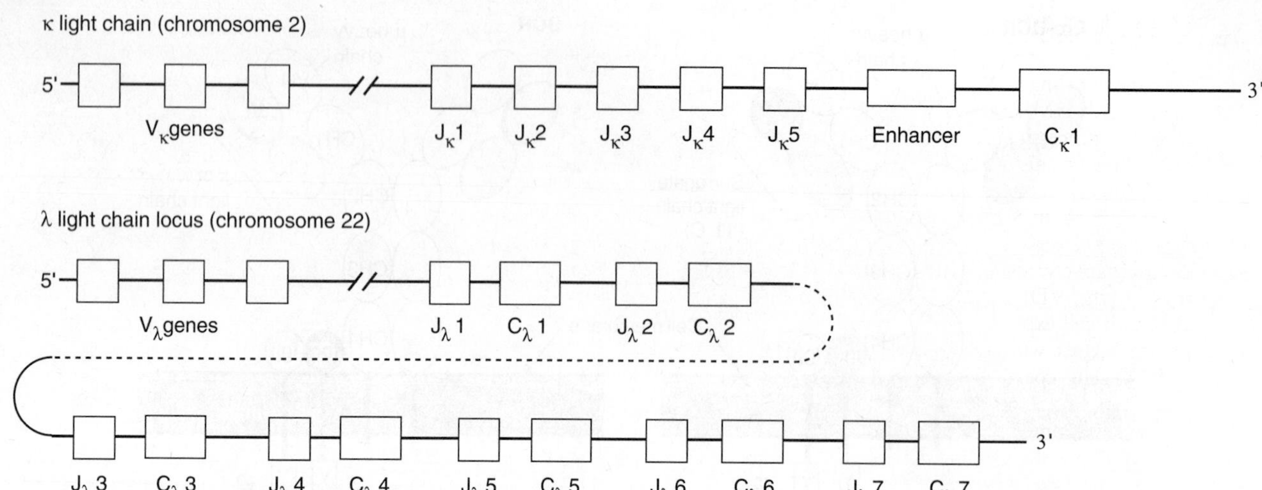

Figure 11–4 Structure of the human immunoglobulin light-chain genes.

gent findings is that different laboratories have used different antibodies to detect surrogate light chain. In addition, the target populations analyzed ranged from normal B-lineage cells to cell lines, some of which were leukemic. These issues aside, expression of the pre-BCR at the pro-B to pre-B-cell transition occurs and is critical in both mice and humans. Disruption of any pre-BCR component, including μ, Igα, and Igβ in both species leads to significant inhibition of early B-lineage development at the pro-B to pre-B-cell transition.[71,72]

One role of the surrogate light chains is to select those heavy chains that will ultimately be capable of pairing with conventional light chains. In fact, those pre-B cells that pair with surrogate light chains to form the pre-BCR have a significant proliferative advantage, thus ensuring that their numbers will increase and that they will generate progeny that will contribute to the B-cell repertoire.[73,74] Another function, as described previously, may be to mediate allelic exclusion.[60] As soon as the pre-BCR is expressed, the genes encoding RAG-1 and RAG-2 are turned off, and the previously synthesized proteins are degraded.[75] These events effectively halt further Ig heavy-chain gene rearrangements.

Lipid rafts that contain mediators of intracellular signaling such as Lyn are constitutively associated with the pre-BCR in human pre-B cells. Cross-linking of the pre-BCR leads to an increase in Lyn kinase activity, phosphorylation of the Igβ chain, and recruitment and activation within the pre-BCR complex of additional signaling intermediates including Syk, BLNK, PI3K, Btk, p85, VAV, and PLCγ2.[76] These events lead to calcium flux and activation of additional signaling cascades within the pre-B cell. Expression and signaling through the pre-BCR result in a marked growth advantage over those pre-B cells that do not express a pre-BCR.[77] A logical assumption is that these events are initiated by binding of the extracellular portion of the pre-BCR to an environmental ligand. However, no definitive pre-BCR ligand has been identified to date. Thus, precisely how these signaling events are initiated in the absence of external cross-linking ligand remains unclear, although it appears likely that constitutive signaling following pre-BCR surface expression may be sufficient.

THE PRE-B TO B-CELL TRANSITION

At some point, pre-BCR-expressing cells cease to proliferate and enter a resting phase. This change occurs coordinately with a cessation of surrogate light-chain expression, reactivation of the recombinatorial machinery, and initiation of conventional light-chain gene rearrangement. The culmination of these latter events is the expression of light-chain protein.

ORGANIZATION OF IMMUNOGLOBULIN LIGHT-CHAIN GENES

Ig light-chain protein can be encoded by the kappa (κ) or lambda (λ) genes (Fig. 11–4). Greater than 90% of murine B cells express κ protein. However, the proportions of human κ and λ proteins are more equivalent, with approximately 60% of human B cells expressing κ light-chain protein. The human κ gene is located on chromosome 2 and includes around 40 $V_κ$ region genes, clustered in up to seven families, five functional $J_κ$ region genes, and one $C_κ$ region gene.[78,79] The human λ locus is located on human chromosome 22. Approximately 30 human $V_λ$ genes exist and are grouped into 10 families. There are seven human $C_λ$ genes, four of which are functional and three pseudogenes. Each $C_λ$ gene is located 3′ of a respective $J_λ$ gene. Light-chain genes do not include D region loci.[80,81]

IMMUNOGLOBULIN LIGHT-CHAIN GENE REARRANGEMENT

Although B cells can express κ or λ light-chain protein, rearrangements initiate at the κ locus, where the initial event is the joining of a $V_κ$ segment to a $J_κ$ segment. The $V_κJ_κ$ complex remains separated from the light-chain C region by an intron, the entire complex is transcribed, and further splicing of the intron between the $J_κ$ and $C_κ$ segment results in formation of a mature $V_κ$–$J_κ$–$C_κ$ transcript. If rearrangements at the first κ allele are unsuccessful, attempts are made to rearrange the second κ gene. If this fails, the λ locus is utilized.[82,83] The regulation of light-chain gene rearrangement is similar to that for heavy-chain gene recombination. For example, the same enzymatic machinery involving the RAG proteins is necessary.

Ig light-chain gene expression is also dependent on the binding of specific transcription factors, which include nuclear factor-κB (NF-κB), to enhancer motifs. For example, an Igκ light-chain enhancer region is located downstream of the $J_κ5$ gene. Analogous to the situation in which the actions of E2A proteins are inhibited by Id, NF-κB is complexed to an inhibitory molecule, inhibitor of NF-κB (I-κB), in the cytoplasm of pre-B cells.[84,85]

IMMUNOGLOBULIN CLASS SWITCHING

At the terminal stage of primary B-cell development, newly produced B cells can express both IgM and IgD. This coexpression occurs by means of alternative processing of a primary RNA transcript. As noted previously, the rearranged V_HDJ_H heavy chain, part of the C region, and the intron separating these exons is transcribed following productive rearrangements in a cell. If the intron is spliced, resulting in association of the Cμ region with the VDJ complex, the B cell expresses IgM. Alternatively, if the Cμ exon is deleted along with the heavy-chain intron, the VDJ complex and the Cδ exon become contiguous and the B cell expresses IgD. The differential processing of heavy-chain transcripts within a single cell explains why some newly produced B cells coexpress both IgM and IgD (see Fig. 11–2).

These primary developmental events are distinguished from Ig class switching that allows the newly produced B cell to express the same VDJ complex associated with additional heavy-chain C regions other than IgM and IgD. Deletion of germline DNA resulting in re-ligation of the VDJ complex to these downstream heavy-chain C region genes, such as γ3, γ 1 γ 2b, γ 2a, ε, and α, is the mechanism by which this takes place. These DNA deletions are believed to occur at or near nucleotide sequences called *switch regions* that are located in the intron 5′ to each C_H exon. As discussed subsequently, these class-switching events are highly regulated, secondary-differentiation events that occur in spleen and lymph nodes and are potentiated by helper T cells and their secreted products.[86,87]

THE B-CELL RECEPTOR

The structure of the B-cell receptor (BCR) is similar to that described earlier for the pre-BCR, except that κ or λ, rather than surrogate light-chain proteins, is associated with the Ig heavy chain. As shown in Fig. 11–3, the BCR consists of the Ig molecule and the associated Igα and Igβ proteins that are required for initiation of the intracellular signaling cascade following binding of antigen to Ig. This requirement exists because even though Ig heavy chains span the cell membrane, their cytoplasmic carboxyl tails are relatively short. For example, the intracellular C terminus of IgM and IgD consists of only three amino acids.

Antigen engagement of the BCR initiates assembly of a lipid raft, BCR-associated "signalosome," composed of multiple signaling molecules that include tyrosine kinases, serine/threonine kinases, lipid kinases, lipases, phosphatases, and linkers and adaptors.[88–91] This signalosome mediates a cascade of intracellular signals that includes the initiation of calcium influx. Additional calcium-dependent and -independent downstream signals that include the mitogen-activated protein kinase cascade (JNK, p38, ERK) and activation of key transcription factors that include JUN, c-fos, NFAT, and NF-κB in turn mediate transcriptional events leading to cell proliferation, survival, and differentiation. The level and duration of receptor activation, and hence transcriptional output, are further modified by a series of cell surface coreceptors or "response modifiers" that bind to complement receptors on the surface of stromal cells, activated T cells, or other populations present in secondary lymphoid organs.

In addition to the critical nature of these signals in mature B cells, these signaling pathways also are crucial in developing pre-B cells. One of the best examples of this requirement is the prototypical humoral immunodeficiency known as X-linked agammaglobulinemia, first described in 1952 by Bruton.[92] X-linked agammaglobulinemia results from mutations within the gene segments that encode the nonreceptor tyrosine kinase, Btk. In males who express a defective Btk protein, pre-B-cell clonal expansion is markedly depressed and there is an almost complete loss of immature B cells in the bone marrow and in secondary lymphoid organs.[91,93] As a result, affected males develop recurrent bacterial infections early in life because of a profound decrease in circulating Ig. A nearly identical clinical phenotype also has been observed in persons with mutations in additional components of the pre-BCR signaling complex, including the μ-heavy chain, λ5, Igα, and the key B-cell adaptor protein BLNK (see Fig. 11–1).

GENERATION AND SELECTION OF THE PRIMARY B-CELL REPERTOIRE

In order for the organism to mount an effective humoral immune response, an array of immunoglobulins with unique antigen-binding specificities, together referred to as the Ig repertoire, must be generated. Several mechanisms have evolved to ensure that this occurs.

First, heavy- and light-chain proteins can be encoded by multiple germline V, J, and, in the case of the heavy chain, D region genes, and the combinatorial diversity among them is enormous.[94–96] Second, nucleotides not encoded in the germline can be added to $D–J_H$ and $V_H–DJ_H$ junctions by a nuclear enzyme known as terminal deoxynucleotidyl transferase (TdT).[97,98] Two splice variants of TdT, encoded by a single gene, have been identified, and it is the short (509-amino acid) variant that catalyzes the addition of nontemplated nucleotides at coding joints. The long (529-amino acid) form is a 3′–5′ exonuclease that catalyzes the deletion of nucleotides at coding joints. Thus, N region diversity catalyzed by TdT may be due to the coordinated activities of short and long forms of that enzyme.[99] Third, the DNA joints that form during recombination are often imprecise and can occur at any of several nucleotides in the germline. This junctional diversity has the potential to generate different amino acid sequences, resulting in added diversity of the Ig repertoire. However, out-of-frame joints that cannot be transcribed also may result.[100] Finally, somatic mutation of V region genes can occur, usually in secondary lymphoid tissues.[101,102] This latter process, which results in an increased affinity of the antibody for antigen, is discussed in more detail in the section on secondary B-cell development.

It is important to recognize that the total number of B-lineage cells in the bone marrow is far greater than the number of mature B cells that are generated.[103,104] The remarkable cell loss that occurs during the process of differentiation of pro-B cells into B lymphocytes is due to a series of selection events. First, *Ig* heavy-chain gene rearrangements are productive in approximately a third of pro-B cells. In addition, functional light-chain gene rearrangements do not occur in all pre-B cells.[105] Those cells with nonproductive *Ig* gene rearrangements undergo apoptosis and are eliminated from the marrow by resident macrophages and stromal cells.[106]

Selection events also are operative on cells that have matured to the surface IgM stage of development. As a result, although approximately 2×10^7 IgM^+ immature B cells are produced daily in murine bone marrow, only 10% to 20% of these cells survive to exit the marrow and enter the spleen as transitional B cells. Some of these surface IgM^+ cells are eliminated because they are potentially self-reactive. Such self-reactive B cells may be generated because the process of Ig gene recombination is random.

Several mechanisms have been proposed to account for the fate of such cells. In some cases, the presence of self-antigen may not activate self-reactive B cells. This scenario may result from weak B-cell affinity for the antigen, or the autoantigen may be present at an extremely low concentration. In other instances, interaction of antigen with the autoreactive B cell may result in anergy. The level of membrane Ig on such anergic B cells may be reduced up to 20-fold, the cell's ability to proliferate may be impaired, and differentiation into Ig-secreting cells may be blocked. Finally, self-reactive B cells may be clonally deleted. Clonal deletion may result from cytolysis by other cells, such as bone marrow macrophages, or autoreactive B cells may undergo a physiologic change resulting in cell death following receptor engagement.[107,108]

The recognition of self-antigen by a B cell may not necessarily result in anergy or deletion but instead may lead to *receptor editing.* In this process, rearranged κ light-chain alleles can be replaced by secondary rearrangements of upstream $V_κ$ genes to downstream,

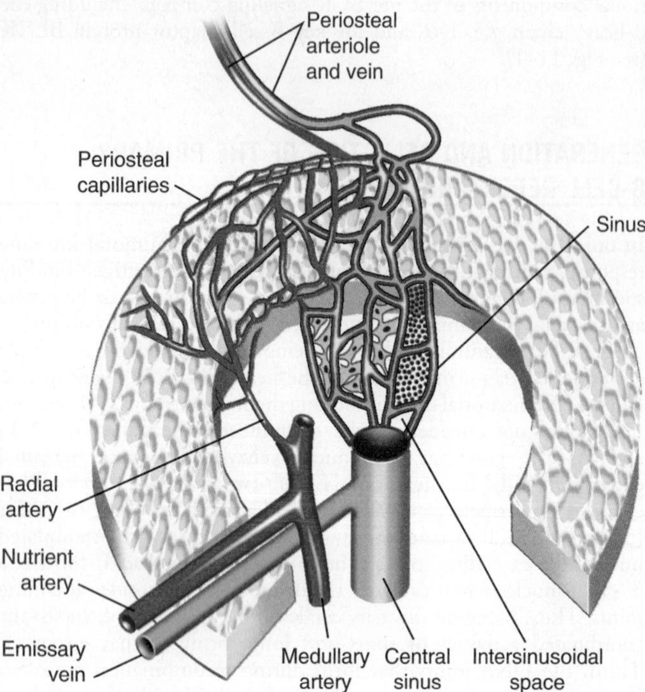

Figure 11–5 Cross section of bone showing elements of the medullary circulation, the marrow sinusoids, and the location of stromal cells. *(From Dorshkind K: Regulation of hematopoiesis by bone marrow stromal cells and their products. Annu Rev Immunol 8:111, 1990. Reprinted with permission from the* Annual Review of Immunology.*)*

unrearranged J_κ segments. These secondary rearrangements, which may delete the primary $V_\kappa J_\kappa$ complex or separate it from C_κ by inversion, are possible because of the continual presence of unrearranged V_κ regions upstream of the joined $V_\kappa J_\kappa$ coding segments.[109] Receptor editing also can occur in peripheral B cells in response to antigen stimulation, as discussed subsequently.

REGULATION OF PRIMARY B-CELL DEVELOPMENT

Hematopoiesis occurs in the intersinusoidal spaces of the medullary cavity in association with a fixed population of stromal cells. Stromal cells are largely sessile and form a three-dimensional hematopoietic microenvironment with which developing blood cells associate (Fig. 11–5).[110–112] Before 1980, little was known about how stromal cells and their secreted products regulate B-cell development. However, advances in molecular biology, the isolation of bone marrow stromal cells, and the development of long-term culture methods for growing B-lineage cells have converged in the last two decades. As a result, considerable insights into the regulation of B-cell development by extracellular signals have been obtained.

CELL–CELL INTERACTIONS

Direct contact between developing B-lineage and stromal cells can be observed on analysis of intact bone marrow or of B lymphopoiesis in long-term bone marrow cultures, and the molecular basis for these associations is being defined in both humans and mice. For example, both murine and human pre-B cells express the VLA-4 integrin that interacts with a stromal cell ligand identified as vascular cell adhesion molecule-1. VLA-4 also promotes binding to fibronectin, an extracellular matrix protein.[113–116] CD44 on developing B-lineage cells also has been implicated in mediating stromal cell–lymphocyte interactions in the mouse through binding to stromal cell-derived hyaluronate.[117] These intercellular interactions presumably would allow B cells to receive proliferative and/or developmental signals from stromal cells. It is important to appreciate that the stromal cells may not be passive populations that constitutively provide these signals. Instead, the binding of the B-lineage cell may stimulate the stromal cell in turn to produce such differentiation or growth-potentiating activities.

CYTOKINES

An additional means by which bone marrow stromal cells regulate the growth and differentiation of B-lineage cells is via the secretion of soluble mediators.[110–112] The literature describing the effects of cytokines on B-cell development is extensive, and a discussion of each one is beyond the scope of this chapter. However, the focus can be narrowed considerably when only those factors with obligate effects on B-cell development are considered.

The critical B lymphopoietic cytokine in mice is IL-7. The gene encoding IL-7 was cloned from a murine stromal cell line, and its product was identified on the basis of its ability to stimulate the proliferation of a pre-B-cell line.[118] IL-7 binds to a cell-surface receptor formed by the IL-7 receptor α chain and the common cytokine γ chain.[119,120] That IL-7 is required for murine B-cell development was demonstrated by studies showing that mice administered antibodies to IL-7 or its receptor exhibit severe lymphopenia. Subsequent analysis of IL-7 and IL-7 receptor knockout mice corroborated these studies.[121,122] These animals also exhibit a severe T-cell depletion, because IL-7 is required for thymopoiesis. Cells that have initiated Ig heavy-chain $D–J_H$ rearrangements are particularly responsive to the growth-stimulating effects of IL-7.[2,35] However, by the time they have matured to the late pre-B-cell stage of development, responsiveness to IL-7 is lost, presumably owing to failure of cells to express the IL-7 receptor.[123] Subsequent murine studies revealed that in addition to its growth-promoting effects, IL-7 acts as a differentiation factor that potentiates the recombination of a V_H region gene segment to an already rearranged DJ_H complex.[124]

In view of these findings, it was expected that IL-7 would function in a similar manner during human B-cell development. Initial reports indicating that human $CD34^+CD19^+$ pro-B cells proliferated in response to IL-7,[125,126] albeit at a lower level than in mice, pointed to the potential for IL-7 to affect human B-cell progenitors. IL-7 is not an obligate human B lymphopoietic factor, however, as indicated by reports of patients with X-linked severe combined immunodeficiency. These patients have mutations in the gene encoding the common γ chain, which is part of the receptor for IL-2, IL-4, IL-9, and IL-15, in addition to IL-7. XSCID patients have severe defects in T-cell development, but B-cell development is normal.[127] Further substantiating the conclusion that IL-7 is not an obligate B lymphopoietic factor is that B-cell development also is normal in patients whose B-lineage cells express a mutated IL-7Rα chain.[128]

Another B lymphopoietic cytokine under current investigation is thymic stromal cell lymphopoietin (TSLP). TSLP was cloned from a murine thymic stromal cell line and has been shown to affect the growth and differentiation of B lineage cells.[129] Similar to IL-7, TSLP can stimulate pro-B-cell proliferation, and there is also evidence that TSLP can potentiate the pre-B to B-cell transition.[130] The TSLP receptor is formed by the IL-7Rα chain and another subunit related to, but not identical with, the common γ chain.[131] Utilization of the IL-7Rα chain in both IL-7 and TSLP signaling indicates that TSLP activity also is unlikely to be essential for human B-lineage development. Thus, at present, the cytokine(s) in humans that mediates the same effects as those mediated by IL-7 in the mouse remains unknown.

SYSTEMIC FACTORS

In addition to regulation by microenvironmental factors, there is a growing appreciation that systemic factors, those of endocrine origin in particular, also regulate B-cell development. For example, B-cell development in mice is dependent on the integrity of the pituitary–

thyroid axis, because mice deficient in the production of thyroid hormone or expression of the thyroid hormone receptor exhibit suppressed bone marrow B lymphopoiesis.[132] Whether or not these events also occur in human B lymphopoiesis has not been established. It also has been demonstrated that hormones can negatively affect B-cell development. In particular, increased levels of estrogens occurring during pregnancy inhibit lymphopoiesis.[133]

FETAL B-CELL DEVELOPMENT

Hematopoiesis initiates during embryogenesis.[134] Developing blood cells in mice are first detected at around day 7.5 of gestation in the murine yolk sac and in the human yolk sac at 3 weeks of gestation.[134] A long-standing model had been that HSC produced in the latter tissue subsequently seed the embryo. However, the analysis of avian chimeric embryos generated by grafting a quail yolk sac onto a chick embryo revealed that definitive blood cell development is derived from embryoid body-derived precursors.[135,136] The precise origin of intraembryonic blood cell development has been localized to the area around the dorsal aorta, developing gonads, and mesonephric kidney, which is referred to as the aorta–gonad–mesonephros (AGM) region.[137,138] The detection of human CD34$^+$CD38$^-$ cells with potent hematopoietic potential on the ventral endothelial wall of the dorsal aorta at day 25 of gestation is consistent with the AGM being a site in which HSC are generated.[139]

The para-aortic splanchnopleura, from which the AGM develops, appears to be the first tissue in the murine embryo that exhibits the potential to generate B lineage cells.[140] Subsequently, additional intraembryonic sites in the mouse embryo, including the fetal liver, the placenta, and the fetal bone marrow, as well as extra-embryonic tissues, such as the yolk sac, and the placenta harbor cells with the potential to generate B lymphocytes. The precise maturational state of the B-cell progenitors in these various intra- and extra-embryonic tissues is unknown, and whether or not they are produced in those sites or migrated into them from another tissue subsequent to the establishment of the fetal circulation remains unclear. Surface Ig-expressing cells develop in the fetus, and in the fetal liver in particular. For example, pre-B cells are present in that tissue by day 13 of gestation in mice, and surface IgM$^+$ cells are detected several days thereafter.

There are numerous parallels between murine and human fetal B-cell development. For example, pre-B cells can also be detected in human fetal liver by week 8 of gestation, and surface IgM$^+$ cells are present at week 9.[141] IgM-expressing cells have also been observed in additional human fetal tissues that include the omentum,[142] the peritoneal cavity, and the spleen.[143]

Many aspects of fetal B lymphopoiesis are similar to those in the adult. Thus, heavy-chain genes rearrange and are expressed before light-chain genes, and the recombinatorial machinery and transcriptional regulators of Ig gene expression are comparable. Nevertheless, murine studies suggest that the processes of fetal and adult B-cell development are not identical. One major difference between fetal and adult B-cell development is that it has been difficult to identify a fetal lymphoid committed progenitor that is devoid of myeloid potential. Instead, fetal B/T/macrophage and B/macrophage progenitors have been defined but not a lymphoid progenitor restricted only to B-cell and T-cell development.[144–146] A second difference between fetal and adult B-cell development is that the intracellular and extracellular signals that regulate growth and development are not identical. For example, although IL-7 is required for adult bone marrow B-cell development in mice, B-1 B-cell progenitors (see below) can develop in an IL-7-independent manner.[147] Also, although it has been thought that B-cell development is blocked completely in PU.1$^{-/-}$ mice, in fact fetal B-cell development occurs, and the cells produced appear to be B-1 B cells.[148] A third difference between fetal and adult B-cell progenitors is that the latter cells tend to express TdT whereas not all fetal B-cell progenitors do so.[149] Thus, the Ig repertoire of fetal-derived B cells is more restricted than that in the adult.[150] Transgenic strains of mice in which TdT is expressed during fetal B lymphopoiesis have altered immune responses to selected microorganisms.[151]

There is a growing appreciation that some fetal-derived B and T cells are functionally distinct from those produced during postnatal life. The fetal-derived cells are part of the innate immune system in contrast to lymphocytes generated during postnatal life that are effectors of adaptive immunity. Included in the former category would be natural killer (NK) cells, selected $\gamma\delta$ T cells, some marginal zone (MZ) cells (defined below), and B-1 B cells.[152]

B-1 B CELLS

The B cells that are produced in adult bone marrow and that constitute the majority of B cells in the peripheral lymphoid tissues, such as the spleen and lymph node, are often referred to as B-2 B cells. This nomenclature serves to contrast them with a distinct population of mature B cells, referred to as B-1 B cells, that constitute around 5% of total B lymphocytes in the mouse.[152] B-1 B cells are found in multiple murine tissues that include various parts of the intestine, the spleen, and serous cavities. Approximately half of the B cells present in these latter tissues, including the pleural and peritoneal cavities, are B-1 B cells. B-1 B cells in serous cavities can be distinguished by their unusual phenotype. For example, peritoneal cavity B-1 B cells can be defined by their expression of high levels of sIgM, low levels of sIgD, and CD11b, a determinant expressed on myeloid cells (sIgM^{high} sIgD^{low} CD11b$^+$). B-1 B cells can be further subdivided according to the differential expression of cell surface CD5 into sIg M^{high}sIgD^{low}CD11b$^+$CD5$^+$ B-1a B cells and sIgM^{high}sIgD^{low}CD11b$^+$ CD5$^-$ B-1b B cells. As noted, B-1 B cells are effectors of innate immunity and generally respond to high-molecular-weight, polymeric T-independent antigens (Table 11–1).[152,153]

Table 11–1 Characteristics of B-Cell Subpopulations

Cells	Immune Function	Phenotype	Properties	Primary Localization
B-1a	Innate Immunity	IgM^{high}IgD^{low}CD11b$^+$CD5$^+$ (in serous cavities)	Secretion of IgM natural antibodies	Serous cavities, spleen, gut
B-1b	Innate Immunity	IgM^{high}IgD^{low}CD11b$^+$CD5$^-$ (in serous cavities)	Antibody production is induced	Serous cavities, spleen, gut
MZ	Innate Immunity	IgM$^+$IgD^{low} (Human MZ B cells also include CD27$^+$IgM$^+$ unswitched memory cells)	Strong response to T-independent antigens	Splenic marginal zone
B-2 (follicular)	Adaptive Immunity	IgM^{low}IgD^{high}	Strong response to T-dependent antigens	Spleen and lymph nodes; recirculate

Adapted from Hardy RR, Hayakawa K: B cell developmental pathways. Annu Rev Immunol 19:595, 2001; Martin F, Kearney J: B1 cells: Similarities and differences with other B cell subsets. Currr Opin Immunol 13:195, 2001; and Martin F, Kearney JF: Marginal zone B cells. Nat Rev Immunol 2:323, 2002.

Recent observations in mice suggest that B-1a and B-1b B cells mediate distinct functions. B-1a B cells spontaneously secrete so-called IgM natural antibodies, whereas antibody production by B-1b B cells is induced following exposure to antigen. Antibodies from both subpopulations of B-1 B cells have been shown to be required for protection against pathogens such as *Streptococcus pneumoniae*.[154,155] The two types of B-1 B cells and B-2 B cells have been proposed to contribute to a "layered immune system." In this regard, the most primitive effectors would be B-1a B cells and the most highly evolved would be B-2 B cells. B-1b cells exhibit properties of both populations and may be an evolutionary link between them.[152]

The origin of B-1 B cells has been a source of considerable controversy. They have been proposed to be a separate B-cell lineage derived from a progenitor distinct from that from which B-2 B cells derive. In addition to this "lineage model," the "selection model" proposes that B-1 cells are conventional B-2 B cells whose characteristics result from selective pressures following antigen exposure.[152,156,157] Classic studies demonstrating that the transplantation of fetal liver most efficiently generated B-1 B cells whereas adult bone marrow most efficiently repopulated B-2 B cells in irradiated murine recipients provided evidence for the lineage model.[158] The recent description of a phenotypically identifiable B-1 B cell-specified progenitor produced during embryogenesis has provided strong support for the lineage model.[159]

This discussion has focused on B-1 B-cell development in mice, because very little is known about the development and role of B-1 B cells in humans. However, some B cells in patients with various autoimmune diseases have properties suggestive of a B-1 B-cell origin, and the role for this population in response to specific infectious challenges makes further studies of human B-1 B-cell development an important area of investigation.[160]

SECONDARY LYMPHOID COMPARTMENTS

Once newly produced B cells exit the bone marrow, they migrate to the spleen, where they undergo further maturation into follicular B cells or MZ B cells. In general, B cells in the follicles are poised to respond to T-dependent antigens, which, as their name implies, require help from T cells. The T cells in the spleen that provide this help are located in the periarterial lymphoid sheath (PALS; Fig. 11–6). The spleen (but not lymph nodes) contains additional B cells located at the outer limit of the splenic white pulp (Fig. 11–6). This area, known as the marginal zone, is where the MZ B cells localize, and the region also contains macrophages and dendritic cells. MZ B cells present in this region play a critical role in the response to T-independent antigens (see below). The development of these populations, known as secondary B-cell development, has been highlighted in recent studies.[161–166]

The first step in secondary B-cell development is the entry of newly arrived bone marrow immigrants into the spleen. These cells, which are now referred to as *transitional 1 (T1) B cells*, localize at the outer edge of the PALS (Fig. 11–6) that surrounds the splenic central artery. The PALS in mice is occupied by a considerable number of T cells but in humans few T cells are present in this region. T1 B cells give rise to a more mature population of splenic B cells, referred to as *T2 or follicular precursor B cells*. The T1 and T2 populations respond differentially to developmental stimuli,[163,164] and a considerable degree of selection occurs during the T1 to T2 transition. For example, T1 cells with BCR specificities for blood-borne self-antigens are deleted by negative selection. Positive selection via BCR signaling must occur, and if it does not, the T2 cells will die by neglect. The survival of T2 cells, but not T1 cells, is also dependent upon the B-cell activation factor BAFF (BLyS, TALL-1, THANK, zTNF4), which is produced by the splenic microenvironment.[165] A significant fraction of T2 cells are no longer in the G_0 phase of the cell cycle, suggesting they are in a more activated state than is the case for T1 cells.

The strength of BCR-mediated signals influences the development of T2 cells. Weaker signaling through the BCR may promote entry into the MZ B-cell compartment. Signaling through Notch2 expressed on T2 cells also determines T2 cell fate. When this occurs, T2 cells are promoted to become MZ B cells, and there is a depletion of MZ B cells when this pathway is blocked.[166] Of note, human MZ B cells are clearly heterogeneous and include a large proportion of $CD27^+IgM^+$ unswitched memory B cells with somatically mutated Ig heavy chains. The origin of this cell population is unclear but is presumed to be antigen driven yet may not require T cell help. While MZ B cells in rodents appear to be a static, nonrecirculating population, cells with an identical $CD27^+IgM^+$ phenotype are clearly present in human peripheral blood as well as other lymphatic tissues. This circulating population becomes detectable in parallel with seeding of the splenic MZ (typically after 2 years of age), increases in number following exposure to polysaccharide antigens, and appears to play an essential role in the rapid response to infection with encapsulated bacteria.[161,167,168]

Strong BCR signals are critical for T2 cells to mature into a follicular B cell. It is estimated on the basis of murine studies that only 1% to 3% of splenic transitional B cells develop into mature, naive B cells.[161,163] Once mature, naive B cells are generated, they recirculate and take up residence in various lymphoid tissues that include lymph nodes, intestinal Peyer patches, and the spleen itself. Within these tissues, mature naive cells localize in clusters of B lymphocytes, and each such cluster is termed a *primary follicle* (see Fig. 11–6). Within those regions, the follicular B cells are poised to respond to antigen and undergo the germinal center reaction described below.

The molecular signals responsible for the intraorgan localization of specific B-cell populations and their migration patterns following antigenic challenge are being identified.[169–173] Proper segregation of splenic B cells in follicles and the MZ is dependent on expression of tumor necrosis factor (TNF) and lymphotoxins α and β (LTα and LTβ). Signaling through LFA-1 and $\alpha_4\beta_1$ integrins also has been implicated in localization and retention of MZ B cells.[174,175] A related TNF family of molecules that includes B-cell activation factor (BAFF) is involved in peripheral B-cell generation, selection, and function. These molecules and their receptors may also transmit signals required for the development of stromal cells that produce chemokines required for movement of cells between different anatomic locations within secondary lymphoid organs. A role for chemokines in B-1 B-cell localization to the peritoneal cavity has also been demonstrated.[174] Further details regarding lymphocyte trafficking can be found in Chapter 16.

T-INDEPENDENT B-CELL RESPONSES

T-independent responses are elicited by polymeric antigens, such as polysaccharides, that are composed of repetitive antigenic epitopes. MZ B cells play a critical role in these responses. On antigen binding, MZ B cells undergo rapid proliferation and maturation into plasma cells that secrete low-affinity IgM.

The rapid response of MZ B cells to antigen has led to the idea that this effector population, like B-1 B cells, constitutes a key element of the innate immune response to bacterial and other selected pathogens. Because they have a low activation threshold, MZ B cells rapidly differentiate into antibody-forming cells in response to antigen. These cells secrete primarily low-affinity IgM and IgG_3 antibodies that provide a first line of defense. This response may be reinforced by B-1 B cells, whose Ig repertoire is designed for responsiveness to the polymeric antigens that characterize the T-independent response. In view of this, it is not surprising that many of the properties of MZ B cells overlap with those of B-1 B cells (see Table 11–1). However, they do not seem to be identical populations, and evidence points to a separate origin.[153,177,178]

The poor response of infants to some types of T-independent antigens correlates with the fact that the MZ is not fully formed until the age of 1 to 2 years.[178] In addition, splenectomized persons are more susceptible to infection with some bacteria, owing to the deficient antibody response to capsular polysaccharides.

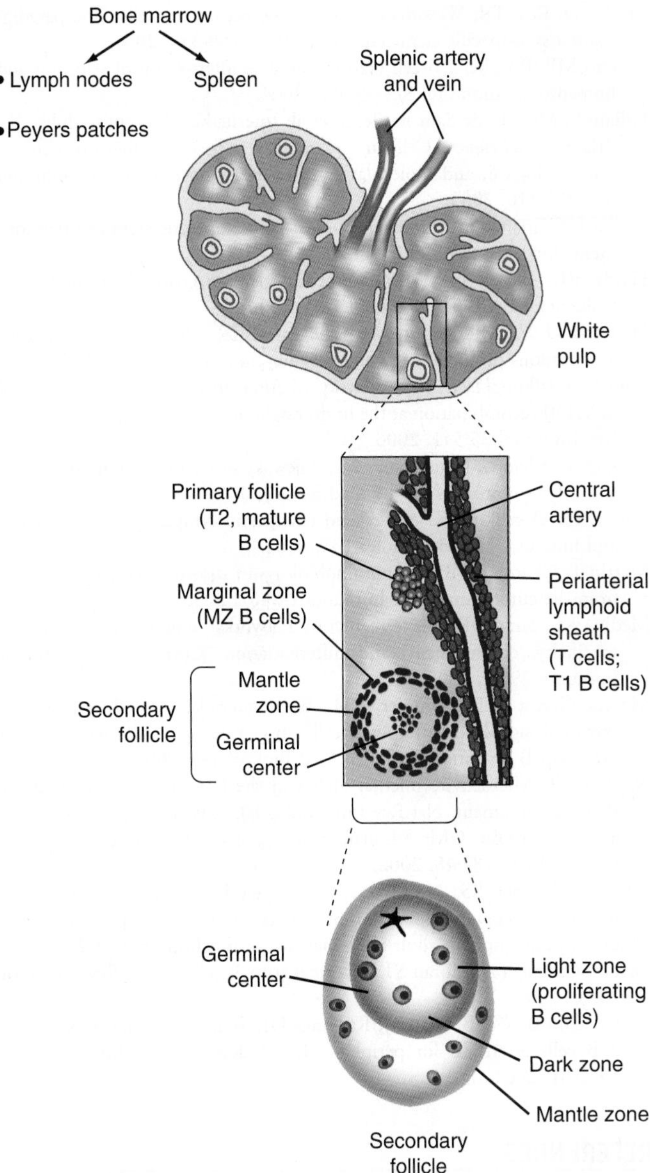

Figure 11–6 Organization of B cells in secondary lymphoid organs, with emphasis on the spleen.

T-DEPENDENT RESPONSES IN SECONDARY LYMPHOID TISSUES

Although some B cells in the MZ can respond to T-dependent antigens, most B cells that do so are the mature, naive B cells located in primary follicles. As described previously, these cells are derived from T2 B cells, and have subsequently migrated into the primary follicle. Following their binding of a T-dependent antigen (as soluble antigen or indirectly via presentation by a local antigen-presenting cell, or, alternatively, as an immune complex), mature, naive B cells in primary follicles undergo a blastogenic response. Some of these cells will immediately mature into plasma cells that secrete low-affinity IgM to provide a rapid initial response to infection.[179–181] In response to T-cell help, however, other B cells will undergo further proliferation and differentiation. The histologic appearance of the follicle changes as these events evolve. The nonresponsive B cells form an outer *mantle zone* surrounding the proliferating, antigen-responsive B cells in a central germinal center.[179,180,182,183]

Germinal center B cells are shielded from soluble antigens and are exposed only to a unique set of antigens presented by follicular dendritic cells.[184,185] Two regions can be distinguished within the germinal center of the secondary follicle. At one pole, the cycling B-cell blasts are referred to as *centroblasts* and form the *dark zone*. The other pole, referred to as the *light zone*, consists of nonproliferating cells referred to as *centrocytes*. Some of these centrocytes will go on to become plasma cells, whereas others will become memory B cells (see Fig. 11–6).[180,186,187] The end result of the germinal center reaction is the formation of plasma cells that secrete high-affinity Ig. Other germinal center B cells convert to memory B cells, which constitute approximately 40% of all B cells and are responsible for the relatively rapid response observed on secondary exposure to the same antigen.

Affinity Maturation and Lymphomagenesis

Following the initial low-affinity IgM response that helps to keep a developing infection in check, the response of B cells in the germinal centers to T-dependent antigens involves Ig class switching and selection of B-cell clones of higher-affinity antigen-binding potential. This process is known as *affinity maturation*.

Affinity maturation results in the selection of B cells estimated to have a 10-fold, or even greater, increase in antigen-binding potential.[188,189] Analysis of Ig gene sequences of pre- and post-germinal center B cells indicates that this increased affinity is secondary to changes in the genes that encode the antigen-binding domain of the Ig molecule. These genomic changes result from three types of modifications.[190] First, as described previously, B cells may undergo receptor editing. Receptor editing usually involves modifications of the existing light chain in which an upstream V region segment joins to a downstream J region gene. As a result, the genetic region encoding the originally expressed light chain is deleted. In order for this process to occur, RAG-1 and RAG-2 expression would be required. It has been proposed that B cells in germinal centers might reactivate *RAG* gene expression in order to mediate events such as receptor editing.[191] However, that this occurs has been questioned in two convincing studies.[192,193] Instead, receptor editing in splenic B cells may be limited to a small subset of recent immature bone marrow immigrants that enter germinal centers before their *RAG* gene expression has been extinguished.

Somatic hypermutation provides a second means to increase antibody affinity. During this process, single-nucleotide exchanges, deletions, and mutations are introduced into the genes encoding the antibody-binding regions of the Ig receptor. Finally, Ig class switching (see earlier) can occur. Class switching results in the replacement of the existing heavy-chain constant region by a downstream constant region gene. Recently, a B cell-specific gene that encodes activation-induced cytidine deaminase (AID), which is expressed in germinal center B cells, has been identified. AID is a putative RNA-editing enzyme that acts as a cytidine deaminase and has been shown to be indispensable for somatic hypermutation and class switch recombination.[194,195] Not all of these changes may increase antigen-binding affinity, however, and some may even result in the generation of autoreactive clones. Thus, a selection process has evolved to delete low-affinity and autoreactive transitional B cells.

Affinity maturation is dependent on signals delivered to the antigen-responsive B cells by antigen-specific T lymphocytes that migrate into the germinal center from the PALS (see Chapter 10).[196,197] T cells mediate their effects on B cells through the secretion of cytokines as well as through direct intercellular contacts, and these stimuli result in B-cell growth, differentiation, and Ig class switching. For example, CD40 is a T cell-surface glycoprotein encoded by a member of the Tumor Necrosis gene family, and its ligand is expressed on B cells.[198,199] CD40 ligand knockout mice do not form germinal centers,[200] and humans who do not express CD40 ligand suffer from X-linked hyperIgM immunodeficiency.[201] Another key T-cell costimulatory signal includes the cytokine IL-10, which is secreted by T cells in response to their activation via the "inducible costimulator" ICOS. Humans lacking expression of ICOS on T cells suffer from adult-onset common variable immune deficiency, leading to a severe deficit in generation of class-switched and memory B cells.[202]

Although the process of affinity maturation is highly efficient, one unintended consequence is thought to be the development of B-cell lymphoma. Lymphomagenesis results in part from the fact that vigorous B-cell proliferation combined with the changes at the DNA level lead to molecular alterations promoting or supporting malignant transformation. Numerous studies have assigned B-cell lymphomas to each of the normal B-cell counterparts (as described).[188] The derivation of the various lymphomas from the normal cellular counterparts and the precise genetic changes that occur in them are described in several chapters in Part VI, Hematologic Malignancies. Events that limit differentiation of immature or activated mature B cells can also promote malignant transformation. For example, disorders leading to defective pre-BCR signaling predispose to development of pre-B acute lymphocytic leukemias.[77]

AGEING AND B-CELL DEVELOPMENT

Studies of both rodents and humans have demonstrated that the quality of the immune response is diminished with age. Such declines are not incompatible with life, but they may become a factor when the individual is required to mount an immune response to a novel pathogen, respond to vaccination, or when considering the potential functional activity of bone marrow derived from older donors. Consequently, defining why aging affects the immune system is critical in order to develop strategies to augment immunity in the elderly.

One contributing factor may be that the production of B cells from HSC is severely reduced with age. For example, the frequency of CLP, pro-B cells, and pre-B cells is significantly reduced in the bone marrow of old mice. Such declines may reflect both age-related defects in HSC as well as in more differentiated lymphoid progeny. In any case, a consequence is that the reduced primary production of B cells results in a lower number of newly produced, naïve B cells that enter secondary lymphoid tissues such as the spleen. Senescence also affects mature B cells resident in peripheral lymphoid tissues. For example, in addition to an accumulation of memory B cells in the spleen of old mice, the immunoglobulins they produce are less protective because of low titer and affinity. Some of these defects may be intrinsic to the B cells while others may be secondary to age-related defects in T cells.[203] Reduced B-cell production may also predispose to alterations in B-cell tolerance. This is because reduced competition for homeostatic signals such a BAFF can lead to an increase in the survival of autoreactive B cells, which are normally outcompeted in nonlymphopenic hosts.[204,205]

SUGGESTED READINGS

Blom B, Spits H: Development of human lymphoid cells. Annu Rev Immunol 24:287, 2006.

Bryder D, Ross DJ, Weissman IL: Hematopoietic stem cells. The paradigmatic tissue-specific stem cell. Am J Pathol 169:338, 2006.

Cancro MP: Peripheral B-cell maturation: The intersection of selection and homeostasis. Immunol Rev 197:89, 2004.

Giliani S, Mori L, de Sain Basile G, et al: Interleukin-7 receptor alpha (IL-7Ralpha) deficiency: Cellular and molecular bases. Analyses of clinical, immunological, and molecular features in 16 novel patients. Immunol Rev 203:110, 2005.

Godin I, Cumano A: Of birds and mice: Hematopoietic stem cell development. Int J Dev Biol 49:2512, 2005.

Hardy RR: B-1 B cells: Development, selection, natural antibody and leukemia. Curr Opin Immunol 18:1, 2006.

Hendriks RW, Middendorp S: The pre-BCR checkpoint as a cell-autonomous proliferation switch. Trends Immunol 25:249, 2004.

Jung D, Giallourakis C, Mostoslavsky R, Alt FW: Mechanism and control of V(D)J recombination at the immunoglobulin heavy chain locus. Annu Rev Immunol 25:541, 2006.

Kuppers R, Klein U, Hansmann M-L, Rajewsky K: Cellular origins of human B-cell lymphomas. N Engl J Med 341:1520, 1999.

Linton PJ, Dorshkind K: Age-related changes in lymphocyte development and function. Nat Immunol 5:133, 2004.

Martin F, Chan AC: B cell immunobiology in disease: Evolving concepts from the clinic. Annu Rev Immunol 24:467, 2006.

Medina KL, Singh HL: Gene regulatory networks orchestrating B cell fate, specificity, commitment, and differentiation. Curr Topics Microbiol Immunol 290:1, 2005.

Moreno-Garcia ME, Sommer KM, Bandaranayake AD, Rawlings DJ: Proximal signals controlling B-cell antigen receptor (BCR) mediated NF-kappaB activation. Adv Exp Med Biol 584:89, 2006.

Nagasawa T: Microenvironmental niches in the bone marrow required for B-cell development. Nat Rev Immunol 6:107, 2006.

Payne KJ, Crooks GM: Human hematopoietic lineage commitment. Immunol Rev 187:48, 2002.

Pelayo R, Welner RS, Nagai Y, Kincade PW: Life before the pre-B cell receptor checkpoint: specification and commitment of primitive lymphoid progenitors in adult bone marrow. Semin Immunol 18:2, 2006.

Pillai S, Cariappa A, Moran ST: Marginal zone B cells. Annu Rev Immunol 23:161, 2005.

Su TT, Guo B, Wei B, Braun J, Rawlings DJ: Signaling in transitional type 2 B cells is critical for peripheral B-cell development. Immunol Rev 197:161, 2004.

REFERENCES

For complete list of references log onto www.expertconsult.com

CHAPTER 12

T-CELL IMMUNITY

Kai W. Wucherpfennig

CENTRAL ROLE OF T CELLS IN ADAPTIVE IMMUNITY

A fundamental understanding of the mechanisms of T cell-mediated immunity is central for an understanding of many hematological diseases. The two branches of the adaptive immune system—B cells and T cells—are specialized in recognizing pathogens in extracellular and intracellular locations, respectively. The essential receptors for B cell- and T cell-mediated immunity—antibodies and T-cell receptors—have related mechanisms for the generation of structural diversity, but distinct recognition mechanisms. Antibodies recognize soluble or cell surface-bound antigens in extracellular spaces and the enormous structural diversity among antibodies permits recognition of virtually any molecular structure: folded proteins, peptides, lipids, carbohydrates, RNA, or DNA. In contrast, T cells sense the presence of intracellular pathogens but do not make direct contact with them. Rather, short proteolytic fragments of pathogen-derived proteins are transported to the cell surface as peptide–major histocompatibility complexes (MHCs) for recognition by the T-cell receptor (TCR). TCR recognition induces clonal expansion, cytokine production, killing of infected cells and other effector functions. Furthermore, activation leads to differentiation into T-cell subsets with defined cytokine profile and function as well as establishment of a long-lived pool of memory T cells. The central role of T cells in immunity against viruses, bacteria, and fungi is illustrated by the severity of the immunodeficiency state that results from destruction of CD4 T cells by the human immunodeficiency virus (HIV).[1] Also, the slow reconstitution of T-cell populations following bone marrow transplantation is responsible for the reactivation of latent viruses, such as cytomegalovirus (CMV).[2]

MOLECULAR MECHANISM OF ANTIGEN PRESENTATION TO T CELLS

Histocompatibility and the Discovery of the Molecular Mechanisms of TCR Recognition

The discovery of the molecular mechanisms of T-cell recognition traces back to the observation that transplanted organs are accepted among identical twins, but not unrelated subjects. The discovery of histocompatibility led Dr Joseph Murray at the Peter Bent Brigham Hospital in Boston in 1954 to perform the first successful solid organ transplant between a patient with end-stage kidney disease and a healthy identical twin.[3] Preceding work had demonstrated that kidney grafts from unrelated donors could function for some time, but were invariably rejected. The major breakthrough in this field occurred several years later when immunosuppressive drugs such as 6-mercaptopurine and the 6-mercaptopurine analog azathioprine were introduced. In 1962, use of azathioprine resulted in the first successful transplant of an unrelated renal allograft, and within several years 1-year survival rates of allografted kidneys from living related donors were approaching 80% and from cadavers 65%. Dr Murray was awarded the Nobel Prize in Physiology or Medicine in 1990 for these landmark contributions.[3] These advances provided a major intellectual stimulus for the discovery of the fundamental role of MHC genes in T-cell function.

Work on the biochemistry of the MHC proteins in the 1970s in Dr Jack Strominger's laboratory at Harvard University identified two major proteins, now known as MHC class I and class II.[4] Sequencing of the proteins demonstrated that each molecule contains four extracellular domains: two membrane-distal domains that contain the polymorphic residues responsible for transplant rejection and two membrane-proximal immunoglobulin domains (Fig. 12–1).[4] Genetic characterization of the MHC locus demonstrated the presence of multiple genes for both MHC class I and class II families: the HLA-A, HLA-B, and HLA-C heavy-chain genes in the human MHC class I region and the HLA-DR, HLA-DQ, and HLA-DP genes in the MHC class II region. These genes are the most polymorphic known genes in the human genome.[5] How do the polymorphic residues contribute to their function?

MHC Molecules Present Peptides to T Cells

The key concept of "MHC restriction" of a T-cell response was established by Drs Rolf Zinkernagel and Peter Doherty through studies of cytotoxic T cells from mice infected with the lymphocytic choriomeningitis virus (Nobel Prize in Physiology or Medicine, 1996).[6,7] They tested T cells from different strains of mice infected with this virus for killing of a particular infected cell line and found that killing only occurred when the MHC haplotype of both T cells and the target cell line were matched. Two models were proposed to explain these results: a single receptor on T cells recognizes a complex formed by the MHC molecule and a viral antigen, or alternatively two receptors on T cells separately recognize MHC and viral antigen. Studies of MHC class I and class II restricted T cells converged on the same answer: MHC class I and class II molecules bind short peptides derived by proteolysis from such antigens.[8,9]

The Structure of MHC Class I Proteins

The classic publication of the crystal structure of the human MHC class I molecule HLA-A2 by Drs Pam Bjorkman, Jack Strominger, Don Wiley, and colleagues established the molecular mechanism of T-cell recognition.[10] The membrane-distal $\alpha1$ and $\alpha2$ domains of the heavy chain form a peptide-binding site (see Fig. 12–1). The floor of this binding site is created by a platform of eight antiparallel β strands and its sides by the two long α-helices of the $\alpha1$ and $\alpha2$ domains. HLA-A2 had been purified from a human EBV-transformed B-cell line and the binding site was filled with a mixture of endogenously processed peptides that were visible in the structure as extra electron density not accounted for by the HLA-A2 protein sequence. The polymorphic residues line this binding site, demonstrating that their biological role is to diversify the repertoire of peptides that can be presented to T cells in different members of a population.[11] This diversification is driven by pathogens, and individuals with rare MHC alleles can have a survival advantage compared to other members of the population because mutations in pathogens that destroy T-cell epitopes occur more frequently for peptides presented by common rather than rare alleles.[12] Transplant rejection is thus a consequence of pathogen-driven diversification of MHC genes.

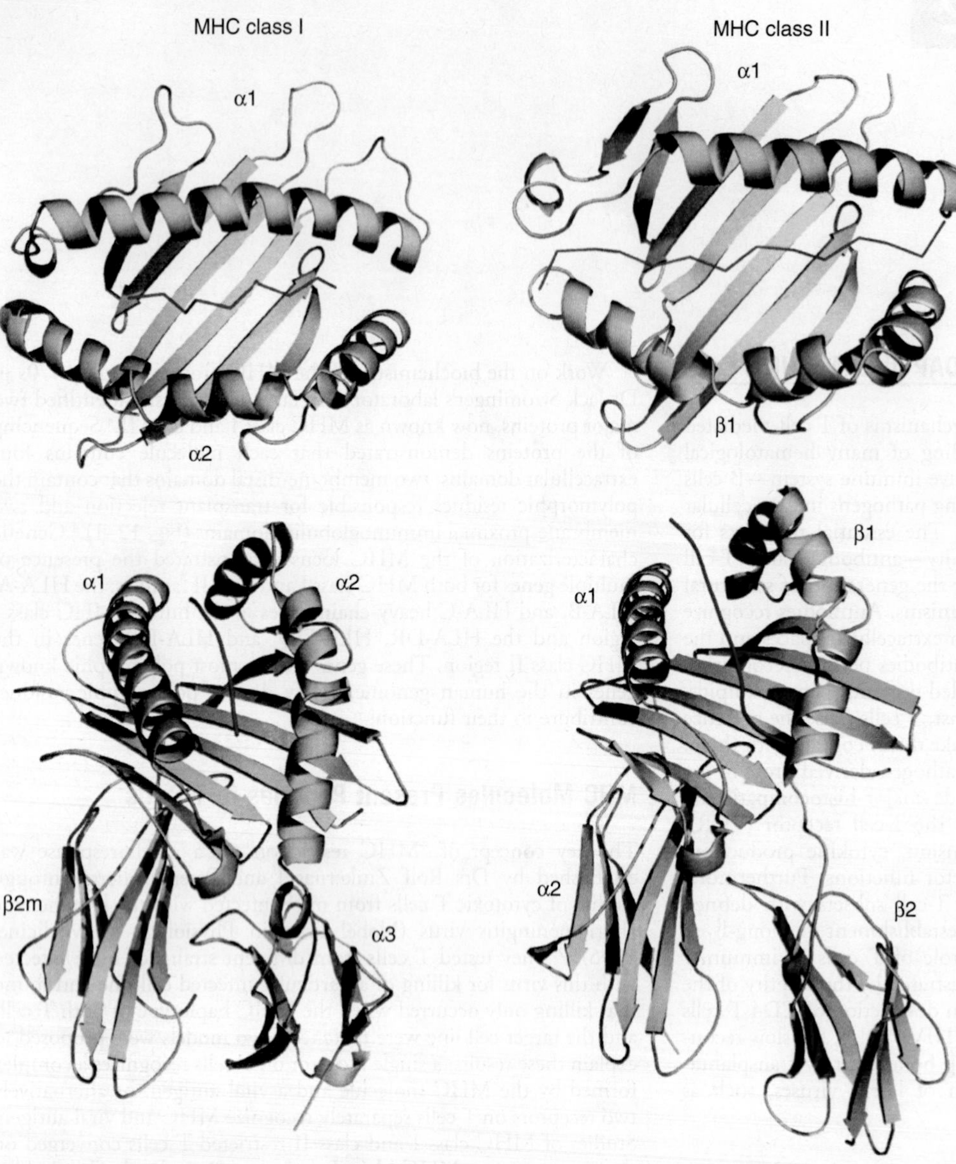

Figure 12–1 Structure of major histocompatibility complex (MHC) proteins. MHC proteins present peptides to the T-cell receptor on T cells. Peptides are bound between the two long helices of the peptide-binding site that sit atop a floor of antiparallel β strands. The α and β chains of MHC class II proteins are both membrane anchored and make equal contributions to the peptide-binding site. In contrast, only the heavy chain of MHC class I is membrane anchored and the α1 and α2 domains of the heavy chain form the peptide-binding site. The MHC class I heavy chain associates in the ER with β2-microglobulin prior to peptide binding. The MHC class II-binding site is open at both ends, permitting the binding of longer peptides compared to MHC class I proteins.

MHC Polymorphisms Determine Peptide-Binding Motifs

The polymorphic residues line six pockets (A–F) of the peptide-binding site. The A and F pockets bind the charged N and C termini of the peptide through a set of conserved hydrogen bonds.[13] The shape and surface properties of the pockets determine which amino acid residues can be accommodated and thus define the repertoire of peptides that can be presented. The majority of peptides that are bound by MHC class I molecules are 8–10 residues in length, but longer peptides have also been identified. Because the N and C termini occupy fixed positions in the A and F pockets, longer peptides "bulge" out in the center.[14] Each MHC molecule has a particular set of preferred amino acids for a given pocket, a peptide-binding motif (Table 12–1). These motifs were first elucidated by elution of peptides bound to MHC class I proteins and sequencing of these peptide pools by Edman degradation.[15] For example, HLA-A2 has a strong preference for hydrophobic amino acids at both positions 2 and 9 (L, M at position 2; V, L at position 9). In contrast, binding to HLA-B27 requires a basic residue at position 2 (R), whereas both basic (R, K, H) and hydrophobic amino acids (L, F, Y) can be accommodated by the P9 pocket.[16] Peptides that bind to HLA-A2 can thus not be presented by HLA-B27 and vice versa. Viral escape mutations that result in loss of MHC binding have been identified for HIV T-cell epitopes, such as mutation of the arginine at position 2 required for binding to HLA-B27.[17] These peptide-binding motifs have proven to be useful for the identification of T-cell epitopes from viral and tumor antigens.

Structural Differences Between MHC Class I and Class II Proteins

MHC class I proteins are expressed by most cell types and present peptides to cytotoxic T cells with the CD8 coreceptor (Fig. 12–2). In contrast, MHC class II proteins are expressed by "professional" antigen-presenting cells, such as dendritic cells, macrophages, and B cells, and present peptides to T cells that express the CD4 coreceptor.[18] The binding site for the coreceptors is located in the membrane proximal domains, the α3 domain of the MHC class I heavy chain for CD8 and the interface between the α2 and β2 domains of MHC class II proteins for CD4.[19,20] The coreceptors recruit the Src kinase Lck during TCR triggering, which phosphorylates tyrosine-based motifs in the cytoplasmic domains of the TCR–CD3 complex.[21,22]

In MHC class I proteins, the peptide-binding site is only formed by the heavy chain (α1 and α2 domains), whereas the peptide-binding groove of MHC class II proteins is created by two chains (α1 and β1 domains; see Fig. 12–1).[13,23] In contrast to MHC class I proteins, the class II-binding site is open at both ends, permitting binding of longer peptides (typically 13–20 residues).[23] Thus, the

Table 12–1 MHC Class I Peptide-Binding Motifs

	HLA-A2 Motif		HLA-B27 Motif
Position	1 **2** 3 4 5 6 7 8 **9**	Position	1 **2** 3 4 5 6 7 8 **9**
Position 2	**L**, **M**	Position 2	**R**
Position 6	V	Position 9	L, F, Y, R, H, K
Position 9	**V**, **L**		
1.	I **L** K E P V H G **V**	1.	G **R** A F V T I G **K**
2.	I **L** G F V F T L T **V**	2.	R **R** I Y D L I E **L**
3.	C **L** G G L L T M **V**	3.	R **R** Y P D A V Y **L**
1.	HIV RT 476-484	1.	HIV gp120 314-322
2.	Influenza A MP 59-68	2.	EBV EBNA-6R
3.	EBV LMP-2 426-434	3.	Measles F protein 323-331

Each MHC class I molecule has a particular peptide-binding motif that specifies the amino acid preferences for peptide side chains in the binding pockets. Motifs and examples of three T cell epitopes are shown for the human HLA-A2 and HLA-B27 proteins.

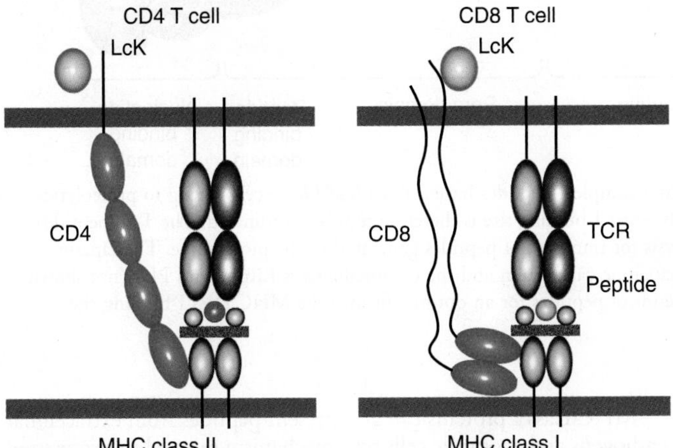

Figure 12–2 The CD4 and CD8 coreceptors bind to the membrane-proximal domains of major histocompatibility complex (MHC) class II and class I proteins, respectively. Coreceptor expression defines the CD4 and CD8 subpopulations of mature T cells. CD8 T cells recognize MHC class I-bound peptides and kill infected cells whereas CD4 T cells recognize MHC class II-bound peptides and coordinate immune responses. CD4 is a single-chain membrane protein with four extracellular Ig domains; CD8 is a homo- or heterodimer (CD8αα or CD8αβ) with an Ig domain and a long, flexible stalk segment. The coreceptors bind to the same peptide–MHC unit as the TCR: the TCR binds to membrane-distal peptide–MHC surface whereas the coreceptors bind to the membrane-proximal Ig domain(s): the CD8 dimer to the α3 domain of MHC class I proteins and CD4 to the interface between the α2 and β2 domains of MHC class II proteins. The coreceptors recruit the Src kinase Lck to the TCR during receptor activation.

peptide termini do not contribute to binding to MHC class II proteins, as described above for MHC class I. Rather, the interaction between the peptide and the MHC protein is stabilized by a set of conserved hydrogen bonds along the peptide backbone and the MHC helices.[24] These conserved interactions provide a peptide sequence-independent binding mechanism and are likely to contribute a substantial fraction of the total binding energy. In addition, pockets of the MHC class II-binding site can accommodate peptide side chains and these interactions contribute sequence specificity to the interaction. Many human autoimmune diseases are associated with particular alleles of MHC class II genes, indicating that the presentation of particular self-peptides to CD4 T cells is important in disease pathogenesis.[25] For example, susceptibility to type 1 diabetes is associated with a polymorphism at position 57 of the HLA-DQβ chain: most alleles carry an aspartic acid at this position, but diabetes-associated alleles have a noncharged amino acid at this site.[26] This polymorphism drastically alters the specificity of one particular pocket of the HLA-DQ binding site (P9 pocket) and enables the binding of certain self-peptides.[27]

Mechanisms of Peptide Generation and Loading

MHC class I and class II proteins sample distinct peptide pools in different subcellular compartments. MHC class I proteins acquire peptides in the endoplasmic reticulum (ER) that are imported from the cytosol through a dedicated peptide transporter (TAP). In contrast, MHC class II proteins traffic to endosomal/lysosomal vesicles and acquire peptides from phagocytosed pathogens. Sampling of these distinct environments is adapted to the lifestyle of the pathogens against which a T-cell response is mounted. CD8 T cells are specialized in detection of pathogens that replicate in the cytosol, viruses as well as intracellular bacteria and parasites, and kill infected cells that display pathogen-derived peptides on the cell surface. CD4 T cells are required for effective immune responses against pathogens that replicate in extracellular environments and induce the production of neutralizing antibodies by B cells, a process referred to as B-cell help (see Chapter 11).[28,29]

The MHC Class I Peptide Loading Complex

In cells infected by viruses and intracellular bacteria, pathogen-encoded proteins are synthesized by ribosomes of the host cell in the cytosol. Peptides loaded onto MHC class I proteins are generated in the cytosol by a large macromolecular complex of approximately 700 kd, the proteasome. The core proteasome is a cylindrical structure composed of four rings, each of which contains seven subunits. The two outer rings contain the α subunits and the two inner rings the catalytically active β subunits that have three different protease specificities. Proteins targeted for degradation thus have to enter the cylinder and are degraded to peptides with a length of approximately 3–22 residues (average of 13–18 residues). Proteins are targeted for proteasomal degradation by attachment of ubiquitin tags, and include misfolded and aging proteins as well as defective ribosomal prod-

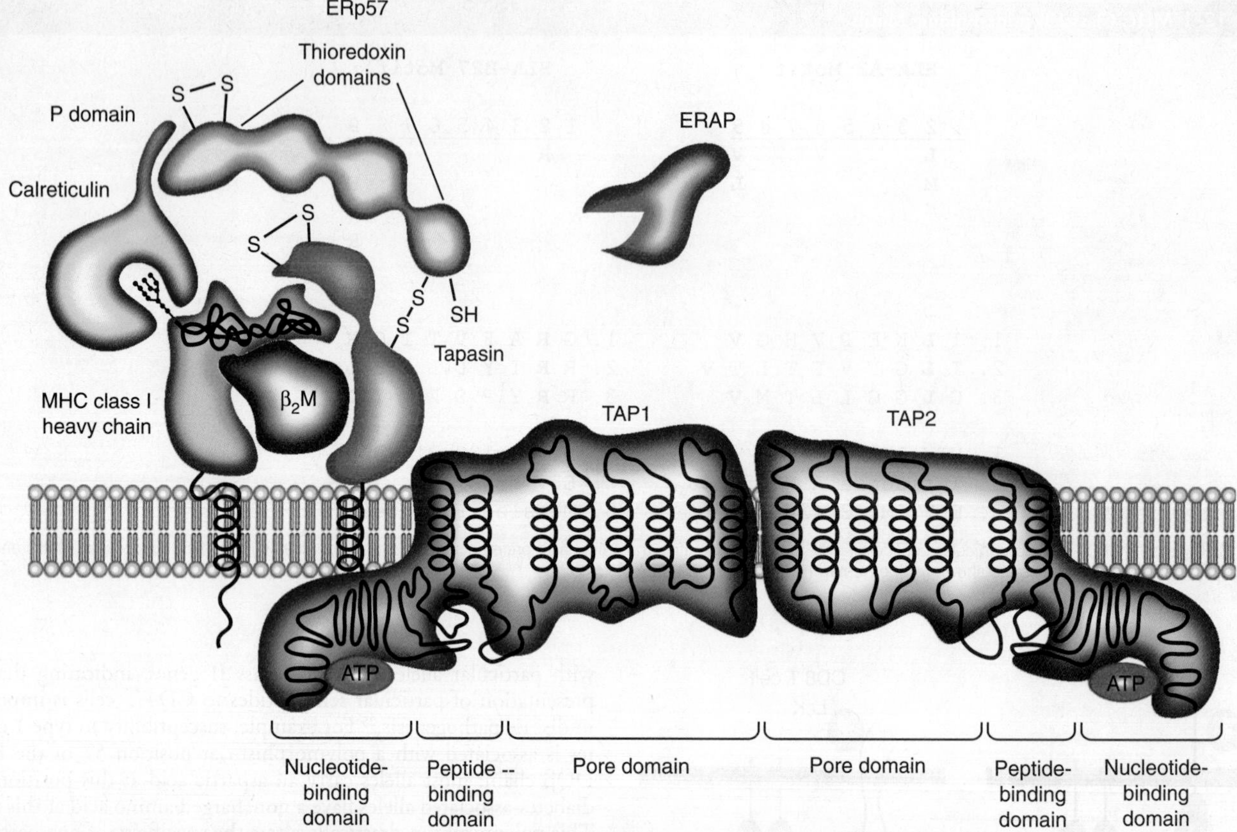

Figure 12–3 The major histocompatibility complex (MHC) class I peptide-loading complex. Peptides have a short half-life in cells owing to proteolytic attack. Translocation of peptides from the cytosol and their loading into the MHC class I-binding site is therefore tightly coordinated. The TAP peptide transporter is a heterodimer composed of TAP1 and TAP2 that uses ATP hydrolysis for transport of peptides generated in the proteasome. The tapasin protein represents the bridge between TAP and the MHC class I protein. The chaperone calreticulin and the oxidoreductases ERp57 and PDI (not shown) participate in peptide loading. The ERAP protease can trim the amino-terminal ends of peptides for an optimal fit into the MHC class I-binding site. Reprinted from *Nature Immunology*.[37]

ucts.[30] Inflammatory mediators (IFNγ and TNFα) enhance expression of immunoproteasome subunits, and the immunoproteasome can degrade proteins that have not been marked with ubiquitin, which accelerates peptide generation from recently synthesized pathogen-encoded proteins.[30,31]

It is important to appreciate that peptides have very short half-lives in cells because they are highly susceptible to degradation by proteases. Translocation of peptides into the ER and loading onto newly synthesized MHC class I molecules are coordinated by a specialized macromolecular protein complex, the MHC class I peptide loading complex (Fig. 12–3).[29] A key component of this complex is the TAP transporter that is responsible for ATP-driven translocation of peptides from the cytosol into the ER lumen.[32,33] MHC class I molecules are recruited to the TAP transporter by the tapasin protein, and this interaction is functionally important, as shown by the defect in MHC class I antigen presentation in tapasin-deficient mice.[34] Four tapasin molecules associate with one TAP transporter, and the complex thus contains four MHC proteins. The presence of four MHC proteins increases the chance that a translocated peptide will bind to one of the different MHC class I proteins (HLA-A, HLA-B, and HLA-C in humans). Three other proteins are associated with this complex: the chaperone calreticulin and the oxidoreductases ERp57 and protein disulfide isomerase (PDI). PDI catalyzes the oxidation of a critical disulfide bond between the floor of the peptide-binding groove and the α2 helix of the MHC class I protein and also transiently binds to peptides. Peptide translocation into the ER lumen, transient binding of peptide to PDI, and transfer of the peptide into the MHC class I cleft are thus closely linked.[35] Following stable binding of peptides, MHC class I molecules dissociate from the peptide-loading complex and are transported to the cell surface.

MHC class I proteins can also present peptides from extracellular pathogens and apoptotic cells by a mechanism referred to as crosspresentation. Proteins or peptides from phagocytosed pathogens or apoptotic cells are transported into the cytosol, and peptides derived from these antigens are then transported into the ER by the TAP transporter.[36,37] The crosspresentation pathway is described in detail in Chapter 14.

The MHC Class II Antigen Presentation Pathway

For MHC class I proteins, assembly and peptide loading occur in the same compartment and are closely linked processes. In contrast, MHC class II molecules assemble in the ER, but acquire peptides in a different compartment (Fig. 12–4). The invariant chain associates with recently assembled MHC class II αβ heterodimers in the ER and plays a critical role in the MHC class II pathway. Invariant chain forms a trimer and can associate with three MHC class II molecules into a nine-chain complex.[38] Invariant chain is a type II membrane protein and its N-terminal cytosolic domain bears an address code that targets the MHC class II-invariant chain complex to the endosomal–lysosomal pathway. Furthermore, the luminal domain of invariant chain protects the hydrophobic MHC class II peptide-binding site from aggregation.[39] The responsible invariant chain segment (CLIP, for class II-associated invariant chain peptide) occupies the groove in the same manner as other peptides and thus prevents binding of peptides to the MHC class II site before these molecules have reached their destination.[40] In the endosomal/lysosomal compartment, the invariant chain is degraded by a series of proteases down to the CLIP peptide segment that occupies the

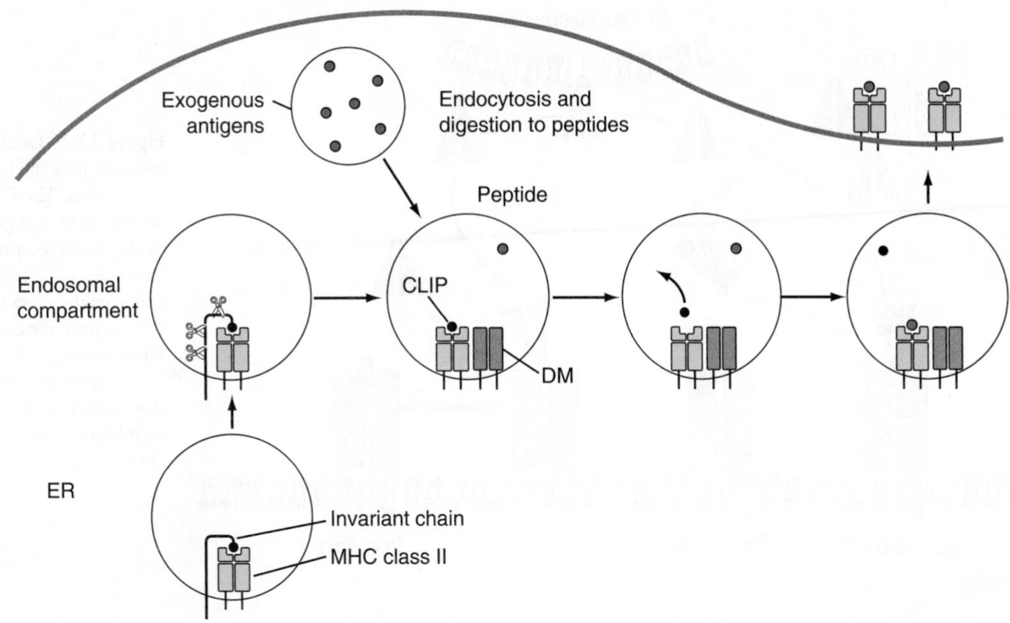

Figure 12–4 The major histocompatibility complex (MHC) class II antigen presentation pathway. MHC class II molecules assemble in the ER with the invariant chain. The class II-associated invariant chain peptide (CLIP) segment of invariant chain occupies the MHC class II groove and prevents binding of irrelevant peptides in the ER. The N-terminal cytoplasmic domain of invariant chain contains a targeting motif that directs the invariant chain–MHC class II complex to the endosomal–lysosomal compartment. In this low-pH compartment, invariant chain is proteolytically degraded down to the CLIP segment. HLA-DM binds to MHC class II–CLIP complexes and catalyzes the exchange of CLIP with peptides generated from endocytosed proteins by limited proteolysis. MHC class II-bound peptides have a long half-life at the neutral pH at the cell surface, resulting in peptide display for extended periods of time.

peptide-binding site. A critical cleavage is performed by the cysteine protease cathepsin S in bone marrow-derived antigen-presenting cells and the related cathepsin L enzyme in thymic cortical epithelial cells.[41,42]

The exchange of the invariant chain remnant CLIP with other peptides is catalyzed by the HLA-DM (DM) protein. DM is a heterodimer with sequence similarity to MHC class II proteins but cannot bind peptide.[43] Rather, it interacts with a lateral surface of MHC class II proteins and destabilizes the MHC class II-bound CLIP peptide.[44] DM also facilitates the dissociation of other peptides and this editing function favors the display of peptides at the cell surface that have a long half-life.[45] The generation of peptides and their loading occur at an acidic pH, and DM is active only in this pH range. The acidic pH in the peptide-loading compartment favors exchange, whereas the high stability of peptide–MHC complexes at a neutral pH favors long-lived display at the cell surface.[46] In fact, high-affinity peptides have exceptionally long half-lives, of several days to weeks, and the half-life of peptides is thus similar to those of the MHC proteins themselves.[47] T-cell epitopes frequently contain protease cleavage sites, and limiting proteolysis can therefore enhance presentation. Key antigen-presenting cells, such as dendritic cells and B cells, have lower levels of lysosomal proteases compared to macrophages that are specialized in rapid pathogen destruction.[48]

Presentation of Lipid Antigens by CD1 Proteins

In addition to the peptide-based surveillance system described above, T cells can also recognize pathogens depending on the recognition of lipid antigens presented by CD1 molecules. The CD1 heavy chains have sequence homology to MHC class I molecules and also assemble with β2-microglobulin. However, the CD1 genes (CD1a, CD1b, CD1c, and CD1d) are nonpolymorphic, which can be explained by the fact that microorganisms cannot readily evade recognition by modification of the lipids presented by CD1 proteins.[49] The ligand-binding site of CD1 molecules is adapted to the presentation of these ligands: it is considerably more hydrophobic than the binding site of MHC class I and class II proteins and also substantially wider.[50] Two large pockets can accommodate the two acyl chains of presented lipids whereas polar groups are positioned in the center for recognition by the TCR. The TCR shows exquisite specificity for these polar groups, such as sugar groups of glycolipids, whereas the length of the acyl chains accommodated in the pockets can vary considerably.[51] CD1 molecules acquire microbial lipid ligands in the endosomal pathway: following biosynthesis they first travel to the cell surface and are then endocytosed through recognition of a cytosolic targeting motif. Different CD1 molecules sample distinct subcompartments of the endosomal–lysosomal pathway and present different microbial lipids.[52] How do lipid groups enter the CD1 groove? Lipid loading is performed in the endosomal–lysosomal pathway by saposins, which are specialized lipid transfer proteins that extract lipids from membranes through specific interaction with their polar head groups (Fig. 12–5). The saposins A–D are generated by proteolytic cleavage of prosaposin and form small homodimers. Analogous to DM, saposins can perform editing of CD1-bound lipids and thus promote presentation of those lipids that form the most stable complexes with CD1 proteins.[53,54] Lipid antigens have been identified for *Mycobacterium tuberculosis*, including mycolic acid and glucose monomycolate, which are presented by human CD1b.[49,55]

MOLECULAR MECHANISM OF T-CELL RECOGNITION

Cloning of the T-Cell Receptor Genes

The physical identity of the TCR was a major question in immunology in the 1970s and early 1980s. Two general approaches were pursued, the generation of T cell-specific mAbs for purification and sequencing at the protein level and the isolation of T cell-specific cDNAs. The genetic studies searched for genes expressed in T cells but not B cells and that are rearranged in T cells to generate receptor diversity. The group led by Dr Mark Davis used subtractive hybridization to remove the cDNAs expressed in both T and B cells, whereas the group led by Dr Tak Mak performed differential hybrid-

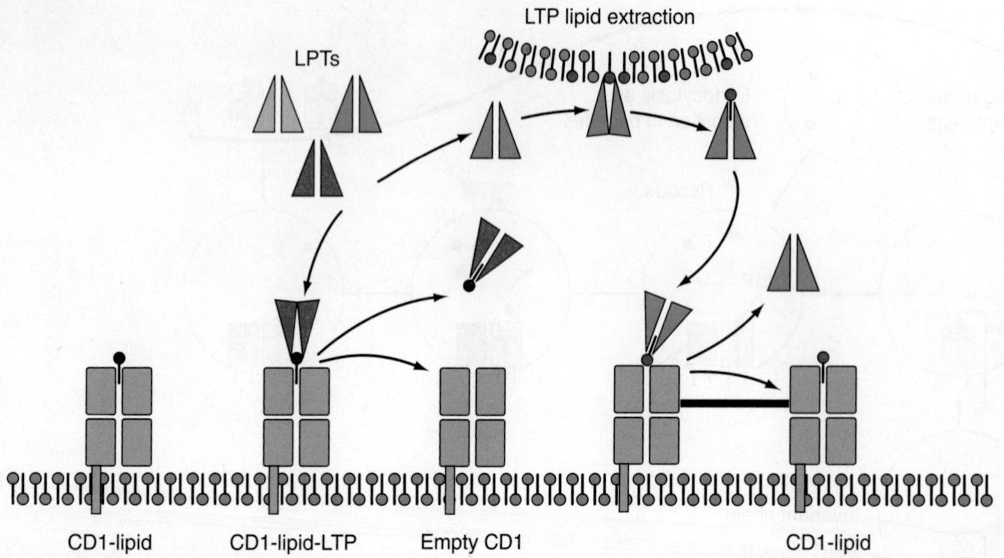

Figure 12–5 Loading of lipid antigens into the CD1 binding site by saposins. The CD1 proteins present lipid and glycolipid antigens to the T-cell receptor. CD1 molecules are targeted to the endosomal–lysosomal pathway, where they acquire exogenous lipid antigens. Lipid loading is facilitated by saposins, small homodimeric proteins that extract lipids from biological membranes. Reprinted from *Science* (53).

ization of T-cell cDNA libraries with T-cell and B-cell mRNA. These studies led to the identification of the TCR β chain in 1984, which was soon followed by isolation of the TCR α chain.[56,57] The availability of both TCR chains enabled an important experiment: transfection of both TCR chains reconstituted both peptide and MHC specificity, unequivocally demonstrating that a single receptor is sufficient for recognition of both components.[58]

These studies demonstrated that the TCR is a member of the immunoglobulin (Ig) superfamily and that each TCR chain possesses a variable and a constant domain with an Ig fold. Diversity is introduced by a molecular mechanism similar to that of antibodies, the rearrangement of variable, diversity, and joining (VDJ) segments. These junctions form the CDR3 loops that are critical for peptide recognition, as described in Structural Basis of TCR Recognition. The V domains encode the CDR1 and CDR2 loops that contribute to MHC recognition. The TCR β chain possesses greater junctional diversity than TCR α because junctions are created by the V, D, and J segments compared to only V and J segments for TCR α. However, a larger number of J segments are present in the TCR α locus, compensating for the absence of the D region.[59]

Further study by the laboratories of Drs Susumu Tonegawa and Michael Brenner led to the identification of a second TCR, the γδ TCR, which is expressed by a distinct T-cell subset.[60,61] γδ T cells have a different tissue distribution than αβ T cells, primarily the epithelial layer of the skin and the mucosal epithelium of the respiratory, intestinal, and reproductive tracts. Their anatomical distribution suggests a specialized role at sites of pathogen entry, but less is currently known about their ligands than for αβ T cells.[62]

The Signaling Subunits of the TCR

Inspection of the TCR α and β chain sequences demonstrated that the cytoplasmic tails are very short and thus not responsible for initiation of signaling. How are activation signals communicated into a T cell? Efforts to identify the TCR based on the monoclonal antibody strategy described above led to the identification of T cell-specific proteins that physically associate with the TCR, the CD3γ, δ, ε, and ζ chains (Fig. 12–6).[63] The CD3γ, δ, and ε chains each contain a single extracellular Ig domain and cytoplasmic domains with an immunoreceptor tyrosine-based activation motif (ITAM). Each ITAM contains two YxxL/I motifs with a tyrosine at the first position and an aliphatic residue (leucine or isoleucine) at the fourth position. These tyrosines are phosphorylated by Lck at an early stage of TCR triggering.[64] The CD3γ, δ and ε chains form two heterodimers, CD3γε and CD3δε. The ζ chain only has a short extracellular domain of nine amino acids, but its cytoplasmic domain is longer and carries three ITAMs. A TCR–CD3 complex is thus composed of a single TCR heterodimer, the CD3δε and CD3γε dimers as well as the disulfide-linked ζζ dimer (see Fig. 12–6).[65,66] Such a complex thus has a total of 10 ITAMs, six in the ζζ dimer and two in each CD3 dimer. The large number of ITAMs may be important for sensitive recognition of peptide–MHC complexes.

Molecular Mechanism for the Assembly of the TCR With Its Signaling Subunits

Inspection of the sequences of the TCR and its signaling subunits revealed an unusual feature: there are three basic residues in the transmembrane domains of the TCR, two in the TCR α chain and one in the TCR β chain, as well as a pair of acidic residues in the transmembrane domains of each of the dimeric signaling subunits. Mutagenesis experiments demonstrated that loss of even a single basic TCR transmembrane residue resulted in loss of surface expression, reflecting the presence of important protein–protein interactions in the membrane.[67] Further studies showed that each of the basic TCR transmembrane residues serves as an attachment site for a particular signaling module: the lysines in the transmembrane domains of TCR α and TCR β interact with CD3δε and CD3γε, respectively, whereas the arginine in the transmembrane domain of TCR α interacts with the ζζ dimer.[68] In each case, both acidic transmembrane residues are required for the interaction with a single basic residue, and the structure of the ζζ transmembrane dimer showed that the two aspartic acids form a single structural unit at the dimer interface.[69] The interaction between these basic and acidic residues stabilizes the receptor because exposure of these polar residues to the hydrophobic interior of the lipid bilayer would be energetically highly unfavorable.[68] This membrane-based assembly mechanism also serves a quality control purpose: unassembled subunits are retained in the ER and rapidly degraded.[70] Export from the ER requires masking of these polar residues at protein–protein interfaces.

Structural Basis of TCR Recognition

Each T cell expresses a distinct rearranged TCR, analogous to B cells that each express one particular BCR. The rearrangement process

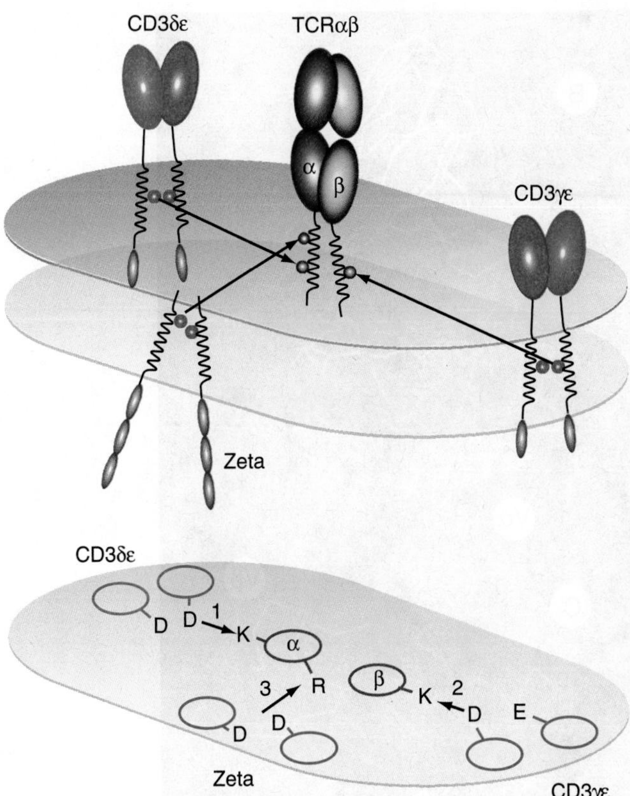

Figure 12–6 Assembly of the T-cell receptor (TCR) with its signaling subunits. The TCR heterodimer is responsible for peptide–major histocompatibility complex (MHC) recognition and assembles in the ER with three dimeric signaling modules, CD3δε, CD3γε, and ζζ. The CD3γ, δ, and ε chains have single extracellular Ig domains and a single immunoreceptor tyrosine-based activation motif (ITAM) motif in the cytoplasmic domain. The ζ chain has a short extracellular domain and a large cytoplasmic domain with three ITAM motifs. There are thus a total of 10 ITAMs in a TCR–CD3 complex that can be phosphorylated following TCR triggering. Each of the dimeric signaling modules carries a pair of acidic residues in the transmembrane domains (red circles) that interact with one particular basic residue (blue circle) in the TCR transmembrane domains. The transmembrane lysine (K) residues of TCR α and TCR β serve as the interaction sites for CD3δε and CD3γε, respectively. The ζζ dimer interacts with the transmembrane arginine (R) residue of TCR α. The lower part of the figure represents a section through the membrane that shows the three-helix interactions required for each of the three assembly steps.

generates a highly diverse TCR repertoire than can recognize virtually any MHC-bound peptide. Infection induces clonal expansion of T cells with specificity for peptides from the respective pathogen, and the maintenance of a subpopulation of these cells over many years represents the cellular basis of T-cell memory. In contrast to antibodies that can be generated against virtually any molecular shape, TCR recognition is limited to recognition of MHC-bound peptides or CD1-bound lipids. How are both peptide and MHC components recognized by the TCR? This question was answered in 1996 by the first crystal structures of TCRs bound to peptide–MHC class I complexes (Fig. 12–7).[71,72] In both structures, the TCR is centered over the peptide–MHC surface in a diagonal orientation that covers most of the MHC-bound peptide. This diagonal orientation appears to maximize the interaction with the MHC-bound peptide and positions the most variable sequence elements of the TCR, the CDR3 loops of TCR α and β chains, over the center of the MHC-bound peptide. The two CDR3 loops form a pocket in the center of the TCR surface that contacts peptide–MHC and this pocket can accommodate a side chain of the peptide. The germline-encoded CDR1 and CDR2 loops are less diverse in sequence and contact the two MHC helices. In all structures that have been determined to date, the CDR1 and CDR2 loops of the TCR α chain are positioned over the α2 helix of the MHC class I molecule, but the precise mechanism for this apparently conserved position is not yet known. The CDR1 loops can also contribute to peptide recognition: the CDR1α loop is positioned close to the peptide N-terminus and the CDR1β loop close to the peptide C-terminus. Four of the six TCR loops can thus read out the side chain specificity of the bound peptide.

Coreceptors and Costimulatory Molecules

The CD8 and CD4 molecules serve as coreceptors for MHC class I and class II restricted T cells, respectively (see Fig. 12–2). Approximately two-thirds of peripheral T cells are CD4 positive and one-third CD8 positive. The CD4 and CD8 molecules represent coreceptors because they bind to the same peptide–MHC unit as the TCR: the TCR binds to the membrane-distal peptide-binding site whereas the coreceptors engage the membrane-proximal Ig domains (see Fig. 12–2). The two coreceptors have a similar function but differ in their organization: CD4 is a single-chain membrane protein with four extracellular Ig domains, and CD8 is a dimer (CD8αβ or CD8αα) with an N-terminal Ig domain and a long extracellular stalk region that is highly glycosylated. The cytoplasmic domains of both CD4 and CD8 bind the tyrosine kinase Lck. The coreceptors thus recruit this Src kinase to the TCR for phosphorylation of the cytoplasmic ITAM domains. The coreceptors are not essential for T-cell activation but substantially increase the sensitivity of TCR activation, because lower peptide concentrations are required for coreceptor-positive T cells compared to coreceptor-loss mutants.[21]

TCR recognition is not sufficient for full T-cell activation. In fact, stimulation of T cells solely through the TCR leads to a state of unresponsiveness, referred to as T-cell anergy. Anergic T cells fail to respond to secondary stimulation with antigen-pulsed antigen-presenting cells, but retain the ability to proliferate in response to IL-2.[73] This observation led to the discovery of the costimulatory receptors, and CD28 was identified as the first member of this group. CD28 binds to CD80 and CD86 on antigen-presenting cells, and expression of these CD28 ligands is upregulated by activated dendritic cells and B cells. The cytoplasmic domains of the CD28 molecule carry a tyrosine-based phosphorylation motif that recruits the p85 subunit of phosphoinositol-3 kinase. Signaling through this receptor induces phosphorylation of c-fos and c-jun, which form the AP-1 transcription factor that binds to the IL-2 promoter. AP-1 also induces expression of the antiapoptotic Bcl-xL gene. CD28 is expressed by resting T cells and thus serves as an important costimulatory receptor of naïve T cells.[74] T-cell activation induces expression of CTLA-4, which also binds to CD80 and CD86, but induces a negative signal. CTLA-4-deficient mice die at a young age because of widespread inflammation, demonstrating the importance of this inhibitory pathway.[75] Blockade of this inhibitory pathway has shown promise in enhancing T-cell responses to tumors, in particular when the CTLA-4 antibody is administered together with a vaccine that induces an antitumor T-cell response.[76]

The inducible costimulatory receptor ICOS represents a third member of this family. In contrast to CD28, it is not constitutively expressed and serves a different function. ICOS-deficient mice have a defect in T cell-dependent antibody production by B cells, which is explained by the fact that stimulation through ICOS by ICOS-L enhances T-cell production of IL-10 and IL-4. Signaling through ICOS also stabilizes the mRNA for CD40L that interacts with the CD40 molecule on B cells.[77] These signals are critical for B-cell isotype switching and germinal center formation (see Chapter 11).

The Immunological Synapse

T-cell activation results in the formation of a highly organized structure at the interface between the interacting T cell and the antigen-presenting cell, the immunological synapse (Fig. 12–8). T cells are

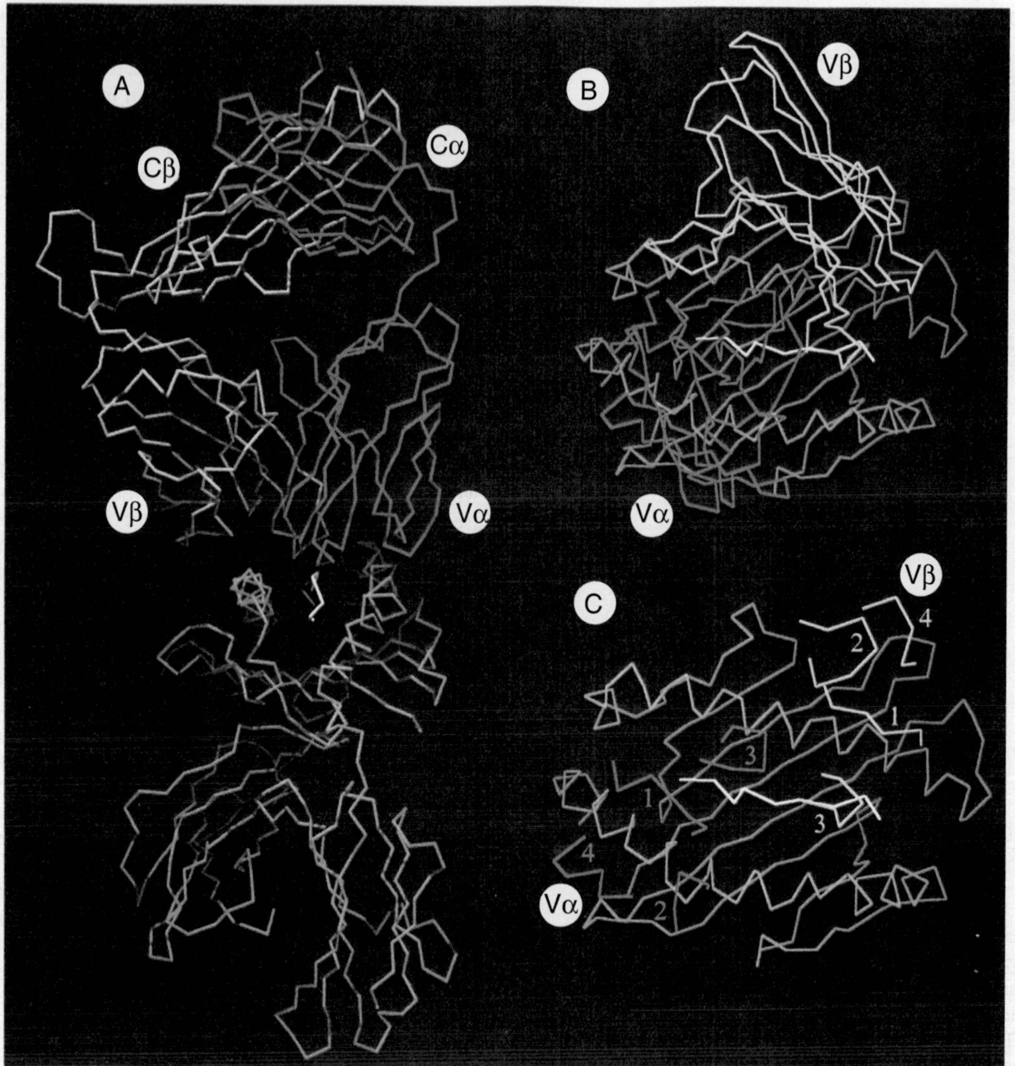

Figure 12–7 Structure of the T-cell receptor (TCR) bound to peptide–major histocompatibility complex (MHC). The TCR binds in a diagonal orientation over the surface created by the peptide and the long α helices of the MHC molecule that flank the bound peptide. This TCR position maximizes the interaction with the peptide. **A**, Overview of the complex composed of the TCR α and β chains (red and yellow, respectively) and the MHC molecule (green) with the bound peptide (white). **B**, The diagonal orientation of the TCR Vα and Vβ domains over the peptide–MHC surface, shown as a top view from the perspective of a T cell. **C**, Position of the TCR loops on the peptide–MHC surface. The hypervariable loops of the TCR α and β chains (CDR3 loops, labeled as 3) are located over the center of the peptide–MHC surface. The V-gene encoded CDR1 and CDR2 loops (labeled as 1 and 2, respectively) contact the MHC helices. The CDR1 loops can also contact the terminal segments of the peptide.

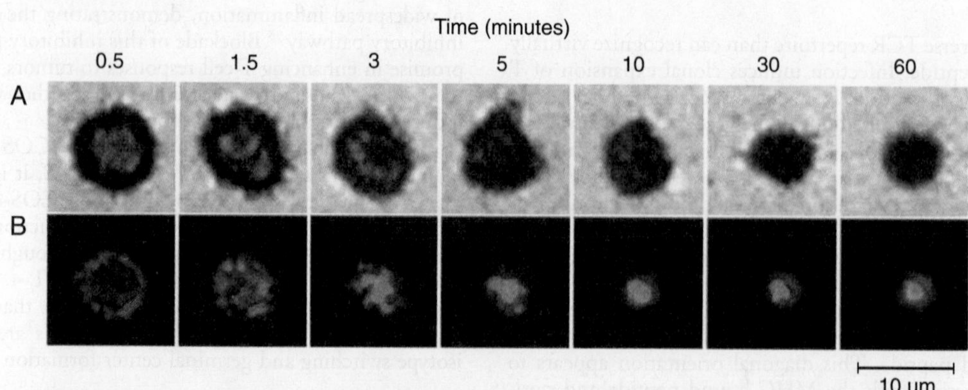

Figure 12–8 The immunological synapse. Recognition of agonist peptide–major histocompatibility complexes (MHCs) leads to the formation of a highly organized interface between the T cell and the antigen-presenting cell, termed the immunological synapse. Peptide–MHC complexes and the adhesion molecule ICAM-1 are labeled with green and red fluorophores, respectively. During initial contact, the peptide–MHC complexes (and corresponding TCRs) are located at the periphery of the interface. The peptide–MHC complexes are then transported into the center of the synapse and surrounded by a ring of ICAM-1 in the "mature" immunological synapse. The upper set of images shows the contact area of the T cell with the lipid bilayer. Reprinted from *Science*.[78]

highly motile and continuously crawl over the surface of antigen-presenting cells. Recognition of agonist peptide–MHC represents a stop signal and leads to the formation of an organized interface with the antigen-presenting cell. During initial contact, the adhesion molecule LFA-1 is located at the center of the interface and engaged TCRs at the periphery. During the next 5 to 10 minutes, this pattern reverses owing to transport of the TCR to the center. A mature immunological synapse is thus characterized by densely clustered TCRs in the center, surrounded by a ring of LFA-1 molecules.[78,79] What is the function of the immunological synapse? Analysis of early signaling events demonstrated the formation of TCR microclusters containing 10 to 20 molecules in the periphery, which are transported within approximately 2 minutes to the synapse center. These microclusters are sites of active signaling based on staining with phosphotyrosine antibodies and contain a number of signaling molecules critical for T-cell function. When these microclusters merge into the central TCR cluster, they are dephosphorylated by the CD45 phosphatase and marked for internalization and degradation by the E3 ubiquitin ligase Cbl. The central TCR cluster thus serves as the site of TCR dephosphorylation and internalization. However, microclusters are continuously formed in the periphery, resulting in sustained TCR signaling.[80]

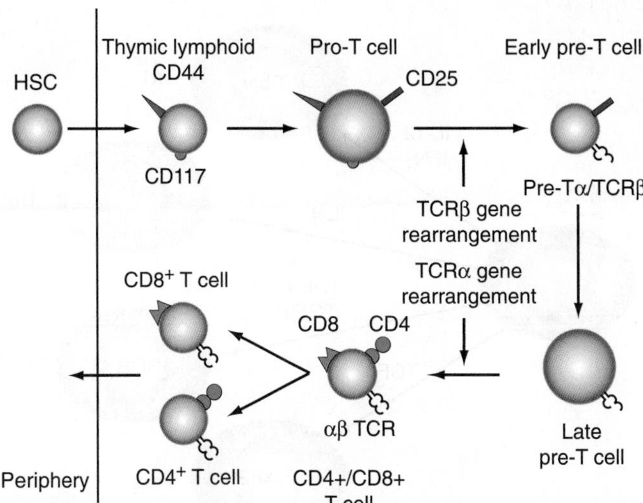

Figure 12–9 Maturation of hematopoietic stem cells in the thymus. (TCR, T-cell receptor.)

Sensitivity of TCR Recognition

Characterization of MHC-bound peptides with mass spectrometry techniques has demonstrated that a given MHC protein can bind several thousands of different peptides.[81] A given TCR has to recognize a particular peptide–MHC complex within a large number of other complexes, even though the complex of interest is present at a low density. Imaging experiments with fluorescently labeled peptides have shown that TCR recognition of only a few peptides is sufficient to induce calcium flux, and that maximum calcium flux is induced by approximately 10 to 20 peptide–MHC ligands.[82] How do T cells achieve such a level of sensitivity? A given TCR not only recognizes one particular agonist peptide–MHC complex but also other endogenous peptide–MHC complexes. The low-affinity interactions with the endogenous peptide–MHC complexes are not sufficient by themselves to trigger T-cell activation, but can amplify the signal induced by agonist peptide–MHC complexes that bind with higher affinity to the TCR.[83] The large number of ITAMs in the cytoplasmic domains of the TCR signaling subunits also contributes to the sensitivity of TCR signaling.

Mechanisms of Positive and Negative Selection of T Cells During Development in the Thymus

A system with the capability to respond to virtually any MHC-bound peptide obviously has the potential to do significant damage owing to attack on self-tissues. Elaborate mechanisms have evolved to eliminate the majority of self-reactive T cells during development in the thymus. Developing thymocytes (Fig. 12–9) first rearrange the TCR β chain, and the functionality of this rearrangement is tested by pairing with a surrogate TCR α chain, the pre-TCR α (pTα) chain.[84] The pTα chain only possesses a single extracellular Ig domain and can thus not form a TCR surface capable of recognizing peptide–MHC. However, it carries the two basic transmembrane residues required for interaction with CD3δε and ζζ and thus enables assembly of complete pre-TCR–CD3 complexes that signal constitutively when they reach the cell surface. preTCR expression prevents rearrangement of the second TCR β locus (allelic exclusion) and allows the cell to survive and rearrange the TCR α locus. Thymocytes that successfully rearrange both TCR loci become "double positive" T cells that express both the CD4 and CD8 coreceptor. Expression of an intact, mature TCR enables the first major selection step referred to as "positive selection." Positive selection requires proper engagement of peptide–MHC complexes on the surface of thymic epithelial cells, and the majority of thymocytes die at this step. The developing T cells then become CD4 or CD8 "single positive" T cells and migrate into the thymic medulla, where they face the second test, referred to as "negative selection."[85] At this stage, T cells are tested for their autoimmune potential and T cells whose TCR binds with too high an affinity to self-peptide–MHC complexes on thymic medullary thymic epithelial cells and dendritic cells die by apoptosis. Thymic medullary epithelial cells express a large variety of peripheral tissue antigens in a promiscuous manner, an unusual property that is in part controlled by the transcription factor Aire.[86] The importance of this pathway for the maintenance of tolerance is shown by the multiorgan autoimmune syndrome in both humans and mice with a defect in Aire expression.[87,88] Proper T-cell development in the thymus thus relies on TCR crossreactivity: T cells that weakly react with self-peptide–MHC complexes are positively selected whereas T cells that react too strongly are deleted. Weak recognition of thymic self-peptide–MHC complexes may set the appropriate recognition threshold for mature T cells and establish the intensity at which endogenous self-peptide–MHC complexes can amplify signaling induced by agonist peptide–MHC complexes without a resulting autoimmunity hazard.

Polyspecificity of TCR Recognition

The finding that endogenous peptides can contribute to TCR activation implies that a given TCR does not have strict specificity for a single peptide. This can be understood by considering the diversity of possible peptide sequences in a 9-mer: $20^9 = 5.12 \times 10^{11}$ sequences. For a given peptide, the precursor frequency in the naïve T-cell pool is in the range of $1:10^5$ to $1:10^7$ T cells, and comparison of the two numbers suggests that a given T cell can recognize a large number of different peptides. This conclusion is supported by experiments with peptide libraries, which demonstrated that a T-cell clone can be stimulated by peptide mixtures in which only one position carried a specified residue whereas all other positions were synthesized with amino acid mixtures. The concentration of an individual sequence in these libraries is thus far too small for activation, implying the existence of a large number of stimulatory sequences.[89] Nevertheless, T-cell activation is highly specific because minor changes in a given T-cell epitope can result in loss of recognition. The observed specificity and crossreactivity can be reconciled: T cells are specific because they recognize a very small subset of peptides but nevertheless cross-reactive because the number of peptides is very large. This finding has implications for the pathogenesis of autoimmune diseases because it raises the possibility that self-reactive T cells can be activated during an infection by a cross-reactive T-cell epitope. A number of examples

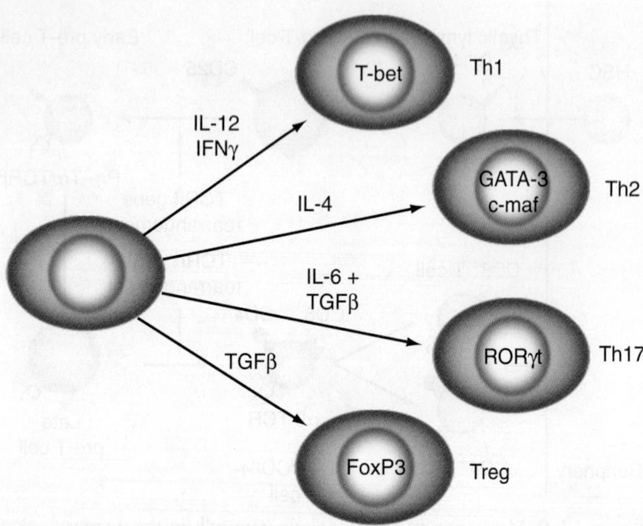

Figure 12–10 Cytokine-dependent differentiation of T cells into distinct subsets. CD4 T cells can differentiate into distinct functional subsets, IFNγ-producing Th1 cells, IL-4-producing Th2 cells, IL-17-producing Th17 cells, and regulatory T cells. The transcription factors that are required for differentiation into these subsets are indicated over the nucleus of the respective cell.

have been identified in which self-reactive T cells from patients with autoimmune diseases were activated by viral or bacterial peptides.[90] The majority of these peptides have only limited sequence similarity with the self-peptide.

T CELL-MEDIATED IMMUNE RESPONSES

CD4 T-Cell Subsets: Th1, Th2, and Th17

Activation of naïve CD4 T cells leads to their differentiation into distinct subsets, depending on the cytokine milieu, that serve specialized roles in the immune response (Fig. 12–10). Early work demonstrated that naïve CD4 T cells can differentiate into either IFNγ-producing cells (termed Th1 cells) or IL-4-producing T cells (Th2 cells).[91] Th1 cells are important in providing immunity to intracellular pathogens, such as viruses, intracellular bacteria, and parasites, whereas Th2 cells regulate immunity to extracellular pathogens through interaction with B cells. Th1 differentiation is favored by IL-12 and IFNγ produced by dendritic cells and macrophages, whereas Th2 differentiation is favored by IL-4. These cytokines also inhibit differentiation into the opposing subset: IL-4 blocks Th1 differentiation and IFNγ Th2 differentiation. The functional properties of Th1 and Th2 cells are controlled by key transcription factors, T-bet for Th1 as well as GATA-3 and c-maf for Th2 cells.[92,93] Expression of T-bet in established Th2 cells results in reversal to a Th1 phenotype, demonstrating the importance of this transcription factor in the biology of Th1 cells. These T-cell subsets also play important roles in particular disease states. For example, allergic diseases and asthma are characterized by accumulation of large numbers of allergen-specific Th2 cells that induce production of allergen-specific IgE antibodies, whereas Th1 cells can predominate in chronic inflammatory diseases.

Recent work has established the presence of another important subset of CD4 T cells that produce IL-17, a proinflammatory cytokine.[94] Such T cells play an important role in the pathogenesis of autoimmune diseases, as shown by studies in the experimental autoimmune encephalomyelitis (EAE) model of multiple sclerosis. Differentiation into this subset requires the coordinated production of two cytokines, IL-6 and TGFβ.[95] IL-23 also plays an important role in the biology of these cells: it is not required for the initial differentiation of Th17 cells, but is essential for their expansion and survival. As a consequence, IL-23-deficient mice are resistant to the induction of EAE. IL-17 induces the production of multiple chemokines and recruitment of other cells of the immune system to sites of inflammation.

CD8 T Cells

CD8 T cells play a central role in protection against infectious agents by killing of infected cells following recognition of microbial peptides presented by MHC class I molecules on the surface of target cells. Major efforts are also under way to harness tumor-specific CD8 T cells for the treatment of cancer. The main pathway for elimination of virus-infected cells is granule exocytosis (Fig. 12–11). After target cell recognition, cytotoxic granules are released into the immunological synapse formed between the killer cell and its target. The granules contain two membrane-perturbing proteins, perforin and granulysin, and a family of serine proteases known as granzymes, complexed with the proteoglycan serglycin. The perforin pore gives granzymes access to the cytosol of the target cells where they induce cell death pathways.[96]

T-Cell Expansion in Response to Infection and T-Cell Memory

The study of T-cell responses to infectious agents has been greatly advanced by the development of techniques that permit quantitative flow cytometric identification of responding T-cell populations. Particularly important has been the introduction of peptide–MHC tetramers as a tool for the visualization of T cells with defined specificity. What are tetramers? The TCR binds with low affinity to peptide–MHC and the off rate is too fast ($t_{1/2}$ of approximately 10 seconds) for TCR labeling with monomeric peptide–MHC complexes. However, the avidity of binding can be substantially enhanced by creation of multivalent ligands. Drs John Altman and Mark Davis created multivalent versions of peptide–MHC complexes by attaching a peptide tag that can be selectively biotinylated to the C-terminus of the MHC class I heavy chain.[97] This approach enables assembly of tetramers through the four biotin-binding sites of streptavidin. Fluorescent tetramers can be used to selectively label T cells with defined peptide–MHC specificity, regardless of their cytokine production profile, and to study the kinetics of T-cell expansion and contraction following viral infection.

T cells against a particular microbial peptide are present at a very low frequency in the naïve T-cell repertoire (approximately $1:10^5$ to $1:10^6$ T cells). Infection triggers massive expansion of these cells and a large fraction of all CD8 T cells can be pathogen-specific at the peak of expansion. The CD8 T-cell response against a viral pathogen can be divided into three distinct phases, as shown by infection of mice with lymphocytic choriomeningitis virus.[98] During the first phase, massive expansion of virus-specific CD8 T cells occurs and 30% to 50% of all CD8 T cells can be specific for a single immunodominant viral peptide on day 8 following infection. These T cells have classical effector properties: they can kill infected target cells by release of granules containing granzyme and perforin, produce cytokines such as IFNγ and TNFα and migrate to nonlymphoid tissues. T-cell proliferation is greatest between days 3 to 5 following infection and T cells increase in frequency approximately 500-fold (9 divisions) during this time window with an estimated doubling time of 6 to 8 hours. In the second contraction phase that follows clearance of the pathogen, 90% to 95% of these effector T cells die by apoptosis. The final phase (after day 30) represents the establishment and maintenance of CD8 T-cell memory. IL-7 provides important survival signals during effector-to-memory cell differentiation through the expression of Bcl-2. Precursors of memory CD8 T cells can be identified within the effector cell population based on high-level expression of the IL-7Rα chain. Memory CD8 T cells rapidly acquire effector function with reexposure to the pathogen and expand rapidly.

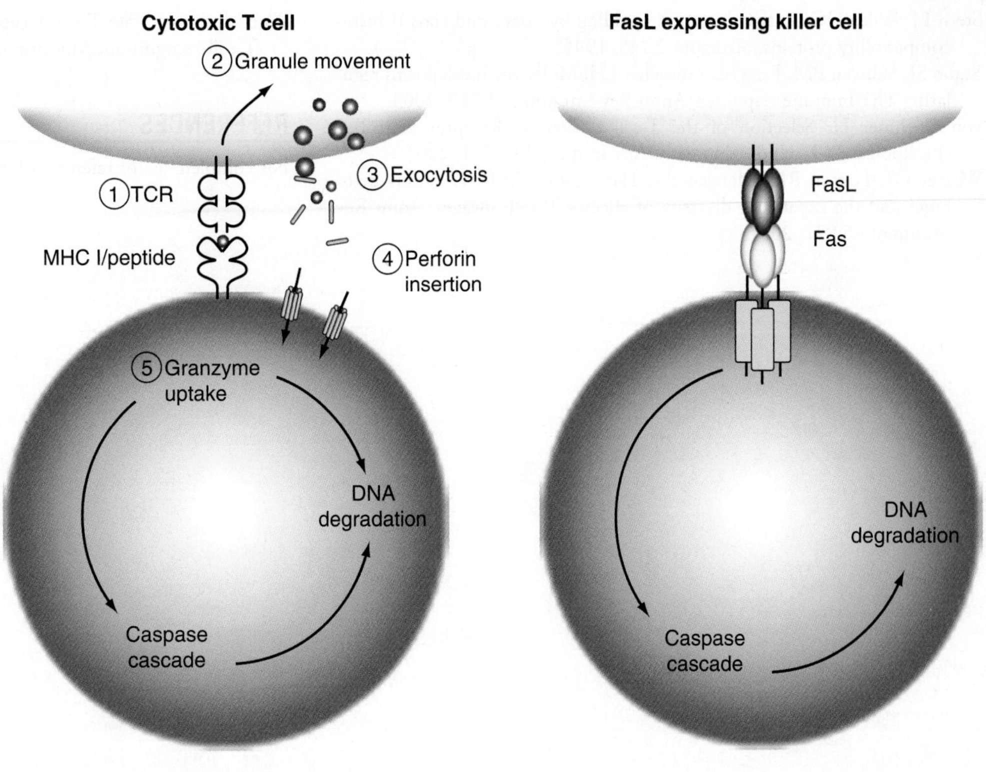

Cytotoxic T cell

FasL expressing killer cell

2 Granule movement

1 TCR

MHC I/peptide

3 Exocytosis

4 Perforin insertion

5 Granzyme uptake

DNA degradation

Caspase cascade

FasL

Fas

DNA degradation

Caspase cascade

Figure 12–11 Apoptosis can be caused by granule exocytosis or Fas–Fas ligand (FasL) pathways. After the interaction of the T-cell receptor (TCR) with major histocompatibility complex (MHC) class I–peptide, granules containing perforin and granzymes localize toward the target cells and are released. Perforin inserts into the plasma membrane, and granzymes move into the target cell. Perforin and granzyme act synergistically to activate the caspase cascade, resulting in apoptosis. Binding of FasL to Fas also activates the caspase cascade, resulting in apoptosis.

Memory CD8 T cells persist for many years at relatively constant numbers owing to homeostatic proliferation that compensates for cell loss. They do not require the continued presence of antigen or expression of MHC molecules and instead depend on the cytokines IL-7 and IL-15; IL-7 promotes their survival and IL-15 induces slow homeostatic proliferation. Memory T cells and B cells provide protective immunity for decades and the rapid and specific response that is induced following reexposure to the pathogen is the basis for vaccination.[99] Vaccination enabled global eradication of smallpox, one of the major achievements of medicine in the past century.

Regulatory T Cells

How are T cell-mediated immune responses regulated? This question had posed a long-standing problem in immunology because it had been very difficult to define precise molecular markers for regulatory T cells. A major breakthrough in this field came when *FoxP3* was identified as the defective gene in a human X-linked multiorgan autoimmune disease.[100] *FoxP3* also represents the defective gene in the Scurfy mouse strain which is characterized by hyperactivation of T cells and overproduction of inflammatory cytokines. Introduction of the *Foxp3* gene into naïve T cells induces a regulatory T-cell (Treg) phenotype and program: these cells express CD25 (the IL-2R α chain), CTLA-4, and GITR and are able to inhibit the activation of other T cells.[101,102] FoxP3 thus represents a key transcription factor for Treg differentiation. IL-2 plays a critical role in the biology of these cells: Tregs do not synthesize IL-2 and instead compete with effector T cells for IL-2 present in the local microenvironment through their high-affinity IL-2 receptor. IL-2 also provides an important signal for production of IL-10 by Tregs, a cytokine that blocks Th1 and Th2 responses. These findings explain why IL-2- and CD25-deficient mice develop a severe inflammatory disease and why neutralization of IL-2 can precipitate autoimmune disease.[103,104] The definitive identification of these regulatory T cells now opens the door to the development of specific therapies for the treatment of autoimmune diseases, allergies, and transplant rejection. Tregs induce local immune suppression, and Tregs with a single specificity are therefore sufficient to inhibit a polyclonal T-cell response by both CD4 and CD8 T cells in a given organ. T cells specific for a myelin peptide could thus inhibit the local immune response in the CNS in multiple sclerosis patients without affecting immune responses at other sites. Furthermore, inhibition of Treg activity at the time of immunization may be useful for enhancement of T-cell responses against tumors.

SUGGESTED READINGS

Bjorkman PJ, Saper MA, Samraoui B, et al: Structure of the human class I histocompatibility antigen, HLA-A2. Nature 329:506, 1987.

Busch R, Rinderknecht CH, Roh S, et al: Achieving stability through editing and chaperoning: Regulation of MHC class II peptide binding and expression. Immunol Rev 207:242, 2005.

Brigl M, Brenner MB: CD1: Antigen presentation and T cell function. Annu Rev Immunol 22:817, 2004.

Call ME, Wucherpfennig KW: The T cell receptor: Critical role of the membrane environment in receptor assembly and function. Annu Rev Immunol 23:101, 2005.

Cresswell P, Ackerman AL, Giodini A, et al: Mechanisms of MHC class I-restricted antigen processing and cross-presentation. Immunol Rev 207:145, 2005.

Dustin ML: A dynamic view of the immunological synapse. Semin Immunol 17:400, 2005.

Garboczi DN, Ghosh P, Utz U, et al: Structure of the complex between human T-cell receptor, viral peptide and HLA-A2. Nature 384:134, 1996.

Gourley TS, Wherry EJ, Masopust D, Ahmed R: Generation and maintenance of immunological memory. Semin Immunol 16:323, 2004.

Greenwald RJ, Freeman GJ, Sharpe AH: The B7 family revisited. Annu Rev Immunol 23:515, 2005.

Irvine DJ, Purbhoo MA, Krogsgaard M, Davis MM: Direct observation of ligand recognition by T cells. Nature 419:845, 2002.

Konig R: Interactions between MHC molecules and co-receptors of the TCR. Curr Opin Immunol 14:75, 2002.

Mowen KA, Glimcher LH: Signaling pathways in Th2 development. Immunol Rev 202:203, 2004.

Sakaguchi S, Ono M, Setoguchi R, et al: Foxp3+ CD25+ CD4+ natural regulatory T cells in dominant self-tolerance and autoimmune disease. Immunol Rev 212:8, 2006.

Stern LJ, Wiley DC: Antigenic peptide binding by class I and class II histocompatibility proteins. Structure 2:245, 1994.

Szabo SJ, Sullivan BM, Peng SL, Glimcher LH: Molecular mechanisms regulating Th1 immune responses. Annu Rev Immunol 21:713, 2003.

von Boehmer H: Selection of the T-cell repertoire: Receptor-controlled checkpoints in T-cell development. Adv Immunol 84:201, 2004.

Weaver CT, Hatton RD, Mangan PR, Harrington LE: IL-17 family cytokines and the expanding diversity of effector T cell lineages. Annu Rev Immunol 25:821, 2007.

Wucherpfennig KW: T cell receptor crossreactivity as a general property of T cell recognition. Mol Immunol 40:1009, 2004.

REFERENCES

For complete list of references log onto www.expertconsult.com

CHAPTER 13

NATURAL KILLER CELL IMMUNITY

Don M. Benson, Jr. and Michael A. Caligiuri

INTRODUCTION

Natural killer (NK) cells are large granular lymphocytes comprising about 10% to 15% of the peripheral circulation.[1,2] First characterized by their ability to lyse targets independent of any prior activating or initiating stimuli,[3] NK cells are a critical cellular component of the innate immune system. In contradistinction to acquired immunity, the innate immune system functions as first line defense, always ready to mount an immediate antigen-independent immune response. Passive components include opsonins, lysozyme and phospholipases found at barriers between host and outside environment. Cellular components of innate immunity include neutrophils, macrophages, eosinophils, and NK cells. In addition, NK cells secrete cytokines that help to marshal and shape the innate and adaptive immune response to infection and malignant transformation. There has been a recent surge of interest in NK cells as new discoveries in both the laboratory and the clinic have characterized the crucial contributions of NK cells in shaping the early immune response.[4] NK cells play a key role in maintaining host defense as exemplified in human NK cell deficiency syndromes (which carry increased susceptibility to overwhelming viral, intracellular, and atypical mycobacterial infections),[5] and animal models of NK cell deficiency (eg, such mice are particularly susceptible to developing cancer).[6,7] The present chapter will review the current understanding of basic NK cell biology, the role of NK cells in human diseases, and the recent clinical applications of NK cells in cancer therapy.

FUNDAMENTAL BIOLOGY

NK Subsets

NK cells are phenotypically recognized by surface expression of CD56 (also called neural cell adhesion molecule, NCAM) and the absence of the T-cell specific surface antigen CD3 as well as the T cell receptor, TCR.[8,9] Based on the intensity of CD56 surface expression, two functional subsets (so called CD56^{bright} and CD56^{dim}) of NK cells may be discriminated from one another. CD56^{dim} NK cells comprise 85% to 90% of the NK cells in peripheral circulation and are potent mediators of cytotoxicity. Ten percent to 15% of NK cells in the circulation are CD56^{bright} and upon activation, this subset is capable of robust cytokine and chemokine production.[2] Fig. 13–1 graphically represents the NK subsets described below, and Table 13–1 summarizes major surface antigens associated with each NK cell subset.

CD56^{dim} NK Cells

CD56^{dim} NK have exquisite natural cytolytic properties, being able to kill infected as well as tumor cell targets without prior sensitization.[10] They constitutively express the IL-2/15 receptor (R) β and common γ receptor chains, which together form a receptor complex through which cells may respond to stimulation by either IL-2 or IL-15.[11,12] CD56^{dim} NK cells can lyse tumor cell targets through at least three distinct mechanisms. First, they can execute cytotoxicity through granule exocytosis of perforin and granzyme.[13,14] Second, cytotoxicity can be mediated through FasL and TRAIL associated with production of cytokines including IFN-γ, TNF-α, and GM-CSF.[15] Third, CD56^{dim} NK cells can mediate antibody dependent cytotoxicity (ADCC) via the high density surface expression of CD16 (the FcγRIII receptor).[2,16] Freshly isolated, unstimulated CD56^{dim} NK cells have intrinsically greater cytotoxicity against NK-sensitive targets such as the K562 cell line in vitro, compared to the CD56^{bright} NK cells.[17]

Other antigens are differentially expressed by CD56^{dim} NK cells and provide insight into their functional role in the immune response. For example, CD56^{dim} NK cells also exhibit relatively high surface density expression of killer immunoglobulin-like receptors (KIR). NK cell KIR expression appears important in preventing autoimmunity and in surveying against malignant transformation.[16,18]

Both CD56^{dim} and CD56^{bright} NK cells express modest levels of the chemokine receptor CXCR3. However, in contrast to CD56^{bright} NK cells, CD56^{dim} NK cells display relatively abundant surface expression levels of CXCR1, CXCR4, and CX_3CR1.[19] CXCR1 binds IL-8, CXCR4 binds SDF-1. These cytokines are associated with local inflammatory response, for example, IL-8 levels are increased in the setting of acute viral infections,[20] and IL-8 and SDF-1 levels are increased with solid[21,22] and hematopoietic malignancies.[23,24] Thus, expression of these chemokine receptors allow NK cells to traffic to local areas of inflammatory response to mediate antiviral and antitumor activity.

CD56^{bright} NK Cells

CD56^{dim} NK cells, with their relatively high density expression of FcγRIII, NKR and KIR, constitutive cytolytic granules and limited proliferative capacity, likely represent the more cytotoxic subset of human NK cells. CD56^{bright} NK cells, conversely play more of an immunoregulatory role. CD56^{bright} NK produce a multitude of cytokines and chemokines, have a relatively high proliferative capacity, reside primarily in the parafollicular T cell rich region of secondary lymphoid tissue (SLT), and have modest cytolytic granules, KIR and FcγRIII expression (Table 13–1).[10] CD56^{bright} NK cells are unique among cytotoxic effector cells in constitutive expression of the high affinity IL-2Rαβγ complex, making them responsive to picomolar concentrations of IL-2 released by activated T cells in the parafollicular T cell rich region of SLT.[25] As noted, CD56^{bright} NK cells comprise only about 10% of the circulating NK population, but predominate almost to the exclusion of the CD56^{dim}NK subset in SLT.[2,26] This likely results from their selective expression of a number of receptors that assist in homing cells to and retaining cells in SLT (eg, CCR7 and CD62L).[10]

The ability of CD56^{bright} NK cells to produce an abundant variety of cytokines and chemokines compared to the CD56^{dim} subset likely relates more to the differential expression of both negative and positive regulators of cytokine/chemokine production and less to constitutive expression of cytokine-activating receptors. For example, CD56^{bright} NK cells have little or no expression of two negative regulators of cytokine/chemokine production, namely SHIP-1 and HLX,[27,28] whereas CD56^{dim} NK lack constitutive expression of a positive regulator of cytokines called SET.[29]

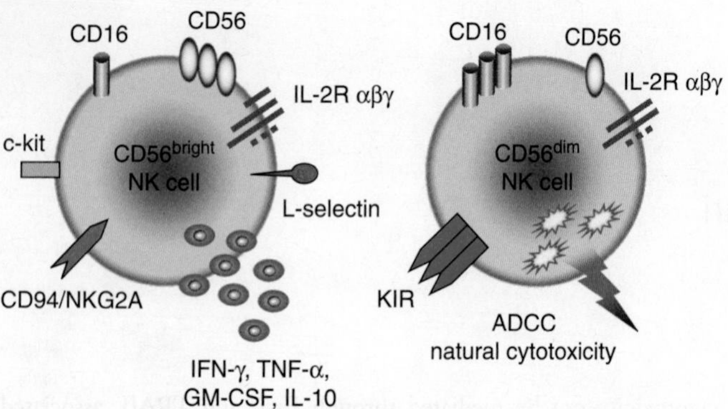

Figure 13–1 Simplified cartoon representation of natural killer cell subsets: CD56[bright] cells have immunoregulatory function whereas CD56[dim] cells have cytolytic function. ADCC, antibody-dependent cellular cytotoxicity; GM-CSF, granulocyte/macrophage-colony stimulating factor; IFN, interferon; IL, interleukin; KIR, killer immunoglobulin receptor; R, receptor; TNF, tumor necrosis factor. *(Adapted from Cooper MA, Fehniger TA, Caligiuri MA: The biology of human natural killer cell subsets. Trends Immunol 22:633, 2001.)*

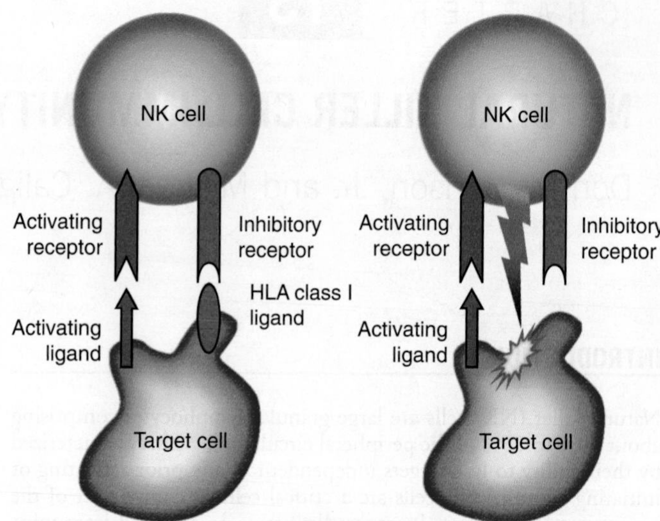

Figure 13–2 Simplified cartoon representation of natural killer cell cytotoxicity mediated through the balance of activating and inhibitory signaling in response to ligands on potential targets. The target cell on the left is spared, whereas the target cell on the right is lysed. *(Adapted from Farag SS, Fehniger TA, Ruggeri L, et al: Natural killer cell receptors: new biology and insights into the graft-versus-leukemia effect. Blood 100:1935, 2002.)*

NK DEVELOPMENT

A series of studies over the past 12 years has demonstrated that IL-15 is required for NK cell development in mouse and humans,[30,31] but until recently, there has been little known about where human NK cells develop. As with B cells and T cells, human NK cells are derived from CD34(+) hematopoietic stem cells in bone marrow (BM), however NK cell precursors in human BM have not been identified, suggesting that maturation may occur elsewhere.[2,32] Freud et al recently identified a CD34[dim]CD45RA(+)$\alpha_4\beta_7$[bright] cell to be the only CD34(+) subset in SLT. Found within the parafollicular T cell rich region of SLT in the same region as the CD56[bright] NK cell, this CD34[dim]CD45RA(+)$\alpha_4\beta_7$[bright] cell can differentiate into a CD56[bright] NK cell in the presence of IL-15.[22] With evidence for a CD34(+) NK precursor and CD56[bright] NK cell in the same region within SLT, Freud et al next hypothesized that NK cells may develop in SLT and thus developmental intermediates should be identifiable. Indeed, four novel, discrete populations representing four stages of NK cell development were subsequently found in situ within the same parafollicular region of SLT, each characterized by their differential expression of CD34, CD117, and CD94.[33] As development proceeds along this continuum, cells acquire the ability to secrete cytokines (eg, interferon-γ),?display natural cytotoxicity, and lose the ability to differentiate into dendritic cells (DC) and/or T cells. Although not yet proven, this orderly development in SLT from a CD34(+) subset to CD56[bright] NK cells suggests that CD56[dim] NK cells represent a terminally differentiated NK stage that follows CD56[bright] NK development and exit into the periphery. The abundance of CD56[dim] NK cells in blood versus SLT, their loss of both CD117 (c-kit) expression and proliferative capacity, along with their acquisition of KIR, FcRγRIII, and cytolytic granules are all consistent with this notion, yet direct evidence to support this is currently not available.[2]

Table 13–1 Human Natural Killer Cell Subsets Display Different Repertoires of Surface Antigens*

Antigen	CD56[dim]	CD56[bright]
CD16 (FcγRIIIa)	+++	–/+
KIR	+++	–/+
CXCR1	+	–
CXCR3	++	–
CX3CR3	+	–
CXCR4	++	–
CD94	–	++
NKG2A	–/+	+
NKG2D	+	+
c-kit	–	+
CCR7	–	++
CD2	++	+++
CD62L (L-selectin)	+	++
CD44	+	++

Adapted from Trends Immunol 22:633, 2001.[2]

NK RECEPTORS

How NK cells recognize infected or neoplastic targets from normal self has been an intense area of research for over two decades.[34] NK cells, as opposed to B and T lymphocytes, do not undergo clonotypic gene rearrangement in order to express antigen receptors; however, through the expression of a complex repertoire of surface molecules, NK cells may efficiently determine nonself from self and rapidly initiate an appropriate response. NK cell receptors may be activating or inhibitory—in other words, binding of the receptor to its ligand expressed on a target cell either activates or suppresses a functional NK response towards the target. Such receptors fall into three general categories: those which are members of the immunoglobulin-like superfamily (KIR), one type which belongs to the C-type lectin receptor (CLR) superfamily,[35] and finally so-called natural killer cell specific receptors (NKR). The complex function of these receptor subsets is still a matter of intense research; however, a model by which NK cell receptors KIR may recognize particular features of MHC class I alleles (eg, HLA-A,[36] HLA-B,[37] HLA-C[38]) or recognize other surface antigens on target cells has been developed.[40] Fig. 13–2 is a simplified, schematic representation of what we currently understand regarding the ability of NK cells and their receptors to survey the immune system.

KIR

KIRs provide one method by which NK cells recognize self from nonself to mediate the appropriate cytotoxic response. There are currently 15 KIRs identified on chromosome 19q13.4.[18,39,40] Structurally, KIRs contain two or three extracellular immunoglobulin like domains and recognize MHC Class I proteins.[18,36,37] KIRs may be either inhibitory or activating, a functional feature associated with the intracellular tyrosine-based motif of the molecule.[18] All of this information may be deduced for a particular receptor through the nomenclature used to identify KIRs. The number of Ig-like domains (2 or 3) is expressed, eg, KIR2D or KIR3D and the length of the intracytoplasmic tail (ie, a long [L] inhibitory tail or a short [S] activating tail) is also incorporated, eg, KIR2DL or KIR2DS. A suffix numeral follows the identification of some KIR to represent polymorphic forms of each receptor; for example, KIR2DS2 and KIR2DS3, each indicating a polymorphic form of an activating KIR that bears the same extra extracellular domains. HLA-C is particularly important in KIR-mediated self/nonself recognition because many well-described KIR have ligand specificity for HLA-C associated antigens. For example, the inhibitory receptor KIR2DL1 (CD158a) recognizes Group 2 HLA-C Asn77Lys80 (HLA-Cw2, w4, w5, w6 and related alleles), and the inhibitory receptors KIR2DL2 and KIR2DL3 recognize Group 1 HLA-C Ser77Asn80 (HLA-Cw1, w3, w7, w8 and related alleles).[40] Activating receptors KIR2DS1 and KIR2DS2 recognize the same Group 2 and Group 1 antigens as the inhibitory counterparts; however, generally, inhibitory receptors bind with greater avidity or attraction for a corresponding HLA antigen than activating receptors.[41] Complementary activating and inhibitory KIRs recognize the same cognate extracellular domains on target cells; thus if an NK cell expresses both activating and inhibitory KIR for an identical ligand, the cell will generally be inhibited from killing.

Understanding of KIRs continues to expand. The KIR family is likely not all inclusive for human classical type I HLA allotypes, for instance, only one inhibitory KIR directed against HLA-A (KIR3KL2) and none towards HLA-B alleles have been found.[40] Additionally, specific KIRs may have particular roles in maintaining host immunity in unique settings. For example, KIR2DL4 recognizes the nonclassical HLA-G molecule that is only expressed on fetal extravillous trophoblasts that invade the maternal decidua during pregnancy.[42] Controversy surrounds the exact nature of this KIR; however, KIR2DL4 is likely not clonally distributed as other KIRs but is present on the surface of most mature NK cells.[43] Interestingly, despite having an inhibitory intracellular signaling moiety, KIR2DL4 serves to promote IFN-γ secretion but not cytolytic activity.[43] It is possible that this KIR functions to facilitate immune tolerance to the developing fetus.[44]

C-Type Lectin Receptors

C-type lectin receptors (CTLRs), located on human chromosome 12p.12.3, share a common subunit (CD94) covalently bonded to one of four closely related gene products of the NKG2 family.[45,46] CTLR represent a second type of NK cell receptor mediating killing and include NKG2A (and splice variant B), NKG2C, NKG2E (and splice variant H), and NKG2F.[46] NKG2D, which does not bind CD94 and shares little sequence homology to other NKG2 proteins, is discussed in next paragraph. All but one of the CTLRs are activating and expressed on NK cells as well as cytotoxic T lymphocytes. CD94/NKG2A is inhibitory and is expressed on NK cells as well as cytotoxic T lymphocytes where they serve to regulate CD8(+) T cell antiviral responses.[47] CD94/NKG2A specifically recognizes the nonclassical HLA-E Class I molecule.[48] Interestingly, HLA-E specifically presents leader peptides from other HLA receptor antigens; thus, sensitivity to HLA-E provides a mechanism for NK cells to sense functional overexpression of class I MHC molecules on cell surfaces. As with KIR, binding between CD94/NKG2A and HLA-E is more avid than binding of activating CTLRs to other epitopes, however, unlike KIR, the target antigens for activating and inhibitory CTLR are not the same.[49]

NKG2D is a CTLR, however, it has only modest sequence homology with other members of the NKG2 family and does not associate with CD94.[48] NKG2D exists as a homodimer and does not have inherent signaling capability, but rather signals via the PI3K pathway as recruited through DAP10[Wu] or KAP10.[50] This unique signal transduction arrangement renders NKG2D signaling privileged from inhibitory, intracellular intermediaries that modulate signal transduction of other CTLR systems. NKG2D is constitutively expressed on all NK cells, γδ T cells, and CD8(+) T cells.[51]

NKG2D mediates killing of cellular targets expressing two antigens associated with viral or neoplastic transformation.[40,52] First, *M*HC class *I* *c*hain-related antigens (MIC) are a family of proteins whose expression correlates with heat shock and viral and neoplastic transformation.[51,53] MICA and MICB expression are under control of promoter elements similar to that of heat shock proteins and have been shown to be upregulated in the setting of CMV infection as well as in a number of epithelial and hematologic malignancies.[53,54] Second, UL16 *b*inding *p*rotein (ULBP) serves as a ligand for NKG2D. UL16 is a type I transmembrane protein ubiquitously expressed in the setting of CMV infection.[55] UL16 binds MICB and two other proteins, ULBP-1 and ULBP-2.[56] (These latter proteins have α1 and α2 domains but lack an α3 domain as MIC and MHC class I molecules have; furthermore, they are expressed via a glycosylphosphatidyl inositol (GPI)-anchor and thus have no requirement for β_2 microglobulin.) In binding MICB, ULBP-1 and ULBP-2, CMV-produced UL16 counteracts cell surface expression of these NKG2D ligands, thus providing a mechanism of immune evasion from NK cell surveillance and cytotoxicity.[57] In similar fashion, some human tumors downregulate expression of NKG2D ligands or release soluble forms of such (eg, MICA or ULBPs), as a mechanism of immune escape from NK cells.[58–60] Although ULBPs are expressed more ubiquitously than MIC proteins, some tissues with high mRNA levels express no protein, implying important posttranscriptional control of these antigens.[56] Interestingly, IL-15 stimulation enhances the NK cell NKG2D-mediated response to tumors expressing ULBP.[61]

Other Activating NK Receptors

A third family of NK receptors that mediate cell killing are called natural cytotoxicity receptors (NCR).[54,62] In addition to NKG2D, NCR comprise an important family of activating NK cell receptors involved in the process of target recognition and elimination. NCR include three receptors called NKp46 and NKp30 which are exclusively and constitutively expressed on NK cells, and NKp44 which is expressed after IL-2 stimulation on NK and some γδ T cells.[54,62,63] Infectious, pathogen-specific ligands for NCR have been identified, eg, NKp46 and NKp44 recognize and engage virus specific hemagglutinin and hemagglutinin-neuraminidase.[64] This provides a mechanistic understanding of how NK cells can target and eliminate cells infected with influenza and parainfluenza virus, for example, although such target cells have not downregulated MHC class I expression.[64] Conversely, endogenous ligands for NCR remain to be identified.[65,66]

THE ROLE OF NK CELLS IN HUMAN DISEASE

NK cells are implicated in an increasingly important role in the immune response to, and in some cases the pathogenesis of, human disease. NK cell deficiencies are rare, however, such conditions provide insight into the role NK cells play in response to infectious pathogens, autoimmune disorders and development of malignancy. For instance, observations gleaned from the study of patients with qualitative or quantitative deficiencies in NK cells have allowed a more complete understanding of this lymphocyte subset's contribution to immunity. Selective NK cell deficiency has not been associated with a particular Mendelian disorder[67]; however, a number of recent studies have shed new light on the genetic mechanisms responsible for proper NK development and function. Many syndromes

Table 13–2 Human Disorders Characterized in Part by Natural Killer Cell Deficiency*

Disease	Gene	Protein	Cell count	Cytotoxicity	ADCC	Cytokine Response
X-linked SCID	IL2Rg	Common g chain	Low/absent	Low/absent	n/a	Reduced
Autosomal recessive severe combined immunodeficiency	JAK3	Janus kinase 3	Low/absent	Low/absent	n/a	n/a
Bloom syndrome	BLM	Bloom helicase	Normal	Low	n/a	Normal
Chediak-Higashi syndrome	LYST	Lysosome trafficking regulator	Normal	Absent	Absent	Reduced
Xeroderma pigmentosum	XPAG	DNA repair enzymes	Normal	Low	n/a	Normal
Familial erythrophagocytic lymphohistiocytosis	PFP1	Perforin	Normal	Absent	Absent	Reduced/absent
X-linked lympho-proliferative syndrome	SH2-DIA	SLAM-associated protein	Normal	Absent	Normal	Normal
Paroxysmal nocturnal hemoglobinuria	PIG-A	Phosphatidylinositol glycan class A	Low	Absent	Normal	Reduced/absent
von Hippel-Lindau syndrome	NKTR	Tumor recognition molecule	Normal	Absent	Normal	Reduced
Wiskott-Aldrich syndrome	WASP	WAS protein	High	Low	Low/normal	n/a
X-linked agammaglobulinemia	BTK	Bruton tyrosine kinase	Normal	Low	Low	n/a
Ectodermal dysplasia with immunodeficiency	IKBKG	NEMO	Normal	Low	Low/normal	Reduced
Common variable immunodeficiency	TACI	TNF receptor family member	Low	Low/normal	Low/normal	Normal

Adapted from Microbes & Infection 4:1545, 2002.[70]

have been linked to increased susceptibility to infection while others may predispose to autoimmune disease as discussed below.

NK Deficiency Syndromes Linked to Increased Infectious Risks

The first gene directly implicated in NK deficiency was FCGR3A which codes for FcγRIIIa (CD16) expressed on NK cells. A "T ◊ A" substitution at position 230 leads to coding of a lysine residue at position 48, normally a histidine. Although the protein expressed appears phenotypically normal, patients present with increased susceptibility to severe and disseminated herpes simplex virus (HSV) infections.[68] Other patients present with progressive Epstein-Barr virus and varicella infections.[69] Patients have variable deficits in NK cytotoxicity and responsiveness to cytokine stimulation. Population studies have subsequently suggested that the H48 allele may be necessary but not sufficient to produce clinical disease.[70]

Clinical examples of patients entirely lacking any CD56$^+$ lymphocyte subsets have been reported. The first report was a young female patient who presented with life-threatening varicella infection. She subsequently developed cytomegalovirus pneumonia and cutaneous HSV infection. Analysis of her lymphocyte subsets demonstrated a striking and selective absolute absence of CD56$^+$ or CD16$^+$ cells.[5] The patient went on to develop aplastic anemia and expired from complications of stem cell transplantation.[70] A second patient has been reported presenting with disseminated *M. avium* who went on to die of disseminated varicella.[71] Other patients have been described with an isolated deficiency of CD56$^+$/CD3$^-$ lymphocytes but with normal or even increased populations of CD56$^+$/CD3$^+$ cells. One such patient presented with severe, recurrent human papilloma virus related condylomatous disease.[72] Although the genetic mechanisms of these diseases remain unknown, they serve to highlight the functional role of NK cells in providing immunity towards a spectrum of infectious pathogens.

NK cell deficiencies have been described as a component of other disease processes affecting multiple hematopoietic and immune lineages, lending some indirect support that this innate immune effector cell is an important component of the immune network. The genetic deficiencies responsible for many of these disorders have been described and can be found in Table 13–2.

The Role of NK Cells in Autoimmunity

Interestingly, NK cells have been implicated in both the regulation and pathogenesis of autoimmune disorders. For example, in a murine experimental autoimmune encephalomyelitis (EAE) model of multiple sclerosis in which disease is induced with myelin oligodendrocyte glycoprotein (MOG), NK depletion leads to enhanced T cell response to MOG. Similarly, in human multiple sclerosis, NK cells have been implicated in the maintenance of disease remission.[73] NK cells have also been shown to control inflammation in an experimental model of autoimmune colitis.[74] NK cells may exert this effect through recognition and elimination of T cells activated against autoantigens.[75]

There are also examples of NK cells promoting autoimmune disorders. For instance, experimental evidence supports the idea that NK cells may promote development of type 1 diabetes mellitus through targeted elimination of pancreatic islet β-cells following viral infection.[76] Other studies suggest that NK cells can promote humorally mediated autoimmune diseases such as myasthenia gravis through potentiation of autoreactive B-cells.[77] Synoviocytes of patients with rheumatoid arthritis (RA) have been shown to express abnormally high levels of MICA, the previously described ligand for NKG2D.[78,79] In fact, NK cells are present in acute RA joint effusions and may perpetuate this autoimmune inflammatory response.[80]

Finally, polymorphisms in receptors expressed on NK cells as well as other immune cell subsets have been implicated in the pathogenesis and progression of autoimmune disease. For example, a T ◊ G substitution at position 559 in the FcγRIIIA (CD16) gene leads to a phenylalanine to valine substitution at residue 176 of the FcγRIIIA protein.[81] Although the receptors are expressed similarly on the cell membrane, the V/V homozygous state is associated with a higher affinity for IgG binding than the F/F state. The low binding state

(F/F) is associated with lupus nephritis.[82] Others have confirmed this observation by genetic linkage studies in patients with systemic lupus erythematosis.[83] Another polymorphism in the FcγRIIIA receptor (158V/F) has been associated with RA in certain ethnic groups.[84] This mutation may also be associated with development of subcutaneous rheumatoid nodules in patients with established RA.[84] As CD16 expressed on a number of immune cells, the specific role of NK cells contributing to pathology is unclear; however, as discussed below, these polymorphisms have also been linked to response to enhanced response to monoclonal antibody therapy of cancer.

THE THERAPEUTIC POTENTIAL OF NK CELLS

T lymphocytes depend on recognition of tumor-specific antigens to affect antitumor immune response, an approach limited by our inability to identify such targets for the vast majority of nonviral neoplasms. NK cells, on the other hand, have long been recognized as being capable of anti-tumor rejection independent of such tumor antigens. As the understanding of how NK cells identify and eliminate targets has advanced, novel roles for the application of NK in clinical anti-cancer therapy have been defined. Three general approaches have been developed.

First, direct infusion of NK cells into patients with therapeutic intent has been performed.[85] This strategy has developed based on observations such as that in the allogeneic peripheral blood stem cell transplant (PBSCT) setting, where higher doses of transplanted NK cells have been associated with better outcomes as evidenced by reductions in posttransplant infections as well as reduction in nonrelapse mortality.[86] Several studies have shown this approach to be safe and associated with at least a modicum of effectiveness in the autologous setting.[87,88] At least one trial evaluating direct NK cell infusion has been reported in the allogeneic setting, correlating successful transfer and expansion of haploidentical NK cells with hematologic remission of leukemia.[89]

Second, NK cells have been successfully expanded in vivo in patients with cancer through the exogenous administration of recombinant human cytokines, such as low, intermediate or high-dose IL-2.[90–94] The tumor nonspecificity of these strategies is being explored by concomitantly administering a tumor-specific monoclonal antibody whose Fc portion can bind to CD16 expressed on the cytokine-expanded NK cells, thus initiating a process called antibody-dependent cellular cytotoxicty.[93,95,96]

A third methodology under development to enhance the antitumor response of NK cells is based on the emerging understanding of KIR biology.[97] Over 20 years ago, an inverse relationship was reported between expression of MHC Class I molecules on target cells and the ability of NK cells to kill such targets successfully.[34] As this "missing self" model was further characterized, three principal, common HLA-Class I allele specificities were identified that serve as ligands for three specific NK cell inhibitory KIR receptors. These have been termed: "Group 1" HLA-C alleles expressing Asn80 (eg, HLA-Cw1, w3, w7, w8, and related alleles), "Group 2" HLA-C alleles expressing Lys80 (eg, HLA-Cw2, w4, w5, w6, and related alleles), and HLA-Bw4 alleles (eg, HLA-B27). As one's NK receptor repertoire, including inhibitory KIRs, is dictated during development by the HLA class I genotype, ultimately every NK cell expresses at least one inhibitory KIR specific to self HLA Class I molecules.[18] Moreover, allogeneic targets sensitive to NK cytotoxicity are identified by their lack of self MHC class I inhibitory KIR ligands.

These principles have been applied in a number of therapeutic settings. Perhaps most dramatically, Velardi and colleagues have demonstrated an impressive improvement in survival following allogeneic stem cell transplantation based therapy for patients with acute myeloid leukemia.[98] Donor-versus-recipient NK cell alloreactivity has been shown to contribute to enhanced survival in this setting, as well as improved engraftment, and protection against graft-versus-host-disease.[99] In a series of patients receiving haploidentical grafts, 68% of patients without NK-alloreactivity had relapsed disease, whereas only 15% of patients with NK-alloreactivity relapsed with a median

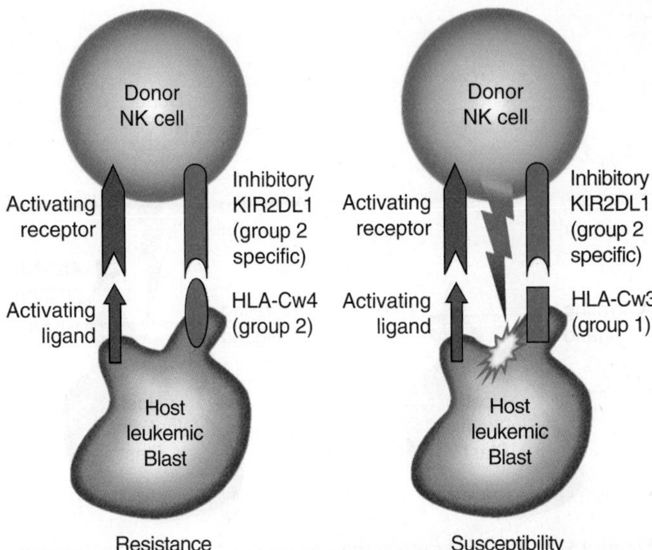

Figure 13–3 Simplified cartoon representation of haplotype mismatched allogeneic stem cell transplant for acute myeloid leukemia: proper MHC class I mismatch can lead to donor natural killer (NK) cell killing host leukemic blasts. As the HLA-C ligand binds to the NK cell inhibitory killer immunoglobulin-like receptor (KIR) on the left, the inhibitory signal interrupts the activation signal, and no killing occurs. However, when the HLA-C ligand does not bind the NK inhibitor KIR on the right, no inhibitory signal is sent, and tumor killing occurs. *(Adapted from Farag SS, Fehniger TA, Ruggeri L, et al: Natural killer cell receptors: new biology and insights into the graft-versus-leukemia effect. Blood 100:1935, 2002.)*

follow-up of 4 years.[99] Similarly, KIR-mismatch has been shown to improve outcome after reduced-intensity chemotherapy followed by allogeneic stem cell transplantation in multiple myeloma patients.[100,101] Fig. 13–3 shows how mismatching KIR epitopes facilitates NK mediated tumor cytotoxicity in a haploidentical setting.

Others have extended on these transplantation-based findings by manipulating the relationship between NK receptors and MHC Class I receptors through the means of monoclonal antibodies. For example, a murine model lends support to the notion that tumor expression of MHC Class I molecules become engaged by inhibitory NK cell receptors and thus mediate NK tolerance.[102] When antibody fragments were introduced to disrupt this ligand-receptor interaction, increased NK cytotoxicity and decreased tumor growth were observed. Furthermore, adoptive transfer of murine NK cells pretreated with an antibody to block inhibitory NK receptor expression into leukemia-bearing mice led to enhanced survival as compared to transfer of untreated NK cells. These findings support the notion that blocking inhibitory NK receptors may be beneficial in increasing the efficacy of cancer immunotherapy.[102] In fact, anti-KIR antibodies are nearing Phase 1 clinical trials in humans. Fig. 13–4 demonstrates this principle.

In complementary fashion, other approaches have sought to enhance activating NK receptors, such as NKG2D. One group has created a novel bivalent protein (ULBP2-BB4) which recognizes NKG2D and CD138, a protein overexpressed in a number of malignancies, including multiple myeloma. Although such an approach is limited by knowledge of particular tumor antigens, the concept of enhancing NK function was demonstrated in this model through increases in NK cytokine secretion as well as abrogation of tumor cell growth in the presence of the molecule.[103]

Finally, the use of monoclonal antibodies directed against tumor cell antigens has significantly advanced treatment of some malignancies. For example, treatment with the monoclonal, IgG, chimeric anti-CD20 antibody rituximab has been shown to improve survival of patients with non-Hodgkin lymphoma. As discussed, genotypic, single nucleotide polymorphisms in the FcγRIIIA (CD16) receptor

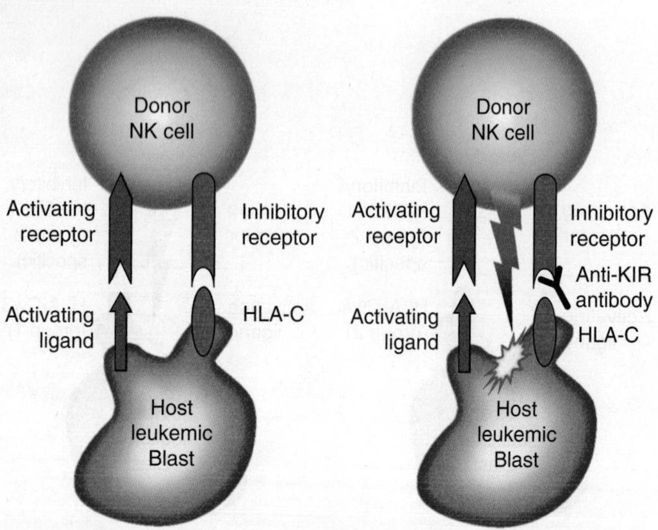

Figure 13–4 Simplified cartoon showing the general equilibrium between activating and inhibitory signaling which favors no killing as shown on the left. However, the introduction of an antibody to the inhibitory receptor tips this balance towards activation and elimination of the target cell, as shown on the right. *(Adapted from Farag SS, Fehniger TA, Ruggeri L, et al: Natural killer cell receptors: new biology and insights into the graft-versus-leukemia effect. Blood 100:1935, 2002.)*

expressed on NK cells and other immune cells may convey functional differences in the receptor that have clinical consequences. Patients with the V/V homozygous state at residue 176 have a higher affinity for the Fc portion of the rituximab, and these patients show enhanced clinical response to the antibody.[104] Such a finding supports the notion that enhanced ADCC function in CD16-bearing cells, including NK cells, is one key mechanism of action of rituximab and suggests that antibody mediated cancer therapies could be advanced by enhancing NK cell numbers and cytotoxic potential in vivo.

CONCLUSIONS

NK cells are a critical cellular component of innate immunity. Rapid secretion of powerful immunomodulatory cytokines and chemokines support the role of NK cells as "first responders" to immune insults, facilitating mobilization and tailoring of the innate and adaptive immune response. Potent natural cytotoxicity, unrestricted by classical antigen presentation, and costimulation required for adaptive immune cells, suggest that NK cells have an important, complementary role to that of cytotoxic T lymphocytes, which provide antigen-specific cytotoxicity and lasting memory. Further understanding of the functional differences between CD56^{dim} and CD56^{bright} subsets, their cytotoxicity and cytokine receptor expression, and their developmental biology will certainly shed more light on the therapeutic potential for NK cells in the pathogenesis, prevention, and treatment human disease.

SUGGESTED READINGS

Becknell B, Caligiuri MA: Interleukin-2, interleukin-15, and their roles in human natural killer cells. Adv Immunol 86:209, 2005.

Borrego F, Masilamani M, Marusina AT: The CD94/NKG2 family of receptors: from molecules and cells to clinical relevance. Immunol Res 35:263, 2006.

Colucci F, Caligiuri MA, Di Santo JP: What does it take to make a natural killer? Nat Rev Immunol 3:413, 2003.

Cooper MA, Fehniger TA, Caligiuri MA: The biology of human natural killer cell subsets. Trends Immunol 22:633, 2001.

Cooper MA, Fehniger TA, Turner SC: Human natural killer cells: a unique innate immunoregulatory role for the CD56(bright) subset. Blood 97:3146, 2001.

Djeu JY, Jiang K, Wei S: A view to a kill: signals triggering cytotoxicity. Clin Cancer Res 8:636, 2002.

Farag SS, Fehniger TA, Ruggeri L, et al: Natural killer cell receptors: new biology and insights into the graft-versus-leukemia effect. Blood 100:1935, 2002.

Freud AH, Yokohama A, Becknell B, et al: Evidence for discrete stages of human natural killer cell differentiation in vivo. J Exp Med 203:1033, 2006.

Jie HB, Sarvetnick N: The role of NK cells and NK cell receptors in autoimmune disease. Autoimmunity 37:147, 2004.

Klingmann HG: Natural killer cell-based immunotherapeutic strategies. Cytotherapy 7:16, 2005.

Lanier L: NK cell recognition. Annu Rev Immunol 2005;23:225–74.

Makrigiannis AP, Anderson SK: Regulation of natural killer cell function. Cancer Biol Ther 2:610, 2003.

Ogasawara K, Lanier LL: NKG2D in NK and T cell-mediated immunity. J Clin Immunol 25:534, 2005.

Orange J: Human natural killer cell deficiencies and susceptibility to infection. Microbes Infect 4:1545, 2002.

Robertson MJ, Ritz J: Biology and clinical relevance of human natural killer cells. Blood 76:2421, 1990.

Sentman CL, Barber MA, Barber A, et al: NK cell receptors as tools in cancer immunotherapy. Adv Cancer Res 95:249, 2006.

REFERENCES

For complete list of references log onto www.expertconsult.com

CHAPTER 14

DENDRITIC CELL BIOLOGY

Olivier Manches, Viswanathan Lakshmanan, Zbigniew M. Szczepiorkowski, and Nina Bhardwaj

INTRODUCTION

Dendritic cells (DC) are a sparsely distributed population of bone marrow derived mononuclear cells that exist in an "immature" form in virtually all tissues in the body.[1] DC serve as professional antigen presenting cells (APC) with an extraordinary capacity to stimulate naïve T lymphocytes (as well as B, NK, and NK-T cells) and initiate primary immune responses. In their immature state DC detect and capture "danger signals" originating from microorganisms or their macromolecular constituents in their resident tissues. Upon encountering such danger signals DC undergo a complex series of events leading to their "maturation."[1] Maturation of DC is characterized by migration of DC to draining lymph nodes and processing and presentation of antigens in the context of antigen presenting molecules such as major histocompatibility complex (MHC) and CD1 to naïve T, B, and NK cells. This chapter attempts to provide a snapshot of our current understanding of DC function as well as their potential clinical applications as immunotherapeutic agents in diseases such as cancer, HIV and autoimmunity.[2]

DENDRITIC CELL SUBSETS AND DEVELOPMENT

Extensive research has demonstrated that DC exist in many "flavors."[3,4] However, our understanding of DC differentiation and the different DC subsets is complicated by the heterogeneity of data, obtained from in vitro human and mouse studies, and in vivo animal studies and limited in vivo human studies. The generation of functionally distinct DC subtypes follows two generally accepted models: (a) the *functional plasticity model* postulating the existence of a single DC lineage possessing functional plasticity, and (b) the *specialized lineage model* postulating the existence of multiple DC lineages displaying functional diversity.[5] Both models assume four stages of DC development namely hematopoietic precursors, DC precursors (pre-DC), immature DC (imDC), and mature DC (mDC) (Fig. 14–1). It is likely, however, that elements of both models are involved in DC subset development. In this short chapter we concentrate on human DC with little reference to murine models. Readers are encouraged to seek additional information in several comprehensive reviews.[5–14]

Most studies on the developmental origin of human DC subsets have used in vitro culture systems. DC precursors and imDC, similar to other cell types in the immune system, are continuously produced in a steady rate and pathogen independent manner from CD34+ hematopoietic stem cells (HSC) within the bone marrow. Fms-like tyrosine kinase-3 ligand (Flt-3-L) and GM-CSF, represent the key DC growth and differentiation factors.[15] The CD34+ HSC differentiate into hypothetical common lymphoid progenitors (CLP) and common myeloid progenitors (CMP) in the bone marrow. Subsequently CMP differentiate into CD34+CLA+ and CD34+CLA– populations (CLA, skin homing receptor cutaneous lymphocyte-associated antigen), which give rise to phenotypically distinguishable CD11c+CD1a+ and CD11c–CD1a+ immature DC, respectively.[16] The former migrate into the skin epidermis and differentiate into Langerhans cells, while the latter localize to skin dermis and other tissues, and become interstitial imDC.[17] The human Langerhans cell DC subset has distinct markers, including the presence of Birbeck granules, the expression of CD1a, and langerin, a member of the C-type lectin family of receptors involved in the uptake of pathogens.[18]

The CD34+ hematopoietic progenitor cells (HPC) and blood monocytes are commonly used as precursor cells for generating DC in culture in vitro for both research and immunotherapeutic purposes. HPC are treated with c-kit ligand and tumor necrosis factor (TNF) α that yield subsets of myeloid DC including Langerhans cells. Monocytes, obtained by simple adherence of HPC to plastic, when exposed to a combination of GM-CSF and IL-4, yield imDC that are comparable to some degree to tissue interstitial DC. Maturation of these different DC can be induced by the addition of various stimuli.

The pre-DC subset expresses several myeloid markers including CD11b, CD11c, CD13, CD14, and CD33, indicating that they may derive from a CMP. In contrast to the blood "myeloid DC" derived from CMP, which we will refer to here as conventional DC (cDC), the "plasmacytoid DC" contain "lymphoid" mRNA transcripts for pre-T α chains, germ line IgK, and Spi-B and are also called interferon (IFN) type I producing cell (IPC). These latter cells display distinct plasma cell morphology, contain abundant endoplasmic reticulum, and express CD4 and high levels of the IL-3αR, but lack myeloid antigens including CD11c and most lineage markers. Plasmacytoid DC are found in peripheral blood, thymus, and many lymphoid tissues. The production of extraordinarily high levels of IFN type 1 by pDC is unique to this cell type and may be important for initiating a strong antiviral innate response and promote maturation of bystander CD11c+ cDC to protect them from the cytopathic effect of viruses.[18–21] It is hypothesized that human cDC and pDC have evolved to recognize and respond to different pathogens in unique ways, owing to their complementary expression of receptors for "pathogen associated molecular patterns" (see Antigen Acquisition section), capacity to secrete either IFN type I or IL-12, antigen presentation, and migration into secondary lymphoid organs. As mentioned, pDC secrete high amounts of IFN-α upon viral infection, but no IL-12, and display poor antigen capture and presentation capacity. Upon activation, pDC differentiate into cells bearing similar characteristics to activated cDC, ie, with a dendritic morphology, high expression of MHC class II molecules, and the capacity to prime naïve T cells,[22,23] but express low levels of CD11c and lack typical myeloid markers. The functional properties of these latter pDC-derived DC is still to be investigated thoroughly,[24] although they may differ from cDC especially in their *cross-presentation*[25] or T cell skewing capacities. Thus, DC derived from pDC upon culture with IL-3 and activation by CD40-L preferentially prime naïve CD4+ T cells towards a Th2 profile, whereas DC derived from pDC by viral/TLR stimulation prime towards a Th1 profile in an IFN-α dependent and IL-12 independent pathway.[20] Upon activation, immature cDC migrate through afferent lymph from nonlymphoid tissues to the T cell rich areas of lymph nodes. Plasmacytoid DC, which also migrate into T cell areas of secondary lymphoid tissues, do so through high endothelial venules (HEV) of lymph nodes and marginal zone of the spleen likely using CCR7 and CD62-L.[26] Both activated blood cDC and pDC can migrate in response to lymph node homing chemokines (CCL19 and CCL21) through expression of CCR7. Although cDC can be found in virtually every peripheral tissues as well as in lymphoid organs, pDC seem to display a more restricted

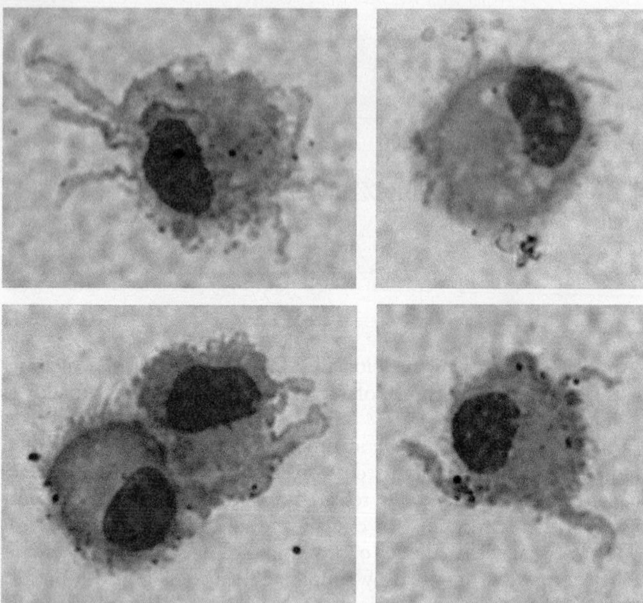

Figure 14–1 Examples of monocyte-derived mature dendritic cells are shown. The mononuclear cells were enriched by adherence, cultured with IL-4 and GM-CSF for 6 days, and underwent maturation with IL-1, IL-6, TNF-α, and PGE2 for 24 hours.

Table 14–1 Agents That Cause DC Maturation

Agent Property	Molecules
Stimulatory agents	TNF family members (TNFα, CD40L, FasL, TRANCE); TLR ligands (dsRNA, LPS, imiquimod, CpG ODNs); Growth factors [thymic stromal lymphopoietin (TSLP)]; Interferons (IFNα); Adhesion molecules [CECAM-1, (CD66a)]; Costimulatory molecules [LIGHT, B7-DC]; Receptors [FcR via Ag-Igs; TREM-2 via Dap-12]; Viruses/microbes (Influenza, bacteria, bacterial products); Chemokines (MCP, MIP1α, RANTES, IP10, IL-8, MDC, TARC); Chemokine receptors (CCR7 and loss of CCR2 and CCR5)
Inhibitory agents	Drugs (Rapamycin, FK506, Cyclosporin A, Dexamethasone, IVIg); Chemokines (IL-10); Viruses (EBV, vaccinia, canarypox, HSV); Others (β2 microglobulin)
Survival signals	CD40 L, TRANCE, B7-DC, BcL-2
Cell-cell interaction	Activated Cells [CD4 and CD8 cells (via CD40L)]; NK cells, NK-T cells; Vδ1+, γδ T cells

Maturation is a complex process tightly linked to antigen acquisition and the surrounding micro-environment. See text for more details.

distribution. They can be found mostly in the T cell area of lymphoid organs (lymph node, tonsils, spleen, thymus, bone marrow, and Peyer patches), blood and some peripheral tissues (liver, nasal mucosa). Although cDC and pDC express a similar array of chemotactic receptors (such as CCR2, CCR5, CXCR2, CXCR4), pDC do not respond to a number of inflammatory chemokines. However, they accumulate in inflamed tissues, such as in systemic lupus erythematosus (SLE) or contact dermatitis, probably through their expression of ChemR23 and CXCR4.

This division of dendritic cells into cDC and pDC subsets is likely to be an oversimplified view of DC heterogeneity. For example splenic DC are heterogenous with regard to expression of CD4, CD11b, and CD11c, whereas most of the thymic DC are CD11c+ but lack other myeloid markers thereby not fitting into either of the classical categories of cDC and pDC in blood.[27] Recently, a new subset of pDC was discovered in mice, which presented functional features of both NK cells and conventional pDC, highlighting the functional diversity of DC.[28,29]

The developmental origin of pDC and cDC is still debated, as pDC and cDC can be derived from both CLP and CMP, suggesting that pDC and cDC may arise during hematopoiesis from progenitors with already distinct and restricted lineage potential.[30] It seems that cDC differentiation is dependent on the transcription factor Ikaros, whereas pDC development is dependent on the Ets family transcription factor SpiB, and probably PU.1. A recent study in mice described the conversion of bone marrow pDC into cDC upon viral infection, again highlighting the complexity and plasticity of DC development.[31]

The migration of myeloid DC and plasmacytoid DC precursors from the bone marrow can be increased by administration of Flt-3-L up to 50-fold for pre-DC and 15-fold for pDC.[32,33] G-CSF is also known to increase the number of pDC in the circulation. With the advent of newer technologies it has also become feasible to generate large numbers of DC subsets in vitro.

THE CONCEPT OF MATURATION

In their resting state, imDC are primed to acquire antigens in situ through a variety of receptors and mechanisms. Upon encountering pathogens or other "activating stimuli," DC undergo a complicated series of phenotypic and functional changes referred here to as "activation" and "maturation," respectively.[1] The process of DC activation is an intricate differentiation process under tight control and closely associated with antigen acquisition. It is induced by various stimuli (Table 14–1) or danger signals (eg, signs of pathogenic infection or cell injury), including cytokines (eg, IFN type I, TNF-α, and IL-1), microbial products (eg, lipopolysaccharide (LPS), flagellin, intracellular products (eg, heat shock proteins), growth factors (eg, thymic stromal lymphopoietin [TSLP]), immune complexes and T cell molecules (eg, CD40). The process of activation is characterized by upregulation of adhesion and costimulatory molecules such as CD54, CD80, CD86, MHC class I and II molecules, cytokines (eg, TNF-α, IL-12, IL-18) and chemokines (eg, RANTES, MIP-1 α, IP-10). The latter enable the recruitment of T cells, monocytes and other DC into the local environment. In their mature state, DC express markers, which distinguish them from imDC such as CD83 (a molecule involved in thymic T cell selection and DC-DC interactions) and DC-LAMP, a lysosomal protein. Maturation also changes the migratory properties of DC. They express CCR7 and acquire responsiveness to the chemokines CCL19 and CCL21 that are expressed in the T cell areas of lymph nodes where mature DC generate immune responses. Concomitantly, DC lose their receptors for CCL3, CCL4, and CCL5, which are produced in sites of inflammation, reduce their capacity for phagocytosis, macropinocytosis, antigen uptake, and processing; but acquire potent immunostimulatory ability through enhanced T-DC immune synapse formation, production of immunoproteosomes and upregulation of unique DC specific costimulatory molecules such as B7-DC.[34] However, although increased expression of costimulatory molecules and migration to secondary lymphoid organs often correlates with their capacity to prime CD4 and CD8 immunity, activated DC may also induce tolerization of T cells, as when CD4+ T cell help is missing[35,36] or on activation by inflammatory cytokines in the absence of TLR engagement,[37] and can potentially induce the generation of regulatory T cell (Treg). Some stimuli, such as TSLP, can induce phenotypic maturation of DC without concomitant secretion of proinflammatory cytokines such as IL-12, IL-6, TNF-α, or IL-1.[38] Therefore, DC maturation is more appropriately used in a functional

Table 14–2 Antigen Recognition and Uptake Receptors Expressed by DC

Receptor	Antigenic Ligand
C type lectins (DC-SIGN, MMR, DEC-205)	Mannosylated molecules, viruses, bacteria, fungi
FcγR (CD32, CD64)	Immune complexes, antibody-coated tumor cells
CD1 a, b, c, d	Biphosphonate moieties in *Mycobacterium tuberculosis*, BCG and *Listeria monocytogenes*; Lipid and glycolipid foreign and self-antigens
Integrins (αVβ5, CR3, CR4)	Opsonized antigens, apoptotic cells
Scavenger receptors (CD36, LOX-1)	Opsonized antigens, apoptotic cells, heat shock proteins
Toll-like receptors (TLR) and other Pattern recognition receptors (PRR)	TLR 2–8 (myeloid DC) peptoglycans, endotoxin, flagellin; TLR 7 (plasmacytoid DC) bacterial DNA; RIG-I, MDA5, PKR, NOD proteins
Heat shock proteins receptor (HSP-R; CD91)	Heat shock proteins
Aquaporins	Fluids

The table lists some of the receptors expressed by DC that are involved in antigen acquisition. The antigen receptor repertoire dictates that range of antigens captured by the DC. Ligation of some of these receptors induces DC maturation.

sense, with mature DC being defined as able to prime naive T cell responses. What makes a phenotypically activated DC capable of priming instead of tolerizing a T cell appears multifactorial and dependent on such factors as the state of the microenvironment and the DC subset in question, although this remains to be clearly defined.

ANTIGEN ACQUISITION

Immature DC sample their environment through several mechanisms, including micropinocytosis, macropinocytosis, receptor mediated endocytosis, and phagocytosis. They display an array of surface receptors, which facilitate acquisition of antigens and pathogens, and at the same time induce differentiation into activated DC. An important class of receptors is the pattern recognition receptors (PRR), which recognize pathogen-associated molecular patterns (PAMP) expressed by many microorganisms. PRR serve as an important link between innate and adaptive immunity as they directly mature DC while also inducing the production of a variety of cytokines and chemokines. PRR consist of several groups of receptors including secreted (eg, MBL, CRP, SAP, LBP), cell-surface (eg, CD14, MMR, MSR, MARCO),[39] and intracellular molecules (eg, RIG-I and MDA5, which are RNA helicases involved in the recognition of nucleic acids upon viral infection; NOD receptors, which recognize peptidoglycan subcomponents or other bacterial molecules; inflammatory caspases, such as caspase-1 and caspase-5, which form an intracellular complex with NALP1 or NALP2 and 3 called the inflammasome that recognize bacterial RNA and other danger signals and induce the production of the proinflammatory cytokines IL1β and IL-18) (Table 14–2). Toll-like receptors (TLR), which constitute another group of PRR, are expressed by imDC, and mediate activation by microbial components such as peptidoglycan, LPS, flagellin, and unmethylated CpG DNA motifs. Ligation of the TLR results in the activation of Rel family members, in particular the transcription factor NF-κB, c-Jun-terminal kinase (JNK) and p38 MAP kinase, leading to the initiation of the maturation process.[40,41] TLR are unevenly distributed among DC, with myeloid DC expressing TLR 2, 3, 4, 5, 8 and plasmacytoid DC strongly expressing TLR 7 and 9 (Table 14–3). Another important feature of some TLR is their capacity to induce secretion of IFN type I for antiviral defense and immune regulation. cDC express TLR3 and 4, mediating recognition of viral double stranded RNA and LPS respectively, and on triggering secrete low amounts of IFN-β through a signaling pathway utilizing the adaptor TRIF and the transcription factor IRF3. Although cDC can also induce IFN type I through RIG-I and MDA-5 upon viral infection, pDC seem to rely mostly on a specialized MyD88-dependent signaling pathway, allowing them to secrete very high amounts of IFN-α upon triggering of TLR7 and 9. This is due to their constitutive high expression of IRF7, a crucial IFN-α gene transcription factor, and to a specialized spatiotemporal regulation of TLR7 and 9 signaling, allowing IRF7 to interact with MyD88 docked onto TLR in the endosomal membrane.[42]

Table 14–3 Toll-Like Receptors Expressed by DCs

mDC	pDC	Ligand(s)
TLR1	TLR1	?
TLR2		Peptidoglycan (*S. aureus*); Lipoproteins and lipopeptides from several bacteria; Glycophopshotidylinositol anchors from *T. cruzi;* Lipoaminomannan from *M. tuberculosis;* Zymosan (yeast)
TLR3		Double-stranded RNA e.g. poly I:C
TLR4		LPS+MD-2, taxol, hsp 60 (?), heparan sulfate (?), RSV, fibronectin
TLR5		flagellin (*S. typhimurium, Listeria*)
TLR6	TLR6	? / Undergoes dimerization with TLR2
	TLR7	Imiquimod (Aldara), R-848 (resiquimod), single-stranded RNA
TLR8	TLR8	Imiquimod (Aldara), R-848 (resiquimod), single-stranded RNA
	TLR9	CpG ODNs, DNA from bacteria and viruses, chromatin-IgG complexes
	TLR10	?

TLRs can form heterodimeric receptor complexes consisting of two different TLRs or homodimers (as in the case of TLR4). The TLR4 receptor complex requires supportive molecules (MD-2) for optimal response to its ligand lipopolysaccharide (LPS). A common feature of the TLR recepors is the cytoplasmic TIR domain that serves as a scaffold for a series of protein-protein interactions which result in the activation of a unique signaling module consisting of MyD88, interleukin-1 receptor associated kinase (IRAK) family members and Tollip, which is used exclusively by TIR family members. Subsequently, several central signaling pathways are activated in parallel, the activation of NF-kB being the most prominent event of the inflammatory response. Recent developments indicate that in addition to the common signaling module MyD88/IRAK/Tollip, other molecules can modulate signaling by TLRs, especially of TLR4, resulting in differential biological responses to distinct pathogenic structures. TLR2 is also involved in cross-presentation.

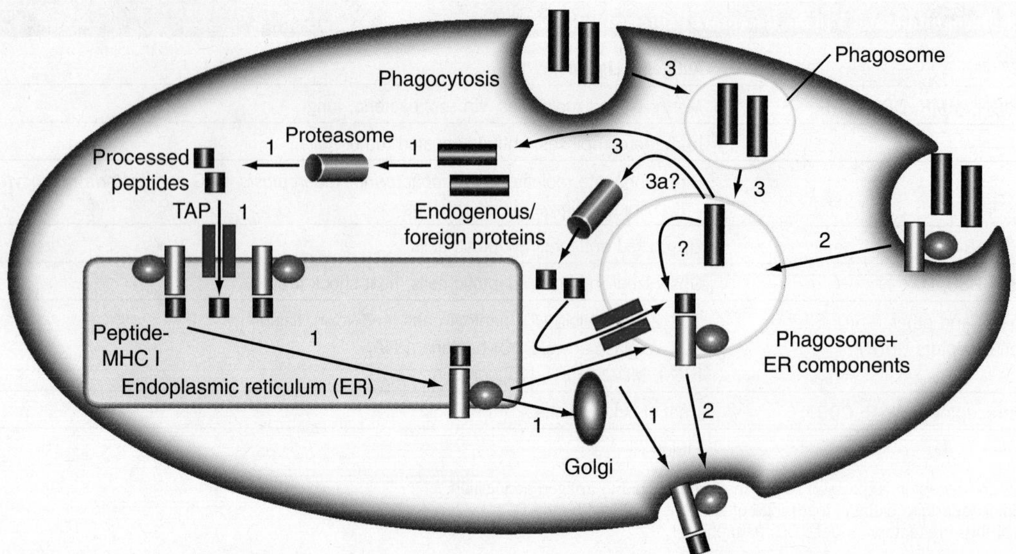

Figure 14–2 PATHWAYS FOR MHC CLASS I PRESENTATION. The classical pathway for MHC class I presentation (1) involves degradation of endogenous or viral antigens into peptides by the proteasome, followed by transport into the endoplasmic reticulum (ER). After further trimming in the ER, the peptides are loaded onto newly synthesized MHC class I molecules and the peptide-MHC class I complexes are transported to the plasma membrane. Two main pathways of cross-presentation (2,3) have been described, which allows presentation of exogenous antigens in association with MHC class I molecules. Antigens endocytosed or phagocytosed can be cleaved into peptides by proteases and loaded onto recycling MHC class I molecules within the same phagosome or on the cell surface (vacuolar pathway) (2). Alternatively, antigens may escape from the phagosome and enter the cytosol (phagosome-to-cytosol pathway) (3) to be processed via the classical MHC class I pathway. It has been suggested recently that elements of ER can be associated with phagosomes, allowing transfer of antigens into the cytosol by the ERAD pathway and degradation by the phagosome-associated proteasome (3a). The importance of each pathway (2,3) for cross-presentation in vivo and the precise mechanisms and location of antigen processing in each model are under investigation.

C-type lectins are calcium-dependent carbohydrate-binding proteins with a broad range of biological functions, many of which are involved in immune responses. They are well represented on dendritic cells and include the following: DC-SIGN, responsible for binding of HIV-1, HIV-2, simian immunodeficiency virus, Ebola viruses, dengue virus, *Candida* species, *Leishmania* species; BDCA-2, potentially responsible for delivering tolerogenic signals; BDCA-4/neuropilin-1, capable of binding VEGF; langerin, responsible for uptake and processing of antigens in Langerhans cells; DEC-205 (CD205) involved in the uptake and processing of antigens in MIIV (vesicles enriched for MHC class II molecules and proteases such as the cathepsins that mediate antigen processing and MHC class II peptide complex formation), and generation of tolerogenic signals; and macrophage mannose receptor (MMR), involved in the processing of microbial organisms.

Other receptors expressed by DC include FcR involved in cross-presentation of immune complexes and antibody opsonized dead cells; integrins such as $\alpha V\beta 5$, scavenger receptors CD36, and Mer-family tyrosine kinases for phagocytosis of apoptotic cells and Lipoxygenase-1 (LOX-1) or CD91 for uptake of HSPs; complement receptors which play a role in uptake of opsonized microbes and apoptotic cells; receptors for viruses (eg, CD4, CCR5, and CXCR4 for HIV, and CD46 for measles virus), and the CD1 family of receptors which activate CD4, CD8, $\gamma\delta$T cells, and NK-T cells through binding and processing of antigens such as sphingolipids, sulfatides, glycosphingolipids GPI-anchored mucin-like glycoproteins (GPI mucins), glycoinositolphospholipids (GIPLs), and their phosphatidylinositol moieties. Altogether, these various receptors provide substantial avenues for DC to efficiently capture multitudes of antigens in their environment.

Antigen capture is tightly coupled to DC activation and antigen presentation, and triggering of TLR or exposure to inflammatory cytokines first induces a transient increase in the macropinocytic uptake, followed by a near complete downregulation of the uptake process. Furthermore, it has been suggested that TLR engagement also enhances microbe-loaded phagosome maturation, potentially discriminating between nonimmunogenic antigens (apoptotic cells) and microbial antigens at the antigen processing level.[43]

ANTIGEN PROCESSING

Dendritic cells have a remarkable ability to process and present antigens restricted by MHC and CD1 molecules. The processing is tightly associated with DC activation.

MHC Class I Antigen Presentation (Endogenous Route)

The process of antigen processing and presentation to CD8+ T cells begins with degradation of proteins synthesized within the cytoplasm, either as mature proteins or as neosynthesized defective proteins (defective ribosomal products or DRiPS), into oligopeptides by the ubiquitin-proteasome pathway. Misfolded proteins are also a source of antigenic peptides after retrotranslocation from the ER to the cytosol through the ER-associated degradation pathway (ERAD). Subsequently, aminopeptidases cleave N-terminal precursors into peptides of appropriate length for presentation on MHC class I molecules. Antigen processing via this route is regulated through activation of the catalytically active subunits of the proteasome, the PA28 proteasome activator and leucine aminopeptidase, which are upregulated by IFN.[44] Mature DC in particular, express immunoproteosomes containing the active site subunits LMP2, LMP7 and MECL-1, which can enhance antigen processing.[45] After transport into the endoplasmic reticulum through the transporter associated with antigen processing (TAP) (Fig. 14–2), long peptides are further trimmed by ER aminopeptidase-1 (ERAP-1) to 8-mer or 9-mer peptides for loading onto MHC class I molecules.

DC also have the capacity to acquire antigens exogenously and process them for presentation on MHC class I molecules. This phenomenon, referred to as cross-presentation allows the immune system to recognize antigens which are not otherwise presented or which may not access DC directly (eg, tumor cells, viruses). DC can acquire such antigens in the form of apoptotic cells, necrotic cells, antibody opsonized cells, immune complexes, and heat shock proteins (intracellular chaperones for antigenic peptides which are released by necrotic cells).[46] DC even acquire antigens via phagocytosis of particles released from intracellular vesicles (referred to as exosomes).[47] Finally, DC may even nibble bits of live cells to acquire antigens.[48] Mechanistically, cross-presentation may involve cathepsin-S dependent processing of antigenic peptides within the endocytic/phagocytic vacuole and subsequent binding to recycling MHC class I molecules within the same organelle (vacuolar pathway) (Fig. 14–2).[49] Alternatively, the antigens may be transferred from the endocytic vacuole to the cytoplasm, followed by processing by the proteasome and loading onto newly formed MHC class I molecules (phagosome-to-cytosol pathway), with a possible recruitment of the endoplasmic reticulum machinery for antigen processing and MHC class I loading (Fig. 14–2).[50–53] Activation of DC through TLR triggering or exposure to fever-like temperatures induces transient formation of large poly-ubiquitinated protein aggregates called dendritic cell aggregosome-like induced structures (DALIS), the role of which might be to temporarily concentrate and store endogenous antigens to reduce self-antigen presentation.[54,55] This phenomenon of cross presentation is especially efficient in, if not unique to, DC as compared to other antigen presenting cells.

MHC Class II Antigen Presentation (Exogenous Route)

Assembly of MHC class II molecules, which present antigen in the form of short peptides to CD4+ T lymphocytes, occurs in the endoplasmic reticulum of DC. Once assembled, these MHC class II molecules are transported to specialized compartments in the lysosomal system involved in the processing of exogenous antigens. These include MIIV which are protease rich compartments containing newly synthesized MHC class II molecules. Epidermal DC or Langerhans cells contain cytoplasmic tubules with internal striations called Birbeck granules. Birbeck granules are rich in langerin (CD205), a C-type lectin necessary for granule formation and possibly for capture of pathogens.[56] Once endocytosed by imDC, antigens are partially retained within lysosomes. Upon receiving a maturation signal, the pH of lysosomes decreases to less than 5 (owing to the activation of a vacuolar H+ ATPase). Concomitantly there is antigen degradation due to activation of proteases such as cathepsins. Cystatin C, a protein which blocks the activity of cathepsin S, is also degraded, thereby allowing the degradation of invariant chain peptide (Ii chain), which normally blocks access of antigenic peptides to MHC class II molecules. These changes occur in late endosomes and lysosomes (the MIIV compartment). Once antigenic peptide is bound to MHC class II molecules, they exit the lysosomes through the formation of long tubular structures, which simultaneously deliver costimulatory molecules such as CD86 to the cell surface.[57,58]

Dendritic cells handle internalized antigens in a specialized way unlike other phagocytic cells such as macrophages which degrade most of the internalized material, leaving only limited amounts of antigenic peptides for presentation onto MHC molecules. On the contrary, internalized antigens in cDC are preserved for longer times, thereby allowing their transport by maturing DC to secondary lymphoid organs, where actual presentation occurs. Mature DC display higher levels of proteolysis than imDC, allowing appropriate degradation of the antigens for loading onto MHC molecules. These differences are accounted for by several features unique to DC, such as low levels of lysosomal proteases in immature stages as compared to macrophages, expression of protease inhibitors (cystatin C), regulation of lysosomal pH (and hence activity of proteases) by regulation of the acidifying V-type H+ ATPase activity and consumption of H+ upon reaction with superoxide radicals generated by NADPH oxidase NOX2 in maturing DC.[59] During maturation, trafficking of MHC class II molecules to the surface is dramatically increased, probably due to degradation of Ii chain (containing endosome-lysosome targeting signal) in acidic compartments, leading to transport of MHC class II via the constitutive secretory pathway to the cell membrane.

T CELL ACTIVATION

T cell activation systematically requires three signals. Signal 1 is generated by the T cell receptor (TCR) after engagement by a peptide-MHC complex on the antigen-presenting cell. Signal 2 or costimulatory signals, determines qualitative and quantitative elements of T cell activation and differentiation and is required for priming of naïve T cells. Signal 3 specifies the type of response to be mounted, inducing either Th1 or Th2 differentiation in CD4 T cells, or promoting a regulatory phenotype. MHC/peptide, costimulatory molecules, and other signaling/adhesion molecules promote DC contact with T cells via formation of an *immunological synapse* that determines the duration and strength of signals transduced to T cells leading to their subsequent activation. The minimum time for productive interaction between naïve T cells and DC is 6 to 30 hours, with lesser time periods required for memory T cell activation.[60,61] Although only a few peptide-MHC complexes (<10) are sufficient to trigger calcium fluxes in T cells,[62] only mature DC can prime naïve CD4 and CD8 T cells.[63] Remarkably, relatively few peptide-MHC complexes (<200) are necessary on mature DC to activate T cells. Compared to other antigen-presenting cells such as B cells and monocytes, DC are up to a thousandfold more efficient in activating T cells.[64]

Costimulatory molecules include the CD80 and CD86 members of the B7 family which ligate to CD28 on T cells and members of the TNF family, such as CD40 (Table 14–4).[12] Notably one new member of the B7 family, B7-DC, is unique to DC, and stimulates naïve T cells highly efficiently.[65] Other molecules play inhibitory roles upon encountering their receptor on T cells. For example, PDL1 on DC interacts with PD1 on T cells to downregulate T cell responses.

Table 14–4 Co-Stimulatory Molecules Involved in the Interaction between DC and T Cells (Signal 2)[8]

Dendritic Cell	T Cell	Signal
B7 Family		
B7-1(CD80)/B7-2(CD86)	CD28	Activating
B7-1(CD80)/B7-2(CD86)	CTLA4	Inhibitory
B7-H1(PDL1)/B7-DC(PDL2)	?	Activating
B7-H1(PDL1)/B7-DC(PDL2)	PD1	Inhibitory
B7-H2 (B7h; B7PR1; ICOSL)	ICOS	Activating
B7H3	?	Activating
B7H4 (B7S1; B7x)	?	Inhibitory
TNF Receptor Family		
4–1BBL	4–1BB	Activating
CD27L	CD27	Activating
OX40L	OX40	Activating
LIGHT	LIGHT-R	Activating
Cytokines		
IL-2	IL-2R	T cell proliferation
IL-12	IL-12R	T cell proliferation
IL-18		

T cell activation requires two signals. The T-cell receptor interaction with a peptide-MHC complex (Signal 1) is accompanied by Signal 2 delivered by one of the mechanisms listed in this table. Formation of the immunological synapse between a DC and a T cell determines the fate of the lymphocyte. The number of identified co-stimulatory molecules responsible for Signal 2 is increasing steadily.

ICOS-L is present on both DC and B cells and is critical for germinal center formation and immunoglobulin class switching.

Signal 3 determines the skewing of the T cell response such that T cells may terminally differentiate towards either IFN gamma producing CD4+ T cells (Th1 cells), which eradicate intracellular pathogens (bacteria or viruses), or into Th2 cells producing IL-4, IL-5 and IL-13, which promote elimination of extracellular infections.

Additionally, cytokines like IL-12 for Th1 or IL-4 for Th2 differentiation are crucial determinants of initiation and/or amplification of Th responses. It has been suggested that DC express the Notch ligands Delta or Jagged under Th1 or Th2 conditions respectively, and that these ligands promote differentiation of naïve T cells towards one or the other Th profile.[66] Thus, factors and pathogens, which stimulate DC maturation and IL-12 production, promote Th1 responses (eg, *Escherichia coli*), whereas inducers of IL-4 production prime Th2 responses (*Porphyromonas gingivalis*).

Furthermore, Th1 polarizing capacity of DC is dependent on a number of variables that include the expression of certain transcription factors, the microenvironment, exposure to various maturation stimuli, the kinetics of maturation, and antigen dose. For example, expression by DC of the transcription factor T-bet which controls IFN-γ expression in CD4+ T cells appears to be required for optimal development of Th1 responses.[67] Epithelial DC in the respiratory tract may by default induce Th2 responses upon production of factors such as TSLP by epithelial cells.[38] The duration of DC activation and antigen dose also determines the direction of T cell skewing. Prolonged activation causes IL-12 depletion and results in "exhausted DC."[34] DC presenting low amounts of antigen skew towards Th2 whereas high doses skew towards Th1, which in turn is dependent upon the maturation state of the DC and consequences of environmental exposure.[68,69]

Recently, a new lineage of effector CD4 T cell was discovered.[70] Named Th17 due to their characteristic secretion of IL17 without IFN-γ or IL-4 secretion, this lineage of cells is implicated in several chronic inflammatory disorders. The IL-12 family member IL-23, and TGFβ have been implicated in the generation of Th17 cells, but the precise role of DC in the formation of these cells remains to be determined.[70] LPS-stimulated DC secrete inflammatory cytokines, notably IL-6, and in combination with TGFβ seem to divert differentiation of Treg into Th17 cells.[71,72]

It is important to note that T cell priming is dependent upon mDC, as immDC may induce immunosuppressive or Treg.[73,74] In fact, antigen presentation by immDC in vivo is an important pathway by which tolerance is maintained at both the CD4 and CD8 T cell level, either through the induction of Treg or through the deletion of autoreactive T cells.[75] Nevertheless, recent data suggest that in some conditions, mDC can also induce the generation of CD4+ CD25+ Treg.[76,77]

CD8+ T cells[78] and generation of effective CD8 memory cells in turn requires CD4 T cell help.[78–80] This help is provided through activation of DC via CD40L-CD40 interactions and the production of cytokines such as IL-2, although some studies have suggested that when cytotoxic T lymphocyte precursor frequencies are high, priming of CD8 T cell responses may be CD4 T cell independent. In these cases though, memory generation is likely to be hampered due to the absence of IL-2 during priming,[81] and primed T cells may commit fratricide through expression of TRAIL,[82] or become functionally tolerant upon receiving signals through the inhibitory receptor PD-1.[83]

Evidence is accumulating that pDC, which were believed to play a role only in the innate immune response due to their ability to produce high levels of IFN type I, can present viral and tumor antigens to initiate both CD4+ and CD8+ T cell responses.[84,85] Plasmacytoid DC mature in response to certain viral infections (eg, influenza and HIV) thereby providing an important link between innate and adaptive arms of the immune response. Like their myeloid counterparts, however, pDC display plasticity, even inducing immunosuppressive responses depending upon their microenvironment or the stimuli they are exposed to.[86] The role of pDC in antiviral responses, autoimmunity and transplant tolerance is discussed below.

B CELL ACTIVATION

In addition to affecting T cell function, DC can also influence B cell proliferation, isotype switching and plasma cell differentiation.[87] DC produce factors that activate and induce B cell proliferation (B-Lys and APRIL).[88] Furthermore, DC stimulate antibody responses in a T cell-independent manner against polysaccharide antigens. The initial interactions between B cells and DC occur in the T cell area of lymph nodes and in the germinal centers of lymph nodes and/or splenic red pulp. Importantly, antigen exposed cDC possess a specialized non-degradative pathway, which allows to present internalized antigens in their native state for the engagement of BCR on B cells. This is mediated by endocytosis of antigenic immune complexes through the inhibitory Fc receptor FcγRIIB and recycling of the endocytic vesicle to the surface without antigen degradation.[89] The follicular DC, which are present in germinal centers of lymph nodes and which constitute a different class of DC, participate in the maintenance of B cell memory by formation of multiple antigen-antibody complexes and continuous stimulation of B cells. The antigen-antibody complexes may remain in the lymph node for an extended period of time (up to months or years).

NK CELL ACTIVATION

The interactions between DC and NK cells are complex and further underscore a role of DC as a link between innate and adaptive immunity.[8] Direct interactions between NK cells and mature DC can result in NK cell activation as well as the potentiation of their cytolytic activity, and conversely, NK cells can induce further DC maturation. NK cells and DC can form an immune synapse, probably helping directional and confined secretion of cytokines as well as facilitating receptor-ligand interactions on one another. Activated NK cells induce DC through both cell contact (involving NKp30) and TNF-α and IFN-γ secretion. In turn, activated DC secrete IL-12/IL-18, IL-15, and IFN-α/β, which enhance IFN-γ secretion, proliferation, and cytotoxicity of NK cells. In some conditions, NK cells can lyse DC through NKp30, although mature DC are protected from cytolysis. This might represent a form of "cellular editing" whereby immature and tolerogenic DC are cleared by NK cells in the course of an ongoing immune response.[90]

It is thus possible that DC and NK cells play complementary roles in sensing pathogens such that DC could be the first to detect microbes through their expression of PRR (TLR, NOD proteins), whereas NK may get activated in the absence of overt inflammation but in the presence of ligands for activating NK-cell receptors, such as in the settings of tumors (which frequently lose MHC class I expression and/or express NKG2D ligands, such as MIC-A/B). In both situations, either DC or NK cells could create an inflammatory environment and induce the integrated activation of other cell types. Thus, in mice, infection by murine cytomegalovirus induces pDC to secrete high levels of IFN-α/β, whereas CD8α+ DC are the major producers of IL-12, and resistance to the virus is associated with expansion of Ly49H+ NK cells, driven by IL-12/IL-18.

The interaction between NK cells and DC is likely to take place early during the course of an immune response. This allows DC to exploit the ability of NK cells to kill tumor or virus/parasite infected cells and to cross-present this material to T cells.[91]

ACTIVATION OF OTHER ELEMENTS OF THE IMMUNE SYSTEM

DC have proven to be quite versatile in their ability to interact with many constituents of the immune system. For example, they can activate NK-T cells by presentation of the synthetic ligand alpha-galactosyl ceramide on CD1, inducing the production of cytokines such as IFN-γ and resistance to tumors.[92] CD1 restricted γδ T cells, which respond to microbial antigens from *Mycobacterium tuberculosis* and other organisms, induce maturation of resting DC, and induce

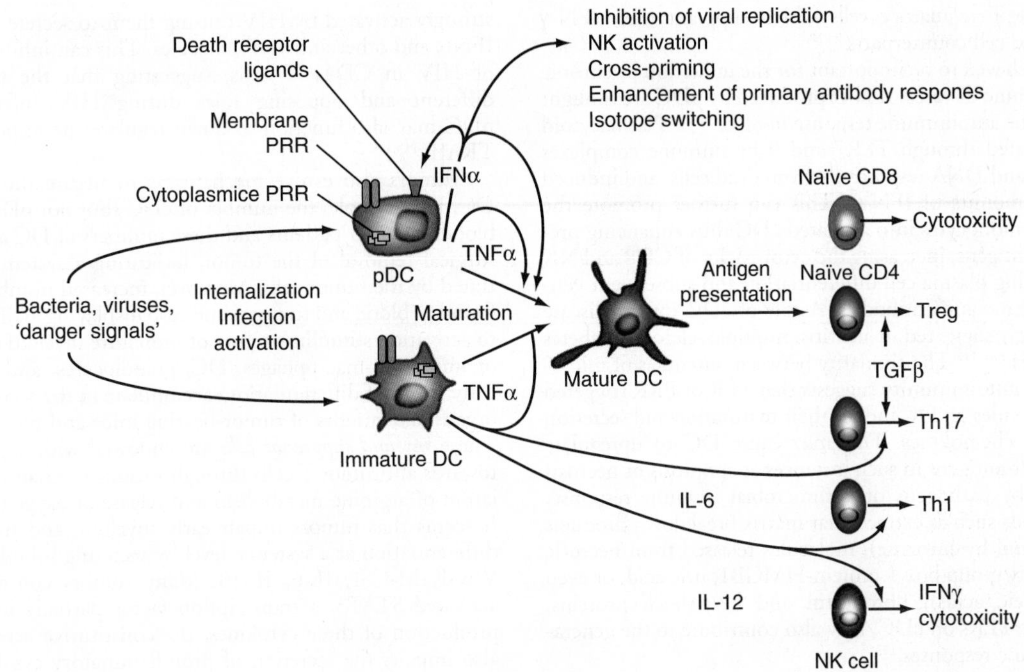

Figure 14–3 DENDRITIC CELLS LINK INNATE AND ADAPTIVE IMMUNITY. Through the expression of pattern-recognition receptors (PRR), like Toll-like receptors, dendritic cells act as sensors of pathogen intrusion. Upon signaling by PRR, they secrete cytokines and express receptors allowing stimulation of the innate immune system. IFN-α or IL-12 stimulate NK cell activation, while also inducing the expression of death-receptor ligands (TRAIL) on dendritic cells, harnessing them for direct killing of infected cells. They take up antigens through direct infection or phagocytosis, undergo a complex program of maturation by up-regulating the expression of costimulatory and MHC molecules, migrate to the secondary lymphoid organs, and stimulate naïve T cells. They secrete cytokines skewing the type of response induced, towards Th1, Th2, Treg, or Th17 differentiation, inducing the generation of cytotoxic CD8 T cells, or participating in the generation of antibody responses.

IL-12 production. This pathway and the IFN-γ secretion by activated γδ T cells, provide the immune system with a source of activated APC, which can polarize Th1 responses.[93]

In summary, the influence of DC on other cell types of the immune system is broad and integrative (Fig. 14–3). Future studies will ascertain the interplay between the myriad of host cells and the innate and adaptive immune response.

TOLERANCE AND AUTOIMMUNITY

DC play a pivotal role in the balance between immunity and tolerance. DC are important in the induction of both central and peripheral tolerance. In the former, DC play a role in deletion of autoreactive T cells in the thymus. In the latter, imDC in their steady state induce T cell deletion, anergy and/or generation of regulatory T cells, which interfere with IL-2 production and proliferation of effector T cells against self.[94] Regulatory T cells are CD4+ or CD8+ in nature, express CD25, CTLA-4 and the transcription factor Foxp3 (a member of the forkhead transcription factor family). These cells exert their tolerogenic effects either via cell contact or through release of immunosuppressive cytokines such as IL-10[95] or TGF-β, preventing proliferation and/or cytotoxicity of activated CD4 or CD8 T cells, and can also inhibit TLR-mediated maturation of cDC, but not pDC.[96] It was recently suggested that a subset of human thymic DC, upon activation by TSLP from epithelial cells of Hassall corpuscles, positively selects CD4+ Treg in the thymic medulla, thereby playing a central role in the generation of naturally occurring Treg.[97] How might DC in peripheral tissues induce tolerance is an open question. One report suggests that uptake of antigens via receptors such as DEC-205, a member of the C type lectin family, can induce T cell deletion and/or generation of antigen-specific Treg.[98]

DC may also be *actively* rendered *tolerogenic* via a number of mechanisms. Resting imDC acquire self-antigens through phagocytosis of apoptotic bodies formed as a consequence of physiological cell turnover. In the absence of a maturation signal, these DC induce tolerance to such self-antigens.[99] Some studies have suggested that ligation of specific receptors on DC such as complement receptors CR3 and CR4[100] by apoptotic cells inhibit their maturation[100] thereby ensuring the delivery of a tolerogenic rather than stimulatory signal. Others include MER, CD91/calreticulin and CD36/αvβ5. External factors such as steroids, IL-10 and/or TGF-β may also compromise DC immunostimulatory function by inhibiting their full maturation.[101] For example, DC isolated from tumor environments are poorly immunostimulatory due to the presence of immunosuppressive cytokines or the induction of costimulatory molecules such as PDL-1 which deliver negative signals.[102] Moreover, there may exist distinct tolerogenic DC subsets. A particular DC subset was recently identified in normal mice that were CD11c-low/CD45RB high), secreted IL-10 after activation, and induced tolerance through induction of Treg.[103] Recently in mice, pDC have been shown to induce tolerance against a vascularized cardiac allograft, upon administration of a tolerizing regimen.[104] After capturing pDC alloantigens from the graft, they migrated to peripheral lymph nodes and induced specific Treg.[104]

Recently, production of indoleamine 2,3 dioxygenase (IDO) has been proposed to account for some of the tolerogenic potential of DC.[105] IDO is an enzyme, which degrades the indole moiety of tryptophan and other molecules, and induces the production of immunoregulatory metabolites known as *kynurenines*. Local depletion of tryptophan and increase in proapoptotic kynurenines affects T cell proliferation and survival. Induction of IDO in DC has been postulated as one means by which deletional tolerance occurs. This is compounded by the observation that Treg may directly act on DC via CTLA-4-B7 interactions to promote IDO production.[105] Moreover, expression of death inducing ligands such as FasL may render DC capable of killing activated T cells.[98,106] Altogether, these properties of DC make them attractive candidates for inducing tolerance in the setting of transplantation or autoimmunity. Indeed, injection of antigen pulsed immature DC in vivo induces antigen specific IL-10-

producing CD8+ T regulatory cells which supplant their IFN-γ producing effector cell counterparts.[74,107]

DC are also believed to be important for the induction or chronic phase of autoimmune diseases. IFN-α produced by pDC are thought to contribute to the autoimmune response in SLE.[108,109] Plasmacytoid DC can be activated through TLR7 and 9 by immune complexes containing RNA and DNA respectively from dead cells, and induced to secrete high amounts of IFN-α. This can further promote the differentiation of monocytes into activated cDC thus enhancing presentation of self-antigens, increasing the cytotoxicity of CD8 and NK cells, and promoting plasma cell differentiation and subsequent generation of pathogenic autoantibodies. A role of cDC during disease onset is also strongly suggested in arthritis, multiple sclerosis, diabetes and atherosclerosis.[110–112] The similarity between outcomes of microbial infection and autoimmunity suggests that TLR or PRR triggered by microbial molecules on DC induce their maturation and secretion of cytokines and chemokines. This may cause DC to upregulate presentation of self-antigens in such instances as apoptosis or necrosis induced directly by pathogens or antimicrobial immune response. Endogenous ligands such as extracellular matrix breakdown products (heparan sulfate and hyaluronate), molecules released from necrotic cells (high-mobility group box 1 protein-HMGB1, uric acid, or even endogenous nucleic acids), fibronectin and heat-shock proteins, which can activate TLRs on cDC, may also contribute to the generation of autoimmune responses.[113]

SUBVERSION OF DENDRITIC CELL FUNCTION BY PATHOGENS AND TUMORS

Several pathogens have evolved different mechanisms to inhibit DC functions, allowing them to downregulate specific immune responses, and hence persist in the host. Numerous viruses, such as measles, vaccinia, herpes simplex, smallpox, and lymphocytic choriomeningitis virus, can impair antigen presentation by infected cells through different mechanisms. Thus, the human cytomegalovirus induces downmodulation of MHC class I or class II molecules, and can inhibit activated T cells through secretion of a virally encoded IL-10 homolog. Directly targeting DC allows viruses to impair the generation and quality of the antiviral immune responses. In mice, the murine cytomegalovirus has been shown to trigger paralysis of infected DC, preventing them from secreting IL-12 or IL-2 upon TLR4 triggering, impairing their capacity to mature, eventually rendering them unable to prime an effective T cell response.[114] Some viral products interfere with IFNα secretion pathways, such as the E6 oncoprotein of human papillomavirus, inhibiting trans-activation of IRF3 or IRF7, or NS3/4A inhibiting RIG-I and MDA5-mediated activation of IRF3.

It is now well documented that in HIV infected patients, not only the number of pDC and cDC in blood is reduced, but also that cDC are less efficient at stimulating primary T cell responses, and may generate IL-10 secreting T cells with a potential regulatory role. DC may be the first cells to encounter HIV in mucosal tissues and may mediate the spread of virus to CD4+ T cells in lymphoid organs. Indeed, cDC can mediate transinfection of CD4+ T cells, through the formation of an *infectious synapse*, carrying the virus with or without infection of the DC itself. DC express the coreceptors CD4, CCR5, CXCR4, and the C-type lectin DC-SIGN necessary for binding and/or entry of HIV, albeit at lower levels than CD4+ T cells, although the expression of DC-SIGN remains to be firmly demonstrated. HIV can infect DC, but its replication is not as efficient as in CD4+ T cells. The viral envelope protein gp120 can bind to CD4 and C-type lectins like DC-SIGN and mannose receptor, but the contribution of each receptor to binding and internalization may vary depending on the particular type of DC encountered by HIV. Thus, although DC are not the main reservoir of HIV, the virus can "highjack" DC to mediate its spread to CD4+ T cells from mucosal tissues to lymphoid organs. Nevertheless, although cDC only get minimally activated by HIV, pDC can get infected and be strongly activated by HIV causing them to secrete high amounts of IFNα and other antiviral molecules. This can inhibit the replication of HIV in CD4+ T cells, suggesting that the two subsets play different and opposing roles during HIV infection. However, pDC may also function to down regulate the response by secreting TRAIL.[115,116]

Tumors also evolve mechanisms to negate the functionality of DC. For example, the number of cDC (but not pDC), is reduced in blood of cancer patients and these numbers of DC are restored upon surgical removal of the tumor, indicating a systemic defect orchestrated by the tumor cells. Moreover, increased numbers of imDC are found in blood and tumor tissue, also displaying an impaired response to activation stimuli. A subset of immature myeloid cells, comprising of immature macrophages, DC, granulocytes, and myeloid cells at early stages of differentiation, accumulate in the secondary lymphoid organs and tumors of tumor-bearing mice and presumably humans. These *myeloid suppressor cells* are endowed with suppressive activity towards antitumor T cells through various mechanisms such as regulation of arginine metabolism and release of oxygen reactive species. It seems that tumors impair early myeloid, and in particular DC, differentiation at a systemic level by secreting soluble factors such as VEGF, M-CSF, IL-6, IL-10. Many tumors constitutively express activated STAT3, a transcription factor partially implicated in the production of these cytokines, the constitutive activation of which also impairs the secretion of proinflammatory cytokines. STAT3 is also responsible for abnormal differentiation of hematopoietic precursor cells, suggesting that inhibition of its activity may be a promising route towards restoring DC function in cancer.

IMMUNOTHERAPEUTIC STRATEGIES AND CLINICAL TRIALS

The last decade has seen an increasing interest in clinical applications of DC, harnessing the growing knowledge about DC biology. It is becoming apparent that any effective vaccine must activate and induce antigen presentation by DC, the most potent cells at stimulating T cell immunity. A number of clinical trials (mostly Phase I and II) have been completed describing the use of DC in cancer immunotherapy (eg, non-Hodgkin lymphoma, malignant melanoma, multiple myeloma, prostate cancer, renal cell carcinoma, breast cancer) and in the immunotherapy of human pathogens such as HIV. Most of these studies have relied on monocyte derived DC while a few have used DC prepared from CD34+ HPC. A critical issue is the antigen delivery to the DC, the nature of the antigen and the vehicle for delivery probably being decisive. DC can be pulsed with defined antigens, in the form of HLA-binding antigenic peptides or whole proteins, or the whole assortment of tumor antigens upon phagocytosis of dying or opsonized autologous tumor cells. Artificial fusion of dendritic cells with tumor cells allows the generation of hybrid cells with characteristic of dendritic cells, but also expressing the whole set of tumor antigens as well. Because autologous tumor cells are not always available from patients with advanced disease, allogeneic tumor cells of the same histological origin expressing shared tumor antigens are also used for loading DC.

DC themselves can also be genetically modified through transfection. However, DC are terminally differentiated nondividing cells and difficult to transfect. Methods using RNA electroporation, and infection by recombinant viruses (lentivirus, poxvirus, herpes virus, and adenoassociated virus) lead to foreign transgene expression in DC. Another strategy is to target DC in situ, using antibodies recognizing DC-specific molecules, such as DEC-205, as demonstrated in mouse models.[117]

Because the activation state of antigen-presenting DC is a determining factor in shaping the ensuing immune response, genetic engineering of DC or triggering activating receptors also allows to enhance their secretion, migration, and antigen presentation capacity. Thus, DC can be activated by artificial TLR ligands (eg, R848, which is a ligand for TLR7, unmethylated CpG oligonucleotides, which are ligands for TLR9, or inflammatory cytokines, such as IL-1β, IL-6, TNF-α) that can be used in a clinical setting to activate DC before injection, or even in vivo.[118] DC can also be transfected for immunostimulatory molecules, like cytokine genes (eg, IL-2, IL-12), or inhibitory siRNA for molecules dampening DC activation (eg, SOCS1).

It is likely that to achieve significant clinical responses upon vaccination for cancer, combining DC vaccination with other strategies will improve the therapeutic outcome. For example, some strategies aim at depleting or inactivating Treg (using a toxin targeting CD25, a molecule expressed by Treg, or cyclophosphamide), alleviating T cell anergy (using antagonistic CTLA-4), differentiating myeloid suppressor cells into nonimmunosuppressive cells (by injection of retinoic acid derivative ATRA), common γ chain cytokines such as IL-7, which have potent effects on T cell survival and function, or adoptive immunotherapy of in vitro activated T cells.[119,120] Finally, it seems that irradiation of the tumor tissue conditions it for enhanced migration of antigen-presenting cells and T cells, augments MHC class I expression on tumor cells, as well as induces apoptotic cells death, thus augmenting delivery of tumor antigens to DC.[121–123] Thus far, DC vaccines have not met the desired endpoints in clinical studies (ie, tumor regression) despite clear evidence that DC vaccination can induce measurable cellular or humoral immune responses in cancer patients.[124–127] In a recent Phase III trial, vaccination of stage IV melanoma patients by DC loaded with multiple peptides could not be demonstrated to be more effective than the standard chemotherapy treatment.[128] However, the optimal DC type, optimal maturation signal(s), mechanism of antigen delivery, nature of antigen, frequency of immunization, and route of administration still remain to be determined. Furthermore, it may be that only a subset of patients may be able to respond to DC vaccination, or in the case of advanced stage cancer patients, to any vaccination. In our opinion, DC immunotherapy will be most efficacious when coadministered with an adjuvant and when tumor burden is low. The timing of vaccination is probably also crucial, and frequent immunizations may dramatically improve the clinical efficacy.[129] In the setting of HIV infection, a recent study in a small group of chronically infected individuals showed that vaccination with DC loaded with chemically inactivated virus allows stabilization and even suppression of viral load for an extended period of time without any other treatment.[130] Vaccination with DC holds great promise in cancer and infectious diseases, but its potential is likely to be best exploited in combination with other strategies manipulating other arms of the immune system.

Although DC are considered the most potent cells in inducing T cell responses, they can also function as tolerizing cells, a function that can be harnessed against autoimmune diseases and in a transplantation setting. Thus it is possible to differentiate in vitro maturation-resistant imDC, or differentially activated DC, using biological agents such as IL-10, TGF-β, or the fusion protein CTLA-4-Ig, and pharmacological agents such as corticosteroids, cyclosporine, rapamycin, mycophenolate mophetil, vitamin D3, or prostaglandin E2. The clinical relevance of some of these strategies is being evaluated. Another way to dampen pathologic immune responses is to use antagonists for TLR or other innate immune sensor participating in amplifying damaging responses. Thus, since the role of DNA-immune complexes has been established as important in the etiology of SLE, synthetic inhibitory oligodeoxyribonucleotides have been developed, that can prevent and/or inhibit activation through TLR9 on pDC and B cells, and block SLE in animal models. Finally, significant challenges remain with respect to DC based immunotherapy ranging from applicability of preclinical models to humans to regulatory and funding hurdles.

SUMMARY

Dendritic cells (DC) are a sparsely distributed population of bone marrow derived mononuclear cells that exist in an immature form in virtually all tissues in the body. DC serve as professional antigen presenting cells with extraordinary capacity to stimulate naïve T lymphocytes (as well as B cells, NK cells, and NK-T cells) and initiate primary immune response. They link innate and adaptive immunity and are responsible for activation and inhibition of effector cells. Their clinical applications in cancer, transplantation, and chronic virus infections are under investigation.

SUGGESTED READINGS

Ackerman AL, Giodini A, Cresswell P: A role for the endoplasmic reticulum protein retrotranslocation machinery during crosspresentation by dendritic cells. Immunity 25:607, 2006.

Akira S, Takeda K, Kaisho T: Toll-like receptors: critical proteins linking innate and acquired immunity. Nat Immunol 2:675, 2001.

Barber DL, Wherry EJ, Masopust D, et al: Restoring function in exhausted CD8 T cells during chronic viral infection. Nature 439:682, 2006.

Cella M, Facchetti F, Lanzavecchia A, et al: Plasmacytoid dendritic cells activated by influenza virus and CD40L drive a potent TH1 polarization. Nat Immunol 1:305, 2000.

Hawiger D, Inaba K, Dorsett Y, et al: Dendritic cells induce peripheral T cell unresponsiveness under steady state conditions in vivo. J Exp Med 194:769, 2001.

Kadowaki N, Antonenko S, Lau JY, et al: Natural interferon alpha/beta-producing cells link innate and adaptive immunity. J Exp Med 192:219, 2000.

Kapsenberg ML: Dendritic-cell control of pathogen-driven T-cell polarization. Nat Rev Immunol 3:984, 2003.

Lu W, Arraes LC, Ferreira WT, et al: Therapeutic dendritic-cell vaccine for chronic HIV-1 infection. Nat Med 10:1359, 2004.

Medzhitov R: Toll-like receptors and innate immunity. Nat Rev Immunol 1:135, 2001.

Moretta A: The dialogue between human natural killer cells and dendritic cells. Curr Opin Immunol 17:306, 2005.

Rapoport AP, Stadtmauer EA, Aqui N, et al: Restoration of immunity in lymphopenic individuals with cancer by vaccination and adoptive T-cell transfer. Nat Med 11:1230, 2005.

Shortman K, Liu YJ: Mouse and human dendritic cell subtypes. Nat Rev Immunol 2:151, 2002.

Skoberne M, Beignon AS, Larsson M, et al: Apoptotic cells at the crossroads of tolerance and immunity. Curr Top Microbiol Immunol 289:259, 2005.

REFERENCES

For complete list of references log onto www.expertconsult.com

CHAPTER 15

REGULATION OF ACTIVATION OF B AND T LYMPHOCYTES

John G. Monroe and Michael J. Lenardo

OVERVIEW

The immune system is composed of different cell types that perform specialized regulatory and effector functions in an orchestrated manner to achieve immunity. Compartmentalization and subspecialization of these cells allow for enormous flexibility in the response to specific types of pathogens. Lymphocytes constitute the effector cells of the adaptive antigen-specific immune response. They are the cells responsible for the characteristics that we often associate with the immune system—namely, memory, specificity, and tolerance to self-antigens. Lymphocytes can be subdivided into two general subpopulations: B lymphocytes and T lymphocytes. B lymphocytes are responsible for antibody production, whereas T lymphocytes are the mediators of cellular immunity: cytotoxic T-lymphocyte responses, delayed-type hypersensitivity, graft-versus-host reactions, and other cellular immune reactions. A secondary role for B lymphocytes is in the major histocompatibility complex (MHC) class II antigen presentation to CD4-expressing T lymphocytes, as discussed in Chapter 12.

Immune responses involve powerful and sometimes destructive mediators that have important effects on normal physiology and anatomy. Therefore, lymphocytes are normally in a quiescent state and only those needed are called forth, or activated, in a particular immune response. Activation includes the initiation of biochemical and metabolic processes that trigger changes in gene expression programs leading to the coordinated production of internal, cell-bound, and soluble proteins that enable the lymphocytes to carry out protective immune functions. The programs of genes expressed differ between B and T cells as well as their subsets and this dictates their distinct immune functions. A crucial effect of these genetic programs is to induce clonal proliferation of the lymphocytes that have been activated. As described throughout this chapter, an elaborate set of positive and negative controls govern the gene-activating signals and thus the levels of the potent mediators and cellular offspring produced.

Activation of lymphocytes requires a means to detect antigens, an immense diversity of molecular structures (termed *epitopes*) on infectious agents or tumor cells that are the targets of immune response. As postulated as long ago as 1900 by Ehrlich[1] and confirmed by numerous studies since then, lymphocytes express clonally distributed receptors on the cell surface that facilitate antigen recognition and serve as signaling molecules to initiate the activation of these cells. Extensive investigation has shown these receptors to be transmembrane protein complexes on the cell surface that link antigen recognition events to the intracellular signaling apparatus. The structure of the antigen-binding component, and hence the specificity of the B- and T-lymphocyte antigen receptors, are determined by a complex recombination process that operates on a large variety of gene segments encoding these regions (see Chapters 11 and 12). The variable regions, which are the amino terminal regions of the receptor proteins that bind antigen, are assembled by mixing and matching assorted genetic segments, thereby generating an enormous diversity of antigen recognition sites. As a consequence of this potential variability, the number of antigenic epitopes that can be recognized has been theoretically calculated to exceed 10^{11}. Because the specificity is determined at the genetic level, the progeny and effector cells derived from a B or a T lymphocyte after antigen activation maintain in many circumstances the identical antigen specificity of the original responding cell. This process ensures the clonality of the immune response. A specific exception to this rule is the somatic hypermutation of the B-lymphocyte antigen receptor gene that occurs during germinal center reactions.[2,3] This alters the DNA sequence of the gene so as to introduce new amino acids in the antigen-combining regions of the receptors, thereby refining it specifically or creating it anew.

For B lymphocytes, antigen recognition and binding is mediated by a surface form of immunoglobulin (sIg). Other proteins that are noncovalently associated with sIg are responsible for generating signals that inform the antigen-bound B lymphocyte to respond. This multimeric protein complex is called the B-cell antigen receptor (BCR) and has separate antigen recognition and signaling components. This compartmentalization of function allows B lymphocytes to maintain maximum diversity in their antigen recognition capability and at the same time trigger identical responses. Along similar lines, the T-cell antigen receptor (TCR) also is a complex of antigen recognition and signal transducer proteins. The largest class of T lymphocytes uses a dimeric protein composed of two disulfide-linked α and β chains as their receptor for antigen recognition (α/β TCRs). A more restricted class of tissue-associated T lymphocytes use separately encoded genome (γ) and delta (δ) receptor chains for antigen recognition ($\gamma\delta$ TCRs).

Although the BCR and, as you will see later, the TCR as well are sufficient for antigen binding and signal initiation, other surface proteins called *coreceptors* can regulate the strength of antigen binding as well as the level of signals generated by this binding. These coreceptor molecules regulate the sensitivity of the antigen receptors for generating activation signals and also play a role in how certain antigens interact with B and T lymphocytes. Coreceptors CD4 and CD8 define the major subsets of T cells and also augment TCR interactions with antigenic peptides in the context of major histocompatibility complex (MHC) class II and class I molecules, respectively, expressed on antigen-presenting cells (APCs). By contrast, the MHC does not influence BCR-dependent interactions, because these receptors can bind native antigen. Distinct B cell-specific coreceptors, including CD22 and the CD19–CD21 complex, regulate BCR signaling. As is discussed in more detail later, CD22 likely modulates receptor sensitivity under defined conditions and CD19–CD21 may regulate responses to specific forms of antigen.

Antigen binding by BCRs or TCRs on fully mature B and T lymphocytes is necessary but not sufficient to generate complete activation responses. Both types of lymphocytes require signals generated through secondary cell-surface proteins called *costimulatory molecules*. For T lymphocytes, signaling through the CD28 coreceptor is required for gene induction controlling growth factor production and proliferation. B lymphocytes require CD40 costimulatory signaling for antibody production and optimal clonal expansion. Finally, for both types of lymphocytes, soluble cytokines amplify and modify the activation responses and determine the effector functions of these cells. Finally, it should be noted that B lymphocytes can be activated in some cases independently of the BCR. B lymphocytes express Toll-like receptors (TLRs) on their surface and in their cytoplasm that recognize common molecular structures or patterns associated with pathogens but not normally expressed by humans and other mammals. Using biochemical pathways different from those used to initiate BCR-induced activation, binding of these pattern-recognition receptors to pathogen-associated molecules triggers the B lymphocyte independently of the BCR. TLRs are described in more detail in Chapter 10 and will not be mentioned further here. Likewise, T cells can also be activated independently of TCR. In this case signals generated through CD2 or the GPI-linked protein Thy-1 can trigger proliferation although the significance of this mechanism of T-cell activation is at present unknown.

This chapter discusses how antigen-induced lymphocyte responses are initiated and the way that the gene-activating signals generated through these receptors are regulated. The focus is on (a) the mechanism and role of the antigen receptor-induced activation signals, (b) the degree to which these signals are necessary for lymphocyte-mediated immune responses, and (c) how they can be modified to adapt the response to different pathogens.

B LYMPHOCYTES

B lymphocytes are the primary effector cells of the antibody-mediated immune response and are APCs for activated and, in some circumstances, resting T lymphocytes. They constitute the cells necessary for the humoral arm of the immune system because the antibody they produce can travel through the blood and lymph (the humor) and have effects at distant sites from the B cells that produced them. Also, humoral immunity can be transferred by serum without cells—a procedure sometimes used as a clinical intervention. Antigen recognition and triggering are accomplished by the BCR expressed on the surface of mature, immunocompetent B lymphocytes. Following antigen binding, the BCR-antigen complex is endocytosed, and protein antigens are processed and re-presented as peptides on the B-lymphocyte surface in association with class II MHC antigens. These peptide–MHC class II complexes are recognized by CD4 T cells. This interaction activates the T cells (see later section on T-lymphocyte activation), and these activated T cells in turn deliver activation and differentiation signals to the B lymphocyte. In this context, the antigen-specific B and T lymphocytes can be viewed as communicating with each other, each providing cues to the other to increase levels of activation and effector cell commitment. This stepwise process makes available multiple levels of regulation, providing the immune system with critical checkpoints to ensure that the appropriate magnitude and effector function are achieved. In addition to its role as a recognition structure and as a mechanism for antigen capture, the BCR also serves as the initiating signaling complex for B cell activation.

B-LYMPHOCYTE ANTIGEN RECEPTOR

The antigen recognition structure of the BCR is a surface form of immunoglobulin (sIg). The basic monomeric structure of sIg is identical to that of the monomeric subunit of the secreted form of this molecule. Each monomer possesses two light-chain proteins (IgLC) disulfide-coupled to two disulfide-linked heavy-chain (IgHC) proteins. The surface and membrane forms of immunoglobulin differ from the secreted form with respect to the carboxyl (C) end of the heavy-chain proteins. Surface immunoglobulin includes additional amino acid residues, comprising a spacer, a transmembrane region, and a cytoplasmic region. The carboxyl-terminal (C-terminal) end of the membrane form is encoded by two additional exons that differ for each immunoglobulin isotype. For sIgM and sIgD, the cytoplasmic region is composed of only three amino acids, whereas IgG and IgA are more extensive, comprising 28 and 14 amino acids, respectively. The reason for the more extensive cytoplasmic domain for IgG and IgA is not established; in IgG, however, this region may be important for optimal expansion of isotype-switched B lymphocytes in the germinal center.[2] In addition the secreted forms of Ig can exist as multimers of the Ig monomeric structure. Such is the case for IgA and IgM. The light chains are linked to the N-terminal domain of the heavy chains and thereby contribute directly to the enormous variability in antigen-binding specificities between individual B lymphocytes. The primary sequence of the heavy- and light-chain variable regions that associate to form the antigen-combining site determines the antigen specificity of a particular B-lymphocyte clone. Importantly, the diversity created by expressing unique antigen recognition elements on every newly created B lymphocyte results in an extremely large repertoire of antigen-reactive B lymphocytes within an individual. Therefore, at any given time an individual has the potential to recognize and react to an enormous universe of potential pathogens that might break through the normal physical barriers of the body.

There are molecularly distinct isotypes of immunoglobulin (IgM, IgD, IgG, IgE, IgA) that all function as antigen receptors on B lymphocytes. These arise from switching of gene segments in the carboxyl-terminal region of the Ig heavy chain via a process called "class switching." For the most part, only one isotype is expressed at any given time. A single exception to this rule occurs in the case of IgM and IgD, which can be coexpressed on resting mature follicular B lymphocytes. For isotypes other than IgM and IgD (ie, IgG, IgA, and IgE), genetic mechanisms similar to those involved in variable region gene rearrangement (see Chapter 11) make it genetically impossible to coexpress these other isotypes.

A genetic process involving the rearrangement of the exons that encode heavy- and light-chain variable regions determines the amino acid sequence of the variable region. Through a process involving stochastic selection of variable region segments, random nucleotide additions, and junctional diversity, the DNA sequence of a rearranged BCR gene has only a 1 in 10^9 to 10^{12} chance of being identical to any other BCR rearrangement. Because this genetic process occurs without antigen selection, the intrinsic antigen specificity of the B lymphocytes produced is quasi-random and highly varied, enhancing the likelihood of clones responsive to new foreign antigens. Although this potential diversity can never be realized in the immune system of a single individual within a group of individuals, it provides a tremendous advantage to a population of individuals because it ensures that the potential exists in the population to respond to a nearly infinite spectrum of antigens. In addition, 2 to 3 million new B lymphocytes are generated daily so that the diversification process constantly generates new specificities and affinities for potential pathogens. This survival advantage must be balanced, however, against the likelihood that many of the BCRs produced may be reactive to self-antigens. Although it is not discussed here, the immune system has evolved mechanisms to identify and remove self-reactive B and T lymphocytes from the repertoire based in part on signals generated through their BCRs.[3–6]

As already mentioned, the BCR exists as a protein complex in the plasma membrane of the B lymphocyte, as illustrated in Fig. 15–1. IgM and IgD are the isotypes expressed on resting B lymphocytes with no prior history of antigen-induced activation (naive or virgin B lymphocytes). However, the short cytoplasmic domain of sIgM or sIgD (three amino acids) is unable on its own to couple cross-linking by antigen to intracellular signal transducers. Consequently, in order to initiate activation signals, sIg exists noncovalently associated with a disulfide bond-coupled heterodimer of two proteins, Igα (CD79a) and Igβ (CD79b).[7,8] These proteins are products of the *mb-1* and *B29* genes, respectively, and constitute the signaling components of the BCR.[9,10] Furthermore, expression of Igα and Igβ is necessary for surface expression of membrane immunoglobulin (mIg).

Igα and Igβ are structurally similar transmembrane proteins with a single immunoglobulin superfamily domain in the N-terminal extracellular portion and a long C-terminal intracytoplasmic domain. As first noted by Reth,[11] within these cytoplasmic domains are regions homologous to other immunologic signaling molecules, such as the γ, ε, and δ chains of the CD3 complex (see later) and the high-affinity IgE receptor β and γ chains in mast cells. These motifs contain two tyrosines (Y) in a pattern of YXXL/I(X 6–8)YXXL/I, where X represents any amino acid. For the BCR and the TCR (see later), it has been shown that these tyrosine-containing motifs—immunoreceptor tyrosine-based activation motifs (ITAMs)—are necessary and largely sufficient for signal transduction.[12] The tyrosines associated with ITAMs are significant because they represent substrates for tyrosine phosphorylation by specific kinases and subsequent docking sites for intracellular signaling molecules, as discussed later.

The earliest detected BCR-triggered event is the activation and phosphorylation of tyrosine-specific kinases, particularly those belonging to the Src, Syk, and Tec families of protein tyrosine kinases (PTKs). The phosphorylation of tyrosines in the Igα and Igβ ITAMs after BCR cross-linking provided the first clue that PTKs were involved in transmembrane signaling. Phosphorylation of these proteins is believed to be accomplished by specific PTKs that exist in noncovalent association with the BCR in an inactive form in resting B lymphocytes. Clustering of the BCR signaling complex, as occurs after binding to multivalent antigen or antigen aggregates, activates the receptor-associated PTKs and the subsequent phosphorylation of the Igα and Igβ ITAM-associated tyrosines. This process facilitates recruitment of signaling proteins containing phosphotyrosine-binding Src homology-2 (SH2) domains, as diagrammed in Fig. 15–2. The

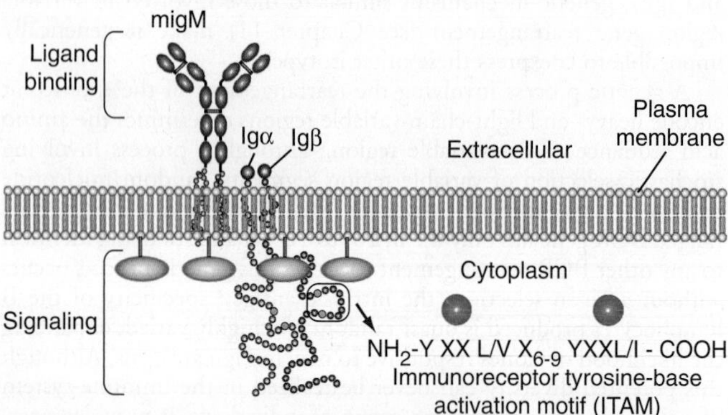

Figure 15–1 Composition of the B lymphocyte (B-cell) antigen receptor complex (BCR) on resting B lymphocytes. Shown are heterodimers of Igα and Igβ in noncovalent association with the membrane form of IgM (mIgM). Also illustrated are BCR-associated Src-family tyrosine kinases because they are believed to associate with the complex in the resting state. These kinases are tethered to the cytoplasmic side of the plasma membrane by a short myristoylated sequence and in noncovalent association with Igα and Igβ by the amino-terminal (N-terminal) portion of the kinase. The specific association of each kinase with either Igα or Igβ is not known and is illustrated here only for convenience. The diagram reflects the known stoichiometric relationship that exists between the number of Igα/Igβ heterodimers and the mIg monomer. The consensus sequence of the immunoreceptor tyrosine-based activation motif (ITAM) associated with Igα and Igβ is depicted.

reader is also referred to several reviews for more details on the regulation of these processes.[13–15] SH2 domains interact with phosphotyrosine residues with characteristic specificities. A common theme for molecules intimately involved in signal transduction is their modular construction, associating different discrete protein–protein interaction domains with domains mediating enzymatic activity. These interaction domains facilitate not only recruitment of enzyme substrates, as in the case of kinases, but also direct the spatial localization of these multiprotein signaling complexes to receptors such as the BCR and TCR.

B-lymphocyte receptor-associated PTKs identified so far are Lyn, Blk, Fyn, and, in a few reports, Lck.[16–18] All are members of the Src family, which is defined by a conserved arrangement of protein–protein interaction domains (Fig. 15–3) as well as a kinase domain and sites for autoregulation by phosphorylation.[19] Kinases of the Src family each have a myristoylation sequence at the N terminus, tethering the kinases to the plasma membrane. Some of these, such as Lyn, also are palmitoylated, which, as discussed later, may influence their association with specific compartments within the plasma membrane. Adjacent to the myristoylation sequence is a unique amino acid sequence that differs for each member of the Src family kinases. This region may be responsible for interactions with the unphosphorylated Igα/Iγβ complex in resting B lymphocytes.[20] At the C terminus of the unique region is a single Src homology-3 (SH3) domain that mediates protein–protein interactions by recognition of proline-rich motifs. C-terminal to the SH3 domain in the protein is the SH2 domain.

For all Src family kinases, the enzymatically active kinase domain is at the C terminus of the protein. All of these family members also share common regulatory mechanisms. One tyrosine residue, near the C terminus of the protein, negatively regulates kinase activity (see Fig. 15–3). If this site is phosphorylated, the enzyme is inactivated, thereby providing a mechanism to turn off the response. Dephosphorylation alters the conformation of the kinase to induce full activity. In B lymphocytes, this inhibitory phosphorylation event is mediated by the Csk tyrosine kinase. This kinase is structurally related to the Src family kinases, containing single SH2 and SH3 domains near the N-terminus of the molecule. Csk is functionally unique, however, in its substrate specificity. The main function of Csk kinase is to phosphorylate Src family kinases, at their C-terminal negative regulatory tyrosines.[21] Thus, the principal function of Csk is to maintain the BCR in the inactive state in the absence of antigen and possibly to downmodulate signaling once antigen is no longer present. Conversely, initiation of signaling requires dephosphorylation at this site.[19] Dephosphorylation is believed to be mediated by coclustering of CD45 (see later) with the aggregated BCR complex. The mechanism by which phosphorylation and dephosphorylation

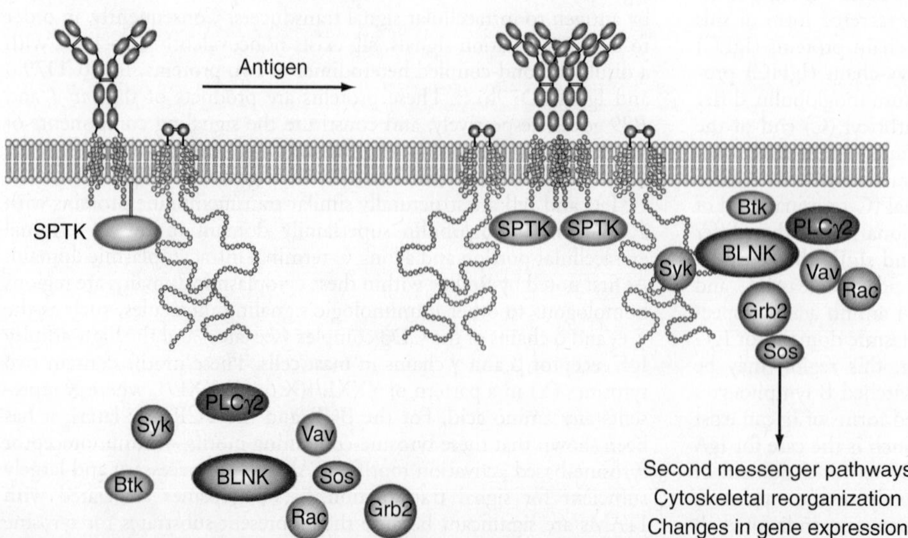

Figure 15–2 Illustrated is the signaling complex formed as a consequence of antigen-induced clustering of B-cell receptor (BCR) complexes. Shown are examples of cytoplasmic signaling effector proteins that are recruited subsequent to the Src kinase-mediated phosphorylation of the Igα/Igβ immunoreceptor tyrosine-based activation motifs (ITAMs). Although this diagram depicts only a selection of the many protein–protein interactions that occur following BCR aggregation, the example serves to illustrate the central role for adapter proteins in the organization of these signaling complexes; B-cell linker protein (BLNK) is used as the example in this figure. Ig, immunoglobulin; PLCγ2, phospholipase Cγ2; SPTK, Src protein tyrosine kinase.

are believed to regulate kinase activity for the Src family protein tyrosine kinases is illustrated in Fig. 15–3.

Subsequent to the initial wave of PTK activation mediated by the BCR-associated kinases, there follows activation of a second set of distinct PTKs. Two of these kinases play unique and critical roles in B-lymphocyte activation: Bruton tyrosine kinase (Btk), which is a member of the Tec PTK family, and Syk. As the name implies, Btk activity is associated with Bruton immunodeficiency. Accordingly, mutations in Btk have been shown to be responsible for X-chromosome-linked B-lymphocyte immune defects in mice and humans.[22–24]

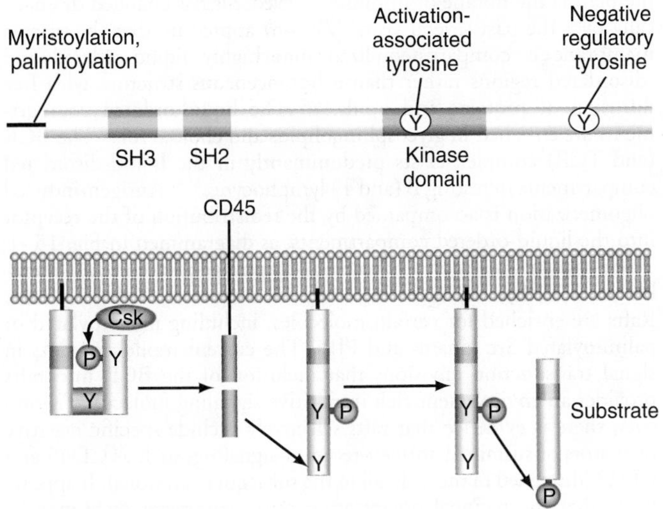

Figure 15–3 Top panel, The modular structure of protein tyrosine kinases belonging to the Src family. Each member of this family contains SH3 and SH2 domains for protein–protein interactions, a kinase domain, and two tyrosine residues that are involved in the regulation of the activity for these proteins (as diagrammed in *bottom panel*). **Bottom panel,** Regulation of the activity of the Src-family protein tyrosine kinases. Illustrated is the model accounting for decreased activity as a consequence of Csk-mediated phosphorylation of the carboxyl-terminal (C-terminal) tyrosine, which then interacts with the SH2 domain (*shaded*) of the kinase, resulting in an inaccessible kinase domain (*cross-hatched*). Cross-linking of the B- or T-lymphocyte receptor is believed to cluster CD45 and the receptor-associated Src family tyrosine kinases. CD45-associated phosphatase-catalyzed dephosphorylation of the C-terminal tyrosine results in an open configuration in which the kinase domain-associated tyrosine is phosphorylated by adjacent tyrosine kinase molecules. This phosphorylated tyrosine serves as a docking site to position substrate proteins near the catalytic domain of the kinase. P, phosphate group; Y, tyrosine.

The Syk kinase bears homology to the zeta-associated protein (ZAP-70; with an Mr of 70,000) PTK that is associated with the ζ chain of the TCR complex (see later).[12] Both ZAP-70 and Syk contain tandem SH2 domains at the N-terminal end of the protein, and a kinase domain in the C-terminal region.[25,26] Syk kinase also is activated and tyrosine phosphorylated following BCR cross-linking, although with slower kinetics than for the Src family PTKs.[27] Src kinase-mediated phosphorylation of the Igα/Igβ ITAMs creates phosphotyrosine docking sites to recruit Syk through its tandem SH2 domains (Fig. 15–4). This docking, coupled with Syk phosphorylation by Src kinases, activates the tyrosine kinase activity of Syk. One of the most immediate substrates of Syk is the cytoplasmic adapter protein BLNK (*B*-cell *linke*r protein; also called SLP-65). BLNK is an example of a rapidly expanding family of intermediate signal-transducing proteins called *adapters*.[28] Adapters lack inherent enzymatic activity but function by recruiting and physically organizing other signal-transducing enzymes. In the case of BLNK, it is phosphorylated on at least five tyrosines by Syk. These phosphotyrosines then interact with the SH2 domains of Btk, PLCγ2, Vav, and potentially other signaling proteins. By so doing, adapters such as BLNK can spatially arrange signaling proteins into organized complexes termed *signalosomes*. The stability of the signalosome and thus the duration of the signal relies entirely on the continued phosphorylation of Igα, Igβ, and BLNK. As a consequence, the strength and duration of BCR signals are critically dependent on the balance of tyrosine kinase and phosphatase activities proximal to the assembled signaling complex.

B-LYMPHOCYTE INTRACELLULAR SIGNALING

Antigen-induced B-cell activation can be separated into two categories depending upon the degree to which antigen–BCR engagement alone is sufficient. Thymus-dependent antigens require secondary signals from activated T cells (as will be discussed later) in addition to BCR signaling for activation of proliferation and IgM secretion, whereas for thymus-independent antigen responses T-cell help can augment BCR-induced responses but are not absolutely required. In either case, following the initiation and transmembrane transduction of BCR signals, the signals are amplified, propagated, and translated by the B lymphocyte into appropriate responses. Many of the events are common to T lymphocytes as well. The linkage of antigen receptor-initiated signals to changes in gene expression necessary to alter the activation state and effector capabilities of the lymphocyte occurs through the generation of cytoplasmic second messengers. All defined second messenger pathways linked to the BCRs and TCRs are triggered by the initial PTK phosphorylation events. As will become evident, the initial two PTK steps are followed by activation of either serine/threonine-directed protein kinases or phosphatases. These pro-

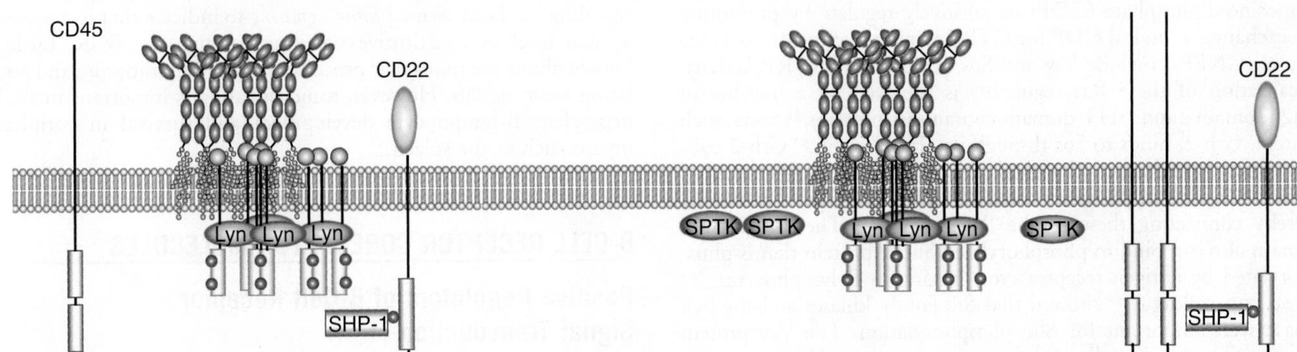

Figure 15–4 Diagram showing the inclusion of the antigen-mediated multimerized B-cell receptor (BCR) into the liquid-ordered plasma membrane compartments (ie, rafts, GEMs, or DIMs; see text) (depicted in *green*). Illustrated here is the proposed model whereby raft compartmentalization excludes negative regulatory protein tyrosine phosphatase complexes (ie, CD45 and CD22/SHP-1) from the multimerized BCR complexes and concentrates positive regulators of BCR signaling (Src protein tyrosine kinases [SPTKs]) to enhance signaling through the antigen-aggregated receptor. DIMs, detergent-insoluble membranes; GEMs, glycosphingolipid-enriched membranes.

teins are directed at the activation of transcription factors that preexist in the resting lymphocyte but in an inactive state.[14]

Three major second messenger pathways have been linked to BCR-mediated signaling. The first is the phosphatidylinositol (PI) hydrolysis pathway, which is initiated by the activation of phospholipase Cγ2 (PLCγ2). In B lymphocytes, Syk and Btk tyrosine kinase activities phosphorylate PLCγ2 to activate its lipase activity, thereby initiating this signaling pathway. The preferred substrate of active PLCγ2 is a plasma membrane phospholipid, phosphatidylinositol-4,5-bisphosphate (PIP_2). PLCγ2 lipolysis of PIP_2 yields inositol-1,4,5-triphosphate (IP_3) and diacylglycerol, each of which in turn generates two second messengers, increasing cytoplasmic free Ca^{2+} and stimulating a serine/threonine protein kinase called protein kinase Cβ (PKCβ), respectively. The rise in intracellular free Ca^{2+} concentration probably triggers a number of changes in cellular physiology; however, at a minimum, it activates calcineurin, an inducible cytoplasmic serine/threonine phosphatase. Calcineurin activity is required for the activation responses of B and T lymphocytes through its ability to activate the nuclear factor of activated T lymphocytes (NFAT).[29] Although the precise role of PKCβ in B-lymphocyte activation is not fully understood, it is critical for normal B-lymphocyte development, survival, and BCR-induced proliferative responses to T cell-independent antigens.[30,31]

Another second messenger pathway linked to BCR signaling is the phosphatidylinositol 3′-kinase (PI3K) pathway. This pathway is initiated by PTK-mediated phosphorylation of the regulatory subunit that induces the enzymatic activity of PI3K.[32,33] Activated PI3K phosphorylates inositol phospholipids converting, in one case, PIP_2 to PIP_3. Although PI3K is important in growth factor-mediated signaling and is known to be activated by BCR-mediated signaling,[34,35] its role in B-lymphocyte responses is not completely clear. One described consequence of PI3K activity is the ability of the PIP_3 product to activate a unique isoform of protein kinase C, PKCζ.[36] PI3K appears to activate another kinase, S6K, which has been shown to facilitate the progression of stimulated cells through the cell cycle.[37–39] An additional downstream kinase that is stimulated by PI3K is Akt (also known as protein kinase B, PKB), which phosphorylates and inhibits the activity of GSK3, another serine/threonine kinase that negatively regulates the transcription factor NFAT.

The third network of regulatory proteins activated by BCR signaling are the small GTPase (or G) proteins of the Ras pathway.[40] In its active state, p21 Ras binds guanosine triphosphate (GTP) and can activate Raf-1, a serine/threonine kinase. Activated Raf-1 is able to phosphorylate and activate mitogen-activated protein kinase kinase (MAPKK), a tyrosine and serine/threonine protein kinase that can then activate mitogen-activated protein kinase (MAPK). MAPKs can in turn phosphorylate and activate transcription factors such as components of activator protein-1 (AP-1), thereby inducing their activity in the nucleus, ultimately leading to specific gene activation. Ras activity is controlled by a number of modulator proteins, which either negatively regulate by promoting GTP hydrolysis to guanosine diphosphate (GDP) or positively regulate by promoting the exchange of bound GDP for GTP. Guanine nucleotide exchange factors (GNEFs) include Vav and Sos, which promote Ras activity. Localization of these Ras regulators is achieved by a number of SH2 domain- and SH3 domain-containing proteins.[41] One such protein, Grb-2, binds to Sos through its SH3 domain.[42] Grb-2 consists of two SH3 domains that flank a single SH2 domain. The Grb-2 SH2 domain binds phosphorylated tyrosines of activated receptors, thereby connecting these to the Ras pathway.[43] The Grb-2 SH2 domain also can bind to phosphorylated Shc, a protein that is phosphorylated by antigen receptor cross-linking in B lymphocytes.[40,44] Nagai and colleagues[44] showed that Src family kinases and the Syk kinase were important for Shc phosphorylation. The Vav protein is expressed only in cells of hematopoietic origin. Vav is tyrosine phosphorylated and GNEF activity is stimulated following BCR cross-linking.[45,46] Deficiencies of Vav in B lymphocytes cause a reduction in the number of peripheral B lymphocytes and the inability to proliferate in response to BCR signaling.[43,47] Downmodulators of Ras such as the Ras-GTPase activating protein (ras.GAP) are inactivated by tyrosine phosphorylation in B cells after antigen receptor stimulation.[48]

In addition to these second messenger pathways, studies of both BCR and TCR signaling (see later) have unveiled other pathways that play more specific activation functions by initiating alterations in cytoskeletal organization and motility. Although we generally describe these pathways as linear sequences of events that operate in parallel, there is considerable cross-talk between them. This cross-talk adds a level of regulation and complexity that makes it difficult to assign a particular pathway to a specific downstream activation-associated event.

Our understanding of the distribution of proteins and lipids in the plasma membrane of immune system cells has changed dramatically over the past several years. We now appreciate that the plasma membrane is compartmentalized into highly liquid-ordered and -disordered regions rather than a homogeneous structure with free diffusion of proteins and lipids.[49,50] The liquid-ordered compartments are enriched in glycosphingolipids and cholesterol.[49] The BCR (and TCR) complex exists predominantly in the liquid-disordered compartments in resting B (and T) lymphocytes.[51,52] Antigen-induced oligomerization is accompanied by the redistribution of the receptor into the liquid-ordered compartments, as diagrammed in Fig. 15–4. These compartments are known as glycosphingolipid-enriched membranes (GEMs), detergent-insoluble membranes (DIMs), or rafts. Rafts are enriched for certain molecules, including myristoylated or palmitoylated Src kinases and PIP_2. The current model for rafts in signal transduction envisions that inclusion of the BCR into rafts provides an environment rich in positive-signaling molecules. Moreover, there is evidence that rafts selectively exclude specific negative regulators of sustained antigen-receptor signaling, such as CD45 and CD22 (discussed in more detail in the subsequent sections). It appears likely that the regional organization on a nanometer scale may be dynamically assembling and dissolving in response to the signaling state of the cell. Thus, the raft concept posits that compartmentalization of oligomerized BCR promotes the ability to sustain a signal and may even enhance, or be required for, assembly of the signalosome. Although attractive conceptually, this remains an area in which there is considerable debate.

The above discussion implies that antigen-induced BCR stimulation causes activation signals in B lymphocytes. This is mainly true for mature follicular and marginal zone B lymphocytes. However, BCR expressing immature B cells in the bone marrow or transitional immature B cells in the spleen are not activated by BCR engagement. Rather, BCR signaling in these B lymphocytes triggers negative responses, resulting in induced apoptotic cell death.[53] Thus, BCR signaling, or at least the cell fates that it triggers, is developmentally regulated. These BCR-triggered negative responses may contribute to the elimination of self-reactive B lymphocytes and immunologic tolerance to self-antigens (see Chapter 18).[53] Finally, it is important to consider data that indicates that to some degree the BCR can signal independently of antigen recognition and receptor aggregation. This signaling has been termed *tonic signaling* to indicate that it represents a basal level of constitutive signaling through the BCR. Little is known about the molecular processes involved in initiating and regulating tonic signals. However, tonic signaling is important in BCR-dependent B-lymphocyte development and survival in peripheral organs such as the spleen.[54]

B-CELL RECEPTOR CORECEPTOR MOLECULES

Positive Regulators of B-Cell Receptor Signal Transduction

Although the BCR is capable of initiating an activation response, its ability to do so is influenced by the selective recruitment of coreceptor molecules by antigen. One of these coreceptors is the CD19–CD21 complex. CD19 is a cell-surface glycoprotein specifically expressed on all B cells. This transmembrane protein has a large (comprising

238 to 242 amino acids) intracellular domain containing nine tyrosine residues. Coligation of CD19 with the BCR dramatically affects the dose response of mature-stage B lymphocytes to antigen by enhancing the BCR signal.[55] The cytoplasmic tail of CD19 interacts with the PI3K p85 regulatory subunit and the Fyn and Lyn tyrosine kinases.[56,57] These interactions as well as the fact that the nine cytoplasmic-region tyrosines are rapidly phosphorylated after BCR cross-linking argue that the CD19 cytoplasmic domain is crucial for signaling. Of particular relevance, although the BCR itself may be capable of triggering the PI3K pathway, optimal triggering occurs through signals initiated by CD19.[58] Loss of CD19 results in impaired preBCR-dependent development, attenuated early BCR signaling, and impaired responses to antigen in vivo.[58,59]

On mature B lymphocytes, CD19 exists on the cell surface as a complex consisting of the complement receptor CD21 as well as Leu-13 and TAPA-1 (*t*arget of *a*nti*p*roliferative *a*ntibody-1) (ie, CD81).[60,61] Each protein brings a unique function in the complex. CD19, with its extensive intracellular domain, is a substrate for tyrosine kinases and can associate with a variety of intracellular signaling proteins. CD21 links this complex with the BCR by binding antigens that are associated with components of the complement cascade. In so doing, CD21 drags CD19 and its cytoplasm-associated signaling molecules into the BCR complex. Thus, this coreceptor enhances the BCR signaling by antigen–complement complexes bound by the B lymphocyte. The roles of TAPA-1 and Leu-13 are less clear, but both mediate homotypical cell adhesion, so they could facilitate cell–cell interaction during the immune response. More recently, it has been suggested that TAPA-1 may stabilize the BCR in lipid raft compartments, thereby sustaining antigen-induced signals under conditions where the CD19–CD21 coreceptor is engaged.[62] Figure 15–5 is a diagram of the BCR–CD19–CD21 coreceptor interaction, illustrating enhanced signaling by an antigen–complement bridge.

Another BCR coreceptor is CD45, which is an abundant, highly glycosylated, leukocyte-specific cell-surface protein. It is estimated to constitute 10% of the total cell-surface glycoprotein in B cells.[63,64] CD45 protein isoforms of various sizes occur on different lymphocyte cell types and on the same cell types during development and differentiation. This variation is due to alternative splicing of three or four exons that encode the N-terminus of the protein. The highest-molecular-weight isoform of the molecule (B220), containing all of the alternately spliced exons, is found primarily on B lymphocytes. The cytoplasmic domain of the CD45 protein contains an active phosphatase domain important for dephosphorylation of a regulatory tyrosine located at the C-terminal end of src kinases during BCR signaling.[12] Dephosphorylation of this tyrosine residue is necessary for full enzymatic acitivity. B-lymphocyte lines as well as B cells from mice lacking CD45 show defects in early BCR-mediated signal transduction.[65] B lymphocytes from mice lacking CD45 are severely compromised in their ability to proliferate in response to BCR cross-linking, although they are able to proliferate in response to the mitogen lipopolysaccharide (LPS).[66] B lymphocytes from CD45-deficient mice showed severe functional defects.[67,68] The population of high-density, IgM^{low}/IgD^{high} B lymphocytes was greatly diminished and B cells exhibited defective extracellular calcium flux, but normal release of calcium from intracellular stores in response to BCR cross-linking. Thus, CD45 expression is necessary for optimal antigen receptor signaling and normal B-lymphocyte development. Whether or not CD45 is a part of the actual signaling complex and therefore functions as a legitimate coreceptor is still unclear. Because of the abundance of the CD45 protein, it might be expected that its association with the BCR may be random and interaction between BCR, CD45, and src kinases may occur even in the absence of antigen. If so, one could predict that signals would be initiated independently of antigen at individual BCR complexes. This stochastic process may in fact represent the mechanism by which tonic signals are generated.[54] Nonetheless, it remains to be established how these tonic signals are terminated to control B-lymphocyte activation in the absence of antigen engagement. Finally, one argument for sufficiency of proximity for CD45 action is that transfection of only the cytoplasmic domain of CD45 in CD45-deficient B lymphocytes restored antigen receptor signaling.[69,70] The tyrosine phosphatase activity of CD45 suggests that it could inhibit the BCR signal by counteracting the antigen-induced ITAM phosphorylation. In this context, CD45 is observed to be excluded from lipid rafts and thus sequestered away from BCR complexes once signals have been initiated.[71,72]

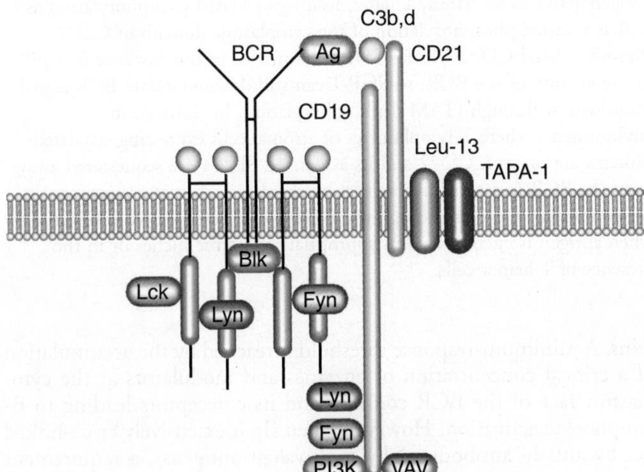

Figure 15–5 Model for antigen–complement C3b,d-mediated coaggregation of the B-lymphocyte receptor (BCR) and the CD19–CD21 coreceptor complex. Coclustering mediated by simultaneous binding of BCR and CD21 serves to recruit the CD19-associated signaling proteins to the BCR signaling complex. As discussed in the text, this is believed to enhance the signal that is generated by BCR aggregation. Ag, antigen; PI3K, phosphatidylinositol 3-kinase; TAPA-1, target of antiproliferative antibody-1.

Negative Modulators of B-Cell Receptor Signal Transduction

The activity and strength of signals generated by the BCR are also tuned or modulated by negative coreceptors. It was observed many years ago that the treatment of B lymphocytes with anti-Ig antibodies that lack the Fc portion of the molecule led to B-lymphocyte proliferation, whereas anti-Ig antibodies with the Fc region intact did not.[73] Furthermore, intact anti-Ig antibodies fail to trigger the signaling pathways leading to PI hydrolysis that is observed when BCR is cross-linked with anti-Ig that does not contain the Fc portion.[74] This effect was presumed to be due to the co-cross-linking of Fc receptors (FcR) with the sIg receptor complex on B lymphocytes. This dual signal would downmodulate a B-lymphocyte response late in an immune reaction, if B lymphocytes encounter an antigen that has been coated with secreted antibody. As illustrated in Fig. 15–6, simultaneous FcR and BCR stimulation would send a signal to shut down production of a specific antibody.

The FcR expressed by B lymphocytes is FcgRIIB1. The region of its cytoplasmic domain that is necessary and sufficient for FcR-negative signaling is a 13-amino acid immunoreceptor tyrosine-based inhibition motif (ITIM). A single tyrosine residue contained in this motif is critical for inhibition of BCR-induced Ca^{2+} flux.[75] Many other transmembrane proteins expressed predominately in hematopoietic cells such as CD22 (see later) and pair immunoglobulin-like receptor B (PIRB), as well as T-lymphocyte cell-surface proteins (see later), also harbor ITIMs. ITIMs interact with protein and lipid phosphatases that can block signaling.[76] In particular, the FcR ITIM is responsible for the interaction of this protein with the SHP-1 and SHIP-1 cytoplasmic phosphatases.[77] The tyrosine residue contained within the putative ITIM is inducibly phosphorylated, and interacts with these phosphatases through their tandem SH2 domains. Tyrosine phosphatase recruitment to the BCR complex allows

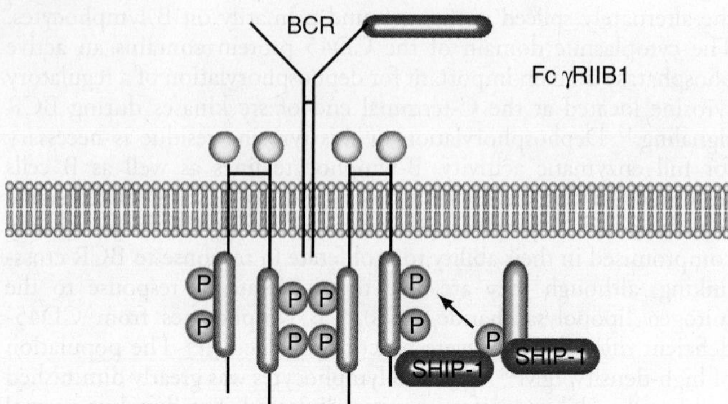

Figure 15–6 Model illustrating modulation of B-lymphocyte receptor (BCR) signal transduction by FcγRII B1. Antigen (*black*)–antibody complexes cocluster the BCR and the FcR. The latter positions the cytoplasmic phosphatases SHP-1 and SHIP-1 in the proximity of the Igα and Igβ ITAMs, thereby dephosphorylating them (note "faded" P) and downregulating their ability to recruit SH2-containing signal transduction proteins. ITAMs, immunoreceptor tyrosine-based activation motifs.

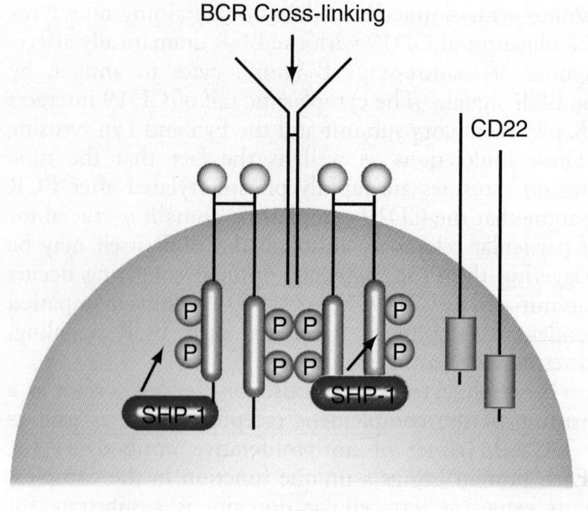

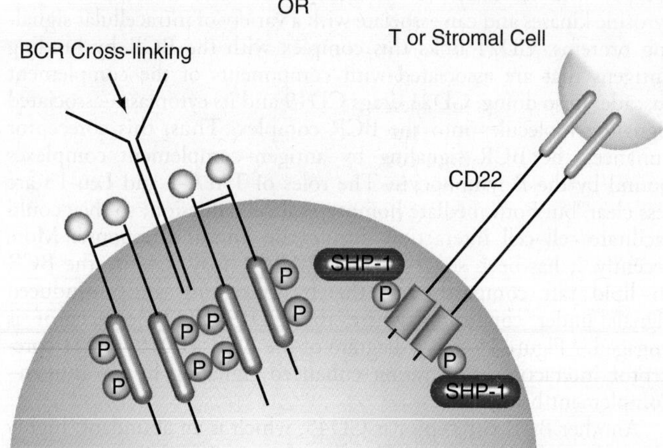

Figure 15–7 One hypothetic model to account for the ability of CD22 clustering to enhance B-lymphocyte (B-cell) receptor (BCR) signal transduction. In the resting B lymphocyte, the cytoplasmic phosphatase SHP-1 is in proximity to the complex either associated with CD22 or perhaps independent of it. In either case, SHP-1 functions to maintain dephosphorylation of the Igα- and Igβ-associated immunoreceptor tyrosine-based activation motifs (ITAMs), thereby decreasing the ability of the receptor to generate signals. Simple cross-linking of the BCR by antigen activates Src family kinases, leading to ITAM phosphorylation as well as tyrosine phosphorylation of the cytoplasmic domain of CD22. Phosphorylated CD22 recruits SHP-1. However, in this instance it is still in the vicinity of the BCR, so SHP-1 can still downmodulate BCR signal transduction through ITAM dephosphorylation. In contrast, in environments where T lymphocytes or stromal cells expressing sialylated proteins are present, CD22 and its associated SHP-1 are sequestered away from the BCR (see text for potential mechanisms). As a consequence, antigen-induced signals through the BCR would be expected to be stronger when antigen is encountered in appropriate anatomic niches or in the presence of T-helper cells.

dephosphorylation of key tyrosine residues in the cytoplasmic domains of Igα and Igβ, and other signaling molecules such as CD22 and molecules associated with it. SHIP-1 is a lipid phosphatase whose activity results in the dephosphorylation of PIP_3 to PIP_2. Because PIP_3 is necessary to initiate the PI3K pathway (see earlier), FcR/SHIP-1 association will inhibit BCR signaling.

CD22 also serves as a negative coreceptor in early BCR signal transduction. CD22 can be coimmunoprecipitated with sIg from B-lymphocyte lysates made in mild detergent, and cross-linking the BCR with anti-Ig leads to phosphorylation of the CD22 cytoplasmic domain.[78–80] CD22 is a single transmembrane-spanning glycoprotein that contains seven immunoglobulin superfamily domains in its extracellular region.[81] A ligand for CD22 has not been defined, although the CD22 extracellular domain can bind sialic acid residues on a variety of proteins and the ectodomain of CD22 is necessary for some but not all of its inhibitory function.[82,83] The intracellular domain of CD22 contains six tyrosine residues, which can be substrates for tyrosine kinases. These two observations led to the inclusion of CD22 into some models of the BCR complex. It seems more likely, because not all sIg has CD22 associated with it,[78] that CD22 only associates transiently with the BCR during an immune reaction. Then, the phosphorylated tail of CD22 brings SH2-containing signaling proteins into the BCR complex, where they can then affect other receptor components. For example, the CD22 cytoplasmic tail associates with a tyrosine-specific phosphatase, protein tyrosine phosphatase 1C SH2-containing tyrosine phosphatase (PTP1C, also known as SHP-1).[82,84] SHP-1 is physically associated with the BCR in resting B cells, where it could dephosphorylate the ITAMs of Igα and Igβ. As depicted in Fig. 15–7, explanation of CD22 enhancement of BCR signaling is that in secondary lymphoid organs, sequestration of CD22 is accomplished by the association of B lymphocytes with sialic acid-modified proteins on the surface of T lymphocytes or stroma. This may involve directed movement of CD22–ligand complexes or, rather, physical displacement of the relatively large CD22 ectodomains as the B lymphocyte and associated cell become physically close.[85] In either model, phosphorylation of the tyrosines in CD22 will partition SHP-1 away from the BCR, thereby enhancing the tyrosine phosphorylation of the Igα/Igβ ITAMs. Other transmembrane proteins that contain ITIMs, including CD72 and CD5, may also modulate BCR signaling by this mechanism.[86,87]

The presence of positive- and negative-acting coreceptors indicates that BCR-mediated signaling is a tightly regulated process. TCR signaling is similarly modulated by coreceptors (eg, CD4, CD8, CD2). The functions of these coreceptors suggest that BCR signaling is not optimal through cross-linking sIg molecules alone but involves a complex orchestration of receptor and coreceptor molecules into a large complex, each element of which brings along associated proteins. A minimum-response threshold is reached by the accumulation of a critical concentration of enzymes and modulators at the cytoplasmic face of the BCR complex and its coreceptors leading to B-lymphocyte activation. However, when sIg is extensively cross-linked (ie, by anti-Ig antibody or by multivalent antigens), a requirement for coreceptor engagement may not be evident.

SECONDARY COSTIMULATORY SIGNALS FOR B-LYMPHOCYTE ACTIVATION

The preceding discussion focused on the process by which antigen through the BCR initiates activation signals in mature, immunocompetent B lymphocytes. However, by themselves, these signals are usually insufficient to promote clonal expansion and antibody secretion. For these processes, secondary signals provided by $CD4^+$ antigen-specific T lymphocytes are necessary. Thus, a humoral immune response involving antibody production usually requires the integration of T- as well as B-lymphocyte activation. Secondary signals for B-lymphocyte activation come in two forms: (a) physical contact between B and T lymphocytes and (b) soluble cytokines secreted by antigen-activated T lymphocytes. CD40 on the surface of resting and stimulated B lymphocytes is the primary receptor for cell contact-mediated secondary signals. CD40 is a 48-kd transmembrane protein belonging to the tumor necrosis factor (TNF) receptor family.[88] CD154 (CD40 ligand), homologous to TNF itself, is induced on antigen-activated $CD4^+$ T lymphocytes and binds to CD40 on nearby B cells. This promotes B-lymphocyte survival and facilitates their proliferation.[88,89] Agents that block CD40–CD154 interactions greatly impair the ability of activated T lymphocytes to interact with and drive B-lymphocyte proliferation. In humans, a genetic deficiency of CD154 causes X-linked hyper-IgM syndrome. Patients with this disorder can make IgM responses to T lymphocyte-independent antigens but fail to generate T lymphocyte-dependent B-lymphocyte responses to protein antigens. Even with T lymphocyte-independent antigens, switching to other Ig isotypes is absent.[90–93] Thus, although BCR signals can initiate B-lymphocyte activation, costimulation through CD40 is necessary for effector-level responses by these cells.

It is generally held that B-cell activation without T-cell costimulation results in an abortive activation response followed by B-lymphocyte death and elimination from the immune cell repertoire.[5,94] This may be the mechanism for deletion of self-reactive mature B lymphocytes. Engagement by self-antigens would provide BCR signals, but the necessary costimulatory signals by antigen-specific T lymphocytes would be absent.

Resting B lymphocytes express CD40, and there is experimental evidence that CD40 triggering together with certain cytokines can activate the B lymphocyte in the absence of BCR signaling. This form of activation could have adverse effects in an immune response, because it could allow activation of B lymphocytes with antibody specificities irrelevant to the pathogen or, worse, of autoreactive B lymphocytes. However, CD40 stimulation does not usually occur in vivo without prior BCR engagement on resting B lymphocytes. The ability of B cells to productively interact with T cells depends on molecules such as MHC class II and B7 that are upregulated after BCR stimulation (see next section).

In addition to CD40–CD154 interactions, other surface ligand-receptor pairs mediate physical interactions between the B and the T lymphocytes. These interactions are diagrammed in Fig. 15–8. Some of these pairs function as signaling molecules; others, such as intercellular adhesion molecule-1 (ICAM-1) and lymphocyte function-associated molecule-1 (LFA-1), are adhesion molecules that increase the strength of the B lymphocyte–T lymphocyte interaction and may also generate signals of their own.

Besides costimulatory signals generated through direct B lymphocyte–T lymphocyte contact, various T lymphocyte-derived cytokines facilitate ongoing regulation of the initial B cell-activation response. Although not completely defined in all cases, certain cytokines have well-characterized effects on the B cell response.[95] For example, interleukin (IL)-4 facilitates isotype switching to IgG1 and IgE, whereas tumor growth factor-β (TGF-β) results in switching to IgA. IL-4 can also augment the early stages of BCR-induced activation, whereas IL-5 may maintain clonal expansion. Because they do not require cell–cell contact for their function, cytokine-mediated effects on B-lymphocyte activation probably are limited to previously antigen- and CD40-activated cells. In this manner, they probably enhance and modify the responses to specific pathogens.

A research area of great recent interest is the involvement of TLRs in costimulation of B cells under specific situations when antigens are associated with certain pathogens. This selectivity comes from the fact that TLR ligands are specific products of microorganisms. As can be deduced from chapters that deal with these receptors and their role in the innate immune system in more detail, the engagement of TLRs during an antigen-specific B-lymphocyte response bridges the innate and adaptive immune systems.

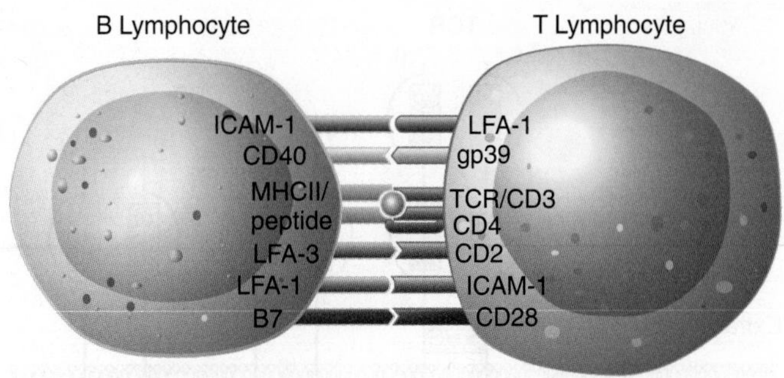

Figure 15–8 Receptor–ligand pairs contributing to association-dependent secondary signals for B- and T-lymphocyte activation. These interactions illustrate the tremendous level of communication between the B and the T lymphocytes during a lymphocyte-mediated immune response. Expression of some of these proteins is enhanced or their signaling capabilities are activated as the B- and T-lymphocyte activation responses proceed. In this way, there is continued reinforcement with checkpoints to ensure that the immune response continues to be appropriate. ICAM, intercellular adhesion molecule; LFA, leukocyte function-associated antigen; MHCII, major histocompatibility complex class II.

T LYMPHOCYTES

T lymphocytes provide the cellular arm of the immune system and characteristically exert effects in situ. There are two main T-cell subsets: those with CD4 surface coreceptors (CD4 T cells) and those with CD8 surface coreceptors (CD8 T cells). CD4 T cells are called helper T cells (T_H) because they help, that is, regulate, immune responses. CD8 T cells are chiefly cytotoxic T cells (CTLs) that directly kill virally infected or transformed cells. These immune responses result from genetic programs initiated by antigen recognition at the cell surface and transmitted to the nuclear genes by an elaborately regulated signaling apparatus (for reviews, see refs 96 and 97). T cells use a structurally unique cell-surface receptor, the TCR, to recognize specific antigen. However, unlike B cells, which recognize foreign antigens in their native conformations, T cells protect against intracellular pathogens and typically recognize a peptide determinant (epitope) or lipid derived from the pathogen. These peptide epitopes or lipids must be bound to an MHC molecule and presented as the antigen on the surface of an APC, such as a dendritic cell or B cell. Most T_H cells utilize the CD4 coreceptor to recognize antigenic peptides displayed on MHC class II molecules, whereas CTLs use the CD8 coreceptor to recognize peptide bound to MHC class I molecules. Lipids typically are presented on the nonclassical, nonpolymorphic MHC molecule CD-I and may involve a special class of αβ-NK T cells with limited TCR diversity.

T-LYMPHOCYTE ANTIGEN RECEPTOR

The antigen-binding component of most TCRs is a heterodimer composed of two glycoproteins, the α chain of 40 to 44 kd and the β chain of 47 to 54 kd, that are selectively expressed on T cells (αβ T cells).[97] The α and β chains are encoded by unique rearranging gene loci resembling Ig gene loci. Enroute to the cell surface, these chains noncovalently associate with nonpolymorphic transmembrane signaling proteins, the CD3γ, δ, ε proteins and the η and ζ chains to form an 8-chain cell-surface TCR holocomplex (Fig. 15–9). Approximately 5% of T cells express γ and δ antigen-binding chains derived from another pair of rearranging gene loci (γδ T cells). The antigen-binding TCR chains have a structural domain called the immunoglobulin fold characteristic of the immunoglobulin gene superfamily which includes immunologically important proteins

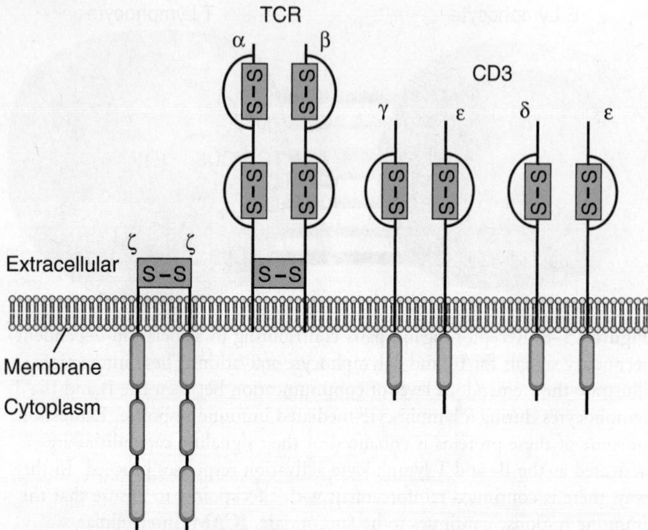

Figure 15–9 Composition of the T-lymphocyte (T-cell) antigen receptor (TCR) complex. Shown are the nonpolymorphic members (CD3γ, δ, ε, and ζ chains) in association with the ligand-binding polymorphic TCR α and β chains. Also illustrated are the immunoreceptor tyrosine-based activation motifs (ITAMs) (*shaded ovals* in the cytoplasmic domains of the CD3 complex and the ζ chain) that are tyrosine phosphorylated on receptor cross-linking and are responsible for the recruitment of other signaling molecules to the TCR complex. S–S, disulfide bonds.

such as Ig, CD4, CD8, and MHC class I and class II molecules.[98] The N-terminal domain of the extracellular portion of each ligand-binding TCR chain contains the polymorphic region that binds antigen in a way that resembles Ig.[99–101] Generally, a unique pair of TCR is expressed by any given T cell and its progeny (constituting a T cell clone), although a fraction of T cells expresses two different α chains of TCRs conferring distinct antigenic specificities.[102] Clonal diversity is generated by variation in the primary amino acid sequence of the TCR (clonal variation) resulting from the specific rearrangement of TCR genetic elements.

The genetic diversification process involves reassortment of TCR gene segments using essentially the same molecular machinery as for Ig genes. Human genetic defects in the V(D)J recombination proteins artemis or recombination activating genes (RAG)-1 or -2 cause severe defects in T (and B) lymphocyte development.[103] TCR genes have variable (V), diversity (D), joining (J), and constant (C) segments as separate genetic elements encoding the antigen-combining portion of each TCR subunit.[100] There are various numbers of V, D, and J segments in the genome that are highly polymorphic, whereas the constant region is invariant and does not contribute to antigen specificity. Each ligand-binding chain contains just one representative family member from each gene segment (V, J, and C for TCR α and γ, and V, D, J, and C for TCR β and δ). Diversity is achieved by the independent, random reassortment of V, D, and J segments that together create the potential for an enormous number of distinct TCRs. Superimposed on this is a process known as *N region addition*, whereby nucleotides not encoded in the germline DNA segments are added at V–D and D–J junctions by terminal deoxynucleotide transferase (TdT).[104,105] Finally, because both chains of the TCR ligand-binding complex contribute to antigen specificity, diversity is increased by the heterodimeric combination of two TCR ligand-binding chains. Although antigen receptor diversity generation is similar in B and T cells, somatic hypermutation of the rearranged TCR gene in peripheral lymphoid organs occurs only rarely if at all.[106] Importantly, the recombination process utilizes slowly evolving elements in the germline-encoded gene segments that predetermine certain range of specificities that function productively within an antigen environment, both internal and external, that the species has encountered during its evolution. However, it also randomly generates new specificities by nucleotide additions and deletions, giving it more adaptive potential. This is perhaps an essential function of the adaptive immune system in an environment of rapidly and continuously evolving threats from emerging infections.

Intracellular signals from the TCR are conveyed by the CD3 polypeptide chains. The C-terminal intracytoplasmic portions of the polymorphic TCR chains are quite small, ranging from 5 to 11 amino acids—a strong indication that they have no intrinsic signaling capacity.[107,108] However, the CD3 polypeptides have long cytoplasmic tails with obvious signaling motifs (ITAMs). Since the CD3 proteins are needed for receptor surface expression and signal transmission, the functional TCR is often called the TCR–CD3 complex (see later). The CD3γ, δ, and ε proteins are 20- to 26-kd structurally related polypeptides (not to be confused with the polymorphic, ligand-binding chains TCR γ and δ).[109,110] The other nonpolymorphic signaling component(s) include the structurally distinct ζ chain and, in the mouse, the η-chain.[111] The significance of the murine η-subunit is uncertain, however, because of the lack of an obvious human analog, its poor conservation across species, and no clear function.[111,112] The stoichiometry of the TCR–CD3 complex reveals four dimers, a disulfide-bonded ligand-binding heterodimer (TCR αβ or γδ), noncovalently coupled to one each of CD3εγ and CD3εδ heterodimers, and a disulfide-linked ζ–ζ homodimer to form an octamer (see Fig. 15–9).

T cell activation is initiated after TCR aggregation by the antigen-laden APCs (see Chapter 12). The resulting biochemical cascade culminates in a coordinated program of gene expression leading to effector functions (eg, cytokine production, proliferation, acquisition of cytotoxicity). Clustering of multiple TCRs on a given T cell apparently potentiates the interaction, because the affinity of individual TCRs with antigen–MHC complexes is low. Coreceptors such as CD4 and CD8 also help by increasing the TCR-antigen-MHC association and recruiting other signaling molecules into the activation complex. The earliest observed biochemical event following TCR cross-linking is tyrosine phosphorylation of the CD3 chains on ITAM motifs (ITAMs are described in the section above on BCR signaling) (Fig. 15–10).[113–115] The CD3γ, δ, and ε components each have one ITAM, whereas each ζ monomer contains three. Two Src-like kinases $p56^{lck}$ (Lck) and $p59^{fyn}$ (Fyn) are involved in phosphorylating CD3ζ[1].[116–120] Gene knockout mice show that Lck plays a more important role than Fyn in T-cell maturation and TCR signaling. Both kinases localize to the plasma membrane by a myristoylation modification. Further associations of Lck with CD4 and CD8 (see later) and Fyn with TCR components promote the phosphorylation of ζ.[121] Phosphorylation of the ζ chain by src family kinases is a pivotal event leading to recruitment of a second family of tyrosine kinases that includes ZAP-70 and Syk. N-terminal tandem SH2 domains in ZAP-70 and Syk bind the phosphotyrosines in the ζ-ITAMs, leading to further phosphorylation events by these kinases (see Fig. 15–10).[122,123] ITAM phosphorylation and the association of ZAP-70 is critical for TCR signaling. In fact, experimental proteins containing ITAMs fused to the transmembrane and extracellular domains of unrelated proteins can, upon cross-linking, transduce signals that mimic early and late signal transduction events characteristic of the intact TCR.[124] It is believed that this reflects essential features of TCR signaling: bringing the surface signaling proteins together so that they can cross-phosphorylate each other and form a scaffold to recruit cytoplasmic signal transducers through phosphotyrosine–SH2 domain associations.

Various inherited immunodeficiencies illustrate the vital role of the invariant TCR components in immunity.[103,125] Genetic deficiency of either CD3δ or CD3ζ severely impairs the development of both αβ and γδ T cells, leading to severe infections.[103,126] Inborn deficiencies of CD3ε and CD3γ are less devastating but still have an adverse effect on T-cell development and immune function. Finally, patients with mutations in ZAP-70 lack peripheral $CD8^+$ T cells and TCR signaling is defective in peripheral $CD4^+$ T lymphocytes, but ostensibly normal in the CD4 thymic precursors, in which Syk kinase compensates.[127,128]

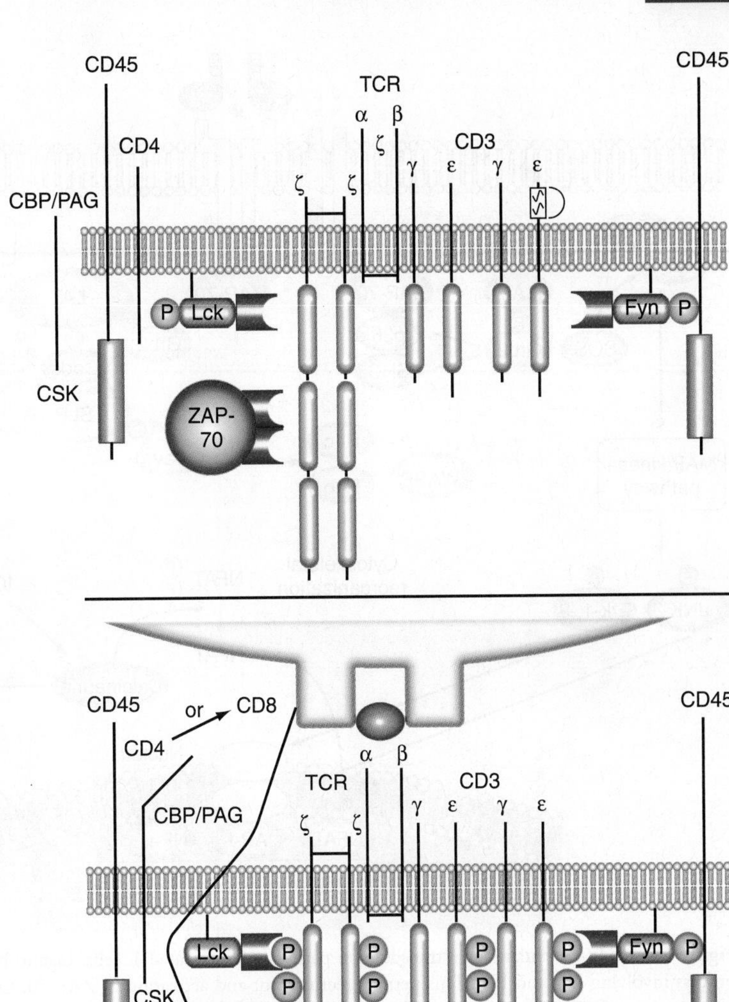

Figure 15–10 The T-cell receptor (TCR) complex and coreceptor molecules in resting and antigen-activated T cells. In the resting T cell, the TCR complex, the CD4 coreceptor, and CD45 are not associated with the membrane. The tyrosine kinase Lck is found associated with CD4, and low levels of the tyrosine kinase Fyn are believed to associate with the TCR complex. However, neither enzyme is activated, because of basal phosphorylation at a negative regulatory site. On receptor ligation, CD45 and CD4 are recruited into the receptor complex. CD45 is believed to be responsible for dephosphorylating the negative regulatory tyrosines on Lck and Fyn (note the *light-colored* P). Activation of Lck or Fyn is believed to lead to phosphorylation of the CD3 complex and the ζ chain, allowing for the association of zeta-associated protein-70 (ZAP-70) via its tandem SH2 domains and its subsequent activation. P, phosphate group.

T-CELL INTRACELLULAR SIGNALING

The initial phase of TCR signaling is completed once ZAP-70 is activated. The secondary signaling events that follow parallel those described for B lymphocytes (vide supra), including: (a) increased intracellular calcium levels and activation of PKC and NFAT as a consequence of PLCγ1 activation, (b) activation of the Ras pathway, (c) activation of PI3K (Fig. 15–11), and (d) NF-κB activation. These culminate in the production of IL-2 and other cytokines. There are two additional T cell-specific tyrosine kinases, RLK and ITK, from the Tec kinase family also involved.[129] Tec kinases can phosphorylate PLCγ1 and modulate downstream effects on Ca^{2+}, the actin cytoskeleton, and T-cell subset accumulation in the periphery. Moreover, PKC-θ has emerged as a crucial early step in the activation process to drive downstream gene regulatory events (see below).

Activation of these three distinct pathways occurs in parallel with lateral integration via cross-talk between them. They are linked by intermediate signaling molecules known as *adapter* proteins, which mediate protein–protein or protein–lipid interactions. As scaffolds, adapters regulate T-cell activation by organizing signaling assemblies and eliminating certain proteins by degradation. The discovery of adapters suggests that lymphocyte activation signals are transmitted by large multifunctional protein complexes that shift in composition and location rather than a series of individual proteins talking to one another in a linear chain. There are several T-lymphocyte adapters that are roughly analogous to the BLNK protein in B cells (see Fig. 15–11): LAT (*l*inker for *a*ctivated *T* lymphocytes), SLP76, Gads, Grb2, and Vav. LAT is a transmembrane protein that contains numerous tyrosine residues in its intracellular domain that are phosphorylated by ZAP-70.[130] These phosphotyrosines recruit Grb2, ITK, PLCγ1, PI3K, and Gads typically through SH2 domain associations. SLP76 can simultaneously bind Gads and PLCγ1, which links SLP76 with LAT. Both LAT and SLP76 are intimately involved in activation of PLCγ1 and therefore have critical roles in T-cell activation. Indeed, mice deficient for one or more of these proteins have defective TCR signaling which prevents thymocyte maturation.[131–133] Another key function of T-cell adapter proteins is to link TCR signaling to cytoskeletal rearrangements. Tyrosine-phosphorylated SLP76 associates with Vav, which activates the GTPases Rac and Rho that control the actin cytoskeleton.[134] These GTPases regulate Wiskott–Aldrich syndrome protein (WASP), which is important for cytoskeletal organization.[135] Gene knockouts in mice show that Vav and WASP play critical roles in T-cell activation and associated cellular changes, perhaps acting in part through the movement of lipid rafts and the immunologic synapse formation (see later).[136–139]

As in B cells, PLCγ1 activation causes hydrolysis of PIP_2, resulting in a rise in intracellular Ca^{2+} levels and PKC activation, which are considered second messengers of T cells. Signaling by increased intra-

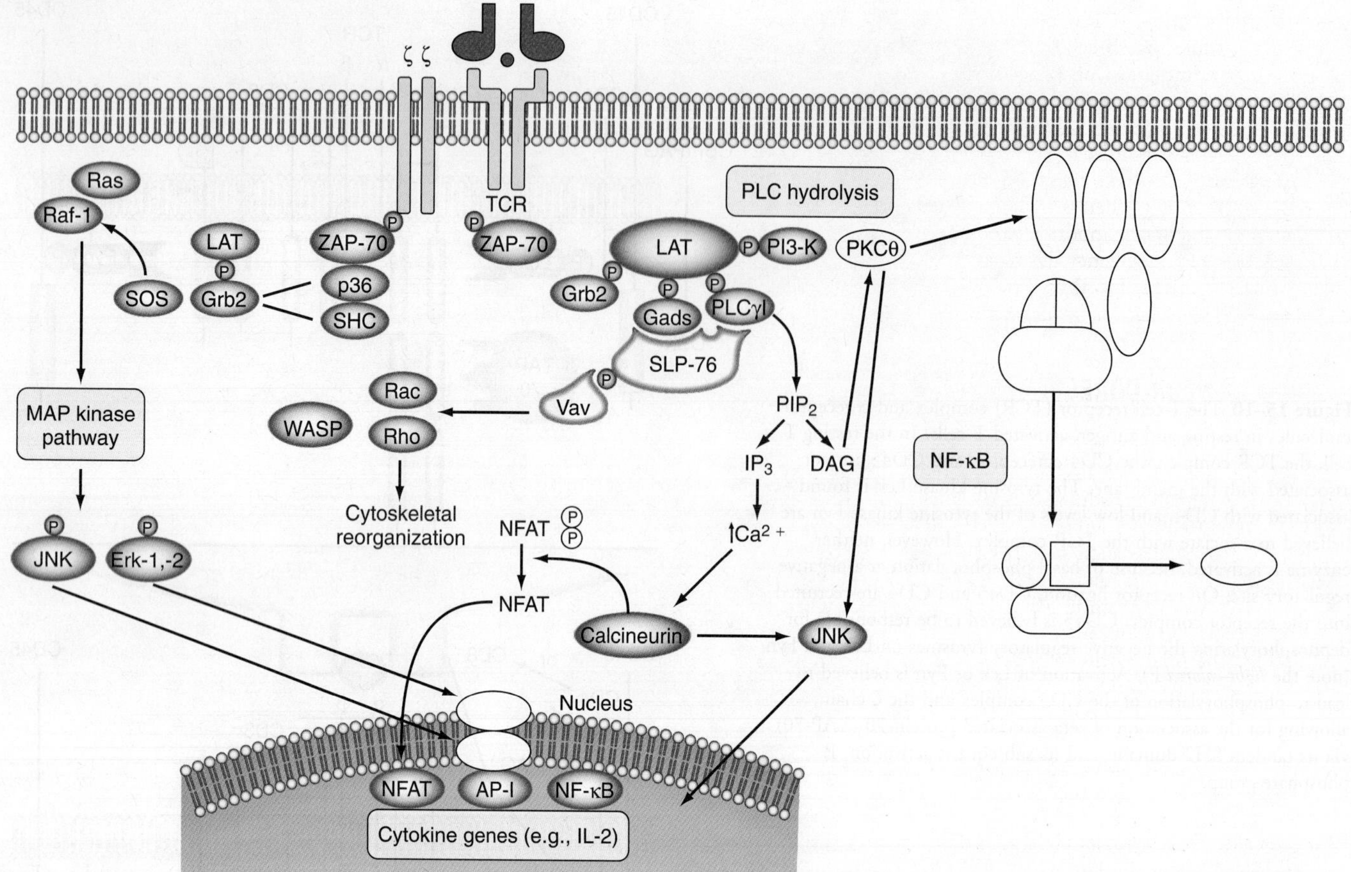

Figure 15–11 Intracellular signal transduction pathways in activated T cells. Ligand binding of the TCR leads to phosphorylation of CD3ζ molecules, a process involving Lck and Fyn. This permits recruitment and activation of ZAP-70. One pathway of downstream signaling is mediated by activation of phospholipase C (PLC) and subsequent activation of protein kinase C (PKC) and a rise in intracellular calcium concentration. Adapter proteins such as LAT, Grb2, Gads, and SLP-76 are critical linkers of CD3ζ and ZAP-70 phosphorylation to inositol phospholipid hydrolysis. Through interactions with Vav, WASP, and the Rac and Rho GTPases, these adapter proteins also serve to link TCR signaling to cytoskeletal rearrangements, which are important for complete T-cell activation. In parallel, TCR stimulation also activates the Ras–Raf–MAPK pathway. Adapter proteins such as LAT, Grb2, and Shc help activate the guanine nucleotide exchange factor SOs to mediate this effect. Together, MAPK activation and inositol phospholipid hydrolysis activate Jnk kinases, Erk kinases, and NF-κB, leading to induction of a series of genes, typified by the encoding cytokines, that characterize the T-cell response. AP-1, activator protein-1; DAG, 1,2-diacylglycerol; IL, interleukin; IP_3, inositol-1,4,5-triphosphate; LAT, linker for activated T lymphocyte; MAP, mitogen-activating protein; NF-κB, nuclear factor-κB; NFAT, nuclear factor of activated T lymphocytes; PI3K, phosphatidylinositol 3-kinase; PIP_3, phosphatidylinositol-4,5-triphosphate; WASP, Wiskott–Aldrich syndrome protein; ZAP-70, zeta (chain)-associated protein.

cellular Ca^{2+} levels is blocked by the immunosuppressive drugs cyclosporine and FK506, which prevents key activation events, especially IL-2 gene transcription.[124,140] Cyclosporine and FK506 bind to distinct proteins, collectively referred to as immunophilins, that form complexes to inhibit a calcium/calmodulin-dependent serine phosphatase calcineurin.[141] Calcineurin's role in TCR-initiated signal transduction is to dephosphorylate and promote nuclear localization of a subunit of the transcription factor NF-AT. NF-AT is a DNA-binding protein and gene activator that is required for IL-2 transcription.[142] Interestingly, T-cell activation can be triggered by the combination of phorbol myristate acetate (PMA) and ionomycin, which are pharmacologic inducers of PKC and Ca^{2+}. This is an oft-used experimental procedure for studying T-cell responses.[96,97,140]

TCR signaling also involves activation of Ras-related G proteins, which causes downstream activation of MAPK pathways (see earlier).[143] Ras activation in T cells involves the guanine nucleotide exchange factor SOS, which is linked to the TCR by the adapter protein Grb2 associated with other adapter proteins, such as p36 or Shc.[144] Stimulation of Ras induces various serine/threonine kinases, leading to the activation of two MAPKs, Erk-1 and Erk-2, among other targets. These kinases are critical for the phosphorylation of transcription factors, including components of the AP-1 complex, that are required for the activation of IL-2 and other genes. In addition to *ras* gene products, other G proteins (small signaling GTPases) expressed in T cells may contribute to TCR-induced signal transduction. For instance, the adapter Crk is linked to the nucleotide exchange factor C3G, which serves to activate the G protein Rap-1. Furthermore, members of the Rho family (Rac and Cdc42) of G proteins may regulate the activation of Jnk, an MAPK, in T cells.[144] These molecules reveal the linkage between the fully assembled adapter complexes and the transcriptional control complexes responsible for the TCR-induced gene activation program.

Although PI3K is activated after TCR engagement, the initial stimulatory effect of antigen is actually quite weak. In T lymphocytes, PI3K is only optimally stimulated after engagement of the costimulatory molecule CD28[144] and after activation by cytokines, such as IL-2, whose receptors contain the common γ chain, γ_c (see later). PI3K may principally participate in T-lymphocyte coreceptor function as discussed next.[145]

The induction of the transcription factor NF-κB is a principal event in the genetic program of T-cell activation because of the many genes it induces through the interplay of DNA-binding complexes.[146,147] Through the activation of PI3K and PLC, the PKC-θ isoform translocates to the cell membrane and becomes active following phosphorylation by Lck.[148] The activated PKC-θ then causes assembly and activation of a triprotein complex containing CARMA-

1, Bcl-10, and MALT-1 (CBM complex), which is essential for NF-κB activation (note that B cells use a different isoform, PKC-β, for this purpose). Stimulation of this pathway causes phosphorylation and activation of the I-κB kinase (IKK) complex composed of IKKα, β, and γ, which, in turn, phosphorylates the inhibitor of κB (I-κB). This leads to I-κB ubiquitination and degradation, which liberates cytoplasm-bound NF-κB to travel into the nucleus and activate specific genes by binding to their promoters and enhancers. Surprisingly, an essential biochemical connection between the CBM complex and IKK is caspase-8.[149] Deficiency of caspase-8 leads to severe immunodeficiency in humans by thwarting NF-κB in T, B, and NK lymphocytes.[150]

T-CELL RECEPTOR CORECEPTOR MOLECULES

The CD4 and CD8 coreceptors define two subsets of αβ T cells and are not expressed on γδ T cells. These transmembrane proteins enhance TCR signal transduction by (a) increasing the affinity of the TCR complex for its MHC–peptide ligand and (b) by recruiting signaling molecules, such as Lck, to the signal complex (see Fig. 15–10). CD4 and CD8 increase TCR affinity for MHC-antigenic peptide complexes by forming a physical bridge by associating with the TCR and MHC molecules.[151] Although the expression of CD4 and CD8 was originally believed to identify functional T-cell subsets (T_H cells being $CD4^+$ and CTLs being $CD8^+$), these functional associations are not mutually exclusive. CD4 CTLs have been described and CD8 cells secrete cytokines that may help immune responses in important ways. Coreceptor expression correlates mainly with the MHC molecule recognized by the TCR: MHC class II for $CD4^+$ T cells and MHC class I for $CD8^+$ T cells. There is also a subset of peripheral αβ T cells that lack CD4 and CD8, called double-negative T cells, that are normally less than 1% but may expand greatly and cause severe autoimmune disease in the autoimmune lymphoproliferative syndrome.[152]

CD4 and CD8 are structurally different. CD4 is a single-chain, type I transmembrane glycoprotein whose extracellular portion contains four immunoglobulin-like domains. By contrast, CD8 is a heterodimer composed of two disulfide-linked type I membrane-spanning glycoproteins, CD8α and CD8β, that each contain a single immunoglobulin-like extracellular domain.[152] Despite these differences, CD4 and CD8 serve analogous coreceptor functions by linking TCRs to MHC class II and I molecules, respectively. The extracellular portion of CD4 binds to a monomorphic element on the β2 domain of MHC class II molecules,[153] a site that is structurally similar to the CD8-binding domain on the MHC class I a3 membrane-proximal domain.[153–155] Coreceptor binding to these monomorphic MHC regions does not sterically interfere with TCR binding to the polymorphic, peptide-binding groove. Indeed, the ability of the coreceptor and the TCR to coengage the same MHC–peptide complex is critical for facilitating TCR-mediated signal transduction.[156]

CD4 and CD8 augment TCR signaling by providing an intracytoplasmic docking site for the Src family kinase Lck. CD4 may be a stronger coreceptor, as it binds more Lck than CD8. In addition, CD4 cross-linking can increase the enzymatic activity of Lck, which is not observed after CD8 cross-linking.[157] CD4 and CD8 interact with a Cys–XX–Cys motif in the N-terminal region of Lck through a Cys–X–Cys motif found in their cytoplasmic tails. During antigen recognition by the TCR, coengagement of the TCR and coreceptor molecules helps draw the coreceptor molecules into the TCR complex, thereby bringing Lck into the signaling complex and enhancing tyrosine phosphorylation of intracellular substrates. Once substrates such as the CD3 components are phosphorylated, the SH2 domain of Lck can interact with the phosphorylated ITAMs, anchoring the coreceptor to the activated TCR complex and further promoting coreceptor function.[158] The importance of CD4 and CD8 in T-cell activation depends on the affinity of the TCR for its peptide–MHC ligand. High-affinity ligands seem to generate enough signal through the TCR to activate T cells without a need for CD4 or CD8 coreceptors, whereas relatively lower-affinity ligands require CD4-CD8 interactions for optimal T-cell stimulation. This difference may be due to the number of TCRs engaged or the duration of engagement, or both.[159]

As in B cells, CD45 also functions as a coreceptor for TCR signaling. CD45 is a highly abundant transmembrane phosphatase required for efficient TCR signaling.[160] In CD45-deficient mice, few mature T cells develop, and those produced have poor TCR responses.[66] CD45 is believed to dephosphorylate the C-terminal inhibitory phosphotyrosine of Lck and Fyn, thereby turning on these kinases.[161] CD45 also has been described to act as a negative regulator of cytokine receptor signaling by dephosphorylating Janus kinases (JAKs), which are important signal transducers through cytokine receptors.[162] Thus, TCR signaling involves an orchestrated addition and removal of regulatory phosphates. There is no known ligand for the extracellular domain of CD45 raising a long-standing question as to whether it is a legitimate coreceptor.[66] However, CD45 has been shown to associate constitutively with the TCR, and expression of the cytoplasmic domain alone in CD45-deficient T cells is sufficient to reconstitute efficient TCR signaling.[69,70,163,164] Mice deficient for CD45 have low T-cell production and those that are produced have defective signaling. Humans with recessive deficiencies of CD45 have defects in T and NK cells leading to severe immunodeficiency.[103] Specific functions have not been ascribed to the various spliced isoforms of CD45, although it has been reported that antibodies against the CD45RB isoform selectively upregulate cytotoxic T cell-associated antigen-4 (CTLA-4).[14,165,166]

LIPID RAFTS AND THE IMMUNOLOGIC SYNAPSE

The plasma membrane of T cells appears to contain highly lipid-ordered compartments termed *lipid rafts* that are selectively enriched in activation molecules, including the TCR–CD3 complex and its attendant signaling molecules. Rafts may provide a membrane structure on which relevant molecules can be mobilized by the cytoskeleton and recruited to the point of T cell–APC contact.[167–169] A huge temporally and spatially regulated assembly of over 20 proteins, termed the *immunologic synapse*, forms where the two cells touch. Synapse formation begins with a central cluster of adhesion molecules (eg, LFA-1) surrounded by a ring of TCRs engaged by MHC (Fig. 15–12). Within 5 to 15 minutes, this orientation reverses, forming the mature synapse. This bull's-eye structure consists of a central supramolecular activation cluster (cSMAC) containing TCRs and their associated signaling machinery, surrounded concentrically by a peripheral SMAC (pSMAC)-containing integrin and adhesion molecules, such as LFA-1 and associated cytoskeletal proteins.[168,170] Synapse formation evidently does not require a live APC, because they are observed when T cells come into contact with artificial phospholipid bilayers containing antigen–MHC complexes. The immunologic synapse, which takes minutes to form, is not a prerequisite for initial TCR signaling, since tyrosine phosphorylation of CD3 proteins and ZAP-70 occurs within seconds.[171] However, optimal T-cell activation apparently requires sustained T cell–APC interactions (and hence continual TCR–MHC ligation) for up to several hours.[172] Current theories suggest that the synapse integrates and amplifies antigen signals by collecting TCRs and signal transduction molecules in a small restricted area of the membrane that synergizes molecular interactions.

Several key observations indicate that T-cell signaling is a highly dynamic process.[172] Cell-surface expression of the TCR is downregulated within minutes following synapse formation and continues for several hours, leaving only 10% to 15% of the basal TCR expression remaining.[159] Downmodulation occurs despite the fact that individual TCR–MHC interactions have half-lives of only seconds, indicating that numerous sequential TCR–MHC binding events take place—a process termed *serial triggering*.[172] In addition, TCR downmodulation following activation are the result of a kinetic equilibrium consisting of TCR reexpression, engagement by ligand, and internalization.[173] This dynamic process can be visualized by

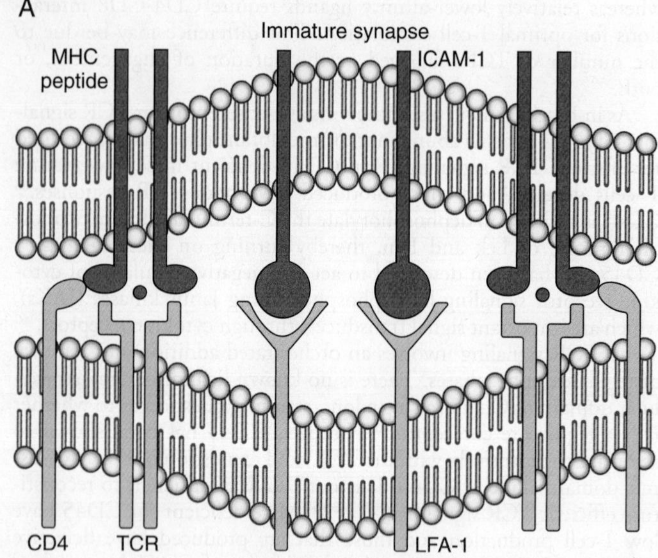

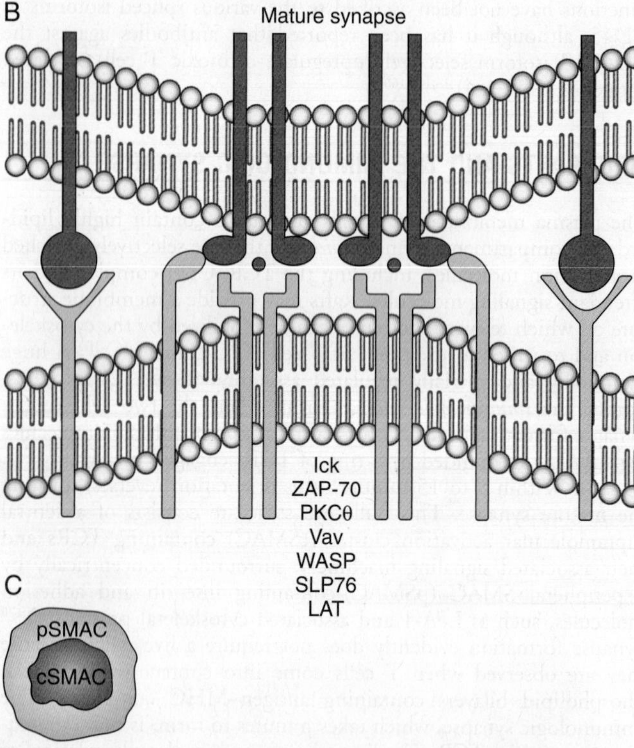

Figure 15–12 Formation of the immunologic synapse. **A**, The immature immunologic synapse consists of a central cluster of adhesion molecules (such as ICAM-1/LFA-1) surrounded by a ring of engaged TCRs. **B**, Within minutes to hours, this orientation is reversed, with a central supramolecular activation cluster (cSMAC) containing TCRs and associated signaling machinery. **C**, A bird's-eye view of the concentric topographic structure. ICAM-1, intercellular adhesion molecule-1; LAT, linker for activated T lymphocyte; LFA-1, leukocyte function-associated molecule-1; MHC, major histocompatibility complex; PKCθ, protein kinase Cθ; TCRs, T-cell receptors; WASP, Wiskott–Aldrich syndrome protein.

removal of T cells from TCR ligand after several hours of activation, which results in a rapid reexpression of surface TCR to levels that far surpass those in the unstimulated cell.[173,174] Thus, low levels of TCR following initial T-cell activation are maintained by continual TCR engagement, explaining how serial triggering is achieved despite TCR downmodulation.[172]

SECONDARY COSTIMULATORY SIGNALS FOR T-CELL ACTIVATION

Costimulation by CD28 and Related Pathways

TCR engagement alone is inefficient for inducing full activation of naive (antigen-inexperienced) T cells. Optimal cytokine production and proliferation require both TCR stimulation and a second signal. The second, or costimulatory, signal is usually delivered through the surface receptor CD28 on T cells from specific ligands on APCs (Fig. 15–13). In fact, without costimulatory signals, strong TCR stimulation of most naive T cells induces a state of long-term functional inactivation (anergy) and apoptosis.[175] CD28 costimulation lowers the antigen threshold of activation and increases the magnitude of the TCR-induced response, including an increase in cytokine gene transcription and mRNA stability.[176] Costimulation may also promote T-cell survival by inducing the antiapoptotic molecule, Bcl-X_L, which engenders more enduring immune responses.[157,177,178] Compared with naive T cells, memory T cells are much less dependent on CD28 costimulation[179] and may receive activation or survival signals through other costimulatory interactions (see below).

CD28 is a member of the immunoglobulin superfamily constitutively expressed on the T-cell surface as either a disulfide-linked homodimer or a monomer.[177] CD28 can be triggered by CD80 or CD86, often called B7-1 and B7-2, respectively, which are expressed on "professional" APC such as dendritic cells (DCs), B cells, and macrophages. CD80 and CD86 are also members of the immunoglobulin gene superfamily, but share relatively little homology with each other or CD28. The CD80 and CD86 genes are strongly induced by various immune stimuli. For example, one hallmark of DC maturation after encountering a pathogen is the upregulation of CD80, CD86 and MHC class II proteins. However, B7-1 and B7-2 are differentially expressed in that B7-2 is weakly constitutively expressed and rapidly induced, followed by slower B7-1 induction. CD80 and CD86 also avidly bind CTLA-4 (CD152), a structural analogue of CD28. However, CTLA-4 engagement downregulates T-cell responses, which is crucial for preventing severe autoimmune reactions (see later).[176]

The mechanism of CD28 costimulatory effects has not been completely elucidated but involves much more than simply causing greater adhesion between the T cell and APC. After CD28 ligation, tyrosine phosphorylation of its cytoplasmic tail promotes the association of Grb-2, Itk, and PI3K.[176] Two key pathways that are important for the substantial boost in IL-2 production involve PI3K and the c-Jun N-terminal kinase (JNK). In fact, PI3K association with CD28 may be more influential than its link to the TCR complex. These signaling mechanisms apparently mediate different functional outcomes. For example, mutation of the tyrosine in the CD28 cytoplasmic tail whose phosphorylation recruits PI3K disrupts Bcl-X_L upregulation (and cell survival) but not IL-2 production or proliferation.[180] By contrast, cytokine synthesis and proliferation require JNK activation which induces the c-Jun-containing AP-1 transcription factors that govern cytokine genes.[181,182] Cytokine gene transcription is also accelerated by cooperative effects of CD28 with the SLP76 and Vav adapters independently of TCR ligation.[183] In addition to internal signals, CD28 also garners lipid rafts and their signaling proteins into immune synapses at the cell surface.[184,185] Within the raft, CD28 invigorates one active isoform of protein kinase C, PKCθ, that stimulates antigen receptor-induced NF-κB, an event that is critical to T-cell responses.[186,187] Therefore, the T-cell reaction to antigen is a product of the convergence of synergistic signals emanating from the TCR and CD28.

T-cell activation is greatly debilitated if CD28–B7 interactions are blocked.[188,189] Mice genetically deficient in CD28 have immune responses hampered by diminished IL-2 production and T-cell proliferation.[190,191] These observations have raised hopes that the approach of B7 manipulation could be used to prevent or abort T cell-mediated immune responses in vivo.[177,188,189,192] The strong avidity of CTLA-4 for B7 ligands has been exploited in a soluble chimeric protein,

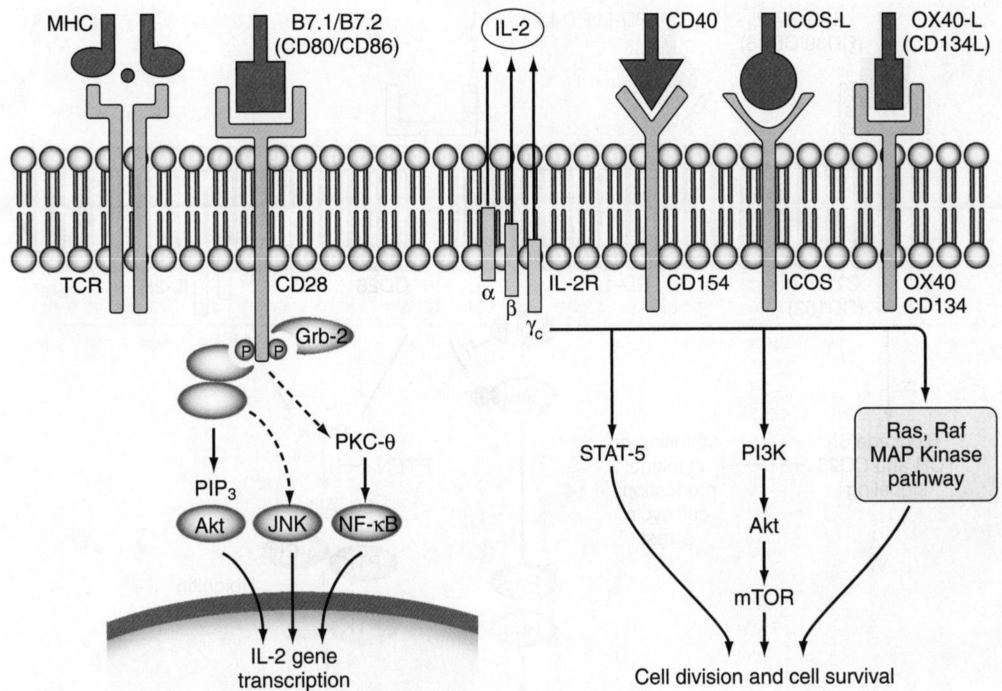

Figure 15–13 Select T-cell costimulatory and cytokine activation pathways. The CD28 receptor is the best-characterized costimulatory molecule on T cells. Ligation of CD28 activates phosphatidylinositol 3-kinase (PI3K), one of whose most important downstream mediators is Akt. Other signals associated with CD28 include activation of JNK and protein kinase Cθ (PKCθ), which in turn may activate nuclear factor-κB (NK-κB). Together these pathways support cytokine gene transcription, such as is represented by IL-2. Once IL-2 binds to its high-affinity receptor (a heterotrimer of an α, a β, and a common γc chain), it activates PI3K and STAT5 signaling pathways. Together these are necessary and probably sufficient to support cell division and promote cell survival. IL-2 signals also may activate the mitogen-activating protein (MAP) kinase pathway, but the importance of these events is unknown. Also shown in the figure are select other costimulatory interactions (CD40/CD154, ICOS ligand [ICOS-L]/ICOS, and OX40-L/OX40; see the text for details on these pathways). ICOS, inducible costimulatory molecule; IL, interleukin; MHC, major histocompatibility complex; PIP_3, phosphatidylinositol-4,5-triphosphate; STAT5, signal transducer and activator of transcription-5; TCR, T-cell receptor.

CTLA-4Ig, that contains the secretory domains of immunoglobulin and the extracellular domains of CTLA-4 (Fig. 15–14; see later).[193] Administration of soluble CTLA-4Ig can prolong allograft survival and ameliorate autoimmune disease in experimental animal models.

ICOS (*i*nducible *co*stimulator) is a distantly related member of the CD28 family.[194] Unlike CD28, which is expressed on all resting T cells, ICOS is expressed following T-cell activation and on memory T cells. The ligand for ICOS, B7-RP1 or B7-H, is expressed on B cells and monocytes.[195] Most initial studies suggested that the primary role of ICOS was to support a T_H2-type differentiation in which an antigen triggers CD4 T cells to secrete cytokines such as IL-4, 10, and 13 which assist B cells in producing antibody.[196] However, ICOS also helps T_H1 responses in which CD4 T cells produce IL-2, gamma-interferon, and lymphotoxin, thereby promoting cellular immunity.[197] The crucial role of ICOS in immunity has been revealed by the identification of mutations in ICOS in common variable immunodeficiency patients.[198] In summary, CD28 is responsible for priming T cells to initiate immune responses whereas ICOS costimulates already activated T cells to further propagate the response.

The Tumor Necrosis Factor / Tumor Necrosis Factor Receptor Superfamily

Costimulatory signals are also delivered through members of the TNF receptor (TNFR) superfamily and their ligands. There are more than 30 distinct receptor–ligand pairs in this family and the majority have either a ligand or a receptor expressed on T cells.[199] These receptors are all structurally related to TNFRs by having variable numbers of cysteine-rich pseudorepeats in their extracellular portion that mediate receptor assembly and ligand binding. Furthermore, their ligands are structurally related to TNF. Although a detailed discussion is beyond the scope of this chapter[199], it is important to highlight a few key regulators of immunity.

A powerful reciprocal interaction between T and B cells is mediated by the interaction between CD154 (CD40 ligand) and CD40.[200] CD154 is strongly induced on all activated $CD4^+$ T cells and some activated $CD8^+$ T cells. Its receptor, CD40, can be found on APCs (dendritic cells, macrophages, and B cells) as well as activated endothelial cells, platelets, and keratinocytes. T-cell engagement of CD40 induces potent pro-inflammatory responses. In the case of myeloid APCs, the responses include induction of B7 molecules that, in turn, powerfully costimulate T-cell activation together with adhesion molecules and cytokines such as IL-12 that promote T-cell immune synapses and differentiation.[201] As discussed above, CD40 stimulation delivered by T cells is required for B cell survival and antibody isotype switching (from IgM to IgE or IgG). Endothelial cells respond to CD40 stimulation by expressing integrins that promote leukocyte binding.[202] These diverse effects make CD154 and CD40 excellent targets for therapeutic intervention in T cell-mediated diseases such as graft versus host disease, transplant rejection, and autoimmunity.[203,204]

Various TNFRs and their cognate ligands have proposed roles in T-cell activation, including OX40/OX40L (CD134/CD134L), CD27/CD70, and 4-1BB/4-1BBL (CD137/CD137L), among others.[199] Others such as Fas, TNF, and LIGHT (the ligand for herpes virus entry mediator [HVEM]) have costimulatory capabilities, but the physiological significance of these effects are unknown.[205] CD134 and its ligand provide signals important for the maintenance of T-cell responses and avoidance of tolerance.[206,207] Gene knockout studies in mice suggest great redundancy in these pathways, and phenotypes are often detectable only when combined with CD28 deficiency. In summary, TNFRs have diverse roles in mediating

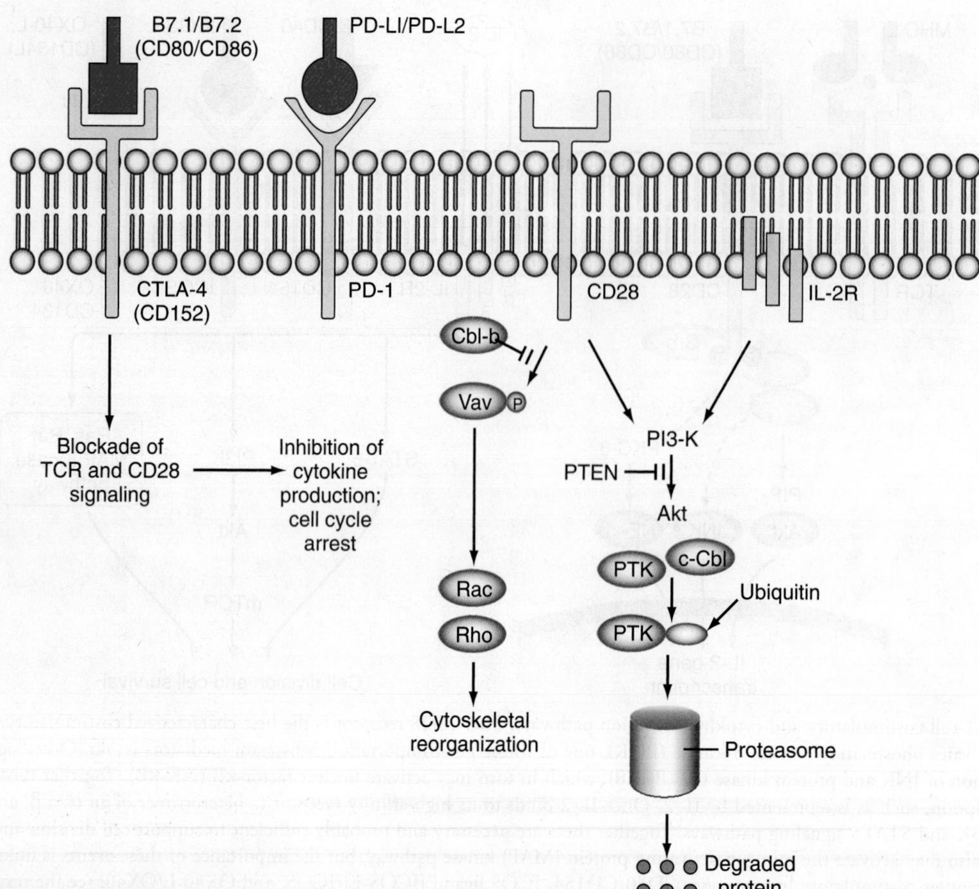

Figure 15–14 Negative signaling pathways that limit T-cell responses. CTLA-4, a homolog of CD28 sharing the same ligands (B7.1 and B7.2), transduces a negative regulatory signal that acts to block TCR- and CD28-mediated signals, leading to inhibition of cytokine production and cell cycle arrest. The inhibitory molecule PD-1 exerts similar effects. CD28 signaling also can be inhibited by Cbl-b, which represses CD28-induced phosphorylation of Vav, thus inhibiting cytoskeletal rearrangements (see text and Fig. 14–11 for further details). A related protein, c-Cbl, promotes ubiquitination of protein tyrosine kinases (PTKs), thereby facilitating proteosomal degradation of signaling molecules. PTEN acts by inactivating lipid mediators of the PI3K pathway, thus preventing activation of downstream kinases such as Akt. IL-2R, interleukin-2 receptor; PD-1, programmed death-1 protein; PI3K, phosphatidylinositol 3-kinase; TCR, T-cell receptor.

intercellular coordination that is critical for memory cell formation, T_H1 versus T_H2 differentiation, and cell survival.

Cytokine Regulation of T-Cell Activation and Function

TCR and costimulatory signals are sufficient for early T-cell activation, but subsequent proliferation and differentiation are governed by cytokines. IL-2, IFN-γ, IL-4, IL-7, and IL-15 are of prime importance.[208] The receptors for IL-2 and IL-15 contain an identical β chain. Although these cytokines are structurally distinct, their receptors share a common γ chain, γc (except IFN-γ), as well as differing, "private" α chains. This explains why human genetic deficiencies of the common γ chain cause profound defects in the production and function of lymphocytes and a near absence of immunity.[209] Genetic deficiencies of the private receptor chains cause more selective immune deficits.

The IL-2 receptor complex was the first identified and remains the most extensively studied of all cytokine receptors on activated T cells. The foundation of signaling by common γ-chain cytokines is the Janus kinase (JAK)–signal transducer and activator of transcription (STAT) proteins, and human deficiencies affecting it can incapacitate the immune system to varying degrees.[209–211] This system, in turn, drives three further signal transduction pathways, mediated by PI3K, STAT-3/5, and Ras/MAPK.[210] PI3K, a signal transducer for many growth factor receptors, typically associates directly with receptors at the cell membrane and becomes activated. However, IL-2R chains lack a PI3K docking motif and instead use adapter proteins such as Grb2 and SHC to recruit PI3K to the IL-2Rβ chain.[212] Downstream targets of activated PI3K include Akt/protein kinase-B, S6 kinase, and mammalian target of rapamycin (mTOR). Cytokine stimulation causes the phosphorylation and recruitment of the JAK kinases, such as JAK 1 and JAK 3 for the IL-2R, to the cytoplasmic domain of the receptor. The activated JAKs then phosphorylate specific STATs (STAT-3 and -5 for IL-2R) within the cytoplasm, causing homodimerization. The dimeric STAT complexes translocate from the cytoplasm to the nucleus, where they bind cognate DNA sites on target promoters, inducing selective gene expression. This enables T cells to traverse the cell cycle and induces critical survival genes such as Bcl-2 and Bcl-xL.[210,211,213] Activated JAKs also phosphorylate the receptor chain that promotes PI3K docking. Finally, the Ras/MAPK pathway also may be activated through IL-2R, although its signaling pathway and physiological role is much less well defined. Each of these pathways is under investigation for developing small-molecule inhibitors that would suppress pathological immune responses or graft rejection.

Negative Modulators of T-Cell Receptor Signal Transduction

To prevent the pathologic consequences of excessive T-cell immune responses, other cell-surface receptors and intracellular molecules serve specifically as negative regulators of responses (see Fig. 15–14). Chief among these is CTLA-4 whose importance was demonstrated by the rapidly fatal lymphocyte infiltrative and inflammatory disease in genetically deficient mice.[214,215] In contrast to the role played by its relative, CD28, CTLA-4 directly inhibits CD28 and TCR signaling, thereby impeding activation and causing cell cycle arrest.[116,216] As with CD28, the extracellular domain of CTLA-4 contains a MYPPPY motif that mediates binding of their shared ligands, CD80 and CD86. The intracellular domain of CTLA-4 also contains an ITIM, which, as discussed above, can shut off activation and signaling events. CTLA-4 inhibits TCR signaling by an associated phosphatase, SHP-2, which dephosphorylates TCRζ, thereby undoing an essential early activation step.[116,217] This action is facilitated by the localization of CTLA-4 to the immunologic synapse following T-cell activation.[218] T cells from mice deficient in CTLA-4 are hyperresponsive to antigenic stimulation and there is uncontrolled proliferation of T cells and lethal autoimmunity in these mice almost certainly in response to self-antigens.[214,215] CTLA-4 is only expressed on activated cells but has a higher affinity for the B7 of ligands. Hence, it becomes influential at a later point in activation by competing with CD28 for its ligands.[177,216,217]

Other distantly related members of the CD28 family, including the programmed death-1 (PD-1) receptor and B- and T-lymphocyte attenuator (BTLA) (see below) have a negative role.[219–221] PD-1 is expressed on activated T, B, and myeloid lineage cells. Unlike CD28 and CTLA-4, which share ligands (CD80 and CD86), PD-1 has unique binding partners, PD-L1 (B7-H1) and PD-L2 (B7-DC), that are B7 family members and displayed on diverse normal and malignant tissues, including activated APCs, lymphocytes, keratinocytes, placenta, and pulmonary and cardiac tissue. Specifically, PD-L1 is widely distributed on various somatic and malignant tissues, including T cells, B cells, macrophages, and DCs. By contrast, PD-L2 is only expressed on macrophages and DCs. Thus, both PD-L1 and PD-L2 may regulate T cells in the lymph nodes, whereas PD-L1 may have additional roles throughout the body, including the CD28 family molecules PD-1. There is some overlap in function, however, because genetic deficiency of both molecules causes a greater elevation in interleukin (IL)-2 and interferon (IFN)-γ following T-cell activation than absence of either one alone. In an experimental mouse model of autoimmune diabetes, double deficiency (PD-L1/PD-L2$^{-/-}$) accelerated diabetes with 100% penetrance in males and females. In control mice, diabetes occurs predominantly in females. On the other hand, ligation of PD-1 inhibits TCR-mediated cytokine production and proliferation (by inducing cell cycle arrest),[222] and mice deficient in PD-1 develop a lupus-like autoimmune syndrome characterized by arthritis and glomerulonephritis.[220] Recent work reveals that PD-1 may mediate exhaustion of CD8 T cells during chronic viral infections, such as HIV, and blockade of this receptor could potentiate antiviral immune responses.[223]

BTLA is structurally similar to CD28, CTLA-4, and PD-1, but the presence of two ITIM motifs in its cytoplasmic region indicates that it is an inhibitory receptor.[205,224] It is selectively expressed in lymphocytes and is induced after T-cell activation, especially on polarized Th1, but not Th2, cells. Remarkably, the ligand for BTLA appears to be the TNFR superfamily member HVEM. A crystal structure of the BTLA–HVEM complex shows that BTLA binds the N-terminal cysteine-rich domain of HVEM using a unique binding surface unlike other CD28-like receptors. Moreover, the structure shows that BTLA recognizes the same surface on HVEM as herpes virus glycoprotein D, which is responsible for viral entry. Immature DCs express high levels of HVEM and as they mature in response to a pathogenic signal, the expression drops, implying that the negative function may correspondingly decrease.

Other B7 family ligands B7-H3 and B7-H4 (also known as B7S1 or B7x) have been shown to inhibit T-cell activation, but their receptors on T cells are not yet known.[221] The newer B7 family members, however, are widely expressed in many different tissues by both hematopoietic and nonhematopoietic cells, suggesting that these molecules may regulate effector T cells that have trafficked to somatic tissues. For instance, it has been shown that PD-L1 is expressed in the maternal part of the placenta during gestation; blockade of PD-L1 increased the spontaneous abortion rate, which indicates that PD-L1 arrests T cells in the placenta to promote fetomaternal tolerance.

Another significant negative regulator is Pten (*p*hosphatase and *te*nsin homolog deleted on chromosome *ten*), which catalyzes the degradation of active phosphatidylinositol lipid intermediates of the PI3K pathway.[225] It can reverse the effects of PI3K and is ubiquitously expressed. Among other effects, Pten negatively regulates Akt and thereby promotes cell death in response to a number of apoptotic stimuli. Targeted deletions of *PTEN* cause an embryonic lethal phenotype, and mice with a single allele of *PTEN* missing (Pten$^{-/-}$) develop lymphoid hyperplasia, autoimmunity, and T-cell lymphomas. Mice with T cell-specific limitation of Pten display defects in thymic and peripheral deletion, and have multiple defects in T-cell apoptosis.[226] A key role of CD28 stimulation may be to overcome the negative regulatory effect of Pten.[227]

Finally, a negative regulator of T-cell and probably B-cell signaling with an interesting mode of action is the protooncogene *c-cbl*, a member of the CBL/SLI family. The c-Cbl protein is an adapter with binding domains for SH2-containing proteins. c-Cbl drives the ubiquitin modification of intracellular proteins, including many involved in T-cell signaling, such as ZAP-70 or other TCR-linked protein tyrosine kinases.[228] As with other proteins, ubiquitination leads to their degradation in the proteasome and thus dampens T-cell signaling. In B cells, Cbl targets Syk for ubiquitination and degradation. A related member of the CBL/SLI family is Cbl-b, which is also a negative regulator.[229] Cbl-b-deficient T cells exhibit hyperresponsiveness to TCR stimuli and do not require CD28 costimulation for optimal IL-2 production or proliferation, effects that has been linked with hyperphosphorylation of Vav1. c-Cbl- and Cbl-b-deficient mice have spontaneous lymphoid proliferation and autoimmune disease. Mice doubly deficient in Cbl-b and Vav1 still have autoimmunity, indicating that at least some of the effects of c-Cbl on T cells must be independent of Vav1. These could be due to the fact that Cbl-b regulates PI3K activity and lipid raft aggregation.[230] In conclusion, there are many ways in which the regulation of phosphorylation—either by inhibiting kinase activity or increasing phosphatase activity[231]—can determine the intensity of the immune activation of T cells.

SUMMARY

The portrait of lymphocyte activation that emerges from a wealth of molecular, biochemical, and cellular investigations over the past 20 years is that a dynamic balance between stimulatory and inhibitory signals is established to govern reactions to antigens. Although this chapter has focused mainly on the intermediary signaling apparatus connecting the cell surface to the nucleus, ultimately, lymphocyte activation involves the successful establishment of a gene expression program appropriate to the specific antigenic challenge. It will therefore be fundamentally important in the future to understand how the balance of positive and negative signals coordinates the nuclear chromatin and transcriptional machinery in lymphocytes for this purpose. Research continues to uncover new molecular determinants of this balance providing hope that specific immune responses can be therapeutically enhanced to generate better vaccines and fight infectious diseases or suppressed to ameliorate autoimmunity, allergies, and allograft rejection.

SUGGESTED READINGS

Bromley SK, Burack WR, Johnson KG, et al: The immunological synapse. Annu Rev Immunol 19:375, 2001.

Buckley RH: Molecular defects in human severe combined immunodeficiency and approaches to immune reconstitution. Annu Rev Immunol 22:625, 2004.

Carter RH, Fearon DT: CD19: Lowering the threshold for antigen receptor stimulation of B lymphocytes. Science 256:105, 1992.

Chung JB, Silverman M, Monroe JG: Transitional B cells: Step by step towards immune competence. Trends Immunol 24:343, 2003.

Jordan MS, Singer AL, Koretzky GA: Adaptors as central mediators of signal transduction in immune cells. Nat Immunol 4:110, 2003.

Koretzky GA, Myung PS: Positive and negative regulation of T-cell activation by adaptor proteins. Nat Rev Immunol 1:95, 2001.

Lee KM, Chuang E, Griffin M, et al: Molecular basis of T cell inactivation by CTLA-4. Science 282:2263, 1998.

Leonard WJ: The molecular basis of X-linked severe combined immunodeficiency: Defective cytokine receptor signaling. Annu Rev Med 47:229, 1996.

Locksley RM, Killeen N, Lenardo MJ: The TNF and TNF receptor superfamilies: Integrating mammalian biology. Cell 104:487, 2001.

Martin-Orozco N, Dong C: New battlefields for costimulation. J Exp Med 203:817, 2006.

Monroe JG: ITAM-mediated tonic signalling through pre-BCR and BCR complexes. Nat Rev Immunol 6:283, 2006.

Niiro H, Clark EA: Regulation of B-cell fate by antigen-receptor signals. Nat Rev Immunol 2:945, 2002.

Pawson T: Protein modules and signalling networks. Nature 373:573, 1995.

Pierce SK: Lipid rafts and B-cell activation. Nat Rev Immunol 2:96, 2002.

Reth M: Antigen receptor tail clue. Nature 338:383, 1989.

Sayegh MH, Turka LA: The role of T-cell costimulatory activation pathways in transplant rejection. N Engl J Med 338:1813, 1998.

Tedder TF, Inaoki M, Sato S: The CD19-CD21 complex regulates signal transduction thresholds governing humoral immunity and autoimmunity. Immunity 6:107, 1997.

Weiss A, Littman DR: Signal transduction by lymphocyte antigen receptors. Cell 76:263, 1994.

REFERENCES

For complete list of references log onto www.expertconsult.com

CHAPTER 16

CELL ADHESION

Rodger P. McEver

Cell adhesion is essential for the development and maintenance of multicellular organisms. Cell–cell and cell–matrix contacts facilitate intercellular communication and define the architecture of organs. The regulated nature of cell adhesion is particularly evident in the hematopoietic system, where cells routinely make transitions between nonadherent and adherent phenotypes during differentiation and in response to stimuli in the circulation or extravascular tissues.

In the bone marrow, proliferation and differentiation of hematopoietic stem cells are controlled not only by soluble growth factors but also by adhesion to stromal cells and matrix molecules. Weakening of these adhesive interactions is required for mature blood cells to enter the circulation. Circulating erythrocytes normally remain nonadhesive until they are finally cleared by the reticuloendothelial system. Other circulating cells often participate in regulated adhesive events during their life span. For example, prothymocytes adhere to components of the thymus, where they undergo further maturation before reentering the circulation. Lymphocytes regularly stick to the specialized high endothelial venules of lymphoid tissues, migrate into these tissues for sampling of processed antigens, and then exit via the lymphatics. During inflammation, specific classes of leukocytes roll on the endothelium, then adhere more tightly, and finally emigrate between endothelial cells into the tissues. There, neutrophils and monocytes phagocytose invading pathogens, whereas lymphocytes adhere to antigen-presenting macrophages. During hemorrhage, platelets stick to exposed subendothelial matrix components, spread, and recruit additional platelets into large aggregates that serve as an efficient surface for thrombin and fibrin generation. Leukocytes also adhere to activated platelets and to other leukocytes, and platelets roll on the endothelium. Endothelial cells express molecules that affect the adhesiveness of platelets or leukocytes. Tight contacts between adjacent endothelial cells also limit access of blood cells to the underlying tissues.

ADHESION MOLECULES

Cells adhere through noncovalent bond formation between macromolecules on cell surfaces with macromolecules on other cell surfaces or in extracellular matrix. These interactions involve either protein–protein or protein–carbohydrate recognition. Although some adhesion molecules are expressed only by blood or endothelial cells, most also are synthesized by other cells. Many adhesion molecules can be grouped into families according to related structural and functional features.

EXTRACELLULAR MATRIX PROTEINS

The principal constituents of the extracellular matrix are adhesive proteins and proteoglycans. The major proteins are von Willebrand factor (vWF), thrombospondin, collagen, fibronectin, laminin, and vitronectin. These proteins are large and often highly extended and consist of multiple domains with different binding functions. In some proteins such as fibronectin, alternative splicing can increase diversity by producing molecules with variable numbers of domains. The many binding domains allow adhesive proteins to interact with each other as well as with cell-surface receptors, resulting in multipoint contacts that stabilize matrix structure. One adhesive protein, fibrinogen, is found predominantly in plasma but also may be deposited in exposed subendothelial matrix following vascular injury. Fibronectin, vitronectin, thrombospondin, and vWF are located predominantly in the extracellular matrix but also are found in plasma. Several adhesive proteins also are stored in α-granules of platelets, where they are secreted following platelet activation at sites of vascular injury.

Proteoglycans contain protein cores to which are covalently attached many glycosaminoglycans-long linear polymers of repeating disaccharides. Most proteoglycans are in the extracellular matrix, but some are anchored on cell surfaces through a core protein that contains a membrane-spanning domain. Hyaluronan is a unique glycosaminoglycan that forms polymers with molecular masses up to several million daltons that are not covalently attached to a protein. Hyaluronan forms noncovalent interactions with globular domains on the protein core of proteoglycans and with a small molecule called *link protein.* The resultant hyaluronan–proteoglycan complexes can become very large, contributing to the structural stability of matrix. Hyaluronan can also bind to cell-surface receptors.

INTEGRINS

Integrins are a broadly distributed group of cell-surface adhesion receptors that consist of noncovalently associated α- and β-subunits (Fig. 16–1 and Table 16–1). There are at least 15 α chains and 8 β chains that pair in many, but not all, of the possible combinations. All blood cells have several different integrins. The four β_2 integrins, each paired with a unique α subunit, are expressed only by leukocytes, and the $\alpha_{IIb}\beta_3$ integrin (glycoprotein IIb–IIIa [GPIIb–IIIa]) is expressed only by megakaryocytes and platelets. Multidomain adhesive proteins of the extracellular matrix are ligands for many integrins. Some integrins bind to specific domains of several different proteins, and some adhesive proteins bind to several different integrins. These interactions generally mediate cell–matrix adhesion. Cell–cell interactions result from integrin recognition of cell-surface members of the immunoglobulin superfamily. Binding of fibrinogen to $\alpha_{IIb}\beta_3$ integrins on adjacent platelets creates a molecular bridge that promotes platelet aggregation. Furthermore, fibrinogen simultaneously binds to the $\alpha_m\beta_2$ integrin on leukocytes and to an immunoglobulin-like receptor on endothelial cells, promoting leukocyte adhesion to the endothelium.

IMMUNOGLOBULIN-LIKE RECEPTORS

Immunoglobulin superfamily members contain a variable number of disulfide-stabilized motifs like those in antibodies, which are linked to transmembrane and cytoplasmic domains (Table 16–2; see also Fig. 16–1). The immunoglobulin-like motif provides a framework on which specific recognition structures for other proteins can be added. Some of these motifs also recognize glycoconjugates. The immunoglobulin-like molecules, intercellular adhesion molecule-1 and -2 (ICAM-1 and ICAM-2) and vascular cell adhesion molecule-1 (VCAM-1), expressed on endothelial cells, as well as ICAM-3, expressed on leukocytes, mediate cell–cell contact through recogni-

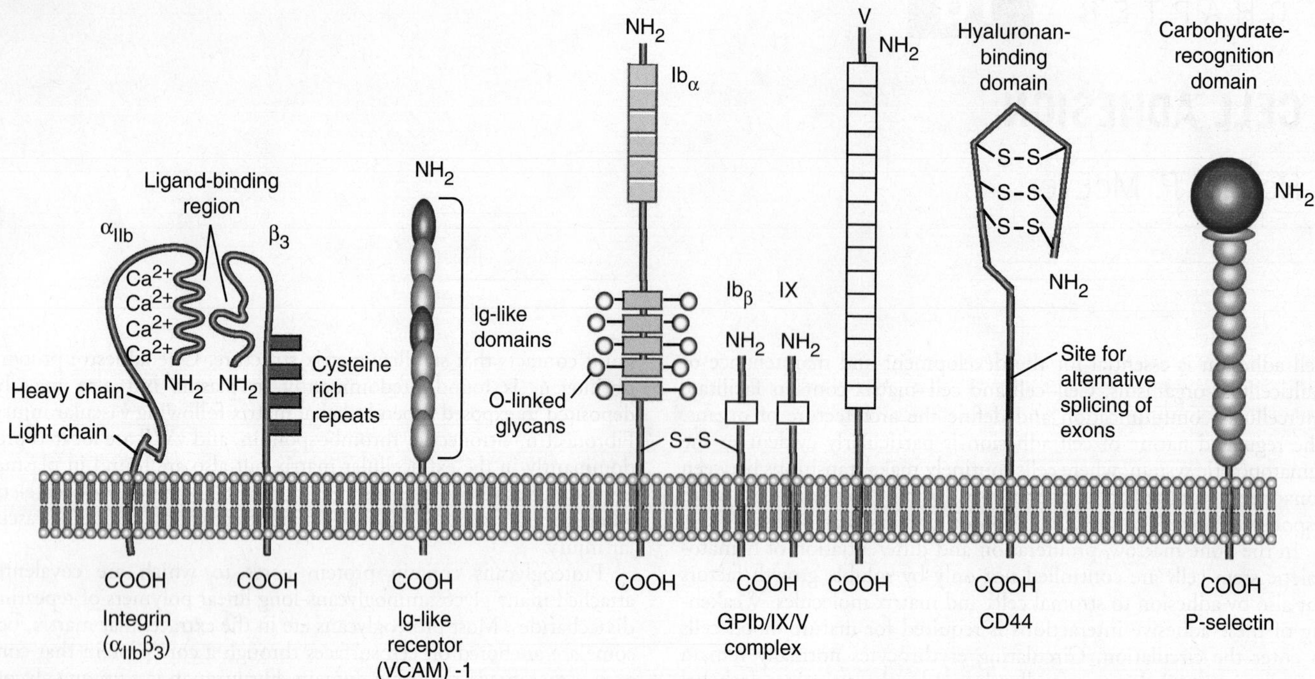

Figure 16–1 Schematic diagrams of several types of cell-surface adhesion receptors. Integrins consist of noncovalently linked α and β subunits, both of which contribute to ligand binding. The platelet $\alpha_{IIb}\beta_3$ integrin is illustrated at *far left.* Immunoglobulin-like receptors contain a variable number of immunoglobulin homology domains, of which some bind ligands and others extend the ligand-binding domains from the membrane. Shown *second from left* is vascular cell adhesion molecule-1 (VCAM-1), which contains seven immunoglobulin domains; the two domains that bind to integrins are *shaded.* The platelet glycoprotein Ib–IX–V (GPIb–IX–V) complex, depicted in the *middle diagram,* consists of several leucine-rich protein subunits. CD44, illustrated next, contains an amino-terminal (N-terminal) domain that binds to hyaluronan. Each of the selectins contains an N-terminal carbohydrate recognition domain that binds sialylated and fucosylated oligosaccharides on specific cell-surface glycoprotein ligands. Illustrated at *far right* is P-selectin, the largest of the three selectins.

tion of specific integrins on leukocytes. ICAM-4, expressed on erythroid precursors, binds to integrins on stromal cells of bone marrow, which may regulate erythropoiesis. The immunoglobulin-like GPVI on platelets promotes cell activation by binding to collagen exposed on damaged blood vessels. Interactions between immunoglobulin-like molecules help to mediate adhesion between T cells and antigen-presenting cells. Thus, the immunoglobulin-like molecules CD8 and CD4 on T cells bind to the conserved membrane-proximal domains of class I and class II major histocompatibility complex (MHC) proteins, respectively, whereas the T-cell receptor (CD3) binds to the polymorphic antigen-presenting domain. In addition, the immunoglobulin-like protein CD2 on T cells binds to the immunoglobulin-like protein leukocyte function-associated antigen-3 (LFA-3) on antigen-presenting cells. The immunoglobulin-like receptor platelet and endothelial cell adhesion molecule-1 (PECAM-1) (CD31) uses homotypical interactions to promote contacts between adjacent endothelial cells and to mediate adhesion of leukocytes to platelets and endothelium. The immunoglobulin-like junctional adhesion molecules (JAMs), expressed on endothelial cells, regulate endothelial cell junctions and leukocyte trafficking between endothelial cells by homotypical interactions or by heterotypical interactions with integrins.

OTHER ADHESION RECEPTORS THAT MEDIATE PROTEIN–PROTEIN INTERACTIONS

Cadherins are cytoskeletally linked membrane proteins that mediate cell–cell contact in many organs through homotypical binding to cadherins on adjacent cells (Table 16–3). Cadherins have not been described on blood cells but are found on endothelial cells, where, like PECAM-1 and JAMs, they help form cell junctions.

The GPIb–IX–V complex on platelets consists of leucine-rich protein subunits (see Fig. 16–1). Under conditions of high shear stress like those found in arterial circulation, this complex promotes the initial platelet adhesion to injured vessels by binding to vWF exposed in the subendothelium. It also may assist interactions with other platelets or with endothelial cells by binding to P-selectin, which normally binds to glycoconjugates, and it may assist platelet adhesion to leukocytes by binding to the integrin $\alpha_m\beta_2$.

CD36 is a receptor with at least two membrane-spanning domains that is expressed on many cell types. On platelets, it has been implicated as a receptor for collagen and perhaps for thrombospondin; both interactions could facilitate adhesion to the subendothelial matrix at sites of hemorrhage.

LECTIN ADHESION RECEPTORS

CD44 is an unusual transmembrane glycoprotein expressed to variable degrees on many subsets of leukocytes (see Fig. 16–1). It has a membrane-distal domain that is structurally related to link protein of extracellular matrix, and, like link protein, can bind to hyaluronan. CD44 also binds to the serglycin, a proteoglycan secreted by hematopoietic cells. The hyaluronan-binding function of CD44 may modulate a number of leukocyte responses. The most clearly demonstrated function is in lymphopoiesis, where maturation of lymphocyte precursors requires contacts with bone marrow stromal cells bearing surface hyaluronan. CD44–hyaluronate interactions also may promote lymphocyte entry to and transit through organized lymphoid tissues. The membrane-proximal regions of CD44 are structurally diverse because of the insertion of variable numbers of domains through alternative splicing. These insertions may regulate the ability of CD44 to bind hyaluronan and may mediate postbinding events that affect cell signaling.

Table 16–1 Integrins on Blood Cells

Integrin Designation	Other Name(s)	Expressed by	Ligand(s)	Function(s)
$\alpha_1\beta_1$	VLA-1	Leukocytes, other cells	Collagens, LM	Adhesion to ECM
$\alpha_2\beta_1$	VLA-2 GPIa/IIa	Leukocytes, platelets, other cells	Collagens, LM	Adhesion to ECM
$\alpha_3\beta_1$	VLA-3	Leukocytes, other cells	Collagens, LM, FN	Adhesion to ECM
$\alpha_4\beta_1$	VLA-4	Monocytes, lymphocytes, eosinophils	VCAM-1, FN	Adhesion to cells, ECM
$\alpha_5\beta_1$	VLA-5 GPIc/IIa	Leukocytes, platelets, other cells	FN	Adhesion to ECM
$\alpha_6\beta_1$	VLA-6 GPIc/IIa	Leukocytes, platelets, other cells	LM	Adhesion to ECM
$\alpha_9\beta_1$		Neutrophils	VCAM-1	Adhesion to ECs
$\alpha_L\beta_2$	LFA-1 CD11a/CD18	Leukocytes	ICAM-1, -2, -3	Leukocyte aggregation and adhesion
$\alpha_M\beta_2$	MAC-1 CR3 CD11b/CD18	Neutrophils, monocytes	ICAM-1, FIB	Neutrophil aggregation and adhesion to ECs
$\alpha_X\beta_2$	p150,95 CD11c/CD18	Neutrophils, monocytes	?	Adhesion to ECs
$\alpha_D\beta_2$	CD11d/CD18	Eosinophils, monocytes, lymphocytes	VCAM-1, ICAM-3	Adhesion to leukocytes and to ECs
$\alpha_{IIb}\beta_3$	GPIIb/IIIa	Platelets	FIB, FN, vWF, VN, TSP	Platelet adhesion and aggregation
$\alpha_V\beta_3$	VN receptor	Platelets, ECs	FIB, FN, vWF, VN, TSP, collagens	Platelet adhesion, angiogenesis
$\alpha_4\beta_7$	LPAM-1	Lymphocytes	VCAM-1, MAdCAM-1, FN	Lymphocyte adhesion to ECs and ECM

CR, complement receptor; ECs, endothelial cells; ECM, extracellular matrix; FIB, fibrinogen; FN, fibronectin; GP, glycoprotein; LFA-1, leukocyte function-associated antigen-1; LM, laminin; LPAM-1, lymphocyte Peyer patch adhesion molecule; MAdCAM-1, mucosal addressin cell adhesion molecule-1; TSP, thrombospondin; VCAM-1, vascular cell adhesion molecule-1; VLA, very late-appearing antigen; VN, vitronectin; vWF, von Willebrand factor.

Table 16–2 Immunoglobulin-Like Receptors

Name	Other Name	Expressed by	Ligand	Function(s)
ICAM-1		Macrophages, EC, other cells	$\alpha_M\beta_2$, $\alpha_L\beta_2$, FIB	T-cell responses, leukocyte adhesion to EC
ICAM-2		EC	$\alpha_L\beta_2$	Leukocyte adhesion to EC
ICAM-3		Leukocytes	$\alpha_L\beta_2$	T-cell responses, leukocyte aggregation
ICAM-4		Erythroid precursors	$\alpha_4\beta_1$, $\alpha_v\beta_3$, $\alpha_{IIb}\beta_3$	Regulate erythropoiesis
GP VI		Platelets	Collagen	Platelet adhesion and activation
PECAM-1	CD31	Leukocytes, platelets, EC	PECAM-1	EC junctions, leukocyte transmigration, cell signaling
VCAM-1		Activated EC, smooth muscle cells	$\alpha_4\beta_1$, $\alpha_4\beta_7$	Mononuclear cell adhesion to EC
MAdCAM-1		EC of Peyer patches	$\alpha_4\beta_7$	Lymphocyte homing
Siglecs		Leukocyte subsets	Sialylated glycans	Regulate B-cell activation, innate immunity? hematopoiesis?
JAMs		EC	JAMs, $\alpha_L\beta_2$, $\alpha_4\beta_1$	EC junctions, leukocyte transmigration
CD2		T cells	LFA-3*	T-cell responses
CD4		T cells	Class II MHC*	T-cell responses
CD8		T cells	Class I MHC*	T-cell responses
CD3	T-cell receptor	T cells	Antigen on MHC*	T-cell responses

ICAM-1, -2, -3, -4, intercellular adhesion molecules; JAMs, junctional adhesion molecules; MHC, major histocompatibility complex; PECAM-1, platelet and endothelial cell adhesion molecule-1. For other abbreviations, see Table 6–1 footnote.
*LFA-3 and classes I and II MHC molecules are also immunoglobulin-like receptors.

Table 16–3 Other Adhesion Receptors

Name	Other Name	Expressed by	Ligand	Function(s)
Cadherins		EC, many other cells	Homotypic binding	Formation of EC junctions
GPIb/IX/V		Platelets	vWF	Platelet adhesion to ECM under shear
CD36	GPIV	Platelets, many other cells	Collagens, TSP	Platelet adhesion to ECM
CD44		Leukocytes, other cells	Hyaluronan, serglycin	Lymphopoiesis, lymphocyte activation
DC-SIGN		Dendritic cells	Mannosylated glycans, other glycans	Regulate T-cell–dendritic cell interactions, recognize pathogens
Natural killer cell receptors		Natural killer cells	MHC molecules	Recognition of virus-infected or other foreign cells

DC-SIGN, dendritic cell-specific ICAM-grabbing nonintegrin; MHC, major histocompatibility complex. For other abbreviations, see Table 16–1 footnote.

Table 16–4 Selectins

Name	Other Names	Expressed by	Ligand*	Ligands Expressed by	Function(s)
P-selectin	CD62P GMP-140 PADGEM	Thrombin-activated platelets and EC, cytokine-activated EC	PSGL-1, GPIbα	Leukocytes, platelets	Leukocyte adhesion to activated EC and platelets
E-selectin	CD62E ELAM-1	Cytokine-activated EC	PSGL-1, other sialylated and fucosylated glycoproteins	Leukocytes	Leukocyte adhesion to activated EC
L-selectin	CD62L LECAM-1 LAM-1	Leukocytes	PSGL-1, also GlyCAM-1, CD34, and other mucins on EC of lymph nodes	Leukocytes, EC of lymph nodes	Leukocyte adhesion to other leukocytes; lymphocyte homing to lymph nodes

EC, endothelial cells; ELAM-1, endothelial leukocyte adhesion molecule-1; Gly-CAM-1, glycosylation-dependent cell adhesion molecule-1; GMP-140, granule membrane protein-140; LAM-1, leukocyte adhesion molecule-1; LECAM-1, leukocyte endothelial cell adhesion molecule-1; PADGEM, platelet activation-dependent granule external membrane protein; PSGL-1, P-selectin glycoprotein ligand-1.

*The selectins bind to sialylated, fucosylated, and (in some cases) sulfated oligosaccharides on specific glycoproteins, of which only some have been identified.

The selectins are a group of three receptors that terminate in a membrane-distal carbohydrate-recognition domain related to those in Ca^{2+}-dependent (C-type) animal lectins such as the hepatic asialoglycoprotein receptor (see Fig. 16–1). L-selectin is expressed on leukocytes, E-selectin on cytokine-activated endothelium, and P-selectin on macrophages, platelets, and endothelial cells exposed to secretagogues such as thrombin or histamine (Table 16–4). The selectins mediate leukocyte adhesion to platelets, endothelium, or other leukocytes through Ca^{2+}-dependent interactions of the carbohydrate-recognition domains with cell-surface carbohydrates on apposing cells. High-affinity binding appears to require specific carbohydrate structures displayed on a limited number of membrane glycoproteins. The best-characterized glycoprotein ligands for selectins are mucins that have large numbers of clustered, sialylated *O*-linked oligosaccharides. Site-specific construction of *O*-glycans with specific sialylated, fucosylated, and, in some cases, sulfated moieties is required for these mucins to bind optimally to selectins. In the case of one mucin, P-selectin glycoprotein ligand-1 (PSGL-1), sulfation of tyrosine residues near a specific *O*-glycan is required for binding to P- and L-selectin.

Dendritic cells and related macrophages express a novel group of C-type lectins, of which the best-characterized is dendritic cell-specific ICAM-grabbing nonintegrin (DC-SIGN). DC-SIGN binds to particular oligosaccharides on ICAMs, thereby regulating T-cell and dendritic cell function during antigen presentation. It also binds to glycans on a variety of pathogens, which may have critical roles in innate immunity. Natural killer cells express a different group of proteins with membrane-distal C-type lectin-like domains. Although these receptors are important for interactions of natural killer cells with target cells, they may bind to proteins rather than to glycoconjugates.

Siglecs are a subgroup of membrane proteins of the immunoglobulin superfamily that bind to carbohydrates instead of to proteins (see Table 16–2). The first two amino-terminal (N-terminal) domains appear to be necessary and sufficient for carbohydrate recognition. The N-terminal domain is a V-type structure that includes an unusual disulfide bond that is not found in the more common C-type immunoglobulin domains. Siglecs bind well to sialylated glycans on some but not all glycoproteins. Different siglecs preferentially recognize sialic acid that is linked α2,6-, α2,8-, or α2,3- to an underlying galactose residue. Siglecs can form *cis* interactions with other glycoproteins on the same cell or *trans* interactions with glycoproteins on another cell. The functions of siglecs have not been fully defined, but increasing evidence suggests that they function as important signaling molecules. The best-characterized example is CD22, which negatively regulates B-cell activation when it engages sialylated glycoproteins. Sialoadhesin, expressed on bone marrow macrophages, may regulate hematopoietic cell differentiation.

LIGAND BINDING VERSUS CELL ADHESION

As with all noncovalent macromolecular interactions, adhesion molecules bind to each other with equilibrium affinities that are defined by their association and dissociation rates. However, the efficiency of cell adhesion is not simply a function of the solution-phase equilibrium affinities of adhesion molecules for one another. Adhesion molecules in cell membranes and matrix are limited primarily to two dimensions, and even low-affinity molecular interactions may stabilize adhesion if there is time for sufficient bonds to form along the plane of cell contact. The efficiency of cell attachment, and the ensuing strength of adhesion, reflects multiple factors that dictate the probability of formation of bonds between adhesion molecules on cell or matrix surfaces. The kinetics of bond formation and dissociation are especially important for certain kinds of cell adhesion. Furthermore, interactions between cell adhesion molecules are

Table 16–5 Regulation of Adhesion Receptors

Mechanism	Example
Synthesis	Erythroid precursor synthesis of $\alpha_5\beta_1$ Lymphocyte synthesis of CD44 Cytokine-induced synthesis of E-selectin, P-selectin, ICAM-1, and VCAM-1 by endothelial cells
Surface expression	Proteolytic cleavage of L-selectin from leukocytes Redistribution of P-selectin from granule membranes to plasma membrane of platelets and endothelial cells Endocytosis of P- and E-selectin on endothelial cells
Ligand affinity	Activation-induced increased affinity of many integrins for their ligands Activation-induced increased affinity of CD44 for hyaluronan

For abbreviations, see Table 16–1 footnote.

subjected to force, which affects the lifetimes of adhesive bonds. This is particularly true in the circulation, where platelets and leukocytes must rapidly adhere to the blood vessel wall and withstand forces applied by the wall shear stresses of flowing blood. Other factors that affect bond formation include the number of adhesion molecules on a cell or matrix surface, the distance the binding domain of an adhesion receptor protrudes from the cell membrane, the lateral mobility of receptors, receptor dimerization, and the clustering of receptors on microvilli or other membrane domains. Cell adhesion can be further stabilized by events that occur after the initial interactions of adhesion molecules. For example, the cytoplasmic domains of many adhesion molecules bind to cytoskeletal components, allowing clustering of receptors into surface patches that strengthen adhesion and promote cell spreading or migration.

REGULATION OF ADHESION RECEPTORS

To prevent inappropriate interactions of cells with each other or with extracellular matrix, the expression and function of adhesion receptors must be tightly controlled. Three primary control mechanisms are used: (a) the rate of synthesis of the receptor, (b) the time during which the receptor is displayed on the cell surface, and (c) the binding affinity/avidity of the receptor for ligands (Table 16–5). All of these mechanisms are used to control interactions of blood and vascular cells.

REGULATION OF SYNTHESIS

The synthesis of many adhesion receptors is regulated. Erythroid precursors synthesize integrins that mediate their interactions with stromal cells and with extracellular matrix in the bone marrow. As the precursors mature, synthesis ceases, resulting in loss of expression of cell-surface integrins by the time a mature erythrocyte enters the circulation. Lymphocyte precursors synthesize CD44 during differentiation in the bone marrow, stop synthesis prior to release, and resume synthesis during maturation in the thymus. On exposure to antigens, immunologically naive lymphocytes synthesize increased amounts of several adhesion receptors during their conversion to the memory phenotype; this process presumably allows these cells to become more adhesive in response to a subsequent antigenic challenge. When exposed to inflammatory cytokines such as tumor necrosis factor-α and interleukin-1, endothelial cells transiently increase synthesis of E- and P-selectin, ICAM-1, and VCAM-1, resulting in an adhesive surface for leukocytes.

REGULATION OF SURFACE EXPRESSION

The surface expression of some adhesion receptors is tightly controlled. L-selectin is present on the plasma membrane of leukocytes, where it is available to bind to ligands on the endothelial cell surface. Stimulation of the leukocyte causes L-selectin to be shed into the plasma by proteolytic cleavage. P-selectin is constitutively synthesized by megakaryocytes (where it is incorporated into platelets) and by endothelial cells. Rather than being directly delivered to the plasma membrane, it is sorted into secretory storage granules: the α granules of platelets and the Weibel–Palade bodies of endothelial cells. On stimulation of these cells by agonists such as thrombin, P-selectin is rapidly transported to the cell surface during fusion of granule membranes with the plasma membrane. Once on the surface of the endothelium, both E-selectin and P-selectin are internalized and delivered to lysosomes for degradation. The cytoplasmic domain of P-selectin contains signals that direct sorting into secretory granules, internalization through coated pits of the plasma membrane, and movement from endosomes to lysosomes; the latter two signals probably also are present in the cytoplasmic domain of E-selectin. The net result of these events is to control the duration of exposure of E- and P-selectin on the endothelium, where they can mediate adhesion of leukocytes. Activation of leukocytes also mobilizes a pool of β_2 integrins from storage compartments to the plasma membrane, although some of these molecules also are constitutively expressed on the cell surface. Finally, platelet activation redistributes a portion of the GPIb–IX–V complexes from ligand-accessible positions on the plasma membrane to sequestered, invaginated membrane domains known as the *surface-connected canalicular system*. This process, which requires interactions of the cytoplasmic domain of GPIb–IX–V with the cytoskeleton, may serve to downregulate GPIb-mediated adhesion of platelets to immobilized vWF.

REGULATION OF BINDING AFFINITY

Regulation of binding affinity is an important control mechanism for other adhesion receptors. Many integrins are constitutively present on the cell surface but interact poorly with their ligands. Cell activation by a number of agonists induces conformational changes in integrins so that they effectively recognize their ligands. An example is the $\alpha_{IIb}\beta_3$ integrin, which requires platelet stimulation to bind fibrinogen; if this binding affinity were not regulated, circulating platelets would indiscriminately aggregate in the fibrinogen-rich plasma milieu. The cytoplasmic domains of integrins can exert both positive and negative influences on binding affinity. Binding of specific cytoplasmic proteins to these domains may propagate structural changes to the extracellular ligand-binding regions of the integrins. Three-dimensional structures of integrins suggest that the integrin "headpiece" faces down toward the membrane in the inactive conformation and rapidly extends upward in a "switchblade"-like opening motion on activation. Low-affinity ligand binding may stabilize some active conformations of integrins, perhaps explaining why integrins on unactivated cells will sometimes bind to immobilized, multivalent adhesive proteins but not to the same proteins in solution. Cellular activation also may regulate the binding avidities of CD44, L-selectin, P-selectin, and some integrins through changes in membrane distribution engineered by interactions of their cytoplasmic domains with the cytoskeleton or with clathrin-coated pits.

CELL SIGNALING THROUGH ADHESION MOLECULES

In addition to their roles in cell–cell and cell–matrix contacts, adhesion molecules may cause cell signaling through indirect or direct mechanisms. Proteoglycans in the extracellular matrix can sequester growth factors that can be released to bind to surface receptors on nearby cells. Some chemoattractants bind to proteoglycans on the surface of endothelial cells, where they can activate adherent leukocytes. Binding of adhesive ligands to cell-surface integrins, GPIb–IX–

V, CD44, cadherins, CD36, PECAM-1, selectins, and perhaps other receptors can directly trigger intracellular events. The consequences of such signaling include changes in affinity/avidity of other adhesion receptors for their ligands, shape change, secretion, proliferation, synthesis of cytokines and other molecules, and migration. In some cases, binding of a monovalent adhesive ligand to a receptor may induce a signal. More commonly, signaling requires cross-linking of several receptors through interactions with multivalent ligands in matrix or on apposing cells.

Many studies of adhesion receptor signaling have focused on integrins. Binding of the same ligand to different integrins can mediate different responses in the same cell. Furthermore, ligand binding to the same integrin expressed in different cells can result in different signals. These data suggest that very specific interactions occur between ligand-occupied integrins and intracellular components. The cytoplasmic domains of integrins are essential for initiating signaling. Tyrosine kinases have been localized at the interaction zones between integrins and the cytoskeleton, and tyrosine phosphorylation of a number of proteins accompanies integrin-mediated cell signaling. Tyrosine phosphorylation initiates a cascade of signaling events, including the activation of serine/threonine kinases, which cause a variety of cellular responses. Ligand binding to integrins also results in generation of lipid second messengers, alkalization of the cytoplasm, and influxes of Ca^{2+}.

COOPERATIVE INTERACTIONS BETWEEN SIGNALING AND ADHESION MOLECULES

Signaling and adhesion molecules frequently function cooperatively in sequential cascades to enhance the specificity of cell adhesion. Three examples of how these cooperative interactions facilitate blood cell responses are described next.

Platelet Adhesion and Aggregation

At sites of blood vessel injury in the arterial circuit, platelets rapidly tether to and then translocate or roll along the damaged vessel through reversible interactions of GPIb–IX–V receptors with immobilized vWF exposed in the subendothelial matrix (Fig. 16–2). These interactions are facilitated by arterial flow, perhaps because of complex effects of high wall shear stresses on the lifetimes of bonds between GPIb and vWF. An important feature of this initial reversible adhesive event is that prior activation of the platelets is not required. After adhesion, however, the interaction of immobilized vWF with GPIb receptors triggers intracellular signals that lead to platelet activation. These signals synergize with those produced by engagement of the collagen receptor GPVI. Platelet activation, in turn, increases the affinity of platelet integrins for collagen and fibronectin, which stabilizes adhesion. Binding of these ligands transduces signals that propagate further activation responses such as spreading, secretion of granule contents, and recruitment of additional platelets through cell–cell contact mediated by binding of fibrinogen to activated $\alpha_{IIb}\beta_3$ integrins. This adhesion cascade allows unstimulated platelets to home to the site of vascular injury and then be activated by locally generated mediators.

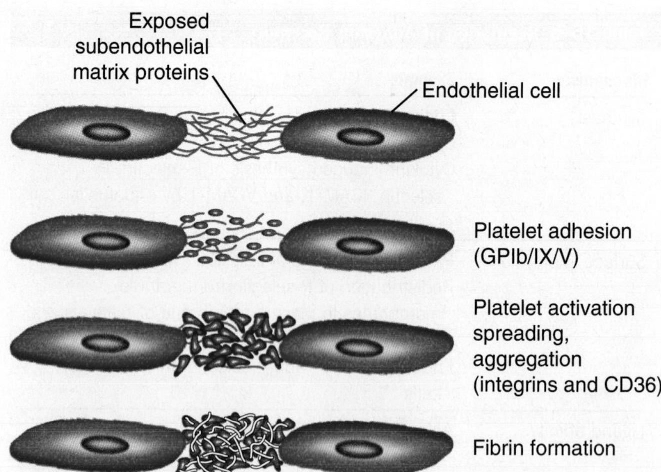

Figure 16–2 Platelet adhesion and aggregation. In response to arterial injury under high shear forces, platelets rapidly adhere to the subendothelial matrix. The initial contacts are made between glycoprotein Ib–IX–V (GPIb–IX–V) on platelets and von Willebrand factor (vWF) in the matrix. These molecular interactions help activate platelets, thereby increasing the affinity of several platelet integrins for other adhesive matrix proteins such as fibronectin, laminin, and collagen. GPVI further activates platelets by binding to collagen. CD36 also interacts with both collagen and thrombospondin. Fibrinogen cross-links activated platelets into aggregates by binding to $\alpha_{IIb}\beta_3$ integrins. The platelet plug then serves as an efficient surface for generation of thrombin and fibrin.

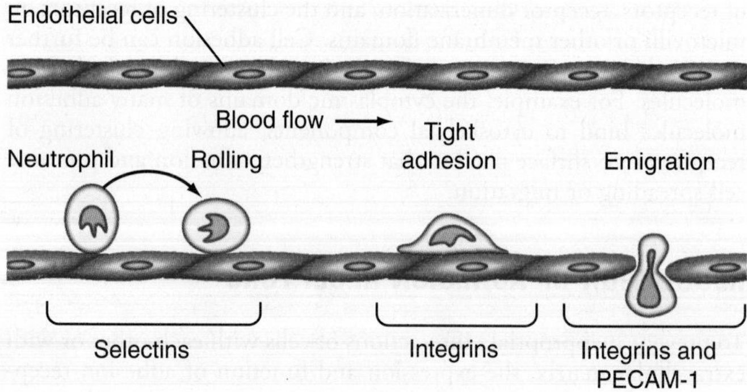

Figure 16–3 Neutrophil rolling, spreading, and emigration. At sites of tissue injury or infection, neutrophils first roll on the endothelial cells in postcapillary venules. These transient adhesive interactions are mediated by activation-induced expression of E- or P-selectin on the endothelial cell surface. E- and P-selectin bind to carbohydrate ligands on the neutrophil. These molecular bonds can form under the shear forces in the venular circulation. The rolling neutrophils are then activated by locally generated inflammatory mediators that increase the affinity of β_2 integrins for immunoglobulin-like receptors such as intercellular adhesion molecule-1 (ICAM-1) on the endothelium. These bonds slow rolling and then promote firm adhesion to the endothelium. Neutrophil migration between endothelial cells into tissues at the site of infection requires disengagement of old adhesive bonds and formation of new bonds between integrins, platelet and endothelial cell adhesion molecule-1 (PECAM-1), and their respective ligands.

Neutrophil Rolling, Spreading, and Migration

Near sites of extravascular bacterial infections, neutrophils first tether to and roll on the endothelial surface of venules through the interactions of selectins with cell-surface carbohydrate ligands (Fig. 16–3). Neutrophil rolling on the endothelium occurs under shear forces, just as platelets adhere to subendothelial matrix under shear forces, although the shear flow in postcapillary venules is lower than that in arteries. Rolling requires a balance between the formation of selectin–ligand bonds at the leading edge of the cell and the dissociation of bonds at the trailing edge of the cell. Shear forces affect the lifetimes of selectin–ligand bonds; lower forces prolong lifetimes (catch bonds), whereas higher forces shorten lifetimes (slip bonds). Catch bonds help explain why a minimum shear force is required to support leukocyte rolling, particularly through L-selectin. Just as the initial adhesion to vWF does not require prior activation of platelets, selectin-mediated rolling does not require prior activation of neutrophils. Instead, locally generated inflammatory mediators induce

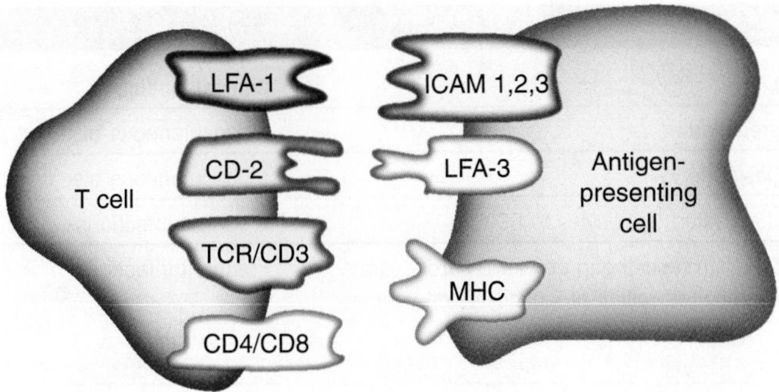

Figure 16–4 Adhesion between T lymphocytes and antigen-presenting cells. The initial contact is mediated by the T-cell receptor (TCR), or CD3, which binds with low affinity but high specificity to a specific antigen presented by a major histocompatibility complex (MHC) molecule. Additional contacts, also of low affinity, are between CD4 (on helper cells) or CD8 (on cytotoxic cells) and MHC, and between CD2 and leukocyte function-associated antigen-3 (LFA-3). These interactions signal the T cell to increase transiently the affinity of the β_2 integrin LFA-1 for the immunoglobulin-like molecules intercellular adhesion molecules ICAM-1, -2, and -3 on the antigen-presenting cell. These bonds strengthen adhesion and transduce further signals to the T cell that cause proliferation and cytokine secretion. Not shown is the redistribution of these adhesion molecules into different regions of the contact zone as adhesion strengthens. Additional signals result from binding of β_1 integrins on the T cell to adhesive proteins in the extracellular matrix.

expression of E- or P-selectin on the endothelial cell surface. The requirement for activation of endothelial cells rather than leukocytes allows the latter to adhere to vessels only at the site of vessel inflammation. Once situated on the vessel wall through selectin-mediated contacts, however, the neutrophils become exposed to activators such as platelet-activating factor, a phospholipid signaling molecule, and interleukin-8, a potent chemoattractant, both of which are presented on the surface of activated endothelial cells. These signals cooperate with others directed by engagement of selectin ligands. Neutrophil activation increases the affinity of β_2 integrins for immunoglobulin counterreceptors on the endothelial cell surface such as ICAM-1. Although flowing cells cannot form these bonds, neutrophils rolling on selectins can do so because of their slower velocities. The integrin-ICAM interactions further slow rolling and then arrest the cells on the endothelium. The leukocytes then migrate, presumably because of disengagement of integrin-ICAM bonds and redistribution of integrins to the leading edge of the cell, where new bonds form. Interactions of leukocytes with JAMs and PECAM-1 in interendothelial cell junctions facilitate transendothelial migration of the neutrophils into the underlying tissues. Adhesion of leukocytes to the endothelium disrupts cytoskeletal tethers to the endothelial cadherins; this disruption leads to dissociation of homotypical cadherin interactions that normally prevent passage of leukocytes. Both the integrin- and the PECAM-1-mediated adhesive events may signal cytoskeletal redistributions in leukocytes that enhance migration toward chemotactic molecules released in the vicinity of the infection. Once leukocytes enter in the tissues, integrin recognition of extracellular matrix protein ligands may trigger secretion of proteolytic enzymes and production of superoxide anions, both required for optimal bactericidal function.

Adhesion of T Lymphocytes to Antigen-Presenting Cells

The initial engagement of T lymphocytes with antigen-presenting cells requires that the T-cell receptor (CD3) recognize antigen presented by the polymorphic domain of MHC molecules (Fig. 16–4). Subsequent interactions include the binding of CD8 or CD4 to MHC class I or II molecules, respectively, plus the binding of CD2 to LFA-3. These molecular contacts are all of low affinity but are highly specific, because they first require specific antigen presentation to the appropriate T cell. The combination of these binding events triggers signals that increase the affinity of LFA-1 ($\alpha_L\beta_2$), a β_2 integrin on T cells, for its ligand, ICAM-1 on antigen-presenting cells, strengthening adhesion. After ICAM-1 binds to LFA-1, the T cell is further activated, resulting in cytokine secretion and proliferation. Additional signaling is mediated through binding of other integrins on T cells to protein ligands in the extracellular matrix.

The first principle of these three responses is that the initial adhesive event, although relatively limited, is highly specific. Thus, platelets bind to exposed subendothelial matrix, neutrophils bind to endothelium near the site of infection, and T cells bind to cells presenting specific antigen. The second principle is that subsequent activation events strengthen cell adhesion and lead to further responses such as secretion, fibrin formation, cellular migration and protein proliferation, or release of cytotoxic mediators. Activation often results from cooperative signaling by soluble agonists and by binding of ligands to adhesion receptors. Costimulation by multiple signals can amplify, and provide specificity to, cellular responses by mechanisms not always feasible for individual mediators. Thus, adhesion and cell signaling are highly interrelated processes.

The process of reversing cell adhesion, although less well understood, is equally important for the control of cell behavior. Some molecules such as the selectins can be proteolytically cleaved or internalized. The activation-induced increases in affinity of integrins and CD44 for their ligands are generally transient, but the mechanisms for return to the inactive conformation are obscure.

ALTERED EXPRESSION OF ADHESION MOLECULES

The highly regulated nature of adhesive events by hematopoietic cells suggests that defects in, or excessive expression of, adhesion molecules may contribute to the pathogenesis of disease. A variety of clinical observations support this hypothesis.

Genetic Deficiencies in Adhesion Molecules

Genetic deficiencies in platelet adhesion receptors such as the GPIb complex (as in Bernard–Soulier syndrome) and the $\alpha_{IIb}\beta_3$ integrin (as in Glanzmann thrombasthenia) result in hemorrhagic symptoms similar to those in patients with thrombocytopenia. Genetic deficiencies in the leukocyte β_2 integrins (as in leukocyte adhesion deficiency-1) are associated with frequent severe bacterial infections and a failure of neutrophils to enter the infected tissues. Similar symptoms are seen in patients with a congenital defect in fucose metabolism that prevents synthesis of the carbohydrate ligands for selectins (leukocyte adhesion deficiency-2) (Table 16–6).

Dysregulated Expression of Adhesion Molecules

Inappropriate expression of adhesion molecules has been implicated in thrombotic and inflammatory disorders and in tumor metastasis. For example, erythrocytes from patients with sickle cell anemia adhere to each other, to leukocytes, and to the endothelium, contributing to vaso-occlusive crises. These adhesive events may reflect, in part, the expression of integrins and selectin ligands not normally found on mature erythrocytes. Inappropriate adhesion and activation of platelets on exposed atherosclerotic plaques may contribute to thrombosis. Dysregulated expression of selectins on the endothelium of ischemic blood vessels during myocardial infarction or shock may contribute to neutrophil-mediated tissue necrosis following reperfusion of the vessel. Mediators released while the neutrophils are adherent in the reperfused vessels may activate integrin function, strengthening adhesion and generating further signals that release destructive oxygen radicals and proteases within the vasculature.

Table 16–6 Genetic Deficiencies in Adhesion Molecules

Molecule	Disease	Laboratory Finding(s)	Clinical Finding
$\alpha_{IIb}\beta_3$	Glanzmann thrombasthenia	Impaired platelet aggregation	Mucocutaneous bleeding
GPIb/IX/V	Bernard–Soulier syndrome	Impaired platelet adhesion to vWF	Mucocutaneous bleeding
β2 integrins	Leukocyte adhesion deficiency-1	Impaired adhesion of activated leukocytes to EC	Frequent infections
Selectin ligands	Leukocyte adhesion deficiency-2	Impaired fucose metabolism resulting in defective carbohydrate ligands for selectins, impaired rolling of leukocytes on venules	Frequent infections

For abbreviations, see Table 16–1 footnote.

Finally, malignant cells appear to utilize molecules normally used for adhesion of blood cells to promote metastatic spread through interactions with platelets, endothelial cells, and extravascular matrix.

These examples underscore the importance of proper regulation of adhesion molecule expression in the physiology of blood cells.

SUGGESTED READINGS

Berndt MC, Shen Y, Dopheide SM, et al: The vascular biology of the glycoprotein Ib-IX-V complex. Thromb Haemost 86:178, 2001.

Bunting M, Harris ES, McIntyre TM, et al: Leukocyte adhesion deficiency syndromes: Adhesion and tethering defects involving β_2 integrins and selectin ligands. Curr Opin Hematol 9:30, 2002.

Cambi A, Koopman M, Figdor CG: How C-type lectins detect pathogens. Cell Microbiol 7:481, 2005.

Carman CV, Springer TA: Integrin avidity regulation: Are changes in affinity and conformation underemphasized? Curr Opin Cell Biol 15:547, 2003.

Chen J, Lopez JA: Interactions of platelets with subendothelium and endothelium. Microcirculation 12:235, 2005.

Crocker PR: Siglecs in innate immunity. Curr Opin Pharmacol 5:431, 2005.

Dustin ML: A dynamic view of the immunological synapse. Semin Immunol 17:400, 2005.

Ginsberg MH, Partridge A, Shattil SJ: Integrin regulation. Curr Opin Cell Biol 17:509, 2005.

Koppel EA, van Gisbergen KP, Geijtenbeek TB, van Kooyk Y: Distinct functions of DC-SIGN and its homologues L-SIGN (DC-SIGNR) and mSIGNR1 in pathogen recognition and immune regulation. Cell Microbiol 7:157, 2005.

Ley K: Integration of inflammatory signals by rolling neutrophils. Immunol Rev 186:8, 2002.

Ley K, Kansas GS: Selectins in T cell recruitment to non-lymphoid tissues and sites of inflammation. Nat Rev Immunol 4:325, 2004.

McEver RP: Adhesive interactions of leukocytes, platelets, and the vessel wall during hemostasis and inflammation. Thromb Haemost 86:746, 2001.

Nourshargh S, Krombach F, Dejana E: The role of JAM-A and PECAM-1 in modulating leukocyte infiltration in inflamed and ischemic tissues. J Leukoc Biol 80:714, 2006.

Ponta H, Sherman L, Herrlich PA: CD44: From adhesion molecules to signalling regulators. Nat Rev Mol Cell Biol 4:33, 2003.

Ruggeri ZM: Platelets in atherothrombosis. Nat Med 8:1227, 2002.

Sperandio M: Selectins and glycosyltransferases in leukocyte rolling in vivo. FEBS J 273:4377, 2006.

Springer TA, Wang JH: The three-dimensional structure of integrins and their ligands, and conformational regulation of cell adhesion. Adv Protein Chem 68:29, 2004.

Tailor A, Cooper D, Granger DN: Platelet-vessel wall interactions in the microcirculation. Microcirculation 12:275, 2005.

Vestweber D: Regulation of endothelial cell contacts during leukocyte extravasation. Curr Opin Cell Biol 14:587, 2002.

CHAPTER 17

CELL TRAFFICKING AND CHEMOKINES

Steffen Massberg, Ulrich H. von Andrian, and Leslie E. Silberstein

The mammalian immune system is designed to prevent infection while preserving self-tolerance and restraining immune-mediated pathology. To accomplish these tasks it involves billions of motile cells that continually travel throughout the body. The migration profiles vary substantially among individual types of leukocytes. Indeed, the distinct traffic patterns of different leukocyte subsets are not random but a precisely organized process that is essential for proper immune surveillance and serves to maximize the likelihood that leukocytes will encounter and eliminate or contain foreign pathogens. During differentiation in the bone marrow (innate immune cells and B cells) or thymus (naïve T cells) leukocytes are equipped with characteristic repertoires of traffic molecules that enable and restrict their migration to certain microenvironments and tissues. In general, naïve lymphocytes are poorly responsive to inflammatory signals but migrate efficiently to lymphoid organs, whereas innate immune cells and antigen-experienced lymphocytes can respond to inflammation-induced traffic cues, although at least some subsets also travel to noninflamed target tissues.[1,2] Notably, not only mature leukocytes migrate to tissues and enter the circulation or lymphatic systems; hematopoietic stem and progenitor cells also travel continuously throughout the body.[3–6]

The characteristic trafficking of each leukocyte subset is coordinated by adhesion molecules, expressed on leukocytes and endothelial cells (see Chapter 15) and through chemokines and chemokine receptors. This chapter first discusses chemokines as master navigators of leukocyte trafficking and then focuses on the specific trafficking pathways on the basis of the type of migration involved.

CHEMOKINES IN CONTROL OF LEUKOCYTE TRAFFICKING

Chemokines are the critical messengers in the complex cellular communication network used by the immune system. At least 47 chemokines have been identified to date (Table 17–1).[7–11] The two major subclasses of chemokines are distinguished as CC- or CXC-chemokines, depending on the arrangement of two canonical cystein residues within the conserved chemokine motif, which are either adjacent (CC) or separated by a single amino acid (CXC). The XC (XCL1 and XCL2) and CX3C chemokines (CX3CL1) constitute two additional structural subfamilies of chemokines. Most chemokines are secreted proteins of 67 to 127 amino acids, only CXCL16 and CX3CL1 possess a transmembrane domain, but also exist in a cleaved soluble form. Traditionally, chemokines were grouped into functional subfamilies termed *inflammatory* chemokines, which are induced by inflammatory signals and control the recruitment of effector leukocytes in infection, inflammation, tissue injury and malignancies; and *homeostatic* chemokines, which navigate leukocytes during hematopoiesis in the bone marrow and thymus, during initiation of adaptive immune responses in secondary lymphoid organs and in immune surveillance of healthy peripheral tissues (eg, CCL19, CCL21, or CXCL12). However, many chemokines cannot be assigned unambiguously to one of these two categories and are, therefore, referred to as dual-function chemokines (eg, CXCL16, CXCL9).

Chemokine messages are decoded through specific cell-surface G protein-coupled receptors (GPCRs) with seven transmembrane domains.[12] The human chemokine receptor repertoire identified at present consists of 20 different GPCRs (Table 17–2).[13] The tremendous specificity and plasticity observed in leukocyte migration and anatomic distribution is largely owed to this system, because each leukocyte subset expresses a distinct repertoire of chemokine receptors, and each chemokine receptor can bind different sets of chemokines with various binding affinities.[14,15] Chemokine receptors function as allosteric molecular relays, where chemokine binding to the extracellular portion modifies the tertiary structure of the receptor. This allows the intracellular domain of the engaged receptor to bind to and activate heterotrimeric G proteins. In response, the activated G proteins exchange guanosine diphosphate (GDP) for guanosine triphosphate (GTP) and in the process, dissociate into Gα and Gβγ subunits. The dissociated Gβγ subunits mediate most chemokine-induced signals by activating different phosphoinositide-3-kinase (PI3K) isoforms, which in turn lead to the formation of phosphatidyl-3,4,5-triphosphate (PIP_3). PI3K and its product PIP_3 then translocate to the pseudopod at the leading edge of migrating leukocytes, where they colocalize with the small GTPase Rac.[16,17] PIP_3 activates Rac through specific guanine nucleotide exchange factors (GEFs).[18,19] Rac in turn acts through the downstream effectors p21-activated kinase (PAK) and the Wiskott–Aldrich Syndrome protein (WASP) homologue WAVE, that stimulate actin-related protein (Arp) 2/3. Together, this process induces focal polymerization, required for the development and forward extension of the pseudopod, a critical step in leukocyte chemotaxis.[20] The importance of PI3K-dependent signaling for leukocyte chemotaxis is evidenced by the lack of migration of myeloid leukocytes to chemokines in mice lacking PI3Kγ.[21] Notably though, distinct signaling pathways or at least other PI3K isoforms appear to be involved in the trafficking of lymphocytes, because lymphocyte chemotaxis is not affected in PI3Kγ-deficient mice,[21,22] but depends on the Rac guanine exchange factor DOCK2.[23]

Different pathways have been identified that can terminate chemokine signaling through GPCRs. The Gα subunit possesses an intrinsic GTPase activity to hydrolyze GTP. In a negative feedback loop this GTPase activity allows the Gα subunits to reassociate with the Gβγ subunits, thereby restoring the heterotrimeric G protein to its inactive state. In addition, another class of molecules, known as regulators of G protein signaling (RGS), also modulates signaling through chemokine GPCRs. RGS are a large and diverse protein family initially identified as GTPase-activating proteins (GAPs) of heterotrimeric G-protein Gα subunits.[24] At least some RGS can also influence Gα activity through either effector antagonism by competing with effector molecules for GTP-bound Gα subunits or by acting as guanine nucleotide dissociation inhibitors (GDIs). To date, over three dozen genes have been identified within the human genome that encode proteins containing an RGS or RGS-like domain. Additional fine-tuning of chemokine communication is achieved by cleavage and inactivation of chemokines and/or chemokine receptors, further adding to the plasticity of the chemokine system.

Proteases, in particular CD26, a surface glycoprotein with intrinsic dipeptidyl peptidase IV enzyme activity, as well as matrix metalloproteases (MMPs), have recently been implicated in the control of chemokine-mediated navigation of leukocyte trafficking.[25] MMPs are a family of more than 20 enzymes with important functions in matrix degradation. They also act on chemokines to regulate varied aspects

Table 17–1 Chemokines and Chemokine Receptors[8,11,36]

Chemokine	Chemokine Receptor*
CC Family	
CCL1 (I309)	CCR8[a]
CCL2 (MCP-1)	CCR2[a], DARC/Duffy[d], D6[d]
CCL3 (MIP-1α)	CCR1[a], CCR5[a], D6[d]
CCL3L1 (MIP-1αP)	CCR1[a], CCR3[a], CCR5[a], D6[d]
CCL4 (MIP-1β)	CCR5[a], D6[d]
CCL4L1 (MIP-1β2)	CCR5[a], D6[d]
CCL5 (RANTES)	CCR1[a], CCR3[a], CCR5[a], DARC/Duffy[d], D6[d]
CCL7 (MCP-3)	CCR1[a], CCR2[a], CCR3[a], CCR5[b], D6[d]
CCL8 (MCP-2)	CCR1[a], CCR2[a], CCR3[a], CCR5[a], D6[d]
CCL11 (eotaxin)	CCR2[b], CCR3[a], CCR5[a], CXCR3A[c], CXCR3B[c], DARC/Duffy[d], D6[d]
CCL13 (MCP-4)	CCR1[a], CCR2[a], CCR3[a], DARC/Duffy[d], D6[d]
CCL14 (HCC1)	CCR1[a], CCR5[a], DARC/Duffy[d], D6[d]
CCL15 (HCC2, MIP-1δ)	CCR1[a], CCR3[a]
CCL16 (HCC4)	CCR1[a], CCR2[a], CCR5[a]
CCL17 (TARC)	CCR4[a], DARC/Duffy[d], D6[d]
CCL18 (PARC)	CCR3[b]
CCL19 (ELC)	CCR7[a], CCX-CKR[d]
CCL20 (MIP-3 β, LARC)	CCR6[a]
CCL21 (SLC)	CCR7[a], CCX-CKR[d]
CCL22 (MDC)	CCR4[a], D6[d]
CCL23 (MPIF-1, SCYA23)	CCR1[a]
CCL24 (eotaxin-2)	CCR3[a]
CCL25 (TECK)	CCR9[a], CCX-CKR[d]
CCL26 (eotaxin-3)	CCR3[a], CCR2[b]
CCL27 (CTACK)	CCR10[a]
CCL28 (MEC)	CCR3[a], CCR10[a]
CXC Family	
CXCL1 (GROα)	CXCR2[a], DARC/Duffy[d]
CXCL2 (GROβ)	CXCR2[a], DARC/Duffy[d]
CXCL3 (GROγ)	CXCR2[a], DARC/Duffy[d]
CXCL4 (PF4)	CXCR3B[a]
CXCL5 (ENA-78)	CXCR2[a]
CXCL6 (GCP2)	CXCR1[a], CXCR2[a]
CXCL7 (NAP-2)	CXCR2[a], DARC/Duffy[d]
CXCL8 (interleukin-8)	CXCR1[a], CXCR2[a], DARC/Duffy[d]
CXCL9 (MIG)	CXCR3A[a], CXCR3B[a], CCR3[b]
CXCL10 (IP-10)	CXCR3A[a], CXCR3B[a], CCR3[b]
CXCL11 (I-TAC)	CXCR3A[a], CXCR3B[a], CXCR7, CCR3[b]
CXCL12 (SDF-1)	CXCR4[a], CXCR7[a]
CXCL13 (BCA-1)	CXCR5[a], CCX-CKR[d]
CXCL14 (BRAK)	?
CXCL16 (SR-PSOX)	CXCR6[a]
CX_3C Familiy	
CX3CL1 (fractalkine)	CX3CR[a]1
XC Family	
XCL1 (lymphotactin, SCM-1α)	XCR1[a]
XCL2 (SCM-1β)	XCR1[a]

[a]agonistic, [b]antagonistic interaction, [c]nonagonist–nonantagonistic interaction, [d]"atypical" interaction, signal transduction as yet undefined.

of inflammation and immunity. In particular, MCPs and CXCL12 [stromal cell-derived factor-1 (SDF-1)] are cleaved and inactivated by several MMPs, including MMP-2. Apart from MMPs, proteases stored in neutrophil granules, in particular cathepsin G and elastase, inactivate chemokines, such as SDF-1 and its receptor CXCR4, that regulate not only the migration of mature leukocytes but also the mobilization and homing of immature hematopoietic stem cells.[26,27] Hence, proteases by means of their chemokine-modifying properties must be regarded as integral components in the control of trafficking of mature leukocytes and their precursors.

In general, leukocyte trafficking can be classified into three distinct patterns of migration: (a) entry into tissues from the circulation; (b) migration within tissues; and (c) exit from tissues. Each of these classes of leukocyte trafficking will be discussed in the following sections.

LEUKOCYTE ENTRY INTO TISSUES

Leukocytes must engage several sequential adhesion steps to be able to leave the circulation and enter target tissues.[2,28–30] Initially, tethers are formed between leukocytes and endothelial cells by adhesion receptors that are characterized by the ability to rapidly bind their ligands with high tensile strength. The most important initiators of leukocyte tethering are selectins, expressed on leukocytes (L-selectin), endothelial cells (E- and P-selectin), and platelets (P-selectin). The bonds formed between selectins and their major ligands, sialomucins decorated with oligosaccharides related to sialyl-Lewis^x, including P-selectin glycoprotein ligand (PSGL)-1 and peripheral-node addressin (PNAd), are transient and do not allow permanent arrest of leukocytes. Selectin-mediated adhesive bonds continuously dissociate at the cell's upstream end whereas new bonds form downstream, resulting in the characteristic rolling motion of tethered leukocytes. To undergo firm adhesion the rolling cell must engage additional adhesion receptors that belong to the integrin family, including CD11a/CD18a (LFA-1) and the α4 integrins, α4β1 and α4β7.

Whereas selectins are constitutively active, integrins need to be activated to promote permanent adhesion. Integrin activation is induced on leukocytes by chemoattractant signals that trigger a reversible change in integrin conformation (leading to enhanced ligand-binding affinity) or in integrin clustering (enhancing avidity), or both. Some (but not all) chemokines presented on the luminal surface of microvascular endothelial cells can trigger rapid integrin activation and efficiently induce leukocyte arrest. Chemokines signal primarily through the $G\alpha_i$ subfamily of G proteins, which can be inhibited by pertussis toxin (PTX). Consequently, intravital microscopy studies have shown that lymphocytes treated with PTX initiate normal tethering and rolling interactions in high endothelial venules in lymph nodes (LN) and Peyer patches (PP), but PTX-treated cells are unable to undergo integrin-dependent firm arrest. Thus, activation of integrins is a mandatory step required to occur before integrins can bind to their ligands. Once arrested, the adherent leukocytes can migrate across the vascular wall and enter their target tissue. Two routes of leukocyte diapedesis have been described so far: a paracellular route that dominates most extravasation processes and a transcellular route, reported for neutrophils and some T cells.[31] Both routes involve the action of apical and junctional endothelial intercellular adhesion molecule-1 (ICAM-1) and, at least in some settings, also vascular cell adhesion molecule-1 (VCAM-1). In inflammatory conditions, additional junctional endothelial ligands such as PECAM-1, CD99, and junctional adhesion molecule (JAMs) can contribute to leukocyte diapedesis.[32,33]

All consecutive steps, (a) leukocyte tethering and rolling, (b) exposure to a chemotactic stimulus, (c) firm arrest, and (d) diapedesis are essential for leukocytes to enter lymphoid tissues and to migrate to sites of inflammation. Correspondingly, in patients suffering from leukocyte adhesion deficiency syndrome, a genetic defect either in β2 integrins (type 1) or in fucosylated selectin ligands (type 2), neutrophils cannot stop or roll, respectively; this syndrome is characterized by marked leukocytosis and frequent and severe soft-tissue infections.[34,35]

Chemokine Control of Lymphocyte Homing to Secondary Lymphoid Organs

Migration of blood-borne lymphocytes to secondary lymphoid organs is the best-characterized example of leukocyte trafficking from the circulation into distinct target tissues.[2,36,37] Lymphocytes constantly survey secondary lymphoid organs, which include the spleen, tonsils,

Table 17–2 Chemokines and Chemokine Receptors[8,11,37]

Receptor	Chemokine Ligands	Cell Types	Disease Association
CC Family			
CCR1	CCL3, CCL3L1, CCL5, CCL7, CCL8, CCL13, CCL14, CCL15, CCL16, CCL23	T cells, monocytes, eosinophils, basophils	Rheumatoid arthritis, multiple sclerosis, kidney disease, cancer
CCR2	CCL2, CCL7, CCL8, CCL11, CCL13, CCL16, CCL26	Monocytes, dendritic cells (immature), memory T cells	Atherosclerosis, rheumatoid arthritis, multiple sclerosis, diabetes mellitus type 2, obesity, asthma
CCR3	CCL3L1, CCL5, CCL7, CCL8, CCL11, CCL13, CCL15, CCL18, CCL24, CCL26, CCL28, CXCL9, CXCL10, CXCL11	Eosinophils, basophils, mast cells, Th2, platelets	Allergic asthma and rhinitis
CCR4	CCL17, CCL22	T cells (Th2), dendritic cells (mature), basophils, macrophages, platelets	Parasitic infection, graft rejection, asthma, skin disease
CCR5	CCL3, CCL3L1, CCL4, CCL4L1, CCL5, CCL7, CCL8, CCL11, CCL14, CCL16	T cells, monocytes	HIV-1 coreceptor, transplant rejection
CCR6	CCL20	T cells (T regulatory and memory), B cells, dendritic cells	Allergic asthma
CCR7	CCL19, CCL21	T cells, dendritic cells (mature), antigen-experienced B cells	Cancer
CCR8	CCL1	T cells (Th2), dendritic cells	Granuloma formation
CCR9	CCL25	T cells, IgA$^+$ plasma cells	Inflammatory bowel disease
CCR10	CCL27, CCL28	T cells	Skin manifestation of lymphoma
CXC Family			
CXCR1	CXCL6, CXCL8	Neutrophils, monocytes	Chronic obstructive pulmonary disease, inflammatory lung disease, sepsis
CXCR2	CXCL1, CXCL2, CXCL3, CXCL5, CXCL6, CXCL7, CXCL8	Neutrophils, monocytes, microvascular endothelial cells	Chronic obstructive pulmonary disease, inflammatory lung disease, tumor growth/angiogenesis
CXCR3-A	CXCL9, CXCL10, CXCL11	Th1 helper cells, mast cells, mesangial cells	Inflammatory skin disease, multiple sclerosis, transplant rejection
CXCR3-B	CXCL4, CXCL9, CXCL10, CXCL11	Microvascular endothelial cells, neoplastic cells	Angiostatic for tumor growth
CXCR4	CXCL12	Widely expressed	HIV-1 coreceptor, tumor metastasis
CXCR5	CXCL13	B cells, follicular helper T cells (T_{FH})	Cancer?
CXCR6	CXCL16	CD8$^+$ T cells, natural killer cells, memory CD4$^+$ T cells	Inflammatory liver disease, atherosclerosis
CXCR7	CXCL11, CXCL12	tumor cell lines, activated endothelial cells, murine fetal liver cells	Cancer?
CX$_3$C Familiy			
CX$_3$CR1	CX3CL1	Macrophages, endothelial cells, smooth-muscle cells	Atherosclerosis
XC Family			
XCR1	XCL1, XCL2	T cells, natural killer cells	Rheumatoid arthritis, IgA nephropathy
Atypical Chemokine Receptors			
CCX-CKR	CCL19, CCL21, CCL25, CXCL13	Widely expressed in tissues, immature dendritic cells	Sarcoidosis?
D6	CCL2, CCL3, CCL3L1, CCL4, CCL4L1, CCL5, CCL7, CCL8, CCL11, CCL12, CCL13, CCL14, CCL17, CCL22	Lymphatic endothelial cells in afferent lymphatics from skin, gut, lung	Experimental autoimmune encephalomyelitis, opposing effects on allergic inflammation and airway reactivity
DARC/Duffy	CCL2, CCL5, CCL11, CCL13, CCL14, CCL17, CXCL1, CXCL2, CXCL3, CXCL7, CXCL8	Vascular endothelial cells, high endothelial venules, erythrocytes	Cancer?

GCP, granulocyte chemotactic protein; GRO, growth-regulated oncogene; ENA, epithelial-cell-derived neutrophil-activating peptide; MIG, monokine induced by interferon-γ; IP-10, interferon-inducible protein 10; I-TAC, interferon-inducible T cell alpha chemoattractant; SDF-1, stromal cell-derived factor-1; BCA-1, B cell chemoattractant 1; SR-PSOX, scavenger receptor for phosphatidylserine-containing oxidized lipids; MIP, macrophage inflammatory protein; MCP, monocyte chemoattractant protein; HCC, hemofiltrate chemokine; TARC thymus and activation-regulated chemokine; MDC, macrophage-derived chemokine; LARC, liver and activation-regulated chemokine; ELC, Epstein–Barr virus-induced molecule 1 ligand chemokine; SLC, secondary lymphoid-tissue chemokine; TECK, thymus-expressed chemokine; CTACK, cutaneous T cell-attracting chemokine; MEC, mammary-enriched chemokine.

appendix, Peyer patches (PPs), and lymph nodes (LNs), to determine whether an antigen is present that poses a threat to the body. This information is provided to T cells by dendritic cells, which collect and trap antigen and then present it to T cells together with costimulatory molecules and cytokines. Mature dendritic cells that have captured antigen in peripheral tissues[38] and some memory cells[39] reach the LNs through afferent lymph vessels. In contrast, circulating T and B lymphocytes gain access to LN and PP through specialized postcapillary microvessels lined with cuboid endothelial cells that are known as *high endothelial venules* (HEV).[40–45] HEV in different secondary lymphoid organs express distinct patterns of trafficking molecules to serve as tethering platforms for defined subsets of lymphocytes. For example, HEV in LN express peripheral node addressin (PNAd), whereas HEV in PP express mucosal addressin-cell adhesion molecule (MAdCAM-1). Other mucosa-associated lymphoid organs, such as mesenteric LNs, express both MAdCAM-1 and PNAd. Although T and B lymphocytes are recruited by similar multistep cascades to home to secondary lymphoid organs, the role of individual traffic molecules is not necessarily identical, even when both subsets interact with the same microvessel.[2,36]

The first step in the homing cascade in LNs is mediated by L-selectin/CD62L expressed on all lymphocytes, except effector/memory cells. PNAd, an O-linked sulfated core 1 carbohydrate moiety that is exclusively found in HEV, is the major endothelial L-selectin ligand.[46,47] Binding of L-selectin to PNAd initiates lymphocyte rolling in HEV and slows down and marginates the free-flowing lymphocytes.[2,28–30] Although the L-selectin–PNAd interaction is required, it is not by itself sufficient to promote firm leukocyte adhesion. The subsequent firm arrest of rolling T and B lymphocytes is mediated by the integrin CD11a/CD18 (LFA-1), which binds intercellular adhesion molecules (ICAM), in particular ICAM-1 and ICAM-2, on high endothelial cells.[44] Like most integrins, LFA-1 needs to be activated before it can promote firm arrest of lymphocytes. Structural studies of LFA-1 indicate that the heterodimeric molecule is folded like a switchblade when it is in a low-affinity state, but opens to an extended, high-affinity configuration upon activation.[48,49]

Chemokines that are present in the lumen of HEV function as triggers of integrin activation.[50,51] On naïve T cells integrin activation is primarily mediated by CCL21 (also called SLC, TCA4, exodus 2 or 6-C-kine), which is constitutively expressed and secreted by HEV. The secreted chemokine is noncovalently bound to glycosaminoglycans on the surface of HEV. Here, it activates rolling lymphocytes through binding to CCR7, which is expressed on naive B and T cells. Another CCR7 ligand, CCL19 (also termed ELC or MIP3β), also supports T cell homing to LNs. CCL19 is not expressed by high endothelial cells themselves. However, CCL19 and other chemokines may be released by extravascular cells in LNs or in tissues that discharge lymph to a local LN. Lymph-borne chemokines can be transported to the luminal aspect of HEV. Correspondingly, chemokines, including CCL2, CCL19, and CCL21, injected under the skin of mice accumulate on the luminal surface of the HEV in draining LNs, where they promote integrin activation on rolling leukocytes bearing the cognate receptors.[52–54]

B cells use largely the same traffic molecules as naïve T cells to home to LN. However, B cell–HEV interactions are only moderately affected by the absence of CCR7 or its ligands. Correspondingly, LNs of mice lacking CCR7 contain few T cells, whereas the B cell compartment (and the memory T cell compartment) is less affected.[55,56] Similar observations were made in *plt/plt* mice, which have a spontaneous genetic defect resulting in deletion of CCL19 and the HEV-expressed form of CCL21 (mice, unlike humans, have a second *ccl21* gene that is only expressed in lymph vessels), demonstrating that B cells are not absolutely dependent on CCR7 to adhere to HEV.[45] In fact, rolling B cells can be induced to arrest in HEVs by either CCR7 agonists or by CXCL12 (also called stromal cell-derived factor [SDF-1]α), the ligand for CXCR4.[57] An additional chemokine pathway involving CXCL13 (also called BLC) and its receptor CXCR5 has also been implicated in B cell homing to secondary lymphoid tissues.[58] Of note, although B cells encounter several distinct integrin-activation signals in HEV, B cell homing to LNs is nonetheless less efficient than that of T cells. A likely reason is that the B cells express only approximately half the number of L-selectin molecules expressed on T cells, which greatly affects their ability to initiate the adhesion cascade in HEV.[59,60]

The requirement for a sequence of at least three distinct molecular steps that each leukocyte must undergo to arrest within microvessels explains why only certain leukocyte subsets gain access to lymphoid tissues, whereas others are excluded. Granulocytes, for example, express LFA-1 and L-selectin but not CCR7. Consequently, although granulocytes can roll in HEV (via L-selectin), these leukocytes do not perceive an integrin-activating stimulus and, therefore, fail to accumulate in LNs or PPs. Likewise, mature dendritic cells express CCR7 and CD11a/CD18, but not L-selectin. Because these cells are thus incapable of rolling in HEV, they fail to home to noninflamed LNs from the blood (although mature dendritic cells readily access LNs via afferent lymph). Hence, the GPCR-mediated integration activation step is critical, for imparting specificity to the process of lymphocyte homing to LNs.

In HEVs of PPs, similar homing mechanisms are encountered as described above for LNs. However, the levels of L-selectin ligands (which are immunologically distinct from PNAd) expressed by HEV in PPs are considerably lower when compared with that in LNs.[61,62] As a result, L-selectin itself is not sufficient to initiate a successful homing cascade for most lymphocytes in PPs.[61] Indeed, HEV in PPs (and also in mucosa-associated LNs) additionally express MAdCAM-1, a ligand for the α4β7 integrin.[62–64] The α4β7 heterodimer, which comprises an α4 integrin chain (CD49d) linked to the β7 integrin chain, is expressed at low levels by naïve T and B cells and is required for the successful homing of these cells in PP HEV.[61,64] Following formation of an initial L-selectin-dependent tether, the α4β7-MAdCAM-1 pathway stabilizes and slows the rolling lymphocytes without requiring chemokine activation. Once a chemokine signal has been transmitted, both α4β7 and LFA-1 become activated and jointly mediate firm arrest.[61]

Of note, α4β7 is strongly upregulated on gut-homing effector or memory lymphocytes but completely absent on skin-homing memory T and B cells; these differential levels of α4β7 integrin expression allow certain antigen-experienced lymphocyte subsets to acquire tissue selectivity.[65] The mechanisms underlying this specificity and plasticity of lymphocyte homing will be addressed in the next section. Like in LNs, chemokines are essentially involved in promoting integrin activation and allowing firm lymphocyte arrest in HEV of PP. Thus, CXCR4, CXCR5, and CCR7 have been implicated in B cell homing, whereas CCR7 seems exclusively responsible for T cell homing. Interestingly, although T and B cells are recruited across the same HEV in LNs, there is segmental segregation of T and B cell recruitment in PPs. HEV supporting B cell accumulation in PPs are concentrated in or near B follicles and present CXCL13, but not CCL21, whereas T cells preferentially accumulate in interfollicular HEV (ie, within the T cell area), which express high levels of CCL21 but not CXCL13.

Trafficking of Leukocytes From Blood Into Nonlymphoid Tissues

As outlined in the above section, naïve lymphocytes migrate most efficiently to secondary lymphoid organs from which innate immune cells are excluded. However, both innate immune cells and subsets of lymphocytes can respond to inflammatory and/or activation signals by modulating the expression and/or activity of traffic molecules in a way that allows them to migrate to nonlymphoid tissues.[1] For example, in response to an inflammatory stimulus, granulocytes, including neutrophils, eosinophils, and basophils, are rapidly recruited to the affected site and provide the first line of defense. Thereafter, additional immune cells, including monocytes, dendritic cells, and effector as well as memory lymphocytes may be recruited. Essentially all of these different recruitment events depend on distinct multistep adhesion cascades.

Many of the inflammation-seeking traffic molecules required for access to nonlymphoid tissues are shared by the different leukocyte subsets. The key receptors that initiate capture of neutrophils, monocytes, natural killer cells, eosinophils, and effector T and B cells at peripheral sites of injury and inflammation are the three selectins, the leukocyte-expressed L-selectin as well as P- and E-selectin, which are induced on both acutely (and in some settings) chronically stimulated endothelial cells.[66,67] In inflamed gastrointestinal venules, the integrin α4β7 and its ligand MAdCAM-1 contribute to leukocyte recruitment. In addition, leukocyte–leukocyte interactions, mediated through PSGL-1 and L-selectin, can also support accumulation of immune cells in inflamed tissues.[68] Subsequent firm arrest of leukocytes in nonlymphoid tissues involves integrins, including CD11a/CD18 (and its ligand ICAM-1 and possibly also ICAM-2), VLA-4 (and its ligand VCAM-1), as well as Mac-1 (and its ligand ICAM-1). As discussed above for lymphoid tissues, chemoattractants, including chemokines and other GPCR agonists, such as formyl peptides, activated complement fragments (particularly C5a), and lipid mediators (eg, PAF and LTB4), contribute essential integrin-activation signals for leukocytes at sites of inflammation. The molecular diversity and selective action of these different chemoattractants on distinct leukocyte subsets as well as their restricted temporal and spatial expression patterns provide a crucial mechanism for the fine-tuning of cellular immune responses.[29,69]

In most innate immune cells the changes that are induced by activation signals are relatively uniform. In contrast, the migratory properties acquired by T and B lymphocytes in response to activation are diverse, depending on the strength, the quality, and the context of the antigenic stimulus.[65] Specifically, antigen stimulation of naïve lymphocytes results in the generation of effector and memory cells that express specific repertoires of trafficking molecules that guide them back to tissues containing the stimulatory antigen.[70–72] Thus, a cutaneous challenge generates preferentially a skin-tropic memory response, whereas oral stimulation induces preferentially gut-homing effector and memory cells. Recent studies have broadened our understanding of the molecular events that induce the generation of tissue-specific memory cells.

In addition to presenting antigen, dendritic cells in different lymphoid organs are endowed with information indicating the tissue from which the antigen was obtained. Dendritic cells in mucosa-associated lymphoid tissues (unlike those in other lymphoid organs) possess the enzymatic machinery to synthesize retinoic acid (RA) from vitamin A.[73] Exposure of activated T cells to RA induces the expression of gut-homing receptors (ie, α4β7 and CCR9) and suppresses skin-homing molecules.[71,74] In the absence of RA, T cell stimulation induces few or no gut-homing molecules, but instead promotes the expression of P- and E-selectin ligands as well as CCR4, which are needed for homing to the skin. Additionally, when activated T cells are exposed to IL-12 and high levels of vitamin D3, which is physiologically induced by sunlight in the skin, they upregulate CCR10, the receptor for the epidermal chemokine CCL27.[75] This organ-specific information can reprogram and "imprint" the tissue-tropic memory cells as they differentiate from naïve lymphocytes.[72]

Like T cells, B-cell subsets also express homing receptors that permit their selective trafficking to specific tissues. For example, distinct B cell subsets produce the immunoglobulin isotype IgA that is present in secreted body fluids, including tears, breast milk, and mucus. IgA$^+$ B cells are characterized by their expression of CCR10.[76,77] The ligand for CCR10, MEC/CCL28, is expressed predominantly in mucosal tissues that secrete IgA.[78] Hence, CCR10 may function as a homing receptor that allows IgA-secreting B cells to migrate to tissues where IgA is required. A large subset among the IgA-secreting B cells are those in the small intestine, which in addition to CCR10 express the gut-homing receptors α4β7 and CCR9. When naive B cells are activated in the presence of intestinal dendritic cells, they upregulate not only these two traffic receptors but also undergo class-switching to IgA. This imprinting effect is dependent upon RA, which is sufficient to induce gut-homing receptors, but must be combined with dendritic cell-derived IL-5 or IL-6 to promote IgA class-switching.[74] At least 50 additional subtypes of lymphocytes have been characterized in human blood and it is likely that multiple similar associations between homing receptors, immunological effector function, and tissue specificity will be revealed in future.

Migration of Hematopoietic Stem Cells to the Bone Marrow

The bone marrow (BM) is the principal site of hematopoiesis in the adult body. Correspondingly, most hematopoietic stem cells (HSCs) are lodged in the BM cavity. Within the BM, maintenance of HSCs and regulation of their self-renewal and differentiation is thought to depend on the specific microenvironment, which has historically been termed *stem cell niche*.[79] The central role of stem cell niches for HSC function has been recognized with the discovery that *Sl/Sl*^{d} (steel-Dickie) mice bearing a mutation in the gene encoding membrane-bound stem-cell factor (SCF, also known as KIT ligand) show failure of bone marrow HSC maintenance.[80] However, the exact localization as well as the composition of BM HSC niches and the molecular crosstalk that controls the retention of HSC within the niches are subjects of intense ongoing research.[81–84]

Notably though, not all HSCs reside within the BM. In fact, it has been known for almost four decades that a small amount of hematopoietic precursors are also present in peripheral blood.[3–6] Blood-borne HSCs continuously migrate back to the BM cavity, presumably to fill any vacant stem cell niches.[6] Although the exact physiological relevance of blood-borne HSCs remains to be determined, the intrinsic capacity of HSCs to home to the BM compartment is the prerequisite for successful clinical bone marrow and stem cell transplantation.

Homing of HSCs to BM is a rapid process, because intravenously injected murine and human progenitors are quickly cleared from the recipient circulation.[6,85,86] Like mature lymphocytes, HSCs and hematopoietic progenitor cells (HPCs) interact through a multistep adhesion cascade with BM microvessels.[86–92] Initially, HPCs tether and roll along BM microvessels. This process involves α4β1 integrin on HSC/HPC, which binds vascular cell adhesion molecule-1 (VCAM-1), as well as E- and P-selectin on BM sinusoidal endothelial cells, which bind α(1–3)-fucosylated ligands including CD44 and PSGL-1 on the surface of HPCs.[86] The subsequent firm arrest is mediated by activated α4β1 and VCAM-1, which is constitutively expressed in BM sinusoids. In addition to α4β1 integrin, the integrins α4β7, α5β1, and α6β1, as well as CD44, have recently been implicated in HSC homing to the BM.[93–95]

The chemokine CXCL12, the ligand for CXCR4 expressed by most hematopoietic cells including HSCs, is thought to play a pivotal role in BM homing of HSC. BM endothelial cells (in addition to immature osteoblasts and other stromal cells) constitutively express and secrete CXCL12.[89,96,97] However, alternate pathways appear to exist because fetal liver-derived mouse HSCs home to the BM of adult recipients independent of CXCR4,[98] and adult HSCs treated with a CXCR4 antagonist are still able to home sufficiently to the BM.[99] This indicates that HSCs may use different receptors and/or respond to distinct integrin-activation signals. In this context, the recent description of CXCR7, an alternate receptor for CXCL12, may explain some of the seemingly contradictory findings.[100]

Of note, the CXCL12/CXCR4 axis is not only involved in the homing process of HSCs to the BM, but (among others) has also been linked to the retention of HSCs within stem cell niches and to the regulation of the maturation of more committed HPCs (in particular B cell progenitor cells).[27,101,102] Correspondingly, disruption of the CXCL12/CXCR4 pathway leads to premature release of HPCs into the peripheral blood.[103,104] HPCs lacking CXCR4 accumulate in the circulation and fail to undergo normal lymphopoiesis and myelopoiesis, most likely because the cells do not receive the required maturation signals. Interestingly, upregulation of metalloproteinases (see above), which cleave and inactivate CXCR4 and CXCL12, has recently been implicated in HSC mobilization.[105] Mechanisms that modulate the CXCR4/CXCL12 axis are also thought to play a role in the coordinated mobilization of HPCs in response to cytokines that are used for this purpose in clinical practice.[26]

LEUKOCYTE MIGRATION WITHIN TISSUES

Trafficking Patterns of Lymphocytes

After a leukocyte has accessed a tissue, it must migrate to specific interstitial positions. As discussed above, homing typically requires that the blood-borne leukocyte completes a complex tissue- and subset-specific multistep adhesion cascade. One exception to this rule is the spleen, where most blood-borne lymphocytes can leave the circulation even when multiple traffic molecules are inhibited. However, chemokines are essential in all lymphoid organs, including the spleen, to guide the newly arrived lymphocytes to their proper position within the organ.

Multiphoton intravital microscopy was recently used as a tool to decipher the mechanisms that control the extravascular traffic patterns of homed lymphocytes within lymphoid and nonlymphoid tissues.[36,106–110] For example, imaging experiments have shown that T cells that have entered an LN move incessantly within the paracortex (T cell area). Here, they query the resident dendritic cells for the presence of antigens that activate their T cell receptor (TCR). B cells that home to LNs migrate to the more superficial B cell-rich follicles, where they may detect antigens presented by follicular dendritic cells. Activated B cells that encounter antigens then move to the margins of the B- and T-cell zones.[108] Here, they can receive help from antigen-specific CD4 T cells. Analogous specific microenvironments for T and B cells exist in the other lymphoid tissues also.

Migration of T Cells to T Zones Within Secondary Lymphoid Organs

After homing to secondary lymphoid organs, T cells migrate within the T zones. They engage in highly motile ameboid movement (average speed ~12 μm/min) guided by a network of fibroblastic reticular cells (FRCs) and undergo multiple brief encounters with resident dendritic cells.[111–114] As a consequence of this high motility, it has been estimated that every dendritic cell in an LN touches as many as 5000 naïve T cells within 1 hour. When T cells encounter a specific antigen, they progressively decrease their motility, become activated, and form long-lasting stable conjugates with DCs. Finally, antigen-experienced T cells start to proliferate and resume their rapid migration while contacting DC only briefly.[113,115]

The positioning and high motility of T cells in the T-cell area is dependent on CCR7 and its ligands CCL19 and CCL21.[55,56,116,117] Both ligands are abundantly expressed in T zones by radiation-resistant stromal cells. Notably, ectopic expression of CCL21 induces the formation of LN-like structures in the pancreas of mice.[118] The expression of CCL19 and CCL21, but also of CXCL13, which attracts B cells to B cell follicles (see below), by lymphoid stromal cells is strongly dependent on the cytokine lymphotoxin (LT)-$\alpha 1\beta 2$ heterotrimers signaling via lymphotoxin β receptor.[119,120] Correspondingly, mice deficient in lymphotoxin have no morphologically detectable LN or PP.[121]

Positioning of B Cells Within Secondary Lymphoid Organs

Similar to T cells, B cells enter secondary lymphoid organs from the blood to search for their specific antigens. As previously outlined, the homing and entry of B cells into secondary lymphoid organs such as the LN and PP depends on chemokine–receptor interactions that finally result in firm adhesion of integrins on the surface of HEV. This adherence is followed by movement into lymphoid tissue.[57] After entering secondary lymphoid organs the naïve B cells travel to B cell-rich areas, the B cell follicles. This migration depends on the presence of CXCR5 on the surfaces of B cells and the localized expression of CXCL13 by follicular stromal cells.[37] Follicular B cells are also highly motile, migrating in a network of follicular dendritic cells (FDC), a process that is thought to be necessary to ensure optimal surveillance of the FDC for surface-displayed antigen. After a period of random migration within follicules, B cells that have not encountered a cognate antigen return to the circulation via the lymph or, in case of the spleen, via the blood. In contrast, B cells that become stimulated by antigen relocate to the B–T boundary area to solicit help from T cells, which is necessary for further differentiation. To achieve this repositioning, activated B cells rapidly upregulate CCR7. This permits their chemotaxis toward CCR7 ligands expressed in the T cell-rich zones of the secondary lymphoid organs.[108] Real-time imaging has been performed to further characterize the timing of this relocalization process. Antigen-engaged follicular B cells initially reduce their migration velocity upon antigen exposure. Approximately 6 hours later the activated B cells move toward the follicle border with the T cell-rich zone and undergo highly dynamic interactions with helper T cells during the following several days.[108]

In the spleen, a subpopulation of B cells is lodged in the marginal zone (MZ) immediately adjacent to the marginal sinus that surrounds the white pulp cords. The exact extent to which chemokine-induced attraction and adhesion affect the positioning of MZ B cells is still unclear. However, recent studies indicate that the lodgment of B cells in the MZ is dependent upon interactions of $\alpha L\beta 2$ and $\alpha 4\beta 1$ on MZ B cells with their ligands (ICAM-1 and VCAM-1, respectively).[122] As with follicular B cells in LNs, antigen encounter of MZ B cells causes their rapid repositioning to the B–T boundary area. The retention of naïve B cells in the MZ and their relocalization to the B–T boundary area upon antigen encounter is thought to involve signaling through the phospholipid sphingosine-1 phosphate (S1P) and its receptor $S1P_1$.[123]

LEUKOCYTE EXIT FROM TISSUES

Although the coordinated role of adhesion molecules and chemokines governing lymphocyte entry into tissues has been examined in great detail, less is known about the exit of these cells from tissues. The final sections of this chapter discuss examples of emerging research on the diverse mechanisms that regulate exit of distinct leukocyte subsets from tissues.

REPROGRAMMING DENDRITIC CELLS TO EXIT TISSUES TOWARD SECONDARY LYMPHOID ORGANS

Lymphocyte homing remains without consequence unless lymphocytes encounter dendritic cells that present their cognate antigen. Dendritic cells capture and present antigen to T cells more efficiently than any other antigen-presenting cell. In general, two routes of antigen delivery to LNs have been described to date: (a) antigenic material becomes lymph-borne and is taken up by dendritic cells that reside in the LN a priori; (b) antigen is acquired by dendritic cells that reside in peripheral tissues and then transport the material to the draining LN. Dendritic cells constitutively patrol all tissues and engulf microorganisms, dead cells, and cellular debris. In the absence of inflammatory stimuli, the cells remain in an immature state that is only weakly immunogenic and often stimulates T cell tolerance, rather than activation. However, multiple signals associated with infection or tissue damage can induce dendritic cell maturation. Immature dendritic cells express a variety of chemokine receptors, including as CCR1, CCR5, and CCR6, which are believed to result in the constitutive homing of immature dendritic cells into tissues, particularly sites of inflammation where ligands for these receptors are abundant.[1,124,125] After exposure to a maturation stimulus, such as Toll-like receptor agonists (eg, LPS, bacterial lipoproteins, peptidoglycans or CpG dinucleotides), which often originate from infectious pathogens,[126,127] dendritic cells lose CCR1, CCR5, and CCR6, whereas expression of GPCRs for lymphoid chemokines, in particular CCR7 and CXCR4, are upregulated.[128] Lymphatic endothelial cells in peripheral tissues express CCL21, the ligand for CCR7.[129] The loss of chemokine receptors that keep the dendritic cells within the tissue together with the increased expression of CCR7 results in the exit of the mature dendritic cells via the lymphatic drainage system.[55] DC migration into the draining lymphatics probably also requires β2 integrin binding to ICAM-1 expressed by lymphatic endothelial cells. While traveling to the draining LN, dendritic cells upregulate the expression of molecules for efficient antigen presentation and T-cell stimulation, and begin to generate chemokines and other cytokines that allow them to attract and stimulate T cells.

EGRESS OF LYMPHOCYTES FROM SECONDARY LYMPHOID ORGANS

When naive lymphocytes do not encounter antigen on antigen-presenting dendritic cells after a period of random walk, they exit secondary lymphoid organs through efferent lymph vessels or, in case of the spleen, by directly returning to the blood. Several adhesion receptors have been implicated in the egress of lymphocytes into lymphoid sinusoids, including PECAM-1 (CD31), the mannose receptor, which interacts with L-selectin, and common lymphatic endothelial and vascular endothelial receptor 1 (CLEVER-1).[130]

We still have very limited information about the signals that determine the dwell time of lymphocytes in secondary lymphoid organs (approximately 12–24 hours for T cells). However, the recent observation that the egress of both T and B cells from LN can be prevented by the immunosuppressant molecule FTY720 has revealed some of the principal mechanisms underlying lymphocyte egress. FTY720 is a synthetic derivative of myriocin, a metabolite of the fungus *Isaria sinclairii*, which has been used in Chinese traditional medicine. FTY720 induces lymphocyte sequestration in LN and causes profound lymphopenia. In animal models of transplantation and autoimmunity FTY720 causes immunosuppression and it has recently been shown to exert significant therapeutic effects in a placebo-controlled clinical trial of relapsing multiple sclerosis.[131,132] Although lymphocyte sequestration in LN and lymphopenia in response to FTY720 have been reported some time ago, the underlying molecular mechanisms were uncovered only recently.[133] Upon in vivo administration, FTY720 becomes rapidly phosphorylated and then binds to four of the five known sphingosine 1-phosphate (S1P) receptors ($S1P_1$and $S1P_{3-5}$).[37,134,135] Naïve B and T cells express substantial levels of $S1P_1$, and it appears to be this receptor that plays a predominant role in lymphocytes' egress from lymphoid tissues into the efferent lymph vessels. Studies using gene-targeted mice have shown that T lymphocytes deficient in $S1P_1$ cannot exit secondary lymphoid organs (and in case of T cells also the thymus).[136] Reports using FTY720 and $S1P_1$-selective agonists also supported a role for S1P–$S1P_1$ signaling in the regulation of lymphocyte egress from secondary lymphoid organs. Notably, $S1P_1$ receptors not only regulate lymphocyte exit from tissues but also modulate lymphocyte homing capacity.[137]

The sphingolipid S1P is abundant in blood and lymph, whereas low levels of S1P are maintained within lymphoid tissues. This S1P gradient is established by the action of the S1P degrading enzyme S1P lyase.[138] On the basis of these findings, it has been proposed that S1P gradients between blood, lymphoid tissue, and lymph fluid together with cyclical ligand-induced modulation of $S1P_1$ on recirculating lymphocytes regulates lymphocyte egress and determines the lymphoid organ transit time of lymphocytes. Indeed, recent observations support that concept by showing that $S1P_1$ on lymphocytes is downregulated in the blood, upregulated in lymphoid organs, and downregulated again in the lymph.[139] Notably, CD69, which is rapidly induced when T cells become activated, negatively regulates $S1P_1$ and thus promotes lymphocyte retention in lymphoid organs.[140]

SUMMARY

In this chapter we have outlined three distinct modes of leukocyte trafficking: (a) leukocyte entry into tissues from the circulation; (b) migration within tissues; and (c) exit from tissues. The constitutive and inducible migration of leukocytes throughout the body is essential for lymphocyte development and warrants proper immune surveillance. The processes involved in leukocyte migration are tightly regulated by chemoattractants and adhesion molecules. Leukocyte migration is characterized by a tremendous level of plasticity and specificity, because different leukocyte subsets express unique patterns of traffic molecules that enable their navigation to target tissues. Our expanding knowledge of the mechanisms that control leukocyte trafficking will likely influence the development of multiple therapeutic strategies, including stem cell mobilization, immunotherapy of cancer, and the treatment of tissue-specific autoimmune, inflammatory, and infectious diseases.

SUGGESTED READINGS

Bonasio R, von Andrian UH: Generation, migration and function of circulating dendritic cells. Curr Opin Immunol 18:503, 2006.

Butcher EC, Picker LJ: Lymphocyte homing and homeostasis. Science 272:60, 1996.

Campbell DJ, Kim CH, Butcher EC: Chemokines in the systemic organization of immunity. Immunol Rev 195:58, 2003.

Charo IF, Ransohoff RM: The many roles of chemokines and chemokine receptors in inflammation. N Engl J Med 354:610, 2006.

Cyster JG: Chemokines, sphingosine-1-phosphate, and cell migration in secondary lymphoid organs. Annu Rev Immunol 23:127, 2005.

Glodek AM, Honczarenko M, Le Y, Campbell JJ, Silberstein LE: Sustained activation of cell adhesion is a differentially regulated process in B lymphopoiesis. J Exp Med 197:461, 2003.

Lapidot T, Petit I: Current understanding of stem cell mobilization: The roles of chemokines, proteolytic enzymes, adhesion molecules, cytokines, and stromal cells. Exp Hematol 30:973, 2002.

Luster AD, Alon R, von Andrian UH: Immune cell migration in inflammation: Present and future therapeutic targets. Nat Immunol 6:1182, 2005.

Massberg S, von Andrian UH: Fingolimod and sphingosine-1-phosphate—modifiers of lymphocyte migration. N Engl J Med 355:1088, 2006.

Parks WC, Wilson CL, Lopez-Boado, YS: Matrix metalloproteinases as modulators of inflammation and innate immunity. Nat Rev Immunol 4:617, 2004.

Rosen SD: Ligands for L-selectin: Homing, inflammation, and beyond. Annu Rev Immunol 22:129, 2004.

Scadden DT: The stem-cell niche as an entity of action. Nature 441:1075, 2006.

Spiegel S, Milstien S: Sphingosine-1-phosphate: An enigmatic signalling lipid. Nat Rev Mol Cell Biol 4:397, 2003.

Sumen C, Mempel TR, Mazo IB, Von Andrian UH: Intravital microscopy: Visualizing immunity in context. Immunity 21:315, 2004.

von Andrian UH, Mackay CR: T-cell function and migration: Two sides of the same coin. N Engl J Med 343:1020, 2000.

von Andrian UH, Mempel TR: Homing and cellular traffic in lymph nodes. Nat Rev Immunol 3:867, 2003.

Zou Y-R, Kottmann AH, Kuroda M, Taniuchi I, Littman DR: Function of the chemokine receptor CXCR4 in haematopoiesis and in cerebellar development. Nature 393:595, 1998.

REFERENCES

For complete list of references log onto www.expertconsult.com

CHAPTER 18

TOLERANCE AND AUTOIMMUNITY

Mark J. Shlomchik

INTRODUCTION

The immune system must balance the capacity to respond to foreign antigens and the need not to respond to self-antigens. A complex and multilayered approach has evolved to successfully handle this problem. However, autoimmune diseases, in which this balance is upset, are remarkably common in the population. The diversity and variable severity of such diseases most likely reflects the various approaches the immune system takes to regulate antiself responses, and thereby, the various points at which this multilayered system can break down. The normal functions that may prevent autoimmune disease are collectively known as "self-tolerance mechanisms."

Autoimmune diseases are relevant to hematology at several levels. Autoimmune hemolytic anemia (AIHA) and idiopathic thrombocytopenic purpura are syndromes in which spontaneous autoimmunity to formed blood components may require transfusion support that is rendered difficult due to the presence of autoantibodies. Some cases of aplastic anemia may also fall into this category. Autoantibodies to red blood cells, whether pathogenic or not, are often problematic in terms of typing and screening. Another class of diseases are those induced by transfusion, but which are nonetheless autoimmune in nature: these include posttransfusion purpura (PTP)[1–3] and possibly AIHA associated with transfused thallasemia.[4–6] Finally, graft-versus-host disease, a common complication of allogeneic stem cell transplantation, although not a classical autoimmune disease, shares many features of autoimmune syndromes.[7,8]

An important principle in understanding the etiology of autoimmune diseases is that no special mechanisms, cells, antibody types, or reactions are specific to autoimmune diseases. Rather, the pathogenesis involves the inappropriate or dysregulated triggering of the normal mechanisms of immunity. Therefore, an understanding of autoimmune disease induction and pathogenesis requires a grounding in the basic immune cell functions and interactions, which can be found in the preceding chapters.

SELF-REACTIVE LYMPHOCYTES: ORIGIN AND CONTROL

Origins

Inevitably, autoreactive lymphocytes are generated as a consequence of the fact that B-cell receptor (BCR) and T-cell receptor (TCR) genes are encoded in pieces that rearrange in the DNA of precursor lymphocytes to ultimately form a complete gene. This process allows for many possible gene segment combinations (eg, 4000 different ones for the human Ig heavy chain alone), and in addition, small deletions and random additions at the sites where the pieces are joined together create additional diversity. There are two implications of this process for self-tolerance. First, it is impossible to prevent the assembly of a self-reactive receptor by filtering these out of the germline gene repertoire. Second, a developing lymphocyte cannot be considered autoreactive until the assembly process is complete and the BCR or TCR is expressed. Thus, autoreactive lymphocytes are produced every day, and it is at this key developmental stage—when the BCR or TCR is first expressed by the cell—that the immune system can first eliminate these potentially harmful cells. For B cells, this occurs in the bone marrow, the primary central lymphoid organ (Fig. 18–1), while for T cells it occurs in the thymus. The process is thus termed "central tolerance."

Regulation: Central Tolerance

Clonal Deletion

The classical experiments of Pike and Nossal were the first to demonstrate that developing autoreactive B cells can be eliminated in the bone marrow.[9–11] The details of this process remained murky until the Goodnow and Nemazee groups each developed a BCR transgenic mouse system for the study of self-tolerance.[12–14] These mice have been genetically altered to carry the preformed Ig variable (V) genes that encode a specific autoantibody. Mice that have undergone this genetic transfer are termed *transgenic* and the gene that is transferred is termed the *transgene* (Fig. 18–2). The presence of this preformed transgene short-circuits and prevents the normal rearrangement process at the natural immunoglobulin (Ig) gene loci. Thus each B cell in the animal expresses only the transgene and has the same specificity. By choosing a target antigen that is carried by only some strains of mice (such as the polymorphic major histocompatibility complex class I genes used by Nemazee), it is possible to render the transgenic B cells autoreactive when crossed onto one strain (Fig. 18–3) but not autoreactive in a different strain. The results of such systems were dramatic. A complete loss or deletion of the B cells was demonstrated in the strain of mice that had the autoantigen, but perfectly good expression of the B cells was observed when the autoantigen was absent. This provided clear proof of B-cell clonal deletion. Furthermore, it was shown that this deletion occurred at the immature B-cell stage, just when the cells first express their BCR.[15–17] It has been since discovered that deletion is just the final step in controlling autoreactive B cells.[15,17–19] B cells which have completed H- and L-chain rearrangement and then recognize self-antigen while still immature in the bone marrow may actually undergo a second round of V gene rearrangement. This most likely occurs at the L-chain loci, which are particularly suited to secondary V to J rearrangements. This process has been termed receptor editing. Evidently, a cell has a certain period of time in which to produce a second L-chain rearrangement that will inactivate the cell's self-reactivity. If this does not occur, the cell fails to mature and is eventually eliminated. The physiologic role of the editing process is still unclear, but it could represent a way to maximize the efficiency of B-cell generation while still maintaining an effective filter against strongly self-reactive B cells.

Clonal Anergy

Another type of self-tolerance mechanism was also revealed by similar experiments. This form, clonal anergy, involves inactivation of the self-reactive cell, but not its elimination.[10,14] Such B cells seem to remain in the peripheral lymphoid circulation, albeit with a shorter life span than normal B cells. In addition, these cells have a lower amount of surface Ig and, moreover, seem much less capable of sensing the presence of antigen when the sIg receptor is triggered. This second form of B-cell tolerance, demonstrated dramatically

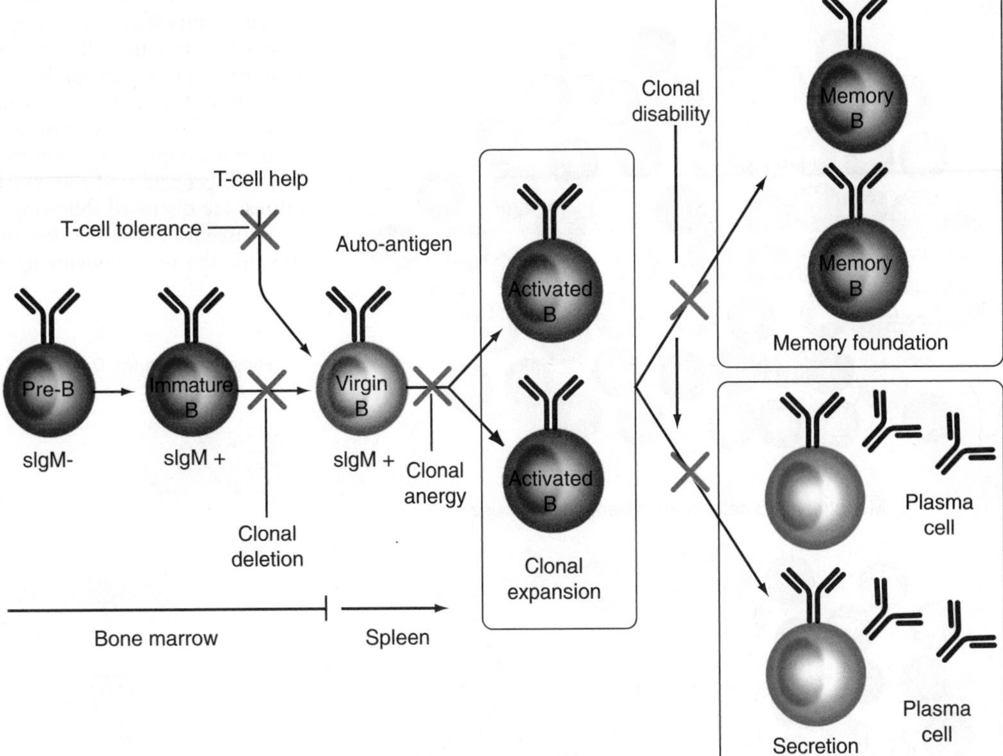

Figure 18–1 Stages at which self-tolerance can block B-cell development. Arrows indicate the normal pathway of development. X indicates where these differentiation steps can be interrupted for self-reactive B cells as a consequence of encountering self-antigen. Each X is labeled with the type of self-tolerance it represents. The clonal disability steps are somewhat more hypothetical than the earlier steps. See text for details.

through the use of Ig transgenic mice, was also anticipated in the experiments of Pike and Nossal.[10] The physiologic advantage of maintaining these anergic cells is unclear. They can be activated by strong stimulation under certain conditions; thus it has been suggested that they are maintained as a secondary repertoire to maintain greater B-cell diversity and thus better protect against a broader spectrum of pathogens. However, the presence of these cells also raises a danger that they may be activated by self-antigens as well, which could represent a source of autoantibodies. Indeed, it has been suggested that autoantibody-secreting B cells can arise by the activation of anergic B cells.

Clonal deletion, receptor editing, and clonal anergy are often referred to as "central" self-tolerance because they can occur in the central lymphopoietic organs and act on immature lymphocytes that have just expressed their antigen receptors. Central tolerance is probably most important in purging or controlling very high-affinity antiself lymphocytes.

Tolerance of Memory B Cells

Figure 18–1 indicates that there are yet other stages of B-cell development at which one could imagine that self-tolerance should occur. The most important of these is development of memory B cells, the long-lasting cells that harbor the ability of the immune system to respond better and faster to antigens that have already been encountered once. An important and unique process occurs during memory cell development—the genes that encode the antibody receptor molecule undergo a process of random mutation.[20–22] This process is thought to provide mutants with an increased affinity for the immunizing antigen, and in fact, the secondary immune response is known to be of higher affinity. However, a side effect of any random process, just as in the receptor rearrangement itself, is the potential to create novel antiself specificities.[23,24] Thus, many have postulated that there should be a screening of cells for self-reactivity during memory B-cell development.[25–27] In fact, some evidence suggests this process exists, but it is much more elusive than clonal deletion or clonal anergy.

T Cells

In many respects, self-tolerance for T cells is similar to that for B cells; both deletion and anergy exist.[28–32] The principle differences reflect the basic differences in B and T development. Deletion for T cells occurs in the thymus (where TCR gene rearrangement occurs), not in the bone marrow. In addition, the self-antigens for T cells consist of self-peptides, just as the foreign antigens for T cells are foreign peptides.

Limitations of Central Tolerance

Although these mechanisms to eliminate or inactivate self-reactive B cells as they first emerge are clearly critical for the viability of an animal, they only account for part of the overall system that protects against autoimmunity. There are many reasons to believe that central tolerance cannot and should not be perfectly efficient. One is that the ability to tolerate self must be balanced against the ability to efficiently respond to a wide variety of foreign antigens. Each cell that is eliminated in the interests of self-tolerance is one that cannot respond to a potential foreign antigen. This concept is illustrated metaphorically in Fig. 18–4. Thus one must suppose that it might be advantageous to allow some (weakly) antiself cells to escape these purging mechanisms. This is indeed the case. A second way to view this same problem is that even if it were desirable to have complete elimination of antiself lymphocytes, it would be impossible. It is unlikely that during development each cell will be exposed to a sufficient quantity of each and every self-antigen in the body to be functionally tested for self-reactivity. Furthermore, some antigens are tissue specific, such as thyroglobulin, and are unlikely to be found in the circulation at appreciable quantities.

Persistence of Self-Reactive Lymphocytes

Despite central tolerance, self-reactive cells nonetheless exist in peripheral lymphoid organs of normal animals. It has been observed

Diversity in B cells from a normal mouse

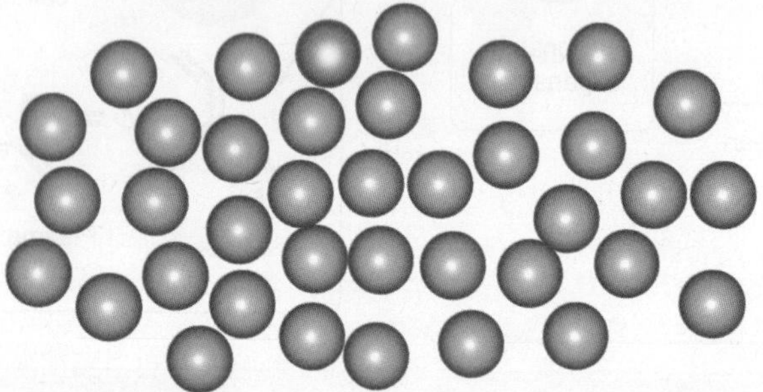

Monotony in B cells in an ig transgenic mouse

Figure 18–2 Clonal diversity in a normal versus transgenic mouse. The great diversity of B-cell specificities found in a normal mouse is indicated by the different patterns in each type of B cell. In contrast, in a transgenic mouse, each B cell expresses the same specificity because each carries the genes for a preformed heavy- and light-chain Ig gene (the transgenes). This is indicated by the same pattern in each B cell. The one B cell with a different pattern signifies that occasional cells will express a unique specificity even in a transgenic because the system is imperfect.

for some time that many immune responses are accompanied by transient antiself antibody responses.[34–38] For example, rheumatoid factors with specificity for self-IgG often accompany strong secondary immune responses to foreign proteins or viruses.[34–36] The simplest explanation for such phenomena is that the B cells that make these autoantibodies already exist in the peripheral lymphoid compartment, but are quiescent until they receive the proper stimulus. (How such cells get activated and why in normal animals this does not pose a threat are discussed following.)

Transgenic mouse models similar to those described above have provided the most convincing evidence of the existence of such B

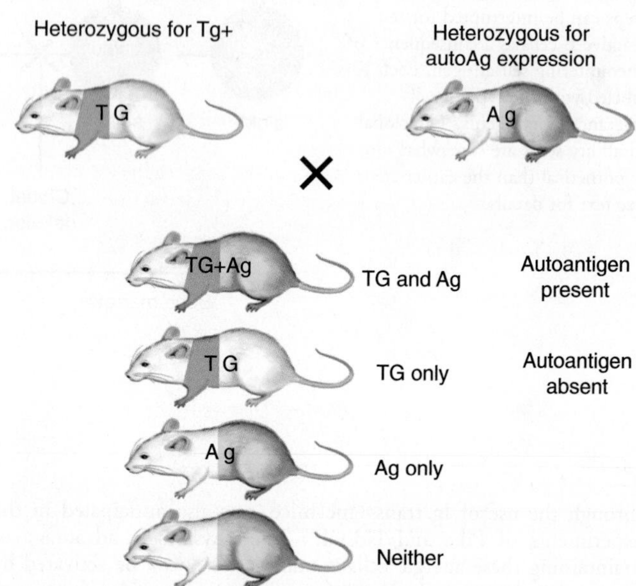

Figure 18–3 Mating strategy to generate transgenic mice with and without a polymorphic autoantigen. Two mice are crossed, each of which is heterozygous: one for the transgene and the other for a polymorphic autoantigen (much as people can be heterozygous for blood group antigens). Shown are the possible resulting progeny of such a cross, each of which would occur at 1/4 frequency. "TG" indicates transgenic and "Ag" indicates presence of the autoantigen. The first two types of mice, one with TG and Ag and the other control with TG and not the Ag are compared in experiments to determine how autoantigen affects the development of the autoreactive B cells.

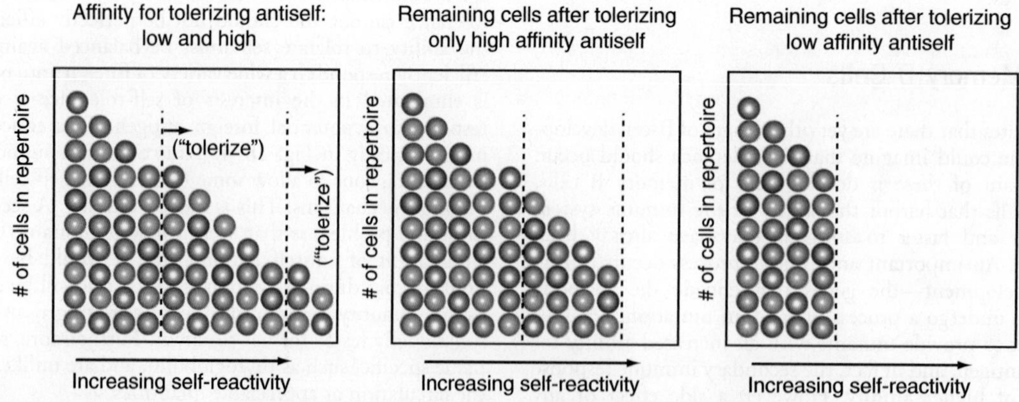

Figure 18–4 How elimination of autoreactive cells affects the repertoire of lymphocytes capable of responding to foreign antigens. A hypothetical population of diverse B cells representing the entire repertoire available to respond to foreign antigen is depicted. The population is arrayed according to increasing self-reactivity (*left panel*). Tolerizing only the high-affinity antiself B cells (*right panel*) leaves most of the potential repertoire intact. However, as the affinity cutoff for self-reactivity increases, fewer B cells will be included. It can be readily seen (*bottom panel*) that a low threshold for inactivation or deletion of self-reactive cells will lead to a small number of competent residual cells available for responses to foreign antigens. Thus, a stringent tolerization of low affinity antiself cells will compromise the ability to respond to nonself.

cells. One of particular relevance to hematology was generated by Honjo and colleagues.[39] These workers isolated the V genes that came from an actual anti-red blood cell autoantibody originally obtained from an NZB mouse with AIHA. Much like Goodnow and Nemazee, they used the transgenic approach to express the anti-red blood cell antibody in a normal nonautoimmune mouse. Although central deletion was seen in most of the transgenic mice studied, many also had some residual autoreactive B cells in spleen and lymph nodes, and some otherwise normal mice even developed frank AIHA. These results were interpreted as follows: central tolerance is not completely efficient even in a nonautoimmune mouse and some autoreactive B cells can be stimulated to cause disease. Shlomchik and colleagues, also using a transgenic approach, demonstrated that a rheumatoid factor autoantibody that was isolated from a diseased mouse was not subject to self-tolerance when expressed in a normal BALB/c mouse.[40] These B cells generally remained quiescent in a normal animal, suggesting that those B cells that are not usually regulated by self-tolerance (perhaps because they recognize the self-antigen only weakly) may be the precursors of pathogenic autoantibodies in disease.

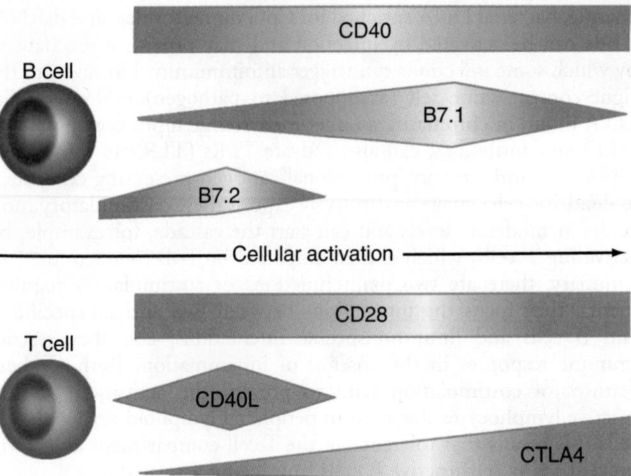

Figure 18–5 Timing of expression of costimulatory molecules. The schematic shows the regulated expression of the CD40–CD40L family (*light red*) and the B7-CD28–CTLA4 family (*dark red*) of molecules. From left to right is depicted increasing cellular activation as time elapses after initial encounter with antigen. The expression level of each molecule over time is indicated by a polygonal shape. The vertical width of the shape at any time reflects the degree of expression at that time. For example, CTLA4 is expressed little at the start and the expression increases continuously over time. The shapes depicting expression of molecules that are thought to deliver signals are outlined in bold, whereas those of molecules thought to receive signals are in fine line. The top three molecules are chiefly expressed on B cells and the lower three on T cells.

Control of Self-Reactive Lymphocytes: Preventing Activation

The recognition that potentially self-reactive lymphocytes exist in the peripheral lymphoid repertoire of normal individuals,[41] despite central tolerance, raises the question of why they do not usually cause disease. One reason is the second layer of immune tolerance that prevents activation of self-reactive lymphocytes that exist in the periphery. This layer consists of several facets, which are described in the following sections.

Absence of Self-Antigen

The simplest explanation for why a self-specific lymphocyte is not spontaneously activated in the peripheral lymphoid compartment is the absence of self-antigen. This may be the reason why it was not eliminated in the first place. This situation has been termed *clonal ignorance*. It is related to the scenario described for rheumatoid factor B cells above in that the cell does not seem to care about the concentration of its autoantigen. In the case of rheumatoid factor, though, this is because the cell has relatively low affinity for self-IgG; in the case of thyroglobulin, for example, this is because the antigen concentration is vanishingly small. However, a change in antigen concentration, such as after thyroid damage from a viral infection, might then precipitate activation of these heretofore ignorant cells, leading to autoimmunity.

This antigen sequestration concept only applies to a limited set of autoantigens. A more general reason that self-specific lymphocytes remain quiescent, despite the ubiquity of self-antigens, is that T and B cells are dependent on each other for activation (Chapter 10).[42–45] It is evident that for this to occur, B and T cells specific for the same self-antigen must be in the same place at the same time. If such cells are rare, then the requisite coexistence of two such cells will happen very infrequently, minimizing the chance of starting an autoimmune reaction. A second consequence of T–B interdependence is that specific inefficiencies of central tolerance in one limb can be compensated for in the other. For example, T cells are probably very efficiently purged of cells that react with thymus-specific antigens, whereas B cells are probably not. However, antithymus B-cell responses are unlikely even though many thymus-specific B cells probably circulate; the cognate T cell with specificity for the same self-antigen simply does not exist.

Costimulation

Even when a B cell and a T cell that do recognize the same self-antigen encounter each other, the result may still not be activation. This is because a positive response by a lymphocyte to antigen encounter also requires a second signal, aside from the stimulus of antigen recognition itself. These signals are transmitted through a series of ligand–receptor molecular pairs known as costimulatory molecules (Chapter 10). The most important of these are: CD80 andCD86[46–51] (expressed on B cells, macrophages, and dendritic cells) and CD28[50,51] (expressed on T cells). Another important pair is CD40[52,53] (expressed on B cells, macrophages, and dendritic cells) and CD40 ligand[54–59] (CD40L, expressed on T cells and missing in patients with X-linked immunodeficiency/hyper-IgM syndrome[60–63]). CD40 stimulation is especially important for B cells, as it is for other antigen-presenting cells as well. Other important costimulatory molecules in T–B interactions include ICOS and ICOS-L (not shown in the figure), which are critical for germinal center responses and isotype switching.[64] Also in this category are lymphokine signals. For B cells, interleukin-4 (IL-4) signaling is important, but other cytokines such as interleukins-5, -6, and -2 (IL-5, IL-6, IL-2) also play roles in growth and differentiation. As shown in Fig. 18–5, some of these molecules are constitutively expressed, whereas others are induced in activated cells. This pattern of expression and induction leads to a cascade of events that occur during immune activation.

In general, for proper transmission of this second signal, one or the other of the lymphocytes must have been previously activated. This concept generates a paradox in that if one lymphocyte must already be activated, how is it possible to start an immune response at all? This is resolved in several ways. First, it is indeed difficult to start immune responses, and this is one of the mechanisms by which nonresponsiveness to self is maintained. However, a strong first signal to a T or B cell may be sufficient for it to induce its costimulatory molecules.[46,65] Second, inflammation of any type is a powerful nonspecific inducer of these same costimulatory molecules.[66–68] Thus, in the presence of ongoing inflammation, such as would occur with infection or trauma, immune responses are much easier to start. Indeed, recent evidence suggests an important role in systemic autoimmunity for Toll-like receptors (TLRs), which recognize molecules specific to pathogens and induce costimulatory molecules and immune system activation. Ligands for TLRs include lipopolysaccharide, bacterial DNA enriched for CpG dinucleotides, and dsRNA. TLRs can be activated by infection and may provide a mechanism by which some infections can trigger autoimmunity. However, in the right context some self (as opposed to pathogen) molecules, like DNA found in chromatin, a target for systemic lupus erythematosus (SLE) autoantibodies, can also activate TLRs (TLR9 in the case of DNA).[69] Third, certain "professional" antigen-presenting cells, such as dendritic cells, may constitutively express these costimulatory molecules at moderate levels and can start the cascade, for example, by activating T cells, which is then amplified by T–B interactions.[68] In summary, there are two main functions of costimulatory requirements: they focus the interactions between two antigen-specific T and B cells and limit nonspecific interactions; and they restrict immune responses in the absence of inflammation. Both of these features of costimulation tend to prevent the activation of self-reactive lymphocytes that exist in peripheral lymphoid organs. For B cells this means that tolerance in the T-cell compartment alone will prevent many self-reactive B cells from being activated.

Even with antigen sequestration and costimulatory regulation, mechanisms that prevent the activation of self-reactive lymphocytes are incomplete at best. For example, it seems likely during infection or trauma that antiself responses could initiate because costimulatory molecules will be nonspecifically induced. Indeed, this is the case. Furthermore, during infection and tissue damage, self-proteins that ordinarily are sequestered can be released. This leads to activation of the ignorant cells circulating in the body.[70–75] In fact (usually) self-limited autoimmune responses after infection are well known, such as poststreptococcal glomerulonephritis or postmycoplasmal cold agglutinins. Although these syndromes can cause serious clinical problems, they are self-limited, unlike autoimmune diseases such as SLE.

Control of Self-Reactive Lymphocytes: Downregulation

The difference between transient autoimmune responses and chronic severe autoimmunity may lie in the third layer of protection against autoimmunity: downregulation of ongoing responses. Again, this layer is a normal part of the immune system, functioning to regulate both normal and autoimmune responses. Initially, in a normal response to a viral pathogen, there is great proliferation of lymphocytes specific for viral antigens. This process leads ultimately to the elimination of the pathogen, which was traditionally thought of as the signal to stop an immune response. However, when the pathogen is eliminated, in the absence of any other regulatory mechanism, there would be many residual cells that had been responding to the pathogen. Although a few such cells could be retained to provide immunologic memory, most of these are no longer useful in the short term. In addition to unnecessarily filling the lymphoid compartment, these cells may be a risk for causing autoimmunity. This is because of the possibility of the generation of newly autoreactive B cells by virtue of random somatic mutation.[24] B cells responding to foreign antigens begin to mutate their antibody V region genes. Mutation is a random process, and thus a mutation could occur that converts a nonautoimmune B cell into a self-reactive B cell.[24] No clear mechanism exists by which the body can discriminate and specifically eliminate these newly self-reactive mutant B cells. However, at a minimum, elimination of most of the reactive B cells regardless of specificity would mitigate this problem.

Over the last several years, several pathways for the elimination of such postexpansion cells have been elucidated. One seems to be an inborn program that causes cells to apoptose after undergoing a certain amount of proliferation.[76–78] Particularly important in this program in lymphocytes are the Bcl2-inhibitable pathways that are activated in large part by Bim.[79,80] In B cells, CD40 signaling in concert with BCR and IL-4 signaling may rescue some cells from this self-destructive fate, and it is believed that these cells become long-lived memory cells.[81–84] There are also active mechanisms that signal cells to apoptose. One receptor–ligand pair called Fas and FasL is central in this process. Generally, when Fas is ligated by FasL, the cell expressing Fas is triggered to die by apoptosis.[85–88] Fas and FasL are not expressed at high levels on unstimulated resting lymphocytes. On activation, T cells express both Fas and FasL, whereas B cells express Fas.[88,89] Sensitivity to the Fas signal may be regulated in the Fas-expressing cell as well. Thus, after a certain degree of activation and proliferation, a T cell (expressing FasL) encountering an activated B cell (expressing Fas) may actually kill that B cell. There are likely other ligand pairs, particularly those in the tumor necrosis factor family, that may serve similar functions, both for B and T cells.

A particularly interesting and instructive receptor ligand pair that downregulates ongoing responses has been elucidated. The receptor, CTLA4, is expressed on activated T cells, and when ligated, causes inactivation or death of the receptive T cell; it is said to therefore transduce a "negative" signal.[90–93] The other ligands in this pair are CD80 and to a lesser extent CD86, the same ligands that gives a positive signal to naive T cells by ligating CD28. Thus, the same molecule can promote activation early on in the immune response while, through a change in the receptive T cell, it can inhibit activation at a later time. An analogous receptor pair of the B7 family are PD-1, an inhibitory receptor similar to CTLA-4, and its ligands PD-L1 and PD-L2. PD-1 is expressed on a number of activated lymphocytes and its ligands are constitutively and inducibly expressed on a variety of parenchymal cells (PD-L1) and dendritic cells (PD-L2).[94] Absence of these molecules leads to exaggerated immune responses and autoimmunity.[95–97] These examples underscore the careful means by which the immune system regulates and dampens activation presumably to prevent autoimmunity.

Recently, attention has turned again to suppressor T cells as potent regulators of autoimmunity. These cells were extensively studied two decades ago but when some of the work could not be reproduced or explained, interest waned and this mechanism was largely ignored by immunologists. These cells have been rediscovered in a sense, and modern tools of immunology have elucidated how they suppress autoimmunity and have left little doubt of their importance. The best-studied regulatory cell expresses CD25, the receptor for IL-2,[98,99] and its development and function is dependent on the expression of a key transcription factor, FoxP3.[100–102] These cells can prevent autoimmune syndromes such as inflammatory bowel disease, diabetes, and autoimmune encephalomyelitis in murine models and can even be used to treat active disease.[103,104] They are also active in preventing transplantation rejection and graft-versus-host disease. These cells may function by secreting suppressive cytokines, like IL-10 and TGF-β, and also by cell–cell contact. Their importance in humans is underscored by a rare and fatal inherited autoimmune disorder, IPEX, that results from a lack of FoxP3, which is needed for the development of $CD25^+$ regulatory cells.[105,106]

How does regulation of ongoing immune responses prevent autoimmunity? In the first place, these normal forms of downregulation undoubtedly prevent common transient autoimmune responses from becoming chronic. More subtly, elimination or control of cells after immune responses will prevent the accumulation of a large number of self-specific memory cells. As long as such cells are rare, it is unlikely for autoreactive T cells and B cells, each specific for the same self-antigen, to wind up in the same place at the same time. Thus, downregulation and elimination of responding cells prevents a critical mass of self-reactive cells from ever forming.

Control of Self-Reactive Lymphocytes: Channeling the Type of Effector Response

A final layer of protection against self-inflicted immune damage involves channeling of responses so they are not harmful. Depending on the context, only certain effector functions will effectively eliminate certain pathogens. For example, antibodies will not be effective against intracellular pathogens. By analogy, only certain effector functions may cause autoimmune disease, depending on the circumstances. It is clear that there are two major types of T-helper cell responses, Th1 and Th2, that in turn lead to very different effector functions.[107–109] The propensity to make these various types of responses depends on a number of ill-understood factors, but these include genetics, route of antigen exposure, and dose of antigen.[110,111] Intriguingly, in certain murine models of autoimmunity such as the NOD diabetes model, experimental manipulations that shift responses away from Th1 and toward Th2 are highly protective against disease.[112–114] This is also relevant to B-cell autoimmunity per se because, through the use of different isotypes of Ig, different effector functions can occur. The cytokines secreted by Th1 and Th2 cells have profound effects on the isotypes of Ig's that are produced during a response. Thus, not only is the T-cell component of the response channeled in this way, but the humoral response is also influenced. Recently, a new subset of T cells that secrete IL-17, thus dubbed Th17, has been recognized as important pathogenic cells in several autoimmune diseases, including experimental autoimmune encephalitis as well as collagen-induced arthritis.[115] At least some of these Th17 cells secrete a related cytokine, IL-22, which in turn may be responsible for their pathogensis in diseases such as psoriasis.[116] Th17 cells depend on IL-6 and TGF-β for their development and IL-23 for their maintenance.[115] The transcription factor ROR-γt is required for these cells to differentiate, which they do to the exclusion of Th1 cells.[117] It is not clear in which diseases Th17 versus Th1 cells will prove to be more important, or how their reciprocal development is controlled. Emerging evidence indicates that Th17 cells are important for resistance to extracellular bacteria as well.[115]

Table 18–1 Patterns of Autoantibody Expression in Systemic Autoimmune Diseases

Autoantigen	Autoimmune Diseases (% of patients *with* autoantibody)			
	Systemic Lupus Erythematosus	Rheumatoid Arthritis	Scleroderma	Sjögren Syndrome
dsDNA	40			
ssDNA	70			
Histones	70			
Sm	30			
nRNP	30			
Ro (SS-A)	35			60
La (SS-B)	15			40
IgG (RF)	5	90		10–20
Scl-70 (Topo I)			70	
Centromere			70	

dsDNA, double-stranded DNA; ssDNA, single-stranded DNA; Sm, Smith ribonucleoprotein; nRNP, native ribonucleoprotein; Scl-70, scleroderma 70-kd antigen (topoisomerase I). Blank space indicates rarely or never detected.

Information derived from Tan EM: Antinuclear antibodies: Diagnostic markers for autoimmune diseases and probes for cell biology. Adv Immunol 44:93, 1989.

BREAKDOWN OF SELF-TOLERANCE IN AUTOIMMUNE DISEASES

Presumably, for autoimmune diseases and autoantibody production to occur, one or more of the multilayered mechanisms to prevent autoimmunity must fail. Surprisingly, the precise nature of these failures is not well understood. The mechanism of failure will differ for the various autoimmune diseases and perhaps even for different patients with similar syndromes. Moreover, it seems likely both from phenomenologic and genetic studies that failures at several levels are required to generate clinically significant autoimmunity. In the following section, examples of the current state of knowledge are given.

This chapter is not meant to review the nature of autoimmune diseases; however, before considering the likely points at which self-tolerance mechanisms break down it is useful to review some basic concepts about these diseases. Grossly, autoimmune diseases have often been divided into organ-specific and systemic autoimmune syndromes. This classification is useful, but as these diseases are becoming better understood, the dividing lines are blurring; pathogeneses of all these diseases are likely to have much in common. In particular, systemic autoimmune diseases are actually much more specific in their antigenic targets than is commonly realized. Table 18–1 shows the types of autoantibodies commonly found in several systemic autoimmune diseases. Certain autoantibodies are diagnostic for specific autoimmune diseases, such as anti-Sm in SLE. Thus, Sm is a specific target in SLE, but other autoimmune patients, such as those with rheumatoid arthritis, do not respond to this autoantigen. In fact, only 30% of all patients with SLE make anti-Sm, meaning that the other 70% are tolerant of their own Sm, despite having a systemic autoimmune disease.[118] Another salient feature of most human autoimmune diseases is adult onset. Both the selective nature of disease and its late onset argue against gross defects in the basic central tolerance mechanisms as being the cause.

Instead, these considerations suggest that most clinical autoimmune diseases are likely to arise from defects in the later stages of self-tolerance, such as preventing the activation of autoreactive cells or downregulating them once they are activated. Because in no case is the primary cause of a polygenic autoimmune disease known, it cannot be excluded that subtle defects in the earlier stages, including central tolerance, may also play a role. However, it does seem clear that a gross defect in central tolerance would lead to a severe syndrome of congenital autoimmunity.

Genetic and Environmental Factors

Genetic Factors

Both genetic and environmental factors help to explain why autoimmunity occurs in some individuals and not others.[119] The most well-known genetic factor is the major histocompatibility complex, known as HLA in the human. Many different autoimmune diseases are more or less associated with specific genotypes at this polymorphic locus. Among these are ankylosing spondylitis (HLA–B27), insulin-dependent diabetes mellitus (HLA–DR3/4), rheumatoid arthritis (HLA–DR4), and to some degree SLE (HLA–DR2/3).[120] It should be emphasized that although individuals with these genotypes are relatively more prone, most will not develop the autoimmune disease. How certain HLA genes predispose to autoimmunity is not very clear. These genes could be involved in the efficiency or specificity of central tolerance in the thymus, but could also be involved in the activation of autoreactive T cells in the periphery.

Inheritance patterns of all systemic autoimmune diseases suggest that multiple genes, in addition to the HLA locus, contribute to susceptibility. Such genes are beginning to be identified in human and in animal models. Some genes associated with a variety of human autoimmune diseases include CTLA-4, PTPN-22, and IRF-5, all of which are known to regulate inflammation.[121,122] Recent work in murine SLE has used genomic scanning with polymerase chain reaction-based polymorphic short simple repeat sequences to identify and map genes that are associated with autoimmune phenotypes. In this type of analysis, an autoimmune strain is crossed with a nonautoimmune strain and then the progeny are back-crossed to the autoimmune strain. Genetic loci segregate in this cross, and for each individual mouse, with the help of the murine genome map, the origin of 100 to 200 genetic locations all along the chromosomes are identified as either from the autoimmune parent or the nonautoimmune parent. Simultaneously, the autoimmune phenotype of each mouse is determined in a variety of assays, most commonly including autoantibody production and glomerulonephritis. By typing a few hundred mice in this way, correlations can be made that link certain genetic loci with certain phenotypic traits. Several genes have been mapped with this approach, and their phenotypes investigated in greater detail.[123–127] Interestingly, most of them seem to have direct

Table 18–2 Genes Involved in Regulation of Autoimmune Responses

Category	Types of Genes[a]	Known Examples[b]
Central and peripheral deletion and anergy	Receptor signaling, MHC genes, receptor V genes	CD45,[128] PTP-1C,[129–131] HLA (certain types),[120] CD3,[132] CD4, CD8, CD28/B7[32]
Initiation of response	Receptor signaling, costimulatory molecules, adhesion molecules	CD45, PTP-1C, FcγRII[130]
Downregulation of response	Apoptosis genes, interleukins, negative costimulatory molecules	Fas,[142,143] TNF,[133,134] CTLA4,[91] CD40, CD3,[135] CD28/B7[50,136]
Channeling of response	Interleukins, interleukin receptors	IL-4, IL-10, IL-12, IFN-γ[113,114]
Autoantigen metabolism and apoptosis	Complement components, apoptosis signaling	C1q, C2, C4, DNAse I, MER[137,138]

PTP-1C, phosphotyrosine phosphatase; IL, interleukin; FcγRII, receptor for IgG-type II; Fas, see text; TNF, tumor necrosis factor, CTLA4, see text; IFN-γ, interferon gamma; MHC, major histocompatibility complex.

[a]Indicates some of the categories of genes that may be involved in regulating autoimmunity at the indicated step.

[b]Some genes in the "Types of Genes" category which have been shown to play a role in the process indicated in the left column. Some have also been directly shown to play a role in autoimmunity.

effects on B-cell function or activity. In the next several years, some of these genes may be identified and cloned and the exact nature of the defects defined. This will in turn permit screening for defects in the homologous genes in human autoimmune disease patients.

Although animal models suggest multigenic inheritance, there are certain instructive cases in which single gene defects play a major role. Table 18–2 lists categories of genes that are likely involved in genetic predisposition to autoimmune disease. Note that these include genes involved in the processes of antigen sequestration, T–B collaboration, and immune response downregulation that were discussed above as key features of the self-tolerance mechanisms that normally prevent autoimmune disease.

The best studied example of mutations in these genes is the *lpr/lpr* mouse, a natural variant originally discovered at the Jackson Laboratories, which carries an inactivated murine Fas.[85,139,140] The *gld* mutation (another natural variant discovered at Jackson), which inactivates murine Fas ligand (FasL),[88] has a very similar phenotype to the *lpr*. Both of these mutations lead to an age-dependent autoimmune syndrome with autoantibody profiles that remarkably resemble human SLE.[140] These mice die prematurely of renal failure. They also have an accumulation of lymphocytes that leads to marked lymphadenopathy.[141] Presumably, this is the result of failure to eliminate postactivation T and B cells by the Fas-based mechanism.[142–144] Exactly how defects in the apoptotic Fas pathway lead to autoimmunity has yet to be elucidated. Interestingly, a rare syndrome in humans with incomplete penetrance, called autoimmune lymphoproliferation syndrome, has recently been traced to mutations in human Fas.[145] Often these patients are misdiagnosed with leukemia or lymphoma and some have even been treated for (and survived) these neoplasms. Clonality and chromosomal studies in autoimmune lymphoproliferation syndrome reveal polyclonal B- and T-cell proliferations with normal karyotypes, in distinction with true lymphoma or leukemia.

The phenotypes of these mutants in the Fas pathway, though more fulminant than most human autoimmune syndromes, illustrate two important points. They demonstrate the critical nature of the late downregulatory controls in preventing autoimmune disease. They also point out pathways in which less severe mutations might be discovered that account for human disease.

A final category of genes regulate the clearance of self-antigens and dead cells, which is particularly important in systemic autoimmune diseases like SLE. These include complement components C4, C3, and C2, C1q, and less-known genes like MER, which plays a role in signaling for the uptake of apoptotic fragments by macrophages.[137,138] Evidently, when self-antigens are not cleared promptly following cell death, they can become targets of the immune system, leading to autoimmunity to intracellular components like chromatin.

As noted, TLRs can recognize some of these molecules when they are present in high concentrations, thus providing proinflammatory signals. In murine models of lupus, it was recently demonstrated in vivo that TLR9 is required to generate antichromatin autoantibodies[146] and that TLR7, which recognizes RNA, is required for the generation of autoantibodies to RNA-related antigens.[147] Indeed, a mutant mouse with a double dose of TLR7 develops spontaneous lupus with high levels of RNA antibodies.[148,149] Stimulation of these TLRs on specialized plasmacytoid dendritic cells leads to release of abundant type I interferon, which itself may be causally linked to lupus in mice and humans.[150] These findings highlight a genetic basis for recognizing self-molecules in autoimmune diseases and suggest new therapeutic targets that are currently being explored. Whether this theme extends to other autoimmune diseases beyond lupus remains to be determined.

Environmental Factors

Environment plays a role that is at least as important as genetics. This is illustrated by the fact that concordance rates among identical twins, even raised in the same household, are surprisingly low. Only 20% of twins of patients with rheumatoid arthritis also get rheumatoid arthritis.[120] There are many examples of environmental factors causing either chronic or transient autoimmune diseases. There are postinfectious syndromes such as postmycoplasmal cold agglutinin disease. The pattern of incidence of multiple sclerosis suggests a viral etiology, although no causative virus has ever been convincingly demonstrated. Another category of infectious associations includes postviral myocarditis, which follows certain coxsackievirus infections.[74] It is sometimes conceptually difficult to draw a line between viral damage and consequent immune system damage; however, if sensitization to self-antigens occurs as a consequence of viral infection, and these later are pathogenic targets independent of viral antigens, it seems reasonable to consider the syndrome as autoimmune.

Infections are not the only source of environmental stimuli for autoimmunity. Toxins, such as mercury, cause autoimmunity in animal models.[151,152] Another form more familiar to those in hematology is drug-induced autoimmunity, as in AIHA. Drugs that cause lupus-like syndromes, such as procainamide, are particularly prominent examples.[153,154] Despite these specific examples, the environmental factors that play a role in promoting common autoimmune diseases such as rheumatoid arthritis or SLE are unknown.

Examples in Hematology: Epitope Spreading in PTP

One potential way to break self-tolerance may be particularly relevant to syndromes found in hematology and is worthy of elaboration. This is a form of environmental stimulation, albeit iatrogenic. In PTP, transfusion with allogeneic platelets that contain a platelet-specific antigen (such as HPA-1[a]) lacking in the recipient (HPA-1[b]) leads to rapid destruction of the transfused platelets and antibody formation to the foreign platelet antigen.[3,155] However, several days later, the recipient becomes severely thrombocytopenic owing to increased destruction of the recipient's own platelets. Although how such destruction of self-platelets occurs secondary to destruction of allogeneic platelets may still be controversial;[3,155,156] the best explanation is an autoimmune response.[1–3] How does this response get stimulated? The probable pathway bears significant parallels to one demonstrated in mice several years ago by Janeway and colleagues.[157,158] These workers immunized normal mice with human cytochrome c, which differed slightly from endogenous murine cytochrome c. The mice made both an antibody response and a T-cell response to the human cytochrome c; however, since the human and mouse cytochromes are so similar, the antibody response (but not the T-cell response) cross-reacted with murine cytochrome c. Presumably, this reflected activation of ignorant B cells with specificity for self-cytochrome c (and also human). However, several weeks later, if the mice were given a dose of self-cytochrome c, now both a vigorous B-cell and T-cell antiself response ensued. These authors suggested that priming with the cross-reactive antigen first induced self-reactive B cells, which in turn could then break tolerance in anergic or ignorant self-reactive T cells.

How does this relate to PTP? Figure 18–6 illustrates the author's hypothetical adaptation of this mechanism to the platelet transfusion situation. The foreign platelets actually share many common antigens with the host, as well as differ at the HPA-1[a] locus. The foreign antigenic difference allows ignorant self-specific B cells (as well as HPA-1[a]-specific B cells) to interact with helper T cells that are specific for the foreign HPA-1[a] antigen and become activated. Moreover, these activated B cells can then present self-platelet antigens along with costimulatory signals to self-reactive T cells. When this happens, the immune response can perpetuate even in the absence of the foreign platelets. This is exactly what is seen in PTP, where a delayed response continues to eliminate self-platelets for many days after the disappearance of the transfused platelets. Thus, a foreign platelet is analogous to foreign cytochrome c in having a few different antigens along with many shared antigens. In the same way as shown experimentally with cytochrome c, it is hypothesized that the few foreign antigens existing on the same particle (in the case of cytochrome c it is the same molecule) allow spreading of autoimmunity from a foreign antigen to self-antigens. The key events are the activation of ignorant B cells that cross-react with both self and foreign molecules, and then the activation by these B cells or T cells that are specific for self.

It is reasonable to question how such antiself responses are ever stopped once started. PTP, for example, is a self-limited syndrome. In fact, the answer is not known; however, both downregulation of antigen as the platelet count falls to near zero and the natural mechanisms that cause apoptosis of responding lymphocytes probably play a role. In the absence of an autoimmune-prone host who has mutations affecting the downregulation of immune responses, these autoimmune reactions will remain transient. It is speculated that when similar events occur in people who do have genetically based problems in downregulating such responses, a chronic autoimmune syndrome can be induced.

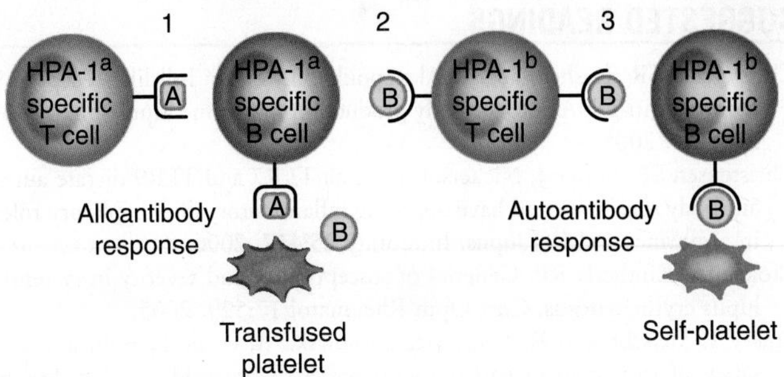

Figure 18–6 Epitope spreading as a possible autoimmune mechanism for PTP. Events are depicted as progressing from left to right. An HPA-1[b] person is transfused with an HPA-1[a/b] platelet product. An alloantibody response ensues as an HPA-1[a]-specific B cell recognizes the platelet, becomes activated to secrete antibody, and presents the HPA-1[a] antigen to an anti-HPA-1[a] T cell (step 1). In addition, the activated B cell may now activate a previously ignorant anti-HPA-1[b]-specific T cell to initiate an autoimmune response (step 2). The activated B cell acquired the self-HPA-1[b] antigen as a passenger on the HPA-1[a/b] allogeneic platelet. This autoreactive T cell can then activate an ignorant anti-HPA-1[b] B cell to make an autoantibody response (step 3) in response to autologous platelets. Note that the sensitization involved in steps 1 and 2 may take place in a primary response during the first transfusion or exposure and that step 3 may take place in a clinically noticeable way only after a secondary exposure to homologous platelets.

IMPLICATIONS AND THERAPY

The significance of this issue to hematology ranges from syndromes such as AIHA and idiopathic thrombocytopenic purpura to iatrogenically induced autoimmunity as in PTP. In the latter case, a phenomenon known as epitope spreading, which is documented in murine models, but little discussed in terms of PTP, is speculated to be a relevant pathogenetic mechanism. A basic understanding of the mechanisms of self-tolerance and their breakdown in autoimmune disease raises the possibility of many types of specific therapeutic interventions. One of the clearest would be to identify initiating factors, such as infections, and to prevent or treat them. A second approach would be to reset tolerance. Some of the previous examples, such as in PTP, illustrate how an initiating event can be amplified, leading to broken tolerance. If the system can be set back to the state before that event, the disease could be cured. At present, it is unclear how to do this; however, an autologous or even allogeneic hematopoietic stem cell transplant may have the desired effect. In fact, this sort of radical therapy has been tried in selected cases of severe SLE and seems to have some efficacy. Another promising area is in channeling the immune response, particularly as the steering mechanisms are becoming better understood at the molecular level. Work in this area is currently active. A third area is to design more specific modulators of inflammation, including interfering with costimulatory signals. These latter approaches have seemed promising in various animal models though issues with unexpected effects on clotting have arisen in clinical trials of CD40L inhibition.

Current therapy is much more crude, and typically involves general nonspecific immunosuppression either with steroids or cytotoxic drugs. Although these therapies can be effective, they have numerous undesirable side effects, not the least of which is increased susceptibility to infection due to immunosuppression. More promising are drugs that inhibit the effects of TNF-α, which have proven successful in modifying progression of rheumatoid arthritis and also in inflammatory bowel disease, psoriasis, and graft-versus-host disease.[159–161] This approach, though a result of modern biotechnology and our understanding of immunopathogenesis, still targets effector function of the immune system and does not modify the root cause of disease. Therapies should ultimately be directed toward either prevention or else specific downregulation of ongoing responses. Recently, rituximab, an antibody to CD20 that depletes B cells and is effective in treating non-Hodgkin lymphoma, has been used to treat a variety of autoimmune syndromes. It is showing great promise[162,163] and it has been approved to treat some rheumatoid arthritis patients.[164] It will be interesting to determine how B-cell depletion leads to long-term remissions, perhaps by interrupting positive feedback loops such as illustrated in Fig. 18–6. Future work will include continuing to define how self-tolerance is imposed and how it is broken in disease, what the critical triggers and autoantigens are, and how to use immunomodulation to treat autoimmune diseases on the basis of a better understanding of the pathogenesis.

SUGGESTED READINGS

Christensen SR, Kashgarian M, Alexopoulou L, et al: Toll-like receptor 9 controls anti-DNA autoantibody production in murine lupus. J Exp Med 202:321, 2005.

Christensen SR, Shupe J, Nickerson K, et al: TLR7 and TLR9 dictate autoantibody specificity and have opposing inflammatory and regulatory roles in a murine model of lupus. Immunity 25:417, 2006.

Croker JA, Kimberly RP: Genetics of susceptibility and severity in systemic lupus erythematosus. Curr Opin Rheumatol 17:529, 2005.

Emery P, Fleischmann R, Filipowicz-Sosnowska A, et al: The efficacy and safety of rituximab in patients with active rheumatoid arthritis despite methotrexate treatment: Results of a phase IIB randomized, double-blind, placebo-controlled, dose-ranging trial. Arthritis Rheum 54:1390, 2006.

Fairhurst AM, Wandstrat AE, Wakeland EK: Systemic lupus erythematosus: multiple immunological phenotypes in a complex genetic disease. Adv Immunol 92:1, 2006.

Graham RR, Kozyrev SV, Baechler EC, et al: A common haplotype of interferon regulatory factor 5 (IRF5) regulates splicing and expression and is associated with increased risk of systemic lupus erythematosus. Nat Genet 38:550, 2006.

Ivanov II, McKenzie BS, Zhou L, et al: The orphan nuclear receptor RORgammat directs the differentiation program of proinflammatory IL-17+ T helper cells. Cell 126:1121, 2006.

Pisitkun P, Deane JA, Difilippantonio MJ, et al: Autoreactive B cell responses to RNA-related antigens due to TLR7 gene duplication. Science 312:1669, 2006.

Subramanian S, Tus K, Li QZ, et al: A Tlr7 translocation accelerates systemic autoimmunity in murine lupus. Proc Natl Acad Sci USA 103:9970, 2006.

Weaver CT, Harrington LE, Mangan PR, et al: Th17: An effector CD4 T cell lineage with regulatory T cell ties. Immunity 24:677, 2006.

Zheng Y, Danilenko DM, Valdez P, et al: Interleukin-22, a TH17 cytokine, mediates IL-23-induced dermal inflammation and acanthosis. Nature 445:648, 2007.

REFERENCES

For complete list of references log onto www.expertconsult.com

PART III

Biology of Stem Cells and Disorders of Hematopoiesis

CHAPTER 19

OVERVIEW OF STEM CELL BIOLOGY

Mervin C. Yoder

INTRODUCTION

Stem cell biology continues to be an area of great interest and debate among scientists, politicians, and the public. In the face of such popularity, stem cell researchers must address new challenges in addition to opportunities. For example, many fundamental principles that define stem cells have not been well described or discussed in a truly detailed fashion in the lay literature and, thus, use of the term *stem cells* in general conversation evokes widely varying responses from engaged parties (some informed, others uninformed, many confused, and occasionally some outrageous). The widespread use of the Internet to gather information (not via physicians or scientists interpreting information from peer-reviewed scientific journals), now educates patients and their families as to the nature and biologic potential of stem cells and the hope for therapeutic application of these cells and their derivatives, and this information influences how physicians and scientist now must communicate with their patients and the public in general. The goal of this chapter is to review some general concepts that apply to all stem cells, to define vertebrate stem cells into two fundamental classes (embryonic and adult stem cells), to compare and contrast stem cells in several different organ systems, and to discuss recent information on the development of stem cell niches in these organ systems.

Defining A Stem Cell

A stem cell may be best defined by the functional properties it displays.[1] For example, many tissues of the fully developed vertebrate require that a mechanism be present for the replacement of aged, injured, or diseased cells. The turnover of blood cells forces such a requirement because 10^8 to 10^9 white blood cells are estimated to be produced every hour in the human bone marrow to replace cells that migrate into tissues and are lost during engagement with invading microbes, become engaged in tissue remodeling and repair, or are programmed to undergo senescence. Likewise, epithelial cells residing in the human small intestine are routinely sloughed into the bowel lumen every 3 to 5 days and are replaced by new epithelium. Although cutaneous epithelial skin cells turn over at different rates depending on the portion of the body being covered, the human skin is renewed on average every 4 weeks. All tissues of the body that have normal cycles of cell replacement and repair are dependent upon resident cells for ongoing cell production, and these "special" cells are termed *stem cells*. The stem cells generally reside in specific locations (niches), are not fully differentiated (may not display the appearance or all of the functions of the mature cells of the tissue), possess controlled but robust proliferative potential (for the lifetime of the host tissue), and have the capacity to divide into daughter cells in which one of the daughter cells retains all the properties of the parental cell (self-renewal) whereas the other daughter cell adopts a differentiated fate specific for the needs of that tissue. Importantly, each stem cell possesses the individual potential to regenerate the stem cells and differentiated cell progeny required to reconstitute the tissue lineage of origin; that is, hematopoietic stem cells should give rise to hematopoietic stem cells and all the progenitors and mature lineage progeny that comprise a functional hematopoietic system upon transplantation. In addition, stem cells can be defined by whether they give rise to multiple types of differentiated cells (multipotent) or a defined number of types of differentiated cells in the host tissue (two distinct cell types within a lineage would arise from a bipotent stem cell, for example). Thus, most tissue stem cells residing in vivo are defined as clonal, self-renewing, multipotent cells sustaining the homeostatic cellular requirements of a tissue or organ for the lifetime of the host.

The current concepts of clonal stem cell properties have been recognized only in the last 40 years. Prior to the 1960s, all proliferating cells in the renewing tissues of the body were thought to possess similar proliferative potential and probabilities for undergoing self-renewal divisions; one daughter cell was always preserved to maintain the proliferative pool while one daughter proceeded to form differentiated progeny. Thus, all dividing cells were thought to contribute to tissue growth and maintenance and were regarded as resident stem cells, and no specific methods were available to determine which daughter cell was specifically retained as a stem cell.

A landmark paper published in 1961 described a method for identifying repopulating cells for the hematopoietic system and established a paradigm for all studies to define stem cells. Till and McCulloch reported that rare bone marrow cells from one mouse could be infused into a lethally irradiated mouse and some of the cells that migrated to the spleen could be demonstrated to give rise to macroscopically visible hematopoietic cell nodules protruding from the spleen within 10 to 14 days posttransplant.[2] These nodules were proven to be derived from a single cell (clone) that had been transplanted from the donor mouse, and the colonies forming the nodules contained further clonogenic, as well as differentiated, hematopoietic cells. The cell clones giving rise to the spleen colonies were called colony-forming units–spleen. Although more recent studies have determined that colony-forming units–spleen are in fact short-term and not long-term repopulating hematopoietic stem cells, the pioneering studies of Till and McCulloch provided the theoretical basis for subsequent bone marrow transplantation studies with proof that the bone marrow contains undifferentiated self-renewing cells with the proliferative potential to generate cells able to differentiate into a variety of lineages with specific properties.[3]

Clonal regeneration methods have subsequently been developed for many other tissues, including epidermis, intestine, kidney, and testis, and have been used to define the resident stem cell populations of a variety of tissues.[4] Many of these approaches require that some form of tissue injury (usually irradiation) be applied to the tissue in order to permit the regenerating clones to emerge. Although there is some concern that this approach may alter the normal cellular interactions that function at homeostasis, these methods have been useful to identify a hierarchal organization of cells within the proliferative pool in these tissues. As noted earlier, stem cells are those cells within the proliferating compartment that remain relatively undifferentiated, maintain their population size when they divide (some of the progeny becoming quiescent stem cells), and produce progeny that go on to further proliferate and differentiate into mature cells comprising the tissue.

TWO CLASSES OF VERTEBRATE STEM CELLS

Vertebrate stem cells can be classified as embryonic stem (ES) cells or adult stem cells (also called somatic or postnatal stem cells). ES cells are derived in vitro from cells removed from preimplantation

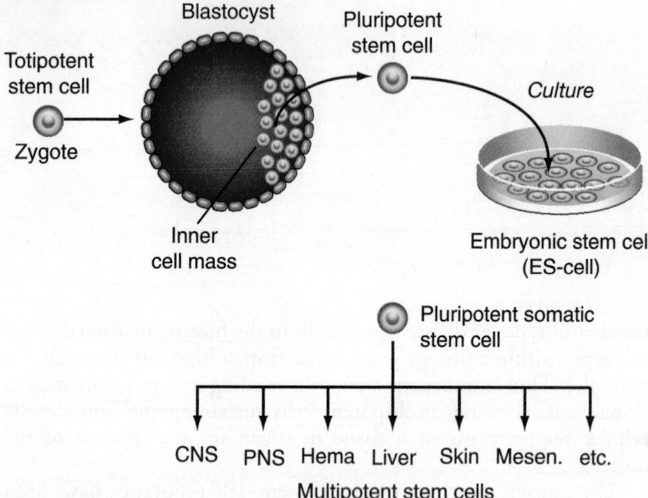

Figure 19–1 The totipotent zygote is formed from the sperm and egg. After several rounds of division, totipotent zygote-derived cells form blastocysts composed of trophoblasts that become the placenta, and the inner cell mass that forms the embryo. The inner cell mass can be collected and expanded in vitro under appropriate conditions to serve as the pluripotent embryonic stem (ES) cells. Proof of pluripotentiality is provided by injecting some of the cultured ES cells into recipient blastocysts and determining the extent of donor ES cell contribution to the cellular composition of tissues and organs throughout the chimeric embryos. The cultured ES cells can also be differentiated into cells of every somatic lineage in vitro. The intermediate stem cells that are formed from the ES cells that are restricted to the lineage of a particular organ are called multipotent stem cells. *(From Anderson DJ, Gage FH, et al: Can stem cells cross lineage boundaries? Nature Med 7:393, 2001 [modified from Fig. 1, p. 394].)*

embryos. Adult stem cells represent the self-renewing populations residing in many tissues and organs including bone marrow, brain, retina, skin, intestine, and perhaps liver, lung, and kidney. The following section will provide a comparative overview of ES cell and adult stem cell biology.

EMBRYONIC STEM CELLS

Introduction

The fertilized oocyte (zygote) is the "mother" of all stem cells (Fig. 19–1). This cell has the potential for forming all the cells and tissues of the body plan, including the placenta and extraembryonic membranes.[5] Thus, the zygote is a totipotent cell. The 3- to 5-day-old embryo is called the blastocyst. The blastocyst is composed of the following structures: the blastocoel, which is the hollow cavity inside the blastocyst; the inner cell mass, which is composed of 30 to 40 cells located at one end of the blastocoel; and the trophoblast, which is the layer of cells that surrounds the blastocyst. The first few cleavage stage divisions also produce blastomere cells, retaining totipotency. The formation of the blastocyst heralds several important changes. One portion of the blastocyst, called the inner cell mass, contains cells that will go on to form the embryo proper (epiblast). The columnar cells of the epiblast are adjacent to the trophoblast, whereas the cuboidal cells of the hypoblast are closer to the blastocoel. Trophectoderm cells comprise the cells forming the outer layer of the blastocoel; these cells will differentiate to form the placenta and some cells of the extraembryonic membranes. The inner cell mass of the blastocyst contains cells that are pluripotent; that is, each cell possesses the potential to give rise to types of cells that develop into each of the three embryonic germ cell layers (mesoderm, endoderm, and ectoderm) and if adoptively transferred into a recipient blastocyst, the donor inner cell mass cells can contribute to formation of all the tissues belonging to the resulting chimeric embryo.[6,7] The inner cell mass cells are no longer totipotent because they have lost the capacity to generate extra embryonic tissues such as a placenta and therefore cannot develop into a fetal or adult animal.

Embryonic Stem Cell Derivation

ES cells were first isolated from cultured murine blastocysts and the murine system continues to be the most amenable among mammalian species for ES cell isolation,[8,9] although precedents may have been established in earlier studies using rabbit blastocysts[10] or murine teratocarcinoma cells.[11] Plating of the pluripotent inner cell mass cells onto a preformed monolayer of mouse feeder cells with or without conditioned medium from teratocarcinoma cells were the tissue culture conditions that ultimately proved successful in promoting emergence of ES cells. In the murine system, cultured ES cells injected into a recipient blastocyst display the potential to repopulate (to some extent) all tissues of the resulting embryo, including germ cells.[12] Because adult stem cell populations are potentially present within these formed tissues and organs, adult stem cells by definition can be derived from ES cells following injection of ES cells into a host blastocyst and transfer of the embryo to a recipient foster female. Although inner cell mass cells develop into ES cells upon plating, the ES cells that emerge are now different from the parental inner cell mass cells. Whereas inner cell mass cells quickly disappear (having a finite lifetime) from the developing embryo as the epiblast develops into the complex array of cells and tissues that comprise the embryo, ES cells in vitro proliferate indefinitely, unless withdrawn from the growth conditions and induced to differentiate. No evidence has yet been presented that inner cell mass cells or ES cells reside within adult tissues, although some stem cells derived in vitro from adult murine tissues display features strikingly similar to ES cells.

Several features distinguish ES cells from resident tissue adult stem cells. Although most adult stem cells reside in specific niches within tissues, ES cells are a derivative of the inner cell mass cells. ES cells can be maintained in vitro as an essentially pure population of stem cells (free from differentiated progeny) for a prolonged period, if not indefinitely.[13] Surprisingly, despite this prolonged period within in vitro culture conditions, ES cells generally retain a normal karyotype and their pluripotentiality. In contrast to most adult stem cells that possess multipotency, ES cells are pluripotent cells and this aspect of murine embryonic stem (mES) cell biology can be demonstrated by injecting these cells into a recipient blastocyst, implantation of the blastocyst into a psuedopregnant dam, and analyzing the resulting reconstituted embryos for the degree of ES cell contribution to tissue chimerism. Thus, the pluripotent mES cells can not only be differentiated in vitro to form multiple cell lineages derived from the mesoderm, endoderm, and ectoderm, but chimeric embryos resulting from the blastocyst injections demonstrate the contribution of the mES cells to tissues derived from each of these germ layers (see Fig. 19–1).[6]

Human ES (hES) cells have also been derived from the inner cell mass of human blastocysts that had been donated for basic research by individuals who had frozen surplus embryos (generated to overcome infertility obstacles to pregnancy). The human inner cell mass cells are cocultured on a feeder monolayer of mouse embryonic fibroblasts under specific growth medium conditions. The hES cells that emerge have been shown to be pluripotent (formed teratomas upon transplantation into immunodeficient mice) with nearly indefinite proliferative capacity and to possess normal karyotypes.[14,15] The hES cells also displayed the ability to form mature cell progeny from all three embryonic germ layers in vitro.[16]

Embryonic Stem Cell Propagation

The capacity to expand ES cells in vitro while maintaining undifferentiated stem cell potential may be the most remarkable attribute of this culture system. As noted above, the earliest successful methods

Recent Advances in Development of ES-Like Cells

Vertebrate stem cells are generally classified into embryonic or adult stem cells. ES cells are derived in vitro from cells removed from preimplantation embryos whereas adult stem cells represent the self-renewing populations residing in many tissues and organs of the fully formed individual. However, there are several recent reports of isolation of cells from newborn or adult tissues that possess ES cell-like proliferative and pluripotent properties and suggest that the general classification of stem cells into embryonic or adult classes may be too simplistic.

Primordial germ cells (PGCs) derived from murine embryos between embryonic day (E) 8.5 and E12.5 display the ability to develop into pluripotent cells upon culture under specific conditions.[82,83] These embryonic germ (EG) cells can be cultured similar to ES cells with near unlimited proliferative potential, contribute to embryonic tissue reconstitution upon injection into recipient blastocysts, and contribution to endoderm, mesoderm, and ectoderm specified cell lineages in vitro. Although these studies have demonstrated that the germline lineage retains the ability to give rise to pluripotent cells, this property has been thought to be lost during gonadal development (beyond E13.5).[84] However, two recent reports suggest that ES-like cells may be derived from newborn or adult testis.

Culture of newborn murine testis cells under specific conditions that included addition of leukemia inhibitory factor (LIF), glial cell line-derived neurotrophic factor, epidermal growth factor, and basic fibroblast growth factor, led to the emergence of germline stem cells (GS) that displayed high proliferative potential, reconstituted the seminiferous tubules of infertile mice to generate normal sperm and produce offspring, and lacked the ability to generate other cell lineages.[85] However, with reproducible frequency, another population of stem cells also emerged in these GS cultures. These ES-like cells displayed higher proliferative potential than the GS cells, differentiated into multiple cell lineages in vitro and formed teratomas following transplantation in vivo.[86] In addition, these ES-like cells contributed to multiple embryonic tissues in embryos upon transplantation into recipient blastocysts including formation of germline chimeras from the living chimeric mice. Thus, ES-like cells could be developed from newborn testis, though this activity was not displayed when adult testis cells were examined.

Recently, derivation of pluripotent cells from adult testis spermatogonial stem cells (SSCs) has been reported.[87] SSCs were enriched using a transgenic mouse expressing a *Stra8* promoter driven–enhanced green fluorescent protein (Stra8-EGFP). The Stra8-EGFP-expressing cells displayed SSC activity, including the ability to reconstitute spermatogenesis in infertile germ cell-depleted mice. Further culture of the Stra8-EGFP-expressing cells in typical ES cell culture conditions (coculture with murine embryonic fibroblasts and LIF) led to emergence of a highly proliferative population of ES-like cells. These cells named multipotent adult germline stem cells (maGSCs) were able to generate differentiated progeny from mesoderm, endoderm, and ectoderm lineages in vitro and produce teratomas upon injection into recipient immunodeficient mice.[87] In addition, maGSCs contributed to multiple tissues of chimeric embryos generated upon transplantation of the maGSCs into recipient blastocysts and transfer into pseudopregnant female mice. Finally, male chimeric mice derived from the chimeric blastocysts were capable of germline transmission when mated. Thus, maGSCs display ES-like activity and suggest that if proven feasible, generation of similar human maGSCs would prove an exciting and noncontroversial source of stem cells, though restricted to male subjects.

A recent series of landmark papers may provide a method to generate induced pluripotent stem cells (iPSCs) from somatic cells of male or female subjects. Mouse embryonic or adult fibroblast cells were reprogrammed to express ES-like properties by retroviral introduction and expression of Oct3/4, Sox2, c-Myc, and Klf4 transcription factors and then selection for cells expressing Fbx15.[88] These cells could commit to differentiate into progeny from multiple germ layers, generate chimeric embryos after blastocyst injection, and form teratomas upon injection into immunodeficient mice. However, the DNA methylation and gene expression patterns were not similar to ES cells and the iPSCs did not form viable chimeric mice. An advance in the procedure with forced expression of the same four fundamental transcription factors but with selection for Nanog expression has led to the isolation of reprogrammed murine fibroblasts that now are ES-like in appearance, proliferation, differentiation potential, and germline competency.[89] A precautionary note from these studies was that nearly 20% of the offspring produced by the chimeric mice developed tumors that appeared to be related to reactivation of c-Myc expression. Finally, a second group of investigators has confirmed that expression of the four transcription factors Oct3/4, Sox2, c-Myc, and Klf4 in mouse fibroblasts resulted in DNA methylation, gene expression, and chromatin states that were similar to those of ES cells.[90] Notably, the cells derived from mouse fibroblasts could generate live chimeric mice when injected into tetraploid blastocysts. Although similar studies have not been conducted in human cells, these data are encouraging that methods are developing that reconstitute an ES-like state from somatic cells. If shown to be feasible, such studies could permit generation of patient-specific iPSCs for cell-based therapies for genetic or acquired disorders. One challenge will be to develop methods of gene insertion without use of retroviral vectors and to ensure that the introduced genes are under strict inducible control to avoid the emergence of tumors that has been observed in some of the above murine studies.[89]

for ES cell derivation required the use of murine feeder cells, suggesting that some feeder cell molecules were required for ES cell survival and/or proliferation. In short time, murine embryonic fibroblasts combined with selected batches of fetal calf serum proved to be a reliable feeder cell system to provide the correct niche for mES cell maintenance. In less than 10 years, culture-derived molecules were identified that have now permitted feeder-free and serum-free culture conditions for routine maintenance of mES cells.[13] Leukemia inhibitory factor (LIF) was reported to be an essential factor for mES cell self-renewal via gp130 activation of the signal transactivator of transcription 3 (STAT 3) signaling pathway.[17,18] Bone morphogenetic protein 4 (BMP4) is a second molecule found to be the critical serum-derived factor important in maintaining mES cell proliferation and its undifferentiated state.[19] Addition of these two molecules is sufficient to replace the original feeder cell niche and fetal calf serum requirements for mES cell maintenance. Thus, it is apparent that the principal factors required for maintaining mES cells are cell-autonomous because few input molecules are required from the feeder cells or as recombinant culture medium supplements. The ability to define the in vitro culture requirements for mES cell maintenance will undoubtedly improve methods for determining specific molecular pathways that define the autonomous self-renewal state of mES cells.

The culture conditions required to maintain hES cell self-renewal and maintenance of pluripotency have been difficult to define because it is now well known that hES and mES cells have different requirements. Whereas mES cells require LIF signaling to maintain pluripotency, hES cells do not.[20] Furthermore, whereas BMP4 is sufficient to maintain mES pluripotent cells by blocking differentiation along the neuroectodermal lineage, hES cells differentiate into trophectoderm cells when exposed to BMP4.[21] Wnt signaling appears to play an important role in maintaining mES and hES cell pluripotency, although activation of this pathway is insufficient for maintaining pluripotent hES cells in vitro.[22] Recent data implicate activin/nodal and fibroblast growth factor (FGF) pathways as the critical molecules for the maintenance of hES cell pluripotency.[23] Further studies to define the culture medium and matrix attachment factor requirements to maintain hES cells in a serum-free media will greatly advance a more widespread study of the biologic potential of these cells.

One recent advance in the field of stem cell biology is the recognition that pluripotent epiblast stem cells (EpiSCs) can be isolated from mice.[24,25] When murine embryonic day (E)5.5–5.75 late epiblast cell layers were dissected from early postimplantation embryos, EpiSCs emerged as flat compact colonies of cells that were morphologically distinct from mES cells. Of interest, EpiSCs only emerged when plated in the presence of irradiated mouse embryonic fibroblast feeder layers or in chemically defined culture medium with added activin A and FGF2. Addition of LIF and/or BMP4, the factors required for mES cell isolation and propagation, failed to support the survival of the EpiSCs. The EpiSCs displayed a pattern of transcription factor expression that is typical of pluripotent cells, maintained normal karyotypes, and gave rise to differentiated progeny of all three embryonic germ layers. Surprisingly, the EpiSCs and hES cells were found to display similar gene expression profiles and signaling responses that correspond to the patterns observed in the epiblast. These novel insights and future study may help to better understand the similarities and differences between mES, hES, and EpiSCs and lead to more focused approaches to maintain hES cells in vitro and differentiate the cells.

Embryonic Stem Cell Differentiation

Removing LIF from the culture medium will induce mES cells to differentiate into progeny belonging to all three embryonic germ layers. Currently, mES cell differentiation is conducted using one of three approaches.[13] If the mES cells are allowed to aggregate, the cells will form three-dimensional spheres called embryoid bodies (EBs). If the mES cells are plated on a feeder cell layer, differentiation will take place as the mES cells and adherent feeder cells interact. Finally, mES cells can be plated on culture dishes coated with a variety of extracellular matrix proteins with or without fetal calf serum and other additives. Obviously, use of these methods differs greatly in the specific mechanisms existent in that system leading to lineage specification and cellular differentiation, and yet each of these approaches strives to address similar principles.[13] First, the differentiation protocol should be reproducible with a robust yield of an enriched cell population. The differentiation protocol should also recapitulate the developmental program that is normally required to establish that particular lineage in the embryo. Finally, the differentiated cells that are derived from the mES cells should display the specific and expected functional properties both in vitro and in vivo known to be representative of the in vivo functions of that particular lineage under investigation. Although great progress has been made in achieving the first two principles, considerable work remains in proving that mES cell-derived cells mimic in entirety the functional properties of their in vivo counterparts. Specific details on the differentiation potential of mES cells and human ES cells can be found in several recent review articles.[13,26–29]

ADULT STEM CELLS

Introduction

Adult stem cells represent the clonal, self-renewing, multipotent cells residing in many tissues and organs that maintain the homeostatic cellular requirements of that tissue or organ for the lifetime of the host. These cells are specified during embryogenesis from one of the primary germ layers. For example, murine hematopoietic cells first emerge from the mesoderm that emigrates from the posterior primitive streak, intestinal stem cells are derived from definitive endoderm, and skin stem cells emerge from an ectoderm origin. We will briefly review some general principles of hematopoietic, intestinal, and skin stem cell functions to highlight some of the similarities and differences among these adult stem cells.

Hematopoietic Stem Cells

Hematopoietic stem cells (HSCs) are characterized by the ability to self-renew and differentiate into all mature blood lineages.[30,31] HSCs are capable of rescuing lethally irradiated hosts by reconstituting the entire repertoire of hematopoietic cells in the host. HSCs are rare cells, occurring at a frequency of 1 in 10,000 to 100,000 murine bone marrow cells with a total pool size estimated at 10,000 to 20,000 cells per mouse.[32] At steady state, the vast majority of HSCs are quiescent with only a fraction of these cells entering into a cycling state to proliferate and give rise to daughter cells that commit to further proliferation and differentiation as progenitors for the mature blood cell lineages. It has been estimated that billions of blood cells are produced each hour in the healthy human adult subject throughout its lifespan and under most circumstances this enormous production is balanced by programmed cell losses so that the circulating number of cells remains unchanged. However, when perturbed by a systemic stress such as an infection, acute bleeding, or chemotherapy, HSCs are called upon and are responsive to proliferate extensively in order to make sufficient progeny to meet the supply of blood cells required.

The stem cell hierarchy theory predicts that the first daughter progeny derived from HSCs are short-term repopulating HSCs with the potential to give rise to both lymphoid and myeloid progeny (Fig. 19–2).[30] Subsequently, daughter cells commit to either the lymphoid lineage via a common lymphoid progenitor or the myeloid lineage via a common myeloid progenitor cell. Common lymphoid progenitors further divide and differentiate into lymphocytes of the T, B, and NK lineages. Common myeloid progenitors give rise to granulocyte–monocyte precursors and megakaryocyte–erythrocyte precursors that subsequently differentiate into granulocytes and monocytes or red blood cells and platelets, respectively.

Evidence that a cell possesses long-term repopulating HSC activity requires transplantation of that cell into a recipient subject. In the murine and human system, HSC transplantation results in complete reconstitution of all blood cell lineages if donor HSCs are injected into hosts following some form of myeloablation (to eliminate the immune system and the endogenous HSC/progenitor cells). Murine HSCs will also engraft in nonablated hosts if very large numbers of HSCs are transplanted or in situations where the vasculature of syngeneic (genetically identical) mice is joined and cells are freely able to circulate from the marrow compartment of one animal through the blood and into the marrow of the parabiotic partner.[33] If the murine donor cells engraft and reconstitute all the blood cell lineages for more than 4 months, the donor cells are confirmed to possess long-term repopulating HSC activity.[34] If the donor cells reconstitute the blood cells for the lymphoid and myeloid lineages, the cells are called long-term multilineage repopulating HSCs. Confirmation of HSC self-renewal activity can be demonstrated by transplanting the reconstituted marrow of the primary recipient animal and determining that secondary myeloablated animals are also fully reconstituted.[3] Despite the fact that HSCs express telomerase activity, replication of HSCs is finite, and donor murine HSCs can be serially transplanted only a certain number of times (four to seven), with eventual stem cell exhaustion.

The HSC repopulating ability can be enumerated by a competitive repopulation assay in the murine system. In this assay, hematopoietic cells from a test mouse are mixed in various proportions with those from a competitor mouse before injection into a lethally irradiated recipient mouse.[35] Using a limiting dilution assay, the frequency of the long-term repopulating HSCs is measured by the ability of these cells to outcompete the competitor cells for engraftment and contributions to all the blood cell lineages in the recipient mouse.[36] In the human system, one cannot perform such a competitive assay. Instead, transplantation of putative human HSCs into sublethally myeloablated immunocompromised mice permits quantitation of human pan-leukocyte antigen CD45-expressing cells residing in the bone marrow of the recipient mice. The combined use of this in vivo assay with several in vitro assays lends experimental support for a stem cell hierarchical organization of human hematopoiesis similar to the mouse model system.

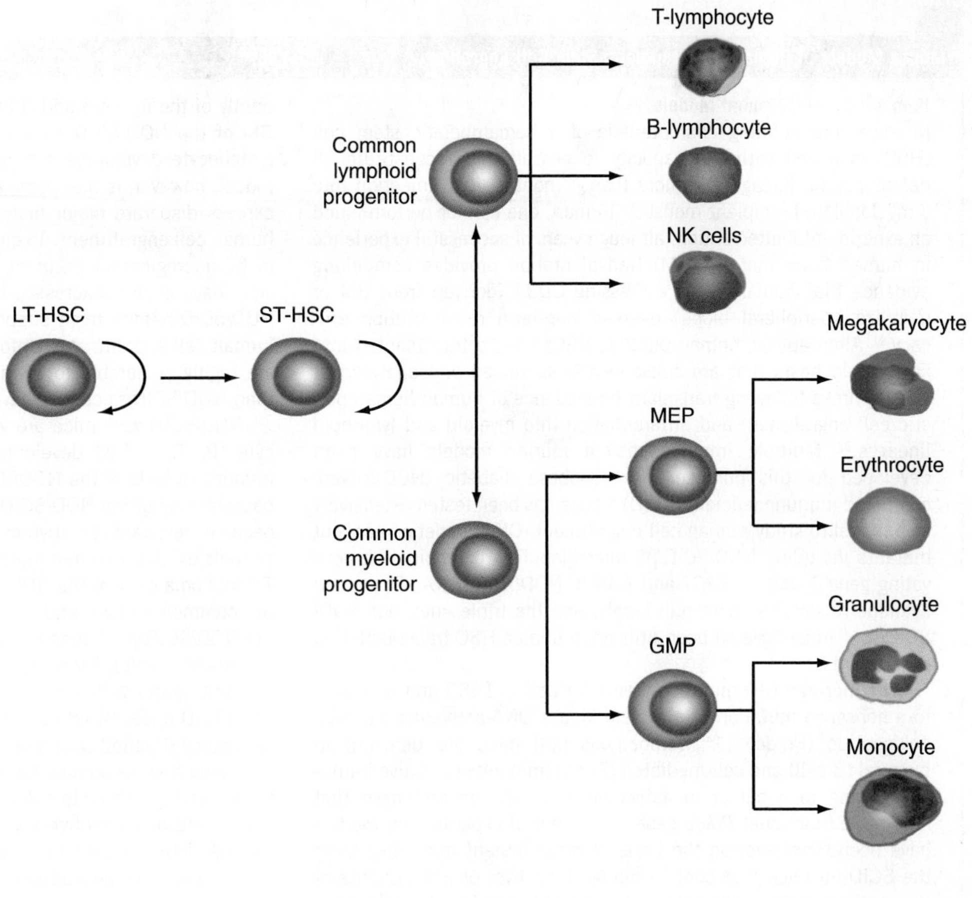

Figure 19–2 The hematopoietic hierarchy. As hematopoietic stem cells divide, they give rise to common lymphoid and common myeloid precursor cells that eventually generate all mature blood lineages of the body. GMP, granulocyte–monocyte precursors; LT-HSC, long-term hematopoietic stem cells; MEP, megakaryocyte–erythrocyte precursors; NK, natural killer; ST-HSC, short-term hematopoietic stem cells. *(From Leung AYH, Verfaillie CM: Stem cell model of hematopoiesis. In 4th Edition of Hematology: Basic Principles and Practice, p. 201, Fig. 17–1 Elsevier, Philadelphia.)*

Intestinal Stem Cells

The intestinal epithelium displays typical epithelial evidence of polarization and organization into discrete units of proliferating and differentiated cells.[37] The small intestine is characterized by complete coverage with finger-like villi protruding into the lumen. The predominant cells covering the villi are columnar epithelium that participate in the uptake of digested food elements, become senescent, and are sloughed from the tip of the villi. Surprisingly, there is no proliferation of cells at the villous tip to replace the lost epithelium, but there is a striking balance between the loss of villous epithelium and proliferation of intestinal epithelial stem cells (ISC) and transient amplifying (TA) epithelial progenitor cells near the base of the villi in regions called crypts.[38] It is estimated that the epithelium covering each villus arises from six adjacent crypts and each crypt can produce cells that migrate onto more than a single villus. More than 50% of the crypt epithelial cells are proliferating with a cell cycle of 12 hours and 200 to 300 epithelial cells are replaced daily. All of the proliferating cells can be traced back to the ISC, which resides four cell diameters from the base of the crypt in the small intestine, near the midcrypt in the ascending colon and in the base of the crypt in the descending colon.[39] Small-intestine ISC display a 24-hour cell cycle and give rise to daughter cells that become TA progenitor cells before giving rise to mature epithelial cells of several different mature cell lineages, including Paneth, goblet, absorptive enterocytes, and enteroendocrine cells (Fig. 19–3).

The highly organized spatial localization of the ISC and TA cells of the small intestine have permitted extensive analysis of villus epithelial regeneration despite the lack of cell surface markers (though some progress in marker identification has been recently reported). In the absence of a transplant assay for ISC identification, several approaches have been used to support the hypothesis of the clonal regeneration of intestinal epithelium from ISC. The crypt microcolony assay utilizes a cytotoxic injury (typically irradiation) to eliminate the villus epithelial cells to induce radioresistant crypt cells to regenerate the entire villus.[40] This assay has provided evidence that a single surviving stem cell can regenerate all of the cell types of a villus.[38] A developmental approach using mouse aggregation chimeras demonstrated that the villus crypts of chimeras were not formed through mixing of readily distinguishable strains but, in fact, were either derived from one strain or the other; that is, each crypt was composed of a clonal population.[41] Similar conclusions have been reached when examining mice carrying somatic mutations at specific loci that permitted tracking clonal succession in the intestinal crypt ISC to replace the villus epithelium.[42] Some human populations carry genetic mutations that also permit analysis of enzymatic activity in the colon, and these studies have provided evidence to support the clonal regeneration of the intestinal epithelium from ISC.[43] In sum, intestinal epithelial cells are regenerated via ISC replication and generation of TA progenitor cells that give rise to the multiple lineages of epithelial cells residing in a villus. This hierarchical organization is quite similar to that of the HSC.

Epidermal Stem Cells

As the outermost protective covering of the body, the epidermis is subjected to a host of challenges. Skin serves as the first line of defense against microbial invasion and prevents the body from dehydrating. Many physical and chemical forces are capable of abrading, cutting, burning, or breaking down the epidermis and, thus, this organ must respond with reepithelialization. Proliferation of cells in the most basal layer of the skin provides the source of cells that migrate outward, differentiate, and mature into the epithelium that produces the keratinized stratum corneum.[44] Cells are routinely sloughed from the interfollicular epidermis; thus, at homeostasis, basal cell proliferation must be balanced to produce sufficient cells to maintain the protective function of the skin but avoid overproduction, as seen in some human disorders such as psoriasis and cancer.[45] The epidermis is replaced in distinct epidermal proliferative units that emerge as

Mouse Models of Human Hematopoietic Stem Cell Engraftment

Human HSC Engraftment Models

In mice, the defining characteristic of a hematopoietic stem cell (HSC) is a cell with the capacity to engraft and reconstitute all hematopoietic lineages for more than 4 months upon injection into a myeloablated recipient mouse.[34] In man, one cannot perform such an experimental intervention, although years of successful experience in human bone marrow (BM) transplantation provides compelling evidence that human HSCs expressing CD34 (derived from BM or mobilized peripheral blood) possess long-term reconstitution efficacy.[91] Alternatively, human putative HSCs can be transplanted into xenogeneic hosts that are subsequently sacrificed and analyzed at varying times following transplant for evidence of human hematopoietic cell engraftment and differentiation into myeloid and lymphoid lineages.[92] Multiple immunodeficient murine models have been developed for this purpose. The nonobese diabetic (NOD)/severe combined immunodeficient (SCID) mouse has been tested extensively as a model to study human cell engraftment. Other genetic knockout mutants including NOD/SCID/β2-microglobulin, recombination activating gene 1 and 2 (*RAG1* and *RAG2*), NOD/*RAG1*, *RAG2*/common cytokine receptor γ chain null (γc^{null}), and the triple knockout NOD/SCID/γc^{null} mice have all been utilized in human HSC transplantation experiments.[92,93]

The murine SCID mutation was described in 1983 and is related to a nonsense mutation of a protein kinase DNA-activating catalytic polypeptide ($Prkdc^{scid}$).[94] Homozygous null mice are deficient in humoral (B cell) and cell-mediated (T cell) immunity (adaptive immunity) owing to a defect in activation of a DNA recombinase that requires a functional *Prkdc* gene. A number of experimental models have been developed on the basis of these mutant mice, including the SCID-hu mice that contain human fetal liver or BM explants of tissue inserted under the host renal capsule to provide "human" sites for human HSC engraftment, triple chimeric mice (normal mice that are lethally irradiated, transplanted with SCID marrow cells, and then transplanted with human BM cells), and the most commonly used model in which sublethally irradiated SCID mice are injected intravenously with human test cells. However, human HSC engraftment in these models remains relatively low because compensatory increases in natural killer (NK) cell, granulocyte, and macrophage cell numbers, and hemolytic complement elevations leads to human graft rejection.[95]

The NOD mouse displays spontaneous autoimmune T cell-mediated, insulin-dependent diabetes mellitus. Defects in innate immunity, including NK and macrophage functions, and diminished complement component C5 activity are also present. Cross-breeding of the NOD and SCID strains generates progeny (NOD/SCID) that are defective in both innate and adaptive immunity but do not develop diabetes. When human HSCs are injected into these animals, significantly greater engraftment is observed compared to human HSC transplantation into the SCID mice.[95] Differentiated cells predominantly of the myeloid and B lymphocyte lineages are observed in the BM of the NOD/SCID mice following transplantation and human T lymphocyte development is lacking. A caveat about the NOD/SCID model, however, is that some animals retain residual NK activity and express disparate major histocompatibility (MHC) loci, limiting the human cell engraftment. To circumvent this limitation, mice deficient in β2-microglobulin ($\beta 2m^{null}$), a protein required for MHC I expression, have been backcrossed into the NOD/SCID mice. The resulting NOD/SCID/$\beta 2m^{null}$ mice support fivefold to tenfold higher levels of human cell engraftment. Unfortunately, these immunodeficient mice are highly vulnerable to thymic lymphoma and more radiosensitive than NOD/SCID mice and have a shorter lifespan.[96]

NOD/SCID/γc^{null} mice are viable and fertile but lack any lymphocyte (B, T, or NK) development in addition to displaying innate immune defects of the NOD/SCID mouse.[95,97] Of interest, during the backcrossing of the NOD/SCID strain with the γc^{null} mice, the animals became resistant to thymic lymphoma and the NOD/SCID/γc^{null} animals exhibit a normal murine lifespan (it became evident that the T lymphoma cells of the NOD/SCID thymus require signaling through the common γ chain and, thus, genetic ablation of this pathway in the NOD/SCID/γc^{null} mice results in thymic lymphoma resistance). As one might predict, these triple knockout mice accept human hematopoietic grafts with significantly higher levels of engraftment than NOD/SCID mice. Of interest, transplantation of these animals during the neonatal period with donor human cord blood cells results in not only bone marrow reconstitution with myeloid and lymphoid cells but thymic and lymph node colonization and circulating T and B cells.[98] The innate and adaptive function of the transplanted human cells can be demonstrated by challenging the engrafted mice with an immunogen and measuring circulating antibody and cytotoxic T-cell responses.

Human Epithelial Stem Cell Engraftment Model

Although transplantation of murine epidermal bulge stem cells (BSCs) into the skin of young mice results in reconstitution of complete hair follicle structures,[99] similar studies have not been conducted with human epidermal stem cells. Likewise, neither murine nor human intestinal stem cells (ISCs) have been demonstrated to reconstitute the intestinal villi in the small or large intestine of a xenogenic model. Development of a small animal transplantation model that permits isolation of BSCs and ISCs that display long-term epithelial reconstitution (including all cell lineages that normally constitute these tissues) upon transplantation would be a great advance in permitting a clearer definition of the key cell types that may be required for therapeutic use in human subjects suffering from epidermal or intestinal epithelial dysfunction. Demonstration of clonal human epithelial reconstitution from a single transplanted epithelial stem cell would also provide an unambiguous assay to permit isolation of the human epithelial stem cells.

hexagonally packed cells.[46] Lineage-marking studies have determined that each epidermal proliferative unit arises from a single basal cell.[47] Clonal regenerative assays developed in mice have revealed that approximately 10% of basal cells function as epidermal stem cells. In the interfollicular epidermis, the self-renewing basal stem cells give rise to a small population of amplifying basal cells that migrate into the spinosum and granular layers of the dermis, differentiate, and give rise to the mature cells and eventually the cornified layer. This cycle of epidermal replenishment is estimated to occur every 4 weeks in human subjects.[44,48]

More recent studies have determined that the hair follicles in the epidermis are also in constant turnover, with specific cycles of degeneration and regeneration, and specific stem cells have been demonstrated to participate in this process (Fig. 19–4).[49] Hair follicles emerge during embryogenesis and undergo a process of follicular cycling after birth. The hair cycle is composed of three phases; anagen, catagen, and telogen (Fig. 19–5). In the murine system, the hair follicles grow synchronously until 2 weeks of postnatal age, when proliferation of cells at the base of the hair shaft ceases, and the follicle enters the destructive catagen phase. This phase is a brief 3 to 4 days in mice but most cells of the follicle undergo apoptosis. During the telogen phase, the follicle lies dormant and the hair becomes a mere remnant; this period can range from 1 to 14 days. To resume the anagen phase, proliferative cells in the follicle must regenerate a new round of hair growth, and this process recurs throughout the life of the animal.[44,49] The lowermost region of the hair follicle during the telogen phase is the site where the stem cells begin proliferating and forming a "bulge" to herald the anagen-phase onset (Fig. 19–4). These follicle stem cells (FSCs) display proliferative kinetics that differ a great deal from other proliferating cells in the basal layer. In

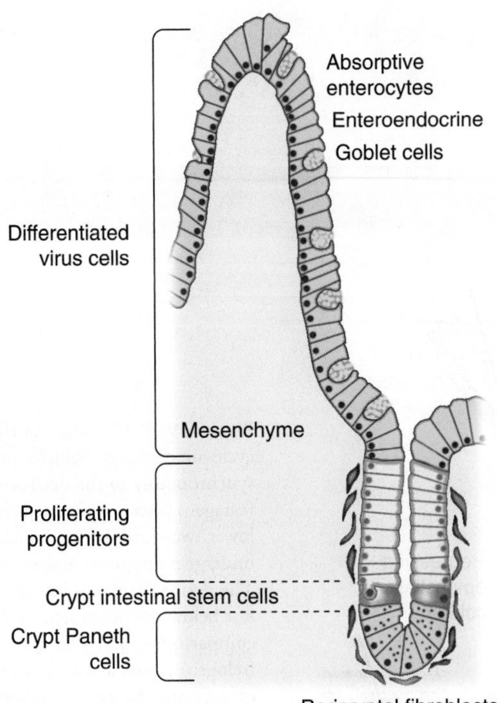

Figure 19–3 Stem cells within their niche in the small intestine. Schematic diagram of the major types and spatial orientations of cells found within the crypt niche and the villus. *(From Moore KA, Lemischka IR: Stem cells and their niches. Science 311:1880, 2006 [modified from Fig. 1A, p. 1881].)*

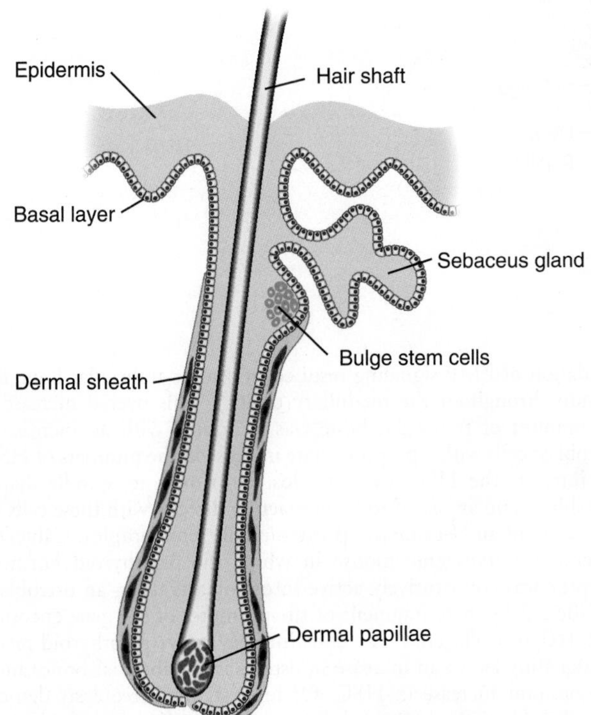

Figure 19–4 Stem cells within their niche in the hair follicle. Schematic diagram of the major types and spatial orientations of cells that make up the hair follicle. Colors correspond to the cell types that mediate the interactive signaling leading to the proliferation and differentiation of the hair follicle cell types. *(From Moore KA, Lemischka IR: Stem cells and their niches. Science 311:1880, 2006 [modified from Fig. 2A, p. 1882].)*

fact, microarray-profiling studies have identified nearly 150 genes that FSCs preferentially express compared to the proliferating basal epidermal cells.[50] Many of the genes that are enriched in FSCs are associated with inducing and maintaining cellular quiescence.[51] Nonetheless, FSCs can be activated and can regenerate the hair follicle and contribute to replace basal cells that may be depleted in response to significant reepithelialization following major cutaneous injury.[52]

Stem cell maintenance of epithelial turnover in another hair follicle appendage, the sebaceous gland, has also recently been demonstrated. Sebaceous glands are located just beneath the orifice of the hair shaft at the surface of the skin and release lipids and sebum that protect the hair canal from microbial overgrowth and invasion. Release of the lipids and sebum occurs with the death of the mature sebocyte, and thus, sebaceous epithelial progenitor cells are constantly producing mature sebocytes to replace the dying cells. Fate-mapping studies using retroviral labeling of epithelial cells in vivo strongly implicated the presence of a sebaceous stem cell population.[53] However, the recognition that cells expressing BLIMP1 can yield sebocyte colonies in vitro and undergo self-renewal provided evidence for the presence of a specific population of stem cells.[54] Surprisingly, during injury to the skin, sebaceous gland homeostasis is altered and BLIMP1-expressing cells are bolstered by an influx of FSCs. Thus, FSCs contribute to regeneration of all the major specialized cells of the epidermis and may serve as a readily accessible source of cells for potential human therapy. Again the hierarchical organization of the FSC, various basal, bulge, and sebaceous stem and progenitor cells, and the mature epidermal lineages derived from each suggest a paradigm very similar to that of the HSC and ISC.

STEM CELL NICHES

Introduction

Stem cells generally reside in specific locations (niches), are not fully differentiated (may not display the appearance or all of the functions of the mature cells of the tissue), possess controlled but robust proliferative potential (at least for the lifetime of the host tissue), and have the capacity to divide into daughter cells in which one of the daughter cells retains all the properties of the parental cell (self-renewal) whereas the other daughter adopts a differentiated fate specific for the needs of that tissue. Although some of the molecular regulation of these stem cell functions may be intrinsic to the stem cells,[55,56] recent evidence highlights the critical role of niche supportive cells that surround the stem cells to form a protective and regulatory microenvironment.[57] Cells that comprise the niche form a highly dynamic interactive system that functions as a physical anchor for the stem cells to regulate their location, generates extrinsic factors that control stem cell fate and number, and protects the stem cells from injurious external stimuli that otherwise might induce stem cell apoptosis. Defining the niche for a variety of tissue-specific stem cells has become a very active area of research. An obvious complication in attempting to dissect the molecular regulation of stem cell activity via the niche is the multicellular nature of many of the tissue resident niches. However, great advances in understanding the molecular mechanisms regulating stem cell development within specific niches in invertebrate species have opened new pathways for discovery in mammalian systems. Several key pathways including Wnt–β-catenin, TGF-β–BMP, and Notch appear to play important roles in the interactions between niche cells and hematopoietic, intestinal, and epidermal stem cells.

Hematopoietic Stem Cell Niche

The concept that hematopoietic progenitors interact with specific cellular elements within a tissue to form a specialized interactive unit (niche) is largely attributed to Schofield nearly 30 years ago.[58] But, as Scadden has recently pointed out, the niche is more of an ecologi-

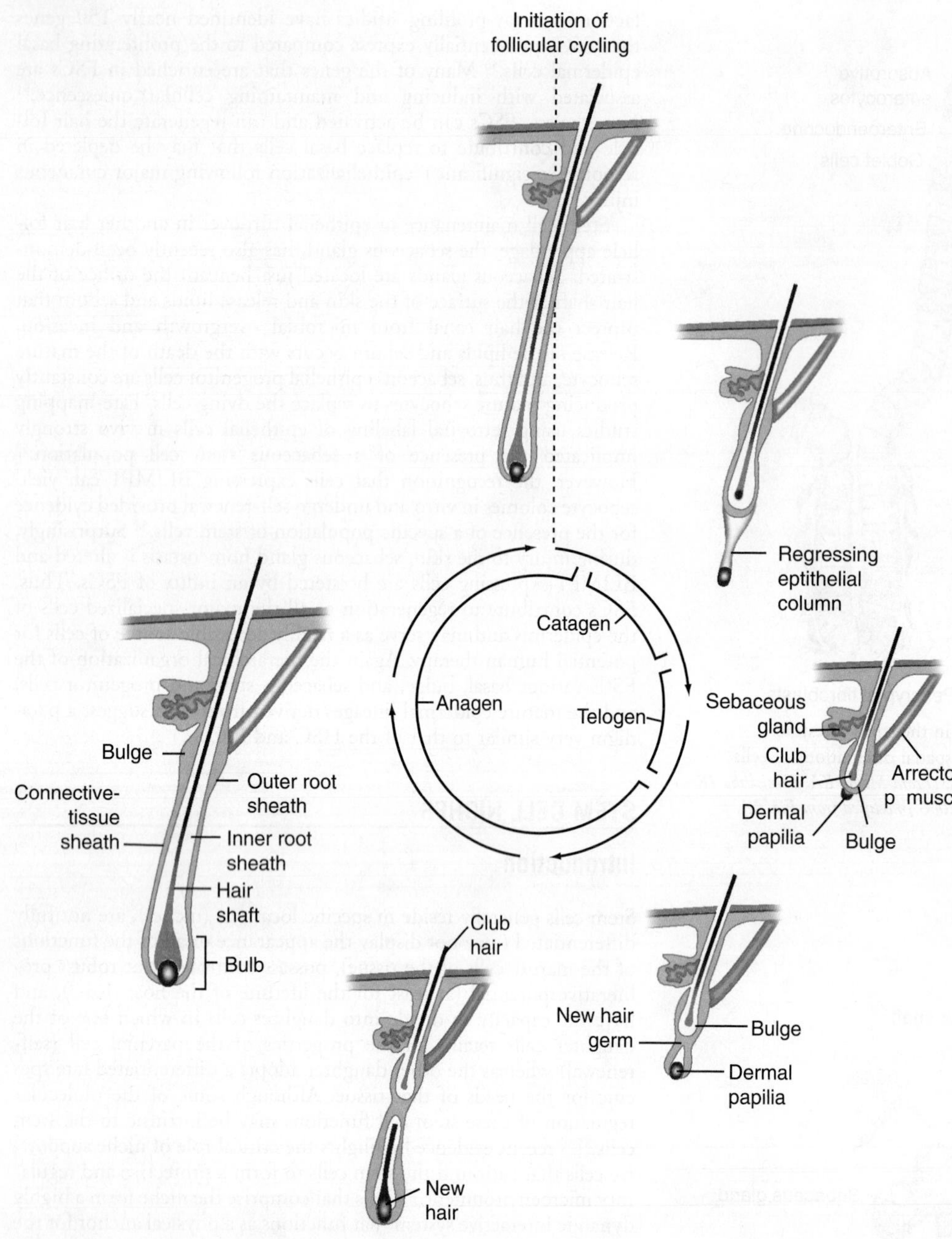

Figure 19–5 The stages of the hair cycle are depicted. Follicles progress synchronously to the destructive (catagen) phase, during which the lower two-thirds of the follicle undergoes apoptosis and regresses. The dermal papilla is brought to rest below the bulge stem cell compartment, and after the resting (telogen) phase, a critical threshold of activating factors is reached and the stem cells become activated to regrow hair. *(From Fuchs E: Scratching the surface of skin development. Nature 445:834, 2007 [modified from Fig. 3, p. 837].)*

cal habitat that requires a sustained interaction between nonhematopoietic cells and the HSCs, rather than an architectural anatomical recess where HSCs merely repose.[59] HSCs are not restricted to the marrow niches but are dynamically entering and traversing the systemic circulation with brief transit times (seconds).[33] The mechanisms for this migration are unknown but, in fact, recapitulate the ontogenic delivery of HSCs from one hematopoietic site to another as gestation progresses. In the adult mouse and man, the bone medullary cavity is the primary residence of the majority of quiescent HSC. In vivo tracking and homing studies have demonstrated a periosteal localization for intravenously injected HSC in mice.[60] The specific interacting cells that comprise the niche have only recently been identified.

Several pieces of evidence suggest that spindle-shaped osteoblasts lining trabecular bone in the marrow cavity play a seminal role in the HSC niche (Fig. 19–6). In vitro culture of osteoblastic cells with HSC promotes progenitor cell expansion, but the documentation of a direct effect of the osteoblast on HSC required in vivo approaches. Using a bone morphogenetic protein (BMP) receptor 1A conditional knockout transgenic mouse model, Zhang et al reported that down-regulation of BMP signaling resulted in ectopic trabecular bone formation throughout the medullary cavity.[61] This overall increase in the amount of trabecular bone was associated with an increase in osteoblast cells with a proportionate increase in the numbers of HSC. Of interest, the HSC were in close proximity to spindle-shaped osteoblasts and appeared to be interacting directly with these cells via formation of an N-cadherin–β-catenin adherens complex. Calvi et al generated a transgenic mouse in which the parathyroid hormone receptor was constitutively active in osteoblasts using an osteoblast-specific 2.3-kilobase fragment of the promoter of the gene encoding type 1α1 procollagen.[62] The constitutively active parathyroid receptor signaling led to an increase in osteoblasts, trabecular bone, and a concomitant increase in HSC. Of interest, the osteoblasts demonstrated an increase in Jagged 1 expression and increased Notch 1 activation in the HSC that could be blocked with γ-secretase inhibition. Whether this is an effect only active in HSC expansion in this transgenic system or plays a role in homeostatic regulation of HSC remains controversial, as Jagged 1-deficient mice have normal hematopoiesis. Support for the specific role of osteoblasts in the regulation of HSC number and function was demonstrated by Visnjic et al, who

Germline Stem Cells: Big Lessons from Small Flies

Introduction

Regulating stem cell divisions to provide for sufficient cells to maintain tissue homeostasis but avoiding overproduction of undifferentiated stem cells (a potential pool of cells susceptible to secondary mutation emergence and tumorigenesis) is a fine balance. Asymmetric stem cell divisions whereby one daughter cell commits to a differentiation pathway whereas the other daughter maintains a stem cell fate, is an obvious strategy to keep stem cell numbers adequate for tissue needs, but a restricted stem cell pool number. *Drosophila* germline stem cells (GSCs) have become well-studied models for understanding the importance of the cellular microenvironment (stem cell niche) in regulating the crucial decision between stem cell maintenance or expansion (self-renewal divisions) and production of differentiated progeny.[100,101]

Male Germ Cells

The adult *Drosophila* testis is a long coiled structure filled with a hierarchically organized arrangement of cells at all stages of spermatogenesis (Fig. 19–7).[102,103] In the apical tip of the testis, 6 to 12 GSCs are arranged in a ring that directly contacts a cluster of postmitotic somatic cells called the hub. The hub cells represent an important microenvironment (niche) that supports the regulation of GSC survival, self-renewal, and differentiation. The GSCs interact with hub cells via adherens junctions and through local signals that are so restricted that stem cells one diameter away are not responsive to the hub cell signals. Division of a male GSC results in the formation of one cell that remains in the niche in contact with the hub cells to retain stem cell activity and a second cell, called the gonialblast, which is moved away from contact with the hub cells and initiates differentiation (Fig. 19–7). The GSC self-renewal decision is mediated via activation of the Janus kinase–signal transducers and activators of transcription (JAK–STAT) pathway in the GSC via a cytokine-like ligand Unpaired (UPD) expressed by the hub cells.[104,105] During GSC division, the daughter cell that is displaced from the hub cell (gonialblast) senses a diminished UPD signal and commences differentiation, whereas the daughter cell remaining in contact with the hub cells retains a strong JAK–STAT signal and a GSC identity. The gonialblast subsequently undergoes four rounds of transient amplifying divisions marked by incomplete cytokinesis to generate a cluster of 16 interconnected spermatogonia. The importance of microenvironmental signals is so crucial to the survival and differentiation of the gonialblast cells that somatic stem cells that lie interposed between the GSCs and in contact with the hub cells divide to form cyst progenitor cells (CPCs) that encircle the gonialblast cells during their proliferation and maturation (Fig. 19–7).[103] Activation of the epidermal growth factor receptor in the CPCs appears essential in limiting the proliferation of the GSCs and promoting gonialblast differentiation.[100]

Female Germ Cells

The *Drosophila* ovarian niche is composed of cap cells (CCs) and escort stem cells (ESCs), a subset of inner germarial sheath cells, which interact with cells comprising the terminal filament of the germarium (Fig. 19–8).[100,101,106] Ovarian GSCs (two to three) directly interact with the cap cells via adherens junctions. Following each GSC division, the posterior daughter cell moves away from the niche and commits to differentiate into a cystoblast cell. The cystoblast cell undergoes four synchronous divisions that are marked by incomplete cytokinesis to form a 16-cell germline cyst. Regulation of female GSC self-renewal requires bone morphogenetic protein (BMP) signaling from the niche cap cells via the ligands decapentaplegic and glass-bottomed boat.[107] The ligand-mediated activation of BMP signaling directly represses transcription of the *bag of marbles (bam)* gene in the GSCs within the niche.[108] Forced expression of the BAM protein in GSCs causes GSCs to differentiate into cystoblast cells. It has been postulated that GSC division in which one daughter loses contact with the niche results in differentiation of that cell via E3 ubiquitin ligase degradation of residual BMP signaling molecules.[100] A subset of the inner sheath cells, called escort cells, encase the newly formed cystoblast cells and remain tightly associated with these cells as they grow into the 16-cell cysts and enter meiosis. At this stage of cyst development, the escort cells undergo apoptosis and a second niche of follicle stem cells produces follicle cells that subsequently encapsulate the passing cysts and participate in the maturation and survival of the cysts.

Stem Cell Polarity in the Niche

In both male and female *Drosophila* GSC niches, there is an apparent elaborate mechanism to constrain the division of the GSCs to ensure that one of the daughter cells is retained in the niche whereas the other daughter is displaced and becomes specified to a differentiated fate. Male and female GSCs divide with mitotic spindles oriented orthogonally to the niche (hub or cap cells).[100,107] This is accomplished in the female GSCs by anchoring the spindle pole to the apical side of the GSC by a subcellular organelle called the spectrosome. In male GSCs, the anaphase-promoting complex 2 protein colocalizes with E-cadherin at the interface between the GSCs and the hub cells. This protein appears to interact with the centrosome to orient the mother centrosome to remain in the GSC near the hub whereas the daughter centrosome is allocated to the displaced daughter cell.[109] Thus, GSC and niche cells directly interact in multiple ways that affect GSC survival, self-renewal, and production of differentiated progeny.

generated a transgenic mouse in which osteoblasts could be specifically ablated.[63] The ablation was achieved using an inducible system in which ganciclovir was administered to activate thymidine kinase specifically expressed in the osteoblast lineage. Loss of osteoblasts in the ganciclovir-treated animals was associated with depressed lymphoid and myelo-erythroid progenitors, HSC number, and an overall lower bone marrow cellularity. If ganciclovir was withdrawn, the animals demonstrated recovery of osteoblast numbers and reappearance of active hematopoiesis. Interactions between angiopoietin-1-expressing osteoblast cells and Tie2-expressing HSCs appears to be required in maintaining HSCs in a quiescent state.[64] Other extrinsic signaling pathways within the niche that may regulate HSC homeostasis include the Wnt–β-catenin pathway, which has been reported to enhance HSC self-renewal.[65] Notch signaling may also play a role in inhibiting cell differentiation in the context of Wnt protein-induced proliferation.[66] However, both of these pathways have been shown to be dispensable for HSC homeostasis in genetic ablation models.[67,68] Nonetheless, these data in aggregate demonstrate an important role for osteoblasts in regulating HSC number and function within the medullary cavity.

As noted above, HSCs display the ability to circulate throughout the systemic circulation without losing potency. Indeed, during murine development, HSCs emerge and maintain a close relationship with the vascular endothelium. Endothelial cells isolated from the yolk sac and embryo proper of the mouse can stimulate adult bone marrow HSC expansion in vitro, and certain adult tissue endothelial cells appear capable of maintaining HSC repopulating ability ex vivo for some time.[69,70] Recent studies have identified HSCs in close association with bone marrow and spleen sinusoidal endothelial cells and have suggested that HSCs may lodge in a vascular niche that provides signals for HSC homeostasis.[71] One concept proposed is that the osteoblastic niche maintains quiescent HSCs and that HSC proliferation and differentiation occur in the vascular niche. Further studies will be required to examine HSC homeostasis using direct

Systems Dependent upon Changing Niches during Development

The hematopoietic system is quite unique in that the primary sites of hematopoiesis change during in utero development. The first blood cell progenitors emerge in the murine embryo on embryonic day (E) 7.0 in the visceral yolk sac.[110,111] These progenitor cells are principally specified to give rise to primitive erythroid cells, named for their expression of embryonic hemoglobin molecules, their large size, and the fact that these red blood cells retain their nucleus for many days (even while circulating) following their emergence.[112] Macrophages and megakaryocyte progenitor cells also emerge during this time and display unique identifying features.[113,114] For the next 24 hours, all three populations increase in number and then differentiate into mature forms within the yolk sac. On E8.25, a second wave of progenitor cells emerge in clusters of cells associated with the yolk sac blood vessel endothelium. These progenitor cells display characteristics of both the myeloid and erythroid lineages and are called definitive progenitors because the erythroid cells that are produced in this site synthesize adult hemoglobin molecules similar to erythrocytes in adult bone marrow.[114] Of interest, although the definitive progenitors emerge in the yolk sac, they do not appear to differentiate into mature cells in the yolk sac. Instead, the yolk sac-derived progenitor cells are hypothesized to migrate via the circulation to engraft the fetal liver, wherein they further expand and differentiate into mature blood cells. At the same time, the emergence of similar progenitor cells can be detected within the embryo proper in the region of the para-aortic splanchnopleure (P-Sp), although the number of progenitor cells emerging from this site is limited.[115] On E10.5 the P-Sp region has differentiated into the aorta–gonad–mesonephros (AGM) region and for the first time, one can isolate HSCs from this region (specifically from mesenchymal cells just beneath or associated with the overlying endothelium of the ventral aorta wall) and these cells will engraft in myeloablated adult recipient mice.[116] The fetal liver is colonized by cells from the systemic circulation at the 28-somite-pair stage of development and by E12.5 becomes the predominant site of hematopoiesis. As noted above, the initial wave of progenitor cell engraftment in the liver has been thought to occur primarily via yolk sac-derived cells. Although the vast majority of progenitor cell differentiation into mature blood cell lineages is occurring in the fetal liver, recent evidence suggests that HSC expansion (and perhaps emergence) is concomitantly occurring in multiples sites, including the yolk sac, placenta, and the AGM in addition to the liver between day E11.0 and E13.5.[117] However, by E13.5, essentially all of the HSC activity becomes restricted to the fetal liver. The next sites of hematopoiesis emerge after E13.5 and include the spleen and finally the bone marrow. Surprisingly, the bone marrow compartment does not become the predominant hematopoietic site until approximately 3 to 4 weeks postnatally. The spleen retains the ability to support some HSC maintenance though not expansion, but serves as an active hematopoietic site throughout the life of the mouse. Thus, the site of emergence and diversity of blood types produced changes dramatically during normal murine development.

It is assumed that multiple hematopoietic niches are established and lost throughout murine ontogeny as the sites of hematopoiesis change; however, very little is known about the specific developmental niches that support blood cell emergence during embryogenesis. Two well-known examples of the importance of HSC interactions with niche cells during fetal development include stromal cell expression of stem cell factor (SCF) and stromal cell-derived factor-1 alpha (SDF-1α, also called CXCL12 for CXC chemokine ligand 12). Homozygous deficiency of SCF in murine fetal liver or bone marrow stromal cells results in profound anemia and dysregulated hematopoiesis, although HSCs are formed and expand in vivo.[118] The hematopoietic defects are generally lethal in utero in the absence of any SCF production. Fetal mice deficient in SDF-1α production in the bone marrow niche fail to establish marrow hematopoiesis, although fetal liver hematopoiesis appears unaffected.[119] Of interest, fetal liver HSCs respond with far greater migration responses to the combined exposure of SCF and SDF-1α than do adult marrow HSCs, suggesting that these stromal cell-derived factors may play a role in HSC-niche establishment in the transition from fetal liver to the marrow compartment. Future studies to identify specific niche-produced factors that are important in the seeding of fetal hematopoietic organs throughout ontogeny will be of great interest, as these sites are generally involved in HSC expansion (fetal HSCs are largely cycling) rather than maintaining the HSCs in quiescence, as is the primary role of the adult bone marrow niche.

The primary sites of hematopoiesis also change throughout human development in utero.[120] Similar to that in the mouse, primitive erythroid cells emerge on day 18 of gestation along with some macrophages in the yolk sac. CD34-expressing progenitor cells are present on day 19. Expansion of the progenitor cells with multipotent and committed progenitor cells for myeloerythroid lineages occurs until day 60 when essentially all hematopoietic progenitor emergence from the human yolk sac ceases. Clusters of hematopoietic cells can be detected in the P-Sp region of the human embryo in contact with the endothelium overlying the ventral wall of the aorta on day 27.[121] The clusters of CD34-expressing cells greatly expand through day 35 and then are abruptly lost by day 40 of human development. Although circulating myeloerythroid cells can be observed in the developing hepatic sinusoids as early as day 23 of development, the first CD34-expressing hematopoietic progenitor cells do not appear before day 30. Subsequently the liver becomes the predominant human hematopoietic site through the 20th week of human gestation. The bone marrow medullary cavity is the final site for establishment of hematopoiesis.[122] Active blood cell production of myeloid and erythroid cells commences around week 11 of gestation, surprisingly without a large preceding pool of CD34-expressing progenitor cells appearing in the organ. These data suggest that committed progenitor cells produced at other sites, most likely the liver, seed the nascent marrow cavity via hematogenous dissemination.[123] Exactly when the long-term repopulating HSCs seed the human marrow cavity is unclear but, certainly, must be established before the fetal liver ceases to function as a hematopoietic site.

imaging approaches to learn more of niche physiology and how the HSCs are recruited for hematopoietic demands. In addition, future studies must address the lineage relationship between the HSCs and endothelial progenitor cells; vasculogenic cells that play an important role in vascular repair and regeneration.

Intestinal Stem Cell Niche

Whereas the location, organization, and function of the ISCs and the TA pool of epithelial progenitor cells are well recognized, the mesenchymal cells that surround the crypt cells are less well characterized. A composite of mesenchymal, endothelial, and myofibroblast cells may comprise the ISC niche.[38] Within this niche, a variety of signaling pathways, similar to those in the HSC niche, are reported to play important roles in regulating ISC proliferation. For example, excessive Wnt–β-catenin signaling can lead to overproduction of ISCs, with associated tumor development.[72] By examining nuclear versus cytoplasmic β-catenin localization, van de Wetering et al[73] have proposed that a gradient of Wnt signaling exists in the epithelium of the villus, and more recent data predict a role for Wnt–β-catenin signaling gradient in both ISCs and surrounding mesenchymal cells of the niche.[74] Evidence for the localized expression of endogenous Wnt inhibitors also contributes to the growing understanding of the complex spatial

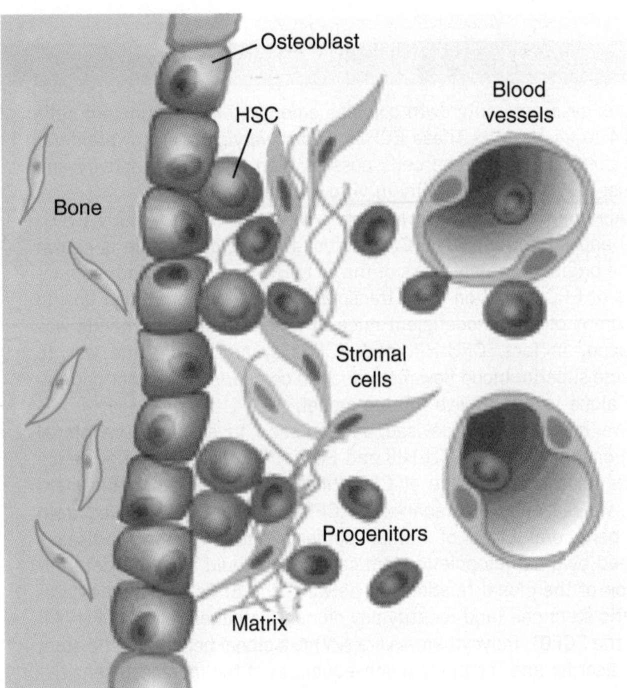

Figure 19–6 Stem cells within their niche in the bone marrow. Schematic diagram of hematopoietic and niche cellular components in the bone marrow. The exact spatial relationships are not well defined. *(From Moore KA, Lemischka IR: Stem cells and their niches. Science 311:1880, 2006 [modified from Fig. 3A, p. 1883].)*

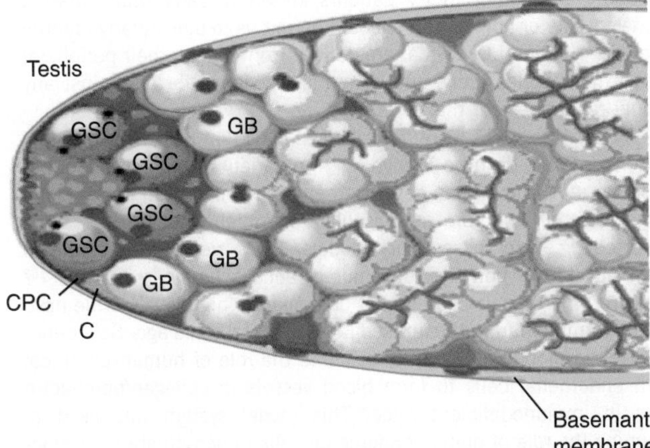

Figure 19–7 Male stem cells in their gonadal niche. Germline stem cells (GSCs) directly interact with hub cells that serve as the stem cell niche within the testis. Differentiated GSC progeny form gonialblast (GB) cells that undergo synchronous incomplete divisions to form germline cysts. Somatic cyst progenitor cells (CPC) associate with GB cells and give rise to daughter squamous cyst (C) cells that surround the differentiating GB cells during the 16-cell germline cyst formation. *(From Fuller MT, Spradling AC: Male and female* Drosophila *germline stem cells: Two versions of immortality. Science 316:402, 2007 [modified from Fig. 1B, p. 403].)*

organization of molecular gradients within the ISC niche.[75] Mesenchymal secreted BMP-4 may play a role in suppressing Wnt signals and thereby participate in balancing Wnt-induced ISC self-renewal.[76] Conditional ablation of the BMP receptor 1A in crypt epithelium results in excessive ISC proliferation. Further evidence to support a role for the BMP pathway in regulating villus epithelial fate comes in the knowledge that mutations in certain BMP receptors and downstream

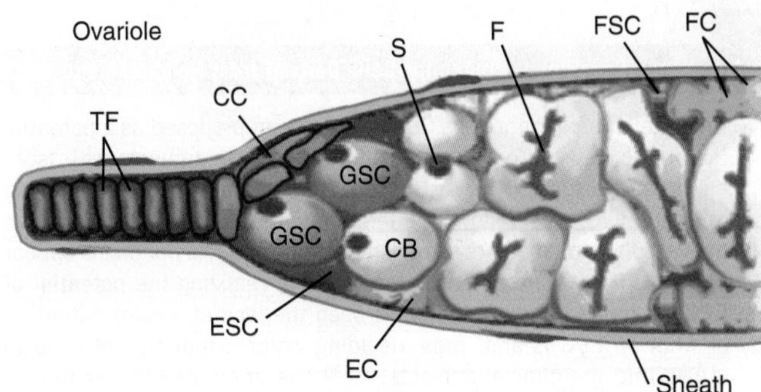

Figure 19–8 Female germline and somatic stem cells in their gonadal niches. Germline stem cells (GSCs) directly interact with cap cells (CC) forming the stem cell niche adjacent to the terminal filament (TF) of the ovariole. Somatic escort stem cells (ESC) associate with the GSC progeny that become cytoblast (CB) cells and the somatic progeny called escort cells (EC) surround the CB that synchronously but incompletely divide to form the 16-cell germline cysts. Follicle stem cells (FSC) differentiate into follicle cells (FC) that further support the differentiation and maturation of the germline cysts. The spectrosome (S) is a protein complex that may play a role in centrosome behavior and asymmetric cell fate decisions. *(From Fuller MT, Spradling AC: Male and female* Drosophila *germline stem cells: Two versions of immortality. Science 316:402, 2007 [modified from Fig. 1A, p. 403].)*

intracellular signaling molecules have been identified in human subjects with juvenile polyposis syndrome.[77] Noggin, an inhibitor of BMP signaling, is expressed by ISCs and may play a role in downregulating BMP signaling during period activation of crypt epithelial regeneration.[76] Further studies to better define the mesenchymal components of the ISC niche may permit tools to develop in vitro models to assist in the study of ISC and the TA progenitor cells of the intestine.

Epidermal Stem Cell Niche

The specific cells comprising the niche for FSCs are not characterized but are likely resident in the bulge area of the hair follicle. FSC maintenance in the niche appears to involve balancing the level of c-Myc expression.[44] Forced c-Myc expression in transgenic mice results in excessive FSC proliferation whereas conditional ablation results in failure of FSC to be maintained and alopecia ensues in the mutant animals. In contrast, LHX2 deficiency results in enhanced FSC proliferation and greater commitment to generation of epithelial progenitor cells than stem cell maintenance. Fuchs has suggested that LHX2 may function as a molecular brake to regulate the balance between FSC maintenance and activation whereas c-Myc functions to accelerate FSC proliferation.[44] Other molecules influencing FSC maintenance include the cell-division cycle 42 (cdc42) and Rac 1 proteins.[78,79] These molecules may impact on FSC maintenance via β-catenin stabilization and negative regulation of c-Myc, respectively.

Like ISCs and perhaps HSCs, FSCs are greatly influenced by the Wnt–β-catenin and BMP pathways. Constitutive expression of an activated form of β-catenin results in skin tumors in transgenic mice.[80] However, transient β-catenin activation is required to activate bulge cells to enter the anagen phase of the hair cycle. Because bulge cells express many proteins typically associated with inhibition of Wnt signaling, Fuchs has proposed that these molecules may facilitate maintaining bulge cells in an undifferentiated state.[44] Only when β-catenin is stabilized and BMP inhibition is achieved in the bulge do the FSCs and participating cells initiate hair follicle regeneration. As expected, mice deficient in expression of the BMP inhibitor Noggin display defects in the functioning of the Wnt pathway and highlight the complex regulation of FSC maintenance in the bulge.

Moore and Lemischka[81] have identified a series of challenges to the comparative study of stem cell niches, including (a) development

Are Human Endothelial Progenitor Cells Derived from Hematopoietic Stem Cells?

Endothelial progenitor cells (EPCs) have been proposed as a potential therapy to improve neovascularization in human subjects with ischemic heart disease.[124,125] At present, the mechanisms for improving myocardial recovery following infarction remain unclear, but improved neovascularization and/or diminished cardiomyocyte apoptosis appear plausible.[126–128] One potential limitation in realizing the potential of EPCs in human clinical trials has been the lack of a clear definition of what an EPC is and, thus, deciding which population of cells to infuse into the clinical subjects.[129,130] The origin of EPCs is further complicated by some evidence that suggest that human EPCs may be derived from human HSCs.

In general, EPCs are thought to represent bone marrow-derived circulating cells that demonstrate the potential to participate in new blood vessel formation (postnatal vasculogenesis).[131,132] New blood vessel formation in adult subjects has long been postulated to occur via sprouting of endothelial cells from preexisting vessels (angiogenesis) or via collateral arterial development (arteriogenesis). In the embryo, blood vessels are first formed from angioblast precursor cells (vasculogenesis) prior to angiogenesis. In 1997, Asahara et al[133] identified circulating CD34+ EPCs from human cord blood that participated in new vessel formation and suggested that these angioblast-like precursor cells form new vessels via postnatal vasculogenesis (because they appeared to be marrow-derived progenitor cells without endothelial commitment at the time of isolation). Subsequently, EPCs have been identified either by cell surface antigen expression profile or through several in vitro colony-forming assays.

Although no single unique cell surface molecule serves to define an EPC, in human subjects, CD34 expression serves as a fundamental marker.[134,135] CD34 is a sialomucin that is expressed by a host of cells throughout the body including hematopoietic stem and progenitor cells, and approximately 1% of human bone marrow mononuclear cells express this cell surface molecule.[31,136] Other antigens such as CD133 and vascular endothelial growth factor 2 receptor (KDR), which are expressed on a rare subset of the CD34+ cells (1%), appear to contain EPC activity.[134] In fact, some investigators propose that the CD133+CD34+KDR+ cells serve as a precursor to the more frequent CD133−CD34+KDR+ circulating EPC.[137] Some evidence has also been presented that EPCs may be derived from the CD34+ hematopoietic stem cell, although analysis of additional informative human patients would be important to support or refute the published work as only a limited number of in vivo studies have been published.[138,139] Numerous papers have correlated the concentration of CD133+CD34+KDR+, CD34+KDR+, or CD34+ cells with the risk for development of adverse cardiovascular outcomes and in general an inverse correlation with each of these EPC subsets and highest risk category exists.[140,141]

EPCs have also been defined using in vitro colony-forming assays, and a comparative analysis of the cells identified in these assays will be the focus of this portion of the present review.[133,141,142] In one assay, peripheral blood mononuclear cells are plated on fibronectin coated tissue culture wells. After a 2-day culture, the nonadherent colony-forming unit–Hill (CFU-Hill) are removed and replated into fresh wells coated with fibronectin. The adherent cells (thought to represent blood monocyte and macrophages or mature endothelial cells) are discarded. Within 5 to 9 days, one can identify colonies emerging from the plated cells. The number of CFU-Hill-derived colonies that are present in the peripheral blood of patients inversely correlates with the severity of cardiovascular dysfunction and with the risk of developing worsening cardiovascular disease.[141]

A second assay identifies another type of endothelial colony-forming cell (ECFC).[143,144] In this assay, peripheral blood mononuclear cells are plated on collagen I coated tissue culture wells in an endothelial growth media that contains several growth factors, including vascular endothelial growth factor, epidermal growth factor, insulin like growth factor 1, and fibroblast growth factor 2.[143,145] Media is changed frequently and the nonadherent cells are discarded. In this case, late outgrowth colonies emerge from the adherent cells at 14 to 21 days.[145] These ECFCs display varying levels of proliferative potential, and some cells possess high telomerase activity and robust vessel-forming ability in vitro and in vivo.[143]

Although there are some obvious differences in the early (CFU-Hill) and late outgrowth (ECFC) colony-forming cells, little is known of the origin and relatedness of the CFU-Hill and ECFC. Both populations of EPCs function upon transplantation, to restore blood flow to the limbs of immunodeficient mice in which hindlimb ischemia was induced; in fact, CFU-Hill and ECFCs synergize in some way to provide superior blood flow restoration in comparison to either population alone in this in vivo murine model.[146]

We have recently devised an approach to examine the clonal relationship between CFU-Hill and ECFC.[147] Because some evidence exists for the emergence of CFU-Hill from the hematopoietic stem cell, we reasoned that analysis of CFU-Hill and ECFC derived from the peripheral blood of human subjects suffering from a disease caused by a hematopoietic stem cell clone should allow for determination of the clonal relationship between the EPCs and the hematopoietic stem cell (and identify any clonal relatedness of the CFU-Hill and the ECFC). Polycythemia vera (PV) is a clonal hematopoietic stem cell disorder and the clinical consequences of the increased sensitivity of hematopoietic progenitors, particularly erythroid progeny, to hematopoietic growth factors has been widely reported.[148] The fundamental etiology for PV remains unclear though uniparental disomy of chromosome 9p is a frequent defect in hematopoietic stem cells in PV patients.[149] Most recently, mutations in the *JAK2* gene (located on chromosome 9p) have been identified in PV patients and some patients with other myelodysplastic syndromes.[150–154] The *JAK2 1849 G > T* mutation leads to a gain of function and erythroid progenitor cells become hypersensitive to erythropoietin. We postulated that isolation of blood from PV patients known to carry this mutation (heterozygote or homozygote) should permit us to molecularly identify the CFU-Hill and ECFCs that are derived from plating their peripheral blood mononuclear cells and determine evidence for or against any clonal relatedness of the EPCs.

By definition, EPCs are described as cells that possess the ability to form vessels de novo in vivo.[155,156] A variety of animal models of vascular injury have been developed and the ability of EPCs to home, engraft, and function as vascular endothelial cells has been reported.[157–160] In these injury models, EPCs clearly play a role in restoring blood flow to the injured and ischemic area.[137,161,162] However, the models used do not demonstrate high levels of de novo vessel formation from the infused EPCs. Several years ago, Schechner et al[163] developed an assay to examine the role of human umbilical vein endothelial cells to form blood vessels in collagen/fibronectin gels in immunodeficient mice. This model system was used to examine the role of human endothelial cells to participate in interactions with immune cells in vivo.[164] We speculated that human EPCs implanted in vivo in the same gel constructs may possess de novo vessel-forming ability. When both CFU-Hill and ECFC were plated in collagen/fibronectin gels and implanted subcutaneously in NOD/SCID mice, ECFC gave rise to numerous human blood vessels that had gained access to murine vessels and were perfused with murine red blood cells. Although CFU-Hill survived in the gels upon implantation, they did not contribute to human–murine chimeric vessel formation. These results suggested that CFU-Hill and ECFC vary widely in their functional capacities.

This comparative analysis set the stage for testing whether there is a clonal relationship between CFU-Hill and ECFC.[147] Peripheral blood mononuclear cells from PV patients were plated in both CFU-Hill and ECFC assays. Clones of each type were isolated and DNA extracted. The *JAK2* genotyping was performed and results compared with the known genotype of the PV patient carrying the mutation (heterozygous or homozygous). All of the CFU-Hill displayed the mutant genotype of the hematopoietic stem cell clone. In contrast,

Are Human Endothelial Progenitor Cells Derived from Hematopoietic Stem Cells?—cont'd

nearly all ECFC displayed the wild-type genotype. Thus, CFU-Hill are hematopoietic progeny that do not display vessel-forming ability, whereas ECFC are not clonally related to the hematopoietic stem cell or CFU-Hill.[147]

These are not the first studies to indicate that CFU-Hill are derived from, or in fact represent, hematopoietic cells. Rehman et al[165] previously reported that the adherent acetylated–low density lipoprotein ingesting and *Ulex Europeus* lectin binding cells derived from human peripheral blood are myeloid cells not EPCs. Rohde et al[166] provided compelling evidence that peripheral blood monocytes cultured under the conditions used to generate EPCs take on the physical appearance and gene expression patterns of classically described EPCs. They interpreted their results as evidence that monocytes and their progeny can phenotypically mimic EPCs including the ability to generate CFU-Hill in vitro. Zhange et al[167] reported that culture of peripheral blood cells from normal human adult volunteer's results in formation of cells with features described as EPCs; however, close examination revealed that the cells maintained typical monocytic function and displayed little proliferative potential.

Summation of these recent data, including the clonal analysis and in vivo vessel-forming capacity, simply illustrates the complexity in defining an EPC. Several recent studies indeed implicate an important role for myeloid cells in initiating the early events to promote changes in the endothelial intima to stimulate endothelial sprouting and neoangiogenesis.[168–175] Further studies will be required to specifically determine the role that the hematopoietic derived angiogenic cells and the ECFC play in neoangiogenesis.

of equivalent definitions and assay systems for stem and progenitor cells, (b) a more comprehensive analysis of niche signaling pathways, (c) creation of in vitro systems that reconstitute the in vivo niches, (d) development and use of real-time imaging to analyze stem cell functions within a niche, (e) description of macromolecular assemblies at cellular interfaces within the niche, (f) elucidation of how niche signals couple to stem cell cell-cycle regulation and/or distinct transcriptional programs that modify cell fate, and (g) elucidation of how niches are altered during stress or pathology. Although some advances have been made in some of these areas, most remain targets to achieve for interested stem cell researchers.

SUMMARY

Stem cells reside in specific locations (niches), are not fully differentiated (may not display the appearance or all of the functions of the mature cells of the tissue), possess controlled but robust proliferative potential (at least for the lifetime of the host tissue), and have the capacity to divide into daughter cells, in which one of the daughter cells retains all the properties of the parental cell (self-renewal) and the other daughter adopts a differentiated fate specific for the needs of that tissue. Although much of the control of the stem cell state may be cell-autonomous, the stem cell niche clearly affects the four major HSC states: quiescence, self-renewal, apoptosis, and differentiation. The recent ability to reprogram somatic cells to exhibit ES cell-like activity is an exciting though preliminary step in development of the methods required to manipulate these stem cell states and raises exciting possibilities for expanding a similar paradigm of research on other stem cell types. One may even hope to contemplate development of tools (small molecules, nanotechnology, etc) to reactivate certain stem cell behaviors in situ in affected patients to repair or regenerate dysfunctional tissues and organs. Thus, the ultimate future for stem cell therapy is to manipulate the stem cells within the host rather than utilize adoptive transplant regimes.

SUGGESTED READINGS

Bryder D, Rossi DJ, Weissman IL: Hematopoietic stem cells: The paradigmatic tissue-specific stem cell. Am J Pathol 169:338, 2006.

Fuchs E: Scratching the surface of skin development. Nature 445:834, 2007.

Keller G: Embryonic stem cell differentiation: Emergence of a new era in biology and medicine. Genes Dev 19:1129, 2005.

Li L, Xie T: Stem cell niche: Structure and function. Annu Rev Cell Dev Biol 21:605, 2005.

Moore KA, Lemischka IR: Stem cells and their niches. Science 311:1880, 2006.

Orlic D, Bodine D: What defines a pluripotent hematopoietic stem cell (PHSC): Will the real PHSC please stand up! Blood 84:3991, 1994.

Pera MF, Trounson AO: Human embryonic stem cells: Prospects for development. Development 131:5515, 2004.

Potten CS, Wilson JW: Development of epithelial stem cell concepts. In Lanza R, Gearhart J, Hogan B, et al (eds.): Handbook of Stem Cells, Vol. 2. Amsterdam, Elsevier, 2004, p. 1.

Preston S, Wright NA, Direkze N, Brittan M: Stem cells in the gastrointestinal tract. In Lanza R, Gearhart J, Hogan B, et al (eds.): Handbook of Stem Cells, Vol. 2. Amsterdam, Elsevier, 2004, p. 521.

Rossant J: Stem cells and lineage development in the mammalian blastocyst. Reprod Fertil Dev 19:111, 2007.

Scadden DT: The stem-cell niche as an entity of action. Nature 441:1075, 2006.

Schofield R: The relationship between the spleen colony-forming cell and the haematopoietic stem cell. Blood Cells 4:7, 1978.

Thomson JA, Itskovitz-Eldor J, Shapiro SS, et al: Embryonic stem cell lines derived from human blastocysts. Science 282:1145, 1998.

Till J, McCulloch E: A direct measurement of the radiation sensitivity of normal mouse bone marrow cells. Radiat Res 14:213, 1961.

Vallier L, Pedersen RA: Human embryonic stem cells: An in vitro model to study mechanisms controlling pluripotency in early mammalian development. Stem Cell Rev 1:119, 2007.

Van der Flier LG, Sabate-Bellver J, Oving I, et al: The intestinal Wnt/TCF signature. Gastroenterology 132:628, 2007.

Weissman I: Stem cells: Units of development, units of regeneration, and units in evolution. Cell 100:157, 2000.

Weissman I: The road ended up at stem cells. Immun Rev 185:159, 2002.

Wright D, Wagers A, Gulati A, Johnson F, Weissman I: Physiological migration of hematopoietic stem and progenitor cells. Science 294:1933, 2001.

REFERENCES

For complete list of references log onto www.expertconsult.com

CHAPTER 20

CELLULAR BIOLOGY OF HEMATOPOIESIS

Hélène Schoemans and Catherine Verfaillie

INTRODUCTION

Hematopoiesis refers to the process of formation, development, and differentiation of the formed elements of blood. This process originates from hematopoietic stem cells (HSCs). These cells are characterized by the ability to self-renew and differentiate into all mature blood cell lineages. They are also capable of rescuing lethally irradiated hosts by reconstituting the entire repertoire of hematopoietic cells in the recipients.[1]

HSCs are rare, occurring at a frequency of 1 stem cell per 10,000 to 100,000 bone marrow (BM) cells. Under steady state, HSCs are quiescent (ie, noncycling), and only a fraction of the HSCs enter into the cell cycle to proliferate and give rise to differentiated progenitors. However, in response to hematopoietic stress (eg, infections, acute bleeding, or chemotherapy), HSCs proliferate extensively. Self-renewal and differentiation are tightly regulated processes which ensure homeostasis. Deregulation of these processes will inevitably manifest as myeloproliferative diseases (such as acute myeloid leukemia) or as bone marrow failure syndromes (such as aplastic anemia). Understanding the cellular biology of HSCs is therefore essential.

HSC studies began in the mid-1950s, when BM transplants were found to rescue lethally irradiated mice by reconstituting ablated hematopoiesis. In the 1960s, similar transplantation experiments identified primitive hematopoietic progenitor cells as BM clonogenic cells which could give rise to discrete colonies in the spleen of irradiated recipient animals. These cells were also capable of forming more spleen colonies in secondary recipients and were therefore referred to as *colony-forming unit-spleen (CFU-S)*. Later, development of in vitro colony assays of hematopoietic myeloid and lymphoid progenitor cells enabled their enumeration. With the advent of monoclonal antibodies and flow cytometry, HSCs and their progenitors have been further characterized by the presence or absence of specific surface markers and by the ability to efflux fluorescent dyes.[2]

In this chapter, we focus on the contemporary concepts regarding the cellular biology of HSCs and its impact on our understanding of early hematopoiesis, and highlight areas relevant to clinicians and transplant physicians. However, as information on HSC behavior is derived from data generated from different species (zebrafish, mice, human and nonhuman primates) and cell sources (BM, umbilical cord blood [UCB], and peripheral blood [PB]), all conclusions should be interpreted with caution because qualitative and quantitative differences in HSCs are bound to exist.

DEFINING HEMATOPOIETIC STEM CELLS

Embryology and Hematopoiesis

Hematopoietic development is highly conserved among frogs (*Xenopus laevis*), zebrafish (*Danio rerio*), and mammals and originates from mesodermal tissue. During gastrulation, mesoderm is induced by the prospective endoderm and is patterned along the dorsal-ventral axis. Two families of proteins seem to play a pivotal role in this process: bone morphogenetic proteins (BMPs) and hedgehog (Hh) proteins.

Cells from the ventral mesoderm then migrate to the extraembryonic yolk sac (in mammals), the tail (intermediate cell mass in zebrafish), and near the liver (ventral blood island in *Xenopus*), where they generate the first wave of hematopoiesis, called primitive hematopoiesis. *Primitive hematopoiesis* is transient and consists primarily of large nucleated erythroid cells that express embryonic hemoglobin and mature macrophages.[3] In mouse and chick embryos, this occurs around embryonic day 7.5 (E7.5). Morphologic analysis of these tissues showed that the site of primitive hematopoiesis comprises erythroid and vascular endothelial cells. Their proximity suggests that they may be derived from a common precursor, known as *hemangioblasts*. The existence of such a precursor in humans, however, remains difficult to establish as the earliest stages of human development are inaccessible for experimentation. However, human embryonic cell (hES) lines provide an interesting alternative to study this, and several groups have recently shown that culture of hES cells with a cytokine cocktail containing either BMP-4 or serum can give rise to a population of cells displaying both endothelial and hematopoietic characteristics, thus providing compelling evidence for the existence of an early human hemangioblastic founder population.[3,4] This finding may be of importance as ES derived hemangioblasts could serve as an unlimited source of both HSCs and endothelial progenitors for human tissue engineering.[4]

Shortly afterward (E8-8.5 in mice), the second wave of hematopoiesis, called *definitive hematopoiesis*, takes place in the aortic-gonad-mesonephros (AGM) region of the embryo (mammals), dorsal aorta (zebrafish), and dorsal lateral plate (*Xenopus*), where HSCs expand and then migrate to the fetal liver and spleen (in mammals) or the kidneys (in zebrafish) to generate hematopoietic cells of all lineages.[5] The origin of HSCs that gives rise to definitive hematopoiesis remains unclear, although evidence suggests that they may be derived from specialized endothelial cells in the dorsal aorta that differentiates to generate hematopoiesis (the *hemogenic endothelium*).[6] During the late fetal stage, HSCs migrate further to BM and thymus in mammals. These definitive hematopoietic progenitors have the unique ability to generate long-term engrafting HSCs and lymphoid populations, thus sustaining lifelong hematopoiesis.[4] Whether the early HSCs that give rise to primitive and definitive hematopoiesis come from one anatomic site and then migrate to the other or the two forms of hematopoiesis are derived from two entirely different HSC pools remains, however, unclear.[7]

From a clinical point of view, understanding the processes by which hematopoiesis shifts during embryonic development may provide insights into the mechanism of HSC mobilization, which is routinely performed to procure HSCs for transplantation. Previous studies have shown that factors, including interaction between stromal cell-derived factor-1 (SDF-1, also called CXC-ligand-12 or CXCL12) and chemokine receptor 4 (CXCR4)[8] or β_1-integrins,[9] are important for HSC migration during embryonic development.[10] In the setting of clinical transplantation, $CD34^+$ cells mobilized by granulocyte colony-stimulating factor (G-CSF) and chemotherapy (eg, cyclophosphamide) express lower levels of CXCR4 with decreased levels or affinity to $\alpha_4\beta_1$-integrin (an adhesion molecule of the very late antigen-4 [VLA-4] adhesion pathway). In fact, G-CSF mediated murine and human HSC mobilization occurs by accumulation of neutrophil serine protease in BM, leading to proteolytic cleavage and inactivation of CXCR4 and SDF-1.[11] Similarly, AMD3100 is a mobilizing agent which reversibly blocks interaction between CXCR4 and SDF-1, in a more direct manner, resulting in very rapid and efficient mobilization of PB HSCs and is currently under clinical investigation.[12] Murine data also suggests that a large subset of HSCs do not only display CXCR4 but also carry CD26 (cluster of differentiation), a cell surface marker with protease activity, which can cleave the N-terminal portion of SDF-1, thereby eradicating its chemotactic potential, without impacting on SDF-1-CXCR4 interactions.[10] Combinations of G-CSF and CD26-agonists could thus be exploited to improve HSC mobilization in vivo. However, use of these alternative mechanisms in the clinic requires further investigation. The process of homing and the hematopoietic microenvironment are discussed further in Chapter 23.

Finally, the migratory nature of HSCs during embryonic development may also explain their existence in adult nonhematopoietic tissues, and the observation that when they migrate to the BM, they can resume hematopoietic properties. This may be one explanation for the phenomenon of stem cell plasticity reported in recent years.[13] The notion is supported by murine studies showing that the ability of adult skeletal muscle to reconstitute hematopoiesis in lethally irradiated recipients could be attributed to $CD45^+$ $Sca1^+$ stem cells residing in muscles.[13] Likewise, it is possible that adult BM may contain, in addition to HSCs, stem cells capable of reconstituting nonhematopoietic tissues (for more details, please refer to Chapter 22).

Definition of Hematopoietic Stem Cells

The two essential attributes of true HSC populations are their "immortality," as characterized by their *self-renewal* potential and their "undifferentiated" state, whilst being able to give rise to multilineage *differentiation*. At the single cell level, this translates into 4 possible fates: self-renewal, differentiation, migration or apoptosis (Fig. 20–1).[1] This means that the HSC compartment will necessarily contain a population of various cell types with specific potentials.

Self-Renewal

The substantial self-renewal capacity of HSCs is essential to provide a continuous lifelong supply of functional hematopoietic cells.

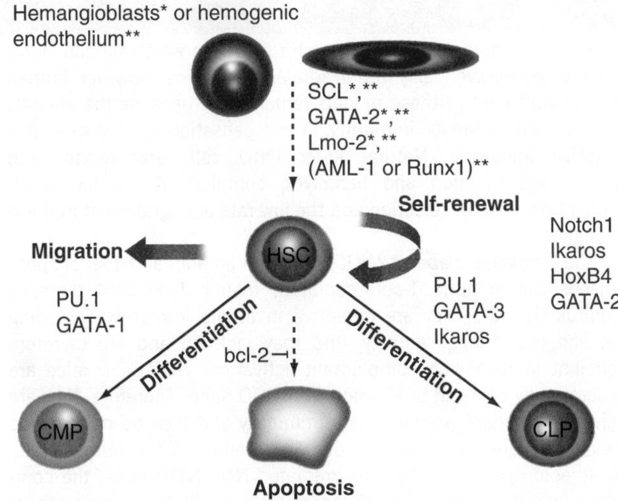

Figure 20–1 DERIVATION AND FATES OF HEMATOPOIETIC STEM CELLS (HSCS). During embryonic development, HSCs may be derived from hemangioblasts (ie, precursors of HSCs and endothelial cells) or hemogenic endothelium (ie, endothelial cells that acquire the potential to generate hematopoiesis). HSCs have one of four fates: self-renewal, differentiation (eventually becoming common lymphoid progenitors or common myeloid progenitors), migration or apoptosis. The cell-fate decision is highly regulated, involving specific transcription factors. *(Adapted from Zhu J, Emerson SG: Hematopoietic cytokines, transcription factors and lineage commitment. Oncogene 21:3295, 2002.)*

From an experimental point of view, this characteristic of HSCs can currently only formally be assessed by evaluating their long-term ability to reconstitute the hematopoietic system of a lethally irradiated host, either in an autologous, allogeneic or xenogeneic setting. In mice, cells capable of unlimited self-renewal are referred to as *long-term repopulating hematopoietic stem cells (LTR-HSC)*. As their self renewal potential decreases, cells are referred to as *short-term-repopulating HSC (STR-HSC)* and *multipotent progenitors (MPP)* respectively (Fig. 20–2).[14] These cells, together with more differentiated progenitor cells, will therefore essentially provide transient hematopoiesis to bridge the aplastic period following lethal irradiation, but will not give rise to long term sustained hematopoiesis.

The earliest description of HSCs was based on studies showing that murine BM transplanted into lethally irradiated mice was able to rescue the recipient by reconstituting donor hematopoiesis. Likewise, human HSCs are characterized by their ability to home to BM and to reconstitute hematopoiesis in xenogeneic transplantation models using sub-lethally irradiated immunodeficient mice or nonirradiated preimmune fetal sheep (Xenogeneic Models of Human Stem Cell Engraftment).

Self-renewing divisions of HSCs can be *symmetric*, in which one HSC gives rise to two identical HSC daughter cells, or *asymmetric*, in which one daughter cell remains as an HSC and the other differentiates or undergoes apoptosis (see Fig. 20–1). The ability of HSCs to self-renew and to maintain hematopoietic homeostasis indicates that, on average, most HSC divisions yield at least one daughter cell which remains as an undifferentiated HSC. However, HSCs must be able to respond to hematopoietic stress by population expansion. Under those circumstances, HSCs probably divide symmetrically into two identical HSCs to replenish the depleted HSC pool. HSCs can also undergo *apoptosis*, because overexpression of *Bcl2* (an anti-apoptotic gene) in transgenic mice increases the number of HSCs and enhances competitive repopulation cell frequency, suggesting that apoptosis is an important mechanism for controlling HSC turnover during steady state conditions.[15]

Finally, the self-renewal potential of HSCs is thought to be partially associated with the activity of telomerase, a reverse transcriptase which makes new telomeric DNA. Telomeric shortening during cell division is secondary to incomplete replication of the lagging strand by the conventional DNA polymerase during chromosomal replication and is associated with replicative senescence.[16] However, despite the fact that HSCs express some telomerase activity, replication of HSCs is finite, as they can be serially transplanted only five to seven times in mice.[17] In humans, HSCs also undergo telomeric shortening after repetitive cell division, particularly when occurring under stress, such as during transplantation,[18] though this does not seem to have clinical relevance to date. These observations suggest that the telomerase activity in HSCs, although endowing them with substantial self-renewing potential, may not be sufficient to prevent telomeric shortening during the stress of replication. Further evidence for this comes from disease states such as dyskeratosis congenita where inherited defective telomerase activity is associated with bone marrow failure. In aplastic anemia and paroxysmal nocturnal hemoglobinuria a correlation between telomere shortening and the degree of pancytopenia has also been found; however, whether this is a consequence of increased HSC turnover or caused by a telomere-mediated replicative exhaustion of the HSC pool remains to be answered.[16]

Multilineage Differentiation

HSCs are capable of differentiating into all mature hematopoietic cell lineages. As HSCs divide, they generate differentiated progenies, which gradually display an increasingly limited capacity to self-renew and much more restricted differentiation options.[19] The first cells committed to lymphoid and myeloid lineages are called *common lymphoid progenitors (CLP)* and *common myeloid progenitors (CMP)* (see Fig. 20–2).

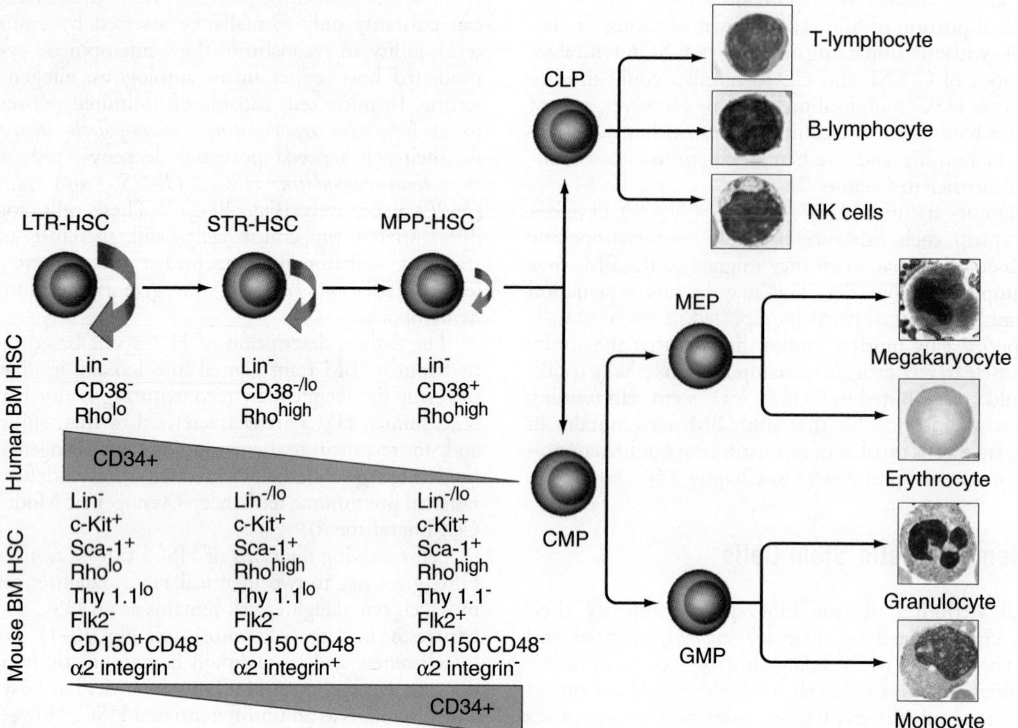

Figure 20–2 THE HEMATOPOIETIC HIERARCHY. As hematopoietic stem cells progressively differentiate, they acquire different phenotypes and are successively referred to as LT-HSC (long term HSC), ST-HSC (short term HSC) and MPP-HSC (multipotent progenitor HSC). The MPP-HSCs then give rise to common lymphoid and common myeloid precursor cells (CLP and CMP respectively) that eventually generate all mature blood lineages of the body (GMP, granulocyte-monocyte precursors; MEP, megakaryocyte-erythrocyte precursors; NK, natural killer). *(Adapted from JA, Negrin RS, Weissman IL: Hematopoietic stem and progenitor cells: clinical and preclinical regeneration of the hematolymphoid system. Annu Rev Med 56:509, 2005.)*

Xenogeneic Models of Human Stem Cell Engraftment

The ability to engraft myeloablated recipients and reconstitute long-term, multilineage hematopoiesis remains of the only definition of HSCs. To study human HSCs, different doses of HSCs from different sources or different culture conditions can be transplanted into xenogeneic hosts, which are sacrificed and analyzed at defined times after transplantation. The key feature of these animals is their immune-incompetence, which allows for xenogeneic engraftment of human HSCs.

Mouse Transplantation Models

Earlier studies, using heavily irradiated mice and mice homozygous for the *nude* gene (*Hfh11^{nu}*), were hampered by low levels of human HSC engraftment. Newer models have been developed, including mice that are null for the *beige*, *nu*, and *X*-linked immunodeficiency loci (ie, *Bnx mice*); mice deficient in *recombination activating genes (Rag1 and Rag2)*, and mice that are homozygous for the *Prkdc^{scid}* (ie, *SCID mice*). The *severe combined immunodeficiency (SCID)* mutation was described in mice in 1983 and is related to a nonsense mutation of a *protein kinase DNA-activated catalytic polypeptide (Prkdc^{scid})*. Homozygous mutation of this gene results in defective activation of a DNA recombinase (which requires a functional *Prkdc* gene) and consequently gives rise to defects in humoral (B-cell) and cell-mediated (T-cell) immunity (ie, adaptive immunity). The latter model has been extensively studied and forms the platform for the development of the *NOD/SCID* model.[165] A number of experimental models have been developed based on these animals, including the *SCID-hu* mice (ie, human fetal liver or bone marrow transplanted under the renal capsule of SCID mice), the *triple chimeric* mice (ie, lethally irradiated normal mice transplanted with BM from SCID mice, followed by a large dose of human BM cells), and a model in which human HSCs are injected intravenously into *irradiated SCID* mice. However, human HSC engraftment in these models remains low because the animals have enhanced innate immunity in compensation for the defective adaptive immunity. Natural killer (NK) cell, granulocyte, and macrophage function and hemolytic complement are increased, accounting for graft rejection and the low rate of engraftment in these animals.

The *nonobese diabetes (NOD)* mouse is an animal model of spontaneous autoimmune T-cell-mediated, insulin-dependent diabetes mellitus (IDDM). They are defective in innate immunity, including NK and macrophage activity, and they lack C5 and are therefore deficient in hemolytic complement activation. *NOD/SCID* mice are generated by crossing SCID mice with NOD mice. Therefore, they are defective in adaptive and innate immunity and they do not develop insulinitis or insulin-dependent diabetes mellitus. When human HSCs are injected intravenously into irradiated NOD/SCID mice, the combined immunodeficiency in these animals facilitates a more robust engraftment compared with the SCID model. Differentiated cells (predominantly of myeloid and B-cell lineages) can be detected in the BM of recipients, but human T-cell development is lacking. A caveat about the NOD/SCID model, however, is that these animals retain some residual NK activity and express disparate *major histocompatibility (MHC) loci*, limiting engraftment of human HSCs. To circumvent this limitation, mice deficient in *β_2-microglobulin (β_2m^{null})*, which is required for MHC I expression, have been backcrossed onto NOD/SCID mice. The resulting *NOD/SCID/β_2m^{null}* mice support fivefold to tenfold higher levels of human cell engraftment. However, because these animals are even more vulnerable to thymic lymphoma and are more radiosensitive than NOD/SCID mice, their lifespan is

Xenogeneic Models of Human Stem Cell Engraftment—cont'd

often shorter. The use of *NOD/SCID/common cytokine receptor γ chain (γc)* triple mutant mice[153] or infusion of antibodies against a sialoprotein or Il-2Rβ can also improve transplantation results by hindering NK response.

Sheep Transplantation Models

In the fetal sheep model, human HSCs are injected in utero into preimmune fetal lambs, and the permissive fetal environment enables long-term HSC engraftment into postnatal life and multilineage differentiation, including myeloid, T, and B cells.[166] Similar to the murine models, only recipients transplanted with $CD34^+CD38^-$ cells (but not those with $CD34^+CD38^+$) exhibit long-term engraftment during serial transplantations. The model does not involve recipient myeloablation or irradiation, and human HSC engraftment can be further enhanced by stimulating the recipients in vivo with human growth factors. The expense of this model, however, has hampered its widespread application.

Nonhuman Primate Transplantation Models

An autologous transplantation model using nonhuman primates, including rhesus macaques (*Macaca mulatta*) and baboons, has begun to shed light on HSC behavior during transplantation. This model is used to provide information on how an individual HSC is related to total hematopoiesis after transplantation.[167] One way to track individual HSCs is by retroviral marking. Because retroviruses integrate randomly into the host genome, the DNA sequence flanking the viral integrant is unique to each host cell, enabling tracking of progeny (clone) from individual cells in vitro or in vivo. There are advantages in using nonhuman primates for this purpose. First, compared with murine models,[40,168] the high genetic and biological similarity within the primate family provides more reliable data regarding human HSCs. Second, the longevity of nonhuman primates (up to 30 years) allows long-term tracking of HSCs after transplantation, which is not possible with small animal models. Third, cross-reactivity of cytokines and antibodies enables the use of human cytokines for peripheral blood mobilization and anti-human antibodies for HSC phenotypic characterization. Autologous transplantation circumvents the problems of homing inherent to the xenogeneic transplantation models when using mice and fetal sheep. Using rhesus macaques and baboons, it has been demonstrated that a single HSC clone is capable of generating mature and functional cells of lymphoid and myeloid lineages, reiterating the multipotency of transplanted HSCs.[169] Moreover, mature progeny from a single HSC clone persists for at least years, demonstrating for each individual HSC the capacity for sustained long-term hematopoiesis after transplantation. More importantly, multiple integration sites can be identified in mature progenies, suggesting that the HSC population that gives rise to hematopoietic reconstitution is highly polyclonal.[169,170] Because of the close resemblance to humans and the advantages described, these primate models may also become a powerful tool to investigate the effect of clinically relevant manipulations such as cytokine stimulation, chemotherapy, and irradiation on hematopoiesis.

$CD34^+$ or $CD34^-$: The Changing Paradigm

CD34 is a sialomucin-like adhesion molecule expressed on 1% to 5% of mononuclear cells, including hematopoietic stem and progenitor cells, vascular endothelial cells, and some fibroblasts. One of the earliest studies supporting the notion that CD34 was a marker of HSCs was reported 15 years ago by Berenson and colleagues.[154] Autologous $CD34^+$-enriched bone marrow (BM) cells were used to engraft lethally irradiated baboons. Two other animals received CD34-depleted marrow; one animal died of nonengraftment on day 29, and the second animal suffered from prolonged pancytopenia. In mice, however, it has become clear that HSCs are $CD34^{-/lo}$ and single $CD34^{-/lo}Kit^+Sca^+Lin^-$ cells transplanted into recipients can reconstitute long-term myelolymphoid hematopoiesis.[155] Murine BM side-population (SP) cells, which are highly enriched in HSCs, are also $CD34^-$.

A model has evolved in which expression of CD34 on murine HSCs varies with HSC activation.[156] Murine HSCs from resting BM of adult mice are $CD34^-$. On activation by 5-fluorouracil (which recruits quiescent HSCs into the cell cycle by depleting marrow of committed progenitors), administration of stem cell factor, or during in vitro culture, some of the $CD34^{-/lo}$ HSCs convert to a $CD34^+$ phenotype. After transplantation, HSCs lose CD34 expression as they become quiescent again in the recipient bone marrow. Interestingly enough, CD34 expression has also been shown to be present in stem cells from neonatal to five-week-old mice, and then to progressively disappear.[157] The same reciprocal relationship is true for CD38 expression, which is typically negative in primitive human HSC and present on steady state murine HSC. Upon activation however, murine HSC can transiently lose CD38 expression.[157]

In humans, $CD34^+$ cells derived from BM, mobilized peripheral blood, and umbilical cord blood (UCB) are able to engraft and repopulate NOD/SCID mice and fetal sheep. It is also clear from clinical observations that such a population of cells contains cells with long-term engraftment ability. A comparison between $CD34^+$ and $CD34^-$ cells showed that the latter made only minor contributions to human cell engraftment in NOD/SCID mice.[158] This has lead to the dogma that human HSCs are $CD34^+$. Consequently, CD34 expression is used clinically to enumerate transplantable cells, since the dose of $CD34^+$ cells can predict the outcome after transplantation.[159] However, there is evidence that human BM $CD34^-Lin^-$ and UCB $CD34^-Lin^-CD38^-$ cells can engraft long term and give rise to multi-lineage differentiation in NOD/SCID mice and fetal sheep.[160,161] $CD34^-Lin^-$ cells are much less clonogenic in vitro but can generate $CD34^+$ cells in vitro and in vivo. The clonogenicity and the ability to engraft in NOD/SCID mice and generate $CD34^+$ cells in liquid culture of $CD34^-Lin^-CD38^-$ cells appears to be confined to a small population that are $CD133^+CD7^-$, suggesting that $CD34^-Lin^-CD38^-CD133^+CD7^-$ may define a very primitive, but also very rare (0.02%), cell population.[41,162] Similar to murine HSCs, the expression of CD34 on human HSCs may be reversible, because $CD34^-CD38^-$ cells transplanted into Bnx mice could give rise to $CD34^-$ progeny, which revert to a $CD34^+$ phenotype upon transplantation into secondary recipients.[163]

The question of whether the most primitive HSCs are $CD34^+$ or $CD34^-$ remains unanswered.[164] The laboratory findings supporting the notion that $CD34^-$ cells are more primitive than $CD34^+$ cells appear at odds with the clinical experience that patients receiving positively selected $CD34^+$ transplants have stable, long-term engraftment. If the most primitive HSC are $CD34^-$, recipients of highly purified $CD34^+$ positively selected transplants may develop late graft failure when these $CD34^+$ progenitors become exhausted, although no evidence has suggested this to be the case.

Common lymphoid progenitors further divide and differentiate into lymphocyte progenitors capable of generating the *T*, *B* and *natural killer (NK)* cells. Common myeloid progenitors give rise to *granulocyte-monocyte progenitor cells* and *megakaryocyte-erythrocyte progenitor cells*. The former develops into granulocytes and monocytes, and the latter develops into platelets and erythrocytes. It was once firmly believed that after a cell was committed to a given lineage, it could no longer change its fate. More recent studies, however, showed that lineage-committed cells (mostly from lymphomatous and transformed cells but also normal murine hematopoietic cells) under specific cytokine stimulation can switch between myeloid and lymphoid fates. This change may even be possible for more differentiated progenitors.[20] Whether and how this reported phenomenon of transdifferentiation between blood lineages contributes to normal hematopoiesis is unknown.

CHARACTERIZING HEMATOPOIETIC STEM CELLS

The study of HSCs is often hampered by their scarcity in hematopoietic tissues and the lack of specific markers and tests for identifying HSCs that fulfill all the defining features of stem cells, including their ability to sustain a long-lasting multi-lineage clone in vivo. Generally speaking, HSC characteristics can be assessed using assays in the in vivo setting, long-term in vitro cultures or based on cell surface and molecular markers. In most circumstances, a combination of tests will need to be used to identify and isolate HSCs, resulting in populations displaying various degrees of purity. The following section describes methods used for HSC characterization.

In Vivo Characteristics

The only true definitive assay for HSCs is based on their ability to reconstitute the entire hematopoietic system of a myeloablated recipient, the two major endpoints being longevity and multi-potentiality. *STR-HSC* have limited self-renewal capacity (they appear after approximately 2 weeks and disappear 4 to 6 weeks later) but can rescue animals from otherwise lethal radiation-induced pancytopenia. These cells can be further divided into day 8 or 12 *colony forming unit spleen (CFU-S)*, according to the time elapsed before they form colonies in a recipient spleen. *Pre-CFU-S* are slightly more primitive cells which are identified in the bone marrow of recipients after 15 days and are defined by their ability to produce *CFU-S* in secondary recipients.[21] *LTR-HSC* have also been identified: they protect against irradiation and give rise to long-term hematopoiesis following serial transplantations.[22] The latter can be enumerated by a *competitive repopulating unit (CRU) assay*. In this assay, hematopoietic cells from a test mouse are mixed with various proportions of those from a competitor mouse before injection into a lethally irradiated recipient mouse. Using a limiting dilution assay, the frequency of LTR-HSCs in the test mouse is measured by their ability to compete for engraftment in the recipient mouse. Typically, Poisson statistics predict that mice are reconstituted by a single LTR-HSC when 33% of transplanted hosts are reconstituted (defined as at least 1% of donor derived cells from both the myeloid and lymphoid lineage identified 3 to 4 months after transplantation).[21]

In humans, HSC enumeration is more difficult because a competitive repopulation assay can clearly not be performed. Instead, *xenogeneic transplantation* models (Red Box 1) have been developed in which human hematopoietic cells are injected into sublethally irradiated, immunodeficient mice or nonirradiated, preimmune fetal sheep. The presence of human hematopoietic cells in BM of recipient animals, characterized by the expression by more than 1% of the cells of the human pan-leukocyte antigen CD45 or the presence of 0.1% to 1% human specific DNA in the bone marrow of mice (in contrast to murine studies where engraftment can be assessed by analysis of the peripheral blood), has been used to determine successful engraftment and the presence of HSCs in the injected cell population. These cells are referred to as human *SCID-repopulating cells (SRC)*. Ideally, identification of not only CD45+ cells but also myeloid as well as lymphoid cells should be used to further demonstrate the presence of SCID-repopulating cells. In all of these models, however, enumeration of transplanted human HSCs is complicated by their xenogeneic nature (leading to homing problems and risk of immunological rejection), and true information on competitive engraftment is not available.

In Vitro Characteristics

There is as yet no in vitro assay that specifically detects HSCs. However, a number of different methods can assess two crucial characteristics of these cells, namely: proliferation and differentiation potential. Experimental conditions should therefore meet the specific requirements of each type of progenitor, while excluding the growth of others. Most of the time, this will require using different methods to avoid underestimating the proliferation and differentiation potential of a given cell. These methods are available for murine and human HSCs and can be categorized according to two different parameters: *short-term* (evaluating approximately 5–10 cell divisions over a maximum of 3 weeks) versus *long-term* assays (evaluating more than 15 cell divisions over a period exceeding 5 weeks) and *clonal* versus *polyclonal* expansions. Clonal assays are single cell cultures, in which each progenitor remains separated and the size of the colony reflects the proliferative potential of the progenitor. The major caveat of these studies is of course that the purified cells are also physically isolated from their normal neighboring cells. Another option is to study cells in their cellular context, inferring the number of progenitor cells with the desired function from statistical methods (law of Poisson, discussed above) based on the maximum likelihood of occurrence of an unlikely event, ie differentiation.[21]

Short-Term Assays

These tests evaluate and quantify lineage restricted progenitors in well-standardized conditions. They are not suitable for identifying very immature progenitors because the lifespan of the viscous medium used typically does not extend beyond three weeks and cannot be renewed. Liquid cultures can also be used, but require clonal cultures and subsequent flow cytometry analysis to identify progeny. Generally speaking, progenitors with different levels of maturity can be recognized from their sensitivity to cytokines, the time required to generated differentiated cells and the size of colonies. These progenitors are then referred to as *CFC (colony forming cells)*, and lead to *CFU (colony forming units)*, referring to their more differentiated progeny, followed by a hyphen and the first letter of the lineage produced (eg, CFU-E for erythroid, etc.).[21]

Long-Term Assays

Extending culture time beyond three to five weeks (typically 5–8 weeks), will allow for differentiation of more immature progenitors, while ruling out any contribution of surviving CFC. All of these assays are performed on feeder layers of supportive cells, mesenchymal bone marrow cells or immortalized murine bone-marrow derived stromal cell lines. Two different cells types can then be identified: *LTC-IC (long-term culture initiating cells)*, whose progeny will be identifiable in the supernatant or feeder and whose myeloid differentiation potential is assessed in subsequent short term assays; and *CAFC (cobblestone area forming cells)*, referring to the appearance of colonies as they integrated into the feeder layer. The interpretation of LTC-IC and CAFC assays is further hindered by the heterogeneous nature of the LTC-IC/CAFC compartment whose progeny can vary widely under identical conditions. When the original culture time on feeder layers is extended to 10 to 12 weeks, these cells are referred to as *ELTC-IC (extended LTC-IC)*. The CAFCs can be counted directly on the initial feeder layer, but this analysis must be performed at limiting dilutions to prevent overlap of cobblestone areas and stromal cells must be prescreened as only some will integrate CAFC. In mice, CAFCs correlate well with numbers of long-term repopulating cells but in humans, these cultures enumerate lineage-committed progenitors, and none of them on their own can predict HSC number.

Secondly, it is essential to realize that these culture conditions in general only give rise to myeloid progenitors. Studying evolution to B, T of NK cell differentiation requires other specific culture systems. While B cells can be generated in liquid media and analyzed by flow cytometry, T-cells ideally require reconstitution of a thymic three-dimensional architecture in *fetal thymus organ culture (FTOC)* (which is possible in mice by using embryonic day 14 thymic lobes depleted from their endogenous T cell populations, but obviously not feasible in humans) to perform quantification of T-cell progenitors using limiting dilutions.[23] Other options include the use of murine stromal lines expressing the Notch ligand Delta-1, however, this simultaneously impairs B cell differentiation and thus precludes simultaneous detection of B and T cells from single progenitors.[24] Specific long term cultures using murine fetal liver cell lines on BM stromal cells, human serum and recombinant interleukin-2 (IL-2) have also been useful in identifying precursors of the natural killer (NK) cell lineage.[25]

Switch Culture Systems

In addition to lineage-specific cultures, *switch culture systems* have been developed in which multipotent human hematopoietic cells can be enumerated. In principle, a switch culture system involves sorting single hematopoietic cells of a primitive cell phenotype into a primary culture system to enable clonal proliferation followed by subculturing its progeny in conditions that facilitate myeloid or lymphoid differentiation. The ability of single-cell–derived progeny to differentiate into myeloid and lymphoid lineages is considered evidence that the initial cell is multipotent. For instance, when single human CD34$^+$CD38$^-$ cells are grown on the murine stromal line S17 for 1 week and progeny that are CD33$^-$CD19$^-$ are then transferred into myeloid-specific conditions, they become CD33$^+$ and give rise to CFCs, but when transferred into B-lymphoid-specific conditions, they become CD19$^+$.[26] When single human BM CD34$^+$Lin$^-$DR^{dim} cells or UCB CD34$^+$CD38$^-$Lin$^-$ cells are cocultured with the murine liver AFT024 cell line for 2 to 4 weeks, followed by re-plating progeny into myeloid and lymphoid systems, they generate primitive myeloid and lymphoid progenitors that are capable of reinitiating long-term myeloid and lymphoid hematopoiesis in vitro and known as *myeloid-lymphoid initiating cells (ML-ICs)*.[27,28] Other studies demonstrated that ML-ICs, in addition to their multi-lineage differentiation capacity, can also self-renew. The ML-IC assay therefore may measure cells that closely resemble true HSCs. A common caveat of all these systems, however, is their inability to measure homing and engraftment of putative HSCs into BM, which can be accomplished only by using transplantation models.

MOLECULAR MARKERS

There is unfortunately no unique unambiguous surface marker that identifies HSCs. However, some combinations of markers are currently being used to define stem cell populations, with various degrees of purity. These markers however differ between species (cf. Fig. 20–2).

Surface Markers

In the mouse, phenotypic analysis of BM and fetal liver cells has identified a population of hematopoietic cells highly enriched for HSCs. This population in BM is *c-Kit$^+$ (receptor for stem cell factor), Thy1^{low} (thymus cell antigen 1), Sca1$^+$ (stem cell antigen)*, and *Lin$^-$ (lineage negative, ie negative for granulocytic, erythroid, and lymphoid antigens)*. This phenotype is often referred to as the *'KTLS' phenotype* and corresponds to about 0.1% of all BM nucleated cells. Since Thy1 is not expressed by all mouse species, cells are sometimes referred to as having a *'KLS'* phenotype, but its use can also be replaced by the absence of *fetal liver kinase 2 (Flk2* also referred to as *Flt3 receptor or fms-related tyrosine kinase 3*[29]*)* on BM cells to identify LTR-HSC.[30] Murine fetal liver HSCs, by contrast, have a slightly different phenotype, expressing other markers such as *AA4.1* and *Mac1$^+$*, while FLK2$^+$ cells will also display some long term repopulating activity.[30,31]

One murine KTLS cell can reconstitute stable long-term multilineage hematopoiesis after transplantation in about 10% of transplanted mice. This suggests either that this population is not totally pure, that some cells transiently lose their engrafting potential, or that only a random proportion of cells properly homes to the bone marrow. Most of these cells will also be CD34$^{-/lo}$ especially in adult mouse BM (this is only the case in 50% of the BM of juvenile mice, and could also be dependent on the activation status of the cell).[32] Combining both phenotypic features, KLS and CD34$^{-/lo}$ identifies a near to homogenous HSC population. The frequency of the latter cells within BM has been estimated to be approximately 0.004%.

It is however possible to further refine this population by using other surface markers such as *signaling lymphocytic activation molecules (SLAM)*, for example, CD150, CD41, and CD48. CD150$^+$CD48$^-$ cells will lead to long term reconstitution of 21% of mice transplanted at the single cell level, whereas combination of these markers with the "KLS CD34$^{-/lo}$" phenotype will yield a 47% reconstitution under similar conditions. However, the CD150$^+$CD48$^-$ KLS CD34$^{-/lo}$ cell population represents only 0.00125% of murine BM.[33,34] These markers are conserved across mice strains and give consistent results in old, reconstituted and cyclophosphamide/GCSF mobilized mice.[34,35] Alternatively, KLS cells have also been sorted according to expression of Tie2, which identifies a subpopulation of quiescent HSCs with long term repopulation ability, shown to be equivalent to side population BM HSCs (see next section on dye exclusion).[36] Finally, the 5% to 15% of KTLS cells expressing low levels of *α2 integrins* also show robust multilineage long term engraftment in contrast to their $\alpha2^+$ counterparts, which are enriched for STR-HSC.[37] This is relatively surprising considering that α2 integrin expression is subsequently lost again by the more differentiated progenitors.[37] Several new positive markers of stem cell populations include *CD201* or *EPCR (endothelial protein C receptor), CD 105* or *endoglin (a component of the TGF-β receptor)* and the *FGFR (FGF receptor)*, which are currently under investigation.[32] Interestingly enough however, it has also been shown that the antigens used to potentially characterize HSCs can vary depending on their cellular activation status, without affecting their regenerative potential, making the marking of "stemness" even more elusive.[38]

In humans, however, the phenotypic features of HSC are less well defined. In contrast to mice, CD34 is expressed on about 1% to 4% of BM cells and contains the majority of cells with in vivo repopulating potential. However, selection of cells based on CD34 expression alone yields a very heterogeneous population of cells of which 20% have CFC activity, 1% LTC-IC and <0.1% SCID-repopulation activity. Based on xenogeneic transplantation into non-obese diabetes/severe combined immunodeficiency (NOD/SCID) mice and on results of in vitro assays, human HSCs can be further characterized by isolating the CD38$^{-/lo}$ fraction of CD34$^+$ cells.[39,40] Alternatively, the subset of CD34$^+$ cells that coexpressed CD133 (also referred to as human homolog of *prominin 5 transmembrane glycoprotein or PROML1*) corresponds to a very primitive population of HSC, as they seem highly enriched for long-term repopulation potential in NOD/SCID mice.[41] Some studies have suggested that CD34$^-$CD38$^-$ Lin$^-$ cells are also capable of engraftment and multilineage differentiation in NOD/SCID mice and that CD34 expression can be acquired from CD34$^-$ cells after in vitro culture, challenging the dogma that human HSCs are CD34$^+$ (cf. Red Box 2). However, the true importance of the CD34- fraction in hematopoietic reconstitution from

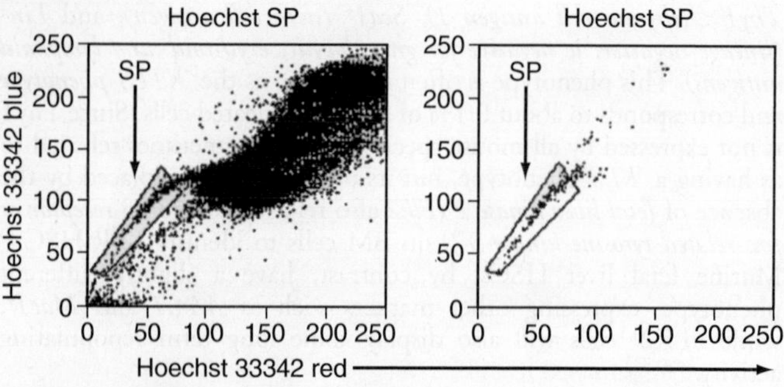

Figure 20–3 Hoechst-33342 side-population (SP) analysis identifies primitive hematopoietic stem cells (HSCs). In the mouse, there is significant overlap between the SP and KTLS phenotype (ie, murine HSC phenotype). SP cells have been identified in hematopoietic and nonhematopoietic tissues from multiple species and are generally considered primitive stem cells. *(Adapted from Bunting KD: ABC transporters as phenotypic markers and functional regulators of stem cells. Stem Cells 20:11, 2002.)*

human BM remains unknown. Other markers used to further define human stem cells are *CDCP1 (Cubdomain containing protein)*, *c-Kit* (which is expressed on about 2/3 of CD34+ cells) and *VEGF receptor 1 and 2* (also called *KDR*) which are expressed on about 5% and 0.1 to 0.5% of $CD34^+$ cells respectively and seem to include the majority of NOD/SCID activity.[32]

Dynamic Methods of HSC Isolation

Another potential strategy to isolate HSC is to make use of detection of enzymatic activity to select for cells which express high levels of specific enzymes. Murine and human HSCs are able to efflux DNA dyes, including *Rhodamine-123 (Rho)* and *Hoechst-33342 (Ho)* dyes, via at least two ATP-binding cassette (ABC) transporters: the *multidrug-resistance P-glycoprotein (MDR1)* and the *breast cancer-resistance protein (BCRP)*, with a certain level of redundancy between these two transporters.[42] These complexes transport Rhodamine-123 and Hoechst-33342 dyes out of the cells through an ATPase-dependent process resulting in a small but distinct subset of cells referred to as *side population cells (SP)*, further characterized as Hoechst or Rhodamine low when a low amount of the fluorescence is displayed simultaneously in two emission wavelengths (Fig. 20–3).[43,44] The physiological function of these transporters in HSCs is unclear, but their ability to efflux dye can be exploited to distinguish HSCs ($Rho^{-/lo}$, $Hoechst^{-/lo}$) from committed progenitors (Rho^{hi}, $Hoechst^{hi}$), as cells exhibiting the highest efflux activity are the most primitive or least restricted in terms of differentiation potential. In mice, SP cells account for about 0.05% of all bone marrow cells, and are enriched 1000 to 3000-fold for stem cell activity.[42] It is however possible to further purify these cells. Selecting only the SP cells with *very low dye efflux* identifies a population referred to as SP^{low} which only comprises 0.005% of all BM cells and overlaps with other phenotypic markers known to identify HSCs (KTLS, $CD34^{-/lo}$, $Tie2^+$ and $Flk2^-$), whilst showing long term repopulating efficiencies of about 35% in lethally irradiated mice.[36,45] It must be noted however, that similarly to antigenic phenotyping, dye efflux has been shown to vary with developmental stage (it is almost absent in fetal liver and bone marrow from young mice, whereas it is present in adult mouse bone marrow) and activation status of HSCs (ie, lost upon activation and differentiation).[38] It is therefore enticing to speculate that both surface markers and dye transporters are mediated by a common pathway involving perhaps cell cycle check points.[38]

In human cord blood, highly purified $CD34^+CD38^-Lin^-$ cells capable of initiating myeloid and lymphoid hematopoiesis are almost exclusively Rho^-.[28] These cells have a high SCID repopulating efficiency (1:30 instead of 1:600 for the total population of $CD34^+CD38^-Lin^-$), thus they can be expected to contain most long-term repopulating cells.[46]

Aldehyde Dehydrogenase (ALDH), an enzyme responsible for oxidizing a variety of aldehydes including vitamin A, is also highly expressed in primitive hematopoietic cells in a number of species and its activity can be detected by supplying cells with polar fluorescent products which will accumulate in cells displaying a high enzymatic activity. This makes it possible to detect potential HSCs which will appear brighter on flow cytometry analysis *($SSC^{lo}ALDH^{br}$ cells)*. *$SSC^{lo}ALDH^{br}$ cells* represent about 1% of UCB cells.[47] Combining this method with conventional CD34 staining, makes it possible to identify two cell populations: the *$ALDH^{br}CD34^+$ cells*, enriched for short term and long term SRC as well as myeloid progenitors, and the *$ALDH^{neg}CD34^+$ cells*, displaying low repopulation activity and possibly enrichment for lymphoid progenitors determined using short term cultures.[48] Hess and colleagues showed that although *$ALDH^{br}CD133^+Lin^-$ UCB cells* contain both the $CD34^+CD38^-$ and the $CD34^-CD38^-$ subsets, they are enriched for HSC as there is a tenfold enhancement of hematopoietic repopulating capacity compared to $CD133^+Lin^-$ cells in a *NOD/SCID/β_2m^{null}* mouse transplantation model.[49] A major advantage of this type of technique is its potential clinical application as the use of toxic DNA intercalating dyes discussed above cannot be used for clinical procedures. In fact, preliminary data already suggests that ALDH activity could be a better predictor of graft quality than $CD34^+$cell content.[50] The actual function of ALDH in HSC metabolism remains unknown, but it was recently demonstrated that addition of ALDH inhibitors to standard cytokine-based human HSC expansion cocktails could potentially lead to preservation of long term repopulating potential of BM and UCB HSCs in a NOD/SCID transplantation model.[51]

A frequent problem with use of dye exclusion and enzymatic activity to identify stem cells, however, is that both are dynamic processes. This implies that slight variations in protocols (eg. tissue dissociation, cell counting, dye concentration, staining time, temperature, FACS gating) can dramatically influence viability, homogeneity and yield of SP cells.[42] Consequently, results from different studies are often difficult to compare and can sometimes considerably differ.

HSC FATE AND REGULATION OF HEMATOPOIESIS

The mechanisms regulating HSC self-renewal, differentiation or apoptosis are intensively studied as it is clear that these cell-fate decisions are responsible for homeostasis. Furthermore, from a clinical point of view, understanding these mechanisms is crucial in many hematopoietic malignant diseases and could be used in developing optimal HSC expansion systems suitable for clinical transplantation.

The first model that attempted to describe cell-fate decisions in hematopoiesis was proposed by Till and McCulloch in 1961.[52] In this model, HSCs would *randomly* commit to self-renew or differentiate: this is called the *stochastic* model. In fact, several studies, where single murine or human HSC clones were followed by viral marking, recently stressed the unpredictability of clonal behavior.[53,54] Results derived from other studies, however, support the *deterministic* model, where the central concept is that the *microenvironment* in which HSCs reside determines whether they self-renew or differentiate.[55] It is possible that the very early decision of HSCs to self-renew or differentiate may be stochastic but that subsequent lineage differentiation and maturation of progenitor cells is instructed by external cues from the microenvironment.[40] However, one could also argue that chance is often the most satisfactory answer for unexplained phenomenon and that stochastic cell decisions simply remain to be understood.

Gene expression in hematopoiesis involves both intrinsic and extrinsic regulation pathways. This has been approached from different angles. Some genes, such as transcription factors and genes involved in epigenetic regulation (including subsets known to be aberrantly expressed in leukemia), have been studied using various loss-of-function (knock-out) and gene overexpression studies (for discussion of transcriptional regulation of hematopoiesis, see Chapter 21). Another approach is to compare the transcriptomes of stem cell populations with variable self-renewal potential, to get a broader picture of the intrinsic regulation at work in determining HSC fate. Finally, cell cycle modifications and signals emanating from the microenvironment are also being investigated to single out important components responsible for preserving stem cell function.

HSC INTRINSIC REGULATION

Transcription Factors

In vertebrates, the stem cell leukemia gene (*SCL*, also known as *TAL1*), Lim-only protein 2 (*LMO2*), *GATA2*, *AML1* (also called *RUNX1*) and *MYB* are all indispensable for hematopoietic specification during embryonic development. Their gene activation profile during hematological ontogeny has been described in vertebrate systems (see Fig. 20–1).[6,7,19] *SCL, LMO2* and *GATA2* are expressed at the hemangioblast and HSC level and are indispensable for primitive and definitive hematopoiesis.[56–58,59] whereas *AML1* and *MYB* are exclusively involved in definitive hematopoiesis in mice and zebrafish.[60–62] Very little is known, however, about the role of these genes and their products during postnatal and adult hematopoiesis or how they may regulate self-renewal or the differentiation decision by postnatal HSCs.

Homeobox genes (HOX) are an evolutionary preserved family characterized by a 60 aminoacid DNA-binding motif called the homeodomain and play a role in normal and malignant hematopoiesis. Additional DNA binding specificity is obtained by interaction between clustered HOX proteins and the non clustered Para-HOX proteins, primarily the *three amino acid loop extension (TALE)* family of transcription factors including *pre-B-cell leukemia homeobox 1 (PBX1)* and *myeloid ecotropic viral integration site 1 (MEIS1)*.[63] The class I HOX family comprises four clusters (A to D) on different chromosomes, and individual genes are numbered in a 3′ to 5′ order in 13 paralog groups, based on sequence homology. HOX genes are expressed in $CD34^+$ cells, and those of the 3′ region, such as *HOXB3* and *HOXB4*, are preferentially expressed in the more primitive $CD34^+CD38^+$ cells.[64] The significance of individual genes has been investigated in loss-of-function and in overexpression studies. Mice homozygous null for *HOXA9* are viable and fertile and have only mild skeletal abnormalities. However, adult mice show significant abnormalities in granulopoiesis and T- and B-cell lymphopoiesis.[65] More importantly, the BM of $HOXA9^{-/-}$ mice shows delayed autologous hematopoietic recovery after sublethal irradiation, and their HSCs engraft poorly when transplanted to wild-type animals.[66] In contrast to *HOXA9*, studies on other *HOX* gene knockouts have been less revealing, because perhaps of redundancy within the multiple HOX dependent pathways. Knocking down both HOXB3 and HOXB4, for example, only resulted in a moderate decrease in cellularity in hematopoietic organs, probably secondary to a limited reduction of primitive fetal liver progenitors.[67] In the transplantation setting, the slightly lower repopulation potential. It seemed to be associated with slower cell cycle kinetics, as demonstrated by the better tolerance of HOXB3/B4 BM cells to pretransplant 5-fluorouracil (5-FU) treatment, which selectively depletes the activated HSC from the BM.[67] The phenotype of $HOXB4^{-/-}$ was in fact strikingly similar to the double knockdown model, but slightly less pronounced, suggesting a potential cooperation between different HOX genes or a dosage effect.[68]

Overexpression of HOX genes however, has repeatedly been shown to impact on HSC turnover. BM cells that overexpress *HOXA9* for instance are leukemogenic,[69] consistent with the clinical observation that *HOXA9* is a fusion partner with *nucleoporin 98kDa (NUP98)* in chromosomal translocation t(7;11), which occurs in about 1% cases of acute myelogenous leukemia (AML). Overexpression of HOXB4, however, appears to increase HSC self-renewal without altering the cell's ability to commit to different lineages.[70–73] Human $CD34^+Lin^-$ cells when overexpressing HOXB4 were transplanted in NOD/SCID mice a threefold to fourfold increase in SRC occurred. Likewise, when murine BM cells overexpressing HOXB4 were cultured in vitro for 10 to 14 days and transplanted into mice, HSC frequency was increased by more than 1000-fold compared with mock-transduced BM cells, without skewing their lymphomyeloid repopulating potential. A possible mechanism for this is suggested by studies with murine yolk sac cells and embryonic stem cells showing that HOXB4 confers definitive hematopoietic potential and facilitates engraftment of hematopoietic cells, possibly by upregulating expression of the chemokine receptor CXCR4 and the transcription factor TEL, both of which are important homing factors for HSCs.[74] Of note, an extra competitive advantage was conferred by concomitantly knocking down the expression of PBX1 cofactors, thereby suggesting that PBX1 acts as a negative regulator of HOXB4-induced HSC proliferation.[75] Leukemic transformation has not occurred in recipients, suggesting that regulated HOXB4 overexpression may be used for ex-vivo HSC expansion suitable for clinical transplantation. In contrast, overexpression of other homeobox genes, such as clustered genes (eg, *HOXB8*, *HOXB3*, and *HOXA10)* or nonclustered genes (eg. *homeobox-like 1 Xenopus laevis (MIXL1) or caudal type homeobox transcription factor 2 (CDX2)*) using retroviral transduction alters lineage-commitment at the progenitor cell level, and can sometimes lead to the development of acute leukemia in recipient animals.[76–78]

Interestingly, several upstream mechanisms regulating expression of HOX genes have been found to be associated with pathological hematological disorders. For instance, *retinoic acid response elements (RARE)* have been identified at the 3′ end of *HOXA* and *HOXB* gene clusters and retinoic acid has been implicated in regulating HOX gene expression during embryonic development.[79] *All-trans-retinoic acid (ATRA)* is used as first-line treatment for *acute promyelocytic leukemia (aPML)*, because it facilitates differentiation of leukemia blasts by degrading the pathological PML-RAR-α fusion protein complex. *HOXC4* expression is in fact typically absent at diagnosis, but appears simultaneously with differentiation markers both in vivo and in vitro after starting ATRA treatment.[80] Another example is the upstream regulation of HOX genes by other highly conserved genes: *mixed-lineage leukemia (MLL)*, a common target of chromosomal translocations in human acute leukemias, which is responsible for positive gene expression during development and its antagonist, the *polycomb gene (PCG)* family. Both of these are believed to regulate gene expression by complex epigenetic mechanisms (see below). Interestingly, while disruption of MLL function generally inhibits growth and differentiation of HSCs, the presence of oncogenic MLL fusion proteins increases their proliferative capacity. Overexpression of HOXA9 and HOXA10 have indeed been observed in patient leukemia cells involving MLL translocations, suggesting an early arrest in hematopoietic differentiation leading to the immature phenotype associated with MLL leukemia.[81] By contrast, expression of some PCG genes, for example *B lymphoma Mo-MLV insertion region 1 (BMI1)*,[82] and in a lesser extent *polyhomeotic-like 1 (PHC1)*[83] and *polycomb group ring finger 2 (PCGRF2)*[84] seem to be necessary for the maintenance and self-renewal of HSC.

Epigenetic Regulation

In addition to gene-specific regulation, the cell-fate decision of HSCs may be regulated by modification of chromatin components, known as *epigenetic regulation*.[85] The basic chromatin unit of a cell, the *nucleosome*, is composed of histone proteins and double-stranded DNA arranged in a beads-on-a-string configuration. Older dogma indicates that such a configuration serves to package the genome within the confines of the cell nucleus. Subsequent data suggest that covalent modification of histone proteins, including phosphorylation, acetylation, methylation, ADP ribosylation and ubiquitination, can affect nucleosomal structure and encode information for gene regulation. Histone modification can be induced locally in a gene-specific manner, in which specific DNA binding proteins activate histone-modifying enzymes to their cognate sites, or induced globally, in which case chromatin is compartmentalized in nuclear subdomains that are enriched with specific modifiers. Such modifications at sites of key lineage-specific genes may be interpreted by HSCs as *restrictive* or *permissive* signals for differentiation. Subsequent protein interaction involving these codes further modulates the activity of the associated genes, thereby restricting differentiation along a chosen lineage.

An example of a candidate gene involved in the epigenetic regulation of HSC cell-fate decision is *Ikaros,* a zinc finger protein that is expressed during primitive and definitive hematopoiesis. Ikaros acts by a bivalent chromatin regulation mechanism, paradoxically either silencing or promoting transcription via specific remodeling.[86] Mice carrying the Ikaros^{null} allele have reduced HSC activity, suggesting that Ikaros may maintain survival and proliferation of HSCs during steady-state hematopoiesis. Furthermore, fetal development of B, T, and NK cells is totally abolished along with a relative increase in myeloid activity, suggesting that Ikaros may be involved in HSC commitment to the lymphoid lineage.[87]

Transcriptome, MRNA Stability Control, and Proteome Analysis

Because the blueprint of the human genome and techniques such as DNA microarray technologies are widely available, it is now possible to study the transcriptional regulation of HSCs on a genome-wide scale. Several studies based on *subtraction hybridization* and *array analyses* have identified classes of genes that are highly expressed in HSCs and other stem cell populations.[88–91] What can be gleaned from these initial studies is that the presence of multiple transcripts, rather than one or a few genes, probably endows stem cells with their unique properties. These observations are in keeping with the multilineage priming model proposed earlier for HSCs.

Several comparisons of LTR-HSC versus STR-HSC and MPP in mice and humans have recently shown the importance of genes associated with quiescence, cell adhesion (with the surrounding environment but also intercellular), and cytoprotection in the long term repopulating cells,[90,92] whereas genes involved in differentiation, proliferation, and chemotaxis seemed to be associated to more differentiated stages.[14] These data also suggest that self-renewal might be more associated with an inhibition of differentiation than an active promotion of self-renewal, but this remains to be proven. Interestingly, HSCs seemed to express several ligand-receptor pairs, suggesting that part of the regulation might be autocrine.[92] Similar pathways could also be detected by comparing stem cells of different origins (fetal versus adult, or neuronal versus hematopoietic) and species subsets, supporting the idea of key stem cell properties needed for stem cell renewal.[90,92] By focusing on differences between human stem cell sources (namely the transcriptomes of Rho^{lo} and Rho^{hi} CD34$^+$Lin$^-$ CD38$^-$ cells from umbilical cord blood (UCB) and bone marrow (BM)) known to have variable bone marrow transplantation outcomes, it was also possible to single out the importance of cell cycle regulators and certain transcription factors, known to play a role in hematopoiesis or leukemogenesis (such as HLF, EVI1), but as for the previous screens, about 40% of genes identified still had an unknown function, suggesting that these may all represent uncharacterized regulators of HSC fate decisions.[90,93]

Apart from the limitations inherent to the choice of genes used for the microarray, the major hurdle of this type of analysis is obviously the technical difficulties of purifying the stem cell population. Selecting them according to their response to transplantation might actually select cells capable of redirecting themselves to the appropriate niche responsible for long-term self renewal (and thus expressing higher amounts of cell-cell and cell-matrix interaction genes) rather than those responsible for the process of self renewal itself.[14]

Furthermore, the amount of protein produced from an mRNA transcript will not necessarily correlate with the amount of mRNA produced, but also will depend on the *stability* of this transcript. Examples of these mechanisms in hematology are still scarce, but cytokine control of GM-CSF and Interleukin 3 (Il-3) signaling for instance are now known to be regulated at least partially by the turnover of *AU-rich elements (ARE)* in physiological circumstances, where the adenosine/uracil (AU) content of the mRNA defines its stability. This also seems to be the case in certain hematological malignancies, where cyclin D1 or BCL2 mRNA stabilization seem to be associated with mantle cell lymphoma and chronic lymphocytic leukemia.[94]

Aside from gene transcription, it has become clear in recent years that mRNA levels are not only determined by transcriptional control alone, but that posttranscriptional events affect mRNA stability. The posttranscriptional regulation is mediated by *micro RNA (miRNA) and small interfering RNA (siRNA).* These small (20–28 base pair) noncoding RNAs, once activated, associate to *miRNA-induced silencing complex (miRISC)* and result in cleavage of their matching target mRNA and/or in more subtle translational repression of target genes when the target contains multiple incomplete matches in the 3′UTR region.[95] Alternatively, they can also mediate gene silencing through chromatin remodeling. Interestingly, the impact of the same miRNA can sometimes differ widely between species.[96] Specific miRNAs are associated with specific hematological cell types and play important regulatory roles in all stages of differentiation: miRNA155 for instance has been shown to negatively regulate normal myelopoiesis and erythropoiesis.[97] They can also function both as oncogenes (eg, miRNA142 translocated in B cell pro-lymphocytic leukemia) and tumor suppressors (eg, miRNA15A deletion in 13q$^-$ chronic lymphocytic leukemia leads to an activation of BCL2), but the fine tuning of their regulation remains largely unknown.[96]

Finally, a gene that is transcribed will not necessarily be translated into an active protein, as some mRNAs will be translated into nonfunctional proteins, which then require posttranslational modifications to become active. Tao and colleagues, for instance, compared the *proteomes* of CD34$^+$ UCB cells versus CD15$^+$ mature granulocytes. This showed that the CD34$^+$ stem/progenitor cells had a much larger proteome than the more terminally differentiated cells, suggesting that lineage choice might occur by shutting down the expression of a specific "stem-cell associated" set of proteins and activating a limited number of lineage-related proteins. Several of the proteins identified to be different between the two populations were also implicated in protein folding and posttranslational quality control systems, further emphasizing the possible impact of this posttranslational remodeling in the self-renewal/differentiation process. Finally, these results also confirmed the hypothesis from the genomic studies that these cells possess attributes of cells under stress.[98]

Cell Cycle Regulation in HSC

Cell cycle regulation (thoroughly discussed in Chapter 7) is crucial in HSC biology, as it regulates the cellular turnover and choice between quiescence and division, leading to self-renewal or differentiation. The critical step for progression to cell division is the transition from *Gap phase 1 (G_1)* to the *Synthesis phase (S),* where DNA is synthesized, as this subsequently commits the cell to cycle progression.[99] The role of several proteins in these fate decisions has recently been elucidated. The *D-type cyclins* (D1, D2, and D3) are the first components to become induced in response to mitogenic stimulation, and are indispensable for hematopoiesis as simultaneous deletion of all D-type cyclins completely suppresses expansion and differentiation of HSC.[100] The roles of these proteins is, however, redundant as Ciemerych and colleagues have shown that the presence of at least one D-type cyclin was sufficient to allow normal development.[101] Interestingly, single knockouts of individuals D-type cyclins resulted in defects in lymphoid development of B and T lymphocytes for cyclin D2 and D3 respectively.[99]

Expectedly, knocking down the preferred catalytic subunits of cyclin D *(cyclin-dependent kinase 4 and 6 (CDK4 and 6)* results in a similar, but milder hematological phenotype as mice lacking D-type cyclins altogether. However, absence of CDK2 (which is normally activated by E-type and A-type cyclins, driving cell proliferation by an alternative pathway) did not seem to impact hematopoiesis.[99]

Cyclin-dependent kinase inhibitors (CDKI) are divided in the *CIP/Kip* (encompassing proteins such as *p21^{cip1}* and *p27^{kip1}*) and *INK4* families which also participate in cell cycle by sequential activation and inactivation of CDKs. For instance, p21 knock-out mice exhibit an increase in HSC cycling and exhaustion upon transplantation,[102] and ex-vivo targeting in UCB also showed relative expansion of HSC, defined by a higher number of CFU colonies, LTC-IC and a higher engraftment in NOD-SCID mice.[103] p27 Knock-out mice, however, have hyperplasia of most organs (hematopoietic organs included), the progenitor cell population is expanded, without impact on the true primitive stem cell function.[104] By contrast, most of the INK4 family proteins do not appear to play essential role in hematopoiesis, except for p15^{INK4b} and p18^{INK4c} which, when knocked down, cause a widespread hyperplasia of the hematopoietic system, demonstrating once more the importance of redundancy of function in these regulatory systems.[99]

HSC EXTRINSIC REGULATION

The cellular proximity in the BM milieu suggests that HSC cell-fate decisions may be subject to the influence of adjacent HSCs and stromal cells in specialized three dimensional niches. Such niches may provide proliferation and differentiation signals to HSCs through direct *cell-cell* or *cell-extracellular matrix (ECM)* interactions or through secretion of cytokines, chemokines, or other extracellular signaling molecules.[105] This concept is supported by observations that HSCs and stromal cells express reciprocal genes encoding for secreted proteins and cytokines that are important for HSC proliferation and differentiation, suggesting that early hematopoiesis is under paracrine or autocrine regulation, or both. Moreover, several cell lines that are capable of maintaining human and murine HSCs in vitro have been generated from the AGM region, yolk sac fetal liver, or BM. The following section describes the roles of early-acting cytokines and embryonic signaling molecules that are implicated in postnatal hematopoiesis and their potential clinical applications. Detailed information on "cell-cell/cell-ECM interactions" and cytokines in the hematopoietic microenvironment can be found in Chapter 23 and 24.

The Stem Cell Niche

Two HSC niches have been identified to date: the endosteal niche and the vascular niche. The *endosteal niche* is situated close to the trabecular bone, where osteoblasts, stromal fibroblasts and CXCL12-abundant reticular cells (CAR cells) appear to play a major role in controlling stem cell number through a number of pathways, such as bone morphogenic pathway (BMP) signaling, Tie2-Angiopoietin 1 signaling, N-cadherin and parathormone (PTH) receptor Notch activation.[33,36,106,107] The concept of a *vascular niche* for HSC arose from the observation of extra-medullary hematopoiesis and the ability of cytokines to mobilize HSCs into the circulation very rapidly. This was further defined by colocalization of HSC expressing a SLAM family signature (CD150$^+$CD48$^-$CD41$^-$) with CAR cells and sinusoidal endothelium both in spleen and bone marrow.[33,34]

The concept of a stem cell niche relies on the effect of this microenvironment on HSC: the factors secreted in the niche ensuring stem cell quiescence or renewal, whereas migration of HSCs out of the niche would result in differentiation.[108] The five major highly conserved pathways thought to play a role in these interactions (*Wnt, Notch, FGF, sHH,* and *BMP* pathways) are briefly reviewed here.

Wnt

The canonical Wnt signaling cascade, thought to play a role in hematopoiesis, is activated by the binding of the Wnt protein to a cell-surface receptor made up of *frizzled* and *low-density lipoprotein receptor related protein (LRP)* 5 and 6. In the absence of Wnt signaling, *β-catenin* is phosphorylated by interacting with an *Axin/GSK3β* (glycogen synthase kinase 3β) complex and thereby targeted for degradation. Wnt signaling blocks this interaction, resulting in accumulation of β-catenin and its translocation to the nucleus, where it binds to *LEF/TCF* transcription factors to activate target genes.[109] Gain of function experiments involving β-catenin overexpression promotes the preservation of a primitive HSC phenotype in vitro despite prolonged culture, and leads to functional expansion of HSC measured in competitive repopulation assays in mice, whereas use of inhibitors of the Wnt pathway (eg, ectopic expression of axin) inhibit HSC growth in vitro and repopulation capacity in vivo.[110] Moreover, gain of function experiments also suggest that activation of this signaling pathway in STR-HSCs or even more committed MPPs may endow these cells, that usually have limited or no self-renewal ability, with the ability to self-replicate.

Notch

The family of Notch receptors encompasses four cell-surface receptors (Notch 1–4) capable of binding two types of ligands: *Delta* (Delta-like 1,3 or 4) and *Jagged* (Jagged 1 or 2). This binding results in proteolytic cleavage of Notch, thus releasing its cytoplasmic intracellular domain and allowing it to translocate to the nucleus where it binds to *CBF-1* and *RBP-Jκ*. Binding converts these transcriptional repressors into activators. Activation of this pathway has repeatedly been associated with cell-fate determination such as self-renewal (both in vitro and in vivo), as they act as a gate-keeper against differentiation signals.[109,111] It must be noted however, that a certain degree of redundancy must exist within this signaling system since selective loss of function experiments, such as blocking of Jagged-1 dependent notch signaling for instance, had no effect on hematopoiesis.[112] Interestingly, Notch signaling is also associated with T-cell cell fate specification, as aberrant expression is seen in several types of T-cell acute lymphoblastic leukemias.[24] This pathway could also be associated with later stages of B cell development, as core binding factor inactivation led to loss of splenic marginal zone B cells, with a moderate increase of follicular B cells, whereas deficiency in *MINT* (a negative regulator of Notch signaling) resulted in the reciprocal phenotype.[24] Expression of Notch receptors and ligands has also been reported in Hodgkin lymphoma, T-cell derived anaplastic large cell lymphoma and B-cell chronic lymphocytic leukemia, but the actual role of this pathway in the pathogenesis of these disorders still needs to be elucidated.[24]

Fibroblast Growth Factors (FGF)

More than 20 different *FGFs* have been identified in mammals, with variable affinity to four different FGF receptor tyrosine kinases (1–4), further modulated by additional binding to *heparin* or *heparin sulfate proteoglycans (HSPG)*. Activation of the pathway takes place by dimerization and phosphorylation of the receptors, leading to transduction of the signal through the *Ras/mitogen activated protein kinase* pathway.[109] There is also growing evidence for the role of this pathway in hematopoiesis. For example, Fgf21 is essential for myeloerythroid progenitor cell fates in zebrafish.[113] Furthermore, murine HSC can be kept in culture in serum free conditions for up to 5 weeks when FGF 1 and/or 2 are added to the medium, while retaining long term repopulating activity.[114]

Bone Morphogenic Proteins (BMPs)

BMPs are members of the *transforming growth factor-β (TGF-β)* superfamily, which play a pivotal role in directing cells toward a ventral mesoderm fate and embryonic hematopoiesis.[115] Binding of BMP ligands to their surface receptor activates the receptor kinase activity, resulting in translocation of complexes of *Smad* proteins to the nucleus to regulate gene transcription.[109] The BMP pathway also involves complex feedback mechanisms via members of the Smad family[115] and zinc finger proteins such as *OAZ*[116] and *Early Hematopoietic Zinc Finger protein (EHZF)* in Xenopus and mice. Precise upstream signals that activate BMP expression are not known, although hedgehog proteins[117] and retinoids[7,118] seem to be involved.

Zebrafish embryos carrying null mutations of genes encoding *BMP2b* and *BMP7* are characterized by with reduced ventral structures, including hematopoietic tissue.[119] Mice that are deficient in *BMP4* die early in utero with defective ventral mesoderm specification and absence of primitive hematopoiesis in the yolk sac.[120] Furthermore, several teams[3,121] have now demonstrated that a combination of *BMP4* and other cytokines promotes hematopoietic differentiation of human ES cells. Components of the BMP pathway, including BMP receptors and intracellular signaling molecules, have also been identified in postnatal human hematopoietic tissues, including BM, UCB, and PB. When exogenous BMP4 is added to in vitro cultures of primitive CD34$^-$CD38$^-$Lin$^-$ cells, SRCs are better preserved as compared with control cultures.[122] The downstream effectors of BMP4 have not been fully elucidated. In rhesus monkey embryonic stem cells, exogenous BMP4 regulates expression of VEGFR, CD34, GATA2, SCL, c-Kit, IL-6R, and EpoR and facilitates differentiation toward hematopoietic cells.[123] An essential question remains whether the effect of BMPs is mediated by pure ventral mesoderm specification (ie, more ventral tissues giving rise to more hematopoietic cells) or whether they induce specific proliferation of HSCs and progenitors, which would have potential implications in the development of ex-vivo culture systems for HSCs to improve clinical transplantation results.

Hedgehog Proteins (HH)

Hedgehog proteins are secreted glycoproteins, which impact on both on tissue specification during embryogenesis and proliferation of adult HSC via cell cycle regulation. Under basal circumstances, the HH transmembrane receptor *Patched (Ptc)* suppresses another transmembrane protein called *Smoothened (Smo)*. However, when HH binds to Ptc, Smo becomes active, and triggers HH target gene transcription via the *Gli* transcription factor family.[124] Three homologs of hedgehog proteins are involved in mammal embryonic and postnatal hematopoiesis through distinct mechanisms: *Sonic (SHH)*, *Indian (IHH)*, and *Desert (DHH)*. IHH seems to be involved in bone formation and in the development of the bone marrow microenvironment. It upregulates BMP-4 expression and leads to induction of primitive hematopoiesis and vasculogenesis in mouse embryos.[125] It has also recently been shown to reversibly increase human cord blood *colony forming units (CFU)* in vitro and lead to greater short term engraftment and higher frequency of NOD-SCID reconstitution by human cord blood cells, when cells were co-cultured with stromal cells overexpressing IHH.[126] On the other hand, SHH, a key signaling component of the notochord, has been shown to be expressed with Ptc, Smo, and Gli in human cord blood CD34$^-$CD38$^-$Lin$^-$ cells and BM stromal cells.[117] When added to in vitro cultures, SHH also enhances proliferation of CD34$^-$CD38$^-$Lin$^-$ cells and supports expansion of SRCs.[117] Although this appeared to improve short term repopulation, the presence of SHH negatively affected long term repopulation results of NOD-SCID mice, possibly due to exhaustion of the HSC compartment.[124]

Cytokines Acting at the Hematopoietic Stem Cell Level

Several cytokines affect the process of self-renewal and differentiation of HSCs. Mice carrying a null mutation for *steel factor* or *stem cell factor (SCF)*, have defects in the HSC microenvironment such that transplantation of HSCs from wild-type mice to SCF$^{-/-}$ animals leads to poor hematopoietic reconstitution. Likewise, bone marrow from mice with a null mutation in the SCF receptor c-Kit (*W* mutants) has reduced long-term repopulating capacity when transplanted to wild-type recipient animals.[127] Murine HSCs deficient in *Flt3 receptor* (also known as *Flk2*, a tyrosine kinase receptor) are defective in lymphoid and myeloid reconstitution when transplanted into wide-type recipient animals.[128] Mice carrying a null mutation for the *Flt3 ligand (FL)* have reduced common lymphoid progenitors, and when wild-type HSCs are transplanted into lethally irradiated FL$^{-/-}$ recipients, reconstitution of common lymphoid progenitors is defective, suggesting that FL is important for cell-fate decisions of HSCs.[129] When Flt3$^{-/-}$ mice are crossed to SCL$^{-/-}$ mice, the double knock-outs have a more severe defect in HSCs, resulting in early postnatal lethality.[128] These results suggest that the *SCF/c-Kit* and *Flt3/FL* pathways interact synergistically in the self-renewal of HSCs.

Another cytokine that acts at the HSC level is *thrombopoietin (Tpo)*, which is also known to enhance megakaryocyte proliferation and differentiation. Mice deficient in genes encoding Tpo, or its receptor, *c-Mpl*, have reduced numbers of megakaryocytes and multilineage progenitors, and Tpo$^{-/-}$ mice poorly support proliferation of transplanted wild-type HSCs.[130,131] The defects in HSC proliferation in these mice are correctible by exogenous Tpo.[130] Moreover, HSCs from mice carrying a null mutation for *c-Mpl* have significantly reduced competitive repopulating cell activity, suggesting that *Tpo* and *c-Mpl* are important in the maintenance of stem and early progenitor cells.[132]

Other important interleukins, growth factors and early-acting cytokines, including *vascular endothelial growth factor (VEGF)* and *angiopoietins*, which act concomitantly on HSCs and endothelial cells, are discussed in Chapter 24. The mechanisms of action of these cytokines are probably multifactorial, involving effects on HSC proliferation, expression of adhesion molecules, and endothelial cell function. Analogous to the use of *granulocyte stimulating factor (G-CSF)* to hasten neutrophil recovery after transplantation, it is possible that early-acting cytokines given to patients may enhance proliferation of HSCs in vivo, thereby facilitating short-term and long-term engraftment, especially in adult patients receiving small UCB grafts.[130] Exogenous *Tpo*, when given to *Tpo*$^{-/-}$ mice receiving wild-type HSC grafts, was able to enhance HSC engraftment and proliferation in vivo.[133] Whether SCF or FL have a similar effect and, more importantly, whether transplant recipients (who already have increased levels of these cytokines) would benefit from such interventions will require further investigation. Another application of these early-acting cytokines is based on their ability to maintain or stimulate the proliferation of HSCs. They constitute an integral part of most laboratory culture systems that aim at expanding HSC ex-vivo. Although many of these factors will stimulate the proliferation of HSC, they induce differentiation at the expense HSC expansion or even maintenance. The challenge today is to develop culture conditions which retain pluripotentiality of HSC while increasing stem cell number.

SOURCES OF HEMATOPOIETIC STEM CELLS

HSCs for clinical transplantation can be derived from BM, peripheral blood after mobilization by chemotherapy and or cytokines (mPB), and UCB. BM grafts have been the classic source of HSCs since the first successful transplantation reported by Thomas in 1959.[32] During the past 2 decades, mPB has become more popular because its collection obviates the need for donors to undergo general anesthesia and because recipients of mPB transplants often have faster neutrophil and platelet recovery. The first UCB transplantation was conducted in 1988, and thereafter, UCB became an alternative source of HSCs for patients without a matched adult donor. Success of UCB transplantation, however, is limited by the cell dose available to patients.[134]

From a biological point of view, these grafts differ quantitatively and qualitatively in stem cell content, as reflected in the kinetics of hematological recovery. In general, patients receiving mPB transplants have a more rapid neutrophil and platelet recovery, BM transplants result in slower recovery, and UCB transplants demonstrate the most delayed recovery. Phenotypically, the percentage of primitive $CD34^+CD38^-$ cells in all three tissues is similar.[135] When the same number of CD34+ cells from mPB or BM are transplanted in fetal sheep, those from mPB engraft faster, but they are more quickly exhausted during serial transplantation.[136] When mononuclear cells from BM, mPB, and UCB were transplanted into NOD/SCID mice at limiting dilutions, the frequency of SRCs in UCB was 1 in 9.3×10^5 and was significantly higher than that in BM (1 in 3.0×10^6) or mPB (1 in 6.0×10^6).[137] The superiority of UCB was also confirmed by more recent ML-IC studies.[138] Although these laboratory results may suggest that mPB $CD34^+$ cells are less potent than BM $CD34^+$ cells, these studies must be interpreted with caution, because there is no clinical evidence to suggest that patients receiving mPB transplants are more susceptible to delayed graft failure. Whether the inferior proliferative and long-term engraftment of HSCs from mPB observed in the laboratory is compensated for by a larger cell dose transplanted into patients is unknown.

EX-VIVO EXPANSION MODELS

The rationale for ex-vivo expansion of hematopoietic cells are either to generate expanded populations of committed cells (to decrease the time to neutrophil and platelet recovery) to generate sufficient HSCs from small grafts such as UCB to be transplanted into adult patients, to enhance proliferation of HSCs as targets for gene therapy to purge autologous transplants of contaminating tumor cells. Several protocols have been developed that expand progenitor cells on a clinical scale, and initial clinical studies suggest that such expanded cell products may shorten the time to neutrophil and platelet recovery after myeloablation.[139] Clinical-scale expansion of HSCs however has not been achieved. Several culture systems have been evaluated.

A number of laboratories have attempted to expand HSCs using early-acting cytokines in the presence of serum without stromal support. These culture systems lead to a massive expansion of committed progenitors but no increase or even loss of HSCs.[140] In a case study, two patients were myeloablated with chemoirradiation, followed by transplantation with autologous mPB grafts alone. The latter were expanded for 8 days in the presence of autologous serum and a cytokine mixture comprising SCF, IL-3, IL-6, IL-1β, and erythropoietin. Both failed to show sustained neutrophil and platelet engraftment after transplantation, suggesting that these culture systems did not maintain HSCs.[141] Similar results were seen in serum-free culture conditions in the presence of a more than tenfold higher concentration of these cytokines. In particular, human UCB $CD34^+$, when cultured in serum-free medium for 14 days in the presence of SCF, TPO, and G-CSF and transplanted into fetal sheep, provide more rapid but only transient engraftment in primary recipients in contrast to uncultured cells that are capable of slower but durable engraftment.[139] In most subsequent clinical trials, expanded UCB HSC grafts were cotransplanted with unmanipulated grafts such that the contribution by expanded grafts alone could not be assessed.[142,143]

Other investigators have evaluated cultures in which hematopoiesis is supported by stromal feeders. The earliest stromal feeders were established from autologous BM mononucleated cells in the presence of horse and bovine serum-containing medium (ie, Dexter cultures). Later, a number of stromal cell lines were developed from murine or human AGM region, yolk sac, fetal liver, or BM. The murine fetal liver AFT024, murine BM MS5, human BM HS27, and human and porcine BM-derived endothelial cells appear to support a twofold to fivefold expansion of HSCs.[144] These stromal cells express specific proteoglycans and ligands for Notch receptors (ie, JAG1 and DLK), which may promote HSC survival and proliferation in vitro.[31,145,146] Because direct contact between HSC and xenogeneic or allogeneic stromal feeders is not suitable for clinical transplantation, investigators have also tested whether HSC can be maintained in *transwells* held above the feeders (ie, noncontact system). Another method to circumvent the problem of direct cell contact is to supplement cultures with media that are *conditioned* by certain stromal feeders. In noncontact and conditioned medium systems, HSCs can be maintained to an extent similar to that achieved with stromal contact systems.[144] Most of these approaches, however, are still at the experimental stage and have not been able to expand HSCs extensively enough to be applicable at a clinical scale.

Why is it so difficult to expand HSCs? To accomplish HSC expansion, the cells must be stimulated to divide repeatedly in a symmetric fashion such that the two daughter cells retain the same stem cell properties as the mother cells. Several factors can cause failure of HSC expansion:

1. Proliferation of HSCs in vitro is limited. In vivo under steady state conditions, HSCs are *quiescent* but they can be recruited into cell cycle (hence, proliferate) upon cytokine stimulation. Thus, it is unlikely that lack of HSC expansion is caused by the inability of HSCs to proliferate.
2. Daughter cells are driven into *differentiation*. One of the biggest problems encountered in the development of ex-vivo HSC expansion culture is that most or all conditions cause lineage commitment. Several advances have pointed to ways to circumvent this problem. A promising method under investigation is the overexpression or in vitro activation of endogenous HOXB4.[73] A second method is the activation of the Notch pathway. Constitutive expression of activated Notch receptors in murine HSCs can redirect them from differentiation to self-renewal.[147] Likewise, culture of UCB $CD34^+CD38^-$ cells with immobilized Delta-1, one of the ligands for Notch, increases the number of multipotent HSCs, as shown by enhanced myeloid and lymphoid engraftment in immunodeficient mice.[148] Finally, modulation of ALDH activity and retinoid signaling might also be a new effective strategy to amplify human HSCs.[51]
3. HSCs or their immediate progenies undergo *apoptosis*. Because apoptosis is involved in the regulation of the HSC pool during steady-state hematopoiesis, ex-vivo expansion of HSCs may be limited by increased apoptosis. Culturing BM $CD34^+$ cells induces expression of *FAS* (CD95, a surface receptor that induces apoptosis when bound to its ligand) and downregulates expression of anti-apoptotic protein BCL2.[46] Although the signals that induce apoptosis are unknown, it is possible that blockade of cell apoptosis may enhance HSC expansion, but carries the risk of leading to uncontrolled cell expansion. This has been shown for murine cells where BCL2 overexpressing cells can be expanded with the simple addition of SCF.
4. HSCs or their progenies fail to *home* to BM. Even though HSCs may persist in the expansion system, the ability to home to BM may be reduced during culture. There is evidence that expression of $\beta_1$integrin and CXCR4 on cultured HSCs may be downregulated, reducing the capacity of HSCs to home and reconstitute hematopoiesis after transplantation.[149] At least in nonhuman primates, there is evidence to suggest that this might be overcome by incubating cells 12 to 24 hours prior to transplantation with SCF alone, which allows cells to reenter G_0/G_1 and enhance homing.[150–152] Whether other methods to reinduce cell cycle quiescence might be developed remains to be determined.

CONCLUSION

The HSC is at the base of the hematopoietic tree. It is defined by its ability to self-renew, to differentiate into all blood lineages, and to reconstitute hematopoiesis in lethally irradiated hosts. HSCs are rare in hematopoietic tissues, and enumeration and characterization of these cells require combinations of laboratory tests, including surface phenotype, dye efflux, in vitro culture, and animal transplantation. Because of the relative ease of procuring HSCs and defining experimental conditions and the availability of knock-out mouse models, murine studies and, to some extent, *Xenopus* and zebrafish studies have provided important information about HSCs that may be extrapolated to their human counterparts. The HSC cell-fate decision is regulated at cell intrinsic (transcriptional and epigenetic) and extrinsic (autocrine or paracrine) levels, and determining how these processes operate in vivo has begun to provide important information that may improve clinical HSC mobilization and transplantation and advance ex-vivo HSC expansion.[153]

SUGGESTED READINGS

Brummendorf TH, Balabanov S: Telomere length dynamics in normal hematopoiesis and in disease states characterized by increased stem cell turnover. Leukemia 20:1706, 2006.

Coulombel L: Identification of hematopoietic stem/progenitor cells: strength and drawbacks of functional assays. Oncogene 23:7210, 2004.

Cumano A, Godin I: Ontogeny of the hematopoietic system. Annu Rev Immunol 25:745, 2007.

Duncan AW, Rattis FM, DiMascio LN, et al: Integration of Notch and Wnt signaling in hematopoietic stem cell maintenance. Nat Immunol 6:314, 2005.

Forsberg EC, Bhattacharya D, Weissman IL: Hematopoietic stem cells: expression profiling and beyond. Stem Cell Rev 2:23, 2006.

Hess DA, Wirthlin L, Craft TP, et al: Selection based on CD133 and high aldehyde dehydrogenase activity isolates long-term reconstituting human hematopoietic stem cells. Blood 107:2162, 2006.

Kiel MJ, Yilmaz OH, Iwashita T, et al: SLAM family receptors distinguish hematopoietic stem and progenitor cells and reveal endothelial niches for stem cells. Cell 121:1109–1121, 2005.

Larsson J, Karlsson S: The role of Smad signaling in hematopoiesis. Oncogene 24:5676, 2005.

Lawrie CH: MicroRNAs and haematology: small molecules, big function. Br J Haematol 137:503 2007.

Myatt SS, Lam EW: Promiscuous and lineage-specific roles of cell cycle regulators in haematopoiesis. Cell Div 2:6, 2007.

Naylor CS, Jaworska E, Branson K, et al: Side population//ABCG2-positive cells represent a heterogeneous group of haemopoietic cells: implications for the use of adult stem cells in transplantation and plasticity protocols. Bone Marrow Transplant 35:353, 2004.

Ng SY, Yoshida T, Georgopoulos K: Ikaros and chromatin regulation in early hematopoiesis. Curr Opin Immunol 19:116–22, 2007.

Ogawa M: Changing phenotypes of hematopoietic stem cells. Exp Hematol 30:3, 2002.

Ross J, Li L: Recent advances in understanding extrinsic control of hematopoietic stem cell fate. Curr Opin Hematol 13:237, 2006.

Steinman RA: mRNA stability control: a clandestine force in normal and malignant hematopoiesis. Leukemia 21:1158, 2007.

Sugiyama T, Kohara H, Noda M, et al: Maintenance of the hematopoietic stem cell pool by CXCL12-CXCR4 chemokine signaling in bone marrow stromal cell niches. Immunity 25:977–88, 2006.

Verfaillie CM: Hematopoietic stem cells for transplantation. Nat Immunol 3:314–7, 2002.

Wilson A, Oser GM, Jaworski M, et al: Dormant and self-renewing hematopoietic stem cells and their niches. Ann N Y Acad Sci 1106:64, 2007.

Wognum AW, Eaves AC, Thomas TE: Identification and isolation of hematopoietic stem cells. Arch Med Res 34:461, 2003.

Zhu J, Emerson SG: Hematopoietic cytokines, transcription factors and lineage commitment. Oncogene 21:3295, 2002.

REFERENCES

For complete list of references log onto www.expertconsult.com

CHAPTER 21

TRANSCRIPTION FACTORS IN NORMAL AND MALIGNANT HEMATOPOIESIS

Richard Dahl and Robert Hromas

INTRODUCTION

The phenotype and function of any given cell is the sum of genes expressed in that cell. Thus, as blood cells mature during hematopoiesis, their gene expression markedly changes. The regulation of gene expression is therefore critical to hematopoiesis. Much of hematopoietic disease, either aplasia or malignancy, occurs when this gene expression is permanently altered. Thus the control of gene expression during hematopoiesis is of utmost importance for survival. Most of gene expression is regulated by transcription factors, whose structural integrity and appropriate function is crucial to proper hematopoiesis. Transcription factors are DNA binding proteins that interact with the regulatory regions in their target genes to activate or repress gene transcription. These regulatory regions may be either immediately adjacent to the transcription start site (promoters) or many kilobases upstream or downstream of the transcribed gene (enhancers or silencers). Cloning of leukemic translocations and gene targeting in mice has identified many transcription factors that are important in the hematopoietic lineage specification and maturation.

Because transcriptional cascades regulate the sum of gene expression in developing hematopoietic cells, and malignancy represents a fundamental change in gene expression, it is not surprising that these factors are often dysregulated in hematologic malignancy. Chromosomal translocations and point mutations involving transcription factors are common in leukemia and lymphoma. In most cases chromosomal translocations result in the creation of an oncogene, which actively promotes hematological malignancy, often by inhibiting differentiation of progenitors. Conversely, point mutations in a transcription factor appear to inactivate tumor suppressor activity, often resulting in uncontrolled proliferation. Perturbing the ability of a transcription factor to direct maturation of a hematopoietic cell leads to a pool of cells that are susceptible to subsequent oncogenic mutations, producing an undifferentiated progenitor with uncontrolled proliferation typical of acute leukemia. Additionally point mutations in transcription factors have been associated with other hematological diseases besides acute leukemia such as thrombocytopenia and neutropenia. These mutations usually lead to an inability of a progenitor in these lineages to turn on critical gene products for mature cell function.

In this chapter we discuss transcription factors that are important in specifying hematopoietic lineages, concentrating on factors that are involved in hematological diseases. Models of how early acting transcription factor interact to direct specific lineage commitment will be discussed.

ORIGINS OF HEMATOPOIESIS

Hematopoietic stem cells (HSCs) give rise to all mature cells of the hematopoietic system for the life of an animal. They have the ability to expand, self renew, and differentiate into multipotential precursors, which have a more restricted developmental potential, and can not proliferate indefinitely. These precursors then give rise to lineage committed progenitors that develop into the mature functional hematopoietic cell.

The first site of hematopoiesis in the developing murine embryo is seen at 7.0 days postcoitus (dpc) in the yolk sac.[1–6] Blood islands appear in the yolk sac, which are made up of proliferating endothelial cells and nucleated erythrocytes. These nucleated erythrocytes contain the embryonic globins. Because these nucleated erythrocytes do not survive long after embryogenesis, and are only produced in the yolk sac, this process is termed primitive hematopoiesis.[1–6] Besides the nucleated erythrocytes, embryonic yolk sac hematopoiesis also generates macrophages.

In contrast to primitive hematopoiesis, definitive hematopoiesis is not restricted in location to the extra-embryonic yolk sac, in lineage to erythrocyte/macrophage lineages, or in time to embryonic blood development, but contains the potential to form all adult hematopoietic lineages.[1–6] Definitive hematopoiesis can be found in several intraembryonic tissues, and survives for the life of the organism. Definitive erythrocytes are not nucleated, and contain fetal and adult globins. Definitive hematopoiesis begins in the yolk sac at 8.75 dpc.[4] Definitive hematopoiesis also initiates in intraembryonic sites such as the Paraaortic Splanchnopleura (PSp) at days 8 to 9.5 pc and the adjacent aorta-gonads-mesonephros (AGM) region at day 10 pc.[7,8]

PSp/AGM hematopoiesis is likely independent of yolk sac hematopoiesis. A definitive hematopoietic stem cell (HSC) that can repopulate ablated adults with long-term hematopoiesis can be found in the PSp as early as 10 dpc.[7,8] In contrast, primitive yolk sac HSC isolated at day 8 to 10 pc can only transiently engraft erythrocytes and some myeloid lineages in ablated adults.[9] However, a day 9 pc yolk sac CD34$^+$/c-kit$^+$ HSC can engraft all hematopoietic lineages when injected into the liver of busulfan-ablated newborn mice.[4,10] Thus, a specific microenvironment is required for long-term complete repopulation by this yolk sac HSC as compared to the PSp HSC. By day 12 pc, the definitive HSC migrates from the PSp/AGM region to the liver, and hematopoiesis shifts to the liver for most of the remainder of embryogenesis. The liver HSC then later seeds the spleen and marrow with HSC by day 16 pc, which are the sites of hematopoiesis for the duration of the life of the mouse.[4,8] The regulation of the complex spatial and temporal shifts in embryonic hematopoiesis is unknown.

DIFFERENTIATION OF HSCS INTO HEMATOPOIETIC PROGENITORS

Weissman and colleagues defined multipotential progenitors downstream of the HSC in mice by the expression of specific proteins on the cell surface (Fig. 21–1).[11–13] Hematopoietic stem cells are negative for cell surface proteins (such as B220, Gr-1, CD3, glycophorin) associated with mature lineage restricted cells (termed Lin$^-$) and are positive for the primitive progenitor markers Sca1 and c-kit. These mouse HSCs can be referred to LSK cells. In the mouse bone marrow HSCs give rise to two distinct multipotential progenitors: the common lymphoid progenitor (termed CLP) and the common myeloid progenitor (termed CMP). The CLP gives rise to B, T, and NK cells, but is unable to generate erythrocytes, megakaryocytes, monocytes, or granulocytes. The CMP in contrast cannot give rise to lymphoid cells but instead generates two more lineage restricted multipotential progenitors, the granulocyte-macrophage progenitor (GMP) and the megakaryocyte-erythroid

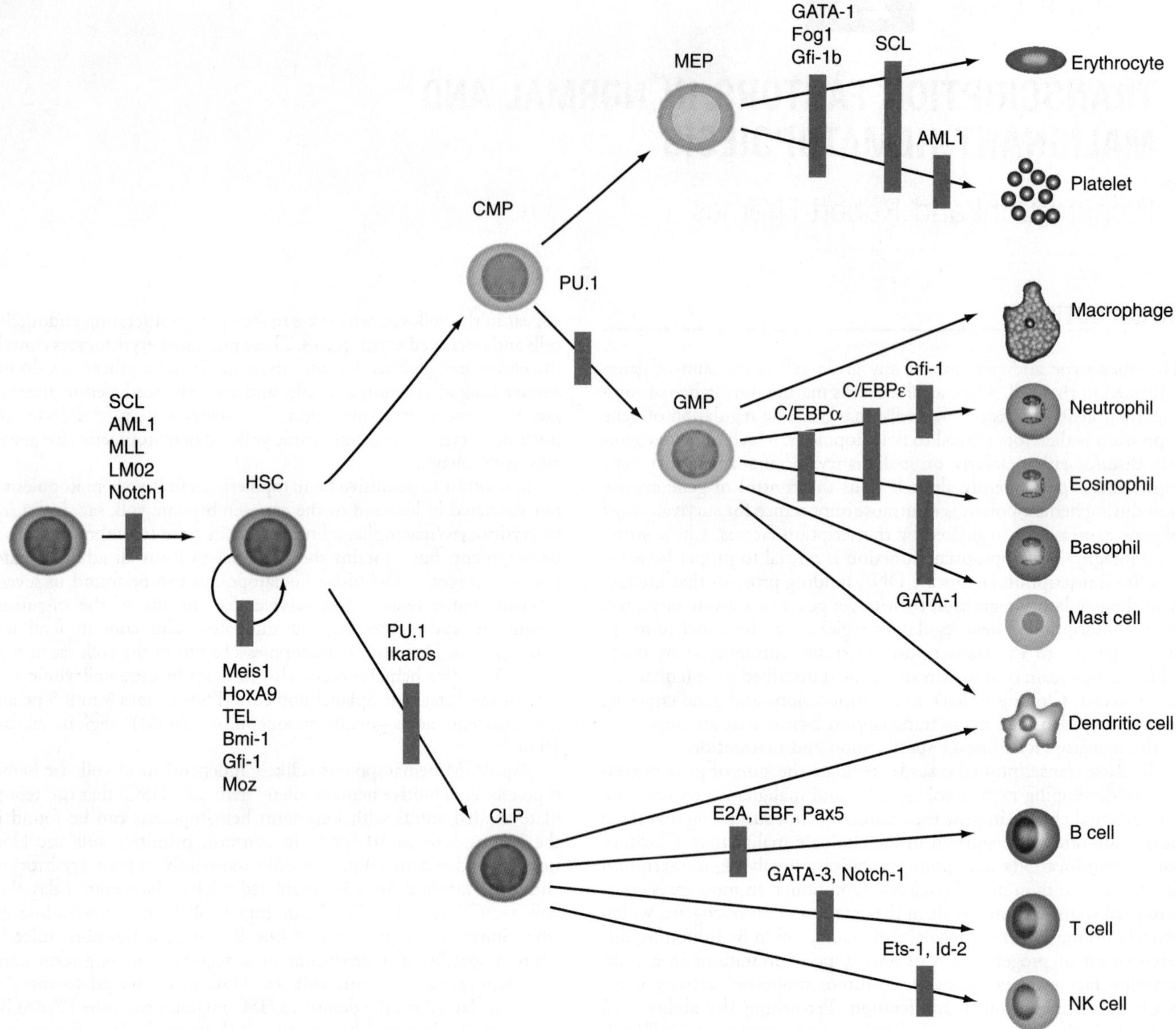

Figure 21–1 THE WEISSMAN-AKASHI MODEL OF HEMATOPOIETIC DIFFERENTIATION. *Red bars* indicate where lack of specific transcription factors discussed in the text affect hematopoietic differentiation. HSC: hematopoietic stem cell, CLP: common lymphoid progenitor, CMP: common myeloid progenitor, GMP: granulocyte-macrophage progenitor, and MEP: megakaryocyte-erythrocyte progenitor.

progenitor (MEP). The GMP gives rise to monocytes and granulocytes only and the MEP is restricted to megakaryocyte and erythroid differentiation.

Dendritic cells are derived from the HSC and are critical antigen presenting cells (APCs) for the immune system. There are probably four different types of dendritic cells, including those derived from myeloid and lymphoid precursors, and Langerhans and plasmacytoid dendritic cells.[14] Interestingly, dendritic cells can be derived from either a CMP or CLP.[15–17] They also can be derived from more mature precursors including the GMP, and pro-T cells but not pro-B cells. The plasticity of the origin of dendritic cells suggests a closer relationship between myeloid and lymphoid cells than one would assume from the model in which monocytes and granulocytes are derived from a precursor with no lymphoid potential.

Although this general differentiation scheme developed in mice is helpful in our understanding of where transcription factor activity is critical in determining lineages decisions, there are important caveats. For example, one must be careful in interpreting results in this model because the progenitors are defined by expression of cell surface proteins which themselves may be 7 targets of a transcription factor of interest. Additionally, there is data to suggest that the barrier between lymphoid and myeloid differentiation is not as stringent in humans as in mice. In humans a subset of bone marrow pro-B cells ($CD34^+$/$CD19^+$), which lacked expression of the chemokine receptor CXCR4 were shown to differentiate into B, cells, monocytes, and granulocytes in vitro.[18] In mice an LSK subset which expressed the tyrosine kinase receptor $Flt3^+$ was shown to have lost the ability to make erythrocytes and megakaryocytes but could produce all other hematopoietic cell types, including lymphoid lineages.[19] These reports suggest that there exists a bone marrow monocyte/granulocyte/lymphoid progenitor. In addition, a fetal liver CLP was shown though to have the ability to differentiate into macrophages, but not erythroid or megakaryocytic cells.[20] Other groups have also described murine fetal liver progenitors that have monocyte/lymphoid potential but not the ability to make erythroid/megakaryocyte potential.[21] Although there is evidence to support the existence of progenitors outside of the Weissman model of hematopoiesis, especially in humans, we use this model to describe the action of transcription factors because this model has been extensively used to characterize the phenotypes of mice lacking various transcription factors.

TRANSCRIPTION FACTOR FAMILIES INVOLVED IN HEMATOPOIESIS

Transcription factors have two requisite domains, a DNA binding domain that confers specificity of target genes regulated, and a transcriptional regulatory domain, that either represses or activates transcription of the target gene. There is a third possible domain that some transcription factors have, and that is a histone modification domain. This domain can mediate methylation or acetylation of the histones packaging DNA, and regulate how accessible the DNA regulatory regions are to other transcription factors. Acetylation of histones usually improves access to DNA, thereby increasing transcription. Methylation of histones can either open or close access to DNA, depending on where on the histone the methylation occurs. Transcription factors fall into families based on shared amino acid sequences, usually in the DNA binding domain. These shared amino acids create the tertiary structure framework necessary to bind the DNA regulatory regions. Not all amino acids within the DNA binding domain of a given family are the same, and differences in the DNA binding domain between transcription factors define which DNA sequences are bound, and transcription of which genes are activated. DNA binding domains often have a high basic amino acid content in order to facilitate DNA interaction, and regulatory domains can have a high acidic amino acid content, which often mediates interaction with other proteins in the transcriptional apparatus. There are five transcription factor families that we describe briefly, and most of the transcription factors discussed in this chapter fall into these families.

Basic Helix-Loop Helix Family

Basic helix loop helix (bHLH) family members have two conserved yet functionally distinct domains, both together make up the approximately 60 amino acid bHLH domain.[22] At the amino-terminal end of this region is the basic domain, which binds the transcription factor to DNA at a consensus hexanucleotide sequence known as the E box: G(or A)CAXXTGG(or A).[23] Different families of bHLH proteins recognize different E-box consensus sequences. At the carboxy-terminal end of the region is the HLH domain, which facilitates interactions with other protein subunits to form homodimeric and heterodimeric complexes. Many different combinations of dimeric structures are possible, each with different binding affinities between monomers. The heterogeneity in the E-box sequence that is recognized and the dimers formed by different bHLH proteins determines how they control diverse developmental functions through transcriptional regulation.

The bHLH motif was first observed by Murre and colleagues in two murine transcription factors known as E12 and E47. With the subsequent identification of many other bHLH proteins, a classification was formulated on the basis of their tissue distributions, DNA-binding specificities and dimerization potential.[24] This classification, which divides the superfamily into six classes, was initially based on a small number of HLH proteins but has since been applied to larger sets of eukaryotic proteins. Examples of bHLH family transcription factors mentioned here include E2A, Id2, and SCL (Tal1).

Leucine Zipper Family

Cytoskeletal proteins, such as myosins and intermediate filaments were noted to dimerize in a coiled-coil motif. This coiled-coil consisted of a 7 amino acid repeats that were termed a heptad. Later, as transcription factors were first being isolated, one group of such factors were also found to use a coiled-coil to dimerize, and these were termed leucine zippers, because of regular repeating leucines.[25] This coiled-coil domain was termed a leucine zipper because of the presence of leucines every heptad (every 7 amino acids). Usually, a minimum of four heptads are required to form a leucine zipper. In leucine zipper transcription factors the amino-terminal portion contains basic amino acids that bind to the major groove of specific DNA sequences. The carboxy-terminal portion makes up the leucine zipper, which mediates the dimerization responsible for DNA binding. There are 53 leucine zipper proteins in the human genome, and homodimerization and heterodimerization can potentially form 1,405 different dimers, generating a huge amount of potential specificity in the number of genes regulated by this family of transcription factors.[26] Examples of leucine zipper proteins mentioned in this chapter include c-Jun C/EBP α and ε.

Ets Family

Ets family transcription factors belong to the winged helix-turn-helix (wHTH) superfamily of DNA-binding proteins.[27] This family also includes other transcription factors such as hepatocyte nuclear factor, heat shock factor, and catabolite activator protein. The family is characterized by the Ets domain, which is composed of 85 amino acids that make up three α-helices and four β-strands.[28] This domain recognizes DNA sequences that have a GGAA/T core.[29] However, the flanking sequences from this core vary widely, and these flanking sequences mediate the DNA binding of the different members of the family. The activation domain of Ets family members is often near the carboxy terminal end, and has a high content of acidic residues. Ets family members also share nuclear localization signatures, and an amino terminal calcium sensitive phosphorylation site. There is occasionally a carboxy terminal auto-inhibitory region as well in this family. Ets family transcription factors discussed in this chapter include PU.1 and Ets-1.

Hox Family

Hox genes were first characterized through the study of mutations that give rise to body segment disruption in Drosophila.[30] These proteins constitute a family characterized by a highly conserved 183-nucleotide sequence encoding a 61 amino acid domain, the homeodomain. These homeodomains are structurally related to the helix-turn-helix motif of prokaryotic DNA-binding proteins and have sequence-specific DNA binding activity. In concert with additional sequences flanking the homeodomain, Hox proteins can serve as transcriptional activators or repressors on their target genes.

During human and murine embryogenesis, *HOX* gene transcription occurs 3′ to 5′ through each paralog group.[31] This is similar to the pattern of *HOX* gene transcription during fly development. The 3′ genes impact development of cephalad structures and the 5′ genes impact caudal structures in the developing human, mouse and fly. Orderly *HOX* gene activation is also essential for normal blood cell development.[32] *HOX* gene activation is also 3′ to 5′ during definitive hematopoiesis. Studies of human and murine hematopoietic stem cells (HSCs) demonstrate the importance of *HOX* genes of the A and B paralog groups for HSC maintenance and expansion.[33] Genes 3′ in the *HOX* clusters are maximally expressed in HSC and Hox7-11 (the Abd B *HOX* genes) are maximally expressed in committed progenitors.[32] Homeobox containing proteins discussed here include Meis1 and HoxA9.

Zinc Finger Family

The zinc finger transcription factor family is by far the largest family of transcriptional regulatory proteins in the genome. The family name comes from the fact that each family member has one to up to thirty multiples of cysteines and histidines that chelate a zinc ion. The first zinc finger protein characterized is the basal transcription factor TFIIIA,[34] and many members of this family are also basal transcription factors, like the well-studied SP1.[35] There are many sub-classes of zinc finger genes, based on the spacing and number of the zinc finger genes.[36] Zinc finger proteins can be also be grouped according to additional shared regulatory domains that mediate interaction with other members of the transcriptional apparatus, such as KRAB, SCAN or BTB domains.[37]

The most common class of zinc finger proteins when grouped according to cysteine-histidine spacing is the C2H2 class (or Kruppel family), where each finger chelates one zinc ion and binds the major groove of DNA, interacting with a specific 3 bp sequence.[38] Thus, the more zinc finger domains, the more specific the sequence bound. The exact amino acids needed to bind specific 3 bp DNA sequences has been worked out, and this is now being exploited to create designer DNA binding transcription factors.[39] These designer transcription factors can be used to block or activate gene expression. In the mouse genome there are 1537 genes that have C2H2 zinc finger motifs, making up approximately 1.5% of all expressed genes.[40] This makes it one of the largest gene families in the genome. Examples of this family of transcription factors mentioned below include Ikaros, Gfi-1 and Gfi-1b, GATA-1 and 3, EGR1 and 2, Bmi1, MOZ, and LMO2.

Another large class of zinc finger transcription factors is the steroid nuclear receptor class. These transcription factors function have two Cys2-Cys2 zinc finger domains that chelate zinc and fold together to mediate DNA binding after interaction with the appropriate steroid ligand.[41] Steroid receptor zinc finger proteins discussed include the RAR α.

MOUSE GENE TARGETING

Much of what we know about the role of transcription factors in hematopoiesis has come from gene targeting in mice.[42] Using homologous recombination in murine embryonic stem (ES) cells, investigators are able to specifically delete genes of interest (Fig. 21–2A).[43] Heterozygous ES cells, which harbor one mutated gene and one normal gene, are then used to generate mice that are heterozygous for the engineered mutation. These mice are then bred to make homozygous mutants, which are examined for the loss of function phenotype.

Gene targeting has been a powerful technique for elucidating the in vivo role of gene products. However, with germline mutations one often only observes defects associated with the earliest developmental requirement for a gene product. If a gene is essential for early developmental processes then one does not know whether the gene may also play a role in later developmental or adult processes. One technique used to examine requirements for a gene product throughout development is to examine chimeric mice.[43] ES cells engineered to have both alleles of a mutated gene are injected into a wild-type blastocyst, and this mixed blastocyst implanted into a foster mother. The resulting mouse will be made up of cells from both the host blastocyst and the injected homozygous ES cells. Investigators then examine what tissues the mutant ES cells are able to contribute to. A modification of this technique has been useful for studying gene contributions to B cell and T cells. For example, chimeric mice can be made with blastocysts derived from RAG2-deficient mice.[44] Immunoglobulin and T-cell receptor gene rearrangements cannot occur without RAG2. Because such rearrangements are critical for the formation of mature B- and T-cells, RAG2 deleted mice do not have any B cells or T cells. Any resulting B or T cells in the mouse derived from the mixed blastocyst must have come from the contributions of the donor ES cells. Contribution of donor ES cells can be assayed by flow cytometry or PCR.

Such chimeric mice will allow one to observe defects in multiple tissues which otherwise would not be observed because of a potential embryonic lethality in germline mice caused by a defect in a single tissue type. However, it will not allow one to see multiple defects in a single lineage. For example, if a gene product is important in HSC survival, and also is involved in the function of monocytes, one would not be able to observe any monocyte defects because monocytes would not be produced. Thus, in chimeric mice one will see that the engineered ES cells do not contribute at all to the hematopoietic system because of the HSC defect, and will never observe the defect in monocytes. A relatively new technique to observe such later defects, below the HSC, is to make conditional knockouts (Figure 21–2B).[45] In this procedure the gene of interest is modified so that it is flanked by 35 bp sequences from a bacteriophage that are called LoxP sites. These LoxP sites are recognized by the enzyme CRE recombinase, which will delete the DNA between the two sites, and then rejoin the gene without the deleted segment. The LoxP sites are placed in introns flanking the exons to be deleted, and therefore do not interfere with normal expression of the gene. Mice homozygous for the LoxP flanked allele will be normal. They can then be bred to several available mouse strains that either have tissue specific expression of CRE, or mice that have an inducible version of CRE. The most popular inducible strain of CRE recombinase for hematopoietic studies is MX-CRE mice.[45] CRE is under control of the interferon-inducible promoter from the MX gene. Injecting mice with interferon or polyIpolyC, which elicits an interferon response in vivo, results in a global deletion of the LoxP flanked allele. This technique has been particular useful for looking at the role of transcription factors that are needed for early progenitor cells but also required in later lineages, as CRE can be induced in cells past the HSC.

TRANSCRIPTION FACTORS SPECIFYING EMBRYONIC HEMATOPOIETIC STEM CELLS

HSCs are specified from the developing mesoderm of the embryo. Gene targeting in mice has defined four pathways that can be disrupted which affect HSCs.[46] In this section we will discuss transcription factors that are critical for specifying HSCs from mesoderm. Interestingly, all the factors to be discussed were initially shown to be essential for initial HSC specification when deleted from the mouse germline, but some are not indispensable for continued HSC activity when deleted in adult mice. CRE-Lox conditional gene targeting in mice was critical for showing the difference in requirements for initial specification and later maintenance of the HSC.[47,48] Transcription factors important in the initial specification of the HSC from mesoderm include SCL, AML1, MLL, LMO2, and Notch1, all of which are genes that appear at sites of translocations in human leukemias.

SCL (TAL1)

Stem cell leukemia factor (SCL) was one of the first transcription factors documented to be required for initial HSC development from mesoderm. SCL was originally identified as a gene frequently translocated in T-cell leukemias.[49,50] It is a basic helix-loop-helix (bHLH) transcription factor. Mice lacking SCL die in utero at approximately 9.5 dpc[51,52] because of a complete absence of yolk sac hematopoiesis. Using *SCL*$^{-/-}$ES cells it was shown both by in vitro differentiation and the generation of mutant ES-derived chimeric mice that SCL was also required for definitive hematopoiesis.[50] Interestingly, SCL is only required for specification of the HSC, but not the maintenance of the HSC. This was shown using a conditional knockout. Using the MX-CRE recombinase system SCL was deleted in adult mice.[48] After CRE deletion of SCL, these mice retained the ability to make both lymphoid and myeloid cells. Additionally SCL deficient HSCs were able to repopulate transplanted mice, indicating stem cell activity was intact. However, adult mice deleted of SCL had defects in maintaining erythropoiesis and megakaryopoiesis. This experiment indicated that SCL functions to specify but not maintain the HSC, and then functions downstream in hematopoiesis to maintain erythroid and megakaryocyte progenitors.

AML1 (RUNX1 or CBF α) and CBF β

Perhaps the most frequently translocated gene in acute leukemia is the transcription factor AML1 (RUNX1 or CBF α), and it is also involved in the initial specification of the HSC. It is highly homolo-

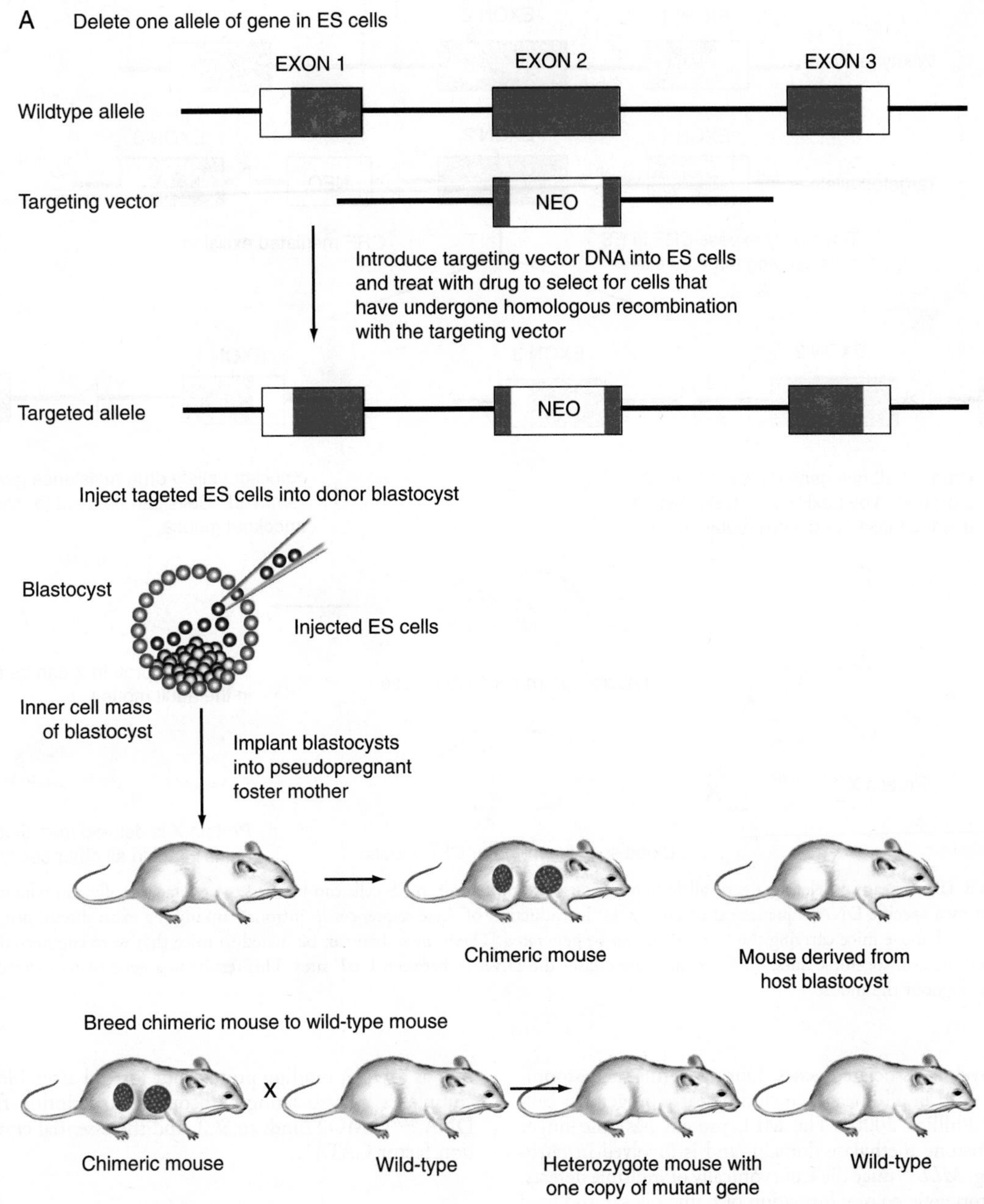

Figure 21–2 GENE TARGETING IN MICE. **(A)** Embryonic stem cells (ES) have one gene allele modified using homologous recombination to disrupt a gene of interest. Heterozygous mutant ES cells are injected into a donor blastocyst. These modified blastocysts are implanted into a recipient mother and allowed to develop. Chimeric mice should result which are made up of cells from the donor blastocyst and the injected ES cells. Chimeric mice are mated to wild-type mice in order to generate mice carrying the mutant allele. Heterozygous mutant mice are mated in order to generate mice that have two mutant alleles.

Continued on page 218

gous to the Drosophila transcription factor runt, and defines its own family of transcription factors.[53] AML1 functions as a heterodimer, complexing with CBF β through its DNA binding domain (which is homologous to the Drosophila Runt DNA binding domain). CBF β does not contact DNA but instead increases the affinity of the heterodimer for DNA.[53,54] AML1 expression is predominantly in the hematopoietic system, whereas CBF β is expressed in most adult tissues. CBF β is also an obligate partner for all other RUNX family members, RUNX2 and RUNX3.

Mice deficient for AML1 die at 12.5 dpc[55,56] Unlike SCL deficient mice, *AML1*$^{-/-}$ mice do undergo yolk sac hematopoiesis. However, they do not have definitive fetal liver hematopoiesis. Like the *SCL*$^{-/-}$ HSC defect, *AML1* deficiency leads to a defect in specifying the definitive HSC but not its maintenance in adults. Inducible gene targeting has demonstrated that deletion of AML1 in the adult animal no longer affects stem cell activity.[47] Similar to SCL, AML1 has essential functions downstream of the HSC as megakaryocyte and lymphoid maturation are perturbed in adult mice deleted of AML1. Mice deficient for CBF β have a very similar phenotype to mice with AML1 deleted, demonstrating its importance for forming a heterodimer with AML1.[56,57]

MLL

Another transcription factor commonly translocated in acute leukemias is the mixed-lineage leukemia gene (MLL). The *MLL* gene is frequently disrupted in both infant acute lymphoblastic leukemia and therapy-induced acute myeloid leukemias. Acute leukemias harboring a MLL translocation are characterized by coexpression of early

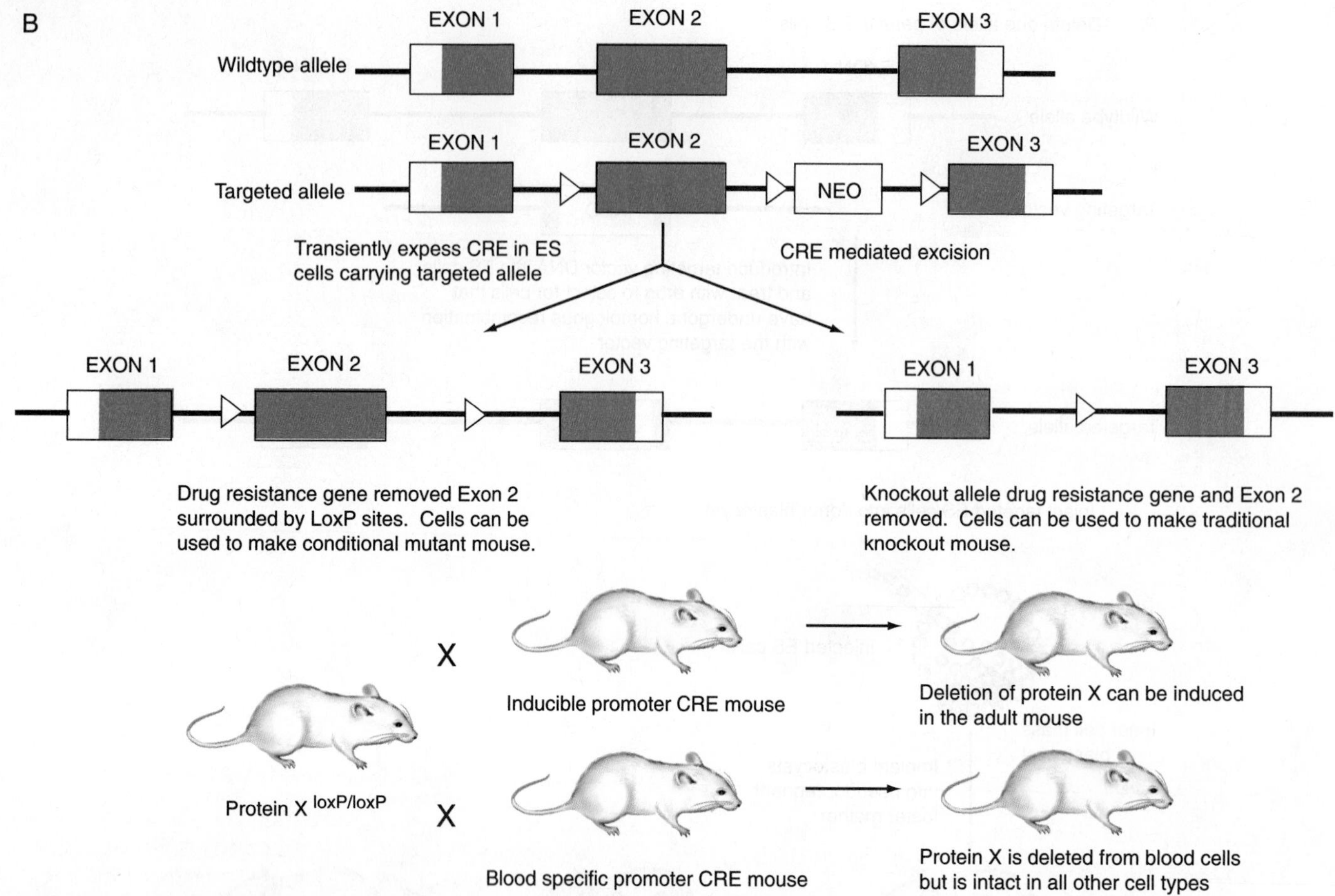

Figure 21–2, cont'd (B) Instead of deleting a gene allele homologous recombination in ES cells can be used to generate an allele in which a critical exon of a gene is flanked by a specific DNA sequence called LoxP sites. Introduction of these sequences in introns flanking the exon should not affect gene expression. As described above mice carrying the LoxP allele can be generated. These mice then can be mated to mice that were engineered to express the enzyme CRE recombinase in specific tissues. CRE recombinase excises the DNA in between LoxP sites. This results in a gene being deleted in a specific tissue instead of throughout the mouse.

lymphoid and myeloid associated genes. During normal hematopoiesis MLL is expressed in all lineages, including early progenitor cells (Kawagee 1999, Phillips 2000). The MLL protein has zinc finger domains and a histone methylase domain, and is involved in chromatin remodeling. *MLL*$^{-/-}$ mice die embryonically of multiple defects. Decreased hematopoietic colony formation of both yolk sac and fetal liver cells was observed, indicating that MLL is important for both primitive and definitive hematopoiesis. However, because of other defects it was not clear if problems in hematopoiesis were caused by an intrinsic cell defect or by other nonhematopoietic defects that might affect the microenvironment.

LMO2 (RBTN2)

LMO2 is a zinc finger LIM domain transcription factor that is indispensable for the initial specification of the HSC from mesoderm.[58,59] It is also frequently a target of chromosomal translocations that lead to human T-cell acute lymphoblastic leukemia.[60,61]

LMO2 knockout mice die around 10.5 dpc because of a lack of yolk sac erythropoiesis.[59] Examination of chimeric mice demonstrated that LMO2 knockout cells could not contribute to any definitive hematopoietic lineages indicating that LMO2 has a role in the HSC. No conditional knockout of LMO2 has been derived, so it is not known if it is required for maintenance of adult HSCs or whether it has a role in more mature cells. Interestingly, LMO2 does not function as a DNA binding protein but instead assembles DNA binding complexes by associating with other transcription factors that bind DNA.[62,63] LMO2 binds to SCL and the essential erythroid transcription factor GATA1.

Notch1 (TAN1)

Notch1 is another nonprototypic transcription regulator involved in definitive HSC specification from mesoderm. It is one of four mammalian homologs of the drosophila Notch protein.[64,65] Notch1 is an unusual transcription factor in that it is initially found at the cell surface. Upon binding to one of its ligands, usually expressed on the surface of a juxtaposed cell, a series of enzymatic cleavages occur, which release the intracellular portion of Notch1, termed ICN1. ICN1 then translocates to the nucleus where it associates with the DNA binding factor RBJ κ to regulate transcription.[66–68] Retroviral expression of ICN1 in HSCs or coculture of HSCs with stromal cells expressing Notch ligands was shown to increase the self-renewal of HSCs.[69–73] Mice that have Notch1 deleted demonstrate an arrest in development at around 9.5 dpc and die within a day afterward as a result of multiple defects, including failure of angiogenesis.[74,75] Hematopoietic colony formation from *Notch1*$^{-/-}$ yolk sacs was observed to be normal. However, when colony formation was examined from the P-Sp region of the early 9.5 dpc embryo there was a severe reduction in colony formation indicating a defect in definitive hematopoiesis. Transplanting P-Sp cells from 9.5 dpc into newborn mice demonstrated that *Notch1*+/− cells could contribute to the hematopoietic system of the recipient mouse, but not *Notch1*−/− cells.[76] However, similar to what is seen with SCL and AML1, conditional disruption of Notch1 in adult mice demonstrated that Notch1-deficient adult HSC could be transplanted without defect.[77] These Notch1 mutant HSCs could differentiate into all mature hematopoietic lineages except for T cells.

TRANSCRIPTION FACTORS MAINTAINING ADULT HEMATOPOIETIC STEM CELL FUNCTION

In contrast to the factors discussed above, there are several transcription factors that do not appear to be involved in initial HSC specification from mesoderm, but are instead required for maintaining the HSC once it arises developmentally. For survival of itself and the organism, an HSC must be able to both self-renew and to differentiate into mature blood cells of all lineages. The transcription factors involved in HSC maintenance after its specification from mesoderm include Meis1, TEL, Gfi-1, Bmi1, and MOZ. These transcription factors can be involved in either self-renewal or lineage differentiation.

Meis1

Meis1 is a transcription factor in the homeobox family, which was originally characterized in Drosophila through the study of mutations that give rise to body segment disruptions.[30,78,79] Homeobox (Hox for mouse and HOX for humans) proteins can serve as transcriptional activators or repressors on their target genes. Although Hox genes were originally identified as master control genes during embryonic development, they also affect various steps in hematopoiesis.[80–82] Meis1 is most related to the Pbx subfamily of homeobox proteins. Pbx1 is a translocation partner for the E2A transcription factor, and the fusion gene E2A-Pbx is observed in human pre-B cell leukemias. Meis1 is expressed in fetal liver stem cells.

Meis1−/− mice die at approximately 13.5 dpc because of extensive hemorrhage.[83] These Meis1-deleted mice also have multiple hematopoietic defects. Hematopoietic progenitors are present but reduced in number in day 13.5 fetal livers in these mutant mice. These mutant fetal liver cells fail to radio-protect lethally irradiated mice, and perform poorly in HSC competitive repopulation assays, indicating a defect in definitive HSC function. Meis1 can partner with Pbx1 to regulate transcription.[84] Pbx1−/− mice share many of the same hematopoietic defects with Meis1−/− mice.[85] Pbx1−/− fetal liver cells form reduced numbers of hematopoietic progenitors. In addition, these fetal liver HSCs perform poorly in competitive repopulation assays. Interestingly, proliferation assays have demonstrated a reduced proliferation capacity of the fetal liver CMP. This suggests that the Meis1- and Pbx1-deficient mice may have defects in HSC proliferation.

HoxA9

The homeobox protein HoxA9 heterodimerizes with Meis1 to activate gene expression, and therefore it is not surprising that it also plays a critical role in maintaining the adult HSC phenotype. Forced overexpression of HoxA9 markedly expands the adult HSC pool.[86] Indeed, continued overexpression of HoxA9 in murine marrow results in a primitive leukemia. This leukemia may require the coexpression of Meis1 to be fully penetrant.[87] Homozygously deleting HoxA9 in mice results in mild defects in both myeloid and lymphoid maturation, indicating that HSC function is partially disrupted.[80] However, these mice are viable and can survive the minor HoxA9 disruption of hematopoiesis, perhaps indicating that another of the many closely related HoxA cluster genes can compensate for the missing HoxA9.

TEL (Etv6)

The TEL (Etv6) gene codes for an Ets family transcriptional repressor. The TEL gene is translocated in several myeloid and lymphoid leukemias. Expression of TEL is not limited to hematopoietic tissue but occurs widely in both embryonic and adult tissues.[88] *TEL*−/− mice die at 10.5 dpc[88] The mice die of defective yolk sac angiogenesis and increased mesenchymal and neural tissue apoptosis. Generation of chimeric mice demonstrated that *TEL*−/− ES cells could contribute to both yolk sac and fetal liver hematopoiesis, indicating that TEL is not required for initial HSC specification from mesoderm.[89] However, TEL−/− ES cells could not contribute to bone marrow hematopoiesis. This indicated that without TEL, the definitive HSC could either not home to the bone marrow or could not be maintained in the bone marrow microenvironment. Conditional disruption of TEL in adult animals leads to a rapid depletion of HSC in the bone marrow.[90] When deleted in more mature hematopoietic progenitors, loss of TEL does not have observable effects on cell differentiation.

Bmi-1

Bmi-1 is a Polycomb family zinc finger protein.[91,92] This group of proteins are involved in epigenetic regulation of gene expression by controlling the accessibility of DNA to transcription factors by regulating chromatin opening.[93] Bmi-1 was originally isolated as a gene which cooperated with the myc oncogene in the induction of murine lymphoid leukemia.[94,95] Bmi-1 is expressed in early hematopoietic progenitors.[96–98] Mice deficient for Bmi-1 are born with severe aplastic anemia caused by a depletion of HSCs.[99,100] Progenitors of all blood lineages are dramatically reduced and mice die within a week from multiple infections. However, the HSC is specified from mesoderm in these mice, rather the proliferative capacity of the HSC and downstream progenitors is greatly reduced. The proliferative defect is observed in the fetal liver HSC but is much worse in the adult bone marrow HSC, indicating that the defect worsens with age. Re-expression of Bmi-1 in HSC by retroviral transduction rescues the cells from this proliferative defect.[98]

Gfi-1

The zinc finger transcriptional repressor Gfi-1 appears to play an opposite role to Bmi-1. Gfi-1 is expressed in the HSC, CLP, GMP, and more mature lineage progenitors such as pro-B cells and pro-T cells.[101] It is also expressed in mature neutrophils.[101] It was originally isolated because of its ability to confer growth factor independence to a rodent T-cell line.[102,103] Additionally, Gfi-1 cooperates with c-myc in the generation of murine T-cell leukemias.[102–104] The major defect seen in *Gfi-1*−/− mice is severe neutropenia.[105,106] Subsequently it was shown that Gfi-1 is essential for proper HSC function.[101,107] Competitive repopulation assays in irradiated mice showed that the mutant HSC failed to compete with normal HSC. Additionally, HSCs that had Gfi-1 deleted were unable to rescue long-term hematopoiesis in a transplant model. When HSCs were isolated from Gfi-1 mutant mice it was shown that these cells had a higher proliferative rate than wild type HSCs. This suggested that the reason Gfi-1 marrow could not rescue irradiated mice was that the mutant HSCs over proliferated and exhausted the stem cell pool. This over-proliferation may occur through the lack of Gfi-1 to induce the cell cycle inhibitor p21.[101,107,108] Gfi-1 associates with the p21 locus and the related protein Gfi-1b, which shares an identical DNA binding domain has been shown to increase p21 expression in a myeloid cell line.[108] P21 levels were decreased in Gfi-1 mutant mice.[101,107]

Normally Gfi-1 represses gene expression so it is unclear how Gfi-1 would up-regulate p21 expression.

MOZ

MOZ (monocytic leukemia zinc finger protein) was first isolated through its involvement with the t(8;16) in acute monocytic leukemia. MOZ functions as a transcriptional coactivator interacting with other DNA binding transcription factors. It has histone acetyl transferase activity, which is involved with activating transcription by opening chromatin and making DNA more accessible to the transcriptional apparatus.

MOZ is widely expressed in embryonic and adult tissues.[109] Its expression is not limited to the hematopoietic system. MOZ, however, does interact with the hematopoietic transcription factors PU.1 and AML1 to augment their transcriptional activity.[110,111]

Two MOZ mutant mouse strains have been generated which have similar defects in the hematopoietic system.[109,111] One strain is considered to be a null mutation of MOZ with homozygotes dying after 14.5 dpc[111] At 14.5 dpc, normal Mendelian frequencies of genotypes were seen, but $MOZ^{-/-}$embryos were pale and the fetal livers were noticeably smaller. The second mouse strain is not characterized by a complete loss of MOZ function.[109] The targeting of the MOZ allele was designed to truncate the MOZ gene in the carboxy terminal portion of the protein, which would be equivalent to the breakpoints involved in t(8;16) translocations. Mice homozygous for the truncation mutation ($MOZ^{\Delta/\Delta}$) died at birth. These mice were not anemic but instead failed to oxygenate the blood because of an aortic arch defect. The mice had deformities including craniofacial defects. It was also observed that the spleen and thymus of these animals developed poorly.

In the $MOZ^{\Delta/\Delta}$ mouse all lineages could mature properly. However, in the $MOZ^{-/-}$ mouse there was an accumulation of erythroblasts caused by a defect in erythroid maturation. Progenitors for all lineages in both mutant models are reduced in number as compared to wild type animals. Cells characteristic of HSCs as determined by flow cytometry could be detected in the fetal livers of both models of mutant MOZ mice. However, these putative HSC could not reconstitute the hematopoietic system of irradiated mice in a transplantation model.[109,111] These results suggested a defect in HSC activity; the exact nature of this defect is not known.

TRANSCRIPTION FACTORS SPECIFYING THE ERYTHROID/MEGAKARYOCYTIC LINEAGES

GATA1

GATA1 is considered the master regulator of erythropoiesis. It was originally identified as a factor that binds to the conserved GATA sequences in the β-globin enhancer.[112–114] It contains two zinc fingers; with the carboxy proximal finger required for high-affinity DNA binding, and the amino terminal proximal finger stabilizing the interaction with DNA.[115–117] It is expressed in erythrocytes, megakaryocytes, mast cells, and eosinophils.[118] It is also detected in early hematopoietic precursors. Outside of the hematopoietic system, GATA1 expression is only detected in the testes. Using ES cells in which GATA1 is deleted, it was shown that GATA1 is essential for the development of erythrocytes.[119] GATA1-deficient mice die at day 10.5 dpc of severe anemia. Erythroid maturation is blocked at the proerythroblast stage. There is also a block in megakaryocyte development. Mice with GATA1 specifically deleted in megakaryocytes had failure of endoredupliction, proliferation, and platelet production.[120] Interestingly, a novel mutation that deleted a GATA binding site in the GATA1 promoter demonstrated that this site was required for GATA1 expression in eosinophils.[121] Without this site, mice were unable to produce eosinophils, demonstrating an essential role for GATA in eosinophil maturation.

FOG1

GATA1 works in cooperation with another transcription factor, Friend of GATA, or FOG1. This factor was identified in a screen for GATA1 interacting partners.[122] GATA1 binds to FOG1 to activate or repress transcription, depending in the target gene. FOG1 does not bind to DNA by itself, but only associates with DNA through its interaction with GATA1. FOG1 contains nine zinc fingers, none of which have been shown to mediate DNA binding but instead mediate protein-protein interactions. FOG1 acts predominantly as a transcriptional repressor, although on certain promoters it has been shown to enhance transcriptional activation with GATA1.[123,124] It is predominantly expressed in erythroid and megakaryocyte precursors.[122] It is also expressed in T cells where it may interact with another GATA family member, GATA3. Homozygous gene disruption of FOG1 results in lethality of mice between 10.5 and 11.5 dpc[125] Similar to GATA1 deleted mice, FOG1 deficient mice die of severe anemia caused by a block at the proerythroblast stage. Distinct from GATA1, FOG1 mice do not make megakaryocytes at all.

Gfi-1b

Another transcription factor involved in the early development of erythrocytes and megakaryocytes is Gfi-1b. Gfi-1b was identified by homology to Gfi-1,[108] and shares nearly identical c-terminal zinc fingers and a repressor domain with Gfi-1. The two proteins are divergent in the sequence between the repressor domain and the carboxyl terminal six zinc fingers. Deletion of Gfi-1 results in embryonic lethality from severe anemia.[126] The embryos do progress further than GATA1 or FOG1 knockouts, with −/− embryos dying at 15 dpc. $Gfi\text{-}1b^{-/-}$ animals specify megakaryocytes but they fail to mature, never becoming functional.

TRANSCRIPTION FACTORS PROMOTING MYELOID LINEAGE SPECIFICATION

There are two major transcription factors are important for specifying monocytes and granulocyte formation from the HSC. These are PU.1 and C/EBP α, both of which may play a role in acute leukemias.

PU.1

PU.1 is an Ets family transcription factor that is also an oncogene upregulated in murine erythroleukemia cells (MEL) infected with Friend virus.[127,128] Forced expression of PU.1 is essential for blocking the differentiation of the infected erythroblasts, and maintaining the erythroleukemia.[129,130] PU.1 is expressed at low levels in early hematopoietic progenitors. As cells mature PU.1 expression is extinguished in erythrocytes, megakaryocytes and T cells, but rises in monocytes, granulocytes and B cells.[131,132] A role for PU.1 in directing myeloid lineage commitment was first established by experiments using the multipotential avian cell line E26-MEPs.[131–133] PU.1 over-expression in these cells redirected the normal megakaryocyte differentiation into monocytes. Gene targeting in mice also confirmed a critical role for PU.1 in myeloid differentiation. Mice lacking PU.1 do not make macrophages, granulocytes or lymphoid cells.[134,135] Examination of bone marrow cells in PU.1 conditional knockout mice showed that $PU.1^{-/-}$ HSCs do not make detectable CLPs or CMPs.[136,137] Deletion of PU.1 in adult GMP cells demonstrated that PU.1 was not required for granulocyte lineage specification, but was still required for proper granulocyte maturation.[136]

PU.1 also has an important role in B-cell development.[134–138] It is essential for specification of the B-cell lineage, but once pro-B cells are specified, PU.1 no longer is critical for further B-cell maturation. Two models of conditional knockout mice were shown to have reduced HSC function as *PU.1*$^{-/-}$ HSCs could not engraft in competitive repopulation transplantation assays.[136,137] Target genes of PU.1 include several crucial cytokine receptor genes, including the receptors for M-CSF, G-CSF and GM-CSF.[139] However, re-expression of G-CSF receptor or M-CSF receptor in *PU.1*$^{-/-}$ hematopoietic cells however does not rescue granulocyte or macrophage differentiation, although it does restore survival and proliferation when precursors are cultured in G-CSF or M-CSF.[140,141]

C/EBP α

C/EBP α is a basic leucine zipper transcription factor that functions as a dimer. It can homodimerize with itself or heterodimerize the related family members C/EBP β, γ, and ε through its carboxy terminal leucine zipper. Within the hematopoietic system C/EBP α is predominantly expressed in monocytes, granulocytes and the progenitors of these cells.[142,143] Ectopically expressing C/EBP α in cells capable of both monocyte and granulocyte differentiation promotes granulocyte differentiation.[142] One of the functions of C/EBP α in granulocyte differentiation is to slow proliferation by inhibiting the transcription of E2F and c-myc, which promote cell cycle progression.[144–146] Mice lacking C/EBP α do not make any mature granulocytes and are also impaired in producing monocytes.[147]

Conditional deletion of C/EBP α in adult mice has demonstrated that it is indispensable for GMP progenitors but not CMP progenitors.[148] This suggests that C/EBP α acts at a later stage than PU.1, which is required to form the CMP.[136,137] However, C/EBP α can regulate PU.1, and if its expression is forced in early B cells, it induces PU.1 transcription, which leads to trans-differentiation of these B cells into monocytes.[149,150]

TRANSCRIPTION FACTORS REQUIRED FOR MYELOID MATURATION

Other transcription factors are needed for the proper maturation of granulocytes and monocytes but not for myeloid lineage specification. These factors include Egr1 and 2 in monocytes; C/EBP ε, Gfi-1, and RAR α in granulocytes.

C/EBP ε

C/EBP ε is a basic leucine zipper transcription factor that is highly related to C/EBP α. It is most highly expressed in granulocytic cells and their precursors, but it is not detected in monocytes.[151,152] Targeted deletions of C/EBP ε demonstrated an essential role in granulocyte differentiation.[153] Although they are viable and fertile, *CEBPE*$^{-/-}$ mice do not produce normal neutrophils or eosinophils. Because of this granulocytopenia, the mice die of opportunistic infection within a few months of birth. C/EBP ε deficient granulocytes do not produce cytoplasmic secondary or tertiary granules. The secondary granule protein lactoferrin has been shown to be a direct C/EBP ε target.[154]

Gfi-1

Gfi-1 is not only important for proper maintenance of adult HSC, but it is also required for granulocyte differentiation. Mice with Gfi-1 deleted suffer from neutropenia.[105,106] The mice make granulocyte progenitors normally, but these progenitors fail to mature. In addition, these granulocytes have aberrant expression of the monocyte genes M-CSFR and Mac3. These granulocytes are functionally compromised, leading to the death of the mice within a few months as a result of systemic infections. One of the critical functions of Gfi-1 in granulocytes may be to downregulate monocyte-specific genes in the GMP as they commit to the granulocyte lineage.[155] Initially myeloid precursors are primed to express genes specific for both lineages, but as cell commit they must turn off the genes corresponding to the other lineage, or they fail to mature properly.

Egr-1 and 2

The zinc finger transcription factors Egr1, and 2 can act as both transcriptional activators and repressors. They are widely expressed outside the hematopoietic system.[156–158] They function opposite of Gfi-1, by turning off granulocyte genes in GMP cells committing to the monocyte lineage.[155] Forcing their expression increases monocytic differentiation at the expense of granulocyte differentiation.[159–161]

Retinoic Acid Receptor α (RAR α)

RAR α is a member of the large nuclear hormone receptor family. These are heterodimeric transcription factors that are regulated by binding to retinoids. RAR α heterodimerizes with the RXR proteins, and binds DNA through its zinc finger DNA binding domains only when retinoic acid (RA) is present.[162] In the absence of RA, this heterodimer binds corepressor complexes and represses transcription. In the presence of RA corepressor complexes are exchanged for coactivator complexes and transcription is induced. RAR α is predominantly expressed in myeloid cells.[163,164] A dominant negative RAR α arrests granulocyte differentiation of a myeloid cell line at a promyelocyte.[165] There are no defects seen in myeloid development of mice lacking RAR α.[164] However, mice lacking both RAR α and γ have neutrophils that are blocked in development at a similar stage as C/EBP ε knockouts.[164]

TRANSCRIPTION FACTORS REGULATING LYMPHOID MATURATION

There are a number of transcription factors that regulate lymphoid maturation. Some act alone, and others act in concert with each other. In some situations ratios of one factor to another may be critical in determining lineage or stage decisions, as will be discussed in a later section (Antagonistic Interactions between Transcription Factors). These transcription factors include PU.1, Ikaros, E2A, EBF, PAX5, Notch1, and GATA3.

PU.1

As discussed, PU.1 is essential for specifying CLP formation. Conditional knockout of PU.1 in the adult marrow leads to a loss of CLPs.[137,166] Germline deleted PU.1 mice have decreased B-cell and T-cell formation.[134,135,138] T-cell development appears to be delayed in PU.1 knockout animals.[135,167] PU.1 is normally expressed in the early stages of T-cell development before expression of the T-cell receptors CD4 and CD8.[168,169] The delayed T lymphopoiesis may be caused by loss of an early proliferative function of PU.1, which is also seen in early erythroblasts that express PU.1.[170,171] Alternatively, the delay may be caused by having to produce T cells through a developmental pathway that does not involve the CLP.

PU.1 is also critical for B-cell maturation, beyond the CLP. Many B-cell specific target genes have been identified for PU.1 including IL7 receptor, the surrogate light chain Mb1, CD45, and immunoglobulin light chains κ and λ.[172,173] Interestingly, in pro-B cells specifically deleted for PU.1 these genes continue to be expressed.[137,166] Similar to the case of SCL and AML1 in HSCs, PU.1 no longer is absolutely required for the B cell lineage once the B-cell precursor is specified from the CLP. There are slight functional defects in *PU.1*$^{-/-}$ B-cells. Additionally, an Ets family member closely related to PU.1, called Spi-B, is also not required to maintain expression of the putative PU.1 target genes in B cells.[166] A potential early target gene of PU.1 that may be involved in committing the CLP to the B-cell lineage may be EBF. PU.1 was shown to regulate EBF and retroviral expression of EBF could overcome the block to B cell development in the absence of PU.1.[174] EBF is discussed more fully below (E2A, EBF, and Pax5).

Ikaros

Along with PU.1, the transcription factor Ikaros is involved in early lymphoid development.[175] Similar to PU.1, it is expressed broadly throughout the hematopoietic system.[176–179] It is a zinc finger DNA binding protein. Its carboxyl terminal zinc fingers are involved in DNA binding and the amino terminal zinc finger mediate partner binding.[177,178,180] Ikaros can function as both a transcriptional repressor and an activator. It also interacts with chromatin remodeling proteins and transcriptional repressor complexes.[181–185] An initial mouse model of Ikaros deletion was found to produce a dominant negative form of Ikaros, which could interfere with the function of Ikaros and the related family members Helios and Aiolos.[186] These mice did not develop T cells, B cells or NK cells. Interestingly, mice with one allele of Ikaros mutated developed T cell leukemia and lymphoma.[187] Null mutations of Ikaros were later engineered, and these mice lack both fetal B cells and T cells.[188,189] In the adult, though, the B cells remain absent but T cells are produced.

E2A, EBF, and PAX5

Other genes involved in B-cell development are E2A, EBF, and PAX5 (also termed BSAP). These transcription factors often work in concert with each other to regulate B-lymphopoiesis. The E2A gene gives rise to two proteins, E12 and E47, by differential splicing of E12- and E47-specific bHLH-encoding exons.[190–192] E12 and E47 are bHLH proteins that dimerize with other bHLH proteins to regulate many genes involved in B-cell antigen receptor arrangement and B cell receptor signaling, often in cooperation with EBF.[193] Deletion of either E2A or EBF results in a block of B cell development at the pro–B-cell stage, before B-cell receptor rearrangement.[194–196] PAX5 acts downstream of E2A and EBF. EBF has been shown to activate the PAX5 promoter.[193,197,198] PAX5-deficient B cells are blocked in development following the rearrangement of the B-cell receptor, yet they express both EBF and E2A.[199] *PAX5*$^{-/-}$ pro-B cells express several myeloid genes, including the cytokine receptors M-CSFR, G-CSFR and GM-CSFR α.[200] These cells have been also shown to be multipotent, with the ability to differentiate into macrophages, erythrocytes and T cells. Similar to Gfi-1 in granulocytes, a critical role of PAX5 may be to turn off inappropriate myeloid gene expression in B cells.[201,202]

Notch1

T-cell development absolutely requires Notch1.[77] In the section on HSC specification we previously discussed Notch1, which not only assists in specifying HSC during embryonic development, but also is crucial for T-cell differentiation. Expressing the transcriptionally active form of Notch1, ICN1, in murine bone marrow induces T-cell development.[203] Similarly, a bone marrow stromal cell line expressing the Notch ligand Delta-like 1 (DL1) induces T-cell differentiation, and blocks B-cell differentiation of fetal liver hematopoietic progenitor cells.[204] Interestingly, low expression of Notch can inhibit B-cell differentiation, but higher levels of expression are required to block NK cell development.[205] Additionally, *Notch1*$^{-/-}$ hematopoietic cells injected into donor mice produce B cells in the thymus, indicating that without Notch1 the CLP is driven towards B lymphopoiesis.[77,206] These experiments suggest that Notch1 is critical in both specifying T-cell development and also promoting T-cell maturation.

As mentioned, Notch1 deficient mice die during embryonic stages of development. *Notch1*$^{-/-}$ bone marrow failed to generate T cells when transferred to irradiated recipients.[77] Closer examination of the blockade of T-cell development indicated that *Notch1*$^{-/-}$ cells had difficulty transitioning the TCR β checkpoint. *Notch1*$^{-/-}$ thymocytes had impaired V-DJ rearrangement and a decreased number of TCR β-expressing cells.[207] This study also showed that although *Notch1*$^{-/-}$ cells could not make α/β T cells, they could generate γ /δ T cells. Notch1 is also thought to be involved in directing CD4 versus CD8 T cell fate cell decisions.[208,209] However, deletion of Notch1 in T cells that had already undergone thymic selection resulted in no defects in the generation of CD4 or CD8 cells.[210] This could be caused by activity from other Notch family members. Thus, Notch1 plays diverse roles at multiple stages of hematopoiesis.

GATA3

GATA3 is a member of the GATA family of zinc finger transcription factors, which includes GATA1 described above.[211] These two proteins are very homologous, and GATA3 can rescue the development of GATA1-deficient erythroblasts.[212,213] GATA3 was originally isolated as a regulator of the TCR α gene enhancer.[214] It is also implicated in the regulation of several other T-cell genes including TCR β, δ and CD8.[215–219] Its expression in the hematopoietic system is limited to T cells and NK cells.[214,220] Mice deficient for GATA3 die between 11.5 and 13.5 dpc of multiple defects, including growth retardation, severe hemorrhage, and neuronal defects.[221] Chimeric mice generated with *GATA3*$^{-/-}$ ES cell demonstrated that GATA3 deficient cells could contribute to all hematopoietic lineages except T cells.[222] *GATA3*$^{-/-}$ *RAG2*$^{-/-}$ chimeric mice had a complete absence of double positive and single positive T cells in the thymus, and no T cells were detected in the periphery.[223] Using a conditional allele of GATA3, it was shown that GATA3 is required at the β-selection point of T-cell development.[224] At this point in T-cell development, CD4/8 double positive thymocytes must rearrange their TCR β chain, and express it on the cell surface in order to proceed to single positive CD4 or CD8 T cells. Surprisingly, TCR-β chain RNA is detected at normal levels in GATA3-deficient CD4/8 double positive T cells.[224] However, they express reduced TCR β protein suggesting that GATA3 is regulating TCR-β through a posttranscriptional mechanism. Later in T-cell development, GATA3 is required for T-cell differentiation into the TH2 helper T-cell subset and is necessary for expression of the cytokine IL4 that partially defines the TH2 subset.

Transcription Factors in NK Cell Development

PU.1 and Ikaros are both required for proper NK development. Transplantation experiments into *RAG2*$^{-/-}$ mice with *PU.1*$^{-/-}$ bone marrow have shown that the *PU.1*$^{-/-}$ cells contributed poorly to the NK progenitor pool, and very few of these progenitors mature and make it to the periphery.[225] The NK cells that did develop had reduced expression of the IL2 receptor, c-kit, and LY49 family receptors. Significantly, *PU.1*$^{-/-}$ NK cells that did make it to the periphery did not seem to be impaired in their cytolytic activity. Therefore, PU.1 may be required for early NK development but may be dispensable in the mature cells, similar to what is observed with B cells.[137,166,225] In addition, *Ikaros*$^{-/-}$ mice also do not make NK cells, and this may be caused by the decreased expression of Flt3 and CD122 in these cells.[226]

Other transcriptions factors required for NK development includes the Ets family member Ets-1 and the inhibitory basic helix loop helix protein Id-2. Deletion of Ets-1 in mice result in functional defects with B cells and T cells, and an absence of functional NK cells.[227] Ets-1 deleted mice have almost a complete absence of NK cells in the bone marrow, spleen and periphery. In vivo, Ets-1-deficient NK cells lacked cytolytic activity. In vivo Ets-1-deficient mice were also susceptible to tumors that are usually cleared by NK cells.[227]

Id-2 is an inhibitory member of the basic-helix-loop-helix family of transcription factors.[228] It lacks the basic domain commonly conserved in this family, but can heterodimerize with other transcription factors, including E2A described above. Because the basic domain interacts with DNA, Id2-containing heterodimers are unable to bind to DNA. Thus, Id-2 appears to function by binding to and inhibiting other helix-loop-helix transcription factors. Mice deficient in Id-2 lack any mature NK cells, and NK cell progenitors are substantially reduced.[229] The ratio of Id-2 to E2A proteins may be critical for determining lymphoid cell fates, where high E2A drives B-cell production, and high Id-2 drives NK cell production. Overexpression of Id-3 in hematopoietic progenitors blocks T cell development, but stimulates NK cell production.[230] The increased production of NK cells by Id-3 may be a result of its mimicking Id-2 activity, because no NK defect has so far been reported for Id-3 deficient mice.[231,232]

Transcription Factors in Dendritic Cell Development

As discussed, dendritic cells (DC) can be derived from cells that come from either the CMP or CLP.[15–17] Because of this many of the same transcription factors involved in myeloid and lymphoid development are required for proper dendritic cell development. There are three major groups of dendritic cells: Langerhans cells, plasmacytoid dendritic cells and conventional dendritic cells, which can be derived from either monocytic or lymphocytic precursors.[233] Requirements for individual transcription factors differ with each subset. The conventional DCs can be further subdivided by expression of cell surface markers. All conventional DCs express both CD11b and CD11c.[233] However, they can be further divided into three subsets: $CD4^+$ or $CD8^+$ DCs (both lymphoid), and CD4/8 double negative (myeloid derived). The lack of either PU.1 or Ikaros produces profound defects in DC development.[234,235] PU.1 is expressed at high levels in conventional DCs, and at lower levels in plasmacytoid DCs.[132] *PU.1*$^{-/-}$ embryos or neonates do not make $CD11b^+/CD11c^+/CD8^-$ (myeloid) or $CD11b^+CD11c^+CD8^+$ (lymphoid) dendritic cells.[234,235] However, using fetal thymus organ culture it was shown that lymphoid DCs could be produced from *PU.1*$^{-/-}$ precursors, and that these DCs were functional.[235] This indicates that the lack of *PU.1*$^{-/-}$ DCs is at least in part caused by a microenvironmental defect. Langerhans and plasmacytoid DCs have not been closely examined in PU.1 null animals. However, PU.1 is upregulated in human myeloid cells differentiated toward Langerhans DCs with TGF β.[236] Additionally, PU.1 retroviral transduction of human $CD34^+$ progenitors promoted Langerhans DC development.[237] The related transcription factor Spi-B has also been implicated in the development of human plasmacytoid cells.[238,239]

PU.1 has been proposed to have an instructive role in DC cell development. Forced expression of PU.1 in monocytes can drive them to differentiate to DCs.[240] The decision between monocyte and dendritic cell fates could be controlled by a balance between the PU.1 and another transcription factor MafB.[240] Exogenous PU.1 expression in monocytes downregulates the expression of MafB. Additionally, PU.1 binds to MafB and inhibits its ability to positively regulate transcription and drive monocyte differentiation of a hematopoietic progenitor cell line.

Ikaros is also critical for DC development. Mice homozygously carrying the dominant negative allele of Ikaros do not generate any of the conventional dendritic cell subsets.[179] However, mice deficient for any expression of Ikaros lack myeloid but not lymphoid DCs.[241] Additionally, expression of a dominant negative form of Ikaros in human CD34+ progenitors blocked their ability to make myeloid but not lymphoid DCs.[242] A role for Ikaros in Langerhans DCs has not been described. Mice expressing a hypomorphic allele of Ikaros lack plasmacytoid DCs.[243] These mice are hindered in their ability to make the antiviral cytokine Interferon γ, and are highly susceptible to viral infection. Ikaros mutant HSC lack the expression of the tyrosine kinase receptor Flt3,[244] which has been shown to be important in dendritic cell development. Thus, the poor DC development in Ikaros mutant mice may be caused by lack of expression of this receptor by DC progenitors.[245,246]

Other factors involved in generating DC subsets that were previously discussed for other lineages are Gfi-1 and Id-2. Gfi-1-deficient mice have a dramatic reduction in myeloid and lymphoid-derived DCs in vivo.[247] Conversely, Langerhans DCs were significantly increased in vivo. In vitro, DCs could not be generated from *Gfi-1*$^{-/-}$ hematopoietic progenitors. Instead, the progenitors had a much greater tendency to differentiate into macrophages.

Id-2 is also required for Langerhans and lymphoid DCs.[248,249] No Langerhans DCs are generated in *Id2*$^{-/-}$ mice, and the $CD11b^+/CD11c^+/CD8^+$ lymphoid DC population is greatly reduced. Id-2, like PU.1, is induced by TGF-β in human hematopoietic progenitors.[236] Forced Id-2 expression alone, or in combination with PU.1, cannot induce Langerhans DC differentiation in the absence of added DC cytokines. However, Id-2 expression does downregulate expression of monocyte genes, and when TGF-β is added, induces Langerhans DC formation.[236]

TRANSCRIPTION FACTOR CONCENTRATIONS IN HEMATOPOIETIC DEVELOPMENT

Several hematopoietic transcription factors have been shown to have concentration dependent effects on lineage specification or stage progression. This concept first arose from work with Oct-4 in ES cells, where different concentrations resulted in distinct cell fates. High expression of Oct-4 in differentiating ES cells promotes mesodermal commitment, whereas low expression of Oct-4 promotes trophoblast commitment.[250] In hematopoiesis, c-myb and PU.1 are the best examples of the principle that different cellular concentrations of transcription factors affect lineage specification.

The presence of PU.1 is needed for the development of monocytes, granulocytes, and B cells.[134,135] In addition, PU.1 is required for proliferation of erythroid precursors.[170,171] However, for erythrocytes to fully mature, PU.1 expression must be extinguished. Similarly, PU.1 is expressed early in T-cell development and may be important for early thymocyte proliferation, but that expression must be extinguished for full T-cell maturation.[169] Because monocytes express higher levels of PU.1 than B cells, it was hypothesized that high levels of PU.1 specified monocyte commitment over B-cell commitment.[131,251] By retrovirally expressing PU.1 in *PU.1*$^{-/-}$ hematopoietic progenitors, it was shown that high concentrations of PU.1 directed the development of $CD11b^+$ macrophages, and low concentrations of PU.1 directed the development of $CD19^+$ B cells.[251] In a later study, it was demonstrated that high levels of PU.1 pushed the GMP towards monocytes rather than granulocytes.[252] *PU.1*$^{+/-}$ ES cells produced more granulocyte precursors and fewer monocytic precursors than normal ES cells compared to wild-type cells. In addition, PU.1 heterozygosity could partially correct the neutropenia of a G-CSF deficient mouse.[252] This observation has implications for leukemogenesis, as both *PU.1*$^{+/-}$ mice and mice with a hypomorphic PU.1 allele have an increased susceptibility to develop AML.[253,254]

The c-Myb gene is abundantly expressed in immature cells of the hematopoietic system. It was originally identified as the transforming gene of the avian retroviruses AMV and E26.[255–257] Mice without c-Myb do not generate definitive hematopoietic cells.[258] In embryos homozygous for deletion of c-Myb, hematopoietic progenitor cells are produced in the AGM. These cells initially migrate to the fetal liver, but do not expand normally there, and the mice ultimately succumb anemia.[259,260] Based on this, it is thought that the major function of c-Myb in early hematopoiesis was to regulate proliferation of hematopoietic progenitor cells, and that loss of c-Myb results in a loss of fetal liver progenitors because of a relative decrease in proliferation versus commitment to terminal differentiation. C-Myb concentrations also play a role in directing distinct lineage fates.[260] Embryos homozygous for hypomorphic c-Myb alleles, resulting in decreased c-Myb expression, had increased numbers of immature cells in the fetal liver. In these embryos, macrophage and megakaryocyte development was increased but erythroid and lymphoid development was compromised.

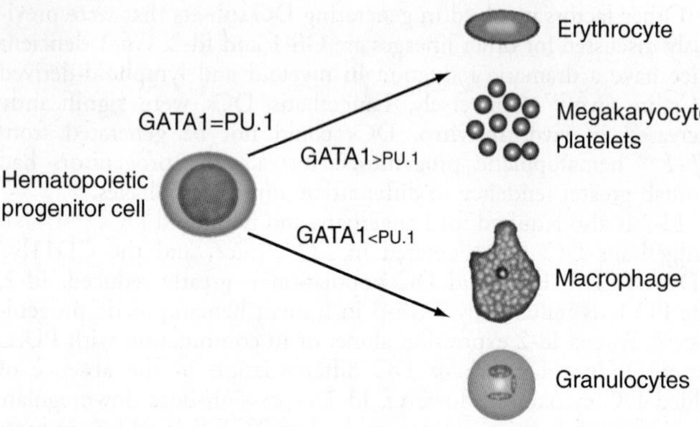

Figure 21–3 Model of how GATA-1 and PU.1 direct hematopoietic differentiation. In an uncommitted progenitor cell the concentrations of PU.1 and GATA-1 are equivalent. PU.1 is able to bind to GATA-1 bound to erythroid target genes and repress transcription and GATA-1 can bind to PU.1 bound to the regulatory elements of myeloid genes, and displace the factor c-Jun which is needed for activation of transcription. By random chance or through environmental signals such as cytokines the levels of GATA-1 could increase allowing it to continue to repress PU.1 targets but also be able to titrate away PU.1 From erythroid genes and allow the activation of the erythroid differentiation program. Similarly levels of PU.1 could increase and drive myeloid development while continuing to repress the erythroid differentiation program.

ANTAGONISTIC INTERACTIONS BETWEEN TRANSCRIPTION FACTORS

Concentrations of transcription factors may play an important role on another level, as a result of antagonistic interactions with other transcription factors. Thus, high levels of one transcription factor may be required to overcome the antagonistic effect of another factor. The interaction between GATA1 and PU.1 demonstrates this principle (Fig. 21–3). Both of these factors are expressed at low levels in the uncommitted CMP.[11,132] In this uncommitted cell, the activities of these factors are thought to be in balance. GATA1 binds to the DNA binding domain of PU.1 through its carboxy proximal zinc finger and inhibits its transcription.[261,262] Likewise, PU.1 also interacts with the GATA1 protein.[261–263] GATA1 interacts with PU.1 and displaces the critical coactivator protein, c-Jun, decreasing the ability of PU.1 to promote transcription.[261,262] Conversely, PU.1 recruits the protein Rb to GATA1, and this in turn recruits a transcriptional repression complex.[264] Several differentiation systems have demonstrated that this cross-antagonism is important in lineage fate choices. The more highly expressed factor turns on its target genes and represses the alternative factor's target genes, which results in distinct lineage commitments—erythroid for GATA1 and granulocyte/monocyte for PU.1. This was demonstrated in murine erythroleukemia cells transduced with a PU.1 retrovirus. Overexpression of PU.1 resulted in the downregulation of endogenous GATA1 expression and switched these cells to a myeloid cell fate, as demonstrated by cell surface markers and the acquisition of phagocytic activity.[265,266] Similarly, manipulating the relative concentrations of PU.1 and GATA1 in *Xenopus* or Zebrafish affected the ratio of macrophage to erythroid differentiation.[267,268]

Another important example of this principle is the ratio of PU.1 to C/EBP α in the GMP, which determines whether the myeloid precursor commits to the granulocyte or monocyte lineage.[252] Both PU.1 and C/EBP α are necessary for proper monocyte and granulocyte differentiation. When PU.1 activity exceeds that of C/EBP α, the expression of PU.1-responsive downstream target genes will direct monocytic differentiation. However, if C/EBP α activity is higher, the GMP will commit to the granulocyte lineage. C/EBP α inhibits PU.1-induced transcription from reporter genes regulated by a multimerized PU.1 binding site.[237] This repression is a result of binding between the leucine zipper domain of C/EBP α and the Ets domain of PU.1. Like GATA1 binding to PU.1, C/EBP α binding results in the dissociation of c-Jun, which blocks PU.1 transactivation.[237] Additionally C/EBP α overexpression had an effect on cell fate decisions. In myeloid progenitors the ratio of PU.1 and C/EBP α to one another may determine whether myeloid progenitors become monocytes or granulocytes.

TRANSCRIPTION FACTORS IN LEUKEMIA

Transcription factors important in hematopoiesis are commonly involved in chromosomal translocations in human leukemias. These translocations alter the function of these transcription factors, often producing blocks in differentiation of hematopoietic progenitors. Indeed, many of these transcription factors were first isolated by cloning of the translocation break point. Thus, defining what has gone wrong in leukemia has greatly assisted in defining what is required for normal hematopoiesis. There are a large number of transcription factors involved in leukemic translocations, but we will focus on Notch1, MLL, SCL, AML1, CBF β, LMO2, E2A, TEL, and MOZ because they have each shed light on crucial characteristics of normal versus malignant hematopoiesis (Table 21–1). Transcription factors can also be altered in acute leukemia by point mutations, and this can lead to inactivation of the function of those transcription factors as well. Examples of this include C/EBP α, GATA1, and PU.1. Alterations in expression of key transcription factors can also promote the development of acute leukemia, and an example of this is Bmi1.

The study of these transcription factors has lead to major advances in understanding leukemogenesis. The fusion oncoproteins resulting from the AML1-ETO and PML-RAR α translocations do not result in the generation of acute leukemia in mice when transduced into bone marrow progenitors.[269,270] An additional genetic lesion was needed in these models to produce acute myeloid leukemia. This additional genetic lesion was often the constitutive activation of a protein that stimulated proliferation, such as the Flt3 internal tandem duplication. This led to the paradigm that two genetic lesions are required for the generation of acute leukemias, one lesion that enhances proliferation and one lesion that blocks differentiation.[271] Translocations involving transcription factors in leukemia most often result in repression of differentiation, by inhibiting the expression of genes normally required for proper maturation. This often occurs because the translocation oncoprotein turns the transcriptional activator into a repressor. Thus, many of the transcriptional activators that are required for proper myeloid or lymphoid differentiation are targets of leukemic translocations. This paradigm has implications for therapy, as both genetic lesions must be targeted for appropriate destruction of the malignancy.

Translocations Involving Transcription Factors Associated with Leukemia

Notch1

In rare cases of T-cell acute lymphoblastic leukemia the t(7;9)(q34;q34.3) translocation occurs. Cloning of this translocation showed that Notch1 (also termed TAN1) located on chromosome 9 was translocated relatively intact to the TCR β locus on chromosome 7, resulting in its constitutive expression.[272] Because Notch1 expression is required for production of early hematopoietic progenitors, it is thought that constitutive aberrantly high expression of Notch1 in a T-cell progenitor maintains the progenitor phenotype and blocks appropriate maturation. Interestingly, although translocations involving Notch1 are very rare, point mutations may be quite common in T-cell ALL. It has been reported that more than 50% of all human T-ALL cases have activating mutations that involve the extracellular heterodimerization domain or the C-terminal PEST domain of

Table 21–1 Transcription Factor Genes Translocated in Leukemia

Transcription Factor	Normal Function	Translocation	Fusion Partner	Disease
Notch1 (TAN1)	HSC specification Lymphoid cell fate decisions T-cell development	t(7;9)(q34;q34.3)	TCR β locus	T-ALL
MLL	HSC specification	t(4;11) t(6;11) t(9;11) t(10;11) t(11;19) t(11;19)	AF4 AF6 AF9 AF10 ELL ENL	ALL AML AML AML AML AML/ALL
SCL (TAL1)	HSC specification Erythropoiesis Megakaryopoiesis	t(1;14)	TCR α/δ locus	T-ALL
AML1 (RUNX1)	HSC specification Megakaryopoiesis	t(8;21)	ETO (MTG8)	AML
CBFb	HSC specification	Inv(16) t(16;16)	MYH11	AML, M4Eo
LMO2	HSC specification	t(7; 11) t(11;14)	TCR δ locus TCR β locus	T-ALL T-ALL
E2A	Lymphopoiesis	t(1;19) t(17; 19)	Pbx HLF	Pre B-ALL Pre B-ALL
TEL	HSC maintenance	t(12;21) t(5;12)	AML1 PDGFR	B-ALL CMML
MOZ	HSC maintenance	t(8;16) t(8;22)	CBP TIF2	AMoL M5 AML

ALL, acute lymphoblastic leukemia; AML, acute myelogenous leukemia; B-ALL, B-cell acute lymphoblastic leukemia; CMML, chronic myelomonocytic leukemia; HSC, hematopoietic stem cells; T-ALL, T-cell acute lymphoblastic leukemia; TCR, T-cell antigen receptor.

NOTCH1.[273] This implies that inappropriate activation of the Notch signaling pathway is a key step in the origin of most T-cell leukemias. Thus, targeting this pathway may be an important new addition to therapy of T-ALL.

MLL (ALL1, HRX)

Recurring translocations involving chromosome 11q23 have been observed that occurred in a wide variety of both ALL and AML. After a prolonged search, several groups cloned the gene at 11q23 disrupted in the t(4;11), t(9;11), and the t(11;19) translocation and termed it variously MLL, ALL1, or HRX.[274,275] MLL gene translocations and subsequent fusion oncoproteins are seen in about 70% of AML and ALL in infants, and are also frequent in treatment-related leukemias, especially in patients treated with drugs inhibiting topoisomerase II.[276,277] There are more than 36 distinct translocation partners of MLL, making it the most promiscuous of the transcription factors disrupted in leukemia.[278] This implies that the critical common element in these leukemias might not be the partner, but rather the loss of the C-terminal regions of MLL. MLL can even be self-rearranged, resulting in a partial tandem duplication of the gene in some cases of AML.[279,280]

The protein has homology to Drosophila trithorax, which regulates homeotic segment formation in development. MLL has amino terminal AT hooks, six zinc finger domains, and a histone methyltransferase domain. MLL normally regulates homeobox gene expression through many mechanisms, including interaction with CBP, histone deacetylases, and TFIID at promoter sequences, and methylating histone H3 lysine 4, which opens chromatin and promotes transcription.[278] In most of the MLL translocations the histone methyltransferase activity is lost, but often the translocation partner provides such methyltransferase activity. The mechanism by which the MLL fusion oncoproteins generate leukemia is complex, and not completely understood.[278] It is thought that MLL transforms hematopoietic progenitors by inappropriately reactivating homeobox gene expression, which prevents differentiation of these progenitors. Constitutive expression of one target of MLL, HoxA9, produces acute leukemia in mice, suggesting a transcriptional mechanism by which MLL generates acute leukemia in humans.[86] In addition, MLL-ENL-transduced mice get leukemia only if HoxA9 and HoxA7 are present, indicating that activation of these homeobox genes is a crucial for MLL leukemogenesis.[281]

SCL (Tal1, TCL5)

Hematopoietic progenitor cell lines were identified from T-cell ALL cases that had a t(1;14) chromosomal translocation. Two groups isolated a gene termed SCL (or TCL5) translocated relatively intact from chromosomes 1 to the TCR δ region on chromosome 14.[282,283] The translocation remaining on chromosome 14 occurred at the TCR δ diversity (D-δ-2) segment, and the reciprocal translocation occurred at the TCR δ diversity segment D-δ-1. The finding that the TCR δ diversity segments were involved in the translocation junctions suggested that the translocation occurred during an attempt at δ-1/δ-2 joining in an early T-cell progenitor as it underwent TCR rearrangement. This implies that aberrant function of the immunoglobulin recombinase proteins may play important roles in the creation of leukemic translocations. Interestingly, rearrangement of the TCL5 locus was also seen in a human melanoma cell line carrying a deletion at 1p32.[282] In this translocation, SCL is not fused to another gene partner, indicating that its abnormal constitutive expression was leukemogenic.

The occurrence of biphenotypic leukemias with both lymphoid and myeloid characteristics, occurring especially frequently in infants, and following chemotherapy administration, is evidence of the stem cell origin of such leukemias. One of the groups isolated SCL from a t(1;14) translocation found it in a leukemic cell line that was capable of differentiating into either myeloid or lymphoid cells, implying that the SCL translocation might occur in the HSC, even though the primary human ALL leukemia had a T-cell phenotype. These data provided evidence for the existence of leukemic stem cells, which are rare, but capable of unlimited proliferation, and giving rise to multiple differentiated progeny. These more differentiated progeny, which make up the bulk of the disease, are capable of only limited proliferation. The finding of SCL in a cell capable of both myeloid and lymphoid differentiation also led to the studies on the essential role of SCL in normal HSC. About a quarter of all T-ALL patients have another abnormality of SCL, a 90-kb deletion of upstream sequences of the first allele of the SCL locus. This fuses the Sil gene promoter to the downstream SCL gene, producing abnormally high expression of SCL.[284] Transgenically overexpressing the Sil-SCL fusion in mice can produce an aggressive form of T-ALL in conjunction with over-expressed LMO1.[285] This study also found that inappropriately expressed SCL interfered with the development of other tissues derived from mesoderm.

AML1

AML1 and CBF β are heterodimeric partners that are critical for the differentiation of myeloid progenitors; translocation of either results in AML. Miyoshi and colleagues isolated and sequenced cDNA clones for a gene they named AML1 on chromosome 21, which was rearranged by the t(8;21) translocation.[286] AML1 is fused to the ETO gene (also termed MTG8) in this translocation. AML1-ETO inhibits transcription of genes important for proper myeloid differentiation, promoting a block of the maturation of a primitive progenitor by several mechanisms. First, AML1-ETO interacts with and inhibits transcriptional activation by E proteins, which precludes recruitment of p300 CREB-binding protein (CBP) coactivators.[287] These interactions occur through the conserved ETO TAF4 domain. Second, AML1-ETO interacts with the nuclear corepressor N-CoR) and histone deacetylase (HDACs) complex, which also inhibits transcription at myeloid differentiation genes. This interaction was found to be required to block hematopoietic differentiation.

Interestingly, AML1-ETO transcripts have been found in patients' hematopoietic cells belonging to many lineages long after they are thought to be cured, indicating that this genetic lesion occurs in a stem cell.[288] It also is evidence that another genetic lesion is required for induction of AML. AML1-ETO was knocked into the mouse AML1 locus to generate a model of the t(8;21) translocation. These mice died before birth from CNS hemorrhage and failure of fetal liver hematopoiesis, identical to the AML1 knock-out discussed above.[289] This indicates that the main function of AML1-ETO fusion protein is to block normal AML1 transcriptional activation. This hypothesis was underscored by the cloning of several translocations in which AML1 was fused out of frame to its partners, demonstrating that it may be disruption of AML1 more than fusion to ETO that is critical for leukemogenesis.[290,291] In addition, a truncated splice variant of AML1-ETO was isolated that had only a small portion of ETO, without the repressor interacting domains, and this truncated version was more leukemogenic that the full length AML1-ETO in mouse models.[292]

There are several other translocation partners of AML1, and they appear to substantiate the hypothesis that disruption of AML1 and perhaps disruption of the partner gene are critical for leukemogenesis.[293,294] Thus, AML1 and its partners may function more as tumor suppressor genes promoting differentiation, compared to the traditional model of fusion products functioning as dominant oncogenes. Although the t(8;21) AML has a good prognosis, all other AML1 translocations occur often in secondary leukemias and have a poor prognosis.

CBF β

Lui and colleagues cloned the breakpoint in the inv[16](p13q22) seen in acute monocytic leukemia with eosinophils.[295] They found that this inversion created a fusion gene between the 5′ portion of CBF β on 16p13 and the myosin heavy chain gene MYH11 on 16p13. A similar fusion occurs in the less common t(16;16)(p13;q22). The result of this is abnormal localization of CBF β, preventing it from forming heterodimers with CBF α, and activating monocyte differentiation.

Like AML1-ETO, transgenic overexpression of this fusion gene in murine marrow progenitors did not produce monocytic leukemia.[296] However, myeloid maturation was impaired, as there were increased numbers of immature myeloid cells in the marrow, and there was less neutrophil differentiation in progenitor colony formation assays. Coexpression of both the fusion gene and activated N-RAS produced a more severe phenotype characterized by myeloid precursor cell dysplasia, somewhat similar to myelodysplastic syndrome. However, acute leukemias were still rare. When the CBF β-MYH11 fusion is expressed during embryonic development leukemia can occur, but with a long latency of approximately five months.[297] These findings led to the search for cooperating genes which might be important in the generation of human acute monocytic leukemia with eosinophils. This search was more successful than in AML1-ETO, and several candidates have been identified.[298]

LMO2

LMO2 is translocated relatively intact to the TCR β region on chromosome 14 in a t(11;14), and to the TCR δ region in a t(7;11) in T-cell acute lymphoblastic leukemia.[299,300] Because it is not fused to a partner gene in these translocations, it is probable that the its constitutive overexpression is leukemogenic. Further evidence of the leukemogenicity of LMO2 in T cells came from a gene therapy study where the IL-2 receptor γ was retrovirally transduced into CD34+ hematopoietic cells in children with X-linked SCID. Three patients ultimately developed T-cell leukemia when the retroviral integration site was in proximity to the LMO2 promoter.[301,302] This led to abnormal constitutive expression of LMO2 in a situation analogous to that of the T-cell ALL cases in which LMO2 was first isolated. By searching the retroviral integration site database (containing more than 3000 sites) cloned from mice with retrovirally-induced leukemias, one leukemia was found to have integration in both the LMO2 and the IL-2 receptor γ sites, similar to the human cases.[303] These integrations were clonal in this leukemia, indicating that they represent an early step in the transformation of a single hematopoietic progenitor that became malignant. Thus, abnormal constitutive expression of LMO2 in T-cell progenitors can be an important step in the transformation of these progenitors to ALL, once again demonstrating the crucial importance of tight transcriptional regulation of the regulators themselves.

E2A

The t(1;19) in the common pre-B ALL was found to translocate the bHLH gene E2A on chromosome 19 to a homeobox gene on chromosome 1 termed Pbx1 (or Prl).[304] This fusion oncogene encodes an 85-kD protein consisting of the N-terminal two-thirds of E2A fused to the carboxy terminal portion of Pbx1. The fusion protein is a chimeric transcription factor with the DNA-binding domain of E2A replaced by the DNA-binding domain of Pbx1. Thus, genes important for B-cell maturation normally activated by E2A no longer are activated, but rather the genes regulated by Pbx1 are now activated.

Rarely B-cell ALL has a t(17;19) translocation involving E2A. Here E2A is fused to the DNA binding portion of a gene on chromosome 17 that encodes a hepatic leukemia factor (HLF). This chimeric transcription factor has the amino-terminal transactivation domain of E2A linked to the carboxyl-terminal DNA binding basic region-leucine zipper domain of HLF.[305]

Transgenically overexpressing E2A-HLF produces acute lymphoid malignancies in mice and disrupts B-cell and T-cell maturation.[306] Overexpressing different structural deletions of the E2A-Pbx1 fusion oncogene in mice resulted in lymphomas after a latency.[307] Interestingly, when the Pbx1 homeodomain of the fusion oncogene was deleted, the remaining fusion oncogene continued to transform.

TEL

In B-cell ALL, there is commonly a t(12;21) translocation associated with a good patient prognosis. Golub and Gilliland cloned this translocation breakpoint, and found that the Ets family gene, TEL, on chromosome 12 was fused to AML1 on chromosome 21.[308] This results in the fusion of the helix-loop-helix dimerization domain of TEL to both the DNA-binding and transactivation domains of the transcription factor AML1. TEL loses its Ets family DNA binding domain, and alters the transcriptional regulatory properties of AML1. This is conspicuously different from AML1 translocations in myeloid leukemia, in which the transactivation domains of AML1 are lost. TEL was first described based on its fusion to PDGF receptor in the t(5;12) translocation seen in CMML.[309] More than 20 other translocation partners of TEL have been described in both lymphoid and myeloid malignancies.[310] These partners appear to fall into two classes. They may be signaling proteins like PDGF receptor, ABL, or ARG, where the HLH domain of TEL enhances inappropriate dimerization and subsequent constitutive activation of the signaling molecule; or they may be transcription factors like AML1, whose activity is altered by fusion to TEL. Interestingly, TEL probably also functions as a tumor suppressor, as its other untranslocated allele is lost in approximately 15% of all B-cell ALL.[311]

Transducing the TEL-AML1 fusion into mouse marrow with a retroviral vector produced ALL in a small fraction of mice.[312] Deletion of the tumor suppressor p16 enhanced the rate of formation of leukemia. Another group transplanted TEL-AML1 transduced progenitors, and this resulted in an accumulation of primitive progenitors, a disruption of B-cell maturation, but normal myeloid development.[313] The low level of leukemogenesis indicates that there are likely other genetic lesions that are required. This hypothesis is supported by the finding that TEL-AML1 transcripts can persist long after ALL patients have obtained a continuous complete remission.[314]

MOZ

MOZ (monocytic leukemia zinc finger protein) was originally isolated as part of fusion protein created by the t(8;16) chromosomal translocation associated with AML with monocytic arrest.[315] This translocation fuses MOZ to another transcription factor CBP (CREB binding protein). MOZ is also involved in another leukemic translocation, t(8;22), which fuses MOZ to the transcription factor TIF2.[316,317] TIF2 is known to interact with CBP, thus providing a common link between leukemogenesis in both translocations.[318] MOZ is the founding member of a group of highly conserved proteins characterized by a single C2HC3 zinc finger next to an acetyltransferase domain. MOZ also contains two C4HC3 zinc finger domains, protein-interaction motifs associated with chromatin-bound proteins. These motifs suggested that MOZ is a histone acetyltransferase and may promote transcription by opening chromatin to allow access by transcription factors to DNA regulatory regions. MOZ was found to be fused to CREB-binding protein (CBP), a transcriptional coactivator in the t(8;16) translocation. Mutation of CBP is responsible for Rubinstein-Taybi syndrome. This inherited disorder is characterized by mental retardation, dysmorphic facial structure, and broad thumbs. Interestingly, these patients have an increased risk for developing benign and malignant tumors including certain kinds of brain tumors.

Overexpressing MOZ-TIF2 in murine marrow produced an acute leukemia with some latency.[318] Induction of this leukemia required the CBP interacting domains of TIF2, further evidence that the two translocations have the same molecular mechanism.

POINT MUTATIONS ASSCOCIATED WITH LEUKEMIA

C/EBP α Mutations in Acute Myeloid Leukemia

C/EBP α is a transcription factor critical for the generation of granulocytes. Because of its essential role in differentiating myeloid cells, it was hypothesized that C/EBP α activity may be perturbed in AML. An initial study of 137 AML patients identified 10 individuals with mutations in the C/EBP α gene (CEBPA).[319] Seven of those 10 samples had no karyotypic abnormalities, and all but one of them contained one normal allele of CEBPA. Five of these mutations were in the region coding for the amino terminus of C/EBP α. Because of the use of an alternative initiating methionine CEBPA normally codes for a 42kD protein and a 30kD form. The 30KD form can acts as a dominant negative and represses transcription. The 42kD C/EBP α isoform but not the 30kD form induces terminal differentiation through cell cycle arrest.[320,321] All five amino terminal mutants had increased production of the 30kD protein compared to the 42kD protein. In addition 4 of the amino terminal mutants produced a shorter 159 amino acid 20kD protein. All mutants demonstrated a reduction in DNA binding with several of carboxy terminal mutants having lost DNA binding ability all together. All of the mutants could inhibit DNA binding of wild-type C/EBP α.

Subsequently, more than a thousand hematologic malignancy patients have been screened for CEBPA mutations.[322] These patients include those with AML, myelodysplastic syndrome, acute lymphoblastic leukemia, and non- lymphoma. CEBPA mutations have been detected only in myeloid malignancies. Approximately 9% of the AML samples examined have CEBPA mutations. Almost 20% of AML samples of the M2 subtype have CEBPA mutations. Along with mutations in the amino terminus that changed the ratio of the p42 to p30 ratio, isolated mutations in the basic leucine zipper region of CEBPA occur.[323–325] These mutations are thought to maintain the ability to dimerize with wild-type C/EBP α protein but with the loss of the ability to efficiently bind DNA.

Altering of C/EBP α activity in AML is not isolated to point mutations. Expression of C/EBP α is downregulated by the AML1-ETO fusion protein (Pabst 2001). AML1-ETO decreased the mRNA and protein expression of C/EBP α in a myeloid cell line. Additionally, exogenous expression of C/EBP α into the AML1-ETO-transformed Kasumi cell line induces granulocytic differentiation. Downregulation of C/EBP α expression by translational silencing has been proposed to occur in chronic myelogenous leukemia.[326] Blasts from p210 BCR-Abl induced CML express CEBPA mRNA but very little C/EBP α protein. Introduction of C/EBP α into CML blasts can induce differentiation.

GATA1 in Down Syndrome Associated with Megakaryocytic Leukemia

Children with Down syndrome (trisomy 21) are prone to develop leukemia, and approximately half of those leukemias are AML. Most of the AMLs in Down syndrome patients are acute megakaryoblastic leukemias (AMKL). In addition, about 10% of children with Down syndrome develop a transient myeloproliferative disorder (TMD). In most patients, TMD spontaneously remits, but in a few cases this develops into a severe myeloproliferative disease, with blasts infiltrating the heart and liver. TMD is considered a preleukemic disorder because more than 20% of children diagnosed with TMD later develop AMKL.

In a study looking for GATA1 mutations associated with AML, it was found that GATA1 was mutated in six of six Down syndrome-associated AMKL.[327] No mutations were discovered in all the other AML subtype samples examined. Subsequent studies have shown that GATA1 is mutated in almost all cases of AMKL in Down syndrome and in the TMD of Down syndrome.[328–332] The mutations that have been identified include missense, nonsense, and splice site mutations, along with insertions and deletions. All of the mutations are in exon 2 or the immediate downstream intron 2. The mutations abrogate expression of the full-length 50 kD protein, and lead to the generation of a truncated 40kD protein (GATA1s), which lacks the domain responsible for activating transcription, but retains both zinc fingers. The importance of the amino terminal transactivation domain is unclear, because in several in vitro assays it is not necessary for the promotion of erythroid development. In vivo a shortened GATA1 still rescues murine GATA1 deficiency.[333–335] Thus, it is unknown how GATA1s promotes leukemia. However, it is assumed that it cooperates with other genetic defects associated with trisomy 21.

PU.1 Mutations and Myeloid Leukemia

PU.1 was originally described as the oncogene in murine erythroleukemia. The SFFV virus integrates into the PU.1 locus and causes PU.1 to be overexpressed in erythroid progenitors,[336] blocking their differentiation. In mice it has been shown that reduction of PU.1 levels can lead to the development of myeloid leukemias.[136,137] Hypomorphic alleles of murine PU.1 also lead to development of leukemia. Deletion of a −14kb enhancer element in the PU.1 locus results in expression of approximately 20% of the normal levels of PU.1 in HSCs and myeloid progenitors.[253] These mice first accumulate of abnormal myeloid progenitors, and then progresses to a fatal AML. Differentiation of these AML blast can be restored by exogenous expression of PU.1 through retroviral transduction.

Further evidence supporting a role for reduced PU.1 concentration in myeloid leukemia comes from murine myeloid leukemias induced by γ irradiation.[254,337] Myeloid leukemias induced by γ irradiation frequently undergo a deletion of a portion of chromosome 2 which harbors the *PU.1* gene. Analysis of the other allele of PU.1 demonstrated that it had undergone point mutations in the DNA binding domain. These mutations reduced but did not completely abrogate the ability of PU.1 to associate with DNA. No malignant cells were ever identified that harbored a null mutation in the remaining *PU.1* allele, suggesting that some PU.1 function is required for maintenance of the leukemic state. To date, PU.1 mutations have not been identified in patients with radiation therapy induced AML.[254]

Loss of one allele of *PU.1* has not been shown to have adverse effects in mice although protein levels are reduced by 50% in hematopoietic tissues examined.[134,138,338] However *PU.1*$^{+/-}$ mice are more susceptible to leukemia development after transduction of PML-RAR α than wild type mice,[339] indicating that reduced PU.1 levels might contribute to the development of acute promyelocytic leukemia.

AML patient samples have been screened for PU.1 mutations. One study observed 10 mutant alleles of *PU.1* in 9 of 126 AML samples examined.[340] These findings are controversial because a subsequent study did not identify any mutations in PU.1's coding region of 77 AML samples.[341] In another study, mutations in PU.1 were discovered in 2 of 60 AML patient samples and 1 of 21 myeloid leukemia cell lines analyzed.[342] The importance of these mutations is unclear because the 2 AML mutations were point mutations in intronic sequence and the one mutation from a myeloid cell line is a silent G-to-A transition at *PU.1*'s codon 65.

Although it is unclear to what extent *PU.1* mutations contribute to leukemia there are additional studies that have demonstrated that PU.1 expression and/or activity is targeted by leukemic oncogenes. The t(8;21) translocation results in the formation of the chimeric oncogene AML1-ETO.[343] Normal AML1 protein has been shown to cooperate with PU.1 in the regulation of myeloid target genes. In contrast, the fusion protein AML1-ETO has been shown to bind to PU.1 and repress the ability of PU.1 to activate transcription.[139] Binding of AML1-ETO displaces c-Jun as a PU.1 coactivator. Additionally, it has been shown the ETO portion of the fusion protein can bind corepressor proteins, and this could also lead to the antagonism of PU.1 transactivation activity.[344] Thus, although mutations within PU.1 itself are unlikely to play much of a role in AML, altering its level of expression may be an important step in leukemogenesis.

Ikaros and Hematological Malignancy

A dominant negative form of Ikaros has severe effects on hematopoietic development. This dominant negative mutant lacks the DNA binding domain of Ikaros, but retains protein-protein interaction domains. The mutant Ikaros forms inactivate dimers with wild-type Ikaros and the related factors Aiolos and Helios. Mice heterozygous for the mutant Ikaros allele do not have any obvious hematopoietic defect in the first month after birth. Soon after the mice develop a lymphoproliferative disorder, which then leads to the development of T-cell leukemias.[187] During the development of this disease the wild-type allele of Ikaros is lost, in a classic tumor suppressor manner.

The Ikaros gene is alternatively spliced in both mice and humans. There are at least 6 different isoforms of Ikaros expressed in hematopoietic cells.[180,345] One of these isoforms, IK6 (lacks the DNA binding domain), is predicted to produce a protein similar to the mouse dominant negative allele. Ectopic expression of IK6 in human CD34^{+} progenitors impairs B cell differentiation.[346] IK6 expression has been detected in several B and T cell malignancies.[346–351] Additionally, the oncogene BCR-Abl has been shown to induce aberrant splicing of Ikaros, increasing the expression of IK6.[352] This implies that aberrant alternative splicing can play a role in leukemogenicity.

Maintenance of Leukemic Stem Cells: Bmi1

It has been proposed that leukemia is a stem cell disease,[353,354] where only a fraction of cells are able to initiate and maintain the leukemia when transplanted. Similar to its role in the HSC, Bmi-1 is dispensable for the initial development of HoxA9-Meis1 induced leukemia.[98] However, Bmi-1-deficient leukemias are not transplantable into secondary hosts. After transplantation, donor cells underwent a cell cycle arrest, differentiation and/or apoptosis. It is possible that leukemic stem cells require Bmi-1 for maintenance in a like manner as normal HSC.

TRANSCRIPTION FACTORS IN OTHER HEMATOLOGICAL DISEASES

GATA1 in Anemia and Thrombocytopenia

Several human hematopoietic diseases have been associated with point mutations in GATA1. Several families have been identified that has missense mutations in GATA1 which damage normal GATA1 function but do not completely ablate it. The first identification of GATA1 mutations was identified in two half brothers that were anemic and thrombocytopenic.[355] The peripheral blood of these siblings contained very few platelets, and their erythrocytes had abnormal size and shape. Their bone marrow was hypercellular, with large multinucleated erythroblasts and dysplastic megakaryocytes. Interestingly the brothers had three unaffected sisters, suggesting that the disorder was X-linked. Because GATA1 is on the X chromosome, it was sequenced for identification of possible mutations. Both boys had a G to A transition mutation in the coding region of GATA1, which leads to amino acid 205 being mutated from valine to methionine. The valine residue is in the highly conserved amino terminal zinc finger of GATA1 which mediates DNA binding and binding to the cofactor FOG1.[122] Interestingly, this mutation is similar to a V205G mutation, which was identified through an in vitro screen to identify mutants of GATA1 that could no longer bind FOG1.[356] It was shown biochemically that the human GATA1 V205G mutant bound DNA as well as the wild-type protein, but was impaired in its ability to bind FOG1. Additionally, the V205G mutant could not promote differentiation of a mouse *GATA1*$^{-/-}$ erythroblast cell line.

Other families have been subsequently identified that carry mutations in the amino terminal finger of GATA1. These mutations include G208S, D218G, and D218Y.[357–359] All of these mutations effect GATA1 binding to FOG1, and severity of their disease appears to correlate with the strength of the interaction with FOG1. An R216Q mutation in the amino terminal finger was also identified in patients with macrothrombocytopenia and β-thalassemia.[360] This mutation interfered with DNA binding but left FOG1 binding intact.

AML1 and Familial Platelet Disorder

Deletion of AML1 in murine adult hematopoietic cells leads to defects in megakaryocytopoiesis. Defects in AML1 can also lead to dysfunctional megakaryopoiesis in humans. Familial platelet disorder (FPD) is an autosomal dominant disorder characterized by a decrease in platelet number and function. Inherited syndromes of leukemia are rare, but when investigated, have led to important insight into leukemogenesis. Two FPD family pedigrees were identified that included members with high propensity to develop AML.[361] The disease-associated region was linked to chromosome 22q22.1-22.2. Subsequent identification of 4 more FPC/AML families delineated the responsible region down to 880 kb on chromosome 21.[362] Based on examining candidate genes in the region, one allele of AML1 was consistently found to be mutated in affected members. Families had either nonsense mutations or intragenic deletions in the AML1 gene, which resulted in loss of function in one allele of AML1. Analysis of bone marrow or peripheral blood demonstrated that affected individuals had defects in megakaryocyte colony formation. The study showed that haploinsufficiency for AML1 can result in defects in megakaryopoiesis and predispose to leukemia. Like PU.1, AML1 concentration appears to have effects on hematopoiesis.

GFI-1 Mutations in Human Neutropenia

Because Gfi-1 mice are neutropenic, a study was performed to determine if mutations in human Gfi-1 are associated with neutropenia.[363] There are two congenital forms of neutropenia: cyclic neutropenia and severe congenital neutropenia (SCN). Mutations in the neutrophil elastase gene ELA2 cause cyclic neutropenia, and are also associated with the majority of SCN cases. More than 200 patient samples from neutropenia patients without known ELA2 mutations were screened for mutations in the Gfi-1 coding region.[363] Two distinct heterozygous missense mutations were discovered. A four-month-old boy with SCN had an A to G transition mutation, which resulted in a change of asparagine to serine at amino acid position 382 of Gfi-1. This mutation is in the fifth zinc finger of Gfi-1. Zinc fingers 3 through 5 are required for DNA binding. Subsequent analysis showed that the patient's brother and father had the same Gfi-1 mutation. The patient lacked neutrophils and monocytes, and there was a reduction in CD4+ T cells and B lymphocytes. In vitro assays detected no defect in production of erythroid progenitors, but did reveal a reduction in the number of myeloid progenitor colonies. Another A to G transition mutation was discovered in a 66-year-old female patient with nonimmune chronic idiopathic neutropenia. This mutation resulted in a change of lysine to arginine at amino acid position 403 in the sixth zinc finger of Gfi-1. The patient had persistent low levels of neutrophils, but elevated numbers of monocytes.

In vitro experiments showed that these mutations interfere with the activity of Gfi-1. Both mutations could inhibit the ability of wild-type Gfi-1 to repress transcription, potentially explaining how the two mutations exert an effect even though heterozygous. DNA binding assays showed that the N382S mutant could not bind DNA, and could inhibit wild-type Gfi-1 binding to DNA. The K403R mutation however does not appear to affect DNA binding of Gfi-1.

C/EBP ε in Severe Granule Deficiency

Neutrophil-specific granule deficiency (SGD) is a rare inherited disorder.[364] Neutrophils from these patients have abnormal nuclei and do not express secondary and tertiary granule proteins.[365] The primary granule proteins myeloperoxidase and lysozyme are expressed but the defensin proteins are not,[366,367] and these neutrophils are functionally defective.[368,369] They have no bactericidal activity potentially caused by the lack of granules, respiratory burst activity and a defect in chemotaxis. Because the secondary granule gene lactoferrin is expressed normally in other cells of the body, it was hypothesized that the defect is caused by a transcriptional regulatory defect in granulocytic cells.[368]

Several transcription factor proteins have been identified as being critical for proper granulocyte differentiation to occur in knockout mice including PU.1, C/EBP α and C/EBP ε. However, the phenotype of CEBPE$^{-/-}$ mice most resembled the phenotype of patients with SGD. Because of this, a study was initiated to determine if SGD patients had mutation in the CEBPE gene.[370,371] Cells from two of the five known patients at the time were examined. One patient was homozygous for a 5-nucleotide deletion in the second exon of CEBPE.[370] This produces a frame shifted protein which lacked the dimerization and DNA binding domains of C/EBP ε. This mutated protein also lost its ability to activate transcription. The second patient had a homozygous A nucleotide insertion into exon 2, which also resulted in a frameshift.[371] The predicted protein from this patient would lack the DNA binding, dimerization, and nuclear localization domains. When the patient's neutrophils were examined, it was determined that mutant C/EBP ε protein accumulated in the cytoplasm and was thus unable to regulate transcription. These two patients and the C/EBP ε mutant mice strongly suggest that CEBPE mutations are causative for SGD. However, other subsequent SGD patients have been shown not to have CEBPE gene mutations.[372] It has not been ruled out that C/EBP ε in these patients may be dysregulated in other ways besides coding sequence mutations.

SUGGESTED READINGS

Akashi K, Traver D, Miyamoto T, Weissman IL: A clonogenic common myeloid progenitor that gives rise to all myeloid lineages. Nature 404:193, 2000.

Friedman AD: Transcriptional regulation of myelopoiesis. Int J Hematol 75:466, 2002.

Georgopoulos K, Winandy S, Avitahl N: The role of the Ikaros gene in lymphocyte development and homeostasis. Annu Rev Immunol 15:155, 1997.

Kelly LM, Gilliland DG: Genetics of myeloid leukemias. Annu Rev Genomics Hum Genet 3:179, 2002.

Laslo P, Spooner CJ, Warmflash A, et al: Multilineage transcriptional priming and determination of alternate hematopoietic cell fates. Cell 126:755, 2006.

Lessard J, Faubert A, Sauvageau G: Genetic programs regulating HSC specification, maintenance and expansion. Oncogene 23:7199, 2004.

Mikkola HK, Orkin SH: Gene targeting and transgenic strategies for the analysis of hematopoietic development in the mouse. Methods Mol Med 105:3, 2005.

Mikkola HK, Klintman J, Yang H, et al: Haematopoietic stem cells retain long-term repopulating activity and multipotency in the absence of stem-cell leukaemia SCL/tal-1 gene. Nature 421:547, 2003.

Pabst T, Mueller BU, Zhang P, et al: Dominant-negative mutations of CEBPA, encoding CCAAT/enhancer binding protein-alpha (C/EBP-alpha), in acute myeloid leukemia. Nat Genet27:263, 2001.

Palis J, Yoder MC: Yolk-sac hematopoiesis: the first blood cells of mouse and man. Exp Hematol 29:927, 2001.

Pevny L, Simon MC, Robertson E, et al: Erythroid differentiation in chimaeric mice blocked by a targeted mutation in the gene for transcription factor GATA-1. Nature 349:257, 1991.

Pui JC, Allman D, Xu L, et al: Notch1 expression in early lymphopoiesis influences B versus T lineage determination. Immunity 11:299, 1999.

Rabbitts TH: Chromosomal translocation master genes, mouse models and experimental therapeutics. Oncogene 20:5763, 2001.

Radtke F, Wilson A, MacDonald HR: Notch signaling in hematopoiesis and lymphopoiesis: lessons from Drosophila. Bioessays 27:1117, 2005.

Rekhtman N, Radparvar F, Evans T, Skoultchi AI: Direct interaction of hematopoietic transcription factors PU.1 and GATA-1: functional antagonism in erythroid cells. Genes Dev 13:1398, 1999.

Roessler S, Grosschedl R: Role of transcription factors in commitment and differentiation of early B lymphoid cells. Semin Immunol 18:12, 2006.

Rosenbauer F, Wagner K, Kutok JL, et al: Acute myeloid leukemia induced by graded reduction of a lineage-specific transcription factor, PU.1. Nat Genet 36:624, 2004.

Scott EW, Simon MC, Anastasi J, Singh H: Requirement of transcription factor PU.1 in the development of multiple hematopoietic lineages. Science 265:1573, 1994.

Ting CN, Olson MC, Barton KP, Leiden JM: Transcription factor GATA-3 is required for development of the T-cell lineage. Nature 384:474, 1996.

Wechsler J, Greene M, McDevitt MA, et al: Acquired mutations in GATA1 in the megakaryoblastic leukemia of Down syndrome. Nat Genet 32:148, 2002.

Zenke M, Hieronymus T: Towards an understanding of the transcription factor network of dendritic cell development. Trends Immunol 27:140, 2006.

REFERENCES

For complete list of references log onto www.expertconsult.com

CHAPTER 22

NONHEMATOPOIETIC STEM CELLS ORIGINATING WITHIN THE BONE MARROW

Magdalena Kucia, Janina Ratajczak, and Mariusz Z. Ratajczak

INTRODUCTION

Bone marrow (BM) was for many years primarily envisioned as the "home organ" of hematopoietic stem cells (HSC). In this chapter we discuss current views of the BM stem cell compartment and present data showing that BM also contains a heterogeneous population of nonhematopoietic stem cells. These cells have been variously described in the literature as (a) endothelial progenitor cells (EPC),[1,2] (b) mesenchymal stem cells (MSC),[3,4] (c) multipotent adult progenitor cells (MAPC),[5] (d) marrow-isolated adult multilineage inducible (MIAMI) cells,[6] (e) unrestricted somatic stem cells (USSC),[7] and (f) very small embryonic-like (VSEL) stem cells.[8] It is likely that in many cases similar or overlapping populations of primitive stem cells in the BM were detected using different experimental strategies and hence were assigned different names. Unexpectedly, it was found that the BM could also be a potential source of precursors of germ cells (oocytes and spermatogonial cells).[9,10] It is still unclear whether BM contains a pluripotent stem cell (PSC). Several attempts have been made to identify such a cell in the BM that at the single cell level in vitro could give rise to cells from all three germ layers (mesoderm, ectoderm, and endoderm). However, the most valuable evidence for pluripotentiality of the stem cell is its contribution to the development of multiple organs and tissues in vivo after injection into the developing blastocyst.

It is hypothesized that the presence of these various populations of stem cells in the BM is a result of the "developmental migration" of stem cells during ontogenesis and the presence of the permissive environment that attracts these cells to the BM tissue. HSC and nonhematopoietic stem cells are actively chemoattracted by factors secreted by BM stroma cells and osteoblasts (eg, stromal derived factor-1, SDF-1, hepatocyte growth factor, HGF); they colonize marrow by the end of the second and the beginning of the third trimester of gestation.[11–14] Accumulating evidence suggests that these nonhematopoietic stem cells residing in the BM play some role in the homeostasis/turnover of peripheral tissues and, if needed, could be released/mobilized from the BM into circulation during tissue injury and stress, facilitating the regeneration of damaged organs.[15–23]

Below is a brief summary of the developmental hierarchy of the stem cell compartment (Fig. 22–1 and Table 22–1). This serves to clarify terms and presents the currently recommended nomenclature for these cells. Next, the mechanisms that lead to the developmental deposition of versatile populations of stem cells in adult BM are discussed, as are the biological consequences of this phenomenon for physiological tissue turnover and regeneration.

Developmental Hierarchy of the Stem Cell Compartment from the Totipotent Zygote to Bone Marrow-Residing Stem Cells

Stem cells are endowed with the property of self-renewal and the ability to differentiate into cells that are committed to particular developmental pathways. The compartment of stem cells is organized in a hierarchical way from the most primitive (totipotent) to already differentiated tissue-committed (monopotent) stem cells. In this context HSC are an example of monopotent stem cells already committed to lympho/hematopoiesis.

In Fig. 22–1 and Table 22–1, the developmental hierarchy of the stem cell compartment is outlined. It begins with the most primitive totipotent stem cell, the zygote, which is the result of the fusion of two germ cells (oocyte and sperm) during the process of fertilization. As a totipotent stem cell, the zygote is able to give rise to both the embryo and the placenta. The "artificial" counterpart of the totipotent zygote is referred to as a *clonote* and can be created in the laboratory with an experimental approach known as somatic nuclear transfer, involving removal of the nucleus from a somatic cell and its insertion/transfer into an enucleated oocyte.[24,25] The first blastomeres are totipotent stem cells that are derived from the first division of the zygote or clonote. In support of this is the well-known fact that the first blastomeres, if separated from each other, can give rise to two independent embryos,[26] as seen in the case of monozygotic siblings.

When the blastomeres have divided into the 32-cell stage the embryo is known as a morula. Cells which form the morula have already lost their totipotentcy and are now pluripotent. The pluripotent stem cell (PSC) is defined as being able to contribute to the development of the embryo but has lost the capacity to form the trophoblast (which gives rise to the placenta). Thus the term PSC refers to the stem cells that contribute to all three germ layers, mesoderm, ectoderm and endoderm, but not to the trophoblast.

During early embryogenesis, the growing morula develops a central cavity and becomes the blastocyst.[27] A fully developed blastocyst contains cells that are precursors for extraembryonic tissues and a distinct group of cells called the inner cell mass (ICM).[28,29] The cells of the ICM are also pluripotent and can give rise to all three germ layers of the developing embryo.[30,31]

Another potential source of PSC are embryonic germ cells (EG), which are derived ex-vivo from primordial germ cells (PGC).[32–35] Precursors of PGC are the first population of stem cells that can be identified in a mouse model at the beginning of gastrulation in the proximal primitive ectoderm (epiblast), a region adjacent to the extraembryonic ectoderm.[36–38] These founder cells subsequently move through the primitive streak and give rise to several extraembryonic mesodermal lineages and to germ cells. From a developmental point of view, PGC are the most important population of stem cells because as precursors of germ cells (sperm and oocytes) they are responsible for passing genetic information to the next generation.[39,40] However, if isolated from the developing embryo and cultured ex-vivo, these cells are mortal and undergo terminal differentiation.[41]

One explanation for this is the fact that PGC are protected from uncontrolled expansion by epigenetic modification/erasure of the somatic imprint on so-called somatic imprinted genes (eg, H19 and Igf2).[42–47] This process occurs very early during development, at a time when the PGC begin to migrate to the genital ridges[48] and it is one of the basic mechanisms that prevents (a) their uncontrolled proliferation, (b) initiation of potential parthenogenesis, and (c) teratoma formation.[49,50] PGC, however, if plated over murine fetal fibroblasts in the presence of selected growth factors (leukemia inhibitory factor[LIF]; basic fibroblast growth factor [bFGF]; and kit ligand),[51,52] may undergo epigenetic changes when maintained within in vitro culture conditions and regain the somatic imprint (and thus become an immortalized population of PSC, the embryonic germ cells [EG]).[32] EG in many aspects are equivalent to ES cells.[53] Both ES

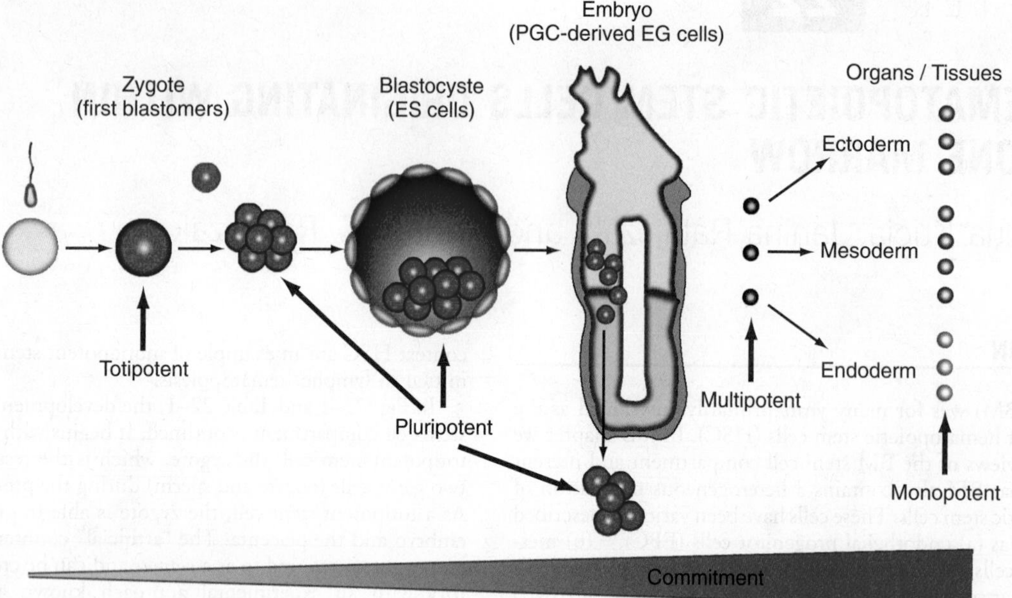

Figure 22–1 Developmental hierarchy of the stem cell compartment. The most primitive stem cell is a totipotent zygote or first blastomere that derives from the first division of the zygote. A totipotent stem cell divides to form both embryo and placenta. Pluripotent stem cells are cells isolated from the inner cell mass (ICM) of a blastocyst or embryonic germ cells (EG) that are in vitro derivatives of primordial germ cells (PGC). These cells contribute to all three germ layers in the developing embryo (ectoderm, mesoderm, and endoderm). Multipotent stem cells give rise to monopotent stem cells that are committed to particular organs/tissues.

Table 22–1 Developmental Hierarchy in Stem Cell (SC) Compartment

Totipotent SC	Give rise to both embryo and placenta. The physiological totipotent stem cell is a fertilized oocyte (zygote) or first blastomere. The artificial counterpart is a clonote obtained by nuclear transfer to an enucleated oocyte.
Pluripotent SC	Give rise to all three germ layers of the embryo after injection to the developing blastocyst. Pluripotent stem cells are cells from the inner cell mass of the blastocyst (ICM), embryonic stem cells (ES), embryonic germ cells (EG) and epiblast-derived stem cells (ESC).
Multipotent SC	Give rise to one of the germ cell layers only, ecto-, meso-, or endoderm.
Monopotent SC	Are tissue-committed stem cells that give rise to cells of one lineage, eg, hematopoietic stem cells, epidermal stem cells, intestinal epithelium stem cells, neural stem cells, liver stem cells, or skeletal muscle stem cells.

Table 22–2 Tissue Contribution of Three Germ Layers

Ectoderm	Brain, sympathetic ganglions, peripheral nerves, eye, epidermis, skin appendices, pigment cells
Mesoderm	Hemato/lymphopoietic cells, endothelium, skeletal muscles, heart, adipocytes, connective tissues (bone, tendon, cartilage), smooth muscles, tubule cells of the kidney
Endoderm	liver, pancreas, lung, gut, thyroid gland

and EG contribute to all three germ layers including the germ cell lineage after injection into a blastocyst. This assay known as blastocyst complementation is a crucial one for confirming in vivo functional pluripotentiality of stem cells.

Next, because during gastrulation three distinct germ layers of cells are established, it is believed that the embryo must possess three stem cell types specific for mesoderm, ectoderm and endoderm. These cells are multipotent stem cells which subsequently give rise to monopotent stem cells specific for tissues/organs that develop from a given germ layer (Table 22–2). For example, multipotent mesodermal stem cells give rise to monopotent hematopoietic, skeletal muscle, heart, endothelial, and mesenchymal tissue-committed stem cells; multipotent endodermal stem cells give rise to monopotent liver, pancreas, and gut epithelium; and ectodermal multipotent stem cells give rise to monopotent brain, peripheral ganglia and nerves, eye, epidermis, and skin tissues.

Looking at this schema of the stem cell developmental hierarchy (Fig. 22–1, summarized in Table 22–1), three questions emerge. First, if the differentiation process is reversible, can monopotent stem cells committed to the given tissue trans-dedifferentiate into other monopotent stem cells? Second, do adult tissues contain, in addition to monopotent tissue-committed stem cells, more primitive populations than pluripotent or multipotent stem cells? Third, if so, are these primitive stem cells, functional not only during ontogenesis but also later on during adult life? These questions are discussed in terms of the BM-derived stem cells.

Bone Marrow Nonhematopoietic Stem Cells—Lessons Learned from the Concept of "Plasticity" of Hematopoietic Stem Cells

Several investigators in the past few years have demonstrated that BM-derived cells can contribute to the regeneration of various organs and tissues.[22,54–62] These observations were mainly explained by the hypothesis that HSC are "plastic" and thus could trans-dedifferentiate into stem cells committed to various nonhematopoietic organs and tissues.[63,64] Occurrence of this phenomenon requires (a) a parallel switch of commitment for HSC in the compartment of monopotent stem cells or (b), as postulated, a step back in the differentiation process of HSC with their dedifferentation into multipotent (one

Table 22–3 Alternative Explanations of the Phenomenon of Trans-Dedifferentiation or Plasticity of HSC

Epigenetic changes	Factors present in the environment of damaged organs induce epigenetic changes in genes that regulate pluripotency of HSC (involvement of changes in DNA methylation, acetylation of histones). More evidence needed that it is a robust and reproducible phenomenon.
Cell fusion	The relatively rare phenomenon by which infused HSC may fuse with cells in damaged tissues and form heterokaryons. Heterokaryons created this way express markers of both donor and recipient cells (pseudochimerism).
Paracrine stimulation	HSC are a source of different trophic and angiopoietic factors that may promote tissue/organ repair.
Microvesicles-dependent transfer of molecules	Some of the plasticity data could be explained by a transient modification of cell phenotype by the transfer of receptors, proteins and mRNA between HSC and damaged cells by membrane-derived microvesicles.
Heterologous population of stem cells in BM	In addition to HSC, BM contains other stem cell populations. Regeneration could be explained by the presence of endothelial progenitors that promote neovasculogenesis and also by the presence of other stem cells including PSC. This could also explain the loss of contribution of BM cells to organ regeneration with use of highly purified populations of HSC.

BM, bone marrow; HSC, hematopoietic stem cells; PSC, pluripotent stem cell.

germ layer-committed) or even pluripotent (three germ layer-committed) stem cells.

This hypothetical possibility that HSC are plastic and able to trans-dedifferentiate raised much hope that HSC isolated from BM, mobilized peripheral blood (mPB) or cord blood (CB) could become a universal source of stem cells for tissue/organ repair. This excitement was bolstered at that time by several reports that demonstrated the remarkable regenerative potential of "HSC" in animal models, for example, after myocardial infarct,[58] stroke,[65] spinal cord injury,[66] and liver damage.[67]

However since these first exciting and promising reports, the role of BM stem cells in the repair of damaged organs has become controversial.[68–70] Further experiments with highly purified populations of HSC showed them not to be effective in regenerating damaged heart[71] or brain.[72] In response to these unexpected results the scientific community became polarized in its view of the concept of stem cell plasticity.

These obvious discrepancies in published results could be explained by differences in the tissue injury models employed and/or problems in detection of tissue chimerism. However, several other possibilities have been proposed to explain these discrepancies (Table 22–3). First, it is possible that, for trans-dedifferentiation of HSC to occur, the appropriate tissue damage models are required which are able to create the permissive "pro-plastic" environment enriched in factors needed to promote this process. Hypothetically such a "permissive" environment could induce epigenetic changes in HSC and thus force them to change lineage commitment.[73,74] Second, it has been postulated that some plasticity data could be explained simply by the phenomenon of cell fusion.[75–79] Accordingly, the donor-derived cells observed in damaged tissues which express nonhematopoietic markers could be in fact heterokaryons, the result of the fusion of BM-derived stem cells with somatic host cells in the damaged organs. Both cell fusion and epigenetic changes, however, are extremely rare and randomly occurring events that certainly could not fully account for all of the positive trans-dedifferentiation data published. Furthermore, fusion as a major contributor to the observed donor-derived chimerism has been excluded in several recently published studies.[80–82]

Another possible explanation of some of the benefits observed in organ/tissue regeneration after infusion of BM-cells is the result of paracrine effects. It is well known that HSC are a source of several trophic cytokines and growth factors and that these factors if released from these cells could promote tissue repair and vascularization.[83] Furthermore, it has been recently shown that cells may transiently modify the phenotype of neighboring cells by transferring surface receptors, intracellular proteins and mRNA by mechanisms that involve exchange of cell-membrane-derived microvesicles.[84,85] Shedding of membrane-derived microvesicles is a physiological phenomenon that accompanies cell growth and cell activation eg, hypoxia or oxidative injury.[86–89] Thus, microvesicle-mediated exchange of receptors, proteins and mRNA between infused BM cells and cells in damaged organs could temporarily modify the phenotype of cells in the damaged organ. An open question is whether microvesicles can also exchange some of the reporter-gene markers employed to detect tissue chimerism (eg, GFP or β-galactosidase).

Surprisingly, during all of these deliberations concerning stem cell plasticity (Table 22–3) and the potential contribution of BM-derived cells to organ regeneration, the concept that BM may contain heterogeneous populations of stem cells was not taken into careful consideration.[69,90] We postulate that regeneration studies demonstrating a contribution of donor-derived BM, mPB or CB cells to nonhematopoietic tissues without addressing this possibility (by including the appropriate controls) has led to misleading interpretations. It is reasonable to assume that the presence of heterogeneous populations of stem cells in BM, mPB, or CB would be considered before experimental evidence is interpreted as examples of plasticity or trans-differentiation of HSC.[91]

Hence the presence of nonhematopoietic stem cells in BM rather than trans-dedifferentiation of HSC, could explain some of the positive results of tissue/organ regeneration as witnessed by several investigators using BM-derived cells.[55,56,67,92] On the other hand, when highly purified HSC were employed for regeneration experiments nonhematopoietic stem cells were likely excluded from these cell preparations. In the current state of knowledge, the phenomenon of trans-dedifferentiation of HSC and their contribution to regeneration of damaged tissues remains questionable.

In summary, the "positive" data supporting stem cell plasticity can be reinterpreted by the assumption that BM-derived stem cells are heterogeneous and that BM tissue contains different types of stem cells including perhaps a rare population of pluripotent stem cells (PSC) (Fig. 22–2). The question remains, however, whether these cells can continuously contribute in adult life to the renewal of other stem cells, including the most numerous population of stem cells in BM, HSC. The mechanisms proposed as responsible for the developmental accumulation of stem cells in BM are discussed below.

Bone Marrow—the Promised Land for Migrating Stem Cells

Early human embryogenesis is the most active period for the developmental migration/trafficking of stem cells. With the beginning of gastrulation and organogenesis, stem cells migrate to places where they establish rudiments for new tissues and organs. Thus at certain points of development, stem cells colonize tissue-specific niches, where they reside as a population of self-renewing cells. These cells supply new cells that effectively replace senescent ones or those undergoing apoptosis. Therefore the role of monopotent tissue residing stem cells during adult life is restricted mainly to cell turnover proper in a given organ or tissue.

The first population of stem cells that are identifiable in the early embryo in the proximal ectoderm (epiblast) are precursors of the PGC already mentioned.[93,94] These cells are endowed from the beginning with robust migratory properties.[95,96] Microscopic analysis of the

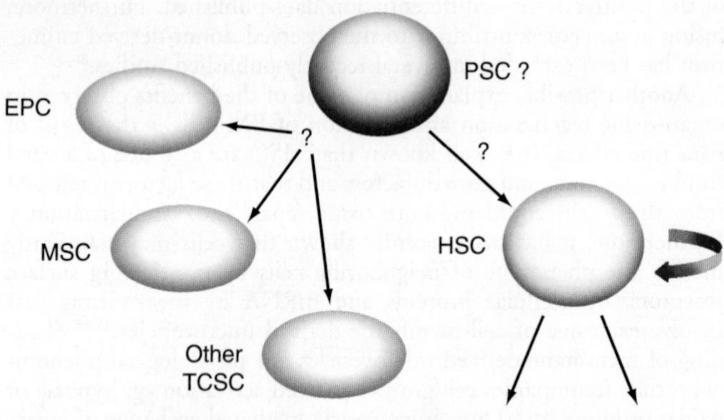

Figure 22–2 Versatile populations of stem cells in bone marrow (BM). BM is traditionally the home of self-renewing hematopoietic stem cells (HSC). BM also contains a small admixture of several nonhematopoietic stem cells such as endothelial progenitor cells (EPC), mesenchymal stem cells (MSC), and perhaps other tissue-committed stem cells (TCSC). The open question is whether BM contains pluripotent stem cells (PSC) and these cells are functional and able to supply all other types of stem cell in BM.

early murine embryo has revealed that by 7.25 days postconception, a distinct cluster of approximately 50 PGC is present at the base of the allantois in the extraembryonic mesoderm close to an area known as the primitive streak.[36] From this place, PGC begin to migrate through the embryo proper towards the gonadal anlagen or genital ridges.[97] Because PGC express the seven-transmembrane span G-protein coupled CXCR4, and because its specific ligand α-chemokine SDF-1 is already expressed in the developing genital ridges, the SDF-1-CXCR4 axis plays a pivotal role in PGC migration and colonization of the developing gonads.[98–101]

It has been proposed that around the same time as PGC are present in the area close to the primitive streak a population of hemangioblasts becomes specified in the same region of the developing embryo.[102,103] Shortly after this in mammals the first primitive HSC are found in the yolk sac and the first definitive HSC can be identified a few days later in the paraaortic splanchnopleura, the aorta-gonad-mesonephros (AGM) region.[104–108] Interestingly, the AGM region is a crossroads through which a population of CXCR4+ PGC migrates to the genital ridges chemoattracted by SDF-1.[96] This association of PGC specification and the appearance of hemangioblasts in the primitive streak and primitive HSC in the yolk sac followed by definitive HSC in the AGM region during the migration of PGC to the genital ridges through the embryo proper gave rise to the hypothesis that PGC could differentiate into HSC and thus could be potential precursors of HSC in the developing embryo.[109,110] This interesting idea, however, requires further study.

Subsequently, HSC from the yolk sac and/or AGM region migrate to the fetal liver which during the second trimester of gestation becomes the major mammalian hematopoietic organ.[111] By the end of the second trimester HSC leave this organ and colonize BM tissue.[106] Signals for the translocation of HSC from the fetal liver to BM are again provided again by SDF-1, which are now being highly secreted by osteoblasts lining the developing marrow cavities, marrow fibroblasts and endothelial cells.[11,12,112] In response to an SDF-1 gradient, CXCR4+ HSC leave the fetal liver and began to home into BM where they finally establish adult hematopoiesis.

It is likely that during these early stages of development the fetal liver and BM are also colonized by other stem cell types that may circulate during organogenesis and rapid body growth/expansion. First, it is possible that during early development epiblast-derived CXCR4+ cells closely related to a population of PGC are deposited in the tissues or even CXCR4+ PGC themselves go astray while migrating through the AGM region to the genital ridges and, together with definitive HSC, follow the same SDF-1 gradient and seed to the fetal liver, subsequently colonizing the BM and perhaps other tissues as well (Fig. 22–3). In support of this hypothesis studies in turtles[113] and more importantly in small and large mammals[114,115] have revealed that during migration to the genital ridges some PGC may stray from the main migration stream and become deposited in various tissues. It is also likely that Oct-4+ cells that were recently identified in several adult organs and tissues could be related to this population of stem cells.[9,10,116–124] Based on this it is possible that the population of Oct-4+ SSEA-1+ CXCR4+ VSEL stem cells recently isolated from adult hematopoietic organs including BM, spleen and thymus are closely related to epiblast-derived cells or migrating PGC that went astray.[8]

Furthermore, it is possible that during later phases of embryogenesis other migrating/circulating stem cells similar to epiblast-derived cells may colonize BM. Supporting this is the fact that all monopotent tissue-committed stem cells (eg, endothelial, neural, skeletal muscle, liver oval, renal tubular endothelium, retina pigment epithelium stem cells) express CXCR4 on their surface and follow an SDF-1 gradient[125–134] thus potentially being able to "home" to the BM. The SDF-1-CXCR4 axis alone or in combination with other chemoattractants could play a crucial role in accumulation of nonhematopoietic stem cells in BM. These cells find a permissive environment in the BM that allows them to survive into adulthood.

It is possible that these BM-residing nonhematopoietic stem cells could play a role as a reserve pool of circulating stem cells for organ/tissue regeneration during postnatal life. Fig. 22–4 shows a schema of stem cell circulation in postnatal life that is supported by several observations.[2,15,16,18,135,136] CXCR4+ HSC, EPC, MSC, skeletal muscle satellite, liver oval, neural, and other monopotent stem cells circulate at low levels in the PB to maintain stem cell pools in distant parts of the body and compete for SDF-1-positive niches in various organs.[15,16,18,21,133] It is also likely that, in addition to these cells, even more primitive PSC (VSEL?) could be released from BM and other tissue niches to circulate in the PB. The number of these cells in the PB increases during tissue damage or pharmacological mobilization.

Further study is required to identify the chemoattractants, besides SDF-1, released from damaged tissues and able to mobilize and chemoattract these cells to these tissues.[17,20,133,137,138] It is postulated that BM, as a source of many stem-cell chemoattractants and survival factors, provides an environment that encourages circulating CXCR4+ tissue-committed stem/progenitor cells to home there.

In this context BM tissue becomes a "home" not only of HSC but also of already differentiated circulating CXCR4+ tissue-committed stem/progenitor cells and more primitive CXCR4+ PSC (VSEL). These cells reside in BM and could play an important role in tissue/organ repair as a mobile reserve pool of tissue-committed stem/progenitor cells. This concept will be discussed in more detail later in this chapter.

Evidence of the Heterogeneity of Bone Marrow Stem Cells

The concept that BM may contain some nonhematopoietic stem cells has been postulated by several investigators and, as previously mentioned, the best evidence that BM stem cells are in fact heterogeneous was provided by experiments showing that BM-derived cells could support the regeneration of various tissues/organs.[69,90,139]

Table 22–4 lists different types of nonhematopoietic stem cells that have been postulated to reside in BM tissue. These cells will be discussed below, and the similarities between these versatile populations of stem cells indicated. It is very likely that several investigators using different isolation strategies described the same populations of stem cells but gave them different names according to circumstance.

Endothelial Progenitor Cell (EPC)

The identification in the BM and PB of cells with endothelial progenitor activities has generated considerable interest in the role of

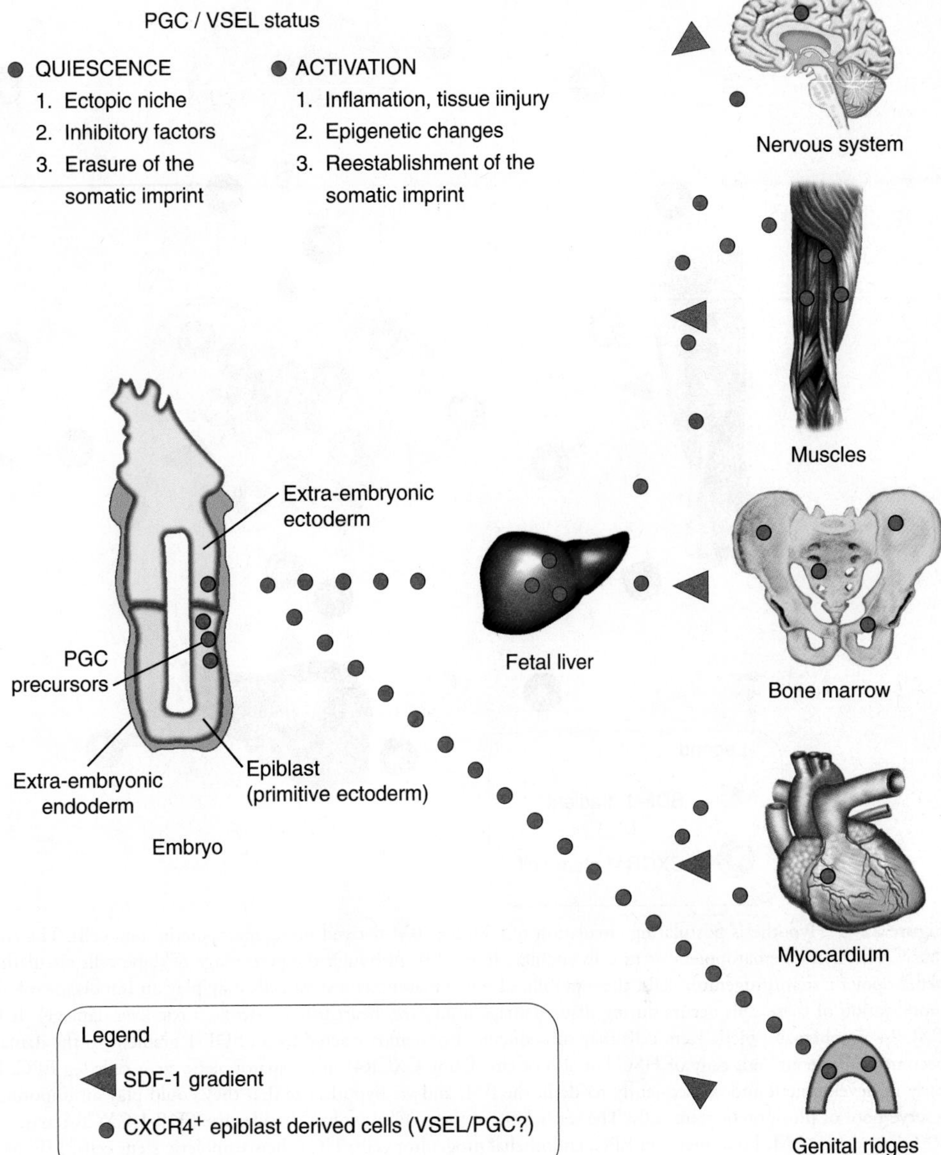

Figure 22–3 Hypothesis of developmental deposition of Oct-4+ epiblast-derived embryonic stem cells (VSELs?) in adult tissues.The presence of Oct-4+ stem cells in the fetal liver, BM and other tissues could be explained by the developmental deposition in different organs (mainly BM) of CXCR4+ epiblast derived stem cells (eg, VSELs) that follow an SDF-1 gradient. The potential relationship of these cells to early epiblast/primordial germ cells (PGC) requires further investigation.

these cells during the maintenance and repair of blood vessels.[140,141] From a historical point of view the close relationship between hematopoiesis and vasculogenesis was postulated almost 2000 years ago by Aristotle. This ancient Greek philosopher came to the conclusion based on his empirical work on development that the heart along with blood vessels were the first structures to appear during embryogenesis in eggs from different species. This notion now appears especially significant because it implies that the heart and the blood have a common origin. Translated into today's language, this means that both descend from a common endothelial and hematopoietic progenitor, the putative hemangioblast in the embryonic mesoderm.[102,103,105] Hemangioblast activity was demonstrated to exist in embryoid bodies formed by embryonic stem cells in in vitro cultures.[142] However, whether hemangioblasts persist in adult life and reside in the adult BM, is not yet clear.[143–145]

Nevertheless, adult BM-derived cells have been shown to contain endothelial precursors in both mice and humans.[1,141] The possible role of these cells in the hierarchy of BM-derived stem/progenitor cells and their potential relationship to PSC and hemangioblasts is shown in Fig. 22–5, panel A. Accumulating evidence suggests that the BM may contain a population of EPCs residing in BM tissues that could be released/mobilized into PB as a source of cells able to play a role in the vascularization of damaged organs.[2,146–148] The phenotype of these cells is shown in Table 22–4. Recently it has been suggested that these cells also express CXCR4 and can be mobilized from the BM.[149–151] While circulating in peripheral blood, they are following an SDF-1 gradient that is deployed at sites of tissue/organ injury, and the ultimate result may be tissue regeneration.

To confirm that BM is a source of endothelial cells, murine HSC ($Kit^+Sca1^+lin^-$ were transplanted into lethally irradiated mice, with the result that these animals were subsequently found to have donor-derived endothelial cells in many tissues, including liver, lung, muscle, gut and heart.[152] Furthermore, a phenotypic and functional evaluation of human HSC subsets revealed that $CD34^+$, KDR^+ (VEGF-R2) HSC can generate both hematopoietic and endothelial cells in vitro and human BM-derived $CD34^+$ cells transplanted into immunodeficient mice can give rise to neovascularization in a retinal ischemia model.[153] Studies in allogeneic sex-mismatched hematopoietic transplants in humans revealed the presence of 2% of donor-derived endothelial cells in the skin and gut.[154] However, although in some experimental models a robust contribution of BM-derived cells in neovascularization was demonstrated, using sophisticated cell-marking strategies other studies indicated that marrow-derived EPC may play minimal or no role in neovasculariza-

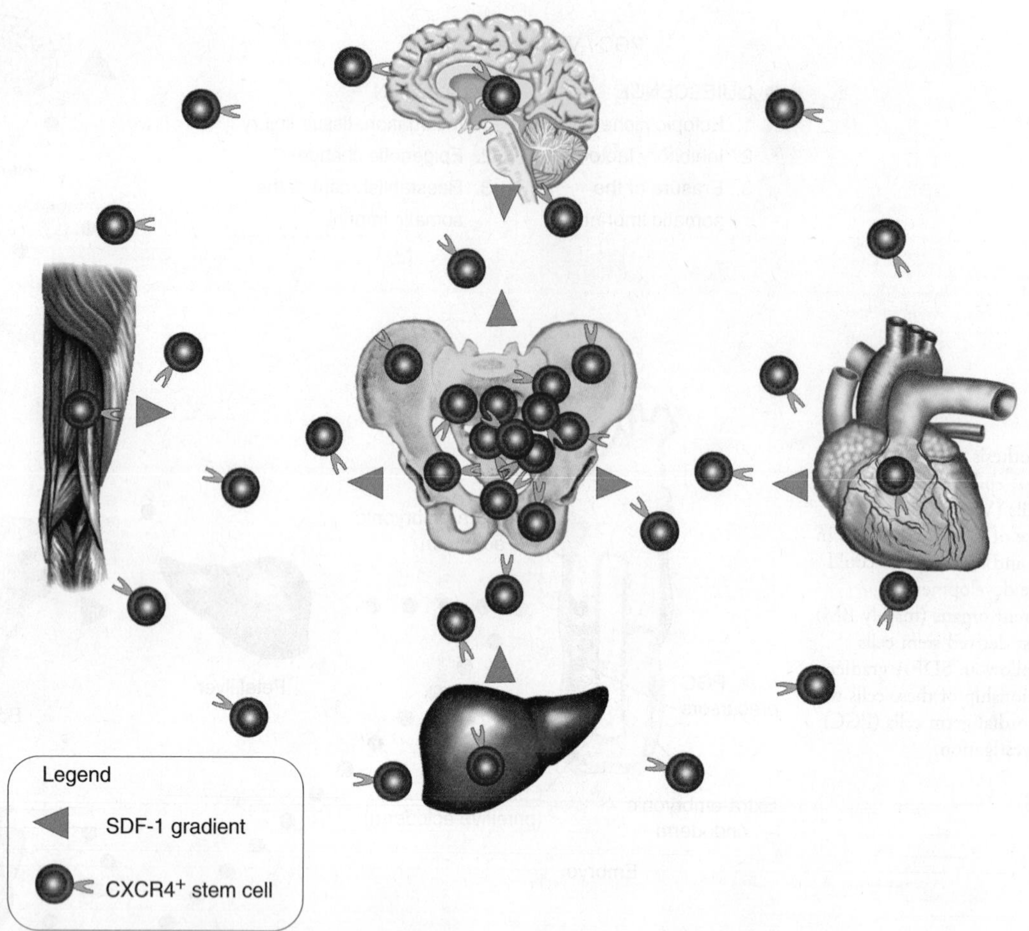

Figure 22–4 Hypothesis postulating circulation of CXCR4+ BM-derived nonhematopoietic stem cells. The concept is presented based on the assumption that CXCR4+ nonhematopoietic stem cells circulate in the PB. Although the percentage of these cells circulating in PB is much lower than that of early hematopoietic stem/progenitor cells, these mobilized nonhematopoietic stem cells may play an important role in tissue repair following injury. The mobilization of these cells occurs during tissue damage/injury (eg, heart infarct, stroke, toxic liver damage). It is postulated that after mobilization into PB CXCR4+ nonhematopoietic stem cells may subsequently be chemoattracted by an SDF-1 gradient to the damaged tissues. In this context BM tissue becomes a "hideout" not only of HSC but also of circulating CXCR4+ nonhematopoietic stem cells (eg EPC, MSC, or VSELs). These cells are deposited early in development and consequently reside in the BM, and we hypothesize that they could play an important role in tissue/organ repair as a mobile reserve pool of pluripotent stem cells. The trafficking of these cells involves, besides the SDF-1-CXCR4 axis, several other motomorphogens such as HGF, VEGF, and LIF. BM, bone marrow; EPC, endothelial progenitor cells; HGF, hematopoietic stem cells; LIF; MSC, mesenchymal stem cells; PB, peripheral blood; VSELs, very small embryonic-like stem cells.

tion of tumors, vessel repair, or normal vessel growth and development.[155,156]

Nevertheless, it was postulated that EPC, which is a rare and very primitive founder population of endothelial cells, may be released during stressed situations and circulate in PB.[1,83,157] Furthermore, BM was also identified as a source of more differentiated circulating endothelial cells (CEC).[2,158] It is not clear whether these cells (Fig. 22–5, panel A) are direct progeny of EPC or can arise from a well-defined population of myeloid lineage-restricted BM progenitors.[159,160] In support of this latter possibility, a recent report has shown that in fact CEC differentiate both from common myeloid progenitors (CMP) and the more mature granulocyte/macrophage progenitors (GMP).[160] In addition, endothelial cells derived from transplanted BM-derived myeloid progenitors expressed CD31, von Willebrand factor and Tie-2 and were CD45−.[152,160] Thus BM-derived CEC probably reside outside the stem cell population consistent with the hypothesis that CEC arise from differentiated progeny of HSC (Fig. 22–5, panel A).

To summarize, it is postulated that the BM is endowed with neoangiogenetic activity and BM in steady state is a source of EPC and CEC that subsequently circulate in PB at very low levels (0.0001% and 0.01%, respectively) and may play a role in the repair of damaged endothelium and contribute to postnatal neoangiogenesis.[161] Although EPC are probably progeny of PSC or perhaps direct descendants of hemangioblasts, the more differentiated CEC originate in the myeloid compartment from a common myeloid progenitor (CMP). The level of contribution of BM-derived cells to organ/tissue vascularization, however, still requires further study.

Mesenchymal Stem Cells (Multipotent Mesenchymal Stromal Cells)

Mesenchymal stem cells (MSC) were identified 40 years ago by Fridenstein as a population of BM-derived adherent bone/cartilage-forming progenitor cells.[162] It was known at the time that BM-adherent cells generate in vitro colonies of fibroblastic-like cells which have a high replating potential.[163] At the same time, it was postulated that among these colonies are some progenitor cells that can generate new fibroblastic colonies and such cells were assigned a functional name, colony-forming units of fibroblasts (CFU-F).[164] If plated at a low density CFU-F grow distinct colonies of spindle-forming cells whereas, by contrast, if they are plated at high a concentration they rapidly establish confluent cell cultures. Of particular interest, if CFU-F-derived cells are implanted in the subrenal capsule or are

Table 22–4 Nonhematopoietic Stem Cells Described in Bone Marrow

Stem Cells	Phenotype
Endothelial Progenitor cells (EPC)	Human: CD133+, CD34+, c-kit (CD117)+, VE-cadherin+, VEGFR2+, CD146+, vWF+, CD31+ Mice: Sca-1+, c-Kit (CD117)+, Lin−, VEGFR2+, VE-cadherin+, Tie2+, CD146+, vWF+, CD31+
Mesenchymal Stem Cells (MSC)*	International Society for Cellular Therapy criteria: CD105+, CD73+, CD90+, CD45−, CD34−, CD14−, CD11b−, CD79a−, CD19−, HLA-DR− Additional markers: Stro-1+, SB-10+ (CD166), SH-2+ (epitope on CD105), SH-3+ (epitope on CD73), SH-4+ (epitope on CD73), CD44+, CD29+, CD31−, vWF− Markers of most primitive MSC: CXCR4, CD133, CD34 (?), p75LNGFR
Multipotent Adult Progenitor Cells (MAPC)*	SSEA-1+, CD13+, Flk-1low, Thy-1low, CD34−, CD44−, CD45−, CD117(c-kit)−, MHC I−, MHC II−
Marrow-isolated Adult Multilineage Inducible Cells (MIAMI)*	CD29+, CD63+, CD81+, CD122+, CD164+, c-met+, BMPR1B+, NTRK3+, CD34−, CD36−, CD45−, CD117 (c-kit)−, HLA-DR−
Unrestricted Somatic Stem Cells (USSC) found in cord blood*	CD13+, CD29+, CD44+, CD49e+, CD90+, CD105+, vimentin+, cytokeratin (CK8/18)+, CD10low, Flk-1low, HLA-Ilow, CD14−, CD33−, CD34−, CD45−, CD49 (b, c, d, f)−, CD50−, CD62 (E, L, P)−, CD106−, c-kit (CD117)−, glycophorin−, DLA-DR−
Very Small Embryonic-Like (VSEL) Stem Cells	CXCR4+, CD133+, CD34+, SSEA-1+ (mouse), SSEA-4+ (human), AP+, c-met+, LIF-R+, CD45−, Lin−, HLA-DR−, MHC I−, CD90−, CD29−, CD105−

*phenotype of expanded/cultured adherent cells.
AP, fetal alkaline phosphatase; BMPR1B, bone morphogenetic protein receptor 1B; c-met, receptor for hepatocyte growth factor; LIF-R, receptor for leukemia inhibitory factor; NTRK3, neurotropic tyrosine kinase receptor 3; vWF, von Willebrand factor.

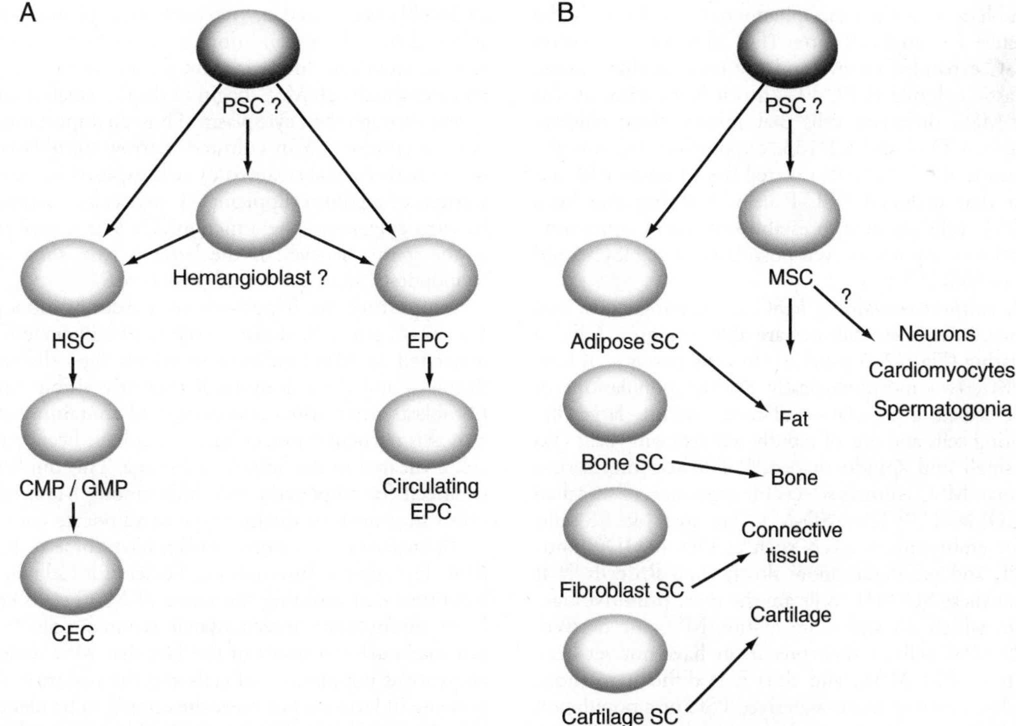

Figure 22–5 Origin of BM-derived EPC and MSC. **(A)** Endothelial progenitor cells (EPC) originate in the BM from the hemangioblast or the even more primitive pluripotent stem cells (PSC). These rare cells may be released from the BM and circulate in the PB (circulating EPC). Another fraction of circulating endothelial cells (CEC) derives directly from descendants of HSC which are common myeloid progenitors (CMP) or granulocyto-monocytic progenitors (GMP). **(B)** MSC are precursors for fat, bone, connective tissues and cartilage. However, it is very likely that separate monopotent stem cells exist for these tissues. The possibility of trans-differentiation of MSC into neurons, cardiomyocytes, and spermatogonia is not clear at this point and requires further studies. BM, bone marrow; MSC, mesenchymal stem cells; PB, peripheral blood.

cultured in differentiating media they are able to accumulate fat and calcium phosphate and grow ectopic bone fragments. Similarly, if they are cultured as a bulk mass in the presence of transforming growth factor (TGF)-β they are able to differentiate into chondrocytes.[165]

It is now widely accepted that MSC cells (Fig. 22–5, panel B) contribute to the regeneration of mesenchymal tissues (eg, bone, cartilage, muscle, ligament, tendon, adipose, and stroma).[166,167] At this point, however, we cannot exclude the possibility that monopotent stem cells specific for all of these tissues exist (Fig. 22–5, panel B). MSC are essential in forming the hematopoietic microenvironment in which HSC grow and differentiate.[166,168,169] In fact it is well known that fresh passages of unpurified MSC always contain a hidden population of HSC.[170] Thus in LTCIC assays, BM-derived stroma cells have to be irradiated before the HSC are plated, not only to inhibit the growth of MSC, but also to eliminate contaminating HSC, which could change conditions for the exogenous HSC to be assayed. However, it is likely that MSC, as well as HSC, may be contaminated by other populations of primitive nonhematopoietic stem cells. This possibility should be considered whenever a trans-dedifferentiation of MSC into cells from other germ layers is demonstrated. Interestingly, MSC engraft very poorly in the BM of recipients of hematopoietic transplants. However, recently a significant degree of chimerism for BM stroma was demonstrated following hematopoietic transplants in pediatric patients.[171]

MSC express several surface markers that could be used for their isolation (Table 22–4), including most importantly Stro-1, SB-10, SH-2, SH-3, SH-4, CD44, CD29, and CD90.[172] They do not express classical hematopoietic (CD34, CD45, CD14) and endothelial markers (CD34, CD31, vWF).[3,173,174] Interestingly some of the MSC were found to express CXCR4 and c-Met receptors and thus may respond to SDF-1 and HGF/SF gradients.[175–177]

The major problem with the exact phenotyping of MSC is the fact that fluorescence activated cell sorter (FACS) analysis is always performed on MSC expanded ex-vivo and not on cells that initiate growth of fibroblastic colonies (CFU-F). Thus it is not clear at this point if the rare MSC precursor cells that initiate these cultures express, for example, CD34 and CD133. Supporting this was the finding of populations of $CD34^+$ cells isolated from human BM and murine fetal liver that included CFU-F cells.[178] It has also been reported that $CD34^+$ cells are able to establish colonies containing BM fibroblasts and recently it was even postulated that HSC could be the precursors of MSC.[179]

As mentioned, cultures containing MSC are heterogenous, and not all the cells present in these cultures are able to regrow CFU-F colonies after replating (Fig. 22–6 panel A). In early passages of low-density plated MSC, two morphologically distinct populations of cells have been described, a population of more mature, large, flat and slowly replicating cells and one of rapidly self-renewing cells (RS cells) which are small and spindle-shaped.[180] Furthermore, serum deprivation of human MSC cultures selects for expansion of so-called serum-deprived (SD) MSC.[181] These SD-MSC are small like RS cells, express mRNA for embryonic markers such as Oct-4, ODC antizyme, and hTERT, and proliferate more slowly than RS cells.[181] It was postulated that these SD-MSC cells are the most primitive fraction of MSC from which RS and more mature MSC are derived. Unfortunately, SD-MSC cells or their precursors have not yet been directly purified from BM MNC and thus it is difficult to judge whether they are derivatives of marrow-derived PSC or a population of MSC that undergoes epigenetic changes caused by the serum-deprived in vitro culture conditions. Nevertheless, these data indicate that cultures containing growing MSC are heterogeneous and contain fibroblastic-like cells at different levels of commitment and maturation.

An unexpected discovery made in recent studies has been that MSC are able to differentiate across germ-layers and give rise to neuronal cells or cardiomyocytes (Fig. 22–5, panel B).[182–186] These phenomena were recently called into question in particular for neural differentiation of MSC,[187] caused by the possibility of some in vitro artifacts.[188,189] Morphological changes of MSC may be induced during their culture by the addition of some components that are included in neural-differentiating media eg, β-mercaptoethanol, dimethylsulfoxide, and butylated hydroxyanisole. Fibroblasts cultured in these conditions could mimic neurons, but in fact it proved to be only an in vitro morphological artifact.[188] These observations raise the question of how much culture conditions may influence the phenotype of MSC, during, for example, osteogenic or adipose differentiation of MSC. Accordingly, MSC cultured in vitro may accumulate special media supplements, for example, calcium phosphate and lipids, according to their osteoblastic or adipocytic differentiation, respectively.

Further work is also needed to explain the actual contribution of MSC to the regeneration of skeleton.[190–193] Relevant to this is evidence suggesting that BM may contain a separate type of monopotent stem cell committed to the skeleton that is distinct from BM-derived MSC.[194] In a recently published paper reporting on the transplantation of BM-derived cells in children suffering from osteogenesis imperfecta, it was suggested that these osteoblastic monopotent stem cells and not marrow fibroblasts were in fact responsible for some of the beneficial therapeutic effects seen.[195] In this context it is not clear whether the process of calcium phosphate accumulation in MSC cultured in high concentrations of ascorbic acid, β-glycerophosphate and dexamethasone is related to the real differentiation process initiated in the stem cell compartment, or is merely an effect of phenotypical changes of fibroblastic cells induced by the in vitro culture conditions.[172] The reported evidence for the presence of an osteoblastic stem cell that resides in BM and differs from the MSC mentioned above, supports this latter concept.

Likewise it is not clear whether accumulation of fat in MSC growing in media containing a cocktail of dexamethasone, isobutyl methyl xanthine, and indomethacin could result from lipoid degeneration of fibroblasts cultured in vitro.[172] The accumulation of lipids in fibroblasts cultured ex-vivo could be explained by fat accumulation induced by culture conditions and not by a process initiated at the level of stem cell differentiation for adipose tissue. In these types of cultures usually all MSC begin to display small lipid droplets that are spread through their cytoplasm. Thus, an important question emerges: is fat accumulation in cultured marrow fibroblasts merely an effect of the pathological steatosis of cells exposed in vitro to high concentrations of medium supplements such as hydrocortisone, or is this an in vitro epigenetic phenomenon? Or is it a process that is initiated at the stem cell level? If the latter is true, then is there a separate monopotent stem cell for adipose tissue?

Supporting the hypothesis of a distinct monopotent stem cell, Fig. 22–6, panel B, shows a colony of adipocyte-like cells that were generated in MSC cultures in which the cells contain large lipid droplets, and the colony itself is clearly visible among BM-derived fibroblasts as a distinct cluster of lipid-containing cells. This suggests that this particular rare colony could have been generated by a stem cell dedicated to the adipocyte lineage. This implies that a primitive stem cell for adipocytes may hide among MSC cells and that such cells can generate a distinct type of adipocyte colony.

Because various inconsistencies have come to light in the field of MSC biology, the International Society for Cellular Therapy recently recommended avoiding the name of MSC stem cells and changing it to multipotent mesenchymal stromal cells.[196] This change in nomenclature is a result of the fact that MSC cultures contain heterogeneous populations of cells and the majority of fibroblastic cells growing in vitro do not meet the criteria to be identified as stem cells (Fig. 22–6 panel A). This name should be reserved for a small population of cells, closely related to CFU-F, RS, or SD cells. More importantly, the abbreviation for mesenchymal stromal cells, MSC remains the same as for mesenchymal stem cells, allowing literature searches using both names.

In addition, the Mesenchymal and Tissue Stem Cell Committee of the International Society for Cellular Therapy proposed minimal criteria to define human MSC.[197] First, MSC must be plastic-adherent when maintained in standard culture conditions. Second, MSC must express CD105, CD73, and CD90 and lack expression of CD45, CD34, CD14 or CD11b, CD79α or CD19, and HLA-DR

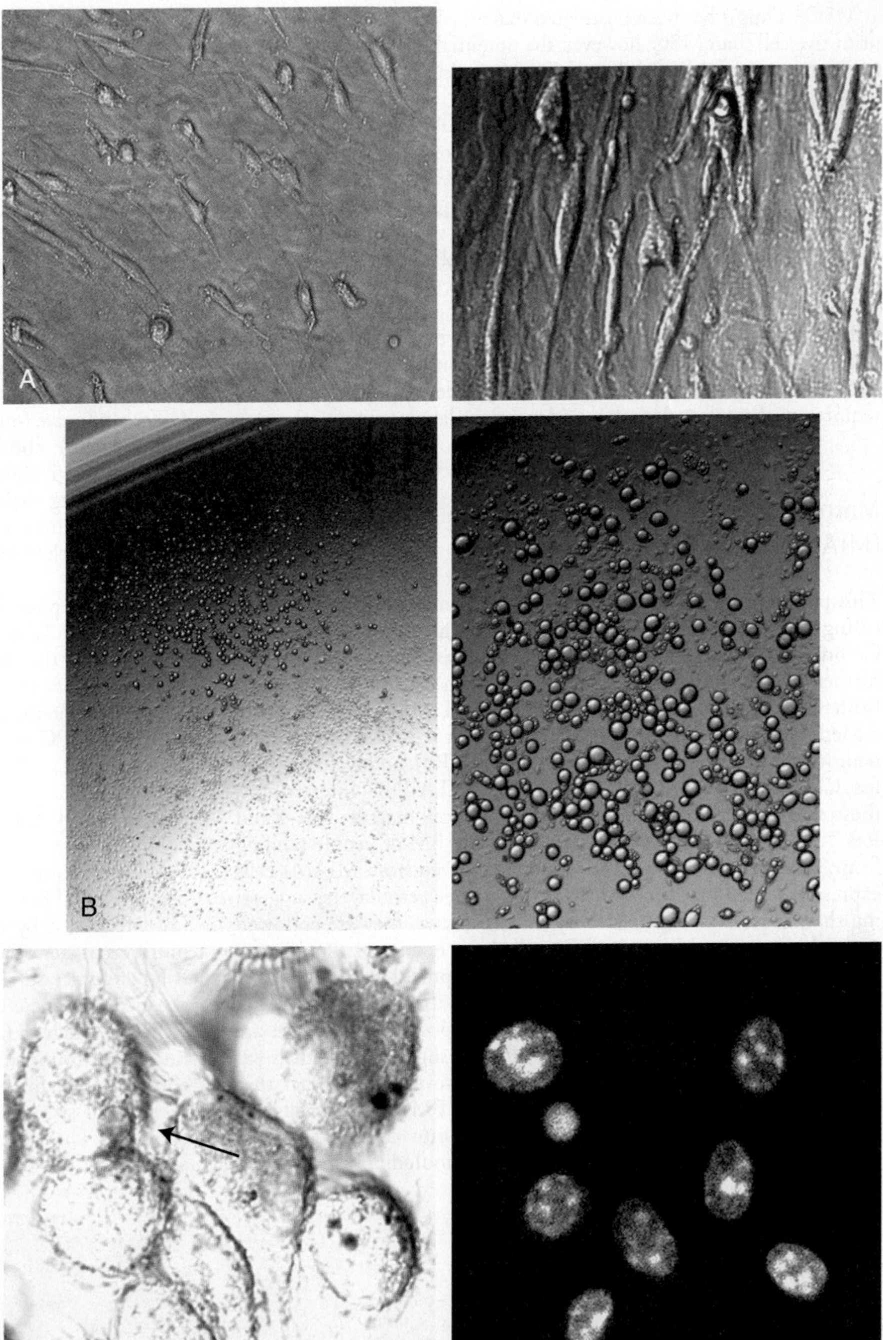

Figure 22–6 Controversies about MSC. **(A)** Low-power and high-power pictures of MSC growing in vitro. These cells look heterogeneous and possess a fibroblast-like morphology. **(B)** A distinct colony containing adipocytes, formed probably by monopotent adipocytic stem cells. Low power (*left*) and high power (*right*). **(C)** *Left:* Confocal analysis of MSC cultures reveals the presence of a very small cell hiding between fibroblastic cells. *Right:* DNA staining of nuclei of cells in these cultures confirms the presence of a small cell hiding among MSC. MSC, mesenchymal stem cells. (VSEL?)

surface molecules. Third, MSC must differentiate into osteoblasts, adipocytes, and chondroblasts in vitro (Fig. 22–5 panel B). This minimal set of standard criteria should foster a more uniform characterization of MSC and facilitate the exchange of data among investigators.[197]

Finally, there are recent reports that a subpopulation of undifferentiated MSC expanded from BM adherent cells could express embryonic stem cell and PSC markers such as Oct-4 and Rex1 or Oct-4 and Nanog.[198] The relationship of these undifferentiated MSC with other populations of putative PSC described in BM requires further study. It is very likely that similar/overlapping populations of stem cells were isolated by employing different strategies and hence assigned different names. Of note, MSC so far have not been shown to be able to complete blastocyst development, and thus they do not fulfill the complete criteria for a pluripotent stem cell.

Furthermore, the reported robust contribution of MSC in regeneration of damaged organs in vivo could be explained by the paracrine effects of these cells affecting angiogenesis in damaged tissues rather than a direct contribution of MSC to supplying tissue-specific functional cells for organ regeneration. Also to be considered is the notion that MSC could serve as scaffolds during regeneration of damaged tissues. Finally, this controversial yet interesting cell type can be successfully employed to modulate Graft-versus host-disease (GvHD) and enhance engraftment in patients after hematopoietic transplants.[171,199]

Multipotent Adult Progenitor Cells (MAPC)

MAPC have been isolated from BM MNC as a population of $CD45^-$ $GPA\text{-}A^-$ adherent cells and display a similar fibroblastic morphology as MSC.[5] Thus it has been postulated that an MAPC could be a more primitive cell than MSC; however, the potential relationship between MSC, in particular RS-MSC and SD-MSC cells and MAPC has yet to be established.

The colonies of cells enriched in murine MAPC express low levels of FLK-1, Sca-1, and CD90, and higher levels of CD13 and SSEA-1.[5] They are also negative for the expression of CD34, CD44, CD45, CD117, and MHC class I and class II.[5,200] The growth of these rare cells depends on selected serum batches and is tightly regulated by oxygen tension. This could explain why several laboratories have had difficulty in establishing cultures of MAPC.

Interestingly MAPC are the only population of BM-derived stem cells that, so far as is known, contribute to all three germ layers after injection into a developing blastocyst, indicating their pluripotency.[5] The contribution of MAPC to blastocyst development, however, requires confirmation by other, independent laboratories.

Marrow-Isolated Adult Multilineage Inducible (MIAMI) Cells

This population of cells was isolated from human adult BM by culturing BM MNC in low oxygen tension conditions on fibronectin.[6] Colonies of small adherent cells were subsequently isolated and further expanded on fibronectin, at low oxygen tension. Cells derived from these cultures expressed CD29, CD63, CD81, CD122, CD164, c-Met, bone morphogenetic protein receptor 1B (BMPR1B), and neurotrophic tyrosine kinase receptor 3 (NTKR3), and were negative for CD34, CD36, CD45, CD117, and HLA-DR. Interestingly, these cells also expressed the embryonic stem cell markers Oct-4 and Rex-1.[201] MIAMI cells were isolated from the BM of people ranging from 3 years to 72 years of age. Colonies derived from MIAMI cells expressed several markers for cells from all three germ layers, suggesting that, at least as determined by in vitro assays, they are endowed with pluripotency. However, these cells have not been tested so far for their ability to complete blastocyst development.

The potential relationship of these cells to MSC and MAPC described above is not clear, although it is possible that these are overlapping populations of cells identified by slightly different isolation/expansion strategies. Lending credence to this is the fact that MIAMI cells are derived from a population of BM-adherent cells like MSC or MAPC and can also differentiate into cells that express markers unique to osteoblasts, chondrocytes and adipocytes.

Unrestricted Somatic Stem Cells (USSC)

Neonatal cord blood (CB) is an important source of nonhematopoietic stem cells. It is well known that CB-derived cells contribute to skeletal muscle,[202,203] liver,[204–206] neural tissue,[61,207] and myocardium regeneration;[208,209] and more importantly, recent multiorgan engraftment and differentiation has been achieved in goats after transplantation of human CB CD34$^+$ in$^-$ cells.[210] Generally, we can envision CB as neonatal PB mobilized by the stress related to delivery. Release of several cytokines and growth factors, as well as hypoxic conditions during labor, may mobilize neonatal marrow cells into circulation. For this reason it is very likely that the population of USSC cells identified in CB originates in neonatal BM.[7]

USSC are very rare cells that are detectable in ~40% of CB units at a frequency 1 to 11 cells/CB unit.[7] These cells were identified in CB as a putative founder cell population that is able to grow adherent colonies with fibroblastic morphology and is present among CB-derived CD45$^-$ adherent cells. USSC can be expanded to 10^{15} cells without losing their potential to differentiate into a variety of cells. In vitro cultures USSC showed homogenous differentiation into osteoblasts, chondroblasts, adipocytes, hematopoietic, and neural cells.

The exact phenotype of cells isolated from USSC-derived colonies is shown in Table 22–4. Unfortunately, the markers which are expressed on the founder cells for these colonies are not described. Further studies are needed to purify USSC and compare these cells with other potentially pluripotent stem cells that could be present in CB (eg, MAPC or, as described next, VSELs).

Very Small Embryonic-Like (VSEL) Stem Cells

Recently a homogenous population of rare (~0.01% of BM MNC) Sca-1$^+$ lin$^-$ CD45$^-$ cells was identified in murine BM. They express (as determined by RQ-PCR and immunhistochemistry) markers of pluripotent stem cells such as SSEA-1, Oct-4, Nanog and Rex-1 and Rif-1 telomerase protein.[8] Direct electron microscopical analysis revealed that these cells display several features typical of embryonic stem cells such as (a) a small size (2–4 μm in diameter), (b) a large nucleus surrounded by a narrow rim of cytoplasm, and (c) open-type chromatin (euchromatin) (Fig. 22–7). Interestingly, these cells despite their small size posses diploid DNA and contain numerous mitochondria. They do not express MHC-1 and HLA-DR antigens and are CD90$^-$ CD105$^-$ CD29$^-$ For the first time a sorting procedure

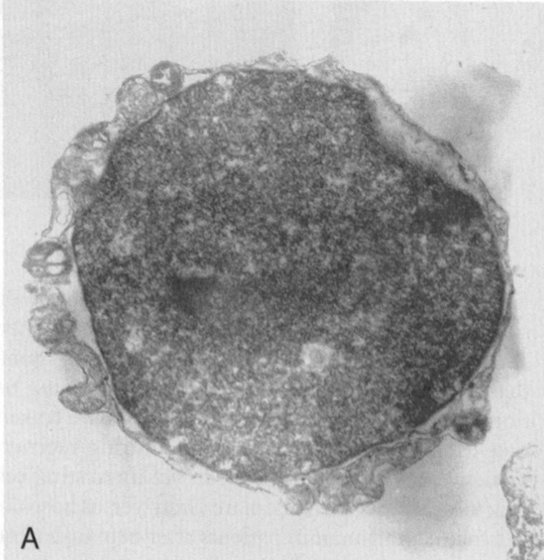

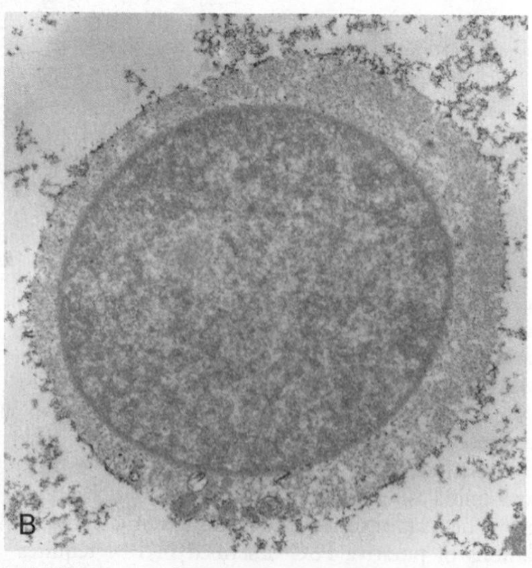

Figure 22–7 TEM of Sca-1$^+$Lin$^-$CD45$^-$ VSEL stem cells. **(A)** Murine BM-derived VSEL stem cells are small, measuring 2–4 μm in diameter. They possess a relatively large nucleus surrounded by a narrow rim of cytoplasm. At the ultrastructural level the narrow rim of cytoplasm can be seen to possess a few mitochondria, scattered ribosomes, small profiles of endoplasmatic reticulum and a few vesicles. The nucleus is contained within a nuclear envelope with nuclear pores. Chromatin is loosely packed and consists of euchromatin. **(B)** CB-VSELs are also small and measure 3–5 μm in diameter. Similarly, they possess a relatively large nucleus surrounded by a narrow rim of cytoplasm. Chromatin is loosely packed and consists of euchromatin.

that indicates how to purify from adult BM a distinct population of very primitive embryonic-like stem cells and, more importantly, the morphology (Fig. 22–7) and the surface markers of these rare cells at the single cell level, have been described.

It is possible that these VSELs may be released from BM and circulate in PB during tissue/organ injury (eg, heart infarct and stroke). Interestingly ~5% to 10% of purified VSELs if plated over a C2C12 murine sarcoma cell feeder layer are able to form spheres that resemble embryoid bodies. Cells from these VSEL-derived spheres (VSEL-DS) are composed of immature cells with large nuclei containing euchromatin, and like purified VSELs are CXCR-4$^+$SSEA-1$^+$Oct-4.$^+$

Furthermore, VSEL-DS, after re-plating over C2C12 cells, may again (up to 5–7 passages) grow new spheres or, if plated into cultures promoting tissue differentiation, expand into cells from all three germ-cell layers. Because VSELs isolated from GFP$^+$ mice grew GFP$^+$ VSEL-DS showing a diploid content of DNA, this confirms that VSEL-DS are derived from VSELs and not from the supportive C2C12 cell line; it also excludes the possibility of cell fusion. Similar spheres were also formed by VSELs isolated from murine fetal liver, spleen, and thymus. Interestingly, formation of VSEL-DS was associated with a young age in mice, and no VSEL-DS were observed in cells isolated from old mice (>2 years).[8,91] This age-dependent content of VSELs in BM may explain why the regeneration processes is more efficient in younger individuals. There are also differences in the content of these cells among BM MNC between long- and short-lived mouse strains. The concentration of these cells is much higher in BM of long-lived (eg, C57Bl6) as compared to short-lived (DBA/2J) mice.[91] It would be interesting to identify genes that are responsible for tissue distribution/expansion of these cells as they could be involved in controlling the life span of mammals.

Because VSELs express several markers of primordial germ cells (fetal-type alkaline phosphatase, Oct-4, SSEA-1, CXCR4, Mvh, Stella, Fragilis, Nobox, Hdac6), they might be closely related to a population of epiblast-derived PGC. VSELs are also highly mobile and respond robustly to an SDF-1 gradient, adhere to fibronectin and fibrinogen, and may interact with BM-derived stromal fibroblasts. Confocal microscopy (Fig. 22–6, panel C) and time "time-lapse studies"[91] revealed that these cells attach rapidly to, migrate beneath and undergo emperipolesis in marrow-derived fibroblasts.[91] Because fibroblasts secrete SDF-1 and other chemottractants they may create a homing environment for small CXCR4$^+$ VSELs. This robust interaction of VSELs with BM-derived fibroblasts has important implications, namely that isolated BM stromal cells may be contaminated by these tiny cells from the beginning. This observation may explain the unexpected "plasticity" of marrow-derived fibroblastic cells (eg, MSC or MAPC).

Recently, a very similar population of cells that show similar morphology and markers to murine BM-derived VSELs has been purified from human CB.[211] Evidence has also mounted that similar cells are also present in the human BM, particularly in young patients. It is anticipated that VSELs could become an important source of pluripotent stem cells for regeneration. At this point, however, it is not clear whether VSELs contribute to blactocyst development.

Bone Marrow-Derived Oocytes and Spermatogonia?

Recently somewhat unexpectedly BM was also identified as a source of oocyte-like and spermatogonia-like cells.[9,10] This observation supports to some extent the concept that during embryonic development some of the primordial germ cells (Fig. 22–3) may go astray on their way to the genital ridges and colonize fetal liver, and subsequently by the end of the second trimester of gestation, together with fetal liver-derived HSC, move to the BM tissue.

Accordingly, oocyte-generating germ line stem cells were found in murine BM in a set of elegant experiments in which BM transplantation restored oocyte production in normal animals sterilized by chemotherapy as well as in ataxia telangiectasia-mutated gene-deficient mice, which are otherwise incapable of making oocytes.[9] Direct sorting analysis revealed in BM the presence of c-kit$^+$Sca-1$^-$lin$^-$ cells that expressed primordial germ cell markers such as Mvh, Dazl, Stella, and Fragilis. Expression of all of these markers correlated with an adherent fraction of BM cells. Based on these observations the authors concluded that BM could be a potential source of germ cells that could sustain oocyte production in adulthood. So far, however, evidence is lacking that these BM-derived oocytes are fully functional, capable of fertilization, and can give rise to embryos.

Another independent group also recently reported that BM cells may also be a source of male germ cells.[10] These cells expressed primordial germ cell markers such as Fragilis, Stella, Rnf17, Mvh, and Oct-4, as well as molecular markers of spermatogonial stem cells and spermatogonia including Rbm, c-Kit, Tex18, Stra8, Piwil2, Dazl, and Hsp90α. Thus BM unexpectedly is emerging as a potential source of cells for reproductive medicine.

This concept, however, recently became somewhat controversial after recent parabiotic experiments excluded BM as a source of oocytes during normal steady state conditions.[212] Nevertheless, the role of BM in supplying oocytes and spermatogonia in stress situations requires further confirmation by other, independent laboratories.

All Roads Lead to the Pluripotent Stem Cell—Does It Really Exist in Bone Marrow?

Above we discussed several types of nonhematopoietic stem cells that have been identified so far in the BM. An important question remains, however: whether a PSC, a founder cell for cells forming all three germ layers, resides in the adult BM. According to definition, these cells ultimately should also give rise to a population of mesoderm-derived HSC. Thus it is likely that such a cell could be related to the so-called long-term repopulating HSC that begins to supply hematopoietic cells a few months after hematopoietic transplantation.[213,214]

Several lines of evidence support the presence of PSC in BM tissue. First, expression of typical PSC markers such as SSEA-1, Oct-4, and Nanog was reported in BM-derived stem cells isolated using various strategies. These early embryonic transcription factors that are characteristic for ES and epiblast-derived cells were demonstrated at the protein and/or mRNA levels in VSEL, MAPC, MSC (in particular the SD fraction), and MIAMI cells.[5,6,8,121,181,198] Second, the contribution of BM-derived cells to regeneration of multiple nonhematopoietic organs and tissues indirectly suggests the existence of pluripotent or multipotent stem cells in BM. Illustrating this are experiments performed at the single cell level with BM-derived stem cells (Fr25 Sca-1(+)Kit$^+$in$^-$ or Fr25SKL cell) that contributed to multiorgan, multilineage engraftment in lethally irradiated mice.[215] These cells were first fractionated by elutriation at a flow rate of 25 mL/min (Fr25), then lineage depleted (lin(−)) and labeled with cell membrane-marking fluorochrome (PKH26) and injected intravenously into lethally irradiated animals. Two days posttransplant, PKH26$^+$ cells were recovered by cell sorting from recipient BM. These single adult BM-derived Fr25SKL cells have a robust capacity to differentiate into epithelial cells of the liver, lung, gastrointestinal tract (endoderm), and skin (ectoderm).[215]

Nevertheless, several questions relating to the presence of a putative PSC in BM remain. First, it is important to elucidate whether this cell is merely a remnant from developmental embryogenesis that resides in a dormant state in the BM tissue, or if it is a rare but mitotically active cell that contributes to the renewal of the pool of other BM-residing stem cells including HSC, EPC, and MSC. Second, what is the relationship of this cell to the cells recently described and purified from BM: (a) SSEA-1$^+$ Oct-4$^+$ Nanog$^+$ VSELs, (b) small Oct-4$^+$ MAPC, (c) Oct-4$^+$ SD-fraction of MSC, and (d) Oct-4$^+$ MIAMI cells? As mentioned, it is likely that each of these versatile BM-derived Oct-4$^+$ on-hematopoietic stem cells, which have been given different operational names, are in fact very closely related to the same type of BM-residing PSC.

As shown in Fig. 22–3, it is possible that these BM-residing PSC, as remnants of embryonic development (eg, derivatives from the epiblast), reside in a dormant state in ectotopic BM niches. The dormant status of these cells could be the result of the fact that these cells are (a) located in a nonphysiologic niche, (b) exposed to inhibitors, (c) deprived of some appropriate stimulatory signals, and finally (d) limited in pluripotency because of the erasure of the somatic imprint on some of the crucial somatically-imprinted genes (eg, H19 and IGF2). These cells, however, could be activated if they are exposed to some appropriate activation signals (eg, upregulated during organ/tissue injury, oncogenesis) or undergo epigenetic changes that change the methylation status of their DNA and acetylation of histones. Finally they may be reactivated if a proper somatic imprint is reestablished (Fig. 22–3).

In summary, there is mounting evidence that BM in fact contains PSC. For example, BM contains a population of VSEL stem cells that express SSEA-1 Oct-4 Nanog and are Lin$^-$ CD45$^-$.[8] These cells display a very primitive morphology and as shown at the single cell level are able in in vitro cultures to differentiate into cells from all three germ layers. Furthermore, Oct-4 and Nanog are also expressed in small MAPC, SD-MSC, and MIAMI cells.[6,121,181]

The most convincing evidence for the pluripotency of BM-derived stem cells would be the demonstration that these cells can complement blastocyst development after injection into a developing blastocyst. Unfortunately, such evidence for pluripotency has so far not been achieved in a reproducible way with any of the BM-derived stem cells.

Bone Marrow as a Source of Circulating Nonhematopoietic Stem Cells

A small number of BM-derived HSC circulates in PB even in steady state conditions as a result of self-renewal of stem cells in BM niches but serves as a way to keep in balance the stem cell pool in stem cell niches in different anatomical locations of the same BM. Stem cells circulating in the PB can also compete for organ/tissue-specific niches (Fig. 22–4). This may explain, for example, why heterogeneous populations of stem cells can also be detected in various organs (eg, HSC in muscle tissue). The number of HSC released/mobilized into PB increases after injection of mobilizing cytokines (eg, G-CSF)[216] or agents (eg, AMD3100)[217] as well as in several stress-related situations (eg, tissue/organ injury, strenuous exercise).[18,133,146]

A similar phenomenon has been described for BM-residing nonhematopoietic stem cells, which are also able to egress from BM tissue and circulate in PB during (a) pharmacological mobilization or (b) stress related to tissue/organ injury (Fig. 22–4). It has been further reported that the number of circulating nonhematopoietic stem cells in PB can be increased after administration of G-CSF alone or in combination with compounds that block the CXCR4 receptor (eg, T140 or AMD3100).[90,218] Hence the process of stem cell mobilization from BM into PB should be envisioned not only as mobilizing HSC but also other BM-residing nonhematopoietic stem cells. Thus pharmacological mobilization could become a means to obtain nonhematopoietic stem cells as well as HSC from the BM.

Table 22–5 shows several clinically relevant situations that lead to an increase of circulating stem cells in PB. Increases in the number of circulating BM-derived cells have been reported in skeletal muscle damage,[16,219,220] heart infarct,[18,19] stroke,[20] multiple bone fractures,[136] liver injury, kidney injury,[133] lung transplantation,[15] cardiac surgery,[221] liver transplant,[222] and limb ischemia.[223] These circulating BM-derived stem cells were identified as endothelial progenitors (EPC and EC), skeletal muscle satellite stem cells,[219] myocardiac,[18] neural and bone tissue-committed stem cells[20,136] and circulating MSC, as well as so-called fibrocytes,[224,225] which are probably a functionally altered subset of MSC.

In summary, mounting evidence suggests that during organ/tissue damage nonhematopoietic stem cells are mobilized from the BM and perhaps other tissue-specific niches into PB where they circulate prior to "homing" to damaged tissues and participating in organ repair. It is well documented that damaged tissues upregulate expression of several potential chemoattractants for these circulating stem cells such as SDF-1, VEGF, HGF/SF, LIF, or FGF-2.[137,226–229] Furthermore, the hypoxia regulated/induced transcription factor (HIF-1) plays an important role in the expression of several of these factors.[230,231] In support of this notion promoters of SDF-1, VEGF, and HGF/SF contain several functional HIF-1 binding sites.[138,230,232,233] Thus hypoxic conditions created by increasing expression of these factors may orchestrate mobilization from BM and subsequently the homing of circulating stem cells to damaged organs/tissues (Fig. 22–4).

Table 22–5 Data Supporting Circulation of Bone Marrow-Derived Nonhematopoietic Stem Cells in Various Clinical Situations

Skeletal muscle damage	Mice: murine BM-derived stem cells were reported to contribute after transplantation to irradiated muscles to skeletal muscle satellite stem cells. These cells subsequently contributed in skeletal muscle regeneration after exercise induced damage
Heart infarct	Human: Increase in circulating CD34$^+$, CXCR4$^+$, c-Met$^+$ cells in peripheral blood after acute myocardial infarction (MI). Increase in mRNA for GATA4, Mef-2C and Nkx.25/Csx in circulating MNC. Mice: Increase in mRNA for GATA-4, Mef-2C and Nkx.25/Csx in peripheral blood MNC in mice after experimental acute MI.
Stroke	Mice: Increase in mRNA for GFAP, Nestin, and βIII-tubulin in peripheral blood MNC in mice after experimental induced stroke.
Multiple bone fractures	Human: Increase in mRNA for bone-related genes (osteocalcin, bone alkaline phosphatase, collagen type I) in peripheral blood MNC in patients with multiple bone fractures.
Liver injury	Human: Increase in homing of human CD34$^+$CXCR4$^+$ in NOD/SCID mice livers damaged by exposure to CCl_4.
Kidney injury	Mice: Increase in circulating CD34$^+$CXCR4$^+$ and Lin$^-$Sca-1$^+$ cells in peripheral blood (PB) during acute renal failure.
Lung transplants	Human: Increase in circulating CXCR4$^+$ cytokeratin-5$^+$ cells in PB.
Cardiac surgery	Human: Increase in circulating CD34$^+$CXCR4$^+$ cells in PB.
Liver transplant	Human: Increase in circulating CD34+ cells and increase in mRNA for GATA4, cytokeratin 19, and α-fetoprotein in PB MNC.
Limb ischemia	Mice: BM-derived Sca-1$^+$ FLK-1$^+$ Tie-2$^+$ CD34$^+$ cells circulate and play a role in neovascularization.

THE ROLE OF BONE MARROW-DERIVED STEM/PROGENITOR CELLS IN HUMAN DISEASE

In parallel, evidence has also accumulated that BM-derived stem cells may play an undesirable role in the development of some pathological disorders.[234] It is likely that if these cells are mobilized at the wrong time and home to the wrong place (eg, into areas of chronic inflam-

Table 22–6 Pitfalls Related to Clinical Application of BM-Derived Nonhematopoietic Stem Cells

- — Isolation of a sufficient number of these cells from BM
- — Proper "repertoire" of homing signals in damaged organs
- — Adequate homing to damaged organs
- — Optimal delivery by systemic or local infusion
- — Effective contribution to organ/tissue regeneration
- — Lack of efficient ex-vivo expansion of stem cells

mation) they may exert unwanted effects.[235,236] For example, BM-derived stem/progenitor cells have been implicated in the pathogenesis of lung fibrosis, ocular pterygia, and diabetic neuropathy.[237–239]

Somewhat unexpectedly, it has been found that BM-derived stem cells may also contribute to the development of some nonhematopoietic tumors. This possibility was recently demonstrated in a model of murine stomach cancer caused by a chronic *Helicobacter pylori* infection.[240] In this model BM-derived cells were identified as a source of developing gastric mucosa adenocarcinomas, and the SDF-1-CXCR4 axis was implicated in the initiation of this tumor.[240] Accordingly, SDF-1 was found to be upregulated in the gastric mucosa affected by chronic inflammation caused by *H. pylori* infection and postulated to be the chemoattractant responsible for attracting CXCR4$^+$ stem cells from the BM. Exposed to the chronic inflammatory environment in the gastric mucosa, these cells transformed into adenocarcinoma initiating cells.[241] A similar phenomenon has recently been postulated in the pathogenesis of colon adenocarcinomas. Mounting evidence also suggests that BM may be a source of EPC and MSC for developing cancer tissue.[242,243] Thus, BM stem cells may in different ways contribute to both initiation and expansion of the growing tumor.

Lending further support to the concept that BM-derived cells may initiate the growth of nonhematopoietic malignancies, was the recent report that BM cells, exposed in vitro to the carcinogen 3-methycholanthrene, could transform into many tumor types, including epithelial, neural, muscular, fibroblastic, blood vessel, endothelial, and poorly differentiated tumors.[244] Moreover, a single transformed BM cell has the ability to self-renew, differentiate spontaneously into various types of tumor cells in vitro, express markers associated with multipotency, and form a teratoma in vivo. These data support the notion that multipotent cancer stem cells originated from transformed BM cells.[244] This provides further evidence that BM stem cells may be the origin of several nonhematopoietic cancers, and that BM is the most likely home of nonhematopoietic stem cells that are susceptible to transformation by carcinogens.

Do Bone Marrow-Derived Nonhematopoietic Stem Cells Hold Promise for Regenerative Medicine?

One can ask the question whether, if BM really contains pluripotent nonhematopoietic stem cells, then why is there so much controversy about the role of BM-derived cells in tissue/organ regeneration? There are several answers to this provocative, but timely, question (Table 22–6), especially in view of the current numerous clinical trials recently performed with BM-derived stem cells in patients with cardiac and neurological disorders.

First, there is the obvious problem of isolating a sufficient number of these cells from the BM. The number of these cells within BM MNC is very low (eg, VSELs represent 1 cell in 10^4–10^5 of BM MNC). Furthermore, there are some indications that these cells are enriched in the BM of young mammals and that their number decreases with age. It is likely that these nonhematopoietic stem cells released from the BM, even if they are able to home to the areas of tissue/organ injury, play a role only in regeneration of minor tissue injuries. Myocardial infarct or stroke, on the other hand, would be considered to involve severe tissue damage beyond the capacity of these rare cells to effectively repair. Second, the allocation of these cells to the damaged areas depends on homing signals that may be inefficient in the presence of other cytokines or proteolytic enzymes released from leukocytes and macrophages associated with damaged tissue. For example, matrix metalloproteinases released from inflammatory cells degrade SDF-1 locally and thus perturb homing of CXCR4$^+$ stem cells.[216,245,246] Third, it is not clear whether the optimal delivery system of these cells is intravenous infusion or direct injection into damaged tissues. Fourth, in order to reveal the full potential of these cells they have to be fully functional. We cannot exclude the possibility that these cells, while residing/being "trapped" in the BM, are not fully functional but remain "locked" in a dormant state and need the appropriate activation signals by unidentified factors (Fig. 22–3). Finally, a major limitation is the lack of effective ex-vivo expansion strategies for the most primitive stem cells. However, when such expansion protocols do become available, they should help resolve the crucial problem of the low numbers of these cells available in the BM.

Humanity continually searches for the holy grail of an end to the suffering caused by illness and a better quality of life in advancing years. There is no doubt that medical science is now looking to stem cells to provide some of milestones in this important quest. However, there is a crucial need for a reliable and noncontroversial source of stem cells. Adult BM stem cells could potentially provide a real therapeutic alternative to the controversial use of human ES cells and therapeutic cloning. Hence, while the ethical debate on the application of ES cells in therapy continues, the potential of BM-derived nonhematopoietic stem cells is ripe for exploration. Researchers must determine whether these cells can be efficiently employed in the clinic or whether they are merely developmental remnants found in the BM that cannot be harnessed for regeneration. The coming years will bring important answers to these questions.

SELECTED READINGS

Asahara T, Murohara T, Sullivan A, et al: Isolation of putative progenitor endothelial cells for angiogenesis. Science 275:964, 1997.

D'Ippolito G, Diabira S, Howard GA, Menei P, Roos BA, Schiller PC: Marrow-isolated adult multilineage inducible (MIAMI) cells, a unique population of postnatal young and old human cells with extensive expansion and differentiation potential. J Cell Sci 117:2971, 2004.

Gomperts BN, Belperio JA, Rao PN, et al: Circulating progenitor epithelial cells traffic via CXCR4/CXCL12 in response to airway injury. J Immunol 176:1916, 2006.

Houghton J, Stoicov C, Nomura S, et al: Gastric cancer originating from bone marrow-derived cells. Science 306:1568, 2004.

Jiang Y, Jahagirdar BN, Reinhardt RL, et al: Pluripotency of mesenchymal stem cells derived from adult marrow. Nature 418:41, 2002.

Johnson J, Bagley J, Skaznik-Wikiel M, et al: Oocyte generation in adult mammalian ovaries by putative germ cells in bone marrow and peripheral blood. Cell 122:303, 2005.

Kogler G, Sensken S, Airey JA, et al: A new human somatic stem cell from placental cord blood with intrinsic pluripotent differentiation potential. J Exp Med 200:123, 2004.

Kollet O, Shivtiel S, Chen YQ, et al: HGF, SDF-1, and MMP-9 are involved in stress-induced human CD34+ stem cell recruitment to the liver. J Clin Invest 112:160, 2003.

Krause DS, Theise ND, Collector MI, et al: Multi-organ, multi-lineage engraftment by a single bone marrow-derived stem cell. Cell 105:369, 2001.

Kucia M, Halasa M, Wysoczynski M, et al: Morphological and molecular characterization of novel population of CXCR4+SSEA-4+Oct-4+ Very small embryonic-like (VSEL) cells purified from human cord blood—preliminary report. Leukemia 21:297, 2007.

Kucia M, Reca R, Campbell FR, et al: A population of very small embryonic-like (VSEL) CXCR4(+)SSEA-1(+)Oct-4+ stem cells identified in adult bone marrow. Leukemia 20:857, 2006.

Kucia M, Zhang YP, Reca R, et al: Cells enriched in markers of neural tissue-committed stem cells reside in the bone marrow and are mobilized into the peripheral blood following stroke. Leukemia 20:18, 2006.

LaBarge MA, Blau HM: Biological progression from adult bone marrow to mononucleate muscle stem cell to multinucleate muscle fiber in response to injury. Cell 111:589, 2002.

Lemoli RM, Catani L, Talarico S, et al: Mobilization of bone marrow-derived hematopoietic and endothelial stem cells after orthotopic liver transplantation and liver resection. Stem Cells 24:2817, 2006.

Liu C, Chen Z, Chen Z, Zhang T, Lu Y: Multiple tumor types may originate from bone marrow-derived cells. Neoplasia 8:716, 2006.

Mann JR: Imprinting in the germ line. Stem Cells 19:287, 2001.

Nayernia K, Lee JH, Drusenheimer N, et al: Derivation of male germ cells from bone marrow stem cells. Lab Invest 86:654, 2006.

Orkin SH, Zon LI: Hematopoiesis and stem cells: plasticity versus developmental heterogeneity. Nat Immunol 3:323, 2002.

Peister A, Mellad JA, Larson BL, Hall BM, Gibson LF, Prockop DJ: Adult stem cells from bone marrow (MSCs) isolated from different strains of inbred mice vary in surface epitopes, rates of proliferation, and differentiation potential. Blood 103:1662, 2004.

Petersen BE, Bowen WC, Patrene KD, et al: Bone marrow as a potential source of hepatic oval cells. Science 284:1168, 1999.

Wagers AJ, Sherwood RI, Christensen JL, Weissman IL: Little evidence for developmental plasticity of adult hematopoietic stem cells. Science 297:2256, 2002.

Wojakowski W, Tendera M, Michalowska A, et al: Mobilization of CD34/CXCR4+, CD34/CD117+, c-met+ stem cells, and mononuclear cells expressing early cardiac, muscle, and endothelial markers into peripheral blood in patients with acute myocardial infarction. Circulation 110:3213, 2004.

REFERENCES

For complete list of references log onto www.expertconsult.com

CHAPTER 23

INTERACTIONS BETWEEN HEMATOPOIETIC STEM/PROGENITOR CELLS AND THE BONE MARROW: THE BIOLOGY OF STEM CELL HOMING AND MOBILIZATION

Ayelet Dar, Orit Kollet, and Tsvee Lapidot

INTRODUCTION

During the final stages of embryo development, hematopoietic stem cells (HSC) migrate from the fetal liver via the circulation, across the physical blood-bone-marrow barrier of endothelial cells and extracellular matrix and home to the bone marrow (BM).[1,2] These progenitor cells repopulate the bone marrow by extensive proliferation and differentiation while maintaining their self-renewal potential and motility, which enables them to egress back to the circulation.[3] Hematopoietic progenitor cells (HPC) in the bone marrow continuously replenish the blood with new maturing myeloid and lymphoid cells with a finite life span throughout life. In parallel, a rare and small subset of stem cells is retained in the bone marrow.[4] Blood forming progenitor cells are retained along the border between the bone and the bone marrow, the endosteum region and are also located in periarterial sites.[5,6] Recent results in mice reveal that certain endosteal osteoblasts are niche-supporting cells.[7] In addition, specific murine bone marrow endothelial regions were also found to support stem cell anchorage and retention.

Bones are dynamic organs, which are continuously remodeled throughout life. Bone remodeling is regulated by interactions between (hematopoietic stem cell derived) bone resorbing osteoclasts and (stromal derived) bone forming osteoblasts.[8] Osteoclasts are multinucleated giant cells, which are formed as a result of fusion of activated myeloid monocytes. Osteoclast precursors are recruited from the circulation to the bone marrow and are activated by osteoblasts via the membrane expressed or secreted cytokines, receptor activator of NF-κB ligand (RANKL), and macrophage colony-stimulating factor (M-CSF).[9] Osteoclast/osteoblast bone remodeling, also takes place in the endosteum region, the site which contains hematopoietic stem cell niches. Stem cell interactions with niche supporting cells maintain their anchorage via adhesion and membrane bound cytokines, which induce retention of quiescent, primitive cells in the bone marrow microenvironment. The bone marrow harbors a reservoir of stem cell derived, immature and maturing lymphoid and myeloid cells with a finite life span, which continuously egress to the circulation as part of homeostasis. Thus, via proliferation, differentiation, and migration, stem cells continuously replenish the blood with new cells throughout life while maintaining a small pool of undifferentiated stem cells in the bone marrow. Some of the circulating leukocytes home back to the bone marrow across the physical blood-bone-marrow-barrier of endothelial and extra cellular matrix. For example, circulating monocyte-derived osteoclast precursors, home back to the bone marrow, fuse in this tissue and transform into bone resorbing osteoclasts in response to signals provided by osteoblasts.[9] Old neutrophils also home back to the bone marrow for their apoptotic cell death.[10] In both cases the chemokine stromal derived factor-1 (SDF-1, also termed CXCL12) and its receptor CXCR4 are involved in this homing process. In addition, very low levels of progenitor cells also egress to the circulation. In mice, intravenously infused progenitors are rapidly cleared from the circulation within a few minutes, yet the low levels of circulating progenitor cells are continuously present in the blood as part of homeostasis.[11] Steady state stem cell proliferation, differentiation and egress to the circulation are dramatically amplified during alarm situations in response to secreted stress signals. These events occur during inflammation induced by viral or bacterial infections, injury, bleeding, ischemia, and DNA damage caused by radiation or chemotherapy. Hence, the transitions between steady state homeostasis egress to massive proliferation and mobilization require the existence of a versatile dynamic mechanism for regulation of the crosstalk between the bone marrow reservoir of leukocytes, peripheral blood and other organs, regulating the need for new blood cells on demand as part of host defense and repair mechanism.

HEMATOPOIETIC STEM AND PROGENITOR CELL HOMING

Homing is a multistep process, which requires directional migration of hematopoietic stem and progenitor cells through the circulation and extravasation across the physical barrier of the blood vessel into the bone marrow or other organs.[12] The bone marrow endothelium is the first anchoring site for homing cells, presenting adhesion molecules and producing stimulating chemokines. The small blood vessels in both human and murine bone marrow, the sinusoids, in which transendothelial migration is thought to take place, are composed of specialized cell structures, which regulate cell trafficking.[10,13] Rolling and firm adhesion of progenitors to endothelial cells in small marrow sinusoids under blood flow is coordinated by signaling via chemokines and cytokines (eg, SDF-1, SCF), resulting in cytoskeleton rearrangement and activation of integrins (eg, VLA-4) and metalloproteinases (eg, MMP2/9, MT1-MMP), followed by trans-migration across the physical endothelium/ECM barrier. Conditioning of the host with ionizing irradiation in the form of total body irradiation (TBI) and chemotherapy (cyclophosphamide) have been shown to disrupt the physical bone marrow endothelium barrier allowing erythrocyte passage from the circulation to the extravascular hematopoietic space of treated, but not control mice[14–16] and irradiated bone marrow endothelium of conditioned patients appears necrotic and disrupted with small gaps.[17] Stem cells finalize their homing uniquely, by selective access and anchorage to their specialized niches in the extravascular space of the endosteum region and in periarterial sites.[5,18,19] The ability of primitive hematopoietic stem and progenitor cells to migrate to specific organs has been identified during early developmental stages. HSC originate in the yolk sac and the aorta-gonadal-mesonephros (AGM) region, migrate to the fetal liver and finally to the BM shortly before birth.[1,2] Autologous or allogeneic transplantation protocols utilize GCSF mobilized cells, umbilical cord blood or adult bone marrow. These cells differ in their BM homing and repopulation properties as demonstrated in the preclinical and functional immunodeficient NOD/SCID mouse model.[17] The biology of human progenitor cell homing has been studied using two main preclinical animal models. The preimmune sheep model, developed by Zanjani and his colleagues, uses preimmune sheep fetuses implanted with immature human $CD34^+$ and $CD34^-$ cells without preconditioning. This model allows one to monitor both short-term and long-term stem cell engraftment in both primary and serially transplanted secondary sheep recipients. In this model, immature human bone marrow $CD34^+$ enriched cells transplanted to sheep fetuses can be detected 24 and 48 hours later in the recipient bone marrow.[20] The second model is based on the use of immune deficient mice preconditioned with sublethal TBI. Transplantation of SCID mice with normal and leukemic human progenitor cells developed by the group of Dick and his colleagues facilitates high levels of multilineage (both myeloid and lymphoid) human hematopoiesis in the murine BM, which is initiated by primitive SCID repopulating cells (SRC), and SCID leukemia initiating cells (SLIC).[21,22] Subsequently, NOD/SCID mice with greater degrees of reduced immunity have been created by Shultz et al and have been used to identify primitive CD34$^+$CD38$^-$ and CD34$^-$CD38$^-$ SRC.[23,24] B2 microglobulin null NOD/SCID (B2mnull NOD/SCID) mice have further reduced innate immunity because of the lack of natural killer cell activity. Definitive stem repopulating cell function of high level multilineage engraftment in primary NOD/SCID mice and serially transplanted B2mnull NOD/SCID mice is dependent on human CXCR4 signaling by murine SDF-1 which is cross-reactive[25] with human SDF-1. Maturing, CD34$^+$CD38$^+$ short term repopulating cells (STRC), which are enriched in mobilized peripheral blood were identified by the group of Eaves et al using B2mnull NOD/SCID mice[26] or by inactivation of natural killer cell activity in NOD/SCID mice by other groups.[27,28] Mechanisms of human stem cell homing have been largely characterized in immune deficient NOD/SCID and B2mnull NOD/SCID mice.[17,29]

A small subset of immature cord blood CD34$^+$ cells, CD34$^+$CD38$^-$ cells, consist of more primitive hematopoietic progenitor cells, which home successfully to the murine bone marrow and spleen while sorted CB CD34$^+$CD38$^+$ maturing progenitor cells, which lack long term repopulation capacity have poor homing capabilities, unless they are prestimulated with cytokines such as SCF in vitro or GCSF introduced for mobilization of adult progenitors in vivo[17] or cotransplanted with mature mononuclear cells.[28,29] Selectins also play a role in regulating HPC trafficking.[30,31] The selectin family of adhesion molecules contains three family members: P- and E-selectin, which are expressed on endothelial cells (and their expression is induced in response to inflammatory signals), and L-selectin, which is constitutively expressed on mature leukocytes and HPC. Previous studies revealed that homing of HPC to the bone marrow of P- and E-selectin deficient mice is defective.[32]

Most clinical protocols use the intravenous administration route for transplantation of hematopoietic cells aimed at reconstituting the bone marrow of patients who have received TBI or chemotherapy. In an attempt to improve the efficiencies of bone marrow homing, seeding and repopulation, transplanted cells have been injected directly into the bone marrow cavity of immune deficient NOD/SCID and normal mice (intraosseous [IO], intra bone marrow [IBM], or intrafemur [IF] transplantation). Studies with enriched human progenitors demonstrate superior seeding efficiencies when the endothelial and extracellular matrix (ECM) barriers are bypassed. IBM injections yielded a 15-fold higher frequency of SRC in sorted cord blood CD34$^+$CD38$^-$ cells in comparison to conventional intravenous (IV) injection. Increased engraftment and improved ability of bone marrow cells obtained from primary recipients to repopulate secondary transplanted recipients have also been documented. Interestingly, neutralization of CXCR4 by antibody treatment similarly abolishes engraftment by human CD34$^+$ enriched cells administrated in both protocols, demonstrating an essential role for this receptor not only in SRC homing to the bone marrow, but also in bone marrow seeding and colonization.[33] Cord blood derived Lin$^-$D34$^-$ primitive cells display limited repopulation potential when transplanted via the tail vein,[24,34] as opposed to high SRC activity when transplanted IO,[35] despite low expression levels of CXCR4 and reduced migration to SDF-1,[35–37] indicating for the crucial role of CXCR4 function in stem cell endothelial transmigration during the course of homing to the BM. Applying intrafemural injection of cord blood CD34$^+$D38(-/low)CD36$^-$ purified cells, Dick and colleagues were able to identify a new short-term SRC subset which is capable of migrating to other bones, and colonizing them with myeloid and erythroid cells.[38] Of interest, when total cord blood mononuclear cells or murine bone marrow cells were transplanted IBM, increased engraftment including a dramatic increase in immature human CD34$^+$ cells was documented transiently about one month post-IF transplantation as compared to IV transplantation, but not two and three months post transplantation.[39] In addition, IF transplanted murine cell levels in the peripheral blood were lower than with IV injected cells, three months posttransplantation.[39]

Despite reduced IF homing in irradiated recipients, donor cell proliferation and repopulation rates are increased as compared to nonirradiated mice. However, retention of undifferentiated donor stem cells in the bone marrow of nonconditioned recipients is evident by transplantation into lethally irradiated secondary recipients,[40] implying that TBI is further needed to reduce competition by host stem cells, and to provide signals which enhance bone marrow reconstitution.[41] Finally, to prevent stress and severe damage to the bone marrow structure associated with IF injection, and to ensure introduction of cells to the blood vessels of the femur rather than to the bone marrow cavity, Scadden and colleagues have examined homing properties of murine bone marrow Lin$^-$ cells injected to the artery of the femur. While homing to the bone marrow and spleen was significantly increased by femoral artery versus tail vein injection in lethally irradiated mice, no differences were found in long-term donor cell repopulation,[42] suggesting that bone marrow repopulation is not enhanced by this approach and that stress and damage caused by the implantation procedure also contributes to the repopulation levels. Preliminary results of clinical, human IBM transplantation of adult BM cells did not lead to improved engraftment,[17] yet iliac crest transplantation of cord blood cells is promising.[43]

Retention of Hematopoietic Stem and Progenitor Cell in the Bone Marrow

The final step for successful homing requires directed migration of homing cells into specialized niches within the bone marrow, which are capable of retaining and promoting the controlled proliferation of the homing primitive hematopoietic stem cells. Of interest, studies conducted with sorted Lin$^-$ murine progenitor and stem cells have revealed that progenitor cells transplanted intravenously specifically home to the endosteum region whereas maturing leukocytes do not.[18] The bone marrow-bone lining cells of the endosteum are known to anchor and support HSCs. However, bone marrow endothelium and extramedullary hematopoiesis, as in the liver and spleen, indicate that the endosteum/osteoblast microenvironment is not the sole supportive niche for HSCs. Murine HSCs, characterized by CD150$^+$D244$^-$D48$^-$ expression were shown to be associated with sinusoidal endothelium in murine spleen and bone marrow. Implying that sinusoidal endothelial cells have the ability to function as specific portals for murine hematopoietic stem cell entry into the marrow space, defining the localization of progenitor cells and serving as stem cell niches throughout hematopoietic tissues.[5,44] In addition, endothelial cells regulate HSC function and are capable of maintaining HSCs in culture.[45–47] Furthermore, ablation of endothelial cells in vivo by administration of anti-VE-cadherin leads to hematopoietic failure.[48] In agreement with these reports, using intravital microscopy studies have shown that murine hematopoietic stem/progenitor cells as well as lymphocytes, that were transplanted IV to recipient mice homed to the bone marrow, adhered to unique bone marrow vascular microdomains, which express SDF-1 after two hours and are retained there as long as two months, documenting the role of these domains as specific portals for the entry of cells into the marrow space.[6]

Intracellular signaling downstream from the chemokine receptor CXCR4, the tyrosine kinase receptor c-kit and ?β1-integrins within HSC and HPC have been shown to be crucial for the migration, homing, and retention of hematopoietic stem cells and progenitors. Each of these receptors signal through Rac-type Rho guanosine triphosphatases (GTPases). Rac GTPases play a major role in the organization of the actin cytoskeleton and also in the control of gene expression and the activation of proliferation and survival pathways. Rac2 regulates the retention of HSC and HPC in the bone marrow microenvironment, and a deficiency of Rac2 is associated with enhanced numbers of circulating hematopoietic stem and progenitor cells. The final localization in the endosteal area of HSC is impaired by the absence of Rac1.[49] Another crucial component in HSC and progenitor cell retention in the endosteal region is the glycosaminoglycan hyaluronic acid (HA), which is synthesized and expressed by endosteal stromal cells.[50] Furthermore, the presence of HA appears to be critical for homing of immature human CD34+ cells via CD44 interactions, and although murine stem cell homing is not dependent on CD44, their spatial distribution in the bone marrow of transplanted mice and their ability to reconstitute hemopoiesis in vivo is correlated with HA expression levels.[51] Together, these results reveal that stem cell directed motility, which includes navigation to target hematopoietic organs and into their specialized niches within these tissues, is essential for their in vivo function, which includes homing to the bone marrow, retention, proliferation, differentiation, and release back to the circulation.

Hematopoietic Stem and Progenitor Cell Mobilization

While most of the stem cell compartment is located within the bone marrow endosteal and endothelial specialized niches, a small and rare population is found in the blood circulation because of steady state homeostatic processes of constitutive release from the bone marrow as part of host defense and repair. Physiological stress, such as injury, and inflammation, or artificial clinical treatments with mobilizing agents (GCSF, chemotherapy), induce massive proliferation of hematopoietic stem and progenitor cells in the bone marrow, which is accompanied with significant increase in progenitor cell egress to the circulation, a process termed *mobilization*. Mobilization is characterized by imbalance of steady state homeostasis, induction of stem and progenitor cell proliferation, differentiation, and massive egress to the circulation. The SDF-1/CXCR4 axis is a pivotal player in this process and is discussed in detail in the following paragraph. Additional major features and dynamic processes involved in HSC mobilization consist of various ligand/integrin or cytokine receptor interactions including VLA-4/VCAM-1, CD62L/PSGL, CD44/HA, and Kit/Kit ligand. Very late antigen-4 (VLA-4 or 41 integrin) is expressed by the majority of HPC in a low-affinity state; however, in response to cytokines such as GM-CSF, interleukin-3, and stem cell factor its function can be rapidly and transiently activated to promote adhesion to fibronectin. The importance of the interactions between VLA-4 with vascular cell adhesion molecule-1 (VCAM-1), which is constitutively expressed by endothelial cells and stromal cells in the bone marrow, to HSC trafficking in the bone marrow has been confirmed by studies using antibodies directed against VCAM-1 or VLA-4 which leads to HPC mobilization.[52,53] Moreover, the inducible deletion of 4 integrins in adult mice results in constitutive HSC mobilization.[54] Anti-VLA-4 induced HSC mobilization is significantly enhanced in CD18 (2-integrin) deficient mice or in wild-type mice treated with anti-2-integrin antibodies, suggesting that both VLA-4 and 2-integrins contribute to the anchoring of HSC in the bone marrow.[55] Mice lacking the receptor for the glycosaminoglycan hyaluronan (HA), CD44, have an impaired mobilization response to GCSF,[56] and treatment of mice with an anti-CD44 antibody results in a modest mobilization of HPC to the blood.[57] Numerous cytokines and growth factors elevation in the plasma induce hematopoietic stem cell mobilization, such as VEGF and angiopoietin-1,[58] SCF, and SDF-1 itself.[8,59] Other factors have been reported to synergize with GCSF to increase mobilization such as, placental growth factor-1 (PlGF-1) in both primate and murine models[60] and the SDF-1 antagonist compound AMD3100, which also induces rapid and massive mobilization when administered solely.[61] Moreover, a combined loss of Racl and Rac2 leads to massive egress of HSC/P, in spite of the inability of these cells to actively migrate in response to in vitro gradients of SDF-1.[49] Of notice, preliminary results demonstrate an essential role for the CD45 phosphatase, which negatively regulates adhesion interactions and secretion of the metalloproteinase MMP-9 in homing and repopulation by human CD34+ cells. Neutralization of this receptor impaired migration to SDF-1, bone marrow homing, and repopulation of NOD/SCID mice.[62]

Proteases and metalloproteinases (extracellular matrix degrading enzymes) also regulate cell migration, facilitating movement across the physical barrier of the ECM and inactivating bone marrow derived growth factors and chemokines, which are responsible for hematopoietic cell adhesion and retention. N-terminal cleavage of SDF-1 associated with its chemotactic inactivation, was demonstrated by several degrading enzymes including CD26/dipeptidylpeptidase IV[63–65] neutrophil elastase, cathepsin G,[66–68] cathepsin K,[8] and matrix metallopeptidase (MMP)-2/9.[69] In addition, membrane-bound SCF (c-kit ligand) is also cleaved by MMP-9[70] and cathepsin K. It was previously shown that this ligand is essential for endosteal lodgment by murine stem cells[71] and that the release of membrane bound SCF from the bone marrow to the peripheral blood caused by proteolytic activity of MMP-9 induces stem cell mobilization.[70] MMP-9 (also termed gelatinase B) accumulates in the plasma and/or bone marrow following mobilization with interleukin-8, GCSF, or cyclophosphamide.[72,73] In line with these observations, human bone marrow CD34+ progenitors in steady state conditions do not secrete the metalloproteinases MMP-2 and MMP-9, which are implicated in cell motility, while circulating CD34+ cells secrete these enzymes, as do GCSF-mobilized progenitors.[74] GCSF treatment in vitro and in vivo in patients or mice preengrafted with human CD34+ cells, increase also the expression of MT1-MMP by hematopoietic human progenitors, which mediates their mobilization.[50,75]

Of interest, by using parabiotic mice with a joint circulation, Abkowitz et al showed a dramatic elevation in the levels of GCSF-mobilized stem cells which efficiently home back to the partner bone marrow as compared to only low homing levels of steady state circulating stem cells.[76] This report demonstrates that during stress-induced mobilization, homing rates are also augmented, confirming that mobilization and homing are sequential, physiological processes.

A recent report suggests that the sympathetic nervous system is involved in a newly recognized pathway by which signals initiated in peripheral organs may reach the bone marrow. Signals from the sympathetic nervous system triggered GCSF or fucoidan-induced mobilization of progenitors. This study demonstrates that while norepinephrine signaling induced a decrease in GCSF induced stem cell mobilization, β2 adrenergic agonists increased mobilization.[77]

Another major component, which plays a role in specifically regulating HSC and progenitor cell mobilization are bone-resorbing osteoclasts.[8,9] Differentiation and activation of osteoclasts are tightly regulated by endosteal bone forming osteoblasts which are derived from mesenchymal stem cells. It is anticipated that conditions, which turn the balance towards osteoblast proliferation and differentiation, would result in the expansion of the size of the stem cell pool and niches within the bone marrow. Indeed, postoperative parathyroid hormone (PTH) administration increased the numbers of endosteal osteoblasts and the number of anchored stem cells in the niche, opposing the situation in PTH-deficient mice.[78] Recent report demonstrates that bone-resorbing osteoclasts are directly involved in mobilization of progenitor cells from the bone marrow to the circulation, both in homeostatic and stress-induced conditions.[8] Physiologic stress, ie, mild bleeding and lipopolysaccharide (LPS) administration mimicking bacterial inflammation or administration of the cytokines SDF-1 or hepatocyte growth factor (HGF), caused robust appearance of bone resorbing TRAP+ active osteoclasts along the endosteum region. This process is associated with mobilization of hematopoietic progenitors to the circulation. Likewise, administration of RANKL, the osteoclast differentiation cytokine, which is presented by osteoblasts to activate osteoclasts, induced in addition to bone resorption also preferential mobilization of immature murine progenitors. In contrast, the hormone calcitonin, which prevents formation of ruffled border and TRAP production by osteoclasts and therefore is used as an anti osteoporotic drug in aging patients, reduced mobilization of progenitors in mice treated with GCSF or LPS; and also lowered the levels of circulating progenitors during homeostasis.[8] A genetic disorder involving osteoclasts caused by protein tyrosine phosphatase ε (PTPε) deficiency in young female mice[79] is accompanied by reduced levels of primitive hematopoietic stem (Lin(−)/Sca-1+c-kit+ cells in the blood in comparison with wild-type phenotype during steady state conditions and also in response to GCSF stimulation. The mechanisms by which bone resorbing osteoclasts induce mobilization includes secretion of the cytokine IL-8 by active human osteoclasts,[80] secretion of MMP-9, cathepsin G and cathepsin K,[81] which cleaves SDF-1 and SCF expressed by endosteal osteoblasts. Another major regulator of the stem cell niche is osteopontin, which is expressed by bone lining osteoblasts during homeostasis. Osteopontin is remarkably reduced in the endosteum of mice treated with RANKL.[8] Taken together these results reveal that the endosteal stem cell niche is dynamic, producing hematopoietic cells on demand. Low level cell production occurs during steady state homeostasis, which is dramatically accelerated in response to alarm signals caused by injury, bleeding and inflammation, which are mimicked by clinical mobilization protocols. Stem cell anchorage and quiescent retention at a nonmotile mode by the stromal niche supporting cells is interrupted in order to induce HSC proliferation, differentiation and recruitment to the circulation as part of host defense and repair. Our view is that the stem cell niche is a negative regulator aimed at preventing stem cell migration and development, maintaining undifferentiated cells in a quiescent nonmotile state. Once these interactions are overcome, stem cells follow signals that determine their tissue localization phenotype and function, involving cytoskeletal rearrangement required for cell motility, proliferation and differentiation, regulation of adhesion interactions within their microenvironment vicinities, and expression of enzymes involved in their active migration, crossing the vasculature endothelium to the bone marrow and other peripheral organs as part of their development.

Chemokine SDF-1 and Its Receptor CXCR4 in Stem Cell Homing and Mobilization

The constitutive egress and induced release of immature and maturing leukocytes as well as rare primitive stem cells to the circulation suggests a regulated active process that has to overcome homing/retention interactions. A major role in regulation of homing and mobilization is attributed to the modulations in the interactions between the G-protein coupled chemokine receptor CXCR4 and its ligand SDF-1. Chemokines are small signaling molecules, which are part of the cytokine super family. These ligands are best known for their ability to attract leukocytes to sites of inflammation by chemotactic signaling via receptors expressed on the migrating leukocytes, as part of host defense. Chemokines are also involved in organ development and angiogenesis, and some chemokines serve as survival factors for immature progenitor cells. The chemokine SDF-1 was first discovered as a pre-B cell growth factor, secreted by the mouse bone marrow stromal cell line, MS5. The major receptor for this chemokine, CXCR4, is expressed by many cell types, including neuronal, endothelial, epithelial, muscle, liver and hematopoietic, and immature and mature lymphoid and myeloid cells. CXCR4 is also used by the HIV virus as a coreceptor to infect human CD4 T lymphocytes. SDF-1 and its receptor are essential for murine embryonic heart and brain development. Of interest, recent data reveal the existence of another receptor on some human leukocytes, named RDC1 (also termed CXCR7), which can bind SDF-1 and respond to adhesion and survival/proliferation mediated by this chemokine,[82,83] revealing a more complex network of interactions between SDF-1 and its receptors. However signaling mediated by this receptor does not induce calcium release and at present it is not clear if or how RDC1 is involved in SDF-1 induced proliferation, migration and/or adhesion. Human and murine SDF-1 are cross-reactive and differ in one amino acid. This ligand is a survival factor for murine myeloid progenitor cells[84] and also for primitive human hematopoietic $CD34^+CD38$(-/low) cells and mesenchymal $Strol^+$ cells.[85] Human and murine bone marrow stromal cells, including bone marrow endothelial and endosteal osteoblasts, express high levels of SDF-1 in vivo and also functionally express its receptor CXCR4. Expression of the receptor RDC1 was documented also on activated endothelial cells.[82] Murine embryos that lack SDF-1, or its receptor CXCR4 have multiple lethal developmental defects, including lack of bone marrow seeding by hematopoietic progenitor cells, migrating from the fetal liver. These results reveal the essential roles that this chemokine and its receptor play in bone marrow seeding during development. However, fetal liver cells isolated from CXCR4 KO embryos can home and engraft the bone marrow of irradiated, adult wild-type mice. These cells have reduced bone marrow homing, preferentially at the more differentiated progenitor stage, and reduced retention of stem cells in the bone marrow. These reduced retention levels can be over come by increasing the transplantation cell dose, leading to normal levels of donor type CXCR4 KO primitive progenitor cells in the bone marrow of primary recipients, but not in the bone marrow of serially, secondarily transplanted wild-type mice. Murine fetal liver cells also express RDC1, which can partially compensate for the lack of CXCR4.[82,86] Currently, SDF-1 is the only known powerful chemotactic factor for human $CD34^+CD38^-$ and murine $Sca1^+ckit^+Lin^-$ (SKL) hematopoietic stem cells. The observation that this ligand is also a survival factor for both human and murine hematopoietic progenitor cells,[84] suggests that it is also involved in cell cycle regulation. In agreement with this concept, SDF-1 was shown to inhibit cycling of long term repopulating human bone marrow hematopoietic progenitors but not of myeloid leukemic CFC cells.[87] In addition, the expression levels of SDF-1 were significantly elevated in the $S/G_2/M$ phase proliferating murine stem cells compared with its levels in G_0/G_1 phase. Of interest, blocking SDF-1 in mice transplanted with cycling progenitors restored their engraftment ability implying that cell cycle progression is SDF-1 dependent and is associated with their potential to successfully reconstitute the bone marrow.[88] Alterations of SDF-1 concentrations also contribute to the delicate balance between the regulation of hematopoiesis and directed motility: low levels of SDF-1 induce directional migration and proliferation, while high levels induce desensitization of the receptor CXCR4, quiescence and inhibition of cell motility.

Cell motility requires shape changes, dramatic cytoskeletal rearrangements and focal adhesion with the ECM components. Activation of HSC bySDF-1 induces signaling pathways that have been shown to be essential for efficient homing of transplanted human and murine HSC in preclinical murine models. SDF-1 activation induces actin polymerization[89] and phosphorylation of focal adhesion molecules such as FAK, RAFTK/Pyk2, p130Cas, Crk, and paxillin. Rho GTPase family members such as RhoA, Rap, and cdc42 and its binding protein WASP are also required for SDF-1 induced morphological changes.[90,91] Functional elevation of CXCR4 expression by immature human $CD34^+$ cells is mediated by the atypical PKCζ upon cAMP stimulation and results in enhanced homing to the bone marrow.[92,93] In the course of mobilization PKC-ζ,[92,93] Rac, RohA, and CDC42 play major roles in CXCR4 mediated migration and proliferation. SDF-1 induces secretion of a number of different proteolytic enzymes, which in turn cleave and inactivate it. For example, CD26 (dipeptidyl peptidase IV), a membrane-bound extracellular serine-protease expressed on a subset of HPC, inactivates SDF-1 through proteolytic cleavage.[94] GCSF induced HPC mobilization is defective in CD26 deficient mice or in wild-type mice treated with a specific CD26 inhibitor[94,95] and CD26-deficient HPC display enhanced homing to the bone marrow and long-term engraftment potential.[94] In addition, SDF-1 signaling induces secretion of MMP-9 by immature human CD34 cells and murine stem cells, which in turn cleaves and inactivates this ligand. Migrating human CD34 cells in the circulation secrete MMP-2 and MMP-9 both during homeostasis and GCSF induced mobilization, while stationary CD34 cells in the bone marrow do not,[74] implicating these enzymes in the regulation of human CD34 progenitors cell motility. Another enzyme, the cell surface protease MT1-MMP, which is expressed by human CD34 cells, is also activated by SDF-1, can cleave this ligand, and is involved in homing and mobilization.[50,75] SDF-1 mediates activation of adhesion molecules such as LFA-1, VLA-4/5, and CD44, which are all part of the motility machinery. Immobilized SDF-1 activates LFA-1 and VLA-4 integrins on immature human CD34 cells under physiological shear flow to bind their respective ligands ICAM-1 and VCAM-1 in vitro. Furthermore, immobilized SDF-1 is also required for development of firm integrin-mediated adhesion and spreading.[96,97] Moreover, the cytoskeleton rearrangement and protrusion formation, as part of immature human CD34+ cell migration, are inhibited by CD44 neutralizing antibodies, revealing a cross-talk between this chemokine and the adhesion machinery, which can veto its chemotactic effect.[50,51,98] These results suggest that immature CD34 progenitors anchored to the bone marrow endosteum, which is rich in hyaluronic acid (the major CD44 ligand) can inhibit MMP-2/9 secretion, proliferation, and migration of progenitor cells, in the presence of SDF-1.

Interestingly, increased SDF-1 expression in injured peripheral organs emerges as a common mechanism that recruits stem cells from the bone marrow reservoir and targets them to the site of injury. SDF-1 expression in ischemic tissues as the skin, which is regulated by the transcription factor hypoxia-inducible factor-1 (HIF-1), increased the adhesion, migration, and homing of recruited CXCR4+ progenitor cells to these ischemic tissues.[99] Myocardial infarction documented in human and animal models is another good example of the importance of SDF-1/CXCR4 interactions in stem cell behavior. Acute myocardial infarction by itself induces progenitor cell mobilization in patients[100] and SDF-1 increased expression in rats.[101] A combination of GCSF administration to increase HSC mobilization, with local upregulation of SDF-1 in peri-infract zone, resulted in enhanced homing of c-kit+ murine progenitors to the injured tissue and improved cardiac function.[101] However, in humans with chronic ischemia of the heart, signals transferred from the damaged organ to the bone marrow, severely affect the function of bone marrow hematopoietic progenitors. Thus, despite a similar frequency of CD34 progenitors in the bone marrow of patients with chronic ischemic cardiomyopathy, these cells demonstrate lower colony formation capacity, which reflects their inferior developmental potential, together with reduced migration to SDF-1 or VEGF.[101] The CXCR4 receptor, expressed by the stationary bone marrow endothelial and other stromal cells but not motile hematopoietic cells, also serves to bind functional SDF-1 present in the blood, which is internalized and transcytosed via special clathrin-coated pits vesicles. SDF-1 is then translocated to the abluminal side of the endothelial cells and secreted into the bone marrow space. The released SDF-1 is able to functionally support and increase the homing of human CD34+ progenitors to the bone marrow of B2mnullNOD/SCID mice.[102,103] Similar mechanisms may explain the extended SDF-1 expression by the endothelium of the injured livers of mice treated with CCL4, or by the bile duct liver epithelium of human individuals infected with hepatitis C virus. Moreover, this increased expression of SDF-1 in the periphery may explain the associated stem cell recruitment and increased liver engraftment by hematopoietic cells.[104] In this case as well, inhibition of CXCR4 or MMP-9, abrogates stem cell recruitment and homing to the injured liver. Additional evidence for the importance of SDF-1/CXCR4 interactions in determining stem cell behavior emerges from studies with the CXCR4 antagonist, AMD3100. A single injection of AMD3100 rapidly induces stem and progenitor cell mobilization to the peripheral blood in mice, humans,[61,100] and primates.[105] AMD3100 mobilized cells exhibit higher expression of CXCR4, which correlates with increased migration to its ligand SDF-1.[61,106] This efficient process may be mediated by binding of AMD3100 to CXCR4 expressed on hematopoietic stem and progenitor cells, to CXCR4 expressed by endothelial cells and other stromal cells, or both. Since AMD3100 synergistically increases G-SCF induced mobilization, additional mechanisms are apparently activated. Preliminary data reveal that AMD3100 induced mobilization is accompanied by increased SDF-1 release from the bone marrow.[107] This finding is consistent with several previous reports demonstrating a correlation between leukocytes and immature hematopoietic cells and an increase in SDF-1 concentrations in the circulation after injection of either fucoidan,[108] SDF-1 overexpressing adenovirus[59] or direct administration of the SDF-1 ligand itself.[8] In addition, inhibition of CXCR4-dependent release of SDF-1 during homeostasis or upon treatment with AMD3100, is correlated with a selective reduction in recruitment of hematopoietic progenitor cells but not mature leukocytes to the circulation. SDF-1 release was mediated by the β-adrenergic receptors of the sympathetic nervous system.[107] Altogether these results imply that homing and recruitment of progenitor cell egress is orchestrated by mutual and reciprocal SDF-1/CXCR4 interactions occurring within the bone marrow stromal and hematopoietic cells as well as between the bone marrow, peripheral blood and distant organs, navigating cell destiny and function in response to stress signals and organ repair and defense requirements.

Leukemic Stem Cells: Migratory Behavior and Immune Regulation

The concept of cancer stem cells was first documented for human leukemia.[21,109] In agreement with this concept, several brain and breast tumor initiating stem cells have been identified recently,[110,111] which can be related to mutations that occur in the normal stem and progenitor cells and lead to malignant transformation and tumor initiation.[112,113] Since leukemic stem cells ultimately are derived from normal hematopoietic stem and progenitor cells, they also express the CXCR4 receptor, which directs the homing of cancer stem cells[113,114] and tumor metastasis (eg, breast, prostate, ovarian) to organs that highly express its ligand SDF-1 (eg, bones, lymph nodes, liver). For example, a positive correlation between SDF-1 expression in a mouse model and human prostate cancer metastatic bone lesions was documented, whereas CXCR4 inhibition reduced the metastatic load.[115] Similarly, CXCR4 expressing human breast cancer cells metastasize to the bone marrow in response to SDF-1 signals from this tissue.[116] In agreement with this concept, prostate cancer cells were found to migrate across bone marrow endothelial cell monolayers in response to SDF-1 in a CXCR4 dependent manner and pretreatment of the prostate cancer cells with SDF-1 significantly increased their adhesion to osteosarcomas and endothelial cell lines.[117] The NOD/SCID mouse model serves also as a preclinical model to study the phenotype of human leukemic stem cells. The SCID leukemia-initiating cells (SLIC), are characterized by primitive nondifferentiated CD34+CD38− expression profile. These cells extensively repopulate the bone marrow of irradiated mice and initiate a disorders, which is similar to the disease in humans.[22,118] Interruptions of CXCR4/SDF-1 interactions prevent homing of pre-B ALL cells[119] and blocking anti-CXCR4 antibodies when administered to chimeric mice previously engrafted with acute myeloids leukemia stem cells, lead to a dramatic reduction in the levels of human AML cells in the BM, blood, and spleen in a dose- and time-dependent manner, revealing that the malignant cells are more dependent on these interactions than are normal human SRC.[113] Similarly, murine leukemic stem cells expressing bcr/abl were found to express higher levels of cell surface CD44 as compared to their normal hematopoietic counterparts and were dependent to a greater extent on CD44 for homing and engraftment than normal HSCs, providing a potential use in autologous transplantation of patients with CML.[120] High levels of cell expression of CXCR4 levels are poor prognostic factors in both human AML and childhood pre-B ALL.[114,119] Recent reports have revealed novel players in CXCR4 mediated spreading and metastasis of tumor cells. Submicron CXCR4 positive vesicles which are shed from the plasma membrane of CD45 positive leukocytes are capable of transferring the CXCR4 molecule to AML cells, enhancing their migration in response to SDF-1 in vitro and increasing their homing to the bone marrow of NOD/SCID mice. These findings indicate for the involvement of CXCR4+ microparticles in cancer progression and reveal their potential as diagnostic tool.[121]

Fibroblast derived SDF-1 has been shown to attract CXCR4-expressing malignant human cells to pre-metastatic niches and to promote invasive breast carcinoma growth.[122] Disruption of CXCR4/SDF-1 interactions inhibits the homing of human Pre-B acute lymphoblastic leukemia cells to the bone marrow. Interestingly, the same bone marrow endothelial domains also define the homing and retention microenvironment for transplanted murine HSC. This vasculature expresses E-selectin and SDF-1 in discrete, discontinuous areas that direct early metastatic cells to those locations.[6] Similarly, human CD34 leukemia cells, transplanted IV into the immunodeficient murine model, were observed using immunohistopathology, and exhibit a similar spatial distribution to cord blood derived CD34+ cells: initially localizing on the surface of osteoblasts and than expanding to the inner vascular and diaphysial regions.[123] In accordance, during the course of preangiogenic niche formation, the retention of recruited bone marrow CXCR4+ myeloid cells, which position and maintain VEGF induced angiogenesis, is mediated by perivascular SDF-1 in the murine liver.[124] Recently, an additional mechanism promoting the establishment of premetastatic sites of human cancer stem cell models in mice has been suggested. Bone-derived hematopoietic progenitor cells expressing vascular endothelial growth factor receptor 1 (VEGFR1, also known as Flt1) home to tumour-specific premetastatic sites and form cellular clusters prior to the arrival of tumour cells. Taken together, these data indicate that SDF-1/CXCR4 interactions anticipate in the migration, repopulation, and development of malignant stem cells in the BM and other organs by regulating the establishment of premetastatic and preangiogenic sites as well as anchorage of malignant cells to the stromal microenvironment and cell survival. Based on differences in reduced sensitivity to blockage of key homing components such as CXCR4 and CD44, neutralization of these molecules may serve as a foundation for potential therapeutic approaches, which may inhibit leukemic stem cell proliferation and migration while only minimally affecting normal stem cells.

SUMMARY

This chapter discusses mechanisms and pathways involved in the regulation of hematopoietic stem and progenitor homing (Fig. 23–1), retention as well as hematopoietic stem cell egress, recruitment and mobilization (Fig. 23–2), emphasizing the major role that the

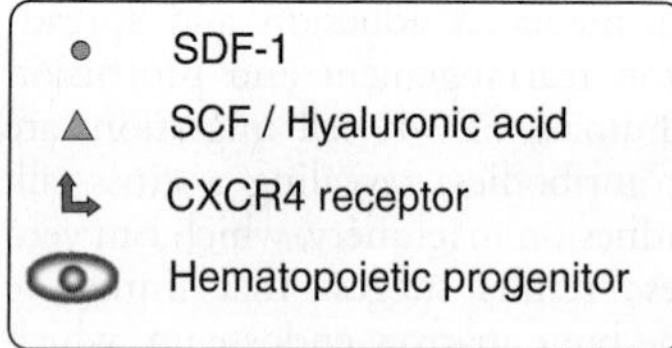

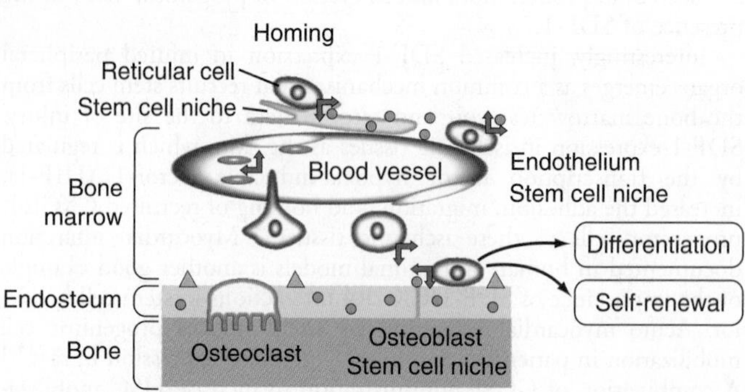

Figure 23–1 Stem and progenitor cell homing into the bone marrow. CXCR4 expressing stem and progenitor cells (*blue cells*) are activated by SDF-1, which is secreted from bone marrow endothelial cells and triggers integrin interactions. The arrested CXCR4+ progenitors, in response to SDF-1, extravasate and migrate through the vessel-marrow barrier. Migrating stem cells eventually reach the "stem cell niches," which consist of stromal cells (reticular cells, endothelial cells, and osteoblasts) that present the proper set of adhesion molecules (eg VCAM-1, hyaluronic acid), SDF-1, and growth stimulatory factors (eg, stem cell factor). SDF, stromal derived factor; VCAM, vascular cell adhesion molecule.

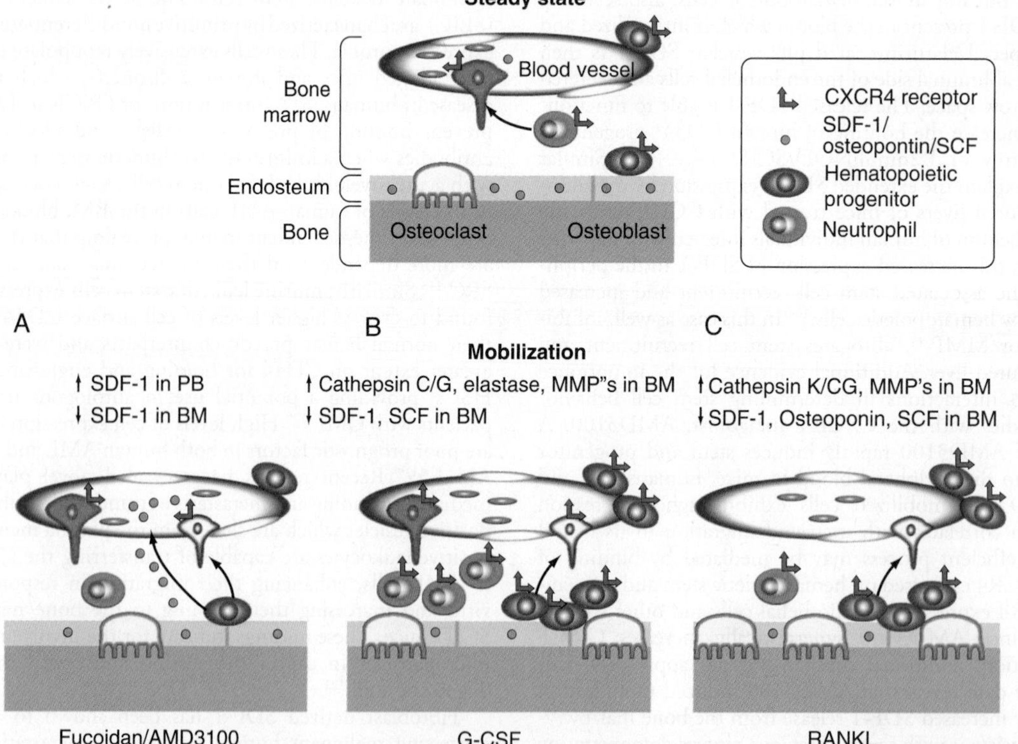

Figure 23–2 Alternative mechanisms of progenitor mobilization. Increased recruitment of hematopoietic progenitors to the circulation upon administration of fucoidan or AMD3100, which induce rapid mobilization (within 1 hour). (**A**) is mediated by massive release of SDF-1 from the bone marrow into the peripheral blood, which in turn chemoattract bone marrow progenitors. The other two mechanisms of mobilization induced by either repetitive administrations of GCSF (**B**) or RANKL (**C**) mediate bone and bone marrow remodeling including: progenitor proliferation and release (**B, C**), bone-resorbing osteoclasts proliferation and activation in the endosteal stem cell niche, and modulation of bone marrow levels of cytokines, growth factors and proteases as indicated (**B, C**). While proliferating mature neutrophils have a fundamental role in GCSF induced mobilization, secreting various proteases (**B**), activated osteoclasts mediate RANKL-induced mobilization preferentially of immature progenitor cells by retraction of bone lining osteoblasts and degradation of components that maintain stem cell retention in the bone marrow endosteal region (**C**). GCSF, granulocyte colony-stimulating factor; RANKL, receptor activator of NF-κB ligand; SDF, stromal derived factor.

Relevance to Clinical Hematology

Most hematopoietic stem and progenitor cells reside in the bone marrow (BM), anchored to specialized niches in the endosteal region and in periarterial sites. However, very low levels of circulating progenitors are continuously present in the blood as part of homeostasis. These low levels are dramatically increased together with maturing leukocytes, which are both recruited from the BM reservoir during situations of stress as part of host defense and repair mechanism. Similarly, clinical protocols, such as repeated GCSF administration, result in stem and progenitor cell proliferation in the BM, differentiation (mostly to myeloid neutrophils), and egress of stem and progenitor cells to the circulation at elevated levels. This process is termed *mobilization* and is used clinically to harvest hematopoietic progenitor and stem cells for transplantation. Successful BM reconstitution requires directed stem cell movement from the circulation, across the blood-marrow barrier into their specialized niches in the BM, a process termed *homing*, wherein stem cells proliferate and differentiate to give rise to multilineage hematopoietic cells while maintaining a small pool of primitive stem cells.

Several cell sources are currently used for BM transplantation: allogeneic umbilical cord blood (CB) from leftover placentas of new born babies, adult BM or mobilized peripheral blood (MPB) cells, which in some cases are enriched for immature CD34 derived cells. While GCSF induced mobilization yields relatively large numbers of immature CD34 cells in the circulation, the numbers of CB MNC and immature CD34 cells is relatively limited. For this reason, the major disadvantage of CB transplantation in adult patients is delayed engraftment. Although children who receive transplants of BM with a cell dose 13 times greater than CB grafts achieve much faster neutrophil and platelet recovery, the levels of progenitors in the BM of such children one year after transplantation with CB were significantly higher, implying that CB has a higher number of long-term repopulating cells. Approaches aimed at overcoming the delayed engraftment with CB transplantation include double CB transplants or together with MPB/BM derived CD34 cell infusion from a matched donor in order to achieve transient engraftment until the CB cells reconstitute the BM. Recently, a pilot study points out the potential of direct intrabone injection of CB cells. This protocol eliminates the step of blood vessel wall transmigration in intravenous infusion to overcome the delayed engraftment. These preliminary results suggest that intrabone transplantation of human CB shortens the time frame for neutrophil and platelet recovery post transplantation and also reduces graft versus host disease initiated by the cord blood cells.

In addition, the CXCR4 chemokine receptor and its ligand SDF-1, the only known powerful chemoattractant for hematopoietic stem and progenitor cells, are major regulators of both stem cell homing, retention, and mobilization processes. Recent studies reveal that the bicyclam AMD3100, a CXCR4 antagonist, induce rapid mobilization of human CD34 cells and synergizes with GCSF, improving clinical progenitor cell mobilization. Since some patients (and also a minority of healthy donors) are poor mobilizers, because of the impact of factors such as aging, heavy prior treatment with chemotherapy, and a diagnosis of AML or ALL in these patients, manipulations of CXCR4/SDF-1 interactions and expansion of primitive hematopoietic stem and progenitor cells ex-vivo prior to autologous transplantation could lead to new perspectives on the development of improved clinical protocols for stem cell mobilization (as well as correcting the release of maturing cells in neutropenic patients and improved homing and repopulation in clinical transplantation protocols).

CXCR4/SDF-1 axis plays in the regulation of these complex interactive processes. The stromal stem cell niche appears to be a dynamic site, which regulates stem and progenitor cell retention proliferation and development by mutual multiple interactions between both cell types and communication with other organs/compartments. The stromal stem cell niche is a negative regulator, which maintains undifferentiated stem cells as quiescent nonmotile cells, which are anchored to the niche supporting stromal cells via adhesion interactions. However, the niche is dynamic and the anchoring interactions can be broken and degraded, allowing the progenitor cells to proliferate, differentiate, and migrate before the niches are reestablished. The findings that are described in this chapter demonstrate fundamental differences between the mechanisms of AMD3100/fucoidan-mediated and GCSF-mediated or RANKL-mediated mobilization (Fig. 23–2). While rapid mobilization induced by AMD3100 or fucoidan within a few hours involves increased release of SDF-1 from the bone marrow into the circulation, which is accompanied by increased release of mature leukocytes and immature progenitors, multiple, daily doses of GCSF and RANKL is mediated by substantial bone and bone marrow remodeling prior to cell egress. Importantly, RANKL administration is unique by inducing massive proliferation and activation of bone-resorbing osteoclasts, which in turn preferentially induce progenitor cell proliferation and mobilization with minor effects on the release of more mature leukocytes. Based on these findings, RANKL should be considered together with other mobilizing agents aimed at selective mobilization of primitive stem and progenitor cells for a broad range of clinical transplantation protocols, in particular for donors who are poor mobilizers: the elderly or heavily chemotherapy-treated patients. Various signals provided during homeostasis versus stress-inducing conditions, provided by the bone marrow tissue and by peripheral organs, determine the fate and localization of the niche residents, the hematopoietic stem cells.

SUGGESTED READINGS

Abkowitz JL, Robinson AE, Kale S, Long MW, Chen J: Mobilization of hematopoietic stem cells during homeostasis and after cytokine exposure. Blood 102:1249, 2003.

Adams GB, Chabner KT, Alley IR, et al: Stem cell engraftment at the endosteal niche is specified by the calcium-sensing receptor. Nature 439:599, 2006.

Broxmeyer HE, Orschell CM, Clapp DW, et al: Rapid mobilization of murine and human hematopoietic stem and progenitor cells with AMD3100, a CXCR4 antagonist. J Exp Med 201:1307, 2005.

Cancelas JA Jansen M, Williams DA: The role of chemokine activation of Rac GTPases in hematopoietic stem cell marrow homing, retention, and peripheral mobilization. Exp Hematol 34:976, 2006.

Christopherson KW 2nd, Hangoc G, Mantel C, Broxmeyer HE: Modulation of hematopoietic stem cell homing and engraftment by CD26. Science 305:1000, 2004.

Dar A, Goichberg P, Shinder V, et al: Chemokine receptor CXCR4-dependent internalization and resecretion of functional chemokine SDF-1 by bone marrow endothelial and stromal cells. Nat Immunol 6:1038, 2005.

Dick JE, Lapidot T: Biology of normal and acute myeloid leukemia stem cells. Int J Hematol 82:389, 2005.

Katayama Y, Battista M, Kao WM, et al: Signals from the sympathetic nervous system regulate hematopoietic stem cell egress from bone marrow. Cell 124:407, 2006.

Kiel MJ, Yilmaz OH, Iwashita T, et al: SLAM family receptors distinguish hematopoietic stem and progenitor cells and reveal endothelial niches for stem cells. Cell 121:1109, 2005.

Kollet O, Dar A, Lapidot T: The multiple roles of osteoclasts in host defense: bone remodeling and hematopoietic stem cell mobilization. Annu Rev Immunol 25:51, 2007.

Kollet O, Dar A, Shivtiel S, et al: Osteoclasts degrade endosteal components and promote mobilization of hematopoietic progenitor cells. Nat Med 12:657, 2006.

Kollet O, Spiegel A, Peled A, et al: Rapid and efficient homing of human CD34(+)CD38(-/low)CXCR4(+) stem and progenitor cells to the bone marrow and spleen of NOD/SCID and NOD/SCID/B2m(null) mice. Blood 97:3283, 2001.

Lapidot T, Dar A, Kollet O: How do stem cells find their way home? Blood;106:1901, 2005.

Lapidot T, Sirard C, Vormoor J, et al: A cell initiating human acute myeloid leukemia after transplantation into SCID mice. Nature 367:645, 1994.

Larochelle A, Krouse A, Metzger M, et al: AMD3100 mobilizes hematopoietic stem cells with long-term repopulating capacity in nonhuman primates. Blood 107:3772, 2006.

Lévesque JP, Hendy J, Takamatsu Y, Simmons PJ, Bendall LJ: Disruption of the CXCR4/CXCL12 chemotactic interaction during hematopoietic stem cell mobilization induced by GCSF or cyclophosphamide. J Clin Invest 111:187, 2003.

Peled A, Petit I, Kollet O, et al: Dependence of human stem cell engraftment and repopulation of NOD/SCID mice on CXCR4. Science 283:845, 1999.

Petit I, Szyper-Kravitz M, Nagler A, et al: GCSF induces stem cell mobilization by decreasing bone marrow SDF-1 and up-regulating CXCR4. Nat Immunol 3:687, 2002.

Sweeney EA, Papayannopoulou T: Increase in circulating SDF-1 after treatment with sulfated glycans. The role of SDF-1 in mobilization. Ann N Y Acad Sci 938:48, 2001.

Wright DE, Wagers AJ, Gulati AP, et al: Physiological migration of hematopoietic stem and progenitor cells. Science 294:1933, 2001.

Yin T, Li L: The stem cell niches in bone. J Clin Invest 116:1195, 2006.

Zhang J, Niu C, Ye L, et al: Identification of the haematopoietic stem cell niche and control of the niche size. Nature 425:836, 2003.

REFERENCES

For complete list of references log onto www.expertconsult.com

CHAPTER 24

THE HUMORAL REGULATION OF HEMATOPOIESIS

Montaser Shaheen and Hal E. Broxmeyer

INTRODUCTION TO HEMATOPOIESIS

Hematopoiesis, a delicately regulated process, results in the production of a variety of cell lineages with diverse functions that range from delivering oxygen to all tissues to immunity, and hemostasis. This highly orchestrated process requires the division of hematopoietic stem cells that give rise to committed progenitors which proliferate and differentiate into functional blood cells. The passage of hematopoietic cells through different stages of stem and progenitor compartments requires the presence of multiple soluble factors known as cytokines.

A major milestone in our understanding of the cellular basis of hematopoiesis was the discovery that intravenously injected marrow cells could save the life and generate hematopoietic colonies in the spleens of lethally irradiated mice.[1] Further analysis revealed that these clusters of cells were clonal progenitors of single hematopoietic cells termed colony forming units-spleen (CFU-S), and that the colonies could mature into hematopoietic populations of multiple lineages.[2] In addition, these colonies contained CFU-S that could generate more splenic colonies in secondary irradiated animals indicating the capacity of these cells for self-generation. Later, CFU-S were found to be distinct from other more primitive bone marrow (BM) cells termed *hematopoietic stem cells* (HSCs) that are able to undergo self-renewal and generate cells of all hematopoietic lineages.[2,3] It has been realized that CFU-S are unable to repopulate irradiated mice on a long-term basis.[4,5] One primitive subset of cells was recognized as repopulating cells that are able to produce all hematopoietic lineages for a long time. These long-term repopulating cells contrast with short-term repopulating cells, which cannot sustain hematopoiesis for the whole animal lifetime, but which are likely responsible for supporting blood formation for the first eight weeks after HSC transplantation in mice.

Identifying the soluble factors regulating hematopoietic functions was hindered by the lack of advanced molecular biology techniques prior to the 1970s and 1980s and was mainly phenomenological and based on detection of biological activities. The interest of immunologists in the 1960s in studying factors mediating various immune reactions was shortly followed by parallel interest to isolate the factors that drive hematopoietic progenitor cells to survive and differentiate into colonies in semi-solid culture systems. The development of such semisolid agar[6,7] or methylcellulose-based[8] systems led to the conclusion that "inducers" required for the formation of these hematopoietic colonies were secreted by the feeder layer cells and could diffuse through the medium. The beginning of 1980s ushered in the molecular cytokine era with the first successful cloning of a cytokine (interferon β1).[9] This type of cloning introduced a unique opportunity to directly and specifically study the cellular and molecular properties of cytokines after producing pure quantities of these factors in a large scale. In this chapter we review the current understanding of hematopoiesis by focusing on cytokines that display hematological activities and that have or are likely in the future to have clinical utility for treatment of malignant and nonmalignant hematopoietic disorders.

CYTOKINES/SOLUBLE FACTORS AND HEMATOPOIESIS

Cytokines may have stimulatory, costimulatory/augmenting, inhibitory, or multiple different activities on hematopoietic progenitor/stem cells. A listing of hematopoietically active cytokines can be found in Table 24–1. Interleukin-4 (IL-4) represents a classic cytokine with a dual activity on hematopoiesis.[10] This activity can be direct, as seen with most cytokines, or indirect and mediated by the induction of other cytokines. IL-17 represents a classic cytokine whose hematopoietic activity is largely indirect.[11] It is oversimplistic to place cytokines into distinct groups, given the overlap and redundancy seen among them (Table 24–2).[12,13]

One group can stimulate colony formation even when added alone to semisolid culture systems. This includes GM-CSF, G-CSF, M-CSF, IL-3, Epo, Tpo, and IL-5. SCF and FL are two important costimulatory factors that have important functions in the hematopoietic system and display significant synergy with other cytokines. IL-6 family members have been demonstrated to be important hematopoietic regulators with overlapping activities that are mediated through the common receptor signal transducer glycoprotein 130 (gp130). Wnt family, Notch ligands, bone morphogenic protein-4 (BMP-4), sonic hedgehog, and the angiogenic factors have been implicated in the regulation of HSC self renewal and differentiation. Other cytokines play an inhibitory role on hematopoiesis. These factors crucially regulate hematopoiesis by influencing different aspects of this process such as self-renewal, cell survival, differentiation, proliferation, mobilization, and homing. These secreted, soluble, membrane or extracellular matrix-bound molecules affect their target cells through high affinity binding of specific receptors that triggers intracellular signaling, leading to the final phenotype or phenotype change.

This chapter starts by briefly discussing current knowledge about the nature of hematopoietic stem and progenitor cells and the different processes that characterize their lifespan. We then discuss the structure and signaling pathway of cytokine receptors and the influence of each cytokine on hematopoiesis.

HEMATOPOIETIC PROGENITOR AND STEM CELLS

The report by Till and McCulloch[1] on CFU-S and subsequent reports by Bradley and Metcalf,[7] and Pluznik and Sachs[6] on in vitro colony forming cells heralded the four-decade search to purify and characterize hematopoietic stem cells as defined by the features of self-renewal and the ability to give rise to all hematopoietic lineages. Direct evidence of these features comes from the observation that single BM cells can repopulate lethally irradiated primary and secondary recipient mice with all hematopoietic lineages.[14,15] Studies of retroviral marketing of HSCs provides data in support of this concept.[16]

The possibility of existence of a precursor cell common to all hematopoietic lineages dates back to 1951 when Dameshek[17] observed that in patients with myeloproliferative disorders affecting one blood cell lineage, other blood lineages were often affected. Subsequently, it was realized that bone marrow of genetically identical mice could rescue recipients exposed to lethal doses of irradiation.[18] CFU-S form splenic colonies 8 to 16 days post transplant. Cells that give rise to colonies in eight days are termed CFU-S_8, which are largely unipotential and form colonies compound erythroid lineage cells. These colonies do not contain cells able to form colonies in secondary recipients. In contrast, CFU-S_{12} colonies contain cells belonging to several hematopoietic lineages including erythrocytes, megakaryocytes, macrophages, and granulocytes. CFU-S_{12} cells represent a more

Table 24–1 Hematopoietic Cytokines

Colony-Stimulating Factors
Granulocyte colony-stimulating factor (G-CSF)
Granulocyte-macrophage colony-stimulating factor (GM-CSF)
Macrophage colony-stimulating factor (M-CSF)
Interleukin-3 (IL-3)
Erythropoietin (Epo)
Thrombopoietin (Tpo)
Interleukin-5 (IL-5)
Costimulatory Cytokines
Classic Growth Factors with Hematopoietic Activities
Stem cell factor (SCF)
Flt3 ligand (FL)
Interleukin-6 (Il-6) Family
IL-6
IL-11
Leukemia inhibitory factor (LIF)
Oncostatin M (OSM)
Other Interleukins with Hematopoietic Activities
IL-1, IL-2, IL-4, IL-7, IL-9, IL-10, IL-12, IL-17
IL-20, IL-31
Candidate Stem Cell Regulators
Wnt family
Notch ligands
Sonic hedgehog
Bone morphogenic protein-4
Vascular endothelial growth factor (VEGF) family
Insulin-like growth factor-1 (IGF-I). IGF-II
Basic fibroblast growth factor (bFGF)
Hepatocyte growth factor (HGF)
Platelet derived growth factor (PTGF)
Angiopoietin-like proteins (AngPtl)
Suppressive Cytokine
Chemokines
Interferons (IFNs)
Tumor necrosis factor α (TNF-α)
Transforming growth factor β (TGF-β)
Lactoferrin (LF)
H-ferritin (HF)

Table 24–2 Redundancy in Cytokine Activities

Hematopoietic Process	Cytokines with Important Enhancing Activity
Erythropoiesis	Epo, SCF, IGF-1, IL-9, IL-3, Tpo, IL-20, SDF-1
Megakaryopoiesis	Tpo, IL-3, IL-6, IL-11, LIF, SCF, Epo, SCF, FL
Mast cell formation	IL-3, SCF, IL-10?
Eosinophil formation	IL-5, IL-3, GM-CSF, SCF
Granulopoiesis	G-CSF, GM-CSF, IL-3, SCF, IL-6, FL, SDF-1
Macrophage formation	M-CSF, GM-CSF, IL-3, FL, SDF-1
Lymphocyte production	IL-7, FL, SCF, SDF-1, IL-2, IL-4, IL-5, IL-10, IL-13, IL-15, notch ligands

Demonstration of the clear redundancy in cytokine activities on every blood lineage maturation process. However, certain cytokines exert more prominent influence on one lineage than the others. For example, Epo is the essential cytokine for erythroid maturation, whereas Tpo deficiency leads to severe thrombocytopenia. IL-5 is the main cytokine driving eosinophil formation. G-CSF is the only cytokine whose deficiency results in neutropenia. IL-7 is essential for both T-cell and B-cell development. Absence of M-CSF results in failure of monocyte maturation into other effector cells such as osteoclasts.

quiescent and primitive population of multipotential cells,[19] and cells taken from these splenic colonies are able to produce colonies in secondary recipients, which attests to their capacity for self-renewal. Subsequent experiments have shown that CFU-S are unable to repopulate recipients on a long-term basis and in essence do not represent true stem cells.[4,5] This led to a conclusion that a smaller subset of repopulating cells exists. Because of lack of a parallel in vivo transplantation system in humans, different in vitro assays have been developed in an attempt to characterize surrogate cells that may be close to true stem cells. A variety of suspension cultures assays indicated that the stromal cells were important for the maintenance and possible expansion of CFU-S and the repopulating cells.[20,21] Later, a cell termed a long-term culture initiating cell (LTC-IC) was characterized.[22–24] This cell is identified in an assay in which BM derived stromal cells or an appropriate mixture of cytokines support the proliferation of hematopoietic cells for at least five weeks. At this time the remaining cells are plated in semisolid culture systems and the colonies are enumerated. These colonies reflect the number of primitive cells that can maintain their colony forming potential for five weeks. These cells are considered more primitive than the colony-forming cells (CFC) that are assayed directly without prior incubation in stromal cell based suspension cultures. The LTC-IC does not necessary represent the most primitive stem cell in vivo. The cobblestone area-forming cell (CAFC) assay[25,26] is another in vitro system in which BM cells are plated on top of a specialized stromal layer. Some cells form colonies of at least five small, nonrefractive cells underneath the stromal layer. These cells can generate progenitors for up to 12 weeks and are considered primitive cells as well. The colony-forming cell with high proliferative potential (HPP-CFC)[27] is a cell that produces a large size colony (>0.5 mm and usually contains >50,000 cells) after a long period of in vitro incubation. It responds to stimulation by a multicytokine cocktail and shows resistance to 5-fluorouracil (5-FU) treatment.

Methods to evaluate the in vivo repopulating potential of human hematopoietic stem cells have been developed. These methods utilize the Non obese diabetic/severe combined immunodeficiency (NOD/SCID) mice that can be repopulated after lethal irradiation with human cells.[28,29] This system provides a quantitative method for what is called the SCID repopulating cell (SRC) through limiting dilution of the injected cells. The NOD/SCID mouse model has been instrumental in the study of the in vivo proliferation of human hematopoietic stem cells and their differentiation into all blood lineages including lymphoid cells.[30] This system has proved the self-renewal capacity of SRC through serial transplantation into secondary and tertiary recipient mice.[31] However, due to the short lifetime of SCID-NOD mice (most of them develop thymoma by age 6 months) the SRC may not represent the true human stem cell that sustains hematopoiesis for longer periods than this. Other SCID mouse models with longer life spans are being evaluated. Another in vivo model of human hematopoiesis utilizes in utero transplantation of stem cells into sheep fetus before the development of the ovine immune system.[32,33] Human HSCs from fetal liver, cord blood, mobilized PB, and BM are able to engraft the ovine BM and undergo multilineage differentiation. In this system, short-term repopulating cells, which give rise temporarily to mature blood cells, can be distinguished from long-term repopulating cells that sustain hematopoiesis in primary and secondary recipients for a long time.[34]

Along with functional characterization of hematopoietic stem/progenitor cells in vitro and in vivo, phenotypical characterization of these cells has been pursued. Extensive screening of murine antibodies against cell-surface molecules elucidated antibodies that could be used to enrich murine BM cells 1000 to 2000-fold for their ability to radioprotect lethally irradiated mice. This subset of BM cells are low for the Thy-1 antigen, negative for mature cell lineage markers (Lin^-), and positive for a stem cell marker called Sca-1; they are termed $Thy\text{-}1^{lo}$ Lin– $Sca\text{-}1^+$.[35] This subset contains all of the repopulating potential of murine BM cells. Twenty to 40 cells belonging to this subset can radioprotect 50% of lethally irradiated mice. Eight percent of $Thy\text{-}1^{lo}$ Lin^- $Sca\text{-}1^+$ cells express the stem cell factor receptor c-Kit. These Kit+ $Thy\text{-}1^{lo}$ Lin^-Sca-1+ (KTLS) cells are highly

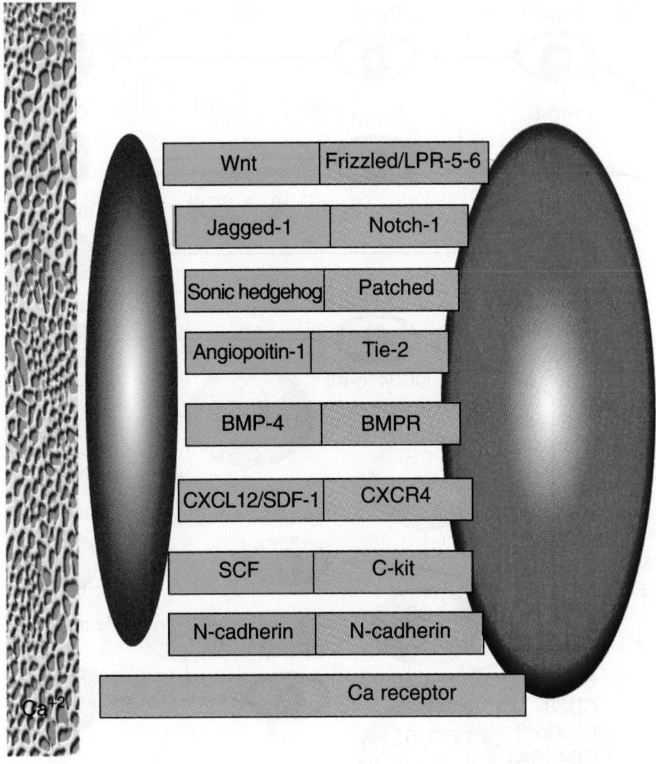

Figure 24–1 The current understanding of HSC in its niche. This figure depicts the currently known regulators through which HSC interacts with the osteoblast. This interaction is thought to determine the stemmness; self-renewal, quiescence, and differentiation of HSC. BMP, bone morphogenetic protein; HSC, hematopoietic stem cells; SCF, stem cell factor.

enriched for self-renewing and repopulating cells.[36,37] One report suggested that the c-Kit$^-$ subset might represent a population of very primitive quiescent cells that do not contribute to hematopoiesis until 40 weeks after transplantation.[38] These cells are heterogeneous for the expression of murine CD34,[15] whereas most human progenitor/stem cells express the sialomucin antigen CD34 on their surface.[39] However only a minority of CD34$^+$ cells have NOD/SCID repopulating potential. The human CD34$^+$ CD38$^-$ fraction is enriched for more primitive cells.[40] It has been found that the CD34$^-$ Lin$^-$ fraction also has SCID- repopulating capacity. These CD34$^-$ Lin$^-$ cells engraft in fetal sheep and form human hematopoietic cell chimeras.[41] However, the exact relationship of CD34$^+$ to CD34$^-$ stem cells remains to be adequately defined, and the presence of CD34 may only define cell activation status.

Another frequently utilized approach to isolate HSCs has been through their ability to efflux fluorescent dyes and to appear as a "side population" on flow cytometric analysis.[42] More recently, novel cell surface markers have been used to isolate a relatively homogenous HSC population. Such markers include endoglin (an ancillary TGF-β receptor),[43] the endothelial protein C receptor (CD201),[44] and SLAM family receptors (see Chapter 20).[45]

Fig. 24–1 represents the current understanding of the hematopoietic hierarchy with emphasis on the principle cytokines that affect each maturation step.

The Interaction of Hematopoietic Stem Cell with Growth Factors Within Its Niche

The concept Of HSC niche was first proposed in 1978.[46] Recent interest in HSC niche was triggered by studies in gonadal tissue of *Drosophila* that identified specific cell-cell interaction between germ stem cells and the niche "cap cells."[47] This interaction determines which of the resulting two cells after germ stem cell division will remain as a stem cell and which will become a differentiating daughter cell. HSC has been proposed to interact closely with the stromal cells within the bone marrow niche.[48] Multiple lines of evidence point to the localization of this niche close to the trabecular bone within BM. Osteoblasts have emerged as principal stromal cells that regulate HSC maintenance and proliferation. Endothelial cells represent an alternative niche.[45,49] Genetically modified mice that overproduce osteoblasts are characterized by an increase in the HSC pool within BM without an increase in the numbers of progenitors.[50,51] Osteoblasts express key cytokines and other surface molecules that are known to play key roles in HSC homing in the BM such as SDF-1/CXCL12, Jagged-1 (notch ligand), SCF, wnt members, angiopoietin-1, and N-cadhern. The angiogenic factor angiopoietin-1 has emerged as a key regulator of HSC quiescence within the niche.[52] Ionic calcium plays an important role in the niche organization since HSCs that lack the Ca^{+2} receptor fail to engraft in the BM.[53] A schematic view of this niche concept with the up-to-date interaction between HSC and the mesenchymal cell is shown in Fig. 24–2.

CYTOKINE REGULATION OF COLONY FORMATION

The first observed biological activity of hematopoietic growth factors was the ability to promote hematopoietic cell colony formation.[6–8] Colony formation is optimal in the presence of multiple cytokines that synergize with each other to increase the number and size of colonies formed by the same seeding dose of progenitor cells. It is important to realize that even though a certain colony-stimulating factor may have a major influence on one blood lineage, it often affects other blood lineages, particularly in the presence of other factors.[54] For instance, G-CSF stimulates the proliferation of granulocyte progenitors but it also augments megakaryocyte colony formation by IL-3.[55] An important theme that has been controversial is the permissive versus instructive role of cytokines in hematopoietic lineage commitment.[56,57] Once the commitment decision has been made, cytokines exert signals for proliferation, survival, and to some extent differentiation that lead to the production of functional hematopoietic cells. We discuss each of the processes that contribute to the observed outcome of cytokines on colony formation.

Instructive Versus Permissive Activity of Hematopoietic Cytokines

The instructive model of cytokine action resembles that of several developmental systems in which secreted factors determine cell fate. The most direct evidence for the operation of such a system in hematopoiesis is the committment decision by bipotential granulocyte-macrophage colony-forming cells (GM-CFC = CFU-GM).[58] In this situation, the daughter cells of GM-CFC are examined for their fate decisions. The addition of M-CSF to cultures results in the formation of macrophage-committed progenitor cells, whereas the addition of GM-CSF results in a higher frequency of granulocyte-committed progenitors. When stem cell factor is used to stimulate early progenitor cells to form blast colonies composed of progenitor cells, the addition of thrombopoietin (Tpo) increases frequency of colonies containing megakaryocyte progenitors, while the addition of IL-5 induces colonies containing eosinophil-committed progenitor cells.[59] Another line of evidence supporting the instructive role of cytokines was generated by a study[60] in which the common lymphoid progenitor cell could change commitment into the myeloid lineage when transduced with IL-2 and GM-CSF receptor genes and transduced cells were cultured in the presence of the corresponding cytokines. This study documented that GM-CSF and M-CSF receptors were expressed at low to moderate levels by primitive hematopoietic cells and were absent on common lymphoid progenitors. These receptors were upregulated with the myeloid lineage induction by IL-2. In

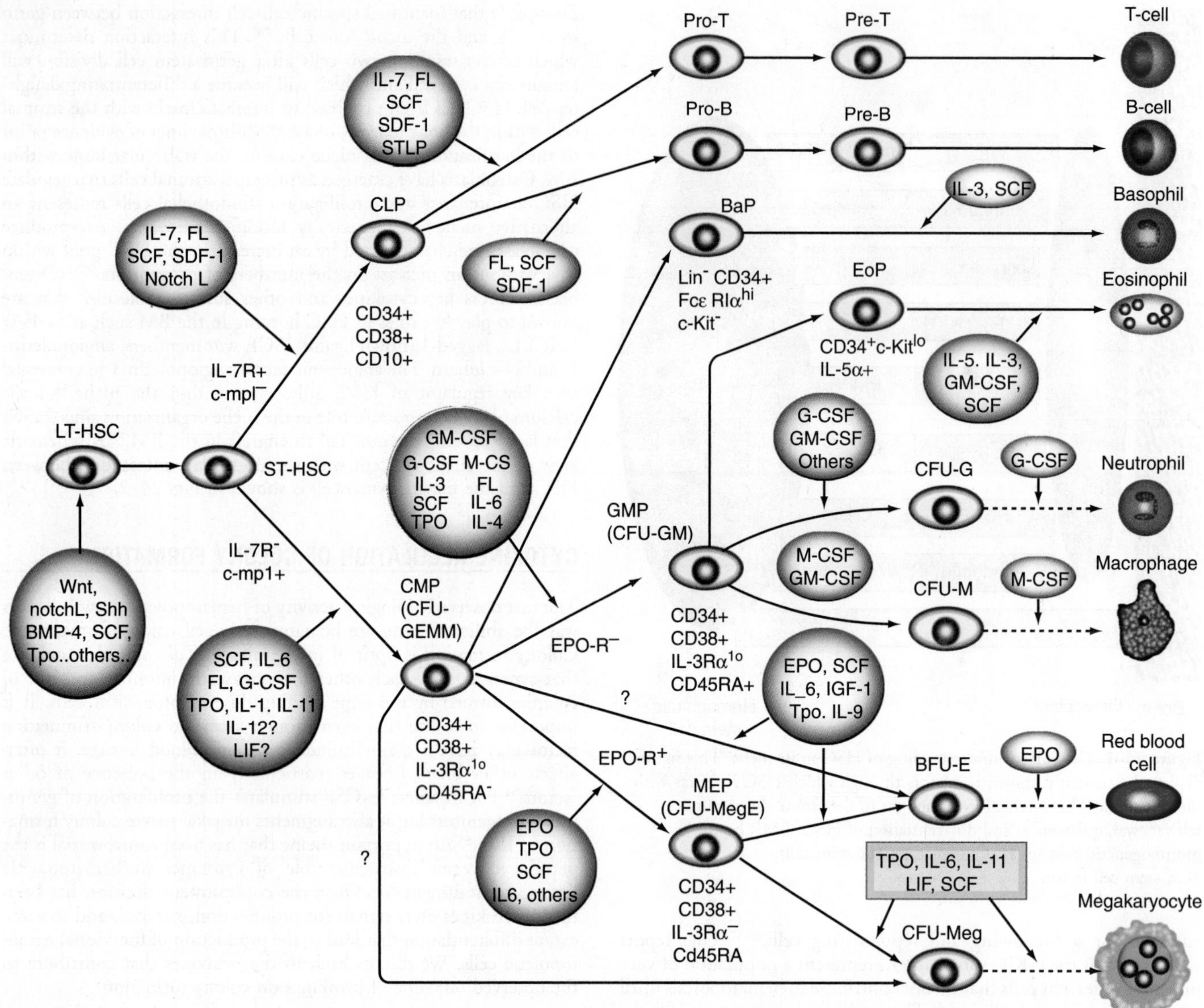

Figure 24–2 Cytokine Activities in Hematopoiesis. The current understanding of hematopoietic hierarchy with the influence of cytokines is indicated. The long-term hematopoietic stem cell (LT-HSC) gives rise to short-term hematpoietic stem cell (ST-HSC). The latter diverges into either common lymphoid progenitor (CLP)[483] or common myeloid progenitor (CMP).[486] CLP harbors transcriptional activity consistent with the lymphoid lineage and gives rise to all lymphoid elements while CMP displays myeloid related gene expression and diverges into granulocyte-macrophage progenitors (GMP) or megakaryocyte-erythroid progenitors (MEP). This progression of maturation associates with suppression of lineage-genes that are not needed. BFU, burst-forming unit; BFU-E, burst-forming unit-erythroid; CFU-MK, colony forming unit megakaryocyte; BMP, bone morphogenetic protein; CSF, colony-stimulating factor; EPO, erythropoietin; IL, interleukin; LIF, leukemia inhibitory factor; SCF, stem cell factor; Tpo, thrombopoietin.

another type of experiment, exogenous erythropoietin receptor (EpoR) expression by the pre-B cell line induced proteins specific to the erythroid progeny in the presence of Epo.[61,62] Ectopic EpoR expression by daughter cells of cord blood CD34+ cells skews the outcome of forming colonies containing more erythroid progeny.[63] Finally the ectopic expression of M-CSFR in an Abelson virus transformed pre-B cell line resulted in a lymphoid to monocytic lineage switch in the presence of M-CSF.[64]

On the other hand, several lines of evidence point to a permissive role of cytokines in the hematopoietic commitment process. In this model the commitment decision is stochastic (random) and independent of cytokine action whose function is to drive proliferation and survival of committed cells that respond to cytokines based on expression of corresponding receptors. The term stochastic was initially utilized by Till et al[65] to explain the mechanism by which a stem cell decides to self-renew or differentiate. Using micromanipulation techniques, Ogawa's group provided evidence in support of a stochastic model of hematopoiesis by analyzing the commitment of cells in the blast colonies.[66,67] The cells of these colonies are characterized by the ability to form secondary multipotential colonies. Analysis of different lineage colonies derived from a single blast cell origin revealed random combinations of lineages.[66] Two daughter cells originating from a single cell origin also gave dissimilar combinations of lineages under identical growth factor conditions.[67] Simulated mathematical models in conjunction with in vivo verification also support a stochastic model of hematopoietic commitment.[68] The most compelling evidence in favor of this model has been obtained from a series of experiments utilizing chimeric cytokine receptors. In one study a chimeric receptor of the extracellular domain of the thrombopoietin receptor (c-mpl) and the cytoplasmic domain of G-CSFR replaced c-mpl in a knock-in model.[69] The homozygous mice had normal platelet levels suggesting that the cytoplasmic domain of the G-CSFR can replace c-mpl to support megakaryocytopoiesis. The cytoplasmic domain of the G-CSFR was replaced with that of the EpoR in a similar approach, without affecting the lineage commitment to neutrophils.[70] The commitment of progenitor cells into a certain lineage seems to be irreversible without converting into cells belonging to other lineages under the influence of cytokines. For example, introducing the EpoR into macrophage precursors results in Epo-stimulated macrophage colonies without development of erythroid cells.[71] Conversely, insertion of the M-CSFR into erythroid precursors results in formation of erythroid colonies under the influence of M-CSF.[72] In other experiments,[73] overexpression of anti-apoptotic gene Bcl-2 in mice deficient in IL-7 receptor reverses the immune dysfunction seen in these mice, which means that a survival signal can compensate for the defect in a cytokine signal, indicating that the specificity in cytokine action may be related to cognate receptor expression on particular cells. Similarly, expression of Bcl-2 restores osteoclast and monocyte deficiencies in M-CSF deficient *op/op* mice.[74] Knock-out models of cytokines and their receptors also support a permissive role of cytokine action. For example, disruption of either Epo or EpoR by gene targeting results in severe anemia.[75] However, the resultant anemia is not due to defective commitment since erythroid progenitors are preserved in these mice.

Cytokines may work though either the instructive or permissive mechanism or both according to the developmental stage of the stem/progenitor cell. It has been clearly demonstrated that multiple lineage genes are transcriptionally active in early progenitors/stem cells and these cells suppress the transcription of irrelevant genes as they progress along the hematopoietic differentiation pathway.[76,77] Certain transcriptional factors are keys in the molecular mechanisms controlling progenitor cell differentiation. The transcriptional factor PU.1 which is an ets family member plays a vital role in myelopoiesis and lymphopoiesis.[78] PU.1 deficient mice lack both myelocytes and lymphocytes. Reintroducing this protein to PU.1 deficient HPCs initially induces mixed myelocyte/macrophage gene expression, but increasing levels of PU.1 promote macrophage differentiation and suppress granulocyte formation.[79] PU.1 (like other transcriptional factors) appears to induce progenitor differentiation at least partly through induction of growth factor receptor expression.[80] The zinc-finger protein GATA1 induces progenitor differentiation into erythroid, eosinophilic and megakaryocyte lineages.[81] There appears to be opposing effects between PU.1 and GATA1 based on their concentrations which direct whether HPC will become myeloid or erythoid cell respectively.[82] In addition, low levels of c-mb favor macrophage and megakaryocyte differentiation, while high levels promote erythropoiesis and lymphopoiesis.[83]

Some of these factors exert negative effects on the development of other lineages. This suppressive activity is released in the absence of such factors. When Pax-5 (a B-cell lymphocyte lineage regulator) is deleted, the knock-out HPCs fail to restrict their lineage choice and differentiate into a variety of cells including macrophages, neutrophils and osteoclasts based on the cytokines added.[84]

Cytokine Regulation of Hematopoietic Progenitor/Stem Cell Proliferation

Progenitor cell proliferation is required for colony formation to occur in vitro and to sustain hematopoiesis in vivo. Lineage-committed progenitors can be triggered to proliferate with the addition of single late acting cytokines such as M-CSF, IL-5, G-CSF, and Epo. On the other hand, triggering proliferation of early progenitors requires stimulation by more than one cytokine. Ogawa divided early-acting cytokines into three groups. One group includes IL-3, GM-CSF, and IL-4, which induce proliferation of multipotential progenitors only after they exit from G_0 and enter cell cycle.[85] A second group includes IL-6, IL-11, IL-12, G-CSF, and LIF and triggers the cycling of dormant early progenitors. A third group includes SCF and FL; this group interacts and synergizes with the factors belonging to the first two groups. Other cytokines have been identified and shown to have activity on HSC/HPC. Cytokine regulation of cell cycle machinery has been studied in detail.[86,87] Cyclin-dependent kinase inhibitors (CDKIs) have stood out as key regulators of HSC/HPC maintenance/proliferation. In knock-out mice of the CDKI $p21^{cip1/waf1}$ the absolute number and proliferation of HSC are increased. HSC self-renewal, as tested by serial transplantation and cyotoxic resistance, was impaired in these mice.[88] It was concluded that $p21^{cip1/waf1}$ controls cell cycle entry of HSCs, and in its absence increased cycling occurs which leads to exhaustion of these cells. Paradoxically $p21^{cip1/waf1}$ plays a role in cytokine-induced proliferation of HPCs and it is upregulated following exposure to synergistic cytokine combinations.[89] In $p21^{cip1/waf1}$ deficient mice, the number and cycling of HPCs appear decreased as compared to wild-type cells.[89,90] This could be due to the association between CDK4 and D-cyclins mediated by $p21^{cip1/waf1}$ and other CDKIs.[91] $p27^{kip1}$ CDKI plays an important role in determining the progenitor pool size and cycling status,[92] where HPC number and cycling is markedly increased in P27 deficient mice. These mice display organomegaly and hyperplasia of different tissues, with tendency to form tumors.[93] HSC cycling and number are not altered in these mice, whereas p27 deficient HPCs dominates hematopoiesis in competitive repopulation experiments.[94] Deletion of the early G_1 phase inhibitor p18 leads to improved long-term engraftment due to improved self-renewal divisions in vivo.[95] Recently, p16 another CDKI was shown to be involved in stem cell aging including HSCs. In its absence, some of the aging qualities such as repopulating defect and apoptosis are reversed.[96] Bim-1 is a polycomb family suppressor gene whose deletion leads to depletion of HSCs and decrease in their self-renewal.[97] This negative effect of Bim-1 loss appears to be largely mediated by derepressing p16 and p19 which are encoded by the same locus.[98] Within the same context another transcriptional repressor; Growth factor independent (Gfi-1) restricts the proliferation of HSCs and enhances their self-renewal and repopulating capacity.[99]

Cytokine Regulation of Hematopoietic Progenitor/Stem Cell Survival

One of the essential functions of cytokines and in general growth factors is to prevent programmed cell death or apoptosis of the target cells.[100] There are few exceptions to this role as seen with some of the suppressive cytokines such as interferons (IFNs) and tumor necrosis factor-α (TNF-α). For example, IFNs increase the expression of pro-apoptotic receptor Fas by hematopoietic progenitors.[101] It is well established that hematopoietic progenitor/stem cells undergo apoptosis upon cytokine withdrawal from culture. This survival enhancing effect of cytokines appears to be independent from the proliferation enhancing action. For example, genistin, a tyrosine kinase inhibitor, blocks IL-3/GM-CSF mediated DNA synthesis but does not affect the action on apoptosis reversal.[102] The GM-CSFR mediates proliferation signals through a cytoplasmic region which is different from that mediating the survival signal.[102] Certain cytokines, such as SCF, can promote hematopoietic progenitor/stem cell survival in the absence of cell division.[103] However, it is too simplistic to consider the processes of proliferation and survival to be mutually exclusive. Quiescent hematopoietic cells are less susceptible to apoptosis inducing stimuli than cycling cells. Variable expression of apoptosis genes occurs during cell cycle progression.[104] Multiple cytokines such as SCF, FL, IL-3 and Tpo suppress apoptosis of $CD34^+$ $CD38^-$ cells in single-cell assays, indicative of a direct effect of these cytokines on progenitor/stem cell survival.[105] Tpo has more potent activity than the other cytokines in this regard. Tpo alone can support the survival of $Sca\text{-}1^+$ Lin^- $c\text{-}kit^+$ cells without stimulating active cell proliferation.[106] Activation of a chimeric receptor that contains the TpoR (mpl) domain results in expansion of BM multipotential progenitors. This effect is not observed with G-CSF or Flt3 fusion receptors, which suggests an essential role for Tpo/mpl in sustaining primitive progenitor survival.[107] Hematopoietic cytokines are selective in their survival enhancing effect. For example, IL-3 enhances $CD34^+$ $HLA\text{-}DR^+$ cell survival more than SCF, while the opposite is true for $CD34^+$ $HLA\text{-}DR^-$ cells.[108] Other nonclassic survival promoting factors have the ability to promote hematopoietic progenitor survival as seen with the chemokine stromal cell-derived factor-1 (SDF-1/CXCL12).[109]

Hematopoietic cytokines and their receptors appear to be essential for the survival of a variety of leukemic cells and may cooperate with oncogenes and tumor suppressor genes to promote leukemogenesis.[110] It is beyond the scope of this chapter to discuss the complex signaling pathways involved in this survival enhancing activity, but there is evidence that more than one survival signal is required. For instance, BCL-2 overexpression can cooperate with c-Kit signaling to prevent primitive progenitor/stem cell apoptosis but neither signal is effective alone.[111]

Synergy among Hematopoietic Cytokines

Another important feature of cytokine activity on hematopoietic progenitors is the synergy seen among cytokines in enhancing colony formation.[112] For example, a combination of Epo, IL-3, GM-CSF, and SCF stimulates the appearance of large colonies of CFU-GEMM, BFU-E, and CFU-GM. Adding Epo alone to BM cells results in the formation of BFU-E derived colonies. CFU-GM derived colonies can form in the presence of GM-CSF as a single cytokine. The size of these single-cytokine induced colonies is smaller and their number is less than those formed in the presence of two or more cytokines. This greater-than-additive effect has been demonstrated with a wide range of cytokine combination. This synergistic activity is explained by several mechanisms including the presence of multiple cytokine receptors on the single progenitor cell,[113] and the induction of the level of some cytokine receptors in the presence of other cytokines.[114] Cytokines may exert their synergy through amplifying the intracellular signals directed towards enhancing survival, and/or proliferation or suppressing differentiation.[115]

Hematopoietic Stem/Progenitor Cell Expansion by the Use of Cytokines

HSCs have the ability to self-renew and divide in vivo to give rise to daughter cells capable of differentiation into all hematopoietic lineages. It is of major clinical interest to expand the pool of HSCs ex-vivo in order to utilize the expanded cells for multiple applications, such as increasing HSCs number in cord blood grafts so that adult recipients can more efficiently undergo cord blood transplantations with single collections. Expanding HSCs and progenitors collected from BM or peripheral blood could potentially shorten or prevent the period of pancytopenia observed after BM ablation. Generating fully functional HSCs from embryonic stem cells is a future goal. Immune-active cells against different tumors might also be produced in adequate quantities from ex-vivo manipulated progenitor/stem cells.

The initial attempts to use cytokines to expand progenitor/stem cells were initiated in the 1980s using crude conditioned media as a source of cytokines.[116] Later, recombinant forms of early-acting cytokines such as SCF, FL, Tpo, Il-6, G-CSF, and IL-3 were used in different combinations in attempts to expand HSCs.[117] Ex-vivo systems that expand committed progenitors have been developed and used with very limited success in clinical settings to shorten the time of pancytopenia following stem cell transplantation.[118,119] Cytokine cocktails have been added to stromal cell-based or stroma-free cultures, in the presence or absence of serum. Many of these systems have resulted in hundreds of fold expansion of the numbers of committed progenitors.[120] However, the major goal is the expansion of primitive stem cells that are capable of engrafting humans. This area of research overlaps with that aimed at understanding the mechanisms of stem cell self-renewal. Several attempts to expand HSCs in cytokine-supplemented conditions have resulted in a modest increase in the numbers of SCID-repopulating cells (SRCs) when culture time is limited to a period of seven days.[121,122] Only a single study has reported a very large expansion of SRC after 9 to 10 weeks of culturing cord blood in vitro.[123] This same group of investigators expanded human adult SRCs sixfold after three weeks of ex-vivo culture.[124] Most other reports have revealed that culturing cord blood HSCs or HSCs from other sources for more than 7 to 14 days results in a loss of long-term engrafting potential as manifested by loss of the capability to engraft secondary or tertiary murine recipients.[125] With the identification of more essential regulators of the HSC self-renewal such as HoxB4, wnt, or notch ligands, it is likely that future efforts may result in more effective expansion of HSCs that could be evaluated in clinical trials.

Cytokine-Mediated Hematopoietic Stem/Progenitor Cell Mobilization and Homing

In mid-1980s it was recognized that hematopoietic cytokines, when administered in vivo, induce elevations of progenitor/stem cell numbers in the peripheral blood.[126] A small percentage of these cells circulates in peripheral circulation during the steady state.[127] Multiple cytokines including certain chemokines exhibit HSC mobilizing activity with variable potency. GROβ, which is a CXCL2 chemokine mobilizes HCS within 15 to 30 minutes of administration in mice and within one hour in rhesus monkeys,[128] whereas cytokine mobilization with factors such as G-CSF occurs days after its administration. G-CSF administration results in degranulation of neutrophils in the BM which release proteases such as neutrophil elastase, cathapsin G, and matrix metalloproteinase-9 (MMP-9). These enzymes cleave essential molecules such as vascular cell adhesion molecule-1/CD106 which is expressed by BM stromal cells and interacts with integrin a4β1 (VLA-4) on HSCs resulting in their release into the circulation.[129] It is of interest that most of the mobilized cells are not cycling and reside in the G_0/G_1 phase of the cell cycle.[130] G-CSF is also an essential regulator of neutrophil trafficking from the BM to peripheral blood.[131] G-CSF administration causes a decrease in the levels of the BM chemokine SDF-1/CXCL12 which has been suggested to play an important role in the mobilization process.[132] SDF-1/CXCL12 is strongly implicated in progenitor/stem cell homing to the BM.[133] SDF-1/CXCL12 is a potent chemoattractant of the progenitor/stem cells.[134,135] Conversely, the hematopoietic stem cell compartment is heterogeneous for CXCR4 (SDF-1 receptor) expression,[136] and CXCR4 null cells from fetal liver engraft normally into BM of wild-type mice. It appears that the SDF-1/CXCL12 pathway is one essential actor, but that other cell surface proteins are also important for homing/mobilization. One strategy that is being pursued is to enhance HSC mobilization is the blockade of the CXCR4-SDF-1/CXCL12 axis, a goal that is achievable with the availability of several CXCR4 antagonists presently being evaluated in clinical trials.[137] Certain cell surface molecules such as the dipeptidylpeptidase CD26 which cleaves SDF-1/CXCL12 play important roles in the homing/mobilization process.[138] Other cytokines may also play a role in HSC homing, such as the membrane form of stem cell factor through interaction with its receptor. A recent report implicates osteoclasts in HSC mobilization in physiologic situations such as bleeding.[139]

Fig. 24–3 illustrates the current understanding of HSC/HPC mobilization.

CYTOKINE RECEPTORS

Cytokine receptors bind their ligands in a specific manner and at low cytokine concentration in order to transduce signals leading to biological responses.[140] These receptors display significant conservation in their structure and activity which allows them to be placed within the cytokine receptor superfamily.[141] There are examples of newly cloned proteins that were determined to be cytokine receptors based on the presence of conserved domains in their structures. For instance, c-mpl was initially cloned as a retroviral oncogene and was promptly designated as an orphan cytokine receptor gene based on its predicted amino acid sequence.[142] This eventually led to the cloning of its ligand, Tpo. Cytokine receptors function as dimeric or oligomeric complexes consisting of two to four chains. Ligand binding results

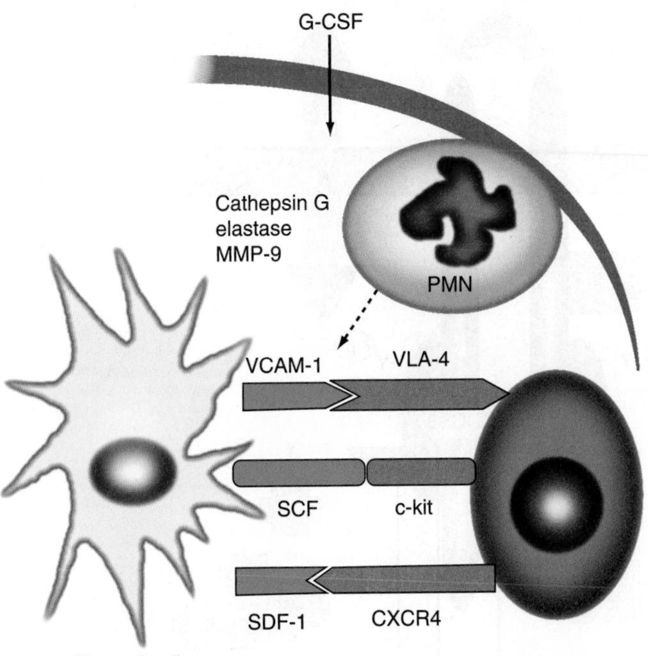

Figure 24–3 Hematopoietic Progenitor/Stem Cell Mobilization. The current understanding of hematopoietic progenitor/stem cell mobilization by growth factor administration is shown. In the model, G-CSF induces proliferation of the progenitor/stem cells and activation of the mature neutrophils. The latter release proteases such as MMP-9, cathepsin G, and Elastase. These disrupt the retention bonds between stromal cells and progenitors/stem cells such as vascular cell adhesion molecule-1 (VCAM-1) on stromal cells and its ligand the integrin VLA-4 on progenitor/stem cell.[129] Other retention signals may include SDF-1/CXCR4,[132,133,135] and SCF/c-kit.These proteases may also contribute by disrupting the extracellular matrix and opening the endothelial gaps. One membrane-bound dipeptidylpeptidase (CD26) is present on progenitor/stem cells, and other cells, and cuts the N-terminal dipeptide of SDF-1 which contributes to producing an inactive SDF-1 which competers with full length SDF-1 for binding to CXCR4.[138]

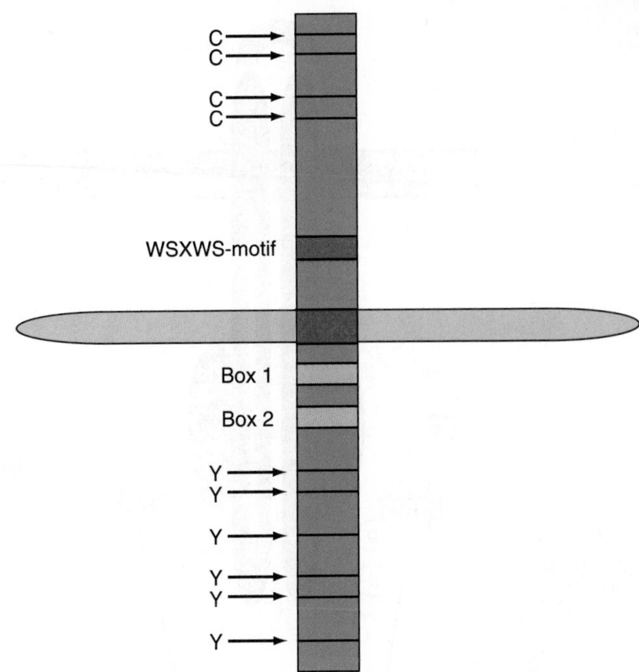

Figure 24–4 Cytokine Receptor Superfamily. The general structure of cytokine receptor superfamily.[141–143] In the extracellular cytokine receptor module (CRM) 4 conserved cysteine residues involved in disulfide bonds. A WSXWS (tre, ser, any, tre, ser) motif that is essential for receptor processing, ligand binding and activation of the receptor. In the intracellular portion, two short domains termed box 1 and box 2 are important for Janus kinases (Jaks) binding. Tyrosine residues are present on the intracellular part to be phosphorylated upon receptor activation.

in dimerization or oligomerization of the receptor chains which causes receptor activation and signal transduction.[143] This mechanism of receptor chain clustering appears to be universal among hematopoietic cytokine receptor and receptor tyrosine kinase families. Other hematopoietic active molecules such as chemokines activate receptors of a different nature.

Cytokine receptor subunit chains can be identical as seen with SCF, Epo, G-CSF, and GH receptors, or different as with IL-6 and IL-3. The cytokine receptor superfamily is generally divided into a few groups based on similarities among members of each group as follows:

Type I Cytokine Receptor Family

The type I cytokine receptor family is also called the hematopoietin receptor family. It contains receptors for most hematopoietic cytokines. The ligands of these receptors have a common four α-helical structure.[144] These receptors exhibit a conserved region of about 200 amino acid residues denoted the cytokine receptor module (CRM) that consists of two β-barrel structural domains. The first domain contains four conserved cyteine residues involved in disulfide bonds and the second domain contains a well-conserved WSXWS motif in its c-terminus.[144] Elucidating the structure of growth hormone receptor (GHR) in complex with GH has provided some explanation of the roles of these conserved residues.[145] Each structural domain within the CRM is related to fibronectin type III domains. These features are present in the extracellular portion of the receptor. Intracellularly, these receptors are more divergent but they have a conserved membrane-proximal domain of two boxes including a hydrophobic α helical segment that serves to bind Janus kinases (Jaks).[146] A general model of type I cytokine-receptor binding comes from a comprehensive evaluation of GH-GHR interaction.[145] In this model, GH binds to one monomer of GHR (which is a homodimer) via a high affinity "site1." After that, the second monomer makes contact with the GH via "site 2." This complex is further stabilized by a receptor-receptor interaction site denoted "site 3." Fig. 24–4 illustrates the general structure of type I cytokine receptors. Fig. 24–5 demonstrates the important signaling molecules that bind to the cytokine receptor and mediate or negatively-regulate its signaling. In the type 1 cytokine receptor family, clusters of receptors share similar components and can be grouped into subfamilies. Fig. 24–6 depicts the cytokine receptor type 1 subfamilies that contain common receptor chains.

IL-3, IL-5, and GM-CSF share a common cytokine receptor β chain (βc) while each receptor has a distinctive α chain.[147] In mice, there is another IL-3 receptor specific chain denoted βIL-3. Targeted disruption of βc results in defective responses to IL-5 and GM-CSF (but not IL-3 due to the presence of βIL-3) with no significant hematological impairment with the exception of reduced numbers of eosinophils due to defective IL-5 signaling.[148] These mice develop alveolar proteinosis.

The IL-6 cytokine subfamily includes IL-6, IL-11, leukemia inhibitory factor (LIF), oncostatin M (OSM), ciliary neurotrophic factor (CNTF), novel neurotrophic-1/B cell-stimulatory factor-3/cardiotrophin-like cytokine (NNT-1/BSF-3/CLC), and cardiotrophin-1 (CT-1). These cytokines exert multiple actions in the hematopoietic, immune, cardiovascular, and central nervous system. They share the gp130 signal transducing molecule as a component of their receptors, whereas the other chains in each receptor contribute to ligand binding.[149] Disrupting gp130 in mice results in embryonic lethality which reflects the importance of gp130 signaling in multiple tissues.[150]

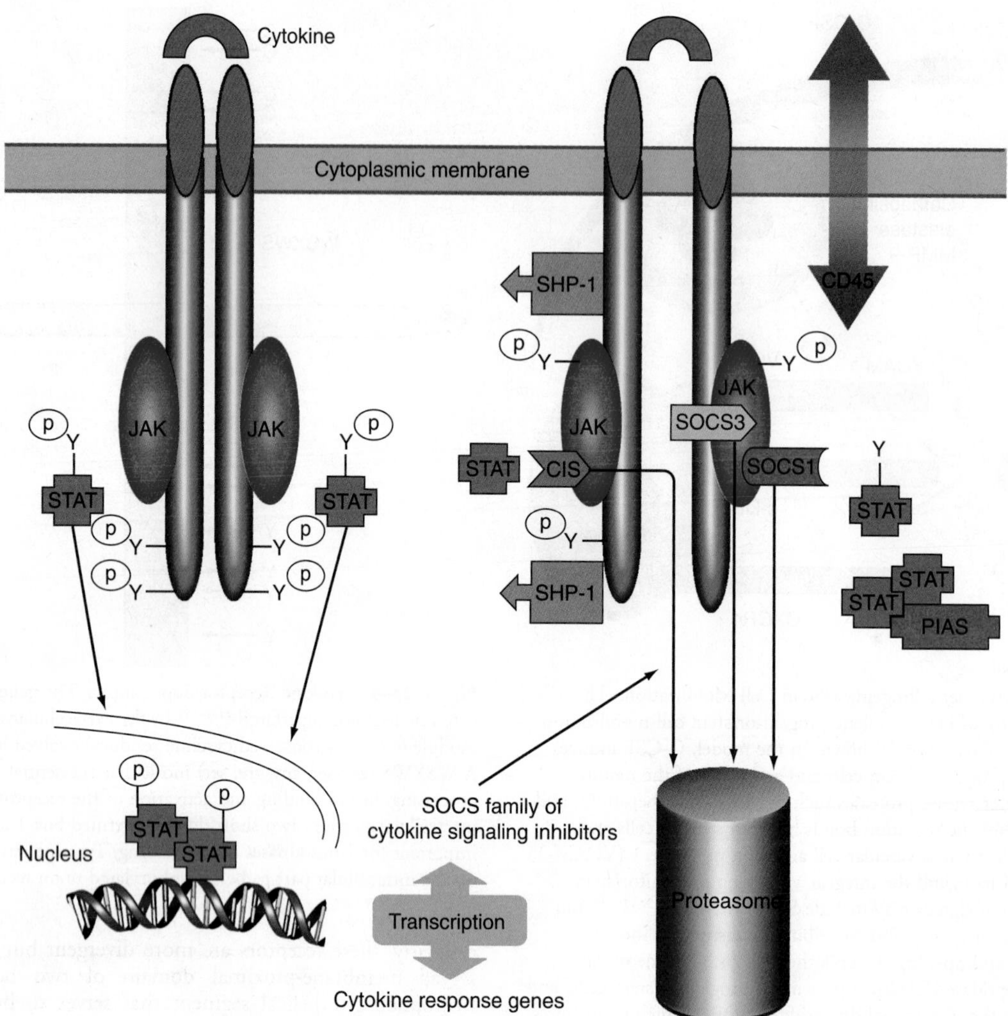

Figure 24–5 Cytokine Activated Signal Transduction. A general depiction of signal transduction by cytokine receptor superfamily. Ligand binding leads to dimerization[143] or oligomerization of the receptor which brings into proximity the associated Janus kinases (Jaks) that phosphorylate tyrosine residues on the receptor and Jaks. This phosphorylation creates docking sites for proteins containing Src-homology 2 (SH2) domains such as signal transducers and activators of transcription (STATs).[156] The latter hetero-or homodimerize and translocate to the nucleus where they affect transcription of target genes by interacting with enhancers/promoters. Several mechanisms exist to reverse this cytokine-activated state. STATs trigger a negative feedback loop by inducing transcription of suppressors of cytokine signaling (SOCSs). There are 8 SOCS members identified. SOCS1 interact directly with Jak and inhibits its catalytic activity. CIS (another SOCS) binds the receptor and blocks binding and phosphorylating STATs. SOCS3 binds the receptor before inhibiting Jak. SOCS proteins contain SOCS box that probably leads to proteosomal degradation of the SOCS associated molecules. SHP-1 is a tyrosine phosphatase that negatively regulates the cytokine transduction process by dephosphorylating Jaks and the cytokine receptors. CD45 is a transmembrane phosphatase that inactivates Jaks as well. PIAS (protein inhibitor of activated STAT) family members bind to STAT dimers and prevent their access to DNA.

The receptors for IL-2, IL-4, IL-7, IL-9, IL-15, and IL-21 share the common cytokine receptor γ chain (γc). This common chain was originally cloned as a third component of the IL-2 receptor and was denoted IL-2Rγ.[151] Mutations in IL-2Rγ result in X-linked severe combined immunodeficiency (X-SCID) in humans.[152] It appears that the severe deficiency in T cells in this disease results from lack of IL-7 signaling, since deletion of IL-7 and IL-7R genes in mice[153] and mutated IL-7R gene in humans[154] results in T-cell deficiency. Defective NK cell function in either IL-15 or IL-15R knock-out mice indicates that NK cell deficiency seen in X-SCID patients is related to defective IL-15 signaling.

Type II Cytokine Receptors

The members of this family are structurally related to typeI receptors and they follow similar patterns of activation and intracellular signaling. This family includes the receptors for IFNs, IL-10 family members, IL-28, IL-29, and the tissue factor (TF or FVIIa) receptor. The extracellular portion contains tandem fibronectin type III domains with other conserved features in analogy with type I receptors.[140] Receptor dimerization or oligomerization results in conformational change in the receptor chains, and the receptor associated Jaks[155] come into opposition with each other. This results in transphosphorylation and catalytic activation of the kinase domain. The activated Jaks in turn phosphorylate the receptor intracellular domain and both phosphorylated receptor and Jaks provide docking sites for a variety of src-homology 2 (SH2) domain containing proteins, particularly the STATs.[156] The latter are then activated by Jak-mediated tyrosine phosphorylation, form homodimers or heterodimers, dissociate from the receptors, and translocate to the nucleus to influence transcription. Table 24–3 demonstrates that cytokines in the same family generally activate the same STAT. IFNs transmit their signals through two types of receptors,[157] type I IFN receptor which binds to type I interferons (IFN-α, IFN-β, IFN-ω, etc). Type I IFNR consists of two components, the IFNAR1 (previously called α

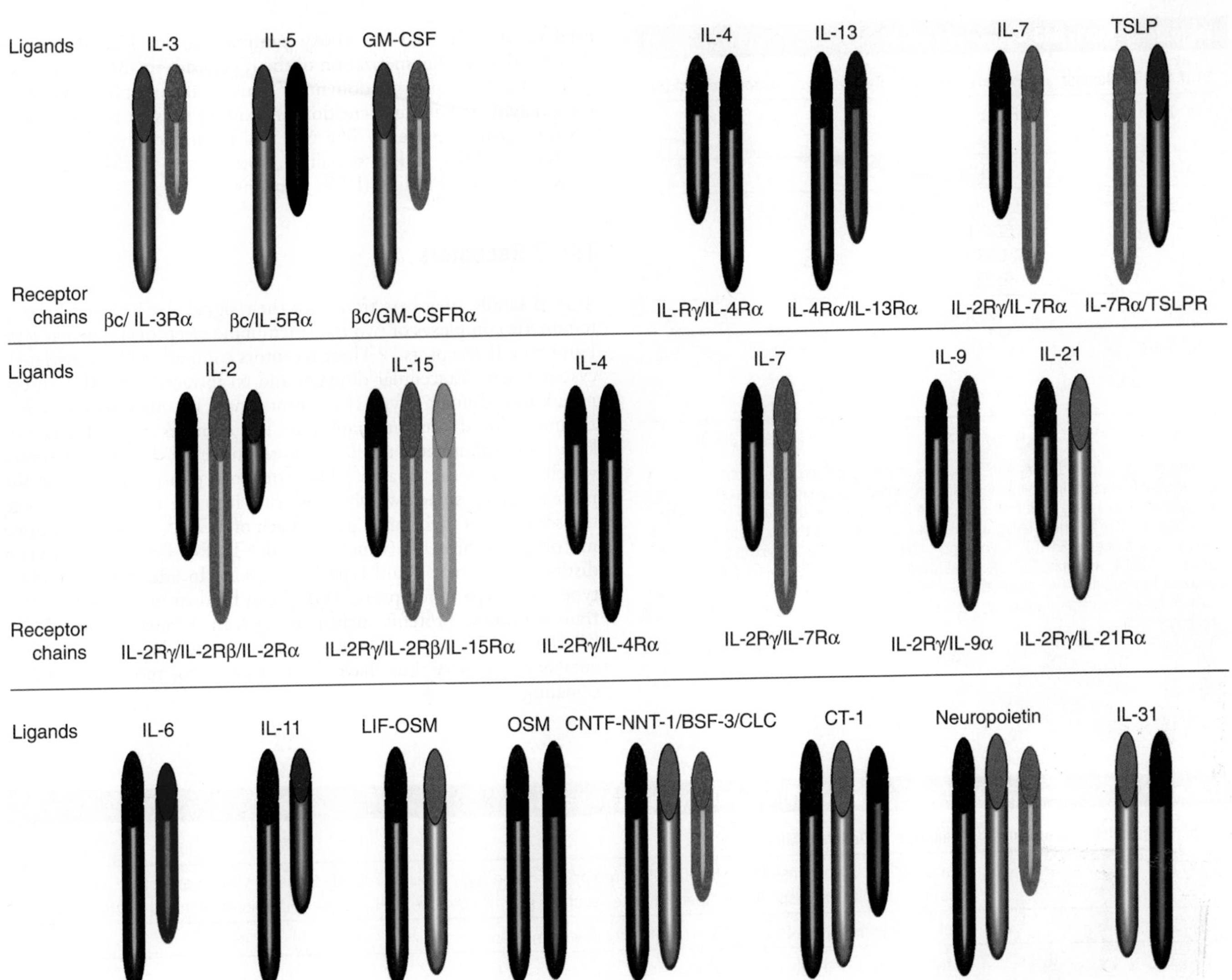

Figure 24–6 Simple depiction of type 1 cytokine receptor subfamilies. IL-3R, IL-5R, and GM-CSFR share a common bc chain that place them in one group. Multiple cytokines (IL-2, IL-4, IL-7, IL-9, IL-15, IL-21) share the IL-2Rg chain, which is mutated in a subset of patients with severe combined immunodeficiency. IL-4R shares a subunit with IL-13R. Both IL-4 and IL-13 drives Th2 response. IL-7R shares one subunit with the thymic stromal lymphopoietin (TSLP). This sharing of receptor subunit may explain why deletion of the gene encoding IL-7R affects the lymphoid system more severely than deleting the IL-7 gene. Finally the IL-6 family includes multiple cytokines that all share the common signal transducer gp130. Deleting gp130 results in embryonic lethality. Some IL-6 family members activate more than one receptor. Oncostatin M (OSM) can work through a heterodimer receptor consisting of gp130 with OSMRb or gp130 with leukemia inhibitory factor-receptor (LIF-R). Ciliary neurotrophic factor (CNTF) shares its receptor with novel neurotrophic-1/B cell-stimulating factor-3/Cardiotrophin-like cytokine (NNT/BSF-3/CLC). Cardiotrophin-1 (CT-1) uses a receptor composed of gp130, LIF-R, and another yet to be identified subunit. Neuropoietin shares the same receptor as CNTF. Il-31 receptor is composed of gp130 like receptor (GLR) and OSMRβ.

subunit) and INFAR2 (previously called β subunit). Type II IFN receptor is also composed of two distinct subunits; IFN-γR1 and IFNγR2. Type II IFN receptor binds to IFN-γ or type II interferon. The receptor chains within a given type II cytokine receptor complex can be divided into two classes denoted R1 and R2. R1 type subunit (eg, IFN-γR1, IL-10 R1) binds its ligand with high affinity, has a long intracellular domain associated with Jak1. IFN-γ and IL-10[158] are homodimers and their binding to R1 subunit leads to homodimerization.[159] However, this event is not sufficient to initiate signaling. The R2 subunit does not bind the ligand and it posses a short intracellular domain which is associated with Jak2 or Tyk2 (IL-10R2).[160] This finally leads to the activation of STATs which translocate to the nucleus. Table 24–4 lists phenotypes of the knock-out mice of the molecules that play important roles in cytokine receptor signalng.

Receptor Tyrosine Kinase Family

The receptor tyrosine kinase family includes c-kit (stem cell factor receptor), flt-3, and c-fms (M-CSF R) in the hematopoietic system. Receptor tyrosine kinases (RTK) act by phosphorylating tyrosine residues on the receptors themselves and on downstream signaling molecules.[161] RTKs consist of an extracellular portion that binds the ligand, a transmembrane helix and a cytoplasmic portion that possesses tyrosine kinase catalytic activity.[162] Most RTKs exist as a single polypeptide chain in a monomeric form in the absence of ligand binding. The extracellular part of RTKs contains a diverse array of globulin domains such as immunoglobulin (Ig)-like domains, fibronectin type III-like domains, cysteine-rich domains and EGF-like domains.[162] In contrast, the cytoplasmic portion is less complicated and consists of a juxtamembrane region followed by tyrosine kinase

Table 24–3 STATs and Associated Jaks

STAT Family Member	Primary Activating Cytokines	Associated Jak(s)
STAT1	IFN-α, β, γ. IL-6, IL-11, OSM, LIF	Jak1, Jak2
STAT2	IFN-α, β	Jak1
STAT3	IL-6, IL-11, LIF, OSM, SDF-1 G-CSF, IL-10, IL20, IL-21, IL-31	Jak1
STAT4	IL-12, IL-23	Tyk, Jak2
STAT5 a/b	Epo, Tpo, FL, GM-CSF, IL-5, IL-3 IL-2, IL-15, IL-7, IL-9, GH	Jak1, Jak2, Jak3
STAT6	IL-4, IL-13	Jak1, Jak3

Listing of signal transducers and activators of transcription (stats), with corresponding activating cytokines and associated Janus kinases (Jaks). Cytokine families tend to activate the same STAT, such as IFN family members that activate STAT1 and STAT2, and IL-6 family members that activate STAT3 and to a less degree STAT1. T-lymphocyte helper (Th)1 cytokines (IL-12, IL-23) activate STAT4, whereas Th2 cytokines (IL-4, IL-13) activate STAT6. STAT5 is activated by multiple hematopoietic-active cytokines such as IL-3, GM-CSF, IL-5 (which share a receptor subunit), Tpo, Epo, and cytokines activating the IL-2 receptor family.

catalytic domain and a carboxy-terminal region. Ligand-induced dimerization or oligomerization of the RTK leads to autophosphorylation of the cytoplasmic domain.[162] This results in enhancement of the catalytic activity and creation of binding sites to recruit downstream signaling proteins. The two well identified phosphotyrosine binding modules within signaling proteins are the SH2 and the phosphotyrosine-binding (PTB) domains.

TGF-β Receptors

TGF-β family members transduce their signals by utilizing heterotetrameric complexes of two transmembrane receptors known as type I and type II receptors.[163] These receptors contain an N-glycosylated, cysteine rich extracellular domain, and an intracellular serine/threonine kinase domain. Type II receptor kinase is constitutively active. Ligand-induced oligomerization of the complex type II receptor kinase phosphorylates typeI receptors on serine/threonine residues which activates the kinase.[163] The latter then phosphorylates specific proteins called smads which translocate into the nucleus to change transcription of their target genes. Each of TGF-β, activins and bone morphogenic proteins (which form the TGF-β family) signal via a distinct set of type I and type II receptors. In addition to binding type I and type II receptors, TGF-β can bind to receptor-associated transmembrane proteins such as betaglycan[164] (also denoted TGF-βR-III) and endoglin. These receptors do not have any intrinsic enzymatic activity but have been shown to modulate TGF-β signaling.

Table 24–4 Consequence of Deficiencies in Genes for Intracellular Signaling Molecules

Signal Transduction Molecule	Phenotype Of Deficient Mice
STAT1	Complete lack of responsiveness to either IFN-α/β or IFN-γ and high sensitivity to infections by viruses and other microbial pathogens. Normal response to other cytokines such as growth hormone (GH), IL-10, and epidermal growth factor (EGF).
STAT2	Lack of responsiveness to IFN-α/β; susceptibility to viral infections
STAT3	Early embryonic lethality prior to gastrulation STAT3 –/+ mice demonstrate decreased HSC/HPCs
STAT4	Defective Th1 response due to defective IL-12 signaling
STAT5a	Defective mammary gland development and lactogenesis; GM-CSF and FL signaling is impaired, but no gross hematopoietic abnormalities
STAT5b	Disrupted sexual dimorphism of body growth rates. Defective GH signaling.
STAT5a/b	Anemic embryos of the double knock-outs with apoptotic erythroid progenitors due to impaired Epo signaling. Adult mouse erythrocyte RBC number is normal. Loss of GH and prolactin signaling. Infertile females. Severe impairment of IL-2 induced T-cell responses
STAT6	Defective Th2 response with eliminated IL-4 signaling
Jak1	Perinatal mortality, defects in IL-6, IL-2, and cytokine receptor type II families.
Jak2	Embryonic lethality due to defective definitive hematopoiesis. Defects in Tpo, IL-2 family, IL-3, and IFN-γ signaling
Jak3	Immunodeficiency due to absent common γ chain signaling. Jak3 expression is restricted to the hematopoietic system
Tyk2	Reduced responses to IFN-α/β, IL-12, and unexpectedly IFN-γ
SHP-1	Natural mutation in *Motheaten* mice results in hair loss, immunodeficiency, autoimmune disorders, enhanced SDF-1 chemotactic activities, enhanced hematopoietic progenitor proliferation in response to cytokines such as GM-CSF.
CD45	Enhanced cytokine and interferon-receptor-mediated activation of Jaks and STATs
SOCS1	Neonatal lethality probably due to excessive IFN-γ responses, with hematopoietic infiltration of multiple organs, lymphopenia, and fatty liver degeneration.
SOCS2	Gigantism due to GH and/or IFG-1 excessive signaling
SOCS3	Embryonic lethality with placental defect. Erythrocytosis in embryos.

This table reveals the phenotypes of mice deficient in the major signaling molecules that directly interact with the cytokine receptors. The phenotype ranges from significant embryonic lethality due to hematopoietic impairment to less remarkable defects in other organ systems. Refer to Figure 24–3 for further information on the functions of these molecules.

Jaks, Janus kinases; SHP-1, Src homology 2 tyrosine phosphatase-1; SOCS, suppressor of cytokine signaling; STAT, signal transducers and activators of signaling.

CHEMOKINE RECEPTORS

Chemokine receptors belong to the superfamily of serpentine seven-transmembrane G-protein coupled receptors. There are 18 chemokine receptors identified which include six CXC, 10 CC, one CX3C, and XC receptors.[165] Each receptor can bind more than one chemokine of the same class, for example, CCR1 binds the chemokines MIP-1α, RANTES and MCP-3 with high affinity.[166] On the other hand, different chemokines can bind a number of receptors such as MIP-1α which binds CCR1, CCR3, and CCR5 with high affinity. Chemokine receptor activation results in conformational change in the trimeric G-proteins which dissociate into α and βγ subunits. These subunits, in turn, activate different targets that lead to the final biological response.[167]

CYTOKINES WITH HEMATOPOIETIC ACTIVITIES

Colony-Stimulating Factors

The colony-stimulating facotrs can induce hematopoietic colony formation in vitro even when used as single factors in the absence of serum. Most of these factors when used alone exert preferential growth-promoting activity on a single blood lineage.

Granulocyte-Macrophage Colony-Stimulating Factor (GM-CSF)

GM-CSF was one of the original four colony stimulating factors identified by its ability to stimulate hematopoietic colony formation in semisolid culture medium systems.[168] The cloning of GM-CSF cDNA led to production of recombinant GM-CSF which provided the opportunity to study its function alone and in combination with other factors.[169] GM-CSF can be produced by a variety of cell types including BM stromal cells, monocytes and T lymphocytes.[170] IL-1 and TNF-α induce the expression of GM-CSF from its source cells.[171,172] GM-CSF induces proliferation and formation of granulocyte-macrophage and eosinophil colonies when added alone to hematopoietic cell cultures.[173] It works in synergy in vitro and in vivo with other cytokines to enhance the proliferation of erythroid, eosinophil, megakaryocyte, and multipotential progenitor cells.[174–176] The concentration of GM-CSF determines myeloid versus monocytic commitment by controlling c-fms (M-CSFR) expression.[177,178] At low concentrations of GM-CSF, macrophage colonies predominate because of the high expression of c-fms, whereas at high concentration mixed (GM) colony formation is favored. When GM-CSF is administered to humans, it enhances the production of neutrophils, monocytes, and eosinophils.[179] Its action on neutrophils production may be indirect and possibly mediated through G-CSF.[180] GM-CSF activates the function of most phagocytes such as neutrophils, macrophages, and eosinophils.[170,181] It can increase their adhesion, chemotaxis, phagocytosis, superoxide production, and their release of other inflammatory cytokines.[182–184] GM-CSF also directs the maturation of dentritic cells from their precursors in combination with other cytokines.[185] The inactivation of GM-CSF in mice does not lead to a significant deficiency of the hematopoietic cells.[186,187] These mice do not display any depletion of mature cells in the peripheral blood. There is also no reduction of BM or spleen cellularity and the progenitor numbers are normal which leads to the conclusion that despite its potent effects in vitro, GM-CSF does not play an essential role in regulating hematopoiesis in vivo at least in mice under basal conditions. Further support of this hypothesis is the observation that the degree of neutropenia in G-CSF knock-out mice is comparable to that of G-CSF and GM-CSF double knock-outs.[188] However, GM-CSF deficient mice are characterized by a deficiency in repopulation by fetal liver stem cells or sorted stem cell, but not by whole BM cells which suggest that GM-CSF production by stromal cells plays a role in radioprotection.[189] The GM-CSF deficient mice develop a characteristic pulmonary pathology that resembles the human disorder alveolar pulmonary proteinosis, since the alveoli contain granular eosinophilic material with peribronchovascular lymphocytic infiltrates.[186,187] These mice acquire multiple bacterial and fungal infections. It is thought that these pulmonary findings are results of hypofunction of alveolar macrophages. GM-CSF receptor is a type I cytokine receptor that is composed of an α chain and a β chain.[190] The latter is shared with IL-3 and IL-5 receptors.[147] One study revealed that the GM-CSFR was not expressed by primitive rhodamine-123 low early progenitor/stem cells but was expressed by more mature progenitor population.[191] GM-CSFR inactivation results in a similar phenotype to that of GM-CSF deficient mice, with the exception that the β-common chain deletion also prevents IL-5 action and causes reduced eosinophil numbers.[192] Conversely, GM-CSF transgenic mice accumulate macrophages and develop blindness and a fatal syndrome of tissue damage.[193]

Granulocyte Colony-Stimulating Factor (G-CSF)

G-CSF was initially purified as a factor that drives the terminal differentiation of a murine myelomonocytic leukemia cell line (WEHI-3B).[194] G-CSF induces the proliferation of granulocyte progenitors and their differentiation into granulocytes.[195] Cloning of the G-CSF gene[196] led to the testing of recombinant G-CSF effects on hematopoietic cells in vitro.[197] G-CSF exerts a proliferative effect on multipotential hematopoietic progenitors[198] that is seen clearly in synergy with other early acting cytokines such as IL-3.[199] Other cytokines that synergize with G-CSF to induce early progenitor proliferation include IL-1, IL-6, and SCF.[200]

G-CSF exerts significant influence on the biological activity of mature neutrophils. For example, it increases neutrophil chemotaxis, adhesion, phagocytic activity, superoxide production, and antibody-dependent cell-mediated cytotoxicity.[201] When a stromal cell feeder line was engineered to produce G-CSF there was an increase in the number of early BM progenitor cells when cultured in the presence of this feeder line.[202] This influence was not observed with a feeder cell line engineered to produce GM-CSF. A role for G-CSF in inducing Th2 and tolerogenic dendritic responses has been suggested.[203] A key role for G-CSF in stem cell mobilization was previously discussed. G-CSF is produced by different mesenchymal cells under the influence of multiple factors such as endotoxin, IL-1[204] and TNF-α.[205] Inactivating the G-CSF gene results in mice with a 70% reduction of circulating neutrophils and a reduced capacity to mount an adequate neutrophil response to infections.[206] In addition, a 50% reduction of progenitors of all lineages is noted, implying the important role of G-CSF in the formation and maintenance of multilineage progenitors from stem cells.[206] Dogs injected with human G-CSF become chronically neutropenic because of the development of neutralizing antibodies to G-CSF.[207] Inactivating mutations of G-CSF receptors can also cause severe congenital neutropenia.[208] The G-CSF receptor is a member of type I cytokine receptor family. It is present on precursor and mature cells of the granulocyte lineage as well as myeloid leukemic cells. It is also expressed on early progenitor/primitive cells.[209] The growth and differentiation signals are mediated by different regions of the cytoplasmic domain of the receptor.[210] Similar to G-CSF knock-out mice, G-CSFR deficient mice have decreased numbers of circulating neutrophils, which are susceptible to apoptosis.[211] In addition there is a decrease in numbers of various hematopoietic progenitors in the bone marrow.

Macrophage Colony-Stimulating Factor (M-CSF)

M-CSF, also known as CSF-1, stimulates macrophage colony growth from hematopoietic progenitors.[212] It is secreted by monocytes/macrophages and BM stromal cells.[213] M-CSF is present in both membrane-bound and soluble forms which are products of alternative splicing.[214] The receptor of M-CSF is the proto-oncogene v-fms which belongs to type III tyrosine kinase receptors.[215] In addition to being a growth factor for monocyte colony formation, M-CSF activates the phagocytic,[216] and respiratory burst activity[217] of these cells. This cytokine is also essential for osteoclast formation[218] and it also affects placental development.[219] Op/op mice, which have a natural M-CSF deficiency, exhibit osteopetrosis and BM failure.[220] The number of hematopoietic progenitors is significantly increased in aorta-gonad-mesonephros (AGM) culture of op/op embryos.[221] The role of M-CSF as a survival factor for monocytes and their derivative cells is nicely demonstrated by the fact that overexpression of the transgenic Bcl-2 gene in these cells corrects the osteopetrosis and marrow failure seen in op/op mice.[74] Finally, certain tumor cell lines secret M-CSF. This implies a possible autocrine or paracrine role in tumor genesis.[222]

Interleukin-3 (IL-3)

Il-3 is a pleiotropic cytokine that is mainly produced by activated T cells although other cell types such as mast cells have been reported to express this cytokine.[223] There is no evidence that BM stromal cells produce IL-3.[171,224] IL-3 has been termed the multi-colony stimulating factor (multi-CSF) due to its wide influence on multiple hematopoietic lineages.[225–227] IL-3 activity is limited when used alone,[228] however, it acts in synergy with multiple cytokines to stimulate the growth of hematopoietic colonies. Such cytokines include SCF, FL, GM-CSF, M-CSF, G-CSF, IL-1, IL-4, IL-5, IL-6, and IL-11.[175,199,229–232] IL-3 stimulates the proliferation of multipotential progenitors[228] and enhances the survival of early hematopoietic progenitors.[108,233] IL-3 exerts a negative effect on lymphoid progenitors.[234] Stromal cell lines have been genetically engineered to produce IL-3.[235,236] These IL-3 producing stromal lines can support sustained hematopoiesis in a murine xenograft model.[235] IL-3 is a direct stimulator of CFU-GM.[229] This cytokine has been reported to promote erythroid burst-colony formation in the absence of detectable Epo.[236] It induces eosinophil formation in synergy with IL-5,[230] and megakaryocyte formation in synergy with IL-11 and SCF.[232] IL-3 can directly promote the differentiation of isolated single megakaryocytes.[237] It is believed that IL-3 may be the main growth and differentiation factor for basophils.[238] This cytokine promotes the differentiation of mast cells from progenitors in murine but not human BM.[239] In humans, mature basophils express IL-3R (CD123) but it is not expressed by mast cells.[240] IL-3 activates basophils and induces them to release histamine. A role for IL-3 in dentritic cell maturation and function has been utilized for generating dendritic cells production in vitro.[241] The IL-3 receptor is a type I cytokine receptor that consists of a specific α chain and a common β chain (βc) that is shared with IL-5 and GM-CSF receptors. In the mouse, a second β chain has been identified that associates exclusively with IL-3Rα and has been termed β IL-3. In mice deficient for βc, the IL-3 response is normal due to compensation by β IL-3.[192] Mice lacking β IL-3 develop normally with normal hematopoiesis.[242] Similarly, hematopoiesis is not impaired in IL-3 deficient mice.[243] This is in contrast to its wide spectrum of in vitro activities.

Erythropoietin (Epo)

Epo was the first hematopoietic cytokine to be cloned[244] and used in a clinical setting: the treatment of the anemia of renal failure. Epo is a hormone in the sense that it is produced by the kidney and to a lesser level by the liver, and it is released to the circulation.[245] VEGF blockade increases hepatic Epo production by more than 40-fold.[246] Hypoxia is the regulator of Epo production.[247] Upon hypoxia, hypoxia-induced factor-1 (HIF-1) enhances production of Epo RNA. HIF-1 participates in the formation of a large protein complex that binds the Epo enhancer.[247] HIF-1 levels are regulated by prolyl hydroxylases (PHDs) which primes HIF-1 for degradation mediated by the Von-Hippel Lindau (VHL) protein.[248] PHD activity is regulated by O_2. Epo does not appear to be required for early progenitor commitment to the erythroid lineage, since both BFU-E and CFU-E are produced in mice lacking either Epo or EpoR.[75] The expression of the EpoR is highest on CFU-E/proerythroblasts and its level decreases with erythroid differentiation.[249] The EpoR is also present on megakaryocytes,[250] endothelial cells,[251] placenta, and cells derived from neuronal tissue. There is an increasing role of Epo in neuronal regeneration and protection from stroke.[252] In the current model of erythropoiesis, Epo appears to rescue EpoR expressing cells from apoptosis[253,254] and it induces erythroid specific proteins such as heme synthesis enzymes and globin. However, there is experimental evidence to indicate that complete erythroid maturation can occur in the absence of Epo. That occurs with the combination of IL-6, SCF, and IL-3.[255] In fact c-kit, the SCF receptor, seems to interact and activate EpoR.[256] Tpo also rescues erythroid colony formation from yolk sac cells of EpoR–/– mice.[257] EpoR is a 66 Kd single chain protein that is a member of the cytokine receptor superfamily.[258] It appears to be activated by homodimerization.

Thrombopoietin (Tpo)

Although suggested to exist more than four decades ago,[259] Tpo is a recently characterized hematopoietic cytokine with a main function of regulating platelet production. Cloning of Tpo was facilitated by identifying the cellular homologue of a retroviral oncogene that causes murine myeloproliferative leukemia.[260] This cellular oncogene termed c-mpl has the amino acid sequence of a cytokine receptor. Three groups cloned the cDNA of the c-mpl ligand.[261–263] Two other groups purified a protein that was found to be identical to Tpo.[264,265] Tpo is produced in the liver, kidney, smooth muscle, and bone marrow among other tissues.[266–268] Its main sources are the liver and kidney. Tpo serum levels are reduced in patients with cirrhosis and increase after liver transplantation.[269] Tpo production is constant, so the increase in its level observed in patients with thrombocytopenia reflects the fact that it is absorbed by platelets by binding to mpl.[270] Tpo levels are relatively low in patients with idiopathic thrombocytopenia (ITP) because of megakaryocytic hyperplasia; megakaryocytes also carry mpl receptors on their surfaces.[270] Certain patients with familial essential thrombocytosis have high levels of Tpo caused by mutations in the 5′-translated region of Tpo gene that causes increased translation of Tpo mRNA.[271] The mpl receptor is expressed by cells belonging to the megakaryocyte lineage from progenitors to platelets[272,273] in addition to being expressed on other lineage committed progenitors.[274] Tpo is the main promoter of megakaryocyte proliferation and differentiation.[274–277] This effect is enhanced by synergistic action of other cytokines.[273,278] There is evidence that Tpo may not enhance the final stage of platelet production.[279]

Tpo effects on hematopoiesis go beyond platelet production into other lineages. Tpo is a well-established stimulant of the proliferation of multipotential progenitor/stem cells both in vitro and in vivo.[280–282] Tpo greatly promotes the in vivo self-renewal and expansion of HSC following BM transplantation.[283] Tpo is an essential cytokine in postnatal stem cell expansion.[284] It synergizes with Epo to expand erythroid progenitors and red cell production.[285,286] The numbers of myeloid progenitors are reduced in Tpo-and c-mpl-deficient mice.[287] C-mpl is a type I cytokine receptor family member. C-mpl deficient mice have been generated.[288] These mice have thrombocytopenia with 100% penetrance. Both megakaryocyte and platelet counts are reduced ≅ 90% while other BM progenitors are reduced from 70% to 90%.[289] Other peripheral blood counts are normal.[288] Tpo deficient mice show a similar phenotype.[290] This phenotype is reversible with administration of Tpo.[287] The remaining platelets are functional in these knock-out mice.[291] The residual megakaryocyte and platelet production in c-mpl deficient animals is not dependent on the action of other active thrombopoietic cytokines such as IL-6, IL-11, IL-3, or LIF.[292,293] Mutations in c-mpl have been identified in children with congenital amegakaryocytic thrombocytopenia.[294]

Interleukin-5 (IL-5)

IL-5 was cloned as an eosinophil differentiation factor.[295] It supports the terminal differentiation and proliferation of eosinophilic precursors.[296] When added alone to untreated BM, it induces the formation of small numbers of colonies, all of which are eosinophilic.[297,298] IL-3 or GM-CSF alone produces similar colonies.[299] These cytokines synergize with each other and with others including SCF and IL-1 in promoting eosinophil colony formation.[299,300] In vivo administration of IL-5 antibodies inhibits eosinophilia in parasitized mice.[301] IL-5 transgenic mice display 65- to 265-fold increases in eosinophil blood counts.[302] Constitutive overexpression of IL-5 in vivo results in a 1.5-fold decrease in BM LTC-IC and 10-fold decrease in fibroblast colony-forming units (CFU-F), with an increase in extramedulary hematopoiesis.[303] Ossification of the spleen has been observed in another transgenic mouse line.[304] Lack of IL-5 severely reduces the eosinophilic response to parasite infection.[304]

Stem Cell Factor and Flt3 Ligand

These two factors demonstrate important costimulatory and synergistic activities with other cytokines, particularly on early hematopoiesis. Mice deficient in these factors or their receptors display significant hematopoietic abnormalities.

Stem Cell Factor (SCF)

The identification of SCF (also known as Steel factor, mast cell-growth factor, and c-kit ligand) and its receptor c-kit culminated years of search for the genetic loci of two naturally occurring mutations in mice: the white (*W*) locus and Steel (*Sl*) locus.[305] The *W* and *Sl* mice have identical phenotypes of hypopigmentation, macrocytic anemia, reproductive difficulties, and defective interstitial cells of Cajal.[305] Transplant studies have demonstrated that the defect in *W* mice is in the hematopoietic stem/progenitor cells, while the defect in *Sl* mice is in the BM microenvironment.[306,307] The *W* locus was identified as encoding the c-kit tyrosine kinase receptor,[308,309] and *Sl* locus was shown to encode the ligand for c-kit that was termed steel factor or stem cell factor.[310–313] Human SCF is present in two isoforms due to alternative splicing.[313] Both forms contain a transmembrane domain that renders them inserted in the cell membrane. The larger form contains a cleavage site that enables a soluble SCF to be released. Both forms are biologically active. However, the cell-bound form appears to be important for in vivo SCF function, since a mutation (Sl^{d}) that eliminates the membrane-bound form without affecting the soluble one results in anemic, sterile, and hypopigmented mice.[314,315] SCF is widely expressed during embryogenesis,[316,317] which suggests that the influence of SCF goes beyond HSC. Germ cells and melanocytes are affected in *W* and *Sl* mutant mice. SCF is expressed on stromal cells,[318] fibroblasts,[319] and sertoli cells.[320] No cytokines have been reported to induce SCF expression, whereas TGF-β represses this expression.[321] C-kit expression has been studied in detail at different stages of the hematopoietic hierarchy.[322] In brief, most murine long-term repopulating stem cells (LTRC) express c-kit,[323–326] although c-kit^{low} LTRC exist. The embryonic AGM progenitor/stem cells of definite hematopoiesis are also characterized by c-Kit expression.[327] Most Thy-1^{lo} Lin$^-$ Sca-1$^+$ cells are c-kit$^+$, however 20% of these cells are negative for c-kit expression.[324] These c-kit$^-$ cells are thought to lack hematopoietic activity. However, one study has suggested that a small population of c-kit$^-$ Sca-1$^+$ BM cells are very primitive HSC which do not contribute to hematopoiesis until 40 weeks after transplantation.[37] With regard to human stem cells, the data are less definitive because of the absence of a comparable transplant assay. In general, CD34$^+$ CD38$^-$ BM cells are highly positive for c-kit.[328] Enrichment of primitive human progenitor cells in the CD34+ c-kit^{low} fraction as compared with the CD34+ c-kit^{high} or CD34+ c-Kit$^-$ fraction has been reported in long-term engraftment studies in fetal sheep.[329] Similarly CD34+ c-kit^{low} cord blood cells contain more cell-cycle dormant and blast cell progenitors than c-kit^{high} or c-kit$^-$ cells.[330]

C-kit is highly expressed by myeloid, erythroid, megakaryocytic, and multipotential progenitors.[331,332] C-kit is also expressed by primary mast cells as well as mast cell lines and primary neoplastic mast cells.[333] It is constitutively activated in a number of mastocytomas.[334] Such gain of function mutations of c-kit are present in human gastrointestinal stromal tumors (GIST).[335] C-kit is frequently expressed by acute myeloid leukemia (AML) blasts of all French-American-British (FAB) subtypes, and activating mutation of c-kit confers a negative prognosis in the subset harboring core binding factor mutations.[336] C-kit expression is restricted to the earliest stages of B-cell progenitors whereas the pre-B cells and subsequent stages are c-kit$^-$.[337] SCF prevents apoptosis of HSC under serum free condition in cooperation with Bcl-2 overexpression.[111] This survival promoting activity can occur in the absence of cell division.[102] SCF sustains HSCs survival in vitro most likely without affecting the self-renewal of these cells.[338,339] There is evidence that this SCF effect on HSC maintenance may be dispensable and other factors may compensate for its loss at least in vitro.[340] Absence of SCF/c-kit axis in vivo results in a partial defect in HSC maintenance and/or self-renewal.[327,341] SCF has little or no effect on colony formation alone, even though it synergizes with other cytokines to promote colony formation.[342–344] This synergy has been reported with almost every known hematopoietic cytokine. This includes, but is not necessarily limited to, IL-3, Epo, GM-CSF, G-CSF, Flt-3, Tpo, IL-9, IL-7, IL-6, IL-4.[343–349] The synergitic activity of SCF is most prominent on the development of mast cell, erythroid, and megakaryocytic lineages. SCF regulates the migration, maturation, proliferation, and activation of mast cells in vivo.[350] Promastocytes proliferate and differentiate in the presence of SCF and IL-3.[351] SCF synergizes with Epo to promote the growth of early erythroid progenitors.[344,345,352,353] Epo overexpression appears to rescue the anemia seen in *W* mice, which suggests a defect in erythroid progenitor cells rather than stem cells.[354] The combination of SCF, IL-6, and soluble IL-6 receptor can support the proliferation, differentiation, and terminal maturation of BFU-E in vitro in the apparent absence of Epo.[346,355] The interaction between c-kit and EpoR may be essential for erythroid precursor response to Epo.[356] SCF synergizes with Tpo to promote megakaryocyte precursor proliferation and maturation.[357,358] Both factors also work in synergy to support multipotential progenitor cell growth.[349,359] The combination of SCF plus other cytokines was used to demonstrate that cord blood contains a higher ratio of immature to mature progenitors than bone marrow.[359] SCF works as adhesion or homing molecule for progenitor/stem cells either directly through its membrane-bound form[360,361] or indirectly by activating the integrins VLA-4 and VLA-5.[362,363] In addition, in vivo administration of SCF causes mobilization of hematopoietic progenitors into peripheral blood.[364–366] It appears that the recruitment of stem and progenitor cells from the quiescent to the proliferative BM niche requires matrix metalloproteinase 9 mediated release of soluble SCF.[367] The molecular defects of c-kit in W mice are heterogeneous but are due to the reduction of tyrosine phosphorylation activity of the protein.[368,369] Such a mutated c-kit is responsible for the human piebald syndrome.[370] Some c-kit activity is needed for postnatal life because homozygous deletion of c-kit or SCF is lethal in mice.[371]

Flt-3 Ligand (FL)

Flt-3 stands for the c-fms (M-CSFR)-like tyrosine kinase 3.[372] Flt-3 as a tyrosine kinase was isolated from a highly purified murine fetal liver progenitor/stem cell pool.[373] Subsequently, its ligand, FL was cloned.[374–376] FL has emerged as an important regulator of hematopoietic progenitor/stem cells.[322] FL is widely expressed by cells in both the murine and human hematopoietic system with the highest level of expression in peripheral blood mononuclear cells.[374–376] Its expression was also reported in the brain and placenta.[377] Flt-3 is expressed on hematopoietic progenitors including 20% to 60% of Lin$^-$ Sca-1$^+$ c-kit$^+$ murine BM cells.[378,379] Flt-3 is expressed by 60% to 80 % of CD34$^+$ BM cells.[380] It is expressed by B- and T-cell precursors, CFU-GM, and HPP-CFC, whereas BFU-E cells appear to be negative for Flt-3.[379–381] Mature hematopoietic cells fractionated from peripheral blood do not express Flt-3.[382] In the Lin$^-$ Sca-1$^+$ c-kit$^+$ pool, only the Flt-3$^-$ fraction supports sustained multilineage hematopoiesis.[379] The Flt-3$^+$ fraction rapidly reconstitutes B and T cell lymphopoiesis in

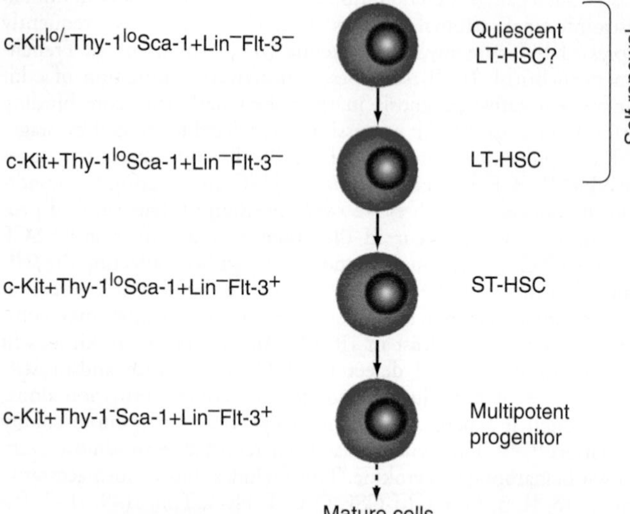

Figure 24–7 Phenotype of Mouse Hematopoietic Stem and Progenitor Cells. C-Kit (SCF receptor) and flt3 expression in early hematopoietic stages.[322] C-Kitlo/- cells used to be called the "mystery cells." Now there is evidence that they may represent quiescent stem cells which require activation before contributing to hematopoiesis.[38] C-Kit expression is seen on the long-term hematopoietic stem cells that give rise to all blood lineages for a lifetime. The latter are negative for Flt3 expression. The appearance of Flt3 corresponds with the short-term repopulating cells that produce multilineage hematopoiesis for the first period (for instance, 8 weeks in mice) after transplantation. The disappearance of Thy-1 antigen indicates maturation into a more restricted stage of multipotent progenitor.

vivo with limited and short-term myeloid reconstitution,[379,383] indicating that Lin⁻Sca-1⁺ c-kit⁺ Flt-3⁺ cells may represent common lymphoid progenitors.[379] Further analysis of this population revealed some myeloid reconstituation with loss of megakaryocye/erythoid potential.[384] The primitive HSC express c-kit but not Flt-3, and it appears that Flt-3 expression is more limited than c-kit expression on committed progenitors by the fact that flt-3 expression is largely limited to the $CD34^+$ $CD38^-$ subset.[385] FL fails to support the survival of the most primitive HSC.[379] However, it promotes the survival of both myeloid and lymphoid progenitors.[386,387] Fig. 24–7 demonstrates the correlation between Flt3 and/or c-kit expression and developmental stage of hematopoietic stem/progenitor cell.

FL has little or no direct in vitro activity on hematopoietic progenitors when used alone. Rather, this cytokine works in synergy with other hematopoietic cytokines, such as SCF, GM-CSF, G-CSF, IL-3, IL-6, Tpo, M-CSF, IL-11, and IL-12 to promote the growth of early progenitor cells.[349,385,388–391] FL promotes the in vitro growth of early B-cell progenitors. Primitive murine ($CD34^+$ $B220^{low}$ $CD24^-$) B cell progenitors do not respond to either FL or IL-7 as single factors, but they do respond to a combination of these cytokines.[392] More differentiated $CD34^+$ $B220^{low}$ $CD24^+$ B-cell progenitors fail to respond to FL.[393] FL synergizes with IL-7 to enhance the production of $B220^+$ cells from $B220^+$ and $B220^-$ murine BM cells. It can promote IL-7 independent B220+ cell development.[394] FL also synergizes with IL-7 to enhance the growth of human $CD34^+$ $CD19^+$ pro B cells.[395] In combination with other cytokines, FL stimulates the growth of $CD4^{low}$ thymic progenitor cells. This effect extends to T-cell production from human CD34+ cells in combination with IL-12.[396] FL enhances the production of dendritic cells (DC) from BM and mobilized $CD34^+$ cells in combination with GM-CSF, TNF-α, and IL-4.[397,398] In vivo administration of FL results in significant increases in a number of both myeloid and lymphoid derived DC in different lymphohematopoietic tissues.[399] This administration results in leukocytosis with mobilization of progenitor/stem cells into peripheral blood.[399,400] Mice with targeted deletion of flt-3 are generally healthy with normal levels of peripheral blood cells.[401] However, these mice have reduced numbers of early B-cell progenitors, plus a defect in repopulating stem cells. Mice homozygous for deletion of both flt-3 and c-kit have markedly reduced hematopoietic progenitor/stem cells and die between days 20 and 50 of age.[401] Further evaluation has revealed that flt-3 deficient mice have a 10-fold reduction in the number of common lymphoid progenitors (CLP) while the numbers of HSCs and common myeloid progenitors (CMP) are normal.[402] FL knock-out mice have a similar phenotype to Flt-3 deficient mice except for decreased cellularity in the peripheral blood, spleen, and BM.[403] This difference has not been convincingly explained. The forced expression of FL in mice results in increased numbers of circulating white blood cell levels with abnormal cellular infiltrates associated with splenic fibrosis.[404]

Interleukin-6 (IL-6) Family

IL-6 family members share multiple characteristics. Most importantly they share the signal transducer gp130 as a component of their receptors. Definite hematopoietic activities have been ascribed to four members of this family: IL-6, IL-11, leukemia inhibitory factor (LIF), and oncostatin M (OSM). These cytokines exert variable effects on and beyond the hematopoietic system. They all share significant stimulating activity on early hematopoietic progenitors, and they all induce the megakaryocyte lineage.

Interleukin-6 (IL-6)

IL-6 was cloned as a novel cytokine that induced B lymphocytes to produce immunoblobulins.[405] It is now realized that IL-6 has a board range of activity on multiple cell types. The IL-6 receptor is a heterodimer consisting of IL-6Rα and gp130.[406] The latter is expressed in cells that do not express IL-6Rα. A soluble form of IL-6R can bind gp130 in the presence of IL-6 and render these cells responsive to IL-6.[407] When used alone, IL-6 has no in vitro hematopoietic activity on human cells even though it induces murine granulocyte-macrophage colony formation.[408] IL-6 synergizes with IL-3 and other early acting cytokines to support the proliferation of early hematopoietic progenitors.[409] It also synergizes with GM-CSF and M-CSF in the formation of granulocyte and macrophage colonies respectively.[410,411] IL-6 stimulates immature megakaryocytes in the presence of other megakaryocytic growth factors.[412] When administered in vivo it stimulates multilineage hematopoiesis and accelerates bone marrow recovery after 5-FU injection or radiation therapy.[413] It increases platelet count in a dose-responsive manner.[414] There is evidence that a significant portion of IL-6 hematopoietic activity is indirect and related to stimulating other cytokines.[415] IL-6 deficient mice display impaired immune and acute-phase responses.[416] In addition, these mice have a decrease in early-multilineage progenitor cell survival.[417] IL-6 is the major cytokine driving myeloma cell proliferation[418] and it is the principal hepatocyte acute phase reactant factor.

Interleukin-11 (IL-11)

IL-11 is a cytokine with a primary hematopoietic function.[419] It was originally cloned from BM stromal cell line.[420] IL-11 exerts minimal influences on hematopoiesis on its own, but it synergizes with multiple cytokines to enhance progenitor cell colony formation. This synergy has been reported with SCF, GM-CSF, IL-3,IL-4, IL-6, and Tpo.[278,421,422] The IL-11 hematopoietic influence is most prominent on the megakaryocytic lineage.[423,424] However, this activity extends to other hematopoietic progenitors such as CFU-GEMM, CFU-GM, BFU-E, CFU-G, CFU-E, and CFU-M.[424,425] When administered in vivo, IL-11 hastens bone marrow recovery after cytotoxic therapy as reflected by increased peripheral blood platelets and neutrophil counts.[424,426] IL-11 stimulates proliferation of multipotential progenitors[425,427] without promoting stem cell self-renewal.[425] IL-11 can maintain early progenitor/stem cell survival in vitro in combination with other cytokines.[428] IL-11 is one of the cytokines that facilitates the entry of dormant hematopoietic cells into the cell cycle.[85,429] IL-11 has activities similar to that of IL-6 in that it promotes the proliferation of immunoglubulin secreting B cells and it enhances the growth of IL-6 dependent plasmacytoma cell lines.[430] It also induces the secretion of hepatic acute phase proteins, but with less potency than IL-6.[431] BM stromal cells, fibroblasts, brain, and testes have been reported to produce IL-11.[432] The receptor for IL-11 consists of two chains, IL-11 Rα[433] and gp 130[434] shared with other IL-6 receptor family members. Despite the tangible influence of IL-11 on in vitro hematopoiesis, IL-11 Rα deficient mice do not display any hematopoietic abnormality.[435]

Leukemia Inhibitory Factor (LIF)

Leukemia inhibitory factor is a pleotropic cytokine with unequivocal hematopoietic activity.[436] It was purified as a factor that induces differentiation of murine myeloid leukemic M1 line.[437] It is a cytokine known for its ability to inhibit the differentiation of mouse embryonic stem (ES) cells.[438] LIF is produced by marrow stromal cells,[439] monocytes, and blastocytes. Cloning[440] and production of pure LIF has shown that it does not stimulate hematopoietic progenitors when used alone, but it induces proliferation of multipotential (CFU-GEMM) and eosinophil (CFU-EO) progenitors when added with serum.[441] BFU-E size is also increased in the presence of LIF.[441] This cytokine is as effective as IL-6 or G-CSF in stimulating IL-3 dependent human blast colony-forming cells that are considered primitive hematopoietic cells.[442] When administered in vivo, LIF expands megakaryocyte mass in mice.[443] LIF induces acute phase proteins and raises platelet counts in primates.[444] Other activities include influencing bone and muscle metabolism, inhibition of lipoprotein lipase, and induction of cytokines production. The LIF receptor shares gp130 with other members of IL-6 family receptors, plus a specific α chain (LIF-Rα) that binds LIF with a low affinity.[445] Targeted disruption of LIF-Rα results in placental, skeletal, neuronal, and metabolic defects, leading to perinatal death.[446] Hematologic and primordial germ cell compartments appear normal in the LIF-Rα knock-out pups.[446]

Oncostatin M (OSM)

OSM was isolated as a growth inhibitor of epithelial cell carcinoma cell lines.[447] It belongs to the IL-6 cytokine family and shares activities, particularly with LIF, such as blocking differentiation of ES cells.[448] T lymphocytes, monocytes, stromal cells, and eosinophils secrete OSM. OSM has no direct effect on hematopoietic progenitors when used alone. Preincubation of BM cells with OSM inhibits cytokine-induced progenitor proliferation.[449] OSM has been implicated in Th1 stimulation of hematopoietic progenitor cell proliferation.[450] OSM, along with SCF and IL-1, is produced by an AGM derived cell line that sustains the survival of SCID-NOD repopulating cells for four weeks.[451] Fetal hepatocyte development is induced in vitro by the addition of OSM and steroids.[452] It is thought that the paracine action of OSM (secreted by hematopoietic cells) is essential for fetal liver development.[453] When fetal hepatic cells are induced to mature by OSM, they lose their hematopoietic supportive capacity.[453] This mechanism is suggested as an explanation for termination of liver hematopoiesis during fetal development. In vivo administration of OSM results in the dramatic accumulation of immature and mature T cells in the lymph nodes that is independent of the presence of the thymus.[454]

OTHER CYTOKINES WITH HEMATOPOIETIC ACTIVITIES

In this section, we discuss a group of classic cytokines that have wide-spectrum regulatory functions on different physiologic and pathologic processes such as immunity and inflammation, and show hematopoietic stimulatory or inhibitory activities as well.

Interleukin-1 (IL-1) Family

IL-1α and IL-1β are the most widely investigated of the IL-1 cytokine family.[455] Although monocytes and macrophages are considered the main source of IL-1,[204] almost every cell type produces and responds to this cytokine. Two IL-1 receptors exist: type I receptors which transmit the intracellular signal[456] and type II receptors which do not signal and may work as a decoy receptor.[457] IL-1 does not induce hematopoietic colony formation when used alone. However, it synergizes with multiple cytokines in this regard. It is thought that most of the hematopoietic activity of IL-1 is indirect and related to its stimulation of cytokine secretion[458] and to a lesser degree cytokine receptor expression. When administered in vivo, IL-1 induces neutrophilia, and a single low dose injection of IL-1 accelerates multilineage recovery after BM ablation.[459] At higher doses IL-1 suppresses myelopoeisis in vivo[460,461] probably due to induction of IFNs, TNF-α and prostaglandin E2 that inhibit progenitor cell proliferation. Chronic administration of IL-1 to mice results in anemia in association with a decrease in the numbers of CFU-E.[461] IL-1 does not appear to be important for normal hematopoiesis since IL-1β deficient mice have no hematopoietic abnormalities.[455] IL-1β and IL-1α double knock-out mice have been created with no disrupted hematopoiesis reported.[462]

Interleukin-2 (IL-2)

IL-2, or T-cell growth factor, was initially isolated from conditioned media that stimulates T-cell proliferation.[463] The main source of IL-2 is the T cells themselves. Apart from its important immunologic activities, IL-2 exerts minimal influence on hematopoiesis. Conflicting reports have described this influence. Some suggested stimulatory functions of IL-2 on in vitro hematopoietic colony formation,[464,465] although others reported inhibition of colony formation by IL-2.[466,467] Most studies indicate that the IL-2 effect on hematopoiesis requires the presence of T cells.[467] IL-2 administration to mice results in enhancement of extramedullary hematopoiesis.[468] The IL-2 receptor is expressed on some hematopoietic cell lines and this expression is induced by IL-3.[469] IL-2 knock-out mice develop autoimmune hemolytic anemia, inflammatory bowel disease, and reduced T-cell response to mitogens.[470] No hematopoietic abnormalities have been reported in these mice.

Interleukin-4 (IL-4)

IL-4 was identified as a T-cell derived B-cell growth factor.[471] The receptors for IL-4 are present on B and T lymphocytes, mast cells, macrophages, and hematopoietic progenitors.[472,473] IL-4 exerts both positive and negative activities on hematopoietic colony formation depending on its target cells and the nature of other cytokines added to the culture media.[10] IL-4 supports the formation of multipotential blast colonies and small GM colonies from BM or spleen cells of 5-FU treated mice.[474] IL-4 is considered to be an intermediate-acting cytokine that acts on early hematopoietic progenitors.[12] It also interacts with lineage specific cytokines, such as G-CSF and Epo to produce neutrophil or erythroid (both CFU-E and BFU-E) colonies, respectively.[475] IL-4 inhibits murine IL-3-dependent colony formation by granulocyte, macrophage, and multipotential progenitors.[476] Some of the IL-4 hematopoietic activity is indirect and related to its induction of other cytokines.[476] IL-4 deficient mice are characterized by reduced hematopoietic progenitor numbers and cycling[477] in addition to having a defect in immunoglobulin production.[477]

Interleukin-7 (IL-7)

IL-7 was cloned as a murine pro-B cell growth factor.[478] Shortly after, it was recognized to have prominent activity on immature and mature T cells.[479] IL-7 is produced by multiple stromal cells particularly the in the thymic stroma. It is also produced by the bone marrow stromal cells.[480] IL-7 is a critical regulator of both T cells and B cells in mice and of T cells in humans.[480] It stimulates the proliferation[481] and prevents the apoptosis[482] of both B- and T-cell progenitors leading to significant increases in B- and T-cell numbers. IL-7R expression has been identified as the earliest phenotypical marker of HSC commitment to the common lymphoid progenitor which gives rise to all lymphoid cell types.[483] IL-7 is also a critical regulator of homeostatic proliferation and survival of naïve T cells.[484] Some reports suggested modest synergistic activity of IL-7 with other cytokines[485] on the myeloid lineage despite earlier reports of absence such activity. However, given the fact that the common myeloid progenitors are present in the IL-7 receptor negative compartment[486] (at least in mice), it is likely that IL-7 myeloid enhancing activity is indirect and mediated by inducing other cytokines. IL-7 knock-out mice have a critical deficiency in the lymphocyte compartment,[487] with 10 to 20-fold reduction in the number of T cells. IL-7Rα deficient mice display a more severe phenotype with massive reduction in thymocytes and peripheral T cells.[488] This may be secondary to a disrupted signaling of the thymic stromal-derived lymphopoietin (TSLP) which utilizes IL-7Rα as a component of its receptor.[489] B-cell development is significantly impaired in both IL-7 and IL-7Rα deficient mice. The IL-7Rα inactivation is seen in subset of patients with severe-combined immunodeficiency.[490] The presence of B cells in these patients indicates different activities of IL-7 in humans compared to mice.

Interleukin-9 (IL-9)

IL-9 was cloned as a cytokine that supports the growth of the human megakaryoblastic leukemia cells line M07E.[491] IL-9 has a positive proliferative activity on the erythroid progenitors.[492] It acts on an early progenitor population of IL-3 responsive BFU-E.[492] This colony-enhancing activity is Epo dependent, although IL-9 alone sustains the survival of erythroid progenitors in vivo as assessed by delayed addition of Epo. SCF and other cytokines enhance the erythroid colony-forming activity of IL-9.[493] IL-9 increases the number of multipotential progenitors in the presence of SCF.[493] Despite its activity on M07E cells, IL-9 has no activity on megakaryocyte colony formation.[491] Transducing $CD34^{++}$ $CD33^{-}$ cord blood cells with retroviral vectors carrying IL-9 or IL-9 receptor resulted in enhanced proliferation of erythroid progenitors.[494] IL-9 deficient mice demonstrate a role for IL-9 in pulmonary mastocytosis and goblet cell hyperplasia.[495] No hematopoietic abnormalities were reported in these mice.

Interleukin-10 (IL-10)

IL-10 was identified as a cytokine synthesis response inhibitory factor that is secreted as a part of Th2 response and that inhibits IL-2 and IFN-γ production by Th1 cells.[496] In contrast to its prominent immunomodulatory effects, IL-10 modestly affects hematopoiesis. It inhibits human BFU-E probably by suppressing other cytokines such as GM-CSF.[497] It also inhibits CFU-GM by the same mechanism.[498] Others reported stimulatory effect of IL-10 on megakaryocytes, mast cells and multilineage colonies in the mouse.[499] IL-10 deficient mice develop chronic enterocolitis if not kept in a germ-free environment.[500]

Interleukin-12 (IL-12)

IL-12 was originally identified as a cytokine that stimulates mature T lymphocytes and NK cells.[501] It promotes the development of Th1 $CD4^{+}$ T cells.[502] IL-12 is a heterodimer of a P40 unit that shows homology to IL-6 receptor, and a P35 unit that is homologous to IL-6 and G-CSF (so it is thought that IL-12 is a complex of a cytokine and a receptor).[503] One monomer of the IL-12 receptor displays high homology to gp130, which is the common signaling chain of IL-6 family receptors.[504] As is the case with costimulatory cytokines, IL-12 requires the presence of other hematopoietic factors to enhance colony formation. It potently and synergistically stimulates murine Lin^{-} $Sca\text{-}1^{+}$ cells to form various hematopoietic colonies in combination with other cytokines such as G-CSF, IL-3, M-CSF, SCF, and FL.[505] It stimulates the proliferation of CFU-GEMM when added with SCF, and supports the growth of progenitors with both myeloid and lymphoid potential indicating an activity on early progenitors.[506] Single-cell experiments suggest that this effect is direct. It is also known that hematopoietic progenitors express the IL-12 receptor. In vivo administration of IL-12 results in enhanced extramedullary hematopoiesis in the spleen and bone marrow hypoplasia with pancytopenia.[507] This in vivo inhibitory effect is secondary to its induction of IFN-γ, because this inhibitory activity is not seen when IL-12 is administered to IFN-γ R–/– mice.[508] IL-12 deficient mice display defective IFN-γ production and type-1 cytokine response.[509] Numbers and cycling of progenitors in the BM are reduced compared to wild-type.[509]

Interleukin-17 (IL-17)

IL-17 was cloned as a CD4 T-Cell secreted cytokine with homology to a herpes virus saimiri gene.[510] IL-17 stimulates epithelial, endothelial and fibroblastic cells to secrete cytokines such as IL-6, IL-8, GM-CSF, Epo, and IL-1.[511] This cytokine is devoid of direct effects on hematopoietic progenitors but works through induction of other cyokine secretion.[511] When cultured in the presence of IL-17, fibroblasts sustain the proliferation of $CD34^{+}$ cells with a preferential maturation into neutrophils.[511] SCF and G-CSF are required for IL-17 mediated granulopoiesis.[512] Overexpression of IL-17 in vivo results in significant granulopoiesis.[513] Other IL-17 family members have been cloned.[514] These display variable activity on hematopoiesis,[515] with mainly inhibitory effects on progenitors.[516]

IL-20

IL-20 stimulates the hematopoietic multipotential progenitors without affecting the more mature progenitors.[517]

IL-31

IL-31 is a recently discovered helical cytokine that is involved in promoting the development of dermatitis. IL-31 R is involved in positive regulation of cycling and numbers of immature subsets of HPCs. IL-31 does not alter in vitro proliferation of HPC, but it enhances the survival of these cells when growth factor addition is delayed.[518]

CANDIDATE STEM CELL REGULATORS

Recent investigations have implicated novel membrane-bound or soluble factors in the regulation of hematopoiesis particularly the early stages of this process. Members of these groups have wide activities outside the hematopoietic system as well.

The Notch Ligands

Four mammalian notch family members have been indentified. These are highly-conserved transmembrane glycoprotein receptors that get activated by binding their ligands such as Jagged-1, Jagged-2, and Delta1-4 which are in turn transmembrane proteins.[519] This binding leads to proteolytic cleavage of the intracellular portion of notch. The latter translocates to the nucleus to influence transcription of target genes. Notch proteins are widely expressed in multiple cell types including the hematopoietic progenitors, T and B lymphocytes, monocytes, and neutrophils.[520] On the other hand, notch ligands are expressed on BM stromal cells, fetal liver and thymus.[520] The first human notch orthologue was discovered as a product of the gene involved in translocation in T-cell lymphoblastic leukemia.[521]

The evidence for a strong involvement in hematopoiesis was inferred when the expression of the constitutively active form of notch1 in murine hematopoietic progenitors resulted in the production of a cell line with the characteristics of primitive cells that can differentiate into lymphoid or myeloid cells in vitro in the presence of relevant cytokines.[522] This cell line can also repopulate lethally irradiated mice. The activation of notch receptors with exogenous ligands presented in soluble or immobilized forms results in an increase in murine progenitor cell numbers with a block in their differentiation. For example, Jagged1 and Jagged2 induce significant amplification of Sca-1$^+$ c-kit$^+$ Lin$^-$ and HPP-CFC cells, respectively.[523,524] A form of Delta1 bound to the Fc portion of immunoglobulin in combination with a cytokine cocktail can cause a massive increase in short-term myeloid and lymphoid repopulating cells.[525] Activated notch1 expression in murine hematopoietic cells resulted in an increase in the number of early progenitor/stem cells in vivo.[526] The effect of notch ligands on the proliferation of human hematopoietic progenitors has been less remarkable. However one report has suggested that an immobilized form of Delta1 is able to remarkably expand human CD34$^+$ cells and SRC again in combination with a cytokine cocktail.[527] There is evidence that Jagged-1 can maintain cord blood NOD/SCID Repopulating Cells (SRCs) in vitro for at least two weeks while these cells lost their repopulating activity in control media.[528] One report has implicated Notch signaling in osteoblast maintance of HSC niche through production of Jagged1.[50] Another report suggested a role of notch signaling in preventing HSC differentiaion, and through the use of Notch/Wnt double reporter mice, the authors revealed the interaction between these pathways. Wnt3a induced notch target genes, and notch signaling had to be intact for Wnt to enhance self-renewal of HSC.[529] Notch signaling has been implicated in cell-fate determination. This has been observed in the hematopoietic system since this system favors lymphoid over myeloid commitment.[525,526] Knock-out mice have been generated for most of the notch receptors and ligands.[519,520] Their embryos die early before E9.5 because of profound developmental defects. No abnormal yolk-sac primitive erythropoiesis is seen.

Wnt Family Members

The Wnt family is a conserved group of proteins with diverse functions in embryogenesis, cell fate, and formation of almost every organ.[530] Wnt proteins are essential for cellular polarity, and they stimulate mammary tumors in mice. Some of them induce axis duplication when ectopically expressed in frog embryos. Wnt proteins are secreted and usually associated with the cell surface or extracellular matrix. Media conditioned with human or murine cells overexpressing these proteins have been used to delineate their roles in the hematopoietic system. Among multiple Wnt members, Wnt-5A and Wnt-10B are expressed in murine yolk sac and fetal liver AA4$^+$ cells.[531] Wnt-10B is expressed in fetal liver AA4$^+$ Sca-1$^+$ c-Kit$^+$ (flASK) primitive cells. Wnt receptors, frizzled 3–7, are also expressed in murine fetal liver. Wnt-1, Wnt-5A, and Wnt-10B stimulate several fold expression of hematopoietic cells after seven days in combination with SCF, compared to a control of SCF alone.[531] Wnt-5A, Wnt-2B, and Wnt-10B are expressed in human fetal bone stromal cells and several hematopoietic cell lines.[532] CD34$^+$ Lin$^-$ cells do not express Wnt proteins even though Wnt-5A may be expressed in some of these cells. Six frizzled genes are expressed in human or fetal CD34+ cells. When conditioned media from stromal cells over-expressing Wnt-5A, Wnt-2B, Wnt-10B are added to CD34$^+$ Lin$^-$ cells, a 20-fold increase in multipotential progenitors is noted. There is also twofold increase in their number compared with SCF or IL-3 containing media.[532] Wnt-11 anti-sense prevents the differentiation of the quail mesoderm stem cell line QCE6 into blood cells in optimized media. Addition of Wnt-11 or Wnt-5A-conditioned media restores the multilineage hematopoietic differentiation of the parent QCE6 cells.[533] Some Wnt proteins are mitogenic for pro-B cells,[534] while Wnt-3A reduces the number of B cells and myeloid-lineage cells produced in long-term bone marrow cultures only in the presence of stromal cells.[535] A lipid modified form of Wnt-3A has been purified and shown to display characteristics of stem cell growth factor.[536] Manipulating molecules of the Wnt signaling pathway affects stem cell expansion as seen with overexpressing β-catenin.[537] Glycogen synthase kinase-3 inhibitors enhance HSC repopulating capacity in vivo.[538] Valproic acid which can work as an histone deacetylase inhibitor was shown to increase the self-renewal potential of mouse stem cells. It was reported to upregulate β-catenin expression.[539] In another experiment conditional inactivation of β-catenin in BM did not affect the self-renewal or the repopulation potential of HSC, which suggests that Wnt may work through a non-canonical pathway.[540] However recent reports utilizing conditional expression of a stable form of β-catenin resulted in blockade in HSC differentiation, loss of repopulating potential and entry into cell cycle.[541,542] This complicates further understanding the exact role of Wnt within the HSC niche and indicates the delicate impact of Wnt signalling dose on HSC response. Mice lacking different Wnt genes display a wide range of abnormalities particularly musculoskeletal, neuronal and kidney defects. Some die perinatally. No specific hematopoietic abnormalities have been reported in these mice.[530]

Sonic Hedgehog

Sonic hedgehog Shh is one of a three member family that is implicated in tissue specification during embryogenesis. Shh was shown to induce HSC proliferation via bone morphogenic protein BMP signaling.[543] Activated Shh pathway induces cycling of HSC but at the expense of self-renewal.[544]

Bone Morphogenic Proteins (BMPs)

BMPs are members of the TGF-β superfamily which also includes Activins. BMP-4 plays a key role in mesoderm induction and hematopoietic commitment.[545] BMPs promote the differentiation of human embryonic stem cells into cells belonging to the hematopoietic lineage in combination with other cytokines.[546] Treatment of human HSCs (CD34$^+$CD38$^-$Lin$^-$) with BMP2 and BMP7 inhibited proliferation while, using relatively high concentrations of BMP4 enhanced survival and increased the engraftment following ex-vivo culture.[547] Mice lacking BMP4 die between E7.5 and E9.5 and exhibit severe defects in mesoderm formation. Embryos that survive up to E9.5 show defective blood islands.[548]

Angiogenic Factors and Angiopoietin-Like Proteins

Multiple angiogenic factors have been identified in different biological systems. We focus on the vascular endothelial growth factor (VEGF) family and angiopoietins (ang-1-4). The VEGF family includes five mammalian members: VEGF-A-D and placental growth factor (PLGF).[549] 4 Receptors have been identified: VEGFR-1 (Flt-1), VEGFR-2 (Flk-1/KDR), VEGFR-3 (Flt-4), and neuropilin-1. Each of these receptors binds more than one ligand which complicates the interpretation of each ligand/receptor function. VEGF family members are essential for regulating various aspects of normal and pathologic angiogenesis. VEGF-A exerts both a stimulatory effect on mature subsets of hematopoietic progenitors and an inhibitory effect on the more immature subsets in the presence of other cytokines.[550] These effects are mediated by both direct and indirect actions on the hematopoietic progenitors.[550] Cells are induced to secrete

VEGF-A by cytokine stimulation.[551] VEGFR-2 (the main receptor for VEGF-A) expression defines a population of early embryonic hematopoietic progenitor/stem cells.[552] NOD/SCID repopulating HSCs were reported to be present in the population of $CD34^+$ $VEGFR2^+$ cells, whereas the $CD34^+$ $VEGFR2^-$ fraction contained no such cells.[553] However, murine BM-derived $VEGFR2^+$ cells could not repopulate lethally irradiated mice in another report.[554] VEGF-A may regulate hematopoietic stem cell survival by an internal autocrine loop mechanism.[555] In vivo over-expression of VEGF-A or angiopoietin-1 results in mobilization of HSCs into peripheral blood and spleen.[556] This is associated with initial enhancement followed by transient suppression of BM hematopoiesis. VEGFR-1 is expressed on human $CD34^+$ and murine $Sca\text{-}1^+$ $c\text{-}Kit^+$ Lin^- repopulating cells.[557] PLGF (which signals through VEGFR-1) restores early and late phases of hematopoiesis following BM suppression.[557] VEGFR-2 deficient mice display failure of blood-island formation and vasculogenesis and die in utero.[558] Both primitive and definite hematopoiesis are disrupted in these mice.[559] Embryonic lethality with vascular and hematopoietic defects are seen in mice lacking even one allele of the VEGF-A gene.[560] Angiopoietins and their receptor Tie2 play significant role in HSC interaction with the stromal cells in the niche.[561] Ang-1/Tie2 signalling regulates HSC quiescence.[561] Tie2 expression is limited to the long-term LT-HSCs.[544] HSCs also express ang-1 which suggests an autocrine/paracrine influence.[562] Tie2 deletion impairs definitive hematopoiesis.[563] Angiopoietin-like (Angptl)2 and Angptl3 molecules were expressed in fetal liver $CD3^+$ cells, and they enhanced net ex vivo expansion of long-term repopulating murine HSC when used in combination with saturating amounts of other growth factors.[564]

CLASSIC GROWTH FACTORS WITH HEMATOPOIETIC ACTIVITIES

There are multiple examples of classic non-hematopoietic growth factors that show some hematopoietic activity both in vitro and in vivo. We elected to discuss three of these: Insulin-like growth factors, Hepatocyte growth factor, and basic fibroblast growth factor.

Insulin-Like Growth Factor (IGF) I and II

IGF-I and IGF-II are well-known growth factors affecting multiple cell types. They mediate their effects through IGF-I R and IGF-II R, which are present in different tissues including the hematopoietic system.[565] IGF-I, whose activity is better delineated, exerts a stimulatory effect on hematopoiesis. BM stromal cells synthesize and secrete IGF-I and IGF-binding proteins.[566] When added to BM cells, IGF-I mediates an Epo-like activity that promotes erythroid lineage differentiation even in the absence of added Epo.[567] Although there is consensus on the hematopoietic effect of IGF-I, there is controversy over whether or not this influence is direct or mediated by other cytokines.[568] It seems that IGF-I is more important than IGF-II for erythroid colony formation by adult hematopoietic progenitors, whereas IGF-II has more significance for colony formation by the cord blood progenitors.[569] IGF-I stimulates granulopoiesis in semisolid culture systems, and IGF-II induces granulocyte-macrophage colony formation.[570] IGF-I can also promote in vitro lymphopoiesis.[571] In vivo administration of IGF-1 stimulates BM B- lymphocyte production and enhances lymphocyte recovery after BM transplantation.[572]

Basic Fibroblast Growth Factor (bFGF)

BFGF is an angiogenic and mitogenic factor for multiple cell types, with an important function in cell differentiation. In the BM environment it is secreted by stromal cells and is a potent mitogen for these cells.[573] It is also expressed by macrophages, megakaryocytes, T lymphocytes, and granulocytes.[574] BFGF enhances the colony stimulating activity of IL-3 and GM-CSF on $CD34^+$ $CD33^-$ progenitors in vitro.[575] It increases the number of $CFU\text{-}S_9$, and $CFU\text{-}S_{12}$ in synergy with GM-CSF.[576] bFGF synergizes with SCF in augmenting committed myeloid progenitor growth.[577] Megakaryocyte progenitors are also targets of bFGF activity.[578]

Hepatocyte Growth Factor (HGF)

HGF was initially purified as a liver regenerating factor from the plasma of a patient with fulminant hepatitis.[579] Shortly after, it was cloned and shown to be the most potent mitogen for mature hepatocytes.[580] HGF exerts wide mitogenic and morphogenic activity on multiple cell types. Both HGF and its tyrosine kinase receptor c-Met proto-oncogene are expressed in BM, fetal liver and yolk sac.[581] In the BM, HGF is predominantly produced by stromal cells, while c-Met is expressed on immature $CD34^+$ $CD38^-$ but not on $CD34^+$ $CD38^+$ cells.[582] It has no colony-stimulating activity when used alone,[582,583] but it synergizes with GM-CSF and IL-3[581,582] with less potency than SCF and FL. HGF promotes proliferation, survival and adhesion of human $CD34^+$ cells.[582] It plays roles in the induction and maintenance of bone marrow stromal cell production of IL-11, SDF-1 α, and stem cell factor.[584] It also increases red blood cells, white blood cells, and platelet counts in SCF/c-Kit deficient mice when given in vivo.[585]

CONSEQUENCES OF CYTOKINE AND/OR CYTOKINE RECEPTOR GENE DEFICIENCY

Table 24–5 reveals the phenotype of mice deficient in the main hematopoietic cytokines and/or their receptor-genes. It is clear that deletion of some genes causes more severe consequences than deletion of others.

Suppressor Cytokines

These cytokines share the ability to suppress hematopoietic colony formation under variable circumstances. Some of them have been implicated in pathologic hypoproliferative processes such as anemia of inflammation and aplastic anemia. We will discuss the chemokine family members, IFNs, tumor necrosis factor (TNF) α, and transforming growth factor (TGF) β family.

CHEMOKINES

Chemokines are small molecules that were originally named for their ability to attract mature leukocytes.[586] Currently, there are more than 45 known chemokines which are classified into four groups according to the position of invariant cystein (c) motifs near the N-terminal portion of the molecule.[587] Table 24–6 is an up-to-date listing of the chemokine groups. The CC and CXC (X indicates any amino acid) groups contain most of the known chemokines. These cytokines have been implicated as negative and to a lesser extent positive regulatory of hematopoiesis. The prototype of the inhibitory chemokines is macrophage inflammatory protein-1α (MIP)-1α, now designated CCL3. MIP1-α was first identified as a suppressor molecule for spleen-CFUs.[588] It was later shown to inhibit multi-cytokine induced growth of CFU-GEMM, BFU-E, and CFU-GM.[589] In vivo administration of MIP-1α results in suppression of hematopoiesis.[590,591] This effect is direct and seen on single cells growing in serum-free medium.[592] The suppressive activity of MIP-1α is initiated during S-phase of cell cycle.[593] The in vivo administration of MIP-1α results in reversible suppression of cycling status and absolute numbers of BM and spleen progenitors.[590,591] MIP-1α also works in opposite fashion by enhancing the proliferation of CFU-GM and CFU-M when stimulated by a single CSF: GM-CSF or M-CSF, respectively.[594] Twenty-three other chemokines demonstrate similar

Table 24–5 Consequences of Cytokine and/or Cytokine Receptor Gene Deficiency

Cytokine	The Hematopoietic Phenotype	Other Important Nonhematologic Defects
SCF/c-kit	Embryonic lethality in homozygous mice Macrocytic anemia in *W* and *Sl* mice which harbor heterozygous mutations of c-Kit and SCF respectively	Hypopigmentation, reproductive defect in *W* and *Sl* mice.
FL/Flt3	Reduced number of early B-cell progenitors and a defect in repopulating stem cells in flt3 knock-outs. FL deficient mice display an additional decrease in peripheral blood, spleen, and BM cellularity.	
G-CSF/G-CSF Receptor (R)	Decrease in number of circulating neutrophils plus in number of BM progenitors of various lineages.	
GM-CSF/GM-CSFR	No obvious hematopoietic defects. Eosinopenia in GM-CSF R deficient mice (caused by IL-5 signaling defect).	Alveolar pulmonary proteinosis
IL-3/IL-3R	Normal hematopoiesis. Eosinopenia in IL-3R deficient mice (caused by IL-5 signaling defect)	
M-CSF/c-fms	BM failure due to osteopetrosis in op/op mice	Osteopetrosis
Epo/Epo	Embryonic lethality due to failure of definite fetal liver erythropoiesis. Committed erythroid progenitors are present.	
TPO/c-mpl	Thrombocytopenia. A decrease in BM progenitors of various lineages	
IL-5/IL-5R	Lack of eosinophilia to allergen challenge in IL-5 deficient mice. Eosinopenia in IL-5R knock-out	
IL-6/IL-6R	Decrease in BM progenitor survival	Impaired immune and acute phase responses Embryonic lethality of gp130 deficient mice (gp130 common to all IL-6 family receptors)
IL-11/IL-11R	Normal hematopoiesis	Embryonic lethality of gp 130 deficient mice
LIF/LIF-R	Perinatal mortality. Hematopoietic system appears normal	Placental, skeletal, neuronal and metabolic defects leading to perinatal mortality
IL-1/IL-1R	Normal hematopoiesis	IL-1R1 deficiency protects against endotoxin-induced lethality
IL-4/IL-4R	Decrease in BM progenitor number and cycling	Defect in immunoglobulin production

Phenotypes observed in mice deficient in the major hematopoietic cytokines. The impact of one cytokine deficiency may be as remarkable as resulting in embryonic lethality as seen with the SCF/c-Kit axis, or as subtle as having no tangible effect on the hematopoietic system as seen with IL-11.

suppressive activities.[595] Table 24–7 lists these known suppressive chemokines. Responsiveness of hematopoietic progenitor cells to suppression by inhibitory chemokines requires the entry of cells to cycle and also the expression of major histocompatibility class II antigens.[596] Chemokines can act in synergy with each other and with other cytokines, such as macrophage stimulatory protein (MSP) and VEGF to inhibit progenitor cell proliferation in vitro.[595] Suppressive chemokines also synergize with each other to inhibit absolute numbers and cycling status of hematopoietic progenitor cells in vivo.[597] A small number of chemokines such as Eotaxin (a CC chemokine) have been shown to exert an enhancing activity on myelopoiesis.[598] Other regulatory roles of chemokines have been uncovered. For instance, MIP-1α has been used in a cocktail of cytokines to maintain myeloid and lymphoid progenitor numbers in long-term marrow culture.[599] Stromal derived factor-1 SDF-1 (or CXCL12) is a chemokine that was isolated from BM stromal cells.[600] It was also cloned as a pre-B cell growth stimulatory factor (PBSF)[601] and recently was shown to regulate the earliest stage of B-cell precursor development.[602] SDF-1 deficient mice die perinatally because of lack of BM hematopoiesis that is thought to be secondary to impaired stem cell migration from fetal liver to the BM.[603] SDF-1 exerts in vitro chemoattracting activity for multipotential (CFU-GEMM), erythroid (BFU-E), granulocyte-macrophage (CFU-GM), and megakaryocyte (CFU-MK) progenitors and for LTC-IC.[134,135] In addtion, there is a strong evidence for an essential role of SDF-1 in stem cell homing to the BM microenvironment when human CD34$^+$ are transplanted into NOD/SCID mice.[16] SDF-1 has also been implicated in hematopoietic progenitor survival.[109,115] It appears that SDF-1 also exert indirect activity on HSC/progenitors by retaining these cells within the niche where other cytokines/GFs are active.[604] SDF-1 is an essential cytokine for early stages of lymphopoiesis.[605] It plays a role in thrombopoiesis as well.[606]

Two other chemokines (CK)β-11/CCL19 and SLC/CCL21 have been shown to be selectively chemotactic for macrophage progenitors.[607] Chemokine receptors are seven transmembrane G-protein-linked receptors.[165] There is redundancy in the chemokine system in that one chemokine may bind more than one receptor and one receptor may bind more than one chemokine. Analysis of mice deficient in some of these receptors has shed light into their roles in hematopoiesis. MIP-1α binds CCR1, CCR5, and CCR9. CCR1 deficient mice display abnormalities in trafficking of myeloid progenitor from BM to spleen particularly in response to bacterial lipopolysaccharide.[608] The inhibitory response is preserved while the enhancing effect on M-CSF and GM-CSF is lost[609] in CCR1 deficient mice. CCR2 is one of the receptors for the myelosuppressive chemokine MCP-1. CCR2 deficient mice demonstrate increased cycling of myeloid progenitors. However the absolute numbers of progenitors are unchanged compared with wild-type, probably because of increased apoptosis in the CCR2–/– mice.[610] IL-8 is another myeloid-inhibitory chemokine. CXCR2 functions as a receptor for IL-8. Deleting CXCR2 results in enhanced myelopoiesis with loss of BM sensitivity to IL-8. This enhanced myelopoiesis is observed in mice bred and raised under a normal environment but not seen in mice kept under germ-free conditions.[611]

Table 24–6 Classification of Chemokines

Chemokine	Other Names	Receptor
	CXC Chemokine/Receptor Family	
CXCL1	GROα/MGSA-α	CXCR2 > CXCR1
CXCL2	GROβ/MGSA-β	CXCR2
CXCL3	GROγ/MGSA-γ	CXCR2
CXCL4	PF4	unknown
CXCL5	ENA-78	CXCR2
CXCL6	GCP-2	CXCR1, CXCR2
CXCL7	NAP-2	CXCR2
CXCL8	IL-8	CXCR1, CXCR2
CXCL9	Mig	CXCR3
CXCL10	IP-10	CXCR3
CXCL11	I-TAC	CXCR3
CXCL12	SDF-1α/β	CXCR4/CXCR7
CXCL13	BLC/BCA-1	CXCR5
CXCL14	BRAK/bolekine	unknown
(CXCL15)	No human ligand identified yet	unknown
CXCL16	No human ligand identified yet	CXCR6
	CC Chemokine/Receptor Family	
CCL1	1–309	CCR8
CCL2	MCP-1/MCAF	CCR2
CCL3	MIP-1α	CCR1, CCR5
CCL4	MIP-1β	CCR5
CCL5	RANTES	CCR1, CCR3, CCR5
(CCL6)	No human ligand identified yet	unknown
CCL7	MCP-3	CCR1, CCR2, CCR3
CCL8	MCP-2	CCR3
(CCL9/10)	No human ligand identified yet	unknown
CCL11	Eotaxin	CCR3
(CCL12)	No human ligand identified yet	CCR2
CCL13	MCP-4	CCR2, CCR3
CCL14	HCC-1	CCR1
CCL15	HCC-2/LKN-1/MIP-1δ	CCR1, CCR3
CCL16	HCC-4/LEC	CCR1
CCL17	TARC	CCR4
CCL18	DC-CK1/PARC/AMAC-1	unknown
CCL19	Mip-3β/ELC/exodus-3	CCR7
CCL20	Mip-3α/LARC/exodus-1	CCR6
CCL21	6Ckine/SLC/exodus-2	CCR7
CCL22	MDC/STCP-1	CCR4
CCL23	MPIF-1	CCR1
CCL24	MPIF-2/Eotamin-2	CCR3
CCL25	TECK	CCR9
CCL26	Eotaxin-3	CCR3
CCL27	CTACK	CCR10
CCL38	MEC	unknown

Table 24-6 Classification of Chemokines—cont'd

Chemokine	Other Names	Receptor
	C Chemokine/Receptor Family	
XCL1	Lymphotactin/SCM-1α/ATAC	XCR1
XCL2	SCM-1β	XCR2
CX3C	Chemokine/receptor family	
CX3CL1	Fractalkine	CX3CR1

Chemokines are divided into two major groups based on the positions of the N-terminal cysteine residues.

CXC family and CC family where X represent an amino acid. Two other smaller groups have been identified. The C chemokine family members contain just one cysteine and the CX3C family single member has three amino acids separating the two cysteine residues. Several chemokines were cloned at the same time by different groups and given different names. A new classification system has been widely utilized in an attempt to simplify dealing with this perplexing system. AMAC, alternative macrophage activation-associated CC chemokine; BCA, B-cell attracting chemokine; BLC, B-lymphocyte chemoattractant; BRAK, breast and kidney-expressed chemokine; CTACK, cutaneous T cell attracting chemokine; DC-CK, dendritic cell-derived CC chemokine; ELC, EBV-induced gene 1 ligand chemokine; GCP, granulocyte chemoattractant protein; Gro, growth-related oncogene; HCC, hemofiltrate CC chemokine; IP, γ-interferon inducible protein; ITAC, interferon-inducible T-cell α-chemoattractant; LARC, liver and activation-regulated chemokine; LEC, liver expressed chemokine; Lkn, leukotactin; MCAF, monocyte chemotactic and activating factor; MCP, monocyte chemoattractant protein; MDC, monocyte derived chemokine; MEC, mucosa-associated epithelial chemokine; MGSA, melanoma growth-stimulatory activity chemokine; Mig, monokine induced by γ-interferon; MIP, macrophage inflammatory protein; MPIF, myeloid progenitor inhibitory factor; NAP, neutrophil-activating peptide; PARC, pulmonary and activation-regulated chemokine; PF, platelet factor; ENA, epithelial-derived neutrophil attractant; RANTES, regulated on activation of normal T cell expressed and secreted; SDF, stromal cell-derived factor; SLC, secondary lymphoid tissue chemokine; STCP, stimulated T cell chemotactic protein; TARC, thymus and activation-regulated chemokine; TECK, thymus expressed chemokine.

Modified from Bacon K, Baggiolini M, Broxmeyer HE, et al: Chemokine/chemokine receptor nomenclature. J Immunol Methods 262, 2002.[662]

Interferons (IFNs)

The term interferon originally referred to a factor produced by virally infected chick cells that on transfer to fresh chick cells could protect against infection by the same virus.[612] IFNs have a wide spectrum of biological effects including antiviral, antiproliferative, and immunomodulatory activities.[613] They are divided into two groups; type I IFNs which include IFN-α, β, and ω, which are molecularly related and probably arose by divergence from a common ancestral gene; and type II IFN or IFN-γ. There are 14 distinct IFN-α genes and four IFN-α pseudogenes, one IFN-β, one IFN-ω, and one IFN-γ gene.[613] Type I interferons bind to the same receptor; type I IFN receptor, whereas IFN-γ binds to the type II IFN receptor. It was noted early on that IFNs inhibit erythroid colony formation.[614] IFNs are well-known inhibitors of hematopoietic progenitors, including CFU-GEMM, CFU-GM, and megakaryocytic (CFU-MK) progenitors.[615–617] IFN-α, β, and γ have equal influence on CFU-GEMM and BFU-E but have differential effect on CFU-GM.[615] IFN-γ is the most studied interferon in this regard and it appears to inhibit to growth of CD34$^+$ CD38$^-$ cells indicating a role in early progenitor/stem cell regulation.[618] In the hematopoietic system, IFNs inhibit cell cycle progression[619] and induce apoptosis.[620] This apoptosis enhancing effect is facilitated by upregulation of Fas expression on CD34+ cells and erythroid colony forming cells.[621] It has been reported that IFN-γ reduces the expression of cytokine receptors such as c-kit and EpoR on hematopoietic progenitors[622] which contributes to its apoptosis-inducing activity. This inhibition on the hematopoietic system is synergistic among IFNs.[623] IFN-γ has been implicated in the pathogenesis of aplastic anemia,[624] and a major role has been suggested for IFN-α/β in virus-induced transient bone marrow aplasia.[625] Despite the well-documented inhibitory function of IFNγ, a few studies reported stimulatory activity on certain hematopoietic cells.[626] No signs of disturbed baseline hematopoiesis have been reported in IFN-γ deficient mice.[627] However, infecting these mice with mycobacteria results in a transition to extramedullary hematopoiesis with expansion of macrophages, granulocytes, and extramedullary hematopoietic tissue.[628]

Tumor Necrosis Factor α (TNF-α)

TNF-α is a potent cytokine produced by many cell types including macrophages, monocytes, lymphocytes, keratinocytes, and fibroblasts in response to inflammation, infection, injury, and other environmental challenges. TNF-α is named for its ability to regress tumor masses when these get infected with bacterial infections. TNF-α was isolated in 1984 and was found to be a pleiotropic cytokine that is expressed as a transmembrane protein that can be cleaved into a soluble form. It belongs to a family of about 20 factors that are grouped together in the TNF superfamily.[629] TNF-α transmits its signal through two receptors: TNFR1 or p55TNFR and TNFR2 or p75TNFR.[630] The influence of TNF-α on hematopoietic progenitor/stem cells is somewhat complex.[630] TNF-α plays a bifunctional role in that it directly inhibits hematopoietic progenitors[631] at least partially by down-regulating CSF receptors.[632] TNF-α also synergizes with IFNγ to inhibit proliferation of hematopoietic progenitor cells.[631] On the other hand, it stimulates proliferation of hematopoietic progenitors probably by inducing secretion of CSFs.[630,633] This differential influence may be related to the particular CSF present in the culture media and the concentration of the added TNF.[632] Retroviral transduction of single hematopoietic progenitors with c-kit decreases the sensitivity to inhibition by TNF-α.[634] One study showed that TNF-α inhibited the development of committed progenitors while stimulating CFU-S in murine long-term BM cultures.[635] TRAIL which belongs to TNF family has a negative regulatory role on erythropoiesis[636] that could be implicated in pathologic states such as multiple myeloma and myelodysplastic syndrome. Study of hematopoiesis in TNF receptor deficient mice has further elucidated the role of the TNF system in this process. P55 TNFR deficient mice display an increase of Sca-1$^+$ Lin$^-$ c-kit$^+$ cells. Increased BM cellularity, and an increase in numbers of myeloid and erythroid colony forming progenitors are seen in p55–/– but not p75–/– deficient mice at age older than six months.[637] This is associated with a fourfold decrease in the number of HSCs, as assayed by quantitating repopulating capacity.[638] These mice also have decreased BM pre-B CFCs and elevated peripheral blood counts compared to the wild-type. Finally Sca-1+ Lin– c-kit+ cells acquire Fas expansion and severely lose their short- and long-term repopulating capacity when cultured in the presence of TNF.[639]

Transforming Growth Factor β (TGF-β)

TGF-β was originally described as a soluble factor that transformed mouse 3T3 fibroblasts.[640] Three mammalian isoforms are recognized with a forth one recently described. TGF-β is present in biologically inactive or latent form that needs to be activated in the extracellular matrix by different mechanisms. TGF-β has no in vitro effect on hematopoietic colony formation when used alone,[641] however it exerts inhibitory[642,643] or stimulatory[644,645] functions in combination

Table 24–7 Suppressive Chemokines

New Designation	Previous Designations
CCL1	1–309
CCL2	MCP-1/MCAF
CCL3	MIP-1α/LD78α
(CCL6)	No human ligand identified yet
(CCL9/10)	No human ligand identified yet
(CCL12)	No human ligand identified yet
CCL13	MCP-4
CCL15	HCC-2/LKN-1/MIP-1δ
CCL16	HCC-4/LEC
CCL19	Mip-3β/ELC/exodus-3
CCL20	Mip-3α/LARC/exodus-1
CCL21	6Ckine/SLC/exodus-2
CCL22	MDC/STCP-1
CCL23	MPIF-1
CCL25	TECK
CXCL2	GROβ/MGSA-β
CXCL4	PF4
CXCL5	ENA-78
CXCL6	GCP-2
CXCL8	IL-8
CXCL9	Mig
CXCL10	IP-10
CXCL11	I-TAC
XCL1	Lymphotactin

This represents a listing of the hematopoietic suppressive chemokines. One can appreciate the large number of suppressive chemokines that may affect the progenitor/stem cells at a variety of physiologic and pathologic states. These suppress HPC colony formation in vitro. Those tested in vivo decrease the absolute number and the cycling status of HPCs. The suppressive chemokines synergize in vitro and in vivo to inhibit HPC proliferation and concentrations below those by which they inhibit HPCs individually.

ELC, EBV-induced gene 1 ligand chemokine; GCP, granulocyte chemoattractant protein; Gro, growth-related oncogene; HCC, hemofiltrate CC chemokine; IP, γ-interferon inducible protein; ITAC, interferon-inducible T-cell α-chemoattractant; LEC, liver expressed chemokine; Lkn, leukotactin; MCAF, monocyte chemotactic and activating factor; MCP, monocyte chemoattractant protein; MDC, monocyte derived chemokine; MEC, mucosa-associated epithelial chemokine; MGSA, melanoma growth-stimulatory activity chemokine; Mig, monokine induced by γ-interferon; MIP, macrophage inflammatory protein; MPIF, myeloid progenitor inhibitory factor; PF, platelet factor; ENA, epithelial-derived neutrophil attractant; STCP, stimulated T-cell chemotactic protein; TECK, thymus expressed chemokine.

with other cytokines. This effect is direct and dependent on the differentiation status of the target cells, the type of the cytokines used, and on TGF-β concentration.[645,646] TGF-β inhibits the proliferation of early progenitor/stem cells but not that of late progenitors.[646] For example, it inhibits the proliferation of CFU-GEMM,[645] and Lin^- Thy-1^{low} (early progenitors) cells while it increases the frequency of Lin^- Thy-1^- (late progenitor) cells.[647] TGF-β completely blocks the cytokine driven proliferation of quiescent Lin^- Hoescht/Rhodamine132^{low} (Ho/Rho) early progenitor/stem cells.[648] Human $CD34^+CD38^-$ cells are highly sensitive to cell-cycle inhibition by TGF-β, whereas more mature $CD34^+CD38^+$ cells are poorly affected or even stimulated.[649] This reversible cell cycle inhibition appears to occur without detectable cell death,[650] and it is augmented by the presence of other inhibitors such as IFNs. Fifty percent of TGF-β deficient mice experience intrauterine mortality due to severe developmental retardation. Dysregulated hematopoiesis is manifested by myeloid hyperplasia, plasmacytosis, reduced number of erythroid cells, and lack of Langerhans dendritic cells.[651,652] These mice develop systemic a massive T-cell inflammatory syndrome and die by five weeks of age. Attempts at isolating the quiescent Ho/Rho^{low} c-kit+ cells from these mice have shown more than 90% reduction in these cells, which suggests a pivotal role of TGF-β in stem cell quiescence. Finally endoglin, an ancillary TGF-β receptor has been found to be a marker that defines long-term repopulating hematopoietic stem cells.[43]

Lactoferrin and H-Ferritin

Lactoferrin and H-ferritin belong to the iron binding family. Members of this family are produced and secreted by a number of different cell types.[653] Lactoferrin in particular has multiple roles in iron homeostasis, innate immunity, inflammation, and differentiation.[653] Both lactoferrin[654,655] and H-ferritin[656–658] suppress hematopoiesis in vitro and in vivo. H-ferritin has direct inhibitory activity on progenitors,[659,660] while lactoferrin has both direct and indirect effects on progenitors.[204,659,661] Major histocompatibility complex class II (MHC II) expression is necessary for these inhibitory effects,[596] as they are for the suppressive chemokines.

CONCLUSION

Hematopoietic cytokines render the suitable milieu for the growth of each hematopoietic lineage that has lead to extensive utilization of a few of these cytokines in variable clinical settings. Multiple challenges still lie ahead, such as translating the ample and overlapping activities of cytokines seen in vitro and in vivo into applications in parallel clinical situations. Another important obstacle is the identification of the environment which permits stem cell division and self-renewal that will lead to a wide range of clinical applications.

SUGGESTED READINGS

Bagby GC: Interleukin-1 and hematopoiesis. Blood Rev 3:152, 1989.

Bradley T, Metcalf D: The growth of mouse bone marrow cells in vitro. Aust J Exp Biol Med Sci 44:287, 1966.

Brandt J, Srour EF, van Besien K, et al: Cytokine-dependent long-term culture of highly enriched precursors of hematopoietic progenitor cells from human bone marrow. J Clin Invest 86:932, 1990.

Broxmeyer HE, Hangoc G, Cooper S, et al: Growth characteristics and expansion of human umbilical cord blood and estimation of its potential for transplantation in adults. Proc Natl Acad Sci U S A 89:4109, 1992.

Broxmeyer HE, Kim CH: Regulation of hematopoiesis in a sea of chemokine family members with a plethora of redundant activities. Exp Hematol 27:1113, 1999.

Broxmeyer HE, Orschell CM, Clapp DW, et al: Rapid mobilization of murine and human hematopoietic stem and progenitor cells with AMD3100, a CXCR4 antagonist. J Exp Med 201:130, 2005.

Broxmeyer HE, Williams DE, Hangoc G, et al: Synergistic myelopoietic actions in vivo after administration to mice of combinations of purified natural murine colony-stimulating factor 1, recombinant murine interleukin 3, and recombinant murine granulocyte/macrophage colony-stimulating factor. Proc Natl Acad Sci U S A 84:3871, 1987.

Broxmeyer HE, Williams DE, Lu L, et al: The suppressive influences of human tumor necrosis factor on bone marrow hematopoietic progenitor cells from normal donors and patients with leukemia: synergism of tumor necrosis factor and interferon-gamma. J Immunol 136:4487, 1986.

Dexter TM, Allen TD, Lajtha LG: Conditions controlling the proliferation of haematopoietic stem cells in vitro. J Cell Physiol 91:335, 1977.

Kaushansky K: Thrombopoietin: the primary regulator of platelet production. Blood 86:419, 1995.

Lyman SD, Jacobsen SE: W: *c-kit* Ligand and flt3 ligand: stem/progenitor cell factors with overlapping yet distinct activities. Blood 91:1101, 1998.

Metcalf D, Begley CG, Johnson GR, et al: Effects of purified bacterially synthesized murine multi-CSF (IL-3) on hematopoiesis in normal adult mice. Blood 68:46, 1986.

Metcalf D: The granulocyte-macrophage colony-stimulating factors. Science 229:16, 1985.

Peled A, Petit I, Kollet O, et al: Dependence of human stem cell engraftment and repopulation of NOD/SCID mice on CXCR4. Science 283:845, 1999.

Piacibello W, Sanavio F, Garetto L, et al: Extensive amplification and self-renewal of human primitive hematopoietic stem cells from cord blood. Blood 89:2644, 1997.

Pluznik D, Sachs L: The induction of clones of normal mast cells by a substance from conditioned medium. Exp Cell Res 43:553, 1966.

Spangrude GJ, Heimfeld S, Weissman IL: Purification and characterization of mouse hematopoietic stem cells. Science 241:58, 1988.

Till JE, McCulloch EA: A direct measurement of the radiation sensitivity of normal mouse bone marrow cells. Radiat Res 14:213, 1961.

Vadhan-Raj S, Buescher S, Broxmeyer HE, et al: Stimulation of myelopoiesis in patients with aplastic anemia by recombinant human granulocyte-macrophage colony-stimulating factor. N Engl J Med 319:1628, 1988.

Williams GT, Smith CA, Spooncer E, et al: Haematopoietic colony-stimulating factors promote cell survival by suppressing apoptosis. Nature 343:76, 1990.

REFERENCES

For complete list of references log onto www.expertconsult.com

CHAPTER 25

BIOLOGY OF ERYTHROPOIESIS, ERYTHROID DIFFERENTIATION, AND MATURATION

Thalia Papayannopoulou, Anna Rita Migliaccio, Janis L. Abkowitz, and Alan D. D'Andrea

Production of erythroid cells is a dynamic and exquisitely regulated process. The mature red cell is the final phase of a complex but orderly series of genetic events that initiates when a multipotent stem cell commits to the erythroid program. Expression of the erythroid program occurs several divisions later in a greatly amplified population of erythroid cells, which have a characteristic morphology, maturation sequence, and function. These maturing cells are termed *erythroid precursor cells* and *reticulocytes*. Terminally differentiated cells have a finite lifespan, and they are constantly replenished by influx from earlier compartments of progenitor cells that are irreversibly committed to express the erythroid phenotype. During ontogeny, successive waves of erythropoiesis occur in distinct anatomic sites. Erythroid cells developing in these sites have distinguishable phenotypes and intrinsic programs that are dependent on gestational time and their microenvironment. At each site, erythroid cells are in intimate contact with other cells (e.g., stromal cells, hematopoietic accessory cells, and extracellular matrix) composing their microenvironment. Within this microenvironment, erythroid development is influenced by cytokines, which are either elaborated by microenvironmental cells or produced elsewhere and then entrapped in the extracellular matrix.

Knowledge of the properties of erythroid progenitor and precursor cells and their complex interactions with the microenvironment is essential for understanding the pathophysiology of erythropoiesis. Aberrations either in the generation and/or amplification of fully mature and functional erythroid cells or in the regulatory influences of microenvironmental cells or their cytokines/chemokines form the basis for various clinical disorders, including aplasias, dysplasias, and neoplasias of the erythroid tissue.

ERYTHROID PROGENITOR CELL COMPARTMENT

The erythroid progenitor cell compartment, situated functionally between the multipotent stem cell and the morphologically distinguishable erythroid precursor cells, contains a spectrum of cells with a parent-to-progeny relationship, all committed to erythroid differentiation. A complete understanding of how erythroid commitment is achieved at the biochemical or molecular level is lacking, although some attempts at determining the molecular basis have been made.[1–4] Evidence from in vitro cultures of single multipotent progenitor cells allowed to differentiate in competent environments as well as evidence obtained by studying the phenotype of leukemic cells suggests that commitment to a specific hematopoietic lineage is accomplished not by acquisition of new genetic information but by restriction (probably on a stochastic basis) to specific programs from a wider repertoire available to pluripotent progenitor cells.[5,6] Molecular evidence supports this view.[6–8] Although all erythroid progenitor cells share the irreversible commitment to express the erythroid phenotype, the properties of these cells progressively diverge as the cells become separated by several divisions.

Erythroid progenitor cells are sparse (Table 25–1) and difficult to isolate in sufficient purity and numbers for study. For these reasons, the existence and characteristics of these cells were inferred from their ability to generate hemoglobinized progeny in vitro in clonal erythroid cultures (Fig. 25–1). Two classes of progenitors have been identified using this approach.[9] The first, more primitive class consists of the burst-forming unit-erythroid (BFU-E), named for the ability of BFU-E to give rise to multiclustered colonies (erythroid bursts) of hemoglobin-containing cells. BFU-E represent the earliest progenitors committed exclusively to erythroid differentiation and a quiescent reserve, with only 10% to 20% in cycle at any given time. However, once stimulated to proliferate in the presence of appropriate cytokines, BFU-E demonstrate a significant proliferative capacity in vitro, giving rise to colonies of 30,000 to 40,000 cells, which become fully hemoglobinized after 2 to 4 weeks, with a peak incidence at 14 to 16 days. They have a limited self-renewal capacity; at least a subset of BFU-E is capable of generating secondary bursts upon replating. In contrast to this class of progenitor cells, a second, more differentiated class of progenitors consists of the colony-forming unit-erythroid (CFU-E). Most (60%–80%) of these progenitors already are in cycle and thus proliferate immediately after initiation of culture, forming erythroid colonies within 7 days. Because CFU-E are more differentiated than BFU-E, they require fewer divisions to generate colonies of hemoglobinized cells, and the colonies are small (8–65 cells per colony).

Although the two classes of committed erythroid progenitors (BFU-E and CFU-E) appear distinct from each other, in reality progenitor cells constitute a continuum, with graded changes in their properties. Only progenitor cells at both ends of the differentiation spectrum have distinct properties. Perhaps the earliest cell with the potential to generate hemoglobinized progeny is an oligopotent progenitor, which is capable of giving rise to mature cells of at least one other lineage (granulocytic, macrophage, or megakaryocytic) in addition to the erythroid. This progenitor, a multilineage colony-forming unit (CFU) called a *colony-forming unit-granulocyte, erythrocyte, macrophage, megakaryocyte* (CFU-GEMM) or *common myeloid progenitor*, and the most primitive BFU-E have physical and functional properties that are shared by both pluripotent stem cells and progenitor cells committed to nonerythroid lineages. These properties include high proliferative potential, low cycling rate, response to a combination of cytokines, and presence of specific surface antigens or surface receptors (Table 25–1). In contrast, the latest CFU-E have many similarities with erythroid precursor cells and little in common with primitive BFU-E. Their proliferative potential is limited, they cannot self-renew, they lack the cell surface antigens common to all early progenitors, and they are exquisitely sensitive to erythropoietin (Epo; Table 25–1).

Although clonal erythroid cultures are indispensable for the study of erythroid progenitors, they do not faithfully reproduce the in vivo kinetics of red cell differentiation/maturation, and many maturing cells have a megaloblastic appearance and lyse before they reach the end stage of red cell development. In vivo, erythropoiesis probably occurs faster than predicted from culture data. For example, studies in dogs with cyclic hematopoiesis, a genetic stem cell defect leading to pulses of hematopoiesis, provide evidence that BFU-E mature to CFU-E over 2 to 3 days in vivo, although this process may require 5 to 6 days in canine marrow cultures.[10]

Erythroid progenitors can be cultured in serum-depleted media[11,12] as well as in serum-containing media. The effects of recombinant growth factors can be studied in serum-depleted cultures without the complicating influences of multiple or unknown factors present in

Table 25–1 Changes in General Properties During Differentiation of Erythroid Progenitors

	CFU-GEMM (CMP)	BFU-E	CFU-E
General Features			
Self-renewal	++	+	0
Differentiation potential	Multipotent	Erythroid committed	Erythroid committed
Cycling status percent suicide with ^{3}H-thymidine	15–20	30–40	60–80
Cell density (g/mL)	<1.077	<1.077	<1.077
Incidence per 10^5 cells	2–5	40–120	200–600
Circulate in blood	+	+	0
Growth Factor Response			
Epo	+	+	++
TPO	+	+	+
KL	+	+	–
GM-CSF, IL-3	+	+	–
FL	+	0	0
G-CSF, IL-6, IL-1	+	0	0
Insulin, insulin-like growth factor, activin	0	0	+
TGF-β1	–	–	++
Hyper–IL-6	+	+	+
Receptor/Antigen			
CD34	++	++	–
CD33	+	+	0
c-kit	++	++	–
HLA-DR (HLA-DP, HLA-DQ)	++	++	+
Epo receptor	+	+	++
gp130	+	+	+
Tumor necrosis factor receptor	+	+	++
Ep-1[108]	+	+	++
23.6[a]			
CD36	0	±	+
Glycophorin A	0	0	+
ABH, il[b]	0	+	+
Adhesion Molecules			
VLA-4 (CD49d/CD29)	++	++	++
VLA-5 (CD49e/CD29)	+	+	++
CD41	+	+	
CD11a/CD18	+	+	
CD44	+	+	
HCAM[c]	+	+	
Transcription Factors			
GATA2	++	+	–
GATA1	+	++	+++
SCL	+	+	+
EKLF	+	+	++
Myb	++	+	–
Id1, Id2	++	+	–

[a]23.6 (SFL 23.6) is a monoclonal antibody reactive with CFU-E, erythroblasts, and erythrocytes.[447]
[b]ABH and il are blood group antigens.
[c]Presence of other cytoadhesion molecules (i.e., CD31, L-selectin, P-selectin, E-cadherin) has been described in progenitors (see text). However, the extent of their presence in BFU-E compared to other cells is not clear.
BFU-E, burst-forming unit-erythroid; CFU-E, colony-forming unit-erythroid; CFU-GEMM (CMP), colony-forming unit-granulocyte, erythrocyte, macrophage, megakaryocyte (common myeloid progenitor); EKLF, erythroid Kruppel-like factor; Epo, erythropoietin; FL, FLT-3 ligand; G-CSF, granulocyte colony-stimulating factor; GM-CSF, granulocyte-macrophage colony-stimulating factor; HCAM, homing-associated cyto adhesion molecule; HLA, human leukocyte antigen; IL, interleukin; KL, kit ligand; SCL, stem cell leukemia; TGF, transforming growth factor; TPO, thrombopoietin.

serum. Conditions that imitate lower oxygen pressures, found in bone marrow in vivo, favorably influence erythroid development in culture and may be advantageous.[13]

BFU-E are generated from multipotent or oligopotent progenitors within the marrow, and their survival and proliferation are dependent on the presence of cytokines, elaborated by either stromal cells or accessory cells within the microenvironment. A number of cytokines influence proliferation and/or survival of early progenitors. Among the cytokines, kit ligand (KL), which is produced by stromal cells, and interleukin (IL)-3, which is produced by a subset of T cells, alone and in synergy, have a profound proliferative effect on BFU-E and its progeny. Other cytokines, such as granulocyte-macrophage colony-stimulating factor (GM-CSF), IL-11, and thrombopoietin (TPO), stimulate a subset of BFU-E.[14–16] Cytokines exert their effects through interaction with specific receptors present on the BFU-E surface. The presence of such receptors also has been documented in

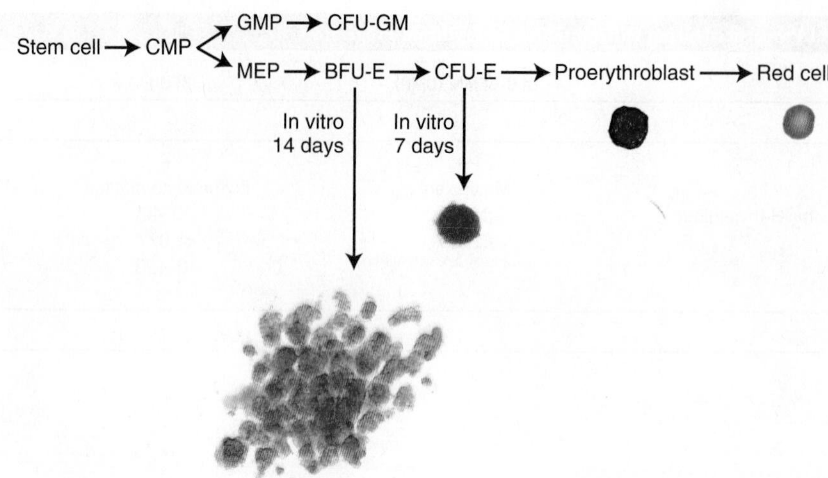

Figure 25–1 Cellular model of erythroid differentiation. Multipotent stem cells generate cellular compartments defined on the basis of their antigenic profile and restricted toward the myeloid differentiation pathway defined common myeloid progenitor (CMP).[64,65] CMP in turn give rise to granulocyte-monocyte progenitor (GMP) and megakaryocyte-erythroid progenitor (MEP), which probably correspond to the burst-forming unit-erythroid (BFU-E). Lastly, MEP generate cells capable of unilineage differentiation toward either the megakaryocytic (colony-forming unit-megakaryocyte [CFU-MK], not shown) or the erythroid pathway (colony-forming unit-erythroid [CFU-E]). These cells occur infrequently in the marrow (approximately 0.3% of mononuclear cells) and are defined on the basis of clonogenic assays. If marrow is placed in semisolid medium (e.g., methylcellulose) to decrease cell motility, with appropriate nutrients and growth factors (e.g., transferrin, insulin, erythropoietin, and interleukin-3), CFU-E (after approximately 7 days) differentiate into small clusters of hemoglobinized or red cells termed *erythroid colonies*. Most BFU-E present in the inoculum differentiate to form multiclustered colonies of hemoglobinized cells, or erythroid bursts, by days 14 to 16. Each erythroid colony or burst derives from one BFU-E or CFU-E, respectively.

the leukemic counterparts of normal BFU-E and in leukemic cell lines.[17] BFU-E in culture cannot survive for more than a few days in the absence of cytokines. If they are deprived of cytokines for more than 6 days, more than 80% of BFU-E are lost.[18] In addition to positive regulators (IL-3, GM-CSF, TPO, KL, and IL-11), substances with negative influences on BFU-E proliferation have been identified. They include tumor necrosis factor α (TNF-α), tumor necrosis factor-related apoptosis-inducing ligand (TRAIL), transforming growth factor β, and interferon γ.[19–21] These negative regulators are responsible, at least in part, for the anemia associated with chronic inflammatory states. The effects of TNF-α and TRAIL are mediated through induction of apoptosis at specific stages of erythroid maturation. In the case of TRAIL, a complex system of signaling and decoy receptor isoforms determines the precise cell window susceptible to TRAIL-induced apoptosis.[21] TRAIL probably induces apoptosis by competing with Epo for activation of Bruton tyrosine kinase. Its effects are counteracted by stem cell factor[22,23] and protein kinase Cε[24] signaling. TRAIL also is involved in determining the anemia associated with multiple myeloma (TRAIL is overproduced by the malignant plasma cells of these patients[25]) and myelodysplastic syndrome (myelodysplastic erythroid progenitors overexpress the adaptor Fas-associated death domain [FADD] of the TRAIL receptor[26]). On the other hand, the negative effects of transforming growth factor β[27] and interferon γ[28] are mainly achieved by accelerating cell differentiation. In addition to the negative growth factors, overexpression of hepcidin, a key regulator of systemic iron homeostasis (see Pathology of iron metabolism[35]), is involved in determining the anemia associated with chronic inflammation.[29] The increased hepcidin synthesis that occurs during inflammation traps iron in macrophages, decreases plasma iron concentrations, and causes iron-restricted erythropoiesis characteristic of the anemia of inflammatory states. Hepcidin deficiency induces iron overload in transgenic mice, whereas hepcidin excess induces iron accumulation in macrophages similar to observations in patients with chronic inflammation.[30] Hepcidin might inhibit proliferation of erythroid progenitors at low Epo concentrations.[31]

BFU-E and immediate progeny (but not CFU-E) are motile cells found in significant numbers in peripheral blood. As with BFU-E, the ability of stem cells and progenitor cells to circulate is physiologically important for the redistribution of marrow cells in cases of local damage to the microenvironment and for reconstitution of hematopoiesis after transplantation. The spectrum of BFU-E in circulation probably is narrower (consisting mostly of early, quiescent BFU-E) than that of BFU-E in the bone marrow; otherwise, their properties are similar to those of marrow BFU-E. The number of circulating BFU-E (along with other progenitors and stem cells) can increase to significant levels after cytokine/chemokine treatments and after chemotherapy, a finding that has been exploited for transplantation purposes.[32] At present, mononuclear cells contained in the blood from subjects mobilized with granulocyte colony-stimulating factor (G-CSF) are routinely used as a source of stem/progenitor cells in autologous and allogeneic transplantation.[33]

In addition to forming colonies in semisolid medium, hematopoietic progenitors from different sources can generate erythroid cells in liquid culture.[34] Liquid cultures do not allow progenitor cell enumeration but may generate more differentiated cells per progenitor cell than do semisolid cultures.[35,36] The number of erythroblasts generated in liquid cultures can be further increased by adding to the media glucocorticoid steroids,[37] which exert a reversible inhibition on proerythroblast maturation.[38,39] Erythroid cells equivalent to one unit of blood can be generated from a quantity of cord blood too small to be stored for transplantation (<50 mL).[40]

Surface antigens of human BFU-E have been defined through the use of monoclonal antibodies.[41,42] The antibodies tested include two broad categories: antibodies raised against leukemic cells or cell lines with progenitor cell properties, and antibodies raised against normal, terminally differentiated red cells. Enrichment in BFU-E (or CFU-E) after labeling with these antibodies, or their loss after complement-dependent lysis, is considered indicative of the presence of test antigens on the BFU-E surface. Reactivities of BFU-E with several antibodies directed against defined surface antigens are listed in Table 25–1. Like other hematopoietic progenitors, BFU-E display human leukocyte antigen (HLA) class I (A, B, C) and class II (DP, DQ, DR) antigens on their surface. Class II antigens (especially the products of the DR locus), in contrast to class I, are variably expressed among BFU-E. This may relate to variations in their cycling status, as myeloid progenitors in S phase have relatively higher expression of class II antigens.[43] The presence of HLA class II antigens (DR and,

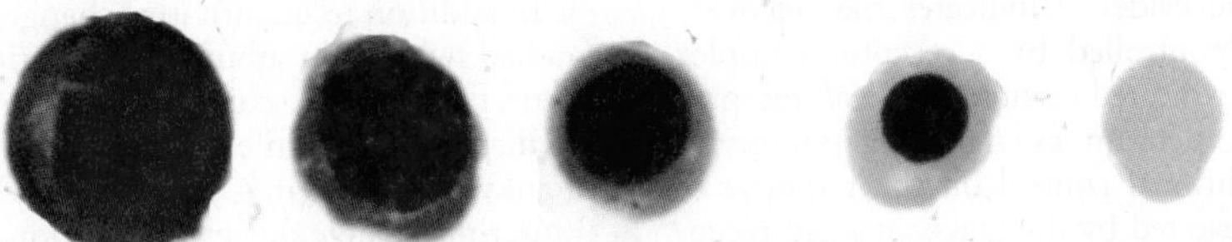

Figure 25–2 Erythroid maturation sequence. As proliferation parameters (i.e., rates of DNA and RNA synthesis) and cell size decrease, accumulation of erythroid-specific proteins (i.e., heme and globin) increases, and the cells adapt their characteristic morphology. (Adapted from Granick S, Levere R: Heme synthesis in erythroid cells. In Moore CV, Brown EB [eds.]: Progress in Hematology, Vol. 4. Orlando, FL, Grune & Stratton, 1964, p 1.[445])

to a lesser extent, DP and DQ) most likely allows BFU-E to recognize and interact with the immunoregulatory cells (e.g., T cells, monocytes), which also express class II determinants.[44] In addition to HLA antigens, several other antigenic structures are found on cells within the BFU-E compartment (Table 25–1). The best representative of these is the CD34 molecule (identified through monoclonal antibodies MY10, 12.8, or HPCA1), which has been successfully exploited for isolation of BFU-E and other progenitors. CD34 is a highly *O*-glycosylated cell surface glycoprotein. It is expressed in all hematopoietic progenitors and vascular endothelial cells.[45] The role of CD34 in hematopoiesis is not clearly defined. The numbers of all hematopoietic progenitors were reduced in CD34 "null" murine embryos and adult animals, but no other abnormalities were identified.[46] Expression of CD34 was low or absent in a population of adult long-term repopulating cells in mouse[47] and in man.[48] However, the clinical significance of this finding is not clear because of the fluctuating expression of CD34[49] and the difference in regulatory mechanisms of CD34 gene expression in mouse and human stem cells.[50] Furthermore, use of antibodies or conjugated ligands determined that BFU-E present in enriched progenitor preparations display receptors for KL, Epo, TPO, GM-CSF, IL-3, IL-6, and IL-11 receptors. However, the majority of BFU-E, in contrast to myeloid progenitors (colony-forming unit granulocyte-macrophage), do not express the restricted hematopoietic phosphatase CD45RA.[51,52] Furthermore, BFU-E appear to share with late colony-forming unit megakaryocyte progenitors the expression of the megakaryocytic receptor c-mpl[52,53] and glycoprotein IIb/IIIa (CD41), a marker of the divergence between definitive hematopoiesis and endothelial cells during development.[54]

As BFU-E mature to the CFU-E stage, they begin to express surface proteins characteristic of erythroblasts, the morphologically recognizable erythroid cells. For example, CFU-E express Rh antigens and the erythroid-specific sialoglycoprotein glycophorin A. Blood group antigens of the ABH Ii type are detectable in a subset of CFU-E. In contrast, CD34 molecules, class II antigens, and certain growth factor receptors (i.e., IL-3R, c-kit) are greatly diminished or virtually absent at the CFU-E stage (Table 25–1). The most important functional difference between BFU-E and CFU-E is the abundance of erythropoietin receptors (EpoRs) on CFU-E and their dependence on Epo for cell survival. CFU-E, in contrast to BFU-E, cannot survive in vitro even for a few hours in the absence of Epo. Although greater than 80% of CFU-E have detectable EpoRs,[55] only a small proportion of BFU-E have receptors[56,57] and can terminally differentiate in culture in the presence of Epo alone.[58] Direct binding studies show that the number of EpoRs peaks at the CFU-E/proerythroblast level and progressively declines when cells mature further (Table 25–1),[55] reflecting the declining influence of Epo. In addition to the abundance of EpoRs, erythroid progenitors are distinguished from other marrow progenitors by the presence of high levels of transferrin receptors (Tfrs).[57,59,60] Peak levels of Tfrs are seen on CFU-E and erythroid precursors, and lower levels are present on reticulocytes.[53,59] (For a detailed review on iron metabolism and heme synthesis in erythroid cells, see references 61–63).

In addition to the functional definition, the hemopoietic compartments in the marrow of a normal adult mouse have been prospectively identified on the basis of expression of specific cell surface antigens and subsequent differentiation in vitro and in vivo.[64] The $Lin^{neg}IL\text{-}7R^{neg}Thy1^{neg}c\text{-}kit^{pos}Sca1^{neg}$ fraction of the marrow of normal adult mice has been subdivided into three populations based on the expression of CD34 and CD16/CD32: $CD16/CD32^{low}$ $CD34^{high}$ representing the common myeloid progenitor, $CD16/CD32^{low}CD34^{low}$ representing the megakaryocyte-erythroid progenitor (MEP), and $CD16/CD32^{high}CD34^{high}$ representing the granulocyte-monocyte progenitor (Fig. 25–1).[64] Many laboratories are prospectively identifying the corresponding human compartments.[65] Whether the correlation between phenotype and function of cells isolated on the basis of these antigenic expression profiles is maintained under conditions of perturbed or stressed erythropoiesis or during ontogenesis remains to be seen.

ERYTHROID PRECURSOR CELL COMPARTMENT

The erythroid precursor cell compartment, also termed the *erythron*, includes cells that, in contrast to the erythroid progenitor cells (BFU-E and CFU-E), are defined by morphologic criteria. The earliest recognizable erythroid cell is the *proerythroblast*, which after four to five mitotic divisions and serial morphologic changes gives rise to mature erythroid cells. Its progeny include *basophilic erythroblasts*, which are the earliest daughter cells, followed by *polychromatophilic* and *orthochromatic erythroblasts*. Their morphologic characteristics reflect the accumulation of erythroid-specific proteins (i.e., hemoglobin) and the decline in nuclear activity (Fig. 25–2). After the last mitotic division, the inactive dense nucleus of the orthochromatic erythroblast moves to one side of the cell and is extruded, encased by a thin cytoplasmic layer. Expelled nuclei are ingested by marrow macrophages, and the resulting enucleated cell is a *reticulocyte*. Although all mammals have enucleated cells in their circulation, the evolutionary advantage of enucleation is not readily apparent. It may allow for more red cell deformability when traveling through the small vasculature, or it may minimize cardiac workload.

Maturation from proerythroblast to reticulocyte likely does not always adhere to a rigid sequence in which each division is associated with the production of two more differentiated and morphologically distinct daughter cells (i.e., basophilic erythroblast gives rise to two polychromatophilic ones). Rather, significant flexibility, both in the number and rate of divisions and in the rate of enucleation, may be allowed. Such deviations from the normal orderly maturation sequence may be dictated by the level of Epo. Thus, in cases of acute demand for red cell production (because of blood loss or hemolysis), the kinetics of formation of new reticulocytes are significantly more rapid. Resulting red cells may be larger (i.e., with increased mean corpuscular volume). This has led to the concept of "skipped" divisions.[66] The orderly unilineage differentiation pathway shown in Fig. 25–1 likely is restricted to conditions of steady-state hematopoiesis. Similar to occurrences in the lymphoid system,[67] alternative routes are taken under conditions of stress. Murine models have been developed to address phenotype–function cell relationships during recovery from acute and chronic erythroid stress. A model for acute stress is represented by the hemolytic anemia induced by phenylhydrazine treatment. Recovery from this acute anemia involves recruitment of the spleen as an additional erythropoietic site and is dependent on Epo. The amount of ^{3}H-thymidine incorporated by splenic erythroblasts produced in response to this stress has long represented the biologic assay for Epo.[68] Genetic evidence indicates that recovery from this hemolytic anemia is controlled by a receptor complex formed between the EpoR and a truncated version of the Stk receptor encoded by $Fv2^s$, a locus that also determines strain susceptibility to Friend virus infection.[69] An additional control on the response to acute erythroid stress in mice is exerted by the glucocorticoid receptor, as mice in which this receptor is targeted recover poorly from phenylhydrazine treatment.[70] On the other hand, experimentally induced mutations in genes involved in the regulation of erythroid differentiation, such as signal transducer and activator of transcription 5 $(STAT5)^{null}$ [71] and $GATA1^{low}$,[72] induce chronic erythroid stress by increasing the rate of erythroblast apoptosis. The spleen also is recruited as a hemopoietic site in response to chronic erythroid stress.[71,72] Several studies in aggregate suggest that the erythron does not respond to stress only by amplifying the normal erythroid progenitor cell compartments (i.e., common myeloid progenitor, MEP, and CFU-E). The erythron also generates alternative routes of differentiation, possibly through cooperation between EpoR and other receptors (e.g., Stk and glucocorticoid receptor) specifically recruited as part of the stress response.[73,74] Genetic heterogeneity in the control of gene expression of these receptors may add another layer of variability in recovery from anemia in humans.

The alterations in cell morphology that occur as erythroid precursor cells mature (Fig. 25–2) are determined by complex biochemical changes, which accommodate the accumulation of erythroid-specific proteins and the progressive decline in proliferation. Compared to erythroid progenitor cells, erythroid precursor cells have been more accessible to study, and considerable information is available about their maturation-related biochemical changes.

The shape and deformability of the red cell are determined by its membrane proteins. Most membrane cytoskeletal proteins (spectrin, glycophorin, band 3, band 4.1, and ankyrin) accumulate after the CFU-E stage (i.e., within the precursor cell compartment). Specifically, expression of membrane glycoproteins such as band 3 and band 4.1 is greatly enhanced at the later stages of erythroid maturation.[75–77] Likewise, the quantity of polylactosaminoglycan, a specific carbohydrate chain that carries blood group ABH and Ii antigenic determinants, is much higher in mature erythrocytes than in erythroblasts.[78] Whereas a linear, virtually unbranched polylactosamine structure is present in fetal and newborn erythroid cells (reflected by i antigenic reactivity), a branched polylactosaminyl structure is present in adult erythroblasts (reflected by I antigenic reactivity), and branching increases further as maturation progresses.[78,79] A correctly assembled cytoskeleton is important for the deformability and dynamic plasticity of red blood cells in circulation. A new player required for actin assembly in red cells, Rac GTPase, has been identified.[80] Glycophorins, especially glycophorin A, are expressed fully at the CFU-E or proerythroblast level just before expression of globin, and few changes occur during maturation.[42] In contrast, the membrane glycoproteins p105 and p95 decline during the later stages of maturation,[78] and yet other membrane glycoproteins, such as vimentin (an intermediate filament protein), are totally lost.[75] Loss of vimentin expression at the late erythroblastic stages most likely facilitates enucleation. The process of erythroblast enucleation involves chromatin reorganization, as evidenced by separation of the nuclei surrounded by plasma and nuclei extrusion from the cell. The expelled nuclei are picked up by macrophages. Sorting of erythroblast plasma membrane components to reticulocytes is regulated by the degree of skeletal linkage,[81] whereas engulfment of nuclei by macrophages occurs only after the nuclei are disconnected from reticulocytes. Phosphatidylserine, the "eat me" flag for apoptotic cells, is also used for engulfment of nuclei expelled from erythroblasts.[82] The enucleation process is caspase independent[83] and erythroblast macrophage protein dependent.[84] Erythroblast macrophage protein is expressed by erythroblast and macrophage and must be expressed by both populations for proper enucleation to occur.[84] The fact that proper enucleation requires interaction with the macrophages explains the old observation that erythroid differentiation in the marrow occurs in discrete sites, the erythroblastic islands, which are composed of erythroblasts surrounding a central macrophage (see Hematopoietic Microenvironment).

In addition to quantitative changes that occur during maturation, gradual switches in subunit composition of some cytoskeletal proteins occur. For example, exclusively erythroid subunits of α and β spectrin are displayed only in end-stage cells.[46] Likewise, multiple transcripts of ankyrin or protein 4.1 have been identified, and the ratios of these transcripts change during maturation.[85] Initial expression of many of these membrane components likely begins at the progenitor cell level. However, in these cells, final assembly may be discouraged because of the higher turnover of these proteins, which minimizes mutual interactions, or because of asynchrony in protein synthesis. Prevention of cytoskeletal assembly at these early stages may secure more membrane fluidity and cell motility needed during this proliferative phase of differentiation. Because molecular probes for many of the red cell cytoskeletal components have been developed, detailed information about the transcription and processing of most of these proteins is beginning to emerge.[77]

Expression of the majority of genes encoding cytoskeletal components is not restricted to red cells. Dissecting hemopoietic from nonhemopoietic consequences of abnormalities in these genes has been difficult, but the development of mouse models that mimic defects found in human diseases has been helpful in this respect.[86]

Gene activity during erythroid maturation is dominated by globin expression. Globin represents less than 0.1% of protein at the proerythroblast level but constitutes 95% of all protein at the reticulocyte level.[87] Globin expression has been extensively studied, and its gene regulation is well understood in molecular terms. Major steps in globin transcription and processing are known in considerable detail and are summarized elsewhere in this text (Chapter 33). The globin type synthesized by adult precursors is hemoglobin A (HbA; $\alpha_2\beta_2$). In addition, two other minor globin components, HbA_2 ($\alpha_2\delta_2$) and HbF ($\alpha_2\gamma_2$), are present. Of significant biologic interest are the low amounts of HbF that continue to be synthesized throughout life.

The small amount of HbF, which is present in all normal individuals, has the following characteristics.[88] (a) It is confined to a small fraction of red cells, called *F cells*, which are detected by sensitive immunofluorescence assays or acid elution techniques and usually constitute 2% to 5% of all red cells. Within each F cell, HbF or γ globin constitutes 14% to 25% of total globin. (b) The number of F cells is genetically determined, and the gene(s) linked or nonlinked to the β-locus is responsible for F-cell formation. (c) F cells do not display other features of "fetalness" because their membrane components and enzymes are characteristically adult. (e) Synthesis of HbF peaks earlier than that of HbA, so the proportion of HbF is higher in immature cells compared with mature, fully hemoglobinized cells. (e) F cells and cells that contain only HbA are not derived from distinct stem cell populations but from a common adult stem cell. Whether this cell will form F or non–F (i.e., A) cells is determined at the BFU-E level and throughout the CFU-E level. In vitro the great majority of BFU-E have the potential to express HbF, whereas in vivo only a very small proportion of red cells contain HbF. This potential appears to be lost during normal cell differentiation and maturation in vivo. This concept links the potential for HbF expression to the pathway of erythroid differentiation and thus may have implications for interpreting the reactivation of HbF that occurs in adults under diverse circumstances (e.g., after chemotherapy or with acute bleeding).[88] Many of these circumstances seem to influence HbF levels by directly or indirectly modifying the kinetics of the normal differentiation/maturation process.[89,90] HbF levels in red cells can be increased by exposing the cells during maturation to chemical inhibitors of histone deacetylase. This class of enzymes nonspecifically suppresses gene transcription by catalyzing histone deacetylation and, consequently, chromatin condensation.[91] Therefore, they can directly activate transcription of γ-globin genes in vitro and in vivo[92–94] and in a number of patients with β-thalassemia.[95,96]

Synthesis of globin appears to be coordinated with synthesis of heme throughout erythroid maturation so that functional hemoglobin tetramers are formed rapidly and spontaneously after release of newly synthesized globins from polysomes. Information about the accumulation of heme and its synthetic intermediaries has been provided by crude biochemical approaches (Fig. 25–2). However, now that the genes for several enzymes in the heme synthetic pathway (e.g., δ-aminolevulinic acid synthetase, porphobilinogen deaminase, and heme synthetase) have been cloned, information about their regulation is rapidly emerging.[61,63]

An important role in coordinating heme and globin chain assembly during hemoglobin production is exerted by alpha hemoglobin-stabilizing protein (AHSP). AHSP is a protein abundantly expressed in erythroid cells[97] whose function is to bind free α-chains, stabilizing their structure and limiting their ability to participate in chemical reactions that generate reactive oxygen species.[98,99] In addition, AHSP binding increases the affinity of α-chains for β-chains, accelerating the formation of Hb tetramers. The essential role exerted by this gene in erythroid development has been demonstrated by the fact that its deletion in normal mice impairs red cell production. $AHSP^{null}$ red cells have a decreased half-life, contain Hb precipitates, and exhibit signs of oxidative damage.[97] The observation that double $AHSP^{null}$ β-thalassemic mutant mice have an exacerbated phenotype[100] suggests that AHSP is a gene modifier that, like the hereditary persistence of HbF mutations, ameliorates the phenotype of thalassemic patients. However, the search for AHSP polymorphisms that might correlate with milder clinical phenotypes in thalassemia has not provided consistent results. Gene mapping, direct genomic sequencing, and extended haplotype analysis did not reveal any mutation or specific association between haplotypes of AHSP in 120 β-thalassemic patients.[101] On the other hand, a polymorphism in the putative AHSP promoter leading to a threefold higher expression of the gene in reticulocytes was observed in the normal population,[102] but any clinical consequences are unknown.

Crucial to the functional response of erythroid precursors is the expression of EpoRs and Tfrs. EpoRs decrease progressively (from approximately 1000 to <300 receptors per cell) as proerythroblasts mature, and they are undetectable at the reticulocyte level.[55,103] Through these receptors, Epo exerts its proliferative influence on proerythroblasts and basophilic erythroblasts, but maturation beyond these stages can proceed in the absence of Epo.

Tfrs are found in characteristic abundance in erythroid cells (300,000–800,000 Tfrs per cell).[104] This composition reflects not only the proliferative needs of erythroid cells but also their extreme requirements for iron uptake for hemoglobin synthesis. For this reason, Tfrs persist in maturing nondividing erythroblasts and in reticulocytes. Tfrs belong to a large group of receptors that internalize their ligand through receptor-mediated endocytosis. This cycle allows for reuse both of the ligand (transferrin) for resaturation with iron and of the receptor for entering an another route of endocytosis.[105] Tfr density decreases with maturation. After the reticulocyte stage, receptors appear to be shed as small lipid vesicles.[106] An inverse relationship exists between receptor density and iron availability. Deprivation of iron results in receptor induction, and excess iron results in receptor suppression.[105] However, the mechanisms that regulate the number of Tfrs throughout the maturation of precursors (even within progenitors) are largely unknown. Erythroid precursor cells differ from nonerythroid cells not only by requiring a higher number and higher occupancy of Tfrs. They also display immunologically distinct receptor isoforms.[60] A second gene for transferrin receptor (TfR2) has been identified,[107] and monoclonal antibodies recognizing distinct receptor isoforms are useful in isolating erythroid cells from bone marrow.[60,108] TfR1 and TfR2 are members of a family of genes encoding at least seven different homologous proteins in primates.[109] TfR1 is a type II membrane glycoprotein that, as a cell surface homodimer, binds iron-loaded transferrin as part of the process of iron transfer and uptake. TfR2 is expressed in two forms—membrane-bound (TfR2-α) and nonmembrane (TfR2-β)—both of which bind transferrin with low affinity. The specific role of TfR2 in hematopoietic cells is unclear. In cells from 67 patients with de novo acute myeloid leukemia (AML), high levels of TfR2-α expression were correlated with better prognosis, and higher levels of both TfR2-α and TfR2-β were associated with longer survival, suggesting that Tfr-independent iron uptake plays a role in in vivo proliferation of AML cells.[110] TfR2 plays its most prominent role in the liver[111] as the key regulator of iron metabolism. Maintenance of stable extracellular iron concentrations requires the coordinate regulation of iron transport into plasma from dietary sources in the duodenum, recycled senescent red cells in macrophages, and storage in hepatocytes. Diferric transferrin is detected in the liver via a complex machinery involving the product of the hereditary hemochromatosis gene HFE (a protein of the major histocompatibility complex class I), TfR2, and the product of the hemojuvelin (HJV) gene (also known as HFE2). Given that the levels of TfR2 expression are exclusively regulated by holotransferrin, TfR2 expressed by hepatocytes likely is the first element of the iron sensory pathway in the liver.[112] Hepatocytes respond to iron sensoring by modulating hepcidin expression and secretion. Hepcidin, a 25-amino-acid disulfide-rich peptide, acts as a systemic iron regulatory hormone that regulates both dietary iron adsorption by the enterocytes and iron recycling by the macrophages. Because ferroportin shuttles iron from the enterocytes to the macrophages and hepcidin is required for ferroportin internalization and degradation, decreased hepcidin expression blocks iron export in the two cell types.[113] Each gene involved in iron metabolism has a role in regulating the expression of the other genes. In particular, reduced expression of HEF, TfR2, and HJV reduces expression of hepcidin. It is not surprising, then, that mutations altering the function of all of these genes have been found associated with hereditary hemochromatosis. The most prevalent form of familial hematochromatosis (type 1; HFE1) involves mutations in HFE.[114] Most families with juvenile hemochromatosis (HFE2) have mutations in the HJV gene.[115] Homozygous nonsense[116] and single-point mutations causing methionine→lysine substitution at position 172 of the protein M172K[117] have been detected in the gene encoding TfR2 in patients with familial hemochromatosis HFE3. Autosomal dominant iron overload is associated with previously unrecognized ferroportin 1 mutations (p.R88T and p.I180T)[118] and with mutations in the divalent metal transporter 1 gene DMT1, which mediates apical iron uptake in duodenal enterocytes and iron transfer from the Tfr endosomal cycle into the cytosol in erythroid cells.[119] The observation that targeted deletions of any of these genes (including TfR2) induce a hematochromatosis-like syndrome in mice provides proof of direct involvement of the mutations in disease development.[120–123] On the other hand, the finding that hepcidin is a gene modifier of the HEF^{null} mouse model of hemochromatosis suggests that heterogeneity at the hepcidin locus mediates the low penetrance of the genetic disease.[124] In addition to its role in determining the pathobiology of hereditary hemochromatosis, hepcidin plays an important role in determining the anemia of chronic diseases. Based on the central involvement of hepcidin in iron regulation and its pathologies, a hepcidin assay has been proposed as a useful tool for diagnosing iron disorders and monitoring their treatment. On the other hand, development of hepcidin agonists and antagonists may provide useful therapeutics for treatment of iron disorders.[125]

The patterns of Tfr and glycophorin A expression during erythroid maturation have been exploited to define flow cytometric criteria that distinguish the different populations of erythroid precursors in mice and men. By coupling size and forward scatter (both progressively reduced) with CD71 (Tfr) and TER-119 (an antibody that recognizes an antigen associated with glycophorin A[126] expression), erythroid precursors were divided into the classes $TER\text{-}119^{med}$ $CD71^{high}$, $TER\text{-}119^{high}CD71^{high}$, $TER\text{-}119^{high}CD71^{med}$, and $TER\text{-}119^{high}CD71^{low}$, which correspond to proerythroblasts and basophilic, chromatophilic, and orthochromatophilic erythroblasts, respectively.[71] However, such distinction is not conserved in all mouse strains. For example, in C57Bl/6 mice, CD71 expression levels remain constant during maturation.[127] Double CD71/glycophorin A staining has been proposed to define human erythroblast precursors by flow cytometry. However, the pattern of CD71 expression during erythroid maturation presents a high level of donor variability. Given that downmodulation of CD36 expression during erythroid maturation is relatively independent of genetic variability, an alternative flow cytometric definition of erythroblast subclasses is proposed by the phenotype $CD36^{high}$/glycophorin A^{medium}, $CD36^{high}$/glycophorin A^{high}, and $CD36^{low}$/glycophorin A^{high}, corresponding to basophilic, polychromatic, and orthochromatic erythroblasts, respectively.[128]

ERYTHROPOIETIN AND EPO-R

Epo, a 35-kd glycoprotein,[129] is the physiologically obligatory growth factor for erythroid development. It is produced mainly in the kidney by peritubular cells.[130] A heme-containing protein senses oxygen need and then triggers the synthesis of Epo and its release into the bloodstream.[131,132] Through the interaction of Epo with receptor-bearing cells within the bone marrow, physiologic oxygen demands are translated into increased red cell production. Thus, Epo is a true hormone, manufactured at one anatomic site and transported through the bloodstream to the site of activity.

According to the prevailing model of hematopoiesis, progenitor cells committed to erythroid differentiation (i.e., BFU-E) are generated in a stochastic fashion from pluripotent stem cells.[4,5] Neither Epo nor other lineage-restricted regulators play any role in determining lineage commitment. According to this model, Epo influences erythroid differentiation by rescuing (from apoptosis) cells that express EpoR and amplifying them further. Whether EpoRs are present on all BFU-E (detectable only in a subset of BFU-E) is not clear.[56] Thus, whether the presence of EpoR in BFU-E is synchronous with the initial commitment event or follows it is not known. In addition to the permissive role of Epo ascribed by the stochastic theory, experiments in vivo, in anemic states, or after pharmacologic doses of Epo suggest that high levels of Epo hasten the transition from BFU-E to hemoglobin-synthesizing cells by decreasing either the number of divisions required for this transition[66] or the resting periods between cell divisions.[133] Autoradiographic studies of purified BFU-E populations indicate that EpoRs increase as BFU-E mature to CFU-E, with the highest level observed at the CFU-E/proerythroblast boundary.[56] That the transition from BFU-E to CFU-E occurs under the influence of Epo suggests ligand (Epo)-induced receptor upregulation. Whether the magnitude of such upregulation is dependent on Epo dose and whether it can modulate the rate of entry of these cells into the maturing compartment is unclear.

BFU-E and CFU-E can be generated in vitro[134] and in vivo,[135] in the absence of Epo or EpoR (in Epo or EpoR^{null} mice), but their survival and terminal maturation normally are dependent on Epo. For CFU-E, Epo seems to stimulate all the biochemical processes characterizing erythroid cells (i.e., heme synthesis, globin synthesis, and synthesis of cytoskeletal proteins). However, the necessity of Epo in these processes is not absolute. In vitro experiments showing complete maturation of BFU-E in the absence of Epo suggest that other factors or combinations of factors can influence red cell maturation. Activation of the gp130 signaling pathway by use of soluble IL-6 receptor and IL-6 leads to full terminal erythroid maturation (in the presence of stem cell factor and IL-3 but in the absence of Epo), suggesting some form of cross-circuiting in signaling pathways among hematopoietic growth factor receptors.[136,137] Furthermore, stimulation by TPO of erythroid colony formation from yolk sac cells in the absence of EpoR (in EpoR$^{-/-}$ embryos)[138] can be explained by the same reasoning and the finding of a very high proportion of bipotent erythroid/megakaryocytic progenitors in yolk sac carrying both Epo and TPO receptors (c-mpl) compared to adult bone marrow.[139–141]

Whatever the precise mode of Epo action, it directly affects the number of CFU-E and the maturation of their progeny. This control is achieved by influencing CFU-E survival and not their cycling status.[142] CFU-E are irrevocably lost after one cycle of DNA synthesis if Epo is not present.[143]

With the availability of radiolabeled recombinant Epo and purified or enriched populations of progenitors and precursors has come information about the characteristics of EpoRs in erythroid cells. Direct binding studies have shown that a progressive decrease in the number of EpoRs as CFU-E and proerythroblasts mature to reticulocytes.[56,57,103] Pure reticulocyte populations show no detectable binding to Epo. The maturation-associated decline in the number of EpoRs parallels the declining influence of Epo on erythroid cells during the terminal phase of maturation. The exquisite role of Epo in determining red cell numbers in the circulation has been clearly established by direct correlations between hematocrit and Epo plasma concentrations in individuals exposed to hypoxia and in patients with compromised kidney functions.[144] However, the variabilities around the mean of hematocrit and Epo plasma levels found in normal individuals under steady-state conditions are not correlated, indicating that other factors (sex and age) cooperate with Epo in determining the fluctuations in red cell mass under steady-state hematopoiesis.[145]

Cloning and expression of EpoR has allowed a better understanding of the role of Epo in the regulation of erythroid development. The EpoR polypeptide is a 66-kd membrane protein that is a member of the cytokine receptor superfamily.[146,147] Many of the structural features of the cell surface EpoR have been previously reviewed.[148] Like other members of the cytokine receptor superfamily, which includes the receptors for IL-3, GM-CSF, and IL-5, the EpoR polypeptide contains four conserved cysteine residues and a WSXWS motif in the extracellular region. Additional extracytoplasmic sequences of EpoR determine the specificity for Epo binding. The cytoplasmic region of EpoR does not contain a tyrosine kinase catalytic domain; instead it interacts with cytoplasmic tyrosine kinases. Cross-linking of radiolabeled Epo to cell surface EpoR results in formation of at least two major cross-linked protein complexes of 140 and 120 kd.[149] The molecular composition of these complexes remains unsolved but suggests that EpoR contains additional subunits or accessory proteins.[150] The extracytoplasmic region of the EpoR polypeptide contains the Epo binding activity of the receptor.[151–153] Therefore, additional EpoR subunits may provide other structural and functional elements of the receptor but are not required for high-affinity Epo binding. The extracytoplasmic region of the EpoR polypeptide has been crystalized.[154–156] The crystal structure confirms the dimeric structure of the activated receptor. Interestingly, small synthetic peptides are capable of inducing EpoR dimerization, suggesting a profitable avenue for Epo-mimetic and Epo-antagonist drug design.[157] Epo-mimetic agents are represented by polypeptides restricted to the portion of the protein that binds the receptor, by forms of the protein molecularly engineered to increase its glycosylation state and therefore its stability in vivo, or by dimeric forms of proteins obtained by genetic introduction of bridging sites or chemical cross-linking.[158] It also is possible that nonpeptide chemicals sharing the same stereo and electric properties of the receptor binding domain of the protein might be identified. As shown for carbamylated Epo, modified isoforms may have biologic activity partially different from, and possible more effective than, the native protein,[159] especially with regard to the activity of the growth factor in nonhematopoietic tissues.[160]

EpoR mRNA, originally isolated from murine erythroblast cell lines (MEL and HCD57)[129] and from a human erythroid cell line (OCIM1),[161] has been found in nonerythroid cells as well. Epo promotes the differentiation of megakaryocytes at physiologic concentrations of hormone, suggesting that megakaryocytes have functional cell surface EpoRs. Rat and mouse placenta also have cell surface EpoR, detected by radiolabeled Epo cross-linking. Epo promotes a chemotactic effect on endothelial cells,[162,163] suggesting the presence of a cell surface receptor in these cells. Other studies suggest that EpoR is expressed in neural cells[164] and smooth muscle cells.[165] Adverse effects in cancer patients treated with Epo have been attributed to the effects of Epo on tumor cells.[166] The functional importance of EpoR expression in nonerythroid cells has been revealed by rescue experiments in EpoR^{null} mice.[167] As EpoR^{null} mutant mice die of severe anemia between days 13 and 15 of embryonic development, the mutant embryos are rescued by transgenic expression of EpoR under the control of the hemopoietic-specific GATA1 regulatory domain. Under steady-state conditions, the rescued animals are normal, as the gene is expressed only in erythroid cells. However, in comparison with normal mice, the increase in plasma Epo concentration in response to induced anemia was delayed in the rescued animals, suggesting that one of the major functions of EpoR expression in nonerythroid cells is fine tuning the regulation of the response to stress (see Alterations in EPOR and its Signalling in Disorders of Erythropoiesis).[167]

The existence of naturally occurring splice variants of the EpoR gene encoding EpoR polypeptides of variable length and activity has been shown.[168–171] The soluble secreted form of EpoR[172] binds Epo and thereby competes with the cell surface receptor isoform. The biologic function of alternative forms of the cell surface EpoR, including a truncated form of EpoR found in early progenitors,[173] remains unknown but may be related either to differential Epo signaling and responses (survival, proliferation, differentiation) at different stages in erythroid development or to the establishment of erythroid-specific versus myeloid-specific niches in the marrow microenvironment.

SIGNAL TRANSDUCTION BY EPO-R

Considerable progress has been made in our understanding of EpoR-mediated signal transduction. Early studies demonstrated that stimulation of EpoR on primary erythroid cells resulted in increased calcium ion flux and increased globin mRNA synthesis.[174] Since the cloning of the EpoR polypeptide and its stable expression in heterologous cell systems, such as the Ba/F3 cell system,[175] considerable molecular insight has been gained.[176] For instance, it now is clear that Epo induces homodimerization of the EpoR polypeptide.[177,178] Following receptor dimerization at the cell surface, a series of tyrosine phosphorylation events occurs, resulting in a mitogenic signal and a differentiative signal.[179,180] Initial studies of the EpoR signal transduction pathway made use of mutant forms of EpoR stably expressed in the indicator cell line Ba/F3. Ba/F3 cells are a murine IL-3–dependent pro–B-lymphocyte cell line. These cells can be readily transfected with the cDNA for EpoR, resulting in stable expression of the receptor on the cell surface. Expression of the full-length, wild-type EpoR polypeptide in these cells resulted in Epo-dependent growth and partial Epo-induced erythroid differentiation.[179,180] Expression of truncated forms of the EpoR polypeptide in these cells resulted in variable growth responses. For instance, truncation of the membrane proximal region of EpoR demonstrated a critical positive regulatory domain of EpoR required for mitogenesis.[175] Furthermore, truncation of the carboxy-terminal 40 amino acids of EpoR resulted in increased Epo-dependent growth, suggesting that the carboxy-terminal region contained a negative regulatory domain normally required for downmodulating EpoR mitogenic signals.[175]

The biochemical basis for these positive and negative regulatory domains has been elucidated. The membrane proximal positive regulatory region of EpoR binds constitutively to Janus kinase 2 (Jak2),[181] a cytoplasmic tyrosine kinase necessary for erythroid differentiation, as evidenced by mice lacking the corresponding gene dying at an early embryonic stage.[182] Upon Epo binding to the receptor, the receptor dimerizes, resulting in activation of prebound Jak2. The Jak2 next tyrosine phosphorylates multiple signaling proteins in the cell, leading to various mitogenic and differentiative responses. The negative regulatory domain of EpoR is required for recruiting the phosphatase SHP1 to EpoR.[183] SHP1 binds to an activated tyrosine phosphate on the EpoR polypeptide and rapidly downregulates Jak2 activity and dephosphorylates the EpoR polypeptide. Failure to recruit the SHP1 phosphatase can result in increased EpoR signaling and a polycythemic state (see Alterations in ERO-R and its Signalling in Disorders of Erythropoiesis).

Jak2 is required for appropriate Golgi processing and cell surface expression of EpoR.[184] Once activated by Epo/EpoR binding on the cell surface, Jak2 initiates several events in EpoR-mediated signal transduction. Jak2 initially activates tyrosine phosphorylation of several tyrosine residues of the cytoplasmic tail of EpoR. These phosphorylated tyrosine residues next serve as docking sites for binding of other cytoplasmic effector proteins containing Src homology 2 (SH2) domains, such as the p85 subunit of phosphatidylinositol 3-kinase,[185] the adaptor protein *Shc*,[186,187] and STAT5.[188,189] (Examples of signal transduction proteins expressed in primary human erythroblasts are given in Table 25–2). Once these proteins have docked on EpoR, they become tyrosine phosphorylated and engage other downstream signaling events. In addition, Jak2 activates the Ras/Raf/MAPK (mitogen-activated protein kinase) pathway, further contributing to the Epo-induced mitogenic signal.[190,191] The molecular mechanism of Ras activation by Jak2 remains unknown but may entail direct binding of the proteins and tyrosine phosphorylation.[191]

Activation of the Jak2/STAT5 signaling pathway has been studied in considerable detail. Upon EpoR tyrosine phosphorylation, STAT5 protein binds to a specific phosphorylated tyrosine residue of the EpoR.[188,192] Binding is mediated by the SH2 domain of STAT5. Following EpoR binding, STAT5 itself becomes tyrosine phosphorylated at amino acid Y694.[193] Activated STAT5 then disengages from EpoR, undergoes homodimerization, and translocates to the cell nucleus, where it activates transcription of Epo-inducible genes. Some Epo-inducible genes, such as *myc* and *fos,* are common to other hematopoietic growth factor signaling pathways. Other Epo-inducible genes are specifically expressed in erythroid cells and are not shared by other growth factor responses.[194]

Other signal transduction pathways downstream from cytokine receptors have been identified. For instance, Epo and IL-3 activate tyrosine phosphorylation of the signaling protein cbl and the subsequent binding and tyrosine phosphorylation of the signal protein CrkL.[195] The mechanism of activation of this pathway by EpoR is not known, and the relative role of this pathway in Epo-induced growth and erythroid differentiation remains largely unexplored. Inositide-specific phospholipases C (PLCs) and the protein kinase C (PKC) pathway also are involved in Epo signaling. PLCs catalyze hydrolysis of phosphatidylinositol 4,5-bisphosphate to generate diacylglycerol and inositol 3,4,5-bisphosphate, a well-known intracellular messenger for PKC activation and intracellular Ca^{2+} mobilization. PLCs are classified into four isoform families (α, β, γ, and δ), and each family has multiple isoforms.[196,197] The involvement of PLCs in erythroid differentiation was suggested by early studies demonstrating that stimulation of EpoR in primary erythroid cells results in increased calcium ion flux.[174] More recent studies demonstrated that primary erythroblasts express only some (i.e., PLC β_1, β_2, β_3, δ_1, γ_1 and γ_2) PLC isoforms. Among these, PLC β_1 most likely is involved in Epo signaling, based on findings that its expression is induced by 6 hours of stimulation with the growth factor.[22,128,198] On the other hand, PKC represents a family of nine different serine-threonine kinases genes, encoding a total of 12 different isoforms, involved in the regulation of many cellular functions.[199] These enzymes exert their biologic functions as a cytoplasmic–nuclear shuttle of the transduction machinery and become phosphorylated, and hence activated, in response to a variety of stimuli. Human multipotent $CD34^+$ progenitor cells express all of the PKC isoforms.[200,201] Commitment of these cells along the erythroid lineage requires suppression of PKCε.[200,202] PKCα exerts a positive control on erythropoiesis, as its inhibitors specifically impair the ability of erythroid cells to respond to Epo[203] and to phosphorylate EpoR, STAT5, GAB1, ERK1/2, and AKT.[204] It also is possible that different PKC isoforms are active at different ontogenic stages, as PKCα and PKCδ are differentially phosphorylated, and hence activated, during differentiation of neonatal and adult erythroblasts.[205]

A critical question in the field of EpoR signal transduction is the mechanism of Epo specificity. Most, if not all, of the signal transduction pathways activated by EpoR (i.e., Ras/Raf/MAPK and Jak/STAT) are shared by other hematopoietic cytokine receptors, such as the receptors for IL-3, GM-CSF, and IL-5. How EpoR triggers a specific growth factor response resulting in erythroid differentiation is unclear. Several models are possible. First, EpoR may activate unique but unknown signaling pathways specific to EpoR and distinct from other cytokine receptors. Alternatively, EpoR may activate identical pathways, activated by other cytokine receptors. In the latter model, the specificity of the Epo signal is derived not from EpoR itself but from interactions with other developmentally programmed events in the erythroid cell, such as expression of erythroid-specific transcription factors.

Activation of EpoR in the murine IL-3–dependent cell line Ba/F3 results in induction of both mitogenesis and β-globin accumulation.[103] In contrast, the murine IL-2–dependent cell line CTLL-2, when engineered to express the heterologous EpoR, grows in Epo but does not differentiate into globin-bearing cells. These data suggest

Table 25–2 Major Transcription Factors/Signaling Molecules Involved in Control of Erythropoiesis

Transcription Factor	Binding Motif	Role in Hematopoiesis	Knockout Phenotype	Mutations/Human Disease
GATA1	(A/T)GATA(A/G)	↑Erythroid differentiation	• No terminal erythropoiesis • Arrest in megakaryocyte development (with hyperproliferation)	• X-linked thalassemia/ thrombocytopenia • Leukemia (Down syndrome)
GATA2	(A/T)GATA(A/G)	↑Proliferation ↓Differentiation	↓Proliferative expansion of primitive and definitive erythropoiesis Absence of mast cells	
FOG1	None	GATA1 cofactor	↓Erythroid maturation Block in megakaryocytopoiesis	
EKLF	CACCC	Promotes terminal erythroid differentiation	Severe anemia β-globin deficiency	β-Thalassemia
SCL	CANNTG (E box)	Specification of hematopoiesis	Absence of prenatal hematopoiesis ↓Erythro/Mk in adults	Translocation in T-ALL
LMO2	LIM domain		Absence of hematopoiesis	T-cell ALL
Myb	(T/C)AAC(G/T)G	↓Definitive erythropoiesis	Block in definitive erythropoiesis	
Fli-1	Winged helix–turn helix	Inhibition of GATA1 expression		
BKLF	CACC		Myeloproliferative disorder	
SHP-1 (BKLF activated?)				Erythroleukemia Polycythemia vera
STAT5	GAS		Transient fetal anemia due to apoptosis of erythroid progenitors Mild anemia exacerbated by stress in adult life	
PU.1	GGAA	↓Erythropoiesis	Absence of myelomonocytic differentiation	
Id		Blocks terminal differentiation of all cell types		
laPI-3 kinase (p85)		↓Proliferation/differentiation	↓Fetal erythropoiesis Perinatal death	
Gfi-1B	Zinc finger domain	↑Proliferation (↑GATA2)		
Sp3			↓Fetal erythropoiesis Perinatal death	
NF-E2	TGAGTCA	Promotes terminal erythroid differentiation in vitro	Thrombocytopenia Absence of erythroid abnormalities (?)	

BKLF, basic Kruppel-like factor; FOG1, friend of GATA1; LMO2, LIM domain only 2. ALL: acute lymphoblastic Leukemia; ↓ erythro/μg: Decrease in erythropoiesis/megakaryocytopoiesis

that expression of EpoR is necessary for erythroid differentiation but is not sufficient alone. Other erythroid-specific markers, such as GATA1 and NF-E2, or erythroid Kruppel-like factor (EKLF), likely are required for cells to differentiate down the erythroid pathway. Other cytokine receptors, such as IL-3R and IL-2R, do not drive β-globin synthesis in these cell lines. Taken together, these results suggest that EpoR generates a differentiation-specific signaling within the context of a proper transcriptional environment.

Regardless of the mechanism of cytokine specificity, each cytokine receptor activates a similar but not identical pattern of signaling events. For instance, EpoR shows a preferential activation of the Jak2/STAT5 pathway in cultured erythroid cells in vitro. In contrast, the IL-2 receptor shows preferential activation of the Jak1/Jak3/STAT6 pathway.[193,206,207] Interestingly, although Epo activates STAT5a and STAT5b in cultured cells, knock-out of the STAT5a or STAT5b gene by homologous recombination results in a mouse phenotype with slightly impaired stem cell activity but apparently normal erythroid development.[208,209] More extensive analysis of this phenotype has revealed that the mice experience increased apoptotic rates at erythroblast levels that are compensated by a cellular compensatory mechanism very similar to that described for GATA1^{low} mutants,[71] involving expansion of hemopoietic progenitors in the marrow and recruitment of the spleen as an additional hemopoietic site. These results suggest that, in vivo, other STAT proteins are at least partially capable of substituting for STAT5 and functioning downstream of the EpoR. These findings emphasize the importance of in vivo studies in confirming the phenotypic relevance of in vitro studies.

Studies have suggested that Epo functions synergistically with other multilineage growth factors, such as KL and IL-3. As discussed in Erythroid Precursor Cell Compartment section, Epo and KL function together, resulting in increased erythroid colony cell growth in methylcellulose culture. Studies with the EpoR polypeptide suggest a molecular mechanism for such synergy.[210] Activation of the kit receptor by KL results in transphosphorylation of EpoR at the cell surface. A direct interaction between EpoR and the kit receptor has been demonstrated.[211] Physical interaction between EpoR and the β common chain of the IL-3 receptor in erythroid cells has been demonstrated.[212] This interaction might be involved in the neuroprotective action exerted by Epo.[213] In fact, a carbamylated derivative of Epo prevents motoneuron degeneration in vitro and in vivo[213] and ameliorates recovery from several in vivo models of brain and heart injuries, such as chronic autoimmunoencephalomyelitis in mice,[214] radiosurgery- or ischemia-induced brain injury,[215] and myocardium ischemia–reperfusion injury[216] in rats. (For a review of the nonhematopoietic activity of Epo, see reference 217.) Taken together, these results suggest that receptor cross-talk at the cell surface may account, at least in part, for the physiologic interaction of some cytokines in controlling hematopoietic versus nonhematopoietic effects of Epo.

ALTERATIONS IN EPO-R AND ITS SIGNALLING IN DISORDERS OF ERYTHROPOIESIS

As discussed earlier in the section of Erythropoietion and EPO-R, the normal role of Epo is to stimulate cell surface EpoR in developing erythroid cells. The latter cells respond to Epo via a proliferative and differentiation response. Epo-activated signal transduction of EpoR is quickly downregulated in the cell, and continuing presence of Epo is required for optimal differentiation.

In some cells, the EpoR may become constitutively activated. In these cases, erythroid progenitor cells are placed into a sustained proliferative state. Interestingly, these mechanisms underlie several murine and human examples of erythrocytosis (erythroid overproduction). Multiple mechanisms exist by which EpoR may become constitutively activated. First, the Friend spleen focus-forming virus of the Friend erythroleukemia complex encodes the glycoprotein F-gp55, which binds and activates murine EpoR.[218–220] F-gp55 appears to bind to EpoR via its transmembrane region. Epo and F-gp55 binding sites are discrete; tertiary complexes of EpoR, Epo, and F-gp55 have been detected on the surface of Friend virus–infected cells.[221] Second, EpoR can be constitutively activated by a point mutation (R129C) in the extracytoplasmic region of the polypeptide.[222] This mutation occurs in the "dimerization domain" of EpoR and results in constitutive homodimerization of the EpoR polypeptide, presumably through a disulfide bond. This mutation further underscores the importance of receptor dimerization in the initiation of a receptor signaling response. Third, EpoR can be constitutively activated in an autocrine manner. Murine erythroleukemia cell lines have been established that coexpress EpoR and Epo. A fourth mechanism of EpoR constitutive activation results from EpoR overexpression. For instance, some murine erythroleukemia cell lines have increased EpoR mRNA, resulting from spleen focus-forming virus proviral integration within the first intron of the murine EpoR gene.[223] Overexpression of the normal murine EpoR polypeptide may thereby contribute to oncogenesis.

Soon after the cDNA of mouse and human EpoR were cloned, the mouse and human genomic structures were identified. The gene for mouse EpoR was found to map to mouse chromosome 9,[224] whereas the human gene was found on human chromosome 19p.[225] Mapping of the EpoR genes led to their implication in various human disease states. For instance, studies demonstrated that a chromosomal breakpoint 3′ to the human EpoR gene results in increased EpoR expression.[226] The rearranged EpoR allele appears to encode a mutated EpoR polypeptide with increased activity, perhaps secondary to loss of the carboxy-terminal negative regulatory domain.

EpoR plays a role in the rare congenital disease familial erythrocytosis. Familial erythrocytosis is a heterogeneous group of hereditary conditions characterized by an increase in red blood cell mass in the setting of low serum Epo levels. A few families that demonstrate autosomal dominant inheritance have been identified.[227] The linkage between the EpoR gene and familial erythrocytosis was first established by the observation that a mutant EpoR allele segregates with the disease in one familial erythrocytosis kindred. This allele contains a nonsense mutation in the coding region of the gene that results in synthesis of a truncated EpoR that lacks the negative regulatory domain of its carboxy-terminal region.[228,229] Since that report, several other frameshift and deletion EpoR gene mutations, all encoding carboxy-terminal–truncated forms of the protein providing Epo hypersensitivity and resulting in familial erythrocytosis, have been reported.[230–234]

Congenital polycythemia may arise not only from gene mutations leading to abnormal Epo/R signaling but also from gene mutations altering Epo production. The T598T mutation in one of the genes controlling oxygen sensoring (von Hippel–Lindau [VHL] gene), which leads to increased Epo production by the kidney, is associated with congenital erythrocytosis, the Chuvash polycythemia.[235,236] The C598T VHL mutation is endemic in Chuvashia, Russia, Federation, and in the small island of Ischia, in southern Italy. The frequency of the mutation on this small island is higher than in Chuvashia (0.07% vs 0.02%), but the haplotype of Italian patients matches that identified in the Chuvash cluster, supporting a single-founder hypothesis.[237]

Acquired mutations in the EpoR signaling pathway have been identified in polycythemia vera (PV), essential thrombocythemia, and idiopathic myelofibrosis, a class of myeloproliferative disorders that do not present the Philadelphia chromosome abnormality (Ph) and, therefore, cannot be cured with inhibitors, such as Gleevec, which are specific for the signaling pathway altered by the Ph abnormality. These diseases originate at the level of the pluripotent hematopoietic stem cell and are characterized by proliferation of one or more of the myeloid lineages but relatively normal hematopoietic cell maturation (see Hematologic Malignancis). Several investigators have reported a mutation in the Jak2 gene resulting in a valine→phenylalanine substitution at position 617 of the protein (^{V617F}Jak2 mutation) in patients with Ph-negative chronic proliferative disorders.[238–241] Since the early reports, the presence of ^{V617F}Jak2 in patients with Ph-negative myeloproliferative disorders has been confirmed by numerous publications. Depending on the study, ^{V617F}Jak2 has been reported in 60% to 90% of patients with PV, 30% to 50% of patients with essential thrombocythemia, and 30% to 60% of patients with idiopathic myelofibrosis. The mutation is harbored at either the heterozygous or, by somatic recombination, the homozygous stage. It is detectable in all myeloid cells up to the clonal hematopoietic stem cells.[242] The mutation affects the domain of the protein that is directly involved in signal transduction but is necessary to return the protein to its resting configuration after signaling. As a consequence, after its first engagement with Epo, EpoR signaling becomes constitutively activated. Because Jak2 is the earliest element of the EpoR pathway, it is conceivable that the high red cell numbers found in patients with PV carrying the ^{V617F}Jak2 mutation is a direct consequence of constitutive Epo signaling in erythroid cells. The extent to which the downstream EpoR signaling pathway is altered as a consequence of this constitutive activation is a debatable issue. The observation that erythroblasts derived in vitro from patients with PV carrying the ^{V617F}Jak2 mutation are highly resistant to TRAIL-induced apoptosis[243] suggests that the mutation exquisitely increases erythroblast survival. However, additional abnormalities induced by the presence of ^{V617F}Jak2 are represented by hypersensitivity to insulin-like growth factor-1[244] and increased EpoR recycling from the Golgi apparatus.[184] Therefore, inhibitors directly targeting the ^{V617F}Jak2 mutation might represent the best candidates for PV therapy. More difficult to understand is why the mutation is also present in some patients with essential thrombocythemia and idiopathic myelofibrosis. Jak2, in addition to EpoR, has an important role in transducing the signal from Mpl, the TPO receptor.[245] The protein has two opposing effects on the intracellular processing of the two receptors after growth factor stimulation: it favors EpoR recycling from the Golgi apparatus,[184] but it determines retention and degradation of Mpl in the cytoplasm.[246] As such, the ^{V617F}Jak2 mutation should increase the number of EpoR on the surface of erythroid cells while reducing that of Mpl on megakaryocytes. This hypothesis explains why the mutation is found preferentially in PV. However, megakaryocytes originating from ^{V617F}Jak2 stem cells might express a reduced number but constitutively active

Mpl, so it can be argued that the mutation manifests itself prevalently in the erythroid or the megakaryocytic lineage, depending on genetic polymorphisms outside the Jak2 locus present in the population. This hypothesis is supported by the observation that mice transplanted with ^{V617F}Jak2 hematopoietic stem cells develop either a PV- or an essential thrombocythemia–like syndrome, depending on their genetic background.[247] Studies on the biology and biochemistry of the ^{V617F}Jak2 mutation are actively being pursued by many investigators. Furthermore, in ^{V617F}Jak2-negative PV or IE patients, several other gain-of-function mutations affecting Jak2 exon 12 with a distinct phenotype (idiopathic erythrocytosis) have been identified.[248] The identification of specific mutations and the availability of the crystal structures of Epo, EpoR, and Jak2 should allow use of computer modeling to design targeted protein-signaling inhibitors for treatment of Ph-negative myeloproliferative disorders.[249]

HEMATOPOIETIC MICROENVIRONMENT

In invertebrates such as worms and sessile marine creatures, erythropoiesis occurs adjacent to peritoneal and endothelial cells. In premammalian species, the spleen is the primary site of erythropoiesis. With evolutionary advancement, the function gradually shifts to the liver and the sinusoidal cavities of bones.[9] These observations suggest that sufficient oxygen, a stagnated flow of blood to avoid dispersion of factors produced locally, and extensive and redundant surfaces for cell–cell interactions are essential to support red cell production. Similar sites support erythropoiesis during human development (see Ontogeny of Erythropoiesis). During both phylogeny and ontogeny, the liver and spleen are primarily erythropoietic organs; granulocytic cells dominate in the bone marrow.[9] Within the bone marrow, hematopoiesis is restricted to the extravascular space, where compact collections of cells are interspersed among venous sinuses. These sinuses originate adjacent to the endosteal bone surface and empty into a central longitudinal vein. Studies in mice demonstrate that BFU-E follow a bimodal distribution with peaks adjacent to the periosteum and mid-cavity, whereas CFU-E and later erythroid cells have a broad distribution with highest incidence toward the axis of the femur, adjacent to the central vein,[9,250] thus suggesting that the local anatomy (specialized niches?) influences the maturation of erythroid cells.

The bone marrow microenvironment consists of three broad components: stromal cells (e.g., fibroblasts, endothelial cells, osteogenic cells), accessory cells (monocytes, macrophages, T cells), and extracellular matrix (a protein–carbohydrate scaffold). Accessory cells are progeny of hematopoietic stem cells; hence, after marrow transplantation, these cells are of donor origin, whereas stromal cells are host derived.[251,252] Extracellular matrix molecules are synthesized and secreted by microenvironmental cells and include collagens (types I, III, IV, and V), glycoproteins (fibronectin, laminins, thrombospondins, hemonectin, and tenascin), and glycosaminoglycans (hyaluronic acid, chondroitin, dermatan, and heparan sulfate).[253,254] Besides providing structure to the marrow space and a surface for cell adhesion, the microenvironment is important for hematopoietic cell homing, engraftment, migration, and the response to physiologic stress and homeostasis.

Although the functional consequences of the microenvironment ultimately must be defined by in vivo studies in mice, dissection of the cellular components of the microenvironment, definition of the cytokines that are produced by individual cells, and the nature of cell–cell interactions have been aided by in vitro models. Long-term bone marrow cultures provide an experimental approach for such studies.[255,256] Under these in vitro conditions, murine hematopoiesis can be maintained for 8 to 10 months and human hematopoiesis for 2 to 3 months.[255] An adherent layer consisting of fibroblasts, adipocytes, and macrophages is a crucial component of the culture system. Progenitor cells adherent to stroma are generally quiescent (dormant), whereas those in the nonadherent cell compartment are in active cell cycle.[256,257]

In vitro studies have demonstrated that stromal cells, including endothelial cells and fibroblasts, elaborate cytokines such as GM-CSF, G-CSF, IL-1, IL-3, IL-6, IL-11, KL, FLT-3 ligand, activin A, and basic fibroblast growth factor, which influence, alone or in combination, the growth of adjacent marrow progenitors.[255–258] In addition to positive regulators of replication and differentiation, stromal cells elaborate factors such as transforming growth factor β, interferon γ, and TNF, which exert a negative influence on proliferation and may help maintain a dormant (noncycling) state.[256,257] Because some regulators inhibit differentiation along certain lineages but not others, there is an intriguing possibility that lineage-specific regulation within the microenvironment can be achieved through negative, rather than positive, factors.[259] Several cytokines are expressed in a transmembrane form as well as a soluble (secreted) product. Others bind extracellular matrix, a mechanism that not only allows for high concentrations of a factor within the microenvironment that metabolically stabilizes these factors but also keeps them adjacent to developing progenitors.

Among the factors elaborated by stromal cells, KL has the most profound effect on erythropoiesis. Mice unable to synthesize KL die in utero because of severe anemia. Steel-Dickie (Sl^d) mice that are unable to make the membrane-restricted form of KL are viable but severely anemic, whereas other lineages in these animals are marginally affected or not affected by this defect.[260] The fact that erythropoiesis is abnormal, despite high levels of circulating Epo and the presence of soluble KL, suggests that normal erythroid differentiation and maturation require both a functional membrane-restricted KL/kit and an Epo signaling pathway. Cross-phosphorylation of EpoR by KL may provide a basis for the predominately erythroid effect.[211] Furthermore, data suggest that tyrosine cross-phosphorylation of EpoR is sustained longer when cells are cultured on steel stromal cells engineered to express the membrane-restricted form of KL than cells expressing the soluble form.[261]

Besides cell–cytokine interactions, (paracrine) cell–cell adhesion and adhesion of cells to the extracellular matrix are important functions of the microenvironment.[262,263] Perhaps most studied are the β_1 integrins VLA-4 and VLA-5, which mediate the adherence of hematopoietic cells to stromal cells, fibronectin, or other components of the extracellular matrix.[263,264] In mice lacking β_1 integrins, hematopoietic stem cells fail to colonize the fetal liver during embryonic development,[265] and cells lacking α_4 integrin fail to contribute to normal hematopoiesis postnatally.[266] Antibodies to VLA-4 or to the vascular cellular adhesion molecule 1 (VCAM-1, a VLA-4 ligand on endothelial cells) impair homing and lead to mobilization of progenitor cells and stem cells in adult mice and primates.[267–270] In in vitro studies, hematopoietic progenitors bind to specific domains of fibronectin in a differentiation-dependent manner (long-term culture-initiating cell and day 12 colony-forming unit-spleen in mice adhere mainly through the heparin-binding domain and CS-1). BFU-E and other progenitor cells adhere to both the cell-binding (RGDS) and heparin-binding domains, whereas CFU-E preferentially bind the RGDS sequence, and reticulocytes fail to adhere to fibronectin.[254,271–274] This differential binding could influence the proliferation and maturation of erythroid progenitor cells as well as the migration of these cells in and out of the bone marrow cavity. Hematopoietic cytokines present in the microenvironment also can modulate the affinity of β_1 integrins for ligand,[275,276] adding complexity to the regulation of erythropoiesis within the marrow microenvironment.

Many observations suggest that hematopoietic progenitor cells at one stage of fetal development may not be supported by a hematopoietic microenvironment of a different ontogenetic stage. For example, cells present in the murine yolk sac are not able to repopulate adult recipients,[277] although they can repopulate newborn recipients with active fetal liver hematopoiesis.[278] Targeted disruption of CXCL12/SDF1, a member of the CXC chemokine family that is constitutively expressed by bone marrow stromal cells (i.e., reticular/endothelial cells or, osteoblasts), leads to inhibition of marrow hematopoiesis, although fetal liver hematopoiesis is unaffected,[279] suggesting that this chemokine has a role in colonization of bone marrow from fetal liver. TEL (translocation-ETS [E26 transformation-specific]-leukemia) transcriptional factor was shown to be critical in

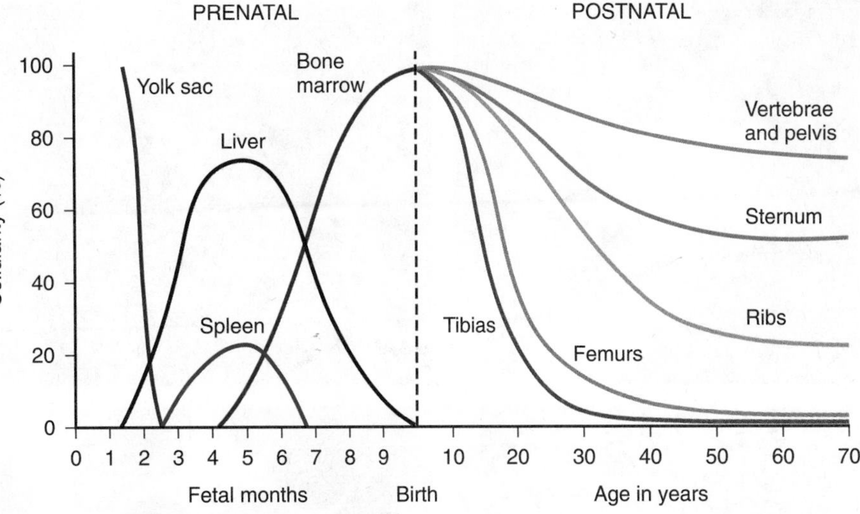

Figure 25–3 Sites of hematopoiesis during fetal development and after birth. Only erythroid cells and possibly lymphocytes are generated by the yolk sac and early embryo. Significant megakaryopoiesis and granulopoiesis develop at 4 to 5 months. After birth, hematopoiesis occurs in the sinusoidal cavities of the tibias, femurs, and axial skeleton. (Adapted from Erslev A, Gabuzda T: Pathophysiology of Blood, 2nd ed. Philadelphia, WB Saunders, 1979.[446])

establishing stable bone marrow hematopoiesis but was not required for embryonic and fetal liver hematopoiesis.[280]

Accessory cells, such as stromal cells, secrete cytokines and express adhesion molecules, and they may influence marrow hematopoiesis by their nonrandom distribution in the marrow cavity. T cells (along with mast cells) are the only source of IL-3 and, through secretion of TNF-α and interferon γ, may negatively impact erythropoiesis. In histologic sections of normal marrow, islands of maturing erythroblasts (erythroblastic islands) often surround a central macrophage, termed a *nurse cell*.[281] Adhesion may be mediated through the binding of VLA-4 (on erythroid cells) to VCAM-1 (on central macrophages).[282] Molecular interactions have been identified as being critical for erythroblastic island integrity. Erythroblast macrophage protein expressed on erythroblasts and macrophages mediates cell–cell attachment through homophilic binding, and erythroblast intercellular adhesion molecule 4 (ICAM-4) links erythroblasts to macrophages by interacting with α_v integrin expressed in macrophages.[283–285] Mice with targeted deletion of erythroblast macrophage protein are severely anemic and die at an embryonic stage,[84] and ICAM-4 kos[284] have markedly reduced erythroblastic islands. Of interest, Rb-deficient macrophages do not bind Rb^{null} erythroblasts,[286] and failure of this interaction may mediate the defect in fetal liver erythropoiesis observed in Rb kos. Rb normally stimulates macrophage differentiation by counteracting inhibition of Id2 (a helix loop-helix protein) on PU-1, a transcription factor crucial in macrophage differentiation. In addition to the aforementioned pathways, macrophage CD163 can serve as an erythroblast adhesion receptor in erythroblastic islands, promoting erythroid proliferation and/or survival.[287] More studies addressing the specific interactions between macrophages and erythroid cells that promote erythroid differentiation are needed for definite conclusions regarding specialized "erythroid niches." Of note, tissue macrophages express RNA for Epo[288] and may influence erythropoiesis through this mechanism.

The microenvironment is not only a passive surface for the adherence of progenitor cells; it exerts a crucial and interactive role in development and maturation. Some interactions are lineage (red cell) specific, whereas other interactions affect hematopoiesis more broadly. Stromal and accessory cells secrete cytokines and/or express them in a transmembrane form on their cell surface. Cytokines are retained via binding to components of the extracellular matrix. All components of the microenvironment are involved in adhesive interactions, some of which maintain quiescence (i.e., interactions of stem cells with endosteal surfaces[289,290]), whereas other cell–cell interactions or interactions of cells with matrix components induce proliferation and/or differentiation.[291–293] An individual progenitor cell, in an anatomic niche adjacent to certain stromal cells, accessory cells, and extracellular matrix molecules, likely responds to the sum of the signals that it uniquely receives. In this way, erythropoiesis, or the entire hematopoiesis, is influenced by the complexity of the interaction network.

ONTOGENY OF ERYTHROPOIESIS

During human development, distinct anatomic areas for production of erythroid cells are recruited sequentially, in a temporal succession that allows overlap (Fig. 25–3). In addition, parallel changes occur in the morphology and functional properties of the erythroid cells themselves.

During the phase of embryonic erythropoiesis in the blood islands of yolk sac, aggregates of immature erythroid cells undergo maturation synchronously as a single cohort. Before their maturation is completed, they begin to circulate, and by gestational week 5 they are found in the vascular spaces of the rudimentary liver (Fig. 25–4). At about the same time, foci of immature erythroid cells emerge within the fetal liver as the fetal (or hepatic) phase of erythropoiesis commences.[294] From week 7 onward, the liver is progressively filled with erythroid precursors and becomes the dominant site of erythroid cell production until approximately gestational week 30. Although some red cell production can be found in the thymus, the spleen, or occasionally in the lymph nodes, these other sites are never dominant. From month 6 onward, the cavities of long bones are invaded by vascular sprouts and become competent to support red cell development. Shortly after birth, all bone cavities are actively engaged in erythroid production, and the hepatic (fetal) phase of erythropoiesis comes to an end, as the final (adult) phase of erythropoiesis unfolds exclusively within the bone marrow.

In addition to the anatomic shifts in the sites of erythropoiesis are associated shifts in the phenotypic characteristics of erythroid cells. Embryonic erythroid cells (derived from the yolk sac) are large (approximately 200 mm), circulate as nucleated cells, and have a megaloblastic appearance (Fig. 25–4). The fact that primitive erythroblasts of mammals, like erythroid cells of lower vertebrates, retain their nuclei at terminal stages of maturation may serve as an example of embryonic recapitulation of the phylogenetic evolution of the erythroid system. However, a study has identified the presence of enucleated megaloblasts in the blood of the mouse embryo at late stages of development, indicating that the enucleation process is at least partially at work.[295] Other studies using genetic reporter models further suggest that embryonic (primitive) cells represent a stable cell population that persists through the end of gestation,[296] but these observations require verification by other independent approaches. Fetal erythroid cells (produced in the fetal liver and later in fetal bone marrow spaces) are smaller than embryonic cells (approximately 125 μm) but have a macrocytic appearance compared with adult normocytic red cells (approximately 80 μm). However,

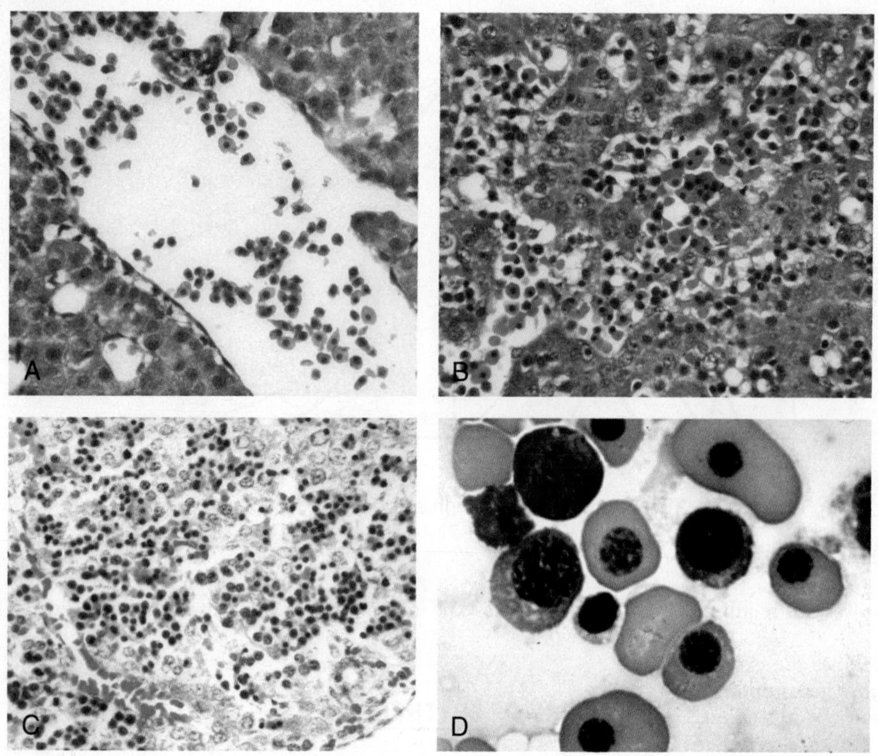

Figure 25–4 **A,** Section of an 8-mm embryo depicting a portion of hepatic parenchymal cells with embryonic erythroblasts present within primitive sinusoidal cavities. **B,** At 6 to 8 weeks, discrete aggregates of definitive erythroblasts appear within the liver parenchyma, whereas mature embryonic erythroblasts persist in well-developed sinusoids. **C,** Definitive erythroblasts are spread throughout the liver (100-day fetus). **D,** Cytologic spread from disaggregated fetal liver cells of a 55-day embryo. Characteristic morphology of embryonic erythroblasts and immature (basophilic) definitive erythroblasts is shown. (A, B, C, hematoxylin-eosin stain; D, Wright-Giemsa stain.)

like adult cells, fetal erythroid cells eject their nuclei during maturation.

Apart from variations in size and morphology, embryonic and fetal erythroid cells differ from each other and from their adult counterparts in several other characteristics, including hormonal or growth factor requirements, proliferative status, and transplantation potential. For example, whereas fetal erythropoiesis is under the control of Epo,[297] the extent of Epo's influence on embryonic erythropoiesis is disputed. Most convincing are the results of Epo/EpoR knock-outs[135] that showed only partial effects on embryonic erythropoiesis, in contrast to fetal erythropoiesis. Evidence suggests that precursor cells from the extraembryonic mesoderm are dependent on Epo for proliferation and erythroid differentiation.[298] Epo levels increase between weeks 9 and 32 of gestation, and fetuses respond to hypoxia or anemia with increased Epo as early as 24 weeks. Fetal erythroid progenitors when studied in vitro appear more sensitive to Epo and KL than adult progenitors. In contrast, their in vitro response to lymphokines (e.g., IL-3 or GM-CSF) is minimal compared to that of adult erythroid progenitors.[299,300] Of note, in the early stages of fetal liver erythropoiesis, mainly erythroid differentiation/maturation is promoted.[187] Progenitors committed to other lineages are abundant in the fetal liver, but few mature cells (granulocytes, megakaryocytes) from other lineages are seen. In addition to their heightened sensitivity to Epo, fetal erythroid progenitors and precursors are characterized by high proliferative potential and shorter doubling times than adult cells when cultured in vitro.[300,301] The dependency of stem/progenitor cells on KL changes during ontogeny. Although generation of repopulating stem cells (c-kit$^+$/Sca1$^+$/Thy1^{lo}/Lin$^-$) and colony-forming unit-spleen is minimally affected during fetal life in mice that cannot produce KL, adult steel-Dickie (Sl/Sl^d) mutant mice (which produce only some soluble KL) display greatly impaired erythropoiesis and hematopoiesis, suggesting that the KL/c-kit pathway plays a role in the recruitment and self-renewal behavior of adult stem cells in vivo.[302,303] The long-term transplantation potential is impaired in cells with mutations of c-kit kinase activity.[303] Transplantable stem cells from the yolk sac, in contrast to fetal liver cells, cannot engraft adult recipients, because of altered homing behavior or inability of bone marrow to support their development,[278] as suggested by their engraftment in neonatal liver.[304] The homing properties of fetal stem cells transplanted into adult irradiated recipients were found to be inferior to those of their adult counterparts.[305] Whether this finding is related to their increased cycling or other reasons is unclear. However, fetal liver stem cells, despite their reduced homing potential,[305] have higher engraftment levels, likely because of their proliferative prowess compared to adult stem cells.[306]

The surface antigenic profiles of erythroid progenitors and precursors are distinct at each ontogenic stage. For example, HLA class I and class II antigens are not detected in embryonic erythroid progenitor cells but reach adult levels at approximately gestational week 9.[307] CD34$^+$ hematopoietic progenitors present in yolk sac express Mac-1 but are negative for stem cell antigen 1 (Sca-1), which is expressed in fetal and adult CD34$^+$ murine progenitor cells.[308] On the other hand, adult CD34$^+$ progenitors lack Mac-1 and AA4.1, which are expressed in fetal CD34$^+$ progenitor cells. Fetal BFU-E and CFU-E express similar levels of HLA class II antigens, whereas adult CFU-E are largely devoid of these antigens.[307,309] β_1 integrins, especially $\alpha_4\beta_1$ and α_5, are expressed widely in all hemopoietic cells, including nucleated erythroid cells. However, in the latter, they display a differentiation-dependent, developmentally segregated pattern of expression, as they are absent in embryonic murine erythroblasts,[310] and among adult cells, stem/progenitor cells express them in a constitutively active form in contrast to more mature cells.[311–313] Fetal red cells display a straight, unbranched polylactosaminyl chain (i antigen) on their surface, whereas in adult cells, this structure, which bears ABH blood group determinants, is highly branched (I antigen).[77] The enzymatic activity of several enzymes in the glycolytic pathway is greater in fetal than in adult red cells.[314] In contrast, carbonic anhydrase levels are very low during intrauterine and early neonatal life.[315] Distinct isozyme patterns for several enzymes (i.e., phosphoglycerate kinase, acetylcholinesterase) also distinguish fetal from adult red cells.[316,317]

The most widely studied changes during red cell ontogeny are the shifts or "switches" in globin types. Embryonic erythroblasts are characterized by their avid accumulation of iron, which is stored as ferritin[318] (0.3–1% of total protein) and by the synthesis of the unique hemoglobins Gower I ($\zeta_2\varepsilon_2$), Gower II ($\alpha_2\varepsilon_2$), and Hb Portland ($\zeta_2\varepsilon_2$). The ζ- and ε-globin chains are embryonic α-like and β-like chains, respectively.[88] These three embryonic types of hemoglobin are most likely synthesized in succession, as the concentration of Gower I is highest in smaller embryos. Thus, a switch from ζ- to α-

and ε- to γ-globin gene production begins during the embryonic phase of erythropoiesis but is not complete until fetal erythropoiesis is well established. During the transition from yolk sac to fetal liver erythropoiesis (6–9 weeks), erythroid precursors within the fetal liver coexpress embryonic (ζ- or ε-) and fetal (α- or γ-) globin both in vivo and in vitro.[319,320] The predominant type of hemoglobin synthesized during fetal liver erythropoiesis is HbF ($\alpha_2\gamma_2$), with a high proportion of γ^G:γ^A (7 : 3). Adult HbA ($\alpha_2\beta_2$), which is detectable at the earliest stages of fetal liver erythropoiesis, is synthesized as a minor component throughout this period. However, HbA_2 ($\alpha_2\delta_2$), which is a minor hemoglobin in the adult, is undetectable in these early stages. From about gestational week 30 onward, β-globin synthesis steadily increases so that, by term, 50% to 55% of hemoglobin synthesized is HbA. By 4 to 5 weeks of postnatal age, 75% of the hemoglobin is HbA. This percentage increases to 95% by 4 months as the fetal-to-adult hemoglobin switch is completed. HbF levels in circulating red cells are in a plateau for the first 2 to 3 weeks (as a result of the decline in total erythropoiesis that follows birth), but the HbF level gradually declines so that normal levels (<1%) are achieved by 200 days after birth.[321]

Several in vitro and in vivo approaches have been used to study the basis of globin switching through development. Beyond its biologic interest, rigorous research in this area was propelled by the possibility of manipulating globin switching to increase HbF production in adults and ameliorate the clinical symptoms of disorders of the β-globin locus (e.g., sickle cell anemia, thalassemia). Transplantation experiments and ablative endocrine maneuvers in the sheep model have failed to provide convincing support for the effects of environmental or humoral factors on the switching process, although some modulation of the rate of switching was seen in these models.[322,323] The most important determinant of fetal-to-adult hemoglobin switching seems to be postconceptual age, with the sharpest period for transition between 30 and 52 weeks. The fetal-to-adult switch appears to be unaffected by the time at which birth occurs or by changes in the kinetics of erythropoiesis induced by perinatal hemolysis.[324] A delay in switching usually is observed in cases of general developmental retardation, in patients with certain chromosomal abnormalities (e.g., trisomy 13), and in diabetic infants because of increased circulating levels of α-aminobutyric acid, which directly affects HbF synthesis.[325] Integration of data from studies using in vitro and in vivo approaches indicates that developmental control of globin switching is intrinsic to erythroid cells. Stage-specific transcriptional forces with negative or positive influences (or both) on specific globin genes may provide the molecular basis for differential transcriptional activity during development. This view is favored by experiments in transgenic mice[326] and in heterokaryons (produced by fusion of human with mouse cells),[327] as well as by isolation of stage-specific transcriptional factors in other erythroid systems (e.g., avian).[328] Furthermore, because β-like and α-like globin genes are activated sequentially in the order of their location in chromosome 11 or 16, respectively, it is possible that polarity of the transcriptional activity and globin promoter competition for the locus control region and developmental stage-specific transcriptional factors contribute to this regulation.[329] Alternatively, specifically for ε globin, direct silencing by factors such as the SOX6 repressor, which operates in definitive erythroid cells, has been shown.[330]

In summary, throughout human development, waves of hematopoiesis are initiated sequentially in newly recruited sites. The first wave of erythropoiesis is seen in yolk sac between days 15 and 18 (7.5 days after conception in mice). In addition to erythroid cells, uncommitted progenitors and progenitors for nonerythroid cells are present in the yolk sac and are thought to be the source of cells colonizing the fetal liver.[141,331–333] However, in addition to yolk sac, foci of hematopoietic activity have been detected within the embryo around the developing aorta (in paraaortic-splanchnopleura [P-Sp] and aorta/gonad/mesonephros [AGM] area).[334–336] In fact, the P-Sp/AGM site in mice was shown to harbor progenitor cells before circulation begins and 1 day before these cells are found in the yolk sac. Long-term repopulating cells after their transplantation in adult recipients were detected only in the AGM area, leading to speculation that this intraembryonic site is the main or only source of fetal liver colonization,[336] in contrast to earlier experiments implicating the yolk sac in that role.[331–333] Presence of mesodermally derived hematopoietic cells in two distinct anatomic sites (extraembryonic and within the embryo proper), one intraembryonic and the other extraembryonic, has been seen in explant studies of *Xenopus* and after analysis of chick-quail chimeras.[337] More recent experiments with human cells have led to similar conclusions.[338] Although the presence of progenitors for definitive hematopoiesis in two independent sites (extraembryonic and within the embryo proper) is indisputable, the extent to which these two sites contribute to fetal liver colonization has been a matter of dispute. The conclusion that only the AGM area contributes to fetal liver colonization was based on transplantation experiments in adult recipients and has been challenged.[278] Transplantation experiments using newborn mice with active fetal liver hematopoiesis as recipients showed that adult long-term repopulating cells are detectable in the yolk sac at day 9 postconception and are 37-fold higher than repopulating cells present in the P-Sp/AGM area at the same time. Therefore, failure of yolk sac cells (or AGM cells before day 10 postconception) to engraft adult recipients may be caused by either compromised homing or impaired survival and proliferation within the adult bone marrow environment (because of positive regulators or inhibition by negative regulators). In light of this information, the 30-year-old theory that yolk sac colonizes the fetal liver has been revived.[331] A question that remains unanswered is whether stem cell activity 9 days postconception in yolk sac and P-Sp/AGM is generated autonomously and independently or is derived from a common precursor cell with migratory properties. Murine studies comparing newborn transplant outcomes before the onset of systemic circulation between the yolk sac site and the intraembryonic AGM site are emerging and promise to resolve this issue.[304]

A common precursor cell giving rise to erythroid cells with either yolk sac or fetal liver characteristics has been identified by culture of murine or human embryonic stem cells in vitro.[339,340] Environmental regulation of specification to the primitive or definitive lineage has been shown in *Xenopus*.[341] However, because BFU-E present in yolk sac, fetal liver, and fetal bone marrow have a definitive-like progeny and these progenitors were not present after ablation of core-binding factor (CBF)β[342] despite the presence of normal embryonic erythropoiesis, the derivation of embryonic erythroblasts from a distinct progenitor, not present in subsequent life, remains a viable hypothesis. Of further interest is the observation that deletion of Mdm2 and Mdm4, two critical negative regulators of p53, exerted distinct outcomes for primitive and definitive hematopoiesis. Whereas Mdm2 is required for primitive erythropoiesis, Mdm4 is required for massive expansion of definitive erythropoiesis in fetal liver and is dispensable for adult erythropoiesis. These data also suggest distinct molecular control between fetal and adult cells.[343]

TRANSCRIPTIONAL FACTORS IN ERYTHROPOIESIS

Lineage-specific transcriptional factors are widely believed to be responsible for regulating the expression of erythroid genes during both ontogeny and the course of erythroid differentiation. The majority of erythroid-specific transcription factors has been identified from cloning of breakpoints or translocations associated with human leukemias or from expression libraries obtained from erythroid cell lines. The precise role exerted by each of these factors in erythropoiesis was later clarified by painstaking experiments with somatic cell fusions and in transgenic mice.[327,344,345] Some of the major transcription factors implicated in the control of erythropoiesis are listed in Table 25–2.

Studies of mice with targeted gene disruption have provided key insights into the complex molecular pathways that regulate hematopoiesis in general and erythropoiesis in particular.[1,2] These studies, complemented by in vitro differentiation of mutated embryonic stem cells into different lineages, have provided clear evidence about distinct regulatory requirements of primitive (yolk sac) versus definitive (fetal liver and bone marrow) erythropoiesis, or of early versus late stages of erythroid differentiation. Because erythropoiesis is the first differentiated lineage in embryonic yolk sac hematopoiesis and the predominant lineage in fetal liver hematopoiesis, factors that affect hematopoiesis in general will disturb erythropoiesis during early stages of development and lead to lethality at different gestational days, depending on the defect. The time in development at which disruption of each specific gene manifests its phenotype is used to establish a hierarchical control among the different transcription factors. The earliest disruption of erythroid differentiation is observed in mice lacking the bHLH factor Tal-1/SCL, which is encoded by a gene initially identified on the basis of its localization in a chromosomal breakpoint region frequently associated with T-cell acute leukemia.[346] SCL^{null} embryos are bloodless and die very early, with abrogation of both yolk sac and fetal liver erythropoiesis.[347] Because of the requirement for SCL in the formation of the transcription complex with the nuclear protein Rbtn2/LMO2 (rhombotin 2/LIM domain only 2) and GATA1 (detailed below), it is not surprising that targeted disruption of Rbtn2 and LMO2 also produces a bloodless phenotype.[348]

Mice lacking expression of GATA2, a member of the GATA family of transcriptional factors, exhibit an early and severe quantitative defect in hematopoiesis that influences all lineages.[349] Other regulatory factors seem to totally spare embryonic (yolk sac) hematopoiesis and have a specific effect only on fetal liver hematopoiesis, with death occurring at later days (12.5 days postconception). In this category are the protooncogene c-myb and the core-binding factors $CBF\alpha_2$/AML-1 and $CBF\beta$.[350–352] Embryonic erythropoiesis is spared in mice with targeted ablation of these genes. Both c-myb, the cellular homologue of v-myb protooncogene, and the heterodimeric transcription factor CBF are abundantly expressed early in normal myelolymphoid cells, with decreasing expression as differentiation proceeds. Their expression pattern and their functional influence on growth factor receptor genes (i.e., IL-3, GM-CSF, CSF-1, T-cell antigen receptor [TCR]α,β) may underlie their importance in the development of all definitive hematopoietic lineages.[1]

Of paramount importance for adult erythropoiesis is the transcription factor GATA1, the founder of the GATA family of factors.[1] The GATA1 protein controls erythroid differentiation at several levels by controlling (in cooperation with GATA2) the proliferative capacity of erythroid progenitor/precursor cells, the apoptotic rate of erythroblasts, and the expression of lineage-specific genes. These effects are mediated through activation of expression of target genes by binding to specific sequences (WGATAR) present in the regulatory domains of virtually any erythroid gene, including EpoR and GATA1 itself. However, WGATAR binding sites also are present in genes specific for megakaryocytic, eosinophilic, and mast cell lineages as well as in genes expressed in testicular Sertoli cells. Insights into the specificity of GATA1 in erythroid differentiation have been provided by studies on the organization of WGATAR sites in erythroid-specific regulatory sequences. A minimal erythroid transcription–activation sequence that consists of a core-binding motif flanked by two canonical GATA1 binding sites has been identified. The core-binding motif is composed of one SCL binding site and one GATA binding site separated by 10 bp.[2] Different domains of the GATA1 protein are responsible for binding to the core and the flanking sequences. At least three functional domains in the GATA1 protein have been identified: two zinc finger domains [amino-terminal finger (NF) and carboxyl-terminal finger (CF)] and an active amino-terminal domain. The NF domain is required for association with friend of GATA1 (FOG1), a protein encoded by a gene identified using GATA1 as bite in the two hybrid yeast assay.[353] FOG1 contains 10 zinc finger domains, only the first of which is required for GATA1 binding. The function of its other nine zinc finger domains is not clear because they appear to be dispensable in structure–function studies but they are well conserved in evolution. The GATA1–FOG1 heterodimeric complex binds to the two flanking sites of the minimal erythroid transcription activation domain. Experimentally induced genetic mutations impairing GATA1–FOG1 interaction in mice lead to impaired megakaryocytopoiesis and absence of definitive erythropoiesis while primitive erythropoiesis is normal.[354] These results indicate that DNA binding of the GATA1–FOG1 complex is necessary for activation of the target genes in definitive erythroid cells but is dispensable for their activation in primitive erythroblasts. It should be emphasized that GATA1–FOG1 interaction, while activating the expression of erythroid genes, inhibits target gene activation in testicular Sertoli cells.[355] This result provides insight into how one factor regulates more than one differentiation program by suggesting that its function, but not its expression, is different depending on the cellular context. Whether GATA1–FOG1 interaction inhibits erythroid gene expression in myelomonocytic cells has not been investigated.

The CF domain, on the other hand, recognizes and binds to the GATA site localized in the core of the minimal erythroid transcription sequence 10 bp downstream to the SCL binding site. SCL and GATA1 bind simultaneously to their respective sites of the core as multimeric complexes formed by SCL/E47/LMO2 on the one hand and by GATA1/LMO2 on the other. Binding of the two complexes to the core is stabilized by Lbd1, which forms a physical bridge between them. The paramount importance of the CF finger for GATA1 function is proved by the fact that GATA1 genes lacking the region encoding this domain are unable to rescue erythroid differentiation in $GATA1^{null}$ embryonic stem cells,[356] whereas mini genes containing only the CF of either GATA1 or GATA2 are sufficient to induce megakaryocytic differentiation of myeloid cell lines.[357] In addition to forming heterodimers with LMO2, CF can form complexes with Sp1 and PU.1, two factors essential for myelomonocytic differentiation. The GATA1–PU.1 complex is unable to bind DNA, so its function might be to establish either an erythroid- or a myeloid-permissive cellular environment depending on which factor is expressed at the highest concentration.[2] The presence of relatively higher concentrations of GATA1 would favor the formation of GATA1–LMO2 complexes leading to activation of erythroid-specific genes, whereas the presence of relatively higher concentrations of PU.1 would lead mainly to the formation of the transcriptionally inactive GATA1–PU.1 complexes.

Although early experiments on cell lines failed to identify any function for the amino-terminal domain of GATA1,[357,358] knock-in experiments in mice indicated that this domain, although dispensable for primitive erythropoiesis, is required for appropriate production of definitive red cells.[356] A truncated GATA1 gene lacking the amino-terminal domain is 10 times less efficient than the full-length gene in rescuing erythroid differentiation in $GATA1^{null}$ mice.[356] This experiment suggests that interaction of the amino-terminal domain of GATA1 with a yet to be identified partner(s) is required for optimal definitive erythropoiesis.

In addition to all the evidence pointing to GATA1 as exerting a predominant but ontogenetic-specific role in the control of erythroid differentiation, other evidence indicates that this gene exerts exquisite control in the differentiation of other hemopoietic lineages, such as megakaryocytes,[1] mast cells,[359] and eosinophils.[360] The mechanism used by one single factor in guiding differentiation along different lineages does not rely on specific domains in the GATA1 protein itself. In fact, the structure of all the GATA proteins is so well conserved among different family members and in evolution that $GATA1^{null}$ embryonic stem cells are rescued not only by reintroduction of the GATA1 gene itself but also by introducing any other member of the GAGA family, such as GATA3.[361] The lineage-specific action of GATA1 in regulating gene expression is achieved through the presence of lineage-specific regulatory sequences in the promoter regions of the target genes. Therefore, the relative concentration of GATA1, as opposed to the levels of a few key regulatory partners, may establish a lineage-permissive microenvironment. Furthermore, the existence of lineage-specific regulatory sequences in the GATA1 gene itself ensures that such concentrations are achieved only in the right cell. Although GATA1 is expressed in erythroid, megakaryocytic, mast, and eosinophilic cells, its level of expression differs greatly among the various cell types, with erythroid cells expressing the most. Three DNase hypersensitive sites (HS) have been recognized within the 8 kb upstream and the first intron of the murine GATA1 gene, defined as HSI, HSII, and HSIII. Targeted deletion mutants in the mouse have shown that each of these sites functions as an enhancer in different cell types. HSI is required for GATA1 expression in megakaryocytes[362] and mast cells[359] and for upregulation of GATA1 expression in erythroid cells.[363] HSIII is capable of sustaining low levels of GATA1 expression in erythroid cells. HSII, which is dispensable for erythroid and megakaryocyte expression, is absolutely required for gene expression in eosinophils.[360] All of the 317 bp of HSI are required for GATA1 expression in megakaryocytes, but only the first 5′ 62 bp are needed for erythroid-specific reporter activity.[364] The HSI region contains a canonical minimal erythroid activation sequence, and point mutations in the GATA site, but not in the E-box, abolish HSI function in both erythroid and megakaryocytic cells. Of note, GATA1 mRNA has an unusually long half-live (>9 hours). Two GATA1 bands, corresponding to the native and processed (acetylated and phosphorylated) forms of the protein, have been detected by Western blot analysis.[365] The processed form binds DNA with higher affinity than the native form. Furthermore, although the half-life of the native form is short (approximately 0.5 hour) and stabilized by Epo, the processed form is extremely stable (half-life >6 hours) and Epo independent.[365] Because the cell cycle of hemopoietic cells in vivo is as short as 6 hours, erythroid cells accumulate GATA1 as mRNA and protein as they proliferate. As maturation is dependent on the levels of GATA1 expressed by cells, the cellular GATA1 content might represent the biologic clock that, by controlling the number of precursors, determines the cellular output of the differentiation process. This hypothesis suggests that Epo-induced GATA1 processing through the ubiquitin–proteasome pathway is an important element in the regulation of erythroid differentiation. On the other hand, the TRAIL–Bruton kinase death pathway has as an endpoint caspase 3, the protein specifically responsible for GATA1 cleavage. However, caspase 3 is unable to cleave GATA1 if the protein is complexed in the nucleus with the chaperone protein Hsp70. Epo-receptor signaling counteracts the apoptotic pathway by favoring Hsp70–GATA1 colocalization in the nucleus.[366] These biochemical studies detailing the biochemical link between Epo and TRAIL from one side and GATA1 from the other are consistent with studies indicating that Epo signaling also induces GATA1 phosphorylation at Ser310 and that this phosphorylation plays an important role in regulating GATA1 function in erythroid cell lines.[367,368] Although GATA1 mutants expressing only the native form of GATA1 do not have a detectable erythroid phenotype under steady-state conditions,[369] more studies on the response of these mice to erythroid stress will clarify the role of GATA1 processing in stress erythropoiesis.

Another gene of the GATA family important for erythroid differentiation is GATA2. Both GATA1 and GATA2 are expressed early in multipotential progenitors; however, their expression ratios change as the cells differentiate (Table 25–1),[370] suggesting that the ratio of these two factors may be important at specific stages of erythroid differentiation. Knock-out experiments with both of these genes have borne this out. Thus, in contrast to GATA2, which is expressed at high levels in early cells and affects expansion of all hematopoietic lineages,[349] GATA1 expression increases as differentiation advances and seems to be the obligatory factor required for survival and terminal differentiation of erythroid cells. In mice with targeted disruption of GATA1, erythropoiesis proceeds only up to the stage of proerythroblasts, which die early and fail to mature further.[371,372] Furthermore, transgenic mice with partial loss of function (knockdown alleles, GATA1^{low}) of GATA1 show that erythroid differentiation is dose dependent with respect to GATA1.[363] High levels of GATA1 are necessary to form complexes with its cofactor FOG1[353] and with the other proteins described above (LM02, SCLor Hsp70 during terminal erythroid differentiation.

The realization that minute differences in transcription factor concentrations are required for lineage specification under physiologic conditions supports the idea that the differentiation system allows more flexibility in both the choice and the reversibility of pathway commitment toward a specific lineage. For example, a CFU-E was thought to have no other choice than to became an erythroid cell or to die.[6] More recently, experiments with forced expression of transcription factors in fully committed or even mature cells have demonstrated that the system has some degree of plasticity and that forced expression of FOG1 into mast cells may turn them into erythroblasts,[373] whereas forced expression of GATA1 into common myeloid progenitor cells induces their transdifferentiation into MEP.[374] All of these manipulations were performed in vitro. Of interest, experimentally decreased expression of GATA1 in progenitor cell compartments in vivo does not alter the frequency of individual compartments (i.e., does not decrease MEP by increasing the granulocyte-monocyte progenitor) but results in alternative differentiation pathways. Although the numbers of cells phenotypically recognizable as MEP in these animals are much higher than normal, MEP with reduced GATA1 expression, unlike normal cells, have the potential also to differentiate into mast cells.[375]

Another factor with special importance in the erythroid lineage is the CACCC binding protein designated EKLF, which is expressed at all stages of erythropoiesis but binds preferentially to CACCC sites in β-globin promoter. Mice lacking EKLF (EKLF^{null}) die of a thalassemic-like defect due to severe deficiency of β-globin expression.[376] Microarray analysis of EKLF^{null} erythroid cells and promoter-specific expression of reported genes in EKLF^{null} cells have identified that the first *Gata1*-dependent molecular control of erythroid differentiation is followed by a second *Eklf*-dependent phase.[377,378] Primarily GATA1-dependent genes include, in addition to EpoR and those involved in the control of apoptosis, α-, and δ-globin. EKLF-dependent genes, in addition to β-globin[379,380] and AHSP, are represented by those required for appropriate membrane assembly, such as β-spectrin, ankyrin, and band 3 (but not α-spectrin). These results are consistent with the notion that, in erythroid differentiation, activation of α-globin gene expression precedes that of β-globin[381] and that loss of GATA1 binding sites in the promoter of the gene is found in α-thalassemia,[382] in the Greek nondeletion hereditary persistence fetal hemoglobin (guanine to adenine at nucleotide position −117 of γ globin),[383] and in δ-thalassemia (point mutation leading to G→A substitution at position +69 of the δ-globin gene),[384] whereas loss of EKLF binding site is present in other forms of hereditary persistence of fetal hemoglobin.

An intrinsic control on erythroid differentiation also is exerted by genes that, until repressed, prevent terminal cell maturation. The most studied of these genes is *Id1*.[385] which, as its name indicates, inhibits differentiation along almost all mesenchymal cell lineages, including the erythroid lineage.[386,387] ID1 appears to act between GATA1 and EKLF by preventing Eklf from executing its program.

As common transcriptional factors are present in erythroid and megakaryocytic cells, and bipotent erythroid/megakaryocytic progenitors exist both in vitro (in the form of cell lines) and in vivo,[52] exciting insights regarding subtleties in the molecular control of these two lineages by the same transcriptional factors have surfaced. Modified gene targeting strategy ("knockdown") of GATA1 uncovered a largely unanticipated role of this transcriptional factor in the control of proliferation and maturation of megakaryocytes.[363] In addition to GATA1, other important transcriptional factors essential for terminal megakaryocytic development are NF-E2[388] and its partner MafG.[389]

Nevertheless, the fact that several regulators are necessary for primitive (yolk sac), as opposed to definitive (fetal liver and bone marrow), erythropoiesis provides evidence that molecular control between these two hemopoietic sites is different and may include both ubiquitous and hematopoietic specific factors. In fact, evidence suggests that GATA1 transcription is differentially regulated in yolk sac cells compared to fetal liver erythroid cells, with alternative promoter use and an additional intron element requirement for promoter activation in fetal liver cells.[390]

In addition to transcriptional factors/oncogenes influencing erythropoiesis, targeted ablation and naturally existing mutations of hematopoietic growth factor receptors, especially of the tyrosine kinase family, have disclosed important insights into the control of erythropoiesis. Whereas deletion of the vascular endothelial growth factor (VEGF)/flk-1 receptor affects both endothelial and hematopoietic development[391] through its presumed presence in the hemangioblast, the common endothelial/hematopoietic stem cell, mutations affecting the tyrosine kinase kit receptor (present in hematopoietic cells) or of its ligand KL (present in stromal cells) seem to predominantly affect erythropoiesis in the fetal liver and the adult animal. Mice with kit mutations (W mutations) leading to absence of or compromised kinase activity and steel mice with mutations of KL have disproportionate and severe abrogation of the late erythroid progenitors, CFU-E, and differentiated erythroid precursors resulting in anemia.[392] Studies showing cross-phosphorylation of EpoR following activation of kit/KL signaling may be relevant to the effect.[210] Mutations or targeted ablations of some downstream signaling substrates for kit or other receptors (i.e., Shp-2 phosphatase or gp130) seem to produce a hematopoietic picture not unlike the one produced by receptor mutations.[393,394]

Taken together, these studies have significantly expanded our understanding of the molecular level of hematopoietic development in general and of erythropoiesis in particular. The emerging picture is that certain genes, such as SCL, are absolutely required for hematopoietic development, whereas other genes, such as GATA2, c-myb, CBF, TEL, and some downstream signal transducing molecules, such as gp30 and Shp-2, are responsible for expansion and maintenance of a normal pool of fetal liver and adult hematopoietic progenitors. The participation of many of these molecules in multicomponent molecular complexes with protein/protein and protein/DNA interactions (i.e., LM02/Lbd1/SCL/E2A/GATA), during the early proliferative stages of hematopoiesis[395] may underlie their role in the proliferation and maintenance of immature progenitor/precursor pools in erythropoiesis. Other genes such as GATA1, its partner FOG1, and EKLF are necessary to direct high levels of function of erythroid-specific genes in cells already committed to terminal differentiation. Thus, a hierarchical requirement in the expression of specific regulators during early versus late erythroid differentiation or during yolk sac versus fetal liver/adult erythropoiesis is demonstrated. However, this does not exclude the involvement of some factors (i. e., SCL, TEL) at both early and late stages of erythropoiesis. In fact, more recent studies on conditional knock-outs have clarified that SCL exerts two different levels of control in the development of the hemopoietic system. First, SCL is required for the determination event that induces one (or few) mesenchymal cell(s) to become a hematopoietic stem cell(s) in the early embryos.[127] After this initial event has taken place, its presence becomes dispensable, as demonstrated by the fact that conditional SCL deletion in the adult animals impairs only erythropoiesis and megakaryocytopoiesis.[127,396] With information from innovative applications of molecular approaches becoming available at a fast pace, the list of regulators with a biologic impact on hematopoiesis/erythropoiesis is continuously expanding.

TRANSCRIPTIONAL AND POSTTRANSCRIPTIONAL FACTOR IMPAIRMENT IN DISORDERS OF ERYTHROPOIESIS

The transcription factor found most frequently altered in inherited and acquired human diseases of the erythroid and megakaryocytic lineage is GATA1. The mutations often involve the region of the gene encoding the NF domain. Mutations in the GATA1 NF domain interrupting its interaction with FOG1, such as V205M and G208S, are responsible for familial dyserythropoietic anemia and X-linked thrombocytopenia, respectively.[397,398] A different mutation at position 208 leading to G→A substitution is associated with dyserythropoietic anemia and macrothrombocytopenia.[399] Mutations in the NF terminal domain of GATA1 responsible for DNA binding, such as A216G[400] and D218G,[401] instead have been found associated with X-linked thalassemia and/or thrombocytopenia. The phenotype of X-linked thrombocytopenia was mimicked in mice by knock-in experiments of the mutant V205G GATA1 gene.[402] However, the same A216G mutation has been found associated with X-linked gray platelet syndrome, a mild bleeding disorder characterized by thrombocytopenia and large agranular platelets.[403] Furthermore, a mutation at codon 216 changing arginine to tryptophan (R216W) was detected in a 3-year-old boy with congenital erythropoietic porphyria, an autosomal recessive disorder usually due to mutations of the uroporphyrinogen III synthase gene (UROS). The boy also presented with microcytic anemia and red cell morphology and globin chain labeling values compatible with β-thalassemia and increased HbF levels (59.5%).[404] The different phenotype expressed by patients carrying mutations either in the FOG1 or the DNA binding portion of NF supported the notion that the two domains influence erythroid versus megakaryocytic maturation.[405] However, the observation that, in certain cases, a mutation in the same codon or even the same mutation results in a different phenotype suggests that the phenotype induced by mutations in the GATA1 gene are extremely sensitive to genetic heterogeneity outside the GATA1 locus. This hypothesis has been demonstrated in mice in which the same mutation induces embryonic lethality, thrombocytopenia, or myelofibrosis, depending on the mouse background in which it is harbored.[406]

On the other hand, frameshift and splice mutations encoding GATA1s, a protein lacking the amino-terminal domain, not only are associated with impaired inherited erythropoiesis[407] but also are found in patients with megakaryocytic leukemia in Down syndrome,[408,409] in newborns with transient myeloproliferative syndromes,[410] and in one adult patient with megakaryocytic leukemia.[411] A mutation equivalent to that found in patients with acute megakaryoblastic leukemia and Down syndrome was created in mice by *N*-ethyl-*N*-nitrosourea mutagenesis screening. The reduced expression of the full-length GATA1 was not compensated in mice by expression of GATA1s. The mutation was embryonic lethal in hemizygous males and induced thrombocytopenia in heterozygous females.[412] However, when introduced in mice the Gata1s mutation increased proliferation of a "unique" fetal stem/progenitor cell extinguished in adult life.[413] The association between mutation of GATA1 and development of leukemia support the concept described that GATA1 exerts an important control on the proliferation of hematopoietic progenitors. Reduced GATA1 expression, by increasing progenitor cell proliferation, may predispose hematopoietic cells to leukemia by favoring accumulation of secondary mutations. Alterations of hematopoietic proliferation appear to be achieved through quantitative, rather than structural, GATA1 alterations. The GATA1s protein is far less efficient than the full-length GATA1 in rescuing the phenotype of Gata-1^{null} embryonic stem cells,[414] and hypomorphic mutations in mice induce either leukemia[415] or a phenotype similar to idiopathic myelofibrosis,[416] depending on the severity of the reduction of the expression. Interestingly, the reduced content of GATA1 in megakaryocytes, through a yet to be identified molecular defect rather than the presence of ^{V617F}Jak2, distinguishes idiopathic myelofibrosis from all the other myeloproliferative abnormalities in humans.[417] (For a more complete review on the role of GATA factors in hematologic diseases, see reference 418.)

Another disease associated with abnormalities in the molecular machinery of red cell differentiation is represented by Diamond-Blackfan anemia, a rare congenital red cell aplasia characterized by anemia, bone marrow erythroblastopenia (lack of late erythroid forms), and congenital anomalies. The disease is associated with heterozygous mutations in the ribosomal protein S19 gene (RPS19) in approximately 25% of probands.[419] In a large cohort of 172 new families with familial history of Diamond-Blackfan anemia, mutations affecting the coding sequence of RPS19 or splice sites were found in 34 cases (19.7%), whereas additional mutations in noncoding regions were found in eight patients (4.6%). Mutations included nonsense, missense, splice sites, and frameshift mutations. More recently, de novo nonsense and splice-site mutations in another ribosomal protein, RPS24 (encoded by RPS24 [10q22-q23]), was identified in approximately 2% of RPS19 mutation-negative probands.[420] The molecular defect of the other families is yet to be uncovered. No correlation between the nature of mutations and the different patterns of clinical expression, including age at presentation, presence of malformations, and therapeutic outcome, has been documented. The lack of a consistent relationship between the nature of the mutations and the clinical phenotype implies that yet unidentified factors modulate the phenotypic expression of the primary genetic defect in families with RPS19 mutations.[421] Two not mutually exclusive hypotheses had been proposed to explain the pathobiologic role of RPS19 (and RPS24) in the pathogenesis of the disease: (a) loss of unknown functions not directly connected with RPS19's structural role in ribosomes and (b) altered protein synthesis because of poor ribosome organization. The first hypothesis was suggested by findings based on a proteomic approach that identified numerous proteins bound to RPS19. In addition to FGF2, complement component 5 receptor 1, a nucleolar protein called RPS19 binding protein, and pim-1, the other RPS19-binding proteins fall in the following Gene Ontology categories: NTPases (ATPases and GTPases; 5 proteins), hydrolase/helicases (19 proteins), isomerases (2 proteins), kinases (3 proteins), splicing factors (5 proteins), structural constituents of ribosome (29 proteins), transcription factors (11 proteins), transferases (5 proteins), transporters (9 proteins), DNA/RNA-binding protein species (53 proteins), other (1 dehydrogenase protein, 1 ligase protein, 1 peptidase protein, 1 receptor protein, 1 translation elongation factor), and 13 proteins with unknown function.[422] However, more recent studies have identified that RPS19 plays an essential role in the biogenesis and maturation of the 40S small ribosomal subunit in human cells[423,424] because of reduced gene expression of clustered ribosomal proteins due to abnormal pre-mRNA processing.[425] Such a defective ribosomal gene expression results in alterations of the transcription, translation, apoptosis and oncogenic pathways.[426] Expression of RPS19 mRNA and protein decreases during terminal erythroid differentiation.[427] A mouse model of the disease has been generated by disrupting the endogenous Rps19 gene.[428] Cellular models of the disease have been established by siRNA technology against RP19 protein.[429–431]

CELLULAR DYNAMICS IN ERYTHROPOIESIS

The primary function of the mature red cell, which is the end product of erythropoiesis, is to transport oxygen efficiently through the circulation to the tissues. To achieve this goal, the adult marrow must release approximately 3×10^9 new red cells, or reticulocytes per kilogram per day.[432] This number of reticulocytes represents {1/100} of the total red cell mass and is derived from an estimated 5×10^9 erythroid precursors per kilogram.[432] In addition to maintaining homeostasis (i.e., a stable hematocrit), the erythron must be able to respond quickly and appropriately to increased oxygen demands, either acute (e.g., following red cell loss) or chronic (e.g., with hypoxia from pulmonary disease or a right-to-left cardiac shunt). It is well established that Epo is responsible both for maintaining normal erythropoiesis and for increasing red cell production in response to oxygen needs. However, the overall marrow response is complex and requires not only the participation of erythroid cells responsive to Epo but also a structurally intact microenvironment and an optimal iron supply within the marrow.

Epo stimulation elicits two types of measurable responses: changes in proliferative activity (including improved survival) and changes in maturation rates. The first detectable response to increased serum Epo is amplification of CFU-E and erythroid precursors, cells that are extremely sensitive to Epo. Because virtually all these cells are already in cycle, increases in their numbers cannot be achieved by increasing their fraction in cycle. Either additional divisions are involved or new cells are recruited to the CFU-E pool (from a pre-CFU-E pool). Additional divisions of CFU-E or precursor cells would increase their transit time within the marrow and potentially delay the delivery of new red cells to the periphery. Because a shortened maturation time has been observed instead and the proliferative potentials of CFU-E and proerythroblasts are finite, high levels of amplification cannot be achieved through this mechanism. Therefore, such needs are met by influx into the CFU-E and precursor pools of newly differentiating cells from earlier progenitor compartments.

Such a surge of newly produced cells has been observed in all previous experiments.[133,433,434] A rapid influx of fresh cells was particularly notable in polycythemic mice that were experimentally depleted of CFU-E and erythroid precursors at the time the stimulus was applied.[105,133] Because of the rapidity of response (i.e., within 24 hours in the polycythemic animals), it appeared that the orderly progression from BFU-E to CFU-E to proerythroblast had been compressed. Such acceleration of differentiation is possible through shortened intermitotic intervals, fewer mitotic divisions, or differentiation without divisions. This short circuiting in differentiation requires high serum levels of Epo and adequate numbers of BFU-E (i.e., these conditions are met in a previously hypertransfused, polycythemic animal stimulated by Epo or in marrow suddenly recovering from acquired pure erythroid aplasia). Once CFU-E and precursors are expanded through this mechanism, most persisting erythropoietic demands can be met through this pool without excess input from pre-CFU-E pools. Thus, acute demands for erythropoiesis are met by influx from pre-CFU-E pools through an accelerated differentiation and maturation sequence. In contrast, chronic demands (i.e., demands in chronic hemolytic anemia) are mainly satisfied through a greatly amplified late erythroid pool and with a minimum distortion in the differentiation sequence.[88,435] The fact that the kinetics of erythroid differentiation/maturation are different in acute versus chronic marrow regeneration is supported by differing qualitative changes in the newly formed red cells. An increase in i antigen and HbF expression as well as an increase in cells with higher mean corpuscular volumes is seen with an acute response, whereas these increases are minimal or less pronounced with chronic responses.[88,436] When severe anemia persists from birth onward, erythroid production can increase up to 10-fold above baseline.[435] This is possible not only because of maximally expanded erythropoietic pools but also because the sites of active erythropoiesis may extend to include those that support red cell differentiation during fetal life. Thus, although the marrow space in axial bones (vertebrae, pelvis, ribs, sternum, clavicles) is sufficient for normal erythropoiesis or for response to moderate anemia, the femur, humerus, spleen and/or liver, and (rarely) thymus may support red cell production in children with congenital hemolytic anemia (e.g., thalassemia major). Expanded erythropoiesis may lead to skeletal deformities, hepatosplenomegaly, or erythropoiesis in the soft tissues adjacent to bone.

Quantitative assessments of changes in erythroid progenitor cell pools in response to Epo stimulation can be made through cultures of bone marrow cells. Despite sampling errors, erythroid cultures can provide rough estimates of relative progenitor abundance within an aspirated marrow specimen and have shown consistent increases in the frequency of CFU-E in proportion to the level of Epo stimulation.[437,438] Conversely, with increases in the hematocrit or in polycythemic animals, a decrease in CFU-E frequency has been observed.[439,440] In contrast to CFU-E, the incidence of BFU-E was found to fluctuate less with either acute or chronic expansion of erythropoiesis, probably because a few BFU-E can generate progeny of several thousand cells. Furthermore, BFU-E can increase their fraction in cycle and thus increase the number of differentiated progeny without a significant change in their total numbers. Most BFU-E detectable in marrow or blood erythroid cultures probably represent a reservoir of progenitors not normally participating in day-to-day erythropoiesis. The parameters needed to maintain a healthy or appropriate BFU-E pool in hematopoiesis are not defined. That hematopoietic expansion is curtailed in mice with steel mutations and anemia develops in mice treated with anti-c-kit Ab antibody[441] suggest that adequate levels of normal KL may be crucial for early erythropoietic expansion.[134]

The rate of red cell production also can be accurately evaluated through ferrokinetics (i.e., study of iron incorporation into developing red cells). In addition, a marrow scan, typically with technetium Tc 99m, can document the extent of active erythropoiesis. However, these approaches seldom are necessary in clinical practice because estimates of erythropoiesis can be obtained from the reticulocyte index.[435] First, the observed percentage of reticulocytes is normalized for the hematocrit to calculate the total marrow output of reticulocytes. Alternatively, the absolute number of reticulocytes per microliter can be counted directly using fluorescent RNA labeling. However, because younger reticulocytes are prematurely released into the circulation under conditions of acute need, the total number of reticulocytes overestimates the true level of red cell production as measured by iron kinetics.[435] Therefore, a second correction is made to account for the maturation of early circulating reticulocytes, or "shift" cells (polychromatophilic red cells) when present in the blood smear. The resulting reticulocyte index gives excellent estimates of effective red cell production.

Although the presence, density, or both of EpoRs on developing erythroid cells determines the responses to Epo, other properties (e.g., surface antigens on BFU-E vs CFU-E vs end-stage red cells) may provide the basis for selective suppression of CFU-E versus BFU-E or selective immune destruction of red cells versus erythroblasts. For example, suppression of CFU-E or erythroblasts can occur in acquired pure red cell aplasia[442] or B19 parvovirus infection,[443] respectively, whereas BFU-E in both these conditions remain largely unperturbed. Thus, the boundary from BFU-E to CFU-E and erythroblast may be biologically important for the pathophysiology of these disease states. Furthermore, in acquired hemolytic anemia, selective destruction at a given stage of maturation (of red cells only or of both erythroblasts and red cells) can be observed depending on the type of antibody produced and the density of its antigen on maturing erythroid cells. Qualitative aberrations in the response of erythroid progenitors to cytokines or Epo may underlie the abnormalities of congenital erythroid aplasia (Diamond-Blackfan syndrome).[278] Analogous qualitative or functional defects can be observed in neoplastic erythropoiesis, as erythroid progenitors from patients with polycythemia vera and other myeloproliferative syndromes have altered sensitivities to Epo.[444] (see Alterations in ERO-R and its Signalling in Disorders of Erythropoiesis)

Detailed knowledge of the structural and functional properties of erythroid cells throughout their differentiation (see Transcriptional and Posttranscriptional Factor Impairment in Disorders of Erythropoiesis above) may provide significant insights into the pathogenesis of hematopoietic disorders affecting the red cell lineage.

SUGGESTED READINGS

Bowie MB, Kent DG, Copley MR, Eaves CJ: Steel factor responsiveness regulates the high self-renewal phenotype of fetal hematopoietic stem cells. Blood 109:5043, 2007.

Bunn HF: New agents that stimulate erythropoiesis. Blood 109:868, 2007.

Choesmel V, Bacqueville D, Rouquette J, et al: Impaired ribosome biogenesis in Diamond-Blackfan anemia. Blood 109:1275, 2007.

Di Baldassarre A, Di Rico M, Di Noia A, et al: Protein kinase C alpha is differentially activated during neonatal and adult erythropoiesis and favors expression of a reporter gene under the control of the A gamma globin-promoter in cellular models of hemoglobin switching. J Cell Biochem 101:411, 2007.

Fabriek BO, Polfliet MMJ, Vloet RPM, et al: The macrophage CD163 surface glycoprotein is an erythroblast adhesion receptor. Blood 109:5223, 2007.

Flygare J, Aspesi A, Bailey JC, et al: Human RPS19, the gene mutated in Diamond-Blackfan anemia, encodes a ribosomal protein required for the maturation of 40S ribosomal subunits. Blood 109:980, 2007.

Fraser ST, Isern J, Baron MH: Maturation and enucleation of primitive erythroblasts during mouse embryogenesis is accompanied by changes in cell-surface antigen expression. Blood. 109:343, 2007.

Ghinassi B, Sanchez M, Martelli F, et al: The hypomorphic Gata1low mutation alters the proliferation/differentiation potential of the common megakaryocytic-erythroid progenitor. Blood 109:1460, 2007.

Lambert LA, Mitchell SL: Molecular evolution of the transferrin receptor/glutamate carboxypeptidase II family. J Mol Evol 64:113, 2007.

Maetens M, Doumont G, Clercq SD, et al: Distinct roles of Mdm2 and Mdm4 in red cell production. Blood 109:2630, 2007.

Orru S, Aspesi A, Armiraglio M, et al: Analysis of the ribosomal protein S19 interactome. Mol Cell Proteomics 6:382, 2007.

Phillips JD, Steensma DP, Pulsipher MA, Spangrude GJ, Kushner JP: Congenital erythropoietic porphyria due to a mutation in GATA1: The first trans-acting mutation causative for a human porphyria. Blood 109:2618, 2007.

Ribeil J-A, Zermati Y, Vandekerckhove J, et al: Hsp70 regulates erythropoiesis by preventing caspase-3-mediated cleavage of GATA-1. Nature 445:102, 2007.

Roy CN, Mak HH, Akpan I, Losyev G, Zurakowski D, Andrews NC: Hepcidin antimicrobial peptide transgenic mice exhibit features of the anemia of inflammation. Blood 109:4038, 2007.

Scott LM, Tong W, Levine RL, et al: JAK2 exon 12 mutations in polycythemia vera and idiopathic erythrocytosis. N Engl J Med 356:459, 2007.

Tober J, Koniski A, McGrath KE, et al: The megakaryocyte lineage originates from hemangioblast precursors and is an integral component both of primitive and of definitive hematopoiesis. Blood 109:1433, 2007.

Tubman VN, Levine JE, Campagna DR, et al: X-linked gray platelet syndrome due to a GATA1 Arg216Gln mutation. Blood 109:3297, 2007.

Wallace DF, Summerville L, Subramaniam VN: Targeted disruption of the hepatic transferrin receptor 2 gene in mice leads to iron overload. Gastroenterology 132:301, 2007.

Zambidis E, Sinka L, Tavian M, et al: Emergence of human angio-hematopoietic cells in normal development and from cultured embryonic stem cells. Ann N Y Acad Sci 1106:223, 2007.

REFERENCES

For complete list of references log onto www.expertconsult.com

CHAPTER 26

GRANULOCYTOPOIESIS AND MONOCYTOPOIESIS

Arati Khanna-Gupta and Nancy Berliner

GRANULOCYTOPOIESIS

Granulocytes-neutrophils, eosinophils, and basophils-are short-lived cells that are critical to both antimicrobial and inflammatory responses. The bone marrow produces granulocytes, especially neutrophils, at a prodigious rate to supply the baseline needs of circulating cells that survive in the peripheral blood only 3 to 6 hours. It also has the capacity to upregulate granulocyte production sharply in response to a wide range of stresses. The regulation of granulocyte production is controlled by a variety of cytokines that induce the myeloid differentiation program through the carefully orchestrated interaction of multiple general and myeloid-specific transcription factors. Understanding this intricate maturation sequence provides important insights into normal neutrophil responses to infectious, inflammatory, and allergic stresses, as well as into the dysregulation of differentiation contributing to myelodysplasia and leukemia.

Granulocyte Ontogeny

Stages of Neutrophil Differentiation

Granulocytes differentiate from early progenitors in the bone marrow in a process that takes 7 to 10 days. The cells pass through several identifiable maturational stages, during which they acquire the morphologic appearance and granule contents that characterize the mature granulocyte.[1,2] The earliest identifiable granulocyte precursor is the myeloblast, a minimally granulated cell with scant cytoplasm and a prominent nucleolus (Fig. 26–1). Transition to the promyelocyte stage is associated with the acquisition of abundant primary granules. Primary granules are found in both granulocytes and monocytes and contain many of the proteins necessary for intracellular killing of microbes. The transition to the myelocyte stage is associated with the acquisition of secondary or "specific" granules, which give the characteristic staining that differentiates neutrophils from eosinophils and basophils.

Neutrophil precursors account for approximately half of the cells in the marrow of normal persons, with a majority of these at the metamyelocyte stage and beyond.[3] Promyelocytes and myelocytes represent the primary proliferative pool of granulocyte precursors in the bone marrow. Beyond the myelocyte stage, cells mature as nondividing cells. Bands and segmented neutrophils constitute greater than 50% of the total granulocyte mass, primarily as a mobilizable pool of cells in the bone marrow. Only 5% of total neutrophils circulate in the periphery, where 60% are marginated in the spleen and on vessel walls. Mature neutrophils circulate in the peripheral blood for 3 to 12 hours and then migrate to the tissues, where they survive 2 to 3 days. Hence, the peripheral blood count reflects roughly 2% of the total neutrophil cell mass during approximately 1% of the neutrophil life span.

Biochemical events that accompany these physical changes include the sequential acquisition of primary granules and their content proteins (eg, myeloperoxidase, lysozyme, neutrophil elastase [NE], defensins, myeloblastin), secondary granules and their content proteins (lactoferrin, neutrophil collagenase, neutrophil gelatinase, neutrophil gelatinase-associated lipocalin [NGAL], transcobalamin 1), and tertiary granules containing neutrophil gelatinase (Table 26–1). The progressive gain of differentiated characteristics is accompanied by a loss of proliferative potential. This carefully coordinated process is disrupted in acute myeloid leukemias (AMLs), in which a block in the myeloid maturation pathway usually results in the circulation of immature blasts in the peripheral blood.

Surface Markers of Granulocytic Maturation

Stem cells have been characterized primarily by their marrow repopulating potential, as outlined in Chapters 19 and 20. Early granulocytic progenitors form hematopoietic colonies in vitro and their more differentiated progeny express specific cell surface proteins that are critically important to myeloid differentiation and function.[4,5] They mediate both the adhesion of precursors within the marrow and the vascular adhesion of mature neutrophils that is critical to normal neutrophil activation. Other proteins serve as receptors that recognize pathogens or as stimulatory peptides that facilitate activation of phagocytosis and killing of organisms. Appropriate expression of these surface proteins plays an important role in normal neutrophil function, and abnormalities of their expression are implicated in a wide range of diseases affecting the neutrophil compartment. For example, congenital abnormalities in the surface expression of integrin proteins are responsible for failure of neutrophil adhesion in leukocyte adhesion deficiency,[6] whereas acquired abnormalities of expression of the same proteins are hypothesized to underlie the abnormal peripheral circulation of immature precursors in myeloproliferative disease.[7] These markers also serve to help distinguish among the stages of myeloid commitment and maturation.

The phenotype of the early hematopoietic stem cells is $CD34^+$/$CD33^-$, with absence of lineage-specific markers. The common myeloid progenitor, colony-forming unit-granulocyte- erythrocyte-macrophage-megakaryocyte (CFU-GEMM), is characterized by the coexpression of CD33. CD33 is expressed at high levels on committed myeloid progenitors and on early precursors of both the granulocytic and monocytic lineages.[8] Expression of CD33 wanes with granulocytic maturation, and it is absent or nearly absent beyond the myelocyte stage. CD33 is a member of the sialic acid-binding Ig-like lectins (siglecs), which generally mediate cell-cell interactions and cell signaling.[9] The precise biologic function of CD33 itself is unknown.

Characteristic granulocyte markers acquired as the early myeloid progenitor cells become committed to the neutrophil lineage include CD45RA,[10–12] myeloperoxidase (MPO), and CD38, all of which are expressed on the myeloblast.[13] Further differentiation beyond the myelocyte stage is associated with acquisition of increased expression of CD16,[11] CD11b/CD18 (Mac-1),[11,14] and leukocyte alkaline phosphatase (LAP), all of which are expressed at high levels in mature neutrophils.

Neutrophil Granules and Their Content Proteins

The acquisition of granules and their content proteins are a critical part of the developmental program of the granulocyte.[15,16] Acquired at specific identifiable stages of neutrophil maturation, these intracellular and secretory organelles contain many of the requisite enzymes that mediate the oxidative and nonoxidative killing functions of the neutrophil (Table 26–1).[17–20]

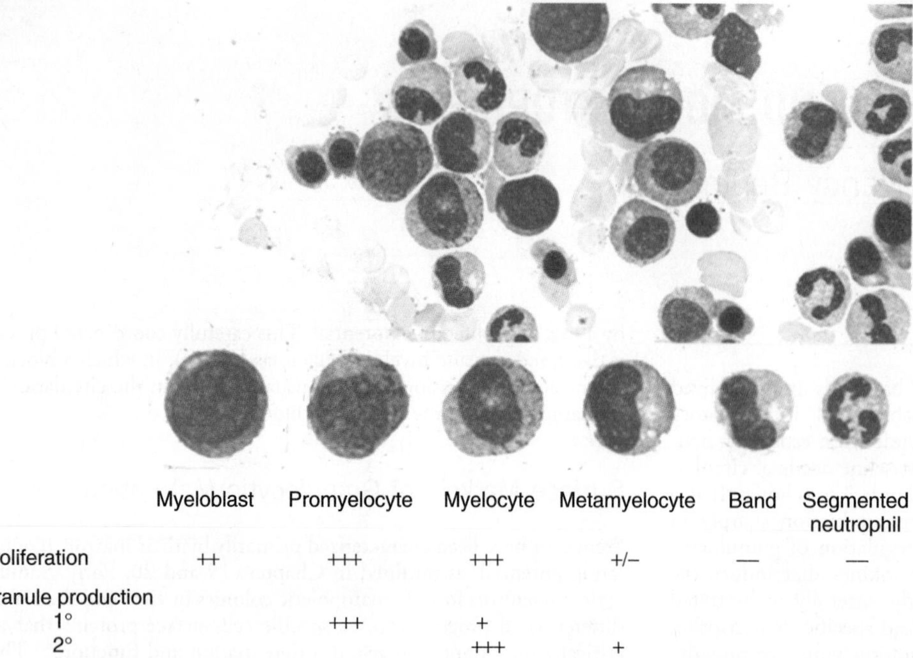

Figure 26–1 Neutrophil maturation stages with associated acquisition of stage-specific granules.

Primary (azurophilic) granules are acquired at the promyelocyte stage and contain a wide array of proteins, including myeloperoxidase, defensins, cathepsins, and elastase.[21,22] *Secondary* granules are secretory granules acquired at the transition to the myelocyte stage. Neutrophil secondary granules contain lactoferrin, the vitamin B_{12}-binding protein transcobalamin I, and the metalloproteinases (neutrophil collagenase and gelatinase), as well as NGAL.[22,23] With the exception of gelatinase, which also is expressed by monocytes, expression of the secondary granule proteins is restricted within the hematopoietic lineage to neutrophils. Secondary granules and the synthesis of their contents therefore constitute a definitive marker of commitment to terminal neutrophil maturation. As discussed later on, characteristic secondary granules are acquired at the same stage by eosinophils and basophils. *Tertiary* granules, containing primarily gelatinase, are formed during later stages of neutrophil maturation.[23,24] *Secretory vesicles* are formed by endocytosis and contain plasma proteins.[25,26]

On stimulation, the neutrophil first mobilizes secretory vesicles, which contribute their membrane proteins, including abundant integrin receptors, to the plasma membrane. They may thus increase cellular adhesion by upregulating surface integrin expression in response to selectin stimulation or inflammatory mediators.[16,27,28] Primary granules fuse with the phagosome and contribute to bacterial killing.[29] Secondary and tertiary granules have a complex function. They are secretory granules, releasing the matrix-modifying metalloproteinases collagenase and gelatinase into the extracellular milieu, enhancing neutrophil penetration into sites of inflammation.[30] The function of lactoferrin and transcobalamin I remains unconfirmed, but they are hypothesized to contribute to the antimicrobial response by sequestering iron and cobalamin, respectively, away from infecting organisms.[31–33] Secretion also results in the contribution of membrane proteins to the plasma membrane and is the source of the prominent upregulation of surface integrin receptor Mac-1 (CD11b/CD18) expression that occurs on neutrophil activation. Finally, they also fuse intracellularly with the phagosome to help promote bactericidal activity.

The fusion of azurophilic and peroxidase-negative granules allows for cross-exposure to their contents within the phagosome. These proteins are carefully sequestered in separate organelles, preventing premature activation and damage to the resting neutrophil; on fusion, the contents of the two granule subtypes cooperate in generating the antimicrobial response. Hydrogen peroxide, a by-product of NADPH oxidase in the secondary granule, in combination with MPO from the primary granules, produces hypochlorous acid, a highly toxic

Table 26–1 Neutrophil Granules: Major Classes and Contents

Primary (Azurophilic)	Secondary (Specific)	Tertiary
Microbial Agents		
Lysozyme	Lysozyme	
Myeloperoxidase		
Defensins		
Cationic proteins		
Bactericidal permeability–increasing agent (BPI)		
Proteases		
Elastase	Collagenase	Gelatinase
Cathepsin G		
Other proteases		
Acid Hydrolases		
N-acetylglucuronidase		
Cathepsins B and D		
β-Glucuronidase		
β-Glycerophosphatase		
α-Mannosidase		
Other		
Kinin-generating enzyme	Lactoferrin	
C5a-inactivating factor	Vitamin B_{12}–binding protein	
	Plasminogen activator	
	Cytochrome *b**	
	CD11/1B complex*	
	Formyl peptide receptor*	
	Histaminase*	
	NGAL	

*These granule constituents are conventionally assigned to the secondary granule, but their exact compartment remains controversial. Some may be located in the tertiary granule or possibly in one of the other, heterogeneous small-granule populations.

Adapted from Boxer LA, Smolen JE: Neutrophil granule constituents and their release in health and disease. Hematol Oncol Clin North Am 2:101, 1988.

microbicidal agent.[34] Additionally, both neutrophil gelatinase and neutrophil collagenase (secondary granule proteins) are produced as zymogens and are converted to their active forms by the action of NE released from the primary granules.[35]

Current evidence largely supports the hypothesis that the content of the neutrophil granules is dictated primarily by the timing of synthesis of their respective content proteins. Recent studies have demonstrated that each distinct granule population is generated not by a sophisticated protein sorting mechanism but rather by a highly regulated transcriptional process that results in sequential gene expression.[36] For example, because myeloperoxidase and the other primary granule proteins are expressed between the promyelocyte and the myelocyte stages of neutrophil development, they are packaged into the primary granules. Secondary granule proteins such as lactoferrin (LF), on the other hand, are expressed between the myelocyte and the metamyelocyte stages and are hence packaged into the secondary granules.[16,36] Overexpression of the secondary granule protein NGAL in HL60 cells, a leukemic cell line that is arrested at the myeloblast stage of differentiation, resulted in its incorporation into primary granules,[37] lending empirical support to the concept that gene expression and protein sorting into granules are coordinate events. This hypothesis may, however, be a somewhat oversimplified view of granule protein sorting, because there is some overlap of expression between certain primary and secondary granule protein genes. Whereas secondary granule protein gene transcription appears to be coordinately regulated, the sequence of primary granule protein gene expression is much less synchronous. The defensins are expressed later than the other primary granule proteins, and defensin transcription appears to be regulated by the same transcriptional regulatory pathway as for the secondary granule proteins gelatinase and lactoferrin.[38] Indeed, the defensins are the only primary granule proteins that are absent in patients with neutrophil-specific granule deficiency. This suggests that defensin regulation would predict targeting to the secondary granule.[39–41] Consequently, how defensins become directed exclusively to the primary granule remains unclear.

CONTROL OF GRANULOPOIESIS

Granulocytes arise from pluripotent hematopoietic stem cells by a process of commitment, proliferation, and differentiation. Stem cells are long-lived cells capable of both self-renewal and differentiation to lineage-specific-committed progenitors. The process governing the cell fate decision that takes a stem cell down the path to lineage commitment and the subsequent factors that regulate lineage- specific differentiation have been the subjects of intense study for many years. Three models of hematopoietic differentiation have been proposed to address the mechanism underlying lineage commitment and differentiation of the pluripotent stem cell. The first or *inductive* model proposes that lineage commitment and differentiation are the results of external stimuli (eg, growth factors, stroma).[42] A second model, the *stochastic* model, emphasizes intrinsic cellular factors as being critical to hematopoiesis[43]; a third model combines the attributes of the first two.[44] It appears likely that the transition from a stem cell to a committed progenitor is largely stochastic, although the subsequent maturation from progenitor to precursor to mature neutrophil requires cytokines. Controversy remains as to whether cytokines and the bone marrow microenvironment play an instructive or a permissive role in influencing stem cell commitment and in inducing the proliferation and maturation of committed progenitors. As discussed subsequently, this complex issue has been elucidated in mice with homologous null mutations in specific cytokines and their cognate receptors, alone or in combination.

Cytokine Regulation of Myeloid Proliferation and Differentiation

Early progenitor cells express receptors for multiple cytokines, but expression becomes more restricted as the cell becomes committed to a specific lineage.[42] As a consequence of this broad range of cytokine receptor expression, early progenitors respond to combined growth factors, many of which show synergy of activity. The "early-acting" cytokines include the interleukins IL-1 and IL-6, stem cell factor (SCF), FLT3 ligand, and several others including granulocyte colony-stimulating factor (G-CSF). IL-3 is important in directing the pluripotent stem cell toward the myelomonocytic lineage, giving rise to the mixed myeloid progenitor (CFU-GEMM). Subsequent stages leading to commitment- and lineage-restricted differentiation are governed by more "late-acting" cytokines (Fig. 26–2).

The major cytokines mediating neutrophil maturation are G-CSF and granulocyte-macrophage colony-stimulating factor (GM-CSF).[45] G-CSF not only supports the survival and proliferation of developing myeloid cells at all stages of differentiation but also increases the functional activity of mature neutrophils. Although the major role of G-CSF is thought to be the induction of neutrophil proliferation and differentiation, the G-CSF receptor (G-CSFR) is expressed on a wide range of cell types. In addition to myeloid progenitors and precursors at all stages of neutrophil differentiation, G-CSFR is expressed on platelets, monocytes, lymphocytes, and several nonhematopoietic cells, including endothelial cells and placenta.[46–49] The role of G-CSF as both an early- and late-acting cytokine is underscored by the successful use of G-CSF to mobilize early progenitors into the peripheral blood for stem cell collection and to speed neutrophil recovery following chemotherapy.[50]

The G-CSFR is a member of the cytokine receptor superfamily that signals through activation of the Jak-STAT (Janus kinase-signal transducer and activator of transcription) pathway and the Ras pathway. Ligand binding induces homodimerization of the receptor, leading to a cascade of downstream phosphorylation events. Dimerization leads to phosphorylation of associated JAK kinases that in turn phosphorylate STAT1 and STAT3. In addition, the activated G-CSFR also phosphorylates mediators of the Ras-mitogen-activated protein (MAP) kinase pathway by tyrosine phosphorylation of Shc.[51]

The importance of G-CSF in myeloid proliferation and differentiation has been studied in G-CSF-null[52] and G-CSFR-null mice.[53] Mice lacking G-CSF[52] or G-CSFR[53] had markedly decreased myeloid progenitors and impaired neutrophil production, with low circulating neutrophil counts. In addition, G-CSF-null mice had impaired neutrophil mobilization, and mature neutrophils from G-CSFR-null mice had increased susceptibility to apoptosis, supporting the role of the G-CSF pathway in sustaining the mobilization, survival, and function of mature neutrophils as well. However, despite all of these profound abnormalities, G-CSF/G-CSFR knock-out mice continued to make some neutrophils, suggesting that there are alternative overlapping cytokine pathways that support granulocyte development.[53]

GM-CSF also induces proliferation and differentiation of myeloid precursors. The GM-CSFR is a heterodimeric protein composed of an α- and a β-subunit. The α-subunit binds GM-CSF. The β-subunit is shared by the GM-CSFR and the receptors for IL-3, IL-5, and IL-6. The β-subunit does not bind ligand but is necessary for the high-affinity ligand binding to the $\alpha\beta$-heterodimer of each receptor. Signaling through the GM-CSFR also depends on the Jak-STAT pathway, signaling through Jak2, and also serves to activate the Ras-MAP kinase pathway.[54] Of interest, however, the GM-CSF-null mouse has no defect in hematopoiesis.[55] Mice with null mutations in both G-CSF and GM-CSF had more profound neutropenia in the perinatal period but the same levels of neutrophils in adulthood as those for mice lacking G-CSF only.[56]

Transcriptional Regulation of Myeloid Differentiation

Lineage-specific maturation of committed hematopoietic progenitors is ultimately driven by transcription factors, which have been hypothesized to be the final common pathway leading to commitment and differentiation of the pluripotent stem cell.[57] The role of transcription factors in cellular proliferation, differentiation, and survival of the stem cell during hematopoiesis in the mammalian bone marrow has

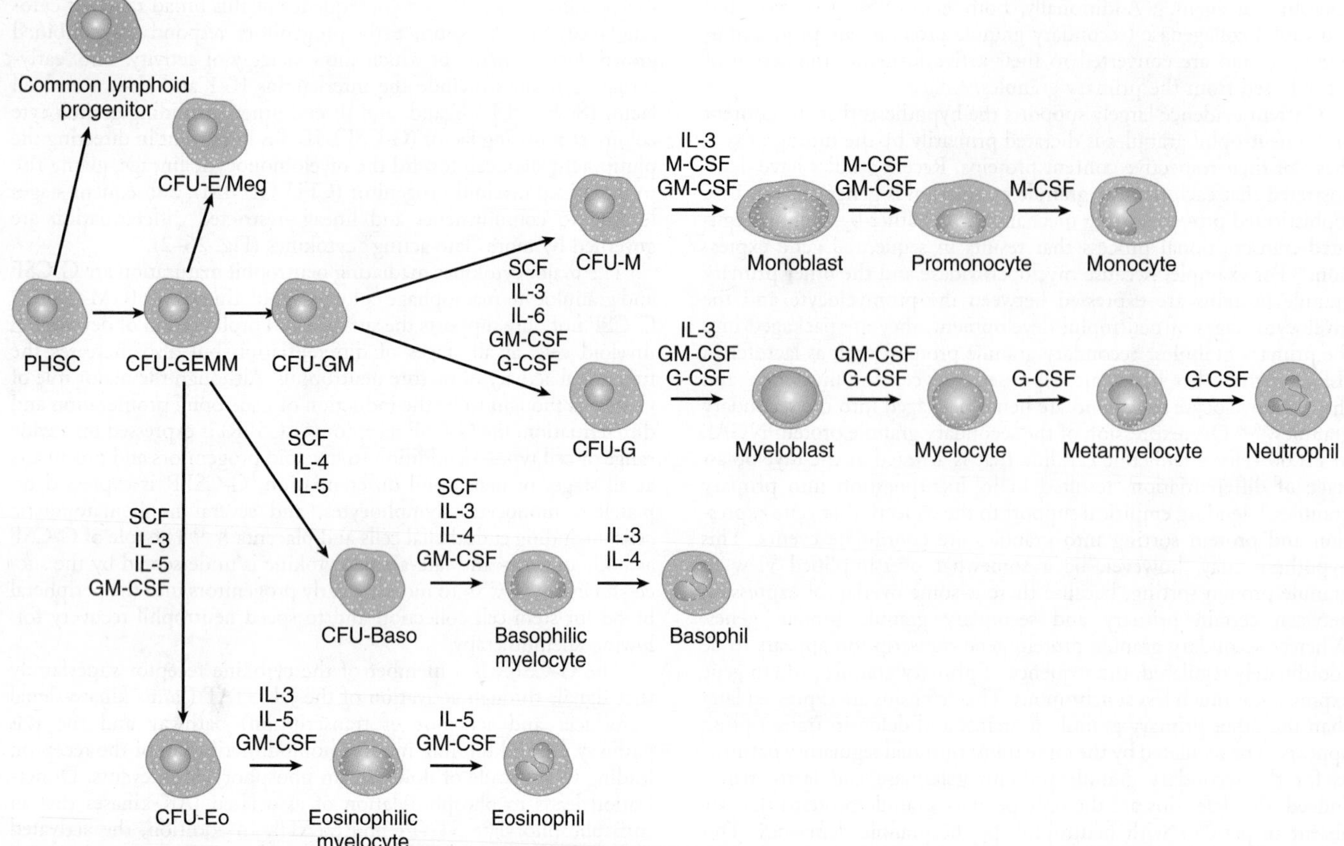

Figure 26–2 Cytokine regulation of granulocytic progenitors. CFU-Baso, colony-forming unit-basophil; CFU-E/Meg, colony-forming unit-erythrocyte/megakaryocyte; CFU-Eo, colony-forming unit-eosinophil; CFU-G, colony-forming unit-granulocyte; CFU-GEMM, colony-forming unit-granulocyte/erythrocyte/macrophage/megakaryocyte; CFU-GM, colony-forming unit-granulocyte/macrophage; CFU-M, colony-forming unit-macrophage; G-CSF, granulocyte colony-stimulating factor; GM-CSF, granulocyte-macrophage colony-stimulating factor; IL, interleukin; M-CSF, monocyte colony-stimulating factor; PHSC, pluripotent hematopoietic stem cell; SCF, stem cell factor.

been well established.[58,59] Studies of the regulation of individual genes that show tissue- and stage-specific myeloid expression have implicated a small number of transcription factors that are responsible for directing both phenotypical myeloid maturation and the expression of functionally important myeloid genes.[57,58,60–62] As described in detail subsequently, this role is underscored by the observations in AML, in which disruption of differentiation and defective myeloid-specific gene expression are linked to pathognomonic chromosomal translocations that result in the dysregulation of transcription factor expression.

Maturation of multipotent progenitor stem cells into specialized blood cells (lymphocytes, erythrocytes, neutrophils, monocytes, and eosinophils, among others) is regulated by a well-orchestrated interplay of transcription factors that are capable of instructing the expression of a specific set of genes within a specified lineage.[57,58,60,63] Gene knock-out technology and overexpression studies, in conjunction with newer techniques that involve the use of multicolor fluorescence-activated cell sorting (FACS), have aided in delineating several transcription factors critical to the development of specific hematopoietic lineages.[58,62,64] On the basis of these studies, critical transcription factors have been classified into two major categories. The first category includes factors such as stem cell leukemia transcription factor (SCL), GATA2, and acute myeloid leukemia transcription factor-1 (AML-1) that influence differentiation to all of the hematopoietic lineages; the second category comprises the master regulators of lineage development, including GATA1, PU.1, and CCAAT enhancer-binding protein-α (C/EBPα).[57] These factors not only promote lineage-specific gene expression but also suppress alternative lineage pathways. Fig. 26–3 summarizes the postulated role of several key transcription factors during hematopoietic development. Myeloid progenitors exhibit multilineage patterns of gene expression. In a recent study Laslo et al[65] elegantly demonstrated that cell fate determination is dependent upon subtle changes in expression levels of transcription factors, which regulate differential lineage maturation. For example, levels of PU.1 expression are increased by Egr-1/Nab-2 in developing macrophages; at the same time, Egr-1 represses the expression of the neutrophil specific Gfi-1 transcription factor, thereby simultaneously repressing the neutrophil development program (See Fig. 26–4).

Transcription Factors Regulating Myeloid Differentiation and Myeloid-Specific Gene Expression

AML-1. AML-1 (Runx 1) belongs to a family of highly conserved transcription factors that harbors a 128-amino-acid motif referred to as the Runt domain. The Runt domain functions in DNA binding, protein-protein interaction, ATP binding and contributes to nuclear localization.[66] This family of transcription factors, also known as the core binding factor (CBF) family, has been implicated in specification of cell fate and has a role in myeloid differentiation and lineage-specific granulocytic function.

AML-1 is the DNA-binding α-subunit of the CBF complex. Together with CBFβ, a widely expressed protein that enhances the DNA-binding affinity of the α-subunit, AML-1 binds the consensus DNA motif 5′ Pu ACCPuCA 3′ as a dimer.[67] Disruption of the

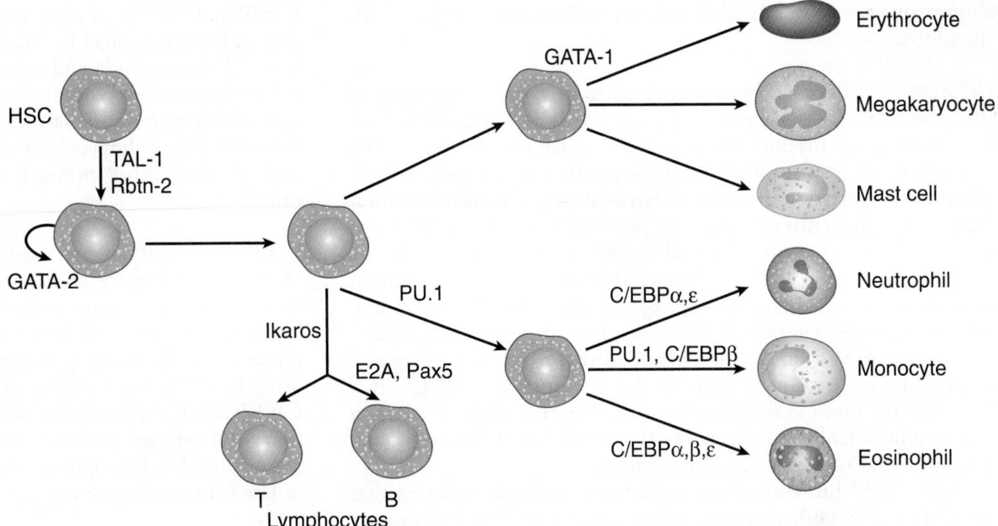

Figure 26–3 Simplified schema of transcriptional regulation of hematopoiesis. C/EBP, CCAAT enhancer-binding protein; HSC, hematopoietic stem cell; SCL, stem cell leukemia transcription factor.

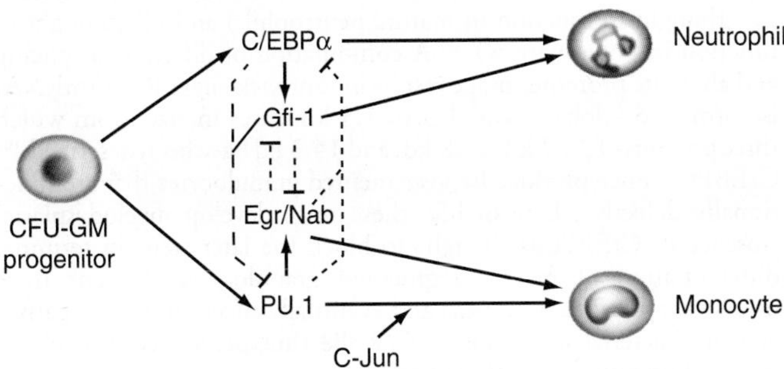

Figure 26–4 Transcription factor cross-talk affecting neutrophil and monocyte development.

AML1 gene in mice results in embryonic lethality resulting from a failure of definitive hematopoiesis in the fetal liver.[68] Although high levels of AML-1 expression have been reported in the early stages of myeloid differentiation, expression levels of AML-1 decrease beyond the promyelocytic stage of differentiation.[69] In concordance with its pattern of expression, AML-1 has been implicated in regulating a number of genes expressed early in the myeloid development pathway, including GM-CSF, macrophage colony-stimulating factor (M-CSF) receptor, myeloperoxidase, NE, and IL-3, among others.[69–72] In addition to activating lineage-specific myeloid markers, AML-1 has been shown to stimulate the G_1 to S transition in myeloid and lymphoid cell lines.[73]

A significant percentage (10%–20%) of human leukemias have been found to be associated with mutations in the *AML1* gene.[74] Most common of these is the t(8;21) translocation, which results in the AML-1-ETO (*e*ight *t*wenty-*o*ne oncoprotein) fusion protein. In AML-ETO, the Runt domain of AML-1 is fused in frame with the ETO transcriptional co-repressor.[75] The fusion protein has been hypothesized to function predominantly as a repressor that inhibits expression of genes that are normally activated by AML-1. For example, the tumor suppressor gene p14/p19(ARF), a critical AML-1 target gene that is necessary for the activation of p53 function, is normally activated by AML-1 but is repressed by AML-1-ETO.[76] The mechanisms underlying AML-1 function through its target genes are not yet fully understood.[77] Recent studies in sea urchins, however, have suggested that AML-1 regulates genes that contribute to chromatin architecture during cell proliferation.[66]

Studies involving mouse knock-in models of AML-1-ETO expression have indicated that the fusion protein alone is not sufficient to cause leukemia.[78] These animals are more susceptible to mutagen-induced AML, however, suggesting that AML-1-ETO is part of a multistep process that contributes to leukemogenesis.[79] Although the fusion partner of AML-1 (eg, ETO) may contribute to the role of the AML-1 fusion protein in leukemogenesis, the primary cause of the disease is thought to be the dysregulation of AML-1-specific target genes that are directly dependent on the Runt domain of AML-1.[80]

CCAAT Enhancer-Binding Protein Family of Transcription Factors. CCAAT enhancer-binding proteins (C/EBPs) are a family of basic region-leucine zipper (b-ZIP) transcription factors that recognize the consensus DNA-binding sequence 5′TKN NGYAAK3′ (Y = C or T; K = T or G) within the regulatory regions of target genes. C/EBP family proteins have been shown to bind DNA as either homo- or heterodimers. This family of transcription factors, which plays a crucial role in hematopoiesis, includes C/EBPα,-β,-γ, -δ,-ε, and -ζ (CHOP-GADD 153), all of which contain highly homologous carboxyl-terminal (C-terminal) dimerization (leucine zipper) domains and DNA-binding (basic region) motifs but differ in their amino-terminal (N-terminal) transactivation domains-with the exception of CHOP-GADD 153, which lacks this domain altogether.[81] Of interest, CHOP-GADD 153 can dimerize with and inhibit transactivation by C/EBPα,-β, and -ε and is found at a breakpoint in liposarcomas resulting in the TLS-CHOP fusion protein.[82]

With the exception of C/EBPε, which is expressed exclusively in the late stages of granulopoiesis and in T lymphocytes, the other C/EBP members are expressed in a wide variety of cells including liver, adipose tissue, lung, intestine, adrenal gland, and peripheral blood mononuclear cells and placenta.[81] Both C/EBPβ and C/EBPδ are expressed at high levels in late-stage granulocytes.[36] The C/EBP family members are known to exert pleiotropic effects in the tissues in which they are expressed. This may be due to their tissue- and stage-specific expression, their ability to dimerize with members of their own family and of the Fos/Jun and ATF/CREB families of transcription factors, and their ability to interact with other transcription factors such as nuclear factor-κB (NF-κB) and specificity protein-1 (Sp-1).[62]

The C/EBP factors have been implicated in regulating the differentiation of a variety of tissues. C/EBPα plays a role in adipocyte differentiation: Inhibition of C/EBPα blocks adipocyte differentiation, and overexpression of C/EBPα induces adipocyte differentiation.[83] Regulation of constitutive hepatic genes as well as acute-phase response genes in the liver involves several C/EBP family members, in particular, C/EBPα.[84] Modulation of myelomonocytic differentiation is also attributed to the activity of C/EBP family members.[81] The importance of this family of transcription factors in myeloid differentiation has been demonstrated by the study of hematopoietic abnormalities observed in mice with targeted disruption of C/EBPα, -β, and -ε.

C/EBPα. C/EBPα has been postulated to be a master regulator of the granulopoietic developmental program. It is expressed at high levels throughout myeloid differentiation and has been shown to bind to the promoters of multiple myeloid-specific gene promoters regulating gene expression at many different stages of myeloid maturation. Although C/EBPα$^{-/-}$ mice die perinatally because of defects in gluconeogenesis that result in fatal hypoglycemia,[85] they also have a selective early block in the differentiation of granulocytes without affecting either monocyte/macrophage maturation or the differentiation of other hematopoietic lineages. Myeloid cells of C/EBPα$^{-/-}$ mice lack G-CSFR, and it has been postulated that lack of mature neutrophils in these mice may be due to the lack of G-CSFR.[86] However, the myeloid defect in C/EBPα$^{-/-}$ mice is more severe than that seen in G-CSFR$^{-/-}$ mice, suggesting that C/EBPα has additional functions vital to granulocytic maturation.

The C/EBP proteins all are expressed in multiple isoforms that are generated by both alternative transcription initiation and alternative splicing. C/EBPα itself is translated from two different start sites, yielding a 42-kd and a 30-kd isoform. Mutations in C/EBPα have been demonstrated in a subset (7%) of patients with AML with normal karyotypes. These mutations result from frameshifts in the N terminus of the C/EBPα gene resulting in the production of a nonfunctional protein. Studies by Tenen and colleagues have shown that the 30-kd isoform of C/EBPα (αp30) is preferentially formed in the setting of AML-associated mutations in C/EBP. In their studies, this isoform showed poor binding to target promoters and was presumed to act by decreasing C/EBPα DNA binding.[87] They concluded that the 30-kd isoform has a dominant negative activity that leads to a loss of C/EBPα function.[57,61] Additionally, the AML-ETO protein associated with the t(8;21) AML physically interacts with C/EBPα, thereby inhibiting the transactivation function of C/EBPα.[88]

The expression of C/EBPα is associated with growth arrest and differentiation of granulocyte precursor cells. This block in proliferation is thought to occur via the interaction of C/EBPα with the cyclin-dependent protein kinases cdk2 and cdk4, resulting in a block in cell proliferation by inhibiting these cell cycle kinases. In addition, C/EBPα inhibits E2F-dependent transcription, which in turn contributes to inhibition of cell proliferation and induction of differentiation associated with C/EBPα-induced granulopoiesis.[89,90]

C/EBPβ. Expression of C/EBPβ increases during myeloid maturation and has been shown to be important for monocyte/macrophage gene expression and development.[91] Mice lacking the C/EBPβ gene demonstrate decreased B-cell levels and defects in macrophage activation and function and are more prone to microbial infections.[92] The C/EBPβ knock-out studies reveal that this transcription factor is not essential for myeloid development per se, but knock-in of C/EBPβ into the C/EBPα locus of C/EBPα$^{-/-}$ mice rescues granulopoiesis.[93] Several monocyte/ macrophage-specific genes are activated by C/EBPβ, including the G-CSF receptor, lysozyme, CD11c, monocyte chemoattractant protein-1 (MCP-1), IL-6, IL-8, and nitric oxide synthase, among others.[60] Three isoforms of C/EBPβ are generated from a single transcript through the use of three translation initiation sites and a leaky ribosome scanning mechanism.[81,94] The shortest of these isoforms, initiated at the most 3′ AUG, results in the formation of LIP (*l*iver-enriched *i*nhibitory *p*rotein), which lacks the N-terminal activation domain present in full-length C/EBPβ and has been implicated as a negative regulator of C/EBPβ function.[93] It has been suggested that the ratio of C/EBPβ to LIP may affect cellular proliferation and differentiation.[95] The activity of C/EBPβ is regulated post-transcriptionally through protein-protein interactions and covalent modifications. For example, in early myeloid progenitor cells, C/EBPβ is found in an unphosphorylated state in the cytoplasm. However, on differentiation, C/EBPβ becomes phosphorylated and translocates to the nucleus.[96]

C/EBPγ. C/EBPγ is a ubiquitously expressed C/EBP family member that was first identified by its affinity for *cis*-regulatory sites in the Ig heavy chain promoter and enhancer. C/EBPγ contains a C/EBP-like b-Zip domain but lacks an N-terminal transactivation domain and can inhibit transcriptional activation of other C/EBP members in some cell types.[97] Impairment of natural killer (NK) cytotoxic activity and of interferon-γ production has been reported in C/EBPγ$^{-/-}$ mice.[98]

C/EBPδ. C/EBPδ is expressed at low or undetectable levels in several tissues of adult mice and humans. Expression has been shown to dramatically increase on induction with bacterial lipopolysaccharide and inflammatory cytokines, suggesting a role for C/EBPδ in acute-phase and inflammatory response. Double-knock-out experiments using C/EBPβ and C/EBPδ suggest a synergistic role for these two C/EBP family members in controlling terminal adipocyte differentiation.[99] Of interest, both C/EBPβ and C/EBPδ are expressed during late neutrophil development and have been postulated to play roles in late neutrophil gene expression.[36]

C/EBPε. CCAAT enhancer-binding protein ε (C/EBPε) is the most recently described C/EBP protein. The human C/EBPε gene resides on chromosome 14 and is transcribed by two alternative promoters, Pα (thought to function in mature neutrophils) and Pβ (thought to function in bone marrow).[100] A combination of differential splicing and alternate promoter usage results in four messenger RNA (mRNA) isoforms 2.6 kilobases and 1.3 to 1.5 kilobases in size, from which three proteins of 32.2 kd, 27.8 kd, and 14.3 kd have been described.[101] C/EBPε$^{-/-}$ mice produce hyposegmented granulocytes that are functionally defective. Late in life, these mice develop myelodysplasia. Absence of C/EBPε is thought to block the later steps in terminal differentiation of mature segmented granulocytes. Mutant mice usually survive 2 to 5 months and eventually succumb to low-pathogenicity bacterial infections.[101] C/EBPε thus plays a crucial role in terminal granulocytic differentiation.[100]

C/EBPε$^{-/-}$ mice have wild-type levels of the G-CSF receptor,[101,102] and the defects manifested in these mice are confined to late-stage gene expression associated with the function of the mature neutrophil. Recently it has been demonstrated that the ability of G-CSF to regulate myeloid differentiation is dependent on the induction of C/EBPε. Verbeek and colleagues[103] showed that the mRNA of several genes including p47 phox (a component of the neutrophil NADPH oxidase complex), as well as the secondary granule protein (SGP) genes, are either absent or abnormal in the bone marrow of C/EBPε$^{-/-}$ mice. These investigators further suggest that C/EBPε plays a critical role in the regulation of host antimicrobial defense.

Neutrophils from C/EBPε$^{-/-}$ mice have morphologic and biochemical features very similar to those observed in patients with neutrophil-specific specific granule deficiency (SGD). SGD is an extremely rare congenital disorder that is characterized by frequent and severe bacterial infections.[104,105] Patients with SGD have defects in neutrophil function including atypical nuclear morphology, impaired bactericidal activity, and abnormalities in neutrophil migration; they also lack both neutrophil and eosinophil secondary granule proteins.[105,106] Recent sequence analyses of genomic DNA from two patients with SGD revealed mutations within the C/EBPε gene, resulting in a mutant protein lacking the dimerization and DNA-binding domains and hence transcriptional activity.[86] Lack of functional C/EBPε activity has been postulated to underlie the observed pathology in these patients.[86,107]

C/EBPζ. C/EBPζ-C/EBP homologous protein (CHOP)-is a C/EBP family member that was originally isolated as the product of a gene induced in response to DNA-damaging agents. It has subsequently been shown to be induced by various extracellular or endoplasmic reticulum stresses. The basic region of CHOP is less well conserved than that of the other C/EBP family members, and CHOP does not seem to bind to canonical C/EBP *cis* elements.[94] CHOP has been shown to interfere with the transcriptional activity of C/EBPβ in a manner dependent on its leucine zipper.[94]

PU.1. PU.1 is a member of the Ets family of transcription factors and is expressed abundantly in B cells and macrophages.[108] Expression of PU.1 has also been reported in granulocytes and eosinophils as well as in CD34$^+$ hematopoietic progenitor cells.[109] High levels of PU.1 expression in fetal livers of mice preferentially directs macrophage development, whereas low levels of PU.1 result in B-cell development.[110] C-Jun, another member of the b-Zip family of transcription factors, serves as a coactivator of PU.1 during macrophage development. It has been demonstrated that overexpression of c-Jun in myeloid progenitor cells results in macrophage development.[111,112] Recent studies have revealed that downregulation of c-Jun by C/EBPα is necessary for granulocytic maturation and appears to be the mechanism through which C/EBPα blocks macrophage development.[111] C/EBPα not only binds to the promoter of the *c-jun* gene and decreases its expression but also binds PU.1, thereby inhibiting its activity.[111]

PU.1-binding sites have been reported in almost all myeloid- specific promoters reported to date, including those for M-CSF, GM-CSF, and G-CSF receptors-all of which play critical roles in myeloid cell development.[60] PU.1 activity is modulated both by covalent modifications and by protein-protein interactions. For example, phosphorylation of PU.1 by casein kinase II or by JNK kinase leads to increased transcriptional activity.[113]

Abrogation of PU.1 expression in PU.1$^{-/-}$ mice results in perinatal lethality accompanied by the absence of mature monocytes/macrophages and B cells and delayed and reduced granulopoiesis.[114] Following in vitro differentiation, embryonic stem (ES) cells derived from PU.1$^{-/-}$ blastocysts fail to express mature myeloid cell markers, suggesting that PU.1 is not essential for the initial events associated with myeloid lineage commitment but is necessary for the later stages of development.

Growth Factor Independence-1 (Gfi-1). The Gfi-1 gene was first identified as a target of proviral insertion following infection with Moloney murine leukemia virus (MoMuLV) resulting in interleukin-2 (IL-2) factor independence in a rat lymphoma cell line (reviewed in[115]).Gfi-1 is a highly conserved gene that encodes a 55kD nuclear proto-oncogene that harbors six C_2H_2 type zinc finger domains at the carboxy terminus and a 20 amino acid stretch at the N-terminus known as the SNAG domain (reviewed in[115]). The SNAG domain which appears to be conserved in the Snail/Slug family of proteins, has been shown to confer transcriptional repressor activity on Gfi-1.[116] The human Gfi-1 gene is located on chromosome 1p22[117]and its closely related paralog Gfi1b maps to chromosome 9q34.[118] Gfi-1 is expressed at high levels in the thymus and bone marrow while Gfi1B expression is confined to the bone marrow and spleen.[119] Homozygous knockout of Gfi-1B results in embryonic lethality at day E15, despite the fact that myelopoiesis is normal. Death in these mice has been attributed to a failure of erythropoiesis and megakaryopoiesis.[120]

The essential role of Gfi1 in neutrophil differentiation became apparent only recently following two reports of gene disruption in mice.[121,122] Gfi1-null mice are severely neutropenic and eventually succumb to bacterial infections. In addition, these mice lack mature neutrophils and their granulocyte precursors are unable to differentiate into mature neutrophils upon induction with G-CSF. These cells also lacked SGP expression reminiscent of C/EBP−/− granulocytes. Gfi-1−/− bone marrow contained an atypical Gr1$^+$Mac1$^+$ myeloid precursor cell that appeared to share characteristics of both granulocyte and macrophage precursors. Ectopic expression of Gfi1 in ex-vivo sorted Gfi1−/− progenitor cells restored G-CSF mediated neutrophil maturation to these cells. These observations provide evidence for the critical role of Gfi1 in the neutrophil maturation program. Recent studies have further demonstrated that Gfi-1 together with C/EBPε synergize to transactivate the promoters of late myeloid genes. This synergy is lost in a patient with specific granule deficiency (SGD), who has a heterozygous substitution mutation in the C/EBPε gene and decreased levels of Gfi-1 in the bone marrow.[123]

Recently, heterozygous dominant negative mutations in the Gfi1 gene have been described in two patients with severe congenital neutropenia (SCN)[124] underscoring the role of Gfi1 in the neutrophil maturation pathway. It has been suggested that mutant Gfi1 in these patients alters the expression of elastase 2 (Ela2), mutations in which are commonly associated with SCN (see below). This observation confirms the vital role Gfi1 plays in human granulopoiesis.

CCAAT Displacement Protein. CCAAT displacement protein/cut (CDP) is a ubiquitously expressed, highly conserved, homeodomain protein with extensive homology to the *Drosophila* cut protein.[125] CDP has been shown to act as a repressor of developmentally regulated genes including the phagocyte-specific cytochrome heavy chain gene (gp91 phox), which is expressed exclusively in differentiating granulocytes.[126,127] Overexpression of CDP in 32Dcl3 myeloid cells blocks G-CSF-induced expression of SGP genes without blocking phenotypical maturation. CDP therefore acts as a negative regulator of stage-specific expression of both early and late neutrophil-specific genes.[128,129]

The CDP homeobox protein contains three highly conserved DNA-binding repeats referred to as *cut repeats* (CR1, CR2, CR3) and a homeodomain (HD), each of which is capable of recognizing and binding specific DNA motifs in target genes.[127,130–132] This may explain why the CDP molecule as a whole does not have a well-defined consensus DNA-binding sequence.[133] A recent study has shown that the cut repeats cannot bind DNA as monomers but in combination exhibit high DNA-binding affinity.[133] It has further been suggested that CDP-binding activity is restricted to proliferating cells, in which CDP target genes are repressed. These targets are upregulated as cells undergo cell cycle arrest and terminal differentiation, in association with a decrease in CDP binding.[126–129,134–136] Target genes of CDP include c-*myc*, c-*mos*, and the thymidine kinase (TK), cdk inhibitor p21(*WAF1/CIP1*), cystic fibrosis transmembrane conductance regulator (CFTR), transforming growth factor-β (TGF-β) type II receptor, gp91 phox, major histocompatibility complex (MHC) class I locus,[135,137–145] and neutrophil SGP genes.[128,129]

During myeloid differentiation, CDP binding has been shown to regulate genes that are expressed at widely disparate stages of differentiation. For example, it represses the gp91 phox gene, which is expressed at a much earlier time in myelopoiesis than is the case for the LF gene. The mechanism by which CDP mediates repression, and the means by which it modulates stage-specific gene expression at different stages of differentiation within a single lineage, are not fully understood. CDP is reported to have repressive activity associated with its ability to be displaced by a positive trans-acting factor involving the CR1 and CR2 cut repeats.[133] However, other modes of repressive activity involving the two active repression domains within the C terminus of CDP also have been reported.[125] Recently, CDP has been shown to function as a repressor of transcription via chromatin modification through recruitment of histone deacetylases (HDACs),[140] consistent with the notion that transcriptional silencing is associated with hypoacetylated histones.[143] Both acetylation and phosphorylation of CDP are post-transcriptional modifications that have been postulated to regulate CDP function.[144,145] Thus, differential modification, by phosphorylation or acetylation, of CDP-DNA complexes binding the promoters of target genes could result in the observed differential repression exerted by CDP during neutrophil development.

ROLE OF DEVELOPMENTALLY IMPORTANT NEUTROPHIL-SPECIFIC GENES IN DISEASE

Our understanding of the role of neutrophil-specific genes has been enhanced by the study of mice in which targeted disruption of a gene

Table 26–2 Differentiation-Specific Genes Implicated in Neutrophil Disorders

Transcription Factors
C/EBPα, PU.1, RARα, AML1, and others in AML
C/EBPε and Gfi-1 in specific granule deficiency
Gfi-1 in neutropenia
Granule and Functional Proteins
Neutrophil elastase in Kostmann syndrome and cyclic hematopoiesis
gp91 phox in chronic granulomatous disease
Adhesion Molecules, Receptors
Common β-chain of integrin receptors in LAD
G-CSF receptor mutations in AML arising in patients with Kostmann syndrome

AML, acute myeloid leukemia; C/EBP, CCAAT enhancer–binding protein; G-CSF, granulocyte colony-stimulating factor; gp91 phox, glycoprotein 91 phagocyte NADPH oxidase; LAD, leukocyte adhesion deficiency.

results in phenotypically important defects in neutrophil differentiation and function. Similarly, the importance of these genes has been underscored by the analysis of naturally occurring genetic events within these genes that result in human disease. The links between some genes and the diseases induced by their dysfunction may be anticipated by their important roles in neutrophil differentiation and function, whereas the pathophysiologic link between others and the diseases they induce remain elusive (Table 26–2).

Disruption of neutrophil transcriptional regulation is a recurring theme in the pathogenesis of leukemia. Nearly half of patients with AML have pathognomonic translocations resulting in the fusion of a transcription factor with a tissue-specific gene. These translocations have been shown to interfere with appropriate myeloid differentiation and emphasize the role of transcription factors in that process.[57,62]

As discussed previously, the same transcription factors that are implicated in the induction of neutrophil differentiation also direct the expression of genes encoding neutrophil-specific functional proteins. The link between morphologic differentiation and synthesis of neutrophil functional proteins is illustrated by the demonstration that disruption of C/EBPε signaling results in SGD, associated with both morphologic abnormalities and increased infections attributable to neutrophil functional defects.[85,99,107] It is intriguing that C/EBPε$^{-/-}$ mice share these abnormalities while also demonstrating a predilection for the development of myelodysplasia (ie, myelodysplastic syndrome [MDS]).[146] Although the development of MDS or AML has not been reported in patients with SGD, the deficiency is a rare disease described in less than a dozen patients, so a tendency to develop MDS/AML could easily be missed.

Other diseases have been linked to defects in functionally important neutrophil proteins. Abnormalities in integrin expression, notably, loss of the common β-chain of the integrin receptors, result in leukocyte adhesion deficiency,[6,147] and absence of any of the components of the reduced nicotinamide adenine dinucleotide phosphate (NADPH) oxidase leads to chronic granulomatous disease.[148]

Abnormalities in granule protein gene expression again underscore the complexity of the granulocyte functional program. Congenital absence of many individual granule proteins, including myeloperoxidase,[149] lactoferrin,[150] and transcobalamin,[151] has been described. In the absence of the more global defects seen in SGD, which presumably reflect more complex abnormalities than simple protein deficiency, these defects tend to be incidental laboratory findings with minimal or no associated pathology.

One prominent exception to that observation is the association between point mutations in the gene encoding NE (ELA2; neutrophil elastase) and severe congenital neutropenia (SCN), or Kostmann syndrome. The pathogenesis of SCN originally was sought in studies of G-CSFR, supported by the observation of a truncation mutation in G-CSFR in select patients with Kostmann syndrome.[152] It was later demonstrated that these were acquired mutations that may predispose the patient to secondary AML but did not constitute the pathologic basis for the neutropenia itself. Subsequent studies have implicated NE in the pathogenesis of SCN. NE is a primary granule protein that digests elastin and has been implicated in the pathogenesis of emphysema.[153] Recent linkage studies have linked heterozygous abnormalities in the NE gene to both SCN (Kostmann syndrome) and cyclic hematopoiesis.[154–156] The link between elastase and the control of neutrophil cell mass remains a mystery.

EOSINOPHIL PRODUCTION

Eosinophil precursors constitute approximately 3% of marrow progenitors, of which about two thirds are myelocyte precursors and the remainder mature eosinophils. Eosinophilic myelocytes are large cells with a single-lobed nucleus. The characteristic specific granules of eosinophils contain major basic protein, eosinophil cationic protein, eosinophil peroxidase, and eosinophil-derived neurotoxin. Eosinophils also contain primary granules that contain Charcot-Leyden crystal protein. Mature eosinophils are released into the marrow, where they circulate up to 18 hours before migrating to the tissues.[157]

Eosinophils proliferate and mature under the influence of IL-3, IL-5, and GM-CSF. Evidence suggests that these cytokines are secreted by T cells as the stimulus to eosinophil production in many disorders associated with eosinophilia. Recent studies of idiopathic hypereosinophilic syndrome have described activating mutations in the platelet-derived growth factor receptor-α (PDGFR-α) that result in constitutive tyrosine kinase activation and eosinophil proliferation.

Transcriptional regulation of eosinophilic differentiation is mediated through PU.1 C/EBPα and -β. Because these same factors serve to induce myeloid differentiation, the modulation of the signals determining the choice between these two lineages is not well defined. It has been proposed that levels of GATA-1 may be important in determining whether C/EBP expression induces the eosinophilic or the myeloid maturation program (see Chapter 45).[158]

BASOPHIL AND MAST CELL PRODUCTION

Basophils and mast cells mediate allergic responses, where they are the central cells involved in IgE-induced immune responses to parasites and other allergens. Both cell types are derived from marrow precursors, but they have a very different ontogeny (see Chapter 73).[159]

Basophils have a bilobed nucleus and characteristic intensely staining purple granules that may cover the nucleus. These granules contain glycosaminoglycans, predominantly heparin. Basophils differentiate from marrow progenitors and are released from the marrow as mature cells, where they circulate briefly, with a lifespan similar to that of neutrophils. Maturation is induced in response to IL-3, which serves both to induce basophilic differentiation and to mediate activation of mature basophils. Although IL-3 is the primary mediator of basophil development, studies of IL-3-null mice have demonstrated that it is not required for baseline production of basophils. It is, however, required for the induction of basophilia in response to parasitic infection.[160]Other cytokines that influence basophil proliferation include GM-CSF, IL-5, and SCF.

Mast cells arise from marrow precursors but are released into the circulation as immature cells. They circulate only briefly in the peripheral blood before migrating to the tissues, where they complete their maturation. There remains some question about whether mast cells and basophils arise from a common precursor.[161] In vitro studies showed that adding SCF to IL-3 to cultured CD34$^+$ cells results in an increased proliferation and maturation of both basophils and mast cells but did not establish a common progenitor cell for the two lineages.[162] It is clear that SCF is especially effective in inducing mast cell proliferation; in fact, activating mutations in c-Kit, the SCF receptor, is the underlying molecular defect in most cases of systemic mastocytosis.

MONOCYTOPOIESIS

Monocyte Ontogeny

Stages of Monocyte Differentiation

Monocytes originate in the bone marrow from promonocytes, which constitute approximately 3% of the total cells in the normal marrow.[3] Promonocytes have round nuclei and basophilic cytoplasm. Differentiation occurs rapidly, with a maturation time of 50 to 60 hours, associated with two rounds of replication and morphologic maturation marked by progressive lobulation of the nucleus.[163,164] Stress-induced release of monocytes occurs primarily through their premature release from the proliferating pool.[152] Survival in the blood is short, approximately 8 to 72 hours.[165] Monocytes then enter the tissues, where they develop into macrophages that may survive 2 to 3 months. Tissue-fixed macrophages are found in the lung (alveolar macrophages), the liver (Kupffer cells), the spleen, and the central nervous system (glial cells).

Monocytes also may serve as precursors to a subset of dendritic cells. Dendritic cells are professional antigen-presenting cells that arise from both myeloid and lymphoid precursor cells.[166] The myeloid subset of dendritic cells arises from a precursor that can alternatively differentiate into macrophages.[167,168] Similar cells have been generated for immunotherapy by exposing peripheral blood monocytes to GM-CSF and IL-4 in vitro.[169]

Markers of Monocyte Maturation

Unique surface markers of monocyte maturation have been difficult to identify. In the mouse, the marker F4/80 was identified as a nearly universal marker of monocytes and macrophages; this antigen has been shown to be homologous to the human EGF module containing mucin-like hormone receptor 1.[170] The function of this receptor is unknown, because the knock-out mouse has no phenotype.[171] Monocyte precursor cells express the M-CSF receptor, lysozyme, the Fcγ receptor (II/III),[172] and the scavenger receptor.[173] Mature monocytes, like neutrophils, show high-level expression of CD11b/CD18. Following differentiation to macrophages, the cells acquire expression of macrosialin (CD68), a glycoprotein of unknown function that may play a role in lipoprotein metabolism.[174] Macrophages also express sialoadhesin, a member of the sialic acid-binding receptor family. Although its precise function has not been proved, sialoadhesin mediates binding to sialic acid moieties on cell surfaces and probably plays a role in macrophage cell-cell interactions and cell-extracellular matrix interactions.[175]

CD14 is a major functional surface protein of the monocyte/macrophage lineage.[176] CD14 is the receptor for lipopolysaccharide (LPS), leading to monocyte/macrophage activation.[177] More recent studies have suggested that CD14 also may have a role in apoptosis.[165]

Monocytes contain both primary (peroxidase-positive) and secondary (peroxidase-negative) granules. The primary granules of monocytes, like those of neutrophils, contain myeloperoxidase.[178] Secondary granule fusion with the membrane on stimulation of monocytes results in upregulation of Mac1 and p150,95 and is thought to play a role in adhesion and diapedesis of stimulated monocytes.[179]

Control of Monocytopoiesis

Cytokine Regulation of Monocyte Proliferation and Differentiation

The effects of colony-stimulating factor 1 (CSF-1), the primary regulator of mononuclear phagocyte production, are thought to be mediated by the high-affinity receptor tyrosine kinase CSF-1 receptor (CSF-1R), encoded by the c-*fms* proto-oncogene.[180] A total of five human or mouse mRNAs resulting from alternative splicing and the alternative use of the 3′ untranslated region resulting in three isoforms of the CSF-1 protein: a secreted proteoglycan, a secreted glycoprotein, and a membrane-spanning cell surface proteoglycan have been described.[181]

The phenotypes of Csfl-null mice and of mice harboring an inactivating mutation in the coding region of CSF-1 ($Csf^{op}/Csf1^{op}$) (osteopetrotic mice) are virtually identical; features include toothlessness, low body weight, low growth rate, and deficient tissue macrophages. Additionally, the mutant mice have defects in both male and female fertility.[180] Compared with their wild-type littermates, splenic erythroid burst-forming unit and high-proliferative-potential colony-forming cell levels in both $Csf1^{op}/Csf1^{op}$ and $Csf1^{-}/Csf1^{-}$ mice were significantly elevated, consistent with a negative regulatory role for CSF-1 in erythropoiesis and in the maintenance and proliferation of primitive hematopoietic progenitors. The circulating CSF-1 concentration in CSF receptor-null ($Csf1R^{-}/Csf1R^{-}$) mice was elevated 20-fold, in agreement with the previously reported clearance of circulating CSF-1 by CSF-1R-mediated endocytosis. Despite their overall similarity, several phenotypical characteristics of the $Csf1R^{-}/Csf1R^{-}$ mice were more severe than those of the $Csf1^{op}/Csf1^{op}$ mice. The results indicate that all of the effects of CSF-1 are mediated via the CSF-1R, but that additional effects of the CSF-1R could result from its CSF-1-independent activation.[182]

Signaling through the CSF-1R appears to be critical for monocyte/macrophage development. Although little is known about the events that lead to stimulation of a monocyte/macrophage specific array of genes, it is clear that several transcription factors, probably stimulated by M-CSF-related signaling events, play vital roles in the development of this lineage. It should be noted, however, that the ability of phorbol esters to induce monocytic differentiation of myeloid cell lines through activation of the protein kinases Cα and Cδ suggests a role for the PKC pathway in monopoiesis.[63]

IL-3, G-CSF, and tumor necrosis factor (TNF) all have been shown to synergize with M-CSF in the proliferation of macrophages.[183] G-CSF also has been shown to induce the increased release of monocytes; this is an indirect effect dependent on the presence of M-CSF.[184] Monocytes also have been demonstrated to have functional G-CSF receptors, although G-CSF appears to function mainly to decrease monokine secretion rather than to increase monocyte proliferation.[185]

Transcriptional Regulation of Monocyte Differentiation

Of the several transcription factors that regulate the development of the monocyte/macrophage lineage, the most well-established is PU.1 (discussed earlier), because abrogation of PU.1 expression in $PU.1^{-/-}$ mice results in perinatal lethality accompanied by the absence of mature monocytes/macrophages and B cells and delayed and reduced granulopoiesis.[114] A number of factors, the most notable of which is c-Jun, cooperate with PU.1 to regulate monocyte-specific genes.

c-Jun. The c-*jun* proto-oncogene encodes the transcriptional activator protein AP-1. As a member of the early response genes, c-*jun* is rapidly and transiently activated in response to external proliferative signals.[186] The expression of c-Jun as well as related family members JunB and JunD is upregulated during monocytic differentiation.[187] In addition, overexpression of c-Jun in M1, U937, or WEHI-B D^+ myeloid cell lines, as well as in myeloid progenitor cells, was found to result in partial monocytic differentiation.[111,112,187] However, $c\text{-Jun}^{-/-}$ fetal liver cells are capable of reconstituting hematopoiesis in syngeneic recipients, suggesting that c-Jun is not required for myeloid development.[188] This finding may reflect a compensatory role played by other Jun family proteins.

As discussed, c-Jun serves as a coactivator of PU.1 during macrophage development. Recent studies have revealed that downregulation of *c-jun* by C/EBPα is necessary for granulocytic maturation and appears to be the mechanism through which C/EBPα blocks macrophage development[111] (Fig. 26–4). C/EBPα not only binds to the promoter of the *c-jun* gene and decreases its expression but also binds to PU.1, thereby inhibiting its activity.[111] Such transcription factor cross-talk resulting in subtle changes in the levels of transcription factors within a given lineage appears to be an emerging paradigm through which master regulators of lineage specification, such as C/EBPα and PU.1, direct lineage-specific development by directly upregulating lineage-specific genes as well as by blocking the progression of alternate lineages.[57]

Other Transcription Factors Modulating Monocyte Development

Egr-1. Egr-1 belongs to a family of zinc finger transcription factors, and is expressed in a number of tissues and at various points in development including the terminal stages of macrophage and neutrophil differentiation.[189,190] Egr-1 is necessary for monocytic differentiation of myeloid cell lines U937 and M1 and prevents factor-induced granulocytic differentiation of HL60 and 32Dcl3 cells.[178,179] Additionally, ectopic expression of Egr-1 in myeloid marrow progenitors was found to result in an increase in the number of CFU-M at the expense of CFU-G.191. However, mice lacking Egr-1 develop normal numbers of macrophages, a phenomenon attributed to the possible compensatory effects of other Egr family members.[181]

C/EBPβ. As discussed, expression of C/EBPβ increases during myeloid maturation and has been shown to be important for monocyte/macrophage gene expression and development.[90]

MafB and c-Maf. The transcription factors MafB and c-Maf belong to a family of basic-leucine zipper (b-Zip) factors that bind DNA as dimers.[193] The Maf proteins can dimerize with members of other b-Zip family proteins including c-Jun, fos, and NF-E2 in erythroid cells.[194,195] Ectopic expression of MafB in myeloblasts directed their expression to macrophages,[196] whereas overexpression of c-Maf in HL60 and U937 myeloid cells resulted in monocytic differentiation.[197]

SUGGESTED READING LIST

Bjerregaard MD, Jurlander J, Klausen P, et al: The in vivo profile of transcription factors during neutrophil differentiation in human bone marrow. Blood 101:4322, 2003.

Buck M, Chojkier M: Signal transduction in the liver: C/EBPβ modulates cell proliferation and survival. Hepatology 37:731, 2003.

Coffman J: Runx transcription factors and the developmental balance between cell proliferation and differentiation. Cell Biol Int 27:315, 2003.

D'Alo F, Johansen LM, Nelson EA, et al: The amino terminal and E2F interaction domains are critical for C/EBPα-mediated induction of granulopoietic development of hematopoietic cells. Blood 109:3163, 2003.

Hattori T, Ohoka N, Hayashi H, Onozaki K: C/EBP homologous protein (CHOP) up-regulates IL-6 transcription by trapping negative regulating NF-IL6 isoform. FEBS Lett 541:33, 2003.

Hock H, Hamblen M, Rooke H, et al: Intrinsic requirement for zinc finger transcription factor Gfi-1 in neutrophil differentiation. Immunity 18:109, 2003.

Horwitz M, Benson KF, Duan Z, et al: Role of neutrophil elastase in bone marrow failure syndromes: Molecular genetic revival of the chalone hypothesis. Curr Opin Hematol 10:49–54, 2003.Jafar-Nejad H, Bellen HJ. Gfi/Pag-3/senseless zinc finger proteins: a unifying theme? Mol Cell Biol 24:8803, 2004.

Jongstra-Bilen J, Harrison R, Grinstein S: Fcgamma-receptors induce Mac-1 (CD11b/CD18) mobilization and accumulation in the phagocytic cup for optimal phagocytosis. J Biol Chem 278:45720, 2003.

Keeshan K, Santilli G, Corradini F, et al: The transcription activation function of C/EBP(alpha) is required for induction of granulocytic differentiation. Blood 102:1267, 2003.

Khanna-Gupta A, Hong S, Zibello T, et al: Growth factor independence 1 (Gfi-1) plays a role in mediating specific granule deficiency (SGD) in a patient lacking a gene inactivating mutation in the C/EBP gene. Blood 109:4181, 2007.

Khanna-Gupta A, Zibello T, Sun H, et al: Chromatin immunoprecipitation (ChIP) studies indicate a role for CCAAT enhancer binding proteins alpha and epsilon (C/EBP alpha and C/EBP epsilon) and CDP/cut in myeloid maturation-induced lactoferrin gene expression. Blood 101:3460, 2003.

Laslo P, Spooner CJ, Warmflash A, et al: Multilineage transcriptional priming and determination of alternate hematopoietic cell fates. Cell 126:755, 2006.

Parfrey H, Mahadeva R, Lomas DA: Alpha$_1$-antitrypsin deficiency, liver disease and emphysema. Int J Biochem Cell Biol 35:1009, 2003.

Person RE, Li FQ, Duan Z, et al: Mutations in proto-oncogene GFI1 cause human neutropenia and target ELA2. Nat Genet 34:308, 2003.

Rangatia J, Vangala RK, Singh SM, et al: Elevated c-Jun expression in acute myeloid leukemias inhibits C/EBPalpha DNA binding via leucine zipper domain interaction. Oncogene 22:4760, 2003.

Tenen DG: Disruption of differentiation in human cancer: AML shows the way. Nat Rev Cancer 3:89, 2003.

Wehrle-Haller B, Imhof BA: Integrin-dependent pathologies. J Pathol 200:481, 2003.

REFERENCES

For complete list of references log onto www.expertconsult.com

CHAPTER 27

THROMBOCYTOPOIESIS

Alan B. Cantor

INTRODUCTION

Platelets, once regarded simply as "blood dust," are now recognized to play essential roles in hemostasis. Not only do they form a hemostatic plug and initiate thrombus formation in the event of vascular injury, but they also repair minute vascular damage that occurs on a daily basis. Platelets are also thought to be involved in wound healing and angiogenesis through delivery of key growth factors, such as vascular endothelial growth factor (VEGF), platelet-derived growth factor (PDGF), and transforming growth factor beta 1(TGF β1) to sites of vascular injury. Disorders associated with platelet production carry significant morbidity and mortality in humans because of hemorrhage, thrombosis, bone marrow fibrosis, bone marrow failure, and/or hematologic malignancy. Platelets are generated from their precursor cells, megakaryocytes, through a complex process. For a long time, the extreme rarity of megakaryocytes significantly hampered studies aimed at understanding the molecular mechanisms underlying platelet biogenesis. However, the purification and cloning of thrombopoietin (Tpo), the major megakaryocyte cytokine, in 1994 has enabled considerable progress to be made. These new insights provide an important foundation for improved diagnosis and treatment of disorders of thrombocytopoiesis. This chapter reviews the current understanding of megakaryocyte biology and platelet production, highlighting connections with human disease.

MEGAKARYOCYTE BIOLOGY

Megakaryocyte Development

Although platelets were described as early as the 1840s, it was not until 1906, in a seminal study by James Homer Wright, that their origin from megakaryocytes was first recognized.[1,2] Megakaryocytes are large polyploid cells that reside predominantly within the bone marrow during postnatal life. They are rare cells, constituting only approximately 0.1% of nucleated cells under normal steady-state conditions.[3] They develop from common bipotential megakaryocyte-erythroid progenitor (MEP) cells, which are themselves derived from common myeloid progenitor (CMP) cells, and ultimately from pluripotential hematopoietic stem cells (HSCs). Once committed to the megakaryocytic lineage, megakaryocyte progenitors undergo a series of dramatic maturational steps ultimately tailored to their final task of platelet production and release. These include changes in proliferative capacity, cell size, nuclear content, organelle biogenesis, membrane development, and cytoskeletal rearrangement. The large increase in cell size is linked to an unusual process termed *endomitosis*, in which cells replicate their DNA but fail to undergo cytokinesis (see Endomitosis discussion below). Mature megakaryocytes reach diameters of approximately 100 microns and contain DNA content as high as 128N.[4–8] They contain a multilobulated nucleus enclosed by a single nuclear membrane. Their abundant cytoplasm is filled with ribosomes, platelet-specific granules, mitochondria, and complex intracellular membrane systems. Although megakaryocytes reside predominantly within the bone marrow, they are also found in peripheral blood, spleen, and lung under normal conditions.[9–15] These extramedullary megakaryocytes release platelets, but their contribution to total thrombocytopoiesis is estimated to account for at most 7% to 15%.[14,16]

Megakaryocyte Progenitors

Like other hematopoietic progenitor cells, megakaryocyte progenitors can be cultured in vitro using semisolid media. Animal studies using these colony assays have allowed delineation of a hierarchal developmental pathway of megakaryocyte progenitor maturation based on proliferative potential, DNA content, morphologic criteria, and gene expression pattern (Fig. 27–1). This pathway can be conceptually divided into three broad stages: proliferating megakaryocytic progenitors, which contain normal DNA content (2N–4N); nonproliferating immature megakaryocytes (4N–8N DNA content); and nonproliferating mature megakaryocytes (DNA content 8N–128N). Within the proliferating megakaryocyte progenitor compartment, the earliest detectable cell is the megakaryocyte high-proliferative-potential colony-forming cell (MK-HPP-CFC), which is capable of generating macroscopically visible colonies containing a few thousand megakaryocytes. This corresponds to a proliferative capacity of approximately 8 to 10 replicative cycles. These cells require interleukin-3 (IL-3) and simultaneous activation of the protein kinase C and cyclic adenosine monophosphate (cAMP) signaling pathway.[17]

The burst-forming unit megakaryocyte (BFU-MK), which is thought to be a direct progeny of MK-HPP-CFC, is more mature than the MK-HPP-CFC, but retains a high degree of proliferative potential, developing "bursts" of individual colony-forming cells. These colonies contain approximately 100 to 500 megakaryocytes, representing approximately 5 to 7 replicative cycles. In humans, BFU-MK cells require mitogenic stimulation with IL-3 or granulocyte-monocyte (GM)–colony-stimulating factor (CSF) and synergistic signaling with stem cell factor (SCF; also called *kit-ligand*), interleukin-11 (IL-11), interleukin-1-alpha (IL-1α), and Tpo.[18–21] They are also resistant to treatment in vitro with 5-fluorouracil (5-FU).[18,20]

The most mature proliferating cell is the colony-forming unit megakaryocyte (CFU-MK), which has very limited proliferative potential, representing only two to five cell divisions (4–32 megakaryocytes per colony).[22] This progenitor responds to a variety of single growth factors, such as IL-3 and GM-CSF, and coregulators such as SCF, fms-like tyrosine kinase 3 (FLT3) ligand, and Tpo.[19,23,24] They express early markers of differentiation such as glycoprotein IIb (GPIIb) and platelet factor 4 (PF4) before initiating endomitotic cell cycles.[5]

Immature Megakaryocytes: Promegakaryoblasts

Promegakaryoblasts are transitional cells intermediate between proliferating progenitor cells and post-mitotic, mature megakaryocytes.[25,26] These cells are not readily observed morphologically in vitro or in bone marrow specimens but can be identified by their expression of megakaryocyte- or platelet-specific markers, such as platelet peroxidase, platelet GPIIb/ glycoprotein IIIa (GPIIIa), and von Willebrand factor (vWF).[27,28] They have DNA content levels intermediate between proliferating progenitors and mature megakaryocytes. Promegakaryoblasts respond to a variety of cytokines in vitro including IL-3, SCF, interleukin 6 (IL-6), and Tpo, to produce large polyploid megakaryocytes.[4,29] At least three distinct subpopulations of promegakaryoblasts have been identified based on different physiochemical characteristics, morphology, antigen expression, and enzyme content.[4,28,30,31]

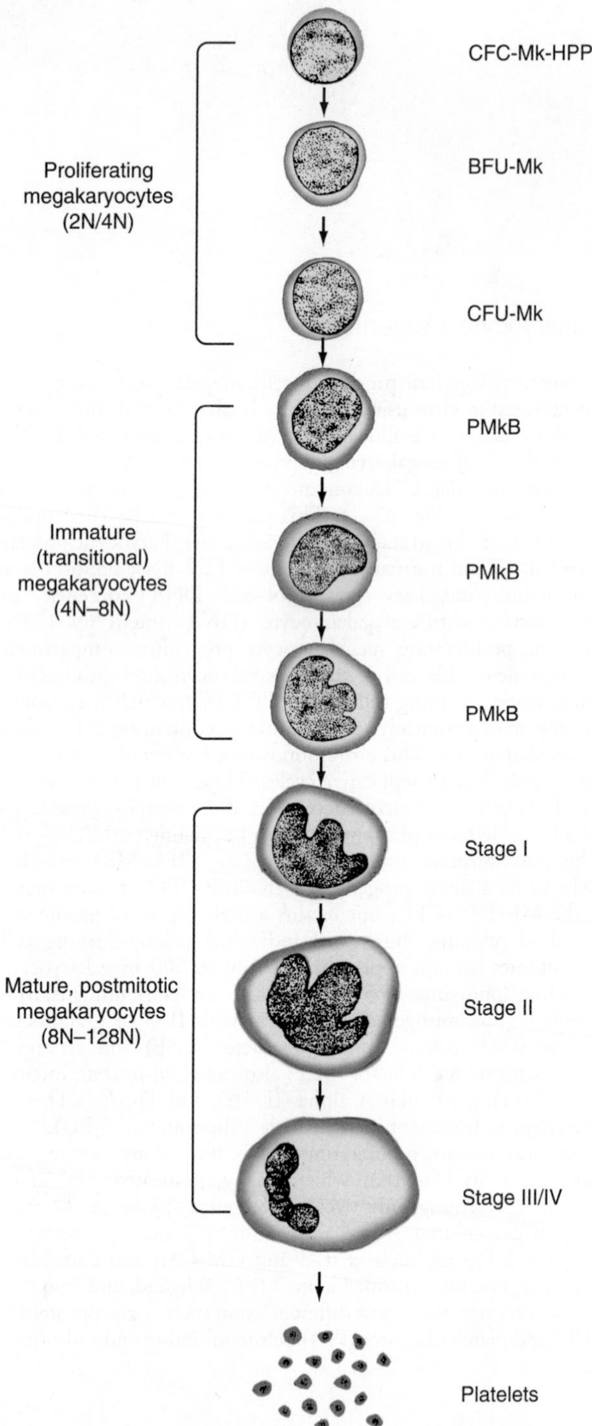

Figure 27–1 Cellular hierarchy of megakaryocyte development. Megakaryocytes can be conceptually divided into three stages: The proliferating progenitor cells, which have the typical 2N/4N DNA content; the immature megakaryocytes, which have an intermediate DNA content and are transitional between the progenitor cells and the more mature cells; and the mature, post-mitotic cells, which have an 8N to 128N DNA content. BFU-Mk, burst-forming unit megakaryocyte; CFC-Mk-HPP, colony-forming unit megakaryocyte high proliferative potential; CFU-Mk, colony-forming unit megakaryocyte; PMkB, promegakaryoblast.

Mature Megakaryocytes

Morphologically recognizable megakaryocytes exist in at least three distinct maturation stages as defined by their morphology (Fig. 27–2). The megakaryoblast (stage I) is characterized by a high nucleus-to-cytoplasm ratio and scanty basophilic cytoplasm, reflecting the large amount of protein synthesis occurring in these cells. The promegakaryocyte (stage II) is the cell in which the cytoplasmic volume and number of platelet-specific granules increase. The granular or "platelet shedding" megakaryocyte (stages III and IV) is the most mature cell. In reality, these stages likely represent a continuum.

Prospective Isolation of Megakaryocyte Progenitor Cells

Weissman and colleagues reported the prospective isolation of clonogenic committed megakaryocyte progenitor cells from the bone marrow of adult C57BLKa-Thy1.1 mice based on selection of a unique cell surface immunophenotype: c-kit^{+}Sca-1^{-}IL7Rα^{-}Thy1.1^{-}Lin^{-}CD9^{+}CD41^{+}FcγR^{lo}CD34^{+}D38^{+}.[32] This fraction represents approximately 0.01% of the total nucleated bone marrow cells and gives rise to CFU-MK and occasionally BFU-MK in colony assays. The ability to prospectively isolate pure populations of committed murine megakaryocyte progenitor cells should facilitate future studies of megakaryocyte development. Identification of a comparable set of surface markers for human megakaryocyte progenitors, if possible, would be of great usefulness.

Structure of Mature Megakaryocytes

Mature megakaryocytes contain a large multilobulated polyploid nucleus often situated toward the periphery of the cell. They have abundant cytoplasm, which contains platelet-specific secretory granules, alpha (α–) granules and dense granules (for more detailed discussion on platelet secretory granule development, see review by King and Reed[33]) (Fig. 27–3). The biogenesis of α-granules and dense granules begins in immature megakaryocytes, and both granule types develop concomitantly.[34] α-Granules are 200 to 500 nm in diameter and have a dense center and fine granular matrix.[35] Megakaryocytes synthesize many of the constituents of α-granules and target them to the granules. These include von Willebrand factor (vWF),[36] fibronectin,[36] P-selectin,[37] fibrinogen receptors, PF4,[38] coagulation factor V,[39] and plasminogen activator inhibitor type 1 (PAI-1),[40] among others. In addition, some constituents, such as fibrinogen, are taken up by megakaryocytes through endocytosis and/or pinocytosis and stored in α-granules.[41,42] Dense granules are 200 to 300 nm in diameter and consist of a halo encircling an electron opaque core.[35] They contain many soluble hemostatic factors such as serotonin, catecholamines, adenosine, adenosine diphosphate (ADP), adenosine triphosphate (ATP), and calcium. Their limiting membranes contain glycoproteins such as αIIbβ3, glycoprotein Ib (GPIb), and P-selectin, which are also present in α-granules, as well as unique membrane proteins such as granulophysin.[43–46] Multivesicular bodies (MVBs) serve as intermediates in the biogenesis of both α-granules and dense granules.[34,41] It has been proposed that they constitute a sorting compartment between α-granule and dense granule components.[34]

The megakaryocyte cytoplasm contains at least two complex membranous systems; the demarcation membrane system (DMS) and the dense tubular system (DTS) (see Fig. 27–3). The DMS consists of an extensive network of tubular and flattened membranous structures that interconnect with one another and communicate with the extracellular space.[47–50] Whole cell patch-clamp studies in living rat megakaryocytes have shown that they are electrophysiologically contiguous with the plasma membrane.[51] The open canalicular system (OCS) of platelets shares many features of the megakaryocyte

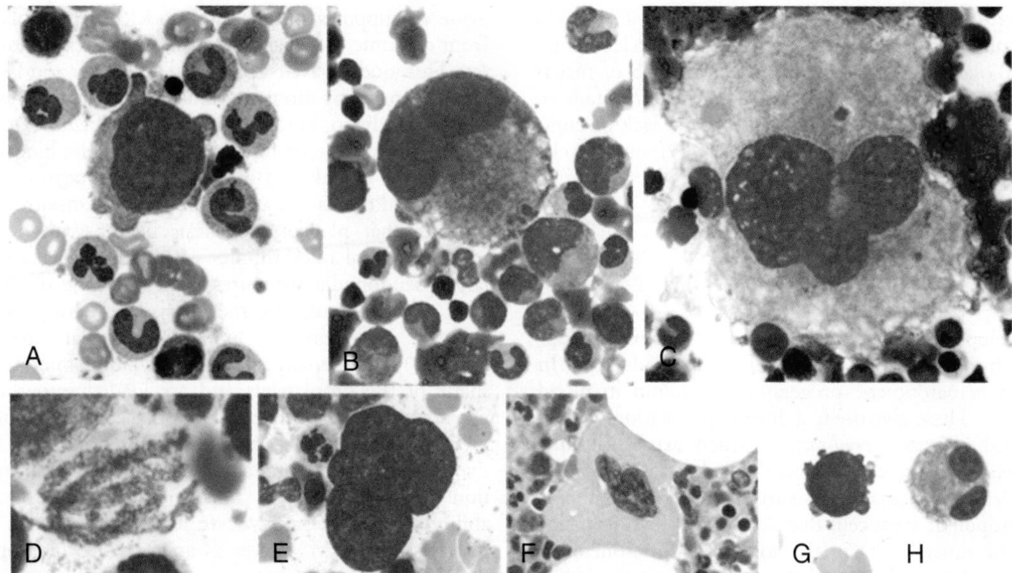

Figure 27–2 Megakaryopoiesis and megakaryocytes. **A,** Megakaryoblast (stage I) with intermediate ploidy level. Cytoplasm is scant. Note prominent cytoplasmic pseudopods. (**B**) Promegakaryocyte with early platelet production (stage II). (**C**) Mature, high ploidy megakaryocyte (stage III or IV) with abundant cytoplasm. Note cells traveling through cytoplasm. This is referred to as emperipolesis and is not uncommonly seen in large megakaryocytes. (**D**) Portion of megakaryocyte cytoplasm in long strand. Fragments of these can sometimes be seen in the blood and are referred to as *proplatelets*. (**E**) Megakaryocyte nucleus denuded of its platelets and cytoplasm. (**F**) Mature megakaryocyte seen in a tissue section of bone marrow biopsy. (**G**) Megakaryoblast from a patient with acute megakaryoblastic leukemia. Note cytoplasmic pseudopods. (**H**) Micromegakaryocyte from a patient with myelodysplasia. Note small, low ploidy (2–4N) nucleus, but mature cytoplasm.

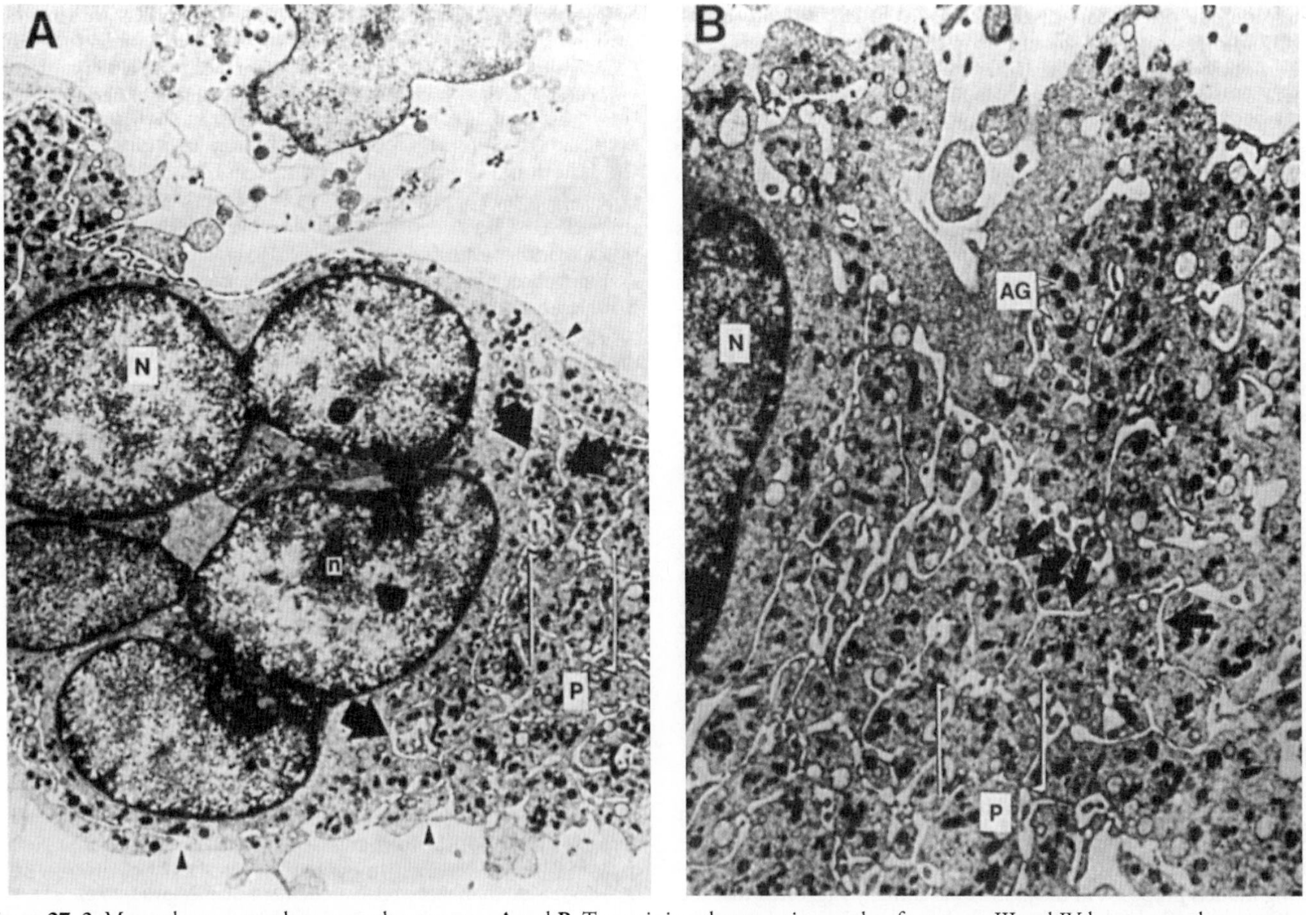

Figure 27–3 Mature human megakaryocyte ultrastructure. **A** and **B**, Transmission electron micrographs of two stage III and IV human megakaryocytes. AG, α-granules; n, nucleolus; N, nucleus; P, a platelet field within the megakaryocyte cytoplasm; *arrowheads*, openings of the demarcation membrane system (DMS). *(Courtesy of Dr. Maryann Weller.)*

DMS, and may represent a remnant of this structure.[35] The DMS serves as a vast membrane reservoir for proplatelet and platelet formation (see Platelet Biogenesis discussion below). The DTS of megakaryocytes is distinct from the DMS. Unlike the DMS, it fails to stain with surface membrane tracer dyes, indicating a lack of communication with the plasma membrane.[52] The DTS is thought to be a site of platelet prostaglandin synthesis.[53]

Ontogeny of Megakaryopoiesis

Hematopoiesis develops in distinct waves during embryonic development (see review by Tavian and Peault[54] for further details). In mammals, the first hematopoietic progenitors are found in blood islands of the yolk sac. These give rise to a distinct population of large erythrocytes, termed *primitive erythrocytes,* which express unique globin genes and retain their nucleus longer than adult-type or *definitive* erythrocytes. Definitive hematopoiesis arises later during embryogenesis from hematopoietic stem cells that develop de novo from the ventral aspect of the dorsal aorta in the aorta-gonad-mesonephros (AGM) region. These then seed the fetal liver, which serves as a major site of hematopoiesis during gestation. Eventually, hematopoiesis shifts to the bone marrow (and spleen in mice) where it is sustained postnatally.

Megakaryocyte progenitors have been detected in yolk sac as early as embryonic day 7.5 (e7.5) of mouse development.[55,56] They are capable of generating proplatelets and platelets after culturing in vitro.[55,56] Circulating platelets have been detected in the mouse embryo as early as e10.5.[56] Megakaryocytes cultured from early yolk sac have features somewhat distinct from those cultured from adult bone marrow, such as lower modal ploidy, smaller size, different cytokine requirements, and faster kinetics of platelet generation.[55] These unique progenitors disappear by e13.5. In addition, mixed erythroid-megakaryocyte colonies derived from the early yolk sac give rise to primitive erythrocytes. It has therefore been suggested that a separate wave of *primitive megakaryocytes,* akin to primitive erythrocytes, exists during early yolk sac stages of hematopoiesis.[55,56] These rapidly maturing megakaryocytes may prevent hemorrhage from the developing vasculature until definitive hematopoiesis is available to provide a steady supply of platelets.

Several pieces of evidence suggest that fetal liver megakaryocytes also have unique features compared to adult bone marrow-derived megakaryocytes. This could be because of either intrinsic differences in the progenitors, or possibly their interactions with different microenvironments. Megakaryocytes that develop from murine neonatal liver progenitors after transplantation into myeloblated mouse recipients are smaller and have lower ploidy levels than those derived from transplanted adult bone marrow.[57] However, these differences disappear by 1 month after transplant. In addition, several congenital disorders of megakaryopoiesis in humans, such as Down syndrome transient myeloproliferative disorder (DS-TMD) and thrombocytopenia and absent radius (TAR) resolve spontaneously after the newborn period, suggesting specific effects on fetal megakaryopoiesis (see GATA Family Transcription Factors discussion below). It is possible that these differences account for the delayed platelet engraftment often observed when umbilical cord blood is used as a source for hematopoietic stem cell transplantation in humans.[57]

Platelet Biogenesis

It has been estimated that each megakaryocyte produces between a few hundred to several thousand platelets.[13,16,58–60] The exact mechanism by which this occurs has been controversial, with several competing models proposed in the past. It was initially suggested that the DMS established platelet fields, which defined territories of prepackaged platelet contents.[61] These fields would generate platelets directly on breakdown of the megakaryocyte cytoplasm. However, prevailing evidence supports an alternate model in which platelets are released from dynamic megakaryocyte pseudopod extensions called *proplatelets.* This model was first proposed by Becker and DeBruyn in 1976,[62] and supported by ultrastructural studies later in the 1980s.[63–65] More recently, Italiano, Hartwig and their associates extended these earlier studies on proplatelet formation and platelet biogenesis using videomicroscopy of cultured murine megakaryocytes[66] (see Chapter 114 for detailed discussion and figures). These in-vitro experiments demonstrate that platelet biogenesis begins with a reorganization of unique cortical microtubules within the megakaryocyte to produce large pseudopodia structures from one pole of the megakaryocyte. This spreads across the megakaryocyte generating extensions that elongate into complex branching tubular proplatelet processes. During this time, organelles travel along microtubules within the shafts of the proplatelets and are loaded into the proplatelet tips where they are captured.[67] It is only at the tips of the proplatelets processes that platelets are shed. During proplatelet formation, extensive remodeling and branching occurs allowing for marked amplification of proplatelet ends. This phenomenon likely accounts for the ability of each megakaryocyte to generate such a large number of platelets. The DMS serves as an extensive membrane reservoir for these processes.[68,69]

Bone Marrow Spatial Cues and Megakaryocyte Maturation

There is mounting evidence that proliferation and terminal maturation of megakaryocyte progenitors occur in distinct spatial compartments within the bone marrow. In a simplified manner, the bone marrow space can be conceptually divided into distinct regions, a space adjacent to the cortical bone (an *osteoblastic niche*), an intermediate zone, and a *vascular niche* containing sinusoidal vessels lined with specialized bone marrow endothelial cells. HSCs are thought to reside in a quiescent state adjacent to the bone. Under appropriate conditions, they are recruited to generate hematopoietic multipotent progenitor cells, which leave the osteoblastic niche, perhaps in part

Inherited Causes of Thrombocytopenia

Although the most common cause of thrombocytopenia is immune thrombocytopenic purpura (ITP), it is important to maintain a high index of clinical suspicion for inherited disorders of thrombocytopoiesis. This is a particular problem as ITP is essentially a diagnosis of exclusion, and many inherited disorders mimic the macrothrombocytopenia seen in ITP. Making the correct diagnosis early is paramount, because it can spare patients unnecessary treatment with corticosteroids, other immunosuppressants, and/or splenectomy. In addition, it can be important in guiding decisions about surveillance for myelodysplasia or leukemia, screening for additional associated clinical problems, and/or possible family planning. Obtaining a careful family history, and sometimes obtaining blood counts on first-degree relatives, is important in fully evaluating patients with chronic thrombocytopenia. Associated abnormalities can provide important clues to the presence of a nonimmune familial thrombocytopenia. For instance, associated erythroid abnormalities and/or an X-linked inheritance pattern (GATA-1 mutations) (obligate females carriers can have dimorphic populations of platelets); leukocyte Dohle bodies, ± nephritis and sensineural hearing loss (Myh9 mutations); family history of myelodysplasia or myeloid leukemia (Runx-1 mutations); developmental delay, congenital cardiac anomalies, hand/face dysmorphogenesis (Paris-Trousseau/Jacobsen syndrome; Fli-1 [Ets-1] mutations); bleeding diathesis out of proportion to degree of thrombocytopenia (Bernard-Soulier syndrome). For a superb review of inherited thrombocytopenias and excellent diagnostic algorithm, see article by Balduini and colleagues.[281]

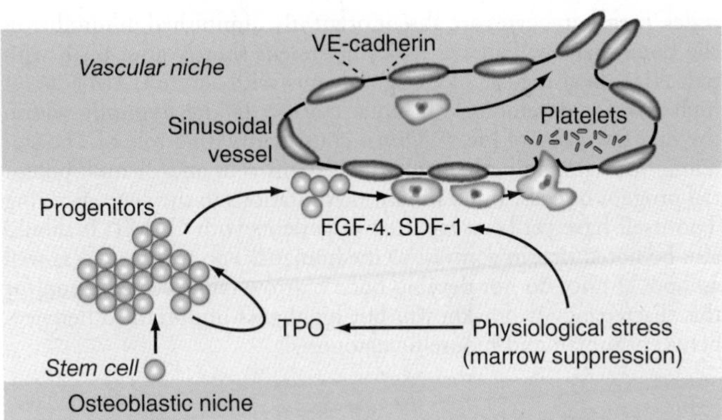

Figure 27–4 Model of terminal maturation of megakaryocytes at the bone marrow vascular sinusoid. Schematic diagram showing hematopoietic stem cells (HSCs) located predominantly adjacent to the cortical bone (osteoblast niche), megakaryocyte progenitors proliferating in the bone marrow space, and migration of progenitor cells to the vascular sinusoid (*vascular niche*) under the influence of chemokines such as stromal derived factor-1 (SDF-1) and fibroblast growth factor 4 (FGF-4). Once attached to the sinusoidal vascular endothelium, megakaryocyte progenitors cease proliferating, undergo terminal maturation and proplatelet formation, and shed platelets into the vascular sinusoidal space. TPO, thrombopoietin. VE, vascular endothelial. *(Reproduced with permission of Avecilla et al.*[70]*)*

under the regulation of metalloproteinases such as matrix metalloproteinase type 9 (MMP-9). The multipotent progenitors are then subject to expansion and lineage commitment under the influence of various cytokines and likely other signaling molecules. This is where Tpo is postulated to affect megakaryocyte progenitor proliferation and survival. Rafii and coworkers have shown that the chemokines stromal derived factor-1 (SDF-1; also called CXCL12) and fibroblast growth factor-4 (FGF-4) promote migration and attachment of murine megakaryocyte progenitor cells (which express the receptor for SDF-1, CXCR4) to the vascular endothelium, where they physically attach, mature, and produce intercalating pseudopod structures.[70,71] In fact, exogenous SDF-1 and FGF-4 restores thrombopoiesis in $Tpo^{-/-}$ or Tpo receptor $(c\text{-mpl})^{-/-}$ mice to near wild type levels. This occurs in the absence of enhanced megakaryocyte progenitor proliferation, and requires direct physical interaction with bone marrow endothelial cells. Based on these findings, Rafii and his colleagues have proposed a model in which megakaryocyte progenitors proliferate in an immature developmental state (in response to Tpo) in a nonvascular niche (Fig. 27–4). However, once the progenitors reach and adhere to the sinusoidal vessels in the vascular niche in response to chemokines, proliferation ceases, and terminal maturation and platelet release ensues. Work from other investigators supports this model. Multiple electron microscopy studies have captured megakaryocytes extending proplatelet processes through vascular endothelium and into bone marrow sinusoids.[62,63,72,73] Isolated megakaryocytes can be induced to form proplatelets after adhering to bovine corneal endothelial cells-derived extracellular matrix[74] or through binding of the megakaryocyte surface integrin $\alpha IIb\beta 3$ to fibrinogen, which is present in bone marrow vascular sinusoids.[75] Conversely, culture of megakaryocytes with bone marrow stromal cells inhibits megakaryocyte differentiation.[76,77]

CYTOKINE REGULATION OF THROMBOCYTOPOIESIS

Thrombopoietin Signaling

Thrombopoietin

It has been estimated that an adult human produces nearly 2×10^{11} platelets per day, and this number can increase four- to eightfold during times of increased demand.[16] The regulation of this process has been the subject of intense investigation. Kelemen first used the term *thrombopoietin* in 1958 to describe a humoral substance responsible for enhancing platelet production following the onset of thrombocytopenia.[78] However, it was not until 1994 that five independent groups succeeded in purifying and cloning the responsible cytokine, now known as Tpo (previously referred to as *c-mpl ligand*, megakaryocyte growth and development factor [MGDF] and megapoietin)[79–85] (see review by Kaushansky[86] for detailed discussion of the Tpo signaling system). The gene for thrombopoietin is located on chromosome 3q27. It encodes a 30 kd glycoprotein of 353 amino acids that can be divided into two structural domains; an amino terminal region with homology to human erythropoietin, and a carboxyl terminal region that contains multiple *N*- and *O*-linked oligosaccharides. The amino terminal 155 residues of human thrombopoietin share 21% sequence identity and 46% overall sequence similarity to human erythropoietin. This region mediates binding to the Tpo receptor (c-mpl). The carboxyl region does not share sequence homology with any known protein. Thrombopoietin is reported to enhance multiple stages of megakaryocyte maturation including cell size, cell ploidy, and platelet production.[79–81] The predominant sites of Tpo production are the liver and kidney, which secrete it constitutively.[80,83,87,88] Inducible expression of Tpo has been detected by more sensitive methods in bone marrow stroma and spleen in the setting of thrombocytopenia, although this likely accounts for only a minor fraction of total Tpo production.[87,89] Low level expression has also been reported in the amygdala and hippocampus of the brain.[90]

Thrombopoietin Receptor (c-mpl)

The receptor for Tpo (Tpo receptor; c-mpl) is the normal homologue of the oncogene v-mpl, the transforming gene of murine myeloproliferative leukemia virus.[91] It is a member of the type I cytokine receptor superfamily. Like the erythropoietin receptor, it is thought to function as a homodimer. The Tpo receptor is expressed on megakaryocyte progenitors, as well as earlier multipotential progenitors including MEPs, CMPs, and HSCs.[92–94] Tpo receptors are present on the surface of platelets at a estimated density of 20 to 200 receptors per platelet and bind Tpo with an affinity of 200 to 560 pM. Binding of Tpo to platelets plays an important role in the regulation of total body platelet mass by the Tpo-Tpo receptor system (see further discussion below). Both Tpo $receptor^{-/-}$ $(c\text{-}mpl^{-/-})$ and $Tpo^{-/-})$ knockout mice contain approximately 85% to 90% lower platelet and megakaryocyte numbers compared to wild type.[95–97] The structure of the megakaryocytes and platelets in these animals is normal, reinforcing the notion that Tpo signaling plays an important role in expansion and development of megakaryocyte progenitors, but not in terminal maturation and proplatelet release.[35] In addition, the residual platelet production in these mice suggests alternate cytokine, or possibly cytokine independent, pathways for thrombocytopoiesis. Interbreeding experiments of Tpo $receptor^{-/-}$ mice with knock-out mice for IL-3, IL-6, IL-11, or leukemia-inhibiting factor (LIF), or their receptors, show that these other cytokines are not responsible for the residual platelet production.[86]

Tpo Receptor Downstream Signaling Pathways

The Tpo receptor lacks intrinsic tyrosine kinase activity. Instead, ligand binding stimulates the cytoplasmic tyrosine kinase JAK2 (Janus-kinase 2) resulting in tyrosine phosphorylation of multiple targets, including STATs (signal transducers for activating transcription), Shc adaptor protein, and the Tpo receptor itself.[98] Additional signaling pathways activated upon Tpo receptor engagement include the mitogen-activated protein kinase (MAPK) p38, p42/p44 extracellular regulated kinase 1 and 2 (ERK1/ERK2), and phosphatidylinositol 3-kinase–Akt (PI3K-Akt) pathways.[98–101]

Several of these downstream signaling pathways have been shown to be functionally important in Tpo-mediated effects on megakaryopoiesis. Double STAT5a/STAT5b deficient mice have impaired platelet production as well as defects in early multipotent progenitor cells.[102] Moreover, megakaryocyte-selective overexpression of a dominant negative mutant STAT3 in transgenic mice reduces platelet recovery following 5-FU–induced myelosuppression.[103] These findings suggest a functional role for STAT family members in thrombopoiesis.

Studies in primary megakaryocytes show a requirement for PI3-Akt signaling in Tpo-induced cell cycling.[99] This involves silencing of the Forkhead O (FOXO) family of transcription factors.[98] Activation of the p42/p44-MAPK plays an important role in Tpo-induced maturation and endomitosis.[101]

Lnk, an adaptor protein implicated in immunoreceptor and cytokine receptor signaling, has recently been shown to negatively modulate Tpo signaling in megakaryocytes.[104] Overexpression of Lnk decreases Tpo-dependent megakaryocyte growth and polyploidization in bone marrow (BM)-derived cultures. Conversely, loss of Lnk expression by gene targeting results in increased numbers of megakaryocytes and accentuated polyploidization compared to wild type controls. This correlates with enhanced and prolonged Tpo-mediated induction of STAT3, STAT5, Akt, and MAPK signaling pathways.

Tpo Signaling in Hematopoietic Stem Cells

It has recently been recognized that the Tpo-Tpo receptor signaling system is not only important for megakaryocyte proliferation and development but also plays a role in hematopoietic stem cell survival, self-renewal, and expansion.[105–108] Tpo receptor$^{-/-}$ HSCs compete poorly with wild type HSCs, even at a ratio of 10 : 1, in murine bone marrow competitive repopulation studies.[108] The role of Tpo signaling in HSC expansion is in part caused by its activation of the homeobox domain containing transcription factor HOXA9, through a mechanism involving phosphorylation and nuclear translocation of its partner protein, MEIS1.[109]

Congenital Amegakaryocytic Thrombocytopenia

A bi-allelic mutation in the thrombopoietin receptor gene causes congenital amegakaryocytic thrombocytopenia (CAMT). In this disorder, megakaryocytes are absent or greatly diminished in number in the bone marrow. Patients typically present shortly after birth with petechiae, bruising, or bleeding. Patients with severe CAMT are at high risk for developing full bone marrow failure, typically within the first few years of life.[110] This is consistent with a role of Tpo signaling in maintaining hematopoietic stems cells and/or multipotential progenitor cells. Interestingly, no mutations in the gene encoding Tpo itself have yet been reported in patients with CAMT. It should also be noted that in contrast to the humans, Tpo receptor$^{-/-}$ (as well as Tpo$^{-/-}$) mice do not develop bone marrow failure. The reason for this discrepancy is not known, but highlights important differences between human and mouse hematopoiesis.

Essential Thrombocythemia

Essential thrombocythemia (ET) is a chronic myeloproliferative disorder associated with sustained megakaryocyte hyperproliferation, thrombocytosis, and abnormal platelet function leading to either hemorrhage or thrombosis (for more complete description, see Chapter 71). In 2005, an acquired activating mutation in the JAK2 gene (V617F JAK2) was identified by four independent groups in a large proportion (23%–57%) of patients with ET[111–114] (see review[115]). The identical mutation has also been identified in several other myeloproliferative disorders including polycythemia vera (65%–97% of patients) and idiopathic myelofibrosis (35%–95% of patients). How the identical mutation leads to distinct clinical entities is not presently understood. Mutations leading to constitutive activation of the Tpo receptor,[116,117] and mutations leading to enhanced translation efficiency of the Tpo gene[86,118] have also been reported in rare cases of familial thrombocytosis.

Regulation of Platelet Mass by Thrombopoietin

Platelet counts are typically held at a relatively fixed level in humans, ranging from 150,000–400,000 platelets/mm.[3] The maintenance of platelet number by the Tpo-Tpo receptor system involves an unusual homeostatic mechanism among hematopoietic cytokine-mediated regulation. This is sometimes referred to as the *Sponge model* (Fig. 27–5). Unlike other cytokines, Tpo is secreted predominantly in a

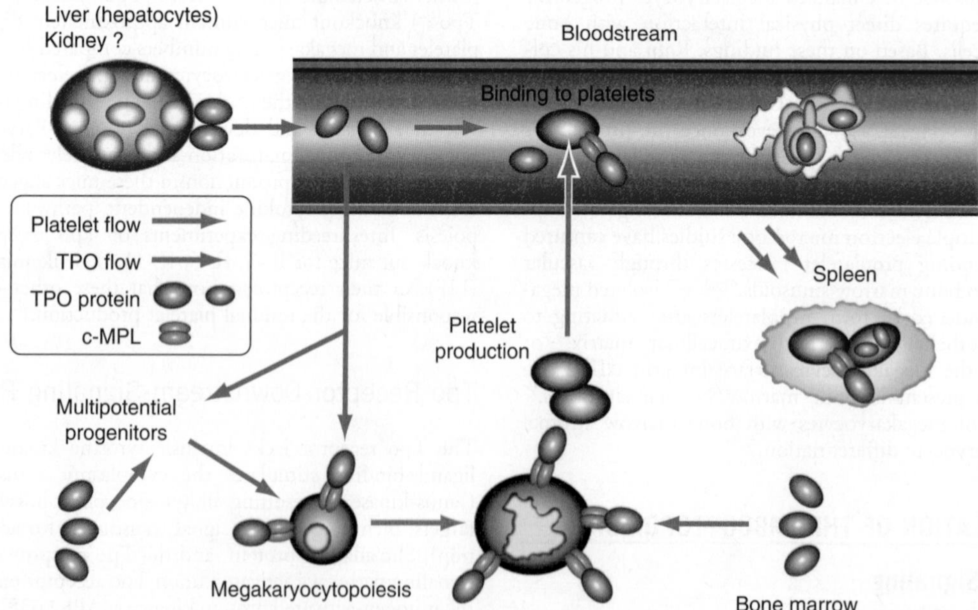

Figure 27–5 Regulation of platelet count by thrombopoietin: the *Sponge* model. Thrombopoietin (Tpo) is secreted at a constitutive rate primarily from liver and perhaps other sources such as the kidney, into the circulation. There, it binds with high affinity to Tpo receptors (c-mpl) present on the surface of platelets. The Tpo is then internalized by the platelets and degraded. Free Tpo (ie, Tpo not bound to platelets) enters the bone marrow and stimulates megakaryopoiesis. Thus, in the presence of high platelet counts, little free Tpo is available to stimulate megakaryopoiesis. Conversely, low platelet numbers lead to increased free Tpo and active megakaryopoiesis. The net result is preservation of total platelet mass.

constitutive manner, mostly from the liver and kidney. High-affinity Tpo receptors present on the platelet surface bind free Tpo and internalize it, where it is degraded.[86,119] Therefore, when platelet counts are low, less thrombopoietin is removed and more is available to stimulate megakaryopoiesis in the bone marrow. Conversely, when platelet counts increase above a given set point, they act as a "sink" for Tpo, binding and destroying it before it can stimulate megakaryopoiesis in the bone marrow. Thus, total platelet mass is preserved, rather than absolute platelet number. This may explain the mild-moderate thrombocytopenia seen in certain large platelet disorders, such as Bernard-Soulier syndrome (BSS).

Several pieces of evidence support this model. First, it has been known for more than 40 years that the peripheral blood platelet count varies inversely with plasma Tpo activity. Second, Tpo receptor deficient mice (c-mpl$^{-/-}$) have elevated levels of circulating Tpo, and this is reduced when the mice are transfused with washed platelets from normal mice.[95,120] Third, in contrast to platelets from Tpo-receptor deficient mice, platelets from normal mice bind purified radiolabeled Tpo and degrade it.[119–121] Fourth, Tpo levels are low to intermediate in normal individuals and in those with idiopathic thrombocytopenic purpura (where the bound Tpo is destroyed along with the platelets).[122] However, following chemotherapy, or in individuals with aplastic anemia, levels are markedly elevated.[122]

Although the model described above likely explains the predominant basal regulation of platelet number by the Tpo-Tpo receptor signaling system, overlying inducible mechanisms also probably exist. It has been shown that the Tpo gene is transcriptionally activated in bone marrow stroma and spleen during times of thrombocytopenia,[87,89] although the degree to which this can contribute to total Tpo levels is uncertain. In addition, IL-6 mediates upregulation of hepatic Tpo mRNA transcripts in inflammation-related thrombocytosis.[123]

Additional Cytokines Involved in Megakaryocytopoiesis

Although Tpo is the major cytokine regulating megakaryocytopoiesis, other cytokines have been shown to be active in vitro, particularly during earlier stages of megakaryocyte development. These include SCF,[19,124–128] IL-3,[124,126,129] IL-6,[124,128] IL-11,[81,129] LIF,[128] granulocyte colony-stimulating factor (GCSF),[128] and erythropoietin (Epo).[129] None of these factors are megakaryocyte-specific but act as synergistic coregulators with Tpo. Only SCF and Tpo have been shown to affect megakaryocyte development and platelet production in vivo using genetic ablation experiments in mice.[95,130] A thrombocytopenia phenotype has not been seen with knockout of IL-3, IL-6, IL-11 receptor, or LIF.

Cytokine Stimulation of Megakaryopoiesis for Clinical Use

Since the identification of Tpo as a major activator of megakaryocyte growth and maturation, there has been considerable interest in developing recombinant forms for clinical use in the treatment of chemotherapy-related thrombocytopenia and immune-mediated thrombocytopenia. Small pilot studies using a polyethylene glycol (PEG)ylated, truncated form of human Tpo (PEG-MGDF) showed activity in stimulating megakaryocyte growth and maturation, resulting in elevated platelet counts. However, some recipients subsequently developed thrombocytopenia because of the generation of a neutralizing antithrombopoietin antibody that cross-reacted with endogenous Tpo. The agent was therefore withdrawn from further testing. Since then, several nonimmunogenic thrombopoietic peptides and small, nonpeptide molecules have been under development (see recent review by Kuter).[131] A recent phase I/II placebo-controlled trial of AMG531, a synthetic molecule consisting of an immunoglobulin crystallizable fragment (Fc) linked to two identical peptide chains that activate the Tpo receptor, has been reported in a small series of adults with chronic, refractory immune thrombocytopenic purpura (ITP).[132] Nineteen of 28 patients (68%) treated at 1-mcg/kg and 3-mcg/kg doses in the combined studies experienced a response with an increase in the platelet count to the target range of 50,000 to 450,000 cells/mm^3 and at least twice the baseline count. The reported adverse effects consisted mostly of mild-moderate headache and transient decrease in the baseline platelet count after discontinuing treatment. No anti-AMG531 or antithrombopoietin antibodies were detected in the recipients. Further clinical study of this agent, as well as others in development, will be required before they can be recommended for clinical use. However, they represent a promising new development for the treatment of certain thrombocytopenic disorders.

IL-11 has multiple effects on in-vivo and in-vitro megakaryocytopoiesis.[21] It affects IL-3-dependent megakaryocyte colony formation and has a potent effect on megakaryocyte maturation. Administration of recombinant IL-11 to mice results in increased numbers of megakaryocyte progenitors, increased megakaryocyte polyploidization, and increased peripheral platelet counts.[133] Recombinant IL-11 has been approved for use in humans for the treatment of chemotherapy-induced thrombocytopenia.

ENDOMITOSIS

Endomitotic Cell Cycle

Megakaryocytes derive their name from their large and complex nuclei. This arises from an atypical cell cycle, termed the *endomitotic* cell cycle (see comprehensive review by Ravid et al [5])(Fig 27–6). Like normal diploid cells, the cycle begins with a G1 phase, followed by an S phase (DNA replication), and a G2 phase. The cells then enter an M phase, but unlike normal diploid mitotic cells, fail to complete anaphase B, telophase, or cytokinesis.[134] Instead they proceed directly to the next G1 phase and subsequent rounds of DNA replication. As DNA ploidy increases, multiple spindle poles and centrosomes form, but chromosome segregation is incomplete and asymmetric.[135,136] During each endomitotic cell cycle, the nuclear envelope breaks down, and later reforms as a single nuclear membrane around all of the sister chromatids.[134,137] The end result is a polyploid cell with a multilobulated nuclei encapsulated by a single nuclear membrane.[6,138] Mature human megakaryocytes have been observed to reach ploidy levels as high as 128N.[5–8] The term *endoreduplication* has at times been used erroneously to describe megakaryocyte polyploidization. Endoreduplication refers to a cell cycle that involves DNA replication but no entry into M phase.[139]

Role of Endomitosis in Thrombocytopoiesis

The advantage of megakaryocytes undergoing endomitosis remains unknown. It has been speculated that it provides a means for generating the abundant membrane, protein, biosynthetic cargo and energy required for the dramatic final stages of proplatelet elaboration and platelet release.[5] Several circumstantial pieces of evidence support this model. First, it is known that megakaryocyte DNA content correlates with megakaryocyte cell size, mRNA content, protein production, and eventual numbers of platelets released.[6,140–142] Second, an increased DNA content of megakaryocytes precedes increases in platelet count during recovery from acute thrombocytopenia.[6] Third, increases in cytoplasmic volume and maturation occur predominantly, if not completely, in stage II and III megakaryocytes, which do not synthesize DNA.[7,6,140,143–145] Fourth, in polyploid megakaryocytes (4N–32N), all alleles of the genes studied (ie, ITGA2B [GPIIb], VWF, ACTB [β-actin], HSPA1 [HSP70], MPL, FLI1, and ZFPM1 [FOG-1]) have been found to be transcriptionally active.[146]

Mechanisms of Endomitosis in Megakaryocytes

The molecular mechanisms mediating endomitosis in megakaryocytes are incompletely understood. Studies investigating endomitosis

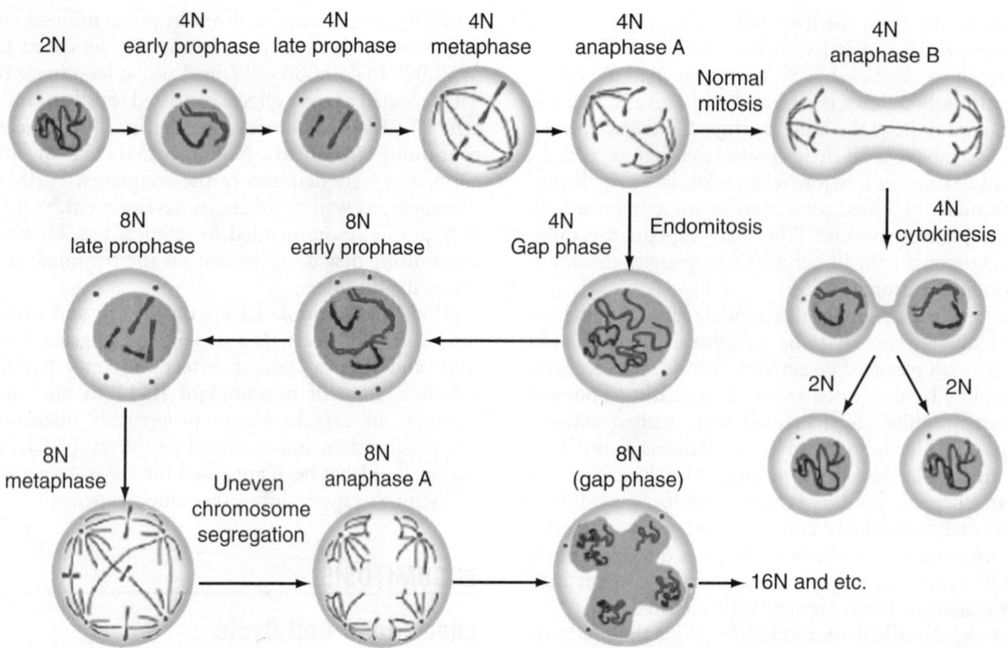

Figure 27–6 The endomitotic cycle in megakaryocytes. Schematic diagram depicting stages of the cell cycle in cells undergoing endomitosis (*bottom left*) versus normal mitosis (*right*). Endomitotic and mitotic cells share all stages of the cell cycle up until Anaphase A. Normal mitotic cells proceed through Anaphase B and complete cytokinesis, yielding two daughter cells each with 2N DNA content. In contrast, endomitotic cells fail to undergo Anaphase B or cytokinesis, and proceed to the next cycle following a Gap phase. Subsequent rounds produce multicentric spindles with uneven chromosome segregation. A single nuclear membrane (*shown in pink*) reforms after each round of endomitosis. Centrosomes are shown as blue dots. *(Reproduced by permission Ravid et al.[5])*

have been hampered by the rarity of megakaryocytes, difficulty separating direct effects from general perturbations of cell maturation, complications associated with synchronizing the cell cycle, use of transformed cell lines, and potential differences between rodent and human megakaryocytes.

Cyclins and Cyclin-dependent Kinases

Two classes of proteins control the cell cycle in mammalian cells. These are the cyclins, so named for their cyclical synthesis and degradation during the cell cycle, and cell division kinases (Cdks) (also known as *cyclin-dependent kinases*). Together these two families of proteins form a protein-kinase complex in which the regulatory unit is the cyclin and the catalytic unit is the Cdk. The role of these kinase complexes in cell cycle control is complex. At least seven members of the cyclin gene family and seven distinct Cdk genes have been identied.[147–149]

Given the importance of cyclins and Cdks in controlling cell cycle, they have been the focus of considerable attention in investigations of the mechanisms underlying megakaryocyte endomitosis. The most evidence probably exists for a role of the D-type cyclins in megakaryocyte endomitosis.[150,151] The D-type cyclins are unique in that their activity can be modulated by extracellular mitogens. Megakaryocytes express cyclin D3 and, to a lesser extent cyclin D1.[5] Levels of both of these factors increase after treatment with Tpo. Overexpression of cyclin D3 results in increased megakaryocyte ploidy in transgenic mouse models.[150] Complexes of cyclin D3 and its major kinase subunit, Cdk2, show high kinase activity in polyploid cells.[152] Antisense knockdown of cyclin D3 levels suppresses endomitosis and abrogates normal development of primary mouse megakaryocytes.[153]

Cyclin D1 is a direct target gene of GATA1, a transcription factor required for megakaryocyte polyploidization and maturation (see Transcriptional Control of Megakaryopoiesis below).[151,154] Overexpression of cyclin D1 in transgenic mice increases megakaryocyte modal ploidy compared to nontransgenic littermates, and the combination of cyclin D1 and CDK4 kinase activity restores polyploidization of GATA1 deficient murine megakaryocytes.[151,154] Conversely, enforced expression of p16(ink4a), a cell cycle inhibitor of Cdk4/6, blocks polyploidization in murine megakaryocytes.[154] p16(ink4a) is also potently repressed by GATA1.

Cyclin $E^{-/-}$ mice have impaired megakaryopoiesis with reduced modal ploidy.[155] These mice also have defective trophoblast development, another tissue dependent on endomitosis. Cyclin B1/CDC2 is a mitotic cyclin complex. Yeast strains deficient in cyclin B1 or CDC2 undergo an additional round of DNA replication without cytokinesis.[156,157] Several studies have shown that low levels of cyclin B1/CDC2 are required for progression of endomitosis in megakaryocytic cells lines.[153,158–160] However, studies of primary megakaryocytes have shown normal cyclin B1 and CDC2 levels and functional mitotic activity during endomitosis.[137]

Other Mitotic Kinases

Aurora-B kinase (also called *AIM1 kinase*) is involved in late anaphase and cytokinesis, and mRNA transcript levels of Aurora-B kinase have been reported to decrease during polyploidization of primary megakaryocytes and megakaryocytic cell lines.[161–163] This suggests that Aurora-B kinase may play a mechanistic role in megakaryocyte endomitosis. However, functional activity of Aurora-B kinase appears normal in late anaphase of endomitotic primary megakaryocytes, indicating that simple deficiency of Aurora-B kinase activation is an unlikely mechanism to explain endomitosis.[164,165] Polo-like kinase (PLK1) is a serine-threonine kinase required for assembly of the mitotic spindle, separation of chromosomes during anaphase, and exit from mitosis.[166–168] PLK1 mRNA and protein levels decrease during polyploidization of murine megakaryocytes, and enforced expression of PLK1 in primary murine megakaryocytes impairs endomitosis.[165] However, the effects of overexpression are modest, preferentially affect lower-ploidy megakaryocytes, and are complicated by alterations in cell cycle kinetics.

Spindle Checkpoint

During mitosis of normal diploid cells, a spindle assembly checkpoint prevents progression of anaphase until all of the chromosomes are aligned with the mitotic spindle and each sister chromatid is properly attached to spindle microtubules originating from the opposing spindle pole. This ensures that each daughter cell receives the proper complement of chromosomes. The anaphase promoting complex (APC) is a multisubunit protein complex with ubiquitin ligase activity that regulates chromosome segregation and anaphase progression by targeting key factors for degradation. As some chromosomal missegregation occurs during megakaryocyte endomitosis, several groups have examined the expression levels and/or activity of certain APC components and associated factors. These studies have shown no significant difference in protein levels of the core APC protein CDC27 or the kinetochore associated signaling protein hsMAD2 in primary murine megakaryocytes undergoing polyploidization compared to nonendomitotic precursors.[165] Haploinsufficiency of BUBR1, a key component of the spindle checkpoint, perturbs megakaryocyte development and polyploidization in mice but does not cause alterations in circulating platelet counts.[169]

Microtubule Regulation

Microtubules play key roles in mitosis. Therefore, factors that regulate their assembly have also been interrogated as candidates involved in megakaryocyte endomitosis. PRC1 is involved in mitotic spindle elongation and cytokinesis. However, no differences in PRC1 levels were detected in primary murine megakaryocytes undergoing polyploidization compared to nonendomitotic precursors.[165] Stathmin is a microtubule depolymerizing factor that plays in important role in regulation of the mitotic spindle.[170] Levels of stathmin are inversely related to the level of ploidy of megakaryocytic cell lines and primary megakaryocytes.[171] Inhibition of stathmin in K562 cells increases their propensity to undergo endomitosis when induced to differentiate into megakaryocytes, and overexpression of stathmin prevents the transition from mitotic to endomitotic cell cycles.[170,171] Together, these findings support a possible role of stathmin in modulating endomitosis. Further studies will be required to fully dissect the molecular pathways involved in megakaryocyte endomitosis.

TRANSCRIPTIONAL CONTROL OF MEGAKARYOPOIESIS

Because platelets do not contain nuclei, all transcriptional regulation of platelet-specific genes must occur at the level of the megakaryocyte. Significant strides have been made recently in identifying key transcription factors involved in megakaryocyte development and platelet-specific gene expression. Importantly, mutations in several of these factors have been linked to various hematologic disorders providing significant new insights into the pathogenesis of these diseases (see Chapter 32 for additional discussion).

GATA Family Transcription Factors

GATA1

GATA transcription factors comprise a family of zinc finger proteins that bind the consensus DNA sequence (T/A))GATA(A/G). There are six known members of the GATA family in vertebrates. GATA1, -2, -3 play roles predominantly, although not exclusively, within the hematopoietic system. GATA4, -5,-6 are expressed in nonhematopoietic tissues and play diverse developmental roles within the cardiac, gastrointestinal, endocrine, and gonadal systems. Functionally important binding sites for GATA factors have been identified in cis-acting regulatory elements of essentially every megakaryocytic and erythroid gene that has been studied.[172] GATA1, the founding member of this family, is highly expressed in erythroid and megakaryocytic cells, and to a lesser extent in eosinophils and mast cells.[173] GATA1 plays an essential role in erythroid development, with loss of function resulting in blocked erythroid maturation and apoptosis of erythroid progenitor cells.[174] GATA1 is also required for megakaryocyte maturation and growth control. Lineage-selective loss of GATA1 in megakaryocytes results in marked thrombocytopenia in mice with platelet counts of only approximately 15% of wild type littermates.[175] Megakaryocytes are present in the mutant animals, but have a disorganized DMS, paucity of platelet-specific granules, reduced expression of multiple megakaryocyte-specific genes including GPIbα, GPIbβ, PF4, c-mpl, and p45 NF-E2, and marked hyperproliferation compared to wild type.[175,176] cDNA microarray studies of GATA1 deficient versus wild type murine megakaryocytes show a large number of potential GATA1 target genes, although evidence for direct targets has only been established for a few.[177] Mice containing reduced megakaryocyte-specific expression of GATA1 ($GATA1^{low}$) develop myelofibrosis as they age,[178] a frequent finding with disorders of megakaryocyte progenitor hyperproliferation. A GATA binding site mutation in the GPIbβ promoter has been described in a patient with BSS, a macrothrombocytopenia disorder characterized by deficiency of the GPIb/IX/V complex and a bleeding diathesis.[179] Taken together, these findings suggest that GATA1 acts as master regulator of megakaryocyte maturation and proliferative control.

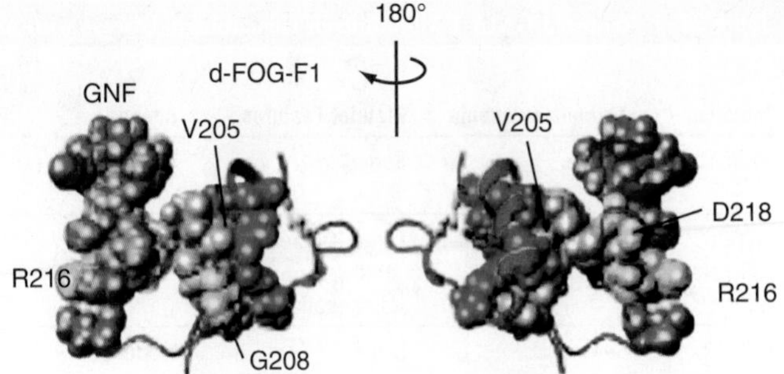

Figure 27–7 Structural basis of GATA1 N-terminal zinc finger mutations associated with familial hematologic disease. Solution nuclear magnetic resonance (NMR)-determined structure of the *N*-terminal zinc finger of murine GATA1 (GNF) complexed with zinc finger 1 of the Drosophila Friend of GATA (FOG) ortholog (U-shaped) (d-FOG-F1). The DNA binding surface of GNF is shown in purple, and the FOG-binding surface is shown in gray. Locations of the residues mutated in GATA1 related cytopenias are shown in yellow. V205 and G208 lie on the FOG contact surface, R216 lies on the GNF/DNA interface, and D218 lies between the two opposing surfaces. *(Reproduced by permission Liew et al,[279] copyright 2005, National Academy of Sciences.)*

Friend of GATA (FOG-1)

All vertebrate GATA factors contain two zinc fingers. The carboxyl zinc finger mediates high affinity DNA binding, whereas the amino zinc finger stabilizes the DNA interaction at certain double GATA sites.[180] Importantly, the amino zinc finger also interacts with Friend of GATA (FOG) proteins, a family of large multitype zinc finger transcriptional cofactors (see review by Cantor and Orkin[181] for more details). This interaction occurs on the surface of the zinc finger opposite to its DNA binding surface (Fig. 27–7).[182] FOG1 (also called *zfpm1*), the founding member, is expressed predominantly within erythroid and megakaryocytic cells.[183] Knockout of FOG1 in mice results in embryonic lethality because of severe anemia from a block in erythroid maturation similar to that observed in $GATA1^{-}$ mice.[184] In addition, $FOG1^{-/-}$ mice have complete failure of megakaryopoiesis, establishing FOG1 as the first identified transcription-associated factor selectively required to generate the entire megakaryocyte lineage. FOG1's role in megakaryocyte and erythroid development requires direct physical interaction with GATA factors.[182,185,186] The discrepancy between the relatively late block in megakaryocyte development seen in GATA1 deficient animals and the complete loss of megakaryopoiesis in $FOG1^{-/-}$ mice is explained by overlapping FOG-dependent roles of GATA1 and GATA2 during early stages of megakaryopoiesis.[186]

Table 27–1 Reported GATA-1 Mutations in Hematologic Disease with Associated Clinical and Biochemical Features

Mutation	Thrombocytopenia	Platelet Features	Anemia	Erythroid Features	Other Features	FOG-1 Binding	DNA Binding	References
V205M	Severe	Large*	Severe, Fetal Hydrops	Dyserythropoiesis	Cryptorchidism	Markedly reduced	Normal	187
G208S	Moderate	Large, Decreased Platelet aggregation	None			Moderately reduced	Normal	188
G208R	Severe	Large*	Moderate	Dyserythropoiesis	Cryptorchidism**	Not Studied	Not studied	189
D218G	Moderate	Large, Decreased platelet aggregation	None	Dyserythropoiesis		Moderately reduced	Normal	190
D218Y	Severe	Large*	Severe		Platelets in carrier female expressed only WT allele	Markedly reduced	Normal	191
R216Q	Moderate	Large, normal platelet aggregation in vitro, but prolonged bleeding time; Gray platelet syndrome	Mild	Mild β-thalassemia	Splenomegaly	Normal	Decreased	192–195
R216W	Moderate	*	Mild	Mild β-thalassemia	Congenital erythropoietic porphyria	Not studied	Not studied	196
G332C***	None	Decreased platelet aggregation, Dysplastic megakaryocytes	Variable	Macrocytosis	Neutropenia	Not studied	Not studied	209

FOG-1, Friend of GATA.
*Function not studied.
**Cryptorchidism also in two siblings with wild type GATA-1.
***Germline splice mutation results in exclusive production of the amino truncated GATA-1s molecule.
Adapted from GATA1 Related X-linked Cytopenia. Available at: http://www.genetests.org/profiles/gata1.

X-linked Dyserythropoietic Anemia and Thrombocytopenia Caused by GATA1 Mutations

Over the past several years, germline GATA1 mutations that impair binding to FOG1 and/or DNA have been identified in several families with X-linked macrothrombocytopenia and/or anemia (GATA1 is located on the X chromosome in humans, as well as in mice). The first case, reported by Weiss and colleagues, involved a woman with mild chronic thrombocytopenia who had two pregnancies with male offspring that were both complicated by severe fetal anemia and thrombocytopenia requiring in-utero transfusions.[187] Bone marrow examination after birth revealed marked dyserythropoiesis and an overabundance of immature-appearing, dysplastic megakaryocytes that share many of the features of GATA1^{low} murine megakaryocytes. Remarkably, sequencing of the GATA1 gene from affected family members identified substitution of valine by methionine at codon 205 within the amino zinc finger. This mutation (GATA1 [V205M]) significantly impairs FOG1 binding but retains normal DNA affinity based on electromobility shift assays using synthetic oligonucleotides. This is consistent with the location of this residue on the surface of the zinc finger opposite the DNA binding face (see Fig. 27–7).

Since the initial report, several other GATA1 mutations have been linked to cases of familial X-linked macrothrombocytopenia with or without anemia (Table 27–1). These substitutions all impair FOG1 binding, although to different degrees. Substitution of glycine by serine at codon 208 (GATA1 [G208S]) results in moderate to severe thrombocytopenia, mild dyserythropoiesis, but no anemia.[188] Substitution of the same residue by arginine (GATA1 [G208R]) results in thrombocytopenia with anemia and severe dyserythropoiesis.[189] Similarly, substitution of aspartic acid by glycine at codon 218 (GATA1 [D218G]) leads only to thrombocytopenia, whereas substitution of this same codon by tyrosine (GATA1 [D218Y]) leads to severe thrombocytopenia, moderate anemia, and marked dyserythropoiesis.[190,191] The severity of the phenotype appears to correlate with the degree of FOG1 binding impairment, suggesting that megakaryocytic development is more sensitive to affinity changes in GATA1:FOG1 interactions than erythroid development.

X-Linked Thrombocytopenia and β-Thalassemia Caused by GATA1 Mutations

Mutations mapping to the DNA binding surface of the amino zinc finger of GATA1 have also been described (GATA1 [R216Q]).[192–194,195] As expected, this reduces DNA affinity to double (palindromic) GATA sites, but not single GATA sites. FOG1 binding is not substantially altered. Affected family members exhibit an X-linked β-thalassemia syndrome characterized by imbalance of α and β globin chain synthesis, reticulocytosis, and hemolysis. They also have mild-moderate thrombocytopenia. In-vitro platelet aggregation studies are normal, but there is a prolonged bleeding time. Substitution of the same residue by tryptophan (R216W) produces thrombocytopenia, β-thalassemia intermedia, and congenital erythropoietic porphyria (CEP).[196] The CEP is likely caused by dysregulation of the GATA1 target gene uroporphyrinogen III synthase.

X-Linked Gray Platelet-Like Syndrome

Gray platelet syndrome (GPS) refers to a disorder of large platelets with absent or markedly reduced α-granules and/or α-granule proteins. Platelets from individuals with GATA1 (Arg261Gln) share some features with classical GPS.[195] Ultrastructural studies of platelets from a different family with GATA1 related X-linked macrothrombocytopenia (GATA1 [G208S]) also demonstrate hypogranular platelets that contain small vacuoles, likely representing membranes of empty α-granules.[197] However, the GATA1 mutant platelets also possess unique features such as masses of dense tubular system channels, dense double membranes, and platelets within platelets, not seen in classical GPS, suggesting a more general disorder of platelet biogenesis.

GATA1 Mutations in Down Syndrome Transient Myeloproliferative Disorders and Acute Megakaryoblastic Leukemia

Approximately 10% of children with Down syndrome (DS) (trisomy 21) are born with a transient myeloproliferative disorder (TMD), which is characterized by an abundance of circulating erythromegakaryocytic precursor cells, pancytopenia, and, in some cases, severe liver fibrosis. Remarkably, this myeloproliferative disorder resolves spontaneously over the first few months of life. In approximately 20% to 30% of cases, acute megakaryoblastic leukemia (AMKL) develops within a few years, sometimes preceded by a myelodysplastic phase. In 2002, Crispino and colleagues reported that DS-AMKL cells harbor acquired mutations in their GATA1 gene.[198] Since then, several groups have reproduced these findings and identified similar mutations in DS-TMD cells.[199–204] Although a wide spectrum of mutations have been found, including missense, deletion, insertion and splice-site mutations, they all involve exon 2 and result in the same outcome: generation of an amino terminal truncated protein (loss of amino acids 1–83) because of translation initiation from a downstream ATG codon (Fig. 27–8). This removes a region that functions as a transcriptional activation domain in transient transfection reporter assays.[205] The mutations are detectable in bone marrow from DS-AMKL patients but disappear when the patients enter remission, indicating a strong correlation between the mutated clone and the leukemic phenotype.[198] Mutations involving exon 2 of GATA1 are highly specific for DS-AMKL and DS-TMD, or AMKL with acquired trisomy 21. There is only one reported case of such a mutation in AMKL without trisomy 21,[206] and no mutations have been detected in DS-acute lymphoblastic leukemia or a large number of healthy individuals.

Analysis of stored neonatal blood spots shows the coexistence of several different GATA1 mutations (all resulting in the generation of GATA1s) in patients who subsequently developed DS-AMKL, suggesting an oligoclonal expansion.[207] In a few cases in which material was available, identical GATA1 mutations have been found in both the DS-TMD and DS-AMKL cells from the same patient. DS-AMKL cells often harbor additional genetics abnormalities, such as trisomy 8 or tetrasomy 21, not observed in DS-TMD cells. Taken together, these findings support a clonal evolution model of DS-AMKL, with GATA1 mutations associated with an early initiating event.

Knock-in mice that recapitulate the truncating GATA1 mutation show unexpected stage-specific effects on megakaryopoiesis.[208] During fetal liver hematopoiesis, the mutant megakaryocytes markedly

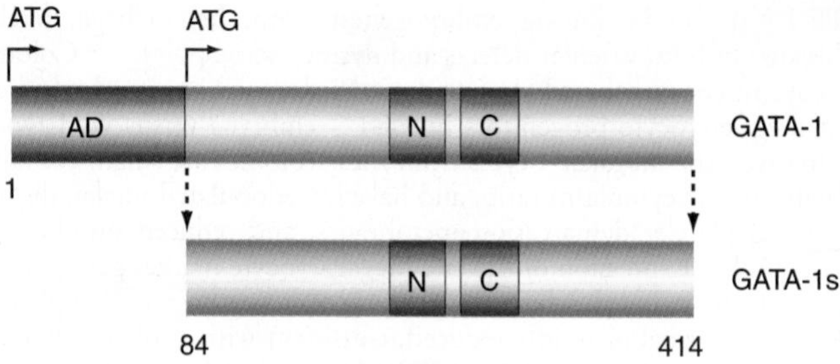

Figure 27–8 Generation of an amino terminal truncated isoform of GATA1 by mutations associated with Down syndrome transient myeloproliferative disorder (DS-TMD) and Down syndrome acute myelogenous leukemia (DS-AMKL). Schematic representation of full-length GATA1 is shown on top, and the truncated form (GATA1s) on bottom. The amino terminal transcriptional activation domain, as defined by reporter assays in transiently transfected cells, is indicated (*AD*). The amino (*N*) and carboxyl (*C*) zinc fingers are shown as gray boxes. In DS-TMD and DS-AMKL, mutations involving exon 2 of GATA1 (point mutations, deletions, insertions, and/or splice-site mutations) lead to exclusive translation from a downstream in-frame methionine at codon 84 producing the amino terminal truncated GATA1 protein (GATA1s). (Reproduced by permission Cantor.[280])

hyperproliferate, similar to what is observed for GATA1 deficient megakaryocytes. However, during adult stage bone marrow hematopoiesis, megakaryopoiesis and thrombocytopoiesis appear normal. This suggests that the fetal liver and bone marrow microenvironments each interact differentially with the GATA1 truncated molecule. This might also explain the restriction of TMD to the neonatal period. Recently, a family was described with members containing a germline GATA1 gene splice site mutation (G332C) that results in exclusive production of a short isoform of GATA1, the GATA1s protein product.[209] Affected individuals exhibit a unique phenotype characterized by trilineage bone marrow dysplasia, macrocytic anemia and neutropenia. None of the family members have developed leukemia, suggesting that trisomy 21 plays a role in DS-TMD progression to DS-AMKL.

Interestingly, Santoro and his colleagues reported nearly 10 years ago that GATA1s is produced naturally at low levels in erythroid cells.[210] They proposed that this might serve a regulatory role during normal hematopoiesis by acting as a dominant negative molecule at specific times/environmental stimuli. Endogenous GATA1s has also been detected in normal mouse fetal liver megakaryocytes and adult human bone marrow megakaryocytes.[198,209] Thus, the ratio of GATA1 and GATA1s may play a role in developmental aspects of megakaryocytopoiesis, and acquired GATA1 mutations observed in DS-TMD and DS-AMKL, or germline mutations in the family described above, may perturb hematopoiesis by altering this ratio.

Ets Family Transcription Factors

A common feature of megakaryocyte-specific genes is the presence of tandem binding sites for GATA and Ets transcription factors in their promoters and enhancers.[211,212] The Ets transcription factor family is comprised of a diverse group of proteins that share a common *Ets* DNA-binding domain, which recognizes a GGAA core sequence.[213] More than 30 different Ets factors have been identified, at least 9 of which (Elf-1, Elf-2, Fli-1, Pu.1, TEL, GABPα, Ets-1, Ets-2, Elk-4) are expressed in megakaryocytes.[214,215] Functional studies have implicated several of these, including Fli-1, Ets-1, TEL, and GABPα, in megakaryocytopoiesis.

Fli-1

The role of Fli-1 has perhaps been best characterized of the Ets factors in terms of its functional role in megakaryocyte development.

Fli-1$^{-/-}$ mice die during embryogenesis from hemorrhage, likely because of both vascular defects and dysmegakaryopoiesis.[216] Colony assays in collagen-based semisolid media show an increased number of megakaryocyte progenitors in Fli-1$^{-/-}$ embryos versus wild type. However, the megakaryocytes from these colonies are small, contain high nuclear/cytoplasm ratio, and have hyperlobulated nuclei, disorganized platelet demarcation membranes, and reduced number of α-granules. Expression of the late megakaryocyte marker gene GPIX is markedly reduced, whereas expression of the early genes c-mpl and αIIb are normal or mildly reduced, consistent with a role of Fli-1 in late megakaryocyte maturation.[216,217] Fli-1 is involved in the synergistic transcriptional activation of several megakaryocyte-specific genes by GATA1 and FOG1.[218] Recent work by Poncz and coworkers shows that different Ets factors act in a stage-specific manner during megakaryocytopoiesis, with GABPα predominantly regulating genes active during early stages of megakaryocytopoiesis, and Fli-1 during later stages.[219]

Fli-1 has been implicated in the lineage commitment of bipotent erythroid-megakaryocyte progenitor cells to the megakaryocyte pathway. Fli-1 expression is downregulated as bipotent cells commit to the erythroid lineage, and its overexpression in the bipotent human erythroleukemia cell line K562 enhances the expression of several megakaryocyte-specific genes and induces a megakaryocyte phenotype.[220] In addition, functional cross-antagonism occurs between Fli-1 and the erythroid-specific transcription factor EKLF.[221,222]

Paris-Trousseau (OMIM 188925) and Jacobsen syndromes (OMIM 147791) are overlapping contiguous gene deletion disorders in humans involving the long arm of chromosome 11 (11q23).[223,224] The constellation of findings in these syndromes includes severe congenital cardiac abnormalities, trigonocephaly, mental retardation, dysmorphogenesis of the hands and face, and macrothrombocytopenia.[225] The etiology of the thrombocytopenia in these patients appears to be related to impaired platelet production, as platelet survival time is normal.[226] Examination of bone marrow reveals significant dysmegakaryopoiesis with an abundance of micromegakaryocytes and death of large numbers of megakaryocytes during late stages of maturation.[227] Peripheral blood platelets contain giant α-granules, which are thought to arise from aberrant α-granule fusion during prolonged residence in the bone marrow.[228] The minimal chromosome regions deleted in Paris-Trousseau and Jacobsen syndromes associated with thrombocytopenia includes the genes for the Ets factors Fli-1 and Ets-1.[216] Lentiviral expression of Fli-1 in CD34+ cells from patients with Paris-Trousseau thrombocytopenia rescues megakaryocyte differentiation in vitro, providing strong evidence that it is deficiency of Fli-1 that is the cause of impaired thrombopoiesis in these patients. Interestingly, Favier and colleagues have shown that in normal individuals expression of Fli-1 is mostly monoallelic in early megakaryocytic progenitors CD41^{+}/CD42^{-} cells), but predominantly bi-allelic in later stages.[229] They propose that the different populations of megakaryocytes seen in patients with Paris-Trousseau disorder arise from expression of the normal allele in the normally differentiating megakaryocytes, and the deleted allele (leading to complete loss of Fli-1 expression) in the dying population of megakaryocytes.

TEL (ETV6)

Generation of a fusion protein between TEL (ETV6) and Runx-1 (formerly called AML-1) is the most frequent chromosome translocation in childhood pre–B-cell acute lymphoblastic leukemia. Although TEL is required for the ontogeny of all definitive hematopoiesis,[230] a recent conditional knock-out study of the TEL gene in mice demonstrates its specific requirement for adult stage megakaryopoiesis.[231]

Runx-1

In 1999, Gilliland and colleagues used positional cloning to identify the genetic cause of a rare dominant disorder characterized by thrombocytopenia, an aspirin-like functional platelet defect, and increased risk of developing acute myelogenous leukemia (FPD/AML; OMIM 601399).[232–234] They identified nonsense mutations, intragenic deletions, or missense mutations on one allele of the gene for Runx-1 (formerly called AML-1 and CBFA2) that cosegregated with the disease in six separate pedigrees. These mutations all resulted in loss-of-function, indicating that haploinsufficiency of Runx-1 plays a causal role in this disorder. Bone marrow or peripheral blood from these patients contained reduced numbers of assayable colonies in megakaryocyte formation, indicating Runx-1 dosage affects megakaryocytopoiesis.

Runx-1 is a member of an evolutionarily conserved family of transcription factors that share a conserved 128 amino acid domain in their amino half with homology to Drosophila *runt* gene. This region mediates binding to DNA (consensus (C/T)G(C/T)GGT)) as well as to its heterodimeric binding partner CBF-β via protein-protein interactions (see review by Speck and Gilliland[235] for additional details). Runx-1 is the most frequently mutated transcription factors in human leukemia. In addition, acquired mutations in Runx-1 have been identified in significant number of patients with myelodysplastic syndrome (MDS), particularly those that progress to acute myelogenous leukemia (AML).[236–238] Homozygous knockout of either Runx-1 or CBF-β in mice is embryonic lethal because of a complete failure of definitive hematopoiesis.[239,240] This is thought to arise from a defect in the ontogeny of hematopoietic stem cells in the AGM region.[241–243] More recent studies using conditional knockout of Runx-1 in adult hematopoiesis demonstrate a specific role of Runx-1 in megakaryopoiesis.[244–246] Deletion of Runx-1 in adult mouse bone marrow results in up to an approximately 80% reduction in peripheral blood platelet numbers, without a bleeding diathesis. Bone marrow megakaryocytes are small, lack lobulated nuclei, have poorly developed demarcation membranes, and reduced polyploidization. These findings are reminiscent of the abnormal *micromegakaryocytes* seen in human myelodysplastic syndromes. Paradoxically, there is an increase in in-vitro megakaryocyte colony plating efficiency suggesting an expansion of early megakaryocyte progenitors. These effects are cell-autonomous. No defects are seen in the erythroid lineage. Reduced dosage of Runx-1's essential cofactor CBF-β also perturbs megakaryopoiesis in vivo.[247] Taken together, these findings indicate a specific role of Runx-1/CBF-β in megakaryocyte terminal maturation.

NF-E2 p45

NF-E2 is a heterodimeric transcription factor composed of two basic region-leucine zipper (bZip) subunits: a hematopoietic-specific 45 kd protein (p45) and a widely expressed 18 kd subunit (p18). NF-E2 p45 is expressed in erythroid, megakaryocytic and mast cell lineages.[248] In-vitro studies implicated NF-E2 p45 as a critical factor for β-globin expression. Unexpectedly, NF-E2 p45$^{-/-}$ mice were found to have only mild perturbations of the erythroid lineage. However, these mice fail to produce platelets secondary to a maturational arrest in the megakaryocyte lineage, and succumb to hemorrhage in the neonatal period.[249,250] Since the initial studies, NF-E2 p45 has been recognized as being a major regulator of late megakaryocyte maturation and platelet release. Interestingly, although NF-E2 p45$^{-/-}$ mice are severely thrombocytopenic, they have normal serum levels of thrombopoietin. In addition, megakaryocytes from these animals proliferate in vivo in response to thrombopoietin administration. These findings suggest that NF-E2 p45 regulates target genes independent of the action of thrombopoietin.

Several important target genes of NF-E2 p45 have been identified, including β-1 tubulin,[251,252] 3β-hydroxysteroid dehydrogenase (3β-HSD),[253] thromboxane synthase,[254] caspase 12,[255] and Rab27b.[256] β-1 tubulin, is a megakaryocyte-restricted isoform of β-tubulin that plays a key role in the marginal band structure of platelets and is essential for their discoid shape.[251,252,257] Deficiency of β-1 tubulin leads to spherocytic platelets. Heterozygosity for a polymorphism (Q43P, because of the double nucleotide substitution AG>CC) in the human β1-tubulin gene is present in approximately 11% of individuals in a white northern European population, and correlates with a reduced risk of cardiovascular disease in men.[258] This can be caused by alterations in platelet structure and function. 3β-HSD catalyzes autocrine biosynthesis of estradiol within megakaryocytes, and plays an important role in proplatelet formation.[253]

p18 (also called mafK) is a member of a family of small maf proteins (mafF, mafG, mafK) related to the chicken v-Maf oncoprotein. Knockout of mafK, and the related mafF, in mice has no discernible phenotypes, whereas deficiency of mafG leads to mild thrombocytopenia.[259–261] Compound mafK::mafG null mice have profound thrombocytopenia, phenocopying NF-E2 p45 mice.[262] This indicates functional redundancy of the small maf family members in megakaryopoiesis.

SCL (Tal-1)

SCL (also known as Tal-1) is a member of the basic helix-loop-helix member of transcription factors and is expressed predominantly in megakaryocytic and erythroid cells. Dysregulated expression of SCL caused by chromosomal translocation is associated with certain cases of T-cell acute lymphoblastic leukemia. SCL forms obligate heterodimers with ubiquitously expressed E proteins (such as E12 and E47), which bind to E-box motifs (sequence CANNTG). It participates in multiprotein complexes that include E2A, GATA1, LM02, ldb1, and the repressor ETO2.[263,264] $SCL^{-/-}$ mice die during embryogenesis because of failure of all hematopoiesis and defective vasculogenesis.[265–267] However, conditional SCL knock-out models show a specific role for SCL in late stages of megakaryopoiesis and stress thrombopoiesis during adult hematopoiesis.[268,269] SCL-null megakaryocytes have disorganized demarcation membrane systems and reduced number of platelet granules. SCL modulates thrombopoiesis, in part, by direct transcriptional activation of NF-E2 p45.[269]

Other Transcription Factors

The transcription factors above have been studied the most in-depth in terms of their roles in megakaryocytopoiesis. Additional factors involved in megakaryocytopoiesis/thrombopoiesis have been identified, although their roles are just beginning to be explored. Gfi-1b is a member of a family of hematopoietic expressed zinc finger transcription factor proto-oncogenes (*Gfi*, for *g*rowth *f*actor *i*ndependent) that contain a unique 20 amino acid amino terminal transcriptional repressor SNAG domain. Knock-out of Gfi-1b in mice results in embryonic lethality because of severe anemia.[270] The fetal liver of mutant mice contains erythroid and megakaryocytic progenitors that are blocked in their maturation. Culture of these cells in the presence of thrombopoietin, in contrast to those from wild type animals, generates only small colonies and the cells are acetylcholinesterase negative (a marker of maturing megakaryocytes in mice). They contain markedly reduced mRNA transcript levels of vWF, NF-E2 p45, c-mpl and GPIIb, compared to wild type, suggesting a requirement for Gfi-1b in at least relatively early stages of megakaryopoiesis. Gfi-1 has been shown to repress target genes by recruitment of histone lysine methyltransferases.[271]

Warren and coworkers performed an N-ethyl-N-nitrosourea (ENU) mutagenesis screen in Tpo $receptor^{-/-}$ mice to identify factors that might influence thrombocytopoiesis. They identified two independent loss-of-function alleles of the transcription factor c-myb (substitution of valine for aspartic acid at residue 152 within the DNA binding domain, and residue 384 within the leucine zipper domain).[272] Both Tpo $receptor^{-/-}$ and wild type mice containing these mutations have supraphysiologic production of platelets because of excessive megakaryocytopoiesis, at the expense of erythroid and lymphocyte development.[273] Megakaryocytes from these animals have a 200-fold increased sensitivity to GM-CSF suggesting dysregulation of signaling pathways. Similar degrees of megakaryocytic hyperplasia and thrombocytosis occur in mice containing germline c-myb mutations that disrupt binding the transcriptional coactivator p300.[274] Thus, c-myb might play an important negative regulatory function in megakaryopoiesis and thrombocytopoiesis.

MICRORNAS IN MEGAKARYOPOIESIS

MicroRNAs are a recently discovered class of small (typically 19–25 nucleotide) noncoding RNAs that interact in a sequence-specific manner with mRNAs (typically in their 3′ untranslated region in mammals) and modulate gene expression through either enhanced mRNA decay or inhibiting translation. There is increasing evidence that they play significant roles in development and differentiation, likely by fine-tuning tissue-specific transcription factor expression. Each microRNA can have multiple target genes, and conversely, each mRNA can be subject to regulation by multiple micro RNA species. In addition, transcription of microRNAs is itself mediated by RNA polymerase II and subject to control by transcription factors. This raises the possibility of complex regulatory networks. Although examination of the functional significance of microRNAs in vivo is still at its infancy, there is some evidence that they play roles in hematopoietic development (see review by Shivdasani[275]). Croce and colleagues recently examined microRNA expression profiles in human CD34+ cells differentiated in vitro into megakaryocytes.[276] They identified a signature set of microRNAs including miR-10a, miR-126, miR-106, miR-10b, miR-17 and miR-20 that are downregulated during megakaryocyte differentiation. When they compared the microRNA expression profile of several megakaryoblastic leukemic cell lines to the differentiated CD34+ set, they found significant upregulation of several microRNAs including miR-101, miR-126, miR-99a, miR-135, and miR-20. Many of the miRs are predicted to target key transcription factors involved in megakaryopoiesis. Further work will be required to fully evaluate the functional significance, and any possible causal relationships, between these changes and altered megakaryocyte differentiation. However, it seems reasonable to speculate that microRNAs may play a role in modulating megakaryocyte differentiation.

CONCLUSION

Although the molecular details regarding the regulation and generation of platelets remain to be fully elucidated, considerable progress has been made over the past decade. This has been significantly facilitated by the isolation of Tpo and its receptor. Important models of thrombocytopoiesis have now been tested rigorously, yielding new insights into the final stages of platelet formation and shedding. These studies highlight the efficient mechanisms that have developed to satisfy the demands for dynamic and high-output platelet production. Several important transcription factors have been identified that regulate different stages of megakaryopoiesis, and mutations in these, and other genes, are beginning to be linked to human disorders of thrombocytopoiesis. The potential role of microRNAs is beginning to be explored. Although mouse models have played important roles in the analysis of these genes, it is becoming clear that they do not always faithfully recapitulate human disease. In addition, several studies have documented important differences between rodent and human platelets including differences in size, circulating numbers, and DMS ultrastructural features.[277] Thus, some caution must be exercised when extrapolating results of mouse studies to human thrombocytopoiesis. The advent of megakaryocyte in-vitro differentiation systems using human embryonic stem (ES) cell and/or $CD34^+$ cells should provide important tools for future studies geared toward dissecting human disorders of megakaryopoiesis and thrombocytopoiesis.[278]

SUGGESTED READINGS

Avecilla ST, Hattori K, Heissig B, et al: Chemokine-mediated interaction of hematopoietic progenitors with the bone marrow vascular niche is required for thrombopoiesis. Nat Med 10:64–71, 2004.

Cantor AB: GATA transcription factors in hematologic disease. Int J Hematol 81:378, 2005.

Garzon R, Pichiorri F, Palumbo T, et al: MicroRNA fingerprints during human megakaryocytopoiesis. Proc Natl Acad Sci U S A 103:5078, 2006.

Harker LA, Finch CA: Thrombokinetics in man. J Clin Invest 48:963, 1969.

Italiano JE Jr, Lecine P, Shivdasani RA, et al: Blood platelets are assembled principally at the ends of proplatelet processes produced by differentiated megakaryocytes. J Cell Biol 147:1299, 1999.

Italiano JE Jr., Shivdasani RA: Megakaryocytes and beyond: The birth of platelets. J Thromb Haemost 1:1174, 2003.

Kacena MA, Kirk J, Chou ST, Weiss MJ, Raskind WH: GATA1-Related X-linked Cytopenia. Available at: http://www.genetests.org/profiles/gata1. Initial posting November 22, 2006. Accessed January 9, 2007.

Kaushansky K: The molecular mechanisms that control thrombopoiesis. J Clin Invest 115:3339, 2005.

Kuter DJ: The promise of thrombopoietins in the treatment of ITP. Clin Adv Hematol Oncol 3:464, 2005.

Kuter DJ, Rosenberg RD: The reciprocal relationship of thrombopoietin (c-Mpl ligand) to changes in the platelet mass during busulfan-induced thrombocytopenia in the rabbit. Blood 85:2720, 1995.

Nakorn TN, Miyamoto T, Weissman IL: Characterization of mouse clonogenic megakaryocyte progenitors. Proc Natl Acad Sci U S A 100:205, 2003.

Nichols KE, Crispino JD, Poncz M, et al: Familial dyserythropoietic anaemia and thrombocytopenia due to an inherited mutation in GATA1. Nat Genet 24:266, 2000.

Ravid K, Lu J, Zimmet JM, et al: Roads to polyploidy: the megakaryocyte example. J Cell Physiol 190:7, 2002.

Richardson JL, Shivdasani RA, Boers C, et al: Mechanisms of organelle transport and capture along proplatelets during platelet production. Blood 106:4066, 2005.

Schulze H, Korpal M, Hurov J, et al: Characterization of the megakaryocyte demarcation membrane system and its role in thrombopoiesis. Blood 107:3868, 2006.

Schulze H, Shivdasani RA: Molecular mechanisms of megakaryocyte differentiation. Semin Thromb Hemost 30:389, 2004.

Song WJ, Sullivan MG, Legare RD, et al: Haploinsufficiency of CBFA2 causes familial thrombocytopenia with propensity to develop acute myelogenous leukaemia. Nat Genet 23:166, 1999.

Wechsler J, Greene M, McDevitt MA, et al: Acquired mutations in GATA1 in the megakaryoblastic leukemia of Down syndrome. Nat Genet 32:148, 2002.

Wright J: The origin and nature of the blood platelets. Boston Med Surg J 23:643, 1906.

REFERENCES

For complete list of references log onto www.expertconsult.com

CHAPTER 28

INHERITED FORMS OF BONE MARROW FAILURE

Melvin H. Freedman

INTRODUCTION

Bone marrow failure is defined as decreased production of one or more of the major hematopoietic lineages on an inherited basis (Table 28–1). The rather outdated term "constitutional" is often used interchangeably with "inherited" and similarly implies that a genetic abnormality causes the bone marrow dysfunction, especially when it occurs in two or more members of the same family or is associated with physical abnormalities. The designation "congenital" has a looser connotation and refers to conditions that manifest early in life, often at birth, but does not connote a particular causation. Congenital marrow failure is not necessarily inherited, therefore, and may be caused by acquired factors such as viruses, drugs, and environmental toxins.

Because hematopoiesis is an orderly but complex interplay of stem and progenitor cells, growth factors, marrow stromal elements, and positive or negative cellular and humoral regulators, marrow failure can potentially occur at a number of critical points in the hematopoietic lineage pathways. For the inherited marrow disorders, current theory holds that genetic mutations interfere with hematopoiesis and cause the marrow failure. The discovery of several abnormal genes, each associated with a specific inherited marrow failure syndrome, gives credence to this theory. Modifying genes and acquired factors may also be operative and interact with the genetic mutations to produce overt disease with varying clinical expression. Hence, the conditions shown in Table 28–1 can be transmitted as a simple Mendelian disorder determined primarily by one or more mutant genes with inheritance patterns of autosomal dominant, autosomal recessive, or X-linked types. Alternatively, some or all of these can be multifactorial disorders caused by an interaction of multiple genes and multiple exogenous or environmental determinants.

The incidence of the inherited marrow failure disorders can be approximated from experience at large centers. For example, data from the Children's Hospital Medical Center, Boston, and the Prince of Wales Hospital, Australia, show that the inherited syndromes comprise about one-third of cases of pediatric marrow failure, and that Fanconi anemia (FA) represents about two-thirds of the inherited forms.[1,2]

BI-LINEAGE AND TRI-LINEAGE CYTOPENIAS

Fanconi (Aplastic) Anemia

Background

Fanconi anemia (FA) is inherited in an autosomal recessive manner in 99% of cases. Rarely, it is transmitted in an X-linked recessive mode, caused by a mutant *FANCB* gene. Its overall prevalence is 1 to 5 cases per million with a carrier frequency of 1:200 to 300 in most populations.[3] It occurs in all racial and ethnic groups. Spanish Gypsies have the world's highest prevalence of FA with a carrier frequency of 1 : 64 to 1 : 70 for a common founder mutation.[4] A founder effect has also been demonstrated in South African Afrikaners in whom one specific mutation is common,[5] as well as in Ashkenazi Jews.

Although the original report in 1927 by Dr. Guido Fanconi described pancytopenia combined with physical anomalies in three brothers,[6] a summary of the large body of published information on 1,206 cases over the ensuing years has underscored the clinical variability of the condition.[7] Basically, FA is a chromosomal fragility disorder characterized by cytopenias, progressive bone marrow underproduction, variable developmental anomalies and a strong propensity for cancer. At presentation patients may have (a) typical physical anomalies but normal hematology; (b) normal physical features but abnormal hematology; or (c) physical anomalies and abnormal hematology, the so-called classic phenotype that fits the original description (Fig. 28–1). There can also be sibling heterogeneity in presentation with discordance in clinical and hematological findings, even in affected monozygotic twins. All patients show abnormal chromosome fragility most easily seen in metaphase preparations of peripheral blood lymphocytes cultured with phytohemagglutinin and enhanced by adding clastogenic agents.

Approximately 75% of patients are between 3 and 14 years of age at the time of diagnosis of Fanconi anemia, with a mean of 6.5 years in males and 8 years in females.[7,8] It is noteworthy that 4% are diagnosed in the first year of life and 9% at 16 years of age or older.

Etiology and Genetics

A breakthrough in the search for FA genes evolved from the important observation that fusion of normal cells with FA cells resulted in correction of the abnormal chromosome fragility, a process known as complementation.[9] It was further demonstrated that cell fusion studies from several unrelated FA patients could also produce the corrective effect on chromosomal fragility by complementation, which led directly to subtyping of patients into discrete complementation groups.[10–13] As of 2008, 13 complementation groups (termed types A, B, C, D1/BRCA2, D2, E, F, G, L, J, M, N, and I) have been distinguished on the basis of these somatic cell hybridization experiments, with Fanconi anemia type A accounting for over 65% of the cases analyzed.[14]

The identification of the 13 subtypes facilitated the cloning of all 13 corresponding FA or *FANC* genes by 2007. The first gene, *FANCC* on chromosome 9q22.3, was discovered in 1992 in Toronto,[15] and then the other genes, corresponding to each of the other complementation groups, were subsequently cloned: *FANCA* on 16q24.3[16]; *FANCB* on Xp22.31[17]; *FANCD1/BRCA2* on 13q12.3[18]; *FANCD2* on 3p25.3[19]; *FANCE* on 6p21.3[20]; *FANCF* on 11p15[21]; *FANCG* on 9p13[22]; *FANCJ/BACH1/BRIP1* on 17q22[23]; *FANCL* on 2p16.1[24]; *FANCM* on 14q21.3[25]; and *FANCI* on 15q26.1.[26] A 13th FA gene, *FANCN* (or *PALB2*), maps to 16p12.[27] Of patients tested, 70% have mutant *FANCA*, 10% *FANCC*, 10% *FANCG*, 5% *FANCE*, and 2% or less for the others.

Knock-out mouse models of FA provide insight into the role of individual mutations. Knockouts of *Fanca*[28] and *Fancg*[29] and two different knockouts of *Fancc*[30] have been generated. The phenotype of these mutant mice is identical and consists of cellular sensitivity to DNA cross-linking agents, abnormal G_2-M progression of the cell cycle similar to FA patients, and hypoplasia of the gonads. Also, hematopoietic progenitor cells from *Fancc* knock-out mice in tissue culture display cytogenetic abnormalities and an increased risk of malignant transformation.[31] *Fancc −/−* progenitor cells are also hypersensitive to inhibitory cytokines and show impaired hematopoietic colony growth and increased apoptosis.[30,32,33] Marrow failure in

Table 28–1 Inherited Bone Marrow Failure Syndromes

Bi-lineage and Tri-lineage Cytopenias
Fanconi anemia
Shwachman–Diamond syndrome
Dyskeratosis congenita
Amegakaryocytic thrombocytopenia
• Other inherited thrombocytopenia disorders (see Table 28–5)
Other genetic syndromes
• Down syndrome
• Dubowitz syndrome
• Seckel syndrome
• Reticular dysgenesis
• Schimke immunoosseous dysplasia
• Noonan syndrome
• Cartilage-hair hypoplasia
• Familial marrow failure (non-Fanconi)
Uni-lineage Cytopenia
Diamond-Blackfan anemia
Kostmann syndrome/Congenital neutropenia
• *ELA2* mutations
• *HAX1* mutations
• *GFI1* mutations
• *WASP* mutations
• Constitutive cell surface G-CSF-R mutations
Other inherited neutropenia syndromes
• Barth syndrome
• Glycogen storage disease 1b
• Miscellaneous (see Table 28–8)
Thrombocytopenia with absent radii
Congenital dyserythropoietic anemias (CDAs)
• Types I, II, III, IV
• Variants
• Non-classifiable CDAs
• Groups IV, V, VI, VII (see reference 551)

Fancc knock-out mice can be induced by treatment with the DNA-damaging agent mitomycin C.[34,35] The stem cells in these mice are intrinsically defective and show impaired ability for long-term reconstitution in recipient mice.[36,37] *Fancd2* knock-out mice serve as an informative murine model of FA-related epithelial cancer.[38]

Cells and cell lines from Fanconi patients are phenotypically similar regardless of the complementation group that they represent. The hypothesis, therefore, that wild-type Fanconi proteins function in a common cellular pathway was substantiated by data showing that proteins A, B, C, E, F, G, and M form a single large nuclear protein complex as an important first step in the DNA damage response pathway.[39–43,17,25] The essence of this elaborate, complicated pathway as it relates to FA is described. For additional details, see the thorough review of the FA pathway of genomic maintenance.[44] Activation of this protein complex by DNA damage or cell cycle progression results in the conversion of the downstream FANCD2 protein from an unubiquitinated (unubiquitinylated) isoform to a monoubiquitinated isoform,[44] a process mediated by FANCL ubiquitin ligase.[24] Monoubiquitination does not occur if the protein complex upstream of FANCD2 is not intact or if FANCL is mutated, and therefore Fanconi cells from patients with these mutations do not show monoubiquitinated FANCD2. In normal cells following monoubiquitination, FANCD2 localizes to nuclear foci where it forms complexes with other DNA-repair proteins such as BRCA1 and RAD51, and interacts with BRCA2[45,46] to complete the final steps of the DNA repair pathway. FANCI protein associates with FANCD2 as a complex and together localize to chromatin in response to DNA damage.[26] Biallelic mutations of *FANCI* cause FA.[47] PALB2 (or FANCN) is a nuclear binding partner of BRCA2. Biallelic mutations of *PALB2* also cause FA.[27]

As summarized,[46] there are important protein-protein interactions between FA proteins and non-FA "binding partners" for cell survival. FANCC and FANCD2 form complexes with members of the STAT family of transcription factors in cytokine-mediated biological responses. Secondy, heat shock proteins serve several cell survival functions, and FANCC specifically facilitates the anti-apoptotic role

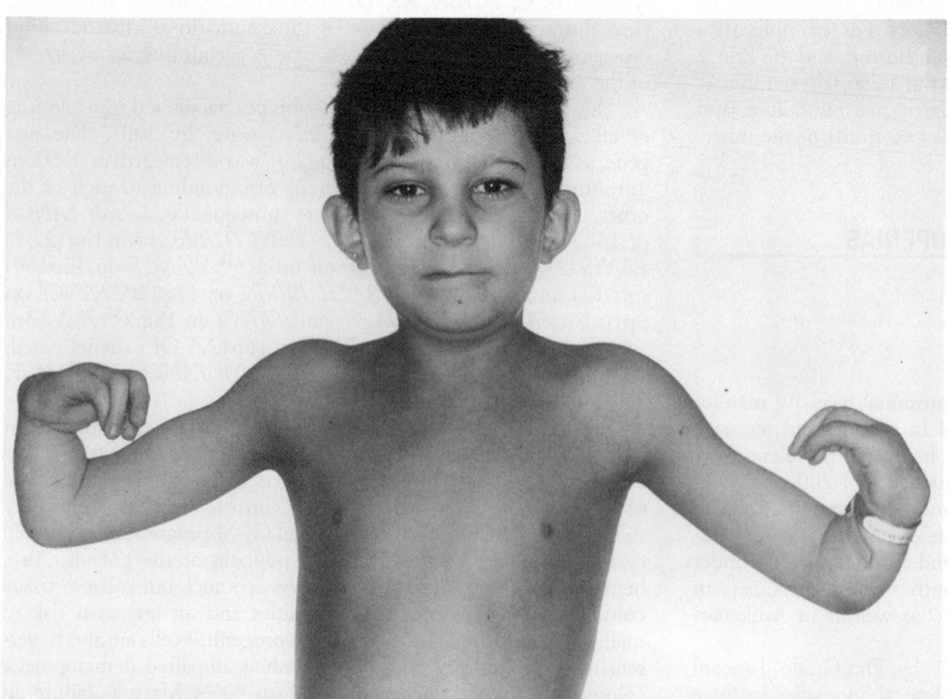

Figure 28–1 Classic phenotype of Fanconi anemia. Patient has pigmentary changes around the neck, shoulders and trunk, short stature, absent radii and absent thumbs bilaterally, microcephaly, and low-set ears.

of hsp 70. Finally, GSTP1 is an enzyme that detoxifies byproducts of redox stress and xenobiotics and FANCC enhances GSTP1 activity in cells exposed to apoptosis inducers.

A genotype-phenotype study examined the consequences of mutations of *FANCC* in patients.[48] Kaplan-Meier analysis showed that IVS4 or exon 14 mutations define poor-risk subgroups clinically and are associated with earlier onset of hematologic abnormalities and poorer survival compared to patients with the exon 1 mutation and to the non-*FANCC* population. This was confirmed in a 20-year follow-up perspective by the International Fanconi Anemia Registry (IFAR).[49] A specific mutation in *FANCC* (IVS4+4A→T) is associated with multiple birth defects and early-onset hematology problems in Ashkenazi Jews[50] but the same mutation results in a mild phenotype in Japanese.[51] Another report showed that FA patients with mutations in the *FANCG* gene are at high risk for a poor hematologic outcome.[52] FA patients with biallelic mutations in *BRCA2* are distinctive in the severity of the physical phenotype, the association with VATER syndrome, and early onset and high rates of leukemia and specific solid tumors.[53] It is clear that FA patients with null mutations are more severely affected than patients with hypomorphic mutations independent of the mutant gene involved.[50]

Pathophysiology

Wild-type FA proteins are part of a cluster of survival signaling molecules that protect against genotoxic insult and suppress apoptosis signaling.[46] Biallelic inactivation of any of the known genes causes FA and the pro-survival benefit is lost. This underlies the phenotype of clinical FA but does not explain or unify the relationship between congenital anomalies, bone marrow failure, the predisposition to cancer, and chromosome fragility.

Two theories of the pathophysiology of FA relate to either defective DNA repair or an inability of FA cells to remove oxygen-free radicals that damage cells. An extensive body of published data was generated mostly in the 1980s, but the data are still relevant today. The strongest evidence supporting an oxygen metabolism deficiency is the G_2 phase cell cycle defect of FA cells, consisting of both a phase transit delay and/or a complete arrest.[54] This finding is reduced when FA cells are grown at low oxygen levels, and a similar defect can be induced in normal cells grown at high oxygen levels.[55,56] This phenotype cannot be induced by treatment with DNA cross-linking agents, suggesting that it is not related to a DNA repair defect. A comprehensive summary of the literature is available,[7] and a more recent interpretation has been published.[57]

The best evidence supporting the theory that the primary defect is in DNA repair comes from our understanding of the critical role of FANC proteins in the DNA damage response pathway. There were also experiments in the 1980s in which the frequency of mutations induced by 8-methoxypsoralen plus near-ultraviolet radiation at the *HPRT* locus was lower in FA cells than in controls.[58,59] These results could indicate that FA cells cannot repair cross-links through the normal pathway involving mismatch repair, or recombinational repair following bypass of the lesion, or both. Similar studies that assayed the repair of cross-linked herpes simplex virus DNA following transfection found that FA cells, unlike controls, were able to repair cross-linked DNA only under conditions of multiple infection.[60] Because multiplicity reactivation is dependent on recombinational repair, it can be inferred that FA cells are defective in an excision repair pathway.

To reconcile the evidence of defective oxygen metabolism with the data demonstrating involvement of the DNA repair system in the pathology of FA cells, we speculate that proteins closely involved in DNA repair are particularly sensitive to oxidative damage. The biallelic gene inactivation in FA could either make the repair pathway sensitive to oxidative damage or cause a transient increase of oxidative damage to which the repair machinery is particularly sensitive. The findings that wild-type FANCA and FANCG proteins are redox-sensitive and are multimerized and/or form a nuclear complex in response to oxidative stress and damage are pertinent.[61]

Hematologic dysfunction in FA is evident at the hematopoietic progenitor level in bone marrow and peripheral blood. The frequencies of CFU-E, BFU-E and CFU-GM colony-forming cells are reduced fairly consistently in almost all patients after aplastic anemia ensues,[62–66] as well as in a few patients before the onset of aplastic anemia.[67] Although FA marrow cells show normal transcripts for the α and β chains of the GM-CSF/IL-3 receptor and for c-kit protein, there is a deficient proliferative response of CFU-GEMM, BFU-E and CFU-GM progenitors in response to GM-CSF plus stem cell factor (c-kit ligand) or IL-3 plus stem cell factor.[68] Because all hematopoietic lineages are affected in these studies, the basic defect is likely at the hematopoietic stem cell level. Cure of FA marrow failure by hematopoietic stem cell transplantation supports this view. Confirmatory data for defective stem cells in FA using long-term bone marrow cultures were reported by one group[69] but not confirmed by another.[70] Decreased colony numbers in these studies can be interpreted as the result of an absolute decrease in progenitors. In support of this, Buchwald documented decreased numbers of $CD34^+$ cells in *Fancc –/–* mice (M. Buchwald, personal communication). Decreased numbers of assayable hematopoietic colonies may also be a result of adequate numbers of progenitors that have faulty proliferative properties and cannot form colonies *in vitro*.

Additional factors are operative in FA bone marrow failure. Telomeres, the non-encoding DNA at each end of chromosomes, shorten with each round of cell division in normal human somatic cells. Their length is a reflection of the mitotic history of the cell. Telomerase, a ribonucleoprotein reverse transcriptase that can restore telomere length, is variably present in hematopoietic progenitors. Leukocyte telomere length is significantly shortened in FA patients but there is increased telomerase activity,[71] suggesting an abnormally high proliferative rate of progenitors, which ultimately leads to their premature senescence. In parallel, apoptosis has surfaced as an important mechanism in some inherited marrow failure syndromes. Increased marrow cell apoptosis has been demonstrated in FA patients[72] and in knockout mouse models[32] and is mediated by Fas, a membrane glycoprotein receptor containing an integral death domain. FA cells exposed to TNF-α, interferon-γ, mip-1α, Fas ligand, and double-stranded RNA undergo exaggerated apoptotic responses.[32,73,74]

Studies of cytokines in FA patients have shown varied abnormalities. Although FA fibroblasts showed no deficiencies in stem cell factor or M-CSF production, variability ranging from diminished production to augmentation of production of IL-6, GM-CSF and G-CSF has been observed in different patients.[75] A consistent finding that may relate directly to pathogenesis is diminished IL-6 production in FA patients and markedly heightened abnormal TNF-α generation.[76]

Clinical Features

History and Physical Examination

The presence of characteristic congenital physical anomalies alone or in combination with signs, symptoms, complications, and laboratory confirmation of bone marrow failure makes a diagnosis of FA straightforward. However, FA patients may lack anomalies. The older historical terms *Estren-Dameshek aplastic anemia* and *constitutional aplastic anemia type II* referred to such patients. With the introduction of clastogenic stress-induced chromosomal breakage analysis as a confirmatory test for FA, data from the IFAR showed that 39% of 202 patients tested had aplastic anemia and anomalies, and 30% had aplastic anemia without anomalies.[77] A summary of 1206 published cases of FA also documented that 25% of patients had no anomalies.[7] Twenty-four percent of patients in the IFAR had anomalies only, and 7% had neither anomalies nor hematologic abnormalities. Hence, the Estren-Dameshek cases that lack anomalies should not be considered as a separate entity but as part of the pleiotropic continuum of FA.

Table 28–2 shows the characteristic physical abnormalities and their approximate frequency. The most common anomaly is skin hyperpigmentation, a generalized brown melanin-like splattering,

Table 28–2 Characteristic Physical Anomalies in 1,206 Fanconi Anemia Patients*

Anomaly	Frequency (%)
Skin pigment changes and/or café au lait spots	55
Short stature	51
Upper limb abnormalities (thumbs, hands, radii, ulnae)	43
Hypogonadal and genitalia changes (mostly male)	35
Other skeletal findings (head/face, neck, spine)	30
Eyes/lids/epicanthal fold anomalies	23
Renal malformations	21
Gastrointestinal/cardiopulmonary malformations	11
Hips, legs, feet, toes abnormalities	10
Ear anomalies (external and internal), deafness	9

Alter BP: "Inherited Bone marrow Failure Syndromes" In Nathan DG, Orkin SH, Look AT, Ginsberg D (eds.): Nathan and Oski's Hematology of Infancy and Childhood, 6th ed. Philadelphia WB Saunders, 2003, p 280.

which is most prominent on the trunk, neck, and intertriginous areas and which becomes more obvious with age. Café-au-lait spots are common alone or in combination with the generalized hyperpigmentation, and sometimes with vitiligo or hypopigmentation. The skin pigmentation should not be confused with hemosiderosis-induced bronzing in transfusion-dependent patients who have not been adequately iron-chelated.

One half of patients are less than the third percentile for height. In some patients, growth failure is associated with endocrine abnormalities. In one report, spontaneous overnight growth hormone secretion was abnormal in all patients tested, and 44% had a subnormal response to growth hormone stimulation.[78] Approximately 40% of patients also have overt or compensated hypothyroidism, sometimes in combination with growth hormone deficiency.[79]

Malformations involving the upper limbs are common—especially hypoplastic, supernumerary, bifid, or absent thumbs. Hypoplastic or absent radii are always associated with hypoplastic or absent thumbs in contrast to the thrombocytopenia with absent radii (TAR) syndrome in which thumbs are always present. Less often, anomalies of the feet are seen including toe syndactyly, short toes, a supernumerary toe, clubfoot, and flat feet. Congenital hip dislocation and leg abnormalities are occasionally seen.

Males often have gonadal and genital abnormalities including an underdeveloped penis or micropenis, undescended, atrophic, or absent testes, hypospadias, phimosis, and an abnormal urethra. Female patients occasionally have malformations of the vagina, uterus, or ovary.

Many patients have a Fanconi "facies," and unrelated patients can resemble each other almost as closely as siblings. The head and facial changes vary but commonly consist of microcephaly, small eyes, epicanthal folds, and abnormal shape, size, or positioning of the ears. Approximately 10% of FA patients are developmentally retarded.

Renal anomalies occur but require imaging for documentation. Ectopic, pelvic, or horseshoe kidneys are detected often, as are duplicated, hypoplastic, dysplastic, or absent organs. Occasionally, hydronephrosis or hydroureter is present.

A scoring system was developed for the probability of an accurate diagnosis of FA using discriminating clinical and laboratory variables in patients enrolled in the IFAR whose diagnosis was confirmed by clastogenic stress-induced chromosomal breakage analysis.[77] The scoring system was useful in proving that diepoxybutane (DEB)-induced chromosomal breakage results could be correlated with common FA findings. DEB testing is considered by the IFAR to be the gold standard for diagnosis, but mitomycin C testing is still used in many laboratories.

Laboratory Findings

Peripheral Blood and Bone Marrow Findings. A cardinal feature is the gradual onset of bone marrow failure usually in the first decade of life, with declining values in one or more hematopoietic lineages. Of 754 FA patients followed prospectively by the IFAR, 80% had hematologic abnormalities other than acute leukemia or MDS.[49] The cumulative incidence of these abnormalities by 40 years of age was 90%. Patients with FANCC mutations appeared to have the earliest onset of changes and the highest incidence.[49] Thrombocytopenia usually develops initially, with subsequent onset of granulocytopenia and then anemia. Severe marrow aplasia eventually ensues in most cases but the full expression of pancytopenia is variable and evolves over a period of months to years. The development of aplastic anemia can be accelerated by intercurrent infections or by drugs such as chloramphenicol. Within families, there is a tendency for the hematologic changes to occur at approximately the same age in affected siblings.

The red cells are macrocytic with mean cell volumes often above 100 fl even before the onset of significant anemia. Erythropoiesis is characterized by increased HbF and increased expression of i antigen, but not necessarily both features in individual cells. The increased HbF production is not clonal and has a heterogeneous distribution. Ferrokinetic studies indicate that most patients have an element of ineffective erythropoiesis as part of the marrow failure. Red blood cell lifespan may be slightly shortened but this is a minor component, if any, of the anemia.

In the early stages of the disease, the bone marrow can show erythroid hyperplasia, sometimes with dyserythropoiesis, myelodysplastic changes, and even megaloblastic-appearing cells. As the disease progresses, the marrow becomes hypocellular and fatty, sometimes in a patchy manner, and shows a relative increase in lymphocytes, plasma cells, reticulum cells, and mast cells. With full-blown marrow failure, the morphology on biopsy is identical to severe acquired aplastic anemia.

A summary of the literature on FA heterozygotes indicates that parents of FA children may have physical abnormalities such as short stature but without hematologic disease.[7] Heterozygote carriers may also have increased levels of HbF, decreased natural killer cell counts and diminished reactivity to mitogen stimulation. In chromosome breakage assays with DEB, FA heterozygotes may have a higher mean breakage value compared to controls but individual testing shows overlap with normal values. Except for FA families with BRCA2 mutations, there is no apparent increased risk of cancer in relatives of FA patients.

Abnormal Chromosome Fragility. A major finding is abnormal chromosome fragility seen readily in metaphase preparations of peripheral blood lymphocytes cultured with phytohemagglutinin. The karyotype shows "spontaneously" occurring chromatid breaks, rearrangements, gaps, endoreduplications, and chromatid exchanges in cells from homozygote FA patients. Cultured skin fibroblasts also show the abnormal karyotype underscoring the constitutional nature of the disorder. The abnormal lymphocyte chromosome patterns and the number of breaks per cell have no direct correlation with the hematological or clinical course of individual patients.

Spontaneous chromosomal breaks are occasionally absent in true cases of homozygote FA.[77] The clastogenic stress-induced chromosomal breakage analysis was introduced, in part, to circumvent this problem and to bring specificity to testing for FA. Chromosomal breakage is strikingly enhanced compared with controls if clastogenic agents (DNA crosslinking compounds) such as DEB or mitomycin C (MMC) are added to the cultures.[80] Indeed, homozygote Fanconi cells are hypersensitive to many oncogenic and mutagenic inducers such as ionizing radiation, SV40 viral transformation, and alkylating and chemical agents including cyclophosphamide, nitrogen mustard, and platinum compounds.[8] For definitive diagnostic purposes, the IFAR has defined FA as increased numbers of chromosome breaks/cell after exposure to DEB[80] with a range of 1.06 to 23.9 compared to the normal control range of 0.00 to 0.05. The abnormal chromosome breakage can be used to make a prenatal diagnosis of FA.[81]

Diagnostic testing can be performed on fetal amniotic fluid cells obtained at 16 weeks' gestation or on chorionic villus biopsy specimens at 9 to 12 weeks. A very high degree of prenatal diagnostic accuracy has been obtained by looking at both spontaneous and DEB-induced breaks in fetal tissue.[81] DEB testing of heterozygote carriers is unreliable for diagnosis because there is overlap of results with the normal range.[7]

Somatic Mosaicism. Ten percent to 15% of patients with clinical FA do not show increased chromosome breakage when tested with DEB or mitomycin C. These patients usually have hematopoietic cell somatic mosaicism as a result of a molecular genetic correction in a stem cell resulting in 1 normal allele.[82–85] The mechanisms for this phenomenon include gene reversion, gene conversion, mitotic recombination and compensatory frameshifts. The end result is mixed populations of somatic cells, some with 2 abnormal alleles and some with 1. If FA is strongly suspected, a skin biopsy is performed to assess chromosomal breakage in cultured fibroblasts.

Immunoblotting for *FANCD2*. An accurate diagnostic and subtyping assay for FA has been introduced.[86] Primary lymphocytes or fibroblasts are assayed after exposure to mitomycin C or radiation for *FANCD2* by immunoblot, which distinguishes the unubiquitinated and monoubiquitinated forms. The testing is useful in 3 situations for screening FA defects.[46] In FA patients with diagnostic mitomycin-induced chromosomal breakage assays, *FANCD2* mutations are presumed if no full-length *FANCD2* is detected by immunoblotting. If *FANCD2* is detected but is not monoubiquitinated, mutations of one of the core complex proteins are predicted. If *FANCD2* is detected and *is* monoubiquitinated, *BRCA2* or *FANCJ* mutations are expected. Monoubiquitination of *FANCD2* is normal in other bone marrow failure syndromes and chromosomal breakage disorders.

Other Findings. Wild-type FA genes can be transfected into FA T cells using retroviral vectors.[87,88] If a specific wild-type FA gene corrects (complements) the abnormal chromosome breakage in an FA patient's T cells on exposure to DEB, the mutant gene is identified. The mutant gene can also be identified by flow cytometry. FA cells exposed to alkylating agents arrest in the G_2/M phase of the cell cycle. The transduced wild-type FA gene that reduces G_2/M arrested cells pinpoints the mutant gene.

A simple, fast, sensitive, and specific biochemical test for FA has also been described,[89] but there are several methods and each requires validation. The vast majority of FA patients have stable, elevated levels of serum α-fetoprotein expressed constitutively that are independent of liver complications and of androgen therapy. Levels are also unchanged after hematopoietic stem cell transplantation.

Predisposition to Malignancy

A major feature of the FA phenotype is the propensity to develop cancer. The chromosome fragility, the defects in DNA repair, the genomic instability, and the cellular damage that occur in FA patients translate into an enormous predisposition for malignancy.[90,91] Since there are at least 13 genetic mutations that are operative in FA, the disorder is a critical human model of the genetic determinants of hematologic cancers and malignant solid tumors. FA is a member of two categories of cancer predisposition syndromes. The first group is comprised of disorders of DNA repair that include ataxia telangiectasia, xeroderma pigmentosum, and Bloom syndrome. The close relationship between FA and ataxia telangiectasia, for example, is underscored by data showing convergence of signaling pathways in both conditions.[92] The second group of predisposition syndromes consists of other inherited marrow failure disorders described herein that show a propensity for malignant myeloid transformation and/or solid tumors.

The magnitude of the risk of malignancy in FA is detailed in two comprehensive reports. The first is a complete survey of literature from 1927 to 2001 that identifies 1301 published cases of FA.[91] Of these, 200 patients had one or more cancers, a crude rate of 17%. The median age for all cancers in these patients was 16 years of age, which is strikingly different from the median age of 68 for the same types of cancer in the general population.

There were 68 patients with a total of 80 solid tumors. The most frequent solid tumors were squamous cell carcinomas of the head, neck, and upper esophagus, followed by carcinomas of the vulva and/or anus, and lower esophagus. Twelve patients were described who developed cancer after bone marrow transplantation. All 12 patients had oral carcinoma, mainly of the tongue, and one case had an additional vulva carcinoma. Liver tumors, benign and malignant, occurred in 37 patients (23 hepatomas, 13 adenomas, and 1 not specified). All of the hepatoma patients and all adenoma cases except one had received androgen therapy for aplastic anemia. Androgen administration has therefore been implicated in liver tumor pathogenesis, as well as in the etiology of peliosis hepatis, which consists of blood-filled hepatic sinusoids in the liver. Indeed, peliosis hepatis is reversible when androgens are stopped, and tumors may regress.

The second report that describes the malignant risk in FA is the 20-year prospective observational study by the IFAR.[49] The findings corroborate the literature survey[91] in terms of type of cancer and site. Of the 754 registered FA patients, 120 (16%) developed hematologic cancer (AML, MDS, or ALL). Based on current data,[49,90,91] the crude risks irrespective of age are about 5% for MDS and up to 10% for leukemia. The cumulative incidence of leukemia by 25 years of age is about 10%. Previous observations by the IFAR showed that the risk of developing MDS and AML was higher for patients in whom a prior clonal marrow cytogenetic abnormality had been detected.[93] Monosomy 7, rearrangement or partial loss of 7q, rearrangements of 1p36 and 1q24-34, and rearrangements of 11q22-25 were the most frequently recurring cytogenetic changes. There is also a high incidence of abnormalities involving chromosomes 2, 6, 8, 5, and 21.

Additional data indicate that patients with partial trisomies and tetrasomies of chromosome 3q in marrow cells also have a high risk of developing MDS and AML.[94] Similar to the literature review[91] and another source,[95] the IFAR verified that the risk of developing hematologic and non-hematologic cancer increased with advancing age, but it did not show an age-related plateau for the risks for MDS and AML, possibly because both diagnoses were analyzed together. When interpreting the significance of cytogenetic clonal abnormalities in FA patients, note that clonal variation is frequent including appearances of new clones, disappearance of established clones, and clonal evolution.[95]

Differential Diagnosis

Patients with hematological abnormalities and characteristic physical anomalies are not difficult to diagnose, especially if there are previously affected siblings. Distinguishing FA from acquired aplastic anemia on clinical grounds can be difficult if the FA patient lacks physical anomalies. In this situation, the clastogenic stress-induced chromosomal breakage analysis using DEB or MMC will specifically identify FA and lead to the correct diagnosis. Although not widely available yet, screening by *FANCD2* immunoblotting or by retroviral-mediated transfer of corrective wild-type *FANC* genes into patient cells is also diagnostic.

Although neutropenia is a consistent feature of Shwachman–Diamond syndrome (SDS), anemia and/or thrombocytopenia is seen in more than 50% of the patients and can be confused with FA. Since growth failure is also a manifestation of SDS, differentiating between the two disorders can initially be difficult. The major difference between them is that SDS is a disorder of exocrine pancreatic dysfunction that produces gut malabsorption. This can be confirmed by fecal fat analysis, by pancreatic stimulation studies using intravenous secretin or cholecystokinin that confirm markedly impaired enzyme secretion, and by showing reduced levels of serum trypsinogen and isoamylase. Computed tomography ultrasonography or magnetic resonance imaging of the pancreas may also demonstrate fatty changes within the body of the pancreas. Other skeletal distinguishing features found in some SDS patients are short flared ribs, thoracic dystrophy at birth, delayed bone maturation, and metaphyseal dysostosis of the long bones. Chromosomes do not show spontaneous breaks in SDS, and there is no increased breakage after clastogenic stress using DEB or MMC. Specific diagnostic confirmation is obtained by demonstrating the mutant *SBDS* gene.

Dyskeratosis congenita (DC) shares some features with FA including development of pancytopenia, a predisposition to cancer and leukemia, and skin pigmentary changes. However, the pigmentation pattern is somewhat different in DC and manifests with a lacy reticulated pattern affecting the face, neck, chest, and arms, often with a telangiectatic component. At some point, usually in the first decade, DC patients also develop dystrophic nails of the hands and feet, and, somewhat later, leukoplakia involving the oral mucosa, especially the tongue. Other findings seen only in DC and not in FA are teeth abnormalities with dental decay and early tooth loss, hair loss, and hyperhydrosis of the palms and soles. Although there are contradictory data regarding chromosomal fragility in DC, DEB testing has not shown any difference between patients and controls, which contrasts sharply with FA patients. In the X-linked form of DC, mutations can be identified in the *DKC1* gene. The *TERC* or *TERT* or *TINF2* gene mutation confirms the dominant form of the disorder. The *NOP10* mutation accounts for autosomal recessive DC.

Congenital amegakaryocytic thrombocytopenia and TAR syndrome both present in the neonatal period with an isolated decrease of platelets. A neonatal hematologic presentation is atypical for FA, as less than 5% of patients are diagnosed in the first year of life. Neither of the thrombocytopenic syndromes shows chromosome fragility, which separates them from FA, and a mutated *MPL* gene is diagnostic of congenital amegakaryocytic thrombocytopenia. In the TAR syndrome, thumbs are always preserved and intact despite the absence of radii, whereas in FA, the thumbs are hypoplastic or absent when the radii are absent.

Schimke immunoosseous dysplasia is characterized by spondyloepiphyseal dysplasia with exaggerated lumbar lordosis, renal dysfunction, hypothyroidism, and cytopenias including lymphopenia. The syndrome is cause by a mutated *SMARCAL1* gene.

The Nijmegen chromosome breakage syndrome is a rare disorder characterized by stunted growth, microcephaly, a distinctive facies, café-au-lait spots, immunodeficiency, and a predisposition to lymphoid malignancy. The genetic defect is a mutant *NBS1* gene whose wild-type protein product is involved in DNA repair. Because these patients show increased chromosomal sensitivity to DEB and MMC, they can mimic and be confused with FA.[96] Genetic testing is diagnostic.

Natural History and Prognosis

The most serious early event for most FA patients is bone marrow failure. The exceptions are patients with biallelic *BRCA2* mutations who manifest early-onset AML, brain tumors, and Wilms tumors. Judging from the literature, the risk for FA patients developing solid malignant tumors, liver tumors, acute leukemia and MDS is at least 15%, but it is likely higher in older patients. Treatment for cancer imposes additional problems and probably increases the risk for additional cancers secondary to therapy.

Despite these major issues, prognosis for FA patients is improving. Older literature describing an early demise of FA patients is flawed because it did not take into account the diversity in clinical and hematological phenotype. Early diagnosis can now be made before the onset of serious marrow failure or malignant transformation, and survival from the time of diagnosis is longer. Also, current management, especially hematopoietic stem cell transplantation (HSCT), has dramatically changed prognosis. From cases reported in the last decade, the projected median survival is greater than 30 years of age.[7] Some middle-aged patients with presumably hypomorphic mutations are not diagnosed as FA until severe complications from treatment in cancer occur.[97] Despite delayed menarche, irregular menses, and early menopause, older female FA patients can be sexually active; at least 20 patients have become pregnant resulting in 21 living infants as well as miscarriages.[7] Four FA males were also reported to be fathers despite the high incidence of underdeveloped gonads and abnormal spermatogenesis reported in FA males overall.[7]

Therapy

Because of their clinical and psychosocial complexity, FA patients should be supervised by a hematologist at a tertiary care center using a comprehensive and multidisciplinary approach. On the initial visit, the following should be performed: a careful physical examination with emphasis on physical anomalies; complete blood counts and chemistries; serum α-fetoprotein level; and diepoxybutane (and/or mitomycin C) chromosome fragility testing on peripheral blood lymphocytes on patients and siblings. When the diagnosis is confirmed, HLA tissue typing on patient and family members should be performed and arrangements made for determining the mutant gene. Imaging studies should also be made to search for internal anomalies described in History and Physical Examination section. When all the results are catalogued, a follow-up visit with the family is arranged to discuss management options and prognosis.

If the patient is stable and has only minimal to moderate hematological changes and does not have transfusion requirements, a period of observation is indicated. Blood counts should be monitored every 1 to 3 months, and bone marrow aspirates and biopsies should be performed annually for morphology and cancer cytogenetics to identify the emergence of a malignant clone or overt transformation to MDS or AML. Spectral karyotyping (SKY), fluorescent in situ hybridization (FISH), and comparative genomic hybridization can enhance the diagnostic capability on marrow cells. Depending on the types of congenital anomalies, subspecialty consultations, for example with orthopedic surgery, can be arranged during this interval.

Growth is followed clinically, and when growth velocity or stature falls below expectations, endocrine evaluation is needed to identify growth hormone deficiency. Impaired glucose tolerance, hyperinsulinemia, and diabetes mellitus occur more commonly in FA[79] and should be screened for annually or biannually depending on the degree of hyperglycemia found on initial testing. Screening for hypothyroidism also should be performed annually. Screening for cancers associated with FA should be initiated at least annually. Dentists, oral surgeons, or head and neck surgeons should be recruited to screen for head and neck squamous cell carcinomas. The risk in untransplanted FA patients is 700-fold that of the general population.[90] After stem cell transplantation, the oral cavity should be examined every 3 months for signs of malignant change, because cancers can occur within a year of the procedure.[98] Beginning at menarche, all women with FA should undergo gynecologic screening annually, because the risk of gynecologic squamous cell carcinoma is 4000-fold that of the general population.[90]

Hematopoietic Stem Cell Transplantation (HSCT)

HSCT is currently the only curative therapy for the hematological abnormalities of FA. The best donor source is an HLA-matched sibling in whom thorough screening has excluded a diagnosis of FA. Initial efforts to transplant FA patients using standard preparative regimens and graft-versus-host prophylaxis were plagued by two serious and often lethal problems: severe cytotoxicity from chemotherapy, and exaggerated graft-versus-host disease (GVHD). HSCT protocols were subsequently modified for FA patients and the outcomes improved substantially. Protocol refinements are ongoing internationally and several approaches are being studied.

Pooled published data on HSCT using HLA-matched sibling donors show a survival of greater than 80% in FA patients less than 10 years of age, and greater than 65% for FA patients of all ages. The multicenter Italian experience reflects these optimistic outcomes.[99] Using a conditioning regimen of low-dose cyclophosphamide (median 20 mg/kg in most patients) and thoracoabdominal or total body irradiation (median dose 500 cGy), survival for 27 consecutive patients at 36 months was 81.5%.

Some transplantation centers have eliminated irradiation in the preparative regimen because of concern for secondary cancer, especially squamous cell carcinoma of the head and neck or genitourinary tract. A retrospective study of 37 FA patients conditioned with low-dose cyclophosphamide plus thoracoabdominal irradiation also identified almost a twofold risk of acute GVHD compared with a cohort of non-FA patients with aplastic anemia transplanted without irradiation conditioning.[100] This risk increased to sevenfold in patients younger than 12 years old.

Reduction in immunosuppression by eliminating radiation is best suited for transplants using genotypically-matched related donors determined by DNA-based molecular methodology. Several reports from 2005 and 2006 reflect this trend.[101–103] Comparable outcomes were seen with protocols using low-dose cyclophosphamide alone (60 or 80 mg/kg),[101] busulfan (6 mg/kg) plus cyclophosphamide (40 mg/kg),[102] and cyclophosphamide (60 mg/kg) plus anti-thymocyte globulin (40 mg/kg/day for 4 doses).[103] There is a growing trend for incorporating fludarabine, a purine anti-metabolite with potent immunosuppressive properties, into conditioning regimens instead of irradiation for FA transplants.[104]

For FA patients who do not have an HLA-A, B, and DRB1-identical sibling donor for HSCT, a search for a matched unrelated donor should be initiated. Because of the heightened graft-versus-host response observed in FA patients, the survivals and cure rates are not as good compared to matched sibling donor HSCT. Even when matched unrelated marrow is fully compatible with the recipient at the DNA level (*molecular match*), these transplants are still problematic. Two reports on outcomes of 69 and 29 FA patients, respectively, transplanted with matched unrelated or alternate donors yielded probabilities of survival of about 33%.[105,106] These outcomes decline sharply to approximately 10% if patients are transplanted with advanced MDS or AML, proven or probable fungal infections, or prior gram-negative infections. Additional risk factors are patients older than 10 years, prior use of androgens, the number of physical anomalies, and female donors.[105] There is evidence that fludarabine-based protocols yield improved outcomes in FA transplantations with unrelated and alternate donors sources.[107–110]

Unless the increased risks associated with alternate donors improve, it is not recommended currently that FA patients undergo this type of HSCT if their clinical and hematological status is stable. Although open to debate, indications to proceed with an alternate donor HSCT include (a) failure to respond adequately to androgen therapy and/or cytokine treatment resulting in severe cytopenia or an impending need for chronic transfusional support; (b) presence of a persistent high risk cytogenetic clone in bone marrow cells, for example, monosomy 7; (c) overt malignant transformation to MDS or AML; and (d) a high risk mutation (FANCC IVS4, FANCC exon 14, or BRCA2).

Cord blood cells, naturally enriched with hematopoietic stem and progenitor cells, are being increasingly used as a donor source. The first cord blood transplantation was reported in 1989 for a FA patient using a matched sibling donor.[111] Since then, cord blood collections and transplants have increased quickly for a variety of indications including more FA patients.[112,113] Using cord cells from related or unrelated donors, engraftment and survival is comparable to related or unrelated bone marrow, although engraftment is slower with cord blood. The incidence of acute and chronic GVHD is reduced with cord blood grafts even in 1 to 2 HLA antigen mismatched transplants.

G-CSF-mobilization and collection of peripheral blood CD34+ cells from FA patients prior to onset of severe pancytopenia[114] has not attained broad application. These cells in theory can be used as targets for gene therapy, or cryo-preserved and infused later when severe marrow failure ensues, or as an autologous rescue after chemotherapy in the event of leukemic transformation.

Molecular technology has led to *preimplantation genetic diagnosis* (PGD) in order to find an HLA-matched donor for transplantation for a FA patient.[115] A couple, both carriers of the IVS4+4A→T mutation in the FANCC gene, had an affected child requiring a hematopoietic stem cell transplantation. Using single-cell PCR technology, isolated cells from several blastomeres fertilized in vitro were each tested for HLA type and for presence of the mutation. HLA- compatible normal blastomeres were then transferred and implanted in utero resulting in one success and the subsequent birth of a matched unaffected sibling. Cord blood from such a PGD-selected healthy sibling has been used successfully for a HSCT of the affected sibling.[116,117] The notion of "designer babies" has sparked ethical debate.[118]

Despite the successes of HSCT in correcting the marrow failure of FA patients, there is a subset of survivors who develop secondary cancers, particularly squamous cell carcinoma of the head and neck.[98] These malignancies reflect the ongoing genetic susceptibility of FA nonhematopoietic tissue to cancer despite successful transplantation for marrow failure.[119] Conditioning regimens clearly play a role in heightening the risk of transformation.

Hematopoietic Growth Factors

The role for recombinant granulocyte colony stimulating factor (G-CSF) therapy for FA has not been defined. A multicenter clinical trial examined the effect of prolonged administration of G-CSF to 12 FA patients with neutropenia.[120] The patients were treated with varying subcutaneous dosages daily or every other day for 40 weeks. By week 8 of the study, all patients had an increase in absolute neutrophil numbers and 4 had an increase in platelet counts. Additionally, four patients who were not being transfused had a significant increment in hemoglobin levels and a fifth patient lost a transfusion requirement. Concurrent with the impressive improvements in hematology, 8 of 10 patients who finished 40 weeks of G-CSF treatment showed increases in the percentage of marrow and peripheral blood CD34+ cells.

Since genomic instability and a marked predisposition to leukemia and cancer are features of FA, the wisdom of using a growth-promoting cytokine on a long-term basis for this disorder continues to be an issue.[121] In the G-CSF study,[120] one patient had a marrow clonal cytogenetic abnormality (48 XXY, +14) without MDS or AML at week 40 of treatment. Therapy was stopped and within 3 months the +X, +14 clone disappeared but monosomy 7 appeared in 11% of metaphases and increased over the ensuing months, prompting bone marrow transplantation. Unlike the monosomy 7, the appearance of the +X, +14 clone while the patient was receiving G-CSF treatment and its disappearance when cytokine was discontinued must be put into the context of FA, per se, in which clones, seemingly unstable, are known to appear and disappear spontaneously.[95]

Another study examined the long term efficacy and safety of G-CSF in 4 FA patients.[121] Three had an increase in neutrophil numbers, a reduction in number and severity of infections, and improvement in clinical status. However two of the responders developed monosomy 7 and showed immature cells in peripheral blood.

Thus, G-CSF when used alone in FA can usually induce an increase in absolute neutrophil numbers and occasionally boost platelet counts and hemoglobin levels. However, there appears to be a heightened risk of developing cytogenetic abnormality such as monosomy 7.

GM-CSF can also induce an increase in neutrophils in FA using a starting dose of 250 $\mu g/m^2$/day subcutaneously. Of 7 patients treated, 6 had a 7- to 25-fold increase in neutrophils that was sustained with minimal side effects.[122]

Combination cytokine therapy consisting of G-CSF 5 µg/kg once daily with erythropoietin 50 units/kg administered subcutaneously or intravenously three times a week was given to patients without a matched donor for transplantation.[123] Androgen therapy was added if the response was inadequate. Of 20 patients treated, all but 1 had improved neutrophil numbers, 20% achieved a sustained rise in platelets, and 33% had an increase in hemoglobin levels. Although more than half of the responders lost the response after one year as a result of progression of marrow failure, the requirement for androgen therapy could be delayed by about a year. A trial of interleukin-11 for patients with inherited marrow failure and thrombocytopenia failed to increase platelet numbers (Dr. James Croop, personal communication).

Androgens

Androgen therapy has been used to treat FA for more than four decades. The overall response rate in the literature is about 50%[7] heralded by reticulocytosis and a rise in hemoglobin within 1 to 2 months. If the other lineages respond, white cells increase next, followed by platelets, but it may take many months to achieve the maximum response. When the response is deemed maximal, the androgens should be slowly tapered but not stopped entirely. Accepted indications for treating with androgens are one or more of the following: hemoglobin level less than 8 g/dL or symptoms from anemia; platelet count less than 30,000/mm^3; and neutrophil count less than 500/mm^3.

Oxymetholone, an oral 17-α alkylated androgen, is used most frequently at 2 to 5 mg/kg once a day with the lower dose preferred initially. Although unproven, corticosteroids are commonly added to offset the androgen-induced growth acceleration and to prevent thrombocytopenic bleeding by promoting vascular stability. For this purpose, 5 to 10 mg of prednisone is given orally every second day. If an injectable androgen is preferred to decrease the risk of liver toxicity and growth of tumors, nandrolone decanoate, 1 to 2 mg/kg/week is given intramuscularly followed by the application of local suitable pressure and ice packs to prevent the development of hematomas. There are insufficient comparative data on the efficacy of the attenuated androgen, Danazol, compared to oxymetholone to make a recommendation. Claims of reduced masculinizing side effects in female FA patients treated with Danazol as compared to oxymetholone have not been substantiated in clinical trials.

Almost all patients relapse when androgens are stopped. Those few who successfully discontinue treatment are often in the puberty age range when temporary "spontaneous hematological remissions" have been observed to occur. A subset of patients on long-term androgens eventually become refractory to therapy as marrow failure progresses. Potential side effects include masculinization, which is especially troublesome in female patients, and elevated hepatic enzymes, cholestasis, peliosis hepatis, and liver tumors. Those receiving androgens should be evaluated serially with liver enzyme profiles every 2 to 3 months and ultrasonography and/or CT scan of liver, every 6 to 12 months. If liver enzymes increase to threefold normal of if abnormalities appear on imaging, the androgen dose should be decreased or stopped.

It is strongly recommended by many transplant centers that an FA patient not receive androgens if it is known that the patient has a matched donor available. Prior use of androgens pre-transplantation adversely affects outcome after the transplantation.[105]

Future Directions

The premise for gene therapy in FA is based on the assumption that corrected hematopoietic cells would have a growth advantage. Strengthening this supposition are FA patients with hematopoietic somatic mosaicism who show spontaneous disappearance of cells with the FA phenotype.[82–85] These patients have two populations of leukocytes, one sensitive to mitomycin C and the other with normal resistance to mitomycin C.[85] These *mosaic* patients may show spontaneous hematologic improvement suggesting that hematopoiesis was derived from stem cells with a normal phenotype. In the context of gene therapy, there is evidence that even one genetically corrected hematopoietic stem cell may be able to repopulate the marrow of a FA patient.[125]

Despite encouraging preclinical studies over a decade ago using retroviral vectors that showed wild-type *FANCC* and *FANCA* could be integrated into normal and FA CD34$^+$ cells,[126–128] the ensuing clinical trials in *FANCC* and *FANCA* patients were disappointing.[129] A central problem is suboptimal wild-type gene integration into FA cells in culture. Because of the apoptotic phenotype, FA cells die rapidly in vitro before efficient gene transfer is accomplished. Lentiviral vectors that can infect noncycling human cells were deemed the solution[130] but obstacles persisted. Recently, there is evidence that FA marrow cell survival in vitro can be ameliorated by using specific culture conditions that limit oxidative stress.[131] Using these conditions, gene-corrected marrow cells using retroviral vectors survived in culture longer than 4 months and showed long term engraftment in NOD/SCID mice.[131] There is also interest in transposons, non-viral vectors that have been used successfully for gene delivery in murine models and may hold promise for human genetic diseases.[132]

Shwachman-Diamond Syndrome

Background

Shwachman-Diamond syndrome (SDS) is an autosomal recessive multisystem disorder characterized by exocrine pancreatic insufficiency and varying degrees of bone marrow failure.[133–138] There may be additional features including short stature and skeletal abnormalities. The mutant gene responsible for this complex, pleiotropic phenotype has been identified[139] and has been confirmed in 90% of patients with the classic presentation. To date, though, no unifying pathogenesis has been able to account for all of the multisystem features of SDS. Chromosomes are normal and there is no increased breakage with clastogenic stress testing in contrast to FA patients. None of these patients have cystic fibrosis; sweat chloride levels are normal. Many families have been identified with at least two affected children, and published studies of segregation ratios and family pedigrees support an autosomal recessive mode of inheritance.

Etiology, Genetics, and Pathophysiology

The identification of SDS-associated mutations on chromosome 7q11 in a previously uncharacterized gene termed "*SBDS*" was the entry point for studies on the molecular basis for SDS.[139] There is an adjoining pseudogene (*SBDSP*) with 97% homology but it contains deletions and nucleotide substitutions that disrupt its coding potential. Recombination occurs whereby segments of *SBDSP* become incorporated into wild-type *SBDS* and interfere with its function.

These recombinational events result in 3 common gene conversion mutations in exon 2 that account for 75% of *SDS* alleles. A nonsense mutation, 183_184TA>CT, introduces an in-frame stop codon (K62X); a splice-site mutation, 258+2T>C, is predicted to result in premature truncation of the SBDS protein by frameshift (C84fs3); and an extended conversion mutation, 183_184TA>TA+258+2T>C, encompasses both mutations. In the Toronto database of 210 SDS families, 89% of unrelated SDS individuals carry a gene conversion mutation on one allele and 60% carry conversion mutations on both alleles. Thus, the vast majority of patients are compound heterozygotes with respect to K62X and C84fs3. Additional rare mutations in the *SBDS* gene have been identified in SDS patients. These include dozens of insertion, deletion, and missense mutations which have not arisen from gene conversion events.

SBDS is a member of a highly conserved protein family of previously unknown function with putative orthologs in diverse species including archaea and eukaryocytes. The gene encodes a 250 amino acid protein product whose phylogeny is shared with proteins that are enriched for RNA metabolism and/or ribosome-associated functions.[140] The SBDS protein can be detected in human cell nuclei and in cytoplasm but is concentrated within nucleoli providing supportive evidence for its role in RNA processing.[141] The pathophysiological link between exocrine pancreatic insufficiency, physical anomalies, partial to complete marrow failure and propensity to myelodysplastic syndromes (MDS) and acute myeloid leukemia (AML) should soon be clarified. SBDS forms a protein complex with nucleophosmin, a multifunctional protein implicated in ribosome biogenesis and leukemogenesis.[142] Biallelic targeted disruption of the mouse ortholog Sbds leads to arrested embryonic development and early lethality.[143]

Regarding the bone marrow failure, initial studies in the 1970s and early 1980s showed reduced CFU-GM and BFU-E colony growth in most patients compatible with a defective stem cell origin

Fanconi Anemia: Hematology and Oncology Details Worth Noting

Because 25% of FA patients do not have physical anomalies, cases may not be recognized until they present with aplastic anemia, MDS, AML, single cytopenias or macrocytic red cells. Thus, FA should be part of the differential diagnosis in children and adults with unexplained cytopenias. Similarly, the diagnosis of MDS or AML in patients less than 1 year to 30 years of age should prompt consideration of FA as the underlying problem. Patients with AML or solid tumors who exhibit excessive sensitivity to chemotherapy or radiotherapy should also be tested for FA. Cases of "acquired" or "idiopathic" aplastic anemia who fail to respond to immunosuppressive therapy with ATG and cyclosporine may also have FA.

The relative risk of AML in FA patients is 800-fold; the frequency of MDS has not been defined in these patients. Although MDS may precede overt transformation to AML, this is not predictable in FA and the temporal relationship between the two is unclear. Data from patients who have annual bone marrow testing for morphology and cytogenetics may show clonal chromosomal abnormalities with or without morphologic evidence of MDS. Isolated cytogenetic clones without signs of MDS in FA are perplexing because they may come and go without progression to leukemia. In some cases, isolated clones have persisted *without* overt marrow transformation for more than 12 years. Findings of clones with cytogenetic abnormalities commonly associated with MDS, however, such as −7 or +8 warrant careful evaluation. There is a striking association between chromosome 3q26q29 amplifications and rapid progression to MDS or AML. The identity of the duplicated material may have to be confirmed by FISH or SKY or by comparative genomic hybridization because G-banding may not be completely informative.

When interpreting marrow morphology and cytogenetic findings the following must be noted. Bone marrow morphology often appears dysplastic in FA patients. Marrow cell dysplasias, such as nuclear/cytoplasmic dyssynchrony, hypolobulated megakaryocytes, and binucleated erythroid cells, are often seen in patients with FA and must be distinguished from MDS. Such marrow dysplasia is commonly seen in the inherited marrow failure syndromes and is not necessarily a sign of impending AML. The distinction between benign and malignant cytology should be established by an experienced morphologist with familiarity of these disorders.

Androgen therapy induces a rise in hemoglobin and sometimes platelets and neutrophils in about 50% of FA patients. A subset of responders becomes refractory over time. MDS and AML are not prevented by androgen treatment. There are 5 complications of androgen therapy that require consideration.

1. *Peliosis hepatis* is a cystic dilation of hepatic sinusoids that fill with blood and can be life-threatening if they rupture. They may be clinically silent or produce right upper quadrant pain. Liver function tests are normal. Imaging is the safest way to diagnose the abnormality. The lesions may regress after stopping the androgens.
2. *Androgens also damage hepatocytes* nonspecifically. This may be manifest as cholestatic jaundice or elevated liver enzymes. Stopping androgen therapy will usually lead to complete resolution. Hepatic cirrhosis may develop in patients on continued androgen therapy. If resolution of enzyme elevation does not occur after androgen withdrawal, a liver biopsy is indicated.
3. *Hepatocellular adenomas* are associated with androgen therapy. These are benign, non-invasive tumors. They can, however, rupture, leading to life-threatening bleeding. FA patients may develop these tumors rapidly but they can be readily detected by imaging. The tumor may regress after stopping the androgens. If persistent, surgical resection or radiofrequency ablation may be necessary.
4. *Hepatocellular carcinoma* (HCC; hepatoma) occurs with androgen use and some studies have suggested that FA patients on treatment may be at increased risk for HCC. The HCC associated with androgens characteristically does not produce α-fetoprotein in serum, distinguishing it from de novo HCC. Patients developing HCC should discontinue androgen therapy.
5. Androgen therapy for FA patients is recognized by hematopoietic stem cell transplanters as an important *adverse prognostic factor* for those receiving a transplant. Several centers with experience in FA transplants firmly recommend that androgens *not* be given to any FA patients unless a suitable donor is not available.

There is up to a 700-fold increase in the incidence of head and neck squamous cell carcinoma in patients with FA. The cumulative risk is 14% for patients surviving to 40 years of age. The biological behavior of these cancers in FA is aggressive with early lymph node metastases and soft tissue invasion. The risk is heightened after hematopoietic stem cell transplantation and is partly related to acute and chronic GVHD. Tobacco and alcohol use, especially together, also increases the cancer risk and total abstinence from both is strongly recommended. Surveillance should begin aggressively by 10 years of age on a semiannual basis by an experienced professional in the field of dentistry, oral surgery, or head and neck surgery.

Similar to the heightened risk of the head and neck sites, there is a 4000-fold risk of genital tract squamous cell carcinoma in women with FA. Cervical, vaginal, vulvar and anal cancers have been recorded. Annual exams for all FA women should begin at age 16 years or at menarche and must include a Papanicolaou (Pap) smear and reactive testing for human papilloma virus (HPV). HPV DNA is detected in 84% of squamous cell carcinoma specimens from various anatomic sites in FA patients compared to 36% of specimens from non-Fanconi controls. Prevention of HPV should become a reality with the availability of the HPV vaccines (example, Gardasil quadrivalent cervical cancer vaccine, Merck Pharmaceuticals).

of the marrow failure.[144] Recent investigations have characterized a much more extensive hematopoietic phenotype (Table 28–3).[145–149] SDS marrow has decreased numbers of CD34$^+$ cells as well as an impaired ability for CD34$^+$ cells to form multilineage hematopoietic colonies in vitro confirming that they are intrinsically defective.[145] The bone marrow stroma is also markedly defective in terms of its ability to support and maintain normal hematopoiesis.[145] Patients' marrow cells over-express Fas, the membrane receptor for Fas ligand, and show increased patterns of apoptosis after preincubation with activating anti-Fas antibody,[146] pinpointing this as a central pathogenetic mechanism for the marrow failure. An additional finding is abnormal telomere shortening in patient leukocytes,[147] reflecting premature cellular aging and likely representing compensatory stem cell hyperproliferation. Lymphoid immune function is also impaired; most SDS patients show decreased numbers or diminished function of B cells, T cells, or NK cells.[148] Marrow microvessel density is increased[149] reflecting neovascularization, a hallmark of malignant tumors, acute leukemia, and MDS. Overexpression of p53 protein

Table 28–3 Hematopoietic Phenotype in Shwachman-Diamond Syndrome

- Decreased marrow CD34+ cells[a]
- Decreased colonies from CD34+ cells[a]
- Abnormal telomere shortening of leukocytes[b]
- Increased apoptosis of marrow cells[c]
- Apoptosis is mediated by Fas pathway[c]
- Marrow stromal cell function is impaired[a]
- Lymphoid immune function is abnormal[d]
- Marrow microvessel density is increased[e]
- Marrow cell upregulation of specific oncogenes[f]

[a]Dror Y, Freedman MH: Shwachman-Diamond syndrome is an inherited preleukemic bone marrow failure disorder with aberrant hematologic progenitors and faulty marrow microenvironment. Blood 94:3048, 1999.

[b]Thornley I, Dror Y, Sung L, et al: Telomere shortening in leukocytes of children with Shwachman-Diamond syndrome. Br J Haematol 117:189, 2002.

[c]Dror Y, Freedman MH: Shwachman-Diamond syndrome marrow cells show abnormally increased apoptosis mediated through the Fas pathway. Blood 97:3011, 2001.

[d]Dror Y, Ginzberg H, Dalal I, et al: Immune function in patients with Shwachman-Diamond syndrome. Br J Haematol 114:712, 2001.

[e]Leung EW, Rujkijyanont P, Beyene J, et al: Shwachman-Diamond syndrome: an inherited model of aplastic anemia with accelerated angiogenesis. Br J Haematol 133:558, 2006.

[f]Rujkijyanont P, Beyene J, Wei K, et al: Leukemia-related gene expression in bone marrow cells from patients with the preleukaemic disorder Shwachman-Diamond syndrome. Br J Haematol 137:537, 2007.

Table 28–4 Clinical Features and Strict Diagnostic Criteria for Shwachman–Diamond Syndrome

Essential Features for Diagnosis	% Patients	References
• Pancreatic insufficiency (decreased digestive enzymes)	100%	151–153
• Hematologic cytopenias:		151,152,155,156
Neutropenia	88%–100%	
Thrombocytopenia	24%–70%	
Anemia	42%–66%	
Pancytopenia	10%–44%	
Supportive Diagnostic Features		
• Short stature	50%	151
• Skeletal abnormalities:		154
Delayed bone maturation	100%	
Metaphyseal dysplasia	44%–77%	
Rib cage anomalies	32%–52%	
• Hepatomegaly/elevated enzymes	<50%	152
• Poor oral health (caries, ulcers, tooth loss)	>50%	*
• Learning and behavioral problems	>50%	*

*Unpublished data.

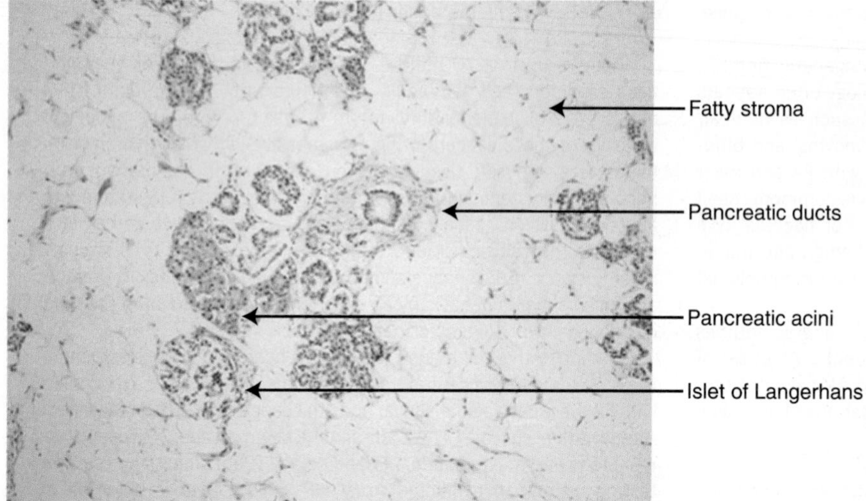

Figure 28–2 Pancreatic tissue pathology in severe Shwachman–Diamond syndrome showing the 2 classic features: deficiency of acinar tissue and fatty replacement. Islets of Langerhans are intact. *(Provided by Dr. Peter Durie, Toronto.)*

has also been demonstrated in bone marrow biopsies from patients[150]; this may represent an early indicator of significant DNA genetic alteration, which is a crucial step in leukemogenesis.

Clinical Features

History and Physical Examination

The many manifestations that occur in varying combinations are shown in Table 28–4; however, the criteria for clinical diagnosis are very specific and strict.[151] Patients must have two essential features for diagnosis: exocrine pancreatic insufficiency *and* one or more hematological cytopenias. Other features like short stature, skeletal abnormalities, hepatic enlargement or impairment, poor oral health, and learning and behavioral problems are supportive of the diagnosis, but cannot substitute for the pancreatic or hematological changes.

The pancreatic pathology is caused by failure of pancreatic acinar development (Fig. 28–2). Pathologic studies reveal normal ductular architecture but extensive fatty replacement of pancreatic acinar tissue, which can be visualized by computed tomography, ultrasonography, or by magnetic resonance imaging. Pancreatic function studies using intravenous secretin or cholecystokinin, confirm the presence of markedly impaired enzyme secretion averaging 10% to 14% of normal but with preserved ductal function.[152] Patients may also have reduced serum trypsinogen and isoamylase levels.[153] Decreased isoamylase levels in children older than three years of age, in particular, are highly sensitive and very specific for the diagnosis.

The vast majority of patients have symptoms of malabsorption from birth caused by the pancreatic insufficiency. The absence of steatorrhea, however, does not exclude a diagnosis of SDS. Approximately 50% of patients appear to exhibit a modest improvement in enzyme secretion with advancing age.[152] Many older patients with SDS actually develop pancreatic sufficiency with normal fat absorption when assessed by 72-hour fecal fat balance studies.

The most conspicuous physical findings relate to the pancreatic insufficiency and malabsorption, especially short stature, which is another consistent feature of the syndrome. When treated with pancreatic enzyme replacement, most patients show a normal growth velocity yet remain consistently below the third percentile for height and weight, indicating an intrinsic growth defect. Some patients have evidence of delayed puberty. The occasional adult achieves the 25th percentile for height. The clinical picture can also be dominated by complications related to the cytopenias. Bacterial and fungal infections, in particular, secondary to neutropenia as well as immune deficiency[148] can be problematic.

Skeletal abnormalities are present in all SDS patients with mutant SBDS.[154] Some patients present at birth with thoracic dystrophy, and others have short, flared ribs. Metaphyseal dysostosis of the long bones is a common radiological abnormality (44%–77% of patients) and is thought to be quite specific, particularly in the femoral head and the proximal tibia. These changes may not be detectable until after 12 months of age. The etiology of the metaphyseal changes is unclear. In most patients these bony lesions fail to produce any symptoms. However, the integrity of the growth plate may be affected which in turn may result in skeletal growth disturbances and joint deformities, particularly in the knees and hips. In 100% of patients, there is delayed appearance of secondary ossification centers resulting in delayed bone maturation.[154]

As summarized,[136] there are additional clinical features that are seen very infrequently in SDS. Endocrine abnormalities include insulin-dependent diabetes, growth hormone deficiency, hypogonadotropic hypogonadism, and hypothyroidism (Dr. Akiko Shimamura, Seattle, unpublished observations). Cardiomyopathies have been noted in some cases. Psychomotor delay of varying severity, urinary tract anomalies, renal tubular acidosis, and cleft palate also occur.

Laboratory Findings

Peripheral Blood and Bone Marrow Findings. Data from 4 publications (Table 28–4) accurately represent the spectrum of hematologic findings.[151,152,155,156] In 1 series,[156] neutropenia was present in virtually all patients on at least one occasion. It can be chronic, intermittent or cyclic although there are no published data on the periodicity of the cycles. Neutropenia has been identified in some SDS patients in the neonatal period during an episode of sepsis. Anemia, usually normochromic-normocytic, was recorded in up to 66% of patients,[156] and thrombocytopenia in up to 70%.[155] Fetal hemoglobin was elevated in 75% of patients at some stage during the disease course.[156] Whether this reflects stress hematopoiesis and/or ineffective erythropoiesis concomitant with chronic infections, or represents MDS in evolution has not been clarified. Reticulocyte responses were inappropriately low for the levels of hemoglobin in 75% of patients.[156]

More than one lineage can be affected, and pancytopenia was observed in up to 65% of cases.[155] The pancytopenia can be severe as a result of full-blown aplastic anemia (Fig. 28–3). However, bone marrow biopsies and aspirates vary widely with respect to cellularity; varying degrees of marrow hypoplasia and fat infiltration are the usual findings, but marrows with normal or even increased cellularity have also been observed.[152,156] The severity of neutropenia does not always correlate with bone marrow cellularity, nor is the severity of the pancreatic insufficiency concordant with the hematological abnormalities.

Patients with SDS are particularly susceptible to severe infections including otitis media, bronchopneumonia, osteomyelitis, septicemia, and recurrent furuncles. Overwhelming sepsis is a well-recognized fatal complication of this disorder, particularly early in life. SDS neutrophils may have a defect in mobility, migration and chemotaxis that does not appear to be caused by malnutrition.[157] Lithium in some manner appears to restore chemotaxis.[158] There appears to be a diminished ability of SDS neutrophils to orient toward a gradient of *N*-formyl-methionyl-leucyl-phenylalanine.[159] An unusual surface distribution of concanavalin A has also been reported that reflects a cytoskeletal defect in SDS neutrophils.[160] Whatever the magnitude of the chemotaxis abnormality is in vitro in SDS, neutrophil recruitment into abscesses or empyemas ensues robustly in vivo.[161]

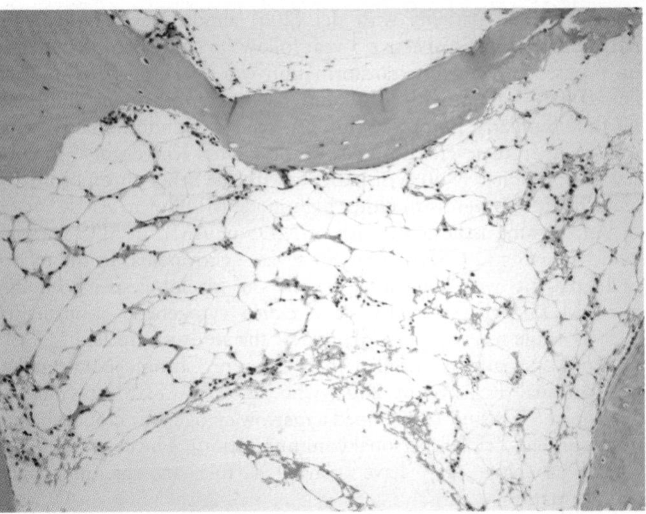

Figure 28–3 Bone marrow biopsy in severe Shwachman–Diamond syndrome showing striking hypocellularity, fatty changes, and tri-lineage aplasia. *(Photomicrograph prepared by Dr. Mohamed Abdelhaleem, Toronto.)*

Immune Dysfunction. Impaired immune function can be significant in SDS and underlie recurrent infections even if neutrophils are at a protective level.[148] Patients have variations of B-cell abnormalities with one or more of the following: low IgG or IgG subclasses, low percentage of circulating B lymphocytes, decreased in vitro B-cell proliferation, and lack of specific antibody production. Patients may also have T-cell abnormalities: low percentage of circulating T lymphocytes or subsets or NK cells, and decreased in vitro T-cell proliferation.

Leukemia, Myelodysplasia, and Clonal Cytogenetic Changes. Like six other inherited bone marrow failure disorders, SDS predisposes patients to MDS and acute myeloid leukemic transformation.[135,138] The crude rate for MDS or acute myeloid leukemia (MDS/AML) in patients with SDS was 8% in one case series (7 of 88 patients)[151] and 33% in a smaller case series (7 of 21).[156] It was 5% in approximately 200 SDS cases reported in the literature prior to 1990, and 10% in more than 300 patients who had not received G-CSF reported through 2000.[162] Of 55 SDS patients followed prospectively in the French Severe Chronic Neutropenia Registry, 7 patients developed MDS or AML with an estimated risk of 19% at 20 years and 36% at 30 years.[163] A literature search revealed 54 SDS cases with MDS/AML of whom 37 developed cytogenetic abnormalities and/or morphologic dysplasia and/or increased numbers of marrow blast cells.[138] Clearly, the propensity for malignant myeloid transformation is very high compared to the general population, but is probably not as high as in Fanconi anemia.

There is an increased frequency of marrow cell clonal cytogenetic abnormalities as an isolated finding in SDS. The incidence is roughly estimated to be 7% to 41% based on pooled published data.[136] In a 2005 review,[138] reports of marrow cytogenetic abnormalities were compiled on 40 SDS patients who showed no evidence of malignant transformation. Isochromosome 7q [i(7q)], an extremely uncommon finding rarely described in MDS or AML in patients without SDS,[164] was seen in 44% of SDS patients. This high occurrence suggests that it is a fairly specific marker for SDS and might be related to the mutant gene on 7q(11).

Other chromosome 7 abnormalities were seen in 33% of the SDS patients and included monosomy 7, i(7q) combined with monosomy 7, and deletions or translocations involving part of 7q. The prognostic significance of the cytogenetic changes requires prospective monitoring for clarification. Of the patients with i(7q), progression to MDS with excess blasts or to AML has rarely been reported.[135,138]

Similarly, SDS patients with del (20q) almost never evolve into MDS/AML. In a prospective 5-year follow-up study of SDS patients, no progression to overt transformation was seen in 2 patients with del (20q), 1 patient with i(7q), and 1 with combined del (20q) and i(7q).[165] Similarly, no progression was seen in six additional patients with i(7q) from several hospitals in the United Kingdom.[166] In contrast, approximately 40% of patients with the other chromosomal 7 abnormalities progress to either high grade MDS or to AML.[138]

An ongoing issue is the risk of MDS or AML in SDS patients while receiving G-CSF therapy for severe neutropenia. In the report of 14 patients with congenital disorders of myelopoiesis who developed MDS/AML (n = 13) or a clonal cytogenetic abnormality (n = 1) while receiving G-CSF, two of the study group had SDS.[167] Of 16 SDS patients enrolled in the Severe Chronic Neutropenic International Registry in 2003 who received G-CSF therapy, 2 developed MDS and 1 developed a marrow cytogenetic clonal change (Dr. Cornelia Zeidler, personal communication). The concern is that G-CSF therapy may have played a role in the malignant transformation.

***SBDS* Gene and MDS/AML.** Wild-type *SBDS* must play a critical role in preventing leukemic myeloid transformation because up to 1/3 of SDS patients develop MDS/AML. To address whether an acquired mutant *SBDS* gene is associated with leukemic transformation in de novo AML, 77 AML marrow samples at diagnosis or relapse were analyzed for *SBDS* mutations and none were identified.[168] To see if a subset of previously undiagnosed SDS patients presented for the first time with AML, 48 AML marrow samples were studied at remission but no *SBDS* mutations were found.[168] SDS patients with MDS/AML have common *SBDS* mutations,[168] and a genotype-phenotype study of 21 cases of SDS with MDS/AML showed no relationship (Linda Ellis, RN, Toronto, personal communication). Thus the link between mutant *SBDS*, hematologic cancer, and upregulated oncogenes[169] including *LARG*, *TAL1*, and *MLL* is undetermined.

Although molecular and cellular parameters do not distinguish SDS patients with clonal cytogenetic changes from SDS patients without clonal changes,[165] it is remarkable that SDS marrows from almost all patients demonstrate many characteristic features seen in MDS.[138] These include impaired marrow stromal support of normal hematopoiesis,[145] increased marrow cell apoptosis mediated by the Fas pathway,[146] p53 protein over expression,[150] telomere shortening of leukocytes,[147] increased marrow neovascularization,[149] and high frequency of cytogenetic clonal abnormalities.[138] It is possible that preleukemia in SDS is established in utero.

Differential Diagnosis

The syndrome of refractory sideroblastic anemia with vacuolization of bone marrow precursors, or Pearson syndrome, is clinically similar to SDS but very different in bone marrow morphology.[170] Severe anemia requiring transfusions rather than neutropenia is often present at birth and by 1 year of age in all cases. In contrast to SDS, the major marrow morphologic findings are ringed sideroblasts with decreased erythroblasts and prominent vacuolation of erythroid and myeloid precursors. The disorder shares clinical similarities with SDS because of exocrine pancreatic dysfunction in both. Malabsorption and severe failure to thrive occurs in approximately one-half of cases within the first 12 months of life. Qualitative pancreatic function tests show depressed acinar function and reduced fluid and electrolyte secretion. Approximately 50% of reported cases die early in life from sepsis, acidosis, and liver failure; the others appear to improve spontaneously with reduced transfusion requirements. At autopsy, the pancreas shows acinar cell atrophy and fibrosis; fatty infiltration as seen in SDS is not a prominent feature. The need for long-term pancreatic enzyme replacement is unclear. These patients have a diagnostic deletion of mitochondrial deoxyribonucleic acid (mtDNA).[171] mtDNA encodes enzymes in the mitochondrial respiratory chain that are relevant to oxidative phosphorylation, including the reduced form of nicotinamide-adenine dinucleotide dehydrogenase (NADH), cytochrome oxidase, adenosine triphosphatase (ATPase), and transfer ribonucleic acids (tRNAs) and ribosomal RNAs.

SDS shares some manifestations with Fanconi anemia such as marrow dysfunction and growth failure, but SDS patients are readily distinguished because of pancreatic insufficiency with a resultant malabsorption syndrome, fatty changes within the pancreatic body that can be visualized by imaging, characteristic skeletal abnormalities not seen in Fanconi patients, and normal DEB clastogenic stress testing. Mutational analysis for mutant *SBDS* is definitive, but 10% of classic clinical SDS cases do not have a mutant *SBDS*.

Natural History and Prognosis

Because of the broad pleiotropy in SDS, the number of undiagnosed patients with mild or asymptomatic disease is unknown. Hence, overall prognosis may be better than previously thought. The majority of *SBDS* mutations represent hypomorphic alleles with reduced but variable protein expression.[172] Also, there is phenotypic heterogeneity in patients carrying identical *SBDS* mutations.[173] Therefore, until more information is forthcoming, the natural history and prognosis are not yet defined.

From a literature review, the projected median survival of SDS patients was calculated as 35 years.[7] During infancy, morbidity and mortality are mostly related to malabsorption, infections, and thoracic dystrophy. Later in life, the major problems are hematological or complications related to their treatment. Cytopenias tend to fluctuate in severity, never fully resolve, and show no genotype-phenotype relationship.[174] Spontaneous remissions do not occur after symptomatic cytopenias ensue or after MDS/AML.

Therapy

Patient management is ideally shared by a multidisciplinary team consisting of a hematologist and a gastroenterologist as core members, and other subspecialists such as a dentist and a psychologist as required. The malabsorption component of SDS responds to treatment with oral pancreatic enzyme replacement with meals and snacks using guidelines similar to those for cystic fibrosis. Supplemental fat-soluble vitamins are also usually required. When monitored over time, approximately 50% of patients convert from pancreatic insufficiency to sufficiency because of spontaneous improvement in pancreatic enzyme secretion.[151,175] This improvement is particularly evident after four years of age. A long term plan should be initiated to monitor changes in peripheral blood counts that require corrective action and to look for early evidence of malignant myeloid transformation. The latter requires serial bone marrow aspirates for smears and cytogenetics, and marrow biopsies. One recommendation is to do marrow testing annually.[135]

Growth Factors and Other Strategies

G-CSF given for profound neutropenia has been very effective in inducing a clinically beneficial neutrophil response.[167,176–179] Cross-over treatment using GM-CSF initially, followed by G-CSF later for a form of childhood neutropenia has shown efficacy from both,[179] but they have not been compared in SDS patients.[179] Of 35 SDS patients enrolled in the Severe Chronic Neutropenia International Registry in 2003, 16 evaluable cases received G-CSF; 14 of the 16 patients had brisk neutrophil responses that were sustained in some cases for more than 11 years (Beate Schwinzer, Hannover, personal communication).

A small number of patients have been treated with corticosteroids with hematologic improvement in 50%. A smaller number received androgens plus steroids in the manner of treating Fanconi anemia and improved marrow function was also noted. Isolated cases treated with androgens alone, cyclosporine, or erythropoietin do not allow broad therapeutic conclusions. Anemia and thrombocytopenia are managed with transfusions of red cells or platelets as needed.

Hematopoietic Stem Cell Transplantation (HSCT)

At present, the only curative option for severe marrow failure in SDS is allogeneic hematopoietic stem cell transplantation. As of mid 2006, 58 patients who had received HSCT were reported in the literature.[180–182] Indications were marrow failure, MDS or leukemia, and there was a mix of sibling and matched unrelated donors. The French Registry reported a 60% overall survival of SDS patients following HSCT.[182] The European Transplantation Group similarly had a 65% overall survival. Analysis[136] of the reported experience[180–182] yielded the following: 21 of 25 transplanted patients for marrow failure were cured, but only 6 of 14 with MDS and 2 of 6 with leukemia survived.

A note of caution is sounded regarding HSCT for SDS. Left ventricular fibrosis and necrosis without coronary arterial lesions have been reported in 50% of SDS patients at autopsy,[183] suggesting that there may be an increased risk of cardiotoxicity as well as other problems with the intensive preparatory chemotherapy used in HSCT. Indeed, 2 pertinent reports[184,185] and a recent literature review[138] emphasized that complications are more common in SDS patients who receive chemotherapy or undergo transplantation than in non-SDS patients with aplastic anemia. Complications include cardiotoxicity, neurological and renal complications, veno-occlusive disease, pulmonary disease, post-transplant graft failure, and severe GVHD. The heightened risk for patients with SDS after transplantation can be explained in three ways; (1) the presence of the SDS marrow stromal defect that is not corrected by the allograft and might be aggravated by the conditioning regimen, (2) increased sensitivity to chemotherapy and radiation resulting in massive apoptosis in various organs, or (3) performing HSCT relatively late and at an advanced disease stage. A reduced-intensity conditioning regimen shows promise for SDS HSCT[186] but has not been extensively used yet.

Future Directions

Mutant *SBDS* causes SDS in 90% of clinically diagnosed patients. The hunt for additional causative mutant genes in the other 10% should demonstrate that SDS is genetically heterogeneous and expand our understanding of pathogenesis. Several other clinical and basic research questions in SDS must be addressed. First, the function of the *SBDS* gene has to be deciphered. How SBDS protein maintains normal hematopoiesis and protects from apoptosis as well as cancer is unclear. The complete clinical phenotype, natural history and risk factors for the development of complications need to be determined. There is also a need to understand the mechanism for the heightened sensitivity of SDS patients to chemotherapy and irradiation and to develop low-intensity regimens for HSCT. Research should continue on the efficacy of innovative drugs such as anti-apoptotic agents in increasing the growth potential of hematopoietic stem cells and relieving the severity of cytopenia. Determining risk factors and molecular events during malignant myeloid transformation might prompt strategies for prevention and screening for complications.

Dyskeratosis Congenita

Background

Dyskeratosis congenita (DC) is an inherited multisystem disorder of the mucocutaneous and hematopoietic systems in association with a wide variety of other somatic abnormalities.[187] The diagnostic ectodermal component invariably consists of the triad of reticulate skin pigmentation of the upper body, mucosal leukoplakia, and nail dystrophy. The skin and nail findings usually become apparent in the first 10 years of life, whereas the oral leukoplakia is seen later. These manifestations tend to progress as patients get older.

DC is also an inherited bone marrow failure syndrome in which aplastic anemia occurs in about 50% of cases, usually in the second decade of life. Patients also have a predisposition to develop cancer and myelodysplastic syndromes. Because of the cluster of abnormalities involving skin and bone marrow and the predilection to cancer, DC resembles Fanconi anemia. However, the genetics, gene mutations, and physical abnormalities of patients with both conditions are quite different and hence the two diseases should be considered as totally discrete entities.

Etiology, Genetics, and Pathophysiology

The inheritance pattern is genetically heterogeneous. Approximately 73% of DC patients in the literature are males, compatible with an *X-linked recessive* trait.[7] Approximately 16% of cases are sporadic female patients, familial cases with affected male and female siblings in one generation, and cases with known parental consanguinity that fit an *autosomal recessive* inheritance pattern. An *autosomal dominant* mode fits the remaining 11% of cases that occur in families with affected male and female members in consecutive generations. The DC Registry at Hammersmith Hospital, London, is less certain about the modes of inheritance.[187] Of 228 DC families, 158 have only a single affected individual (123 male, 35 female) and it is not possible to infer the inheritance pattern.[188]

From the literature, the autosomal dominant group seems to have clinically milder manifestations, and the autosomal recessive group appears to have more physical anomalies and a higher incidence of aplastic anemia and cancer. In one series, the actuarial probability of male patients developing aplastic anemia was 94% by 40 years of age.[189]

The X-linked recessive form of DC maps to Xq28 and many mutations have been identified in the *DKC1* gene, which codes for the nuclear protein dyskerin.[190] Dyskerin is critically involved in the telomere maintenance pathway. It is a component of small nucleolar particles that are important in ribosomal RNA processing. The autosomal dominant form of DC is caused by germline mutations in the *TERC* gene, the *TERT* gene, or the *TINF2* gene. *TERC* encodes the RNA component of telomerase that is also involved in telomere maintenance.[191] Indeed, very short telomeres have been demonstrated in peripheral blood cells of all patients with autosomal dominant, autosomal recessive, and X-linked recessive forms of the disorder[192] and is a marker for the genetic abnormalities.[193] Defective telomere maintenance leading to heightened cellular apoptosis is a central pathogenetic mechanism for these 3 forms of DC.[194,195] The *TERT* gene encodes a reverse transcriptase that adds telomere repeats of the ends of each chromosome. *TERT* and *TERC* work together in telomere maintenance. *TINF2* encodes a component of the shelterin telomere protection complex and when mutated impairs telomere maintenance and causes DC.[196] Autosomal recessive DC has been linked to mutations in the telomerase-associated protein NOP10.[197]

Most studies of the pathogenesis of the aplastic anemia in DC have shown a marked reduction or absence of CFU-GEMM, BFU-E, CFU-E and CFU-GM progenitors.[62,63,198,199] Long-term bone marrow cultures were used to study hematopoiesis in three patients with DC[199]; hematopoiesis was severely defective in all with a low frequency of colony-forming cells and a low level of hematopoiesis in long-term cultures. The function of DC marrow stromal cells was normal in their ability to support growth of hematopoietic progenitors from normal marrow in all 3 cases, but generation of progenitors from DC marrow cells seeded over normal stroma was reduced, strongly suggesting that the defect in DC is of stem cell origin.

Thus, the marrow failure in this disorder may be a result of a progressive attrition and depletion of hematopoietic stem cells which manifests as pancytopenia when patients are in their mid-teens. Alternatively, the marrow dysfunction may not be a simple conse-

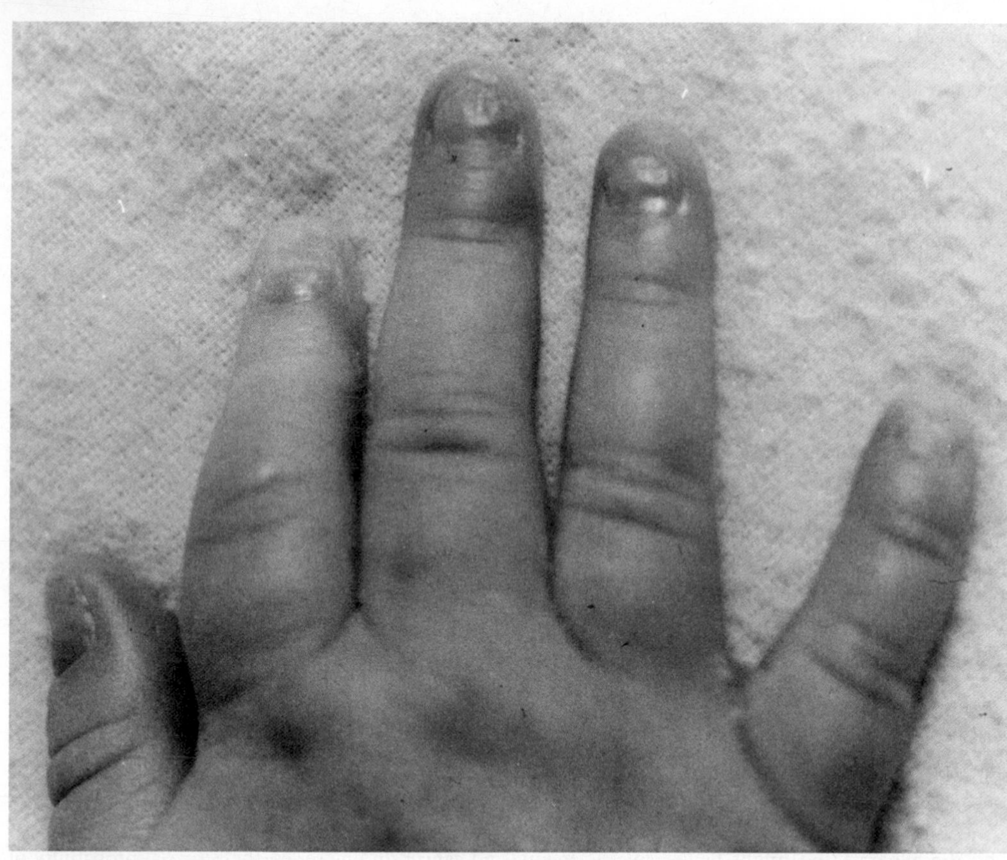

Figure 28–4 Dystrophic nails in dyskeratosis congenita.

quence of a limited stem cell pool but may represent a failure of replication and/or maturation.

Clinical Features

History and Physical Examination

Clinical manifestations in DC often appear during childhood. The skin pigmentation and nail changes typically appear first, mucosal leukoplakia and excessive ocular tearing appear later, and by the midteens the serious complications of bone marrow failure and malignancy begin to develop. In rare cases the marrow abnormalities may appear before the skin manifestations. The main causes of death relate either to bone marrow failure or to malignancy with an additional risk of fatal pulmonary complications. The actual median age at death is 20 years for males with X-linked and sporadic DC and those with autosomal recessive DC.[7] Autosomal dominant DC patients have a milder disease and survive longer.

The DC Registry data show the prevalence of somatic abnormalities in families with classic DC.[187,189] The phenotype in female cases varies considerably but many share the same features as male cases. Cutaneous findings are the most consistent feature of the syndrome. Lacy reticulated skin pigmentation affecting the face, neck, chest, and arms is a common finding (89%). The degree of pigmentation increases with age and can involve the entire skin surface. There may also be a telangiectatic erythematous component. Nail dystrophy of the hands and feet is the next most common finding (88%) (Fig. 28–4). It usually starts with longitudinal ridging, splitting, or pterygium formation and may progress to complete nail loss. Leukoplakia usually involves the oral mucosa (78%), especially the tongue (Fig. 28–5), but may also be seen in the conjunctiva, anal, urethral, or genital mucosa. Hyperhidrosis of the palms and soles is common, and hair loss is sometimes seen. Eye abnormalities are observed in approximately 50% of cases.[200] Excessive tearing (epiphora) secondary to nasolacrimal duct obstruction is common. Other ophthalmologic manifestations include conjunctivitis, blepharitis, loss of eyelashes, strabismus, cataracts, and optic atrophy. Abnormalities of the teeth, particularly an increased rate of dental decay and early loss of teeth, are common. Skeletal abnormalities such as osteoporosis, avascular necrosis, abnormal bone trabeculation, scoliosis, and mandibular hypoplasia are seen in approximately 20% of cases.[201,202] Genitourinary abnormalities include hypoplastic testes, hypospadias, phimosis, urethral stenosis, and horseshoe kidney. Gastrointestinal findings, such as esophageal strictures, hepatomegaly, or cirrhosis, are seen in 10% of cases.[203] A subset of patients develop pulmonary complications with reduced diffusion capacity and/or a restrictive defect.[189] In fatal cases, lung tissue shows pulmonary fibrosis and abnormalities of the pulmonary vasculature.

Laboratory Findings

Peripheral Blood, Bone Marrow, and Immunological Findings. Approximately 50% of the X-linked male DC patients and 70% of the autosomal recessive patients develop aplastic anemia, usually in the teenage years. It occurs in the autosomal dominant patients as well but much less frequently. Most of these patients already have manifestations of DC, but some younger patients can develop marrow failure before the clinical onset of the mucocutaneous manifestations. The initial hematological change is usually thrombocytopenia or anemia, or both, followed by full-blown pancytopenia caused by aplastic anemia. The red cells are often macrocytic and the fetal hemoglobin can be elevated. Oddly, early bone marrow aspirations and biopsies may be hypercellular; however, with time the cellular elements decline with a symmetrical decrease in all hematopoietic lineages. Ferrokinetic studies at this point are consistent with aplastic anemia. Some patients with DC have immunologic abnormalities including reduced or elevated immunoglobulin levels, reduced B- and/or T-lymphocyte numbers, and reduced or absent proliferative responses to phytohemagglutinin.[189]

Chromosome Fragility Findings. There is a large body of contradictory information regarding chromosomal fragility and instability in DC. Spontaneous chromosome breaks in patients' lymphocytes were

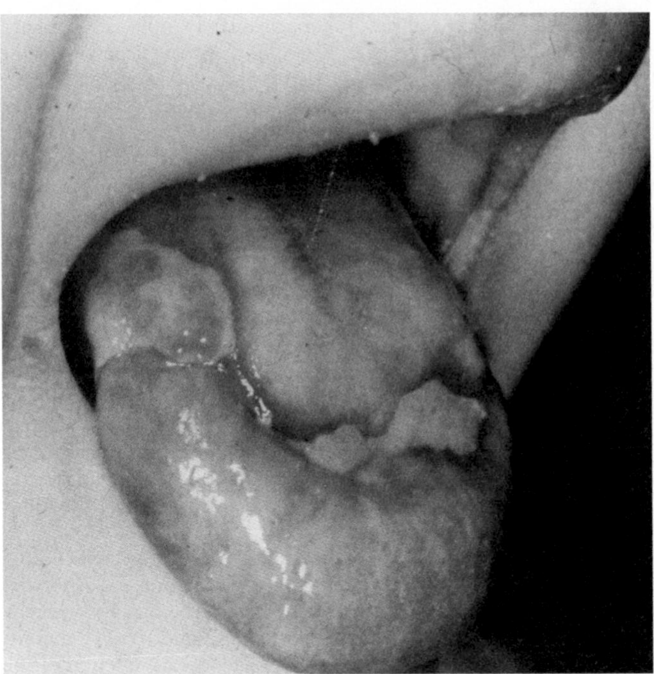

Figure 28–5 Leukoplakia of the tongue in dyskeratosis congenita.

reported in some studies but were not confirmed. Similarly, excessive spontaneous and clastogenic-induced sister chromatid exchange in patient lymphocytes were observed by some investigators but not by others. Finally, a definitive study demonstrated that there was no significant difference in chromosomal breakage between patient and normal lymphocytes with or without exposure to bleomycin, diepoxybutane, MMC, and γ radiation.[204] This contrasts sharply with Fanconi anemia cells and distinguishes one disorder from the other.

However, Dokal argues that DC is a chromosome "instability" disorder of a somewhat different type than Fanconi anemia.[189] Primary skin fibroblasts in culture are abnormal in morphology and doubling rate and show numerous unbalanced chromosome rearrangements such as dicentrics, tricentrics and translocations in the absence of clastogenic agents. These findings provide evidence for a defect that predisposes patient cells to developing chromosomal rearrangements and possibly DNA damage.

Predisposition to Cancer and Myelodysplasia

Cancer develops in about 10% to 15% of patients, usually in the third and fourth decades of life. Similar to Fanconi anemia in which malignant tumors and MDS or AML are seen, DC patients are predisposed to MDS as well as to solid tumors but much less so. The literature was summarized on cancers in 43 DC patients including 35 X-linked and sporadic males, 6 autosomal recessive cases, and 2 autosomal dominant patients.[7] Most of the cancers were squamous cell carcinoma or adenocarcinoma, and the oropharynx and gastrointestinal tract were involved most frequently. One patient had three separate primaries in the tongue, nasopharynx, and rectum, one had esophageal and cheek carcinomas, and one had separate nasal and tongue malignancies.[205] Thus, the sites of most of the cancers involve areas known to be abnormal in DC, such as mucous membranes and the gastrointestinal tract. Four male patients were identified with MDS of 148 in the DC Registry.[189] Two had refractory anemia and 2 had refractory anemia with excess blasts.

Differential Diagnosis

Several physical findings can be used to distinguish Fanconi anemia from DC clinically. The following abnormalities are seen only in DC and not Fanconi anemia: nail dystrophy, leukoplakia, abnormalities of the teeth, hyperhydrosis of palms and soles, and hair loss. There are overlap syndromes that share some of the features of DC. The Hoyeraal–Hreidarsson syndrome is a multisystem disorder affecting mostly boys who manifest aplastic anemia, immunodeficiency, microcephaly, growth retardation, and cerebellar hypoplasia. The syndrome is caused by mutations in *DKC1* and hence is a severe variant of X-linked DC. The Revesz syndrome consists of dystrophic nails, leukoplakia, aplastic anemia, cerebellar hypoplasia, growth retardation, microcephaly, and bilateral exudative retinopathy. Mutant *TINF2* was identified in revese syndrome[196] and hence is an autosomal dominant variant of DC.

Natural History and Prognosis

In classical DC, nail dystrophy and skin pigmentation present first, often in the first 10 years of life. Bone marrow failure usually follows in the teenage years and twenties. The primary cause of death is either from hemorrhage secondary to thrombocytopenia or sepsis from severe neutropenia. In the 10% of cases who develop cancer or MDS, the disease or its treatment can prove fatal. Pulmonary complications can develop in 20% of cases and be life-threatening. However, considerable clinical heterogeneity exists even within the same family, and some patients live into their forties with only moderate nail changes and mild cytopenias.

Therapy

Management of aplastic anemia is similar to that for Fanconi anemia. Androgens, usually combined with low-dose prednisone, can be expected to induce improved marrow function in about 50% of patients. If a response is seen and deemed to be maximal, the androgen dose can be slowly tapered but not stopped. As in Fanconi anemia, patients can become refractory to androgens as the aplastic anemia progresses. There is no evidence that immunosuppressive therapy is effective for this disorder. A small number of patients were reported who responded to G-CSF therapy with significant increases in absolute neutrophil counts.[206–209] Similarly, two other patients received GM-CSF therapy which resulted in improved neutrophil numbers.[210,211] G-CSF with erythropoietin resulted in a trilineage hematologic response in one patient.[212] G-CSF plus androgens has led to splenic peliosis and rupture in DC and is not recommended.

Although the reports are scanty, cytokine therapy appears to offer potential benefit, at least in the short-term, especially for improving granulopoiesis.

Hematopoietic Stem Cell Transplantation

A relatively small number of patients with DC have undergone HSCT using standard myeloablative protocols, mostly with matched related donors.[7] Of these patients, approximately 50% survived longer than 3 years after HSCT. Vascular lesions and fibrosis involving various organs occurred in these patients in both early and late periods after transplantation and carried a high mortality rate. DC patients may be more susceptible to endothelial damage,[189,213,214] which occurs after HSCT as a result of various factors including the conditioning regimen, cyclosporine A, infectious disease, GVHD, and cytokine storm. Another striking complication for DC patients after HSCT is bronchopulmonary disease. An inherent propensity for pulmonary disease[189] explains the high incidence (up to 40%) of early and late fatal pulmonary complications after HSCT. These unusual complications, uniquely seen in DC,[213] have not been reported in other inherited bone marrow failure syndromes such as Fanconi anemia. DC is a disorder involving a subtle degree of chromosomal instability with a predisposition to chromosomal rearrangements,[189] rather than to gaps and breaks as seen in Fanconi anemia. Flawed telomere maintenance in virtually all cases of DC sheds additional light on the hypersensitivity to irradiation and chemotherapy found in these patients. The increased hypersensitivity of DC patients to transplant conditioning can be related to the telomere shortening from DC combined with the accelerated telomere shortening that occurs after HSCT.[215]

The increased predisposition to posttransplant complications, especially pulmonary and vascular, the chromosomal instability, and the tendency to develop tumors highlight the need to avoid certain conditioning agents such as busulfan and irradiation. The strategy of using low-intensity fludarabine-based protocols for HSCT has produced encouraging results for DC patients.[216–218] These regimens appear to be well tolerated and allow prompt engraftment without significant complications. The long-term risk of the conditioning regimen inducing cancer in predisposed DC transplant survivors is still to be determined.

Future Directions

Although 5 mutated genes for the three forms of dyskeratosis congenita are known, prospects for gene therapy are not imminent. The identification of other DC genes should clarify how the activity, transport, and stability of telomerase and other ribonucleoprotein complexes interact and influence hematopoietic stem cell function.

Amegakaryocytic Thrombocytopenia

Background

Amegakaryocytic thrombocytopenia or congenital amegakaryocytic thrombocytopenia (CAT or CAMT) is an autosomal recessive syndrome that presents in infancy with isolated thrombocytopenia caused by reduced or absent marrow megakaryocytes with preservation initially of granulopoietic and erythroid lineages.[219] Aplastic anemia subsequently ensues in approximately 45% of patients, usually in the first few years of life. The diagnosis depends on the exclusion of all other specific causes for thrombocytopenia in early life. The mutant gene has been identified and confirms that sporadic and familial cases are inherited in an autosomal recessive manner. *CAMT* is a distinct genetic entity, but mutations in several other genes have been described in a number of inherited thrombocytopenias that must be considered in the differential diagnosis (Table 28–5).

Etiology, Genetics, and Pathophysiology

The defect in *CAMT* is directly related to mutations in *MPL*, the gene for the thrombopoietin receptor that maps to 1p34.[220–222] Carriers of the mutant gene have normal blood cell counts; affected individuals have mutations in both alleles. Some patients have inherited two different *MPL* mutations resulting in a compound heterozygous state.[220,223,224] Inheritance of homozygous *MPL* mutations also occurs.[223]

Mutations have been found throughout the *MPL* gene including nonsense, missense, frameshift, and splicing mutations. A genotype-phenotype correlation was identified in 23 CAMT patients whereby two prognostic groups were established, types I and II.[225] Frameshift and nonsense mutations produce a complete loss of function of the thrombopoietin receptor in type I with persistently low platelet counts and a fast progression to pancytopenia. Since thrombopoietin also has an anti-apoptotic effect on hematopoietic stem cells,[226] impaired stem cell survival explains the evolution of type I CAMT into aplastic anemia. Type II CAMT with missense and splicing mutations is characterized by a milder course, a transient increase in platelet counts during the first years of life, and delayed onset, if any, of pancytopenia, indicating residual receptor function.

Table 28–5 Inherited Thrombocytopenia Disorders

Disorder	Genetics*	Mutant Gene	Platelet Size†	Features	References
Amegakaryocytic thrombocytopenia	AR	*MPL*	Normal	± physical anomalies	222
Thrombocytopenia absent radii	AR	Unknown	Normal	Physical anomalies	219
MYH9-related thrombocytopenia					238
May–Hegglin anomaly	AD	*MYH9*	Large	Neutrophil inclusions	
Fechtner syndrome	AD	*MYH9*	Large	Neutrophil inclusions, hearing loss, nephritis	
Epstein syndrome	AD	*MYH9*	Large	Absent inclusions, hearing loss, nephritis	
Sebastian syndrome	AD	*MYH9*	Large	Neutrophil inclusions	
X-linked macrothrombocytopenia	X-linked	*GATA1*	Large	Anemia, dyserythropoiesis, thalassemia	239
Wiskott–Aldrich syndrome	X-linked	*WAS*	Small	Immune deficiency, eczema	238
X-linked thrombocytopenia	X-linked	*WAS*	Small	No associated features	238
Thrombocytopenia and radioulnar synostosis	AD	*HOXA11*	Normal	Fused radius, limited range of motion	240
Familial platelet disorder—AML	AD	*AML1* (*RUNX1; CBFA2*)	Normal	MDS, AML	238
Familial dominant thrombocytopenia	AD	*FLJ14813*	Normal	No associated features	241
Paris–Trousseau thrombocytopenia	AD	*FLI1*	Large	Psychomotor retardation, facial anomalies (Jacobsen syndrome)	242
Bernard–Soulier syndrome	AR	*GP1BA*	Large	No associated features	243
Bernard–Soulier carrier/ Mediterranean macrothrombocytopenia	AD	*GP1BA*	Large	No associated features	244

*AD = autosomal dominant; AR = autosomal recessive.
†Platelet size: small, MPV <7 fL; normal, MPV 7–11 fL; large/giant, MPV >11 fL.

Informative serial studies of hematopoiesis using clonogenic assays were performed in a female infant with CAMT.[227] Initially, when the only hematologic abnormality was isolated thrombocytopenia, the number of clonogenic hematopoietic progenitors was comparable to controls, including the number of megakaryocyte precursors, CFU-MK (CFU-Meg). As the disease evolved into aplastic anemia over an 11-month period, the peripheral blood counts declined, and colony numbers from four classes of progenitors also declined in parallel. When added to the marrow cultures, patient plasma was not inhibitory to control or to patient colony growth. Similarly, no cellular inhibition of hematopoiesis was observed when the patient's marrow was cultured after depleting the sample of T lymphocytes or after adding them back. Stromal cells established in short-term and long-term cultures of the patient's marrow showed normal proliferative activity and yielded a "fertile" marrow microenvironment for patient and control marrow colony growth. The data suggested that the central problem in CAMT was an intrinsic hematopoietic stem cell defect rather than an abnormality of the marrow milieu. The findings are consistent with current knowledge about *MPL* mutations.

Another study demonstrated measurable numbers of CFU-MK progenitors in vitro from five patients with CAMT in response to IL-3, GM-CSF, or a combination of both.[228] The identification of megakaryocyte progenitors in these patients agrees with the data described above when patients are studied early in the course of the disease. Another report described the effect of recombinant human thrombopoietin on CFU-MK colony formation from a patient with CAMT in which there was a defective response.[229] The patient's serum thrombopoietin level was significantly elevated as compared to controls, and the patient's marrow cells did not express mRNA for *MPL*. The pathophysiology of CAMT in this case was directly attributable to these findings and consistent with current evidence.

Plasma thrombopoietin levels in patients with CAMT are always elevated and are amongst the highest seen in any patient population.[221,230] The detectable immunoreactive material retains full biological activity.[230]

Clinical Features

History and Physical Examination

Almost all patients present with a petechial rash, bruising, or bleeding in the first year of life. Most cases are obvious at birth or within the first 2 months. Roughly 30% of the patients have characteristic physical anomalies that do not fit with other specific syndromes; the other patients have normal physical and imaging features. Some affected sibships manifest both normal and abnormal physical findings in the same family. As in Fanconi anemia, CAMT patients with and without anomalies should be considered as part of the clinical spectrum of one entity.

The commonest manifestations in those with anomalies are neurologic and cardiac. Findings related to cerebellar and cerebral atrophy are a recurrent theme and developmental delay is a prominent feature in this group. Patients may also have microcephaly and an abnormal facies. Congenital heart disease with a variety of malformations can be detected, including atrial septal defects, ventricular septal defects, patent ductus arteriosus, tetralogy of Fallot, and coarctation of the aorta. Some of these occur in combinations. Other anomalies include abnormal hips or feet, kidney malformations, eye anomalies, and cleft or high-arched palate.

Laboratory Findings

Thrombocytopenia is the major laboratory finding with normal hemoglobin levels and white blood cell counts initially. Although there are usually measurable but reduced platelet numbers, peripheral blood platelets may be totally absent. Those that can be identified are of normal size and appearance. Similar to other inherited bone marrow failure syndromes, red cells may be macrocytic. HbF can be increased and there may be increased expression of i antigen. Bone marrow aspirates and biopsies show normal cellularity with markedly reduced or absent megakaryocytes (Fig. 28–6). In patients who develop aplastic anemia, marrow cellularity is decreased with fatty replacement, and the erythropoietic and granulopoietic lineages are symmetrically reduced.

Predisposition to Leukemia

Some patients with CAMT have developed MDS or acute myeloid leukemia.[7,223] One male with a normal physical appearance had amegakaryocytic thrombocytopenia from day 1 of life, developed aplastic anemia at 5 years of age, responded poorly to androgens and steroids, and then evolved into AMML at age 16 with death at age 17. A female had thrombocytopenia at 2 months of age, pancytopenia at 5 months, and thereafter developed a preleukemic picture with clonal abnormalities involving chromosome 19. The patient described herein[227] had thrombocytopenia at 6 months of age, developed progressive aplastic anemia over the next 2 years, acquired monosomy 7 in marrow cells at 5 years of age, and then evolved into MDS with an activating *ras* oncogene mutation in hematopoietic cells. Hence, the current evidence shows that CAMT is another inherited marrow failure disorder that is preleukemic. The risk or incidence of malignant conversion is difficult to determine because of the rarity of the disease and paucity of published data dealing with this issue.

Differential Diagnosis

If CAMT presents beyond the neonatal age group, a marrow aspirate and biopsy will point to the diagnosis, and mutational analysis will confirm it. (Certified mutation analysis for *MPL* can be obtained at Gene Dx, Gaithersburg, MD.) If CAMT presents at birth or shortly after, it must be distinguished from other causes of severe neonatal thrombocytopenia. Usually, these are caused by increased peripheral destruction of platelets and marrow sampling is not the customary first step.

Passive transplacental passage of IgG antiplatelet antibodies into fetal circulation can cause rapid destruction of fetal platelets. This occurs in two circumstances: a maternal autoimmune disease such as idiopathic thrombocytopenic purpura (ITP) or systemic lupus erythematosus (SLE); and in neonatal alloimmune thrombocytopenia by alloimmunization of the pregnant mother to fetal antigens inherited from father but absent in the mother. In the former situation, mother has thrombocytopenia or a past history of such; in the latter

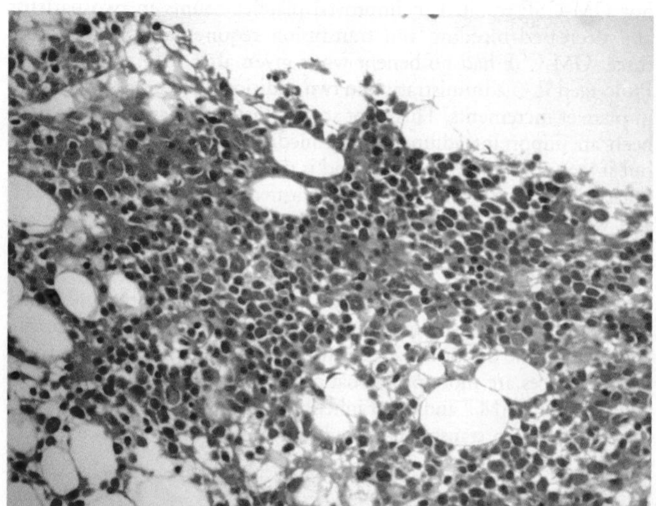

Figure 28–6 Low-power view of a bone marrow aspirate from a newly diagnosed patient with congenital amegakaryocytic thromobocytopenia. The 3 findings are normal celllularity, normal granulopoiesis and erythropoiesis, and absent megakaryocytes. *(Photomicrograph prepared by Dr. Mohamed Abdelhaleem, Toronto.)*

situation, mother has a normal platelet count and serum antibodies to human platelet alloantigens.

TAR syndrome is distinguished from CAMT because in TAR the radii are absent. Peripheral blood chromosomes are not characterized by increased fragility with DEB or MMC clastogenic stress testing in CAMT, which distinguishes it from Fanconi anemia. Several severe systemic neonatal infections collectively designated as the TORCH syndrome are associated with thrombocytopenia but are usually obvious clinically. Increased platelet destruction also occurs in newborns with giant benign hemangiomas of skin, liver or spleen, the so-called Kasabach-Merritt syndrome.

In an infant or young child with a CAMT clinical diagnosis but without mutant *MPL*, other inherited forms of thrombocytopenia have to be addressed (Table 28–5). These can generally be classified according to inheritance pattern (autosomal dominant, autosomal recessive, or X-linked), size of the platelets (small, normal, or large/giant), and presence or absence of associated clinical features. Identification of the specific mutant gene for each disorder confirms the diagnosis.

Therapy and Prognosis

Historically, treatment has been unsatisfactory and the mortality rate from thrombocytopenic bleeding, complications of aplastic anemia, or from malignant myeloid transformation has been very close to 100%. For that reason, HLA typing of family members should be performed as soon as the diagnosis is confirmed to see if a matched related donor for a HSCT exists. If not, a search for a matched unrelated donor or for cord blood cells should ensue as soon as the seriousness of the clinical picture dictates. The need for transfusional support is a cogent indication.

Platelet transfusions should be used discretely. Platelet numbers should not be a sole indication; clinical bleeding is a more appropriate trigger for the use of platelets. Single-donor filtered platelets are preferred to multiple unfiltered random donor platelets in order to minimize sensitization, and if HSCT is a realistic possibility all blood products should be free of cytomegalovirus.

Corticosteroids have been used for thrombocytopenia with no apparent efficacy. For aplastic anemia, androgens in combination with corticosteroids may induce a temporary partial response but the effect is short-lived and does not prevent mortality.

Based on the in vitro augmentation of megakaryocyte progenitor colony growth in response to IL-3, GM-CSF, or both, a phase I/II clinical trial was initiated for five patients with CAMT.[228] IL-3 but not GM-CSF resulted in improved platelet counts in two patients and decreased bleeding and transfusion requirements in the other three. GM-CSF had no benefit when given after IL-3 pretreatment. Prolonged IL-3 administration in two additional patients also resulted in platelet increments. This pilot study illustrates that IL-3 may have been an important adjunct to the medical management of CAMT but it was not adopted broadly and is no longer available. Thrombopoietin has not been tried for the treatment of severe Type I CAMT and would likely fail because endogenous thrombopoietin levels are markedly increased and the mutated thrombopoietin receptor is nonfunctional.

CAMT can be cured by HSCT.[223,231–236] Most of the published cases have had successful outcomes. Matched sibling donor sources are best, even if the donor is a carrier with one mutant allele.[235] Alternate donor sources are more problematic. Reduced-intensity conditioning regimens for CAMT and other inherited marrow failure disorders hold promise to lessen transplant-related morbidity and mortality.[237]

Future Directions

As summarized,[219] novel therapy may be available shortly for type II CAMT patients who retain some MPL function. MPL agonist antibodies can be engineered in the laboratory that bind and activate partially functional thrombopoietin receptors. CAMT is also a candidate disease for gene therapy as restoration of wild-type *MPL* would provide in vivo selection of corrected hematopoietic stem cells.

Other Genetic Syndromes

Bone marrow failure can occur in the context of several specific nonhematologic syndromes, and also in familial settings that do not exactly correspond with the entities already described.

Down Syndrome

Down syndrome, or constitutional trisomy 21, has a unique association with aberrant hematological abnormalities. Three seemingly related events can occur.[245] In the neonatal period, a myeloproliferative blood picture with large numbers of circulating blast cells has been observed in approximately 10% of these infants. The blasts show somatic *GATA1* mutations[246] and apparently are clonal but, remarkably, disappear spontaneously over several weeks in most cases. The term "transient leukemia" is often used to reflect this unusual natural history.

Secondly, in 20% to 30% of these cases, "true" acute megakaryoblastic leukemia (AMKL) appears later and requires oncologic management. Acute lymphoblastic and myeloblastic leukemias are also seen in Down syndrome, but AMKL is the most common form of the myeloblastic leukemias and is estimated to be 500 times greater in children with Down syndrome than in normal children.[245]

Thirdly, the onset of AMKL is frequently preceded by an interval of MDS characterized by thrombocytopenia, abnormal megakaryocytopoiesis, megakaryoblasts in the marrow, and an abnormal karyotype, commonly trisomy 8.[247,248] In addition to the propensity for leukemia, a few patients have been reported with aplastic anemia. Alter summarized five of these aplastic cases,[7] three of whom died of marrow failure and two who responded to androgen therapy.

Dubowitz Syndrome

This is an autosomal recessive disorder characterized by a peculiar facies, infantile eczema, small stature, and mild microcephaly. The face is small with a shallow supraorbital ridge, a nasal bridge at the same level as the forehead, short palpebral fissures, variable ptosis, and micrognathia.[249] This is a rare disorder and incidence rates for complications are difficult to establish, however, there appears to be a predilection to cancer as well as hematopoietic disorders in Dubowitz syndrome.[250] Patients have developed acute leukemia, neuroblastoma, and lymphoma.[250–252] Approximately 10% of patients also develop hematopoietic abnormalities varying from hypoplastic anemia, moderate pancytopenia, and full-blown aplastic anemia.[250,253]

Seckel Syndrome

Sometimes called "bird-headed dwarfs," patients with this autosomal recessive developmental disorder have marked intrauterine and postnatal growth failure and mental deficiency, severe microcephaly, a hypoplastic face with a receding forehead and chin, a prominent curved nose, and low-set and/or malformed ears.[254] These patients can be distinguished from those with Fanconi anemia on the basis of a negative DEB clastogenic chromosome stress test. About 25% of cases develop aplastic anemia or malignancies.[7,255–257] One form of Seckel syndrome is caused by a mutant *ATR* gene, and another by a mutant *PCNT2* gene. Different loci for 2 additional forms have also been identified demonstrating genetic heterogeneity.

Reticular Dysgenesia (Dysgenesis)

This is an immunologic deficiency syndrome coupled with congenital agranulocytosis.[258] The mode of inheritance is probably autosomal recessive but an X-linked mode is also possible in some cases. The disorder is a variant of severe combined immune deficiency (SCID) in which cellular and humoral immunity are absent and patients also have severe lymphopenia and neutropenia. Because of profoundly compromised immunity, the syndrome presents early with severe infection at birth or shortly thereafter. A striking feature is absent lymph nodes and tonsils and an absent thymic shadow on radiograph. In addition to lymphopenia and neutropenia, anemia and thrombocytopenia may be present. Bone marrow specimens are hypocellular with markedly reduced myeloid and lymphoid elements. Clonogenic assays of hematopoietic progenitors consistently show reduced to absent colony growth, indicating that the disorder has its origins at the pluripotential lympho-hematopoietic stem cell level.[259–262] The only curative therapy is HSCT.[261–263]

Schimke Immunoosseous Dysplasia

Schimke immunoosseous dysplasia is an autosomal recessive disorder caused by mutations in the chromatin remodeling protein SMARCAL1.[264,265] Patients manifest spondyloepiphyseal dysplasia with exaggerated lumbar lordosis and protruding abdomen.[266] There are pigmentary skin changes and abnormally discolored and configured teeth. Renal dysfunction can be problematic with proteinuria and nephrotic syndrome. The R561C missense mutation in the *SMARCAL1* gene is associated with a mild phenotype.[266] Approximately 50% of patients have hypothyroidism, 50% have cerebral ischemia, and 10% have bone marrow failure with neutropenia, thrombocytopenia, and anemia. Lymphopenia and altered cellular immunity are present in almost all patients. One case underwent a successful bone marrow transplantation.[267]

Noonan Syndrome

Noonan syndrome (NS) is a development disorder characterized by the "Noonan facies" (hypertelorism, ptosis, short neck, low-set ears), short stature, congenital heart disease, and multiple skeletal and hematologic abnormalities. NS is an autosomal dominant disorder with genetic heterogeneity. Heterozygous mutations in *PTPN11* which encodes SHP-2 cause about 50% of NS cases.[268] There is a resultant gain of function of SHP-2, a protein tyrosine phosphatase that positively modulates RAS signaling. Germline *KRAS* mutations also cause NS.[269,270] A variant of neurofibromatosis type 1 caused by mutations in the *NF1* gene results in a phenotypic overlap disorder with NS, the so-called neurofibromatosis-Noonan syndrome.[271] Remarkably, mutations of *PTPN11*, *RAS*, and *NF1* also are found in children with juvenile myelomonocytic leukemia (JMML), an aggressive hematologic cancer requiring hematopoietic stem cell transplantation.[272] JMML also occurs in NS patients but it regresses spontaneously without treatment. As summarized,[7] several NS patients developed amegakaryocytic thrombocytopenia, and one other patient manifested pancytopenia and a hypocellular marrow.

Cartilage-Hair Hypoplasia

Cartilage-hair hypoplasia (CHH) is an autosomal recessive syndrome characterized by metaphyseal dysostosis, short-limbed dwarfism, and fine, sparse hair. Additional skeletal findings include scoliosis, lordosis, chest deformity, and varus lower limbs. Aganglionic megacolon and other gastrointestinal abnormalities have been reported.[7] Most cases in the literature are Finnish or Amish. Mutations in the RNA component of RNase MRP cause CHH.[273,274] Macrocytic anemia is seen in over 80% of cases.[275] Most are mild and self-limited but some patients show a severe, persistent anemia resembling Diamond–Blackfan anemia. Neutropenia has been reported in 25% of CHH cases[7,276] and lymphopenia in 65%. Lymphomas and other cancers also occur at an increased frequency.[7]

Familial Forms of Marrow Failure

Bone marrow failure can cluster in families, but many of these cases cannot be readily classified into discrete diagnostic entities such as Fanconi anemia. Baseline chromosome breakage is almost always normal in these non-Fanconi syndromes but clastogenic stress testing with DEB or MMC is required for clarification. The phenotype of these conditions can be complex with varying combinations of cytopenias, macrocytosis, elevated levels of HbF, hypocellular bone marrows, immunologic deficiency, physical malformations, and predisposition to leukemia. The marrow failure is the result of a complex interplay of genetic and environmental influences that are likely specific to each affected family. Alter's practical approach to nosology is to divide the disorders into inheritance patterns, and then subdivide them into those with and without physical anomalies.[7]

Some families show an **autosomal dominant** mode of inheritance of marrow dysfunction associated **with physical anomalies**. The *WT syndrome* is characterized by successive generations of affected family members who have radial-ulnar hypoplasia, abnormal thumbs, short fingers, and fifth finger clinodactyly.[277,278] Pancytopenia or thrombocytopenia, sometimes with leukemia, occurs in some of the affected. The *IVIC syndrome*[279–281] or oculo-oto-radial syndrome[282] manifests with radial ray hypoplasia, absent thumbs or hypoplastic radial carpal bones, impaired hearing, strabismus, mild thrombocytopenia in about 50% of cases, and sometimes imperforate anus. The *ataxia-pancytopenia syndrome* is a combination of cerebellar atrophy and ataxia associated in affected family members with varied manifestations of anemia, aplastic anemia, MDS, AML, monosomy 7 in marrow cells, and immune deficiency.[283–285] Other autosomal dominant syndromes with anomalies include a family with marrow failure, ALL, skin pigmentation, warts, immune dysfunction, and multiple spontaneous abortions[286]; successive generations of family members with unilineage cytopenia or pancytopenia with vascular occlusions[287]; and proximal fusion of the radius and ulna, and aplastic anemia or leukemia.[288] The latter syndrome was associated with a mutation in a gene involved in bone marrow morphogenesis, *HOXA11*.[240,289]

Autosomal recessive inheritance **with physical anomalies** and marrow dysfunction also occurs. Consanguinity can result in a syndrome of microcephaly, mental retardation, skin pigmentation, short stature, and pancytopenia, possibly with a clonal cytogenetic marker in bone marrow cells.[290] A second example of this inheritance mode presents with central nervous system anomalies such as the Dandy–Walker syndrome or ventricular dilatation and asymmetry, and aplastic anemia.[291] Two cousins had oculocutaneous albinism, microcephaly, facial dysmorphia, immunodeficiency, neutropenia, and thrombocytopenia.[292] Three siblings with consanguineous parents had facial dysmorphia, steatorrhea, increased skin folds, congenital heart disease, vesicoureteral reflux, decreased cellular immunity, and severe neutropenia but normal chromosomes.[293] Seven families with a specific pattern of inheritance have been reported: five sporadic, one consanguineous, and one with affected siblings. Diaphyseal dysplasia and anemia were observed in all of the families.[294–296]

Autosomal dominant inheritance of a wide-ranging pattern of disordered marrow function can be seen **without physical anomalies**. Successive generations have been described with the following: "acquired" aplastic anemia in 4 families comprised of 9 patients with an affected parent, aunt, or uncle[297]; aplastic anemia in a mother and neutropenia and thrombocytopenia in her offspring[298]; aplastic anemia, AML and monosomy 7 in various family members[299]; and hypoplastic anemia in a parent and offspring with either myelofibrosis, AML, MDS, or pancytopenia, all associated with the acquired Pelger-Huet anomaly.[300]

Marrow dysfunction can also be inherited in an **autosomal recessive mode without physical anomalies.** One example encompasses pancytopenia, immune deficiency, multiple cutaneous basal cell and squamous cell carcinomas, oral telangiectasias, and neck and chest poikiloderma.[301] Another pattern includes immune deficiency, pure red cell aplasia and/or neutropenia, and unusual crystalloid structures seen by electron microscopy in neutrophils.[302] In one generation of a large maternal kindred, there were 8 members with aplastic anemia, AML and monosomy 7.[303] Thrombocytopenia was reported in 2 adult siblings with a Robertsonian translocation t (13;14).[304] Xeroderma pigmentosum can be associated with aplastic anemia,[305] as well as MDS,[306] and AML.[307,308]

An **X-linked inheritance without physical anomalies** is suggested by a syndrome affecting males in successive generations with one or more of pancytopenia, AML, ALL, and light chain disease but without physical anomalies.[309] The X-linked lymphoproliferative syndrome is a well-documented genetic disorder associated with the Epstein-Barr virus that causes malignant infectious mononucleosis and fatal aplastic anemia.[310,311] In most patients a mutant *SH2D1A* gene can be demonstrated. A mutant *XIAP* gene accounts for other cases.

Therapy for Familial Marrow Failure

Because these disorders are rare, broad conclusions about management are difficult to formulate. For full-blown aplastic anemia with a hypocellular, fatty marrow, curative therapy with HSCT remains the first choice if a suitable donor is identified. In the familial cases, potential stem cell donors must be thoroughly assessed clinically, hematologically and by marrow morphology, clonogenic activity, and cytogenetics to ensure that latent or masked marrow dysfunction is not present. If a matched donor is not available, principles of medical management used for Fanconi anemia and for acquired aplastic anemia should be used.

UNI-LINEAGE CYTOPENIAS

Diamond-Blackfan Anemia

Background

Diamond-Blackfan anemia (DBA), or congenital hypoplastic anemia, is an inherited form of pure red cell aplasia.[312,313] The syndrome is heterogeneous with respect to inheritance patterns, clinical and laboratory findings, in vitro data, and therapeutic outcome. Although it was formerly believed that 80% of DBA cases were sporadic, molecular studies in conjunction with data on family members for red cell adenosine deaminase levels, red cell macrocytosis, and congenital anomalies suggest that approximately 45% of cases[314,315] are autosomal dominant with variable penetrance.[316,317] Recessive inheritance was inferred in more than 30 families published in the literature in which there were affected siblings with normal parents, affected cousins, or consanguinity.[7] However, these cases have not been confirmed as autosomal recessive.[314] Some of these may be autosomal dominant with non-penetrance[318] or from gonadal mosaicism.[319] DBA likely represents a family of disorders with different genetic and molecular etiologies that share the common hematological phenotype of pure red cell aplasia. Based on data from a European registry of DBA patients, the suspected incidence of the disorder in Europe is approximately 7 cases per million live births.[317]

The uniform diagnostic criteria for all cases are (a) normochromic-macrocytic anemia presenting in 90% of cases in the first 12 months of life; (b) profound reticulocytopenia; (c) normocellular marrow with a selective, marked deficiency of red cell precursors; (d) increased serum levels of erythropoietin; (e) normal or slightly decreased white cell counts; and (f) normal, decreased, or increased platelet counts. Fetal hemoglobin is usually increased with a fetal G-γ/A-γ pattern, is distributed heterogeneously, and is associated with increased expression of red cell i antigen as well as with fetal levels of red cell glycolytic and hexose monophosphate shunt enzyme activities.

Etiology, Genetics, and Pathophysiology

In most DBA cases, cytogenetic findings are normal although alterations of chromosomes 1 and 16 have been reported.[320,321] Discovery of a balanced reciprocal translocation t(x;19) in a sporadic female case of DBA[322] and the identification of microdeletions on chromosome 19 in some other DBA patients[323] localized a gene responsible for DBA to 19q13.2. Cloning of the 19q13 breakpoint region revealed a mutated gene encoding ribosomal protein (RP) S19 associated with the ribosomal 40S subunit.[324] Subsequent studies identified mutations in one allele for the gene in 25% of patients.[325–327]

The exact function of this protein in ribosome biogenesis is still poorly understood. The yeast homolog of RPS19 is required for the maturation of the 3′ end of 18S rRNA, failure of which results in the accumulation of faulty pre-40S ribosome subunits.[328] Extra-ribosomal functions have been ascribed to RPS19 in addition to the post-apoptotic mediation of monocyte chemotaxis.[329] RPS19 has been shown to interact with a novel nucleolar protein S19-binding protein (S19BP),[330] fibroblast growth factor 2,[331] and the PIM-1 oncoprotein.[332] PIM-1 is an ubiquitous serine-threonine kinase whose expression can be induced in erythropoietic cells by several growth factors including erythropoietin. Thus, for the first time, a link between erythropoietic growth factor signaling and RPS19 was identified.

In 25% of cases with mutant *RPS19*, the prevailing opinion is that the disorder results from protein haploinsufficiency.[333] In support of this, two classes of *RPS19* mutations have been described: quantitative defects resulting in undetectable protein, and hotspot mutations leading to loss of function.[333] Additional links between *RPS19* and erythropoiesis have now been clearly established. When *RPS19* is knocked down in cellular models,[334–336] defective erythropoiesis results. In addition, wild-type gene transfer corrects the defective erythropoiesis in *RPS19*-deficient DBA CD34$^+$ cells resulting in a 3-fold increase in erythroid colony growth.[337] In yeast, the introduction of *RPS19* mutations found in DBA results in a defect in the processing of pre-rRNA similar to that observed in DBA cells with decreased expression of *RPS19*.[328]

There is recent evidence that *RPS19* mutations lead to downregulation of multiple ribosomal protein genes as well as downregulation of genes involved in translation in DBA cells.[338] These data coupled with earlier reports establish the important relationship between *RPS19* and erythroid proliferation and maturation.[339,340]

In DBA patients without *RPS19* mutations, a second DBA locus has been mapped to chromosome 8p22-p23 in approximately 35% of cases,[341] but a candidate gene, tentatively called *DBA2*, has not been identified. There are DBA patients with neither mutant RPS19 nor linkage to 8p22-p23. In approximately 2% of *RPS19* mutation-negative probands, de novo nonsense and splice-site mutations can be identified in another ribosomal protein, RPS24. The gene *RPS24* (*DBA3*) maps to 10q22-q23.[342] A third mutant ribosomal protein gene, *RPS17*, has also been decribed[343] strengthening the theory that impaired translation may be the pathogenetic explanation for DBA. At the 9th annual DBA International concensus conference in 2008, two additional ribosomal protein gene mutations were described, *RPL5* and *RPL11*.[344] Thus, at least 6 genetic mutations account for DBA.

Initial reports of humoral, cellular, or microenvironmental inhibitors of erythropoiesis in DBA could not be confirmed. Claims for immune-mediated erythroid suppression in DBA would need to satisfy strict criteria: patients must be newly diagnosed, untreated, and not previously transfused; the in vitro testing system must be completely autologous using only patient cells and serum; and any degree of inhibition must be totally selective for the erythroid lineage. Since almost none of the reports met these criteria, the notion of an immune pathogenesis of DBA shifted to alternate possibilities.

A large body of evidence indicates that the erythroid progenitor compartment is intrinsically defective in DBA.[345–350] Cultures of DBA marrow using standard clonogenic assays for CFU-E and BFU-E progenitors consistently have shown reduced or absent colonies in most DBA patients, and intermediate, normal, or occasionally increased numbers in the rest. The DBA erythroid progenitors are relatively insensitive to Epo in vitro[348] and to burst-promoting activity,[351] but the hyporesponsiveness to Epo can be corrected in some cases by the addition of glucocorticoids in vitro[352] or by clinically administering prednisone.[353] A recent report localized the DBA defect down-stream of the erythropoietin receptor.[354]

The data underscore the fact that the intrinsic defect of DBA erythroid progenitors is an inability to respond normally to inducers of erythroid proliferation and/or differentiation. Confirmation of the overall defect was demonstrated by showing that $CD34^+$ DBA progenitors differentiated normally along megakaryocytic and granulocytic pathways but aberrantly along the erythroid lineage.[355] Accelerated programmed cell death (apoptosis) plays a central role in this pathogenesis[356] as it does in many if not all inherited marrow failure disorders. A role for induction of apoptosis by the Fas-Fas ligand system in DBA was suggested because of elevated serum soluble Fas ligand in patients compared to controls.[357] Based on the various patterns of erythroid colony growth seen with DBA patients, a model for the aberrant erythropoiesis was developed that proposes maturational arrests at varying sites along the differentiation pathway.[313]

Recombinant interleukin-3 (IL-3)[358] and Steel factor (SCF) in combination with Epo[359–361] may increase the in vitro clonogenicity of DBA bone marrow progenitors from unfractionated cell preparations. The size and number of DBA BFU-E colonies are dramatically increased by adding IL-3 to the cultures.[358] One study showed a growth response of BFU-E from 4 patients to SCF alone or in combination with IL-3, GM-CSF, or conditioned media.[359] Another study described a lack of response of enriched $CD34^+$ progenitors to IL-3, GM-CSF and erythroid potentiating activity (EPA) in 10 DBA patients, but SCF in combination with IL-3 promoted BFU-E colony growth in 3 patients.[355] A further report described heterogeneity in vitro in 10 patients with normal, intermediate or absent responses to SCF.[360] Additional data showed that 15 of 16 DBA marrow cultures had increased erythropoiesis, often to normal levels, in the presence of SCF compared to cultures lacking SCF.[361] The human ligand for flt-3 apparently has no effect on DBA marrow colony growth. However, addition of IL-9 to SCF, IL-3, and Epo does potentiate DBA BFU-E growth.[362]

There are significant age-related changes in erythroid and granulopoietic progenitors in DBA patients.[363] Despite profound anemia, 7 of 10 patients studied within 1 year of diagnosis had normal numbers of CFU-E and BFU-E that showed a normal response to cytokines. In contrast, 12 of 14 patients followed more than 3 years had decreased erythroid progenitors and, in 7 cases, decreased CFU-GM. The data are consistent with the idea that the DBA defect involves other hematopoietic lineages and worsens with time.

Strong support for this conclusion comes from a detailed study that examined the interaction between DBA $CD34^+$ cells and the hematopoietic microenvironment using long-term bone marrow cultures.[364] Stromal adherent layers from DBA patients did not show evidence of any morphological, phenotypic, or functional abnormality and the stroma sustained the proliferation of normal $CD34^+$ cells. A major finding was an impaired capacity of DBA $CD34^+$ cells in the presence of normal stromal cells to proliferate and differentiate along not only the erythroid pathway but also along the granulocytic-macrophage pathway. These results indicate an intrinsic defect of a hematopoietic progenitor with at least bi-lineage potential that places it earlier than previously suspected and which was only unmasked by testing in long-term cultures. These findings were extended with evidence in long-term culture initiating assays for a trilineage defect in DBA refractory to treatment.[365] The data broaden the definition of DBA and explain generalized marrow dysfunction and hypoplasia in some cases of DBA that have puzzled investigators for years.

The in vitro findings raised speculation that DBA is caused by one or more receptor-ligand abnormalities involving various growth-promoting cytokines such as Epo, IL-3, and SCF. Studies have failed to identify any of these putative abnormalities. DBA lymphocytes produce high levels of IL-3, DBA marrow stromal cells express mRNA for SCF, and DBA patients have measurable serum levels of SCF and have SCF receptors on marrow cells.[366] Moreover, molecular studies have not disclosed mutations in genes for c-kit (SCF receptor) or SCF.[367–369] Thus, current thinking based on cases with mutant *RPS19* is that haploinsufficiency of RPS19 protein either quantitatively or qualitatively accounts for DBA. A second theory in DBA without mutant *RPS19* is that an intracellular defect exists in signal transduction or in a transcription factor acting early in differentiation. Such anomalies could account for the increased tendency of DBA erythroid progenitors to undergo apoptosis upon Epo deprivation in vitro.[356]

Clinical Features

History and Physical Examination

DBA registries with longitudinal data,[315,317,370–374] and a summary of published cases[7] provide comprehensive information about clinical aspects of the disorder. Aside from findings associated with anemia, about one-half of infants at presentation look healthy and are normal physically. Unless the patient develops cardiac failure as a result of anemia, hepatosplenomegaly and edema are absent.

Both sexes are equally affected. Although the majority of published patients are white, DBA has been recognized in several ethnic groups, including African blacks, Arabs, East Indians, and Japanese. Pregnancy, birth history, or both are often abnormal. In a survey from the French and German DBA registries of 64 pregnancies in 26 women with DBA,[375] complications were seen in 42 pregnancies (66%) and included abortion, preeclampsia, in utero fetal death, in utero growth retardation, retroplacental hematoma, and preterm delivery. Thirteen of 34 children born alive had DBA.

From 30% to 47% of patients present with one or more congenital defects.[315,317,370–374] Most of these phenotypic abnormalities belong to the following categories: (a) craniofacial dysmorphism, including hypertelorism, microcephaly, microphthalmos, congenital cataract or glaucoma, strabismus, microretrognathism, and a high-arched palate or cleft palate; (b) prenatal or postnatal growth failure, independent of steroid therapy; (c) neck anomalies; these may consist of a pterygium coli, or the fusion of cervical vertebrae with flaring of the trapezius muscle (Klippel-Feil syndrome) giving a Turner syndrome appearance; there may also be the Sprengel deformity (congenital elevation of the scapula) as an isolated anomaly, or a combination of the two anomalies; and (d) thumb malformations, such as bifid thumb (Fig. 28–7), duplication, subluxation, hypoplasia, or absence of the thumb. There is a characteristic association of triphalangeal thumbs with DBA (Fig. 28–8) commonly referred to as "Aase syndrome II" or "Aase-Smith syndrome." In addition, some patients have a flat, hypoplastic thenar eminence, weak or absent radial pulses, or both, which probably represent variations of the thumb malformations.

Some patients have a characteristic facial appearance. The facies of DBA is said to consist of tow-colored hair, snub nose, wide set eyes, thick upper lip, and an intelligent expression.[376] Another facies observed in two unrelated girls of markedly different ancestries consists of small heads, almond-shaped eyes with a slight antimongoloid slant, a "carp-like" smile, and pointed chins.[313] These patients resemble each other more than they resemble their own family members (Figs. 28–9A and 28–9B). Some patients with DBA have a phenotype indistinguishable from Treacher-Collins syndrome, a disorder of ribosome biogenesis caused by *TCOF1* mutations.[314,377,378]

Various other anomalies are occasionally reported in association with DBA. There may be urogenital malformations, such as dysplastic or horseshoe kidneys, duplication of ureters, or renal tubular acidosis. There may also be congenital heart disease, mainly ventricular and atrial septal defects, or hypogonadism, ear malformations, mental retardation, congenital hip dislocation, cartilage-hair hypoplasia with T-cell dysfunction, or tracheoesophageal fistula.

Laboratory Findings

Peripheral Blood and Bone Marrow Findings. The main hematological findings in DBA are summarized in Table 28–6. The anemia is usually profound at the time of diagnosis. Hemoglobin levels average 6.5 g/dL in patients diagnosed in the first 2 months of life

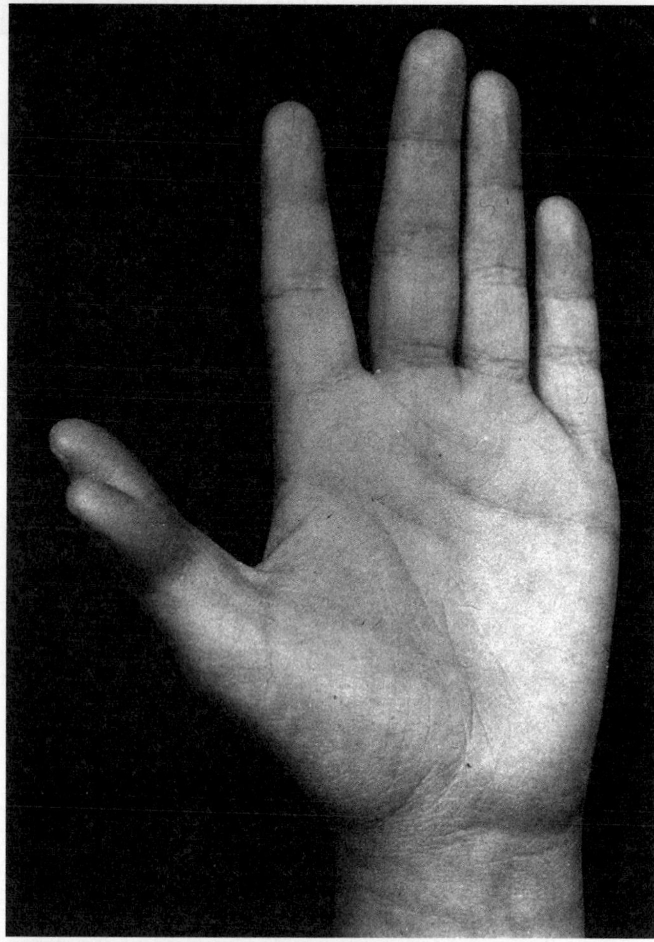

Figure 28–7 Bifid thumb in Diamond-Blackfan anemia.

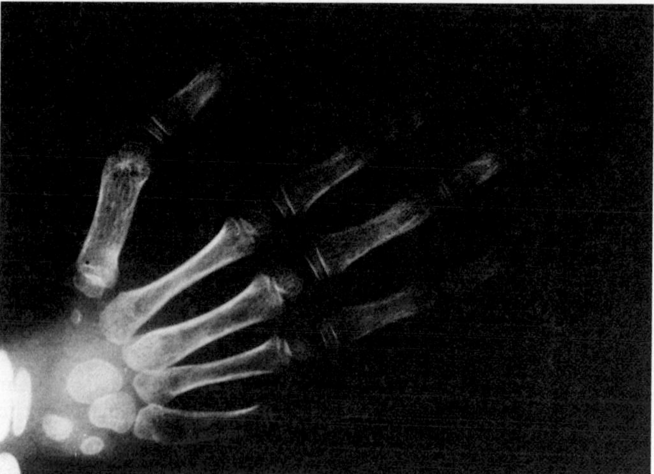

Figure 28–8 Radiograph of a triphalangeal thumb in Diamond-Blackfan anemia.

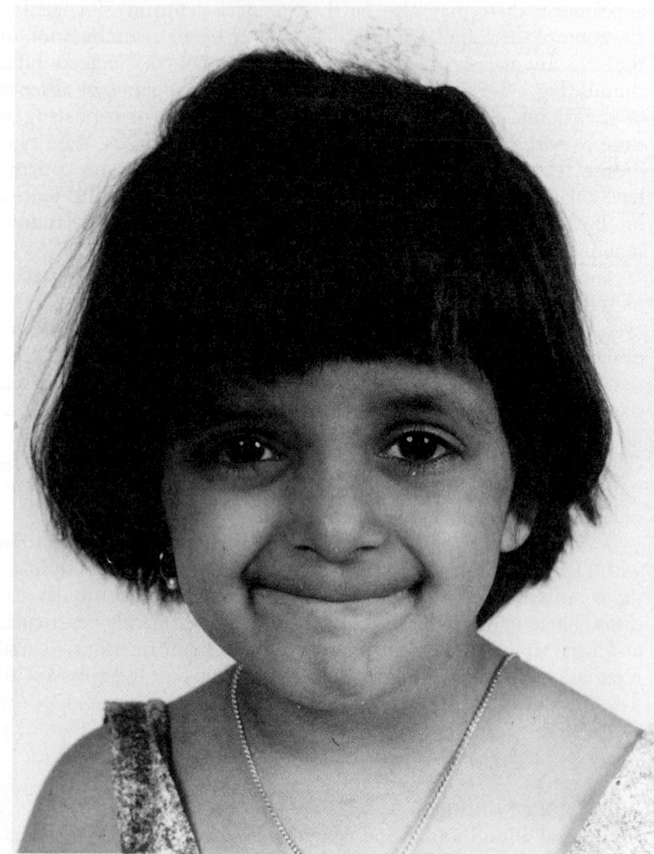

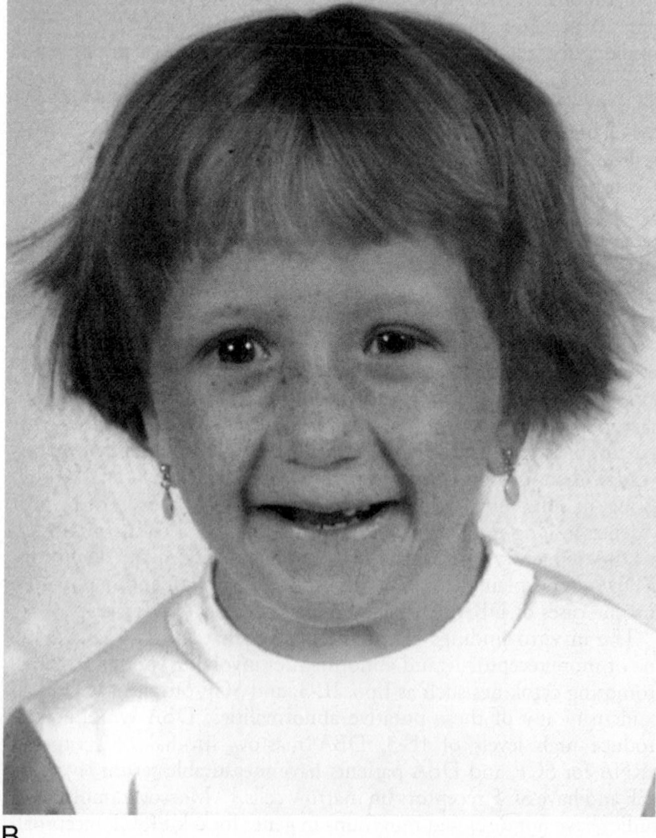

Figure 28–9 Similar Diamond-Blackfan facies in two unrelated girls of different ancestries consisting of a small head, almond-shaped eyes with slight antimongoloid slant, a "carp-like" smile, and a pointed chin.

Table 28–6 Hematological Features of Diamond-Blackfan Anemia at Diagnosis

Hematologic Parameters	Lab Findings
Mean hemoglobin value (range):	
Newborns under 2 months of age[a]	6.5 g/dL (1.7–9.1 g/dL)
Children 2 months of age or older[a]	4.0 g/dL (1.8–7.4 g/dL)
Mean corpuscular volume (MCV)	Usually increased for age
Reticulocytes	Markedly decreased (<1%)
White cell count	Normal or slightly decreased
Platelet count	Normal or increased
Fetal hemoglobin	Increased (>5% after 6 months of age)
Red cell i antigen	Expression increased beyond first year of life
Red cell enzymes	Fetal pattern
Red cell adenosine deaminase activity	Elevated in 40%–90% of cases
Bone marrow morphology:	
In >90% of cases	Marked reduction or absence of erythroid precursors
In 5–10% of cases	Slightly reduced or normal number of proerythroblasts with or without maturation arrest
In all patients	Normal cellularity; normal myeloid and megakaryocytic lineages

[a]Toronto series (n = 21). See reference 313.

(range of 1.7–9.1 g/dL) and 4.0 g/dL (range of 1.8–7.4 g/dL) in those diagnosed later. Macrocytosis is seen in the vast majority of patients with the mean corpuscular volume (MCV) being above the expected values for age. The peripheral blood smear may show, in addition to macrocytes, a mild degree of nonspecific anisocytosis and poikilocytosis. The aregenerative component of the anemia is reflected by the absence of both polychromasia and nucleated red cells on the blood film. Decreased red cell production is confirmed by absence of a reticulocyte response and by characteristic findings on bone marrow examination.

In more than 90% of patients, the bone marrow aspirate is normocellular, but erythroblasts are markedly decreased or absent. Proerythroblasts, if present, account for less than 3% of all nucleated elements, with a myeloid:erythroid ratio of >10 : 1 (Fig. 28–10). In 5% to 10% of cases, proerythroblasts may be present in normal numbers, with or without a maturation arrest. The other cell lines are normal. White cell counts and platelet counts are usually normal at diagnosis, but platelets may be decreased, or increased and with normal function. Mild to moderate neutropenia, thrombocytopenia, or both may occur later in the course of the disease, particularly in multitransfused patients who have hemosiderosis and secondary hypersplenism. Progression of the single-lineage erythroid deficiency of DBA into pancytopenia and severe aplastic anemia is rare but occurs.[365,379] Of 36 deaths reported to the American DBA Registry (DBAR), 1 died from severe aplastic anemia.[314]

Erythrocyte Findings. Erythrocytes in DBA express a number of fetal characteristics.[380] The level of hemoglobin F (HbF) is increased persistently even during remission. It remains at a level of 5% to 10% after the age of 6 months and has a heterogeneous distribution in red cells. The HbF has a specifically fetal amino-acid profile, with a high glycine:alanine ratio (G-γ:A-γ). Similarly, the i antigen, which normally disappears from the erythrocyte surface by 1 year of age, is expressed at near fetal levels in older patients with DBA.

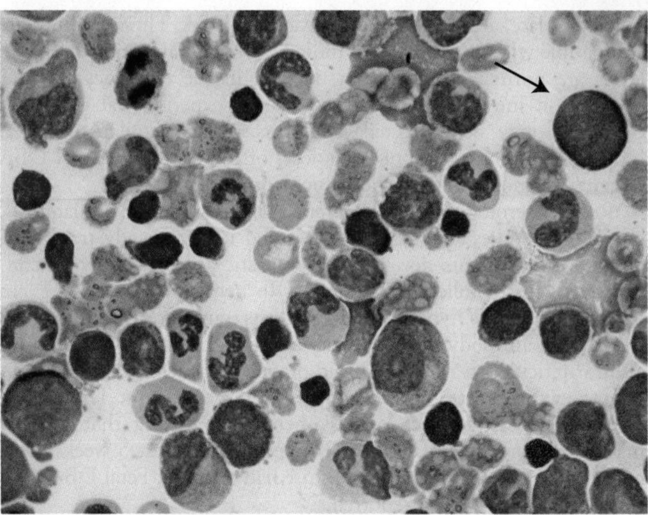

Figure 28–10 High-power view of a bone marrow aspirate from a newly diagnosed infant with Diamond-Blackfan anemia. The findings are active granulopoiesis, normal lymphoid activity for age, and an isolated pronormoblast (*arrow*) with total absence of early-, intermediate-, and late-stage nucleated red cells. *(Photocmicrograph prepared by Dr. Mohamed Abdelhaleem, Toronto.)*

The precise cause of this fetal-like erythropoiesis is unclear.[381,382] It is clearly distinct from the fetal erythropoiesis implicated in various types of leukemia, notably in juvenile myelomonocytic leukemia in which the fetal red cells presumably arise from the leukemic clone. The situation in DBA may be analogous to that in other forms of bone marrow failure and in the hematological recovery phase following bone marrow transplantation.[381] In all of these conditions, the fetal (or "stress") erythropoiesis may represent an accelerated recapitulation of red cell ontogeny in the face of an increased demand for new red cells in peripheral blood.

Red cell enzymes often display an abnormal pattern of activity.[383] Enzymes, such as enolase, glyceraldehyde-3-phosphate dehydrogenase, phosphofructokinase, and glutathione peroxidase, have increased activity in patients with DBA compared to those in normal children and adults or in patients with transient erythroblastopenia of childhood. For some enzymes, this increased activity is comparable to cord blood red cells. In apparent contradiction, carbonic anhydrase isoenzyme B, which is not normally present in fetal red cells, was detected in hemolysates from three patients with DBA.[380] Also, the red cells of two of the three patients had adult hexokinase isoenzyme distribution by isoelectric focusing.

Abnormalities in purine and pyrimidine metabolism are reflected by increased activity of red cell adenosine deaminase (ADA) in many patients with DBA.[384–387] Also, increased orotidine decarboxylase (ODC) activity is seen in some patients.[387] ADA activity is raised in DBA erythrocytes, but not in cord blood red cells from normal newborns or from patients with any of several hematologic conditions associated with "stress" erythropoiesis. Thus, this enzymatic abnormality cannot be due simply to a "reversion" to fetal erythropoiesis. Red cell ADA activity was initially reported to be elevated in up to 90% of patients with DBA and to be elevated occasionally in some of their nonanemic relatives. However, in subsequent studies, ADA levels were found to be raised in only 40% of patients. Raised ADA activity may also be detected in some hemolytic anemias and acute leukemias which limits the utility of this assay as a specific diagnostic marker for DBA. However, increased ADA activity does appear to be useful in differentiating DBA from transient erythroblastopenia of childhood on a biochemical basis,[383–387] and for epidemiologic testing of DBA pedigrees to identify family members with a mild phenotype.[315]

Miscellaneous Laboratory Findings. Serum levels of various factors involved in red cell production, such as erythropoietin, iron, vitamin

B_{12}, and folate, are appropriately elevated in DBA. These findings are compatible with any form of chronic hypoplastic anemia. Riboflavin levels are normal in the serum but not in the erythrocytes. This observation initially aroused interest since experimental riboflavin deficiency may be corrected by corticosteroids similar to DBA. However, administration of large doses of riboflavin to several DBA patients did not result in a hematopoietic response.

Red cell serology is usually unremarkable at the time of diagnosis, but alloantibodies are frequently detected in chronically transfused patients. Two infants developed hypoplastic anemia, either in conjunction with or following a bout of Rh hemolytic disease.[388,389] In one of them,[388] the hypoplastic anemia was transient. It was proposed that the Rh antibody had specificity not only for mature red cells but also for reticulocytes and erythroid progenitors thereby causing temporary erythropoietic suppression of the bone marrow. The second patient[389] presented with a brisk hemolytic anemia that initially masked the presence of DBA. DBA became manifest 5 weeks postnatally when the Rh hemolytic disease had resolved. Fetal DBA with hydrops fetalis has been reported.[390]

Differential Diagnosis

Transient Erythroblastopenia of Childhood

In clinical practice, after excluding a viral etiology, particularly parvovirus B_{19}, transient erythroblastopenia of childhood (TEC) is usually the only diagnosis that is confused with DBA (Table 28–7). Both entities share the same morphologic findings in the bone marrow. However, TEC is a self-limited disorder with an excellent prognosis and needs no specific therapy except for red cell transfusions in the most profoundly anemic patients.[391] The definition of TEC includes the following features: (a) gradual onset of pallor in previously healthy children usually 1–4 years of age (85% of cases); (b) normochromic-normocytic anemia with varying reticulocytopenia unless recovery has already ensued; (c) marrow erythroid hypoplasia (60% of cases), or aplasia (10% of cases), or a recovery picture (30% of cases); (e) spontaneous recovery usually within 4 to 8 weeks without recurrence, with rare exceptions.[392]

There are some additional important features of TEC. It can occur in siblings simultaneously and in seasonal "clusters" from June to October and from November to March. Of concern are the transient neurologic changes that can accompany TEC and which appear to be linked to the disorder. Affected children may have one or more of the following: hemiparesis, papilledema, abnormal extraocular movements, seizures, and unsteadiness of gait. The affected patients in the published reports recovered without sequelae, and the precise relationship of these neurologic changes to the pathogenesis of TEC has not been determined.

It was claimed initially that only the erythroid lineage was affected in TEC and all other hematopoietic lineages were normal. Although the mechanism is not clear, significant neutropenia also occurs in many patients with TEC, being associated in some with hypocellular marrows or with a granulopoietic maturational arrest. The neutropenia may be caused by a common pathogenetic mechanism that produces anemia. Increased numbers of $CD10^+$ lymphoid cells have been observed in bone marrow of some TEC patients but the interpretation of this finding is not clear.[393,394] An unusual presentation of TEC as a leukoerythroblastic anemia has been recorded.[395]

Although one case of TEC was caused by parvovirus B19,[396] there are no data that firmly incriminate other infectious agents in the etiology of TEC, although a history of a preceding viral-like illness can be obtained in more than half of the patients. The most plausible explanation proposed to date is that TEC is caused by transient immunosuppression of erythropoiesis,[397] and possibly of granulopoiesis in those with neutropenia. Most supportive evidence for this thesis comes from in vitro studies. Two reports described an inhibitory effect of TEC serum and fractionated IgG on erythroid colony growth that disappeared as TEC improved.[398,399] An IgG inhibitor of erythropoiesis was discovered in one case, and an IgM inhibitor in a second patient.[397] A summary of other published studies[400] suggests that over 60% of TEC patients have autologous or allogeneic serum inhibitors of erythroid colony formation. Autologous or allogeneic cell-mediated immune suppression of erythropoiesis has also been identified in about 25% of cases.[397,400,401] All of the in vitro studies have generated varying patterns of erythroid colony growth in TEC. Colony numbers can be normal, but reduced numbers of BFU-E and CFU-E progenitors have been recorded in 30% and 50% of cases, respectively.

Therefore, TEC has an autoimmune pathogenesis. There are data that indicate that TEC cases are allelic with DBA on chromosome 19q13.2 but are not caused by mutations of the *RPS19* gene.[402] The transient nature of TEC is similar to other autoimmune hematologi-

Table 28–7 Distinguishing Features Between Diamond–Blackfan Anemia (DBA) and Transient Erythroblastopenia of Childhood (TEC)

	DBA	TEC
Etiology	Genetic	Acquired
Immune-mediated	None	Common
Family history	About 10%	Occasional siblings with concurrent TEC
Antecedent history	None	Viral infection
Age at diagnosis	90% by 1 year	6 months–4 years
Physical anomalies	About 50%	None
Neurologic findings	None	Occasional
Transfusion dependence	Yes, if steroid-refractory	None
Course	Chronic	Full recovery
Risk of cancer	Increased	Not increased
Risk of MDS/leukemia	Increased	Not increased
Laboratory findings at diagnosis:		
RBC size	Macrocytic	Normocytic
HbF	Increased	Normal[a]
i antigen	Increased	Normal[a]
RBC enzyme activities	Fetal levels	Adult levels[a]
RBC adenosine deaminase	Increased in 40%–90%	Normal

[a]During recovery, values may be increased.

cal disorders of childhood, such as idiopathic thrombocytopenic purpura and some cases of autoimmune hemolytic anemia. The decreased activities of virtually all red cell enzymes in TEC compared to controls probably relate to the aged population of peripheral blood erythrocytes being tested.[391]

Viral Etiologies of Erythroid Failure

Regarding viral causes of non-DBA red cell aplasia, Epstein-Barr virus, hepatitis virus, human T-cell leukemia virus-1, and human immunodeficiency virus-1 have all been implicated and should be excluded if the etiology of the anemia remains unclear. Parvovirus B_{19} stands out as a major causal agent of red cell aplasia in the context of an underlying chronic hemolytic anemia in infants and children with chronic congenital and acquired forms of immunosuppression. The fetus is uniquely susceptible to parvovirus infection and in utero transmission is a well-documented cause of nonimmune hydrops fetalis. Parvovirus infection should be ruled out in every case of childhood red cell aplasia by serial measurements of serum IgM and IgG, and by bone marrow examination for the characteristic giant pronormoblasts. Parvovirus may also be detected in marrow by gene amplification using the polymerase chain reaction and confirmed by direct in situ hybridization.

Predisposition to Malignancy

Although not generally regarded as a preleukemic or precancerous condition, DBA is clearly associated with hematologic cancer and with solid tumors. The link between DBA and hematologic cancer is more understandable from the data described herein that implicate an early pluripotent marrow progenitor in the pathobiology of DBA.[364,365] As summarized,[314] 10 DBA cases developed acute myeloid leukemia, 2 developed MDS, 1 had acute lymphoblastic leukemia, and 1 had non-Hodgkin lymphoma. There have also been reports of neoplasms including three cases of osteogenic sarcoma, two cases each of hepatocellular carcinoma, breast carcinoma, and Hodgkin disease, and one case each of gastric carcinoma, vaginal melanoma, and malignant fibrous histiocytoma. Although the actuarial risk of cancer in DBA is unknown, the risk exists and hence DBA is considered to be a cancer predisposition syndrome. The published cases implicate several possible operative factors including transfusional iron overload, use of androgens, immunosuppression from corticosteroids, thymic and skeletal irradiation during childhood as "therapy" for DBA in one case, and cyclophosphamide "treatment" in another. Although some DBA patients with mutant *RSP19* developed cancer,[314] there are insufficient data to predict a cancer genotype.

Natural History and Prognosis

Historically, the only treatment for DBA was blood transfusions. Without this, patients died of anemia. When corticosteroids were introduced as an effective therapy for DBA, all patients were assigned to one of the two therapeutic interventions and the "natural history" of the disorder took on a different dimension. A notable example is the phenomenon of spontaneous remission that occurs in about 20% of cases that allows patients to discontinue whatever treatment they are receiving, either chronic transfusion therapy or corticosteroids. The DBAR has some actuarial data showing that 75% remit prior to their 10th birthdays, and in most cases the remission is sustained.[403] It appears that an equal number of patients remit from either corticosteroids or transfusions. A relapse of DBA requires reintroduction of treatment.

The overall actuarial survival for DBA patients greater than 40 years of age is 75% ± 4.8%.[403] For those in sustained spontaneous remission, it is 100%; for corticosteroid responders it is 57% ± 8.9%; and for transfusion-dependent patients it is 8.9%. Causes of death mostly relate directly to the development of cancer or its treatment, complications from corticosteroid-induced immunosuppression, stem cell transplant-related complications, and transfusional hemosiderosis.

Therapy

In younger children and infants, it is important to determine whether the red cell aplasia is DBA or TEC (Table 28–7). Until a firm diagnosis is established, the initial treatment in children is almost always the use of transfusions. This allows the flexibility to complete the viral work-up and other investigations, and to await a spontaneous remission if the anemia is caused by TEC or another self-limited condition. The principle to follow if transfusions are used is to aim for a moderate but not full correction of anemia so that erythropoiesis is not suppressed and recovery from TEC not delayed. Most patients with TEC usually recover within a few weeks after receiving only one transfusion. Occasionally, recovery from TEC is slow and starts to mimic DBA in chronicity. If there is confusion about the proper diagnosis, it is appropriate to withhold corticosteroids in favor of a further transfusion in order to allow more observation time. Demonstration of a mutant ribosomal protein gene would clinch the diagnosis, but only in about 25% of patients.

Transfusions

Before the first transfusion, it is recommended that a full red cell phenotype be performed on the patient. This information will be valuable for prevention and management of alloantibody formation caused by sensitization. For patients in whom corticosteroids are either ineffective or excessively toxic, a regular program of red cell transfusions is usually required. During the course of this program, a small number of steroid-resistant patients may show sensitivity to corticosteroids when re-treated, or even proceed to a spontaneous transient or prolonged remission. If not, leukocyte-depleted packed red cells are given monthly to keep the hemoglobin concentration at a level compatible with normal activity. CMV-negative packed cells should be used if stem cell transplantation is contemplated. The nadir should not be less than 6 g/dL. Several complications may arise from transfusions such as blood-borne infections and sensitization, but the major long-term threat is iron overload, which causes delayed puberty, growth retardation, diabetes mellitus, hypoparathyroidism, and eventually liver cirrhosis and cardiac failure. These complications can be delayed, and possibly prevented, by the early administration of an iron chelator. Deferoxamine (Desferal), administered with a battery-powered pump as a daily 12-hour subcutaneous infusion, has been the main chelator for the past 3 decades. However in a randomized trial of Desferal or deferasirox (Exjade), a once-daily oral iron chelator, in patients with transfusional iron overload, the two chelators showed similar efficacy.[404] It is predicted that Exjade will replace Desferal as the chelator of choice. The oral iron chelator deferiprone (L1) has caused significant neutropenia and death in one case[405] in DBA and is not recommended (Dr. Jeffrey Lipton, public communication).

As long as Desferal remains the main chelator, there are uncertainties about the optimal age at which to start it for patients with transfusion-dependent anemia. There have been reports of abnormal linear growth and metaphyseal dysplasia in thalassemia major patients treated with deferoxamine before the age of 3 years.[406] This adverse event has prompted recommendations for starting therapy later. However, a progressively rising serum ferritin level or, more accurately, excessive hepatic iron concentration obtained by biopsy after 1 year of regular transfusions would be appropriate indications to commence chelation. The daily starting subcutaneous infusion dose of Desferal should not exceed 50 mg/kg. Ascorbate supplementation should be considered if there is sustained loss of efficacy of Desferal, especially if tissue ascorbate concentrations are reduced.[407]

Corticosteroids

Steroid responsiveness is present in 50% to 75% of DBA patients. Upon administration of prednisone at a dose of 2 mg/kg/day in three divided doses, reticulocytosis is usually seen within 1 to 4 weeks, and is followed by a rise in hemoglobin concentration. Once the hemoglobin level reaches 9.0 to 10.0 g/dL, prednisone can be slowly tapered by reducing the number of daily doses. If a single daily dose of prednisone maintains the desired hemoglobin level, the dose can be doubled and given on alternate days but this may not prevent significant steroid toxicity.

The dose of prednisone can be further reduced by small decrements on a weekly basis, or more slowly, until the minimal effective dose is determined. This dose is extremely variable. A few patients can be maintained on minute, nonpharmacologic doses, whereas other patients need large doses that preclude long-term therapy because of serious side effects like cushingoid features, pathologic fractures, cataracts, growth failure, diabetes, and avascular necrosis of the femoral or humeral heads. There is no known predictor of steroid responsiveness, nor any way to anticipate the type of individual responses. In general, a corticosteroid dose-equivalent of prednisone, 0.5 mg/kg/day, is suggested as a maximum "maintenance" dose after the initial dose of 2 mg/kg/day.[314]

There are several patterns of response to corticosteroid therapy, some of which may occur at different times in the same patient.[317] Most children who respond to steroids cannot be completely weaned off the medication and become steroid dependent. About one-third of these patients, however, enter steroid-free remission after a prolonged period of treatment.[317] Between 1% and 5% of responders immediately enter a durable steroid-independent remission. However, late relapses, sometimes precipitated by an infectious illness or by hormonal changes such as in pregnancy or with the use of birth control pills, are not uncommon. In other cases, a progressive resistance to steroids occurs, requiring escalating doses of prednisone or alternative therapy. Following a relapse, some patients are responsive to steroids again, whereas others are refractory to subsequent trials. Initial insensitivity to steroids is observed in 36% of cases.[317] In over 60% of patients long-term steroid therapy is hampered by the development of resistance or by side effects of the treatment. In adolescent responders on long-term steroids, an option is to stop prednisone temporarily to allow a normal growth spurt. Infants with DBA on steroids are at risk for pneumocystis pneumonia and should be given prophylactic antibiotics.

High-Dose Methylprednisolone. Megadose steroid therapy for patients refractory to conventional prednisone induced a sustained erythroid response leading to transfusion independence in 8 of 13 DBA patients.[408] Eleven had been treated with 100 mg/kg/day intravenously, and 2 additional patients with 30 mg/kg/day orally. Another report showed only a transient response in 1 of 8 patients after intravenous treatment with 30 mg/kg/day and a sustained response after a higher dosage (100 mg/kg/day) in 3 of 8 patients, but side effects were weight gain, oral moniliasis, increase in hepatic transaminases, transient hyperglycemia, and bacteremia related to central venous access.[409] A conclusive study[410] of nine refractory DBA patients using megadose oral methylprednisolone showed no response in five cases, and a partial or complete response in the other four in the initial 4 to 8 weeks of therapy, but all of these relapsed with a taper and became transfusion-dependent. Thus, none of the cases exhibited a clinically significant or durable response.[410]

Cytokine Therapy

Because of the "corrective" effect on erythropoiesis by IL-3 in vitro, clinical trials were introduced for steroid-refractory and steroid-dependent DBA patients and for those in whom BMT was considered too risky.[411–415] The early enthusiasm generated by sustained remissions in some patients was tempered by the realization that IL-3 is effective in only a very small number of cases of steroid-refractory, transfusion-dependent DBA. Of 49 patients treated with IL-3 in a European multicenter compassionate-need study, only 3 children had a significant response with sustained remissions off therapy.[414] A comparison of individual patient characteristics confirmed that patients who had never achieved significant in vivo erythropoiesis in response to steroids or during a spontaneous remission were highly unlikely to respond to IL-3. Thus, the overall response rate in all published studies averages 10–20%. Currently, there are no IL-3 or other growth factor clinical trials in North America for DBA. Serum Epo levels are elevated in DBA and attempts at treatment with high-dose Epo have been ineffective.

Hematopoietic Stem Cell Transplantation (HSCT)

HSCT is a therapeutic option for DBA but risks must be weighed against benefits on a case-by-case basis. The fundamental issue centers on the defined mortality rate with HSCT when used for a non-lethal medical disorder, at least a disorder that is non-lethal in the short-term. In steroid-responsive patients on low-dose maintenance, and in properly transfused and adequately chelated patients, quality of life is not threatened by life-threatening complications. Thus, the decision for intervention with HSCT in this setting is difficult.

Nevertheless, experience has broadened since the first BMT was performed for DBA in 1976.[416] Preparative regimens, supportive measures, and graft-versus-host disease management have progressively become more refined thereby reducing overall risks of the procedure. For consideration in the decision-making, though, there are still lethal risks[417,418]: interstitial pneumonia, cardiac failure, fatal complications associated with chronic graft-versus-host disease, graft failure, graft rejection and sepsis. Results from the International Bone Marrow Transplant Registry show a 64% 3-year probability of overall survival of 61 transplanted DBA patients.[419] The American DBA Registry[420] and the Aplastic Anemia Committee of the Japanese Society of Pediatric Hematology[373] report an 87.5% and an 85% survival, respectively, but with a caution that alternative donors pose a much higher risk than matched sibling donors.[420] From the DBAR database, the survival rate for patients under the age of 10 years receiving matched related HSCT is greater than 90%.

This success has sparked a big interest in preimplantation genetic diagnosis (PGD) with in vitro fertilization to "create" HLA-matched, non–*RPS19*-mutated sibling donors, and a number of patients worldwide have been successfully transplanted using umbilical cord-derived stem cells from donors produced in this way. The religious, ethical, and economic questions generated by PGD to find a healthy matched donor for DBA and other inherited marrow failure transplantations is ongoing.[116–118,429–432] Related and unrelated umbilical cord blood as a stem cell source has been used for DBA HSCT with favorable results.[314,421–426]

Other Therapeutic Options

Two options deserve consideration. The first, cyclosporin-A (CSA), has been reported to produce remission in some DBA patients in whom standard prednisone therapy had failed.[433–436] In one report, 4 of 8 steroid-refractory patients responded to CSA and remained transfusion-independent for a 12-month follow-up.[436] The second option arose from a report of an adult DBA patient whose anemia remitted during pregnancy and was sustained during breast feeding, suggesting that prolactin effected the improvement. Metoclopramide, an inducer of prolactin release, was subsequently administered and sustained the hemoglobin for several years.[437] A subsequent case report confirmed efficacy of metoclopramide for DBA.[438]

A number of other uncontrolled therapeutic trials have been performed in steroid-refractory patients using various medications and treatments with varying success in a few patients. The medications include: androgens, riboflavin, vitamin B_{12}, folate, iron and other "hematinic" agents, 6-mercaptopurine, cyclophosphamide with anti-lymphocyte globulin, and antithymocyte globulin alone. Administration of the amino acid leucine was effective in a DBA patient (D. D. Pospisilova, public communication). There is a case report claiming efficacy of valproic acid for DBA,[439] and another report of an 8-month transfusion-free remission after rituximab therapy.[440] Plasmapheresis has also been tried. Splenectomy, employed in the past, shows no effect on erythropoiesis but may be helpful in transfused patients with proven hypersplenism.

Future Directions

Registries and DBA patient databases will continue to broaden our understanding of the genetic origins and epidemiology of DBA. Specimen collection and distribution to qualified research laboratories globally will identify the remaining DBA genes. Genetically-based DBA diagnosis and pedigree analysis will underscore the broad dimensions of the DBA phenotype, from clinically silent to life-threatening severe. Genotype-phenotype correlations will facilitate HSCT donor selection, allow counseling for reproductive options, and predict for cancer risk.

Kostmann Syndrome/Congenital Neutropenia

Background

Severe chronic neutropenia (SCN) and recurrent serious infections are features of a heterogeneous group of disorders of myelopoiesis including congenital neutropenia, cyclic neutropenia, and idiopathic neutropenia. Kostmann syndrome (KS) is an inherited subtype of congenital neutropenia with onset in early childhood of profound neutropenia (absolute neutrophil count <200/µL), recurrent life-threatening infections, and a maturation arrest of myeloid precursors at the promyelocyte-myelocyte stage of differentiation. The initial description of KS included several neutropenic patients in a large intermarried Swedish kinship.[441,442] An autosomal recessive mode of inheritance in 24 cases was deduced by inference because of hematologically normal parents with two or more neutropenic children in several families. It is now clear that KS and congenital neutropenia are genetically heterogeneous despite a shared hematologic phenotype. The cloning of the neutrophil elastase 2 gene (*ELA2*) and the identification of heterozygous mutations in patients with the KS phenotype support an autosomal dominant inheritance in many cases.[443] Homozygous germline *HAX1* mutations have been identified in autosomal recessive patients, including some from Kostmann's original pedigree.[444]

Congenital neutropenia and KS are indistinguishable hematologically. "Congenital neutropenia" is a term that usually refers to a single "sporadic" case in a family, and may or may not be inherited in the same mode as KS. Many sporadic cases, though, have heterozygous mutations of *ELA2*.[445] The option to "lump" or "split" the two disorders is debatable, but in this chapter, the terms "KS" and "congenital neutropenia" are used interchangeably. These disorders are rare with an estimated frequency of one to two cases per million with equal distribution for gender.

The Severe Chronic Neutropenia International Registry (SCNIR) was established in 1994 to catalogue the clinical features and to monitor the clinical course, treatment, and disease outcomes in patients with SCN.[446] The Registry is a valuable resource for clinical data because of the large numbers of patients entered into its worldwide database. Patient data are submitted internationally to the coordinating centers at the University of Washington, Seattle, and the Medizinische Hochschule, Hannover. As of 2004, short-term and long-term information dating back to 1987 on a total of 1,163 patients was available for analysis. Of the total, 422 patients were classified as having congenital neutropenia including KS.

Etiology, Genetics, and Pathophysiology

The discovery of heterozygous mutations in the ELA2 gene encoding neutrophil elastase in 22 of 25 sporadic and dominantly-inherited patients with congenital neutropenia was the entry point for understanding the molecular basis of the disorder in many patients.[443] As experience with genetic testing has broadened it appears that 60% to 80% of cases have spontaneously-occurring or inherited point mutations in ELA2 and, less commonly, mutations in other genes.[445] ELA2 encodes neutrophil elastase, a glycoprotein synthesized in the promyelocyte/myelocyte stages and packed in the azurophilic cytoplasmic granules. It is released in response to infection and inflammation. The wild-type neutrophil elastase diffusely localizes throughout the cytoplasm but the mutated protein in cases of congenital neutropenia abnormally concentrates in the nucleus and plasma membrane. Mutant *ELA2* also occurs in all cases of classical cyclic neutropenia, but the mutations cluster in exon 4 or 5 on the gene on chromosome 19p13.3 or at the junction of exon 4 with intron 4. Patients with congenital neutropenia have mutations more widely distributed over exons 2, 3, 4, and 5.[443,447]

In congenital neutropenia, mutant *ELA2* results in impaired survival of myeloid progenitor cells.[447] Neutrophil elastase mutations alone may not be sufficient to cause the congenital neutropenia phenotype. This conclusion is based on 2 siblings with congenital neutropenia who inherited the same heterozygous mutation from their unaffected, hematologically normal father. In contradiction, in vivo confirmation of the pathogenic role of the mutations in neutropenia was demonstrated in a healthy father of a congenital neutropenia patient; he was mosaic for his daughter's mutation, and his myeloid precursors with the mutation were selectively lost during myelopoiesis or failed to mature to neutrophils.[448]

The exact mechanism by which mutant *ELA2* causes neutropenia is under intense study.[449–454] There are several lines of evidence that mutant ELA2 protein triggers accelerated apoptosis of developing neutrophil precursors.[450] Mutant protein leads to cytoplasmic accumulation of non-functional protein, disturbance of cellular trafficing, and activation of unfolded protein response in congenital neutropenia neutrophils.[454] Downregulation of lymphoid enhancer-binding factor 1 (LEF-1), a feature of KS, interferes with myeloid maturation and imposes additional interference on granulopoiesis.[455] In addition, decreased expression of Bcl-2 was observed in Kostmann myeloid progenitor cells along with constitutive mitochondrial release of cytochrome C, and excessive cellular apoptosis.[454] Of note, administration of G-CSF restored Bcl-2 expression and improved survival of myeloid progenitor cells.

In autosomal recessive KS patients caused by mutant *HAX1*, there is a deficiency of the mitochondrial protein HAX1 which normally functions in signal transduction and cytoskeletal control. Normal HAX1 protein is critical for maintaining the inner mitochondrial membrane potential and protecting against apoptosis in myeloid cells.[444]

A constitutively activating mutation in the Wiskott-Aldrich syndrome protein encoded by the *WASP* gene was discovered in 5 males from a three-generation family.[456] The phenotype of the resulting X-linked immunodeficiency syndrome was comprised of severe neutropenia from birth, bacterial infections, monocytopenia, and shifts of lymphocyte subsets. Bone marrow morphology showed a selective maturation arrest at the promyelocyte/myelocyte stage similar to KS. Mutant *WASP* leads to constitutive activation of the WASP protein because of disruption of an autoinhibitory domain in the wild-type protein. This increased WASP protein activity produces marked abnormalities of cytoskeletal structure and dynamics.[457]

Mutations in the protooncogene *GFI1* also cause congenital neutropenia with the Kostmann syndrome phenotype.[458] Wild-type *GFI1* is a transcriptional repressor of *ELA2* and when mutated, repressor activity is disabled and *ELA2* is overly expressed. This leads to premature apoptosis and reduced proliferation of granulopoietic cells.[459]

A constitutive point mutation was discovered in the extracellular domain of the G-CSF receptor in a patient with congenital neutropenia who also had a mutant *ELA2* gene.[460] The receptor mutation affected ligand-receptor complex formation with severe consequences for intracellular signal transduction; the patient was totally unresponsive to G-CSF therapy. As demonstrated in vitro and then clinically, corticosteroids combined with G-CSF produced a corrective action through synergistic activation of STAT5 and the patient responded to G-CSF therapy.[461] Three subsequent reports of patients with cell-surface G-CSF receptor mutations were also refractory to G-CSF therapy and suggest that this may be a common finding in cases unresponsive to treatment.[462–464]

In patients with KS who are treated with G-CSF, transformation to MDS and/or AML (MDS/AML) is associated in most cases with *acquired* G-CSF receptor (CSF3R) point mutations.[465–468] These CSF3R nonsense mutations result in the truncation of the C-terminal cytoplasmic region, a subdomain that is crucial for G-CSF induced maturation.[469,470] The acquired mutation is directly operative in the conversion to MDS/AML. In murine models, the mutation results in impaired ligand internalization, defective receptor downmodulation, and enhanced growth signaling that produces an exaggerated hyperproliferative effect in response to G-CSF.[471,472–474] This also confers resistance to apoptosis and enhances cell survival[475] that favors clonal expansion in vivo.[473] The clinical interplay between G-CSF and the receptor mutation was underscored in the report of a patient with congenital neutropenia on G-CSF who developed the receptor mutation and AML.[476] When G-CSF was stopped, the blast count in blood and in marrow fell to undetectable levels on two occasions without giving chemotherapy although the mutant receptor was persistently detectable during the remissions. These acquired receptor mutations appear at varying time points after G-CSF therapy is started.[468,477]

Regarding the cellular pathology of KS, many cell culture studies performed in the 1970s and 1980s provided clonogenic data that pointed to intrinsically defective granulocytic progenitors.[478] Further reports confirmed this and excluded other possible pathogenetic factors.[477,479–482] To summarize: (1) KS marrow myeloid colony growth is defective,[481,482] (2) Western blot and in vitro bioassays show that KS serum contains normal or increased levels of G-CSF,[479,480] (3) endogenous KS G-CSF has normal biologic activity,[477] (4) G-CSF receptors are expressed in slightly increased numbers on myeloid cells from KS patients,[480] and (5) the binding constant for G-CSF to its receptor in KS is normal.[477]

Clinical Features

History and Physical Examination

Approximately half the patients develop clinically impressive infections within the first month of life and almost all others develop them by 6 months. Skin abscesses are common but deep-seated tissue infections and septicemia also occur. SCNIR data illustrate examples of every conceivable form of bacterial and fungal infection in the pre-cytokine era. Especially troublesome in survivors were recurrent episodes of otitis media and pneumonia, advanced gingival-stomatitis sometimes with tooth loss, and in the extreme, gut bacterial flora overgrowth leading to malabsorption requiring total parenteral nutritional therapy. In contrast to some of the other inherited bone marrow failure syndromes, physical malformations are not a feature. Birth weights are generally unremarkable and physical examination is normal. There are a small number of reports of short stature, microcephaly, mental retardation, and cataracts but the association with KS does not appear to be strong. Data from the SCNIR indicate that some patients with KS develop bone demineralization that may be an intrinsic component of the disorder[445,480]; it has been observed before and during G-CSF therapy. The underlying pathogenesis is unclear but patients can develop bone pain and unusual fractures.

Laboratory Findings

Peripheral Blood and Bone Marrow Findings. Neutropenia is profound and persistent in KS, usually less than 200/μL, but often absolute. A small number of patients appear to have intermittent cycling patterns with regular periodicity that mimic classic cyclic neutropenia.[443] A compensatory two to four-fold increase in monocytes is seen, sometimes accompanied by eosinophilia. At diagnosis, platelet numbers are normal or increased, and hemoglobin values are usually normal. In survivors in the pre-cytokine era, anemia of chronic disease associated with recurrent infections and inflammation were common. Aside from neutropenia, humoral and cellular immunity is completely normal.

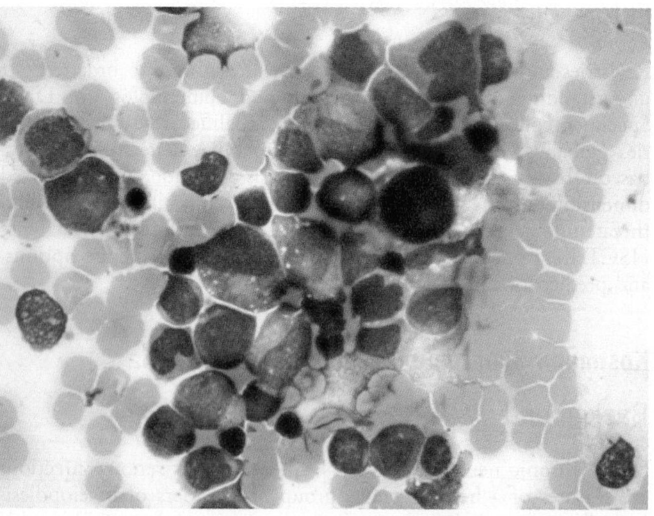

Figure 28–11 High-power view of a bone marrow aspirate from a patient with Kostmann syndrome (congenital neutropenia) prior to a G-CSF therapy. The findings are a "maturation arrest" with recognizable myeloblasts, promyelocytes, myelocytes, occasional metamyelocytes, but total absence of band forms and neutrophils. *(Photomicrograph prepared by Dr. Mohamed Abdelhaleem, Toronto.)*

Bone marrow specimens are usually normocellular. The striking classical finding is a maturation arrest at the promyelocyte or myelocyte stage of granulocytic differentiation with a paucity of more mature elements. Promyelocytes may have atypical nuclei and the cytoplasm may be vacuolated. Neutrophils and bands are usually absent (Fig. 28–11). Marrow eosinophilia and monocytosis is common. The other hematopoietic lineages are normal, active, and undisturbed.

Predisposition to Leukemia and MDS

In 1997, the SCNIR provided its first report on patients with congenital neutropenia on G-CSF therapy who developed MDS/AML.[484] Since then, there has been progressive enrollment of new patients into the SCNIR from North America, Europe, and Australia and there has also been in parallel an annual accrual of new patients with congenital neutropenia and Shwachman-Diamond syndrome on G-CSF that evolved into MDS/AML.[485] From 1987 to year-end 2005, data at the SCNIR confirmed that 65 patients with congenital neutropenia and 5 with Shwachman-Diamond syndrome developed MDS/AML while taking G-CSF.[445] The crude rate of MDS/AML conversion was 11.5% for the 70 patients (70 cases among 611 exposed), with an average follow-up of 5 to 6 years. The leukemic transformation occurred in patients with *ELA2* mutations, in unclassified congenital neutropenia cases, and in Shwachman-Diamond syndrome, but not in patients with *GFI1* mutations, *WASP* mutations, Barth syndrome, or in glycogen storage disease type 1b.

To determine if the incidence of MDS/AML in the SCNIR patients is related to G-CSF dosage or duration of therapy, or to other patient demographics, a detailed analysis was conducted on data received up to December 31, 1998, on 352 patients with congenital neutropenia treated with G-CSF,[485] and then again on data received up to 2000 on 374 patients.[486] In the second more recent analysis, the hazard of MDS/AML increased significantly during the period of observation on G-CSF, from 2.9% per year after 6 years to 8.0% per year after 12 years. The cumulative incidence of MDS/AML was 21% after 10 years. The risk of MDS/AML increased with the dose of G-CSF. Less responsive patients, defined as those requiring greater than 8 μg/kg/d of G-CSF, had a cumulative incidence of MDS/AML of 40% after 10 years, compared to 11% of more responsive patients. The data were interpreted as indicating that a poor response to G-CSF defines an "at-risk" population and predicts an adverse outcome. The data do no necessarily support a cause-and-effect relationship between development of MDS/AML and G-CSF therapy; the results may only mean that patients requiring higher G-CSF therapy have a more severe disease phenotype. A report from the French Severe Chronic Neutropenia Study Group confirmed that increased exposure to G-CSF with respect to dose and duration in congenital neutropenia patients was associated with a heightened risk of MDS/AML[487] but they do not speculate on the mechanism.

Conversion to MDS/AML in congenital neutropenia patients receiving G-CSF is associated with one or more cellular genetic abnormalities that provide insight into the pathobiology of the transformation, and may be useful in identifying patients who are at high risk. The cellular genetic changes are acquired after starting G-CSF and occur singly or in combinations. Remarkably, the abnormalities have predictably similar characteristics in most patients and underscore a fairly specific multistep pathogenesis in the evolution into MDS/AML. As summarized herein, 60% to 80% of patients with congenital neutropenia (but not with SDS) have a heterozygous mutation in the gene encoding neutrophil elastase.[445] At varying time points after starting G-CSF therapy, about half of the congenital neutropenia patients who transform acquire the same activating RAS oncogene mutation, namely a GGT (glycine) to GAT (aspartic acid) substitution at codon 12.[488] More than 90% of patients who transform also show an acquired cytogenetic clonal alteration in bone marrow cells, usually −7 or 7q-, but also +21.[484–489] Occasionally chromosome 7 and 21 abnormalities occur in the same cell. Over 80% of patients develop one or more G-CSF receptor point mutations. The detection of these mutations places patients at high risk for malignant conversion, but the time course from detection of mutations to overt MDS/AML varies considerably and may take years.[445]

The role of G-CSF in myeloid transformation in these patients is obscured because of their predisposition to AML as a component of the natural history. There were three case reports of patients who developed AML prior to the use of hematopoietic growth factors[490–492] and one more recent patient diagnosed with acute leukemia prior to starting G-CSF.[493] Because most patients with congenital neutropenia died at a young age from bacterial sepsis or pneumonia in the pre-cytokine era, the true risk of patients with congenital neutropenia developing MDS/AML was not clearly defined. As a rough estimate, in the literature there were 128 cases of congenital neutropenia reported and the 3 cases of AML[490–492] up to 1989, the first year that G-CSF was available for general use, leading to a crude estimated risk of leukemia of 2%.

Although patients requiring greater than 8 μg/kg/day of G-CSF to attain safe neutrophil levels are an "at risk" group for MDS/AML, there is no definitive evidence that G-CSF directly causes malignant transformation. G-CSF may simply be an "innocent bystander" that corrects the neutropenia, prolongs patient survival, and allows time for the malignant predisposition to declare itself. Alternatively, G-CSF may accelerate the propensity for MDS/AML in the genetically altered stem and progenitor cells in congenital neutropenia. G-CSF may rescue malignant clones that would otherwise be destined for apoptosis. An axiom of oncogenesis is that rapidly dividing cells are more susceptible to mutational events. Since therapeutic G-CSF provides a powerful proliferative signal for marrow cells, it is a reasonable hypothesis that congenital neutropenia marrow progenitors acquire new mutations. From the evidence cited herein, acquisition of a G-CSF receptor mutation in the face of therapeutic G-CSF in congenital neutropenia can provide the hyper-responsive replicative scenario[471,472–474,494] that can relentlessly evolve into MDS/AML. Is recombinant human G-CSF a carcinogen? This would seem highly unlikely. As a physiologic regulator of hematopoiesis, it would be unexpected for G-CSF to break molecular bonds and cause DNA damage, even when used in therapeutic dosages. It is noteworthy that MDS/AML has rarely been seen in other categories of SCN patients on long-term G-CSF therapy.

Differential Diagnosis

The commonest cause of isolated neutropenia in very young children is viral-induced marrow suppression. An antecedent history of good health, the occurrence of a viral illness, and the transient nature of the neutropenia distinguishes this disorder from KS/congenital neutropenia. Autoimmune neutropenia of infancy is recognized as a fairly specific syndrome of early childhood. Low neutrophil numbers are often discovered during the course of routine investigation for a benign febrile illness. The illness abates but the neutropenia persists, sometimes for months and occasionally for years. A marrow biopsy is normocellular and an aspirate shows active granulopoiesis up to the band stage; neutrophils may be normally represented, reduced or absent. The neutropenia is caused by increased peripheral destruction and the diagnosis is confirmed serologically by demonstrating anti-granulocyte antibodies.[495] The prognosis is good, the neutropenia is self-limited albeit protracted, and patients seldom develop serious bacterial infections as a result of it. Other infrequent acquired causes of severe, isolated neutropenia in this age group include marrow suppression from a drug or toxin, and neutrophil sequestration as part of a hypersplenism syndrome.

Of the inherited forms of neutropenia, Shwachman-Diamond syndrome can also manifest as isolated neutropenia but can be identified because of growth failure, the malabsorption component caused by pancreatic insufficiency, fatty changes in the pancreas seen on computed tomography scanning, and characteristic skeletal abnormalities. Glycogen storage disease type 1b and Barth syndrome are also in the differential diagnosis. Neutropenia can also be a prominent part of antibody deficiency syndromes and/or cellular immunodeficiency disorders (Table 28–8); investigation of chronic neutropenia of childhood should include an immunoglobulin electrophoresis, T-cell proliferative studies, and quantitation of T-cell subsets and NK cell activity. Cyclic neutropenia is distinguished by predictable symptomatology, especially mouth sores every 21 days in classic cases, often associated with chronic gingivitis. A complete blood count 2 or 3 times a week for 4 to 8 weeks will demonstrate the diagnostic oscillation pattern with the 21-day nadir. Familial cases of neutropenia with an autosomal dominant mode of inheritance also occur; parents and siblings of all cases should be screened with a complete blood count. When severe neutropenia is diagnosed in the newborn period, the cause may be passive transfer transplacentally of IgG anti-neutrophil antibodies from mother. This can occur if mother has an autoimmune disorder with neutropenia, or by alloimmunization caused by feto-maternal incompatibility for a neutrophil-specific antigen.

Therapy and Prognosis

Before the introduction of G-CSF as a specific therapy of KS and other forms of severe chronic neutropenia, there was limited treatment. Antibiotics were the mainstay of management for active infection and for prophylaxis. Attempts to mobilize neutrophils in KS with lithium had limited application.[496]

Cytokine Therapy

G-CSF has supplanted all other forms of management since more than 90% of KS patients respond. The SCNIR has consistently recommended that it should be initiated as front-line treatment when the diagnosis is established.[480,497] GM-CSF in crossover trials with G-CSF for KS is not as effective and does not induce a neutrophil response consistently. If the ANC remains below 1.0×10^9/L after initiation of G-CSF at 5 μg/kg/dose once a day subcutaneously, the dose should be escalated to 10 μg/kg/dose and then by increments of 10 μg/kg/dose at 14-day intervals until a response is seen. As soon as the ANC can be maintained at 1.0×10^9/L or above, the G-CSF dose does not have to be increased further since the occurrence of bacterial infection is reduced dramatically with an ANC at this level. The G-CSF dose can be reduced if the ANC increases to 5.0×10^9/L or above in order find the lowest dose necessary for maintaining a neutrophil count at 1.0×10^9/L or greater. Nonresponders are defined as patients who do not respond to G-CSF levels exceeding 120 μg/kg/dose. Partial responders show an increase of their ANC to 0.5 to 1.0×10^9/L, with the highest dose, but they still suffer bacterial infections. In these patients the dose of G-CSF cannot be increased because of the large volume and frequency of injections required. In some of these patients a combination of G-CSF with stem cell factor (SCF) can induce a further increase in the ANC, but the potential allergic side effects of SCF have limited the use of this treatment combination to hospitalized patients with severe infections who also receive concomitant antihistaminic medication.[498] The only currently available treatment for patients who do not respond to G-CSF treatment alone or in combination with SCF is HSCT.

All patients on G-CSF therapy should be seen by a physician every 3 to 6 months. Patients requiring more than 8 μg/kg/day are at higher risk for MDS/AML and should be reviewed more often. Blood counts (white blood cells, hemoglobin, platelets, and differential blood counts) should be obtained and a physical examination performed at least every three months, including assessment for weight and height in pediatric patients, and documentation of intercurrent infections. Bone marrow examination for morphology and cytogenetics is recommended once a year to search for acquired cytogenetic abnormalities such as monosomy 7 or trisomy 21.

In the SCNIR report in 2003, a sustained hematological response in patients treated with G-CSF for more than 12 years was confirmed.[480] With therapy, neutrophil counts rise in more than 90% of SCN patients and are maintained at a plateau for protracted periods resulting in vast clinical benefits. In no instance has there been marrow or hematopoietic lineage "exhaustion" or depletion with G-CSF therapy. The overall safety of long-term administration of G-CSF is reviewed in detail.[477,480,484,497]

Hematopoietic Stem Cell Transplantation (HSCT)

Prior to the use of G-CSF, HSCT was tried in a small number of KS patients with mixed success. Data from the International Bone Marrow Transplantation Registry are limited and series is heterogeneous with regard to donor source and clinical status of patients at the time of the procedure.

A report from the SCNIR summarizes its experience with HSCT for KS.[499] Of 29 who were transplanted, 18 had transformed to MDS and/or AML and the dual goal was to cure the malignancy and the neutropenia. Only 3 of the 18 were successful. The causes for failure included mismatched transplants, progressive refractory AML, serious illness at the time of the procedure, and transplants performed in desperation. The other 11 patients underwent HSCT for reasons other than malignant transformation, mostly because of no response or only partial response to G-CSF. Eight patients received stem cells from an HLA-matched sibling after conditioning mainly with busulfan/cyclophosphamide alone or with additional immunosuppression. In sharp contrast to the MDS/AML group, 9 of the 11 were cured with resolution of neutropenia.

Since the SCNIR report in 2000, there have been several additional publications describing experiences with single or multiinstitutional HSCT for a variety of indications using matched-related or MUD marrow or cord blood with variable outcomes.[476,500–505] In general, the best scenario for a curative HSCT is when the procedure is performed prior to developing MDS/AML, using a matched-related donor, and when the patient is in good physical condition. In a small series of 6 transplanted patients for MDS or AML, 2 with MDS who underwent the procedure without being given induction chemotherapy survived, whereas 4 with AML given induction chemotherapy had significantly more morbidity and died post-transplant, raising questions about conditioning strategies for these patients.[504]

The discovery of an isolated marrow clonal cytogenetic abnormality without other evidence of MDS or AML in patients with congenital neutropenia raises management issues. One option is to perform HSCT if there is a matched donor as soon as feasible. This has generally been recommended for patients with −7, 7q-, or +21. The a priori argument is that the chance for cure is higher when the patient is well and with a low burden of malignancy. The problem with this decision centers on not knowing the tempo of progression from the cytogenetic change to clearcut MDS or AML. Thus, there may not be a need to rush to transplant in all patients. Instead, one recommendation is to lower the G-CSF to the lowest dose that maintains neutrophil counts greater than 0.5×10^9/L and to monitor the patient regularly for change with blood counts and by serial marrow testing.

Opinions vary about the best way to manage patients with non-cytogenetic evidence of clonal disease but without overt hematologic malignancy. This would include acquisition of a G-CSF receptor mutation or an activating RAS oncogene mutation in marrow from a patient with congenital neutropenia taking G-CSF who shows no other signs of MDS or AML. In one patient with an isolated G-CSF receptor mutation, a hematopoietic stem cell transplant was performed to eliminate the risk of leukemic conversion.[499] Debate about this form of management remains open, and watchful waiting is an acceptable option.

Bisphosphonates for Osteoporosis

Bone density measurements of congenital neutropenia patients on G-CSF show varying degrees of osteopenia or osteoporosis in about 50% of cases. Most of these are subclinical and asymptomatic, but some patients complain of bone pain and have fractures. In a small series of 5 congenital neutropenia cases treated with bisphosphonates, 4 remodeled and re-expanded fractured vertebrae during treatment and no side effects were seen on follow-up.[506] Bisphosphonates appear to be effective treatment for these patients.

Future Directions

Mutational analysis of congenital neutropenia patients will continue to be informative. Thus far, genotype-phenotype relationships have not been possible and will require further accrual of data. It is also not yet clear if there is an association between specific mutations and the risk of evolution to MDS and acute leukemia, but studies are ongoing to try to answer this clinical question. At present, diagnosis of cyclic and congenital neutropenia still depends primarily upon observations of serial blood cell counts, but it is expected that mutational analysis of the *ELA-2* gene will become a routine part of diagnosis and prognosis for these patients in the years ahead. Since apoptosis is a central mechanism of neutropenia in these patients, it is expected that the term "maturation arrest" will soon be replaced by "accelerated apoptosis" as a descriptive term for the marrow findings. It appears that cellular models involving transfection of the mutant genes into human myeloid cell lines provide evidence of how neutropenia occurs. Potentially, these models can also be used to examine new approaches to preventing apoptosis and serve to provide clues to new and more effective therapies. Considerable data now suggest that the effectiveness of G-CSF in the treatment of various forms of severe chronic neutropenia is related to anti-apoptotic effects in addition to its effects on stimulating and expanding myeloid cell production.

Other Inherited Neutropenia Syndromes

Barth Syndrome

Barth syndrome is a rare multisystem metabolic disorder inherited in an X-linked recessive mode.[507] It is the first human disease in which the primary causative factor is an alteration in cardiolipin remodeling. Cardiolipin is a component of the inner mitochondrial membrane necessary for proper functioning of the electron transport chain. The findings in typical cases are cardiomyopathy of the dilated type, skeletal myopathy, growth failure, 3-methylglutaconic aciduria, and neutropenia. The neutropenia has been termed "classic cyclic neutropenia" but documentation is lacking. Absolute neutrophil counts are variable, but total agranulocytosis has been recorded.[508] Marrow morphology shows a maturation arrest at the myelocyte stage.[507] By

Table 28–8 Miscellaneous Inherited Neutropenia Disorders*

Diagnosis	Genetics†	Mapping	Mutant Gene	Additional Features
WHIM syndrome	AD	2q21	*CXCR4*	Warts, ↓IgG, myelokathexis
Hyper IgM syndrome, type 1	X-L	Xq26	*CD40L*	↓IgG, IgA, IgE, autoimmune cytopenias
Hermansky-Pudlak syndrome, type 2	AR	5q14.1	*AP3B1*	↓IgG, partial albinism, platelet dysfunction
Griscelli syndrome, type 2	AR	15q21	*RAB27A*	Hemophagocytosis, partial albinism
Chediak-Higashi syndrome	AR	1q42.1-q42.2	*LYST(CHS1)*	Immunodeficiency, neurologic dysfunction, partial albinism

*Data compiled from Online Mendelian Inheritance in Man (OMIM; ncbi.nlm.nih.gov/omim) 193670, 308230, 608233, 607624, and 214500 and reference 520.
†Genetics: AD, autosomal dominant; AR, autosomal recessive; X-L, X-linked recessive.

electron microscopy, mitochondria show concentric, tightly packed cristae and occasional inclusion bodies; these are seen in various tissues including granulocyte precursors. Female carriers are healthy and hematologically normal, likely because of extreme skewing of X-inactivation.[509] The initial impression that Barth syndrome is a lethal infantile disease has to be modified. Age distribution in 54 living patients ranges from 0 to 49 years and peaks around puberty.[510]

The Barth syndrome gene was mapped to Xq28 which led to the cloning of the *G4.5* (*TAZ*) gene[511] and the various mutations that account for the phenotype. The *TAZ* gene produces several different mRNAs which predict resultant proteins called *tafazzins*. The role of the tafazzins is under study. Mutations in *TAZ* result in a decrease in tetralinoleoyl species of cardiolipin and an accumulation of monolysocardiolipin within cells.[512] This is a sensitive and specific marker for Barth syndrome.[513] Clinically, the cardiomyopathy dominates the clinical picture, but gingivitis, oral problems, and bacterial sepsis can be problematic. The mechanism of neutropenia has not been characterized. There are anecdotal reports that G-CSF is highly effective in correcting the neutropenia.

Glycogen Storage Disease Type 1b

Glycogen storage disease (GSD) type 1b is an autosomal recessive disorder that results from a deficiency of the glucose-6-phosphate translocase enzyme caused by mutations in the *G6PT1* gene. This enzyme transports glucose-6-phosphate into the lumen of the endoplasmic reticulum where it is hydrolyzed into glucose and inorganic phosphate.[514] Absence of the translocase, therefore, results in an inability to liberate glucose from glucose-6-phosphate. Consequently, patients with GSD type 1b are susceptible to fasting hypoglycemia and lactic acidosis, and have hepatomegaly, poor linear growth, delayed pubertal development, and other systemic complications.[515]

Depending on the type of mutations of *G6PT1*, patients with GSD 1b may or may not be neutropenic. Neutrophil dysfunction with defective chemotaxis and an impaired respiratory burst is an additional feature. Patients are consequently susceptible to recurrent infections and to inflammatory bowel disease. Infections most commonly involve the skin, perirectal area, ears, and urinary tract; however, severe or life-threatening infections, such as sepsis, pneumonia, and meningitis, may also occur. The most frequently isolated organisms include *Staphylococcus aureus*, group A streptococci, *Streptococcus pneumoniae, Escherichia coli,* and *Pseudomonas* species.

Neutropenia is often[516] but not always[514] associated with a hypocellular marrow and a maturation arrest at the myelocyte stage. Neutrophil apoptosis appears to be a central mechanism of the granulop oietic failure.[517] G-CSF therapy is extremely effective in almost all GSD 1b patients.[514,518] Marrow cellularity increases, the ANCs increase exuberantly, and impaired oxygen radical formation is corrected. The SCNIR has long-term prospective data on 29 GSD 1b patients receiving G-CSF therapy.[514] Forty percent had splenomegaly prior to starting G-CSF, with 81% developing splenomegaly by the first year of treatment and 100% by 3 years. Hypersplenism occurred in 5 patients, two of whom required splenectomy; in the other 3, hypersplenism resolved by reducing the G-CSF dose. Histology of the removed spleens showed extramedullary hematopoiesis. None of the SCNIR patients developed leukemia, but AML was reported in one non-registry case of GSD 1b while on G-CSF therapy.[519]

Kostmann Syndrome/Congenital Neutropenia: G-CSF versus HSCT as First-line Therapy

Therapeutic options for newly-diagnosed patients with KS must be constantly reevaluated. Since the inception of the Severe Chronic Neutropenia International Registry (SCNIR) in 1994, the recommendation for treating new KS patients with G-CSF has not wavered.[446,480] This opinion was underscored in a recent review[445] because more than 90% of KS patients show a robust neutrophilic response to G-CSF treatment. HSCT has been regarded as "salvage" therapy for patients who acquire G-CSF receptor mutations, clonal cytogenetic abnormalities, RAS mutations, or overt MDS/AML, or who fail to respond to G-CSF altogether.

This opinion requires ongoing review in light of the startling annual accrual of KS patients on G-CSF who transform to MDS/AML, usually with a fatal outcome regardless of treatment. The hazard of MDS/AML has increased over time from 2.9% per year after 6 years of therapy to 8% per year after 12 years on G-CSF.[486] After 10 years of therapy the cumulative incidence is 21% for MDS/AML. Remarkably, for those patients requiring 8 micrograms/kg/day of G-CSF or greater the cumulative incidence for MDS/AML after 10 years is 40%. Clearly, this is a strategic issue.

Discussions with stem cell transplant physicians have centered on the following. For KS patients transplanted with a fully matched donor *prior* to transforming to MDS/AML and in stable health, the chance for cure is at least 85%, possibly higher. The SCNIR data support this estimate.[499] Not only is the neutropenia fully corrected by HSCT, but the risk of MDS/AML is also eliminated. The onerous burden of daily subcutaneous injections is removed, the financial expense is relieved, and the side effects of G-CSF are prevented. Clearly, an 85% cure rate stacks up favorably against the 21% to 40% cumulative incidence of incurable MDS/AML in those on G-CSF over time. HSCT is a reasonable option as front-line therapy for these patients instead of G-CSF, and the option should be discussed fairly and sensibly with newly diagnosed patients and families.

Other Inherited Neutropenias

There are other inherited neutropenia disorders associated with specific mutant genes but they do not necessarily have the Kostmann marrow phenotype, nor is their pathophysiology necessarily similar (Table 28–8). Immune deficiency appears to be an important component of these syndromes. Unlike congenital neutropenia, these miscellaneous forms tend to have distinguishing physical abnormalities such as partial albinism, and are not predisposed to MDS/AML.

Thrombocytopenia With Absent Radii (TAR)

Background

TAR syndrome was first described in 1929,[521] defined by Hall et al. in 1969,[522] and subsequently reviewed.[219,523,524] The two essential features of TAR syndrome are hypomegakaryocytic thrombocytopenia and bilateral radial aplasia with thumbs present. It is one of a group of inherited hematologic disorders that include Fanconi anemia and Diamond-Blackfan anemia with radial ray anomalies. The manifestation of the phenotype vary widely and patients can manifest with abnormalities involving skeletal, skin, gastrointestinal, brain, renal and cardiac systems. Most of the genetic evidence supports an autosomal recessive mode of inheritance for TAR syndrome because many families have been observed with more than one affected sibling. Each child in 2 sets of identical twins had TAR[525,526] whereas one of a pair of fraternal twins had the syndrome.[527] The possibility of autosomal dominant inheritance with variable penetrance for TAR syndrome has also been raised.[523,524,528] Almost always, parents of TAR patients are phenotypically normal. Females with TAR syndrome can conceive and give birth to hematologically and phenotypically normal offspring.

Three cases of acute myeloid leukemia[529–231] and one case of acute lymphoid (*lymphoidic*) leukemia[532] in TAR syndrome patients have been reported. Using a denominator of about 250 published cases of TAR,[7] four leukemic episodes (1%–2% crude rate) suggests a predisposition to hematologic cancer.

Etiology and Pathophysiology

Thrombocytopenia in TAR syndrome is the result of a defect in megakaryocytopoiesis and thrombocytopoiesis.[533] The gene responsible for the disorder has not been identified. However, an interstitial deletion of 200 kb on chromosome 1q21.1 in 30 TAR patients and 25% unaffected parents has been identified.[534] Whereas targeted disruptions of several *Hox* genes result in abnormal development of the mouse radius, the normal genomic sequences for human *HoxA10*, *HoxA11* and *HoxD11* were determined and sequenced in 10 TAR syndrome patients and the results were identical to normal controls.[535] In contrast to congenital amegakaryocytic thrombocytopenia, mutational screening of coding and promoter regions of the *MPL* gene by sequence analysis was normal in 10 TAR syndrome patients.[536,537]

Thrombopoietin levels in plasma or serum are consistently elevated in TAR syndrome thereby excluding a cytokine production defect as a cause for thrombocytopenia in this disorder.[537–539] Marrow CFU-Meg (CFU-Mk) progenitors are either absent,[533] or are present in low to normal frequencies[537,539] but are composed of small colonies in vitro[539] with abnormal morphology.[534] CFU-GM and BFU-E colony growth is often increased.

In a detailed study of $CD34^+$ cells, the thrombocytopenia of TAR syndrome was associated with a dysmegakaryocytopoiesis characterized by cells blocked at an early stage of differentiation.[537] Cells expressing CD41 without CD42 accumulated behind the block, and there was a decrease in c-mpl transcripts and mpl protein. The response of platelets to adenosine diphosphate or to the thrombin receptor agonist peptide, SFLLRN (TRAP), is normal in TAR patients.[538] However, in contrast to controls there is no in vitro reactivity of platelets from TAR patients to recombinant thrombopoietin as measured by testing thrombopoietin-synergism to ADP and TRAP in platelet activation.[538] Thrombopoietin-induced tyrosine phosphorylation of platelet proteins in this setting is completely absent or markedly decreased. The results indicate that there is a lack of response to thrombopoietin in the signal transduction pathway of c-mpl.

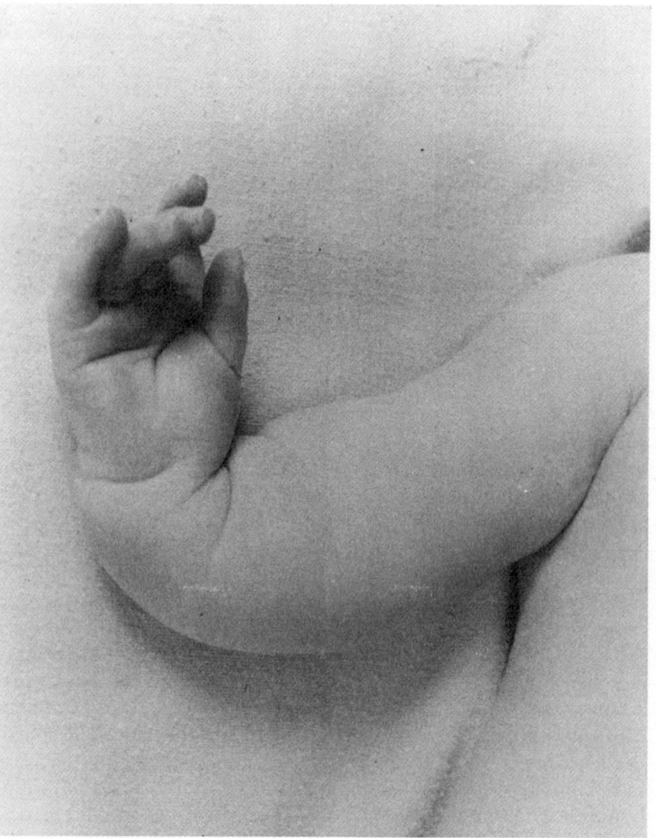

Figure 28–12 Radial aplasia with preservation of the thumb in a newborn with TAR syndrome.

No recurrent chromosomal changes are seen in TAR syndrome. Some karyotypic abnormalities found in a few patients are of unclear significance.[524] Despite one report of non-hematologic cancer in a presumed TAR patient whose lymphocytes demonstrated radiation hypersensitivity,[540] abnormal chromosomal breakage is not seen in TAR syndrome.[524]

Clinical Features

History and Physical Examination

The diagnosis is made in the newborn period because of the absent radii, and in about half of patients because of a petechial rash and overt hemorrhage such as bloody diarrhea. Patients have bilateral radial aplasia (Fig. 28–12) with preservation of thumbs and fingers on both sides. Additional upper extremity deformities include radial clubhands, hypoplastic carpals and phalanges, and hypoplastic ulnae, humeri, and shoulder girdles. Syndactyly and clinodactyly of toes and fingers are also seen. Characteristic findings include a selective hypoplasia of the middle phalanx of the fifth finger and altered palmar contours. Upper extremity involvement ranges from isolated absent radii to true, often asymmetric, phocomelia. The lower extremities are involved in about half of cases.[524] Malformations include hip dislocation, coxa valga, femoral torsion, tibial torsion, abnormal tibiofibular joints, small feet, and valgus and varus foot deformities. Abnormal toe placement is commonly seen, especially the fifth toe overlapping the fourth. Like upper limb involvement, lower extremity deformities range from minimal involvement to complete phocomelia. An asymmetric first rib, a cervical rib, cervical spina bifida, and a fused cervical spine can occur, but trunk involvement is usually minimal. Micrognathia has been associated with the TAR syndrome in up to 65% of cases.

Cardiac abnormalities occur in 15% of the patients.[219] The commonest are atrial septal defect, tetralogy of Fallot, and ventricular septal defect. Capillary hemangiomas are common (24%) as well as redundant nuchal folds. Genitourinary tract malformations are detected in 23% of cases. About 95% of patients have short stature, 76% have macrocephaly, and 53% show facial dysmorphism. Two recent reports highlight structural brain abnormalities.[541,542] Additional findings are dorsal pedal edema, hyperhydrosis, and gastrointestinal disturbances such as diarrhea and feeding intolerance; almost one-half of patients are intolerant of cow's milk.[524]

Prenatal diagnosis can be made by ultrasound imaging of absent radii with thumbs present[543] and by quantitating platelet numbers obtained by fetoscopy or cordocentesis. In one case after the diagnosis was made, a prenatal in utero platelet transfusion was given to effect a safe delivery.[544]

Laboratory Findings

Thrombocytopenia as a result of bone marrow underproduction is a consistent finding. Marrow specimens show normal to increased cellularity with decreased to absent megakaryocytes. The erythroid and myeloid lineages are normally represented. When a few megakaryocytes can be identified in biopsies, they are small, contain few nuclear segments, and show immature nongranular cytoplasm. If platelet counts increase spontaneously in patients after the first year of life, megakaryocytes increase in parallel and appear more mature morphologically. At diagnosis, leukocytosis is seen in the majority of patients and is sometimes extreme to over 100,000/μL with a "left shift" to immature myeloid forms. The cause of this leukemoid reaction is unclear but it is usually transient and subsides spontaneously. If anemia is present, the likeliest etiology is from blood loss caused by thrombocytopenia. When platelet numbers are adequate for study, their size is generally normal and routine testing of function is unremarkable,[545] although some patients may show abnormal platelet aggregation and storage pool defects.[546–548] Unlike some of the other inherited marrow failure syndromes, red cell size and fetal hemoglobin levels are normal.

Differential Diagnosis

There are important clinical differences that distinguish TAR syndrome from Fanconi anemia. In Fanconi patients, when radii are absent, the thumbs are hypoplastic or absent. Fanconi patients do not have skin hemangiomas like some TAR patients, whereas TAR patients do not show abnormal skin pigmentation like 55% of Fanconi patients. Confirmation of Fanconi anemia is made by the clastogenic chromosome stress test showing increased fragility and by mutational analysis. TAR patients do not have increased chromosomal breakage.

Some infants with trisomy 18 have absence or hypoplasia of radii and thrombocytopenia. Similar to Fanconi anemia, however, thumbs are absent in trisomy 18 if radii are absent, and the disorder can also be distinguished from TAR syndrome cytogenetically. As summarized,[219] there are several syndromes with radial abnormalities but with *normal* platelet counts that can be diagnosed by mutational gene analysis. These include Roberts syndrome (mutant *ESCO1*), Holt-Oram syndrome (mutant *TBX5*), and the clinical spectrum of three disorders caused by mutant *RECQL4* (Rothmund-Thomson syndrome, Baller-Gerold syndrome, and the RAPADILINO syndrome).

Therapy and Prognosis

The risk of hemorrhage is greatest in the first year of life. Deaths are usually caused by intracranial or gastrointestinal bleeding. If patients survive the first year, platelet counts spontaneously increase inexplicably to levels that are hemostatically safe and which do not require platelet transfusional support. A minority of patients have sustained, profound thrombocytopenia that does not improve spontaneously. A summary of published cases of TAR syndrome[7] shows an actuarial survival curve plateau of 75% by age 4 years. Many of these publications antedated the modern use of platelet transfusions so the survival is likely much better currently. TAR patients do not evolve into marrow failure with pancytopenia but may develop acute leukemia in 1% to 2% of cases.

Platelet Transfusions

As in other inherited marrow failure disorders associated with thrombocytopenia, platelet transfusions should be used judiciously. Clinical bleeding or prophylaxis for orthopedic surgical procedures is an appropriate indication. Persistent platelet counts below 10,000/μL may require preventative platelet transfusions on a regular basis, especially in the first year of life when the expectation is that a spontaneous improvement in platelet number will ensue with time in most infants. Single donor platelets are preferred to multiple random donor platelets to minimize the risk of alloimmunization. HLA-partially-matched or fully-matched donors for platelets may be required if patients become refractory to transfusions.

Other Therapies

Supportive management is the mainstay but in exceptional situations profound, persistent life-threatening thrombocytopenia can be successfully treated by HSCT.[549] The role of thrombopoietin therapy in the management of TAR patients is unclear. Elevated serum thrombopoietin levels at baseline[538] may predict for a poor response to the cytokine therapy. IL-11, another thrombopoietic cytokine, has not been studied in clinical trials; however, endogenous IL-11 serum levels in TAR patients are also elevated.[538] One child had a moderate, increase in platelet numbers while receiving IL-6,[550] but its use causes fevers and chills and its clinical development has been halted. Androgens, corticosteroids, and splenectomy are ineffective therapies for TAR syndrome.

Congenital Dyserythropoietic Anemias

Background

The designation *congenital dyserythropoietic anemia* (CDA) refers to a family of inherited refractory anemias characterized by marrow erythroid multinuclearity, ineffective erythropoiesis, and secondary hemosiderosis. The ineffective erythropoiesis is reflected by marrow erythroid hyperplasia, inappropriately low reticulocyte counts for the level of hemoglobin, and intramedullary red cell destruction. Splenomegaly and chronic or intermittent jaundice are additional features. Granulopoiesis and thrombopoiesis are normal. Although these disorders are not bone marrow failure syndromes per se, they are genetically transmitted and result in anemia with a blunted erythropoietic response.

Three forms of CDA have been described as well as a number of variants.[551] An arbitrary classification used in practice is based on the inheritance pattern, the peripheral blood and bone marrow morphology, and the serologic findings in each case. The distinguishing features of the three classical types of CDA are as follows:

Type I: Autosomal recessive; macrocytosis; megaloblastic erythroid precursor cells; 2% to 5% binucleated erythroid precursor cells; internuclear chromatin bridges; negative Ham test.

Type II: Autosomal recessive; normocytosis; normoblastic erythroid maturation; 10% to 35% binucleated late normoblasts; positive Ham test.

Type III: Autosomal dominant; macrocytosis; megaloblastic erythroid maturation; giant multinucleated erythroid precursors with up to 12 nuclei per cell; negative Ham test.

The designation "type IV" has been used for decades to classify cases of morphologic type II CDA with a negative Ham acidified

Inherited Marrow Failure and Malignant Hematopoietic Transformation

Historically, the inherited marrow failure syndromes were classified as "benign" hematology in order to contrast sharply with hematologic cancer. Patients with Kostmann syndrome/congenital neutropenia, Shwachman-Diamond syndrome, Fanconi anemia, dyskeratosis congenita, congenital amegakaryocytic thrombocytopenia, Diamond-Blackfan anemia, or TAR syndrome often died early in life from complications of cytopenias. However, in the current era of advanced supportive care and availability of recombinant cytokines and other effective therapeutics, patients with these conditions usually survive the early years of life and beyond. With the extended life span of patients, a new natural history for some of these disorders is evident. One of the most sobering observations is that the seven disorders cited above confer an inordinately high predisposition to MDS and AML. Thus, the distinction between "benign" and "malignant" hematology in the context of the inherited marrow failure disorders has become blurred, and a new clinical and hematologic continuum is evident.

Carcinogenesis occurs as a multistep sequence of events that is driven by genetic damage and by epigenetic operative factors. In the traditional view, the initiation of cancer starts in a normal cell through mutations from exposure to carcinogens. In the proliferative phase that follows, the genetically altered, initiated cell undergoes selective clonal expansion that enhances the probability of additional genetic damage from endogenous mutations or DNA-damaging agents. Activation of protooncogenes, inactivation of tumor-suppressor genes, or inactivation of genomic stability genes may be central in this process. Finally, during malignant conversion and cancer progression, malignant cells show phenotypic changes, gene amplification, chromosomal alterations, and altered gene expression.

With respect to the seven inherited marrow failure syndromes that are predisposed to develop hematologic cancers, there is reason to believe that leukemogenesis is also a multistep process. The first genetic "hit" or leukemia-initiating step may be the syndrome-specific inherited genetic abnormality itself, which initially manifests as the single- or multiple-lineage marrow failure state. The "predisposed" progenitor, already initiated, could conceptually develop decreased responsiveness to the signals that regulate homeostatic growth, terminal cell differentiation, or programmed cell death. Leukemic promotion and progression with clonal expansion leading to MDS or AML could then ensue readily. Since many of the mutant genes that produce the inherited marrow failure syndromes have been discovered, the nature of the leukemogenic-initiating events in these conditions should become evident.

Three of the syndromes illustrate the point. The best example is the multistep evolution of leukemic transformation over time in patients with congenital neutropenia while taking G-CSF. The acquisition of activating RAS oncogene mutations, cytogenetic abnormalities involving primarily −7, 7q- and +21, and G-CSF receptor mutations in the majority of patients who transform is remarkable.

Other than clonal cytogenetic changes, we know little about the timeline or sequence of events that characterize the malignant phenotype of Shwachman-Diamond syndrome. It is striking, though, that the syndrome from early age already shares many of the findings of de novo adult MDS including abnormal hematopoietic colony growth, abnormally short leukocyte telomeres, elevated apoptotic index mediated by FAS/FAS ligand, an abnormal immune system, an aberrant marrow microenvironment that shows impaired support of normal hematopoiesis, and marrow neoangiogenesis. Many if not all of these findings may evolve in utero.

Finally, Fanconi anemia has a "short cut" mechanism to leukemic conversion. Biallelic mutant genes from conception result in genomic instability, compromised DNA repair and chromosome breakage. The opportunities for hematologic cancer in this setting are infinite. Actuarial data from the IFAR[93] showed that the risk of acquiring clonal cytogenetic abnormalities was 67% by 30 years of age in patients with bone marrow failure. The actuarial risk of MDS or AML was 52% by 40 years of age. This steady tempo of leukemic evolution implies a stepwise acquisition over time of additional, critical genetic "hits" prior to overt MDS/AML.

serum test.[552,553] There are also several other forms of CDA that are distinct from CDA types I, II, III, and IV. These other forms have been identified in 3 or more families and have been tentatively classified into CDA groups (not types) IV, V, VI, and VII.[554,551] The growing number of variants[555–562] underscore the complex nature of CDA and the need to reclassify these disorders accurately when the molecular basis for the various types and groups becomes clear.

Etiology, Genetics, and Pathophysiology

The gene for CDA I was mapped to chromosome 15q15 using homozygosity linkage mapping in a cluster of highly inbred Israeli Bedouins.[563] The gene responsible, *CDAN1*, was then identified.[564] The gene product, codanin-1, may be involved in nuclear envelope integrity, conceivably related to microtubule attachments. The gene for CDA II (*CDAN2*) has not been identified but it maps to 20q11.2.[565] Nor has the gene for CDA III (*CDAN3*) been discovered, but there is close linkage of the locus at 15q21.[566]

The defect that accounts for each type of CDA is found in all of the erythroid progenitors rather than in a subpopulation of cells.[567,568] Some pertinent biochemical abnormalities are related to the etiology of CDA I,[569–573] but little more is known about pathogenesis. In comparison, the pathogenesis of CDA II has been almost completely clarified. At the stem cell level, in vitro culture of CDA II erythroid progenitors produces CFU-E and BFU-E colonies with erythroblast multinuclearity.[567] Initially, studies of peripheral blood CDA II red cells identified a number of chemical abnormalities including unbalanced globin chain synthesis,[571] increased membrane glycolipids,[574] and altered red cell membrane protein patterns demonstrated by two-dimensional electrophoresis.[573] Furthermore, glycoproteins on CDA II red cells were found to have an abnormal carbohydrate structure leading to aberrant reactivity with anti-i sera.[575] Additional data suggested that the IgM antibody responsible for hemolysis in the acidified-serum lysis test (Ham test) recognizes an abnormal glycolipid structure sharing homology with the i and I antigens.[576] Thus, a variety of data predicted that abnormalities in the glycosylation pathway were involved in the etiology of CDA II.

Indeed, there are two distinct defects in the glycosylation enzymatic pathway that occur in CDA II:[577,578] α-mannosidase II deficiency and *N*-acetylglucosaminyl transferase II deficiency, although the genes encoding these proteins were excluded as the CDA II mutation.[579] As a result of the former abnormality, addition of new sugar moieties to the oligosaccharide core structure is impaired. A defect, probably in the promoter region of the gene encoding for α-mannosidase II, has been identified. There is also a report that multinucleated erythroblasts are formed in vitro when normal bone marrow is cultured with an inhibitor of α-mannosidase II.[577] Also, low levels of *N*-acetylglucosaminyl transferase II, the enzyme responsible for addition of an *N*-acetylglucosamine residue to one of the arms of the core, result in glycoproteins with truncated oligosaccharides.

A third enzymatic defect has been described in a variant case of CDA II.[580] Low levels of the membrane-bound form of galactosyl transferase, involved at various stages of oligosaccharide synthesis, severely affect processing and lead to the presence of primitive high-mannose core structures on glycoproteins.[580]

All three of these enzymatic deficiencies lead to abnormal oligosaccharides on major erythrocyte proteins such as the anion transporter, Band 3.[581,582] In addition to its other functions, this glycoprotein plays a critical role in the organization of the membrane skeleton that determines normal red cell strength, flexibility, and shape. Abnormal glycosylation of Band 3 may cause it to cluster on the cell surface.[583] Such clustering could cause disruption of the structural network of the erythrocyte and its precursors, thereby leading to their premature demise.

Defective glycosylation on the red blood cell surface may also affect the regulation of complement on the surface of erythrocytes. Enhanced functional activity of the alternative pathway C3 convertase and of the membrane attack complex may result from the improper glycosylation of glycophorin A, which has been proposed to serve as a complement regulatory protein.[584]

CDA III is the rarest of the three classical forms of CDA and little is known about its pathophysiology. However, in some dominantly inherited and sporadic cases of CDA III, electron microscopy reveals that an occasional erythroblast section contains stellate or branching electron-dense intracytoplasmic inclusions.[585–587] These are morphologically indistinguishable from those in HbH disease and consists of precipitated β-globin chains. In one sporadic case with such inclusions, the α:β globin chain synthesis ratio was 0.76 and DNA studies demonstrated the presence of four α genes and excluded two of the common mutations of nondeletion α thalassemia.[585]

Clinical Features

History, Physical Examination, and Laboratory Findings for Each CDA Type

Some features are shared by all forms of CDA and some features are specific for each type. In general, for all types there is a wide variation in age of onset of clinical problems related to CDA. Most patients are diagnosed in late childhood or adolescence; however, a few CDA cases have been reported in newborn infants presenting with hydrops fetalis.[588–590] Clinical manifestations may include intermittent jaundice and dark urine caused by increased hemoglobin catabolism, or signs and symptoms of anemia. Rarely, hyperbilirubinemia without anemia may be the initial presentation of CDA patients. The degree of splenomegaly and hepatomegaly is quite variable. Cholelithiasis may be present as a consequence of chronic hyperbilirubinemia. In some older patients, evidence of hemosiderosis (skin hyperpigmentation, diabetes mellitus, hypogonadism, or delay of secondary sexual characteristics) is often present. It is noteworthy that hemosiderosis occurs in both transfused and nontransfused CDA patients. In the latter, iron overload is a direct consequence of high plasma iron turnover and low iron utilization by normoblasts caused by ineffective erythropoiesis. Gastrointestinal absorption of iron is also increased. Large series of patients with CDA I and CDA II, respectively, illustrate the spectrum of clinical manifestations of these disorders.[591–594]

CDA Type I. CDA I is inherited in an autosomal recessive manner. The disorder is caused by biallelic mutant *CDAN1*. In several reported families, more than one sibling was affected, and the disorder has been seen in fraternal and identical twins. The onset of anemia, jaundice, or other symptoms may be noted at any age especially in neonates. Eighty percent of infants in a recent large series required blood transfusions during the first month of life.[595] One case was reported with fetal anemia requiring intrauterine exchange transfusions at 28 and 30 weeks' gestation.[596] Affected patients often manifest some degree of icterus and splenomegaly.

CDA I has been associated with a variety of congenital anomalies. As summarized,[551] the following have been catalogued: patches of brown skin pigmentation, syndactyly in the feet, absence of phalanges and nails in the fingers and toes, an additional phalanx, duplication or hypoplasia of metatarsals, short stature, pigeon chest deformity, varus deformity of hips, flattened vertebral bodies, a hypoplastic rib, congenital ptosis, Madelung deformity, and deafness. The pigmentation, syndactyly and absence of phalanges and nails are not common in CDA I patients but appear to be quite specific for this subtype. Dysmorphic features are seen in up to 65% of patients. Three siblings from a Bedouin family presented with neonatal pulmonary hypertension.[597] In a French family, three siblings had sensorineural deafness and a lack of motile sperm cells.[564]

The degree of anemia is usually mild to moderate (hemoglobin in the range of 6.6 to 11.6 g/dL), and red cells appear macrocytic. Peripheral blood red cell morphology is characterized by anisocytosis and poikilocytosis, and occasionally Cabot rings are seen. Cabot rings appear to be unique to CDA I and are not seen in types II and III. White blood cells and platelets are normal. Examination of the bone marrow reveals erythroid hyperplasia with some megaloblastic erythropoiesis, and a small number of erythroblasts with dyserythropoietic features. The unique morphologic abnormality seen in CDA I is the presence of chromatin bridges between nuclei of two separate erythroblasts, a reflection of impaired cellular division (Fig. 28–13). This internuclear bridging of erythroblasts seen with light microscopy is also a common feature in myelodysplastic syndromes. Electron microscopy reveals additional abnormalities that include widening of the nuclear membrane pore space with cytoplasmic invagination into the nucleus, separation of nuclear chromatin, and chromatin condensation, all of which give the general appearance of a spongy nucleus (Fig. 28–14). Dyserythropoiesis seems limited mostly to more mature red cell precursors. In contrast to CDA II, there are no unique serologic features.

The defect in CDA I is at the stem cell level. The numbers of CFU-E and BFU-E colonies are normal but they contain a mixture of normal and abnormal cells when examined by electron microscopy.[598] This suggests that the abnormality is expressed variably in the mature progeny of each stem cell. Erythroid precursors also demonstrate S phase arrest and morphologic features of apoptosis.[599] In some CDA I patients, hemoglobin A_2 levels are increased. Also, some cases show unbalanced globin chain synthesis. Patients do not have thalassemia and the cause of these findings is not known.[551]

CDA Type II (HEMPAS). CDA II is commonly known as HEMPAS, an acronym for *H*ereditary *E*rythroblastic *M*ultinuclearity with a *P*ositive *A*cidified *S*erum test.[600] It is inherited in an autosomal recessive manner but the mutant gene is not known. There is overlap of some clinical and laboratory manifestations between CDA I and CDA II, but there are three major differences. The first is that the magnitude of anemia is usually more severe and patients, especially children, often require red cell transfusions.[593] Peripheral blood red cells are usually normocytic but show anisocytosis and poikilocytosis (Fig. 28–15). The second difference is that the bone marrow in CDA II reveals more abnormal erythroblasts with binuclearity in up to 35% late erythroblasts, as well as multinuclearity, and abnormal lobulation (Fig. 28–16). These nuclear abnormalities are seen only in the late erythroblasts, not in basophilic erythroblasts. Karyorrhexis is commonly observed, and pseudo-Gaucher cells may be present representing the ingestion of debris by histiocytic cells from ineffective erythropoiesis. Electron microscopy of late erythroblasts also reveals an excess of endoplasmic reticulum parallel to the cell membrane, giving the appearance of a double cell membrane (Fig. 28–17).[601,602] A third difference, which is also a pathognomonic finding, is that CDA II red cells are lysed by acidified (pH 6.8) sera obtained from approximately 30% to 60% of fresh ABO-compatible sera from normal persons (Ham test), but there is no lysis when red cells are incubated with the patient's own acidified serum. This lysis is a result of a naturally occurring IgM antibody that recognizes an antigen on CDA II cells and binds complement; this antibody can be removed by preincubating normal sera with HEMPAS erythrocytes. However, the specific HEMPAS antigen recognized by this antibody is not known. In contrast to HEMPAS, the erythrocytes of patients with paroxysmal nocturnal hemoglobinuria (PNH) undergo lysis when the acidified serum is from the PNH patient or from

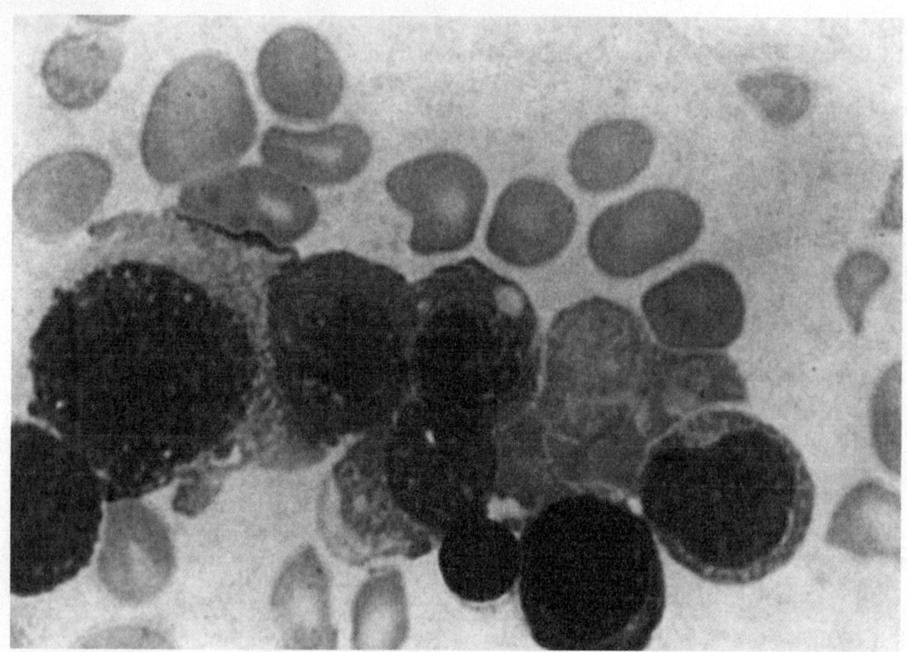

Figure 28–13 Bone marrow from patient with type I CDA. Erythroblasts are connected by internuclear bridges between two cells. *(Provided by Dr. Jean Shafer, Rochester, NY).*

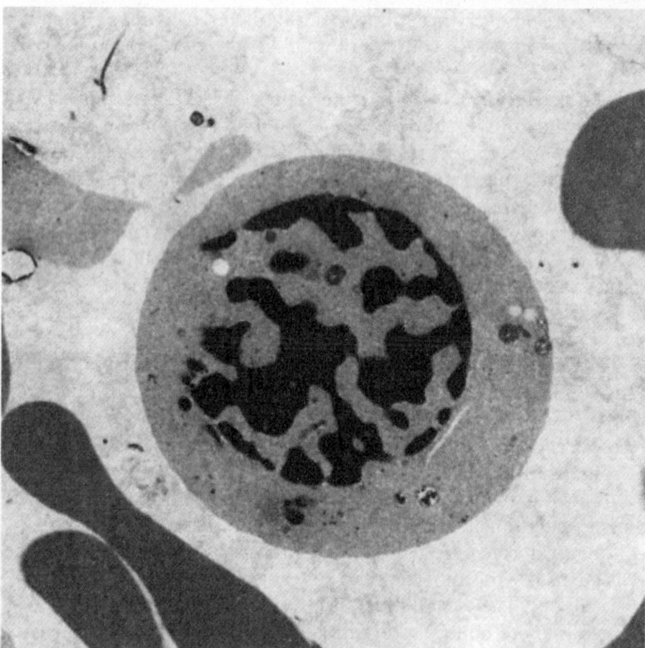

Figure 28–14 Electron microscopy of bone marrow from CDA type I. Note the "spongy" appearance of the nucleus resulting from uneven chromatin with cytoplasmic invagination into the nucleus. *(Provided by Dr. Raoul Fresco, Maywood, IL.)*

normal donors. Another difference is that PNH erythrocytes undergo lysis in isotonic sucrose, (sugar water test), whereas HEMPAS red cells do not lyse in isotonic sucrose.

The erythrocytes from patients with CDA II also exhibit an increased agglutinability and lysis to anti-i and anti-I sera and manifest increased expression of both antigens. These surface antigens are complex carbohydrate structures found predominantly on fetal and adult red cells, respectively. Increased expression of i antigen can be demonstrated on all red cells in CDA II using fluorescent labels. Relatives of patients with CDA II who have normal marrows but increased agglutinability to anti-i appear to be heterozygote carriers of this disorder.[603] HEMPAS erythrocytes bind a normal amount of complement (C1), but more antibody and less C4 than normals.[604] This causes binding of an excess of C3 and hemolysis.

The number of erythroid progenitors is probably normal in marrow and blood. Although one study found only normal morphology of the erythroblasts produced in culture,[605] subsequent studies reported multinuclearity similar to that seen in the bone marrow.[606] As in CDA I, the defect in CDA II is in the erythroid progenitor cell and is expressed variably in more mature erythroblasts.

CDA II patients may develop progressive, lifelong iron overload even in the absence of transfusions,[533] and approximately 20% develop cirrhosis as a consequence. Splenomegaly is a feature in the majority of CDA II cases. A number of other clinical associations with CDA II have been reported such as mental retardation, Sweet syndrome, von Willebrand disease, and Dubin-Johnson syndrome, among others.[607–609] Rather than true associations, it is likely that the majority represent coincidental occurrences. An adult patient was reported with an extramedullary hematopoietic mass in the posterior mediastinum that was a result of marrow expansion associated with ineffective erythropoiesis.[610] In a retrospective study of 41 patients, coinheritance of Gilbert syndrome was associated with a significantly increased risk of hyperbilirubinemia and early-onset gallstone formation.[594]

CDA Type III. Based on reported CDA cases, type II is the most common, type I is next, and CDA III is the rarest of the three major forms. In contrast to the other major forms, CDA III is inherited as an autosomal dominant disorder[611–614] although sporadic cases have also been described.[615,616] These latter cases with hematologically normal parents and relatives may represent autosomal recessive inheritance, or may have been caused by spontaneous dominant mutations.[617] In a Swedish family with 31 cases inherited in an autosomal dominant mode, an excess number of cases of monoclonal gammopathy and myeloma have occurred.[618] Also, an adult patient with CDA III was described with T-cell non-Hodgkin lymphoma.[619] These cases, plus a case of Hodgkin disease occurring in an additional patient,[620] may indicate an increased incidence of lymphoproliferative disease in CDA III.

In CDA III, splenomegaly is usually minimal or absent. The anemia is usually mild to moderate, but transfusion-dependent patients have been observed.[621] The circulating red cells can be normal or mildly macrocytic. Bone marrow examination shows erythroid hyperplasia. Giant erythroblasts with up to 12 nuclei are the most distinctive feature of CDA III observed on light micro-

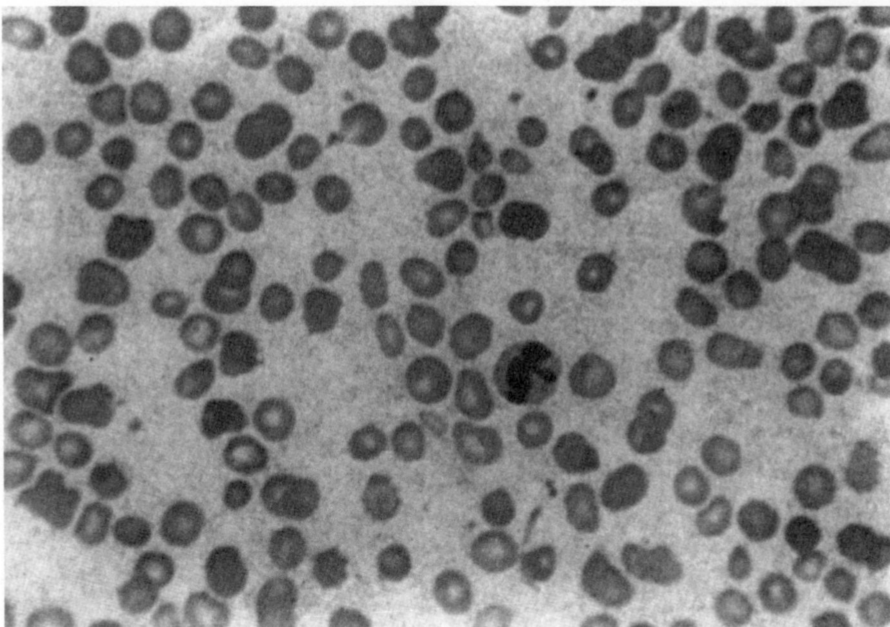

Figure 28–15 Peripheral blood smear from a patient with CDA type II. Note the marked variation in size and shape.

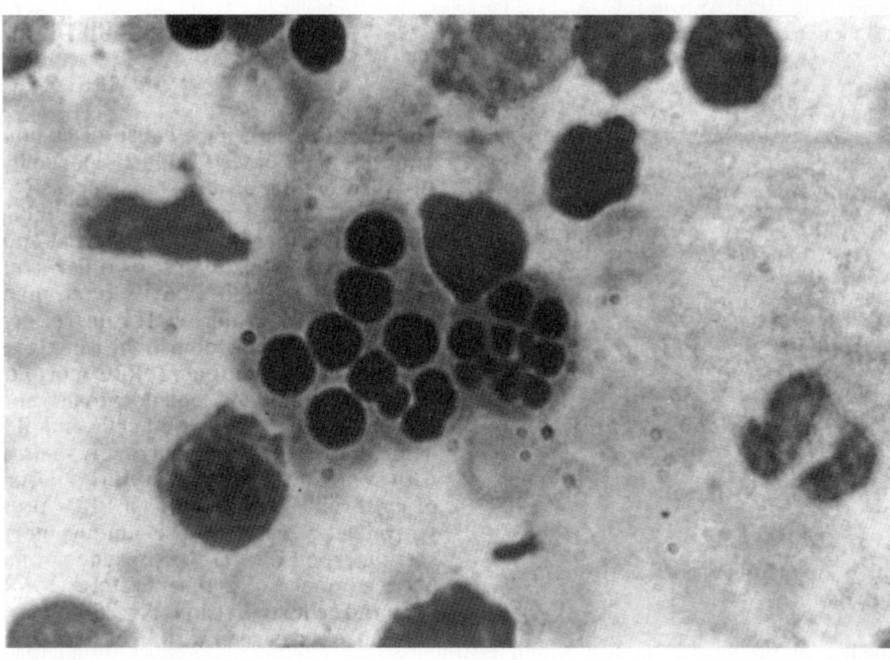

Figure 28–16 Bone marrow aspirate from a patient with HEMPAS (type II CDA) showing erythroid hyperplasia and multinucleated erythroblasts. *(Provided by Dr. Jean Shafer, Rochester, NY.)*

scopic examination of the bone marrow. These may appear similar to some of the large multinucleated cells seen in CDA II (Fig. 28–16). Abnormally large lobulated nuclei and discordance in nuclear maturation are also found. Although they are hallmarks of CDA III, these findings are not pathognomonic and may be seen in erythroleukemia. Electron microscopy demonstrates nuclear clefts and blebs, autolytic areas within the cytoplasm, and iron-filled mitochondria.

The acidified-serum lysis test is negative in CDA III. Agglutination and lysis of erythrocytes to anti-i antibody has only been examined in a few cases of CDA III with conflicting findings.[615,617] Serum thymidine kinase was measured in 20 CDA III patients and 10 healthy siblings.[622] Elevated thymidine kinase was found in all 20 cases but was normal in the siblings. It is suggested that measuring thymidine kinase levels can allow clinicians to discriminate between affected individuals and healthy siblings without performing a marrow aspirate.

Other CDAs, Nonclassifiable and Classifiable. Dozens of cases of CDA have been reported that do not conform with the classification of types I, II, III, and IV (Ham test-negative type II).[556,623] The major features of some of the earlier variant cases were reviewed[624] and representative findings are summarized here. In two kindreds, apparent CDA IV was inherited in an autosomal dominant mode. Long-lasting erythroblastosis occurring after splenectomy of type IV patients has been attributed to impairment of the denucleation of erythroblasts.[624] Unbalanced globin-chain synthesis with excess production of α-chains was documented in several patients. In one kindred, a disorder with features of both thalassemia and hereditary erythroid multinuclearity was dominantly transmitted.[625] In other cases there were also differences in the degree of agglutination by anti-i antibodies and in the concentrations of hemoglobins F and A_2.

Possible cases of CDA have been observed with lifelong anemia, which were probably inherited.[626] These were characterized by marked aniso- and poikilocytosis and occasional teardrop and fragmented

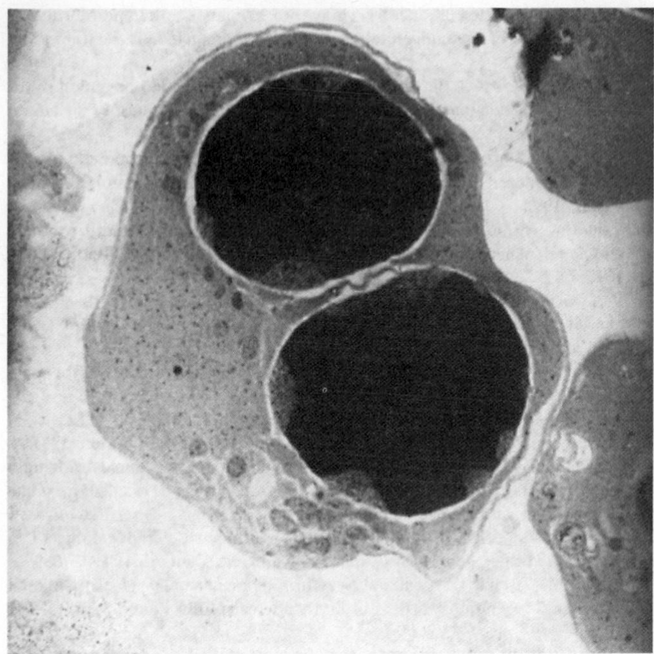

Figure 28–17 Electron microscopy of a bone marrow erythroblast from a patient with HEMPAS (type II CDA). Note the appearance of a double cell membrane reflecting an excess of endoplasmic reticulum. *(Provided by Dr. Raoul Fresco, Maywood, IL.)*

erythrocytes in the peripheral blood. Hyperplastic marrows showed megaloblastoid features without multinuclearity or ringed sideroblasts,[626] but a case with prominent ringed sideroblasts was also described.[627] Neutropenia or thrombocytopenia has been observed in some of these patients. Cytogenetic studies of marrow revealed no clonal chromosomal abnormalities. Reticulocyte response to anemia was absent or inappropriately low in all. Most case studies of parents failed to reveal abnormalities, suggesting an autosomal recessive mode of transmission.

In an attempt to sort out some of these CDAs, a phenotypebased classification was proposed that assigns patients to 1 of 4 groups (not types) designated group IV, V, VI, and VII.[551] To qualify for inclusion in this classification, each group contains cases from three or more unrelated families. The features of each are as follows:

CDA group IV. This group has severe anemia, transfusion dependence from birth, marked erythroid hyperplasia, normoblastic or mild to moderate megaloblastic changes, up to 8.0% marrow erythroblasts with markedly irregular or karyorrhectic nuclei, and an absence of precipitated protein within erythroblasts by electron microscopy. An infant with group IV CDA presented with hydrops fetalis. The spleen is enlarged. The inheritance is not clear.

CDA group V. Patients have normal or near-normal hemoglobin levels, a normal or slightly elevated MCV, and an increased serum unconjugated bilirubin. The marrow shows marked erythroid hyperplasia, and normoblastic or mild to moderate megaloblastic changes. The spleen may be palpable. The condition has been previously described as "primary shunt hyperbilirubinemia." Inheritance is variable and appears to be autosomal recessive in some cases but possibly autosomal dominant or X-linked in others. In CDA group V, the bone marrow macrophages phagocytose morphologically normal but functionally abnormal erythroblasts.

CDA group VI. This group is characterized by marked macrocytosis (MCV 119–125 fL) with little or no anemia and grossly megaloblastic erythropoiesis. There may be mild jaundice and an increased serum bilirubin. The differential diagnosis includes orotic aciduria and thiamine-responsive anemia. Vitamin B_{12} and red cell folate levels are normal.

CDA group VII. These patients have severe transfusion-dependent anemia from birth, marked erythroid hyperplasia, normoblastic or nonspecific dysplastic changes, markedly abnormal nuclear shapes in many erythroblasts, and intraerythroblastic inclusions resembling precipitated α globin chains. The inclusions do no react with monoclonal antibodies against α and β globin chains. The diagnosis requires the exclusion of β-thalassemia trait in the parents.

Differential Diagnosis

Dyserythropoiesis with erythroblast multinuclearity is seen with other hematologic disorders but these can be readily distinguished from CDA. The megaloblastic anemias have a different clinical presentation and are identified in the laboratory by the presence of hypersegmented neutrophils, decreased red cell folate values, or reduced serum levels of vitamin B_{12}. The myelodysplastic syndromes may manifest as an isolated refractory anemia but they often present with bi- or tri-lineage cytopenias that contrast sharply with CDA. The FAB and WHO myelodysplastic syndrome subsets may also show marrow granulocytic and megakaryocytic morphologic abnormalities, the presence of myeloblasts, ringed sideroblasts, and clonal cytogenetic changes. Erythroleukemia (AML, M6) is another cause of marked dyserythropoiesis but typically there is pancytopenia, the erythroblasts are avidly positive for the periodic acid-Schiff stain, and the marrow cells may show a clonal cytogenetic marker. The β-thalassemia syndromes differ from CDA by the presence of marked microcytosis with elevated levels of hemoglobin A_2, fetal hemoglobin, or both.

Therapy and Prognosis

In general, the CDAs are associated with a favorable long-term prognosis. For example, CDA I can be diagnosed late in life.[628] One case was associated with a relatively benign course over a 30-year follow-up.[629] Anemia is typically mild in most cases of CDA and requires no intervention, but in more severe presentations, especially those requiring transfusional support, splenectomy may be beneficial. Most of the experience showing an improvement in hemoglobin levels after splenectomy has been in CDA II; the benefit of splenectomy in CDA I is less clear.[621,630,631] Splenectomy may cause a persistent thrombocytosis in CDA types I and II and contribute to the development of Budd-Chiari syndrome[551] and to portal vein thrombosis.[552]

Treatment of all forms of CDA with androgens, corticosteroids, vitamin E, vitamin B_{12}, folic acid, pyridoxine, or iron is ineffective in ameliorating the anemia. Iron therapy is also contraindicated because of the underlying propensity for hemosiderosis secondary to ineffective erythropoiesis, transfusional iron overload, and increased gut iron absorption. Even if regular red cell transfusions are not initiated, patients should be routinely monitored for evidence of iron overload. Iron chelation with daily subcutaneous infusions of deferoxamine (Desferal) has been underused in CDA even though deaths have been recorded from hemochromatosis. The value of the oral iron chelators deferiprone (L1) and deferasirox (Exjade) has not been defined yet for the CDAs.

Phlebotomy has been carried out to remove iron in CDA patients but this could result in a worsening of the anemia and theoretically enhance gut iron absorption. An additional concern is that CDA patients seem predisposed to hepatic cirrhosis irrespective of body iron burden.[632] The pathogenesis of this is unclear.

Interferon α-2a, interferon α-2b, and peg-interferon α-2a increase hemoglobin levels in CDA I patients who require repeated transfusions for moderately severe anemia.[551,633,634] Erythrokinetic studies demonstrate a striking reduction of ineffective erythropoiesis in patients receiving interferon, and electron microscopy shows a reduction in nuclear structural abnormalities. Interferon therapy should also be considered in moderately anemic CDA I patients prior to treatment of iron overload by phlebotomy. CDA type II patients do not respond to interferon α.[551]

Hematopoietic stem cell transplantation has been curative in a few severe cases of CDA including transfusion-dependent CDA type I,[635] CDA type II,[636] Ham test–negative CDA type II,[637] and an unclassified CDA.[638]

Asymptomatic extramedullary hematopoiesis may mimic tumors of the mediastinum, abdomen, and vertebral column.[610,639,640] Because of the increased red cell production that occurs, the development of sites of extramedullary hematopoiesis may result in an amelioration of the degree of anemia.[641] Technetium-99m sulfur colloid scintigraphy is useful in delineating the extent of these regions.[640]

Future Directions

Identification of the various mutant genes for the CDA types will facilitate a more precise classification than the phenotype-based system used currently. The wild-type protein product of *CDAN1* requires further research to clarify its function in health, and its role in producing CDA type I when mutant. CDA types I and II mimic thalassemia and show unbalanced globin chain synthesis; this requires explanation. Strategies are required for managing iron overload similar to those for Diamond-Blackfan anemia and thalassemia major. In this regard, the therapeutic benefit of the oral iron chelators deferiprone and deferasirox should be explored fully.

ANNOTATED BIBLIOGRAPHY

General

Alter BP: Inherited bone marrow failure syndromes. In: Nathan DG, Orkin SH, Look AT, Ginsburg D (eds.): Nathan and Oski's Hematology of Infancy and Childhood, 6th edition, W B Saunders, Philadelphia, 2003, p 280.

Bagby, GC (Guest Editor): Constitutional marrow failure. Semin Hematol 43:145, 2006.

Alter BP: Diagnois genetics, and management of inherited bone marrow failure syndromes. In: Gewirtz AM, Winter JN, Zuckerman K (eds): Hematology 2007, Education Program Book, American Society of Hematology 2007, p 29.

Fanconi Anemia

Levitus M, Joenje H, de Winter JP: The Fanconi anemia pathway of genomic maintenance. Cell Oncol 28:3, 2006.

Owen J, Frohnmayer L, Eiler ME (eds.): Fanconi Anemia Standards for Clincial Care, 2nd edition, Fanconi Anemia Research Fund, Eugene, Oregon, 2003 (fanconi.org/pubs/StandardsCare.htm).

Taniguchi T, D'Andrea AD: Molecular pathogenesis of Fanconi anemia: recent progress. Blood 107:4223, 2006.

Shwachman-Diamond Syndrome

Dror Y, Freedman MH: Shwachman-Diamond syndrome. Br J Haematol 118:701, 2002.

Dror Y: Shwachman-Diamond syndrome. Pediatr Blood Cancer 45:892, 2005.

Dyskeratosis Congenita

Dokal I: Dyskeratosis congenita in all its forms. Br J Haematol 110:768, 2000.

Congenital Amegakaryocytic Thrombocytopenia

Drachman JG: Inherited thrombocytopenia: When a low platelet count does not mean ITP. Blood 103:390, 2004.

Germeshausen M, Ballmaier M, Welte K: MPL mutations in 23 patients suffering from congenital amegakaryocytic thrombocytopenia: the type of mutation predicts the course of the disease. Hum Mutat 27:296, 2006.

King S, Germeshausen M, Strauss G, et al: Congential amegakaryocytic thrombocytopenia: A retrospective clinical analysis of 20 patients. Br J Haematol 131:636, 2005.

Diamond-Blackfan Anemia

Lipton JM, Atsidaftos E, Zyskind I, Vlachos A: Improving clinical care and elucidating the pathophysiology of Diamond-Blackfan aneumia: an update from the Diamond-Blackfan Anemia Registry. Pediatr Blood Cancer 46:558, 2006.

Willing T-N, Niemeyer CM, Leblanc T, et al: Identification of new prognosis factors from the clinical and epidemiologic analysis of a registry of 229 Diamond-Blackfan anemia patients. Pediatr Res 46:553, 1999.

Daniella Maria Arturi Foundation, Proceedings of the 9th Annual Diamond-Blackfan Amemia International concensus conference, 2008 (contact Foundation Director, Lauren Carroll: lcarroll@dmaf.org).

Kostmann Syndrome/Congenital Neutropenia

Dale DC, Cottle TE, Fier CJ, et al: Severe chronic neutropenia: Treatment and follow-up of patients in the Severe Chronic Neutropenia International Registry. Am J Hematol 72:82, 2003.

Welte K, Zeidler C, Dale DC: Severe congenital neutropenia. Semin Hematol 43:189, 2006.

Rosenberg PS, Alter BP, Bolyard AA, et al: The incidence of leukemia and mortality from sepsis in patients with severe congenital neutropenia receiving long-term G-CSF therapy. Blood 107:4628, 2006.

Congenital Dyserythropoietic Anemias

Wickramasinghe SN, Wood WG: Advances in the understanding of the congenital dyserythropoietic anaemias. Br J Haematol 131:431, 2005.

REFERENCES

For complete list of references log onto www.expertconsult.com

CHAPTER 29

APLASTIC ANEMIA

Neal S. Young and Jaroslaw P. Maciejewski

Aplastic anemia (AA), the paradigm of bone marrow failure syndromes, is most simply defined as peripheral blood pancytopenia and a hypocellular bone marrow (Fig. 29–1). From epidemiologic and clinical features, pathophysiologic studies, and response to therapy, AA is a distinctive disease. However, the diagnosis of AA requires excluding other causes of pancytopenia (Table 29–1). AA can occur as a primary hematologic disorder, most often idiopathic, or apparently result from various proximate causes, including obvious physical and chemical toxins but also drugs and viruses that can act indirectly. Although AA is usually characterized by a severe diminution in bone marrow function that affects all the hematopoietic lineages, granulocyte, platelet, and red blood cell (RBC) levels may not be depressed uniformly, and less severe degrees of marrow hypoplasia and odd combinations of bicytopenias and monocytopenias can occur. AA can be especially difficult to distinguish from hypocellular forms of myelodysplasia, a diagnostic dilemma that can rest on real biologic similarities. Even typical AA can vary in its clinical presentation and course, from a fulminant illness marked by continuous or recurrent hemorrhage and major infections to an indolent process manageable by transfusion therapy alone.

HISTORY

The study of bone marrow failure dates to 1888, when Paul Ehrlich described a young woman who died after an explosive short illness marked by severe anemia, bleeding, and high fever. As a pathologist, Ehrlich was struck by the absence of nucleated RBCs and the fatty quality of the femoral marrow.[1] Vaquez and Aubertin, in a 1904 case report of "pernicious anemia with yellow marrow," named the disease and emphasized a pathophysiology of "*anhematopoiesis*."[2] Cabot stressed the marrow's distinctive pathology and the need for its examination in making the diagnosis.[3] Tissue from patients with early cases of AA could only be examined at autopsy, and in practice, pancytopenia was often equated with AA. The etymologic root of the term *aplastique* is the Greek verb πλ¿ϑω, to create and give shape to(¿πλαζτκ⟨, the adjective, unformed). Inferences about the cause of the disease were made from the bone marrow appearance. The aplastic variety of pancytopenia was distinguishable from secondary cellular or regenerative pernicious anemias, and AA was recognized as primary and caused by failed blood cell production.[2] Pathologically, the watery, yellow marrow seen at autopsy uniquely characterized the aplasia, but the limited and rather general clinical signs were less helpful in distinguishing this type of aregenerative marrow failure from other anemias.[4]

CLASSIFICATION

AA is a major sequela of irradiation and exposure to cytotoxic chemotherapy. It has been associated with the use of chemicals and drugs, viral infections, and other diseases (Table 29–2). Most patients have an idiopathic form of the disease, meaning that the cause is unknown. Too strict a division of cases into categories can obscure important pathophysiologic relationships. Historically, the relation between clinical associations and causation can be neither direct nor reliable. Thus the basis for assigning a particular case to a particular cause has depended on the history. How closely is the patient questioned? How biased are the inquiries? How conscientiously is a possibly significant but distant toxic exposure sought? How exaggerated is a brief episode?

EPIDEMIOLOGY

Incidence

The largest and most comprehensive study of the epidemiology of bone marrow failure was the International Aplastic Anemia and Agranulocytosis Study (IAAAS), conducted in Europe and Israel from 1980 to 1984.[5] This study was performed prospectively and applied strict case definition to pathologically confirmed cases. Using stringent criteria, the overall annual incidence of AA was 2 cases per 1 million people. Other subsequent studies of similar design have confirmed this figure.[6] The incidence rates reported in the IAAAS are threefold to fourfold lower than rates reported in many earlier, mainly retrospective, and far less well-designed surveys.

A remarkable feature of the epidemiology of AA is the unexplained geographic variation in its incidence. The incidence of AA in Bangkok and two rural regions of Thailand has been accurately determined using the same methods as employed by the IAAAS researchers in Europe and Israel; the annual incidence was 4.0 cases per 1 million people in the capital and 5.6 cases per 1 million people in the northeastern province of Khonkaen.[7] The incidence in 21 Chinese provinces has been estimated to be 7.4 cases per 1 million people annually,[8] and in the Sabah province of Malaysia, a retrospective analysis suggested a rate of 5 cases per 1 million people.[9] From published, hospital-based series, personal communications, and first-hand observations, AA appears most prevalent in less developed specific regions of the world, including Vietnam, Indonesia, Russia, the former Soviet republics, Iran, Iraq, Pakistan, India, Mexico,[10] certain regions of Latin America,[11] and Africa, where it is probably underdiagnosed.[12] There are no major sex or racial differences in the occurrence of AA.[5,7,13]

Geographic and Age Distribution

AA is a disease of the young. (Fig. 29–2) Most patients present between 15 and 25 years of age or older than 60 years of age.[14,15]

Epidemiologic Clues to Causality

Population-based studies have investigated possible causal associations. Drugs are implicated in only approximately 25% of cases of AA[5] in the west; in Thailand, AA was attributed to drug exposure in only approximately 15% of cases.[16,17] There are associations with chemical exposures, exposures to viruses, hepatitis, and occupation.[18] There is evidence that geographic variation in AA might result from environmental causes[17,19,20] and also genetic predisposition.[21]

Genetic Aspects

More than one case of acquired AA in a single family is a rare occurrence. In children and young adults, acquired AA should be distin-

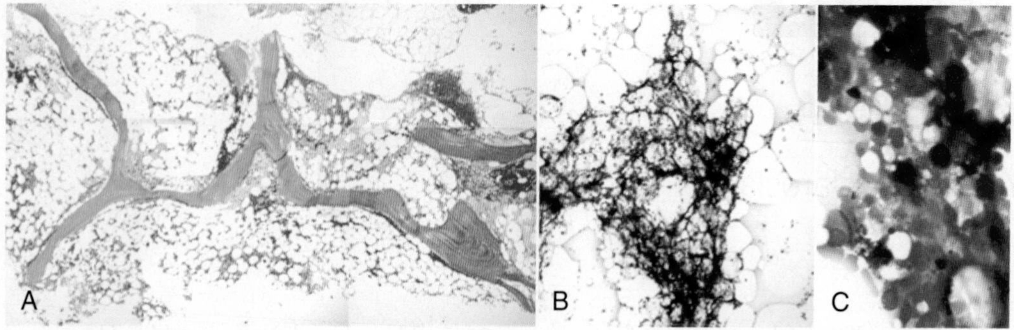

Figure 29–1 BONE MARROW MORPHOLOGY IN SEVERE APLASTIC ANEMIA (A–C). Bone marrow biopsy specimen, of sufficient length (**A**) shows severe hypocellularity. The corresponding aspirate (**B, C**) shows empty marrow spicules and residual stoma including lymphoid cells, plasma cells, histiocytes and mast cells.

Table 29–1 Differential Diagnosis of Pancytopenia

Pancytopenia with Hypocellular Bone Marrow
Acquired aplastic anemia
Inherited aplastic anemia (Fanconi anemia and others)
Some myelodysplasia syndromes
Rare aleukemic leukemia (acute myelogenous leukemia)
Some acute lymphoblastic leukemias
Some lymphomas of bone marrow
Pancytopenia with Cellular Bone Marrow
Primary bone marrow diseases
Myelodysplasia syndromes
Paroxysmal nocturnal hemoglobinuria
Myelofibrosis
Some aleukemic leukemias
Myelophthisis
Bone marrow lymphoma
Hairy cell leukemia
Secondary to systemic diseases
Systemic lupus erythematosus, Sjögren syndrome
Hypersplenism
Vitamin B_{12}, folate deficiency (familial defect)
Overwhelming infection
Alcohol
Brucellosis
Ehrlichiosis
Sarcoidosis
Tuberculosis and atypical mycobacteria
Hypocellular Bone Marrow ± Cytopenia
Q fever
Legionnaires disease
Mycobacteria
Tuberculosis*
Anorexia nervosa, starvation
Hypothyroidism

*Pancytopenia in tuberculosis only rarely is associated with a hypocellular bone marrow at biopsy or autopsy. Marrow failure in the setting of tuberculosis is almost always fatal; exceptional patients probably had underlying myelodysplasia or acute leukemia.

Table 29–2 A Classification of Aplastic Anemia

Acquired Aplastic Anemia
Secondary aplastic anemia
Irradiation
Drugs and chemicals
Regular effects
Cytotoxic agents
Benzene
Idiosyncratic reactions
Chloramphenicol
Nonsteroidal antiinflammatory drugs
Antiepileptics
Gold
Other drugs and chemicals
Viruses
Epstein-Barr virus (infectious mononucleosis)
Hepatitis virus (non-A, non-B, non-C, non-G hepatitis)
Parvovirus (transient aplastic crisis, some pure red cell aplasia)
Human immunodeficiency virus (acquired immunodeficiency syndrome)
Immune diseases
Eosinophilic fasciitis
Hyperimmunoglobulinemia
Thymoma and thymic carcinoma
Graft-versus-host disease in immunodeficiency
Paroxysmal nocturnal hemoglobinuria
Pregnancy
Idiopathic aplastic anemia
Inherited Aplastic Anemia
Fanconi anemia
Dyskeratosis congenita
Shwachman-Diamond syndrome
Reticular dysgenesis
Amegakaryocytic thrombocytopenia
Familial aplastic anemias
Preleukemia (eg, monosomy 7)
Nonhematologic syndromes (eg, Down, Dubowitz, Seckel)

guished from the inherited forms of bone marrow failure such as Fanconi anemia and dyskeratosis congenita. Identification of patients with Fanconi anemia has important therapeutic implications. Patients with constitutional AA can lack typical physical anomalies, and the pancytopenia can develop after childhood (see Chapter 28), mimicking the acquired disease.

A few histocompatibility types have also been associated with AA, most consistently human leukocyte antigen (HLA)-DR2.[22–24] HLA-DR subtypes have proved useful in predicting response to immunosuppressive therapy; in a large cohort of US AA patients, HLA-DR15 was associated with the presence of the paroxysmal nocturnal hemoglobinuria (PNH) clone and responsiveness to immunosuppression.[24] In Japanese patients, the presence of the *DRB*1501* allele was strongly associated with hematologic responses to cyclosporine[25] and with the probability of relapse[22] and cyclosporine dependence.[26] Haplotypes associated with clozapine-induced agranulocytosis have been linked to the heat-shock protein variants encoded within the large major

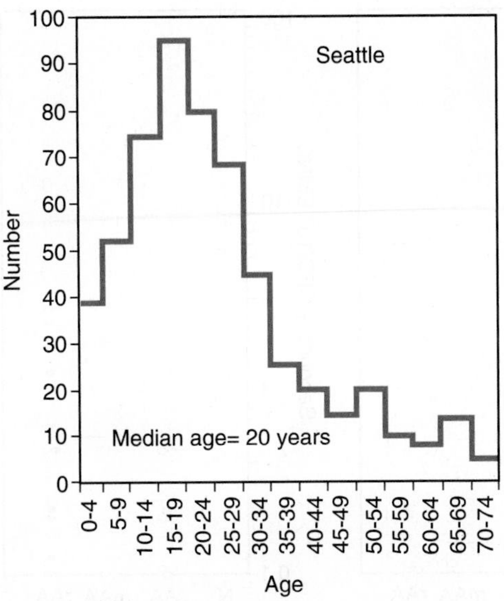

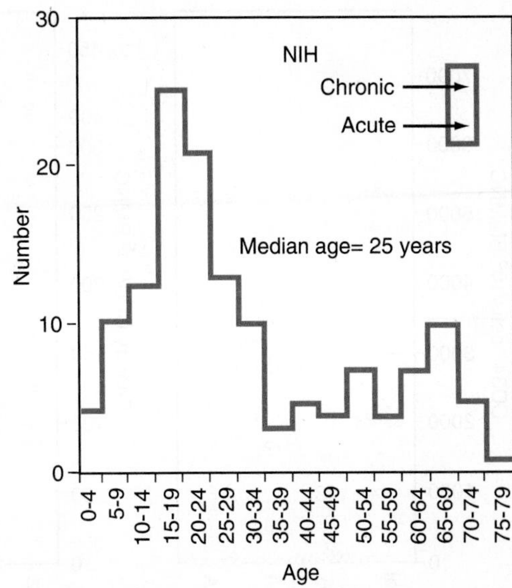

Figure 29–2 Distribution of aplastic anemia by age. For the patients at the University of Washington, a major transplantation center, the age given is at the time of first treatment. For the patients at the National Institutes of Health (NIH), where immunosuppressive therapy is offered, the age given is at the time of diagnostic bone marrow biopsy. Acute disease is defined as less than 3 months between diagnosis and presentation at NIH, and chronic disease is defined as more than 3 months. *(Seattle statistics are courtesy of Rainer Storb, University of Washington.)*

histocompatibility gene region.[27] Genetic predisposition may be responsible for some idiosyncratic reactions to drugs and chemicals leading to the development of AA. Polymorphisms in cytokine genes, associated with an increased immune response, also are more prevalent in AA: a nucleotide polymorphism in the tumor necrosis factor α (TNF-α; *TNF2*) promoter at −308,[26,27] homozygosity for a variable number of dinucleotide repeats in the gene encoding γ-interferon (IFN-γ), and polymorphisms in the interleukin 6 (IL-6) gene.[28] Genome wide transcriptional analysis of T cells from aplastic anemia patients has implicated components of innate immunity in aplastic anemia, including Toll-like receptors and natural killer cells,[29] for which there is some preliminary experimental support.[30,31]

ETIOLOGY AND PATHOGENESIS

Hematopoiesis in Bone Marrow Failure

Stem Cells

A consistent laboratory finding for patients with AA is a very low number of hematopoietic progenitor cells.[28,32,33] Colony formation by bone marrow cells of AA patients remains unresponsive, even to high levels of hematopoietic growth factors.[29,34] The total number of progenitors in a marrow sample is reduced, and the number of colony progenitor cells assayed from a purified CD34 population is low.[32] In humans, a stem-cell surrogate assay that assesses cells capable of colony formation after more than 1 month in long-term bone marrow culture is available; these long-term culture-initiating cells (LTC-ICs) share the frequency, phenotype, and kinetic properties of true stem cells. Studies indicate a profound deficiency in LTC-IC numbers in all patients with severe AA.[30,31,35] At clinical presentation, the number of LTC-ICs is usually less than 10% of normal; combined with a reduction in total marrow cellularity to 10% or less, the stem-cell number is estimated to be reduced to 1% or less than normal in patients with AA (Fig. 29–3).

One peculiar feature of white blood cells in AA is short telomeres.[36,37] Telomere shortening was initially most easily attributed to stem-cell exhaustion. However, the discovery, first by linkage analysis in large pedigrees, that the X-linked form of dyskeratosis congenita was caused by mutations in *DKC1* and subsequently purposeful identification of mutations in *TERC* in some autosomal dominant patients with this constitutional marrow failure syndrome indicated a genetic basis for telomere deficiency. Central to the repair machinery is an RNA template, encoded by *TERC*, on which telomerase, a reverse transcriptase encoded by *TERT*, elongates the nucleotide repeat structure; other proteins, including the *DKC1* gene product dyskenin, are associated with the telomere repair complex. Systematic surveys of DNA disclosed first *TERC*[38,39] and later *TERT* mutations[40] in some patients with apparently acquired AA, including older adults. Family members who share the mutation, despite normal or near normal blood counts, have hypocellular marrows, reduced CD34 cell counts and poor hematopoietic colony formation, increased hematopoietic growth factor levels, and of course short telomeres; however, their clinical presentation is much later than in typical dyskeratosis congenita, and they lack typical physical anomalies.[38,40] Chromosomes are also protected by several proteins that bind directly to telomeres, and polymorphisms in their genes (*TERF1, TERF2*) are also more or less prevalent in AA compared to healthy controls.[41] A few patients also have heterozygous mutations in the Shwachman-Bodian-Diamond syndrome (*SBDS*) gene. Almost all children with this form of constitutional AA are compound heterozygotes for mutations in *SBDS*, and their white cells have extremely short telomeres;[42] however, the *SBDS* gene product has not been directly linked to the telomere repair complex or to telomere binding. A parsimonious inference from all these data is that inherited mutations in genes that repair or protect telomeres are genetic risk factors in acquired AA, probably because they confer a quantitatively reduced hematopoietic stem cell compartment that may also be qualitatively inadequate to sustain immune-mediated damage.[43] However, telomeres are short in one-third to one-half of AA patients,[36,37] but mutations have only been identified in less than 10% of cases.

Stromal and Hematopoietic Growth Factors

Stromal cell function is usually not defective in cases of AA.[28] Adherent cells from patients support hematopoiesis by normal CD34 cells, whereas no hematopoietic colonies develop when patients' CD34 cells are cultured in the presence of normal stroma[36,44] (Fig. 29–4). Stromal cells cultured from patients' bone marrow generally produce normal quantities of hematopoietic growth factors.[37] Serum levels of erythropoietin,[39] thrombopoietin,[40] granulocyte colony-stimulating factor (GCSF),[41] and granulocyte-macrophage colony-stimulating

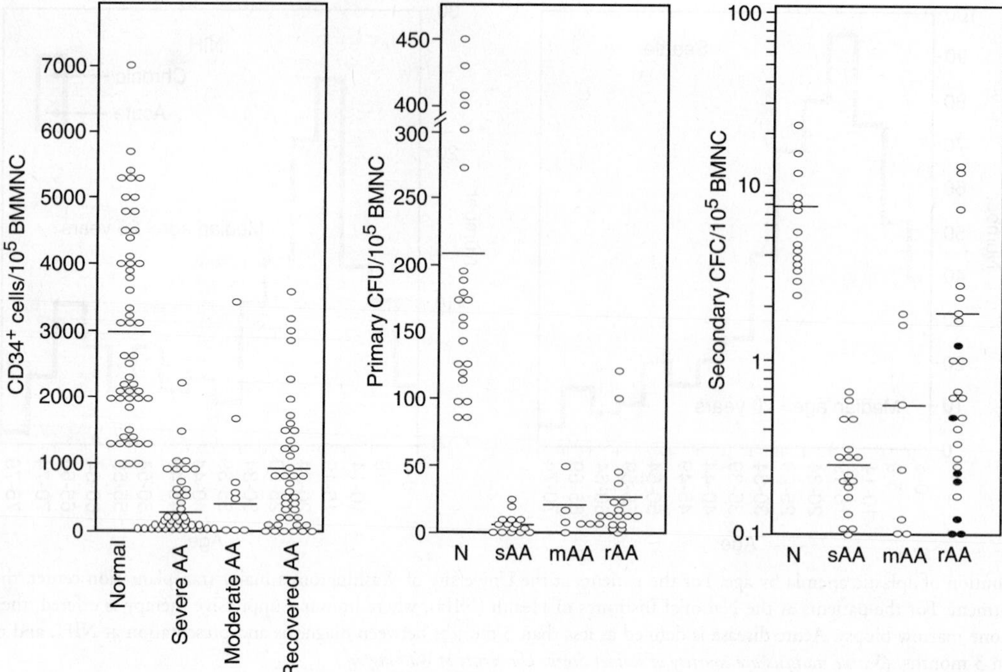

Figure 29–3 The numbers of CD34 cells, primary colony-forming cells (CFC), and long-term culture-initiating cells (LTC-ICs) were measured in the bone marrow of aplastic anemia patients. Each dot represents an individual patient's sample studied. Severe aplastic anemia (sAA) includes patients at presentation, cases refractory to immunosuppressive therapy, and patients who relapsed after a period of recovery. Primary CFC were measured in short-term methylcellulose cultures. Secondary CFC after long-term bone marrow cultures reflect LTC-IC numbers. BMNC, blood mononuclear cell; CFU, colony-forming unit; mAA, moderate aplastic anemia; N, normal; rAA, recovered from aplastic anemia.

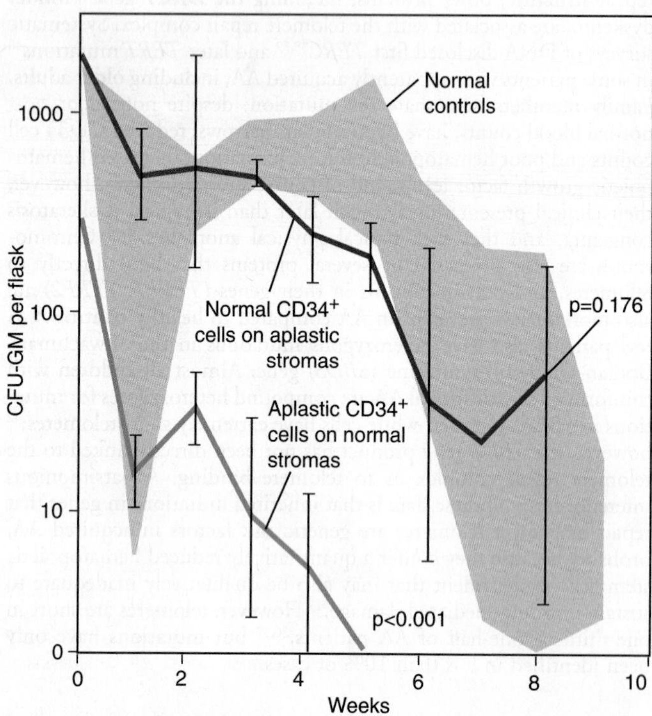

Figure 29–4 Normal stromal cell function in long-term culture of aplastic anemia bone marrow. AML, acute myelogenous leukemia; MDS, myelodysplastic syndrome. *(Courtesy of Dr. Judith Marsh, St. George's Hospital Medical School, London.)*

factor (GM-CSF) are almost always normal or elevated.[42] Cytokines that act at very early stages of hematopoiesis have been studied as possible etiologic factors in the pathobiology of AA. Blood levels of FLT3 ligand are highly elevated in AA,[43] stem cell factor (SCF) levels are modestly decreased,[45] and SCF stromal cell production is normal.[45]

Adequate stromal function is implicit in the success of marrow transplantation in AA because important stromal elements remain of host origin.

PATHOPHYSIOLOGIC PATHWAYS LEADING TO APLASTIC ANEMIA

Direct Hematopoietic Injury

The most common form of AA is iatrogenic; transient marrow failure often follows treatment with cytotoxic chemotherapeutic drugs or irradiation (Fig. 29–5). Certain chemical or physical agents directly injure proliferating and quiescent hematopoietic cells. However, patients with community-acquired AA rarely have a history of exposure to such physicochemical agents. Even benzene, which can act as a particularly inefficient cytotoxic chemical, is an infrequent cause of AA in developed countries.[5] Therapeutic drugs are associated with acquired AA, and in some instances, they can directly cause marrow damage. However, compared with chemotherapeutic agents, which are delivered in high doses, relatively low total quantities of ingested drug apparently cause idiosyncratic hematologic reactions. In addition to their direct toxic effects, chemicals and viruses can induce complex immune reactions leading to bone marrow failure in persons with AA (see Fig. 29–5).

Immune-Mediated Marrow Failure

In the 1970s, Mathé and colleagues[46] observed unexpected improvement of pancytopenia after failed marrow transplantation. They speculated that the immunosuppressive conditioning regimen, intended to allow engraftment of the donor marrow, might instead have promoted the recovery of host marrow function.[46] The effectiveness of diverse treatments that reduce lymphocyte number or block T-cell function, and the superior results obtained when agents are

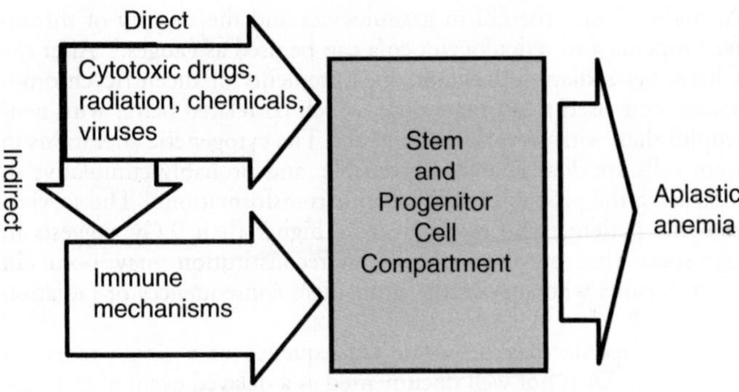

Figure 29–5 Possible causes of direct and indirect bone marrow failure in patients with aplastic anemia (AA).

combined strongly suggest that such therapeutic success is caused by the immunosuppressive effects of the drugs employed. AA shares numerous clinical and pathophysiologic features with other autoimmune disorders that all are characterized by T-cell–mediated, tissue-specific organ destruction. Like AA, these disorders tend to occur in younger persons and show geographic variation in incidence. The late immune events that dominate at the time of clinical presentation—cytotoxic lymphocyte activation, cytokine production, and specific target cell elimination—are common to many autoimmune disorders.

Immune system destruction of marrow occurs in animal models of graft-versus-host disease (GVHD) and in humans with transfusion-associated GVHD, in which AA is the invariable cause of death.[47] Very small numbers of effector cells, which have been conveyed by residual lymphocytes contained within the transfusion product[48] or with solid organ transplants,[49] are sufficient to mediate GVHD under these conditions. AA is associated with rheumatologic syndromes, such as eosinophilic fasciitis,[50] and with systemic lupus erythematosus, which can appear or worsen with pregnancy.[51] AA occasionally occurs in individuals with hypogammaglobulinemia or congenital immunodeficiency syndrome,[52] thymoma, thymic hyperplasia,[53] and thymic carcinoma.[54]

Laboratory support for the immune hypothesis first came from coculture experiments in which mononuclear cells from AA patients' blood or bone marrow were shown to suppress in vitro colony formation by hematopoietic progenitor cells. Removal of T cells from the patient samples sometimes improved colony formation in vitro.[55] Peripheral blood and bone marrow samples from patients were shown to produce a soluble factor that inhibited hematopoiesis,[56–58] ultimately identified as IFN-γ.[59] Patients' T cells[60,61] overproduced IFN-γ and tumor necrosis factor (TNF), two cytokines that inhibit hematopoietic proliferation.[62] Increased expression of IFN-γ was detected in samples from most AA patients.[63,64] Constitutive expression of Tbet, a transcriptional regulator that is critical to Th1 polarization, was present in a majority of AA patients[33] Patients' blood and marrow also contained elevated numbers of activated cytotoxic lymphocytes.[65] The activity and levels of these cytotoxic cells decreased appropriately with antithymocyte globulin (ATG) therapy.[66,67] Cytotoxic T lymphocytes (CTLs) that contain IFN-γ can be measured by flow cytometry and correlate with disease activity.[68]

The lymphokines IFN-γ and TNF suppressed proliferation of early and late hematopoietic progenitor and stem cells.[62] These effects were far more potent when these lymphokines are secreted into the marrow microenvironment than when they were simply added to the cultures,[69] consistent with their localization in the marrow of patients. Although IFN-γ and TNF can suppress hematopoiesis by effects on cell proliferation, an important component of their inhibitory activity is cell death by induction of apoptosis: Both lymphokines induced expression of the Fas receptor on CD34 progenitor cells; triggering of the Fas receptor by its ligand initiates a fatal process of apoptosis.[70,71] Apoptosis of hematopoietic cells in AA is suggested by the findings of high Fas receptor expression[72] and increased numbers of apoptotic cells[73] in patients' bone marrow. Immune-mediated cell cycle blockade and apoptosis can lead to the dramatic elimination of hematopoietic progenitor and stem cells in patients with AA.

The early immune system events that must precede the global destruction of hematopoietic cells are not clear. Involvement of CD4 lymphocytes has been suggested and a more specific class II haplotype has been identified among Japanese patients.[26] Clones of HLA-DR–restricted T cells derived from a few patients have been shown to proliferate in response to marrow cells.[74,75]

Molecular analyses of the T-cell receptor repertoire have been used to study the T-cell responses in AA.[76] Oligoclonal skewing of a large number of CTL repertoire consistent with the presence of expanded immunodominant clones has been observed, suggesting the presence of an ongoing CTL response.[77–79] Using the unique region of the variable portion of the β-chain of the T-cell receptor, immunodominant CTL clones have been identified and their levels correlated with the hematologic parameter.[79] Similar clonotypic sequences have been observed in patients matched for certain HLA restriction elements, a finding suggestive of the response to common or closely related antigens. Clonotypic sequences derived from the T-cell receptor may serve in the future as a molecular marker for the activity of disease and indicate the presence of specific antigens driving the immune response.[76,80]

Radiation

Marrow aplasia is a major acute toxic effect of radiation;[81,82] both stem and progenitor cells are damaged (Fig. 29–6). The dose-related occurrence of pancytopenia 2 to 4 weeks after exposure to radiation is caused by injury of actively replicating progenitor cells. Mortality from hematologic toxicity is a function of the marrow's ability to tolerate depletion of hematopoietic cells and damage to the stem cell. The capacity for recovery of hematopoietic function after even massive single irradiation exposures is considerable, reflecting the resistance of the quiescent stem cell to damage and the enormous marrow repopulating potential of even a greatly reduced stem cell pool. At intermediate radiation doses around the median lethal dose (LD_{50}), at which marrow toxicity limits survival, supportive efforts can drastically alter outcome. Autopsies of atomic bomb victims in Japan showed acellular bone marrows in the first weeks of the explosion, but there frequently was regenerating bone marrow in those who survived longer.[83] The histologic picture of radiation-mediated aplasia includes necrosis, nuclear pyknosis and karyorrhexis, nuclear lysis, and ultimately cytolysis; the associated phagocytosis, marked congestion, and hemorrhage are rapidly followed by fatty replacement.[84] Bone marrow hypoplasia occurs with radiation doses higher than 1.5 to 2 Gy to the whole body. Precise LD_{50} figures for humans do not exist, and estimates are based on the limited direct human data and extrapolation from animal experiments. The LD_{50} is highly dependent on the quality of medical care, and improved support may double the tolerated radiation dose.[85] From assessment of the outcome of radiation accidents and high-dose therapeutic irradiation, the LD_{50} has been estimated at approximately 4.5 Gy,[86,87] an almost mythical figure sometimes called the Shields Warren number (see Fig. 29–6).

Although the principles of management of pancytopenia after a single large dose of irradiation are similar to those for treating AA in general, some unique points should be made concerning immediate evaluation and long-term prognosis. The type and intensity of the source of radiation and the distance and shielding of the subject are the major determinants of radiation injury; because of the nature of the exposure, these factors are often difficult to assess. Early recognition of the nature of the accident provides the best opportunity for dosimetry by accident reconstruction and can allow employment of blocking, displacement, or chelation agents. Exposure correlates well with the degree of pancytopenia.[88] Because lymphocytes are particularly sensitive to radiation, their rate of decline can be used to estimate the dose of total body exposure to a level of approximately 3 Gy.[88]

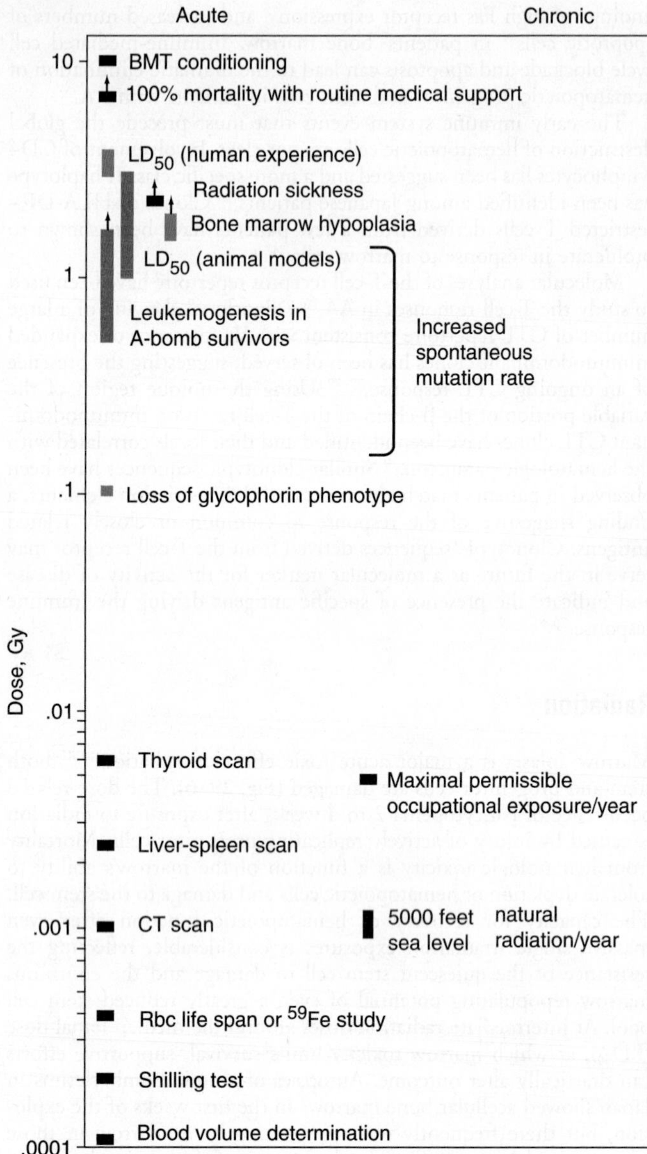

Figure 29–6 Scale of whole-body radiation doses. A Gray (Gy) is a measure of absorbed dose equivalent to 1 J/kg unit mass, and 1 Gy equals 100 rads. Radiation represents radiant energy. When absorbed by biologic tissue, radiant energy causes release of electrons and molecular ionization, which result in further energy release. Radiant energy can directly break chemical bonds and indirectly damage macromolecules through generation of high-energy free radical forms. The relationship between increased mutation rate and radiation dose is very approximate *(hatched bars)*. Measurement of the phenotype of an autosomal recessive gene such as for glycophorin would be expected to be a very sensitive indicator. Because malignant transformation is almost certainly a two-step process, increased leukemogenesis is probably an underestimation of the effect of radiation on a single gene. Even the extensive data on the atomic bomb survivors of Hiroshima are subject to statistical errors because of the small number of cases; a linear or exponential curve fit gives various results, and very high doses of radiation may not be associated with as high a risk of leukemia because of stem cell death. Other data that can bear on mutation frequency lie outside the range shown. In a patient with ankylosing spondylitis who underwent irradiation of the spine, leukemogenesis was observed at relatively low doses (doubling of the leukemia rate can be extrapolated to approximately 7 Gy), but such individuals can be predisposed to leukemia. An increased risk of thyroid cancer after irradiation of the mediastinum in childhood occurred at approximately 4 Gy. BMT, bone marrow transplantation; CT, computed tomography; LD_{50}, median lethal dose; Rbc, red blood cell.

At higher doses, the fall in granulocytes and the severity of thrombocytopenia and reticulocytopenia can be used as gauges.[89] After the Chernobyl radiation accident, measurements of dicentric chromosomes were used to estimate dose, which correlated better with neutrophil than with lymphocyte kinetics. The cytogenetic alterations in stem cells are dose related, irreversible, and probably cumulative in increasing the probability of leukemic transformation.[90] The survival of some patients who received doses higher than 9 Gy suggests in retrospect that autologous marrow reconstitution may occur in most persons who survive the immediate consequences of radiation exposure.[91]

Pancytopenia may be a late consequence of a single radiation dose,[92] but AA is not well documented as a delayed event after radiation exposure. Of 156 cases of AA in Japan in the 20 years after the atomic bomb explosions, only 13 individuals had received more than a 1-rad dose, and of the 3 individuals who had been heavily irradiated, only 1 had typical AA.[93]

A variety of hematologic abnormalities are associated with chronic low-level radiation exposure, most commonly lymphocytosis, neutropenia, immature or dysmorphic white blood cells (WBCs), and giant platelets (see Fig. 29–6). Cytogenetic abnormalities accumulate with time after chronic exposure, but they may not be reliably related to dose.[94] Repeated low doses of radiation can damage bone marrow and have been associated with AA in special circumstances,[95] but even in these circumstances, only a small proportion of exposed individuals developed hematologic disease.[96] AA does not appear to be more frequent among nuclear power plant or thorium processing factory workers or among residents living close to the plants.[97] Excessive numbers of deaths from AA were reported after therapeutic irradiation of the spine for ankylosing spondylitis,[98] although later analysis has suggested that the risk may have been overestimated.[99] Despite occasional instances in which marrow failure developed years after radiation therapy and chemotherapy,[100] AA was not found in unexpected numbers in a large population of cancer patients who had received therapeutic irradiation.[101] Bone marrow failure has not been observed with abnormally high frequency among persons exposed to higher natural background radiation.[102] Excessive deaths from AA did occur among North American radiologists who died between 1948 and 1961.[103]

Drugs and Chemicals

AA is frequently associated with medical drug use (Table 29–3).[104] At the end of the 19th century, chemicals were linked to marrow function through observations of benzene effects on workers. Establishment of a relationship between the analgesic amidopyrine and agranulocytosis in the early 20th century and an apparent epidemic of AA after the introduction of chloramphenicol in the 1960s also supported this concept. Initially suggested by the accumulation of case reports, drug associations have been established in formal case-control population-based epidemiologic studies. In the IAAAS, relative risks were estimated for individual drugs and large classes of pharmaceutical agents, including nonsteroidal antiinflammatory drugs (NSAIDs), drugs affecting thyroid function, certain cardiovascular agents, some psychotropics, and sulfa-based antibiotics (Table 29–4).[5] Approximately 25% of the cases of AA identified in the IAAAS could be attributed to drug use. Drug use as a risk factor was also assessed by similar methods in Thailand,[105] where the incidence of AA is higher than in the West.[7] Surprisingly, chloramphenicol was not shown to be a risk factor; only sulfonamide exposure reached statistical significance, and the etiologic fraction for drugs in AA was only approximately 15%.[105]

Associations between drug exposure and AA can be divided into two classes. Drugs used in cancer chemotherapy are selected for their cytotoxicity, and their regular, dose-dependent induction of marrow aplasia is an expected effect. Most AA associated with medical drug use in the community is described as idiosyncratic, meaning that its occurrences are unexpectedly rare. Many of the drugs implicated in AA also appear to cause other, milder forms of marrow suppression

Table 29–3 Classification of Drugs and Chemicals Associated with Aplastic Anemia

I. Agents that regularly produce marrow depression as a major toxic effect when used in commonly employed doses or normal exposures

Cytotoxic drugs used in cancer chemotherapy
Alkylating agents (busulfan, melphalan, cyclophosphamide)
Antimetabolites (antifolic compounds, nucleotide analogs) antimitotics (vincristine, vinblastine, colchicine)
Some antibiotics (daunorubicin, doxorubicin [Adriamycin])
Benzene (and less often benzene-containing chemicals: kerosene, carbon tetrachloride, Stoddard solvent, chlorophenols)

II. Agents probably associated with aplastic anemia but with a relatively low probability relative to their use

Chloramphenicol
Insecticides
Antiprotozoals (quinacrine and chloroquine)
Nonsteroidal antiinflammatory drugs (including phenylbutazone, indomethacin, ibuprofen, sulindac, diclofenac, naproxen, piroxicam, fenoprofen, fenbufen, aspirin)
Anticonvulsants (hydantoins, carbamazepine, phenacemide, ethosuximide)
Gold, arsenic, and other heavy metals such as bismuth and mercury
Sulfonamides as a class
Antithyroid medications (methimazole, methylthiouracil, propylthiouracil)
Antidiabetes drugs (tolbutamide, carbutamide, chlorpropamide)
Carbonic anhydrase inhibitors (acetazolamide, methazolamide, mesalazine)
D-Penicillamine
2-Chlorodeoxyadenosine

III. Agents more rarely associated with aplastic anemia

Antibiotics (streptomycin, tetracycline, methicillin, ampicillin, mebendazole and albendazole, sulfonamides, flucytosine, mefloquine, dapsone)
Antihistamines (cimetidine, ranitidine, chlorpheniramine)
Sedatives and tranquilizers (chlorpromazine, prochlorperazine, piperacetazine, chlordiazepoxide, meprobamate, methyprylon, remoxipride)
Antiarrhythmics (tocainide, amiodarone)
Allopurinol (can potentiate marrow suppression by cytotoxic drugs)
Ticlopidine
Methyldopa
Quinidine
Lithium
Guanidine
Canthaxanthin
Thiocyanate
Carbimazole
Cyanamide
Deferoxamine
Amphetamines

Table 29–4 Drugs Associated with Aplastic Anemia in the International Aplastic Anemia and Agranulocytosis Study*

Drug	Stratified Risk Estimate (95% CI)	Multivariate Relative Risk Estimate (95% CI)
Nonsteroidal analgesics		
Butazones	3.7 (1.9–7.2)	5.1 (2.1–12)
Indomethacin	7.1 (3.4–15)	8.2 (3.3–20)
Piroxicam	9.8 (3.3–29)	7.4 (2.1–26)
Diclofenac	4.6 (2.0–11)	4.2 (1.6–11)
Antibiotics		
Sulfonamides†	2.8 (1.1–7.3)	2.2 (0.6–7.4)
Antithyroid drugs	16 (4.8–54)	11 (2.0–56)
Cardiovascular drugs		
Furosemide	3.3 (1.6–7.0)	3.1 (1.2–8.0)
Psychotropic drugs		
Phenothiazines	3.0 (1.1–8.2)	1.6
Corticosteroids	5.0 (2.8–8.9)	3.5 (1.6–7.7)
Allopurinol	7.3 (3.0–17)	5.9 (1.8–19)
Gold	29 (9.7–89)	

CI, confidence interval.
*The multivariate model included the following factors: age, gender, geographic area, date of interview, reliability of the patient, person interviewed, transfer from another hospital, history of blood disorder or tuberculosis, exposure to benzene and related chemicals, and use of other suspected drugs.
†Other than trimethoprim-sulfonamide combination.
From Kaufman DW, Kelly JP, Levy M, Shapiro S: The Drug Etiology of Agranulocytosis and Aplastic Anemia. New York, Oxford University Press, 1991.

such as neutropenia. Although difficult to prove, some dose relationship probably does exist even for idiosyncratic reactions. In most case reports, patients received normal or high doses of the agent, usually for a period of weeks to months. Drug-induced aplasia cannot be distinguished by history from idiopathic forms of the disease; the clinical course, including the favorable response to immunosuppressive therapy, of patients with histories of drug exposure are the same as in idiopathic disease.[106]

The low probability of developing AA after a course of drugs may be a reflection of the gene frequency for metabolic enzymes (for direct chemical effects) or immune response genes (for immune-mediated marrow failure) in the population. The rarity of idiosyncratic drug reactions could then arise from the infrequent combination of unusual circumstances: exposure, genetic variations in drug metabolism, the physical properties of the agent, enzymatic pathways that chemically alter the drug, and the susceptibility of the host to the action of a toxic compound. Many drugs and chemicals, especially if they have limited water solubility, must be enzymatically degraded before conjugation and excretion. Degradative pathways for xenobiotics are complex, specific, redundant, and interrelated. Intermediate metabolites in complex degradation pathways can be toxic, highly reactive, and responsible for some adverse effects of the primary agents. Examples of detoxifying enzyme systems directly applicable to bone marrow failure and that also demonstrate genetic variability include arylhydrocarbon hydroxylase (eg, benzene toxicity), epoxide hydrolases (eg, phenytoin toxicity), *S*-methylation (eg, 6-mercaptopurine, 6-thioguanine, azathioprine) and *N*-acetylation (eg, sulfa drugs). The role of genetic background was shown in experiments using cells of a patient with carbamazepine-associated AA. Only after generation of reactive metabolites from the incriminated agent by rat microsomes were the patient's lymphocytes killed in a dose-dependent, drug-specific pattern.[107] These metabolites were not toxic to normal donors' cells and displayed intermediate toxicity toward cells of the patient's mother.

Benzene

Benzene is convincingly linked to AA.[108–111] Benzene myelotoxicity can be placed between the predictable effects of chemotherapeutic agents and idiosyncratic drug reactions. Industrial emissions add greatly to the biologic sources of ambient benzene. Significant benzene exposure can also occur outside of industry. Although the concentrations of benzene to which consumers are exposed are orders of magnitude lower than those observed in industrial workers, the effect of low-dose chronic exposure is uncertain, but genetic variations in the metabolizing enzymes may influence susceptibility to marrow suppression at these levels.[109] Benzene metabolites are also generated from the diet.[110]

Water-soluble products of benzene metabolism such as phenols, hydroquinones, and catechols mediate the toxicity to the marrow. Benzene and its intermediate metabolites covalently and irreversibly bind to bone marrow DNA, inhibit DNA synthesis, and introduce DNA strand breaks. Benzene acts as a "mitotic poison" and as a mutagen. Acutely, the more mature, actively cycling marrow precursor cells are preferentially damaged over the more primitive progenitors.[111] Intermittent exposure may be more damaging to the stem cell compartment than is continuous exposure.[111] Marrow stroma can also be damaged by benzene.[112]

The range of hematologic disease attributable to benzene is broad, from relatively frequent mild alterations in blood counts to AA or leukemia. Studies of exposed North American workers earlier in the 20th century suggested that the risk of AA was 3% to 4% in men exposed to concentrations higher than 300 ppm and that 50% of individuals exposed to 100 ppm developed some blood cell count depression.[113] The prevalence of some form of marrow suppression with heavy exposure can be high; more than 10% of workers developed leukopenia, and with improved hygiene, the figure was lowered to 0.5%.[114] Leukopenia, anemia, thrombocytopenia, and lymphocytopenia are common consequences of benzene; other manifestations include macrocytosis, acquired Pelger-Huet anomaly, eosinophilia, basophilia, and less often, polycythemia, leukocytosis, thrombocytosis, or splenomegaly. The marrow is usually normocellular but can show hypocellularity or hypercellularity;[113] a hypercellular phase can precede complete aplasia. In addition to hypocellularity, chronically exposed workers can have marrow necrosis, fibrosis, edema, and hemorrhage.[115] AA and acute myelogenous leukemia (AML) have occurred in the same person,[116] and pancytopenia preceded acute leukemia in one-fourth of industrial workers.[117] Marrow failure and leukemia in benzene workers can manifest decades after exposure.

Aromatic Hydrocarbons

The common perception that other molecules resembling benzene or containing a benzene ring can also cause marrow suppression is not well supported. Neither the closely related alkylbenzenes nor pure toluene or xylene are established marrow toxins. Often, an aromatic hydrocarbon has been implicated by the clinician as a causative agent for AA for lack of another apparent cause. For some substances, toxicity can result from the presence of benzene as a contaminant of the synthesis of the molecule or in the petroleum distillates used to dissolve the compound. However, the total number of AA cases reported with aromatic hydrocarbon exposures is small when the large populations exposed to this heterogeneous group of chemicals are considered. For example, surveys of AA patients found that only 2% to 6% of cases were associated with insecticide exposure.[17,118,119] The significance of a handful of case reports associated with insecticide exposure in the context of the vast use of these compounds is questionable. However, the very high prevalence of aromatic hydrocarbons in daily life would greatly amplify even a small individual risk. Pesticides and insecticides have been associated with AA for decades, with almost 300 medical case reports appearing in the medical literature.[120] The most frequently cited insecticides are chlordane, lindane, and dichlorodiphenyltrichloroethane (DDT). For the miscellaneous aromatic hydrocarbons, case reports also greatly outnumber series of patients, and systematic epidemiologic surveys have shown mixed results. Significant excesses of cases of AA were found in workers in the printing industry (odds ratio [OR] = 6.2), in lumber and wood products industries (OR = 3.7), in agriculture workers (OR = 2.4), and in construction workers (OR = 2.0).

Chloramphenicol

Structural similarity of chloramphenicol to amidopyrine, a drug known to cause agranulocytosis, led to early prediction of possible hematotoxicity.[121,122] During the period of its unrestrained use, chloramphenicol was considered the most common cause of AA in the United States,[123] accounting for 20% to 30% of total cases and 50% of drug-associated cases.[124–126] Estimates of the risk of AA after a course of chloramphenicol ranged from 1 case per 20,000[125] to 1 case per 800,000 people.[127] Based on these figures, a course of chloramphenicol was estimated to increase the risk of AA 13-fold. Although the introduction of chloramphenicol into the American market was perceived as having increased the total number of cases of AA,[123,128] this assumption was only weakly supported by epidemiologic data, and the mortality from AA remained essentially constant during the period of chloramphenicol's introduction and extensive use and after the withdrawal of chloramphenicol from the market. In series reported from the United States and Europe, of a total of 394 patients, only 1 was found to have ingested the drug.[18,129] Chloramphenicol has not been associated with AA in Thailand, despite its high rate of use there. In Hong Kong, where the use of chloramphenicol is almost 100 times higher than in the West, drug-associated AA occurs infrequently.[130] The early epidemiologic surveys stressed excessive dosage, high blood levels, repeated or intermittent courses, young age, and oral route of administration as particular risks for chloramphenicol marrow toxicity. However, in a series of 600 cases, most patients had received a dose of less than 10 g.[131]

At ordinary doses, a pattern of reversible alterations in erythropoiesis occurs in most patients treated with chloramphenicol.[132] In vitro, chloramphenicol can decrease hematopoietic colony formation[133] or diminish colony size,[134] although usually at doses greater than those achieved in patients. Inhibition of marrow stromal cell proliferation[135] and the production of growth factors[136] have also been reported. There is no consistent evidence of abnormal marrow sensitivity to the drug in affected individuals. Chloramphenicol was also claimed to produce marked chromosome abnormalities in WBCs.[137] Others have proposed that chloramphenicol toxicity is the result of covalent binding of the drug to reactive oxidative metabolites, such as an oxalic acid derivative produced by P450 cytochrome-mediated oxidative dehalogenation to produce a chloramphenicol-free radical and hydroxylamine intermediate, all capable of acylating proteins.

Nonsteroidal Antiinflammatory Drugs

Compared with chloramphenicol, it took far longer to associate phenylbutazone with AA.[138] Mortality estimates have ranged from 1 case per 100,000 to 1 case per 1 million treatment courses.[139] The use of other NSAIDs is associated with case reports of AA. A large case-control led investigation in Europe confirmed the risk of AA with phenylbutazone use and identified even higher probabilities with other NSAIDs.[140] There was a suggestion of increased risk with drugs taken regularly for a prolonged period at very high doses, and in some cases, hematologic reactions were reproduced on repeat exposure.

Neuroleptics and Psychotropic Drugs

A variety of drugs used to treat disorders of the central nervous system have been associated with AA: the hydantoins and carbamazepine, antidepressants, tranquilizers, and felbamate. The marketing of felbamate was severely affected by the occurrence of aplasia in more than 30 patients.[141] Monitoring of drug blood levels and peripheral blood counts in patients receiving carbamazepine was recommended despite fewer than two dozen AA cases reported by 1982.[142] Doubt about the validity of many cases reported in the literature, as well as several large series of patients who did not develop hematologic toxicity[143] and an estimated AA case rate of approximately 1 in 200,000 treated patients,[144] have led to questions concerning the relationship between carbamazepine and AA.

Gold and Heavy Metals

Gold salts have an extraordinarily high frequency of fatal adverse reactions, estimated at 1.6 cases per 10,000 prescriptions. Dose-dependent leukopenia is common, but several dozen cases of AA have been reported.[145] In the IAAAS, exposure to gold salts was the most

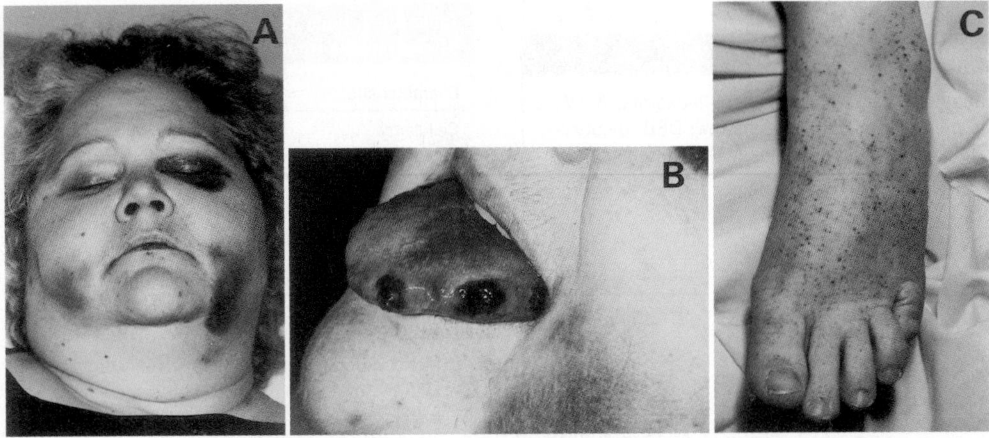

Figure 29–7 Clinical presentations of aplastic anemia. (**A**) Ecchymosis in pancytopenic women. (**B**) Submucosal hematomas. (**C**) Petechial eruptions in a thrombocytopenic patient.

Table 29–5 Presenting Symptoms of Aplastic Anemia

Symptoms	Number of Patients
Bleeding	41
Anemia	27
Bleeding and anemia	14
Bleeding and infection	6
Infection	5
Routine examination	8
Total	101

Adapted from Williams DM, Lynch RE, Cartwright GE: Drug induced aplastic anemia. Semin Hematol 10:195, 1973.

Table 29–6 Severity of Aplastic Anemia as Defined by Laboratory Studies

Severe aplastic anemia
Bone marrow cellularity <30%
Two of three peripheral blood criteria:
Absolute neutrophil count <500 cells/mm^3
Platelet count <20,000 cells/mm^3
Reticulocyte count <40,000 cells/mm^3
No other hematologic disease
Moderate aplastic anemia
Patients with pancytopenia who do not fulfill the criteria of severe disease

significant drug association for developing AA, with a relative risk of 29 and an excess risk of 23 cases per 1 million users in 1 week.[5] Spontaneous recovery rarely occurs.[146] Patients have been successfully treated with stem-cell transplantation or immunosuppressive therapy; chelation therapy usually has not been helpful.[147] High concentrations of gold salts inhibit hematopoietic colony formation in vitro.[148] There is some evidence for a dose relationship.[149]

Arsenic poisoning can result in neutropenia, anemia, and thrombocytopenia.[150] Organic arsenicals, originally used in the treatment of syphilis (arsphenamine) and now as antihelminthic (arsenamide), have also been associated with AA.[151]

TYPICAL AND ATYPICAL PRESENTATIONS

Most patients with AA seek medical attention for symptoms that occur as a result of low blood counts (Fig. 29–7 and Table 29–5). All of the blood elements can be depressed, or a decrease in a single lineage can dominate the clinical picture. However, the differential diagnosis of pancytopenia includes a variety of diseases (see Table 29–1). Except for complaints related to the blood counts, most patients do not have systemic symptoms. Weight loss, persistent fever, pain, and loss of appetite point to an alternative diagnosis.

Bleeding is the most alarming manifestation of pancytopenia and most frequently sends the patient to a doctor. Thrombocytopenia usually does not cause massive bleeding. Instead, the patient reports easy bruisability and the appearance of red spots, especially over dependent surfaces; gum bleeding with tooth brushing and episodic nosebleeds are common. Heavy menstrual flow or irregular vaginal bleeding can occur in younger women. In AA associated with PNH, there are reports of red or dark urine that is caused by free hemoglobin, but visible bleeding from the genitourinary and gastrointestinal tracts is rare on presentation in AA. Extensive hemorrhage from any organ can occur but usually late in the course of the disease and almost always associated with infections, drug therapy (eg, corticosteroids), or invasive procedures.

The ability to adapt to a gradual reduction in hemoglobin concentration is remarkable. The anemic patient might mention fatigue, lassitude, shortness of breath, or ringing in the ears, but some individuals can tolerate astonishingly low hemoglobin levels without complaint. Even abrupt cessation of erythropoiesis leads to only a slow decline in hemoglobin (approximately 1 g/dL each week).

Infection is an uncommon presentation in patients with AA. The sore throat of agranulocytosis is not often observed, presumably because other alarming symptoms appear earlier.

Retrospective studies of AA associated with drugs and viruses and the observation of the occasional patient with serially monitored blood counts suggest a latent period of 6 to 8 weeks between the inciting event and the onset of pancytopenia.[152] The interval can be more prolonged when pancytopenia is well tolerated or moderate. For purposes of diagnosis and management, a history of blood diseases in other family members is very important and should trigger appropriate genetic tests for constitutional causes.

Findings on physical examination usually reflect the severity of the pancytopenia (Table 29–6). However, patients with severe disease can look remarkably well. The patient can present with subtle variations from normal or with a dramatic, even toxic appearance. Petechiae are often present over the pretibial surface of the lower leg and the dorsal aspects of the forearm and wrist; a few petechiae can be seen in the oropharynx and on the palate. Scattered ecchymoses typi-

Diagnostic Algorithm in Aplastic Anemia

AA, aplastic anemia; AML, acute myelogenous leukemia; AMM, agnogenic myeloid metaplasia; BM, bone marrow; DEB, diepoxybutane; MDS, myelodysplastic syndrome; MMC, mitomycin C; PB, peripheral blood.

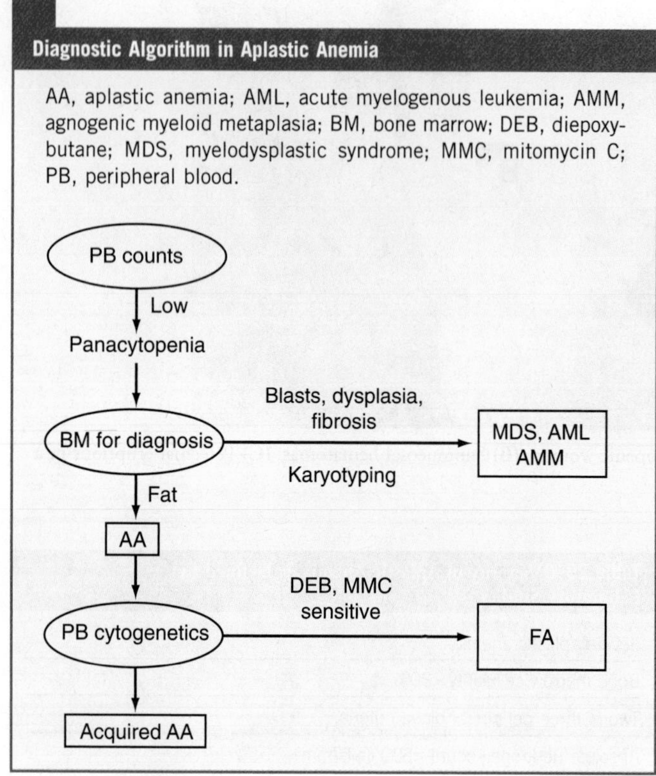

Table 29–7 Bone Marrow Morphologic Findings that Discriminate Myelodysplasia from Aplastic Anemia

Characteristic*	Myelodysplasia	Aplastic Anemia
Cellularity	Usually normal to increased	Decreased
Erythropoiesis		
Megaloblastic	Very common	Common
Dyserythropoietic	Very common	Unusual
Maturation defects	Common	Not found
Ringed sideroblasts	Common	Not found
Myelopoiesis		
Monocyte prominence	Very common	Unusual
Mid-myeloid predominance	Very common	Unusual
Increased blasts	Yes	Not found
Megakaryocytes		
Atypical morphology	Very common	Not found

*Ringed sideroblasts and myeloblasts are observed by definition in some of the myelodysplastic syndromes. Dyserythropoietic red blood cell precursors show bizarre forms with multiple or irregular nuclei. Megakaryocytes can show defective nuclear polyploidization and increased internuclear spaces, or they can be small with only a few nuclei and peculiar granulation.

Adapted from Bagby GC: The preleukemic syndrome (hematopoietic dysplasia). In Shahidi NT (ed): Aplastic Anemia and Other Bone Marrow Failure Syndromes. New York, Springer-Verlag, 1990, p 199, which provides percentages for myelodysplasia.

cally appear in areas exposed to minor trauma. With severe thrombocytopenia, retinal hemorrhages can be present on funduscopic examination, there can be gingival oozing or blood in the nares, and hemorrhage can be apparent at the uterine cervical os. The stool can contain traces of heme. Pallor is common and is best appreciated on the mucosal membranes and palmar surfaces. The new patient can be febrile, but specific or localizing signs of infection are uncommon on presentation. Cachexia, splenomegaly, and lymphadenopathy are not associated with AA, and these findings should strongly suggest another diagnosis. The examiner should look carefully for café au lait spots and other physical anomalies of Fanconi anemia and for leucoplakia and nail changes of dyskeratosis congenita in children *and* adults. Acquired AA is usually a diagnosis of exclusion, and evidence from the history or physical examination of another major disease suggest secondary pancytopenia; an exception is drug-associated aplasia, as in the patient with chronic rheumatoid arthritis.

Several atypical presentations of AA should be pointed out. A physician might encounter an elderly patient with pancytopenia in whom subsequent bone marrow examination reveals dysplastic features (box on Diagnostic Algorithm in Aplastic Anemia and Table 29–7). Although the history of the illness in a newly diagnosed patient is short—in the range of months—a few patients recall a long history of bruisability, anemia, and low blood-cell counts reported to them by previous physicians during routine examinations. These patients can have a moderately severe, chronic disease that is stable for years. Pancytopenia from childhood should suggest a constitutional AA. Some patients can be diagnosed incidentally and show remarkable few symptoms despite severely depressed blood counts.

CLINICAL ASSOCIATIONS

A number of clinical syndromes, usually revealed through a careful history and physical examination, are associated with AA (see box on Diagnostic Algorithm in Aplastic Anemia and Tables 29–2 and 29–3).

Posttransfusion Graft-Versus-Host Disease

Almost uniformly fatal AA is a constant feature of transfusion-associated GVHD, produced by the transfusion of competent lymphocytes into immunodeficient hosts, including children with congenital syndromes, cancer patients receiving high-dose chemotherapy, and patients with adoptive cellular immunotherapy for leukemia.[47] Rarely, posttransfusion GVHD occurs in an apparently immunocompetent recipient in the special circumstance in which the donor is homozygous for an HLA haplotype also shared by the recipient, as can occur among first-degree family members. Small numbers of lymphocytes are sufficient to produce the syndrome, which is surprisingly resistant to immunosuppressive therapy. Pancytopenia with marrow hypoplasia is an almost constant feature of posttransfusion GVHD. Runt disease in animals is a model of this immune-mediated marrow failure syndrome.[153,154]

Pregnancy

Pregnancy is common in the age groups most susceptible to marrow failure, and in many cases, its association is probably only coincidental. The true frequency of AA in pregnancy is unknown, but from the number of cases reported it appears rare,[155–157] although bone marrow hypoplasia may be relatively common during pregnancy. A causal relationship is suggested by the temporal relationship between the onset of pancytopenia and that of pregnancy and by resolution after delivery and spontaneous or induced abortion; some patients have developed AA that remitted after each delivery. Survival rates for AA in pregnancy have been relatively high for the mother (83%) and baby (75%), with most pregnancies successful (69%).[157] Hemorrhage is the most common cause of death from AA during pregnancy. The published data are insufficient to guide the management of the pregnant woman with AA, especially because it is clear that AA in some cases is serendipitously diagnosed and can persist beyond parturition. However, in one series,[158] successful pregnancies were reported, and the mortality rate was low. A woman who desires a child can be maintained with transfusions, with the understanding that any clinical deterioration is a criterion for interruption or termination of the pregnancy. The hazard of pregnancy to the woman who has recovered from idiopathic AA is unknown, but most hematologists, recognizing the risk of relapse, advise patients not to become pregnant, especially if thrombocytopenia and a PNH clone are present.[158]

Post Hepatitis Aplasia Anemia

The association of AA and acute, apparently viral hepatitis is not rare. Several hundred cases have been reported.[159–162] A prior history of hepatitis is recognized in 2% to 9% of AA patients in Western series.[163,164] Uncomplicated viral hepatitis is frequently associated with mild blood cell count depression, but severe pancytopenia with marrow aplasia is a rare sequela, estimated at less than 0.07% of total pediatric hepatitis cases[165] and 2% of patients with non-A, non-B hepatitis.[166] However, in patients, usually children, who develop hepatic failure after fulminant seronegative hepatitis, approximately one-third develop AA at the time of liver transplantation.[167]

Hepatitis-associated AA has several peculiar features.[160–162,168,169] Typically, an uneventful episode of apparent viral hepatitis in a young man is followed in 1 to 2 months, during convalescence from the liver inflammation, by very severe pancytopenia. Depression of blood cell counts during the course of hepatitis is common; leukopenia, atypical lymphocytosis, erythroid macrocytosis, and thrombocytopenia mimic in milder forms the hematologic changes of AA. However, posthepatitis AA has a very poor prognosis, with early estimates of mortality of 90% at 1 year,[160] and a history of hepatitis in AA has been considered an indication for early marrow transplantation. Patients with posthepatitis AA can successfully undergo marrow transplantation without an increased risk of veno-occlusive disease.[170] Patients with hepatitis-associated aplasia have markers of immune system activation and respond well to intensive immunosuppressive therapy.[161,171]

The putative viral agent in posthepatitis AA is unknown. Almost all cases have been non-A, non-B, non-C,[172,173] and non-G hepatitis by serology;[161] nor have hepatitis E or B19 parvovirus been convincingly associated.[174] Posthepatitis AA is linked to fulminant hepatitis of childhood and acute seronegative hepatitis. Acute viral hepatitis that is seronegative differs clinically from hepatitis C disease; parenteral exposure is not a risk factor, liver functions abnormalities are more severe during the acute phase, and late complications are more common.[175]

Postmononucleosis Aplastic Anemia

Acute infection with Epstein-Barr virus (EBV) causes infectious mononucleosis that is commonly associated with neutropenia and other hematologic abnormalities[176–178] but, like acute hepatitis, is only rarely complicated by AA.[179–181] However, EBV can be involved in the cause of AA more frequently than originally appreciated, because a large number of primary EBV infections are unrecognized.[180,182,183] Pancytopenia can be first observed during the acute mononucleosis syndrome or shortly after disappearance of symptoms. Some patients have recovered spontaneously, and others have recovered after therapy with corticosteroids or ATG. EBV can occasionally be demonstrated in the bone marrow cells of patients with apparently idiopathic AA, in association with serologic evidence of a primary or reactivated viral infection. Some patients with EBV-associated AA can respond to antiviral therapy.[180,184–186] For those with severe disease, conventional therapeutic interventions should be implemented early.

Hemophagocytic Syndrome

The marrow is hypocellular in approximately one-third of cases with hemophagocytic syndrome. In this disorder, there can be progression from marrow hypercellularity to aplasia; myelofibrosis is also common. Pancytopenia occurs in 74% of cases. Anemia is a universal finding; thrombocytopenia (91%) and neutropenia (65%) are also common.[187] In contrast to typical AA, these patients appear systemically ill, with fever and constitutional symptoms, and peripheral blood-cell count depression is often associated with abnormalities of other organ systems: hepatosplenomegaly, lymphadenopathy, cutaneous eruptions, and pulmonary infiltrates.[187–189] Hemophagocytic syndrome is associated with a large variety of diseases, including immunodeficiency, malignancy, and infections. In the infectious category, viral infections are most common and include EBV, cytomegalovirus, herpes simplex, and herpes zoster.[187,190] B19 parvovirus, HIV-1, and bacterial and parasitic infections also have been associated with hemophagocytosis. Hemophagocytosis is often observed on supravital[191] or Wright-Giemsa staining[152] of the marrow of patients with idiopathic AA, and it is also a morphologic feature of graft rejection after marrow transplantation.[192] In virus-associated hemophagocytosis, there is evidence of immune system activation. The sera of patients contain high levels of IFN-γ, TNF-α, IL-6, soluble CD8, and soluble interleukin 2 (IL-2) receptor, and T cells overproduce IFN-γ in vitro.[193] The clinical response to cyclosporine is consistent with a T-cell–mediated pathophysiology of hematopoietic failure.[194]

Paroxysmal Nocturnal Hemoglobinuria and Aplastic Anemia

There is a strong association between AA and PNH (see Chapter 30).[195] These diseases frequently are diagnosed concurrently or sequentially in the same individual, and they share similar clinical and pathologic features (ie, pancytopenia and marrow hypocellularity). The presence of an expanded PNH clone is associated with HLA-DR15 and has been reported as a good prognostic factor for the responsiveness to immunosuppressive therapy.[24,196–199] Marrow failure can be present at the onset of PNH or can develop after diagnosis. In a retrospective review, marrow failure was especially prevalent among young patients, occurring in 58% of them.[200] In a cooperative study from France of 220 patients with PNH (defined by a positive Ham test), there was a previous history of AA in 30%, and for the remainder, the actuarial risk of developing pancytopenia was estimated at 14% at 4 years.[201] Conversely, AA can evolve into PNH months or years after successful immunosuppressive treatment; many patients have only a positive Ham test or a population of granulocytes lacking glycophosphoinositol-linked proteins. In one study, a presumptive diagnosis of PNH based on flow cytometry was made in almost 50% of AA cases at presentation,[202] and at least one-third of all AA cases probably contain PNH clones.[203–205] Longitudinal studies of patients with de novo PNH[206] or PNH developing from AA[207] indicate a low probability of spontaneous remission, and in many patients, the contribution of the PNH clones remains stable for years. Hemolytic disease can develop in approximately one-third of these patients or 10% of AA patients.[203]

In the setting of marrow failure, PNH could develop as a result of an intrinsic growth or survival advantage for the somatically mutated cell or because of extrinsic selection of cells bearing the *PIGA* defect; most evidence favors the latter possibility. Supporting an extrinsic mechanism are the presence of multiple genetically different *PIGA* mutations in a single patient;[208] apparent in vivo selection for the development of PNH-like lymphocytes occurs in lymphoma patients treated with alemtuzumab (Campath-1), a monoclonal antibody that incidentally recognizes a glycophosphoinositol-linked protein;[209] and lack of a growth advantage for *PIGA* knock-out cells in vitro[210] and in vivo.[211] Increased rates of apoptosis within phenotypically normal, compared with PNH CD34, cells derived from the same patient are consistent with selective escape of the mutated cells from an immune attack.[212,213]

Collagen Vascular Diseases

AA is a component of the collagen vascular syndrome called eosinophilic fasciitis.[214–216] This severe, scleroderma-like disease is characterized by fibrosis of subcutaneous and fascial tissue, localized skin induration, eosinophilia, hypergammaglobulinemia, and an elevated erythrocyte sedimentation rate. The rheumatologic symptoms of fasciitis respond to corticosteroids, but the associated AA has a very poor prognosis. A few patients have survived after bone marrow transplantation or immunosuppressive therapy. More rarely, AA has complicated systemic lupus erythematosus and rheumatoid arthritis, but in many cases, the role of concomitant drug therapy is confounding.[217] Rarely, AA can accompany Sjögren syndrome,[218] multiple sclerosis,[219] and immune thyroid disease.[219] AA occasionally occurs in individuals with hypogammaglobulinemia or congenital immunodeficiency syndrome,[52] thymoma, or thymic hyperplasia.[53,54]

LABORATORY EVALUATION

Peripheral Blood

In typical cases of AA, all the blood cell counts are depressed. The blood smear usually shows obvious paucity of platelets and leukocytes but normal RBC morphology; toxic granulations can be present in neutrophils. Automated cell counting shows erythrocyte macrocytosis and a normal red cell distribution of width. Platelet size is normal and not increased as in immune peripheral destruction, but the low number can cause greater heterogeneity of size. Prior transfusions alter platelet numbers, relative reticulocyte counts, and hemoglobin values. Although relative lymphocytosis is very common, most patients also have decreased absolute numbers of monocytes[220] and lymphocytes. The severity of AA can be graded based on the peripheral blood cell counts (see Table 29–6 and box on Diagnostic Algorithm in Aplastic Anemia).

DIAGNOSIS OF APLASTIC ANEMIA

Although the ultimate diagnosis of AA rests on the interpretation of an adequate bone marrow biopsy specimen, important clues to the cause of pancytopenia can be obtained from the history, physical examination, and laboratory data. Pancytopenia that is not primarily hematologic in origin but secondary to other disease processes is usually an obvious diagnosis. Patients with severe liver disease and splenomegaly, systemic lupus erythematosus, or overwhelming sepsis can have low blood cell counts, but their clinical presentation is not subtle. Similarly, bone marrow aplasia follows cytotoxic drug therapy for cancers and is an anticipated and transient toxic effect for a variety of nonmalignant diseases. In the challenging case, obvious medical causes of pancytopenia usually have already been excluded. Pancytopenia almost never results from peripheral blood cell destruction alone. In AA, the blood smear does not show reticulocytes, band forms, or the large platelets typical of increased compensatory bone marrow efforts.

Acquired AA is a disease of the young, as is constitutional aplasia. Patients with Fanconi anemia often, but not always, have physical abnormalifies. In the absence of a suggestive family history or the presence of physical anomalies, the distinction between acquired and constitutional disease depends on the results of a clastogenic-stress culture of peripheral lymphocytes (for Fanconi anemia) and increasingly on genetic testing for mutations in the fanconi anemia (FA), telomere repair, and other genes.

In most older patients, the major differential diagnosis is between AA and myelodysplasia. There is a gray area between hypocellular myelodysplasia and moderate aplastic anemia, and competent hematologists might not agree on the final diagnosis. Bone marrow cytogenetics can help in establishing the proper diagnosis.

Myelofibrosis can also produce pancytopenia, but the bone marrow is not aspirable, the spleen is often enlarged, and the peripheral blood smear shows characteristic abnormalities. Acute leukemia in children and the elderly can manifest as bone marrow hypocellularity, requiring a careful search for lymphoblasts or myeloblasts, including phenotypic analysis by flow cytometry. Peripheral blood flow cytometry for glycophosphoinositol-anchored proteins should be performed to diagnose PNH (see Chapter 30).

The patient's history can provide clues, such as benzene exposure for myelodysplasia and acute leukemia or a suspicious drug history for AA. Discontinuation of exposure to the incriminated drugs or chemicals is mandatory, and in some instances, patients may then recover. However, given the difficulty of assigning blame with absolute certainty to environmental agents, we treat all patients similarly and do not advocate protracted observation for possible spontaneous recovery. For patients with severe disease (see Table 29–6), suitable and early preparation for bone marrow transplant should be undertaken or immunosuppression begun, whereas for those with moderate disease, the clinical status should be evaluated, and serial blood cell counts are required to assess progression of the disease.

BONE MARROW

The marrow must be assessed quantitatively and qualitatively for cellularity and the morphology of residual cells (Fig. 29–8 and see Fig. 29–1). Marrow aspiration and biopsy should always be performed, and the core specimen should be at least 1 cm long. There should be no compromise in obtaining adequate specimens and no hesitation in performing a second procedure if required.

Bone marrow cellularity is best estimated from the core biopsy. Point counting under microscopic cross hairs in many parts of a histologic section[221] is the most accurate method of determining cellularity, but hematologists commonly rely on visual estimation only.[222] A crude "eyeball" approximation is almost always adequate in severe aplasia, because the hematopoietic content of the marrow specimen is usually close to zero. Estimates of marrow cellularity based on examination of the aspirate smear and biopsy specimen are correlated, but dilution of the aspirate by sinusoidal blood often occurs, and the aspirate can be hypocellular when the biopsy specimen is hypercellular[223] or can show focal areas of active hematopoiesis.[224] Normal marrow cellularity decreases considerably with age, a variation that is of some importance in assessing the older patient with aplasia or myelodysplasia. In autopsy samples from normal, young children, approximately 80% of the marrow space of the iliac crest is cellular (range, 60% to 100%);[225] marrow from the sternum, vertebrae, and long bones is usually 100% cellular in infants;[226] for sternal aspirates, cellularity ranges from 35% to 80%.[227] Marrow cellularity gradually decreases from age 20 to 70 years and more precipitously in the very elderly, to approximately 30% in the eighth decade of life.[225] For practical purposes, the lower limit of normal marrow cellularity in adults is accepted at approximately 30%, but the differences at the extremes of life should be recalled when evaluating infants and the elderly. In most patients with AA, total marrow cellularity is extremely low, but there can be significant residual lymphocytosis. The increase in marrow fat in aplasia is caused by increases in the size and number of individual fat cells. "Hot pockets" of hematopoiesis can be present.[228] The marrow tends to contract centripetally with age, and a similar process can be observed in pathologic states, so the sternal bone marrow can be more cellular than iliac crest samples.

Examination of the bone marrow (Figs. 29–8 and 29–9 and see Fig. 29–1) is basic for the diagnosis of most primary hematologic causes of pancytopenia (see Table 29–1 and box on Diagnostic Algorithm in Aplastic Anemia). Information can be gained by observing the marrow aspirate itself. A fatty, even watery specimen can usually be aspirated without difficulty from an aplastic patient, whereas a truly dry tap is more typical of a packed or fibrotic bone marrow. The morphology of individual cells is best seen in the Wright-Giemsa–stained aspirate smear, and the architecture of the marrow is appreciated in a biopsy section. In acellular specimens, the only cells visible are usually lymphocytes, plasma cells, and stromal elements—fibroblastoid and histiocytic cells. Some degree of dyserythropoiesis is common, usually the megaloblastoid features of macrocytosis and some nuclear-cytoplasmic maturation asynchrony, but sometimes more complex degenerative changes in nuclei and cytoplasm can be

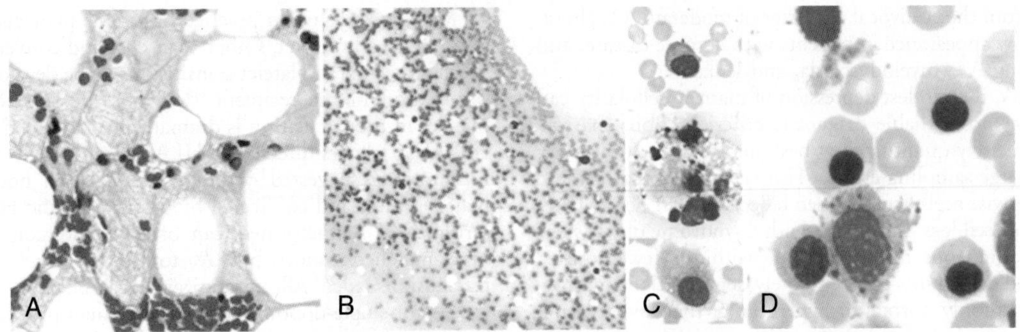

Figure 29–8 SOME MORPHOLOGIC FEATURES OCCASIONALLY OBSERVED IN PATIENTS WITH APLASTIC ANEMIA. (A–D). Empty marrow with eosinophilic ground substance consistent with serous atrophy or stomal injury (**A**), possibly indicative of marrow damage. Scanty marrow aspirate in severe disease (**B**) showing only rare nucleated elements many of which are from blood. Presence of plasma cells, histiocytes and osteoblasts (**C**) confirms marrow nature of aspirate. Note: sometimes the histiocytes can show hemophagocytosis. Megaloblastoid erythropoiesis (**D**) is sometimes seen in aplastic anemia and in recovery.

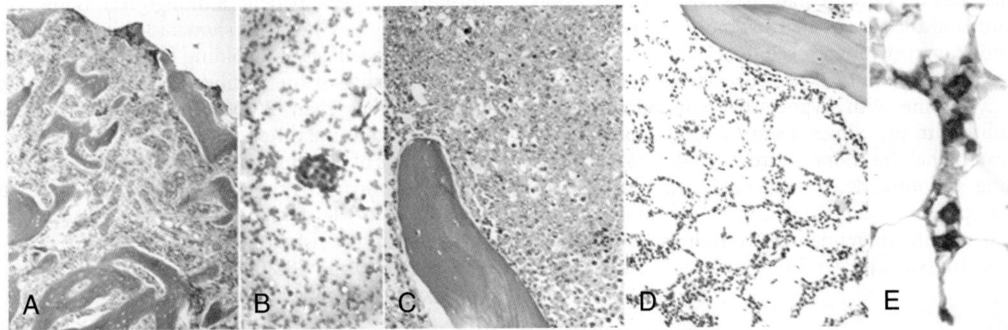

Figure 29–9 MORPHOLOGY OF OTHER DISEASES THAN MAY MANIFEST WITH PANCYTOPENIA. (A–E). Bone marrow biopsy from patient with pancytopenia showing myelofibrosis and osteosclerosis associated with metastatic prostate cancer (**A**). The aspirate was hypocellular but did show occasional tumor clusters (**B**). Another case where the patient presented with pancytopenia and was found to have a bone marrow packed with lymphoma cells (**C**). Hairy cell leukemia can present with pancytopenia and with a hypocellular bone marrow (**D**) difficult to distinguish from aplastic anemia. The diagnosis rests on identifying a B-cell infiltrative process with immunohistochemical stains (**E,** CD20).

observed by light[229] and electron[230] microscopy (see Fig. 29–8). These features are common to AA and myelodysplasia (see Table 29–7), which can be very difficult to distinguish.[231] Hemophagocytosis of RBCs can also be seen in AA. Examination of the cells close to the spicules of a sparse aspirate smear can disclose a distinctive population of leukemic blasts; increased numbers of myeloblasts are not seen in AA and are evidence of aleukemic leukemia or herald the evolution of leukemia from pancytopenia.[232] Lymphoid aggregates, nests of tumor cells, granulomas, and infectious particles can be apparent on examination of the fixed biopsy specimen.

Karyotyping of marrow cells is diagnostically important. Unfortunately, the yield of cells from a hypocellular marrow can be inadequate to perform cytogenetic analysis. Chromosome analysis is usually normal in AA[231] but frequently reveals a clonal abnormality in myelodysplasia.[233,234]

Radiographic Measures of Bone Marrow Function

Magnetic resonance imaging (MRI) with spin-echo sequences can be useful in the study of bone marrow disease. On T1-weighted spin-echo images, fatty marrow appears bright and cellular marrow exhibits a lower density signal (see Fig. 29–9). The high fat content of aplastic bone marrow can be readily appreciated on MRI. Magnetic resonance (MR) spectroscopy, which detects the type of fat signal, has shown diverse patterns among AA patients.[235] MRI is complementary to tissue sampling, allowing a large area of marrow to be visualized and fat content to be roughly quantified. The technique appears to be worthwhile in diagnosis, because the patterns of fat and cell distribution appear to differ between aplasia and hypocellular myelodysplasia, and in prognosis, to monitor improvements in hematopoiesis after treatment.[236]

DIFFERENTIAL DIAGNOSIS OF PANCYTOPENIA

AA is not the most common cause of pancytopenia (see Table 29–1). In one study of 100 pancytopenic cases, a diagnosis of AA could be made in only 19, despite prescreening for systemic or malignant diseases.[237] A rational diagnostic algorithm can be very helpful in establishing a correct diagnosis (see box on Diagnostic Algorithm in Aplastic Anemia). Pancytopenia is unlikely to be the presenting feature of hypersplenism in cirrhosis or of Evans syndrome in systemic lupus erythematosus. Findings on physical examination can point strongly toward another diagnosis. For example, the patient with myelofibrosis usually has splenomegaly, whereas a large spleen is very unusual in AA. Although vitamin B_{12} and folate deficiencies have been reported to be associated with erythroid hypoplasia,[238] this must be an exceedingly rare event. For the practicing hematologist, the most important and difficult choice of diagnoses in pancytopenic patients is among the primary bone marrow disorders. An empty bone marrow is usually obvious, but diagnostic confusion arises from the equivocal character of moderate AA, alterations in the marrow appearance in patients with chronic disease, and real overlaps among AA, myelodysplasia, and leukemia.

In moderate AA, the modest depression of marrow cellularity can muddle the single most reliable diagnostic criterion. Bone marrow cellularity is imprecisely quantitated at best, and further uncertainty is introduced by large sampling errors. "Hot spots" of hematopoietic activity in an otherwise acellular specimen reflect biologic heterogeneity in the pattern of cell loss. In patients with a syndrome of transient pancytopenia, spontaneous recovery occurs within a few months; although the blood cell counts can be severely depressed, the marrow is much more commonly normal or hypercellular than hypoplastic. In patients with chronic bone marrow failure, serial bone marrow specimens may not be identical because of sampling error or because the original disease was misdiagnosed or has changed its character. Some patients with AA are not pancytopenic; they do not have uniform depressions of RBC, WBC, and platelet production, despite an empty bone marrow, and their clinical course is dominated by failure in two cell lines or a single hematopoietic lineage. Related conditions such as pure red cell aplasia, amegakaryocytic thrombocytopenia, and agranulocytosis, although usually distinctive in their clinical presentation, can evolve into more generalized marrow failure. In the absence of better markers, sometimes the only accurate diagnosis is a description of the clinical features and the specific marrow morphology.

A hypocellular bone marrow often precludes the proper morphologic diagnosis. This problem can be especially evident in the case of a myelodysplastic syndrome with hypoplastic bone marrow (see Table 29–7). In addition to the clinical features, more sophisticated laboratory studies can be helpful. Bone marrow cytogenetics, if positive for chromosome abnormalities, can facilitate the diagnosis of leukemia or myelodysplastic syndrome. Conventional bone marrow examination is not helpful in differentiating AA from Fanconi anemia or dyskeratosis congenita (see Chapter 28).

TREATMENT

AA should be considered a medical emergency. Lives are lost, mainly because the grave consequences of severe pancytopenia go unrecognized. The ultimate benefits of definitive therapies such as transplantation or immunosuppression will be unrealized if the patient succumbs to an early clinical catastrophe. A haphazard transfusion policy increases the risk of graft rejection after marrow transplantation, but an overly conservative approach to transfusion can jeopardize the patient's life and increase morbidity. Supportive management therefore requires meticulous attention to the daily problems that occur as a consequence of pancytopenia and appreciation of their impact on the ultimate possibilities for cure or amelioration of AA. AA can be cured by replacement of stem cells, by bone marrow transplantation, and by immunosuppressive therapy. Androgens and hematopoietic growth factors have secondary roles (box on Treatment Algorithm in Aplastic Anemia).

Supportive Management

Bleeding

Bleeding was historically a common symptom in AA, and death from hemorrhage occurred frequently in the premodern era. Platelet transfusions have substantially improved survival in patients with this disease. Measurable correction of the platelet count by transfusion almost always alleviates the minor mucocutaneous bleeding common in thrombocytopenic patients. Major bleeding usually is not caused by thrombocytopenia alone, and ancillary explanations for massive hemorrhage should be sought. The bleeding time improves after erythrocyte transfusion in patients with anemia, and there is a strong inverse correlation between the hematocrit and bleeding.[239] The treatment of serious hemorrhage should include correction of severe anemia and RBC transfusions.

Modern transfusion practice has made platelets readily available and safe to administer. Other than cost and convenience, the major problem related to platelet transfusions is the development of alloimmunization in the recipient.[240,241] The life span of the transfused platelet in the circulation is dramatically shortened by host antibodies, almost always directed to HLA-A and HLA-B antigens. Alloimmunization is suggested by poor recovery of the 1-hour posttransfusion platelet count and confirmed by finding specific HLA antibodies in serum.[242,243] Refractoriness can often be overcome by selection of HLA-matched donors, but 6% to 39% of perfectly HLA-matched transfusions fail.[243] Alloimmunization can be prevented or delayed by the use of single-donor platelets rather than pooled platelets,[244] and by physical leukocyte depletion by filtration or ultraviolet treatment of blood products[245–247] Avoidance of platelet transfusions except when there is active bleeding is another alternative to prevent alloimmunization, but the dose relationship between exposure to different donors' platelets and the probability of developing refractoriness are not clearly established,[243] and only after more than 40 units have been administered does the risk of alloimmunization clearly increase.[248]

Prophylactic transfusion of platelets is not standard.[249,250] The primary indication for platelet prophylaxis is to prevent intracranial hemorrhage, but the risk of this complication in the chronically thrombocytopenic patient, although real, is low. Prophylactic platelet transfusions have not been shown to alter survival.[249–251] Nevertheless, the beneficial effects of avoiding bleeding complications and improving the quality of life justifies their use.[252] Maintenance of platelet counts higher than 20,000 platelets/μL decreases bleeding episodes,[253,254] but the threshold is based on an old study showing reduction in days of bleeding and serious hemorrhage among children with acute leukemia.[255] Although the 20,000 platelets/μL value has long been used to trigger transfusion, many reports have suggested little difference in the risk of bleeding over a wide range of platelet counts between 5000 and 100,000 platelets/μL.[256,257] In one study of a rigorous transfusion policy during induction therapy, fatal or severe bleeding episodes were rare and did not occur in patients with platelet counts higher than 10,000 platelets/μL; the worst bleeding episodes in these cases were associated with refractoriness to platelet transfusions.[258] In a randomized trial of patients with AML, the risk of major bleeding was no different when 10,000 or 20,000 platelets/μL was chosen as the threshold, whereas the lower value led to a 20% reduction in platelet use.[259] Any prophylaxis program must be modified to address the individual patient, but a goal of maintaining platelet counts higher than 5000 platelets/μL is reasonable.

Major surgery can be accomplished in the setting of thrombocytopenia. In one study, blood loss and morbidity rates were low even at platelet counts of less than 30,000 platelets/μL.[260]

Anemia

Other than to reduce the risk of graft rejection after receiving an allogeneic transplant, there is no reason to allow a patient to suffer the symptoms of anemia. After equilibrium is achieved, a constant amount of blood will be required to maintain a given hemoglobin concentration. Physically fit individuals are usually not symptomatic at hemoglobin concentrations higher than 7 g/dL; patients with underlying cardiovascular disease should be maintained at a higher level (≥9 g/dL). Iron chelation should be used in patients with unresponsive chronic anemia who have a reasonable expectation of survival.

Alloimmunization as a result of blood product administration increases the probability of graft rejection and mortality after marrow transplantation. Blood products from a potential marrow donor such as a sibling or a parent (who share histocompatability antigens) should be avoided. Small numbers of transfusions do not have a major deleterious effect on survival. The 5% risk of graft rejection after transplantation in entirely untransfused patients was increased to 15% with receipt of 1 to 40 units and to higher than 25% only in more heavily transfused patients.[261] An increased rate of graft rejection was observed in patients who had received more than 10 units

Treatment Algorithm in Aplastic Anemia

Algorithm-based selection of treatment for patients with aplastic anemia. ATG, antithymocyte globulin; BMT, bone marrow transplantation; CSA, cyclosporine A; HLA, human leukocyte antigen; IS, immunosuppression, TX, treatment.

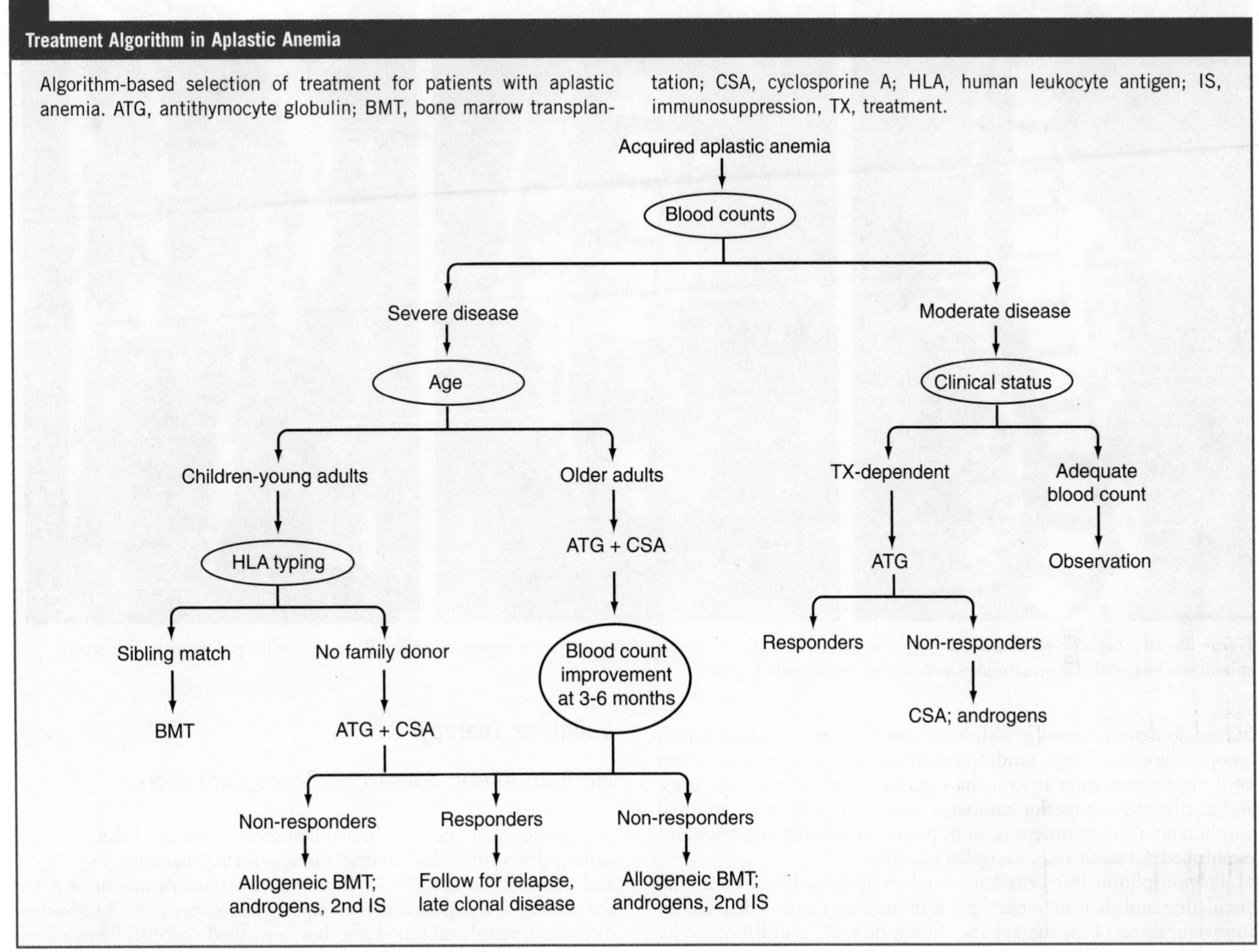

of erythrocytes or 40 or more units of platelets and would be anticipated to be lower with leucocyte-depletion methods of platelet preparations.[262] Speed in arranging tissue typing and transfer to an appropriate center has a greater impact on the survival of the patient than the judicious transfusion of a few units of RBCs to a severely anemic patient or platelets to a bleeding patient. Transfusions should not be withheld in an older patient in whom immunosuppressive therapy will be the first-line therapy.

Infection

There are very few specific reports of infections and their therapy in patients with AA.[220,263] The duration of neutropenia is the major difference between the neutropenia of bone marrow failure and that induced by cytotoxic chemotherapy. With longer periods of neutropenia, the probability of serious bacterial or fungal infection increases. A second major difference is that neutropenia is part of a complex of problems associated with malignant disease and its therapy. In AA, the immune system is activated, and with the exception of intravenous catheter placement, the integument is preserved. Studies of cancer patients have usually identified a low-risk category of neutropenia, determined by the relatively brief period of neutropenia; by this criterion, almost all unresponsive patients with AA are at high risk.

In classic studies of leukemic children, neutropenia was shown to increase susceptibility to bacterial infections, and the number of infectious episodes was quantitatively correlated with the degree and duration of neutropenia.[264,265] Susceptibility to infection is extremely high with an absolute neutrophil count of less than 200 platelets/μL, and this value has been used to define a category of very severe AA.[266] As severe granulocytopenia becomes prolonged, infection is inevitable.

Recommendations for initiation of empirical antibiotic therapy are similar for AA patients and other patients with neutropenia. The cardinal rule is, if the absolute neutrophil count is less than 500 cells/μL and infection is suspected, broad-spectrum parenteral antibiotic therapy should begin immediately. Any regimen can need modification based on results of cultures, new symptoms or signs, or a deteriorating clinical course. Bacteremia is present in only 20% of febrile neutropenic episodes, and in only approximately 40% of those can a microbiologic cause or localizing physical findings be identified.[267,268] Early discontinuation of antibiotics when cultures are unrevealing in persistently neutropenic patients is dangerous.

Patients often remain febrile despite antibiotic therapy, or fever reappears. In the absence of additional microbiologic data or clinical clues from the patient's complaints or physical examination, antifungal therapy should be instituted in patients who have remained febrile despite adequate antibacterial therapy. Current infectious disease guidelines recommend introduction of antifungal therapy after five days,[269] but earlier addition can be advisable in the AA patient, especially if there are findings on chest tomography and a positive test for galactomannan protein. Fungemia during an initial febrile episode is rare, but fungal infection becomes more likely with repeated courses of antibiotics and ultimately is the major cause of death in AA patients in whom definitive therapy fails.[270] *Candida* and *Aspergillus* species account for almost all fungal diseases in AA.[270] Early aggressive treatment of neutropenic patients can reverse fungal

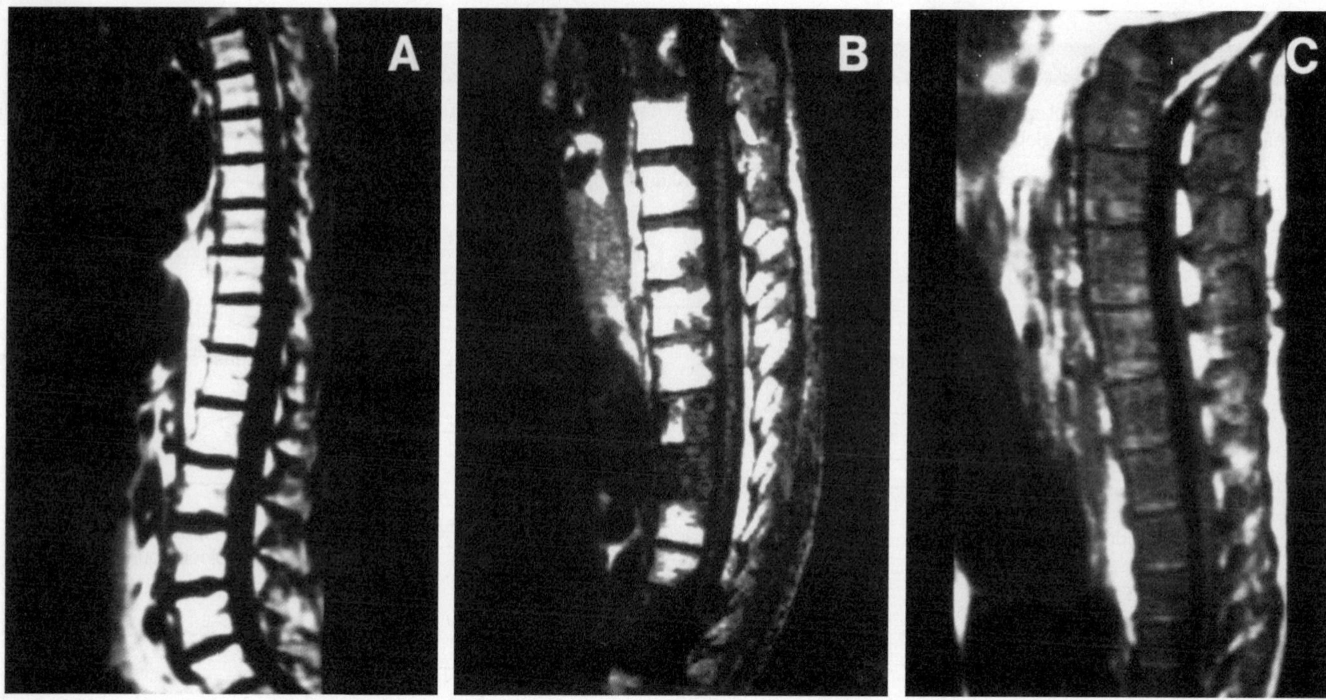

Figure 29–10 Magnetic resonance imaging of bone marrow (**A**) in a young man with severe aplastic anemia, (**B**) in a middle-aged woman with severe aplastic anemia, and (**C**) in a middle-aged woman with myelodysplasia.

disease, as demonstrated in individual cases[271] and by comparison of autopsy series.[272] Large randomized trials have shown that newer antifungal agents such as voriconazole and caspofungin are less toxic and as effective or superior compared to amphotericin and liposomal amphotericin for treatment of both persistent neutropenic fever and established *Candida* and *Aspergillus* infection.[273–276]

Polymorphonuclear cells have a relatively brief life span in the circulation and their major activity is in infected tissue. There are no simple measures of the therapeutic efficacy of WBC transfusions. The absolute neutrophil count is not measurably increased by standard transfusions. Nonetheless, several controlled trials performed in the 1970s reported improved survival in patients who received granulocyte transfusions; the negative studies were criticized because of the relatively low numbers of granulocytes transfused ($<10^{10}/m^2$/day).[277–279] Granulocyte transfusions are expensive and associated with serious toxicity: severe febrile reactions, pulmonary capillary leak syndrome, an increased risk of infection, and inevitable alloimmunization. A meta-analysis of published studies suggested that granulocyte transfusions helped in patients with sepsis unresponsive to antibiotics if adequate cell numbers were administered (2 to 3×10^{10}/day), donor and recipient were compatible, and the patients treated were unlikely to have imminent improvement in marrow function.[280] Later studies suggested that if sufficient numbers of granulocytes can be harvested, granulocyte transfusions could be beneficial in the management of refractory infections in neutropenic patients.[281]

Cytokines offer a strategy for increasing the efficiency of donor harvests. Administration of GCSF to normal donors greatly increases the yield of leukapheresis without adverse effects on the volunteers.[282,383] The addition of dexamethasone to GCSF results in granulocyte yields higher than GCSF or dexamethasone alone.[284,285] Excellent results can be obtained from community donors,[286] and the use of allocompatible granulocytes (as determined by lymphocytotoxicity screening assay) can further improve clinical results of granulocyte transfusions.[286] Large numbers of neutrophils can be obtained, allowing dramatic increases in the absolute granulocyte levels in neutropenic recipients, which can improve clinical outcomes; case reports and phase I and II studies have suggested that GCSF (GCSF plus dexamethasone)-mobilized granulocyte transfusions can be helpful in the treatment of life-threatening fungal infections in severely neutropenic patients.[287–291]

Definitive Therapy

Hematopoietic Stem Cell Transplantation

Allogeneic bone marrow transplantation from an HLA-matched sibling donor provides curative therapy for AA patients (Fig. 29–10 and Tables 29–8 and 29–9). Bone marrow transplantation in AA is the subject of a large number of reports and reviews.[292–296] Cytokine-mobilized peripheral blood also has been used successfully as a stem cell graft.[297–299] The convenience of this method probably has led to its substitution for marrow harvesting as the major method of stem cell collection in many circumstances, but whether results for patients with AA for both sources are equivalent remains uncertain[300] (see box on Treatment Algorithm in Aplastic Anemia).

The first studies of allogeneic bone marrow transplants conclusively demonstrated their value compared with conventional supportive therapy. In a controlled trial reported by the International Aplastic Anemia Study Group, patients with severe disease who received transplants early had an actuarial survival rate of more than 60%, compared with approximately 20% in patients who received androgens and blood transfusions only.[301] Results with marrow transplantation have improved over time because of a combination of factors: progressive modification of conditioning regimens and lower procedure-related early mortality, improved transfusion support and antibiotic regimens, and the introduction of cyclosporine as prophylactic therapy for GVHD. Analysis of the International Bone Marrow Transplant Registry data showed that 5-year survival rates climbed from 48% in the years 1976 to 1980 to 66% is 1988 to 1992.[302] Some hospitals now report very high rates of survival: 89% in Seattle at 8 years,[303,304] 79% in Baltimore,[305] 89% and 95% at Viennese centers.[306,307] Registry data indicate lower survival values as the general experience for the same period, with 64% of patients who received transplants during the period of 1985 to 1991 alive at 5 years after the procedure.[308] Between 1990 and 1994, the European Group for Bone Marrow Transplantation (EGBMT) reported a 72% survival rate at 3.5 years.[309] In the latest update of the EGBMT, the long-term survival had further improved over the past 5 years to 80%[310,311] In the most favorable subgroup—untransfused or minimally transfused, young, uninfected patients—survival rates of 80% to 90% should be routinely achieved (see Fig. 29–10).[312] Overall,

Table 29–8 Results of Matched Sibling Donor Allogeneic Marrow Transplantation for Aplastic Anemia

Institution/Study	Years of Study	N	Age (median in years)	Graft Rejection/Failure	Acute GVHD	Chronic GVHD	Actuarial Survival
IBMTR[91]	1988–1992	471	20 (1–51)	16%	19%	32%	66% at 5 years
Vienna[307]	1982–1996	20	25 (17–37)	0%	26%	53%	95% at 15 years
EBMT[337]	1991–1998	71	19 (4–46)	3%	30%	35%	86% at 5 years
Seoul[215]	1990–1999	22	22 (14–43)	5%	10%	33%	95% at 5 years
Seoul[105]	1990–2001	64	28 (14–43)	18%	31%	19%	79% at 6 years
Hamburg[106]	1990–2001	21	25 (7–43)	5%	5%	5%	86% at 5 years
Paris[107]	1994–2001	33	20 (8–42)	6%	0%	42%	94% at 5 years
Sao Paulo[531]	1993–2001	81	24 (3–53)	22%	37%	39%	56% at 6 years
Taipei[532]	1985–2001	79	22 (4–43)	8%	7%	35%	74% at 5 years
Tunis[533]	1998–2001	31	19 (4–39)	16%	11%	3%	86% at 2 years
Seoul[534]	1995–2001	113	28 (16–50)	15%	11%	12%	89% at 6 years
London[111]	1989–2003	33	17 (4–46)	24%	14%	4%	81% at 5 years
Seattle[85,89]	1988–2004	94	26 (2–59)	4%	24%	26%	88% at 6 years
Mexico City[86]	2000–2005	23	25 (4–65)	26%	17%	26%	88% at 4 years

EBMT, European Group for Bone Marrow Transplant; GVHD, graft-versus-host disease; IBMTR; International Blood and Marrow Transplant Registry.
GVHD results are generally for grades II–IV and in patient at risk.
Only studies reporting ≥20 patients are tabulated.
In contrast to Table 29–1, response rates are not provided because, in surviving patients who do not experience primary graft rejection or secondary graft failure, full hematologic recovery with donor hematopoiesis is anticipated.

Table 29–9 Alternative Donor Stem Cell Transplantation for Severe Aplastic Anemia

Study	Year of Publication	N	Donor Source	Conditioning	Age (median in years)	Acute GVHD*	Chronic GVHD	Survival
Nagoya[360]	2001	15	MUD—11 MMUD—4	Cy/ATG/TBI	11 (3–19)	33%	13%	100% at 4 years
Great Britain[113]	2001	8	MUD—7 MMUD—1	Cy/CP/TBI	7 (0–10)	25%	0%	100% at 3 years
Japan Marrow Donor Program[358]	2002	154	MUD—79 MMUD—75	Cy ± TBI or LFI; Cy/ATG ± TBI or LFI	17 (1–46)	29%	30%	56% at 5 years
Memphis[114]	2004	9	MUD—4 MMUD—5	High CD34+ cell dose, TCD, Cy/ATG/TLI or TBI ± thiotepa	11 (6–16)	0%	0%	89% at 4 years
Gyeonggi-do[115]	2004	5	MUD	Cy/Flu/ATG	13 (7–18)	0%	0%	80% at 2 years
Guangzhou[98]	2004	6	UCB	Cy/ATG	26 (22–37)	0%	33%	66% at 2 years
Genova[95]	2005	38	MUD—33 MMRD—5	Cy/Flu/ATG	14 (3–37)	11%	24%	73% at 2 years
Philadelphia[116]	2005	12	MUD—4 MMUD—8	Partial TCD, TBI + Cy/Ara-C or Cy/TT or ATG	9 (1–20)	33%	25%	75% at 4 years
Seoul[117]	2005	13	MUD—12 MMUD—1	Cy/ATG	22 (15–34)	31%	62%	75% at 3 years
IBMTR[91]	2006	318	MUD—181 MMRD—86 MMUD—51	Various	16 (1–55)	48% for MUD	29% for MUD	39% at 5 years for MUD
Seattle[94]	2006	87	MUD—62 MMUD—25	Cy/ATG/TBI	19 (1–53)	70% for MUD	52% for MUD	61% at 5 years for MUD

ATG, anti-thymocyte globulin; CP, Campath; Cy, cyclophosphamide; Flu, fludarabine; GVHD, graft-versus-host disease; IBMTR, International Blood and Marrow Transplant Registry; LFI, limited field irradiation; MMRD, mismatched related donor; MMUD, mismatched unrelated donor; MUD, matched unrelated donor; TBI, total body irradiation; TCD, T-cell depletion; TLI, total lymphoid irradiation; TT, thiotepa; UCB, umbilical cord blood.
*GVHD results are generally for grades II–IV and in patient at risk.
Only studies reporting ≥5 patients are tabulated.

Therapy for Aplastic Anemia

After the diagnosis of acquired AA has been established, treatment options must be identified, considered carefully, and chosen with alacrity (see box on Treatment Algorithm in Aplastic Anemia). For patients with moderate disease (see Table 29–6), an expectant approach can be chosen based on a stable course and adequate blood counts, or for patients dependent on transfusion support, ATG (40 mg/kg/day for 4 days) can be given. Intradermal sensitivity testing with 50 ng/mL of ATG solution should be performed, and patients showing an immediate reaction should be desensitized. After assessment of the response, patients who improve should be monitored for hematologic signs of relapse, and nonresponders can be offered alternative therapy, such as androgens or cyclosporine. Daclizumab, a humanized monoclonal antibody to the IL-2 receptor, improved blood counts and relieved transfusion requirements in 6 of 16 patients who were able to be evaluated; this outpatient regimen had little toxicity.[82] In severe disease for which the prognosis with blood transfusion and antibiotic support alone is very poor, bone marrow transplantation from a histocompatible sibling or immunosuppression are accepted and effective therapies. Although large, retrospective analyses have shown that long-term survival rates from transplantation or immune therapy are equivalent, each has its own advantages and disadvantages. For children, bone marrow transplantation remains the treatment of choice if an appropriate family donor is available, because these patients have a low rate of GVHD, and the marrow disease is cured by stem cell replacement. The risk of therapy-related cancers can be increased, especially in children, after marrow transplantation. Adults with AA also successfully receive transplants, although the risk and severity of chronic GVHD and other treatment-related complications increase with age. Bone marrow transplantation has been performed in patients older than 50 years of age, and it is a reasonable approach in a younger adult, especially with more severe degrees of neutropenia.

Most patients with AA do not have an HLA-matched sibling donor, and immunosuppression is the treatment of choice in these cases. Patients with severe disease should receive a combination of ATG and cyclosporine. We recommend a regimen consisting of 40 mg/kg/day of horse ATG on days 1 to 4, followed by cyclosporine for 6 months at a dose of 12 mg/kg. Corticosteroids are added in moderate doses (1 mg/kg of prednisone or methylprednisolone) during the first 2 weeks to ameliorate serum sickness. Improvement should be expected within 6 months. This regimen has produced hematologic responses in approximately 70% of treated patients, who then have an excellent 5-year survival rate.

Although immunosuppressive therapy is relatively nontoxic, patients frequently relapse and require further treatment; however, relapse is not associated with a poor prognosis. A more serious problem is the development of late-onset hematologic clonal diseases, PNH (which may not be clinically significant), myelodysplastic syndrome, and rarely, acute myeloid leukemia. Immunosuppression can be considered ameliorative therapy in which bone marrow destruction may continue and abnormal stem cell clones develop.

For patients in whom immunosuppressive therapy fails, there are a number of options. For children, alternative donor bone marrow transplantation should be seriously considered; at the best centers, survival rates now are almost as good as with sibling donors. Adults do less well, primarily because of transplant-related mortality from the intensive conditioning regimen. Some patients respond to androgen therapy, and others to combinations of growth factors. Repeated immunosuppression in a patient in whom a first course of ATG and cyclosporine has failed is successful in about 30% of cases. High-dose cyclophosphamide can also be effective therapy for AA at presentation and in those patients refractory to ATG.

Patients with severe AA should not be subjected to useless early trials of corticosteroids or hematopoietic growth factors as the primary treatment. For the occasional patient who must decide between bone marrow transplantation and immunosuppression, the advice of experts familiar with this disease and careful counseling of the patient are advisable. Age and severity of neutropenia are decisive factors. A limited number of transfusions can be necessary to optimize the patient's condition before definitive therapy and are acceptable. Single-donor platelets should be given and can be obtained from HLA-compatible donors. In severely neutropenic patients, GCSF therapy can decrease the risk of life-threatening infections. In the absence of overt bleeding, platelet counts as low as 5000 cells/μL appear to be safe.

the survival rates reported from major centers are approximately 70%.[313,314]

Graft rejection and GVHD are the major complications of allogeneic transplantation in AA. Graft rejection is a major predictor of posttransplantation survival. In one study of transplantations performed between 1981 and 1986, 29% of deaths resulted from graft rejection, the single most common cause of mortality.[315] The rate of graft rejection decreased with intensification of the immunosuppressive conditioning regimen from 15% to 4% in Europe[315] and from 35% to between 10% and 15% in Seattle[316] and has remained stable in the past decade.[317] Graft rejection can be caused by the pathophysiology of AA, a finding supported by the unexpectedly high proportion of failures in unprepared patients receiving syngeneic transplants[318–321] and even in adequately preconditioned patients receiving syngeneic transplants.[322,323] In a group of untransfused patients who received allogeneic stem cells, the incidence of graft rejection was 10%, indicating that AA patients may be particularly sensitive to alloimmunization.[324] Nevertheless, the influence of the number of transfusions on graft rejection is relative, and modest numbers of blood donations (<40 units in the International Bone Marrow Transplant Registry experience[261] and less than 10 units of erythrocytes or 40 units of platelets in Seattle[262]) did not greatly increase the risk of graft rejection.

Matched Sibling Donor (Hematopoietic Stem Cell Transplantation [see Table 29–8])

Intensification of immunosuppressive conditioning regimens with the use of total-body[261,325,326] or lymphoid irradiation,[327,328] cyclosporine,[261,305] or ATG[303] reduces the risk of graft rejection. Such measures, however, have not been shown to influence long-term survival.[261,329,330] The effect of the conditioning program on graft rejection probably is achieved through elimination of the recipient's lymphocytes and of subsequent mixed hematologic chimerism, which is associated with rejection.[331,332] More rapid regeneration of bone marrow grafts has been observed when cyclosporine[3] was used,[333] and second transplantations have been successful when ATG was added to the conditioning regimen.[334] The effect of ATG or cyclosporine in the conditioning regimen on the rate of graft rejection has been tested in randomized studies.[303,335,336] Conditioning regimens that do not include irradiation now regularly achieve engraftment and avoid many of irradiation's long-term complications, especially late cancers. In a recent series of 81 patients who were prepared by cyclophosphamide plus ATG, sustained engraftment was achieved by 96%, and three of the four patients who rejected were successfully retransplanted; 88% of patients survived long-term.[85] The combination of cyclophosphamide plus fludarabine, with or without ATG, has achieved high rates of graft acceptance and survival even in heavily transfused patients who were transplanted with mobilized peripheral blood stem cells, months after proving refractory to immunosuppressive drugs.[86,87] The use of methotrexate and cyclosporine has not improved rates of GVHD compared with cyclosporine, but surprisingly, methotrexate was associated with a better survival rate for patients with AA transplanted from matched sibling donors.[337] Overall, the reported rejection rates range between 10% and 15%, account for 14% of deaths in the first 100 days after transplantation and 23% of deaths therafter.[313]

Rates of chronic GVHD vary and are related to patient selection and treatment regimens. Historically, age is the major risk factor for the development of chronic GVHD. The incidence of chronic GVHD ranged from 19% for patients between 0 and 10 years old to 46% for those between 11 and 30 years old and to 90% for patients older than 31 years in an older Seattle series.[338] With improved treatment regimens, patients have fared better, but additional studies have confirmed a higher incidence and more serious consequences of GVHD in older patients.[339,340] Children have a lower probability of suffering and dying from chronic GVHD.[341] In an EGBMT analysis, a significant survival difference was observed between those younger than 20 years of age (65%) and those older than 20 years of age (56%), but there was no survival difference between patients 21 to 30 years old and those 31 to 55 years old.[329] Young adults have fared better in other series,[342,343] although morbidity from severe GVHD disease was far more prevalent in the young adults than in children (43% versus 10%).[342,343] Overall, the acute GVHD rate between 1991 and 1997 was approximately 20% for patients younger than 20 years of age and 40% for those older than 40 years of age. In general, similar numbers were cited for chronic GVHD.[313]

In summary, excellent survival rates and low morbidity in younger patients make allogeneic bone marrow transplantation the treatment of choice for children and adolescents. Older adults have a higher risk of transplant-related morbidity and mortality. Younger adults have a good opportunity for cure with transplantation but face more complications than children. In addition to age, a prolonged interval between diagnosis and transplantation, multiple transfusions, and serious infections before transplantation are poor risk factors.

Matched Unrelated and Nonhistocompatible Family Donors (see Table 29–9)

Until recently, the lack of an HLA genotypically identical sibling donor has precluded marrow transplantation, excluding approximately 70% of patients with AA from access to this therapeutic option. Alternative potential donors include relatives who are phenotypically matched or partially matched and HLA phenotypically matched but unrelated volunteers. Although phenotypically identical family donors are occasionally available, mismatched family members and matched but unrelated donors represent a much larger pool.[344]

Haplotype sharing between parents occasionally has allowed identification and successful transplantation between phenotypically matched relatives.[345,346] Long-term survival after even one-locus-mismatched family donation is inferior to genotypically matched transplants, mainly because of graft rejection and GVHD. In the large European experience, for phenotypically identical family matches, the actuarial survival rate was 45%; for patients with a single-locus mismatch, it was 25%; and for those with two to three loci mismatched, the survival rate was 11%.[347,348] In a report from Seattle,[346] although all patients who received fully HLA-matched transplants survived, those with mismatches at one or more loci had a much poorer outcome, and even with total-body irradiation added to the conditioning regimen, the survival rate was only 50%. Most large studies of unrelated donors have shown inferior long-term survival and higher rates of complications such as graft rejection,[349] GVHD,[350,351] and delayed immune system reconstitution.[352] Even more than in standard sibling transplants, age is a crucial risk factor in unrelated transplants and probably more important than the level of match, conditioning regimen, or use of T-cell depletion.[344,348,353–355] For patients with AA who received unrelated transplants and who were enrolled in the National Marrow Donor Program, the survival rate at 2 years was 29%.[356] In the EGBMT's 1994 report, the survival rate for 110 recipients of marrow grafts from other than a matched sibling was 34%, approximately one-half of the rate of standard transplantation.[309] Superior results were obtained at Children's Hospital in Milwaukee, where T-cell depletion of the donor graft was combined with a rigorous conditioning program of cytosine arabinoside, cyclophosphamide, and total-body irradiation. For 28 transfused and previously treated children with severe AA, a survival rate of 54% was reported at a median follow-up of almost 3 years, with no incidence of chronic GVHD.[357] Similar results have been reported in a series of 154 transplantations performed in patients between the ages of 1 and 46 years of age (median, 17 years of age), with delayed transplantation (>3 years after diagnosis), HLA-A or HLA-B mismatch, and age being poor risk factors.[358] In a meta-analysis,[359] for fully matched, unrelated recipients, the survival rate was 25% to 50%, with rates of graft failure and GVHD of 0% to 50% and 28% to 100%, respectively. The degree of match clearly impacts the outcome of the unrelated bone marrow transplantation.

Despite progress, matched but unrelated transplantation is associated with a high mortality rate, and perhaps refractory, high-risk patients are therefore often selected for this procedure. It is likely the poor results may be a consequence of this referral bias. However, alternative-donor transplantation is feasible; the rare phenotypic match from within the family may be equivalent to a sibling donor, but with other family members or unrelated donors, there is a high risk of transplantation-related mortality. Because unrelated-donor transplantation takes months to arrange, it should be considered early. At the best centers, alternative-donor transplantation represents an option, especially for the young patient with very severe pancytopenia in whom immunosuppressive therapy has failed. In Japan, an unrelated but matched transplant has been reported to produce better results in refractory pediatric cases when used early rather than after repeated courses of immunosuppression.[360] In an analysis from Seattle, patients who failed one or more courses of immunosuppression had an overall survival rate of 36% at 3 years.[361]

Introduction of transplantation with less intense conditioning (ie, nonmyeloablative transplantation) and cord blood transplantation are promising therapeutic concepts that can help to improve the results of unrelated transplantation in AA and make the procedure available to a higher number of patients.

Late Complications of Bone Marrow Transplantation

Very late complications after transplantation include effects on growth and development, as well as on the function of endocrine, neurologic, and other organ systems.[362,363] A high rate of secondary malignancies has been recorded after transplantation. In a National Cancer Institute retrospective analysis of almost 20,000 transplantations, the risk of late-onset cancer was eightfold higher at 10 years than in the general population and even higher for young patients, for whom the risk of malignancy was increased approximately 40-fold.[364] Multivariate analysis suggested that high-dose radiation was a risk factor for the development of malignancies. For AA, among 320 patients who received transplants in Seattle, 4 developed cancer, leading to a calculated risk 7 times higher than for normal controls.[365] In a recent update, 12% of patients who survived more than 2 years after transplantation developed solid tumors.[366] In a French survey, 4 of 147 AA patients developed solid tumors, an 8-year cumulative incidence rate of 22%.[367] In an analysis of 700 transplantation patients with AA and Fanconi anemia, the risk of developing a secondary malignancy was 14% at 20 years. The hazard of lymphoid malignancies decreased with the time after transplantation, whereas the risk of solid tumors progressively increased.[368] Secondary solid tumors developed in the radiation fields of 5 of 147 AA patients whose conditioning regimens included irradiation of the thorax and abdomen.[369] In general, the rates of secondary malignancies after bone marrow transplantation for AA and other diseases are similar.[370] Immune events such as acute GVHD, treatment with ATG or monoclonal antibodies, and total-body irradiation have been related to the development of secondary malignancies.[370] Patients with these secondary cancers have a poor prognosis.[371] The risk of cancer after bone marrow transplantation must be evaluated in the context of other therapeutic options, especially immunosuppression, because a significant risk of late malignancy exists in AA patients independent of transplantation therapy. The risk of malignancy in the large registry of the EGBMT was equivalent for patients who received immunosuppression and those who underwent transplantation. Compared with the general European population, the relative risk of malignancy was calculated at 5.15 for AA patients treated with immunosuppression (confidence interval [CI]: 3.26–7.94) and at 6.67 (CI: 3.05–12.65) for patients receiving transplants.[372] Overall, the rate of malignancy after bone marrow transplantation has been calculated to be 3.8-fold higher than in the age-matched population.[373]

Immunosuppression

Antithymocyte Globulins

Immunosuppressive therapy is an effective alternative treatment for patients who are not candidates for bone marrow transplantation (Table 29–10 and see box on Treatment Algorithm in Aplastic Anemia). Immunoglobulin preparations made from the sera of horses (less frequently from rabbits) immunized against human thymocytes are the mainstays of current regimens.[374–378] Rabbit and horse ATGs are licensed for use in the United States as ATGAM (Pfizer) and Thymoglobulin (Genzyme), respectively.

The efficacy of antilymphocyte globulin (ALG) in marrow failure was discovered serendipitously in the late 1960s, when Mathé[46] observed recovery of autologous hematopoietic function in patients who received antilymphocyte serum as conditioning for marrow transplantation. In a collection of European cases from Basel, Paris, and Leiden in which patients were treated with different serum preparations and with a variety of dose regimens, sustained hematologic improvements occurred in 12 (41%) of 29 patients with severe AA, and the 1-year survival rate of the entire group was 55%.[379] In a multicenter study, Swiss ALG was clearly superior to androgen treatment, with a significantly better response rate (70% versus 18%) and 1-year survival rate (76% versus 22%).[380] Similar results were also obtained in a randomized study of ATG versus supportive care.[381] In a large multicenter American trial, 47% of patients improved.[382] Review of published results from Europe and North America suggests that approximately one-half of patients treated with ATG and ALG show hematologic improvement, broadly defined as an end to transfusion dependence and an improvement in a neutrophil number to a level protective against infection.[374] Response rates vary from 20% to 85%.[374]

The putative cause of AA is not a factor that predicts response. Virus-associated[161,180] and drug-induced aplasia[383,384] respond similarly as compared to idiopathic disease. Cytogenetic abnormalities do not preclude a response because AA with chromosome abnormalities[385–387] and some cases of frank myleodysplasia[388] can be responsive to immunosuppressive therapy. The response rate to ATG or ALG is not improved by the addition of androgens[389] or very high doses of corticosteroids.[390]

A hematologic response to ATG is usually apparent within several months of therapy; in some cases, all blood counts rise dramatically, and in others, increases in platelets or RBCs can be delayed (see box on Treatment Algorithm in Aplastic Anemia). The average time to improvement in neutrophil number is 1 to 2 months.[382] Transfusion independence occurs approximately 2 to 3 months after initiation of treatment.[391,392] Continued improvement without further therapy commonly occurs after 3 months; nevertheless, clinical status by 3 months is strongly correlated with long-term survival. Blood cell counts above the critical values for severity and platelets and reticulocyte counts of more than 50,000 cells/μL are highly prognostic.[382,393,394] Patient selection is important; in general, survival correlates with disease severity,[395,396] and in particular, with a low neutrophil count.[266,329,393] Patients who develop trisomy 8 frequently maintain responsiveness to immunosuppression.[397]

ATG has three major toxic effects: immediate allergic phenomena, serum sickness, and transient blood cell count depression (see Fig. 29–10). Fever, rigors, and an urticarial cutaneous eruption are common on the first or second day of ATG therapy, and these symptoms respond to antihistamines and meperidine therapy. Anaphylaxis is rare but can be fatal.[398] A positive immediate wheal-and-flare reaction to the cutaneous application of a 50 mg/mL of stock solution of horse ATG can be predictive of massive histamine release on systemic infusion, and desensitization with gradually increasing doses of horse ATG administered intradermally, subcutaneously, and then intravenously has permitted use in allergic individuals.[398] Corticosteroids are administered in moderate doses (1 mg/kg of prednisone or methylprednisolone) during the first 2 weeks to ameliorate the symptoms of serum sickness. Doses of ATG and ALG have varied from 5 to 50 mg/kg, and the duration of administration has varied from 4 to 28 days. It is more rational to administer equivalent doses of horse ATG by the schedule originally employed in Europe (40 mg/kg/day for 4 days); antiserum will then have reached low levels in the circulation by the time host antibody appears.[399] A short course of therapy is easier to administer, associated with less serum sickness, and equally effective as the same dose given over a more prolonged course. Thymoglobulin, rabbit ATG, has been approved for use in the United States. Rabbit ATG is more potent by weight than horse

Table 29–10 Intensive Immunosuppression in Severe Aplastic Anemia

Study	N	Median Age (years)	Response	Relapse	Clonal Evolution	Survival
German[448]	84	32	65%	19%	8%	58% at 11 years
EGMBT[63]	100	16	77%	12%	11%	87% at 5 years
NIH[62]	122	35	61%	35%	11%	55% at 7 years
Japan*[64]	119	9	68%	22%	6%	88% at 3 years
NIH**[73]	104	30	62%	37%	9%	80% at 4 years

*With androgens and ± granulocyte colony-stimulating factor (G-CSF).
**With mycophenolate mofetil.
Only studies of >20 enrolled patients are tabulated. Responses to immunosuppressive therapy are usually partial; blood counts may not become normal, but transfusions are no longer required, and the neutrophil count is adequate to prevent infection. Relapse is usually responsive to further immunosuppressive therapies. Clonal evolution is to dysplastic bone marrow changes and/or cytogenetic abnormalities. For details, see accompanying text.

ATG, and the dose used is in the range of 2 to 5 mg/kg daily for 4 to 5 days (Thymoglobulin at 3.5 mg/kg for five days). Rabbit ATG may cause more leukopenia.

Antilymphocyte globulins are immunosuppressive. ATGs contain a heterogeneous mix of antibody specificities for lymphocytes, including reactivity to antigens such as CD2, CD3, CD4, CD8, CD25 (the receptor for IL-2), and HLA-DR.[400–402] Horse sera fix human complement efficiently, and all preparations are T-cell cytotoxic in vitro, with little difference among ATGs or among lots for lymphocyte killing in vitro.[401] In vitro, antilymphocyte globulins efficiently inhibit T-cell proliferation and block IL-2 and IFN-γ production and IL-2 receptor expression.[403] ATG induces Fas-mediated apoptosis of T cells, especially after activation.[404] In monkeys, ATG suppresses cutaneous allograft rejection.[402] Studies of rabbit ATG in rhesus monkeys undergoing kidney transplantation have indicated that persistence of specific antibodies may be responsible for a chronic anergic state and tolerance induction.[405] In patients, the administration of ATG results in rapid reduction in the number of circulating lymphocytes, usually to less than 10% of starting values, and lymphocytopenia persists for several days after discontinuing therapy. Although lymphocyte numbers return to pretreatment values by 3 months, reductions in activated lymphocyte numbers in recovered patients persist.[66,406–408] It seems likely that these inhibitory effects on T cells are responsible for the efficacy of antilymphocyte globulins in AA. Nevertheless, the ability of ATG to stimulate lymphocyte function by acting as a mitogen may also have a role in their therapeutic efficacy. ATG provoked IL-2 nd hematopoietic growth factor production by peripheral blood mononuclear cells,[409] later identified as GM-CSF[61,409,410] and IL 3 (IL-3).[405] T cells cloned after stimulation produced GM-CSF or IL-3 (or both), and less frequently, they produced IL-2 and IFN-γ.[411] Administration of ATG after human marrow transplantation is associated with increased serum levels of IL-3.[412] ATG also binds to bone marrow precursor[413] and progenitor[414] cells[415] and may modestly directly enhance hematopoiesis, possibly through binding to CD45RO, a molecule capable of promoting tyrosine phosphatase signaling.[416]

Reliable methods to predict which patients will respond to ATG are lacking. In some cases, inhibitory activity of lymphocytes on hematopoiesis is no longer detected after successful ATG therapy.[417,418] In one study, CD8 T cells obtained from patients before treatment inhibited autologous hematopoietic colony formation, whereas CD8 lymphocytes isolated from the same patients after recovery were not active.[419] Good correlations were reported between the clinical response to immunosuppression and improvement in hematopoietic colony formation in vitro after T-cell depletion.[57,417] These findings have not been confirmed by others.[191,394,420–422] The lymphocyte stimulatory effects of ATG have been associated with positive clinical outcomes by some[423] but not by others.[409] Flow cytometric detection of intracellular IFN-γ expression in lymphocytes correlates with the responsiveness to ATG.[68]

Cyclosporine

Several groups[424–431] reported success with cyclosporine therapy combined with androgens in individual patients with AA, in many of whom other therapies had failed. Several studies suggested efficacy of cyclosporine in patients refractory to ALG or ATG alone, with salvage rates of approximately 50%.[432–437] The use of cyclosporine as initial therapy was promoted by a large French cooperative randomized study in which low but equivalent response rates were observed compared with standard ATG therapy.[438] However, in a randomized German trial,[404] cyclosporine was clearly inferior to ATG as measured by response and survival rates.

The optimal regimen has not been determined. In the United States, cyclosporine has usually been employed in high doses (12 mg/kg/day for adults and 15 mg/kg/day for children), with adjustment according to plasma drug concentrations and serum creatinine levels. In Europe, lower doses (3 to 7 mg/kg/day) have been reported to be equally efficacious.[439,440] Hematologic improvement can occur in a few weeks or months. A 6-month trial is warranted. Remissions, when achieved, usually have been durable, but some patients experience relapse when cyclosporine is discontinued. Most patients who relapse will respond to the reinstitution of cyclosporine.[439–442] Some patients require maintenance treatment.[429,432]

Cyclosporine has considerable toxicity. Hypertension and azotemia are the most common serious side effects; hirsutism and gingival hypertrophy are also frequent complaints. Increasing serum creatinine levels are an indication for dose reduction. Chronic cyclosporine nephropathy characterized by interstitial fibrosis and tubular atrophy can be irreversible. The risk of nephropathy is increased by high doses and longer duration of therapy and occurs more commonly in older than in younger patients. Cyclosporine, especially in combination with corticosteroids, converts patients with AA to a temporary immunodeficiency state and puts them at high risks for opportunistic infections. Monthly aerosolized pentamidine prophylaxis can prevent *Pneumocystis carinii* pneumonia in patients receiving cyclosporine. Convulsions, possibly related to hypomagnesemia, are another serious complication of cyclosporine therapy.

Combined or Intensive Immunosuppressive Therapy

The combination for the treatment of AA of an agent that lyses lymphocytes (ATG) with a drug that blocks lymphocyte function is rational (see Table 29–10). The strategy resulted in a striking increase in the response rate to immunosuppressive therapy observed in a German randomized trial in which patients were treated initially with a combination of ATG and cyclosporine or ATG only. The addition of cyclosporine led to higher hematologic response rates and more complete responses than were observed with ATG alone: 65% versus 39% and 70% versus 46% at 3 and 6 months, respectively.[443] In the European randomized trial of ATG and cyclosporine versus cyclosporine alone for nonsevere AA, a superior response rate was achieved with the combination regimen.[444] In a National Institutes of Health (NIH) study of combination ATG and cyclosporine therapy[393,445] and in a multicenter European study of ATG and cyclosporine,[446,447] the hematologic response rates at 1 year were 60% to 80%. In a long-term follow-up report from NIH, although the responses plateaued, few late deaths were reported.[393] In all the trials, the 5-year survival rates for responding patients have been between 80% and 90%. In the 11-year follow-up of the German randomized ATG versus ATG plus cyclosporine trial, patients who received the combination showed a better response rate and failure-free survival, but overall survival, perhaps linked to the efficacy of salvage regimens, was not different in both groups.[448] In elderly patients, the response rates to cyclosporine alone, ATG alone, and a combination were higher than 50%, but there was no difference in the outcome between regimens.[449]

Immunosuppressive therapy has been intensified in other regimens. In Europe, repeated courses of ATG are commonly given in an effort to induce hematologic improvement.[395,450–452] A longer course of ATG (28 days versus 10 days) appeared to produce more complete responses in a North American multicenter trial.[382] The addition of high-dose methylprednisolone to ATG has been associated with very high response rates in some trials.[45,453,454] In patients refractory to the initial therapy with ATG and cyclosporine, a repeat course of ATG is often administered as a salvage regimen and can rescue a proportion of patients. Rabbit ATG for patients refractory to the first course of ATG. In addition to inducing a response in 30% of patients, their survival was excellent (97% within the median follow-up of more than 900 days), unexpected for refractory disease.[455]

Cyclophosphamide

Since the initial pilot series of 11 patients who received high doses of cyclophosphamide (45 mg/kg/day for 4 days) without stem cell rescue,[456] a larger cohort ($n = 19$) of newly diagnosed AA patients has been reported with an overall response rate similar to that achieved with ATG therapy.[457] After cyclophosphamide therapy, blood cell counts were reported to be normal, and there was no evidence of relapse or late complications. These favorable but uncontrolled, single-institution, phase II results prompted a randomized trial in which ATG plus cyclosporine was compared with cyclophosphamide and cyclosporine. However, because of the excess toxicity in the cyclophosphamide-treated patients (invasive fungal infections or death in 6 of 15 versus 0 of 16[458]), the study was terminated. In an update of the results, although the response rate was comparable, the development of clonal disorders was observed in the cyclophosphamide arm, and relapses were observed.[459] Cyclophosphamide has been associated with a lower relapse rate, but comparison with ATG is difficult because most of the cyclophosphamide-treated patients may not achieve normal counts for 2 years after the therapy—a period in which a significant proportion of relapses occurs with ATG.[457]

Corticosteroids

Methylprednisolone in modest doses (1 mg/kg/day) is usually administered during ATG and ALG therapy to ameliorate the symptoms of serum sickness. Very-high-dose ("industrial strength") steroids are delivered boluses of 6-methylprednisolone given intravenously in dosages of 20 mg/kg/day on days 1 to 3, 10 mg/kg/day on days 4 to 7, 5 mg/kg/day on days 8 to 11, 2 mg/kg/day on days 12 to 20, and 1 mg/kg/day until day 30, followed by a maintenance regimen. Such high-dose regimens can be effective, especially in recently diagnosed patients.[191,452,460] High-dose methylprednisolone also has been added to ATG therapy, with inconsistent results. ATG therapy is associated with better response rates and many fewer associated toxic effects than high-dose steroid therapy and is generally preferable as initial therapy. Modest doses of corticosteroids do not have roles in the treatment of AA except in combination with ATG. There is little evidence of their effectiveness in reversing marrow failure or improving hemostasis, and even limited courses of steroids can contribute to the development of aseptic vascular necrosis and the increase in the rate of fungal infections.[461]

Late Complications of Immunosuppressive Therapy

Relapse after immunosuppressive therapy is common. In the European experience, in 719 patients treated with immunosuppressive therapy, the actuarial rate of relapse among 358 responders was 35% at 14 years; relapse was more common among patients who had initial rapid responses.[462] Approximately one-half the patients who relapsed responded to a second course of immunosuppression, but survival rates were lower for patients who experienced relapse than for those who did not. In the large NIH cohort of 112 patients, relapse, defined as a need for treatment, was even more common, with a risk estimated at 35% at 7 years for responders; however, survival was unaffected by the occurrence of relapse. Pancytopenia occurred in a minority of patients, and most patients responded to further therapy, usually reinstitution of cyclosporine.[207,393] These observations are consistent with a view of AA as a chronic immunologic disease that might not be cured by a single course of immunosuppressive therapy.

A much more serious complication is the development of late-onset clonal hematologic disorders. The syndromes include PNH, myelodysplasia, and AML.[463–485] Some of these events can represent part of the natural history of AA. Before recent improvements in treatment, leukemia was considered an unusual complication,[466] but late-onset clonal disorders do not appear to simply be the result of the introduction of immunosuppressive therapy. In a series of 156 patients treated with androgens, there was a 10% actuarial probability of developing PNH; in addition, five cases of late-onset myelodysplasia and one of non-Hodgkin lymphoma were observed.[467] In retrospective analyses performed by the EGBMT, of 223 long-term survivors after immunosuppression, 19 developed PNH (13% risk at 7 years), and 11 developed myelodysplastic syndrome, which in 5 years later evolved to AML (combined risk of 15% at 7 years).[468] In single-center series, estimated rates of late-onset clonal disease have ranged from 9% (at 6 years)[390] to 57% (at 8 years).[469] Children appear to be at similar risk for the development of clonal complication as adults, and evolution to myelodysplastic syndrome can occur in responders and in refractory patients.[470,471] Myelodysplastic syndrome that develops after AA can transform to acute leukemia[463] but can also be surprisingly indolent.[472] In a series from the NIH, in 29 patients with AA who developed a chromosome abnormality, monosomy 7 and trisomy 8 were the most common defects observed. Clinically, monosomy 7 was more likely to occur in primarily refractory patients and had a poor prognosis, whereas patients with trisomy 8 remained responsive to cyclosporine and had excellent survival.[473] Similarly, AA patients who develop 13q− appear to have a good prognosis and retain responsiveness of their counts to continued immunosuppression.[474] Overall, the frequency of the development of a new chromosome abnormality was estimated to be approximately 15% at 7 years.

A PNH clone can be detected in up to 50% of patients on their presentation. Approximately 10% to 15% of patients will develop the hemolytic or thrombotic form of PNH;[203] and in most, the proportion of PNH cells remains stable and low. Immunosuppressive therapy does change the size of the PNH clone. In an analysis of a large cohort of PNH patients, those with a history of AA constituted a larger group than those with primary hemolytic PNH.[203]

Immunosuppression Versus Bone Marrow Transplantation

Immunosuppression and transplantation are both effective therapies for AA (Figs. 29–11 and 29–12). Lack of a matched sibling donor, the expense and availability of transplantation, and risk factors such as active infections, advanced age, or a heavy transfusion burden lead most patients to automatically undergo treatment with ATG and cyclosporine.[475] For a few patients with AA, a choice does exist between transplantation and immunosuppressive therapy. Marrow transplantation offers a permanent cure. Its disadvantages are cost, procedure-related morbidity and mortality (especially GVHD in older patients), and an increased incidence of solid organ malignancies. Immunosuppressive therapy is easier and initially cheaper. However, many patients do not achieve normal blood cell counts and remain at high risk for relapse and the more serious complications of late-onset clonal hematologic disease, especially myelodysplasia.

Retrospective analyses of the large number of European patients reported to the EGBMT show consistently improved results with both therapies but have repeatedly failed to demonstrate a survival advantage for transplantation over immunosuppression.[329,476–478] The latest 5-year survival rate quoted was higher than 80% for both treatments.[479] Single-center studies are similar. Certain categories of patients, defined by neutrophil number and age, probably benefit from one therapy or the other. In the EGBMT analyses, marrow transplantation yielded superior results in children younger than 10 years old and in younger patients with a neutrophil count of less than 400 cells/μL, whereas immunosuppressive therapy was superior for adults 40 years old or older. For patients of intermediate age and a neutrophil count of less than 300 cells/μL, transplantation results in a more favorable outcome compared with immunosuppressive therapy.[315] Superior results with matched sibling transplantation in children have been reported by others.[266,473–483]

Much improved results with matched sibling and with unrelated matched transplantation were reported from Seattle.[484] However, older individuals are likely to fare less well than children undergoing transplantation.[293,484] A cutoff of 40 years of age was adopted for consideration of transplantation in one review. In some cases, an unsuccessful trial of immunosuppression can be followed by stem cell

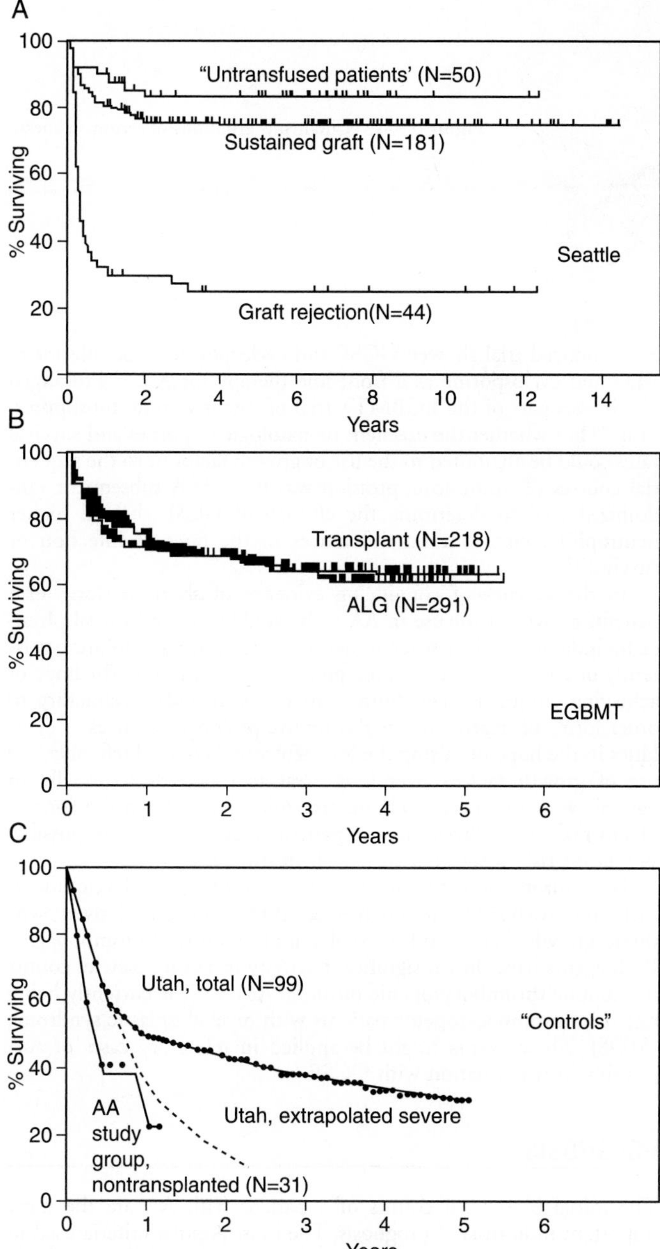

Figure 29–11 Actuarial survival rates for patients with aplastic anemia (AA). (**A**) Data on bone marrow transplantation from the University of Washington. (**B**) Data from the European Group for Bone Marrow Transplantation on bone marrow transplantation versus immunosuppression with antilymphocyte globulin (ALG). (**C**) Natural history as indicated by survival with supportive and other treatments. Two groups are illustrated. Extrapolated survival curves for patients with severe disease are derived from retrospective reviews from the University of Utah of 101 records collected from the late 1940s to early 1970s. The patients received blood transfusions and, later in this period, also received platelets. Almost all were treated with corticosteroids, and one-half were also treated with androgens. Data for patients who did not receive transplants come from a multicenter study of the efficacy of marrow transplantation performed in the early 1970s; this control group was treated with androgens.

transplantation from a sibling donor.[485] For the more risky matched unrelated donor transplant, the decision to undergo this procedure can be difficult, but outcomes are improving. Increasingly children who have failed a single course of immunosuppression and adults refractory to multiple courses of ATG are offered this procedure.

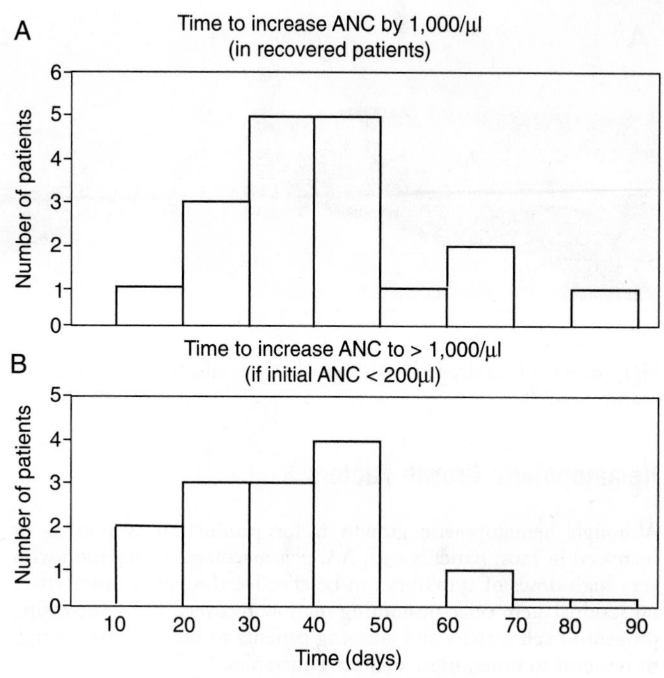

Figure 29–12 Time to response after treatment with antilymphocyte globulin (ATG). (**A**) Distribution of patients with severe aplastic anemia by time to achieve an increase in the absolute neutrophil count of 1000 cells/mm^3. (**B**) Distribution of patients with an initial absolute neutrophil count of less than 200 cells/mm^3 by time to achieve an absolute neutrophil count of 1000 cells/mm^3. ANC, absolute neutrophil count.

Androgens

Testosterone and synthetic anabolic steroids appeared to be major advances in the treatment of AA when they were introduced in the 1960s.[239,486] The high response rates in some early series may be retrospectively attributed to the inclusion of patients with moderate acquired and constitutional AA. For severe AA, controlled trials in general have not demonstrated efficacy, as measured by survival rates[487] or hematologic improvement.[382] When added to immunosuppressive therapies, androgens failed to result in any increase in response rates.[389] In Europe, a modest survival advantage was observed only in women with severe neutropenia who received combined therapy.[488]

Although marrow transplantation or immunosuppressive therapy is generally preferred, certain androgen regimens have their advocates. These investigators have reported response rates and prolonged survivals[467] similar to those observed with ATG.[489] Androgens continue to be helpful in some patients when used as a second-line therapy. Most hematologists have observed patients who appeared to respond or even to develop hormone dependence.[490,491] Androgen therapy is popular in Asia[492–495] and Mexico[496] because it is inexpensive and seemingly effective. Various preparations of androgens in different doses have resulted in virtually identical response rates of 35% to 60% after 6 months of therapy.[497]

Useful androgens include nandrolone decanoate, oxymetholone, and danazol; unfortunately, their popularity and abuse by athletes has led to restrictions of their availability and manufacture. The hemoglobin response frequently is more impressive than improvements in granulocyte or platelet levels. An adequate trial is considered to be a full dose given for at least 3 months. Complications occur infrequently, although some are serious and can limit effective therapy, especially in the elderly.[498] The associated liver cholestasis is usually reversible. Hepatotoxicity (eg, bile duct proliferation, peliosis, atypical hepatocyte hyperplasia, tumors) can occur but is less common with parenteral formulations.[499] Children appear to tolerate

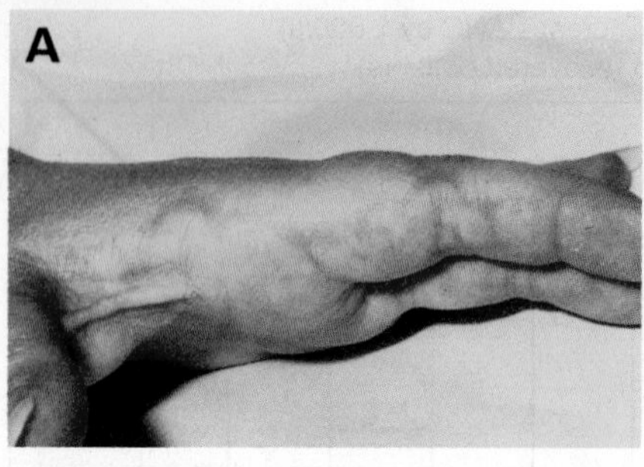

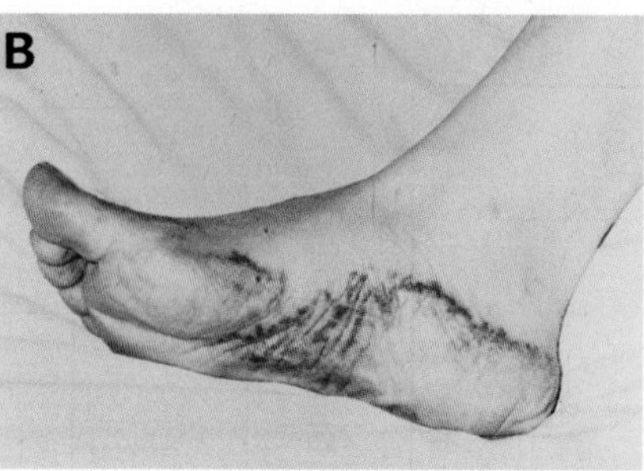

Figure 29–13 Cutaneous eruptions of serum sickness.

high doses of androgens without lasting effects on growth or maturation.[500]

Hematopoietic Growth Factors

Although hematopoietic growth factor production is normal or increased in most patients with AA, pharmacologic stimulation with very high doses of cytokines can be effective through a direct effect on residual stem cells, promoting marrow recovery, or by increasing progenitor cell activity and allowing patients to survive long enough to respond to other, more definitive therapies.[501,502]

Neutropenia most often leads to serious and life-threatening infections. GCSF and GM-CSF are capable of increasing neutrophil counts in patients with AA.[503–505] Controlled trials with these agents have not been performed, and data demonstrating that growth factor administration alone decreases the incidence of serious infections or improves survival are lacking. In general, neutrophil responses to growth factors are transient, dependent on their continuous administration, and usually restricted to patients with quantitatively less severe forms of AA. Nevertheless, occasional bilineage and trilineage responses have been observed.[506] Children can be more sensitive to the effects of prolonged administration of GCSF.[504,507]

A concern has been the possibility that prolonged administration of GCSF might increase the probability of late clonal disease, especially monosomy 7. In retrospective analyses of Japanese children and adults[508,509] with severe AA, this syndrome appeared to occur most frequently among patients who had received growth factor.[510,511] Although not initially observed among European patients in GCSF protocols, a recent retrospective analysis has suggested a higher risk of myelodysplasia associated with GCSF use.[512] The mechanism of GCSF's relationship to monosomy appears to be selection of aneuploid cells bearing an isoform of GCSF; these cells are less sensitive to GCSF, but once triggered by the cytokine proliferate and do not differentiate.[513] Regardless of toxic or late effects, growth factors, often are inappropriately employed as the first-line therapy in AA, for which they have not been shown to be useful. Such practices lead to unfortunate delays in the institution of definitive therapy.[514]

Anemia and pancytopenia in rare patients have responded to prolonged administration of high doses of erythropoietin. Clinically meaningful hematologic responses to the administration of single cytokines have been limited in marrow failure syndromes, but combinations of growth factors might be more effective because of physiologic or pharmacologic synergism. Some complete remissions have been reported with GM-CSF and erythropoietin[386] and with IL-3 and GCSF.[515] In a large, randomized protocol, the combination of GCSF and high doses of erythropoietin improved hemoglobin values, mainly in patients with moderate disease.[516]

Growth factors have also been combined with definitive medical therapy for the purpose of improving neutrophil counts during the early phase of immunosuppression. Often, therapy with GCSF or GM-CSF is instituted because the neutropenic patient is febrile and unresponsive to antibiotics; its value in these circumstances is unknown. A brief course of GM-CSF before or concurrent with ALG has not added appreciable benefit in two small trials.[517,518] A few case reports have suggested that the combination of a growth factor with cyclosporine might rescue patients with refractory disease,[519–521] but a randomized trial showed GCSF and cyclosporine to be inferior to ALG and cyclosporine as a front-line therapy for AA.[522] Prolonged GCSF was part of the EGBMT's trial of intensive immunosuppression,[446] but whether the excellent hematologic responses and survival rates could be attributed to the use of growth factor or to the sequential courses of immunosuppression was unclear. A subsequent randomized trial to determine the efficacy of GCSF showed higher neutrophil counts but no differences in the rates of infection or survival.[523]

In the absence of convincing evidence of short- or long-term benefit, growth factor use in AA is dictated by the individual physician's judgment. Most severely neutropenic patients who are persistently or seriously infected undergo a therapeutic trial in the hope of achieving clinical benefit. Some patients with disease refractory to other forms of treatment can also receive prolonged courses of cytokines in the hope of raising the low neutrophil count. Preferably, the use of growth factors over long treatment periods, especially in patients who are not severely neutropenic, should be in the context of a formal study. Physicians and patients should be aware of possibly significant risks associated with such treatment.

New thrombopoietic factors are currently under development, including AMG531, an engineered thrombopoietin-derived synthetic growth factor, and an oral c-mpl agonist, elthrombopag.[524] Both agents have shown significant activity in raising platelet counts in immune thrombocytopenic purpura. AMG531 is currently being tested in thrombocytopenic patients with myelodysplastic syndrome (MDS). These agents might be applied in refractory cases of AA, possibly in combination with GCSF.

PROGNOSIS

The initial blood cell counts of a patient with AA are the most important indicators of prognosis. The most popular criteria used to define severe disease are the presence of two of the following three: neutrophil count of less than 500 cells/μL, platelet count of less than 20,000 cells/μL, and corrected reticulocyte level of less than 1% (<40,000 cells/μL).[301] More complicated formulas are less easy to use and often only quantitate the obvious.[525] In a comparative study of prognostic indices, decreasing blood cell counts during the first 3 months of therapy were uniformly associated with death within 5 years, and stable or improved blood cell counts correctly predicted long-term survival for 75% of patients. Of the prognostic indices, the simple criteria described previously were the most accurate at 6 months, correctly predicting poor survival for 85% of patients with 100% sensitivity after 6 months.[526] In a long-term follow-up study of 122 patients treated with an ATG plus cyclosporine combination at the NIH, blood count improvement (no longer meeting severity criteria) and the robustness of the platelet and reticulocyte response correlated with long-term survival.[393] One modification to the standard criteria is useful. Although bleeding was a major cause of death in the past, infection kills the overwhelming proportion of patients today. In the large European cooperative trials, a category of *supersevere* AA has been defined by an extremely low absolute neutrophil count (<200 cells/μL).[266] Relapse does not appear to affect the probability of survival;[393] clonal evolution, especially monosomy 7, is a poor prognostic factor.[473]

Bone marrow examination is subject to sampling error, and cellularity is not usually quantitated; for these reasons, blood cell counts have been more readily correlated with survival than gross marrow appearance.[527] A predominance of lymphoid cells in the bone marrow has been associated with a bad prognosis in some studies,[229] and the presence of residual hematopoiesis, particularly erythropoiesis, with a good outlook in others.[528,529]

The rate of spontaneous recovery is difficult to estimate, but most observers believe it to be low. Untreated severe disease is almost invariably fatal. In contrast, moderate AA has a good prognosis, and some patients with minimal blood cell count depression recover normal blood cell counts with limited or no therapy.[530] Nevertheless, in an older series of pediatric patients treated mainly with transfusions, only 3% of 334 were judged to be cured,[128] and among African patients who received transfusions, corticosteroids, and androgens, the mortality rate was 56% at 1 year and 72% after 18 months.[12] Interpretation of older publications is complicated by uncertainties concerning diagnosis and the inclusion of a large proportion of patients with moderate disease. In a randomized study from the contemporary era, none of 21 patients assigned to supportive care improved during 3 months of observation.[381]

SUGGESTED READINGS

Adkins DR, Goodnough LT, Shenoy S, et al: Effect of leukocyte compatibility on neutrophil increment after transfusion of granulocyte colony-stimulating factor-mobilized prophylactic granulocyte transfusions and on clinical outcomes after stem cell transplantation. Blood 95:3605, 2000.

Brodsky RA, Sensenbrenner LL, Smith BD, et al: Durable treatment-free remission after high-dose cyclophosphamide therapy for previously untreated severe aplastic anemia. Ann Intern Med 135:477, 2001.

Chen J, Lipovsky K, Ellison FM, Calado RT, Young NS. Bystander destruction of hematopoietic progenitor and stem cells in a mouse model of infusion-induced bone marrow failure. Blood 104:1671, 2004

Deeg HJ, Leisenring W, Storb R, et al: Long-term outcome after marrow transplantation for severe aplastic anemia. Blood 91:3637, 1998.

Heckman KD, Weiner GJ, Davis CS, et al: Randomized study of prophylactic platelet transfusion threshold during induction therapy for adult acute leukemia: 10,000/microL versus 20,000/microL. J Clin Oncol 15:1143, 1997.

Herbrecht R, Denning DW, Patterson TF, Bennett JE, et al: Voriconazole versus amphotericin B for primary therapy of invasive aspergillosis. N Engl J Med 347:408, 2002.

Horowitz MM: Current status of allogeneic bone marrow transplantation in acquired aplastic anemia. Semin Hematol 37:30, 2000.

Hughes WT, Armstrong D, Bodey GP, Bow EJ, et al: 2002 Guidelines for the use of antimicrobial agents in neutropenic patients with cancer. Clin Infect Dis 34:730, 2002.

International Agranulocytosis and Aplastic Anemia Study: Risks of agranulocytosis and aplastic anemia: A first report of their relation to drug use with special reference to analgesics. JAMA 256:1749, 1986.

Kojima S, Matsuyama T, Kato S, et al: Outcome of 154 patients with severe aplastic anemia who received transplants from unrelated donors: The Japan Marrow Donor Program. Blood 100:799, 2002.

Marsh J, Schrezenmeier H, Marin P, et al: Prospective randomized multicenter study comparing cyclosporin alone versus the combination of antithymocyte globulin and cyclosporin for treatment of patients with nonsevere aplastic anemia: A report from the European Blood and Marrow Transplant (EBMT) Severe Aplastic Anaemia Working Party. Blood 93:2191, 1999.

Morgan GJ, Alveres CL. Benzene and the hemopoietic stem cell. Chem Biol Interact 30;153, 2005

Rosenfeld SJ, Follman D, Nunez O, Yuong NS. Antithymocyte globulin and cyclosporine for severe aplastic anemia. Association between hematologic response and long-term outcome. JAMA 289:1130, 2003.

Socie G, Stone JV, Wingard JR, et al: Long-term survival and late deaths after allogeneic bone marrow transplantation. Late Effects Working Committee of the International Bone Marrow Transplant Registry. N Engl J Med 341:14, 1999.

Tichelli A, Socie G, Marsh J, et al: Outcome of pregnancy and disease course among women with aplastic anemia treated with immunosuppression. Ann Intern Med 137:164, 2002.

Tisdale JF, Dunn DE, Geller N, et al: High-dose cyclophosphamide in severe aplastic anaemia: A randomised trial. Lancet 356:1554, 2000.

Walsh TJ, Teppler H, Donowitz GR, et al: Caspofungin versus liposomal amphotericin B for empirical antifungal therapy in patients with persistent fever and neutropenia. N Engl J Med 351:1391, 2004.

Young NS, Calado R, Scheinberg P: Current concepts in the pathophysiology and treatment of aplastic anemia. Blood 108:2511, 2006.

REFERENCES

For complete list of references log onto www.expertconsult.com

CHAPTER 30

PAROXYSMAL NOCTURNAL HEMOGLOBINURIA

Robert A. Brodsky

INTRODUCTION

Paroxysmal nocturnal hemoglobinuria (PNH) is a clonal hematopoietic stem-cell disorder that has fascinated hematologists for more than a century because of its protean clinical manifestations and captivating pathophysiology. One of the earliest descriptions of PNH was by Dr. Paul Strübing, who in 1882 described a 29-year-old cartwright who presented with fatigue, abdominal pain, and severe nocturnal paroxysms of hemoglobinuria that were exacerbated by excess alcohol, physical exertion, and iron salts.[1] Strübing deduced that the hemolysis was occurring intravascularly as the patient's plasma turned red following severe attacks of hemoglobinuria. Decades later his prescient deduction was confirmed. Later reports by Marchiafava and Micheli led to the eponym, Marchiafava-Micheli syndrome, but it was Enneking, in 1925, who introduced the term *paroxysmal nocturnal hemoglobinuria.*[2]

In 1937, Thomas Ham found that PNH erythrocytes were hemolyzed when incubated with normal, acidified serum.[3] This seminal discovery resulted in the first diagnostic test for PNH, the acidified serum or Ham test. The cell lysis following acidified serum appeared to be complement dependent because heat inactivation abrogated the reaction; however, it was not until 1954, with the discovery of the alternative pathway of complement activation, that complement was formally proven to cause the hemolysis of PNH red cells.[4] Following the emergence of specific diagnostic tests, additional disease manifestations such as venous thrombosis, bone marrow failure, and development of myelodysplastic syndromes and acute leukemia were associated with PNH. These nonerythroid manifestations of the disease foreshadowed the discovery that PNH results from the clonal expansion of a mutated hematopoietic stem cell.

In the 1980s, roughly 100 years after Strübing's initial description of the disease, it was discovered that PNH cells display a global deficiency in a group of proteins affixed to the cell surface by a glycosylphosphatidylinositol (GPI) anchor. Interestingly, several of the missing proteins (eg, CD55 and CD59) are important complement regulatory proteins. A few years later, the genetic mutation (*PIGA*) responsible for the GPI-anchor protein deficiency was discovered,[5] and most recently, a humanized monoclonal antibody that inhibits terminal complement activation has been shown to ameliorate hemolysis and disease symptoms in PNH patients.[6] Although the pathophysiology of many of PNH's clinical manifestations are now understood, the mechanism of thrombosis, the mechanism of clonal dominance, and the close association with aplastic anemia continue to be areas of intense investigation. PNH is an extremely rare condition; however, the risk for developing PNH in patients with acquired aplastic anemia is 20% to 30%. In addition, 20% to 65% of patients with aplastic anemia harbor a small to moderate PNH population at diagnosis.[7,8] Understanding the factor(s) that promote the clonal outgrowth of diseases such as PNH should give insight into the genesis of other clonal hematologic malignancies.

PATHOPHYSIOLOGY

The Glycosylphosphatidylinositol Anchor

Covalent linkage to GPI is an important means of anchoring many cell-surface glycoproteins to the cell membrane.[9–11] Alkaline phosphatase was the first GPI-anchor protein recognized after it was discovered that cell surface alkaline phosphatase could be removed by a bacterial enzyme, phosphatidylinositol-specific phospholipase C (PIPLC).[12] PIPLC cleaved the phosphate from phosphatidylinositol and left the enzyme with full activity after its release, suggesting that the protein structure was unperturbed. This fundamental observation led to the discovery of dozens of GPI-anchored proteins.

The GPI anchor consists of a highly conserved glycan core (ethanoloamine-*P*-6Manα1-2Manα1-6Manα1-4GlcN) linked to the 6-position of the D-*myo*-inositol ring of phosphatidylinositol (Fig. 30–1). The anchor is synthesized in a stepwise manner in the endoplasmic reticulum membrane involving at least 9 reactions and more than 20 different genes (Table 30–1).[11] The first step in GPI anchor biosynthesis is the transfer of *N*-acetylglucosamine (GlcNAc) from uridine diphosphate (UDP)-GlcNAc to phosphatidylinositol (PI) to yield GlcNAc-PI. This step is catalyzed by GlcNAc-PI α1-6 GlcNAc transferase, an enzyme whose subunits are encoded by seven different genes: *PIGA,*[5] *PIGC,*[13] *PIGH,*[14] *GPI1,*[15,16] *PIGY,*[17] *PIGP,* and *DPM2.*[18] In the second step, GlcNAc-PI is deacetylated by the gene product of *PIGL* to form glucosamine (GlcN)-PI.[19] GPI anchor assembly continues in the endoplasmic reticulum with acylation of the inositol and stepwise addition of mannosyl and phosphoethanolamine residues. The preassembled GPI is linked to nascent proteins that contain a C-terminal GPI-attachment signal peptide, displacing it in a transamidase reaction.[20] The GPI-anchored protein (AP) then transits the secretory pathway to reach its final destination at the plasma membrane. If the GPI anchor is not attached to the protein, it is degraded intracellularly, probably in lysosomes.[21,22]

Given the numerous gene products involved in GPI anchor assembly, it seemed improbable that PNH would be the consequence of a single genetic mutation. However, after intense scrutiny of this pathway, it became apparent that in all PNH cases, the defect could be attributed to mutations in the *PIGA* gene, whose product is essential for the first step of GPI anchor biosynthesis. Later it was determined that the *PIGA* gene is on the X chromosome and that its product is part of a complex that transfers *N*-acetylglucosamine to phosphatidylinositol to form GlcNAc-PI.[16] Thus, a single "hit" will generate a PNH phenotype because males have only one X chromosome, and in females one X chromosome is inactivated through lyonization. Conceivably a mutation in any one of the genes in this pathway would cause the disease; however, other genes involved in GPI anchor biosynthesis are located on autosomes (see Table 30–1). Inactivating mutations in these genes would have to occur on both alleles to produce the PNH phenotype. Recently, a rare autosomal recessive disease that manifests with seizures and venous thrombosis was found to be caused by a point mutation near the start codon of *PIGM.*[23] The mutation resulted in a partial but severe deficiency of GPI-anchored proteins.

Acetylcholinesterase from erythrocytes and alkaline phosphatase from leukocytes were the first GPI-anchored proteins shown to be missing in PNH. Since then, more than a dozen GPI-anchored proteins with heterogeneous expression on hematopoietic cells have been found to be missing in PNH (Table 30–2). The functions of these cell surface GPI-anchored proteins are manifold; they can serve as complement regulatory proteins, enzymes, blood group antigens, receptors, and adhesion molecules. Membrane inhibitor of reactive lysis (CD59) and decay accelerating factor (CD55)—both complement regulatory proteins—are the most widely expressed GPI-

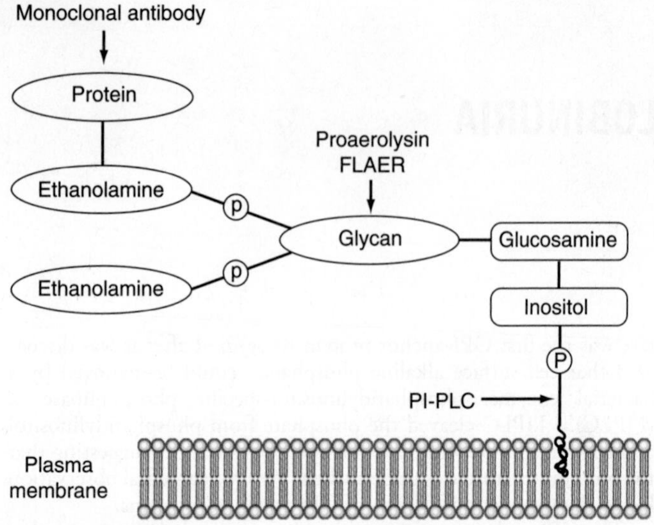

Figure 30–1 Structure of the glycosylphosphatidylinositol (GPI) anchor. Phosphatidylinositol is inserted into the lipid bilayer of the plasma membrane. The glycan core, which serves as the binding site for aerolysin, proaerolysin, and FLAER, consists of a molecule of *N*-glucosamine, three molecules of mannose, and a molecule of ethanolamine. The representative protein (eg, CD55, CD59, etc.) is covalently attached through an amide bond to an ethanolamine on the terminal mannose. Individual monoclonal antibodies used for the diagnosis of PNH (eg, CD55, CD59, etc.) bind to the protein, but not the GPI anchor. Phosphatidylinositol-specific phospholipase C (PIPLC) cleaves the phosphate from phosphatidylinositol and leaves the enzyme with full activity after its release.

Table 30–1 Genes Involved in GPI Anchor Biosynthesis

Number	Gene	Location
1	PIG-A*	Xp22.1
2	PIG-C*	1q23.3
3	PIG-H*	14q11-q24
4	PIG-P*	21q22.2
5	GPI1 (PIG-Q)*	16p13.3
6	PIG-L	17p12
7	PIG-M	1q22
8	PIG-N	18q21
9	PIG-B	15q21-q22
10	PIG-F	2q16-p21
11	PIG-O	9
12	GPI8 (PIG-K)†	1p22.2-p22.3
13	GAA1 (GPAA1)†	8q24.3
14	PIG-S†	17
15	PIG-T†	20q12-q13
16	DPM1	20q13.1
17	DPM2	9q33
18	DPM3	1q21.2
19	SL15 (MPDU1)	17p13.1
20	PIG-U†	20q11
21	PIG-V	1p36.11
22	PIG-W	17p12
23	PIG-X	3q29
24	PIG-Y*	4q21

GPI, glycosylphosphatidylinositol.
Note: *Indicates genes involved in the first step of GPI anchor biosynthesis.
†Denotes genes involved in the transamidase reaction.

Table 30–2 Cell Surface GPI-Anchored Protein Absent on PNH Blood Cells

Antigen	Hematopoietic Lineage	Classification
CD55—decay accelerating factor	All blood cells	Complement regulator
CD59—membrane inhibitor of reactive lysis	All blood cells	Complement regulator
CD58—lymphocyte function associated antigen-3	All blood cells	Adhesion molecule
Acetylcholinesterase	Red cells	Enzyme
CD14—monocyte differentiation antigen	Granulocytes, monocytes, macrophages	Endotoxin-binding receptor
CD16—Fcγ receptor III	Granulocytes, NK cells	Receptor
CD66b	Granulocytes	Adhesion
Neutrophil alkaline phosphatase	Granulocytes	Enzyme
CD87—urokinase (plasminogen activator) receptor	Monocytes, granulocytes	Receptor
Leukocyte alkaline phosphatase	Granulocytes	Enzyme
CDw52—Campath-1 antigen	Lymphocytes, monocytes	Unknown
CD24	B lymphocytes, granulocytes	B cell differentiation
CD48	All leukocytes	Adhesion molecule
CD73—ecto-5′-nucleotidase	Some B and T lymphocytes	Enzyme
Dombrock-Holley/Gregory-bearing protein	Red cells	Blood group antigen
Folate receptor	Myeloid and erythroid cells	Receptor

anchored proteins and can be found on all hematopoietic lineages including CD34⁺CD38⁻ progenitor cells.[24] Certain proteins, CD58 (LFA3) and CD16 (FcγRIII), may exist in both GPI-linked and transmembrane forms.

PIGA Gene

Investigators in Osaka, Japan, first identified the gene that was defective in PNH.[5] The gene was isolated by expression cloning and named *PIGA* (**p**hosphatidyl**i**nositol-**g**lycan complementation class **A**). *PIGA* was then cloned into an expression vector and transfected into GPI-deficient cell lines derived from PNH patients; cell surface expression of all the missing GPI-anchored proteins was restored, confirming that *PIGA* mutations are responsible for causing PNH.[25,26] Since this seminal discovery, somatic mutations of the *PIGA* gene have been found in all PNH patients to date.[27–31] Little to no GPI anchor is made when the *PIGA* gene is mutated. Consequently, the translated protein (eg, CD59, CD55, etc.) residing in the cisterna of the endoplasmic reticulum cannot be attached to the GPI anchor and is degraded in situ.[32]

The human *PIGA* gene contains 6 exons, 5 introns, and extends over 17 kb (Fig. 30–2); it encodes for a protein that contains 484 amino acids (60 kd). In humans, there is a single copy of the gene located on the short arm of the X chromosome (Xp22.1), although an intronless pseudogene has been found on chromosome 12q21.[33,34] A wide range of somatic mutations interspersed throughout the entire coding region of the *PIGA* gene have been described in PNH patients. There are no true mutational "hot spots," although exon 2, which contains almost half of the coding region, is the exon where most mutations occur. Most *PIGA* mutations are small insertions or deletions, usually one or two base pairs, which result in a frameshift in the coding region and consequently a shortened, nonfunctional product. Although *PIGA* function is abolished by these frameshift mutations, missense mutations, where the product of the mutated *PIGA* gene has some residual activity, have also been described. In most patients studied, a single (monoclonal) *PIGA* mutation has been discovered. However, two different mutations (biclonal) and in one case four separate *PIGA* mutations have been found in PNH patients.[35]

PNH Stem Cell

PNH is a clonal hematopoietic disorder similar to myelodysplastic syndrome (MDS), chronic myelocytic leukemia, and acute myeloid leukemia. The first evidence to support the notion that PNH arises through the mutation of an abnormal multipotent hematopoietic stem cell was derived from glucose 6-phosphate dehydrogenase studies on the red cell of women with PNH.[36] Subsequently, flow cytometric analyses revealed that all hematopoietic lineages—myeloid, erythroid, and lymphoid—were involved. Furthermore, *PIGA* mutations found in granulocytes match those found in other lineages,[25,37] and CD34⁺CD38⁻ progenitor cells have been shown to be missing GPI-anchored proteins in PNH patients.[38] Thus, the "hit" in PNH clearly involves a multipotent hematopoietic stem cell and may even involve an earlier stem cell than diseases such as chronic myelocytic leukemia, MDS, or acute leukemia. In the latter disorders, B cells are sometimes derived from the leukemia clone, but T cells are seldom involved. In PNH, both B cells and T cells have been shown to be derived from the malignant clone.

PNH Red Cells

PNH cells can display one of three phenotypes (Fig. 30–3): cells with normal expression of GPI-anchored proteins (type I cells), cells with intermediate expression of GPI anchor proteins (type II cells), and cells with no expression of GPI anchor proteins (type III cells). These three populations are most easily seen in the erythrocyte and granu-

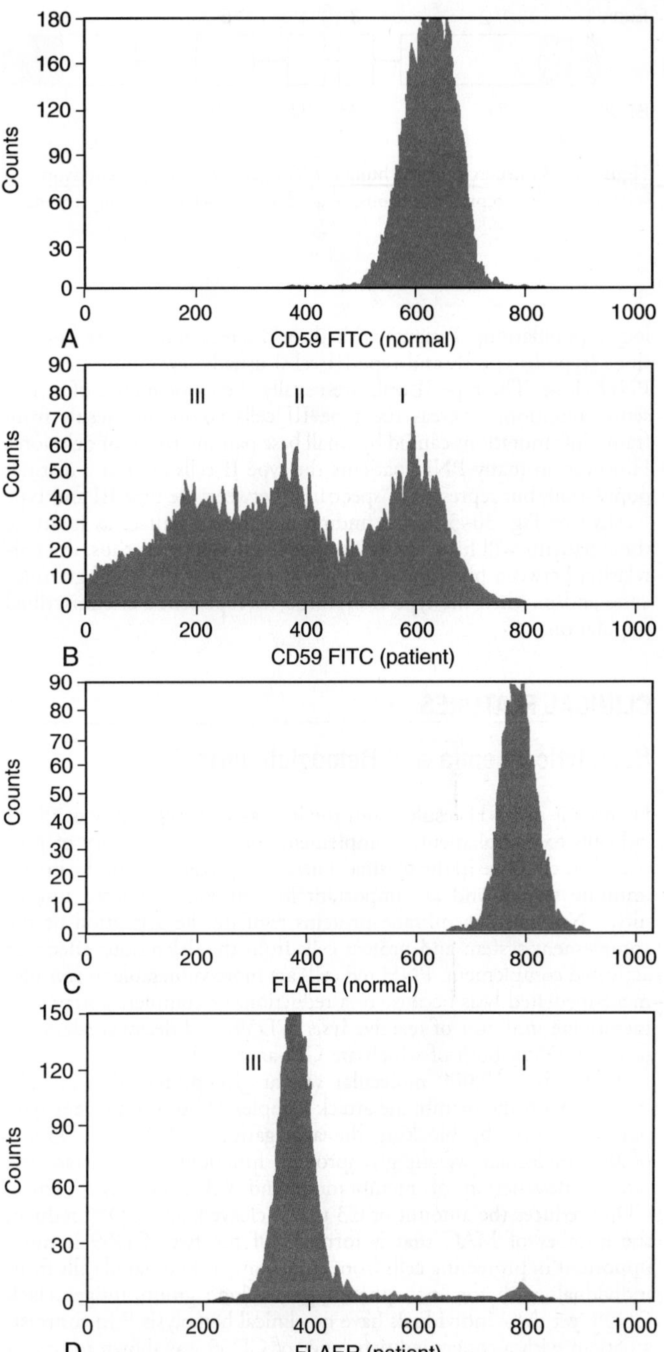

Figure 30–2 Flow cytometric analysis or peripheral blood cells from a paroxysmal nocturnal hemoglobinuria (PNH) patient. (**A**) Fluorescence intensity of erythrocytes from a healthy control after staining with anti-CD59. (**B**) Fluorescence intensity of erythrocytes from an untransfused PNH patient after staining with anti-CD59. Type II cells are "blended" between the type I (normal) and type III cells. (**C**) Fluorescence intensity of granulocytes from a healthy control stained with FLAER. (**D**) Fluorescence intensity of granulocytes from the same PNH patient as **B** following staining with FLAER. Note that the granulocytes are almost exclusively type III cells. A small population of type I granulocytes is present.

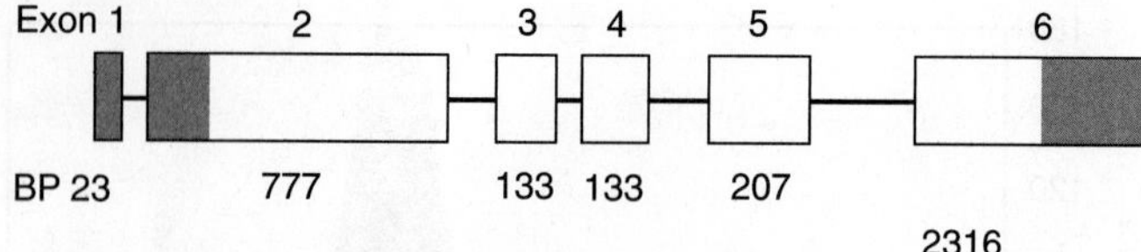

Figure 30–3 Structure of the human *PIGA* gene. Boxes represent exons; intervening lines represent introns. Shaded areas show noncoding regions.

locyte populations. Patients with three discreet granulocyte populations (type I, type II, and type III cells) usually have more than one PNH clone. The type II cells are usually the consequence of a missense mutation, whereas the type III cells commonly result from frameshift mutations caused by small base pair insertions or deletions. However, in many PNH patients the type II cells are not a distinct population, but represent a "spectrum" between the type III and type I cells (see Fig. 30–3). This finding may be an artifact as many of these patients will have few to no type II granulocytes; thus, the correlation between phenotype and genotype is best for PNH granulocytes and/or when the type II erythrocytes represent a circumscribed population.

CLINICAL FEATURES

Hemolytic Anemia and Hemoglobinuria

Hemolysis in PNH results from the increased susceptibility of PNH red cells to complement. Complement consists of a battery of proteins that circulate in the plasma. These proteins are part of the innate immune system and are important for antibody-mediated immunity.[39] Normally, membrane proteins regulate the activation of the complement system and protect cells from the deleterious effects of activated complement. PNH red cells are more vulnerable to complement-mediated lysis because of a reduction, or complete absence, of membrane inhibitor of reactive lysis (CD59) and decay accelerating factor (CD55), both of which are GPI-anchored.

CD59 is a 19,000 molecular weight glycoprotein that directly interacts with the membrane attack complex (MAC) to prevent lytic pore formation by blocking the aggregation of C9.[40,41] CD55, a 68,000 molecular weight glycoprotein, functions to accelerate the rate of destruction of membrane-bound C3 convertase. Hence, CD55 reduces the amount of C3 that is cleaved, and CD59 reduces the number of MAC that is formed. Of the two, CD59 is more important in protecting cells from complement. Red blood cells from individuals with the Inab phenotype, a blood group antigen, lack CD55, yet these individuals have no clinical hemolysis.[42] In contrast, a patient with a congenital deficiency of CD59 was shown to have a compensated hemolytic anemia.[43] Furthermore, incorporation of CD59 onto PNH erythrocytes was shown to ameliorate acidified serum lysis to a greater extent than incorporation of CD55.[44]

The classic manifestation from which PNH derives its name—paroxysmal bouts of reddish, brownish, or "cola-colored" urine that strikes predominantly overnight—is described by a minority of PNH patients. Most PNH patients have no noticeable hemoglobinuria or have intermittent episodes of hemoglobinuria with no relation to the time of day. Early speculation that the nocturnal hemoglobinuria was a function of a mild drop in pH that occurs with sleep has not been validated. Patients with a history of hemoglobinuria are more likely to have a large PNH clone and less likely to have a markedly hypocellular bone marrow.

Although hemolysis is often the most conspicuous feature in patients with classical PNH, many patients, particularly those with coexisting bone marrow failure, exhibit mild to barely detectable hemolysis. The hemoglobin concentration can range from normal to severely depressed. The reticulocyte count is often elevated but usually lower than expected for the degree of anemia. Patients with PNH manifest all the usual clinical and laboratory signs of chronic hemolytic anemia: weakness, fatigue, pallor, and dyspnea on exertion. In patients with prominent hemolysis, the magnitude of fatigue can be out of proportion to the degree of anemia. Morphologically, the red cells appear normal, although some cases display mild to moderate poikilocytosis and anisocytosis. The haptoglobin levels are usually low, and the lactate dehydrogenase (LDH) is frequently elevated, sometimes greater than 3000 IU/L, depending on the degree of hemolysis.

Multiple factors influence the degree of hemolysis in PNH, including the size and type of the PNH clone and the degree of complement activation. In general, the percentage of PNH erythrocytes correlates with the degree of hemolysis. However, the type of PNH erythrocytes may also influence the degree of hemolysis. Type III erythrocytes are more readily lysed than type II erythrocytes and almost always constitute a larger percentage of the PNH red cells. Thus, patients with a large percentage of type III erythrocytes tend to have more hemolysis than patients with a large percentage of type I or type II cells. Finally, hemolysis is frequently exacerbated by infections (especially gastrointestinal infections), surgery, strenuous exercise, excessive alcohol intake, blood transfusions, and anything else that initiates complement activation.

Smooth Muscle Dystonia and Nitric Oxide

Many clinical manifestations of PNH are readily explained by hemoglobin-mediated nitric oxide scavenging.[45,46] Failure of complement regulation on the PNH erythrocyte membrane leads to intravascular hemolysis resulting in the release of large amounts of free hemoglobin into the plasma. Free plasma hemoglobin leads to increased consumption of nitric oxide resulting in manifestations that include fatigue, abdominal pain, esophageal spasm, erectile dysfunction, and possibly thrombosis. Indeed, hemoglobinuria, thrombosis, erectile dysfunction, and esophageal spasm are more common in patients with large PNH populations (>60% of granulocytes) than in patients with relatively small PNH populations. In a study of 49 PNH patients diagnosed using flow cytometry, Moyo and colleagues demonstrated that large PNH clones were associated with an increased risk for thrombosis, hemoglobinuria, abdominal pain, esophageal spasm, and male impotence.[47] Thus, many of the clinical manifestations of PNH appear to be a direct consequence of intravascular hemolysis, leading to the release of free hemoglobin, scavenging of nitric oxide, and smooth muscle dystonias.

Renal Manifestations

PNH patients can experience renal manifestations that resemble those observed with sickle cell anemia.[48] Perturbed tubular function and declining creatinine clearance are found in a high percentage of patients. Radiologically, patients can exhibit large kidneys, cortical infarcts, cortical thinning, and papillary necrosis. PNH patients display marked hemosiderin deposition in the proximal tubules; however, microvascular thrombosis can be responsible for many of the renal abnormalities in PNH.[48] Acute renal failure following massive hemolysis occurs infrequently and usually resolves in days to weeks.

Thrombosis and PNH

Thrombosis is an ominous complication of PNH and the leading cause of death from the disease. It occurs in approximately 40% of PNH patients and almost invariably involves the venous system. Patients with a large percentage of PNH cells and classical symptoms (hemolytic anemia and hemoglobinuria) have a greater propensity for thrombosis than patients with a small percentage of PNH cells.[47,49–51] According to logistic regression modeling, for a 10% change in PNH clone size, the odds ratio for risk of thrombosis is estimated to be

1.64.[47] Patients with PNH granulocyte clones of greater than 60% appear to be at greatest risk for thrombosis. The mechanism of thrombosis in PNH is not entirely understood and probably multifactorial, but similar to other manifestations of the disease, it is probably related to the GPI anchor protein deficiency. Indeed, nitric oxide depletion has been associated with increased platelet aggregation, increased platelet adhesion, and accelerated clot formation.[46] In an attempt to repair damage, PNH platelets undergo exocytosis of the complement attack complex.[52] This results in the formation of microvesicles with phosphatidylserine externalization, a potent in-vitro procoagulant. These prothrombotic microvesicles have been detected in the blood of PNH patients.[53] Fibrinolysis can also be perturbed in PNH given that PNH blood cells lack the GPI-anchored urokinase receptor.[54] Lastly, tissue factor pathway inhibitor (TFPI), a major inhibitor of tissue factor, has been shown to require a GPI-anchored chaperone protein for trafficking to the endothelial cell surface.[55] Although the mechanism of thrombosis in PNH is not entirely clear, the sites of venous thrombosis in PNH are manifold with the abdominal veins and the cerebral veins being the most commonly involved regions.

Liver

Hepatic vein thrombosis (Budd-Chiari syndrome) is the most common site of thrombosis in PNH and is frequently a fatal complication.[47,56,57] Moreover, PNH is probably the condition that confers the highest risk for developing hepatic vein thrombosis.[58] The clinical manifestations of hepatic vein thrombosis include abdominal pain, hepatomegaly, jaundice, ascites, and weight gain.[59] The onset of symptoms can be abrupt or insidious. Hepatic vein thrombosis in PNH tends to inexorably progress with periodic exacerbations followed by intervals of relatively stable disease. Although some patients live many years with the condition, it frequently results in death. The best noninvasive tests to confirm the diagnosis include computed tomography scanning, magnetic resonance imaging, and ultrasonography. Thrombosis can involve the small hepatic veins, large-sized hepatic veins, or both. Thrombolytic therapy has been used successfully to restore venous patency and reverse the hepatic congestion; however, because of the potential danger of this approach, it should be used judiciously.[60] Patients with acute onset disease, preserved platelet counts (>50,000 cells/mm^3), and large vessel involvement are the best candidates for thrombolysis. For patients with massive ascites who are not suitable candidates for thrombolytic therapy, transjugular intrahepatic portal-systemic shunting or surgical shunting can successfully palliate some patients. Orthotopic liver transplantation has also been performed in a few cases; however, this is not routinely recommended as the underlying disease leads to prompt relapse.[61]

Portal vein thrombosis is also common in PNH and can occur with or without hepatic vein thrombosis.[47,57,62,63] Patients frequently present with nausea, vomiting, abdominal pain, and liver dysfunction. Management is similar to that of hepatic vein thrombosis.

Other Abdominal Veins

Venous thrombosis in PNH has been described in all abdominal and retroperitoneal venous systems including the splenic veins,[64] mesenteric veins, renal veins, and the inferior vena cava.[65] Thrombosis of minor veins can also occur and can be difficult to diagnose because of the protean manifestations and their relapsing and remitting nature.[66] Often such patients present with recurrent, severe abdominal pain crises sometimes mimicking intestinal obstruction. The consequence of these microthromboses can sometimes be visualized with esophagogastroduodenal endoscopy or colonoscopy. Patients with intestinal thromboses can present with ischemic colitis and can be misdiagnosed as having Crohn's disease. Upper gastrointestinal bleeding can be caused by esophageal or gastric varices that develop as a consequence of portal hypertension or splenic vein thrombosis.

Cerebral Veins

Cerebral veins, particularly the sagittal veins and sinuses, are also highly prone to thrombosis in PNH.[47,57,63,67] Patients can present with severe headaches and/or focal neurologic deficits depending on the location of the thrombosis. Similar to hepatic vein thrombosis, cerebral vein thrombosis is an ominous complication that can result in substantial morbidity and mortality. Magnetic resonance imaging to carefully examine the cerebral blood flow is helpful in establishing the diagnosis.

Other Sites

Dermal venous thrombosis can occur virtually anywhere on the body but seem to have a predilection for the face and upper extremities. Patients usually complain of pain, discolorations and swelling. The lesions can reach several centimeters in diameter and are firm and tender. Necrosis and the formation of a black eschar can occur. Anticoagulation and warm compresses can ameliorate the attacks. Pulmonary emboli and deep venous thrombosis have also been reported in PNH but are uncommon; arterial thrombosis is rare.

CLONALITY AND BONE MARROW FAILURE

PIGA Mutations in Aplastic Anemia and Myelodysplastic Syndrome

Small to moderate PNH clones are found in up to 70% of patients with acquired aplastic anemia, demonstrating a pathophysiologic link between these disorders.[7,8,68,69] Typically, less than 20% GPI anchor protein-deficient granulocytes are detected in aplastic anemia patients at diagnosis, but occasional patients can have larger clones.[8] DNA sequencing of the GPI anchor protein-deficient cells from aplastic anemia patients reveals clonal *PIGA* gene mutations.[29] Moreover, many of these patients exhibit expansion of the *PIGA* mutant clone and progress to clinical PNH. Although it was once thought that PNH evolving from aplastic anemia is more benign than classical PNH, this observation can be a consequence of lead time bias, as many of these patients eventually develop classical PNH symptoms.

GPI anchor protein-deficient cells have also been reported in patients with MDS,[7,69] but sequencing of the *PIGA* gene to establish clonality has not been performed in most of these studies. MDS patients reported to have small PNH populations tend to be classified as refractory anemia and often have the following characteristics: a hypocellular marrow, human leukocyte antigen (HLA)-DR15 positivity, normal cytogenetics, moderate to severe thrombocytopenia, and a high likelihood of response to immunosuppressive therapy.[69,70] Thus, it is possible that many of these patients have moderate aplastic anemia rather than MDS. Distinguishing hypoplastic MDS from aplastic anemia is often difficult; however, quantitative analysis of bone marrow CD34 positive cells is useful for discriminating between these two entities.[71]

PIGA Mutations in Healthy Controls

PNH is an uncommon disease, with only two to five new cases per million US inhabitants annually; however, *PIGA* mutations can be found in the blood from virtually all healthy controls.[37,72,73] Araten and coworkers used flow cytometric analysis of blood from 9 healthy controls and found an average of 22 GPI anchor protein-deficient granulocytes per 10^6 cells, yet none of these subjects developed PNH. GPI anchor protein-deficient lymphocytes have also been detected in patients with lymphoid malignancies or rheumatoid arthritis after treatment with alemtuzumab (Campath-1H). Alemtuzimab is a monoclonal antibody that recognizes CD52, a GPI-anchored protein expressed on monocytes, B cells, and T cells.[74–77] None of these patients developed PNH; furthermore, when the alemtuzimab was discontinued, the GPI anchor protein–deficient cells regressed.

How can such a common mutation, *PIGA,* be so specific for PNH, yet so rarely result in disease? One hypothesis to explain the close relationship between PNH and aplastic anemia, and the mechanisms whereby the PNH clone achieves dominance, involves a "two-step" model. This model proposes that hematopoietic stem cells randomly and spontaneously acquire *PIGA* mutations at a very low frequency (step one). Step two in this model proposes that the immunologic attack that targets hematopoietic stem cells in aplastic anemia spares PNH cells, ostensibly because they lack GPI-anchored proteins.[78,79] Indeed, *PIGA* mutant cells are found at low frequency in most healthy controls.[37,72,73,76] More recent data suggest that most, if not all, *PIGA* mutations in healthy controls arise from colony-forming cells rather than hematopoietic stem cells[37]; thus, the relevance of these mutations is unclear. Furthermore, there is no direct evidence to support a GPI-anchored protein being the target of the immune attack in aplastic anemia. Importantly, this two-step model does not explain the similarly high incidence of MDS in aplastic anemia patients.[80,81]

An alternative hypothesis that could explain the predisposition of patients with aplastic anemia to develop both PNH and MDS has been proposed. MDS and PNH evolving in the setting of aplastic anemia could be analogous to the *field cancerization effect* described in aerodigestive and other solid tumors to explain second primary tumors in the affected tissue.[82,83] That is, a single insult to the marrow, such as generalized toxic damage or a genetic predisposition, may be responsible for bringing about different forms of marrow disorders; these disorders can occur alone, simultaneously, or sequentially.[84,85] In aplastic anemia, the bone marrow injury may primarily trigger an autoimmune attack on the hematopoietic stem/progenitor compartment, perhaps by exposing cryptic epitopes through molecular mimicry, or by sending a "danger" signal. In primary PNH or MDS, the injury may primarily produce a genetic mutation that leads to clonal dominance of the affected clone.[86–88] In other patients, bone marrow injury may induce both an autoimmune hematopoietic attack and a clonal genetic mutation that present either simultaneously or sequentially. Examples of simultaneous presentation are the aplastic anemia/PNH overlap and hypoplastic MDS. Lastly, a third hypothesis proposes that additional mutations occurring in *PIGA* mutant stem cells are required for clonal expansion PNH.[89–91] These hypotheses may not be mutually exclusive; thus, further investigation is needed to fully understand the mechanism of clonal dominance in PNH.

Clinical observations also provide clues to understanding clonal dominance in PNH and the relationship between aplastic anemia and PNH. Up to 30% of aplastic anemia patients treated with conventional immunosuppressive therapy (antithymocyte globulin and cyclosporine) will develop PNH or MDS, usually several years after therapy.[81,92] In contrast, allogeneic bone marrow transplantation appears to eliminate the risk for developing PNH in patients with aplastic anemia. These data suggest that secondary clonal disorders (PNH and MDS) are part of the natural history of aplastic anemia. Although immunosuppressive therapy unequivocally prolongs survival, it does not prevent these late complications. High-dose cyclophosphamide therapy for severe aplastic anemia appears to result in more durable and complete remissions than conventional immunosuppression, but it is premature to conclude that this approach eliminates the risk for developing PNH.[93–95]

Clonal Transformation

PNH patients, similar to aplastic anemia and MDS patients, are at increased risk for clonal transformation;[96] however, the incidence of leukemic transformation in PNH is less than that of MDS. Abnormal cytogenetics can be found in up to 20% of PNH patients.[97] MDS and acute myeloid leukemia are the most common malignancies to evolve from PNH; the leukemic cells arise from the GPI anchor-deficient clone in most, but not all cases.[98,99]

NATURAL HISTORY

The natural history of PNH ranges from indolent to severely debilitating and life-threatening.[47,56,57] Females and males are equally affected with the median age of diagnosis being 40 years old. The median survival from time of diagnosis is 10 to 15 years. Thrombosis, severe pancytopenia, evolution to MDS or leukemia, older age, and thrombocytopenia at diagnosis portend a poor prognosis. Older literature, where patients were diagnosed with PNH based on the Ham test or sucrose hemolysis test, reported on the occurrence of spontaneous long-term remissions in up to 10% of PNH cases[57]; however, in patients diagnosed with PNH based on flow cytometric assays, spontaneous remissions are extremely rare.[47]

LABORATORY EVALUATION

Blood

Peripheral blood counts in PNH patients vary from severe pancytopenia to normal. Virtually all patients will present with anemia, frequently with mild macrocytosis. Thrombocytopenia and/or neutropenia are also common. A mild to moderate reticulocytosis is usually present in patients with the classical form of the disease; however, in patients with hypoplastic PNH (also known as *aplastic anemia/PNH overlap*), the reticulocyte count can be reduced. Similarly, in patients with hypoplastic PNH, the biochemical profile can be normal, but in patients with large PNH clones the indirect bilirubin and LDH are significantly elevated. In patients with vigorous hemolysis, it is not uncommon for the laboratory to report the specimen as "hemolyzed."

Bone Marrow

Bone marrow cellularity can be hypocellular, normocellular, or hypercellular. In patients with classical PNH (not arising from or coinciding with aplastic anemia), the marrow is usually normocellular to hypercellular with erythroid hyperplasia. Mild to moderate dyserythropoiesis is common. Stainable iron is frequently absent because of iron loss associated with the intravascular hemolysis. Cytogenetic abnormalities can be found in up to 20% of patients.

DIAGNOSIS

Complement-Based Assays

The Ham test and the sucrose hemolysis test (sugar water test) were two of the first assays used to diagnosis PNH. Both assays are performed on erythrocytes and discriminate PNH cells from normal cells based on a differential sensitivity to the hemolytic action of complement. In the Ham test, complement is activated by acidification of the serum. This results in lysis of PNH erythrocytes but not normal erythrocytes.[3] The Ham test is relatively specific for PNH, but is not very sensitive.

Complement is also activated in a low ionic strength sucrose-containing medium. Preferential lysis of PNH erythrocytes through the activation of complement in this sucrose-containing medium forms the basis for the sugar water test.[100] This assay is easier to perform and is more sensitive than the Ham test but not as specific; other hemolytic anemias and even leukemias can produce false positive results. The complement lysis assay in which complement is activated with antibody will also detect PNH erythrocytes.[101] These complement-based red cell assays are important from a historical perspective, but should no longer be used to establish the diagnosis of PNH.

GPI Anchor-Based Assays

Most laboratories use monoclonal antibodies against specific GPI-anchored proteins in conjunction with flow cytometry to diagnose PNH. Anti-CD59 is most commonly used because it is widely expressed and is displayed on all hematopoietic lineages. Anti-CD55, anti-CD14, anti-CD16, anti-CD67, and a variety of other monoclonal antibodies can also be used to establish the diagnosis. Flow cytometry offers several advantages over complement-based assays for diagnosing PNH: It measures the size of the PNH clone in the various cell lineages, it is more sensitive and specific, and it is less affected by blood transfusions. It is noteworthy that rare congenital deficiencies of CD59 and CD55 can lead to a false positive test for PNH if only one monoclonal antibody is used. This, coupled with the variable expression of GPI-anchored proteins on different hematopoietic lineages, accounts for the recommendation that at least two different monoclonal antibodies, directed against two different GPI-anchored proteins, on at least two different cell lineages, should be used to diagnose a patient with PNH. Solely screening patients' red cells for PNH can lead to falsely negative tests, especially in the setting of a recent hemolytic episode or a recent blood transfusion. As granulocytes and monocytes have a short half-life and are not affected by blood transfusions, the percentage of PNH cells in these lineages best reflects the size of the PNH clone.

Aerolysin Assays

A fluorescein-labeled proaerolysin variant, 5 *Fl*ourescent *Aer*olysin FLAER, is increasingly being used as a flow cytometric assay to diagnose PNH.[102,103] Aerolysin is the principal virulence factor of the bacterium *Aeromonas hydrophila*. It is secreted as an inert protoxin termed, proaerolysin, that binds selectively and with high affinity to the GPI anchor.[104,105] After binding to its receptor (the glycan portion of the GPI anchor), the C-terminal peptide of proaerolysin is cleaved by cell proteases. This activates the toxin and leads to the formation of heptameric channels that insert into the membrane and kill the cell.[106] PNH cells are resistant to aerolysin and proaerolysin because PNH cells lack GPI-anchored proteins. FLAER binds to the GPI anchor without forming channels and gives a more accurate assessment of the GPI-anchor deficit in PNH than anti-CD59.[102] Because the GPI anchor is the major determinant for binding FLAER, it allows for the direct assessment of GPI anchor expression on virtually all cell lineages.[8,102,103] Red cells are a notable exception; this may be because both normal and PNH red cells express large amounts of glycophorin, a protein shown to bind aerolysin weakly.[107] Nevertheless, in mononuclear cells FLAER eliminates the need for multiple lineage-specific monoclonal antibodies. These properties make FLAER more reliable for detecting the diminutive PNH populations often found in patients with aplastic anemia.[8]

THERAPY

Introduction

Some PNH patients can be managed conservatively with supportive care alone. The major exceptions are patients with hypoplastic PNH (especially those who also meet criteria for severe aplastic anemia) and patients with life-threatening thromboses or debilitating hemolysis and smooth muscle dystonias. Cytopenias in patients with hypoplastic PNH are usually caused by immune suppression of hematopoiesis; thus, the management of these patients should be similar to those with acquired aplastic anemia. Classical PNH patients manifesting with recurrent thrombosis and/or severe intravascular hemolysis are particularly challenging to manage. For these patients, eculizumab or bone marrow transplantation are reasonable therapeutic options.

Immunosuppressive Therapy

PNH patients with a hypoplastic bone marrow, low reticulocyte count, and pancytopenia (hypoplastic PNH) will frequently respond to immunosuppressive therapy.[108,109] The response rate in this group is more than 50%. In fact, finding a minor population of PNH-like cells in severe aplastic anemia may predict for response to immunosuppressive therapy.[110] The impaired hematopoiesis that occurs in hypoplastic PNH may respond to antithymocyte globulin and/or cyclosporine, but the PNH clone is not affected.[109] In some cases, immunosuppressive therapy has ameliorated the aplasia but with preferential expansion of the PNH clone.[111] Immunosuppressive therapy does not appear to benefit patients with classical PNH.

Management of Anemia

The cause of anemia in PNH is often multifactorial. In patients with hypoplastic PNH, bone marrow failure, usually because of autoimmunity, is the major etiologic factor for anemia. Patients with hypoplastic PNH may respond to immunosuppressive therapy. However, in patients with cellular bone marrows, elevated reticulocyte counts, and a high LDH (classical PNH), intravascular hemolysis is the major mechanism of anemia. Traditionally, these patients were given a trial of adrenocorticosteroids. Prednisone therapy (0.5 mg to 1 mg/kg/day) can reduce hemolysis and increase hemoglobin levels in some patients. If possible, the prednisone dose should be tapered to 10 mg to 20 mg on alternate days to reduce the toxicities from chronic steroid therapy. If no salutary effect is observed after 1 to 2 months of therapy, prednisone should be discontinued. Danazol can also be effective in some patients with classical PNH.[112] Erythropoietin is rarely beneficial. Iron deficiency caused by intravascular hemolysis can also contribute to the anemia of PNH; thus, in patients with absent iron stores, iron replacement therapy is indicated. Folic acid supplementation is also recommended in PNH because of the high red cell turnover. Some patients are refractory to therapy and can require periodic red cell transfusions. These patients should receive group-specific blood and blood products. Washing the red cells with saline, once advocated to minimize hemolysis after transfusion in PNH, is unnecessary.[113]

Eculizumab

Eculizumab is a humanized monoclonal antibody against C5 that inhibits terminal complement activation (Fig. 30–4) and will likely become the treatment of choice in patients with classical PNH. A 12-week open-labeled trial of eculizumab in 11 PNH patients demonstrated that the drug reduced intravascular hemolysis and transfusion requirements.[6] A recent international double-blind, randomized, controlled trial in PNH patients demonstrated that eculizumab was effective in stabilizing hemoglobin levels and reduced transfusion requirements in patients with classical PNH.[114] Blockade of the complement cascade at C5 preserves the early activity of the complement cascade that is necessary for the opsonization of microorganisms and clearance of immune complexes;[39] however, as terminal complement blockade can be associated with an increased risk for *Neisserial* infections, all patients in this study were vaccinated against *Neisseria meningitides* 2 weeks before receiving the study drug. The study randomized 87 PNH patients to receive either placebo ($n = 44$) or eculizumab ($n = 43$) administered intravenously at 600 mg weekly for 4 weeks, 900 mg the following week, and then 900 mg every 2 weeks for a total of 6 months. The primary endpoints were hemoglobin stabilization and reduction in units of transfused blood. Eligible PNH patients were required to be red cell transfusion dependent with a platelet count of >100,000 per mm^3 and an LDH level >1.5 times

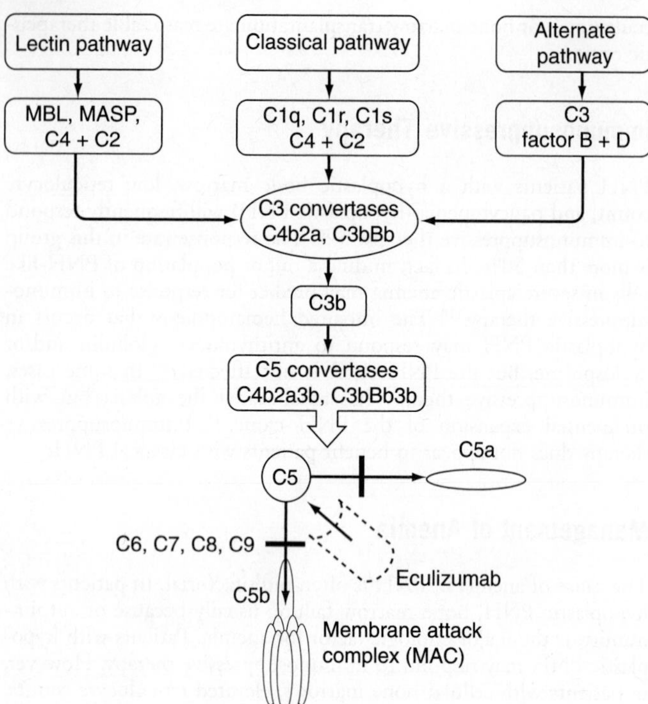

Figure 30–4 Overview of the complement cascade. Classic, alternative, and lectin pathways converge at the point of C3 activation. The lytic pathway is initiated with the formation of C5 convertase and leads to the assembly of the C5, C6, C7, C8, (*n*) C9 membrane attack complex. Eculizumab is a monoclonal antibody that binds to C5, thereby preventing the formation of C5a and C5b. C5b is the initiating component of the membrane attack complex (MAC). FITC, fluorescein isothiocyanate.

the upper limit of normal. Hemoglobin stabilization was maintained by 48.8% patients in the eculizumab-treated group and 0% in the placebo-treated group ($P < 0.001$). A median of 0 units of packed red cells were transfused in the eculizumab-treated group compared with a median of 10 units in the placebo-treated group ($P = 0.001$). The eculizumab-treated group also showed significant improvements in quality of life and a significant decrease in LDH levels. The most common adverse events reported for eculizumab-treated patients were headache, nasopharyngitis, back pain, and upper respiratory tract infections. Thus, in patients with classical PNH, eculizumab is highly effective in decreasing intravascular hemolysis; the drug greatly improves quality of life and reduces or eliminates the need for blood transfusions. Importantly, eculizumab also mitigates the smooth muscle dystonias that are often associated with PNH by reducing plasma free hemoglobin levels. Eculizumab is not yet approved by the FDA; however, on approval and further investigation, it is likely that eculizumab will become the recommended initial therapy for patients with classical PNH. Patients with hypoplastic PNH are less likely to respond to eculizumab, because bone marrow suppression, rather than complement-mediated hemolysis is the major mechanism of anemia. Whether eculizumab will decrease the risk for thrombosis and improved survival in PNH remains to be determined.

Thrombosis

Thrombosis is often the most pernicious complication of PNH and usually represents an indication for long-term anticoagulation. In patients with acute onset abdominal vein thrombosis, thrombolytic therapy has been successfully employed.[60] However, in some patients, thrombolytic therapy and/or anticoagulation is relatively contraindicated because of severe thrombocytopenia. Managing PNH patients on chronic warfarin therapy is often challenging. Platelet counts are usually mildly to moderately reduced and sometimes erratic. Furthermore, maintaining a therapeutic international normalized ratio (INR) is difficult in some patients because of frequent PNH attacks that can be associated with anorexia, nausea, and vomiting. The use of oral contraceptives and pregnancy can exacerbate the proclivity for thrombosis in PNH and should be considered high risk.

Bone Marrow Transplantation

Allogeneic hematopoietic stem cell transplantation is the only curative therapy for PNH.[115–117] Because of the substantial morbidity and mortality of this procedure and the sometimes indolent natural history of PNH, bone marrow transplantation (BMT) should only be offered to patients with more severe forms of the disease. Younger patients with severe pancytopenia or life-threatening thrombosis who have an HLA-identical sibling are the best candidates for this approach. The International Bone Marrow Transplant Registry (IBMTR) reported a 2-year survival probability of 56% in 48 recipients of HLA-identical sibling transplants between 1978 and 1995. The median age was 28 years. The majority of the deaths in this study occurred within 1 year of transplantation. One of seven recipients of alternative donor allogeneic transplants reported to the IBMTR during this period was alive 5 years after transplant. Both nonmyeloablative syngeneic BMT and nonmyeloablative stem cell transplants from HLA-matched siblings have been performed in PNH patients.[115,116,118] Interestingly, the latter approach, but not the former, appears to cure the disease, suggesting that there is an important *graft-versus- PNH* effect with bone marrow transplantation. Future use of bone marrow transplantation to treat PNH may be curtained once eculizumab becomes more widely available.

APPROACH TO DIAGNOSING PNH

PNH has an estimated incidence of 2 to 5 per million in the United States. This, coupled with its protean manifestations, make diagnosing PNH a challenge for even the most astute diagnostician. However, given the ease and specificity of modern diagnostic assays, the most important attribute a physician can possess in diagnosing PNH is to maintain a high level of suspicion and to be cognizant of the various presentations of the disease. A small sample of peripheral blood sent to an experienced flow cytometric laboratory is usually sufficient to establish or exclude the diagnosis of PNH. These assays are fast, reliable, and inexpensive. If monoclonal antibodies are used to establish the diagnosis, it is imperative that two or more antibodies be used on at least two different lineages. Assaying granulocytes is the most reliable method to diagnose PNH as they are not affected by blood transfusions. I prefer to use FLAER over monoclonal antibodies on granulocytes and monocytes because of the improved sensitivity and specificity; anti-CD59 is the most reliable marker on erythrocytes.

Classical PNH is usually more conspicuous than hypoplastic PNH. Patients typically present with a direct antiglobulin negative hemolytic anemia, hemoglobinuria, and mild to moderate cytopenias. Obscure paroxysms of back pain, abdominal pain, fatigue and/or headaches are often present. The bone marrow is typically normocellular to mildly hypercellular with intense erythroid hyperplasia and mild to moderate dyserythropoiesis. Bone marrow iron stores are frequently, but not always, absent. PNH patients can also present with abrupt, severe abdominal pain and jaundice caused by thrombosis. All patients presenting with unexplained hepatic vein, portal vein, mesenteric vein, or portal vein thrombosis should be screened for PNH.

It is important to distinguish PNH from MDS. Most patients with refractory anemia should be screened for PNH, especially those with moderate to severe cytopenias and a hypocellular bone marrow. In addition, all patients diagnosed with aplastic anemia should be screened for PNH. In rare instances idiopathic myelofibrosis or autoimmune hemolytic anemias can mimic PNH. Patients with a history of aplastic anemia—especially those managed with immunosuppressive therapy—should be monitored closely for the outgrowth of PNH.

APPROACH TO TREATMENT

Classification of PNH: Classical PNH Versus Hypoplastic PNH

I find it useful to classify PNH patients as either "classical" or "hypoplastic." This can usually be accomplished by ordering a complete blood count, reticulocyte count, LDH, peripheral blood flow cytometry for PNH, and a bone marrow aspirate, biopsy, and cytogenetics. Patients with classical PNH tend to have mild to moderate cytopenias, a normocellular to hypercellular bone marrow, an elevated reticulocyte count, a markedly elevated LDH, and a relatively large PNH granulocyte population (>30%). In contrast, hypoplastic PNH patients present with manifestations similar to that of aplastic anemia or hypoplastic MDS. These patients typically present with moderate to severe cytopenias, a hypocellular bone marrow (<25% cellularity), a decreased corrected reticulocyte count, a normal or mildly elevated LDH, and a relatively small (<20%) PNH granulocyte population. Most, but not all, patients can be readily subdivided into classical versus hypoplastic PNH, a distinction that aids with therapeutic decisions.

Hypoplastic PNH

Because bone marrow failure is the major risk for patients with hypoplastic PNH, I direct my therapy toward the pancytopenia. If, in addition to the PNH, the patient fulfills criteria for severe aplastic anemia (see Chapter 29), appropriate therapeutic options include allogeneic bone marrow transplantation, high-dose cyclophosphamide, or antithymocyte globulin and cyclosporine. Young patients (ie, <30 years of age) with an HLA-matched sibling should be transplanted; for older patients and for those without an HLA-matched sibling, high-dose cyclophosphamide or antithymocyte and cyclosporine is appropriate. I prefer to use high-dose cyclophosphamide because of the improved quality and duration of remissions. If the patient's cytopenias do not fulfill criteria for severe aplastic anemia, supportive care or a trial of immunosuppressive therapy is appropriate.

Classical PNH

Symptoms in patients with classical PNH vary from mild, to severely debilitating, to acutely life-threatening. Hence, therapy should be directed toward the specific manifestations (eg, anemia, thrombosis, etc). Allogeneic bone marrow transplantation, preferably from an HLA-matched sibling, is appropriate for patients with severely debilitating or acutely life-threatening disease. In general, these are patients with recurrent thrombosis or those with clonal evolution to either MDS or acute leukemia. Patients with less severe disease should not be transplanted because of the relatively high morbidity and mortality of the procedure. Antithymocyte globulin (ATG) and cyclosporine or high-dose cyclophosphamide does not appear to benefit patients with classical PNH.

Anemia

All patients with classical PNH should be placed on folic acid (1 to 2 mg/day). Patients with absent iron stores, usually because of chronic intravascular hemolysis, should be treated with oral iron supplementation. Pending FDA approval, eculizumab is likely to become the standard-of-care to treat patients with classical PNH. It is the only drug demonstrated in a randomized study to benefit PNH patients. Eculizumab has been shown to decrease the need for transfusions, decrease paroxysms, and improve quality of life in patients with classical PNH; however, it has not been shown to benefit patients with hypoplastic PNH.

If eculizumab is unavailable, a trial of prednisone (0.5 to 1.0 mg/day) can occasionally decrease hemolysis and increase hemoglobin levels. If a salutary effect is not achieved within 6 to 8 weeks, the steroids should be discontinued. In responding patients the steroids should be tapered to the lowest dose that still provides a beneficial effect. Alternate day steroids can help decrease the risk of deleterious long-term side effects. Danazol (400 mg/day) can also decrease hemolysis; if no response is observed after 8 weeks, the drug should be discontinued.

Thrombosis

Patients who present with acute life-threatening or organ-threatening thrombosis should be considered for thrombolytic therapy. In patients with chronic, insidious thrombosis, anticoagulation with heparin followed by long-term warfarin anticoagulation should be initiated. Meticulous monitoring of warfarin levels in PNH patients is warranted, as the risk for bleeding complications is high. Erratic oral intake during PNH attacks, and underlying liver dysfunction can lead to volatility in the INR. In addition, most PNH patients have thrombocytopenia. Thus, the potential risks and benefits of anticoagulation must be scrupulously considered, especially in patients with platelet counts below 50,000 cells/mm^3.

SUGGESTED READINGS

Araten DJ, Nafa K, Pakdeesuwan K, et al: Clonal populations of hematopoietic cells with paroxysmal nocturnal hemoglobinuria genotype and phenotype are present in normal individuals. Proc Natl Acad Sci U S A 96:5209, 1999.

Bessler M, Mason PJ, Hillmen P, et al: Paroxysmal nocturnal haemoglobinuria (PNH) is caused by somatic mutations in the PIG-A gene. EMBO J 13:110, 1994.

Brodsky RA, Mukhina GL, Nelson KL, et al: Resistance of paroxysmal nocturnal hemoglobinuria cells to the glycosylphosphatidylinositol-binding toxin aerolysin. Blood 93:1749, 1999.

Chen R, Nagarajan S, Prince GM, et al: Impaired growth and elevated fas receptor expression in PIGA(+) stem cells in primary paroxysmal nocturnal hemoglobinuria. J Clin Invest 106:689, 2000.

Ham T: Chronic hemolytic anemia with paroxysmal nocturnal hemoglobinuria. A study of the mechanism of hemolysis in relation to acid-base equilibrium. N Engl J Med 217:915, 1937.

Hillmen P, Lewis SM, Bessler M, et al: Natural history of paroxysmal nocturnal hemoglobinuria. N Engl J Med 333:1253, 1995.

Hillmen P, Young NS, Schubert J, et al: The complement inhibitor eculizumab in paroxysmal nocturnal hemoglobinuria. N Engl J Med 355:1233, 2006.

Hu R, Mukhina GL, Piantadosi S, et al: PIG-A mutations in normal hematopoiesis. Blood 105:3848, 2005.

Inoue N, Izui-Sarumaru T, Murakami Y, et al: Molecular basis of clonal expansion of hematopoiesis in two patients with paroxysmal nocturnal hemoglobinuria (PNH). Blood 108:4232, 2006.

Miyata T, Takeda J, Iida Y, et al: The cloning of PIG-A, a component in the early step of GPI-anchor biosynthesis. Science 259:1318, 1993.

Moyo VM, Mukhina GL, Garrett ES, et al: Natural history of paroxysmal nocturnal hemoglobinuria using modern diagnostic assays. Br J Haematol 126:133, 2004.

Nagarajan S, Brodsky RA, Young NS, et al: Genetic defects underlying paroxysmal nocturnal hemoglobinuria that arises out of aplastic anemia. Blood 86:4656, 1995.

Rollins SA, Sims PJ: The complement-inhibitory activity of CD59 resides in its capacity to block incorporation of C9 into membrane C5b-9. J Immunol 144:3478, 1990.

Rosse WF, Dacie JV: Immune lysis of normal human and paroxysmal nocturnal hemoglobinuria (PNH) red blood cells. I. The sensitivity of PNH red cells to lysis by complement and specific antibody. J Clin Invest 45:736, 1966.

Rother RP, Bell L, Hillmen P, et al: The clinical sequelae of intravascular hemolysis and extracellular plasma hemoglobin: A novel mechanism of human disease. JAMA 293:1653, 2005.

Saso R, Marsh J, Cevreska L, et al: Bone marrow transplants for paroxysmal nocturnal haemoglobinuria. Br J Haematol 104:392, 1999.

Schrezenmeier H, Hertenstein B, Wagner B, et al: A pathogenetic link between aplastic anemia and paroxysmal nocturnal hemoglobinuria is suggested by a high frequency of aplastic anemia patients with a deficiency of phosphatidylinositol glycan anchored proteins. Exp Hematol 23:81, 1995.

Socie G, Henry-Amar M, Bacigalupo A, et al: Malignant tumors occurring after treatment of aplastic anemia. N Engl J Med 329:1152, 1993.

Takeda J, Miyata T, Kawagoe K, et al: Deficiency of the GPI anchor caused by a somatic mutation of the PIG-A gene in paroxysmal nocturnal hemoglobinuria. Cell 73:703, 1993.

Watanabe R, Inoue N, Westfall B, et al: The first step of glycosylphosphatidylinositol biosynthesis is mediated by a complex of PIG-A, PIG-H, PIG-C and GPI1. EMBO J 17:877, 1998.

REFERENCES

For complete list of references log onto www.expertconsult.com

CHAPTER 31

ACQUIRED DISORDERS OF RED CELL AND WHITE CELL PRODUCTION

Jaroslaw P. Maciejewski and Ramon V. Tiu

PURE RED CELL APLASIA

Acquired pure red cell aplasia (PRCA) is characterized by the presence of an acquired severe normochromic, most frequently normocytic, anemia associated with a complete disappearance of reticulocytes and erythroid precursors in the marrow and normal production of myeloid cells and platelets. Consequently, it is presumed that the defect lies within erythroid precursors and not within stem cells as seen in aplastic anemia. Initially described by Kaznelson in 1922,[1] PRCA is a rare bone marrow failure disorder without geographic or racial predilection. All ages can be affected but, if present in children, it is called transient erythroblastopenia of childhood (TEC) and may be difficult to distinguish from congenital causes of anemia, mainly Diamond–Blackfan anemia (DBA). Former nosology included various terms such as erythrophthisis, chronic hypoplastic anemia, pure red cell agenesis, and primary red cell anemia.

ETIOLOGY AND CLASSIFICATION

Acquired forms of PRCA must be distinguished from congenital forms of PRCA, which usually manifest themselves early in life (see Chapter 28). Acquired PRCA occurring in childhood may be difficult to distinguish from DBA. As an acquired disease, PRCA may be a primary disorder or secondary to a variety of systemic diseases, including a number of hematologic diseases (Table 31–1).

Pathogenesis

The inciting events in the development of PRCA are not known. However, as with idiopathic aplastic anemia, viruses or exposure to chemicals can serve as potential triggers (Fig. 31–1). Theoretically, a viral infection could lead to depletion of erythroid precursors. Studies of B19 parvovirus (see later) suggest such an etiology. Because hematopoietic stem cells are not affected by B19 parvovirus, myeloid cells and platelets are normally produced and upon clearance of the virus, normal erythroid production can resume. Similarly, in immune-mediated PRCA, the mechanism of erythroid inhibition may vary and may include (a) antibodies to proteins specific to erythroblasts, (b) direct cytotoxic T-lymphocyte (CTL)-mediated killing of erythroid precursors, and (c) production of soluble products by CTLs such as inhibitory or proapoptotic cytokines that directly affect the erythroid series.

Historically, initial studies concentrated on examining the effects of soluble serum inhibitors of erythropoiesis. These investigations revealed a decline in erythroid colony formation in the presence of patient serum or failure to induce erythroid colony formation in the presence of erythropoietin.[2,3] Such serum inhibitors can be found in 40% of patients with PRCA.[2–4] In 60% of patients, erythroid colony formation can be induced in vitro with hematopoietic growth factors.[2–4] The inhibitory activity is localized to the immunoglobulin (IgG) fraction and disappears upon achieving a clinical remission. The antigenic targets for autoantibodies have not been well characterized, but various stages of erythroid differentiation can be affected (also called PRCA type A) as seen in the reduction of BFU-E or CFU-E.[5,6] In certain cases of antibody-mediated PRCA, the involvement of the complement system is a prerequisite to disease causation.[7] Perhaps, the exception and a model for antibody-induced red cell aplasia is the identification of PRCA associated with antierythropoietin antibodies (also called PRCA type B) in rare cases.[8,9] Consistent with the specificity of the antibodies, myeloid colony formation is not impaired, making it unlikely that a more ubiquitous inhibitory cytokine mediates the specific erythroid inhibition.

In recent years, experimental and clinical observations have suggested that PRCA may be mediated by CTLs, which specifically recognize and kill erythroid precursors similar to CTL-mediated killing of cells in aplastic anemia.[10–12] Although such a T cell-mediated antierythroid response is likely to be polyclonal, rare instances of T-cell large granular lymphocyte (T-LGL) leukemia associated with PRCA or erythroid inhibition may represent an extreme form of the clonal continuum of CTL responses (see T-Cell Large Granular Lymphocyte-Associated). In addition to CTLs expressing α/β TCR, T cells with a γ/δ TCR can mediate PRCA.[13,14] The antigens/antigenic peptides triggering such a response have not been well described.[15,16] Similarly, natural killer (NK) cells have also been implicated in mediating cytotoxicity directed against erythroid precursors.[17,18] NK cells like γ/δ T-lymphocytes and unlike α/β CTL do not rely on MHC-restricted cytotoxicity, but may utilize killer-cell inhibitory receptors (KIRs).[19,20] KIRs inhibit cytolysis when they encounter a cell bearing HLA class I molecules. A lack of appropriate KIRs may predispose cells to increased attack by NK cells or γ/δ CTL. Physiologic down-regulation of KIR has been implicated in the pathogenesis of PRCA in a patient with concomitant γ/δ T-LGL clonal proliferation.[13,21] An alternative NK-cell cytotoxic mechanism independent of KIR has been reported in healthy individuals.[22]

Peripheral T-helper lymphocyte polarization has been implicated in the pathogenesis of PRCA.[16,23] Polarization toward the Th2 functional subtype (IL-4) during disease relapse and normalization of Th1/Th2 ratio after effective treatment has been reported in both monoclonal gammopathy of undetermined significance (MGUS) and thymoma-associated PRCA. Further studies have shown increased *C-MAF* gene expression in relapsed PRCA associated with Th2 polarization, a mechanism that may help explain the alteration in Th1/Th2 balance.[16]

PRIMARY PURE RED CELL APLASIA

Primary PRCA occurs in the absence of any underlying disorder. It may be acute and self-limited or may be a chronic and refractory condition. Acute forms are uncommon. Most cases are protracted and chronic, unlike TEC, which is an acute and self-limited disorder. Most of the cases of classical primary PRCA are autoimmune in origin, but a significant proportion will remain idiopathic in origin in spite of an exhaustive workup.

Table 31–1 Classification of Pure Red Cell Aplasia

Congenital (DBA)		
Primary	Autoimmune Idiopathic	
Secondary	Thymoma[8,9,32–34]	
	Hematologic malignancies	CLL[24,25] T-LGL/chronic NK-LGL leukemia[10,11,17,18,28–31] Myeloma[435] NHL[436,437] MDS[438] ALL[439–441]
	Solid tumors	Renal cell carcinoma[442] Thyroid cancer[443] Various adenocarcinomas[444,445]
	Infections	Parvovirus B19[50] EBV,[59] Mumps HIV,[61] HTLV-1[28] CMV[60] Viral hepatitis (Hep A,[55,56,446] Hep C[57,58]) Leishmaniasis[240] Gram+ systemic infections eg, staphylococcemia Meningococcemia
	Autoimmune conditions	SLE[74] RA[69] Sjögren's syndrome[71,72] Mixed connective tissue disease[66] Autoimmune hepatitis[447] Anti-Epo antibodies[448,449] ABO-incompatible BMT Minor incompatibility[93–98]
	Drugs and chemicals	
	Pregnancy[43,44]	
	Severe nutritional deficiencies[450,451]	
	Renal failure[452]	

ALL, acute lymphoblastic leukemia; BMT, bone marrow transplantation; CLL, chronic lymphocytic leukemia; CMV, cytomegalovirus; DBA, Diamond–Blackfan anemia; EBV, Epstein–Barr virus; HTLV-1, human T-lymphotrophic virus; MDS, myelodysplastic syndrome; NHL, non-Hodgkin lymphoma; NK-LGL, natural killer large granular lymphocyte; RA, refractory anemia; SLE, systemic lupus erythematomus; T-LGL, T-cell large granular lymphocyte.

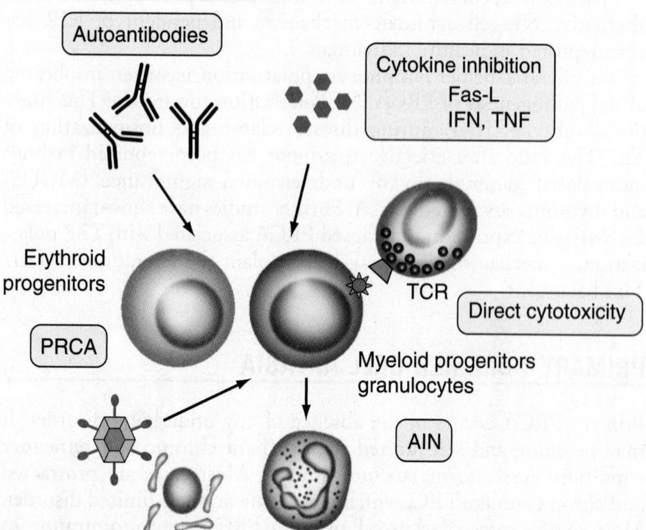

Figure 31–1 Pathogenesis of pure red cell aplasia.

SECONDARY FORMS OF PURE RED CELL APLASIA

Clinical Associations

B-Cell Chronic Lymphocytic Leukemia-Associated PRCA

In B-cell chronic lymphocytic leukemia (CLL), PRCA can be observed in up to 6% of cases.[10,24,25] The underlying pathogenetic mechanisms are not clear and the inhibition of the erythroid series does not appear to be mediated by a soluble factor.[26,27] The distinction between whether the PRCA is a result of the primary B-cell CLL disease or its therapy becomes difficult in circumstances when PRCA presents as a late event. In most cases, PRCA cannot be attributed simply to infiltration of the marrow by the lymphoma.

T-Cell Large Granular Lymphocyte-Associated PRCA

Although neutropenia is a typical finding in T-LGL leukemia, PRCA with varying degrees of erythroblastopenia can also be observed in 10% to 15% of patients with T-LGL leukemia.[11,28–31] In such a setting, PRCA is often accompanied by red cells with an increased mean corpuscular volume. T-LGL leukemia with PRCA may respond to oral cyclophosphamide, cyclosporine A (CsA), methotrexate, and in refractory cases therapy to antithymocyte globulin (ATG). It is possible that PRCA associated with T-LGL leukemia represents an extreme form of the T-cell–mediated disease that, if polyclonal, might be classified as idiopathic PRCA.

Thymoma-Associated PRCA

Thymoma is associated with PRCA; thus a chest x-ray or CT scan should be included in the workup for PRCA. Antibodies with direct inhibitory effects against erythroid precursors may be present,[8,9,32–34] T cell-mediated inhibition of erythropoiesis has also been implicated in the pathogenesis of PRCA associated with either benign or malignant thymomas.[35–38] Thymectomy is the usual initial treatment approach[34]; however, incomplete responders, nonresponders, and patients who relapse are common,[38] necessitating additional therapies in the form of azathioprine,[39] intravenous immunoglobulins (IVIg),[40] and CsA.[41]

Pregnancy-Associated PRCA

Pregnancy-associated PRCA is a self-limited syndrome that may occur at any age of gestation.[42] It has a high risk for relapse during subsequent pregnancies and can be safely managed with either blood transfusions or corticosteroids.[43,44] Patients with other forms of PRCA may also be more prone to relapse during pregnancy.[45]

Parvovirus B19 and Other Viral-Induced PRCA

Parvovirus B19 is a single-stranded DNA virus, which in normal individuals causes fifth disease (erythema infectiosum) in children and arthropathy in adults.[46–49] The cellular receptor for the virus is the P antigen, a blood group antigen also responsible for the agglutination reaction that occurs in the presence of the virus. Detection of parvovirus B19–specific IgM without anti–parvovirus B19 IgG supports the diagnosis of acute infection whereas the parvovirus–B19 specific IgG suggests immunity.[50] Addition of parvovirus B19 in vitro to cultures of erythroid progenitor cells completely abolishes erythroid colony formation.[47,48] Primary infection causes life-long immunity; however, it is possible that a latent virus may persist in a healthy individual for years.

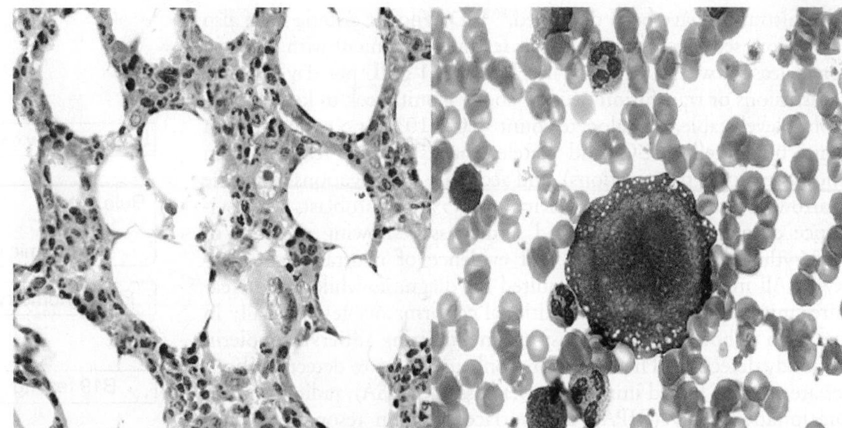

Figure 31–2 Parvovirus B19–mediated pure red cell aplasia.

A transient aplastic crisis is a typical complication of a primary parvovirus B19 infection in patients with increased red cell turnover (usually chronic hemolysis, eg, hemoglobinopathies, and hereditary disorders of red blood cell [RBC] membrane, eg, hereditary spherocytosis).[51–53] In typical cases, the occurrence of acute reticulocytopenia results in a sudden drop in hemoglobin (Hgb)/hematocrit (Hct) levels as RBC destruction continues but is unsupported by a suppressed marrow. Occasionally, characteristic giant pronormoblasts may be seen in marrow aspirates (Fig. 31–2). This disorder is often self-limiting with the evolution of a protective IgG response. Viral titers in the serum of affected patients may be high. Supportive transfusions may be needed during the acute phase of the disease.

A more chronic form, parvovirus B19–related PRCA, may develop in immunocompromised patients as, for example, in AIDS. In such cases, IVIg can produce remarkable responses. High doses of IVIg are required (>2 g/kg) as an insufficient dose may not produce the desired effect. DNA dot blot hybridization is the best diagnostic test for the detection of viremia. Parvovirus B19 can also be detected by polymerase chain reaction (PCR), a routinely available test, but this method may provide a high rate of false positive results. However, if negative, it excludes B19 parvovirus–mediated disease.[50] Improved tests have been developed that allow for the detection of neutralizing antibodies and infectivity of parvovirus B19.[54]

Several other viral infections including viral hepatitis (A[55,56] and C[57,58]), Epstein–Barr virus (EBV),[59] cytomegalovirus (CMV),[60] human T-lymphotrophic virus–1 (HTLV-1),[28] and HIV[61] have been implicated as causative agents of PRCA. Little is known about the exact mechanisms underlying these disorders but they likely involve T cell-mediated suppression as observed during HTLV-1 infection[28] and EBV or antibody-mediated destruction of red cell precursors, as in hepatitis C-induced PRCA.[57,58] Frequently, the presence of multiple comorbidities and medications makes it difficult to pinpoint the exact causative agent.[61,62]

Connective Tissue Disease-Associated PRCA

The majority of connective tissue diseases associated with PRCA are autoimmune in nature. Several rheumatologic diseases have been associated with PRCA including adult-onset Still disease,[63,64] dermatomyositis,[65] mixed connective tissue disease,[66] polymyositis,[67] rheumatoid arthritis,[68,69] Sjögren syndrome,[70–72] and systemic lupus erythematosus.[73–75] The pathogenesis of the PRCA in this setting may vary and includes (a) autoantibody-mediated erythroid inhibition,[76] (b) autoantibody directed against erythropoietin,[77] and (c) CTL-mediated killing of erythroid precursors.[73]

Drug-Induced PRCA

Various chemical agents and drugs have been associated with PRCA. The mechanisms responsible for erythroid inhibition may be diverse depending on the offending agent (Table 31–2) but may include induction of antibodies targeting the drugs or drugs bound to cellular and plasma proteins. Another possible mechanism involves drug-mediated triggering of T-cell responses, or direct toxicity to the erythroid series as seen with diphenylhydantoin.[78]

Table 31–2 Drugs and Chemicals Implicated in Pure Red Cell Aplasia

Alemtuzumab[151]	Erythropoietin[448,449]	Phenytoin[78,482,483]
Allopurinol[453,454]	Estrogens[468]	Procainamide[484–486]
α-Methyldopa[455]	Fludarabine[469]	Ribavirin[487,498]
Aminopyrine[456]	FK506[470]	Rifampicin[489]
Azathioprine[457,458]	Gold[471]	Sulfasalzine[490,491]
Benzene[459]	Halothane[472]	Sulfathiozole[492]
Carbamazepine[460]	Interferon-α[473,474]	Sulindac[493]
Cephalothin[461]	Isoniazid[475–477]	Tacrolimus[494]
Chloramphenicol[462]	Lamivudine[62]	Mycophenolate mofetil[487]
Chlorpropamide[463,464]	Linezolid[478]	Thiamphenicol[495]
Cladribine[465]	Maloprim[479]	Ticlopidine[496,497]
Cotrimoxazole[466]	Penicillin[480]	Valproic acid[194,498]
D-Penicillinamine[467]	Phenylbutazone[481]	Zidovudine[499]

Erythropoietin Antibody-Associated PRCA

Erythropoietin is produced mainly by the kidneys and to a limited extent by the liver. Recombinant erythropoietin is used in the treatment of anemias of various origins, including, for example, anemia of chronic disease, renal disease, and a variety of bone marrow failure syndromes, particularly MDS. Cases of PRCA have developed as a consequence of antibody formation against endogenous erythropoietin[79] or while receiving treatment with recombinant erythropoietin.[80–82] The latter condition has been referred as to epoietin-induced PRCA or epo-PRCA. The first three cases of epo-PRCA were reported between 1988 and 1998,[81,83] with 13 cases subsequently reported in France between 1998 and 2000 mainly related to exposure to epoietin-alpha (Eprex; 92%) and epoietin-beta (NeoRecormon; 8%).[84] The exact pathogenesis remains unclear but may be related to the formation of neutralizing antierythropoietin antibodies. There are several risk factors to the development of epo-PRCA, including subcutaneous route of administration, use of epoietin-alpha stabilized in a human serum albumin (HAS)-free formulation, use of silicone oil as lubricant in prefilled Eprex syringes, and use in patients with chronic renal disease.[85,86] All these factors increase the immunogenic potential of the antierythropoietin antibodies. This observation has lead to the modification in the storage, handling, and administration of Eprex favoring IV administration, especially with Eprex stabilized with HAS-free formulation and avoidance of the subcutaneous (SQ) non-HAS stabilized Eprex for patients with chronic renal disease. Of note is that cases of epo-PRCA occurring after intravenous epoietin administration have been described.[80,87] Diagnostic criteria have also been proposed incorporating major features (treatment with epoietin for at least 3 weeks, decrease in Hgb by 0.1 g/dL per day without transfusions or transfusion need of about 1 unit/week to keep hemoglobin level stable, reticulocyte count $<10 \times 10^9$/L, no major drop in white blood cell [WBC] and platelet counts), minor features (skin and systemic allergic reactions), and accessory investigations (eg, bone marrow showing normal cellularity and <5% erythroblasts with evidence of maturation block, and serum assay showing presence of antierythropoietin antibodies and evidence of neutralizing capacity).[80] All major criteria are required for diagnosis while minor features must be confirmed by additional confirmatory tests, usually in the form of bone marrow biopsy and neutralizing antierythropoietin antibody detection. The most commonly used tests to detect antibodies are enzyme-linked immunosorbent assay (ELISA), radioimmunoprecipitation assay (RIPA), and surface plasmon resonance. Once antibodies are detected, their neutralizing ability is tested using in vitro bioassay. Following establishment of diagnosis, management should include discontinuation of exogenous erythropoietin, administration of immunosuppressive agents, or, in cases of anemia secondary to renal insufficiency, renal transplantation. It is possible to use and regain response to recombinant erythropoietin once antierythropoietin antibodies have disappeared.[88]

PRCA Post Allogeneic Stem Cell Transplantation

In contrast to HLA matching, ABO-blood group incompatibility plays a minor role in the success of allogeneic hematopoietic stem cell transplantation. However, PRCA may be associated with major ABO incompatibility between the donor and recipient, leading to inhibition of donor erythroid precursors by residual host isoagglutinins. This complication is more commonly observed following the use of nonmyeloablative conditioning regimens. PRCA may also be resistant to the withdrawal or decrease of immunosuppression, or donor-lymphocyte infusions. Responses to rituximab,[89,90] erythropoietin,[91] and azathioprine[91] have been reported. A case responsive to purified CD34+ cell infusion has also been reported.[92] Resolution of PRCA is generally associated with decrease and subsequent disappearance of host isoagglutinins.[93–98]

PRCA Post Radiation Therapy

In rare circumstances, PRCA may be associated with prior radiation therapy. The cases described usually involve radiation therapy being administered to a patient with an underlying thymoma not previously associated with PRCA.[99,100]

CLINICAL MANIFESTATIONS OF PRCA

Anemia is the leading symptom of PRCA and can be severe at diagnosis as the fall in hemoglobin occurs over a protracted period of time and patients often exhibit a good degree of adaptation. Arrest of erythropoiesis is obvious with a profound reticulocytopenia. In children, TEC is usually diagnosed during evaluation of a febrile illness. In primary, idiopathic PRCA, physical signs other than those of anemia are usually absent. In secondary PRCA, the physical findings are consistent with the underlying primary disease.

LABORATORY EVALUATION

A complete blood count with differential, peripheral smear review, reticulocyte count, and a bone marrow examination remain the cornerstone in the diagnosis of PRCA. The classic hematologic picture of PRCA includes a complete blood count showing a normocytic, normochromic anemia (anemia associated with T-LGL leukemia is often macrocytic) with normal WBC and platelet count. The reticulocyte count is significantly reduced to less than 1% (a reticulocyte level >2% is not compatible with the diagnosis of PRCA) (Fig. 31–3). The bone marrow examination generally shows absence of the erythroid lineage and normal appearance of granulocytic and monocytic precursors and megakaryocytes. Erythroid precursors, if present, are usually less than 1%, and only a few residual proerythroblasts or basophilic erythroblasts may be seen. Blast cell numbers and cellularity are within normal limits. There are no dysplastic changes, ringed sideroblasts, or reticulin fibrosis. Cytogenetics is normal. In some cases, neutropenia,[101] mild thrombocytopenia, eosinophilia,[16] thrombocytosis,[16] leukocytosis, or relative lymphocytosis may be seen. Cytogenetic abnormalities, if present, may indicate concomitant myelodysplasia and is a poor prognostic marker for both response to treatment and propensity to leukemic transformation.[102,103] In the natural history of PRCA, ineffective erythropoiesis characterized by maturation arrest at the proerythroblasts or basophilic erythroblast stage may be observed and signifies either partial response to treatment or initial recovery from treatment or a prelude to the development of full-blown PRCA.[104]

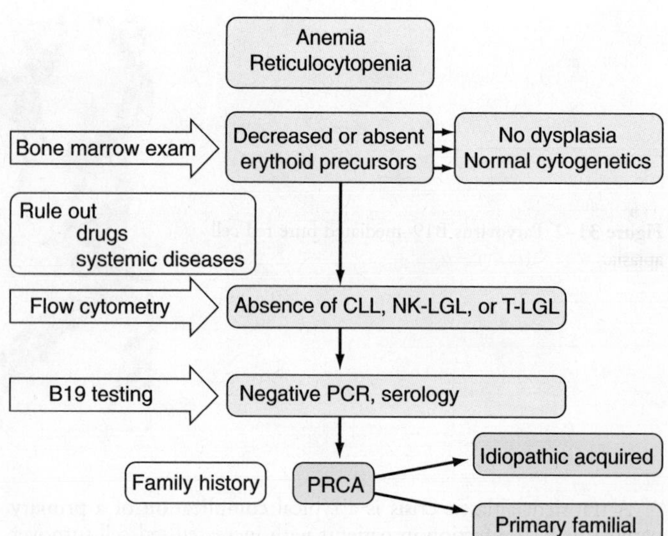

Figure 31–3 Diagnostic algorithm in pure red cell aplasia.

It is important to exclude vitamin B_{12} and folate deficiencies, and depending on the etiology and associated disease, other blood and bone marrow findings may be seen. The presence of giant and vacuolated pronormoblasts in the bone marrow examination should raise the suspicion for parvovirus B19 infection.[50] The presence of large granular lymphocytosis, neutropenia and/or thrombocytopenia, expansion of CD3+CD8+CD57+ T cells, clonal cytotoxic T-cell receptor (TcR) gene rearrangement, expansion of specific TcR Vβ region family gene segment, and splenomegaly may point toward concomitant T-LGL leukemia,[105,106] B cell lymphocytosis, especially of the CD5+/CD19+/CD20+/CD23+/cyclinD−/SmIg−dim phenotype with concomitant lymphadenopathy, hepatosplenomegaly, hypogammaglobulinemia, and thrombocytopenia, may be very suggestive of a B-cell CLL. Other laboratory findings that may help point to a secondary cause of PRCA includes the presence of monoclonal gammopathy.[16] Parvovirus B19 DNA titers (DNA hybridization and amplification techniques) may show high levels of the virus at 10^{12} genome copies per milliliter but it is important to note that serologic (IgM and IgG) titers are usually absent.[50] Erythropoietin antibodies,[84] antinuclear antibodies,[107,108] and/or complement consumption may point toward a specific disease mechanism.[109] A radiographic workup may also be useful in the clinical workup as chest x-ray or CT scan may show evidence of a thymoma.

Table 31–3 Therapy of Pure Red Cell Aplasia and Its Results

	Study								
Agent	***Chikkappa***[142]	***Means***[144]	***Au***[152]	***Dessypris***	***Zecca***[500]	***Lacy***[103]	***Charles***[102]	***Sloand***[148]	***Abkowitz***[146]
Steroids				18/41		9/29	9/36	—	
Cytotoxic agents				24/54		14/29	8/27	—	
Antithymocyte globulin				2/6		0/1	8/12		6/6
Cyclosporine A	6/7	6/9		3/4		4/5	2/3		
Splenectomy				4/23		0/1	0/1		
Daclizumab								6/15	
Rituximab					1/1				
Campath			2/2						
Methotrexate							2/37		

DIFFERENTIAL DIAGNOSIS

PRCA can be easily differentiated from aplastic anemia and other types of bone marrow failure syndromes. A distinction between MDS with erythroid hypoplasia and idiopathic PRCA may be more difficult. In childhood, TEC has to be distinguished from DBA but a history of normal blood counts, late onset of manifestation, and transient disease course are characteristic of TEC.

THERAPY

The distinction between primary and secondary forms of PRCA is essential as many secondary types have specific and very effective therapies (Table 31–3). All potentially offending drugs should be discontinued and drug-associated PRCA should remit within 3 to 4 weeks. Nutritional deficiencies (B_{12} and folic acid) should be excluded and treated if present. The therapy of primary and secondary forms of PRCA refractory to the treatment of an underlying disease may be challenging and should include a sequential trial of various immunosuppressive agents until a response is achieved. Spontaneous remissions have been reported.

Surgery or Radiation

In cases associated with thymoma, thymectomy is the usual initial treatment of choice prior to immunosuppression and may induce remission with return of erythropoiesis 4 to 8 weeks in about 30% to 40% of patients.[110–112] Patients who remain refractory following surgery should be treated as patients with idiopathic PRCA. The removal of a thymoma may improve responsiveness to immunosuppressive therapy.[111] Thymectomy in the absence of a thymoma in other forms of PRCA is not recommended. In circumstances where surgical resection of thymoma is contraindicated, radiation therapy with or without chemotherapy may be administered.[113]

Medical

Supportive

Supportive care includes blood transfusions and iron chelation with deferasirox (Exjade). Deferasirox is a new once-daily, oral iron chelator developed for treating transfusional iron overload syndromes used in a variety of hematologic disorders, including thalassemia and sickle cell anemia, and works primarily by promoting fecal excretion of iron. Side effects may include diarrhea, renal failure, and, rarely, agranulocytosis.[114,115]

Immunosuppression

Prednisone therapy at a dose of 1 mg/kg is associated with significant response rates (approximately 40%) and should constitute the initial therapeutic approach.[103] Initial responses are generally observed after 4 to 6 weeks.[102,116] A slow taper of prednisone is suggested over a period of 3 to 4 months. The disease may relapse and the minimal maintenance dose of corticosteroids may need to be established to maintain the desired hemoglobin levels.[117] Trials of prednisone therapy without clinical response longer than 8 weeks are not warranted.[102,103,116]

Alternative therapies may include cyclosporine, oral cyclophosphamide, azathioprine, antithymocyte globulin (ATG), rituximab, and alemtuzumab (Table 31–3). Erythropoietin and darbepoietin[118,119] are usually not effective as a sole agent but may hasten recovery following an adequate trial of cyclophosphamide. No randomized trials exist to favor a particular treatment based on efficacy. The choice of therapy may be influenced by clinical clues. For example, the presence of large granular lymphocytes may suggest the use of CsA, hypogammaglobulinemia may be corrected with IVIg, whereas detection of hypergammaglobulinemia or monoclonal protein may suggest a choice of rituximab. Most refractory cases may require administration of ATG. The age of the patient may influence a choice of the cytotoxic agent, which may pose a significant risk for the development of secondary leukemias, especially with a prolonged administration.

Danazol is a synthetic attenuated androgen that has been used for many years for the treatment of a variety of hematologic disorders mainly myelofibrosis.[120] Usually given at 200 mg PO BID, the maximum dose per day is 600 mg. It has been used to treat PRCA either as a single agent or in conjunction with steroids or other agents and have shown efficacy in PRCA of various etiologies.[121–124] The main adverse events reported include liver transaminitis and vascular liver tumors.

IVIg (Gammagard, Octagam, Panglobulin) given at 1 to 2 g/kg IV for 5 days is also effective in several types of PRCA.[125–128] Higher doses of usually 2 g/kg of IVIg for 5 days are necessary for the treatment of parvovirus B19 virus-induced PRCA. In AIDS patients with parvovirus B19 virus-induced PRCA, a regimen consists of induction therapy with 1 g/kg daily for 1 to 2 days followed by 1 g/kg for 2 days. If the patient relapses, then maintenance therapy with IVIg 0.4 to 1.0 g/kg q 4 weeks is recommended.[129]

Azathioprine is an imidazolyl derivative of mercaptopurine that inhibits DNA synthesis by inhibition of purine metabolism. In PRCA, it may be given at a dose of 2 to 3 mg/kg/day IV and has been found to be effective in patients nonresponsive to cyclophosphamide.[39,130]

Oral cyclophosphamide may be started at a dose of 50 mg PO daily, with a maximal dose of no more than 150 mg daily. Blood counts should be monitored and the dose may be escalated accordingly. Trials of therapy longer than 3 months without signs of response are not warranted. Monitoring of the reticulocyte count may allow for the early assessment of response. Often, a delayed response may be seen when cyclophosphamide is withdrawn, which reflects the fine balance between adequate immunosuppression and cytotoxicity.[3,4,103,116,131,132]

Rituximab given at 375 mg/m^2 intravenous infusion weekly for 4 weeks has been found to be efficacious in PRCA. PRCA in a variety of settings, including B-cell CLL, EBV-associated posttransplant lymphoproliferative disorder (EBV-PTLD), ABO-incompatible allogeneic hematopoietic stem cell transplantation for acute myeloid leukemia, and hairy cell leukemia variant, has been successfully treated.[89,133–136] Owing to the fact that it is specific for B cells alone, cases of nonresponders to rituximab have been reported and attributed to an alternative T-cell–mediated pathogenesis.[137] In cases refractory to immunosuppressive agents affecting T-cell function, rituximab or low-dose alemtuzumab constitutes reasonable options. Rituximab is effective in patients with PRCA owing to ABO incompatibility following bone marrow transplantation.[89,90]

CsA can be administered at a dose of 5 to 10 mg/kg orally (PO) daily in divided doses. CsA can be combined with prednisone at doses of 20 to 30 mg PO. The trough levels of CsA should be monitored and the dose adjusted to achieve a level between 200 and 300 µg/mL. An adequate trial of therapy is considered 3 months of therapy. The response rates may be as high as 60% to 80%. After a response is achieved, the therapy should be continued for 6 months followed by a slow taper.[102,103,138–144]

Horse ATG may be given to refractory cases at a dose of 40 mg/kg IV daily × 4 days with prednisone at 1 mg/kg. Rabbit ATG (thymoglobulin) may be given a dose of 2.5 to 3.5 mg/kg daily IV for 4 or 5 days with prednisone at 1 mg/kg. Concomitant prednisone should be administered and then tapered over 2 to 3 weeks. A therapeutic response should occur within 3 months post therapy, although responses at or beyond 6 months may be observed.[8,102,103,116,145–147]

Daclizumab, an anti–interleukin 2 receptor antibody (Zenapax, anti-CD25 mAb), may constitute a good alternative to ATG as it does not require hospitalization and is well tolerated. In a recent trial, a dose of 1 mg/kg IV was administered every 2 weeks. The therapy should be given for at least 3 months. It is possible that combination with CsA may increase the response rate but no data exist as to the observed response rates.[148,149]

Methotrexate, an antimetabolite, at low doses (7.5–15 mg/week PO) is useful in treating PRCA, especially in patients with concomitant LGL leukemia. The responses are generally sustained and therapy is well tolerated. Methotrexate may be given in conjunction with other therapies like CsA.[12,102]

Alemtuzumab (Campath, anti-CD52 mAb) is a recombinant DNA-derived humanized monoclonal antibody directed against the cell surface glycoprotein CD52, which is expressed on the surface of normal and malignant B- and T-lymphocytes. It can be given IV or SQ every other day with an initial dose of 3 mg, and subsequent doses can be increased until response is obtained. The usual cumulative dose before response is usually between 200 and 400 mg. Alemtuzumab has been tested in a variety of lymphoproliferative disorders including diffuse large B-cell lymphoma, B-cell CLL, and T-cell LGL leukemia. Similarly, PRCA occurring in the context of these conditions previously unresponsive to therapy with steroids, CsA, and even cytoxan has been shown to be responsive to this agent. Alemtuzumab can be given either intravenously or subcutaneously.[150–152]

Hematopoietic Stem Cell Transplantation

Despite advances in immunosuppressive regimens, subsets of patients with PRCA remain refractory and are very difficult to treat. As with other bone marrow failure disorders with autoimmune pathogenesis like aplastic anemia, hematopoietic stem cell transplantation (HSCT) is an important treatment option especially for refractory and relapsed PRCA cases. Matched sibling donor allogeneic HSCT results in restoration of normal hematopoiesis in patients with refractory PRCA.[153–155] In another case, a patient with relapsed PRCA underwent matched sibling donor allogeneic HSCT combined with donor lymphocyte infusions resulting in full donor engraftment and subsequent return of normal hematopoiesis, suggesting a graft-versus-autoimmunity effect as the likely mechanism for response.[156]

PROGNOSIS

The prognosis of secondary PRCA depends upon the underlying disease. Idiopathic PRCA may be very refractory to treatment. Ultimately, remission may be achieved in a significant proportion (approximately 68%) of patients, especially when sequential regimens are used. Spontaneous remissions are observed in 5% to 10% of cases. Relapses are common especially during the first year postremission but are usually responsive to the same regimen that induced remission.[102,116] Chronic, low-dose immunosuppressive therapy may be needed in certain cases that have relapsed. In one study, median survival was reported to be 14 years.[116] Unlike a megakaryocytic thrombocytopenic purpura, evolution to aplastic anemia is rare[111,157] in PRCA and, moreover, very few patients (3%–5%) evolve into acute leukemia.[102,116]

DISORDERS OF NEUTROPHIL PRODUCTION

Neutropenia is a common condition. The majority of cases are secondary to a variety of etiologies, including systemic or hematologic diseases. In this chapter we will describe a primary, isolated form of neutropenia in which other hematopoietic lineages are not affected. In such a setting, neutropenia may be the result of peripheral destruction or perhaps less frequently, the result of the absence of myeloid progenitors in the marrow. Neutropenia may be initially noted during workup for fever and infections or may be an incidental finding on a routine CBC. The cut-off value for the diagnosis of neutropenia is an absolute neutrophil count (ANC) of less than 1500 cells/µL. This value is generally accepted as a definition for neutropenia for all ages and ethnic backgrounds except for newborn infants.[158] Clinically, the most concerning consequence of neutropenia is the propensity to develop infections. ANC is the best parameter to assess the severity of neutropenia; however, the correlation between ANC and the propensity for infection is variable in different circumstances and determined by marrow neutrophil reserves, duration of neutropenia, and clinical context.[159–162] This is best illustrated in patients with chronic benign neutropenia of childhood and infancy, where patients may have ANC as low as less than 250 cells/µL and yet they may be devoid of infections or only have mild infections.[163–165] Instead of ANC, it is the bone marrow neutrophil pool reserve that serves as the most suitable determinant of risk for infection, best evaluated through a bone marrow biopsy. In the setting of neutropenia, should the bone marrow examination reveal depleted neutrophil reserves, the ANC level correlates with the risk of infection. In contrast, if bone marrow shows adequate neutrophil reserves, then ANC levels are not predictive of the risk of developing a serious infection.

CLASSIFICATION OF ACQUIRED NEUTROPENIAS

Neutropenia as a primary disease should be distinguished from inherited forms of neutropenia, which commonly present during early childhood (see Chapter 28), and secondary forms of neutropenia associated with systemic disorders. In addition, idiopathic neutropenia is distinct from the constitutional or familial benign neutropenia frequently seen in African Americans,[166,167] Yemenites, and Falashah Jews or black Bedouins.[168] The degree of neutropenia is often mild and there is no propensity to develop infections. This condition is described in Chapter 50. Most cases of neutropenia are secondary to

Table 31–4 Classification of Neutropenia

Congenital	
Primary	Autoimmune neutropenia
	Pure white cell aplasia
	Idiopathic
	Thymoma
	Hematologic malignancies, eg, T-LGL leukemia
	Infections/postinfectious
	Viral
	Measles,[215] mumps, roseola,[216,217] rubella,[501] RSV, influenza[214]
	Hepatitis A,[209] B,[209,210] and C[58]
	CMV,[218,219,502] EBV,[211–213] HIV[224,225]
	Parvovirus[221–223]
	Bacterial
	Tuberculosis[235,236]
	Brucellosis[232–234]
	Tularemia[231]
	Typhoid fever [230]
	Rickettsial
	Rocky Mountain spotted fever[503]
	Ehrlichiosis.[242,243]
	Fungal
	Histoplasmosis[237,238]
	Parasitic
	Malaria,[239] leishmaniasis[240,424]
	Autoimmune conditions, eg, SLE[504,505], RA[506]
	Drugs and chemicals
	Neutropenia associated with immunodeficiency[314,320]
	Severe nutritional deficiencies[247,248]
	Neutropenia due to increased margination
	Iatrogenic, eg, hemodialysis[321,322]

CMV, cytomegalovirus; EBV, Epstein–Barr virus; RA, refractory anemia; RSV, respiratory syncytial virus; SLE, systemic lupus erythematomus; T-LGL, T-cell large granular lymphocyte.

a variety of disorders. Primary autoimmune neutropenia (AIN) and idiopathic neutropenia are less common. We will limit our description to isolated forms of neutropenia (Table 31–4).

Primary Neutropenia

Most neutropenias are secondary to various hematologic conditions and systemic diseases. However, in a small proportion of cases, an inciting cause cannot be identified despite intensive testing. Such idiopathic cases are most likely autoimmune in nature.

Chronic Idiopathic Neutropenia in Adults

Chronic idiopathic neutropenia in adults compared to those in infancy and early childhood has lesser tendency toward spontaneous remission although it does generally remain clinically benign. There may be concomitant anemia or thrombocytopenia that may portend a higher incidence of splenomegaly, infectious complications, and antineutrophil antibodies (ANAs) that are complement fixing.[169] The bone marrow biopsy may show evidence of arrest in myeloid maturation and mild hypercellularity. ANAs may be seen in 36% of patients, suggesting an immunologic pathogenesis.[169]

Idiopathic neutropenias may be chronic and benign in nature or may be associated with significant morbidity. In certain instances immune neutropenia may be associated with hemolytic anemia or with immune thrombocytopenia, but these forms likely represent a distinct nosologic entity. Idiopathic neutropenia can occur at any age, including early childhood. Such cases may be difficult to distinguish

Table 31–5 Human Neutrophil Alloantigens and Autoantigens

		Nomenclature
Integrin α M chain	CD11b	HNA-4a (MART)
Integrin α L chain	CD11a	HNA-4a (OND)
Gp50–64	CD177	HNA-2a (NB1) PRV-1
Gp70–95		HNA-3a/5b
Integrin β2 chain	CD18	
FcγIII	CD16	
FCGR3B-01		HNA-1a (NA1)
FCGR3B-02		HNA-1b (NA2)
FCGR3B-03		HNA-1c (SH/NA3)

from hereditary neutropenia syndromes. AIN may be associated with moderate and severe depression of neutrophil counts. Monocytosis is frequently present.[160,161] Some cases present with splenomegaly, which is to be distinguished from cytopenias associated with hypersplenism in Felty syndrome.[170] The frequency of infectious complications does not correlate with the severity of neutropenia, and patients with severe depletion of neutrophils may remain asymptomatic for long periods of time.

Conceptually, AIN may be due to peripheral autoimmune destruction of neutrophils due to lineage-specific inhibition of myeloid precursors, with its extreme form being pure white cell aplasia (Fig. 31–3). Consequently, increased peripheral destruction is associated with marrow hypercellularity and an increased number of myeloid precursors or, if myeloid progenitors are the targets, decreased myeloid precursors and a myeloid maturation arrest. Autoimmune ANAs have been implicated in the pathogenesis of AIN and could be mediated by both peripheral destruction of neutrophils and inhibition of myelopoiesis.[171,172] The antigens involved in these processes include neutrophil antigens NA1, NA2, ND1, ND2, and NB1 (Table 31–5). Both IgG and IGM antibodies have been implicated. Neutrophil-specific antibodies can be detected using many assays, including specific ELISA, opsonization,[173,174] leukoagglutination,[175] and direct antibody binding.[176] There are several proposed effector mechanisms as to how ANA can result in neutropenia or affect neutrophil integrity. For example, ANA may act as opsonins and directly enhance neutrophil destruction.[174] Alternatively, ANA can indirectly activate, complement, and facilitate opsonization.[177] Immune complexes may also bind to the neutrophil Fc portion, leading to increased neutrophil clearance by the reticuloendothelial system,[178] and finally, ANA may recognize and damage myeloid precursors.[179] The currently available diagnostic assays used to detect ANA are generally based on immunofluorescence and agglutination assays. The former allows for the detection of IgM and IgG antibodies from a suspected patient that are attached to normal donor neutrophils detected by flow cytometry performed with patient's serum and antihuman IgG. The results may be reported as strongly positive, weakly positive, or absent. The second technique, called agglutination assay, utilizes serum that leads to agglutination of normal neutrophils into either small or large clumps. These tests may help suggest an underlying immunologic process but cannot establish the definite. If there is a high index of suspicion that ANA is the causative factor, some authors suggest that a minimum of two methods be used to detect ANA, namely granulocyte agglutination test (GAT) and granulocyte immunofluorescence test (GIFT).[180]

In addition to antibodies, T-cell responses may be associated with neutropenia. The most extreme example of such responses is T-cell LGL leukemia associated with neutropenia and polarized proliferation of CTL (see later). In AIN, CTL responses are polyclonal and are often accompanied by the simultaneous presence of antibodies. It is likely that specialized CTL clones are capable of recognizing and killing myeloid precursors, interrupting granulocyte production. Consequently, some of the cases of AIN may be amenable to therapy with immunosuppressive agents directed against T cells.

Chronic Benign Neutropenia of Infancy and Childhood

Chronic benign neutropenia of infancy and childhood is considered the most common cause of chronic neutropenia in the pediatric age group. The majority of cases are autoimmune in nature and show clinical overlap with childhood idiopathic thrombocytopenic purpura and autoimmune hemolytic anemia. It is therefore considered a type of AIN.[181–186] An incidence of 1:100,000 has been reported in a childhood population in Scotland.[185] This form of neutropenia typically presents in children less than 3 years of age, with a median age of 8 to 11 months and with a predominance of females.[181,183,184] The CBC usually shows an ANC of less than 250 cells/μL with normal morphology and normal hemoglobin and platelet count. Occasionally monocytosis, eosinophilia, and mild thrombocytopenia may be present. In this condition, neutropenia is due to chronic depletion of mature granulocytes and is accompanied by a compensatory myeloid left shift in the marrow.[163–165] Most frequent clinical signs and symptoms are oral infections, including bothersome ulcers, but these are often associated with additional functional defects of neutrophils, and cellulitis of the labia majora. Of importance is the normal neutrophil count at birth and absence of a history of familial forms of neutropenia. The etiology of this condition is unknown but the pathogenesis involves ANAs, detectable in the majority of patients.[183,164,181] The antibodies are generally directed against similar antigens seen in adult AIN, especially those involving NA, NB, and ND loci. In about 25% of cases, the antibody is against an allele of neutrophil FcγRIII opsonin receptor called NA1.[181,183,184] Immunosuppressive therapy leads frequently to responses supporting the immune pathogenesis of this disease. Although the neutrophil count can be severely depressed, serious infectious complications are uncommon and therefore treatment to raise the ANC is generally not indicated except if recurrent infections occur. Antibiotics are useful to treat infections and G-CSF has been shown to be effective in elevating neutrophil counts.[187]

SECONDARY FORMS OF NEUTROPENIAS

Clinical Associations

Drug-Induced Neutropenia/Agranulocytosis

Drug-induced neutropenia is common.[188] The association was first described by Kracke in 1931 when agranulocytosis was observed in patients taking aminopyrine. The incidence in various studies is 1.0 to 3.4 cases/million per year.[188–193] Drugs may induce granulocytopenia by (a) direct toxicity leading to inhibition of myelopoiesis frequently observed in drugs like valproic acid,[194] carbamazepine,[195] and β-lactam antibiotics[196,197]; (b) immune-mediated (either antibody/complement-mediated) as seen with penicillin and antithyroid drugs[198–200] or immune complex mediated (quinidine)[201] destruction of myeloid progenitors and mature neutrophils; and (c) induction of CTL responses.[202] Genetic predisposition due to polymorphisms in various genes coding for cytokine and cytokine receptors as demonstrated for clozapine with tumor necrosis factor (TNF) and HLA polymorphisms as well as possibly variants of genes coding for a variety of metabolizing enzymes also plays a role.[203,204] Of interest are drugs that directly antagonize important vitamin cofactors necessary in normal bone marrow development. Neutropenia observed in patients treated with trimethoprim-sulfamethoxazole is due to the inhibitory effects on granulopoiesis by trimethoprim, owing to its antifolate action, which is reversed by folinic acid.[205] A similar finding can be seen with methotrexate owing to its antifolate action.

Most patients present with either asymptomatic neutropenia discovered on routine examination or symptomatic neutropenia with infectious complications including fever, angular stomatitis, or pneumonia. The reported mortality rates vary from 1% to 25%. Most patients recover without further complications. It has been estimated that drugs account for 72% of cases of agranulocytosis. The usual time to development of overt neutropenia is around 1 to 2 weeks and it resolves upon discontinuation of the offending drug within 10 to 14 days,[206] although time to recovery may vary depending on whether bone marrow hypoplasia is present (10 days) or not (14 days).[207] The recovery in neutrophil counts is usually preceded by increases in peripheral blood monocytes and immature granulocytes.[208] The International Aplastic Anemia and Agranulocytosis Study (IAAAS) has identified the most commonly associated agents and the relative odds ratios for developing agranulocytosis (Table 31–6).[193] In some instances, the severity of neutropenia is related to the dose and duration of the therapy. The therapy includes discontinuation of the potentially offending agents. In some instances associated with infections or prolonged recovery, G-CSF may be administered.

Table 31–6 Drugs Associated With Agranulocytosis

	Etiologic Fraction	
	Agranulocytosis	Aplastic Anemia
Overall	64%	62%
IAAAS	12%	27%
US	72%	17%
Thailand	70%	2%

Drugs associated with agranulocytosis (IAAAS and other drugs of interest)

Acetyldigoxin[507]	Mefloquine[525]
ACE inhibitors[508,509]	Nifedipine[526]
Allopurinol[510–512]	Phenytoin[527,528]
Amodiaquine[513]	Procainamide[529,530]
Benzafibrate[514]	Salicylates[531]
β-Lactam antibiotics[189]	Sulfasalazine[532,533]
β-Blockers[507,515]	Sulfonylureas[179,534]
Carbamazepine[516]	Tetracyclines[193]
Cinepazide[415,517]	Thenalidine[418,419]
Corticosteroids[518]	Thyrostatics[535–537]
Cotrimoxazole[205] Other sulfonamides	Troxerutine[193]
Dipyridamole[507]	
Deferasirox (Exjade)[519]	
Dypirone[408,193]	
Histamine-2 receptor antagonist[520]	
Indomethacin[188]	
Isoniazid[521,522]	
Macrolides[523,524]	

Neutropenia as a Manifestation of Systemic Diseases

Postinfectious Neutropenia

Neutropenia is commonly associated with viral infections, particularly in children. Various mechanisms have been implicated in neutropenia associated with systemic viral infections, including inhibition of hematopoiesis, granulocyte sequestration, margination, and peripheral destruction. Neutropenia generally improves when the viremia resolves. Neutropenia has been associated with hepatitis A,[209] B,[209,210] and Cvirus,[58,209] EBV,[211–213] influenza,[214] measles,[215] roseola,[216,217] CMV,[218–220] and parvovirus B19 infections.[221–223] Neutropenia is also frequently encountered in patients with AIDS, with approximately 70% of patients being neutropenic during their illness.[224,225] The mechanisms vary and may include antibody formation against neutrophils,[226–228] direct viral inhibition of hematopoietic progenitor cells, abnormal expression of growth factors and other cytokines, and inhibitory effects exerted by HIV-infected accessory cells.[229] The HIV virus not only suppresses hematopoiesis but also increases the risk of acquiring other infections. Furthermore, therapy with antiretroviral agents may dramatically decrease neutrophil counts (Table 31–4).

Systemic bacterial, fungal, and parasitic infections can be accompanied by neutropenia, including typhoid fever,[230] tularemia,[231] brucellosis,[232–234] mycobacterial infections,[235,236] histoplasmosis,[237,238] malaria,[239] leishmaniasis,[240,241] and ehrlichiosis.[242,243] The pathogenesis include margination and sequestration of leukocytes as observed in malaria, where there is reduction in the circulating polymorphonuclear neutrophil (PMN) pool and enlargement of the marginating PMN pool, primarily in the spleen and lung. Neutropenia can be present during sepsis, especially in newborns or debilitated individuals.[244,245] In such situations, neutropenia may be due to inhibition of hematopoiesis by inflammatory cytokines, exhaustion of marrow reserves, or redistribution.[246]

Neutropenia in Nutritional Deficiency and Nutritional Excess

Malnutrition, dietary restrictions, malabsorptive states, and concomitant intake of inhibitory drugs are just a few common causes of nutritional deficiencies that may lead to neutropenia. Vitamin B_{12} and folate deficiency frequently associated with megaloblastic anemia can also manifest with neutropenia. Lack of these essential vitamin cofactors results in the impairment of normal DNA synthesis, leading to abnormal granulopoiesis. A frequently observed morphologic feature is the presence of hypersegmented neutrophils.

Copper deficiency may also be associated with neutropenia.[247,248] Possible mechanisms may include arrest in maturation of neutrophil development as shown in studies in mice,[249] and increased antineutrophil antibody formation.[250,251] Most cases have been found in malnourished infants, in patients with zinc intoxication[252,253] and malabsorption states,[254,255] and in persons receiving total parenteral nutrition without adequate copper supplementation.[256,257] Copper deficiency is often accompanied by a normocytic anemia while platelet counts are invariably normal.[258] Other clinical and laboratory manifestations associated with copper deficiency include presence of ringed sideroblasts in the bone marrow,[259,260] macrocytic anemia,[261] low ceruloplasmin levels,[259] myeloneuropathy,[262] and skeletal abnormalities.[263]

Zinc intoxication in the absence of concomitant copper deficiency has also been associated with neutropenia generally in conjunction with severe anemia. A dysregulation in calprotectin metabolism has been suggested as a mechanism. Calprotectin, also known as the S100A8/A9 or MRP8/14 complex, is a major calcium-binding protein present in the cytosol of neutrophils, monocytes, and keratinocytes that increases during inflammatory states.[264]

Neutropenia Associated With Metabolic Disorders

Various acquired or inherited metabolic conditions may be associated with neutropenia. For example, neutropenia has been observed in patients with ketoacidosis and hyperglycemia, orotic, or methylmalonic aciduria.[265–268] Similarly, glycogen storage disease type Ib is commonly associated with neutropenia responsive to myeloid growth factors.[269–272]

Acquired Neonatal Neutropenias

Neutropenia has been described in infants of hypertensive mothers. In this syndrome, the ANC can be severely depressed for 1 to 30 days postpartum.[273–275] This type of neutropenia is associated with an increased risk of early-onset sepsis in neonates,[276] a prolonged duration of neutropenia, and an increased risk of neonatal nosocomial infections.[277] Granulocyte kinetic investigations suggested that the neutropenia is the result of diminished neutrophil production. An inhibitor released by the placenta and present in cord blood serum has been shown to play a role in this syndrome.[273,278]

Moderate to severe neutropenia has been also observed secondary to IgG antibodies transferred from mother to infant. This is a condition called isoimmune neonatal neutropenia or neonatal alloimmune neutropenia. In most cases, antibodies are directed against antigens on neutrophil FcγRIIIb (anti-NA1, anti-NA2, and anti-SH)[279] and NB1,[280,281] but in rare circumstances, maternal neutrophil-specific isoantibodies are also produced when there is deficiency of the FcγRIIIb gene.[282–286] The incidence of this condition can be as high as 2:1000 live births.[287] In both neutropenia occurring in hypertensive mothers and isoimmune neonatal neutropenia, differentiation from congenital forms of neutropenia may be difficult. Treatment with G-CSF is usually effective in neutropenia of infants of hypertensive mothers but higher doses may be needed as preeclampsia-associated inhibitor of rhG-CSF may be present.[275,288,289] IVIg[290] and G-CSF[279,291] are both effective for treatment of isoimmune neonatal neutropenia.

Neutropenia and Hypersplenism

Hypersplenism may be associated with neutropenia, but in most instances other cytopenias will also be present. However, hypersplenism may be a sign of diseases that can result in neutropenia, such as in T-LGL leukemia[105,106,292] and Felty syndrome.[293,294] Other than direct sequestration, another potential mechanism leading to neutropenia may be increased neutrophil apoptosis that normalizes after splenectomy.[295] Recently a high incidence of *Helicobacter pylori* infection has been noted among individuals with neutropenia and splenomegaly. A potential role for the bacterium in the pathogenesis of the splenomegaly is being explored. Conversely one can hypothesize that the bacterium may be the culprit in the development of the neutropenia.[296] Splenectomy either laparoscopically[297] or through laparotomy[298] may be effective in most cases. Although in situations precluding splenectomy, intraoperative splenic artery embolization is also effective.[299,300]

Pure White Cell Aplasia

Pure white cell aplasia (PWCA) is a rare condition with pathophysiologic overlap with some forms of AIN associated with myeloid suppression. Similar to PRCA, the pathogenesis may vary and includes antibody-mediated suppression of granulopoiesis,[198,301] T-cell–mediated suppression of granulopoiesis, direct myelotoxicity as seen with certain drugs,[302] opsonization of neutrophil precursors in the bone marrow leading to its destruction by macrophages within the bone marrow,[302] and formation of antibody–drug complex that may damage myeloid progenitors.[303] A bone marrow examination reveals either a total absence of myeloid precursors or arrest at the promyelocyte stage, with megakaryocytes and the erythroid series remaining quantitatively and qualitatively normal. In many cases, a thymoma is present.[304,305] PWCA, if associated with thymoma, has a variable clinical outcome. The complete absence of granulocytic precursors portends a poor response to both immunosuppression and thymectomy and is often fatal, whereas the presence of a maturation arrest at the promyelocyte stage may respond to immunosuppressive therapy.[301,305–308] PWCA has been described in connection with imipenem-cilastatin,[309] ibuprofen,[310] and chlorpropramide.[179] The discontinuation of the offending drug leads to rapid improvement. Recently, PWCA has also been associated with primary biliary cirrhosis.[311]

Therapeutic options may include azathioprine,[301] G-CSF combined with plasmapheresis especially if the disease process is antibody mediated,[312] methylprednisolone,[309] IV cyclophosphamide combined with plasmapheresis and G-CSF,[313] and thymectomy.[304] Severe depression of counts may require ATG therapy (see later).

Neutropenia Associated With Immunologic Abnormalities

Acquired and inherited defects of the cellular and humoral immune system may be accompanied by secondary neutropenias. In the inherited immunodeficiency syndromes, the initial presentation is in children and may be associated with failure to thrive. X-linked agammaglobulinemia (XLA) is a primary immunodeficiency disorder caused by mutations in the gene for Bruton tyrosine kinase (BTK) expressed in both myeloid and B cells that result in the absence of development of B lymphocytes and hypogammaglobulinemia. Neutropenia is seen in 15% to 26% of patients with X-linked agammaglobulinemia and most suffer from upper respiratory tract infection.[314–316] The exact pathogenetic mechanism is not clear but is believed to be related to the crucial role of BTK in myeloid survival under stress.

Neutropenia is seen in 40% to 50% of patients with X-linked hyper-IgM syndrome,[317] and has been associated with defects of myelopoiesis. The most common form of hyper IgM syndrome is due to mutations in the CD40 gene. This defect also leads to a decrease in IgG and IgA. In addition to chronic anemia, children suffer from various infectious complications. They typically lack ANAs and show an arrest at the promyelocyte–myelocyte stage of neutrophil development.[318] Allogeneic HSCT has been curative in some instances.[319]

Common variable immunodeficiency is also frequently associated with neutropenias that can be either chronic or episodic.[320] In addition, hyper- and hypogammaglobulinemia and T- and NK-cell abnormalities of various etiologies (both inherited or acquired) can also be associated with neutropenia.

Other Iatrogenic Forms of Neutropenia

Hemodialysis, which is critical in the care of end-stage renal disease patients, can result in neutropenia.[321,322] One important mechanism postulated is through activation of the plasma complement pathway by dialyzer cellophane membranes and generation of C5a (desarg) that causes reversible neutrophil aggregation, resulting in transient neutropenia.[321,323] Similar mechanisms to explain neutropenia have been noted in other clinical settings, including leukapheresis[324] and cardiopulmonary bypass surgery.[325]

LABORATORY EVALUATION

Laboratory studies aim at the identification of the primary causes of neutropenia, as outlined in Figure 31–4. Idiopathic and autoimmune neutropenia remains, in most instances, diagnoses of exclusion. A careful history, including family history and initial age of first abnormal counts, help to distinguish familial neutropenias (see Chapter 28). Should primary causes such as drugs or systemic diseases be identified, the diagnostic evaluation will concentrate on disease-specific tests. In addition to a complete blood count and differential, which will help establish the severity of neutropenia and tests to diagnose a specific disorder such as T-LGL leukemia, a bone marrow examination may be required. Lack of morphologic or cytogenetic signs of primary hematologic diseases (eg, myelodysplastic syndromes or aplastic anemia) and peripheral destruction will be supported by the observation of left shift and myeloid predominance. Inhibition of myeloid production is exemplified by an increased E:M ratio.

In some instances, auxiliary tests may help identify the cause of the neutropenia, including vitamin B_{12}, zinc, folate, or copper levels. Determination of immunoglobulin levels may be helpful to establish the presence of immunodeficiency. Detection of ANAs has a limited significance as most of the currently available routine tests are not very sensitive and may not be specific. The presence of antibodies, however, may be helpful and support the diagnosis of autoimmune forms of neutropenia.

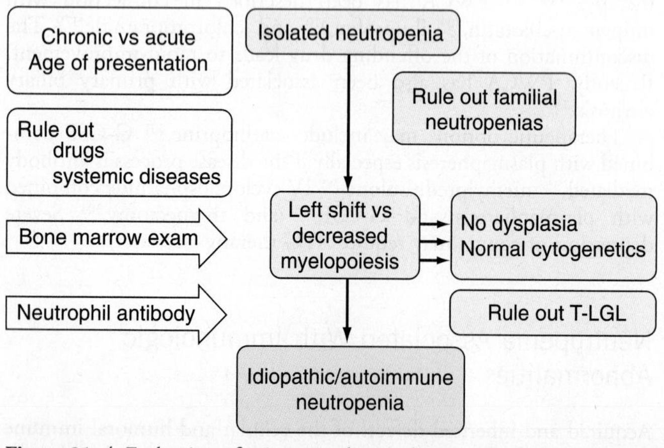

Figure 31–4 Evaluation of primary and secondary neutropenia.

DIFFERENTIAL DIAGNOSIS

Differential diagnostic consideration aims to distinguish primary from secondary forms of neutropenia and to exclude familial hematologic diseases. Suspicion of neutropenia secondary to a primary hematologic disorder requires a bone marrow examination that may be consistent with early form of aplastic anemia or myelodysplastic syndrome (MDS).

THERAPY

In secondary neutropenias, the therapy is aimed at the primary disease. If potentially offending drugs are present, they should be discontinued. G-CSF (4–10 μg/kg SQ per day until ANC is above 500 cells/μL) may be used for both severe cases of primary and secondary neutropenias.[272,326,327] It may help to speed up recovery but if the primary cause persists, it will have only a temporary effect. The use of antibiotics may be useful for the treatment of certain infections. Primary or idiopathic neutropenias most often have an autoimmune cause. Prednisone (1 mg/kg PO QD for 3 months) may be used as first-line therapy,[311] but other B-cell–targeted agents may be needed, including rituximab (375 mg/m^2 IV every week for 4 weeks).[328,329] IVIg (2 g/kg IV for 5 days) is effective in certain cases of PWCA.[330] Cytotoxic therapies like cytoxan (50–100 mg PO QD for 3–6 months) may be difficult to administer owing to their inherent myelotoxicity. In cases of neutropenia secondary to lupus or rheumatoid arthritis, such agents may be effective but the distinction between neutropenia due to the myelosuppressive effects of previous or concurrent treatments for increased activity of the autoimmune disease is necessary. Finally, similar to the treatments applied for T-LGL leukemia, T-cell–targeted approaches, such as CsA, can be used (1–1.5 mg/kg PO BID and titrated to maintain a trough level of 250–400 ng/mL).[331,332] A trial of at least 6 weeks is recommended. Similarly use of ATG has also been effective for cases of PWCA[333] and other idiopathic forms of neutropenia.[334] Methotrexate is effective in treating neutropenia related to Felty syndrome (5–7.5 mg/week for 1–2 months)[335] and T-LGL leukemia.[172,336] Of note is that in many instances isolated neutropenias may be asymptomatic and therapy may not be needed. Alemtuzumab has been used with success in treating thymoma-associated PWCA and other cases of neutropenias.[337–339]

LARGE GRANULAR LYMPHOCYTE LEUKEMIA

Large granular lymphocyte leukemia is a chronic clonal lymphoproliferation of cytotoxic T cells (T-LGL) or NK cells (NK-LGL), often associated with cytopenias, including neutropenia, red cell aplasia, and thrombocytopenia. Pancytopenia is less frequently encountered and may be related to splenomegaly. T-LGL leukemia may be an indolent disorder and present with leukopenia or with lymphocytosis. LGLs observed on a peripheral smear are characteristic of LGL but their frequency can vary.

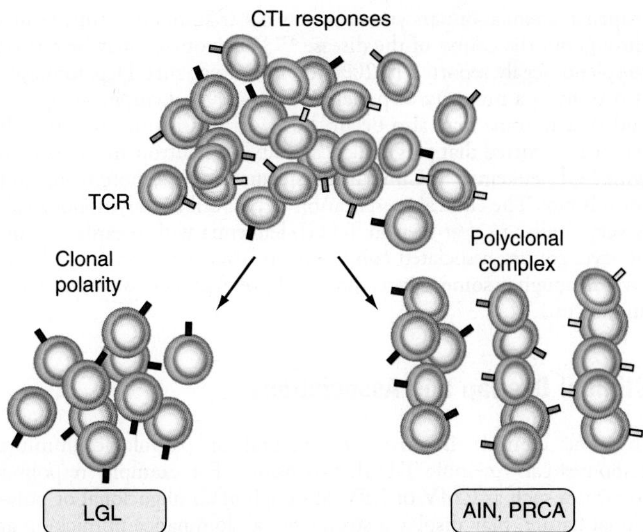

Figure 31–5 Pathophysiology of cytotoxic T-lymphocyte responses.

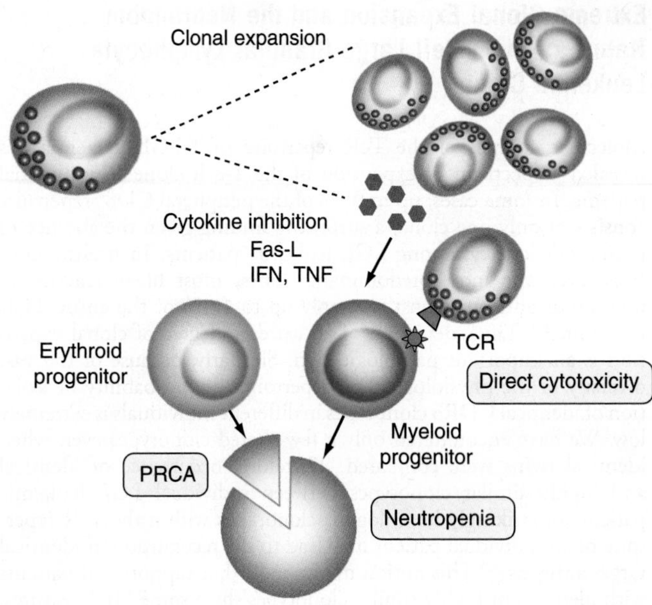

Figure 31–6 Pathophysiology of cytopenias in T-cell large granular lymphocyte leukemia.

T-LGL leukemia results from a proliferation of cytotoxic T cells (CTL) and often resembles reactive CTL expansion. It is frequently associated with other autoimmune disorders, including rheumatoid arthritis, Crohn disease, multiple sclerosis, and many hematologic conditions including MDS. Most reactive processes are polyclonal but immunodominant CTL clones may be present making a distinction between true T-LGL and reactive process difficult (Fig. 31–5). A reduction in the variability of the CTL repertoire can occur in the elderly, and clonal or oligoclonal CTL expansions may be more frequent in older individuals. If asymptomatic, this disorder has been termed monoclonal clonopathy of unclear significance (MCUS).

PATHOGENESIS

Inciting Events

T-LGL leukemia frequently arises in the context of a reactive polyclonal CTL expansion undergoing transformation in a manner similar to that proposed for CLL.[340,341] It is possible also that in T-LGL leukemia, one of the effector CTL clones may be initially driven by an exciting antigen, may transform and consequently the cells fail to undergo apoptosis. The initial or initiating polyclonal response may be a component of the pathophysiologic process associated with infectious agents, rheumatoid arthritis, or other autoimmune disorders.

An initial T cell-mediated process may be responsible for cytopenias in the absence of clonal predominance. In concurrence with this hypothesis, the clinical spectrum of T-LGL is determined by the specificity of the TcR: for example, if myeloid precursors are targets of clonal CTL, neutropenia will be a clinical manifestation. Conversely, if erythroid progenitors are affected, patients will present with anemia (Figs. 31–1 and 31–6). However, unlike the cytopenias that resolve following immunosuppression, the CTL clone may persist at a certain level, suggesting that other disease mechanisms involving soluble factors play a role in the development of the cytopenias. Various soluble agents including Fas-ligand (Fas-L), and perforin have been implicated in the pathophysiology of the cytopenias in T-LGL leukemia.[342–344]

Clonal Transformation

Clinically, T-LGL leukemia does not behave as a typical leukemia: excessive accumulation of malignant cells is often absent and progression to a more malignant phenotype is rare (for clinical review, see references 105 and 345). Instead, the expanded clone in T-LGL leukemia resembles a normal antigen-activated CD8$^+$CD57$^+$ effector-cell; both normal and malignant LGL constitutively express perforin and Fas-L and can suppress neutrophil development in vitro.[343,346–348] Gene expression studies have shown that the T-LGL leukemia clone exhibits upregulation of cytotoxic proteases and adhesion molecules and downregulation of protease inhibitors.[346,347] Typical clonal LGL cells seem to be terminally differentiated and cannot be effectively expanded in vitro by polyclonal mitogens (unpublished observations).

It is likely that a polyclonal CTL response predates the outgrowth of the immunodominant T-LGL leukemia clone (see Fig. 31–3). The putative transforming event most likely involves a memory cell that feeds into the mature effector CTL compartment.[349] Under normal physiologic circumstances, activated effector T cells are deleted after antigen-driven expansion by Fas-mediated apoptosis. The failure of an activated memory and/or effector clone to undergo apoptosis may result in its persistent expansion.[350–353] LGL leukemia cells express high levels of Fas/Fas-L, yet themselves are resistant to Fas-mediated apoptosis.[354] It is conceivable that persistent LGL leukemia cell expansion may result from this resistance to homeostatic apoptosis. In addition to the high surface expression of Fas/Fas-L, soluble Fas-L has been detected in sera from T-LGL leukemia patients and may contribute to the induction of apoptosis of neutrophil precursors in the bone marrow.[336]

An LGL clone persists mostly in the G_0/G_1 phase of cell cycle[348] and clonal transformation may also be due to a constitutive overexpression of prosurvival and antiapoptotic transcription factors. STAT3 has been shown to be involved in cellular transformation along with an active Src family kinase[355] and appears to be constitutively activated in T-LGL leukemia cells.[356,357] In addition, a constitutive activation of an Src family kinase in T-LGL leukemia (likely Lck or Fyn) has been reported that may be related to this increased STAT phosphorylation.[358] It has been proposed that STAT3 activation in T-LGL may inhibit apoptosis downstream of Fas receptor signaling by induction of MCL-1, a member of the BCL-2 family of antiapoptotic proteins.[356] This finding is further supported by data showing that blockade of STAT signaling in T-LGL cells leads to the reversal of Fas resistance. Similarly, constitutive activation of the ERK mitogen activated protein kinase pathway seem to play a role in survival of NK-LGL leukemia cells.[359] ERK was found to be constitutively activated in T-LGL as well.[358]

Extreme Clonal Expansion and the Nonrandom Nature of the T-Cell Large Granular Lymphocyte Leukemia Clone

Molecular analysis of the TcR repertoire in T-LGL leukemia has revealed a spectrum of expansion of the T-cell clone in individual patients. In some cases, up to 98% of the peripheral CD8$^+$ repertoire consists of only one clone, a surprising finding given the absence of immunodeficiency among LGL leukemia patients. In healthy controls, even the most predominant clones, most likely reactive to ubiquitous antigens, constitute only up to 1.4% of the entire TCR repertoire.[360] Thus, detection of an extreme degree of clonal expansion is an important pathologic sign. Similarly, because of the vast diversity of the physiologic TcR repertoire, the probability of isolation of identical CDR3 clonotypes in different individuals is extremely low. We have encountered only a few shared clonotypes even when identical twins were compared. Therefore, occurrence of identical and highly similar clonotypes between individual LGL leukemia patients or strikingly homologous clonotypes within the TcR repertoire of an individual patient may lead to the recognition of identical target antigens.[360] This notion might be further supported if patients with identical or highly similar clonotypes share some HLA features, leading to the display of identical antigenic peptides. It is possible that structurally similar clonotypes present in some patients with T-LGL arise in the context of initial polyclonal CTL response and the initial transformation step is not random (see Fig. 31–3). Once a pathogenic immunodominant clonotype is identified and characterized, its sequence can be used for the design of clonotypic Taqman PCR. This quantitative method may be employed to track the immunodominant clone throughout the course of therapy and thus may potentially predict an impending relapse.[360]

Putative Viral Culprits

While no particular virus has been singled out, according to evidence to date, HTLV-1 (or a related retrovirus) and/or a member of the γ-herpesvirus family are interesting candidates implicated in the pathogenesis of LGL leukemia.[361–365] For instance, patients with NK-cell LGL are often seropositive for the p21e envelope protein of HTLV-1, known to activate the ERK pathway. HTLV epitope mapping has demonstrated a strong reactivity against env p21e protein, with particular specificity for the BA21 epitope. However patients seroreactive for this epitope were negative for HTLV. Consequently, it has been hypothesized that a cellular or retroviral protein with homology to BA21 may play a major role in LGL etiology.[361] In addition, rabbit and bovine LGL infected with alcelaphine herpes virus-1 or bovine herpes virus-2, respectively, have been shown to display several properties of human T-LGL, such as poor proliferation after mitogen stimulation, constitutive ERK activation, and constitutive Lck and Fyn kinase activity.[366]

CLINICAL PRESENTATION AND PHYSICAL FEATURES

Patients with T-LGL leukemia present at a median age of about 55 years, with an equal male/female distribution. The clinical course may be indolent and chronic. Patients are asymptomatic in one-third of cases. The most common clinical presentation is neutropenia (observed in approximately 85% of patients) often accompanied by infections or neutropenic fever.[105,106,292,345,367–369] However, in contrast to neutropenia associated with other hematologic disorders, LGL leukemia patients may remain surprisingly free of infectious complications for extended periods of time regardless of the depressed ANC. Despite the extreme clonality within the T-cell population (suggesting a decreased antigen recognition spectrum), opportunistic infections are rare. Other single-lineage cytopenias, including PRCA and immune-mediated thrombocytopenia, accompany T-LGL leukemia less frequently than neutropenia.[12,367,368,370,371] In some patients, neutropenia, anemia, or pancytopenia may occur at different time points throughout the course of the disease.[372] Pancytopenia may be related to splenomegaly reported in 20% to 50% of patients. Hepatomegaly is present in a minority of patients (10%–20%). Lymphadenopathy and B symptoms may also occur; however, this is uncommon.[345] It has been reported that pregnancy can improve neutropenia in women with LGL leukemia.[373] Clinical transformation to a more malignant form is rare. The clinical presentation of NK-cell LGL lymphocytosis is very similar to that seen in T-LGL leukemia with regards to lymphocyte counts, associated conditions, treatment responses, and survival although in some reports there is a lower incidence of neutropenia and anemia.[374]

Clinical Overlap and Associations

In some clinical circumstances, natural or pathologic immune responses can resemble T-LGL expansions. For example, responses to viruses such as CMV or EBV, although of an oligoclonal or polyclonal nature, may display a strong clonal dominance mimicking at times a true clonal process.[377] Consequently, polarized CTL responses in the context of infections have to be distinguished from true LGL leukemia.

T-LGL leukemia can occur concomitantly with several autoimmune diseases. Rheumatoid arthritis is likely the most common association occurring in one-third of patients with T-LGL leukemia, but other diseases such as ulcerative colitis, Sjögren syndrome, SLE, multiple sclerosis, and a number of other (auto)immune conditions have been described.* Felty syndrome is characterized by neutropenia with rheumatoid arthritis and splenomegaly; 80% of cases express the *HLA-DR4* allele, a finding also observed in T-LGL leukemia.[386] This common immunogenetic link and similar patterns of cytotoxic clonal expansion with T-cell infiltration suggest that Felty syndrome and T-LGL represent components of the same disease process.[378,387–389] In addition, PRCA and immune-mediated thrombocytopenia may also be associated with LGL lymphoproliferation.† Clonal expansions that characterize T-LGL leukemia can appear similar to oligoclonal CTL responses elicited by strong immunodominant antigens, including certain viruses[389–392]—thus the distinction between T-LGL leukemia and a reactive lymphoproliferative process. LGL leukemia has also been described after bone marrow and solid organ transplantation, perhaps initiated by an alloantigen or an infectious agent such as EBV.[393–398]

LGL-like expansions may also be present in other hematologic disorders, including MDS, aplastic anemia, and paroxysmal nocturnal hemoglobinuria,[369,399–403] and may coincide with a number of lymphoproliferative disorders as well.[379,404–406] In MDS, the prognosis is usually determined by the presence of MDS, but the presence of LGL may provide a rational target for immunosuppressive therapy. In MDS, T-LGL leukemia has been reported to negatively impact the outcome of therapy directed against the CTL clone.[402] LGL leukemia has also been described in conjunction with hemolytic anemia following bone marrow transplantation, perhaps a process initially driven by an alloantigen or infectious agent such as EBV.[31] As with infections, distinction between an LGL leukemia and reactive lymphoproliferation may be blurred. For example, neutropenia may be associated with various degrees of clonality, with an LGL leukemia representing the most extreme form of this process.

LABORATORY DIAGNOSIS

Diagnostic criteria remain a subject of considerable discussion (Table 31–7). Traditionally, LGL lymphocytosis (identified by morphology and flow cytometry) is a significant diagnostic criterion.[292,379] However, not all clonal cells display the typical morphology and some

*See references 105, 106, 292, 368, 372, and 376–383.

†See references 12, 13, 367, 368, 370, 371, and 388.

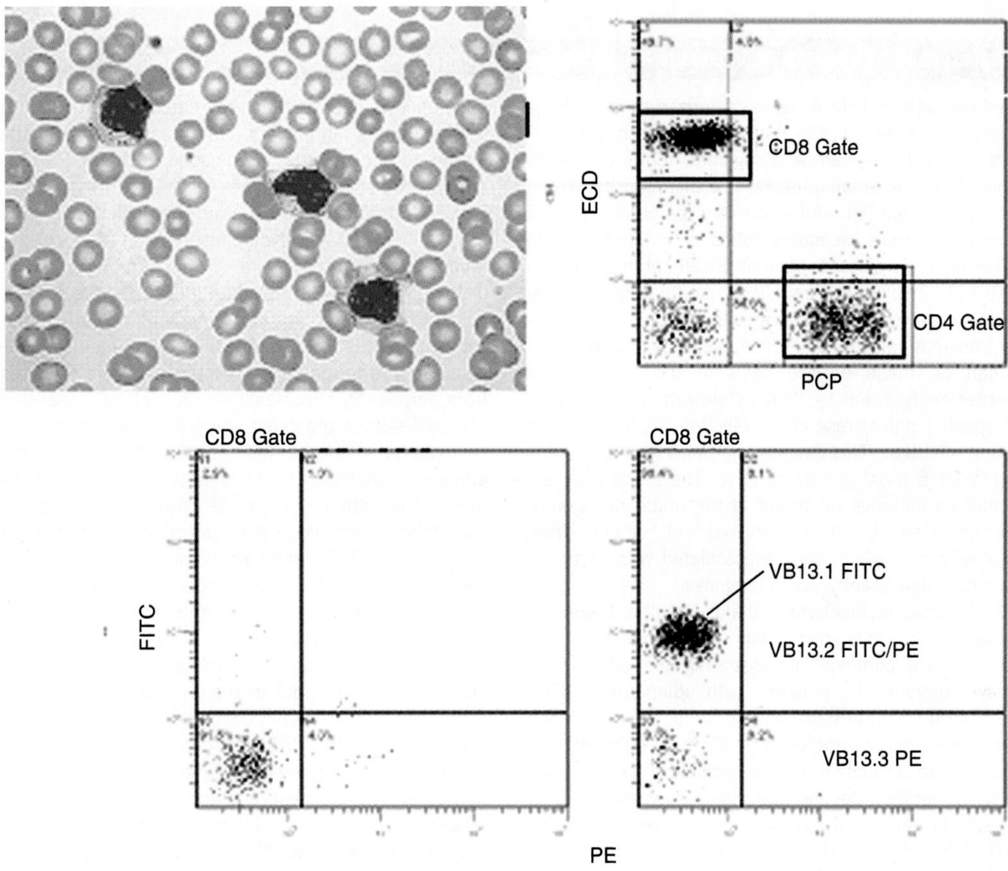

Figure 31–7 Morphology and flow cytometry of T-cell large granular lymphocyte.

Table 31–7 Immunophenotype and Laboratory Features of T-Cell Large Granular Lymphocyte Leukemia

Laboratory features	
Relative/absolute lymphocytosis	
LGL on peripheral blood smear	
CD4/CD8 ratio reversed	
Vβ family skewing (flow cytometry)	
Immunophenotype	$CD2^+$, $CD5^+$, $CD3^+$ Majority $CD8^+$, few $CD4^+/CD8^+$ or $CD4^+$ $CD27^+CD28^-$ $CD57^+CD16^+$ perforin/granzyme+ $CD56^+$ associated with more aggressive forms
TcR rearrangement	TCR-γ PCR Southern blot

patients present with leukopenia. Consequently, an LGL count of greater than 2000/μL of blood has been abandoned as a strict diagnostic requirement, and lower numbers such as 0.400/μL of blood have been proposed.[105,407] Most investigators consider the presence of an expanded homogeneous $CD3^+$, $CD16^+$, $CD28^-$, $CD57^+$ cell population as diagnostic of LGL leukemia; in almost all patients the expanded clone is $CD8^+$ (only very rarely $CD4^+$)[105,408–410] and in the majority of cases this population also expresses CD57, but LGL cases without this marker have been observed.[105,410] In addition, clinically aggressive T-LGL leukemia is characterized by expression of CD26.[411] In most cases of LGL leukemia, CD94 is expressed at increased levels and other receptors for class I MHC molecules are abnormally expressed.[412–414] Some investigators have suggested that a pool of $CD8^+$ memory cells exists that lack CD57 expression but feed into the mature CD57 effector compartment.[408,415] The size of the abnormal clone defining T-LGL leukemia remains controversial. It is likely that the size of the leukemic T-cell population influences the detection of the clonal TCR γ-chain (G) rearrangement by PCR or Southern blotting; thus, such tests are considered mandatory for diagnosis.[416,417] These methods may detect a clonal population that represents 15% of the cell population but it is also likely that smaller CTL expansions may be consistent with latent T-LGL detected only if more precise methods are used. T-LGL can express CD4, but both $CD4^+$ as well as double positive $CD4^+/CD8^+$ cases are rare. Cytogenetic analyses are not useful although cases with chromosomal aberrations have been described.[418,419]

Flow cytometric analysis of Vβ utilization pattern with antibodies directed against most of the Vβ-chain types may be helpful in making the diagnosis. The Vβ family expansion by flow cytometry does not prove clonalily but it may help assess the contribution of the F-LGL clone to the $CD8^+$ or $CD4^+$ population (Fig. 31–7).

Rare immunophenotypic variants of T-LGL exist that coexpress CD4 and CD8, lack both of these markers, or utilize γ/δ TCR instead of α/β TCR chains. Vβ flow cytometry has been used to assess the size of the LGL clone and its Vβ utilization; Vβ usage can be identified in 80% of patients. The current Vβ antibody panel does not cover 25% to 35% of the Vβ spectrum. In usual cases, T-LGL does not express CD56 antigen; the presence of this marker has been associated with a more aggressive clinical phenotype.[420] A monotypic expression pattern of KIR can be found with monoclonal antibodies to CD157b, CD158a, and CD158e (corresponding to the most prevalent KIR genes) in about 50% of patients.[421]

Additional supportive tests include a reticulocyte count, which is low in cases presenting with red cell aplasia. The MCV is usually

Approach to the Diagnosis and Treatment of Acquired Pure Red Cell Aplasia, Acquired Neutropenia, and T-LGL Leukemia

Acquired pure red cell aplasia (PRCA) is characterized by reticulocytopenia but diagnosis is based on the morphologic absence of erythroid precursors in the bone marrow. Congenital forms of PRCA, including Diamond–Blackfan anemia, need to be distinguished when presenting in young children. In adults, primary idiopathic disease has to be differentiated from secondary forms of red cell aplasia associated with hematologic diseases such as B-cell chronic lymphocytic leukemia (CLL), myeloma, T-cell large granular lymphocyte (T-LGL) leukemia, and parvovirus B19–associated chronic reticulocytopenia or acute transient aplastic crisis. The diagnosis of parvovorus B19 infection can be made on the basis of the presence of parvovirus B19–specific IgM and by DNA hybridization techniques. Parvovirus B19–specific polymerase chain reaction (PCR) can help rule out an ongoing infection. This diagnosis is important as therapy with IVIg (2 g/kg IV for 5 days) can be curative. The therapy of secondary red cell aplasia includes treatment of the underlying condition. It is also important to distinguish red cell aplasia from myelodysplastic syndromes, which can be associated with erythroid hypoplasia but carry a significantly worse prognosis.

In cases with thymoma, thymectomy is the usual initial treatment approach; however, incomplete responders, nonresponders, and patients who relapse are common, necessitating the addition of immunosuppressive therapy. In patients with idiopathic PRCA, therapy includes immunosuppressive agents such as prednisone (1 mg/kg PO for 3 months), cyclosporine A (CsA; 5–10 mg/kg PO daily in divided doses for 3 months), or oral cyclophosphamide (50–150 mg PO QD for 3 months). Second-line therapies include ATG (if horse ATG, 40 mg/kg IV daily for 4 days with prednisone at 1 mg/kg, and if rabbit ATG, 2.5–3.5 mg/kg daily IV for 4 or 5 days with prednisone at 1 mg/kg) or rituximab (375 mg/m^2 IV every week for 4 weeks).

Neutropenia may be associated with severe infections, but the risk associated with neutropenia depends on its clinical context, severity, and duration. The management of neutropenia must account for its clinical presentation and the risk of possible life-threatening complications and includes supportive care, clinical monitoring, and implementation of prophylactic antibiotics and/or hematopoietic growth factors. Neutropenia in childhood may be due to congenital diseases, be associated with viral infections, or be immune mediated. These three etiologies are usually self-limiting. In adults, most neutropenias are secondary to other conditions, including hematologic or systemic diseases. In general, drug reactions are a very common cause of neutropenia. Idiopathic or autoimmune neutropenia as a primary disease is a diagnosis of exclusion. The pathogenesis involves T-lymphocyte/natural killer–mediated inhibition of myelopoiesis or antineutrophil antibodies. Immunosuppressive therapy may be employed and includes prednisone (1 mg/kg PO QD for 3 months), methotrexate (5–7.5 mg/week for 1–2 months), CsA (1–1.5 mg/kg PO BID and titrated to maintain a trough level of 250–400 ng/mL), IVIg (2 g/kg IV for 5 days), cyclophosphamide (50–100 mg PO QD for 3–6 months), or rituximab alone (375 mg/m^2 IV every week for 4 weeks) or in conjunction with myeloid growth factors.

T-LGL is a chronic, often indolent clonal lymphoproliferation of cytotoxic T cells associated with immune-mediated cytopenias. It may be a part of a continuum of reactive cytotoxic T-cell responses ranging from polyclonal, oligoclonal, to monoclonal expansions as seen in T-LGL. Persistent antigenic drive or dysfunction of the homeostatic termination of clonal T-cell expansion may be involved, and the abnormal cytotoxic T lymphocyte (CTL) in LGL is not entirely autonomous. The pathophysiology of cytopenias includes cytokine effects and direct antigen-specific cytotoxicity. Most patients present with neutropenia. PRCA and pancytopenia are less common. Hemolytic anemia and pancytopenia may be the result of splenomegaly present in a significant minority of patients. B symptoms and lymphadenopathy are uncommon and many patients remain asymptomatic. The diagnosis is established according to the presence of characteristic LGL lymphocytosis, but in some patients the LGL count may not be very high. The immunophenotype is CD3$^+$, CD8$^+$, CD57$^+$, CD16$^+$, CD56$^-$, and CD28$^-$. CD56 antigen-expressing LGL may be characterized by a more aggressive course. Some cases may coexpress CD4 and CD8. The diagnosis includes detection of T-cell receptor rearrangement. In most instances, expansion of the involved Vβ family may be detected using Vβ flow cytometric clonotyping. T-LGL is often associated with autoimmune diseases, including rheumatoid arthritis and Felty syndrome. T-LGL can accompany myelodysplasia and, in rare instances, aplastic anemia or paroxysmal nocturnal hemoglobinuria. Reactive, often viral infection–associated, CTL proliferation may be difficult to document. Asymptomatic cases are monitored, and development of systemic symptoms or symptomatic cytopenias may prompt therapy. Current treatments include immunosuppressive agents such as prednisone, CsA (1–1.5 mg/kg PO BID then adjusted to maintain a trough level of 250–400 ng/mL for 8–10 weeks), oral methotrexate (10 mg/m^2 week for 21 months), or cyclophosphamide (50–100 mg/day for 3–6 months). Chronic long-term therapy may be more effective than high-dose combination chemotherapy applied in B-cell lymphomas. Second-line treatments may involve alemtuzumab or ATG. The prognosis is generally good and transformation to a more aggressive lymphoproliferative disorder is rare.

high. Serologic studies or DNA titer to detect evidence of EBV infection is usually not needed but may be helpful to distinguish reactive immunologic responses. The rheumatoid factor is frequently positive. Antinuclear antibodies and ANAs may also at times be positive.[422,423]

Unless additional hematologic diseases, such as MDS, are suspected, bone marrow examination may not be required. Bone marrow biopsy and aspirate should be obtained in cases of pancytopenia or involvement of several lineages. Morphologic hallmarks of MDS and cytogenetic analysis may help establish a diagnosis of MDS.

DIFFERENTIAL DIAGNOSIS

Differential diagnostic considerations include reactive processes such as viral infections. Occasionally, MDS may be present simultaneously or serve as an alternative diagnosis; T-cell oligoclonality may accompany MDS.

THERAPY

A significant proportion of patients will be asymptomatic and the diagnosis may be totally coincidental. Should the patient be asymptomatic, therapy may be delayed. Lymphocytosis may be significant but absolute lymphocyte counts more than 40,000/μL are unusual. Symptomatic splenomegaly may be an indication for splenectomy. Pancytopenia may be a result of splenomegaly and the procedure aids in the treatment of a hemolytic anemia that can be present in some patients.

Patients may tolerate significant degrees of neutropenia for many years. Indications for treatment include neutropenic complications or transfusion-dependence (Fig. 31–8). G-CSF therapy will increase counts in some patients, but a significant proportion of patients will be refractory or would have delayed response.[225,424–426] Of interest is the observation that high-dose therapy with typical lymphoma regimens such as CVP or CHOP may be ineffective and therefore should not be used. Cases refractory to bone marrow transplantation have

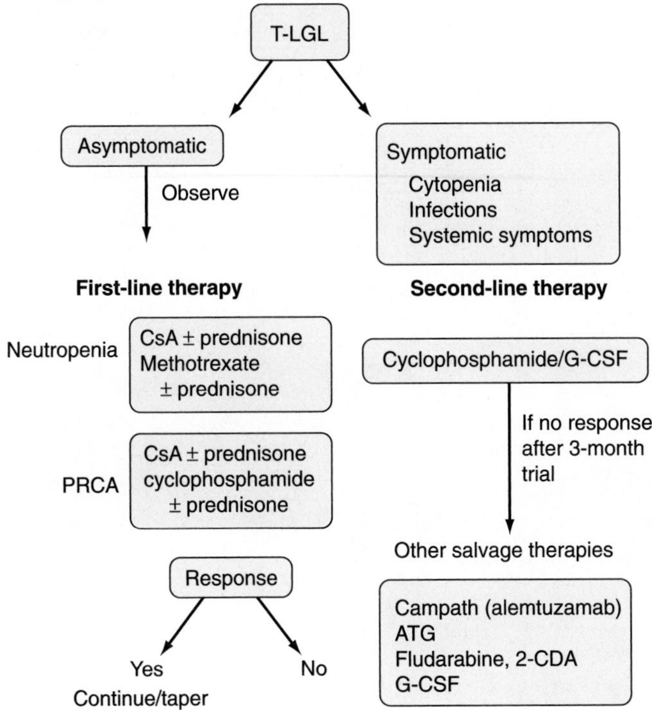

Figure 31–8 Therapy of T-cell large granular lymphocyte leukemia.

been described.[427] Monotherapy with prednisone may relieve some of the symptoms and improve neutropenia but remissions are usually not durable. CsA given at 1 to 1.5 mg/kg PO BID then adjusted to maintain a trough level of 250 to 400 ng/mL represents a reasonable first-line therapy; however, a course of sufficient duration has to be given, with a response expected after 8 to 10 weeks of therapy.[331,428] Weekly oral methotrexate given at 10 mg/m^2 PO weekly has been used successfully.[428,429] Patients with LGL leukemia–associated PRCA may be better treated with oral cyclophosphamide instead of methotrexate with a dose between 50 and 100 mg/day. In LGL leukemia with associated PRCA, responses may be delayed and the PRCA may recur after discontinuation of cyclophosphamide therapy, or if insufficient treatment (<6–8 weeks) was administered. Therapy with cyclophosphamide in neutropenic patients may be difficult due to myelosuppression. In most refractory cases, ATG has been also used with success.[430] In recent years, successful therapy with alemtuzamab has been reported.[431] Allogeneic HSCT has also been used successfully in some cases.[432,433]

Relapses are frequent but usually responsive to the previously effective therapy. Certain patients may require low-dose maintenance therapy with CsA. In some cases, remarkable improvement of cytopenia can be achieved with splenectomy.[434]

PROGNOSIS

LGL leukemia is a chronic condition and may be indolent. In general, mortality is low. Transformation to more aggressive forms of lymphomas or leukemias is uncommon. In cases of T-LGL leukemia associated with a primary hematologic disease such as MDS, the prognosis is dependent on the therapy of the underlying problem.

SUGGESTED READINGS

Boxer LA, Stossel TP: Effects of anti-human neutrophil antibodies in vitro. Quantitative studies. J Clin Invest 53:1534–1545, 1974.

Bux J, Behrens G, Jaeger G, Welte K: Diagnosis and clinical course of autoimmune neutropenia in infancy: analysis of 240 cases. Blood 91:181–186, 1998.

Casadevall N, Nataf J, Viron B, et al: Pure red-cell aplasia and antierythropoietin antibodies in patients treated with recombinant erythropoietin. N Engl J Med 346:469–475, 2002.

Cines DB, Passero F, Guerry D, et al: Granulocyte-associated IgG in neutropenic disorders. Blood 59:124–132, 1982.

Clark DA, Dessypris EN, Krantz SB: Studies on pure red cell aplasia. XI. Results of immunosuppressive treatment of 37 patients. Blood 63:277–286, 1984.

Conway LT, Clay ME, Kline WE, et al: Natural history of primary autoimmune neutropenia in infancy. Pediatrics 79:728–733, 1987.

Dale DC, Bonilla MA, Davis MW, et al: A randomized controlled phase III trial of recombinant human granulocyte colony-stimulating factor (filgrastim) for treatment of severe chronic neutropenia. Blood 81:2496–2502, 1993.

Doron MW, Makhlouf RA, Katz VL, Lawson EE, Stiles AD: Increased incidence of sepsis at birth in neutropenic infants of mothers with preeclampsia. J Pediatr 125:452–458, 1994.

Greer JP, Kinney MC, Loughran TP Jr: T cell and NK cell lymphoproliferative disorders. Hematology (Am Soc Hematol Educ Program) 259–281, 2001.

Handgretinger R, Geiselhart A, Moris A, et al: Pure red-cell aplasia associated with clonal expansion of granular lymphocytes expressing killer-cell inhibitory receptors. N Engl J Med 340:278–284, 1999.

Koenig JM, Christensen RD: Incidence, neutrophil kinetics, and natural history of neonatal neutropenia associated with maternal hypertension. N Engl J Med 321:557–562, 1989.

Lalezari P, Khorshidi M, Petrosova M: Autoimmune neutropenia of infancy. J Pediatr 109:764–769, 1986.

Lamy T, Loughran TP Jr: Current concepts: large granular lymphocyte leukemia. Blood Rev 13:230–240, 1999.

Liu JH, Wei S, Lamy T, et al: Chronic neutropenia mediated by Fas ligand. Blood 95:3219–3222, 2000.

Loughran TP Jr: Clonal diseases of large granular lymphocytes. Blood 82:1–14, 1993.

Perzova R, Loughran TP Jr: Constitutive expression of Fas ligand in large granular lymphocyte leukaemia. Br J Haematol 97:123–126, 1997.

Risks of agranulocytosis and aplastic anemia. A first report of their relation to drug use with special reference to analgesics. The International Agranulocytosis and Aplastic Anemia Study. JAMA 256:1749–1757, 1986.

Scadden DT, Zon LI, Groopman JE: Pathophysiology and management of HIV-associated hematologic disorders. Blood 74:1455–1463, 1989.

Sood R, Stewart CC, Aplan PD, et al: Neutropenia associated with T-cell large granular lymphocyte leukemia: long-term response to cyclosporine therapy despite persistence of abnormal cells. Blood 91:3372–3378, 1998.

Young NS, Brown KE: Parvovirus B19. N Engl J Med 350:586–597, 2004.

REFERENCES

For complete list of references log onto www.expertconsult.com

CHAPTER 32

THROMBOCYTOPENIA DUE TO DECREASED PLATELET PRODUCTION

Alan M. Gewirtz

In this chapter we consider the diagnosis, pathogenesis, and treatment of platelet production (thrombopoiesis) abnormalities. To accomplish this goal, it is useful to first briefly review the biology of megakaryocyte development, a topic that is treated in much greater detail in Chapter 27 of this book. Platelets are the direct progeny of megakaryocytes; as such, disorders of megakaryocyte development are important causes of thrombocytopenia.

In 1906, J. Homer Wright, using only a microscope and histochemical stains, formulated the seminal hypothesis that platelets were derived from bone marrow megakaryocytes.[1] His insightful observations proved correct and were the beginning of a long, technically difficult, and still incomplete investigation into the processes that control megakaryocyte development and the production of platelets. Having said this, however, it is still clear that the study of thrombopoiesis has come a very long way and much has been revealed about the cellular, biochemical, and molecular aspects of this process.[2]

Megakaryocytes, like all formed elements of the peripheral blood, are ultimately derived from undifferentiated hematopoietic stem cells that exist in a developmental continuum (see Chapter 20).[3] Through a series of still incompletely understood events, stem cells undergo an asynchronous division that gives rise to two daughter cells. One daughter cell remains a stem cell, fulfilling the requirement for self-renewal of the stem cell compartment, and the other commits to developing within a given lineage, likely through the induction of specific transcription factors such as GATA-1, FOG-1, and FLI-1, in the case of megakaryocytes,[4,5] and perhaps by downmodulation of other transcription factors, such as c-myb.[6,7] Lineage-committed *progenitor cells* are characterized by a loss of "plasticity" and a remarkable capacity for proliferation. The latter is required because approximately 15×10^6 megakaryocytes/kg body weight must be available to produce the roughly 100×10^9 new platelets that are needed daily to maintain a normal platelet count of 150 to 400×10^9/L.[8] As progenitor cell divisional activity proceeds, maturation, as defined by the acquisition of lineage-specific proteins, ensues, largely under the control of the hematopoietic cytokine thrombopoietin.[2,9,10] After a variable number of mitoses, proliferative activity eventually declines, giving rise to many daughter cells, which are known as *precursors*. Precursor cells are essentially postmitotic and are capable of one or two additional cell divisions at most. They are often morphologically identifiable as belonging to a given lineage and are primarily engaged in the terminal maturation steps that allow them to function as competent members of their lineage. In the case of megakaryocytes, precursor cells undergoing nuclear endoreduplication to increase their ploidy (to a mean of approximately 16 N), a characteristic unique to cells of the megakaryocyte lineage.[4,11–17] Nuclear endoreduplication is accompanied by an increase in megakaryocyte cytoplasm and thereby the number of platelets that an individual megakaryocyte can produce.[14]

As discussed in Chapter 27, the process of platelet formation, or thrombopoiesis, occurs during megakaryocyte terminal maturation.[18,19] It is initiated by the development of the demarcation membrane system in the megakaryocyte's cytoplasm.[20] Among the functions of the demarcation membrane system is delineation of platelet fields. These fields are filled with the granules and proteins that ultimately make up the contents of mature platelets. The latter are shed from pseudopods that mature megakaryocytes extend through endothelial cell junctions into the lumen of marrow capillaries. The pseudopods fracture, because of shear stress in the lumen of these capillaries, and release shards of megakaryocytic cytoplasm, or proplatelets, that are the immediate antecedents of circulating platelets. A fully mature megakaryocyte is estimated to produce approximately 1 to 1.5×10^3 platelets. The molecular regulation of this process is beginning to be better understood. It has been shown, for example, that the apoptosis-stimulating gene Bax promotes platelet production.[21] Interestingly, very recent evidence suggests that the lifespan of circulating platelets is also regulated by the apoptosis proteins. Using the strategy of ethylnitrosourea (ENU)-inducted mutations, Mason and colleagues have recently demonstrated that mutations in the Bcl-x_L gene lead to synthesis of a form of the protein that no longer inhibits Bax, and that this in turn leads to accelerated platelet death and a heritable form of thrombocytopenia (Fig. 32–1).[22]

Failure in the process of either megakaryocytopoiesis or thrombopoiesis will result in thrombocytopenia. Under either circumstance, platelet production is characterized as "ineffective," either because there is an absolute decrease in available megakaryocyte cytoplasm (failure of megakaryocytopoiesis) or because cytoplasmic development is defective (failure of thrombopoiesis). Selective impairment of megakaryocytopoiesis may also result from damage to the progenitor cell compartment (the burst-forming units–megakaryocyte [BFU-MK] or colony-forming units–megakaryocyte [CFU-MK]; see Chapter 27) or, rarely, from a compromised ability to synthesize thrombopoietin, the chief cytokine regulator of this compartment (Fig. 32–2).[23] Inherent or acquired defects in megakaryocyte precursor cells may lead to ineffective thrombopoiesis.[23,24] The relative effectiveness of platelet production can be calculated by measuring platelet mass turnover, which is defined as the product of the mean megakaryocyte cytoplasmic volume multiplied by the total number of marrow megakaryocytes.[8,25–27] A disparity between cytoplasmic mass and platelet delivery to the peripheral blood (platelet count divided by platelet survival, corrected for splenic pooling) is the hallmark of ineffective platelet production (Fig. 32–3). Table 32–1 shows the typical kinetic characteristics of diseases characterized by ineffective platelet production.

An examination of the peripheral blood smear is the first step in the initial assessment of patients who present with thrombocytopenia. The presence of platelet clumps, indicative of pseudothrombocytopenia, or abnormally large, or small, platelets can be very useful in generating a differential diagnosis, as can the presence of inclusion bodies in neutrophils. Nevertheless, the current gold standard for diagnosing thrombocytopenia due to ineffective platelet production is a bone marrow aspirate and biopsy. At the moment, direct visualization of the marrow and its cellular contents is the only way to judge the quantity and quality of the megakaryocyte population (Fig. 32–4). However, noninvasive methods for making a diagnosis of ineffective platelet production are being developed. For example, the concentration of serum glycocalicin, the soluble fragment of glycoprotein (GP) Ib, has been shown to be significantly diminished in patients with platelet production abnormalities when compared with normal control subjects.[28] Reticulated platelets, like red blood cell reticulocytes, contain RNA. It has been suggested that as is true for red blood cell reticulocytes, the presence of residual RNA in platelets indicates that they have been newly formed.[28,29] Thus, they may be

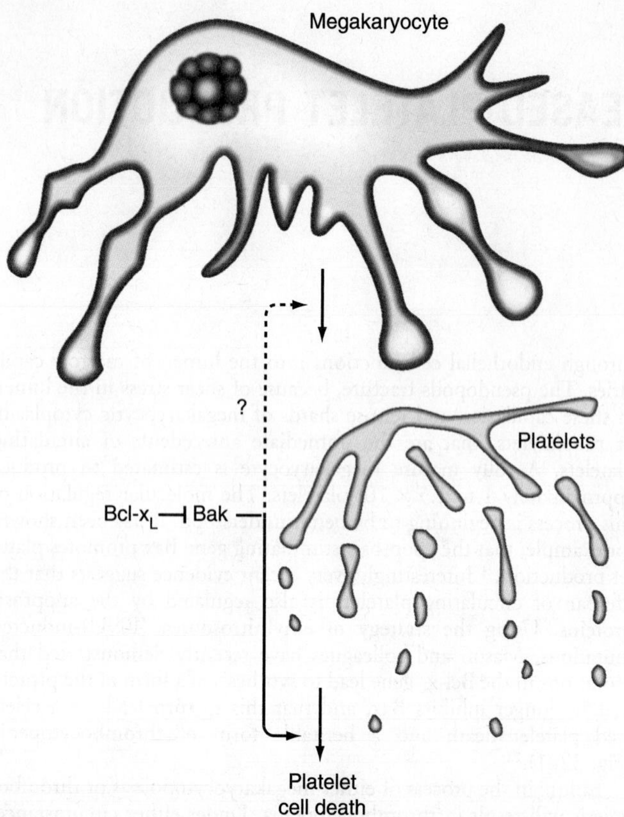

Figure 32–1 Bcl-x$_L$ and platelet life span. Mason et al[22] subjected mice to ethylnitrosourea (ENU) mutagenesis and screened their first-generation offspring for platelet deficiency. They identified two mutations in the gene encoding the antiapoptotic factor *Bcl-x$_L$* that give rise to a dominantly inherited reduction in platelet count. Bcl-x$_L$ appears to promote platelet survival through inhibition of the proapoptotic activity of Bak. Bax promotes production of platelets,[21] and overexpression of antiapoptotic Bcl-xL impairs the fragmentation of megakayocytes.[289] *(Adapted from Qi B, Hardwick JM: A Bcl-xL timer sets platelet life span. Cell 128(6):1035, 2007.)*

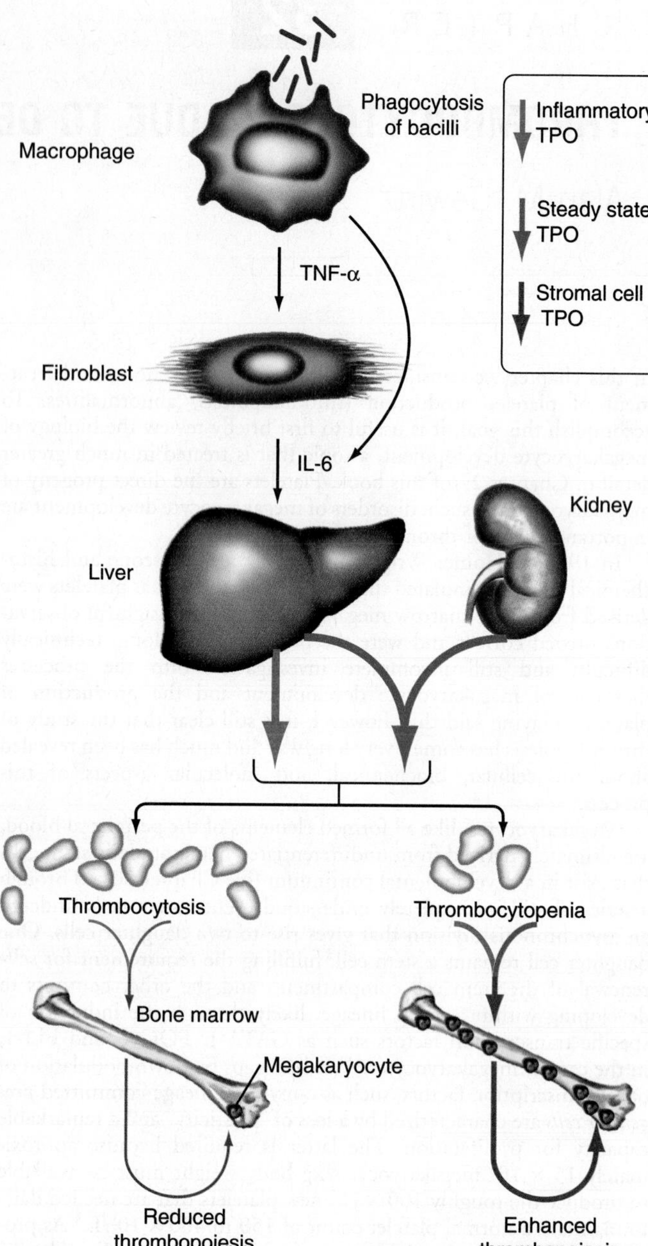

Figure 32–2 The regulation of thrombopoietin levels. A steady-state amount of hepatic thrombopoietin (TPO) is regulated by platelet c-Mpl receptor–mediated uptake and destruction of the hormone. Hepatic production of the hormone is depicted. Upon binding to platelet c-Mpl receptors, the hormone is removed from the circulation and destroyed, which reduces blood levels. In the presence of inflammation, IL-6 is released from macrophages and, through TNF-α stimulation, from fibroblasts and circulates to the liver to enhance thrombopoietin production. Thrombocytopenia also leads to enhanced marrow stromal cell production of thrombopoietin, although the molecular mediator(s) of this effect is not yet completely understood. *(Adapted from Kaushansky K: The molecular mechanisms that control thrombopoiesis. J Clin Invest 115(12):3339, 2005.)*

useful for assessing the dynamics of platelet production, under baseline conditions and after marrow insults such as chemotherapy or irradiation.[30–33] Platelet RNA can be detected by staining with dyes such as thiazole orange,[29] and it has been suggested that assessing the mean thiazole orange staining can be used to construct a reticulated platelet maturation index.[30] Although appealing in concept, the ultimate usefulness of this assay remains to be determined, because staining artifacts[34] and paradoxically low reticulated platelet counts in cases of disorders characterized by peripheral destruction may complicate the interpretation of such results.[29,34] Yet another approach to assessing platelet production is the measurement of serum thrombopoietin levels. Thrombopoietin is synthesized constitutively in the liver and then binds to its receptor c-MPL on megakaryocytes and platelets. Accordingly, in patients with disorders in which megakaryocytes are reduced in the marrow, thrombopoietin levels rise.[29,34–37] However, the wide variation in "normal" thrombopoietin concentrations in serum make this determination somewhat problematic as well. Some of this variability may be attributed to the fact that TPO synthesis is inducible in marrow stromal cells, perhaps by platelet α-granule proteins.[38,39] Reports attesting to the increased reliability and precision of measuring several of these parameters at once have appeared,[30,40] but it remains unclear whether the expense and time involved will prove cost-effective when compared with the relative simplicity of a bone marrow examination.

CONGENITAL OR HEREDITARY PLATELET PRODUCTION DISORDERS

Once thought rare, congenital or hereditary thrombocytopenias are becoming increasingly recognized and their molecular genetic bases more clearly understood. They vary in severity as an indirect function

Table 32–1 Typical Kinetic Profiles in Patients With Thrombocytopenia Due to Production Abnormalities

	Megakaryocytes			Platelets			
Category	**Cell No. (×10⁶/kg)**	**Cytoplasmic Volume (fL)**	**Cytoplasmic Mass (×10¹¹ fL/kg)**	**Concentration (Platelets/mm³)**	**Volume (fL)**	**Survival (Days)**	**Mass Turnover (×10⁵ fL/mm³/day)**
Normal	15 ± 4	12,000 ± 1,700	1.8 ± 0.4	250,000 ± 40,000	8.7 ± 0.8	9.6 ± 0.6	3.2 ± 0.5
Decreased Megakaryocytopoiesis —Damaged marrow	2	14,000	0.3	22,000	9.1	5.2	0.7
Ineffective production							
Autosomal dominant	49	9,400	4.6	64,000	8.9	8.4	1.1
Wiskott-Aldrich syndrome	20	9,000	1.8	40,000	4.0	5.0	0.4
Vitamin B_{12} deficiency	51	8,900	4.5	62,000	8.5	8.4	0.8
Preleukemia	18	13,300	2.4	16,000	9.0	6.7	0.4

Adapted from Thompson A, Harker L: Quantitative platelet disorders. In Manual of Hemostasis and Thrombosis. Philadelphia, FA Davis, 1983, p 65.

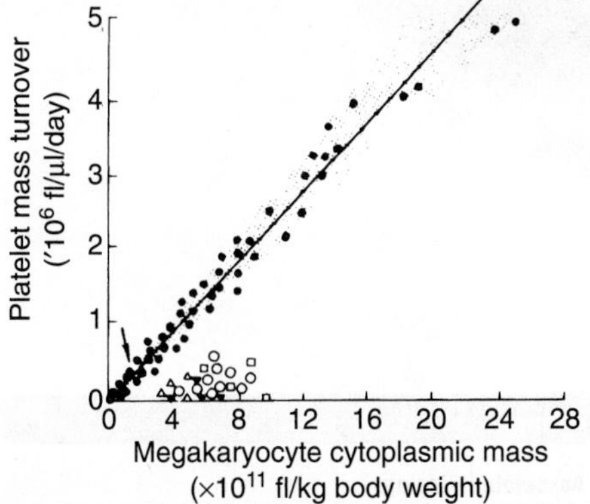

Figure 32–3 Ineffective platelet production. In thrombocytopenia, the relationship between marrow megakaryocyte cytoplasmic mass and the turnover of platelet mass in the peripheral blood is usually direct. Platelet mass turnover represents the product of the mean megakaryocyte cytoplasmic volume multiplied by the total number of marrow megakaryocytes. The results in normal subjects are indicated by the *arrow*, and the *stippled area* represents 95% of confidence limits in thrombocytopenic patients with effective production. Ineffective thrombocytopoiesis is identified as a disparity between available marrow substrate (megakaryocyte cytoplasmic mass) and delivery of platelet mass to the peripheral blood (platelet mass turnover). Results in patients with autosomal dominant thrombocytopenia (*open circles*), Wiskott–Aldrich syndrome (*open triangles*), megaloblastic anemia (*open squares*), and preleukemia (*closed triangles*) are characterized by ineffective platelet production. *(Data from Thompson A, Harker L: Quantitative platelet disorders. In: Manual of Hemostasis and Thrombosis. Philadelphia, FA Davis, 1983, p 65.)*

of age, so that the most severe forms are diagnosed, not surprisingly, in newborns and infants, whereas the least clinically significant are diagnosed in adults. The congenital thrombocytopenia syndromes have been the subject of a number of authoritative reviews.[41,42] Because profound thrombocytopenia is a common problem in sick newborns, it is important to note that in this population, thrombocytopenia is typically due to sepsis, viral infections, perinatal asphyxia, or immunologic causes.[43,44] It has been estimated that less than 5% of cases of neonatal thrombocytopenia are due to inherited or congenital disorders of platelet production.[45] It is also worth noting that Fanconi anemia, congenital aplastic anemia, and other marrow failure syndromes involving multiple lineages may also manifest initially, though uncommonly, as an isolated thrombocytopenia (see Chapter 28).

Congenital thrombocytopenias can be classified in a number of ways, including clinical features (e.g., age of onset and severity of bleeding), platelet size (large, normal, small),[41] or by mode of inheritance and genetic mutation (Table 32–2).[42] The latter may be considered the most modern approach and perhaps ultimately the most informative with regard to etiology.

AUTOSOMAL DOMINANT THROMBOCYTOPENIA

Autosomal dominant thrombocytopenia can be encountered with or without other congenital abnormalities.[46–51] Patients with isolated thrombocytopenias usually have only modest reductions in their platelet counts, with normal platelet morphology and normal numbers of megakaryocytes. These individuals rarely have clinical symptoms related to their thrombocytopenias.

Patients with autosomal dominant thrombocytopenia may be relatively more common than previously believed. Many cases are not diagnosed until adulthood, again because these patients usually are asymptomatic, although exceptions have been reported.[52] The most important reason for recognizing these disorders is that patients may be misdiagnosed as having immune thrombocytopenic purpura (ITP) and treated for that disorder.[42,46] A detailed family history may be useful, as family studies of 54 patients referred with the diagnosis of refractory ITP showed that these patients had autosomal dominant thrombocytopenia with large platelets, normal megakaryocytes, and normal platelet survival.[49] Treatment is usually not indicated. Corticosteroids are ineffective, although splenectomy occasionally results in a modest response.[53]

THROMBOCYTOPENIA SYNDROMES ASSOCIATED WITH *MYH9* GENE MUTATIONS

The nonmuscle myosin heavy-chain IIA gene, *MYH9*, is found on chromosome 22q.[14,16,52,54] *MYH9* is expressed in platelets and upregulated during granulocyte differentiation.[52,55,56] Quite recently, May–Hegglin anomaly (Online Mendelian Inheritance in Man [OMIM] 155100), Fechtner syndrome (OMIM 153640), Sebastian syndrome (OMIM 605249), and Epstein syndrome (OMIM 153650) have all been found to be associated with mutations of this gene. These disorders share a characteristic triad of thrombocytopenia, macrothrombocytes, and neutrophil inclusions termed *Döhle-like bodies*.

The May–Hegglin anomaly, also called familial thrombocytopenia with leukocyte inclusions, was the first of these syndromes to be recognized and was in fact described almost 100 years ago. The thrombocytopenia associated with May–Hegglin anomaly is usually mild to moderate and, as just noted, is associated with giant platelets whose volumes may actually exceed those of red blood cells.[57] Up to one-third of platelets have volumes between 30 and 80 fL. Although

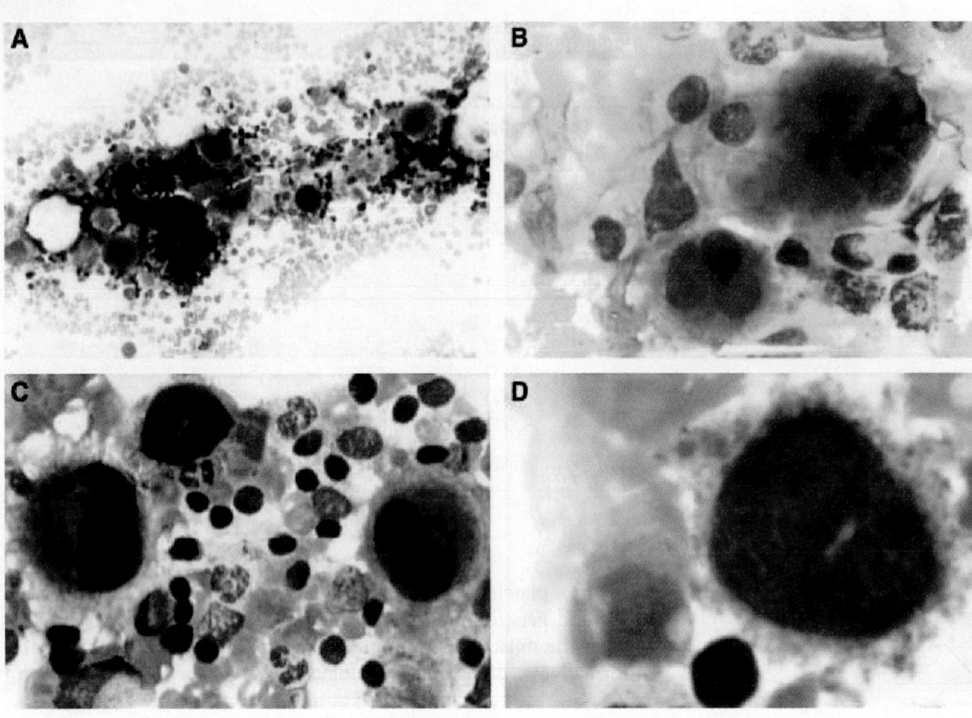

Figure 32–4 Marrow aspirate obtained from a child with thrombocytopenia and dysmegakaryocytopoiesis. The megakaryocytes are small and hypolobular, with diminished cytoplasm. Cells are viewed at magnifications of 250× (**A**), 1000× (**B**), 200× (**C**), and 1600× (**D**). *(From van den Oudenrijn S et al: Three parameters: Plasma thrombopoietin levels, plasma glycocalicin levels, and megakaryocyte culture, distinguish between different causes of congenital thrombocytopenia. Br J Haematol 117:390, 2002.)*

Table 32–2 Inherited Thrombocytopenias Classified by MYH9 Mutations and Associated Findings

Syndrome	Gene Mutation	Chromosome Location	Associated Findings
MYH9-related thrombocytopenia			
May–Hegglin anomaly	MYH9	22q11	Neutrophil inclusions, sensorineural hearing loss, nephritis, cataracts
Fechtner syndrome	MYH9	22q11	
Epstein syndrome	MYH9	22q11	
Sebastian syndrome	MYH9	22q11	
Mediterranean thrombocytopenia Bernard–Soulier carrier	GPiBB possibly others	17pter-pt2	None
Bernard–Soulier syndrome	GP1BA, GP1BB	17pter-pt2	None
Velocardiofacial/DiGeorge syndrome (CATCH22)	?GP1BB	22q11	Cancer facial, parathyroid, and thymus anomalies, cognitive learning impairment
Familial platelet discordant/acute myeloid leukemia	AML1	21q22.2	Myelodysplasia, acute myeloid leukemia
Chromosome 10THC22	?FL/14813	lop12-11.2	None
Paris–Trousseau thrombocytopenias/ Jacobsen syndrome	?FLIt	11q23	Psychomotor retardation, facial anomalies (Jacobsen syndrome)
Gray platelet syndrome	Unknown	Unknown	None
Congenital amegakaryocytic thrombocytopenia	MPL	1p34	Marrow failure during second decade
Thrombocytopenia and absent radii	Unknown	Unknown	Shortened absent radii bilaterally
Thrombocytopenia and radial synostosis	*HOXA11*	7prs-p14.2	Fused radius, incomplete range of motion
Wiskott–Aldrich syndrome	*WAS*	Xp11.23-p11.22	Immunodeficiency, eczema, lymphoma
X-linked thrombocytopenia	*WASI*	Xp11.23-p11.22	None
GATA-1 mutation	*GATA1*	Xp11.23	Anemia, dyserythropoiesis, thalassemia

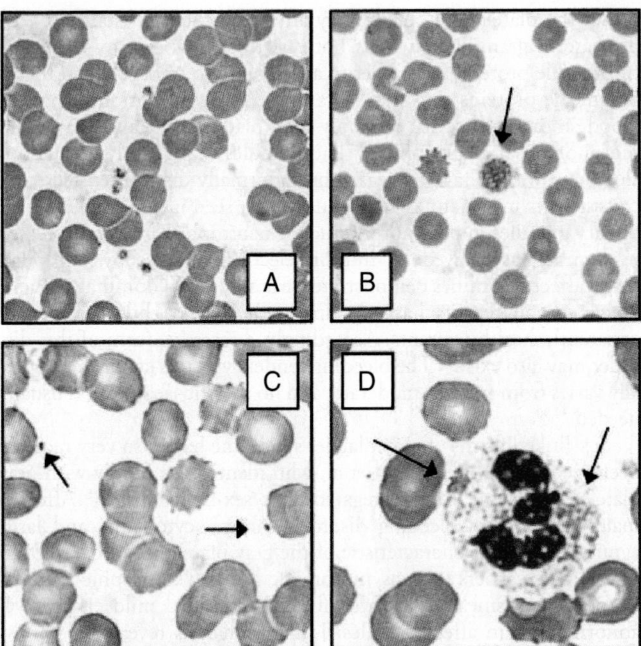

Figure 32–5 Peripheral blood platelets. **A**, Normal blood smear. **B**, Macrothrombocyte. The platelet depicted (*arrow*) is larger than the average erythrocyte. **C**, Microthrombocytes (*arrows*) are typical of those seen in Wiskott–Aldrich syndrome or X-linked thrombocytopenia. **D**, Döhle-like bodies in the cytoplasm of neutrophils (*arrows*) are seen in the May-Hegglin anomaly. All photomicrographs originally made at a magnification of 100× (Wright–Giemsa stain). *(From Drachman JG: Inherited thrombocytopenia: When a low platelet count does not mean ITP. Blood 103:390, 2004.)*

the platelets are large, they exhibit no intrinsic structural abnormalities and have normal surface membrane proteins.[58] Because marrow megakaryocytes are morphologically normal and platelet survival has been shown to be normal or modestly decreased in most cases,[59,60] ineffective production is the likely cause of the thrombocytopenia. The mechanism by which the giant platelets are formed in May–Hegglin anomaly and in other macrothrombocytopenias is not known with certainty, but recent studies suggest that abnormalities in the Rho-ROCK-myosin-IIA signaling pathway play a role.[61] Abnormal fragmentation of megakaryocyte pseudopods may also be involved.[59] The other characteristic of May–Hegglin anomaly is the presence of cytoplasmic inclusions in the patient's neutrophils, eosinophils, and, less commonly, monocytes. Morphologically, the inclusions resemble the classic Döhle bodies found in neutrophils from patients with acute inflammatory conditions, but unlike Döhle inclusions, they are present throughout the lifespan of affected individuals (Fig. 32–5). The inclusions appear bright blue on Wright–Giemsa staining and are composed largely of mutated nonmuscle myosin heavy-chain IIA, an important cytoskeletal contractile protein in hematopoietic cells.[55] Because the thrombocytopenia is modest and bleeding times are variable, treatment is usually not required.[62] Platelet transfusions have been given for thrombocytopenia, but their role is not clear.[63,64] Pregnancy is not difficult to manage and normal vaginal deliveries in these patients should be possible.[65]

May–Hegglin-like variants have also been described (Fechtner, Sebastian, and Epstein syndromes). All have mild macrothrombocytopenia.[51] They are distinguished according to whether the individual's neutrophils contain the Döhle-like inclusion bodies and whether the patient manifests abnormalities similar to Alport syndrome, such as nephritis, sensorineural hearing loss, and cataracts.[66,67] The clinical distinction of these syndromes can be quite difficult because within the same family and indeed the same individual, expressions of nephritis and hearing loss can be variable as a result of other as yet unidentified environmental factors. Fortunately, the bleeding tendency in affected individuals is mild, likely because the platelet mass in these patients is nearly normal, and functional defects are equally mild.

Macrothrombocytopenia is frequently discovered during routine testing of an asymptomatic individual. Diagnosis can be aided by examination of the peripheral blood smear, and identification of neutrophilic inclusions and giant platelets. As noted, individuals with mutations of *MYH9* and associated syndromes do not have life-threatening bleeding events. Nevertheless, genetic counseling should be offered to affected kindreds, if for no other reason than that platelet function-compromising drugs should be avoided as well as potentially dangerous treatments for presumed ITP.[42,66] For periods of hemorrhagic stress, such as trauma or surgery, platelet transfusions would be useful for uncontrolled bleeding.

MEDITERRANEAN MACROTHROMBOCYTOPENIA (OMIM 153670)

Not every macrothrombocytopenia is caused by mutations in the *MYH9* gene. Mediterranean macrothrombocytopenia,[68] common in people of Southern European extraction, has been assigned to an as yet unidentified gene mutation on the short arm of chromosome 17 through linkage analysis of affected families.[69] The degree of thrombocytopenia in affected individuals is generally mild to moderate, with platelet counts ranging from 70,000 to 150,000/μL. Flow cytometric analysis of platelets has shown decreased expression of the GPIb/IX/V complex in a high percentage of affected individuals, and sequencing of the *GPIBA* gene has revealed an Ala156Val mutation in the GP1b in almost all families examined.[69] Functional defects, if any, are minor, so bleeding is not a problem in these individuals. In virtually all respects, the clinical phenotype and the molecular genetics of the condition are essentially identical to what is observed in carriers of the Bernard–Soulier syndrome, an autosomal recessive thrombocytopenia described below. Because there is no bleeding tendency related to the thrombocytopenia, no therapy is required. Nonetheless, recognition of this entity is in the patient's interest, because it will avoid interventions that are potentially harmful, such as platelet transfusions. In addition, genetic counseling is suggested for couples in which both mother and father are affected, because of the possibility of having a child with Bernard–Soulier syndrome.

MACROTHROMBOCYTOPENIA ASSOCIATED WITH VELOCARDIOFACIAL SYNDROME (OMIM 192430) AND DIGEORGE SYNDROME (OMIM 188400)

Patients with the velocardiofacial and DiGeorge syndromes have a host of congenital abnormalities affecting their skeletal, cardiac, endocrine, neurologic, and immune systems.[70,71] Collectively, these disorders are known by the acronym CATCH22 (*c*ardiac *a*bnormality, *T*-cell deficit, *c*left palate, *h*ypocalcemia due to a chromosome *22* deletion).[4,72,73] Mild thrombocytopenia, unassociated with a bleeding diathesis, is frequently observed in affected individuals. Similar to Mediterranean macrothrombocytopenia, the platelet abnormality found in these conditions appears to be due to a deletion in one of the four genes that comprise the von Willebrand receptor locus (*GP1BA*, *GP1BB*, *GP5*, and *GP9*) on chromosome 22q11.[74] Whereas *GP1BA* is affected in the Mediterranean variant, in these cases *GP1BB* is deleted.[74] As of today, thrombocytopenias due to deletions or mutations of *GP5* and *GP9* have not been described; it is possible that mutations in one or both of the other two genes will be identified, causing similar disorders (ie, *GP9* and *GP5*). No therapy is necessary for the thrombocytopenias seen in these patients. Genetic counseling considerations are the same as those for patients with Mediterranean macrothrombocytopenia.

FAMILIAL PLATELET DISORDER WITH ASSOCIATED MYELOID MALIGNANCY (OMIM 601399)

The autosomal dominant thrombocytopenia known as familial platelet disorder with associated myeloid malignancy was first described in 1985.[47,74] Its genetic basis has only recently been deciphered.[75] Patients with this disorder have mild to moderate thrombocytopenia. The platelets appear normal morphologically, but an aspirin-like aggregation defect has been documented, and bleeding times are prolonged. Linkage analysis narrowed the defect to an interval on human chromosome 21q22.1–22.2.22 which greatly assisted in identification of the responsible genetic abnormality; a gene identified as *AML1*, now known as *CBFA2*.[75] *CBFA2* is a hematopoietic transcription factor that plays an important role in regulating cell development. Nonsense mutations, or an intragenic deletion of one *CBFA2* allele, are now known to be responsible for the condition. It is of interest that in mice, similar lesions of *CBFA2* cause a more global disruption of hematopoiesis.[76,77] In humans, the numbers of assayable CFU-MK are diminished, but not the progenitors of other lineages.[75] Why the defect results only in thrombocytopenia in humans is not certain. It is also unclear why these defects predispose patients to developing acute myeloid leukemia.[78] Bleeding in these patients can be treated in the usual manner, but the high likelihood of leukemic transformation has led some investigators to suggest that these patients should undergo bone marrow transplantation.[42] This could be problematic in an affected family because, if unrecognized, a sibling HLA-matched donor might transmit the disease again. At least one case has been reported of a transplant from a sibling in which the donor and recipient subsequently developed donor-derived leukemia.[79]

PARIS–TROUSSEAU SYNDROME (OMIM 188025) AND JACOBSEN SYNDROME (OMIM 147791) MACROTHROMBOCYTOPENIA

The autosomal dominant macrothrombocytopenias Paris–Trousseau and Jacobsen syndromes are associated with deletions of the distal portion of chromosome 11,11q23–24.[78–82] In children with Jacobsen syndrome, in addition to the platelet abnormalities, psychomotor retardation and facial and cardiac abnormalities are also seen.[79] Affected individuals have only a mild bleeding diathesis. Platelets in patients with this disorder are larger than normal and are characterized by giant granules that stain red with Giemsa. Megakaryocytes are increased in the marrow but are dysplastic; micromegakaryocytes with small hypolobulated nuclei are present.[78,81] It is believed that the paucity of larger, more mature cells is due to their spontaneous lysis. Mutations of the Ets family transcription factor gene, *FLI1*, have been implicated in the etiology of Paris–Trousseau thrombocytopenia. This association has been made because of morphologic similarities observed in the megakaryocytes of mouse embryos in which *fli1* has been genetically deleted,[78] and because the *FLI1* gene has been mapped to the region deleted in Paris–Trousseau and Jacobsen syndrome thrombocytopenia. Very recently, Wenger and colleagues reported a female patient with an approximately 10 Mb interstitial deletion involving chromosome 11 and with many of the features of Jacobsen syndrome.[83] The karyotype of the patient was 46,XX,del(1 1)(q24.1q24.3). The interstitial deletion was found to be in the distal portion of 11q, and included FLI-1 but not JAM-3, a finding that should assist in determining the critical genes involved in these syndromes.

GRAY PLATELET SYNDROME (OMIM 139090)

The gray platelet syndrome is a rare congenital bleeding disorder in which thrombocytopenia is associated with increased platelet size and decreased α-granule content.[79,84,85] It is the latter phenomenon that causes the platelets to appear gray after histochemical staining. The decrease in granule content is not due to an inability to synthesize the granule proteins but rather to an inability to transport and incorporate the proteins into the α granules.[86–88] Examination of patient blood smears will reveal not only gray platelets but also gray polymorphonuclear neutrophils.[89] The granules of the polymorphonuclear neutrophils have decreased or abnormally distributed secretory constituents in a manner analogous to that seen in the platelets. Secondary granules in polymorphonuclear neutrophils are also decreased in number, as assayed by immunoelectron microscopy. Although many affected families demonstrate clear autosomal dominant inheritance, several reports have documented affected children born of apparently healthy parents. Accordingly, a recessive form of this disorder may also exist.[89] The bleeding tendency in this syndrome generally varies from mild to moderate, and no specific treatment is usually needed.[84,90]

Sex-linked forms of gray platelet syndrome have also very recently been recognized by Tubman et al, who identified a family with gray platelet syndrome that segregated as a sex-linked trait.[91] Affected males had a mild bleeding disorder, thrombocytopenia, and large agranular platelets characteristic of the gray platelet syndrome. Obligate female carriers were asymptomatic but had dimorphic platelets on peripheral smear. Associated findings included mild erythrocyte abnormalities in affected males. Linkage analysis revealed a 63 cM region on the X chromosome between markers G10578 and DXS6797 which segregated with the platelet phenotype and included the GATA1 gene. Sequencing of GATA1 revealed a G-to-A mutation at position 759 corresponding to amino acid change Arg216Gln. Interestingly, this mutation has been previously described as a cause of X-linked thrombocytopenia with thalassemia (XLTT) but not of gray platelet syndrome. These investigators hypothesized that XLTT is within a spectrum of disorders constituting the gray platelet syndrome, and further proposed that GATA1 is an upstream regulator of the genes required for platelet α-granule biogenesis. Other formes frustes of this disease have also been reported.[92–94]

AUTOSOMAL RECESSIVE THROMBOCYTOPENIAS

Congenital Amegakaryocytic Thrombocytopenia (OMIM 604498)

Profound thrombocytopenia in an otherwise well newborn (<10,000 platelets/L) should always raise the question of whether the baby has congenital amegakaryocytic thrombocytopenic purpura (CAMT).[95–97] The diagnosis is first entertained when an apparently well newborn develops easy bruising or bleeding soon after birth. Milder forms are sometimes discovered in the course of routine screening examinations. As with any recessive disorder, neither parent will have an abnormality of platelet count or function, and the family history is likely to be negative as well. A bone marrow examination will reveal markedly diminished or absent megakaryocytes. CAMT is a progressive disorder, so even children with milder forms will develop worsening thrombocytopenia, as well as leukopenia and anemia, toward the end of the first decade of life. By the second decade, pancytopenia is likely to have developed. Other marrow failure syndromes, such as Fanconi anemia, aplastic anemia, or dyskeratosis congenita might be confused with CAMT.

The differential diagnosis for severe congenital thrombocytopenia includes thrombocytopenia with absent radii syndrome (TAR)[98] and Wiskott–Aldrich syndrome (WAS). These conditions can often be distinguished from CAMT on the basis of associated skeletal hypoplasia of the arms, in the case of TAR, and microthrombocytes, in the case of WAS. Neonatal alloimmune thrombocytopenia, which may present with profound thrombocytopenia due to the transfer of maternally derived antiplatelet antibodies at the time of delivery, should also be included in the differential diagnosis.[9] Neonatal alloimmune thrombocytopenia is most often due to the maternal absence of an epitope on GPIIIA (PlA1).[99] Typically, alloimmune thrombocytopenias are self-limited and resolve as the maternal antibodies degrade. In addition, these children will have normal numbers of megakaryocytes in their bone marrows.

The molecular lesions responsible for CAMT have been identified as composite mutations affecting both alleles of the thrombopoietin receptor gene, c-*MPL* (chromosome 1p34).[100–103] HOXA11 mutations have also recently been described.[104] The definitive diagnosis of CAMT is based on identification of one of these mutations. Many *MPL* mutations have been described in CAMT patients. New mutations are recognized with some frequency.[105] They are located in exons 2, 3, 4, 5, 6, 10, and 12 and a splice-junction mutation of intron 10. Some of these mutations, such as nonsense or frameshift types, will completely abrogate receptor function. Single amino acid substitutions may allow some receptor function to remain. The severity of the disease correlates directly with the degree of receptor impairment. The evolution of CAMT into complete marrow failure can be explained by the recognition that, in addition to being required for megakaryocyte maturation, thrombopoietin, and of course its receptor, are required for maintenance of the stem cell compartment.[9,106] Accordingly, even milder forms of CAMT will evolve, because minimal MpL function is apparently insufficient to maintain the integrity of the stem cell compartment.[9]

Treatment options for children with CAMT are limited. For acute bleeding episodes, platelet transfusions are indicated and effective. Over time, however, platelet alloimmunization is likely to be a problem. For this reason, and because this is ultimately a disease of stem cells, allogeneic stem cell transplantation is the only potentially curative, long-term solution.[107] The disease would clearly be a good candidate for genetic therapies that would either replace or correct the defective gene.

Thrombocytopenia With Absent RADII Syndrome (OMIM 274000)

Thrombocytopenia with absent radii (TAR) syndrome is typically an autosomal recessive disorder, though other forms of transmission have been recorded, including dominant transmission from an affected parent to offspring (Chapter 28).[108,109] In one recent report, all of 30 patients examined manifested a common interstitial microdeletion of 200 kb on chromosome 1q21.1, which was detected using microarray-based comparative genomic hybridization. Analysis of the parents revealed that the deletion occurred de novo in 25% of affected individuals. Inheritance of the deletion along the maternal as well as the paternal line was also observed. Because the deletion was not detected in a cohort of control individuals, it was argued that this microdeletion could play an important role in the pathogenesis of TAR syndrome. It was further hypothesized that TAR syndrome is not only associated with a deletion on chromosome 1q21.1 but that the phenotype develops only in the presence of an additional, as-yet-unknown modifier (mTAR).[110]

Patients typically are of short stature, but the syndrome's most striking physical manifestation is a pathognomonic absence of radii with intact thumbs (Fig. 32–6). In affected individuals, muscles that normally attach to the radius are inserted instead onto the carpal bones of the hands. Other skeletal malformations, including absence or malformation of the ulnar bones and abnormalities of the humerus, shoulder joint, and lower extremities, are also frequent. Cardiac malformations, in particular the tetralogy of Fallot and atrial septal defects, occur in one-third of patients. Mental retardation has also been reported in approximately 7% of affected individuals, presumably on the basis of cerebral hemorrhage. Single case reports of TAR-associated hypoplasia of the cerebellum, horseshoe kidney, and both of the abnormalities have been reported.[111] Symptomatic milk allergy has been observed frequently and may cause severe bloody diarrhea.[112]

Thrombocytopenia of TAR patients is most severe perinatally, with counts ranging from 15,000 to 30,000/mm^3. The low platelet counts may be further exacerbated by any significant intercurrent stress, including infection, surgery, or even the gastrointestinal disturbances that accompany milk allergies. Such episodes are often accompanied by a myeloid leukemoid reaction. Eosinophilia is noted in approximately 50% of patients and is particularly common, not surprisingly, in patients with milk allergies. Anemia related to bleeding, or hemolysis, is typical in the first year of life. Interestingly, the thrombocytopenia improves with age, so that children who survive the first year or two of life are believed to have normal life spans.[109,113]

A bone marrow aspirate will show decreased or absent megakaryocytes. Those megakaryocytes that are present are often small, basophilic, and vacuolated. Erythroid hyperplasia is sometimes observed, presumably in anemic patients. Recent studies on the megakaryocyte progenitor cell compartment and c-*MPL* expression in six patients have found CFU-MK numbers to be markedly reduced and very primitive progenitor cells to have increased, suggesting an inability

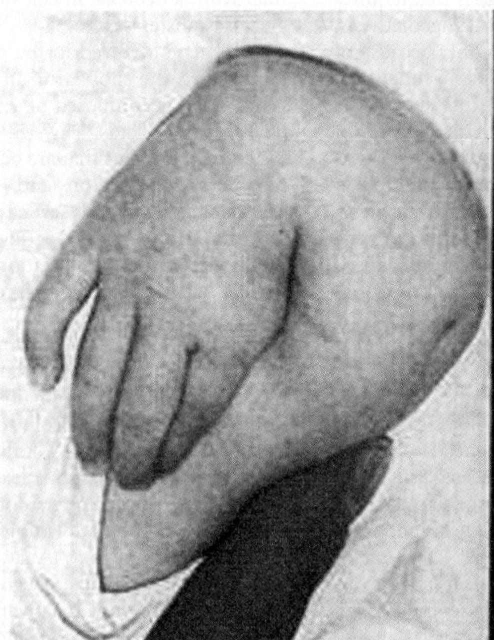

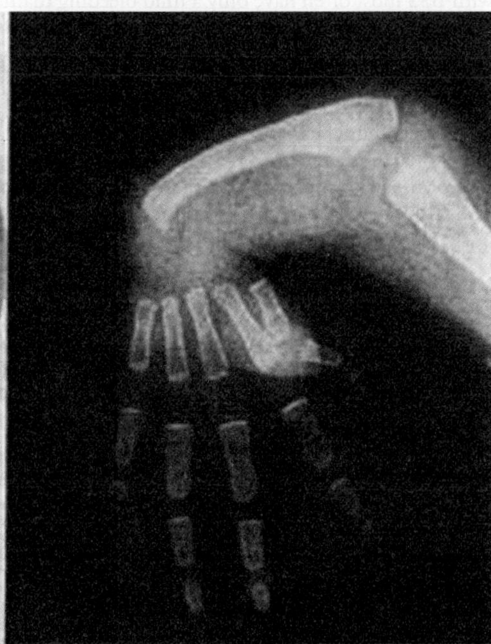

Figure 32–6 Thrombocytopenia with absent radii syndrome. *Left*, A typical upper extremity deformity. *Right*, Radiograph showing complete absence of the radius. *(Adapted from Hoffbrand A, Pettit J: Sandoz Atlas of Clinical Hematology. London, Gower Medical, 1988.)*

of primitive cells to differentiate into the megakaryocyte lineage.[114] This was found not to be secondary to c-*MPL* genetic abnormalities in any of the patients, as no mutation or rearrangement in the c-*MPL* gene, or its promoter, was found by Southern blotting or gene sequencing. Western blot and RNA analyses revealed decreased levels of *MPL* RNA and protein in the platelets of these same patients compared with normal control subjects, but other studies have found normal *MPL* receptor level expression and structure in TAR patients.[115] Abnormalities in thrombopoietin signaling in TAR patients have been suggested.[115]

The molecular cause of TAR remains unknown, as does the link between osteodysgenesis and thrombocytopenia. Recently, however, an intriguing link between these two seemingly disparate abnormalities was uncovered. The homeobox (HOX) transcription factors have long been considered candidate genes for TAR syndrome because of their well-established function in limb development.[116] In support of the possible involvement of the *HOX* genes, two families were recently reported with radial-ulnar synostosis and amegakaryocytic thrombocytopenia (OMIM 605432) caused by a mutation of the *HOXA11* gene.[98] However, the autosomal dominant inheritance pattern, mild forearm deformities of the patients, and persistence of severe thrombocytopenia all distinguished this condition from a typical TAR syndrome.[98] Complete sequencing of the coding regions of *HOXA10*, *HOXA11*, and *HOXD11* failed to detect any abnormalities in ten individuals with TAR syndrome.[117]

The diagnosis of TAR is suspected when the typical skeletal malformations are encountered. Prenatal diagnosis is possible using ultrasonography, skeletal radiography, and fetal blood sampling.[115,118] TAR is distinguished from Fanconi syndrome by the presence of the thumbs and by the lack of genetic instability. There is no specific treatment for TAR except for platelet transfusions when necessary. Steroids, splenectomy, or intravenous IgG treatments are usually ineffective.[113,119] Orthopedic surgery to correct skeletal defects is best postponed during the first few years of life. On rare occasions, thrombocytopenia may first manifest itself in adulthood. Splenectomy has been reported to be useful under such circumstances.[120] In the unusual case in which the disease does not remit, stem cell transplantation may be considered for children who suffer from recurrent significant bleeding episodes.[121]

Bernard–Soulier Syndrome (OMIM 231200)

Bernard–Soulier syndrome (BSS) is characterized by mild to moderate, though occasionally severe, macrothrombocytopenia. Patients with BSS most often have only a mild bleeding diathesis that requires no treatment.[122] Others may have a significant bleeding diathesis, often out of proportion to the thrombocytopenia alone, because of the functional defects displayed by BSS platelets.[119] The functional defect of BSS platelets is due to decreased or absent expression of the von Willebrand factor (vWF) receptor.[123] WF receptor consists of four polypeptide chains: GP1b-a, GP1b-b, GPV, and GPIX. Mutation of the gene encoding GP1b-a (*GP1BA*) is the most common in BSS. Mutant GP1b-b has also been reported.[74,124] Recently, a previously reported A-to-G mutation in nucleotide 1826 of the *GPIX* gene was found in several German patients who had been misdiagnosed with ITP. This mutation results in an Asn-to-Ser substitution. Because this mutation had been described previously, it is now the most commonly identified molecular defect causing BSS in Caucasian subjects.[125]

Why a seemingly isolated defect in the vWF receptor would lead to macrothrombocytopenia remains unclear. Although shortened platelet survival has also been reported in BSS patients,[126,127] many others are reported to have normal platelet survival, suggesting that production defects contribute to the thrombocytopenia in some patients. A candidate mechanism for disordered thrombopoiesis would be dysfunctional internal membrane formation.[128] The role of this abnormality in causing large platelets is uncertain. It is also conceivable that deficiencies or mutations of the GPIb-IX complex may be important in the formation of platelet territories.[129]

The presence of large platelets in decreased numbers may at times suggest a diagnosis of ITP. In patients who bleed out of proportion to their thrombocytopenia, or who do not respond to the usual ITP treatments, platelet function studies will suggest the correct diagnosis. Significant bleeding is usually managed by platelet transfusions, but success with the use of recombinant factor VIIa has also been reported.[130] For particularly difficult cases, with severe recurrent bleeding, hematopoietic stem cell transplantation has also been employed.[131]

X-LINKED DISORDERS

Wiskott–Aldrich Syndrome and X-Linked Thrombocytopenia (OMIM 301000 and 313900)

The Wiskott–Aldrich syndrome is a rare X-linked disorder characterized by microthrombocytopenia, immunodeficiency, and eczema.[132,133] The platelets of WAS patients, and those with related disorders, are reduced in number and size. Typically, platelet counts are in the 5000 to 50,000 μL range, with a volume approximately 50% that of normal platelets (MPV 3.5–5.0 fL). It has been estimated that the combined reduction in platelet volume and number results in an effective platelet mass approximately 1% of that found in normal individuals. Biochemical abnormalities are also present that variably compromise platelet function.[134–137] An abnormality of GPIb, for example, has been observed in some, but not all, patients.[138,139] The protease calpain is reduced in the platelets of WAS patients relative to normal subjects as well, although, interestingly, calpain levels are normal in affected lymphocytes.[140] It has been speculated that decreased platelet calpain leads to inappropriate platelet stimulation and subsequent increased clearance from the circulation.[132] WAS patients will have a rise in their platelet counts after a splenectomy. Nevertheless, whereas platelet survival time is approximately half of normal,[141] this finding has proved insufficient to explain the degree of thrombocytopenia seen in all patients. In this regard, platelet turnover has been estimated to be approximately 25% of normal, and the mass of megakaryocyte cytoplasm has been found to be normal.[142] Therefore, ineffective platelet production also makes an important contribution to the thrombocytopenia observed in WAS patients.[136] The immune defects are due to dysfunctional T lymphocytes. The T cells of WAS patients manifest decreased responsiveness to mitogenic stimuli. Ultrastructural and biochemical defects have been noted in the T cells of WAS patients, including a decrease in the surface microvilli, a decrease in cell surface sialoglycoproteins, and abnormal glycosyltransferases.[133,143]

The gene involved in the pathogenesis of the syndrome has been localized to the short arm of the X chromosome (Xp11.22).[144] The gene, *WAS*, is composed of 12 exons and encodes a protein (WASP) of 502 amino acids.[145] WASP (WAS protein) contains a number of functional domains that are believed to provide a critical link between the cell's cytoskeleton and signal transduction pathways.[146] For example, WASP and several related proteins are involved in the reorganization of the actin cytoskeleton by activating Arp2/3-mediated actin polymerization.[147] This function is controlled by the small GTPase Cdc42, which regulates the autoinhibitory loop formation of WASP. In addition, WASP is involved in cytoplasmic signaling through its interaction with a variety of adaptor molecules. There are src homology 3 (SH3) domains for interacting with GTPases, the Pleckstrin homology domain for membrane phospholipid interactions, Cofilin and Verprolin domains for polarized cytoskeletal elements, and the unique WASP-interacting protein.[148]

How WASP mutations lead to the development of microthrombocytes is still not understood. Megakaryocytes from patients with WAS are capable of forming proplatelet processes and platelets of normal sizes in vitro.[149] Analysis of the X-chromosome inactivation pattern in female heterozygotes (who have no abnormalities) has revealed nonrandom inactivation of WASP in multiple hematopoietic lineages, including $CD34^+$ progenitors, suggesting that WASP plays a crucial function in hematopoietic cell development.[150] Quite recently, Sabri and colleagues have reported mechanistic studies that might shed light on this phenomenon. Using a murine model, these workers identified a critical role for WASP during murine platelet biogenesis. By electron microscopy, WASP-deficient MKs appeared to have shed platelets ectopically within the bone marrow space. WASP-deficient megakaryocytes (MKs) also displayed defects in response to fibrillar collagen I in vitro, the major matrix component of bone. These included a loss of normal $\alpha_2\beta_1$ integrin-mediated inhibition of proplatelet formation, a marked abrogation of SDF-1-induced chemotactic migration of $CD41^+$ MKs adherent to fibrillar collagen I, and an almost complete lack of actin-rich podosomes, normally induced by interaction between fibrillar collagen I and its receptors GPVI or $\alpha_2\beta_1$ integrin. On the basis of these results, these investigators postulated that WASP plays an important role in platelet biogenesis, at least in mice, and might also be important in explaining the platelet abnormalities characteristic of patients with WAS.[151] In addition to these studies, it has also been reported that gene silencing-induced loss of PIP4Kα impaired demarcation membrane system development, actin fiber assembly, as well as enlargement of megakaryocyte size. On this basis, they suggested that a perturbation of the signaling pathway employing PI-4,5-P(2) might contribute to the abnormal platelets found in Wiskott–Aldrich syndromes.[20]

There are a variety of mutations involving the WASP gene, leading to either absent or mutated protein.[141,142,144,145,152] To a large extent, the phenotypic variation of WAS can be explained by the location and nature of the genetic mutations.[153] Frameshifts, nonsense mutations, and large deletions generally cause classic WAS, whereas single amino acid substitutions, especially of exons 1 to 3, cause the milder X-linked thrombocytopenia. When WASP is completely absent, the disease is more severe likely for the reasons just discussed above. When WASP is present at even low-moderate levels, the disease is frequently milder.[153]

The diagnosis of WAS should be considered in any male child with thrombocytopenia and immunodeficiency.[133] Classic WAS is usually recognized in the first year of life as a result of the affected child's hemorrhagic tendencies, typified by easy bruising, epistaxis, bloody diarrhea, and even intracranial hemorrhage. Intercurrent infections, usually bacterial in origin, are also typical. The classic triad of infections, thrombocytopenia, and eczema is only seen in approximately 25% of patients at diagnosis, perhaps because infections and eczema, unlike the thrombocytopenia, are not present at birth. The latter are usually problematic after the first 6 to 12 months of life.[154] One-third of cases have no family history. In such instances, it has been suggested that confirmatory sequencing of the *WAS* gene be carried out.[42] Beyond the complications of infections and bleeding, there is a significant risk of the development of a malignancy. These are most often lymphoid, and patients with autoimmune manifestations of this disease are at highest risk.[154] Acute myeloid leukemia may also complicate this syndrome, as well as other malignancies that are not hematopoietic in origin.[155] Enlarged lymph nodes and hepatosplenomegaly resulting from lymphoid hyperplasia occur commonly and must be distinguished from the development of a lymphoid malignancy. Fifty percent of the deaths associated with this syndrome are infectious, 25% related to hemorrhage, and 5% related to malignancy.[156] Life expectancy is usually less than 10 years.

The thrombocytopenia of WAS has been reported to respond to anti-CD20 monoclonal antibody treatment, though relapse rates were as high as 80%. For that reason, multiple treatment courses would likely be required.[157] Such treatments will not prevent the development of leukemia or other marrow failure syndromes. Accordingly, as with many disorders affecting stem cells, hematopoietic stem cell transplantation, either in the form of an HLA-matched marrow or cord blood donor is probably the most effective treatment for WAS.[146,158–161] Corticosteroids are not indicated, because they do not ameliorate the thrombocytopenia and only contribute to the propensity for infection. Some recent studies suggest that patients who exhibit significant bleeding may benefit from splenectomy.[158,162–164] Median survival times in 39 untransplanted, splenectomized patients have been reported to be 25 years, but many patients are now living into their third and fourth decades, thanks primarily to advances in support therapy, in particular antibiotics and intravenous gamma globulin.[158,162]

Wiskott–Aldrich Syndrome Variants and Other X-Linked Recessive Thrombocytopenias

Girls have occasionally been noted to have microthrombocytes, with or without other components of WAS.[165] In one such patient, a spontaneous mutation in one *WAS* allele, coupled with skewed X inactivation among hematopoietic cells, was shown to be responsible.[166] However, in other families more than one female has been affected, and no *WAS* gene mutations could be found.[167] A mutation in a gene that encodes a WASP interacting protein might conceivably cause a similar disease phenotype.

A number of families with an isolated X-linked thrombocytopenia, or with a WAS-like condition consisting of variable immune deficiencies and eczema, have been described.[168,169] Family studies of patients with WAS-like disorders have suggested both autosomal recessive and autosomal dominant modes of inheritance.[165,167] The thrombocytopenia usually is mild in these families, and most cases have been discovered incidentally. Marrow megakaryocytes are normal or increased.[149,170,171] As noted earlier, in those few patients in whom thrombocytopenia was severe and bleeding was a significant clinical issue, splenectomy was found to be useful. Because it is now felt that WAS and, aside from the rare exceptions noted earlier, most of the X-linked isolated thrombocytopenias are caused by *WAS* mutations, sequencing of the gene should prove a reliable molecular diagnostic tool. At institutions where such molecular diagnostics are not available, a diminished lymphocyte mitogenic response to periodate may be useful as a diagnostic test, because WAS variants as well as classic WAS have such defects in lymphocyte function.[172] This fact could also prove useful for distinguishing variant WAS from other congenital thrombocytopenias.

GATA1 Mutation: A Recently Recognized X-Linked Thrombocytopenia (OMIM 305371)

A thrombocytopenic disorder accompanied by mild to moderate dyserythropoiesis and an X-linked pattern of inheritance was recently described in five separate families.[173–177] This disorder was distinguishable from WAS by the fact that the platelets were of normal to large size, and none of the affected individuals developed eczema, immunodeficiency, hematologic malignancies, or aplastic anemia over time. The degree of thrombocytopenia was moderate to severe (10,000–40,000/L) and platelet function defects were detectable.[174] The associated bleeding diathesis was often severe. In contrast, the anemia was of variable severity. The bone marrow of these individuals was typically hypercellular, with dysplastic erythropoiesis and megakaryopoiesis.[176]

Mutations in the *GATA1* gene, which encodes a transcription factor required for normal megakaryocyte and erythroid development, has been found in each of the five families. The mutations are clustered in the highly conserved N-zinc finger domain. They result in single amino acid substitutions at four positions (Val205Met,[65] Gly208Ser,[68] Arg216Gly,[69] Asp218Gly,[66] and Asp218Tyr[69]). Four of these mutations disrupt the ability of *GATA1* to associate with a known cofactor, *FOG1* (friend of *GATA1*).[178,179] Interestingly, the severity of the thrombocytopenia correlates with the degree to which the *GATA1–FOG1* interaction is impaired.[166,174,176] In contrast, Arg216Gly results in impaired binding of *GATA1* to palindromic DNA-binding sites.[177] This mutation also causes a moderate globin chain imbalance (thalassemia).[180] *FOG1* gene mutations, which would be expected to yield a similar clinical phenotype, have yet to be described. More disruptive *GATA1* mutations are unlikely to be compatible with survival of the embryo, because the gene is required for normal hematopoietic cell development.

GATA1 mutations should now be suspected in male children with severe thrombocytopenia, normal to large platelets, and absence of immunodeficiency and eczema. Mild anemia and a hypercellular bone marrow with dyserythropoiesis and megakaryocytopoiesis are supportive of the diagnosis as well. *GATA1* gene sequencing, available only in a specialized reference laboratory, would be required to confirm this diagnosis. Bleeding episodes in these patients can be treated with platelet transfusions, which, for reasons already discussed, should be kept to the minimum necessary to control this problem. If life-threatening thrombocytopenia or anemia intervenes, stem cell transplantation is a potentially curative option. The development of an effective gene therapy, though likely a long way off, would be a very acceptable alternative to hematopoietic stem cell transplant.

ACQUIRED THROMBOCYTOPENIAS DUE TO INEFFECTIVE THROMBOPOIESIS

As is true for the congenital thrombocytopenias, acquired thrombocytopenia can be caused by a failure of either megakaryocytopoiesis or thrombopoiesis. Of these two possibilities, ineffective thrombopoiesis is the more likely cause, as pure megakaryocyte aplasia or hypoplasia is quite rare. Indeed, thrombocytopenia secondary to decreased marrow megakaryocytes is much more likely to be a prodrome of aplastic anemia, or an early myelodysplastic syndrome. Clues to these conditions can be found in the marrow, where often subtle abnormalities of other hematopoietic lineages, such as macrocytosis or dyserythropoiesis, can be observed.[181]

SELECTIVE MEGAKARYOCYTE APLASIA

Acquired selective amegakaryocytic thrombocytopenia is quite rare. It is almost always due to an autoimmune mechanism, either antibody or cell mediated. Autoantibodies reacting with megakaryocytes or their progenitor cells, presumably leading to their destruction, have been described.[182] Antibodies directed to cytokines that regulate megakaryocyte development, in particular thrombopoietin, might also play a role in the biogenesis of such disorders. An unusual case of cyclic amegakaryocytic thrombocytopenia due to an antibody to granulocyte–macrophage colony-stimulating factor (GM-CSF) was documented in one patient. Cases of cell-mediated suppression of megakaryocytopoiesis leading to a complete selective megakaryocyte aplasia have also been described.[183] In these cases, suppression was shown in one case to be due to autoreactive T lymphocytes, whereas a macrophage-derived "factor" was implicated in the other. In the latter case, suppression was shown to be specific for megakaryocytes, because no significant effect on blast-forming units–erythrocyte (BFU-E) or colony-forming units–erythrocyte (CFU-E) derived colony formation by autologous marrow mononuclear cells was reported.

Patients in whom an autoimmune mechanism is operative may respond to treatment with cyclosporine and antithymocyte globulin, achieving durable remissions.[184] Cytotoxic antibodies directed toward the CFU-MK may be treated with corticosteroids, plasmapheresis, intravenous IgG, danazol, cyclosporine, or cyclophosphamide.[185] In a patient in whom an IgG antibody was found to be blocking GM-CSF action, a complete response to cyclophosphamide was observed.[186] Patients with T-cell–mediated inhibition of megakaryocytopoiesis may respond to antithymocyte globulin, cyclosporine, or hematopoietic growth factors.[185] If a particular drug or toxin exposure is believed to be responsible, for example ethanol or a thiazide diuretic, then withdrawal of the offending agent is obviously indicated. If the cause is viral, intravenous IgG or anti-human immunodeficiency virus (HIV) therapies are indicated.[185] Despite the various etiologies of ineffective thrombopoiesis, immunosuppressive therapy was found to be effective in 8 of 30 patients in one series.[187] Therefore, although worth trying, most patients do not respond to this form of therapy, and for these individuals, hematopoietic stem cell transfer remains an option. Treatment with intensive immunosuppressive therapy may not prevent progression to aplastic anemia.[188]

INFECTION

Many infectious diseases are associated with thrombocytopenia, and it is likely that infection is the greatest noniatrogenic cause of ineffective platelet production.[189] Infectious agents associated with decreased platelet counts include mycoplasma,[107] mycobacteria,[190] ehrlichiosis,[191] and malaria.[192] In these disorders, the cause of the thrombocytopenia is believed to be diminished platelet production,[193] although immune-mediated thrombocytopenia has also been described in some patients.[190]

Viral infections are by far the most common infectious agents associated with thrombocytopenia due to ineffective megakaryocyte or platelet production. Thrombocytopenia has been reported in cases of mumps, rubella, measles, varicella, cytomegalovirus, infectious mononucleosis, chickenpox, dengue and other hemorrhagic fevers, hepatitis, and parvovirus infections.[180,194–196] Live measles virus vaccination can also induce thrombocytopenia due to decreased production.[197] The mechanism responsible for viral suppression of platelet counts is not completely clear. It is known that megakaryocytes are capable of being infected by a variety of viruses. Infected cells may appear dysplastic, with inclusion bodies, vacuoles, or degenerating nuclei. Naked megakaryocyte nuclei may be seen in particular after HIV infection.[193] That such cytopathic cells might have trouble producing platelets is not difficult to imagine.

Perhaps the best studied virally induced thrombocytopenia is that associated with HIV infection.[198] Mild to moderate reduction in platelet counts are quite common in patients with this disease. In a large study (738 patients) of HIV-positive patients with hemophilia, the cumulative frequency of thrombocytopenia 6 years after seroconversion was 16% for children and 18% for adults. At 10 years, the frequency increased to 27% in children and 43% in adults.[199] In another study, the frequency of thrombocytopenia was 16% among 103 homosexual men and 37% among 182 intravenous drug users with a new diagnosis of HIV infection.[200] Thrombocytopenia was also reported to be relatively common in HIV-negative homosexual men (3%) and intravenous drug users (9%). It was speculated that this might be due to the high rates of hepatitis in these patient groups.[200] Except for patients who acquire HIV in the background of hemophilia, bleeding secondary to thrombocytopenia is unusual, as the counts are rarely less than 50,000/µL. Thrombocytopenia may precede frank immunodeficiency, but does correlate with viral load and depletion of the CD4 T-cell population.[185,201]

The principal cause of thrombocytopenia appears to vary with the stage of disease. A retrospective study of 85 patients with HIV and thrombocytopenia suggested that in the early stages of infection, platelet destruction is predominant, whereas in patients with full-blown acquired immunodeficiency syndrome, thrombocytopenia is more often due to a production defect.[202,203] Thrombocytopenia due to platelet production abnormalities may be related directly to an HIV infection, to adverse effects of drug therapy, or to secondary malignancy or myelodysplasia. Platelet kinetic studies have shown that patients infected with HIV have a moderate reduction in platelet survival, but all have decreased platelet production regardless of the degree of thrombocytopenia.[202,204] On the basis of the finding of HIV mRNA and p24 antigen in megakaryocytic cytoplasm, HIV has been shown to infect megakaryocytes directly, as evidenced by finding HIV mRNA and p24 antigen in megakaryocyte cytoplasm.[205–207] The portal of entry might be through megakaryocyte surface CD4,[208,209] but more recent studies suggest that CXCR4, which is expressed on megakaryocytes[210] and is a critical coreceptor for viral uptake, is more likely involved.[211] In these studies, infection with HIV-1 Env-pseudotyped luciferase reporter viruses indicated that X4 Env

Table 32–3 Infiltrative Marrow Disorders Associated With Thrombocytopenia

1. Metastatic cancer	6. Gaucher disease
2. Leukemia	7. Osteopetrosis
3. Lymphoma	8. Histiocytosis
4. Myeloma	9. Infectious processes
5. Myelofibrosis	

(CXCR4-using) pseudotypes infected megakaryocytic cells whereas R5 Env (CCR5-using) pseudotypes did not.

Examination of a bone marrow aspirate and biopsy specimens may be required to assess whether infiltration by granulomatous infection or a malignancy is contributing to, or causing, the thrombocytopenia in an HIV patient (Table 32–3). Assuming no other obvious cause of the thrombocytopenia, and the presence of typical megakaryocytic morphologic abnormalities, antiretroviral therapy is the principal treatment. Zidovudine was the mainstay in the past,[201] but current combination antiretroviral regimens will likely be more effective in increasing platelet counts as well as enhancing CD4 cell counts and reducing HIV viral loads.[197,212,213] For patients with severe and/or symptomatic thrombocytopenia, ITP regimens may well be effective. These include prednisone (1 mg/kg per day) or short courses of dexamethasone.[198] IVIgG may be effective in low weekly doses (0.04 g/kg per week),[214] and anti-D has been used extensively in these patients.[198] Splenectomy is quite effective therapy when the above therapies are either ineffective or contraindicated, and it appears to have no adverse effect on HIV progression.[215]

CHEMOTHERAPY AND IRRADIATION

Chemotherapy and irradiation reliably damage bone marrow in a dose-dependent fashion. Megakaryocytes and their progenitors seem to be particularly sensitive to the effects of these agents. As a result, thrombocytopenia is one of the most frequent adverse effects of total body irradiation[216] and chemotherapy. Allogeneic or autologous marrow transplantation is often complicated by prolonged thrombocytopenia, which may persist long after restoration of neutrophil and red blood cell counts. Transplantation of umbilical cord stem cells is also associated with delayed platelet recovery. In one study of 39 pediatric patients receiving such transplants, the median time to platelet count recovery was 49 days (range, 15–117 days).[217] The explanation for the tardiness of platelet recovery in these instances is not always clear, but ineffective thrombopoiesis has been shown to be important in at least some cases.[218] Various strategies to ameliorate this problem have been tried, including the use of peripheral blood "stem cells," which may lead to a faster rate of platelet recovery when compared with marrow transplantation. More recently, attempts have been made to expand megakaryocyte progenitor cells, either with a recombinant form of thrombopoietin[219] or other cytokines.[220] The clinical utility of this approach, or the simple administration of recombinant thrombopoietin after transplantation, remains uncertain[221] but might eventually prove useful.[222] Accordingly, posttransplantation thrombocytopenia remains a problem.[223]

Isolated thrombocytopenia with decreased megakaryocytes has been reported after chemotherapy for acute myeloid leukemia. Cyclosporine was reported to augment the platelet count in such patients.[224] Recombinant thrombopoietin has not been shown to be useful in this setting and appears to induce marrow changes suggestive of a myeloproliferative disorder, which is reversed when the thrombopoietin is discontinued.[225]

Alkylating agents in general produce more prolonged thrombocytopenia than antimetabolites. It has been claimed that some alkylating agents spare megakaryocytes (eg, cyclophosphamide), but this is a relative phenomenon. Agents such as busulfan, the nitrosoureas, or platinum may cause cumulative damage of the more primitive progenitor cells. Other chemotherapeutic agents, such as the vinca alkaloids, may not decrease the platelet count significantly.

Potential mechanisms for the relative sparing of platelets production by certain chemotherapeutic regimens have been investigated.[226] In one study, for example, potential platelet sparing mechanisms of chemotherapy regimens containing paclitaxel and carboplatin has been explored by examining (a) normal donor and chemotherapy patient-derived erythroid (BFU-E), myeloid (CFU-GM), and megakaryocyte (CFU-MK) progenitor cell proliferation in vitro; (b) P-glycoprotein protein and glutathione *S*-transferase (GST) messenger RNA expression; (c) serum thrombopoietin, stem cell factor, interleukins (IL)-6, IL-11, IL-1b, IL-8, and tumor necrosis factor-α levels in patients treated with paclitaxel and carboplatin; and (d) stromal cell production of thrombopoietin and stem cell factor after paclitaxel and carboplatin exposure. It was found that CFU-MK was more resistant to paclitaxel alone, or in combination with carboplatin, than CFU-GM and BFU-E. Although all progenitors expressed P-glycoprotein protein and GST mRNA, verapamil treatment significantly, and selectively, increased the toxicity of paclitaxel and carboplatin to CFU-MK, suggesting an important role for P-glycoprotein in megakaryocyte drug resistance. Compared with normal controls, serum thrombopoietin levels in patients receiving paclitaxel and carboplatin were significantly elevated 5 hours after infusion and remained elevated at day 7 (287% ± 63% increase; $P < 0.001$). Marrow stroma was shown to be the likely source of this thrombopoietin. It was concluded that P-glycoprotein-mediated efflux of paclitaxel, and perhaps GST-mediated detoxification of carboplatin, results in relative sparing of CFU-MK, which may then respond to locally high levels of stromal cell-derived thrombopoietin. The confluence of these events was hypothesized to bring about the platelet-sparing phenomenon observed in patients treated with this form of combination chemotherapy.

For patients who suffer from severe or prolonged thrombocytopenia, reducing the intensity of the chemotherapy is the most appropriate approach to management. It had been anticipated that the use of recombinant thrombopoietin might significantly ameliorate this problem, but unfortunately this has not yet been demonstrated.[227] The formation of antibodies to a thrombopoietin derivative, with resulting profound thrombocytopenia, has significantly slowed clinical investigations of this cytokine.[228] Administration of the compound intravenously instead of subcutaneously might avoid at least some of this immunogenicity observed.[227] A number of other cytokines have also been reported to raise platelet counts in this setting, including IL-1, IL-3, IL-6, and IL-11, but most are no longer available and their clinical utility was not clearly demonstrated.[229–235] Only IL-11 is currently approved for the treatment of thrombocytopenia following chemotherapy. Newer thrombopoietin mimetic drugs have recently entered clinical trial. It is thought that they will be less immunogenic, and in disorders such as ITP they appear to have activity.[236] Whether they will be of help in patients with impaired thrombopoiesis is undetermined but this will no doubt be evaluated in the near future.

At the present time, supportive therapy with platelet transfusions and drugs such as ε-aminocaproic acid for patients who have become refractory to platelet transfusions remain the mainstays of therapy. Amifostine, a phosphorylated aminothiol agent used primarily in the treatment of myelodysplastic syndromes, has been reported to have cytoprotectant value and to ameliorate the neutropenia and thrombocytopenia in patients being irradiated or receiving various types of chemotherapy in a phase III study.[237] Nevertheless, differences in the degrees of thrombocytopenia and neutropenia were not dramatic, and the investigators suggested that confirmatory studies needed to be carried out.

NUTRITIONAL DEFICIENCIES

Thrombocytopenia of various degrees can be observed in patients with either folate or vitamin B_{12} deficiency.[238–240] In some cases, it can be severe.[241,242] The mechanism of thrombocytopenia is ineffective platelet production.[11] Megakaryocyte numbers are normal or increased in the marrow, and platelet survival is normal or slightly shortened.[243] Vitamin B_{12} deficiency was reported to cause a case of amegakaryocytic thrombocytopenia.[244] Folate deficiency is frequently associated with ethanol abuse, and the etiology of the thrombocytopenia in patients who abuse ethanol is often complex.

Examination of a peripheral blood smear will typically show macrocytosis and hypersegmented neutrophils in addition to thrombocytopenia. The bone marrow often, but not always, shows megaloblastic changes in the erythroid and myeloid lineages.[245] Megakaryocytes are normal in number. Some may appear large, and in some cells multiple disconnected nuclear lobulations have been described. Often, however, distinctive morphologic abnormalities of the megakaryocytes are not seen. Rapid recovery of the platelet count can be achieved with administration of the appropriate vitamin.

IRON DEFICIENCY

Patients with iron deficiency typically exhibit thrombocytosis, but rare patients may become thrombocytopenic.[246] In some instances, decreased megakaryocytes are seen in the marrow,[247] but in a very recent study of six children with severe iron deficiencies when bone marrow examinations were performed in three patients, all showed increased numbers of megakaryocytes. After treatment with therapeutic doses of oral iron, each of the patients showed rapid increases in their platelet counts. The increased numbers of megakaryocytes and the extremely rapid increase in platelet counts after initiation of iron therapy suggested an essential role for iron in a late stage of thrombopoiesis.[248] Curiously, thrombocytopenia has been caused by iron therapy in a patient with severe iron deficiency. It was suggested, but not addressed experimentally, that the profound anemia caused preferential development of erythroid cells with a consequent decrease in megakaryocytes because they share a common progenitor.[249]

MARROW INFILTRATION

It is not rare for marrow infiltrative diseases of any type to cause ineffective hematopoiesis. Blood cell production disorders are commonly observed when the marrow is involved with metastatic cancer, lymphoma, or leukemia. Table 32–3 categorizes the infiltrative processes associated with thrombocytopenia. Physical replacement of marrow is the cause of the thrombocytopenia in many cases; it is also possible that inhibitory factors produced by the infiltrating cells are toxic to the cells of the megakaryocytic lineage or interfere with normal regulatory mechanisms. The diagnosis of infiltrative disease is made by marrow examination, although diagnostic clues are usually provided by history, physical examination, and a leukoerythroblastic blood smear. The marrow shows decreased megakaryocytes, which may be larger than normal because of a compensatory physiologic response to the thrombocytopenia. The treatment approach is specific to the infiltrative process.

ETHANOL-RELATED DISORDERS

Ethanol abuse is very commonly associated with thrombocytopenia, which may result from several different mechanisms.[240,250–255] These include, most commonly, increased splenic pooling as a result of portal hypertension and ineffective production related to folate deficiency (which may lead to severe thrombocytopenia). Ethanol itself can be directly toxic to the marrow.[253,256,257] In vitro studies have shown that alcohol concentrations achievable in vivo inhibit megakaryocyte maturation but do not inhibit CFU-MK.[253,256] Megakaryocyte numbers usually are normal, but markedly decreased megakaryocytes have been observed.[253] In one such case, labeling with platelet-specific antibodies demonstrated that numerous, small, unidentifiable cells were immature megakaryocytes.[253] Rarely, marrow panhypoplasia has been observed in association with alcohol ingestion.[257] Anemia and macrocytosis accompanied by megaloblastic changes and ringed sideroblasts in the erythroid marrow are typically observed in the marrows of patients who abuse ethanol. The severity of the anemia shows no correlation with the thrombocytopenia. Treatment consists of withdrawal of ethanol and administration of a normal diet. Recovery of the platelet count, often with a rebound thrombocytosis, usually occurs within 2 weeks.

OTHER DRUG-RELATED DISORDERS

A variety of drugs and toxins have been implicated in isolated platelet production defects. Estrogen, for example, has been reported to decrease platelet counts through an unknown mechanism.[258] Thrombocytopenia due to thiazide diuretics has been reported frequently.[259] Although the cause of the thrombocytopenia in most cases is probably increased clearance, decreased marrow megakaryocyte numbers have been noted.[260] Interferons and IL-2 may induce thrombocytopenia.[261,262] The most likely explanation is an inhibition of CFU-MK. Anagrelide is a very useful drug for lowering platelet counts in patients with myeloproliferative disorders and appears to work by reducing megakaryocyte size and ploidy and by disrupting maturation.[263]

Paroxysmal Nocturnal Hemoglobinuria

Paroxysmal nocturnal hemoglobinuria (PNH) is a clonal disorder resulting from mutations in the X-linked gene *PIG-A* that encodes for an enzyme required in the initial step of biosynthesis of glycosylphosphatidylinositol anchors (PNH is discussed in Chapter 30).[264] Approximately 25% of patients with PNH have significant marrow aplasia.[265] Thrombocytopenia at diagnosis is a poor prognostic indicator.[74] Because platelet survival is usually normal in cases of PNH,[266] thrombocytopenia is due to decreased or ineffective platelet production. Megakaryocyte progenitors have a decreased proliferative activity and exhibit increased sensitivity to complement.[4,267,268] Treatment with antithymocyte globulin or granulocyte colony-stimulating factor and cyclosporine has ameliorated the thrombocytopenia in some patients,[269,270] whereas marrow transplantation has resulted in long-term remissions in patients with aplasia associated with PNH.[271]

Refractory Thrombocytopenia Due to Myelodysplasia

Myelodysplastic syndromes may present as isolated thrombocytopenias in a very small number of cases (<1%).[272] The diagnosis of myelodysplasia should be considered when there are clonal chromosome abnormalities. Typically, they involve chromosomes 3, 5, 8, or 20, but partial deletions of other chromosomes have also been reported.[273] The usual laboratory findings include macrocytosis of platelets and red blood cells. Small dysplastic megakaryocytes, sometimes present in increased numbers, are the most typical abnormalities observed.[272,274,275] Dysplastic erythroblasts or myeloid cells may also be noted.

The clinical course of patients with this type of disorder is progressive. Additional cytopenias invariably develop so that the patient then has a typical myelodysplastic syndrome. A significant number of cases will evolve into an acute myeloid leukemia.[272] Therapy has not been shown to be beneficial. Some patients with a full-blown myelodysplastic syndrome associated with marked thrombocytopenia and less than 10% blasts have been reported to experience increases in platelet counts after androgen therapy.[276] As noted earlier, amifostine may be beneficial for some patients. It has been reported that some of these patients have been misdiagnosed as having ITP and treated for this disease. Because such therapy is not useful or helpful, it is important to recognize this entity.

Cyclic Thrombocytopenia

Cyclic oscillations in the platelet count have been reported many times in the literature.[186,277–282] The fluctuations in platelet count can be extreme, with thrombocytopenic bleeding being the result.[283] Women are often affected and in such patients the cycling occurs in association with the menstrual cycle. A study of 10 patients with cyclic thrombocytopenia suggested various causes of the thrombocytopenia, with cyclic variations in platelet production being responsible for some cases, including the two male patients in that group.[284] A case with antibodies toxic to megakaryocytes has also been reported.[37] The possibility that fluctuating cytokine levels may contribute to the pathogenesis of the disorder has been raised by several studies, although it is difficult to distinguish cause from effect.[184,285,286] Cyclic thrombocytopenia may rarely be a presenting manifestation of myelodysplasia.[287] Treatment has been variable; responses to low-dose contraceptives and intravenous gamma globulin have been reported.[279,288]

DIAGNOSING THROMBOCYTOPENIA DUE TO IMPAIRED THROMBOPOIESIS

Compiling a thorough patient history is the first step in a complete workup of a thrombocytopenic patient. Many potential causes will be revealed by a good history, including obtaining a family history of thrombocytopenia, recent infection, medication or substance ingestion, or radiation or chemotherapy.

A careful physical examination could also contribute to making a diagnosis. For example, physical findings suggesting any of the inherited disorders described earlier might be discerned, as might findings suggestive of malignancy such as enlarged lymph nodes. Splenomegaly itself is not indicative of a platelet production abnormality, but is often found in patients with lymphoma, or other processes associated with marrow infiltration and damage that might cause impaired thrombopoiesis.

The peripheral blood smear is next examined and this is needed to rule out pseudothrombocytopenia. Moreover, the blood smear provides additional clues to both the pathophysiologic mechanism of the thrombocytopenia and the diagnosis. For example, giant platelets suggest a hereditary or myelodysplastic syndrome; oval macrocytosis and hypersegmented neutrophils suggest a folate or vitamin B_{12} deficiency; and a leukoerythroblastic smear points to an infiltrative process.

Examination of the bone marrow is also required to evaluate megakaryocyte number and morphology. A biopsy is more reliable than an aspirate to determine whether megakaryocytes are decreased in number. However, an aspirate showing abundant megakaryocytes in the presence of thrombocytopenia is sufficient to suggest platelet destruction or ineffective production. Megakaryocytes are not evenly distributed throughout the marrow so examination of many fields is required in order to determine if adequate numbers of cells are present. Megakaryocyte morphology is also useful to observe. The normal compensatory response to thrombocytopenia is enlargement of the cells with increased ploidy. Small, microlobulated or hypolobulated megakaryocytes may be seen in myelodysplastic syndromes. Dysmorphic megakaryocytes may be also observed in viral infections, including human immunodeficiency virus. In the future, flow cytometry[61] may provide a more objective analysis of megakaryocytes.

Ultimately, a diagnosis of ineffective thrombopoiesis is made by exclusion. The marrow examination reveals quantitatively normal megakaryocytes, and the apparent absence of peripheral platelet destruction together with the appropriate clinical circumstances (eg, folate or vitamin B_{12} deficiency) often point to this mechanism. Platelet function tests may be helpful in distinguishing ineffective production from platelet destruction. In destructive processes such as immune thrombocytopenia, function is normal, whereas in ineffective platelet production impaired function is not uncommon, as noted above. In complex cases, platelet survival studies may be necessary to show that consumption or splenic pooling are not significant contributors to the thrombocytopenia; however, survival studies are rarely required for clinical purposes. In the future, flow cytometric estimation of platelet production rate and measurement of thrombopoietin levels may permit a more facile approach to the differential diagnosis of thrombocytopenia.

SUGGESTED READINGS

Bussel JB et al: AMG 531, a thrombopoiesis-stimulating protein, for chronic ITP. N Engl J Med 355(16):1672, 2006.

Carbonara S et al: Response of severe HIV-associated thrombocytopenia to highly active antiretroviral therapy including protease inhibitors. J Infect 42(4):251, 2001.

Gewirtz AM et al: Cell-mediated suppression of megakaryocytopoiesis in acquired amegakaryocytic thrombocytopenic purpura. Blood 68(3):619, 1986.

Hoffman R et al: An antibody cytotoxic to megakaryocyte progenitor cells in a patient with immune thrombocytopenic purpura. N Engl J Med 312(18):1170, 1985.

Horvat-Switzer RD, Thompson AA: HOXA11 mutation in amegakaryocytic thrombocytopenia with radio-ulnar synostosis syndrome inhibits megakaryocytic differentiation in vitro. Blood Cells Mol Dis 37(1):55, 2006.

Imai K et al: Clinical course of patients with WASP gene mutations. Blood 103(2):456, 2004.

Kaushansky K: The molecular mechanisms that control thrombopoiesis. J Clin Invest 115(12):3339, 2005.

Klopocki E et al: Complex inheritance pattern resembling autosomal recessive inheritance involving a microdeletion in thrombocytopenia-absent radius syndrome. Am J Hum Genet 80(2):232, 2007.

Kurata Y et al: Diagnostic value of tests for reticulated platelets, plasma glycocalicin, and thrombopoietin levels for discriminating between hyperdestructive and hypoplastic thrombocytopenia. Am J Clin Pathol 115(5):656, 2001.

Locatelli F, Rossi G, Balduini C: Hematopoietic stem-cell transplantation for the Bernard-Soulier syndrome. Ann Intern Med 138(1):79, 2003.

Mason KD et al: Programmed anuclear cell death delimits platelet life span. Cell 128(6):1173, 2007.

Notarangelo LD, Ochs HD: Wiskott-Aldrich syndrome: A model for defective actin reorganization, cell trafficking and synapse formation. Curr Opin Immunol 15(5):585, 2003.

Nurden AT, Nurden P: The gray platelet syndrome: Clinical spectrum of the disease. Blood Rev 21(1):21, 2007.

Qi B, Hardwick JM: A Bcl-xL timer sets platelet life span. Cell 128(6):1035, 2007.

Pertusini E et al: Investigating the platelet-sparing mechanism of paclitaxel/carboplatin combination chemotherapy. Blood 97(3):638, 2001.

Ramasamy I: Inherited bleeding disorders: Disorders of platelet adhesion and aggregation. Crit Rev Oncol Hematol 49(1):1, 2004.

Shivdasani RA: Molecular and transcriptional regulation of megakaryocyte differentiation. Stem Cells 19(5):397, 2001.

Song WJ et al: Haploinsufficiency of CBFA2 causes familial thrombocytopenia with propensity to develop acute myelogenous leukaemia. Nat Genet 23(2):166, 1999. (see comments)

van den Oudenrijn S et al: Mutations in the thrombopoietin receptor, Mpl, in children with congenital amegakaryocytic thrombocytopenia. Br J Haematol 110(2):441, 2000.

White JG, Nichols WL, Steensma DP: Platelet pathology in sex-linked GATA-1 dyserythropoietic macrothrombocytopenia I ultrastructure. Platelets 18(4):273, 2007.

REFERENCES

For complete list of references log onto www.expertconsult.com

PART

IV

RED BLOOD CELLS

CHAPTER 33

PATHOBIOLOGY OF THE HUMAN ERYTHROCYTE AND ITS HEMOGLOBINS

Martin H. Steinberg, Edward J. Benz, Jr., Adeboye H. Adewoye, and Benjamin L. Ebert

Anemia, polycythemia, and functional derangements of the human erythrocyte together represent a particularly important group of human disorders. Although sickle cell disease, hemoglobin E (HbE)-associated disorders and the thalassemias are humankind's most common single gene diseases, the relevance of red cell disorders to general medicine extends beyond their individual clinical severities or the number of patients affected. A critical added dimension of erythrocyte disorders is the extraordinarily detailed knowledge available about the basic biochemistry, physiology, and molecular biology of the human red blood cell and its membrane, enzymes, and major component, hemoglobin. Red blood cells are especially abundant, relatively simple, and readily accessible for repeated testing in individual patients. These features have facilitated rapid application of the techniques of cellular and molecular biology to studies of the red blood cell, its component molecules and structures, and syndromes resulting from abnormalities of these entities. Taken as a group, erythrocyte disorders are better understood at the molecular and cellular levels than disorders of any other cell or tissue. It is for this reason that these conditions merit particularly careful scrutiny by students of hematology.

This chapter reviews concepts about normal red blood cell homeostasis that form the essential knowledge base for understanding anemias, polycythemias, and functional erythrocyte disorders. The primary focus and the object for detailed discussion within this chapter is hemoglobin, the major component, both quantitatively and qualitatively, of the erythrocyte. Hemoglobin molecules dominate the pathophysiology of many red blood cell disorders and modulate most of the others, in part because of their sheer quantitative predominance in red blood cell cytoplasm. The other major relevant aspects of human red blood cells—the membrane, the enzymes used for intermediary metabolism, differentiation and development, and the process of destruction—are discussed in detail in the introductory portions of other chapters. This chapter surveys these areas only briefly. Detailed descriptions of the red blood cell membrane can be found in Chapter 46. Red blood cell enzymes and enzymopathies are described in Chapter 45; differentiation and development are described in Chapter 25; regulation of the red blood cell mass by erythropoietin is discussed in Chapter 25; and the necessary aspects of red blood cell destruction are considered in Chapters 33, 47, and 48.

ESSENTIAL FEATURES OF RED BLOOD CELL HOMEOSTASIS

As discussed in Chapter 25, the mature red blood cell is the product of a complex and orderly set of differentiation and maturation steps beginning with the pluripotent stem cell. By incompletely understood mechanisms involving hierarchic networks of cytokines, a portion of these cells becomes committed to differentiate along the erythroid pathway. Commitment to erythropoiesis provokes a progressively increasing sensitivity to the stimulatory actions of the hormone erythropoietin. As differentiation proceeds there is preprogramming of certain genes whose expression at high levels will be required during the maturation phase of erythropoiesis. Genes coding for molecules defining the red blood cell phenotype (eg, globin) are poised for activation at later maturation steps.

Intermediate progenitor cells arising during differentiation have been characterized experimentally, including the burst-forming unit-erythroid (BFU-E) and the colony-forming unit-erythroid (CFU-E) stages. BFU-Es are progenitor cells that in culture produce bursts or clusters of erythroid colonies, are relatively less sensitive to erythropoietin, and are more plastic with respect to important gene expression parameters, such as the synthesis of adult or fetal hemoglobin by their descendants. CFU-Es produce single colonies, exhibit considerably higher sensitivity to erythropoietin, and appear to be more fixed in their potential to express a particular subset of globin genes. As discussed in Chapter 25, CFU-Es appear to give rise to the first morphologically recognizable erythroid cells, the proerythroblasts. At this "primitive" morphologic stage, the program of erythroid cell expression has already been essentially predetermined. The cell is predestined to undergo only a limited additional number of cell divisions, culminating in formation of the enucleate reticulocyte. The terminal maturation stages are morphologically recognizable as erythroblasts exhibiting progressive hemoglobinization of the cytoplasm, condensation and eventual ejection of the nucleus, and remodeling of the plasma membrane. Actual expression of the preprogrammed genes occurs during the 5- to 7-day period of erythroblast maturation.

As discussed in Chapter 25, the actual reconfiguration of chromatin for activation of the genes and activation itself appear to require the concerted and complex interaction of a diverse but limited group of transcription factors. These regulatory proteins recognize a specific array of promoter and enhancer sequences that are embedded as recurrent motifs in and around the appropriate target genes. Even though an enormous amount of information has been gathered about sequences such as the GATA enhancers and their cognate transcription factors (eg, GATA, FOG, ETS), the precise means by which these sequences and factors cause erythroid differentiation remains mysterious. At this time, this information is of limited clinical relevance to anemias or polycythemias. The orderly 14- to 21-day sequence of differentiation and maturation becomes progressively influenced by the levels of erythropoietin available to the progenitor cells, possibly because of increasing density and affinity of erythropoietin receptors on their cell surfaces. Cytokines such as fibroblast growth factor (FGF) can affect erythroid and myeloid development. In the Zebrafish, knockdown of FGF expression alters normal development of erythroid and myeloid elements. Although the exact role of FGF has not been fully elucidated in humans, these observations suggest that FGF-related pathways might play a role in aplastic anemia and pure red cell aplasia. Within 24 hours after enucleation, the reticulocyte traverses the bone marrow–blood barrier membrane and enters the circulation as an immature erythrocyte. These cells retain remnants of nucleated precursors in the form of a relatively small number of polyribosomes actively translating messenger RNA (>90% of which is globin messenger RNA), a cell membrane that retains some molecules and structures reminiscent of its earlier stages of differentiation, and the only complement of enzymes, phospholipids, and cytoskeletal proteins that the cell will possess throughout its remaining life span.

During its first 24 hours in the circulation, the reticulocyte spends considerable amounts of time in the spleen, during which its membrane is "polished." This is a poorly understood remodeling process by which some lipids and proteins, including adhesive molecules such as fibronectin, are removed. The content of polyribosomes and other nucleic acids progressively declines so that stainability with methylene blue, until recently the standard method used for clinical enumeration of reticulocytes, is lost by the end of the first day. At this time, the red blood cell is regarded as a mature erythrocyte, and it circulates largely unchanged for the remainder of its 120-day life span.

Perhaps the most remarkable feature of the human red blood cell is its durability, given that it is an enucleated cell devoid of organelles that appear to be critical for the survival and function of most other cell types. The red blood cell has no mitochondria available for efficient oxidative metabolism, no ribosomes for regeneration of lost or damaged proteins, a very limited metabolic repertoire that largely precludes de-novo synthesis of lipids, and no nucleus to direct regenerative processes, adaptation to circulatory stresses, or cell division to replenish itself. Given these handicaps, the 120-day survival of these cells is even more striking considering the multiple and often exceedingly hostile environments they must traverse. Mechanical stresses of the circulation include high hydrostatic pressure and turbulence and the shear stresses inherent in a microcirculation networked with many capillaries having diameters only one-third to one-half that of the normal red blood cell. Biochemical stresses include osmotic and redox fluxes associated with travel through the collecting system of the kidney; the sluggish vascular beds of the spleen, muscle, and bone; and the rapid changes in ambient oxygen pressures occurring in the lungs. All conspire to damage red blood cells. Their 4-month survival is truly remarkable.

The ability of the red blood cell to persist in the circulation depends on its simple but exquisitely adaptive membrane structures, its pathways of intermediary energy metabolism and redox regulation, and its ability to maintain its largest cytoplasmic component, hemoglobin, in a soluble and nonoxidized state. The membrane and enzymes of the red blood cell appear to be exquisitely crafted to protect the cell from the external ravages of the circulation and the potential internal assaults of the massive amount of iron-rich and potentially oxidizing protein represented by its complement of hemoglobin molecules. For these reasons, a few basic features of these membrane and enzyme systems merit comment before considering the hemoglobin molecule itself.

MAJOR FEATURES OF THE RED BLOOD CELL MEMBRANE

Chapter 45 describes the red blood cell membrane in considerable detail, using it as a model for understanding membrane structure in general. Only a few major aspects of that discussion bear repeating for the purposes of this chapter. The red blood cell membrane and its underlying cytoskeleton have evolved to provide mechanical strength and the necessary pliability and resilience to withstand the mechanical, osmotic, and chemical stresses of the circulation. Because the lipid bilayer membrane essentially has the physical properties of a soap bubble, it would rapidly be emulsified in the circulation. Strength and order are provided to the lipid bilayer by the hexagonal arrays of the highly helical protein spectrin, which forms a latticework underlying the membrane.

The spectrin meshwork is held together by adaptor molecules, such as protein 4.1, adducin, p55, and ankyrin, arrayed at defined points along the highly coiled, rod-like structure of the spectrin oligomers. These protein-protein interactions appear to be critical for holding the latticework together in what has been described as the "horizontal" dimension that permits resistance to shear stress (see Chapter 46). The involvement of intermediate-length actin fibers and the variability of binding affinities by phosphorylation state appear to provide some flexibility and pliability at these points of interaction. Strength in the "vertical" dimension is provided by additional molecules or additional binding functions of the same molecule, whereby the latticework is attached to the lipid bilayer. For the most part, the physiologically important attachments appear to be indirect. Linkage is mediated through the interaction of the adaptor proteins, such as ankyrin and protein 4.1, with the cytoplasmic domains of abundant transmembrane proteins. These proteins traverse and are embedded in the lipid bilayer, providing a firm anchor. The two most critical of these molecules appear to be band 3 (ie, the anion transport channel) and a glycophorin, probably glycophorin C/D. A possible additional stabilizing role for the Rh protein complex has been suggested. The construction of these attachments by multiple "hinge" or coupling molecules appears to provide for the flexibility and distensibility of the red blood cell membrane, a property essential to its ability to flow through small capillaries.

As described in Chapter 46, the complex structure of the membrane is exquisitely sensitive to perturbations impinging on any of its components. In particular, the membrane cytoskeleton and phospholipid structures are each highly susceptible to oxidation, particularly by partially proteolyzed molecules of hemoglobin, which denature to form highly toxic compounds called *hemopyrroles*. This interaction of denatured hemoglobin with the red blood cell membrane is clinically important, as illustrated by its impact on the pathophysiology of sickle cell anemia (see Chapter 42) or of oxidized and precipitated globin inclusion bodies in thalassemia. In this chapter, it is sufficient to note that alterations of proteins of the red blood cell membrane can contribute to shortening the life span of the red blood cell. Damage can result from direct defects in the cytoskeletal proteins themselves or from susceptibility of these proteins to direct oxidation or attack by oxidized or denatured hemoglobin molecules. The reader is referred to the aforementioned chapters for detailed descriptions of the relevant phenomena.

ENZYMES OF RED BLOOD CELL INTERMEDIARY

Metabolism

Mammalian erythrocytes possess a highly specialized but remarkably simplified set of metabolic pathways. As discussed in Chapter 45, there are essentially three relevant sets of pathways. The first two are interconnected by the enzyme glucose-6-phosphate dehydrogenase (G6PD). Glucose entering the red blood cell is metabolized by an anaerobic pathway, the Embden-Meyerhof pathway, which terminates with the enzyme lactic dehydrogenase, forming lactate. Despite its inefficiency (a net of only two adenosine triphosphate [ATP]/ glucose molecule), this pathway is the sole source of usable ATP in the cell. Moreover, the pathway generates reduced nicotinamide adenine dinucleotide (NADH), a molecule necessary for driving the reduction of methemoglobin to hemoglobin (see Chapter 45). A shunt within this pathway, the Rapoport-Luebering shunt, generates the compound 2,3-bisphosphoglycerate (bis[phosphoglyceric acid]) (2,3-BPG), an important cofactor that, when bound to hemoglobin, reduces the affinity of hemoglobin for oxygen (see "Hemoglobin Function). The ATP generated is necessary for kinase reactions controlling phosphorylation of membrane and signaling components, for fueling ion pumps and channels, and for maintaining phospholipid levels.

The anaerobic metabolic pathway generates, as one of its intermediates, glucose-6 phosphate, which is the substrate for G6PD. G6PD appears to be the rate-limiting enzyme for a linked pathway called the *oxidative hexose monophosphate shunt*. This pathway involves a cascade of reactions culminating in the reduction of oxidized glutathione to reduced glutathione. Reduced glutathione is used to reverse oxidation of critical structures, including hemoglobin, cytoskeletal proteins, and membrane lipids. Anaerobic glycolysis generates NADH for methemoglobin reduction, 2,3-BPG for modulation of hemoglobin oxygen affinity, and ATP for metabolic energy requirements. Its end product is lactate. The oxidative glycolysis pathway generates nicotinamide adenine dinucleotide phosphate (NADPH) and reduced glutathione for use as the major erythrocyte antioxidant.

During the past decade, most of the enzymes (or at least the erythroid isoforms of these enzymes) involved in red blood cell intermediary metabolism have been characterized at the molecular level by cloning of their cDNAs or genomic loci, or both. Some of the more relevant information arising from this progress is discussed in Chapter 45. The erythrocyte possesses membrane-based signaling receptors and cytoplasmic signal transduction elements similar, although perhaps less elaborate, than those of nucleated cells. The relevance of these systems to the pathophysiology of red blood cell disorders is just becoming apparent.

RED BLOOD CELL SENESCENCE AND DESTRUCTION

Erythrocytes, despite their impressive adaptations to circulatory stresses, eventually wear out and are destroyed. Red blood cell survival in humans appears to be remarkably uniform under normal circumstances, spanning approximately 120 days from release of the reticulocyte into the circulation to sequestration of the senescent red blood cell in the reticuloendothelial cells of the liver and spleen. The precise signal, or signals, marking red blood cells for destruction remain unknown, as does the underlying pathophysiology within the red blood cell or on its surface. However, several interrelated theories have emerged; these are discussed only briefly because they are mentioned in other chapters.

Red blood cells accumulate surface blemishes during their lives in the circulation. These appear to result in part from the accumulation of small amounts of oxygen damage to membrane structures. The altered regions are sensed by the reticuloendothelial cells during passage of the erythrocytes through the liver and spleen. Removal or pitting of these damaged regions from red blood cell membranes can be documented microscopically; small amounts of normal membrane are also lost during the process.

The biconcave disk shape of the red blood cell, so important to its distensibility, depends on a high ratio of surface area to volume. This requires redundant membrane surface area. The membrane surface area of the normal biconcave disk is approximately 140 μm^2. To enclose a sphere containing a normal red blood cell volume (approximately 90 fL), only approximately 95 μm^2 would be needed. Progressive loss of membrane surface by means of the pitting phenomenon should ultimately cause the aging erythrocyte to assume a more rigid spherical shape. A sphere is inevitably far less distensible and far less capable of passing through small apertures than a disk, especially in the sluggish and torturous circulation of the spleen. This geometric mechanism can lead to the eventual destruction of the red blood cell.

Red blood cells progressively lose some of the critical enzymes needed for intermediary metabolism and antioxidant capacity. G6PD levels, for example, progressively decline during the circulating life span, as do levels of several other enzymes. The decline of certain enzymes can be used as a crude means of estimating the relative age of different red blood cell populations. The biochemical or oxidative mechanism of destruction postulates that aged red blood cells are eventually depleted of critical enzymes needed for maintenance of redox status. Oxidation of critical membrane proteins, lipids, and hemoglobin would then ensue, causing distortion and rigidity of the red blood cell membrane, with accelerated loss as previously described. The end product would be spherocytes incapable of traversing the splenic vascular bed and escaping engulfment by the reticuloendothelial cell.

It has been proposed that an immune-type mechanism can contribute to normal and pathologic red blood cell senescence. This hypothesis is based on the observation that oxidative damage, regardless of cause, promotes a clustering, or *capping*, of oligomers of band 3 on the red blood cell surface. Under normal circumstances, band 3 molecules form monomers, dimers, or tetramers. Higher-order aggregates appear to be recognized by an endogenous isoantibody possessed by all people. Any red blood cell accumulating oxidative damage from wear and tear in the circulation, from depletion of enzymes, or from internal pathologic processes such as denaturation of hemoglobin in certain hemoglobinopathies can accumulate these aggregates. The aggregates would then be bound by antibody and be removed by the reticuloendothelial cells as antigen-antibody complexes, employing the same means used by reticuloendothelial cells to recognize any immune complex. This mechanism could also provide for the pitting or polishing of damaged red blood cell membranes. All three of the proposed mechanisms are interrelated by their inception with oxidative damage.

Other membrane-related changes might influence red cell destruction. Bcl-X_L (also designated BCL2L1), a suppressor of apoptosis, is present in erythrocyte membranes and its antagonization may promote cell death. This may be mediated by calcium accumulation and phosphatidylserine exposure. Cholesterol and fatty acids accumulate on the aging red cell membrane and might be targets for oxidation induced by reactive oxygen species. Red cells are removed from the circulation by splenic macrophages, probably by several mechanisms. SHPS-1, a surface glycoprotein and a member of the immunoglobulin superfamily that interacts with red cell membrane CD47, is abundant in macrophages. Studies using mice expressing a mutant SHPS-1 suggested that this molecule might negatively regulate phagocytosis influencing cell lifespan. Increasing phosphatidal serine exposure and reduced aminophospholipid translocase activity during aging might induced oxidative damage to the cell. It is probable that these mechanisms leading to cell destruction are not mutually exclusive, that no single effect predominates, and these events occur at different times at different sites of red cell damage.

Regardless of the mechanism(s) fostering eventual senescence and destruction of red blood cells, the process itself involves components clinically useful for assessment of anemias associated with accelerated destruction. Chief among these is the generation of indirect or unconjugated bilirubin, the by-product of heme catabolism occurring within the reticuloendothelial cells. In markedly accelerated states of red blood cell destruction, hypertrophy of the liver and spleen can also occur, providing a useful physical indicator of hemolytic anemia. These indirect clinical features, coupled with the reticulocyte count, remain more useful for detecting clinical hemolysis than complicated studies of red blood cell kinetics.

HEMOGLOBIN SYNTHESIS, STRUCTURE, AND FUNCTION

Basic Features

Hemoglobins are the major oxygen-carrying pigments of the body. They are packaged into red blood cells in quantities sufficient to carry enough oxygen from the lungs to the tissues to meet the needs of those cells for oxidative metabolism. These quantities are enormous– almost two pounds of hemoglobin are present in the body of a reasonably sized human at any given time. Because free hemoglobin in the bloodstream is catabolized and excreted renally in a matter of minutes, packaging in erythrocytes is essential to preserve the newly synthesized molecules for the entire 4-month life span of the red blood cell. Otherwise, the caloric and biosynthetic resources needed to replace daily losses of hemoglobin would be prohibitive. The red blood cell's major function is to encase hemoglobin and protect it so it can function as an oxygen transporter for a prolonged period. An additional function of hemoglobin is to modulate vascular tone by its transport of nitric oxide (NO), and, possibly nitrous oxide.

The cellular content of blood influences its viscosity; in particular, the hemodynamics are adversely compromised by the presence of too many circulating erythrocytes, because blood viscosity correlates especially with hematocrit. To provide for adequate oxygen transport (ie, enough hemoglobin molecules) in a number of red blood cells compatible with tolerable viscosity, each cell must enclose a high concentration of hemoglobin (32 to 35 g per 100 mL of cytoplasm). This concentration is close to the solubility limit of hemoglobin in physiologic solutions. It follows that even minor perturbations within these molecules (eg, oxidation) or in the milieu (eg, changes in pH or ionic strength) can have potentially devastating effects on the solubility of hemoglobin. Because polymerized or precipitated hemoglobins derange intracellular viscosity, trigger proteolytic reactions that lead to oxidative damage of erythrocytes, and compromise oxygen transport, it is not surprising that the fate of the red blood cell is inextricably interwoven with the state of its enormous complement of hemoglobin molecules.

Hemoglobin Structure

The hemoglobin tetramer consists of two pairs of unlike globin polypeptide chains, each associated with a heme group. Normal hemoglobin has two α- and two non-α-globin chains; the interaction of these chains is responsible for the quaternary structure of the hemoglobin molecule and normal oxygen transport. Functionally, the second exon of each globin gene encodes the major component of the heme-binding pocket, and the α and non-α contacts are regulated by the third exon.

The behavior of hemoglobin is determined by its primary structure, the covalent linking of amino acids to form the polypeptide globin. The higher-order structures of hemoglobin depend on the sequence of amino acid residues that make up the globin chain. The α-globin chains contain 141 residues, and the β-globin–like chains are 146 amino acids long (Fig. 33–1). There is considerable homology among these globins, especially among the non–α-globin chains. Whereas the α-globin genes (*HBA2, HBA1*) result from a very ancient gene duplication, the non–α-globin genes (*HBE, HBG2, HBG1, HBD, HBB*) are the result of more recent gene duplications and are more akin to each other than they are to the α-like globin genes. Gene conversion events also ensure the similarity of duplicated genes.

Elements of the secondary structure of globin are shown in Figs. 33–1 and 33–2. Approximately 75% of the globin polypeptide chain forms an α-helix. There are eight helical segments, A through H, separated by short stretches from which the α-helix is absent. These nonhelical segments permit folding of the polypeptide on itself and are often dictated by the presence of prolyl residues, which are generally unable to participate in the formation of α-helices. Although the helical segments of the α- and non–α-globin chains do not exactly correspond, it is possible to align amino acid residues in all globin peptides by their helical and nonhelical residue numbers, as indicated in Fig. 33–1. This permits greater appreciation of the homology among globins. Some of the amino acids of globin are invariant, or conserved, in the sense that they are preserved during phylogeny. These residues occur at portions of the molecule that are critical for its stability and function, such as heme binding residues, hydrophobic amino acids of the interior of the molecule, and certain subunit contacts at the α_1-β_2 interface. The introduction of prolyl residues into α-helical segments by mutation leads to interruption of the α-helix and instability of the resulting hemoglobin molecule.

The poorly understood laws that govern the folding of proteins are responsible for the tertiary structure of globin, shown in Fig. 33–2. This folding pattern places polar residues exteriorly and provides a hydrophobic niche for the heme ring between the E and F helices. Numerous noncovalent bonds are formed between the heme and surrounding amino acid residues of globin. An iron atom in the center of the porphyrin ring forms an important bond with the F8 or proximal histidine and through the linked oxygen with the E7 or distal histidine residue. Oxygenation and deoxygenation of hemoglobin occur at the heme iron. Folding of globin and association of chains into dimers and tetramers was once thought to occur spontaneously. However, it is now clear that these processes are assisted by chaperone proteins, which are described in Chapters 3, 4 and 5.

Two α-globin chains and two non–α-globin chains fit together specifically to form a hemoglobin tetramer with a molecular mass of approximately 64,000 daltons and with the quaternary structure shown in Fig. 33–3. The motion of individual globin chains, as well as the movement of globin chains relative to each other during oxy-

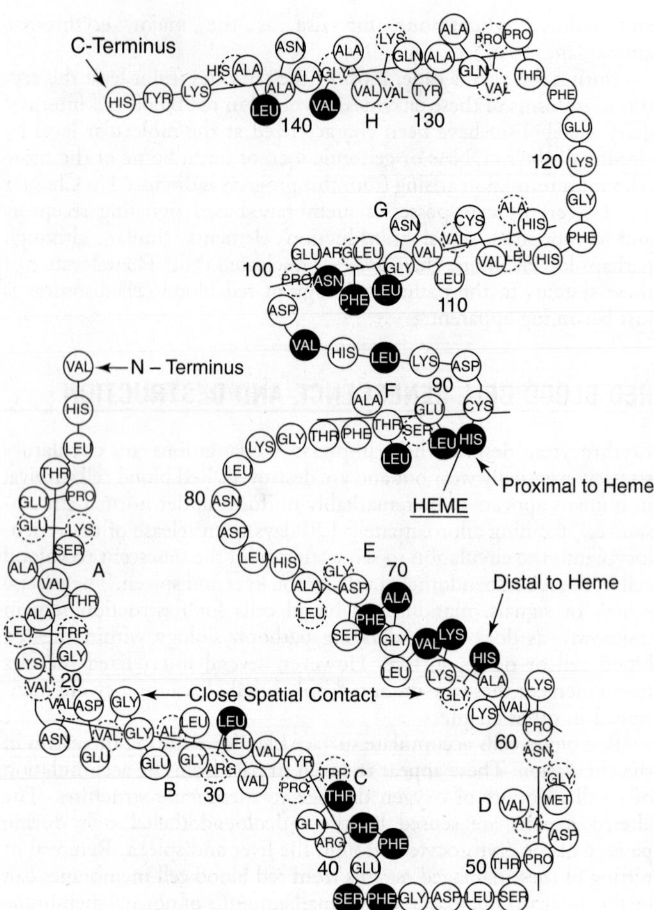

Figure 33–1. The β-globin chain, showing helical and nonhelical segments. The helical segments are labeled A through H, and nonhelical segments are designated NA for residues between the N terminus and the A helix, CD for residues between the C and D helices, and so forth. *(From Huisman THJ, Schroeder WA: New Aspects of the Structure, Function, and Synthesis of Hemoglobin. Boca Raton, FL, CRC Press, 1971.)*

genation and deoxygenation, gives hemoglobin its unique usefulness as a respiratory protein.

Hemoglobin Function

Evolution has honed the hemoglobin tetramer into a molecule ideally suited for its tasks. Because human hemoglobin must behave differently than that of altitude dwelling species or species inhabiting hypoxic locales, many different variants of the same basic molecular design have evolved. Because of the exigencies of molecular evolution, we find in the genome of all animals, including humans, attempts by nature to propagate a variety of different globin genes. The crystallographic studies of Perutz and coworkers defined the oxygenated and deoxygenated structures of hemoglobin at Ångström-unit resolution and provided an exquisitely detailed picture of how the globin chains and individual amino acid residues respond to the loading and unloading of oxygen. All of these, however, share the properties of highly reversible oxygen binding, and high solubility in cytoplasm. We know more about the function of hemoglobin than about virtually any other protein, and the knowledge of this mechanism provides a beautiful and intellectually satisfying culmination to decades of study by many investigators.

The oxygen dissociation curve of hemoglobin, shown in Fig. 33–4, describes the percent saturation of hemoglobin with oxygen at

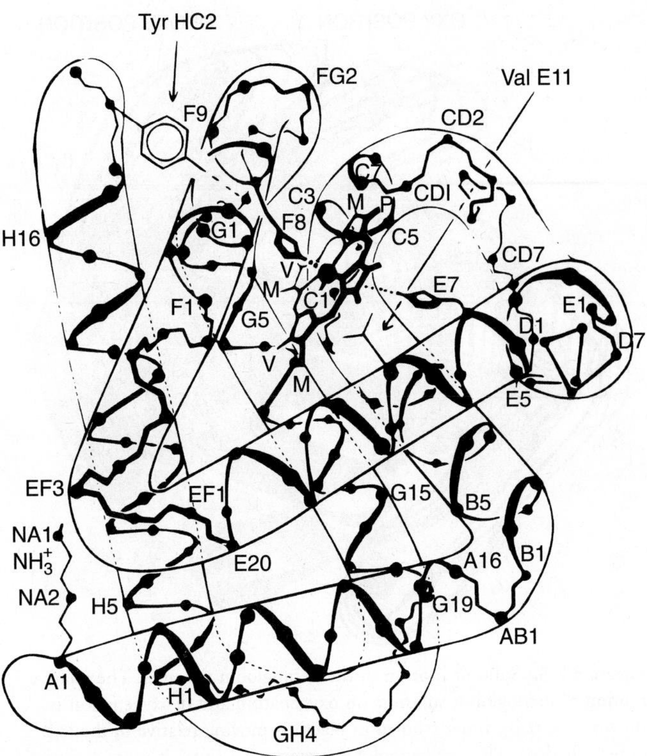

Figure 33–2. Tertiary structure of a globin chain. Globin folds into a tertiary structure such that polar or charged amino acids are located on the exterior of the molecule and the heme ring resides in a hydrophobic niche between the E and F helices. Linked to the heme are the proximal (F8) histidine and the distal (E7) histidine. *(From Perutz MF: Molecular anatomy, physiology, and pathology of hemoglobin. In Stamatoyannopoulos G, Neinhuis AW, Leder P, Majerus PW [eds]: The Molecular Basis of Blood Diseases. Philadelphia, WB Saunders, 1987, p 127.)*

different oxygen tensions. The sigmoidal shape of this curve is a result of interaction among the subunits of hemoglobin. Communication within the tetramer is called heme-heme interaction or cooperativity. This implies that the four heme groups do not undergo simultaneous oxygenation or deoxygenation, but rather that the state of each heme unit with regard to the presence or absence of bound oxygen influences the binding of oxygen to other heme groups. Myoglobin, a heme-containing protein with virtually the same tertiary structure as globin, exists in muscle as a monomer. The oxygen equilibrium curve of myoglobin is a rectangular hyperbola; in physiologic terms, it rapidly becomes fully saturated at low oxygen tensions and remains saturated as the oxygen tension plateaus. The difference in the oxygen equilibrium curves of myoglobin and hemoglobin lies in the tetrameric nature of the hemoglobin molecule and the cooperativity permitted by the association of similar but unlike subunits. Compared with hemoglobin, myoglobin has a very low P_{50} (ie, oxygen partial pressure at which the molecule is one-half saturated). It therefore has an extremely high oxygen affinity and would not be useful for delivering oxygen to tissues. The oxygen in myoglobin is passed on to the mitochondria, where oxidative metabolism occurs. The sigmoidal shape of the oxygen dissociation curve of hemoglobin indicates that the totally deoxygenated hemoglobin tetramer is slow to become oxygenated, but as oxygenation proceeds, the reaction of heme with oxygen accelerates. Perutz has drawn an analogy in which the "appetite" of heme for oxygen grows with the "eating," and conversely, loss of oxygen by heme lowers the oxygen affinity of the remaining heme groups. The Hill coefficient, *n*, which can be calculated from plots of oxygen equilibrium curves, is a description of heme-heme interaction or cooperativity that explains in part the oxygen-binding properties of hemoglobin and myoglobin. The Hill coefficient for myoglobin is 1, indicating no cooperativity; *n* is approximately 3 for the normal human hemoglobin A molecule.

The oxygen affinity of hemoglobin within the erythrocyte does not depend solely on the intrinsic properties of the tetramer. The position of the hemoglobin oxygen dissociation curve, and therefore the P_{50}, can be influenced by a number of heterotropic modifiers,

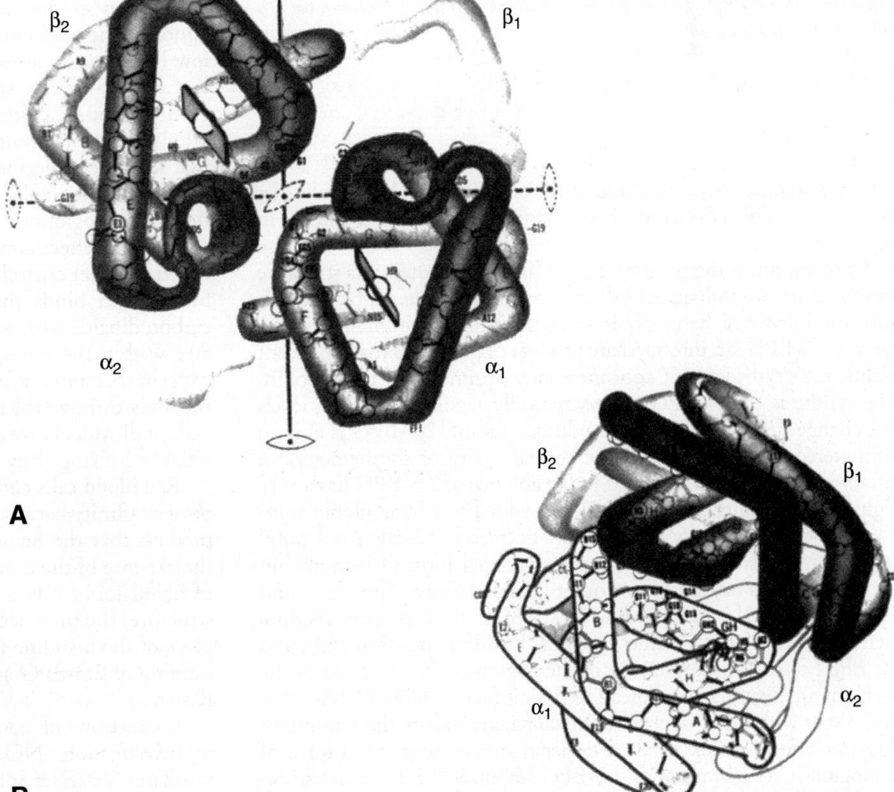

Figure 33–3. Quaternary structure of hemoglobin. The contacts between subunits are shown as circled amino acids. In the front view (A), α1-β2 contacts are shown, and in the side view (B), α1-β1 contacts are depicted. *(From Dickerson RE, Geis I: Hemoglobin: Structure, Function, and Evolution Pathology. Menlo Park, CA, Benjamin-Cummings, 1983.)*

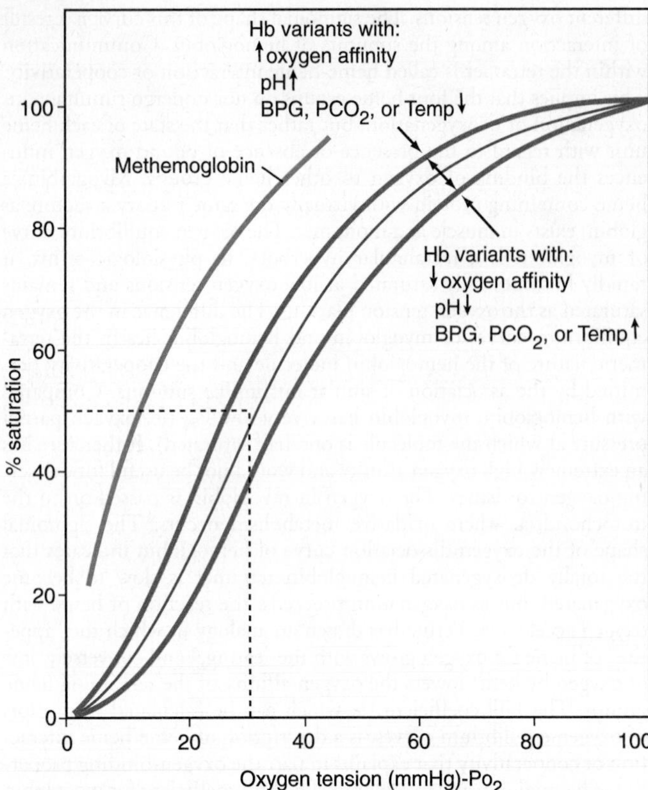

Figure 33–4. Oxygen dissociation curve of hemoglobin. The percent saturation of hemoglobin with oxygen at different oxygen tensions is depicted by the red sigmoidal curve. The P_{50} (ie, oxygen tension at which the hemoglobin molecule is one-half saturated) is approximately 27 mm Hg in normal erythrocytes (dotted lines). Heterotopic modifiers of hemoglobin function can shift the curve leftward by increasing or rightward by decreasing its oxygen affinity. PCO_2, partial pressure of carbon dioxide. *(From Benz EJ Jr: Synthesis, structure, and function of hemoglobin. In Kelly WN, DeVita VT [eds]: Textbook of Internal Medicine, vol 1. Philadelphia, JB Lippincott, 1989, p 236.)*

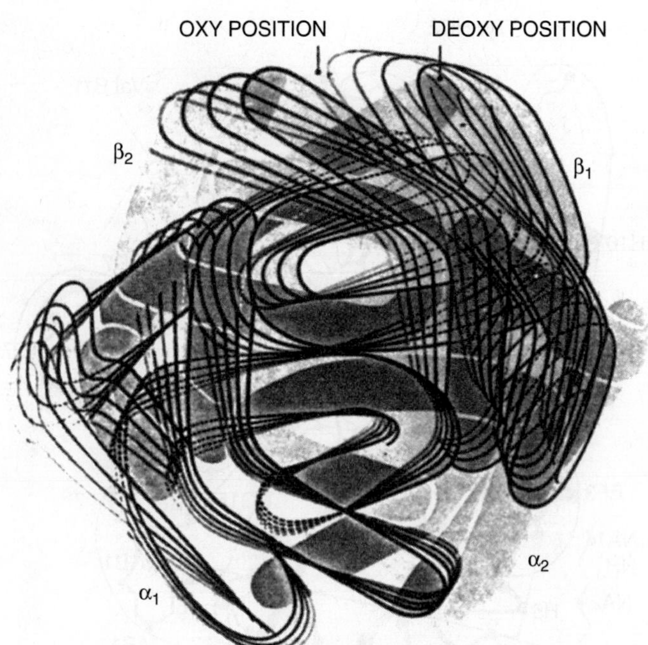

Figure 33–5. Subunit motion in the hemoglobin tetramer. The relative motion of hemoglobin subunits on oxygenation and deoxygenation is shown. The $\alpha_1\beta_1$ dimer (shown in black) is moving relative to the $\alpha_2\beta_2$ dimer (shaded). The oxyhemoglobin tetramer (R state) is more compact than the deoxyhemoglobin configuration (T state). *(From Dickerson RE, Geis I: Hemoglobin: Structure, Function, and Evolution Pathology. Menlo Park, CA, Benjamin-Cummings, 1983.)*

including temperature, pH, and small organic phosphate molecules in the cell. The effects of these modifiers on P_{50} are shown in Fig. 33–4.

Hemoglobin is the prototype of an allosteric protein; its structure and function are influenced by other molecules. The major intracellular modulator of hemoglobin-oxygen affinity in human erythrocytes is 2,3-BPG, an intermediate product of glycolysis that is present within the erythrocyte at concentrations equimolar to hemoglobin. The synthesis of 2,3-BPG is enzymatically regulated, and its levels can change depending on the conditions extant. 2,3-BPG is able to bind stereospecifically within the central cavity of the hemoglobin tetramer. Hemoglobin prepared in the absence of 2,3-BPG has a very high oxygen affinity, but as 2,3-BPG is added to a hemoglobin solution, the oxygen affinity progressively decreases. 2,3-BPG is a polyanion that binds strongly to the deoxygenated form of hemoglobin but poorly to its oxygenated or other liganded forms. Specific amino acids are involved in the binding of 2,3-BPG; these β-chain residues include the N-terminal valines, the H21 histidine (position 143), and the EF6 lysine (position 82). In oxyhemoglobin, the H helices of the β-chains are insufficiently spread to permit firm binding of 2,3-BPG; this, along with other conformational changes, favors the binding of this anion to the deoxygenated rather than the oxygenated form of hemoglobin. The binding of 2,3-BPG stabilizes the T (tense) structure of the deoxygenated form at the expense of the R (relaxed) structure of the oxyhemoglobin tetramer.

Transition from the deoxy (T) to the oxy (R) form of hemoglobin is accompanied by rotation of the αβ dimers along the α_1-β_2 contact region (Fig. 33–5). The T structure is stabilized by salt bridges, which are broken as the molecule switches into the R structure. Some abnormal hemoglobins with an intrinsically high oxygen affinity, or low P_{50}, occur as a result of an amino acid substitution that leads to loss of bonds that stabilize the tetramer in the T conformation. Hydrogen ions, chloride ions, and carbon dioxide all decrease the affinity of hemoglobin for oxygen by strengthening the salt bridges that lock the molecule into its T conformation. The corollary of the lowering of hemoglobin oxygen affinity by protons is the combination of hemoglobin with protons on deoxygenation. This is known as the Bohr effect and is responsible for carbon dioxide transport in blood, another critical function of the hemoglobin molecule. Deoxyhemoglobin binds the hydrogen ion liberated by the reaction of carbon dioxide with water, increasing the concentration of bicarbonate. Within the lungs, hydrogen ions are lost as hemoglobin binds oxygen; therefore, carbon dioxide leaves solution and is excreted from the body through the lungs. Deoxyhemoglobin can also directly bind carbon dioxide; however, this process involves the minority of carbon dioxide exchanged by the red blood cells.

Red blood cells containing high levels of hemoglobin F have high oxygen affinity because it binds 2,3-BPG poorly. Physiologically, this predicts that the hemoglobin of the fetus should be oxygenated at the expense of the maternal hemoglobin A. The high oxygen affinity of hemoglobin F is accounted for by a single change in its primary structure, the presence of a serine residue at helical position H21 in place of the histidine found in the β-globin chain. This weakens the binding of 2,3-BPG and leads to stabilization of the molecule in its R state.

Interactions of hemoglobin with NO have been a recent focus of investigation. NO, generated from L-arginine by nitric oxide synthases, activates soluble guanylate cyclase to produce the second messenger cyclic guanosine monophosphate (cGMP). As a potent vasodilator, NO is an important regulator of vascular tone. The

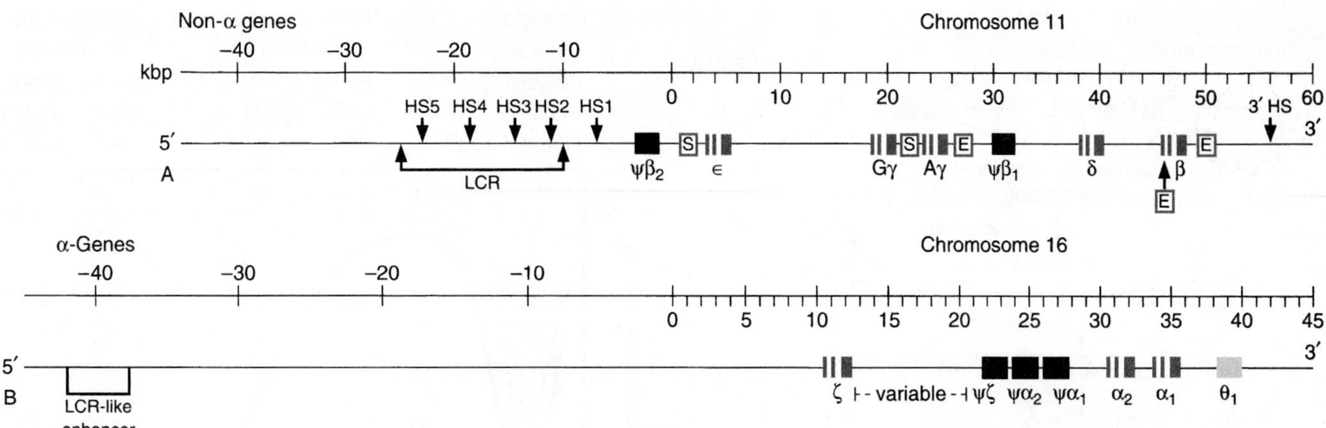

Figure 33–6. Maps of the β-like and α-like globin gene clusters located on chromosome 11 (**A**) and chromosome 16 (**B**). Within each gene cluster are pseudogenes, which are remnants of previously expressed globin genes that have become inactivated as a result of mutation. Active genes are shown in *red boxes* filled with clear introns; inactive or pseudogenes genes are shown in *solid boxes*, and the θ-globin gene is shown as a *pink box*. Although this gene is transcribed, it is not clear whether it is represented in a cellular protein. The distance between the functional ζ-globin and pseudo-ζ-globin gene is variable because of the presence of repeated elements. E, enhancer; HS, DNase hypersensitive site; LCR, locus control region; S, silencer.

reaction of free NO with erythrocytes is diffusion-limited. Normally, the primary NO-hemoglobin adduct is nitrosyl (heme) hemoglobin (HbFe[II]NO). Within the erythrocyte, β93 cysteine is reduced and seems incapable of NO storage and delivery by *S*-nitrosohemoglobin as originally proposed. NO was thought to form *S*-nitrosylhemoglobin in the lungs, where hemoglobin is in its R or oxygenated state, and liberate NO in the microcirculation, where the transition of the R to T conformation induced by deoxygenation released NO from hemoglobin. However, studies suggest that NO binding to heme groups is physiologically a rapidly reversible process. This view supports a model of hemoglobin delivery of NO distinct from its dissociation from the β93 cysteine residues. Small nitrosothiol molecules could also be involved in NO transfer. The thiol groups of hemoglobin can exchange NO with small nitrosothiols derived from free cysteine and glutathione. Accordingly, the thiol groups of hemoglobin could bind and transfer NO or exchange NO with small shuttle molecules, increasing perfusion of hypoxic tissues. It has been suggested that cytoskeletal and other erythrocyte proteins slow NO influx into the cell and, coupled with NO heme binding, preserve NO bioactivity. NO-hemoglobin interactions, whether through *S*-nitrosohemoglobin formation at the β93 cysteine or the formation of nitrosointermediates are likely to be physiologically important. Hemoglobin liberated from the intravascularly hemolyzed red cells rapidly inactivates NO. As the red cell lyses, arginase is also released and destroys the substrate for NO synthases, L-arginine. Together, this leads to a reduction in biologically active NO. With hemolysis as in sickle cell disease or thalassemia, reduced NO bioavailability is associated with disease complications such as pulmonary hypertension, leg ulcers, priapism, and perhaps increased risk of stroke. Lactic dehydrogenase also released from the red cell in hemolytic anemia is an excellent marker of these complications.

In summary, the primary amino acid structure of α- and non–α-globin chains dictates the inevitable quaternary structure in which resides the ability of hemoglobin to serve as a respiratory protein. Cooperativity ensures rapid binding of oxygen in the lungs and unloading in tissues. Similarly, carbon dioxide is transported from tissues to lungs. The function of hemoglobin may be influenced by mutation and by heterotropic effectors such as protons and 2,3-BPG. The molecule itself changes shape as it provides oxygen for metabolism; it is a lung in miniature, breathing as it allows the body to respire.

Globin Gene Clusters

The amounts and types of human hemoglobin produced at any given age are determined primarily by the selective expression of the individual genes encoding each globin chain. The globin genes of humans are located in two clusters (Fig. 33–6): α-like genes in approximately 30 kb of DNA on the short arm of chromosome 16 between band p13.2 and the telomere and β-like genes in approximately 70 kb of DNA on the terminal portion of the short arm of chromosome 11 (p15). Each gene shares certain basic organizational features. Each contains three exons separated by two introns. Both introns of the α-gene are small (100 to 300 bp); non–α-genes have one small and one large (1000 to 1200 bp) intron. The second exon of each globin gene encodes the major components of the heme-binding pocket, and the third encodes the α- and non-α contact points.

Flanking each gene at the 5′ and 3′ ends are groups of conserved nucleotides. In conjunction with protein factors, these influence the promotion of gene transcription, ensure the fidelity of the transcript and its translatability, specify sites for the initiation and termination of translation, and improve the stability of the newly synthesized mRNA (Fig. 33–7). Also encoded within the genes are signals that permit the enzymatic machinery within the nucleus to excise precisely the introns from the mRNA precursor and splice together the exons to form a contiguous “mature” mRNA. The spliced mRNA is transported to the cytoplasm and translated into protein. These conserved signals lie at the junction of the exon and intron and within the introns themselves. They are recognized by small nuclear ribonucleoprotein (RNP) particles, which participate in the formation of a spliceosome, or splicing complex. Their preservation is critical for the splicing process to occur. When mutations occur within splice signal sites, globin synthesis is often impaired. The 5′ end of the mRNA contains a cap structure, and the 3′ end contains a poly(A) tail, as described in Chapter 1.

Conserved nucleotide clusters 5′ to the coding portion of each globin gene in aggregate act as promoters (see Fig. 33–7). Globin promoters are modular. Some modules are located relatively close to the initiation site of mRNA translation, and some are more distally placed. Promoters ultimately form the binding sites for the RNA polymerase complexes that catalyze gene transcription. Mutations within the promoter can affect the level of gene transcription and the amount of globin made. Surrounding and within each gene are other sequence elements that play important roles in its transcriptional

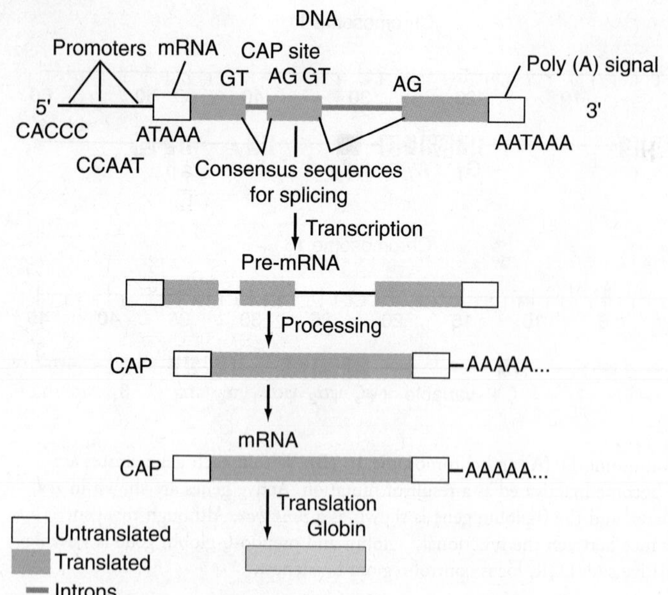

Figure 33–7. Pathway of globin biosynthesis. Transcription of the globin gene results in a large pre-mRNA molecule containing intervening sequences. During intranuclear processing of this molecule, the intervening sequences are excised and the coding sequences ligated to form a contiguous stretch of RNA, which codes for the globin protein. The message is further processed by the addition of a CAP and a poly(A) tail. The mature message is transported from the nucleus to cytoplasm, where it is translated on polyribosomes by the addition of activated amino acids to a growing polypeptide chain. Globin acquires heme and α: non-α dimers are formed and a hemoglobin tetramer is assembled. *(From Steinberg, MH: Hemoglobinopathies and thalassemias. In Stein JH [ed]: Internal Medicine, 4th ed. St. Louis, Mosby-Year Book, 1994, p 852.)*

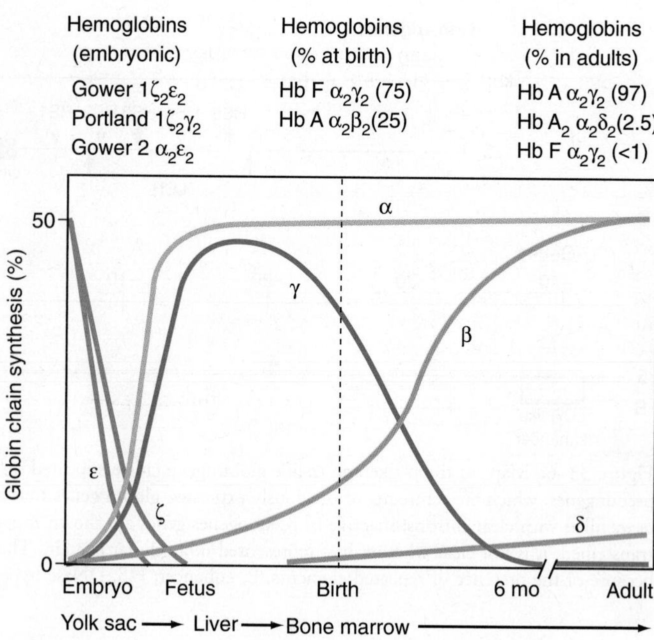

Figure 33–8. Hemoglobin (Hb) switching during embryonic, fetal, and adult development. The ζ and ε genes are transcribed during embryonic development and are soon replaced by the fetal γ- and adult α-globin gene. At birth, fetal hemoglobin (HbF) forms approximately 75% and hemoglobin A forms 25% of the total. Transcription of the γ gene begins to decrease before birth, and by 6 months of age, this gene is expressed only at very low levels. Expression of the δ-globin gene begins near birth. In adults, hemoglobin A makes up approximately 97%, hemoglobin A_2 approximately 2.5%, and HbF less than 1% of the total. *(From Steinberg MH: Hemoglobinopathies and thalassemias. In Stein JH [ed]: Internal Medicine, 4th ed. St. Louis, Mosby-Year Book, 1994, p 852.)*

regulation (see Fig. 33–6). These clusters, called *enhancers* and *silencers* (see Chapter 1) may lie within introns or 5′ and 3′ to the coding sequences; in some instances, they are quite remote from the gene. The higher-order structure of DNA in chromatin may permit close approximation of these remote enhancers to the gene during transcription. Enhancers play important roles in the tissue-specific regulation of globin gene expression. Representative regulatory sequences near the globin genes are shown in Fig. 33–6 (locus control region [LCR], LCR-like enhancer). DNA elements controlling globin genes are described in more detail later.

The α-like and β-like globin genes are ordered in the 5′ to 3′ direction in the same sequence expressed during embryonic, fetal, and adult development (Fig. 33–8). The functional significance of this arrangement is unclear. However, evidence suggests that the ordering of the ε, γ, δ, and β genes could be an important factor influencing the ability of each locus to interact with distant control elements at different developmental stages.

The α-like and β-like gene clusters probably are the result of an ancient duplication of a primordial globin gene that existed early in the history of vertebrates, approximately 500 million years ago. Each gene cluster probably developed from the duplication of ancestral genes and subsequent divergence through eons of evolution. Within the α-like gene cluster, the δ-globin gene is expressed only very early in embryogenesis and participates in the formation of embryonic hemoglobins. A μ, α-like globin gene (*HBM*), that codes for a 141 amino acid α-globin–like chain has been recently detected and is expressed in erythroid cells in a highly regulated fashion however, an associated protein has not been found.

The α-globin genes are duplicated, a characteristic of most globin genes, and their encoded amino acid sequences are identical; therefore, only a single α-globin polypeptide results. Minor differences within the second intervening sequence and the 3′ flanking regions of the α-globin gene permit identification of transcripts from each gene. The 5′ or α_2-gene is expressed more efficiently than the 3′ or α_1-gene, so that abnormalities of this gene are more likely to be clinically apparent. Both clusters contain genes that are actively transcribed, as well as pseudogenes whose defective structures prohibit expression at any time.

The gene 3′ to the α_1-gene is the θ-gene, a somewhat mysterious element of the α-gene cluster. Although θ-gene transcripts are found in fetal tissue and adult erythroid marrow, it is unclear whether this gene's translation product is able to participate in the formation of a functional tetramer. The θ-globin protein has been found in vivo, but deletion of the θ-globin gene does not appear to have any implications for the developing fetus. In vitro, θ-globin mRNA is correctly spliced, and θ-globin cDNA can direct synthesis of a translatable mRNA and a θ-globin protein.

The β-like–globin gene cluster consists of the embryonic ε-gene, transcribed only during the first 6 to 11 weeks of life; the duplicated γ-globin genes that code for the dominant non–α-globin of fetal life; and the δ- and β-globin genes that code for the hemoglobins of the adult. The coding sequences of the two γ-globin genes are identical, except at codon 136, where the 5′ or Gγ-gene codes for glutamic acid; the 3′ or Aγ-gene encodes an alanine residue. These genes are unequally expressed during fetal development. A switch in their relative rates of expression leads to a similar disparity between the amounts of Gγ and Aγ chains in adults. Although the Gγ/Aγ switch is interesting from the standpoint of the control of gene expression, it is of little clinical importance. Hemoglobin F in the fetus and the adult contains a mixture of Gγ and Aγ chains; the functional qualities of these hemoglobins are identical.

The δ- and β-globin genes are probably the result of a duplication event that occurred more than 40 million years ago. The β-globin gene has become the predominant gene, coding for most non–α-globin chains of the adult. The δ-globin gene has undergone mutation in several critical areas, and its expression is greatly curtailed. Its product, a minor fraction of adult hemoglobin (HbA_2), has become functionally insignificant by virtue of its very low level in the erythrocyte. It is likely that the δ-globin gene is a "pseudogene in evolution." HbA_2 is clinically useful however, for characterizing hemoglobinopathies such as β-thalassemia. In time, its expression may be totally abolished as it acquires an inactivating mutation. The pseudogenes dispersed within both globin gene clusters provide interesting glimpses into the evolutionary history of globin genes. Pseudogenes are inactive remnants of previously expressed genes. As a result of relaxed selection, their mutation rates are higher than those of surrounding active genes.

The expression of the human globin genes is highly regulated. Globin is synthesized in only one tissue—erythroid cells—and only during a narrowly defined stage of erythroid progenitor cell differentiation—the 5 to 7 days that commence with the proerythroblast stage and end when the enucleated reticulocyte loses the last traces of its RNA. Within the confines of these strict tissue-specific and differentiation stage-specific boundaries, the globin genes are extraordinarily active. By the late normoblast and reticulocyte stages, 90% to 95% of all protein synthesis in these cells is globin synthesis.

Individual globin genes are expressed at different levels in developing erythroblasts of the human embryo, fetus, and "adult" (ie, 37 to 38 weeks of gestation and beyond). Different subsets of α- and non–α-genes are expressed and silenced at each developmental stage. Moreover, the overall balance of non–α-globin, α-globin, and heme production is maintained throughout each of these complex switching events. The complex mechanisms ensuring the proper tissue-specific, differentiation stage-specific, and ontologic stage-specific expression are incompletely defined. Much information about relevant DNA control elements and transcription factors is emerging. These topics are discussed after a review of the ontogeny of hemoglobin.

Ontogeny of Hemoglobin

The hemoglobin composition of the erythrocyte depends on when in gestation or postnatal development it is measured. This is a result of sequential activation and inactivation (i.e., switching) among genes within the α- and non–α-globin gene clusters (see Fig. 33–8). What controls these switches in globin gene transcription is not understood. The two early embryonic hemoglobins consist of ζ- and ε-globin chains (Hb Gower-1) and α- and ε-globin chains (Hb Gower-2). The ζ-globin gene is akin to the α-globin genes but is expressed only during early embryogenesis. The ε-embryonic globin chain is a β-like element. The combination of ζ- and γ-globin chains forms hemoglobin Portland. These early hemoglobins are made primarily in yolk-sac erythroblasts and are detectable only during the very earliest stages of embryogenesis except in certain pathologic states, in which they may persist until gestation is complete. The major hemoglobin of intrauterine life is fetal hemoglobin (HbF), which consists of two α- and two γ-globin chains. Expression of the γ-globin gene begins early in embryogenesis, peaks during midgestation, and begins a rapid decline just before birth. By 6 months of age in normal infants, only a remnant of prior γ-globin gene expression remains. The level of HbF in the blood declines rapidly thereafter to less than 1% of the total. Expression of the α-globin gene starts early in the first trimester, peaks quickly, and is sustained for life. Expression of the β-globin gene also commences early in gestation and reaches its zenith within a few months after birth. The combination of α-globin with β-globin chains forms hemoglobin A (HbA) the predominant hemoglobin of postnatal life. Adult cells also contain Hb-A_2. The δ-globin gene, which directs synthesis of the non–α-globin chain of HbA_2, is very inefficiently expressed. Only low levels of HbA_2 are present; defects in the δ-globin gene are of no clinical consequence. In adult blood, HbF is not evenly distributed among erythrocytes and is present in only a very small number of red blood cells, called *F cells*. HbA_2 is present in all red blood cells, albeit at levels less than 3.5% of the total hemoglobin in adult life.

Hemoglobin Biosynthesis and Its Regulation

Throughout development, genes coding for α-globin, non–α-globin, and heme exhibit coordinated expression. Almost equal amounts of each of the moieties that ultimately constitute the hemoglobin tetramer are made. Excess unpaired globin chains and mutant globins are removed from the cell by ATP-dependent proteases, ensuring a balance between accumulation of α- and non–α-globin chains. Balanced chain synthesis and coordination of globin chain production with synthesis of heme are important because hemoglobin tetramers are highly soluble, whereas the components of hemoglobin (ie, unpaired chains, protoporphyrin, and iron) are not. Precipitation of any of these is deleterious to cell survival. Erythroblast proteases are not efficient enough to eliminate the substantial excesses of unpaired chains that accumulate when an α- or non–α-gene is selectively impaired by severe thalassemia mutations. The mechanisms regulating heme production and some of the interactions between heme and globin synthesis are discussed in Chapter 38.

The proper production of the individual globin chains within erythroid tissues at the appropriate states of differentiation and development is predominantly ensured by regulation at the level of transcription. The onset of phenotypic maturation at the proerythroblast stage is marked by the onset of globin mRNA biosynthesis in dramatically increasing quantities. Expression of α- and non–α-globin genes begins at essentially the same time, although some studies suggest a slightly earlier onset for α-globin gene expression. Transcription persists at a high level throughout most of the remainder of erythropoiesis, declines as the nucleus condenses, and is eventually lost in late erythroblasts. Even as the absolute rates of globin gene transcription begin to decrease, however, the relative percentage of total transcriptional activity devoted to globin gene expression continues to increase; this reflects the silencing of transcription of almost every other gene in the erythroblast.

The transcriptional activation of the globin genes is the major event that must be understood to define and manipulate the regulation of hemoglobin biosynthesis and hemoglobin switching. However, posttranscriptional mechanisms contribute to the final distribution of globin and nonglobin mRNAs and to the balance of α- and non–α-globins within the erythroblasts. When compared with many other mRNAs, such as cytokine mRNAs, globin mRNAs are extraordinarily stable. Their half-lives have been estimated at 30 to 50 hours. Most other mRNAs have turnover rates, or half-lives, measured within the range of a few minutes to 5 or 6 hours. The increase in the percentage of total mRNA that is globin mRNA is greatly accentuated because the newly transcribed globin mRNAs accumulate and remain quite stable in the cell, whereas nonglobin mRNAs, which are no longer being produced, are also disappearing at a faster rate. Consequently, the mRNA content of the reticulocytes consists of 90% to 95% globin mRNA.

The transcription rates of the α- and non–α-globin genes are not precisely equal. (This phenomenon has been studied in detail only in adult erythroid cells expressing the α- and β-globin genes.) A slight, but reproducibly detectable, excess of α-globin mRNA is present in erythroblasts. However, β-globin mRNA is translated somewhat more efficiently than α-globin mRNA. These counterbalancing forces result in almost equal syntheses of α- and β-globin polypeptide chains. There is a very slight excess of α-globin production, resulting in a small pool of free α-globin chains.

Alpha hemoglobin-stabilizing protein (AHSP), a small protein present at high concentrations in red cells, binds specifically to the α-globin polypeptide protecting the unstable free α-globin chain by inhibiting heme loss, and oxidant-mediated chain precipitation. It remains unclear whether mutations of this protein can modify the phenotype of β-thalassemia by increasing the imbalance in globin chain synthesis. Some α-globin chain variants, because the mutations alter AHSP binding, are associated with mild thalassemia-like features.

Newly synthesized β-globin chains are rapidly and completely incorporated into αβ dimers, that spontaneously associate as tetramers. Hemoglobin tetramers are remarkably stable throughout the life span of the circulating red blood cell by virtue of their long half-lives. Only small amounts suffer oxidative or proteolytic damage.

Hemoglobin molecules are exposed for prolonged periods to chemically active compounds in the milieu of the bloodstream. They often become nonenzymatically modified by such processes as glycosylation, acetylation, and sulfation. Glycosylation occurs more extensively during periods of hyperglycemia and leads to elevated levels of the glycosylated form of HbA, HbA_{1c}. This phenomenon is the basis of a useful test for control of the blood sugar in diabetics. Other posttranslational modifications are of little clinical importance, except as already noted for 2,3-BPG, carbon dioxide (CO_2), and NO.

Transcriptional Regulation of Globin Gene Expression

Precise regulation of the globin gene clusters involves a complex interplay between *trans*-acting proteins, such as transcription factors, and *cis*-acting sequences that act as promoters, enhancers, and silencers of gene activity. DNA-binding proteins interact with sequences in regulatory regions of the globin gene cluster and with other proteins through specific protein-protein interactions, forming DNA-protein complexes that regulate gene transcription. Chapter 21 provides background information about the basic features and properties of transcription factors. *Trans*-acting factors mediate the remodeling of chromatin structure, influencing gene expression for the entire globin gene clusters. Mutations in the *cis*-acting sequences or *trans*-acting proteins cause dysregulated expression of globin genes, resulting in thalassemia-like syndromes. Elucidating the full extent of sequences required for appropriate expression of globin genes will inform the development of constructs for gene therapy.

Requisite for the expression of the globin genes is a local chromatin structure that supports transcription. "Open" chromatin, or (EO) euchromatin, generally appears cytogenetically uncondensed and is associated with hyperacetylated histones, unmethylated CpG dinucleotides, and active transcription. ATRX is a protein that has been implicated in the modulation of chromatin structure at the α-globin locus. Mutations in the *ATRX* gene, located on the X chromosome, cause a syndrome of α-thalassemia, severe mental retardation, facial dysmorphism, and urogenital abnormalities. ATRX, a member of the SNF2 family of helicase/ATPases, localizes to pericentromeric heterochromatin during interphase and mitosis and contains a plant homeodomain (PHD)-like domain that is found in chromatin-associated proteins. Cells with a mutated *ATRX* gene have altered patterns of DNA methylation. The ATRX protein therefore exemplifies the connections between DNA methylation, chromatin remodeling, and expression of the α-globin genes.

Chromatin structure can be manipulated pharmacologically through the influence of drugs on methylation and histone acetylation. Cytidine analogs such as 5-azacytidine and its less toxic derivative, decitabine, inactivate DNA methyltransferases, inducing γ-globin gene expression and increasing HbF levels in patients with sickle cell anemia. Histone deacetylase inhibitors such as butyric acid are being studied as agents to increase γ-globin expression.

The regions of the globin gene clusters with essential regulatory sequences and erythroid-specific chromatin remodeling extend far beyond the coding sequences of the globin genes. The key regulatory element for the α-globin gene (HS −40) lies in an erythroid-specific DNase I hypersensitive site 40 kb from the α-globin gene. The LCR is critical for high level expression of the β-globin gene cluster, consisting of five sites that are hypersensitive to DNase I (HS 1–5) (see Chapter 1). Patients with deletion of the HS −40 site exhibit α-thalassemia, and patients with deletions of the β-globin LCR develop β-thalassemia; however, the thalassemia can be a result of changes in chromatin caused by the large deletion. Similarly, transgenic mice bearing deletions of these critical regulatory regions have severely restricted expressions of the respective globin genes.

Mini-chromosome constructs, in which globin genes are attached directly to the LCR in the absence of most intervening DNA sequences, are expressed at rates approaching those of endogenous globin genes in cultured erythroid cells and transgenic mice. Some nonglobin genes are also expressed at very high levels in erythroid cells when attached to these LCR sequences. The LCRs contain binding sites for the major erythroid transcription factors, GATA1 and NFE2, as well as sites for transcription factors found more widely distributed in many cell types. One site in the β-globin LCR is believed to act as an insulating element, which protects expressed genes from gene silencing through the regulation of chromatin structure. The interrelationships among the LCR and individual promoters, enhancers, and silencers during erythroid differentiation and hemoglobin switching remain incompletely understood despite extraordinary experimental scrutiny. The LCR might have its effects by multiple mechanisms that include chromatin looping between the enhancer and promoters, by tracking or scanning along chromatin until a competent promoter is encountered, a combination of the two mechanisms or by binding of facilitator proteins between an enhancer and its cognate gene defining an activation domain. Modification of chromatin histones by acetylation and other mechanisms might determine which genes are activated by the LCR.

The LCR is unquestionably essential for the quantitatively high rates of β-globin gene expression during erythroid differentiation. The role of the LCR in dictating tissue specificity (ie, shutdown of globin gene expression in other tissues) or the sequential activation of silencing of genes during hemoglobin switching is less clear. Studies suggest that tissue specificity and qualitatively proper switching of γ- and β-globin gene expression in transgenic mice could be obtained with DNA constructs lacking the LCR. However, these genes were invariably expressed only 0.5% to 5% as actively as the endogenous globin genes of the host cell. The degree and fidelity of tissue-specific expression also appeared to depend on several factors, such as the site of transgene integration.

Shutdown of the embryonic genes late in the first trimester and, possibly, the decline of γ-gene expression during the perinatal period may also require the participation of active silencing mechanisms. The predominance of β-globin gene expression over γ-gene expression in adult life is not merely the result of preferential stimulation of β-gene expression. Active repression of the γ-genes may also be relevant; these mechanisms, if they exist, may have to be reversed to manipulate hemoglobin switching therapeutically.

The nuclei of erythroid cells contain numerous proteins that have been identified as transcription factors. Many of these are found in a wide variety of tissues. At least two factors, GATA1 and NFE2, are much more restricted in their ranges of expression and have been implicated as particularly important for globin gene expression. Mutations in GATA1 or its required coactivating protein (FOG1, also known as ZFPM1) can cause β-thalassemia and thrombocytopenia in patients.

GATA1 is named on the basis of the DNA sequence motif (T/A) GATA (A/G), the GATA motif that it recognizes and binds. It is a zinc finger class DNA-binding protein (see Chapter 21). GATA1 has been shown to activate promoters containing the cognate DNA sequence motif, even when placed in nonerythroid cells. Activity of GATA1 requires binding to a zinc finger protein cofactor called FOG1 (named for Friend of GATA1, but renamed ZFPM1 for zinc finger protein, multitype 1). NFE2 recognizes the DNA sequence motif (T/C) GCT GA (C/G) TCA (T/C). It is a member of the B-zip class of transcriptional activators. GATA1 and NFE2 were originally identified and cloned on the basis of their interactions with their cognate sequences in the globin genes. Initially, each was thought to be present only in erythroid cells. However, further work has demonstrated that each protein has a wider range of tissue expression. For example, GATA1 is also present in other hematopoietic cell lineages, whereas NFE2 consists of two subunits, one that is widely expressed and one that is expressed in several hematopoietic lineages and the intestine. Erythroid Kruppel-like factor (EKLF, also called KLF1) may be the most specific of the erythroid transcription factors yet discovered. EKLF interacts specifically with the β-globin gene promoter and may influence the γ-β switch. Mice homozygous for disruption of the EKLF gene have lethal β-thalassemia.

Neither GATA1, NFE2, EKLF, nor FOG1 alone can be the sole determination of tissue specificity of the globin genes; otherwise, globin gene expression should occur at some level in other tissues in which these proteins are present. However, there is no doubt that each of these proteins is indispensable for globin gene expression and erythropoiesis. Gene knock-out studies have shown that absence of each protein results in greatly impaired erythropoiesis. Several other proteins have been identified as binding to various control elements in the globin gene cluster. Some of these appear to be stage-specific selector elements that bind predominantly to the γ- or β-globin gene enhancers and promoters. Others are generic transcription factors. Regulation at these sites is probably hierarchic, depending on the appropriate combination of DNA-binding proteins, the types of proteins that interact with them, and the activation state of the bound proteins through such processes as ribosylation and phosphorylation. It is also possible that the same sequence element may interact with different combinational sets of proteins, with a different resulting effect on transcriptional activity, depending on the stage of differentiation and embryonic, fetal, or adult development.

The precise molecular machinery necessary for regulation of transcription of individual globin genes is beginning to be defined. The globin genes are also subject to regulation by cellular, microenvironmental, and humoral influences affecting the proliferation and differentiation state of primitive erythroid stem cells in yolk sac, fetal liver, or bone marrow. Overwhelming evidence supports the hypothesis that the potential for expression of γ- or β-genes, or both, is determined in primitive erythroid stem cells (ie, BFU-E) long before actual expression of the globin genes is initiated at a later stage of differentiation. The relative percentage of maturing erythroblasts that will ultimately express HbF or HbA, or both, can be altered by factors such as cytotoxic drugs or bone marrow stress that alter the relative percentages of HbF-potent or HbA-potent stem cells undergoing cell cycle events, differentiation, and so forth. Drugs used to manipulate HbF switching seem to work primarily through these cellular mechanisms (see Chapter 25).

Posttranscriptional, Translational, and Posttranslational Mechanisms

Processed globin mRNA is exported from the nucleus to the cytoplasm by a mechanism that is not clearly defined. mRNA translation occurs in the cytoplasm (see Fig. 33–7). The triplet codons or mRNA are recognized by the anticodons of specific tRNAs that bring activated amino acid residues to the nascent polypeptide chains. The process of translation, in which an mRNA template directs the synthesis of protein, is typically divided into three phases: initiation, elongation, and termination (see Chapter 1). Each phase is regulated by a variety of protein factors.

The globin mRNA molecule becomes associated with four to six ribosomes, forming the polyribosome. At least 11 eukaryotic translation initiation factors interact with the polyribosome. They mediate stabilization of a preinitiation complex, binding of the initiator methionine tRNA to ribosomal subunits, binding of mRNA to the preinitiation complex, stabilization of mRNA binding, recognition of the cap site at the 5′ end of mRNA, and release of initiation factors from the preinitiation complex. Several elongation and termination factors have also been defined. Initiation or an early step in the elongation process is the rate-limiting factor.

The first posttranslational step in tetramer formation is the combination of α- and non–α-globin chains to form dimers, an event that appears to depend on the relative charge of each globin subunit. The dimers then form tetrameric hemoglobin. Because of charge differences among non–α-globin chains, there is a hierarchy or affinity of these chains for α-globin chains. The combination of α- and β-globin chains is most favored, followed by a combination of α-, γ-, and δ-globin chains. Certain mutant hemoglobins that have gained or lost a charge may alter this hierarchic arrangement. This may influence the proportion of variant hemoglobin present, especially when the patient also inherits an α-thalassemia syndrome, in which the synthesis of α-globin chains is reduced. The supply of available α-globin chains is then limited, and non–α-globin chains compete with one another to form tetramers with the limiting α-globin chain pool.

Globin chain biosynthesis and heme synthesis are mutually important. Heme plays a role in the regulation of the initiation complex. A deficiency of heme (eg, in iron deficiency) is associated with the accumulation of a repressor of translation initiation factors. Translation of β-globin mRNA appears to be initiated more efficiently than α-globin mRNA, conferring on the associated anemia some of the features of mild α-thalassemia. This phenomenon occurs

Table 33–1. Classification of Hemoglobinopathies and Thalassemias

Structural hemoglobinopathies—mutations altering the amino acid sequence of a globin chain and altering physical or chemical properties of the hemoglobin tetramer in such a way that function is deranged
Abnormal hemoglobin (Hb) polymerization—sickle cell hemoglobin (HbS); hemolysis, vasoocclusion
Abnormal hemoglobin crystallization (eg, HbC)
High oxygen affinity—polycythemia (Hb Zurich)
Low oxygen affinity—cyanosis (Hb Kansas)
Hemoglobins that oxidize or precipitate too readily—unstable hemoglobins (Hb Köln)
M hemoglobins—methemoglobinemia, cyanosis (eg, Hb Milwaukee)
Thalassemia—defective production of globin chains with hypochromia, anemia, hemolysis, altered erythropoiesis
α-Thalassemia
β-Thalassemia
δβ-Thalassemias, γδβ-thalassemias, αβ-thalassemias
"Thalassemic" hemoglobinopathies and dominantly inherited thalassemias—mutations altering the synthesis and structure or function of the hemoglobin gene products (eg, HbE, Hb Terre Haute, Hb Lepore, Hb Constant Spring)
Hereditary persistence of fetal hemoglobin—persistence of high levels of fetal hemoglobin (HbF) into adult life
Pancellular—high HbF levels in all red blood cells
Nondeletion forms
Deletion forms
Hb Kenya
Heterocellular—inherited increases in the percentage of F cells
Acquired hemoglobinopathies
Methemoglobinemia caused by toxic exposures
Sulfhemoglobinemia caused by toxic exposures
Carboxyhemoglobinemia caused by toxic exposures
HbH in erythroleukemias
Acquired elevations in F cells and HbF
Erythroid stress (eg, recovery from bone marrow suppression)
Bone marrow dysplasias
Exposure to agents altering stem cells or gene expression (eg, hydroxyurea, butyric acid)

because heme deficiency depresses the availability of initiating factors for which the less efficient α-mRNA must compete with the more efficient β-mRNA.

NOSOLOGY OF HEMOGLOBINOPATHIES

Inherited abnormalities of the hemoglobin molecules that cause morbidity are called *hemoglobinopathies* and *thalassemias*. Many of these conditions produce diseases (eg, sickle cell anemia, thalassemia, unstable hemoglobins, M hemoglobins) that are especially important to hematologists. A few acquired conditions lead to modifications of hemoglobin (eg, carbon monoxide exposure, producing carboxyhemoglobinemia, nitrite exposure causing methemoglobinemia) that produce clinical abnormalities. These situations are summarized by the term *acquired hemoglobinopathies* or *dyshemoglobinemias*.

Most of the more than 1200 mutations of the globin gene that have been described produce no disease or only trivial clinical effects. The remainder can be classified according to the hematologic and clinical phenotypes that cause reduced solubility with hemolytic anemia (unstable hemoglobins and polymerizing hemoglobins, such as sickle hemoglobin), hemoglobins with altered oxygen affinity, hemoglobins predisposing to methemoglobin formation, and the thalassemias involving abnormal synthesis of one or more globin chains with anemia, hemolysis, and alterations of erythropoiesis. Some mutations, such as that responsible for HbE, can alter the structure and synthesis of the molecule. A classification of hemoglobinopathies and thalassemias is provided in Table 33–1. Individual conditions are discussed in the chapters already cross-referenced in earlier sections of this chapter.

SUGGESTED READINGS

Bank A: Regulation of human fetal hemoglobin: New players, new complexities. Blood 107(2):435, 2006.

Boas FE, Forman L, Beutler E: Phosphatidylserine exposure and red cell viability in red cell aging and in hemolytic anemia. Proc Natl Acad Sci U S A 95:3077, 1998.

Burgess-Beusse B, Farrell C, Gaszner M, et al: The insulation of genes from external enhancers and silencing chromatin. Proc Natl Acad Sci U S A 99(Suppl 4):16433, 2002.

Cantor AB, Orkin SH: Transcriptional regulation of erythropoiesis: An affair involving multiple partners. Oncogene 21(21):3368, 2002.

Chakalova L, Carter D, Debrand E, et al: Developmental regulation of the beta-globin gene locus. Prog Mol Subcell Biol 38:183, 2005.

Chiu CH, Schneider H, Slightom JL, et al: Dynamics of regulatory evolution in primate β-globin gene clusters: *cis*-Mediated acquisition of simian gamma fetal expression patterns. Gene 205:47, 1997.

Dzierzak E: The emergence of definitive hematopoietic stem cells in the mammal. Curr Opin Hematol 12(3):197, 2005.

Feng L, Zhou S, Gu L, et al: Structure of oxidized alpha-haemoglobin bound to AHSP reveals a protective mechanism for haem. Nature 435(7042):697, 2005.

Gibbons RJ, Picketts DJ, Villard L, Higgs DR: Mutations in a putative global transcriptional regulator cause X-linked mental retardation with α-thalassemia (ATR-X syndrome). Cell 80:837, 1995.

Gladwin MT, Wang X, Reiter CD, et al: *S*-nitrosohemoglobin is unstable in the reductive erythrocyte environment and lacks O_2/NO-linked allosteric function. J Biol Chem 277:27818, 2002.

Gow AJ, Stamler JS: Reactions between nitric oxide and haemoglobin under physiological conditions. Nature 391:169, 1998.

Hardison R, Riemer C, Chui DH, et al: Electronic access to sequence alignments, experimental results, and human mutations as an aid to studying globin gene regulation. Genomics 47:429, 1998.

Higgs DR, Garrick D, Anguita E, et al: Understanding alpha-globin gene regulation: Aiming to improve the management of thalassemia. Ann N Y Acad Sci 1054:92, 2005.

Jenuwein T, Allis CD: Translating the histone code. Science 293:1074, 2001.

Kato GJ, McGowan V, Machado RF et al: Lactate dehydrogenase as a biomarker of hemolysis-associated nitric oxide resistance, priapism, leg ulceration, pulmonary hypertension, and death in patients with sickle cell disease. Blood 107(6):2279, 2006.

Kihm AJ, Kong Y, Hong W, et al: An abundant erythroid protein that stabilizes free alpha-haemoglobin. Nature 417:758, 2002.

Li Q, Peterson KR, Fang X, Stamatoyannopoulos G: Locus control regions. Blood 100:3077, 2002.

Miller IJ, Bieker JJ: A novel erythroid cell-specific murine transcription factor that binds to the CACCC element and is related to the Kruppel family of nuclear proteins. Mol Cell Biol 13:2776, 1993.

Rother RP, Bell L, Hillmen P, Gladwin MT: The clinical sequelae of intravascular hemolysis and extracellular plasma hemoglobin: A novel mechanism of human disease. JAMA 293(13):1653, 2005.

Stamatoyannopoulos G: Control of globin gene expression during development and erythroid differentiation. Exp Hematol 33(3):259, 2005.

Stamler JS, Jia L, Eu JP, et al: Blood flow regulation by *S*-nitrosohemoglobin in the physiological oxygen gradient. Science 276:2034, 1997.

Steinberg MH, Forget BG, Higgs DR, Nagel RL: Disorders of Hemoglobin: Genetics, Pathophysiology, and Clinical Management. Cambridge, Cambridge University Press, 2001.

Viprakasit V, Tanphaichitr VS, Chinchang W, et al: Evaluation of alpha hemoglobin stabilizing protein (AHSP) as a genetic modifier in patients with beta thalassemia. Blood 103(9):3296, 2004.

Walsh M, Lutz RJ, Cotter TG, O'Connor R: Erythrocyte survival is promoted by plasma and suppressed by a Bak-derived BH3 peptide that interacts with membrane-associated Bcl-X(L). Blood 99:3439, 2002.

Weatherall DJ, Clegg JB: The Thalassaemia Syndromes, 4th ed. Oxford, Blackwell Science Limited, 2001, p 818.

Weiss MJ, Zhou S, Feng L et al: Role of alpha-hemoglobin-stabilizing protein in normal erythropoiesis and beta-thalassemia. Ann N Y Acad Sci 1054:103, 2005.

CHAPTER 34

APPROACH TO ANEMIA IN THE ADULT AND CHILD

Peter W. Marks and Bertil Glader

Anemia is among the most common hematologic problems in both adults and children.[1–3] A systematic approach to the patient with anemia can rapidly lead to the appropriate diagnosis of the most common entities with minimal diagnostic testing. It also facilitates the specialized investigation necessary to identify some of the less commonly encountered congenital and acquired anemias.

OVERVIEW OF ERYTHROPOIESIS

Erythropoiesis is an orderly process that leads to the production of mature erythrocytes.[4] Proliferation and differentiation of stem cells in the bone marrow are driven by a variety of factors, most notably erythropoietin. Reticulocytes are ultimately released into the circulation (Fig. 34–1). Within one day, reticulocytes transition into mature red blood cells that circulate for 100 to 120 days, at which time they are removed from the circulation by macrophages in the spleen and other reticuloendothelial tissues.[5] Under normal conditions, the process is regulated such that an equivalent number of erythrocytes are produced to replace those lost through senescence. In the event of anemia (defined by a decline in the circulating red blood cell mass), decreased oxygen delivery to the kidney drives the production of erythropoietin, which then stimulates red blood cell production in the bone marrow (Fig. 34–2).[6] Provided that there is an adequate supply of folate, vitamin B_{12}, iron, and other nutrients, the marrow responds by increasing the production and release of erythrocytes into the circulation.[7]

MECHANISMS OF ANEMIA

In the setting of acute or chronic blood loss, increased red blood cell production occurs in response to erythropoietin, provided that adequate nutrients are present for the formation of new cells.[8] Aside from hemorrhage, anemias can be categorized as either hypoproliferative or hemolytic (hyperproliferative). Hypoproliferative anemias are due to impaired red blood cell production and often result from acquired nutritional deficiencies or systemic diseases. Hemolytic anemias may be either congenital or acquired, the former being more common in children and the latter in adults.[9]

Hypoproliferative Anemias

The inability to produce an adequate number of erythrocytes in response to the appropriate stimulus defines the hypoproliferative anemias. Nutritional deficiencies are the most common causes of hypoproliferative anemia worldwide and affect both adults and children (Table 34–1).[10] It is estimated that 4% of women in the United States between the ages of 20 and 49 years have iron deficiency anemia.[11] Other common causes include the anemia of acute or chronic inflammation[12,13] and the anemia of renal disease (essentially a deficiency in erythropoietin).[12] Hematologic malignancies and solid tumors infiltrating the bone marrow (myelophthisis) may be encountered in adults and, to a lesser extent, in children. Acquired and congenital red blood cell hypoplastic disorders frequently are encountered in children and much less so in adults.[14]

Hemolytic Anemias

The hemolytic anemias are a consequence of the premature destruction of erythrocytes and are due to a broad array of disorders that may be congenital or acquired (see Table 34–1).[15] Congenital causes of hemolytic anemia may lead to severe problems in early childhood (eg, β-thalassemia major, sickle cell anemia), or may remain silent until a stressor is encountered later in life, provoking a crisis (eg, glucose-6-phosphate dehydrogenase deficiency).[16] Alternatively, some hereditary hemolytic anemias may go unrecognized throughout much of childhood and adult life (eg, mild hereditary spherocytosis).[17] Acquired hemolytic anemias due to stem cell disorders (paroxysmal nocturnal hemoglobinuria) occur primarily in adults. Acquired hemolytic disorders resulting from immune dysregulation (autoimmune hemolytic anemia) and those caused by the mechanical destruction of the erythrocyte (microangiopathic hemolytic anemia) occur in both children and adults.[18,19]

NORMAL RED BLOOD CELL VALUES IN THE ADULT AND CHILD

Modern laboratory instruments provide a wealth of diagnostic information for interpretation.[20] Using these data thoughtfully in combination with information from review of the peripheral blood smear can often lead directly to the correct diagnosis without additional diagnostic testing.

It is important to recognize that the normal ranges for hemoglobin, hematocrit, and red blood cell indices are different for infants, children, and adults (Table 34–2).[21] In addition, with the aging process, modest changes in red blood cell mass occur in adults.[22,23] Knowledge of age- and sex-appropriate normal values is important in the evaluation of anemia. For instance, in healthy men, there is a modest decline in hemoglobin with age of about 1 g/dL between the ages of 70 and 88 years, in part due to the decreased production of androgens. Only a minimal decrease in hemoglobin occurs between these ages in healthy women (about 0.2 g/dL).[24] Physician awareness of the expected change in hemoglobin in older men and its relative stability in older women can help avoid unnecessary laboratory investigations in older men and correctly initiate further diagnostic evaluations in older women with mild anemia.

SYSTEMATIC APPROACH TO THE EVALUATION OF ANEMIA

The correct diagnosis of anemia can often be determined by combining a thorough history and physical examination with reviews of the complete blood cell count, reticulocyte count, and peripheral blood smear.

History and Physical Examination

Because anemia can be a primary disorder or secondary to other systemic processes, a careful history and physical examination will provide valuable insight into the potential cause. Fatigue often

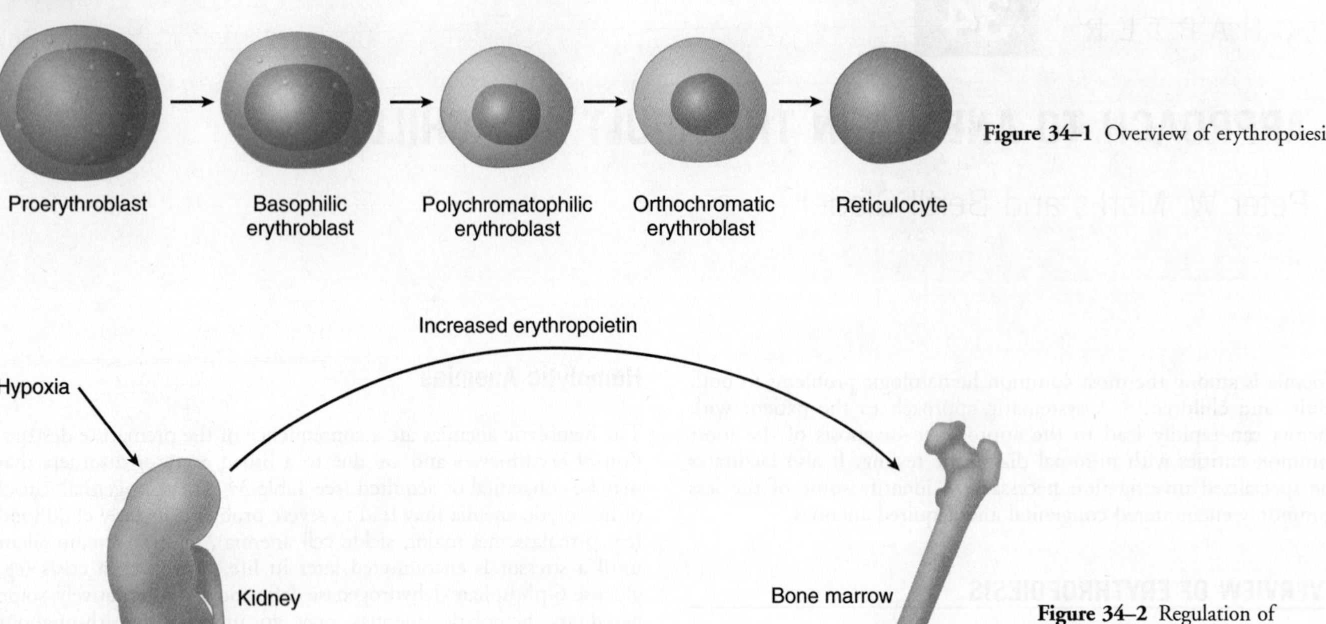

Figure 34–1 Overview of erythropoiesis.

Figure 34–2 Regulation of erythropoiesis.

Table 34–1 Common Causes of Newly Diagnosed Anemia

Iron deficiency
Acute or chronic inflammation
Renal disease
Folate or vitamin B_{12} deficiency
α- or β-thalassemia syndromes
Sickle cell disease
Enzymopathies (G6PD, others)
Hereditary spherocytosis
Autoimmune hemolytic anemia
Myelodysplastic syndromes
Myelophthisic processes
Leukemia
Congenital or acquired red cell aplasia

G6PD, glucose-6-phosphate dehydrogenase.

accompanies anemia, but it is very nonspecific and may be related to systemic illness. Nonetheless, determining the concomitant presence of a systemic inflammatory disorder, infection, or malignancy associated with fatigue may be critical in determining the underlying causes of anemia in both adults and children.[25] Past medical history may also be quite informative. For example, a history of diabetes mellitus can be associated with significantly impaired renal production of erythropoietin even in the setting of only a mildly elevated creatinine level.[26] Because certain medications may be associated with bone marrow depression or, alternatively, the development of autoimmune hemolytic anemia, all pharmacologic agents, prescribed and over-the-counter, including alternative medicines, should be reviewed.[27] Occupational history is occasionally relevant, as in the case of individuals, such as welders, who might have been exposed to lead or other potentially marrow toxic agents.[28,29] Social history can be important. Thus, a history of intravenous drug use might suggest the possibility of virally transmitted diseases, such as HIV, which may be associated with anemia.[30] Dietary history is very important, particularly in the young and the elderly with anemia. The finding of pica in adults (most commonly ice chips or cornstarch) is well known to be associated with iron deficiency anemia.[31] Ingestion of paint chips may suggest the need to investigate the possibility of toxic lead ingestion. Family history of anemia is particularly important in the evaluation of children with anemia. However, it is also relevant in adults because certain congenital anemias, such as hereditary spherocytosis, occasionally first become clinically apparent in adulthood.[32]

The significance of pallor on physical examination is in many ways similar to the historic feature of fatigue: it is a common but nonspecific finding. More specific findings may be found in certain types of anemias. For example, angular cheilitis (cracking at the edges of the lips) and koilonychia (spooning of the nails) may accompany iron deficiency anemia.[33] Splenomegaly may be present in patients with anemia arising from a wide variety of different causes.[34] When present early in life, it is suggestive of a congenital hemolytic anemia, such as thalassemia, sickle cell disease, or hereditary spherocytosis. When found for the first time later in life, splenomegaly may indicate an acquired disorder, such as autoimmune hemolytic anemia, lymphoproliferative disease, or agnogenic myeloid metaplasia. Other physical findings can also sometimes provide insight into the investigation of anemia when combined with historic features and laboratory data. Although anemia itself may lead to the presence of systolic cardiac murmurs, the finding of an increased cardiac murmur in an anemic patient with a prosthetic aortic valve and new microangiopathic change on peripheral smear may indicate that investigation into the possibility of perivalvular leak or prosthetic dysfunction is in order.[35] Finally, because neurologic manifestations can accompany or even predate the anemia associated with vitamin B_{12} deficiency, findings

Table 34–2 Normal Red Blood Cell Values

	Hemoglobin g/dL		Hematocrit (%)		Red Cell Count (10^{12}/L)		MCV (fL)		MCH (pg)		MCHC (g/dL)	
Age	***Mean***	***−2SD***	***Mean***	***−2SD***	***Mean***	***−2SD***	***Mean***	***−2SD***	***Mean***	***−2SD***	***Mean***	***−2SD***
Birth (cord blood)	16.5	13.5	51	42	4.7	3.9	108	98	34	31	33	30
1–3 days (capillary)	18.5	14.5	56	45	5.2	4.0	108	95	34	31	33	29
1 week	17.5	13.5	54	42	3.1	3.9	107	88	34	28	33	28
2 weeks	16.5	12.5	51	39	4.9	3.6	105	86	34	28	33	28
1 month	14.0	10.0	43	31	4.2	3.0	104	85	34	28	33	29
2 months	11.5	9.0	35	28	3.8	2.7	96	77	30	26	33	29
3–6 months	11.5	9.5	35	29	3.8	3.1	91	74	30	25	33	30
0.5–2 years	12.0	11.0	36	33	4.5	3.7	78	70	27	23	33	30
2–6 years	12.5	11.5	37	34	4.6	3.9	81	75	27	24	34	31
6–12 years	13.5	11.5	40	35	4.6	4.0	86	77	29	25	34	31
12–18 years												
Female	14.0	12.0	41	36	4.6	4.1	90	78	30	25	34	31
Male	14.5	13.0	43	37	4.9	4.5	88	78	30	25	34	31
18–49 years												
Female	14.0	12.0	41	36	4.6	4.0	90	80	30	26	34	31
Male	15.5	13.5	47	41	5.2	4.5	90	80	30	26	34	31

Data from Oski FA: Pallor. In Kaye R, Oski FA, Barness LA (eds): Core Textbook of Pediatrics, 3rd ed. Philadelphia, Lippincott, 1989, p 62.

such as loss of vibration or position sense in the extremities may be relevant.[36]

Reticulocyte Count

As a marker of red blood cell production, the reticulocyte count provides important information in directing the initial investigation of anemia. Modern flow cytometers accurately determine the reticulocyte count using fluorescent probes that bind to the residual ribonucleic acid present in newly released red blood cells.[37] These measurements are useful, are accurate, and reflect the state of erythropoiesis. However, when significant numbers of nucleated red blood cells or nuclear debris are present in the peripheral blood, this diagnostic accuracy declines, and manual counting methods are generally preferable.

When the reticulocyte count is reported as a percentage, it needs to be adjusted for the total number of red blood cells present. This correction can be made by multiplying the reticulocyte count by the patient's hematocrit divided by an age- and sex-appropriate normal hematocrit. No such correction is necessary when the reticulocyte count is reported as an absolute number or when it is converted to an absolute number by multiplying the percentage by the red blood cell number (in RBC/μL).

In the absence of anemia, the normal absolute reticulocyte count is between 25,000 and 75,000/μL. In the presence of anemia, an absolute reticulocyte count of less than 75,000/μL is indicative of a hypoproliferative process, whereas an absolute reticulocyte count of greater than 100,000/μL is indicative of hemolysis or an appropriate erythropoietic response (Table 34–3). Reticulocyte counts between 75,000 and 100,000/μL require interpretation in the context of other available clinical data including the severity of anemia present.

Table 34–3 Usefulness of the Reticulocyte Count in the Diagnosis of Anemia

Diagnosis	Value
Hypoproliferative anemias	***Absolute reticulocyte count <75,000/μl***
Anemia of chronic disease	
Anemia of renal disease	
Congenital dyserythropoietic anemias	
Effects of drugs or toxins	
Endocrine anemias	
Iron deficiency	
Marrow replacement	
Maturation abnormalities	***Absolute reticulocyte count <75,000/μl***
Vitamin B_{12} deficiency	
Folate deficiency	
Sideroblastic anemia	
Appropriate response to blood loss or nutritional supplementation	***Absolute reticulocyte count >100,000/μl***
Hemolytic anemias	
Hemoglobinopathies	
Immune hemolytic anemias	
Infectious causes of hemolysis	
Membrane abnormalities	
Metabolic abnormalities	
Mechanical hemolysis	

Mean Corpuscular Volume and Red Blood Cell Distribution Width

Automated cell counters provide a wealth of information regarding the size, shape, and hemoglobin content of red blood cells. The two parameters most useful in classifying anemia are the mean corpuscular volume (MCV) and the red blood cell distribution width (RDW). MCV is reported in femtoliters (fL) and reflects average cell size. RDW is a dimensionless quantity (actually the standard deviation of red blood cell volume divided by the mean volume) that reflects the variation in cell size in the population of red blood cells.[38] These parameters are useful because relatively reproducible changes in the MCV and RDW are associated with certain types of anemia (Table 34–4). Particularly when combined with the reticulocyte count, the MCV and RDW can significantly narrow the differential diagnosis (Table 34–5).

Examination of the Peripheral Blood Smear

Despite the availability of automated cell counters and sophisticated diagnostic testing, review of a well-made peripheral blood smear remains one of the most informative and rewarding diagnostic procedures. It offers the chance to confirm the findings of the automated complete blood cell count, which can be inaccurate in the presence of nucleated red blood cells or rouleaux formation. Review of the blood smear also allows for evaluation of other cell lineages, which might suggest a primary marrow or infiltrative disease. The finding of hypersegmented neutrophils suggests a megaloblastic process, and this morphologic abnormality can be seen in the blood smear before there are significant changes in the hemoglobin or MCV (see box on the Systematic Approach to the Diagnosis of Anemia). Also, only the blood smear reveals the unique morphologic changes occurring with various hemolytic disorders.

There are several commonly encountered findings that can be seen in red blood cells on the peripheral blood smear (Table 34–6, and Fig. 34–3). Microcytic, hypochromic red blood cells are suggestive of iron deficiency anemia or thalassemia (Fig. 34–3F); whereas macrocytic red blood cells with ovalocytes (oval red blood cells) are suggestive of megaloblastic anemias (Fig. 34–3G). Some findings reflect organ dysfunction, such as echinocytes (burr cells) in uremia (Fig. 34–3R), or acanthocytes (spur cells) in severe liver disease (Fig. 34–3S), although acanthocytes may also be seen in rare conditions such as abetalipoproteinemia. Target cells may be seen in cases of liver disease but may also be present in hemoglobinopathies, including sickle cell disease or thalassemia (Fig. 34–3W). The presence of schistocytes or red blood cell fragmentation often reflects systemic disease, such as disseminated intravascular coagulation, thrombotic thrombocytopenic purpura, or the hemolytic uremic syndrome (Fig. 34–3P). Finding spherocytes on a smear is suggestive of autoimmune hemolytic anemia or hereditary spherocytosis (Fig. 34–3H). Occasionally, the clue to the correct diagnosis of a systemic illness comes in the form of the observation of intraerythrocytic inclusions, such as malarial (Figure 34–3O) or babesial forms, and examination of a thick blood smear may be useful for the diagnosis of these disorders when a low parasite burden is suspected.

Systematic Approach to the Diagnosis of Anemia

Integration of historic features and physical findings with thoughtful review of the results of the automated complete blood cell count and of the peripheral smear often serves to narrow down the differential diagnosis significantly. For example, a patient status post-gastric bypass eating a normal diet who presents with gradual onset of fatigue accompanied by the more recent onset of distal paresthesias and a finding of decreased vibration sense, in the setting of anemia with significantly elevated MCV and RDW values and numerous six-lobed polymorphonuclear leukocytes on peripheral blood smear, almost certainly has a vitamin B_{12} deficiency. This is suggested even before the return of specific laboratory testing because of the relatively narrow differential diagnosis for megaloblastic anemia and the fact that neurologic abnormalities are not associated with folate deficiency. For the purposes of diagnostic efficiency, the rewards of correlation of historic features and physical findings with a careful review of the peripheral blood smear cannot be overstated.

Special stains of the peripheral blood smear can be helpful in elucidating the cause of anemia. If there is significant nuclear debris present, the reticulocyte count obtained by automated methods can be inaccurate. In such cases, manual counting after staining with new methylene blue, which stains residual RNA in reticulocytes, permits accurate enumeration. If bite cells are detected on peripheral smear, supravital staining with methyl crystal violet can reveal Heinz bodies. These are aggregates of denatured hemoglobin reflecting an oxidative insult, most commonly due to glucose-6-phosphate dehydrogenase deficiency or, less frequently, to the presence of an unstable hemoglobin (Fig. 34–3H).

Table 34–5 Combining the Reticulocyte Count and Red Blood Cell Parameters for Diagnosis

MCV, RDW	Reticulocyte Count <75,000/μL	Reticulocyte Count >100,000/μL
Low, Normal	Anemia of chronic disease	
Normal, Normal	Anemia of chronic disease	
High, Normal	Chemotherapy/antivirals/alcohol Aplastic anemia	Chronic liver disease
Low, High	Iron deficiency anemia	Sickle cell-β-thalassemia
Normal, High	Early iron, folate, vitamin B_{12} deficiency Myelodysplasia	Sickle cell anemia, sickle cell disease
High, High	Folate or vitamin B_{12} deficiency Myelodysplasia	Immune hemolytic anemia Chronic liver disease

MCV, mean corpuscular volume; RDW, red blood cell distribution width.

Table 34–4 Usefulness of the Mean Corpuscular Value (MCV) and Red Blood Cell Distribution Width (RDW) in the Diagnosis of Anemia

	Low MCV (<80 fL)	Normal MCV (80–99 fL)	High MCV (>100 fL)
Normal RDW RDW	Anemia of chronic disease α- or β-Thalassemia trait Hemoglobin E trait	Acute blood loss Anemia of chronic disease Anemia of renal disease	Aplastic anemia Chronic liver disease Chemotherapy/antivirals/alcohol
Elevated RDW RDW	Iron deficiency Sickle cell-β-thalassemia	Early iron, folate, or vitamin B_{12} deficiency Dimorphic anemia (for example, iron + folate deficiency) Sickle cell anemia Sickle cell disease Chronic liver disease Myelodysplasia	Folate or vitamin B_{12} deficiency Immune hemolytic anemia Cytotoxic chemotherapy Chronic liver disease Myelodysplasia

Table 34–6 Features of the Peripheral Blood Smear

Red Blood Cell Morphology	Definition	Interpretation
Polychromasia	Large, bluish red blood cells lacking normal central pallor on peripheral blood smear; bluish stain is the result of residual ribonucleic acid.	Rapid production and release of red blood cells from marrow; elevated reticulocyte count; most commonly seen in hemolytic anemia.
Basophilic stippling	Many small bluish dots in portion of erythrocytes; comes from staining of clustered polyribosomes in young circulating red blood cells.	Seen in a variety of erythropoietic disorders, including acquired and congenital hemolytic anemias and occasionally in lead poisoning (lead inhibits pyrimidine 5′-nucleotidase, which normally digests the residual RNA).
Pappenheimer bodies	Several grayish, irregularly shaped inclusions in a portion of erythrocytes visible on peripheral smear; composed of aggregates of ribosomes, ferritin, and mitochondria.	Erythropoietic malfunction in congenital anemias such as hemoglobinopathies, particularly with splenic hypofunction or acquired anemias such as megaloblastic anemia.
Heinz bodies	Several grayish, round inclusions visible after supravital staining with methyl crystal violet of the peripheral blood smear, often in the context of bite cells; represent aggregates of denatured hemoglobin.	Indicative of oxidative injury to the erythrocyte, such as occurs in G6PD deficiency, or less commonly of unstable hemoglobins.
Howell-Jolly bodies	Usually one or at most a few purplish inclusions in the erythrocyte visible on the routine peripheral blood smear; represent residual fragments of nuclei containing chromatin.	Associated with states of splenic hypofunction or after splenectomy.
Schistocytes	Red blood cells that are fragmented into a variety of shapes and sizes, including helmet-shaped cells; indicative of shearing of the erythrocyte within the circulation.	Associated with microangiopathic hemolytic anemias, including DIC, TTP/HUS, as well as other mechanical causes of hemolysis, such as prosthetic valves.
Spherocytes	Red blood cells that have lost their central pallor and appear spherical; indicative of loss of cytoskeletal integrity due to internal or external causes.	Associated with hereditary spherocytosis, autoimmune hemolytic anemia; may also be observed in addition to schistocytes in the presence of microangiopathic hemolytic anemia.
Teardrop cells	Pear-shaped erythrocytes visible on peripheral blood smear; indicative of mechanical stress on the red blood cell during release from the bone marrow or passage through the spleen.	Seen in a variety of conditions, including congenital anemias such as thalassemia and acquired disorders such as megaloblastic anemia; may also suggest a more ominous process such as myelophthisis (marrow replacement).
Burr cells (echinocytes)	Red blood cells that have smooth undulations present on the surface circumferentially; pathogenesis unknown.	Indicative of uremia when present on a properly made peripheral blood smear.
Spur cells (acanthocytes)	Red blood cells that have spiny points present on the surface circumferentially; reflective of abnormal lipid composition of red blood cell membrane.	Most commonly indicative of liver disease when present in significant numbers; also seen in abetalipoproteinemia and in red blood cells lacking the Kell blood group antigen.

DIC, disseminated intravascular coagulation; G6PD, glucose-6-phosphate dehydrogenase; HUS, hemolytic uremic syndrome; TTP, thrombotic thrombocytopenic purpura.

Bone Marrow Examination

Bone marrow aspiration and biopsy permit evaluation of cellular morphology and marrow architecture, respectively. Special stains, flow cytometry, cytogenetics, fluorescence in situ hybridization (FISH), and molecular testing that can be performed on the marrow also can provide a wealth of diagnostic information.[39] Because of the discomfort involved in the procedure, however, careful consideration should be given to determining the array of tests required, so that repeated marrow aspirates or biopsies need not be performed. If there is any consideration of the possibility of myelodysplasia, leukemia, or lymphoma, an aliquot of anticoagulated aspirate should be set aside at the time of the initial procedure that can be sent, if necessary, for flow cytometry or cytogenetics after review of the aspirate smear.

Diagnostic uncertainty in the setting of hypoproliferative anemia is an indication for bone marrow biopsy. Hematologic disorders such as myelodysplasia, leukemia, lymphoma, or myeloma may be identified. Myelodysplasia in the marrow classically includes megaloblastic change and nuclear budding in maturing erythroblasts, as well as morphologic abnormalities in other lineages, such as hypolobated megakaryocytes and hypogranulation of the myeloid lineage.[40] A variety of infiltrative (myelophthisic) processes may be observed. These include malignancies such as small cell lung, breast, and prostate cancers, which not infrequently can appear in advanced stages with marrow involvement. Alternatively, granulomas may be present, suggesting the possible presence of mycobacterial disease. In children, disseminated neuroblastoma and rhabdomyosarcoma occasionally can appear as a myelophthisic anemia.

Even when properly performed, difficulty obtaining a bone marrow aspirate is commonly observed in certain situations, such as myelofibrosis, erythroblastic leukemia (M6), and hairy cell leukemia.[41] In these cases, touch preps of the bone marrow biopsy may help expedite diagnosis.

DIFFERENCES IN THE EVALUATION OF ANEMIA BETWEEN PEDIATRIC AND ADULT PATIENTS

There are several features that distinguish evaluation of pediatric patients, the most important being that the normal ranges for red blood cell parameters are significantly different in infants and chil-

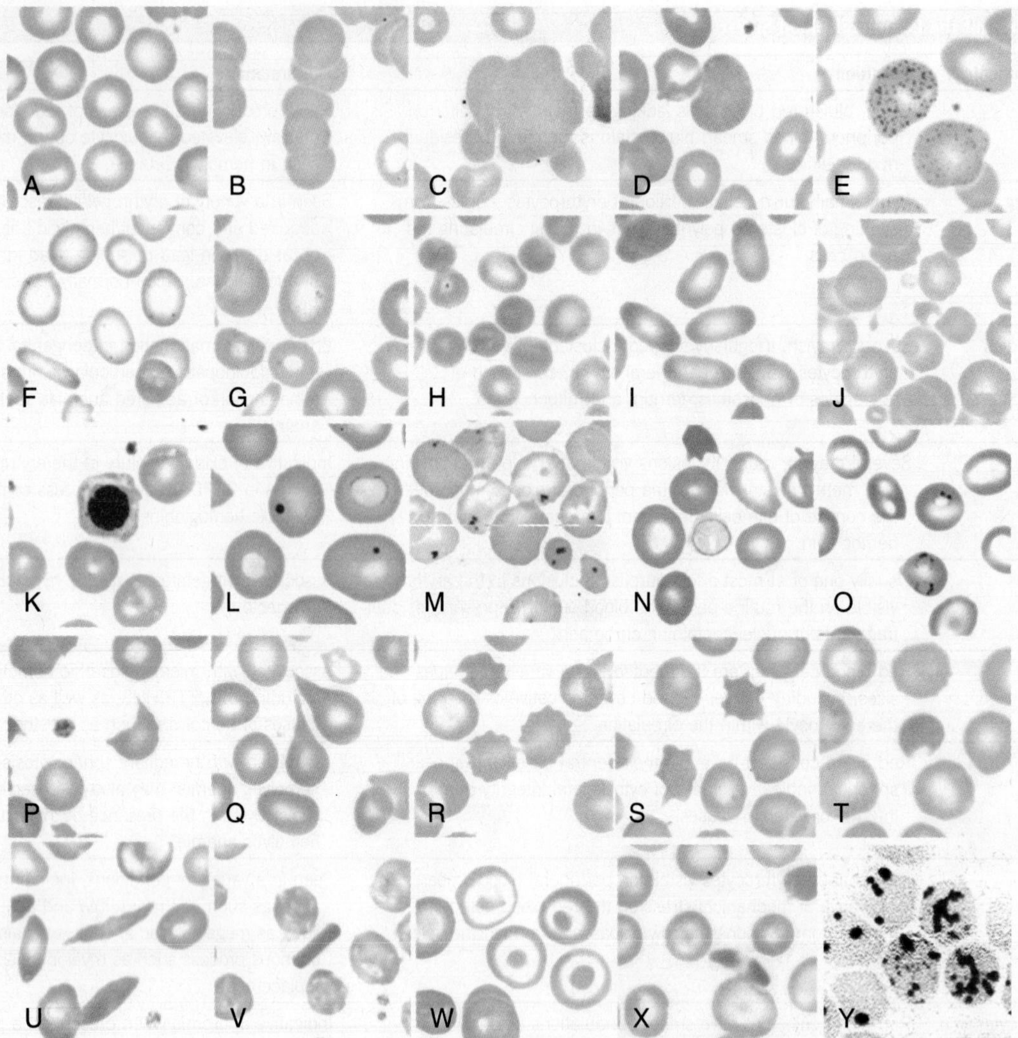

Figure 34–3 Useful peripheral blood and red blood cell features in the evaluation of anemia: A–Y. **A.** Normal red blood cells. Note the central pallor is one-third the diameter of the entire cell. **B.** Rouleaux formation is indicative of increased plasma protein. **C.** Agglutination indicates an antibody-mediated process such as cold agglutinin disease. **D.** Polychromatophilic cell. The gray-blue color is due to RNA and the cell is equivalent to a reticulocyte, which must be identified with a reticulocyte stain. **E.** Basophilic stippling. This also is due to increased RNA due either to a left shift in erythroid cells or to lead toxicity. **F.** Hypochromic microcytic cells typical of iron deficiency anemia. Note the widened central pallor, and the "pencil" cell in lower left. **G.** Macroovalocyte as can be seen in either megaloblastic anemia or MDS. **H.** Microspherocytes typical of hereditary spherocytosis. **I.** Elliptocytes (ovalocytes) from a patient with hereditary elliptocytosis. **J.** Red blood cell fragments from thermal injury (burn patient). **K.** Nucleated red blood cell. **L.** Howell-Jolly bodies indicative of splenic dysfunction or absence. **M.** Pappenheimer bodies from patient with sideroblastic anemia. **N.** Cabot ring, as can be seen in megaloblastic anemia or MDS. **O.** Malarial parasites (*Plasmodium falciparum*). **P.** Schistocyte typical of a microangiopathic hemolytic anemia. **Q.** Tear-drop form indicates marrow fibrosis and extramedullary hematopoiesis. **R.** Echinocyte (Burr cell) with rounded edges. **S.** Acanthocyte (spur cell) with more irregular pointed ends. This was from a patient with neuroacanthocytosis. They can also be seen in patients with liver disease and lipid abnormalities. **T.** "Bite" cell from a patient with G6PD deficiency. **U.** Sickle cell, from a patient with HbSS disease. **V.** Hemoglobin C crystal. **W.** Target cells. **X.** Hemoglobin SC. Note red blood cell in center has condensed hemoglobin at each pole. **Y.** Heinz body preparation (supravital stain) from a patient with G6PD deficiency. Note cells to right have increased precipitated hemoglobin. G6PD, glucose-6-phosphate dehydrogenase; HbSS, homozygous sickle cell; MDS, myelodysplasia syndrome.

dren and do not reach adult levels until adolescence. Thus, the determination of whether anemia is present must be based on age-appropriate normal values (see Table 34–2). Upon identification of anemia, the likelihood of certain diagnostic entities is different in infants, children, and adults. In infants and children, anemia often represents a nutritional deficiency or a primary hematologic process, whereas in adults anemia more commonly is an indicator of systemic disease or malignancy.

Approach to Hypoproliferative Anemia in the Adult

Hypoproliferative anemia is reasonably common in adults. Except in the setting of acute blood loss, the new onset of anemia in an adult is more commonly associated with a hypoproliferative process rather than a hemolytic one. A systematic approach integrating historic features with laboratory findings can often lead to a short differential diagnosis list (Fig. 34–4).

Microcytic anemia with an MCV of less than 70 fL is most commonly associated with iron deficiency anemia or thalassemia. MCV values between 70 and 80 fL may be associated with the anemia of chronic disease or endocrine causes such as hyperthyroidism. MCV values above the upper limit of normal suggest the possibility of increased ethanol intake, liver disease, myelodysplastic syndrome, and also megaloblastic anemia due to folate or vitamin B_{12} deficiency. When the MCV is greater than 120 fL, however, this most often is associated with folate or vitamin B_{12} deficiency.

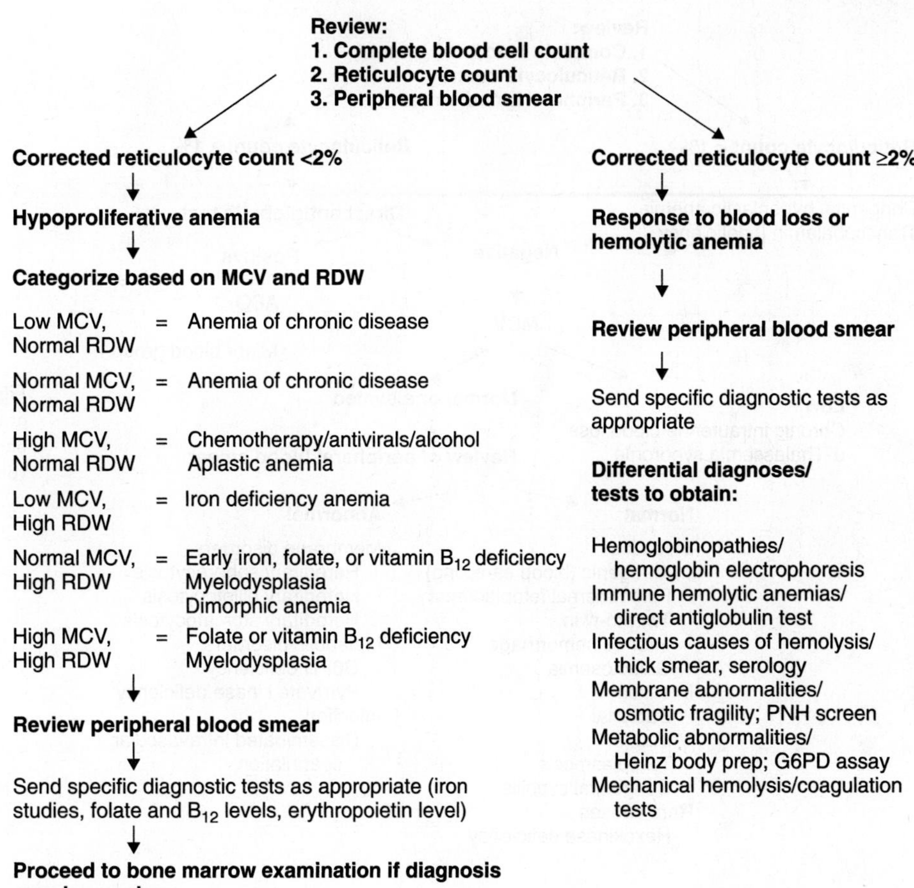

Figure 34–4 Approach to the differential diagnoses of anemia in the adult and child. G6PD, glucose-6-phosphate dehydrogenase; MCV, mean corpuscular volume; PNH, paroxysmal nocturnal hemoglobinuria; RDW, red blood cell distribution width.

The most commonly encountered normocytic hypoproliferative anemia in adults is due to chronic disease, which, when broadly defined, includes anemias due to renal disease and inflammatory causes. Mild or early iron deficiency anemia is also a common cause of normocytic anemia. In such cases, erythropoietin levels may be of value in the diagnostic evaluation, before proceeding to bone marrow examination.[42] Occasionally, a normocytic anemia represents the result of averaging two populations of red blood cells: one microcytic and one macrocytic. Such cases of dimorphic anemia are encountered in combined nutritional deficiencies, such as when iron and folate deficiencies are present. The RDW is usually markedly elevated in such cases, and review of the peripheral blood smear confirms the diversity in red blood cell size.

Approach to Hemolytic Anemia in the Adult

Newly diagnosed hemolytic anemia is less common in adults than hypoproliferative anemia. Because the differential diagnosis is relatively broad, historical factors, such as information regarding the onset of anemia, and physical findings, such as splenomegaly, may help to narrow the diagnostic entities under consideration (see Fig. 34–4). Review of the peripheral blood smear is essential and potentially more useful than bone marrow examination in providing valuable diagnostic information.

Hemolytic anemia in the adult may represent an inherited condition that has gone previously undiagnosed. For example, mild to moderate hereditary spherocytosis or sickle/β^+-thalassemia sometimes may not manifest until adulthood. Alternatively, hemolysis may be due to a new acquired disorder such as autoimmune hemolytic anemia (AIHA) or a microangiopathic process. Autoimmune hemolytic anemia is occasionally associated with lymphoproliferative and rheumatologic disorders, so these potential underlying conditions should routinely be considered when the diagnosis of AIHA is made. Similarly, the cause of a microangiopathic hemolytic anemia is often clear from the clinical setting, although it sometimes is a clue to the diagnosis of an occult malignancy, such as metastatic prostate cancer.

Approach to Hypoproliferative Anemia in the Child

A systematic diagnostic approach, similar to that used in the adult, is most productive in children (see Fig. 34–4). Nutritional anemias due to iron deficiency are a particularly common cause of low hemoglobin in the first 2 years of life. Often the cause of this anemia is excessive intake of cow's milk to the exclusion of other sources of calories, and this information is often obtained from the medical history. Anemia due to iron deficiency often is quite severe, and characteristically has a very low MCV (50–65 fL). Hypoproliferative anemia in childhood also occurs in association with leukemia, and in these cases, other characteristic clinical and laboratory features also are present. Two other causes of hypoproliferative anemia are congenital and acquired red blood cell aplasia. The former, also known as Diamond-Blackfan anemia, is a lifelong disorder manifesting in the first year of life, usually with persistent macrocytosis beyond infancy; it is also associated with a variety of congenital abnormalities. Transient erythroblastopenia of childhood is an acquired immunologic red blood cell aplasia, lasting a few weeks, and occurring in the first 3 years of life in otherwise normal children. The MCV in children with transient erythroblastopenia of childhood is normal for age, thus distinguishing them from children with iron deficiency (low MCV) or Diamond-Blackfan anemia (high MCV).

Approach to Hemolytic Anemia in the Child

Hemolytic anemia in children most commonly reflects an inherited disorder. However, acquired causes of hemolysis also occur, such as autoimmune hemolysis or microangiopathic hemolytic anemia as

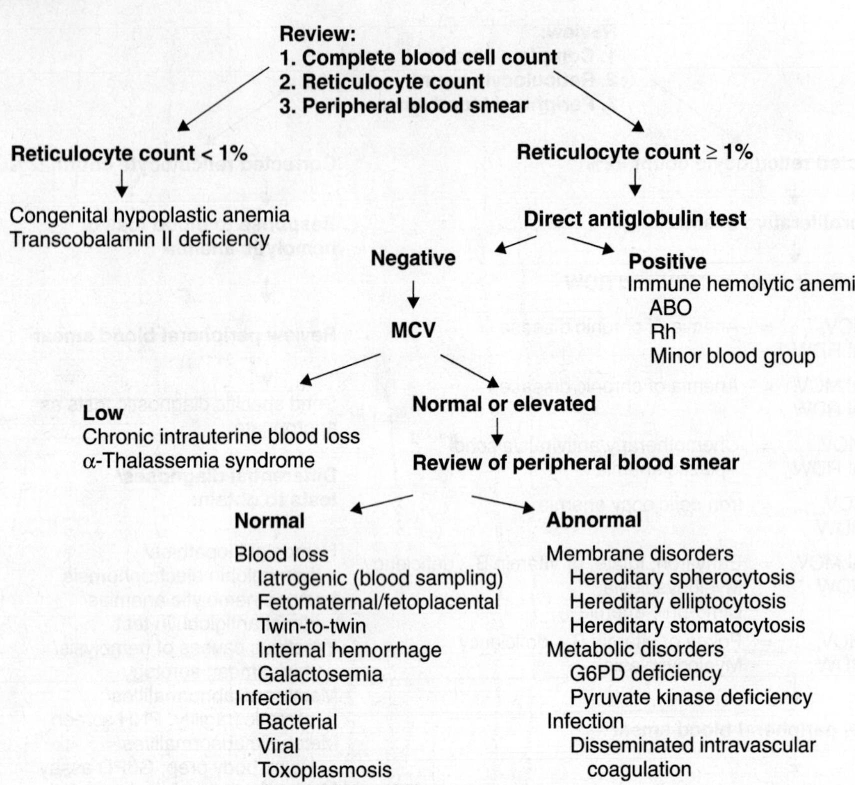

Figure 34–5 Approach to the differential diagnosis of anemia in the newborn. G6PD, glucose-6-phosphate dehydrogenase; MCV, mean corpuscular volume.

seen in the hemolytic uremic syndrome. In newborns, the major clinical finding suggestive of hemolysis often is a marked exaggeration of the normal physiologic hyperbilirubinemia, thus causing significant jaundice that requires specific therapy. Once it is ascertained that a neonate has a hemolytic anemia, the differential diagnosis is limited. The most important consideration is immune-mediated hemolysis, although hemolytic anemias caused by red blood cell membrane and metabolic disorders also occur (Fig. 34–5). Of interest, the anemias caused by sickle cell disease and β-thalassemia are not associated with clinical manifestations in the newborn period. These disorders become significant only after 4 to 6 months of age when β-globin production is established. Review of family history and ethnic background of the parents often is highly informative. Physical findings may include splenomegaly, such as those observed in patients with hereditary spherocytosis. In addition to careful review of the peripheral blood smear, hemoglobin electrophoresis is of utility when a hemoglobinopathy is suspected. In the United States, however, some of this information may be available as a result of newborn hemoglobin screening programs.

CONCLUSION

Anemia may represent a primary hematologic disorder or may represent the manifestation of a systemic process. In the pediatric population, the former tends to be somewhat more common than the latter, and in adults the converse is true. However, in both children and adults, a systematic approach to the evaluation of anemia that includes careful review of historic features, the complete blood cell count, and peripheral smear facilitates an efficient diagnosis and minimizes unnecessary testing.

SUGGESTED READING LIST

Centers for Disease Control and Prevention: Iron deficiency-United States 1999–2000. MMWR Morb Mortal Wkly Rep 51:897, 2002.

Dikow R, Schwenger V, Schomig M, Ritz E: How should we manage anaemia in patients with diabetes? Nephrol Dial Transplant 17(Suppl 1):67, 2002.

Fishbane S: Anemia treatment in chronic renal insufficiency. Semin Nephrol 22:474, 2002.

Gehrs BC, Freidberg RC: Autoimmune hemolytic anemia. Am J Hematol 69:258, 2002.

Perry C, Soreq H: Transcriptional regulation of erythropoiesis: Fine tuning of multi-domain elements. Eur J Biochem 269:3607, 2002.

Roy CN, Weinstein DA, Andrews NC: 2002 E. Mead Johnnson Award for Research in Pediatrics Lecture: The molecular biology of the anemia of chronic disease: A hypothesis. Pediatr Res 53:507, 2003.

Sullivan P: Associations of anemia, treatments for anemia, and survival in patients with human immunodeficiency virus infection. J Infect Dis 185(Suppl 2):S138, 2002.

Tefferi A: Anemia in adults: A contemporary approach to diagnosis. Mayo Clin Proc 78:1274, 2003.

REFERENCES

For complete list of references log onto www.expertconsult.com

CHAPTER 35

PATHOLOGY OF IRON METABOLISM

Nancy C. Andrews

INTRODUCTION

Iron is an essential metal for all mammalian cells, serving as a mediator of enzymatic electron exchange (in cytochromes, peroxidases, ribonucleotide reductases, and catalases) and a carrier of oxygen (in hemoglobin and myoglobin). However, its flexible redox state and its interactions with oxygen can also promote cellular damage when the reactivity of iron is not restrained by protein binding. Excess iron potentiates the formation of reactive oxygen species that attack cellular lipids, proteins and nucleic acids. In normal individuals, iron homeostasis is meticulously regulated to avoid deleterious extremes of iron deficiency and iron overload. All known disorders of iron metabolism can be considered abnormalities of iron balance or distribution.

Iron normally enters the body through dietary absorption, at a rate that balances small losses caused by bleeding and exfoliation of skin and mucosal cells. Neither the liver nor the kidney has a mechanism for excretion of iron that is not needed. In fact, no regulated pathway for iron excretion has been identified, making it likely that iron balance is determined primarily by the absorptive capacity of the intestinal epithelium. This is modulated in response to various conditions, as discussed in Regulation of Iron Homeostasis in the Entire Organism. Iron homeostasis is challenged when intake and losses are not matched. Iron deficiency occurs when the dietary iron supply is inadequate, when losses are increased (usually because of bleeding) or when both of these circumstances act to put the body into iron deficit. Iron overload results when iron absorption is constitutively increased because of genetic defects perturbing normal regulation, or when repeated blood transfusions create an iron surfeit.

Normal adult men usually absorb approximately 0.5 to 1 mg of iron on a daily basis. This amount is doubled in menstruating women, and approximately quadrupled during pregnancy, to balance the high iron cost of carrying and delivering an infant. On average, each pregnancy results in maternal iron losses of approximately 680 mg, and an additional 450 mg is used transiently to support increased maternal blood volume, although this latter amount is returned to maternal stores after delivery. Lactation results in a daily iron loss of approximately 0.5 to 1 mg. The iron content of human breast milk is minimally affected when maternal iron stores are depleted. Because normal menstruation is usually inhibited while breast-feeding continues, iron requirements in the lactating mother approximate those of the menstruating woman.

Full-term infants are born with an iron endowment of approximately 350 mg. Over the course of a lifetime this increases to a total of 3 to 5 g in normal individuals. Patients with genetic hemochromatosis can have iron burdens greater than 15 g. Approximately 2.7 g of iron is normally dedicated to the erythron in adults, distributed between bone marrow precursors and circulating erythrocytes. Packed red blood cells contain approximately 1 mg/mL iron. Iron not required by other tissues is stored in hepatocytes and macrophages. In adult men, iron stores gradually increase throughout life. In contrast, iron stores are small in prepubertal children and menstruating women, because of the demands of rapid growth and menstrual blood loss, respectively.

Our understanding of the molecular processes of iron metabolism has advanced considerably over the last decade, as new techniques in genetics and molecular biology have been applied to problems in iron biology. The study of animal models has been particularly valuable, owing to the existence of both spontaneous and induced mutations affecting key genes. Mechanisms of iron transport and regulation are highly conserved among mammalian species, allowing information from experiments in rodents to be extrapolated to humans.

MECHANISMS OF IRON TRANSPORT

General Concepts

Iron cannot freely diffuse across cellular membranes; therefore, transmembrane transfer requires specialized transport mechanisms. Some cells, including intestinal epithelial cells, hepatocytes and macrophages, are equipped both to take in (import) iron and to release (export) it. These cells play roles in the acquisition, storage, and mobilization of iron. Other cells, particularly erythroid precursors, use most or all of the iron they import and do not need to export it. These cells are the major consumers of iron.

Each day, normal adults need 25 mg of iron to support hemoglobin production in maturing erythrocytes. This amount is much greater than the 1 to 2 mg absorbed daily through the intestine. Obviously, iron needed for erythropoiesis must be acquired from supplies already existing in the body. The primary source of plasma iron is the reticuloendothelial macrophage system, which recovers iron from senescent and damaged erythrocytes. In normal individuals, nearly all circulating iron is bound to transferrin (Tf), an abundant plasma protein with the capacity to bind two iron atoms per molecule. Because macrophages both supply iron to erythroid precursors and recover it from effete erythrocytes, much of the body's iron metabolism can be considered to be a closed loop (Fig. 35–1). Other significant sites of iron exchange are the intestine, as discussed earlier, and the liver, whose iron stores can be expanded or mobilized as needed.

Several distinct iron uptake (import) mechanisms have been described in mammals. Intestinal absorptive cells express plasma membrane transporters that carry ferrous (Fe^{2+}) ions directly across the membrane. They may also have mechanisms for transport of intact heme. Erythroid precursors meet their large iron needs by accumulating diferric (Fe_2)-Tf within intracellular vesicles prior to transmembrane transport of the metal into the cytoplasm (the Tf cycle, see The Transferrin Cycle). Some embryonic cells may use an analogous uptake mechanism, involving receptor-mediated endocytosis of iron bound to a lipocalin molecule.[1] Cardiac cells may, under conditions of iron overload, take up iron through co-opted *L*-type calcium channels.[2] Hepatocytes may use all of these strategies. Finally, reticuloendothelial macrophages acquire much of their iron through phagocytosis of aged or damaged erythrocytes, destruction of the phagocytosed cells, and enzymatic degradation of their hemoglobin. Other iron transport mechanisms, including receptor-mediated uptake of the iron-containing ferritin, have also been postulated. Furthermore, it is possible that molecules transporting other transition metals (eg, copper, zinc) can also carry iron across cellular membranes.

Intestinal Iron Absorption

Dietary iron is absorbed in the first segment of the duodenum, just beyond the gastric outlet. The duodenal epithelium is organized into

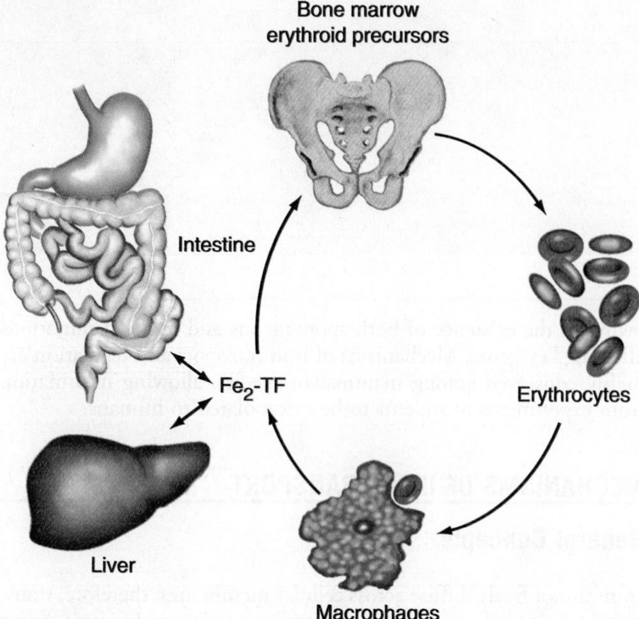

Figure 35–1 The iron cycle. To a first approximation, mammalian iron metabolism can be thought of as a closed loop involving circulating diferric transferrin, the erythroid bone marrow, circulating erythrocytes, and reticuloendothelial macrophages. Most iron in the body can be found in this cycle. However, a small amount is absorbed and lost through the intestinal mucosa. Additionally, iron in excess of tissue needs is stored in the liver. For simplicity, other sites of iron use are not shown here. The most important of these is muscle, where iron is incorporated into myoglobin. Iron homeostasis is markedly affected by pregnancy, when the developing fetus draws iron out of this system in the mother. Fe_2-TF, diferric transferrin.

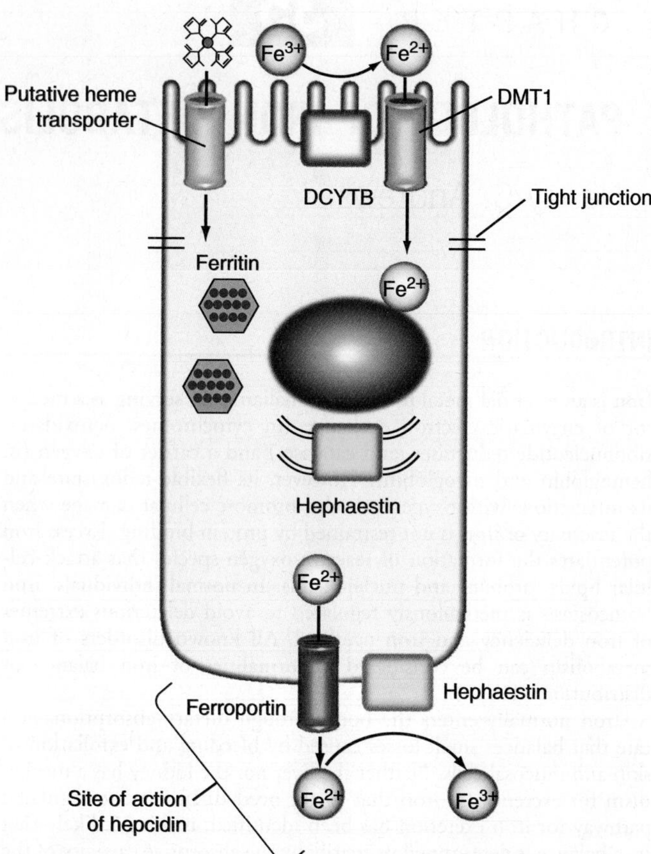

Figure 35–2 Intestinal nonheme iron transport. This diagram summarizes our current understanding of iron transport through enterocytes in the duodenal epithelium. The apical brush border of the cell, facing the gut lumen, is shown at the top, and the basolateral surface on the bottom. The mechanism of heme iron uptake has not yet been worked out, but a transmembrane heme transporter has been postulated to exist. Dietary nonheme iron is primarily in the ferric (Fe^{3+}) form. Fe^{3+} must be reduced to the Fe^{2+} form, probably by the ferrireductase DCYTB. The reduced iron is a substrate for the transporter DMT1, which is located in the apical membrane. Iron entering the cell is partitioned between storage (ferritin) and export across the basolateral membrane. Ferroportin serves as the basolateral transporter, most likely requiring Fe^{2+} as its substrate. Hephaestin, a ferroxidase, appears to aid ferroportin, although some investigators have reported that it localizes to a perinuclear compartment rather than the basolateral surface. For that reason, it is shown in both sites in this diagram. Regardless, iron must be oxidized to the Fe^{3+} form to bind transferrin (Tf). Hepcidin regulates basolateral iron export by binding to ferroportin to trigger its internalization and lysosomal degradation.

fingerlike villi, lined by absorptive cells. The apical brush border of this epithelium is bathed in gastric acid, which solubilizes iron in food and provides a low pH environment necessary for the function of membrane transporters. Most nonheme dietary iron is in the ferric (Fe^{3+}) form. It can be reduced to ferrous (Fe^{2+}) iron by a cytochrome b-like ferrireductase, DCYTB[3]. Expression of DCYTB is induced by iron deficiency. Fe^{2+} ions are carried across the apical membrane by divalent metal transporter 1 (DMT1, also called NRAMP2, DCT1, SLC11A2), an integral membrane protein that bears no resemblance to other classes of membrane transporters.[4,5,6] DMT1 is not specific for iron—it also transports divalent forms of manganese, cobalt, copper, zinc, and lead.[4] Metal transport is dependent on cotransport of protons in the same inward direction. Animals lacking DMT1 activity have profound iron deficiency, indicating that it is a major carrier for nonheme iron entering through the brush border.[7] However, human patients with mutations in DMT1 have been reported to have hepatic iron overload and iron-deficient erythropoiesis.[8] The increased hepatic iron may be attributable to multiple transfusions or to increased heme iron absorption through an alternative pathway.

Within intestinal epithelial cells, some of the imported iron is incorporated into ferritin and other storage forms. A fraction of the iron taken up from the intestinal lumen passes through the cell, and is exported across the basolateral membrane to enter the body. Ferroportin (also called IREG1, MTP1, SLC40A1), a metal ion transporter that bears no structural homology to DMT1, serves as the basolateral iron exporter.[9] Like DMT1, ferroportin is an integral membrane protein that transports ferrous ions. It may work in conjunction with a multicopper oxidase protein, hephaestin, which is believed to oxidize Fe^{2+} to Fe^{3+} to allow it to bind to plasma Tf.[10] Our current understanding of enterocyte nonheme iron transport is depicted in Fig. 35–2.

The mechanisms controlling the rate of iron flux through this enterocyte transport system determine overall iron absorption. It is important to consider that only some of the dietary iron taken up by enterocytes transits both the apical and basolateral membranes to enter into the plasma. Iron that is retained within enterocytes is lost from the body when those cells senesce and are sloughed into the gut lumen. Thus, absorption can be regulated simply by controlling how much iron is retained and how much is exported to the plasma. As discussed in Regulation of Iron Homeostasis in the Entire Organism, the peptide hormone hepcidin modulates iron absorption in this way.

Uptake of heme iron occurs through a distinct pathway, but the details have not been worked out. A membrane transporter that was recently postulated to be a heme importer was subsequently shown to be a folate transporter instead. Heme iron absorption is important, because 10% to 15% of iron in nonvegetarian Western diets is in this form. It is more efficient than absorption of inorganic iron, and it appears to be less sensitive to the regulatory mechanisms that govern nonheme iron absorption.

Iron absorption is affected by the presence of other substances in the intestinal lumen. It is enhanced by dietary meat proteins and ascorbate, but inhibited by phytates, tannins, phosphates, antacids, and competing metals (eg, zinc). Although milk components generally inhibit iron absorption, extraction of iron from human breast milk is highly efficient, allowing young infants to acquire a very large proportion of the limited iron present in that fluid.

The Transferrin Cycle

In normal individuals, almost all iron in the circulation is carried by Tf, which is present at concentrations of 2 to 3 g/L. Tf binds iron with extremely high affinity to prevent precipitation of Fe^{3+} ions, which are almost insoluble in aqueous fluids. It prevents the iron from reacting with other molecules and allows it to be delivered to the tissues in a safe, non-toxic form. Tf molecules carrying one or two iron atoms bind to specific cell surface Tf receptors (Tfrs), which have a preference for the diferric form. Mature, differentiated cells express few, if any Tfrs. In contrast, they are highly expressed on the surfaces of cells with exceptional need for iron, including erythroid precursors, tumor cells, and activated lymphocytes. Erythroid precursors have the greatest demand for iron, to support the large scale production of hemoglobin. They express as many as 800,000 Tfr molecules per cell at the time that they are taking up maximal amounts of iron. Tfrs are cleared from the cells as they complete maturation, and few if any are found on circulating, fully differentiated erythrocytes. Tumor cells and activated lymphocytes presumably express Tfrs to optimize iron uptake to support rapid proliferation. Serum or soluble Tfr (sTfr) is a proteolytic cleavage product of Tfr that contains the entire extracellular portion of the molecule. It is found in the circulation in proportion to the erythroid cell mass.[11] Measurement of elevated sTfr concentration is useful in the diagnosis of iron deficiency, although sTfr levels also increase in conditions associated with ineffective erythropoiesis.[12]

When iron-loaded Tf binds to Tfr, portions of the cell membrane bearing the Tf-Tfr complex invaginate into the cytoplasm and bud off as intracellular vesicles. The vesicular pH drops to approximately 5.5, leading to conformational changes in the Tf-Tfr complex and liberation of the bound iron. Released iron is reduced to the ferrous form by the ferrireductase Steap3 protein[13] and transported across the endosomal membrane into the cytoplasm by DMT1, taking advantage of the acidic milieu within the endosome for the same type of proton-dependent transport process as occurs at the apical membrane of the intestine.[14] Different isoforms of the DMT1 protein appear to be used for intestinal iron uptake and endosomal iron transport, but they are highly similar and are encoded by the same gene.[15] Concurrently, apoprotein (apo)-Tf and Tfr proteins return to the cell surface to participate in further cycles of iron delivery. This process is summarized in Fig. 35–3.

Within the cytoplasm, iron is sequestered by proteins and small molecules, and shuttled to sites of use and storage. Most stored iron is present in ferritin, a polymeric protein basket that can hold up to 4500 atoms of iron (see Cellular Iron Storage below). There is less ferritin in erythroid precursors, because most iron is destined for the mitochondria where it is incorporated into heme.

Considering the fact that cells can take iron up directly, why should they need the complicated Tf cycle? There are at least two likely answers. First, tight binding of iron to Tf is advantageous while iron is in the circulation, but it complicates the matter of bringing iron into cells. The pH-dependent release of iron, occurring in a controlled intracellular environment, solves the problem of liberating the iron. Second, receptor-mediated endocytosis of diferric Tf serves to concentrate iron, achieving high local concentrations in the vicinity of DMT1. It thus allows more efficient iron uptake by cells with substantial needs without exposing other cells to unnecessary iron. Studies of animals lacking either Tf[16] or Tfr[17] indicate that erythroid

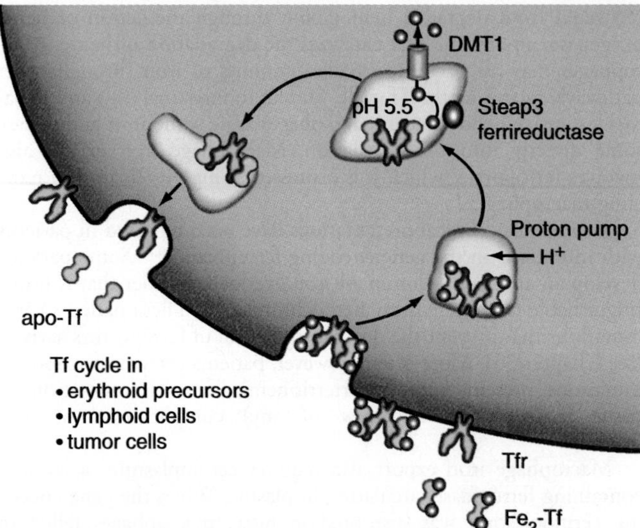

Figure 35–3 The transferrin cycle. Erythroid precursors, lymphoid cells, tumor cells and perhaps others rely on the transferrin (Tf) cycle to augment cellular iron uptake. Diferric-Tf (Fe_2-Tf) binds to a specific cell surface receptor, Tfr, to initiate receptor-mediated endocytosis. Within the cell the Tf-containing endosomes are acidified through the action of a proton pump, resulting in dissociation of iron from the proteins. The iron is reduced by Steap3, a ferrireductase located in the endosomal membrane. The reduced iron exits the endosome through DMT1 to enter the cytoplasm. The Tf-Tfr protein complex recycles to the cell surface where the ambient pH leads to dissociation of Tf and availability of both protein components for further cycles of iron delivery. Tfr, transferrin receptor.

precursors are highly dependent on the Tf cycle, but most other cell types assimilate iron efficiently without it.

Iron Transport in Other Cells

Hepatocytes serve as a major storage depot for body iron in excess of immediate needs. They express Tfr but also express high levels of a related molecule designated transferrin receptor 2 (Tfr2).[18] Like Tfr, Tfr2 can bind and internalize Tf, although it does so much less efficiently, and Tf-mediated iron uptake is probably not its primary physiological role. Importantly, Tfr2 forms a molecular complex with HFE, the protein mutated in patients with classical hemochromatosis,[19] and mutations in the gene encoding Tfr2 also cause hemochromatosis. Over the past few years the molecular basis of hemochromatosis has been worked out in detail (see Chapter 36).

Hepatocytes are also capable of taking up non-Tf-bound iron directly when the plasma iron concentration exceeds the binding capacity of Tf. This is an abnormal situation, because there is normally enough Tf in the plasma to bind approximately three times more iron than is present (ie, plasma Tf is normally approximately 30% saturated with iron). But patients with genetic or transfusional iron overload disorders can have fully saturated Tf, and excess iron is rapidly removed from circulation by the liver. The molecular details of hepatic non-Tf-bound iron uptake are not yet understood, but this process appears to involve a transport mechanism distinct from DMT1.

Hepatocyte iron stores act as a reserve that can be mobilized when the plasma iron supply becomes insufficient for erythropoiesis and other needs. Ferroportin, the iron exporter thought to function in basolateral intestinal iron transport, may also mediate iron export from hepatocytes, but this has not yet been established experimentally. To date, no other transmembrane iron exporters have been identified in mammals.

As discussed earlier, reticuloendothelial macrophages recycle iron from phagocytosed red blood cells. After they lyse the cells, iron is recovered from degraded hemoglobin through the action of heme oxygenase, an enzyme that catalyzes the degradation of heme. Macrophages may also acquire smaller amounts of iron through other pathways, including the Tf cycle. Similar to intestinal cells and hepatocytes, reticuloendothelial macrophages store some iron and release some directly into the circulation. Macrophage iron export also involves ferroportin, which it is expressed at high levels in iron recycling macrophages.[9]

Two distinct clinical presentations have been reported in patients with mutations in the gene encoding ferroportin.[20,21] Some patients develop an autosomal dominant iron overload disorder that is indistinguishable from hereditary hemochromatosis. These patients carry mutations that prevent the normal regulation of ferroportin's activity (see Chapter 36). More often, however, patients carrying ferroportin mutations present with hyperferritinemia, iron accumulation in tissue macrophages, and few (if any) complications of iron overload.

Macrophage iron export also requires ceruloplasmin, a copper-containing ferroxidase circulating in plasma. When the gene encoding ceruloplasmin was disrupted in mice, macrophages failed to release their iron at a normal rate, leading to hypoferremia in the presence of normal iron stores.[22] The abnormality was promptly corrected by administering exogenous ceruloplasmin. A similar phenomenon was noted in aceruloplasminemic human subjects.[23] Ceruloplasmin probably acts by catalyzing the oxidation of ferrous iron to the ferric form, which is a prerequisite for iron binding by apo-Tf. This function is analogous to that proposed for hephaestin, a highly related intestinal protein.

The capacity for macrophage iron storage is regulated in response to the iron needs of the body, through the action of the peptide hormone hepcidin (see Regulation of Iron Homeostasis in the Entire Organism). The concentration of plasma iron (and hence the Tf saturation) is predominantly determined by two factors—macrophage iron release (allowing iron to enter the plasma) and erythroid iron use (extracting iron from the plasma). Intestinal iron absorption and hepatocyte iron mobilization both contribute to the amount of plasma iron too, but to a lesser extent. When erythropoiesis occurs at a steady rate, Tf saturation is determined primarily by the amount of iron entering the plasma, that is, the amount of iron exported from macrophages, enterocytes and hepatocytes. When erythroid demand increases, plasma iron concentrations decrease unless release from stores is accelerated. Serum Tf saturation is calculated as the ratio of serum iron to total iron-binding capacity (TIBC; binding sites for iron available on plasma Tf) expressed in the same units. In clinical practice, Tf saturation is a useful indicator of how much iron is available for erythropoiesis.

Serum ferritin concentration, also used for clinical evaluation of iron status, reflects the amount of storage iron in the body. The origin of serum ferritin is not known, but it appears to be derived primarily from hepatocytes and reticuloendothelial macrophages. It differs from the ferritin used to store iron within cells—it is glycosylated (suggesting that it is actively secreted) and iron-poor. Serum ferritin is not a very accurate indicator of iron stores, however, because levels are increased when there is inflammation or tissue damage and in rare, congenital hyperferritinemia disorders. Nonetheless, a low serum ferritin value invariably indicates depleted iron stores. The ratio of sTfr to the log of the serum ferritin concentration has been touted as an index to distinguish pure iron deficiency anemia from the anemia of chronic disease. When this ratio is greater than 1.5, iron deficiency is usually present, with or without inflammation.[24]

The Iron-Copper Connection

It has long been known that copper deficiency is associated with abnormalities in iron metabolism and iron deficiency anemia. It is now clear that this is caused, at least in part, by the importance of the copper-containing ferroxidases ceruloplasmin and hephaestin. Both molecules are glycoproteins containing six to seven copper atoms. Ceruloplasmin has been shown to act as an oxidase for a variety of substrates. Hephaestin functions similarly. As discussed earlier, there is evidence that each of these molecules is required for the optimal mobilization of iron from cells to plasma.

Cellular Iron Storage

Intracellular storage iron is mostly found in ferritin, a large polymer composed of two types of polypeptide subunits (L and H ferritins), each approximately 20 kilodaltons in size. The H ferritin polypeptide has an enzymatic ferroxidase activity that is lacking in the L polypeptide. Each ferritin multimer is made up of 24 of these subunits, with changeable proportions of L and H chains. The L to H ratio varies among different cell types, but it is not known how it is determined. The interior of the ferritin molecule contains mineralized iron in a solid form. Ferritin prevents iron from reacting with other cellular constituents and allows for controlled iron release in response to increased cellular needs. Hemosiderin is a conglomerate composed of partially degraded ferritin, remnants of organelles and other proteins associated in an amorphous particle. The iron in hemosiderin is difficult to mobilize, and the conglomerate probably serves little purpose other than to keep iron from causing harm. Both ferritin and hemosiderin are abundant in iron-overloaded tissues.

As discussed earlier, the liver serves as the major depot for iron in excess of immediate needs. Hepatocytes and macrophages have a very large capacity for accumulating and holding iron, although this capacity is ultimately exceeded in iron overload disorders. The liver is an early site of iron accumulation in iron overload, owing to the fact that hepatocytes avidly take up non–Tf-bound iron from the plasma. Although other tissues (myocardium, pancreas) also accumulate excess iron, liver damage is often the first major clinical complication in adult-onset hemochromatosis. In contrast, juvenile hemochromatosis and transfusional (secondary) iron overload frequently present with relatively insignificant liver damage but prominent cardiomyopathy and endocrinopathies. The heart and endocrine tissues seem to be more susceptible to damage when iron loading occurs rapidly, particularly in young patients who develop significant iron overload before puberty.

Regulation of Cellular Iron Balance

Iron balance is regulated at many levels. The most fundamental level is iron-regulated expression of intracellular proteins of iron metabolism. There is evidence for transcriptional regulation in response to cellular or organismal iron status, but the mechanisms responsible for this effect have not been elucidated in mammals. Regulation at the level of translation is better understood. Several mRNA molecules encoding proteins of iron metabolism contain similar RNA stem-loop structures in their non-coding segments. These RNA stem-loop structures are iron responsive elements (IREs), which are specifically recognized and bound by iron regulatory proteins (IRPs).[25]

IRPs bind to IREs when iron is scarce, and dissociate from IREs when iron is plentiful. There are two known IRPs, IRP1 and IRP2. IRP1 has two distinct activities—in addition to binding to IREs, it can function as a cytoplasmic aconitase enzyme. The IRP1 polypeptide incorporates an iron-containing functional group, termed an iron-sulfur cluster. When present, the iron-sulfur cluster is important for aconitase activity, but it precludes binding to IREs. When it is absent, IRP1 no longer functions as an aconitase, but it gains the ability to bind to IREs. IRP2 is a similar protein, but it is regulated differently—it is stable under low iron conditions but rapidly degraded when iron is abundant. IRP2 has no aconitase activity.

IRPs are known to mediate translational effects in two distinct ways, depending on the location of the IRE stem-loop structure in the mRNA. When the IRE is located within the 5′ untranslated region of an mRNA (as in the mRNAs encoding L- and H-ferritin, ferroportin, and the heme biosynthetic enzyme aminolevulinic acid synthase), IRP binding is known[26] or expected to disrupt translational initiation by preventing assembly of initiation factors at the initiator

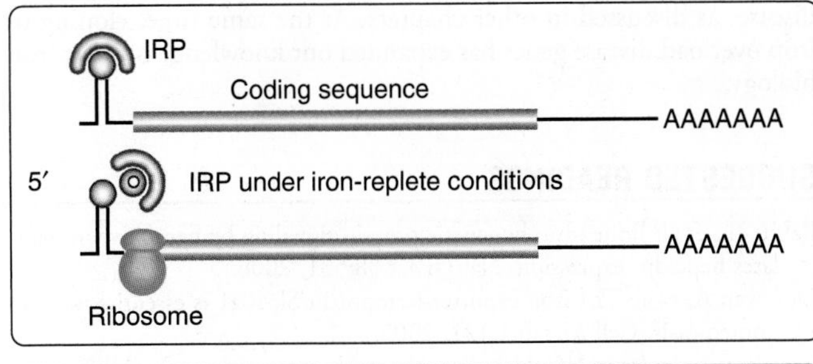

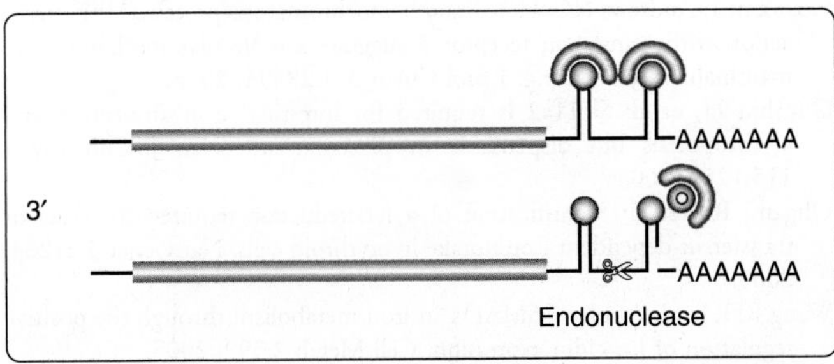

Figure 35–4 Regulation of gene expression by iron regulatory proteins (IRPs). Translation is regulated by iron through at least two distinct activities of iron responsive elements (IREs) and IRPs. When IREs are located in the 5′ untranslated regions of mRNAs (eg, ferritin mRNAs) binding of IRPs blocks the initiation of translation, thereby preventing protein expression (*top panel*). This blockade is relieved in the presence of iron, as described in the text. In contrast, the IREs located in the 3′ untranslated region of the mRNA encoding transferrin receptor (Tfr) are involved in regulating message stability. IRP binding prevents degradation by cellular endonucleases, resulting in increased protein expression in the absence of iron. Under iron replete circumstances the IRPs do not bind, and the mRNA is unstable (*bottom panel*). IREs located in the 3′ untranslated region of other mRNAs are believed to act through a similar mechanism, though this has not been validated experimentally.

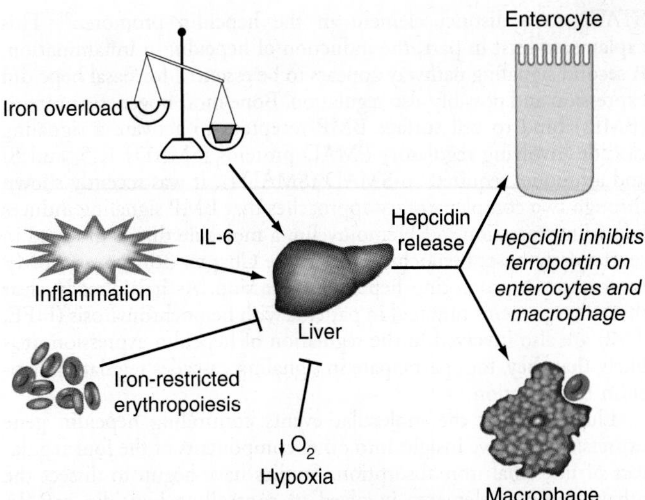

Figure 35–5 Regulation of hepcidin expression. At least four circumstances modulate hepcidin expression by the liver. Expression is increased in response to iron overload and inflammation. Interleukin-6 (IL-6), and possibly other inflammatory cytokines, induces hepcidin transcription in inflammation. Hepcidin expression is decreased in response to iron-restricted erythropoiesis and hypoxia, but the molecular details of those regulatory pathways have not yet been elucidated. In the effector arm of these multiple pathways, hepcidin produced by the liver has two actions: It blocks intestinal iron transport and inhibits export of iron from macrophages. Both can be explained by its regulatory interaction with ferroportin. O_2, oxygen.

methionine codon. In contrast, when IREs are found within the 3′ untranslated region of mRNAs (such as the mRNAs encoding Tfr and DMT1) IRP binding is known[27] or expected to confer stability to messages that would otherwise undergo rapid endonucleolytic digestion. Thus, in contrast to the effect mediated by 5′ IREs, 3′ IREs increase translation in the absence of iron. The current model is that binding of IRPs to IREs controls and coordinates translation of iron-related mRNAs in two ways—it inhibits production of proteins involved in iron storage (and probably iron export) and it promotes production of proteins necessary for iron uptake. These activities should contribute to the maintenance of intracellular iron homeostasis in response to iron levels. This is summarized in Fig. 35–4.

Regulation of Iron Homeostasis in the Entire Organism

Just as individual cells must have mechanisms for coordinated regulation of iron transport and iron storage to maintain adequate amounts to meet their needs but avoid iron overload, so must whole tissues. Regulation involves control of cellular iron uptake, retention and export. Recently, new insights have emerged that are leading to a comprehensive understanding of regulation at each of these steps.

In the absence of medical intervention, iron can only enter the body through the intestine. Dietary iron absorption is enhanced in response to insufficient iron stores, increased erythropoietic demand or hypoxia. It is diminished in response to iron surfeit and inflammation. Based on these observations, four different "regulators" have been defined functionally, although they are incompletely understood at a molecular level. The *stores regulator* modulates absorption several fold, increasing it in iron deficiency and decreasing it in iron overload. The *erythroid regulator* is more potent—it can increase iron absorption 6- to 10-fold when erythropoiesis becomes iron-restricted. Iron-restricted erythropoiesis can result either from iron deficiency (linking the stores and erythroid regulators) or from accelerated production of erythroid precursors, outstripping the capacity of Tf to supply adequate iron for hemoglobin synthesis. The *hypoxia regulator* appears to be distinct from the erythroid regulator, although it has overlapping function. It mediates an increase in iron absorption in response to hypoxia, to allow for production of hemoproteins that bind and carry oxygen. Finally, there is compelling evidence that an *inflammatory regulator* also exists, which acts to decrease iron absorption in response to inflammation associated with a wide variety of medical conditions. The inflammatory regulator comes into play in the anemia of chronic disease, as discussed in Chapter 37.

It is now clear that all of these regulators act through a common, humoral effector that coordinates intestinal iron absorption and macrophage iron recycling. Hepcidin (also called HAMP) is a 25 amino acid peptide that has intrinsic antimicrobial activity, similar to defensins, but also plays a major role in iron metabolism. It is produced in the liver, cleaved from a larger precursor molecule and secreted into the plasma. The amino-terminal portion of the preprotein has no known function, although there have been several studies attempting unsuccessfully to relate serum levels of this remnant to iron homeostasis. Hepcidin itself is rapidly cleared by the kidneys, allowing for dynamic regulation at the level of its production. Over the past few years, the biologic activity of hepcidin has been elucidated. Circulating hepcidin attaches to ferroportin expressed on enterocytes and macrophages, causing ferroportin to be internalized into the cell and degraded in lysosomes.[28]

Expression of hepcidin is modulated in response to all of the regulators described earlier (Fig. 35–5). Hepcidin is induced in response to iron overload and inflammation. It is turned off in response to iron deficiency, ineffective erythropoiesis and hypoxia. Although it has become clear that much or all regulation of hepcidin expression takes place at the level of transcription, the signals that turn on and turn off hepcidin production are incompletely understood. Two cellular signaling pathways have clearly been shown to regulate hepcidin transcription. In the setting of inflammation, the inflammatory cytokine interleukin-6 (IL-6) binds to hepatocyte IL-6 receptors, triggering a JAK/STAT3 signaling cascade that leads to binding of activated

STAT3 to a distinct element in the hepcidin promoter.[29] This explains, at least in part, the induction of hepcidin in inflammation. A second signaling pathway appears to be essential for basal hepcidin expression and possibly also regulation. Bone morphogenetic proteins (BMPs) bind to cell surface BMP receptors to activate a signaling cascade involving regulatory SMAD proteins (SMADs 1, 5, and 8) and a unique, required co-SMAD (SMAD4). It was recently shown through two complementary approaches that BMP signaling induces hepcidin expression.[30,31] Hemojuvelin, a molecule that is mutated in severe, early onset hemochromatosis (see Chapter 36) acts as a BMP coreceptor in promoting hepcidin expression. As it is already clear that other proteins mutated in patients with hemochromatosis (HFE, Tfr2) are also involved in the regulation of hepcidin expression, it is likely that they, too, participate in signaling cascades regulating hepcidin transcription.

Elucidation of the molecular events controlling hepcidin gene expression will give insight into other components of the four regulators of intestinal iron absorption. Studies have begun to dissect the other promoter elements involved in controlling hepcidin mRNA expression.[32]

CONCLUSIONS

Many details of iron transport and homeostasis have been elucidated over the past decade, but much remains to be learned. Identification and characterization of the genes and proteins involved has given insight into human iron overload disorders and the anemia of chronic disease, as discussed in other chapters. At the same time, cloning of iron overload disease genes has expanded our knowledge of basic iron biology.

SUGGESTED READINGS

Babitt JL, et al: Bone morphogenetic protein signaling by hemojuvelin regulates hepcidin expression. Nat Genet 38:531, 2006.

Donovan A, et al: The iron exporter ferroportin/Slc40a1 is essential for iron homeostasis. Cell Metab 1:191, 2005.

Goswami T, Andrews NC: Hereditary hemochromatosis protein, HFE, interaction with transferrin receptor 2 suggests a molecular mechanism for mammalian iron sensing. J Biol Chem 281:28494, 2006.

Gunshin H, et al: Slc11a2 is required for intestinal iron absorption and erythropoiesis but dispensable in placenta and liver. J Clin Invest 115:1258, 2005.

Ohgami RS, et al: Identification of a ferrireductase required for efficient transferrin-dependent iron uptake in erythroid cells. Nat Genet 37:1264, 2005.

Wang RH, et al: A role of SMAD4 in iron metabolism through the positive regulation of hepcidin expression. Cell Metab 2:399, 2005.

Wrighting DM, Andrews NC: Interleukin-6 induces hepcidin expression through STAT3. Blood 108:3204, 2006.

REFERENCES

For complete list of references log onto www.expertconsult.com

CHAPTER 36

DISORDERS OF IRON METABOLISM: IRON DEFICIENCY AND IRON OVERLOAD

Gary M. Brittenham

Iron is an essential nutrient required by every human cell. Both decreases and increases in body iron are often clinically important. If too little iron is available (iron deficiency), limitations on the synthesis of physiologically active iron-containing compounds can have deleterious consequences. If too much iron accumulates (iron overload) and exceeds the body's capacity for safe transport and storage, iron toxicity may produce widespread organ damage and death.

Remarkable progress in our understanding of the molecular mechanisms underlying iron homeostasis is described in Chapter 35. This chapter focuses on the clinical applications of these advances and improvements in the diagnosis and management of both iron deficiency and iron overload.

LABORATORY EVALUATION OF IRON STATUS

The major routes of iron movement are shown in Fig. 36–1. The continuum of changes in iron stores and distribution in the presence of increased or decreased body iron content is illustrated in Fig. 36–2, along with characteristic values for clinically available indicators of iron status. The general usefulness of these measures is considered in this section, and their specific applications in the diagnosis of iron deficiency and iron overload are described in Iron deficiency laboratory evaluation and in Iron overload: laboratory evaluation.

Body iron supply and stores can be evaluated by both direct and indirect means, but no single indicator or combination of indicators is ideal for evaluation of iron status in all clinical circumstances. As body iron content decreases from the iron-replete normal to the amounts found in iron-deficiency anemia or as it increases to the magnitudes found in the various forms of iron overload, each available measure reflects in a different manner the continuum of changes shown in Fig. 36–2. In addition, each indicator may be affected by coexisting conditions, such as infection, inflammation, ineffective erythropoiesis, hypoxemia, liver disease, malignancy, and malnutrition. Recognizing that these coexisting conditions act principally through a common pathway that modulates the expression of hepcidin (see Chapter 35 and box on Control of Iron Homeostasis by Hepcidin and Ferroportin) greatly assists in the interpretation of the patterns of changes found in specific clinical conditions.

Direct Measures

The direct measures of body iron status yield quantitative, specific, and sensitive determinations of body or tissue iron stores. Quantitative phlebotomy provides a direct measure of total mobilizable storage iron.[1] Quantitative phlebotomy is inapplicable to most anemic disorders but occasionally is useful in the diagnostic evaluation of some forms of iron overload (e.g., in patients with hereditary hemochromatosis who do not undergo liver biopsy). Bone marrow aspiration and biopsy can provide information about (a) macrophage storage iron, by semiquantitative grading of marrow hemosiderin stained with Prussian blue or, if needed, by chemical measurement of nonheme iron; (b) iron supply to erythroid precursors, by determining the proportion and morphology of marrow sideroblasts (i.e., normoblasts with visible aggregates of iron in the cytoplasm); and (c) general morphologic features of hematopoiesis. Bone marrow aspiration and biopsy are useful in studies of iron deficiency[2] but of limited applicability in the evaluation of iron overload because no information about the extent of parenchymal iron deposition is provided. In the evaluation of iron overload, liver biopsy is the best direct test for assessing iron deposition, permitting quantitative measurement of the nonheme iron concentration and histochemical examination of the pattern of iron accumulation in hepatocytes and Kupffer cells.[1,3–5]

Direct methods for assessing iron status have the disadvantages of being invasive procedures, with their attendant discomfort, lack of acceptability to patients, and, in the case of liver biopsy, risk. A variety of noninvasive means of measuring tissue iron stores have been developed and applied in clinical studies,[6,7] including determination of hepatic magnetic susceptibility, computed tomography, and magnetic resonance imaging.[8–12] When available as appropriately calibrated and validated techniques, these new noninvasive methods are helpful in the diagnosis and management of iron overload[13] but lack the accuracy required for measurements to detect iron deficiency.

Indirect Measures

Indirect measures of body iron status have the advantages of ease and convenience, but all are subject to extraneous influences and lack specificity, sensitivity, or both. When used to estimate body iron stores, all of the available indirect measures are influenced not only by total body iron stores but also by the effects of acute or chronic changes in plasma hepcidin (see box on Control of Iron Homeostasis by Hepcidin and Ferroportin). Assays for urinary and plasma hepcidin are under development[14,15] and likely will be helpful in the clinical evaluation of patients with disorders of iron metabolism.

Measurement of plasma ferritin provides the most useful indirect estimate of body iron stores. Ferritin is secreted into the plasma in small amounts, but its physiologic role is obscure.[16,17] Whereas intracellular ferritin is produced by the smooth endoplasmic reticulum, plasma ferritin is synthesized by the rough endoplasmic reticulum and glycosylated by the Golgi apparatus. Under normal circumstances, the amount of plasma ferritin synthesized and secreted seems to be proportional to the amount of cellular ferritin produced in the internal iron storage pathway so that the plasma ferritin concentration is related to the magnitude of body iron stores. The small amounts of ferritin secreted into the circulation can be measured by immunoassay and have a logarithmic relationship to body iron stores in healthy persons. In the absence of complicating factors that alter plasma hepcidin, plasma ferritin concentrations decrease with depletion of storage iron and increase with storage iron accumulation. A maximum glycosylated plasma ferritin concentration of approximately 4000 mg/L has been postulated, perhaps representing an upper physiologic limit of the rate of synthesis.[18] Higher concentrations are believed to be due to release of intracellular ferritin from damaged cells.

Measurement of plasma transferrin receptor concentration provides a useful new means of detecting tissue iron deficiency.[19–21] The soluble transferrin receptor is a truncated form (relative molecular mass [M_r] 85,000) of the tissue transferrin receptor that consists of the amino (N)-terminal cytoplasmic domain that probably has been proteolytically released from the cell membrane. Immunoassays that

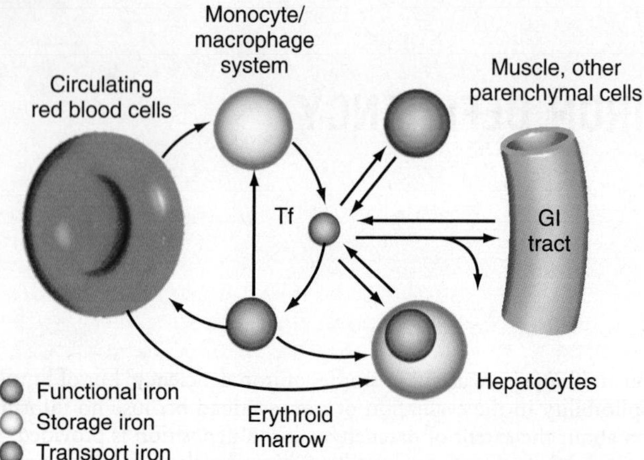

Figure 36–1 Body iron supply and storage. Schematic representation of the routes of iron movement. The major pathway of internal iron exchange is a unidirectional flow from plasma transferrin (Tf) to the erythron to the macrophage and back to plasma transferrin. Storage iron in the macrophages of the liver, bone marrow, and spleen is derived almost entirely from phagocytosis of senescent erythrocytes or defective developing red cells. The macrophage takes up little iron from plasma transferrin, whereas the hepatocyte may either donate iron to or receive iron from plasma transferrin. Other pathways of iron movement involve approximately equal exchanges for iron absorption and losses, for transfer between the plasma and extravascular transferrin compartments, and for movement between extravascular transferrin and parenchymal tissues. Increases in hepcidin decrease macrophage release of iron derived from senescent red blood cells, diminish delivery of iron from duodenal enterocytes absorbing dietary iron, and inhibit release of iron stored in hepatocytes. *(Modified from Finch CA, Huebers H: Perspectives in iron metabolism. N Engl J Med 306:1520, 1982.*[230]*)*

Control of Iron Homeostasis by Hepcidin and Ferroportin

Hepcidin functions as the chief controller of body iron supply and storage by interacting with ferroportin, a transmembrane protein that is the only known iron exporter in humans (see Chapter 35). Hepcidin binds to ferroportin, inducing its internalization and degradation, thereby inhibiting iron efflux from the principal sources of plasma iron: macrophages, duodenal enterocytes, and hepatocytes (see Fig. 36–1). Under physiologic conditions, hepatic hepcidin production coordinates body iron supply with iron need. If body iron stores expand, hepcidin production increases. Increments in plasma hepcidin reduce the amount of ferroportin in cell membranes, causing a prompt fall in plasma iron concentration by decreasing macrophage release of iron derived from senescent red blood cells, diminishing delivery of iron from enterocytes absorbing dietary iron, and inhibiting release of iron stored in hepatocytes. Conversely, if body iron stores contract, hepcidin production decreases. Decrements in plasma hepcidin concentration increase the amount of ferroportin, producing a rise in plasma iron concentration as a consequence of enhanced delivery from macrophages, increased dietary iron absorption from enterocytes, and mobilization of storage iron from hepatocytes. In addition to these effects of body iron stores, hepcidin production is stimulated by inflammation and inhibited by increased erythropoiesis. Depending on clinical circumstances, the effects of inflammation or increased erythropoiesis on hepatic hepcidin synthesis may predominate over the effects of body iron stores.

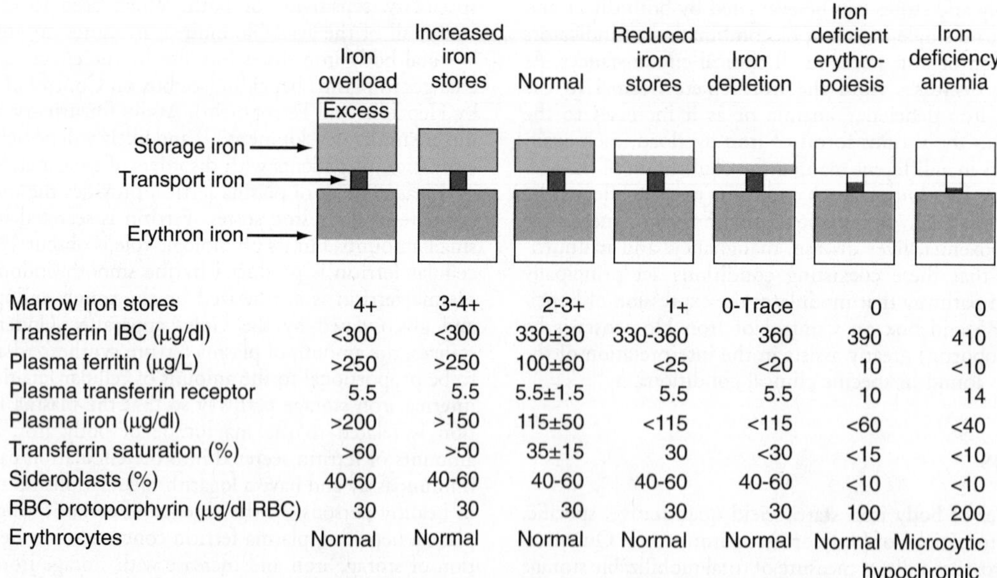

	Iron overload	Increased iron stores	Normal	Reduced iron stores	Iron depletion	Iron deficient erythropoiesis	Iron deficiency anemia
Marrow iron stores	4+	3-4+	2-3+	1+	0-Trace	0	0
Transferrin IBC (μg/dl)	<300	<300	330±30	330-360	360	390	410
Plasma ferritin (μg/L)	>250	>250	100±60	<25	<20	10	<10
Plasma transferrin receptor	5.5	5.5	5.5±1.5	5.5	5.5	10	14
Plasma iron (μg/dl)	>200	>150	115±50	<115	<115	<60	<40
Transferrin saturation (%)	>60	>50	35±15	30	<30	<15	<10
Sideroblasts (%)	40-60	40-60	40-60	40-60	40-60	<10	<10
RBC protoporphyrin (μg/dl RBC)	30	30	30	30	30	100	200
Erythrocytes	Normal	Normal	Normal	Normal	Normal	Normal	Microcytic hypochromic

Figure 36–2 Continuum of changes in iron stores and distribution in the presence of increased or decreased body iron content. Abnormalities indicating the onset of specific stages of negative iron balance are enclosed in boxes. In iron overload, excess storage iron may increase from the normal range of 1 g or less to as much as 40 to 50 g. Marrow iron stores are increased as shown only in disorders of iron overload with reticuloendothelial iron loading, such as transfusional iron overload. Marrow iron stores may be normal or even absent in hereditary hemochromatosis. *(Adapted from Herbert V: Anemias. In Paige DM [ed.]: Clinical Nutrition. St. Louis, CV Mosby, 1988, p 593,*[231] *with permission.)*

can detect the soluble truncated form of the transferrin receptor in human plasma are clinically available.[22] A majority of plasma transferrin receptors are derived from the erythroid marrow, and their concentration is determined primarily by erythroid marrow activity. Decreased levels of circulating soluble transferrin receptor are found in patients with erythroid hypoplasia (aplastic anemia, chronic renal failure), whereas increased levels are present in patients with erythroid hyperplasia (thalassemia major, sickle cell anemia, anemia with ineffective erythropoiesis, chronic hemolytic anemia). Iron deficiency also increases soluble transferrin receptor concentrations. The plasma transferrin receptor concentration reflects the total body mass of tissue receptor; thus, in the absence of other conditions causing erythroid hyperplasia, an increase in plasma transferrin receptor concentration provides a sensitive, quantitative measure of tissue iron deficiency.[19] In particular, measurement of plasma transferrin receptor concentration may help differentiate between the anemia of iron deficiency and the anemia associated with chronic inflammatory disorders. Although the plasma ferritin concentration may be disproportionately elevated in relation to iron stores in patients with inflammation or liver disease, the plasma transferrin receptor concentration seems to be unaffected by these disorders and appears to provide a more reliable laboratory indicator of iron deficiency.[20]

The erythrocyte zinc protoporphyrin level provides an indicator of iron supply to erythroid precursors.[20,23] In heme biosynthesis, the final reaction is chelation of a ferrous ion by protoporphyrin IX. If no iron is available, zinc is chelated instead to form zinc protoporphyrin. Because zinc protoporphyrin formed during development persists throughout the lifespan of the red cell, the blood concentration changes only as new cells are formed and old cells are destroyed, providing a retrospective view of iron supply over the preceding several weeks. An elevated erythrocyte zinc protoporphyrin concentration (sometimes measured as the zinc protoporphyrin-to-heme ratio) lacks specificity because concentrations increase not only with absent iron stores in iron deficiency but also with other conditions that increase plasma hepcidin and restrict iron availability, such as infection, inflammation, and malignancy. Levels also are increased in many sideroblastic anemias and especially with chronic lead poisoning.[20,24] The test is useful for detecting lead poisoning but is of no value in detecting iron overload.

Measurements of the proportion of hypochromic circulating red cells and the hemoglobin content of reticulocytes are possible with some hematology analyzers[25,26] and offer new means of detecting restriction of iron supply for erythropoiesis. The proportion of hypochromic red cells provides information similar to that derived from the erythrocyte zinc protoporphyrin level and becomes abnormal only after weeks of iron-restricted erythropoiesis. Measurements of the mean cellular hemoglobin content of reticulocytes or the reticulocyte hemoglobin equivalent permit earlier detection of iron-restricted erythropoiesis[25] but are unable to distinguish between the absent iron stores of iron deficiency and decreased iron availability due to increases in plasma hepcidin associated with infection, inflammation, and malignancy.

Measurement of urinary iron excretion with chelating agents, usually either deferoxamine or diethylenetriamine pentaacetic acid, offers another means of assessing body iron stores.[7,27] This test is not helpful for detecting iron deficiency because of the overlap between values in persons with normal and those with decreased iron stores; it is used primarily for the evaluation of iron overload. The usefulness of the measurement of chelated iron in the urine is limited by a lack of correlation between chelatable iron excretion and the results of quantitative phlebotomy with parenchymal iron overload and by the susceptibility of the effects of increases in plasma hepcidin associated with inflammatory states.

Examination of peripheral blood by measurements of hemoglobin concentration, hematocrit, red cell indices, red cell volume distribution, and reticulocyte count and by inspection of erythrocyte morphology reveals abnormalities only after depletion of iron stores restricts the availability of iron for erythropoiesis. The changes are not specific for iron deficiency and may be found in other conditions with defective hemoglobin synthesis, such as thalassemia, infection, inflammation, liver disease, and malignancy. Iron overload does not produce any diagnostic abnormalities in the peripheral blood.

IRON DEFICIENCY

Iron deficiency denotes a deficit in total body iron resulting from a sustained increase in iron requirements over iron supply. The continuum of decreased body iron is shown in Fig. 36–2. Three successive stages of iron lack can be distinguished. A decrement in storage iron without a decline in the level of functional iron compounds is termed *iron depletion* (see Fig. 36–2). After iron stores are exhausted, lack of iron limits the production of hemoglobin and other metabolically active compounds that require iron as a constituent or cofactor. *Iron-deficient erythropoiesis* (see Fig. 36–2) develops, although the effect on hemoglobin production may be insufficient to be detected by the standards used to differentiate normal from anemic states. Further diminution in the body iron produces frank *iron-deficiency anemia* (see Fig. 36–2).

Epidemiology

Iron deficiency is the most common cause of anemia in the United States and worldwide.[28–30] In the United States, adequacy of bioavailable iron in the diet, together with food fortification and the widespread use of iron supplements, has reduced the overall prevalence and severity of iron deficiency, but iron nutrition remains a problem in some subpopulations, especially toddlers, adolescent girls, women of childbearing age, and some minority groups.[28,31,32] Without iron supplementation, most women will become iron deficient during pregnancy. Globally, 30% to 70% of the populations in developing countries are iron deficient, with the highest prevalence among persons who have diets low in bioavailable iron, or who suffer from chronic gastrointestinal blood loss as a result of helminthic infection, or both.[28–30,33]

Etiology and Pathogenesis

The foremost task in the evaluation of patients with iron deficiency is identifying and treating the underlying cause of the imbalance between iron requirements and supply that is responsible for the lack of iron (Table 36–1). Overall, the *iron requirement* for an individual includes not only the iron needed to replenish physiologic losses and meet the demands of growth and pregnancy but also any additional amounts needed to replace pathologic losses. Physiologic iron losses generally are restricted to the small amounts of iron contained in the urine, bile, and sweat; shedding of iron-containing cells from the intestine, urinary tract, and skin; occult gastrointestinal blood loss;

Table 36–1 Causes of Iron Deficiency

Increased Iron Requirements
Blood loss
Gastrointestinal tract
Genitourinary tract
Respiratory tract
Blood donation
Growth
Pregnancy and lactation
Inadequate Iron Supply
Dietary insufficiency of bioavailable iron
Impaired absorption of iron
Intestinal malabsorption
Gastric surgery
Impaired iron transport

and, in women, uterine losses during menstruation and pregnancy.[34–36] In normal men, the daily basal iron loss is slightly less than 1.0 mg/day. In normal menstruating women, the daily basal iron loss is approximately 1.5 mg/day. The median total iron loss with pregnancy is approximately 500 mg, or almost 2 mg/day over the 280 days of gestation. Genetic factors may influence the risk of iron deficiency, but the mechanisms responsible have not been identified.[35,36]

The most common pathologic cause of increased iron requirements leading to iron deficiency is blood loss. In men and postmenopausal women, iron deficiency almost inevitably signifies gastrointestinal blood loss.[20,37] Within the gastrointestinal tract, any hemorrhagic lesion may result in blood loss, and the responsible lesion may be asymptomatic. Iron deficiency often is the first sign of an occult gastrointestinal malignancy[38,39] or other unrecognized conditions such as coeliac disease,[40] or autoimmune, atrophic, or *Helicobacter pylori* gastritis.[41,42] Chronic ingestion of drugs such as alcohol, salicylates, steroids, and nonsteroidal antiinflammatory drugs may cause or contribute to blood loss. Worldwide, the most frequent cause of gastrointestinal blood loss is hookworm infection, but other helminthic infections, such as *Schistosoma mansoni* and *Schistosoma japonicum,* and severe *Trichuris trichiura* infection also may be responsible.

In women of childbearing age, genitourinary blood loss with menstruation adds to iron requirements.[43] Menstrual losses tend to decrease with use of oral contraceptives but increase with use of intrauterine devices. Other, less frequent causes of genitourinary bleeding should be considered, including chronic hemoglobinuria and hemosiderinuria resulting from paroxysmal nocturnal hemoglobinuria[44] or from chronic intravascular hemolysis.

Uncommonly, respiratory tract blood loss resulting from chronic recurrent hemoptysis of any cause produces iron deficiency. In two rare conditions, Goodpasture syndrome and idiopathic pulmonary siderosis, hemoptysis and intrapulmonary bleeding may be inapparent but lead to sequestration of iron in pulmonary macrophages.[45] Although still within the body, the sequestered iron is "lost" from systemic use, and severe iron-deficiency anemia may develop. Recurrent blood donation may lead to iron deficiency, particularly in menstruating women.[46]

In infants, children, and adolescents, the need for iron for growth may exceed the supply available from diet and stores.[47] Premature infants, who have a lower birth weight and a more rapid postnatal rate of growth, are at high risk for iron deficiency unless given iron supplements.[48] With rapid growth during the first year of life, the body weights of term infants normally triple, and iron requirements are at high levels. Iron requirements decline as growth slows during the second year of life and into childhood but rise again with the adolescent growth spurt.[49]

Without supplemental iron, pregnancy entails the net loss of the equivalent of 1200 to 1500 mL of blood. After delivery, resumption of menstruation usually is delayed for months. If the infant is breast-fed, lactation necessitates an intake of approximately 0.5 to 1.0 mg of iron daily.

In some instances, an insufficient supply of iron may contribute to the development of iron deficiency. In infants or in women who have experienced heavy menstrual losses or multiple pregnancies, the risk of iron deficiency may be further increased by diets with insufficient amounts of bioavailable iron, such as those with little or no heme iron and with small amounts of enhancers or large amounts of inhibitors of nonheme iron absorption.[37] For older children, men, and postmenopausal women, the restricted availability of dietary iron is almost never the sole explanation for iron deficiency, and other causes, especially blood loss, must be considered.[20,37]

Impaired absorption of iron in itself infrequently produces iron deficiency. Intestinal malabsorption of iron may occur as a manifestation of more generalized syndromes.[50] Atrophic gastritis and the attendant achlorhydria may impair iron absorption.[42] In persons of all ages and both genders, but particularly in pregnant women and children, pica, the compulsive chewing or ingestion of food or nonfood substances, may contribute to iron deficiency if the material consumed inhibits iron absorption.[51] Iron deficiency frequently complicates gastric surgery, such as partial or total gastric resection or gastroenterostomy for bypass of the duodenum.[52]

Increased iron requirements and an inadequate supply of iron often work in concert to produce iron deficiency. Infants fed cow's milk receive a diet that not only contains small amounts of iron of low bioavailability but also increases iron losses by causing gastrointestinal bleeding.[47] Menstruating women, who have some of the highest iron requirements, may consume diets that have a low content of iron and contain inhibitors of iron absorption, such as calcium.[43] Patients with ulcer disease and increased gastrointestinal blood loss may habitually take antacids, which diminish dietary iron absorption.

Clinical Presentation

Patients with iron deficiency may present with (a) no signs or symptoms, coming to medical attention only because of abnormalities noted on laboratory tests; (b) features of the underlying disorder responsible for the development of iron deficiency; (c) manifestations common to all anemias; or (d) one or more of the few signs and symptoms considered highly specific for iron deficiency, namely, pagophagia, koilonychia, and blue sclerae. In addition, a high prevalence of iron deficiency with or without anemia has been reported among patients with the restless legs syndrome (Ekbom syndrome), a neurologic disorder characterized by a distressing need or urge to move the legs (akathisia).[53,54]

An uncomplicated depletion of storage iron generally is not associated with signs or symptoms, although patients without iron reserves will not respond as rapidly to an increased need for iron resulting from blood loss, growth, or pregnancy. Greater deficits in body iron, which restrict the synthesis of functional iron compounds and cause anemia, either may be asymptomatic or may produce a variety of clinical manifestations. Iron-deficiency anemia produces the signs and symptoms common to all anemias: pallor, palpitations, tinnitus, headache, irritability, weakness, dizziness, easy fatigability, and other vague and nonspecific complaints. The prominence of these signs depends on the degree and rate of development of the anemia. Because iron deficiency often is of insidious onset and prolonged duration, adaptive circulatory and respiratory responses may minimize these manifestations, permitting a surprising tolerance of low hemoglobin concentrations. With greater severity, anemia becomes increasingly debilitating as work capacity and tolerance of physical exertion are restricted and eventually can produce cardiorespiratory failure and even death.

Iron deficiency may produce clinical manifestations independent of anemia. The abnormalities seem to result from depletion of functional iron compounds in nonerythroid tissues, resulting in impaired proliferation, growth, and function. Epithelial tissues have high iron requirements due to rapid rates of growth and turnover and thus are affected in many patients with chronic iron deficiency. Glossitis, angular stomatitis, postcricoid esophageal web or stricture (which may become malignant), and gastric atrophy may develop. The combination of glossitis, a sore or burning mouth, dysphagia, and iron deficiency is called the Plummer-Vinson or Paterson-Kelly syndrome.[55] The prevalence of these abnormalities seems to vary geographically, which suggests that environmental or genetic factors are involved.

Determining whether gastric atrophy is the cause or the consequence of iron deficiency may be difficult,[42] particularly in older patients. In some patients, pernicious anemia and iron deficiency coexist. Changes in the lingual or buccal mucosa have been suggested as factors causing or contributing to the pica that develops in many patients with iron deficiency.[51] Pagophagia, a variant of pica in which ice is the substance obsessively consumed, is a behavioral abnormality that is considered to be a highly specific symptom of iron deficiency, resolving within a few days to 2 weeks after beginning iron therapy.[56] Other types of pica involving a variety of nonfoods, such as clay, starch, paper, and dirt, or an assortment of foods may occur in iron

Iron Deficiency and Coexisting Disorders

Detection of iron deficiency in the presence of chronic infectious, inflammatory, or malignant disorders is more problematic than in the absence of such disorders. Even if iron lack contributes to the anemia of chronic disease, the transferrin concentration (or total iron-binding capacity) will be decreased and the plasma ferritin concentration will be increased. Because the serum transferrin receptor concentration is not affected by inflammation, its measurement usually can determine whether iron stores are absent.[20,22,65] If uncertainty remains, bone marrow examination is definitive. If iron deficiency is present, iron stores are absent; if the anemia of chronic disease alone is responsible, iron stores are present and typically increased.

deficiency but are not as clearly linked to a lack of iron or as frequently responsive to iron therapy. In *koilonychia*, the fingernails are thin, friable, and brittle, and the distal half of the nail is a concave or "spoon" shape resulting from impaired nail bed epithelial growth. This condition is considered virtually pathognomonic of iron deficiency but occurs in a small minority of patients.[57] Blue sclerae, a condition in which the sclerae have a definite or striking bluish hue, were recognized in 1908 by Osler as being associated with iron deficiency[58] and have been reported to be a highly specific and sensitive indicator of iron deficiency.[59] The bluish tinge is believed to result from thinning of the sclera, which makes the choroid visible. This thinning has been postulated to result from impairment of collagen synthesis by iron deficiency. Iron deficiency has been postulated to have other nonhematologic consequences associated with impaired immunity and resistance to infection,[60] diminished exercise tolerance and work performance,[61] and a variety of behavioral and neuropsychological abnormalities.[62]

Laboratory Evaluation

A characteristic sequence of changes in the clinically useful indications of iron status occurs as body iron decreases from the iron-replete normal to the levels found in iron-deficiency anemia. This sequence is illustrated in Fig. 36–2. The patterns shown develop in the absence of complicating factors, such as infection, inflammation, liver disease, malignancy, or other disorders (see box on Iron Deficiency and Coexisting Disorders). Initially, as a result of any of the causes listed in Table 36–1, iron requirements exceed the available supply of iron. Iron is mobilized from body stores, and iron absorption is increased. If the amounts of iron available from body reserves and absorption are inadequate, depletion of storage iron follows. At this stage, bone marrow examination shows absent, or nearly absent, hemosiderin iron. The serum ferritin level falls while the total iron-binding capacity rises. Exhaustion of iron reserves then results in an inadequate supply of iron to the developing erythroid cell, and iron-deficient erythropoiesis commences. Plasma transferrin receptor concentrations increase as the total body mass of tissue receptor expands. The plasma ferritin level decreases to less than 12 mg/L (see box on Plasma Ferritin Concentrations), reflecting the absence of storage iron, and the total iron-binding capacity continues to rise. The plasma iron level declines, and, in combination with the increase in total iron-binding capacity, transferrin saturation falls to less than 16% (see box on Plasma Iron and Transferrin Saturation). Marrow examination shows, in addition to the absence of hemosiderin iron, a decrease in the proportion of sideroblasts because too little iron is available to support siderotic granule formation. The erythrocyte zinc protoporphyrin level progressively increases with reduction of the amount of iron available for heme formation. Measurement of reticulocyte cellular indices, such as the reticulocyte hemoglobin content or the reticulocyte hemoglobin equivalent, seems to provide an nearly means of detecting iron-restricted erythropoiesis,[25] both in uncomplicated iron deficiency and in the "functional" lack of iron in patients receiving recombinant erythropoietin.[63,64]

Plasma Ferritin Concentrations

Decreased plasma ferritin concentrations are of great value in the detection of iron deficiency. Plasma ferritin concentrations decline with storage iron depletion; a plasma ferritin concentration less than 12 mg/L is virtually diagnostic of absence of iron stores. The only known conditions that may lower the plasma ferritin concentration independently of a decrease in iron stores are hypothyroidism and ascorbate deficiency,[66] but these conditions only rarely cause problems in clinical interpretation. Increased plasma ferritin concentrations may indicate increased iron stores, but a number of disorders may raise the plasma ferritin level independently of the body iron store. Plasma ferritin is an acute-phase reactant, with increased ferritin synthesis a nonspecific response that is part of the general pattern of the systemic effects of inflammation. Thus, fever, acute infections, rheumatoid arthritis, and other chronic inflammatory disorders elevate the plasma ferritin concentration. Both acute and chronic damage to the liver, as well as to other ferritin-rich tissues, may increase plasma ferritin concentration through an inflammatory process or by releasing tissue ferritins from damaged parenchymal cells; these tissue ferritins are not glycosylated. Plasma ferritin concentrations in individuals of Asian or Pacific Island ancestry have been found to be higher than in other populations,[67] but the basis for this difference is unknown.

Plasma Iron Concentration and Transferrin Saturation

Plasma iron concentration and transferrin saturation, which equals the ratio of plasma iron to total iron-binding capacity, provide a measure of current iron supply to tissues. After storage iron is depleted, the serum iron concentration falls; a transferrin saturation less than 16% often is used as the criterion for iron-deficient erythropoiesis. In contrast, plasma iron concentration and transferrin saturation are not reliably elevated with increased iron stores within macrophages, as occurs initially with transfusional iron overload, although the transferrin saturation may increase with parenchymal iron loading. Interpretation of the transferrin saturation is complicated by substantial circadian fluctuations in plasma iron concentration as day-to-day variations of 30% or greater. Furthermore, plasma iron concentration is decreased by infection, inflammation, malignancy, and ascorbate deficiency but increased by iron ingestion, aplastic and sideroblastic anemias, ineffective erythropoiesis, and liver disease.

As hemoglobin production becomes restricted, frank iron-deficiency anemia develops. The normocytic, normochromic red cells previously formed under iron-replete circumstances gradually are replaced by a microcytic hypochromic population. Both the time needed to replace the normal population and the extent of the disparity between erythroid needs and available iron supply determine the rate and degree of change in erythrocyte morphology and red cell indices, such as mean corpuscular volume, mean corpuscular hemoglobin, and measures of the distribution of red cell volumes such as red cell volume distribution width. Chronic, long-standing iron-deficiency anemia may produce severe microcytosis and hypochromia, with very pale, distorted red cells and dramatic reductions in the mean corpuscular volume and mean corpuscular hemoglobin (Fig. 36–3). In contrast, some patients with mild iron-deficiency anemia may have erythrocyte morphology and indices indistinguishable from values found in normal, iron-replete individuals.

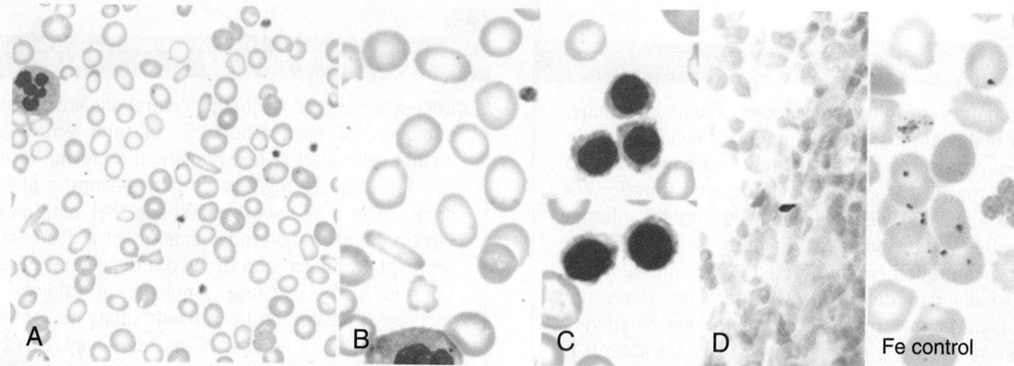

Figure 36–3 Iron-deficiency anemia. Peripheral blood smear (**A, B**), bone marrow aspirate (**C**), and Prussian blue stain of bone marrow aspirate (**D**) with control from a 16-year-old girl with hemoglobin 6.7 g/dL, hematocrit 22.6%, and mean corpuscular volume 59.2 fL. Peripheral smear shows hypochromic microcytic red blood cells (**A**), with widening of the central pallor and "pencil" cells (**B**). Polychromatophilic erythroid precursors in the aspirated specimen have scanty cytoplasm that is irregular and vacuolated (**C**). The Prussian blue–stained aspirate shows no iron stores in multiple spicules (**D**). Care must be taken not to overinterpret positive staining debris on top of cells (center). Lack of staining on the bone marrow biopsy sample can be misleading because the decalcification process is known to "leach-out" iron. An appropriate control should be similar to the patient material. Peripheral blood smears made from a patient with increased iron-containing Pappenheimer bodies and fixed with 100% methanol can serve as an easily accessible control.

Table 36–2 Differential Diagnosis of Microcytic Hypochromic Anemia

Decreased Body Iron Stores
Iron-deficiency anemia
Normal or Increased Body Iron Stores
Impaired iron metabolism
Anemia of chronic disease
Defective absorption, transport, or use of iron
Disorders of globin synthesis
Thalassemia
Other microcytic hemoglobinopathies
Disorders of heme synthesis: sideroblastic anemias
Hereditary
Acquired

Nonetheless, laboratory evaluation of uncomplicated iron deficiency in otherwise healthy persons usually is not difficult, and the characteristic patterns of indicators of body iron status shown in Fig. 36–2 typically are diagnostic. The diagnostic point is that early or mild iron deficiency must be considered in the workup of normocytic as well as microcytic anemia.

Therapeutic Trial of Iron

The diagnosis of iron deficiency often is confirmed by the outcome of a therapeutic trial of iron. A specific orderly response to, and only to, treatment with iron constitutes the final definitive proof that a lack of iron is the cause of an anemia. The unequivocal diagnostic response consists of (a) a reticulocytosis, which begins approximately 3 to 5 days after adequate iron therapy is instituted, reaches a maximum on days 8 to 10, and then declines; and (b) a significant increase in hemoglobin concentration, which should begin shortly after the reticulocyte peak, is invariably present by 3 weeks after iron therapy is begun, and persists until the hemoglobin concentration is restored to normal. The result of a therapeutic trial of iron must be evaluated for possible confounding factors, such as poor compliance with iron therapy, malabsorption of therapeutic iron, continuing blood loss, and the effects of coexisting conditions, especially infectious, inflammatory, or malignant disorders. The therapeutic trial merely aids in establishing the presence of iron deficiency. The search for underlying causes must continue despite a positive response to iron therapy.

Differential Diagnosis

Iron deficiency is the only microcytic hypochromic disorder in which mobilizable iron stores are absent; in all other disorders, storage iron is normal or increased (Table 36–2). Early or mild iron deficient anemia may be normocytic. In these cases, the hematocrit usually is greater than 30, but the serum iron and iron saturation levels usually are low. Difficulties in the evaluation of microcytic hypochromic disorders usually arise when direct assessment of marrow iron is unavailable and the diagnosis depends on indirect indicators of iron status (see boxes on Iron Deficiency and Coexisting Disorders and on Therapeutic Trial of Iron). Of the indirect indicators, the plasma ferritin level is most useful if the concentration is less than 12 mg/L, because in the absence of hypothyroidism or ascorbate deficiency, such a low ferritin level is highly specific for iron deficiency. In contrast, a plasma ferritin concentration within the normal range does not necessarily indicate the presence of storage iron, because ferritin concentrations may be increased independently of iron status by infectious, inflammatory, or malignant disorders, liver disease, and other conditions. Measurement of the plasma transferrin receptor concentration may be useful in differentiating the anemia of iron deficiency from the anemia associated with chronic inflammatory disorders. The ratio of serum transferrin receptor to serum ferritin concentration may provide an even better means of identifying iron deficiency.[19]

Specific entities to be considered in the differential diagnosis of hypochromic microcytic disorders are listed in Table 36–2; in all of these disorders, body iron stores are normal or increased. The anemia of chronic disease (see Chapter 37) is the most common cause of anemia in hospitalized patients and generally is mild to moderate, typically developing over several weeks in patients with chronic infectious, inflammatory, or malignant disorders.[68] Microcytic hypochromic anemias resulting from disorders of heme synthesis (sideroblastic anemias, congenital and acquired) and disorders of globin synthesis (thalassemias, microcytic hemoglobinopathies) are discussed in Chapters 38 and 41, respectively. Other rare congenital or acquired defects with microcytic hypochromic anemias are atransferrinemia[69] (or hypotransferrinemia; see Table 36–4) and a variety of other uncommon disorders.[69–78]

Oral Iron Therapy

Oral iron therapy should begin with a ferrous iron salt, taken separately from meals in three or four divided doses and supplying a daily total of 150 to 200 mg of elemental iron in adults or 3 mg of iron per kilogram of body weight in children. Simple ferrous preparations are the best absorbed and least expensive. Ferrous sulfate is the most widely used, either as tablets containing 60 to 70 mg of iron for adults or as a liquid preparation for children. Administration between meals maximizes absorption. In patients with a hemoglobin concentration less than 10 g/dL, this regimen initially will provide approximately 40 to 60 mg of iron daily for erythropoiesis, permitting red cell production to increase to two to four times normal and the hemoglobin concentration to rise by approximately 0.2 g/dL/day. An increase in the hemoglobin concentration of at least 2 g/dL after 3 weeks of therapy generally is used as the criterion for an adequate therapeutic response. For milder anemia, a single daily dose of approximately 60 mg of iron per day may be adequate. After the anemia has been fully corrected, oral iron should be continued to replace storage iron, either empirically for an additional 4 to 6 months or until the plasma ferritin concentration exceeds approximately 50 μg/L.

Therapy

The goal of therapy for iron-deficiency anemia is to supply sufficient iron to repair the hemoglobin deficit and replenish storage iron. Oral iron is the treatment of choice for almost all patients because of its effectiveness, safety, and economy and should always be given preference over parenteral iron for initial treatment (see box on Oral Iron Therapy).[20,37] The risk of local and systemic adverse reactions restricts the use of parenteral iron to the small number of patients who are unable to absorb or tolerate adequate amounts of oral iron. Rarely, red cell transfusions are needed to prevent cardiac or cerebral ischemia in patients with severe anemia or to support patients whose chronic rate of iron loss exceeds the rate of replacement possible with parenteral therapy.[79]

Most patients are able to tolerate oral iron therapy without difficulty, but 10% to 20% may have symptoms attributable to iron.[20,37] The most common side effects are gastrointestinal. The development of either diarrhea or constipation usually can be treated symptomatically, because alterations in bowel habits do not appear to be related to the dose of iron and seldom necessitate a change in the oral regimen. Upper gastrointestinal tract symptoms do seem to be dose related, reflecting the concentration of ferrous iron in the stomach and duodenum. These side effects occur within approximately 1 hour of iron ingestion and may be mild, with nausea and epigastric discomfort, or severe, with abdominal pain and vomiting. Often, upper gastrointestinal side effects can be managed by administering the iron with or immediately after meals. If symptoms persist, reductions in the amount of iron in each dose may be helpful, either by changing to tablets that contain smaller amounts of iron or by using a liquid preparation of ferrous sulfate. Decreasing the amount of iron in each dose usually is effective in controlling side effects, but if symptoms persist, a reduction in frequency to a single daily dose may be helpful. After a time at lower doses, patients subsequently may be able to tolerate more iron. With persistence and patience, an acceptable oral iron regimen can be devised for virtually all patients. Costly iron preparations with other additives, polysaccharide–iron complexes, or enteric coatings or in sustained-release forms do not appear to offer any advantages that cannot be achieved by simply reducing the dose of plain ferrous salts.[80] Administering iron with food and decreasing the dose will diminish the amount of iron absorbed daily and thereby prolong the period of treatment, but haste in the correction of iron deficiency is rarely needed.

Parenteral Iron Therapy

Four parenteral iron preparations are approved for use in the United States: higher- and lower-molecular-weight iron dextran, sodium ferric gluconate complex, and iron sucrose.[82] Each has been widely used, often in hemodialysis patients receiving recombinant human erythropoietin, but prospective, randomized controlled comparisons among the four agents are lacking. Immediate life-threatening anaphylactic reactions constitute the most serious risk associated with use of either intramuscular or intravenous iron preparations and may have a fatal outcome. Delayed but severe serum sickness-like reactions may develop, with fever, urticaria, adenopathy, myalgias, and arthralgias. Data from the U.S. Food and Drug Administration from 2001 to 2003 found that the absolute rates of reported *life-threatening* adverse drug events were 11.3, 3.3, 0.9, and 0.6 per million for higher- and lower-molecular-weight iron dextran, sodium ferric gluconate complex, and iron sucrose, respectively.[84]

Parenteral iron therapy (see box on Parenteral Iron Therapy), with the risk of adverse reactions, should be reserved for the exceptional patient who (a) remains intolerant of oral iron despite repeated modifications in dosage regimen, (b) malabsorbs iron, or (c) has iron needs that cannot be met by oral therapy because of either chronic uncontrollable bleeding or other sources of blood loss, such as hemodialysis, or a coexisting chronic inflammatory state.[20,81,82] A screening test for iron malabsorption is the administration to the fasting patient of 100 mg of elemental iron as ferrous sulfate in a liquid preparation, followed by measurements of plasma iron concentrations 1 and then 2 hours later. In an iron-deficient patient with an initial plasma iron concentration less than 50 mg/dL, an increase in plasma iron concentration of 200 to 300 mg/dL is expected. An increase in plasma iron concentration less than 100 mg/dL suggests malabsorption and is an indication for a small-bowel biopsy.[83]

Prognosis

The prognosis for iron deficiency itself is excellent, and the response to either oral or parenteral iron also is excellent. Frequently, both clinical and subjective indications of constitutional improvement are seen within the first few days of treatment, with the patient reporting an enhanced sense of well-being and increased vigor and appetite. Pica may resolve, and soreness and burning of the mouth abate. Mild reticulocytosis begins within 3 to 5 days, is maximal by days 8 to 10, and then declines. The hemoglobin concentration begins to increase after the first week and usually returns to normal within 6 weeks. Complete recovery from microcytosis may take up to 4 months. With oral iron dosage totaling 200 mg/day or less, the plasma ferritin concentration remains less than 12 mg/dL until the anemia is corrected and then gradually rises as storage iron is replaced over the next several months. Although epithelial abnormalities begin to improve promptly with treatment, resolution of glossitis and koilonychia may take several months. The overall prognosis depends on the underlying disorder responsible for the iron deficiency.

Failure to obtain a complete and characteristic response to iron therapy necessitates a review of findings and reevaluation of the patient. A common problem is an incorrect diagnosis, with the anemia of chronic disease mistaken for the anemia of iron deficiency. Coexisting conditions, such as other nutritional deficiencies, hepatic or renal disease, or infectious, inflammatory, or malignant disorders, may impede recovery. Occult blood loss may be responsible for an incomplete response. With oral iron therapy, the adequacy of the form and dose of iron used should be reconsidered, compliance with the treatment regimen reviewed, and, finally, the possibility of malabsorption considered.

IRON OVERLOAD

Iron overload denotes an excess in total body iron resulting from an iron supply that exceeds iron requirements. Because requirements are limited and humans lack a physiologic means of excreting excess iron, any sustained increase in intake eventually may result in accumulation of iron. The continuum of increased body iron is shown in Fig. 36–2. Whatever the source and the sites of excess iron deposition, when the accumulation overwhelms the cellular capacity for safe storage, potentially lethal tissue damage is the result. The toxic manifestations of iron overload vary with the precise pathogenic defect responsible but are dependent on the amount of excess iron, rate of iron accumulation, cellular pattern of deposition, and presence of complicating factors such as hepatitis or drug or alcohol use.

Epidemiology

The most common form of iron overload in the United States is a genetically determined disorder, the homozygous state for hereditary hemochromatosis, which occurs in approximately 0.26% of the total population, or approximately 1:385 persons.[85] In the United States, other forms of iron overload are less frequent but affect thousands of patients with iron-loading or chronically transfused anemias, such as thalassemia major, sickle cell disease, and acquired refractory anemias. Globally, hereditary hemochromatosis is the most common genetic disorder in populations of northern European ancestry.[86–89] Thalassemia major and other iron-loading anemias are important public health problems in countries bordering the Mediterranean and in an area extending from southwest Asia and the Indian subcontinent to southeast Asia.[90] Dietary iron overload resulting from intake of iron in brewed beverages is a common problem affecting many populations in sub-Saharan Africa and may have a genetic component.[91,92] Other inherited types of systemic iron overload, the various forms of perinatal iron overload,[93] and the syndromes associated with focal sequestration of iron are uncommon or rare disorders.

Genetic Aspects

The varieties of iron overload known to be genetically determined are listed in Table 36–3, and their cardinal features are summarized in Table 36–4 (see Chapter 35 for a description of the genes involved). By far, the most common form of inherited iron overload is hereditary hemochromatosis, a disorder of autosomal recessive inheritance. In populations within Europe or of European ancestry, 64% to 100% of cases clinically diagnosed as hemochromatosis are due to mutations in the *HFE* gene and are classified as HFE-associated hemochromatosis.[94] The great majority of affected persons are homozygous for the mutation designated C282Y (i.e., C282Y/C282Y) or are "compound" heterozygotes for the C282Y mutation and either the mutation identified as H63D (C282Y/H63D) or, in a smaller proportion of cases, S65C (C282Y/S65C). In most of the other patients, the disorder is classified as non–HFE-associated hemochromatosis.[95,96] A subset of these patients have a disorder of autosomal recessive inheritance associated with mutations in the gene for transferrin receptor 2 (see Chapter 35)[97]; the genetic basis for the remaining patients is unknown.

Juvenile hemochromatosis is a rare disorder of autosomal recessive inheritance that produces a pattern of iron loading like that seen in hereditary hemochromatosis but becomes clinically manifest much earlier, in the second decade of life.[98] Most cases seem to be due to mutations in the gene *HJV* at chromosome 1q21, but a severe form is caused by mutations in *HAMP*, the gene for hepcidin.[99]

Autosomal dominant forms of hemochromatosis have been found to be caused by mutations in the gene for ferroportin.[95,100] Homozygous or compound heterozygous mutations in divalent metal transporter 1 (*DMT1, SCL11A2*) have been found to be associated with severe microcytic anemia and hepatic iron overload; three patients have been identified.[70,75,101] Mutations in the genes for transferrin[69] and ceruloplasmin[102] produce rare autosomal recessive disorders with distinctive syndromes of iron overload. Many of the genetically determined forms of iron overload are rare, but their characterization has made fundamental contributions to the understanding of the control of iron metabolism (see Chapter 35).

Several of the acquired forms of iron overload involve disorders with a genetic origin or component. The genetically determined iron-loading anemias include the inherited sideroblastic anemias (see Chapter 38), some of the hereditary disorders of globin synthesis (see Chapter 41), and some chronic hemolytic anemias (see Chapters 44, 45, and 46). Similarly, some forms of chronic liver disease and porphyria cutanea tarda are inherited disorders. African dietary iron overload[103] and, possibly, susceptibility to iron accumulation with prolonged medicinal iron ingestion may have genetic components.[104] Many of the disorders necessitating chronic red cell transfusion are hereditary, including thalassemia major (see Chapter 41), sickle cell disease (see Chapters 42 and 43), and other chronic refractory anemias. Although the precise etiology of many of these conditions are unknown, subsets of the disorders leading to perinatal iron overload[93] or focal sequestration of iron[105] have an established genetic basis.

Table 36–3 Causes of Iron Overload

Hereditary Iron Overload
Hereditary hemochromatosis
HFE-associated (type 1)
Non–HFE-associated:
Transferrin receptor 2–associated (type 3)
Juvenile hemochromatosis (type 2)
Hemojuvelin-associated (type 2A)
Hepcidin-associated (type 2B)
Autosomal dominant hemochromatosis
Ferroportin-associated (type 4)
DMT1-associated hemochromatosis
Atransferrinemia
Aceruloplasminemia
Acquired Iron Overload
Iron-loading anemias (refractory anemias with hypercellular erythroid marrow)
Chronic liver disease
Porphyria cutanea tarda
Insulin resistance–associated hepatic iron overload
African dietary iron overload[a]
Medicinal iron ingestion[a]
Parenteral iron overload
Transfusional iron overload
Inadvertent iron overload from therapeutic injections
Perinatal Iron Overload
Neonatal hemochromatosis
Trichohepatoenteric syndrome
Cerebrohepatorenal syndrome
GRACILE[b] (Fellman) syndrome
Focal Sequestration of Iron
Idiopathic pulmonary hemosiderosis
Renal hemosiderosis
Associated with neurologic abnormalities
Pantothenate kinase–associated neurodegeneration (formerly called Hallervorden-Spatz syndrome)
Neuroferritinopathy
Friedreich ataxia

[a]May have a genetic component.
[b]GRACILE, growth retardation, aminoaciduria, cholestasis, iron overload, lactic acidosis, and early death.

Table 36–4 Hereditary Iron Overload Disorders

Disorder	Gene, Chromosome Location	Inheritance	Plasma Transferrin Saturation	Plasma Ferritin	Iron Deposition Sites	Clinical Manifestations
Hereditary hemochromatosis, HFE-associated	*HFE*, 6p21	Autosomal recessive	Early increase; >45%	Later increase after third decade	Parenchymal iron overload affecting liver, heart, pancreas, other organs	Liver and heart disease, diabetes, gonadal failure, arthritis, skin pigmentation
Hereditary hemochromatosis, TfR2-associated	*TFR2*, 7q22	Autosomal recessive	Early increase; >45%	Later increase after third decade	Parenchymal iron overload affecting liver, heart, pancreas, other organs	Liver and heart disease, diabetes, gonadal failure, arthritis, skin pigmentation
Juvenile hemochromatosis, hemojuvelin-associated	*HJV*, 1q21	Autosomal recessive	Early increase; >45%	Increased by second decade	Parenchymal iron overload affecting liver, heart, pancreas, other organs	As for hereditary hemochromatosis, but liver involvement less prominent
Juvenile hemochromatosis, hepcidin-associated	*HAMP*, 19q13	Autosomal recessive	Early increase; >45%	Increased by second decade	Parenchymal iron overload affecting liver, heart, pancreas, other organs	As for hereditary hemochromatosis, but liver involvement less prominent
Hemochromatosis, ferroportin-associated	*SLC11A3*, 2q32	Autosomal dominant	Remains normal or low	Early increase	Some mutations show selective reticuloendothelial; others also show parenchymal (liver, heart, pancreas)	None with only reticuloendothelial iron; others as for HFE-associated hemochromatosis
DMT1-associated hemochromatosis	*SCL11A2*, 12q13	Autosomal recessive	Early increase; >45%	Normal to moderately elevated	Hepatic iron overload, predominantly parenchymal	Severe microcytic anemia, liver dysfunction
Atransferrinemia	*TF*, 3q21	Autosomal recessive	No plasma transferrin	Increased	Parenchymal iron overload affecting liver, heart, pancreas; no iron in bone marrow or spleen	Transfusion-dependent iron deficiency anemia, growth retardation, poor survival
Aceruloplasminemia	*CP*, 3q23-q24	Autosomal recessive	Decreased	Increased	Marked iron accumulation in basal ganglia, liver, pancreas	Diabetes, progressive neurologic disease, retinal degeneration

Etiology and Pathogenesis

Iron overload is caused by conditions that alter or bypass the normal control of body iron content by adjustment of intestinal iron absorption (see Table 36–3). Genetic characterization of patients with disorders listed in Table 36–3 and studies of animal models of disorders of iron homeostasis (see Chapter 35) are helping to decipher the intricate regulatory pathways involved.[89,96,100,106–108] A major advance has been the recognition that the known forms of hereditary iron overload (see Table 36–3) have a common pathogenic origin in genetically determined abnormalities in the interaction of hepcidin and ferroportin[109] (see box on Common Pathogenic Origin of Hereditary Iron Overload: The Interaction of Hepcidin and Ferroportin).

The exact mechanisms whereby iron produces cellular injury are not established, but lipid peroxidation of membrane lipids of subcellular organelles, iron-induced lysosomal disruption, or both may be involved.[113] Whatever the precise mechanisms responsible for the harmful effects of iron, the pattern of the organs affected, the timing of the onset of toxic manifestations, and the severity of tissue damage are known to be influenced by a variety of factors in both hereditary and acquired varieties of systemic iron overload. Within the systemic circulation, these factors include (a) the specific underlying genetic or acquired abnormality, (b) the magnitude of iron excess, (c) the rate of iron loading, (d) the distribution of iron load between more innocuous storage deposits in reticuloendothelial macrophages and potentially injurious accumulations in parenchymal cells of the liver, pancreas, heart, and other organs, and (e) the extent of internal redistribution of iron between macrophage and parenchymal sites. Twin studies suggest that still unidentified genes have substantial effects on iron accumulation and toxicity.[114] In other forms of iron overload, another level of complexity is introduced because the central nervous system, the testes, and the fetus are functionally separate from the systemic circulation and cannot acquire iron directly from plasma transferrin.[115] Instead, iron must be taken up from the systemic circulation by barrier cells and then exported across the blood–brain and blood–cerebrospinal fluid barriers into the brain interstitial and cerebrospinal fluids, across the blood–testis barrier, and across the placenta to the fetus. As a consequence, disorders affecting the proteins responsible for iron supply to these compartments have distinctive manifestations.

Hereditary Iron Overload

Within the systemic circulation, the specific patterns of iron deposition and damage found in the hereditary disorders of iron overload can be characterized by reference to the pathways of internal iron exchange shown in Fig. 36–1 and the classification of disorders given in Table 36–4. For the specific defects in the interaction between hepcidin and ferroportin responsible for each form of iron overload, see the box on Common Pathogenic Origin of Hereditary Iron Overload: The Interaction of Hepcidin and Ferroportin.

In *hereditary HFE-associated hemochromatosis*, an autosomal recessive disorder, the underlying genetic defect in the regulation of hepcidin production results in an inappropriately elevated iron absorption at any level of body iron, with a chronic progressive increase in body iron stores accompanied by enhanced release of iron from reticuloendothelial macrophages. The means whereby mutations in *HFE* produce these effects are unknown but involve an impaired increase in production of hepcidin in response to iron loading (see Chapter 35). Patients seem unable to effectively upregulate hepcidin expression as iron stores increase.[116] Of importance, intestinal iron absorption, although inappropriately high in hereditary HFE-associated hemochromatosis, still is regulated by body iron levels.[117] As the body iron level rises as a consequence of increased absorption, circulating transferrin becomes fully saturated. The excess iron is deposited predominantly within the parenchymal cells of the liver (Fig. 36–4), but subsequently the iron accumulates in the pancreas, heart, and other organs. By the time symptoms of organ damage develop, usually in the fourth or fifth decade of life, body iron stores typically have increased from the normal range of 1 g or less to 15 to 20 g or more.[118] Further increments in body iron stores may be fatal, although some patients are able to tolerate a total iron accumulation of as much as 40 to 50 g.

Patients with autosomal recessive *hereditary non–HFE-associated hemochromatosis* due to mutations in the gene for transferrin receptor 2 seem to be clinically similar to those with the HFE-associated form.[107,109] This clinical resemblance and observations in vitro suggest that these two proteins are involved in a common pathway regulating hepcidin synthesis.[119]

Patients with autosomal recessive *juvenile hemochromatosis* have the same pattern of tissue iron deposition found in hereditary HFE-associated hemochromatosis but develop severe iron overload much earlier, with hypogonadism and cardiac disease manifesting in the second decade of life.[120] The rate of iron accumulation is increased substantially and is estimated to be three to four times greater than that in HFE-associated disease. The gene responsible for most cases of juvenile hemochromatosis has been identified as *HJV* with the protein product hemojuvelin.[121,122] A subgroup of patients with juvenile hemochromatosis with null mutations in the hepcidin gene has been identified.[99] The consequent loss of all hepcidin-mediated regulation of intestinal iron absorption may explain the great acceleration in the rate of iron loading in this form of juvenile hemochromatosis. Interestingly, digenic inheritance of mutations in both the *HFE* genes (C282Y/H63D heterozygote) and the transferrin receptor 2 genes (Q317X homozygote) results in a phenotype like that of juvenile hemochromatosis.[123]

Patients with *autosomal dominant hemochromatosis* resulting from mutations in the ferroportin gene share the characteristic of reticuloendothelial iron overload, in contrast to the relative sparing of reticuloendothelial macrophages seen in patients with hereditary HFE-associated hemochromatosis.[95] Some mutations (i.e., those resulting in ferroportins that are unable to reach the cell surface to interact with hepcidin) produce an exclusively reticuloendothelial pattern of iron overload that is devoid of clinical manifestations and apparently does not require treatment.[100,124] Other mutations (i.e., those resulting in ferroportins that reach the cell surface but do not respond to hepcidin) are implicated not only in reticuloendothelial iron deposition but also in parenchymal iron loading associated with hepatic fibrosis, diabetes, impotence, arthritis, and arrhythmias. Affected patients may have a reduced tolerance for phlebotomy and become anemic with therapy, despite persistently elevated serum ferritin concentrations.[125,126] Another form of autosomal dominant iron overload reported in a single family has been attributed to a mutation in the gene for the iron responsive element of the H-subunit of ferritin.[127]

The three patients reported with *DMT1-associated hemochromatosis* have in common a severe microcytic anemia with high transferrin saturation, marked hepatic iron deposition, but normal to moderately elevated serum ferritin concentration.[70,75,101]

Congenital *atransferrinemia* (hypotransferrinemia) is a rare disorder of autosomal recessive inheritance in which plasma transferrin is nearly absent; only 10 cases have been reported.[69,128] Hepcidin levels are extremely low[107] and iron absorption is increased, but the absorbed

Common Pathogenic Origin of Hereditary Iron Overload: Interaction of Hepcidin and Ferroportin

The known forms of hereditary iron overload (Table 36–3) all involve defects in the interaction of hepcidin and ferroportin. Hepatic hepcidin production is inappropriately low in the autosomal recessive disorders HFE-associated and transferrin receptor 2–associated hereditary hemochromatosis and hemojuvelin- and hepcidin-associated juvenile hemochromatosis.[107] In autosomal dominant ferroportin disease, mutations produce ferroportins that either are unable to reach the cell surface to interact with hepcidin or reach the cell surface but do not respond to hepcidin.[100,110] In DMT1-associated hemochromatosis, urinary hepcidin is low.[75] In atransferrinemia, hepcidin levels are extremely low.[107,111] In aceruloplasminemia, the lack of ceruloplasmin prevents stable expression of ferroportin on the cell surface, leading to its internalization and degradation.[112] In each form, the resultant homeostatic dysregulation leads to excessive intestinal iron absorption and body iron excess. The rate, distribution, and harmful effects of tissue iron loading depend on the specific abnormality in the interaction between hepcidin and ferroportin produced by each mutation.

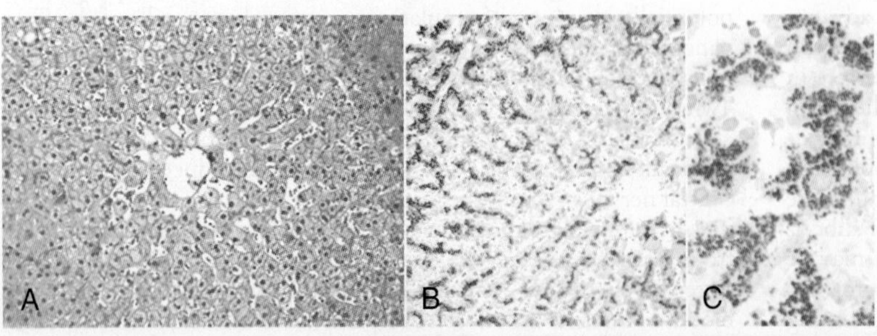

Figure 36–4 Hemochromatosis. Liver biopsy sample from a 46-year-old man with homozygous hemochromatosis. Hematoxylin and eosin stain of the liver (**A**) shows intact hepatic architecture. Iron stain (**B,C**) shows marked diffuse iron deposits in the hepatocytes throughout the lobules. A normal liver would show essentially no iron in the hepatocytes.

iron circulates as non-transferrin-bound plasma iron and, lacking a physiologic means of entry into erythroid precursors, cannot be used for erythropoiesis. Patients have a severe hypochromic microcytic anemia and die without transferrin infusion or blood transfusions. The circulating non-transferrin-bound plasma iron is progressively deposited in the liver, pancreas, heart, and other parenchymal tissues, but deposits are scant or absent in the bone marrow and spleen.[69,128] The distribution of iron deposits with atransferrinemia suggests the importance of non-transferrin-bound plasma iron as a mediator of iron accumulation by parenchymal tissues in hereditary and acquired forms of iron overload.[129]

Hereditary *aceruloplasminemia* (hypoceruloplasminemia) is a rare disorder of iron metabolism inherited as an autosomal recessive trait, resulting from absence or severe deficiency of ceruloplasmin occurring as a consequence of mutations in the ceruloplasmin gene.[102] Ceruloplasmin has an essential role in iron metabolism as a multicopper ferroxidase[102] catalyzing the oxidation of ferrous to ferric iron, a prerequisite for iron binding by apotransferrin (see Chapter 35). A glycosylphosphatidylinositol-anchored form of ceruloplasmin is expressed in the central nervous system and is required for iron efflux.[115,130] It appears to help protect the brain against iron-mediated oxidant damage. The lack of ceruloplasmin prevents stable expression of ferroportin on the cell surface, leading to its internalization and degradation[112] and intracellular accumulation of iron. Patients with ceruloplasminemia typically present in the fourth or fifth decade of life with a triad of diabetes mellitus, progressive neurologic disease (dementia, dysarthria, and dystonia), and retinal degeneration.[102] Marked iron accumulations are evident in the liver, pancreas, and brain, with smaller amounts of excess iron found in the spleen, heart, kidney, thyroid, and retina. Despite a degree and distribution of hepatic iron deposition comparable with those found in hereditary HFE-associated hemochromatosis, liver injury or fibrosis is not seen. The serum iron concentration is low, the serum total iron-binding capacity is normal, the serum ferritin concentration is moderately elevated, and a mild normochromic normocytic anemia usually is present.[102] Phlebotomy does not mobilize hepatic iron, but iron chelation with deferoxamine is effective and can ameliorate neurologic symptoms.[112,131]

Acquired Iron Overload

Iron-loading anemias may be associated with excessive absorption of dietary iron that can produce severe iron overload. The postulated *erythroid regulator*[132] can increase iron absorption dramatically when accelerated erythropoiesis exceeds the ability of transferrin to provide sufficient iron for hemoglobin production (see Chapter 35). The iron-loading anemias are characterized by the combination of erythroid hyperplasia with marked ineffective erythropoiesis.[133,134] These refractory disorders include thalassemia major and intermedia, hemoglobin E/β-thalassemia, congenital dyserythropoietic anemia, pyruvate kinase deficiency, a variety of sideroblastic anemias, and other anemias associated with blocks in the incorporation of iron into hemoglobin. The rate of iron loading is related not to the severity of the anemia but rather to the extent of ineffective erythropoiesis, and patients with nearly normal hemoglobin concentrations may develop massive iron overload. Any red cell transfusions will add to the iron burden.[135] Clinical manifestations include liver disease, diabetes mellitus, endocrine disorders, and cardiac dysfunction. Diminished hepcidin production as a result of ineffective erythropoiesis is believed to be responsible for increased iron absorption.[135,136]

Chronic liver disease with increased absorption of dietary iron may produce mild iron overload in some patients,[137,138] including individuals with alcoholic cirrhosis or portacaval shunts. Patients with alcoholic liver disease are more commonly iron deficient as a result of repeated episodes of gastrointestinal blood loss, but storage iron is increased in a minority of patients. The *HFE* gene is not responsible. The cause(s) of the increased absorption is not established with certainty, but alcohol metabolism–mediated oxidative stress downregulates hepcidin transcription, leading to increased intestinal iron absorption.[139–141] Alcohol-induced folate and sideroblastic abnormalities with ineffective erythropoiesis and hyperferremia also may contribute. Patients with chronic hepatitis C have been reported to have decreased hepatic hepcidin expression.[142] Storage iron usually is increased modestly, to only 2 to 4 g, but in patients with alcoholic cirrhosis, the higher the liver iron, the shorter the survival.[143] The pattern of iron distribution is seen predominantly in Kupffer cells rather than in parenchymal cells.

Porphyria cutanea tarda (see Chapter 38), the most common type of human porphyria, is caused by iron-dependent oxidation of uroporphyrinogen to uroporphomethene, a competitive inhibitor of uroporphyrinogen decarboxylase.[144] In this disorder, the liver produces excessive amounts of photosensitizing porphyrins, which circulate in the skin.[145] Mild hepatic iron overload is found in most patients, and iron depletion by phlebotomy produces clinical and biochemical remission of the disease.[146] *HFE* mutations are common in patients of European origin and seem to contribute to the pathogenesis of both the familial and sporadic forms of the disorder.[147] The mechanism for iron loading in patients without mutations in *HFE* is unknown.

Insulin resistance–associated hepatic iron overload (also known as "dysmetabolic hepatosiderosis") is a syndrome of iron overload in which the combination of an increased serum ferritin level with a normal transferrin saturation is found in association with glucose or lipid metabolic abnormalities.[148,149] The iron overload typically is mild or moderate, and there is no evidence of familial transmission. On histologic examination, a mixed pattern of iron deposits in hepatocytes and sinusoidal cells is seen that is distinct from that of HFE-associated hemochromatosis.[150] The clinical value of phlebotomy in removing the modest iron excess in these patients is under study.[151,152]

African dietary iron overload occurs in sub-Saharan Africa in association with greatly increased dietary iron intake from a traditional fermented beverage with high iron content; however, a genetic component not linked to *HFE* also may be involved.[92,103,153] Iron burdens of magnitudes comparable to those found in hereditary hemochromatosis may accumulate, and liver disease with cirrhosis and hepatoma, pancreatic disease with diabetes mellitus, endocrine disorders, and cardiac dysfunction may develop.[91] On histologic examination, iron deposits are prominent in both macrophages and hepatic parenchymal cells,[91] in contrast with the predominantly parenchymal iron loading found in HFE-associated hemochromatosis. A ferroportin mutation (Q248H), unique to African populations, has been identified but does not seem to account for the condition.[92,103]

Medicinal iron ingestion can add to the body iron burden of patients with iron-loading disorders, especially iron-loading anemias.[104] In persons without abnormalities affecting iron homeostasis, the extent to which orally administered iron can increase the body iron stores is uncertain. Although case reports have described iron accumulation in patients who have taken medicinal iron for long periods, the potential involvement of an unrecognized iron-loading mutation in these patients cannot be excluded.

Parenteral iron overload usually is the result of repeated red cell transfusions in patients with chronic anemia, but occasionally it is unintentionally produced by repeated injections of iron dextran or other parenteral iron preparations in patients with anemias unresponsive to iron therapy, such as patients undergoing chronic hemodialysis.[154]

Transfusional iron overload progressively develops in patients with chronic refractory anemia who require red cell support.[155] In patients with severe congenital anemias such as thalassemia major (Cooley's anemia) or Blackfan-Diamond syndrome, transfusional iron loading begins in infancy.[156,157] Severe iron loading may develop in transfusion-dependent anemias that appear later in life, namely, aplastic anemia, pure red cell aplasia, hypoplastic or myelodysplastic disorders, and the anemia of chronic renal failure. Patients with sickle cell anemia or sickle cell/β-thalassemia also are at risk for iron overload if chronically given transfusions for prevention of recurrent complications such as stroke, severe infections and incapacitating painful crises.[158] If ineffective erythropoiesis and erythroid hyperplasia complicate the underlying anemia, increased absorption may contribute to the iron burden. The greater the extent of ineffective erythropoiesis, the greater the suppression of hepcidin synthesis and the greater the magnitude of the increase in iron absorption.[135,159,160] An adequate transfusion regimen will help suppress erythropoiesis and contribute to iron loading, resulting in relatively higher hepcidin levels, which in turn will decrease dietary iron absorption.

Perinatal iron overload develops in some rare or uncommon metabolic disorders of the newborn, presumably as the result of disturbances in the regulation of fetal or maternal–fetal iron balance and in some instances as a result of severe intrauterine liver disease producing severe hypotransferrinemia.[93] *Neonatal* (or *perinatal*) *hemochromatosis* is a diverse collection of disorders associated with severe congenital hepatic disease and deposits of iron in the liver and pancreas, heart, and other extrahepatic sites, with evidence of autosomal recessive inheritance in some cases and an alloimmune etiology in others.[161,162] The *trichohepatoenteric syndrome* is an apparently distinct disorder with hepatic hemosiderosis, facial dysmorphism, hair abnormality, failure to thrive and intractable diarrhea.[163,164] The *cerebrohepatorenal syndrome* (or Zellweger syndrome) is a fatal disorder of peroxisomal biogenesis with an autosomal recessive mode of inheritance, characterized by abnormal facies, hypotonia, and polycystic kidneys. Parenchymal iron deposits are found in the liver, spleen, kidney, and lungs.[165,166] *GRACILE* (*g*rowth *r*etardation, *a*minoaciduria, *c*holestasis, *i*ron overload, *l*actic acidosis, and *e*arly death) *syndrome* is a recessively inherited lethal disease characterized by fetal growth retardation, lactic acidosis, aminoaciduria, cholestasis, and abnormalities in iron metabolism.[167] A mutation in *BCS1L*, a gene that encodes a mitochondrial protein that functions as a chaperone in the assembly of complex III (cytochrome bc1 complex) of the mitochondrial respiratory chain, is responsible,[168] but the mechanism of the effects on iron metabolism has not been identified.

Focal sequestration of iron in other rare disorders produces various patterns of localized iron deposition. In *idiopathic pulmonary hemosiderosis*, repeated episodes of alveolar hemorrhage are followed by uptake and sequestration of iron in pulmonary macrophages.[169] The excess iron is not available for use elsewhere, and iron stores in the liver and bone marrow may be decreased or absent.[45,170] In conditions with chronic hemoglobinuria, *renal hemosiderosis* may develop and, in some cases, can cause or contribute to renal failure.[171] Finally, remarkable progress is being made in elucidating the bases for disorders with specific patterns of brain iron deposition in association with neurologic abnormalities,[105,115] including *Friedreich ataxia*,[172] *pantothenate kinase-associated neurodegeneration*[173] (formerly called Hallervorden-Spatz syndrome), and *neuroferritinopathy*.[174]

Clinical Presentation

Clinical manifestations of iron toxicity generally develop only in patients with forms of systemic parenchymal iron overload in which the magnitude of iron accumulation is sufficient to produce tissue and organ damage. Individuals at risk include homozygotes for the types of hereditary and juvenile hemochromatosis listed in Table 36–3, some forms of ferroportin-associated hemochromatosis, aceruloplasminemia, and patients with iron-loading anemias, African dietary iron overload, transfusional iron overload, and, apparently, insulin resistance-associated hepatic iron overload. Patients with forms of iron overload restricted to reticuloendothelial tissue do not seem to develop clinical complications.[124] Specific patterns of neurologic signs and symptoms occur in patients with aceruloplasminemia,[102] pantothenate kinase-associated neurodegeneration,[173] Friedreich ataxia,[172] and neuroferritinopathy that reflect the brain distribution of the excess iron.[174]

In patients with systemic parenchymal iron loading, similar clinical features eventually develop with sufficient iron accumulation to produce organ dysfunction and damage. At earlier stages, with lower body iron burdens, no distinctive signs or symptoms may be present, and patients may come to attention only because of abnormal laboratory test results. Symptomatic patients may present with any of the characteristic manifestations of parenchymal iron deposition: liver disease, diabetes mellitus, gonadal insufficiency and other endocrine disorders, cardiac dysfunction, arthropathy, and increased skin pigmentation. The rate of iron deposition also seems to influence the pattern of organ dysfunction that develops. For example, the mean body iron burdens as determined by phlebotomy were almost identical in a group of patients homozygous for juvenile hemochromatosis and a comparison group of patients with hereditary hemochromatosis (all homozygous for the C282Y mutation in *HFE*).[120] In the patients with juvenile hemochromatosis, the iron load had accumulated by a mean age of 23.3 ± 6.2 years, and the major manifestations were hypogonadism in 96%, reduced glucose tolerance in 58%, and cardiomyopathy in 35%. In the patients with hereditary HFE-associated hemochromatosis, the nearly identical mean body iron burden had accumulated significantly later, by a mean age of 44.8 ± 10.7 years, and the corresponding prevalences for these complications were significantly lower: hypogonadism was present in only 18%, reduced glucose tolerance in 27%, and cardiomyopathy in 7%. The prevalences of cirrhosis (42% vs 52%) and arthropathy (27% vs 12%) did not differ significantly between the two groups.[120]

Characteristic manifestations of iron toxicity are found in specific organ systems. Liver disease is the most common complication of systemic iron overload.[137,138] In all varieties of systemic parenchymal iron overload, the development and severity of liver damage are closely correlated with the magnitude of hepatic iron deposition. On an intriguing note, the sole exception seems to be aceruloplasminemia, in which liver damage and fibrosis do not develop despite hepatic iron accumulations of the magnitudes found in hereditary hemochromatosis.[175] Otherwise, whether derived from increased absorption of dietary iron or from transfused red cells, progressive parenchymal iron accumulation eventually produces hepatomegaly, functional abnormalities, fibrosis, and, finally, cirrhosis. Hepatocellular carcinoma seems to be the ultimate complication of cirrhosis in iron overload. The development of cirrhosis increases the risk of hepatoma by more than 200-fold.[176]

Diabetes mellitus is another common complication of all forms of systemic parenchymal iron overload[151,177,178] (including aceruloplasminemia[102,175]). The risk may be greater in patients with a family history of diabetes. Virtually all of the secondary manifestations of diabetes may develop, including retinopathy, nephropathy, neuropathy, and vascular disease.

Gonadal insufficiency and other endocrine abnormalities occur.[151,178,179] Hypogonadism may result from primary testicular failure or may be hypogonadotropic in origin. Abnormalities in pituitary and end-organ functions may develop; hypothyroidism, hypoparathyroidism, and adrenal insufficiency are infrequent complications. During the second decade of life, both growth and sexual maturation usually are retarded in untreated patients with transfusional iron overload.

Iron-induced cardiac disease, occurring as a cardiomyopathy with heart failure, arrhythmias, or both, may be a fatal complication of all varieties of systemic parenchymal iron overload. Heart disease is the most frequent cause of death in patients with transfusional iron overload.[177,180] Severe cardiac disease in particular may be the presenting manifestation in young patients with juvenile hemochromatosis.[120]

Increased skin pigmentation, with a bronze hue in some patients and a slate-gray coloration in others, often accompanies iron overload, although the change in pigment may be too slight to be readily evident clinically. Massive iron overload sometimes produces "reverse freckling," with small pigment-free areas scattered over a conspicuous slate-gray discoloration of the skin. Chondrocalcinosis and other forms of arthropathy are common complications of hereditary hemochromatosis and may occur in other forms of systemic parenchymal iron overload.[151,181–183] An increased susceptibility to infectious disease may be found in patients with transfusional and other forms of iron overload. Clinical reports suggest that an increased availability of iron may be related pathogenetically to infections with certain organisms, including *Vibrio vulnificus*, *Listeria monocytogenes*, *Yersinia enteroco-*

litica, Escherichia coli, Candida species, and *Mycobacterium tuberculosis.*[184–188]

Laboratory Evaluation

The typical sequences of changes in clinically useful indicators of iron status, as body iron increases from the iron-replete normal to the amounts found in hereditary hemochromatosis and transfusional iron overload, are shown in Fig. 36–2. Characteristic changes in laboratory measures of iron status in the disorders of hereditary iron overload are listed in Table 36–4.

Population-based screening for iron overload has been widely discussed.[189–192] However, after review of the available evidence,[193] the U.S. Preventive Services Task Force presently recommends against routine genetic screening for hereditary HFE-associated hemochromatosis in the general population.[194] Uncertainty about the penetrance of the most common form of iron overload has been a major consideration.[88] Large studies have suggested that the penetrance of hereditary HFE-associated hemochromatosis is low.[195–197] One of the studies concluded that a "best estimate is that less than 1% of homozygotes develop frank clinical hemochromatosis."[195] These interpretations, based on cross-section surveys that did not include thorough evaluation of hepatic function with liver biopsy, have been challenged,[87,198] but large-scale population-based screening seems unlikely to be adopted in the near term.

In contrast, screening for iron overload is clearly indicated for patients with any of the symptoms and signs associated with iron overload, including chronic liver disease, cardiomyopathy, diabetes, endocrine disorders, arthropathy, increased skin pigmentation, and porphyria cutanea tarda.[94,151] Screening can use phenotypical methods, genotypical methods, or both. Phenotypical screening can provide biochemical evidence of iron overload in patients with hereditary or juvenile hemochromatosis but will not identify all persons genetically at risk for iron loading.[195] In populations of northern European ancestry, genotypical screening for the C282Y and H63D mutations in *HFE* can identify most persons at risk for developing hereditary hemochromatosis but gives no information about the presence or magnitude of iron overload. Genotyping the spouse of a C282Y homozygote provides the best guide for assessing children for *HFE* mutations. Despite these advantages, testing solely for the C282Y and H63D mutations of *HFE* will not identify other mutations associated with iron loading. In populations not of northern European ancestry, many persons at risk will not be identified.[199,200] In most clinical circumstances, a combination of phenotypical and genotypical methods is the best strategy for screening.

In individuals of northern European ancestry, measurement of the serum transferrin saturation usually is the best method for initial phenotypical screening for systemic parenchymal iron overload. A persistent value of 45% or greater often is recommended as a threshold value for further investigation. In the absence of complicating factors, elevated concentrations of serum ferritin provide biochemical evidence of iron overload. Genetic testing then should be considered in persons with abnormal transferrin saturation, serum ferritin concentration, or both. If a persistently elevated transferrin saturation is found in a person who is homozygous for the C282Y mutation (i.e., C282Y/C282Y), the diagnosis of hereditary hemochromatosis can be considered established. In most such patients, liver biopsy is no longer needed to confirm the diagnosis. Liver biopsy is indicated for prognostic purposes to detect cirrhosis if the serum ferritin concentration is greater than 1000 μg/L and may be contemplated in the presence of hepatomegaly or abnormalities on liver function testing, or in patients older than 40 years.[151,178,201,202] Bone marrow examination is of limited usefulness in the evaluation of patients for hereditary or juvenile hemochromatosis because no information about the extent of parenchymal iron deposition is provided.

Heterozygotes for the C282Y mutation (C282Y/wild-type) have serum transferrin saturations and serum ferritin concentrations that are similar to those of wild-type homozygotes, and clinically meaningful iron overload does not develop.[35,196] In heterozygotes for the C282Y and H63D mutations (C282Y/H63D), mild–to-moderate iron overload may develop, but the penetrance of this genotype is even less than that of C282Y/C282Y homozygotes.[196,203,204] Heterozygotes for H63D (i.e., H63D/wild-type) may have elevated transferrin saturations,[203] but iron overload does not develop. Homozygotes for H63D (i.e., H63D/H63D) also may have elevated transferrin saturations but have little risk of iron overload.[203] Less common mutations of the *HFE* gene have been identified. In S65C heterozygotes with either C282Y (i.e., S65C/C282Y) or H63D (i.e., S65C/H63D), mild iron overload may develop.[205,206]

Persons with phenotypical evidence of iron overload who are neither C282Y/C282Y homozygotes nor C282Y/H63D heterozygotes can be considered for further genetic testing for less common *HFE* mutations and for non-*HFE* mutations associated with iron loading, for noninvasive assessment of the liver iron concentration,[6,7] or for diagnostic liver biopsy.

Liver biopsy can establish a definitive diagnosis of hereditary and juvenile hemochromatosis regardless of genotype and can demonstrate the reticuloendothelial pattern of iron loading found with ferroportin mutations and the characteristic histologic appearance of insulin resistance-associated hepatic iron overload (see box on Testing for Iron Overload).[150,151,178,201] A quantitative determination of the nonheme iron concentration in the liver sample should be made, the pattern of iron deposition examined histochemically, and the extent of tissue injury assessed histopathologically. In patients found to have an increased body iron concentration, additional clinical and laboratory studies should seek evidence of complications of iron overload. Further investigation may include liver function testing, testing for diabetes mellitus, evaluation of hormonal function, cardiac examination, joint and bone x-ray examination, and, especially if cirrhosis is present, screening for hepatocellular carcinoma.[151,178,201] Liver biopsy with quantitative determination of iron stores remains the reference method for assessing the extent of iron overload in patients with transfusional iron overload.[1,6,7,13]

Patients with autosomal dominant forms of iron overload generally display an early increase in the plasma ferritin concentration that precedes a rise in the transferrin saturation.[204] A mild hypochromic anemia may be present, especially among young women. Liver biopsy demonstrates predominantly reticuloendothelial iron overload; a lesser degree of parenchymal iron deposition is found in some but

Testing For Iron Overload

A direct measure of body iron avoids the uncertainties inherent in the interpretation of indirect indicators of iron status. Liver biopsy is the definitive direct test for assessing iron deposition and tissue damage in iron overload, permitting measurement of the nonheme iron concentration, histochemical determination of the cellular distribution of iron between hepatocytes and Kupffer cells, and pathologic examination of the extent of tissue injury. When available as appropriately calibrated and validated techniques, new noninvasive methods using hepatic magnetic susceptibility and magnetic resonance imaging[9–12,207,208] may replace liver biopsy when only determination of the liver iron concentration is needed. Magnetic resonance imaging studies of the heart are particularly useful in patients at risk for cardiac iron deposition.[180,208,209] In patients with hereditary hemochromatosis undergoing therapeutic venesection, quantitative phlebotomy provides an accurate retrospective determination of the amount of storage iron that can be mobilized for hemoglobin formation. When liver biopsy is contraindicated in a patient, quantitative phlebotomy occasionally is useful in establishing the diagnosis of hereditary hemochromatosis. Bone marrow aspiration and biopsy provide no information about the extent of parenchymal iron loading and are of limited value in the evaluation of iron overload. Iron overload produces no specific abnormalities in the peripheral blood.

not all patients.[110,204] Atransferrinemia or hypotransferrinemia is readily demonstrable by measurement of the plasma transferrin concentration.[69,128] Similarly, aceruloplasminemia or hypoceruloplasminemia can be diagnosed by measurement of the plasma ceruloplasmin concentration.[102,210] At diagnosis, the plasma ferritin concentration is increased, often to 1000 to 2000 μg/L, but the transferrin saturation is decreased. A mild normochromic, normocytic anemia usually is present. Liver biopsy shows iron accumulation in hepatocytes and Kupffer cells. Magnetic resonance imaging examination shows low-intensity signals on T1- and T2-weighted studies of the basal ganglia.

For detection and diagnosis of iron-loading anemias, measurement of the plasma transferrin receptor and examination of the bone marrow may be helpful in demonstrating ineffective erythropoiesis in combination with the erythroid hyperplasia characteristic of these disorders.

Differential Diagnosis

Detection and diagnosis of iron overload are most problematic in the hereditary forms of iron overload (see Table 36–3). The combination of phenotypical and genotypical screening described in the preceding section should lead to a definitive diagnosis in most patients. Practice guidelines for the detection, diagnosis,[211] and management of hereditary hemochromatosis have been published.[151,178,193,194,201,211] Aceruloplasminemia is a rare disorder, but distinguishing this form of iron overload from hereditary hemochromatosis is important in guiding effective therapy that can prevent or arrest neurologic damage.[140,151,210]

In patients with iron-loading anemias who are not transfusion dependent, the severity of anemia provides no indication of the risk of iron loading from increased dietary iron absorption. Patients with only minor degrees of anemia may accumulate major iron loads.[133,136,212] In the diagnostic evaluation of these patients, examination of the peripheral blood may show changes indicative of the underlying hematologic disorders. Either morphologic techniques or measurement of the plasma transferrin receptor concentration can be used to estimate the extent of ineffective erythropoiesis and of erythroid marrow hyperplasia and may be useful in assessing the risk of iron loading.[213] The differential diagnosis directed at the remaining causes of iron overload listed in Table 36–3 poses few problems. Porphyria cutanea tarda is discussed more fully in Chapter 38 and is readily diagnosed by the measurement of urinary porphyrins. The source of iron overload in patients with parenteral iron loading is evident, whether from transfusion or from repeated injections of therapeutic iron. The various causes of perinatal iron overload are clearly distinguished by clinical and pathologic findings. The diagnosis of idiopathic pulmonary hemosiderosis should be considered whenever iron-deficiency anemia develops with coexisting pulmonary abnormalities. Previously, the demonstration of iron deposits in the brain of patients with Friedreich ataxia, pantothenate kinase-associated neurodegeneration (formerly called Hallervorden-Spatz syndrome), and neuroferritinopathy was possible only at autopsy, but magnetic resonance imaging now provides a means for detecting localized brain iron deposits during life.[214]

Patients with hyperferritinemia but no clinical manifestations or elevated transferrin saturations may have mutations in the ferroportin gene (Table 36–4) or in the gene for the iron responsive element in L-ferritin messenger RNA.[100,215–217] The latter mutations are responsible for hereditary hyperferritinemia with cataract, a newly recognized disorder of autosomal dominant inheritance in which affected family members present with early-onset bilateral nuclear cataracts and moderately elevated plasma ferritin concentrations due to increased concentrations of L-ferritin. Serum iron concentration and transferrin saturation are normal or low, body iron level as evaluated by phlebotomy is not increased, and no hematologic or biochemical abnormalities are evident in affected persons.[216] Molecular studies have identified mutations in the iron responsive element of the L-ferritin messenger RNA as responsible. The only sign of the mutation seems to be an accumulation of L-type ferritin in the lens, resulting in cataract formation.[218]

Therapy

The goal of therapy for iron overload is reduction and maintenance of body iron at normal or near-normal levels. If possible, phlebotomy is the treatment of choice for hereditary hemochromatosis,[151,178] iron-loading anemia if the hemoglobin concentration is high enough to permit venesection,[134] porphyria cutanea tarda,[146] and African dietary iron overload.[91] Once the diagnosis of iron overload is established, phlebotomy therapy should begin promptly because any delay extends exposure to potentially toxic iron accumulations.

For most patients, phlebotomy should remove 500 mL of blood, containing 200 to 250 mg of iron, once weekly, until storage iron is depleted. The regimen should be individualized. For patients with iron-loading anemia, smaller amounts of blood will need to be withdrawn weekly, whereas for heavily iron-loaded patients with hereditary hemochromatosis, an even more vigorous program of twice-weekly phlebotomy can be used. The hematocrit or hemoglobin concentration should be measured before each phlebotomy procedure. After an initial fall in the hemoglobin concentration as erythropoiesis accelerates to keep pace with venesection, the hemoglobin will remain at approximately 90% of its initial value. The progress of iron removal can be followed by periodic measurements of plasma ferritin and iron concentrations and transferrin saturation. The plasma ferritin concentration declines progressively as iron is removed, but the plasma iron concentration and transferrin saturation remain elevated until iron stores near depletion. In a patient with porphyria cutanea tarda, a few weeks of phlebotomy will suffice, whereas in a patient with hereditary hemochromatosis and an initial body iron burden of 25 g, removal of the iron burden may require 2 years or more of phlebotomy.

Occasionally, plasma iron concentration falls and hemoglobin regeneration is temporarily delayed despite incomplete removal of excess iron, as indicated by continued elevation of the plasma ferritin concentration. A brief halt in the phlebotomy regimen, which presumably allows mobilization of the remaining iron, usually is all that is needed before resumption of weekly venesection. Eventually, when iron stores are exhausted, the ferritin will decline to less than 12 mg/L, the plasma iron concentration and transferrin saturation will be decreased, and the hemoglobin concentration will fall to less than 10 g/dL for 2 weeks without further phlebotomy. After complete removal of the iron load, lifelong maintenance therapy is needed, usually necessitating phlebotomy of 500 mL every 3 to 4 months or, in some patients, even less frequently. Maintenance phlebotomy should preserve a plasma ferritin concentration less than 50 mg/L. Although well-controlled studies are lacking, phlebotomy generally is not recommended for patients with the modest iron overload that sometimes develops with chronic liver disease; removal of the iron load in these cases seems to have no clinical benefit. In aceruloplasminemia, phlebotomy cannot remove the excess iron,[219] but iron chelation therapy with deferoxamine can provide effective treatment.[131,220]

For patients with transfusion-dependent refractory anemias, most patients with iron-loading anemias, and rare patients with hereditary hemochromatosis in whom phlebotomy is impossible, treatment with an iron chelator is the only means of preventing or removing toxic accumulations of iron (see box on Timing of Chelation Therapy). In patients with hereditary hemochromatosis and cardiac failure, a combination of phlebotomy and chelation therapy has been recommended. In the United States, two iron-chelating agents are available: deferoxamine, given parenterally, and deferasirox, administered orally.

For the past 3 decades, deferoxamine, a hexadentate bacterial siderophore purified from *Streptomyces pilosus*, has been regarded as the drug of choice for treatment of transfusional iron overload. It is a generally safe and efficacious means of controlling body iron that can prolong survival and prevent or ameliorate organ dysfunc-

Timing of Chelation Therapy

In patients who are transfusion dependent from early infancy (i. e., those with thalassemia major or other congenital refractory anemias), chelation therapy is best started after 10 to 20 transfusions, usually at approximately 3 years of age. In older patients with acquired refractory anemias who become transfusion dependent, it seems advisable to begin chelation early, after transfusion of 10 to 20 units of blood. In patients with iron-loading anemias and those with sickle cell disease who are chronically transfused for prevention of complications, early therapy also seems prudent, beginning when the hepatic iron concentration or the serum ferritin concentration increases to about two or three times the upper limit of normal. In each of these disorders, delay in beginning chelation therapy only exposes the patient to greater risk of iron toxicity.

tion.[207,221–223] Unfortunately, deferoxamine given orally is poorly absorbed. To be effective, the drug must be administered by prolonged subcutaneous or intravenous infusion with a small portable syringe pump, ideally each day, making compliance a demanding task. In patients with modest iron loads and no evidence of iron toxicity, slow subcutaneous infusion of deferoxamine for 9 to 12 hours daily usually provides adequate therapy.[223] In severely iron-loaded patients and in patients with evidence of iron toxicity, particularly those with cardiac complications, chronic slow intravenous infusions given through an indwelling central venous catheter may permit more rapid reduction of the body iron burden.[224] Deferoxamine is a generally safe and nontoxic drug for iron-loaded patients, but systemic complications have been reported, including allergic anaphylactoid reactions, infectious complications, visual abnormalities, auditory dysfunction, and growth retardation. The risk of many of these complications may be minimized by adjusting the deferoxamine dose to the magnitude of the body iron load.[223] Adequate deferoxamine therapy should produce a progressive decrease in the body storage iron of almost any patient with iron overload. If no decline is observed, blood and deferoxamine use, compliance, ascorbate status, and other features of the therapeutic regimen should be thoroughly reassessed.

Deferasirox, a synthetic orally active tridentate iron chelator, was approved for use by the U.S. Food and Drug Administration in 2005 for treatment of transfusional iron overload in adults and children older than 2 years.[225] Deferasirox has a long plasma half-life, making possible once-daily dosing. Extensive systematic clinical trials in patients with thalassemia major,[226] sickle cell disease,[227] and other transfusion-dependent anemias have provided evidence that the effectiveness of deferasirox in the management of iron overload is comparable to that of deferoxamine.[228] The most common adverse events have been rash, gastrointestinal disturbances, and abnormalities in renal function. Additional clinical studies examining the long-term safety and efficacy of deferasirox are in progress, but the initial experience suggests that this orally active iron-chelating agent is a well-tolerated, once-daily treatment for control of transfusional iron overload.

Prognosis

The prognosis in patients with iron overload is influenced by many factors, including the magnitude, rate, and route of iron loading; distribution of iron deposition between macrophage and parenchymal sites; amount and duration of exposure to circulating nontransferrin-bound iron; ascorbate status; and coexisting disorders, especially alcoholism. The magnitude of iron accumulation seems to be a critical determinant of the risk of cirrhosis of the liver and, in turn, of hepatocellular carcinoma, now the two major causes of death in hereditary hemochromatosis.[118] The development of cirrhosis increases the risk of hepatocellular carcinoma more than 200-fold.[118] Hepatomas, the ultimate cause of death in 20% to 30% of patients with hemochromatosis, occur almost exclusively in patients with hepatic cirrhosis.[229] If the disease is diagnosed before tissue injury occurs, phlebotomy therapy to remove the excess iron can prevent all of the complications of hemochromatosis, including cirrhosis, and return the patient's life expectancy to normal.[118] Even if organ damage is present, phlebotomy prevents further progression, and amelioration of some features of the disease is possible. Skin pigmentation diminishes; hepatic function may improve while fibrosis is arrested or sometimes regresses;[87] and cardiac abnormalities, including even cardiac failure, may resolve. Diabetes and other endocrine abnormalities usually are ameliorated only slightly, if at all, although reversal of hypogonadism has occurred. Arthropathy usually does not subside and may even continue to progress despite phlebotomy.

In patients with iron overload who cannot be treated by phlebotomy, chelation therapy is effective in reducing the body iron burden and improving the prognosis. Chronic infusion of parenteral deferoxamine decreases the hepatic iron concentration, improves hepatic function, promotes growth and sexual maturation, and helps protect against cardiac disease and early death. Early experience suggests that orally administered deferasirox may be similarly effective in many patients. In all forms of iron overload, the most effective means of preventing complications is prevention of iron accumulation, either by early identification and phlebotomy treatment of homozygotes for hereditary hemochromatosis or by early institution of chelation therapy in patients with iron-loading or transfusion-dependent anemias.

SUGGESTED READINGS

Allen RP: Controversies and challenges in defining the etiology and pathophysiology of restless legs syndrome. Am J Med 120:S13, 2007.

Anderson GJ, Darshan D, Wilkins SJ, et al: Regulation of systemic iron homeostasis: How the body responds to changes in iron demand. Biometals 20:665, 2007.

Auerbach M, Ballard H, Glaspy J: Clinical update: Intravenous iron for anaemia. Lancet 369:1502, 2007.

Batts KP: Iron overload syndromes and the liver. Mod Pathol 20(Suppl 1): S31, 2007.

Boelaert JR, Vandecasteele SJ, Appelberg R, et al: The Effect of the Host's Iron Status on Tuberculosis. J Infect Dis 195:1745, 2007.

Camaschella C, Campanella A, De Falco L, et al: The human counterpart of zebrafish shiraz shows sideroblastic-like microcytic anemia and iron overload. Blood 110:1353, 2007.

De Domenico I, Ward DM, di Patti MC, et al: Ferroxidase activity is required for the stability of cell surface ferroportin in cells expressing GPI-ceruloplasmin. EMBO J 26:2823, 2007.

De Domenico I, Ward DM, Langelier C, et al: The molecular mechanism of hepcidin-mediated ferroportin down-regulation. Mol Biol Cell 18:2569, 2007.

Domellof M: Iron requirements, absorption and metabolism in infancy and childhood. Curr Opin Clin Nutr Metab Care 10:329, 2007.

Dweikat I, Sultan M, Maraqa N, et al: Tricho-hepato-enteric syndrome: A case of hemochromatosis with intractable diarrhea, dysmorphic features, and hair abnormality. Am J Med Genet A 143:581, 2007.

Farrell DE, Allen CJ, Whilden MW, et al: A new instrument designed to measure the magnetic susceptibility of human liver tissue in vivo. IEEE Trans Magn 43:3543, 2007.

Fujita N, Sugimoto R, Takeo M, et al: Hepcidin expression in the liver: Relatively low level in patients with chronic hepatitis C. Mol Med 13:97, 2007.

Gardenghi S, Marongiu MF, Ramos P, et al: Ineffective erythropoiesis in β-thalassemia is characterized by increased iron absorption mediated by down-regulation of hepcidin and up-regulation of ferroportin. Blood 109:5027, 2007.

Goodnough LT: Erythropoietin and iron-restricted erythropoiesis. Exp Hematol 35:167, 2007.

Harris EL, McLaren CE, Reboussin DM, et al: Serum ferritin and transferrin saturation in Asians and Pacific Islanders. Arch Intern Med 167:722, 2007.

Hershko C, Ianculovich M, Souroujon M: A hematologist's view of unexplained iron deficiency anemia in males: Impact of Helicobacter pylori eradication. Blood Cells Mol Dis 38:45, 2007.

Hershko C, Patz J, Ronson A: The anemia of achylia gastrica revisited. Blood Cells Mol Dis 9:178, 2007.

Karam LB, Disco D, Jackson SM, et al: Liver biopsy results in patients with sickle cell disease on chronic transfusions: Poor correlation with ferritin levels. Pediatr Blood Cancer 50:62, 2008.

Kemna EH, Tjalsma H, Podust VN, et al: Mass spectrometry-based hepcidin measurements in serum and urine: Analytical aspects and clinical implications. Clin Chem 53:620, 2007.

Killip S, Bennett JM, Chambers MD: Iron deficiency anemia. Am Fam Physician 75:671, 2007.

Koorts AM, Viljoen M: Ferritin and ferritin isoforms I: Structure-function relationships, synthesis, degradation and secretion. Arch Physiol Biochem 113:30, 2007.

Kratovil T, Deberardinis J, Gallagher N, et al: Age specific reference intervals for soluble transferrin receptor (sTfR). Clin Chim Acta 380:222, 2007.

Lambrecht RW, Thapar M, Bonkovsky HL: Genetic aspects of porphyria cutanea tarda. Semin Liver Dis 27:99, 2007.

McCann JC, Ames BN: An overview of evidence for a causal relation between iron deficiency during development and deficits in cognitive or behavioral function. Am J Clin Nutr 85:931, 2007.

Murphy AT, Witcher DR, Luan P, et al: Quantitation of hepcidin from human and mouse serum using liquid chromatography tandem mass spectrometry. Blood 110:1048, 2007.

Ohtake T, Saito H, Hosoki Y, et al: Hepcidin is down-regulated in alcohol loading. Alcohol Clin Exp Res 31:S2, 2007.

Origa R, Galanello R, Ganz T, et al: Liver iron concentrations and urinary hepcidin in beta-thalassemia. Haematologica 92:583, 2007.

Phillips JD, Bergonia HA, Reilly CA, et al: A porphomethene inhibitor of uroporphyrinogen decarboxylase causes porphyria cutanea tarda. Proc Natl Acad Sci U S A 104:5079, 2007.

Poitou Bernert C, Ciangura C, Coupaye M, et al: Nutritional deficiency after gastric bypass: Diagnosis, prevention and treatment. Diabetes Metab 33:13, 2007.

Rao R, Georgieff MK: Iron in fetal and neonatal nutrition. Semin Fetal Neonatal Med 12:54, 2007.

Rivers CA, Barton JC, Gordeuk VR, et al: Association of ferroportin Q248H polymorphism with elevated levels of serum ferritin in African Americans in the Hemochromatosis and Iron Overload Screening (HEIRS) Study. Blood Cells Mol Dis 38:247, 2007.

Taher A, Nathan D, Porter J: Evaluation of iron levels to avoid the clinical sequelae of iron overload. Semin Hematol 44:S2, 2007.

Valenti L, Fracanzani AL, Dongiovanni P, et al: Iron depletion by phlebotomy improves insulin resistance in patients with nonalcoholic fatty liver disease and hyperferritinemia: Evidence from a case-control study. Am J Gastroenterol 102:1251, 2007.

Vichinsky E, Onyekwere O, Porter J, et al: A randomised comparison of deferasirox versus deferoxamine for the treatment of transfusional iron overload in sickle cell disease. Br J Haematol 136:501, 2007.

Walker SP, Wachs TD, Gardner JM, et al: Child development: Risk factors for adverse outcomes in developing countries. Lancet 369:145, 2007.

REFERENCES

For complete list of references log onto www.expertconsult.com

CHAPTER 37

ANEMIA OF CHRONIC DISEASES

Lawrence B. Gardner and Edward J. Benz, Jr.

Anemia is commonly associated with many diverse systemic inflammatory conditions, including infection, rheumatologic disorders, and cancer. The cause of the anemia of chronic disease (ACD) is multifactorial and includes a mildly decreased life span of erythrocytes coupled with deregulated iron absorption and transport, a direct inhibition of hematopoiesis, and a relative deficiency of erythropoietin. Research over the past decade has delineated the important role of inflammatory cytokines in each of these causes and the emerging role of the iron regulator hepcidin in the pathogenesis of ACD. Clinical trials have led to effective treatment options for patients with ACD.

DESCRIPTION AND EPIDEMIOLOGY

ACD is an anemia of underproduction that usually is normocytic, normochromic, and relatively mild, with a hemoglobin level greater than 10 g/L.[1] However, the anemia can be severe, and the mean corpuscular volume may be reduced, sometimes dramatically, in approximately 30% of patients. ACD is one of the most common causes of anemia. Over a 2-month period of observation, 52% of hospitalized patients with anemia who were not iron deficient, hemolyzing, or suffering from a hematologic malignancy met the laboratory criteria for ACD.[2] Although anemia is extremely common in cancer patients undergoing chemotherapy, up to 30% of patients with a variety of nonhematologic cancers have anemia before treatment. The presence of anemia may correlate with survival.[3] ACD has been diagnosed in up to 27% of outpatients with rheumatoid arthritis.[4] Although most hospitalized patients with ACD have active infection, an inflammatory condition, or a malignancy, other reported precipitating illnesses include alcoholic liver disease, congestive heart failure, thrombosis, chronic pulmonary disease, diabetes, trauma, and a variety of other medical conditions.[2,5] Because of the lack of standard for the diagnosis of ACD (as discussed in Diagnosis), such epidemiologic studies may be suspect. However, it is intriguing that some of the diverse diseases that have not been thought to be inflammatory in nature, such as congestive heart failure, have been associated with many of the cytokine abnormalities found to play a causative role in ACD.[6]

ETIOLOGY AND PATHOGENESIS

ACD is marked by low serum levels of iron. However, in contrast to iron-deficiency anemia, total iron stores are normal or elevated, and these findings appear to parallel disease activity.[7] Because of the well-established serum markers in ACD, initial theories on the etiology of ACD emphasized the role of iron. Subsequent models focused on a direct suppression of hematopoiesis and a relative deficiency of erythropoietin. With the observations that hepcidin levels are elevated in ACD and that hepcidin plays an important role in iron utilization (see Biology and Molecular Aspects), models of ACD again are focusing on the role of iron metabolism. Interestingly, evidence also suggests that hepcidin has a direct effect on erythroid progenitor proliferation and survival.[8,9] It is clear that the pathogenesis of ACD is multifactorial and complex (Table 37–1).

Although a variety of studies demonstrate that red cell survival in ACD is only mildly decreased, even a small decrease in erythrocyte half-life may have an impact on hemoglobin concentrations when erythropoiesis is concomitantly suppressed, as has been demonstrated in ACD (see Biology and Molecular Aspects). Rats given endotoxin have a reduced erythrocyte half-life,[10] and a mildly shortened erythrocyte half-life has been observed in patients with rheumatoid arthritis and ACD.

It has long been established that iron metabolism is deregulated in ACD. Early studies in a variety of animal models demonstrated that radiolabeled iron absorption and half-life were diminished with concomitant systemic inflammation.[10,11] Other studies using trace quantities of labeled iron showed no direct impairment of iron incorporation into red blood cells, suggesting that inflammation impairs iron release from storage sites, decreasing plasma iron concentrations and decreasing iron available for hemoglobin synthesis. Sterile inflammation in a dog model impairs only the reuse of iron from senescent red cells, further suggesting that inflammation leads to a defect in iron release from tissues to the plasma transferrin pool.[12] Studies in patients with rheumatoid arthritis and a diagnosis of ACD also demonstrate decreased iron turnover in comparison to normal or iron-deficient control subjects.[13]

Abnormal iron turnover in ACD may occur via several mechanisms. Decreased transferrin receptors in the serum[14] and on erythroblasts[15] have been found in patients with ACD. Other investigators have suggested that increased release of lactoferrin from neutrophils[16] or increased synthesis of apoferritin[17] leads to a pool of iron trapped in storage form, unavailable for hemoglobin synthesis. More recently, hepcidin, originally characterized as a small, circulating antimicrobial, has been implicated in ACD. Hepcidin binds, internalizes, and degrades the iron export channel ferroportin, thus blocking iron release from macrophages, hepatocytes, and the duodenum and leading to a decrease in available iron.[9,18,19] Overexpression of hepcidin leads to a fatal anemia in mice, with a decrease in iron absorption and an increase in reticuloendothelial stores of iron.[20] Hepcidin is increased in inflammatory conditions in mice (see Biology and Molecular Aspects later)[21] and is elevated in a variety of diseases associated with ACD. Together, these data suggest that hepcidin is a major mediator for many of the iron changes seen in ACD.

In addition to a decrease in an important hemoglobin precursor (i.e., iron), a direct inhibition of hematopoiesis and a relative deficiency of erythropoietin are found in ACD. Inhibition of hematopoiesis found in ACD is thought to be caused by soluble factors present in the perturbed bone marrow microenvironment (see Biology and Molecular Aspects later). Studies have shown that removal of bone marrow–adherent cells (mostly macrophages and monocytes) from patients with ACD leads to increased erythroid colony formation. This process can be reversed by coculture of ACD-adherent cells but not by adherent cells from control marrow.[22] In a study of patients with rheumatoid arthritis with ACD, the numbers of erythroid progenitors in control and in anemic patients were similar (not accounting for the difference in anemia between the two groups). Serum from patients with rheumatoid arthritis with anemia produced decreased burst-forming unit-erythroid (BFU-E) proliferation, whereas serum from nonanemic arthritic patients did not.[23] Peripheral blood mononuclear cells from patients with rheumatoid arthritis also suppress BFU-E growth.[24]

Most of the supporting data for direct inhibition in hematopoiesis are derived from in vitro studies. Data from more clinically relevant studies have clearly documented a *relative* deficiency of erythropoietin in many chronic diseases associated with anemia. Although serum

Table 37–1 Suspected Causes of Anemia of Chronic Disease

Shortened erythrocyte survival
Block in reuse of iron by erythrocyte
Direct inhibition of erythropoiesis
Relative deficiency of erythropoietin

erythropoietin levels may be increased, they are not as elevated as they should be for the degree of anemia present. In a study of 81 patients with solid tumors who exhibited laboratory data compatible with ACD and who did not have marrow involvement by tumor, erythropoietin levels were higher than in control subjects without anemia, but they were only half the values typical of subjects with similar hematocrits caused by iron deficiency. The normal inverse relationship between hemoglobin and erythropoietin levels also was not seen.[25] In 41 anemic patients with rheumatoid arthritis, 14 of whom had plentiful iron on bone marrow aspirate, serum erythropoietin levels for all rheumatoid patients were lower than for those with simple iron-deficiency anemia and comparable hemoglobin levels.[26] Serum erythropoietin levels have been shown to be inappropriately low in human immunodeficiency virus (HIV)-positive patients with normochromic normocytic anemia[27] and in lung transplant recipients.[28]

Patients with diabetes with anemia, normal renal function, and lower-than-expected erythropoietin levels have been reported. This condition is hypothesized to be caused by diabetic neuropathy,[29] although there also may be a direct role of insulin on stem cells.[30] Up to 40% of patients with chronic liver disease are anemic. Although this anemia is clearly multifactorial, some studies have found a blunted erythropoietin response to anemia in patients with cirrhosis.[31] However, at least one study of veterans with anemia and alcoholic liver disease found a serum erythropoietin level appropriate for the degree of anemia.[32] Of note, the observation that hepcidin synthesis may be altered in liver disease may provide further insight into ACD in this setting.[33]

BIOLOGY AND MOLECULAR ASPECTS

The role of inflammatory cytokines in many of the underlying diseases associated with ACD has suggested a mechanistic link for much of the pathophysiology of anemia, including decreased erythrocyte survival, decreased access to available iron through upregulation of hepcidin and other mechanisms, direct inhibition of hematopoietic progenitor growth, and inadequate erythropoietin response to anemia.

Increased serum levels of cytokines, particularly interleukin (IL)-1, IL-6, IL-10, tumor necrosis factor (TNF), interferon (IFN)-α, and IFN-β, have been observed in many inflammatory diseases, including acquired immunodeficiency syndrome (AIDS), hepatitis C, tuberculosis, bacterial and fungal infection, rheumatoid arthritis, inflammatory bowel diseases, and both solid and hematologic malignancies.[34–36] Erythrocytes infected with various strains of malaria or with peptides of *Plasmodium falciparum* stimulate macrophages to secrete TNF. Elevated levels of several cytokines have been found in patients with malarial infections.[37] TNF-α synthesis is increased in mucosal T cells in patients with Crohn disease[38] and in blood mononuclear cells from patients with rheumatoid arthritis.[39] High levels of inflammatory cytokines may be concentrated in the bone marrow milieu. Bone marrow of patients with rheumatoid arthritis has increased levels of IL-6 and TNF-α.[40] Bone marrow stromal cells in patients with giant cell arteritis may produce less stem cell factor and granulocyte-macrophage colony-stimulating factor than do controls.[39]

The fact that cytokines are thought to play such an important role in many of the diseases associated with anemia and that levels of many of these cytokines often correlate with the degree of anemia suggests an association between inflammatory cytokines and anemia. Indeed, serum TNF-α levels correlate with both disease activity and the degree of anemia in rheumatoid arthritis.[41] Trials of cytokine antagonists in inflammatory diseases have shown them to improve anemia.[42,43] Many molecular mechanisms by which cytokines directly or indirectly affect hematopoiesis have been described.

Cytokine-Induced Decreases in Red Cell Survival

Several studies suggest a role for decreased erythrocyte survival in the pathogenesis of ACD. Early in vivo and in vitro experiments suggested that fever itself can induce rheologic changes in erythrocytes within a few days, leading to increased destruction and up to 15% decline in red cell mass.[44] Later studies suggested that cytokines, the cause of fever in many of the diseases associated with ACD, also may alter red cell kinetics. For example, rats receiving chronic intraperitoneal injections of IL-1 and TNF showed a twofold decline in ^{59}Fe radioactivity, suggesting decreased erythrocyte survival. This effect has been postulated to involve cytokine-induced macrophage and reticuloendothelial system activation.[10]

Cytokine-Induced Abnormalities in Iron Metabolism

Many of the cytokines implicated in ACD appear to have effects on iron metabolism. Nude mice inoculated with Chinese hamster ovary cells that had been engineered to secrete TNF-α show an almost 60% decline in serum iron levels after 3 weeks while maintaining normal bone marrow stores of iron.[45] Rats injected with IL-1 or TNF experienced a 40% drop in serum iron levels; TNF also caused a significant decrease in iron incorporation into erythrocytes.[10] These findings are consistent with the observation that iron reuse is defective in ACD.[12] TNF has been shown to increase radiolabeled iron uptake by peritoneal macrophages without an increase in iron release,[46,47] suggesting that macrophage sequestration of iron is cytokine induced. In clinical trials, IL-10 led to anemia in patients with Crohn disease and to an increase in ferritin levels, decreasing iron availability to red blood cell precursors.[35]

Molecular evidence suggests a direct cytokine effect on iron metabolism. Even though IL-1β has no effect on ferritin transcription, it increases the synthesis of ferritin in human hepatoma cells by an increase in mRNA translation.[48,49] Increased translation depends on a 5′ untranslated region, distinct from the well-known iron responsive element but similar to a 38-nucleotide consensus sequence found in other IL-sensitive acute-phase reactants.[49] The increase in ferritin synthesis occurs without increased cellular transferrin receptor transcription or expression and involves no new iron influx.[48] IL-1 could lead directly to the creation of an intracellular iron pool that is not available for hemoglobin synthesis. IL-10 also appears to increase ferritin translation.[35]

More recent data demonstrate that inflammatory cytokines upregulate hepcidin, which, as previously noted, may mediate many of the iron changes seen in ACD. IL-1α, IL-1β, and other inflammatory cytokines have been demonstrated to upregulate hepcidin,[50,51] but the best described inducer, and perhaps the only direct inducer, of hepcidin is IL-6.[52] The transcription factors STAT3[53] and SMAD4,[54] both of which are upregulated by IL-6 and other inflammatory cytokines, have been found to activate the hepcidin promoter and induce hepcidin mRNA. In humans injected with lipopolysaccharide, IL-6 increases dramatically after 3 hours, followed by an increase in urinary hepcidin by 6 hours.[55] Direct administration of IL-6 to humans also leads to increased urinary hepcidin and decreased serum iron.[19] In patients with ACD, increased pro-hepcidin serum concentrations are associated with decreased expression of ferroportin in circulating monocytes along with increased ferritin accumulation in these cells.[56]

Cytokines Leading to Direct Inhibition of Hematopoiesis

Although data demonstrate that cytokines, including IL-1, IFN, and TNF, can have a direct inhibitory effect on hematopoiesis, almost all of the evidence supporting such a role for cytokines is derived from in vitro experiments, and the clinical relevance is unclear. The role of IL-6 in the direct inhibition of hematopoiesis is controversial. Exogenous IL-6 given to monkeys causes a dose-dependent, mild, short-lived anemia within 4 weeks.[57] Some studies have shown that IL-6 has direct inhibitory effects on stem cells.[58] However, other studies have demonstrated that IL-6, which is elevated in rheumatoid arthritis, has no direct effect on bone marrow hematopoiesis.[59] Juvenile-onset chronic arthritis is associated with increased IL-6 levels and anemia, but this anemia is one of iron deficiency.[60] IL-6 has been shown to cause bleeding in the rat intestinal wall.[40] As discussed, several cytokines, including IL-6, can upregulate hepcidin. In vitro studies have demonstrated that colony-forming unit-erythroid (CFU-E) formation is diminished at low erythropoietin conditions when hepcidin was added. Some evidence suggests that this effect may be due to proapoptotic functions of hepcidin.[8]

There is much better evidence for the role of IFN in the direct inhibition of erythropoiesis. IFN-γ can inhibit highly purified CFU-E from mice spleens in a dose-dependent manner.[61–63] Marrow stromal cells retrovirally engineered to secrete IFN-γ inhibit hematopoiesis in long-term bone marrow cultures by blocking cell cycle progression and inducing apoptosis in CD34 cells to a much greater degree than exogenous IFN.[64] IFN inhibition can be reversed by exogenous addition of murine IFN-γ receptors.[61] Inhibition by IFN-γ can be reversed in a dose-dependent manner by erythropoietin, a phenomenon also seen in ACD,[61,65,66] and partial reversal can be achieved by stem cell factor.[67] The concentration of IFN-γ required to suppress BFU-E was less than that needed to suppress CFU-E, suggesting the suppression occurs at the earlier stages of erythroid development.[63] Like IFN-γ, IFN-β appears to act directly on CFU-E, and inhibition does not require accessory T cells or adherent bone marrow cells.[61,68] Inhibition by IFN-α appears to work indirectly. Inhibition by IFN-α or IFN-β is not reversed by erythropoietin.[68]

TNF serum levels correlate with the degree of anemia in ACD. Erythroid growth is increased in the bone marrow of control and chronically anemic patients by monoclonal antibodies against TNF.[41] Transplantation of a Chinese hamster ovary cell line transfected with the human TNF gene led to anemia in nude mice within 3 weeks, with a significant decrease in BFU-E and CFU-E.[45] Exogenous TNF decreases erythroid colony formation.[41] For example, the inhibition of BFU-E growth sustained by normal bone marrow cultured in the presence of peripheral blood mononuclear cells of patients with rheumatoid arthritis can be reversed by antibodies to TNF-α.[24] However, evidence indicates that the effect of TNF on hematopoiesis is indirect, mediated by the local release of other cytokines, including IFN from accessory cells.[66] The inhibitory effect of TNF on CFU-E was completely abated by neutralizing antibodies against IFN-β but not by antibodies to IFN-γ or IL-1.[34] The effects of IL-1 also appear to be indirect. Growth of purified CFU-E is inhibited by recombinant IL-1 only in the presence of adherent T lymphocytes. The inhibition can be reversed by antibodies to IFN-γ, suggesting that IL-1 leads to lymphocyte secretion of IFN.[68]

Cytokines Leading to Decreased Erythropoietin Secretion

Cytokines have been implicated in the blunted, inappropriately low erythropoietin levels seen in ACD. In the erythropoietin-producing human hepatoma cell line HepG2 grown in diffusion-limited oxygen conditions, IL-1α, IL-1β, and TNF-α significantly lowered erythropoietin production. IL-1β also inhibited erythropoietin production in perfused rat kidneys. These effects were not accompanied by alterations in α-fetoprotein, showing that the effect was specific and not secondary to a generalized inhibitory growth effect.[69] Using another hepatoma cell line, Hep3B, hypoxia-driven erythropoietin production was inhibited with IL-1α, IL-1β, and TNF-α (with IL-1β being the most potent inhibitor) in a dose-dependent, additive manner.[58] Other soluble factors, in addition to cytokines, may play a role in directly inhibiting erythropoiesis in ACD. Animal models have suggested that vascular endothelial growth factor, which is commonly elevated in cancer, wounds, and ischemia, may act as a negative regulator of erythropoietin synthesis,[70] thus suggesting a potential link between diverse systemic illnesses and erythropoietin deficiency.

Perhaps one of the strongest arguments for a role of erythropoietin in causing ACD is that exogenous erythropoietin can at least partially reverse ACD. However, supraphysiologic levels of erythropoietin may simply overcome a direct inhibition of erythropoiesis (see Treatment later). Inhibition by IFN-γ can be reversed by erythropoietin.[65] Moreover, the capacity of monocytes from patients with inflammatory bowel disease to secrete TNF predicts therapeutic response to exogenous erythropoietin.[71]

DIAGNOSIS

Because ACD is a multifactorial disease and is seen in many clinical settings, an unequivocal diagnosis often is difficult. Many chronic illnesses are associated with other factors leading to anemia, including iron and nutritional deficiency, bleeding, hemolysis, renal failure with absolute erythropoietin deficiency, and marrow fibrosis or infiltration. Up to 70% of the anemia associated with rheumatoid arthritis may be multifactorial.[72] From 25% to 70% of patients with rheumatoid arthritis whose iron study results are consistent with ACD also are iron deficient.[73,74] Of 184 patients admitted to intensive care units, most anemic patients were found to have erythropoietin levels and iron study results consistent with ACD; however, 13% also had iron, folate, or B_{12} deficiency.[75] The role of frequent phlebotomy in hospitalized patients should be fully appreciated[76] (see box on Diagnosis of Anemia of Chronic Diseases).

ACD often is not diagnosed, although it plays an important role in anemia. For example, the anemia of renal failure traditionally has not been thought of as an ACD but rather as an anemia of absolute erythropoietin deficiency. However, efficient dialysis leads to an improved response to erythropoietin,[77,78] which suggests that other factors, perhaps including cytokines, play a role. Anemic hemodialysis patients may have occult infections of nonfunctioning arteriovenous grafts with markers of inflammation and erythropoietin resistance; removal of these grafts may correct the anemia.[79] Fifty percent of adults with chronic idiopathic neutropenia have an anemia consistent with ACD.[80] Remarkably, multiply traumatized patients have increased inflammatory cytokines and inappropriately low erythropoietin levels consistent with ACD.[5] In patients with congestive heart failure, TNF is elevated, cytokines levels are proportional

Diagnosis of Anemia of Chronic Diseases

The diagnosis of ACD is primarily one of exclusion and often is difficult. Various laboratory tests have been suggested as helpful, but few have proven value in the general population. However, because ACD occurs in too large a variety of acute and chronic illnesses. The best way to diagnose ACD, at least provisionally, is to document an anemia of underproduction (i.e., low reticulocyte index) with low serum iron and transferrin levels and elevated serum ferritin level in the setting of a systemic, usually inflammatory, illness. A thorough search may be necessary to document the precise underlying illness.

Other causes of anemia, such as hemolysis, nutritional deficiency, or sequestration, should be ruled out, and a component of iron deficiency should be strongly considered in a patient with systemic inflammation and a low or "normal" serum ferritin concentration. These other causes of anemia often accompany ACD. Bone marrow examination usually is not helpful but may be necessary to rule out malignancy (including a myelodysplastic syndrome), infection, or iron deficiency.

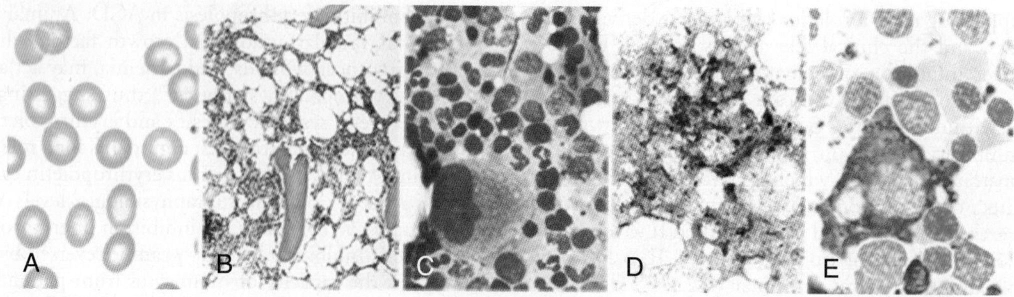

Figure 37–1 Anemia of chronic disease. **A,** Peripheral blood typically exhibits a normochromic, normocytic anemia. **B, C,** Bone marrow examination is sometimes performed to rule out other causes of anemia. Typically the marrow is morphologically normal. **D, E,** Prussian blue iron stain shows increased iron stores with increased histiocytic iron but decreased sideroblastic iron.

to the severity of anemia, and erythropoietin level is not elevated in proportion to the degree of anemia,[6,81,82] all consistent with ACD playing a role in the anemia commonly found in patients with heart failure.

The clinical setting in which the anemia is found helps with the diagnosis; however, in 30% of cases, no chronic illness can be identified. Acute illnesses can lead to anemia.[2] Some authorities argue that a normocytic, normochromic anemia may occur in otherwise healthy people; normal elderly people can have mild anemia.[83] One major problem with prevalence studies is that ACD is primarily a diagnosis of exclusion. This often necessitate evaluation of the bone marrow to ensure adequate iron stores, rule out infiltration by tumor, fibrosis, or infections, and exclude a myelodysplastic syndrome (Fig. 37–1). It should be noted, however, in a study of mostly older patients with an idiopathic mild anemia (10 ± 0.6 g/dL), a bone marrow aspirate with biopsy was found to add little to an extensive negative serologic workup and physical examination.[77]

The diagnosis of ACD usually is made on the basis of elevated marrow iron stores (usually assessed by serum ferritin) and low serum iron level, transferrin level, and total iron-binding capacity. Because ACD is a hypoproliferative and sometimes microcytic anemia, the differential diagnosis often includes iron deficiency. A low serum ferritin level associated with anemia suggests iron deficiency. A normal or elevated ferritin level is more difficult to interpret because ferritin is an acute-phase reactant. Some investigators argue that a ferritin level higher than 50 ng/mL excludes any component of iron deficiency, even in inflammatory states.[84] Nomograms correcting ferritin for the degree of inflammation present have been published.[85] Other researchers have shown that, in acute inflammation, serum ferritin levels greater than 3500 ng/mL can exist with absent bone marrow iron stores tested by aspirate.[86] Most investigators maintain that serum iron studies cannot predictably rule out iron deficiency.[87]

The concentrations of erythroblast and serum transferrin receptors are elevated in iron-deficiency anemia. Several studies have shown that the numbers of transferrin receptors on erythroblasts are lower in rheumatoid arthritis patients with ACD than in patients with iron-deficiency anemia,[15] and some may be decreased even below those without inflammatory conditions.[88] Although erythroblast transferrin studies are primarily a research tool, several studies have shown that the levels of serum transferrin receptors in rheumatoid arthritis and ACD are normal or slighter higher than normal, although generally lower than those with iron-deficiency anemia.[89,90] Patients with rheumatoid arthritis and elevated concentrations of serum transferrin receptors have responded to iron therapy.[90]

Several algorithms have been generated to diagnose or exclude ACD. In 120 anemic patients with inflammatory, infectious, or malignant diseases in whom bone marrow aspirates were obtained for assessment of iron stores, the serum ferritin level was significantly lower in patients who were iron deficient but still was elevated (63.7 vs 212 ng/mL). The combination of a serum ferritin level less than 70 ng/mL and a red cell ferritin level of 4 ng or less per erythrocyte had specificity of 0.97 and positive predictive value of 0.82, although these values were not validated in a prospective study.[74] A three-step algorithm has been derived for patients with rheumatoid arthritis and serologic evidence of ACD. Male patients with hemoglobin levels less than 11.0 g/dL and serum ferritin concentration less than 40 μg/L have iron deficiency, and those with a mean corpuscular volume greater than 85 fL or an iron saturation level greater than 7% have ACD. This formula led to a correct diagnosis in 89% of patients, but this finding was not independently validated.[73] Combining assessment of serum ferritin and plasma transferrin receptor concentration with the erythrocyte sedimentation rate has been suggested as an algorithm for differentiating iron deficiency and ACD in elderly women.[91] However, the specificity for any individual test and even for complex algorithms is relatively poor. Although hepcidin currently is measured in the urine, studies have demonstrated that urinary hepcidin levels mirror hepatic hepcidin mRNA concentrations in patients with a variety of inflammatory diseases.[92] The finding that hepcidin levels are elevated in ACD and parallel both IL-6 and ferritin levels[93] may make the assessment of hepcidin levels helpful in diagnosing ACD, although the sensitivity, specificity, and clinical utility of this assay in a wide patient population is unknown (see Summary and Future Directions later). Therefore, the diagnosis of ACD remains a clinical one.

TREATMENT

The anemia associated with chronic illness usually is mild. Correction often is unnecessary, especially if as many contributing factors as possible can be reversed. There may be a teleologic reason for ACD; the fever associated with infections has been shown to inhibit bacterial growth, and decreased iron concentrations (as seen in ACD) act synergistically with pyrexia to inhibit bacterial growth.[94] The attempt by hosts to withhold iron from invaders, called *nutritional immunity*, has been postulated to be an adaptive factor of ACD.[95] However, ACD can be severe, and almost by definition patients with ACD have comorbidities. Optimizing any reversible process, including hemoglobin and oxygen content and delivery, may have a dramatic beneficial effect. Unfortunately, few randomized, well-controlled, blinded studies are available to support anecdotal observations (see box on Treatment of Anemia of Chronic Diseases).

Optimal treatment of ACD is correction of the underlying disease process, if one can be clearly documented. ACD mirrors laboratory[59,72] and clinical[7] correlates of disease activity and duration of disease in rheumatoid arthritis. HIV patients receiving highly active antiretroviral therapy have a mean increase in hemoglobin concentration of more than 3 g/L compared with a decrease in hemoglobin concentration in patients not receiving these medications.[96] Treatment of underlying inflammatory diseases using cytokine antagonists has often led to improvements in anemia.[42,43] Definitive treatment of chronic diseases usually is difficult. Iron chelators such as deferoxamine have been shown in some animal studies to have mild effects on ACD, perhaps by decreasing free radicals and inflammation, but other studies have not duplicated this finding.[97,98]

Treatment of Anemia of Chronic Diseases

Treating ACD often is unnecessary if the patient is asymptomatic. However, the anemia may be severe, and quality of life may be greatly improved with treatment, even in patients who believed they felt well with their anemia. A trial of therapy may be indicated.

The first priority should be to correct any reversible contributors to the anemia (e.g., iron deficiency, absolute erythropoietin deficiency). Because the extent of ACD mirrors the activity of the underlying disease, all efforts should be made to treat the underlying disease. Although transfusion is the fastest way to reverse ACD, many studies have shown responses to erythropoietin. High doses of erythropoietin may be necessary. A starting dose of 20,000 to 40,000 units given subcutaneously each week can be initiated. If a hemoglobin response is seen, the dose can be decreased and the duration prolonged to titrate the hemoglobin to an asymptomatic level. Not only does this minimize expense and the number of injections needed, but it also may minimize any potential detriments of high hematocrits and/or high levels of exogenous erythropoietin. This response may take 4 to 8 weeks and should be monitored with objective symptomatic improvements (e.g., exercise tolerance). Although oral iron may not be absorbed or may be poorly tolerated and intravenous iron may be inconvenient and potentially dangerous, iron administration should be considered in poor responders, even in individuals with normal iron stores.

If the anemia is symptomatic or severe, treatment of the anemia itself may be indicated. Transfusion therapy may be the most common form of treatment of symptomatic ACD. Unfortunately, red blood cell transfusions are costly, have the potential detriments of infection, alloimmunization, and graft-versus-host disease, and are a limited resource. Serum levels of erythropoietin, although often elevated in ACD, are not elevated appropriately for the degree of anemia. Moreover, inhibition of hematopoiesis by cytokines is reversed in model systems by erythropoietin.[65] These observations have led to several successful trials of recombinant erythropoietin in the treatment of ACD. This strategy may be more cost effective than transfusion but erythropoietin must also be used cautiously . A relatively small, multicenter, placebo-controlled trial monitored the effects of erythropoietin in patients with rheumatoid arthritis and laboratory data consistent with ACD. The results showed a dose-dependent response to 50 to 150 U/kg of erythropoietin three times each week; 11 of 17 patients had a response rate of almost six hematocrit points.[99] Anemic patients with AIDS who were treated with recombinant erythropoietin had a significantly decreased transfusion requirement, especially if their endogenous erythropoietin level was less than 500 IU/L; however, all of these patients were also receiving zidovudine, a potential bone marrow suppressant.[100] Recombinant erythropoietin raised the hemoglobin level in patients with a variety of nonhematologic malignancies, including squamous cell cancer, breast cancer, and colon cancer.[101–104] Large trials enrolling patients undergoing chemotherapy have suggested that once-weekly injections of recombinant erythropoietin are as effective as thrice-weekly injections.[105] Injections of long-lasting erythropoietin analogues have been effective in treating the anemia that occurs with chemotherapy administration[106] and in animal models of ACD[107] and can be used to decrease the frequency of administration.

Responses by patients with ACD to erythropoietin range from 40% to 80% and can take up to 4 weeks.[98,99,108] Studies suggest that if no effect is seen by 3 months, further treatment likely will not be effective.[109] The response of ACD to erythropoietin is predicted by a low pretreatment erythropoietin level.[101,104] Although baseline duration of malignant disease, previous and current cancer treatment, bone marrow involvement, and type of tumor (hematologic vs solid tumor) were found to be negative predictors of response to erythropoietin treatment, only the absolute hemoglobin value, serum erythropoietin level, and ferritin level were found to be independent predictors in a multivariate analysis of 80 patients with chronic anemia of cancer.[109] Median survival of patients who responded was 12.6 months, compared with 4.3 months for nonresponders. This finding does not necessarily causally link correction of anemia to survival, because ability to respond, like baseline hematocrits, may be a marker for improved survival.[3] If after 2 weeks the serum erythropoietin level is higher than 100 mU/mL and the hemoglobin concentration has not increased by at least 0.5 g/dL or if after 2 weeks of treatment the serum ferritin level is higher than 400 ng/mL, a response is very unlikely.[109]

Functional iron deficiency is one possible reason for a failed response to erythropoietin.[110] It may be caused by a baseline iron deficiency, depletion of iron stores during hematopoiesis, or inability to mobilize stored iron; the latter is a hallmark of ACD. Intravenous iron decreased erythropoietin requirements, even compared with oral iron, in several cohorts, including hemodialysis patients[111] and those with inflammatory bowel disease.[112] Intravenous iron improves erythropoietin responses and is a cost-effective measure in dialysis patients, even in those with elevated ferritin levels.[113]

Although erythropoietin administration often leads to an increased hemoglobin concentration, this does not a priori ensure an improvement in morbidity, mortality, or quality of life. Reversal of anemia with erythropoietin in randomized and nonrandomized, open-label studies has been correlated with improvements in functional status, pain, nausea, anxiety, level of activity, and fatigue in large cohorts of patients receiving chemotherapy and smaller studies of cancer patients not undergoing chemotherapy.[102,104,105,114] However, these studies have limitations.[115] A thorough examination of the literature led to the suggestion that in cancer patients receiving chemotherapy, the hemoglobin level should be maintained at 12 g/L, and further rigorous studies on the impact on quality of life are necessary.[115] Many studies have shown that pretreatment anemia is a poor prognostic factor for a wide variety of patients with solid tumors undergoing chemotherapy and irradiation, it is unclear whether correction of this anemia can improve survival.[3]

Most studies and consensus statements on the efficacy of correcting anemia have derived from cancer patients receiving chemotherapy. However, the acute anemia and symptoms associated with myelosuppressive chemotherapy have limited similarities to ACD. Small and preliminary studies of cancer patients with ACD who were not receiving cytotoxic therapy suggest that performance and quality of life may improve with increased hemoglobin concentrations.[104] In a large study of critically ill patients, no change in a variety of outcomes were observed when patients were transfused when the hemoglobin level was 10 g/L, as opposed to a control group in whom the transfusion trigger was a hemoglobin level of 7 g/L.[116] Although administration of erythropoietin to critically ill patients decreased the number of transfusions, no change in clinical outcome was observed.[117] Moreover, increasing the hematocrit to 42% in a large number of hemodialysis patients with cardiac disease led to an increased number of deaths, and the number of cardiac events was increased in patients with chronic renal disease treated with erythropoietin with a goal of complete normalization of hemoglobin (12.0–15.0 g/dL) as opposed to partial normalization (10.5–11.5 g/dL).[118,119] Although low pretreatment hemoglobin levels have been demonstrated repeatedly to be a predictor of good response to chemotherapy and radiation,[120] two studies have demonstrated that patients with breast cancer or head and neck cancer treated with erythropoietin have increased disease progression and worse survival than placebo-treated patients.[121,122] This finding may reflect a direct antiapoptotic effect of erythropoietin on tumors.[123] Not all studies have demonstrated increased risks associated with aggressive erythropoietin treatment in patients with kidney disease or cancer.[124,125] However, based on these studies and interim analyses of several additional studies, in early 2007 the United States Food and Drug Administration warned that erythropoietin should be given only in the lowest possible doses necessary to avoid blood transfusions.

In summary, although treatment of ACD often increases the hemoglobin level and may improve quality of life and function, data from formal, well-controlled studies are pending, especially for patients not receiving cytotoxic chemotherapy. In particular, high doses of erythropoietin and/or high hemoglobin levels may be associated with increased risk for cardiac events, thromboses, and tumor progression.

SUMMARY AND FUTURE DIRECTIONS

Anemia is common in many chronic inflammatory, infectious, and malignant conditions, and often it is multifactorial. Anemia is exacerbated by inflammatory cytokines, which are thought to be the most important causative factors in ACD. ACD is difficult to diagnose but usually can be strongly suspected based on clinical findings, elimination of other causes of anemia, low serum iron and transferrin levels, and elevated ferritin level.

Cytokines such as IFN and TNF have wide-ranging effects, including both direct and indirect inhibition of hematopoiesis. Direct inhibition of hematopoiesis is mediated by both a relative decrease in erythropoietin as well as a decrease in iron available for hemoglobin synthesis. Many of the abnormalities of iron metabolism in ACD are caused by cytokine-induced increases in hepcidin. An understanding of the role of hepcidin in ACD may lead to improvements in both the diagnosis and treatment of ACD. Additional studies are required to delineate better the role of cytokine antagonists in treating ACD and its underlying causes. Controlled studies, clearly revealing the impact of correction of anemia on quality of life, medical outcomes, and survival of patients with ACD, particularly in those not undergoing chemotherapy, could provide insight into the role of hypoxia on tumors and other disease.

SUGGESTED READINGS

Bohlius J, Wilson J, Seidenfeld J, et al: Recombinant human erythropoietins and cancer patients: Updated meta-analysis of 57 studies including 9353 patients. J Natl Cancer Inst 98:708, 2006.

Canon JL, Vansteenkiste J, Bodoky G, et al: Randomized, double-blind, active-controlled trial of every-3-week darbepoetin alfa for the treatment of chemotherapy-induced anemia. J Natl Cancer Inst 98:273, 2006.

Dallalio G, Law E, Means RT Jr: Hepcidin inhibits in vitro erythroid colony formation at reduced erythropoietin concentrations. Blood 107:2702, 2006.

Detivaud L, Nemeth E, Boudjema K, et al: Hepcidin levels in humans are correlated with hepatic iron stores, hemoglobin levels, and hepatic function. Blood 106:746, 2005.

Drueke TB, Locatelli F, Clyne N, et al: Normalization of hemoglobin level in patients with chronic kidney disease and anemia. N Engl J Med 355:2071, 2006.

Ganz T: Hepcidin—A peptide hormone at the interface of innate immunity and iron metabolism. Curr Top Microbiol Immunol 306:183, 2006.

Inamura J, Ikuta K, Jimbo J, et al: Upregulation of hepcidin by interleukin-1beta in human hepatoma cell lines. Hepatol Res 33:198, 2005.

Kemna E, Pickkers P, Nemeth E, et al: Time-course analysis of hepcidin, serum iron, and plasma cytokine levels in humans injected with LPS. Blood 106:1864, 2005.

Lee P, Peng H, Gelbart T, et al: Regulation of hepcidin transcription by interleukin-1 and interleukin-6. Proc Natl Acad Sci U S A 102:1906, 2005.

Okonko DO, Van Veldhuisen DJ, Poole-Wilson PA, et al: Anaemia of chronic disease in chronic heart failure: The emerging evidence. Eur Heart J 26:2213, 2005.

Opasich C, Cazzola M, Scelsi L, et al: Blunted erythropoietin production and defective iron supply for erythropoiesis as major causes of anaemia in patients with chronic heart failure. Eur Heart J 26:2232, 2005.

Roy CN, Andrews NC: Anemia of inflammation: the hepcidin link. Curr Opin Hematol 12:107, 2005.

Singh AK, Szczech L, Tang KL, et al: Correction of anemia with epoetin alfa in chronic kidney disease. N Engl J Med 355:2085, 2006.

Tam BY, Wei K, Rudge JS, et al: VEGF modulates erythropoiesis through regulation of adult hepatic erythropoietin synthesis. Nat Med 12:793, 2006.

Theurl I, Mattle V, Seifert M, et al: Dysregulated monocyte iron homeostasis and erythropoietin formation in patients with anemia of chronic disease. Blood 107:4142, 2006.

Tomosugi N, Kawabata H, Wakatabe R, et al: Detection of serum hepcidin in renal failure and inflammation by using ProteinChip System. Blood 108:1381, 2006.

Wang RH, Li C, Xu X, et al: A role of SMAD4 in iron metabolism through the positive regulation of hepcidin expression. Cell Metab 2:399, 2005.

Wrighting DM, Andrews NC: Interleukin-6 induces hepcidin expression through STAT3. Blood 108:3204, 2006.

REFERENCES

For complete list of references log onto www.expertconsult.com

CHAPTER 38

HEME BIOSYNTHESIS AND ITS DISORDERS: Porphyrias and Sideroblastic Anemias

James S. Wiley and Michael R. Moore

The porphyrias and the sideroblastic anemias are metabolic disorders that involve defects in heme biosynthesis. Most forms of porphyria are inherited in a Mendelian autosomal dominant pattern, but some types are recessive and others are acquired through exposure to porphyrinogenic drugs and chemicals. A linked group of diseases, the porphyrinurias, are not porphyrias but have in common alterations of heme biosynthesis. Porphyrins are tetrapyrroles, which are ubiquitous in nature and exhibit characteristic red fluorescence on exposure to ultraviolet light. The iron-porphyrin complex, called *heme*, is central to all biologic oxidation reactions. In plants, the porphyrin molecule is combined with magnesium to form chlorophyll. Porphyrin biosynthesis is one of the most essential biochemical processes in most life forms.

In humans, mutations affecting the first enzyme of the heme biosynthetic pathway produce sideroblastic anemia. Inborn errors that occur at subsequent sites in this pathway usually result in metabolic disorders known as the *porphyrias* (Fig. 38–1). Historical analysis of the potential presence of acute porphyria in the British Royal family has been published,[1–3] as well as a study of the family of Vincent van Gogh.[4]

HEME BIOSYNTHESIS

Biosynthetic Pathways

Heme biosynthesis is an essential pathway and occurs in all metabolically active cells that contain mitochondria. It is most active in erythropoietic tissue, where it is required for hemoglobin synthesis, and in hepatic tissue, where the heme forms the basis of various heme-containing enzymes such as the cytochromes P450, catalase, cytochrome oxidase, and tryptophan pyrrolase. The synthetic pathway starts with the condensation of glycine and succinyl CoA to form 5-aminolevulinate (ALA) under the control of the mitochondrial enzyme ALA synthase (ALAS). This enzyme requires pyridoxal phosphate as a cofactor. A series of enzymes then controls the conversion of ALA first to the monopyrrole porphobilinogen (PBG) and then to the various porphyrins. Iron is inserted into protoporphyrin by the enzyme ferrochelatase to form heme (see Fig. 38–1). During the past 10 years, cDNA clones have been obtained for all of the enzymes of heme biosynthesis, and the structures of the corresponding genes have been determined. These advances are certain to improve understanding of the pathogenesis of the porphyrias and methods for identification of carriers. The enzymes of the biosynthetic pathway have all been mapped to specific chromosomes (Table 38–1). Heme synthesis and its disorders have been the subject of reviews[5–9] and included in a volume covering the history and biological diversity of the tetrapyrroles.[10]

Control of Heme Biosynthesis

The overproduction of porphyrins and their precursors in the different porphyrias is mainly hepatic or erythropoietic in origin. In the acute porphyrias and in porphyria cutanea tarda, the liver is the main source of overproduction; in congenital porphyria, the marrow is the main source; and in erythropoietic protoporphyria, porphyrins are overproduced by the liver and marrow.

Control of hepatic heme biosynthesis is regulated by the rate of the initial enzymatic step, ALAS (now designated ALAS1) which is under negative-feedback control by heme. This occurs by more than one mechanism. Heme represses transcription of the *ALAS1* gene and increases the rate of degradation of the mRNA (Fig. 38–2A). At the posttranslational level, heme blocks the translocation of pre-ALAS1 into the mitochondrion.[11] In the mitochondrion, the molecular mass of ALAS is smaller than that of the cytosolic pre-ALAS[11] because of the removal of the mitochondrial targeting sequence.

The erythroid bone marrow is the major heme-forming tissue in the body, producing 85% of the daily heme requirement. Heme synthesis in erythroid cells varies from that in hepatocytes; it is linked to tissue differentiation, and the half-life of the same end product of the two is quite different. Heme complexed with globin is preserved in circulating red blood cells for approximately 120 days, whereas heme produced in liver for cytochromes and enzymes, such as catalase, is subject to much more rapid turnover, measurable in hours. Regulation in the liver is exquisitely sensitive to fluctuations in intracellular heme levels[12] and responds rapidly to the requirements for synthesis as described in Fig. 38–2A. However, heme synthesis in the bone marrow shows a more leisurely response. This fundamental difference is explained by the finding of two different tissue-specific isoenzymes and two different cDNAs for human liver or "housekeeping" ALAS (ALAS1) and an erythroid ALAS (eALAS or ALAS2), which is expressed exclusively in erythroid cells.[13] The gene for ALAS2 has been mapped to the X chromosome and that for the hepatic enzyme to chromosome 3.[13] The *ALAS2* gene has 11 exons; exons 5 to 11 encode the catalytic domain of the enzyme and include a lysine residue that forms a Schiff base with the pyridoxal phosphate cofactor. Exon 1 contributes to the 5′-untranslated region whose structure allows iron to regulate ALAS2 mRNA translation, whereas exons 1 and 2 contribute the sequence that targets the enzyme to the mitochondria and is cleaved after import. Succinyl CoA synthetase associates specifically with ALAS2 within the mitochondrion, which helps promote the first step of heme synthesis.[14]

Enzyme levels of ubiquitous and erythroid isoenzymes of ALAS are controlled by different mechanisms. Ubiquitous ALAS1 levels in liver are regulated by negative feedback by heme that inhibits gene transcription and import of pre-ALAS1 (see Fig. 38–2A). More recently ALAS-1 has been shown to be upregulated by PPAR γ-coactivator 1α which regulates mitochondrial biogenesis and oxidative metabolism. Transcription of this coactivator 1α is controlled by glucose availability. Coactivator 1α production increases when glucose levels are low leading to increased levels of ALAS-1 and heme. These conditions are conducive to an acute attack of porphyria. However the relative contribution of heme and PGC-1α in regulating ALAS-1 expression remains to be resolved.[15,16] In contrast, heme does not affect transcription of the *ALAS2* gene, which is under the control of erythroid-specific promoters such as GATA1, a globin transcription factor. Whether heme inhibits import of pre-ALAS2 into the mitochondrial matrix remains to be unequivocally established. Heme may possibly also prevent the accumulation of intracellular iron by controlling the acquisition of iron from transferrin (Fig. 38–2B). In addition to transport of iron from plasma to the cytosol by the transferrin receptor, a second transport step is required for mitochondrial uptake of iron. This step is fulfilled mitoferrin (mfrn), a 333 residue polypeptide recently cloned from zebrafish.[17] Levels of intracellular iron regulate the translation of ALAS2 mRNA. A specific repressor protein interacts with an iron-responsive element in the 5′ untranslated region of the ALAS2 mRNA and prevents translation, and this repression is relieved by high iron levels.[12] Iron uptake by erythroid cells has a positive effect on the enzymatic step catalyzed by ALAS2 (see Fig. 38–2B). This effect ensures that protoporphyrin synthesis is coupled to iron availability.

A second rate-limiting step in the overall heme synthetic pathway lies at the level of porphobilinogen deaminase (PBGD), which has a low endogenous activity and is inhibited by protoporphyrinogen and coproporphyrinogen. There are also two forms of PBGD. The PBGD gene *(HMBS)* encodes two enzymes; the 10-kb-long gene with 15 exons has two overlapping transcription units. The upstream promoter works in all cell types and produces a protein with a molecular mass of 42 to 44 kd, whereas the downstream promoter is only active in erythroid cells and by differential splicing produces a smaller protein with a mass of 40 to 42 kd.[18]

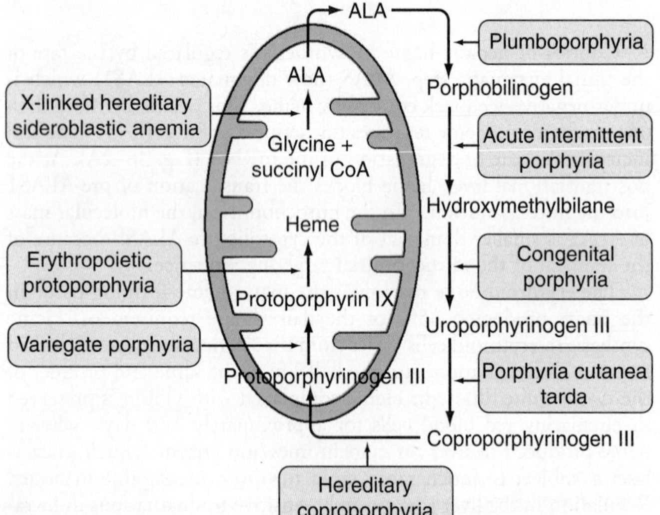

Figure 38–1 Pathway of heme biosynthesis in mammalian cells. The first step in the pathway is catalyzed by aminolevulinate synthase (ALAS) and occurs within the mitochondrion using pyridoxal 5′-phosphate as a cofactor. 5-Aminolevulinate (ALA) then leaves the mitochondrion and is converted by ALA dehydratase to give a monopyrrole, porphobilinogen. Four molecules of this compound are converted by porphobilinogen deaminase to a linear tetrapyrrole, hydroxymethylbilane. This molecule is then cyclized by uroporphyrinogen III synthase to uroporphyrinogen III, which is decarboxylated to coproporphyrinogen III. This molecule enters the mitochondrion and is oxidized in succession by coproporphyrinogen III oxidase and protoporphyrinogen III oxidase. The product is protoporphyrin IX, a substrate for ferrochelatase, which catalyzes the insertion of Fe^{2+} to form heme. The defective steps associated with specific porphyrias and X-linked hereditary sideroblastic anemias are shown.

Erythroid porphobilinogen deaminase (ePBGD) is stimulated by erythropoiesis in vitro and may play a regulatory role in heme biosynthesis during differentiation. Studies of the erythroid promoter for ePBGD have found that two major erythroid transcription factors, GATA1 and NFE2, may bind to sequences in the PBGD promoter.[19]

HMBS, the human PBGD gene, has attracted extensive investigation because of the practical importance of detecting carriers of the gene for acute intermittent porphyria.[20] Studies of the genetic locus of PBGD on chromosome 11 show great molecular heterogeneity,[21] as is also found in the parents of a homozygous case of acute intermittent porphyria.[22] This heterogeneity results in several phenotypic subtypes of the enzyme at the protein level. Most are cross-reacting immunologic material (CRIM)-negative subtypes, but some are CRIM-positive types.[23] There is a high interspecies conservation of structure of the enzyme. Most human mutations have been described on exons 10 and 12,[24] which is consistent with alteration of the binding sites for the dipyrromethane cofactor for the enzyme.[25] The three-domain structure of porphobilinogen deaminase has been defined by x-ray crystallography. The active site is located between domains 1 and 2. The dipyrromethane cofactor linked to cysteine protrudes from domain 3 into the mouth of the cleft. Flexible segments between domains 1 and 2 are thought to have a role in a hinge mechanism, facilitating conformational changes. Biochemical and x-ray crystallographic studies have shown that the enzyme from *Escherichia coli, Euglena gracilis,* rats, and humans has 12 conserved arginine residues in the cleft between the three protein domains. This structure fits well with the need to bind six PBG molecules each with two carboxyl groupings.

PORPHYRIAS

Biologic and Molecular Aspects

The porphyrias are classified as acute or nonacute (cutaneous) according to their clinical and biochemical features (Table 38–2).

Table 38–1 Porphyrias: Clinical Involvement, Enzymatic Etiology, and Chromosomal Location

Porphyria (Synonym)	Acute Attack, Skin and Organ Involvement	Enzyme of Heme Biosynthesis Affected	Chromosome Location
—	—	Hepatic aminolevulinate synthase-1 (ALAS1)	3p21
X-linked sideroblastic anemia	Bone marrow	Erythroid ALA synthase (ALAS2)	Xp11.21
ALA dehydratase deficiency porphyria (plumboporphyria)	Acute liver	ALA dehydratase (porphobilinogen synthase)	9q34
Acute intermittent porphyria (intermittent acute porphyria)	Acute liver	Porphobilinogen deaminase (hydroxymethylbilane synthase)	11q24.1–q24.2
Congenital erythropoietic porphyria (Günther disease)	Skin, red cells, bone marrow	Uroporphyrinogen III synthase	10q25.2–q26.3
Porphyria cutanea tarda (symptomatic porphyria, cutaneous hepatic porphyria)	Skin, liver	Uroporphyrinogen decarboxylase	1p34
Hereditary coproporphyria	Acute skin, liver	Coproporphyrinogen oxidase	3q12
Variegate porphyria (porphyria variegata)	Acute skin, liver	Protoporphyrinogen oxidase	1q21–q23
Erythropoietic protoporphyria (erythrohepatic protoporphyria)	Skin red cells, liver	Ferrochelatase (heme synthase)	18q21.3

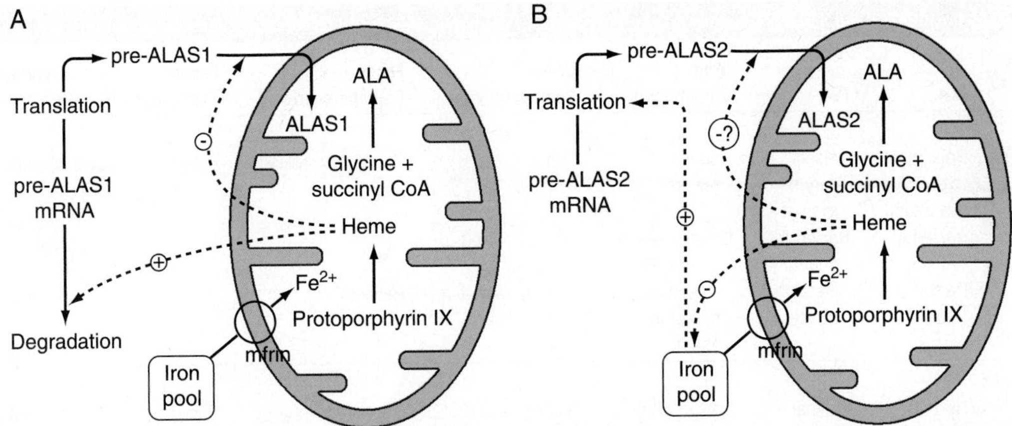

Figure 38–2 **A,** Control of heme synthesis in hepatic and other tissues. The rate of heme synthesis depends on the first and rate-limiting enzymatic step catalyzed by aminolevulinate synthase-1 (ALAS1). Heme represses transcription of the *ALAS1* gene, increases the rate of degradation of its mRNA, and blocks the translocation of the ALAS1 isoenzyme into the mitochondrion. **B,** Control of heme synthesis in erythroblasts. Cytosolic iron enhances the translation of mRNA of the pre-ALAS2 by inhibiting the interaction of a repressor protein with an iron-responsive element in the mRNA. The product of the last step, heme inhibits the uptake of iron from transferrin into the cytosol. Heme also may inhibit translocation of ALAS2 into the mitochondrion. The overall result is that the rate of heme synthesis is tightly linked to the availability of iron for the ferrochelatase reaction. Mfrn-mitoferrin transports Fe^{2+} into the mitochondrial matrix.

Table 38–2 Classification of Porphyrias

Classification	Disease	Biochemistry	Clinical Features
Acute porphyria	Acute intermittent porphyria	Increased ALA and PBG	Acute attack
	Variegate porphyria	Increased ALA and PBG; increased porphyrin	Acute attack; photosensitivity
	Hereditary coproporphyria	Increased ALA and PBG; increased porphyrin	Acute attack; photosensitivity
Nonacute porphyria	Porphyria cutanea tarda	Increased porphyrin	Photosensitivity
	Erythropoietic protoporphyria	Increased porphyrin	Photosensitivity
	Congenital porphyria	Increased porphyrin	Photosensitivity
Porphyrinurias	Lead, alcohol, iron-deficiency anemia, liver disease	Various biochemical manifestations	Various clinical presentations

ALA, 5-aminolevulinate; PBG, porphobilinogen.

Each of the different types of porphyria is linked to a reduced activity or deficiency of a specific enzyme in the heme biosynthetic pathway (see Fig. 38–1). The enzyme deficiency impairs the production of the end product heme, and there is overproduction and increased excretion of the heme precursors formed by the steps before the enzyme defect. There is also a compensatory increase in activity of the initial and rate-controlling enzyme ALAS. In the acute porphyrias, there is overproduction of all the porphyrins and porphyrin precursors (eg, ALA, PBG) formed proximal to the enzyme defect. The increased excretion of porphyrin precursors in the acute porphyrias is caused by decreased activity of PBGD in these conditions. The decrease can be caused by genetic mutation of the enzyme (in acute intermittent porphyria) or by inhibition of PBGD by protoporphyrinogen and coproporphyrinogen in variegate porphyria and hereditary coproporphyria, respectively.[26]

In the nonacute porphyrias, there is overproduction of all porphyrins formed before the enzyme defect but no overproduction of porphyrin precursors. The cause of this lack of overproduction of porphyrin precursors in the nonacute porphyrias is unclear, but it may result from a compensatory increase in the activity of the enzyme PBGD in addition to increased activity of ALAS and to site-specific heme synthesis.[29] The pattern of overproduction and excretion of porphyrins and porphyrin precursors in the various porphyrias is shown in Table 38–3. A consequence is that each of the different porphyrias is characterized by a different excretion pattern. Quantitative studies of the different porphyrins and precursors in the urine and feces usually identify the particular type of porphyria. The porphyrin precursors ALA and PBG and the more water-soluble porphyrins (with multiple carboxyl groups) are excreted mainly in the urine. Other porphyrins are mainly excreted in the feces by way of the bile (see box on Measurement of Porphyrins and Precursors).

The clinical manifestations of an acute attack of porphyria can be explained by dysfunction of the central, peripheral, and autonomic nervous systems. The mechanism by which altered heme synthesis results in dysfunction is unknown.

Perhaps the most likely hypothesis is that the clinical manifestations of acute porphyria arise as a result of heme deficiency within the nerve cells, although this does not exclude the possibility that ALA may also act as a pharmacologic agent in these diseases, compounding the effects of heme deficiency.[30] ALA has a prooxidant

Measurement of Porphyrins and Precursors

Diverse techniques such as high-pressure liquid chromatography,[27] extraction, and various forms of fluorometry are used to measure porphyrins and precursors. A recent addition has been fluorescence emission scanning to differentiate variegate porphyria, erythropoietic protoporphyria, and other photocutaneous porphyrias.[28] The International Federation for Clinical Chemistry presents diagnostic information on the Internet (www.ifcc.org).

Table 38–3 Changes in Porphyrins and Their Precursors in the Porphyrias, Porphyrinurias, and Hereditary Sideroblastic Anemia

Porphyrias and Other Conditions	ALA	PBG	Urine Uroporphyrin	Urine Coproporphyrin	Feces Coproporphyrin	Feces Protoporphyrin	Erythrocyte Protoporphyrin
ACUTE PORPHYRIAS							
Acute intermittent porphyria	Raised, very high in attack	Raised, very high in attack	Usually raised*	Sometimes raised	Sometimes raised	Sometimes raised	Normal
Variegate porphyria	Raised in attack	Raised in attack	Usually raised in attack	Usually raised in attack	Raised	Raised	Normal
Hereditary coproporphyria	Raised in attack	Raised in attack	Sometimes raised in attack	Usually raised, always in attack	Raised	Usually normal	Normal
NONACUTE PORPHYRIAS							
Porphyria cutanea tarda	Normal	Normal	Raised (7-/8-carboxylate porphyrin levels very high in attack)	Slightly raised	Isocoproporphyrin raised in remission	Raised in remission	Normal
Erythropoietic protoporphyria	Normal	Normal	Normal	Normal	Normal	Usually raised	Raised, usually very high
Congenital porphyria	Usually normal	Usually normal	Raised, isomer 1	Raised, isomer 1	Normal	Usually raised	Usually raised
OTHER CONDITIONS							
Hereditary sideroblastic anemia	Normal	Normal	Normal	Normal	Normal	Normal	Occasionally raised
Lead poisoning	Raised	Normal	Normal	Sometimes raised	Normal	Normal	Raised when blood lead level > 2 μm
Hereditary tyrosinemia	Raised	Normal	Normal	Normal	Normal	Normal	Normal
Iron-deficiency anemia	Normal	Normal	Normal	Normal	Normal	Normal	Raised

* PBG may cyclize to uroporphyrin nonenzymatically. ALA, 5-aminolevulinic acid; PBG, porphobilinogen.

effect on rat brain tissues and generates free radical species during its autooxidation.[30,31] The concept of autooxidation or oxidative stress is supported by the hypothesis that manganese excess could contribute to induction of superoxide dismutase[32] and increased indicators of such stress in lead exposure.[33] There is evidence that ALA enters cells by a pathway common to it and γ-aminobutyric acid (GABA).[34]

Genetic Aspects

The enzymatic links and genetic loci in each of the hereditary porphyrias are shown in Table 38–1. Nearly all are inherited as autosomal dominant traits. Few carriers of the abnormal gene show clinical signs of the disease, but most can be identified by intensive biochemical investigation. The rare congenital porphyria shows autosomal recessive inheritance. The mutations producing each of the acute porphyrias are heterogeneous at the molecular level and include complete or partial gene deletions, alterations of splicing or stability of mRNA, and missense mutations. An exception is variegate porphyria in South Africa, in which the founder effect ensures a predominance of the Arg59Tryp mutation.[35,36] Homozygotic or compound heterozygotic inheritance has been found in a number of the porphyrias, as has concurrent inheritance of more than one defect. This may present as two types of porphyria in one family[37] or as two types in one patient.[38] Examples of this "concurrent" porphyria are the Chester porphyria (ie, acute intermittent porphyria and variegate porphyria)[37] and dual porphyria (ie, variegate porphyria and porphyria cutanea tarda).[39]

The prevalence of the different forms varies widely. For example, in northern Europe and North America, approximately 1 of 10,000 individuals carries the gene for acute intermittent porphyria, although only about 10% of the affected persons will present with clinical features. It has been suggested that spontaneous mutation accounts for 3% of acute intermittent porphyria cases.[40] Variegate porphyria occurs in 1 of 400 white South Africans. There is a reduction in gene frequency in variegate porphyria from generation to generation that suggests that the allele associated with it is selectively deleterious.[41] The same is probably true of the other porphyrias. The pedigree of Chester porphyria is shown in Fig. 38–3.

Acute Intermittent Porphyria

Clinical and Laboratory Manifestations

Acute intermittent porphyria is the most severe of the acute porphyrias. During an attack, patients display abdominal and neuropsychiatric or neurovisceral disturbances. Onset occurs in puberty; female patients exhibit a fourfold greater incidence of attacks than males. Attacks occur mainly in young adults and become less frequent after menopause. It is uncommon to see attacks in children.[42] Crises may vary in duration from several days to months. They are most commonly followed by complete remission, although deaths are still reported, especially with acute intermittent porphyria[43] (see box on Precipitating Factors in Acute Porphyria).

Gastrointestinal symptoms occur in 95% of cases; most patients present with acute colicky central abdominal pain. Examination reveals tenderness but little rigidity, and patients may also experience limb pain or generalized muscular aches. Severe vomiting may occur, and constipation is usual. Hyponatremia occurs in severe attacks.

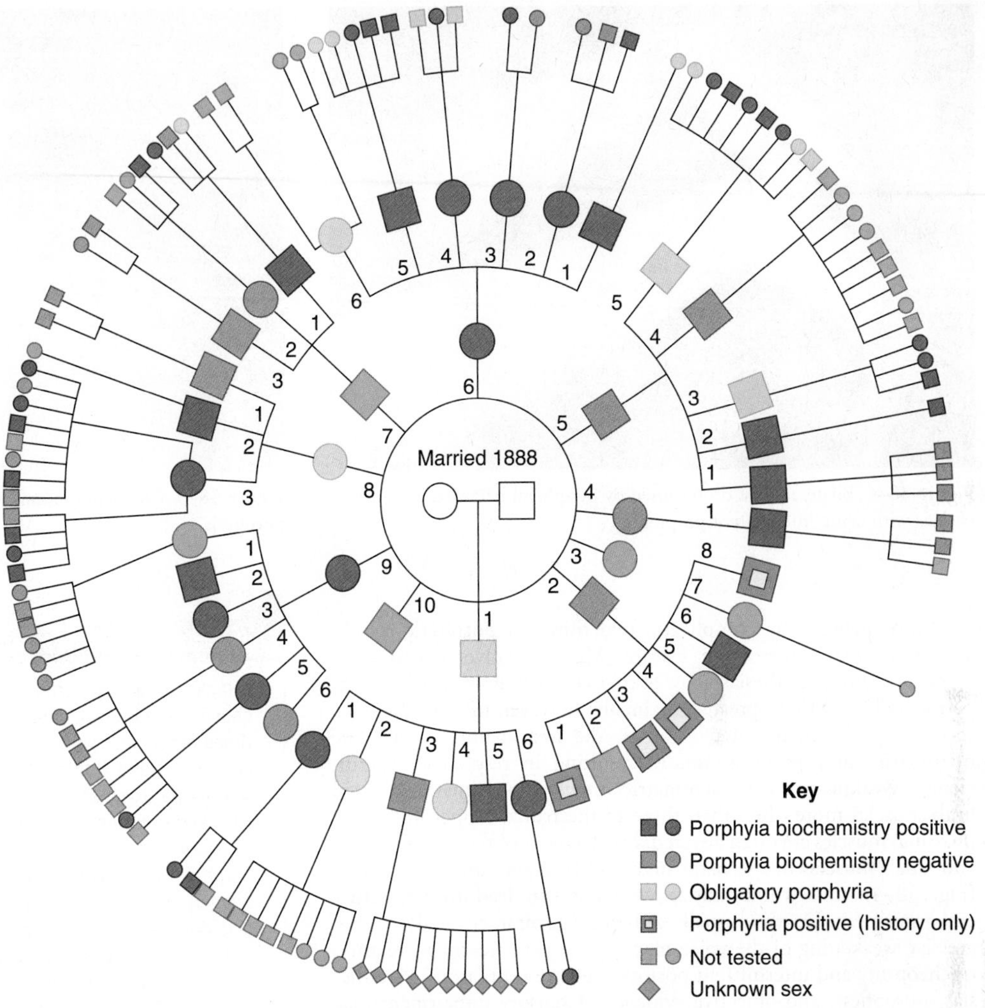

Married 1888

Key
Porphyia biochemistry positive
Porphyia biochemistry negative
Obligatory porphyria
Porphyria positive (history only)
Not tested
Unknown sex

Figure 38–3 The Chester family pedigree. The propositus, Peter Dobson, was a salmon fisherman from a close-knit community living on the bank of the River Dee, which runs through the city of Chester, U.K. Most of the 330 descendants of his marriage in 1888 still live in the city. Many suffered disabling illnesses and psychiatric upsets, which often went unrecognized as porphyria. The family called their illness *Dobson's complaint. (Courtesy Giles R. Youngs.)*

Precipitating Factors in Acute Porphyria

Most patients who have inherited acute porphyria enjoy normal health and go through life without any knowledge of their disorder or ever experiencing an acute attack. All porphyrics, however, are at risk of developing an attack if exposed to various precipitating factors. Drugs are the most common precipitating agents. Other factors that may trigger attacks include alcohol ingestion, reduced caloric intake (from fasting or dieting), and infection. Smoking can cause more frequent attacks.

Hormonal status is also important. Attacks are more common in females, and rarely, they occur before puberty or after menopause. Pregnancy and oral contraceptives may also precipitate attacks. Some women experience regular attacks, commencing in the week before the onset of menstruation. These may require luteinizing hormone–releasing hormone (LHRH) antagonists for control (see Table 38–4).

Drugs for Porphyria

Before prescribing any medication to a porphyric patient, advice must be sought from an appropriate specialist. Full drug lists are available on the Internet (www.drugs-porphyria.org). It should be borne in mind that such lists are far from encyclopedic, that new drugs are constantly being introduced to the pharmacopoeia, and that any form of combined preparation must be viewed with suspicion, because little is known about metabolic interactions in these diseases.[48] More details of such use and side effects of drugs can be sought from the literature.[49]

Table 38–4 PRECIPITATING FACTORS IN ACUTE PORPHYRIA

Drugs	Other Stimuli
Alcohol	Fasting or dieting
Barbiturates	Hormones, stress
Angiotensin-converting enzyme (ACE) inhibitors	Smoking
Anticonvulsants	
Antidepressants	
Calcium channel blockers	
Cephalosporins	
Ergot derivatives	
Erythromycin	
Steroids or anabolic steroids	
Contraceptives, hormone replacement therapy	
Sulfonamides	
Sulfonylureas	

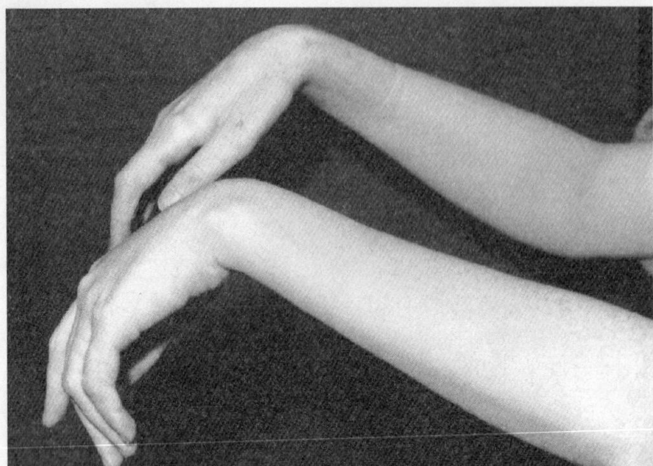

Figure 38–4 Bilateral wrist drop caused by peripheral neuropathy in a patient with acute intermittent porphyria.

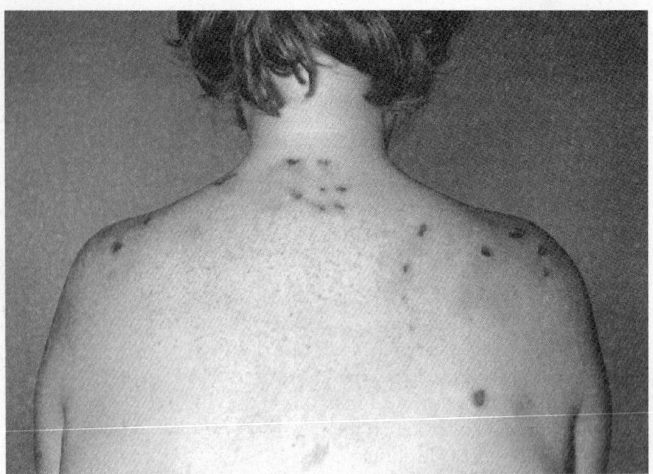

Figure 38–5 Cutaneous lesions and scarring in a patient with variegate porphyria.

Motor neuropathy complicates two thirds of porphyric attacks and may be the presenting feature. Motor involvement is most common, but paresthesias may also occur. Paralysis usually starts peripherally and then spreads proximally; however, in some patients, shoulder girdle involvement may be the first manifestation. The neuropathy may progress rapidly, resulting in respiratory insufficiency. Weakness, usually symmetric, involves proximal and distal limb muscles more often than those of the trunk. Upper limbs and proximal muscles are often affected. Involvement of the wrists, ankles, and small muscles of the hand may lead to a permanent deformity (Fig. 38–4), and trunk muscle weakness can lead to respiratory embarrassment. Death is usually caused by respiratory paralysis. Progressive weakening of the voice may suggest this; treatment requires tracheotomy and intermittent positive pressure ventilation. Paresthesias, numbness, and objective evidence of sensory impairment may occur with loss of pinprick sensation, which is most marked around the shoulder and hip areas; generalized tonic-clonic seizures occasionally occur.

Severe anxiety, depression, and frank psychosis are the main psychiatric manifestations of porphyric attacks. These psychiatric manifestations may result in a patient being misdiagnosed as suffering from a primary psychiatric disorder. Agitation, mania, depression, hallucinations, and schizophrenic-like behavior may occur. Psychiatric manifestations may persist between attacks.[44] Quality of life is severely affected in those suffering from repeated attacks of acute porphyria.[45]

The cardiovascular system is involved in approximately 70% of attacks. Sinus tachycardia (to 160 beats/min) and hypertension can occur; these elevations usually revert to normal after an attack. There is evidence that hypertension may occasionally be permanent, even in latent cases of acute intermittent porphyria (see box on Differential Diagnosis of Acute Intermittent Porphyria).

Other Acute Porphyrias

Hereditary Coproporphyria

Hereditary coproporphyria (HC) combines the clinical features of acute porphyria with photosensitive skin manifestations. It results from mutations in the gene encoding coproporphyrinogen oxidase, whose activity is decreased,[46,47] leading to overproduction of coproporphyrin.

The porphyrin precursors ALA and PBG and the more water-soluble porphyrins (with multiple carboxyl groups) are excreted mainly in the urine. Other porphyrins are mainly excreted in the feces by way of bile.

Differential Diagnosis of Acute Intermittent Porphyria

Attacks of acute porphyria must be distinguished from other causes of acute abdominal pain or peripheral neuropathy sometimes associated with psychosis. Heavy metal poisoning (ie, lead or arsenic) and Guillain-Barré syndrome must be considered, as well as paroxysmal nocturnal hemoglobinuria with its characteristic early morning hemoglobinuria and abdominal pain.

During an attack, all patients excrete a massive excess of the porphyrin precursors, 5-aminolevulinic acid (ALA) and porphobilinogen (PBG), in their urine. Urine, when first voided, is clear and darkens on exposure to light as the hexa-hydroporphyrins, the porphyrinogens, are oxidized to porphyrins.

A rapid screening test during an acute attack is to mix equal volumes of urine and Ehrlich's aldehyde reagent and observe for the pink color of porphobilinogen. The differential diagnosis of porphyrias uses qualitative and quantitative measurement of porphyrins and precursors, with subsequent use of enzymatic assay and identification of familial genetic alterations.[50]

Variegate Porphyria

Variegate porphyria is similar to hereditary coproporphyria, except that there are more severe skin lesions, sometimes with scarring (Fig. 38–5). Protoporphyrinogen oxidase is the affected enzyme, and protoporphyrin is the major circulating porphyrin. Conventionally, variegate porphyria is most readily diagnosed by measurement of fecal porphyrin concentrations. However, it has been reported[51] that biliary porphyrin levels may provide a better discriminator from normal patients in the asymptomatic phase. As in erythropoietic protoporphyria, there is a tendency toward cholelithiasis. The mechanism by which gallstones form is not certain, but some studies have suggested that porphyrins are cholestatic.[52] In hereditary coproporphyria and variegate porphyria, the pathway intermediates produced in excess, coproporphyrinogen and protoporphyrinogen, respectively, are inhibitors of the secondary rate-controlling enzyme PBGD.[26,53] Numerous mutations in the protoporphyrinogen oxidase gene have been described leading to 50% reduction in enzyme activity. In a few cases homozygosity or compound heterozygosity has been described.[54,55]

ALA-Dehydratase Deficiency Porphyria

In this porphyria (also known as plumboporphyria), the ALA dehydratase activity is depressed, as occurs in lead poisoning. The clinical

Management of Acute Porphyria

Treatment of Acute Attack

A carbohydrate intake of 1500 to 2000 kcal/24 hours should be maintained throughout the attack to reduce porphyrin synthesis; give this orally or, for more severe attacks, through a fine-bore Teflon nasogastric tube. If this cannot be tolerated, intravenous dextrose (eg, 20% solution, 2 L/day) should be given. If early in the attack (2 to 4 days from onset), give intravenous hematin as heme arginate (Normosang, Leiras) at 2 to 4 mg/kg over 30 minutes once or twice each day to further reduce the overproduction of porphyrin and precursors.[63,64] Hematin (Panhematin, Abbott) in similar doses may also be used, although it should be reconstituted in human albumin solution to avoid phlebitis and mild transient prolongation of coagulation times. No renal complications have occurred with the standard recommended dosages, and even patients with renal insufficiency tolerate hematin well, although the dosage should be reduced slightly. The action of heme therapy may be extended by heme oxygenase blockers such as tin protoporphyrin.[63]

Prophylaxis

Many drugs are contraindicated, and the patient must be warned to avoid precipitating factors. Alcohol should be restricted and smoking discouraged. Dieting (<800 kcal/day) must be avoided. Pregnancy should also be avoided if the disease is active. If a patient requires an anesthetic, nitrous oxide, ether, and cyclopropane are safe, and suxamethonium appears to be a safe muscle relaxant. The opiates and belladonna derivatives can be used for premedication and propofol for maintenance of anesthesia. Infection can precipitate an attack and should therefore be sought and treated. Blood relatives of patients should be screened to see if they carry the gene.

Luteinizing hormone-releasing hormone (LHRH) antagonists that suppress ovulation are a valuable form of prophylaxis in menstrually related attacks.[65] Estrogens and progestogens such as those in the contraceptive pill must be avoided in acute porphyria. The same applies to most steroids and receptor antagonists such as mifepristone.[66]

Management of Nonacute Porphyria

Patients should avoid exposure to sunlight and use sun block and physical barriers such as cotton gloves.

Porphyria Cutanea Tarda

The clinical features are reversed by removing any precipitating agent such as alcohol, halogenated hydrocarbons, and drugs. The patient should be screened for hepatic neoplasm and hepatitic viral infection. The mainstay of treatment is to remove liver iron by venesection of 500 mL of blood weekly until clinical remission occurs or until the hemoglobin level falls below 12 g/dL. Chloroquine, at low doses of 125 mg twice per week for several months, has also been helpful because it enhances urinary clearance of porphyrin. When venesection is difficult, desferrioxamine can be used to reduce liver iron stores. It is of value to screen the patient and first-degree relatives for hereditary hemochromatosis.

Erythropoietic Protoporphyria

Oral β-carotene offers effective protection in EPP against solar sensitivity. It does so by quenching the radical formation that is a feature of the skin damage. Yellowing of the skin (ie, carotenemia) is one side effect. Interruption of the enterohepatic protoporphyrin circulation by bile salt sequestering agents such as cholestyramine reduces plasma protoporphyrin levels and may retard the development of the liver disease. Liver transplantation has been reported to be an effective measure in preventing the progression of this disease,[67] and sequential liver and bone marrow transplantation has been described in one patient.[68]

Congenital Porphyria

Erythropoiesis should be reduced by means of erythrocyte hypertransfusion and by hematin or heme arginate infusion.[69] Bone marrow transplantation has given encouraging biochemical and clinical results but insufficient numbers of patients have been treated to be certain of the future prospects of this therapy.[70] Splenectomy and chloroquine therapy (125 mg twice weekly) have an ameliorating effect, as does hypertransfusion, but life expectancy is usually severely shortened.

picture resembles acute intermittent porphyria, but very few cases have been described, and the disease only manifests in homozygous cases when there is a precipitating factor.[56,57]

Concurrent Porphyrias

The concurrent porphyrias are a rare group of conditions in which there is concurrent inheritance of two different defects within the heme biosynthetic pathway. There is good precedent for more than one defect within the pathway. Previous descriptions[39–42] have shown the presence of concurrent porphyria within a family, and toxicologically, there is good evidence that exposure to poisons such as lead can induce multiple changes within the pathway.[58] Chester porphyria, for example, combines the clinical features of acute and cutaneous porphyria. PBGD and protoporphyrinogen oxidase activity are reduced, leading to overproduction of PBG and protoporphyrinogen.[37] In another patient, dual genetic defects involving 5-aminolevulinate dehydratase and coproporphyrinogen oxidase have been described.[659,60]

Nonacute or Cutaneous Porphyrias

In all cutaneous porphyrias, porphyrins (which are photosensitizing) are deposited in the upper layers of the skin, and they are responsible for the characteristic skin lesions.[61] In the development of these lesions, reactive oxygen species and other radicals are formed and probably induce oxidative membrane damage, particularly to mast cells, which enables complement activation as one part of the inflammatory reaction[62] (see box on Management of Acute Porphyria).

Porphyria Cutanea Tarda or Cutaneous Hepatic Porphyria

Biologic and Molecular Aspects

Porphyria cutanea tarda (PCT) exists in inherited and acquired forms. An inherited, more severe form of this disease, hepatoerythropoietic porphyria (HEP), has been described.[71,72] Mutations in the uroporphyrinogen decarboxylase are found in around one-third of patients with PCT. In inherited and acquired forms, there is diminution in the activity of hepatic uroporphyrinogen decarboxylase, which converts uroporphyrinogen to coproporphyrinogen by the stepwise decarboxylation of the acetyl groups to methyl groups. Most carriers of mutant uroporphyrinogen decarboxylase are not clinically evident unless precipitating factors are present. Iron alone or chlorinated hydrocarbons can diminish activity of uroporphyrinogen decarboxylase, and this effect is greatly potentiated when both are given

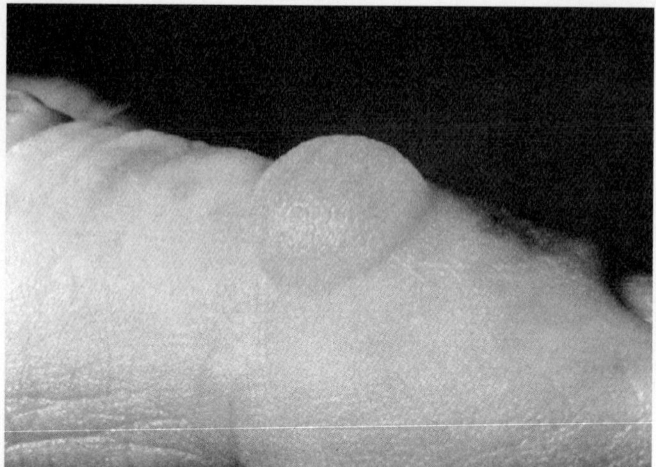

Figure 38–6 A bullous skin lesion of porphyria cutanea tarda.

together.[72,73] A genetic mouse model has been developed for familial PCT, and a zebrafish model is available for HEP, which should enhance our understanding of these diseases.[74,75]

Patients may have clinical and biochemical evidence of liver disease. Hepatic siderosis invariably occurs, and iron is one of the causative agents in acquired PCT. An association of PCT with hereditary hemochromatosis has been documented, with about 20% of PCT patients being homozygous for the Cys282Tyr mutation in the *HFE* gene, a defect that characterizes hereditary hemochromatosis.[76–78] These results strongly implicate the *HFE* gene as a genetic susceptibility factor in acquired PCT. An apparent association has emerged between HIV infection, hepatitis C infection, and PCT.[79] The etiologic role of viral infection in PCT is not yet clear. It is possible that therapy for HIV with zidovudine precipitates the disease, but it is more likely that the association is merely coincidental or that the viral infection unmasks the preexisting uroporphyrinogen decarboxylase defect.[80]

Genetics

Whereas familial PCT is inherited in an autosomal dominant mode, HEP is inherited in an autosomal recessive pattern.[72] As in the other genetic lesions in the porphyrias, there is heterogeneity in the mutations causing PCT and HEP phenotypes.[81,82] In the inherited form, more than 40 different mutations (mainly missense) have been identified in uroporphyrinogen decarboxylase, many of which lie near the dimer interface resulting in an unstable protein and reduced enzyme activity.[83] In different population groups, it is difficult to find the relative numbers of acquired and familial disease. In one analysis in Hungary, 77.5% of patients were found to suffer from the acquired form, and of the patients with the familial disease, females were affected more than males, suggesting that inheritance may predispose patients to estrogen-precipitated disease.[84]

Clinical Features

The most striking clinical feature of both forms of PCT is a bullous dermatosis on light-exposed areas. This starts as erythema and progresses to vesicles that become confluent to form bullae (Fig. 38–6), which may hemorrhage and leave scars; pruritus is often troublesome. Milia are common and may precede or follow vesicle formation. Increased fragility of the skin is important and, in less severe cases, may be the only clinical sign. In severe cases, photomutilation can result, usually because of infection of slowly healing lesions.

The thickening and scarring with calcification has been described as pseudoscleroderma. Hyperpigmentation is common, and women often complain of hirsutism. Neurologic change is not observed.

Pseudoporphyria and Renal Dialysis

The term *pseudoporphyria* has been used to describe a bullous dermatosis associated with a number of dermatologic conditions that bear some resemblance to porphyria.[85] This photosensitivity is often induced by drugs such as the tetracyclines, naproxen, furosemide, voriconazole, oxaprozin, and many others. In these conditions, there is no alteration in porphyrin metabolism or excretion. It is therefore incorrect to name any of them porphyria; the term pseudoporphyria should not be applied to them, but only to conditions in which alterations of porphyrin metabolism can be found such as the bullous dermatosis of hemodialysis.[86]

Patients with renal failure can present with many biochemical features of porphyria before hemodialysis. These abnormalities normalize after dialysis, especially when electrolyte abnormalities such as zinc deficiency are also corrected.[86] In a considerable proportion of patients with chronic renal failure, skin changes resembling porphyria cutanea tarda (PCT) develop some months to years after the onset of maintenance hemodialysis. In a minor proportion, genuine PCT can be diagnosed.[87] In such cases, there are elevated total porphyrin levels in plasma and in urine if the patient is not anuric. These patients present a therapeutic dilemma because they are normally anemic and unsuitable for phlebotomy therapy.

Patients may have clinical and biochemical evidence of chronic liver disease, sometimes with cirrhosis. There is an association with hepatocellular carcinoma. Hepatomegaly is particularly common when alcohol intake is excessive.

Precipitating Factors

Many patients with PCT have multiple precipitating factors, including mutations of the *HFE* gene, hepatitis C infection, or exposure to estrogen.[76,77] Excessive alcohol intake is an important precipitating agent, perhaps because of increased hepatic iron deposition in alcoholics. However, certain halogenated hydrocarbons are sometimes implicated. PCT may also develop in people treated with hemodialysis for kidney failure. An outbreak of cutaneous hepatic porphyria in southeast Turkey in 1956 was traced to seed wheat dressed with the fungicide hexachlorobenzene. A neoplastic subgroup has been identified in which PCT is associated with benign or malignant liver tumors.

Differential Diagnosis

Other causes of bullous or vesicular skin lesions should be excluded, such as a drug reaction (see box on Pseudoporphyria and Renal Dialysis) or chronic renal failure. The distinction between PCT, variegate porphyria, and hereditary coproporphyria rests on biochemical testing of urine and feces, with the highest levels of urinary uroporphyrin found during attacks of PCT (see Table 38–3).

Erythropoietic Protoporphyria

Biologic and Molecular Aspects

Although not described until 1961, this form of erythropoietic porphyria (EPP), also known as erythrohepatic protoporphyria, is much more common than congenital porphyria. Ferrochelatase activity is reduced in peripheral blood, liver, bone marrow, and skin, and protoporphyrin is synthesized in excess.[88] The erythroid progenitor cells (ie, burst-forming units-erythroid [BFU-E]) in EPP patients show intense fluorescence when viewed under 405 nm light. The gene

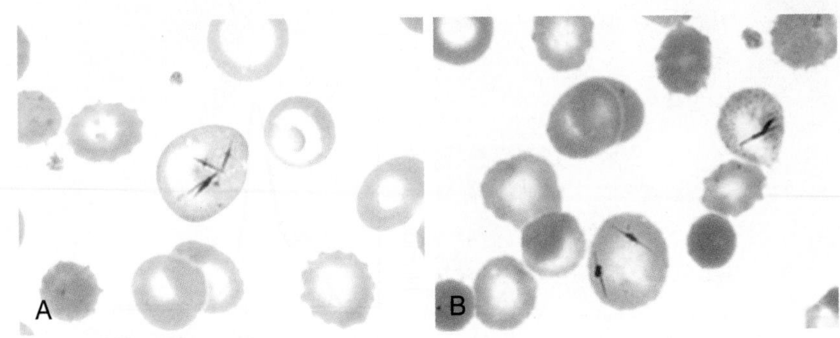

Figure 38–7 Needle like inclusions of porphyrin in the circulating red cells of a patient with congenital porphyria after splenectomy *(Merino A, To-Figueras J, Herrero C: Atypical red cell inclusions in congenital erythropoietic porphyria. Br J Haematol 132:124, 2006.)*

mutation in EPP shows heterogeneity as in other porphyrias.[89] The last enzyme of the biosynthetic pathway, ferrochelatase, is important because its endogenous activity is relatively low, and it could act as a control point in the pathway. Ferrochelatase ligates iron bound to three cysteine residues in an iron-sulfur cluster,[90] the mutation of which leads to decreased enzyme activity.[91] A multiple-enzyme complex spanning the mitochondrial membrane would allow for channeling of substrate from the cytoplasm to the mitochondrial matrix.[92] Immunologic studies on human protoporphyria show that immunologically reactive ferrochelatase is present, but that enzyme activity in three subjects was on average only 17% of normal.[93]

Genetics

EPP is inherited as an autosomal dominant disorder with incomplete penetrance, although recessive inheritance has been described.[94,95] Haplotype segregation analysis has shown intronic nucleotide polymorphisms in the ferrochelatase gene (FECH) that produces aberrant splicing of mRNA to a form that degrades more rapidly resulting in enzyme deficiency.[96] Although these disease associated polymorphisms are common,[97] there is heterogeneity of the molecular defect, including aberrant splicing and loss of function of the mitoferrin protein.[14,88,89,98]

Clinical Features

The clinical features are mainly cutaneous on exposure to sunlight and can occur at any age, including infancy and childhood.[94] They include pruritic urticarial swelling and redness of the skin on exposure to sunlight. The most distressing symptom is an unbearable burning sensation on the affected parts. Remarkably, such features are ameliorated during pregnancy, which has been linked to lowered protoporphyrin levels.[99] Hepatic involvement, which occurs in later life, involves deposition of hepatotoxic protoporphyrin in the liver and can lead to fatal liver failure from an active chronic hepatitis with cirrhosis.[100] Such protoporphyrin deposition may also cause cholelithiasis; the gallstones contain high concentrations of protoporphyrin. The liver disease of EPP seems to correlate with erythrocyte protoporphyrin concentrations.[101] Mild microcytic anemia has been reported,[102,103] as well as mitochondrial iron accumulation and ring sideroblasts, in about 30% of patients.[104] Late onset of EPP has been reported in patients with myelodysplastic syndrome or overlap myelodysplasia/myeloproliferation. In one patient EPP has been acquired as a result of expansion of hemopoietic cells containing only one allele of the FECH gene. Inactivation of one allele by deletion involving chromosome 18 thus appears to be sufficient for overproduction of protoporphyrin.[104,105]

Differential Diagnosis

EPP should be distinguished from other causes of a photosensitive rash. The distinction can be made by demonstrating fluorescence in a proportion of red cells (ie, fluorocytes) in the peripheral blood and confirmed by measurement of greatly increased erythrocyte and fecal protoporphyrin. Patients with EPP have a relatively high incidence of ring sideroblasts in the marrow.[104] This can lead to diagnostic difficulty because some patients with idiopathic sideroblastic anemia have increased levels of erythrocyte protoporphyrin.[107–110] However, EPP can be distinguished by the autosomal dominant inheritance pattern, dermal photosensitivity, normal or low serum levels of iron, and levels of protoporphyrin in red blood cells and feces.

Congenital Porphyria (Gunther Disease)

Biologic and Molecular Aspects

Congenital porphyria, or Günther disease, although extremely rare, was the first porphyria to be described in 1874.[111] Unlike the other porphyrias, it is inherited in a Mendelian autosomal recessive pattern causing reduced activity of uroporphyrinogen III synthase. The onset of solar photosensitivity results from gross overproduction of porphyrins, caused by deficiency of uroporphyrinogen III synthase. Like other porphyrias, the defective enzyme results mainly from point mutations at multiple sites within the gene.[112] Other enzymes are largely normal, although there is an increase in ALAS activity.[113] Excess porphyrins, particularly uroporphyrin-1, accumulate in the normoblasts of the bone marrow and are excreted in the urine and feces. They are also deposited in bones and in the teeth, resulting in a pink-brown discoloration that fluoresces bright red in light of wavelengths around 400 nm. Dental restoration has been used to correct the esthetic appearance of the teeth. There are frequently profound changes in bone structure in patients with congenital porphyria. This has been linked to vitamin D deficiency because of light avoidance.[114] However, bone changes can be seen when vitamin D levels are adequate, and it is reasonable to speculate that the porphyrins deposited in bone are cytotoxic because similar bone changes are features of homozygous variegate porphyria and hepatoerythropoietic porphyria.[115]

Clinical Features

Typically, the onset of congenital porphyria is from birth, but occasionally, late-onset cases have been reported.[116] The skin reaction is severe and can be devastating, and the teeth become brownish pink because of their high porphyrin content. Severe cutaneous photosensitivity is manifested by blistering of light-exposed areas and fragility of the epidermis. Skin thickening occurs, and there is extensive scarring and hypertrichosis. The recurrent damage associated with scarring on the hand may produce a claw-shaped deformity and loss of digits. Dystrophic nails may curl up and drop off. Lenticular scarring may lead to blindness. Hemolytic anemia often occurs and is associated with increased erythrocyte fragility and splenomegaly. Dyserythropoiesis may contribute to the anemia.[117] One patient who underwent splenectomy at five years of age has been described with needle-like inclusions of porphyrin in the circulating red cells (Fig. 38–7).[118]

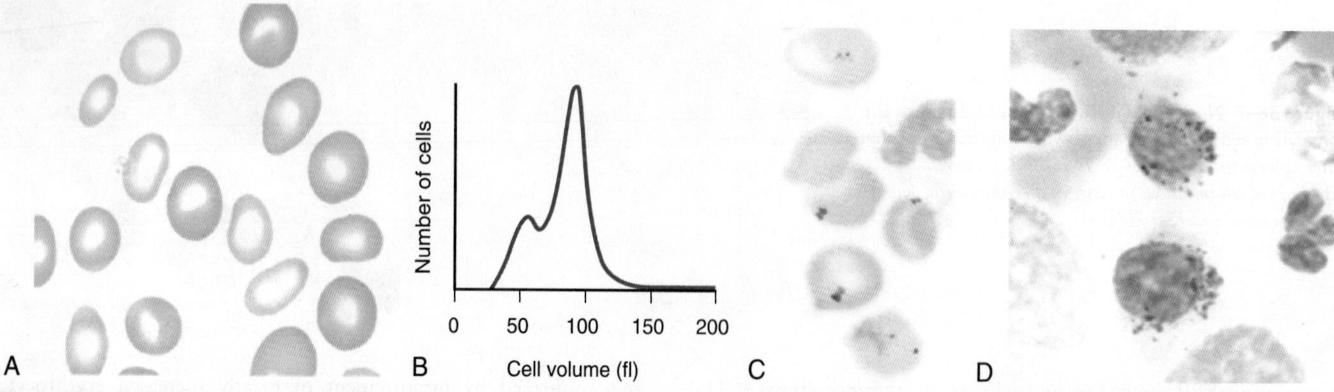

Figure 38–8 **A,** Peripheral blood smear from a patient with hereditary sideroblastic anemia shows a population of hypochromic and microcytic erythrocytes. **B,** Erythrocyte volume distribution curve of a patient with hereditary sideroblastic anemia. A dimorphic size distribution is evident. **C,** Peripheral blood showing Pappenheimer bodies (Prussian blue stain). **D,** The bone marrow smear stained with Prussian blue shows ring sideroblasts.

Differential Diagnosis

The most characteristic feature of congenital porphyria is the excess production of series 1 porphyrins rather than series 3 isomer produced in the other porphyrias. Red blood cells fluoresce in ultraviolet light, as do the brown-stained teeth, because of high porphyrin content (see box on Pseudoporphyria and Renal Dialysis).

SIDEROBLASTIC ANEMIAS

Sideroblastic anemias are a heterogeneous group of disorders characterized by anemia of varying severity and diagnosed by finding ring sideroblasts in the bone marrow aspirate. The peripheral blood shows hypochromic red cells, which are microcytic in the hereditary forms (Fig. 38–8A) but are often macrocytic in the acquired forms of the disease. The red blood cell parameters from automated cell counting may show bimodal volume distribution curves or widened range of cell sizes (see Fig. 38–8B); however, this dimorphic size distribution is not always present. Tiny inclusions may be visible in the red blood cells; these can be confirmed as iron-containing Pappenheimer bodies by Prussian blue staining of the blood smear (see Fig 38–8C). The diagnostic test is bone marrow examination together with Prussian blue staining of the bone marrow smears.

The presence of ring sideroblasts (see Fig. 38–8D) is defined as erythroblasts containing iron-positive (siderotic) granules arranged in a perinuclear collar distribution around one-third or more of the nucleus. Electron microscopic examination has shown that these siderotic granules are mitochondria containing amorphous deposits of ferric phosphate and ferric hydroxide. Iron is also bound to mitochondrial ferritin, a molecular form of ferritin that can be distinguished from cytoplasmic ferritin and that accumulates in large amounts in the erythroblasts of subjects with impaired heme synthesis.[119,120]

Iron overload is a common clinical feature of refractory sideroblastic anemia and, in severe cases, may lead to complications that characterize secondary hemosiderosis (eg, diabetes, cardiac failure). Marrow examination shows prominent erythroid hyperplasia, which is a sign of the ineffective erythropoiesis and is responsible for increased iron absorption. The sideroblastic anemias have diverse causes but have in common an impaired biosynthesis of heme in the erythroid cells of the marrow. Most sideroblastic anemias are acquired as a clonal disorder of erythropoiesis, with various degrees of myelodysplastic features (Table 38–5). The inherited forms are uncommon and occur predominantly in males with an X-linked pattern of inheritance. A number of drugs have been associated with reversible sideroblastic anemia, and ring sideroblasts may be found in patients who abuse alcohol (see Table 38–5). The first descriptions of ring sideroblasts in association with chronic refractory anemias appeared in the late 1950s,[121,122] after an earlier description of familial X-linked hypochromic microcytic anemia.[123]

Table 38–5 Classification of Sideroblastic Anemias

Hereditary
X-linked*
Autosomal dominant or recessive
Acquired
Idiopathic acquired* (refractory anemia with ring sideroblasts)
Associated with previous chemotherapy, irradiation, or in "transitional" myelodysplastic or myeloproliferative diseases
Drugs
Alcohol
Isoniazid
Chloramphenicol
Other drugs
Rare causes
Erythropoietic protoporphyria
Pearson syndrome
Copper deficiency or zinc overload
Thiamine-responsive megaloblastic anemia
Hypothermia

*Trial of pyridoxine indicated.

Hereditary Sideroblastic Anemia

Biologic and Molecular Aspects

Erythroid cells from patients with X-linked forms of hereditary sideroblastic anemia generally exhibit low activity of ALAS.[8,124] A defect in this enzyme is firmly established in patients whose anemia responds to pyridoxine therapy, because pyridoxal phosphate is an essential cofactor for ALAS. However, even affected female patients with moderate anemia unresponsive to pyridoxine have been documented to have low levels of ALAS in bone marrow lysates. In some male patients with X-linked pyridoxine-responsive sideroblastic anemia, the low ALAS activity in bone marrow increased to levels above the normal range when the patient took pyridoxine supplements and

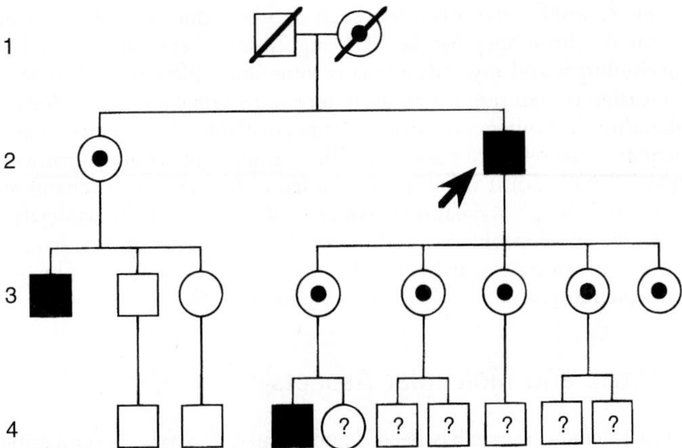

Figure 38–9 Pedigree of a family with pyridoxine-responsive sideroblastic anemia showing X-linked recessive inheritance. Affected *(filled box)*, carrier *(filled circle within open circle)*, and unknown status *(question mark within circle or box)* are indicated. *Diagonal lines* indicate deceased members. This pedigree[125] has been abbreviated to show only the affected branches of the family. The *arrow* indicates the proband.

recovered from the anemia.[125] There are several possible explanations for this enhancement of ALAS activity by dietary pyridoxine supplements. The most likely is that pyridoxine (or its phosphate) may stabilize the ALAS during folding of the mutant enzyme after its synthesis.[124] The gene for the ALAS2 isoenzyme has been localized to the X chromosome, and this gene is known to be the site of most mutations giving rise to X-linked pyridoxine-responsive sideroblastic anemia.[9,126] Approximately three dozen different mutations have been identified in individuals or families with hereditary sideroblastic anemia, and nearly all have resulted from single base alterations in DNA. A frequent mutation affects arginine at residue 452 of ALAS-2, which occurs in a quarter of all pedigrees but does not affect enzyme activity measured in vitro.[127] All known mutations lie between exons 5 and 11 of *ALAS2*, the region that codes for the catalytic domain, with most lying within exon 9, which contains the lysine at which binding of pyridoxal 5′-phosphate occurs.[7] A mutation, Asp190Val, has been described in a pyridoxine-refractory patient and appears to affect the proteolytic processing of the ALAS2 during or after import into the mitochondrion.[128] The variety of different mutations in the erythroid *ALAS2* gene responsible for X-linked sideroblastic anemia and their pyridoxine responsiveness have been reviewed recently.[9]

An inherited deficiency of flavin monooxygenase has been suggested as a rare cause of sideroblastic anemia.[129]

Genetic Aspects

In most families with hereditary sideroblastic anemia, males are affected with an X-linked pattern of inheritance (Fig. 38–9). However female carriers, although usually normal, can develop erythrocyte dimorphism or varying degrees of anemia. The assignment of the gene for erythroid *ALAS2* to the X chromosome[126] and the many mutations documented in erythroid *ALAS2* provide the genetic basis for this X-linked disease. In several families, coinheritance of other X-linked traits (eg, glucose-6-phosphate dehydrogenase [G6PD] deficiency, ataxia with sideroblastic anemia) has been described.[130,131] In X-linked sideroblastic anemia with ataxia, a mutation has been described in the *ABCb7* gene, which leads to a limitation of competent heme synthesis from protoporphyrin and iron, possibly through diminished availability of Fe^{2+} iron,[132,133] There are well-documented families in which the sideroblastic anemia was inherited as an autosomal dominant trait, as well as rare cases that are autosomal recessive.[134] Sporadic and familial cases have been described that affect only females, which has been shown to represent skewed X-chromosome inactivation ("unfortunate skewing") affecting the normal allele for the *ALAS2* gene.[135] The absence of affected male members in these pedigrees suggests that the *ALAS2* defects identified are lethal in hemizygous males.

Clinical and Laboratory Evaluation

Typically, the anemia manifests in infancy or childhood, but the milder forms of anemia may not be found until midlife. Even elderly patients have been diagnosed with this anemia.[136] Some cases may be discovered only during family surveys, which should always be undertaken when hereditary sideroblastic anemia is diagnosed. Still other patients may present with features of iron overload, such as diabetes or cardiac failure. Iron overload occurs commonly even with mild anemia and may occasionally be seen with female carriers. Enlargement of the liver and spleen may occur with mild abnormalities of liver function tests.

Anemia is extremely variable, but even when little or no anemia is present, the mean corpuscular volume (MCV) is low, and the red cell volume distribution width may be increased. When anemia is severe, the MCV may be as low as 50 fL (μ^3). The blood smear shows a population of cells with hypochromic, microcytic morphology (see Fig. 38–8), which contrasts with the other normochromic, normocytic cells (ie, dimorphism). Anisocytosis, poikilocytosis, elongated cells, and siderocytes may also be seen. The characteristic erythrocyte dimorphism is most prominent in patients with milder anemia, in female carriers, and in patients in whom pyridoxine has corrected the anemia but not restored the MCV to normal. In some pedigrees with only affected females macrocytosis may be present which contrasts with the typical microcytosis of male hemizygotes.[110,135] Leukocyte values are normal, whereas the platelet count is normal or increased.

Serum iron concentration is increased, and transferrin shows an increased percentage of saturation with iron. Serum ferritin levels are invariably increased. Ineffective erythropoiesis can be confirmed by ferrokinetic measurements showing that plasma iron clearance is rapid, with subnormal retention of the iron isotope in erythrocytes after 10 to 14 days. Other features of ineffective erythropoiesis may be variably present: a mild increase in bilirubin concentration, decrease in haptoglobin levels, mild increase in lactate dehydrogenase levels, and normal or slight increase in reticulocyte numbers. The magnitude of iron overload correlates poorly with the degree of anemia in patients who are not transfused. The degree of ineffective erythropoiesis is a better predictor of the amount of iron overload. When ferrokinetics are unavailable, the extent of erythroid hyperplasia relative to normal acts as a rough measure of the magnitude of ineffective erythropoiesis. Several studies have shown that the relative increase in erythroid activity multiplied by the patient's age shows a good correlation with the degree of iron overload as measured by plasma ferritin.[137,138] The iron overload does not result from mutations in the *HFE* gene[139] (see box on Therapy for Hereditary Sideroblastic Anemia).

Differential Diagnosis

Hereditary sideroblastic anemia should be distinguished from idiopathic hemochromatosis, because both have biochemical evidence of iron overload and a similar tissue pattern of iron deposition. Careful hematologic assessment of patient and family members should make the distinction, because the hemoglobin level and MCV are normal in idiopathic hemochromatosis.

Acquired Idiopathic Sideroblastic Anemia

Acquired sideroblastic anemia may be idiopathic or occur after chemotherapy or irradiation (see Table 38–5). The clonal nature of hemopoiesis in this condition was first suggested by Dacie and col-

Therapy for Hereditary Sideroblastic Anemia

A trial of pyridoxine (100 to 200 mg/day taken orally) is indicated for 3 months for all patients with hereditary sideroblastic anemia. Response is variable and ranges from complete correction of hemoglobin levels to no effect. Even when pyridoxine completely corrects the anemia (Fig. 38–10), the increase in MCV may not reach normal values, and a population of hypochromic, microcytic cells remains.

About 25% to 50% of patients with hereditary sideroblastic anemia show a full or partial response to pyridoxine, and this vitamin should be continued on a lifelong basis in the responders. A lower maintenance dose should be determined for each responding patient by progressive dose reduction, because long-term therapy with pyridoxine at 100 to 200 mg/day has been associated with peripheral neuropathy.[140] The adult nutritional requirement for pyridoxine is 1 to 2 mg/day; some patients have been maintained on as little as 4 mg/day as a supplement.[125] Folic acid supplements should also be administered because the erythroid hyperplasia increases demand for this vitamin.

There is one report of successful allogeneic peripheral blood stem cell transplantation in a 19-year-old man with transfusion-dependent hereditary sideroblastic anemia.[141] Transfusions are the mainstay of treatment for severe anemia unresponsive to pyridoxine. Regular administration of packed red cells using white blood cell filters are given to relieve symptoms and permit normal childhood development. Iron overload and secondary hemosiderosis rapidly progress after transfusions begin; chelation therapy with desferrioxamine or oral deferasirox should be initiated from the onset.

Iron removal may be of great benefit for patients who have mild or moderate anemia and evidence of iron overload.[137,138] These patients can often tolerate intermittent phlebotomy, which is preferable to chelation therapy for iron removal, and should be continued to reduce ferritin levels to less than 300 ng/mL. All patients with iron overload should avoid ingestion of ascorbic acid supplements, which enhance iron absorption and increase the tissue toxicity of elemental iron. Alcohol should also be avoided. Splenectomy is contraindicated in this disease.

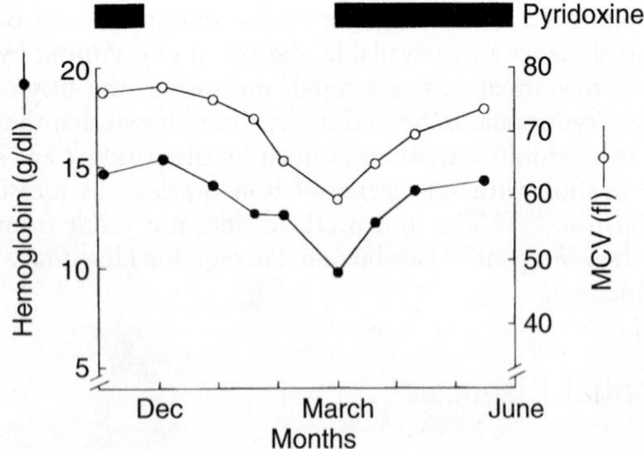

Figure 38–10 Response of the hemoglobin concentration and mean corpuscular volume (MCV) to withdrawal and reinstitution of pyridoxine in a patient with responsive hereditary sideroblastic anemia.

leagues.[122] Nearly all cases show evidence of dyserythropoiesis in the marrow, and there may also be dysplastic changes in the myeloid precursors or megakaryocytes, or both. Acquired idiopathic sideroblastic anemia falls within the diagnostic category of refractory anemia with ring sideroblasts as defined by the French-American-British group.[142] Acquired sideroblastic anemia has also been a rare finding in myeloproliferative disorders such as idiopathic myelofibrosis or essential thrombocythemia. Distinguishing between idiopathic myelofibrosis and myelodysplasia is sometimes difficult, and there is increasing recognition for an overlap or transitional entity, myelodysplasia/myeloproliferative disease, unclassifiable.[143,144] Thus many patients with refractory anemia with ring sideroblasts and thrombocytosis have a point mutation in the Janus Kinase 2 gene (changing valine-617 to phenylalanine), which is a feature usually associated with the myeloproliferative disorders.[145] This latter group have a clinical phenotype which includes normal MCV, marrow fibrosis, and splenomegaly (See Chapters—37 and 67).[145]

Biologic and Molecular Aspects

Clonal hematopoiesis has been demonstrated in acquired idiopathic sideroblastic anemia and in the related myelodysplastic syndromes. Specific evidence was first provided by finding a single G6PD isoenzyme in erythrocytes, granulocytes, platelets, and B lymphocytes in a woman who was heterozygous for G6PD and carried two isoenzymes in her skin and T lymphocytes.[146] This technique is applicable only to the few women who have G6PD heterozygosity, but restriction fragment length polymorphism analysis can be applied to most women using probes directed at other X-chromosome genes such as that for phosphoglycerate kinase or to an X-linked, variable-copy-number tandem repeat sequence (see Chapter 1).[147] The results show uniform monoclonality of hematopoiesis in acquired sideroblastic anemia with or without associated myelodysplastic features. Initial reports of low levels of ALAS in bone marrow of acquired idiopathic sideroblastic anemia have not been confirmed, and the cause of the defective heme synthesis in the abnormal clone is unclear. Some indirect evidence exists for a primary mitochondrial lesion, perhaps in the mitochondrial respiratory chain, which impairs the reduction of Fe^{3+} because Fe^{2+} is essential for heme synthesis.[148–150]

Etiology

Clonal chromosomal changes are found in bone marrow cells in approximately 60% of patients with acquired sideroblastic anemia. Characteristic changes are monosomy 7; trisomy 8; deletions involving chromosomes 5, 7, 11, or 20; and a number of balanced translocations.[151] When sideroblastic anemia is acquired after chemotherapy or irradiation, chromosomal changes are usually found and tend to be multiple.[151] Among these changes, the loss of an entire chromosome (5 or 7, or both), deletion of a long arm [del(5), del(7), or del(13)], and an unbalanced translocation are typical.[152,153] When karyotype shows loss of material from chromosomes 5 or 7, or both, a detailed occupational history may show exposure to potentially mutagenic chemical agents in a proportion of patients.[154] However, the development of visible chromosomal changes is probably a late event in acquired sideroblastic anemia and may be preceded by the expansion of a clone of genetically unstable stem cells. This concept is in accord with the view that multiple genetic events underlie the pathogenesis of other myelodysplastic syndromes and acute myeloid leukemia[146,155](see box on Clinical and Laboratory Evaluation of Sideroblastic Anemia).

Differential Diagnosis

Ring sideroblasts are not limited to acquired sideroblastic anemia; they also occur in other myelodysplastic conditions, such as refractory anemia with excess blasts, in which the blast count is higher than 5%.[156] Careful examination of peripheral blood and bone marrow can distinguish acquired idiopathic sideroblastic anemia from these related myelodysplastic conditions. Family surveys are very useful in distinguishing acquired from hereditary forms of sideroblastic anemia, because the latter may present in late adult life.

Clinical and Laboratory Evaluation of Sideroblastic Anemia

Typically, sideroblastic anemia develops insidiously in a middle-aged or elderly patient with normal or increased MCV and a blood smear showing a population of hypochromic red cells. Hepatosplenomegaly may be present. Leukocyte and platelet counts are usually normal, but some patients have thrombocytosis that occasionally exceeds 1000×10^9/L.[157] If leukopenia or thrombocytopenia is present, a careful search should be made for myelodysplastic features, which lead to the more descriptive term of *refractory cytopenia* for the condition.[158,159] An iron stain of the bone marrow aspirate shows ring sideroblasts, which should total more than 15% of all erythroblasts to make the diagnosis of acquired sideroblastic anemia.[142,159–161] Iron cannot be assessed in the marrow trephine biopsy core because it may leach out during decalcification.

The bone marrow also shows erythroid hyperplasia. Although mild dyserythropoiesis (eg, multinuclearity, nuclear budding) and megaloblastoid changes are present, myelopoiesis and megakaryopoiesis are usually normal. When changes are confined to dyserythropoiesis, the condition has been called *pure sideroblastic anemia*.[159,162] However, dysplasia of myelopoietic and megakaryopoietic elements may be present (ie, trilineage dysplasia) with the following features: Pelger-Huët–like anomaly, hypersegmentation or hypogranularity of neutrophils, micromegakaryocytes, large mononuclear megakaryocytes, and megakaryocytes with multiple small nuclei (see Chapter 67).[159] Dysmegakaryopoiesis is more easily detected in trephine biopsies than in marrow smears, although the trephine may also show unsuspected islands of myeloblasts characteristic of myelodysplasia.[163] The overall blast count in marrow smears is, by definition, less than 5%, and the peripheral blood monocyte count is less than 1.0×10^9/L. Cytogenetic analysis of marrow aspirates provides important information, because a normal karyotype predicts long survival in any type of acquired sideroblastic anemia.[164]

Prognosis

Acquired idiopathic sideroblastic anemia and the related entity of refractory anemia have the most favorable outlook among the myelodysplastic syndromes, with a median survival of 42 to 76 months and 3% to 12% incidence of leukemic progression in different series.[151,165,166] The prognosis can be correlated with three factors. First is the severity of the anemia, because repeated transfusions markedly increase iron overload and invariably lead to the organ dysfunction characteristic of secondary hemosiderosis (eg, heart and liver failure, diabetes). The second factor is whether neutropenia and thrombocytopenia are associated with the anemia. These cytopenias form the basis of a simple prognostic scoring system in which two or more of the following place the patient in a poor prognostic category: hemoglobin level less than 10 g/dL, neutrophil count less than 2.5×10^9/L, platelet count less than 100×10^9/L, and blasts more than 5% of the total.[165,166] Thirdly, karyotypic analysis of marrow aspirates provides valuable information, because a normal karyotype carries a more favorable prognosis. Conversely, monosomy 7 or a partial loss of the long arm of chromosome 7 as a single defect imparts a high probability of transformation to acute myeloid leukemia. Multiple chromosomal abnormalities and del(20q) are also associated with an increased risk of progression to leukemia; in contrast, trisomy 8 has no adverse prognostic significance.[151] Evolution of acquired idiopathic sideroblastic anemia to other myelodysplastic conditions, such as refractory anemia with excess blasts, has been described[167] (see box on Therapy for Acquired Sideroblastic Anemia).

Therapy for Acquired Sideroblastic Anemia

Transfusions are indicated for relief of symptomatic anemia. A trial of pyridoxine at 100 to 200 mg/day for 3 months is worthwhile in patients who have anemia but who do not display neutropenia or thrombocytopenia. However, few patients with acquired idiopathic sideroblastic anemia respond to this vitamin. If any response is achieved, maintenance therapy with pyridoxine at lower dosage is indicated. Cyclosporin (5 to 6 mg/kg/day) has been reported to benefit the anemia of the closely related myelodysplastic condition of refractory anemia, although the response appeared limited to those with hypoplastic bone marrows.[168]

SIDEROBLASTIC ANEMIA AND PORPHYRINURIA CAUSED BY DRUGS

Alcohol

Ring sideroblasts may be found in the bone marrow of malnourished anemic alcoholics, usually in the presence of associated folate deficiency.[169–171] In contrast, binge drinking or chronic alcohol ingestion in subjects with good nutrition is not associated with sideroblastic abnormality. Sideroblastic change is never the sole cause for the anemia of alcoholism. Alcohol has a direct toxic effect on hematopoiesis.[172] An increased or high-normal MCV and vacuolation of red blood cell precursors is often seen in addition to the ring sideroblast abnormality. Red blood cells show dimorphic morphology; evidence in the marrow of folate deficiency is present in half of cases.[172] Transferrin saturation and marrow iron stores tend to be increased but may be low if gastrointestinal bleeding is present. The ring sideroblasts gradually disappear over 4 to 12 days when alcohol is withdrawn[171]; during this period, there may be a rebound erythroid hyperplasia, reticulocytosis, and thrombocytosis. Folic acid should be given for the associated megaloblastic changes after blood is taken for vitamin B_{12} and folate assays.

Alcohol consumption lowers the plasma concentration of pyridoxal phosphate, a cofactor for ALAS, needed in the first step in heme synthesis.[173] Conversion of ethanol to acetaldehyde is necessary for this effect, and acetaldehyde acts by accelerating the degradation of intracellular pyridoxal phosphate in the liver, lowering plasma levels of this coenzyme.[174]

Chronic alcoholics have an altered heme metabolism with increased urinary excretion of coproporphyrin, mainly isomer 3, but normal urinary excretion of uroporphyrin, ALA, and porphobilinogen. Acute and chronic ethanol ingestion markedly depresses the activity of ALA dehydratase in peripheral blood. Ethanol administration to normal subjects results in increased activity of leukocyte ALAS and erythrocyte PBGD, the two rate-controlling enzymes of the pathway. The activities of each of the other four enzymes are depressed. Ferrochelatase, the enzyme that inserts iron into protoporphyrin to form heme, shows the most marked depression, and in alcoholism there is prolonged depression of uroporphyrinogen decarboxylase, which provides a rationale for the role of ethanol in the etiology of porphyria cutanea tarda.[175,176] As above, ethanol is a major precipitating factor in acute porphyria.[177]

Isoniazid

Administration of the antituberculous drug isoniazid occasionally has been associated with development of a sideroblastic anemia after 1 to 10 months of therapy. The anemia is hypochromic and microcytic, with a dimorphic blood smear and ring sideroblasts in the marrow. This complication is thought to occur only in slow acetylators of isoniazid, allowing this drug to react nonenzymatically with pyridoxal and to form a hydrazone that is rapidly excreted in the urine. The anemia can be fully reversed by coadministration of pyridoxine (25 to 50 mg/day) with isoniazid or by withdrawing isoniazid.[178]

Chloramphenicol

Chloramphenicol is an antibiotic that produces a reversible suppression of erythropoiesis after several days of therapy (plasma levels of 10–15 μg/mL). This effect is predictable and separate from the rare idiosyncratic side effect of aplastic anemia in approximately 1 of 20,000 exposed persons. Nearly all patients given chloramphenicol (>2 g/day) develop vacuolation of the erythroid precursors and ring sideroblasts. These effects are thought to arise from suppression of mitochondrial respiration. Chloramphenicol inhibits mitochondrial protein synthesis and reduces cytochrome $a + a_3$ and b levels.[179] Serum iron concentrations are increased, and reticulocyte numbers are subnormal; these changes revert on stopping the antibiotic.

Other Drugs

A reversible acquired sideroblastic anemia has been described with penicillamine therapy and with the use of triethylene tetramine hydrochloride, a copper-chelating agent used in the treatment of Wilson disease.[180] Acquired sideroblastic anemia has also been precipitated by progesterone given to a patient on two separate occasions 15 years apart, and this anemia promptly reversed on withdrawal of the drug.[181]

Presentations Associated with Sideroblastic Anemia or Porphyrinuria

Mitochondrial Myopathy and Sideroblastic Anemia (Pearson Syndrome)

Pearson syndrome is a rare entity that manifests in early infancy with anemia and exocrine pancreatic dysfunction. The anemia is normocytic or macrocytic, reticulocyte counts are low, and variable degrees of neutropenia and thrombocytopenia are present. The bone marrow shows a striking vacuolation and ring sideroblasts.[182] Although usually fatal, milder forms of the anemia are consistent with survival into adult life. The syndrome, which is related to the Kearns-Sayre syndrome, is thought to result from deletions, mutations, or duplications of mitochondrial DNA, variably affecting multiple tissues of the body.[183,184] A missense mutation of mitochondrial DNA (in the PUS1 gene coding for pseudouridine synthase) has been associated with mitochondrial myopathy and sideroblastic anemia.[185]

Copper Deficiency or Zinc Overload

The copper content of a Western diet averages 0.9 to 1.6 mg each day, which is only a few times greater than the amount needed to maintain homeostasis of this essential element.[186] Copper deficiency has been described in malnourished premature infants,[187] in patients receiving long-term parenteral or enteral hyperalimentation,[188] after gastrectomy,[189] with copper-chelating agents,[180] or on an idiopathic basis.[190] The syndrome of copper deficiency consists of sideroblastic anemia with hypochromic cells in the blood smear, accompanied by ring sideroblasts and vacuolated erythroid and myeloid precursors in the marrow, and of neutropenia with an absence of late myeloid forms in the marrow. In some reports, patients present with neurologic symptoms such as paresthesias, weakness, or ataxia; and demyelination is seen on the magnetic resonance image of the brain.[190] In infants, additional features may be seen, such as osteoporosis and long bone changes, depigmentation of skin and hair, and central nervous system abnormalities. The platelet counts remain normal. Serum copper and ceruloplasmin levels are low, whereas serum iron and transferrin saturation levels are normal. The serum zinc concentration may be increased.[190] Prompt reversal of the hematologic changes follows therapy with 2 to 5 mg per day of copper sulfate taken orally or 100 to 500 μg per day of copper supplement to the intravenous alimentation formula.

Large quantities of ingested zinc interfere with copper absorption and produce the neutropenia and sideroblastic anemia characteristic of copper deficiency.[191] Zinc sulfate is freely available from health food stores, and as little as 450 mg per day for 2 years is sufficient for this effect. Sideroblastic anemia has also been ascribed to zinc toxicity arising from the ingestion of coins over a period of many years.[192] Serum zinc levels are high, whereas serum copper and ceruloplasmin levels are low. Zinc must be discontinued for 9 to 12 weeks for full reversal of the anemia and neutropenia.

Iron-Deficiency Anemia

In iron-deficiency anemia, there is an accumulation of protoporphyrin in erythrocytes that rarely reaches the level found in EPP. The zinc complex of protoporphyrin is produced, because ferrochelatase uses Zn^{2+} during iron-deficient erythropoiesis.[193] Erythrocyte protoporphyrin may be raised before changes appear in peripheral blood and may be helpful in diagnosing iron deficiency when serum iron and ferritin levels are rising as a result of patients having started iron therapy. In iron-deficient erythropoiesis, erythroid ALAS activity is reduced below normal.[194]

Hypothermia

Thrombocytopenia, erythroid hypoplasia, and ring sideroblasts have been described in patients with hypothermia associated with neurologic disease.[195] These changes reverse slowly as body temperature returns to normal.

Thiamine-Responsive Megaloblastic Anemia

A triad of megaloblastic anemia with ring sideroblasts, diabetes mellitus, and progressive neural deafness has been described as a rare autosomal recessive disorder.[196] The anemia responds to high doses of thiamine and is thought to result from a defect in the cell-membrane transporter for thiamine.[197]

Other Conditions

In hereditary tyrosinemia, excess urinary ALA is excreted because ALA dehydratase is inhibited by succinyl acetone. Like acute porphyria and lead poisoning, this disease is associated with neurobehavioral disturbance (see box on Lead Poisoning). In liver disease, there may be increased urinary excretion of coproporphyrin, predominantly isomer I.[10] In the Dubin-Johnson syndrome, the ratio of coproporphyrin isomer I to isomer 3 is markedly increased in the urine (>80%), possibly as a result of deficiency of hepatic uroporphyrinogen III cosynthase and increased activity of PBGD. In Rotor syndrome, total urinary excretion of coproporphyrin is markedly increased and consists predominantly of coproporphyrin isomer I. In the unconjugated hyperbilirubinemia of Gilbert syndrome, depressed activity of protoporphyrinogen oxidase and increased activity of ALAS has been found in peripheral leukocytes.[198]

Environmental Intolerances

It has been hypothesized that several otherwise-unexplained chemical-associated illnesses, such as multiple chemical sensitivity (MCS) syndrome, may represent mild chronic cases of porphyria or other acquired abnormalities in heme synthesis. However, evidence for this concept is lacking.[200,201]

Lead Poisoning

It has been known for some time that patients suffering from lead poisoning have an accumulation of protoporphyrin in erythrocytes and increased urinary excretion of ALA and coproporphyrin.[199] There are sex-related differences in the porphyrin synthetic response to lead, with females showing a more profound coproporphyrinuria than men.[200] The elevated protoporphyrin chelated by zinc is retained in the erythrocyte, which may explain the absence of photosensitivity. This accumulation of porphyrins and precursors is caused by the inhibition by lead of the heme biosynthetic enzymes: ALA dehydratase, coproporphyrinogen oxidase, and ferrochelatase. An increase in the activity of the rate-controlling enzyme ALAS results.

Many of the clinical manifestations of lead poisoning may be the result of altered heme biosynthesis.[58] A mild to moderate anemia that can be hypochromic and microcytic occurs in a minority of patients, whereas basophilic stippling is prominent due to inhibition of pyrimidine 5′- nucleotidase in the maturing reticulocyte. Ring sideroblasts have not been reported. The abdominal pain, constipation, and peripheral neuropathy that occur in lead poisoning are also seen in acute attacks of hepatic porphyria. Neuropathy, seen in lead poisoning, may also be the result of disorders of heme biosynthesis, as in the porphyrias.[199] Alterations in porphyrin metabolism have provided a useful means of detecting and assessing the severity of lead exposure and poisoning. The diminution in activity of erythrocyte ALA dehydratase and elevated erythrocyte protoporphyrin levels are the most sensitive measures.

SUGGESTED READING LIST

Aivado M, Gattermann N, Rong A, et al: X-linked sideroblastic anemia associated with a novel ALAS2' mutation and unfortunate skewed X-chromosome inactivation patterns. Blood Cells Mol Dis 37:40, 2006.

Anderson KE, Collins S: Open-label study of hemin for acute porphyna. Clinical practice implications. Amer J Med 119, U19, 2006.

Bottomley SS: Congenital sideroblastic anaemias. Curr Hematol Rep 5: 41, 2006.

Furuyama K, Harigae H, Heller T, et al: Arg-452 substitution of the erythroid-specific 5—aminolaevulinate synthase, a hot spot mutation in X-linked sideroblastic anaemia, does not itself affect enzyme activity. Eur J Haematol 76:33, 2006.

Goodwin RG, Kell J, Laidler P, et al: Photosensitivity and acute liver injury in myeloproliferative disorder secondary to late-onset protoporphyria caused by deletion of a ferrochelatase gene in hematopoietic cells. Blood 107:60, 2006.

Kadish KM, Smith KM, Guilard R. The Porphyrin Handbook. Vol 14: Medical aspects of Porphyrins. Academic Press, 2006.

Macours P, Cotton F: Improvement in HPLC separation of porphyrin isomers and application to biochemical diagnosis of porphyrias. Clin Chem Lab Med 44:1438, 2006.

Merino A, to-Figueras J, Herrero C: Atypical red cell inclusions in congenital erythropoietic porphyria. Br J Haematol 132:124, 2006.

Nakano H, NakanoA, Toyomaki Y, et al: Novel ferrochelatase mutations in Japanese patients with erythropoietic protoporphyria: high frequency of the splice site modulator IVS3–48C polymorphism in the Japanese population. J Invest Dermatol 126:2717, 2006.

Pondarre C, Campagna DR, Antioches B, et al: Abcb7, the gene responsible for X-linked sideroblastic anemia with ataxia, is essential for hematopoiesis. Blood 109:3567, 2007.

Rand EB, Bunin N, Cochran W, et al: Sequential liver and bone marrow transplantation for treatment of erythropoietic protoporphyria. Pediatrics 118:1896, 2006.

Sarkany RP, Ross G, Willis F: Acquired erythropoietic protoporphyria as a result of myelodysplasia causing loss of chromosome 18. Br J Dermatol 155:464, 2006.

Shaw GC, Cope JJ, Li L, et al: Mitoferrin is essential for erythroid iron assimilation. Nature 440:96, 2006.

Szpurka, H, Tiu R, Murugesan G, et al: Refractory anemia with ringed sideroblasts associated with marked thrombocytosis (RARS-T) another myeloproliferative condition characterized by JAK2 V617F mutation. Blood 108, 2173, 2006.

Thunell S, Pomp E, Brun A: Guide to drug porphyrogenicity prediction and drug prescription in the acute porphyrias. Br J Clin Pharmacol 64:668, 2007.

REFERENCES

For complete list of references log onto www.expertconsult.com

CHAPTER 39

MEGALOBLASTIC ANEMIAS

Aśok C. Antony

GENERAL CONCEPTS

The term *megaloblastic anemia* is used to describe a group of disorders characterized by a distinct morphologic pattern in hematopoietic cells. A common biochemical feature is a defect in DNA synthesis, with lesser alterations in RNA and protein synthesis, leading to a state of unbalanced cell growth and impaired cell division. Most megaloblastic cells are not resting but vainly engaged in attempting to double their DNA, with frequent arrests in the S phase and lesser degrees of arrest in other phases of the cell cycle. An increased percentage of these cells have DNA values between $2N$ (N = amount of DNA in the haploid genome) and $4N$ because of delayed cell division. This increased DNA content in megaloblastic cells is morphologically expressed as larger than normal "immature" nuclei with fine particulate chromatin, whereas the relatively unimpaired RNA and protein synthesis results in large cells with greater "mature" cytoplasm and cell volume. The net result of megaloblastosis is a cell whose nuclear maturation is arrested (immature) while its cytoplasmic maturation proceeds normally independently of the nuclear events. The microscopic appearance of this nuclear–cytoplasmic asynchrony (or dissociation) is morphologically described as megaloblastic. Each cell lineage has a limited but unique repertoire of expression of defective DNA synthesis. This is significantly influenced by the normal patterns of maturation of the affected cell line. Additional variables that affect RNA and protein synthesis can lead to the attenuation or modification of megaloblastic expression (see Masked Megaloblastosis).

Megaloblastic hematopoiesis commonly manifests as anemia, but this feature is only a manifestation of a more global defect in DNA synthesis that affects all proliferating cells. The peripheral blood picture is characteristic and reflective of megaloblastic hematopoiesis within the bone marrow. The diagnosis is therefore usually straightforward, but because any condition that specifically perturbs DNA synthesis may lead to megaloblastosis, determination of the precise cause is necessary before institution of therapy. Inappropriate therapy can lead to disastrous consequences for the patient. The biochemical basis for megaloblastosis needs to be understood within the context of evaluation of potential and real variables affecting DNA, RNA, and protein synthesis in a given patient. The most common causes of megaloblastosis are true cellular deficiencies of vitamin B_{12} (cobalamin) or folate, vitamins that are essential for DNA synthesis. The pathophysiology of cellular deficiency is most readily discerned by the clinician who approaches megaloblastosis with a clear understanding of the physiology of these vitamins. A detailed discussion of cobalamin and folate therefore follows.

COBALAMIN

The term *cobalamin* refers to a family of compounds with the structure shown in Fig. 39–1; cobalamin itself lacks a ligand in the cobalt beta-position. Vitamin B_{12} is called *cyanocobalamin* because when it was originally isolated from the liver, this position was occupied by a cyano group (an artifact generated in vitro). Details of the chemistry, nomenclature, and in vivo substitutions of cobalamin are shown in Figs. 39–1 to 39–3, and excellent reviews are available on the history, chemistry, and biology of cobalamin.[1,2] Cobalamin is synthesized and used by some microorganisms (eg, bacteria, fungi). Some strains produce cobalamin in excess of their requirements, making them excellent and cheap commercial sources for cobalamin used in therapy. Cobalamin analogs with cobalamin-like or anticobalamin-like effects are produced by microbes through purely chemical interactions of cobalamin in nature or as by-products of cobalamin metabolism in vivo.[2]

Nutrition

Cobalamin is only produced in nature by cobalamin-producing microorganisms, and humans receive cobalamin solely from the diet.[3] Although cobalamin is produced by bacteria in the large bowel of humans, this is at a site that is too distal for physiologic cobalamin absorption. Herbivores obtain their dietary quota of cobalamin from plants contaminated with cobalamin-producing bacteria that grow in the roots and nodules of legumes. Exogenous contamination of plants by feces (eg, manure used in fertilization) may also be a source of cobalamin, so in theory organically grown leafy vegetables may have higher cobalamin than those exposed to nonorganic (chemical) fertilizers. Moreover, insecticides could render such vegetables free of minute insects that could otherwise be inadvertently consumed and be a contributory source of cobalamin.[4] Lower animals receive their cobalamin by eating insects and other animals and by coprophagy, and the ingested cobalamin is then used for cobalamin-dependent reactions in muscular and parenchymal tissues that are then consumed by higher animals.

Animal protein is the major dietary source of cobalamin for nonvegetarians. Meats from parenchymal organs are richest in cobalamin (>10 μg cobalamin per 100 g wet weight); fish and animal muscle, milk products, and egg yolks have 1 to 10 μg per 100 g of wet weight. An average nonvegetarian Western diet contains 5 to 7 μg of cobalamin per day, which adequately sustains normal cobalamin equilibrium. A vegetarian diet supplies between 0.25 and 0.5 μg cobalamin daily, so most vegetarians do not receive adequate dietary cobalamin and are at risk for cobalamin deficiency.[5] The recommended daily allowance is 2.4 μg for men and nonpregnant women, 2.6 μg for pregnant women, 2.8 μg for lactating women, and 1.5 to 2 μg for children 9 to 18 years old.[4]

Although food cobalamin is stable at high-temperature cooking processes, it can readily be converted to inactive cobalamin analogs by ascorbic acid. Cobalamin is exceptionally well stored in tissues in its coenzyme forms. Of the total-body content of 2 to 5 mg in adults, approximately 1 mg is in the liver. There is an obligatory loss of 0.1% per day (1.3 μg) regardless of total-body cobalamin content. It takes approximately 3 to 4 years to deplete cobalamin stores when dietary cobalamin is abruptly malabsorbed, but it may take longer to develop nutritional cobalamin deficiency, because of an efficient enterohepatic circulation, which accounts for the turnover of 5 to 10 μg/day of cobalamin.[1]

Absorption

Cobalamin in food is usually in coenzyme form (5′-deoxyadenosyl cobalamin [adenosylcobalamin] and methylcobalamin), nonspecifically

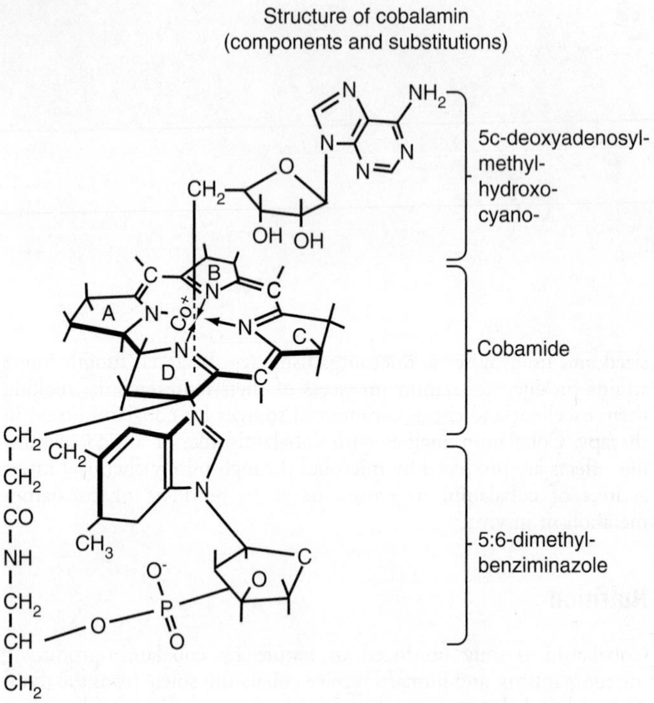

Structure of cobalamin
(components and substitutions)

5c-deoxyadenosyl-
methyl-
hydroxo-
cyano-

Cobamide

5:6-dimethyl-
benziminazole

Figure 39–1 Cobalamin chemistry and nomenclature. Vitamin B_{12} (ie, cyanocobalamin) is a complex molecule consisting of two major portions. A planar group consisting of four reduced pyrrole rings (ie, the corrin nucleus) is attached at right angles to an unusual nucleotide. Three of the four reduced pyrrole rings (designated A to D) are connected to one another by methylene carbon bridges; the alpha-carbons of rings A and D are, however, directly linked. The pyrrole rings are linked to a central cobalt atom. One coordinate position of cobalt (above the plane of the corrin nucleus) occupied by CN in cyanocobalamin can be occupied by various anionic group ligands (–R) in vitro and in vivo. Substitution at this position forms the basis for the specificity of the molecule as a coenzyme in vivo. The second coordination position of the central cobalt atom (below the plane of the corrin nucleus and almost perpendicular to it) is a linkage with the glyoxalinium nitrogen atom of the imidazole ring of the nucleotide. The nucleotide consists of a base, 5,6-dimethylbenziminazole, attached to ribose phosphate by alpha-glycoside linkages. The ribose is phosphorylated at C3; the nucleotide is connected to ring D of the corrin nucleus through an ester linkage. Compounds containing a corrin nucleus are given the generic name *corrinoid.* The addition of cobalt to the corrin nucleus containing standard side chains gives rise to cobyrinic acid. Additional substitutions in terminal carboxyl groups or modified carboxyl groups (designated *a* to *g*) give rise to various compounds such as cobamic acid, cobinic acid, cobinamide, and cobamide. Cobamide is found in vitamin B_{12}, whose systematic name is therefore alpha-(5,6-dimethylbenziminazolyl)cobamide cyanide (Adapted from Chanarin I: The Megaloblastic Anemias. Oxford, UK, Blackwell Scientific Publications, 1979.)

bound to proteins (see Fig. 39–2). In the stomach, peptic digestion at low pH is a prerequisite for cobalamin release from food protein.[1] This is of clinical significance in the 70- to 80-year-old population among whom hypochlorhydria is frequently present (in 25% to 50%) leading to inadequate release of protein-bound cobalamin by proteolysis with pepsin (because pepsin requires a low pH for optimum activity); these individuals can therefore develop cobalamin deficiency, resulting in what is known as food-cobalamin malabsorption. Although they can absorb crystalline cobalamin well, such individuals exhibit abnormalities in absorption when crystalline cobalamin is bound to proteins before ingestion (in the research setting).[2]

Once released by proteolysis, cobalamin preferentially binds a high-affinity, 150-kd, cobalamin-binding protein called R protein (also called haptocorrin) from gastric juice and saliva that has higher affinity for cobalamin than the gastric intrinsic factor (IF). The cobalamin–R protein (holo-R protein) complex, along with excess unbound (apo)-R protein and IF, passes through into the second part of the duodenum where pancreatic proteases degrade holo-R and apo-R proteins (but not IF). This results in the transfer of cobalamin to IF, a 45-kd glycoprotein with high-affinity binding ($K_a = 1.5 \times 10^{10}\ M^{-1}$), 1 : 1 molar stoichiometry, stability, and resistance to proteolysis over a pH range of 3 to 9.[1] Failure to degrade holo-R proteins by pancreatic protease precludes the involvement of IF in cobalamin absorption, because ileal IF–cobalamin receptors are specific for IF-bound cobalamin and not for R-bound cobalamin.[1] Although R proteins bind cobalamin and most cobalamin analogs with comparably high affinity, IF only binds cobalamin.

IF is produced in parietal (oxyntic) cells in the fundus and cardia of the stomach,[1] and released by membrane-associated vesicular transport.[1] IF has two binding sites: one for cobalamin and another for the ileal IF–cobalamin receptor. IF is produced in far greater excess than is actually required for absorption[1] and the IF in 2 to 4 mL of normal gastric juice is all that is necessary to reverse cobalamin deficiency in adults who lack IF. In the absence of IF, less than 2% of ingested cobalamin is absorbed, whereas in its presence approximately 70% is absorbed.

IF is secreted in response to food in the stomach in a manner analogous to secretion of acid (ie, by vagal and hormonal stimulation); IF release can be inhibited by long-term intake of H_2 blockers. Addition of proton pump inhibitors can reduce the absorption of protein-bound cobalamin, which can eventually lead to food-cobalamin malabsorption.[2] IF binds biliary cobalamin and newly ingested cobalamin following its transfer from R protein.[1,2] Because biliary cobalamin analogs are not transferred from R protein to IF, this appears to be an efficient method for fecal excretion of cobalamin analogs while allowing for reabsorption of biliary cobalamin. The stable IF–cobalamin complex passes through the jejunum to the ileum, where specific membrane-associated IF–cobalamin receptors for IF–cobalamin are located on the microvilli of the mucosal cells of the ileum.[1]

The functional IF–cobalamin receptors are composed of a complex of two proteins collectively known as cubam—composed of cubilin (encoded by the *CUBN* gene)[6] and amnionless (encoded by the *AMN* gene)[7]—that are essential to complete transport of the IF–cobalamin complex from the intestinal lumen into the enterocyte. Dysfunction of cubam is the basis for Imerslund–Gräsbeck syndrome. These IF–cobalamin receptors (cubam) require Ca^{2+} for binding at pH above 5.4; they do not bind free IF, cobalamin, or R-cobalamin and are therefore highly specific for IF–cobalamin ($K_a = 10^9\ M^{-1}$). The human ileum contains enough IF–cobalamin receptors to bind up to 1 mg of IF-bound cobalamin; this is the rate-limiting factor in cobalamin absorption.[1] Parenthetically, cubam is also responsible for the reabsorption of several vitamin carrier proteins (ranging from the transcobalamin–B_{12} complex, vitamin D–binding protein, retinol-binding protein) and a laundry list of other carrier proteins (albumin, myoglobin, hemoglobin, lactoferrin, transferrin), hormones (insulin, parathyroid) enzymes, drugs, and toxins (aminoglycosides).[8]

The events following the binding of the IF–cobalamin complex to IF–cobalamin receptors on enterocytes have not been fully delineated. Although transport into the cells requires energy, some studies suggest that the IF–cobalamin complex is first internalized by endocytosis and then released from cobalamin by lysosomal digestion, whereas others suggest that only cobalamin, but not IF, is internalized.[1] Transcobalamin II (TC II) is secreted unidirectionally across the basolateral surface and cobalamin apparently binds TC II within or at the basal surface of the ileal enterocyte.[1] Cobalamin bound to IF is transcytosed from the apical to the basal direction, and during transcytosis, a transfer to TC II is accomplished.[2] After a delay of 3 to 5 hours, cobalamin appears in the portal blood largely (>90%) bound to TC II. Although some cobalamin in the enterocyte is converted to adenosylcobalamin, most is destined for the portal blood and reaches peak levels in approximately 8 hours.[1]

Cobalamin in large doses can also passively diffuse through buccal, gastric, and jejunal mucosa so that less than 1% of a large dose of

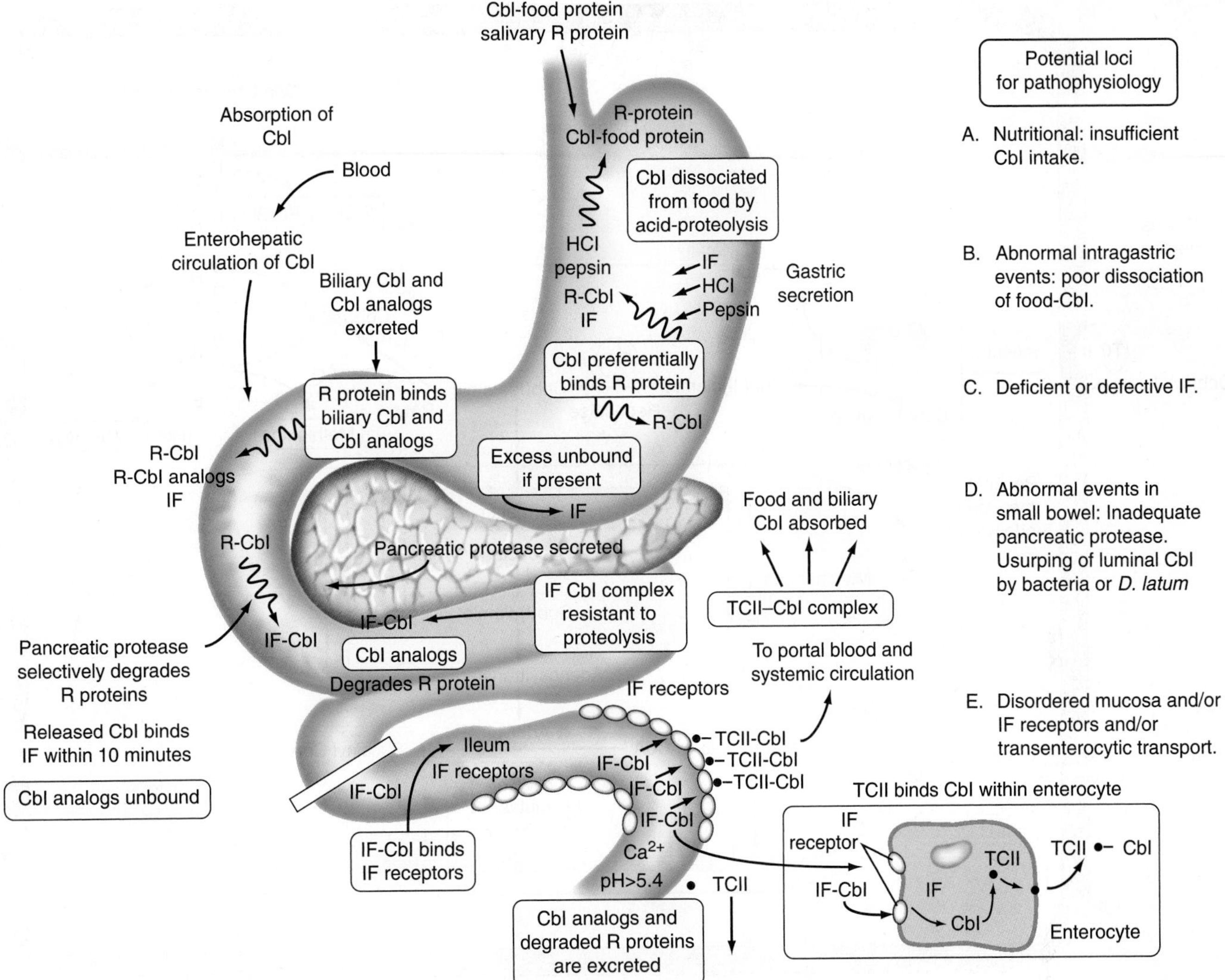

Figure 39–2 Components and mechanism of cobalamin absorption. Cbl, cobalamin; HCl, hydrochloric acid; IF, intrinsic factor; R, protein ligand; TCII, transcobalamin II.

oral cobalamin appears in the circulation within minutes. This property is used to advantage in some individuals with cobalamin malabsorption in lieu of parenteral replacement (discussed later).[1]

Transport

More than 90% of recently absorbed or injected cobalamin is bound to TC II, which is a specific transport protein for delivery of cobalamin to tissues. TC II, a 38-kd polypeptide synthesized in many tissues, binds cobalamin with 1 : 1 molar stoichiometry and high affinity ($K_a = 1 \times 10^{11}\ M^{-1}$).[2] Unlike IF, it can also bind a variety of cobalamin analogs (as R protein does). However, it does not belong to the R protein family and is immunologically distinct from two other plasma cobalamin-binding R proteins, TC I and TC III. The TC II–cobalamin complex is cleared so rapidly from the circulation (half-life of 6–9 minutes)[1] that 98% of TC II in plasma is unsaturated. TC II–cobalamin is rapidly bound to specific surface receptors for TC II present on several cells.[1] High-affinity TC II–cobalamin binding to TC II receptors is specific only for holo- and apo-TC II ($K_a = {\sim}5 \times 10^{10}\ M^{-1}$). Because some cobalamin analogs can bind TC II with high affinity, these also have the same potential for cellular uptake as cobalamin.[1] Once bound to TC II receptors, the TC II–cobalamin complex is internalized by receptor-mediated endocytosis.[1] At the low pH extant in lysosomes, TC II dissociates from cobalamin; it is then degraded and the cobalamin is reduced and converted to coenzyme forms (see Fig. 39–3). The importance of the transport function of TC II is underscored by the fact that TC II deficiency leads to life-threatening cellular cobalamin deficiency.[1]

Cobalamin is not found free in plasma. Binding to TC II accounts for 10% to 30% of the total serum cobalamin, and most of the remaining cobalamin is bound to another R protein, TC I. TC I is not a transport protein and cobalamin-bound TC I has a slow clearance rate (half-life of 9–12 days). Despite the fact that TC I binds approximately 75% of the circulating cobalamin (present predominantly as methylcobalamin) in fasting plasma, approximately one-half of the total TC I is in apo-form.

Neither the origin nor the physiologic importance of TC I in blood has been defined. Hereditary deficiency of TC I is apparently of no clinical consequence.[1] TC I may be a plasma-storage form of cobalamin, because it accounts for less than 0.5% of total cellular cobalamin uptake. TC I and TC III are found in secondary granules of mature polymorphonuclear leukocytes (PMNs).[2] TC III appears to have a transport function, because it is cleared from plasma within 3 minutes exclusively by hepatic asialoglycoprotein receptors, a mechanism common to a variety of asialoglycoproteins whose terminal beta-galactosyl end groups are intact. Conversely, desialation of TC I results in hepatic clearance identical to that of TC III,[1] which because of its rapid clearance is predominantly unsaturated. Functionally, TC III binds a wide spectrum of cobalamin analogs that are

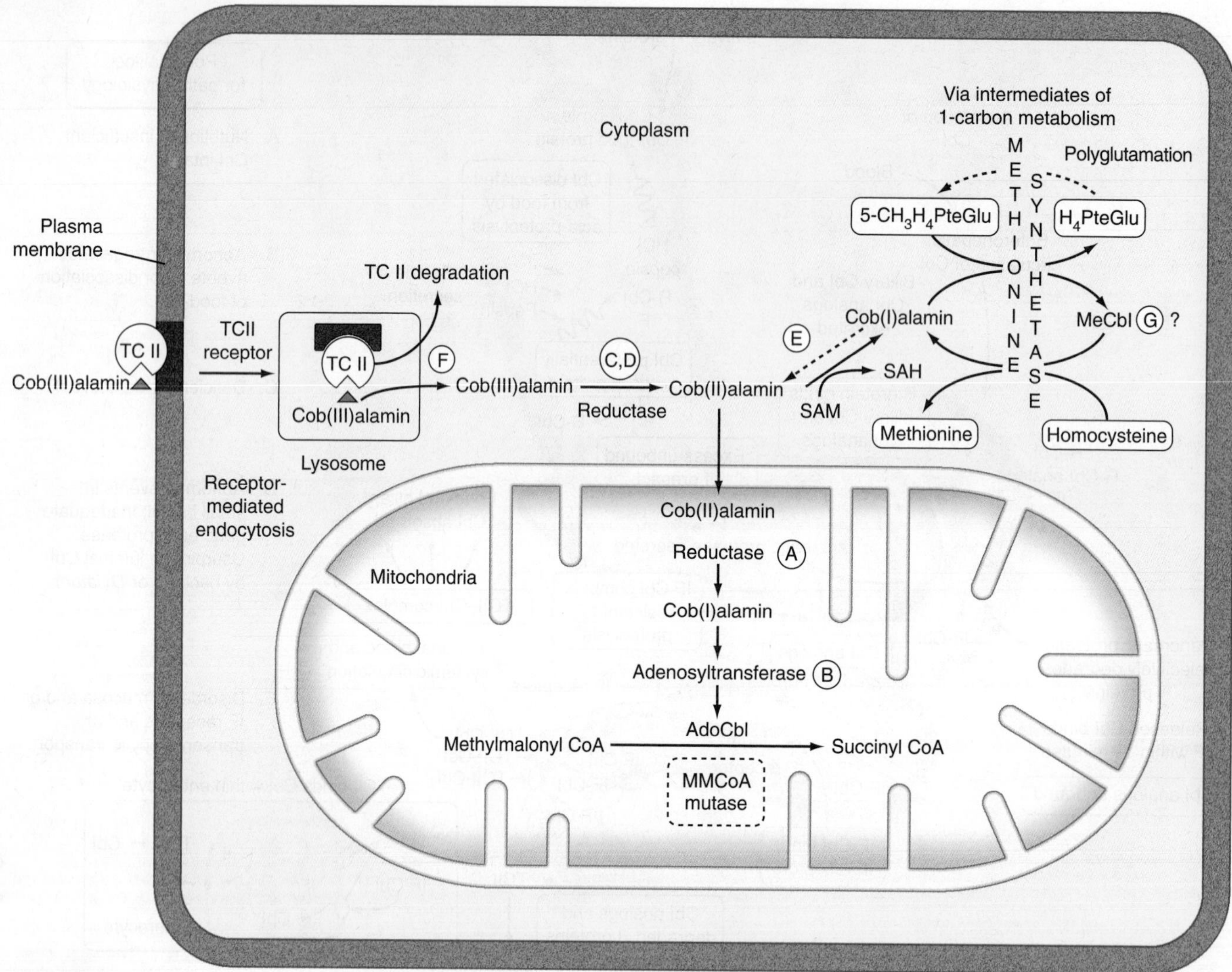

Figure 39–3 Cellular uptake and intracellular reactions involving cobalamin. A large family of natural and synthetic cobalamins can be generated when the cyanide (CN) moiety (upper axial ligand in cyanocobalamin) is replaced. On exposure to light, CN is gradually lost from cyanocobalamin, with the production of hydroxocobalamin. In vivo substitutions include the replacement of hydroxocobalamin or cyanocobalamin by a 5′-deoxyadenosyl group attached by a covalent bond, giving rise to adenosylcobalamin (AdoCbl). Methylcobalamin (MeCbl) is the main form in plasma. In vivo, 5-methyl-tetrahydrofolate readily donates its methyl group to cob(I)alamin in a reaction involving methionine synthase to form methylcobalamin. The loci for defects in cobalamin mutants *cblA* through *cblG* are indicated.

rapidly cleared by the liver into bile for fecal excretion. In contrast, between 0.5 and 9 μg of cobalamin taken up by hepatic TC II receptors is secreted into the bile, of which approximately 75% is reabsorbed, analogous to food cobalamin.[1]

Cellular Processing

After TC II receptor-mediated endocytosis (see Fig. 39–3) into lysosomes, the release of cobalamin by lysosomal degradation of TC II is an obligatory process for further intracellular metabolism.[1] After transport across the lysosome into the cytoplasm by a specific transport system,[2] more than 95% of intracellular cobalamin is bound to two intracellular enzymes, methylmalonyl-CoA mutase and methionine synthase.[1] Cob(III)alamin, the most "oxidized" form of cobalamin, must be converted to cob(II)alamin and cob(I)alamin by two sequential reductase steps (see Fig. 39–3).

In mitochondria, cob(I)alamin is subsequently converted to its coenzyme form adenosylcobalamin, which acts as a coenzyme in the intramolecular exchange of a hydrogen atom attached to one carbon atom with a group attached to an adjacent carbon atom. Methylmalonyl-CoA mutase in the presence of adenosylcobalamin converts methylmalonyl-CoA to succinyl-CoA, thereby converting the products of propionate metabolism (ie, methylmalonyl-CoA) into easily metabolized products. In the cytoplasm, cobalamin, as methylcobalamin, functions as a coenzyme for the reaction involving methionine synthase, which catalyzes the transfer of methyl groups from methylcobalamin to homocysteine to form methionine.[2] In this process methylcobalamin is converted to cob(I)alamin. The methyl group of 5-methyl-tetrahydrofolate (5-methyl-H_4PteGlu) is donated to cob(I)alamin, regenerating methylcobalamin, and 5-methyl-H_4PteGlu is converted to tetrahydrofolate (H_4PteGlu). Thus, folates and cobalamin are required together for normal one-carbon metabolism. After methionine is formed, it can get adenylated to *S*-adenosyl-methionine that can, in turn, donate its methyl group in a critical series of biologic methylation reactions involving more than 80 proteins, phospholipids, neurotransmitters, RNA and DNA. Methionine synthase also catalyzes the conversion of *S*-adenosyl-methionine to *S*-adenosyl-homocysteine, during which process the methyl group of *S*-adenosyl-methionine may also be used for remethylation of cob(I)alamin. Spontaneous oxidation of cob(I)alamin to the catalytically inactive cob(II)alamin form requires reduction back to cob(I)alamin before it can accept a methyl group because the cobalt atom in methylcobalamin has a 1+ valence. There is a redox regulator known as *methionine synthase reductase* that restores enzyme activity in the presence of *S*-adenosyl-methionine and NADPH.[9] This enzyme is clinically significant in that mothers with a polymorphism in methionine synthase reductase (A66G) and the common *MTHFR* (C677G) polymorphism are at increased risk of producing offspring with Down syndrome.[10] The physiologic importance of the key cofactor roles of the two forms of cobalamin, adenosylcobalamin and methylcobalamin, in methylmalonyl-CoA mutase and methionine synthase, respectively, is that the products and by-products of these enzymatic reactions are critical for DNA, RNA, and protein biosynthesis (discussed later).

Methionine synthase is a modular protein with four distinct and separate regions for binding homocysteine, 5-methyl-tetrahydrofolate (5-methyl-H_4PteGlu), the cobalamin prosthetic group, and *S*-adenosyl-methionine.[2] This explains how this enzyme plays a central role in catalyzing the transfer of a methyl group from bound methylcobalamin to homocysteine, yielding enzyme-bound cob(I)alamin and methionine, after which the free cofactor, cob(I)alamin, is remethylated by the methyl group from 5-methyl-H_4PteGlu, thereby completing the cycle (see Fig. 39–3).

Renal conservation of cobalamin is poorly understood. A 550-kd membrane protein called *megalin*, which interacts with cubulin and is found in renal proximal epithelial cells, functions as a multiligand receptor for a variety of macromolecules.[11] Megalin also specifically binds to and mediates the endocytosis of TC II–cobalamin complexes in kidney proximal tubules.[2]

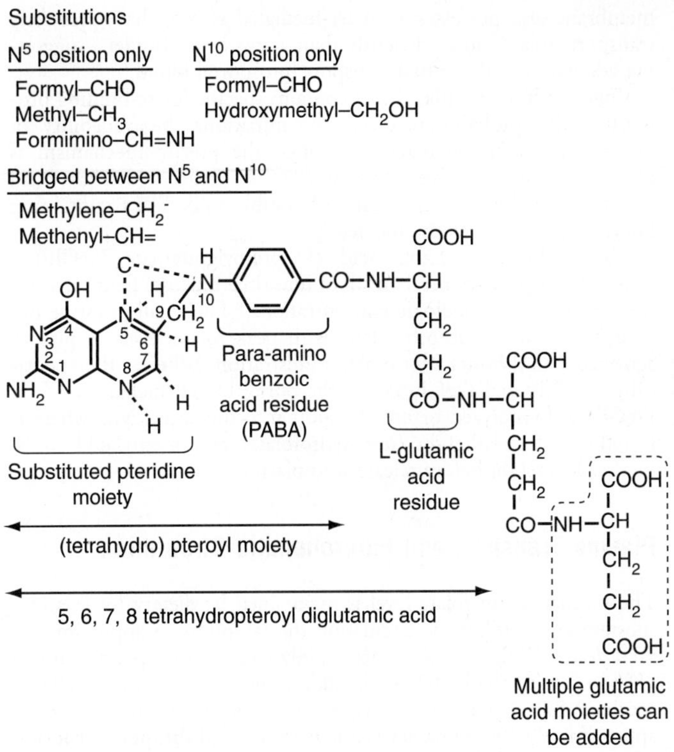

Substitutions

N⁵ position only: Formyl–CHO; Methyl–CH_3; Formimino–CH=NH

N¹⁰ position only: Formyl–CHO; Hydroxymethyl–CH_2OH

Bridged between N⁵ and N¹⁰: Methylene–CH_2; Methenyl–CH=

Substituted pteridine moiety — Para-amino benzoic acid residue (PABA) — L-glutamic acid residue

(tetrahydro) pteroyl moiety

5, 6, 7, 8 tetrahydropteroyl diglutamic acid

Multiple glutamic acid moieties can be added

Figure 39–4 Folate chemistry and nomenclature. Folic acid (pteroylmonoglutamate [PteGlu]) is the commercially available parent compound for more than 100 compounds collectively referred to as *folates*. PteGlu consists of three basic components: a pteridine derivative, a *p*-aminobenzoic residue, and an L-glutamic acid residue. Before PteGlu can play a role as a coenzyme, it must first be reduced at positions 7 and 8 to dihydrofolic acid (H_2PteGlu) and then to 5,6,7,8-tetrahydrofolic acid (H_4PteGlu), and one to six additional glutamic acid residues must then be added by means of gamma-peptide bonds to the L-glutamate moiety (for which the subscripted *n* in $PteGlu_n$ denotes polyglutamation). Folate coenzymes donate or accept one-carbon units in numerous reactions in amino acid and nucleotide metabolism. The various substitutions in $H_4PteGlu_n$ occur at position 5 or 10, or both; position 5 can be substituted by methyl (CH_3), formyl (CHO), or formimino (CHNH), and position 10 can be substituted by formyl or hydroxymethyl (CH_2OH). Positions 5 and 10 can be bridged by methylene (–CH_2–) or methenyl (–CH=).

FOLATES

Nutrition

Folates, which are widely distributed in nature in reduced and polyglutamated forms, are synthesized by microorganisms and plants; Fig. 39–4 shows the chemistry and nomenclature, and Hoffbrand and Weir[12] provide an engaging review of the rich history of folic acid. Leafy vegetables (eg, spinach, lettuce, broccoli), beans, fruits (eg, bananas, melons, lemons), yeast, mushrooms, and animal protein (eg, liver, kidney) are rich sources of folate.[1] Folates are highly susceptible to breakdown during cooking for >15 minutes, so cultural and ethnic cooking practices that often involve prolonged boiling of lentils or beans in spices for over 30 minutes in large volumes of water,[2] or frying foods in an open pan, can result in loss of 50 to 95% of folate. In many cultures, it is also not common to eat fresh raw or stir-fried vegetables or salads that are rich in folate. Oxidation of food folate by nitrites (used in curing meats) reduces its bioavailability.[2] The recommended daily allowance of folate is as follows: adult men and nonpregnant women, 400 μg; pregnant women, 600 μg; lactating women, 500 μg; children aged 9 to 18 years, between 300 and 400 μg.[4] A balanced Western diet contains adequate amounts of folate, but the net dietary intake of folate in many developing countries is often insufficient to sustain folate balance.[1,2,13,14]

Absorption

Dietary folates, which are in the form of pteroyl*poly*glutamates ($PteGlu_n$), are absorbed less efficiently than pteroyl*mono*glutamate (PteGlu; folic acid). Although folates in some foods (eg, cabbage, lettuce, orange) are not well absorbed,[1] most other dietary folates are nutritionally available (ie, bioavailable). Pteroylpolyglutamates must be hydrolyzed to pteroylmonoglutamate derivatives before absorption by pteroylpolyglutamate hydrolase, an enzyme present in the brush border membranes of small intestinal cells.[1] This enzyme has maximal exopeptidase activity at pH 5.5 in the presence of zinc, with equal affinity for $PteGlu_n$ of different glutamate chain lengths. Luminal pteroylglutamate interacts with brush border membrane-associated reduced-folate carriers (RFCs), which exhibit rapid equilibrium binding (<5 minutes), pH dependency (pH 5 optimal), high affinity (K_d approximately 0.08 mM), and transport of reduced folates within seconds.[15,16] *RFC* gene expression (encoding a 58-kd protein) is developmentally regulated, showing higher maximum capacity for 5-methyl-H_4PteGlu influx in mature (absorptive) rather than proliferative crypt cells.[2] RFC can be upregulated in response to dietary folate deficiency in mice, which would presumably allow maximizing the transport of folate under conditions of dietary folate deficiency.[17] The simultaneous upregulation in the activity of pteroylpolyglutamate hydrolase[18] and cell surface folate receptors[17,19] allows folate-deficient luminal cells to maximize their own uptake and maintain cellular integrity under folate-deficient states. However, the key experimental studies designed to distinguish transenterocytic folate transport from the transport of folate that is only destined for the enterocyte remain to be conducted to clarify the functional basis for upregulation of these two folate transporters.

Considerable gaps still exist in our knowledge of the structure and functional interrelationships of the human intestinal folate transport carrier proteins, the precise mechanism of passage of folate within the enterocyte, and interaction with lysosomal pteroylpolyglutamate hydrolases. This 75-kd enzyme is maximally active at pH 4.5 and cleaves terminal and internal gamma-glutamate linkages with greatest affinity for $PteGlu_n$ with longer glutamate chains.[1] The basolateral membrane also possesses a carrier-mediated system that apparently transports folate more efficiently than across brush borders, suggesting adaptation for eventual transport into portal blood.[1]

Ingested human milk, which contains specific folate-binding proteins (FBP), probably regulates the nutritional bioavailability of ingested folate in neonates.[2] Although the precise mechanism is obscure, it could involve interaction with megalin, which can bind and mediate the cellular uptake of soluble milk FBPs containing bound folate into the enterocytes.[20]

Passive diffusion of folic acid (aka pteroylglutamate, PteGlu) is probably the primary mechanism of intestinal mucosal folate absorption at high pharmacologic concentrations.[1] The small intestine has a large capacity to absorb folate, with peak folate levels in plasma achieved 1 to 2 hours after oral administration. Whereas therapeutically administered PteGlu enters the portal blood unchanged, food $PteGlu_n$ is hydrolyzed before transport into the enterocyte, where it is reduced to H_4PteGlu (tetrahydrofolate) and methylated to 5-methyl-H_4PteGlu before release into plasma.

Plasma Transport and Enterohepatic Circulation

The normal serum folate level is maintained by dietary folate and a substantial enterohepatic circulation that amounts to approximately 90 µg/day of folate.[1] Folates are rapidly cleared from plasma (up to 95% in 3 minutes) by tissues, including the liver, by an RFC-related species.[15] Biliary drainage results in a dramatic fall in serum folate (to approximately 30% of basal levels in 6 hours), and abrupt interruption of dietary folate leads to a fall in serum folate levels in approximately 3 weeks. In the plasma, one-third of the folate is free, and two-thirds is nonspecifically and loosely bound to serum proteins. A small amount of folate is specifically bound to high-affinity, intrinsically soluble hydrophilic 40-kd FBPs; the physiologic significance of this interaction is not clear.[21] In contrast to cobalamin uptake, there is no specific *serum* transport protein that enhances cellular folate uptake.

Cellular Folate Uptake

Folate transport involves translocation of the ligand into cells from the extracellular compartment (ie, cellular uptake mechanisms) or across cellular barriers from one compartment to another (ie, transcellular mechanisms).[2,21] Two distinct components are involved in cellular folate transport. The RFC is a low-affinity, high-capacity system that mediates the uptake of physiologic and other reduced folates into a variety of cells.[15] Folate transport into cells is also mediated by 44-kd membrane-associated FBPs or folate receptors (FRs) (these terms are synonymous) that bind physiologic folates (ie, serum 5-methyl-H_4PteGlu) with high affinity in the nanomolar range (ie, the range needed for binding serum folates).[21]

The pathways for entry of folates and antifolates are likely to be distinct in different cells depending on the relative efficiency of FR- and RFC-mediated mechanisms, as well as the intracellular and extracellular concentration of folates and antifolates. There are probably other determinants in some malignant human cells; for example, despite high FR expression, the RFC was the preferential carrier of antifolates in some cells.[2]

Transcellular folate transport systems are operative in placental[22] and renal tubular cells.[2] Although choroid plexus contains a significant amount of FR, their role in folate transport across the blood–brain barrier and blood–cerebrospinal fluid barrier is still unclear.[21] A third pathway for folate transport by passive diffusion[21] is also integrally involved (in concert with FR) in transplacental folate transport (discussed later).[22]

Folate Receptors

FRs mediate the cellular uptake of the physiologic folate, 5-methyl-H_4PteGlu, in several malignant and normal cells.[21,23] Of the three human FR isoforms, FR-alpha and FR-beta are attached to the cell surface through a glycosyl-phosphatidylinositol membrane anchor, whereas the third (FR-gamma) is constitutively secreted.[2]

FR transfers folate intracellularly by endocytosis by means of clathrin-coated pits[2] or by caveolae.[2] In the latter model (which is controversial),[2,21] folate is dissociated from the FR at acid pH generated within caveolae by a proton pump and is transported through a putative folate transporter into the cytoplasm, whereas apo-FRs recycle back to the surface to bind more folate (Fig. 39–5). More recent studies on this issue have been reviewed.[24] FR-alpha are expressed in most normal and many malignant epithelial tissues.[2] The expression of FR-beta in normal tissues is restricted to the placenta and hematopoietic cells.[2,25]

The FR- and RFC-mediated folate transport systems do not communicate with one another (ie, there is no cross-talk), and both RFC and FR are efficient in the transport of methotrexate and function independently of one another.[2] When enough FRs are expressed, they can mediate the uptake of methotrexate and 5-methyl-H_4PteGlu with comparable rates to cells expressing only the RFC, so FRs have physiologic and pharmacologic importance.

There is an inverse relationship between cell proliferation and FRs,[2,26] but the underlying mechanism of this relationship is still unclear. FRs are upregulated in response to extracellular and intracellular folate concentrations in some cells[2] through transcriptional, translational, or posttranslational mechanisms. Posttranslational downregulation of FRs (ie, FBPs) in rat kidney during folate deficiency occurs through preferential proteolysis of apo-FR by a kidney metalloprotease called *meprin*, but the precise triggering mechanism is unclear.[27] In human cervical cancer, translational upregulation of FR-alpha in folate deficiency is mediated by homocysteine, which increases interaction between an 18-base *cis*-element in the 5′-untranslated region of FR-alpha mRNA and a heterogeneous nuclear ribonucleoprotein E1 *trans*-factor.[28,29] On replenishment of folate and reduction in intracellular homocysteine, there is reversal of this interaction leading to downregulation. This is an example of linkage between perturbed folate metabolism and coordinated upregulation of FRs.[29] Perturbation of plasma membrane metalloprotease,[2] cholesterol,[2] and sphingolipids[2] can also modulate the expression of FRs in various tissues through poorly understood mechanisms.

The functional role of FRs, which are expressed in several normal tissues,[2] has been demonstrated in the placenta, proximal renal tubular cells, and hematopoietic progenitor cells. Because FR-α are overexpressed in some malignancies (eg, most cervical[26] and ovarian cancers[2]), they are potential targets for exploitation as Trojan horses for the delivery of folate-tethered liposomes bearing various cargos (ie, chemotherapy, imaging reagents, genes, or other agents).[2,30,31] Induction of FR-beta expression in AML with retinoic acid is another possible therapeutic strategy under investigation.[2,32]

Reduced-Folate Carriers

The second mechanism for folate uptake is a carrier-mediated, pH- and energy-dependent process that transports reduced folates equally efficiently at higher than physiologic concentrations.[15] The RFC gene[33,34] encodes a 58-kd polypeptide and resembles the mammalian glucose transporter (GLUT1), which is a member of the 12-transmembrane domain-spanning membrane transporter family. The acquisition of methotrexate transport deficiency in some cells results from inactivating mutations of RFC gene alleles,[2] and acquired transport resistance in relapsed acute lymphocytic leukemia is also associated with decreased RFC expression.[2]

Cellular Retention and Excretion

Polyglutamation of folate is the major factor for intracellular retention (see Fig. 39–5).[2] As a corollary, human malignant cells with reduced folylpolyglutamate synthase are resistant to antifolates, which

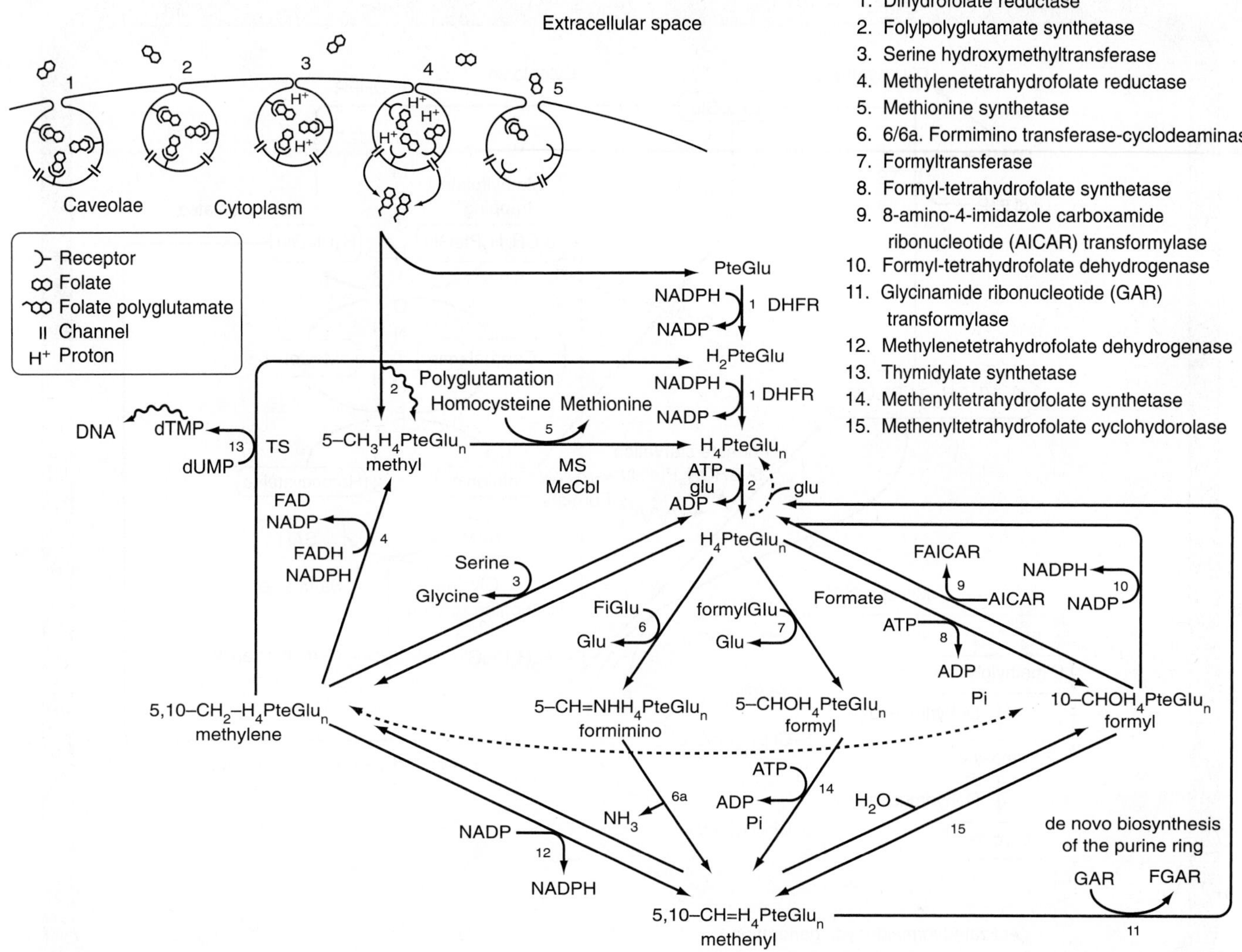

Figure 39–5 Folate receptor (FR)-coupled folate uptake and intracellular one-carbon metabolism involving folates. See text for details. The contribution of the reduced-folate carrier (RFC)-mediated transport and passive diffusion of folate into cells is not shown. (Adapted from Shane B, Stokstad EL: Vitamin B_{12}–folate interrelationships. Annu Rev Nutr 5:115, 1985, and from Rothberg KG, Ying Y, Kolhouse JF, et al: The glycophospholipid-linked FR internalizes folate without entering the clathrin-coated pit endocytic pathway. J Cell Biol 110:637, 1990.)

cannot be (polyglutamated and) retained intracellularly.[2] In human erythrocytes (RBCs), folate is accumulated at earlier stages within the marrow by FRs[1]; on maturation, more than 90% of $PteGlu_n$ molecules interact with hemoglobin, which, because of its high capacity, assists in intracellular folate retention.[1]

Folate turnover and catabolism can be accelerated by the activity of heavy-chain ferritin,[35] which limits the amount of newly imported (unbound) folate monoglutamates before they are polyglutamylated and can function as cofactors with intracellular enzymes; indeed, increased ferritin expression can deplete cellular folate concentrations in cells cultured with folate-rich medium.[35] However, approximately 50% of intracellular folates appear protected, possibly because of sequestration in mitochondria.

After glomerular filtration, luminal folate binds FR in the brush border membranes of proximal renal tubular cells[2] and is internalized rapidly by FR-mediated endocytosis; in the low pH of endocytotic vesicles, there is dissociation of folates and slow transport across basolateral membranes into the blood, with recycling of apo-FR back to the luminal brush border membrane.[1] Both megalin and cubulin cooperate to mediate the uptake of several other ligands via receptor-mediated endocytosis including reabsorption of filtered folate bound to soluble FBPs via kidney proximal tubules.[20]

INTRACELLULAR METABOLISM AND COBALAMIN–FOLATE RELATIONSHIPS

Pteroylpolyglutamates are the natural substrates for the various enzymes involved in one-carbon metabolism (Figs. 39–5 and 39–6). Pteroyl*mono*glutamates must be *poly*glutamated by folylpolyglutamate synthase before they participate in one-carbon metabolism.[1] Tetrahydropteroylglutamate ($H_4PteGlu$) is the preferred physiologic substrate for folylpolyglutamate synthase, and the polyglutamyl form ($H_4PteGlu_n$) plays a central role in one-carbon metabolism.[1] Factors that limit the supply of $H_4PteGlu$ or regulate folylpolyglutamate synthase influence polyglutamation and cellular retention of folates. $H_4PteGlu_n$ can be converted to formate as 10-formyl-$H_4PteGlu_n$ (used in de novo biosynthesis of purines) and formaldehyde as 5,10-methylene-$H_4PteGlu_n$ (for synthesis of thymidylate). Moreover, 5,10-methylene-$H_4PteGlu_n$ and 10-formyl-$H_4PteGlu_n$ can be interconverted by intermediates (see Fig. 39–5).

To understand the functions of folate coenzymes (see Figs. 39–5 and 39–6), it is important to recognize at the outset that 5,10-methylene-$H_4PteGlu_n$ can be used in the *thymidylate cycle* by thymidylate synthase for thymidine and DNA synthesis or in the *methylation cycle* after its conversion to 5-methyl-$H_4PteGlu_n$, which by means of

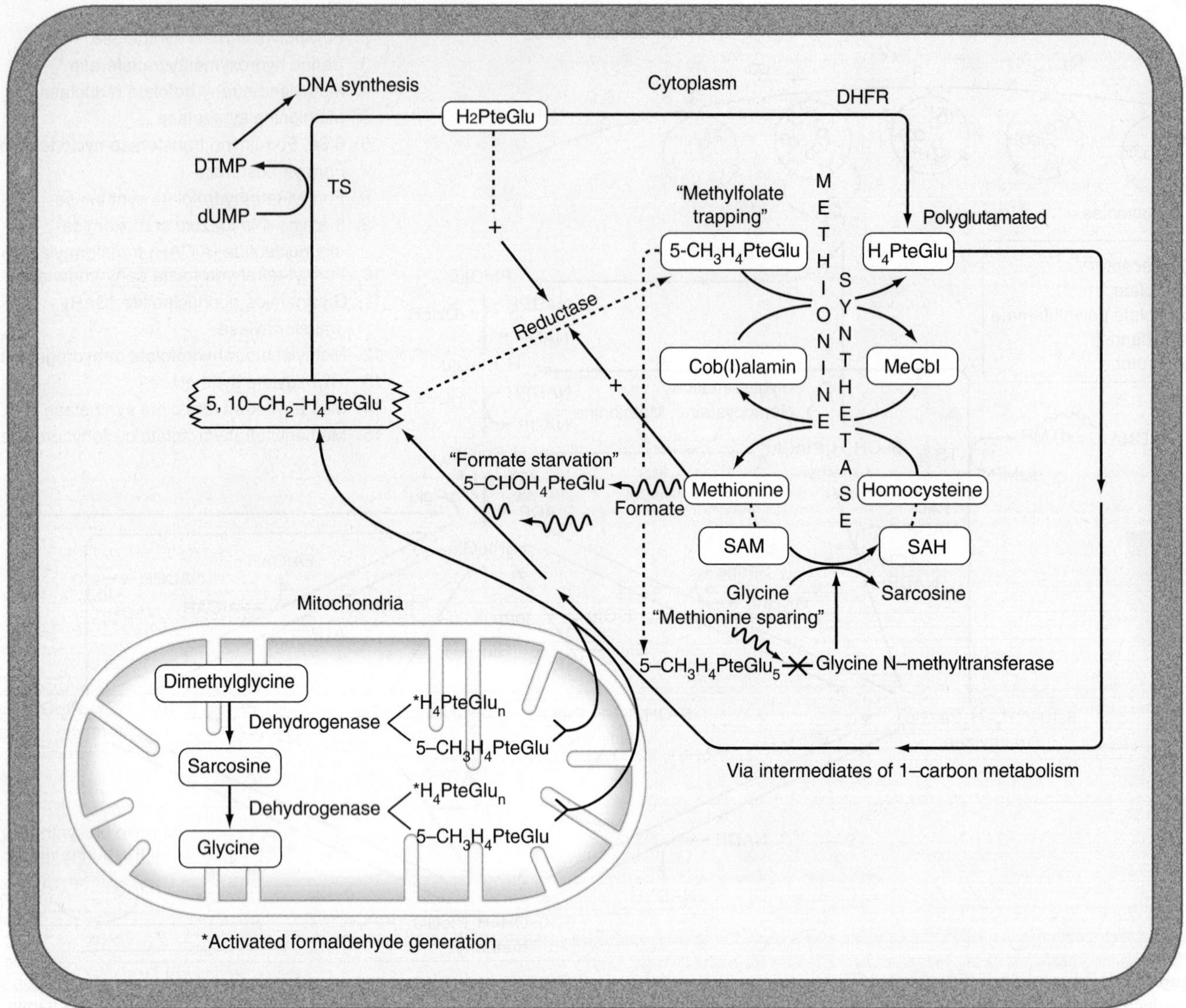

Figure 39–6 Major pathways involving cobalamin–folate interrelationships. Intramitochondrial dehydrogenases that preferentially bind $H_4PteGlu_5$ provide activated formaldehyde (by means of dimethylglycine to sarcosine to glycine). The activated formaldehyde nonenzymatically reacts with the enzyme-bound tetrahydrofolate pentaglutamate ($H_4PteGlu_5$) to form 5,10-methylene-$H_4PteGlu_n$ for methionine synthase and thymidylate synthase. Another cytosolic dehydrogenase (glycine *N*-methyltransferase) that synthesizes sarcosine in the presence of *S*-adenosyl-methionine from glycine (with conversion of *S*-adenosyl-methionine to *S*-adenosyl-homocysteine) is activated on phosphorylation but is allosterically inhibited (trapped and polyglutamated) by 5-methyl-$H_4PteGlu_5$ in cobalamin deficiency. This effect of 5-methyl-$H_4PteGlu_5$ may lead to methionine-sparing, and the methionine could inhibit the formation of more 5-methyl-$H_4PteGlu_5$ from 5,10-methylene-$H_4PteGlu_n$ and channel the latter for DNA synthesis.[2]

methionine synthase leads to the formation of methionine and $H_4PteGlu_n$.

Pteroylmonoglutamate (PteGlu, folic acid) is not a biologically active form of folate; when given therapeutically, it requires reduction to $H_4PteGlu$ by dihydrofolate reductase (a 20-kd enzyme) in a two-step reaction (pteroylglutamate [PteGlu] to *dihydro*pteroylglutamate [$H_2PteGlu$] to *tetrahydro*pteroylglutamate [$H_4PteGlu$]). The major form of folate transported into the cell by FR and RFC is 5-methyl-$H_4PteGlu$ (see Fig. 39–5). Evidence suggests that folate-mediated one-carbon metabolism is compartmentalized among intracellular organelles, leading to substrate channeling along folate coenzymes.[2,36] For example, some of the enzymes distal to $H_4PteGlu_n$ are multifunctional, allowing sequential channeling of folate coenzyme forms (eg, $H_4PteGlu_n$ to 5-formino-$H_4PteGlu_n$ to 5,10-methenyl-$H_4PteGlu_n$). Thymidylate synthase catalyzes the transfer of the formaldehyde from 5,10-methylene-$H_4PteGlu_n$ to the 5 position of deoxyuridylate; in this process 5,10-methylene-$H_4PteGlu_n$ is also reduced to dihydrofolate, which inhibits 5,10-methylene-$H_4PteGlu_n$ reductase. Because methionine, the product of the methionine synthase reaction, also inhibits this enzyme, this illustrates that modulation of 5,10-methylene-$H_4PteGlu_n$ reductase by levels of dihydrofolate and methionine can determine the degree of channeling of 5,10-methylene-$H_4PteGlu_n$ into the methylation and thymidylate cycle (Figs. 39–5 and 39–6).

Folate metabolism and folate-dependent enzymes are compartmentalized in the mitochondrial matrix and cytoplasm (with each compartment containing near equal concentrations of folate cofactors),[37] and there are homologs of the major cytosolic enzymes (see Fig. 39–5) within mitochondria. Folate monoglutamates are transported from the cytoplasm into the mitochondria by a reduced-folate carrier that is specific for mitochondria,[38] within which they are converted to polyglutamylated forms. Most of the one-carbon units, in the form of formate, are derived from mitochondria and are used for the synthesis of formate, glycine, and f-met-tRNA. A new model[36] suggests a smooth unidirectional flow of one-carbon units from the mitochondria to the cytosol. In the mitochondria, 5,10-methylene-$H_4PteGlu$ is first generated primarily from the conversion of serine to glycine (with other contributions from the catabolism of glycine and choline) followed by sequential transfer of one-carbon units to 10-formyl-H_4PteGlu and then on to formate, which then leaves the mitochondria. In the cytosol, formate is coupled to H_4PteGlu to form 10-formyl-H_4PteGlu, which constitutes the major pool of cytosolic folate and the primary source of one-carbon units for the synthesis of thymidylate, methionine, and purines.

The mechanism whereby cobalamin deficiency produces its megaloblastic effects is not precisely known. It is generally agreed that cobalamin deficiency causes a functional intracellular deficiency of 5,10-methylene-H_4PteGlu$_n$ (see Figs. 39–5 and 39–6). The methylfolate trap hypothesis was originally formulated in an attempt to explain why cobalamin deficiency resulted in a functional folate deficiency. Under normal conditions, 5-methyl-H_4PteGlu is converted by the cobalamin-dependent methionine synthase to H_4PteGlu, which is subsequently polyglutamated and then used in one-carbon metabolism. With cobalamin deficiency, methionine synthase is inactive, leading to buildup of 5-methyl-H_4PteGlu, which is a particularly poor substrate for folate polyglutamate synthase. With no alternative metabolic pathway but this cobalamin-dependent reaction, the "trapped" 5-methyl-H_4PteGlu leaks out of the cell, leading to a progressive deficiency of polyglutamated folate intracellularly. The formate starvation hypothesis centers on the relatively greater merit of formate (in the form of 10-formyl-H_4PteGlu$_n$) and the precursor of formate, methionine, which is also decreased when methionine synthase is inhibited by cobalamin deficiency.[1] When methionine is in excess intracellularly, its methyl group is oxidized to formate, which can be used to generate 5-formyl- and 10-formyl-H_4PteGlu$_n$ (Fig. 39–5, reactions 7 and 8). There are articles that support either hypothesis.[2]

CONSEQUENCES OF PERTURBED ONE-CARBON METABOLISM

Thymidylate and DNA Synthesis

In cobalamin or folate deficiency, a net decrease in 5,10-methylene-H_4PteGlu$_n$ interrupts the reaction mediated by thymidylate synthase, which converts deoxyuridine monophosphate (dUMP) to deoxythymidine monophosphate (dTMP). Although there is a salvage pathway using thymidine kinase that normally accounts for 5% to 10% of thymidine synthesis, this pathway cannot meet the remaining 90% demand for dTMP generation. (Salvage pathways for purine synthesis can be activated to compensate for diminished generation of purines through folate coenzyme-mediated reactions.) The resulting thymidine deficiency causes a marked increase in the dUMP/dTMP ratio. Because of the decrease in dTMP (and eventually dTTP), dUMP and therefore deoxyuridine triphosphate (dUTP) increase. Because DNA polymerase cannot distinguish between dUTP and dTTP, the elevated dUTP level promotes misincorporation of uridine residues into DNA.[2] An editorial enzyme, DNA uracil glycosylase, recognizes this faulty misincorporation. It excises dUTP, but the inadequate supply of dTTP leads to failure to repair the break in this DNA strand. Repeated DNA strand breaks lead to significant fragmentation of DNA, with consequent leakage of DNA fragments out of the cell.[2] The foregoing considerations form the basis for the dU suppression test that is occasionally employed as a research tool clinically to differentiate cobalamin from folate deficiency and when inborn errors of cobalamin or folate metabolism are suspected.[1]

Chromosome and Cell Cycle Defects

Defective DNA synthesis is reflected by numerous chromosomal abnormalities. There is excessive chromosomal elongation with despiralization associated with random breaks and exaggerated centromere constriction, expression of folate-sensitive fragile sites in hematopoietic cells, and reduced biosynthesis, acetylation, and methylation of arginine-rich histone.[1,2] All this leads to perturbation of the cell cycle, with an increased proportion of cells in the prophase of the mitotic cycle and G_2. In an in vitro model of folate-deficient erythroblastosis, apoptosis of erythroblasts in the late stages of differentiation apparently led to decreased erythrocyte production and anemia.[2]

MORPHOLOGIC EXPRESSION OF MEGALOBLASTOSIS

There is widening disparity in nuclear–cytoplasmic asynchrony as a cobalamin- or folate-deficient cell divides, until the more mature generations of daughter cells die in the marrow or are arrested (as megaloblastic cells) at various stages in the cell cycle.[1] The plethora of bone marrow morphologic changes may lead the untrained observer to the diagnosis of acute leukemia.[2] All proliferating cells exhibit megaloblastosis, including epithelial cells lining the gastrointestinal tract (buccal mucosa, tongue, small intestine), cervix, vagina, and uterus.[1] However, megaloblastic changes are most striking in the blood and bone marrow (see Fig. 39–7). Ineffective hematopoiesis extends into the long bones, and the bone marrow aspirate (which is better than the biopsy for observing megaloblastosis) exhibits trilineal hypercellularity, especially in the erythroid series. The appearance of exuberant cell proliferation with numerous mitotic figures is misleading because these cells are actually very slowly proliferating.

Erythroid hyperplasia reduces the myeloid-to-erythroid ratio from 3 : 1 to 1 : 1. Proerythroblasts are not as obviously abnormal as later forms; they may simply be larger (promegaloblasts). Megaloblastic changes are most strikingly displayed in intermediate and orthochromatic stages, which are larger than their normoblastic counterparts. In contrast to the normally dense chromatin of comparable normoblasts, megaloblastic erythroid precursors have an open, finely stippled, reticular, sievelike pattern. The orthochromatic megaloblast, with its hemoglobinized cytoplasm, continues to retain its large sievelike immature nucleus, in sharp contrast to the clumped chromatin of orthochromatic normoblasts. The nucleus is often eccentrically placed in these large oval or oblong cells and lobulation or indentation of nuclei with bizarre karyorrhexis is often seen. In cells destined for the circulation as macroovalocytes, the nucleus may occasionally not be completely extruded. Of the potential progeny of proerythroblasts that develop into later megaloblastic forms, 80% to 90% die in the bone marrow. Marrow macrophages effectively scavenge dead or partially disintegrated megaloblasts. This is the basis for ineffective erythropoiesis (intramedullary hemolysis).

Morphology in Megaloblastosis from Cobalamin and Folate Deficiency is the Same

Peripheral Smear

- Increased mean corpuscular volume (MCV) with macroovalocytes (up to 14 μm), which is variously associated with anisocytosis and poikilocytosis
- Nuclear hypersegmentation of polymorphonuclear neutrophils (PMNs) (one PMN with six lobes or 5% with five lobes)
- Thrombocytopenia (mild to moderate)
- Leukoerythroblastic morphology (from extramedullary hematopoiesis)

Bone Marrow Aspirate

- General increase in cellularity of all three major hematopoietic elements
- Abnormal erythropoiesis-orthochromatic megaloblasts
- Abnormal leukopoiesis-giant metamyelocytes and "band" forms (pathognomonic), hypersegmented PMNs
- Abnormal megakaryocytopoiesis-pseudohyperdiploidy

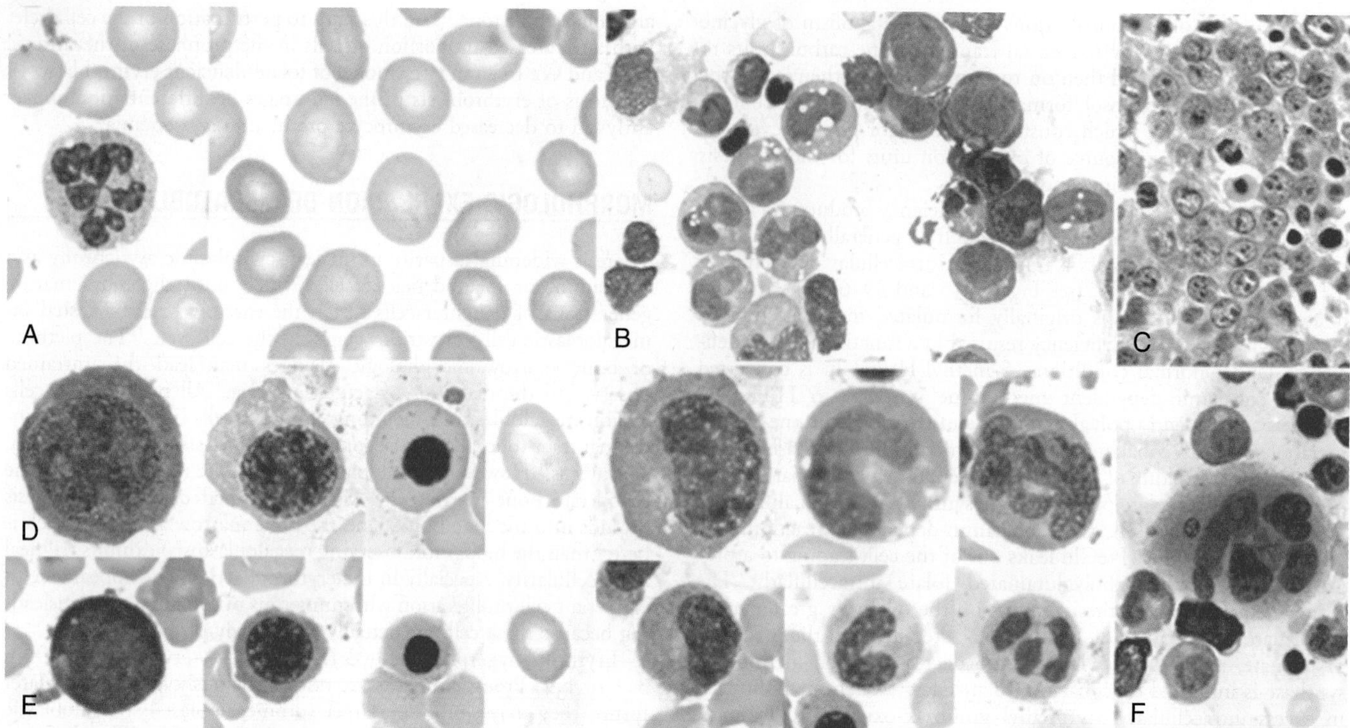

Figure 39–7 Megaloblastic anemia: peripheral blood (**A**), bone marrow aspirate (**B**), and biopsy **C**. The peripheral smear (**A**) exhibits macroovalocytosis, and hypersegmented polys (inset). The bone marrow aspirate (**B**) shows megaloblastic changes in both granulopoiesis and erythropoiesis. The biopsy (**C**) is hypercellular and shows sheets of immature erythroid precursors with a high mitotic rate. These can mimic acute erythroleukemia or even metastatic tumor cells. Details from the cells in the aspirate (**D**) compared with normal hematopoiesis at same magnification (**E**). Note the giant metamyelocyte and band form. In megaloblastic anemia, megakaryocytes also have nuclear atypica including abnormal nuclear segmentation (**F**).

Leukopoiesis is also abnormal. There is an absolute increase in these cells, which are large and have similar sievelike chromatin. Spectacular giant (20–30 μm) metamyelocytes and "band" forms that are often seen are pathognomonic for megaloblastosis. There may be bizarre nucleoli with small cytoplasmic vacuoles. It is probable that giant metamyelocytes cannot easily traverse marrow sinuses, and their maturation into circulating hypersegmented polymorphonuclear neutrophils (PMNs) is unlikely. Granulation of the cytoplasm remains unaffected.

Megakaryocytes may be normal or increased in numbers and may exhibit additional complexities in megaloblastic expression. The process of complex hypersegmentation (ie, pseudohyperdiploidy) is associated with liberation of fragments of cytoplasm and giant platelets into the circulation. The net output of platelets is invariably decreased in severe megaloblastosis and abnormal but reversible platelet dysfunction has been documented.[2]

In early cobalamin or folate deficiency, normoblasts may dominate the marrow, with only a few megaloblasts seen. Complete transformation to megaloblastic hematopoiesis is observed in florid cases and is reflected by various degrees of pancytopenia.

The earliest manifestation of megaloblastosis is an increase in mean corpuscular volume (MCV) with macroovalocytes (up to 14 μm). Because these cells have adequate hemoglobin, the central pallor, which normally occupies approximately one-third of the cell, is decreased. In severe anemia, poikilocytosis and anisocytosis are evident. Cells containing remnants of DNA (ie, Howell–Jolly bodies), arginine-rich histone, and nonhemoglobin iron (ie, Cabot rings) may be observed. Extramedullary megaloblastic hematopoiesis may also result in a leukoerythroblastic picture.

Ineffective use of iron results in an increased percentage of saturation of transferrin and increased iron stores. If there is associated iron deficiency, the MCV may be normal, and only iron therapy can unmask the megaloblastic manifestations in the peripheral blood. In thalassemia, the entire erythrocyte morphology normally expected in megaloblastosis is masked[1]; however, megaloblastic leukopoiesis is still observed. Significant intramedullary hemolysis (ineffective erythropoiesis) involving more than 90% of megaloblastic precursors is reflected by a lowered absolute reticulocyte count, increased bilirubin (up to 2 mg/dL), decreased haptoglobin, and increased lactate dehydrogenase (often above 1000 units/mL). There is also a modest decrease in the circulating RBC life span.

Nuclear hypersegmentation of DNA in PMNs strongly suggests megaloblastosis when associated with macroovalocytosis. Normally, less than 5% of PMNs have more than five lobes, and no cells have more than six lobes in the peripheral blood. If megaloblastosis is suspected (greater than 5% PMNs with more than five lobes or a single PMN with more than six lobes), a formal lobe count per PMN (ie, lobe index) above 3.5 may be obtained.

Megaloblastosis in rapidly proliferating cells of the gastrointestinal tract leads to a variable degree of morphologic changes and atrophy of the epithelial cells of the luminal lining. This leads to functional defects, which include a failure in secretion of IF and malabsorption of cobalamin and folate in certain subsets of patients. A vicious cycle whereby megaloblastosis begets more megaloblastosis is established that can be interrupted only by specific therapy with cobalamin or folate. This fact must be recognized when interpreting diagnostic tests involving cobalamin absorption (Table 39–3). Similar hematopoietic changes have been induced in a folate-deficient mouse model.[2]

NEUROLOGIC DYSFUNCTION WITH COBALAMIN DEFICIENCY

Because megaloblastosis due to folate or cobalamin deficiency leads to a functional folate coenzyme deficiency, the morphologic mani-

Clues for Distinguishing Cobalamin and Folate Deficiencies

Although the megaloblastic manifestations of cobalamin and folate deficiencies are clinically indistinguishable, certain distinct patterns in mode of presentation provide clues to the type and cause of deficiency. In general, the cause of folate deficiency can be found in the patient's recent past (within 6 months), primarily discerned from the history and physical examination. In contrast, the cause of cobalamin deficiency can remain obscure until specific tests to define the cause (eg, Schilling test) are carried out. In the past, by the time anemia was symptomatic, more than 80% of patients had neurologic manifestations, and in 50%, this led to some incapacity. Perhaps as a result of widespread use of multivitamins containing folic acid among patients and even in the food given livestock in the West, the hematologic expression of cobalamin deficiency is often substantially attenuated, leading to pure neurologic presentations. Studies highlight the apparent inverse correlation between hematologic and neurologic presentations such that in a third of patients with cobalamin deficiency, the earliest signs are often purely neurologic, and symptoms related to paresthesias and diminished proprioception cause the patient to see the physician. On the basis of the multiple potential causes, the warning that "what the mind does not know, the eyes do not see" is a caveat that cannot be taken lightly; failure to recognize cobalamin deficiency as the cause of neurologic disease and treatment of cobalamin deficiency with folate or misdiagnosis of megaloblastosis as erythroleukemia represent significant extremes of deviation from the dictum *primum non nocere.* Areas of overlap in the symptoms of cobalamin or folate deficiency are related to megaloblastosis (ie, common cardiopulmonary and some gastrointestinal manifestations). Although pure folate deficiency in the alcoholic with thiamine deficiency (ie, Wernicke encephalopathy) and peripheral neuropathy is almost indistinguishable from and may mimic cobalamin deficiency, the remainder of the neurologic manifestations are uniquely characteristic of cobalamin deficiency. Folate deficiency in adults has not been unequivocally shown to give rise to neurologic findings. Coexistence of folate deficiency with neurologic disease should prompt investigations to rule out cobalamin and other nutrient deficiencies arising from dietary insufficiency or malabsorption.

festations of both deficiencies are understandably indistinguishable. However, only cobalamin deficiency results in a patchy demyelination process, which is expressed clinically as cerebral abnormalities and subacute combined degeneration of the spinal cord.[1] The precise role of cobalamin in maintaining the integrity of the central nervous system has not been completely defined. Reviews have presented balanced views on various arguments.[2]

The demyelinating process involves patchy swelling of the myelin sheath followed by its breakdown (demyelination), leading to axonal degeneration. Microscopic foci coalesce with one another, giving the surface of the spinal cord (on cross-section) a spongy appearance; later there is secondary Wallerian degeneration of long tracts. Patchy demyelination usually begins in the dorsal columns in the thoracic segments of the spinal cord and then spreads *contiguously* to involve corticospinal tracts. These lesions spread throughout the length of the cord and ultimately involve spinothalamic and spinocerebellar tracts. There is also degeneration of the dorsal root ganglia, celiac ganglia, and Meissner and Auerbach plexus. Although demyelination may also extend to the white matter of the brain, it is unclear whether the peripheral neuropathy is caused by a distinct lesion or results from spinal cord disease; the clinical manifestations may be extremely varied.[1,2]

OTHER EFFECTS OF COBALAMIN AND FOLATE DEFICIENCY

Cobalamin deficiency more often than folate deficiency can also result in sterility from the effects on the gonads. An unexplained finding is generalized melanin pigmentation that is reversible by specific nutrient replenishment. Defective bactericidal activity and increased susceptibility to *Mycobacterium tuberculosis* occurs in cobalamin deficiency for poorly understood reasons.[1] The associations of folate deficiency with increased susceptibility to carcinogenesis, neural tube defects (NTDs), and hyperhomocysteinemia are discussed later in this chapter.

BIOCHEMICAL INDICATORS OF EVOLVING DEFICIENCY

Early clinically evaluable manifestations of negative cobalamin balance are increased serum methylmalonic acid (MMA) and total homocysteine levels.[2] This occurs when the total cobalamin in serum is still normal. Continued negative cobalamin balance leads to an absolute decrease in serum cobalamin level. Likewise, metabolic evidence for folate deficiency (ie, increased homocysteine level) is often found when serum folates are still in the low normal range. Metabolite tests reflective of decreased intracellular nutrient availability are also reflected by biochemical evidence of abnormal thymidylate synthesis (impaired conversion of dUMP to dTMP), morphologic expression of perturbed DNA in PMNs (lobe index), macroovalocytosis, and anemia. The biochemical basis for selective nutrient deficiency in various tissues (eg, cervical[2] or hematopoietic but not gastrointestinal cells[1]) is still unclear.

BIOCHEMICAL EVALUATION OF COBALAMIN AND FOLATE DEFICIENCIES

Total Serum Homocysteine and Methylmalonic Acid Levels

Cellular nutrient *deficiency* of cobalamin or folate is reflected by decreased intracellular concentrations. *Defective use* of cobalamin or folate because of intracellular cobalamin- or folate-dependent enzyme deficiency may allow normal intracellular coenzyme levels. Deficient coenzyme and enzyme levels are both reflected by perturbation of the major cobalamin- or folate-dependent enzyme-catalyzed reactions. The activity of methionine synthase is reduced, leading to substrate (homocysteine) buildup and to elevated serum levels of homocysteine, which can be measured by a sensitive assay.[2] In a classic series of studies, 77 of 78 patients with clinically confirmed cobalamin deficiency had elevated values of homocysteine, correlating with clinical parameters of cobalamin deficiency.[2] In this patient group, 74 of the 78 also had increased serum methylmalonic acid (MMA) levels, indicating reduced activity of the second cobalamin-dependent enzyme, methylmalonyl-CoA mutase, which converts methylmalonyl-CoA to succinyl-CoA. Similarly, 18 of 19 patients with folate deficiency had elevated levels of homocysteine due to reduced activity of the methionine synthase-catalyzed reaction.[2]

Both homocysteine and MMA levels are elevated in patients with dehydration and renal failure; propionic acid derived from anaerobic fecal bacterial metabolism can also contribute substantially to methylmalonate production.[4] In this setting, the gut flora contribution to MMA can be reduced by treatment with metronidazole.

Total homocysteine concentration, which comprises the sum of all homocysteine species in the plasma and serum, including free and

Total Serum Homocysteine and Methylmalonic Acid Levels in Cobalamin and Folate Deficiencies

The combined use of homocysteine and methylmalonic acid (MMA) levels can differentiate cobalamin from folate deficiency, because most patients with folate deficiency have normal MMA levels, and the remainder have only mild elevations.[2] These two tests are useful diagnostically. The abnormally high levels of metabolites return to normal only when the patient receives replacement with the appropriate (deficient) vitamin. A positive response to cobalamin, documented by falling levels of homocysteine and MMA, is evidence of cobalamin deficiency. Conversely, therapy with folate results in a decrease in the isolated homocysteine level if folate deficiency is present.[2] Indeed, because of several non–vitamin deficiency-related variables (such as age, mild renal dysfunction) that can falsely elevate serum homocysteine and MMA levels, proof of vitamin deficiency requires clear-cut demonstration of a reduction in metabolite levels after specific vitamin supplementation.[2,40]

If the serum cobalamin test is broadly used as a screening test, by virtue of the way *normalcy* is defined, 2.5% of nondeficient individuals will have low levels. Because many millions of individuals probably have serum cobalamin tests done every year, several thousand are found to have "low" cobalamin levels, which reflects our definition of the lower limit of normal for this test.[2]

The serum cobalamin concentration is less than 300 pg/mL in 99% of patients with clinical hematologic or neurologic manifestations of cobalamin deficiency.[2] Conversely, a cobalamin level of more than 300 pg/mL predicts folate deficiency or some other hematologic disease (Table 39–2). However, if the serum folate levels are borderline or normal and the patient has megaloblastic anemia with cobalamin levels more than 300 pg/mL, metabolite tests or a therapeutic trial may be necessary to rule out underlying folate deficiency.

How often do patients with cobalamin deficiency have normal cobalamin levels? Among 173 unambiguously cobalamin-deficient patients,[2] approximately 5% had normal cobalamin levels and up to 10% of adults with true cobalamin deficiency have cobalamin values in the low normal (200–300 pg/mL) range. Although traditionally such patients would have been regarded as not having cobalamin deficiency, they should be tested with the more sensitive metabolite tests (MMA and homocysteine), (Table 39–2). Studies have again highlighted the need to be vigilant for clinical and biochemical evidence of cobalamin deficiency in the elderly at "normal" cobalamin concentrations.[2] A study of 548 surviving members of the original Framingham Study revealed a prevalence of cobalamin deficiency of approximately 12%.[2] Nevertheless, approximately 90% of older patients with serum cobalamin levels less than 150 pmol/L show evidence of true tissue cobalamin deficiency.[2]

protein-bound forms, can be measured in the plasma or serum.[2,39] In general, plasma levels are slightly lower. The normal value for serum homocysteine is 5.1 to 13.9 μM and serum MMA is 73 to 271 nM, and in general, the higher the values, the more severe the clinical abnormalities.[2] However, there is a fairly wide range of "normalcy" in homocysteine values because of age-, creatinine-, gender-, diet-, and race-dependent variables.[39] Homocysteine is a continuous (progressive) risk factor for occlusive vascular disease (ie, higher levels predict higher risk) that is modifiable and likely causal; therefore, the lower the level, the better. Basal levels of MMA are usually less than 500 nM, and in renal failure, it rarely increases by more than 1000 nM.[2] If unseparated blood stands at room temperature, homocysteine levels will *increase* over 4 to 24 hours, but frozen serum (from measurements of serum folate or cobalamin) can be used for serum MMA and homocysteine determinations (See box on left and Table 39–2).

Table 39–1 Serum Cobalamin: False-Positive and False-Negative Test Results

Falsely Low Serum Cobalamin in the Absence of True Cobalamin Deficiency
Folate deficiency (one-third of patients)
Multiple myeloma
Transcobalamin I (TC I) deficiency
Megadose vitamin C therapy
Patient's serum contains other radioisotopes (^{99m}Tc or ^{67}Ga and other radiopharmaceuticals used in organ scanning)
Falsely Raised Cobalamin Levels in the Presence of a True Deficiency*
Cobalamin binders (TC I and II) increased (eg, myeloproliferative states, hepatomas, and fibrolamellar hepatic tumors)
TC II-producing macrophages are activated (eg, autoimmune diseases, monoblastic leukemias and lymphomas)
Release of cobalamin from hepatocytes (eg, active liver disease)

*Although a low serum cobalamin is not synonymous with cobalamin deficiency, 5% of patients with true cobalamin deficiency have low-normal cobalamin levels, a potentially serious problem because the patient's underlying cobalamin deficiency will progress if uncorrected.

Among 1160 elderly participants in the original Framingham Heart Study cohort, almost one-third had high plasma homocysteine levels that inversely correlated most with plasma folate levels and, to a lesser extent, with cobalamin and vitamin B_6 (ie, pyridoxine; pyridoxal-5′-phosphate is the active form).[2] Most cases of high homocysteine levels in the elderly can probably be attributed to low vitamin status.

Serum Cobalamin Levels

Serum cobalamin levels previously measured by microbiologic assay using the cobalamin-dependent organism *Lactobacillus leichmannii* have been replaced by a simpler assay method that relies on the competitive inhibition by serum cobalamin of the binding of CN-[^{57}Co]cobalamin (cyanocobalamin) to IF. Earlier, the use of R protein (which measures cobalamin analogs in addition to cobalamin) led to misleadingly higher serum cobalamin values that masked the presence of true cobalamin deficiency.[1,2] For the most part, serum cobalamin is an established biochemical indicator of cobalamin deficiency. However, a report of neuropsychiatric disorders attributed to cobalamin deficiency in some patients, despite the absence of anemia and normal or minimally depressed cobalamin levels, underscores the caution with which clinicians should proceed when interpreting this test.[2] A low serum cobalamin is not synonymous with cobalamin deficiency and several associated diseases and conditions can falsely raise or lower cobalamin levels (Table 39–1). Studies have also identified patients with true cobalamin deficiency who have cobalamin levels in the low normal range (see discussion in box on left).

Serum Folate Levels

Microbiologic assays of folate using *Lactobacillus casei* suffer from the same limitations as microbiological assays for cobalamin,[1] and these have been supplanted, primarily for convenience, by various radioisotope dilution or other biochemical assays. However, the clinical validity of these modifications has in many cases not been adequately documented.[1] There is also significant discrepancy in folate levels when a variety of kits are used on the same sample, raising questions about the reliability of these assays for clinical use, especially compared with microbiologic assays.[2]

Diagnosing Folate Deficiency

When combined with a clinical picture of megaloblastic anemia and additional results of low cobalamin levels, the serum folate concentration is the cheapest and most useful initial biochemical test to diagnose folate deficiency (Table 39–2).[2] The serum folate level is highly sensitive to folate intake, and a single hospital meal may normalize it in a patient with true folate deficiency. Rapidly developing nutritional folate deficiency first leads to a decline in the serum folate level below normal (less than 2 ng/mL) in approximately 3 weeks; it is a sensitive indicator of negative folate balance.[1] However, isolated reduction of serum folate in the absence of megaloblastosis (ie, false-positive result) occurs in one-third of hospitalized patients with anorexia, after acute alcohol consumption, during normal pregnancy, and in patients on anticonvulsants[2]; unfortunately, these are the very groups at high risk for folate deficiency and the people who exhibit low serum folate levels when they become folate deficient.[1] Conversely, in 25% to 50% of cases (predominantly alcoholics) with folate-deficient megaloblastosis, the serum folate levels may be low normal or borderline (2–4 ng/mL by radioisotope dilution assay).[2] The serum folate level alone should never dictate therapy. It is important to consider the clinical picture, peripheral smear, and bone marrow morphology and to rule out underlying cobalamin deficiency.

When negative folate balance continues, hepatic folate stores are depleted in approximately 4 months.[1] This leads to tissue folate deficiency, which was clinically correlated with a decrease in RBC folate (less than 150 ng/mL) by a microbiologic assay in the 1960s.[1] Thus, a reduction in serum and RBC folate in the setting of megaloblastic anemia was consistent with the diagnosis of folate deficiency using the older microbiologic RBC folate assays.[1] However, current RBC folate tests have major limitations in sensitivity and specificity and are notoriously unreliable in alcoholics and in pregnancy; furthermore, a reduction of RBC folate also occurs in approximately 60% of patients with cobalamin deficiency. By contrast, the serum folate level is falsely low less often (<10%) with cobalamin deficiency.

Other compelling evidence argues against the use of RBC folate in the diagnosis of folate deficiency. The original microbiologic assays for RBC folates have been replaced by radioassays currently used for measurement of *serum* folate levels. However, unlike the serum folate (which is entirely 5-methyl-tetrahydrofolate), RBC folates are a heterogeneous mixture of different coenzyme forms with various polyglutamate chain lengths that have different affinity for the FBP used in the radioassay kit for folates; whether this can affect net measurement of RBC folate content has not been experimentally clarified. Moreover, apart from a lack of clinical validation of the use of *radio*assays for measuring RBC folates (ie, they have not been adequately validated against actual patients with normal and deficient folate status), the assays themselves have had a long history of being unreliable.[2] A quality assurance study from Australia involving 134 laboratories identified nine operator-controllable factors that could also lead to poor RBC folate results.[2] An analysis of its clinical value led to the conclusion that RBC folate tests added little useful information to that provided by serum folate levels.[2] Together, these clinically relevant issues have considerably dampened the enthusiasm for use of RBC folate tests and have led several experts in the United States to entirely avoid their use pending a resolution of these multiple problems (see Table 39–2).[2] Parenthetically, it should be noted that the large clinical trials that rely on measurement of RBC folates use a single commercial kit for their studies that allows for direct comparison of RBC folate values among study subjects; however, this is not the real-world situation, where a variety of RBC folate kits are available and where there has been proven inaccuracy among several of them. This is the reason why the measurement of serum folate is preferred over RBC folates as the initial test for evaluation of folate deficiency.

Summary of the Clinical Usefulness of Tests for Cobalamin and Folate Deficiencies

The greater sensitivity of MMA and homocysteine test results (than of cobalamin) are best illustrated in patients with pernicious anemia who do not receive cobalamin for some time; the levels of MMA and homocysteine progressively increase much earlier than the drop in cobalamin levels.[2] Overlooking true cobalamin deficiency is highly unlikely when the two metabolites are measured, because one or both metabolites was increased in 99.8% of more than 400 patients with proven cobalamin deficiency.[2] These serum tests (MMA and homocysteine) are the gold standard for the diagnosis of cobalamin deficiency.

On the basis of the lower costs of serum cobalamin and folate compared with serum MMA and total serum homocysteine levels, it is recommended (see Table 39–2) to first use the cheaper tests that can assist in the diagnosis of the most obvious cases of cobalamin and folate deficiency.[2] Clinicians should also restrict the use of serum MMA and homocysteine to patients with borderline cobalamin and folate levels; to patients with existing conditions associated with difficulties in the interpretation of test results; to situations in which cobalamin and folate levels are low, when a high MMA level is useful in confirming cobalamin deficiency (rather than attributing the condition to folate deficiency alone); and to patients with clearly low serum levels but for whom there is an alternative explanation for the findings that caused an unusual serum cobalamin level to be obtained (eg, a diabetic or alcoholic with peripheral neuropathy, an alcoholic with a high MCV and a low serum cobalamin without anemia). In these cases, serum levels of metabolites can assist in the diagnosis of vitamin deficiency.

Diagnostic algorithms consistently stress the value of clinical data to improve the pretest probability of serum cobalamin and serum folate tests.[2] Without detailed clinical information, the combined test results for serum cobalamin, folate, and metabolites (homocysteine and MMA) are not sufficiently unambiguous to diagnose and distinguish cobalamin deficiency from combined cobalamin-plus-folate deficiency. In combined cobalamin-plus-folate deficiency, both vitamins would be needed to restore baseline values particularly of homocysteine.[2] In the context of diagnosing a subclinical deficiency of cobalamin (or folate) based on increased serum levels of MMA or homocysteine, or both, despite normal serum cobalamin (or folate) levels, positive attribution can be confidently made only after the demonstrated reversal of laboratory values after treatment with cobalamin or folate, or both.[2] This is similar in principle to that used to confirm clinically significant nutrient deficiency.[2,40,41]

Other Tests

The use of low holo-transcobalamin II (holo-TCII) levels to diagnose cobalamin deficiency is still under evaluation to identify its proper niche within the diagnostic algorithm for cobalamin deficiency.[42] Although holo-TCII is an early marker of cobalamin homeostasis,[43] it cannot be used as a marker to diagnose cobalamin malabsorption or as a surrogate for the Schilling test,[44] neither can it be used to displace the use of metabolite measurements to define the cause of cobalamin deficiency in routine clinical use. There is insufficient clinical data to support the routine use of a urinary MMA test.[2]

Table 39–2 Approach to the Diagnosis of Cobalamin and Folate Deficiencies

Megaloblastic Anemia or Neurologic–Psychiatric Manifestations Consistent with Cobalamin Deficiency Plus Test Results for Serum Cobalamin and Serum Folate

Cobalamin[†] *(pg/mL)*	*Folate*[‡] *(ng/mL)*	*Provisional Diagnosis*	*Proceed with Metabolites?*
>300	>4	Cobalamin or folate deficiency is unlikely	No
<200	>4	Consistent with cobalamin deficiency	No
200–300	>4	Rule out cobalamin deficiency	Yes
>300	<2	Consistent with folate deficiency	No
<200	<2	Consistent with (1) combined cobalamin plus folate deficiency or (2) isolated folate deficiency	Yes
>300	2–4	Consistent with (1) folate deficiency or (2) an anemia unrelated to vitamin deficiency	Yes

Test Results for Metabolites: Serum Methylmalonic Acid and Total Homocysteine[§]

Methylmalonic Acid (Normal = 70–270 nM)	*Total Homocysteine (Normal = 5–14 μM)*	*Diagnosis*
Increased	Increased	Cobalamin deficiency is confirmed; folate deficiency still possible
Normal	Increased	Folate deficiency is likely; <5% may have cobalamin deficiency
Normal	Normal	Cobalamin and folate deficiency is excluded

[†]Serum cobalamin levels: abnormally low, <200 pg/mL; clinically relevant low-normal range, 200–300 pg/mL.
[‡]Serum folate levels: abnormally low, <2 ng/mL; clinically relevant low-normal range, 2–4 ng/mL.
[§]Any frozen-over sample from a serum folate or cobalamin determination can be subjected to metabolite tests.

PATHOGENESIS OF COBALAMIN DEFICIENCY

Nutritional Cobalamin Deficiency Because of Insufficient Intake

Vegetarian diets can be classified as lacto-vegetarian, ovo-vegetarian, lacto-ovo-vegetarian, or vegan, respectively, if they include dairy products, eggs, dairy products and eggs, or no animal products at all.[5] Vegan diets contain a very low cobalamin content, warranting routine cobalamin supplementation. Studies over the past five decades have consistently demonstrated that asymptomatic lacto-ovo-vegetarians and lacto-vegetarians[5] also have low cobalamin levels when compared with nonvegetarians, but it was difficult to characterize this as a cobalamin-deficient state (implying disease). However, new evidence[45] suggests that such individuals have increased blood total homocysteine and MMA levels consistent with biochemical evidence for cobalamin deficiency. Ultimate proof of deficiency must be based on complete normalization of abnormal test results after specific vitamin replacement.[40] Nevertheless, all of the earlier studies using cobalamin levels as an indicator of cobalamin status raise the likelihood (confirmed recently)[45] that those "normal" asymptomatic subjects would have been found to be cobalamin deficient had more sophisticated metabolite tests been employed.[5] Because one-half or more of those with metabolically defined mild, preclinical cobalamin deficiency[2] have abnormalities in electroencephalographic, evoked potential, and electrophysiologic markers of cognitive ability, this strongly supports a causal relationship between subtle neurologic problems associated with otherwise "asymptomatic" cobalamin deficiency.

There are two closely related groups whose diets are quite similar and who exhibit clinical and biochemical evidence of dietary cobalamin deficiency: voluntary vegetarians who base their dietary preferences on religious or philosophical grounds (many among the Indian population) and poverty-imposed near-vegetarians who live in developing countries worldwide. The latter are nonvegetarians who consume meat infrequently (because it is more expensive than plant protein) and when consumed, the serving portions of meat are also meager. These poverty-imposed near-vegetarians have a cobalamin status that is only marginally better than lacto-ovo-vegetarians.[5] Thus, as many as 700 to 800 million Indians who are life-long vegetarians or near-vegetarians could have low cobalamin status in addition to the untold millions of poor in two parts of the developing world subjected to poverty-imposed near-vegetarianism. Thus worldwide, the commonest cause of cobalamin deficiency among all ages is likely to be nutritional insufficiency. But in the West, where regular consumption of cobalamin-rich foods such as meat is common, food-cobalamin malabsorption especially among the elderly is probably the commonest cause of cobalamin deficiency [Inadequate Dissociation of Cobalamin From Food Protein (Food-Cobalamin Malabsorption)].

Infants born of cobalamin-depleted vegetarian mothers are at risk for cobalamin deficiency, especially if they receive prolonged breast-feeding. An "infantile tremor syndrome" is found exclusively among breast-fed infants of mothers who come from extremely low socioeconomic conditions in developing countries.[5] Within a background of apparently adequate general nutrition, these infants exhibit apathy, megaloblastic anemia, skin pigmentation, involuntary movements, and developmental regression that is rapidly corrected by cobalamin. Similar cases have been described in the West. Whereas the fetus depends on the mother for cobalamin,[1,2] the longer the mother has been vegetarian, the greater the likelihood she will have low maternal serum and breast milk cobalamin concentrations that closely correlate with cobalamin insufficiency in the infant.[46]

A longitudinal cohort study has documented that infants fed a macrobiotic (vegan-like with occasional servings of fish) diet[2] must be rapidly replenished with supplemental cobalamin before switching to a cobalamin-rich diet. Otherwise, up to 20% continue to have low cobalamin status.[2] This can lead to impaired psychomotor functioning well into youth and later adolescence with compromise in faculties related to reasoning, abstract thinking, and learning ability.[47]

Reports on nutritional macrocytic anemia identified cobalamin deficiency as the basis for anemia in up to 50% of cases of Indian children 6 months to 12 years old,[5] and 20% of anemic children 3 months to 3 years old in an urban Indian slum had cobalamin deficiency by serum levels.[2] It is likely that metabolite testing would have picked up many more asymptomatic cobalamin-deficient children. Parallel results come from studies on Guatemalan women.[2] Further evaluation of Guatemalan children indicates that they too continue to have low cobalamin status through dietary insufficiency alone or combined with as yet uncharacterized gastrointestinal cobalamin malabsorption.[48] The risk of a lower cognitive and neuromotor performance is real among children with low cobalamin status.[2,22] Reasoning, short-term memory, and perception were poorer than in the adequate-cobalamin group.[2,22] Guatemalan children represent the category of poverty-imposed near-vegetarianism that is prevalent throughout the developing world. Therefore cobalamin deficiency in children fed vegetarian diets, as with poverty-imposed near-vegetarianism, has very significant worldwide health implications. The fact that there is clear-cut biochemical evidence of perturbed cobalamin metabolism in vegetarians[45] and that hyperhomocysteinemia is a risk factor for several diseases (discussed later) suggests that vegetarians should be routinely taking inexpensive (generic) cobalamin supplements.[5]

Poverty afflicts approximately one-third of the Indian subcontinent,[2] and a World Bank report[2] on the crisis of malnutrition in India highlighted the fact that one-half of all children younger than 4 years are malnourished, 30% of all newborns are underweight, and 60% of all women are anemic. Any discussion of vegetarianism and cobalamin deficiency in developing countries immediately raises the question of whether folate deficiency—which consistently accompanies poverty and malnutrition—has become an uncommon cause of megaloblastic anemia. Although some studies suggest this is the case,[2] there remain nagging questions as to whether such patients had combined cobalamin-plus-folate deficiency.[2,40] This remains unresolved because testing using metabolites before and after cobalamin replacement has not been carried out in these populations.[5]

INTRAGASTRIC EVENTS LEADING TO COBALAMIN MALABSORPTION

Inadequate Dissociation of Cobalamin From Food Protein (Food-Cobalamin Malabsorption)

Dietary cobalamin is bioavailable only after proteolytic digestion of food by gastric acid and pepsin. Failure to release cobalamin from food protein can present as cobalamin deficiency even though gastric analysis reveals the presence of IF.[2] Some older patients (over 50 years of age) with atrophic gastritis or partial gastrectomy with hypochlorhydria have low serum cobalamin levels and normal absorption of crystalline cobalamin. Although they have poor absorption of CN-[^{57}Co]cobalamin that is incorporated into food as a "food cobalamin" absorption test,[2] this test is not standardized for general clinical use.

Among a cohort of patients (median age 76 years) with food-cobalamin malabsorption (who had normal stage I Schilling tests),[49] the clinical spectrum included neurologic or psychologic impairment with mild sensory polyneuropathy (nearly among one-half), with confusion or impaired mental functioning and physical asthenia (among one-fifth). There were mild hematologic changes (in one-third). Although there was improvement in hematologic changes among two-thirds, only one-third had improved peripheral neuropathy.

Congenital Intrinsic Factor Deficiency

Congenital IF deficiency, transmitted as an autosomal recessive trait and expressed in homozygotes by the age of 2 years, is characterized by a pure IF deficiency without other gastric abnormalities. Only approximately 40 cases have been described; affected children present with irritability, vomiting, diarrhea, and loss of weight with megaloblastic anemia. Except for the absence of IF in gastric juice, gastric histology and function are normal.[1] Mutations in the gastric IF are the basis for hereditary intrinsic factor deficiency (less than 100 cases reported).[50]

Loss or Atrophy of Gastric Oxyntic Mucosa

IF deficiency arising from atrophy of gastric parietal (oxyntic) mucosal cells must be associated with parallel insufficient HCl secretion and can be caused by total or partial gastrectomy; autoimmune destruction as observed in adult addisonian pernicious anemia or, rarely, in a similar disease in children (juvenile pernicious anemia); and destruction of gastric mucosa by caustic (lye) ingestion.

Total gastrectomy that results in removal of IF-producing cells invariably leads to cobalamin deficiency in approximately 5 years (range 2–10 years). This condition is often associated with iron deficiency (dimorphic anemia),[1] warranting routine cobalamin and iron replacement prophylactically.

Cobalamin deficiency is observed in only 10% to 20% of patients 8 years after partial gastrectomy, although 30% have cobalamin malabsorption[1]; up to 6% of these cobalamin-deficient patients will develop frank clinical manifestations of cobalamin deficiency with megaloblastic anemia. The cause is multifactorial, and contributing factors include decreased IF secretion, hypochlorhydria (from atrophy of residual oxyntic mucosal cells), intestinal bacterial overgrowth of cobalamin-consuming organisms, associated nutritional folate deficiency in 20%, and iron deficiency in approximately 50%. The degree of cobalamin deficiency depends on the size of the remaining gastric remnant. It is more common in Bilroth II than in Bilroth I surgery, in subtotal than in partial gastrectomy, and in gastric rather than duodenal peptic ulcer disease. Morbidly obese patients treated surgically with gastric bypass also have more food-cobalamin malabsorption than patients treated with vertical banded gastroplasty.[2]

Absent Intrinsic Factor Secretion and Pernicious Anemia

The most common cause of cobalamin malabsorption is pernicious anemia, a disease of unknown origin in which the fundamental defect is atrophy of the gastric (parietal cell) oxyntic mucosa eventually leading to the absence of IF and HCl secretion. Because cobalamin is only absorbed by binding to IF and uptake by ileal IF–cobalamin receptors, the net consequence is severe cobalamin malabsorption leading to cobalamin deficiency.

The annual incidence of pernicious anemia is approximately 25 new cases per 100,000 persons older than 40 years. Although the average age of onset is approximately 60 years, it is increasingly encountered in persons 5 to 10 years younger.[1] Pernicious anemia is not a respecter of age, race, or ethnic origin. The predisposition to developing pernicious anemia may have a genetic basis but neither the mode of inheritance nor the initiating event or primary mechanism is precisely understood. There is a positive family history for approximately 30% of patients, among whom the risk of familial pernicious anemia is 20 times as high as in the general population; approximately 20% of siblings of patients are projected to develop pernicious anemia by the age of 90 years. Pernicious anemia developing concordantly in identical twins has been documented.

There is a significant association of pernicious anemia with other autoimmune diseases[1] (ie, the polyglandular autoimmune syndrome characterized by multiple endocrine hypofunction with antibodies to endogenous endocrine glands). Pernicious anemia is associated with Graves disease (30%), Hashimoto thyroiditis (11%), vitiligo (8%), Addison disease, idiopathic hypoparathyroidism, primary ovarian failure, myasthenia gravis, insulin-dependent diabetes, and adult hypogammaglobulinemia.[1,2] Autoimmune gastritis (leading to chronic atrophic gastritis) associated with pernicious anemia involves the fundus and body of the stomach. The histologic appearance of the gastric mucosa (infiltration with plasma cells and lymphocytes) is also strongly reminiscent of autoimmune-type lesions. There is also a high incidence of anti–parietal cell IgG antibodies in the serum of 90% of patients with pernicious anemia. The major antigen to which antibodies from patients with autoimmune gastritis and pernicious anemia are directed is the acid-producing enzyme H^+/K^+ ATPase (a 92-kd protein, the target of proton pump inhibitors), found on the membrane of parietal cells.[2] The precise interplay of the various mechanisms for anti–parietal cell IgG-mediated dysfunction of parietal cells remains to be shown in vivo. Anti-IF antibodies are found in the serum of approximately 60% of patients with pernicious anemia and in the gastric juice of 75%; approximately 90% of patients with pernicious anemia have anti-IF antibodies in serum or gastric juice.[1] Similar IF antibodies are quite rare in the general population. Thus, anti-IF antibodies are highly specific and confirmatory for pernicious anemia, but their absence does not rule out the condition. The assay for anti-IF blocking antibodies depends on the displacement of CN-[^{57}Co]cobalamin binding to IF in vitro. This can be significantly affected by prior injection of cobalamin (as given with a Schilling test) or by radioactive isotopes from other diagnostic tests.

There are two types of IF antibodies. Type I antibodies are directed to the cobalamin-binding site on IF and are usually of IgG subclass in the serum. In gastric secretions, they may be both IgG and secretory IgA subclasses. Type II IF antibodies bind to the IF–cobalamin complex and prevent binding to ileal IF–cobalamin receptors. Type II antibodies, usually not seen in the absence of type I antibodies, are found in approximately 35% of patients with pernicious anemia, although studies using a technique that detects both antibodies indicates a higher prevalence than previously documented.[2] Because of their functional properties, these intraluminal anti-IF antibodies may hasten development of pernicious anemia and interfere with tests for cobalamin absorption.[1]

The corticosteroid responsiveness in some patients with pernicious anemia (ie, regeneration of atrophic gastric mucosa and increased IF secretion antedating a decrease in anti-IF antibodies) also implicates an autoimmune pathogenesis of pernicious anemia.[1] The clustering of parietal cell dysfunction among first-degree relatives of patients with pernicious anemia (in inbred populations), the fact that some individuals (96% of African American women with pernicious anemia) have high titers of blocking anti-IF antibodies but lack anti–parietal cell antibodies,[1] and the fact that neither antibody may be detected in patients with pernicious anemia and acquired agammaglobulinemia all suggest that the pathogenesis of pernicious anemia is heterogeneous.

Juvenile pernicious anemia manifests in the second decade with severe cobalamin deficiency in conjunction with many of the associated endocrinopathies and autoantibodies observed in adults.[1] Why these patients present so much earlier with an apparently identical disease is unknown. Taken together, these facts suggest that although there is a genetic predisposition to pernicious anemia, the full expression of the disease, which appears to have an autoimmune basis, may be modified by acquired environmental influences.

Undiagnosed pernicious anemia is common among the free-living elderly (over 60 years)[2] who have only minimal clinical manifestations of cobalamin deficiency (ie, 1.9% of the survey population had unrecognized and untreated pernicious anemia). The prevalence was 2.7% in women and 1.4% in men, but 4.3% of the African American women and 4.0% of the white women had pernicious anemia. If these findings can be extrapolated, approximately 800,000 elderly people in the United States may have undiagnosed pernicious anemia.

In the absence of a Schilling test (which is currently not available in the United States), one-half of those with pernicious anemia can be diagnosed using serum anti-IF antibodies. The other half with pernicious anemia and negative antibodies and those with suspected food-cobalamin malabsorption (with no other obvious causes of malabsorption) are clinically indistinguishable. Fortunately, both these types of individuals can be successfully treated with oral cobalamin (over 1000 μg/day) in the long term (discussed later in Therapy).

Abnormal Intrinsic Factor Molecules

In three siblings, a defective IF molecule was identified by age 2 years that was identical to IF in all but one respect: it was markedly susceptible to acid and proteolytic enzyme (pepsin or trypsin) digestion, resulting in defective cobalamin absorption by ileal IF–cobalamin receptors and megaloblastic anemia.[1] In another case, an abnormal IF molecule having a 60-fold lower binding affinity for ileal IF–cobalamin receptors resulted in lower (but not absent) cobalamin absorption, probably accounting for the delayed clinical presentation with cobalamin deficiency at the age of 13 years.[1]

ABNORMAL EVENTS IN THE SMALL BOWEL LUMEN: IMPAIRED TRANSFER OF COBALAMIN FROM R PROTEIN TO INTRINSIC FACTOR

Insufficient Pancreatic Protease

Because approximately 30% of patients with severe pancreatic insufficiency fail to degrade R proteins, there is no transfer of food cobalamin to IF and consequent cobalamin malabsorption (R-cobalamin does not bind ileal IF–cobalamin receptors). R proteins are highly susceptible to proteolysis by even small quantities of pancreatic protease released in response to food. In partial insufficiency, there is abnormal absorption of CN-[^{57}Co]cobalamin on an empty stomach but normal absorption when the CN-[^{57}Co]cobalamin is given with food. Administration of pancreatic extract normalizes cobalamin malabsorption in those with complete pancreatic insufficiency.[1]

Inactivation of Pancreatic Protease

Pancreatic protease can be inactivated by massive gastric hypersecretion arising from a gastrinoma in Zollinger–Ellison syndrome.[1] The continued low pH of the luminal contents reaching the ileum may also perturb interaction of the IF–cobalamin complex with IF–cobalamin receptors (which requires a pH above 5.4).

Usurpation of Luminal Cobalamin

The near-sterile condition of the small bowel is maintained by a combination of the mechanical cleansing action of peristalsis and the chemical action of gastric acid. Disorders conducive to relative stasis, impaired motility, and hypogammaglobulinemia are predisposing factors favoring colonization by bacteria. Many of these bacteria take up free cobalamin, whereas the uptake of IF-bound cobalamin is markedly diminished. However, if colonization extends proximally to the locus at which IF and cobalamin interact, significant cobalamin may be usurped before it can bind to IF.[1] This cobalamin malabsorption can be corrected to some extent by a 7- to 10-day course of antibiotic therapy; definitive surgical correction may be indicated if the patient has significant symptoms (weight loss and diarrhea) that are only partially relieved by antibiotics. The malabsorption of food cobalamin in patients with atrophic gastritis has also been normalized with antibiotics, thereby incriminating bacterial usurpation of food cobalamin at a very proximal level.[2]

Approximately 3% of individuals infested with the fish tapeworm *Diphyllobothrium latum* develop frank cobalamin deficiency. In the life cycle of this parasite, tapeworm eggs passed in human feces embryonate in cool freshwater; the ciliated embryos are then swallowed by cyclops, which are the first intermediate host. After burrowing into the body cavity of the cyclops, they mature into the procercoid larval stage. The hapless cyclops (now infected with procercoids) are then swallowed by freshwater fish (eg, pike, perch, trout, and salmon found in lakes in Russia, Japan, Switzerland, Germany, and North America), and procercoids then migrate into the fish's flesh (ie, second plerocercoid larval stage). Humans become infected when they eat partially cooked or raw fish containing plerocercoids that develop into adult worms in approximately 6 weeks, growing to a length of 10 m, with up to 4000 proglottids[1]; when these worms lay eggs, the life cycle is repeated. In a given patient, the degree of cobalamin deficiency is probably related to the number and extent to which worms lodge proximal to ileal IF–cobalamin receptors. They are commonly found in the jejunum; poised in this strategic location, they avidly usurp cobalamin for growth.[1] After ova have been identified in the stools, expulsion of the worms by praziquantel (10–20 mg/kg as a single dose taken orally) and cobalamin replenishment is invariably curative.

DISORDERS OF ILEAL INTRINSIC FACTOR-COBALAMIN RECEPTORS OR MUCOSA

Absence of Intrinsic Factor–Cobalamin Receptors

The distal ileum has the greatest density of IF–cobalamin receptors, and removal of only 1 to 2 feet of terminal ileum by resection or bypass can reduce ileal IF–cobalamin receptor numbers or interaction with IF–cobalamin, respectively, to result in cobalamin malabsorption.[1,2] Ileal bypass or diseased ileal architecture may lead to reduction in transenterocytic transport of cobalamin, which is treatable with parenteral cobalamin replacement.

Defective Intrinsic Factor–Cobalamin Receptors or Post-Intrinsic Factor–Cobalamin Receptor Defects

Imerslund–Gräsbeck syndrome is a term used collectively for a heterogeneous group of congenital disorders in children involving selective cobalamin malabsorption that cannot be corrected by the administration of IF and that lead to megaloblastic anemias and low serum cobalamin associated with mild, persistent, benign, proteinuria (in 90% of cases). There have only been approximately 250 cases described worldwide. There is recessive inheritance, early onset (between 3 and 10 years), pallor, fatigue, anorexia, and failure to thrive, associated with frequent infections and bruising (from pancytopenia). In addition, there have also been variable neurologic symptoms such as cognitive problems, peripheral neuropathy, and dementia among these patients. These children have normal IF. It has now been shown that biallelic mutations in either the cubulin (*CUBN*) or amnionless (*AMN*) genes—whose gene products combine tightly to form the functional IF–cobalamin receptor[51] (now also called cubam)—are the cause of Imerslund–Gräsbeck syndrome. Because cubam also participates in the renal tubular absorption of several other proteins, this is the basis for proteinuria found in Imerslund–Gräsbeck syndrome. Interestingly, in Finland, all cases of Imerslund–Gräsbeck syndrome were found to be due to mutations in cubulin, whereas in Norway, the cases involved mutations in amnionless.[52] Because the radiocobalamin (Schilling) test is not available in many countries and without this test hereditary IF deficiency is indistinguishable from Imerslund–Gräsbeck syndrome, the only way to distinguish between these is through the analysis of mutational status of *CUBN* and *AMN* genes.[53]

Drug-Induced Defects

H_2 antagonists, but not proton pump inhibitors, inhibit IF secretion.[2] However, malabsorption of food-cobalamin from long-term omeprazole has been reported.[2] Biguanides (ie, metformin) appear to decrease IF and acid secretion in healthy volunteers; they also inhibit transenterocytic transport of cobalamin in 7%.[1] The latter is presumed to be caused by the displacement of calcium, which is required for the normal interaction of IF–cobalamin with the IF–cobalamin receptor. Because many diabetics take metformin, this could lead to a significant problem; fortunately, increased intake of calcium (1.2 g/day) can reverse the cobalamin malabsorption.[54] Other drugs (eg, Slow-K, cholestyramine, colchicine, neomycin) probably also impair transepithelial transport of cobalamin[1]; these drugs can interfere with the Schilling test.

DISORDERS OF PLASMA COBALAMIN TRANSPORT

Absence of Transcobalamin I and Transcobalamin III

Congenital R-protein deficiency is not associated with cellular cobalamin deficiency. However, because approximately 80% of serum cobalamin is bound to TC I, the serum cobalamin levels are invariably low with normal MMA and homocysteine levels. Two of six patients in one study developed a biochemically uncharacterized neurologic syndrome, which led to speculation that TC III deficiency might result in the inability to clear cobalamin analogs that may have a pathogenic role in the neurologic dysfunction.[1]

Deficiency of Transcobalamin II

Megaloblastic anemia in infancy associated with normal cobalamin levels is the characteristic clinical presentation when TC II is absent or markedly deficient. The impairment in intestinal absorption of cobalamin in such patients is also caused by the absence of TC II, which plays an important role in binding cobalamin within the enterocyte before its entry into the circulation. In all, approximately 30 patients have been described.[2] They can be successfully treated by daily or biweekly injections of 1 mg of cobalamin, which ensures passive cobalamin delivery into cells.

Defective Transcobalamin II

Defective TC II can be diagnosed when the amount of TC II measured by radioimmunoassay is normal but there is a qualitative abnormality based on its inability to bind cobalamin.[1] Conversely, in another patient with normal amounts of TC II by radioimmunoassay, the TC II was functionally active in binding cobalamin but unable to facilitate the uptake of cobalamin into cells.[1]

Clinical correlations of various polymorphisms among proteins involved in cobalamin metabolism are still under scrutiny to define if there are populations who are more susceptible to cobalamin deficiency and who may benefit from cobalamin supplementation. In most instances, these polymorphisms result in minor elevations in homocysteine that are clinically insignificant.[55]

DISORDERS OF INTRACELLULAR COBALAMIN USE

Congenital Metabolic Defects of Cobalamin Metabolism: Cobalamin Mutants A–F

The combination of megaloblastic anemia with increased levels of homocysteine or MMA, or both, in serum and urine despite normal cobalamin and folate levels should suggest an inborn error of cobalamin metabolism.[2,50] The inherited defects of cobalamin use (see Fig. 39–3) are heterogeneous and are empirically defined as cobalamin mutations A to G (*cblA* to *cblG*) through the use of complementation studies involving in vitro fusion of cultured mutant fibroblasts obtained from skin biopsies. Mutants involving the synthesis of adenosylcobalamin within the mitochondria involve defects in the reduction of cob(II)alamin to cob(I)alamin (*cblA*) and of cob(I)alamin to adenosylcobalamin by adenosylcobalamin transferase (*cblB*). These defects result in an accumulation of excess MMA. The clinical picture in infancy is dominated by acidosis and ketosis associated with lethargy, failure to thrive, vomiting, dehydration, respiratory distress, hepatomegaly, and coma. Biochemical evidence of methylmalonic acidemia, ketonemia, and ketonuria without megaloblastosis is found. Because some of these defects are incomplete, treatment with large doses of cobalamin may alleviate the defect.[2,50] Defects involving conversion of cob(III)alamin to cob(II)alamin (*cblC, cblD*) present with combined evidence of reduced activity of methylmalonyl-CoA mutase and methionine synthase (ie, with increased homocysteine and MMA in blood and urine).[2,50] These patients have prominent neuropsychiatric problems with mental retardation, microcephaly, psychosis, delirium, and retinopathy with megaloblastosis. The *cblC* mutants have hemolytic uremic syndrome as an integral manifestation of the spectrum of this disorder.[2] Although the disorder usually manifests in infancy, some patients manifest problems in later childhood. Hydroxocobalamin [cob(III)alamin] appears to be more effective than cyanocobalamin in these patients. *cblE* (distinguished by the lack of increase in MMA) is thought to be a defect arising from the inability to maintain cobalamin bound to methionine synthase in its reduced state.[1] The *cblF* mutation is caused by an inability of cobalamin to be transported from the lysosome into the cytoplasm.[2] *cblG* patients have defects in methionine synthase activity.[2] Among patients with mutant *cblG* defects, one patient presenting at the age of 21 years with a multiple sclerosis-like syndrome was initially undiagnosed simply because the serum cobalamin level and studies of cobalamin absorption were normal.[2] This suggests that adults presenting with cerebral, myelopathic, or neuropathic disturbances (occasionally masquerading as multiple sclerosis) should be screened for such defects in specialized laboratories. The retardation of myelination in a small series of infants with congenital disorders of cobalamin metabolism[56] and dramatic reversal with cobalamin on cranial MRI indicates the possibility of reversibility with early diagnosis and treatment with cobalamin.

Functional Cobalamin Deficiency after Nitrous Oxide Exposure

Nitrous oxide (N_2O) inactivates coenzyme forms of cobalamin by oxidizing the fully reduced cob(I)alamin to cob(III)alamin; this results in a state of functional intracellular cobalamin deficiency. This syndrome was first identified in patients with tetanus given N_2O for up to 6 days.[1] Subsequently, persons exposed to N_2O for open heart surgery and through chronic (surreptitious, accidental, or occupational) exposure have been recognized as being at a high risk for developing megaloblastosis and cobalamin-deficient neuromyelopathy.[1] Although megaloblastosis develops within 24 hours and lasts less than 1 week after a single exposure, the neurologic syndrome is usually seen with chronic intermittent exposure. However, severe neurologic deficits have been reported after prolonged intraoperative exposure to N_2O in patients with unsuspected cobalamin deficiency.[2] The integrity of the methionine synthase-catalyzed reaction can be tested by measuring the serum homocysteine concentration, even after 75 minutes of exposure during surgery.[2] Reduced enzyme activity explains the metabolic block, which can be bypassed by 5-formyl-tetrahydrofolate (ie, leucovorin). No screening is routinely carried out for elderly patients who are placed under anesthesia with N_2O, despite the fact that subclinical cobalamin deficiency exists among 15% to 20% of them in some series, and despite the recognition that those with frank cobalamin deficiency can suffer adversely with postoperative cognitive and other neurologic dysfunction following exposure to N_2O.[2,57] Whether individuals with subclinical cobalamin deficiency are indeed at risk for postoperative cognitive dysfunction remains to be defined.

CLINICAL EVALUATION OF COBALAMIN ABSORPTION

The Schilling Test

With rare exceptions, adults with cobalamin deficiency have cobalamin malabsorption (from pernicious anemia, food-cobalamin malabsorption, infestation with *D. latum*, bacterial overgrowth, or ileal malabsorption) or, in vegetarians, dietary cobalamin insufficiency. All of these conditions can be treated similarly with monthly parenteral cobalamin or daily oral cobalamin (discussed later in this chapter in Therapy). Because information on the cause and locus of cobalamin deficiency does not appear to alter or direct therapy with cobalamin, does the identification of the locus of cobalamin malabsorption make any difference to the outcome in adults? (That is, should a Schilling test be done at all?) Two compelling arguments in favor of the Schilling test are that the test results can suggest additional diagnostic tests (eg, intestinal biopsy, examination of stool for malabsorption, *D. latum* infestation) and specific therapy (eg, gluten-free diet, folate, antibiotics, antihelminthics) and that it can identify the potential for reversibility and thereby dictate the duration of cobalamin replacement.

Etiopathophysiologic Classification of Cobalamin Deficiency

I. Nutritional cobalamin deficiency (ie, insufficient cobalamin intake)
   A. Vegetarians, poverty-imposed near-vegetarians, breast-fed infants of mothers with pernicious anemia
II. Abnormal intragastric events (ie, inadequate proteolysis of food cobalamin)
   A. Atrophic gastritis, partial gastritis with hypochlorhydria, proton-pump inhibitors, H_2 blockers
III. Loss or atrophy of gastric oxyntic mucosa (ie, deficient intrinsic factor [IF] molecules)
   A. Total or partial gastrectomy, pernicious anemia, caustic destruction (lye)
IV. Abnormal events in small bowel lumen
   A. Inadequate pancreatic protease (eg, R-cobalamin not degraded, cobalamin not transferred to IF)
      1. Insufficient pancreatic protease (ie, pancreatic insufficiency)
      2. Inactivation of pancreatic protease (ie, Zollinger-Ellison syndrome)
   B. Usurping of luminal cobalamin (ie, inadequate cobalamin binding to IF)
      1. By bacteria, during stasis syndromes (eg, blind loops, pouches of diverticulosis, strictures, fistulas, anastomosis), impaired bowel motility (eg, scleroderma), hypogammaglobulinemia
      2. By *Diphyllobothrium latum* (fish tapeworm)
V. Disorders of ileal mucosa/IF–cobalamin receptors (ie, IF–cobalamin not bound to IF–cobalamin receptors)
   A. Diminished or absent IF–cobalamin receptors (eg, ileal bypass, resection, fistula)
   B. Abnormal mucosal architecture/function (eg, tropical or nontropical sprue, Crohn disease, tuberculosis ileitis, infiltration by lymphomas, amyloidosis)
   C. IF-/post-IF–cobalamin receptor defects (eg, Imerslund–Gräsbeck syndrome, transcobalamin II [TC II] deficiency)
   D. Drug effects (eg, slow K, metformin, cholestyramine, colchicine, neomycin)
VI. Disorders of plasma cobalamin transport (ie, TC II–cobalamin not delivered to TC II receptors)
   A. Congenital TC II deficiency, defective binding of TC II–cobalamin to TC II receptors (rare)
VII. Metabolic disorders (ie, cobalamin not used by cells)
   A. Inborn enzyme errors (rare)
   B. Acquired disorders (eg, cobalamin functionally inactivated by irreversible oxidation, N_2O inhalation)

Nevertheless, given the current lack of availability of the Schilling test, the default option is to give cobalamin replacement at a dose of 2000 μg/day (orally) for adult cobalamin deficiency from any cause. (If there are clinical or metabolic abnormalities arising from longstanding cobalamin deficiency, the patient would be best served by initial parenteral therapy with cobalamin to rapidly replenish stores.) The same approach may not be appropriate in the case of children with congenital cobalamin deficiency where it is important to know the basis for cobalamin deficiency, and how best to aggressively reverse congenital metabolic defects of cobalamin metabolism, as well as which type of cobalamin preparation should be used. Such children should be referred to specialized centers for further evaluation.[50]

A promising alternative to the Schilling test that is currently under investigation involves oral administration of ^{14}C-cobalamin and measurement of absorbed ^{14}C-cobalamin in a capillary-sized blood sample by accelerator mass spectrometry.[58] This method can measure attomole (10^{-18} mol) amounts of ^{14}C-cobalamin in milligram or microliter amounts without need of a flushing dose or collection of urine and with negligible exposure of subjects to radioactivity (equivalent of 1.1 millirem, which is comparable to the solar radiation dose sustained by passengers during a 2-hour commercial airline flight). Although the principles of the Schilling test would still be applicable to any new cobalamin absorption test, this method using accelerator mass spectrometry still requires additional clinical validation.

The Schilling Test

If cobalamin absorption is intact, CN-[^{57}Co]cobalamin administered orally will first bind R-protein in the stomach. In the duodenum, the R-protein of the R-CN-[^{57}Co]cobalamin complex is degraded by pancreatic protease, resulting in rapid transfer of released CN-[^{57}Co]cobalamin to the patient's own intrinsic factor (IF). The CN-[^{57}Co]cobalamin–IF complex travels to the ileum, where it interacts with specific IF–cobalamin receptors. After it is taken up by the enterocyte, CN-[^{57}Co]cobalamin is transported into the portal blood while bound to transcobalamin II (TC II). If the blood contains an excess of cobalamin (eg, from a flushing injection of exogenously administered cobalamin), more than 8% of the CN-[^{57}Co]cobalamin will be excreted in the urine within 24 hours (ie, a normal stage I test). If there is a decrease in endogenous IF, as in pernicious anemia, less than 8% will ultimately be excreted; however, if IF is given exogenously with the CN-[^{57}Co]cobalamin, the abnormality will be corrected (ie, a corrected stage II test). When CN-[^{57}Co]cobalamin is usurped by bacterial overgrowth, resulting in decreased absorption of CN-[^{57}Co]cobalamin plus IF, prior therapy with antibiotics for 7 to 10 days can correct cobalamin malabsorption (ie, a corrected stage III test)[1]; however, antibiotics cannot correct cobalamin malabsorption caused by fish tapeworm infestation or defects involving net deficiency of IF–cobalamin receptors, such as ileal resection, fistulas, or diseases of the ileal mucosa, including TC II deficiency (Table 39–3 and Fig. 39–2). The most common cause of an abnormal Schilling test[1] is incomplete collection of urine. Patients with renal impairment also excrete less than normal amounts of radioactive cobalamin. A significant titer of IF antibodies of the blocking type in gastric juice can lead to an abnormal stage II Schilling test. False normal values in the presence of true cobalamin deficiency can arise from contamination of urine with stool containing unabsorbed CN-[^{57}Co]cobalamin and the presence of another isotope used in diagnostic tests (such as ^{99m}Tc, ^{67}Ga, ^{123}NaI, ^{131}I-MIBG, and ^{201}thallous chloride); delaying the Schilling test by 4 months will avoid interference with radiopharmaceuticals.[2] The flushing dose of unlabeled cobalamin administered during the Schilling test invalidates further testing of serum cobalamin and initiates a hematologic response in cobalamin-deficient patients. Because cobalamin or folate deficiency causes megaloblastosis of intestinal cells, the stage I Schilling test (with CN-[^{57}cobalamin] alone) may be abnormal in folate deficiency, or a patient with IF deficiency (eg, pernicious anemia) may be diagnosed as having an abnormal stage II test result because of an intestinal disorder.[1] This phenomenon occurs often enough (25% to 75% of cases) to warrant a repeat stage II Schilling test in patients diagnosed as having cobalamin malabsorption (from an intestinal cause) after 2 months of cobalamin replacement; only patients with pernicious anemia show correction in the stage II test (see Table 39–3).

Gastric Analysis

Gastric analysis for achlorhydria in adults is valuable only in the single situation in which the presence of gastric acidity in response to maximal stimulation (eg, Histalog) helps exclude the diagnosis of pernicious anemia. In children, however, gastric analysis for IF and acid can differentiate between congenital IF deficiency (acid present), juvenile pernicious anemia (acid and IF absent), and Imerslund–Gräsbeck syndrome (acid and IF present).

PATHOGENESIS OF FOLATE DEFICIENCY

Folate deficiency is usually recognized in the course of certain clinical presentations that predispose to negative folate balance and subsequent deficiency. It is instructive, therefore, to conceptualize cellular folate deficiency as arising from etiologic categories of *decreased supply*

Table 39–3 Results of Schilling Tests

	Material Administered				
Condition	***CN-[^{57}Co]Cbl Plus H_2O (Stage I Test)***	***CN-[^{57}Co]Cbl Plus IF (Stage II Test)***	***CN-[^{57}Co]Cbl After 7–10 Days of Antibiotics (Stage III Test)***	***CN-[^{57}Co]Cbl Plus Pancreatic Extract***	***CN-[^{57}Co]Cbl Food-Cbl Absorption Test (Research Tool)***
Normal	N				
Lack of IF	Low	N			
Usurping of Cbl by bacteria	Low	Low	N		
Pancreatic insufficiency	Low	Low	Low	N	
Lack/bypass of ileal IF-Cbl receptors or defective transenterocytic Cbl transport	Low	Low	Low	Low	
Inadequate dissociation of food Cbl	N				Low

Cbl, cobalamin; IF, intrinsic factor; Low, results indicate less than normal absorption; N, results indicate normal absorption.

Table 39–4 Similarities of Clinical Manifestations and Megaloblastic Sequelae of Folate and Cobalamin Deficiency*

System	Manifestations
Hematologic	Pancytopenia with megaloblastic marrow
Cardiopulmonary	Congestive heart failure
Gastrointestinal	Beefy-red tongue and added stigmata of broad-spectrum malabsorption in folate deficiency†
Dermatologic	Melanin pigmentation and premature graying
Genital	Cervical or uterine dysplasia
Reproductive	Infertility or sterility
Psychiatric	Depressed affect and cognitive dysfunction
Neuropsychiatric‡	Unique to cobalamin deficiency with cerebral, myelopathic, or peripheral neuropathic disturbances, including optic and autonomic nerve dysfunction

*However, the neurologic spectrum of dysfunction in cobalamin deficiency is distinct. Inadequate hemoglobinization (from inadequate iron stores or globin synthesis) can mask the expected erythroid megaloblastic morphology in the bone marrow and peripheral smear, and only specific therapy (ie, iron) can unmask classic megaloblastic manifestations (ie, masked megaloblastosis). Megaloblastic leukopoiesis is unchanged.

†If folate deficiency is uncorrected for 2 to 3 years, cobalamin deficiency will supervene.

‡Dorsal tract involvement is earliest manifestation in more than 70% of patients with cobalamin deficiency. Neuropsychiatric manifestations are not associated with megaloblastosis in up to 30% of patients.

(ie, reduced intake, absorption, transport, or use), or *increased requirement* (ie, metabolic consumption, destruction, or excretion). However, in the same patient more than one mechanism may result in net folate deficiency. The precise contribution of one mechanism over the other is often not obvious. And specific tests to define each mechanism are not routinely available for clinical use. Thus, the clinical context is especially important for interpreting test results for folate supply and function. Manifestations of folate deficiency may be hematologic (pancytopenia with megaloblastic marrow), cardiopulmonary, gastrointestinal (megaloblastosis with or without malabsorption), dermatologic (skin pigmentation), genital (megaloblastosis of cervical epithelium), infertility (sterility), and psychiatric (Table 39–4). These manifestations are discussed within the context of the history and physical examination (see Clinical Presentations and Evaluation for Floate and Cobalamin Deficiency). Cases of neuropathy in adults attributed to folate deficiency are rarely encountered; when they are, the possibility of alcoholism with thiamine deficiency must be considered. In any case, every patient with neuropathy, myelopathy, or psychiatric manifestations associated with megaloblastosis must be investigated in detail to rule out cobalamin deficiency. It must be remembered that gastrointestinal megaloblastosis begets further folate malabsorption, which propagates a vicious cycle of folate deficiency in the short term and cobalamin deficiency in the long term. With the exception of drug-induced defects or inborn errors of folate metabolism that result in decreased use of intracellular folates, all causes, irrespective of mechanism, result in reduced net delivery of folates to normal proliferating cells. In pursuing the causes of folate deficiency in a given patient, efforts should be directed toward obtaining positive evidence for all possible conditions predisposing to negative folate balance and deficiency.

NUTRITIONAL CAUSES OF FOLATE DEFICIENCY

The body stores of folate are adequate for approximately 4 months only.[1] Folate stores are probably depleted much earlier in individuals who are chronically in negative folate balance or who have additional conditions that can "tip" them into true folate deficiency. The incidence of folate deficiency in the setting of general malnutrition in developing countries is very high and is invariably a problem of multiple vitamin deficiencies when associated with protein-calorie malnutrition.[2] Decreased availability of folate-rich foods (in winter, after natural disasters, or the wet season in central Africa), poverty, various cultural or ethnic diets (consisting of maize, rice or well-cooked beans and vegetables), and cooking techniques that destroy food folate, coupled with the anorexia that accompanies chronic illnesses, are just a few of the reasons for rapid development of folate deficiency.[1,2]

Etiopathophysiologic Classification of Folate Deficiency

I. Nutritional causes
   A. Decreased dietary intake
      1. Poverty and famine
      2. Institutionalized individuals (eg, psychiatric, nursing homes), chronic debilitating disease
      3. Prolonged feeding of infants with goat's milk, special slimming diets or food fads (ie, folate-rich foods not consumed), cultural or ethnic cooking techniques (ie, food folate destroyed)
   B. Decreased diet and increased requirements
      1. Physiologic (eg, pregnancy and lactation, prematurity, hyperemesis gravidarum, infancy)
      2. Pathologic (eg, intrinsic hematologic diseases involving hemolysis with compensatory erythropoiesis, abnormal hematopoiesis, or bone marrow infiltration with malignant disease and dermatologic disease such as psoriasis)
II. Folate malabsorption
   A. With normal intestinal mucosa
      1. Some drugs (controversial)
      2. Congenital folate malabsorption (rare)
   B. With mucosal abnormalities (eg, tropical and nontropical sprue, regional enteritis)
III. Defective cellular folate uptake
   A. Familial aplastic anemia (rare)
   B. Acute cerebral folate deficiency
IV. Inadequate cellular use
   A. Folate antagonists (eg, methotrexate)
   B. Hereditary enzyme deficiencies involving folate
V. Drugs
   A. Multiple effects on folate metabolism (eg, alcohol, sulfasalazine, triamterene, pyrimethamine, trimethoprim-sulfamethoxazole, diphenylhydantoin, barbiturates)
VI. Acute folate deficiency
   A. Intensive care unit setting
   B. Uncertain origin

The rapidly proliferating tissues in children have an absolute requirement for exogenously supplied folate. Although human or cow's milk is barely adequate to maintain folate balance in breast-fed infants, superimposition of associated illnesses that lead to anorexia or folate malabsorption readily shifts them into negative folate balance. Infants fed powdered milk formulas, goat's milk (which contains only 6 μg/L folate), or milk that has been boiled (approximately 50% of folate may be destroyed) are at high risk in this regard, as are those on restricted formulas for phenylketonuria and maple syrup urine disease. In Western countries food faddism, alcoholism, and slimming diets usually lead to decreased folate intake in young to middle-aged individuals.[1] Although beer has a higher folate content than other alcoholic beverages, alcoholism may lead to neglect of healthy dietary practices in favor of the high calories and "high" of alcohol. The edentulous, infirm, or neglected elderly who are too ill to prepare their meals, as well as psychiatric patients, are particularly at risk for nutritional folate deficiency.[1]

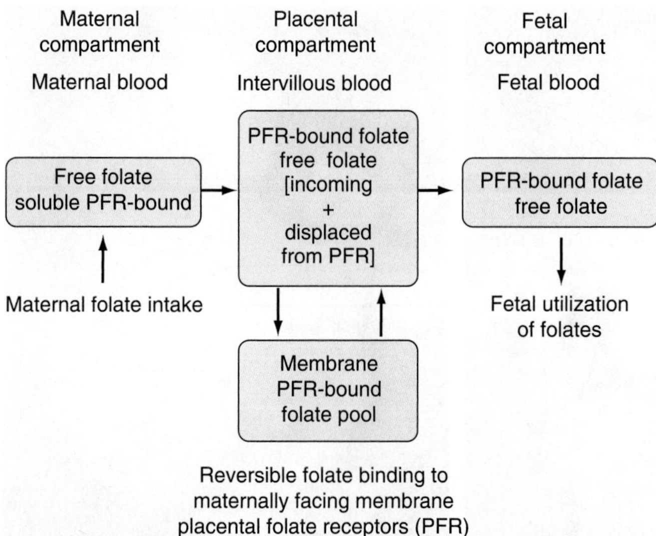

Figure 39–8 Diagrammatic representation of maternal-to-fetal transplacental folate transport involving placental folate receptors (PFRs). (Adapted from Henderson GI, Perez T, Schenker S, et al: Maternal-to-fetal transfer of 5-methyltetrahydrofolate by the perfused human placental cotyledon: Evidence for a concentrative role by placental folate receptors in fetal folate delivery. J Lab Clin Med 126:184, 1995.)

PREGNANCY AND INFANCY

Except for malnutrition in children, pregnancy with poor folate intake is the most common cause of megaloblastic anemia in the world. Pregnancy and lactation are associated with significantly higher folate requirements (over 400 μg/day) for growth of the fetus, placenta, breast, and other maternal tissues[59]; studies have identified increased catabolism of folate during pregnancy as another cause of deficiency.[2] This demand for folate must be met by adequate dietary intake. The placenta has a large number of folate receptors (FRs)[2,23] that facilitate binding and transport of folates to the developing fetus.[22] Preferential delivery of folate to the fetus can cause or aggravate folate deficiency in the mother.[1] This is observed clinically when a mother with severe folate deficiency gives birth to a baby who has normal folate stores. Folate deficiency in the pregnant mother can nevertheless lead to decreased placental weight and premature, low-birth-weight infants.[1] In this context, it is significant that (folate-responsive) hyperhomocysteinemia is recognized as a risk factor for women with unexplained recurrent early pregnancy loss[2] as well as in placental abruption or infarction[2]; thus, the very significant protective role of folates for the fetus.[22]

Placental FRs have a major role in transplacental folate transport (Fig. 39–8).[2,22] Net maternal-to-fetal folate transfer is a process consisting of two steps. First is the concentrative component in which circulating 5-methyl-tetrahydrofolate (5-methyl-H_4PteGlu) is bound to (ie, captured by) placental FR on the maternally facing chorionic surface. Although kinetics favor binding, a dynamic state exists wherein a gradual release of 5-methyl-H_4PteGlu from this pool adds to incoming circulating folates to generate an intervillous blood level approximately three times that in the maternal blood. In the second step, folates are transferred to the fetal circulation along a downhill concentration gradient. It turns out that the prodigious, reversible, high-affinity binding of maternal folates by placental FRs[2,22] is the key modulator of transplacental folate transport. Once captured, placental FR-bound folates are predestined for transplacental folate transport, because incoming (dietary) folates displace placental FR-bound folates, which then passively diffuse down a concentration gradient to the fetus.[2,22] This elegant cycle ensures continued unidirectional transplacental folate transport (Fig. 39–8).

Before the advent of routine folate supplementation during pregnancy, the incidence of megaloblastic marrows in the United States, Canada, and the United Kingdom during late pregnancy was approximately 25%, but in southern India, it was approximately 55%.[1] Folate deficiency is eight times as high in twin pregnancies. Multiparity (multiple frequent pregnancies with a prolonged state of negative folate balance) and hyperemesis gravidarum commonly lead to folate deficiency. Because the anemia of pregnancy is most frequently caused by iron deficiency, combined iron and folate deficiency (dimorphic anemia) is the more frequent clinical presentation. Increased use of folates in newborns leads to a drop in folate levels by approximately 6 weeks. This drop is exaggerated in premature infants, who because of feeding difficulties, infection, or hemolytic disease often develop pure folate deficiency.[1]

Recent studies of low socioeconomic status groups from North India[13,14] have estimated that the daily intake of folic acid range between 75 and 167 μg, which is far lower than the 400 μg necessary to prevent birth defects. Experimental studies to define the influence of gestational folate deficiency on the fetus (conducted on dams) using controlled dietary folate restriction—which was similar in principle to the extant diet of women in North India[13,14]—have identified adverse effects on reproductive performance, implantation, fetal growth, and other defects in murine fetal development; these defects included increased cell loss and subtle architectural anomalies that were traced in some tissues to megaloblastosis and in some cells apoptosis and severe dysplasia.[19] The folate-deficient murine fetuses exhibited an impressive net loss of cortical cells (by ~20%) in various regions of the brain, as well as a major alteration in white matter,[19] findings consistent with decreased progenitor cell proliferation and increased apoptosis in fetal mouse brain.[60] Because cobalamin deficiency leads to a functional intracellular folate deficiency and apoptosis, these findings of a loss of brain cell mass in folate deficiency in utero can explain the profound anatomic abnormalities noted on magnetic resonance imaging of the brains of infants and children with cobalamin deficiency.[2,61] Longitudinal follow-up identified that gestational folate deficiency also resulted in behavioral changes—an anxiety phenotype—during adulthood in these mice,[62] thereby supporting the fetal origins of disease hypothesis; the extent to which these important findings are relevant to humans remain to be determined.

FOLATE-RESPONSIVE NEURAL TUBE DEFECTS AND NEUROCRISTOPATHIES

NTDs are the most common major congenital malformation of the central nervous system. They arise from disturbances in neurulation that involve incomplete closure of neural tissues leading to major midline defects. The neural tube, which begins as a tiny ribbon of tissue, normally folds inward to form a tube by the 28th day after conception. Thus, NTDs originate in the first month of pregnancy (before many women know they are pregnant). Embryonic neural tube and neural crest cells have critical bursts of proliferative activity (with occasional doubling times as fast as 5 hours!), so it is not surprising that cellular folate deficiency has profoundly adverse effects on cells of the neural tube and neural crest that are responsible for midline closure during embryogenesis.[63] It is critical for a woman to have enough folic acid in her system before conception (periconceptionally) to ensure availability for the embryo.

The delivery of an optimum physiologic amount of folic acid to developing neural tube and neural crest cells appears to be the critical determinant to prevent NTD.[22,63] Genetic susceptibility, as occurs with the thermolabile *MTHFR* polymorphism, can explain only a small proportion (<15%) of the incidence.[2,64] A recent review[65] concluded that definitive conclusions about the precise role of specific folate pathway gene variants (polymorphisms) in causing spina bifida cannot be made at this time. However, a transgenic mouse model with a targeted inactivation of the murine FR-alpha gene resulted in homozygous mice that had NTDs and died by the 10th gestation day; these embryos could be rescued by very large doses of folinic acid.[2] Studies using mouse embryos cultured in vitro have demon-

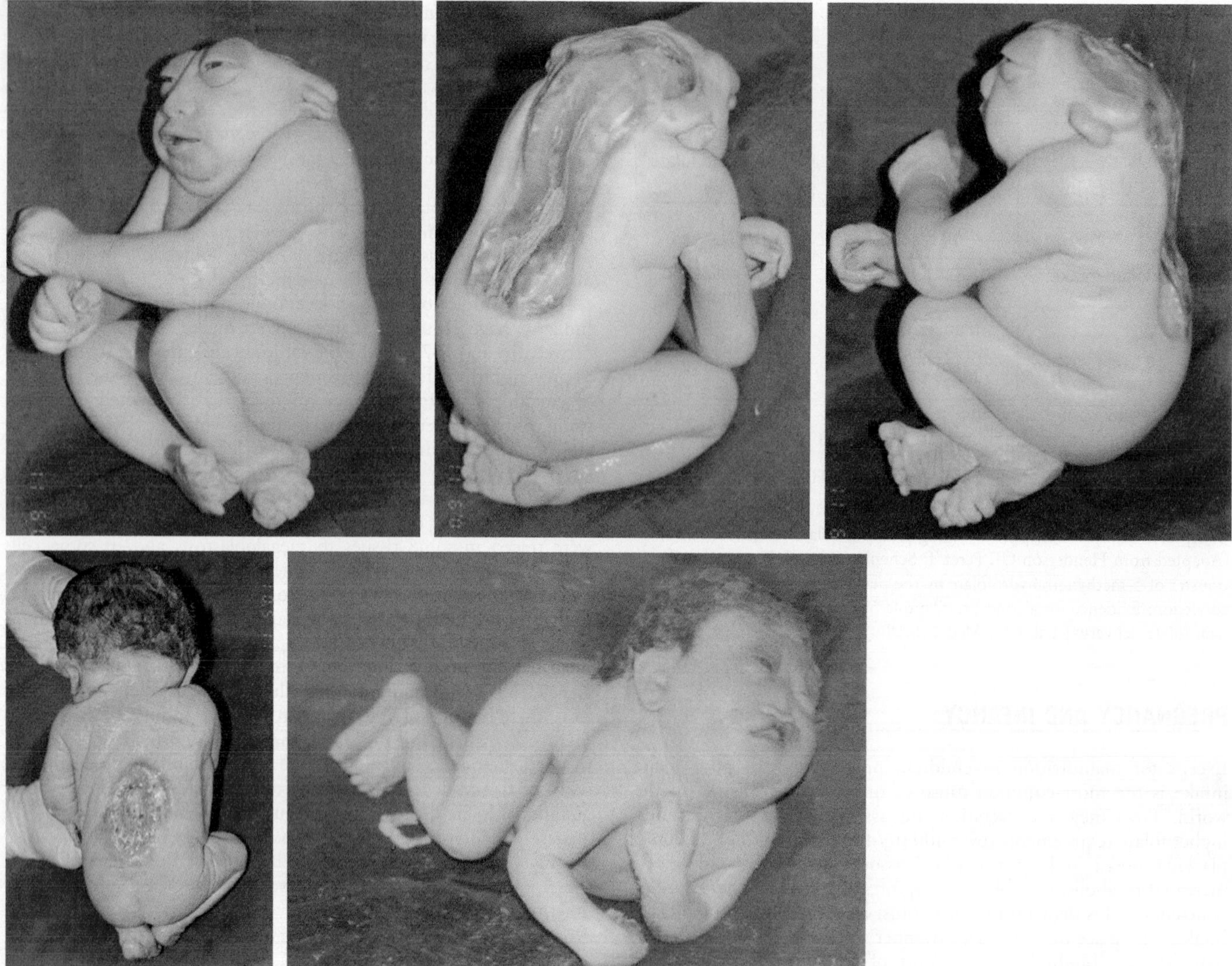

Figure 39–9 Folate-responsive neural tube defects: anencephaly with complete rachischisis (*top panel*); open infected meningomyelocele (*bottom left*); and iniencephaly with cleft lip (*bottom right*). (Courtesy of Prof Molly Paul, Anatomy Department Museum, Christian Medical College and Brown Memorial Hospital, Ludhiana, Punjab, India.)

strated that alterations in FR by perturbing the coding sequences or a critical regulatory *cis*-element can play a role in NTDs.[66] So whether defects in regulatory proteins involved in translation of FR can lead to reduced expression of FR and NTD is now under investigation. In parallel with experimental studies involving exposure of pregnant rats to anti-FR antisera[67] which induced NTD, blocking autoantibodies against FR have been detected in women with a pregnancy that was complicated by a NTD[68] and orofacial clefts.[69] In addition to induction of NTD, knockout of FR and knock-down of FR have given rise to neurocristopathies that have now provided more support to the observational clinical studies which suggested that many of these—including cleft lip/palate,[2] conotruncal heart defects,[2] urinary tract defects[2] and limb reduction defects,[2] and omphalocele[70]—may be prevented by periconceptional folate supplements.[2,22]

Anencephaly and spina bifida, the commonest NTDs, are important factors in fetal mortality (Fig. 39–9). Worldwide, the risk in the general population ranges from less than 1 to 9 cases per 1000 births; for example, a recent population-based study in the least developed area in India identified that the incidence of NTDs was up to 8.21 per 1000 live births, which is among the highest worldwide.[71] By contrast, with less than 1 case per 1000 each year in the United States, approximately 4000 fetuses are affected, and at least one-third are lost through spontaneous or elective abortions when an affected fetus is detected; 100% of fetuses with anencephaly are stillborn or die shortly after birth. An association between folate and NTDs was conclusively established by a randomized, controlled study that investigated mothers with a history of delivery of a child with an NTD; these women have a 10-fold higher risk of having a second and subsequent baby with an NTD. This study showed that periconceptional folate supplementation (4000 μg/day) reduced NTD recurrence by 72%.[2] Periconceptional folate supplementation (800 μg/day) was then shown to dramatically reduce the first-time occurrence of NTD,[2] a result confirmed by a large study (with over 100,000 subjects in each arm) in which periconceptional folates (400 μg/day) also led to a dramatic prevention of NTDs in China.[2] There is some (nonrandomized) evidence that periconceptional folate deficiency also leads to oral clefts, conotruncal heart defects, and urinary tract abnormalities and limb reduction defects.[2] Conversely, the use of folic acid antagonists (trimethoprim, triamterene, carbamazepine, phenytoin, phenobarbital, and primidone) during pregnancy increases the risk of these birth defects by twofold.[72] Collectively, these studies confirm that folic acid has multiple salutatory effects during human development and that major abnormalities can be prevented by periconceptional folate supplementation.[59]

Can a young woman get enough folic acid by eating a "balanced Western diet"? The answer found in a controlled study[2] was a definitive no. Only those who received folic acid supplements or had folate-fortified foods improved their folate status (this is explained by the lower bioavailability of folate in foods). Because 50% of pregnancies in the United States are unplanned and compliance with taking folic and supplements to preventing NTD is only at approximately 50%, this led to a consensus that fortification of food with folic acid in the United States was the best way to improve overall folate status in women at risk for NTD occurrence. By January 1998, fortification of foods (ie, rice, flour, pasta, macaroni, breads, and cake at 140 μg of folic acid per 100 g of food) was part of American Law. This level was chosen to ensure that women of childbearing age would have an increase in folic acid intake of 100 μg a day, which is approximately 25% of the recommended daily intake.

Assessment of folate status in the Framingham Offspring Cohort before and after fortification has indicated that food fortification with folate does not give the expected 100 μg a day; instead the estimate is between 1.5 and 3 times more than originally estimated.[2] As a consequence, after fortification the prevalence of folate deficiency (based on a plasma folate level less than <3 ng/mL) has been reduced in the United States from approximately 20% to 1%.[2] Independent studies have confirmed a near doubling of serum folate after fortification—from 12 to 20 ng/mL in a managed care setting.[73] This is suspected to be caused by manufacturers' overages (ie, addition by the manufacturer of a greater amount than specified) in folate fortification.

Although typical intakes of folic acid from fortified foods are more than twice the level originally predicted,[74] there remain questions about the effectiveness of the folic acid fortification program for women in the 15- to 35-year age group in preventing NTDs. Because of an incomplete knowledge base among some women,[2,75] and the tendency to consume low-carbohydrate foods (which are the very foods that are fortified), there is continued concern that this group is still not getting adequate amounts of dietary folate. This is the basis for recommendations to continue to educate women in the childbearing age to take folate supplements at 400 μg/day (beyond what they are already receiving through food folate fortification).

What impact has folic acid fortification of the US food supply had on the occurrence of NTDs? The birth prevalence of NTDs reported on birth certificates has decreased by 19%,[76] but the use of birth certificate data[77] might have led to underreporting. In Ontario, Canada, the prevalence of open NTDs also has declined from 1.13 per 1000 pregnancies before fortification to 0.58 per 1000 pregnancies thereafter.[78] Another recent study from Canada has identified that the prevalence of NTDs decreased from 1.58 per 1000 births before fortification to 0.86 per 1000 births during the full fortification period (a 46% reduction), with the decrease greatest in areas in which the baseline rate was high.[79]

Despite recommendations to increase folic acid to prevent NTDs, there has been no detectable impact in the trends of incidence of NTD worldwide.[80] This has led to calls to redouble efforts to quickly integrate food fortification with fuller implementation of recommendations on supplements. Even in the USA, it has been the position of some authorities that the majority of women in the childbearing age are not receiving the optimum amount of folate (400 μg folic acid per day). This has led to calls to increase the current fortification levels (140 μg/100 g of flour) to levels such as those used in Chile using 220 μg/100 g of flour[81]; however, this has been resisted with cogent arguments by others.[82] Moreover, based on a recent analysis of high quality studies from Canada that has a similar fortification program as the USA, it appears that the food fortification program is achieving near maximal outcomes, in that it appears to be preventing approximately 50% of NTDs.[79,83]

The potential masking of the hematologic manifestations of cobalamin deficiency by food fortification with folic acid remains a valid concern.[84] Those at greatest risk for receiving too much folate are the elderly with biochemical evidence of cobalamin deficiency.[2] This concern is amplified by a recent study that identified an increase in cognitive impairment among those with low cobalamin status who have high serum folate levels.[85] Another group who could potentially be inadvertently affected are children who consume large amounts of folate-fortified cereal and thereby exceed their recommended daily allowance of folate (ie, greater than 300 μg/day); the long-term consequence of persistently higher-than-normal folate levels is an unknown entity.

Among cultures in which most pregnancies are well planned, supplementation in the form of folic acid tablets is considered best.[2] Moreover, in places where food production and distribution is generally local, centralized fortification does not reach the masses, as is the case in developing countries such as India, where approximately 80% live in villages and small towns. There is no formal program in most developing countries for prevention of NTDs. In these settings, the methods employed to educate the educated minority need to be different from those used to educate the less educated. However, there is no information on which is the best method to reach these groups of women from the behavioral research standpoint.

INTRINSIC HEMATOLOGIC DISEASE

Because folate is necessary for hematopoiesis, folate requirements are increased when there is significant compensatory erythropoiesis in response to peripheral RBC destruction, abnormal hematopoiesis, or infiltration by abnormal cells in the marrow. The recognition that folate deficiency developing in hemolytic disorders can lead to an acute aplastic crisis has led to routine prophylactic administration of folate. An unexpected increase in transfusional requirement or a fall in platelets should also suggest folate deficiency.[1] The case of a patient with sickle cell disease on long-term folate who developed cobalamin malabsorption and presented with neuropsychiatric dysfunction is a valuable reminder that those on folate prophylaxis need periodic follow-up for signs and symptoms of supervening cobalamin deficiency.[86]

Folate Malabsorption With Normal Intestinal Mucosa

The enzyme folylpolygamma-glutamate carboxypeptidase that is expressed by the *GCP2* gene (also called *FOLH1*) is responsible for breakdown of polyglutamated folates to monoglutamated forms before absorption. The extent of [poly]glutamylation of folate in natural food folates is not the limiting factor in the extent of absorption of food folates,[87] and there appears to be little effect of an earlier described polymorphism[88] in the catalytic region of GCPII (resulting in 50% enzyme activity) on intestinal absorption of dietary folates.[89]

Congenital Folate Malabsorption

Patients with this disorder (usually the progeny of consanguineous marriages) present in the first 3 months with failure to thrive; diarrhea; sore mouth; megaloblastic anemia with low levels of serum, RBC, and cerebrospinal fluid folates; normal cobalamin levels; progressive mental retardation; seizures; cerebral calcification; athetosis; and ataxia. They do not respond to oral folate or 5-formyl-H_4PteGlu (5 mg) because of specific intestinal folate malabsorption as well as defective folate transport into the central nervous system.[1] Parenteral therapy in high concentrations is necessary to ensure passive folate transport. To establish the diagnosis, it is necessary to document that the patient has normal gastrointestinal absorption of other nutrients, intact pancreatic function, and normal mucosa on small intestinal biopsy. The differential diagnosis includes congenital IF deficiency, Imerslund–Gräsbeck syndrome, TC II deficiency, and inborn errors of cobalamin metabolism.

Folate Malabsorption With Intestinal Mucosal Abnormalities

Tropical Sprue

Residents of, and visitors to, endemic areas in the tropics can acquire a disorder of unknown cause characterized by small intestinal malabsorption.[1] Generalized, nonspecific small bowel malabsorption leads to a wide spectrum of clinical manifestations arising from defective absorption of fat, carbohydrate, albumin, calcium, folate, and in later stages, cobalamin.[1] The endemic nature of this disorder in the tropics (and in certain households)[1] and the beneficial response to antibiotics all suggest an infectious origin. However, the dramatic response to folate, which is curative in the first year in approximately 60% of cases (this cure is cited to be almost diagnostic of the disease), has not been explained.[1] It is unlikely that pure folate deficiency is the primary cause, because nutritional folate deficiency does not result in tropical sprue; the clinical response to antibiotics suggests a close interplay between a pathogenic infectious agent, endogenous flora, and the folate status of the enterocyte.

There is some degree of villous atrophy and loss of intestinal functional surface. Although less severe than in nontropical sprue, it is more extensive, involving the entire small intestine. There is abrupt onset of explosive, intermittent, or continuous diarrhea, abdominal distention, and pain associated with anorexia, vomiting, and extreme fatigue. Stools are fluid or semisolid and frequently contain mucus and blood. This stage is followed weeks to months later by nutrient deficiency. Later, as steatorrhea continues, megaloblastosis dominates the clinical picture. In the short term, malabsorption leads to folate deficiency, but later in the chronic (longer than 3-year) phase of the disease, cobalamin malabsorption contributes additional clinical manifestations of cobalamin neuropathy.[1]

Coexisting iron deficiency (common in these areas) leads to a dimorphic blood picture; pellagra and beri-beri may also coexist in these patients. Treatment of the chronic phase with folate can cure the hematologic manifestations but exacerbate cobalamin-deficient neurologic disease. In South India, among 64 patients with megaloblastic anemia from tropical sprue, 21% were caused by cobalamin deficiency, 33% by folate deficiency alone, and 44% by combined cobalamin and folate deficiency.[1] After investigations for associated iron, cobalamin, and folate deficiencies, therapy with folate and a broad-spectrum antibiotic (eg, tetracycline) is indicated together with symptomatic treatment of diarrhea, vomiting, fluid, mineral and electrolyte imbalance, and associated additional nutritional deficiencies.[1]

Nontropical Sprue

Nontropical sprue (ie, celiac disease, gluten-induced enteropathy) is the most common cause of intestinal malabsorption in temperate zones. It results from a possibly inherited sensitivity to gluten (a glutamine-rich protein found in wheat, barley, rye and other grains) and a related substance, gliadin.[1] The precise mechanism for induction of sensitivity is not known. The intestinal lesion (ie, villous atrophy with hypertrophied crypts and lymphocytic and plasma cell infiltrate of the lamina propria) is more florid than that seen in tropical sprue but occurs to a greater extent in the proximal small intestine with relative ileal sparing; as a result, cobalamin malabsorption is less common. The consequences of malabsorption are otherwise the same. Patients present between the ages of 30 and 50 years with intermittent or persistent diarrhea (abrupt in 20%), weight loss, abdominal distention with discomfort, glossitis, and megaloblastic anemia. Diagnosis is established by demonstration of sensitive and specific serum antiendomysial antibodies IgA type or antitissue transglutaminase antibodies, malabsorption, and jejunal biopsy. The symptoms are exacerbated after a challenge with gluten, and institution of a gluten-free diet not only is curative but also decreases the risk of subsequent malignancy (small intestinal lymphoma or gastrointestinal carcinoma, especially esophageal). Iron deficiency is prominent, especially in children. The megaloblastosis responds well to folate therapy.[1]

Regional Enteritis and Other Small Intestinal Disorders

The distal small intestine is involved in 80% of individuals with Crohn disease, but folate is efficiently absorbed in other more proximal areas. Only with extensive involvement or fistulas do these patients develop folate deficiency. Even in this case, the blood picture is more that of an iron deficiency or anemia of chronic disease. Frank, pure megaloblastic anemia occurs rarely enough in this setting to suggest another cause for folate or cobalamin malabsorption. HIV infection results in an enteropathy, in the absence of opportunistic infection, which leads to the malabsorption of folates.[2]

INFANTILE ACUTE CEREBRAL FOLATE DEFICIENCY SYNDROME

Infantile-onset cerebral folate deficiency[90] that develops 4 to 6 months after birth is characterized by marked irritability, slow head growth, psychomotor retardation, cerebellar ataxia, pyramidal tract signs in the legs, dyskinesias (such as choreoathetosis and ballismus), and in some cases, seizures. Untreated, central visual disturbances can become manifest and lead to optic atrophy and blindness by the third year. Because there is a low level of 5-methyl-$H_4PteGlu_n$ in the cerebrospinal fluid, with normal folate levels in the serum and erythrocytes, a blood-to-CSF folate transport defect was suspected. Further analysis has demonstrated that a high number of children (25 of 28) had high-affinity blocking FR-autoantibodies that could react against membrane-bound FR that are normally present on the choroid plexus. Oral folinic acid normalized 5-methyl-$H_4PteGlu_n$ levels in the cerebrospinal fluid and led to clinical improvement. It is therefore speculated that anti-FR antibodies prevented the transfer of folate from the plasma to the cerebrospinal fluid via the choroid plexus, thereby depriving the developing brain of folate. Although plausible, this hypothesis has not been rigorously proven experimentally. Nevertheless, this experiment of nature may point to a situation where normal physiology involving the blood-to-CSF folate transport has gone awry.

INBORN ERRORS OF FOLATE METABOLISM

Knowledge of the intracellular metabolic pathways involving folates can help predict the net effect of deficiency of a single enzyme (see Fig. 39–5). Substrate buildup or product deficiency leads to the clinical manifestations. The precise biochemical defects can be proved by specific enzyme assays of the patient's fibroblasts. Deficiency of 5,10-methylene-tetrahydrofolate reductase (MTHFR) is the most frequent of these rare disorders and manifests with excess homocysteine in the serum and urine and with hypomethioninemia. The disease is recognized in infancy because of developmental delay or mental retardation, with motor abnormalities and disturbance in gait. It has, however, occasionally remained undiagnosed until the teenage years. Serum folate levels are normal or low, but the cobalamin concentration is normal. There is no megaloblastosis, TC II levels are normal, and there is often a poor response to folic acid (PteGlu). Despite a variety of treatments administered, no consistent pattern of response has emerged (which likely reflects significant genetic heterogeneity within this disorder).[2,50] Excellent reviews of these and other inborn errors of folate metabolism are available.[2,50] Thermolabile MTHFR is discussed later in Hyperhomocysteinemia and Folate and Carcinogenesis.

ACUTE FOLATE DEFICIENCY

The cause of acute folate deficiency in some patients in intensive care units is not known. Clinically the presentation is acute megaloblastic arrest of hematopoiesis with thrombocytopenia. These patients are often acutely ill and in subclinical negative folate balance. The combination of additional insults (decreased intake, total parenteral nutrition containing ethanol, dialysis, surgery, sepsis, drugs) appears to provoke frank folate deficiency. The serum folate is often normal in the face of megaloblastosis in the bone marrow without obvious peripheral blood abnormalities. The dU suppression test[2] has documented intracellular folate deficiency, but there are no data on MMA and homocysteine levels in this condition. Empirical therapy with 5-formyl-H_4PteGlu (leucovorin) is recommended. Exposure to N_2O should also be considered in the differential diagnosis.[2]

MEGALOBLASTIC ANEMIA NOT CAUSED BY FOLATE OR COBALAMIN DEFICIENCY

Several chemotherapeutic agents (eg, antimetabolites, alkylating agents) kill malignant cells primarily by interfering with DNA synthesis; megaloblastosis is therefore an expected side effect. Hereditary orotic aciduria usually manifests in the first year of life because of a deficiency or absence of enzymes that convert orotic acid to uridine monophosphate via orotidine monophosphate. The net cellular deficiency of uridine monophosphate leads to perturbed synthesis of DNA as well as RNA.[1] Thiamine-responsive megaloblastic anemia is an early-onset, autosomal recessive disorder defined by the occurrence of megaloblastic anemia, diabetes mellitus, and sensorineural deafness (ie, the DIDMOAD syndrome: *d*iabetes *i*nsipidus, *d*iabetes mellitus, *m*egaloblastosis, *o*ptic *a*trophy, and sensorineural *d*eafness) that responds to various degrees to thiamine treatment; it is caused by a single gene disorder involving the thiamine transporter.[2]

CLINICAL PRESENTATIONS AND EVALUATION FOR FOLATE AND COBALAMIN DEFICIENCY

Clinical presentations and evaluations for folate and cobalamin deficiency are shown in Table 39–4.

INTERVIEW

The patient's general demeanor and answers to questions may reveal a blunted affect with evidence of depression, irritability, forgetfulness, and sleep deprivation (common in pure folate deficiency). Alternatively, cobalamin deficiency may present with paranoid ideation (mimicking paranoid schizophrenia), dementia, cognitive dysfunction, delusions, or lack of energy manifested by slowed responses. Hallucinations or even obtundation may preclude obtaining an adequate history. The family may indicate the progressive evolution of a marked personality change and may be able to help trace the evolution of symptoms and deviations from the time when the patient was last well. Intermittent therapy with multivitamins, liver pills, or injections (often given by a well-meaning family member or unregistered practitioner) is a common quick fix in many cultures. The family is a good source for details on the patient's dietary habits (food faddism, vegetarianism, alcohol intake) and family history of medical problems (blood diseases, gluten sensitivity, autoimmune diseases).

A medical history of epilepsy or alcoholism with seizure disorder (anticonvulsant therapy) is important. Rarely, patients with autoimmune hemolytic anemias may be lost to follow-up and return with acute aplastic crises when they run out of folate. A surgical history of total or partial gastrectomy, anastomosis, fistula, or bowel resection can reveal the potential for perturbation of physiologic absorption (loss of IF, bypassing or loss of absorptive surface, blind loop syndromes). Surreptitious or accidental inhalation of N_2O in an occupational setting (dental or anesthesiology professionals) and deliberate inhalation of N_2O (cartridges attached to whipped-cream dispensers or visits to "houses of laughter," where N_2O can be inhaled for a small fee) can be revealed only on direct questioning. Visits to tropical countries and the development of intermittent episodic diarrhea may give a clue to tropical sprue; prolonged (over 3 years) chronic gastrointestinal symptoms followed by insidious development of neurologic problems predicts a combined (folate followed by cobalamin) deficiency.

Systemic review of symptoms may range from none (ie, incidental increased MCV or PMN hypersegmentation) to severe (ie, unstable angina from severe anemia). With slow development of anemia, the patient often does not develop cardiopulmonary symptoms until there is a 50% reduction in hemoglobin concentration, which leads to dyspnea on exertion, palpitation, and generalized fatigue or lethargy. Only when the hemoglobin concentration is below 5 g/dL does the patient develop dyspnea at rest and angina on modest exertion or even at rest. Congestive heart failure is heralded by pedal edema, nocturia, orthopnea, and tender hepatomegaly.

Upper gastrointestinal symptoms with anorexia associated with intrinsic gastrointestinal disease or anemia with heart failure must be distinguished from symptoms due to glossitis. The latter may lead to inability to wear dentures, tolerate hot drinks or spicy foods because of burning, and even odynophagia, which may further compromise food intake (seen in cobalamin and folate deficiencies). The patient may volunteer that glossitis is relieved by multivitamin ingestion. Weight loss in cobalamin deficiency is not as severe as in folate deficiency arising from intrinsic gastrointestinal disease. Episodic or chronic diarrhea with steatorrhea is commonly caused by tropical sprue, although it may be brought on by gluten-containing foods. Although these symptoms may be accompanied by abdominal pain, pain in the absence of diarrhea could be caused by tabetic crisis (vomiting, abdominal rigidity, absence of leukocytosis, or fever) accompanying spinothalamic involvement in cobalamin-deficient myelopathy.

The patient with pernicious anemia may have two or three semisolid bowel movements per day; although this may be construed as a normal pattern, it may represent a change since the last time the patient was well. Constipation may be related to obstipation arising from the involvement of Meissner and Auerbach plexus within the gastrointestinal tract. Similarly, incipient loss of bladder or bowel control due to cobalamin myelopathy may present with urgency or nocturia.

In contrast to musculoskeletal symptoms (arthralgia or frank arthritis) of autoimmune diseases, nocturnal cramps or pain in upper and lower extremities may indicate spinothalamic tract involvement. Hypoparathyroidism or systemic lupus erythematosus, alone or associated with pernicious anemia, leads to significant overlap of cerebral, musculoskeletal, and neurologic presentations.

Review of skin symptoms may elicit a history of increased diffuse or blotchy generalized brownish skin pigmentation, especially of nail beds and skin creases. This is common in cobalamin and folate deficiency; associated vitiligo suggests autoimmune disease.

Although symptoms related to neurologic dysfunction may be volunteered, a complete detailed questionnaire should be formulated during the interview. Questions should be directed to perversions in taste or smell, decreased visual acuity, changes in color vision, and eye pain (neuritis), tinnitus, or headache. Dizziness with orthostatic hypotension and "blacking out" may be related to severe anemia.

Miscellaneous Megaloblastic Anemias Not Caused By Cobalamin or Folate Deficiency

I. Congenital disorders of DNA synthesis
   A. Orotic aciduria
   B. Lesch–Nyhan syndrome
   C. Congenital dyserythropoietic anemia
II. Acquired disorders of DNA synthesis
   A. Deficiency (ie, thiamine-responsive megaloblastic anemia [DIDMOAD syndrome])
   B. Malignancy (ie, erythroleukemia)
      1. Refractory sideroblastic anemias
      2. All antineoplastic drugs that inhibit DNA synthesis (and antinucleosides used against HIV and other viruses)
   C. Toxic sources, including alcohol

Drugs That Perturb Folate Metabolism

Ethanol in amounts of more than 80 g/day is toxic to hematopoietic precursors and can directly lead to megaloblastosis with abnormal vacuolization of normoblasts and to sideroblastic anemias. These toxic changes seen in severe alcoholics are usually associated with significantly higher alcohol consumption and revert to normal with alcohol withdrawal. Patients who have one nutritious meal each day tend to stave off the eventual development of folate deficiency. Alcohol consumption leads to a relatively rapid (2- to 4-day) fall in serum folate levels. This is a result of the combined effects of increased urinary folate excretion[2]; interruption of the enterohepatic circulation (resulting from an effect on hepatic pteroylpolyglutamate synthesis and reduced release of tissue folates into plasma and bile); formation of acetaldehyde–H_4PteGlu adducts (5,10-(CH_3-CH)-H_4PteGlu$_n$); increased catabolism of folate by ethanol to acetaldehyde/xanthine oxidase-generated superoxide[2]; malabsorption of folate by inhibition of jejunal folate pteroylpolyglutamate hydrolase[2]; perturbation of methionine synthase activity[2]; and increased urinary excretion of formate, which is normally metabolized by folate-requiring enzymes.[1] The relative degree to which each of these mechanisms contributes to folate deficiency remains to be determined. Excess alcohol consumption is probably the most common cause of folate deficiency in the United States.[1]

Trimethoprim and *pyrimethamine* bind to bacterial and parasitic dihydrofolate reductase with much greater affinity than to human dihydrofolate reductase, but patients with underlying folate deficiency appear to be more susceptible to the effects of these drugs. The ensuing megaloblastosis can be reversed by 5-formyl-H_4PteGlu.

Methotrexate binds to human dihydrofolate reductase ($K_i = 7 \times 10^{-10}$ M) and leads to trapping of folate as a metabolically inert form (dihydrofolate, H_2PteGlu). This leads to a true depletion of H_4PteGlu$_n$ within hours and consequently to functional deficiency of 5,10-methylene-H_4PteGlu$_n$ and reduced thymidylate synthesis. Although megaloblastosis can develop rapidly, the toxic effects of methotrexate can be avoided by rescue with 5-formyl-H_4PteGlu (ie, leucovorin). However, the effects of repletion on tumor with 5,10-methylene-H_4PteGlu$_n$ presents a problem. Folate receptors take up methotrexate at lower doses, but reduced-folate carrier-mediated and passive diffusion appear to be the main routes of cellular uptake at high doses. Once in the cell, methotrexate is polyglutamated, which determines its cytotoxicity. The maintenance of a gradient between the extracellular and intracellular compartment appears to determine polyglutamation and efficiency of cytotoxicity.

Sulfasalazine produces megaloblastosis in up to two-thirds of patients taking full doses (over 2 g/day) by decreasing absorption of folates (ie, decreasing conversion of H_4PteGlu$_n$ to H_4PteGlu) and induction of Heinz body hemolytic anemia (ie, increased requirements).

It is still not clear whether cases in which megaloblastic anemia develops while patients are receiving *oral contraceptives* represent a cause-and-effect relationship. Oral contraceptives may increase folate catabolism (ie, metabolic consumption) or may weakly interfere with DNA synthesis. It is significant that the megaloblastosis of cervical epithelium often reverses with folate therapy alone.

Reduction of serum folate levels by *anticonvulsants* during prolonged therapy probably results from the combined action on reduced absorption and through induction of microsomal liver enzymes.[2] It is unclear how folates provoke a return of seizures in some patients receiving anticonvulsants, but this effect may be mediated by glutamate (or related) receptors.[2] Despite this potential risk, consensus guidelines have stressed the importance of ensuring that pregnant women[2] and children[91-94] with epilepsy be prescribed folates together with anticonvulsants.

Although *antineoplastics* and *antiretroviral antinucleosides* such as azidothymidine lead to megaloblastosis, the temporal sequence and investigations to rule out cobalamin or folate deficiency should easily lead to a correct causal assignment.

Vertigo or difficulty in walking in the dark (loss of proprioception and position sense), difficulty in ambulation (which may feel like "walking on cotton wool"), stiffness of extremities (corticospinal tracts), or ataxia (spinocerebellar tracts) may be indicative of a serious cobalamin myelopathy. Early symptoms are symmetrical tingling ("pins and needles"), extending from the tips of the toes to a glove and stocking distribution in later stages. "Burning feet" syndrome, or more commonly, complaints of difficulty in performing simple tasks such as buttoning clothes, may also be a presenting symptom. When loss of bladder and bowel control brings the patient to the physician, advanced neurologic dysfunction is invariably present.

Other genitourinary symptoms such as recurrent cystitis from bladder dysfunction, impotence (ie, cobalamin neuropathy), or a recent Pap smear indicative of cervical dysplasia rarely may be presenting symptoms. Multiple pregnancies with short intervals between delivery and conception predispose to a high risk for overt folate deficiency (cobalamin deficiency is more often associated with infertility).

PHYSICAL EXAMINATION

Physical examination may reveal different features in well-nourished patients (cobalamin-deficient vegetarians or pernicious anemia patients) and poorly nourished (folate-deficient) individuals. The latter show evidence of significant weight loss or other stigmata of multiple deficiencies due to "broad-spectrum" malabsorption. Associated deficiency of vitamins A, D, and K and protein-calorie malnutrition may give rise to angular cheilosis, bleeding mucous membranes, dermatitis, osteomalacia, and chronic infections. Various degrees of pallor with lemon-tint icterus (ie, a combination of pallor and icterus best observed in fair-skinned individuals) are common features of megaloblastosis.

When anemia is severe, the patient may have a low-grade fever. The skin may reveal a diffuse, brownish pigmentation or abnormal blotchy tanning. Special emphasis should be given to pigmentation of skin creases and nail beds. (Mucous membrane pigmentation is not observed, in contrast to Addison disease.) Premature graying is observed in light- and dark-haired individuals.

A blunted masklike facies is extremely common in folate deficiency. Alternatively, there may be evidence of classic hyperthyroid or hypothyroid facies (associated with pernicious anemia). Special attention should be given to the eyes and eyebrows for signs of thyroid dysfunction.

Examination of the mouth may reveal glossitis with a smooth (depapillated), beefy red tongue with occasional ulceration of the lateral surface. The neck may reveal thyromegaly (diffuse or with nodules) if there is associated disease. Increased jugular venous distention should alert the examiner to cardiovascular failure, with its attendant gallop, cardiomegaly (with or without pericardial effusions), pulmonary basal crepitations, and pleural effusion, tender hepatomegaly, and pedal edema. Nontender hepatomegaly, but more often mild splenomegaly, may rarely be caused by extramedullary hematopoiesis in severe anemia, but a midepigastrium mass raises the ominous possibility of gastric carcinoma, which is three times as likely in patients with pernicious anemia.

An inverse correlation has been identified between the extent of anemia and neurologic dysfunction. Patients with normal complete blood count values often have neurologic signs and symptoms. In prolonged cobalamin deficiency, the neurologic examination reveals clear-cut evidence of involvement of posterior and pyramidal, spinocerebellar, and spinothalamic tracts. Among the earliest signs of posterior column dysfunction are loss of position sense in the index toes (before great toe involvement), which is elicited by passive movement, and loss of the ability to discern vibration of a high-pitched (256 Hz) tuning fork (a very early elicitable, objective sign), which invariably precedes by many months the loss of ability to sense the vibration of a lower-pitched (128 Hz) tuning fork. Usually, the patient loses vibration sense to 256 Hz from toe to hip before the loss of 128 Hz vibration sense even begins. Because of the slow coalescence of contiguous spinal cord lesions, a constellation of elicitable signs may be obtained. Upper motor neuron disease is indicated by weakness and progressive spasticity with increased muscle tone, exaggerated deep tendon reflexes with clonus, extensor plantar response, and incoordinate or scissor gait, which may progress to spastic paraplegia. The involvement of peripheral nerves may markedly modify these signs to include flaccidity and the absence of deep tendon reflexes. A positive Romberg sign is not uncommon and a positive Lhermitte sign may be elicited. Loss of sphincter and bowel control, altered cranial nerve dysfunction with altered taste, smell, and visual acuity or color perception, and optic neuritis (unexplained predominance in males) may be other physical signs indicating cobalamin deficiency. Inability to carry out serial subtraction of 7 from 100 is a valuable test to document reduced cerebral function (the electroencephalogram often reveals slow wave frequency) in pernicious anemia.

INSIGHTS INTO THE CHANGING SPECTRUM OF COBALAMIN DEFICIENCY

The biochemical and clinical spectrum of presentations of cobalamin deficiency has changed dramatically compared with earlier descriptions. For instance, earlier in developing countries, most cases with nutritional cobalamin deficiency presented in the second and third decades with pancytopenia, mild hepatosplenomegaly, fever, and thrombocytopenic bleeding, all of which are in keeping with the concept of ineffective hematopoiesis of megaloblastosis.[2] Implicit in the earlier literature was the dictum that the neurologic and psychiatric syndrome uniquely associated with cobalamin deficiency usually developed in approximately 80% by the time anemia was symptomatic, and in approximately 50% of patients, this led to some incapacity. However, from southern Africa among 144 consecutive adults (who were not vegetarian, pregnant, or lactating) with megaloblastic anemia[2] and similar presentations of megaloblastosis as reported from India, there was a high incidence of neurologic disease among patients with mild to moderate anemia due to cobalamin deficiency (in 86%). (How many of these subjects had nutritional cobalamin deficiency from poverty-imposed near-vegetarianism is unclear.) This report nevertheless reversed previous presumptions that the primary cause of megaloblastic anemia in this population in developing countries is invariably folate deficiency.

That such classic hematologic presentations are infrequently observed in the West was initially recognized when anemia and macrocytosis were not invariably associated with cobalamin deficiency.[2] When the clinical spectrum and diagnosis of cobalamin deficiency was reevaluated among a cohort of unselected consecutive patients in New York and Colorado who fulfilled criteria for unambiguous cobalamin deficiency, normal values in hematocrit, mean cell volume, and LDH were found in more than one-third of the patients, and approximately 80% had normal white blood cells and platelets and serum bilirubin levels.[2] Strikingly, 33% of the patients' blood smears were not identified as diagnostic when evaluated by laboratory personnel, compared with 94% when evaluated by the investigators themselves. This fact is important because most physicians in general practice rely heavily on laboratory personnel to identify an abnormal blood smear. Equally striking was the important finding that neuropsychiatric abnormalities were observed in nearly one-third of patients often in the absence of anemia, macrocytosis, or both.[2] These data formed the basis for reevaluating the diagnostic sensitivity and specificity of serum homocysteine and MMA in clear-cut cobalamin deficiency (406 patients) or folate deficiency (119 patients).[2] In patients with cobalamin deficiency, serum MMA levels were elevated in 98.4% and serum homocysteine in 95.9%; both metabolites were normal in only one patient (0.2%). For patients with folate deficiency, the serum homocysteine was increased in 91% and MMA was elevated in 12.2%, but in all but one this was attributed to renal insufficiency or dehydration, conditions that are known to falsely raise concentrations of this metabolite. These data allowed for the conclusion that normal levels of MMA and homocysteine rule out clinically significant cobalamin deficiency with virtually 100% certainty.[2]

The changing pattern of neurologic presentations also deserves special mention. From a classic review of 153 episodes of cobalamin deficiency involving the nervous system, the following facts emerged[2]: First and foremost, in over a quarter of these patients, there was no reduction in the hematocrit level despite neurologic disease, and only a minority of patients had combined hematologic and neurologic disease. The inclusion of anemic and nonanemic patients who were cobalamin-deficient led to the dramatic conclusion that the higher the hematocrit, the more severe is the neurologic disorder. (This has its experimental correlates in monkeys and fruit bats, which have severe neurologic disease in the absence of anemia![1,2]) Profoundly anemic patients frequently had no neurologic deficits, and the level of cobalamin had no correlation with the existence or severity of neurologic disease. Although simultaneous consumption of folate may have negated the development of potential hematologic abnormalities in cobalamin deficiency, this could not be documented. Among patients studied, 65% had mild, approximately 25% had moderate, and approximately 10% had severe neurologic deficits. Paresthesias or ataxia were most commonly the first symptoms and diminished vibratory sensation and proprioception in the lower extremities were the most common objective early signs. Although multiple neurologic syndromes were often seen in the same patient, the spectrum of objective signs could include loss of fine or coarse touch, decreased or increased deep tendon reflexes with spasticity or muscle weakness, urinary or fecal incontinence, orthostatic hypotension, amaurosis, dementia, psychosis, or mood disturbances.[2] Overall, although the neurologic deficits were mild in most cases, the severity was judged relative to the duration of symptoms before diagnosis; not unexpectedly, those with a shorter duration of symptoms responded most to appropriate replacement. The demonstration of cognitive improvement in 11 of 18 geriatric subjects with low cobalamin and quantitative cognitive dysfunction treated with cobalamin, and the observation that there is a limited window of opportunity for effective intervention, also highlights the importance of early diagnosis for this population.[2]

Although the basis for these changes in clinical presentation is speculative, it may reflect heightened awareness of cobalamin deficiency, better diagnostic tools, or supplementary folates taken by humans and given to livestock (which corrects megaloblastosis but aggravates neuropsychiatric disease). As a result of food fortification with folic acid, hyperhomocysteinemia in the United States is most frequently caused by cobalamin deficiency.[2,95]

Among the elderly population, it is estimated that 40% to 50% of cases with subclinical cobalamin deficiency (diagnosed by elevations in both metabolites) are caused by food-cobalamin malabsorption, with only a minority having pernicious anemia; the cause among the remaining 50% to 60% cases of subclinical cobalamin deficiency is not known. These individuals would respond to daily replacement with 1000 μg of cobalamin orally.[96] In developing countries, because of widespread vegetarianism or poverty-imposed near-vegetarianism, the predominant cause is probably dietary deficiency of cobalamin,[5] but an additional gastrointestinal basis for cobalamin malabsorption is also suspected.[48] Classical presentations of cobalamin deficiency are still not uncommon in developing countries, where cobalamin deficiency may be accompanied by folate and iron deficiency.

DIAGNOSTIC ISSUES RELATED TO INFORMATION FROM THE PERIPHERAL SMEAR AND BONE MARROW ASPIRATE

Although not specific for megaloblastic anemia, macroovalocytes are the hallmark of megaloblastosis (Table 39–5). This distinction is important because only 55% of 109 patients with MCV values greater than 105 fl had vitamin deficiency (this percentage may be lower or higher depending on the population under study). In almost one-half of all cases, macrocytosis per se is not associated with megaloblastosis (see Table 39–5) and additional tests are necessary for a complete diagnosis.

The frequency of hypersegmented PMNs (5% with 5 lobes or 1% with six-lobed PMNs) in patients with megaloblastic hematopoiesis is 98%. The sensitivity decreases to only 78% in alcoholics although the specificity of this finding is approximately 95%. With a combination of hypersegmented PMNs and macroovalocytosis, the specificity is 96% to 98%, and the positive predictive value of folate or cobalamin deficiency is approximately 94%.[2] Hypersegmentation of PMNs is insufficiently sensitive, when compared with metabolite levels, to be used as a clinical tool in the diagnosis of mild cobalamin deficiency.[2]

MASKED MEGALOBLASTOSIS

The term *masked megaloblastosis* is reserved for conditions in which true cobalamin or folate deficiency with anemia is not accompanied by classic findings of megaloblastosis in the peripheral blood and bone marrow. This occurs when there is a coexisting condition that neutralizes the tendency to generate megaloblastic cells (usually involving reduction in RBC hemoglobinization, as in iron deficiency or thalassemia). Among the 123 episodes of folate deficiency in 119 patients, the MCV was normal in 25%.[2] A wide RBC distribution width (RDW) on the Coulter counter readout in the presence of a "normal" mean corpuscular hemoglobin (MCH) or MCV may reflect megaloblastic anemia[2] or dimorphic (macroovalocytes plus microcytic hypochromic RBCs) anemia. Because megaloblastic white blood cells and precursors are unaffected by deficient hemoglobinization, these pathognomonic findings (giant myelocytes and metamyelocytes, and hypersegmented PMNs) remain; the latter may persist for up to 2 weeks after replacement with cobalamin or folate.[1] The recognition of masked megaloblastosis should initiate investigations to rule out iron deficiency, anemia of chronic disease, or hemoglobinopathies. Appropriate replacement with cobalamin or folate elicits a maximal therapeutic benefit only when iron deficiency is corrected. Conversely, if combined iron and cobalamin deficiency (total gastrectomy) or iron and folate deficiency (pregnancy) is treated with iron alone, megaloblastosis will be unmasked.

Diagnostic Bone Marrow Aspiration

Is bone marrow aspiration always necessary to diagnose cobalamin- or folate-deficient megaloblastosis? With the addition of highly sensitive serum tests for the specific diagnosis of cobalamin and folate deficiency, the need for a bone marrow test is often dictated by the urgency to diagnose megaloblastosis (with results available in an hour). For example, in the case of florid hematologic disease with or without neurologic disease suggestive of cobalamin or folate deficiency, bone marrow aspiration carried out as soon as possible is invaluable in assisting the rapid diagnosis of megaloblastosis. However, in the outpatient setting, when the patient has a characteristic peripheral smear, or for a patient with a primary neuropsychiatric presentation, a case can be made to initiate the sequence of diagnostic tests without bone marrow aspiration by proceeding with measurement of serum levels of vitamins or metabolites (see Table 39–2). In pregnant patients with pancytopenia with macroovalocytes, hypersegmented polymorphonuclear neutrophils, and reticulocytopenia with a history of noncompliance with prenatal supplements (and no neurologic findings suggestive of cobalamin deficiency), bone marrow aspiration may not be necessary to initiate therapy for a strong presumptive diagnosis of folate deficiency. If there is no evidence of response within 10 days, bone marrow aspiration is indicated.

APPROACH TO DIAGNOSIS AND THERAPY OF MEGALOBLASTOSIS

In general, there are three stages in approaching a patient: *recognizing* that megaloblastic anemia is present; *distinguishing* whether folate or cobalamin or combined folate and cobalamin deficiencies have led to the anemia; and diagnosing the *underlying disease* and *mechanism* causing the deficiency. Establishing that the patient does have megaloblastosis is, in theory, straightforward. This is easily done by first evaluating the complete blood count, the mean corpuscular volume and the peripheral smear, followed by a bone marrow aspiration. Clues to whether cobalamin or folate deficiency is responsible for megaloblastosis can be obtained by serum cobalamin and serum folate levels; additional testing of serum MMA and serum homocysteine can define the true nature of the deficiency.[2,97] However, this ideal and orderly workup is not always feasible in clinical practice, because the patient may present for the first time with or without associated neurologic disease, be referred after a variable workup has already been initiated for possible megaloblastosis, present with symptoms primarily attributed to a disease predisposing to cobalamin or folate deficiency (in which case anemia or neurologic dysfunction may only be a minor symptom), present with isolated neurologic disease in the absence of anemia, or be referred after empirical therapy has been given for presumed cobalamin or folate deficiency. The immediate question therefore pertains to the overall status of the patient.

If the patient is decompensated or decompensation is imminent, obtain serum folate and cobalamin levels and bone marrow aspiration to confirm megaloblastosis and proceed with transfusion of 1 unit of packed RBCs *slowly*, with vigorous diuretic therapy to obviate further congestive heart failure from fluid overload. The serum potassium

Table 39–5 Clinical Conditions Not to Be Confused With Megaloblastosis

Macrocytosis* Without Megaloblastosis†
Reticulocytosis
Liver disease
Aplastic anemia
Myelodysplastic syndromes (especially 5q−)
Multiple myeloma
Hypoxemia
Smokers
Spurious Increases in Mean Corpuscular Volume Without Macroovalocytosis‡
Cold agglutinin disease
Marked hyperglycemia
Leukocytosis
Older individuals

*The central pallor that normally occupies about one-third of the normal red blood cell is decreased in macroovalocytes. This contrasts with the finding of thin macrocytes, in which the central pallor is increased.

†Although megaloblastosis implies that a bone marrow test has been performed, with the addition of highly sensitive tests for the specific diagnosis of cobalamin and folate deficiency, the need for a bone marrow test is often dictated by the urgency to make the diagnosis.

‡When the Coulter counter readings of a high MCV are not confirmed by looking at the peripheral smear.

level must be carefully monitored. Cobalamin and folate should be administered simultaneously in full doses. Tests for cobalamin absorption can be deferred until the patient is more stable. Transfusion does not apparently alter serum folate or cobalamin levels but can alter red cell folate levels.[2]

If the patient is moderately symptomatic (but not in heart failure), the strong likelihood of a dramatic response (in the sense of well-being and relief of sore tongue) within 2 to 3 days before hematologic improvement argues against immediate blood transfusion.[2] Therefore, proceed with appropriate diagnostic workup as for the well-compensated patient.

If the patient is well compensated, and in the outpatient setting, the physician has time to develop an orderly sequence of diagnostic tests. First, check the peripheral smear and rule out other macrocytic anemias (thin macrocytes with a normoblastic marrow in contrast to macroovalocytes). Draw blood for cobalamin and folate levels (*before* the patient's first hospital meal) to sort out whether the problem is caused by a deficiency of folate or cobalamin, or both, or some other deficiency (see Table 39–2). Assuming that there is no urgency to make the diagnosis, the physician can elect to wait for the results of these tests before proceeding with the next test in the diagnostic workup. If making the diagnosis is urgent, a cost-effective test is the bone marrow aspirate; results indicating megaloblastosis (or not) can be available within an hour. If bone marrow aspiration is performed, samples are sent for special stains and flow cytometry (megaloblastic erythropoiesis can resemble erythroleukemia) and cytogenetic analysis (myelodysplastic syndromes can exhibit some megaloblastic changes in the erythroid series but megaloblastic granulopoiesis is not seen). If the marrow is not obviously megaloblastic but the iron stain reveals absent stores, review the morphology again with special emphasis on granulocytic precursors and promegaloblasts, and look for more subtle megaloblastic changes.

If the patient refuses bone marrow aspiration and serum cobalamin and folate levels are equivocal (ie, in the low normal range), a strong case can be made to test for serum homocysteine and MMA. Serum MMA and homocysteine are ordered together (the same sample remaining from the serum sent for cobalamin and folate may be used if they were frozen away). Integrating the results for serum MMA and homocysteine levels (which will be available after a week or more) with those for serum cobalamin and folate levels can help distinguish cobalamin and folate deficiencies (see Table 39–2). A normal MMA and homocysteine level eliminates cobalamin deficiency with 100% confidence, and normal homocysteine levels suggest that megaloblastic anemia is not caused by folate deficiency. These tests are particularly useful if the patient has pure neurologic disease or if there are associated conditions such as iron deficiency or thalassemia that can mask megaloblastosis. Administration of folate or cobalamin will reduce elevated serum homocysteine and MMA levels to basal values by 1 week, so there is only a narrow window to clinch the diagnosis using metabolite tests.[2] In the rare situation when a defect in cobalamin or folate metabolism is suspected, early consultation with experts who have published in this area is advised.[50]

A reticulocyte count is useful to follow the patient's response to appropriate replacement therapy. Additional supporting studies documenting increased serum lactate dehydrogenase, haptoglobin, and bilirubin (evidence for intramedullary hemolysis) may be performed. Later, studies to define the mechanism for cobalamin malabsorption can be carried out.

When the megaloblastic state is established, try to determine the underlying mechanism of cobalamin or folate deficiency. The cause of folate deficiency is usually sorted out by this time from the history, physical examination, and the clinical setting. If pure folate deficiency has been prolonged, expect associated cobalamin deficiency to ensue (special emphasis should be given to identifying subtle manifestations of neurologic disease). If cobalamin deficiency is suspected, test for serum anti-IF antibodies (highly specific for pernicious anemia). After this, proceed with the Schilling test (see Table 39–3) to differentiate pernicious anemia from other causes of cobalamin deficiency. (The Schilling test can initiate a reticulocytosis by the second or third day in patients with pure cobalamin deficiency and may also demonstrate a partial response in cases of pure folate deficiency.) Additional tests for associated autoimmune diseases should be made (if indicated) by this time. If serum IF antibodies are negative, gastric analysis for Histalog-fast achlorhydria need not be performed, except in children, for whom it is necessary to differentiate congenital IF deficiency from juvenile pernicious anemia and Imerslund–Gräsbeck syndrome. In adults, a strong presumptive diagnosis of pernicious anemia can usually be made with the Schilling test (see Table 39–3).

THERAPY

Routinely, treatment with full doses of parenteral cobalamin (1 mg/day) and oral folate (folic acid) (1–5 mg) before knowledge of the type of vitamin deficiency is established should only be reserved for the severely ill patient. An appropriate regimen for conditions in which cobalamin replenishment can correct cellular cobalamin deficiency (but not correct the underlying problem that led to the deficiency, such as pernicious anemia) is 1 mg of intramuscular cyanocobalamin per day (week 1), 1 mg twice weekly (week 2), 1 mg/week for 4 weeks, and then 1 mg/mo for life (approximately 15%, or 150 μg, is retained 48 hours after each 1-mg cobalamin injection).

Modified Therapeutic Trials

The traditional therapeutic trial using physiologic doses of vitamins (100 μg of folate or 1 μg of cobalamin given daily while monitoring the reticulocyte response)[1] has given way to a modified therapeutic trial. Rather than making the diagnosis of a deficiency, the intention is often to confirm the clinical suspicion that the patient does not have deficiency.[2] This can be demonstrated by lack of response to full replacement doses of both vitamins (1 mg of folic acid orally for 10 days and 1 mg of cobalamin intramuscularly for 10 days). Clinical scenarios in which such trials may be applicable (after drawing blood for serum cobalamin and folate) are as follows:

1. There is a clinical suspicion that the underlying disease is not caused by a vitamin deficiency, but this idea is not supported by results of clinical, morphologic, and biochemical evaluations. Such conditions include anemia with a megaloblastic bone marrow that may be secondary to chemotherapy, myelodysplastic syndromes, or acute myeloid leukemia; when time is of the essence in making the diagnosis; when the levels of cobalamin are likely to be falsely abnormal because of these diseases; or when there is underlying dehydration or renal dysfunction that predictably gives falsely high levels of metabolites.
2. In other situations (ie, pregnancy, acquired immunodeficiency syndrome [AIDS], or alcoholism) with a multifactorial basis for anemia, the response or lack thereof to full doses can eliminate cobalamin or folate deficiency and thereby narrow the (often extensive) differential diagnosis.
3. In instances when severe anemia with megaloblastosis is clinically obvious and so serious that the physician cannot wait for the results of specific tests for deficiency. Full doses of both vitamins are administered, and if there is a response manifested by brisk reticulocytosis by days 5 to 7, retrospective assignment of the deficiency is based on the results of blood samples drawn before beginning the trial.

In all therapeutic trials, if there is no evidence of response within 10 days, bone marrow aspiration is indicated to identify another primary hematologic disease.

Because the doses of cobalamin are much greater than that required physiologically, any theoretical advantage of OH-cobalamin over cyanocobalamin (greater binding to cobalamin-binding proteins, greater serum levels, and less renal excretion) is of little significance in general clinical practice. A randomized study has demonstrated equivalence between 2 mg cobalamin tablets daily and traditional parenteral treatment for those with relatively replete cobalamin stores.[2] For patients who refuse monthly parenteral therapy or prefer daily oral therapy or in those with disorders of hemostasis, cobalamin (1–2 mg/day as tablets) can be recommended for patients with cobalamin malabsorption (where cobalamin is passively absorbed at high doses).[1,2] This is applicable for patients with pernicious anemia and patients with the inability to absorb food cobalamin. It is important to emphasize that the physician must ensure that the patient's depleted cobalamin stores are rapidly repleted by parenteral cobalamin *before* switching to oral cobalamin in the long term and that the patient is compliant and demonstrates adequate cobalamin levels and resolution of hematologic and neurologic abnormalities on follow-up. For nutritional cobalamin deficiency (eg, vegetarians) when the entire circuitry in cobalamin absorption is intact, oral cobalamin of 5 to 10 μg (found in conventional multivitamin tablets in the United States) taken for a lifetime of vegetarianism will suffice, but only after initially replenishing exhausted cobalamin stores with higher doses. However, if there is malabsorption of food-bound cobalamin, higher doses of cobalamin (greater than 1000 μg/day) are required for elderly patients.[96]

Oral folate (folic acid) at doses of 1 to 5 mg per day results in adequate absorption (even where intestinal malabsorption of physiologic food folate is present). Therapy should be continued until complete hematologic recovery is documented. If the underlying cause leading to folate deficiency is not corrected, folate may be continued. Folinic acid (ie, 5-formyl-H_4PteGlu [leucovorin]) should be reserved *only* for rescue protocols involving antifolates (methotrexate or trimethoprim-sulfamethoxazole) or for 5-fluorouracil modulation protocols, in the rare acute folate deficiency syndrome or after N_2O toxicity. It is too expensive for conventional repletion in folate-deficient states.

RESPONSE TO REPLENISHMENT

The response of the patient to appropriate replacement is reversion of megaloblastic hematopoiesis to normal hematopoiesis (probably initiated at the stem cell level) within the first 12 hours; by 48 hours normal hematopoiesis is reestablished, and the only evidence for a prior megaloblastic state may be the persistence of a few giant metamyelocytes. Because megaloblastosis caused by cobalamin or folate deficiency can be reversed in 24 hours by administration of folate (ie, a nutritious hospital meal), delay of a diagnostic bone marrow aspirate is to be avoided for this reason. Clinically, the first 36 to 48 hours are often highlighted by the awakening of an occasional semistuporous individual whose "chief complaint" is amazement at the remarkably improved sense of well-being experienced, with increased alertness and appetite and reduced soreness of the tongue. The ongoing normoblastic hematopoiesis is evidenced by decreases in plasma iron and potassium (1–2 mEq/dL drop in 48 hours), MMA, homocysteine, and phosphate excretion. The patient must be given supplemental potassium if borderline or low potassium levels are found *before* therapy is initiated to obviate potentially fatal arrhythmias. The elevated serum MMA and homocysteine levels will return to normal by the end of the first week.

Accelerated turnover of normal DNA in erythroid precursors is associated with an increase in serum urate, which usually peaks by the fourth day, and with increased cellular phosphate uptake for nucleotide synthesis. This may precipitate an attack of gout if the patient has a "gouty predisposition." The reticulocyte count increases by the second to third day and peaks by the fifth to eighth day (the peak reticulocyte count is directly proportional to the degree of preexisting anemia). This is followed by a rise in RBC count, hemoglobin, and hematocrit by the end of the first week, which normalizes in approximately 2 months, regardless of the initial degree of anemia. By the end of the third week, the RBC count should be above 3×10^6 mm^3; if it is not, additional causes of underlying iron deficiency, hemoglobinopathy, chronic disease, or hypothyroidism should be considered (Table 39–6).

Table 39–6 Causes of Megaloblastosis Not Responding to Therapy with Cobalamin or Folate

Wrong Diagnosis
Combined folate and cobalamin deficiencies being treated with only one vitamin
Associated iron deficiency
Associated hemoglobinopathy (eg, sickle cell disease, thalassemia)
Associated anemia of chronic disease
Associated hypothyroidism

Hypersegmented PMNs continue to remain in the blood for 10 to 14 days; however, the number of normal PMNs and platelets rises and normalizes within the first week. During this process, there may be a transient left shift to include myeloid precursors. The reduced intramedullary hemolysis (as a result of normalized hematopoiesis) leads to a gradual reduction in the serum bilirubin by the end of the first week, and LDH levels will drop concomitantly.

In response to cobalamin, progression of neurologic damage and dysfunction is inhibited. In general, the degree of functional recovery (reversal of neurologic damage) is inversely related to the extent of disease and duration of signs and symptoms. As a rough estimate, signs and symptoms that have been present for less than 3 months are usually completely reversible; with longer duration, there is invariable residual neurologic dysfunction. The reversibility of neurologic damage is slow (a maximal response may take 6 months). Substantial increments (in recovery) are unlikely to be gained after the first 12 months of appropriate therapy, which indicates irreversibility at this point. However, most neurologic abnormalities have improved in up to 90% of patients, with documented subacute combined degeneration.

FOLLOW-UP

Patients with neurologic dysfunction from cobalamin deficiency have traditionally been given more frequent doses of cobalamin (biweekly rather than monthly therapy for the first 6 months), despite the lack of evidence that this form of therapy is more beneficial. This approach, nevertheless, serves a purpose in that improvement in neurologic status can be carefully documented. Once maximal responses have been established, most patients can be treated with life-long cobalamin with a dose that is appropriate for the underlying cause of cobalamin deficiency. Follow-up outpatient visits every 6 months should be instituted to ensure adequate maintenance of hematopoiesis, as well as early diagnosis of other diseases commonly associated with the cobalamin- or folate-deficient state. Follow-up of 95 patients with pernicious anemia indicates that individuals older than 60 years are prone to developing iron deficiency that arises from poor iron absorption from achlorhydria.[2] All patients with pernicious anemia, especially the elderly, should be screened for iron deficiency at the beginning and during follow-up.

Although patients with pernicious anemia have a twofold increase in proximal femur and vertebral fractures and a threefold increase in distal forearm fractures, it is unclear whether this is reduced by therapy with cobalamin. Because cobalamin stimulates proliferation of bone marrow stromal osteoprogenitors and osteoblastic cells, the suppressed activity of osteoblasts may contribute to osteoporosis and fractures in patients with pernicious anemia.[2]

Studies of a cohort of 5072 patients with pernicious anemia registered in Denmark (1977–1989) revealed that in addition to the well-established increased risk for stomach cancer, there was also a twofold increase in the relative risk for cancer of the buccal cavity and pharynx; however, previously reported elevated risks for other digestive tract cancers were not confirmed. Because of the excess risk of gastric cancer and carcinoid tumors in patients with pernicious anemia,[2] the value of endoscopic surveillance was studied prospectively; in 56 patients, two patients each with early gastric cancer and gastric carcinoids were identified. Gastric carcinoids associated with pernicious anemia are clinically indolent tumors, particularly when they are smaller than 2 cm.[2] This information can be used to formulate general guidelines for more frequent surveillance of a patient with pernicious anemia who has larger gastric carcinoids.

ROUTINE SUPPLEMENTATION OF COBALAMIN AND FOLATE

Routine *periconceptional* supplementation of folate for normal women[2] and in higher doses for women at risk for delivery of babies with NTDs[2] provides effective prophylaxis against the development of NTDs. Supplementation with folate throughout pregnancy also helps to prevent premature delivery of low-birth-weight infants,[1] and routine supplementation for premature infants and lactating mothers is also recommended. There remains a great discrepancy between increasing knowledge of the value of folic acid for birth defect prevention (which is directly related to educational status of women), and actual intake of folic acid supplements[98]; currently, it is estimated that less than one-third of reproductive aged American women take folic acid supplements daily. Because only half of US obstetricians regularly discuss folic acid with their patients,[99] apart from food fortification (which is intended to provide only one-quarter of the recommended dietary allowance of folate), other innovative methods have been investigated. A recent randomized controlled trial has demonstrated that very brief physician advice combined with a booster phone call and starter bottle of folic acid tablets can markedly increase women's regular intake of folic acid (increase by 68% vs 20% in the control group).[100]

In addition to hematologic diseases leading to increased folate requirements (eg, autoimmune hemolytic anemia, beta-thalassemia), folic acid supplements appear to reduce the toxicity of methotrexate in psoriasis.[2] A recent review[101] concluded that despite the paucity of studies, it appears that folate supplementation is appropriate for all patients receiving methotrexate for psoriasis to reduce hepatotoxicity and gastrointestinal intolerance without impairing the efficacy of methotrexate.

Whether folic acid administered to patients with rheumatoid arthritis reduces the efficacy of methotrexate has been raised, but analysis of the data reveals that these conclusions are far from definitive and none of the studies have been without flaws.[102] It is also not clear whether folate fortification in the USA has negated the need for additional folic acid supplements for patients receiving methotrexate. Supplementation with folic acid protects against the development of colorectal neoplasia in high-risk patients with ulcerative colitis.[2]

Between 15% of Austrian children (average age approximately 13 years)[91] and up to 40% of Spanish children[92] who are on long-term antiepileptic drug therapy (carbamazepine, phenytoin, phenobarbital, and valproate) have hyperhomocysteinemia that is easily reversed by 1 mg folic acid per day.[93] Because hyperhomocysteinemia can be induced within a year of initiation of carbamazepine or valproate in adolescents, and homocysteine is directly neurotoxic leading to DNA damage and hypersensitivity to excitotoxicity,[94] this underscores the importance of prophylactic therapy of all children receiving antiepileptic drugs with folic acid.

Whether cobalamin should be added to food that is fortified with folate is still under consideration; it has been demonstrated that cobalamin added to breakfast cereals can reduce plasma homocysteine concentrations.[103] This could serve two needs: (a) there would be less chance that fortified food folate would mask the neurologic signs of underlying cobalamin deficiency in vulnerable populations (those with undiagnosed clinical or subclinical cobalamin deficiency); and

Table 39–7 Indications for Prophylaxis with Cobalamin or Folate

Prophylaxis with Cobalamin
Infants of mothers with pernicious anemia*
Infants on specialized diets*
Vegetarians and poverty-imposed near-vegetarians*
Total gastrectomy†
Prophylaxis with Folic Acid‡
All women contemplating pregnancy (at least 400 μg/day)§
Pregnancy and lactation, premature infants
Mothers at risk for delivery of infants with neural tube defects††
Hemolytic anemias/hyperproliferative hematologic states
Patients with rheumatoid arthritis or psoriasis on therapy with methotrexate¶

*For vegetarians, prophylaxis with cobalamin (5- to 10-μg tablet/day) orally should suffice. In food-cobalamin malabsorption from an inability to cleave food cobalamin by acid and pepsin, replacement therapy should be with daily tablets of more than 100 μg taken orally. In these and other conditions involving any abnormality of cobalamin absorption, cobalamin tablets of 1000 μg/day should be administered orally to ensure that cobalamin transport by passive diffusion across the intestine is sufficient to meet daily needs.

†Consider late development of cobalamin deficiency and iron malabsorption (prophylaxis with oral cobalamin and iron).

‡Ensure that the patient does not have a cobalamin deficiency before initiating long-term folate prophylaxis.

§For prevention of first occurrence of neural tube defects.

††Previous delivery of a child with neural tube defects (eg, anencephaly, spina bifida, meningocele) imparts a 10-fold greater risk for subsequent delivery of infant with neural tube defects.

††Folic acid (4 mg/day) is administered periconceptionally and throughout the first trimester.

¶To reduce toxicity of the antifolate.

(b) the cobalamin that is present in fortified food will supply those populations who subsist on low cobalamin stores with adequate cobalamin; this latter need is the far greater worldwide, where several hundred million in the developing world do not obtain adequate dietary cobalamin as a result of vegetarianism or poverty-imposed near-vegetarianism.[5] The role of topical cobalamin in atopic dermatitis (presumed through a scavenger role of nitric oxide by cobalamin) requires confirmation.[104] Table 39–7 summarizes conditions that warrant routine folate or cobalamin supplementation.

HYPERHOMOCYSTEINEMIA

Normally in cells, homocysteine is metabolized by a methylation and a transsulfuration pathway.[105] In the methylation pathway, homocysteine is methylated to methionine in a reaction involving the cobalamin-dependent enzyme (methionine synthase) and 5-methyltetrahydrofolate (5-methyl-H_4PteGlu), which donates its methyl group to homocysteine (see Figs. 39–3, 39–5, and 39–6). Cellular 5-methyl-H_4PteGlu is generated by the enzyme 5,10-methylene-tetrahydrofolate reductase (MTHFR). The critical nature of the function of this MTHFR (to provide 5-methyl-H_4PteGlu to drive the methylation cycle) is highlighted by evidence that in some adults with hyperhomocysteinemia, a polymorphism within its folate-binding pocket (involving a C-to-T substitution at nucleotide 677, which converts an alanine to valine) results in a dysfunctional thermolabile MTHFR.[106] This leads to a pathologic buildup of homocysteine, which exits from cells into the circulation where it predisposes the patient to premature occlusive vascular disease. In the transsulfuration pathway, cystathionine beta-synthase catalyzes the condensation of homocysteine with serine in the presence of pyridoxyl phosphate (vitamin B_6) to form cystathionine, which is further cleaved by a vitamin B_6-dependent gamma-cystathionase to form cysteine and alpha-ketobutyrate. The cysteine can be used for synthesis of the antioxidant glutathione, a key component that defends against oxidative stress within cells. A limiting reagent in the synthesis of glutathione is cysteine, and approximately 50% of the cysteine in the liver is generated from the transsulfuration pathway. There is a metabolic link between homocysteine metabolism and the redox pool of glutathione, and there appears to be reciprocal oxidative sensitivity between methionine synthase activity and cystathionine beta-synthase. Oxidative stress inactivates methionine synthase, whereas homocysteine flux is increased through the transsulfuration pathway, which generates more cysteine and glutathione; conversely, antioxidants can generate the opposite effect.[107] Based on these considerations, the level of plasma homocysteine depends on genetically regulated levels of essential enzymes and the intake of folic acid, vitamin B_6 (pyridoxine), and cobalamin, as well as other conditions (renal dysfunction, increased age, nitrous oxide, and antifolates).

Chronic hyperhomocysteinemia is established as a major risk factor in occlusive vascular diseases.[2] These include myocardial infarctions from coronary atherosclerosis,[2] extracranial carotid artery stenosis,[2] and stroke,[2] vascular disease in end-stage renal failure,[2] thromboangiitis obliterans, aortic atherosclerosis,[2] venous thromboembolism,[2] placental abruption or infarction, and recurrent stillbirths.[2] An increment of 5 μmol/L of homocysteine elevates coronary artery disease risk by as much as cholesterol increases of 20 mg/dL.[2] Hyperhomocysteinemia is also associated with increased incidence of bone fracture,[108] dementia and Alzheimer disease,[109] a higher prevalence of chronic heart failure in adults without prior myocardial infarction,[110] and left ventricular mass and wall thickness only among women.[111]

The strong correlation between homocysteine and occlusive vascular disease has been identified primarily through retrospective studies.[112] Although daily oral cobalamin (2500 μg/day), folic acid (400 μg/day), and vitamin B_6 (2 mg/day) can lower elevated homocysteine and MMA levels in elderly persons with hyperhomocysteinemia,[95] prospective studies intended to test the hypothesis that reduction of homocysteine levels results in beneficial vascular outcomes in patients with a prior stroke or venous thromboembolism have been disappointing.[113–115] A recent meta-analysis concluded that folic acid supplementation has not been shown to reduce risk of cardiovascular diseases or all-cause mortality among participants with a prior history of vascular disease.[116] These results cannot however ignore or discount the substantial body of evidence that homocysteine is a factor that promotes oxidant stress, inflammation, cell proliferation, thrombosis, and endothelial dysfunction.[117] It should also be noted that all the current studies related to prevention of disease by homocysteine-lowering maneuvers relate to *secondary* prevention, and it may well be that primary prevention is the more worthwhile target. Hovering over these large negative clinical trials is the fact of a lack of statistical power (to demonstrate the 10%–20% improvement in clinical outcome that might be expected from homocysteine-lowering treatment) arising from mandatory fortification of food by folate.[118]

A notable study among 365 individuals in the NHLBI Family Heart Study[2] raises issues of a gene–environment interaction. Among subjects with lower plasma folate concentrations (less than 15.4 nmol/L), those with the homozygous thermolabile *MTHFR* genotype had fasting homocysteine levels that were 24% greater than those with the normal genotype. Because a difference between genotypes was not seen among individuals with folate levels higher than 15.4 nmol/L, this suggested that a gene–environment interaction might increase the risk by elevating homocysteine, especially when folate intake is low. A similar issue may be relevant to other polymorphisms involving folate and cobalamin metabolism.

How does hyperhomocysteinemia contribute to atherogenesis? There are several plausible mechanisms, among which platelet activation, hypercoagulability, altering expressivity of multiple genes,[2] increased smooth muscle cell proliferation,[2] induction of endothelial cytotoxicity or dysfunction, stimulation of low-density lipoprotein oxidation and apoptosis in various cell types,[2] have all been suggested.[117] In addition, direct molecular targeting by homocysteine of various proteins can occur through the ability of homocysteine to form stable disulfide bonds with target protein cysteine residues even in the presence of other thiols. This is because of the greater stability of a protein–cysteine–S–S–homocysteine mixed disulfide bond than a protein–cysteine–S–S–cysteine disulfide bond based on higher sulfhydryl pK_a's (because the pK_a of the sulfhydryl of homocysteine is 10.0, whereas that of cysteine is 8.3, this results in greater disulfide bond stability for homocysteine in comparison to cysteine).[119] The current thinking is that such homocysteinylation of a target protein can somehow impair its function (eg, fibronectin, metalloproteases, annexin II), but in other cases homocysteinylation can also result in a gain of function in the target protein. Thus, identification of the entire spectrum of target proteins may begin to explain the myriad of effects of homocysteine.

Recent animal models further support the concept that homocysteine causes atherosclerosis and is not merely associated with the disease.[120] However, whether *smaller* concentrations of homocysteine in the human body (intracellularly or in the blood) such as found in folate or cobalamin or vitamin B_6 deficiency can lead to the same plethora of adverse effects (as noted with animal models) remains to be resolved.

Hyperhomocysteinemia is also linked to osteoporotic fractures; indeed, there is a higher incidence of fractures in those with pernicious anemia, and a lower bone mineral density in those with low cobalamin status.[121] A recent randomized double-blind trial among Japanese patients following stroke who were treated with folate and cobalamin had a five times lower risk for hip fracture over a follow-up period of 2 years compared with a placebo group.[122] Although there are inherent problems with this study,[123] it remains to be demonstrated if other populations with high fracture risk and mechanistic studies at a more fundamental level can unravel a causal relationship between homocysteine and bone.

Several clinical trials[124,125] that have employed a variety of vitamin (cobalamin, vitamin B_6, folate) cocktails to successfully reduce plasma homocysteine levels to normal also found no detectable effects on (improvement in) cognitive function. However, because these trials included too few participants, the duration of treatment was too short, and cognitive-function scores in controls remained intact throughout the trial, they lack the statistical power to refute the "homocysteine hypothesis of dementia."[126]

RENAL FAILURE AND COBALAMIN REPLENISHMENT

When coupled with a predisposition to chronic disease anemia, the demonstration of a borderline or low cobalamin level arising from increased cobalamin clearance during high-flux hemodialysis is a matter of some concern,[2] especially because MMA and homocysteine levels are elevated in patients with renal dysfunction and because elevated homocysteine represents an independent risk factor for vascular events in patients on peritoneal dialysis and hemodialysis.[2] Should such individuals be treated during hemodialysis with cobalamin, pyridoxine, and folate? Administration of supraphysiologic-dose folic acid (15 mg/day), B_6 (100 mg/day), and cobalamin (1 mg/day) can lead to a significant reduction in homocysteine without toxicity, and one-third may correct to normal values.[2] Large trials are under way to define whether lowering the elevated homocysteine found in patients with chronic kidney disease can result in reduced cardiovascular disease.[127]

FOLATE AND CARCINOGENESIS

There appears to be gathering evidence that low folate status can predispose to carcinogenesis. The epidemiologic evidence linking low folate status and cancer, the "soft" evidence from intervention studies, and evidence from animal and in vitro studies, and possible mechanisms have been critically assessed.[128] The mechanisms could involve alterations in methylation of DNA, instability of DNA through strand breaks, or misincorporation of uracil into DNA. Methylation of cytosines (as 5-methyl-deoxycytidine) in DNA can involve the coding region of genes (where it could be the initiator of mutations in tumor suppressor genes) or within cytosines of CpG islands within promoters (where methylation can lead to silencing of tumor suppressor genes, or hypomethylation can lead to activation of protooncogenes). Studies suggest that methylation silences gene expression through the acetylation of histone, which is involved in transcriptional repression.[2] Conversely, hypomethylation of DNA relieves the repression, leading to activation of genes. Of significance, such epigenetic changes (hypomethylation) have been observed experimentally in the white blood cells of humans and in carcinogenesis, when adenomas progress to colon cancer. Equally important, there appears to be a field defect involving normal rectal mucosa adjacent to adenomas also. The high frequency of the thermolabile MTHFR in the general population has allowed further study of risk related to carcinogenesis as related to altered folate flux. MTHFR is involved in the unidirectional generation of 5-methyl-H_4PteGlu.[129] When it is thermolabile, there is a preferential rerouting of the one-carbon group through the 5,10-methylene-H_4PteGlu pathway to generate more thymidylate for DNA synthesis (as verified in erythrocytes) provided folate status is normal (see Fig. 39–5). As a consequence, some studies suggest that those who are homozygous for MTHFR have one-half of the risk for colon cancer (provided they have adequate amounts of folate, which optimizes the rerouting). This suggests that preferential flux of folate through the thymidylate synthesis pathway at the expense of the methylation pathway protects DNA. But in individuals with homozygous thermolabile MTHFR who have low folate status, 5,10-methylene-H_4PteGlu fails to stabilize the flavin adenine nucleotide cofactor within the binding pocket of the MTHFR leading to its reduced enzyme activity.[2] The folate deficiency predisposes to hypomethylation of DNA, which can lead to a procarcinogenic risk.[129] This (among other possibilities) can explain the conflicting data on thermolabile MTHFR and risk for cancer.[128]

Overall it appears that there may be a reduction in risk in those with highest dietary intake of folate and indeed small intervention studies have demonstrated some improvement or reversal in surrogate end-point markers. However, it has also been observed in animals that folate supplementation may increase colorectal cancer risk and accelerate progression after neoplastic foci are established. Hence the need for caution and for careful monitoring of populations in the long term in populations that have food fortification programs. However, the jury is still out on the issue of folates and colorectal cancer risk.

Although there is a wealth of animal data and some human studies[130] on a role of folate in DNA hypermethylation of CpG islands resulting in transcriptional silencing of tumor suppressor genes or global hypomethylation, there is insufficient information to conclude that physiologic folate deficiency induces significant enough changes in genomic DNA hypomethylation and/or site and gene-specific aberrant DNA methylation in the colorectal mucosa. Moreover, because of a variety of animal models employed, extrapolation to the human condition must be made with caution. Thus, despite a plethora of experimental evidence that folate deficiency or excess can influence the transformation of normal cells to cancer, and several retrospective and a few prospective epidemiologic studies linking folate deficiency with cancer risk, there is still insufficient data in humans to make conclusions on the role of diet and cancer.

CONCLUSIONS

In this age of spiraling costs for health care delivery and the ongoing debate on ways to reduce these costs, few instances in internal medicine yield more satisfying dividends than diagnosing and treating cobalamin and folate deficiency. These conditions are devastating when undiagnosed, misdiagnosed, or when cobalamin deficiency is treated with folate alone. Recognition of changes in the clinical presentation of cobalamin deficiency and availability of sensitive and specific tests should reduce uncertainty in diagnosis. The studies on folate supplementation during pregnancy that identified new folate-responsive NTDs and neurocristopathies are a paradigm for identification of hitherto unrecognized roles for other nutrients in human development. The significant impact of supplemental folates in relieving human suffering consonant with reducing costs for intensive- and long-term care of infants with prematurity or NTDs is a major achievement and outstanding example of cost-effective preventive medicine. As a result of parallel research in the veterinary sciences, folate supplements have also profited the meat industry. Decisions on the optimum amount of folates needed for fortification of food to prevent this devastating complication in newborns must also respect the dictum of *primum non nocere* for the millions of elderly people with cobalamin deficiency, who could be adversely affected from folate supplementation alone. However, consideration of any adverse effects on these cobalamin-deficient individuals also needs to be tempered by the projected beneficial effects in correction of hyperhomocysteinemia and occlusive vascular disease in many more subjects. Resolution of this very complex debate will establish yet another paradigm for fortification of foods with nutrients that can be beneficial for some but harmful for other population groups.

Dedication

This chapter is dedicated to the memory of Professor Victor Herbert (1927–2002), whose sustained investigations on clinically relevant issues related to vitamin B_{12}, folate, and one-carbon metabolism earned him respect, admiration, and the status as one of the giants in this field.[131]

SUGGESTED READINGS

Andres E, Affenberger S, Vinzio S, et al: Food-cobalamin malabsorption in elderly patients: clinical manifestations and treatment. Am J Med 118:1154, 2005.

Antony AC: Vegetarianism and vitamin-B12 (cobalamin) deficiency. Am J Clin Nutr 78:3, 2003.

Antony AC: In utero physiology: Role of folic acid in nutrient delivery and fetal development. Am J Clin Nutr 85:598S, 2007.

Botto LD, Lisi A, Robert-Gnansia E, et al: International retrospective cohort study of neural tube defects in relation to folic acid recommendations: Are the recommendations working? Brit Med J 330:571, 2005.

Carmel R, Green R, Rosenblatt DS, Watkins D: Update on cobalamin, folate, and homocysteine. Hematol Am Soc Hematol Educ Program 62, 2003.

Chitambar CR, Antony AC: Nutritional aspects of hematologic diseases. In Shils ME, Shike M, Ross AC, Caballero C, Cousins RJ (eds.): Modern Nutrition in Health and Disease, 10th ed. Philadelphia, Lippincott Williams & Wilkins, 2005, p 1436.

Clarke R: Vitamin B12, folic acid, and the prevention of dementia. N Engl J Med 354:2817, 2006.

He Q, Madsen M, Kilkenney A, et al: Amnionless function is required for cubilin brush-border expression and intrinsic factor-cobalamin (vitamin B12) absorption in vivo. Blood 106:1447, 2005.

Kim Y-I: Nutritional epigenetics: Impact of folate deficiency on DNA methylation and colon cancer susceptibility. J Nutr 135:2703, 2005.

Lentz S: Mechanisms of homocysteine-induced atherothrombosis. J Thromb Haemost 3:1646, 2005.

Mills JL, Signore C: Neural tube defect rates before and after food fortification with folic acid. Birth Defects Res A: Clin Mol Teratol 70:844, 2004.

Rader JI, Schneeman BO: Prevalence of neural tube defects, folate status, and folate fortification of enriched cereal-grain products in the United States. Pediatrics 117:1394, 2006.

Ramaekers VT, Hansen RS, Sequeira JM, et al: Autoantibodies to folate receptors in the cerebral folate deficiency syndrome. N Engl J Med 352:1985, 2005.

Refsum H, Smith AD, Ueland PM, et al: Facts and recommendations about total homocysteine determinations: An expert opinion. Clin Chem 50:3, 2004.

Rothenberg SP, da Costa MP, Sequeira JM, et al: Autoantibodies against folate receptors in women with a pregnancy complicated by a neural-tube defect. N Engl J Med 350:134, 2004.

Selhub J: The many facets of hyperhomocysteinemia: Studies from the Framingham Cohorts. J Nutr 136:1726S, 2006.

Stabler SP, Allen RH: Vitamin B12 deficiency as a worldwide problem. Annu Rev Nutr 24:299, 2004.

Tamura T, Picciano MF: Folate and human reproduction. Am J Clin Nutr 83:993, 2006.

Tanner SM, Li Z, Perko JD, et al: Hereditary juvenile cobalamin deficiency caused by mutations in the intrinsic factor gene. Proc Natl Acad Sci USA 102:4130, 2005.

Whitehead V: Acquired and inherited disorders of cobalamin and folate in children. Br J Haematol 134:125, 2006.

REFERENCES

For complete list of references log onto www.expertconsult.com

CHAPTER 40

LABORATORY DIAGNOSIS OF HEMOGLOBINOPATHIES AND THALASSEMIAS

David H. K. Chui and Martin H. Steinberg

INTRODUCTION

Hemoglobin is a tetramer of two pairs of dissimilar globin chains, each containing an identical heme group. Normal adult hemoglobin (Hb A; $\alpha_2\beta_2$) is made of two α- and two β-globin chains. A minor adult hemoglobin (Hb A_2; $\alpha_2\delta_2$) has two α- and two δ-globin chains. Fetal hemoglobin (Hb F; $\alpha_2\gamma_2$) is made of two α- and two γ-globin chains. The α-globin gene cluster, 5′-ζ_2-α_2-α_1-3′, is located on chromosome 16pter-p13.3. The β-globin gene cluster, 5′-ε-$^G\gamma$-$^A\gamma$-δ-β-3′, is located on chromosome 11p15.5.[1]

More than 1300 natural mutations have been found in the α (>400 mutations), β (>700), δ (>70), and γ (>100) globin genes. These can be reviewed through the World Wide Web (globin.cse.psu.edu). Additional novel globin gene mutations are still being discovered.

More than 900 of the globin gene mutations result in changes of the amino acid composition of the corresponding globin chains, resulting in variant hemoglobins. Most of these mutations are clinically insignificant; however, a small number cause some of the most common hereditary diseases in humans, such as Hb S (*HBB* codon 6 GAG → GTG or Glu6Val), which causes sickle cell disease; Hb C (*HBB* codon 6 GAG→AAG or Glu6Lys), which in combination with Hb S causes a sickling disorder; and Hb E (*HBB* codon 26 GAG→AAG or Glu26Lys), which is a major contributor to severe β-thalassemia syndromes.[2–4]

Almost 400 globin gene mutations can cause either α or β thalassemia. These mutations downregulate or abolish either the transcription of the corresponding globin genes or the translation of the globin mRNA. There are about 50 mutations such as Hb E, Hb Lepore caused by a δ–β fusion globin chain, or Hb Constant Spring (*HBA2* codon 142 TAA→CAA or Term142Gln), which can result in both a variant hemoglobin and a thalassemia phenotype.

Other globin gene mutations can cause hemoglobins with either increased or decreased oxygen affinity (nearly 100 mutations); produce unstable hemoglobins and hemolysis (more than 100 mutations); or allow hemoglobin to be oxidized, causing methemoglobins and cyanosis (9 mutations).

DIAGNOSIS

Collectively, hemoglobin mutations form the most common human single gene disorders. Their detection and correct diagnosis are clinically important. There are several indications for investigation of hemoglobinopathy and thalassemia:

1. Clinical suspicion of sickle cell disease or thalassemia syndromes
2. Hemoglobinopathy and/or thalassemia carrier screening in couples from high-risk populations, for genetic counseling and reproductive decisions
3. Confirmation and follow-up of an abnormal neonatal hemoglobin screening result
4. Investigation of the family members of an individual known to have a hemoglobinopathy or thalassemia
5. Preoperative screening for Hb S and other relevant mutations in high-risk populations
6. Laboratory evidence of hemoglobinopathy and/or thalassemia such as
   a. unexplained or familial polycythemia, hemolytic anemia, or cyanosis
   b. positive Hb S solubility test
   c. hemoglobin variant detected during Hb A_{1C} determination
   d. microcytosis, not due to iron deficiency or chronic disease
   e. abnormal erythrocyte morphology of unknown cause
7. Follow-up studies on patients with severe hemoglobinopathies and/or thalassemia to determine their therapeutic response (eg, Hb F level)

Correct diagnosis of these hereditary hemoglobin disorders and their carrier state is important for several reasons:

1. Planning for appropriate medical treatment program, such as transfusion and iron chelation therapy in β-thalassemia major
2. Instituting appropriate preventive health care measures, such as penicillin prophylaxis and pneumococci vaccination in infants diagnosed to have sickle cell disease, or avoidance of oxidant drugs and prompt treatment of infections and fever in children diagnosed to have Hb H disease
3. Predicting prognosis of affected infants, thus helping parents and families to cope with future disease burdens
4. Preventing an incorrect diagnosis that might lead to invasive investigations such as endoscopy to look for gastrointestinal bleeding, and potentially harmful treatment such as long-term iron therapy for people who have thalassemia trait
5. Detecting carriers of globin gene mutations, which is essential for proper genetic counseling and future reproductive decisions.
6. Determining parental mutations for use in prenatal diagnosis, when appropriate and requested
7. Elucidating complex cases and family studies

Initial Workup

Sickle cell disease and α- and β-thalassemias are the three major and severe hemoglobin disorders. Originating in subtropical and tropical regions of the world where malaria was and might still be endemic, these diseases are now found throughout the world, caused by voluntary and forced population migrations and genetic admixture with indigenous populations over the past two and more centuries. Furthermore, sporadic globin gene mutations are encountered in all populations, including northern Europeans. Thus, an individual's ethnicity is helpful but should not be the sole criterion to determine if a search for a hemoglobin disorder is indicated.[5]

A positive family history such as anemia, erythrocytosis, painful sickle cell crises, hydrops fetalis, or repeated transfusions should alert the physician to the possibility of hereditary hemoglobin disorders. However, for most globin gene mutations like those causing sickle cell disease and β-thalassemia, heterozygous carriers are clinically well. Therefore, the lack of a relevant family history does not in any way exclude the possibility that globin gene mutation(s) might be present.

Consideration of age, gender, ethnicity, reproductive plans, and concomitant medical conditions is also important for the workup of

Hemoglobin Bart Hydrops Fetalis Syndrome

A 22-year-old woman of Asian ethnic background was seen by her physician at the 9th week of her first pregnancy. Blood was sent for blood counts and hemoglobin electrophoresis. The laboratory reported the following: "Hb 12.0 g/dL; MCV 68 fL; Hb A_2 2.6%; Hb F <2%; No abnormal hemoglobin detected."

At a later date, she was sent for consultation at the genetic clinic, because her maternal serum triple screening for α-fetoprotein, estriol, and β-human chorionic gonadotropin was positive for possible neural tube defect or Down syndrome. At the 21st week of pregnancy, an amniocentesis was done. At the same time, the blood sample of her husband was sent for testing. The laboratory reported: "Hb 13.1 g/dL; MCV 62 fL; Hb E 22%; Hb H inclusion bodies positive; Consistent with Hb E trait and α-thalassemia trait; Suggest molecular studies to confirm."

At the 25th week of pregnancy, blood samples from the couple were sent for DNA-based globin genotyping. Both were found to be carrier of deletion of two α-globin genes in *cis* of the Southeast Asian type ($- -^{SEA}/\alpha\ \alpha$).

At the 27th week of pregnancy, the cultured amniocytes were sent for DNA analysis. The fetus was diagnosed to have inherited both parental α-thalassemia deletion ($- -^{SEA}/- -^{SEA}$). Counseling was provided to the couple at the 30th week. Delivery of a stillborn infant with the Hb Bart hydrops fetalis syndrome occurred at the 34th week.

α-Thalassemia deletion of two α-globin genes in *cis* of the Southeast Asian type is prevalent in southern China and Southeast Asia. Up to 14% of the general population are heterozygous carriers of this deletion in parts of Thailand, for example. This deletion causes almost all hydrops fetalis due to α-thalassemia in southeast Asia, and also contributes to most cases of Hb H disease.[15,16]

Heterozygotes for this deletion are clinically well, have near-normal Hb level, significant microcytosis, and no abnormal hemoglobin. The correct diagnosis, which is necessary for family counseling and prenatal diagnosis, can only be confirmed by relatively simple DNA-based gap-PCR procedures. Affected homozygous stillborn has been variously misdiagnosed to have congenital heart disease or unusual genetic syndrome. Incorrect assessment of the reproductive risk of the at-risk couple can result in recurrence of the same devastating syndrome in subsequent pregnancies, and medical and psychological ordeals for the affected parents. This syndrome is encountered in increasing numbers in North America and ought to be recognized by both clinical and laboratory physicians.[16]

Hb S/Hb S-South End Mimicking Hb S/β^+-Thalassemia

A 28-year-old woman from Uganda presented with a history of monthly "painful crises" that required on average hospital admission five or six times a year. She also had avascular necrosis of the right femoral head. Her hemoglobin levels varied between 8 and 10 g/dL, MCV was 79 fL, and reticulocyte count 10%. Her serum ferritin was 210 ng/mL. Hemoglobin analysis by cation HPLC was interpreted to show Hb A 36.8%, Hb S 52.7%; Hb A_2 4.4%; and Hb F 5.4%. Based on these results, she was diagnosed to have Hb S/β^+-thalassemia. Her physician was puzzled by her severe symptoms in view of her having more than 35% Hb A.

She was referred for molecular diagnosis. Her β-globin genes were amplified and sequenced. There was homozygosity for the Hb S mutation in codon 6 (GAG→GTG or Glu6Val). In addition, there was heterozygosity for a single-nucleotide mutation in codon 132 (AAA→AAC or Lys132Asn). These results indicate that one of her β-globin gene alleles had the Hb S mutation. The other β-globin gene allele had two mutations, the Hb S in codon 6 plus another mutation in codon 132. The variant hemoglobin made up of the abnormal β-globin chain with amino acid substitutions in both residues 6 and 132 eluted on HPLC like Hb A, and was named Hb S–South End (Fig. 40–4).[53]

The variant hemoglobin with Lys132Asn alone has been previously described as Hb Yamagata and has a low oxygen affinity. It is surmised that Hb S–South End might have similarly low oxygen affinity, and that in combination with Hb S will impart a relatively severe clinical phenotype as exhibited in this patient.

The patient was also a heterozygous carrier of the single α-globin gene of the rightward type ($-\alpha^{3.7}/\alpha\ \alpha$) that might account for her borderline low MCV.

There are nine known sickle hemoglobin variants, each of which has Hb S mutation plus another mutation in the same β-globin gene.[53] Some of these can bring about sickling symptoms even in heterozygotes, such as Hb S-Antilles (Glu6Val, Val23Ile), Hb Jamaica Plain (Glu6Val, Leu68Phe), and Hb S-Oman (Glu6Val, Glu121Lys). Furthermore, the electrophoretic mobility or HPLC retention time of these variant hemoglobins can mimic that of either Hb A (eg, Hb S-South End), Hb S (eg, Hb Jamaica Plain), or Hb C (eg, Hb S-Oman). There was a 1½-year-old child initially thought to have sickle cell trait based on hemoglobin analysis results who developed a life-threatening splenic sequestration syndrome during her first airplane flight. Subsequently DNA-based diagnostics were carried out. The Hb S fraction eluted from HPLC was actually Hb Jamaica Plain, which can cause sickling symptoms in heterozygotes.[54]

There are other variant hemoglobins of clinical importance that mimic Hb A on HPLC or electrophoresis. There was another child initially diagnosed to have sickle cell trait on the basis of hemoglobin analysis results who developed sickle cell disease complications. Further investigation revealed that she was compound heterozygous for Hb S and Hb Quebec–Chori (*HBB* Thr87Ile).[36,55] Hb Quebec–Chori behaves like Hb A on electrophoresis and HPLC, and in combination with Hb S can cause sickle cell disease. Mixture of Hb Quebec–Chori with Hb S has the same delay time of polymerization as pure sickle hemoglobin. The isoleucine at codon 87 could stabilize a lateral contact between Hb S polymer strands and accelerate sickle hemoglobin polymerization.

Hb C (*HBB* Glu6Lys) and Hb O-Arab (*HBB* Glu121Lys) cannot be separated by HPLC or alkaline electrophoresis but can be resolved by IEF or citrate agar electrophoresis. The distinction between these two variant hemoglobins is clinically important because although Hb O-Arab is much less common than Hb C, when coinherited with Hb S, Hb O-Arab can facilitate the polymerization of Hb S and is associated with more severe disease than Hb SC disease.[56]

Hb Malay (*HBB* Asn19Ser) and Hb Volga (*HBB* Ala27Asp) both behave like Hb A on HPLC or electrophoresis. Hb Malay is common in parts of Southeast Asia, and causes a β-thalassemia phenotype because of the creation of a cryptic RNA splice site. Patients with β-thalassemia intermedia due to compound heterozygosity for Hb Malay and a β^+- or β^0-thalassemia mutation may be misdiagnosed as having β-thalassemia trait.[57] Hb Volga is an unstable variant hemoglobin and causes hemolytic anemia. A person who is heterozygous for Hb Volga and has hemolysis would appear to have only Hb A.[58]

Variant hemoglobins have abnormal HPLC eluting profile or electrophoretic mobility largely because of different surface charge caused by amino acid substitution. As illustrated by this case report and other examples, there are variant hemoglobins of clinical importance that cannot be identified by hemoglobin analytical techniques used in clinical laboratories. These observations illustrate the importance of correlation between clinical and laboratory findings to ensure that correct diagnosis is made. DNA-based globin genotyping is the only way to provide correct and definitive diagnosis.

Hb E/β⁰-Thalassemia with Concomitant α-Thalassemia

A baby boy of Asian ancestry presented to pediatric clinic because of growth retardation. Both parents were healthy, and the full term pregnancy was uneventful. Neonatal hemoglobin screening showed Hb FE. At 9 months, he was seen by a pediatrician for failure to thrive. His Hb was 7.4 g/dL. Iron supplements were prescribed.

At 14 months, hemoglobin investigation revealed Hb F 48% and Hb E 52%, consistent with the diagnosis of Hb E/β⁰-thalassemia. By 20 months, he was pale, mildly icteric, and noted to have frontal bossing. Both his weight and height were far below the 5th percentile. Marked splenomegaly was present. Blood counts are shown in the table.

He was transfused, subsequently underwent splenectomy, and later started on a regular transfusion program. He gradually improved substantially, and regained appropriate developmental milestones.[7]

Results of hematologic studies and DNA-based diagnostics of both parents and their infant son are summarized as follows:

	Father	*Mother*	*Infant son*
Age	29 years old	23 years old	1½ year old
Hb (g/dL)	11.6	13.0	4.7
MCV (fL)	51	74	61
Reticulocyte (%)	1.5	1.0	15
Hb A (%)	—	65	—
Hb E + A_2 (%)	95	34	52
Hb F (%)	4	<1	48
β-Globin genotype	Compound heterozygous for Hb E, and codon 17 AAG→TAG or Lys17Term β⁰-thalassemia mutation.	Heterozygous for Hb E	Identical β-globin genotype as father's
α-Globin genotype	(– – SEA/αα)	(αα/αα)	(αα/αα)

Coinheritance of a single α-globin gene deletion has been reported to ameliorate the severity of β-thalassemia major or intermedia, likely due to lesser imbalance of the β/α-globin chain synthesis.[59] This beneficial effect, however, does not always hold true. In this family, the coinheritance of deletion of two α-globin genes (– – SEA) in the father might account for his relatively mild phenotype, in contrast to his son who was severely affected.[7] But there could be other yet unknown genetic modifiers that are responsible for the phenotypic dichotomy found between the father and son.[50,60] It should also be pointed out that unlike the father in this family, many patients with Hb E/β-thalassemia have Hb E varying from 40% to 70% and Hb F varying from 30% to 60%.

Hb S/β⁰-Thalassemia

A 25-year-old African American man had been relatively well except for occasional painful episodes in his extremities. His Hb was 10.7 g/dL and MCV 71 fL. At age 23 following a febrile illness, he had one occurrence of splenic sequestration from which he recovered without the need for transfusion. He had a 32-year-old sister with identical hematologic findings, who also was well, and had two uneventful pregnancies.

DNA-based diagnostics revealed that both the proband and his mother were heterozygous for β⁰-thalassemia due to a 1.4 kb deletion from nt –486 to nt +909 relative to the β-globin gene mRNA cap site that removes the promoter region as well as the 5′-coding regions of the β-globin gene and ends in IVSII.[61] The proband also inherited Hb S from his father.

	Father	*Mother*	*Son (age 25 years)*
Hb A (%)	50	90	Absent
Hb S (%)	44	Absent	84
Hb A_2 (%)	3.4	8.8	4.9
Hb F (%)	0.1	2.2	16.2
β-Globin genotype	Heterozygous for Hb S	Heterozygous for 1.4 kb deletion β⁰-thalassemia	Compound heterozygous for both parental mutations
α-Globin genotype	(αα/αα)	(αα/αα)	(αα/αα)

The sum of this patient's Hb F and Hb A_2 adds up to more than 20%, which may be sufficiently high to interfere with intracellular Hb S polymerization and thereby lead to a relatively mild phenotype, unlike most other patients with Hb S/β⁰-thalassemia.

Point mutations in the γ-globin gene promoter region known to cause hereditary persistence of fetal hemoglobin were looked for in the proband, and none was found. In addition, he did not have the T→C polymorphism at nt –158 5′ to the ᴳγ-globin gene, the so-called *XmnI* polymorphism associated with elevated Hb F in some patients with sickle cell disease. The proband had another sister who inherited the same β⁰-thalassemia deletion, but not Hb S mutation. Her Hb A_2 was 8.4% and Hb F 3.4%, similar to her mother.

It is now known that carriers of several relatively small deletions removing β-globin gene promoter regions have much higher Hb A_2 and/or Hb F levels than carriers of most other β-thalassemia mutations due to point mutations. The absence of the β-globin gene promoter sequences may conceivably increase the likelihood that transcription factors bind the remaining δ and/or γ-globin gene promoters, thus enhancing gene transcription and expression.[62]

The differential diagnosis of patients found to have only Hb S, no Hb A, slightly elevated Hb A_2 and microcytosis includes homozygosity for Hb S and concomitant inheritance of α-thalassemia. Approximately 30% of African Americans are carriers of α-thalassemia due to either heterozygosity or homozygosity for single α-globin gene deletion that can account for the microcytosis. Therefore, α-globin genotyping ought to be included in the diagnostic schema for these patients.

hemoglobin disorders. In particular, when a pregnant woman is referred for hemoglobin studies, it is imperative to make the correct diagnosis in a timely manner, and to perform a diagnostic evaluation of her partner at the same time.

Some individuals might have inherited two or more globin gene mutations. For example, a person harboring β-thalassemia mutations affecting both β-globin genes on chromosome 11 may also have inherited an α-thalassemia deletion involving two α-globin genes in *cis* on one chromosome 16.[6,7] Correct deciphering of these complex genotypes often can be done only by DNA-based diagnostics.

Physical findings, such as splenomegaly, and clinical history can be very helpful when correlated with laboratory results in pointing to the appropriate diagnosis. In some cases, the possibility of nonpaternity or de novo mutation can be confounding factors in arriving at the correct diagnosis.[8,9]

Table 40–1 Mean Cell Volume (MCV) during Development

Age	Mean Cell Volume (fL)
At birth	110–128
1 week	107–129
1 month	98–112
2 months	87–113
3 months	80–96
1 year	70–84
4 years	73–86
10 years	75–90
15 years	77–92
Adult	80–96

Data from Segal GB, Palis J: Hematology of the newborn. In Beutler E, Lichtman MA, Coller BS, et al (eds.): Williams Hematology, 6th ed. New York, McGraw-Hill, 2001, p 77; and from Hord JD, Lukens J: Anemias unique to infants and young children. In Lee GR, Foerster J, Lukens JN, et al (eds.): Wintrobe's Clinical Hematology, 10th ed. Baltimore, Williams & Wilkins, 1999, p 1518.

Hematologic Parameters

Hemoglobin level and erythrocyte indices are readily available through automated electronic cell counters. Mean corpuscular volume (MCV) is a highly reliable measurement. One potential source of error is that erythrocytes tend to swell after being stored for 2 to 3 days in vitro, and thus have a higher MCV. MCV varies considerably during infancy and adolescence years (Table 40–1). Low MCV, that is, microcytosis, is usually indicative of iron deficiency, thalassemia, or anemia of chronic disease. MCV can be within normal range in heterozygous carriers of α^+-thalassemia or the Hb E mutation.[10]

Iron deficiency usually is characterized by low serum ferritin, low serum iron, high total iron-binding capacity (transferrin), and low serum transferrin saturation. People who have inherited either an α- or a β-thalassemia trait usually have normal iron stores. However, the presence of iron deficiency does not necessarily preclude the person also having inherited thalassemia mutations, or vice versa. In chronic inflammatory disorders, high serum ferritin and low transferrin saturation might be accompanied by mild microcytosis.

The MCV of poorly deformable sickle erythrocytes may be overestimated by cell counters that measure the electrical resistance of cells passing through a small orifice (Coulter principle). Analyzers using light scattering (Mie principle) are more accurate for this determination.[11] This latter method can determine the distribution of red cell density that may be useful for evaluating treatments and clinical course of sickle cell anemia.

Mean corpuscular hemoglobin (MCH) is a calculated value derived from other direct cell counter measurements. This test result remains relatively stable even in blood samples that have been kept at room temperature for 2 to 3 days, and some advocate the use of this parameter instead of MCV.[12]

Red cell distribution width (RDW) index is often normal in thalassemia trait and high in iron deficiency. Several "discriminant functions" using blood counts and erythrocyte indices have been proposed to distinguish iron deficiency from thalassemia trait. These cannot be recommended for reliable diagnostic purposes.

Reticulocyte count reflects erythrocyte production, and when persistently elevated is suggestive of hemolysis. Reticulocytes can be enumerated rapidly by automated blood cell analyzers. However, it should be noted that these instruments are unable to discern reticulocytes from erythrocytes containing Heinz bodies, and therefore yield spuriously high reticulocyte counts in hemolytic anemia caused by unstable variant hemoglobins.[13,14]

Peripheral blood smear morphology can provide clues to the diagnosis of hemoglobin disorders, as in sickle cell disease and thalassemia. In Hb C and Hb SC disease, there is microcytosis, target cells, irregularly contracted cells, and intracellular Hb C crystals. The presence of "bite cells" and irregularly contracted erythrocytes is suggestive of a hemolytic disorder.

In α-thalassemia, there is an excess of β-globin chains. These form β_4 tetramers (Hb H) that precipitate within red blood cells. The formation of these precipitates, Hb H inclusion bodies, is enhanced under the influence of oxidants such as brilliant cresyl blue, and these inclusion bodies can be visualized by light microscopy. When carried out and examined by experienced laboratory personnel, this is a specific screening test for α-thalassemia. But it is time consuming and its accuracy is highly observer-dependent.[15] In Hb H disease, there are many erythrocytes with these inclusion bodies. However, concomitant inheritance of Hb H disease and heterozygosity for β-hemoglobinopathies such as β-thalassemia or Hb E would lead to markedly decreased amount of Hb H and inclusion bodies, and may confound the correct diagnosis of the underlying Hb H disease.[15]

In general, heterozygous carriers of β-thalassemia mutations have microcytosis and elevated Hb A_2 levels. In α-thalassemia carriers, there is microcytosis but Hb A_2 level is normal. A person who is heterozygous for both α- and β-thalassemia mutations has microcytosis and elevated Hb A_2 level, often indistinguishable from a person with β-thalassemia trait alone.[16] For genetic counseling and assessment of potential reproductive risks, DNA-based diagnostics are necessary to determine the correct α- and β-globin genotypes.[17]

HEMOGLOBIN ANALYSIS

High-Performance Liquid Chromatography

High-performance liquid chromatography (HPLC) has become the standard analytical procedure for the initial evaluation of hemoglobin variants and thalassemia in clinical laboratories. It is rapid, automated, capable of resolving most of the common and many uncommon variants, and provides reliable quantitative measurements of hemoglobin fractions like Hb A_2 and Hb F.[18,19] In cation-exchange HPLC, hemolysate is injected into a chromatography column containing a negatively charged resin onto which the positively charged hemoglobins are adsorbed. Hemoglobins are eluted by passing through a carefully calibrated developing solution containing an increasing concentration of cations (Fig. 40–1).[20] The rate of hemoglobin elution, or the retention time, corresponds to the affinity of each hemoglobin for the column matrix, and is continuously monitored by an optical detector. The chromatogram is stored in and analyzed by a microcomputer.

One caveat with HPLC analysis is that Hb A_2 level measurement is often high in the presence of Hb S. Recent improvement in HPLC and also capillary electrophoresis have largely rectified this problem.[21,22] Furthermore, Hb E and Hb Lepore have similar retention time as Hb A_2, and these hemoglobins cannot be positively separated. Hb C and Hb O^{Arab} also cannot be definitively distinguished by cation-HPLC (Fig. 40–2).

Isoelectric Focusing

In isoelectric focusing (IEF), an electric current is passed through a supporting medium such as a precast agarose or polyacrylamide gel containing carrier ampholytes. These ampholytes migrate through the medium to form a stable pH gradient ranging from pH 6.0 at the anode to pH 8.0 at the cathode. Hemolysate is applied to the gel at the cathode end, and hemoglobin fractions migrate through the pH gradient until they are "focused" into a sharp, distinct band at the pH equal to the isoelectric point (pI) at which the hemoglobin is neutrally charged.[23–25] It has better resolving power than many other electrophoretic techniques as it can distinguish variant hemoglobins on the basis of their minute differences in pI. However, Hb

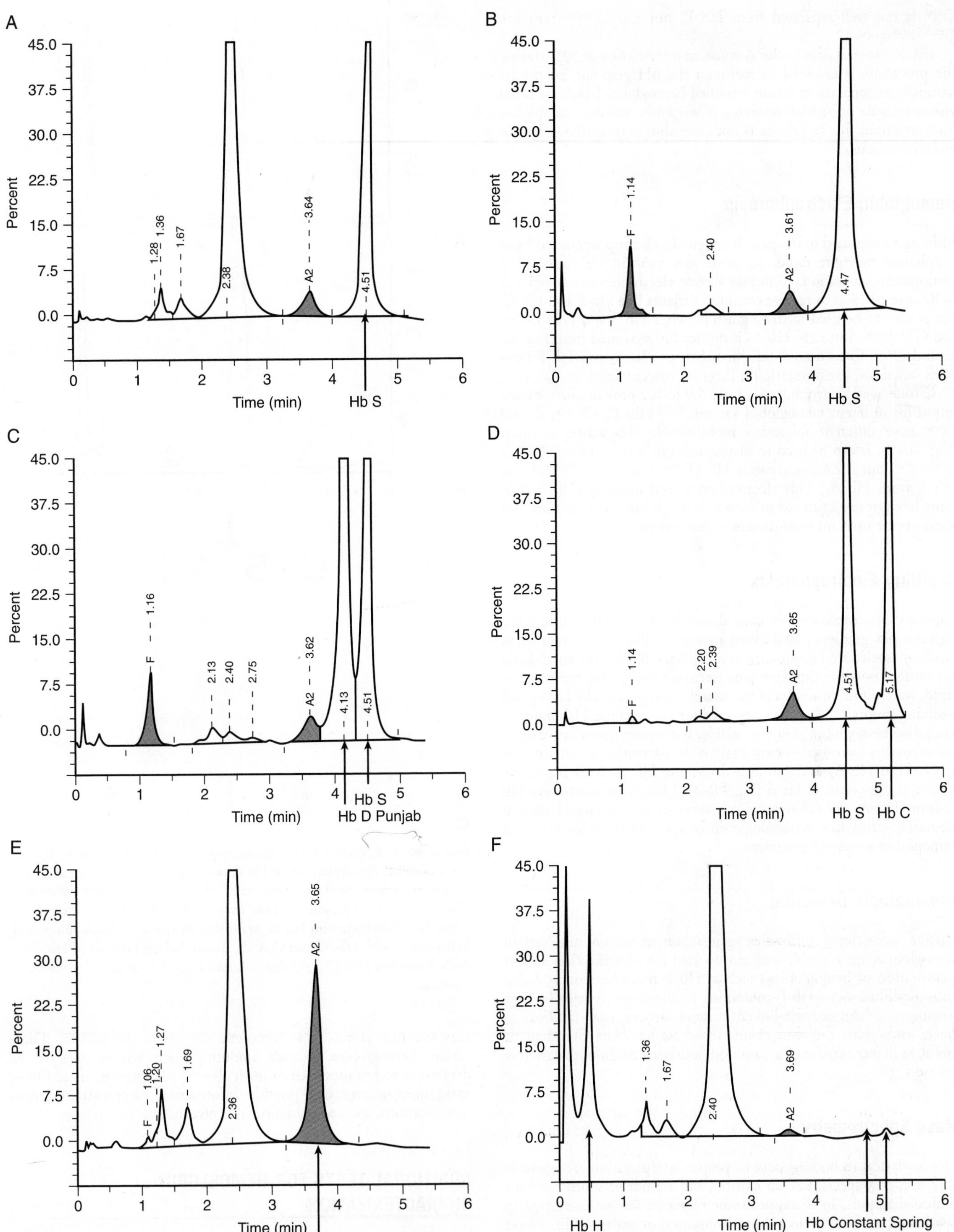

Figure 40–1 Representative tracings from the output of the Biorad Variant II high-performance liquid chromatography analysis of selected hemoglobin variants using the β-thalassemia short program. **A**, Sickle cell trait. **B**, Sickle cell anemia. **C**, Compound heterozygote for Hb D Punjab and Hb S. **D**, Hb SC disease. **E**, Hb E trait. **F**, Hb H disease with Hb Constant Spring. Notice the clear separation of HbA_2 from Hb C (**D**) but the failure to distinguish HbA_2 from Hb E (**E**). Associated with each hemoglobin peak is the elution time from the chromatography column. Hb F and Hb A_2 peaks are shaded. Other peaks represent hemoglobin fractions that have been modified by glycosylation and other posttranslational events. *(Courtesy of Andrew G. McFarlane.)*

O^{Arab} is not well separated from Hb E, nor Hb D^{Punjab} from Hb $G^{Philadelphia}$.

IEF has several drawbacks: A constant temperature at 59°F during the procedure is essential to maintain the pH gradient for proper hemoglobin separation; minor modified hemoglobin bands are often visible because of its high resolving power and these may complicate interpretation; this technique is not amenable to quantifying hemoglobin fractions.

Hemoglobin Electrophoresis

Although a standard in the past, hemoglobin electrophoresis has been supplanted by more rapid, sensitive, and quantitative methods of hemoglobin separation. Cellulose acetate electrophoresis at pH 8.2 to 8.6 can be used to resolve common variants like Hb S and Hb C, but it cannot be used to distinguish between Hb S and Hbs D^{Punjab} and $G^{Philadelphia}$. Similarly, Hb A_2 is not readily separated from Hbs C, E, and O^{Arab}. Quantitative measurements of Hb A_2 and Hb F fractions based on densitometric readings are inaccurate.

Citrate agar electrophoresis at pH 6.0 to 6.2 provides better resolution for different hemoglobin variants.[26–28] Hbs C, C^{Harlem}, E, and O^{Arab} have different migrating mobilities in this acidic medium (Fig. 40–2). It can be used to distinguish Hb S from Hbs D^{Punjab} or $G^{Philadelphia}$, but it cannot separate Hb D^{Punjab} from Hb $G^{Philadelphia}$, or Hb A from Hb A_2. This electrophoretic technique is still used in some laboratories as an aid to variant hemoglobin identification, but it cannot be used for quantitative measurements.

Capillary Electrophoresis

Capillary electrophoresis is carried out by hemoglobin migrating through pH gradients established in fine capillary tubes known as capillary isoelectric focusing or in a capillary filled with an alkaline salt buffer known as capillary zone electrophoresis. This technique is rapid, uses minute amounts of test sample, and potentially has a good resolving power.[29,30] A system designed for use in clinical laboratories to analyze hemoglobin is now available. It provides quantitative measurements and automated data analysis. In particular, it can separate Hb E from Hb A_2 and can also determine Hb A_2 level accurately even in the presence of Hb S (Fig. 40–3).[31] But it cannot resolve Hb C from Hb A_2. These systems can serve as an automated clinical laboratory procedure for hemoglobin analysis, and also for newborn hemoglobin screening programs.

Immunologic Detection

Murine monoclonal antibodies against human normal and variant hemoglobins are available and can be used for identification and/or quantitation of hemoglobins, such as Hb F measurement by radial immunodiffusion, or Hb F-containing erythrocytes (F-cells) by flow cytometry.[32,33] An enzyme-linked immunosorbent assay (ELISA) to detect embryonic ζ-globin chains in adults has been found to be useful to detect carriers of a common Southeast Asian α-thalassemia deletion.[34,35]

Mass Spectrometry

This analytical technology and its proper interpretation are available only in highly specialized laboratories and are not presently used for clinical diagnosis. In mass spectrometry, molecules are converted to gaseous ions, often by electrospray ionization or matrix-assisted laser desorption/ionization. As an accelerating voltage is applied, these particles are separated according to their mass-to-charge ratio. The determination of molecular weight is exquisitely accurate and thus can be reliably used to decipher variant hemoglobins.[36,37] Mass spectrometry can be used to identify highly unstable hemoglobins that may manifest clinically as hemolytic anemia or thalassemia. These variant hemoglobins in trace amounts might not be detected by diagnostic techniques used in most clinical laboratories. In addition, mass spectrometry can provide information on posttranslational modifications, such as oxidation and glycation.

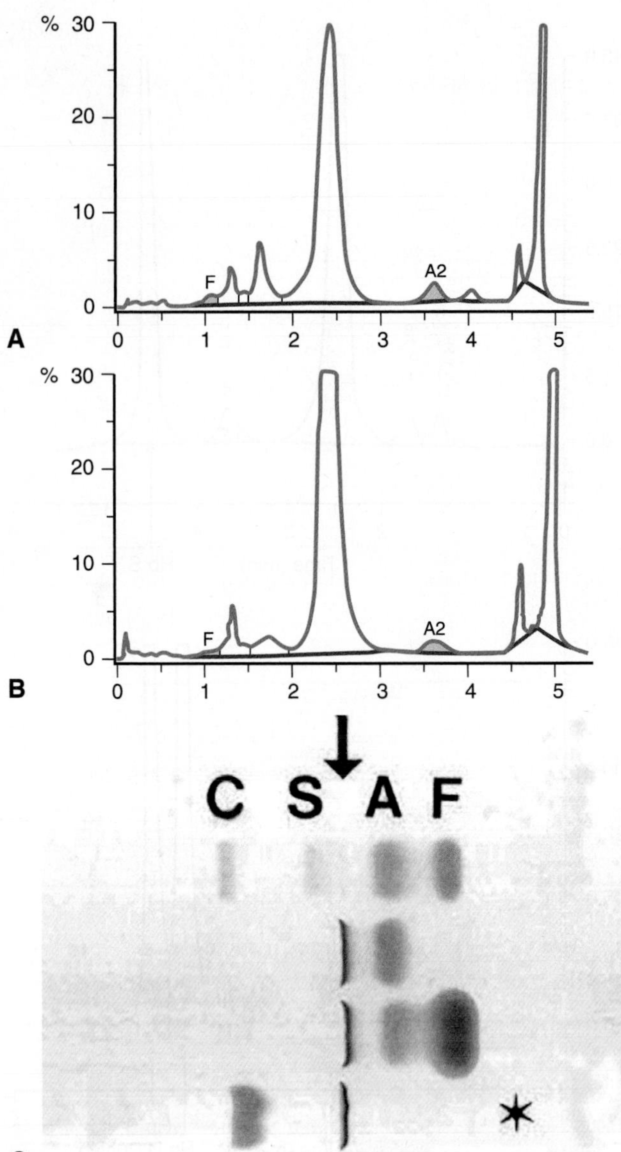

Figure 40–2 A, Cation-HPLC chromatogram of Hb O-Arab trait. **B**, Cation-HPLC chromatogram of Hb C trait. Note that Hbs O-Arab and C cannot be distinguished by cation-HPLC. **C**, Citrate agar electrophoresis. *Top lane:* Hbs C, S A, and F. *Second lane:* Adult with Hb O-Arab trait. *Third lane:* Newborn with Hb O-Arab trait. *Bottom lane:* Adult compound heterozygote with Hbs C and O-Arab. Arrow denotes position of Hb O-Arab. Note that Hbs C, S, O-Arab, A, and F can be separated by this technique.

ADDITIONAL TESTS FOR HEMOGLOBIN CHARACTERIZATION

The Hb S Solubility Test

When reduced with sodium dithionite, Hb S is insoluble and precipitates in high-molarity phosphate buffer at neutral pH. This forms the basis for the simple Hb S solubility test.[38] It is also positive in

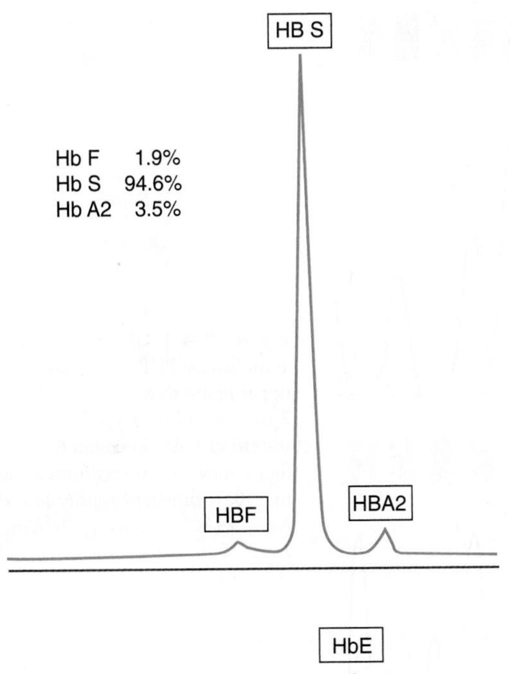

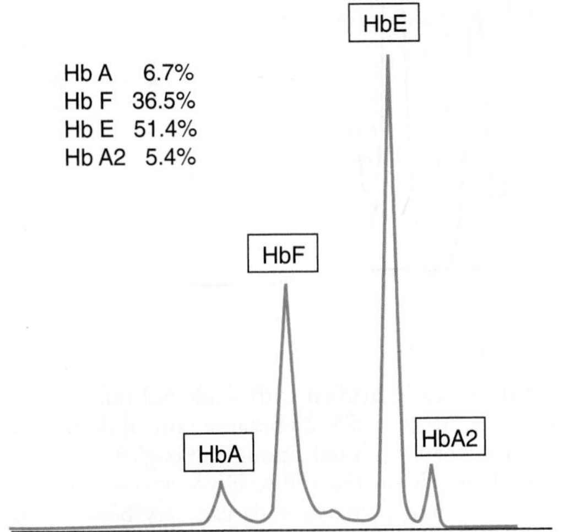

Figure 40–3 Tracings from capillary electrophoresis of hemolysate from homozygous sickle cell anemia (upper figure), and Hb E/IVSI-5 G→C β^{+}-thalassemia (lower figure). *(Courtesy of Andrew G. McFarlane.)*

other variants that have the Hb S mutation plus an additional amino acid substitution, such as Hb S-Antilles, C-Ziquinchor, C-Harlem, S-Providence, S-Oman, and S-Travis.

The Hb S solubility test has very limited applicability: (a) as a screening test for Hb S in patients preparing for emergency surgery under general anesthesia; and (b) as a confirmatory test when Hb S is detected by either electrophoresis, IEF, HPLC, or capillary electrophoresis to distinguish Hb S from other variants with similar migrating mobility as Hb S.

This solubility test cannot distinguish between sickle cell trait, sickle cell disease, or Hb S/β-thalassemia. The test is negative when the concentration of Hb S is less than 15%, and thus is not suitable for testing blood samples from infants or patients who have been transfused. More important, the test cannot detect hemoglobin variants such as Hbs C, D^{Punjab}, and O^{Arab}. These variant hemoglobins in combination with Hb S can cause a sickling disorder. Thus, Hb S solubility tests should not be used for assessment of potential reproductive risk, for genetic counseling or as a primary diagnostic test.

Hemoglobin Functional Investigations

1. Determination of the P_{50} or oxyhemoglobin dissociation curve is necessary to document variant hemoglobins with either high or low oxygen affinity, including those that might have similar electrophoretic mobility as Hb A.
2. Detection of hemoglobin instability by exposure to heat or isopropyl alcohol, and also by Heinz body detection.
3. Identification of methemoglobins is done by studying their unique absorption spectrum.
4. α- and β-globin chain synthetic studies can be helpful to determine whether a patient might have either α- or β-thalassemia mutation but are rarely used clinically.

Iron Studies

Serum ferritin, or serum iron, total iron-binding capacity, and transferrin saturation determinations are helpful to determine if an individual is iron deficient. Most patients with thalassemia trait are not iron deficient, but there are some who have both thalassemia trait and iron deficiency. Measurement of free erythrocyte protoporphyrin or zinc protoporphyrin are other adjunctive tests that are useful to detect iron deficiency or erythrocyte heme synthetic abnormalities.

DNA-Based Globin Gene Analysis

DNA-based mutational analysis is the only method to provide specific genotyping on hemoglobinopathies and thalassemias, and is essential for family counseling and reproductive decision making. Recent advances in molecular genetics and diagnostic innovations have made it possible to carry out these tests rapidly and efficiently. Increasingly, this technology is now accepted and incorporated into the clinical laboratory diagnostic repertoire for both hereditary and acquired disorders.

Gap-PCR (polymerase chain reaction) tests are now often employed to diagnose common deletions, either singly or in mutliplex form for several deletions.[39,40] Southern blot analysis is still used to detect large or novel deletions. For small deletions/insertions, PCR-based heteroduplex analysis is a reliable and simple test.[41]

To detect single-nucleotide mutations, dot blotting or reverse dot blotting with allele-specific oligonucleotide probes are used.[42] To detect several commonly found mutations in a specific population, one can resort to multiplex PCR using allele-specific primers, or multiplex amplification refractory mutational analysis.[43] Other diagnostic alternatives such as minisequencing, denaturing HPLC, or array testing using allele-specific arrayed primer extension have been proposed to be applicable in different locales and laboratories.[44–46]

For the uncommon mutations, nucleotide sequencing of the PCR-amplified globin gene is necessary. This can now be readily carried out for α-, β-, δ-, and γ-globin genes (Fig. 40–4). Other methods are single-strand conformation polymorphism, denaturing gradient gel electrophoresis, and restriction endonuclease analysis of mutations. Except for the common variant hemoglobins, such as Hbs S, C, and E, variant hemoglobin detection based on hemoglobin analysis is primarily a screening test, and ought to be confirmed definitively by DNA-based diagnostics if clinically indicated.

DNA-based mutational analysis is used for prenatal diagnosis on fetal DNA extracted from either primary chorionic villi samples, amniocytes, or their respective cultured cells. Recent reports of success in analyzing fetal DNA in maternal circulation provide a potential method for noninvasive prenatal diagnosis in the future.[47,48]

Interpretation of Laboratory Results

No single hemoglobin analytical procedure available in clinical laboratories can distinguish definitively all common and clinically

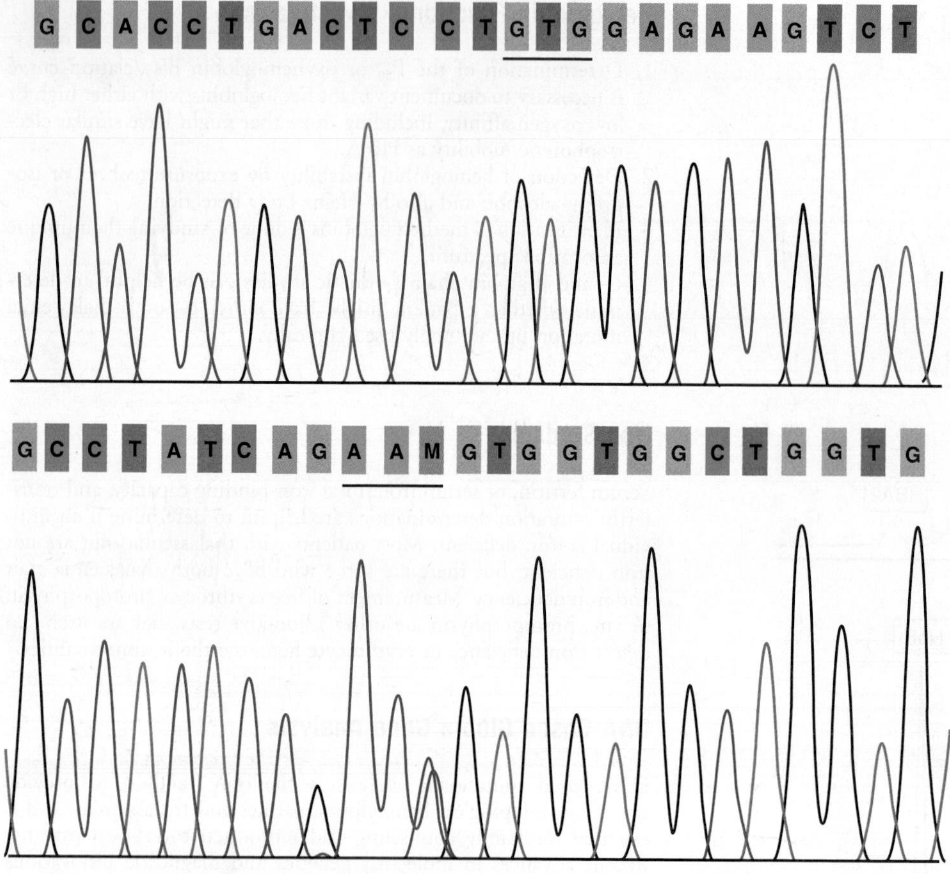

Figure 40–4 β-Globin genes were amplified by PCR and sequenced. The upper figure shows sequences from codons 2 to 9, with homozygosity for GTG instead of GAG in codon 6. The lower figure shows sequences from codons 129 to 136, with heterozygosity in codon 132 AAA→AAC. *(Courtesy of Dr. Hong-Yuan Luo.)*

important variant hemoglobins such as Hb S, C, D[Punjab], E, and O[Arab]. Currently, cation HPLC is the method of choice (Fig. 40–1). It is advisable to have a different diagnostic method, such as IEF or citrate agar electrophoresis, available for confirmation.

Most variant hemoglobins do not cause disease. As the worlds' populations mix, coinheritance of mutations for hemoglobinopathies and thalassemias which alone are innocuous may lead to severe disease.[49] Therefore, careful clinical–laboratory correlation is required to determine if additional investigations are needed to precisely characterize globin gene mutations.

Heterozygotes for β-globin gene mutations usually have one major variant hemoglobin fraction ($\alpha_2\beta^{Variant}{}_2$), which is often slightly less in amount to the normal Hb A ($\alpha_2\beta_2$). However, heterozygotes for α-globin gene mutations usually have one major variant hemoglobin fraction ($\alpha^{Variant}{}_2\beta_2$) of approximately 20% of the normal Hb A ($\alpha_2\beta_2$) plus a minor variant hemoglobin made up of two mutant α-globin chains and two normal δ-globin chains forming a variant Hb A_2 fraction ($\alpha^{Variant}{}_2\delta_2$), in addition to the normal Hb A_2 ($\alpha_2\delta_2$).

Quantitation of Hb A_2 is vitally important, as an elevated value is a diagnostic criterion for β-thalassemia carriers. Care should be exercised to be aware of δ-globin mutations that may cause variant Hb A_2 with a different migration mobility from normal Hb A_2 or δ-thalassemia. Their disregard might lead to an erroneous conclusion that the individual under study is not a β-thalassemia carrier.

Quantitation of Hb F is important for the diagnosis of thalassemia syndromes and hereditary persistence of fetal hemoglobin. It is also often used as a marker for treatment response in sickle cell disease and thalassemias. Hb F can be reliably measured by HPLC or CE, or can be determined by immunologic methods using specific anti-γ-globin chain antibodies.

The accumulation of different hemoglobin in vivo depends on the expression of individual globin genes, the stability of the globin produced, and on the posttranslational assembly of hemoglobin dimers. As an illustration, the Hb A : Hb S ratio in uncomplicated sickle cell trait is 60 : 40. In an individual with sickle cell trait and α-thalassemia, this ratio is 70 : 30 to 75 : 25 because normal β-globin chain has a greater affinity for the limited amounts of α-globin chain than does the sickle β-globin chain. The Hb A : Hb S ratio in a person who has coinherited Hb S and β^+-thalassemia can vary between 30 : 70 and 10 : 90 depending on the nature of the β^+-thalassemia mutation that affects the amount of β^A-globin produced (Table 40–2).

Also as illustrated in Table 40–2, there are considerable overlaps in hematologic findings in sickle cell anemia, Hb S/β^0-thalassemia, and also sickle cell anemia with concurrent α-thalassemia. In all three conditions, the major hemoglobin present is Hb S, with variable amounts of Hb F, and Hb A is absent. Molecular or family studies often are needed to distinguish among these possibilities. Transfusion can provide yet another confounding factor in arriving at the correct diagnosis.

There are genetic modifiers that play critical roles in determining the phenotypic expression of hemoglobin disorders.[50–52] The highly variable clinical manifestations of sickle cell disease and of Hb E/β-thalassemia are but two examples. As these genetic modifiers are characterized, they will have to be included into the future laboratory diagnostic repertoire as they become clinically relevant for predicting prognosis and planning for therapeutic strategies.

There are more than 1300 natural globin gene mutations. In today's multicultural societies in North America and elsewhere, there can be a vast number of different globin genotypes. In some countries, high carrier frequencies of β- and α-thalassemias and variant hemoglobins are present. The common hemoglobin disorders such as homozygous sickle cell anemia can be diagnosed in most clinical laboratories. More complicated and unusual cases should be studied in a reference laboratory capable of carrying out more sophisticated investigations including DNA-based procedures and having both clinical and laboratory expertise in order to provide the best possible diagnostic and consultative advice to the physicians and genetic counselors caring for these patients and their families.

Table 40–2 Hematologic and Hemoglobin Findings in Hemoglobin S, Hemoglobin C, and Hemoglobin E Syndromes

Diagnosis	α-Globin Genotype	Hb (g/dL)	MCV (fL)	Reticulocytes (%)	Variant Hemoglobin (%)	Hb A (%)	Hb A_2 (%)	Hb F (%)
Sickle cell syndromes								
β^A/β^S (sickle cell trait)	$\alpha\alpha/\alpha\alpha$	13–15	80–90	Normal	Hb S 40	60	2.5	<1
β^A/β^S (sickle cell trait)	$-\alpha/\alpha\alpha$	13–14	75–85	Normal	Hb S 30–35	65–70	2.5	<1
β^A/β^S (sickle cell trait)	$-\alpha/-\alpha$	12–13	70–75	Normal	Hb S 25–30	70–75	2.5	<1
β^A/β^S (sickle cell trait)	$--/-\alpha$	7–10	50–55	Normal	Hb S 17–25	75–80	2.5	<1
β^S/β^S (sickle cell disease)	$\alpha\alpha/\alpha\alpha$	8.1	92	12	Hb S >85	0	2.9	2–20
β^S/β^S (sickle cell disease)	$-\alpha/\alpha\alpha$	8.7	84	9	Hb S >85	0	3.3	2–20
β^S/β^S (sickle cell disease)	$-\alpha/-\alpha$	9.1	72	6	Hb S >85	0	3.7	2–20
β^S/β^+-thalassemia	$\alpha\alpha/\alpha\alpha$	8–12	65–75	4	Hb S 70–90	5–30	3.5–6	1–15
β^S/β^0-thalassemia	$\alpha\alpha/\alpha\alpha$	7–11	60–80	4	Hb S 80–95	0	3.5–6	1–15
β^S/HPFH	$\alpha\alpha/\alpha\alpha$	11–14	80–90	2	Hb S 70–80	0	1–3	20–30
β^S/β^C (Hb SC disease)	$\alpha\alpha/\alpha\alpha$	8–13.5	75–90	4–5	Hb S 50; Hb C 50	0	Normal	1–7
Hb C syndromes								
β^A/β^C (Hb C trait)	$\alpha\alpha/\alpha\alpha$	Normal	Normal to low	Normal	Hb S 40–45	55–60	Normal	Normal
β^A/β^C (Hb C trait)	$-\alpha/\alpha\alpha$	Few cases reported			Hb S 35–40	60–65	Normal	
β^A/β^C (Hb C trait)	$-\alpha/-\alpha$	Few cases reported			Hb S 25–35	65–75	Normal	
β^C/β^C (Hb C disease)	$\alpha\alpha/\alpha\alpha$	10–15	60–90	2–7	Hb C 95	0	Normal	2–4
β^C/β^0-thalassemia	$\alpha\alpha/\alpha\alpha$	8–12	55–70	5–20	Hb S 90–95	0	Elevated	3–10
Hb E syndromes								
β^A/β^E (Hb E trait)	$\alpha/\alpha\alpha$	11–14	80–90	Normal	Hb S 27–32	66–70	Unable to determine	0.5–1.5
β^A/β^E (Hb E trait)	$-\alpha/\alpha\alpha$	12–15	84–92	Normal	Hb S 27–32	66–70	Unable to determine	0.5–1.5
β^A/β^E (Hb E trait)	$-\alpha/-\alpha$	11–14	72–82	Normal	Hb S 20–22	76–80	Unable to determine	0.5–1.5
β^A/β^E (Hb E trait)	$--/-\alpha$	8–10	57–63	High	Hb S 12–16	85	Unable to determine	2–4
β^E/β^E (homozygous Hb E)	$\alpha\alpha/\alpha\alpha$	10–13	66–74	Normal	Hb E 95	0	Unable to determine	5
β^E/β^+-thalassemia	$\alpha\alpha/\alpha\alpha$	6–12	60–70	High	Hb E 44–70	5–25	Unable to determine	10–55
β^E/β^0-thalassemia	$\alpha\alpha/\alpha\alpha$	5–10	60–70	High	Hb E 46–70	0	Unable to determine	30–70

These laboratory results represent ranges in general for adults, and adapted from data from several recent book chapters.[2–4] Individual patient's values might vary and be significantly different from figures in this table. Blood counts and hemoglobin fractions show developmental changes so that a patient's age must be considered in their interpretation.

Considerable overlap of hematologic values and hemoglobin fractions in sickle cell anemia with α thalassemia and Hb S/β^0-thalassemia make family and molecular studies imperative for genetic counseling.

Older methods of measuring Hb A_2, such as hemoglobin electrophoresis, were unable to separate this minor hemoglobin fraction from Hb C and Hb E. Newer techniques like HPLC or CE are able to do this. Whether or not concurrent α-thalassemia changes Hb A_2 in Hb C or Hb E heterozygous carriers is not known.

One caveat with HPLC analysis was that Hb A_2 levels were spuriously elevated in the presence of Hb S.[21] Newer design for HPLC or capillary electrophoresis now allow accurate measurement of Hb A_2 when Hb S is present.[22,31]

SUGGESTED READINGS

Chui DHK, Fucharoen S, Chan V: Hemoglobin H disease: not necessarily a benign disorder. Blood 101: 791–800, 2003.

Chui DHK, Waye JS: Hydrops fetalis caused by α-thalassemia: An emerging health care problem. Blood 91:2213–2222, 1998.

Hardison RC, Chui DHK, Giardine B, Reimer C, patrinos GP, Anagnou N, Miller W, Wajcman H: Hb Var: A relational database of human hemoglobin variants and thalassemia mutations at the globin gene server. Human Mutation 19:225–233, 2002. http://globin.cse.psu.edu

Harteveld CL, Voskamp A, Phylipsen M, Akkermans N, den Dunnen JT, White SJ, Giordano PC: Nine unknown rearrangements in 16p13.3 and 11p15.4 causing α- and β-thalassaemia characterized by high resolution multiplex ligation-dependent probe amplification. Journal of Medical Genetics 42:922–931, 2005.

Old JM: Screening and genetic diagnosis of haemoglobinopathies. Scandinavian Journal of Clinical and Laboratory Investigation 67:71–86, 2007.

Steensma DP, Gibbons RJ, Higgs DR: Acquired α-thalassemia in association with myelodysplastic syndrome and other hematologic malignancies. Blood 105:443–452, 2005.

Steinberg MH: Predicting clinical severity in sickle cell anaemia. British Journal of Haematology 129:465–481, 2005.

Thein SL: Is it dominantly inherited β-thalassaemia or just a β-chain variant that is highly unstable? British Journal of Haematology 107:12–21, 1999.

Thein SL: Genetic modifiers of the β-haemoglobinopathies. British Journal of Haematology 141:357–366, 2008.

Wild BJ, Bain BJ: Detection and quantitation of normal and variant haemoglobins: an analytical review. Annals of Clinical Biochemistry 41:355–369, 2004.

REFERENCES

For complete list of references log onto www.expertconsult.com

CHAPTER 41

THALASSEMIA SYNDROMES

Patricia J. Giardina and Bernard G. Forget

The thalassemia syndromes are a heterogeneous group of inherited anemias characterized by defects in the synthesis of one or more of the globin chain subunits of the hemoglobin tetramer. The clinical syndromes associated with thalassemia arise from the combined consequences of inadequate hemoglobin production and imbalanced accumulation of globin subunits. The former causes hypochromia and microcytosis; the latter leads to ineffective erythropoiesis and hemolytic anemia. Clinical manifestations are diverse, ranging from asymptomatic hypochromia and microcytosis to profound anemia, which can be fatal in utero or in early childhood if untreated. This heterogeneity arises from the variable severities of the primary biosynthetic defects and coinherited modifying factors, such as increased synthesis of fetal globin subunits or diminished or increased synthesis of α-globin subunits. Palliative treatment of the severe forms by blood transfusion is eventually compromised by the concomitant problems of iron overload, alloimmunization, and blood-borne infections.

As a group, the thalassemias represent the most common single genetic disorder known. In many parts of the world, they constitute major public health problems. Laboratory analysis of these disorders has been one of the most productive and enlightening endeavors of biomedical research. Study of the molecular defects underlying the thalassemia syndromes has led to fundamental advances in our understanding of eukaryotic gene structure and function. For each of these reasons, a thorough understanding of thalassemia and its related disorders is essential to the hematologist. This chapter reviews the major features of these syndromes. Readers wanting more detailed information than can be included here are referred to more comprehensive monographs elsewhere.[1,2]

The classification, genetic basis, and pathophysiology of the thalassemia syndromes are based on a thorough understanding of the human hemoglobins, their biosynthesis, their encoding globin gene families, and their roles as soluble oxygen-carrying molecules. Therefore, the readers of this chapter should first familiarize themselves with the material presented in Chapter 33. The material presented in this chapter is also substantially clarified by prior reading of Chapters 35 and 36, because the principles underlying the pathophysiology of and therapy for thalassemia draw heavily on knowledge of iron metabolism.

DEFINITIONS AND NOMENCLATURE

The term *thalassemia* is derived from a Greek term that roughly means "the sea" (Mediterranean) in the blood.[1] It was first applied to the anemias frequently encountered in people from the Italian and Greek coasts and nearby islands.[3–5] The term is now used to refer to inherited defects in globin-chain biosynthesis. Individual syndromes are named according to the globin chain whose synthesis is adversely affected. Thus, α-globin chains are absent or reduced in patients with α-thalassemia, β-globin chains in patients with β-thalassemia, δ-globin and β-globin chains in patients δβ-thalassemia, and so forth. In some contexts, it is also useful to subclassify the syndromes according to whether synthesis of the affected globin chain is totally absent (eg, β^o-thalassemia) or only partially reduced (eg, β^+-thalassemia).

The most common forms of thalassemia arise from total absence of structurally normal globin chains or a partial reduction in their synthesis. In contrast to the "structural" hemoglobinopathies (eg, sickle cell anemia), which are characterized by the production of normal amounts of mutant globin chains having deranged physical or chemical properties, thalassemias are quantitative disorders: the primary lesion lies in the amount of globin produced. However, some rare forms of thalassemia are characterized by the production of structurally abnormal globin chains in reduced amounts. These thalassemic hemoglobinopathies share features of thalassemia as well as those of structural hemoglobinopathies.[6]

Some mutations alter the patterns of fetal to adult hemoglobin switching. These conditions, called *hereditary persistence of fetal hemoglobin*, are not generally associated with clinical symptoms; nonetheless, they merit consideration in this chapter. Their importance lies in their role as modulating factors when coinherited with other hemoglobinopathies, in their usefulness as models for investigating the molecular basis for globin gene regulation during human development and as paradigms for rational therapy for the major β-chain hemoglobinopathies, namely, sickle cell anemia and β-thalassemia.

ETIOLOGY, EPIDEMIOLOGY, AND PATHOPHYSIOLOGY

The thalassemias are inherited as pathologic alleles of one or more of the globin genes located on chromosomes 11 and 16 (see Chapter 33). These lesions range from total deletion or rearrangement of the loci to point mutations that impair transcription, processing, or translation of globin mRNA. The precise nature of the defects is summarized in a later section.

Thalassemias have been encountered in virtually every ethnic group and geographic location. They are most common in the Mediterranean basin and tropical or subtropical regions of Asia and Africa. The "thalassemia belt" extends along the shores of the Mediterranean and throughout the Arabian peninsula, Turkey, Iran, India, and southeastern Asia, especially Thailand, Cambodia, and southern China.[7–10] The prevalence of thalassemia in these regions is in the range of 2.5% to 15%. Like sickle cell anemia, thalassemia is most common in those areas historically afflicted with endemic malaria. Malaria seems to have conferred selective survival advantage to thalassemia heterozygotes, in which infection with the malarial parasite is believed to result in milder disease and less impact on reproductive fitness.[1,2,11] Therefore, the gene frequency for thalassemia has become fixed and high in populations exposed to malaria over many centuries.

PATHOPHYSIOLOGY: GENERAL PRINCIPLES

The pathophysiology and molecular genetics of individual forms of thalassemia are closely intertwined. Therefore, detailed consideration of these syndromes is best deferred to their individual subsections. This section considers only mechanisms common to the pathogenesis of all of these syndromes.[1–5,12]

The primary lesion in all forms of thalassemia is reduced or absent production of one or more globin chains. For all practical purposes, the major impact on clinical well-being occurs only when these lesions affect the α- or β-globin chains necessary for the synthesis of hemoglobin (Hb A; $\alpha_2\beta_2$). (Severe impairment of γ-, ε-, or ζ-globin production is presumably lethal in utero.) One consequence of reduced globin-chain production is immediately apparent: reduced production of functioning hemoglobin tetramers. As a result, hypochromia and microcytosis are characteristic of virtually all patients with thalassemia. In the milder forms of the disease, this phenomenon may be barely detectable.

The second consequence of impaired globin biosynthesis is unbalanced synthesis of the individual α- and β-subunits. Hemoglobin tetramers are highly soluble and have reversible oxygen-carrying properties exquisitely adapted for oxygen transport and delivery under physiologic conditions. Free or "unpaired" α-, β-, and γ-globin chains are either highly insoluble or form homotetramers (Hb H and Hb Bart) that are incapable of releasing oxygen normally and are relatively unstable and precipitate as the cell ages. For poorly understood reasons, no compensatory regulatory mechanism exists whereby impaired synthesis of one globin subunit leads to a compensatory downward adjustment in the production of the other (partner) globin chain of the hemoglobin tetramer. Thus, useless excess α-globin chains continue to accumulate and precipitate in β-thalassemia, whereas excess β-globin chains form Hb H in α-thalassemia. During uterine development, excess γ-globin chains form Hb Bart in α-thalassemic individuals.

The abnormal solubility or oxygen-carrying properties of these chains lead to a variety of physiologic derangements. Indeed, in the severe forms of thalassemia, it is the behavior of the unpaired globin chains accumulating in relative excess that dominates the pathophysiology of the syndrome, rather than the mere underproduction of functioning hemoglobin tetramers. The precise complications of this pathophysiologic phenomenon are diverse and depend on the amount and the identity of the globin chain accumulating in excess. For the moment, the fundamental principle that must be appreciated is that thalassemias cause symptoms by underproduction of hemoglobin and by accumulation of unpaired globin subunits. The unpaired subunits are usually the major sources of morbidity and mortality.

The predominant circulating hemoglobin at the moment of birth is fetal hemoglobin (Hb $F^{\alpha_2\gamma_2}$) (see Chapter 32). Although the switch from γ- to β-globin biosynthesis begins before birth, the composition of hemoglobin in the peripheral blood changes much later because of the long life span of normal circulating red blood cells. Hb F is thus slowly replaced by adult hemoglobin (Hb A), so that infants do not depend heavily on normal amounts and function of Hb A until they are between 4 and 6 months old. The pathophysiologic consequences of these considerations are that α-chain hemoglobinopathies tend to be symptomatic in utero and at birth, whereas individuals with β-chain abnormalities are asymptomatic until 4 to 6 months of age. These differences in the onset of phenotypic expression arise because α-chains are needed to form Hb F and Hb A, whereas β-chains are required only for Hb A.

β-THALASSEMIA SYNDROMES

Nomenclature

Many different mutations cause β-thalassemia and its related disorders, such as δβ-thalassemia and the silent carrier state. They are inherited in a multitude of genetic combinations responsible for a heterogeneous group of clinical syndromes. β-Thalassemia major, also known as Cooley's anemia or homozygous β-thalassemia, is a clinically severe disorder that results from the inheritance of two β-thalassemia alleles, one on each copy of chromosome 11. As a consequence of diminished Hb A synthesis, the circulating red blood cells are very hypochromic and abnormally shaped; they contain markedly reduced amounts of hemoglobin. Accumulation of free α-globin chains leads to the deposition of precipitated aggregates of these chains to the detriment of the erythrocyte and its precursor cells in the bone marrow. The anemia of thalassemia major is so severe that long-term blood transfusions are usually required.

The term β-*thalassemia intermedia* is applied to a less severe clinical phenotype in which significant anemia occurs but chronic transfusion therapy is not absolutely required. It usually results from the inheritance of two β-thalassemia mutations, one mild and one severe; the inheritance of two mild mutations; or, occasionally, the inheritance of complex combinations, such as a single β-thalassemia defect and an excess of normal α-globin genes, or two β-thalassemia mutations coinherited with heterozygous α-thalassemia (in this last form, known as αβ-thalassemia, the α-thalassemia allele reduces the burden of unpaired α-chains).[13–15] Simple heterozygosity for certain forms of β-thalassemic hemoglobinopathies can also be associated with a thalassemia intermedia phenotype, sometimes called dominant β-thalassemia.[16,17]

Thalassemia minor, also known as β-thalassemia trait or heterozygous β-thalassemia, is caused by the presence of a single β-thalassemia mutation and a normal β-globin gene on the other chromosome. It is characterized by profound microcytosis with hypochromia but mild or minimal anemia.

β-Thalassemia is also called by several other names, including Cooley's anemia, Mediterranean anemia, von Jaksch anemia,[1] target cell anemia, erythroblastic anemia, and familial microcytosis.

Molecular Pathology

Forms of β-thalassemia arise from mutations that affect every step in the pathway of globin gene expression: transcription, processing of the mRNA precursor, translation of mature mRNA, and post-translational integrity of the β-polypeptide chain (Fig. 41–1 and Table 41–1).[18–20] Large deletions removing two or more non-α-genes are found in rare cases, as are smaller partial or total deletions of the β-gene alone (see Fig. 41–1). Most types of β-thalassemia are caused by point mutations affecting one or a few bases. (The original literature for this section is extensive; it is summarized in various publications and databases.[18–25] Of the more than ~200 mutations causing β-thalassemia, approximately 15 account for the vast majority of affected patients, with the remainder responsible for the disorder in only relatively few patients. It has been determined that five or six mutations usually account for more than 90% of the cases of β-thalassemia in a given ethnic group or geographic area (see Table 41–1).[22]

Table 41–1 Common β-Thalassemia Mutations in Different Racial Groups

Racial Group	Description
Mediterranean	IVS-1, position 110 (G → A) Codon 39, nonsense (CAG → TAG) IVS-1, position 1 (G → A) IVS-2, position 745 (C → G) IVS-1, position 6 (T → C) IVS-2, position 1 (G → A)
Black	–34 (A → G) –88, (C → T) Poly(A), (AATAAA → AACAAA)
Southeast Asian	Codons 41/42, frameshift (–CTTT) IVS-2, position 654 (C → T) –28 (A → T)
Asian Indian	IVS-1, position 5 (G → C) 619-bp deletion Codons 8/9, frameshift (++G) Codons 41/42, frameshift (–CTTT) IVS-1, position 1 (G → T)

Data from Kazazian HH Jr, Boehm CD: Molecular basis and prenatal diagnosis of beta-thalassemia. Blood 72(4):1107, 1988; and Kazazian HH Jr, Boehm CD: personal communication, 1993.

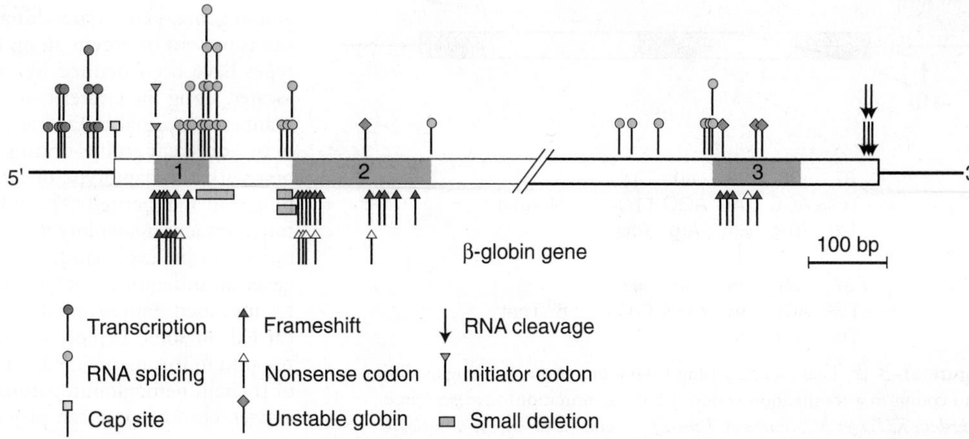

Figure 41–1 Model of the human β-globin gene showing sites and types of various mutations causing β-thalassemia. *(Adapted from Kazazian HH Jr: The thalassemia syndromes: Molecular basis and prenatal diagnosis in 1990. Semin Hematol 27:209, 1990.)*

Transcription

Several mutations alter the promoter region upstream of the β-globin mRNA-encoding sequence, impairing mRNA synthesis, whereas mutations that derange the sequence used as the signal for the addition of the poly-(A) tail of the mRNA (polyadenylation signal; see Chapter 33)[21] have been shown to result in abnormal cleavage and polyadenylation of the nascent mRNA precursor, with resulting reduced accumulation of mature mRNA.[19–21]

Processing

Many forms of β-thalassemia are caused by mutations that impair splicing of the mRNA precursor into mature mRNA in the nucleus or that prevent translation of the mRNA in the cytoplasm. The molecular pathology of splicing mutations is complex (see Fig. 41–1). Some base substitutions ablate the donor (GT) or acceptor (AG) dinucleotides (see Chapter 33), which are absolutely required at the intron–exon boundaries for normal splicing, and thereby completely block production of mature functional messenger RNA. Thus, no β-globin can be synthesized (β^0-thalassemia). Other mutations alter the consensus sequences that surround the GT- and AG-invariant dinucleotides and decrease the efficiency of normal splicing signals by 70% to 95%, resulting in β^+-thalassemia; some consensus mutations even abolish splicing completely, causing β^0-thalassemia. A third type of splicing aberration results from mutations that are not in the immediate vicinity of a normal splice site. These alter regions within the gene, called *cryptic splice sites*, which resemble consensus splicing sites but do not normally sustain splicing (Fig. 41–2). The mutations activate the site by supplying a critical GT or AG nucleotide or by creating a sufficiently strong consensus signal to stimulate splicing at that site 60% to 100% of the time. The activated cryptic sites generate an abnormally spliced, untranslatable mRNA species. Only 10% to 40% of the mRNA precursors are thus spliced at the normal sites, which causes β^+-thalassemia of variable severity. The mutation responsible for the most common form of β-thalassemia among Greeks and Cypriots (see Fig. 41–2) activates a cryptic splice site near the 3′ end of the first intron (position 110).[26,27] The determinants that dictate the degree to which each mutation alters splice site use remain largely unknown.

Translation

Mutations that abolish translation occur at several locations along the mature mRNA and are very common causes of β^0-thalassmia (see Fig. 41–1 and Table 41–1). The most common form of β^0-thalassemia in Sardinians results from a base substitution in the gene that changes the codon encoding the 39th amino acid of the β-globin chain from CAG, which encodes glutamine to TAG, whose equivalent (UAG)

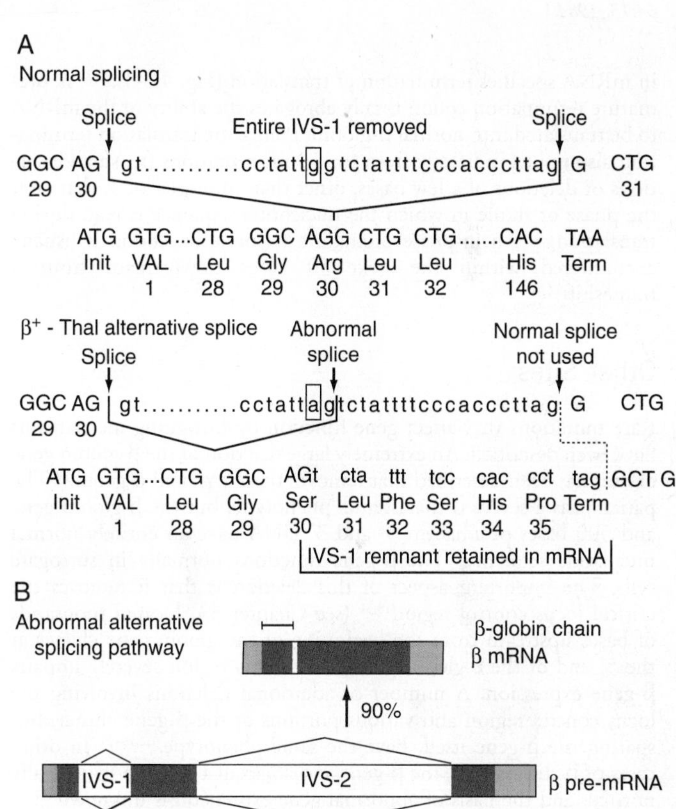

Figure 41–2 β^+-Thalassemia arising from alternative mRNA splicing due to a mutation activating a cryptic splicing site. **A**, The G→A mutation is shown enclosed in squares, located near the 3′ end of intron 1 (IVS-1); it creates a sequence motif closely mimicking a pre-mRNA acceptor splice site. The product of the alternative splicing event is also shown. Note that use of the activated cryptic site generates a mature mRNA that contains an in-frame termination codon and therefore does not encode a functional β-globin chain. *(From Benz EJ Jr: The hemoglobinopathies. In Kelly WN, DeVita VT [eds.]: Textbook of Internal Medicine. Philadelphia, JB Lippincott, 1988, p 1423.)* **B**, Diagram of the means by which use of the cryptic splice site 90% of the time results in only 10% of the mRNA precursor molecules to be spliced normally into translatable mature mRNA, thus causing β^+-thalassemia. *(Adapted from Bunn HF, Forget BG: Hemoglobin: Molecular, Genetic and Clinical Aspects. Philadelphia, WB Saunders, 1986.)*

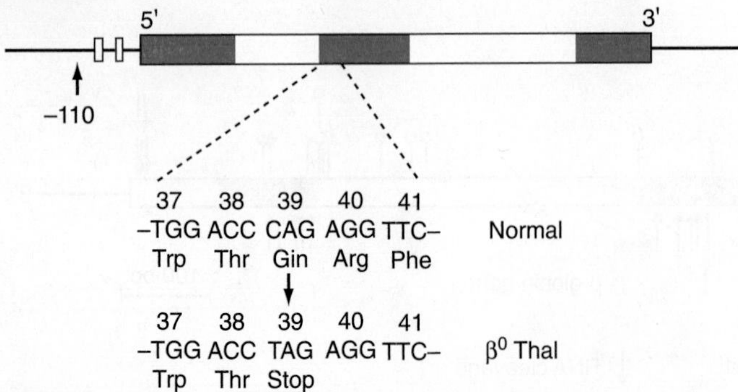

Figure 41–3 β^0-Thalassemia arising from a mutation changing an amino acid codon to a termination codon (nonsense mutation). *(Adapted from Takeshita K, Forget BG, Scarpa A, Benz EJ Jr: Intranuclear defects in b-globin mRNA accumulation due to a premature translation termination codon. Blood 64:13, 1984.)*

in mRNA specifies termination of translation (Fig. 41–3).[28,29] A premature termination codon totally abrogates the ability of the mRNA to be translated into normal β-globin. Premature translation termination also results indirectly from frameshift mutations (ie, small insertions or deletions of a few bases, other than multiples of 3, that alter the phase or frame in which the nucleotide sequence is read during translation).[29] An in-phase premature termination codon is usually encountered within the next 50 bases downstream from a frameshift.

Other Sites

Rare mutations that affect gene function by intriguing mechanisms have been described. An extremely large deletion of the β-globin gene cluster has been described that removes the ε-, γ-, and δ-genes.[30] The patient has a severe β-thalassemia phenotype, but the β-globin gene and 500 bases of adjacent 5′ and 3′ DNA have an entirely normal nucleotide sequence. The β-gene functions normally in surrogate cells. The important aspect of this deletion is that it removes the critical locus control region[18,31] (see Chapter 33) located thousands of bases upstream from the beginning of the globin gene cluster at the 5′ end of the ε-globin gene; loss of this region severely impairs β-gene expression. A number of additional deletions involving the locus control region and various portions of the β-gene cluster, but sparing the β-gene itself, have the same phenotype.[1,2,19–21] In other cases of β-thalassemia, the β-gene and adjacent DNA are structurally normal, and the basis of abnormal gene expression is unknown.[22]

Relationship between Specific Mutations and Clinical Severity

The relationship between an individual mutation and the clinical severity of the β-thalassemia phenotype associated with that particular mutation is complex.[22] For example, the A to G mutation at position −34 of the β-gene promoter commonly encountered in black patients is associated with a different clinical severity than that found in Chinese patients inheriting the same mutation.[32] Clearly, the genetic "context" of the mutation is different in the two populations. The mutant β-globin gene in the two different racial groups probably arose in different chromosome backgrounds that have different potentials for γ-gene expression, as discussed in the following paragraph.

Multiple forms, or haplotypes, of normal non-α-globin gene clusters exist in various human populations. These are defined by the patterns of restriction fragment length polymorphisms[28] detected when DNA is digested with restriction endonucleases and analyzed by Southern gene blotting for the fragments bearing the non-α-globin genes. Haplotypes differ according to whether each restriction site is present or absent along the gene cluster. More than 12 haplotypes have been defined by examination of several restriction sites located along the cluster that are present or absent in a polymorphic manner in normal individuals.[28] The clinical variability encountered in two different groups bearing identical primary mutations correlates best with the haplotype or chromosome background on which the mutation is inherited. The differences in physiologically important functions among haplotypes that modulate severity remain unknown, but a possible explanation lies in the variable abilities of the γ-globin genes on different chromosomes to respond to severe erythroid stress by increased expression during postnatal life. The β-globin genes carried on some haplotypes differ in the degree to which they can respond in this manner.[33] Because Hb F synthesis reduces the severity of β-chain hemoglobinopathies,[1] the level of γ-gene expression from a given chromosome can play an important modulating role.

Pathophysiology

The biochemical hallmark of β-thalassemia is reduced biosynthesis of the β-globin subunit of Hb A ($\alpha_2\beta_2$). In β-thalassemia heterozygotes, β-globin synthesis is about half-normal (β/α synthetic ratio 0.5–0.7). In homozygotes for β^0-thalassemia, who account for approximately one-third of patients, β-globin synthesis is absent. β-Globin synthesis is reduced to 5% to 30% of normal levels in β^+-thalassemia homozygotes or β^+/β^0-thalassemia compound heterozygotes, who together account for approximately two-thirds of cases.[1]

Because the synthesis of Hb A ($\alpha_2\beta_2$) is markedly reduced or absent, the red blood cells are hypochromic and microcytic. γ-Chain synthesis is partially reactivated, so that the hemoglobin of the patient contains a relatively large proportion of Hb F.[1] However, these γ-chains are quantitatively insufficient to replace β-chain production.

In heterozygotes (β-thalassemia trait), relatively little α-globin accumulation occurs. Output from the single normal β-globin gene supports substantial Hb A formation, thus preventing harmful accumulation of excess α-globin chains. Thus, one encounters hypochromia with microcytosis but relatively little evidence of anemia, hemolysis, or ineffective erythropoiesis.

Individuals inheriting two β-thalassemic alleles experience a more profound deficit of β-chain production. Little or no Hb A is produced; more importantly, the imbalance of α- and β-globin production is far more severe (Fig. 41–4). The limited capacity of red blood cells to proteolyze the excess α-globin chains, a capacity that probably exerts a protective effect in heterozygous β-thalassemia, is overwhelmed in homozygotes. Free α-globin accumulates, and unpaired α-chains aggregate and precipitate to form inclusion bodies, which cause oxidative membrane damage within the red blood cell[34] and destruction of immature developing erythroblasts within the bone marrow (ineffective erythropoiesis).[35] Consequently, relatively few of the erythroid precursors undergoing erythroid maturation in the bone marrow survive long enough to be released into the bloodstream as erythrocytes. The occasional erythrocytes that are formed during erythropoiesis bear a burden of inclusion bodies. The reticuloendothelial cells in the spleen, liver, and bone marrow remove these abnormal cells prematurely, producing a hemolytic anemia.

Defective β-globin synthesis exerts at least three distinct yet interrelated effects on the generation of oxygen-carrying capacity for the peripheral blood (see Fig. 41–4): (a) ineffective erythropoiesis, which impairs production of new red blood cells; (b) hemolytic anemia, which shortens the survival of the few red blood cells produced; and (c) hypochromia with microcytosis, which reduces the oxygen-carrying capacity of those few red blood cells that do survive. In the most severe forms of the disorder, these three factors conspire to produce a catastrophic anemia, complicated by the effects of exuberant hemolysis.

The profound deficit in the oxygen-carrying capacity of the blood stimulates production of high levels of erythropoietin in an attempt to promote compensatory erythroid hyperplasia. Unfortunately, the

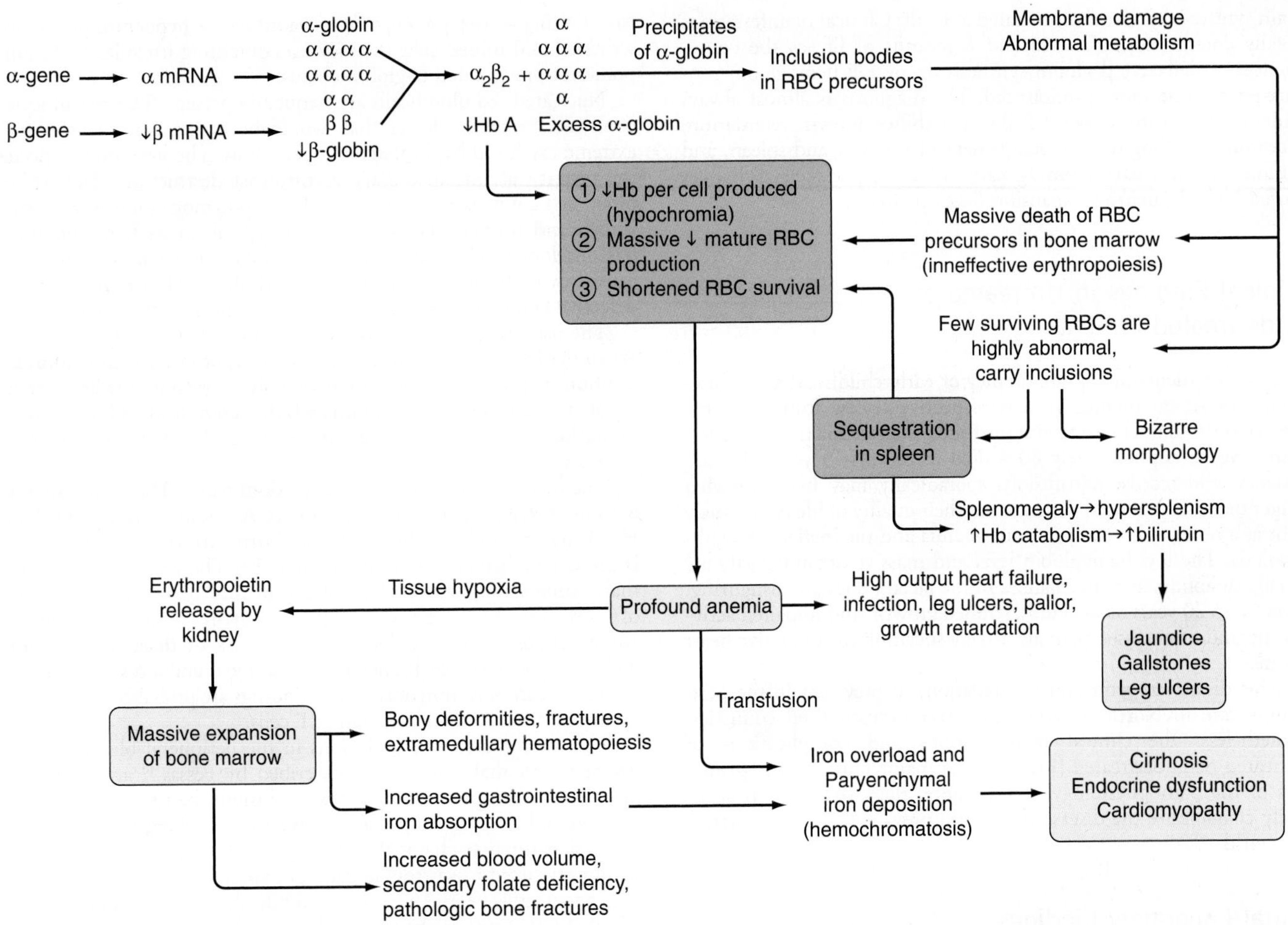

α-gene → α mRNA → α-globin αααα αααα αα → $\alpha_2\beta_2$ + ααα ααα α → Precipitates of α-globin → Inclusion bodies in RBC precursors → Membrane damage Abnormal metabolism
β-gene → ↓β mRNA → ββ ↓β-globin
↓Hb A Excess α-globin

① ↓Hb per cell produced (hypochromia)
② Massive ↓ mature RBC production
③ Shortened RBC survival

Massive death of RBC precursors in bone marrow (inneffective erythropoiesis)

Few surviving RBCs are highly abnormal, carry inciusions

Sequestration in spleen

Bizarre morphology

Splenomegaly→hypersplenism
↑Hb catabolism→↑bilirubin

Jaundice
Gallstones
Leg ulcers

Erythropoietin released by kidney

Tissue hypoxia

Profound anemia

High output heart failure, infection, leg ulcers, pallor, growth retardation

Transfusion

Massive expansion of bone marrow

Bony deformities, fractures, extramedullary hematopoiesis

Increased gastrointestinal iron absorption

Increased blood volume, secondary folate deficiency, pathologic bone fractures

Iron overload and Paryenchymal iron deposition (hemochromatosis)

Cirrhosis
Endocrine dysfunction
Cardiomyopathy

Figure 41–4 Pathophysiology of severe forms of β-thalassemia. The diagram outlines the pathogenesis of clinical abnormalities resulting from the primary defect in β-globin chain synthesis. RBCs, red blood cells.

ability of the marrow to respond positively is markedly impaired by ineffective erythropoiesis. Massive bone marrow expansion does occur, but very few erythrocytes are actually supplied to the circulation. The marrow becomes packed with immature erythroid precursors, which die from their burden of precipitated α-globin chains before they reach the reticulocyte stage. Profound anemia persists, driving erythroid hyperplasia to still higher levels. In some cases, erythropoiesis is so exuberant that masses of extramedullary erythropoietic tissue form in the chest, abdomen, or pelvis.

As described in the following section, massive bone marrow expansion exerts numerous adverse effects on the growth, development, and function of critical organ systems and creates the characteristic facies caused by maxillary marrow hyperplasia and frontal bossing (Fig. 41–5). Hemolytic anemia results in massive splenomegaly and high-output congestive heart failure. In untreated cases, death occurs during the first two decades of life. Treatment with red blood cell transfusions sufficient to maintain hemoglobin levels above 9.0 to 10.0 g/dL improves oxygen delivery, suppresses the excessive ineffective erythropoiesis, and prolongs life. Unfortunately, as discussed in more detail later, complications of chronic transfusion therapy, including iron overload, usually proved to be fatal before 30 years of age. The addition of iron chelation therapy to regular transfusion therapy now prolongs survival and improves the quality of life.

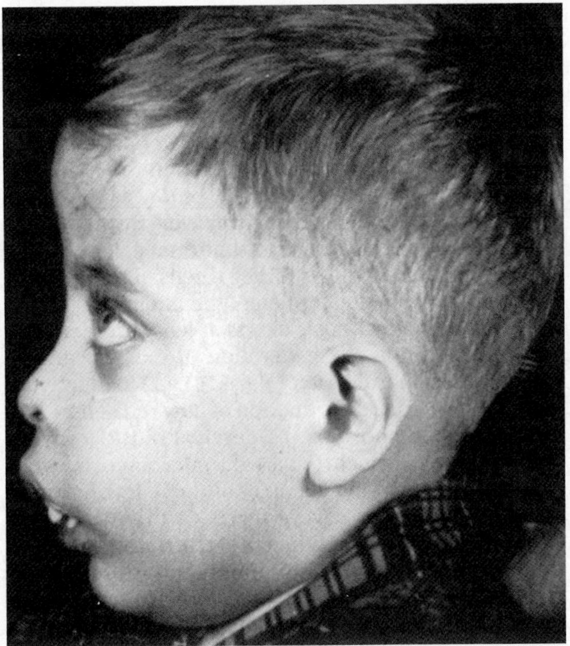

Figure 41–5 Thalassemic facies. See text for description. *(From Jurkiewicz MJ, Pearson HA, Furlow LT Jr: Reconstruction of the maxilla in thalassemia. Ann N Y Acad Sci 165:437, 1969.)*

Clinical Manifestations

Clinical Findings at Diagnosis

Protected by prenatal Hb F production, the infant with β-thalassemia major is born free of significant anemia. Nevertheless, deficient β-chain synthesis can be demonstrated at birth. Clinical manifestations usually emerge during the second 6 months of life as the consequences of defective β-globin synthesis on overall hemoglobin production become more pronounced. The diagnosis is almost always evident by 2 years of age.[36] Pallor, irritability, growth retardation, abdominal swelling due to enlargement of the liver and spleen, and jaundice are the usual presenting features.[37] Facial and skeletal changes caused by bone marrow expansion develop later.

Clinical Findings in Untreated or Undertreated Patients

Untreated patients die in late infancy or early childhood as a consequence of severe anemia. In a retrospective review from Italy, the average survival of children with untreated thalassemia major was less than 4 years; approximately 80% died in the first 5 years of life.[38] Patients who receive transfusions sporadically may live somewhat longer than untransfused patients, but their quality of life is extremely poor as a result of both the chronic anemia and the ineffective erythropoiesis. The low hemoglobin level and massive organomegaly are usually disabling, and the changes in the facial bones are disfiguring. After 10 to 20 years of weakness, stunted growth, and impaired activity, the undertransfused patients usually succumb to congestive heart failure.

This disastrous symptom constellation, so prevalent in the past, is now rare in North America and most industrialized countries. Nonetheless, the clinical manifestations and complications of untreated or undertreated β-thalassemia major illustrate the principles of the pathophysiology. Furthermore, these descriptions accurately characterize the disease that is still prevalent in many parts of the world.

Initial Laboratory Findings

The anemia of thalassemia major is characterized by severe hypochromia and microcytosis. The hemoglobin level decreases progressively during the first months of life. When the child becomes symptomatic, the hemoglobin level may be as low as 3 to 4 g/dL. Red blood cell morphology is strikingly abnormal, with many microcytes, bizarre poikilocytes, teardrop cells, and target cells (Fig. 41–6). A characteristic finding is the presence of extraordinarily hypochromic, often wrinkled and folded cells (leptocytes) containing irregular inclusion bodies of precipitated α-globin chains.

Nucleated red blood cells are frequently present. The reticulocyte count is 2% to 8% lower than would be expected in view of the extreme erythroid hyperplasia and hemolysis. The low count reflects the severity of intramedullary erythroblast destruction. The white blood cell count is elevated. A moderate polymorphonuclear leukocytosis and normal platelet count are typical unless hypersplenism has developed. The bone marrow exhibits marked hypercellularity caused by erythroid hyperplasia. The red blood cell precursors show defective hemoglobinization and reduced amounts of cytoplasm.

The osmotic fragility is strikingly abnormal. The red blood cells are so markedly resistant to hemolysis in hypotonic sodium chloride solution that some are not entirely hemolyzed even in distilled water. Before transfusion therapy is initiated, the serum iron and transferrin saturation are already increased as a result of increased iron absorption.[39]

The hemoglobin profile reveals predominantly Hb F. In patients with homozygous β^0-thalassemia, no Hb A is found throughout life. Hb A may be undetectable in the newborn with β^+-thalassemia and is present in reduced amounts in later life. The levels of Hb A_2 in thalassemia major are variable, probably because of increased numbers of F cells that have a decreased Hb A_2 content.[1] Other biochemical abnormalities of the red blood cell in cases of thalassemia major include a postnatal persistence of the i antigen and a decrease of red blood cell carbonic anhydrase; these findings are probably also caused by the elevated levels of circulating F cells.

The intraerythrocytic inclusions in the peripheral blood cells of patients with thalassemia, first described by Fessas,[40] are especially prominent after splenectomy. These inclusions, best seen by staining with methyl violet or by phase microscopy, are aggregates of precipitated, denatured α-chains.[41] They are also found in large numbers within erythroid precursors in the bone marrow.

The serum is icteric; unconjugated bilirubin levels are in the range of 2.0 to 4.0 mg/dL at the time of diagnosis but may rise substantially as the anemia worsens in the absence of transfusion. Red blood cell

Clinical Heterogeneity of Thalassemia

The severity of β-thalassemia is remarkable for its variability in different patients. Two siblings inheriting identical thalassemia mutations sometimes exhibit markedly different degrees of anemia and erythroid hyperplasia. Many factors contribute to this clinical heterogeneity. Individual alleles vary with respect to severity of the biosynthetic lesion. Other modifying factors ameliorate the burden of unpaired α-globin. High levels of Hb F expression persist to widely various degrees in β-thalassemia. As γ-globin can substitute for β-globin, simultaneously generating more functional hemoglobins and reducing the α-globin inclusion burden, this is a powerful modulating factor. Theoretically, patients may also vary in their ability to solubilize unpaired globin chains by proteolysis. Occasional heterozygous patients have had more severe anemia than expected, possibly because of defects in these proteolytic systems, or because of the type of thalassemic mutation. Inheritance of more than the usual complement of α-globin genes may also increase with severity of β-thalassemia because of additional production of unpaired α-globin chains. All these factors emphasize the essential role of α-globin inclusions in the pathophysiology of β-thalassemia.

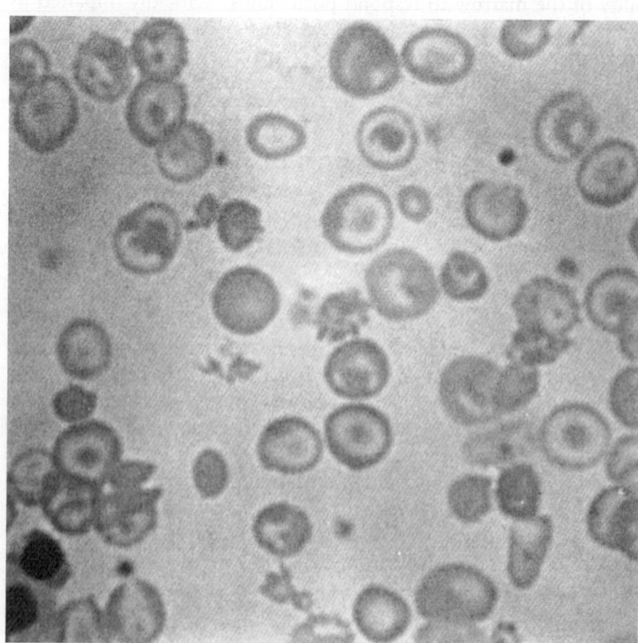

Figure 41–6 Morphologic appearance of the peripheral blood film in a case of severe β-thalassemia. Note the many bizarre cells, the hypochromia, nucleated red blood cells, target cells, and leptocytes. *(From Pearson HA, Benz EJ Jr: Thalassemia syndromes. In Miller DR, Baehner RL, McMillan CW [eds.]: Smith's Blood Diseases of Infancy and Childhood, 5th ed. St. Louis, CV Mosby, 1984, p 439.)*

survival in cases of thalassemia major is variable but usually markedly decreased. The ^{51}Cr half-life ranges between 6.5 and 19.5 days, compared with the normal half-life of 25 to 35 days.[35] Increased plasma iron turnover and poor use of radiolabeled iron indicate ineffective erythropoiesis.[35] Serum aspartate aminotransferase levels are frequently increased at diagnosis because of hemolysis. Alanine aminotransferase levels are usually normal prior to transfusion therapy but may rise subsequently because of iron-induced hepatic damage or viral hepatitis. Lactate dehydrogenase levels are markedly elevated as a consequence of ineffective erythropoiesis. Haptoglobin and hemopexin are reduced or absent.[42]

Later Laboratory Findings

Serum zinc levels may fall to abnormally low levels. A relationship between this finding and growth failure has been postulated but not established.[43,44] Low levels of plasma and leukocyte ascorbic acid are common in thalassemic patients because of increased metabolism of the vitamin to oxalic acid in the presence of iron overload.[45,46] Biochemical evidence of folic acid deficiency may occur as a result of excessive consumption secondary to increased requirements.[47,48] The serum levels of α-tocopherol are often reduced to less than 0.5 mg/dL, and increased red blood cell membrane lipid peroxidation has been described.[49–51]

Coagulation abnormalities consistent with liver disease (ie, lowered levels of factors II, V, VII, IX, and X) may occur in older patients with hepatitis or iron-induced hepatic injury.[52] Only rarely are the abnormalities sufficient to require specific therapy. However, the combination of mild thrombocytopenia due to hypersplenism and low coagulation factors and platelet dysfunction due to liver disease may cause or aggravate bleeding.[53]

Numerous laboratory abnormalities reflect the accumulation of excessive iron and the consequences of iron-induced organ damage, and they are described in the following sections.

Treatment

The advent of modern therapy has had a major impact on the clinical and laboratory features of thalassemia major. Transfusion and chelation therapy, described subsequently in detail, have ameliorated many of the most striking manifestations of the disease. Bone marrow transplantation has allowed for the cure of a select few. However, these therapies have created their own complications, and therefore this section addresses the treatment of the complications of thalassemia and its therapy. Current clinical management and associated clinical manifestations and complications have been reviewed in a number of publications.[54–59]

Transfusion Therapy

Transfusion therapy for thalassemia was once used sparingly administered as a palliative measure when patients became symptomatic. These periodic transfusion regimens were unsatisfactory even for those limited purposes, symptoms of anemia and the cosmetic and other consequences of overgrowth of erythropoietic tissue rendered life unpleasant and uncomfortable for patients. Consequently, several centers initiated transfusion programs in which patients received regular transfusions to keep their hemoglobin levels high enough to ameliorate these symptoms[60,61] but the median survival of patients transfused to maintain hemoglobin levels of 7 to 8 g/dL in the USA in the 1960s was only 17 years of age.[61,62] These "hypertransfusion" programs were designed initially to maintain hemoglobin levels above 8 g/dL. In the more modern application of hypertransfusion therapy, hemoglobin levels are usually maintained above 9 to 10.5 g/dL.

The clinical benefits of hypertransfusion programs are dramatic. The growth of younger children follows normal percentiles for height and weight.[63] Erythropoiesis is partially but substantially suppressed,

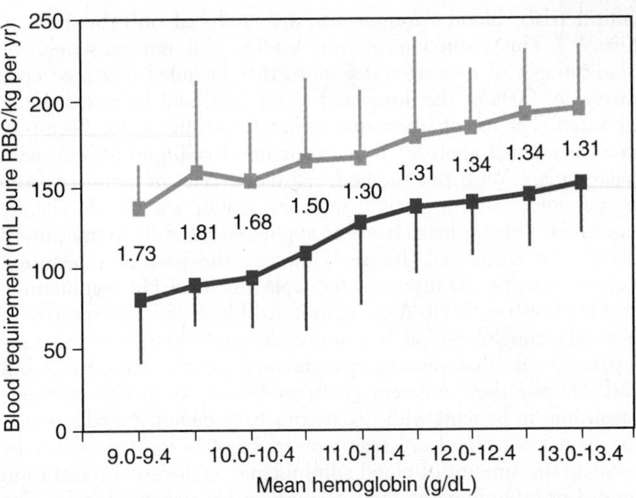

Figure 41–7 Relationship between transfusion requirements and mean hemoglobin level maintained by patients with thalassemia major. *(Adapted from Rebulla P, Modell B: Transfusion requirements and effects in patients with thalassaemia major. Lancet 337:277, 1991.)*

Guidelines for Transfusion Therapy

Although some of the details of a transfusion program for patients with thalassemia major vary from center to center, the following guidelines are important for achieving the benefits while controlling the risks of a transfusion program. The rationales for these guidelines are discussed in the text.

1. Obtain a complete red blood cell antigen profile before the first transfusion.
2. Administer 10 to 15 mL/kg of red blood cells every 2 to 4 weeks to maintain the pretransfusion hemoglobin level above 9 to 10.5 g/dL.
3. Use leukoreduced washed red blood cells that have been stored for less than 7 to 10 days.
4. Avoid the use of first-degree relatives as blood donors.
5. For patients who come to a new center after receiving transfusions elsewhere, contact the previous blood bank for information about alloantibodies.

as evidenced by decreased numbers of reticulocytes and normoblasts, and transferrin receptor levels.[64,65] Hypertransfusion reduces or prevents the enlargement of the liver and spleen. Abnormal facies and bone fractures occur less frequently. The overall sense of well-being allows normal age-appropriate activities.[66,67]

A more vigorous transfusion program (supertransfusion) aimed at keeping hemoglobin levels above 12.0 g/dL has been recommended.[68] This approach rests on the assumption that the benefits of further suppression of erythropoiesis and gastrointestinal iron absorption will offset the increased need for red blood cells. However, several, though not all, studies have demonstrated that transfusion requirements (and therefore the rates of transfusional iron loading) increase as the hemoglobin level is raised (Fig. 41–7).[63,69,70] As a result, the consistent maintenance of hemoglobin levels above 11 or 12 g/dL is generally reserved for patients with poor tolerance of lower hemoglobin levels due to cardiac disease or other reasons.

Alternative approaches to conventional transfusion therapy have been proposed in an effort to reduce the rate of transfusion iron loading. These approaches have generally relied on the concept that younger red blood cells (neocytes) will circulate longer in the recipient than older red blood cells. Preclinical experiments based on the difference in density between younger and older red blood cells established the validity of this approach.[71,72] However, in prospective clinical trials, blood requirements were reduced only by 13% to 20%.[73–75] This reduction in iron loading did not outweigh the disadvantages of neocyte transfusions that included increased cost, wastage of 50% of the donor red blood cells, and increased donor exposures. The use of automated exchange transfusion has been proposed as another approach to reducing iron loading in patients with thalassemia.[76] With this method, red blood cells are removed from the patient at the same time that new donor red blood cells are transfused. This approach has been applied successfully to transfusion therapy for sickle cell disease. However, the goal of transfusion therapy in sickle cell disease is the replacement of Hb S-containing red blood cells with Hb A-containing red blood cells, irrespective of the total hemoglobin level. In contrast, the goal of transfusion therapy in patients with thalassemia is to maintain a specific total hemoglobin level. Despite these different goals, studies of automated exchange transfusion in patients with thalassemia have demonstrated a reduction in net red blood cell requirements of 30% to 50%, either by reducing the amount of blood administered at the usual transfusion interval or by prolonging the interval between transfusions.[76,77] The benefits of this approach are probably due to the removal of previously transfused red blood cells from the patients and replacement with younger, recently donated red blood cells, reducing the overall age of the circulating red blood cell population. Further clinical trials of automated exchange transfusion in thalassemia are currently underway.

The decision to initiate transfusion therapy should take into account the overall clinical condition of the patient as well as the hemoglobin level. Patients with severe and persistent anemia (hemoglobin level of less than 6–7 g/dL) will usually also have failure to thrive, decreased activity level, and irritability. For these patients, transfusion therapy should begin after confirmation of the diagnosis of thalassemia and after demonstration that acute factors such as a febrile illness or folic acid deficiency are not confounding the assessment of the severity of anemia. For patients with higher hemoglobin levels, the decision to begin transfusion depends on the careful assessment of the child's clinical findings. For example, some children with thalassemia will have early and pronounced facial bone deformities caused by bone marrow expansion despite a hemoglobin level of 8 g/dL or higher. For such children, the benefits of transfusion therapy may outweigh the risks. In contrast, some patients with thalassemia have little or no clinical difficulty despite a persistent hemoglobin level of 7 to 8 g/dL, and the benefits of transfusion therapy may be small. Determination of genotype may provide some guidance by distinguishing patients with more severe defects in β-globin production from those with less severe defects, but the overlap between genotype and phenotype in thalassemia still requires reliance on clinical assessment.

Deciding to Begin Transfusion Therapy in Patients with Thalassemia

The decision to initiate regular red blood cell transfusions is one of the most important—and sometimes most difficult—steps in the management of thalassemia. Regular red blood cell transfusions not only distinguish thalassemia major from thalassemia intermedia but also commit the patient to long-term chelation therapy to control the transfusional iron loading. The decision should include consideration of both clinical and laboratory findings. Children who are growing poorly and developing disfiguring bone changes will benefit from regular transfusions even if their hemoglobin levels are 8 to 9 g/dL. On the other hand, children who are asymptomatic at hemoglobin levels of 7 to 8 g/dL may have little to gain from transfusions. Hemoglobin levels below 7 g/dL are usually associated with problems related to both the anemia and the compensatory erythropoiesis. When the hemoglobin level is consistently less than 7 g/dL, there is usually little to be gained from delaying transfusion.

Before the first blood transfusion is given to a child with thalassemia major, a complete red blood cell antigen profile should be obtained. This information is valuable for identifying minor blood group incompatibility if alloimmunization develops later and also helps to distinguish alloantibodies from autoantibodies. The value of extended matching of donor red blood cells has not been established in cases of thalassemia, but experience with sickle cell disease suggests that matching for the full Rh system as well as the Kell antigen may reduce the rate of alloimmunization.

In practice, the goal of maintaining the hemoglobin level above 9 to 10.5 g/dL is usually achieved by administration of approximately 15 mL/kg/month or 1 to 2 units of donor red blood cells every 2 to 5 weeks. Patients with heart disease may need smaller aliquots of red blood cells at more frequent intervals to prevent problems related to volume overload. In general, patients can receive whole units of donor red blood cells. However, fractional units may be appropriate for small patients and for older patients with heart disease. At present, the blood product of choice for patients with thalassemia is filtered red blood cells. Although some centers use filtered washed red cell transfusions, others reserve washed red blood cells to prevent febrile reactions despite filtration of the blood product. Frozen-thawed red blood cells are primarily useful for patients with multiple antibodies who require donor red blood cells with rare phenotypes that must be collected and stored well in advance of the actual transfusion.

With the use of current additive solutions, the duration of storage of donor red blood cells has only a small effect on the 24-hour recovery and the survival of the red blood cells in each transfused unit. However, for patients with thalassemia major who undergo transfusion every 2 to 5 weeks, these small differences may have a significant impact on the annual consumption of blood. Consequently, the use of donor red blood cells that have been stored for less than 7 to 10 days strikes a reasonable balance between the potential reduction in transfusion iron loading and the efficient use of the blood bank inventory. The use of volunteer blood donors remains the standard for patients with thalassemia. Although some families of children with thalassemia prefer directed donations, this approach has not reduced the rate of transfusion-transmitted infections among blood recipients in general and has not been shown to reduce the rate of alloimmunization in thalassemia. If directed donations are used, close relatives should be avoided, because stem cell transplantation may be a later therapeutic option.

Other complications of transfusion therapy include those that are annoying as well as those that can be life threatening. Febrile reactions occur less commonly than in the past as a result of the use of leukoreduced donor red blood cells. If such reactions occur despite the use of filtered blood products, additional measures include pretransfusion therapy with acetaminophen and the use of washed or frozen-thawed red blood cells. Urticarial and other allergic reactions can usually be managed with antihistamine therapy or, when persistent, pretransfusion administration of corticosteroids.

Red blood cell alloimmunization occurs in 3% to 23% of patients with thalassemia major.[70,78–80] If blood donors and recipients come from different ethnic backgrounds with different red blood cell antigen profiles, as in some North American thalassemia centers, the risk of alloimmunization is increased.[81] New alloantibodies may be clinically silent, associated with increasing transfusion requirements, or accompanied by signs of active hemolysis such as increasing jaundice and dark urine. As noted earlier, the use of extended antigen matching may help prevent alloimmunization. Initiation of transfusion therapy before the age of 3 years may also be associated with a lower risk of this complication.[70,80,82] Patients with a history of alloantibodies require particular attention when receiving a transfusion at a new hospital because the serologic studies may fail to detect a clinically significant antibody that is present in low amounts. A review of the blood bank records from the previous institutions is essential in choosing the appropriate red blood cell product.

Autoantibodies also occur in patients with thalassemia major, usually, but not always, after the development of an alloantibody.[83] A subset of patients with autoantibodies has a clinically important autoimmune hemolytic anemia that leads to the premature destruction of donor cells as well as destruction of the patient's own red blood cells. Transfusion requirements are markedly increased, and further transfusion therapy may be impossible for some patients. Treatment with corticosteroids, other immunosuppressive therapy, or intravenous gamma globulin may improve red blood cell survival in some cases.

A syndrome of posttransfusion hypertension, convulsions, and cerebral hemorrhage has also been reported.[84] The mechanism underlying this complication is uncertain but is possibly related to large changes in hemoglobin level at the time of transfusion. These reactions are uncommon in conventional transfusion programs.

The potential impact of transfusion-transmitted infections on patients with thalassemia major is demonstrated by the high prevalence of human immunodeficiency virus infection in certain thalassemia centers during the 1980s and the nearly universal problem with hepatitis C infection in patients who began transfusion therapy before the 1990s. A 1987 study found that 17% of patients with thalassemia major in one center in New York City were positive for human immunodeficiency virus antibody.[85] The prevalence of hepatitis C infection among patients with thalassemia major is 12% to 91%, with a higher rate among older patients.[86,87] Improvements in donor screening and testing have markedly reduced the risk of transmission by transfusion of known viruses,[88] but patients with thalassemia, because of the frequency of their transfusions, remain at risk not only for viruses that are transmitted infrequently but also for new agents such as Hepatitis A, Babesiosis, and West Nile virus.[89] Hepatitis B vaccine, if not administered as part of the routine childhood immunization program, should be given to patients with thalassemia before transfusion therapy begins.[90] Hepatitis A vaccine should also be administered when age appropriate. The cytomegalovirus status of patients who are potential candidates for stem cell transplantation should be ascertained prior to transfusion and every attempt should be made to provide them with cytomegalovirus-negative blood products. Current studies of pathogen-inactivated red blood cell products hold forth the promise of a means for preventing transfusion-transmitted infections even when the donor's infection escapes detection or when new agents enter the blood supply.[91,92]

Progressive iron overload is the life-threatening complication of transfusion therapy that accounts for the most important long-term morbidity and mortality in patients with thalassemia major.

Chelation Therapy

The clinical effects of iron overload in patients with thalassemia major depend on the amount and the duration of excessive iron accumulation. Transfusion hemosiderosis is the major cause of late morbidity and mortality in patients with thalassemia major. Establishment of therapeutic strategies to achieve iron balance should lead to improved survival. Various strategies to reduce the rate of transfusion iron loading have included modifying the pretransfusion hemoglobin level, adjusting the intervals between transfusions and splenectomy as well as with methods to enhance the rate of iron removal through chelation therapy. Historically efforts were focused on identifying methods to enhance parenteral iron chelation, by adjusting the frequency of daily use, the hours of administration and the route of parenteral administration. These have optimized the use of iron chelation with deferoxamine (Desferal). More recently, efforts are focused on addressing the safety and efficacy of new oral iron chelators, deferasrox (Exjade) and deferiprone (L1), and new ways to assess iron excess.

Each unit of packed red blood cells contains approximately 200 to 250 mg of iron. Based on usual blood requirements in patients with thalassemia major, the rate of transfusional iron accumulation is approximately 0.30 to 0.60 mg/kg/day. The massive ineffective erythropoiesis associated with the intermedia and major thalassemias leads to excessive gastrointestinal iron absorption that adds to the transfusional iron burden, although absorption is reduced when a hemoglobin level above 9 g/dL is maintained.[93,94] Humans have no physiologic mechanism to induce significant excretion of excess iron.

Benefits of Iron Chelation Therapy

More than 30 years of experience using iron chelation therapy with deferoxamine in thalassemia major patients have demonstrated that

1. Liver iron concentrations can be maintained at normal or mildly elevated levels.
2. Hepatic fibrosis is slowed or prevented.
3. The risk of iron-induced cardiac disease, including heart failure and serious arrhythmias, is markedly decreased.
4. Normal growth and sexual development are common although not universal.
5. Long-term survival is substantially improved.

These benefits are directly related to compliance and generally require the prolonged administration of deferoxamine at least five times per week.

6. Long-term safety and efficacy studies of oral iron chelators, deferiprone and deferasirox, are on-going.

Phlebotomy, the most efficient method of removing iron in other situations, is precluded in severely anemic patients with thalassemia owing to transfusion dependence. Phlebotomy may be only applicable in a very few select patients with thalassemia intermedia, and constitutes an important part of the management of patients with thalassemia major who have successfully undergone stem cell transplantation.

A pharmacologic approach using specific iron-chelating agents remains the only strategy for removing excess iron in transfusion-dependent patients.

Several drugs with chelating properties have been synthesized or recovered from microorganisms. Many lack iron specificity or are inefficient; others cause significant toxicity. To chelate iron, the chelating agent must complex with all of the iron atom's six available coordination sites. Three general classes of iron chelators occur or have been synthesized: hexadentate (deferoxamine), bidentate (deferiprone), and tridentate (deferasirox). Only one hexadentate molecule is necessary to bind one atom of iron whereas three molecules of a bidentate iron chelator bind one iron atom and two molecules of a tridentate chelator are required to bind one atom of iron.

Chelatable iron is thought to be derived from the intracellular "labile iron pool"[95,96] and from non-transferrin-bound plasma iron.[97,98]

Deferoxamine

Deferoxamine mesylate (Desferal, DFO) is a naturally occurring hexadentate siderophore isolated from cultures of *Streptomyces pilosus* introduced in 1960. Deferoxamine has a high molecular weight of approximately 600, is poorly absorbed by the gastrointestinal tract, and is rapidly removed from the plasma. It has a relatively short half-life of 8 to 10 minutes, which necessitates intravenous or subcutaneous parenteral administration. It is a hexadentate iron chelator that binds iron in a 1-to-1 complex. It is highly specific for iron and is associated with relatively low toxicity.[99] Deferoxamine enters cells, chelates iron and appears in the serum and bile as the iron chelate product, ferroxamine.[100] Deferoxamine chelates iron released by the reticuloendothelial systems following the catabolism of senescent red blood cells and is excreted in the urine.[101] Unbound deferoxamine is absorbed by the hepatic parenchymal cells and chelates iron from the intracellular pool which is excreted in bile. Approximately one-half to two-thirds of the iron excreted in response to deferoxamine is in the stool, with the remainder in the urine.[102] These proportions vary from patient to patient and at different levels of iron overload, dose of deferoxamine, and endogenous erythropoietic activity.[103]

Iron excretion after the administration of deferoxamine is proportional to body iron stores. To achieve negative iron balance, the chelating agent must cause the daily excretion of 0.3 to 0.6 mg/kg of iron. In the 1960s, deferoxamine was initially administered by daily intramuscular injections of 0.5 g, which led to reduced rates of hepatic iron accumulation and hepatic fibrosis in patients with thalassemia.[104,105] However, intramuscular injections proved to be too painful and were insufficient to achieve negative iron balance. In the mid 1970s it was demonstrated that iron excretion with deferoxamine was markedly enhanced and negative iron balance was attained by continuous, prolonged 24-hour intravenous or 8- to 12-hour subcutaneous infusions administered via a lightweight battery-operated or balloon-driven pump.[106,107] In addition, maintaining normal ascorbic acid levels optimizes iron excretion because it increases tissue iron turnover in the plasma.

Continuous, slow deferoxamine infusions allows for a longer exposure of the drug to the relatively small nontransferrin iron or labile iron pool that is in equilibrium with a nearly nonchelatable iron pool.[108]

A pump infuses an aqueous solution of DFO through a small 27-gauge butterfly needle placed under the skin of the abdomen, thigh, or extremities. Most patients use the pump during sleep.[109] Bolus subcutaneous injections of deferoxamine used twice daily induce levels of urinary iron excretion comparable with subcutaneous infusions and may prove helpful as a respite from overnight infusions in some patients not adherent to prolonged infusions.[110,111] In patients who are poorly compliant with subcutaneous therapy, administration of DFO in normal or higher doses can be accomplished intravenously by means of a deep line indwelling catheter, an externalized venous catheter or a subcutaneous port. Continuous intravenous administration of DFO is particularly useful for rapidly lowering the total iron burden and is used for reversal of cardiac morbidity, for example, cardiac arrhythmias or left-ventricular dysfunction. Complications of indwelling catheters including infection and thrombosis rates have been reported at 1.2 and 0.5 per 1000 catheter days respectively in patients treated over 1 to 5 years.

Prolonged infusions of deferoxamine achieve negative iron balance in most transfusion-dependent patients older than 4 or 5 years of age.[62,112–116] This approach to chelation therapy involves daily 8- to 12-hour subcutaneous infusions of 20 to 60 mg/kg of deferoxamine that should result in 20 to 50 mg/day of iron loss in the urine and stool.[62]

The optimal age for beginning parenteral or oral iron chelation therapy in patients with thalassemia has not been established with certainty. The surprisingly high liver iron concentrations that have been found in some patients with thalassemia within the first 2 to 3 years of transfusion therapy, occasionally accompanied by histologic finding of fibrosis, provided the rationale for the early initiation of deferoxamine iron chelation.[117,118] On the other hand, iron excretion in response to deferoxamine is relatively low during the first few years of iron accumulation and the pharmacokinetics and clearance of iron chelators in children is being further evaluated. Regular deferoxamine chelation therapy begun after the age of 3 to 5 years seems capable of removing previously stored iron and preventing iron-induced liver disease.[62] Data show that deferoxamine started by the age of 3 or 4 forestalls significant iron overload. However, it also promotes elimination of excess iron in patients if started after significant transfusional iron burden has already developed.[119–129] Moreover, deferoxamine may adversely affect bone development and growth in some young patients and the effect newer oral chelators on growth has yet to be addressed.[130–132] Some investigators have recommended the annual assessment of liver iron concentration as a guide for determining the appropriate time to begin iron chelation therapy[118] or a test infusion of DFO to determine if mobilizable iron is present.[133] Others have based this decision on the number of transfusions administered to the patient, that is, approximately 20 to 25 units of blood. Still others wait until the patient is 3 to 5 years old, when significant iron excretion can be accomplished and patient cooperation is better.[62,132]

Assessment of Iron Stores

Because excess transfusional iron cannot be actively excreted it is deposited in the macrophages of the reticuloendothelial system (RES). When the RES is overwhelmed, iron spills over into parenchymal tissue, generating free radical damage with cellular membrane lipid peroxidation and leading to end organ dysfunction, especially of the liver, endocrine system, and myocardium.

The best strategy for monitoring iron accumulation in patients with thalassemia remains controversial. Before chelation therapy is begun, careful recording of transfusion volumes provides an accurate assessment of iron loading. Each milliliter of red blood cells contains approximately 1.1 mg of iron. Therefore, each unit of blood contains approximately 200 mg of iron. The total transfusional iron intake can be calculated from the transfusion record and should be as useful in determining the need to begin chelation therapy as indirect or direct measures of body iron stores, if not more useful. Chelation therapy is initiated after approximately 20 to 25 units of blood have been transfused. However, once chelation therapy has been initiated, iron is going out as well as coming in. Under these circumstances, regular assessment of iron stores is needed to determine the severity of iron overload and to achieve an optimal treatment program.

Measurement of liver iron concentration by biopsy provides a direct assessment of tissue iron loading and reflects total body iron stores. Recent experiences with hepatic resonance imaging suggests that changes in R2 reflects liver iron concentration comparable to that on liver biopsy. Levels between 3 and 7 mg/g dry weight appear to be associated with minimal toxicity. Levels greater than 15 mg/g dry weight are associated with an increased risk of heart disease. Liver biopsy requires a skilled technician, at least 1 mg of tissue at least 2.5 cm in length with 5 portal tracts and has the risk of hemorrhage.

Serum ferritin levels are safe, inexpensive, and readily available and serial measurements are predictive both of critical complications such as iron-induced heart disease and of adverse effects of chelation therapy such as impairment of vision and hearing. However, single ferritin levels may correlate poorly with liver iron concentration, because it is an acute phase reactant, and may be influenced by inflammation, vitamin C deficiency, hepatitis, and other infectious states. Transferrin saturation is not very useful in evaluating the severity of iron overload in patients with thalassemia because the massive ineffective erythropoiesis usually results in a transferrin saturation greater than 60% even in the absence of iron overload.[515]

Noninvasive hepatic magnetic resonance imaging of liver iron by R2 changes correlates with liver iron concentration by biopsy but cannot be used in patients with pacemakers or those who are claustrophobic.

Recent experience with cardiac magnetic resonance imaging suggests that changes in T2* reflect levels of iron in the heart and may predict adverse changes in cardiac function.

Unfortunately, no measure of iron stores has been thoroughly and prospectively studied in patients with thalassemia major or intermedia to establish levels predictive of iron-related complications. Most guidelines are based on retrospective analyses, experience with other diseases, or limited outcome data.

The most common side effect of subcutaneous deferoxamine therapy is inflammation and induration at the site of infusion. Painful lumps may occur despite rotation of infusion sites, appropriate dilution of the drug, and proper placement of the needle. Some investigators have recommended the addition of small amounts of hydrocortisone to the infusion to prevent local reactions. Patients receiving aggressive chelation therapy with lower iron burdens may be more susceptible to toxicity. Neurosensory toxicity of DFO is dose related and inversely correlated with body iron burden. Impairments of visual and auditory acuity are associated with high doses of deferoxamine relative to the iron load.[134] The ototoxicity is characterized by bilateral high-frequency hearing loss. The retinal toxicity is characterized by the loss of night and color vision, retinal atrophy, and cataract formation.[135] Patients receiving deferoxamine should undergo baseline and annual audiograms and ophthalmologic examinations. Deferoxamine should be discontinued if such abnormalities arise, with cautious reinitiation at lower doses when abnormalities improve or resolve. The risk of visual and auditory side effects can be minimized by adjusting the daily deferoxamine dose to the patients' serum ferritin level.[134] Impaired growth associated with growth plate deformities or metaphyseal rickets-like changes in the long bones and histologic evidence of cartilage dysplasia may occur in young children receiving deferoxamine.[130–132] Regular monitoring with plain radiographs of the extremities and vertebral column allows early detection of this complication and reduction in the dose of deferoxamine or temporary interruption of chelation therapy.

Other, less common complications of deferoxamine include anaphylaxis, hypotension, allergic reactions, acute pulmonary disease, impairment of renal function, and infection.[136–142] Severe allergic reactions are rare and desensitization has been achieved successfully in some patients.[138,139] Acute pulmonary disease and renal failure have occurred in a few patients receiving unusually high doses of deferoxamine by intravenous infusion.[140] The mechanism of this toxicity is unclear. One of the most serious complications of deferoxamine is an increased risk of infection with *Yersinia* and mucomycosis, which uses the deferoxamine iron chelate as a siderophore, whereby enhancing their growth and presenting as colitis, abdominal abscess, or sepsis.[141,142] The safety of deferoxamine during pregnancy has been inferred from case reports rather than formal studies. A summary of these case reports identified 11 women who received deferoxamine beginning in the first trimester and 33 women who used the chelator beginning in the second or third trimester.[142] None of the infants showed evidence of drug-related toxicity.[143]

Regular chelation with deferoxamine has proven remarkably effective in reducing the transfusional iron burden of thalassemia patients. There is increasing evidence that endocrine dysfunction is improved and cardiac disease is delayed or prevented with standard deferoxamine regimens.[144] Cardiac arrhythmias and congestive heart failure have reversed in some patients with standard or aggressive deferoxamine regimens and life expectancy is significantly prolonged.* Intense 24-hour intravenous deferoxamine regimens of more than 15 mg/kg/hour have been reported to reverse early cardiac hemosiderosis whereas even more conventional doses of 50 mg/kg/day have improved left ventricular ejection fractions and prevented death in some patients.[148,149]

Prior to subcutaneous DFO therapy, estimated survival was approximately 16 to 17 years of age, with rare patients surviving into their mid-20s.[62,146,150,151] Since regular subcutaneous deferoxamine regimens have been in use, life expectancy has extended into the fourth decade.[152–154] The increasing widespread use of deferoxamine has steadily increased survival probabilities worldwide.[153,154] However, long-term European studies have demonstrated that improved survivals are clearly related to the degree of compliance with chelation regimens and are associated with lower serum ferritin levels (<1000 mg/mL).[155] Deferoxamine chelation regimens are clearly cumbersome, inconvenient, and costly. More tolerable approaches are required and investigations for alternative oral iron-chelating agents have been ongoing and recently more successful.

Although the prevalence of endocrine disturbances, for example, glucose intolerance and diabetes have reduced since the regular use of subcutaneous deferoxamine,[55,58,144] they persist especially in those who initiated deferoxamine late in their first decade.[124] Growth hormone deficiency, hypothyroidism, hypoparathyroidism, vitamin D deficiency, diabetes, and osteoporosis are still observed and there is little evidence that DFO can reverse established endocrine dysfunctions. The North American Thalassemia Clinical Research Network Registry reported that 96% of thalassemia patients with median age of 20 years were free of hypoparathyroidism, 91% had no thyroid disease, 90% were free of diabetes mellitus, and overall 62% free of any endocrinopathy.[156]

It remains to be determined if starting chelation at a very young age or more easily administered use of oral iron chelation will diminish the endocrine morbidities and further prolong survival associated with iron overload. Direct and indirect measures of iron stores reflect the progress of chelation therapy and help determine appropriate changes in the dose or frequency of chelator use. The serum ferritin level generally declines during regular chelation therapy and may decline rapidly in the first year of treatment in patients with very large iron stores.[112,114] Serum ferritin levels measured over time with use of deferoxamine have predicted the risk of iron-induced heart disease in patients with thalassemia major, and the ratio of the dose of deferoxamine to the ferritin level has identified patients at risk for auditory and visual complications of chelation therapy.[134,147] Although easy to obtain and relatively inexpensive, the serum ferritin level may be increased in the presence of inflammation and may be decreased when iron overload is accompanied by vitamin C deficiency.[157] For these and other reasons, serum ferritin levels frequently correlate poorly with liver iron concentrations, and clinicians and patients may have a false sense of security when the ferritin level is below 2000 μg/L. Some studies using deferoxamine suggest ferritin levels lower than 1000 μg/L are associated with better survival and less cardiac disease as well as hepatic histology and pathology.[155,158,159]

Liver biopsy with biochemical measurement of iron concentration provides a more direct assessment of iron overload, and some investigators recommend such testing yearly. Hepatic iron levels of 15 mg/g dry weight have been associated with a greater risk of iron-induced heart disease.[119] The meaning of lower hepatic iron levels has generally been inferred from experience with primary hemochromatosis.[160] Further studies are needed to determine the clinical usefulness of liver iron concentration in the overall management of thalassemia. Noninvasive techniques for assessing tissue iron offer the possibility of serial measurements without substantial risk to the patient. The noninvasive measurement of iron in the liver, heart, and other target organs are in development. Measurements of liver iron concentration by magnetic susceptometry using a superconducting quantum interference device (SQUID) correlate well with biochemical measurements of tissue iron.[161,162] At present, measurement of tissue iron by SQUID is limited to the liver, and the instruments are available in only two sites in the United States and two sites in Europe. The ability to use magnetic resonance imaging to measure iron stores would dramatically extend the availability of noninvasive tissue iron measurements. Investigators have reported success using proton transverse relaxation rates (R2) with spin-echo imaging, signal intensity ratios, and gradient-echo T2* to assess liver iron concentration.[163–167] The latter two techniques also yield information that appears to reflect cardiac iron loading. Direct comparisons with hepatic tissue samples demonstrate significant correlations ($r = 0.97$ vs 0.95) with biopsy-measured liver iron concentrations in two separate studies.[164,166–170] These noninvasive technologies to measure liver, cardiac, and other tissue iron concentration may prove useful in the future to refine therapeutic strategies. Current needs include the further refinement of magnetic resonance imaging techniques and a better understanding of the relationship between liver iron, iron in other organs (in particular the heart), and clinical complications of iron overload.

A relationship between iron overload and ascorbic acid depletion, first suggested by the epidemiology of scurvy among the Bantu, exists in thalassemia major.[45,157] For thalassemia patients with low levels of ascorbic acid, daily supplementation with 100 to 200 mg of this vitamin increases urinary iron excretion in response to deferoxamine by approximately twofold.[46,108] Ascorbic acid may retard the conversion of ferritin to hemosiderin and therefore allow more iron to remain in the chelatable form.[171,172] However, it can also enhance iron-mediated peroxidation of membrane lipids[173,174] as well as membrane damage in cultured myocardial cells.[175] Cardiac toxicity

*References 55, 61, 119, 120, 123, 125, and 145–147.

manifested as arrhythmias and decreased ventricular contractility has been attributed to vitamin C therapy.[176] Ascorbic acid should be used only while deferoxamine is being administered and only in patients who are ascorbate depleted. Chelation therapy with deferoxamine is expensive and cumbersome because of the need for daily or nightly subcutaneous infusions. Regular infusions require a great deal of dedication and persistence from the patient and family. Noncompliance is common, particularly in the teenage and young adult years, and failure to follow prescribed treatment regimens is the major cause of mortality in patients with thalassemia major.[155] The cost and complexity of deferoxamine administration prevents its availability worldwide, especially in developing countries. The search for a less expensive iron chelator that can be more easily orally administered led to the identification of compounds such as deferiprone and deferasirox.

Deferiprone

One such oral agent is 1,2-dimethyl-3-hydroxypyrid-4-one (L1, deferiprone), a synthetic compound with a low molecular weight of approximately 200. It is an orally active bidentate iron chelator that requires three molecules to bind one iron atom. Deferiprone is absorbed by the gastrointestinal tract, has a plasma half life of approximately 90 minutes (2–3 hours). Chelated iron is excreted predominantly in the urine (90%) and far less in the stool (10%). It was synthesized in the late 1980s and was first tested in uncontrolled clinical trials at the Royal Free Hospital in London, hence the eponym L1.[177,178] Subsequent clinical efficacy studies appeared initially encouraging[179–181] but its long-term efficacy and safety have not been totally established.[180,182–186] Unfortunately, deferiprone was not subjected to Phase III studies wherein its safety and efficacy were directly compared to deferoxamine. Nonetheless, at doses of 75 mg/kg/day, deferiprone administered in three divided doses with meals reduces or maintains iron stores in many regularly transfused patients, for the most part, particularly those with more severe transfusional iron overload.[179,180,182–188] However, some patients continue to accumulate iron during long-term therapy with this dose of deferiprone.[180,184,189] Regimens using higher doses up to 100 mg/kg/day of deferiprone or combination regimens with deferoxamine reduce iron stores or have proved effective in restoring negative iron balance in some of these patients.[190–192] Enhanced urine and stool iron excretion in thalassemia patients using both deferoxamine and deferiprone have suggested an additive effect postulated by the shuttle hypothesis, that is, deferiprone may chelate intracellular labile iron and shuttle it to deferoxamine.[193] Some studies have also suggested that deferiprone alone or in combination with deferoxamine may be more effective than deferoxamine in removing iron from the heart, improving cardiac function, and preventing iron-induced cardiac disease.[170,188,194–197] Schedules for combination therapy vary but have usually included 5 to 7 days of deferiprone and 2 days of subcutaneous deferoxamine weekly.

Side effects of deferiprone include gastrointestinal complaints, mostly nausea and some vomiting that occur in approximately 33% of patients and usually resolve without specific intervention. Arthropathy with arthalgias and some joint effusions occur in approximately 15% of patients. The incidence of joint symptoms varies widely among various studies but may be severe enough to require reduction or interruption of chelation therapy. Abnormal liver function tests may occur gradually or suddenly and in the absence of other causes of hepatic dysfunction. These elevations may return to baseline values with the interruption of deferiprone followed by reinitiation beginning with lower doses and close monitoring of liver function tests. Progressive liver disease attributed to deferiprone has not been reported and concerns about drug-induced hepatic fibrosis have not been substantiated by subsequent studies.[180,183,198,199] However, there is in vitro evidence that deferiprone may potentiate oxidative DNA damage in iron-loaded liver cells that could occur when the concentration of iron is low relative to the iron chelator (Fig. 41–8).[200] Agranulocytosis occurs in 1% of patients and, although rare, remains

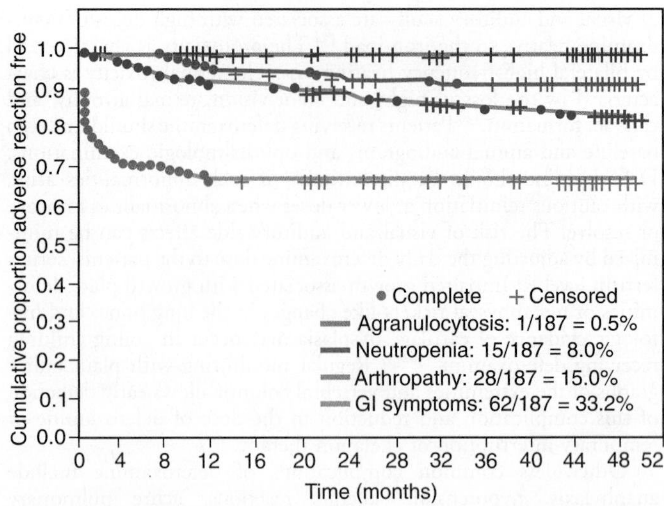

Figure 41–8 Kaplan–Meier curves showing the time to first occurrence of important adverse events in patients treated with deferiprone. The only case of agranulocytosis occurred in the first year, and gastrointestinal complaints were very uncommon after the first year. Neutropenia and joint problems occurred throughout the 4-year study period but were more common in the first year than in each of the subsequent years. *(Adapted from Cohen AR, Galanello R, Piga A, et al: Safety and effectiveness of long-term therapy with the oral iron chelator deferiprone. Blood 102:1583, 2003.)*

the principal concern for patients receiving deferiprone. Milder neutropenia is more common and occurs in approximately 8% of patients. Severely depressed neutrophil counts represents a significant risk of sepsis, hospitalizations, and in some cases administration of G-CSF is required. Some reported deaths have been related to deferiprone-induced agranulocytosis and/or neutropenia. Regular weekly monitoring of blood counts during deferiprone therapy is essential to detect the rare but important deferiprone-induced complications of neutropenia and agranulocytosis.[184–186,201]

Several clinical studies of deferiprone speak to its relative safety and utility demonstrated by a decline in serum ferritin levels in the majority of patients.[170,183–188,194,195,197] Retrospective studies have suggested that deferiprone might be more effective than deferoxamine in chelating cardiac iron. Two multicenter studies have futher supported the theory that combination therapy increases total iron excretion and selectively reduces organ iron burden.[195,197] Longitudinal clinical studies using innovative magnetic resonance imaging technology to measure cardiac (T2*) and liver iron concentration have demonstrated higher estimated liver iron concentration but lower myocardial iron concentration in deferiprone-treated thalassemia patients in comparison to those treated with deferoxamine.[194] In another study, thalassemia patients using deferiprone did not experience any cardiac events nor any cardiac-related deaths in comparison to thalassemia patients on deferoxamine who experienced both cardiac events and some deaths.[195] In another 1-year prospective trial of cardiac iron and function, thalassemia patients treated with deferiprone or deferoxamine had improved myocardial T2* values but more so in the deferiprone-treated group, who also showed a greater improvement in left ventricular ejection fraction. Liver iron concentration fell significantly in the deferoxamine-treated patients but not in the patients receiving deferiprone. A prospective randomized study comparing the combination of deferiprone at 75 mg/kg/day and deferoxamine at 40 to 50 mg/kg/day with deferoxamine alone demonstrated that the combination therapy more rapidly reduced hepatic and cardiac iron stores than deferoxamine alone.[202] Further prospective studies are warranted, especially with the combination of deferiprone with deferoxamine. Deferiprone may play a role in shuttling iron from within intracellular pools and enhance the available iron pool to bind with deferoxamine.[183,203–205] Deferiprone continues to be tested in clinical trials alone and in combination with deferoxamine to address its impact on cardiac function.[197] The safety profile of deferiprone has been largely defined by single-center studies, multicenter trials, and postmarketing surveillance largely in European and Asian continents. Deferiprone is currently licensed only in Europe as alternative iron chelation therapy for those who are unable to be successfully treated with deferoxamine.

Deferasirox

Deferasirox (ICL670, ExJade) is an orally active iron chelator that was identified by computer technology at Novartis Pharmaceuticals in the 1990s. It is a tridentate compound known as 4-(3,5-bis(2-hydroxyphenyl)-1*H*-1,2,4-triazol-1-yl)-benzoic acid,[206] wherein two molecules of deferasirox are required to bind one atom of iron. It has a high affinity for iron and a much lower affinity for copper and zinc. Deferasirox is orally bioavailable with a low molecular weight of 373 and is absorbed by the gastrointestinal tract. It has a dose-dependent plasma half-life of 12 to 18 hours that allows for once-daily oral administration after fasting on an empty stomach.[207] Deferasirox is given as a suspension in water or apple or orange juice.[208] Iron excretion in response to deferasirox is largely in the stool (90%) and far less in the urine (10%).[208] The pharmacodynamic effects of deferasirox tested in a Phase I clinical iron balance metabolic study measuring stool and urine iron excretion demonstrated increasing iron excretion at doses of 10, 20, and 40 mg/kg/day, which induced a mean net iron excretion (0.119, 0.329, and 0.445 mg Fe/kg/day, respectively) within the clinically relevant range of the rate of transfusion iron loading for most patients. No significant acute side effects occurred other than gastrointestinal disturbances that were generally mild and a diffuse rash in some cases.[208]

Utility and safety of deferasirox have been also shown in short-term toxicity and pharmacokinetic studies.[208,209] Initially, a 1-year Phase II randomized multicenter study of transfusion-dependent thalassemia patients receiving deferasirox at doses of 20 mg/kg in comparison to deferoxamine at 40 mg/kg used subcutaneously 5 nights per week showed that deferasirox induced a 10% greater reduction in liver iron concentration by SQUID measurement than that of deferoxamine.[210] The Phase III worldwide multicenter open-label randomized active comparator control study of deferasirox in comparison to deferoxamine was conducted in 65 sites with 586 regularly transfused patients 2 years or more of age with β-thalassemia. Results indicated that chronic daily use of deferasirox, via a single oral dose of 20 to 30 mg/kg/day, induced decreases in liver iron concentration by biopsy comparable to that achieved with deferoxamine. Patients with liver iron concentrations greater than 7 mg/g dry weight receiving deferasirox at 20 to 30 mg/kg/day had a mean decrease of 5.3 mg/g dry weight that did not differ significantly from a mean decrease of 4.3 mg/g dry weight in patients receiving 35 mg/kg/day or more deferoxamine. Changes in serum ferritin were dose dependent in both treatments paralleling trends in liver iron content.[209] Doses of 5 and 10 mg/kg per day of deferasirox were unlikely to achieve negative iron balance and did not maintain or reduce absolute liver iron concentration and serum ferritin levels increased at these lower doses. The rate of transfusional iron loading may also influence the effectiveness of deferasirox in controlling liver iron concentration, and maintaining a transfusional iron requirement of 0.5 mg/kg/day or less may benefit reduction in liver iron concentration using 20 mg/kg/day of deferasirox.[211] Deferasirox was given Orphan Drug status and was approved by the FDA in 2005 and is commercially available in the United States. Long-term extension clinical studies using deferasirox are in progress.

Deferasirox was generally well tolerated in these clinical trials. Mild gastrointestinal complaints and skin rashes were the most common adverse events. Discontinuation of deferasirox was rarely required but abdominal discomfort occurred in 14% of patients, 12% with diarrhea, 10% nausea, and 9% vomiting. Mild increases in serum creatinine occurred in 38% of patients and a small number exceeded the upper limits of normal; intermittent proteinuria was also observed in 19% of patients. Duplicate serum creatinine level should be assessed prior to initiating therapy. Close monthly monitoring of serum creatinine needs to be maintained because of nephropathy in animal studies and cases of acute renal failure that were reported following postmarketing use of deferasirox. Severe renal complications may occur in patients with preexisting renal disease. Dose reduction, interruption, or discontinuation should be considered for elevations in serum creatinine. Elevations in serum transaminases also occurred in a small number of patients (6%). Recommendations to monitor liver function closely at monthly intervals with interruptions or discontinuations of deferasirox if unexplained or progressive transaminase increases occur. Skin rashes also occurred in 15% of patients usually within the first 2 weeks of treatment. The maculopapular eruptions often resolved spontaneously but severe rashes may require interruption of deferasirox with antihistamine support and possible steroid administration, following which deferasirox may be reintroduced at a lower dose with gradual dose escalation. Minimal (<1%) auditory and ophthalmologic toxicity occurred in the preliminary 1-year safety and efficacy trial. No agranulocytosis was observed in thalassemia subjects during the 1-year primary efficacy trial. Reports of pancytopenia have occurred in postmarketing reports, however, mostly in other patients with preexisting hematologic disorders such as myelodysplastic syndromes that are frequently associated with bone marrow failure. Four-year extension trials of deferasirox are ongoing after licensing by the FDA.

Other approaches to improved chelation therapy have focused on parenteral therapy. The compound HBED, originally developed as a potential oral agent, has been shown in primate studies to be more effective when administered as a subcutaneous injection than deferoxamine administered by subcutaneous infusion.[212] The attachment of deferoxamine to a backbone of starch (S-DFO) extends the circulation time of the chelator, and early studies suggest that this novel form of deferoxamine may reduce the frequency of infusions required to achieve negative iron balance.[213] Another promising oral desferithiocin derivative, Deferitrin (GT56–252), is under study because early phase I safety and efficacy studies have demonstrated tolerability and efficacy.[214]

Specific Complications and Their Management

Skeletal Changes

Skeletal abnormalities (Fig. 41–9) are less common in patients receiving regular red blood cell transfusions but may still occur as a result of partially unchecked ineffective erythropoiesis and expansion of the erythroid marrow.[215] These cause widening of the marrow space and thinning of the cortex, with consequent osteoporosis.[216,217] Changes in the skull and facial bones, including expansion of the frontal bone with prominent frontal bossing, may occur prior to the initiation of transfusion therapy. Radiographs reveal the diploic spaces to be widened. At first, the skull has a granular appearance, but later perpendicular bony trabeculae appear, giving the classic "hair on end" or "crewcut" appearance. Marked overgrowth of the maxilla results in severe malocclusion, jumbling of the upper incisors, and prominence of the molar eminences.[218] These bone changes produce the classic facies. Additional skeletal changes are observed in the metacarpals, metatarsals, and phalanges, where expanded medullary cavities produce a rectangular and then a convex shape (see Fig. 41–9). Irregular fusion of the epiphyses of the proximal humerus results in characteristic shortening of the upper arms.[219,220] Marked osteoporosis and cortical thinning may predispose to pathologic fractures of the extremities and compression fractures of the vertebrae. (Fig. 41–10)

Several abnormalities in the ribs may occur, including notching and osteolytic lesions.[215,221] The ribs become very wide, especially at the points of their attachment to the vertebral column. Marrow masses may extrude from these sites, creating the appearance of paravertebral masses and compressing the spinal cord.[222] Although bone deformities and extramedullary hematopoiesis is uncommon in properly transfused patients with β-thalassemia major, it is not

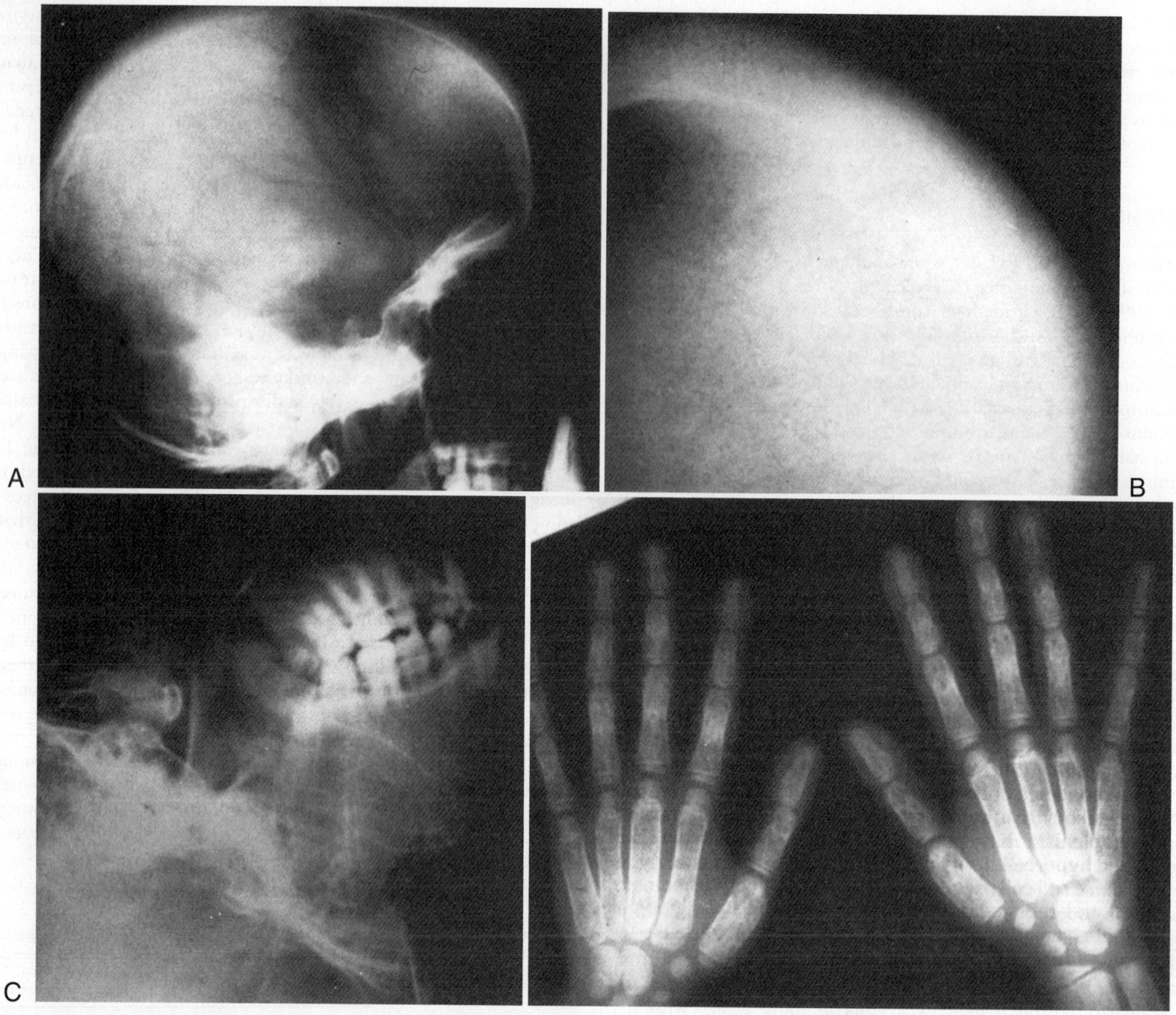

Figure 41–9 Bony abnormalities in a patient with severe β-thalassemia. **A** and **B**, "Hair-on-end" appearance of the skull, especially obvious in the close-up view shown in part **B**. **C**, Distortion of the maxillary bones, as well as poor development of the sinus cavities due to opaque masses of extramedullary erythropoiesis. **D**, Squaring and convexity abnormalities of the hands. *(From Pearson HA, Benz EJ Jr: Thalassemia syndromes. In Miller DR, Baehner RL, McMillan CW [eds.]: Smith's Blood Diseases of Infancy and Childhood, 5th ed. St. Louis, CV Mosby, 1984, p 439.)*

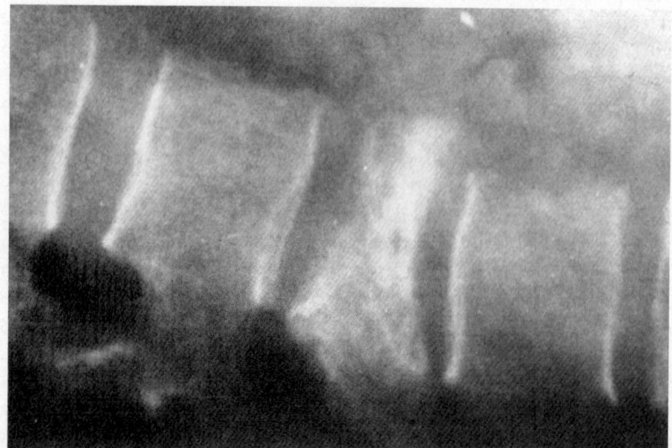

Figure 41–10 Compression fracture of L2 vertebra in a patient with severe β-thalassemia. *(From Pearson HA, Benz EJ Jr: Thalassemia syndromes. In Miller DR, Baehner RL, McMillan CW [eds.]: Smith's Blood Diseases of Infancy and Childhood, 5th ed. St. Louis, CV Mosby, 1984, p 439.)*

infrequently observed in patients with thalassemia intermedia whose marrow is not suppressed by regular transfusions (see the section Thalassemia Intermedia).

The character and degree of the bone lesions change significantly with age. In older children, the bone lesions regress in the more distal portions of the skeleton (hands, arms, and legs), a feature correlating with the normal developmental replacement of red marrow by fatty marrow. The characteristic changes of the hands and other peripheral areas are thus diminished and may disappear in later life.[55,223] However, in the skull, spine, and pelvis (which are sites of active, persistent erythropoiesis), the radiographic changes become more conspicuous.[75]

Growth and Endocrine Status

Growth retardation, including skeletal and dental deformities,[224] was common even in young children until the use of hypertransfusion regimens restored relatively normal growth during the first decade. Without iron chelation therapy, the adolescent growth spurt is often delayed or absent; most patients, even those well maintained by transfusion, may not attain normal stature, in part because of iron-induced damage to the hypothalamic–pituitary axis.[36,225,226] Menarche is frequently delayed. Breast development may be poor, and many female patients have primary or secondary amenorrhea. Boys are frequently immature, with sparse facial and body hair. Although spermatogenesis may be normal, libido is often decreased. A multicenter study of 250 adolescent patients in northern Italy showed that despite hypertransfusion and 7 to 10 years of deferoxamine iron chelation therapy, two-thirds of male patients and one-third of female patients older than 14 years of age were 2 SDs or more below the mean for height.[227] Many adolescents between 12 and 18 years of age lacked any secondary sexual changes of puberty. However, the mean serum ferritin level in the entire group was 3500 ng/mL, indicating persistence of a high level of excess iron burden in most of this group.

Regular chelation therapy started early in the first decade of life frequently will allow normal onset of puberty and development of secondary sexual changes.[228] Administration of recombinant human growth hormone in conventional doses increases height velocity in patients with growth hormone deficiency.[229,230] Normal or higher doses of recombinant human growth hormone increase growth velocity in patients with normal growth hormone reserve but low levels of insulin-like growth factor I.[231,232] For patients with a functional hypothalamic–pituitary axis, treatment with gonadotropin-releasing hormone may induce pubertal changes.[233] In others, administration of sex steroids is necessary to induce secondary sexual characteristics.

More than 100 pregnancies either have been achieved spontaneously in patients with normal menstrual function or have been induced in patients with primary or secondary amenorrhea.[234–239] Transfusion requirements frequently increase during pregnancy, especially during the third trimester.[234] Diminished ventricular contractility during pregnancy and the death from heart disease of at least one mother within a year of delivery argue strongly for the careful consideration of the overall clinical condition and degree of iron loading before planning a pregnancy.[237,240] The safety of chelation therapy during pregnancy is discussed above. At least one successful pregnancy has occurred in a woman with thalassemia after bone marrow transplantation that included ablative therapy with busulfan and cyclophosphamide.[241]

Abnormal carbohydrate metabolism is common in older patients with thalassemia major. Prepubertal children usually have normal glucose metabolism, but pubertal patients exhibit impaired responses to glucose load. Higher than normal insulin levels despite normal glucose levels are also encountered during puberty.[242] The defect in these patients appears to be related to insulin resistance, with insulin deficiency developing later in the progression to diabetes. Rates of diabetes are reported close to 6% to 8%.[154] Diabetes occurs more frequently in patients with hepatitis C and hepatic dysfunction.[243–245] Oral hypoglycemic agents have been used to regulate hyperglycemia and may reduce the rate of further deterioration of glucose metabolism.[246]

Laboratory findings of hypothyroidism and hypoparathyroidism are present in approximately 14% of patients with thalassemia major.[247–251] Clinical findings associated with these deficiencies are uncommon.[252]

Low Bone Mass

With improved survival in patients with thalassemia major, the problem of osteoporosis has assumed greater importance. The widespread prevalence of osteoporosis in thalassemia major patients was first observed across all ages in 1995.[253] Subsequently, others reported a high frequency of abnormal *Z* scores in pediatric, adolescent, and adult patients. Abnormal bone mineral density has been reported in pediatric and adolescent thalassemia major patients.[254–256] The Thalassemia Clinical Research Network has identified the prevalence of fractures in a contemporary sample of 702 patients with α-and β-thalassemia. The overall fracture prevalence was 12%, with fractures occurring more frequently in thalassemia major (17%) and intermedia (12%) compared to β-E (7%) and α-thalassemia (2%). Facture prevalence increased with age and with sex hormone replacement therapy.[257] More recently an observational study by the Thalassemia Clinical Research Network has demonstrated a high prevalence of low bone mass across all the thalassemia syndromes, including β-thalassemia major, intermedia, β-E, hemoglobin H, H-Constant Spring, and homozygous α-thalassemia, which progresses with aging. Low bone mass is associated with high prevalence of fractures, hypogonadism, and increased bone turnover.[254,257,258] Bone resorption is usually increased and new bone formation is decreased.[259] Treatment with some but not all bisphosphonates improves bone mineral density.[260–263] Vitamin D and calcium supplementation with age-appropriate hormone replacement therapy are important preventive measures, although low bone mass may still occur in treated patients. Gonadal steroid replacement of hypogonadal patients has been shown to improve bone mass in some studies.[258,264]

Liver and Gallbladder

Hepatomegaly occurring prior to the initiation of transfusion therapy in severely affected patients is primarily a consequence of extramedullary hematopoiesis. With the amelioration of the anemia, the liver diminishes in size. However, as transfusion therapy continues, iron accumulation provides a new reason for hepatomegaly and resultant liver injury. Iron deposition, first present in the Kupffer cells, ultimately engorges the parenchymal cells, resulting in an appearance that is indistinguishable from that of idiopathic hemochromatosis.[265–267] The hepatocellular injury of iron overload may be due to the liberation of hydrolases resulting from initiation by the ferrous form of iron and peroxidative damage of lysosomal membrane lipids.[268] Fibrosis is usually followed by cirrhosis and an increased risk of hepatocellular carcinoma. The risk of liver damage and the rate of progression may be increased by the concomitant presence of excessive iron with viral hepatitis. The concentration of liver iron that constitutes a threshold for liver damage in patients with thalassemia is similar to that found in patients with hereditary hemochromatosis. In contrast to hereditary hemochromatosis, however, death from liver failure or liver cancer is much less common than death from cardiac failure in patients with thalassemia.[153]

Regular chelation therapy is the key to maintaining normal or near-normal hepatic iron concentrations and preventing iron-induced hepatic fibrosis and cirrhosis. Treatment with deferoxamine slows or prevents iron-induced liver damage and may reduce the severity of preexisting fibrosis in some cases.[104,124,269] Results of treatment of hepatitis C in patients with thalassemia major are similar to those found in other patients. Sustained viral responses occur in 28% to 40% of patients treated with interferon alone and, in two smaller series, 46% to 72% of patients treated with interferon and ribavirin.[270–274] Transfusion requirements increase by 30% to 40% in patients treated with ribavirin as a result of drug-induced hemolysis.[271,273,274] Lower levels of viral RNA and non-1 genotypes are associated with better responses. Higher iron levels adversely affect the response to antiviral therapy in some studies but not in others.[270,272,275] The Thalassemia Clinical Research Network studied the use of pegylated interferon and ribavirin in 16 thalassemia patients. Fifty percent genotype 1 patients had sustained viral response as well as 25% of genotype 2 and 3 patients; median transfusion requirements increased by 44% after 24 weeks of treatment and liver iron concentration increase of more than 5 mg/g dry weight occurred in 29% of patients, but overall liver iron concentration remained stable over the course of the study. In addition, neutropenia occurred in 52% of patients.[274] Interferon therapy in patients with hepatitis C who have previously undergone bone marrow transplantation is as effective and safe as in nontransplanted patients.[276]

Pigmentary gallstones caused by high levels of bilirubin production are found in an increasing number of patients over 4 years old. Two-thirds of patients have multiple calcified bilirubinate calculi after the age of 15 years.[277] Gallbladder surgery is not usually indicated unless biliary colic or obstructive jaundice has occurred.

Heart

Cardiac abnormalities are important causes of morbidity and mortality in patients with thalassemia major. Cardiac enlargement secondary to anemia is almost always present in untransfused children (see Fig. 41–9). Before the availability of chelation therapy, myocardial hemosiderosis and serious iron-induced cardiac diseases were inevitable during the second decade. These problems still occur often in older patients with thalassemia who are poorly compliant with chelation therapy, and heart disease, usually in the form of cardiac failure or serious arrhythmias, remains the most common cause of death in patients with thalassemia major.[153,155]

Left-sided heart failure predominates in patients with thalassemia major and is characterized by dyspnea and orthopnea.[278] Right-sided heart failure is less common but may be the presenting cardiac finding in older patients with more severe iron overload. Symptoms include hepatic pain, abdominal discomfort, and peripheral edema. Acute myocarditis, which occurs in approximately 5% of patients with thalassemia, is frequently followed by acute or chronic heart failure.[279]

Early electrocardiographic abnormalities include a prolonged P–R interval, first-degree heart block, and premature atrial contractions. Later, ST-segment depression and ventricular ectopic beats constitute ominous indicators of myocardial damage. Periodic evaluation of cardiac function is essential to detect iron-induced heart disease and to identify patients who will benefit from more intensive chelation therapy (see later). Unfortunately, by the time cardiac studies such as echocardiography and 24-hour rhythm monitoring become abnormal, clinical heart disease is imminent. Whether assessment of cardiac iron by MRI using T2* or other measures can better anticipate the development of clinical heart disease is currently under investigation.

In the absence of intensified chelation therapy, ventricular dysfunction progresses rapidly to chronic refractory congestive heart failure, and arrhythmias become increasingly difficult to control. In the past, death usually occurred within 1 year of onset of heart failure. More recent data demonstrate a survival rate of 48% at 5 years.[278] Survival is notably poorer in patients with heart failure after myocarditis or with heart failure accompanied by arrhythmias.[279]

In addition to standard therapy for heart failure and arrhythmias, including angiotensin-converting enzyme inhibitors, β blockers, diuretics, and antiarrhythmic agents, the pretransfusion hemoglobin level should be maintained between 10 and 12 g/dL. The volume of transfused red blood cells should be reduced as needed to prevent acute fluid overload. Because the iron-overloaded myocardium has little capacity to improve its performance unless excess iron is removed, intensive chelation therapy is a critical part of the management of heart disease in patients with thalassemia. Several studies have shown that heart failure can be reversed in many patients with the use of continuous treatment with deferoxamine.[145,280,281] The benefits of this approach may derive from the reduction in cardiac iron stores, the prevention of acute toxicity from non-transferrin-bound iron, or a combination of these two mechanisms. Recent data suggest that deferiprone may be more effective than deferoxamine in reducing the cardiac iron load and treating iron-induced cardiac disease, perhaps because of deferiprone's ability to enter cardiac cells more rapidly than deferoxamine.[170,194] Different iron chelators seem to have different accessibility to hepatic and extrahepatic iron stores. Deferoxamine works more rapidly and efficiently in removing liver iron than cardiac iron.[149,281] Deferiprone seems to remove iron from the heart effectively[282] despite its relative inefficiency in controlling hepatic iron content.[170,194] In the gerbil animal model, deferasirox and deferiprone were equally effective in removing cardiac iron and deferasirox removed even more hepatic iron for a given cardiac iron burden.[283] Deferasirox treatment for 1 to 2 years has also been shown to reduce cardiac iron and improve cardiac MRI T2* in patients with transfusional iron overload.[284,285] Additional studies are needed to confirm these observations and to establish the relative roles of deferiprone, deferasirox and deferoxamine or a combination thereof in the management of patients with established iron-related heart disease.[286] In patients who have undergone bone marrow transplantation, improvements in left ventricular contractility and diastolic function accompany the removal of excess iron by phlebotomy.[287] Heart transplantation and combined heart–liver transplantation have been performed successfully in patients with end-stage cardiac disease.[288–290]

Sterile pericarditis occurs in some patients with massive iron overload.[291] Although pericarditis is most often attributed to hemosiderosis, an association with β-hemolytic streptococcal infection and other infectious agents has also been suggested.[292] Therapy usually consists of bed rest, treatment of infection, management of superimposed congestive heart failure, and the use of salicylates or corticosteroids. Occasionally, pericardiectomy may be indicated.

Lungs

Mild abnormalities of pulmonary function are common in patients with thalassemia but rarely cause clinical problems. Some patients exhibit primarily restrictive defects[293,294]; others experience mild to moderate small-airway obstruction and hyperinflation.[295–297] Most patients have a decreased maximal oxygen uptake and anaerobic threshold; these do not normalize after transfusion.[298] Postsplenectomy thrombocytosis and other prothrombotic changes can predispose to pulmonary vascular occlusion and pulmonary hypertension.[299–302] Treatment with high doses of the iron chelator deferoxamine may also be associated with acute deterioration of pulmonary function.[140,141]

Kidneys

The kidneys are frequently enlarged, due in part to extramedullary hematopoiesis and in part to marked dilation of the renal tubules.[303] The urine is often dark brown, reflecting the excretion of products of heme catabolism.[304] The urine also contains large amounts of urates and uric acid.

Spleen and Splenectomy

Massive splenomegaly is unusual in regularly transfused patients, but moderate splenomegaly may be associated with findings of hypersplenism. Thrombocytopenia and neutropenia are usually mild, and infection and bleeding are distinctly unusual in the absence of other risk factors. The usual indication for splenectomy is a progressive increase in transfusion requirements due to hypersplenism. The transfusion requirements, and therefore the rates of iron loading, of splenectomized patients are often considerably less than those of patients whose spleens are intact.[69,70,305,306] A transfusion requirement of more than 180 to 200 mL/kg/year of packed red blood cells usually represents excessive red blood cell requirements.[305,306] For such patients, a 25% to 60% reduction in transfusion requirements after splenectomy is generally predictable. Before attributing increased transfusion requirements to hypersplenism, it is important to look for other causes, such as red blood cell alloimmunization or a change in the hematocrit of the units of donor blood. Red blood cell survival studies using ^{50}Cr-labeling are not usually of value for predicting response to splenectomy. Because of the greater risk of postsplenectomy sepsis in younger patients, surgery should be deferred until after 5 years of age whenever possible. For well-transfused and well-chelated patients, splenectomy may have little benefit, and some centers have noted a significant decline in the number of patients undergoing splenectomy in recent years.

Laparoscopic splenectomy has proved safe for patients with thalassemia and has dramatically shortened the recovery time compared with open procedures.[307] Partial splenectomy and partial dearterialization of the spleen have been suggested as alternative approaches to reducing blood requirements without incurring the risk of sepsis.[308–310] The long-term benefits of this approach remain uncertain. Therapeutic embolization of the spleen avoids the need for surgery,[311–313] but this approach is frequently associated with postprocedure pain and fever and does not permit the removal of accessory spleens.

After splenectomy, striking thrombocytosis may occur. Increased numbers of nucleated red blood cells appear in the blood, and the presence of many red blood cells containing inclusion bodies composed of precipitated α-globin chains can be demonstrated by staining with methyl violet or brilliant cresyl blue.

A period of observation without transfusion after splenectomy may be helpful in identifying those patients who can now maintain an acceptable hemoglobin level without regular transfusions. This approach may be particularly useful for patients whose thalassemia mutations would predict a milder clinical course. Hemoglobin levels should be monitored weekly to determine whether transfusion therapy should be reinstituted.

Patients with thalassemia major are at significant risk for the development of overwhelming, often fatal, infection after splenectomy (postsplenectomy sepsis syndrome).[314] The problem is most common in young children. *Streptococcus pneumoniae* causes two-thirds of cases; *Hemophilus influenzae* type B and *Neisseria meningitidis* account for most of the remaining infections. Typically, there is a fulminant clinical course, proceeding from mild fever and headache to hyperpyrexia, prostration, shock, and death within 6 to 12 hours. Immunization against the most common pathogens before splenectomy, prophylaxis with antibiotics, and early assessment of fever after splenectomy have dramatically reduced the incidence of fatal post-splenectomy sepsis.

Splenectomy should generally be reserved for patients with excessive transfusion requirements due to hypersplenism and difficulty controlling iron overload. A large spleen alone does not usually cause significant clinical problems and should rarely, if ever, be the sole reason for splenectomy. If possible, splenectomy should be delayed until children with thalassemia are at least 5 years old. By this time, children are more likely to have developed humoral immunity to a broad range of bacteria. Before splenectomy, polyvalent pneumococcal, meningococcal, and *H influenzae* vaccines should be administered if they have not been given earlier in life.[315,316] Oral penicillin therapy, 250 mg twice daily, is generally used as prophylaxis against postsplenectomy infection in patients with thalassemia. However, the optimal duration of penicillin prophylaxis remains unknown, and compliance is frequently inadequate.[317] Although the risk of postsplenectomy sepsis decreases with age, it does not disappear, and fatal pneumococcal sepsis has occurred many years after removal of the spleen.[318]

Pneumococcal sepsis is not totally preventable, because not all pneumococcal strains are represented in the available vaccines. In addition, penicillin-resistant strains of *S pneumoniae* have emerged with a prevalence in the United States of 5% to 10%, or even higher in some localities. Therefore, it is particularly important that patients and families be instructed to seek medical attention immediately if significant fever or other signs of infection develop.

Vitamin Supplementation

Although folic acid deficiency is uncommon in patients receiving regular transfusions, daily supplementation with 1.0 mg of folic acid is reasonable, especially if dietary intake is not optimal. Therapy with large doses of vitamin E neither improves survival of transfused red blood cells nor decreases transfusion requirements.[319] Whether vitamin E supplementation decreases the toxic effects of iron overload on specific tissues remains uncertain. Zinc supplementation is appropriate for patients with clinical or laboratory findings of zinc deficiency, usually a result of intensive iron chelation therapy. One center has reported an enhancement of linear growth in children with thalassemia receiving zinc for 1 to 7 years.[320]

Table 41–2 Survival by Birth Cohort at Different Ages of Patients With Transfusion-Dependent Thalassemia

	Cohort		
Patient Age (Years)	1970–1974	1975–1979	1980–1984
10	98% (96–99)	98% (96–99)	99% (95–100)+
15	95% (92–97)	97% (94–98)	98% (93–100)
20	89% (85–92)	96% (93–98)	
25	82% (77–86)		

Data from Borgna Pignatti C, Rugolotto S, De Stefano X, et al: Survival and disease complications in thalassemia major. Ann N Y Acad Sci 850:227–231, 1998.

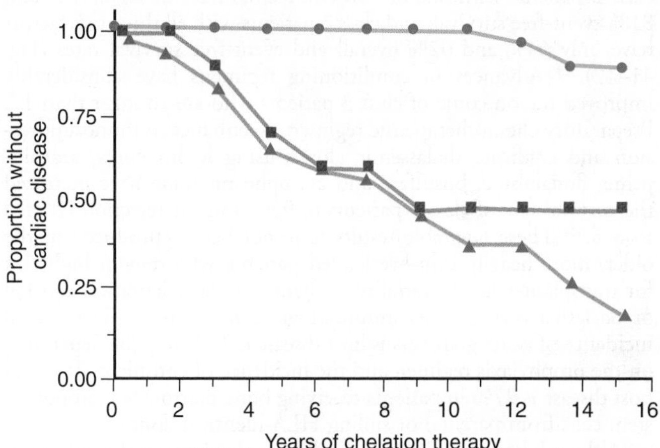

Figure 41–11 Survival without cardiac disease in patients with thalassemia major treated with deferoxamine according to the proportion of serum ferritin measurements greater than 2500 ng/mL. The *circles* show cardiac disease-free survival among patients in whom less than 33% of ferritin measurements exceeded 2500 ng/mL; *squares* show survival among patients in whom 33% to 67% of ferritin measurements exceeded 2500 ng/mL; and *triangles* show survival among patients in whom more than 67% of ferritin measurements exceeded 2500 ng/mL. *(Adapted from Olivieri NF, Nathan DG, MacMillan JH, et al: Survival in medically treated patients with homozygous beta-thalassemia. N Engl J Med 331:574, 1994.)*

Survival in Patients with Thalassemia Major

Improved transfusion therapy and the consistent use of iron chelation therapy have extended the life span of patients with thalassemia major.[61,153,155,321] In a multicenter study of 1079 patients in Italy, the probability of survival to age 20 was 96% for patients born between 1975 and 1979, the time at which chelation therapy became a regular part of the overall management of thalassemia major (Table 41–2).[153] In contrast, the probabilities of survival at 20 years of age were only 61% and 69% for those born in the periods of 1960 through 1964 and 1965 through 1969, respectively. Other investigators have shown that survival or prevention of life-threatening complications is strongly related to good chelation therapy, assessed either by compliance or by control of iron stores (Fig. 41–11).[119,147,155] The importance of good compliance with chelation therapy is further demonstrated by data from the United Kingdom showing that the probability of survival for the 1975 through 1984 birth cohort is to date not substantially different than the probability of survival for the 1965 through 1974 birth cohort.[321] The researchers attribute this poorer than expected survival rate, despite the availability of deferoxamine, to a lack of adherence to the recommended schedule of treatment with this chelator.

Hematopoietic Stem Cell Transplantation

The first transplantation of allogeneic hematopoietic stem cells derived from the bone marrow of an HLA-identical sibling donor was reported in 1982.[322] There is now extensive experience with transplantation, with well over 1000 patients having undergone transplantation. The pioneering work of Lucarelli's group in Pesaro, Italy, has allowed for the prognostic classification of patients under the age of 17 years who receive an HLA-identical sibling donor with a preparative regimen including busulfan, cyclophosphamide, and cyclosporine. This risk classification is based on hepatomegaly, the degree of portal fibrosis, and the regularity of prior iron chelation therapy.[323] In class 1 without adverse factors, overall survival rate is 95% and the event-free survival rate (without thalassemia) is 90%; class 2 patients with one or two risk factors have 85% survival and 81% event-free survival; and class 3 patients with all three risk factors have only 64% and 62% overall and event-free survival rates (Fig. 41–12).[323] Advances in conditioning regimens have considerably improved the outcome of class 3 patients who are younger than 17. Preparatory chemotherapeutic regimens to enhance immunosuppression and eradicate thalassemic clones using hydroxyurea, azathioprine, fludarabine, busulfan, and cyclophosphamide have increased the survival rate of class 3 patients to 93% and the rejection rate fell to 8%.[324] These favorable results have not been reproduced in the older, more heavily iron-overloaded patients who remain high risk for transplant-related mortality.[325] Stem cell transplantation can fail or be lethal owing to its immunologic complications. The overall incidence of acute graft versus host disease is 17% to 32% depending on the prophylaxis regimen and the incidence of chronic graft versus host disease is 27% in patients receiving bone marrow hematopoietic stem cells from parental or sibling HLA-identical donor.[326]

Although hematopoietic stem cell transplantation is the only curative therapy available, its use has been limited by cost and the rarity of HLA-identical related donors.

Building on the success of bone marrow transplantation for patients with thalassemia major using HLA-identical related donors, investigators have explored alternative strategies to increase the safety and availability of transplantation. In pediatric patients, transplantation of stem cells from umbilical cord blood has been associated with a reduced risk of graft-versus-host disease compared with bone marrow transplantation.[327,328] Stem cells derived from sibling umbilical cord collections have increased in part the safety and availability of HLA-identical related donor transplantation. The probabilities of acute and chronic graft versus host disease are decreased to 11% and 6%, respectively, in patients who receive allogeneic related cord blood transplantation.[327] However, despite the 100% overall probability of survival, disease-free survival was only 79%.[328]

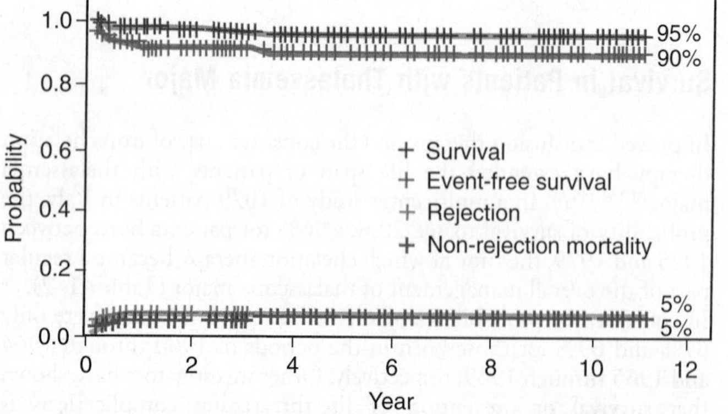

Figure 41–12 Kaplan–Meier probabilities of survival, event-free survival, rejection, and nonrejection mortality for 121 class 1 thalassemic patients younger than 17 years, receiving bone marrow transplants from HLA-identical donors after preparation with busulfan (14 mg/kg), cyclophosphamide (200 mg/kg), and cyclosporine alone, from January 2, 1986, through April 10, 1997, and calculated on May 15, 1997. *(Adapted from Lucarelli G, Galimberti M, Giardini C, et al: Bone marrow transplantation in thalassemia. Ann N Y Acad Sci 850:270, 1998.)*

Reports of graft rejection and mixed chimerism using cord stem cells have occurred as well as a high rate of nonengraftment with secondary rejection at a median follow-up of 49 months.[328] The size of the cord blood collection and small number of cord stem cells transplanted relative to the number required to allow engraftment, sustain hematopoiesis, and prevent graft rejections are most likely responsible for failures. Rare case reports describe successful outcome with nonrelated cord blood transplantation.

Successful use of cord blood transplantation has led to the development of the Sibling Cord Blood Donor Program in the United States and 1617 cord blood collections have been processed for families with thalassemia. Some patients have received cord blood transplantation either alone or in combination with bone marrow or peripheral progenitor cells.[329] In addition, bone marrow donor registries have also developed worldwide to identify HLA-compatible unrelated donors with more that 10 million volunteers registered.

In an effort to increase the pool of potential recipients of stem cell transplantation for thalassemia, investigators have also explored the use of matched unrelated donor bone marrow transplantation. Extended haplotype and family segregation studies may identify suitable unrelated donors using HLA closely matched unrelated donor transplantation in thalassemia using high resolution molecular HLA typing. LaNasa reported 79% disease free and 66% event free survival, but 19% died of transplant related complications, 41% developed grade II–IV acute graft versus host disease and 25% had chronic graft versus host disease.[330] Most of the deaths occurred in patients with heavy iron overload or hepatic complications. The results suggested that engraftment and less graft versus host disease occurred when the recipient and donor were identical for one or two extended haplotypes.[330] Other reports also using unrelated hematopoietic stem cells selected according to stringent criteria of compatibility and using high-resolution molecular typing have indicated that unrelated donor transplantation may offer results comparable to those obtained with HLA-identical family donors for patients with limited iron overload.[331,332] Otherwise, the overall disease-free survival rate is only 60%, with a significant risk of chronic graft versus host disease. The results obtained with cord blood stem cell transplantation are encouraging but too little experience exists for definitive conclusions.[333]

Alternative unrelated matched or mismatched related donor transplantation is associated with greater risk of immune complications. The only well-established curative therapy is allogeneic stem cell transplantation from a matched related donor. Transplantation is an important consideration in management for the young thalassemia patient who has yet to accumulate excessive iron or those who have successfully controlled iron stores with chelation and who have an HLA-identical matched related donor.

The options of cord blood stem cell collection and cord blood or bone marrow transplantation discussions with families of the newly diagnosed are warranted as is a discussion of the long-term outcomes.

After a successful stem cell transplantation, some patients remain iron overloaded and require phlebotomy to prevent the risks of progressive hepatic fibrosis; other previously affected patients with hepatitis C require antiviral treatment[160,334] that may improve hepatic fibrosis and cirrhosis.[335]

Posttransplantation, some patients develop a state of mixed chimerism that may persist 10% to 30% of patients with a predominance of host cells in the marrow even though transfusion dependence may have dissipated.[336] However, 30% of patients with early mixed chimerism subsequently reject their graft.[337] Those patients with mixed chimerism and falling hemoglobin who require supportive transfusion may successfully undergo a second transplant with nonmyeloablative conditioning to restore normal hemoglobin levels.[338]

Subsequent investigations to evaluate the effect of nonmyeloablative conditioning regimens as a primary approach to transplantation with the objective of causing a chimeric outcome have been attempted and are of questionable benefit.[331,339,340]

Allogeneic hematopoietic stem cell transplantation from a partially HLA-matched relative has also been investigated, with much less encouraging results. Gaziev has reported early or late graft-versus-host and graft failure in 55% of partial HLA familial matched without significant correlation between the degree of antigen disparities and graft failure. Graft-versus-host disease was a major factor contributing to death (50%) followed by infection (30%). The probability of overall survival and transfusion dependence were 65% and 21%, respectively, with a median follow-up at 2.5 years for surviving patients.[325]

In view of the available evidence, stem cell transplantation from a partially HLA-matched relative is not routinely advisable although it may be considered in extreme situations where transfusion support is impossible or life threatening when a patient is completely noncompliant with any type of iron chelation therapy.

The excellent results of bone marrow transplantation in young patients with thalassemia who have yet to accumulate excessive iron or who have successfully controlled iron stores have made transplantation an important consideration in their management. The option of bone marrow or umbilical cord blood transplantation should be discussed with families of newly diagnosed patients with thalassemia major and should be compared with long-term transfusion and chelation therapy. Both approaches should be addressed in terms of currently identified risks and benefits, the likelihood of future improvements, and the potential for new treatments such as gene therapy. In some centers, tissue typing of immediate family members is undertaken routinely, whereas in others this evaluation is performed only if the family wishes to consider transplantation as a treatment option. On the basis of the positive results with umbilical cord blood transplantation, parents of children with thalassemia should be encouraged to collect and store cord blood with future pregnancies.[329] The use of preimplantation diagnosis to identify an HLA-identical embryo unaffected with the sibling's blood disorder poses significant ethical dilemmas but has been used to create suitable donors for cord blood or bone marrow transplantation in cases of other hematologic diseases.[341–345] A related and also controversial approach is the use of both fetal and family HLA typing in pregnancies at risk of homozygous thalassemia to determine whether an HLA-identical sibling is available as a potential bone marrow donor if the fetus is affected and carried to term.[346,347]

The rate of success for bone marrow transplantation in children with more significant iron overload, in adults, and in patients without an HLA-identical sibling or parent suggests caution in the use of this approach. Transplantation has been recommended for such patients if they show progressive deterioration with conventional transfusion and chelation therapy. The availability of new chelating agents may significantly affect this balance, as may improvements in transplantation.

Some patients with thalassemia develop a state of mixed chimerism after transplantation. Approximately one-third of patients with early mixed chimerism subsequently reject their graft.[337] However, mixed chimerism may persist in 10% to 30% of patients, and the dependence on transfusion therapy often disappears despite a predominance of host cells in the bone marrow.[336] For patients with falling hemoglobin levels and renewed need for transfusion, a second transplant with nonmyeloablative conditioning may restore normal hemoglobin levels.[338] The clinical outcomes in patients with mixed chimerism have prompted the ongoing investigation of nonmyeloablative conditioning as the primary approach to transplantation for thalassemia.

Long-term complications of stem cell transplantation have also been reported, including gonadal dysfunction and fertility as well as growth failure and other endocrinopathies.[348,349]

In conclusion, hematopoietic stem cell transplantation with the use of matched related or unrelated donors is an alternative to standard transfusion and chelation therapy and generally results in excellent outcomes for low-risk patients. However, there are small risks of serious complications including death, graft failure or rejection, graft-versus-host disease as well as growth failure, infertility, and other endocrinopathies. Stem cell transplantion should be considered for class 1 and 2 children who have suitable donors. Unrelated HLA-matched donors, although an acceptable source of allogeneic stem cell for other conditions, are not yet considered suitable for children with thalassemia because of the relatively long-term survival associated with conventional therapy. Owing to the considerable risks and experiences of transplantation as well as the prospect of two or three decades of life with conventional management, discussions with the families of children who are potential candidates for transplant should be thorough.

Transplantation for those class 3 older patients and adults fare less well[350–352] and should be considered only for those who have a suitable donor or deteriorate with conventional treatment.[59]

Experimental Therapies

Enhancement of β and γ Gene Expression

Much recent effort has focused on stimulation of γ-globin gene expression or replacement of defective β-globin genes. Enhanced γ-globin gene expression would ameliorate the unbalanced globin chain synthesis and replace the missing adult hemoglobin with fetal hemoglobin. Normal β-globin genes, if introduced into stem cells in such a way as to allow them to function normally, would directly correct the β-globin chain deficit.

Active γ-globin genes are hypomethylated in utero but are methylated and inactive after birth. Hypomethylation of the γ-globin genes can be induced by the drug 5-azacytidine; indeed, short-term administration of this drug produced the predicted effect in vivo.[353–355] Despite much subsequent experimental work, it remains unclear whether the effect was due to direct stimulation of fetal genes by demethylation or to recruitment and accelerated differentiation of primitive burst-forming unit–erythroid (BFU-E) progenitor cells, which have greater potential to produce Hb F.[356–358] Hydroxyurea has an effect on BFU-E similar to that of 5-azacytidine and is a safer drug for long-term use.[357,359] Short-term as well as longer trials with hydroxyurea have been reported in a number of patients with thalassemia.[360–367] Hb F levels frequently increase without a proportionate increase in total hemoglobin level. A small improvement in total hemoglobin level occurs in some patients with thalassemia intermedia but usually does not exceed 1 to 2 g/dL.[364,365] Some patients report improvement in their overall sense of well-being even in the absence of an improvement in the anemia.[364] This may be a result of suppression of abnormal erythropoiesis, an effect that may also explain the value of hydroxyurea in the treatment of extramedullary hematopoietic masses (see later).[368] Although one patient with thalassemia major had sufficient improvement in his hemoglobin level to end his dependency on regular transfusions,[366] most transfusion-dependent patients have shown no clinical benefit. In a review of hydroxyurea therapy, Steinberg and Rodgers identified 52 patients with β-thalassemia who were treated with a variety of regimens.[367] They concluded that hydroxyurea alone had only a modest effect in thalassemia intermedia and did not look promising for thalassemia major.[369]

Recombinant erythropoietin has produced inconsistent responses in patients with thalassemia intermedia.[370–374] When the series are combined, approximately 40% of patients have an increase in hemoglobin level of 2 to 3 g/dL. Fetal hemoglobin levels are unchanged. The potentially adverse consequences of further stimulation of an already hyperactive bone marrow are uncertain. Erythropoietin has shown little benefit overall in patients with thalassemia major, although there are occasional reports of patients whose transfusion requirements were reduced or eliminated.[373,375]

Butyrate and other short-chain fatty acids have been demonstrated to augment Hb F production in various animal model systems as well as in humans.[376–378] These compounds are believed to act by altering chromatin configuration, perhaps due to inhibition of histone deacetylatase.[379–383] Short-term treatment with intravenous infusions of arginine butyrate in a limited number of patients resulted in increased levels of γ-globin chain production that were quite striking in some cases and resulted in a marked increase in γ/α-globin chain synthetic ratios.[379] One patient who was homozygous for Hb Lepore and could not be transfused because of alloimmunization was treated on a compassionate basis for a longer period of time, with a resulting rise in the total hemoglobin level (virtually all Hb F) from less than 5.0 g/dL to approximately 10.0 g/dL over approximately 60 days and healing of a leg ulcer.[379,384] In a subsequent longer-term trial, five patients with various other forms of severe β-thalassemia did not have a sustained hematologic response.[385] In yet another trial, administration of arginine butyrate intravenously in pulsed fashion to patients with sickle cell anemia and thalassemia resulted in favorable hematologic responses, raising the possibility of hematologic toxicity and suboptimal responses with continuous infusions of the drug.[386] Orally absorbable butyric acid compounds including sodium phenylbutyrate and isobutyramide also have been reported to result in an increase in F-cell and γ-globin chain production, but the effect was not as sustained or as quantitatively comparable to that originally obtained with intravenous arginine butyrate.[359,368,387–445] Total hemoglobin levels of patients with thalassemia intermedia showed little or no change,[444] although a study of isobutyramide in cases of thalassemia major found a reduction in transfusion requirements in two of eight patients.[445] No severe toxic side effects were observed in these relatively short-term trials in humans, but the infusion of high doses of butyrate into baboons did result in significant neurologic toxic effects.[446] Further studies will be required to assess the long-term safety and efficacy of therapy with butyrate.

Various combinations of hydroxyurea, butyrate, and erythropoietin have been used to try to achieve hematologic benefits that cannot be achieved with a single agent.[379–381,447] The addition of hydroxyurea to therapy with sodium phenylbutyrate led to a further increase in hemoglobin level in a patient with homozygous Lepore.[448] However, the combination of sodium phenylbutyrate and hydroxyurea was no better than hydroxyurea alone in other patients with thalassemia intermedia.[365] Combined therapy with hydroxyurea and erythropoietin produced marginally higher hemoglobin levels than either drug alone in only two of seven patients with thalassemia intermedia.[371] A more dramatic rise in hemoglobin level occurred in a patient with thalassemia major, but the relative contributions of pharmacologic therapy and splenectomy are unclear.[449]

Decitabine has been shown to result in a considerable sustained increase of Hb F and total hemoglobin in patients with sickle cell disease with the low likelihood of neutropenia and may have a similar effect in thalassemia but its therapeutic efficacy remains to be proven.[450,451]

Although the pharmacologic enhancement of fetal hemoglobin production remains an attractive strategy in the management of thalassemia, the results to date strongly suggest the need for new agents or new combinations of agents. At present, the primary clinical application of this approach is in the management of the severely affected patient who is unable to be transfused because of multiple alloantibodies or because of autoantibodies. This approach might also be used for patients with thalassemia intermedia who develop a need for frequent transfusions. However, studies suggest that the current approaches to fetal hemoglobin enhancement will usually be unsuccessful in either of these situations.

β-Globin Gene Therapy

Cure of thalassemia by genetic transfer of the normal β-globin gene into the pluripotent hematopoietic stem cell awaits further advances in molecular biology but is a goal of the foreseeable future.[396] β-Globin gene transfer and expression has been accomplished in thalassemia murine models, which have demonstrated that retroviral vectors are capable of transferring the human β-globin gene sequences and its promotor regions into murine stem cells[400,452] and into long-term repopulating hematopoietic cells of primates and humans.[453,454] Studies of a safe and efficient specific targeting vectors in humans are ongoing.[455] Techniques for obtaining long-term expression of human globin genes after transfer into murine hematopoietic stem cells have been developed.[394,395] Thus, there has been remarkable success in the use of globin gene transfer for "therapy" of murine models of β-thalassemia and sickle cell anemia.[396–401] However, clinical trials have suffered from problems of vector instability, low viral titers and variable expression of globin genes.[456] These formidable problems must be solved before it becomes routinely possible to transfer and effectively express globin genes in human hematopoietic stem cells, ensure their safe and active expression at effective levels, and preserve normal growth, differentiation, and proliferation of the genetically transformed stem cell. Nevertheless, protocols have been developed to carry out gene transfer experiments in humans and it is likely that there will be attempts to do so in the not-too-distant future.

Thalassemia Intermedia

Approximately 10% of patients with homozygous β-thalassemia exhibit a phenotype characterized by intermediate hematologic severity.[1–4] The balance of globin chain synthesis is better than in typical thalassemia major because of a less severe defect in β-globin chain synthesis, a decrease in α-globin chain synthesis as well as β-globin chain synthesis, or an increase in γ-globin chain synthesis. For example, homozygous β-thalassemia in African Americans, Portuguese, and other populations may be relatively mild, at least for the first two decades of life.[402,403] Homozygotes or mixed heterozygotes for forms of β-thalassemia associated with normal Hb A_2 and normal Hb F (silent carrier state) also tend to have mild to moderate disease.[404,405] Certain patients have a milder clinical phenotype because they have coinherited a form of α-thalassemia,[13–15] or because they carry one (or two) β-thalassemia chromosome(s) with a greater than usual potential for high levels of γ-globin gene expression.

The ability to maintain a hemoglobin level compatible with comfortable survival in the absence of regular transfusions is the generally accepted criterion for the diagnosis of thalassemia intermedia. In other words, distinguishing between thalassemia major and thalassemia intermedia, which in turn is the distinction between initiating a regular transfusion program or not, requires consideration of the hemoglobin level and the quality of life. These two parameters do not have a predictable relationship. Patients with thalassemia and hemoglobin levels of 7 g/dL may be relatively symptom-free, whereas patients with hemoglobin levels of 9 g/dL may have numerous problems related to ineffective erythropoiesis. Thus, the assessment of the patient rather than the hemoglobin level alone is essential in deciding who does not require regular transfusions and therefore, by definition, has thalassemia intermedia. Some nontransfused patients have normal growth and sexual development, few medical problems, and normal or near-normal survival rates. However, others develop disfiguring facial changes, markedly delayed growth and sexual maturation, heart failure, severe osteoporosis, repeated fractures, arthritis, and massive splenomegaly. Calling the condition of this latter group thalassemia intermedia implies a milder disease than thalassemia major but, in fact, the patients' quality of life does not compare favorably with the quality of life of patients with thalassemia major. Nonetheless, many families and physicians are reluctant to initiate a chronic transfusion program because of concern about the risks of long-term transfusion therapy and the inevitable need for iron chelation therapy. If the decision is made to manage the patient initially without regular transfusions, regular reassessments of the patient's clinical condition, including appearance, growth, and development, and bone expansion are crucial.[406] Short-term transfusion therapy may be useful during pregnancy or in the management of cardiac and other serious complications. The need for regular transfusions often develops in adults with thalassemia intermedia because of a further decline in the hemoglobin level or a growing intolerance of the anemia.

Even in the absence of regular transfusions, many patients develop progressive iron overload because of increased absorption of dietary iron induced by ineffective erythropoiesis and, in many cases, the intermittent administration of red blood cell transfusions. By the third or fourth decade, the total iron burden may attain the levels seen in transfusion-dependent patients.[407] Ferritin levels may underestimate the degree of tissue iron loading in thalassemia intermedia, and assessment of liver iron concentration is more helpful in determining the need for chelation therapy. Deferoxamine as well as the orally active iron chelator deferiprone (L1) has proved effective in thalassemia intermedia.[408,409]

Splenectomy raises the hemoglobin level by 1 to 3 g/dL in many patients with thalassemia intermedia.[410,411] Removal of the spleen should receive careful consideration as a potential alternative to beginning transfusion therapy. As noted earlier, for patients who undergo splenectomy while on a chronic transfusion program, a period of careful monitoring of the hemoglobin level after surgery may occasionally identify individuals who are no longer transfusion-dependent and who can therefore be reclassified as having thalassemia intermedia.

Thromboembolic events represent a major complication of thalassemia intermedia, occurring in 10% to 34% of patients.[302,412] These events include stroke, pulmonary embolism, portal vein thrombosis, and deep vein thrombosis of the legs. A hypercoagulable state may also contribute to the pulmonary hypertension that commonly occurs in patients with thalassemia intermedia and is the primary cause of congestive heart failure.[413] Splenectomy is a risk factor for thromboembolic events in patients with thalassemia intermedia, resulting in thrombocytosis and allowing the prolonged circulation of damaged red blood cells that generate increased amounts of thrombin.[302] Some investigators consider the risk of thromboembolic events after splenectomy for thalassemia intermedia to be sufficiently high to warrant short-term anticoagulation in the perioperative period and during pregnancy.[302] Oral contraceptives should be used with extreme caution, if at all.

Extension of hematopoietic tissue beyond the confines of the bones occurs in patients with thalassemia intermedia as a result of the intense erythropoiesis. This complication occurs less frequently in patients with thalassemia major because of the partial suppression of erythropoiesis by regular transfusions. Masses of extramedullary hematopoietic tissue develop in the spinal epidural space, thorax, cranium, pelvis, and elsewhere.[368,414–424] These masses may be detected as incidental findings on imaging studies of the chest or abdomen.[415–421] In other instances, the masses produce symptoms by compressing neighboring structures. For example, patients with extramedullary hematopoietic masses may develop paraplegia from spinal cord compression or loss of visual acuity or visual fields caused by optic nerve compression.[414,417,423,424] Additional clinical presentations of hematopoietic masses include pleural effusions and upper airway obstruction.[419,420,422] Initiation of regular transfusions for patients with thalassemia intermedia or intensification of the ongoing transfusion program for patients with thalassemia major reduces the size of extramedullary hematopoietic masses and helps to prevent recurrences. Therapy with hydroxyurea has also been associated with shrinkage of hematopoietic masses.[368] Low-dose radiation therapy provides more immediate relief and may be particularly useful for acute neurologic complications.[425]

Reconstruction of the maxilla may be needed for some patients with thalassemia intermedia to provide cosmetic improvement of facial asymmetry and malocclusion.[426] Gallstones regularly occur by the second decade of life.[427] Leg ulcers often occur in late adolescence or afterward and may require red blood cell transfusions as well as local measures for healing. Because of the marked marrow hyperplasia, supplementation with folic acid is necessary to prevent megaloblastic anemia. Aplastic crises associated with parvovirus or other infections may result in exacerbations of the anemia.

Some patients with heterozygous β-thalassemia will have a moderately severe clinical disorder, with anemia, hemolysis, and splenomegaly. Some of these patients carry a greater than normal number of α-globin genes as a result of triplication of one of the α-globin gene loci: ααα/αα.[34,335,428,429] However, most heterozygous patients with triplicated α-globin gene loci are clinically similar to those with the simple β-thalassemia trait. Most patients with severe heterozygous β-thalassemia have so-called dominant β-thalassemia, which is due to the inheritance of a gene for a β-thalassemia hemoglobinopathy associated with a structurally abnormal, unstable, β-globin chain that may form inclusion bodies.[16,17] For those heterozygotes with disease of unusual clinical severity, splenectomy may be beneficial.

β-Thalassemia Minor (Thalassemia Trait)

Inheritance of a single β-thalassemia allele usually results in a mild hypochromic microcytic anemia. The hemoglobin level averages 1 or 2 g/dL lower than that seen in normal persons of the same age and gender. Hb F levels decline more slowly than usual in the first year of life and the diagnostic elevated Hb A_2 levels are established by approximately 6 months of age.[432–434] Strong intrafamilial correlations of both Hb A_2 and mean corpuscular volume (MCV) are noted.[435] Osmotic fragility is decreased; indeed, a one-tube osmotic fragility test has been used in the past for mass screening.[433] The red blood cell count is increased or normal. The red blood cells are characteristically hypochromic (mean corpuscular hemoglobin <26 pg) and microcytic (MCV <75 fL). The smear shows varying numbers of target cells, poikilocytes, ovalocytes, and basophilic stippling (Fig. 41–13). The reticulocyte count is normal or slightly elevated. Red blood cell survival is normal, iron utilization is decreased, and slight ineffective erythropoiesis is present.[434] Most patients are asymptomatic. Many patients who have thalassemia trait are erroneously believed to have iron deficiency. Testing to distinguish these two disorders is important for genetic counseling of carriers of thalassemia trait, for the avoidance of unnecessary investigations in patients incorrectly assumed to have iron deficiency and to prevent unwarranted supplementation with iron. Although a variety of indices calculated from blood count parameters have been suggested to differentiate thalassemia from iron deficiency, each has some degree of inaccuracy; most are no better than the MCV alone.[435,436] In general, the MCV is rarely greater than 75 fL or the hematocrit less than 30 in patients with β-thalassemia trait. In cases of iron deficiency, the hematocrit level usually falls to less than 30 before the MCV falls to less than 80 fL. Free erythrocyte porphyrin levels are normal in patients with thalassemia trait but are elevated in patients with iron deficiency (see Chapter 36).[1] Specific studies for iron deficiency, such as the serum iron level and total iron-binding capacity or the serum ferritin level, help to prevent misdiagnosis.

During pregnancy, the anemia of thalassemia trait often becomes more severe, but transfusions are rarely necessary. Because iron deficiency may occur during pregnancy, iron supplementation has been advised to avoid compounding the causes of anemia.[437,438]

There may be characteristic racial differences in the hematologic severity of β-thalassemia trait. In African Americans, the condition is invariably milder, red blood cell morphologic abnormalities are less marked, and β/α synthetic ratios are higher than in whites and Asians with the trait.[439]

The diagnosis of β-thalassemia trait is established in most instances by the demonstration of altered proportions of Hb A_2. The level of Hb A_2 in β-thalassemia trait averages 5.1% (range, 3.5%–7.0%), approximately twice the normal level (1.5%–3.5%); the Hb A_2/Hb A_1 ratio is 1:20 instead of the normal 1:40. This increase is probably due to a posttranslational (assembly) phenomenon with increased opportunity for δ-globin chains to combine with α-globin chains in the face of β-globin chain deficiency. If concomitant iron deficiency anemia occurs, Hb A_2 levels may fall, sometimes into the normal range.[440]

The Hb F levels are inconsistently elevated in β-thalassemia. In approximately one-half of cases, Hb F is within the normal range (<2.0%); in the remainder, it is moderately elevated (2.1%–5.0%). However, in almost every instance, a minor population of red blood

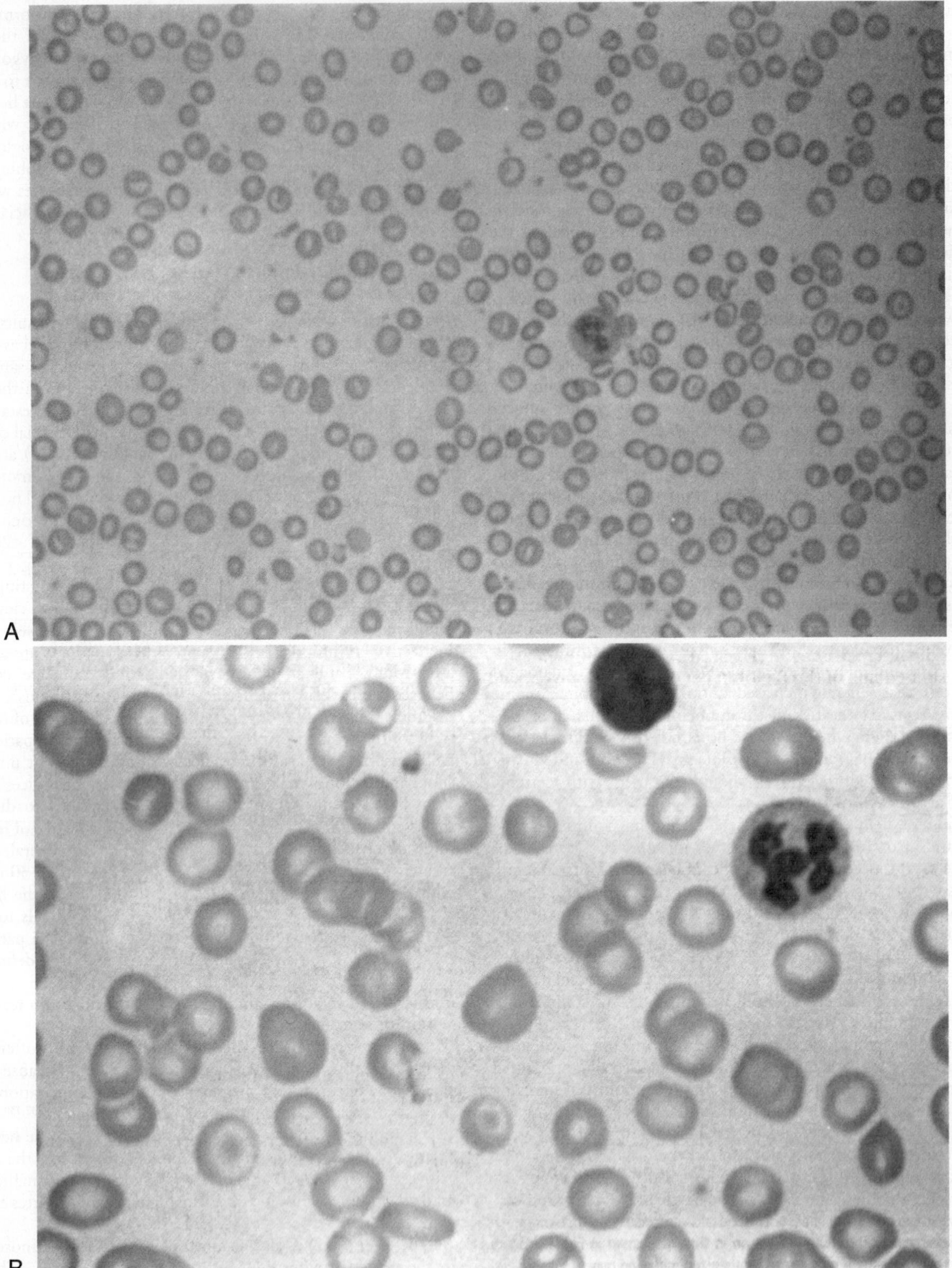

Figure 41–13 Morphology of the peripheral blood film in a case of heterozygous β-thalassemia (**A**) and a case of heterozygous α-thalassemia (**B**). Note the profound hypochromia and microcytosis and the many target cells. *(From Pearson HA, Benz EJ Jr: Thalassemia syndromes. In Miller DR, Baehner RL, McMillan CW [eds.]: Smith's Blood Diseases of Infancy and Childhood, 5th ed. St. Louis, CV Mosby, 1984, p 439.)*

cells (F cells) containing substantial amounts of Hb F can be demonstrated by the Kleihauer technique.[1] Rarely, an individual with heterozygous thalassemia, as evidenced by a reduced β/α synthetic ratio or by virtue of having a child with thalassemia intermedia or major, has normal Hb A_2, Hb F, and hemoglobin electrophoresis, with minor (quiet carrier) or no (silent carrier) hematologic changes.[405] Rare individuals have been encountered who exhibit characteristically abnormal red blood cell morphology but normal levels of Hb A_2 and Hb F.[1] Such individuals are probably carriers of γδβ-thalassemia.[1] Iron deficiency must be excluded and globin-chain synthesis or molecular studies done to establish a diagnosis with certainty.

The diagnosis of thalassemia trait assumes particular importance in women who are pregnant or considering pregnancy because of the potential for having a child with thalassemia major. The presence of a low MCV should be investigated further with levels of Hb A_2 and Hb F, as well as a hemoglobin electrophoresis to look for thalassemic variants such as Hb E and Hb Lepore (see later). If either the father or the mother is known to have thalassemia trait, the other person should be assessed using these more definitive studies rather than the MCV alone.

Prenatal Diagnosis of β-Thalassemia

Thalassemia mutations can now be routinely and reliably diagnosed by using fetal DNA obtained between the 8th and 18th weeks of gestation. The most reliable methods are based on identification of the abnormal gene by direct DNA analysis.[22,441,442] Both amniocentesis and chorionic villus sampling have been used with success. In experienced hands, the latter method is preferable because adequate amounts of DNA can be obtained safely at an earlier gestational age. New techniques have been developed for obtaining fetal DNA for prenatal diagnosis either directly from maternal plasma or by the isolation of fetal nucleated red blood cells from maternal peripheral blood.[438,444] The DNA is analyzed by a variety of polymerase chain reaction (PCR)-based or other methods for the presence of the thalassemia mutation.

The heterogeneity of thalassemia mutations complicates the approach to antenatal diagnosis. More than 175 independent mutations can cause β-thalassemia. However, a number of factors have improved the speed, efficacy, and reliability of DNA diagnosis. Extensive surveys of most populations in which these alleles are frequent have revealed that approximately 15 β-thalassemia mutations account for more than 90% of individuals afflicted worldwide. Within any given ethnic group, three to six mutations usually account for the vast majority of severe cases (see Table 41–1).[22] One can thus customize the search for mutations according to the ethnic origins of the family at risk. PCR techniques and exquisitely precise hybridization assays (allele-specific oligonucleotide hybridization), which detect single-base changes with great reliability, can now be combined to permit screening of minute DNA samples for several mutations very rapidly (Fig. 41–14). This procedure can also be done using nonradioactive oligonucleotide probes immobilized to filters, so-called reverse dot blot analysis.[445,446] Single-base mutations can also be detected by the PCR technique called amplification refractory mutation system (ARMS).[442,457] An amplification and direct sequencing of the β-globin genes (in cases in which the mutation is unknown) can also be carried out rapidly by use of PCR techniques.

Genetic counseling and antenatal diagnosis should be offered to all families at risk for severe α- or β-thalassemia. Prenatal diagnosis is one component of large-scale screening, education, and genetic counseling programs that are active in Italy, Greece, Cyprus, and other areas where the frequency of thalassemia is very high.[448] In some countries, particularly those with a high rate of consanguineous marriages, screening efforts can be refined to gain further efficiency in identifying at-risk couples.[449] Comprehensive programs of education, screening, and diagnosis have dramatically decreased the incidence of thalassemia major births in several countries (Fig. 41–15),[448,458,459] but they require a critical mass of expert professionals and laboratory back-up. Voluntary informed participation, confidentiality of results, and meaningful counseling must be ensured.

α-THALASSEMIA SYNDROMES

The α-thalassemias are more difficult to diagnose, because characteristic elevations in Hb A_2 or Hb F, seen in many cases of β-thalassemia, do not occur. However, the gene deletions responsible for the most common varieties are readily detectable by molecular biology methods.

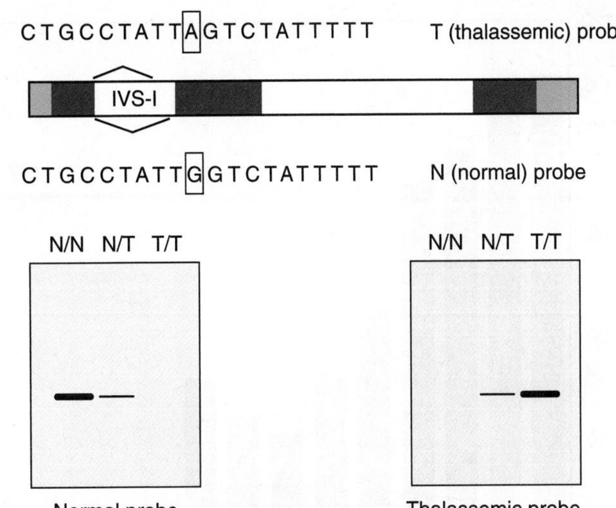

Figure 41–14 Example of the use of allele-specific oligonucleotide probes for diagnosis of a common form of β-thalassemia. The mutation shown is that discussed in Figure 35–2 and the text. Two oligonucleotide probes are synthesized, differing only at the position of the mutation. When hybridized under sufficiently stringent conditions, each probe will anneal only to the gene that is perfectly complementary by Watson–Crick base-pairing. Thus, a homozygous normal fetal DNA sample (N/N) will anneal only to the normal probe, homozygous β-thalassemic DNA (T/T) only to the thalassemic probe, and DNA from a heterozygote (N/T) to both probes, but with a reduced intensity to each. *(Adapted from High KA, Benz EJ Jr: The ABCs of molecular genetics: A haematologist's introduction. In Hoffbrand AV [ed.]: Recent Advances in Haematology. New York, Churchill Livingston, 1985, p 25.)*

Molecular Pathology and Pathophysiology

The four classic α-thalassemia syndromes are α^+-thalassemia trait, in which one of the four α-globin genes fails to function; α^o-thalassemia trait, with two dysfunctional genes; Hb H disease, with three affected genes; and hydrops fetalis with Hb Bart, in which all four genes are defective. In the older literature, α^o- and α^{++}-thalassemia are referred to as α-thalassemia-1 and α-thalassemia-2, respectively. These syndromes are usually caused by deletion of one, two, three, or all four of the α-globin genes, respectively (Fig. 41–16). Nondeletional forms of α-thalassemia, which account for 15% to 20% of patients, arise from mutations similar to those described for β-thalassemia.[460,461] Figure 41–17 illustrates the different α-thalassemia mutations and phenotypes. Structurally abnormal hemoglobins have also been associated with α-thalassemia. The Quong Sze α-globin chain ($\alpha^{125Leu\rightarrow Pro}$) is exceedingly labile and is destroyed so rapidly after its synthesis that no hemoglobin tetramers containing the mutant α chain can be formed.[462]

α^+-Thalassemia trait is an asymptomatic silent carrier state that is commonly associated with the deletion of a single α-globin gene. Offspring of an individual with α^+-thalassemia whose spouse has α^o-thalassemia trait can inherit a form of α-thalassemia more severe than either of these, namely Hb H disease.

α^o-Thalassemia trait results from deletion or nonfunction of two α-globin alleles. In Asian and Mediterranean populations, a deletion that removes both loci from the same chromosome (*cis* deletion) is common[460,461]; homozygosity for α^+-thalassemia (*trans* deletion) is also seen. In African Americans, both α-globin genes are only rarely deleted in *cis*, whereas homozygosity for α^+-thalassemia (*trans* deletion) is quite common.[463] Both genotypes produce asymptomatic hypochromia and microcytosis. Hb H disease usually results from coinheritance of the *cis* α^o-thalassemia deletion and α^+-thalassemia trait. α-Globin chain production is only 25% to 30% of normal; excess γ-globin chains accumulate during gestation and excess β-globin chains during adult life (Fig. 41–17). The unpaired β-globin

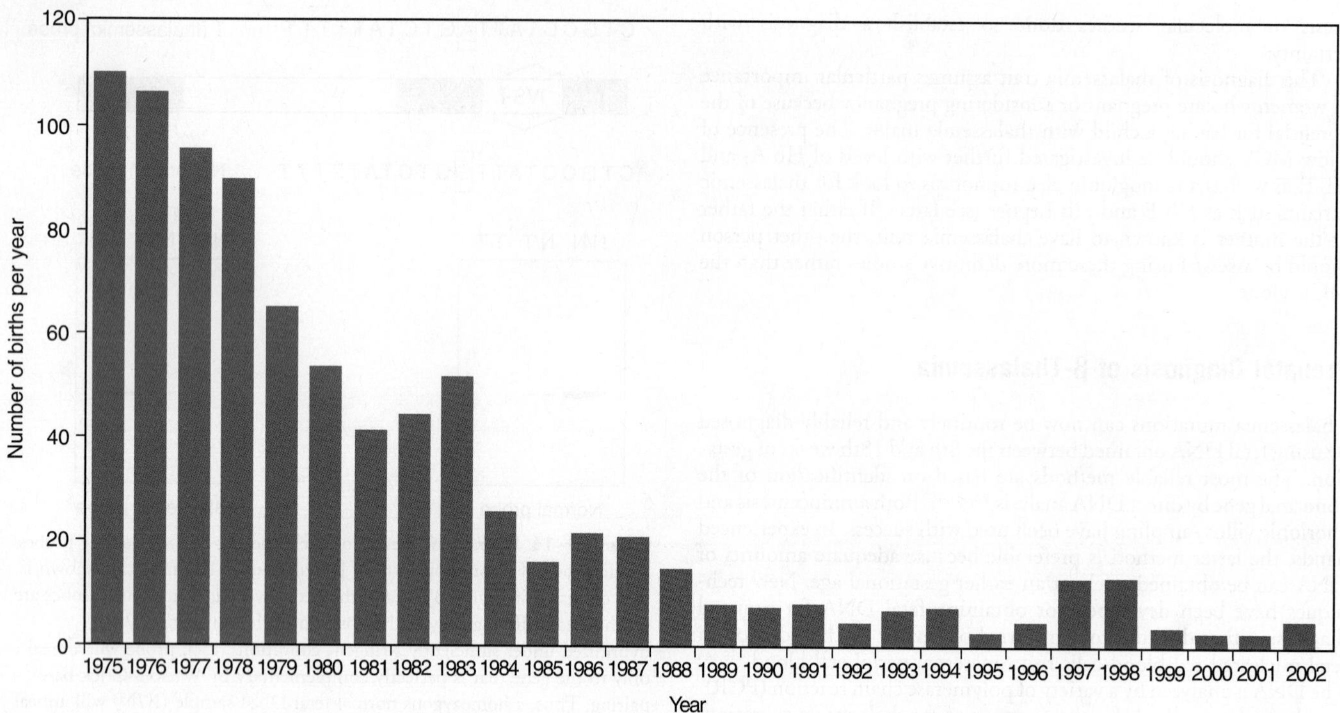

Figure 41–15 Declining rate of birth of infants homozygous for β-thalassemia in Sardinia since 1975, when a comprehensive screening program began. *(Adapted from Cao A, Galanello R: Effect of consanguinity on screening for thalassemia. N Engl J Med 347:1200, 2002.)*

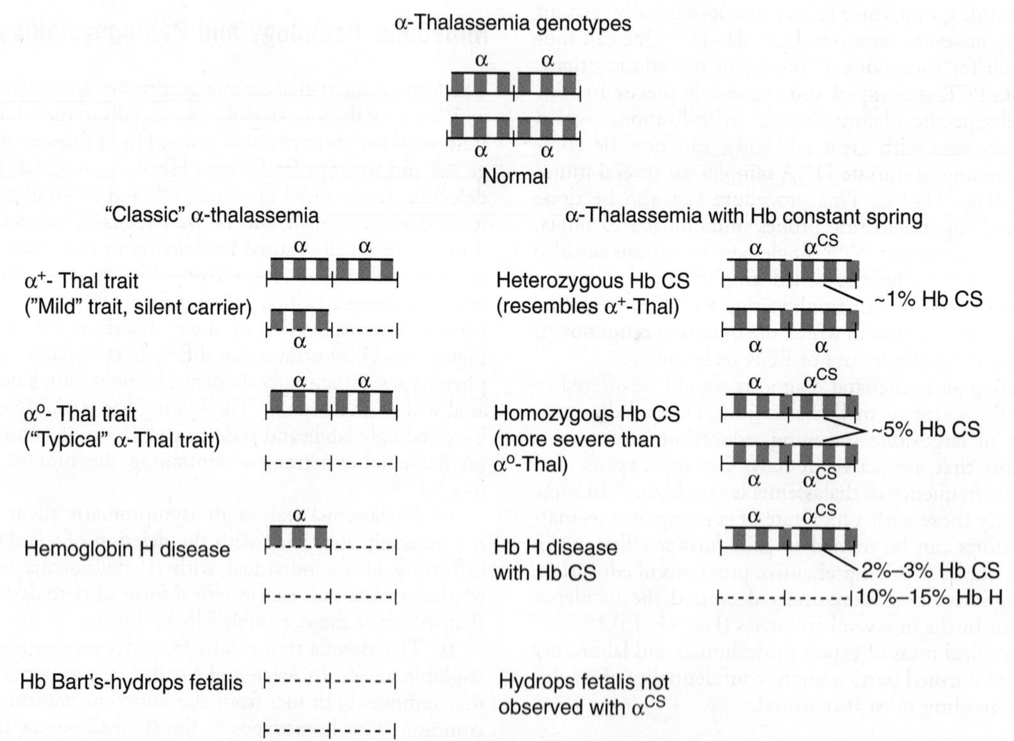

Figure 41–16 Genetic origins of the "classic" α-thalassemia syndromes due to gene deletions in the α-globin gene cluster. Hb Constant Spring (Hb CS) is an α-globin chain variant synthesized in such small amounts (1%–2% of normal) that it has the phenotypic impact of a severe nondeletion α-thalassemia allele; however, the α^{cs} allele is always linked to a functioning α-globin gene, so it has never been associated with hydrops fetalis.

A
Hydrops fetalis with Hb Bart's in fetus
α genes absent → α mRNA absent → α globin absent → No Hb F
γ genes → γ mRNA → γ_4 (Hb Bart's)
Extremely high O_2 affinity → Profound tissue hypoxia → Heart failure, Liver failure (↓albumin) → Massive edema (hydrops), Hypoxic death in utero
Mildly unstable → Hemolysis → Anemia

B
Hb H disease in adult
1 of 4 α gene loci present → ↓α mRNA → ↓α globin
β gene → β mRNA → β globin
↓Hb A ← → Excess β globin → β_4 (Hb H) → Moderately unstable
Moderate hypochromic hemolytic anemia with splenomagaly, bizarre morphology
N.B.: During fetal life, similar syndrome but with accumulation of Hb Bart's

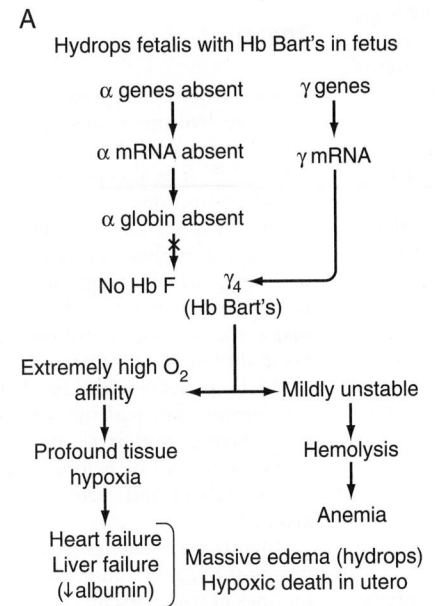

Figure 41–17 Pathophysiology of Hb H disease and hydrops fetalis with Hb Bart. *(Adapted from Benz EJ Jr: The hemoglobinopathies. In Kelly WN, DeVita VT [eds.]: Textbook of Internal Medicine. Philadelphia, JB Lippincott, 1988, p 1423.)*

chains are somewhat more soluble than the excess α-globin chains that accumulate in cases of β-thalassemia, forming recognizable β4 tetramers designated as Hb H. Hb H forms relatively few inclusions in erythroblasts; rather, it precipitates slowly within mature circulating red blood cells. Patients with Hb H disease thus have a moderately severe hemolytic anemia but relatively little ineffective erythropoiesis. Patients usually survive into adult life. These clinical observations illustrate the central role of unpaired globin chains and ineffective erythropoiesis as determinants of clinical severity.

Hydrops fetalis with Hb Bart results from the homozygous state for the α°-thalassemia *cis* deletion. The α-globin genes are totally absent; no α-globin is produced, so no physiologically useful hemoglobin accumulates beyond the embryonic stage. Free γ-globin chains accumulate, forming γ_4 tetramers called Hb Bart (see Fig. 35–13). Hb Bart has an extraordinarily high oxygen affinity, comparable with that of myoglobin. It binds oxygen delivered to the placenta but releases almost none of it to fetal tissues. Severe hypoxia occurs at the tissue level, causing profound edema (hydrops), congestive heart failure, and, in most cases, death in utero. These fatal complications do not occur in fetuses with Hb H disease because enough Hb F is made to sustain life.

α^+-Thalassemia trait is very common in black patients, having a genetic frequency of 20% to 30% in some populations. However, the *cis* α°-thalassemia deletion is rare in black patients. Thus, even though α^+-thalassemia trait and the *trans* deletion form of α°-thalassemia are very common, Hb H disease is rarely encountered, and hydrops fetalis has not yet been reported in black patients.[463,464]

Clinical Manifestations

Silent Carrier (α^+-Thalassemia Trait)

α^+-Thalassemia trait has no consistent hematologic manifestations. The red blood cells are not microcytic, and Hb A_2 and Hb F are normal. During the newborn period, small amounts (≤3%) of Hb Bart (γ_4) can be seen by electrophoresis or other techniques. This condition is most often recognized when an apparently normal individual becomes the parent of a child with Hb H disease after mating with a person with α°-thalassemia trait. The mild excess of β-globin chains is probably removed in erythroblasts by proteolysis.[465] α^+-Thalassemia is particularly common in Melanesia, as well as in Southeast Asia and in African Americans, reaching a prevalence of more than 80% in north coastal Papua New Guinea. At the molecular level, α^+-thalassemia has been found to be associated with two common gene deletions resulting from different nonhomologous crossing-over events between the two linked α-globin genes: a 3.7-kb rightward deletion ($-\alpha^{3.7}$) resulting in a fused α2α1-globin gene, and a 4.2-kb leftward deletion ($-\alpha^{4.2}$) resulting in loss of the 5′ (α2) gene.[460,461,466] The level of α-globin gene expression differs in the two conditions, as discussed in the following section.

α-Thalassemia Trait (α°-Thalassemia Trait)

Levels of Hb A_2 in the low to low normal range (1.5%–2.5%) and β/α synthetic ratios averaging 1.4 : 1 characterize α°-thalassemia trait. During the perinatal period, elevated amounts of Hb Bart are noted (3%–8%). Microcytosis is present in cord blood erythrocytes.

Studies of newborns from the archipelago of Vanuatu in the southwest Pacific and from Papua New Guinea indicate that homozygotes for the rightward $-\alpha^{3.7III}$ deletion (where only a fused α2α1-globin gene, mostly of the α2 type, remains) have lower Hb Bart levels (3.5% ± 0.8%) than those of infants homozygous for the leftward $-\alpha^{4.2}$ deletion (where only the α1-globin gene remains) (6.0% ± 1.4%). These results suggest that the 5′ α2-globin gene has a higher output than the 3′ α1-globin gene, a conclusion supported by direct measurement of α2/α1 mRNA ratios.[467,468]

Hb H is not detected in hemolysates of peripheral red blood cells, probably because of rapid proteolysis of Hb H or free β-globin chains. However, approximately 1% of erythroblasts and marrow reticulocytes have inclusions. When an α-thalassemia gene occurs in persons who are also heterozygous for β-globin chain variant hemoglobins, such as Hb S, Hb C, or Hb E, the proportion of the abnormal hemoglobin is lower than that seen in simple heterozygotes.[469] The lower level of the abnormal hemoglobin is due to posttranslational control because of higher affinity of β^A chains for a limited pool of α-globin chains,[470] coupled with proteolysis of the uncombined $\beta^{variant}$ chains.

Hb H Disease

Hb H disease is associated with a moderately severe but variable anemia resembling thalassemia intermedia, with osseous changes and splenomegaly.[471] However, the clinical phenotype may be considerably milder in some patients and severe enough to cause hydrops fetalis in others.[472,473] It occurs predominantly in Asians and occasionally in whites (Mediterraneans) but is rare in blacks. Exacerbations of anemia during febrile illnesses are common and are usually characterized by increasing fatigue and jaundice.

Because Hb H is unstable and precipitates within the circulating red blood cells, hemolysis occurs. Hb H can be demonstrated by incubation of blood with supravital oxidizing stains such as 1% brilliant cresyl blue. Multiple small inclusions form in the red blood cells (see Fig. 41–17). Electrophoresis of a freshly prepared hemolysate at alkaline or neutral pH demonstrates a fast-moving component amounting to 3% to 30% of the total hemoglobin. Concomitant iron deficiency may reduce the amount of Hb H in the patient's red blood cells.[474] A syndrome of Hb H disease associated with mental retardation, other congenital anomalies, and large deletions on chromosome 16 has been noted in several white families.[475,476]

Hydrops Fetalis With Hb Bart

Hydrops fetalis with Hb Bart occurs almost exclusively in Asians, especially Chinese, Cambodians, Thais, and Filipinos. Affected fetuses usually are born prematurely and either are stillborn or die shortly after birth.[1–4] Marked anasarca and enlargement of the liver and spleen are present. Severe anemia usually is present, with hemoglobin levels of 3 to 10 g/dL. The red blood cells are markedly microcytic and hypochromic and include target cells and large numbers of circulating nucleated red blood cells. These morphologic abnormalities and a negative Coombs test result exclude hemolytic diseases due to blood group incompatibility. Hemoglobin electrophoresis reveals predominantly Hb Bart, with a smaller amount of Hb H. A minor component identified as Hb Portland ($\zeta_2\gamma_2$) migrating in the position of Hb A is also seen. Normal Hb A and Hb F are totally absent.[477]

Hydropic infants have massive hepatosplenomegaly. Extreme extramedullary erythropoiesis occurs in response to the profound hypoxia and hemolytic anemia characteristic of this disease. The universal edema characteristic of the hydrops fetalis syndrome is a reflection of severe congestive heart failure and hypoalbuminemia in utero. This is partly a consequence of anemia, but the strikingly abnormal oxygen affinity of the tetrameric Hb Bart is probably the most important determinant of the severe tissue hypoxia. The oxygen dissociation curve of Hb Bart lacks the normal sigmoid form because of noncooperativity during oxygen loading and unloading and is markedly shifted to the left. The shift is so great that little oxygen is released under conditions of low oxygen concentration in the tissues.

Infants with this syndrome do not die in an earlier trimester of pregnancy because of the presence of Hb Portland ($\zeta_2\gamma_2$). This hemoglobin does display cooperativity in a manner similar to that of Hb F and therefore has a much more favorable oxygen dissociation pattern than that of Hb Bart. A high incidence of toxemia of pregnancy has been described in women carrying severely affected infants, providing an increased rationale for prenatal diagnosis of this condition.

Prenatal Diagnosis of α-Thalassemia

Using molecular hybridization technology, Dozy and associates detected the complete absence of α-globin genes in fetal fibroblasts obtained by amniocentesis in a pregnancy at risk of homozygous α°-thalassemia and the hydrops fetalis syndrome.[478] A quantitative PCR method provides similar information rapidly and accurately.[479] The presence of hydrops can also be detected by ultrasonography. DNA studies or globin synthesis evaluation may be used to confirm the diagnosis in utero. PCR-based assays are available for the detection of the common α-thalassemia deletions.[479–482]

Therapy

Fetuses with homozygous α°-thalassemia usually die in utero because of severe hydrops fetalis and are stillborn. However, some infants have had successful blood exchange transfusion immediately after birth.[483–487] It is also possible to salvage affected fetuses by in utero blood transfusions.[488,489] Limb and urogenital defects are present in a substantial portion of infants with homozygous α°-thalassemia who are rescued by these measures, and some infants have developmental delay or other neurologic abnormalities. Management after the perinatal period is similar to the management of patients with thalassemia major and includes transfusion and chelation therapy as well as the possibility of bone marrow transplantation.[490]

Many patients with Hb H disease do not require red blood cell transfusions. For patients with more severe disease, characterized by lower hemoglobin levels or frequent exacerbations of the anemia, splenectomy can be helpful. Oxidant drugs can accelerate precipitation of Hb H and exacerbate hemolysis; they should therefore be avoided.

Infants with heterozygous α°-thalassemia trait lose their Hb Bart during the first few months of life and are left with the hematologic findings of α-thalassemia trait, a mild hypochromic microcytosis that persists throughout life.[1] The degree of morphologic abnormality varies greatly among different individuals. That α-thalassemia can be easily diagnosed by hemoglobin electrophoresis at birth gives some impetus to cord blood screening studies. Confusion between heterozygous α°-thalassemia trait and iron deficiency may lead to unnecessary evaluations for possible blood loss or unnecessary supplementation with iron unless the overlap in hematologic findings is recognized and more specific diagnostic studies are performed.

De Novo and Acquired Forms of α-Thalassemia

Two distinct α-thalassemia syndromes have been described that are due to acquired or de novo mutations: (a) α-thalassemia associated with mental retardation and (b) Hb H disease associated with myelodysplastic syndromes.

α-Thalassemia Associated With Mental Retardation

α-Thalassemia or Hb H disease can occur as a de novo abnormality in a rare disorder called the α-thalassemia with mental retardation syndrome (or ATR).[475–476] In this disorder, affected patients have mental retardation and a number of other developmental abnormalities in association with α-thalassemia trait or Hb H disease that is inherited in a nontraditional manner. Two distinct types of the ATR syndrome have been identified. In some cases, there is the de novo appearance of large (2000 kb or so) deletions involving the entire α-globin gene cluster and adjacent DNA at the tip of chromosome 16, the so-called ATR-16 syndrome. In some of these patients, the deletion produces detectable cytogenetic abnormalities of chromosome 16, indicating that a very large segment of the chromosome is deleted, sometimes because of unbalanced chromosomal translocations involving the telomeres of the affected chromosomes. In some cases, one parent is heterozygous for α⁺-thalassemia by various criteria and the other parent is completely normal; in such cases, the child has Hb H disease (—/–α). In other cases, both parents are normal and the affected child has the hematologic phenotype of heterozygous α°-thalassemia (—/αα) without Hb H disease. In this form of ATR, the clinical findings, such as the degree of mental retardation and associated congenital abnormalities, are variable.

The second type of ATR syndrome is not associated with detectable deletions of the α-globin gene complex. The molecular basis of the disorder consists of mutations of a gene on the X chromosome and the condition has been called the ATR-X syndrome.[491] In contrast to patients with the ATR-16 syndrome who have a varied phenotype of developmental abnormalities, patients with the ATR-X syndrome have a more uniform or consistent phenotype, in particular, severe mental retardation (with IQs of 50–70) and a characteristic dysmorphic facial appearance.[476]

The affected gene in this syndrome encodes a *trans*-acting factor, called ATRX, that is thought to influence the expression of the α-globin genes as well as that of other genes.[492,493] The structure of this large (280 kd) DNA-binding protein is complex and contains two major functional domains: an N-terminal cysteine-rich zinc finger–containing domain, called the ADD domain, that has structural features similar to those of DNA methyl transferases; and a C-terminal helicase/ATPase domain. The majority of the mutations associated with the ATR-X syndrome are located in the ADD domain or the helicase domain. The ATRX protein is widely expressed in many different tissues and its intracellular localization is within three different nuclear subcompartments: heterochromatin, ribosomal DNA arrays, and PML bodies. It has been shown to interact with other proteins such as the heterochromatin-associated protein HP1 and Daxx, one of the proteins localized in PML bodies. The prevailing opinion is that the ATRX protein is part of a large chromatin-remodeling complex of the SWI2/SNF2 family. It also has ATPase activity and has translocase activity, that is, it can move along DNA as a "molecular motor." The precise mechanism(s) by which ATRX influences the expression of α-globin (and other) genes remains unknown.

Acquired Hb H Disease Associated With Myelodysplastic Syndrome or ATMDS

Hb H disease has occasionally been observed to develop during the course of different types of myelodysplastic syndrome (MDS) and more rarely in patients with other hematologic malignancies.[494] The disorder usually affects elderly males over the age of 60. The degree of imbalance of globin chain synthesis and of α-globin mRNA deficiency in erythroid cells of affected patients is greater than that observed in the hereditary type of Hb H disease. It is conceivable that erythroid cells of the abnormal clone synthesize no α-globin chains at all and that the expression of all four α-globin genes is suppressed or silenced,[495] but this phenomenon is difficult to document in total blood as long as some normal erythroid cells are being produced.

Until recently, the molecular basis of this fascinating disorder remained unknown. Cytogenetic, gene mapping, gene sequencing, and gene or chromosome transfer studies failed to detect any deletion or mutation in the α-globin gene cluster or functional abnormality of α-globin gene of affected patients. The results of all of these prior studies suggested that the defect responsible for this disorder probably involved the abnormal expression or function of a *trans*-acting factor capable of influencing α-globin gene expression and, indeed, such a factor was recently identified. The discovery of the factor responsible for Hb H disease in MDS results from cDNA microarray analysis of RNA isolated from granulocytes of an affected patient. One of the genes that was found to be markedly underexpressed, when compared to results obtained with RNA of normal granulocytes, was the ATRX gene,[496] the same gene that is mutated in the α-thalassemia with mental retardation syndrome of the ATR-X type. Sequence analysis of the ATRX gene in the DNA of blood cells of affected individuals has identified a number of different mutations. It is noteworthy that the mutations of the ATRX gene associated with acquired Hb H disease associated with MDS (ATMDS) occur in the same regions of the gene as the mutations associated with the ATR-X syndrome, that is, in the ADD or helicase domains. In fact, some of the ATRX gene mutations identified in ATMDS are identical or similar in expected functional consequences to various mutations found in the ATR-X syndrome.

The hematologic features in the syndrome are characterized by the presence on blood smear of a dimorphic red cell population, one of which is hypochromic, microcytic, hypochromic, and poikilocytic. Incubation of the blood with the supravital stain brilliant cresyl blue results in the detection of typical Hb H inclusions. Hemoglobin electrophoresis or HPLC detects the presence of Hb H, usually in greater quantities than that typically observed in inherited Hb H disease. In typical MDS, the MCV of the erythrocytes is normal or elevated, frequently higher than 100 fL. However, in ATMDS, the MCV and MCH are low: MCV usually less than 80 fL and MCH usually less than 26 pg.[494] The amount of Hb H usually remains stable, but may actually decrease during the course of the disease and no longer persists after transformation of MDS to acute leukemia. This finding suggests that the Hb H-producing clone does not have a selective survival or growth advantage.

The hematologic phenotype, as reflected by the amount of Hb H present in blood, of ATMDS is much more severe than that of the ATR-X syndrome.[492] Some of this difference in severity may be due to the nature of the ATMDS mutations, some of which are null mutations that are likely to be lethal when present in germline DNA of ATR-X embryos. However, the difference in severity is also observed in the case of mutations found in both syndromes that are identical or similar in expected functional consequences. This finding suggests that additional abnormalities in gene expression in ATMDS contribute to the severity of the deficit in α-globin gene expression observed in this syndrome. Perhaps the responsible defective cofactor(s) is one or more of the proteins that interact with the ATRX protein to produce a fully functional macromolecular complex that can act as a transcriptional cofactor or that can influence the epigenetic control of α-globin gene expression.

THALASSEMIC STRUCTURAL VARIANTS

Certain structural hemoglobin variants are characterized by the presence of a biosynthetic defect as well as abnormal structure.[6] Thalassemic hemoglobinopathies are unusual forms of thalassemia caused by such structural variants.

Hb Lepore

Hb Lepore ($\alpha_2\beta\delta$) is the prototype of a group of hemoglobinopathies characterized by fused globin chains.[1–4] The chains begin with a normal δ-chain sequence at their N-terminus and end with the normal β-chain sequence at their C-terminus. These hemoglobinopathies arise by unequal or nonhomologous crossover or recombination events that fuse the proximal end of one gene with the distal end of a closely linked structurally homologous gene (Fig. 41–18). During meiosis, mispairing and crossover of the highly homologous δ- and β-globin genes can occur, resulting in a Lepore chromosome, which contains (in addition to γ-globin genes) only the fused δβ gene, and an anti-Lepore chromosome, which contains the reciprocal fusion product (βδ), as well as intact δ- and β-globin genes.[1]

Lepore globin is synthesized in low amounts, presumably because it is under the control of the δ-globin gene promoter, which normally sustains transcription at only 2.5% the level of the β-globin gene.[497] Patients with Hb Lepore have the phenotype of β-thalassemia, distinguished by the added presence of 5% to 15% Hb Lepore. In contrast, the anti-Lepore globin (Miyada) is not associated with a β-thalassemia phenotype because of the presence of an intact and functionally normal β-globin gene on the same chromosome.

Heterozygotes for Hb Lepore have the clinical phenotype of β-thalassemia trait; homozygotes are usually similar to patients with homozygous β-thalassemia. Compound heterozygotes for Hb Lepore and a "classic" β-thalassemia allele usually have severe thalassemia. Hb Lepore thus interacts with thalassemia in the same way that a severe β-thalassemia gene does, although occasional cases have a milder phenotype of the thalassemia intermedia variety, perhaps because of an associated higher than usual level of γ-globin gene expression. The presence of Hb Lepore should be suspected in individuals with a microcytic, hypochromic anemia who also have a small amount of an abnormal hemoglobin migrating in the position of Hb S on routine hemoglobin electrophoresis. Hb Lepore accounts for

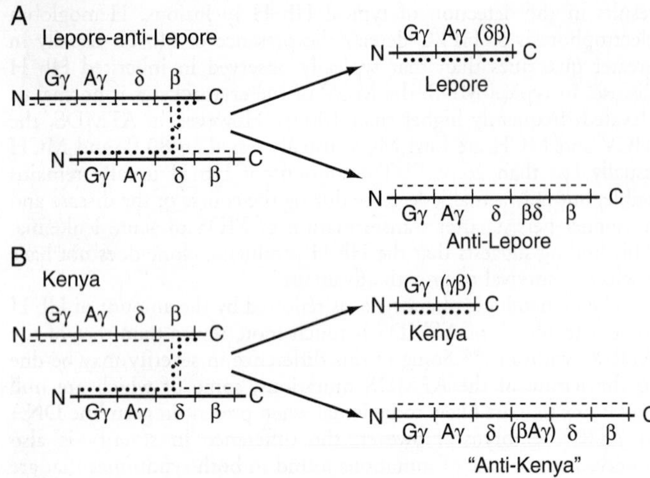

Figure 41–18 Genetic origins of Hb Lepore, anti-Lepore Hb, and Hb Kenya. *(Adapted from Benz EJ Jr: The hemoglobinopathies. In Kelly WN, DeVita VT [eds.]: Textbook of Internal Medicine. Philadelphia, JB Lippincott, 1988, p 1423.)*

5% to 10% of the β-thalassemias seen in Greek and Italian populations. Several forms of Hb Lepore have been described that differ in the position at which the transition from δ to β DNA and amino acid sequence occurs.

An analogous but rare variant, Hb Kenya [$\alpha_2(^{A}\gamma\beta)_2$], arises from nonhomologous crossing over between the $^{A}\gamma$- and β-globin genes[498] (see Fig. 41–14) and is associated with the phenotype of $^{G}\gamma$ HPFH. A DNA sequence approximately 600 bases downstream from the β-globin gene acts as a strong enhancer, promoting the erythroid-specific expression of the β-globin genes in adult cells.[3,4,21] The fused $^{A}\gamma\beta$ gene as well as the linked upstream $^{G}\gamma$ gene are believed to come under the influence of the enhancer, because of its abnormal proximity, and thus are expressed at high levels in adult life.

Hb E

Hb E ($\alpha_2\beta_2^{26Glu\rightarrow Lys}$) is a common variant (15%–30% of the population) in Cambodia, Thailand, parts of China, and Vietnam. Hb E is very mildly unstable, but this instability does not significantly alter the life span of red blood cells. Hb E trait resembles very mild β-thalassemia trait. Homozygotes exhibit more microcytosis but are still asymptomatic.[499] Compound heterozygotes for Hb E and a β-thalassemia gene (Hb E–β-thalassemia) resemble patients with β-thalassemia intermedia or β-thalassemia major. However, some problems such as infection and pulmonary hypertension may occur more commonly in Hb E–β-thalassemia than in homozygous β-thalassemia.[500]

The only nucleotide sequence abnormality found in the β^E-gene is a base change in codon 26 that causes the amino acid substitution. This mutation, which occurs in a potential cryptic RNA splice region, alters the consensus sequence surrounding a potential GT donor splice site and thus activates the cryptic site. Alternative splicing at this position occurs approximately 40% to 50% of the time, generating a structurally abnormal globin mRNA that cannot be translated appropriately.[501] The other mRNA precursors are spliced at the normal site, generating functionally normal mRNA, which is translated into β^E-globin because the mature mRNA retains the base change that encodes lysine at codon 26.

Hb E is important because it is so common in Southeast Asian populations. With increased emigration of Southeast Asians to North America, Hb E syndromes are being seen there with increased frequency.[502,503] Genetic counseling of these individuals should emphasize the potential consequences of the interaction of Hb E with β-thalassemia. Hb E is also an instructive example of the pleiotropic effects that point mutations can have on the amounts and types of gene products derived from a single mutant gene.

Hb Constant Spring

Hb Constant Spring (see Fig. 41–16) is an elongated α-globin variant resulting from a mutation that alters the normal translation termination codon.[504] Polyribosomes read through the usual translation stop site and incorporate an additional 31 amino acids until another in-phase termination codon is reached within the 3′ untranslated sequence. The amount of α^{cs} mRNA is markedly reduced, and α^{cs}-globin is synthesized in only minute amounts.[466,505] Six possible mutations of the normal translation termination codon (UAA) in α-globin mRNA could result in the generation of a "sense" codon.[506] Of these, five variants have been identified, each having a markedly underproduced abnormal variant, indicating that disruption of normal translation termination is in some way associated with abnormal mRNA accumulation, presumably due to instability of the mRNA.[466] The output of α-globin from the α^{cs} allele is only approximately 1% of normal, and the gene is thus rendered α-thalassemic. The α^{cs} allele has been identified only on chromosomes containing a *cis*-linked functionally normal α-globin gene.[1–4] Thus, α^+-thalassemia trait and Hb H disease ($-/\alpha^{cs}\alpha$) associated with Hb Constant Spring are common, but hydrops fetalis due to four abnormal α-globin genes cannot occur in association with this variant. Homozygosity for the variant is associated with a relatively mild form of Hb H disease.[1]

EXTRAORDINARILY UNSTABLE HEMOGLOBINS

Rare cases of α-thalassemia (eg, Hb Quong Sze[462]) and β-thalassemia (eg, Hb Indianapolis, recently renamed Hb Terre Haute[507,508]) arise from mutations that produce extremely labile globin chains. The chains fail to pair with the complementary chain, or they precipitate and are degraded so rapidly that they never form tetramers. These posttranslational lesions have the same pathophysiologic effects on hemoglobin biogenesis as reduction of globin mRNA production or function. Another group of β-globin chain variants, usually due to mutations in exon 3 of the β-globin gene, are associated with inclusion body formation and a phenotype of dominant β-thalassemia intermedia.[16,17,509]

HEREDITARY PERSISTENCE OF FETAL HEMOGLOBIN

Hereditary persistence of fetal hemoglobin (HPFH) consists of a group of rare conditions characterized by continued synthesis of high levels of Hb F in adult life.[1,510–512] No deleterious effects on patients are observed, even when 100% of the hemoglobin produced in HPFH homozygotes is Hb F. These patients thus demonstrate convincingly that prevention or reversal of the Hb F–to–Hb A switch would provide efficacious therapy for β-thalassemia.

Two major types of HPFH have been described. Very high levels of fetal hemoglobin synthesis and uniform distribution of Hb F among all red blood cells characterize pancellular HPFH. Heterocellular HPFH results from inherited increases in the number of F cells (see Chapters 25 and 33).

HPFH shows ethnic differences. In black patients with heterozygous pancellular deletional HPFH, the Hb F is within a range of 15% to 35% and contains $^{G}\gamma$ and $^{A}\gamma$ chains in a ratio of 2:3. In Greeks with pancellular nondeletional HPFH, Hb F levels are lower, 10% to 20%, and the Hb F is 90% of the $^{A}\gamma$ type. Hb A_2 levels are lower than normal. There are usually no other hematologic abnormalities in these persons, although β/α-globin chain synthesis ratios may be lower in some black heterozygotes.

A few black patients have been described with homozygous HPFH. All hemoglobin within the red blood cells of these patients is Hb F. Mild microcytosis and hypochromia of the red blood cells are present without anemia. In fact, hemoglobin levels are mildly elevated, presumably due to increased erythropoiesis stimulated by the left-shifted oxygen dissociation curve of red blood cells rich in Hb F. Globin chain synthesis reveals a γ/α synthetic ratio of approximately 0.5.

Pancellular HPFH can be divided into two classes. The deletional forms arise from large deletions within the β-globin gene cluster that remove the δ- and β-globin genes, part of the γδ intergenic DNA, and DNA downstream (to the 3′ side) from the β-globin genes.[1,510–512] The deletions appear to bring enhancer sequences into the proximity of the remaining γ-globin genes, promoting their high expression. Homozygotes for this condition produce only Hb F. In nondeletional HPFH, the β- and δ-globin genes are present. Single-base changes have been shown to occur in the promoter regions of either the $^{A}\gamma$- or $^{G}\gamma$-globin gene, resulting in overexpression of that form of Hb F.[1,510–512] In these individuals, Hb F levels rarely account for more than 20% of total hemoglobin.

A case of HPFH/β-thalassemia resembles β-thalassemia trait except for a higher proportion and regular distribution of Hb F in the red blood cells.[1]

In δβ-thalassemia and HPFH patients, persistence of Hb F after the period of perinatal Hb F to Hb A switching is more marked than in patients with the "classic" (high Hb A_2) forms of thalassemia. Indeed, δβ-thalassemia and HPFH represent various degrees of the same genetic phenomenon. Both conditions frequently arise from deletions of DNA that remove or inactivate the β-globin gene.[1,510–512]

Heterocellular HPFH appears to result in many cases from mutations outside the β-globin gene cluster.[512] One controlling locus resides on the X chromosome.[513,514] Patients with these conditions probably represent the extreme end of a distribution of polymorphic capacities to produce F cells in adult life. Hb F levels are usually much lower than those in the pancellular forms. In some situations, elevated levels of Hb F are seen in otherwise normal individuals. In others, the high levels of Hb F become apparent only when other factors producing erythroid stress are present.

SUGGESTED READINGS

Angelopoulos NG et al: Hypoparathyroidism in transfusion-dependent patients with beta-thalassemia. J Bone Miner Metab 24(2):138, 2006.

Borgna-Pignatti C et al: Cardiac morbidity and mortality in deferoxamine- or deferiprone-treated patients with thalassemia major. Blood 107(9):3733, 2006.

Boulad F: Hematopoietic stem cell transplantation for the treatment of beta thalassemia. In Kline R (ed.): Pediatric Hematopoietic Stem Cell Transplantation. New York, Informa Healthcare, 2006, p 383.

Cappellini MD et al: A phase 3 study of deferasirox (ICL670), a once-daily oral iron chelator, in patients with beta-thalassemia. Blood 107(9):3455, 2006.

Cohen A, Glimm E and Porter JB: Effect of transfusional iron intake on response to chelation therapy in β-thalassemia major. Blood 111:583–587, 2008

Dodd RY: Current safety of the blood supply in the United States. Int J Hematol, 80(4):301–305, 2004.

Eleftheriou P et al: Response of myocardial T2* to oral deferasirox monotherapy for 1 year in 29 patients with transfusion-dependent anaemias: A subgroup analysis. Haematologica 91(Suppl 1):366, 2006.

Gilfillan CP et al: A randomized, double-blind, placebo-controlled trial of intravenous zoledronic acid in the treatment of thalassemia-associated osteopenia. Calcif Tissue Int 79(3):138, 2006.

Harmatz P et al: Safety and efficacy of peginterferon alfa-2a and ribavirin for hepatitis C in thalassemia. Blood 108:558, 2006.

Harmatz P et al: Phase Ib clinical trial of starch-conjugated deferoxamine (40SD02): A novel long-acting iron chelator. Br J Hematol, 2007.

Hongeng S et al: Outcomes of transplantation with related- and unrelated-donor stem cells in children with severe thalassemia. Biol Blood Marrow Transplant 12(6):683, 2006.

Kattamis A et al: Iron chelation treatment with combined therapy with deferiprone and deferioxamine: A 12-month trial. Blood Cells Mol Dis 36(1):21, 2006.

Kolnagou A et al: Low serum ferritin levels are misleading for detecting cardiac iron overload and increase the risk of cardiomyopathy in thalassemia patients. The importance of cardiac iron overload monitoring using magnetic resonance imaging T2 and T2*. Hemoglobin 30(2):219, 2006.

Kolnagou A, Kontoghiorghes GJ: Effective combination therapy of deferiprone and deferoxamine for the rapid clearance of excess cardiac iron and the prevention of heart disease in thalassemia. The Protocol of the International Committee on Oral Chelators. Hemoglobin 30(2):239, 2006.

Neufeld EJ: Oral chelators deferasirox and deferiprone for transfusional iron overload in thalassemia major: New data, new questions. Blood 107(9):3436, 2006.

Pennell DJ et al: Randomized controlled trial of deferiprone or deferoxamine in beta-thalassemia major patients with asymptomatic myocardial siderosis. Blood 107(9):3738, 2006.

Tanner M et al: A randomized placebo controlled double blind trial of the effect of combination therapy with deferoxamine and deferiprone on myocardial iron in thalassemia major using cardiovascular magnetic resonance. Blood 106:1017A, 2006.

Vogiatzi MG et al: Prevalence of fractures among the thalassemia syndromes in North America. Bone 38(4):571, 2006.

Voskaridou E et al: Zoledronic acid for the treatment of osteoporosis in patients with beta-thalassemia: Results from a single-center, randomized, placebo-controlled trial. Haematologica 91(9):1193, 2006.

Wood JC et al: Deferasirox and deferiprone remove cardiac iron in the iron-overloaded gerbil. Transl Res 148(5):272, 2006.

REFERENCES

For complete list of references log onto www.expertconsult.com

CHAPTER 42

PATHOBIOLOGY OF SICKLE CELL DISEASE

Robert P. Hebbel

Since it was identified as the first molecular disease in 1949,[2] sickle cell disease which is caused by the mutant sickle cell hemoglobin (HbS), has provided the classic paradigm for understanding single-gene disorders. The predominant clinical features of this condition include hemolytic anemia, episodic painful events, chronic organ deterioration, and various acute complications.[1] However, the genesis of clinical sickle cell disease is exceedingly complicated, and an understanding of its pathophysiology integrates concepts from multiple disciplines, includes contributions from the red blood cell (RBC) membrane and the vascular wall endothelium, and recognizes the likely participation of multiple genetic influences. This chapter addresses the pathophysiology that underlies the sickle cell disease syndromes described in Chapter 43.

EARLY YEARS OF SICKLE CELL DISEASE RESEARCH

Sickle cell disease probably was recognized for centuries in some parts of Africa,[3] but it was first reported in the medical literature in 1910, when Herrick described a young Grenadan man with recurrent pain, anemia, and sickle-shaped red corpuscles in the blood (Fig. 42–1).[4] Early milestones in elucidating the basis of this disorder included demonstration that reversible sickling is induced by deoxygenation (Fig. 42–2), recognition of a carrier state, and observation that sickled RBCs contain protein having unusual properties.[5] In 1940, Ham and Castle[6] described a PO_2 threshold for concomitant induction of sickling and hyperviscosity, from which they postulated that sickle cell pathophysiology resulted from a "vicious cycle of erythrostasis" involving mutually promotive sickling and viscosity changes. In 1949, Neel[7] recorded the Mendelian genetics of sickle cell anemia, and Pauling and colleagues[2] used protein electrophoresis to directly demonstrate the presence of abnormal hemoglobin in patients and carriers. This was followed by observation of the reversible sol-gel transformation[8] and the insolubility[9] of deoxygenated HbS solutions. In 1957, Ingram[10] identified the molecular basis of the mutant HbS. Thereafter, increasingly detailed investigations began to reveal the striking complexities of sickle cell disease pathobiology.[1]

GENETIC CONSIDERATIONS

Molecular Context

The sickle mutation in the β-globin gene is a GAG→GTG conversion that creates a $\beta^{6Glu\rightarrow Val}$ substitution and thereby forms β^S globin chains. The β-globin gene is represented by a single copy on each chromosome 11, and other β-globin disorders can be allelic to the sickle gene and have a codominant impact on the clinical phenotype. Examples include the gene for the normal β chain (β^A), β mutants (eg, β^C), β°- or β^+-thalassemia, and hereditary persistence of fetal hemoglobin (HPFH). Compound heterozygosity for β^S and each one of these forms results in well-defined clinical syndromes, such as HbAS (ie, sickle trait), HbSC disease, HbS β-thalassemia, and HbS HPFH. Eight percent of African Americans have a β^S gene, 3% have β^C, 1.5% have β-thalassemia, and 0.1% have HPFH.[11] Among African Americans, about 1 in 600 births results in the homozygous state, sickle cell anemia (HbSS), and about 1 in 400 results in a form of sickle cell disease.

Residing within a cluster of β-like genes, the β-globin gene is in linkage disequilibrium with multiple nearby polymorphic sites. Different combinations can be identified by restriction endonuclease cleavage, which thereby defines discrete β-locus haplotypes. This approach has revealed that the β^S gene tends to reside on one of several distinct chromosomal patterns, referred to as the Senegal, Benin, Bantu, Cameroon, and Arab-India haplotypes (Fig. 42–3A).[12] Each designation refers to an ethnographic region in which the sickle gene achieved polymorphic frequency (see Fig. 42–3B), with gene frequency peaking at 0.10 to 0.15 (perhaps even 0.20 in West Africa)[3] and diminishing as distance from the regional center increases.[12] Gene frequency is stated as fraction of all chromosomes, and the proportion of individuals with the mutation is about twice the gene frequency. The Cameroon haplotype occurs within a single ethnic group, beyond which expansion did not occur, and the India-Arab haplotype has two centers of high gene frequency, one in India and one in the eastern Arabian Peninsula. In most cases, the sickle gene resides on one of these five major haplotypes. Other haplotypes occur uncommonly, but these are largely explained by recombination events at a "hot spot" near the ψβ gene.[12]

Origin, Selection, and Dispersion of the Sickle Gene

Within the ethnographic regions defined by major β haplotypes, β^A and β^S alleles tend to reside on the distinct regional type of chromosome 11, suggesting that the sickle mutation arose independently in the five locations.[12] The β^C mutation arose only once. Historical and biologic data argue that frequency of the β^S gene greatly expanded in Africa 2000 to 3000 years ago and in Asia about 4000 years ago.[13] Its high prevalence suggests positive selection, and it is proposed that the introduction of iron tools led to adoption of an agricultural system that promoted increased human habitation density and favorable breeding conditions for the mosquito vector, *Anopheles*.[14,15] This allowed development of endemic *Plasmodium falciparum*, the most virulent of human malarias. In this context, high β^S gene frequencies were reached because of a balanced polymorphism, such that heterozygotes (HbAS) have an adaptive advantage over homozygotes (HbAA or HbSS). Consistent with this scenario, there is a remarkable concordance of geographic distributions of the sickle gene and of historical endemic malaria in the Old World (see Fig. 43–2B). Thus, it has been suggested that the sickle gene represents "a biologic solution to a cultural problem."[15]

In hyperendemic areas, *falciparum* malaria uniformly infects the young and is the primary killer of children with sickle cell disease. However, those with sickle trait are less likely to develop high-level parasitemia, to have severe malaria, or to die.[13,16] At the level of the RBC, this protection probably reflects steps after successful initial invasion, and a number of mechanisms have been proposed.[13] One that seems particularly plausible links protection to the instability of HbS (discussed later) and splenic function.[17] In support, infection of normal RBCs with *P. falciparum* leads to hemoglobin denaturation, clustering of membrane protein band 3, opsonization by band 3 autoantibody, and enhanced erythrophagocytosis, even of the early ring forms.[18] This scenario presumably would be augmented for infected HbS-containing trait cells, leading to their clearance by the spleen. In mice, the protective effect of HbS is lost after splenectomy,[13] indicating that an autosplenectomized state may contribute

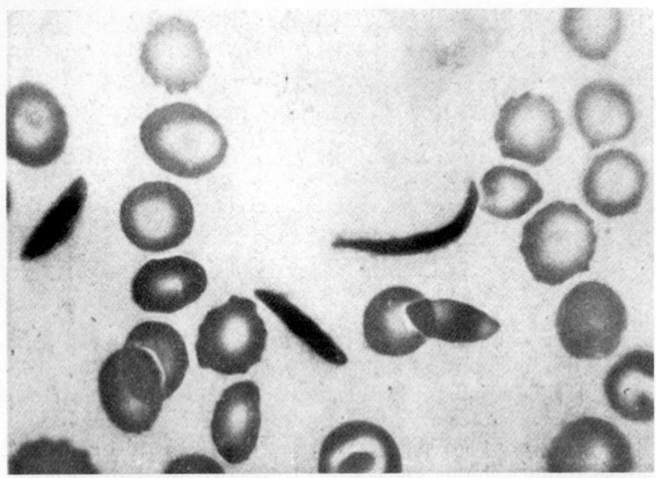

Figure 42–1 Blood smear from the first description of sickle cell disease. *(From Herrick JB: Peculiar elongated and sickle-shaped red blood corpuscles in a case of severe anemia. Arch Intern Med 5:517, 1910.)*

to malarial virulence in HbS homozygotes. However, the timing of appearance of anti-band 3 autoantibodies in childhood is not defined, and the relationship of this scenario to the appearance of immune mechanisms of protection at about 2 years of age[19] is not known. Additional factors may be involved. Truncation mutations of CD36, a molecule implicated in the endothelial adhesion exhibited by sickle and *falciparum*-parasitized RBCs, exist at allelic frequencies in Gambians and may predispose them to severe malaria.[20]

Eventually, the sickle gene spread geographically by means of commerce, slave trading, and migration. This dispersion has been tracked by analyses of regional β haplotypes, a biologic marker that largely corroborates expectations of gene flow derived from known historical records.[12] As a generalization, it spread on the Benin haplotype to North Africa and then across the Mediterranean. All three major African haplotypes are present in the western Arabian Peninsula, but on the eastern side, the sickle gene tends to be on the Arab-India haplotype, as it is in south Asia. The gene arrived in the Americas mostly through the Atlantic slave trade, with Benin, Senegal, and Bantu haplotypes accounting for most β^S genes in the United States.

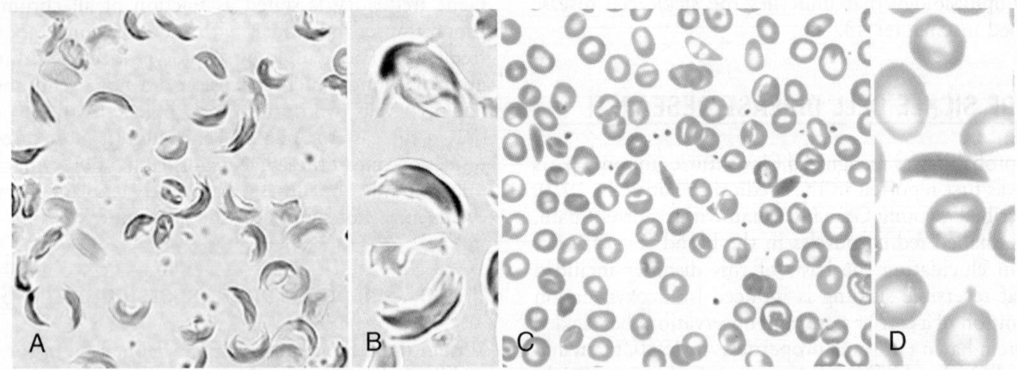

Figure 42–2 Sickle cells in deoxygenated sickle cell preparation compared to peripheral smear. Sickle cell preparation using sodium metabisulfate **(A, B)** to illustrate the marked degree of sickling of the majority of the cells in a deoxygenated state. Note the pointed ends of the sickle cells distorted due to the polymers of sickle hemoglobin. Some forms are called "holly-leaf" forms. In comparison, on the Wright-stained peripheral blood smear from same patient **(C, D)**, the few sickle cells present are only those that remain irreversibly sickled due to membrane damage. These are referred to as "irreversibly sickled" cells.

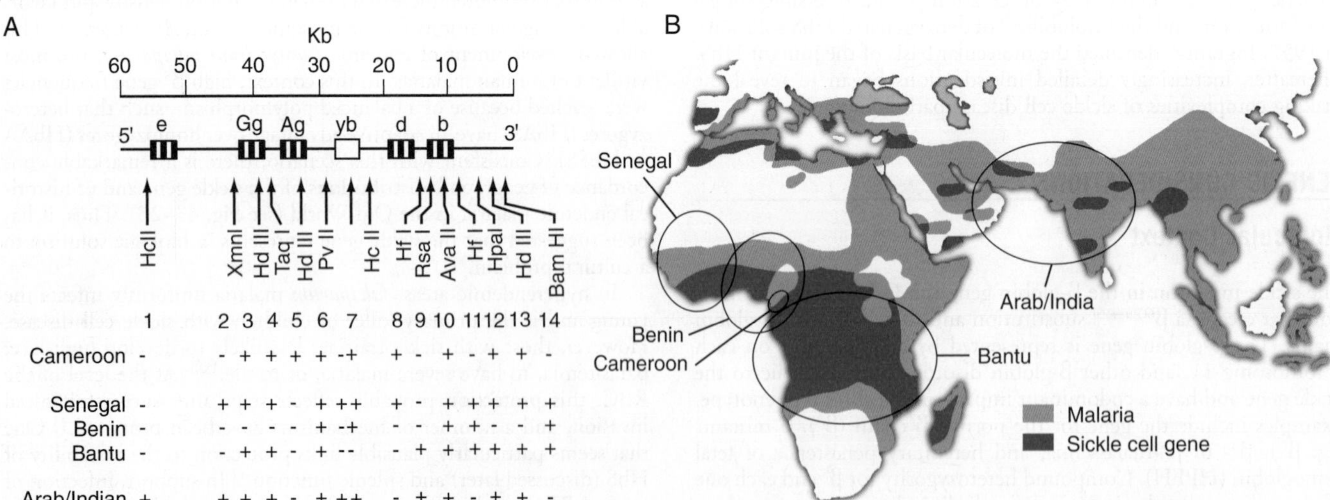

Figure 42–3 **A,** The β haplotypes are defined by polymorphic sites in the β-globin cluster. **B,** The corresponding regions in which the sickle gene achieved polymorphic frequency are superimposed on shading that identifies the Old World distribution of the sickle gene and of historical, endemic malaria. *(**A,** Adapted from Lapoumeroulie, Dunda O, Ducrocq R, et al: A novel sickle cell mutation of yet another origin in Africa: The Cameroon type. Hum Genet 89:333, 1992; **B,** adapted from Friedman MJ, Trager W: The biochemistry of resistance to malaria. Sci Am 244:154, 1981 and from Nagel RL, Steinberg MH: Genetics of the β^S gene: Origins, epidemiology, and epistasis in sickle cell anemia. In Steinberg MH, Forget BG, Higgs DR, Nagel RL [eds]: Disorders of Hemoglobin: Genetics, Pathophysiology, and Clinical Management, Cambridge, Cambridge University Press, 2001, p 711.)*

Clinical Consequences of the Abnormal Molecular Behaviors of HbS

Tetramer assembly → RBC Hb composition
Genotype and diagnosis
Effect on sickling, therefore vasoocclusion
Hb stability → membrane defects
Hemolysis
Malaria resistance
Adhesion, therefore vaso-occlusion
Hb polymerization → sickling
Hemolysis
Vaso-occlusion

ABNORMAL MOLECULAR BEHAVIORS OF SICKLE HEMOGLOBIN

Because of its $\beta^{6Glu \rightarrow Val}$ substitution, entailing a loss of negative charge and gain in hydrophobicity, HbS exhibits three abnormal molecular behaviors of direct relevance to pathophysiology. (See box on Clinical Consequences of the Abnormal Molecular Behaviors of HbS.)

Hemoglobin S Charge and Tetramer Assembly

Formation of hemoglobin tetramers requires proximate assembly of stable dimers from unlike monomers (eg, $\alpha + \beta \rightarrow \alpha\beta$), which is governed by electrostatic attraction.[21] The normal α and β chains are positively and negatively charged, respectively. In heterozygous states for β-globin mutants, β-chain competition for dimer assembly is a determinant of the relative proportions of HbA versus non-HbA variants. Mutant β chains with lowered negative charge form αβ dimers more slowly, and the relative rates for dimer association are $\alpha\beta^A > \alpha\beta^S > \alpha\beta^C$, with $\alpha\beta^A$ dimers formed about twice as rapidly as $\alpha\beta^S$ dimers.[21] This explains why individuals with sickle trait typically have only 40% rather than 50% HbS and why the proportion of HbS is higher in HbSC disease than in HbAS disease. It also explains the effect of concurrent α-thalassemia on the proportion of HbS in sickle trait; as availability of α chains becomes limiting, the percentage of HbS typically drops from 40% to 35% (one α deletion), 30% (two α deletions), or less than 25% (three α deletions).

Hemoglobin S Stability and Oxidant Formation

HbS is modestly unstable, observed in vitro as instability to various applied stresses,[22] but the underlying mechanism varies. Precipitation of HbS by mechanical agitation does not depend on hemoglobin oxidation, but rather reflects a surface denaturative tendency related to the hydrophobicity of the β^6 amino acid and tetramer-to-dimer dissociation. In contrast, the stresses that are more clearly physiologic depend on hemoglobin oxidation as a proximate event. HbS has an abnormal redox potential compared with HbA[23] that may underlie its increased autoxidation rate,[24] and it is unstable in response to oxidant drugs, adventitious iron, and interaction with aminophospholipids characteristic of the membrane's inner leaflet.[22] Although the physical-chemical basis for the destabilizing role of the β^6 valine in HbS is not known, this instability leads to accumulation of hemoglobin and iron on the RBC membrane and contributes to abnormal oxidative biochemistry at the cytosol-membrane interface.

Hemoglobin S Solubility, Hemoglobin S Polymerization, and Red Blood Cell Sickling

Oxy-HbS, oxy-HbA, and deoxy-HbA have very high solubilities, but deoxy-HbS aggregates into densely packed polymers, a process that is fully reversible on reoxygenation. This abnormal property forms the fundamental basis for the sickling disorders, the eponymous RBC shape change caused by polymer-mediated distortion.

Polymer Structure

Deoxygenation causes transformation of soluble HbS to a highly viscous and semisolid gel that behaves thermodynamically like a crystal in equilibrium with a solution of individual tetrameric Hb molecules.[25] Even complete deoxygenation does not convert all deoxy-HbS to polymer. The insoluble phase is a collection of domains of aligned polymers, the basic unit of which is a double strand in which two strings of deoxy-Hb tetramers make multiple contacts with each other (Fig. 42–4).[26] In the physiologic form of the polymer, the component strings of hemoglobin molecules in a double strand are half-staggered and have a slight twist, creating a fiber that is approximately 21 nM in diameter and is composed of one central and six peripheral double strands.[27] The crystal formed in vitro lacks the twist, but its molecular structure is known in detail.[28] Each HbS tetramer has two β chains, the β_1 and β_2 subunits. Deoxy-HbS undergoes a slight structural shift so that the A helix β^{6Val} "donor" site of the β_2 subunit in one tetramer can contact an EF helix "acceptor" site (formed mainly by β^{85Phe}, β^{88Leu}, and β^{70Ala}) in the β_1 subunit of a tetramer in the neighboring single string.[28] This critical, lateral association can be made only when HbS is in its deoxy conformation; the EF helix hydrophobic pocket is not a favorable acceptor site for the charged β^{6Glu} of Hb A. The β^{6Val} in the β_1 subunit is located so it cannot participate in such contacts. However, the β_2 subunit of the second single string can form chemically similar β^{6Val}-dependent contacts with the β_1 subunit of the first single string. There are multiple additional axial and lateral contacts, but these are largely the same for deoxy-HbA and deoxy-HbS and are not themselves sufficient to stabilize a polymeric structure.

Role of Hemoglobin S Solubility

The abnormal dehydration of sickle RBCs dominates the physiologic chemistry of HbS.[25,26] Because the solubility of deoxy-HbS, approximately 16 g/dL, is much lower than the mean corpuscular hemoglobin concentration (MCHC), deoxygenation can result in a deoxy-HbS concentration that would exceed its solubility limit. Macromolecular crowding confers nonideal behavior on cytoplasmic constituents (boosting activity above that predicted from concentration alone), and high total hemoglobin concentration helps promote deoxy-HbS polymerization even during partial deoxygenation.

In vitro studies of polymerization carried out under equilibrium conditions (i.e., stable oxygen tension and long time scale) corroborate crystallographic data on critical amino acids involved in atomic contacts by revealing the effect of other hemoglobins on HbS solubility.[26] When different hemoglobins are mixed together, the constituent dimers dissociate and intermix randomly to form hybrid tetramers. A mixture of 50% HbS and 50% HbX yields three types of tetramers: 25% $\alpha\beta^S/\alpha\beta^S$, 50% $\alpha\beta^S/\alpha\beta^X$, and 25% $\alpha\beta^X/\alpha\beta^X$. The impact of naturally occurring hemoglobin mixtures can be understood with this information in mind. In mixtures of HbS and HbA, overall solubility is improved because the hybrid $\alpha\beta^S/\alpha\beta^A$ tetramer integrates into polymer only one half as well as the $\alpha\beta^S/\alpha\beta^S$ tetramer. Addition of HbF to HbS has an even greater sparing effect because the hybrid $\alpha\beta^S/\alpha\gamma$ tetramer cannot be incorporated into polymer. In this regard, HbC has the same effect as HbA, and HbA_2 has the same effect as HbF (Fig. 42–5A). As studied under equilibrium conditions, this sparing effect of HbA is such that much lower hemoglobin oxygen saturation is required for polymer to form in HbAS than in HbSS RBCs (see Fig. 42–5B). A curiosity is that the oxygen dissociation curve of sickle RBCs is right shifted, which increases in proportion to the MCHC. This is caused by the extremely low oxygen affinity of extant deoxy-HbS polymer, and it should promote neither hemo-

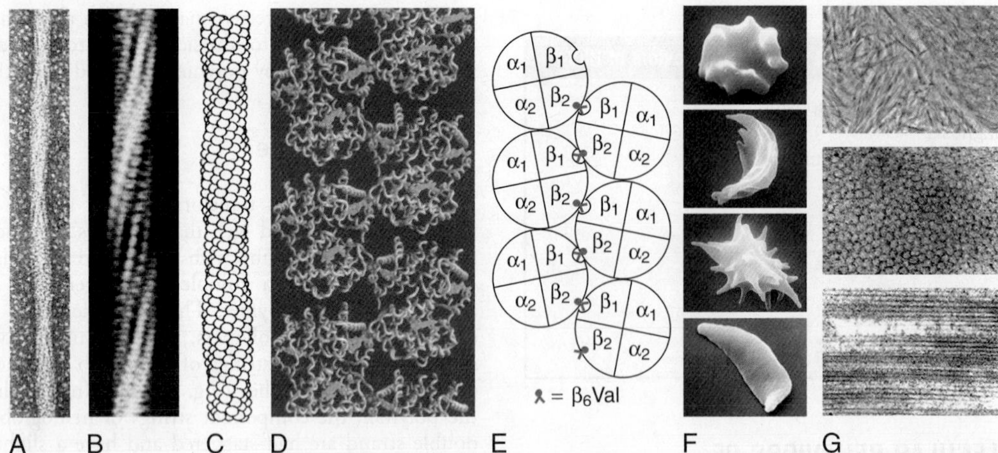

Figure 42–4 Deoxygenated hemoglobin S polymer. **A,** Electron micrograph of a fiber of polymerized hemoglobin S (HbS) obtained from a sickled red blood cell. **B,** Electron density surface map, modeled from authentic HbS fibers, shows pairings that create double strands plus a helical twist. **C,** Model of the HbS fiber, with Hb tetramers rendered as solid spheres. **D,** Protein backbone shows tetramer staggering in the HbS crystal. **E,** Schematic, two-dimensional representation of a double strand, demonstrating that only one of the two β^6 valine residues in each given tetramer participates in critical lateral contacts. **F,** Sickled red blood cells, showing various morphologies *(top to bottom)*: granular, holly shaped, classically sickled, and smoother and irreversibly sickled. **G,** Electron microscopy of sickled red blood cells reveals highly ordered polymer domains, as seen from the side *(bottom)* and on end *(middle)*, or highly disorganized domains *(top)*. *(**A** and **C**, From Dykes G, Crepeau RH, Edelstein SJ: Three-dimensional reconstruction of the fibres of sickle cell hemoglobin. Nature 272:506,1978; **B,** from Carragher B, Bluemke DA, Becker M, et al: Structural analysis of polymers of sickle cell hemoglobin. J Mol Biol 199:315,1988; D, from Harrington DJ, Adachi K, Royer WE Jr: The high resolution crystal structure of deoxyhemoglobin S. J Mol Biol 272:398, 1997; **F** and **G**, courtesy of Dr. James G. White and from White JG: Ultrastructural features of erythrocyte and hemoglobin sickling. Arch Intern Med 133:545, 1974.)*

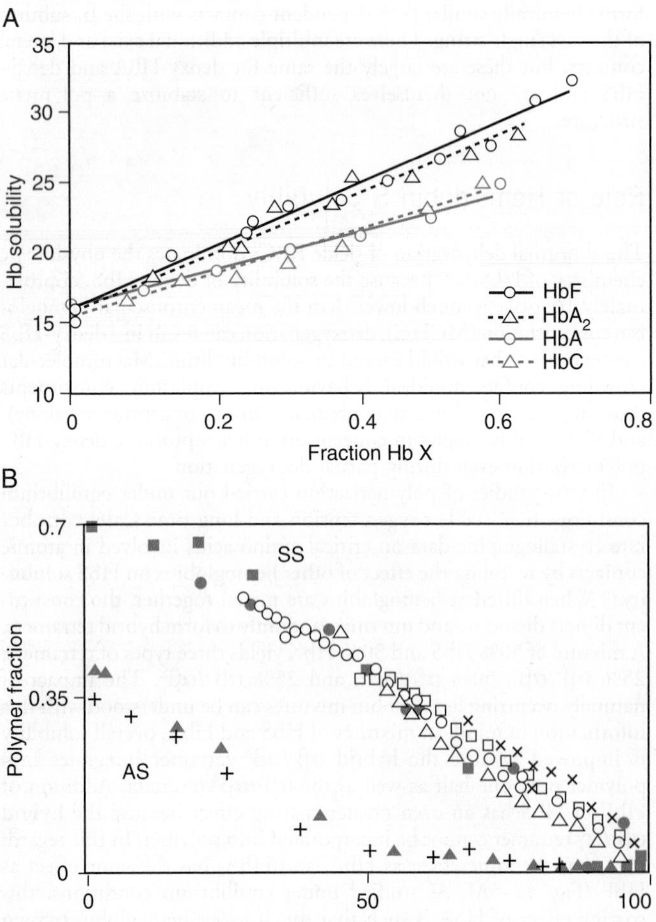

Figure 42–5 Deoxyhemoglobin S solubility, defined by studies at equilibrium (ie, constant oxygen tension and long times). **A,** Admixture of other hemoglobins with hemoglobin S raises overall solubility in absence of oxygen. **B,** The hemoglobin oxygen saturation required to initiate intracellular polymer formation (ie, polymer fraction) is much lower for sickle trait than for normal red blood cells. *(**A,** Data from Poillon WN, Kim BC, Rodgers GP, et al: Sparing effect of hemoglobin F and hemoglobin A_2 on the polymerization of hemoglobin S at physiologic ligand saturations. Proc Natl Acad Sci U S A 90:5039, 1993; **B,** Data from Schechter AN, Noguchi CT: Sickle hemoglobin polymer: Structure-function correlates. In Embury SH, Hebbel RP, Mohandas N, Steinberg MH [eds]: Sickle Cell Disease: Basic Principles and Clinical Practice, New York, Raven Press, 1994.)*

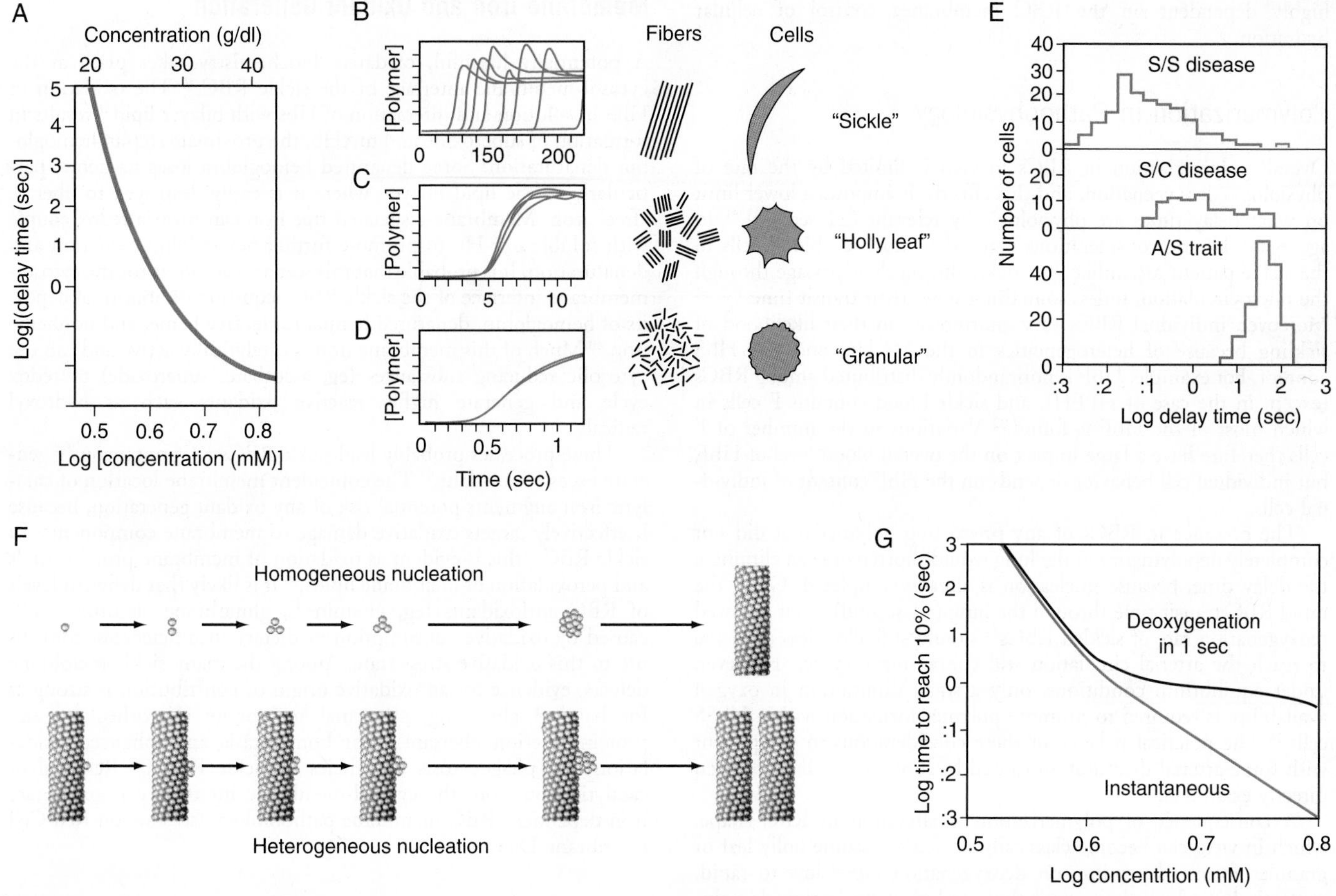

Figure 42–6 Kinetics of hemoglobin S polymerization, studied by near-instantaneous and complete deoxygenation. **A,** Extreme dependence of delay time on hemoglobin concentration. **B-D,** Kinetic progress curves for polymer formation show that long delay times are highly variable (**B**), but very short delay times are highly reproducible (**D**). *To the right* is a representation of domains and corresponding red blood cell morphology postulated to result from these different scales of polymerization rate (see Fig. 42–3F). **E,** Delay times for individual red blood cells are influenced by substituent hemoglobins. **F,** A double nucleation process is hypothesized to underlie polymer formation. **G,** Physiologically, the finite rate of deoxygenation effectively "caps" the polymerization rate and eliminates the relevance of delay times that are short relative to deoxygenation rate. *(A-E, Data From Eaton WA, Hofrichter J: Hemoglobin S gelation and sickle cell disease. Blood 70:1245, 1987; F, Adapted from Ferrone FA, Hofrichter J, Eaton WA: Kinetics of sickle hemoglobin polymerization II. A double nucleation mechanism. J Mol Biol 183:611, 1985; G, Data from Ferrone FA: Oxygen transits and transports. In Embury S, Hebbel RP, Mohandas N, Steinberg MH [eds]: Sickle Cell Disease: Basic Principles and Clinical Practice, New York, Raven Press, 1994.)*

globin polymerization (it results from it) nor tissue oxygenation (polymer would be virtually nonfunctional in oxygen delivery).

Kinetics of Polymerization

In normal physiologic conditions, sickle RBCs are not at equilibrium with a constant oxygen tension, and venous blood typically contains only about 20% sickled cells instead of the 90% predicted by equilibrium studies.[25] Measurements of polymerization kinetics, using nonphysiologic methods that create instantaneous and complete conversion of HbS from R (oxy) to T (deoxy) state, reveal a delay before onset of polymerization, which then occurs explosively.[25,26] Under in vitro conditions, this delay time is inversely related to an extremely high power of the initial Hb concentration; it is approximately 10 milliseconds at Hb of 40 g/dL, but it is 100,000 seconds at 20 g/dL (Fig. 42–6A). HbS solutions and sickle RBCs behave similarly in this regard. Delay times must then vary enormously from cell to cell because they are dominated by marked heterogeneity in the MCHC (ie, shorter delay for more dehydrated cells) and are influenced by presence of any non-S Hb (ie, longer delay for presence of HbA or C or F) (see Fig. 42–6E). Admixture of 20% to 30% HbA with HbS (simulating HbS-β^+-thalassemia) increases delay time 10^1- to 10^2-fold, and admixture of 20% to 30% HbF with HbS (simulating HbS-HPFH) increases it by 10^3- to 10^4-fold.[29]

Actual polymer formation is hypothesized to proceed by a two-step, double-nucleation mechanism (see Fig. 42–6F).[25,26] Accordingly, the initial *homogeneous nucleation* takes place in bulk solution, during which small numbers of tetramers associate, with accumulation not favored until a critical nucleus size develops (estimated to be 30 to 50 tetramers). Then, new tetramers can be added lengthwise to form a very large polymer. After this occurs, *heterogeneous nucleation* of new fibers takes place on the surface of the preexisting polymers, resulting in explosive, autocatalytic polymer formation. It is believed that the striking irreproducibility of long delay times (see Fig. 42–6B) reflects a stochastic formation of a single homogeneous nucleation event (or at least very few events) in cells that slowly polymerize and that very short delay times (see Fig. 42–6D) reflect simultaneous formation of multiple nucleation sites in cells that polymerize rapidly.[25,26,30]

An unresolved issue is whether the RBC membrane has any influence on polymerization. The good qualitative correspondence between polymerization in solution and in RBCs[25] argues that the fundamental mechanism is not altered by membranes, but it remains possible that the abnormal sickled cell membrane could contribute nucleation sites.[26] The two central features of the polymerization process, governance by MCHC and the delay time, are highly dependent on the RBC membrane's control of cellular hydration.

Polymerization in Pathophysiology

Overall polymerization in RBCs in vivo is limited by the rate of physiologic deoxygenation, and this effectively imposes a lower limit on what delay times are physiologically relevant (≥1 second).[31] In aggregate, kinetic considerations argue that most red blood cells in the sickle patient are unlikely to sickle during their passage through the microcirculation, unless something slows their transit time.[25,26,31] Moreover, individual RBCs vary enormously in their likelihood of sickling because of heterogeneities in the MCHC and non-HbS content. For example, HbF is nonrandomly distributed among RBCs (except in the case of HPFH), and sickle blood contains F cells in which most of the HbF is found.[32] Variations in the number of F cells therefore have a large impact on the overall blood level of HbF, but individual cell behavior depends on the HbF content of individual cells.

The presence in RBCs of any preexisting polymer that did not completely depolymerize in the lung would shorten or even eliminate the delay time, because nucleation is already completed. Given the rapid RBC transit time through the lung (<1 second), even a slowed reoxygenation rate of sickled RBCs[33] should still allow less than 1% to reach the arterial circulation still containing polymer. However, under equilibrium conditions, only a small diminution in oxygen availability is required to promote polymer formation within HbSS cells.[34] The practical balance of these considerations in the patient with some arterial desaturation caused by lung disease has not been directly examined.

A consequence of polymerization is alteration in RBC shape, which in vitro can become classically sickled or assume holly leaf or granular forms, depending on deoxygenation rate (slow to rapid, respectively), which determines the number of nucleation domains created (see Fig. 42–6).[25,26,30,31] However, physiologic oxygen transits are rapid relative to those typically used in vitro, and granular cells seem most likely to be the dominant type to develop in vivo. The RBC shape is not particularly important (ie, shape is not a determinant of RBC deformability), but the corresponding presence of polymer causes cells to lose their deformability. This is critical for unimpeded passage through the microvasculature.[35,36]

Alternative Ligands: Nitric Oxide and Carbon Monoxide

Nitric oxide (NO) does not materially alter HbS solubility or oxygen affinity,[37] but it can promote conversion of oxy-Hb to met-Hb.[23] This species cannot carry oxygen, and its formation is the initial step in oxidative denaturation of hemoglobin.[22] NO reaction with hemoglobin may be important for its role in vasoregulation. Hemoglobin that is partially liganded with carbon monoxide (CO) is shifted to the R state, and the CO eliminates a portion of the oxygen carrying capacity and renders the remaining available hemoglobin as a high-affinity protein. Patients with sickle cell disease have elevated COHb levels (as high as 7.6% in children) because of their hemolytic anemia.[38] Notably, the possible effects of second hand smoke exposure on sickle pathobiology have not been evaluated.

ABNORMALITIES OF SICKLE RED BLOOD CELLS

Even oxygenated sickle RBCs exhibit a variety of membrane abnormalities that contribute to pathophysiology.[39] Some are the consequence of proximate polymer formation, and others result from oxidative biochemistry. Several of these defects present attractive targets for development of novel therapeutics.

Membrane Iron and Oxidant Generation

A potentially harmful, oxidative biochemistry takes place at the cytosol-membrane interface of the sickle RBC.[40] The oxidation of HbS in solution and interaction of Hbs with bilayer lipid[22] results in formation of superoxide and metHb, the proximate step in hemoglobin denaturation. Some denatured hemoglobin loses its heme, particularly to the lipid bilayer, where it is easily destroyed to liberate "free" iron. Membrane-associated free iron can form a redox couple with soluble oxy-Hb to promote further hemoglobin oxidation and denaturation. It is probable that this scenario accounts for the cytosol-membrane interface of the sickle RBC acquiring its abnormal deposits of hemoglobin, denatured hemichrome, free heme, and nonheme iron.[40] Much of this membrane iron is catalytically active and can use cytosolic reducing substances (eg, ascorbate, superoxide) to redox cycle and generate highly reactive oxidants such as hydroxyl radicals.

These processes probably lead sickle RBCs to spontaneously generate excessive oxidant.[41] The coincident membrane location of catalytic iron augments potential risk of any oxidant generation, because it effectively targets oxidative damage to membrane components. In sickle RBCs, this is evident as oxidation of membrane protein thiols and peroxidation of membrane lipids.[40] It is likely that deficient levels of RBC antioxidants (eg, vitamin E, glutathione, ascorbic acid), caused by oxidative consumption or dietary insufficiencies, contribute to this oxidative stress state. Among the many sickle membrane defects, evidence for an oxidative origin or contribution is strongest for band 3 clustering, abnormal membrane microrheology and protein function, aberrant cation homeostasis, and enhanced vesiculation and phagocytosis tendencies of sickle RBCs.[40] Removal of catalytic iron from the cytosol-membrane interface can ameliorate iron-dependent RBC membrane pathobiology (see box on Red Cell Membrane Defects).[42]

Cation Homeostasis and Dehydrated Cells

For normal RBCs, the MCHC averages about 32 g/dL and varies from 27 to 38 g/dL, with fewer than 1% of cells having an MCHC greater than 38 g/dL. In contrast, the MCHC for sickle RBCs averages about 34 g/dL and varies from 23 to 50 g/dL, with up to 40% of cells having an MCHC greater than 38 g/dL.[43] This extreme heterogeneity results from reticulocytosis (low-density, low-MCHC cells) and dehydrating mechanisms (high-density, high-MCHC cells) (Fig. 42–7).

The most dramatic ion-handling abnormality of the sickle RBC is a loss of monovalent cation content induced by sickling.[44] This depends on cell deformation[45] and may partly reflect an enhanced mechanosensitivity of the sickle membrane because of the presence of lipid hydroperoxides.[46] Experimental data[44] and mathematical modeling[47] suggest that the initial membrane permeability caused by sickling results in increased calcium ion (Ca^{2+}) influx and a slight acidification, occurring stochastically and only in some cells at any one time.[48] This is followed by net potassium ion (K^+) and water loss, mediated mostly by activation of a Ca^{2+}-activated K^+ channel and K–Cl cotransport. The latter can be activated by lowered pH, endo-

Red Cell Membrane Defects

- Abnormal microrheology → ↓ deformability → occlusion, hemolysis
- PS flip flop → coagulation acceleration → thrombotic risk
- Abnormal cation homeostasis → ↑ RBC density → sickling, occlusion
- Ig opsonization → hemolysis
- Membrane oxidation → ↑ fragility, ↓ deformability → ISC shape, hemolysis

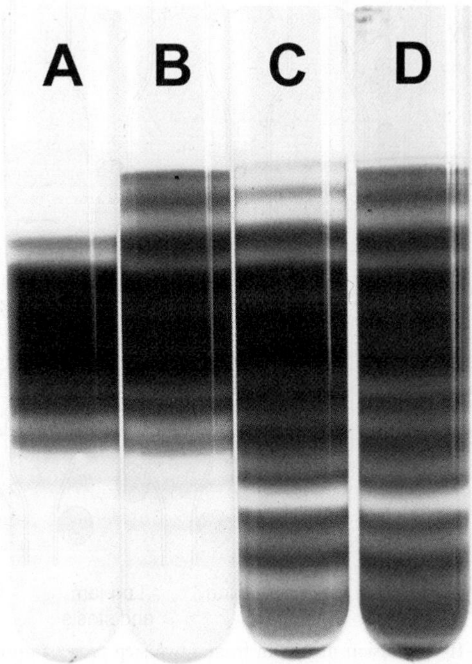

Figure 42–7 Marked heterogeneity in sickle red blood cell hydration. Compared with normal red blood cells (**A**) studied by discontinuous density-gradient centrifugation, red cells from a sickle subject with four α genes (**D**) include cells of unusually low density (usually reticulocytes) and abnormally high density (dehydrated cells). Sickle subjects with three and two α genes are shown in **C** and **B**, respectively. *(From Embury SH, Clark MR, Monroy G, Mohandas N: Concurrent sickle cell anemia and a-thalassemia. J Clin Invest 73:116, 1984.)*

thelin-1,[49] thiol oxidation (part of the reason in sickle cells[44]), and the presence of a relatively positively charged hemoglobin such as HbS or HbC (indicating an effect of a hemoglobin-membrane interaction).[44] It probably is influenced by macromolecular crowding of cytosolic proteins caused by the high MCHC.[50] Even at steady state, sickle RBCs contain increased Ca^{2+} because it is sequestered in cytoplasmic inside-out membrane vesicles,[51] providing evidence of prior cytosolic Ca^{2+} transients. Dense RBCs are not necessarily older cells, but rather can develop through these mechanisms very rapidly from young RBCs, with the cells having lower HbF levels being particularly susceptible.[52,53]

Dehydrated RBCs have decreased deformability[43] and increased propensity for sickling,[25] and the mutually promotive effects of dehydration and sickling constitute a vicious cycle. RBC dehydration is particularly likely to be exaggerated by the hypoxic and acidotic renal medullary environment, virtually the only focus of disease in persons with sickle trait, and very probably by nocturnal arterial desaturation.[54]

Deformability, Fragility, and Vesiculation

Even oxygenated sickle RBCs are poorly deformable.[43] The dominant cause of this is the high MCHC that entails increased cytoplasmic viscosity and a poorly understood, hemoglobin-induced effect on membrane stiffness. There may also be a smaller oxidation-related component to membrane stiffness.[40] On RBC deoxygenation in vitro, there is a temporal correspondence between appearance of polymer-induced shape change and deterioration of deformability, as measured by micropipette[35] and laser diffractometer.[36] On the other hand, filtration studies found decreased deformability before morphologic change,[55] and viscometry reveals a large deterioration in bulk viscosity caused by deoxygenated dense discocytes that show little shape change.[56]

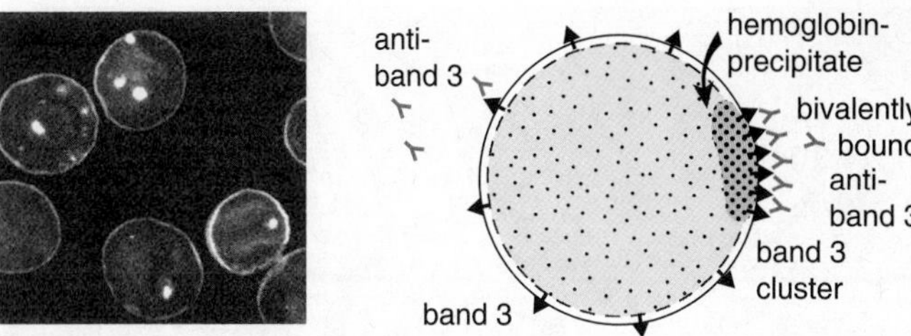

Figure 42–8 Colocalization of denatured hemoglobin on the membrane, clumping of band 3, and opsonization by naturally occurring anti-band 3 antibody. Clusters of band 3 are colocalized with immunoglobulin on the membranes of sickle red blood cells *(left)*. The drawing shows the colocalization scheme *(right)*. *(From Schluter K, Drenckhahn D: Co-clustering of denatured hemoglobin with band 3: Its role in binding of autoantibodies against band 3 to abnormal and aged erythrocytes. Proc Natl Acad Sci U S A 83:6137, 1986.)*

Sickle RBCs are somewhat mechanically fragile,[43] which may be a consequence of dehydration and a weakening of critical skeletal associations caused by oxidative protein damage. The tendency of sickle RBCs to lose membrane vesicles after sickling[57] may reflect separation of the bilayer from the underlying skeleton by spicules of polymerized hemoglobin[58] and enhanced susceptibility caused by protein thiol oxidation and dysfunction.[40]

Membrane Proteins

Abnormality of membrane proteins in sickle RBCs is dramatically illustrated by the fact that the membranes of irreversibly sickled cells (ISCs) are locked into that shape, irrespective of polymer content.[59] Sickle membrane ankyrin interactions with spectrin[60] and band 3[61] are abnormal; glycophorin and band 3 exhibit decreased mobility[62]; and β-actin from ISCs is abnormal and causes slow dissociation of the spectrin-actin-4.1 complex.[63] These abnormalities are most likely caused by oxidative damage, because sickle membranes exhibit abnormal thiol oxidation.[40] Band 3 is abnormally clumped because of binding of denatured HbS to its cytosolic portion, which causes sickle RBCs to attract opsonizing, naturally occurring anti-band 3 immunoglobulin and complement (Fig. 42–8).[64]

Membrane Lipids

The processes that normally enforce bilayer phospholipid asymmetry (ie, a scramblase that can move phosphatidylserine outward and be activated by calcium transits and a translocase that moves phosphatidylserine inward but can be inhibited by thiol oxidation) are impaired in sickle RBCs.[65] RBC sickling promotes externalization of phosphatidylserine, perhaps by separating lipid bilayer from the underlying protein skeleton.[58] This externalization is permanent for membranes of ISCs,[66] but a substantial portion of reticulocytes also exhibits this because of impaired translocase activity,[67] perhaps from thiol oxidation.[40] Other changes include presence of peroxidation by-products such as malondialdehyde, which can modify and cross-link proteins, and increased bilayer lipid hydroperoxides.[40]

Endothelial Adhesivity

Oxygenated sickle RBCs are abnormally adhesive to vascular endothelial cells in vitro[68] and in vivo (Fig. 42–9).[69] A number of mechanisms can underlie this, involving adhesogenic plasma proteins (eg, thrombospondin, high-molecular-weight von Willebrand factor, fibrinogen), adhesive structures specific to reticulocytes (eg, CD36, $\alpha_4\beta_1$) or present on all RBCs (eg, IAP, BCAM/Lu, exposed phosphatidylserine, glycated molecules), adhesion molecules on endothelium (eg, CD36, $\alpha_v\beta_3$, GPIb, vascular cell adhesion molecule [VCAM],

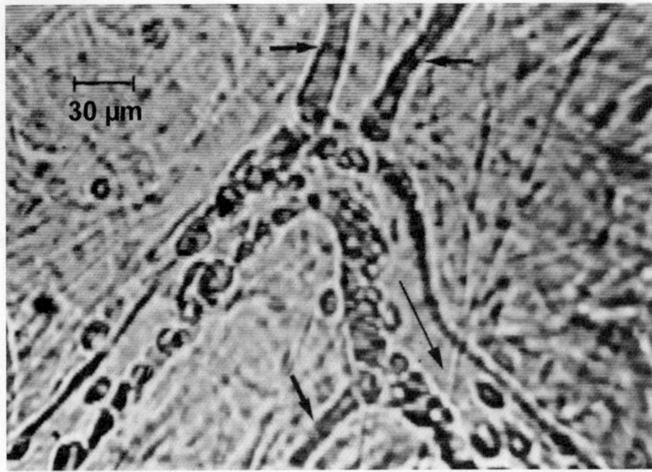

Figure 42–9 Sickle red blood cells adhere to the vascular wall endothelium under flow conditions in the microcirculation of a rat infused with human cells. Notice the two feeder microvessels *(arrows)* that have no flow because of the logjam of red blood cells. *(From Kaul DK, Fabry ME, Nagel RL: Microvascular sites and characteristics of sickle cell adhesion to vascular endothelium in shear flow conditions: Pathophysiological implications. Proc Natl Acad Sci U S A 86:3356, 1989.)*

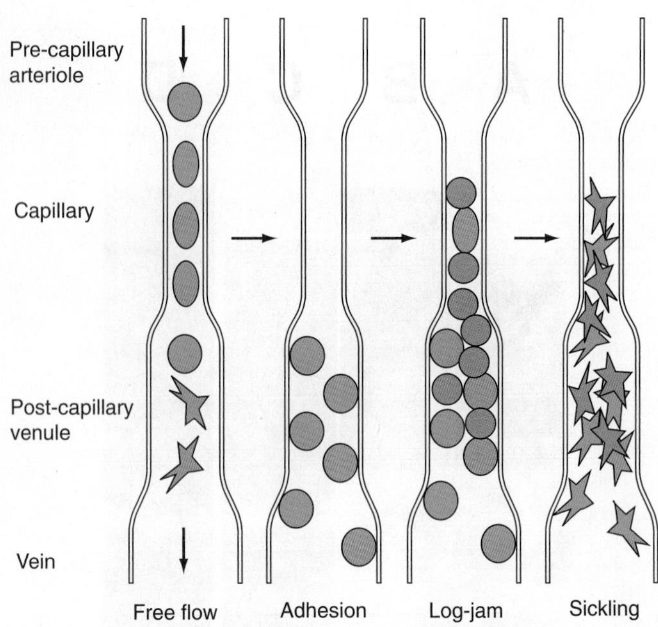

Figure 42–10 Occlusion may stem from a two-step process: initiation due to endothelial adherence and propagation caused by the logjam of poorly deformable cells.

P-selectin, glycated molecules, phosphatidylserine receptor), and possibly immobilized subendothelial matrix molecules (eg, thrombospondin, laminin, fibronectin). It seems probable that there is no single, most important mechanism. Rather, it is likely that multiple mechanisms participate, and mechanisms may vary between patients, from time to time within a single patient, and perhaps even with organ-to-organ or other regional differences.[68] For example, the role of adhesogenic plasma proteins can vary dramatically, depending on concurrent biology; for example, platelet activation can promote release of thrombospondin from α granules, and patient dehydration can elevate von Willebrand factor by means of vasopressin stimulation of endothelium.

A number of these mechanisms are high affinity and demonstrable under flowing conditions, but in the biologic context of tiny vessels in the microcirculation, even low-affinity adhesive mechanisms probably can be relevant.[68] The physiology may be governed to a significant extent by biologic modifiers of endothelial activation state, such as hypoxia, thrombin, interleukin-1 (IL-1), tumor necrosis factor (TNF), endotoxin, leukotriene B_4, endothelial injury (eg, viral infection), and other factors. Some adhesion mechanisms (eg, mediated by VCAM or P-selectin) are relevant only if the endothelium is activated. Others are activated if internal RBC signaling is triggered. It also is possible that biologic adhesivity involves mixed RBC interactions with adhesive leukocytes or platelets, or both, activated by inflammation and hemostatic activity.[70] Additional governing factors include the RBC hydration state, reticulocyte count, flow and shear rates, vessel diameter and geometry, and disturbances of flow regimens because of marginated white blood cells (WBCs). RBC adhesion can slow microvascular flow, providing the time extension needed to overcome the delay time requirement for HbS polymerization to occur.[25] Work in experimental animals suggests that occlusion is a two-step process in which adhesive RBCs initiate vasoocclusion, after which more dense and stiff cells provide propagation through a logjam effect (Fig. 42–10), all of which eventually results in RBC sickling.[69,71]

MACROPHAGE INTERACTION

Sickle RBCs are ingested abnormally readily by macrophages[72,73] because of membrane modification by malondialdehyde, externalization of phosphatidylserine, and opsonization by immunoglobulin. The latter process is triggered mainly by clustering of membrane protein band 3 because of the presence of denatured hemoglobin at the cytosol-membrane interface (see Fig. 42–8).[64] Because the densest cells have greater surface immunoglobulin[74] and high phosphatidylserine externalization,[67] they have the greatest interaction with macrophages.[72]

Irreversibly Sickled Cells

The sickled RBCs seen on a blood smear are mostly ISCs. Except for having membranes locked into an elongated shape,[59] the characteristics of ISCs are similar to other equally dense but not elongated cells: high MCHC, poor deformability, externalized phosphatidylserine, and lower-than-average HbF content. Although still adhesive to endothelium, they are less so than other sickle subpopulations,[68] probably because of their lack of deformability, but they exhibit greater adherence to macrophages.[72] ISC counts on average are higher in male patients, perhaps reflecting their average lower levels of HbF. Most significantly, ISCs are very short lived.[75] The two fundamental requirements for ISC formation seem to be RBC dehydration and assumption of an elongated and fixed membrane shape. The elongation implies prior prolonged sickling, perhaps caused by a "conditioning" period caused by residence of adhesive but deoxygenated cells in the postcapillary venules. The locked-in shape probably derives from membrane protein thiol oxidation.[156] The clinical importance of ISCs lies in their ability to prompt diagnosis of a sickling disorder when seen on blood smear and their contribution to hemolytic rate. They probably contribute to the logjam in areas of partial obstruction (see Fig. 42–10), but there is soft evidence both for and against a correlation between ISC number and vasoocclusive manifestations.

ENDOTHELIAL BIOLOGY OF SICKLE CELL DISEASE

The vascular endothelium serves multiple critical functions in physiology,[76] and it is likely that many of these roles are involved in the pathobiology of sickle cell disease.[68]

Inflammation

Sickle cell disease is an inflammatory state with abnormal endothelial cell activation.[68] Evidence for this in humans includes the persistent increase in leukocyte counts; ongoing activation of granulocytes and monocytes; chronic elevation of multiple proximate inflammatory mediators (eg, IL-6, TNF-α), acute-phase reactants (eg, C-reactive protein), and soluble adhesion molecules (eg, sVCAM-1); persistent activation of hemostatic systems; presence of nitrotyrosine-modified proteins in tissues; and exhibition of an activated, proadhesive and procoagulant phenotype for circulating endothelial cells. Clinically, leukocytosis in sickle cell disease is a risk factor for mortality,[77] clinical and silent stroke,[78,79] and acute chest syndrome,[80] and it helps predict which babies will develop a severe clinical course.[81] Acute vasoocclusive crises have been precipitated by growth factor induction of granulocytosis. In a large clinical trial demonstrating the efficacy of hydroxyurea, a drug that lowers the WBC count (among many other effects), the pain crisis rates correlated strongly with leukocyte counts.[82] Sickle transgenic mice seem to share with humans an inflammatory phenotype.[68]

Multiple mechanisms can underlie this inflammatory pathobiology. Infections and an iron-rich state may contribute. However, the pathobiology of sickle cell disease probably includes reperfusion injury physiology,[68,83–85] a postocclusive vascular pathobiology in which a cascade of events causes oxidative stress and induces inflammation.[86] This may involve a shift of xanthine oxidase from liver to plasma, with consequent deposition of this oxidant-generating enzyme on and in the vessel wall.[85] Reperfusion injury would damage the vascular wall and could lead to chronic vasculopathy. Adhesion of sickle RBCs itself incites an injury-like response by endothelial cells that may contribute to vascular pathobiology.[68] Another likely, but untested, possibility is that adherent sickle RBCs could directly activate blood monocytes and thereby incite inflammation. Regardless of proximate mechanism, the inflammatory phenotype of endothelium in sickle cell disease would highly promote RBC and WBC adhesion to the vessel wall.

Coagulation Activation

The coagulation system is chronically activated in sickle subjects, but more so during acute vasoocclusive episodes.[87] Described abnormalities include activation of plasmatic coagulation, platelets, and fibrinolysis, accompanied by thrombin generation and consumption of anti-thrombotic proteins. Tissue factor is abnormally expressed not only on blood monocytes, stimulated by C-reactive protein and other biologic mediators,[88] but also on circulating endothelial cells,[89] suggesting expression by vascular wall endothelium. Indeed, there are tissue factor positive endothelial cells in the sickle mouse.[90] Sickle blood contains tissue factor-positive microparticles derived from endothelial cells and monocytes, supporting the concept of an activation state. Correlative data indicate that the abnormally externalized phosphatidylserine on sickle RBCs plays a very significant accelerating role by providing a favorable surface template for lipid-dependent coagulation reactions.[91] About one half of sickle patients have antiphospholipid antibodies.[92] The role of thrombosis in sickle stroke and probably in pulmonary arteriopathy constitutes the most obvious involvement of the hemostatic system in sickle cell disease, but a contributory role for hemostatic activation in other clinical aspects of the disease has not been specifically excluded (see box on Coagulation Activation in Sickle Cell Anemia).

Vasoregulation

Sickle cell disease is a state of diminished NO bioavailability,[93] as evidenced by abnormal functional flow dynamics.[94,95] This may derive in part from abnormal consumption of NO by plasma hemoglobin,[96] the levels of which tend to be elevated early in crisis,[97] although it is not known whether such elevations precede the crisis. Other factors may play a role, such as endothelial dysfunction, consumption of NO by myeloperoxidase,[98] or exaggerated superoxide generation derived from vessel wall xanthine oxidase[85] or oxidation-induced uncoupling of NO synthase.[99] NO bioavailability seems to be higher for females than males, who exhibit substantial non-NO regulation of flow.[95] A role has been proposed for heme-oxygenase-1,[100,155] which has vasoprotective and vasoregulatory functions.[93] It has been suggested that sickle cell disease constitutes a state of enhanced instability of vascular tone,[93] and sickle patients are observed to exhibit abnormal capillary flow dynamics in the skin.[101] Systemic blood pressure in subjects with sickle cell disease is lower than in nonanemic, race-matched controls but higher than in comparably anemic, race-matched β-thalassemic patients.[102] Experimental interference with NO generation precipitated acute vasoocclusion and stroke in a rodent model of sickle cell disease.[103] Diminished NO bioavailability would also be expected to harmfully augment endothelial expression of VCAM-1, inflammatory effectors, and tissue factor (see box on Endothelial Biology of Sickle Cell Anemia).[68]

Coagulation Activation in Sickle Cell Anemia

Conversion of prothrombin to thrombin
Increased F 1.2 fragment
Thrombin generation
Increased thrombin : antithrombin complexes
Proteolysis of fibrinogen
Increased fibrinopeptide A
Degradation of cross-linked fibrin
Increased D-dimer
Formation and subsequent degradation of fibrin
Increased fragment E[a]
Activation of "intrinsic pathway"
Reduced factor levels
Activation of "extrinsic pathway"
Increased factor VII turnover
Inhibitor consumption
Reduced protein C, S, ATIII
Increased platelet activation
Activation antigen expression

Endothelial Biology of Sickle Cell Anemia

Coagulation activation →?thrombosis
Inflammation chronic →?vasculopathy
Abnormal vasoregulation → blood pressure, blood flow
Adhesion of WBC and RBC →?occlusion, inflammation
Abnormal NO bioavailability →?effects on coagulation and inflammation

PATHOGENESIS OF CLINICAL DISEASE

Hemolytic Anemia

At least three fundamental, proximate destructive mechanisms underlie the accelerated removal of sickle RBCs, which causes the anemia of sickle cell disease.

Poor Deformability

Deformability[43] and survival[75] are most abnormal for the very dense cell population, perhaps indicating some degree of causality.

Opsonization

Sickle RBCs are coated with immunoglobulin, which promotes their erythrophagocytosis.[72] Proximate triggers for this are mostly clustering of band 3 by means of denatured hemoglobin on the membrane[64] (see Fig. 42–8) and perhaps modification by malondialdehyde.[72] Externalized phosphatidylserine also promotes interaction with phagocytic cells.[74,104] The densest cells, including ISCs, have greater surface immunoglobulin[74] and high phosphatidylserine externalization,[67] and they exhibit greater erythrophagocytosis.[72]

Mechanical Fragility

Fragility plays some role, because it is estimated that about one third of RBC destruction takes place within the intravascular space.[105] The greatest stressor in this regard is likely to be cell sickling. A substantial portion of free hemoglobin in sickle plasma is encapsulated in microvesicles released from RBCs,[90] probably caused by sickling-induced perturbation of the bilayer[58] and augmented by protein oxidation[40] and dysfunction. The inverse relationship between (calculated) RBC polymer content and blood hemoglobin concentration is reported to be robust[106] or weak,[107] depending on rigor of the assumptions made. Hemolytic rate clearly is proportional to ISC count,[108] and life span is shortest for dense cells with low levels of HbF.[75] Improved RBC hydration caused by concurrent α-globin gene deletion improves survival and elevates the hemoglobin level.[109] The change in HbF levels in patients taking hydroxyurea is strongly associated with a change in RBC survival.[110]

Vasoocclusion

Vascular occlusion is believed to underlie the major clinical manifestations of sickle cell disease, particularly the most frequent event, the acute painful episode.[111] Notwithstanding the conceptual simplicity of the sickling phenomenon, it is likely that vasoocclusion is a complex and evolutionary process that involves multiple mechanisms and cell types. The likely roles of inflammation and reperfusion injury establish the probability that ongoing endothelial perturbation and activation may participate in disease genesis.[68] The endothelial biology of sickle cell disease can be influenced by concurrent illness. The long-held concept of a steady state of relative wellness between acute episodes can perhaps be more accurately described as an interlude in which the patient's symptoms do not reach the rather arbitrary threshold of requiring medical attention.[111] That steady state does not necessarily mean an absence of ongoing pathophysiology is supported by elevations and fluctuations of acute-phase reactants[68,112] and hemostatic markers[87] during the period. What is most striking in patients is a high level of clinical phenotypic diversity within a given genotype (eg, HbSS, HbSC).[1] It seems probable that this reflects the pathogenic participation of multiple biologic systems, even though HbS polymerization forms the fundamental, genetic basis for the clinical sickle syndromes.

Sickling

Intense sickling in the venous circulation probably contributes to the pathobiology of the pulmonary arterial system. Whether RBCs sickle elsewhere depends on the relationship between their inherent delay time and the degree and rate of deoxygenation.[25,26,31] Supporting the importance of polymerization are the facts that HbSC disease is clinically more severe than sickle trait (because the former has very dehydrated RBCs[44]) and that patients with Hb AS develop disease specifically in the hypoxic-acidotic renal environment. An inverse relationship between HbF and pain[113] and mortality[77] is supportive, but this is seen largely at the population level, and there is no such preventive effect for stroke.[114] Although the calculated polymer fraction is reported to correlate modestly with self-reported clinical severity,[115] more thorough analysis of polymer fraction using multiple physiologic variables showed no correlation with hospitalization rate.[107] Although α-gene deletion improves RBC hydration (and lowers ISC number), it does not improve clinical severity,[109] perhaps because of a resulting elevation of blood viscosity.

Adhesion and Inflammation

The fact that acute painful episodes often include multicentric pain[1] and are associated with distant flow changes in conjunctival vessels[116] perhaps indicates that the pain crisis is a systemic, rather than a strictly local, event. The ability of adherent WBCs or RBCs, or both, to slow the microvascular transit of RBCs may allow polymerization and occlusion.[25,26,31] Determinants of endothelial adhesivity, inflammation, and endothelial activation are probably important in this process. Supportive evidence from humans includes a clinical benefit from hydroxyurea,[82] which lowers RBC adhesivity[117,118] and WBC count.[82] Animal studies have been interpreted to suggest that adhesion-triggered occlusion occurs in the postcapillary venule,[69] but there are no confirmatory data from humans. Clinical vasoocclusive severity correlates with the endothelial adhesivity of sickle RBCs.[119]

Deformability

Deficient deformability[43] of RBCs can impede microvascular transit and even hinder the ability to enter the microvasculature in the first place. It has been proposed that precapillary arteriolar blockage might cause occlusion, but there is little evidence for this. Clinical vasoocclusive severity correlates with good deformability rather than the absence thereof.[120,121] There is no correlation between the fraction of cells having the highest density and crisis frequency,[122] and the least deformable cells seem to not correlate with clinical vasoocclusive severity.[123] However, in animals, poorly deformable cells begin to create a logjam and participate in occlusion after adhesive cells have initiated partial obstruction (see Fig. 42–10),[69,71] and there are changes of observable cell density associated with acute crisis.[43]

Other Factors

Activation of the coagulation system[87] may contribute to development of ischemic stroke and to pulmonary arterial disease, but the extent to which it contributes to other occlusive manifestations is insufficiently tested. A role for diminished NO bioavailability[93] and concomitant impairment of endothelial function[68] is beginning to be explored. Nonetheless, an acute change in NO bioavailability is an interesting candidate precipitant for occlusive events.

CHRONIC VASCULOPATHY

It is not clear whether the pathogenesis of the organ-specific clinical syndromes in sickle cell disease is the same or different from genesis of the acute painful episode. Development of complicating syndromes does not necessarily occur in those having the highest pain crisis frequency; for example, a low pain rate is a risk factor for silent stroke.[79] Sickle cell disease includes a component of chronic vasculopathy,[68,124] although this is an incompletely evaluated concept. The most information is available for disease in the large or medium vessels at the circle of Willis, where some children develop occlusive pathology characterized by intimal hyperplasia, fibrotic and proliferative changes, and damage to internal elastic lamina.[103] Similar pathologic changes have been observed in large vessels in the spleen in children,[125] in umbilical vessels,[126] and in the pulmonary arterial tree.[127] The accompanying clinical syndromes in these four high-flow organs are, respectively, ischemic stroke,[128] autosplenectomy,[129] fetal wastage and growth retardation,[130] and pulmonary hypertension.[131] Sickle vasculopathy shares with atherosclerotic disease a nonrandom-ness of location, a likely proximate role for inflammation, and a fundamental pathologic change (ie, intimal hyperplasia). Although sickle vasculopathy does not include a fatty streak (sickle patients have low blood lipid levels[132]), in vitro stimulation of endothelial cells by an inflammatory mediator, IL-1β, promotes formation from the membrane of the same oxidized lipid species implicated in early development of the atherosclerotic lesion.[133] Other contributing factors may be persistently increased shear rates, chronic hypoxia, and ongoing perturbation by sickled or adherent RBCs. Thrombosis probably is a late aspect of this process in the brain,[103,128] but the timing of its development in lung[134] is unclear. It is not known whether the occurrence of vasculopathy in one organ correlates with its appearance in others, and the pace of its temporal development is not well defined. However, it recently has been suggested that the commonality of hemolypsis (and NO consumption) may link the various vasculopathy events.[157] Thus, the presence of the vasculopathy suggests that novel therapeutic approaches, such as use of statins and other antiinflammatory drugs, should be tested experimentally. Because NO and CO inhibit development of experimental intimal hyperplasia, the deficient NO and excessive CO in sickle cell disease may affect vessel wall biology.

MORTALITY

Adult patients with higher pain crisis rates (ie, three or more per year) have a higher mortality rate.[77] This relationship is not evident for children, possibly because time-dependent disease effects have not fully accumulated. It seems likely, but has not been demonstrated, that extent of presumed subclinical disease activity would be proportional to severity of clinically evident disease. Approximately one-third of deaths occur during acute complications such as pain, stroke, or acute chest syndrome, and many are caused by overt organ failure (usually renal). Infection continues to contribute. Notable risk factors for mortality are low HbF levels and a WBC count higher than 15,000 per μL.[77] A decade ago in the United States, the median age at death was 42 years for men and 48 years for women with sickle cell anemia; the comparable ages were 60 and 68 years, respectively, for HbSC disease.[77] This statistic improved markedly after the introduction of prophylactic penicillin for children,[135] indicating the dramatic loss of dominance for pneumococcal sepsis in disease natural history.

Stroke

Clinical and silent strokes are a frequent complication of sickle cell disease.[103,114,128] Ischemic stroke develops in early childhood and is particularly associated with large- and medium-vessel occlusive changes at the circle of Willis that involve hyperplastic intimal changes in the vessel wall.[128] However, a significant portion of patients also have small-vessel disease.[136] Identified risk factors include low blood levels of hemoglobin, high WBC counts, relatively high blood pressure, acute development of hypoxia, a prior neurologic event, presence of moyamoya, low pain crisis rate, and concurrent or antecedent inflammatory conditions.[79,114,128] The fact that a history of acute chest syndrome is a (see Chapter 43) notable antecedent event is of particular interest, in view of the relatively common role of *Chlamydia* infection in this syndrome[137] and the contrasting hypothesized role for this agent in atherosclerotic disease.[138] The classic inherited risk factors for thrombosis seem not to be associated with stroke in the sickle context, but concurrent α-thalassemia or HbSC disease lower the risk. However, the HbF level is not protective.[114] There is a familial tendency[139] and a relationship to human leukocyte antigen (HLA) type.[140]

For the most part, identified risk factors are those for any acute stroke event. It is not entirely clear whether the same or different risk factors account for the underlying vessel wall disease. Known facets of sickle cell disease that could play an etiologic role include activation of the coagulation system and antiphospholipid antibodies, inflammation and endothelial cell activation, RBC or WBC adhesion to the vascular wall, and disturbances of NO bioavailability.[68] It is possible that inherited differences in endothelial gene expression influence this clinical phenotype,[68] as has recently been shown for inflammation signalling.[158] The relationship of sickle stroke to the background of increased risk for stroke in the general African American population is not established. It is not clear whether ischemic stroke in adults involves exactly the same process as in children or additional processes supervene over time. Among persons with sickle cell disease, young adults have the highest rates of hemorrhagic stroke.[114]

Pulmonary Disease

Sickle pulmonary disease includes multiple pathologies, including fibrosis, pulmonary hypertension, infection, in situ and embolic thrombosis, and acute chest syndrome.[78,131,134,141,142] The lung is a common target organ of inflammation biology in general, and it seems likely that endothelial perturbation from the persistent flooding of the pulmonary arterial tree with sickled cells from the venous circulation plays a role in some pulmonary syndromes.[68]

Acute chest syndrome is particularly important as a life-threatening event and as a predictor of chronic lung disease[143] and stroke.[114] Risk factors include[80,142,159] leukocytosis, lower hemoglobin levels, and a lower level of HbF, implying etiologic roles for inflammation, deficient NO bioavailability, and RBC sickling, respectively. Infection plays a greater role in children, whereas in adults, acute chest syndrome often is associated with acute painful episodes.[142] Fat embolism is commonly associated with acute chest syndrome,[142] probably as a consequence of marrow infarction and accompanying elevation of blood phospholipase A_2 activity,[144] which can generate fatty acids that permeabilize pulmonary endothelium and augment the endothelial perturbing effects of hypoxia.[145] Additional contributing processes may include rib pain causing atelectasis, a tendency toward pulmonary endothelial permeability caused by elevated levels of vascular endothelial growth factor (VEGF)[68] and high-dose opioid administration, hypoxemia and sickling, RBC adhesion to endothelium, and even iatrogenic fluid overload. Deficient NO bioavailability[93,95] is implicated in pulmonary hypertension,[159] and it allows augmented tissue factor and VCAM expression, which are likely participants in the acute chest syndrome. It appears that multiple proximate triggering events (eg, rib pain, infection, fat embolism) lead to a syndrome in which inflammation, NO deficiency, and endothelial permeability conspire to augment the deleterious effects of hypoxia on the pulmonary endothelium.

Retinopathy

Sickle cell disease is associated with neovascularizing retinopathy; the risk is higher in HbSC disease than in sickle cell anemia.[146] Although this difference is postulated to be a consequence of higher blood viscosity in HbSC disease, the risk for retinopathy seems to be greater with a higher hemolytic rate (ie, higher reticulocyte count and lower hemoglobin concentration).[147] Greater anemia and increased numbers of adhesive RBCs can increase hypoxia, which stimulated the generation of VEGF, a major angiogenesis-promoting growth factor. VEGF has been found in human sickle retinopathy lesions,[148] and the blood concentration tends to be elevated in sickle cell disease.[149]

BASIS OF PHENOTYPIC DIVERSITY

The remarkable diversity of clinical phenotypes in sickle cell anemia is largely unexplained. This disease provides a dramatic illustration of a paradigm in which a single-gene disorder is exceedingly complex and produces a "polygenic" disease. The phenotype can be significantly influenced by geography, infectious disease, and other environmental factors.[3] In countries with lower infant mortality and childhood infection rates, phenotypic variability is especially evident. An emerging story is a gender difference in apparent NO bioavailability,[93,95] which is unexplained but corresponds to the gender difference in longevity.[77] The benefits of coinherited genetic influences are probably understood virtually entirely by their impact on hemoglobin polymerization, the sickling phenomenon, and hemolysis.

Level of Hemoglobin F

After the fall in HbF level occurring during the first 6 months of life,[150] most of the protection from RBC sickling that derived from the high HbF level at birth is lost, but the HbF level still varies among adults over a 20-fold range. Viewed from a population level, protection from pain and mortality is conferred as a continuous function of the Hb F level,[77,113] but some clinical complications are forestalled by HbF (eg, acute chest syndrome[80]) and others are not (eg, stroke[114]). The HbF level reflects the number of F cells, the amount of HbF per F cell, and the preferential survival of F cells compared with cells containing low levels of Hb F.[32,53] The known determinants of the HbF level probably account for only about one half of its variance: the polymorphic *Xmn*I site 5′ to the Gγ gene (about 10% of the variance) in the Senegal and Arab-India β^S haplotypes (see Fig. 42–3A) and female gender (about 40% of variance).[109] The effect of gender may result in part from greater NO bioavailability,[95] because NO promotes HbF production.[151]

α-Thalassemia

Because of duplication of the α-globin gene, the normal genotype is αα/αα. About 30% of people in the United States with West African ancestry have a single α deletion (–α/αα),[109] so concordance with sickle cell disease is common, and homozygosity for the allele is seen (–α/–α). α-Thalassemia is uncommon in Greeks with sickle cell disease, but in eastern Saudi Arabia and India, α-thalassemia occurs in more than 50% of the sickle population.[12] An α-gene deletion has minimal effect on the HbF level but results in improved RBC hydration (see Fig. 42–7), a lower ISC count, improved RBC survival, and high blood levels of hemoglobin.[109] Surprisingly, there is no parallel amelioration of clinical severity, and some complications (eg, osteonecrosis, retinopathy) increase,[109] possibly because of increased blood viscosity. However, α-thalassemia may ameliorate HbSC disease somewhat.[152]

β-Globin Alleles

Compound heterozygosity for the sickle gene and another β allele can affect the clinical phenotype.[153] In deletional HPFH, coinheritance of a pancellular high level of HbF results in about 20% to 30% HbF (but no HbA) and a dramatic amelioration of disease severity. Benefit from concurrent β^+-thalassemia can be quite variable, depending on level of HbA (which ranges from approximately 10% to 30%). In contrast, concurrent β^o-thalassemia has no HbA and manifests a typical sickle cell anemia-like syndrome. HbSC disease presents a unique case that should be clinically similar to sickle trait (see Fig. 42–5A), but interaction of HbC with the RBC membrane causes a striking stimulation of K–Cl cotransport and consequent RBC dehydration.[154] Combined with the somewhat higher HbS concentration (about 50% versus about 40% in HbAS) and higher blood hemoglobin level, this yields a clinical sickling disorder only somewhat less severe than sickle cell anemia and having an increased propensity for retinopathy and osteonecrosis.[152]

Other interesting situations are created by concurrence of HbS and HbD-Los Angeles ($\beta^{121Glu\rightarrow Gln}$) or HbO-Arab ($\beta^{121Glu\rightarrow Lys}$), which have unusually severe phenotypes that are hypothesized to result from heightened polymer stability (and reduced solubility) caused by β^{121} substitutions. An even more remarkable example is provided by the unique double mutation in HbS-Antilles ($\beta^{6Glu\rightarrow Val}$ and $\beta^{23Val\rightarrow Ile}$), which has such reduced solubility that it causes clinical sickle cell disease in the heterozygous state.[153]

Unexplained Phenotypic Diversity

Notwithstanding these well-defined influences, affected individuals still exhibit enormous unexplained variability in clinical phenotype. The complex diversity of physiologies that potentially participate in the vasoocclusive disease, chronic vasculopathy, and specific complicating syndromes predicts a variety of possibilities. It is likely that this complexity is influenced by underlying genetic variations in adhesion molecule biology, determinants of RBC cation homeostasis, inflammatory signaling or negative-feedback loops, propensity for angiogenesis or vessel wall injury, oxidant-antioxidant biology, hemostasis, or regulation of vascular tone and blood flow. It remains to be seen how substantial the influence of such differences may be.

It is likely that the contribution of such additional genetic influences will begin to be identified now that modern genomic approaches are being applied to the problem of phenotypic diversity in sickle cell disease. In this regard, studies of stroke are the most advanced.[158,160] Sadly, factors such as environment, nutrition, socioeconomic status, endemic infection rates, and availability of medical care also remain contributors.

SUGGESTED READINGS

Ballas SK, Mohandas N: Sickle Red cell microrheology and sickle blood rheology. Microcirculation 11:209, 2004.

Browne P, Shalev O, Hebbel RP: The molecular pathobiology of cell membrane iron: the sickle red cell as a model. Free Radic Biol Med 24:1040, 1998.

Embury SH: the not-so-simple process of sickle cell vasoocclusion. Microcirculation 11:101, 2004.

Ferrone FA: Polymerization and sickle cell disease: a molecular view. Microcirculation 11:115, 2004.

Francis, Jr. RB, Hebbel RP: Hemostasis. In Embury SH, Hebbel RP, Mohandas N and Steinberg MH (eds): Sickle Cell Disease: Basic Principles and Clinical Practice. New York, Raven Press, 1994, p 299.

Goodman SR: The irreversibly sickled cell: a perspective. Cell Mol Biol 50:53, 2004.

Hebbel RP, Osarogiagbon R, Kaul D: The endothelial biology of sickle cell disease: inflammation and a chronic vasculopathy. Microcirculation 11:129, 2004.

Kaul DK, Fabry ME: In vivo studies of sickle red blood cells. Microcirculation 11:153, 2004.

Lew VL, Bookchin RM: Ion transport pathology in the mechanism of sickle cell dehydration. Physiol Rev 85:179, 2005.

Lubin B, Kuypers F, Chiu D: Red cell membrane lipid dynamics. Prog Clin Biol Res 319:507, 1989.

Nagel RL, Steinberg MH: Genetics of the β^S gene: Origins, epidemiology, and epistasis in sickle cell anemia. In Steinberg MH, Forget BG, Higgs DR, Nagel RL (eds): Disorders of Hemoglobin: Genetics, Pathophysiology, and Clinical Management. Cambridge, Cambridge University Press, 2001, p 711.

Nath KA, Katusic ZS, Gladwin MT: The perfusion paradox and vascular instability in sickle cell disease. Microcirculation 11:117, 2004.

Steinberg MH, Adewoye AH: Modifier genes and sickle cell anemia. Curr Opin Hematol 13:131, 2006.

REFERENCES

For complete list of references log onto www.expertconsult.com

CHAPTER 43

SICKLE CELL DISEASE—CLINICAL FEATURES AND MANAGEMENT

Yogen Saunthararajah and Elliott P. Vichinsky

INTRODUCTION

Sickle cell disease is an inherited disorder in which patients inherit specific mutated variants of the β-globin gene that lead to hemoglobin polymerization. The sickle mutation of the β-globin gene results in the production of an abnormal hemoglobin called sickle hemoglobin (Hb S). The sickle mutation has undergone positive selection during human evolution because individuals with one copy of the sickle gene and one normal β-globin gene (sickle cell trait) have a survival advantage in malaria-endemic regions. In individuals with two copies of the sickle gene (Hb SS or sickle cell anemia) or the sickle mutation and another mutated β-globin gene, for example, sickle cell–β° thalassemia (Hb S–β thal) or Hb SC disease (Hb SC), the less soluble Hb S can polymerize in deoxygenated regions of the circulation, resulting in hemolysis, red-cell rigidity, and red-cell adhesion to endothelium with consequent inflammatory and coagulation pathway activation and vasoocclusion.[1] The cardinal clinical manifestations of these processes are chronic hemolytic anemia, recurrent painful episodes, and chronic organ damage. A comprehensive approach directed at preventing pain crises, chronic organ damage and early mortality while effectively managing acute complications, offers the best method of management. The further exigency of living with a painful, life-threatening chronic disease in an ethnically diverse society provides additional complexity to the psychosocial aspects of this illness. This chapter presents the diagnosis and natural history and describes overall clinical management as well as specific management by organ complications. Clinical interventions are founded on an understanding of the pathophysiologic processes that underlie the disease. For a full discussion of the fascinating history and molecular pathology of this disease, please see Chapter 42. Normal hemoglobin synthesis, structure, and function are described in Chapter 33; the thalassemias are considered in Chapter 41.

Prevalence

The distribution and frequency of the sickle cell gene in different areas of the world have been influenced by evolutionary pressures[2] and transmission of the gene via trade routes and the slave trade.[3] Among African Americans, the prevalence of sickle cell trait is 8% to 10% among newborns,[4] and in this population the frequencies of the sickle cell (0.045), Hb C (0.015), and β thalassemia (0.004) genes[4] indicate that there are 4000 to 5000 pregnancies a year at risk for sickle cell disease. The burden of this disease in the United States is dwarfed by that in the rest of the world, as evidenced by a prevalence of the sickle cell gene as high as 25% to 30% in western Africa and an estimated annual birth of 120,000 babies with sickle cell disease in Africa.[5]

DIAGNOSIS

The diagnosis of a sickle cell syndrome is suggested by characteristic findings on the complete blood count and peripheral smear which then require confirmation with hemoglobin electrophoresis. If a diagnosis of sickle cell disease is confirmed, evaluation of the various organ systems at risk is required. These evaluations are outlined and discussed later in this chapter in the section on clinical management.

Complete Blood Count and Peripheral Blood Smear

The chronic hemolytic anemia of sickle cell disease is usually associated with mild to moderately low hematocrit and hemoglobin levels and a reticulocytosis of approximately 3% to 15%, accounting for high or high-normal MCV. If the age-adjusted MCV is not elevated, the possibility of sickle cell–β thalassemia, coincident α thalassemia, or iron deficiency must be considered. Additional laboratory findings of hemolysis are unconjugated hyperbilirubinemia, elevated lactate dehydrogenase, and low haptoglobin levels.

In the peripheral smear (Fig. 43–1), there may be sickled forms, target cells, polychromasia indicative of reticulocytosis, and Howell–Jolly bodies demonstrating hyposplenia. The red cells are normochromic unless there is coexistent thalassemia or iron deficiency. Sickled forms (ISCs) occur in the peripheral smear only in the sickle cell diseases and not in sickle cell trait. In Hb SS disease, ISCs predominate and target cells may be few; in sickle cell–β thalassemia, ISCs, target cells, and hypochromic microcytic discocytes are prominent; in Hb SC disease, target cells predominate and ISCs are rare.

White cell counts are higher than normal in Hb SS disease, particularly in patients under age 10 years. Mean white cell counts tend not to be elevated in Hb SC disease or sickle cell–β^+ thalassemia. Mean platelet counts are elevated in Hb SS disease, particularly in patients under age 18 years, but are usually normal in those with Hb SC disease and sickle cell–β^+ thalassemia.

Solubility Tests and Hemoglobin Electrophoresis

Solubility tests (eg, Sickledex) are positive in both sickle cell disease and sickle cell trait. All patients require definitive diagnosis with hemoglobin electrophoresis (which separates hemoglobin species according to amino acid composition) (Fig. 43–2) or DNA testing. Cellulose acetate electrophoresis at pH 8.4 is a standard method of separating Hb S from other variants. However, Hb S, G, and D have the same electrophoretic mobility with this method. Using citrate agar electrophoresis at pH 6.2, Hb S has a different mobility than Hb D and G, which comigrate with Hb A in this system (see Chapter 40).

Results from electrophoresis or thin-layer isoelectric focusing are similar in Hb SS disease and sickle cell–β° thalassemia: nearly all the hemoglobin consists of Hb S. Although differences in the Hb F (see Variant Sickle Cell Syndromes) and Hb A_2 levels may be useful in distinguishing these syndromes, the presence of microcytosis or of one parent without sickle cell trait is a more useful indicator of sickle cell–β° thalassemia. The diagnosis of Hb SC disease is straightforward; nearly equal amounts of Hb S and Hb C are detected. Sickle cell–β^+ thalassemia and sickle cell trait both have substantial amounts of Hb A and Hb S. This superficial electrophoretic similarity does not provide an obstacle to diagnosis: sickle cell trait is associated with neither anemia nor microcytosis and has an Hb A fraction more than 50%,[6] whereas sickle cell–β^+ thalassemia is associated with anemia, microcytosis, and an Hb A fraction that ranges from 5% to 30%.

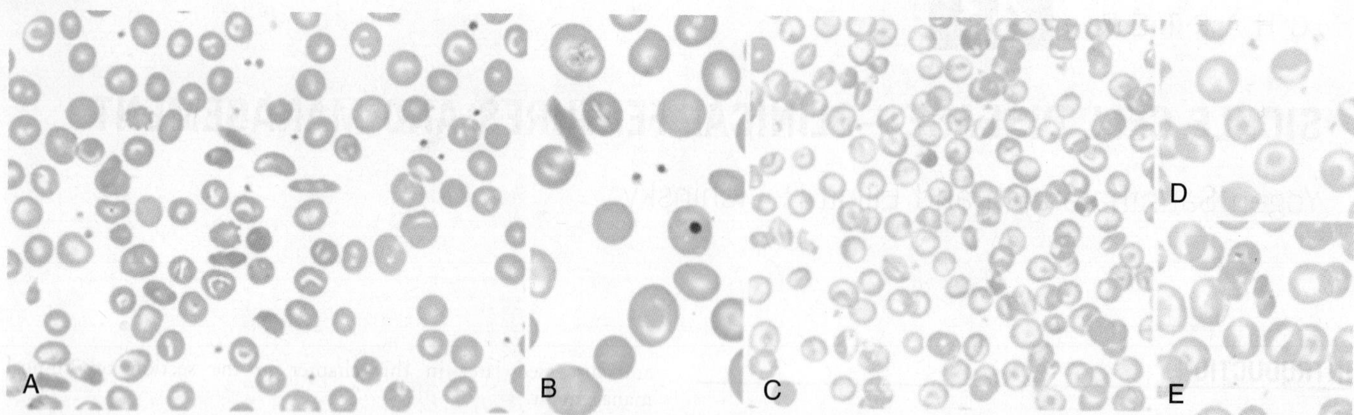

Figure 43–1 Sickle cell disease and Hb SC, peripheral blood smears (**A–E**). The peripheral smear in sickle cell disease (**A**) shows sickle cells that are mostly irreversibly sickled, and sometimes referred to as "cigar-forms." Higher power detail (**B**) shows sickle cell (upper left), red blood cell containing a Howell–Jolly body (middle right), and polychromatophilic cell (lower center). These indicate sickle cell anemia, splenic dysfunction, but marrow response with reticulocytosis, respectively. Peripheral smear of a patient with Hgb SC (**C**) shows no sickled cell, but there are target forms (**D**) and occasional cells (**E**) with hemoglobin condensed at each pole of the cell.

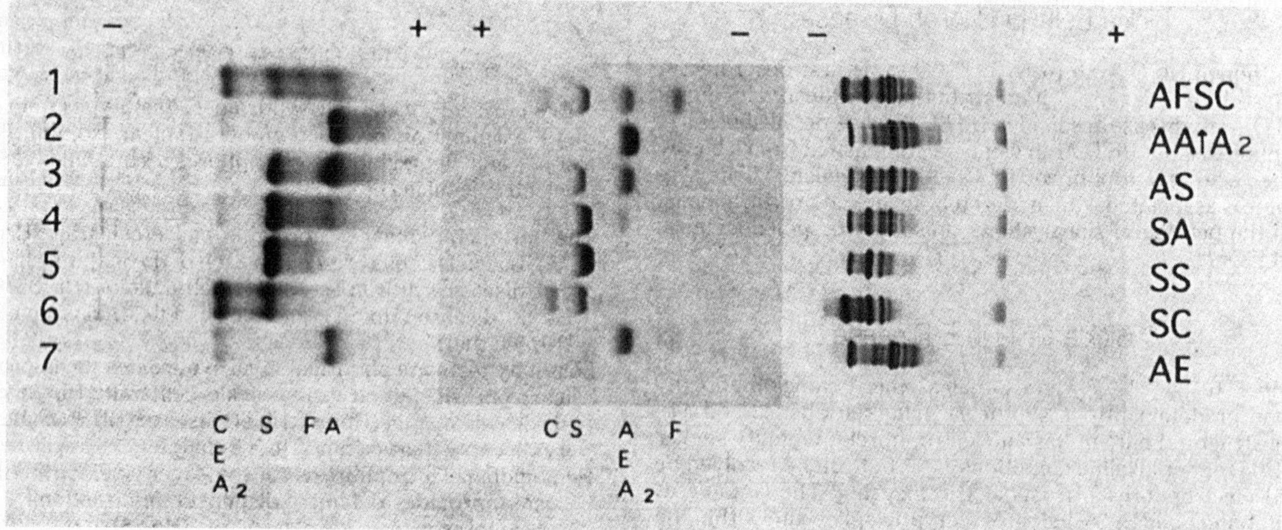

Figure 43–2 Comparative analyses of several mutant hemoglobins using alkaline electrophoresis, acid electrophoresis, and thin-layer isoelectric focusing. On the right are shown the components of the standard (at the top) and the phenotypes of the other six samples. Their analyses are shown by alkaline hemoglobin electrophoresis in the left panel, acid electrophoresis in the center panel, and thin-layer isoelectric focusing in the right panel. Locations of the various hemoglobin bands are shown below the left and center panels. *(Kindly provided by M. H. Steinberg.)*

The Hb F level is usually slightly to moderately elevated; the degree varies among patients. The amount of Hb F present is a function of the number of reticulocytes that contain Hb F, the extent of selective survival of Hb F-containing reticulocytes to become mature Hb F-containing erythrocytes (F cells), and the amount of Hb F per F cell.[7] The Arab–Indian and Senegal haplotypes are associated with higher levels of Hb F than the others.[8]

Newborn Screening

The use of prophylactic penicillin[9] and the provision of comprehensive medical care during the first 5 years of life have reduced mortality from approximately 25% to less than 3%, thereby providing impetus for early identification of infants with sickle cell disease. Based on its economy and superiority of detection, universal screening of all newborns is preferred over ethnically targeted approaches.[10,11] Blood samples for testing are obtained by heel stick and spotted onto filter paper for stable transport and subsequent high-performance liquid chromatography.[12] Results of solubility testing may be invalid because of the large amount of Hb F present.

Characterization of adult hemoglobins is challenging in the fetal and newborn periods because of the predominance of Hb F, which confounds reliable detection of Hb S by solubility testing. In infancy, the diagnosis of sickle cell disease is also influenced by the absence of anemia. As Hb S increases and Hb F declines in the first months of life (Fig. 43–3), the clinical manifestations of sickle cell disease emerge.[13] ISCs can be seen on the peripheral blood smear (Fig. 43–4) of children with sickle cell anemia at 3 months of age, and by 4 months of age moderately severe hemolytic anemia is evident.

A requirement for tests used in newborn screening is the capability to distinguish Hb F, S, A, and C. The patterns of hemoglobins present are described in descending order according to the quantities detected. Therefore, a newborn with sickle cell anemia who has predominantly Hb F, with a small amount of Hb S and no Hb A, is described as having an FS pattern. An FS pattern is obtained also in newborns who have sickle cell–β° thalassemia, sickle cell–hereditary persistence of fetal hemoglobin (HPFH), and sickle cell–Hb D or sickle cell–Hb G (ie, Hb D and E have the same electrophoretic mobility as Hb S). The newborn with sickle cell trait will have Hb F, Hb A, and Hb S (FAS pattern). The quantity of Hb A is greater than that of Hb S. If the quantity of Hb S exceeds that of Hb A, the

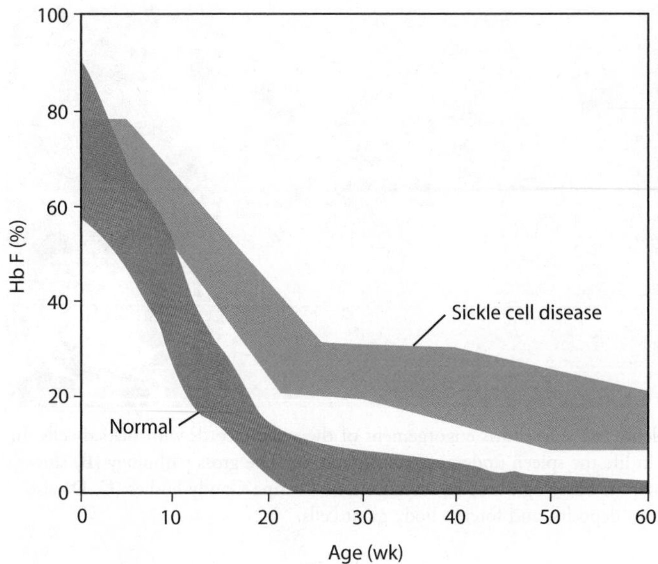

Figure 43–3 Hb F decline in children with hemoglobins AA and SS. *(Data from O'Brien, Mclatosh S, Aspnes AT, et al: Prospective study of sickle cell anemia in infancy. J Pediatr 89(2):205, 1976.)*

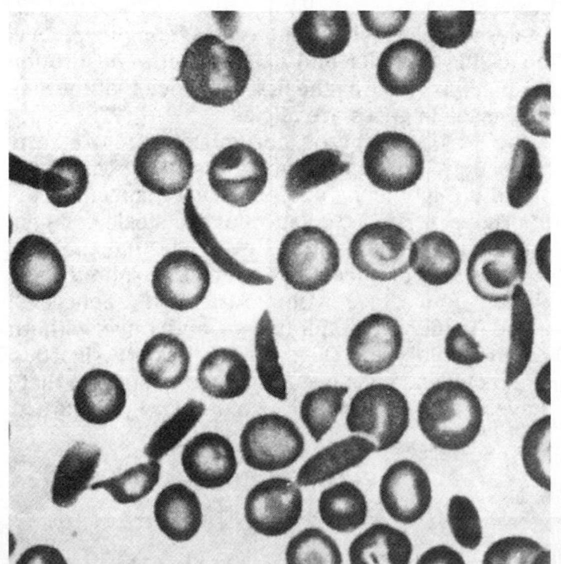

Figure 43–4 Peripheral blood smears showing the peculiar elongated forms of the red corpuscles (originally seen by Herrick). (*With permission from Herrick JB: Peculiar elongated and sickle-shaped red blood corpuscles in a case of severe anemia. Arch Intern Med 6:517, 1910.*)

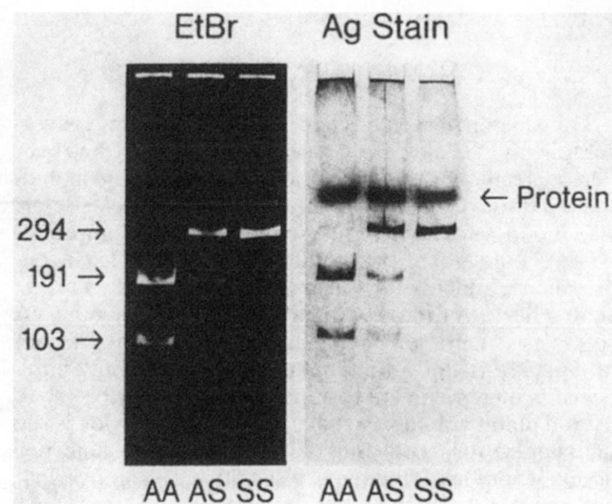

Figure 43–5 PCR-based restriction analysis for the sickle cell gene. The genotypes of the DNA samples tested are shown below. The size in base pairs for the undigested PCR product and the products resulting from Oxa Nl are shown at left in base pairs. The fragments from normal β-globin DNA (AA) shows complete Oxa Nl cleavage, from sickle cell trait DNA (AS) shows partial cleavage, and from sickle cell anemia (SS) shows no cleavage.

presumptive diagnosis is sickle cell–β^+ thalassemia (FSA pattern). It may not be possible to distinguish FAS and FSA patterns in newborns, so DNA-based testing or repeat hemoglobin testing at age 3 to 6 months is recommended.

Prenatal Diagnosis

One large survey found that parents at risk for having a child with sickle cell disease were interested in prenatal diagnosis and would consider termination of pregnancy for an affected fetus.[14] Community acceptance of reproductive genetic services depends on the effectiveness of education and counseling. One major ethical issue pertains to our diagnostic skills' having outstripped our ability to predict the severity of diagnosable conditions.

Fetal DNA samples are obtained by chorionic villus sampling at 8 to 10 weeks' gestation. Polymerase chain reaction (PCR)-based methods for detecting the sickle gene include restriction analysis (Fig. 43–5), allele-specific hybridization, reverse dot-blotting, and allele-specific fluorescence PCR. PCR-based diagnosis for Hb SC disease is possible using specific molecular methods for detecting the Hb C gene, and the diagnosis of sickle cell–β thalassemia can be made using reverse dot-blot methodology to screen the many African American β thalassemia mutations, as well as the Hb S and Hb C mutations, in a single hybridization reaction.

CLINICAL PRESENTATION AND MANAGEMENT

The cardinal clinical manifestations of sickle cell disease are chronic hemolytic anemia, recurrent painful episodes, and chronic organ damage, particularly of the spleen, bones, brain, kidneys, lungs, skin, and heart. The pattern of disease varies among the major genotypes of Hb SS, Hb SC, and Hb S–β thalassemia but also within the same genotype. Some of this variability results from additional inherited genotypes, for example, α thalassemia or HPFH (discussed at the end of this chapter). Typically, patients are anemic but lead a relatively normal life punctuated by painful episodes. However, it is important to realize that chronic organ damage and decreased survival occur even in patients who do not have recurrent pain. This section begins with a brief overview of natural history and survival followed by a discussion of basic management that has as its aim improving this natural history (disease modification). This is followed by a discussion of organ-specific complications and their management.

Natural History and Life Expectancy

The manifestations of disease begin after the first few months of life as Hb F levels decline and Hb S levels increase. Certain complications predominate in particular age groups: between the ages of 1 and 3, splenomegaly and splenic sequestration (see Fig. 43–6), and pneumonia and meningitis from *Streptococcus pneumoniae* and other encapsulated organisms (because of functional hyposplenism), as well as a hand–foot syndrome; in early childhood, stroke, acute chest syndrome, and osteonecrosis; in midchildhood, pain crises, osteonecrosis, and acute chest syndrome; between ages 12 and 20, strokes, priapism, and pain crises; between ages 20 and 30, renal insufficiency, pulmonary hypertension, disabling osteonecrosis, retinopathy, leg

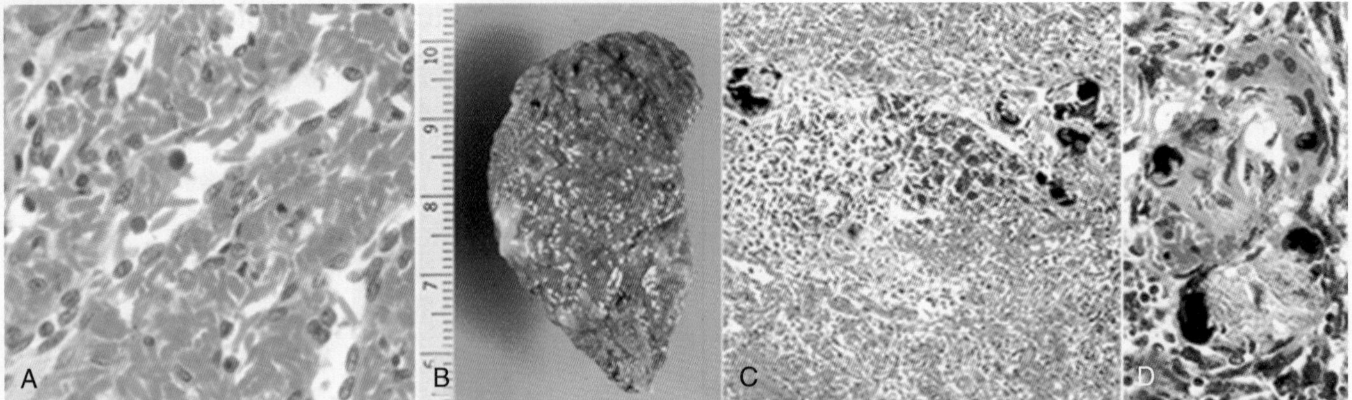

Figure 43–6 Spleen in sickle cell disease (**A–D**). Histologic section (**A**) of the splenic red pulp shows engorgement of the splenic cords with sickled cells. In infants, excessive pooling in cords can lead to a splenic sequestration crisis. Later in life the spleen undergoes autoinfarction. The gross pathology (**B**) shows a tiny 4.5-cm spleen with rough external surface due to scarring from repeated infarcts. Histologic section reveals classic Gamna-Gandy bodies (**C, D**) also due to repeated infarction. These comprise hemosiderin-laden macrophages, calcium deposits, and foreign body giant cells.

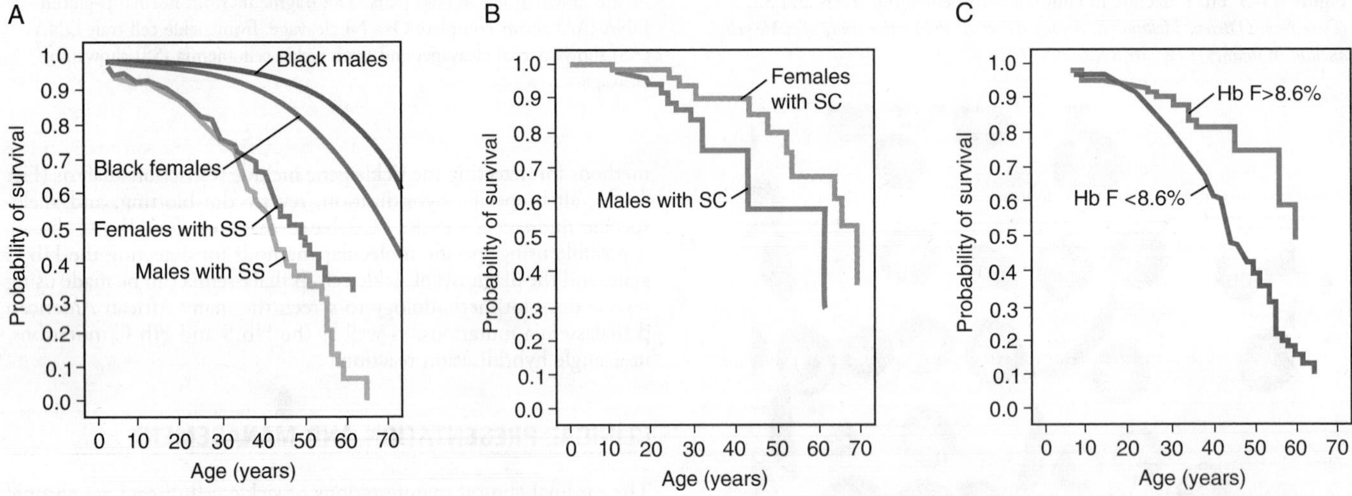

Figure 43–7 Life expectancy. *(From Platt OS, Brambilla DJ, Rosse WF, et al: Mortality in sickle cell disease. Life expectancy and risk factors for early death. N Engl J Med 330(23):1639, 1994.)*

ulcers, and pain crises; and at age more than 30, congestive heart failure, renal failure, and pain crises.

Patients have decreased life expectancy, although in the past 30 years, this has dramatically improved for patients in the West. In 1973 Diggs reported that the mean survival was 14.3 years[15]; in 1994 Platt et al reported that life expectancy was 42 years for men and 48 years for women with sickle cell anemia (Fig. 43–7).[16] This improvement in survival is most likely the result of improved general medical care, including prophylactic penicillin therapy and vaccination against *S pneumoniae*.[9] These survival profiles are likely to be relevant even today, although a cohort of patients followed since 1975 show improvement in the probability of survival to age 20 compared with patients born before 1975 (89% vs 79%).[17] The poor survival and litany of chronic organ damage in survivors emphasizes the need for disease-modifying interventions to prevent vasculopathy.[17] There are indications that disease-modifying agents such as hydroxyurea can improve survival.[18]

Predictors of Disease Severity

The ability to predict clinical course would allow more rational tailoring of therapy to individual patients (e.g., selection of patients for high-risk but effective options such as stem cell transplant). Higher HbF levels and the coinheritance of an α thalassemia trait have been identified as favorable disease modifiers in multiple studies (Table 43–1).[19–21] The level of chronic anemia (which is influenced by the presence of an α thalassemia trait and by Hb F levels) is of considerable predictive value. Patients with more severe anemia are more likely to develop infarctive and hemorrhagic stroke,[22] to have glomerular dysfunction,[23,24] and perhaps to give birth to low-birthweight babies.[25,26] Conversely, they have fewer episodes of acute chest syn-

Table 43–1 Effect of α Thalassemia on the Level of Anemia in Sickle Cell Anemia

Reference	αα/αα*	–α/αα	–α/–α
Embury et al[240]	7.8† (*n* = 25)‡	9.7 (*n* = 18)	9.2 (*n* = 4)
Higgs et al[241]	7.8 (*n* = 88)	8.1 (*n* = 44)	8.8 (*n* = 44)
Steinberg et al[242]	8.0 (*n* = 73)	9.0 (*n* = 39)	9.5 (*n* = 13)
Felice et al, age 5 years[243]	8.6 (*n* = 88)	8.4 (*n* = 52)	8.3 (*n* = 50)
Felice et al, age 11 years[243]	7.9 (*n* = 40)	8.5 (*n* = 34)	9.6 (*n* = 2)

*The different α-globin genotypes indicate the presence of four (αα/αα), three (–α/αα), or two (–α/–α) α-globin genes.
†The mean Hb level (g/dL) for each group is shown.
‡The number of subjects in each group is denoted by n.

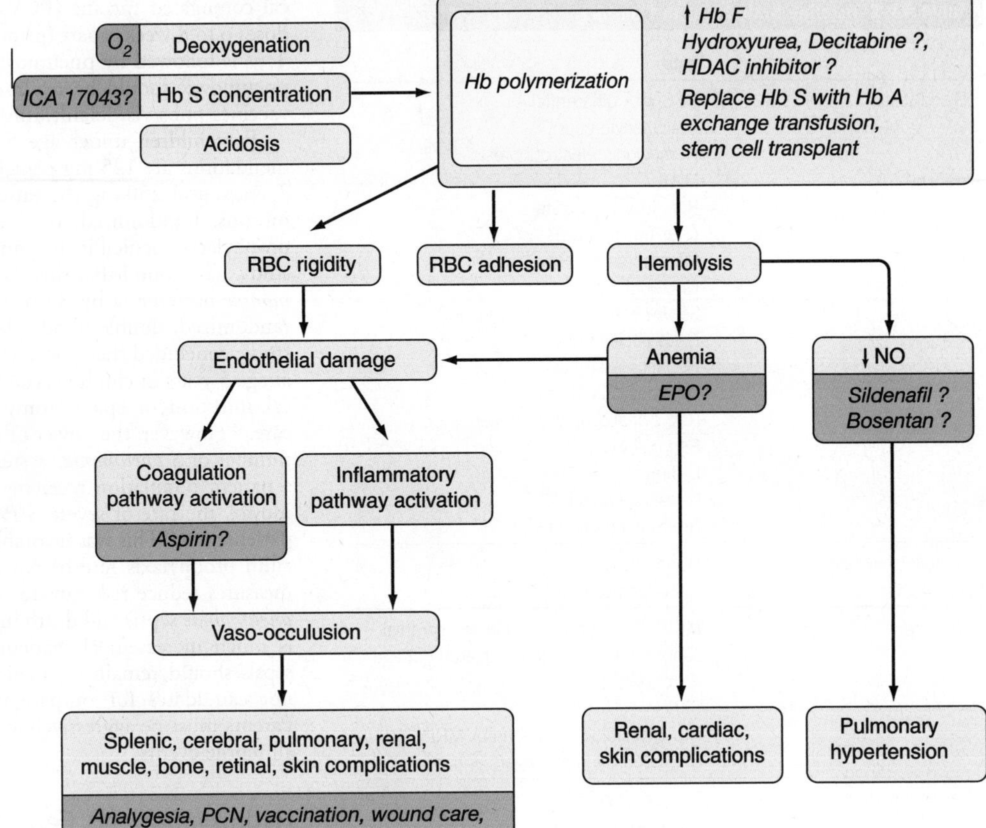

Figure 43–8 Where therapeatics intervene in the pathophyrsiological cascade.

drome,[27] and (after age 20 years) a lower mortality rate.[27] Progressive anemia from renal endocrine deficiency and/or decrease in bone marrow function from vasoocclusion is associated with early death.[18]

There are a number of other genetic polymorphisms that may be relevant to disease severity, for example, with regards to the risk of stroke. However, most of these markers are not widely used to guide decision making.[20]

Principles of Management

The twin pillars of therapy are disease modification (prevention of crises, complications, chronic organ damage, and early mortality) and compassionate, prompt, effective and safe relief of acute crises, including pain episodes. Therefore, outpatient clinic management is mostly directed at initiating measures to prevent pain crises, prevent organ complications and improve survival. An effort should be made to identify existing organ complications and initiate measures to prevent further deterioration. Outpatient management can thus be divided into baseline evaluations, basic treatment or disease modification, and additional treatment dictated by the organ complications that are identified. The suggested treatments are based on current understanding of sickle cell disease pathophysiology. As shown in Fig. 43–8, some treatments address only one aspect of pathophysiology whereas others may have a broader impact. Inpatient management is directed at effective and safe relief of acute crises.

Baseline Evaluations

Baseline blood, urine, and other evaluations are directed at quantifying the chronic hemolytic anemia and organ-specific complications (Table 43–2). They also provide baseline parameters that can be followed to assess response to therapeutic interventions.

In pediatric patients, at least annual assessment of cerebral blood flow in the internal carotid artery and the middle or anterior cerebral artery using transcranial Doppler ultrasonography (TCD) is recommended. This evaluation is a validated predictor of stroke risk. Primary prevention with chronic transfusion is effective in such patients.[28] In adults, magnetic resonance imaging (MRI)/ magnetic resonance angiography (MRA) of the brain should be used instead of TCD[29] to assess thrombotic or hemorrhagic stroke risk, especially those with a previous history of stroke or seizure. The recognition of pulmonary hypertension as a cause of early mortality in sickle cell disease warrants evaluation for this condition with either echocardiogram or brain natriuretic peptide (BNP) levels; potential interventions for this condition are being evaluated in clinical trials. Retinal evaluation is begun at school age and continued on an annual basis. More frequent retinal evaluations will be necessary if retinopathy is noted.

Basic Management and Disease Modification

There is sufficient evidence to suggest that a number of treatments should be considered in all patients. These treatments have been demonstrated to decrease symptoms/complications, increase survival, or both (Table 43–3) (disease modification). There are other treatments for which there are sufficient scientific grounds and/or clinical data to suggest a potential impact on disease natural history. However, there is presently insufficient clinical data to make firm recommendations (Fig. 43–8, Table 43–3). Although treatments such as vaccination and penicillin prophylaxis do not directly affect the sickling process or vasculopathy, they have had an impact on survival and therefore are included under the umbrella of disease-modifying therapies.

Therapeutic options are further discussed in the sections describing organ specific complications.

Table 43–2 Baseline Evaluations to Consider

	Tests
Blood tests	-CBC with differential -Reticulocyte count -Hemoglobin electrophoresis -LDH -Renal function tests -Liver function tests -Mineral panel -Uric acid -Serum iron, ferritin, TIBC -Erythropoietin level -Hepatitis B sAg -Hepatitis C antibody -Red cell alloantibody screen -Red cell typing -D-dimer* -C-reactive protein* -Brain natriuretic peptide†
Urine/kidney tests	-Urinalysis -Renal ultrasound‡
Radiology	-MRI/MRA brain (adults) or transcranial Doppler ultrasonography starting at age 2 (children) -CXR§ -Hip or shoulder x-ray and/or MRI§ -Bone density in teenagers and adults
Cardiology/Pulmonary	-Echocardiogram -Right heart catheter† -Six-minute walk test†
Neurocognitive	-Neurocognitive testing¶

Key: *Consider following as a surrogate marker after initiation of disease modifying intervention; †to further evaluate pulmonary hypertension; ‡if hematuria with red blood cells in urine; §as clinically indicated; ¶if poor school performance, abnormal memory, or abnormal MRI.

Table 43–3 Disease Modifying Treatments to Consider (See Text for Specific Indications and Limitations)

Robust clinical data	-Penicillin prophylaxis -*S pneumoniae* vaccination -Hydroxyurea -Chronic exchange transfusion -Iron chelation for chronic iron overload*
Limited clinical data	-Folate supplementation† -H. influenzae vaccination -Influenza vaccination -Erythropoietin -Phlebotomy
Experimental	-ICA 17043 (decreasing Hb S concentration) -Decitabine (Hb F reactivation) -Nutritional supplements (eg, glutamine, zinc, multivitamins)

*Best data from thalassemia patient experience; †risks minimal (however, can mask B12 deficiency), therefore it is generally done.

Vaccination and Penicillin Prophylaxis

Children should be immunized against *S pneumoniae, H influenzae*, hepatitis B, and influenza.[30] Vaccination and penicillin prophylaxis can reduce the risk of serious pneumococcal infections.[9,31] Vaccination schedules recommend inoculation with heptavalent pneumococcal conjugated vaccine (PCV_7) at 2 months followed by two more doses 6 to 8 weeks apart (primary series) and a booster at 12 months. This is followed by pneumovax at age 2 and 5 years. In adults, the pneumovax should be readministered every 5 years (www.cdc.gov/vaccines/pubs/vis/default.htm).

For children under age 5 years, prophylactic penicillin recommendations are 125 mg penicillin V orally twice daily until age 2 to 3 years, and 250 mg thereafter.[30] Penicillin prophylaxis begins at 2 months. Randomized, double-blind, placebo-controlled studies of prophylactic penicillin beginning in infancy, including the PROPS study, have found that this therapy reduced the incidence of *S pneumoniae* bacteremia by 84% in children younger than 3 years.[9,31] A randomized, double-blind, placebo-controlled study, the PROPS II study, concluded that it is safe to stop prophylactic penicillin therapy at age 5 years in children who have not had prior severe pneumococcal infection or splenectomy and are receiving regular follow-up care.[32] However, the power of the study was restricted by the limited number of *S pneumoniae* systemic infection events. In an analysis of a patient population receiving penicillin prophylaxis and the pneumovax, the rate of severe *S Pneumoniae* infections was 2.4 per 100 patient-years. This was favorable compared to the historical pre-penicillin prophylaxis rate of 3.2 to 6.9 per 100 patient-years.[33] These measures reduce risk but do not remove it. The risk of recurrent *S pneumoniae* sepsis and death in patients who have had previous sepsis is much increased; all patients having a history of pneumococcal sepsis should remain on penicillin prophylaxis indefinitely and are not candidates for outpatient management of febrile episodes.[34] Parents must be aggressively counseled to seek medical attention for all febrile events.

Hydroxyurea and Fetal Hemoglobin (Hb F) Reactivation

The level of HbF in erythrocytes plays a critical role in determining patient outcomes. Individuals who have sickle cell disease and another condition called HPFH have 70% hemoglobin S (HbS) in their red blood cells, but are neither anemic nor symptomatic.[35] The uniform distribution of HbF among their red cells interferes with HbS polymerization, increases its solubility, and prevents red cell sickling.[36,37] Even at lower levels of HbF seen in patients without HPFH, crisis rate and mortality are inversely proportional to HbF level.[18–21] These findings prompted the idea that pharmacologic reactivation of HbF production might be of benefit to patients.

Hydroxyurea (HU) is an inhibitor of ribonucleotide reductase and a cytotoxic agent that can elevate Hb F levels. A double-blind, placebo-controlled, intention-to-treat multicenter study of HU as treatment of pain crisis in sickle cell disease found that HU produced definite hematologic changes. Hydroxyurea was started at 0.15 mg/kg/day and escalated to 0.30 mg/kg/day as tolerated and to maintain an absolute neutrophil count no lower than $2000 \times 10^9\ L^{-1}$. There were significant increases in the levels of hemoglobin, Hb F, F cells, F reticulocytes, PCV, and MCV and declines in the mean level of leukocytes, PMN, reticulocytes, and dense sickle cells (Table 43–4).[38] The significant clinical changes were decreased rate of acute painful episodes, longer interval to first and second acute painful episode, fewer episodes of acute chest syndrome, and diminished number of subjects and units transfused (Table 43–5).[39] In follow-up analysis, higher pre- or posttreatment Hb F levels were associated with a reduction in mortality (although no significant changes were observed in the incidence of stroke, hepatic sequestration, or death in the initial study).[18] No short-term toxicity due to HU was observed. One child born to a subject taking HU and two born to partners of subjects taking HU were normal at birth. Although the follow-up analyses suggest the importance of induced Hb F to the improved outcomes produced by HU, some HU-induced changes in sickle cell erythrocytes, such as reduced neutrophil count, increased water content, and decreased HbS concentration,[40] may be independent of Hb F.

In the original study, only patients with two or more pain crises per year requiring hospitalization were eligible. However, other at-

Table 43–4 Hematologic Effects of Hydroxyurea Therapy

Variable	Hydroxyurea	Placebo	P
Leukocytes (10^3 cells/μL)	9.9	12.2	0.0001
PMN (10^3 cells/μL)	4.9	6.4	0.0001
Reticulocytes (10^3 cells/μL)	231	300	0.0001
Hemoglobin (gm/dL)	9.1	8.5	0.0009
PCV (%)	27.0	25.1	0.0007
MCV (fl)	103	93	0.0001
Hb F (%)	8.6	4.7	0.0001
F-cells (%)	48	35	0.0001
F-Reticulocytes			
(10^3 cells/μL)	17	15	0.0036
Dense sickle cells (%)	11	13	0.004

Shown are mean values after 2 years of study. Baseline values, which were not significantly different, are not shown.
Adapted from Charache et al,[255] with permission.

Table 43–5 Clinical Effects of Hydroxyurea Therapy

Variable	Hydroxyurea	Placebo	P
Acute pain crisis rate	2.5/year	4.5/year	<0.001
Hospitalization rate for acute pain crisis	1.0/year	2.4/year	<0.001
Interval to first pain crisis	3.0 months	1.5 months	<0.001
Interval to second pain crisis	8.8 months	4.6 months	<0.001
Acute chest syndrome	25	51	<0.001
Subjects transfused	48	73	0.001
Blood units transfused	336	586	0.004

Adapted from data in Charache et al.[253]

risk patients should be considered for hydroxyurea therapy. These include patients with evidence of chronic organ damage, patients with severe anemia (<9 g/dL, consider erythropoietin if the reticulocyte count is <250,000 μL^{-1}), and patients with indications for chronic transfusion but who have alloantibodies. After obtaining the baseline evaluations per Table 43–2, hydroxyurea is usually started at 500 to 1000 mg/day with monitoring of the complete blood count every 4 to 8 weeks to ensure that neutropenia (absolute neutrophil count $<2 \times 10^9\ L^{-1}$) is not produced. The dose is increased to a stable maximum NGF response or neutropenia, but most patients receive between 1000 and 2000 mg/day. Response is defined clinically and by a persistent and significant (>0.5 g/dL) increase in total hemoglobin/fetal hemoglobin and a decrease in the LDH. These improvements in symptomatology and hematologic indices may take 3 to 4 months of therapy to manifest but can be seen after approximately 6 weeks. Lower doses may be required in patients with renal insufficiency. If the reticulocyte count is less than 250,000 μL^{-1}, then the possibility of erythropoietin deficiency should be considered (see section on erythropoietin).

In studies of HU as a therapy for children with sickle cell disease, the drug was well tolerated and produced favorable hematologic changes similar to those seen in the adult population.[41] In approximately 10% of the children treated, the increase in Hb F was less than 2%. Baseline Hb F levels, baseline total hemoglobin levels, and compliance were associated with the final Hb F level.[42] Other studies in children have documented a decrease in the number of days of hospitalization and suggest a decreased incidence of vasoocclusive crises.[43] The favorable changes in hematologic indices suggest that HU therapy might be an alternative to blood transfusions for the prevention of recurrent stroke in children with sickle cell disease.[44,45] HU therapy appears to lower transcranial Doppler velocities in children with sickle cell disease.[46] Studies in the United States and in Belgium support the potential role of hydroxyurea in the prevention of cerebral vascular accidents.[45,47,48] HU was found to improve, but not correct, the abnormal cerebral oxygen saturation associated with sickle cell disease.[49]

A persistent concern pertaining to the use of HU in sickle cell disease is its putative leukemogenic effect. This concern derives from reports on HU treatment of myeloproliferative diseases, conditions associated with an inherent propensity for leukemic conversion. Although the use of HU combined with ^{32}P or alkylating agents is associated with increased leukemic conversion in patients with myeloproliferative disease,[50] reports claiming a leukemogenic effect for HU alone in polycythemia vera either lacked controls[51] or were not designed to assess this issue.[52] In children with the nonmalignant underlying condition of erythrocytosis secondary to inoperable cyanotic congenital heart disease, no leukemic conversion was observed.[53]

Vitamin or Nutritional Supplementation

Chronic hemolysis results in increased utilization of folic acid stores. Megaloblastic crises from folic acid deficiency have been reported.[54,55] Pediatric patients with sickle cell disease had higher homocysteine levels than age-matched control African American patients.[56] Folic acid, 1 mg orally per day, is administered as a standard of care.[57] B_{12} deficiency can also be seen in sickle cell disease patients. Folate replacement can mask and possibly exacerbate B_{12} deficiency.[58]

A growing body of research indicating that sickle cell patients have widespread mineral and vitamin deficiencies, including zinc, vitamin C, vitamin E, acetylcysteine, calcium, vitamin D, vitamin A, and others.[59] Fifty percent of children with sickle cell disease have evidence of osteoporosis or osteopenia that is associated with inadequate calcium and vitamin D intake.[60–62] Recently, zinc supplementation in a prospective trial documented significant improvement in linear growth and weight gain in children with sickle cell disease.[63]

Despite increased intestinal absorption of iron in sickle cell disease, the combination of nutritional deficiency and urinary iron losses results in iron deficiency in 20% of children with sickle cell disease.[64] The diagnosis of iron deficiency may be obscured by the elevated serum iron levels associated with chronic hemolysis, necessitating the detection of a low serum ferritin level or an elevated serum transferrin level for the diagnosis.

Transfusion Therapy

There are two main approaches to transfusion in sickle cell disease—simple transfusion and exchange transfusion. These transfusions can be administered in an episodic fashion or in a chronic fashion. Therefore, transfusion therapy in sickle cell disease is of the following types: episodic simple, episodic partial exchange, or chronic partial exchange. In both simple and exchange transfusion, the target hemoglobin level is 10 to 11 g/dL (hematocrit 30%).[65,66] Transfusing to a higher hemoglobin or hematocrit level is avoided because a hematocrit level greater than 30% is associated with hyperviscosity if there is a substantial proportion of Hb S in the blood. In exchange transfusion, an additional objective is to achieve an HbS percentage of less than 30% (or sometimes <50%). In partial-exchange transfusion, a proportion of the patient's diseased red cells are removed before transfusion of normal donor red blood cells; this can be done manually through phlebotomy followed by transfusion or concurrently using an automated device. In those patients who need chronic transfusion, partial exchange is recommended because of the reduced iron burden

Table 43–6 Transfusion Formulas

A. Simple transfusion
PRBC volume (PRBCV) (mL) = $(Hct_d - Hct_i) \times TBV \times Hct_{rp}$B. Dilutional effects of transfusion on Hb S
Hb $S_f = 1 - (PRBCV \times Hct_{rp})(TBV \times Hct_i) + (PRBCV \times Hct_{rp}) \times$ Hb S_iC. Manual partial-exchange transfusion*
Exchange volume (mL) = $(Hct_d - Hct_i) \times TBVHct_{rp} - (Hct_i + Hct_d)$2D. Automated exchange transfusion
RBC volume (mL) = $Hct_i \times TBV$

TBV, estimated total blood volume in mL (children 80 mL/kg, adults 65 mL/kg, nomograms are available)†; Hct_d, desired hematocrit; Hct_i, initial hematocrit; Hct_{rp}, hematocrit of replacement cells (usually 0.75); Hb S_i, initial Hb S; Hb S_f, final Hb S.

In these formulas Hct and Hb S are fractions (eg, 40% = 0.4).

*From Nieburg and Stockman,[826] with permission. Copyright 1977, American Medical Association.

†From Linderkamp et al,[827] with permission. Copyright 1977 by Springer-Verlag GmbH & Co, KG.

of this approach. Partial exchange is also indicated if the baseline hemoglobin level is more than 10 g/dL. Simple transfusion in this context risks exacerbating the clinical condition through increased viscosity. For critical illness, exchange transfusion is also preferred. Although the target Hb S level should be less than 30% in exchange transfusion, decreasing Hb S levels to less than 50% may suffice depending on the severity of the complication being treated.

The volumes required for simple and exchange transfusions (Table 43–6) are particularly important for transfusing children. For normal-size adults, the general rule is that each unit of red cells infused increases the hemoglobin level approximately 1 g/dL. One approach to manual partial-exchange transfusion in adults is to phlebotomize 500 mL, infuse 300 mL normal saline, phlebotomize another 500 mL, then infuse 4 to 5 units of packed red cells.[67]

Episodic simple transfusion should be considered for blood volume replacement in aplastic crisis and splenic sequestration crisis, and protection during severe illness such as septicemia or severe vasoocclusive crisis/hyperhemolysis associated with a more than 20% decrease in hemoglobin from baseline or hemoglobin levels of less than 5 g/dL. Episodic simple or exchange transfusion should be considered for acute chest syndrome, priapism, and preoperatively. The choice of simple versus exchange transfusion is determined by the pretransfusion total hemoglobin level and the severity of the illness.

In the preoperative setting, simple transfusion to increase the total hemoglobin level to 10 g/dL was as effective in preventing perioperative complications and was associated with fewer transfusion-associated complications than an aggressive exchange transfusion regimen to decrease Hb S levels to less than 30%.[68] The efficacy of preoperative partial-exchange transfusion in patients with Hb SC disease undergoing abdominal surgery suggests that this type of transfusion be performed preoperatively in this group of patients.

Chronic partial-exchange transfusion is indicated in primary and secondary prevention of cerebral thrombosis as discussed in the section on neurologic complications.

Transfusion complications include alloimmunization, delayed hemolytic transfusion reactions (discussed in Exacerbations of Anemia), iron overload, and transmission of viral illness. The incidence of alloimmunization is between 19% and 30% and usually occurs with less than 15 transfusions.[69] Some patients seem to tolerate multiple transfusions without developing alloantibodies whereas others are readily allosensitized. The high rate of alloimmunization in transfused sickle cell patients is due in part to minor blood group incompatibilities between the recipient and donor pool, which often differ in ethnicity.[69,70] Antibodies against the C and E antigens of the Rh group, Kell (K) and Lewis, Duffy (Fya, Fyb), and Kidd (Jk) are common.[69] In the Stroke Prevention Trial in Sickle Cell Anemia, the routine use of WBC-reduced RBCs matched for E, C, and Kell decreased the allosensitization rate compared to historical data from 3% to 0.5% per unit transfused and decreased the rate of hemolytic transfusion reactions by 90%.[71] Therefore, the recommended approach to preventing alloimmunization is to reduce leukocytes and perform limited phenotype matching for all patients (ABO, C, D, E, and Kell) and extended phenotype matching for patients with alloantibodies.[66] The management of a delayed hemolytic transfusion reaction and transfusional iron overload are discussed under Exacerbations of Anemia below.

Transmission of HIV, hepatitis B and C, and human T-cell leukemia/lymphoma virus-1 has diminished with improved screening of banked units but remains an issue. In addition to better screening programs, the use of leukocyte-depleted red cell transfusions can reduce this hazard.[72]

Stem Cell Transplantation

At this time, allogeneic stem cell transplantation remains the only curative option for sickle cell disease. The largest series to date has been in a pediatric population with severely symptomatic sickle cell disease failing to respond to hydroxyurea. Using myeloablative conditioning and HLA-matched or one-mismatch (two cases) sibling donors, with bone marrow as the source of stem cells in the majority, there was a 10% mortality rate with 90% overall survival and 82% event-free survival at a median follow-up of 54 months.[73] Similar results were obtained when related, HLA-matched umbilical cord blood was used as the source of stem cells.[74] According to these results, stem cell transplant is a therapeutic option for the severely symptomatic child with an HLA-matched sibling donor. Non-myeloablative conditioning approaches may allow a further decrease in transplant-related mortality. Extended molecular phenotyping may decrease the risks of matched unrelated stem cell transplantation for those patients without matched sibling donors.[75] The issue of the cost-effectiveness of BMT gains perspective from the comparative costs in the United States of $150,000 to $200,000 for an uncomplicated BMT versus up to $112,000 annually for conventional medical care of a chronically transfused, iron-overloaded patient.[76]

Education

Education regarding the nature of the disease, genetic counseling, and psychosocial assessments of patients and their families are best accomplished during routine visits. Parents of small children are instructed regarding early detection of infection and palpating enlarging spleens.

Phlebotomy

As mentioned, a hemoglobin level of more than 10 to 11 g/dL (hematocrit 30%) in the presence of substantial amounts of Hb S (>30%) is associated with hyperviscosity. There are some data to indicate that phlebotomy, to reduce the hematocrit and viscosity (and which may also address iron-overload), can decrease the frequency of crises in Hb SC or Hb S–β^+ disease.[77] In Hb SS disease, phlebotomy has successfully been used in combination with hydroxyurea (which increases the hemoglobin level) in secondary stroke prevention in patients previously treated with chronic transfusion.[78] Phlebotomy alone has also been used in Hb SS disease with baseline Hb levels of more than 9.5 g/dL with favorable results on the frequency and duration of pain crises. This benefit may have resulted from decreased hematocrit and viscosity and also from a decrease in intracellular hemoglobin concentration from iron deficiency.[79] One approach to phlebotomy is to remove approximately 10 mL/kg of blood over 20 to 30 minutes followed by infusion of an equal volume of normal saline. This is repeated every 2 weeks until the target hemoglobin level of 9 to 9.5 g/dL is achieved.

Erythropoietin or Darbepoietin

Generally low erythropoietin levels are seen in sickle cell disease,[80] one contributing factor could be increased uptake by the massive compensatory reticulocytosis. Therefore, erythropoietin levels in isolation are difficult to interpret in sickle cell disease. However, inappropriately low erythropoietin levels are more severe in adults than in children,[80] and relative reticulocytopenia (reticulocyte count $<250{,}000 \times 10^9\ L^{-1}$) is associated with evidence of renal damage such as proteinuria, suggesting that erythropoietin deficiency should be considered in cases of progressive anemia or relative reticulocytopenia, even if the creatinine levels are within the normal range. Relative reticulocytopenia is a risk factor for early death,[81] and reversing the resulting progressive anemia may have benefits. The cumulative published experience of erythropoietin use in sickle cell disease is limited (52 patients).[82] Although erythropoietin by itself has been reported to increase HbF levels, the most important role for erythropoietin may be as replacement therapy for erythropoietin deficiency that results in relative reticulocytopenia and progressive anemia. As noted above, erythropoietin deficiency may be clinically significant even when creatinine levels are in the normal range. Erythropoietin replacement can also facilitate enhanced hydroxyurea dosing and HbF augmentation.[82] In using recombinant human erythropoietin, caution must be exercised not to elevate the hematocrit to levels that result in hyperviscosity. Also, the reticulocyte fraction is the most adhesive, and it is possible that erythropoietin could exacerbate or trigger sickle cell crises.[82] Sickle cell patients may be relatively resistant to erythropoietin and require doses higher than those used in other patients with chronic renal failure. The reasons for erythropoietin resistance are unclear but may include increased inflammation-mediated suppression of erythropoiesis.[83]

Erythropoietin therapy is probably not indicated in patients receiving chronic transfusion therapy in whom encouraging endogenous HbS containing erythropoiesis may be counterproductive.

Iron Chelation

Early death is well described in association with iron overload from β-thalassemia and hereditary hemochromatosis.[84,85] Similarly, iron overload is likely to be a problem in chronically transfused sickle cell disease patients although the clinical significance may critically depend on the degree and duration of overload. Chelation guidelines for patients with sickle cell disease are similar to those for other chronically transfused, iron-overloaded patients; iron chelation indicated when the total body iron level is elevated (ferritin >2000, quantitative liver iron by dry weight of 2000, transfusion history >1 year of monthly transfusions).[86] Notably, the serum ferritin level may underestimate clinically significant iron overload.[87,88] Iron chelation options in the USA are deferoxamine (via continuous IV or SQ infusion) or deferasirox (orally), both of which appear to have similar efficacy although the oral route of administration and toxicity profile may favor deferasirox.[20,89,244]

Newer FDA-approved methods of quantitating iron burden by Ferriscan of the liver[90] can avoid the need for liver biopsies. T2* MRI of the heart indicates hemosiderosis of cardiac tissue, and when it is abnormal, aggressive chelation is mandated.[91]

Alternatives to HU for HbF Induction

Alternatives to HU for pharmacologic induction of HbF that are being studied in clinical trials include the methyltransferase inhibitor 5-aza-2′-deoxycytidine (decitabine) and histone deacetylase inhibiters.[92] These classes of agents act on chromatin processes that regulate gene transcription.

The methyltransferase inhibitors 5-azacytidine and 5-aza-2′-deoxycytidine have produced the largest increases in HbF of any of the pharmacologic reactivators of HbF that have been tested.[93,94] Responding patients include those who did not respond to hydroxyurea, consistent with a different mechanism of action for decitabine. Although improvements in a number of surrogate clinical endpoints have been demonstrated, larger studies to confirm safety and clinical effectiveness with chronic use are required. In the United States, decitabine has been approved by the Food and Drug Administration (FDA) for the treatment of myelodysplastic syndrome.

The efficacy of the class of agents known as histone deacetylase inhibitors in HbF reactivation has been reviewed.[95,96] However, the absence of large clinical trial data, practical issues with administration and stability of some agents, and the lack of FDA approval for many drugs in this class are limitations.

Preventing Red Cell Dehydration With Ion Channel Inhibitors

Polymerization of HbS is related to the HbS concentration within the cell. Therefore a therapeutic strategy could be to reduce the intracellular HbS concentration by improving cellular hydration. Potential therapeutic options to maintain red-cell hydration for which there is preliminary clinical data include cetiedil citrate, imidazole inhibitors of the Gardos pathway,[97] novel Gardos channel inhibitors[98] or magnesium supplements, which inhibit potassium chloride cotransport.[99]

It also is possible to reduce the hemoglobin concentration by reducing the hemoglobin content with iron deficiency. It has been observed that spontaneous or induced iron deficiency (see Phlebotomy above) sufficient to reduce the serum ferritin, mean corpuscular volume (MCV), and mean cell hemoglobin concentration (MCHC) resulted in variably improved HbS polymerization, red cell survival, level of anemia, and clinical status.[100]

Anticoagulation or Antiplatelet Therapy

Although there is clear evidence of activation of the coagulation system in sickle cell disease, the role of thrombogenesis in vasoocculsive crisis remains unclear.[101] D-dimer levels (a degradation product of cross-linked fibrin) increase during acute vasoocclusive crisis.[102]

Heparin

Minidose heparin, 5000 to 7500 units every 12 hours, administered to four patients for 2 to 6 years, reduced hospitalization and emergency room time by 75%, and pretreatment pain frequency recurred after heparin was discontinued.[103] Larger clinical studies will be required to better understand the risks and benefits of heparin therapy for acute vasoocclusive crisis in sickle cell disease. Heparin has not been studied for acute arterial stroke in patients with sickle cell disease but has a role in sickle cell-associated dural venous sinus thrombosis.[104] The management of stroke is fully discussed under Specific Complications and Their Management.

Oral Anticoagulants

Acenocoumarol was administered in low doses that achieved a mean INR of 1.64 and reduced the elevated levels of prothrombin activation fragment (fragment 1+2) to 50% of pretreatment levels.[105] Clinical endpoints were not measured. In a crossover study, 29 patients were treated with acenocoumarol to target an INR of 1.6 to 2.0. No effect on crisis frequency was noted, although again, there were significant reductions in markers of coagulation system activation.[106] In 37 acutely ill sickle cell patients with elevated D-dimers, the effect of low-dose warfarin therapy (1 mg without a target INR) in 12 of them was examined. In multivariate analysis, low-dose warfarin was the only variable associated with a significant decrease in D-dimer levels, suggesting a warfarin-induced decrease in thrombin activity.[102] Therefore, oral anticoagulation, even at low doses, is associated with

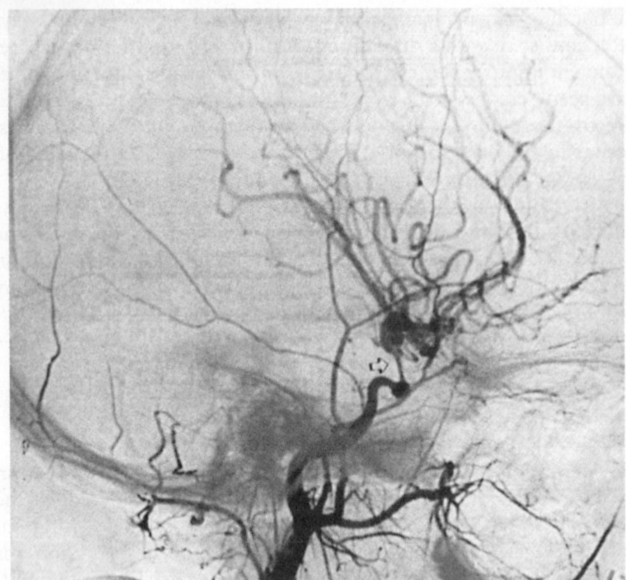

Figure 43–9 Right common carotid arteriogram taken in anteroposterior projection, demonstrating complete occlusion of the origin of the right anterior cerebral artery (arrowhead). *(From Stockman JA, Nigro MA, Mishkin MM, Oski FA: Occlusion of large cerebral vessels in sickle-cell anemia. N Engl J Med 287(17):846, 1972.)*

a decrease in laboratory markers of coagulation pathway activation in sickle cell disease; however, further clinical trials are required to understand the clinical risks and benefits.

Aspirin

Aspirin was compared with placebo in 49 pediatric sickle cell disease patients in a double-blind crossover study. The frequency and severity of crises were not affected by aspirin therapy.[107] Cerebral thrombosis, which accounts for 70% to 80% of all cerebrovascular accidents (CVAs) in sickle cell disease, results from large-vessel occlusion (Fig. 43–9) rather than the more typical microvascular occlusion of sickle cell disease. In the United States, there is an ongoing clinical trial testing the safety and efficacy of aspirin in diminishing the incidence and progression of cognitive defects and overt or silent stroke in pediatric patients.

The management of stroke risk and stroke is fully discussed under Specific Complications and Their Management.

Experimental Therapies

A number of therapies are in early stages of clinical evaluation and could have a role in disease modification of sickle cell disease. These include agents that directly address sickle erythrocyte adhesion to endothelium (recombinant PSGL–IgG conjugate), agents that increase the production of nitric oxide (NO) (glutamine), and herbal extracts with unknown mechanisms of action (niprisan).[108]

Specific Complications and Their Management

Pain Crisis

Acute Pain Episode or Crisis

Acute pain is the first symptom of disease in more than 25% of patients and is the most frequent symptom after age 2 years.[109] Pain is the complication for which patients with sickle cell disease most commonly seek medical attention.[110] An episode of acute pain was originally called a "sickle cell crisis" by Diggs, who used the expression "crisis" to refer to any new rapidly developing syndrome in the life of a patient with sickle cell disease.[111] The basic mechanism is believed to be vasoocclusion of the bone marrow vasculature causing bone infarction, which in turn causes release of inflammatory mediators that activate afferent nociceptors.[112]

Although a general correlation of vasoocclusive severity and genotype has been posited,[113] there is tremendous variability within genotypes and in the same patient over time. In one large study of patients with Hb SS disease, one-third rarely had pain, one-third were hospitalized for pain approximately two to six times per year, and one-third had more than six pain-related hospitalizations per year.[114] Over a 5-year period in the National Cooperative Study of Sickle Cell Disease, 40% of patients had no painful episodes and 5% of patients accounted for one-third of the emergency room visits. Pain is more frequent with the Hb SS genotype, low levels of Hb F, higher Hb levels[27] and sleep apnea.[115] The frequency of pain peaks between ages 19 and 39 years. After the age of 19 years, more frequent pain correlates with a higher mortality rate.[27] Medical personnel who see patients only in the emergency department gain a biased view of sickle cell disease skewed by a frequently afflicted minority with severe disease.[116,117]

Pain may be precipitated by events such as cold, dehydration, infection, stress, menses, and alcohol consumption. Any underlying cause should be searched for and corrected, but the majority of painful episodes have no identifiable cause. It can affect any area of the body, most commonly the back, chest, extremities, and abdomen, may vary from trivial to excruciating, and is usually endured at home without a visit to the emergency department. There may be premonitory symptoms.[117] The duration averages a few days, with hospital admissions typically lasting between 4 and 10 days. Painful episodes are biopsychosocial events caused by vasoocclusion in an area of the body having nociceptors and nerves.[112] Pain is an affect and, as such, consists of sensory, perceptual, cognitive, and emotional components. Frequent pain generates feelings of despair, depression, and apathy that interfere with everyday life and promote an existence that revolves around pain. This scenario may lead to a chronic debilitating pain syndrome; fortunately, this is rare.

There is no specific clinical or laboratory finding pathognomonic of pain crisis. The diagnosis is established by history and physical examination. Changes in steady-state Hb values, sickled cells on blood smear, WBC counts, etc, are not reliable indicators. Numerous laboratory tests, leukocytosis, D-dimer fragments of fibrin, and markers of platelet activation have been found to lack specificity as indicators of acute vasoocclusion. Often patients can tell if it is a typical pain crisis or something more sinister. It is thus good practice to ask the patient if it feels like usual pain crisis pain.

Initial medical assessment should focus on detection of triggers or medical complications requiring specific therapy: infection, dehydration, acute chest syndrome (fever, tachypnea, chest pain, hypoxia, and chest signs), severe anemia, cholecystitis, splenic enlargement, neurologic events, and priapism.[118] Pain management should be aggressive to make the pain tolerable and enable patients to attain maximum functional ability. To make the patient pain-free is an unrealistic goal and risks oversedation and hypoventilation, which must be avoided. A pain chart should be started, and analgesia titrated against the patient's reported pain together with medical assessment of their overall clinical status, paying particular attention to avoiding oversedation. When clinicians consistently observe a disparity between patients' verbal self-report of their pain and their ability to function, further assessment should be performed to ascertain the reason for disparity. Patients are often undertreated for pain because many physicians and other health care providers are overly concerned with the potential for addiction. Undertreatment of pain is no more desirable than overtreatment and oversedation; undertreatment can prolong the duration of a painful episode and can poison the relationship between the patient and the health care system. In assessing patient responses to conventional doses of analgesia, it must be remembered that those with sickle cell disease metabolize narcotics rapidly.[119]

The pain pathway should be targeted at different points with different agents, avoiding toxicity with any one class (Table 43–7). The

Table 43–7 Recommended Dose and Interval of Analgesics Necessary to Obtain Adequate Pain Control in Sickle Cell Disease

	Dose/Rate	Comments
Severe/moderate pain		
1. Morphine	Parenteral: 0.1–0.15 mg/kg q 3–4 h. Recommended maximum single dose 10 mg PO: 0.3–0.6 mg/kg q 4 h	Drug of choice for pain; lower doses in the elderly and infants and in patients with liver failure or impaired ventilation
2. Meperidine	Parenteral: 0.75–1.5 mg/kg q 2–4 h. Recommended maximum dose 100 mg PO: 1.5 mg/kg q 4 h	Increased incidence of seizures. Avoid in patients with renal or neurologic disease or those who receive monoamine oxidase inhibitors.
3. Hydromorphone	Parenteral: 0.01–0.02 mg/kg q 3–4 h PO: 0.04–0.06 mg/kg q 4 h	
4. Oxycodone	PO: 0.15 mg/kg/dose q 4 h	
5. Ketorolac	Intramuscular: Adults: 30 or 60 mg initial dose, followed by 15–30 mg. Children: 1 mg/kg load, followed by 0.5 mg/kg q 6 h	Equal efficacy to 6 mg MS; helps narcotic-sparing effect; not to exceed 5 days. Maximum 150 mg first day, 120 mg maximum subsequent days. May cause gastric irritation.
6. Butorphanol	Parenteral: Adults: 2 mg q 3–4 h	Agonist-antagonist. Can precipitate withdrawal if given to patients who are being treated with agonists.
Mild pain		
1. Codeine	PO: 0.5–1 mg/kg q 4 h. Maximum dose 60 mg	Mild to moderate pain not relieved by aspirin or acetaminophen; can cause nausea and vomiting
2. Aspirin	PO: Adults: 0.3–6 mg q 4–6 h. Children: 10 mg/kg q 4 h	Often given with a narcotic to enhance analgesia. Can cause gastric irritation. Avoid in febrile children.
3. Acetaminophen	PO: Adults 0.3–0.6 g q 4 h. Children: 10 mg/kg	Often given with a narcotic to enhance analgesia
4. Ibuprofen	PO: Adults: 300–400 mg q 4 h. Children: 5–10 mg/kg q 6–8 h	Can cause gastric irritation
5. Naproxen	PO: Adults: 500 mg/dose initially, then 250 q 8–12 h. Children: 10 mg/kg/day (5 mg/kg q 12 h)	Long duration of action. Can cause gastric irritation.
6. Indomethacin	PO: Adults: 25 mg q 8 h. Children: 1–3 mg/kg/day given 3 or 4 times	Contraindicated in psychiatric, neurologic, renal diseases. High incidence of gastric irritation. Useful in gout.

Adapted from Charache et al,[330] with permission.

mainstays are NSAIDs, acetaminophen, and opioids. NSAIDs can be used to control mild to moderate pain and may have an additive role in combination with opioids for severe pain. The most potent NSAID is ketorolac. NSAIDs should be used with caution in those with a history of peptic ulcer, renal insufficiency, asthma, or bleeding tendencies. Within limits, use the agents that the patients know work for them—avoid meperidine (Demerol), which should only be used under very exceptional circumstances. Sedatives and anxiolytics alone should not be used to manage pain, because they can mask the behavioral response to pain without providing analgesia.

Treatment of persistent or moderate to severe pain should be based on increasing the opioid strength or dose.[118] One approach is to administer morphine 0.1 mg/kg intravenously or subcutaneously every 20 minutes until pain is controlled. The patient should be checked at 20-minute intervals for pain, respiratory rate, depth and quality, and sedation until the patient is stable with adequate pain control. Subsequently, the patient should receive a maintenance dose of 0.05 to 0.15 mg/kg intravenously or subcutaneously every 2 to 4 hours. A rescue dose of 50% of the maintenance dose can be considered on an as-needed basis every 30 minutes for breakthrough pain.

During maintenance with opioids, pain control, respiratory rate, depth and quality, and oxygen saturation should be monitored approximately every 2 hours. If respiratory depression is noted, omit the maintenance dose of morphine. For severe respiratory depression or oxygen desaturation, administer naloxone. Incentive spirometry and mandatory time out of bed are helpful in patients with chest pain to decrease the risk for hypoventilation. Adjuvant medications to consider include NSAIDs, acetaminophen, antiemetics, and antihistamines. Laxatives or stool softeners should be prescribed in keeping with close monitoring for constipation.

After 2 to 3 days, consider decreasing the dose and switching from parenteral to oral administration of opioids. For adult patients whose pain requires several or many days to resolve, a sustained-release opioid preparation is appropriate and provides a more consistent analgesia.

Hydration is a critical part of management. However, cardiac function may be significantly impaired, especially in adult patients, and standard discipline must be followed with IV fluid management to avoid iatrogenic fluid overload. Sickle cell patients cannot concentrate their urine and are at risk for dehydration when not taking adequate fluids (60 mL/kg/24 h in adults). Intravenous hydration is indicated when the patient is not taking oral fluids adequately. Ideally the urine specific gravity should be kept under 1.010 by daily testing when in hospital. Hemoglobin may decrease by 1 to 2 g/dL in an uncomplicated pain crisis, blood transfusion is not routinely indicated for an uncomplicated pain crisis.

Equianalgesic doses of oral opioids should be prescribed for home use when necessary to maintain the relief achieved in the emergency department or hospital ward. Care should be taken to appropriately taper opioids in patients who have received daily opioids over many days. In these patients, there may be physical opiate dependence, which is characterized by the onset of acute withdrawal symptoms upon cessation of opioid administration. For patients at risk for physical dependence, opiates should be titrated downward by 15% to 20% per day to zero. Physical dependence is a physiological problem, addiction is a psychological problem characterized by craving—behavior that is overwhelmingly directed at obtaining drug, use of the drug for purposes other than pain control, and use of the drug despite negative physical, social, legal, or psychological consequences.

If the patient is not on a disease-modifying agent such as hydroxyurea, consideration should be given to initiating such therapy either as an inpatient or during follow-up in the outpatient setting.

Table 43–8 Hematologic Variables Associated With Sickle Cell Anemia and the Different Sickle Cell-β Thalassemia Syndromes

Genotype	Hb*	%Hb A†	%Hb F†	%Hb A_2*	MCV*	Reticulocytes*	No.
Hb SS‡	7.83	0	4.56	2.87	85.9	10.18	~123
Hb S-β° thal‡	8.85	0	5.86	5.02	69.3	7.2	~41
Hb S-β+ thal, type I§	8.37	3–5	6.8	4.90	63.7	9.7	3
Hb S-β+ thal, type II§	10.28	8–14	5.2	4.68	70.0	6.6	14
Hb S-β+ thal, type III‖	11.55	18–25	5.1	4.66	73.3	1.27	76
Hb S-HPFH¶	14.6	0	25.8	1.95	81.7	2.4	4

*The mean data for each variable are shown. Units of measure are g/dl for Hb, percentage of total hemoglobin for Hb F and A2, fl for MCV, and percentage of total red cells for reticulocytes.
†Percentage Hb A that defines the Hb S-β+-thalassemia type.[245]
‡Data from Serjeant et al.[247]
§Data from Christakis et al.[246]
‖Data from Serjeant et al.[248]
¶Data from Friedman et al.[249]

Chronic Pain

Chronic pain in sickle cell disease usually (but not always) has an identifiable basis such as vertebral fractures, femoral head necrosis, early degenerative changes/osteoarthritis, or chronic skin ulcers. Most patients without such identifiable complications will not require chronic pain medications similar to those used for terminal cancer because the pain from a typical vasoocclusive crisis is episodic. Inappropriately maintaining patients without chronic musculoskeletal degeneration on long-acting opiates can impair their overall psychosocial functioning. On the other hand, adequate analgesia with long-acting opiates (such as long-acting morphine preparations similar to those used in cancer patients) is important to maintain the psychosocial functioning of patients who do have complications that cause chronic pain. Also consider agents such as amitriptyline or antiseizure medications[120] that can address neuropathic components and help decrease the sleep impairment and depression that can occur with chronic pain. If the patient is not on a disease-modifying agent such as hydroxyurea, consideration should be given to initiating such therapy.

Chronic Anemia

Chronic hemolytic anemia is one of the hallmarks of sickle cell disease. Sickle erythrocytes are destroyed randomly, with a mean life span of 17 days.[121] The overall hemolytic rate reflects the number of ISCs.[122] The degree of anemia is most severe in sickle cell anemia and Hb S–β° thalassemia, milder in Hb S–β+ thalassemia and Hb SC disease,[123] and, among patients with sickle cell anemia, less severe in those who have coexistent α thalassemia (Tables 43–8 and 43–1).[124]

As already noted, erythropoietin deficiency, from otherwise subclinical chronic renal damage, may also contribute to a decline in Hb levels below baseline. The level of chronic anemia is a significant prognostic marker.

The treatment options for the chronic anemia of sickle cell disease have already been mentioned. These strategies attempt to decrease hemolysis by increasing HbF (HU and the experimental approaches with erythropoietin, decitabine and histone deacetylase inhibitors) or decreasing the intracellular Hb S concentration by preventing red cell dehydration (Gardos channel inhibitors).

Exacerbations of Anemia

The rather constant level of hemolytic anemia may be exacerbated by additional events such as aplastic crises, acute splenic sequestration, acute hepatic sequestration, chronic renal disease or renal endocrine deficiency that may be present without overt renal failure, bone marrow necrosis, deficiency of folic acid or iron, delayed hemolytic transfusion reactions, autoimmune hemolytic anemia, or hyperhemolysis (hemolytic exacerbations) of unknown etiology. Laboratory evaluations that are very useful in the evaluation of a patient with anemia exacerbation are the reticulocyte count, the LDH, alloantibody screening, the direct antiglobulin (Coombs) test, and an erythropoietin level.

Aplastic Crises

Aplastic crises are transient arrests of erythropoiesis characterized by abrupt falls in hemoglobin levels, reticulocyte number, and red cell precursors in the marrow without necessarily an increase in the LDH. Although these episodes typically last only a few days, the level of anemia may be severe because the hemolysis continues unabated in the absence of red cell production. Although the mechanisms that impair erythropoiesis in inflammation are operative in infections of all types (see Chapter 24), human parvovirus B19 specifically invades proliferating erythroid progenitors, which accounts for its importance in sickle cell disease (see Chapters 19 and 24).[125] Parvovirus B19 (Fig. 43–10) accounts for 68% of aplastic crises in children with sickle cell disease,[126] but the high incidence of protective antibodies in adults makes parvovirus a less frequent cause of aplasia in this age group (see also Infections later in this chapter). Other reported causes of transient aplasia are infections by *S pneumoniae*, salmonella, streptococci, and Epstein–Barr virus. Bone marrow necrosis, which too may be the result of parvovirus infection, characterized by fever, bone pain, reticulocytopenia, and a leukoerythroblastic response, also causes aplastic crisis.[127,128]

Inhaled oxygen therapy also causes transient red cell hypoproduction; supraphysiologic oxygen tensions curtail erythropoietin production promptly and suppress reticulocytosis within 2 days.[129]

The mainstay of treating aplastic crises is red cell transfusion. When transfusion is necessitated by the degree of anemia or cardiorespiratory symptoms, a single transfusion usually will suffice, because reticulocytosis resumes spontaneously within a few days. Transfusion may be avoided by keeping severely anemic patients at bed rest to prevent symptoms and by avoiding supraphysiologic oxygen tensions. A useful guideline for transfusion in the context of an aplastic crisis is the reticulocyte count. A patient having an aplastic crisis with a reticulocyte count that is recovering is less likely to require urgent transfusion than one with a normal or low absolute reticulocyte count.

Sequestration Crisis (Spleen or Liver)

Acute splenic sequestration of blood is characterized by acute exacerbation of anemia, persistent reticulocytosis, a tender, enlarging spleen, and sometimes hypovolemia.[130] The LDH may remain stable

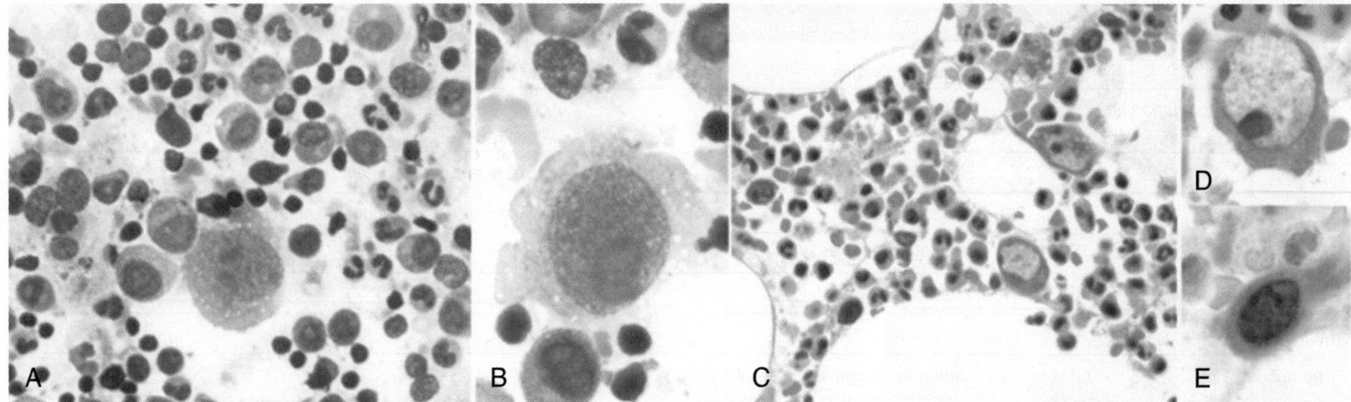

Figure 43–10 Parvovirus (**A–E**). Bone marrow aspirate in a patient with sickle cell disease and aplastic crisis (**A**). Note the absence of red blood cell precursors except for the single, large degenerating pronormoblast (lower center). Such pronormoblasts contain large nuclear inclusions (**B**) as a result of replication of parvovirus B19. The same can be seen in the tissue sections of a bone core biopsy (**C, D**). The parvovirus can now be recognized immunohistochemically with an immunostain (**E**).

or increase. Patients susceptible to this complication are those whose spleens have not undergone fibrosis—young patients with sickle cell anemia and adults with Hb SC disease or sickle cell–β^+ thalassemia. Sequestration may occur as early as a few weeks of age and may cause death before sickle cell disease is diagnosed. In one study, 30% of children had splenic sequestration over a 10-year period and 15% of the attacks were fatal.[131]

The basis of therapy is to restore blood volume and red cell mass. Because splenic sequestration recurs in 50% of cases, splenectomy is recommended after the event has abated. Alternatively, chronic transfusion therapy is used in young children to delay splenectomy until it can be tolerated safely. Because recurrence is possible during transfusion therapy, parents should be trained to detect a rapidly enlarging spleen and to seek immediate medical attention in this event. Less common sites of acute sequestration include the liver and possibly the lung.[132,133]

Delayed Hemolytic Transfusion Reaction and Autoimmune Hemolytic Anemia

Approximately 30% of patients are predisposed to develop alloantibodies, in part because of minor blood group incompatibilities in racially mismatched blood.[69,70] The corollary is that the other patients can receive multiple transfusions without demonstrating alloantibodies. Following alloimmunization, there is a subsequent decrease in antibody titer that can fall below serologically detectable levels. Therefore, antigen-positive red blood cells appear compatible in cross-matching and are transfused. This can result in a delayed hemolytic transfusion reaction produced by the amnestic response of the immune system (as opposed to the immediate hemolytic reaction that occurs with preformed antibody). The delayed hemolytic transfusion reaction consists of an unexplained fall in Hb, elevated LDH, elevated bilirubin above baseline, and hemoglobinuria, all occurring between 4 and 10 days after the red cell transfusion. Delayed hemolytic reactions and hyperhemolysis have been shown to occur in 11% of pediatric patients with sickle cell disease and a history of alloantibodies.[134] In sickle cell disease, the delayed hemolytic transfusion reaction can be particularly devastating because it can be accompanied by reticulocytopenia, which together with a bystander effect of destruction of recipient blood (not just donor blood) can result in unanticipated worsening of anemia to levels below that seen before transfusion.[135] In addition to the manifestations of a delayed hemolytic transfusion reaction as listed above, patients may develop acute congestive heart failure, acute renal failure, or acute chest syndrome (accompanied by vasoocclusive pain crisis). Subsequent transfusions may further exacerbate the anemia.

Resolution of severe anemia may only occur after withholding further transfusions with subsequent reticulocyte count recovery. Corticosteroids at high doses (eg, intravenous methylprednisolone 500 mg QD for 2 to 3 days) should be considered if the anemia is life-threatening or if further transfusion is deemed necessary to save life. Intravenous immunoglobulin can also be considered, with proper attention paid to avoiding iatrogenic fluid overload. Approaches to minimizing this complication include transfusing extended-matched (see Basic Management and Disease Modification), phenotypically compatible blood.[69–71] This syndrome may or may not recur with further transfusions after a recovery period.[136]

Hyperhemolytic Crisis

Hyperhemolytic crisis is the sudden exacerbation of anemia with increased reticulocytosis and bilirubin level. If suspected, the approach to management should first be to look for an underlying etiology which may be one of the events listed above: aplastic crisis (during the recovery phase when the reticulocyte count may not be decreased), sequestration crisis, delayed hemolytic transfusion reaction or autoimmune hemolysis. Another possible cause is G6PD deficiency.[137]

Erythropoietin Deficiency

This entity is discussed under Basic Management and Disease Modification.

Nutritional Deficiencies: Folate, Iron, or B_{12} Deficiency

This entity is discussed under Basic Management and Disease Modification.

Hypothyroidism

Iron overload in sickle cell disease can result in hypothyroidism.[138] Therefore, hypothyroidism is another etiology to consider in a sickle cell disease patient with an otherwise unexplained decrease in hemoglobin below baseline.

Infections

Immune Deficit

The propensity of children with sickle cell disease to contract *S pneumoniae* infection is related to impaired splenic function[139] and diminished serum opsonizing activity. Even before the anatomic autoinfarction of the spleen in patients with sickle cell anemia, defective splenic function is demonstrable by Howell–Jolly bodies on the peripheral blood smear, visible "pits" on the surface of red blood cells, and abnormal results of radionuclide spleen scanning.[140] Specific

Table 43–9 Bacteria and Viruses That Most Frequently Cause Serious Infection in Patients With Sickle Cell Disease

Microorganism	Type of Infection	Comments
Streptococcus pneumoniae	Septicemia	Common despite prophylactic penicillin and pneumococcal vaccine
	Meningitis	Less frequent than in years past
	Pneumonia	Rarely documented except in infants and young children
	Septic arthritis	Uncommon
Haemophilus influenzae, type b	Septicemia	
Meningitis		
Pneumonia	Much less common in recent years because of immunization with conjugate vaccine	
Salmonella species	Osteomyelitis	
Septicemia	Most common cause of bone and joint infection	
Escherichia coli and other gram-negative enteric pathogens	Septicemia	
Urinary tract infection		
Osteomyelitis	Focus sometimes inapparent	
Staphylococcus aureus	Osteomyelitis	Uncommon
Mycoplasma pneumoniae	Pneumonia	Pleural effusions; multilobe involvement
Chlamydia pneumoniae	Pneumonia	
Parvovirus B19	Bone marrow suppression (aplastic crisis)	High fever common; rash and other organ involvement infrequent
Hepatitis viruses (A, B, and C)	Hepatitis	Marked hyperbilirubinemia

From Buchanan,[431] with permission.

syndromes exhibiting greater rates of hemolysis cause loss of splenic function at earlier ages—sickle cell anemia → Hb SC disease → sickle cell-β^+ thalassemia.

Infectious complications of sickle cell disease are a major cause of morbidity and mortality,[141] even with current vaccination and prophylactic antibiotic regimens. The infections caused by particular organisms are shown in Table 43–9 and the specific organisms affecting different target organs are shown in Table 43–10. By 5 years of age, almost all patients are functionally asplenic, contributing to infectious susceptibility. Historically, pneumococcal sepsis has been the predominant cause of death in those less than 20 years of age.[142]

Evaluation

The most critical aspect of infectious illness in sickle cell disease is the evaluation and treatment of the febrile child. Routine evaluation includes a physical examination, a complete blood count, blood and urine cultures, a lumbar puncture if meningitis is suspected, and a chest x-ray to evaluate for pneumonia. Results of the complete blood count are compared to baseline values. A left shift in the differential count suggests bacterial infection.

Penicillin Prophylaxis and Pneumonia Vaccination

Data and recommendations regarding penicillin prophylaxis and pneumonia vaccination are discussed under Basic Management and Disease Modification.

S pneumoniae, H influenzae, Atypical Mycobacteria, and Acute Febrile Illness

S pneumoniae bacteremia is accompanied by leukocytosis, a left shift, aplastic crisis, sometimes disseminated intravascular coagulation, and a 20% to 50% mortality rate.[141] Although concerns about *S pneumoniae* sepsis are largely for young children, this complication also occurs in adults, often with devastating results.[143] *S pneumoniae* is the major cause of meningitis in infants and young children with sickle cell disease, and occurs in the setting of bacteremia.

The second most common organism responsible for bacteremia in these children, *Hemophilus influenzae* type b, accounts for 10% to 25% of episodes. *H influenzae* bacteremia affects older children and is less fulminant than *S pneumoniae* bacteremia, but it may be fatal.[141] Conjugated *H influenzae* type b vaccines produce excellent antibody responses in children with sickle cell disease and now are administered in early infancy (www.cdc.gov/vaccines/recs/schedules/child-schedule.htm).

Owing to the high mortality rate of bacteremia, hospitalization, blood and CSF cultures, and parenteral antibiotics has been the standard of care for children with fevers higher than 38.5°C. Prompt attention to fever can reduce the risk of severe pneumococcal sepsis. Rapid administration of antibiotics has resulted in a lower incidence of meningitis among bacteremic patients than 20 years ago, when the incidence was 50%.[144] The efficacy of ceftriaxone therapy for *S pneumoniae* and *H influenzae* infection[145] has led to new treatment algorithms that recommend outpatient therapy for most patients. However, resistant *S pneumoniae* have emerged, necessitating a thorough knowledge of local resistance patterns to guide the choice of alternate antibiotics (in particular, vancomycin, to which resistance has not been observed).

Table 43–10 Organ-Related Infection in Sickle Cell Disease

Primary Sites of Infection	Most Common Pathogen(s)	Other Pathogens	Pathophysiology	Prevention	Management
Septicemia	*Streptococcus pneumoniae*	*Haemophilus influenzae* type b *Escherichia coli* *Salmonella* sp.	Defective splenic function; deficiency of opsonic antibody	Vaccines* Prophylactic penicillin	Empiric intravenous antibiotics for fever
Meningitis	*S pneumoniae*			Same as for septicemia	
Osteomyelitis and septic arthritis	*Salmonella* species *S pneumoniae*	*E coli* *Proteus* species *Staphylococcus aureus*	Ischemic or infarcted tissue, prolonged course	—	Surgical drainage, intravenous antibiotics
Pneumonia	*Mycoplasma pneumoniae* Respiratory viruses	*Chlamydia pneumoniae* *S pneumoniae*	Concomitant infection and intrapulmonary vasoocclusion leading to infarction and/or sequestration	Vaccines[a]	See Pulmonary and Therapy sections for management of acute chest syndrome.

*Against *S pneumoniae* and *H influenzae* type b.
From Buchanan,[431] with permission.

Please see Pulmonary Complications for further discussions regarding pneumonia and acute chest syndrome.

Meningitis

Meningitis therapy should cover *S. pneumoniae* and probably *H. influenzae* type b and should be continued for at least 2 weeks.

Salmonella and Osteomyelitis

In this patient population, osteomyelitis is commonly caused by *Salmonella* species.[146] *Staphylococcus aureus*, the most common etiology in patients without sickle cell disease, accounts for less than 25% of sickle cell disease cases. Infection usually affects long bones, often at multiple sites.

Diagnosis is confirmed by culture of blood or infected bone. Parenteral antibiotics that cover *Salmonella* and *S. aureus* are given, and antibiotic therapy is based on culture results. Parenteral antibiotics are continued for 2 to 6 weeks.[146] Surgical drainage or sequestrectomy may be required. Most patients are cured by this approach, but there may be recurrences.[146]

Articular infection is less common and is often due to *S. pneumoniae*.[146]

Parvovirus B19 (see also Aplastic Crisis)

The specificity of the parvovirus B19 for erythroid precursor cells, coupled with the accelerated erythropoiesis in hemolytic anemias, leaves sickle cell patients vulnerable to infection by this agent.[147] In sickle cell disease, parvovirus infection is a common cause of aplastic crisis, especially in children. It has been reported to cause bone marrow necrosis, acute chest syndrome, pulmonary fat embolism, hepatic sequestration, and glomerulonephritis.[125–128]

Urinary Tract Infections

Patients with sickle cell disease are at a higher risk for urinary tract infections and pyelonephritis than the general population. *Escherichia coli* is the most common uropathogen and can cause septicemia in these patients. Persistent urinary tract infections may be secondary to renal papillary necrosis. All urinary tract infections in this patient population should be considered complicated, requiring 10 to 21 days of appropriate antibiotic therapy.

Neurologic Complications

Neurologic complications occur in 25% or more of patients with sickle cell disease.[148] Neurologic complications include cerebrovascular accidents (CVAs: consisting of transient ischemic attacks [TIAs], overt and silent cerebral infarction, cerebral hemorrhage), seizures (which can be a presenting feature of CVA), unexplained coma, spinal cord infarction or compression, central nervous system infections, vestibular dysfunction, and sensory hearing loss.[149]

Cerebrovascular Accidents, Pathophysiology, Incidence, Risk Factors, and Presentation[150]

Histopathologic evaluation of large-vessel involvement in sickle cell disease shows a pattern of smooth muscle proliferation with overlying endothelial damage and fibrosis. Smaller arterioles and capillaries demonstrate distension, thrombosis, and vessel wall necrosis.[151,152] Aneurysmal dilation associated with hemorrhagic stroke occurs at regions of intimal hyperplasia.[153] The vessel wall changes are likely multifactorial in origin related to endothelial injury from high and turbulent flow, RBC adherence, and hypoxia. But in addition, it has been speculated that depletion of nitric oxide (NO) by the free hemoglobin released through intravascular hemolysis may also play a role.[153] The age-specific pattern of stroke risk in sickle cell disease may be related to the higher cerebral flow rates in early childhood.[153] Cerebral thrombosis, which accounts for 70% to 80% of all CVAs in sickle cell disease, results from large-vessel occlusion (Fig. 43–9) rather than the more typical microvascular occlusion of sickle cell disease.[154] Silent infarcts are thought to result from microvascular vasoocclusion or thrombosis or chronic hypoxia in the periphery stemming from large-vessel disease.[155] In 30% of patients with sickle cell disease, major-vessel stenosis results in the formation of friable collateral vessels that appear as puffs of smoke (*moyamoya* in Japanese) on angiography.[156] Moyamoya disease predisposes to thrombotic and hemorrhagic strokes, seizures, and cognitive disability.[157]

The relative risk for stroke is 200 to 400 times higher in children with sickle cell disease compared to the children without sickle cell disease. The prevalence of clinically overt stroke is 11%. Clinically silent infarction detectable by MRI affects 17% to 20% of patients by age 20.[158] Silent infarcts are associated with cognitive impairment. Even in patients without silent or overt cerebral infarction, cognitive functioning can be impaired.[159] Almost 50% of the children with "silent" infarcts eventually require lifelong support or custodial care because of neuropsychologic deficits.[160] Infarctive strokes were common in children and those more than 30 years of age, whereas hemorrhagic stroke was most common between ages 20 and 30 years.[22]

Sickle cell-specific risk factors for CVA include increased cerebral blood flow velocity[161] (discussed further under Primary Prevention of Cerebrovascular Accidents), a previous history of overt or silent cerebral infarction,[162] nocturnal hypoxemia,[163] more severe anemia, higher reticulocyte counts, lower Hb F levels, higher white cell counts, the Hb SS genotype (rather than Hb SC disease or sickle cell–β thalassemia), nocturnal hypoxemia or sleep apnea, migraines, elevated homocysteine levels, "relative" systolic hypertension (ie, those at the high end of the lower-than-normal range characteristic of sickle cell disease).[22,164,477] Genetic markers of increased risk are the Central African Republic haplotype and the absence of α thalassemia.[153,165] Both small-vessel and large-vessel thrombosis can occur. Specific HLA alleles separately correlate with small- versus large-vessel stroke risk, suggesting that different pathologic processes may be involved.[153]

In addition to these sickle cell-specific predictors of stroke, one must also consider the well-documented modifiable risk factors for stroke that are operational in the general population; these are hypertension, exposure to cigarette smoke (active smoking or passive exposure), diabetes, atrial fibrillation, dyslipidemia, carotid artery stenosis, postmenopausal hormone therapy, poor diet, physical inactivity, obesity, and fat distribution. Less well-documented but potentially modifiable risk factors include alcohol or drug use, oral contraceptive use, and sleep-disordered breathing.[158]

CVAs are heralded by focal seizures in 10% to 33% of cases and by TIAs in 10%. CVAs are fatal in approximately 20% of initial cases, recur within 3 years in nearly 70%, and are the cause of motor and cognitive impairment in the majority. Intracranial hemorrhage results in the same signs as thrombosis, but in addition neck stiffness, photophobia, severe headache, vomiting, and altered consciousness may occur. Coma suggests hemorrhage rather than thrombosis. A typical presentation is coma and seizures without hemiparesis. Although the mortality rate may be as high as 50%, the morbidity of survivors is low. Hemorrhage may be subarachnoid, intraparenchymal, or intraventricular, which can be differentiated by angiography. The favorable neurosurgical outcome in subarachnoid hemorrhage due to ruptured aneurysm justifies an aggressive approach to diagnosis, transfusion, vasodilatory therapy, and surgery.

Primary Prevention of Cerebrovascular Accidents

The overall risk of stroke in pediatric patients with sickle cell disease is 1% per year; however, in the subset of patients with transcranial Doppler evidence of a high (>200 cm/s) cerebral blood flow velocity in the internal carotid artery or middle cerebral artery the stroke risk is in excess of 10% per year (although this is still much lower than the risk of recurrent stroke in a sickle cell patient after a first event, which is approximately 70%). In the Stroke Prevention Trial in Sickle Cell Disease (STOP), 130 children diagnosed as having clinically silent cerebral artery stenosis on the basis of high cerebral flow rates were randomized to receive chronic transfusion therapy or not. Over a period of more than 2 years, the risk of stroke was reduced to less than 1% per year in the transfused group[161] (a risk reduction of >90%). The ability of transfusion to curtail progression of large-vessel stenosis has also been proven with angiography.[166]

Because of the risks of iron overload and allosensitization with chronic transfusion, a randomized controlled trial of withdrawal of transfusion was conducted (STOP 2). This trial evaluated discontinuation of transfusion after at least 30 months in children who had not had an overt stroke and in whom the cerebral flow rates decreased to low risk (<170 cm/s) with transfusion. This study was terminated early because of a high rate of reversion to high-risk TCD flow rates (34%) and stroke (5%) in the patients taken off transfusion compared to the group who continued transfusion.[167]

In children, MRI can also be used to assess stroke risk: 8.1% of children with an asymptomatic MRI lesion versus 0.5% of those with a normal MRI had a stroke during the ensuing 5 years.[162] A randomized trial of MRI-guided prophylactic transfusion is in progress (Silent Infarct Treatment Trial [SITT]). In adults, MRI/MRA of the brain should be used[29] to assess thrombotic or hemorrhagic stroke risk.

Chronic transfusion is associated with a significant complication rate. Therefore, there is a need for alternatives, especially because some patients and physicians feel that the 10% annual stroke risk does not warrant the risks and burdens of chronic transfusion.[150] The role of aspirin in ischemic stroke prevention in sickle cell disease is being evaluated (see Basic Management and Disease Modification). Hydroxyurea significantly lowered the TCD velocity values in a group of 24 children with Hb SS disease compared to an age-matched control group.[46] The role of hydroxyurea is being formally evaluated in secondary stroke prevention (see Secondary Prevention below). Stem cell transplantation has resulted in stabilization of cerebral vasculopathy[168] but there is a mortality risk with this procedure of between 6% and 10%.

Other modifiable risk factors for stroke (see Cerebrovascular Accidents, Pathophysiology, Incidence, Risk Factors, and Presentation above) should be identified and treated. Notably, in the general population, hypertension is particularly associated with a risk for hemorrhagic stroke, and effective treatment of hypertension can produce a relative risk reduction of 26% for ischemic stroke and 49% for hemorrhagic stroke.[169] In patients with sickle cell disease followed through the Cooperative Study of Sickle Cell Disease, both diastolic and systolic blood pressures were noted to be lower than for matched controls. Patients with systolic pressures in the higher range for the sickle cell group, even with systolic pressures less than 140 mmHg, had an increased risk of first ischemic stroke (there were insufficient events to make firm conclusions regarding hemorrhagic stroke).[164] Therefore, at a minimum, it seems reasonable to follow population-wide recommendations for blood pressure control in patients with sickle cell disease.

Evaluation and Management of Acute Cerebrovascular Accidents

Patients with symptoms and signs of CVA should be evaluated immediately using computed tomographic (CT) scanning or magnetic resonance imaging to distinguish TIA, cerebral thrombosis, and hemorrhage. In those with hemorrhage, angiography or magnetic resonance angiography is indicated, after partial-exchange transfusion is performed to avoid complications associated with the injected contrast material. In both thrombosis and hemorrhage, prompt partial-exchange transfusion is performed, and chronic direct transfusion to maintain the Hb S level below 30% is instituted to prevent recurrent events (see also Basic Management and Disease Modification) and promote resolution of arterial stenoses.[166]

Secondary Prevention of Cerebrovascular Accidents

The risk of recurrent stroke is approximately 70%, a risk that is reduced to around 13% with chronic transfusion.[170] Although recurrent CVAs during chronic transfusion have been reported, this therapeutic modality provides the best means of preventing recurrence (Fig. 43–11). This treatment also provides incidental protection against pain crises, bacterial infections, acute chest syndrome, and hospitalization.

Based on the data from STOP 2 (see Primary Prevention of Cerebrovascular Accidents above), chronic transfusion is continued

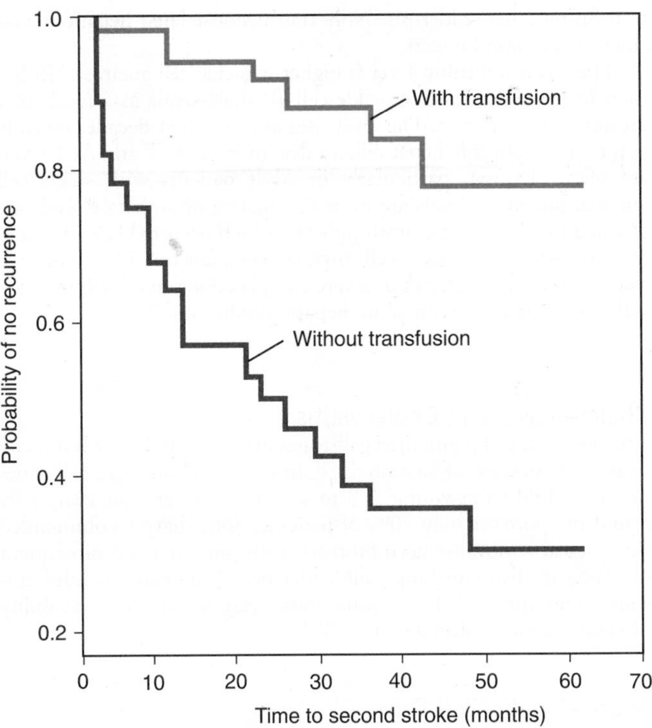

Figure 43–11 Comparison of stroke recurrence over 62 months in a transfused group and in untransfused historical control groups.[467,823] *(Adapted from Pegelow et al, with permission.)*

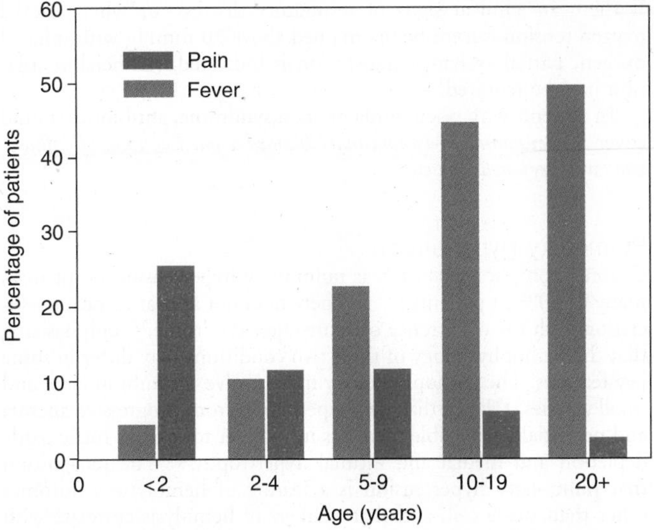

Figure 43–12 Age-specific associated events within 2 weeks preceding acute chest syndrome. *(Adapted from Vichinsky et al with permission.)*

indefinitely. This may not be feasible for administrative reasons or because of allosensitization or iron overload for which the patient is unable or unwilling to undergo treatment. Therefore, clinical trials to determine if disease modifiers such as hydroxyurea or decitabine can reduce stroke risk are indicated. In patients with a history of CVA transitioned from chronic transfusion to hydroxyurea, the recurrent stroke rate remained stable and in the range seen with continued transfusion.[78]

Per primary prevention, all other identified modifiable risk factors for stroke should be identified and treated.

In patients with moyamoya disease, surgical approaches to therapy, such as extracranial–intracranial bypass, have been useful in improving the perfusion of affected regions of the brain.

Stem cell transplantation has resulted in stabilization of cerebral vasculopathy,[168] but the risk of a second neurologic event is higher in the peritransplant period and mortality with this procedure is between 6% and 10%.[168]

Seizures

Seizures occur more commonly among patients with sickle cell disease. In one study, 21 of 152 patients in a pediatric clinic had seizures, 4 of which were related to meperidine therapy. Most had nonfocal CT and MRI studies but focal electroencephalographic changes.[171] CVAs are heralded by focal seizures in 10% to 33% of cases. Therefore, seizures in sickle cell disease ultimately may be related to the underlying vasculopathy.

Pulmonary Complications

Pulmonary disease is the leading cause of death in sickle cell disease.[16] Both acute and chronic pulmonary complications are common. The common acute complications are pneumonia and acute chest syndrome, and the common chronic complication is pulmonary hypertension.

Pneumonia

Pneumonia is defined as chest infiltrates on chest x-ray or chest CT scan associated with fever and an identified infectious etiology.

The risk for and increased frequency of *S pneumoniae* infections is discussed under Infections above. In addition, *Mycoplasma pneumoniae*, *Chlamydia pneumoniae*, and *Legionella* are also relatively common causes of pneumonia in sickle cell disease. Antibiotic therapy for pneumonia or acute chest syndrome should cover these agents in addition to pneumococcus and *H influenzae*.

When antibiotics are used to treat the acute chest syndrome, they should cover *S pneumoniae*, *H influenzae* type b, *M pneumoniae*, and *C pneumoniae*. The combination of cefuroxime and erythromycin is recommended.

Acute Chest Syndrome

Acute chest syndrome occurs in approximately 30% of patients.[172] Acute chest syndrome is defined as a new infiltrate on chest x-ray or chest CT scan associated with one or more new symptoms: fever, chest pain, cough, sputum production, dyspnea, or hypoxia. This entity is included in discussions of sickle cell disease because processes other than infection, such as vasoocclusion, could also lead to pulmonary symptoms, signs, and chest x-ray changes. However, it should be borne in mind that the usual etiology might be both vasoocclusion and infection simultaneously, and in almost all cases of chest syndrome, antibiotics should be administered. Many episodes in which common pathogens are not cultured are due to "atypical" agents (*Mycoplasma*, *Legionella*, and *Chlamydia*), suggesting that antibiotic therapy include agents directed at atypical agents. Pulmonary fat embolus, evidenced by stainable fat in pulmonary macrophages obtained by bronchoalveolar lavage or sputum induction, is found in 44% to 60% of cases of acute chest syndrome.[173] Acute chest syndrome due to pulmonary fat embolus is associated with more severe hematologic and clinical abnormalities. In adults the mortality rate is four times higher than in children.[3,174]

Acute chest syndrome is often preceded by febrile episodes in children and by vasoocclusive pain crisis in adults (Fig. 43–12).[174] Elevation of serum phospholipase A2 (sPLA2) was detected in patients admitted with vasoocclusive pain crisis 24 to 48 hours before acute chest syndrome was clinically diagnosed.[175] Pulmonary fat embolus is often preceded by an acute painful episode. Some patients have a rapidly progressive course associated with a precipitous decrease in arterial oxygen tension; they may require intensive care treatment.

If there are clinical signs of respiratory distress, or when arterial oxygen tension cannot be maintained above 70 mmHg with inhaled oxygen, partial-exchange transfusion is indicated. Artificial ventilation may be required.

In patients with pneumonia or chest syndrome, antibiotics should cover *S pneumoniae*, *Mycoplasma/Chlamydia pneumoniae*, *H influenzae*, and *Legionella* species.

Pulmonary Hypertension

Chronic complications such as pulmonary hypertension occur in as many as 60% of patients.[176–178] There does not appear to be an association with the occurrence of acute chest syndrome,[177] emphasizing that the pathophysiology of these two conditions may differ in some key features. The pathophysiology may involve thrombi in large and small arteries,[179,180] cardiac decompensation from progressive anemia and potentially reversible increases in vascular tone from nitric oxide depletion and medial and intimal hypertrophy.[180] The recognition that pulmonary hypertension is a feature of hemolytic syndromes other than sickle cell, and that markers of hemolysis correlate with the risk of pulmonary hypertension, supports the idea that depletion of nitric oxide (NO) through scavenging by free hemoglobin may have an important role in the pathophysiology of this disease.[177,181] Pulmonary hypertension usually occurs in adults and carries a poor prognosis.[182]

The association with early death and the emerging availability of candidate treatments suggest that efforts should be made to diagnosis this condition in all patients with sickle cell disease.[176,181] Routine clinical exam and routine tests like the CXR are not sufficient to make the diagnosis, because changes in these assessments may be evident only in very late stages of chronic lung damage. The feasibility of an echocardiogram determined tricuspid regurgitant jet (TR-jet) velocity measurement of 2.5 m/s to make the diagnosis was suggested by selective cardiac catheterization in a cohort of 195 patients[176]; however, the sensitivity and specificity of this test may have limitations.[181] Elevations in brain natriuretic peptide (BNP) levels correlate with an increased TR-jet and risk of early death. The gold standard for diagnosing pulmonary hypertension remains right heart catheterization.

Although there have been no completed definitive treatment trials of pulmonary hypertension in sickle cell disease, there are a number of options that have demonstrated efficacy in other populations with pulmonary hypertension and for which there is pilot data and/or ongoing trials in sickle cell disease. These options include sildenafil, arginine, and bosentan.[183–186] These patients should also be considered for disease modification (see Basic Management and Disease Modification).

Other Pulmonary Complications

Other findings include restrictive and obstructive lung disease and hypoxemia.[187] High-resolution, thin-section CT scanning of the lungs may show chronic interstitial fibrosis. Airway hyperreactivity occurs in nearly two-thirds of children with sickle cell disease not diagnosed as having asthma. Thirty-six percent of 53 children with sickle cell disease were found to have sleep-related upper-airway obstruction, 16% had hypoxemia, and all 15 who underwent adenotonsillectomy were symptomatically improved and had improved hypoxemia.[188] Sleep apnea may be associated with surgically reversible exacerbations of painful episodes and strokes. Blood gas and pulmonary function measurements should be obtained as baseline data for all patients.

Hepatobiliary Complications

Hepatobiliary complications in sickle cell disease include cholelithiasis, cholecystitis, acute hepatic cell crisis, acute hepatic sequestration crisis, and sickle cell intrahepatic cholestasis.[189] Chronic transfusion also places patients at risk for infection with hepatitis viruses and for transfusional hemasiderosis. Non–transfusion-related hepatic hemasiderosis can also be seen.

The serum bilirubin level is higher in sickle cell anemia (Hb SS) than in Hb SC disease or sickle cell–β^+ thalassemia as a result of a greater hemolytic rate. The level rises after the first decade, possibly as a result of chronic hepatobiliary dysfunction. AST and ALT levels are often elevated, particularly in adult patients with sickle cell anemia, but mean levels are normal. Alkaline phosphatase levels are elevated in all genotypes until puberty, which occurred later in males and in those with sickle cell anemia. Percutaneous liver biopsy is associated with a high risk of severe complications and death in sickle cell disease patients with acute hepatic syndromes.[190]

Cholelithiasis and Cholecystitis

The prevalence of pigmented gallstones in sickle cell disease is directly related to the rate of hemolysis.[191] In sickle cell anemia, gallstones occur in children as young as 3 to 4 years of age and are eventually found in approximately 70% of patients. Some have recommended the surgical removal of asymptomatic gallstones to avoid subsequent difficulty in distinguishing gallbladder pain from acute painful episodes. This approach has become more feasible with the availability of laparoscopic cholecystectomy.[192]

Acute Hepatic Cell Crisis

Acute hepatic cell crisis presents with tender hepatomegaly, worsening jaundice, and fever.[189] The likely etiology is hepatocellular cell ischemia. The AST and bilirubin are elevated, but rarely above 300 IU/L and 255 μM, respectively. This syndrome usually resolves within 3 to 14 days with supportive care alone but can progress to liver failure and fatal outcome; therefore, patients should be monitored closely and exchange transfusion initiated if there are signs of progressive liver dysfunction (eg, increasing AST).

Acute Hepatic Sequestration Crisis

Acute hepatic sequestration crisis presents with acute hepatic enlargement and a dramatic fall in hemoglobin concentration, the most likely mechanism being sequestration of sickled erythrocytes in the liver. Management is with supportive care and transfusions.

Intrahepatic Cholestasis

Sickle cell intrahepatic cholestasis results in severe, asymptomatic hyperbilirubinemia without fever, pain, leukocytosis, hepatic failure, or death.[193] Asymptomatic hyperbilirubinemia without signs of progressive liver dysfunction (eg, increasing AST) does not require specific therapy. Evidence of progressive liver dysfunction should prompt consideration of acute hepatic cell crisis and exchange transfusion.

Hepatitis C Infection

Chronic hepatitis C infection in sickle cell disease occurs with a prevalence that is related to the number of transfusions received; it may be a leading cause of cirrhosis. Liver transplantation has been used successfully as therapy for this complication.[194] If indicated, interferon-ribavarin can be used to treat hepatitis C in sickle cell disease patients.[195]

Obstetric and Gynecologic Issues

Gynecologic complications (delayed menarche, dysmenorrhea, ovarian cysts, pelvic infection, and fibrocystic disease of the breast) are more common in women with sickle cell disease. Pregnancy entails increased risks to mother and child compared to the general population.

Pregnancy

Pregnancy in patients with sickle cell disease is associated with increased risks to both the mother and fetus, although these risks are not so great as to prohibit continuation of pregnancy.[196,197] The fetal complications of pregnancy, most of which are related to compromised placental blood flow, are the increased incidence of spontaneous early abortion, intrauterine growth retardation, low birthweight, and fetal death. Maternal complications include increased rates of painful episodes, severe anemia due to iron or folate deficiencies, exaggeration of the physiologic "anemia of pregnancy," increased infections (urinary tract, pneumonias, endometritis), preeclampsia, and death.[197] It is controversial whether the degree of anemia predicts the birth of babies with low birthweight. The occurrence of a perinatal death in a previous pregnancy and the presence of twins in the present pregnancy are two major risk factors for an unfavorable outcome. The course of pregnancy is more benign in Hb SC disease than in sickle cell anemia.

Better fetal and maternal outcomes in recent years are largely due to generally improved antenatal and obstetric care. The patient should be followed in a high-risk obstetric clinic in addition to the hematology clinic and receive the usual vitamin, mineral, and folate supplements. A high-calorie, high-protein diet can be considered. There is no specific therapeutic or preventive treatment for intrauterine growth retardation. Some experts recommend prophylactic transfusion, but a large controlled study showed no improvement in fetal outcome from this management option although maternal symptoms are reduced. In addition to the usual indications for transfusion therapy in sickle cell disease, transfusion therapy is indicated for patients with cardiac or respiratory compromise, in preparation for C-section, preeclampsia, twin pregnancy, acute chest syndrome, hemoglobin levels more than 20% below steady state or less than 5 g/dL, and previous history of perinatal mortality. If the hemoglobin is between 8 and 10 g/dL, and transfusion is indicated for any of the reasons above, partial exchange should be performed (eg, phlebotomy of 400–500 mL and transfusion of 2 units PRBC).[196] The type of delivery does not appear to represent a problem, and both spontaneous delivery and cesarean section are well tolerated.

Some experts advise that hypertonic saline injections are contraindicated for elective termination of pregnancy because of the risk of sickling-induced vasoocclusion. However, most methods of abortion are well tolerated. There are anecdotal reports of a higher incidence of acute painful episodes after therapeutic abortion; inpatient intravenous hydration before and for the 24 hours after the procedure is recommended.

Birth Control

Modern non–estrogen-containing intrauterine devices should be considered. Although depot injections of medroxyprogesterone (Depo-Provera) given every 3 months may be safe with regards to stroke risk,[198] there is a risk of bone loss, a consideration in patients with sickle cell disease and their propensity to skeletal complications. Oral contraceptives containing low doses of estrogen can be considered with no clear evidence of increased stroke demonstrated to date, although the patients' overall stroke risk should probably still be taken into consideration until there is more phase IV follow-up on the clinical experience. Another caution with low-dose estrogen oral contraception is the risk of contraceptive failure with less than excellent compliance. There may be risks to contraception, but against this must be weighed the risks of unintended pregnancy. Sexually active women should have routine pelvic exams and birth control instructions.

Renal Complications

Hypertension, proteinuria, hematuria, increasing anemia, and nephrotic syndrome reliably predict progression to renal failure, clinical indices to pay attention to because the serum creatinine may be misleading. Patients with sickle cell anemia exhibit an increased proximal tubular secretion of creatinine. Thus, patients may have a significant decline in renal function before it is detectable by measuring creatinine clearance.[199] The mean age at presentation with end-stage renal disease is 41 years.[200] Serum creatinine levels are low in all genotypes until age 18 years, when males experience a rise, apparently related to increasing muscle mass. Creatinine levels increase with age in all genotypes, presumably due to declining renal function (see also organ-specific complications, kidney).

Other risk factors for the development of chronic renal failure include use of nonsteroidal antiinflammatory drugs[201] and genetic predisposition associated with the CAR β-globin haplotype; the latter has been suggested as an indication for bone marrow transplantation to prevent this outcome.[202] Acute renal failure from infarction may result from hypovolemia, sepsis, hepatorenal syndrome, cardiac failure, renal vein thrombosis, and rhabdomyolysis. These patients typically survive and recover their renal function with no increased risk of developing chronic renal failure.

There are seven well-described nephropathies that affect patients with either sickle cell trait or disease. These are gross hematuria, papillary necrosis, nephrotic syndrome, renal infarction, inability to concentrate urine, pyelonephritis, and renal medullary carcinoma.[199]

Renal transplantation is recommended for patients with sickle cell and end-stage renal diseases.

Renal Endocrine (Erythropoietin) Deficiency

This is discussed under Basic Management and Disease Modification.

Gross Hematuria

Hematuria may result from microthrombi formation in the peritubular capillaries of the renal medulla or from frank papillary necrosis. Significant hematuria may resolve with high urinary flow through oral hydration and bed rest. Hematuria that lasts longer than 1 to 2 weeks or the need for transfusion may require maintenance of a high urinary flow using a combination of hypotonic fluids and loop diuretics and urinary alkalinization using sodium bicarbonate and acetazolamide. These therapies are aimed at changing the acidic, hypertonic environment of the renal medulla that favors erythrocyte dehydration, increased HbS concentrations, and HbS polymerization. If bleeding persists for 72 hours despite these measures then alternative treatment should be considered. These may include oral urea,[203] ε-aminocaproic acid, and vasopressin. Embolization or nephrectomy should be reserved for prolonged, life-threatening cases of hematuria that require multiple transfusions.

Increased hematuria can also be seen as a consequence of delayed hemolytic transfusion reactions (discussed in Exacerbations of Anemia).

Papillary Necrosis

Papillary necrosis is most often detected incidentally by imaging or microscopic examination of urine in asymptomatic patients. Sloughed papilla may cause ureteral obstruction and urinary tract infection. In addition to broad-spectrum antibiotics, this occurrence requires emergent relief of the obstruction with a retrograde ureteral stent or placement of a percutaneous nephrostomy tube. Nonsteroidal anti-inflammatory agents should be avoided in patients with papillary necrosis. Otherwise treatment is as for hematuria.

Proteinuria

Proteinuria has been found in 20% to 30% of patients with sickle cell disease. Increasing age and low hemoglobin levels correlate with proteinuria. Proteinuria can progress to nephrotic syndrome characterized by proteinuria, hypoalbuminemia, edema, and hyperlipidemia. Angiotensin-converting enzyme inhibitors produce a significant

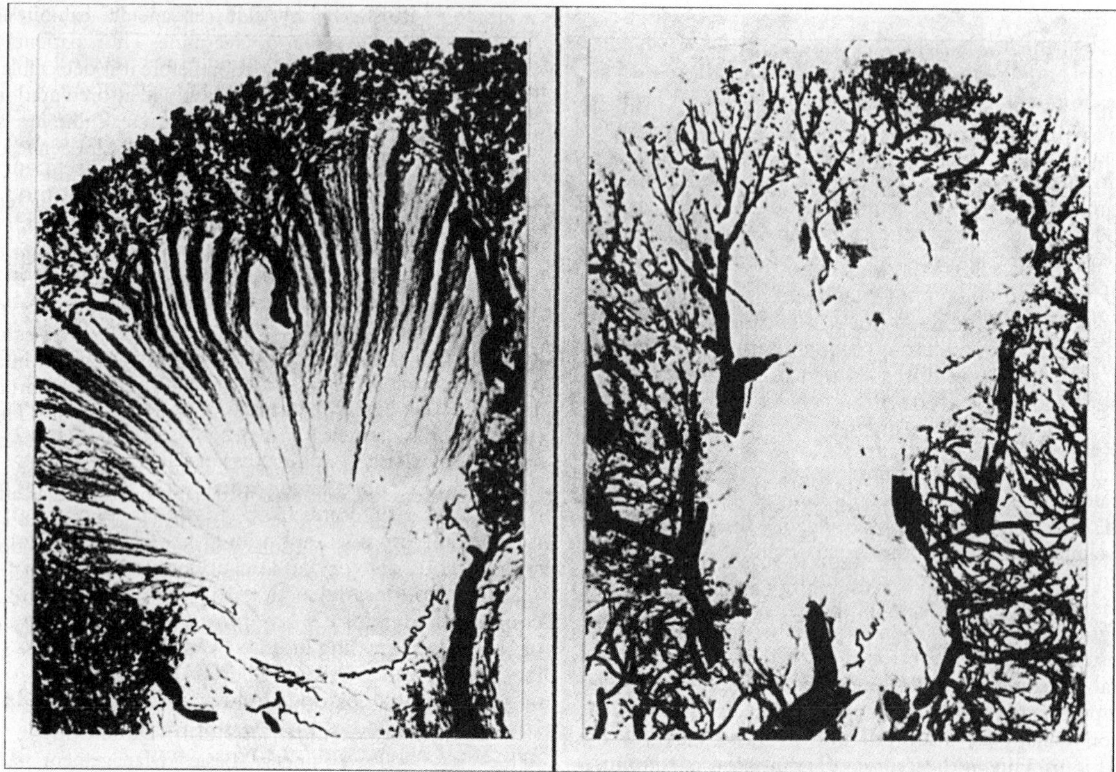

Figure 43–13 Postmortem microangiographic studies of the vasa recta in a normal individual (left) and a patient with sickle cell anemia (right). *(From Bertles JF, Döbler J: Reversible and irreversible sickling: A distinction by electron microscopy. Blood 33:884, 1969, with permission.)*

reduction in sickle proteinuria although it is unclear if ACE inhibitors might slow or halt the progression of proteinuria to nephrotic syndrome and renal failure.[204,205] Angiotensin II inhibitors are being studied for a potential role in decreasing sickle cell-related proteinuria and renal function deterioration.

Hyposthenuria and Other Abnormalities of Tubular Function

The inability to maximally concentrate urine (hyposthenuria) in response to water deprivation is an early finding of sickle cell nephropathy. Both sickle cell trait and disease patients may be affected. Hyposthenuria is the cumulative result of recurrent micro-infarcts in the vasa recta due to sickling (Fig. 43–13). When water-deprived, these patients cannot maximally concentrate their urine, developing hypovolemia and dehydration.

Other abnormalities of renal tubular dysfunction found in sickle cell anemia include an incomplete form of distal renal tubular acidosis with hyperchloremic metabolic acidosis and hyperkalemia.[206] The hyperkalemia may respond to oral sodium bicarbonate.

Urinary Tract Infections

Urinary tract infections and pyelonephritis are discussed under infectious complications.

Renal Medullary Carcinoma

Sickle cell trait has been reported to be associated with renal medullary carcinoma.[207] Presentation is with gross hematuria, abdominal and or flank pain, or significant weight loss. The disease may be metastatic at diagnosis and the prognosis is poor. There is a weak association of renal medullary carcinoma with Hb SC disease but no identified association with sickle cell anemia. The reason for these patterns of disease are not known.

Priapism

Priapism is a condition that is characterized by sustained erection that does not result from sexual desire and is not relieved by sexual activity. Stuttering priapism is a separate entity that is characterized by multiple, brief episodes of sustained unwanted erection. It has been reported to affect 6.4% to 42% of males with sickle cell disease[208] and can also occur in sickle cell trait. Its peak frequencies are between ages 5 and 13 years and 21 and 29 years. Priapism is most likely to develop in patients with lower Hb F levels and reticulocyte counts, increased platelet counts, and the Hb SS genotype. Priapism caused by sickle cell disease is usually ischemic, or low-flow, priapism (high-flow priapism is caused by unregulated arterial flow and can be distinguished from low-flow priapism by a blood gas obtained from the corpora). Most likely, priapism begins with a physiologic erection. The relative stasis of blood within the corpora leads to a decrease in oxygen tension and development of acidosis, predisposing to HbS polymerization in the corporal sinusoids, venous occlusion, and low-flow priapism. Pain develops as the corpora become increasingly ischemic after approximately 4 hours of erection. In a minority of patients, usually postpubertal, the engorgement also affects the corpus spongiosum and glans. The mild acidosis that accompanies hypoventilation during sleep may also contribute to the pathophysiology. Impotence is the primary complication of priapism although patients with a history of multiple episodes of priapism and significant corporeal fibrosis may report fair erections and maintain active sex lives. Corporeal ischemia during priapism may induce local inflammation, causing the fibrosis responsible for impotence.

The goal of treatment is to relieve priapism and maintain potency. Patients should be educated to seek medical attention for unrelenting erection of more than 2 hours' duration. Detumescence within 12 hours is optimal to retain potency. After 72 hours, impotence is more likely. The strategy is prompt initiation of supportive medical therapy with intravenous hydration and analgesia, and involvement by a urology consultant if the priapism persists for more than 4 hours;

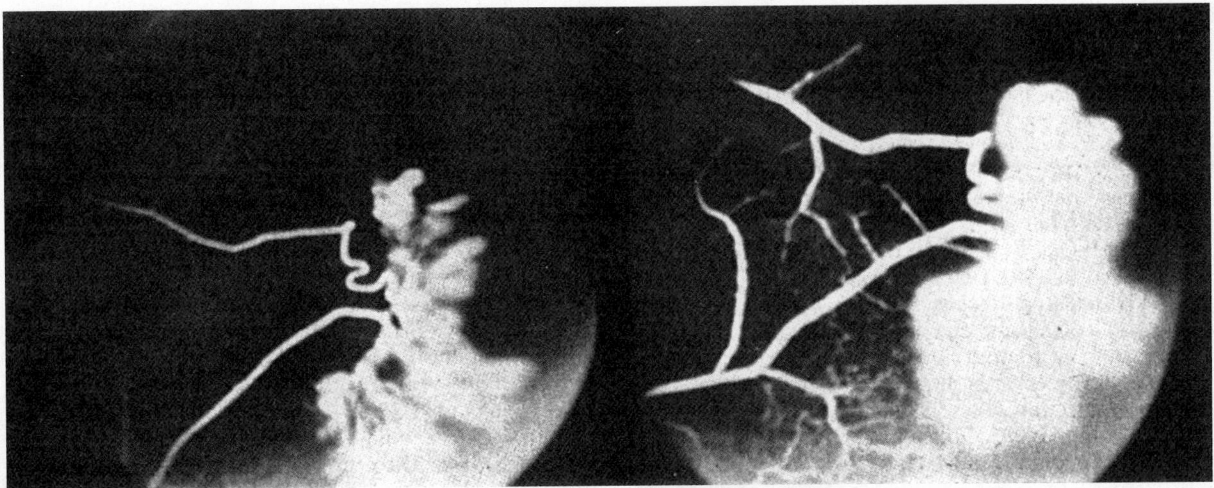

Figure 43–14 Fluorescein angiography demonstrating a "sea fan" appearance of sickle proliferative retinopathy. *(Kindly provided by WC Mentzer.)*

aspiration of blood from the corpora with or without irrigation and injection of an α-adrenergic agonist should be considered (Guidelines of the American Urological Association, www.guideline.gov). If priapism persists 12 hours, options include partial-exchange transfusion to reduce the Hb S level to less than 30% with a total hemoglobin of less than 10 g/dL and/or irrigation as outlined above. The latter procedure is less effective after 36 hours of priapism. Irrigation should be performed using penile anesthesia (dorsal nerve block, circumferential penile block, or subcutaneous, local, penile shaft block). All pediatric irrigation should be performed under conscious sedation. There is anecdotal evidence for the use of hydralazine to treat acute priapism.[209]

Preventing recurrent priapism is an important component of management. Strategies include hydroxyurea administration, chronic transfusion, the antiandrogen bicalutamide,[210] self-administration of the α-adrenergic agent etilefrine orally and, for episodes lasting over an hour, by intracavernous injection, and monthly administration of intramuscular gonadotropin-releasing hormone analogue.[211,212] Prophylactic pseudoepinephrine (Sudafed) appears beneficial in preventing recurrent mild episodes.

Surgical creation of shunts is reserved for severe cases resistant to the above interventions. As many as 45% of patients who have priapism develop some degree of impotence.[213] When impotence persists 12 months, a semirigid penile prosthesis may be implanted.

Ocular Complications[214]

The retina is particularly vulnerable to vasoocclusion, and annual retinal examination is part of routine health care maintenance for patients with sickle cell disease. Superficial retinal hemorrhages have a pink "salmon patch" appearance. Deeper retinal hemorrhages have a "black sunburst" appearance. Other manifestations of sickle cell retinopathy include iridescent spots, retinal neovascularization, and retinal detachment. More subtle signs of sickle cell retinopathy are optic nerve head vascular changes, vascular tortuosity, macular changes (eg, microaneurysms and vascular loops), and peripheral arteriovenous anastamoses. Other ophthalmologic complications are anterior chamber ischemia, tortuosity of conjunctival vessels, retinal artery occlusion, and angioid streaks. Sickle cell retinopathy is best seen by fluorescein angiography (Fig. 43–14). The earlier onset and greater frequency of proliferative retinopathy in Hb SC disease and sickle cell–β^+ thalassemia compared to sickle cell anemia and sickle cell–β° thalassemia suggest that retinal vessels are more susceptible to occlusion by more viscous blood than by more rigid individual cells. Peripheral sickle retinopathy may require vision-saving therapy with laser photocoagulation. Orbital compression syndrome due to vasoocclusion of the periorbital marrow space and subperiosteal hemorrhage has been observed to result in headache, fever, and palpebral edema. In this situation, culture, CT scan, and MRI should be used to rule out infectious, neoplastic, and other hemorrhagic etiologies. Conservative therapy, including local measures, analgesia, fluids, transfusion, and careful ophthalmalogic surveillance, is recommended, unless compression of the optic nerve ensues, in which case surgical decompression should be considered.

Bone Complications

Chronic tower skull, bossing of the forehead, and fish mouth deformity of vertebrae are the result of extended hematopoietic marrow, causing widening of the medullary space, thinning of the trabeculae and cortices, and osteoporosis. Osteonecrosis may cause a steplike depression of vertebrae, selected shortening of the cuboidal bones of the hands and feet, and acute aseptic or avascular necrosis. The excruciating pain of bone infarction in the "hand–foot syndrome" that occurs around age 2 years is often the first symptom of sickle cell disease (Fig. 43–15).[215] This dactylitis resolves spontaneously and is treated with hydration and analgesia. Bone infarcts are demonstrable using nuclear medicine scintigraphy or MRI. Serial scans specific for bone osteoclasts, bone marrow macrophages, and inflammatory cells may be useful adjuncts for distinguishing bone marrow infarction from osteomyelitis, but it is essential to obtain cultures directly from the affected tissue before starting antibiotics. Treatment of osteomyelitis was addressed in the Infection sections.

Bone necrosis occurs with equal frequency in the femoral and humeral heads, but the femoral heads more commonly undergo progressive joint destruction as a result of chronic weight bearing. The process is associated with increased intraosseous pressure, and is most sensitively detected by MRI. Aggressive physical therapy appears to prevent progression in mild cases and should be considered in the therapy of avascular necrosis. Core decompression surgery to relieve increased intraosseous pressure can be used in early-stage osteonecrosis (ie, no radiographic evidence of bone collapse) to prevent disease progression. In more advanced disease, joint replacement can be considered. There is a 30% likelihood that a second hip revision will be required within 4 to 5 years of prosthetic hip placement in patients with sickle cell disease.[216]

Arthritic pain, swelling, and effusion may be related to periarticular infarction or gouty arthritis.

Bone marrow infarction causes reticulocytopenia, exacerbation of anemia, a leukoerythroblastic picture, and sometimes pancytopenia.[127,128] Pulmonary fat embolism is a rare complication of marrow infarction.[217] It is associated with fat globules in the sputum and refractile bodies visible in the optic fundi. It is a life-threatening event

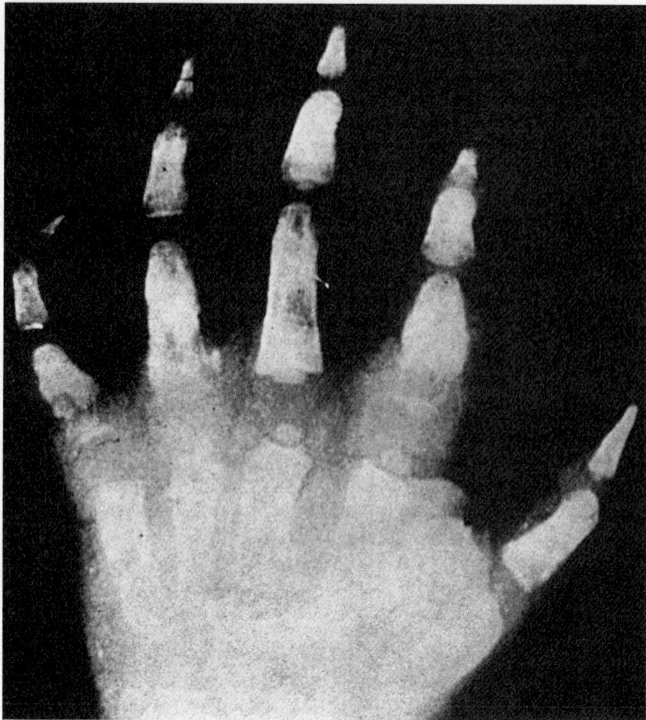

Figure 43–15 Radiogram showing the bone infarctions in the hands of a child with the "hand–foot syndrome" dactylitis. *(Kindly provided by WC Mentzer.)*

that may require prompt exchange transfusion and perhaps the use of heparin and corticosteroids.[217]

Dermatologic Complications

Leg ulcers are major causes of morbidity in sickle cell disease as a result of their frequency, chronicity, and resistance to therapy. Most occur near the medial or lateral malleolus (Fig. 43–16), may be associated with venous hypertension[218] and hemolytic rate,[219] and are frequently bilateral.[220] They may begin spontaneously or as a result of trauma and may become infected, most commonly by *S aureus*, *Pseudomonas*, streptococci, or *Bacteroides*. Systemic infection, osteomyelitis, and tetanus are rare complications. Ulcers are resistant to healing and tend to be recurrent in well over half the cases. Their incidence has been reported to vary from 25% to 75%.[221] Ulcers rarely occur in patients younger than age 10 years and are most common in sickle cell anemia, less common in sickle cell–β° thalassemia, and nonexistent in Hb SC disease and sickle cell–β^{+} thalassemia.[220] The incidence in sickle cell anemia patients declines substantially in those who have coexistent α thalassemia.[220] Low steady-state Hb levels and low fetal hemoglobin levels are associated with an increased risk of leg ulceration.[222] Males have a threefold greater risk for developing leg ulcers than females. Treatment of leg ulcers requires persistence and patience; healing usually takes weeks. Therapy[223] begins with gentle debridement to remove nonviable, superficial tissue from more vital areas. Wet-to-dry dressings and Duoderm hydrocolloid dressings facilitate devitalization. Once debridement is complete, zinc oxide-impregnated Unna boots are used to promote healing. Bed rest speeds healing,[224] and topical antibiotics may be required. It may be necessary to use elastic wraps or leg elevation to control edema. Rapid healing of leg ulcers has been reported in patients treated with intravenous arginine butyrate.[225] Oral zinc, local hyperbaric oxygen, chronic transfusion, recombinant erythropoietin, propionyl-L-carnitine, skin grafts, pentoxifylline, and becaplermin (platelet-derived growth factor) may have therapeutic roles and should be considered in individual cases but have not been

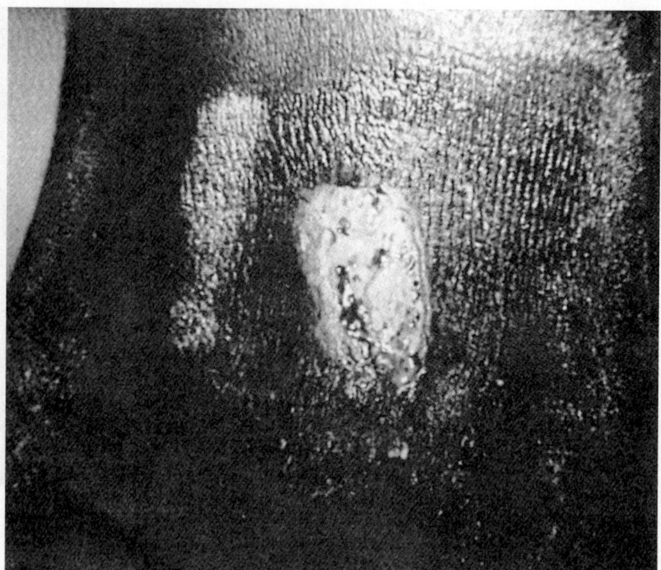

Figure 43–16 Chronic leg ulcer near the medial malleolus. *(Kindly provided by WC Mentzer.)*

formally tested for their effectiveness in accelerating resolution of sickle cell-associated leg ulcers.

Myofascial syndromes consist of soft-tissue swelling in subcutaneous edema that may have a *peau d'orange* appearance. These may be large or discrete lesions a few centimeters in diameter. These lesions are probably the result of dermal or subdermal vasoocclusion. Treatment is symptomatic.

Cardiac Complications

The chronic anemia of sickle cell disease is compensated by high cardiac output, which results in chronic chamber enlargement and cardiomegaly, and mild to moderate mitral and tricuspid regurgitation, even in young children. The electrocardiogram shows evidence of left ventricular hypertrophy, and less often first-degree block and nonspecific ST-T wave changes. Left ventricular dilation correlates with age and inversely correlates with total hemoglobin.[226] An age-dependent loss of cardiac reserve may predispose to heart failure in adult patients stressed by fluid overload, transfusion, exacerbation of anemia, hypoxia, or hypertension. Cardiac function can be improved by transfusion.[227] Acute myocardial infarction in the absence of coronary disease has been reported, and in one autopsy series 9.7% of 72 consecutive patients with sickle cell disease had myocardial infarction.[228] It appears that myocardial infarction may occur with normal coronary arteries as a result of increased oxygen demand exceeding limited oxygen-carrying capacity, or as a result of microcirculatory impairment. As mentioned earlier, pulmonary hypertension (>30 mmHg) is a relatively common finding in sickle cell disease and can be associated with right ventricular hypertrophy. It has been suggested that the increased rate of sudden death observed in sickle cell disease may be related to cardiac autonomic dysfunction, as detected by abnormal heart rate variability in response to selected postural maneuvers.[229]

Multiorgan Failure

This disastrous acute event involves multiple organ systems, including the lungs, brain, kidneys, liver, hematologic system, and heart, and usually leads to death.[230] It may be precipitated by infection, vasoocclusion, or fat embolus and consists of a constellation of life-threatening processes, including hypoxemia, acidosis, inflammation, vascular permeability, severe anemia, disseminated intravascular coagulation, renal failure, and hepatic failure. In addition to therapy specific for these processes, exchange transfusion, plasma infusion or exchange, and corticosteroids should be considered.

Psychosocial Issues

Modern insights into the psychosocial adjustment of patients with sickle cell disease have provided a level of understanding that allows interventional therapy. Although most patients with sickle cell disease are generally well adjusted,[231] there are risks of depression, low self-esteem, social isolation, poor family relationships, and withdrawal from normal daily living.[231] Particular stressors are recurrent and unpredictable pain and the response to it, curtailed activity due to pain, misinterpretation of the meaning of pain, and depression leading to learned helplessness. Although some patients with sickle cell disease become addicted to narcotics, this is uncommon and usually is the result of social influences rather than pain therapy. Well-adjusted patients have active coping strategies, family support, and support from the extended family unit common in African American society. Interventional approaches should emphasize recognizing and reinforcing individual strengths, confronting pathologic behavior, and establishing coping skills through reinterpreting pain, diverting attention from pain, and using support systems.[232] Attention to psychosocial concerns is vital to the psychosocial well-being and integration into society of patients with sickle cell disease (see Chapter 93).

Growth and Development

By age 2 years, children with sickle cell disease have detectable growth retardation that affects weight more than height and has no clear gender difference.[233] By adulthood, normal height is achieved, but weight remains lower than that of controls. More severe growth delay is noted in children with sickle cell anemia and sickle cell–β° thalassemia; Hb SC disease is associated with a less severe growth delay. Girls with sickle cell disease have retarded sexual maturation that is greater in those with sickle cell anemia and sickle cell–β° thalassemia than those with Hb SC disease and sickle cell–β^{+} thalassemia[233]; it is associated with elevated gonadotropin levels for the stage of sexual development and delayed menarche. Boys also have delayed sexual maturation, which is more severe in those with sickle cell anemia than those with Hb SC disease.[233] Retarded sexual maturation in males can be due to primary hypogonadism, hypopituitarism, or hypothalamic insufficiency. The etiology of these multiple endocrine deficiencies may relate to underlying sickle cell pathophysiology and/or iron overload and emphasizes the importance of a comprehensive basic management and disease modification approach as outlined earlier in this chapter. Improved growth has been reported with hydroxyurea,[234] transfusion,[234] folic acid supplementation, zinc supplementation,[235] and nutritional supplementation.[236] When children have both sickle cell disease and hypersplenism, splenectomy may result in improved protein turnover, metabolic rate, and growth parameters.[237]

VARIANT SICKLE CELL SYNDROMES

The sickle cell syndromes that result from inheritance of the sickle cell gene in simple heterozygosity or in compound heterozygosity with other mutant β-globin genes are sickle cell trait, Hb SC disease, and sickle cell–β thalassemia. These and other less common compound heterozygosity syndromes are reviewed.

Sickle Cell Trait

The prevalence of sickle cell trait is approximately 8% to 10% in African-Americans and as high as 25% to 30% in certain areas of western Africa.[4] There are approximately 2.5 million people in the United States and 30 million in the world who are heterozygous for the sickle cell gene. Sickle cell trait is largely a benign carrier condition with no obvious laboratory hematologic manifestations under basal conditions: red cell morphology, red cell indices, and the reticulocyte count are normal, and sickle forms (ISCs) are not seen on the peripheral blood smear. The usual partition of Hb A and Hb S in sickle cell trait is 60:40 owing to a greater posttranslational affinity of α chains for β^A than for β^S chains.[6] When α thalassemia is coinherited with sickle cell trait, the preferential affinity results in a decreased percentage of hemoglobin S relative to the number of α-globin genes deleted (ie, αα/αα 40% Hb S; –α/αα 35% Hb S; –α/–α 29% Hb S; – –/–α 21% Hb S).[124]

There are a few clinical complications of sickle cell trait: splenic infarction occurs at high altitude.[238] It is a cause of hematuria and hyposthenuria.[239] The frequency of urinary tract infection may be increased. There is an association with renal medullary carcinoma.[207] There is an increased risk for venous thrombosis with an approximately twofold increase in risk and sickle trait explaining 7% of thrombotic episodes in African Americans.[240] Recruits in basic training with the sickle-cell trait have a substantially increased, age-dependent risk of exercise-related sudden death.[241]

Despite the known complications, past experiences with discrimination in the employment market and health insurance industry provide reminders that the rare clinical events in sickle cell trait provide no real justification for regarding it as anything but a benign carrier condition.[242] Newborn screening programs detect a large number of infants with sickle cell trait; for these parents, genetic counseling is essential. Parents should understand that their child has a benign hereditary condition with some risks as above, but that there is a risk for a subsequent child to be born with sickle cell disease.

In individuals who appear to have sickle cell trait but are symptomatic, the laboratory diagnosis must be verified. Hemoglobins other than S that polymerize may account for reports of "sickle cell trait" associated with clinical problems. Examples are heterozygous Hb S Antilles and Hb Quebec-CHORI. In the latter case, the hemoglobin variant was distinguished from Hb A using mass spectroscopy.

Hb SC Disease

The gene for Hb C ($\alpha_2\beta_2{}^6$Glu→Lys) is approximately one-fourth as frequent among African Americans as the sickle cell gene.[8] Although oxygenated Hb C forms crystals, Hb C does not participate in polymerization with deoxy-Hb S. However, HbC sustains potassium chloride cotransport and red cell dehydration, raising the intraerythrocytic concentration of Hb S to levels that support polymerization, sickling, and clinical symptoms. As a result of a longer circulatory survival of Hb SC red cells compared to Hb SS cells (ie, 27 vs 17 days),[121] the degree of anemia and reticulocytosis is frequently mild: 75% of the patients have a milder level of anemia (hematocrit level >28%) than is usually seen in sickle cell anemia. The predominant red cell abnormality on the peripheral smear is an abundance of target cells; folded ("pita bread") cells, ISCs, "billiard ball" cells, and crystal-containing cells also may be seen.

Splenomegaly may be the only physical finding, and the frequency of acute painful episodes is approximately half that in Hb SS disease, with a life expectancy two decades longer.[16] Nonetheless, significant morbidity can occur. The incidence of fatal bacterial infection is less than in sickle cell anemia, but there is still an increased risk of *S pneumoniae* and *H influenzae* infection. Osteonecrosis occurs in approximately 15% of patients.[243] There is a higher incidence of peripheral retinopathy in Hb SC disease than in sickle cell anemia. Coexistent α thalassemia reduces risk of chronic organ complications.[243] There is an association between renal medullary carcinoma and Hb SC disease.

Sickle Cell–β Thalassemia

The gene frequency of β thalassemia among African Americans is 0.004, one-tenth that of the sickle cell gene,[8] and hence there is one-tenth the prevalence of compound heterozygous sickle cell–β thalassemia in this population. Sickle cell–β thalassemia is divided into sickle cell–β^+ thalassemia and sickle cell–β° thalassemia, which have, respectively, reduced or no amounts of Hb A present. Most β thalassemia mutations among African Americans result in β^+ thalassemia. Sickle cell–β^+ thalassemia is subclassified according to the percentage of Hb A present: type I has 3% to 5%; type II has 8% to 14%; and type III has 18% to 25%. Eighty percent of African American α-thalassemia mutations are due to the promoter region mutations [−88 (C to T) and −29 (A to G)] that result in a type III phenotype. Compound heterozygous sickle cell–β° thalassemia occurs infrequently.

In sickle cell–β thalassemia, the red cells are hypochromic and microcytic. The ISCs present on the peripheral blood smear are more numerous in sickle cell–β° thalassemia than in sickle cell–β^+ thalassemia. The hematologic and clinical severity is a function of the amount of Hb A inherited (Table 43–8).

Additional mitigating influences in sickle cell–β thalassemia are elevated levels of Hb A_2 and, in sickle cell–β^+ thalassemia, levels of Hb A up to 30%. These affect both the solubility and polymerization of Hb S. Hb F is a more active inhibitor of polymerization than Hb A, as shown by Hb S solutions with 15% to 30% Hb A (resembling sickle cell–β^+ thalassemia) having delay times 10 to 100 times longer than pure Hb S solutions, and Hb S solutions with 20% to 30% Hb F (resembling Hb S–HPFH) having delay times 1,000 to 1,000,000 times longer. A further influence mitigating the polymerization, sickling, and clinical aspects of sickle cell–β thalassemia is the reduced MCHC, which retards Hb S polymerization. Hematologic values for sickle cell anemia, the sickle cell–β thalassemias, and Hb S–HPFH are found in Table 43–8.

Sickle Cell–Hb Lepore Disease[244]

The Hb Lepore gene is a crossover fusion product of the δ- and β-globin genes, the product of which, in the case of Hb Lepore Boston, has the same alkaline electrophoretic mobility as Hb S. Therefore, patients with the Hb Lepore trait can appear to have sickle cell trait, but with only 12% Hb S from thalassemic expression of the abnormal fusion gene. Again, because of the electrophoretic similarity with HbS, compound heterozygous Hb S–Hb Lepore Boston resembles sickle cell anemia or sickle cell–β° thalassemia electrophoretically but clinically have less severe anemia, resembling that of sickle cell–β^+ thalassemia. The diagnosis is also suggested by the low to low-normal Hb A_2 levels that result from the incapacitation of one δ-globin gene by the crossover. Hb F levels vary. The peripheral smear shows microcytosis, hypochromia, and ISCs. Vasoocclusive complications occur, and splenomegaly is common.

Sickle Cell–Hb D Disease[245]

Because Hb D Punjab or Hb D Los Angeles ($\alpha_2\beta_2{}^{121}$Glu→Gln) has a similar electrophoretic mobility to Hb S under alkali conditions, Hb SD disease was first reported as an unusual case of sickle cell anemia. Hb D can be distinguished from Hb S by acid electrophoresis or isoelectric focusing. There is moderately severe hemolytic anemia, and the peripheral smear shows marked anisocytosis and poikilocytosis, target cells, and ISCs. The clinical manifestations of this syndrome are similar to those of sickle cell anemia (see Chapter 40).

Sickle Cell–Hb O Arab Disease[246]

Although Hb O Arab ($\alpha_2\beta_2{}^{121}$Glu→Lys) was first described in an Israeli Arab family, its distribution is widespread. Sickle cell–O Arab disease resembles Hb SC disease on alkaline electrophoresis, but Hb O Arab can be distinguished from Hb C by acid electrophoresis or isoelectric focusing. This syndrome is associated with moderately severe hemolytic anemia, and the peripheral smear shows anisocytosis, poikilocytosis, and ISCs (see Chapter 40).

Sickle Cell–Hb E Disease[247]

Hb E ($\alpha_2\beta_2{}^{26}$Glu → Lys) is a β-thalassemic hemoglobinopathy found predominantly in southeast Asia (see Chapter 41). The structural mutant has an electrophoretic mobility similar to Hb C under alkaline conditions but can be resolved by acid electrophoresis or isoelectric focusing. The GAG→AAG mutation in codon 26 activates a cryptic splice site within the first intron of the β^E gene, causing alternate splicing and decreased expression of the structural mutant. As a result, Hb E makes up only 30% of the total hemoglobin in compound heterozygosity for the sickle cell and Hb E genes. Hb SE disease is essentially benign in at least 50% and possibly most patients, with only mild hemolysis, no vasoocclusive complications, and no remarkable abnormality of red blood cell morphology. However, vasoocclusive complications and manifestations of chronic hemolytic anemia such as pain crisis, splenic infarction, recurrent pneumonia, and frontal bossing have been reported.

Coinherited Hemoglobin Abnormalities That Interact With Sickle Cell Disease: Hereditary Persistence of Fetal Hemoglobin and α-Thalassemia Trait

Sickle Cell–Hereditary Persistence of Fetal Hemoglobin

Adult hemoglobin (or in the case of sickle cell anemia Hb S) replaces Hb F as a result of the switch from γ- to β-globin synthesis that occurs in the fetus. Because of the inhibitory effect of Hb F on Hb S polymerization and cellular sickling (please see Chapter 42), the high fraction of Hb F at birth masks the expression of sickle cell disease until Hb S levels increase to 75% at approximately 6 months of age (Fig. 43–3). Conditions that preserve elevated levels of Hb F into adulthood similarly modulate the course of sickle cell disease. The compound heterozygous conditions sickle–hereditary persistence of fetal hemoglobin (Hb SS–HPFH) and sickle cell–β° thalassemia–HPFH both have higher Hb F levels and milder clinical courses than are characteristic of sickle cell anemia.[113]

Hereditary persistence of fetal hemoglobin results from one of several large deletions of the δ- and β-globin genes that retard the switch from the production of Hb F to adult hemoglobin (see Chapters 22 and 29). A more recently discovered variety of HPFH is not due to a deletion but to one of many point mutations that upregulate the expression of the γ-globin gene. The clinical expression of deletional and nondeletional HPFH differs in that the 15% to 35% Hb F in the former is distributed in a pancellular fashion, the 1% to 5% Hb F in the latter is distributed in a heterocellular fashion, and certain mild types of nondeletional HPFH express high Hb F levels not in simple heterozygosity but only in conditions of erythropoietic stress, such as compound heterozygosity with the sickle cell gene. It is likely that many cases of apparent sickle cell anemia with unexplained elevations of Hb F are the result of a nondeletion HPFH mutation.

The gene frequency of the deletional HPFH locus is 0.0005 among African Americans, resulting in a calculated incidence for compound heterozygous sickle cell–deletional HPFH of 1/100 that of sickle cell anemia. Sickle cell–deletional HPFH provided the first evidence that Hb F was a potent inhibitor of Hb S polymerization: individuals with pancellular distribution of 25% Hb F were generally neither anemic nor afflicted with vasoocclusive manifestations (Table 43–8).[248] Hemoglobin electrophoresis revealed only Hb S, F, and A_2, which resembles sickle cell anemia, sickle cell–β° thalassemia, and sickle cell–δβ° thalassemia. Notable differences, however, are the pancellular distribution of 15% to 35% Hb F, Hb A_2 levels less than 2.5%, and the absence of anemia.[249] The generally benign course of sickle cell–deletional HPFH is uncommonly associated with vasoocclusive complication.

Sickle Cell Anemia With Coexistent α Thalassemia

Prevalences of the silent carrier of α-thalassemia syndrome (genotype -α/αα) and α-thalassemia trait (genotype –α/–α) among African Americans are approximately 30% and 2%, respectively.[250] The peripheral blood smear contains less polychromasia and fewer sickle forms and more hypochromia and microcytosis, commensurate with the numbers of α-globin genes deleted. There are increased Hb A_2 levels associated with increasing α-globin gene deletions; the Hb F levels are not consistently affected.

Clinically, the impact of α-globin gene deletions on sickle cell is not as consistent as that of high Hb F.[20] Because of the powerful effect of Hb S concentration on the kinetics and extent of Hb S polymerization (please see Chapter 42), the lower MCHC from α-globin gene deletions decreases the hemolytic rate, and anemia is milder in subjects with both α-thalassemia syndrome (genotype -α/αα) and trait (genotype –α/–α) (Table 43–1). There is a decreased incidence of leg ulcers but an increased incidence of osteonecrosis. The frequency of retinal vessel closure is higher, but not the incidence of retinopathy. Complications related to hemolysis (eg, leg ulcers, chronic renal damage) may be decreased, but the heterogeneity of the patients in previous studies and mixed results make conclusions difficult. Similarly, the influence of α-gene deletions on survival in patients with sickle cell disease is not well understood.[20]

SUGGESTED READINGS

Austin H, Key NS, Benson JM, et al: Sickle cell trait and the risk of venous thromboembolism among blacks. Blood 110(3):908, 2007.

Goldstein LB, Adams R, Alberts MJ, et al: Primary prevention of ischemic stroke: A guideline from the American Heart Association/American Stroke Association Stroke Council: Cosponsored by the Atherosclerotic Peripheral Vascular Disease Interdisciplinary Working Group; Cardiovascular Nursing Council; Clinical Cardiology Council; Nutrition, Physical Activity, and Metabolism Council; and the Quality of Care and Outcomes Research Interdisciplinary Working Group. Circulation 113(24):e873, 2006.

Karam LB, Disco D, Jackson SM, et al: Liver biopsy results in patients with sickle cell disease on chronic transfusions: Poor correlation with ferritin levels. Pediatr Blood Cancer 2007.

Knox-Macaulay HH, Ahmed MM, Gravell D, Al Kindi S, Ganesh A: Sickle cell-haemoglobin E (HbSE) compound heterozygosity: A clinical and haematological study. Int J Lab Hematol 29(4):292, 2007.

Machado RF, Anthi A, Steinberg MH, et al: N-terminal pro-brain natriuretic peptide levels and risk of death in sickle cell disease. JAMA 296(3):310, 2006.

Maggio A: Light and shadows in the iron chelation treatment of haematological diseases. Br J Haematol 138(4):407, 2007.

Manchikanti A, Grimes DA, Lopez LM, Schulz KF: Steroid hormones for contraception in women with sickle cell disease. Cochrane Database Syst Rev (2):CD006261, 2007.

Pakbaz Z, Fischer R, Fung E, Nielsen P, Harmatz P, Vichinsky E: Serum ferritin underestimates liver iron concentration in transfusion independent thalassemia patients as compared to regularly transfused thalassemia and sickle cell patients. Pediatr Blood Cancer 49(3):329, 2007.

Schleucher R, Gaessler M, Knobloch J: Rapid healing of a late diagnosed sickle cell leg ulcer using a new combination of treatment methods. J Wound Care 16(5):197, 2007.

Zimmerman SA, Schultz WH, Burgett S, Mortier NA, Ware RE: Hydroxyurea therapy lowers transcranial Doppler flow velocities in children with sickle cell anemia. Blood 110(3):1043, 2007.

REFERENCES

For complete list of references log onto www.expertconsult.com

CHAPTER 44

HEMOGLOBIN VARIANTS ASSOCIATED WITH HEMOLYTIC ANEMIA, ALTERED OXYGEN AFFINITY, AND METHEMOGLOBINEMIAS

Edward J. Benz, Jr. and Benjamin L. Ebert

Hemoglobinopathies are inherited diseases caused primarily by mutations affecting the globin genes. Nearly 1000 mutations that alter the structure, expression, or developmental regulation of individual globin genes, and the hemoglobins they encode, have been described; most do not produce clinical disease. Many are highly instructive for students of gene structure, function, and regulation, but further consideration of most is not warranted in a clinically oriented textbook. The gene mutations that cause sickle cell anemia and the thalassemia syndromes are by far the most important mutations that cause clinical morbidity, in terms of both the complexity of the clinical syndromes they cause and the number of patients affected. These conditions are considered in detail in other chapters (see Chapters 42 and 43). This chapter reviews other abnormalities of the hemoglobin molecule that produce clinical syndromes. Each variant is uncommon. In the aggregate, however, hemoglobinopathies represent important problems for hematologists because they must be considered as possible causes for conditions about which hematologists are often consulted: hemolytic anemia, cyanosis, polycythemia, jaundice, rubor, splenomegaly, and reticulocytosis.

The major hemoglobinopathies producing clinical symptoms, other than sickle cell anemia and thalassemias, can be classified as those hemoglobins exhibiting altered solubility (unstable hemoglobins), hemoglobins with increased oxygen affinity, hemoglobins with decreased oxygen affinity, and methemoglobins (Table 44–1). A few acquired conditions in which toxic modifications of the hemoglobin molecule are important (eg, carbon monoxide poisoning) are also considered briefly.

The sections that follow emphasize hemoglobinopathies that produce the most severe or dramatic alterations in clinical phenotype and those in which a single clinical abnormality (eg, hemoglobin precipitation) predominates. It is important to emphasize at the outset, however, that although more than 100 mutations affect solubility or affinity, only a few are clinically important. The abnormal functional properties of most mutant hemoglobins can be detected readily in sophisticated research laboratories, but only a few mutant hemoglobins produce laboratory or clinical abnormalities relevant to clinical practice. Moreover, many mutations are pleiotropic, affecting several functional properties of the hemoglobin molecule. Thus, a single mutation can increase oxygen affinity and reduce solubility, or produce methemoglobinemia and reduce solubility.

Table 44–2 summarizes the major forms of structurally abnormal hemoglobin, with examples. This table serves as a point of reference for the remaining sections of the chapter.

UNSTABLE HEMOGLOBINS

The term *unstable hemoglobins* refers to hemoglobins exhibiting reduced solubility or higher susceptibility to oxidation of amino acid residues within the individual globin chains. More than 100 unique unstable hemoglobin mutants have been documented. Most exhibit only mild instability in in vitro laboratory tests and are associated with minimal clinical manifestations. Both α- and β-globin variants can cause this condition. Approximately 75% of the mutations described, however, are β-globin variants. This probably reflects the potential for α-globin variants to exert pathologic effects in utero. Clinical symptomatology of unstable hemoglobins also depends in part on the quantitative proportion of the abnormal hemoglobin. Because the α-globin genes are duplicated, mutations in an individual locus generally produce only 25% to 35% abnormal globin. By contrast, a simple heterozygote at the single β-globin locus usually produces approximately 50% of the abnormal variant.

The mutations that impair hemoglobin solubility usually disrupt hydrogen bonding or the hydrophobic interactions that either retain the heme moiety within the heme-binding pockets or hold the tetramer together (Fig. 44–1). Some alter the helical segments (eg, Hb Geneva [$\beta^{28Leu\rightarrow Pro}$]), others weaken contact points between the α and β subunits (eg, Hb Philadelphia [$\beta^{35Tyr\rightarrow Phe}$]), and still others derange interactions of the hydrophobic pockets of the globin subunits with heme (eg, Hb Köln [$\beta^{98Val\rightarrow Met}$]). The common pathway to reduced solubility invariably involves weakening of the binding of heme to globin. Actual loss of heme groups can occur, for example, in Hb Gun Hill, in which five amino acids, including the F8 histidine, are deleted. In other cases, mutations that introduce prolines into helical segments disrupt the helices and interfere with normal folding of the polypeptide around the heme group. Another feature of these mutations is disruption of the integrity of the tetrameric structure of globin chains. Only the intact hemoglobin tetramer can remain dissolved at the high concentrations that must be achieved within the circulating red blood cell (see Chapter 33).

Pathophysiology of Unstable Hemoglobin Disorders

The mechanisms by which unstable hemoglobin mutations produce hemoglobin precipitation remain incompletely understood. However, the major outlines of the process have been described (Fig. 44–2). The fundamental step in pathogenesis appears to be derangement of the normal linkages between heme and globin. Loss of appropriate globin chain folding and interaction may ultimately destabilize the heme–globin linkage or lead to partial proteolysis of the chain, thereby releasing heme from that linkage. Once freed from its cleft, heme probably binds nonspecifically to other regions of the globin molecule, forming precipitated hemichromes, which lead to further denaturation and aggregation of the globin subunits. These form a precipitate containing α- and β-globin chains, globin fragments, and heme, called the *Heinz body*.

Heinz bodies interact with delicate red blood cell membrane components (see Chapter 33), thereby reducing red blood cell deformability. These rigid cells tend to be detained in the splenic microcirculation and "pitted," reflecting attempts by the splenic macrophages to remove the Heinz bodies. Red blood cell damage can be aggravated by the release of free heme into the red blood cell. Several biochemical perturbations correlate with the presence of free heme, such as generation of reactive oxidants (ie, hydrogen peroxide, superoxide, and hydroxyl radicals). The end result of this process is premature destruction of the red blood cell, producing the hemolytic anemia.

Individual unstable hemoglobins vary in their propensity to generate Heinz bodies and hemolysis. For example, Hb Zurich exhibits relatively mild insolubility. Hemolysis is virtually absent in patients with this variant. Hemolysis may become clinically apparent only in the presence of additional oxidant stresses, such as infection, fever, or the ingestion of oxidant agents. Because of the propensity of these

Table 44–1 Classification of Hemoglobinopathies

Structural hemoglobinopathies—hemoglobins with altered amino acid sequences that result in deranged function or altered physical or chemical properties
Abnormal hemoglobin polymerization—Hb S
Altered oxygen affinity
High affinity—polycythemia
Low affinity—cyanosis, pseudoanemia
Hemoglobins that oxidize readily
Unstable hemoglobins, hemolytic anemia, jaundice
M hemoglobins—methemoglobinemia, cyanosis
Thalassemias—defective production of globin chains
α Thalassemias
β Thalassemias
δβ, γδβ, αβ Thalassemias
Structural hemoglobinopathies—structurally abnormal Hb associated with coinherited thalassemia phenotype
Hb E
Hb Constant Spring
Hb Lepore
Hereditary persistence of fetal hemoglobin—persistence of high levels of Hb F into adult life
Pancellular—all red blood cells contain elevated Hb F levels
Nondeletion forms
Deletion forms
Hb Kenya
Heterocellular—only specific subpopulation of red blood cells contain elevated levels of Hb F
"Acquired hemoglobinopathies"
Methemoglobin due to toxic exposures
Sulfhemoglobin due to toxic exposures
Carbonoxyhemoglobin
Hb H in erythroleukemia
Elevated Hb F in states of erythroid stress and bone marrow dysplasia, usually heterocellular

Table 44–2 Mutations Producing Abnormal Hemoglobin Molecules*

Residue	Mutation	Common Name(s)	Molecular Pathology
Abnormal solubility			
β6	Glu→Val	S	Polymerization
β6	Glu→Lys	C	Crystallization
β121	Glu→Gln	D-Los Angeles, D-Punjab	Increases polymer in S/D heterozygote
β121	Glu→Lys	O-Arab	Increases polymer in S/O heterozygote
Increased oxygen affinity			
α92	Arg→Gln	J-Capetown	Stabilizes R state
α141	Arg→His	Suresnes	Eliminates bond to Asn 126 in T state
β89	Ser→Asn	Creteil	Weakens bonds in T state
β99	Asp→Asn	Kempsey	Breaks T state intersubunit bonds
Decreased oxygen affinity			
α94	Asp→Asn	Titusville	Alters R state intersubunit bonds
β102	Asn→Thr	Kansas	Breaks R state intersubunit bonds
β102	Asn→Ser	Beth Israel	Breaks R state intersubunit bonds
Methemoglobin			
α58	His→Tyr	M-Boston, M-Osaka	Heme liganded to Tyr not His
α87	His→Tyr	M-Iwate	Heme liganded to both His and Tyr
β28	Leu→Gln	St. Louis	Opens heme pocket
β63	His→Tyr	M-Saskatoon	Tyr ligand stabilizes ferri-heme
β67	Val→Glu	M-Milwaukee-I	Negative charge stabilizes ferri-heme
β92	His→Tyr	M-Hyde Park	Bond of His to heme disrupted
Unstable			
α43	Phe→Val	Torino	Loss of heme contact
α94	Asp→Tyr	Setif	Alters subunit contacts
β28	Leu→Gln	St. Louis	Polar group in heme pocket
β35	Tyr→Phe	Philadelphia	Loss of dimer bond favors precipitation
β42	Phe→Ser	Hammersmith	Loss of heme
β63	His→Arg	Zürich	Opens heme pocket
β88	Leu→Pro	Santa Ana	Disrupts helix
β91	Leu→Pro	Sabine	Disrupts helix
β91-95	Deletion	Gun Hill	Shortens F helix
β98	Val→Met	Köln	Alters heme contact

*Partial list includes some of the most widely studied hemoglobin structural mutations.

Adapted from Dickerson RE, Geis I: Hemoglobin: Structure, Function, Evolution, and Pathology. Menlo Park, CA, Benjamin-Cummings, 1983. Copyright Irving Geis.

molecules to be hypersensitive to oxidation, some patients with unstable hemoglobins can exhibit episodic hemolysis in response to many of the same oxidative stressors as those exacerbating the clinical phenotype of glucose-6-phosphate dehydrogenase (G6PD)-deficient patients (see Chapter 45).

Patterns of Inheritance and Clinical Manifestations

Unstable hemoglobins are usually inherited as autosomal dominant disorders. However, the rate of spontaneous mutation appears to be high, so the absence of affected parents or siblings does not rule out the presence of an unstable hemoglobin in an individual family. Nonetheless, the presence of a positive family history can be a useful adjunct to diagnosis and should provoke consideration of an unstable hemoglobin as the cause of the familial hemolytic diathesis.

The clinical syndrome associated with unstable hemoglobin disorders is often called *congenital Heinz body hemolytic anemia.* This term derives from the fact that only the most severe cases were detected before the widespread availability of sophisticated methods for detecting and characterizing abnormal hemoglobins. Clinical manifestations are highly variable, ranging from a virtually asymptomatic state in the absence of environmental stressors to severe hemolytic anemia manifesting at birth. Patients with chronic hemolysis present with variable degrees of typical symptoms, including anemia, reticulocytosis, hepatosplenomegaly, jaundice, leg ulcers, and a propensity toward premature biliary tract disease.

For hemoglobin variants with a given degree of reduced solubility, the degree of anemia may fluctuate because some of these variants also exhibit altered oxygen affinity. Thus, Hb Köln has increased oxygen affinity, resulting in relatively higher levels of tissue hypoxia and erythropoietin stimulation at any given level of hematocrit (see next section); therefore, patients with Hb Köln tend to have higher hematocrit levels than expected on the basis of hemolytic severity because of increased erythropoietin stimulation. By contrast, Hb Hammersmith exhibits decreased oxygen affinity, improving oxygen delivery and allowing patients to function at a lower hematocrit level.

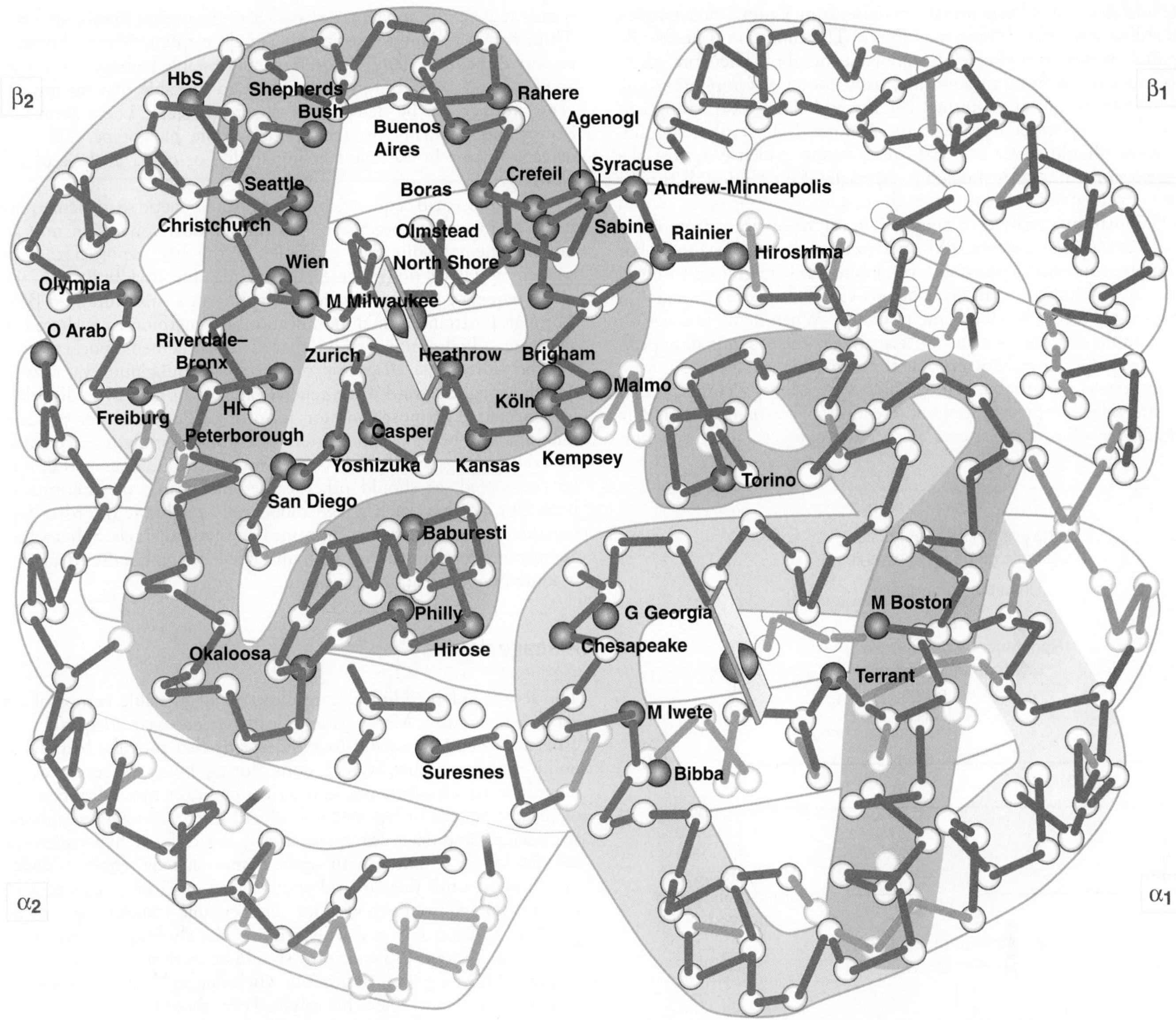

Figure 44–1 Hemoglobin tetramer showing the position of the more common, clinically significant hemoglobin mutants. Most of those that have been described occur on the β chain at invariant residue sites, near critical intermolecular contacts, or in proximity to the prosthetic heme-binding site. *(Modified from Dickerson RE, Geis I: Hemoglobin: Structure, Function, Evolution, and Pathology. Menlo Park, CA, Benjamin-Cummings, 1983. Copyright Irving Geis.)*

Hb Zurich possesses, for complex molecular reasons, a higher-than-normal affinity for carbon monoxide. A high hemoglobin carbon monoxide level develops in patients with Hb Zurich who also smoke. Binding of carbon monoxide protects Hb Zurich from denaturation, thus reducing hemolysis, so these people tend to exhibit lesser degrees of hemolytic anemia than do nonsmoking relatives.

Diagnosis

> The presence of an unstable hemoglobin should be suspected in patients with one or more stigmata of accelerated red blood cell destruction: chronic or intermittent hemolytic anemia or jaundice, premature development of bilirubin gallstones or biliary tract disease (as a result of accelerated red blood cell turnover), unexplained reticulocytosis, or bouts of intermittent symptoms that can be related to exposure to oxidant drugs or infections. Other suggestive symptoms include dark urine, transient jaundice, and leg ulcers.

Laboratory diagnosis depends on identification of a mutant hemoglobin that precipitates more easily than normal hemoglobin. The peripheral blood smear may or may not show evidence of hemolysis (ie, poikilocytosis, polychromasia, or shift cells; see Fig. 44–3A). The morphologic evidence for precipitated hemoglobin is the Heinz body, the intraerythrocytic inclusion body detected by staining the peripheral blood smear with a supravital dye, such as brilliant cresyl blue or new methylene blue (see Fig. 44–3B,C). The spleen removes Heinz bodies efficiently, especially if hemolysis is not particularly acute or brisk. Thus, Heinz bodies may not be demonstrable at all times. Two provocative laboratory maneuvers are used to aid detection, both of which unmask the tendency of unstable hemoglobins to precipitate: the heat instability test (heating of a hemoglobin solution to 50°C) or the isopropanol instability test (insolubility in 17% isopropanol).

Hemoglobin electrophoresis should be performed but *should not be relied on as the major diagnostic criterion for ruling in or ruling out a hemoglobinopathy.* Many amino acid substitutions that have a profound effect on solubility do not change the overall charge on the hemoglobin molecule. For example, Hb Köln, the most common of the unstable hemoglobin mutations, arises from a mutation changing the valine at position 98 to a methionine. This mutation is electrically neutral; it does not alter electrophoretic mobility. Therefore, these variants do not form an abnormal band on an electrophoresis gel. Demonstration of an abnormal band would clearly add strong evidence in support of the diagnosis. A normal electrophoretogram, however, should never be regarded as strong evidence against the presence of a mutant hemoglobin, especially if the clinical picture or family history otherwise supports the diagnosis.

Sophisticated analyses of hemoglobin can be obtained from reference laboratories if detailed characterization seems warranted. For example, abnormal hemoglobin or globin bands migrating to novel positions on an isoelectric focusing gel can result from hemoglobin or globin moieties lacking heme in groups. When heme is added to the sample and the proteins are reanalyzed, these bands disappear. This behavior is nearly diagnostic of an unstable variant.

Detection of unstable hemoglobins is occasionally compromised by the selective precipitation of the unstable variant into Heinz bodies. Because most patients are heterozygotes, this phenomenon greatly reduces the apparent percentage of the variant in soluble form. Thus, even a variant possessing altered electrophoretic mobility may be very difficult to detect. Indeed, some unstable hemoglobins, such as Hb Geneva or Hb Terre Haute, are so unstable that no mutant gene product can be detected in the steady state. These abnormal hemoglobins actually produce a thalassemic phenotype. They are detectable only by isotope labeling studies or direct analysis of the globin genes.

The amino acid sequence predicted from genetic sequencing may rarely be inaccurate because of posttranslational conversion into an unstable hemoglobin. For example, in the first reported case of congenital Heinz body hemolytic anemia due to Hb Bristol, the DNA sequence predicts a valine-to-methionine substitution at β67. Through posttranslational modification, the methionine is altered to aspartate, a hydrophilic residue that disrupts the heme pocket.

The differential diagnosis of unstable hemoglobin variants is usually straightforward if the general category of hemolytic disorders is suspected. The most common form of G6PD deficiency can also manifest with bouts of intermittent or chronic hemolysis exacerbated by oxidant drugs or infection (see Chapter 45). This diagnosis should be considered, as should other causes of chronic or intermittent hemolytic anemia, such as red blood cell membrane disorders (eg, hereditary spherocytosis) or immune hemolytic anemias. Spherocytes are relatively rare in patients with unstable hemoglobin disorders; this is sometimes a useful discriminant.

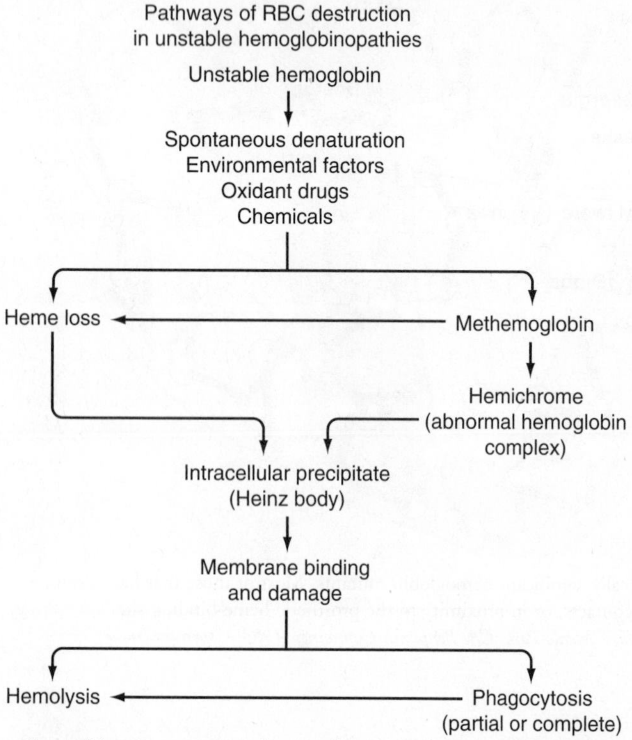

Pathways of RBC destruction
in unstable hemoglobinopathies

Unstable hemoglobin
↓
Spontaneous denaturation
Environmental factors
Oxidant drugs
Chemicals
↓
Heme loss ← Methemoglobin
Methemoglobin ↓ Hemichrome (abnormal hemoglobin complex)
Heme loss, Hemichrome ↓
Intracellular precipitate (Heinz body)
↓
Membrane binding and damage
↓
Hemolysis ← Phagocytosis (partial or complete)

Figure 44–2 Presumed mechanisms by which denaturation of hemoglobin leads to erythrocyte destruction. The rate of travel through the various pathways probably differs for the different hemoglobin variants and for a variety of stresses to which the protein is subjected. RBC, red blood cell. *(From Wynngaarden JB, Smith LH Jr, Bennett JC [eds.]: Cecil Textbook of Medicine. Philadelphia, WB Saunders, 1992.)*

Management

The severity of the clinical complications of unstable hemoglobins varies enormously. Many patients can be managed adequately by observation and education to avoid agents that provoke hemolysis. Some patients require transfusions during bouts of severe acute hemolytic anemia. Patients who have significant morbidity because of chronic anemia or repeated episodes of severe hemolysis should be considered candidates for splenectomy, especially if hypersplenism has developed. Children with severe hemolysis may require transfusion support until they are old enough (at least 3 or 4 years of age) to undergo splenectomy without unacceptable immunologic compromise. Splenectomy is usually effective for abolition or reduction of anemin. However, splenectomy should be used only as a last resort because of the long term risks of out whelming sepsis and thrombosis. Infection often exacerbates hemolysis. Fever should therefore prompt close monitoring of patients for evidence of hemolysis or anemia.

HEMOGLOBINS WITH INCREASED OXYGEN AFFINITY

Efficient oxygen delivery by hemoglobin depends on the sigmoid shape of the hemoglobin–oxygen affinity curve. During the transition from the fully deoxygenated to the fully oxygenated state, the initial oxygenation steps occur with difficulty. In fact, the act of binding the first oxygen molecule increases the affinity of the molecule for subsequent oxygen-binding events, thus creating the sigmoid shape of the curve. The necessary intramolecular reorganization occurs only when the precise arrangement of hydrogen bonds, hydrophobic inter-

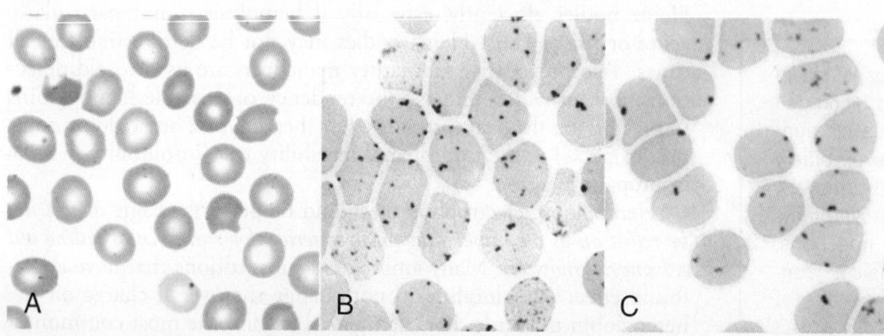

Figure 44–3 Unstable hemoglobins; peripheral blood smear and Heinz body preparation: **A–C**. The peripheral smear (**A**) shows "bite" cells with pitted out semicircular areas of the red blood cell membrane as a result of removal of Heinz bodies by macrophages in the spleen. The Heinz body preparation (**B**) shows increased Heinz bodies in the same specimen, when compared to a control (**C**).

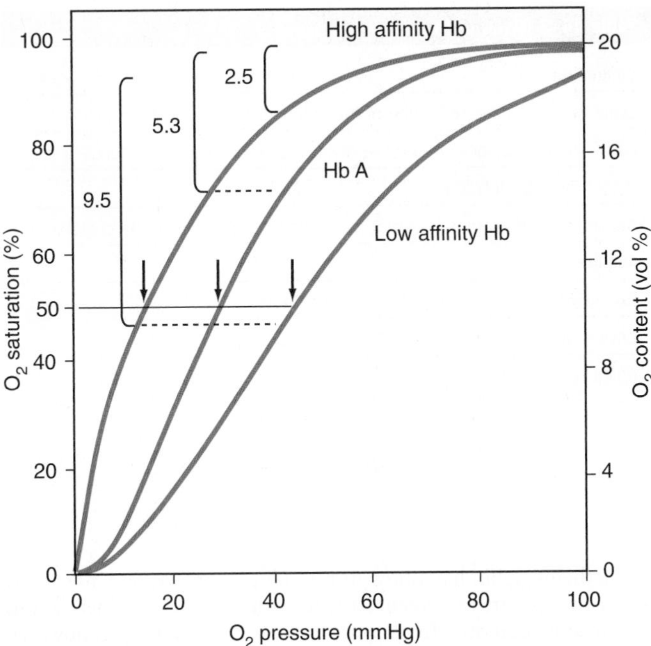

Figure 44–4 Hemoglobin–oxygen dissociation curves are illustrated for normal hemoglobin (Hb A) and for model abnormal hemoglobins with high and low oxygen affinities. On the abscissa, the partial pressure of oxygen is indicated in millimeters of mercury. On the left ordinate, the saturation of hemoglobin with oxygen is indicated as a percentage; on the right ordinate, the oxygen content of the hemoglobin is expressed as volumes percent. The three inverted arrows show the P_{50} for the three hemoglobins (the Po_2 at which the hemoglobin is 50% saturated). This value is lowest for the high-affinity hemoglobin. As the Po_2 drops from 100 (arterial) to 40 (tissues), hemoglobin desaturates, giving up a portion of its bound oxygen; the numbers on the brackets indicate the amount of oxygen unloaded by the three hemoglobin types expressed as volumes percent. Note that the high-affinity hemoglobin delivers less than one-half the oxygen that Hb A gives to the tissues, resulting in tissue anoxia, increased erythropoietin secretion, and erythrocytosis. Conversely, the low-affinity hemoglobin is even more efficient than Hb A in supplying tissues with oxygen, resulting in diminished erythropoietin production and anemia. *(From Wynngaarden JB, Smith LH Jr, Bennett JC [eds.]: Cecil Textbook of Medicine. Philadelphia, WB Saunders, 1992.)*

actions, and salt bridges are broken and formed in the proper sequence.

Mutant hemoglobins exhibiting altered oxygen affinity arise from amino acid substitutions at the interface between α and β chains or in regions affecting the hydrogen bonds, hydrophobic interactions, or salt bridges that influence the interaction of heme with oxygen. A second major class of mutations alters binding to 2,3-diphosphoglycerate (2,3-DPG), which in turn alters oxygen affinity when bound to hemoglobin.

Pathogenesis and Pathophysiology

High-affinity hemoglobins exhibit higher avidity for oxygen, causing the oxygen dissociation curve to shift to the left; an example is Hb Kempsey ($\beta^{99Asp\rightarrow Asn}$) (Fig. 44–4). These hemoglobins bind oxygen more readily than normal and retain more oxygen at lower Po_2 levels. They thus deliver less oxygen to tissues at normal capillary oxygen pressures. The Po_2 in the normal lung (Po_2 = 90–100 mmHg) is well above that needed to saturate hemoglobin fully with oxygen (60 mmHg). These variant hemoglobins cannot acquire any additional oxygen in the lung despite their higher affinity. At capillary Po_2 (35–45 mmHg), however, high-affinity hemoglobins deliver *less* oxygen. At normal hematocrit levels, a mild tissue hypoxia results, triggering increased production of erythropoietin and red blood cells, thus resulting in polycythemia. In extreme cases, hematocrit levels of 60 to 65% can be encountered.

Many types of mutations can increase oxygen affinity. Some alter interactions within the heme pocket, others disrupt the Bohr effect or the salt-bond site, and still others impair the binding of Hb A to 2,3-DPG. Loss of 2,3-DPG binding results in increases in oxygen affinity. These and numerous other examples that have been analyzed at the molecular level have greatly aided our understanding of the molecular basis for reversible oxygen binding.

Diagnosis

High-affinity hemoglobins are a cause of familial unexplained erythrocytosis (see Chapter 30). Functional testing of the hemoglobin is the key to diagnosis. Oxygen affinity is usually measured as P_{50}, the partial pressure of oxygen at which hemoglobin is 50% saturated with oxygen (see Fig. 44–4). The hemoglobin preparation is exposed to increasing oxygen pressures and the relative percentages of oxyhemoglobin and deoxyhemoglobin are determined. The values are plotted on a curve, and the 50% saturation point is determined. A shift to the left means that the hemoglobin reaches 50% saturation at a lower partial pressure of oxygen. High-affinity variants are thus associated with a lower-than-normal P_{50} value. Hemoglobin electrophoresis can, but may not, reveal an abnormal band.

The most common cause of a low P_{50} value is carbon monoxide. Carbon monoxide stabilizes hemoglobin in the R "oxy" state without the need for oxygen binding. The oxygen affinity curve is therefore extremely left-shifted and is hyperbolic, rather than sigmoidal, in shape. The clinical consequences of mild chronic CO poisoning are the same as those seen with high-affinity hemoglobin variants. The most common cause of carbon monoxide toxicity is cigarette smoking, although chronic carbon monoxide exposure can elevate the hematocrit level in people such as caisson workers or tunnel toll collectors. Severe acute CO poisoning can cause rapid death as a result of tissue hypoxia.

Management

Most patients with high-affinity hemoglobins have mild erythrocytosis; they do not require intervention. Very rarely, the hematocrit level is very high (>55–60%). The blood viscosity is then sufficiently elevated to require therapeutic phlebotomy. Carbon monoxide poisoning is treated with supplemental oxygen. When a patient breathes room air, the half-life of carboxyhemoglobin is 4 to 6 hours, but the half-life is 40 to 80 minutes with the use of normobaric oxygen and 15 to 30 minutes with the use of hyperbaric oxygen. Carbon monoxide detectors, designed to detect occult CO poisoning, are now required in many municipalities and are predicted to prevent numerous fatalities from occult carbon monoxide poisoning.

HEMOGLOBINS WITH DECREASED OXYGEN AFFINITY

Pathogenesis

Low-affinity hemoglobin variants, such as Hb Kansas ($\beta^{102Asn\rightarrow Thr}$), arise from mutations that impair hemoglobin–oxygen binding or reduce cooperativity. In cases of Hb Kansas, the threonine position, β^{102}, cannot form a hydrogen bond with aspartic acid at position α^{94}. Because this aspartate residue stabilizes the R (oxy) state, Hb Kansas binds oxygen less well and exhibits a right-shifted P_{50} value (see Fig. 44–4).

Most low-affinity variants possess enough oxygen affinity to become fully saturated in the normal lung. At the low capillary PO_2 in other tissues, these hemoglobins deliver *higher* than normal amounts of oxygen. They become more desaturated than normal hemoglobins. Two abnormalities result from this high level of oxygen delivery. First, because tissue oxygen delivery is so efficient, normal oxygen requirements can be met by lower than normal hematocrit levels. This situation produces a state of "pseudoanemia," in which the low hematocrit level is deceiving because both oxygen delivery and the patients are completely normal. Second, the amount of desaturated hemoglobin circulating in capillaries and veins can be greater than 5 g/dL. Cyanosis may thus be associated with these variants. This usually ominous finding is entirely misleading in these individuals, because it reflects no morbidity.

Diagnosis

Patients with unexplained anemia or cyanosis who appear to be entirely well in all other respects should be evaluated, especially if there is a positive family history. Testing for the abnormal variant follows the same reasoning as that just described for high-affinity variants. The O_2 dissociation curve will be shifted to the right, and the numeric value of the P_{50} will be higher than normal.

Management

Patients with low-affinity hemoglobins are usually asymptomatic. No treatment is required. It is important to document that a low-affinity hemoglobin is the cause of an apparent anemia or cyanosis to preempt inappropriate workups and provide reassurance to the patient. Cyanosis in some patients can pose a cosmetic problem, but correction with transfusions is rarely justified.

METHEMOGLOBINEMIAS

Methemoglobin results from oxidation of the iron moieties in hemoglobin from the ferrous (Fe^{2+}) to the ferric (Fe^{3+}) state. Normal oxygenation of hemoglobin causes a partial transfer of an electron from the iron to the bound oxygen. Iron in this state thus resembles ferric iron and the oxygen resembles superoxide (O_2-). Deoxygenation returns the electron to the iron, with release of oxygen. Methemoglobin forms if the electron is not returned. Methemoglobin constitutes 3% or less of the total hemoglobin in normal humans. Under normal circumstances, these levels in humans are maintained at 1% or less by the methemoglobin reductase enzyme system (nicotinamide adenine dinucleotide [NADH]-dehydratase, ADH-diaphorase, erythrocyte cytochrome b_5).

Pathogenesis and Clinical Manifestations

Methemoglobinemias of clinical interest arise by one of three distinct mechanisms: (a) globin chain mutations that result in increased formation of methemoglobin, (b) deficiencies of methemoglobin reductase, and (c) "toxic" methemoglobinemia, in which normal red blood cells are exposed to substances that oxidize hemoglobin iron to such a degree that normal reducing mechanisms are subverted or overwhelmed (see Chapter 45; Table 44–3).

Abnormal hemoglobins producing methemoglobinemia (M hemoglobins) arise from mutations that stabilize the heme iron in the ferric state. Classically, a histidine in the vicinity of the heme pocket is replaced by a tyrosine; the hydroxyl group of the tyrosine forms a complex that stabilizes the iron in the ferric state (Fig. 44–5). The oxidized heme iron is relatively resistant to reduction by the methemoglobin reductase system.

Table 44–3 Types of Methemoglobinemia

Congenital
Defective enzymatic reduction of Fe^{3+}-hemoglobin to Fe^{2+}-hemoglobin
NADH-methemoglobin reductase (cytochrome b_5 reductase) deficiency
Cytochrome b_3 deficiency
Abnormal hemoglobins resistant to enzymatic reduction (M hemoglobins)
Acquired
Excessive (toxic) oxidation of Fe^{2+}-hemoglobin
Environmental chemicals
Drugs

Methemoglobin has a brownish to blue color that does not revert to red on exposure to oxygen. Patients with methemoglobinemia thus appear to be cyanotic. In contrast to truly cyanotic people, however, PaO_2 values are usually normal. Patients with these hemoglobins are otherwise asymptomatic because methemoglobin is rarely greater than 30 to 50, the levels at which symptomatology becomes apparent.

Hereditary methemoglobinemia resulting from methemoglobin reductase deficiency (cytochrome b_5 reductase deficiency) is very rare. Mutations in the b_5 reductase gene cause two distinct phenotypes. In cases of type I methemoglobin reductase deficiency, patients suffer solely from cyanosis; in cases of type II disease, patients manifest both cyanosis and severe mental retardation. One isoform of the b_5 reductase gene is expressed in diverse tissues for participation in a variety of cellular processes. A second isoform, produced by alternative splicing, is expressed in erythrocytes, producing a soluble protein that reduces methemoglobin. Mutations causing type I methemoglobin reductase deficiency occur throughout the gene and result in an unstable protein. Such mutations are primarily significant in erythrocytes that, without nuclei, cannot replace the degraded protein. Mutations causing type II disease occur in the critical NADH or FAD binding domains, causing inactivation of the protein in all tissues and the more severe clinical phenotype.

Like patients with M hemoglobins, patients with methemoglobin reductase deficiency exhibit slate-gray "pseudocyanosis." Even homozygotes, however, rarely accumulate more than 25% methemoglobin, a level compatible with minimal symptoms. Heterozygotes can have normal methemoglobin levels but are especially sensitive to agents causing methemoglobinemia.

A third toxic form of methemoglobinemia is caused by exposure to certain chemical agents and drugs that accelerate the oxidation of methemoglobin (Table 44–4). Some compounds directly oxidize hemoglobin, whereas other compounds produce reactive oxygen intermediates that oxidize hemoglobin. Nitrite compounds are especially notorious and common. Some of these compounds also have a propensity to exacerbate G6PD deficiency and the precipitation of unstable hemoglobins.

Nitrates are a frequent environmental cause of toxic methemoglobinemia. Nitrates do not directly interact with either hemoglobin or the reductase pathway but are converted to nitrites in the gut. Well water is a frequently encountered source of excessive nitrates. In general, substantial intake of these agents is required before significant amounts of methemoglobin are generated. Very young infants have lower levels of methemoglobin reductase in erythrocytes and are therefore more susceptible to these agents than are adults. However, all age groups are at risk, given sufficient exposure. Systemic acidosis, particularly in young infants suffering from diarrhea and dehydration, can also cause clinically significant methemoglobinemia.

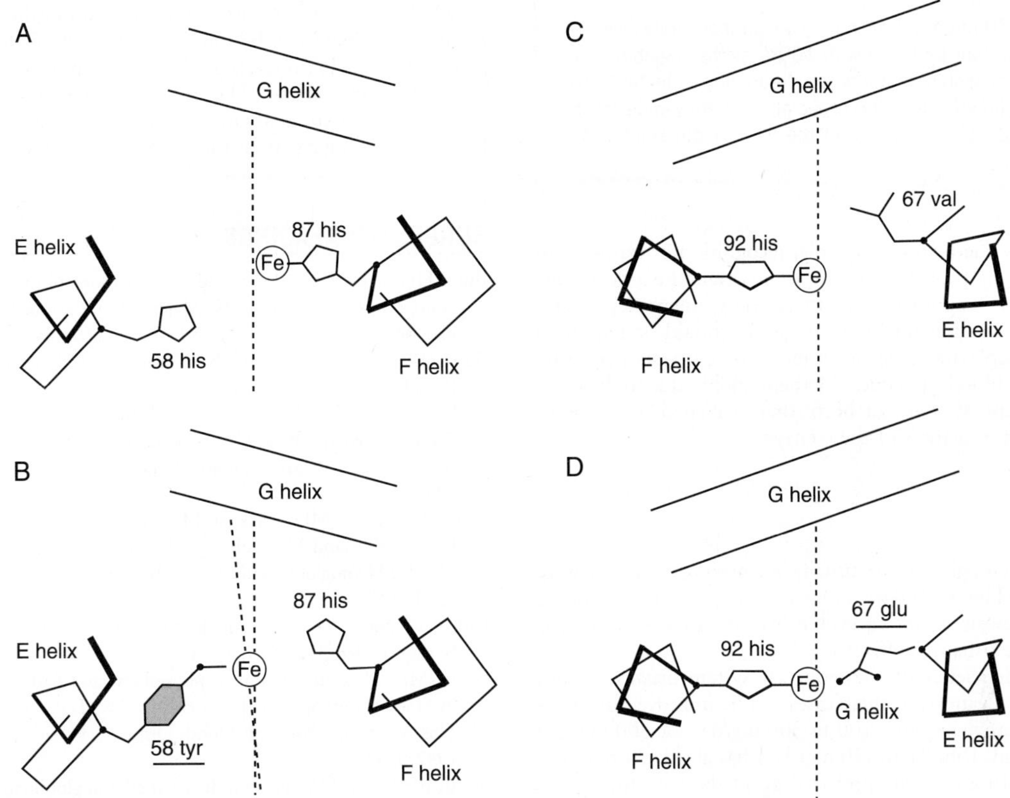

Figure 44–5 Modifications of the heme and its environment that account for two common M hemoglobins. **A**, Hemoglobin A has a His residue at the α58(E7) position. **B**, In hemoglobin M-Boston, the histidine is replaced by a tyrosine, the phenolic side chain of which is capable of covalently binding to the heme iron, resulting in stabilization in the oxidized form. **C**, Hb A has a Val residue at position β67(E11). **D**, Hb M-Milwaukee has a glutamic acid substitution for the β67 valine. The carboxylic side chain of the Glu forms a bond with iron, shifting the equilibrium toward the ferric state. *(Modified from Dickerson RE, Geis I: Hemoglobin: Structure, Function, Evolution, and Pathology. Menlo Park, CA, Benjamin-Cummings, 1983. Copyright Irving Geis.)*

Table 44–4 Drugs and Chemicals Having Toxic Effects on Hemoglobin Molecule

	Observed Hemoglobin-Derivative	
Agent	***Methemoglobin***	***Sulfhemoglobin***
Acetanilid, phenacetin	+	+
Nitrites (ferryl, amyl, sodium, potassium, nitroglycerin)	+	+
Trinitrotoluene, nitrobenzene	+	+
Aniline, hydroxylamine dimethylamine	+	+
Sulfanilamide	+	+
p-Aminosalicylic acid	+	
Dapsone	+	
Primaquine, chloroquine	+	
Prilocaine, benzocaine, lidocaine	+	
Menadione, naphthoquinone	+	
Naphthalene	+	
Resorcinol	+	
Phenylhydrazine	+	+

Acquired methemoglobinemia is virtually the only situation in which life-threatening amounts of methemoglobin accumulate. In general, the only symptom produced when methemoglobin comprises less than 30% of total hemoglobin is the cosmetic effect of cyanosis. As levels of methemoglobin rise to greater than 30%, however, patients begin to exhibit symptoms of oxygen deprivation, such as malaise, giddiness, and other alterations of mental status. The symptoms reflect a true lack of oxygen availability at the tissue level. Methemoglobin is a markedly left-shifted hemoglobin that delivers little oxygen to the tissues. When methemoglobin accounts for more than 50% of total hemoglobin, loss of consciousness, coma, and death can rapidly ensue. At this level, the blood is chocolate brown.

Diagnosis

Methemoglobinemia should be suspected in patients with unexplained cyanosis. It is obviously a medical emergency when any patient has cyanosis and altered mental status; a normal PaO_2 should trigger a consideration of methemoglobinemia. The ingestion of nitrites as a suicidal gesture, especially in people knowledgeable with respect to chemistry, medicine, or pharmacology, should be considered. Methemoglobinemia can be suspected from the brownish color of blood when it is drawn. Laboratory detection is simple; methemoglobin exhibits characteristic peaks of absorption at 630 and 502 nm, rendering it easily distinguishable from normal hemoglobin. Pulse oximetry, utilizing a ratio of absorption at 660 nm and 940 nm, gives an inaccurate reading of 85% O_2 saturation for blood with 100% methemoglobin. The inherited M hemoglobin mutants are frequently detectable by altered electrophoretic mobility, especially if ferricyanide treatment in vitro is used to convert all the hemoglobin solution to methemoglobin.

In the case of toxic methemoglobinemia, recognition of exposure to an appropriate agent provides the most important historical clue. Acute poisoning can represent a life-threatening emergency; therefore, laboratory evaluation for methemoglobin should be requested for any person displaying atypical cyanosis or cyanosis occurring along with normal blood gas values. Methemoglobin due to deficiencies of the reductase system can be further evaluated in reference laboratories by direct analysis of these enzymes.

Management

Patients with M hemoglobins are usually asymptomatic and require no management. The secondary cyanosis can present a cosmetic problem. The cyanosis is not reversible because ascorbic acid and methylene blue are usually ineffective.

Patients with deficiency of the reductase system usually do not require treatment. Cyanosis in these cases can be improved by treatment with oral methylene blue, 100 to 300 mg/day, or 500 mg/day of oral ascorbic acid. Riboflavin (20 mg/day) has also been reported to be effective and may be the preferred agent, because methylene blue produces discolored (blue) urine, and ascorbic acid can cause sodium oxalate stones.

Emergency treatment of high levels of toxic methemoglobinemia begins with 1 to 2 mg/kg of intravenous methylene blue as a 1% solution in saline. It is usually infused rapidly (over 3–5 minutes); the dose can be repeated at 1 mg/kg after 30 minutes if necessary. This treatment is usually effective. Methylene blue acts through the NADPH reductase system, which in turn requires G6PD activity. The method is therefore ineffective in patients who also have G6PD deficiency. These patients, or patients who are severely affected, may require exchange transfusion. Oral ascorbic acid is not useful for emergency situations because it acts too slowly. Follow-up maintenance management, however, can be accomplished with either ascorbic acid or oral methylene blue.

Mild cases of methemoglobin intoxication do not require treatment. The patient can be monitored for 1 to 3 days, during which time methemoglobin levels gradually return to normal if the offending agent is eliminated. The most important follow-up therapy for patients with toxic methemoglobinemia involves a thorough search for the offending agent and its removal from the environment.

SUGGESTED READINGS

Bunn HF: Sickle hemoglobin and other hemoglobin mutants. In Stamatoyannopoulos G, Nienhuis AW, Majerus PO, Varmus H (eds.): The Molecular Basis of Blood Disease, 2nd ed. Philadelphia, WB Saunders, 1993.

Bunn HF, Forget BG: Hemoglobin: Molecular, Cellular and Clinical Aspects. Philadelphia, WB Saunders, 1985.

Dickerson RE, Geis I: Hemoglobin: Structure, Function, Evolution, and Pathology. Menlo Park, CA, Benjamin-Cummings, 1983.

Ernst A, Zibrak J: Carbon monoxide poisoning. N Engl J Med 339:1603, 1998.

Fermi G, Perutz MF: Atlas of Molecular Structures in Biology. Vol. 2: Hemoglobin and Myoglobin. Oxford, Oxford University Press, 1981.

Ho C (ed.): Hemoglobin and Oxygen Binding. New York, Elsevier Biomedical, 1982.

Park CM, Nagel RL: Sulfhemoglobinemia: Clinical and molecular aspects. N Engl J Med 310:1579, 1984.

Perutz MF: Molecular anatomy, physiology, and pathology of hemoglobin. In Stamatoyannopoulos G, Nienhuis AW, Leder P, Majerus PW (eds.): The Molecular Basis of Blood Diseases. Philadelphia, WB Saunders, 1987, p 127.

Smith RP, Olson MV: Drug-induced methemoglobinemia. Semin Hematol 10:253, 1973.

Wishner BC, Ward KB, Lattman EE, Love WE: Crystal structure of sickle-cell deoxyhemoglobin at 5Å resolution. J Mol Biol 98:179, 1975.

Wright RO, Lewander WJ, Woolf AD: Methemoglobinemia: Etiology, pharmacology, and clinical management. Ann Emerg Med 34:646, 1999.

Wynngaarden JB, Smith LH Jr, Bennett JC (eds.): Cecil Textbook of Medicine. WB Saunders, Philadelphia, 1992.

CHAPTER 45

RED BLOOD CELL ENZYMOPATHIES

Xylina T. Gregg and Josef T. Prchal

Clinically significant abnormalities of red blood cell enzymes cause diverse clinical abnormalities, including hemolytic anemia, polycythemia, and methemoglobinemia. Deficiencies of some red cell enzymes may also provide a protective advantage to external challenges. Common mutations of glucose-6-phosphate dehydrogenase (G6PD) likely reached their prevalence by providing some protection against lethal malarial complications. In other instances, although there is no detectable red blood cell phenotypic abnormality, enzymes from easily accessible red blood cells can be assayed to diagnose systemic disorders such as galactosemia, adenosine deaminase deficiency, and deficiencies of some vitamins, for example, riboflavin. In addition, the study of red blood cell enzymes has helped to uncover important biologic principles, such as X-chromosome inactivation, and provided the groundwork for important principles of population genetics, biochemistry, and molecular biology.

Mature erythrocytes are the product of a highly specialized cellular process involving loss of the nucleus prior to release from the bone marrow and loss of mitochondria and ribosomes after 1 to 2 days in circulation. Unable to carry out oxidative phosphorylation and protein synthesis, the erythrocyte still has to sustain an active metabolism to maintain its viability and to preserve hemoglobin in its functional form to ensure adequate oxygen delivery to tissues.

Red blood cell enzymes allow erythrocytes to accomplish these tasks by supporting glycolysis and the pentose shunt, and by providing protection against oxidants by maintaining a high ratio of reduced (GSH) to oxidized (GSSG) glutathione (Fig. 45–1). Glycolysis and the pentose shunt generate four important metabolic intermediates: NADH; NADPH; 2,3-BPG; and adenosine triphosphate (ATP). Under physiologic conditions, approximately 90% of glucose is consumed in the glycolytic pathway and approximately 10% is utilized in the pentose shunt. Under conditions of increased oxidant stress, however, the contribution of the pentose shunt may be significantly increased.

To provide proper oxygen delivery, the erythrocyte must (a) maintain a high ratio of NADH to NAD for continuous reduction of methemoglobin to reduced hemoglobin; (b) maintain a high ratio of NADPH to NADP (generated in the pentose shunt from the glycolytic intermediate glucose-6-phosphate) for reduction of glutathione and protection against oxidant damage; (c) maintain a high concentration of 2,3-BPG generated in the Rapoport–Luebering shunt of glycolysis to ensure optimal oxygen delivery to the tissue; and (d) maintain the flexibility and integrity of the red blood cell membrane using ATP from glycolysis.

Glycolytic enzymes also have diverse, nonenzymatic functions, including stimulation of cell movement, control of apoptosis, and modulation of oncogene regulation. These other roles of glycolytic enzymes may explain some of the nonerythroid effects of mutations of the glycolytic enzyme genes.

Other erythrocyte enzymes such as pyrimidine 5′ nucleotidase participate in nucleotide degradation and salvage and are essential for the removal of nucleotide precursors that may be toxic to erythrocytes. In addition, erythrocytes contain enzymes, such as glutamine-oxaloacetic transaminase, with no obvious physiologic function; these may be remnants of its nucleated past.

RED CELL ENZYMOPATHIES CAUSING METHEMOGLOBINEMIA

Methemoglobin Formation

Methemoglobin is a derivative of hemoglobin in which the ferrous (Fe^{2+}) irons are oxidized to the ferric (Fe^{3+}) state. Oxygen binds easily to the ferrous form of iron present in deoxyhemoglobin. In the formation of oxyhemoglobin, one electron is partially transferred from iron to the bound oxygen, forming a ferric–superoxide (Fe^{3+}–O_2^-) anion complex.[1] During deoxygenation, some of the oxygen leaves as a superoxide (O_2^-) radical. The partially transferred electron is not returned to the iron moiety, thus leaving the iron in the ferric state and forming methemoglobin (Fig. 45–2). This autoxidation of hemoglobin occurs spontaneously at a slow rate, creating 0.5% to 3% methemoglobin per day.[2]

Methemoglobin is also formed from the oxidation of hemoglobin in other reactions with endogenous compounds and free radicals, including hydrogen peroxide (H_2O_2), nitric oxide (NO), O_2^-, and hydroxyl radical (HO^-).[3] Exogenous compounds can oxidize hemoglobin to methemoglobin directly, by a metabolic derivative, or by generating O_2^- and H_2O_2 during their metabolism.

A balance to methemoglobin formation is antioxidant protein 2 (AOP2), which is present in high concentrations in human and mouse red cells. This member of the peroxiredoxin protein family binds to hemoglobin and prevents spontaneous as well as oxidant-induced methemoglobin formation.[4] Mutations of this gene or its acquired deficiency are theoretical candidates responsible for congenital and acquired methemoglobinemia.

The ferric hemes of methemoglobin are unable to bind oxygen. In addition, the oxygen affinity of the accompanying ferrous hemes in the hemoglobin tetramer is increased.[5] As a result, the oxygen dissociation curve is left-shifted and oxygen delivery is impaired.

Methemoglobin Reduction

Although several potential mechanisms exist to reduce methemoglobin back to hemoglobin, only the NADH-dependent reaction catalyzed by cytochrome b_5 reductase (b5R) is physiologically important. Cytochrome b5R, previously known as diaphorase[6] and methemoglobin reductase,[7] contains a noncovalently bound prosthetic flavin adenine dinucleotide (FAD) group that acts as an electron acceptor.[8,9] NADH generated from glycolysis reduces FAD to $FADH_2$, which then reduces the heme protein cytochrome b_5. Electrons from the reduced cytochrome b_5 are in turn transferred to methemoglobin, reducing iron back to the ferrous state (Fig. 45–3).

An alternative pathway mediated by NADPH-flavin reductase uses NADPH generated by glucose-6-phosphate dehydrogenase (G6PD) in the hexose monophosphate shunt as a source of electrons to reduce redox dyes, such as methylene blue, and flavin (Fig. 45–4).[10] Reduced methylene blue, or leukomethylene blue, then reduces methemoglobin. Because these electron acceptors are not physiologic, this electron transfer is not significant under normal conditions, and NADPH-flavin reductase deficiency does not cause

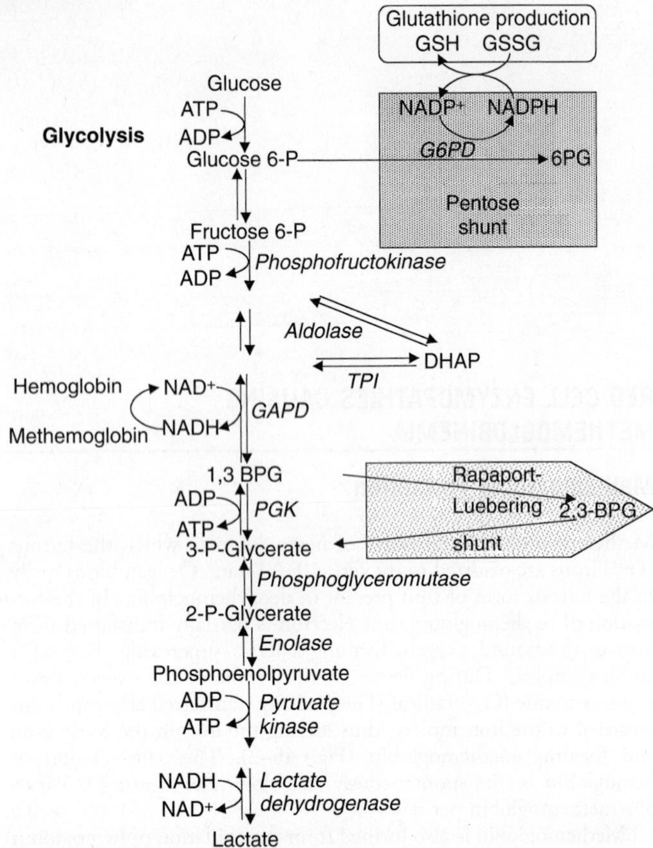

Figure 45–1 Glycolysis (Embden–Meyerhof pathway). 2,3-BPG, 2,3-bisphosphoglycerate; DHAP, dihydroxyacetone-P; GAPD, glyceraldehyde phosphate dehydrogenase; G6PD, glucose-6-phosphate dehydrogenase; GSH, reduced glutathione; GSSG, oxidized glutathione; 6PG, 6-phosphogluconate.

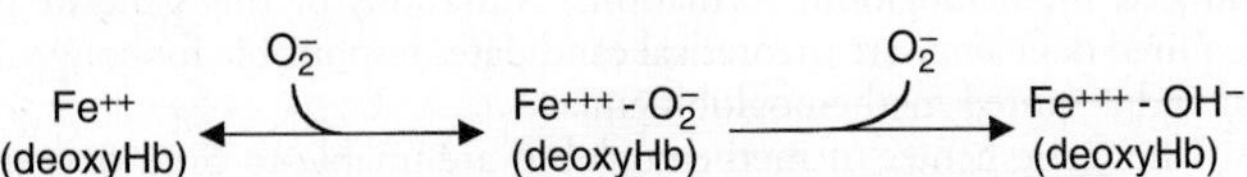

Figure 45–2 Autoxidation of hemoglobin. Iron is in the ferrous state (Fe^{2+}) in deoxyhemoglobin. When oxygen is bound, an electron is partially transferred from the iron moiety to the bound oxygen, forming a ferric–superoxide anion complex (Fe^{3+}–O_2^-). During deoxygenation, some of the oxygen leaves as a superoxide (O_2^-) radical. The partially transferred electron is not returned to the iron moiety, leaving the iron in the ferric state (Fe^{3+}) and forming methemoglobin (metHb).

methemoglobinemia.[11] However, methylene blue is useful in the treatment of acute toxic methemoglobinemia by providing an alternative to an overwhelmed cytochrome b_5 reductase pathway. Because the reduction of methemoglobin by methylene blue is dependent on NADPH generated by G6PD, methylene blue may be ineffective in the treatment of methemoglobinemia in individuals with G6PD deficiency.[12] In addition, the use of methylene blue in these patients is potentially dangerous because it may produce hemolysis.[12]

Methemoglobin can also be reduced directly by ascorbic acid, reduced glutathione, and reduced flavin; however, these reactions occur slowly and play a minor role in methemoglobin reduction.

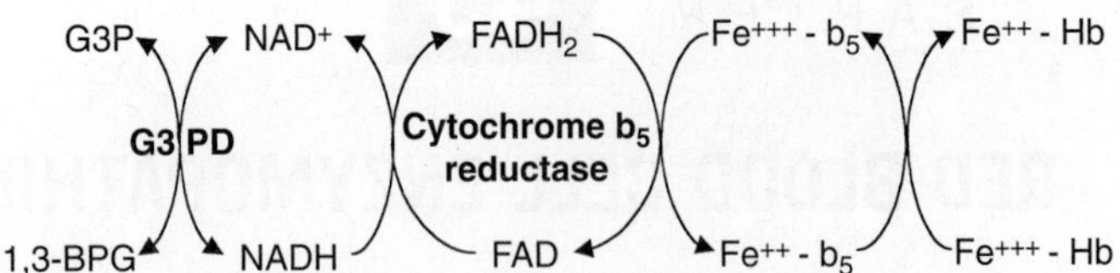

Figure 45–3 NADH-dependent methemoglobin reduction. NADH is generated during glycolysis in the reaction mediated by glucose-3-phosphate dehydrogenase (G3PD). A pair of electrons from NADH is transferred to the FAD prosthetic group of cytochrome b_5 reductase, reducing it to $FADH_2$. Two molecules of ferric (Fe^{3+}) cytochrome b_5 are then sequentially bound and reduced, forming ferrous (Fe^{2+}) cytochrome b_5. An ionic complex between ferrous (Fe^{2+}) cytochrome b_5 and a ferric (Fe^{3+}) subunit of a hemoglobin (methemoglobin) tetramer is formed and an electron transferred between the two hemes, creating ferrous (Fe^{2+}) hemoglobin. 1,3-BPG, 1,3-bisphosphonate glyceraldehyde; G3P, glyceraldehyde-3-phosphate.

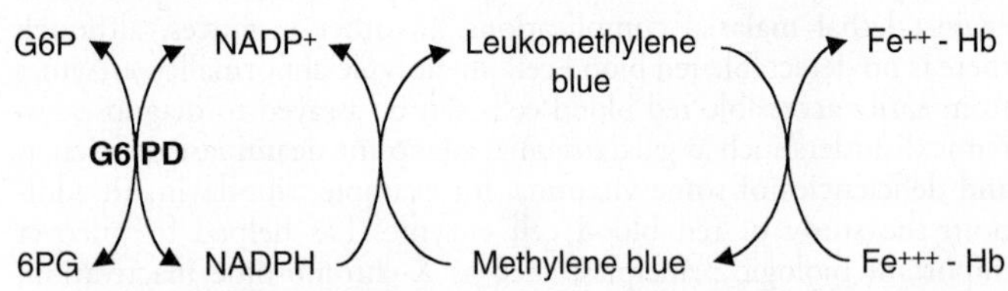

Figure 45–4 NADPH-dependent methemoglobin reduction. NADPH methemoglobin reduction can be activated by exogenously administered methylene blue. G6P, glucose-6-phosphate; G6PD, glucose-6-phosphate dehydrogenase; 6PG, 6-phosphogluconate.

METHEMOGLOBINEMIA

Normally, the formation and reduction of methemoglobin by the mechanisms described act to maintain a steady-state level of methemoglobin of 1% or less of total hemoglobin. Methemoglobinemia occurs when an imbalance due to either increased methemoglobin production or decreased methemoglobin reduction is present.

Acquired or Acute Toxic Methemoglobinemia

Most cases of methemoglobinemia are acquired, resulting from increased methemoglobin formation by various exogenous agents. Many drugs and toxins have been implicated.[13–17] Benzocaine, a topical anesthetic, is a frequently reported cause of acquired methemoglobinemia. The estimated incidence in a population undergoing transesophageal echocardiography was 0.115%.[18] The true incidence of drug-induced methemoglobinemia due to less frequently used agents is not known. Although flutamide has been reported to cause methemoglobinemia, in 50 consecutively studied patients with prostate cancer treated with flutamide, none developed clinically significant methemoglobinemia.[19] Furthermore, it is unknown whether the development of methemoglobinemia is dose related or idiosyncratic. In a retrospective review of 138 cases of acquired methemoglobinemia,[20] 42% were caused by dapsone. Topical benzocaine was responsible for five severe cases of methemoglobinemia, including one fatality. However, a cause could not be identified in 56 cases of mild methemoglobinemia; many of these cases were detected incidentally during intraoperative monitoring. Methemoglobinemia occurred equally between males and females and over a wide range of ages. The vast majority (94%) of the patients who developed methemoglobinemia were anemic.

Substances Associated with Methemoglobinemia

Acetaminophen (nitrobenzene derivative)
Acetanilide
Aniline dyes
Local anesthetics
- Benzocaine
- Lidocaine
- Prilocaine

Celecoxib
Dapsone
Flutamide
Ifosfamide
Metoclopramide
Nitric oxide
Nitrites
- Amyl nitrite
- Isobutyl nitrite
- Sodium nitrite
- Nitrates (bacterial conversion to nitrites)

Nitrobenzenes/nitrobenzoates
Nitroethane (nail polish remover)
Nitrofurans
Nitroglycerin
Paraquat/monolinuron
Phenacetin
Phenazopyridine (Pyridium)
Primaquine
Rasburicase
Sulfamethoxazole

In some instances, methemoglobinemia clearly occurs in the setting of overdoses or poisoning, but it may also occur at standard doses of drugs, particularly in individuals with partial deficiencies of b5R.[21,22] Infants are more susceptible to the development of methemoglobinemia because their erythrocyte b5R activity is normally 50% to 60% of adult activity.[23,24] Activity in the premature infant is even lower. Although b5R levels rise to those of an adult within months of birth, young infants are unusually vulnerable to developing toxic methemoglobinemia upon ingestion of nitrates.[25] Nitrates do not oxidize hemoglobin directly but are converted to nitrites by intestinal bacteria. Methemoglobinemia caused by nitrates in well water continues to be a problem in infants in rural areas.[26] Infants fed homemade preparations of vegetables with high nitrate content have developed methemoglobinemia.[27] Topical lidocaine used as an anesthetic for circumcision is another reported cause of methemoglobinemia in infants.[28]

Methemoglobinemia has also been associated with diarrheal illnesses in infants without known toxin exposure.[29] The exact mechanism leading to methemoglobinemia is unknown but may involve increased endogenous nitrite production.[30] An association with weight in the lower percentiles has been reported.[31,32]

Although individuals with congenital, chronically elevated methemoglobin concentrations are generally asymptomatic, acute acquired methemoglobinemia can be associated with symptoms at similar methemoglobin levels. The "cyanosis" or slate-blue color of the skin and mucous membranes results from the different absorbance spectrum of methemoglobin compared to oxyhemoglobin. Cyanosis is clinically discernible when the absolute level of methemoglobin exceeds 1.5 gm% (10%–15% methemoglobin at normal hemoglobin concentrations).[33] Symptoms of methemoglobinemia are related to impaired O_2 delivery to tissues. Early symptoms include headache, fatigue, dyspnea, and lethargy. At higher levels, respiratory depression, altered consciousness, shock, seizures, and death may occur.[13]

Hereditary Methemoglobinemia

There are three types of hereditary methemoglobinemia. In our experience, most cases are due to a deficiency of the red blood cell enzyme b5R (see section on cytochrome b_5 reductase deficiency). This enzyme deficiency is inherited in an autosomal recessive pattern and was the first hereditary condition in which an enzyme deficiency was identified.[7]

Deficiency of cytochrome b_5 is a rare disorder that also causes congenital methemoglobinemia. Only one well-documented case of cytochrome b_5 deficiency has been described,[34] as compared with more than 500 reported cases of b5R deficiency. This patient, a product of an Israeli consanguineous marriage, was also a male pseudohermaphrodite. Further analysis revealed that he was homozygous for a splicing mutation in the cytochrome b_5 gene, resulting in a premature stop codon and truncated protein.[35] Another family with probable cytochrome b_5 deficiency, as other causes of methemoglobinemia were excluded, was described prior to the recognition of this entity.[36] However, the inheritance pattern in this family was autosomal dominant.

The third type of hereditary methemoglobinemia, hemoglobin M (Hb M) disease (see Chapter 44), is caused by an abnormal globin and is autosomal dominant. It is associated with an abnormal pattern of spectrophotometric absorbance and sometimes with abnormal migration on hemoglobin electrophoresis.

Owing to the relative rarity of hereditary methemoglobinemia, it is unknown which type is the most common. However, even if we do not consider endemic Navajo, Athabascan, and Yakutsk congenital methemoglobinemia due to b5R deficiency, the literature over the last several decades suggests that congenital methemoglobinemia is far more frequently due to b5R deficiency than to hemoglobin M. Furthermore, in the experience of one of the authors supervising a red blood cell disorder reference laboratory, more than 20 new cases of hereditary methemoglobinemia were due to b5R deficiency, compared with only one case with hemoglobin M.

CYTOCHROME b_5 REDUCTASE DEFICIENCY

Function of Cytochrome b_5 Reductase

b5R, a housekeeping enzyme and a member of the flavoenzyme family of dehydrogenases–electron transferases, is involved in the transfer of electrons from the NADH generated by glyceraldehyde 3-phosphate in the glycolytic pathway to cytochrome b_5.[37] b5R exists in both cytosolic and membrane-bound forms, which participate in a variety of reactions. In erythrocytes, b5R transfers electrons to methemoglobin to reduce it to hemoglobin. In other cells, b5R transfers electrons from cytochrome b_5 to stearyl-CoA in the endoplasmic reticulum.[38] This reaction plays an important role in cholesterol biosynthesis, fatty acid elongation and desaturation, and drug metabolism.[39–41] The crystal structure of erythrocyte b5R has been solved[42]; this information should be useful to understand the differences between ubiquitously and erythrocyte-restricted b5R deficiency states and their radically different clinical outcomes.

b5R Gene and Isoforms

The b5R gene locus (*DIA1*) has been mapped to chromosome 22.[43] Multiple isoforms of b5R are generated from a single gene by a combination of alternative promoters and alternative initiation of translation.[44,45] Both a cytosolic isoform and a membrane-bound isoform are found in erythrocytes; the cytosolic isoform is involved in methemoglobin reduction.[46,47] Although the membrane-bound isoform contributes only 20% to 25% of erythrocyte b5R activity in adult humans, it represents a greater proportion in infants owing to a decreased cytosolic form.[48] Other isoforms have been described; however, there are significant interspecies differences in the structure of isoforms, so findings from animal studies may not be applicable to humans.[49]

b5R Gene Mutations

To date, more than 30 mutations have been described that result in b5R deficiency.[50] The mutations occur in all racial and ethnic groups. Although most of the mutants have been found in white populations, five unique mutations were found in Chinese,[51] at least three in Thai,[52,53] and two in African Americans.[54] The b5R mutations that cause endemic autosomal recessive congenital methemoglobinemia in Yakutsk, Navajo, and Athabascans have not been defined. Furthermore, an additional mutation of *b5R (116 T > S)* is not a disease-causing mutation but a high-frequency African-specific polymorphism that does not cause any appreciable disruption of the b5R secondary structure.[55]

There are two clinical types of b5R deficiency. The inheritance pattern is autosomal recessive, and a history of consanguinity is often present in sporadic cases. Mutations in cases of type I b5R deficiency are usually missense mutations leading to decreased stability of the enzyme. Thus, although b5R is abnormal in all cells, only mature red blood cells, which cannot synthesize proteins and replace the enzyme, are significantly affected in patients with type I b5R deficiency. On the other hand, type II mutations affect the catalytic site or lead to marked structural changes because of aberrant splicing, generation of premature stop codons, or partial gene deletions and all cells have decreased b5R activity.[56,57]

Clinical Features of b5R Deficiency

Type I b5R Deficiency

The majority of cases of enzymopenic congenital methemoglobinemia are type I, in which the functional deficiency of b5R is limited to erythrocytes. Homozygotes or compound heterozygotes[58] have methemoglobin concentrations of 10% to 35% and appear cyanotic but are usually asymptomatic, even with levels up to 40%.[33] Some patients have reported nonspecific symptoms of headache and easy fatigability. Life expectancy is not shortened and pregnancies occur normally. Significant polycythemia (erythrocytosis) is only rarely observed. The cyanosis is of cosmetic significance only but can be treated with methylene blue or ascorbic acid, both of which facilitate the reduction of methemoglobin through alternate pathways.[59]

In contrast to the chronically methemoglobinemic homozygotes (or compound heterozygotes) who are asymptomatic, heterozygous individuals are normal under basal conditions, but at risk for developing acute, symptomatic methemoglobinemia after exposure to exogenous methemoglobin-inducing agents. The report from Cohen and colleagues[21] of acute toxic methemoglobinemia in US military personnel receiving malarial prophylaxis in Vietnam is a classic description of this phenomenon.

Type I b5R deficiency is distributed worldwide but is endemic in Athabascan Alaskans,[60,61] Navajo Indians,[62] and Yakutsk natives of Siberia.[63,64] The Navajo Indians and the Athabascan Indians of Alaska are known to share a common ancestor, and the high frequency of b5R deficiency in these groups suggests a common origin for all three of these populations. However, it remains to be determined whether the molecular defect resulting in b5R deficiency is identical in these populations. In other ethnic and racial groups, the defect occurs sporadically. Although cyanosis is difficult to detect because of skin pigmentation, type I deficiency has been reported in two unrelated African American families.[65]

Type II b5R Deficiency

In type II b5R deficiency, b5R is deficient in all cells. Type II b5R deficiency represents 10% to 15% of cases of enzymopenic congenital methemoglobinemia and has a sporadic distribution. In addition to methemoglobinemia and cyanosis, patients exhibit mental retardation and developmental delay with failure to thrive.[66] Other neurologic symptoms may be present, including microcephaly, opisthotonus, athetoid movements, strabismus, seizures, and spastic quadriparesis. Life expectancy is significantly shortened, and death in infancy is typical. The mechanism resulting in the neurologic problems is currently unknown but it has been suggested that it may involve abnormal lipid elongation and desaturation in the central nervous system.[67] Another possible molecular basis for the neurotoxicity and failure to thrive may be failure to keep the heme iron in hemoglobin-related globins, including neuroglobin, cytoglobin, and myoglobin, in the ferrous state.[68–70]

Methylene blue or ascorbic acid improves the cyanosis, as in type I b5R deficiency; however, this therapy has no effect on the neurologic and other systemic defects in type II b5R deficiency. Theoretically, a bone marrow or liver transplant would alleviate the neurologic problems of individuals with type II deficiency if they are caused by a problem with circulating fatty acids. Nevertheless, these approaches have not yet been tested, and because the aberrantly elongated fatty acids may not be the primary cause of the pathophysiology, they may not work. In addition, because the enzyme defect is found in fibroblasts, analysis of b5R activity in cultured amniotic cells for prenatal diagnosis is possible.[71,72]

Assays of Enzyme Activity

Types I and II b5R deficiency are distinguished by their clinical phenotype and by analysis of enzymatic activity in erythroid and nonerythroid cells. Reports of decreased b5R activity are difficult to compare because several different assays of b5R activity, varying in their substrate and in their normal values, have been used.[58,60,64,65,73,74] These assays also vary in their technical difficulty.[75] Currently, the most prevalent assay uses ferricyanide as an enzyme substrate.[76] Although not as rigorous as previous assays, it is simple and has proved to be reliable. Type I and type II b5R deficiencies can be readily differentiated because patients with type I deficiency have normal enzyme activity in platelets, fibroblasts, Epstein–Barr virus-transformed lymphocytes, and granulocytes, whereas in type II deficiency the activity in nonerythroid tissues is markedly to moderately decreased.[54,65,76]

Two families with type III deficiency, in which b5R activity was decreased not only in erythrocytes but also in platelets and leukocytes, have been described.[77] However, the existence of this entity is difficult to accept because these individuals did not exhibit the neurologic abnormalities characteristic of type II deficiency. Reevaluation of one of the patients with a rigorous assay using recombinant cytochrome b_5 confirmed b5R activity in the platelets, leukocytes, and fibroblasts consistent with type I deficiency.[78]

DIAGNOSIS OF METHEMOGLOBINEMIA

Methemoglobinemia can be clinically suspected when cyanosis occurs in the presence of a normal partial arterial pressure of oxygen (Pa_{O_2}), as obtained by assessment of arterial blood gases. Methemoglobinemia causes clinically discernible cyanosis when the absolute level of methemoglobin exceeds 1.5 gm%; this correlates with approximately 10% to 15% methemoglobin.[33] Sulfhemoglobin in concentrations greater than 0.5 gm% also causes cyanosis with a normal Pa_{O_2} and may be erroneously measured as methemoglobin. The laboratory diagnosis of methemoglobinemia is based on analysis of its absorption spectra. A fresh specimen should always be obtained because methemoglobin levels tend to increase with storage. Methemoglobin has peak absorbance at 631 nm. The standard method of assaying methemoglobin utilizes a microprocessor-controlled, fixed wavelength co-oximeter. This instrument interprets all readings in the 630 nm range as methemoglobin; thus, false-positive readings may occur in the presence of other pigments, including sulfhemoglobin and meth-

Suspecting, Detecting, and Treating Methemoglobinemia

Methemoglobinemia should always be suspected when cyanosis is present with normal oxygen saturation. Methemoglobin levels interfere with the measurement of oxygen saturation by conventional pulse oximetry; thus, an oxygen saturation discrepancy between values obtained from pulse oximetry and from arterial blood gas may be a diagnostic clue. The initial screening for methemoglobinemia can be performed in the arterial blood gas laboratory, which uses a cooximeter to detect the different absorption spectrum of methemoglobin. Methemoglobin detected by cooximetry should be confirmed by the specific Evelyn–Malloy method.

If the patient is symptomatic, acute toxic methemoglobinemia is likely and, after the diagnosis is confirmed, treatment with methylene blue 1 mg/kg over 5 minutes should be initiated. However, methylene blue should not be used in patients with known or suspected G6PD deficiency (including heterozygous females who may not be detected by routine G6PD screening tests). Instead, the preferred treatment for these patients is ascorbic acid, although the rate of response to this therapy is considerably slower than for methylene blue.

Because cooximetry detects methylene blue as methemoglobin, it cannot be used in following methemoglobin levels after treatment with methylene blue; however, the specific Evelyn–Malloy method can be used for this purpose.

Treatment is not indicated for patients with asymptomatic chronic methemoglobinemia, except for cosmetic reasons.

ylene blue.[79,80] Methemoglobin detected by cooximeter should be confirmed by the specific Evelyn–Malloy method.[81] In this assay, cyanide (CN^-) is added and binds to the positively charged methemoglobin, eliminating the peak at 630 to 635 nm in direct proportion to the methemoglobin concentration. The subsequent addition of ferricyanide converts the entire specimen to cyanomethemoglobin for measurement of the total hemoglobin concentration. Methemoglobin is expressed as a percentage of the total concentration of hemoglobin.

Distinguishing the hereditary forms of congenital methemoglobinemia requires interpretation of family pedigrees as well as biochemical analyses. Cyanosis in successive generations suggests the presence of the autosomal dominant Hb M disease, whereas having normal parents but possibly affected siblings implies autosomal recessive b5R deficiency or the very rare cytochrome b_5 deficiency. Incubation of blood with methylene blue distinguishes b5R deficiency from Hb M disease, because this treatment results in the rapid reduction of methemoglobin through the NADPH-flavin reductase pathway in cases of b5R deficiency but not in cases of Hb M disease.[82,83] Measurement of the level of b5R activity in erythrocyte and nonerythroid cells is required to distinguish type I from type II b5R deficiency; however, these assays are not commercially available. Differentiating b5R deficiency from cytochrome b_5 deficiency is usually based on measurement of b5R activity, because currently only one or two research laboratories can perform cytochrome b_5 quantitation.

TREATMENT

Offending agents in cases of acquired methemoglobinemia should be discontinued. No other therapy may be required, but if the patient is symptomatic, which is often true in cases of deliberate or accidental overdoses or toxin ingestion, specific therapy is indicated. Methylene blue, 1 to 2 mg/kg over 5 minutes, provides an artificial electron acceptor for the reduction of methemoglobin via the NADPH-dependent pathway. Response is usually rapid; the dose can be repeated in 1 hour, but frequently this is unnecessary. Caution should

When to Suspect a Red Blood Cell Enzymopathy

The following clinical situations should raise suspicion for a red blood cell enzymopathy:

1. Chronic hemolytic anemia without specific morphologic red blood cell abnormalities.
2. Chronic hemolytic anemia with basophilic stippling (pyrimidine 5′ nucleotidase deficiency).
3. Acute hemolysis occurring after exposure to oxidant drugs (G6PD deficiency)
4. Whenever Heinz bodies are observed on the blood film, although the absence of Heinz bodies does not exclude a red blood cell enzymopathy (G6PD, glutathione synthase, and reductase deficiencies).
5. Chronic hemolytic anemia in association with other congenital disorders such as myopathy, mental retardation, and metabolic acidosis.

be exercised to avoid overdosage because large (>7 mg/kg) cumulative doses have been reported to cause dyspnea, chest pain, and hemolysis.[84] Because co-oximetry detects methylene blue as methemoglobin, it cannot be used in following methemoglobin levels after treatment with methylene blue; however, the specific Evelyn–Malloy method[81] allows discrimination of methemoglobin from methylene blue. Methylene blue should not be administered to patients with G6PD deficiency. If methylene blue is contraindicated, ascorbic acid can be given. Red blood cell exchange transfusion has also been reported to be an effective treatment in symptomatic methemoglobinemic patients with coexistent G6PD deficiency.[85]

Treatment of the cyanosis in individuals with types I and II b5R deficiency is indicated for cosmetic reasons only. Treatment options include methylene blue (100–300 mg/day orally) or ascorbic acid (300–1000 mg/day orally in divided doses), although this therapy has been associated with renal calculi formation. The use of riboflavin (20–30 mg/day) has also been reported.[86] Unfortunately, there is currently no effective therapy for the neurologic disorder associated with type II deficiency.

RED BLOOD CELL ENZYMOPATHIES ASSOCIATED WITH HEMOLYTIC ANEMIA

The red blood cell enzyme deficiencies causing hemolytic anemia can be divided arbitrarily into those directly or indirectly involved with the maintenance of a high ratio of reduced to oxidized glutathione, those participating in the glycolytic (Embden–Meyerhof) pathway, and, lastly, one enzyme in the nucleotide degradation and salvage pathway (pyrimidine 5′ nucleotidase).

INHERITANCE

G6PD and phosphoglycerate kinase are encoded on the X chromosome and are subject to dosage compensation by X chromosome inactivation. The remaining enzymes are present on the autosomal chromosomes; deficiencies of these enzymes can cause a clinical phenotype if the subject is either homozygous or doubly heterozygous for separate defects affecting both alleles.

CLINICAL AND LABORATORY MANIFESTATIONS

The hemolysis associated with a red blood cell enzyme deficiency may be chronic or acute intermittent. Acute intermittent hemolysis is typically seen in patients with enzyme disorders affecting glutathione metabolism, such as G6PD. During the hemolytic episodes, either normal red blood cell morphology or nonspecific abnormalities (anisocytosis, polychromasia) can be observed. In defects of enzymes affecting glutathione metabolism, the morphologic sequelae of the oxidative denaturation of hemoglobin, Heinz bodies, can be seen either directly on microscopic evaluation of the blood film or after the red blood cells are preincubated with oxidants such as phenylhydrazine.[87] Although "bite cells" are reported in many textbooks as pathognomonic for G6PD deficiency, the authors of this chapter have never observed bite cells during acute hemolytic episodes in G6PD-deficient subjects nor in patients with severe G6PD enzyme defects causing rare chronic hemolytic anemia (G6PD Dothan, G6PD Birmingham). The only enzyme deficiency associated with hemolysis that causes consistent morphologic abnormalities is pyrimidine 5′ nucleotidase deficiency wherein basophilic stippling is observed. Although laboratory screening tests such as the "autohemolysis test"[88] were previously advocated to detect enzyme disorders causing hemolysis, they do not have a sound physiologic basis and should play no role in modern hematology practice.[89]

ENZYMOPATHIES OF GLUTATHIONE METABOLISM

Glutathione Metabolism

Erythrocytes contain a remarkably high concentration of glutathione (approximately 2 mM),[90] more than any other cell in the body. Oxidant damage converts reduced glutathione (GSH) to the oxidized form (GSSG) and also forms mixed disulfides of proteins (such as hemoglobin) containing free –SH groups. A high GSH to GSSG ratio is the major mechanism protecting the red blood cell proteins from oxidant damage. Enzymes involved in this metabolic pathway (Fig. 45–5) include γ-glutamyl cysteine synthase and GSH synthase, which synthesize glutathione; glutathione reductase, which reduces GSSG to GSH; and G6PD, which generates the NADPH needed for the reduction of GSSG.

An additional protective mechanism against oxidant damage involves unidirectional active transport of oxidized glutathione out of the erythrocyte.[91,92] GSH is actively synthesized in the red blood cells, but its half-life is only 3 to 4 days because of the efflux of oxidized glutathione by an active transport mechanism. This transport mechanism provides additional protection from severe oxidative stress; thus far, no disorder involving this pathway has been described.

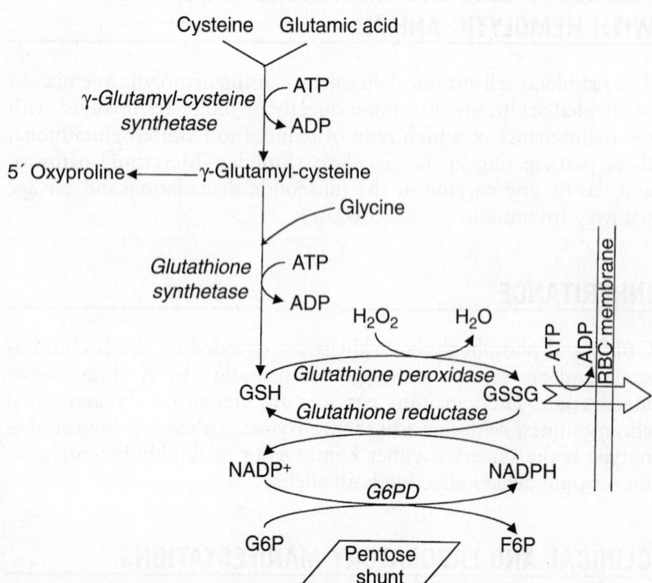

Figure 45–5 Glutathione pathway. G6P, glucose-6-phosphate; G6PD, glucose-6-phosphate dehydrogenase; GSH, reduced glutathione; GSSG, oxidized glutathione; 6PG, 6-phosphogluconate.

G6PD deficiency is very common, but deficiencies of other enzymes of the glutathione pathway are rare. Deficiencies of these enzymes are expected to resemble G6PD deficiency with precipitation of hemolysis and formation of Heinz bodies after exposure to certain drugs, infections, and other oxidant stresses. However, these enzyme defects can also be associated with additional clinical manifestations.

G6PD Deficiency

History

The discovery of G6PD deficiency represents a legendary example of clinical investigation that led to the delineation of important biochemical and genetic principles. During the investigation of a newly developed malaria drug, primaquine, Beutler and colleagues[93,94] noted that although the drug was tolerated by the majority of the male volunteers, some developed acute hemolytic episodes. These episodes were short-lasting and typically did not recur after immediate reintroduction of the drug but could recur when the drug was reintroduced after a period of several months. These drug-induced reactions were seen in subjects of particular ethnic groups, including African Americans and individuals of Mediterranean extraction. Biochemical analysis of erythrocytes during an acute hemolytic episode revealed a decrease in reduced glutathione (GSH).[94] Shortly thereafter, Carson[95] found that the cause of the GSH decline was a deficiency of the first step of pentose shunt-G6PD. Subsequent studies of carrier females led to the codiscovery of X chromosome inactivation.[96–98] Further investigations of this phenomenon have played a pivotal role in our understanding of the hierarchy of hematopoiesis,[99–101] clonality of malignant neoplasms,[102] and the mechanism of X chromosome inactivation.[96,103]

Biology and Molecular Aspects

G6PD is a housekeeping enzyme that plays an essential role not only in the reduction of NADPH from NADP but also in the generation of five-carbon sugars. In the reaction catalyzed by G6PD, electrons generated by the conversion of glucose 6 phosphate to 6-phosphogluconate are transferred to NADP. The *G6PD* gene spans approximately 20 kilobases with 13 exons.[104,105] G6PD activity decreases significantly as erythrocytes age, with a half-life of approximately 60 days.[106] Reticulocytes have five times higher enzyme activity than the oldest erythrocyte subpopulation.[107]

G6PD-Deficient Variants

More than 300 G6PD variants have been defined; most are sporadic but some occur at a high frequency. G6PD variants can be divided into three categories, based on the type of hemolysis they cause. Most common are those variants associated with acute intermittent hemolytic anemia; some of these variants are endemic (Mediterranean, A-, some Southeast Asian variants). In contrast, the variants associated with chronic hemolytic anemia are very rare. The third type of variant is associated with no obvious risk of hemolysis and is also uncommon. A detailed list of these variants is continuously updated and can be found elsewhere.[108,109]

In the past, new variants were defined by their enzyme activity, thermal stability, K_M for normal (G6P, NADP) and artificial (2-deoxy G6P, deamino-NADP) substrates, K_i for NADPH, and electrophoretic mobilities under various conditions.[110] When the nucleotide sequence variations for the wild-type G6PD enzyme, designated G6PD B, were established,[105] some of these previously described variants were found to represent identical mutations.[111] Interestingly, they arose independently in some cases on different haplotypes of the *G6PD* gene.[112]

The vast majority of the *G6PD* mutations are missense. Mutations associated with chronic hemolysis tend to cluster in the vicinity of the NADP-binding domain of the *G6PD* gene, whereas those associated with acute intermittent hemolysis or no hemolysis are scattered throughout the gene. Unlike disease-causing mutations of other genes, deletions and insertions causing frame shift and stop codon mutations are not observed; these null mutation events would be expected to be fatal, because *G6PD* is a housekeeping gene essential for basic cellular functions.[113] One intronic mutation of the *G6PD* gene (G6PD Varnsdorf) has been described[114]; this mutation is associated with chronic hemolysis, but the molecular consequences of this mutation have not been fully elucidated.[115]

Of the G6PD-deficient variants that occur at a high frequency, the best known are African G6PD A$^-$ and the Mediterranean variants; several variants are also present in Southeast Asia. All of these variants cause acute intermittent hemolysis. African G6PD A$^-$ and the Mediterranean variant of G6PD deficiency have been particularly well studied. G6PD A$^+$, another well-studied isoenzyme variant, is associated with no obvious hematologic phenotype and has a gene frequency similar to that of G6PD A$^-$ among African Americans.[116] The *G6PD A$^-$* mutation (G202A) arose on a *G6PD A$^+$* chromosome (A376G).[117]

Epidemiology

G6PD deficiency is one of the most prevalent disease-causing mutations worldwide, affecting hundreds of millions of people.[114,118] Most of the G6PD isoenzymes with decreased activity are associated with only moderate health risks without a significant effect on longevity.[90,119]

In the United States, G6PD deficiency is seen frequently among African Americans (G6PD A$^-$), affecting approximately 10% of males. The Mediterranean variant of G6PD deficiency is common in the southern part of Italy, Greece, Spain, and Corsica, and among Arabs and Sephardic Jews. In some populations of Kurdish Jews, the gene frequency exceeds 50%. This variant is heterogeneous at the nucleotide level and is composed of several distinct mutations.[120,121] Several variants are pandemic in Asia. G6PD Mahidol is common in Thailand and India[122]; G6PD Chinese-1, G6PD Chinese-2, G6PD Chinese-3, and G6PD Canton are frequent in China and Southeast Asia.[123] G6PD Viangchan (871G > A) is the most common mutation among Cambodians and is also found in Thais and Laotians.[124] It is assumed that malaria provided a positive selection pressure, accounting for the high gene frequency of these G6PD variants (see discussion following), whereas mutations that arose in parts of the world not plagued by malaria are sporadic.

Acute Hemolysis and G6PD Deficiency

Hemoglobin is maintained in solution in a high concentration in the cytoplasm of the erythrocyte. Oxidant damage leads to the oxidation of free –SH groups of hemoglobin, forming disulfide bridges that in turn lead to decreased hemoglobin solubility. The precipitated hemoglobin may be morphologically recognized as Heinz bodies. The high ratio of reduced-to-oxidized glutathione represents the major defense against the oxidative damage of hemoglobin. The enzymatic activity of G6PD generates NADPH that is utilized for glutathione reduction (see Fig. 45–5). Reduced glutathione (GSH) reconstitutes –SH groups of hemoglobin, maintaining the solubility of hemoglobin.

In cases of G6PD deficiency, this process is variably impaired, depending on the type of the G6PD mutation. In a subject with an acute hemolytic G6PD deficient variant, there is no clinical or laboratory evidence of hemolysis unless the individual is exposed to certain clinical situations. The severity of hemolysis in those inheriting the rare chronic hemolytic G6PD variants ranges from mild to transfusion dependent. Predictably, exposure to the oxidants that cause hemolysis in the acute hemolytic G6PD variants further exacerbates hemolysis.

An acute insult, most commonly drugs, infections, or fava bean ingestion, typically precipitates hemolysis. In spite of continuation of the drug or persistence of infection, hemolysis is short-lasting, presumably because of the elimination of a subpopulation of red blood cells with very low G6PD activity. The younger red blood cells and reticulocytes, which have higher G6PD activity, are typically not hemolyzed. The Mediterranean variant is more severe than the African A$^-$ G6PD-deficient variant and is thus prone to more severe hemolytic episodes.

Pharmaceutical agents are the best-defined precipitants of hemolysis. Although many drugs have been alleged to precipitate hemolysis in G6PD-deficient subjects, relatively few have withstood scrutiny.[125] Many of these agents are now obsolete and unlikely to be used. A discussion of a selected number of these agents follows.

Methylene blue administration to subjects with acute toxic methemoglobinemia is a well-known cause of severe hemolysis[125] that may be life-threatening in a subject with already compromised oxygen delivery due to methemoglobinemia (see section on methemoglobinemia earlier in this chapter). Infections have been widely recognized as a cause of hemolysis in G6PD-deficient subjects. It is assumed that diffusion of oxidants from neutrophils undergoing oxidative bursts leads to the formation of disulfide bridges of hemoglobin.

Fava beans are a staple food in many parts of the world where G6PD deficiency is found at a high gene frequency. The hemolysis precipitated by fava bean ingestion, favism, has been widely recognized in the Mediterranean region[130,131] and occurs only in subjects who are also G6PD deficient. However, not all G6PD-deficient variants are prone to favism. Subjects with the G6PD A$^-$ variant are typically not susceptible (although a rare exception to this rule was reported),[132] and not all subjects with the more severely deficient Mediterranean variant of G6PD deficiency are sensitive. It is assumed that the hemolytic risk of fava beans depends on the source and preparation of the beans[133] as well as individual variation due to an additional genetic component that has not yet been characterized.[134] Two fava bean metabolites, divicine and isouramil, are presumed oxidants and have been reported as possible causes of favism.[133]

In infants, a large study from Taiwan showed that neonatal jaundice is far more common in G6PD-deficient infants.[135] Furthermore, those G6PD-deficient subjects who also coinherit a promoter variant of uridine-5²-diphosphate-glucuronyl transferase have an even greater risk of neonatal hyperbilirubinemia.[136,137]

Nonerythroid Effect of G6PD Deficiency

Although patients with the common endemic G6PD variants are not at increased risk for infections, neutrophil dysfunction has been described in patients with some rare, severely deficient G6PD variants.[138,139]

Substances to Be Avoided in Cases of G6PD Deficiency

- Acetanilid
- Doxorubicin[126]
- Isobutyl nitrite[127]
- Methylene blue
- Naphthalene[128]
- Nitrofurantoin (Furadantin)
- Phenazopyridine (Pyridium)[129]
- Phenylhydrazine
- Primaquine
- Sulfacetamide
- Sulfamethoxazole (Gantanol)
- Sulfanilamide
- Sulfapyridine

Evolutionary Benefit of G6PD Deficiency

Shortly after the discovery of G6PD deficiency, it became apparent that the geographic distribution of populations with a high gene frequency of deficient variants overlapped closely with the prevalence of malaria. On the basis of this association, it was suggested that G6PD deficiency might be protective against malaria.[140,141] Unexpectedly, in the initial studies of acutely infected subjects, no protective effect of the G6PD deficiency was found for hemizygous G6PD-deficient males.[142] However, an apparent protection was found for heterozygous females[142] who, because of X-chromosome inactivation, are mosaics for deficient and nondeficient cells. This led to elegant studies demonstrating that although the malarial parasite does not initially thrive in a G6PD-deficient environment,[119] it adapts after several days of residence in a G6PD-deficient erythrocyte by increased production of malarial G6PD.[143,144] This strategy counteracts the evolutionary defense of G6PD deficiency in males; however, when the parasites infect the variably deficient and nondeficient erythrocytes of heterozygous females, malarial G6PD production is not efficient.[144] However, more recent epidemiologic and population genetic studies indicate that even G6PD-deficient males have some protection against malarial virulence[145,146] and suggest that the G6PD A^- variant arose only recently in human evolution and presumably spread rapidly as a result of positive selection by malaria infection.[146,147] Increased removal of G6PD-deficient erythrocytes containing ring-stage parasites was shown to be a likely mechanism of malarial protection.[148]

Diagnosis

The diagnosis of G6PD deficiency is based on the generation of NADPH from NADP as detected by either quantitative spectrophotometric analysis[149] or, more conveniently, by a rapid fluorescent screening test.[150] False-negative results are not unusual, especially if enzymatic analysis is performed shortly after resolution of acute hemolytic episodes.[90] After acute hemolysis, reticulocytes and young erythrocytes, which have much higher enzymatic activity, predominate. These false-negative test results are more likely to occur when a screening test rather than a quantitative spectrophotometric analysis of the enzyme activity is used. A high proportion of young red blood cells, which could contribute to a falsely "normal" result, can be conveniently estimated by concomitant spectrophotometric analysis of hexokinase, another red blood cell enzyme whose activity is markedly dependent on red blood cell age.

G6PD-deficient erythrocytes of heterozygous females are also prone to hemolysis, but because of the natural mosaicism for X-chromosome enzymes in females, females heterozygous for G6PD deficiency are particularly difficult to diagnose.[90] In populations of African ancestry, the faster electrophoretic mobility of G6PD A^- discriminates it from the wild-type G6PD B isoenzyme, but electrophoresis does not differentiate G6PD A^- from the other African polymorphic nondeficient isoenzyme G6PD A^+.[90] However, now that the nucleotide substitutions of many G6PD-deficient isoenzymes have been established, molecular diagnostic methods can be more reliably used for the accurate diagnosis of females who are heterozygous for G6PD deficiency.[90]

Therapy

Drugs that are known to precipitate hemolysis in G6PD-deficient subjects should be avoided. In subjects with G6PD A^- deficiency, hemolysis is typically short-lasting in spite of continuous use of the offending agent. This is not always the case in patients with the more severe Mediterranean variant of G6PD deficiency, and the precipitating agent should be always withdrawn. When anemia is severe and symptomatic, blood transfusion may be necessary.

γ-Glutamyl Cysteine Synthase Deficiency

γ-Glutamyl cysteine synthase catalyzes the first metabolic step of glutathione synthesis. Only two families with a defect of this enzyme have been reported.[151,152] The first family had hemolytic anemia and progressive neurologic defects; the other family had hemolytic anemia but was neurologically normal.[152]

Glutathione Synthase Deficiency

Glutathione synthase deficiency is an autosomal recessive disorder; patients are homozygous or compound heterozygotes for mutations in the glutathione synthase gene. The clinical presentation is variable; classification into mild, moderate, or severe phenotypes has been proposed.[153] Mildly affected patients have only hemolytic anemia, whereas moderately affected individuals have both hemolytic anemia and severe metabolic acidosis because of the accumulation of 5-oxoproline (see Fig. 45–5). Severely affected patients also have neurological symptoms (seizures, psychomotor retardation), which are progressive. Although mutations causing frameshifts, premature stop codons, or aberrant splicing are associated with the moderate or severe phenotype, other factors including environmental factors and other modifier genes likely affect the clinical phenotype because there may be considerable phenotypic variability even among the siblings affected by the same mutations.[154] High levels of 5-oxyproline in the urine (found in all severely and moderately affected but in only some of the mildly affected patients) suggests the diagnosis, which is confirmed by documenting deficiency of the enzyme.

Deficiency of this enzyme in neutrophils has also been alleged to cause intermittent neutropenia in some families,[155] and recurrent bacterial infections have been described.[153] One affected African American patient was also an albino,[156] suggesting the participation of this enzyme in melanin metabolism. Therapy with vitamins E and C has been recommended[153] but is not always effective.[156]

Glutathione Reductase Deficiency

Glutathione reductase requires the riboflavin-derived cofactor FAD for full activity. Its in vitro activity with and without exogenously added FAD can be conveniently used for diagnosing riboflavin deficiency.[149] The first reported case of an inherited deficiency of this enzyme was a Dutch family with two affected siblings who had unstable GSH and developed a hemolytic crisis after eating fava beans[157]; their disease resulted from a homozygous large glutathione reductase gene deletion. In the second reported family, which was also Dutch, the propositus had severe neonatal jaundice and was a compound heterozygote for two different mutations than that found in the first family.[158] Acquired deficiency of this enzyme secondary to riboflavin deficiency does not appear to have any hematologic phenotype.

Glutathione Peroxidase Deficiency

Glutathione peroxidase contains selenium. Selenium deficiency is particularly common in New Zealand, where many individuals with decreased enzyme activity have been found.[159] This acquired decreased activity has not been associated with a recognizable phenotype, and no clear-cut congenital deficiency of this enzyme has been reported. Knockout of this gene in mice results in only a mild defect with propensity to cataracts.[160]

ENZYMOPATHIES OF THE GLYCOLYTIC PATHWAY

The enzyme deficiencies of the glycolytic pathway differ from those enzyme abnormalities of glutathione pathway metabolism in several ways: (a) they do not have any characteristic morphologic abnormalities such as Heinz bodies; (b) they are not subject to hemolytic crises after exposure to oxidants; and (c) their mechanism of hemolysis is not clearly understood. Furthermore, the clinical phenotypes are highly variable and appear to be specific for each enzymatic defect. Diagnosis of these disorders depends on the quantitation of enzyme activity in a hemolysate prepared from leukocyte- and platelet-depleted washed red blood cells.[149]

Pyruvate Kinase Deficiency

Pyruvate kinase (PK) deficiency is the most common genetic defect causing congenital enzymopathic hemolytic anemia. Although this disorder is far less common than G6PD deficiency, the vast majority of patients with G6PD deficiency never suffer an acute hemolytic episode and those G6PD variants associated with chronic hemolytic states are rare. PK deficiency, in contrast, exhibits high penetrance of the hemolytic phenotype.

Pyruvate Kinase Isoenzymes and Molecular Biology

The PK isoenzymes, M_1, M_2, L, and R, are products of two distinct genes. The *PK-M* gene, which is expressed in muscle, leukocytes, platelets, brain tissue, and other cells, is located on chromosome 15q22.[161] The M_1 and M_2 isoforms result from differential processing of a single transcript of this gene.[162] PK-M_2 is the dominant fetal form of PK (including fetal erythroid cells). In adult life it is largely replaced in muscle and brain by PK-M_1 but persists in leukocytes, platelets, and early erythroid progenitors.[163]

A gene on chromosome 1q21 encodes the L and R PK isoenzymes.[164] This gene utilizes two different tissue-specific promoters initiating transcription at different exons.[165] The L isoform is found in hepatocytes, the renal cortex, and the small intestine. The R form is present in two isoforms; the smaller of the two is the result of proteolytic degradation. These two PK peptides are unique to erythrocytes and gradually replace the M_2 isoform as erythroid cells mature. The crystal structure of the R form composed of the larger R peptides was published,[166] but it is not clear how relevant it is to in vivo red cell PK, which exists in two different forms. The complexity of PK isoforms is further accentuated by the fact that the functional enzyme is a tetramer and that heterotetramers exist.

An allosteric enzyme with one substrate-binding site, PK converts phosphoenol pyruvate to lactate, generating ATP in the process. PK also interacts with fructose diphosphate (FDP). Similar to the interaction of hemoglobin with 2,3-BPG, this interaction changes the conformational structure of PK and decreases its Michaels enzymatic constant (K_M) for its substrate phosphoenol pyruvate, thus dramatically increasing the activity (V_{max}) of the enzyme.[167,168] PK-M_1 is the only isoform that does not allosterically interact with FDP. The PK M variants also have quite different kinetic properties than the adult erythrocyte PK isoform R.

PK Mutations

More than 150 mutations of *PK* have been reported.[169,170] There appears to be some correlation with the location of the mutation and the severity of the hemolytic anemia.[170] Affected individuals are either homozygous for the same mutation or doubly heterozygous for two different PK defects. PK deficiency is distributed worldwide, but it has been reported that the gene is more common among people of northern European extraction[171] and perhaps among Chinese[172] and certain other ethnic and racial groups. In these populations, the frequency of heterozygosity may exceed 1% and the affected subjects are more likely homozygous for common mutations.[171,172] Single nucleotide substitutions have been described as well as intronic mutations, deletions, and insertions.[173] The three most prevalent mutations are 1456T, 1468T, and 1529A; 1529A is the most common mutation in the United States and Northern and Central Europe. 1456T is most common in Spain, Portugal, and Italy whereas 1468T is more frequent in Asia.[170]

An additional molecular mechanism for PK deficiency has been reported.[174] Combined heterozygosity for the common 1529A PK mutation and a unique promoter mutation on the other allele that markedly reduced its allelic transcription resulted in a severe hemolytic variant.

Malaria protection

PK deficiency is associated with protection against malaria in mice.[175] A similar effect in humans has not yet been established, and there is no indication of a positive selection pressure in the geographic distribution of human PK deficiency.

Mechanism of Hemolysis and Physiologic Implications of PK Deficiency

The mechanism of hemolysis is not clear. Although it has been postulated that the defect in ATP generation contributes to the hemolytic process,[176] this explanation is insufficient because ATP deficiency is difficult to demonstrate in many patients,[177] and other disorders with more severe ATP deficiency are not associated with significant hemolysis.[178]

It has been suggested that the anemia of PK deficiency is better tolerated than a comparable level of anemia seen in patients with hexokinase deficiency, because the block in glycolysis occurs after the Rapoport–Luebering shunt (see section on 2,3-BPG deficiency). The accumulation of 2,3-BPG in this downstream glycolytic defect leads to higher 2,3-BPG concentrations and thus better oxygen delivery to the tissue and superior tolerance of anemia.[179]

Patients with hemolytic anemia who undergo splenectomy, with a resultant decrease in the hemolytic process and improvement of anemia, have a higher number of reticulocytes than they did before the splenectomy.[180,181] This perplexing observation indicates that our knowledge of the regulation of erythropoiesis and reticulocyte kinetics remains incomplete.

PK deficiency may affect both the survival of red cells and the maturation of erythroid progenitors, although this has only been studied in splenic erythroid progenitors. This results in premature cell death, that is, apoptosis, as demonstrated in a splenectomized PK-deficient patient,[182] and more conclusively in the splenic erythroid progenitors of a PK-deficient mouse.[183]

However, it remains to be established whether the apoptosis of erythroid progenitors in PK deficiency extends to marrow erythroblasts, whether this observation accounts for the previously unexplained postsplenectomy reticulocytosis, and whether PK activity has any role in the apoptotic pathway in other tissues.[184]

Indications for Splenectomy in a Patient with Enzymopathy-Induced Hemolysis

The only proven benefit of splenectomy is in patients with severely hemolytic (ie, significantly anemic, or transfusion dependent) variants of pyruvate kinase deficiency and glucose phosphoisomerase deficiency, and possibly in pyrimidine 5′ nucleotidase deficiency. Although splenectomy will decrease the biochemical parameters of hemolysis such as lactate dehydrogenase and total bilirubin and decrease or eliminate transfusion requirements, the reticulocyte count will rise in pyruvate kinase deficiency and in pyrimidine 5′ nucleotidase deficiency.

Diagnosis

There are no specific clinical findings or morphologic abnormalities in patients with PK deficiency. No routinely available laboratory measurements aid in diagnosis.

A screening test, using crude hemolysate with one concentration substrate, has been employed for detection of pyruvate deficiency.[149] However, this screening test misses the PK variants characterized by increased K_M and those with abnormal FDP interaction. Furthermore, because leukocytes have much higher PK activity than red cells, care must be taken to rigorously remove the leukocytes by reliable means such as filtration of the blood by special leukocyte- and platelet-retaining columns.[149] Specialized laboratories can perform quantitative PK enzyme analysis with various concentrations of substrate with and without FDP (the native FDP must first be removed by dialysis).[149] The mutant enzyme can be further analyzed by comprehensive kinetic and electrophoretic studies of the partially purified enzyme.[178] However, these studies have now been largely replaced by the detection of specific mutations of the enzyme at the cDNA or genomic level.[185] Because most sporadic cases of PK deficiency are compound heterozygotes, testing of obligate heterozygote family members facilitates the diagnosis.[170]

Clinical Presentation and Therapy

The severity of hemolysis in PK-deficient patients is highly variable. It ranges from rare hydrops fetalis due to homozygosity for PK null mutations, to life-threatening transfusion-requiring hemolytic anemia present at birth, to a mild, fully compensated hemolytic process without anemia. The degree of severity is typically similar among siblings of a given family.[170] Hemolysis may be exacerbated in acute infections and during pregnancy.

Patients with severe hemolysis may be chronically jaundiced and may develop the clinical complications of chronic hemolytic states, including gallstones, transient aplastic anemia crises (often due to parvovirus infection), folate deficiency, and, infrequently, skin ulcers. As with any autosomal recessive disorder, the defect is more common in a group with a history of inbreeding or consanguinity. A high frequency of this disorder has been well documented among Pennsylvania Amish.[186]

Splenomegaly is frequently seen but is not invariable. The beneficial effect of splenectomy on hemolysis is well documented; typically, the degree of hemolysis and anemia is ameliorated and in severe cases the transfusion requirement is generally abolished or markedly decreased. The increase in hemoglobin concentration in non–transfusion-requiring patients after splenectomy ranges from 1 to 3 gm%.[170] However, as stated earlier, reticulocytes invariably rise after splenectomy. Unless the patient is transfusion dependent, it is advisable to delay splenectomy until after the age of 3 years when the risk of pneumococcal, *Haemophilus influenzae*, and meningococcal infections declines. Furthermore, in most cases the degree of hemolysis declines after infancy, by a not fully understood pathophysiologic mechanism. In severely affected subjects, who are typically transfusion dependent, iron overload has been reported.[170] Although folic acid replacement is frequently used, it may not always be necessary; however, it is inexpensive and safe. One PK-deficient boy with severe hemolysis was apparently cured by an allogeneic marrow transplant.[187]

Glucose Phosphoisomerase Deficiency

Glucose phosphoisomerase deficiency is one of the three most common red blood cell enzyme defects causing chronic hemolytic anemia (including pyruvate kinase deficiency and pyrimidine 5′ nucleotidase deficiencies). More than 100 families have been described. In some families, the hemolysis is severe enough to necessitate chronic blood transfusions.[188] Very severe hemolysis was seen in a girl who also coinherited a mild G6PD deficiency, suggesting an additive role of these two defects.[189] Neonatal jaundice is common in patients with this disorder,[190] and hydrops fetalis has also been reported.[191] Although no specific therapy is available, it has been suggested that splenectomy provides a moderate benefit.[192]

Hexokinase Deficiency

Hexokinase catalyzes the initial step of glycolysis and produces glucose 6-phosphate, which is utilized in both glycolysis and the pentose pathway (see Fig. 45–1). Fewer than 50 cases have been reported. Most are of individuals of northern European extraction,[193] although one case was found in a Chinese individual.[194] Because the metabolic defect is proximal to the generation of 2,3-BPG, it has been suggested that the resultant decreased level of 2,3-BPG leads to a left-shifted hemoglobin–oxygen dissociation curve and a more symptomatic anemia than comparable levels of anemia seen in patients with other red blood cell disorders.[195]

Phosphofructokinase and Aldolase Deficiencies

Deficiencies of phosphofructokinase and aldolase are rare causes of glycogen storage disease and chronic nonspherocytic hemolytic anemia. As in the cases of patients with other rare autosomal recessive disorders, consanguinity is frequent.

Phosphoglycerokinase Deficiency

Deficiency of this X-chromosome-encoded enzyme is associated with hemolytic anemia, mental retardation, and myoglobinuria. The cDNA for the phosphoglycerokinase gene has been cloned[196] and several mutants described.

Triosephosphate Isomerase Deficiency

Triosephosphate isomerase deficiency is a rare red blood cell defect reported to cause congenital hemolytic anemia and other severe organ dysfunctions, including progressive neurologic abnormalities and early death.[197] An increased susceptibility to bacterial infections has also been described.[198] No specific therapy for this disorder is available. In a single reported case, splenectomy did not ameliorate hemolysis.

PYRIMIDINE 5′ NUCLEOTIDASE DEFICIENCY

Enzyme Classification and Function

Red cell pyrimidine 5′ nucleotidase is a member of a family containing at least seven genes encoding 5′ nucleotidases.[199] Other members of this family play a role in activation of antiviral compounds (cN-II) and in T cell activation and cell adhesion (ecto-5′ nucleosidase, also known as CD73). Previously thought to be a single entity, red cell 5′ nucleotidase is composed of two enzymes encoded by two different genes.[200] Pyrimidine 5′N type 1 (P5′N-1), also designated cytosolic 5:nucleosidase II (cN-III), participates in degradation of pyrimidine ribonucleotides, whereas pyrimidine 5′N type 2, more efficiently degrades deoxyribonucleotides. Only P5′N-1 deficiency has been associated with a clinical syndrome of hemolytic anemia. P5′N-1 activity is much higher in reticulocytes than mature red cells, and its activity rapidly declines during the first few days of red cell maturation.

The accumulation of pyrimidines in the red blood cells due to a deficiency of P5′N-1 is presumed to be toxic and a cause of hemolysis. However, deficiency of P5′N-1 is at least partly compensated in vivo by other nucleosidases or other nucleotide metabolic pathways.[201]

P5′N-1 Mutations

The P5′N-1 gene is localized to chromosome 7p15-14. Three transcripts are produced by alternative splicing; one transcript is ubiquitously expressed, but two are predominantly expressed in reticulocytes.[200] More than 20 different mutations in *P5′N-1* have been reported; all but two patients are homozygous.[200]

Clinical Features and Differential Diagnosis

Deficiency of P5′N-1is the third most common enzymatic deficiency resulting in hemolysis. Inherited in an autosomal recessive manner, it is the only congenital hemolytic anemia due to a red blood cell enzyme deficiency that has a specific, consistent morphologic abnormality, that is, basophilic stippling.[202] Thus, morphologic examination of the peripheral blood smear provides simple and inexpensive screening. Basophilic stippling is also found in cases of hemolytic anemia due to acute lead toxicity. Lead is a powerful inhibitor of P5′N-1,[203] and determination of lead levels should be included whenever the constellation of acquired hemolytic anemia, P5′N-1 deficiency, and basophilic stippling is found.

The degree of hemolysis in hereditary P5′N-1 deficiency is generally constant but may be exacerbated by infection and pregnancy; the severity ranges from compensated hemolysis without anemia to transfusion-dependent anemia. In several reported instances, splenectomy was beneficial, with an average improved hemoglobin concentration of approximately 3 gm%, and curiously their reticulocyte count also increased after splenectomy.[200]

The coinheritance of P5′N-1 deficiency and hemoglobin E was reported to be associated with severe hemolytic anemia, suggesting that this enzyme is particularly susceptible to oxidative damage resulting from the instability of hemoglobin E.[204] However, pyrimidine 5′ nucleotidase deficiency may increase oxidative stress on its own because it partially inhibits G6PD activity and reduces GSH by an as yet unknown mechanism.

POLYCYTHEMIA DUE TO CONGENITAL RED BLOOD CELL ENZYME DEFICIENCY

The polycythemias (also known as *erythrocytosis*) comprise a group of etiologically different disorders.[205] Absolute polycythemias may be primarily due to an intrinsic defect of hematopoietic progenitors or, more commonly, secondarily due to stimulation of normal hematopoietic progenitors by extrinsic factors such as erythropoietin. Although most polycythemias are acquired, some are congenital.[206] One rare cause of congenital secondary polycythemia is familial 2,3-bisphosphoglycerate (2,3-BPG, previously known as 2,3-DPG) deficiency, which results from a deficiency of the red blood cell enzyme bisphosphoglyceromutase (BPGM). Present in a very high concentration in red blood cells, 2,3-BPG binds hemoglobin, allosterically changing hemoglobin conformation and modulating its ability to bind oxygen. A decreased 2,3-BPG level shifts the hemoglobin oxygen dissociation curve to the left (increases hemoglobin affinity for oxygen), resulting in decreased delivery of oxygen into the peripheral tissues and compensatory polycythemia.

Biochemistry

The formation of 2,3-BPG constitutes the Rapoport–Luebering shunt,[207] which is often called an *energy switch* because it bypasses the formation of ATP in the reaction mediated by the glycolytic enzyme phosphoglycerate kinase (Fig. 45–6). A single multifunctional enzyme, BPGM, with both synthase and phosphatase activity, controls this shunt. BPGM is a homodimer of two identical 258-amino-acid subunits. The *BPGM* gene has been mapped to 7q34-7q22; transcripts of the gene have been detected in higher levels in erythroid cells than in nonerythroid cells, although no erythroid-specific promoter region has been identified.[208]

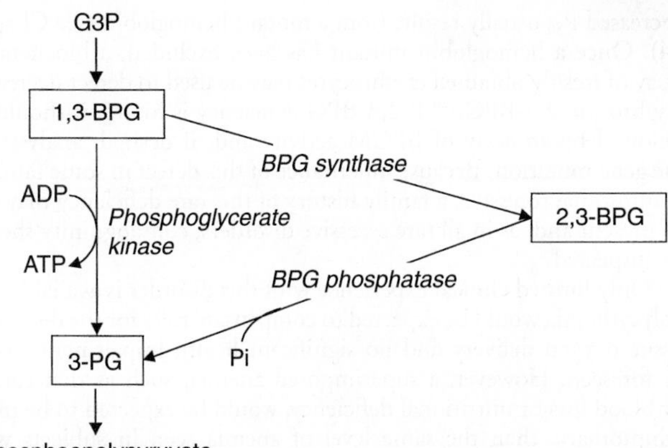

Figure 45–6 Rapoport–Luebering shunt. 2,3-BPG metabolism is regulated by a multifunctional enzyme, bisphosphoglycerate mutase, with both synthase (BPG synthase) and phosphatase (BPG phosphatase) activity. This reaction bypasses the formation of ATP in the glycolytic pathway. 1,3-BPG, 1,3-bisphosphoglycerate; 2,3-BPG, 2,3-bisphosphoglycerate; G-3-P, glyceraldehyde-3-phosphate; 3-PG, 3-phosphoglycerate; Pi, inorganic phosphate.

The conversion of 1,3-bisphosphoglycerate to 2,3-BPG is catalyzed by the synthase activity of BPGM. 2,3-BPG is then metabolized to 3-phosphoglycerate (3-PGA), an intermediate of the glycolytic pathway, by BPGM-phosphatase activity residing in the same protein molecule.[209–213] The synthase activity of BPGM is activated by alkalosis, whereas the phosphatase activity of BPGM is enhanced by acidosis.[214]

Clinical Manifestations and Inheritance

Deficiency of BPGM leads to a marked decrease in 2,3-BPG levels. The resultant increased hemoglobin oxygen affinity decreases the amount of oxygen released peripherally, leading to a compensatory polycythemia. Only one family with this deficiency has been well studied. The propositus and his sister were compound heterozygotes for two different BPGM mutations and had complete deficiency of BPGM synthetase activity and marked polycythemia. Some of their heterozygote relatives had a milder decrease of 2,3-BPG levels and a mild polycythemia.[215–219]

Other reports of reduced BPGM activity and decreased 2,3-BPG levels are difficult to interpret or do not pass rigorous biochemical and molecular biologic scrutiny.[220–223] In some of these reports, the phenotype included hemolysis; however, other causes of hemolysis were not definitively excluded. Because of the rarity of complete BPGM deficiency, it is not possible to predict the phenotype of heterozygous individuals; however, it is likely that some individuals heterozygous for this enzyme deficiency will have a mild to moderate polycythemia and in these families an apparent autosomal dominant pattern of inheritance may be observed.[216,218,219,224]

Diagnosis and Therapy

Determination of hemoglobin–oxygen association kinetics is the best initial-screening laboratory test for congenital secondary polycythemia If a cooximeter is not available, the P_{50} can be estimated from a venous blood gas measurement using a relatively complex mathematical formula.[225] An Excel spreadsheet formula that rapidly obtains the PSO value from venous blood gases by entering venous Po_2, O_2 saturation and PN has been published[225a] providing that both the venous Pao_2 and the hemoglobin oxygen saturation are measured. A decreased P_{50} usually results from a mutant hemoglobin (see Chapter 44). Once a hemoglobin mutant has been excluded, a biochemical assay of freshly obtained erythrocytes may be used to detect decreased erythrocyte 2,3-BPG.[149] If 2,3-BPG deficiency is found, it should be followed by an assay of BPGM activity and, if desired, analysis for the gene mutation. Because inheritance of this defect in some families is autosomal recessive, a family history of this rare deficiency may not be present and, as in all rare recessive disorders, consanguinity should be suspected.

Only limited clinical experience with this disorder is available; the polycythemia would be expected to compensate fully for the decreased tissue oxygen delivery and no significant health impairment would be foreseen. However, a superimposed anemia, such as that caused by blood loss or nutritional deficiency, would be expected to be more symptomatic than the same level of anemia seen in subjects with normal enzyme activity and normal levels of 2,3-BPG.

NONENZYMATIC FUNCTIONS OF RED CELL ENZYMES

It is increasingly recognized that enzymes of the glycolytic pathway also have nonenzymatic functions. Many of these discoveries stemmed from the work of Otto Warburg on respiration and energy metabolism of cancer cells and the different regulation of cancer cells by hypoxia, which is now partially explained by the constitutive upregulations of hypoxia-inducible factor HIF-1. Glycolytic enzymes play a role in tumor metastasis and cell motility. Glucose-6-phosphate isomerase acts as an autocrine motility factor in cell migration and appears to be important in cancer metastasis.[226,227] Other glycolytic enzymes help regulate apoptosis. Mitochondrial hexokinase appears to inhibit apoptosis via interaction with the proapoptotic protein BAD, whereas glyceraldehyde phosphate dehydrogenase appears to have a proapoptotic function.[226,228] Other glycolytic enzymes, including hexokinase, GAPD, enolase, and lactic dehydrogenase, have important roles in the regulation of the transcription of an array of genes by multiple mechanisms.[226]

DIAGNOSTIC AND OTHER USES OF BLOOD CELL ENZYMOPATHIES

Deficiencies of some erythrocyte enzymes, such as lactate dehydrogenase or catalase, have no discernible phenotypes. Even when red blood cell enzymopathies do not cause abnormalities of the erythrocyte, they can be useful diagnostically. Easily obtainable red blood cells can serve as a convenient source of material for diagnosing systemic diseases. The red blood cell is capable of metabolizing galactose, but abnormalities of galactose metabolism do not have any hematologic phenotype. Galactose kinase deficiency is associated with cataracts, and galactose uridinyl-1-transferase is associated with classic galactosemia (ie, cataracts, congenital deafness, and mental retardation). Adenosine deaminase deficiency is associated with profound immunologic disturbance, but no red blood cell abnormalities. Measurement of adenosine deaminase in erythrocytes is a convenient diagnostic tool. The activity of erythrocyte glutathione reductase, which requires the riboflavin-derived coenzyme FAD, can be measured with and without FAD, serving as a convenient indicator of riboflavin deficiency.

SUGGESTED READINGS

Aizawa S, Harada T, Kanbe E, et al: Ineffective erythropoiesis in mutant mice with deficient pyruvate kinase activity. Exp Hematol 33:1292, 2005.

Ash-Bernal R, Wise R, Wright SM: Acquired methemoglobinemia: A retrospective series of 138 cases at 2 teaching hospitals. Medicine (Baltimore) 83:265, 2003.

Beutler E, Vuillamy TJ: Hematologically important mutations: Glucose-6-phosphate dehydrogenase. Blood Cells Mol Dis 28:93, 2002.

Beutler E: DNA-based diagnosis of red cell enzymopathies: How we threw out the baby with the bathwater. Blood 97:3325, 2001.

Beutler E: Red Cell Metabolism: A Manual of Biochemical Methods, 2nd ed. New York, Grune and Stratton, 1975.

Burmester T, Weich B, Reinhardt S, et al: A vertebrate globin expressed in the brain. Nature 407:520, 2000.

Gregg XT, Prchal JT: Recent advances in the molecular biology of congenital polycythemias and polycythemia vera. Curr Hematol Rep 4:238, 2005.

Kim J, Dang CV: Multifaceted roles of glycolytic enzymes. Trends Biochem Sci 30:142150, 2005.

Leroux A, Junien C, Kaplan J-C, Bamberger J: Generalized deficiency of cytochrome b5 reductase in congenital methaemoglobinaemia with mental retardation. Nature 258:619, 1975.

Leroux A, Mota Vieira L, Kahn A: Transcriptional and translational mechanisms of cytochrome b5 reductase isozyme generation in humans. Biochem J 355:529, 2001.

Min-Oo G, Fortin A, Tam MF, Nantel A, Stevenson MM, Gros P: Pyruvate kinase deficiency in mice protects against malaria. Nat Genet 35:357, 2003.

Ruwende C, Khoo S, Snow R, et al: Natural selection of hemi- and heterozygotes for G6PD deficiency in Africa by resistance to severe malaria. Nature 376:246, 1995.

Shimizu T, Uehara T, Nomura Y: Possible involvement of pyruvate kinase in acquisition of tolerance to hypoxic stress in glial cells. J Neurochem 91:167, 2004.

Zanella A, Bianchi P, Fermol E, Valentini G: Hereditary pyrimidine 5′-nucleotidase deficiency: From genetics to clinical manifestations. Br J Haematol 133:113, 2006.

Zanella A, Fermo E, Bianchi P, Valentini G: Red cell pyruvate kinase deficiency: Molecular and clinical aspects. Br J Haematol 2130:11, 2005.

REFERENCES

For complete list of references log onto www.expertconsult.com

CHAPTER 46

RED BLOOD CELL MEMBRANE DISORDERS

Patrick G. Gallagher and Petr Jarolim

Progress in the characterization of the structure and function of red blood cell membrane proteins and their genes has led to considerable advances in the understanding of the molecular pathology of red blood cell membrane disorders. This has led to the definition and characterization of mutations of membrane proteins as a well-defined cause of hereditary hemolytic disease. Likewise, knowledge of the molecular mechanisms underlying changes in red blood cell deformability, structural integrity, and shape has advanced. Red blood cell shape abnormalities often provide a clue to the pathobiology and diagnosis of the underlying disorder. This chapter categorizes red blood cell membrane disorders according to the following morphologic and clinical phenotypes: (1) hereditary spherocytosis (HS); (2) hereditary elliptocytosis (HE), hereditary pyropoikilocytosis (HPP) and related disorders; (3) Southeast Asian ovalocytosis (SAO); (4) hereditary and acquired acanthocytosis; and (5) hereditary and acquired stomatocytosis (Tables 46–1 and 46–2). The structure and function of the normal red blood cell membrane are described in Chapter 33; a review of that chapter will facilitate understanding of the material in this chapter.

VERTICAL AND HORIZONTAL INTERACTIONS OF MEMBRANE PROTEINS AND DISORDERS OF RED BLOOD CELL SHAPE

Palek and colleagues first proposed dividing membrane protein-protein and protein-lipid interactions into two categories, vertical and horizontal interactions.[1] Vertical interactions, which are perpendicular to the plane of the membrane, stabilize the lipid bilayer. These interactions include spectrin-ankyrin-band 3 interactions, spectrin-protein 4.1R-junctional complex proteins linkage, spectrin-ankyrin-Rh multiprotein complex linkage, and the weak interactions between the skeletal proteins and the negatively charged lipids of the inner half of the membrane lipid bilayer. Horizontal interactions, which are parallel to the plane of the membrane, support the structural integrity of erythrocytes after their exposure to shear stress. Horizontal interactions involve the spectrin heterodimer association site, where spectrin heterodimers assemble into tetramers, the principal building blocks of the membrane skeleton, and the contacts of the distal ends of spectrin heterodimers with actin and protein 4.1R within the junctional complex. Although interactions between proteins of the erythrocyte membrane are more complex than can be classified by this model of horizontal and vertical interactions,[2] the model serves as a useful starting place for understanding erythrocyte membrane protein interactions, particularly in reference to membrane-related disorders.

According to the vertical/horizontal model, HS is considered a disorder of vertical interactions (Fig. 46–1). Although the primary molecular defects in HS are heterogeneous (including deficiencies or dysfunctions of α- and β-spectrin, ankyrin, band 3, and protein 4.2; see Etiology and Pathobiology), one common feature of HS red blood cells is a weakening of the vertical contacts between the skeleton and the overlying lipid bilayer membrane together with its integral proteins.[3] Consequently, the lipid bilayer membrane is destabilized, leading to release of bilayer lipids from the cells in the form of skeleton-free lipid vesicles. This lipid loss, in turn, results in membrane surface area deficiency and spherocytosis.

In most patients with HE and the related disorder HPP (see Hereditary Elliptocytosis and Related Disorders), the principal lesion involves horizontal membrane-protein associations, primarily spectrin dimer-dimer interactions. In a subset of HE patients with a deficiency or a dysfunction of protein 4.1R or glycophorin C, the horizontal defect resides in the junctional complex, where the distal ends of spectrin tetramers connect to actin, with the aid of the 4.1R protein. In patients with severely dysfunctional spectrin mutations, the weakened spectrin dimer-dimer self-association disrupts the skeletal lattice, leading to a marked skeletal instability and cell fragments. In patients with mildly dysfunctional spectrins, red blood cell shape is that of biconcave elliptocytes. It is speculated that elliptocytes are permanently deformed cells because the weakened horizontal interactions facilitate a shear stress-induced rearrangement of skeletal proteins, precluding recovery of the normal biconcave shape (for details, see the discussion under Hereditary Elliptocytosis and Related Disorders). This hypothesis is not applicable to all forms of elliptocytosis. For example, in SAO, the elliptocytic/ovalocytic cells containing mutant band 3 protein are rigid and "hyper-stable" rather than unstable.

Acanthocytosis, Stomatocytosis, and the Bilayer Couple Hypothesis

The mechanism of acanthocytosis and stomatocytosis associated with defects of membrane proteins is much less clear. Most forms of acanthocytosis are associated with either acquired or inherited abnormalities of membrane lipids (eg, acanthocytosis in end-stage liver disease or abetalipoproteinemia). In rare subjects with acanthocytosis, membrane protein abnormalities have been detected, but the mechanism whereby they lead to acanthocyte formation is unknown. These abnormalities occur in the McLeod phenotype, the chorea-acanthocytosis syndromes, and other rare disorders. In acanthocytosis erythrocytes, agents that interact with the lipids of the inner lipid bilayer leaflet normalize the shape. These studies suggest that the shape abnormalities reflect an asymmetry in the distribution of membrane lipids between the two halves of the red blood cell lipid bilayer as predicted by the bilayer couple hypothesis (Fig. 46–2). This hypothesis is based on the well-established idea that the lipid bilayer is highly asymmetric, with phosphatidylcholine and sphingomyelin the main phospholipids of the outer face of the bilayer leaflet.[4] According to the bilayer hypothesis, the shape of the red blood cell reflects the ratio of the surface areas of the two hemileaflets of the bilayer. The preferential expansion of the outer leaflet leads to red blood cell crenation (echinocytosis or acanthocytosis), whereas expansion of the inner lipid bilayer produces a cup shape (stomatocytosis) and surface invaginations.

Hereditary Spherocytosis

Definition, Prevalence, and History

The typical features of HS include a dominantly inherited hemolytic anemia of mild to moderate severity, spherocytosis on the peripheral blood film, and a favorable response to splenectomy.[1,3–6] The

Table 46–1 Erythrocyte Membrane Abnormalities in Hereditary Spherocytosis, Hereditary Elliptocytosis, and Related Disorders

Gene	Disorder	Comment
α Spectrin	HS, HE, HPP, NIHF	Location of mutation determines clinical phenotype. α–Spectrin mutations are most common cause of typical HE.
Ankyrin	HS	Most common cause of typical, dominant HS.
Band 3	HS, SAO, NIHF, HSt	In HS, pincerlike spherocytes on smear presplenectomy. SAO erythrocytes have transverse ridge or bar
β Spectrin	HS, HE, HPP, NIHF	Location of mutation determines clinical phenotype. In HS, acanthocytic spherocytes on smear presplenectomy.
Protein 4.2	HS	Common in Japanese HS.
Protein 4.1	HE	
Glycophorin C	HE	Concomitant protein 4.1 deficiency is likely basis of HE in glycophorin C defects.

HE, hereditary elliptocytosis; HPP, hereditary pyropoikilocytosis; NIHF, nonimmune hydrops fetalis; HS, hereditary spherocytosis; HSt, hereditary stomatocytosis; SAO, Southeast Asian ovalocytosis.

Table 46–2 Peripheral Blood Film Evaluation in a Patient With Red Cell Membrane Disorder

Shape	Pathobiology	Diagnosis
Microspherocytes	Loss of membrane lipids leading to a reduction of surface area resulting from deficiencies of spectrin, ankyrin, or band 3 and protein 4.2. Removal of membrane material from antibody coated red cells by macrophages. Removal of membrane associated Heinz bodies, with the adjacent membrane lipids, by the spleen	HS Immunohemolytic anemias Heinz body hemolytic anemias
Elliptocytes	Permanent red cell deformation resulting from a weakening of skeletal protein interactions (such as the spectrin dimer-dimer contact). This facilitates disruption of existing protein contacts during shear stress induced elliptical deformation. Subsequently, new protein contacts are formed that stabilize elliptical shape.	Mild common HE Iron deficiency, megaloblastic anemias, myelofibrosis, myelophthisic anemias, myelodysplastic syndrome, thalassemias
Poikilocytes/Fragments	Weakening of skeletal protein contacts resulting from skeletal protein mutations	Hemolytic HE/HPP Iron deficiency, megaloblastic anemias, myelofibrosis, myelophthisic anemias, myelodysplastic syndrome, thalassemias
Schistocytes, fragmented red cells	Red cells "torn" by mechanical trauma (fibrin strands, turbulent flow)	Microangiopathic hemolytic anemia associated with disseminated intravascular coagulation, thrombotic thrombocytopenic purpura, vasculitis, heart valve prostheses
Acanthocytes	Uptake of cholesterol and its preferential accumulation in the outer leaflet of the lipid bilayer Selective accumulation of sphingomyelin in the outer lipid leaflet	Spur cell hemolytic anemia in severe liver disease Abetalipoproteinemia Neuroacanthocytosis, chorea-acanthocytosis syndrome, McLeod phenotype, malnutrition, hypothyroidism
Echinocytes	Expansion of the surface area of the outer hemileaflet of lipid bilayer relative to the inner hemileaflet	Hemolytic anemia associated with hypomagnesemia and hypophosphatemia in malnourished patients, pyruvate kinase deficiency; in-vitro artifact of low blood storage (ATP depletion), contact with glass or elevated pH Hemolysis in long-distance runners, renal failure
Stomatocytes	Expansion of the surface area of the inner hemileaflet of the bilayer relative to the outer leaflet	Exposure of red cells to cationic anesthetics in vitro; in vivo, the drug concentrations may not be sufficient to produce similar effect Alcoholism, inherited disorders of membrane permeability (hereditary stomatocytosis)
Target cells	Absolute excess of membrane lipids (both cholesterol and phospholipids: "symmetric" lipid gain), followed by an increase of cell surface area Relative excess of surface area because of a decrease in cell volume	Obstructive jaundice, liver disease with intrahepatic cholestasis Thalassemias and some hemoglobinopathies (C, D, E)

HE, hereditary elliptocytosis; HPP, hereditary pyropoikilocytosis; HS, hereditary spherocytosis.

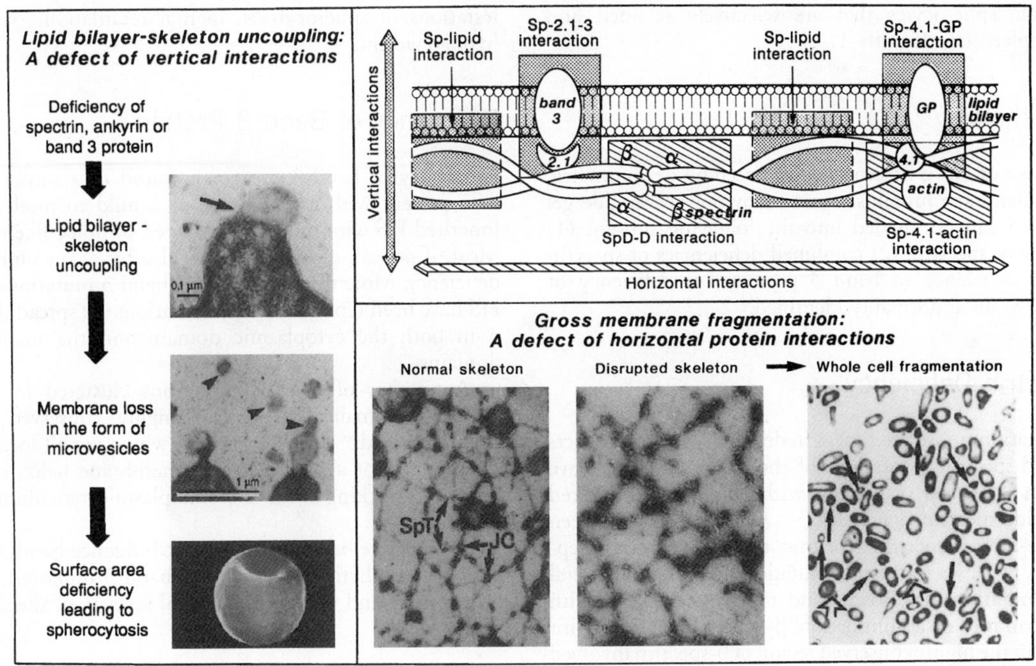

Figure 46–1 The red blood cell membrane lesion in hereditary spherocytosis (HS). (*Left*) Partial deficiencies of spectrin, ankyrin, or band 3 protein lead to uncoupling of the membrane lipid bilayer from the underlying skeleton (*arrow*), followed by a formation of spectrin-free microvesicles of approximately 0.2 to 0.5 mm in diameter (*arrowheads*). These vesicles can be visualized by transmission electron microscopy, but they are not seen on examination of a peripheral blood film. The subsequent loss of cell surface area and a decrease in the surface/volume ratio lead to spherocytosis. (*Right*) Two distinct pathways lead to reduced membrane surface area in HS. (**A**) Primary defects of spectrin, ankyrin, or protein 4.2 lead to reduced density of the membrane skeleton (*solid rectangles*). This causes destabilization of the lipid bilayer with the resultant loss of band 3-containing microvesicles. (**B**) Primary defects of band 3 (*black ovals*) result in band 3 deficiency. This leads to the loss of the lipid-stabilizing effect of band 3 with the release of band 3-free microvesicles from the membrane. Both pathways ultimately result in the loss of membrane material with a reduction in membrane surface area. The ensuing decrease in membrane surface area with the formation of spherocytes is paralleled by a decrease in erythrocyte deformability that predisposes the cells to splenic entrapment and conditioning. The spleen plays a secondary, but important, role in the pathobiology of HS. Splenic destruction of abnormal erythrocytes with decreased deformability is the primary cause of hemolysis experienced by HS patients.

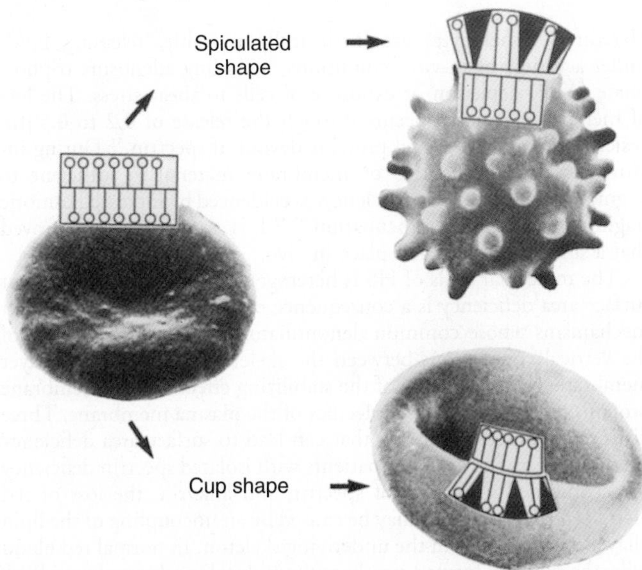

Figure 46–2 Bilayer couple hypothesis and the discocyte-echinocyte-stomatocyte transformation. Red blood cell shape is determined by the ratio of the surface areas of the two hemileaflets of the lipid bilayer. Compounds (*black triangles*) that preferentially accumulate in the outer hemileaflet produce its expansion, followed by red blood cell crenation (echinocytosis or acanthocytosis). In contrast, expansion of the inner lipid bilayer leaflet leads to a cup shape (stomatocytosis) and surface invaginations.

clinical spectrum of HS is variable and includes both mild and asymptomatic forms as well as severe forms that appear in infancy. The previously reported HS prevalence in Western populations of 1 in 5000 persons is an underestimation, because milder forms of HS might be asymptomatic, suggesting a prevalence of 1 in 2000 individuals.[7,8] HS has been reported worldwide, particularly in Japanese and African populations, but its prevalence in other ethnic groups is unknown.[9]

Hereditary spherocytosis was first described in 1871 by Vanlair and Masius and rediscovered 20 years later by Wilson and Minkowski. The next major contributions were Chauffard's description of increased osmotic fragility, reports of correction of hemolysis by splenectomy, and the studies by Ham and Castle implicating the spleen in the conditioning of hereditary spherocytes.[10] Soon thereafter, HS membranes were found to be leaky to sodium and to exhibit a loss of lipids, leading to surface area deficiency. An abnormality of the erythrocyte membrane was suspected; subsequently, molecular defects of membrane proteins and their genes were identified. A historic overview of HS is available.[11]

Etiology and Pathobiology

Two major factors are involved in HS pathophysiology (1) an intrinsic red blood cell defect, and (2) an intact spleen that selectively retains and damages abnormal HS erythrocytes. An inherited deficiency or dysfunction of proteins of the erythrocyte membrane leads to a multistep process of accelerated HS red blood cell destruction. Destabilization of the lipid bilayer facilitates a release of lipids from the membrane, leading to surface area deficiency and formation of poorly deformable spherocytes that are selectively retained and damaged in the spleen (see Fig. 46–1).

Molecular Pathology

The molecular basis of HS is heterogeneous. Based on densitometric quantitation of membrane proteins separated by polyacrylamide gel electrophoresis, HS can be divided into the following subsets: (1) isolated deficiency of spectrin, (2) combined deficiencies of spectrin and ankyrin, (3) deficiency of band 3 protein, (4) deficiency of protein 4.2, and (5) no abnormality identified.

Isolated Spectrin Deficiency

The reported mutations of isolated spectrin deficiency include defects of both α- and β-spectrin. Mutations of the β-spectrin gene have been identified in a number of patients with dominantly inherited HS associated with spectrin deficiency.[12,13] A few cases have been associated with de-novo β-spectrin gene mutations.[14] With the exception of β-spectrin^{Houston},[13] a frameshift mutation identified in several kindreds, these mutations are private and may be associated with decreased β-spectrin mRNA accumulation. β-Spectrin^{Kissimmee}, a point mutation located in the highly conserved region of β-spectrin involved in the interaction with protein 4.1R, is dysfunctional in its in-vitro binding to protein 4.1R and thereby the linkage of spectrin to actin.[12]

In nondominantly inherited HS associated with isolated spectrin deficiency, the defect involves α-spectrin.[14,15] In normal erythroid cells, α-spectrin is synthesized in large excess of β-spectrin. Thus, subjects with one normal and one defective α-spectrin allele are expected to be asymptomatic, because α-spectrin production remains in excess of β-spectrin synthesis, allowing normal amounts of spectrin heterodimers to be assembled on the membrane. Patients who are homozygotes or compound heterozygotes for α-spectrin defects will suffer from severe HS. Wichterle and associates described a patient with severe HS who was a compound heterozygote for two different α-spectrin gene defects: in one allele, there was a splicing defect associated with an upstream intronic mutation, α^{LEPRA}; in the other allele, there was another mutation, α^{PRAGUE}. The α^{LEPRA} allele produces approximately six times less of the correctly spliced α-spectrin transcript than the normal allele.[16] Further studies have shown that in many patients with nondominant, spectrin-deficient HS, including a number of the patients originally described by Agre and associates, α-spectrin^{LEPRA} is in linkage disequilibrium with α-spectrin$^{Bug\ Hill}$, which carries an amino acid substitution in the αII domain.[17] Thus, it appears that the combination of the α^{LEPRA} allele with other defects of α-spectrin in *trans* leads to significant spectrin-deficient spherocytic anemia.[18]

Combined Deficiency of Spectrin and Ankyrin

The biochemical phenotype of combined spectrin and ankyrin deficiency is the most common abnormality found in the erythrocytes of HS patients.[19] Ankyrin represents the principal binding site for spectrin on the membrane; thus, it is not surprising that ankyrin deficiency is accompanied by a proportional decrease in spectrin assembly on the membrane despite normal spectrin synthesis. Similar to HS associated with β-spectrin mutations, most ankyrin defects are private point mutations in the coding region of the ankyrin gene associated with decreased messenger RNA accumulation.[3,20] In some cases, mutations of the ankyrin promoter leading to decreased ankyrin expression have been found.[21,22] Approximately 15% to 20% of ankyrin gene mutations reported are de-novo mutations.[23]

A number of patients with atypical HS associated with karyotypic abnormalities involving deletions or translocations of the ankyrin gene locus on chromosome 8p have been described.[24] Ankyrin deletions may be part of a contiguous gene syndrome with manifestations of spherocytosis, mental retardation, typical facies, and hypogonadism.

Deficiency of Band 3 Protein

Deficiency of band 3 protein is found in a subset of HS patients who present with a phenotype of a mild to moderate dominantly inherited HS with mushroom-shaped or pincerlike red blood cells.[25] Most, if not all, of these patients also have concomitant protein 4.2 deficiency. More than 50 different band 3 mutations associated with HS have been reported. These mutations are spread throughout band 3 in both the cytoplasmic domain and the membrane-spanning domains.

A number of band 3 mutations clustered in the membrane-spanning domain that replace highly conserved arginines have been described.[26] These arginines, which are all located at the cytoplasmic end of a predicted transmembrane helix, exhibit defective cellular trafficking from the endoplasmic reticulum to the plasma membrane.[27]

Alleles have been identified that influence band 3 expression and that, when inherited in *trans* to a band 3 mutation, aggravate band 3 deficiency and worsen the clinical severity of the disease.[28]

Deficiency of Protein 4.2

Recessively inherited HS caused by mutations in protein 4.2 is relatively common in Japan.[29] In these cases, an almost total absence of protein 4.2 from the erythrocyte membranes of homozygous patients is detected. Protein 4.2-deficient erythrocytes can also have a decreased content of ankyrin and band 3. Protein 4.2 deficiency also occurs in association with band 3 mutations, probably as a result of abnormal binding of protein 4.2 to the cytoplasmic domain of band 3.[30]

A detailed listing of HS mutations can be found at the Human Gene Mutation Database Web site (www.hgmd.cf.ac.uk/ac/index.php) maintained by Institute of Medical Genetics in Cardiff.

Molecular Basis of Surface Area Deficiency

Hereditary spherocytes are intrinsically unstable, releasing lipids under a variety of in-vitro conditions, including adenosine triphosphate (ATP) depletion or exposure of cells to shear stress. The loss of membrane material occurs through the release of 0.2 to 0.5 μm vesicles containing integral proteins devoid of spectrin.[31] During in-vitro incubation, the loss of membrane material is sufficient to augment the surface area deficiency, as evidenced by increased osmotic fragility of the cells after incubation.[31,32] It is assumed but not proved that a similar process takes place in vivo.

The molecular basis of HS is heterogeneous; thus, it is likely that surface area deficiency is a consequence of several distinct molecular mechanisms whose common denominator is either a weakening of the vertical connections between the skeleton and the lipid bilayer membrane or a weakening of the stabilizing effect of transmembrane proteins on adjacent lipid molecules of the plasma membrane. Three distinct hypothetic pathways that can lead to surface area deficiency are depicted in Fig. 46–1. In patients with isolated spectrin deficiency or a combined deficiency of spectrin and ankyrin, the loss of red blood cell (RBC) surface may be caused by an uncoupling of the lipid bilayer membrane from the underlying skeleton. In normal red blood cells, the skeleton forms a nearly monomolecular submembrane layer occupying more than one-half of the inner surface of the membrane. Consequently, spectrin deficiency leads to a decreased density of this network. As a result, areas of the lipid bilayer membrane that are not directly supported by the skeleton are susceptible to release from the cells in the form of microvesicles.

In HS associated with a deficiency of band 3 protein, two hypothetic pathways may lead to a loss of surface area. One mechanism may involve a loss of band 3 protein from the cells. Because band 3 protein spans the lipid bilayer membrane many times, it is likely that a substantial amount of "boundary" lipids are released together with the band 3 protein, thus leading to surface area deficiency. Another possible mechanism may involve a formation of band 3-free domains in the membrane, followed by the formation of membrane blebs, which are subsequently released from the cells as microvesicles. Such a hypothesis is based on the observation that aggregation of intramembrane particles (composed principally of band 3) in ghosts leads to the formation of particle-depleted domains from which membrane lipids bleb off as microvesicles. Additional evidence supporting the latter model comes from the band 3 knockout mouse model and from human, cow, and zebrafish cases of complete band 3 deficiency.[33–36] Erythrocytes lacking band 3 spontaneously shed membrane vesicles, leading to severe spherocytosis and hemolysis.

Alterations in Cation Content and Permeability

HS red blood cells, particularly those collected from the spleen, are somewhat dehydrated and abnormally permeable to monovalent cations, presumably as a consequence of the underlying membrane defect. The cellular dehydration may be caused by activation of pathways causing a selective loss of potassium and water or a hyperactive Na+/K+ pump.[37,38]

Entrapment of Nondeformable Spherocytes in the Spleen

The importance of the spleen in the pathophysiology of hemolysis in HS was appreciated in the original description of the disease and has been substantiated by subsequent studies. HS cells are selectively destroyed in the spleen because of their poor deformability and because of the unique anatomy of the splenic vasculature that acts as a microcirculation filter.

The poor red blood cell deformability is principally a consequence of a decreased cell surface-to-cell volume ratio resulting from the loss of surface material.[39] Normal discocytes have an excess surface, which allows them to deform and pass through narrow microcirculation openings. In contrast, HS red blood cells lack this extra surface, and their poor deformability may be further impaired by cellular dehydration.[38,39]

The principal sites of red blood cell entrapment in the spleen are fenestrations in the wall of splenic sinuses, where blood from the splenic cords of the red pulp enters the venous circulation.[40] In the rat spleen, the length and width of these fenestrations, 2 to 3 μm and 0.2 to 0.5 μm, respectively, are approximately one-half the red blood cell diameter. Electron micrographs of spleen show that very few HS red blood cells traverse these slits. Consequently, the nondeformable spherocytes accumulate in the red pulp, which becomes grossly engorged.[41]

Splenic Conditioning and Destruction

Once trapped in the spleen, HS red blood cells undergo additional damage or conditioning marked by further loss of surface area and an increase in cell density, as is evident in cells removed from the spleen at splenectomy.[42,43] Some of these conditioned red blood cells reenter the systemic circulation, as revealed by the "tail" of the osmotic fragility curve, indicating the presence of a subpopulation of cells with a markedly reduced surface area. After splenectomy, this red blood cell population disappears.

Contributions to conditioning may include a relatively low pH in the spleen as well as in the sequestered red blood cells that may further compromise the poor HS red blood cell deformability, and contact of red blood cells with macrophages that may inflict additional damage on the red blood cell membrane. The conditioning effect of the spleen appears to represent a cumulative injury. The average residence time of HS red blood cells in the splenic cords is between 10 and 100 minutes compared to 30 to 40 seconds for normal red blood cells, and only 1% to 10% of blood entering the spleen is temporarily sequestered in the congested cords, whereas the remaining 90% of blood flow is rapidly shunted into the venous circulation.

Inheritance

The HS genes are assigned to several chromosomes, including chromosome 1 (α-spectrin), chromosome 8 (ankyrin), chromosome 14 (β-spectrin), chromosome 15 (protein 4.2), and chromosome 17 (band 3). In approximately two-thirds of HS patients, inheritance is autosomal dominant.[3] In the remaining patients, inheritance is nondominant. In many of these patients, HS is caused by a de-novo mutation,[14,23] which is inherited in an autosomal recessive fashion in subsequent generations.[10,42] Recessively inherited HS cases manifesting with severe hemolytic anemia have been reported. The majority of the affected patients were found to be severely deficient in red blood cell spectrin, associated with α-spectrin defects. The remaining cases characterized by a recessive inheritance pattern are caused by a defect in protein 4.2,[29] deficiency which is associated with relatively mild hemolysis.

Only a few cases of homozygous HS have been reported.[36,44,45] These patients have a severe hemolytic anemia, whereas their mostly consanguineous parents have a mild to moderate form of the disease or are asymptomatic.

Although the clinical severity of HS is highly variable among different kindreds, in general it is relatively uniform within a given family, in which HS is typically inherited as an autosomal dominant disorder. However, HS kindreds have been described in which there was great variability in the clinical severity of affected family members. Several explanations might account for these observations, including variable penetrance of the genetic defect, a de-novo mutation, presence of a mild recessive HS in the kindred, presence of a modifier allele that influences the expression of a membrane protein, or a tissue-specific mosaicism of the defect.[3]

Clinical Manifestations

Typical Forms

The typical HS patient is relatively asymptomatic. As noted in the earliest descriptions of HS, mild jaundice can be the only symptom of the disease. Splenomegaly gradually develops in most patients, with the spleen occasionally reaching large dimensions. Anemia is usually mild to moderate but can occasionally be absent because of compensatory bone marrow hyperplasia.

Mild Forms and Carrier State

In some families, anemia is absent, the reticulocyte count is normal or only minimally elevated, laboratory evidence of hemolysis is minimal or absent,[46–48] and the changes in red blood cell shape can be mild, escaping detection on the peripheral blood film. The presence of HS is detected only by osmotic fragility testing or during evaluation of a relative with a more symptomatic form of the disease. Some patients are first diagnosed during transient viral infections such as infectious mononucleosis or parvovirus infection, during pregnancy, or even in the seventh to ninth decades of life as the bone marrow's ability to compensate for hemolysis wanes.

Severe and Atypical Forms

The relatively uncommon patients with nondominant forms of HS can present with a severe life-threatening hemolysis early in life.[1,3,6]

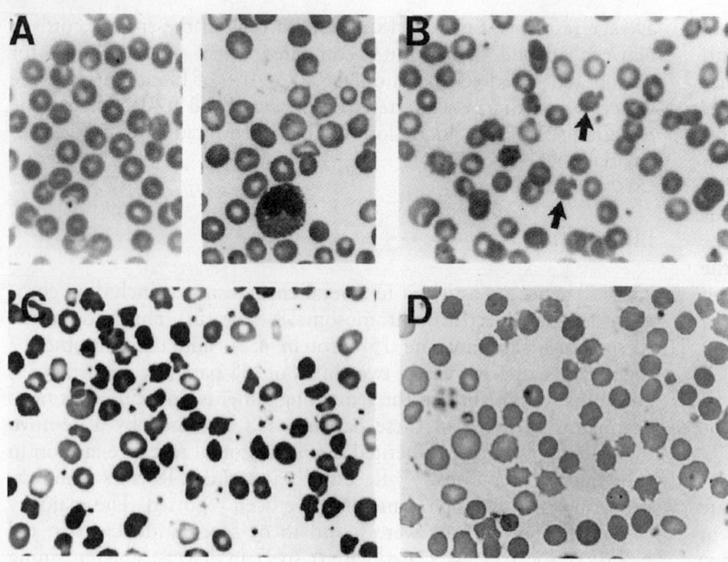

Figure 46–3 Blood films from patients with hereditary spherocytosis (HS) of varying severity. (**A**) Two blood films of typical moderately severe HS with a mild deficiency of red blood cell spectrin and ankyrin. Although many cells have a spheroidal shape, some retain a central concavity. (**B**) HS with pincerlike red blood cells (**arrows**), as typically seen in HS associated with band 3 deficiency. Occasional spiculated red blood cells are also present. (**C**) Severe atypical HS caused by a severe combined spectrin and ankyrin deficiency. In addition to spherocytes, many cells have irregular contour. (**D**) HS with isolated spectrin deficiency caused by a β-spectrin mutation. Some of the spherocytes have prominent surface projections resembling spheroacanthocytes.

Some patients can be transfusion dependent during early infancy and childhood. The underlying molecular defects include severe spectrin or band 3 deficiency.

Hereditary Spherocytosis and Nonerythroid Manifestations

In most HS cases, the clinical manifestations are confined to the erythroid lineage, probably because many of the nonerythroid counterparts of the red blood cell membrane proteins (eg, spectrin and ankyrin) are encoded by separate genes or because some proteins (eg, protein 4.1R, β-spectrin, ankyrin) are subject to tissue-specific alternative splicing. However, several HS kindreds have been reported with a cosegregating neurologic or muscular abnormality, such as a degenerative disorder of the spinal cord, cardiomyopathy, or mental retardation. The observation that both erythrocyte ankyrin and β-spectrin are also expressed in muscle, brain, particularly the cerebellum, and spinal cord raises the possibility that these HS patients may have a defect in one of these proteins. This hypothesis is further supported by studies of *nb*/*nb* mice, a mouse model of HS caused by an ankyrin mutation.[42] These mice develop a neurologic syndrome with a progression that coincides with the loss of ankyrin from the Purkinje cells of the cerebellum.[49]

Mutations of band 3 without HS have been described in patients with distal renal tubular acidosis.[50] Most patients with heterozygous mutations of band 3 and HS have normal renal acidification. The exceptions are two kindreds with co-inherited HS and renal acidification defects because of band 3 mRNA processing mutations, band 3^{Pribram}, and band 3^{Campinas}.[51,52] The pathogenesis of the renal tubular acidosis in these cases is unknown.

Laboratory Evaluation

Most HS patients have either a mild to moderate anemia or no anemia at all, reflecting the facts that the hemolytic rate can be very mild and that the hemolysis is fully compensated for by increased red blood cell production, as evidenced by reticulocytosis. Some patients, however, particularly those with nondominantly inherited HS, are severely anemic, with hemoglobin concentrations as low as 4 to 6 g/dL.

Despite the increased percentage of reticulocytes with a larger volume than mature red blood cells, the mean corpuscular volume (MCV) of HS red blood cells is often low normal or even slightly decreased, and the mean corpuscular hemoglobin concentration (MCHC) is usually increased (>35 g/dL), together reflecting mild cellular dehydration.

The finding of an MCHC > 35.4 g/dL combined with an elevated red blood cell distribution width (RDW) >14% has been found to be an excellent screening test for HS.[50] Another screening method measures MCV by light scattering and provides a histogram of hyperdense erythrocytes (MCHC > 40 g/dL) claimed to identify nearly all HS patients.[53–55] These hyperdense erythrocytes can be detected with newer laser-based blood counters or using aperture impedance analysis available in many clinical laboratories.

Evidence of accelerated red blood cell destruction, as indicated by increased lactate dehydrogenase and unconjugated bilirubin levels and by decreased haptoglobin, as well as by reticulocytosis, is present in typical HS patients. However, these abnormalities can be absent in individuals with a mild form of the disease.

Blood Film

In a typical case of HS, spherocytes are readily identified by their characteristic shape on the peripheral blood film (Fig. 46–3). They lack central pallor, their mean cell diameter is decreased, and they appear more intensely hemoglobinated, which reflects both altered red blood cell geometry and increased cell density. In a three-dimensional view, some spherocytes have a spherostomatocytic shape that is occasionally appreciated on the peripheral blood film. In mild forms of the disease, the peripheral blood smear can appear normal because the loss of surface area can be too small to be appreciated by blood smear evaluation; the cells appear as "fat" disks rather than as true spherocytes.

Additional morphologic features have been described in some HS patients (see Fig. 46–3). A subset of HS patients whose red blood cells are deficient in band 3 protein have some pincerlike red blood cells on the peripheral blood film, a finding that is both sensitive and specific for this HS subset.[25] However, pincerlike cells disappear after splenectomy. Surface spiculations or acanthocytic spherocytes have been described in cases of HS associated with defects in β-spectrin.[12,13] Frequent sphero-ovalocytes and stomatocytes were reported in Japanese patients with protein 4.2 deficiency.[29]

Osmotic Fragility

The osmotic fragility test (Fig. 46–4) measures the in-vitro lysis of red blood cells suspended in solutions of decreasing osmolarity. The

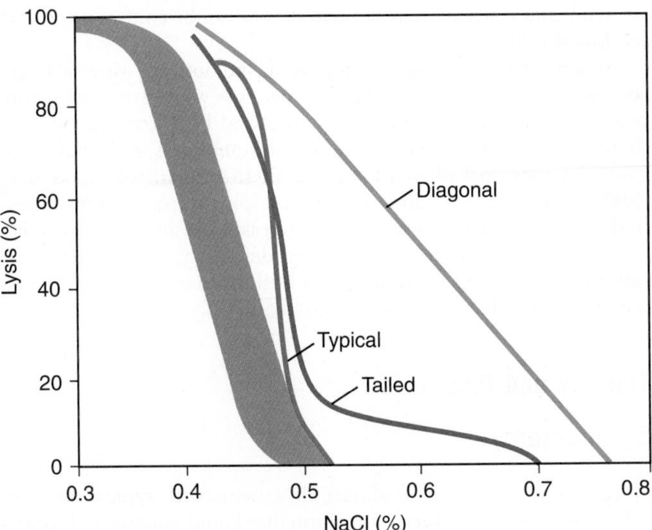

Figure 46–4 Characteristic osmotic fragility curves in hereditary spherocytosis (HS). The typical curve of increased osmotic fragility is the most common finding. The tailed curve reveals a second population (a tail) of very fragile erythrocytes conditioned by the spleen. This tail disappears after splenectomy. The diagonal curve is seen in patients with severe HS. *(Modified from Dacie J: Hereditary spherocytosis (HS). In The Haemolytic Anaemias, 3rd ed, vol 1. Edinburgh, Churchill Livingstone, 1985, p 134.)*

normal red blood cell membrane is unstretchable and is virtually freely permeable to water. Thus, the cell behaves as a nearly perfect osmometer in that it increases its volume in hypotonic solutions progressively until a "critical hemolytic volume" is reached. At this point, the red blood cell membrane ruptures, and hemoglobin escapes into the supernatant solution. As a result of the loss of membrane and the ensuing surface area deficiency, the critical hemolytic volume of spherocytes is considerably lower than that of normal red blood cells. Consequently, these cells hemolyze more than normal red blood cells when suspended in hypotonic sodium chloride (NaCl) solutions. However, a finding of increased osmotic fragility is not unique to HS and is also present in other conditions associated with spherocytosis on the peripheral blood film, such as autoimmune hemolytic anemia.

The slight dehydration of hereditary spherocytes (which in other conditions is associated with decreased osmotic fragility) has no appreciable effect on HS osmotic fragility because of the overriding effect of the markedly diminished cell-surface area. In fact, the densest, most dehydrated cells exhibit the greatest increase in osmotic fragility.

The osmotic fragility curve often reveals uniformly increased osmotic fragility. A "tail" of the osmotic fragility curve can be present in nonsplenectomized HS subjects, indicating a subpopulation of particularly fragile red blood cells conditioned by splenic stasis. This subpopulation of cells disappears after splenectomy.[48] In subjects with mild HS, osmotic fragility can be normal and abnormalities can only be found after incubation that further augments the loss of surface area; however, the sensitivity of the incubated osmotic fragility test can be outweighed by a loss of its specificity. The relative contributions of cell dehydration and surface area deficiency can be accurately determined by osmotic gradient ektacytometry, available only in specialized laboratories.

Autohemolysis and Other Tests

Red blood cell autohemolysis, the spontaneous hemolysis of red blood cells incubated under sterile conditions without glucose, was previously advocated as a sensitive test for the detection of HS. This test is being used less frequently and is probably no more sensitive than the incubated osmotic fragility test. Other tests described in the literature such as the glycerol lysis test, the pink test, hypertonic cryohemolysis, and the skeleton gelation test, are not widely used in the United States. The former two tests, which employ glycerol to retard the osmotic swelling of red blood cells, are preferred by some laboratories because they are easy to perform and can be adapted to microsamples. Cryohemolysis testing remains popular in Europe.[56]

The observations that most spherocytes are deficient in band 3 (see Fig. 46–1) and that eosin-5'-maleimide (EMA) covalently binds band 3 and Rh-related proteins with a 1:1 stoichiometry have been used in a screening test in which binding of fluorescently-labeled EMA to erythrocytes is followed by flow cytometric quantitation. This method is fast and simple and appears to have both high sensitivity and specificity.[57] Like osmotic fragility (OF) and cryohemolysis, other erythrocytes abnormalities such as abnormalities of erythrocyte hydration and variants of dyserythropoietic anemia can also yield abnormal results.

Detection of the Underlying Molecular Defect

Because the most common finding in erythrocytes of patients with HS is a deficiency of one or more of the membrane proteins, initial studies often include sodium dodecyl sulfate-polyacrylamide gel electrophoresis (SDS-PAGE) solubilized red blood cell membrane proteins followed by densitometric quantitation. The results are expressed as ratios of individual red cell membrane proteins to band 3. This technique reveals abnormalities in approximately 70% to 80% of patients, defining the distinct biochemical phenotypes discussed previously. Direct quantitation of membrane proteins by radioimmunoassay is superior to densitometric quantitation and permits accurate measurement of the copy number of the individual proteins per red blood cell. The importance of the latter approach is heightened by the fact that the loss of band 3 can overestimate the spectrin/band 3 or ankyrin/band 3 ratios and, consequently, underestimate the extent of protein deficiencies. As less band 3 is lost after splenectomy, densitometric measurements are more reliable in splenectomized patients.

Subsequent strategies to search for the underlying defect are complex. Studies of protein function, readily employed in the detection of spectrin mutations in cases of HE and HPP (see Pathobiology of the Red Blood Cell Lesion), have been disappointing in detecting abnormalities in HS, with the exception of HS characterized by a weakened β-spectrin-protein 4.1R interaction. Studies of membrane protein synthesis and assembly, using either reticulocytes or erythroblasts derived from peripheral blood burst-forming units in vitro, have been used but they are insensitive in detecting mild to moderate abnormalities in membrane protein synthesis and assembly and are technically cumbersome to perform.

Genetic linkage analysis has been employed in cases of HS, but it suffers from the disadvantages of the need to study large kindreds and its lack of usefulness in studying patients with de-novo mutations. Because of the large sizes of the HS genes, mutation-screening techniques have been developed. Polymerase chain reaction–based mutation screening techniques include single-strand conformational polymorphism analysis and denaturing high-performance liquid chromatography.[20,44] Both techniques identify candidate regions in HS genes of affected patients. These regions are then subjected to nucleotide sequence analysis for detection of the precise genetic defect. Combinations of techniques have been employed in the search for ankyrin gene mutations.[58]

Complications

Gallstones

Bilirubin stones are found in approximately 50% of patients with HS, often even in those with a very mild form of the disease.[3] Gallstones have occasionally been detected during infancy, but they are most likely to occur in children and young adults.[59] The co-inheritance of Gilbert syndrome markedly increases the risk for gallstones in HS patients.[60] Because of the high incidence of gallstones, HS patients should be periodically examined by ultrasonography for the presence of gallstones, beginning early in childhood.

Crises

True hemolytic crises are relatively rare and only occasionally reported in association with infections. Aplastic crises during viral infections are largely attributable to infection by parvovirus B19.[61] This infection (erythema infectiosum, fifth disease) manifests with fever, chills, lethargy, malaise, nausea, vomiting, abdominal pain with occasional diarrhea, respiratory symptoms, muscle and joint pains, and a maculopapular rash on the face (slapped cheek appearance), trunk, and extremities. The virus selectively infects erythroid precursors and inhibits their growth.[62] The ensuing anemia, often profound, can be the first manifestation of HS.[63] Multiple family members with undiagnosed HS who are infected with parvovirus have developed aplastic crises at the same time. Infection with parvovirus is a particular danger to susceptible pregnant women because it can infect the fetus, leading to fetal anemia, hydrops fetalis, and fetal demise.

Rarely, at least in developed countries, patients present with megaloblastic crises caused by folate deficiency. This typically occurs in patients with increased folate demands, such as those recovering from an aplastic crisis, pregnant women, and the elderly. Megaloblastic crisis in pregnancy has been reported as the first manifestation of HS. Folate supplementation (1 mg/day) is recommended for all patients with HS.

Other Complications

In patients with more severe forms of HS, other complications include gout, leg ulcers, or chronic dermatitis of the legs that heal after splenectomy and symptoms of expanded erythroid space, including paravertebral or renal pelvic masses of extramedullary hematopoiesis, which can mimic an underlying neoplasm. Several cases of hemochromatosis in HS patients have been reported. In some, iron overload resulted from repeated transfusions; in others, the patients had two genetic defects, one involving HS and the other involving a hemochromatosis carrier state.[64] Other rare complications include thrombosis, spinocerebellar degenerative syndromes, movement disorders, myopathy, and hypertrophic cardiomyopathy.

More than a dozen cases of HS and hematologic malignancy, including myeloproliferative disorders, multiple myeloma, and leukemia, have been reported. It is unknown if long-standing hematopoietic stress predisposes to the development of these secondary disorders or if they occurred randomly.

Differential Diagnosis

Because of the relatively asymptomatic presentation of HS, this diagnosis should be considered during an evaluation for unexplained splenomegaly, unconjugated hyperbilirubinemia of unknown cause, gallstones at a young age, severe anemia during pregnancy, or transient anemia during acute infections. The diagnosis of HS can be missed in mild forms of the disease, because spherocytosis might not be apparent on the peripheral blood film. An osmotic fragility test of incubated red blood cells usually provides a diagnostic answer. Autoimmune hemolytic anemia (AIHA) should be ruled out by a negative Coombs test.

More typical forms of HS, characterized by relatively uniform spherocytosis with increased MCHC, are usually easily distinguished from other disorders manifesting with spherocytosis, such as immune hemolytic anemias and unstable hemoglobins. In some patients, the spherostomatocytes in the rare Rh null syndrome and the intermediate syndromes of hereditary stomatocytosis can be confused with HS red blood cells.

Spherocytosis is transiently improved, and both the osmotic fragility and hemolysis are normalized in patients with obstructive jaundice. This is because of an expansion of red blood cell surface area that follows an increased uptake of phospholipids and cholesterol from the abnormal plasma lipoproteins. In normal red blood cells, this leads to target cell formation; in HS, spherocytes are transformed to discocytes. Spherocytosis and the increased osmotic fragility of HS red cells are likewise improved by iron deficiency, but the red blood cell life span remains shortened. In addition, coexistence of β-thalassemia trait and HS partially corrects the HS phenotype.

Therapy and Prognosis

Splenectomy

Splenectomy is curative in almost all patients with typical forms of HS, as red blood cell survival is normalized, and anemia and hyperbilirubinemia are corrected. Spherocytosis and the increase in osmotic fragility persist, but the tail of the osmotic fragility curve, indicating the presence of a subpopulation of cells conditioned by the spleen, disappears. In patients with severe, nondominantly inherited HS, splenectomy produces a dramatic clinical improvement, but hemolysis is only partially corrected.[14,15]

Several weeks to months before splenectomy, patients should be immunized with polyvalent vaccine against pneumococcus as well as vaccines against *Haemophilus influenzae* type b and meningococcus.

Indications for Splenectomy

Risks and benefits should be considered carefully in HS patients before splenectomy is performed. A multitude of factors influence the decision for splenectomy in HS patients, including the risk of overwhelming postsplenectomy sepsis, the emergence of penicillin-resistant pneumococci, and the potentially increased risk of cardiovascular disease and pulmonary hypertension later in life.[65–69] Indications for splenectomy include growth retardation, skeletal changes, symptomatic hemolytic disease, anemia-induced compromise of vital organs, the development of leg ulcers, or the appearance of extramedullary hematopoietic tumors. Whether to perform splenectomy in patients with moderate HS without any of the above factors remains controversial.

Because of an increased frequency of postsplenectomy infection in young children, splenectomy should not be performed earlier than 3 to 5 years of age.

Operative Considerations

When splenectomy is warranted, laparoscopic splenectomy has become the procedure of choice in many centers.[70,71] Laparoscopic splenectomy has been associated with less postoperative discomfort, a quicker return to preoperative diet and activities, a shorter hospitalization time, decreased costs, and smaller scars. Early complications of splenectomy include local infection, bleeding, and pancreatitis. In general, the morbidity rate of splenectomy is lower in patients with HS than with other hematologic diseases. However, the benefits of surgery must be weighed against possible complications, such as postsplenectomy infections, including the postsplenectomy sepsis syndrome. Although these complications are rare and their frequency is likely to diminish further with appropriate vaccinations, the indiscriminate performance of splenectomy in all HS patients with splenomegaly is unwarranted.

Subtotal (Partial) Splenectomy

Partial splenectomy has been suggested for infants and young children with severe HS, anemia, and poor growth with the goals of palliating anemia and decreasing transfusion requirements while preserving splenic function.[72–74] The goal of this operation is to decrease hemolysis while maintaining splenic phagocytic function. It has been so far performed in a few hundred patients with stable increase in hemoglobin levels and decrease in reticulocyte counts. The volume of splenic tissue left behind ranges from 10 to 30 mL. Although initial data are promising, it is not clear whether the remaining splenic tissue will effectively prevent postsplenectomy sepsis. In addition, regrowth of the splenic remnant has been reported in most patients, which can eventually lead to recurrence of HS and another operative procedure.[75]

After splenectomy, prophylactic antibiotics for at least 5 years are recommended by some practitioners, and for life by others.

Postsplenectomy Failures

Postsplenectomy failures are caused either by the presence of an accessory spleen missed during surgery (accessory spleens were found in 17%–39% of all patients)[76] or by the presence of another superimposed red blood cell disorder such as pyruvate kinase deficiency. The recurrence of hemolytic anemia several years after splenectomy should raise the suspicion of development of splenunculi, resulting from autotransplantation of splenic tissue during surgery. The presence of an accessory spleen or splenunculus is suggested by the absence of both Howell-Jolly bodies and the "pitted" cells with crater-like surface indentations readily seen by interference contrast microscopy.[77] A definitive confirmation of splenosis is made by a radiocolloid liver-spleen scan or by a scan using chromium (Cr)-labeled heated red blood cells, which are taken up by the ectopic splenic tissue.

Genetic Counseling

After a patient is diagnosed with HS, family members should be examined for the presence of HS. A history, physical examination for splenomegaly, complete blood count with indices, reticulocyte count, examination of the peripheral blood smear for spherocytes, and biochemical evaluation including bilirubin and haptoglobin levels should be obtained for available close relatives.

HEREDITARY ELLIPTOCYTOSIS AND RELATED DISORDERS

Definition, Prevalence, and History

Hereditary elliptocytosis designates a group of inherited disorders that have in common the presence of elliptical red blood cells on peripheral blood films.[78] Elliptocytosis was first described by Dresbach in 1904,[79] and its heritability was firmly established by Hunter.[80] Subsequent reports have revealed a considerable heterogeneity of clinical expression and have defined several distinct syndromes, including HPP and SAO.[1,6]

Hereditary elliptocytosis is common in people of African and Mediterranean ancestries. In the US population, the prevalence of HE is approximately 3 to 5 per 10,000.[81] The true incidence of HE is unknown because its clinical severity is heterogeneous and most patients are asymptomatic without anemia.[82] HE is considerably more frequent in areas of endemic malaria. In equatorial Africa, the prevalence of common HE has been estimated at between 0.6% and 1.6%. Worldwide, HE appears to be more common among people of African origin. In Southeast Asian populations, the prevalence of SAO, a variant of HE, is as high as 30%.[83]

The molecular basis of HE remained obscure until a defect of membrane skeletal proteins was suggested. Subsequently, defects in the erythrocyte membrane proteins α-spectrin, β-spectrin, protein 4.1R, glycophorin C, and band 3 were described.

On the basis of red blood cell morphology, HE can be divided into three major groups (Fig. 46–5). Common HE, a dominantly inherited condition, is morphologically characterized by biconcave elliptocytes and, in some patients, rod-shaped cells. The clinical severity of common HE is highly variable, ranging from an asymptomatic condition to a severe recessively inherited hemolytic anemia, including hemolytic HE and HPP, in which the blood film reveals numerous red blood cell fragments, microspherocytes, and poikilocytes. Spherocytic HE, also called hemolytic ovalocytosis, is a much less common condition in which both round "fat" ovalocytes and spherocytes are present on the blood film. SAO, a disorder highly prevalent in the malaria-belt of Southeast Asia and the Pacific, is characterized by rigid, spoon-shaped cells that have either a longitudinal slit or a transverse ridge.

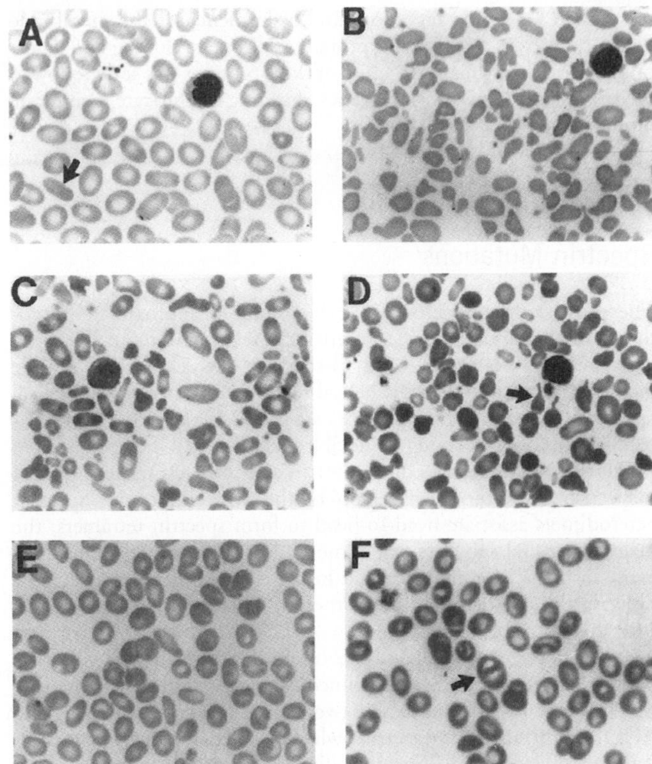

Figure 46–5 Blood films of subjects with various forms of hereditary elliptocytosis (HE). **(A)** Simple heterozygote with mild common HE. Note the predominant elliptocytosis with some rod-shaped cells (*arrow*) and virtual absence of poikilocytes. **(B)** Simple heterozygote with severe common hemolytic elliptocytosis. Note the numerous small fragments and poikilocytes. **(C)** "Homozygous" common HE because of doubly heterozygous state for two mutant α-spectrins. Both parents have mild HE. Note the many elliptocytes as well as numerous fragments and poikilocytes. **(D)** Hereditary pyropoikilocytosis. The patient is a double heterozygote for a structural α-spectrin mutant and a presumed α-spectrin synthetic defect. Note the prominent microspherocytosis, micropoikilocytosis, and fragmentation. Only few elliptocytes are present. Some poikilocytes are in the process of budding (*arrow*). **(E)** Spherocytic HE (hereditary ovalocytosis). Most red blood cells are oval rather than truly elliptical. Many oval cells are "fat," lacking a central concavity, the feature distinguishing spherocytic HE from common HE. **(F)** Southeast Asian ovalocytosis (Melanesian). Most cells are oval, some containing either a longitudinal slit or a transverse ridge (*arrow*).

Common Hereditary Elliptocytosis

The possibility that the primary lesion of HE and HPP erythrocytes resides in the proteins of the red blood cell membrane skeleton was first raised by the findings of thermal instability of HPP spectrin, retention of the elliptical shape in HE membrane skeletons, disintegration of membrane skeletons after exposure to shear stress, defective self-association of spectrin dimers to tetramers, altered susceptibility of spectrin to tryptic digestion, and a deficiency of the membrane skeleton proteins spectrin and protein 4.1R. Gene cloning and determination of the primary structure of these proteins was soon followed by reports of mutations in the genes encoding erythrocyte membrane proteins.

Etiology

Spectrin Mutations

The most common defects in HE, found in approximately two-thirds to three-quarters of all patients, are mutations of α- or β-spectrin.[1,6,78,84] Both α- and β-spectrin are elongated flexible molecules consisting of triple helical repeats connected by nonhelical segments. These polypeptides are associated side-to-side in an antiparallel position, forming a flexible, rod-like αβ heterodimer in which the NH_2-terminus of α-spectrin and the COOH-terminus of β-spectrin form the head region of the heterodimer.[84,85] Spectrin heterodimers associate head-to-head to form spectrin tetramers, the major structural subunits of the membrane skeleton. Spectrin tetramers, in turn, are interconnected into a highly ordered two-dimensional lattice through binding, at their distal ends, to actin oligomers with the aid of protein 4.1R.[86]

The contact site between the α- and β-spectrin chains of the opposed heterodimers is a combined "atypical" triple helical repetitive segment in which the first two helices are contributed by the COOH-terminus of β-spectrin, whereas helix 3 is the first helical segment of α-spectrin. Spectrin dimer-tetramer interconversion is governed by a simple thermodynamic equilibrium that under physiologic conditions strongly favors spectrin tetramers.[87,88] Most α-spectrin defects are at or near the NH_2-terminus of α-spectrin, which is involved in the heterodimer contact (the so-called αI domain defined by limited tryptic peptide mapping; see the discussion under Laboratory Evaluation),[84] and impair the self-association of spectrin into tetramers. Most α-spectrin mutations are point mutations.[78,84] These mutations create abnormal proteolytic cleavage sites that typically reside in the third helix of a repetitive segment and give rise to abnormal tryptic peptides on two-dimensional tryptic peptide maps of spectrin.

Elliptocytogenic β-spectrin mutations are COOH-terminal point mutations or truncations that disrupt the formation of the combined β triple-helical repetitive segment and consequently the self-association of spectrin heterodimers to tetramers.[78,84] All of these mutations open a proteolytic cleavage site residing in the third helix of the combined repetitive segment, which gives rise to a 74-kd αI peptide.

Although most spectrin mutations reside in the vicinity of the αβ-spectrin self-association site, a few mutations remote from the self-association site have been described. These mutations are asymptomatic in the simple heterozygous state but cause hemolytic anemia, which can be severe, in homozygous patients.[89–91] Unlike mutations located in the self-association contact site which are predicted to disrupt the conformation of the local protein structure,[92] mutations outside this region are predicted to perturb long range protein-protein interactions, disrupting the positively coupled, cooperative interactions of αβ spectrin self-association, spectrin-ankyrin interactions, and ankyrin-band 3 interactions.[93,94] One HE-associated mutation in a linker region remote from the self-association contact site disrupted the stability propagated from one spectrin repeat to the next.[93,94]

Protein 4.1R Mutations

Another group of elliptocytogenic mutations, although much less common than spectrin mutations, are quantitative or qualitative defects of protein 4.1R.[78] Protein 4.1R is a multifunctional protein that contains several important sites of protein interactions, including the spectrin-binding domain, where 4.1R binds to the distal end of the spectrin αβ heterodimer, markedly increasing the binding of spectrin to oligomeric actin, and the basic NH_2-terminal domain, where 4.1R interacts with glycophorin C, phosphatidylinositol, and phosphatidylserine, facilitating the attachment of the distal end of spectrin to the membrane.[85,86]

Studies of 4.1R mRNA from normal red blood cells revealed 4.1R isoforms resulting from complex tissue and developmental-stage specific patterns of alternate mRNA splicing.[95–99] Alternate translation initiation sites are present in the protein 4.1R mRNA. When an upstream AUG is used, isoforms greater than 80 kd are synthesized. During erythropoiesis, this upstream AUG is spliced out and a downstream AUG is used, leading to the production of the 80-kd mature erythroid protein 4.1R isoform.[96] On SDS-PAGE, protein 4.1R is resolved into two bands of different sizes: 4.1a and 4.1b. The larger band, 4.1a, is typically found in normal red blood cells, whereas the shorter one, 4.1b, represents the major isoform of reticulocytes. The 4.1b isoform is converted into the 4.1a isoform by deamidation of Asn 502.

A partial deficiency of protein 4.1R is associated with mild, dominantly inherited HE, whereas a complete deficiency (a homozygous state) leads to a severe hemolytic disease.[100,101] Homozygous 4.1R(–) erythrocytes fragment more rapidly than normal at moderate sheer stresses, an indication of their intrinsic instability.[102] Membrane mechanical stability can be restored by reconstituting the deficient red blood cells with protein 4.1R or the protein 4.1R/spectrin/actin-binding site.[103] Homozygous protein 4.1R(–) erythrocytes also lack p55 and have only 30% of the normal content of glycophorin C. These homozygous 4.1R(–) erythrocytes, as well as glycophorin C(–) Leach erythrocytes, demonstrate decreased invasion and growth of *Plasmodium falciparum* in vitro.

Mutations associated with protein 4.1R deficiency have included deletions that include the exon encoding the erythroid transcription start size and mutations of the transcription initiation codon.[78] Qualitative defects of protein 4.1R protein include deletions and duplications of the exons encoding the spectrin-binding domain, leading either to truncated or elongated forms of protein 4.1R. Electron microscopic studies of homozygous 4.1R(–) erythrocyte membranes revealed a markedly disrupted skeletal network with disruption of the intramembrane particles, suggesting that protein 4.1R plays an important role in maintenance not only of the skeletal network but also of the integral proteins of the membrane structure.[104]

Glycophorin C Deficiency

Glycophorin C (GPC) has been found absent because of a variety of molecular defects.[105] In contrast to other forms of HE, which are dominantly inherited, heterozygous carriers are asymptomatic, with normal red blood cell morphology, and homozygous subjects have no anemia and only mild elliptocytosis apparent on the peripheral blood film.

GPC deficiency with elliptocytosis, the so-called Leach phenotype,[106] caused by reduced expression of GPC, should be distinguished from the immunochemically defined phenotypes Gerbich and Yus, in which abnormal glycoproteins are formed that can functionally substitute for normal GPC and preserve the normal red blood cell shape. The Leach phenotype is usually caused by a large deletion of genomic DNA (~7 kb) that removes exons 3 and 4 from the GPC/GPD locus. In one patient, the Leach phenotype was caused by a frameshift mutation.

GPC-deficient subjects are also partially deficient in protein 4.1R and lack p55, presumably because these proteins form a complex and recruit or stabilize each other on the membrane.[107] It has been speculated that the protein 4.1R deficiency in Leach erythrocytes is the cause of the elliptocytic shape. In contrast, subjects deficient in glycophorin A, the major transmembrane glycoprotein, are asymptomatic.

Pathobiology of the Red Blood Cell Lesion

Most of the elliptocytogenic mutations of spectrin reside within, or in the vicinity of, the spectrin heterodimer self-association site, dis-

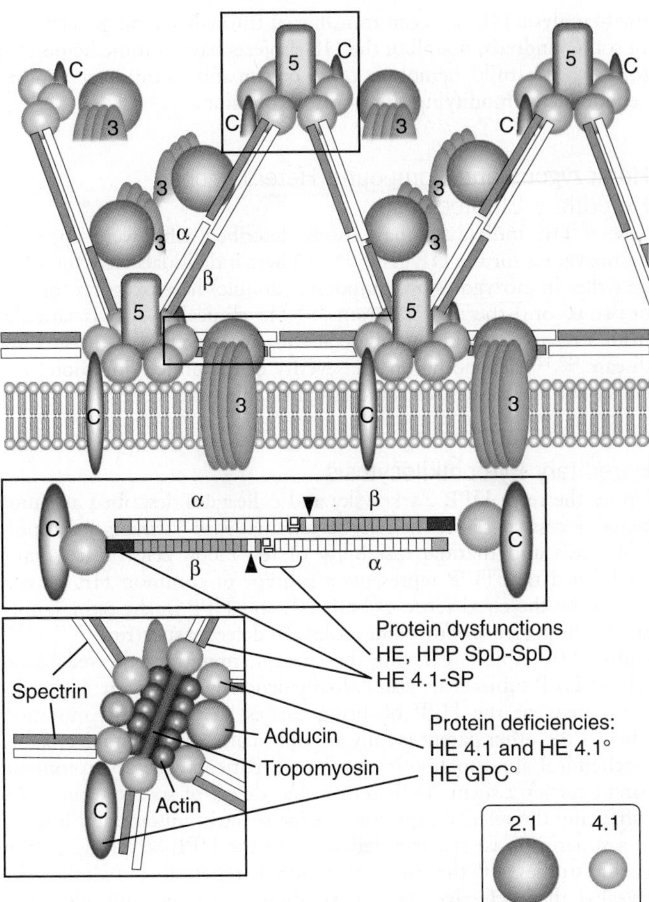

Figure 46–6 Schematic representation of the molecular assembly of the membrane skeleton and the molecular defects in hereditary elliptocytosis HE and hereditary pyropoikilocytosis (HPP). Spectrin is composed of α- and β-spectrin heterodimers (SpD) that associate in their head regions into tetramers. At their distal ends, SpD bind to the junctional complexes of oligomeric actin (band 5) and protein 4.1. Additional proteins found in the junctional complex, such as adducin, tropomyosin, and protein 4.9, are shown in the lower enlarged area. The membrane skeleton is attached to transmembrane proteins by interactions of β-spectrin with ankyrin (protein 2.1; [*black arrow*] designates the ankyrin-binding site in β-spectrin), which in turn binds to the cytoplasmic domain of band 3, and by linkage of protein 4.1 to glycophorin C. The known protein dysfunctions in HE and HPP include (1) defects of the SpD head region because of a mutation of either α- or β-spectrin, causing impaired assembly of SpD into tetramers, and (2) defects of proteins of the junctional complex such as a qualitative or quantitative defects of protein 4.1R or glycophorin C.

rupting this region and consequently disrupting the two-dimensional integrity of the membrane skeleton (Fig. 46–6). These defects are detected by ultrastructural examination of the membrane skeleton, which reveals disruption of a normally uniform hexagonal lattice. Consequently, membrane skeletons are mechanically unstable, as are whole cell membranes and the cells.[108] In patients with severely dysfunctional spectrin mutations or patients homozygous or doubly heterozygous for spectrin mutations, the membrane instability is sufficient to cause red blood cell fragmentation with hemolytic anemia under conditions of normal circulatory shear stress.

The pathobiology of the elliptocytic shape is less clear. Red blood cell precursors in common HE are round, and the cells become progressively more elliptical as they age in vivo.[109,110] Red blood cells subjected to shear stress in vitro, or red blood cells flowing through microcirculation in vivo, have an elliptical or parachute-like shape, respectively. It is possible that elliptocytes and poikilocytes are permanently stabilized in their abnormal shape because the weakened spectrin heterodimer contacts facilitate skeletal reorganization, which follows axial deformation of cells resulting from application of a prolonged or excessive shear stress. This reorganization is likely to involve breakage of the unidirectionally stretched protein connections followed by the formation of new protein contacts that preclude the recovery of a normal biconcave shape.[87] This process has been shown to account for permanent deformation of irreversibly sickled cells.[111]

In HPP, the recessively inherited form of HE characterized by severe hemolysis, red blood cells have two abnormalities.[112,113] They contain a mutant spectrin that characteristically disrupts spectrin heterodimer self-association, and they are also partially deficient in spectrin, as evidenced by a decreased spectrin/band 3 ratio. In some HPP cases, this biochemical phenotype is a consequence of a double heterozygous state for an elliptocytogenic α-spectrin mutation and a defect involving reduced α-spectrin synthesis. Such synthetic defect of α-spectrin is fully asymptomatic in the heterozygous carrier, because under normal conditions, the synthesis of α-spectrin is approximately three to four times greater than that of β-spectrin.

When present in conjunction with an elliptocytogenic mutation of α-spectrin, such a synthetic defect augments the expression of the mutant spectrin. Because the elliptocytogenic α-spectrin mutants are often unstable, the combination of the two defects leads to spectrin deficiency in the cells. Other HPP subjects are homozygous or doubly heterozygous for one or two elliptocytogenic spectrin mutations, respectively.[84] In such cases, the spectrin deficiency may be a consequence of spectrin instability that reduces the amount of spectrin available for membrane assembly. Furthermore, in red blood cells containing a high fraction of unassembled dimeric spectrin, the spectrin deficiency may in part be related to the stoichiometric ratio of one ankyrin copy per one spectrin tetramer (ie, two spectrin heterodimers). Consequently, only approximately one-half of spectrin heterodimers succeed in attaching to the ankyrin-binding sites. The phenotype of HPP, characterized by the presence of fragments and elliptocytes, together with evidence of red blood cell surface area deficiency (as reflected by the presence of microspherocytes on the peripheral blood film), suggests that the membrane dysfunction involves both vertical interactions (a consequence of spectrin deficiency) and horizontal interactions involving the elliptocytogenic spectrin mutation.

The red blood cell lesion in protein 4.1R deficiency shows similarities in regard to cell shape and membrane stability to the above elliptocytogenic mutations of spectrin, suggesting that the deficiency principally affects the spectrin-actin contact (see Fig. 46–6) rather than the skeleton attachment to glycophorin C via protein 4.1R (a vertical interaction).[108]

The molecular basis of elliptocytosis and the mechanical instability of glycophorin C-deficient red blood cells are not fully understood. However, recent studies suggest that the deficiency of glycophorin C is not directly responsible for the altered mechanical properties. Instead, the mechanical instability appears to be related to a concomitant partial deficiency of protein 4.1R, as evidenced by a full correction of membrane instability by introduction into the cells of protein 4.1R or its spectrin-binding peptide, which facilitates the contact of β-spectrin to actin. The superimposed deficiency of protein 4.1R is likely to be related to the fact that glycophorin C serves as an attachment site for protein 4.1R to the membrane, recruiting protein 4.1R to the red blood cell membrane. The effects of these defects on the mechanical stability of glycophorin C-deficient cells appear to be relatively minor, because glycophorin C-deficient subjects have no detectable hemolytic anemia and the mechanical properties of the red blood cells are normal when tested by micropipette aspiration.

Inheritance

In most patients, HE is inherited as an autosomal dominant disorder. The clinical severity is highly variable among different kindreds (reflecting heterogeneous molecular lesions) and, to a lesser extent, within a given kindred, presumably because of other genetic or acquired defects that modify disease expression.[6,78] Occasionally, HE is inherited as an autosomal recessive condition from an asymptomatic parent who carries the same molecular defect of spectrin as the HE offspring. In one kindred with a submicroscopic chromosome X deletion, inheritance was X-linked.[114]

The inheritance of the related disorder HPP is autosomal recessive: one of the parents carries the α-spectrin mutation and either is asymptomatic or has mild HE, whereas the other parent is fully asymptomatic and has no abnormalities detectable by current biochemical approaches. However, several HPP patients have recently been studied who were doubly heterozygous for two α-spectrin mutations; in the heterozygous parents, these mutations were either silent or expressed as mild HE.

Clinical Manifestations

In view of the striking molecular heterogeneity of common HE, it is not surprising that the clinical spectrum of this disorder is variable, ranging from an asymptomatic trait without hemolysis to a life-threatening hemolytic anemia.

Mild Hereditary Elliptocytosis and Asymptomatic Carrier State

In most of these subjects, HE is found accidentally during evaluation of the peripheral blood film. Although some HE subjects have a mild compensated hemolytic anemia, others do not have any evidence of hemolysis, their red blood cell survival is normal, and the peripheral blood film may reveal only modest (≥15%) elliptocytosis. The molecular basis of mild HE is heterogeneous, and the reported molecular defects include both α- and β-spectrin mutations, partial deficiency of the 4.1R protein, and the absence of glycophorin C. Some individuals carrying the spectrin mutation are completely asymptomatic, including normal red blood cell morphology; this is often the case in one of the parents of a patient with HPP.

Hereditary Elliptocytosis with Sporadic Hemolysis

Worsening of hemolysis together with the appearance of poikilocytes on the peripheral blood film has been reported in patients with hypersplenism, infections, or vitamin B_{12} deficiency, as well as in those with microangiopathic hemolysis such as disseminated intravascular coagulation or thrombotic thrombocytopenic purpura.[115] In the latter two conditions, worsening hemolysis can be caused by microcirculatory damage superimposed on the underlying mechanical instability of the red blood cells.

Hereditary Elliptocytosis with Neonatal Poikilocytosis

Neonatal offspring of parents with mild HE present with symptomatic hemolytic anemia and a marked poikilocytosis.[116,117] During the first year of life, the hemolysis and poikilocytosis abate, and the clinical picture transforms into that of mild HE. Such patients typically carry one mutant α-spectrin allele. The severity of the molecular defect, in terms of the percentage of spectrin dimers and the amount of mutant spectrin in the cells, is the same in the neonatal period as it is later in life. The worsening of hemolysis in the neonatal period has been attributed to the presence of fetal hemoglobin, which binds poorly to 2,3-diphosphoglycerate (2,3-DPG).[118] The ensuing elevation of free 2,3-DPG levels has a marked destabilizing effect on the spectrin-protein 4.1R-actin interaction, thereby further destabilizing the membrane skeleton.

Hereditary Elliptocytosis with Chronic Hemolysis

Patients with HE with chronic hemolysis present with moderate to severe hemolytic anemia with elliptocytes and poikilocytes on peripheral blood film; some require splenectomy. In some of the kindreds, the hemolytic HE has been transmitted through several generations. In some kindreds, not all of the HE subjects have chronic hemolysis; some have a mild hemolysis only, presumably because of another genetic factor modifying the disease expression.

Homozygous and Compound Heterozygous Hereditary Elliptocytosis

Several HE individuals have been described who were apparent homozygotes for the HE gene.[116–120] These individuals were found to be either homozygotes or compound (double) heterozygotes for one or two α- or β-spectrin mutations.[6,78] The clinical severity is variable, from a relatively mild hemolytic anemia to a severe, life-threatening disease,[119–121] depending on the severity of the underlying molecular defect and in some cases is indistinguishable from HPP.

Hereditary Pyropoikilocytosis

Under the term HPP, Zarkowsky and colleagues described an autosomal recessive severe hemolytic anemia with striking micropoikilocytosis and thermal instability of red blood cells.[122] It is now established that HPP represents a subtype of common HE, as evidenced by the coexistence of both HE and HPP in the same family and by the presence of the same molecular defect of spectrin.[112,113,123,124] Unlike HE subjects carrying the spectrin mutation, the red blood cells of HPP subjects are also partially deficient in spectrin. Typically, one parent of the HPP offspring carries an α-spectrin mutation whereas the other parent is fully asymptomatic and has no detectable biochemical abnormality. In many such patients, the asymptomatic parent carries a silent "thalassemia-like" defect of spectrin synthesis, enhancing the relative expression of the spectrin mutant and leading to a superimposed spectrin deficiency in the HPP offspring. Subsequent studies of the original kindred reported by Zarkowsky revealed that defective spectrin synthesis from the null allele was caused by a splicing mutation of the α-spectrin gene.[125] Some HPP subjects inherited two α-spectrin mutations; either their parents were hematologically normal or one had mild HE. In these HPP subjects, spectrin deficiency may be related to instability of the mutant spectrin. The thermal instability of spectrin originally reported as diagnostic of HPP is not unique for this disorder;[122] it is also found in HE subjects carrying this α-spectrin mutation, in the homozygous and in the heterozygous states. HPP is seen predominantly in black subjects, but it has also been diagnosed in Arabs and whites.

Molecular Determinants of Clinical Severity

The severity of hemolysis in common HE often varies not only among different kindred but within a given family as well. The two principal determinants of severity of hemolysis are the spectrin content of the cells and the percentage of dimeric spectrin in the crude spectrin extract. The fraction of dimeric spectrin in such extracts in turn depends on several factors. The first of them is the degree of dysfunction of the mutant spectrin. Typically, mutations that are either within or near the combined αβ triple helical repetitive segment representing the spectrin heterodimer self-association site produce a more severe clinical phenotype and a more severe defect of spectrin function than those seen with point mutations in the more distant triple helical repeats.[100] Second, the percentage of the dimeric spectrin depends on the fraction of the mutant spectrin in the cells, which in turn is determined by the gene dose (eg, simple heterozygote versus homozygote or double heterozygote) or the presence of other genetic defects such as the presence, in *trans*, of a defect leading to a reduced α-spectrin synthesis in some subjects with HPP.

The low-expression α-spectrin allele α^{LELY} is the best-characterized abnormality affecting spectrin content and clinical severity. Initially, a polymorphism of the αV domain, $\alpha^{V/41}$, was identified in HE patients who, when they inherited $\alpha^{V/41}$ in *trans*, had more severe HE than expected. Subsequently, an amino acid substitution of exon 46,

Leu1857Val, and partial skipping of exon 46, linked to the $\alpha^{V/41}$ polymorphism, were identified as the characteristics of the α^{LELY} allele.[126] These abnormalities are located within the site at which spectrin monomers assemble into heterodimers (the spectrin heterodimer nucleation site). In-vitro studies suggest that the inability of α-spectrin chains to assemble into the mature membrane skeleton is because of a combination of decreased αβ dimer-binding affinity and increased proteolytic cleavage of the mutant α-spectrin chains.[127] The presence of α^{LELY} in *trans* diminishes the propensity of the otherwise normal allele to associate with the corresponding β-chain, favoring the attachment of the elliptocytogenic α-spectrin allele. Conversely, coexistence of the α-spectrin mutation in *cis* and the mutation involving the α-spectrin nucleation site diminishes the propensity of the mutant allele to be incorporated into the spectrin heterodimer, thereby ameliorating the clinical severity of this mutation. The α^{LELY} allele is clinically silent by itself, even when inherited in the homozygous state, probably because α-spectrin is normally synthesized in three- to fourfold excess.

Laboratory Evaluation

Blood Film and Laboratory Evidence of Hemolysis

A careful blood smear evaluation is essential for the diagnosis of HE and for the classification of the disorder into the three major subtypes outlined earlier (see Hereditary Elliptocytosis and Related Disorders, Definition, Prevalence, and History and Fig. 46–5). In patients in whom elliptocytosis is the only morphologic abnormality, hemolysis is characteristically minimal or absent, with the exception of spherocytic elliptocytosis, in which the presence of round "fat" ovalocytes is associated with accelerated red blood cell destruction. In patients with hemolytic forms of common HE, poikilocytosis is characteristically found on the blood film. In severe forms of HE, particularly in homozygous HE, many red blood cells circulate as cell fragments, producing a marked decrease in MCV. The finding of red blood cell fragments together with a striking microspherocytosis and often only occasional elliptocytes is characteristic of HPP (see Fig. 46–5).

Osmotic, Thermal, and Mechanical Fragility

Osmotic fragility is increased in HPP, in spherocytic elliptocytosis, and in HE subjects with poikilocytosis apparent on the peripheral blood film.[128] In patients with a mild common HE without poikilocytosis on the peripheral blood film, osmotic fragility is normal.

Thermal instability of red blood cells was originally reported by Zarkowsky and colleagues as a characteristic feature of HPP.[122] It reflects thermal instability of the mutant spectrin: In normal red blood cells, spectrin is denatured and red blood cells fragment at 50°C (122°F). HPP red blood cells fragment and their spectrin denatures at 41°C (105.8°F). However, the diagnostic value of this test is limited, because thermal instability of red blood cells is also noted in HE red blood cells containing mutant spectrin. In contrast, an occasional patient with otherwise typical HPP may have normal thermal stability of red blood cells and spectrin. Red blood cells in common HE have unstable membranes and membrane skeletons when subjected to shear stress.

Electrophoretic Separation of Solubilized Membrane Proteins

In HE and HPP, SDS-PAGE can reveal proteins of abnormal mobility, the origin of which can be subsequently identified by Western blotting (eg, truncated α- or β-spectrins in HE and HPP, or elongated or truncated forms of the 4.1R protein, and a partial or, rarely, complete deficiency of the 4.1R protein in HE).[84] In HPP, SDS-PAGE reveals a partial deficiency of spectrin, as indicated by a decreased spectrin/band 3 ratio. Spectrin deficiency, in conjunction with an elliptocytogenic spectrin mutation affecting the spectrin heterodimer contact, is invariably found in cases of HPP.

Nondenaturing Gel Electrophoresis of Low Ionic Strength Spectrin Extract

Analysis of the ratio of tetrameric and dimeric spectrin in the low ionic strength extracts reveals the most common functional abnormality in HE (ie, weakened self-association of spectrin heterodimers into tetramers).[111] Because the spectrin dimer-tetramer interconversion has a high activation energy, it is kinetically immobilized at near 0°C (32°F). Consequently, the percentage of spectrin dimers and tetramers in the 0°C (32°F) crude spectrin extract reflects the relative distribution of these species in the red blood cell membrane in situ. Mutations of α- or β-spectrin residing within or near the αβ-spectrin heterodimer self-association site invariably lead to an increase in the fraction of dimeric spectrin (normal range, 5 ± 2.5%) in the crude 0°C (32°F) spectrin extract.

Tryptic Peptide Mapping of Spectrin and the Detection of the Underlying DNA Defect

As reviewed elsewhere,[84] tryptic digestion of spectrin under controlled conditions followed by electrophoretic separation gives rise to highly reproducible tryptic peptide patterns. Among these peptides, the 80-kd αI domain peptide representing the self-association site of the normal α-spectrin is the most prominent one. Nearly all α- or β-spectrin mutations reported are associated with a formation of tryptic peptides of abnormal size and mobility that are generated instead of the normal 80-kd αI domain peptide. The cleavage sites of the most common abnormal tryptic peptides were mapped and found to reside in the third helix of a given triple helical repetitive segment. The reported mutations reside in the vicinity of these cleavage sites either in the same helix or, less commonly, in helix 1 or 2 of a given repetitive segment. Consequently, tryptic peptide mapping remains a powerful tool with which to map the site of the underlying spectrin mutation, which can be subsequently defined by polymerase chain reaction amplification and sequencing of the respective region of the genomic DNA or cDNA.

Differential Diagnosis

Various acquired and inherited conditions can be associated with elliptocytosis and poikilocytosis, including iron deficiency, thalassemias, megaloblastic anemias, myelofibrosis, myelophthisic anemias, myelodysplastic syndromes, and pyruvate kinase deficiency. The percentage of elliptocytes in these conditions is seldom greater than 60%. However, this is not diagnostically useful, because some HE subjects can have a relatively low percentage of elliptocytes. In normal subjects, the percentage of elliptocytes is not greater than 5%, although in earlier reports it was listed as high as 15%. Previous diagnostic criteria of HE, based on the percentage of elliptocytes, such as 25%, 33%, or 40%, and their axial ratio, do not appear useful. The most reliable differentiation of HE from the above-mentioned conditions is based on a positive family history rather than on the percentage of elliptocytes.

Treatment and Prognosis

As in the case of HS, red blood cells from patients with more severe forms of HE are retained by the spleen, producing a marked engorgement of splenic pulp. Consequently, patients with symptomatic hemolysis benefit from splenectomy.[128] This procedure is virtually never indicated in heterozygotes with autosomal dominant HE because most do not have clinically significant hemolytic anemia. If hemolysis is still active after splenectomy, folate should be administered daily. Recommendations for antibiotic prophylaxis, immunizations, and monitoring for intercurrent illnesses are similar to those noted earlier for HS patients before and after splenectomy. Serial interval ultrasonographic investigations to detect gallstones should be performed in patients with significant hemolysis.

Spherocytic Elliptocytosis

Spherocytic elliptocytosis, which shares features of HS and HE, has been designated spherocytic HE, HE with spherocytosis, or hereditary hemolytic ovalocytosis. The diagnosis is based on the simultaneous presence of elliptical red blood cells and spherocytes or "fat," round sphero-ovalocytes in the peripheral blood film (see Fig. 46–5). In contrast to common HE, cells of other shapes, such as rod-shaped cells, poikilocytes, and fragments, are absent. Importantly, hemolysis, despite relatively mild alterations in red blood cell morphology, and increased osmotic fragility are the main diagnostic features distinguishing this disorder from common HE.

The molecular basis of classic spherocytic HE is unknown. However, patients with mutations, particularly truncations at the C-terminus of β-spectrin, have many of the clinical features of spherocytic HE and probably represent an example of this disorder.[84,129] Patients who lack glycophorin C have rounded, smooth elliptocytes and could be classified as having a mild, recessively inherited variant of spherocytic HE. Finally, some patients with recessively inherited defects of protein 4.2 can display some features of spherocytic HE, particularly mild ovalostomatocytosis.[29]

Southeast Asian Ovalocytosis

Southeast Asian ovalocytosis is characterized by the presence of oval red blood cells, many containing one or two transverse ridges or a longitudinal slit (see Fig. 46–5). The condition is widespread in certain ethnic groups of Malaysia, Papua New Guinea, the Philippines, and Indonesia.[83,130] Numerous functional abnormalities of ovalocytes have been reported, including increased red blood cell rigidity, decreased osmotic fragility, increased thermal stability, resistance to shape change by echinocytogenic agents, and a reduced expression of many red blood cell antigens. A remarkable feature of ovalocytes is their resistance to in-vitro invasion by several strains of malaria parasites, including *Plasmodium falciparum* and *Plasmodium knowlesi*. Moreover, in areas of endemic malaria, the ovalocytic subjects have reduced numbers of intracellular parasites in vivo.[83,131,132] In these regions, there is a decrease in the prevalence and in the disease severity of malaria in patients with SAO compared with control subjects.[133]

All SAO individuals are heterozygotes for two band 3 gene mutations in *cis*: the deletion of nine codons encoding amino acids 400 through 408 from the boundary of the cytoplasmic and membrane domains of band 3, and the 56 Lys to Glu substitution. The 56 Lys to Glu substitution represents an asymptomatic polymorphism known as band 3 Memphis. The SAO phenotype is associated with a tighter binding of band 3 to ankyrin, increased tyrosine phosphorylation of the band 3 protein, inability to transport sulfate anions, and a markedly restricted lateral and rotational mobility of band 3 protein in the membrane.[134–138]

Laboratory Evaluation

The finding of 30% or greater of oval red blood cells on the peripheral blood film, some containing a central slit or a transverse ridge, in the context of a notable absence of clinical and laboratory evidence of hemolysis in a subject from the above-noted ethnic groups is highly suggestive of the diagnosis. A useful screening test is the demonstration of the resistance of ovalocytes or their ghosts to changes in shape produced by treatments that produce spiculation in normal cells, such as metabolic depletion or exposure of ghosts to salt solutions. In contrast to normal red blood cells, which form spicules in response to such stimuli, SAO red blood cells or ghosts do not change shape after these treatments. The mechanism of this resistance to changes in shape is not clear, and it may reflect the high rigidity of the red blood cell membrane.

Because the underlying cause of SAO is the deletion of 27 bases from the band 3 gene, isolation of genomic DNA or reticulocyte cDNA with subsequent amplification of the deletion-containing region appears to be the most specific test for establishing the diagnosis of SAO.[136] Interestingly, this mutation appears to be lethal in the homozygous state, as large screens of individuals from indigenous areas have only identified heterozygotes.[139]

Molecular Basis of Southeast Asian Ovalocytosis Membrane Rigidity and Malaria Resistance

The red blood cells of SAO are unique among axially deformed cells in that they are rigid and hyperstable rather than unstable. The SAO mutation is the first example of a defect of an integral membrane protein leading to red blood cell membrane rigidity, an observation previously attributed to properties of the membrane skeleton. The basis of the increased rigidity is unclear.

The molecular basis of malaria resistance of SAO red blood cells is likely related to altered properties of the band 3 protein, which serves as one of the malaria receptors, as evidenced by the inhibition of in-vitro invasion by band 3-containing liposomes. In normal red blood cells, the invasion process is associated with a marked membrane remodeling that involves redistribution of intramembrane particles that contain band 3 protein. Such particles cluster at the site of parasite invasion, forming a ring around the orifice through which the parasite enters the cell. The invaginated red blood cell membrane, which surrounds the invading parasite, is free of intramembrane particles. The reduced lateral mobility of band 3 protein in SAO red blood cells may preclude band 3 receptor clustering, thereby preventing the attachment of the parasites to the cells. Decreased exchange of anions across the red blood cell membrane has also been proposed to contribute to the resistance of ovalocytes to malaria invasion. In addition, SAO red blood cells consume ATP at a higher rate than normal cells, and the partial depletion of ATP levels in ovalocytes has been suggested to account, at least in part, for the resistance of these cells to malaria invasion in vitro.

Acanthocytosis and Related Disorders

Acanthocytes (from the Greek *acantha*, "thorn") or spur cells are red blood cells with prominent thorn-like surface protrusions that vary in width, length, and surface distribution. Spur cells must be distinguished from echinocytes (Greek *echinos*, "urchin") or burr cells, characterized by multiple small projections that are uniformly distributed throughout the cell surface (Fig. 46–7). Acanthocytes should also be distinguished from keratocytes ("horn" red cells) that have few massive protuberances.

Acanthocytosis was first described in cases of abetalipoproteinemia and subsequently in severe liver disease, the chorea-acanthocytosis syndrome, the McLeod blood group phenotype, and other conditions. The molecular mechanisms leading to acanthocytosis in abetalipoproteinemia and severe liver disease have been extensively studied and have been attributed to changes in composition of membrane lipids and their altered distribution between the two hemileaflets of the lipid bilayer.

Spur Cell Hemolytic Anemia of Severe Liver Disease

Spur cell hemolytic anemia is an uncommon ominous complication of severe liver disease that is manifested by rapidly progressive hemolytic anemia and acanthocytes on the peripheral blood smear.

Pathobiology

The human red blood cell membrane contains nearly equal amounts of free (unesterified) cholesterol and phospholipids.[140] The free cholesterol in the plasma readily equilibrates with the red blood cell

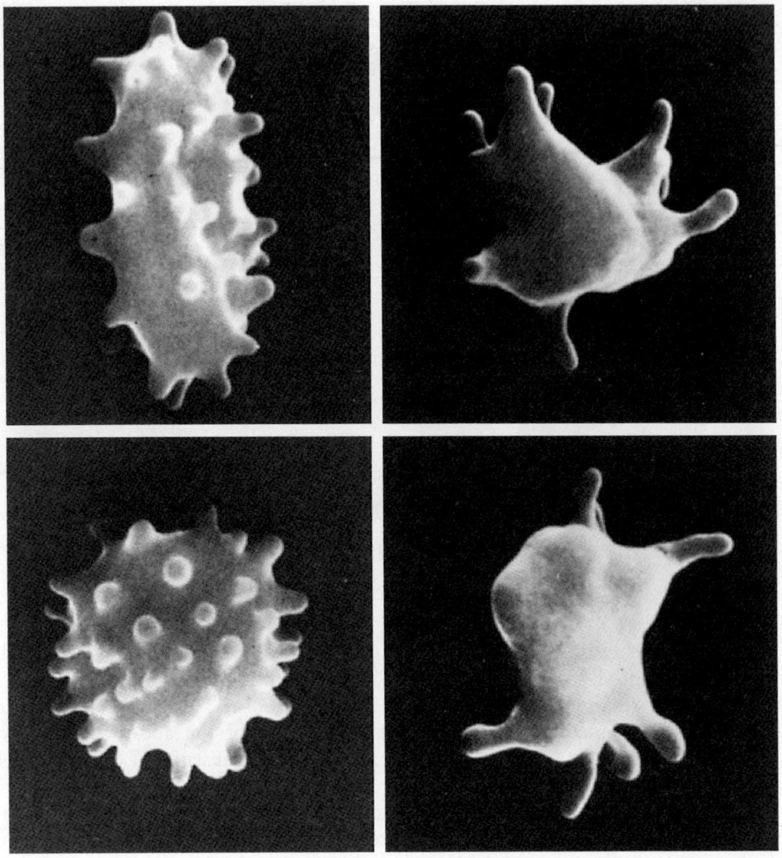

A

B

Figure 46–7 Morphologic differences between acanthocytes (**A**) and echinocytes (**B**) as demonstrated by scanning electron microscopy. *(Adapted from Bessis M: Red Cell Shapes: An Illustrated Classification and Its Rationale. New York, Springer-Verlag, 1973.)*

membrane cholesterol pool. This is in contrast to esterified cholesterol, which cannot be transferred from plasma into the red blood cell membrane. The plasma of patients with severe liver disease contains abnormal lipoproteins that have a high free cholesterol/phospholipid ratio. The excess free cholesterol readily partitions into the red blood cell membrane, leading to a marked increase in free cholesterol in the cells. Consequently, normal cells can develop a spur cell shape after their transfusion into a patient with severe liver disease or after incubation with the liver disease patient's plasma or cholesterol-enriched liposomes.

Spur cell formation involves two steps (Fig. 46–8). The first step is evident in red blood cells of splenectomized subjects with spur cell hemolytic anemia: Red blood cells have an expanded surface area with irregular contour and targeting, reflecting accumulation of free cholesterol in the membrane. This extra cholesterol accumulates preferentially in the outer bilayer leaflet, as suggested by findings of increased accessibility of cholesterol to cholesterol oxidase and a selective decrease in lipid fluidity of the outer hemileaflet of the lipid bilayer.

The second step in acanthocyte formation involves red blood cell remodeling by the spleen. As a result, red blood cells become spheroidal, and the surface projections are considerably longer and more irregular (see Fig. 46–8). The end result of these processes is poorly deformable red blood cells with long bizarre projections that are readily trapped in the spleen, which is often markedly enlarged because of passive congestion because of underlying portal hypertension.[141] Cholesterol also alters membrane permeability and interacts with several membrane skeletal proteins, but the role of these changes in spur cell lesions is unclear.

Clinical Manifestations

Most patients with chronic liver disease have a mild to moderate anemia related to gastrointestinal blood loss, iron and folic acid deficiencies, or hemodilution or as a direct effect of alcohol on red blood cell precursors.[142] Peripheral blood smears from these patients often reveal target cells that are particularly prominent in obstructive jaundice.

In some patients, particularly those with end-stage liver disease, anemia rapidly worsens and spur cells appear in high percentage in the peripheral blood. This is accompanied by worsening jaundice, rapid deterioration of liver function, hepatic encephalopathy, and hemorrhagic diatheses. A similar clinical syndrome has been described in patients with advanced metastatic liver disease, cardiac cirrhosis, Wilson disease, fulminant hepatitis, and infantile cholestatic liver disease. The development of spur cell hemolytic anemia is an ominous sign in most patients, predicting a survival seldom exceeding weeks to months.[143] In theory, splenectomy could provide a marked improvement, because the spleen is the major sequestration site of nondeformable acanthocytes; in reality, splenectomy is seldom considered because of severity of the underlying liver disease.

Abetalipoproteinemia

Definition and History

Bassen and Kornzweig first described an association of acanthocytosis with atypical retinitis pigmentosa, progressive ataxic neurologic disease, and a "celiac disease" later attributed to fat malabsorption. Subsequently, several investigators reported a congenital absence of β-lipoprotein, accounting for the diverse manifestations of the disorder.

Pathobiology

This autosomal recessive disorder has been detected in people of diverse ethnic backgrounds. The primary molecular defect involves a

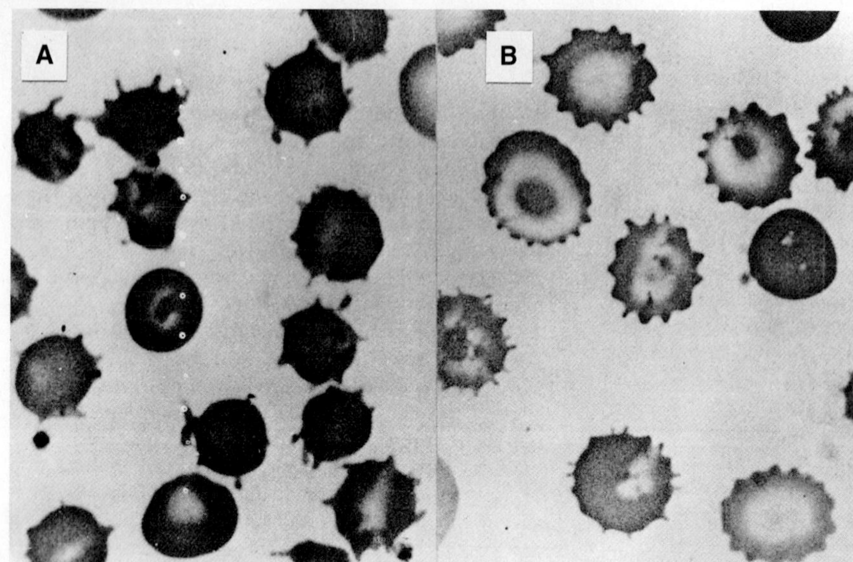

Figure 46–8 Blood film of a patient with liver cirrhosis and spur cell anemia before (**A**) and after (**B**) splenectomy. The latter smear demonstrates the effect of cholesterol acquisition leading to targeting (indicating increase in surface area) and irregularities in cell contour. The conditioning effect of the spleen (smear A) is demonstrated by the spheroidal shape of the cells and the remodeling of the spicules. *(From Cooper RA, Kimball DB, Durocher JR: The role of the spleen in membrane conditioning and hemolysis of spur cells in liver disease. N Engl J Med 290:1279, 1974.)*

congenital absence of β-apolipoprotein in plasma.[144] The B apoproteins (B100 and B48) are generated by alternate transcription of a single gene residing on the short arm of chromosome 2. Their deficiency is secondary to defective cellular secretion of the apoprotein by liver cells, caused either by aberrant posttranslational processing or by defective aposecretion. In some patients, this is because of qualitative or quantitative defects in the microsomal triglyceride transfer protein, which catalyzes the transport of triglyceride, cholesterol ester, and phospholipid from phospholipid surfaces. Microsomal triglyceride transfer protein is the only tissue-specific component, other than apolipoprotein B, required for secretion of apolipoprotein B-containing lipoproteins. As a result, apoprotein B is absent in plasma, as are the individual lipoprotein fractions that contain this apoprotein. These lipoprotein fractions include chylomicrons and very-low-density lipoproteins that transport triglycerides, as well as the low-density lipoproteins that are products of very-low-density lipoproteins and transport cholesterol. Consequently, preformed triglycerides are not transported from the intestinal mucosa, and they are nearly absent in the plasma. Plasma cholesterol and phospholipids are markedly reduced, with a relative increase in sphingomyelin at the expense of lecithin.

As is the case in acanthocytosis of liver disease, the acanthocytic lesion is acquired from the plasma. Erythrocyte precursors are of normal shape, and the acanthocytic lesion develops as the cells mature and age in the circulation.[145] Normal cells acquire this shape when transfused into the recipient.

The most striking abnormality of red blood cell membrane lipids involves a net increase in sphingomyelin. Because plasma lipids readily exchange with the lipids of the red blood cell membrane, it is likely that this change simply mirrors the alterations in plasma lipid composition. In contrast to red blood cells in spur cell anemia of severe liver disease, the content of membrane cholesterol is normal or only slightly increased.[146]

The role of membrane lipids in the acanthocyte shape transformation was first established by findings of restoration of biconcave shape after extraction of lipids from the cell membrane by detergents.[147] The molecular basis of the acanthocytic shape is unknown, but several indirect observations suggest that it is related to an increase of the surface area of the outer hemileaflet of the lipid bilayer relative to the inner leaflet. Several other abnormalities have been noted in abetalipoproteinemia, including a decrease in plasma lecithin cholesterol transferase activity and an increased susceptibility of membrane and plasma lipids to oxidation as a result of malabsorption-induced deficiency of vitamin E. The contributions of these abnormalities to the acanthocyte red cell lesions are unknown.

Clinical Manifestations

This autosomal recessive disease can become evident in the first few months of life, manifested by fat malabsorption with normal absorption of other nutrients. Intestinal biopsy is diagnostic, revealing engorgement of mucosal cells with lipid droplets. Other features include retinitis pigmentosa and a progressive ataxia with intention tremors that usually develops at 5 to 10 years of age, progressing to death in the second or third decade of life. The hematologic manifestations are mild and include mild normocytic anemia with acanthocytosis (50%–90%) and normal or slightly elevated reticulocyte counts. Occasional patients can have more severe anemia resulting from the nutritional deficiencies (iron and folate) that accompany fat malabsorption. The treatment includes dietary restriction of triglycerides and supplementation with the lipid-soluble vitamins A, K, D, and E. Vitamin E can stabilize or even improve both the retinal and neuromuscular abnormalities.

Autosomal recessive abetalipoproteinemia should be distinguished from the homozygous form of familial hypobetalipoproteinemia. Although the clinical presentation of both disorders is similar, the latter disorder is milder, and the parents have occasional acanthocytes on the peripheral blood film, and their plasma low-density lipoproteins are decreased. The molecular lesions in familial hypobetalipoproteinemia involve a variety of apoprotein B gene mutations, leading to aberrant apoprotein B gene transcription or translation.

Varying degrees of acanthocytosis without anemia have also been described with isolated deficiency of apoprotein B100.

Neuroacanthocytosis Syndromes

The neuroacanthocytosis syndromes are a group of degenerative neurologic disorders with phenotypic and genetic heterogeneity that share the feature of acanthocytes on peripheral blood smear.[148] These disorders include chorea-acanthocytosis (ChAc), the X-linked McLeod syndrome (see McLeod Phenotype below) and several other neurodegenerative diseases including Huntington disease-like 2 (HDL2) caused by mutations in junctophilin-3 and pantothenate kinase-associated neurodegeneration (formerly known as Hallervorden-Spatz syndrome and its allelic variant syndrome—hypobetalipoproteinemia, acanthocytosis, retinitis pigmentosa, pallidal degeneration [HARP]) caused by mutations in pantothenate kinase 2 (PANK2).[149,150]

Chorea-acanthocytosis syndrome is an autosomal recessive syndrome of adult onset that is manifest by multiple neurologic abnormalities, including limb chorea, progressive orofacial dyskinesia with tics, tongue-biting neurogenic muscle hypotonia, and atrophy. The hematologic manifestations are minimal and include a variable percentage of acanthocytes on the peripheral blood film without anemia and normal or only slightly decreased red blood cell survival.[151] The mechanism of acanthocytosis in this syndrome is unknown. Studies of plasma and red blood cell membrane lipids have revealed a high content of unsaturated fatty acids, presumably accounting for reduced red blood cell membrane fluidity. Additional abnormalities of uncertain significance include an uneven distribution of intramembrane particles, impaired phosphorylation of the erythrocyte actin-bundling protein dematin, abnormal accumulation of transglutaminase products, and altered function and structure of band 3.

Recently, the chorein gene (also known as CHAC or VPS13A-vacuolar protein sorting 13 homolog A) was cloned and mutations identified in affected patients.[152–154] Chorein does not belong to any known human gene family, and computer searches have not identified any known structural motifs or domains. The function of the chorein gene product remains unknown in either erythrocytes or the brain. In yeast, a chorein homologue is involved in protein sorting and transport.

McLeod Phenotype

The McLeod syndrome is characterized by a mild compensated hemolytic anemia with a variable percentage of acanthocytes on the peripheral blood film and, in some patients, late-onset myopathy or chorea.[155,156] The McLeod blood group phenotype is an X-linked anomaly of the Kell blood group system in which red blood cells, white blood cells, or both react poorly with Kell antisera. The affected cells lack Kx, the product of the *XK* gene, which appears to be a membrane precursor of the Kell antigens. The *XK* gene encodes a novel 444-amino acid integral membrane transporter. As expected, Kx is defective in McLeod patients. Male hemizygotes who lack Kx have variable acanthocytosis (8%–85%) and mild, compensated hemolysis. Because of the red blood cell mosaicism predicted by the Lyon hypothesis of X chromosome inactivation, female heterozygote carriers can have occasional acanthocytes on the peripheral blood film.[157] Lyonized women with more severe symptoms have been described.[158] Because of the susceptibility to alloimmunization, it is important to diagnose affected patients because if they are transfused, they can develop antibodies compatible only with McLeod red cells.

The McLeod syndrome has been reported in association with chronic granulomatous disease of childhood, retinitis pigmentosa, and Duchenne muscular dystrophy.[159] This association is caused by the close proximity of the genetic loci for these disorders in the p21 region of the X chromosome (Xp21), suggesting the occurrence of various manifestations because of contiguous gene syndromes. This may explain the occasional findings of either echinocytes or stomatocytes in Duchenne dystrophy, or a choreiform disorder in some subjects with the McLeod phenotype.

The Kell antigen consists of two protein components: a 37-kd protein that carries the Kx antigen, a precursor molecule necessary for the Kell antigen expression, and a 93 kd protein that carries the Kell blood group antigen.[156] Red blood cells with the McLeod phenotype have no detectable Kx antigen, and they have a marked deficiency of the 93 kd protein that carries the Kell antigen. McLeod red blood cells should be distinguished from Kell null (K_0) red blood cells, which have a normal shape. In K_0 cells, only the Kell antigen carrying the 93 kd glycoprotein is absent, whereas these cells have twice the amount of the Kx antigen. As in the other acanthocytic disorders, the surface projections of acanthocytes may be related to asymmetry of the surface area of the two lipid bilayer hemileaflets, as indicated by correction of the acanthocytosis by agents that expand the inner lipid layer, as well as the finding of an increased rate of exchange of phosphatidylcholine (localized preferentially in the outer lipid hemileaflet) with an exogenous source.

Acanthocytosis in Other Conditions

Two of eight subjects carrying the In phenotype, characterized by decreased expression of the Lutheran P1, I, and Aua blood group antigens, were reported to have acanthocytes on their peripheral blood smears. In one report, a dominantly inherited acanthocytosis was found in association with structural alterations of band 3 protein involving increased molecular size, restricted rotational diffusion, and a decrease in high-affinity binding sites for ankyrin.

Acanthocytes have also been noted in malnourished patients, including those with anorexia nervosa and cystic fibrosis. In these patients, red blood cell shape normalizes after restoration of the nutritional status. Likewise, a small number of cells with long spicules resembling acanthocytes are found in patients with hypothyroidism, after splenectomy, and with myelodysplasia.

Differentiation of Acanthocytes from Other Spiculated Red Blood Cells

Echinocytes (Burr Cells)

In contrast to acanthocytes, echinocytes, also called burr cells, have rather uniform surface projections. Although early echinocytic forms have a regularly scalloped cell contour, advanced forms of echinocytes have a spheroidal shape and the surface projections appear as short, narrow spikes (see Fig. 46–7). Although the finding of echinocytes on a peripheral blood film is often an artifact related to blood storage, contact with glass, or an elevated pH, several hemolytic anemias have been reported in association with echinocytosis on peripheral blood films. These conditions include mild hemolytic anemia in long-distance runners and in patients with hypomagnesemia and hypophosphatemia (presumably because of decreased intracellular ATP stores), uremia because of an unknown plasma factor, and pyruvate kinase deficiency.

Inspection of wet blood preparations (but not dried blood films) reveals echinocytosis in most patients with liver disease. In contrast to spur cells in patients with severe liver disease, these echinocytes have a normal cholesterol content, and the molecular abnormality may be related to the binding of abnormal echinocytogenic high-density lipoproteins to the red blood cell surface.

The mechanisms of echinocytosis in these diverse disorders are likely to be heterogeneous, as suggested by findings that many diverse factors, such as exposure of red blood cells to certain drugs, calcium loading, or ATP depletion, can induce the transformation of discocytes to echinocytes in vitro. However, in-vitro studies of the discocyte-echinocyte-stomatocyte equilibrium have suggested a possible common denominator. As discussed earlier, the lipid bilayer of normal red blood cells is asymmetric in lipid composition: The outer half of the lipid bilayer is relatively enriched in sphingomyelin and phosphatidylcholine, whereas the inner half is preferentially enriched in the negatively charged phosphatidylserine and phosphatidylethanolamine. Agents that preferentially bind to one or another class of these phospholipids dramatically influence red blood cell shape. Consequently, agents that preferentially accumulate in the outer half of the red blood cell lipid bilayer, expanding this lipid bilayer, produce an echinocytic shape, presumably by creating an asymmetry between the two surface areas of the two halves of the lipid bilayer (see Fig. 46–2). Conversely, agents that asymmetrically expand the inner half of the lipid bilayer, such as chlorpromazine, lead to stomatocytic shape transformation. In the case of echinocytes produced by ATP depletion or calcium loading, the altered phospholipid distribution between the two bilayer hemileaflets may be a consequence of calcium-induced phospholipid scrambling or a decrease in the activity of aminophospholipid translocase, an ATP-dependent enzyme that actively translocates aminophospholipids from the outer leaflet to the inner hemileaflet.

Keratocytes, Bizarre Poikilocytes, and Schistocytes

Mechanical trauma of circulating red blood cells has occasionally produced bizarre shapes resembling acanthocytes, such as cells with horny projections (keratocytes). Some acanthocyte-like cells are also seen in splenectomized HE and HS subjects. Similar shape changes are seen in heated red blood cells, in which spectrin has been damaged by thermal denaturation, suggesting that these cells are bizarre poikilocytes rather than true acanthocytes.

RED BLOOD CELL MEMBRANE DISORDERS MANIFESTED BY TARGET CELL FORMATION

The common feature of target cells is an increase in the ratio of the cell surface area to cell volume. In microcytic red blood cells of patients with various forms of thalassemia and hemoglobinopathies, the increased surface-to-volume ratio, and consequently the target cell shape, reflect, at least in part, the relative abundance of cell-surface area. In liver disease and other disorders discussed subsequently, the target cell formation reflects an absolute expansion of the cell-surface area because of a net accumulation of membrane phospholipids and cholesterol.

Liver Disease

The presence of target cells in association with either normal or slightly increased cell volume is characteristically found in patients with obstructive jaundice, including various forms of liver disease associated with intrahepatic cholestasis. These target cells have a normal survival in the peripheral circulation and do not typically account for the anemias often encountered in patients with liver disease.

In these patients, target cell formation is a consequence of a net uptake of both free cholesterol and phospholipids into the red blood cell membrane from the plasma because of abnormalities in the cholesterol/phospholipid/protein ratios of low-density lipoproteins. Target cells have a decreased osmotic fragility, as the excess of membrane surface area leads to an increase in the critical hemolytic volume.

Lecithin Cholesterol Acyltransferase Deficiency

The lecithin-cholesterol acyltransferase (LCAT) enzyme catalyzes the transfer of fatty acids from phosphatidylcholine to cholesterol. It circulates in plasma as a complex with components of high-density lipoproteins.[160] LCAT deficiency is a rare autosomal dominant disorder manifested by hyperlipidemia, premature atherosclerosis, corneal opacities, chronic nephritis, proteinuria, mild anemia, and the presence of target cells on the blood film. The anemia is caused by mild hemolysis together with a diminished compensatory erythropoiesis. As in obstructive jaundice, the target cells in LCAT deficiency have a marked increase in both cholesterol and phospholipids. In addition, the membrane phosphatidylcholine is increased at the expense of sphingomyelin and phosphatidylethanolamine. Bone marrow aspiration and biopsy reveal the presence of sea blue histiocytes. Analysis of plasma lipoproteins reveals multiple abnormalities secondary to the underlying enzyme deficiency. Inherited LCAT deficiency should be distinguished from an acquired deficiency of this enzyme, which is found in patients with severe liver disease.

Stomatocytosis and Related Disorders

Stomatocytes were first described in a girl with dominantly inherited hemolytic anemia.[161] On blood films, her red blood cells contained a wide transverse slit or stoma (Fig. 46–9). In a three-dimensional view, these cells have a shape of a cup or a bowl. The slit-like appearance is an artifact that results from folding of the cells during blood smear preparation.

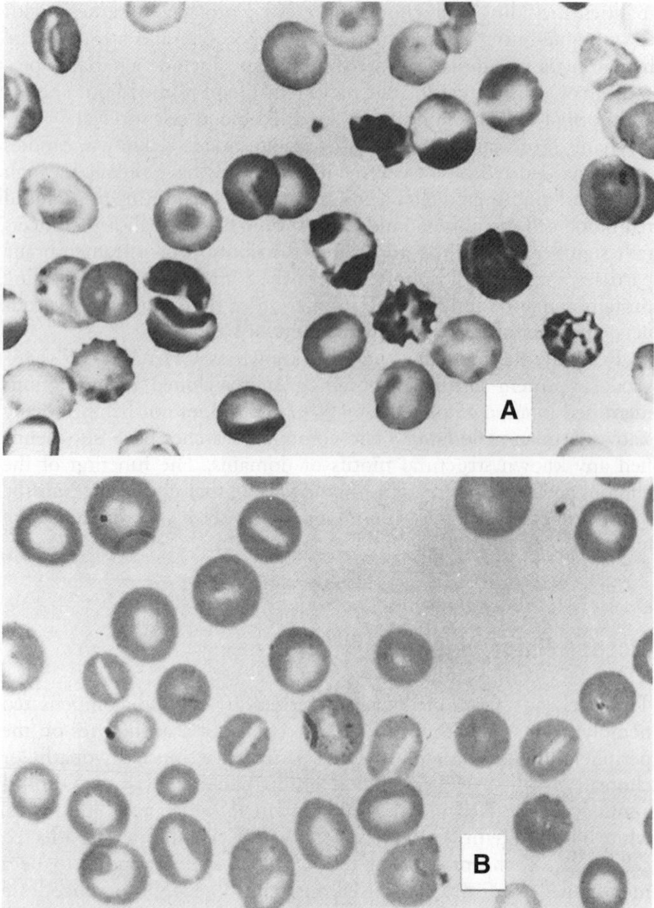

Figure 46–9 Peripheral blood smear of a patient with hereditary xerocytosis (desiccytosis) (**A**) and stomatocytosis (hydrocytosis) (**B**). *(From Lande WM, Mentzer WC: Haemolytic anaemia associated with increased cation permeability. Clin Haematol 14:89, 1985.)*

Stomatocytes are seen in a variety of acquired and inherited disorders. The latter are often associated with abnormalities in red blood cell cation permeability that lead to changes in red blood cell volume, which can be either increased (hence the designation hydrocytosis) or decreased (desiccytosis or xerocytosis), or, in some cases, near normal.[162–164]

There is no unifying theory to explain this morphologic abnormality. In vitro, stomatocytes can be produced by drugs that preferentially intercalate into the inner half of the asymmetric lipid bilayer, expanding its surface area relative to that of the outer half of the bilayer.

Hereditary Stomatocytosis-Hydrocytosis

Hereditary hydrocytosis designates a seemingly heterogeneous group of hereditary hemolytic anemias that are transmitted in an autosomal dominant mode in most patients.[163,164] The disorder is characterized by a moderate to severe hemolytic anemia with 10% to 30% stomatocytes (see Fig. 46–9), an elevated MCV, and a reduced MCHC. Osmotic fragility of red blood cells is markedly increased, as some of the swollen red blood cells approach their critical hemolytic volume. For unexplained reasons, red blood cell membrane lipids and, consequently, membrane surface area are also increased, but this increase in surface area is insufficient to correct the osmotic fragility of the red blood cells. Red blood cell deformability is decreased.

The principal cellular lesion involves a marked increase in intracellular sodium and water content with a mild decrease in intracellular potassium as a result of a marked sodium influx into the red blood cells. Despite a marked compensatory increase in active transport of sodium (Na) and potassium by the Na^+/K^+-ATPase (which normally maintains the low sodium and high concentrations in the cells) and an ensuing increase in glycolysis, the pump hyperactivity is unable to compensate for the vastly increased sodium leak. The molecular basis of this permeability defect is unknown. Stomatin (also known as band 7.2b), an integral membrane protein, is decreased or absent from the erythrocyte membranes of affected patients. This deficiency appears to be a maturational loss in the bone marrow and in the circulation, perhaps because of a defect in cellular trafficking.[165,166] Stomatin gene mutations have not been found in unrelated stomatocytosis patients deficient in this protein.[165]

Splenectomy can improve, but not fully correct, the hemolysis. In some patients, splenectomy can be deleterious or even contraindicated (see later),[167] perhaps because of altered endothelial cell adherence and membrane phospholipid asymmetry.[168]

Hereditary Xerocytosis and the Intermediate Syndromes

Hereditary xerocytosis or desiccytosis describes an autosomal dominant hemolytic anemia characterized by red blood cell dehydration and decreased osmotic fragility.[162,164] Affected individuals have characteristically moderate to severe hemolysis with an increased MCHC, reflecting cellular dehydration. Hydrops fetalis with fetal anemia or fetal ascites has been reported in a number of xerocytosis kindreds. Frequently, the MCV is mildly increased. In Coulter-type electronic counters, the conversion of pulse height (from the resistance of a cell passing through an electric field) to a cellular volume is dependent on cell shape. Xerocytes do not deform to the same degree as normal cells, which causes the MCV to be approximately 10% too high. The peripheral blood film (see Fig. 46–9) does not always reveal stomatocytes (which are more prominent on wet films), but frequently target cells, desiccocyte, and spiculated cells are seen. In some of the cells, hemoglobin is concentrated ("puddled") in discrete areas on the cell periphery.

The mechanism of cellular dehydration is unclear and complex, involving a net potassium loss from the cells that is not accompanied by a proportional gain of sodium. Consequently, the net intracellular cation content and cell water are decreased. In some reports, a decrease in red blood cell 2,3-DPG has also been noted. The gene for xerocytosis has been mapped to 16q23–q24.[169] A clinical syndrome of xerocytosis, perinatal ascites, and pseudohyperkalemia has been described.[162] Genetic studies of patients with this constellation of disorders and with isolated pseudohyperkalemia also show linkage to this region.

Some of the reported cases of hereditary stomatocytosis share features of both hereditary stomatocytosis and xerocytosis categorized as "intermediate" syndromes. These patients characteristically have both stomatocytes and some target cells on the peripheral blood smear. Osmotic fragility is either normal or slightly increased. Sodium and potassium permeability is somewhat increased, but the intracellular cation concentration and the red blood cell volume are either normal or slightly reduced. These cells were reported to have subnormal glutathione content. In some patients, red blood cells undergo in-vitro hemolysis at 5°C (41°F), hence the designation cryohydrocytosis.[170] A similar susceptibility to cold-induced cation permeability in which potassium and water loss predominates, and xerocytes instead of hydrocytes are present has also been described.

A study of stomatocytosis, spherocytosis, and spherostomatocytosis patients whose erythrocytes demonstrated significant cation leaks at 0°C (32°F)and in some cases, band 3-deficient membranes, revealed a series of missense mutations located in an intramembrane domain of band 3.[171] In-vitro studies suggest that these mutations convert band 3 from an anion exchanger to a nonselective cation leak channel.[171,172]

Several investigators have also reported a dominantly inherited hemolytic anemia with stomatocytosis, occasional target cells, spherocytes, and a decreased osmotic fragility in which the main red blood cell membrane abnormality involved a nearly 50% increase in phosphatidylcholine and a corresponding decrease in phosphatidyl-ethanolamine.[173] Because abnormalities in membrane phospholipid composition have not been systematically investigated, it is uncertain whether the disorder represents a distinct disease entity.

The results of splenectomy in this group of disorders are variable. In some patients the hemolytic anemia is improved, although often not fully corrected, by splenectomy, whereas in others the severity of the hemolysis is unchanged. Splenectomy should be carefully considered in patients with hereditary stomatocytosis. Several patients with stomatocytosis (both hydrocytosis and xerocytosis) have developed hypercoagulability after splenectomy, leading to catastrophic thrombotic episodes or chronic pulmonary hypertension.[167] Fortunately, the majority of persons with hereditary stomatocytosis are able to maintain an adequate hemoglobin level, so that splenectomy is not required.

Rh Deficiency Syndrome

Rh deficiency syndrome designates rare individuals who have either absent (Rh_{null}) or markedly reduced (Rh_{mod}) Rh antigen expression, mild to moderate hemolytic anemia associated with the presence of stomatocytes, and occasional spherocytes on the peripheral blood film. Hemolytic anemia is improved by splenectomy.

The Rh antigens are present in approximately 20,000 to 30,000 copies per cell and reside on minor transmembrane proteins with an electrophoretic mobility of 28 to 33 kd on SDS-PAGE. The Rh gene locus encodes two closely linked genes, one encoding the D polypeptide and the other encoding the Cc,Ee proteins, the antigenic expression of which is a consequence of alternate splicing of their pre-mRNA.[174]

Rh proteins are part of a multiprotein complex that includes two Rh proteins and two Rh-associated glycoproteins (RhAG). Other proteins that associate with this complex include CD47, LW, glycophorin B, and protein 4.2.[175] The Rh-RhAG complex interacts with ankyrin to link the membrane skeleton to the lipid bilayer. The Rh proteins share sequence homology to the Mep/Amt family of ammonium transporters in lower organisms and may participate in ammonium transport.[176]

Rh_{null} erythrocytes have no Rh antigen and have reduced or absent LW, Fy5, Ss, U, and Duclos antigens. Rh, RhAG, LW, glycophorin B, CD47, and protein 4.2 are also reduced or absent. Rh_{null} erythrocytes have increased osmotic fragility, reflecting a marked reduction in membrane surface area.[177] These cells are also dehydrated, as indicated by decreased cell cation and water content and increased cell density. The potassium transport and the Na^+/K^+ pump activity are increased, possibly because of reticulocytosis. Phospholipid asymmetry is also altered.

Although the clinical syndromes are the same, the genetic basis of the Rh deficiency syndrome is heterogeneous, and at least two groups have been defined. The *amorph type* is caused by defects involving the *RH30* locus encoding the RhD and RhE polypeptides. The *regulatory type* of Rh_{null} and Rh_{mod} phenotypes results from suppressor or *modifier* mutations at the *RH50* locus. When one chain of the Rh-RhAG complex is absent, the complex either is not transported to or is assembled at the membrane.

Familial Deficiency of High-Density Lipoproteins

Familial deficiency or absence of high-density lipoproteins (Tangier disease) because of mutations in ABCA1, a protein involved in cellular export of cholesterol, leads to accumulation of cholesterol esters in many tissues. Clinical manifestations include large orange tonsils, hepatosplenomegaly, lymphadenopathy, cloudy corneas, and peripheral neuropathy.[178] Reported hematologic manifestations include a moderately severe hemolytic anemia with stomatocytosis and thrombocytopenia. Erythrocyte membrane lipid analyses reveal a low free cholesterol content, leading to a decreased cholesterol/phospholipid ratio and a relative increase in phosphatidylcholine at the expense of sphingomyelin.

Sitosterolemia

Sitosterolemia or phytosterolemia is a recessive disorder associated with elevated plasma levels of plant sterols.[179] Affected patients exhibit xanthomatosis and early onset premature cardiovascular disease. Reported hematologic manifestations include hemolytic anemia with stomatocytosis and macrothrombocytopenia.[180] Mutations in the transporters ABCG5 or ABCG8 lead to gastrointestinal hyperabsorption and decreased biliary elimination of plant sterols as well as altered cholesterol metabolism. Plant sterols are not synthesized endogenously in humans, but are passively absorbed in the intestine.[181] ABCG5 and ABCG8 actively pump plant sterols out of the intestinal cells back into the intestine and out of liver cells into bile ducts. It has been suggested that the stomatocytic phenotype is caused by intercalation of plant sterols into the inner leaflet of the lipid bilayer.

Acquired Stomatocytosis

Stomatocytes have been noted in diverse acquired conditions, including neoplasms, cardiovascular and hepatobiliary disease, alcoholism, and therapy with drugs, some of which are known to be stomatocytogenic in vitro. In some of these conditions, the percentage of stomatocytes on the peripheral blood smear can approach 100%. However, the clinical significance of this observation is unclear because stomatocytes are absent in most patients with the conditions listed. Furthermore, some stomatocytes can be found in normal individuals (3%–5%). The most consistent association is that of stomatocytosis and heavy alcohol consumption.

RED CELL MEMBRANE VARIANTS AND INFECTIOUS DISEASE

Viral, bacterial, and parasitic infection can all cause anemia. Multiple mechanisms leading to hemolysis have been described. As mentioned earlier in this chapter, parvovirus B19 selectively infects erythroblasts through interaction with globoside, which encodes the P blood group antigen and temporarily shuts down erythropoiesis.[62] Although this infection is tolerated well by healthy subjects, it can lead to severe, at times life-threatening, aplastic crises in patients with anemias because of premature erythrocyte destruction. As one might predict, parvovirus cannot invade erythroblasts of the rare p-negative individuals.[182]

Most infections cause hemolytic anemias triggered by several distinct, and at times overlapping, mechanisms. *Plasmodium, Babesia,* and *Bartonella* species directly attack the membrane and lyse the red cells. Some bacteria, such as *Clostridium perfringens,* elaborate hemolytic toxins or phospholipases that damage the membrane. Other infectious agents trigger occasional production of autoantibodies against red cell membrane components, which in turn leads to autoimmune hemolytic anemia. Finally, many sepsis syndromes are associated with anemia because of disseminated intravascular coagulation.

Malaria and the Erythrocyte Membrane

The red cell membrane defects described earlier in this chapter cause mild to severe hemolytic anemias. At the same time, many red cell membrane alterations have developed as a defense against microorganisms and parasites invading and lysing red cells. This is especially true for malarial parasites. Although four different species of the malaria parasite *Plasmodium*, including *P. falciparum, P. ovale, P. vivax*, and *P. malariae*, infect humans, almost all of the 1.5 to 2 million annual deaths caused by malaria are attributable to *P. falciparum*.

Because malaria coexisted with humans over the course of human evolution, it comes as no surprise that multiple erythroid genotypes were selected that confer some level of resistance to infection or mitigate disease severity. The ensuing heritable phenotypes include, among others, resistance to red cell adhesion and/or invasion, slower intraerythrocytic growth, decreased or increased adhesion of infected red cells to vascular endothelium or increased phagocytosis of parasitized red cells.

Malaria and other infections causing hemolytic anemias are described in more detail in chapters (37, 44) that also discuss hemoglobinopathies and red cell enzyme variants that reduce invasion and/or retard parasite growth. Consequently, we focus here on the heritable erythrocyte membrane alterations that developed as a defense against malaria.

Erythrocyte Preference

Two parasites, *P. vivax* and *P. ovale*, selectively infect reticulocytes, whereas *P. malariae* infect older erythrocytes. In contrast, *P. falciparum* infects red cells of all ages. This fact and the tendency of *P. falciparum*-infected erythrocytes to sequester in circulation explain the markedly higher severity of *P. falciparum* malaria.

Attachment and Invasion

Duffy Antigen

The *P. vivax* merozoite is completely dependent of attachment to the Duffy blood group antigen (also know as the Duffy antigen receptor for chemokines [DARC]) for erythrocyte invasion and, consequently, it cannot invade Duffy-negative red blood cells.[183] It has been hypothesized this is why the Duffy-negative phenotype is common in large areas of Africa. The Duffy-negative phenotype is caused by mutation in a GATA1 motif in the Duffy antigen gene promoter, preventing its expression in erythroid cells,[184] leaving its expression in other tissues intact. Elucidation of this mutation explained a longstanding conundrum of transfusion medicine: why individuals with the Duffy-negative phenotype never develop antibodies against the Duffy antigen.

Glycophorins

All major erythrocyte glycophorins, A, B, and C/D, are involved in attachment of *P. falciparum* to the red blood cell membrane. Consequently, invasion of *P. falciparum* into red cells from subjects lacking glycophorin A (En(a–)), glycophorin B (S-s-U-), or glycophorins C and D (Gerbich negative, Ge–) is diminished. As noted above, the Gerbich-negative phenotype is associated with mild, asymptomatic ovalocytosis.

Protein 4.1R and Spectrin

Deficiency of protein 4.1R or self-association defects of spectrin are associated with elliptocytosis of varying severity. Both phenotypes appear to reduce the red blood cell invasion.[185]

Band 3 and Southeast Asian Ovalocytosis

Conflicting explanations of the basis of the protective phenotype of Southeast Asian ovalocytosis (described above) from malaria have been described. Initial reports suggested that SAO erythrocytes were resistant to malarial invasion. These results were repeatedly questioned until recent studies demonstrated SAO cells to be resistant to invasion by the more virulent *P. falciparum* strains. This may explain the apparent contradiction with the reports of comparable parasitemias in SAO carriers and subjects with a normal red cell phenotype from Papua, New Guinea.

The protection from cerebral malaria afforded by SAO erythrocytes is likely because of reduced cytoadherence of SAO red cells to the cerebral vasculature. Under conditions of flow, *P. falciparum*-infected ovalocytes adhere more strongly than normal infected red cells to the endothelial receptor CD36.[186] As this receptor is not expressed in the brain, this raises a possibility that ovalocytosis protects from cerebral malaria by diminishing the number of parasitized red cells available for adhesion to the cerebral vasculature via alternative receptors. Moreover, ovalocytes appeared resistant to invasion by parasite strains that tend to bind to ICAM-1, the likely receptor for cytoadherence in the brain,[187] but the exact mechanism is not yet known.

Knops Blood Group System

Severe malaria, particularly cerebral malaria, has been associated with the formation of rosettes, clumps of cells formed by the adhesion of malaria-infected erythrocytes to complement receptor 1 (CR1) on uninfected erythrocytes. Identification of the Knops blood group antigens on CR1, followed by observations that frequencies of various Knops antigens varied significantly in whites and individuals of African ancestry, led to the hypothesis that some Knops group antigens might be protective from rosetting and severe malaria.[188] Case control studies with genotyping and/or flow cytometry have yielded conflicting results, but several have linked low-expression CR1 alleles with malaria resistance. Further studies have shown that the expression of CR1 and other complement proteins increase with age. Together, these data suggest that genetic and age-related differences in complement protein expression contribute to the variability observed in individuals with severe malaria.[189]

Although these erythrocyte membrane polymorphisms offer fascinating insight into natural defenses against one of the most serious diseases affecting humans, the mechanism of resistance to malaria has not been fully elucidated for any of them. Malaria has clearly had a profound impact on the genetic makeup of populations living in endemic areas and provided us with multiple clues about the host-parasite relationship. Better understanding of these natural defenses might eventually be converted into effective therapeutic interventions.

SUGGESTED READINGS

Dhermy D, Schrevel J, Lecomte MC: Spectrin-based skeleton in red blood cells and malaria. Curr Opin Hematol 14:198, 2007.

Edelman EJ, Maksimova Y, Duru F, Altay C, Gallagher PG: A complex splicing defect associated with homozygous ankyrin-deficient hereditary spherocytosis. Blood 109:5491, 2007.

Guizouarn, H, Martial S, Gabillat N, Borgese F: Point mutations involved in red cell stomatocytosis convert the electroneutral anion exchanger 1 to a non-selective cation conductance. Blood 2007.

Jenkins N, Wu Y, Chakravorty S, et al: Plasmodium falciparum intercellular adhesion molecule-1-based cytoadherence-related signaling in human endothelial cells. J Infect Dis 196:321, 2007.

Johnson CP, Gaetani M, Ortiz V, et al: Pathogenic proline mutation in the linker between spectrin repeats: Disease caused by spectrin unfolding. Blood 109:3538, 2007.

Peng J, Redman CM, Wu X, et al: Insights into extensive deletions around the XK locus associated with McLeod phenotype and characterization of two novel cases. Gene 392:142, 2007.

Perrotta S, Gallagher PG, Narla M: Hereditary spherocytosis. Lancet in press 371: In press, 2008.

Smedema JP, Louw VJ: Pulmonary arterial hypertension after splenectomy for hereditary spherocytosis. Cardiovasc J S Afr 18:84, 2007.

Walker RH, Jung HH, Dobson-Stone C, et al: Neurologic phenotypes associated with acanthocytosis. Neurology 68:92, 2007.

Wang DQ: Regulation of intestinal cholesterol absorption. Annu Rev Physiol 69:221, 2007.

REFERENCES

For complete list of references log onto www.expertconsult.com

CHAPTER 47

AUTOIMMUNE HEMOLYTIC ANEMIA

Amy Powers and Leslie E. Silberstein

Autoimmune hemolytic anemia (AIHA) represents a spectrum of disorders in which antibodies against self-antigens on the erythrocyte membrane cause a shortened red blood cell (RBC) lifespan. The antigens targeted often have a high incidence so that both native and transfused RBCs are destroyed.[1] Three types of AIHA can be distinguished based on their serologic properties and clinical characteristics (Table 47–1). IgG warm autoantibodies bind to erythrocytes at 37°C (99°F) but fail to agglutinate the cells; cold agglutinins, almost always of the IgM isotype, clump RBCs at cold temperatures and occasionally lead to hemolysis; and the IgG Donath-Landsteiner antibody binds to RBC membranes in the cold and activates the hemolytic complement cascade when the cells are warmed to 37°C (99°F). All three can occur as an idiopathic (primary) disorder or can coexist with another disease (secondary). AIHA can follow administration of certain drugs (drug induced). This chapter refers to the hemolytic diseases associated with warm-reactive IgG autoantibodies as *warm autoimmune hemolytic anemia* (WAIHA), to the hemolytic anemias caused by cold-reactive IgM autoantibodies as *cold agglutinin disease*, and to the syndromes associated with the Donath-Landsteiner antibody as *paroxysmal cold hemoglobinuria* (PCH).

HISTORICAL BACKGROUND

PCH was the first recognized form of hemolytic anemia, probably because its clinical manifestation, the passage of black urine after exposure to the cold, was so striking. Descriptions of patients with attacks of hemoglobinuria after exposure to cold temperatures, including the case of a 10-year-old boy with chromaturie,[2] began to appear between 1854 and 1865 in the medical literature.[2,3]

The association of PCH with syphilis was first noted in 1884 by Gotze,[4] but nothing else of the cause of the disease was known until 1904, when Donath and Landsteiner[5] reported their landmark work. They described three cases of PCH in which an autolysin bound to the patient's RBCs in the cold, and a heat-labile serum factor (now known to be hemolytic complement components) lysed the sensitized erythrocytes when the temperature was raised to 37°C (99°F). They later proved the P antigen of RBCs to be the target in cases of both syphilitic and nonsyphilitic PCH.[6]

In 1908, Moreschi[7] developed the equivalent of the antiglobulin test, or what is now referred to as the *Coombs test.* He developed and tested it on animal RBCs. His animal studies were ignored for almost 40 years. The antiglobulin test, designed to detect nonagglutinating antierythrocyte antibodies on human cells, was introduced by Coombs et al.[8] in 1945. Within 1 year it was applied to the clinical diagnosis of AIHA.[9] Recognition of both idiopathic and secondary forms occurred early. In one of the first collections of 175 cases retrospectively studied by Dacie,[10] 71% were described as idiopathic, a number not very different today.

EPIDEMIOLOGY

The incidence of AIHA is estimated to be approximately 1:100,000 in adults[1] and less than 0.2:100,000[11] in children. It is less common than immune thrombocytopenia.[12] AIHA in teenagers and adults is more common in women than in men. The peak incidence in pediatric patients occurs in preschool-age children.[11] Boys are 2.5 times more likely to be affected than are girls.[13] In children, occurrences in patients younger than 2 years and older than 12 years are more likely to have a chronic unremitting course.[11] However, the majority of pediatric cases are acute in onset and self-limiting. Often these cases resolve within 6 months without treatment,[11] and the decision to treat is based on the degree of anemia and physiologic compromise. Approximately 50% to 70% of cases are idiopathic,[14] occurring at all ages, but the highest prevalence occurs in midlife. Some cases of AIHA are induced by drugs; others occur simultaneously with another autoimmune disease, particularly systemic lupus erythematosus. A substantial proportion of cases develop in patients with B-cell lymphoma or chronic lymphocytic leukemia (CLL). Treatment of the underlying malignancy often can resolve the AIHA.[15] In other instances, presumably by affecting T cells more than B cells, medications used to treat malignancies trigger the onset of hemolytic anemia.[16]

A retrospective analysis of 83 adult patients reviewed the epidemiology.[17] Sixty-seven percent of cases of AIHA occurred in women. Warm-reactive antibodies were the causative agent in 87% and cold-reactive in 13%. Of the WAIHA cases, 43% of antibodies were reactive with complement and IgG, 32% against IgG, and 25% against complement alone. Fifty-one percent of cases were secondary; systemic lupus erythematosus and non-Hodgkin lymphoma were each the primary diagnosis in 38% of those cases. The presence of hypogammaglobulinemia was significantly associated with non-Hodgkin lymphoma and prompted further workup, including chest and abdominal computed tomographic scans. The onset of hemolysis in this review preceded the diagnosis of lymphoma by a range of 22 to 66 months. No cases of PCH were reported in the review of these cases occurring between 1980 and 2000. Of the 15.6% of patients who died, 38% died of infectious complications and the same percentage of non-Hodgkin lymphoma, but none directly due to physiologic compromise of decreased oxygen-carrying capacity.

Few large studies of AIHA in children have been undertaken. A retrospective review of 100 cases of childhood AIHA (age range 6 months to 16 years) diagnosed over a 20-year period revealed a peak incidence in the first 4 years of life.[1] No sex predilection was observed. The majority of patients (64%) were diagnosed with WAIHA, whereas cold agglutinin disease and PCH accounted for 26% and 6% of children, respectively. A mixed type of AIHA was observed in four subjects. Overall, 54% of children had coexisting disease, including hematologic disorders, autoimmune disease, infection, and neoplasia. All cases of PCH were associated with a recent viral illness.[18]

WARM AUTOIMMUNE HEMOLYTIC ANEMIA

Pathophysiology

Immune Clearance of Erythrocytes

The serologic specificities of the autoantibodies that cause RBC destruction in patients with AIHA can be identical to the autoantibodies causing no discernible signs of hemolysis in healthy persons. Therefore, the pathogenicity of anti-RBC autoantibodies must depend on additional factors, including the amount of autoantibody, its avidity for the erythrocyte autoantigen, and its ability to fix complement.[19] Each of these factors may contribute independently and cumulatively to the erythrocyte lesion.

Table 47–1 Characteristics of Autoimmune Hemolytic Anemia

	Type of Autoimmune Hemolytic Anemia		
Characteristic	**Warm Autoimmune Hemolytic Anemia**	**Cold Agglutinin Disease**	**Paroxysmal Cold Hemoglobinuria**
Antibody isotype	IgG, rare IgA, IgM	IgM	IgG
Direct antiglobulin test (DAT) result	IgG and/or C3	C3	C3
Antigen specificity	Multiple, primarily Rh	i/I, Pr	P
Hemolysis	Primarily extravascular	Primarily extravascular	Intravascular
Common disease associations	B-cell neoplasia/lymphoproliferative, collagen–vascular	Viral, neoplasia	Syphilis, viral

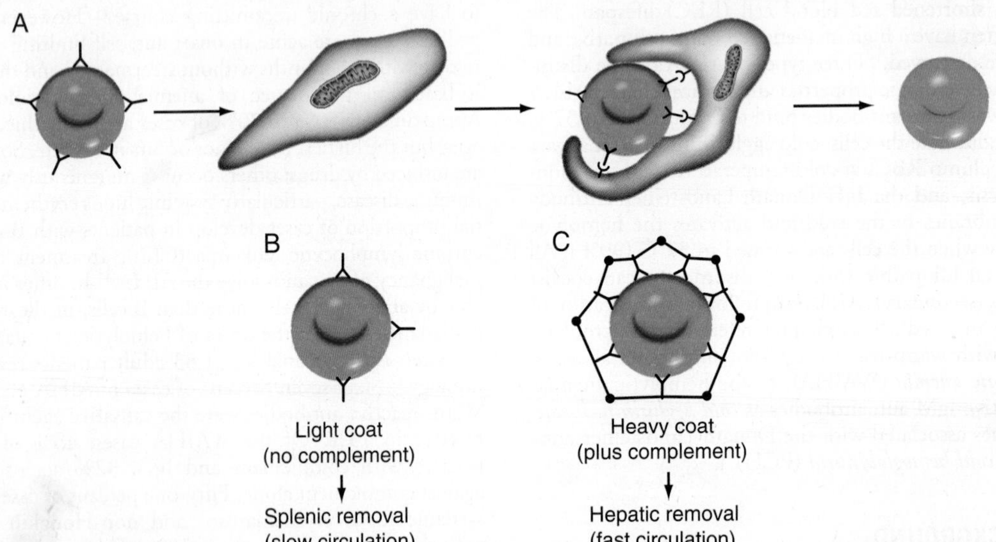

Figure 47–1 Mechanism of extravascular hemolysis in autoimmune hemolytic anemia. **A,** Macrophage encounters an IgG-coated erythrocyte and binds to it via its Fc receptors. Thus entrapped, the red blood cell (RBC) loses bits of its membrane as a result of digestion by the macrophage's ectoenzymes. The discoid erythrocyte transforms into a sphere. **B,** RBC lightly coated with IgG (and therefore incapable of activating the complement cascade) is preferentially removed in the sluggish circulation of the spleen. **C,** RBC with a heavy coat of IgG; thus, C3b (black circles) can be removed by both the spleen and the liver.

Immune hemolysis in vivo begins with opsonization by autoantibodies. The terminal effect can be destruction of the RBC directly within the circulation (intravascular hemolysis), removal of the cell from the circulation by tissue macrophages in the liver or spleen (extravascular hemolysis; Fig. 47–1), or both. The interaction of macrophages with RBCs coated with IgG and/or C3b occurs through receptors specific for the Fc portion of IgG (especially IgG1 and IgG3) and for C3b.[20,21] The presence of both IgG and C3b accelerates immune clearance,[22] suggesting that Fc and C3b macrophage receptors act synergistically.

Red Blood Cell Destruction

The macrophage may ingest an opsonized RBC entirely. More likely, proteolytic enzymes on its surface digest bits of the erythrocyte membrane producing a spherocyte, an RBC with the lowest possible surface area-to-volume ratio.[21] Spherocytes are less deformable and more susceptible to osmotic lysis than disk-shaped RBCs and thus are especially susceptible to hemolysis during their travels through the sluggish circulation of the splenic sinusoids. This is why the predominant mechanism of destruction of erythrocytes coated with IgG with or without C3b occurs extravascularly in cases of AIHA.

Macrophage-mediated mechanisms predominate in causing the lesion of AIHA, but the participation of cytotoxic lymphocytes (natural killer cells), which cause antibody-dependent cell lysis, has not been excluded. The efficiency of reticuloendothelial function probably also contributes to the degree of immune clearance and may account for exacerbations concurrent with viral or bacterial infections.[23,24]

Isotype Influence

Attachment of antibody to the surface of the RBC may lead to intravascular, extravascular, or no hemolysis. The degree of hemolysis is influenced by both the antigen and the antibody. The density and expression of the target antigen are important, as are the quantity, specificity, thermal amplitude, and ability to fix complement and bind tissue macrophages of the antibody.[1] Thus, the class or subclass of antibody attached is a crucial determinant of pathology. IgA, IgM, IgG1, and IgG3 can fix complement. If complement is activated through the C5 to C9 membrane attack complex, intravascular hemolysis occurs. Regulatory mechanisms at the level of C4b/C3b can arrest the cascade and prevent hemolysis.[25] IgG1 and IgG3 are recognized by Fc receptors of phagocytes and therefore can cause extravascular hemolysis.[1] RBCs coated with simply antibody or C3b are phagocytized by macrophages and destroyed extravascularly in the spleen and liver, respectively. IgG-coated cells are destroyed primarily in the spleen and IgM-coated cells in the liver.[14]

Under certain circumstances, IgM can activate complement and cause severe intravascular hemolysis. However, extravascular hemolysis predominates because the pathogenic effect is modulated by the RBC regulatory proteins decay accelerating factor (CD55) and membrane inhibitor of reactive lysis (CD59), which can eliminate hemolysis.[1] Complement components remain attached to the RBC membrane after incomplete intravascular activation and cytolysis and are targets of the extravascular reticuloendothelial phagocytes.[1] IgM antibodies reacting optimally at 37°C (99°F) in the absence of IgG antibodies are exceedingly rare, yet they occur in 2% to 73% of cases of AIHA in conjunction with IgG antibodies. Although IgM antibodies usually mediate cold agglutinin disease and often have a more indolent course, cases of warm-reactive fatal IgM-mediated hemolysis have been reported in the literature.[26,27] These cases warrant very aggressive intervention. The reported surviving patient was treated with high-dose prednisone, intravenous Ig, and exchange transfusion.[27] Warm IgA hemolytic antibodies are reported in 14% to 21% of cases in combination with IgG antibodies.[28] Alone, their incidence is less than 0.2%.[28] This finding underscores the need to perform further testing for IgA or IgM autoantibodies in cases that are negative by the direct antiglobulin test (DAT) but clinically appear to be AIHA so that appropriate prompt management can be instituted.

The mechanism of IgA-mediated intravascular hemolysis is not completely understood. Complement activation by the classic and alternative complement pathways can be caused by IgA. In addition, Fc receptors for IgA have been discovered on human lymphocytes, granulocytes, and monocytes[29] and presumably mediate extravascular hemolysis.

Pathophysiology of Secondary AIHA

A CTLA-4 exon polymorphism has been associated with autoimmune diseases and was demonstrated to be present at a statistically significant increased prevalence in patients with AIHA, especially in cases secondary to CLL.[16,30] The CTLA-4 molecule is an important downregulator of T-cell antigen responses. The polymorphism with the substitution (Thr→Ala) at codon 17 appears to confer susceptibility to autoimmunity. AIHA occurs in patients with primary immune deficiencies, more commonly in patients with antibody defects such as common variable immunodeficiency and IgA deficiency. A number of other diseases also are complicated by AIHA (Table 47–2).[31]

As more diseases are treated with bone marrow and peripheral blood stem cell transplantation, the number of cases of posttransplant autoimmune hemolysis is expected to increase. A study of adult patients who received T-cell–depleted allogeneic bone marrow transplants revealed a 5% incidence of AIHA in patients surviving 6 months.[32] In a more recent study, the 3-year cumulative incidence of AIHA in a series of 272 adult hematopoietic stem cell transplant patients was 4.44%.[33] Factors associated with the development of AIHA in this population included transplant from an unrelated donor and the development of chronic extensive graft-versus-host disease.[33] The incidence in children is similar, with AIHA occurring in 6% of pediatric recipients undergoing unrelated donor hematopoietic cell transplantation.[34] The timing of development of AIHA after bone marrow transplantation depends on the antibody mediating the hemolysis, possibly because IgM reconstitutes earlier than IgG. In the posttransplant setting, three distinct mechanisms can account for hemolysis: true autoimmune hemolysis, immune hemolysis mediated by passenger lymphocytes, and immune hemolysis in the setting of chimerism and major blood group mismatch (Table 47–3).[35] Investigations to determine the cause of hemolysis will appropriately direct therapy, expected duration, and prevention.[35]

Clinical Findings

The clinical findings in WAIHA are variable. They are determined by the rate of hemolysis and the ability of the body to process breakdown products and mount a reticulocytosis. Some signs are associated with hyperdynamic circulation secondary to anemia and concomitant decreased oxygen-carrying capacity. They include hepatomegaly and, in more severe cases, pulmonary edema, lethargy, and obtundation. Splenomegaly can occur due to an increase in white pulp. Jaundice and fever are caused by cytokines and breakdown products. Rather than injury due to free hemoglobin, vasoconstriction and decreased renal perfusion lead to renal insufficiency.

Table 47–2 Diseases Rarely Associated with Autoimmune Hemolytic Anemia

Collagen vascular disease
Rheumatoid arthritis
Scleroderma
Polyarteritis nodosa
Serum sickness
Sjögren syndrome
Lymphoreticular malignancy
Macroglobulinemia
Hodgkin lymphoma
Multiple myeloma
Mycosis fungoides
Other malignancy
Acute leukemia
Thymoma
Carcinoma (colon, kidney, lung, ovary)
Miscellaneous diseases
Myelofibrosis with myeloid metaplasia
Ulcerative colitis
Pernicious anemia
Thyroid disease
Ovarian cysts
Mucocutaneous lymph node syndrome (Kawasaki disease)
Evans syndrome (thrombocytopenia and hemolytic anemia)
Congenital immunodeficiency syndromes
Guillain-Barré syndrome
Primary biliary cirrhosis
Multiply transfused patients with hemoglobinopathies

The disease can occur acutely, with symptoms caused by rapidly developing anemia, or it can develop gradually in a relatively asymptomatic form. Occasionally, the blood bank provides the diagnosis through a positive antiglobulin test in a patient referred for transfusion therapy. Lymphadenopathy, fever, hypertension, renal failure, rash, petechiae, or ecchymoses should alert the physician to the possibility of a secondary AIHA and warrant a search for an underlying disease.

Laboratory Evaluation

Differentiating AIHA from other forms of hemolytic anemia based on laboratory data alone may be difficult. The DAT, also known as the *Coombs test,* is considered pathognomonic of immune-mediated hemolysis. This assay detects the presence of IgG or complement bound to the RBC membrane (Fig. 47–2). In patients with severe AIHA, the DAT results may be strongly positive, but the strength of the reaction and titer of the autoantibody do not always predict the severity of disease. A false-negative result may be observed in some situations, including cases attributed to low-affinity autoantibodies and rare patients with IgA- or IgM-mediated hemolysis.

Rapid destruction of erythrocytes leads to other laboratory changes that are not specific for AIHA. These changes include increased serum levels of unconjugated bilirubin and lactate dehydrogenase and a reduction in plasma haptoglobin levels. Rare intravascular destruction of erythrocytes elevates the plasma free hemoglobin level and results in hemoglobinuria. In this situation, hemosiderinuria will follow in approximately 7 days when renal tubular epithelial cells containing absorbed iron exfoliate into the urine.

A positive DAT, confirmed with a specific anti-IgG reagent, is occasionally found in healthy people; approximately 1:10,000 blood donors has a positive antiglobulin test result without anemia or evi-

Table 47–3 Posttransplant Immune Hemolysis

	AIHA	Passenger Lymphocyte	ABO Rh mismatch
Mediated by	Donor lymphocytes	Donor memory B cells in solid organ or stem cells	Recipient Ab
Directed against	Donor RBCs	Recipient RBCs	Donor RBCs
Cause	T-cell dysfunction; immunomodulatory medications	GVHD-like reaction with production of Ab	Preformed Ab or Ab formed in response to donor tissue
Onset	2–25 months posttransplant	5–17 days	Acute-timing depends on preformed or newly formed Abs
Duration	Variable, depending on response to therapy	Usually resolves in 3 months	
Treatment options	Same as idiopathic AIHA	Compatible RBC transfusions, plasma or RBC exchange	Compatible RBC transfusion; immunosuppression
Prevention	None known	Prophylactic donor-compatible RBC transfusions	Removal of recipient Ab by plasma exchange or donor RBC purge

Ab, antibody; AIHA, autoimmune hemolytic anemia; GVHD, graft-versus-host disease; RBC, red blood cell.

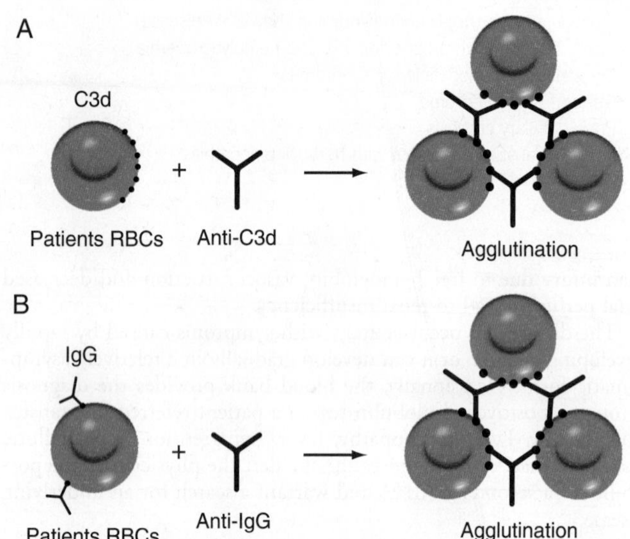

Figure 47–2 Direct antiglobulin test for detection of (**A**) erythrocyte-bound C3d or (**B**) IgG. Hemagglutination occurs when anti-C3d or anti-IgG can create a lattice structure by bridging sensitized red blood cells.

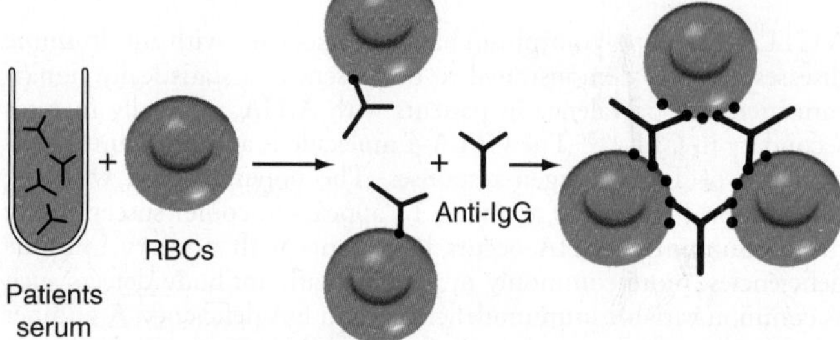

Figure 47–3 Indirect antiglobulin test for detection of antierythrocyte antibodies in serum. The patient's serum is mixed with a panel of normal red blood cells, some (or all) of which express the antigen(s) recognized by the serum antibodies. After the antibody-coated erythrocytes are washed, an anti-IgG reagent is added and hemagglutination occurs.

dence of increased hemolysis.[36] In approximately 10% of cases of AIHA, erythrocyte-bound C3b occurs in the absence of erythrocyte-bound IgG.

The unexpected report of a negative antiglobulin test result in a patient suspected of having AIHA is uncommon but may have several explanations. Technical errors are infrequent but can occur. Other rare causes are IgA and IgM autoantibodies or low-affinity IgG autoantibodies.[37] More commonly, the test is not sufficiently sensitive to detect small numbers of erythrocyte-bound IgG molecules; this occurs most often in cases of AIHA associated with a lymphoma or CLL. If the DAT result is positive, specific reagents are required to identify the erythrocyte-bound protein.

In approximately 80% of patients with AIHA, the autoantibodies are present in the serum as well as on the RBC membrane.[38] The indirect antiglobulin test (indirect Coombs test) detects the presence of these serum antibodies in the patient's serum (Fig. 47–3). The indirect antiglobulin test also detects alloantibodies induced by blood transfusion or maternal–fetal incompatibility. Alloantibodies have specificity for RBC antigens not present on the patient's native erythrocytes. Therefore, the DAT result is negative in cases of alloimmunization, unless the patient has been recently transfused. In this setting, alloantibodies may bind to the recently transfused RBCs and yield a positive DAT result. Therefore, an accurate transfusion history is essential in differentiating alloimmune from autoimmune hemolysis.

Laboratory findings also reflect the intensity of the hemolytic process, the ability of the body to process the RBC breakdown products, and the ability of the bone marrow to respond to the anemia. In fulminant cases, in which the RBC lifespan is less than 5 days, the anemia is severe, and erythropoiesis increases eightfold to 10-fold. As a result, the reticulocyte count rises, sometimes to levels greater than 40%. If the regenerative capacity of the bone marrow lags only slightly behind the rate of RBC destruction, a mild anemia with an elevated reticulocyte count occurs. If the gap is greater, severe anemia ensues. Inspection of the blood smear in a typical case reveals polychromatophilia, spherocytes, a few fragmented RBCs, nucleated RBCs, and occasionally erythrophagocytosis. Examination of the bone marrow, rarely indicated, shows erythroid hyperplasia, often with megaloblastoid features. Occasionally, RBC autoantibodies cause reticulocytopenia and dyserythropoiesis, thereby contributing to the severity of anemia.[39]

Patients with severe hemolytic anemia and markedly increased erythropoiesis occasionally develop folate deficiency and frank megaloblastosis. Growth of hematopoietic tissue in the bone marrow also leads to moderate increases in the white blood cell and platelet counts. The absence of reticulocytosis does not exclude the diagnosis of AIHA but portends a serious prognosis.[40,41] The low count may be due to destruction of young erythrocytes by the autoantibody or a concurrent parvovirus B19 infection. This reticulocytopenia impairs the compensatory response, aggravates the severity of the anemia, and increases the need for RBC transfusions.

Therapy

General Principles

AIHA ranges from indolent to life threatening. Initiation of treatment and selection of the intervention (immediate transfusion vs attempts to modulate the immune system's production of autoantibody and destruction of antibody-coated RBCs) must begin with a thorough appraisal of symptoms and extent of the clinical compromise. The earliest historical records of treatment of acquired hemolytic anemia include splenectomy performed in 1911.[42] In 1950, the beneficial effect of corticotropin on AIHA in two patients with lymphoma was reported by Dameshek[43] and in a 5-year-old girl by Gardner.[44] Up until the last several years, treatment options changed little from these initial therapies.

Rapidly developing anemia with a hematocrit less than 20 requires urgent management. However, in the less aggressive forms of the disease, allowing physiologically compensated anemia rather than instituting treatment may be prudent. Management of AIHA depends in part on whether the disease is primary or secondary to disorders such as B-cell malignancies and systemic lupus erythematosus.[45] This also demands careful assessment before any treatment begins. In some cases of AIHA secondary to lymphoma or CLL, the pathogenic autoantibody (usually monoclonal) is secreted by neoplastic B cells. Combination chemotherapy or irradiation of the underlying malignancy often brings the hemolytic anemia under control.[46,47] In other cases, however, the autoantibodies (usually polyclonal) do not originate from the B-cell neoplasm but probably result from abnormal immune regulation instigated by the neoplastic B cells. Treatment of the latter type of secondary AIHA with immunosuppressive agents may improve the anemia, but it also can trigger an exacerbation.[48] Some chemotherapeutic agents and immunosuppressive medications interfere with T-cell function and thus can trigger autoimmune processes, including AIHA. Fludarabine and cladribine given as therapy for CLL precipitate autoimmune processes by interfering with the delicate balance between T- and B-cell functions.[16]

The ultimate goal of therapy is controlling the B-cell populations that secrete pathogenic autoantibodies. However, so little is known about such cells[49,50] that the currently available therapy is, by default, nonspecific. The desired therapeutic effect is eradication of the abnormal hemolytic process, not reversal of the serologic abnormalities. Indeed, the DAT result often remains positive in the face of hematologic recovery.

Transfusion

Some cases of AIHA are life threatening and necessitate transfusion with RBCs.[51] Severe anemia can cause high-output cardiac failure and subsequent pulmonary edema, somnolence, and even obtundation, which require immediate intervention with RBC transfusion. The hemoglobin at which these symptoms occur varies based on the rate of fall of hemoglobin, degree of cardiac compensation, and other underlying clinical features. Oxygen therapy can be prescribed but is no substitute for transfusion.

The clinician must recognize that the presence of autoantibodies will complicate and prolong the pretransfusion evaluation performed by the blood bank and that, despite a complete blood bank workup, the patient often will receive "cross-match incompatible" blood. In situations where transfusion is required, blood should not be withheld simply because it is not fully compatible.[52] However, transfusion should be administered with particular care and close monitoring.

Occasionally (1%–2% of cases), the relative specificity of autoantibodies can be demonstrated. This usually occurs within the Rh system, and RBCs lacking the corresponding Rh antigen survive better in vivo than those that express the antigen.[53] Specificities of IgG autoantibodies for other blood groups have been described.[54] Whether such relative specificity should be respected in the selection of donor units is controversial, as exposure to RBCs lacking the implicated antigen may increase the risk of alloimmunization in these patients.[55] An important practical point is that, with rare exceptions, the implicated autoantigens are present on all normal erythrocytes. Thus, in practice, all RBCs will be "incompatible." In addition, the blood bank must screen for alloantibodies that may be obscured by autoantibody reactions. Alloantibodies, usually with specificity for the Rh or Kell blood group system, occur in approximately 30% of patients with AIHA who have a history of blood group immunization by maternal–fetal incompatibility or previous transfusions.[56,57] These alloantibodies can escape notice in a patient with a positive result on the indirect antiglobulin test because of the concomitant presence in the serum of autoantibodies that react with virtually all normal RBCs. To detect suspected alloantibodies, adsorption techniques that use either the patient's own cells (autologous adsorption) or cells of known phenotype (heterologous adsorption) to remove autoantibodies from the serum are available.

A pretransfusion sample should be obtained for RBC phenotyping if possible. When available, some centers will provide these patients with RBCs that are phenotypically matched for common clinically significant antigens. Providing matched units decreases the rate of subsequent alloimmunization and prevents delayed hemolytic transfusion reactions.[58]

The preceding techniques should not be required as pretransfusion tests in patients with AIHA. Transfusions should never be delayed if the tests are not readily available or completed (see box on Hazards of Transfusion Therapy). However, standard antibody detection and identification tests with both the patient's serum and an eluate prepared from the patient's cells should be performed whenever possible. Titration of the eluate and the serum against RBCs of various Rh phenotypes can indicate an autoantibody specificity (or preference) within the Rh system. Some experts recommend that any such specificity be respected in selecting donor units.[59] RBC substitutes have been transfused in a few situations of severe hemolytic anemia and demonstrate benefit to the patients.[60] However, no RBC substitutes are approved by the United States Food and Drug Administration for routine clinical use.

Hazards of Transfusion Therapy

The idea that transfusion therapy represents a special hazard in patients with autoimmune hemolytic anemia has been overemphasized. Nevertheless, transfusions are not to be undertaken lightly in such patients. The decision to transfuse requires that the clinician and the blood bank work together. The clinician must supervise the transfusions and insist on close observation of the patient. An adverse reaction dictates additional laboratory tests, but even sophisticated serologic techniques do not ensure uneventful transfusions. Acute intravascular hemolysis can occur with no evidence of serologic incompatibility. In vivo compatibility testing with ^{51}Cr-tagged RBCs is of no value in the management of most patients.

Transfusion is warranted without delay and, if necessary, before all serologic tests are completed when cardiac or cerebral function is threatened. Alleviation of signs and symptoms of anemia usually can be accomplished with relatively small quantities of RBCs, as little as 0.5 to 1 units. Overtransfusion in the presence of high-output cardiac failure can easily lead to circulatory overload, another reason to justify careful observation of the patient during the transfusion.

Corticosteroids

Corticosteroids are first-line treatment for most patients with symptomatic unstable AIHA of either the idiopathic or the secondary form. The clinical response to prednisone results primarily from its ability to disable macrophages from clearing IgG, inactivated C3b, or C3b-coated erythrocytes. Corticosteroids interfere with both the expression and the function of macrophage Fc receptors. This probably is the earliest, and perhaps even the primary, mechanism of the ability of steroids to diminish the immune clearance of blood cells.[61–63] Prednisone can reduce autoantibody production but only after several weeks of therapy (see box on Prednisone Therapy).

The side effects of corticosteroids often preclude long-term use of high-dose therapy. The cushingoid features that develop can lead to patient noncompliance, especially in the adolescent population. The associated osteoporosis, myopathies, psychiatric changes, immunosuppression, and risk of gastric bleeding can warrant discontinuation.

Intravenous γ-Globulin

Intravenous γ-globulin has been found effective in managing selected cases of AIHA. The soluble IgG in the material may increase the lifespan of IgG-coated RBCs by saturating Fc receptors on macrophages. In a study of patients with AIHA associated with lymphoproliferative disorders, a long-term benefit was observed with a maintenance dose schedule of intravenous IgG given every 21 days. A decrease in antiglobulin titer found in these patients suggests a mechanism other than blockade of Fc receptors by intravenous IgG.[64]

Prednisone Therapy

Therapy can begin with prednisone (there is no clear advantage to alternative forms of corticosteroids) at a dose of 1 to 2 mg/kg/day in divided doses, depending on the severity of the disease. The physician can consider beginning with a lower dose (e.g., 0.6 mg/kg/day) in elderly patients, especially those who are immobilized or who already have osteoporosis, or in patients with infection or other mitigating complications. Whatever the amount selected, it should be continued until a response becomes evident, usually within 3 weeks, by a rise in the hematocrit and a fall in the reticulocyte count.

Autoimmune hemolytic anemia in children is likely to respond to prednisone with a durable remission. By contrast, permanent remissions are infrequent in adults. Therefore, therapy for adults requires a plan to manage (or prevent) relapse. Essential elements to consider in formulating the long-term management of a patient with autoimmune hemolytic anemia are the duration of treatment with the initial dose of prednisone and the rate of dosage reduction after a response has been achieved. The tapering schedule depends, in part, on the severity of the initial presentation and the prominence of side effects of treatment. In the absence of contraindications, prednisone is continued at the initial dose until the hemoglobin level reaches 10 g/dL or greater, by which time transfusions should no longer be necessary. Thereafter, the dose can be gradually reduced, usually at a rate of 5 to 10 mg/week. During this second phase of treatment, the divided daily prednisone dose can be consolidated into a single daily dose. If the remission remains stable after a dose of 10 mg/day is reached, further tapering over a 3- to 4-month period can proceed with caution. Some hematologists continue treatment for many months at low doses (e.g., 10 mg every other day), but the efficacy of this practice has not been established.

The mechanism of action of intravenous Ig was further elucidated in a murine model of immune thrombocytopenia.[59,65] The model demonstrated that the inhibitory Fc receptor FcγRIIB was necessary for intravenous Ig to confer protection against platelet destruction. This suggests that modulation of inhibitory signals is involved in other autoimmune diseases and could be investigated as a therapeutic target in AIHA.

Although intravenous γ-globulin Ig may be effective in managing selected cases of AIHA, it currently is not recommended for routine use in either acute or chronic treatment of AIHA. Intravenous Ig may be considered for treatment of severe life-threatening AIHA, in cases where AIHA is refractory to conventional treatment with corticosteroids, or possibly as a temporizing measure prior to splenectomy.[66,67] Although no controlled trials have been performed, published reports of intravenous Ig use in AIHA suggest a dose as high as 400 to 1000 mg/kg/day for successful clinical response.[67]

Splenectomy

For many years splenectomy has been used as therapy for AIHA.[68] Successful techniques for laparoscopic splenectomy have improved this therapeutic modality.[69] Indications for splenectomy include failure to respond to prednisone, dependence on prednisone dosages larger than 20 mg/day, or intractable side effects of the corticosteroid. The procedure can be highly effective, presumably by removing the major reticuloendothelial site of RBC destruction. An animal model demonstrated that IgG-coated RBCs are removed almost exclusively by the spleen.[70] In addition, the procedure eliminates many phagocytosing macrophages and autoantibody-producing B cells.

In most young adults with chronic AIHA, the question of splenectomy arises almost inevitably. However, in elderly patients with stable but incomplete remission, maintenance therapy with prednisone at a dose of 10 mg/day for an indefinite period may be the preferred alternative. There is a slight risk that overwhelming sepsis by encapsulated organisms can develop immediately or up to 25 years after splenectomy.[69] This risk is increased in the pediatric population, especially in patients younger than 6 years at the time of splenectomy, and a conservative approach to splenectomy in this age group is prudent. The risk of sepsis is lessened by immunization with pneumococcal and meningococcal vaccines, optimally administered at least 2 weeks preoperatively, and by prompt use of antibiotics for febrile illness.[71] Pediatric patients should complete the *Haemophilus influenzae* series of vaccines prior to undergoing splenectomy.

The response to splenectomy does not correlate with the age of the patient, presence or absence of an underlying B-cell disorder, strength of the antiglobulin test, prior response to prednisone, or pattern of sequestration of ^{51}Cr-labeled RBCs. Approximately 50% to 60% of patients with classic AIHA have a good-to-excellent initial response to splenectomy. They need less than 15 mg/day of prednisone to maintain an adequate level of hemoglobin.[72] Information regarding the clinical implications of an accessory spleen in patients with AIHA is meager. Faced with such a rare finding in a patient with relapse, many hematologists recommend its removal. The role of splenectomy in patients with mixed IgG, IgM, or mixed cold- and warm-reactive IgG antibodies is unclear.

Immunomodulatory Therapy

Most experience with immunosuppressive drugs for treatment of AIHA has been with alkylating agents (cyclophosphamide and chlorambucil) and thiopurines (azathioprine and 6-mercaptopurine; see box on Cytotoxic Drug Therapy).[73] The basis for the clinical use of these drugs is their inhibitory effect on the immune system, possibly affecting both B cells and T cells.[74] High-dose cyclophosphamide 50 mg/kg/day for 4 days induced durable remission (median follow-

Cytotoxic Drug Therapy

Administration of cytotoxic drugs is best reserved for refractory cases: symptomatic patients who have not responded to splenectomy, those in whom splenectomy is an unacceptable medical risk, patients who refuse the operation, and those who have serious side effects from corticosteroids. Cyclophosphamide (2 mg/kg/day) or azathioprine (1.5 mg/kg/day) should be continued for 3 months or more to ensure maximal inhibition of autoantibody synthesis. Less than half of patients treated with these drugs will respond with a rise in the hemoglobin that can be maintained in the face of substantially reduced doses of prednisone. This estimate may be overly optimistic, as negative or unfavorable results seldom are reported. Unfortunately, no controlled clinical trials of cytostatic agents for treatment of autoimmune hemolytic anemia have been conducted.

Cyclophosphamide and azathioprine, like prednisone, can induce numerous side effects. Early side effects include bone marrow suppression and impairment of the immune response (particularly T-cell–mediated immunity) and can occur concomitantly with therapy. After sustained administration, cyclophosphamide can damage ovarian function, inhibit spermatogenesis,[76–78] and cause bladder fibrosis.[79] Acute myeloid leukemia can develop years after administration.[80] By contrast, prolonged use of azathioprine has not been associated with a statistically significant increase in malignant diseases. All these considerations mandate careful monitoring of any patient treated with either cyclophosphamide or azathioprine.

Cyclosporine, a powerful T-cell modulator, has been used alone and in combination to elicit successful and sometimes durable remission in patients with AIHA and Evans syndrome.[81] Three of three patients with AIHA treated with cyclosporine achieved complete remission on initial doses of 2.5 mg/kg twice daily for 6 days then 3 mg/kg/day and 5 mg/day of prednisone for a median follow-up period of 49 months.[81] Mycophenolate mofetil successfully induced remission of AIHA complicating myelodysplastic syndrome.[82]

up 15 months) in 66% of patients treated.[75] This small refractory group of patients had been treated with a median of three other treatment regimens (range 1–7 other regimens).[74]

Rituximab Therapy

Rituximab is a chimeric anti-CD20 monoclonal antibody with a well-established favorable safety profile that has exciting possibilities for widespread clinical application in patients with autoimmune disease in general and AIHA specifically.[83,84] Several large trials of adult patients with non-Hodgkin lymphoma have demonstrated the efficacy and safety of rituximab.[84] Infusion-related side effects, including fever, respiratory distress, and hypotension, in a small population of lymphoma patients have been reported.[85,86] Massive cytokine release leads to this complication of infusion and is associated with high tumor burden.[87,88] No side effects have precluded completion of planned therapy in patients with autoimmune disease.[89] The occurrence and severity of side effects seem to be related to B-cell, and thus tumor, burden.[88] It has been anticipated and demonstrated that the side-effect profile is even more favorable in autoimmune disease patients with a lower level of B cells.[90] Other complications include long-term impairment of humoral immunity, which may be obviated with monthly infusions of intravenous Ig. Reactivation of hepatitis B[91] and parvovirus[92] and cases of some autoimmune diseases have been reported.

The mechanism of action of rituximab is multifaceted, complex, and incompletely understood. Rituximab induces cell death through complement-dependent lysis; antibody-dependent cellular toxicity; antibody-dependent phagocytosis mediated by Fc, complement, and phosphatidylserine receptors; direct antibody effects of CD20 ligation leading to inhibition of proliferation; apoptosis and sensitization to chemotherapy; and induction of active immunity.[83] Plasma cells are $CD20^-$. The response rate of patients with AIHA and thrombocytopenia suggests that earlier, $CD20^+$ B cells are producing antibody or that other as yet not clearly delineated mechanisms are affecting the disease remission. Reports that rituximab induces remission in patients with AIHA within 1 week to 3 months of first infusion suggest that the mechanism of action involves more than elimination of B cells. Table 47–4 summarizes selected case reports and small case studies of patients with both idiopathic and secondary AIHA treated with rituximab. The safety profile and response rate of this medication in patients with AIHA is favorable, which has prompted some experts in the field to attempt a trial of rituximab prior to splenectomy. A few cases of serious side effects, including *Pneumocystis carinii* pneumonia, varicella pneumonia,[93] *Escherichia coli* pyelonephritis,[94] and neutropenia.[95,96] have been reported.

Alemtuzumab Therapy

Use of alemtuzumab, a monoclonal antibody to the CD52 antigen, has been reported in idiopathic and secondary therapy-refractory AIHA.[97] Alemtuzumab binds both normal and malignant T and B lymphocytes and can cause cell death via complement fixation, antibody-dependent cell-mediated cytotoxicity, and apoptosis induction. Administration results in prolonged lymphocytopenia, and the resultant immunosuppression leads to increased susceptibility to infections for several months following cessation of therapy, requiring antiinfective prophylaxis.[98] Although experience with alemtuzumab for treatment of AIHA is limited, alemtuzumab may be beneficial for patients refractory to first-line treatments, including rituximab. In a recent study, five patients with CLL and AIHA were treated with alemtuzumab (30 mg three times weekly for 3–12 weeks) after not responding to conventional therapy; two patients were previously treated with rituxan.[99] All patients responded with a ≥2 g/dL rise in hemoglobin concentration and did not require further RBC transfusion requirement after a median of 5 weeks (range 4–7 weeks). They remained clinically stable without AIHA after a median of 12 months (range 2–13 months). Due to the demonstrated efficacy of alemtuzumab in the treatment of B-cell CLL, use of alemtuzumab may be considered before use of rituximab in patients with AIHA and progressive CLL in need of cytoreduction.[99] Further prospective studies of alemtuzumab in both idiopathic and secondary AIHA are needed.

Plasma Exchange

Because a single-volume plasma exchange replaces approximately 60% of the patient's plasma volume, the therapeutic advantage comes from removal of the IgG and/or IgM plasma antibodies mediating the hemolysis. Unfortunately, continuous antibody production and the large extravascular distribution of IgG limit the long-term efficacy of plasma exchange in patients with IgG-mediated AIHA. On cessation of therapy, the rate of return to pretreatment levels of autoantibody depends on the rate of autoantibody production.[100] A small retrospective case-control study showed no benefit from RBC transfusion following plasma exchange compared to RBC transfusion alone.[101] However, efficacy in IgG-mediated disease has been reported.[102] Occasional dramatic responses have been reported in patients being prepared for surgery or when plasma exchange was used as a temporizing measure after initiation of immunosuppressive therapy.[102,103] Therefore, this therapy should be reserved for patients who are unresponsive to transfusion and in critical condition because of rapid clearance of RBCs.

Table 47–4 Summary of Selected Studies and Case Report Data for Rituximab for Autoimmune Hemolytic Anemia

No. of Patients/Disease	Rituximab Dose (mg/m²)	Dosing Schedule	Response [% (n/N)]	Previous Regimens[a]	Splenectomy (n/N)	Follow-up Period (months)
15 Pediatric/idiopathic[171]	375	Weekly × 2–4	87 (13/15)	Two or more S, C, I, CyA, Az	2/15	7–28
1 Pediatric/SLE,[172] idiopathic[173]	375	Weekly × 2	100 (2/2)	S, C, I, CyA	0/2	5–7
6 Pediatric/idiopathic[94]	375	Weekly × 4 Weekly × 12 (2 patients)	100 (6/6)	S, I, Ph, CyA, Az	2/6	15–22
4 Pediatric/idiopathic[93]	375	Weekly × 4–6	100 (4/4)	S, V, CyA, Az, I, C, T	2/4	3–14
1 Pediatric/idiopathic[174]	375	Weekly × 4 then repeat	100(1/1)	S, I, C, CyA, ATG, Ph, Az	Yes	19
1 CAD, 2 WAIHA[175]	375	Weekly × 4	33 (1/3)	S, C, Az	0/4	96
6 Adult/5 lymphoma;	375	Weekly × 4	17 (1/6)	3 untreated	1/6	6–14
1 idiopathic[96]			PR in 4/6	S, C, Cl, Chl		
1 Pediatric/Hurler post BMT[176]	375	Weekly × 3	100 (1/1)	I, S, CyA	0/1	21
1 Pediatric post BMT/ β-thalassemia,[177] WAS[178]	375	Weekly × 2 Weekly × 4	100 (2/2)	S, I	0/2	3–12
1 Adult/idiopathic CAD + WAIHA[179]	375	Weekly × 4 then 1 month later Weekly × 4	100 (1/1)	S × 2 long tapers	No	7
9 Adult/CAD ± lymphoma/CLL[110,140,180–186]	375	Weekly × 4	100 (9/9)	S, CyA, Chl, Az, C, MM, CHOP for lymphoma	1/9	9–36
8 Adult/CLL[95]	375	q4weeks Given with C and D	100 (8/8)	S, F, C, Chl	0/8	7–23
27 Adult/CAD[130]	375	Weekly × 4 ± IFN	1 CR, 19 PR	S, C, MP	—	2–42
14 Adult/CLL[187]	375	Weekly × 4	72% (3 CR, 7 PR)	S, C, V	—	3–49
20 Adult/CAD[188]	375	Weekly × 4	45% (1 CR, 8 PR)	S, C, Chl 9 untreated	—	12

ATG, antithymocyte globulin; Az, azathioprine; BMT, bone marrow transplantation; C, cyclophosphamide; CAD, cold agglutinin disease; Chl, chlorambucil; CHOP, cyclophosphamide, doxorubicin, vincristine, prednisone; Cl, cladribine; CLL, chronic lymphocytic leukemia; CR, complete remission; CyA, cyclosporine; D, dexamethasone; I, intravenous Ig; IFN, interferon; F, fludarabine; MM, mycophenolate mofetil; MP, mercaptopurine; Ph, plasmapheresis; PR, partial remission; S, corticosteroids; SLE, systemic lupus erythematosus; T, tacrolimus; V, vincristine; WAIHA, warm autoimmune hemolytic anemia; WAS, Wiskott–Aldrich synodrome.

Other Therapies

A few therapies for AIHA have been reported but are rarely used. They include infusion of vincristine-laden IgG-coated platelets,[9] use of danazol, an attenuated synthetic androgen,[104] and splenic irradiation.[105,106] In addition, B- and T-cell–depleted, allogenic and autogenic[107,108] bone marrow transplantation have been performed in extreme refractory cases of AIHA, with limited success. Erythropoietin has been used in some cases to increase RBC production in an attempt to decrease transfusion needs.

COLD AGGLUTININ DISEASE

Cold agglutinin disease refers to a group of disorders caused by antierythrocyte autoantibodies (e.g., cold agglutinins) that preferentially bind RBCs at cold temperatures (4°C–18°C [39°F–64°F]) and may or may not induce hemolysis. Virtually all sera from healthy individuals contain low-titer cold agglutinins, regarded as benign or harmless RBC autoantibodies and considered polyclonal. Similarly, cold agglutinins that arise after certain infections are polyclonal and usually benign. In rare cases, a transient form of cold agglutinin disease ensues and is thought to be produced as a result of random rearrangement of immunoglobulin gene segments and molecular mimicry of antigens on the surface of infective agents.[109] By contrast, monoclonal cold agglutinins are generally pathogenic and are derived from clonal B-cell expansions (as in idiopathic/chronic cold agglutinin disease), which may progress to frank lymphoma. Cold agglutinin disease develops in 1.1% to 4.9% of all cases of non-Hodgkin lymphoma.[110]

Pathophysiology

Immune Clearance of Erythrocytes

The pathogenic IgM autoantibody in cold agglutinin disease is highly efficient in activating the classic complement pathway on the erythrocyte membrane.[111,112] However, the thermal dependency of the antibody constrains its pathogenic effects. The autoantibody rapidly elutes off RBCs at the 37°C (99°F) temperature of the visceral circulation, but in the cool peripheral circulation of the hands and feet, the cold agglutinin remains on the erythrocyte membrane for at least a few seconds. That amount of time is sufficient to activate the complement cascade to the stage of C3b, which adheres to the RBC after it reenters the central circulation. In the hepatic circulation, C3b-coated RBCs encounter macrophages with receptors specific for C3b[113]; however, C3b sensitization is only a weak signal for activation of phagocytosis. Hepatic clearance of C3b-coated RBCs requires 500 to 800 C3b molecules per RBC.[114] Thus, many C3b-coated cells escape into the systemic circulation, where the C3b inactivator system degrades C3b into C3dg, C3d, or both. The result is a cohort of erythrocytes coated with C3d, but not with the IgM autoantibody,[115] which have a near-normal survival in vivo, as macrophages bind to C3d with low avidity.[116] The DAT result remains positive, but little if any hemolysis occurs.[114]

These limits on the pathogenicity of cold agglutinins account for the subdued hematologic picture in most patients with cold agglutinin disease. However, if the regulatory C3b inactivator proteins are impaired, cleavage of RBC-bound C3b is limited, which permits completion of the complement cascade in the visceral circulation and results in severe extravascular hemolysis. Several patients with high titers of IgA cold agglutinins have been reported. These cases are not associated with cold agglutinin disease, which may relate to the lack of complement activation by IgA antibodies.[117]

Targets of Cold Agglutinin Disease

The antigenic specificity of cold agglutinins usually is identified by their degree of reactivity with RBCs from adults (blood group I) and cord blood (blood group i) (Fig. 47–4). The cold-reactive autoantibody produced after some cases of *Mycoplasma pneumoniae* infection has anti-I specificity,[118] whereas the antibody associated with infectious mononucleosis frequently, but not always, has anti-i specificity.[119,120] Antibody that agglutinates adult Group O cells with titers fourfold or greater than CORD RBCs at 4°C (39°F) is anti-I. The opposite results demonstrate anti-i.[121] Additional specificities have been identified by tests with rare adult RBCs that lack the I antigen or with enzyme-treated erythrocytes. Rarely cold agglutinins are specific for the A blood group antigen.[122]

Clinical Findings

The most common type of cold agglutinin disease, a chronic form characterized principally by a stable anemia of moderate severity and attacks of acrocyanosis precipitated by exposure to cold, constitutes approximately one third of all cases of immunohemolytic anemia. Cold agglutinins cause the cardinal abnormalities of the disease. The acrocyanosis stems from intraarteriolar agglutination of erythrocytes in the relatively cool tips of the fingers, feet, earlobes, and nose. Hemolytic anemia depends on the capacity of the cold agglutinins to initiate activation of the complement cascade on the surface of the RBC. Most patients with chronic cold agglutinin disease are in the fifth to eighth decades of life, and many of them have a B-cell neoplasm-lymphoma, Waldenström macroglobulinemia, or CLL. The cold agglutinin in those latter cases is monoclonal, almost always IgM-κ, and may manifest as a monoclonal band in the serum protein electrophoretic pattern. In the absence of a B-cell neoplasm, the spleen and lymph nodes are rarely enlarged; such findings warrant a search for the neoplasm. Some studies demonstrate that these patients have a relative paucity of complement. In the setting of intercurrent viral or bacterial illness, complement levels, and thus the degree of hemolysis, are increased.[123,124]

A second type of cold agglutinin disease, usually acute and always self-limited, occurs as a rare complication of several infectious diseases, most notably *M. pneumoniae* infection and infectious mononucleosis. Patients with this form of cold agglutinin disease are much younger than those with chronic cold agglutinin disease. Onset is abrupt, appearing as the infection wanes, and the anemia can be severe. Evaluation for *M. pneumoniae* infection should be considered in all cases of cold agglutinin–mediated hemolysis because prompt treatment of the pneumonia will resolve the hemolysis.[125] Most often, however, *M. pneumoniae* infections are not associated with pathologic hemolysis. The cold agglutinin titers are moderately elevated and are polyclonal.

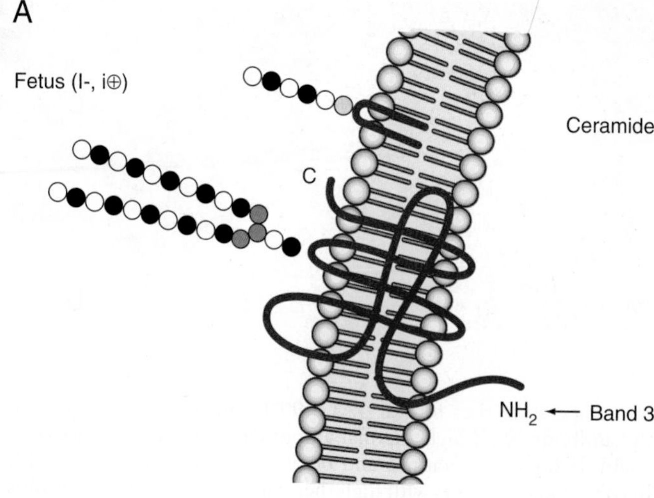

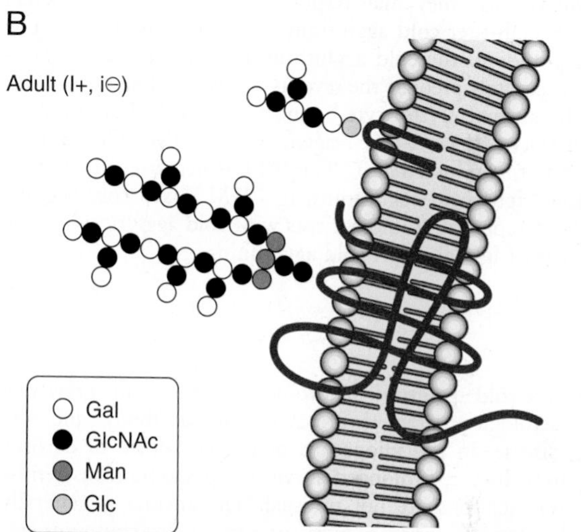

Figure 47–4 The I/i blood group system in (**A**) fetus and (**B**) adult. The fetus lacks the enzymes (branching enzymes) required to produce the branched forms of ceramide and the I antigen. The unbranched (fetal) and branched (adult) variants of the I antigen are immunochemically distinct structures. Shaded structure represents the erythrocyte membrane. The modified N-terminus of band 3 faces the interior of the red blood cell. *(From Hakomori S: Blood group ABH and Ii antigens of human erythrocytes: Chemistry, polymorphism, and their developmental change. Semin Hematol 18:39, 1981.)*

Laboratory Evaluation

The usual laboratory findings of hemolytic anemia (i.e., anemia, reticulocytosis, polychromatophilia, spherocytosis, erythroid hyperplasia in the bone marrow, and elevated serum bilirubin and lactate dehydrogenase levels) are generally not striking in patients with chronic cold agglutinin disease. Hemagglutination may be visible to the unaided eye in blood drawn from a patient with cold agglutinin disease and can interfere with automated blood counts. The agglutination usually can be seen on the peripheral blood smear (Fig. 47–5). The anemia often is mild and stable because the C3b inactivator in serum limits the extent of cold agglutinin–induced complement activation and phagocytosis. However, exposure to cold may greatly augment the binding of cold agglutinins, exceeding the restraints of the inactivator system. This can result in a sudden drop in hematocrit with complement-mediated intravascular hemolysis and renal failure.

In typical cases of chronic cold agglutinin disease, the cold agglutinin titer is very high (>1:10^5 and occasionally >1:10^6). The antibodies are most reactive in the cold, and hemagglutination disappears as

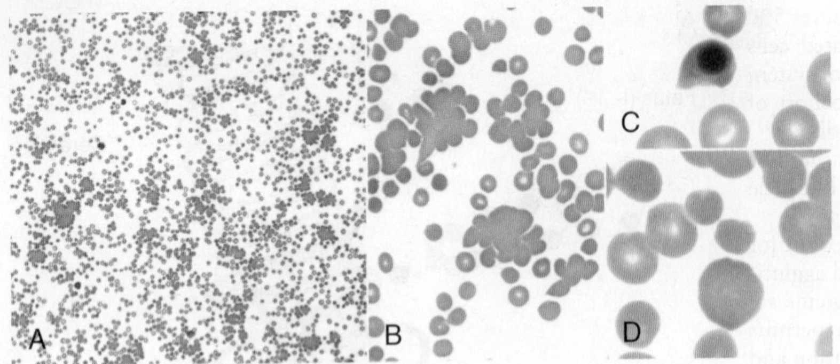

Figure 47–5 Peripheral smear in cold agglutinin disease. Low-power scan shows uneven distribution of red blood cells (**A**), which at slightly higher power (**B**) shows the red blood cells to be clumped together or agglutinated. This must be distinguished from rouleaux formation. High–power scan shows nucleated red blood cells (**C**), polychromatophilia, and microspherocytes (**D**).

the temperature rises toward 37°C (99°F). In some cases, however, the antibody has a high thermal amplitude, that is, it is reactive at relatively high temperatures and occasionally even at 37°C (99°F). Recognition of patients with high thermal amplitude cold agglutinins is important because they may respond to prednisone,[126] whereas patients with high-titer cold agglutinin disease usually do not. The thermal amplitude of the cold agglutinin, not the titer of the antibody, most accurately predicts the severity of disease. The DAT result is positive because of erythrocyte-bound C3d (see Pathophysiology above), but tests with anti-IgG reagents are negative. The indirect antiglobulin test, conducted at 37°C (99°F), is negative. In addition to monoclonal IgM cold agglutinins, IgG/IgM mixed cold agglutinins have been reported. Some patients with cold agglutinin disease have low titers of IgG and IgA cold agglutinins.

Transfusions and Cold Agglutinin Disease

Transfusion in a patient with cold agglutinin disease requires the same prudent safeguards observed with transfusions in patients with autoimmune hemolytic anemia. All compatibility tests must be performed at 37°C (99°F) and IgG-specific antiglobulin reagents used to avoid confusion with the serum cold agglutinin and the erythrocyte-bound C3d. Use of "inline" blood warmers is advisable, and more elaborate measures for performing the entire transfusion process at 37°C (99°F) occasionally are required. Hypothermia during cardiac surgery must be prevented, and special techniques must be used to avoid lowering the temperature of blood in the coronary arteries.

Therapy

Therapy for the cold agglutinin syndromes depends on the gravity of symptoms, serologic characteristics of the autoantibody, and any underlying disease. In the idiopathic, or primary, form of chronic cold agglutinin disease, prolonged survival and spontaneous remissions and exacerbations are not unusual. The anemia is generally mild, and the simple measure of avoiding exposure to cold temperatures can avoid exacerbations, especially when the cold agglutinin has a low thermal amplitude.

The purine analogue fludarabine has proved to be of therapeutic benefit in patients with chronic cold agglutinin disease.[127] However, WAIHA and immune thrombocytopenia purpura are documented side effects of this modality. Prednisone has been beneficial in rare cases showing relatively low titers of cold agglutinins of a high thermal amplitude or in which an IgG cold-reactive antibody is produced. However, prednisone is not useful therapy in most patients with primary IgM-induced cold agglutinin disease, and its administration should not be undertaken lightly, given the chronicity of the disease.[128] Plasma exchange may help as a temporary measure in acute situations.[129] Because 95% of IgM is intravascular and up to 80% of Igm can be removed by plasma exchange, plasma exchange should theoretically offer optimal and effective therapy. However, if the thermal amplitude of the antibody is such that agglutination occurs at room temperature, RBC agglutination within the cell separator and tubing can occur. In these situations, therapy may need to be initiated in a controlled, very high temperature setting of 37°C (99°F).[116] Splenectomy usually is ineffective because the liver is the dominant site of sequestration of RBCs heavily sensitized with C3b. In rare cases, however, patients with an enlarged spleen have responded to splenectomy. In some of these patients, a localized splenic lymphoma was found, whereas in others only lymphoid hyperplasia was evident. Rituximab, an anti-CD20 monoclonal antibody, has demonstrated some clinical effectiveness in cases of cold agglutinin disease (see Table 47–4). A prospective phase II study of patients with primary cold agglutinin disease reported a 54% response rate in 27 patients treated with 37 courses of rituximab.[13] Some of the patients who did not respond to the first course of four weekly doses of rituximab were treated with a combination of rituximab and interferon-α. Among the responses, one patient achieved complete remission and 19 partial remission. The complete remission was sustained at 42 months, although all but one of the patients with partial remission relapsed at a mean of 11 months.[130] It is essential to seek evidence of a B-cell neoplasm before initiating therapy for chronic cold agglutinin disease. Oral alkylating agents (chlorambucil or cyclophosphamide) help many patients with the secondary form of cold agglutinin disease because of their effect on the B-cell neoplasm, but only occasionally do they benefit patients with the primary form of the disease.[118,119,131,132] When cold agglutinin disease is part of an established B-cell malignancy, the severity of hemolysis often waxes and wanes in parallel with the activity of the neoplasm.

Transient cold agglutinin disease is a rare form that is always self-limited. Supportive measures, including transfusions and avoidance of cold, may suffice (see box on Transfusions and Cold Agglutinin Disease). Treatment of the *Mycoplasma* infection, if detected, shortens the duration and severity of hemolysis. Corticosteroids usually are not helpful, and splenectomy almost never is indicated.

PAROXYSMAL COLD HEMOGLOBINURIA

Epidemiology

PCH historically was associated with tertiary syphilis. This syphilitic variant is rarely seen today. PCH now is more commonly seen primarily in children after a viral or, much less commonly, a bacterial illness. Most commonly, the viral cause is not identified but the condition is associated with an upper respiratory tract infection. Case reports of PCH secondary to varicella infection[133] in adults and children have been reported.

In a review of 52 cases of PCH over a 37-year period, the median age at presentation was 5 years.[134] In a study of 100 children with onset of AIHA before age 16 years, six (6%) had PCH as defined by a positive Donath-Landsteiner test.[18] All six cases were associated with symptoms suggestive of an acute viral illness.

Pathophysiology

The IgG antibody responsible for PCH is found in the patient's serum by incubation of normal erythrocytes, fresh normal serum as a source of complement, and the patient's serum, first at 4°C (39°F)and then at 37°C (99°F), with appropriate controls. The target usually is the P blood group system,[135] which is a tetraglycosyl ceramide called *globoside*, although other targets have been reported.[136] The Donath-Landsteiner antibody fixes the first two components of complement in the cold and completes the cascade on warming to 37°C (99°F).[137]

Clinical Findings

Although the pathognomonic Donath-Landsteiner antibody often occurs in cases of tertiary or congenital syphilis, it generally does not cause hemolytic disease in this situation. On exposure to cold, an occasional patient experiences paroxysms of hemoglobinuria and constitutional symptoms: fever, back pain, leg pain, abdominal cramps, and rigors, followed by hemoglobinuria. In contrast, the postviral form of PCH[138,139] is characterized by constitutional symptoms with fulminant intravascular hemolysis and its associated signs of hemoglobinemia, hemoglobinuria, jaundice, severe anemia, relative reticulocytopenia,[134] and sometimes renal failure. The disease is self-limited, usually lasting 2 to 3 weeks, although it can be life threatening because of the degree of hemolysis and consequent anemia.

Laboratory Evaluation

The DAT finding almost always is negative, but occasionally weak reactions for erythrocyte-bound complement are manifested. The indirect antiglobulin test result is negative. The diagnosis depends on recognition of the clinical picture because tests for the Donath-Landsteiner antibody are not routinely performed.

Therapy

No specific treatment of PCH is available. Unlike the positive response to steroids of most IgG-mediated autoimmune diseases, prednisone is not useful. The best approach is supportive care, transfusions to alleviate symptoms, and avoidance of cold temperatures. The patient should be kept in a warm room, and transfusions should be given through a blood warmer. Unlike patients with cold agglutinin disease in whom the pathogenic antibody is IgM, PCH IgG antibody is less amenable to removal via plasma exchange. However, the literature reports a child with severe hemolysis secondary to the Donath-Landsteiner antibody in whom intravenous Ig, corticosteroids, and warming of the patient had failed, but in whom daily single-volume plasma exchange for 3 consecutive days immediately eliminated the need for further transfusions.[140]

DRUG-ASSOCIATED IMMUNE HEMOLYTIC ANEMIA

Drug-associated hemolytic anemia can be drug induced or drug dependent. The antibodies can be specific for RBC antigens alone or for RBC-bound drug.[1] Four distinct mechanisms are associated with the disorder. The first involves drug that can bind to the RBC membrane. The patient makes antibodies against the drug (e.g., penicillin) that combine with the erythrocyte-bound drug, opsonizing and preparing the RBC for destruction. Discontinuation of the drug brings the hemolytic anemia to a rapid halt because the antibodies have no specificity for antigens on the RBC membrane. Clues to the diagnosis are the appropriate clinical findings, a positive result on the DAT, a negative result on the indirect antiglobulin test, and failure of antibodies eluted from the patient's RBCs to bind to normal erythrocytes. The diagnosis is established when both the eluate and the patient's serum contain antibodies directed against the drug-coated cells. In the case of penicillin,[141] hemolytic anemia occurs only when large amounts are administered; in patients treated with lower doses, a positive DAT result without hemolytic anemia is not unusual because production of low-avidity IgG antipenicillin antibodies is a common event.

The second mechanism involves immune complexes. The offending drug, or drug metabolite, binds to a plasma protein, forming an immunogenic conjugate. An antibody to the conjugate, if one develops, usually is IgM. The antibody then binds to the immunogenic conjugate, forming an immune complex that adheres to RBCs. Through efficient activation of complement on the erythrocyte membrane, this process causes a clinical picture of intravascular hemolysis and concomitant hemoglobinemia, hemoglobinuria, and possible renal failure. This chain of events accounts for most reported examples of drug-induced immune hemolytic anemia. Reports on the nonsteroidal drug diclofenac have shown that AIHA is induced by sensitization to the glucuronide conjugate of the drug.[142]

Serologic findings with erythrocyte-bound immune complexes are similar to those of the first mechanism, except that the DAT reveals complement bound only to the RBC. The IgM antibody is presumed to be no longer present after complement activation. The patient's serum reacts with RBCs (lacking antidrug antibody) in the presence of the offending drug, and the eluate from the patient's RBCs generally does not react with normal erythrocytes.

The third mechanism involves in vivo sensitization to drugs by the formation of immunogenic drug–RBC complexes. In these cases, the specificity of the drug-induced antibodies not only is contributed by the drug (or its metabolites) but also is by defined RBC antigens, particularly of the Rhesus and I/i systems.[143]

The fourth mechanism involves the induction of authentic autoantibodies against RBCs by a drug. α-Methyldopa is the classic example.[144] The DAT result turns positive in as many as 20% of patients treated with α-methyldopa, but few of these patients develop hemolytic anemia. The antiglobulin test result may take several months to 1 year or more after the start of drug therapy to become positive. In patients with hemolytic anemia, discontinuation of the drug results in gradual cessation of the hemolytic anemia and disappearance of the autoantibody because the drug itself is not required for the hemolytic process but only for the initiation of antibody production. Curiously, the autoantibody usually is specific for antigens of the Rh system. The serologic findings are indistinguishable from those of primary AIHA and include a positive DAT result, usually a positive result on the indirect antiglobulin test, and an eluate that reacts with normal erythrocytes. Patients taking α-methyldopa often have other antibodies in addition to the RBC autoantibodies. The mechanism by which α-methyldopa induces autoantibodies is unknown but may involve effects on immunoregulatory T cells.

Drug-induced immune hemolytic anemia was commonly seen when penicillin was administered in large doses (i.e., >20 million units/day) and when α-methyldopa was widely used for treatment of hypertension.[59,145] The disease now is less common in clinical practice. Numerous drugs can induce hemolytic anemia. A 20-year retrospective review of 71 cases referred to an immunohematology reference laboratory revealed that 51% were due to cephalosporins and 15% were due to nonsteroidal antiinflammatory drugsS.[146] The remainder of cases included examples due to penicillin or penicillin derivatives, quinine, quinidine, probenecid, levofloxacin, cefoxitin (Mefoxin), carboplatin, and oxaliplatin.

UNUSUAL FORMS OF IMMUNE HEMOLYTIC ANEMIA

In certain cases, hemolytic anemia due to heteroantibodies or alloantibodies may be confused with AIHA. Some lots of antithymocyte globulin contain heterologous antihuman RBC antibodies, which can precipitate attacks of immune hemolysis.[147] Anti-A alloantibodies in some preparations of intravenous human γ-globulin have resulted in RBC destruction,[148] and synthesis of alloantibodies by passenger B cells in transplanted livers and kidneys can cause a hemolytic anemia that masquerades as AIHA.[149]

IN VITRO AND ANIMAL MODELS OF POTENTIAL THERAPEUTIC INTERVENTIONS

Complement receptor 1 (CR1) negatively regulates B-cell antigen receptor–mediated activation.[82] The human recombinant soluble form of complement receptor 1 (sCR1) has been investigated in vitro and in vivo.[150] The in vitro alloimmune incompatibility model demonstrated inhibition of complement activation and abrogated hemolysis. In murine models, 10 mg/kg of sCR1 administered with human group O RBCs prevented alloimmunization and, in mice with preexisting anti-A antibodies, improved posttransfusion survival by 50%, reduced intravascular hemolysis, and decreased complement deposition. Further study is warranted to determine the appropriateness of phase I trials of human AIHAs resistant to standard therapies.

In vitro data suggest that an imbalance in T_H1/T_H2 cytokine production plays a role in AIHA. Decreased production of T_H1 cytokines, particularly interleukin (IL)-12, and increase in T_H2 cytokines, particularly IL-10, may play a role in the pathogenesis of AIHA.[151] Statistically significant differences in levels of T_H1/T_H cytokines were demonstrated in a study of 13 patients with AIHA compared with 13 control subjects.[152] Manipulation of the IL-10/IL-12 balance may offer potential therapeutic benefit.

NZB Mice

The inbred NZB mouse is genetically programmed to develop AIHA at approximately age 6 to 8 months (lifespan of a normal mouse is approximately 2 years). Antierythrocyte autoantibodies begin to appear at approximately age 3 months, and by 9 months the DAT result is positive in 60% to 80% of the animals. Typical signs of hemolytic anemia develop, with reticulocytosis, spherocytosis, shortened RBC survival time, and splenomegaly.[153]

Okamoto et al.[154] developed a transgenic murine model of AIHA. The symptoms in this model are variable, ranging from unaffected to severe anemia. The B1 cells have been demonstrated to mediate AIHA.[155] They are activated in both T-cell–dependent and T-cell–independent fashion.[156] B1 cells are distinct from B2 cells, the more prevalent B cells, in several ways. They preferentially locate in the peritoneal and pleural cavities, produce 50% of the natural serum IgM, and escape clonal deletion. IL-10 influences T-cell–proliferation of B1 cells, and continuous administration of anti–IL-10 monoclonal antibody depletes B1 but not B2 cells in murine models. B1 autoantibody production, but not spontaneous proliferation, is upregulated by IL-5.[155] The influence of T_H2 cytokines on the behavior of B1 cells in vivo[157] suggests possible avenues for treatment.

ORIGINS OF ANTIERYTHROCYTE ANTIBODIES

The vast improvement in our understanding of what prevents autoimmunization has not yet informed us of the mechanism that causes autoimmunization. Virtually nothing is known of the origins of warm-reactive IgG antierythrocyte autoantibodies, despite the availability of a thoroughly investigated, spontaneous animal model of the disease (the NZB mouse) and stocks of pathogenic autoantibodies, readily obtained from patients with the disease. A major impediment to advances in our perceptions of how AIHA originates is that the autoantigens are mostly unknown. Even in cases in which blood group specificity of the autoantibodies has been identified, the relevant structures have not been elucidated. Leddy et al.[158] succeeded in identifying four proteins on the RBC membrane that bind to antierythrocyte autoantibodies: the band 3 anion transporter, glycophorin A, and two polypeptides, probably related to the Rh family of antigens. Various combinations of these four autoantibody specificities were found in a group of 20 patients with AIHA.

The association of AIHA with systemic lupus erythematosus and immune thrombocytopenia (Evans syndrome), the induction of the disease by drugs that seem to perturb immune regulation, and the graft-versus-host model of AIHA all suggest, at least in some cases, antigen-independent activation of clones of B cells with the capacity to produce IgG anti-RBC autoantibodies. Such polyclonal B-cell activation may account for the production of antierythrocyte autoantibodies in patients with the acquired immunodeficiency syndrome.[118,159] Hypergammaglobulinemia and other signs of nonspecific activation of B cells are prominent in patients with human immunodeficiency virus infection.[160]

The immunologic basis of AIHA in patients with CLL or B-cell lymphoma is equally obscure.[161] In malignant diseases, there is indirect evidence that AIHA may be caused by immune dysregulation and not strictly malignant B-cell clone production of autoantibody. Malignancies can be complicated by AIHA prior to onset of disease or during remission and may not recur with relapse of the same malignant clone. In cases of CLL, the autoantibodies are IgG and often polyclonal,[162] whereas the malignant $CD5^+$ B cells of that disease generally produce only IgM antibodies that are monoclonal. Therefore, B cells other than those constituting the leukemia likely produce the autoantibodies. The large mass of $CD5^+$ B cells in patients with CLL might induce nonneoplastic $CD5^-$ B cells to produce IgG autoantibodies, perhaps by disturbing immunoregulatory idiotypic networks. Demonstration of the simultaneous presence of autoantibodies and antiidiotypic antibodies on RBCs in cases of AIHA[163] suggests that such networks may have a role in the disease.

In contrast to the antigens that incite warm autoantibodies, the structures of the autoantigens of cold agglutinin disease, the I/i system, are known (see Fig. 47–4).[164] This information has clarified our thinking about the immunology of this group of disorders. There is little reason to doubt that the very high levels of monoclonal cold agglutinins found in some patients with B-cell neoplasms are produced by the malignant cells. The demonstration that an idiotypic marker on monoclonal cold agglutinins could be detected not only on the patient's neoplastic B cells but also on 3% to 10% of normal B cells[165] supports the view that these autoantibodies are part of the normal immune repertoire. Malignant transformation of a cold agglutinin-producing B cell results in a lymphoma complicated by chronic cold agglutinin disease.

The basis of the association of PCH with syphilis may be antigenic mimicry, in which structural similarities between a microbial antigen and a self-antigen trigger an autoantibody response. In the case of PCH, the infecting organism, *Treponema pallidum*, should possess two antigenic determinants (epitopes): one recognized by T cells (the foreign epitope) and the other by self-reactive B cells (mimicking epitope). Donath-Landsteiner antibodies would be produced only by syphilitic patients whose class II major histocompatibility complex glycoproteins could present the foreign epitope in an immunogenic form to T cells. A similar mechanism could apply to postinfectious acute cold agglutinin disease, in which a cross-reaction involving antigenic determinants of *M. pneumoniae* and the I blood group substance has been incriminated.[166]

Structural analyses of monoclonal anti-I and anti-i autoantibodies from patients with B-cell neoplasms are beginning to yield important clues about the origins of chronic cold agglutinin disease. A striking observation is the repetitive use of the same immunoglobulin V_H gene, V_{H4-34}, in monoclonal IgM cold agglutinins, regardless of the anti-I or anti-i specificity of the autoantibody.[167,168]

From these results it appears that (a) the germline V_{H4-34} heavy chain encodes the dominant specificity of monoclonal cold agglutinins, (b) the somatic mutations of the light chain genes of the cold agglutinins are the result of an immune response, and (c) the V_H CDR3 and the light chain confer fine specificity (e.g., for I or i) on the cold agglutinin and influence its affinity. These data make a convincing case that monoclonal cold agglutinins arise as the result of an immune response, perhaps an autoimmune response to an autoantigen on erythrocytes. The results of these molecular studies of cold agglutinins complement other evidence favoring a role for antigen-mediated clonal selection in some types of B-cell neoplasms.

In contrast to monoclonal cold agglutinins associated with chronic cold agglutinin disease, the naturally occurring IgM cold agglutinins that are present in low titers in normal serum are not restricted to the $V_{H4\text{-}34}$ gene segment. Thus, naturally occurring low-titer cold agglutinins are associated with different genes of the V_{H3} family as well as the $V_{H4\text{-}34}$ gene.[169] Therefore, it appears that B-cell neoplasia is an important, but not exclusive, element in the association between $V_{H4\text{-}34}$ and cold agglutinins. The correlation with lymphomas has added interest because $V_{H4\text{-}34}$ has been independently linked to B-cell lymphomas that do not secrete cold agglutinins.[170] Both kinds of $V_{H4\text{-}34}$-related B-cell tumors may originate from an uncontrolled autoimmune response against I or i RBC antigens, one type lacking the capacity for secreting the cold agglutinin and the other able to secrete it as a monoclonal IgM immunoglobulin.

SUGGESTED READINGS

Carstairs KC, Breckenridge A, Dollery CT, Worlledge SM: Incidence of a positive direct Coombs test in patients on alpha-methyldopa. Lancet 2:133, 1966.

Coombs RRA, Mourant AE, Race RR: A new test for the detection of weak and incomplete Rh agglutinins. Br J Exp Pathol 26:255, 1945.

Ness P: How do I encourage clinicians to transfuse mismatched blood to patients with autoimmune hemolytic anemia in urgent situations? Transfusion 46:1859, 2006.

Okamoto M, Murakami M, Shimizu A, et al: A transgenic model of autoimmune hemolytic anemia. J Exp Med 175:71, 1992.

Petz LD, Fudenberg HH: Coombs-positive hemolytic anemia caused by penicillin administration. N Engl J Med 274:171, 1966.

Petz LD, Garratty G: Acquired Immune Hemolytic Anemias. New York, Churchill Livingstone, 1980.

Rosenfield RE, Schmidt PJ, Calvo RC, McGinniss MH: Anti-i, a frequent cold agglutinin in infectious mononucleosis. Vox Sang 10:631, 1965.

Sokol RJ, Stamps R, Booker DJ, et al: Posttransplant immune-mediated hemolysis. Transfusion 42:198, 2002.

Schreiber AD, Herskovitz BS, Goldwein M: Low-titer cold-hemagglutinin disease: Mechanism of hemolysis and response to corticosteroids. N Engl J Med 296:1490, 1977.

Shirey RS, Boyd JS, Parwani AV et al: Prophylactic antigen-matched donor blood for patients with warm autoantibodies: An algorithm for transfusion management. Transfusion 41:1435, 2002.

REFERENCES

For complete list of references log onto www.expertconsult.com

CHAPTER 48

EXTRINSIC NONIMMUNE HEMOLYTIC ANEMIAS

Stanley L. Schrier and Elizabeth A. Price

By definition, extrinsic causes of hemolysis are abnormalities in the environment in which the red blood cells (RBCs), usually normal themselves, circulate. These abnormalities can be acute or chronic in nature. They can arise from congenital lesions but usually result from acquired lesions. Inherited anomalies of glucose-6-phosphate dehydrogenase (G6PD) deficiency which reduces the red cell's ability to deal with oxidative insults can leave red cells more vulnerable to environmental insults. Determination of hemolysis with various levels of compensation as the cause of an anemia is accomplished using the approaches described in Chapter 34. Signs of extrinsic hemolysis with minimal or no anemia can be valuable clues to diseases of other organ systems. Among the most important forms of extrinsic hemolytic anemia are those caused by immune mechanisms; these are discussed in Chapter 47.

Clinical and morphologic findings suggest the many misfortunes that can befall RBCs in their travels. They can be trapped in an abnormal marrow stroma network, sheared by jets in an abnormal heart, cut and fragmented by fibrin strands stretched across damaged areas in the microvasculature, or attacked by parasites. They can undergo stasis and perhaps metabolic depletion in giant hemangiomas or in an enlarged spleen. An abnormally functioning liver or kidney can cause a buildup of substances in plasma that alter RBC shape and metabolism. Drugs can cause oxidation or other metabolic damage. Oxidant injury provokes degradation of hemoglobin with the formation of hemichromes (see Drug-Induced Oxidative Hemolysis below). Degraded hemoglobin and hemichromes bind avidly to the cytoplasmic tail of the major transmembrane protein band 3 (see Chapter 46) and cause clustering of band 3 oligomers.[1] Immunoglobulins and complement then bind to the external membrane face over clusters of band 3, promoting immune destruction. Other membrane proteins may be subject to oxidative attack. Toxins, venoms, heat, and mechanical trauma can directly destroy the membrane. These agents may cause an alteration in the asymmetry of the phospholipid bilayer, causing phosphatidylserine to move from the inner leaflet of the membrane bilayer to the outer leaflet, where it can be recognized by macrophages.

In general, only the most devastating damage leads to direct intravascular destruction. Usually, the initial insult leads to an eventual change in the external portion of the RBC membrane, which causes macrophages to retard, hold, remove, or otherwise modify RBCs. Infection or inflammation can activate these macrophages. Some RBC changes are accompanied by a decrease in RBC deformability, which retards flow and thereby facilitates the action of macrophages on the affected RBC. All of these changes lead to extravascular hemolysis.

FRAGMENTATION HEMOLYSIS: MICROANGIOPATHY

Clinical Manifestations

Patients present with various degrees of hemolytic anemia and compensation, with evidence of RBC fragmentation on smear (Fig. 48–1 and see box on Differential Diagnosis of Extrinsic Nonimmune Hemolytic Anemias). RBC removal is generally extravascular, with minimal or moderately decreased levels of haptoglobin. If RBC damage is sufficiently severe, signs of intravascular hemolysis may be present. Because of the underlying pathology, some of these syndromes show evidence of platelet removal, leading to thrombocytopenia. Occasionally, the underlying cause produces activation and depletion of procoagulant factors with consequent activation of the fibrinolytic system, consistent with disseminated intravascular coagulation (DIC; see box on Causes of Red Blood Cell Fragmentation Hemolysis).

Pathophysiology

Fragmentation hemolysis occurs when mechanical forces disrupt the physical integrity of the RBC membrane. Brain et al.[2] observed a possible relationship between vascular lesions and RBC fragmentation. They postulated that lesions produced shearing forces sufficiently strong to fragment RBCs or incited inflammation of small vessel walls, which generated fibrin strands that cut the passing RBCs into irregular pieces. Subsequent studies documented that in vitro shear stresses in excess of 3000 dynes/cm^2 cause RBC fragmentation. In vivo studies in patients with mitral prosthetic regurgitation and hemolysis show high peak shear stresses of 4500 dynes/cm^2, very rapid acceleration or deceleration, or both.[3]

Research suggests alternative mechanisms of producing microangiopathic hemolysis that involve platelets and small-vessel thrombi. Taylor et al.[4] described a baboon model in which injection of C4b-binding proteins and *Escherichia coli* produced a picture of DIC with microangiopathic hemolysis and thrombocytopenia. Treatment with the F(ab)$'_2$ monoclonal antibody against platelet glycoprotein (GP) IIb/IIIa complex reduced the microangiopathic hemolysis and renal disease. The platelet-rich, fibrin-poor microvascular thrombi found in many patients with thrombotic thrombocytopenic purpura (TTP) now are thought to be caused by abnormally decreased ADAMTS-13 activity. This metalloprotease is responsible for converting the highly thrombogenic large multimers of von Willebrand factor made by platelets and endothelial cells into the smaller forms normally found in circulation. Mutations in or antibodies against ADAMTS-13 result in unusually large multimers of von Willebrand factor attached to endothelial cell surfaces, where platelets may excessively aggregate, leading to formation of microvascular thrombi even in the absence of endothelial damage.

Whatever the mechanism of mechanical trauma, the RBC membrane is viscoelastic and has self-sealing properties (see Chapter 46) so that little hemoglobin leaks out as the cell is being cut. However, prolonged distortion of the membrane produces a plastic change; therefore, the smaller RBC fragments usually do not become microspheres or microdisks but continue to display evidence of the shearing event or distortion in the form of typical irregular shapes. These irregular shapes and the rigidity that they reflect subsequently interfere with the ability of RBCs to fold, elongate, and deform sufficiently to pass through 3-μm capillaries and even smaller slits in the walls of the sinusoids of the reticuloendothelial system. This sequence leads to their destruction.

Differential Diagnosis

Generally, the differential diagnosis of fragmentation hemolysis can be deduced from the clinical findings. The presence of a prosthetic heart valve or a regurgitant jet that fragments or accelerates[5] (i.e.,

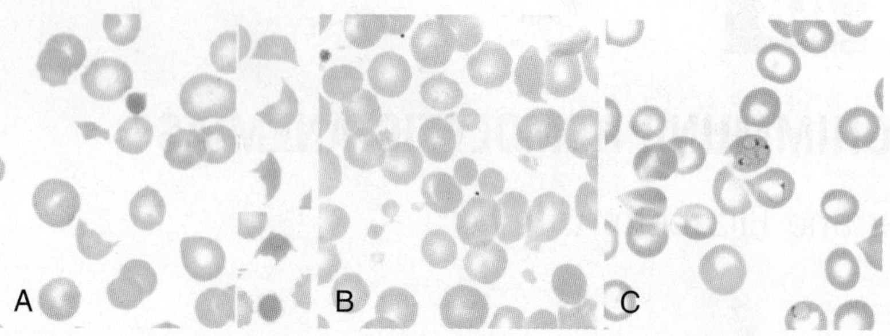

Figure 48–1 Peripheral blood smears from examples of extrinsic nonimmune hemolytic anemia. **A,** Microangiopathic hemolytic anemia. Note the schistocyte, fragmented cells, spherocyte, and polychromasia. More examples of damages red cells, including classic "helmet cell" (*top*), are seen to the immediate *right*. **B,** Thermal injury from burn. Thermally damaged red blood cells from numerous microspherocytes and tiny red cell fragments. **C,** Malaria infestation. Red cells contain *Plasmodium falciparum* malaria. Note the high rate of infestation, the presence of only ringed forms, and the multiply infested red cell (*center*).

Differential Diagnosis of Extrinsic Nonimmune Hemolytic Anemias

There is no simple approach to the differential diagnosis of hemolysis caused by extrinsic nonimmune hemolytic anemia. The physician must pay close attention to the clinical finding. Useful clues come from a determination of whether RBC breakdown is predominantly extravascular or intravascular, but most important in the analysis is the observation of RBC morphology, which can focus the differential diagnosis. Unhelpful terms such as *aniso* and *poik* should be discarded. RBCs are spherocytic, stomatocytic, fragmented, echinocytic, acanthocytic, spurred, or bite cells or can be mixtures of these types.

Causes of Red Blood Cell Fragmentation Hemolysis

Damaged microvasculature
Thrombotic thrombocytopenic purpura–hemolytic uremic syndrome (TTP–HUS)
Associated with pregnancy: Preeclampsia or eclampsia; hemolysis plus elevated liver enzymes plus low platelets (HELLP syndrome)
Associated with malignancy, with or without mitomycin C treatment
Vasculitis: Polyarteritis, Wegener granulomatosis, acute glomerulonephritis, or *Rickettsia*-like infections
Abnormalities of renal vasculature: Malignant hypertension, acute glomerulonephritis, scleroderma, or allograft rejection, with or without cyclosporine treatment
Disseminated intravascular coagulation
Malignant hypertension
Catastrophic antiphospholipid antibody syndrome
Atrioventricular malformations
Kasabach–Merritt syndrome
Hemangioendotheliomas
Atrioventricular shunts for congenital and acquired conditions (e.g., stents, coils, transjugular intrahepatic portosystemic shunt, Levine shunts)
Cardiac abnormalities
- Replaced valve, prosthesis, graft, or patch
- Aortic stenosis or regurgitant jets (e.g., in ruptured sinus of Valsalva)

Drugs: Cyclosporine, mitomycin, ticlopidine, tacrolimus, or cocaine

Waring blender syndrome) can be readily discerned. The clinical picture of thrombotic thrombocytopenic purpura–hemolytic uremic syndrome (TTP–HUS) is generally dramatic and acute (see Chapter 139). Atrioventricular malformations may be associated with DIC and platelet removal; the diagnosis requires a high index of suspicion and imaging studies. The presence of preeclampsia in a pregnant woman with microangiopathic hemolysis usually is obvious, but the HELLP (hemolysis, elevated liver enzymes, and low platelet count) syndrome is a serious complication of pregnancy that can occur without other signs of preeclampsia or hypertension.[6] This syndrome can produce hepatic rupture, visual failure, DIC, seizures, and congestive heart failure and requires treatment by prompt delivery of the fetus (see Chapters 140 and 161). Cancer can be an underlying cause of microangiopathy. Vessels supplying malignant tumors are thought to be structurally abnormal. They exhibit the same sort of fibrin stranding that produces fragmentation hemolysis in DIC and TTP–HUS.

Continued use of invasive diagnostic and therapeutic procedures with insertion of foreign bodies into the circulation has been complicated by microangiopathic hemolysis. A transjugular intrahepatic portosystemic shunt can cause the syndrome in approximately 10% of patients.[7] The hemolysis usually disappears after 12 to 15 weeks. Similarly, use of coil embolization to seal off a patent ductus arteriosus produced a fall in hemoglobin from 11.6 to 6 g in one patient.[8] Vasculitis also has been implicated as a cause.[9]

Several drugs are associated with microangiopathic hemolysis. Cyclosporine, tacrolimus, and mitomycin C have been implicated as causing an HUS picture that typically develops within weeks to months of exposure. Total body irradiation, combination chemotherapy, and bone marrow transplantation also are associated with microangiopathic hemolysis.[10] The antiplatelet agents ticlopidine and clopidogrel are capable of producing a TTP-like syndrome.[11] Quinine attaches to platelet glycoproteins and may induce antibodies against the altered glycoprotein epitopes. In one series, quinine exposure was implicated in 11% of 132 patients presenting with TTP–HUS.[12] Other reported exposures associated with TTP include use of cocaine,[13] the herb echinacea,[14] imatinib,[15] and gemcitabine.[16] The mechanisms of drug-induced TTP are not well understood but likely include direct toxicity to the endothelium.[16]

Therapy

Management is primarily directed toward the underlying disease or event. Compensation of RBC production should be optimized by replacing iron or folic acid if the patient is deficient in these nutrients. Occasionally removal or repair of a damaged native or prosthetic heart valve is necessary when the hemolysis produces a disabling transfusion requirement. Treatment of TTP–HUS with plasma exchange has been found to be superior to plasma infusions, with fresh frozen plasma and cryo-free plasma appearing to have equal efficacy.[17] The HUS of mitomycin C use in adenocarcinoma has been

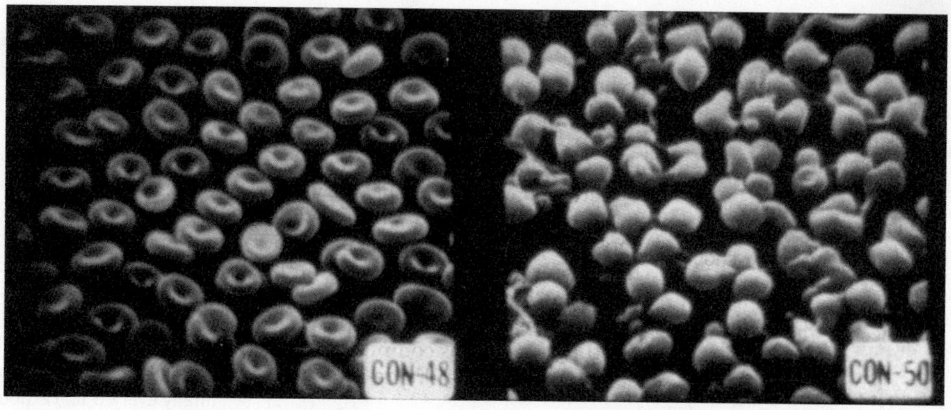

Figure 48–2 Morphologic changes are produced by heating normal red blood cells at the indicated temperatures. Budding begins abruptly at 50°C (122°F)and eventually leads to spherocytosis.

reported to respond reasonably well to use of the staphylococcal protein A immunoperfusion column[18] or to vincristine,[19] but apheresis with fresh frozen plasma replacement still may be needed. Thrombotic microangiopathy associated with cyclosporine often is reversible with cessation of cyclosporine.[20]

OTHER FORMS OF MECHANICAL DAMAGE TO RED BLOOD CELLS

Heat Denaturation

Normal RBCs undergo budding and fragmentation when exposed to a temperature of 49°C (120°F) in vitro (Fig. 48–1B). In some of the hereditary hemolytic anemias, this process occurs at temperatures as low as 46°C (115°F; see Chapter 46). Under some clinical circumstances, temperatures sufficient to cause heat denaturation of RBCs have been generated. Occasionally, cell warmers used with transfusions in cold agglutinin disease have malfunctioned and cooked the RBCs about to be transfused. In one case, a patient's mother warmed the RBCs with a hot water bottle, reasoning that such cells would cause less vein irritation to her child. Such transfusion was followed by evidence of intravascular and extravascular hemolysis, and the peripheral smear showed RBC budding and fragmentation (Fig. 48–2). Presumably, similar events can lead to hemolysis in patients who have sustained very extensive burns. In patients suffering from heat stroke, the temperature usually is below 42°C (108°F), a temperature at which little RBC denaturation occurs.

Mechanical Trauma

The classic example of RBC damage due to mechanical trauma is march hemoglobinuria, which occurs in soldiers after a long march, in joggers after running on a hard road, or in karate or conga drumming enthusiasts after practice. Anemia is rare, and reticulocytosis is uncommon. Evidence of typical intravascular RBC destruction is present and is thought to be caused by direct trauma to RBCs in the vessels of the feet or hands. Switching jogging paths or using better footwear often relieves the problem. Some cases show evidence of an underlying RBC membrane abnormality.[21] Strenuous exercise may induce oxidant stress, as evidenced by increased levels of malonyldialdehyde, a marker of lipid peroxidation, in marathon runners after a race.[22] Occasionally, malfunction of the cell savers used during abdominal or thoracic surgery mechanically injures RBCs.

Cardiopulmonary Bypass

Postperfusion syndrome occurs in some patients after cardiopulmonary bypass. The syndrome includes acute intravascular hemolysis and leukopenia as part of a febrile, inflammatory clinical picture. Affected patients may develop pulmonary distress and even adult/acute respiratory distress syndrome. Visible hemoglobinemia occurs, with rising plasma hemoglobin levels, and is associated with an increase in lysed RBC ghosts seen in the whole blood and plasma. These ghosts are coated with the complement complex C5bC9 (see Chapter 49). Presumably, the complement pathway is activated as the blood passes through the oxygenator. The reason why complement activation results in lytic attack on RBCs (and granulocytes) is unknown. Treatment involves knowledge of the process and requisite support[23] until the situation corrects itself.

Osmotic Attack

Abrupt changes in osmolality can cause hemolysis. Freshwater drowning may be associated with so much water in the lungs that the RBCs swell as they undergo an in vivo osmotic fragility test in the pulmonary vasculature. Conversely, saltwater drowning can cause profound dehydration of RBCs, producing a situation analogous to xerocytosis (see Chapter 46). Rarely, acute hemolysis occurs from mistaken infusion of, or exposure to, concentrated hypertonic solutions such as those used in hemodialysis. To manage such an event, the physician must recognize its cause, appreciate the shrunken RBCs on a peripheral smear, and restore isotonicity as quickly as possible. In this case, use of a hemodialysis device, if available, may be helpful.[24]

Hypersplenism

In all organs of the monocyte–macrophage system (i.e., reticuloendothelial system), blood cells leaving the arterial bed are generally unloaded into channels such that the RBCs must pass through the wall of the sinus to reenter the circulation. The sinusoidal wall has slits 2 to 3 μm long and usually is endothelialized on one side and has a macrophagic lining on the other side. The normal human adult RBC is a discocyte with a surface area 40% larger than a sphere of that volume (see Chapter 33). This excess surface area allows an RBC with a diameter of approximately 8 μm to twist, elongate, and deform sufficiently to squeeze through these 2- to 3-μm slits. The excess surface area, occasionally referred to as the *ratio of surface area to volume* (SA:V), is critical and normally is approximately 1.4. Any condition that reduces SA:V reduces the ability of RBCs to traverse these sinusoidal slits because plump spheres cannot deform sufficiently.

Factors that interfere with interaction of the cytosol and the membrane also impair the ability of the RBC to deform. Oxidant attack may produce Heinz bodies that come to lie adjacent to the membrane. They interfere with the smooth movement of the membrane over the cytosol, a process called *tank treading*. Such cells are selectively blocked from leaving the splenic cords and entering the sinuses.[25] Inflammation or infection may enhance the ability of splenic macrophages to attack and ingest RBCs. Although not strictly a mechanism of hypersplenism, Kupffer cell erythrophagocytosis is a prominent finding in patients undergoing graft-versus-host hemolysis seen after liver transplantation.[26]

Table 48–1 Causes of Splenomegaly

Cause	Example
Neoplasia	Lymphoma, hairy cell leukemia
Infection	Bacterial endocarditis, malaria, schistosomiasis, tuberculosis
Portal bed obstruction	Alcoholic cirrhosis, splenic vein thrombosis
Collagen vascular disease	Systemic lupus erythematosus, malignant phase of rheumatoid arthritis
Chronic inflammatory disease	Rheumatoid arthritis
Chronic hereditary or acquired hemolytic anemia	Severe β-thalassemia, autoimmune hemolytic anemia
Lipoidosis	Gaucher disease
Amyloidosis	AL and AA types
Tropical splenomegaly syndrome	Hyperreactive malarial splenomegaly syndrome

The spleen is more complicated than other reticuloendothelial organs in that the afferent arterioles pass through lymphoid nodules (i.e., white pulp) and then terminate in the cords of Billroth (i.e., red pulp), into which blood cells are discharged. In the slow flow of the cords of Billroth, blood cells are selectively attacked by macrophages and are in direct contact with several classes of lymphocytes. The blood cells then must pass through the cordal walls before they can approach the sinus wall, which they must pass through to reenter the circulation. The spleen provides a double filter, and the blood cells must be remarkably deformable to pass through it. This slow passage permits highly selective action by macrophages, which have receptors that can detect several sorts of alterations in these blood cells. These receptors include the Fc receptor for the appropriate portion of the immunoglobulin molecule, receptors for complement components such as C3b, and perhaps receptors that detect alterations in the outer portion of the phospholipid bilayer or in the externally oriented glycopeptides. The macrophage then holds, retards, modifies (i.e., pitting function), or removes (i.e., culling function) the blood cells identified. Normally, the pitting function of the spleen allows it to remove Howell-Jolly bodies and normally occurring endocytic vacuoles (called *pocks* because of their appearance on phase interference or Nomarski microscopy). The normal culling function of the spleen is exemplified by its removal of senescent RBCs.[27]

All the activities of the spleen presumably are markedly accentuated in a large spleen, and if the increased activity is sufficiently extensive, hypersplenism ensues. It is the size of the spleen, not the portal pressure, that is important in determining the degree of RBC sequestration.[28] Other factors that may play a role are the state of activation of the splenic macrophages and the size of the small slits between the splenic cords and sinuses. The macrophages and slits seem to be under a degree of control, as evidenced by variations in splenic removal of RBCs in patients with malaria.[29]

The clinical picture of hypersplenic hemolysis is dominated by the specific cause of the splenomegaly. Although the causes of splenomegaly are legion, there are several general mechanisms (Table 48–1). Usually some degree of anemia is seen, with evidence of a compensatory increase in RBC production. Because stasis and trapping in the spleen are associated with macrophagic attack and remodeling of the RBC surface, the reduction in SA:V leads to spherocytosis. If the RBCs undergo a prolonged period of distortion when traversing the cordal–sinus barrier, tailed RBCs will be present as the RBC membranes undergo a plastic change (see Chapter 46 and box on Therapy for Lead-Related Hemolysis). Because the enlarged spleen can trap and remove platelets and white blood cells, variable thrombocytopenia and leukopenia may occur. The bone marrow may show normal to increased cellularity with erythroid hyperplasia.

Therapy for Lead-Related Hemolysis

In an acute situation with multiple organ malfunctions and hemolysis, lead ingestion is stopped immediately, and therapy is begun inadults with edetate calcium disodium 30 to 50 mg/kg/day by either deep IM or slow intravenous infusion divided twice daily for up to 5 consecutive days. The chelator–lead complex is nephrotoxic, and urine output must be monitored. Dimercaprol is also started at least 4 hours prior to starting edetate calcium disodium in order to prevent worsening CNS toxicity with increased blood lead levels. Dimercaprol is given intramuscularly for a total of 11 days. It is dosed initially at 4 mg/kg every 4 hours for the first 48 hours, then at 6-hour intervals for the next 48 hours, and finally every 6 to 12 hours for 7 days.[36] If symptoms improve and urine lead levels fall satisfactorily, the patient can be started on a regimen of oral penicillamine, given at a dose of 1 to 1.5 grams/day for 1 to 2 months given 2 hours before or 3 hours after meals. If symptoms do not improve satisfactorily, another course of edetate calcium disodium is given. Dimercaprol is pregnancy category C, and penicillamine is pregnancy category D.

Management depends on the cause of splenic enlargement. The anemia or pancytopenia usually is not profound; however, splenectomy may be contemplated if the anemia is severe. In most situations, recognition of the possibility of hypersplenism is most important in guiding the approach to diagnosis of an unexplained anemia. Massive splenomegaly frequently is associated with expansion of the plasma compartment, and measurement of hemoglobin, hematocrit, or RBC levels may give a falsely low value of the RBC mass present. In that circumstance, the true RBC mass can be determined by ^{51}Cr assay.

A good example of massive splenomegaly causing plasma volume expansion is tropical splenomegaly syndrome, which has been renamed *hyperreactive malarial splenomegaly syndrome*. Diagnostic criteria include massive splenomegaly more than 10 cm below the costal margin, with no other cause identified; immunity to malaria; elevated serum IgM levels; and clinical response to treatment with antimalarial drugs such as chloroquine, proguanil, or pyrimethamine and folic acid.[30] The pathophysiology of the splenomegaly seems to be poorly controlled B-lymphocytic production of antibodies, and IgM stimulation may be a response to malarial antigens or an unidentified mitogen. Malarial parasites are almost never found. The apparent anemia is in large part caused by plasma volume expansion, although RBC survival is reported to be slightly attenuated. Antimalarial therapy for several months reduces spleen size, so splenectomy is unnecessary.

Infection

Infection can cause hemolytic anemia via several pathophysiologic mechanisms (Table 48–2).

Parasite Infections

The classic example of direct parasitization is infection by *Plasmodium falciparum* (Fig. 48–1C), *Plasmodium vivax*, or *Plasmodium malariae*. Infection with malaria, primarily *P. falciparum*, is a major health problem in the developing world, causing an estimated 300 to 500 million infections and one to three million deaths annually.[31,32] The burden of disease rests most heavily on young children and pregnant women. Falciparum malaria can cause a life-threatening anemia, with severe anemia defined as hemoglobin less than 5 g/dL.[31] Although malaria is primarily a disease of the tropical developing world, since the 1950s sixty-three outbreaks due to locally acquired mosquito-borne transmission have occurred in the United States.[33]

Table 48–2 Mechanisms by Which Infection Can Cause Hemolysis

Mechanism	Example
Direct parasitization of red cells	Malaria, babesiosis
Immune mechanisms	Cold agglutinin hemolysis after infectious mononucleosis or mycoplasmal pneumonia (see Chapter 47)
Induction of hypersplenism	Malaria, schistosomiasis
Altered red cell surface topology	*Haemophilus influenzae* infection
Release of toxins and enzymes	Clostridial infection causing thrombotic thrombocytopenic purpura–hemolytic uremic syndrome, *Escherichia coli* 0197, human immunodeficiency virus infection (?)

In each of the malarias, sporozoites injected by the mosquito in its saliva make their way to liver cells. After 1 to 2 weeks, they become merozoites, which burst out of the liver cells and into the bloodstream. Then, in a remarkable process, the parasite, by means of its apical end and related organelles called *rhoptries*, attaches to a specific receptor on the RBC surface. For *P. vivax,* the Duffy blood group antigen appears to be involved, making it a promising target for vaccine-based prevention.[34]

Plasmodium falciparum binds to sialic acid residues on the RBC surface that are on glycophorin A. After specific attachment, a convulsive movement occurs during which the RBC engulfs the parasite by a process resembling receptor-mediated endocytosis. The parasite then immediately recruits the RBC's metabolic machinery, degrades and ingests hemoglobin, and grows, eventually bursting out of the RBC, and the cycle begins again. The RBCs are lysed intravascularly as a consequence of direct parasitic destruction, extravascularly as a consequence of changes in the splenic microvasculature, and in the activation state of the monocyte–macrophage system. Treatment consists of the use of appropriate antimalarials and the support of erythropoiesis, including the use of RBC transfusion and/or exchange when indicated.[35]

The anemia of malarial infections also involves mechanisms distinct from lysis of parasitized RBCs. Erythropoiesis is suppressed, leading to suppression of erythroid precursors[37] and inadequate reticulocytosis during acute infection.[38] Bone marrow suppression may continue with persistent infection that is no longer demonstrable microscopically.[39] This inadequate hematopoietic response may be exacerbated by underlying iron deficiency, hemoglobinopathies, or concomitant infection (e.g., HIV), all potential contributors to the severity of anemia.[31] In addition, loss of uninfected erythrocytes plays a major role in the development of anemia, with an eight-fold to 10-fold greater loss of unparasitized red cells compared to parasitized cells.[40,41] Uninfected red cells have reduced deformability, and the degree of reduced deformability correlates with the severity of infection.[42,43] Poorly deformable red cells likely are cleared by the spleen. Evidence of in vivo removal of immature malarial forms prompts the question of whether "uninfected" cells that are lost represent previously infected cells that nevertheless remain abnormal. Insertion of a merozoite rhoptry protein, ring surface protein 2, on red cells in which infection was aborted has been implicated in the clearance of unparasitized erythrocytes and erythroid progenitors.[44] In addition, uninfected RBCs demonstrate increased binding of immunoglobulins that probably are nonspecific immune complexes.[45] Acute malarial infection, particularly with *P. falciparum,* also leads to alteration in splenic function that incites premature destruction of uninfected red cells.[29] Children with severe malarial anemia have low levels of complement regulatory proteins CR1 and CD55 in comparison to children with uncomplicated malaria or asymptomatic children,[46] suggesting a contribution of complement-mediated destruction of red cells. Oxidative stress may occur, as indicated by decreased α-tocopherol in RBC membranes of infected patients.[47]

The lifespan of transfused RBCs is likewise decreased. ^{51}Cr-Labeled normal RBCs infused into patients infected with malaria demonstrate a shorter lifespan than in normal controls; this effect may persist after clearance of the parasitemia.[48]

Alternatively, parasites can be removed from red cells along with red cell membrane by the process of pitting, producing parasite-free spherocytes.[49] This mechanism potentially explains the observed disparity between anemia and parasitemia.

Other infections that have somewhat similar pathophysiologies include Carrión disease (i.e., bartonellosis), in which a bite from the sandfly injects *Bartonella bacilliformis,* which attaches to the RBC surface of up to 80% of erythrocytes and causes lysis, leading to the massive hemolysis that characterizes acute infection. It appears that invasion of RBCs partly depends on the flagella of *Bartonella*. Incubation with antiflagellin antiserum reduces invasion of RBCs.[50] The bacteria also secrete deformin, a factor that leads to deep pitting on the surface of RBCs,[51] presumably providing a portal of entry into the erythrocyte. There also may be a role for splenic clearance of infected cells, and prior splenectomy appeared to protect a patient from hemolysis during acute infection.[52]

Babesia organisms also directly invade RBCs, producing fever and hemolytic anemia. The parasite is transmitted by ticks and transfusions of infected blood products[53] and can be transmitted vertically.[54] Most tick-borne cases occur on the West Coast, particularly in Washington and California, and in the northern portion of the Midwest; cases occurring on the East Coast are concentrated in Massachusetts and Nantucket Island.[55] The organisms can be seen invading RBCs on smear examination, somewhat like *P. falciparum* malaria, but these organisms produce no pigment. The highest risk of death from babesiosis occurs in individuals who are older than 50 years or are immunocompromised due to acquired immunodeficiency syndrome (AIDS), drugs, or asplenism. Sporadic reports indicate that acquired chronic toxoplasmosis occasionally is associated with hemolytic anemia.[56]

Alteration of the Red Blood Cell Surface by Bacterial Products

Infection can produce hemolysis by altering the RBC surface. An example is the hemolysis caused by *Haemophilus influenzae* type b.[57] Severely affected patients, particularly those with meningitis, have developed hemolytic anemias requiring RBC transfusions. The capsular polysaccharide of the bacterium, composed of polyribosyl ribitol phosphate (PRP), is released during infection and binds to the RBC surface. Infected patients develop antibodies to PRP. When the balance between PRP-coated RBCs and anti-PRP antibodies is correct, an immune-type hemolysis occurs and requires complement. RBC destruction is thought to be both intravascular and extravascular.

Bacterial Products Causing Hemolysis by Direct Damage to Red Blood Cells

The most dramatic example of hemolysis due to bacterial action is clostridial infection, during which the organism releases enzymes that acutely degrade the phospholipids of the membrane bilayer and the structural membrane proteins. The resulting spherocytes are extremely sensitive to osmotic lysis. In one case, the serum phospholipase C level increased fivefold over 4 hours and the patient died.[58] The setting can be any infection, but my experience is limited to acute cholecystitis, surgery of the biliary tree, and infections surrounding an obstetric event, including criminal or self-induced abortion or other infection of the gravid uterus. Patients may also have an underlying malignancy, such as a gastrointestinal, genitourinary, neuroendocrine, or hematologic malignancy.[59] The signs of infections may be obvious, but fever may be unimpressive. Signs of collapse appear acutely, and the clue is profound intravascular hemolysis, with a spherocytic anemia developing with shocking suddenness. The blood smear characteristically has numerous spherocytes with little evidence of microangiopathy, may be tinged red due to marked hemoglobinemia, and may have ghost cells.[59,60] A clue to the severity of the process may be the inability of the laboratory to perform chemical determinations or to type and cross-match the blood because the sample is hemolyzed. With even the slightest suspicion of hemolysis due to bacterial action, the physician immediately starts full doses of penicillin and clindamycin, evaluates the patient for DIC (see Chapter 132), and prepares to support the patient for shock, DIC, acute renal failure, and hemolytic anemia. Whether hysterectomy is lifesaving in the case of septic abortion is unclear.[61]

Hemolysis Caused by Less Well Understood Infections

HIV infection can cause Coombs-positive autoimmune hemolytic anemia, a TTP-like syndrome, and microangiopathic hemolysis. Cytomegalovirus infection was reported to cause hemolysis associated with thrombocytopenia by unknown mechanisms in an immunocompetent woman.[62] Case reports of autoimmune hemolytic anemia and HUS associated with cytomegalovirus infection have emerged. The hemolytic anemia in visceral leishmaniasis may be caused in part by generation of oxidative metabolic products.[63] Severe microangiopathic hemolytic anemia has been described for two cases of cutaneous anthrax.[64]

Hemolysis Associated with Liver Disease

Hemolysis in liver disease by itself usually is not of overwhelming clinical importance, but it may contribute to the severity of anemia when coupled with defects in RBC production and the type of gastrointestinal blood loss that occurs in several forms of liver disease. Hemolysis in patients with liver disease has several causes. The spleen may be enlarged as a consequence of portal hypertension and produce a hypersplenic picture, a phenomenon seen commonly in hepatic cirrhosis.

The literature on RBC shape change in liver disease is considerable. The target cell in cirrhosis has an increased SA:V that appears to be a consequence of increased cholesterol and phospholipid content of the membrane bilayer. The cholesterol increase usually is proportionately greater, resulting in an increased cholesterol-to-phospholipid ratio. This increase in lipid probably accounts for the increased RBC surface area, such that more membrane than usual is present in relation to cellular contents. These RBCs probably circulate as bell-shaped RBCs called *codocytes.* However, on dried blood films, they assume the appearance of target cells. Target cells do not have a shortened survival. The RBCs of patients with liver disease frequently are echinocytes when wet preparations are examined, but these echinocytes are not easily apparent on dried blood smears. The echinocytes seem to be produced by a material in the patient's plasma that causes normal RBCs to become echinocytic; this material is an abnormal echinocytogenic high-density lipoprotein. Echinocytes do not necessarily have a shortened survival. Some forms of echinocytic RBCs are normally deformable when studied in the ektacytometer or rheoscope.[65]

A brisk, clinically important hemolysis can occur in some patients with severe liver disease. The peripheral smear in these individuals usually shows acanthocytes (i.e., distorted RBCs). Extreme forms are called *spur cells,* which probably are acanthocytes additionally remodeled by an enlarged spleen (see box on Reduction of Dangerous Methemoglobin Levels) and are considerably enriched in cholesterol.[66] They are rapidly removed in the spleen, which usually is enlarged.

Increased RBC membrane proteolytic activity may be a partial explanation for the differences between acanthocytosis and spur cells,[67] and additional pathophysiologic mechanisms may be involved. Although the adult RBC cannot synthesize phospholipids de novo, it can identify and remove peroxidized fatty acid chains that interfere with normal membrane lipid fluidity.[66] When the fatty acid is removed, a lytic lysoderivative remains; therefore, the missing fatty acid chain must be replaced. A store of acyl groups in the form of acylcarnitine exists in RBC membranes. When needed, the fatty acid (i.e., acyl group) is transferred to acyl-coenzyme A and then inserted into the potentially lytic lysophospholipid by the enzyme lysophosphocholine acyltransferase. Lysophosphocholine acyltransferase is inhibited in spur RBCs, and the same inhibition can be produced by heavily loading RBCs with cholesterol in vitro.[66]

In spur cell anemia, the RBCs have an abnormal membrane SA:V ratio, their membrane fluidity is impaired, and they are unable to remove and repair peroxidatively damaged fatty acids. Occasionally, spur cell hemolytic anemia is severe enough to necessitate consideration of splenectomy. Operative morbidity in such cases is considerable because the underlying liver disease usually produces problems with thrombocytopenia and leukopenia as well as with procoagulants and intolerance to anesthesia.

Acute alcoholism can be associated with hypophosphatemia, defined as levels less than 0.2 mg/dL. Such hypophosphatemia presumably interferes with RBC intermediary metabolism (see Chapters 33 and 45), and RBC ATP levels fall. Very low ATP levels are associated with RBC rigidity, which leads to fragmentation, loss of surface area, and spheroidicity. The RBCs then are further trapped in the spleen. This hypophosphatemia syndrome can also cause neuromuscular disorders, including weakness, paresthesias, tremors, and seizures. It should be treated aggressively with orally and intravenously administered phosphate supplements. Hypophosphatemia also occurs in cirrhotic patients, patients receiving total parenteral nutrition whose phosphate intake is not carefully monitored, and patients taking large amounts of phosphate-binding antacids.[69–71]

Stomatocytosis can occur in severe liver disease and is thought to be a sign of acute alcoholic intoxication. The change in RBC shape can also be seen in acute pancreatitis. The stomatocyte is a cell well on its way to becoming a spherocyte. The reduction in SA:V leads to trapping in the microvasculature of the spleen and other organs of the monocyte–macrophage system, producing various degrees of hemolysis.

Reduction of Dangerous Methemoglobin Levels

Levels of methemoglobin in excess of 20% to 30% can be dangerous, but they can be easily treated with methylene blue (1–2 mg/kg) infused intravenously over 5 minutes as 0.1 to 0.2 mL/kg of a 1% solution. In the presence of a functioning, intact NADPH-methemoglobin reductase system, methylene blue is reduced to leukomethylene blue, which reduces methemoglobin to hemoglobin.

In a case of almost fatal oxidative hemolysis, hydrogen peroxide was injected directly into the Hickman catheter of a patient with AIDS because some persons infected with HIV had circulated a pamphlet suggesting that hydrogen peroxide could be used therapeutically to control HIV infection. We now are seeing AIDS patients with dapsone-induced methemoglobinemia and hemolytic anemia (see Chapters 44 and 45). Methemoglobinemia, if severe, is treated as described in the preceeding paragraph and in Chapter 44. One study suggests that the severity of the oxidative attack can be partially ameliorated by administration of 800 units per day of vitamin E, an antioxidant agent.[68]

Renal Disease

The anemia in renal disease is multifactorial. A major component is impaired RBC production, which can be well controlled with erythropoietin. Renal disease also impairs platelet function, which may lead to occult blood loss. However, hemolysis also can occur and is multifactorial. Disease of the small renal arterioles can produce fragmentation hemolysis of the sort seen in TTP–HUS, preeclampsia, and malignant hypertension (see box on Causes of Red Blood Cell Fragmentation Hemolysis). In the past, some patients undergoing chronic hemodialysis were exposed to unusual concentrations of chloramine in tap water and underwent acute oxidative hemolysis.[72] This occurrence has become rare or nonexistent. Otherwise, whether uremia produces significant shortening of RBC survival is not clear. Patients with chronic renal failure who are undergoing hemodialysis may be particularly susceptible to oxidative damage to their RBCs. RBC glutathione (GSH) is reduced in some patients, and the activity of the enzymes G6PD and glutathione peroxidase is relatively low. The ability of these RBCs to deal with generation of peroxides probably is impaired.[73]

Venoms, Bites, Stings, and Toxins

The best-known example of toxin-caused hemolysis was discussed in the earlier section on Bacterial Products Causing Hemolysis by Direct Damage to Red Blood Cells.

Insect, Spider, and Snake Bites

Hemolysis occurs after bee and wasp stings, snake bites, and spider bites. Isolated cases of acute intravascular hemolysis after bee and wasp stings have been reported. Two kinds of dangerous spiders live in the United States: the southern black widow and the brown recluse spider. Both sexes of the black widow produce the venom, but only the female has fangs capable of penetrating human skin. Black widow spider bites produce generalized muscle pain and muscular rigidity. Hemolysis is not common. Brown recluse spider bites cause a considerable local reaction, called the *volcano lesion*. DIC and hemolysis may occur after a lag of 24 to 48 hours. Envenomation results in cleavage of RBC glycophorins, presumably making the RBCs more susceptible.[74] Corticosteroids may be beneficial. The hemolysis appears to be self-limiting, but RBC transfusion support may be needed.

In some parts of the world, cobra bites can cause intravascular hemolysis because the venom contains phospholipases. In the United States, the two classes of venomous snakes are pit vipers (e.g., rattlesnakes, cottonmouths, moccasins, and copperheads) and coral snakes. Pit viper venom affects hemostasis and may produce DIC with bleeding but rarely hemolysis. Coral snake venom produces severe neurologic impairment. Therapy consists of support and use of the appropriate antivenin and prophylactic antimicrobials and tetanus injections.

Drugs and Chemicals Exclusive of Those Producing Oxidative Hemolysis

Potassium Chlorate

Potassium chlorate ingestion is listed as a cause of hemolysis, but this compound is no longer available in hospital pharmacies and has no currently recognized medical use. Arsine gas (AsH_3) is generated in industrial plants that engage in lead plating, galvanizing, etching, and soldering. Inhalation of a toxic amount produces a severe intravascular hemolysis[75] of unknown pathogenesis and may require urgent RBC and plasma exchange.[76]

Copper

The idea that copper can produce human hemolytic disease is best supported by observations of episodes of severe hemolysis in patients with Wilson disease. The patient usually is a child, adolescent, or young adult for whom the diagnosis of Wilson disease has not yet been made.[77,78] The initial clinical presentation usually is dominated by the hemolytic anemia, accompanied by weakness and dark urine. The RBC morphology has not been well described, but reticulocytosis is present, with an increased serum bilirubin level partly attributable to the underlying liver disease. A clue to the underlying diagnosis is the presence of liver failure with low alkaline phosphate levels. Because of the hereditary deficiency in the copper-binding protein ceruloplasmin, urine and serum non–ceruloplasmin-bound copper levels in patients with hemolysis are very high. Curiously, in one report hemoglobin A_2 levels also were elevated.[77]

Free copper can interfere with glucose metabolism by hexokinase inhibition and alternatively can generate oxidative hemolysis, perhaps by acting as a Fenton reagent. It is important to establish the diagnosis promptly. When this condition is suspected, look for Kayser–Fleischer rings on physical examination and measure serum and urine copper and ceruloplasmin levels. Treatment with penicillamine reduces the serum copper level and stops the hemolysis. Plasmapheresis and hemofiltration may be beneficial in reducing the copper level and can serve as a bridge to transplant.[79–81] Other forms of copper poisoning may cause hemolysis in patients who do not have underlying Wilson disease. The amount of copper ingested would have to exceed the copper-binding capacity of normal ceruloplasmin levels.

Lead

There are at least two general forms of lead intoxication. One type is *chronic, slow cumulative poisoning* (i.e., saturnism). An example is occupational exposure. Symptoms are predominantly neurologic and nephrologic, with variable degrees of anemia, which may be caused by a production defect combined with hemolysis. *Relatively acute poisoning* occurs when lead inadvertently finds its way into a food source[82] or is consumed as part of an exotic medication. Subacute lead poisoning leads to central nervous system symptoms, hepatitis, nephrotoxicity, hypertension, and abdominal colic, along with seizures and severe hemolytic anemia. Physical examination may reveal the lead line on the gums. Peripheral smear shows extensive coarse basophilic stippling and reticulocytosis; however, RBC morphology is not otherwise characteristic. Some researchers state that intravascular destruction occurs, but no proof has been provided. Bilirubin levels are not significantly elevated.

The diagnosis of lead-related hemolysis can be made from the history and findings on physical examination finding: lead line on the gingiva and coarse basophilic stippling on RBCs, which reflects the pathologic aggregation of ribosomes. The diagnosis is confirmed by measuring blood and urine lead levels. The level of acuity determines the therapy.

The cause of the anemia is complex. Lead interferes with several steps in heme synthesis, particularly those involving heme synthetase and δ-aminolevulinic acid dehydratase (see Chapter 39). The inhibition of heme synthetase probably accounts for the elevation in free erythrocyte protoporphyrin, which provides a useful corroborative diagnostic test for lead toxicity. Inhibition of heme synthesis also probably accounts for the elevated urinary levels of δ-aminolevulinic acid and coproporphyrin. Lead poisoning mimics the basophilic stippling and accumulation of pyrimidines seen in hereditary deficiency of the enzyme pyrimidine 5′-nucleotidase, probably because lead attacks the enzyme (see Chapter 45).[83,84]

Ribavirin

Current treatment of chronic hepatitis C virus (HCV) infection consists of combination therapy with pegylated interferon and ribavirin, a nucleoside analogue. Ribavirin's activity against HCV includes inhibition of inosine monophosphate dehydrogenase, a key step in de novo guanine synthesis. Treatment with ribavirin may produce a dose-dependent hemolytic anemia, which typically is reversible 1 to 2 months after discontinuing treatment.[85] The hemoglobin drops by an average of 2 to 3 g/dL and may fall below 11 g/dL in one third or more of patients.[86] Although the anemia may necessitate a dose reduction in a substantial number of patients, decreases in hemoglobin can be treated with recombinant erythropoietin at 40,000 units weekly.[87] Ribavirin is transported into the erythrocytes and accumulates as ribavirin monophosphates, diphosphates, and triphosphates.[85] The steady-state concentration of ribavirin in erythrocytes is approximately 100-fold higher than that of plasma, and higher erythrocyte ribavirin levels correlate with worsened anemia during therapy.[88] Accumulation of phosphates leads to a decrease in ATP levels in comparison to control erythrocytes.[89] Because ATP is required to generate the glucose-6-phosphate needed for glycolysis and the hexose monophosphate shunt, reduced levels of ATP may lead to oxidative damage, as evidenced by increased aggregates of band 3, which bind anti-band 3 IgG and complement.[89] Newer inosine monophosphate dehydrogenase inhibitors, which spare the erythrocyte, include the drug viramidine, which currently is in clinical trials.[90] The anemia in patients treated with ribavirin may be exacerbated by concomitant treatment with pegylated interferon, which suppresses hematopoiesis. In addition, treatment with pegylated interferon has been associated with autoimmune hemolytic anemia.[91]

DRUG-INDUCED OXIDATIVE HEMOLYSIS

General Concepts

The potential for normal RBCs to undergo auto-oxidative destruction is great because the cell is loaded with 20 mM hemoglobin, most of which is bonded to oxygen at the iron(II) atom in heme. The bond that allows the reversible association and dissociation of oxygen from the heme moiety of hemoglobin involves partial transfer of an electron from iron(II) to oxygen. That oxygen then has an extra electron, which makes it a superoxide radical. Ordinarily, when oxygen leaves hemoglobin, it returns the electron. If it does not, a highly reactive superoxide ion is released, leaving behind it an iron(III) moiety called *methemoglobin.*

$$\text{Hb Fe}^{2+}\,O_2 \rightarrow \text{Hb Fe}^{3+} + O_2^{-1}$$

Methemoglobin cannot reversibly bind oxygen. Methemoglobin in itself is not harmful to RBCs, but if the oxidative assault persists, methemoglobin is converted to hemichromes, which are variably denatured hemoglobin intermediates in which the distal histidine unit binds to the oxidized heme. This step is associated with conversion from a high to a low spin state, as measured by electron spin resonance. Continued oxidation leads to irreversibility of hemichrome oxidation, precipitation, and eventually formation of Heinz bodies. Hemichromes and Heinz bodies can destroy membrane function directly or by causing oxidation of membrane proteins and lipids.[92] Approximately 3% of hemoglobin is converted to methemoglobin each day, but the finding that only 1% of hemoglobin normally is in the form of methemoglobin indicates that a mechanism preventing oxidation in RBCs is in effect. These mechanisms are limited, as RBCs lack the ability to either efficiently generate ATP or synthesize enzymes. The primary means for preventing or addressing oxidant injury are the generation of the reduced form of nicotinamide adenine dinucleotide (NADH) via the Embden-Meyerhof glycolytic pathway and the generation of nicotinamide adenine dinucleotide phosphate (NADPH) via the hexose monophosphate shunt. NADH is used to reduce methemoglobin by cytochrome b5 reductase, and NADPH is used to reduce glutathione and for catalase activity.[93] Defects in this defense system against oxidation lead to an enhanced tendency to oxidative hemolysis. Examples are G6PD deficiency states. G6PD catalyzes the initial rate-limiting step in the hexose monophosphate shunt. Deficiencies lead to a reduced ability to generate NADPH in response to oxidant stress. Any agent or event that interferes with the smooth offloading of oxygen enhances the generation of O_2^{-1} and methemoglobin, as indicated in the equation. If the reducing power of the RBC is inadequate, hemichromes and Heinz bodies are generated. Many agents appear to cause oxidative hemolysis by interfering with the smooth functioning of the heme cleft.

Hemolytic Anemia in Chronic Large Granular Lymphocytic Leukemia

Although large granular lymphocytic leukemia usually manifests as neutropenia and a rheumatoid-like picture, several patients with a severe Coombs-negative hemolytic anemia in the absence of splenomegaly have been described. Large granular lymphocytic leukemia has occurred in a splenectomized subject. The mechanism is unknown, but one report identified direct cytotoxicity against RBCs by the large granular lymphocytic cell lines.[102]

There are no formal studies on therapy for large granular lymphocytic leukemia-related hemolysis. One patient had a partial response to therapy with 60 mg/day of prednisone, and two patients responded well to weekly doses of methotrexate started at 5 mg/week.[103]

Pathophysiology

After the oxidative attack has been initiated, the sequence proceeds along a recognizable track. The oxidative attack is directed at hemoglobin and the RBC membrane. However, these structures are not clearly separable because the precipitated hemichrome and Heinz bodies come to lie against the cytosolic face of the membrane. Methemoglobin may be detectably elevated, with levels as high as 50% to 60% of total hemoglobin. The hemichromes, by themselves or with their iron portions acting as a Fenton reagent, mediate the generation of hydroxyl free radicals, which add their effect to that of superoxide and hydrogen peroxide. Lipid peroxidation may take place, leading to membrane blebbing and cell lysis as well as loss of asymmetry of the phospholipid membrane bilayer. Movement of phosphatidylserine and phosphatidylethanolamine to the outer bilayer of the membrane[94] results in increased recognition by macrophages in the reticuloendothelial system.[95] Membrane proteins may be cross-linked, with binding of denatured, oxidized hemoglobin to the membrane cytoskeleton,[96,97] which may increase splenic macrophage recognition.[98] In addition, the RBCs are rigid and susceptible to trapping in sinusoidal structures, whether or not they have Heinz bodies lying against the membrane. In vitro evidence suggests that oxidized RBCs are increasingly susceptible to phagocytosis by macrophages. These features may account for extravascular destruction. The oxidative lesions can be severe enough to cause intravascular destruction as well, producing hemoglobinemia and hemoglobinuria.

The smear may show bite cells, which look as if a macrophage had taken a bite, removing a Heinz body-containing segment of membrane. RBC rigidity may result in irregularly shaped cells because these undeformable cells are unable to undergo elastic recoil after fighting their way through the sinus wall. Recurrent loss of membrane material may produce spherocytes. Severe hemolysis may produce the kind of circulating ghost or hemighost called a *blister cell* or *bite cell.* These RBCs have an empty veil of membrane on one side and puddled hemoglobin on the other.[99,100] A Heinz body preparation may be positive. However, the absence of bite cells does not rule out the diagnosis.

The clinical picture is determined by the specific agent used. Screening for G6PD deficiency or a related disorder using an enzyme assay or the ascorbate cyanide test may be useful. Although any defect in the antioxidant defense mechanisms, such as G6PD deficiency, considerably increases the susceptibility to hemolysis, many agents can produce oxidant hemolysis even in persons with normal defense mechanisms (see box on Agents That Cause Oxidative Hemolysis). Paraquat ingestion has occurred inadvertently and in suicide attempts.[101] Profound cyanosis with methemoglobinemia can occur within hours, with levels of 120% or higher. The condition may be succeeded by hemolysis, with Heinz bodies seen in appropriate preparations of RBCs.

Toxic ingestion or inhalation of nitrites may occur in suicide attempts,[104] from industrial exposures, via diets high in pickled or smoked foods,[105] through intentional recreational use,[104] or, in

Agents That Cause Oxidative Hemolysis

Therapeutic agents
- Nitrofurantoin (Furadantin)
- Sulfasalazine (Azulfidine)
- *p*-Aminosalicylic acid
- Phenazopyridine (Pyridium)
- Phenacetin
- Dapsone and other sulfones
- Primaquine

Recreational drugs
- Isobutyl nitrate
- Amyl nitrite

Miscellaneous agents
- Naphthalene mothballs
- Paraquat
- Hydrogen peroxide

infants, from formulas prepared using well water high in nitrates, which are reduced to nitrites in the infant gut.[106] The nitrite may be sold in sex shops under the names *locker room, sweat,* or *rush*. Nitrites bind to hemoglobin, producing methemoglobinemia, which may be so profound as to produce coma. If methylene blue infusion does not quickly turn the chocolate color of blood back to normal, the physician must consider the possibility that the patient is G6PD deficient and therefore unable to generate adequate amounts of NADPH (discussed earlier under Drug-Induced Oxidative Hemolysis; General Concepts). In that case, exchange transfusion may be lifesaving.[107,108] Benzocaine topical anesthesia in the form of a spray or cream can cause methemoglobin levels of 23% or more, with cyanosis and dyspnea requiring methylene blue treatment.[109,110]

Pyridium (phenazopyridine) can cause oxidative hemolysis,[111] even in the absence of renal disease.[112] This agent is commonly used for treatment of bladder irritation. The *Physician's Desk Reference* recommends maximum therapy of 2 days. However, patients not uncommonly are given a prescription for 1 to 4 weeks of therapy.

It has been recognized for more than 130 years that therapy with dapsone causes oxidative hemolysis.[113] In the past, dapsone was used primarily to treat leprosy and dermatitis herpetiformis and was not often encountered as a cause of oxidative hemolysis. Dapsone has come into more widespread use in some communities as a very effective prophylactic agent against *Pneumocystis carinii* pneumonia in patients with AIDS. The reduced levels of GSH reported in patients with AIDS may enhance dapsone toxicity. Some clinics screen potential recipients for G6PD deficiency (see Chapter 45) and, if negative, proceed with dapsone therapy. However, dapsone can cause oxidative attack on normal RBCs, leading sequentially to methemoglobinemia, Heinz bodies, and hemolysis, all occurring at generally accepted standard doses.[114] Dapsone is metabolized to a hydroxylamine derivative that is directly toxic to RBCs.[115]

MISCELLANEOUS, POORLY CHARACTERIZED CAUSES OF EXTRINSIC HEMOLYTIC ANEMIAS

Interferon-α as a Cause of Hemolytic Anemia

Both microangiopathic and autoimmune hemolysis have been reported with interferon-α use. Zuber et al.[116] reported eight patients with chronic myeloid leukemia who developed thrombotic microangiopathy confirmed by renal biopsy. Seven of these patients had identifiable hemolysis, and three had thrombocytopenia. They also reviewed 13 other cases of microangiopathy associated with interferon–α reported in the literature and observed that most cases occurred in the setting of prolonged therapy in chronic myeloid leukemia. Two cases of chronic hepatitis with microangiopathy were notable for having received unusually high doses of interferon for this indication. Cases of autoimmune hemolysis have been reported with interferon-α therapy in the setting of chronic myeloid leukemia or chronic hepatitis C.

Hemolysis With Intravenous Immunoglobulin G

Strictly speaking, hemolysis with intravenous immunoglobulin G (IgG) is a form of immune hemolysis. However, preparations of IgG contain anti-A and anti-B antibodies and rarely cause an alloimmune hemolytic anemia, as described in two young women undergoing treatment for idiopathic thrombocytopenic purpura. If this situation occurs and more intravenous IgG is needed, performing a minor cross-match and choosing a preparation of intravenous IgG that gives no reaction is recommended.[117] In addition to isoantibody production, anemia has been reported with intravenous IgG because of immune complex-mediated complement activation.[118]

For hemolytic anemia with large granular lymphocyte leukemia, see box on Hemolytic Anemia in Chronic Large Granular Lymphocytic Leukemia.

SUGGESTED READINGS

Casals-Pascual C, Roberts DJ: Severe malarial anaemia. Curr Mol Med 6:155, 2006.

Chiu D, Lubin B: Oxidative hemoglobin denaturation and RBC destruction: The effect of heme on red cell membranes. Semin Hematol 26:128, 1989.

Coleman MD, Coleman NA: Drug-induced methaemoglobinaemia: Treatment issues. Drug Saf 14:394, 1996

Forman SJ, Kumar KS, Redeker AG, Hochstein P: Hemolytic anemia in Wilson disease: Clinical findings and biochemical mechanisms. Am J Hematol 9:269, 1980.

George JN: Clinical practice. Thrombotic thrombocytopenic purpura. N Engl J Med 354:1927, 2006.

Hasegawa S, Rodger GP, Shio H, et al: Impaired deformability of Heinz body-forming red cells. Biorheology 30:275, 1993.

Kojouri K, Vesely SK, George JN: Quinine-associated thrombotic thrombocytopenic purpura-hemolytic uremic syndrome: Frequency, clinical features, and long-term outcomes. Ann Intern Med 135:1047, 2001.

Krause PJ: Babesiosis. Med Clin North Am 86:361, 2002.

McArthur HL, Dalal BI, Kollmannsberger C: Intravascular hemolysis as a complication of clostridium perfringens sepsis. J Clin Oncol 24:2387, 2006.

McHutchison JG, Manns MP, Longo DL: Definition and management of anemia in patients infected with hepatitis C virus. Liver Int 26:389, 2006.

Miller LH, Baruch DI, Marsh K, Doumbo OK: The pathogenic basis of malaria. Nature 415:673, 2002.

Owen JS, Brown DJC, Harry DS, et al: Erythrocyte echinocytosis in liver disease. J Clin Invest 76:2275, 1985.

Poyart C, Wajcman H: Hemolytic anemias due to hemoglobinopathies. Mol Aspects Med 17:129, 1996.

Zakarija A, Bennett C: Drug-induced thrombotic microangiopathy. Semin Thromb Hemost 31:681, 2005.

REFERENCES

For complete list of references log onto www.expertconsult.com

PART V

HOST DEFENSE AND ITS DISORDERS

CHAPTER 49

COMPLEMENT AND IMMUNOGLOBULIN BIOLOGY

Robert Mandle, Robert A. Barrington, and Michael C. Carroll

This chapter is divided into two parts. The first part details the current understanding of the activation and biology of the complement system and how it links innate and adaptive immunity. The second part focuses on immunoglobulins and their importance in protecting against disease. The goal of this chapter is to impart to the reader the underlying role of the complement system and antibody in protecting the host from microbial insult and disease.

THE COMPLEMENT SYSTEM: AN OVERVIEW

Complement refers to a family of distinct proteins that play a pivotal role in host defense against infection. In the 1880s, the serum factors involved in host response to pathogens were placed into two categories based on sensitivity to heat. The *heat-stable* component, antibody, was recognized as being specific for the invading pathogen and arose after immunization, whereas the *heat-labile* (>56°C [133°F]) fraction displayed nonspecific killing activity. The heat-labile fraction acted to *complement* the antibody-mediated killing of targeted organisms.[1–3]

In addition to its role in the effector arm of the antibody response, the complement system serves several other functions. First, components of the complement system are involved in clearance of targeted microorganisms by the process of opsonization. *Opsonization* is coating of a particle with proteins that facilitate phagocytosis of the particle by tissue macrophages and activated follicular dendritic cells (FDCs) as well as binding by receptors on peripheral blood cells.[4,5] Second, complement promotes inflammation by releasing small peptide fragments from complement proteins. These peptides cause mast cell degranulation, smooth muscle contraction, and directed migration (chemotaxis) of motile cells to sites of inflammation.[6,7]

Complement can be activated via three distinct pathways: classical, mannan-binding lectin, and alternative. Although all depend on different molecules for their initiation, eventually they converge to generate the same set of effector molecules. Each of these pathways is described here (Fig. 49–1).

Classical Pathway

The classical pathway (CP), so called because it was the earliest studied arm of the complement system, directly links the innate and acquired immune systems. There are nine proteins in the CP. As a matter of terminology, each CP component protein is designated with an uppercase C followed by a number. Fragments of these proteins generated by cleavage during the complement cascade are designated with a lower case letter suffix (e.g., C3a, C3b).

C1, the first component of the CP, binds and is activated by the Fc portion of the antibody molecule. C1q is a macromolecule complex composed of three individual protein subunits: C1q, C1r, and C1s.[8–12] The largest of these subunits, C1q, is a 18-chain molecule with six copies each of three chains: A, B, and C. Structurally C1q consists of a central core with six radiating arms. Each arm possesses a triple helical structure similar to collagen, capped at the end with a globular domain. C1q is responsible for forming an ionic bond that links the C1 complex to the antibody molecule. In addition to its capacity for binding to antibody molecules, C1q possesses the capability to bind directly to the surfaces of some microorganisms and apoptotic cells, not unlike mannan-binding lectin (see Mannan-Binding Lectin below).

Associated with C1q are two molecules each of C1r and C1s. In unactivated C1, C1r and C1s are proenzyme serine esterases. Upon binding of C1q with Fc or pathogen, a conformational change occurs that leads to activation of an C1r. The active form of C1r then cleaves its associated C1s to generate an active serine protease.

Activated C1s is responsible for cleaving C4 and C2, the next two proteins in the complement pathway. Cleavage of C4 yields two fragments: C4a and C4b. C4b possesses a highly reactive thioester group that allows it to bind covalently to molecules in the immediate vicinity of its active site. Only a small proportion of the C4b produced binds to proteins or carbohydrates on the targeted surface; the rest is inactivated by reaction with water in the surrounding milieu. This helps to prevent inadvertent C4b binding to surrounding host cells.

C2, the next substrate in the CP cascade, is susceptible to cleavage by C1s only when it is bound by C4b. This helps to prevent serum-phase activation of C2. Upon association with C4b, C2 is cleaved by activated C1s into two fragments: C2a and C2b. C2a remains bound to C4b, thereby confining C2a to the targeted surface. C4bC2a is termed the *C3 convertase*, an enzymatic complex that is responsible for binding and cleaving C3, the next component in the cascade. The function of the C3 convertase is to cleave large numbers of C3 molecules to produce C3b, which coats the targeted surface (opsonization of the target) and marks it for phagocytosis, and C3a, which initiates a local inflammatory response.

An Ig-independent mechanism for activation of C1q has been identified.[13] The lectin protein Sign R1, which is expressed on a subset of macrophages within the outer marginal zone sinus of the spleen and upon uptake of bacteria, binds C1q and activates the CP. This novel pathway provides an alternative innate recognition of pathogens leading to activation of the CP of complement.

Mannan-Binding Lectin

Before continuing with the discussion of the complement cascade at the point of C3 cleavage by convertase, we turn our attention to the other two complement-activating pathways: the mannan-binding lectin (MBL) pathway and the alternative pathway. What will become evident is that all of these pathways converge at C3.

The MBL pathway is a recently described pathway for complement activation.[14,15] MBL, like C1q, is a triple helical structure with six collagen-like arms coupled to globular domains, which form carbohydrate recognition domains that bind repeating polysaccharides present on the surfaces of many microorganisms. MBL attaches to the terminus of polymeric carbohydrate chains in the following order: mannose > GlcNAc > fucose > glucose. The greatest avidity appears to be for repeating mannose-based structural patterns typical of microbial surfaces. On vertebrate cells, these sugars often are covered by sialic acid residues, thus limiting recognition by MBL. Upon binding to polysaccharides on a pathogen surface, MBL activates the serine proteases MBL-associated serine protease (MASP)-1 and MASP-2. MASP-2 acts similar to C1s, cleaving C4 and C2 and

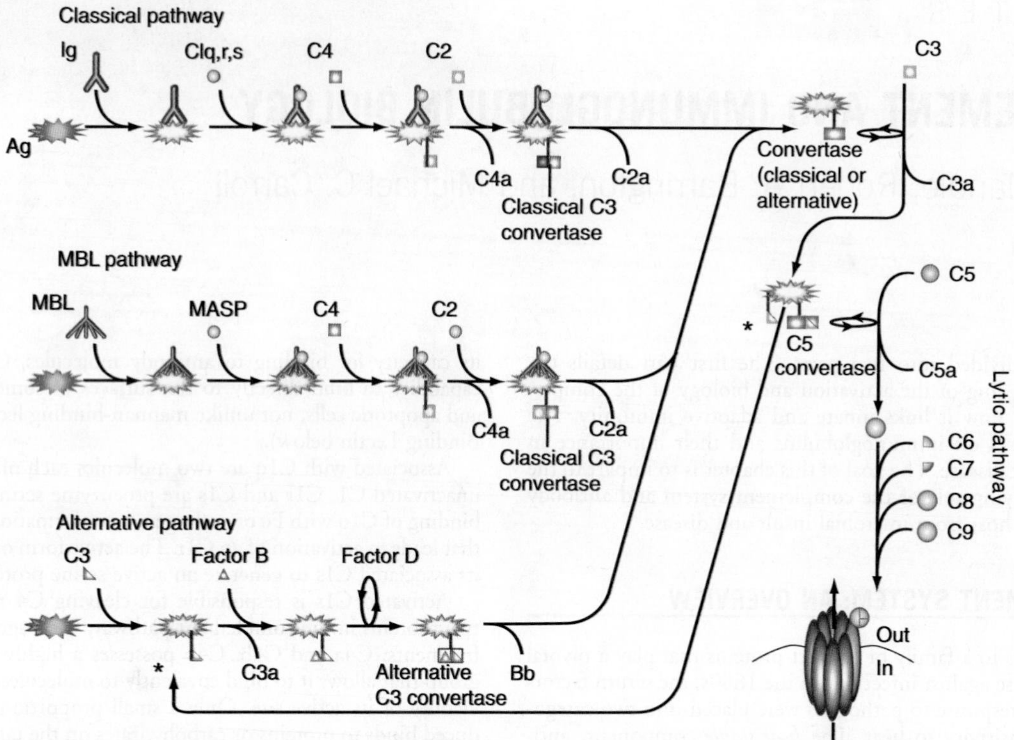

Figure 49–1 Schematic overview of the complement cascade. Classical, mannan-binding lectin, and alternative pathways commence from the left side of the figure, leading to the converging point of C3 activation (top right). In every subsequent proteolytic step, the position of the new addition to the antigen complex is shown in black for clarity. From the central C3 activation step downward, the C3 amplification loop through the alternative pathway is indicated by asterisks. The lytic pathway is initiated with the formation of C5 convertase and leads to the assembly of the C5,C6,C7,C8,(n)9 membrane attack complex, which interferes with the target's structural integrity by penetrating the cellular membrane (bottom right).

thereby forming a C3 convertase with C4bC2a, as found in the CP.[16]

MBL serum concentration can differ by up to 1000-fold among individuals, with those having low circulating MBL apparently more vulnerable to infections. MBL insufficiency appears to be a particular risk factor for infections in infants or individuals undergoing chemotherapy or immunosuppression treatment.[17]

Given the relatively recent discovery of the MBL pathway in the 1990s, progress into fully understanding this pathway is now just beginning. Gene-targeted knock-out mouse models deficient in MBL components have been described. Interestingly, mice rendered deficient for MBL appear to have resistance to infection compared to sufficient cohorts when challenged with microbial pathogens such as *Candida albicans* and *Plasmodium yoelii*.[18] Further study is needed to determine the role of MBL in host protection.

Alternative Pathway

The alternative pathway (AP) may represent the earliest form of innate immunity. Unlike the CP or MBL pathway, the AP can be fully activated in the absence of specific pathogen binding.[19] In fact, the AP is always "on" at a low level. In addition, the AP forms and uses the distinct C3 convertase C3bBb.[20]

Complement C3 is a two-chain protein with an apparent molecular weight of approximately 200 kd. The crystal structure of native C3 identified 12 distinct domains, including the thioester domain (TED).[21–23] Most recently, solution of the atomic structure of the activated form of C3 (i.e., Cb) demonstrated a dramatic shift in the location of the TED. Proteolytic cleavage releases the C3a anaphylatoxin peptide and the TED becomes fully exposed to engage potential targets. Thus, the dramatic shift in structure also exposes potential binding sites for factor B of the AP and competing sites for regulators of C3b, such as factor H (FH), membrane cofactor protein (MCP), complement receptor type 1 (CR1), and decay accelerating factor (DAF; all described later in this section). At a low level, the thioester bond undergoes spontaneous hydrolysis, forming C3(H_2O). This conformationally altered form of C3 allows for binding to factor B, a plasma protein. Factor B is a serine protease that is approximately 30% homologous to C2. The binding of factor B by C3(H_2O) allows factor D, another protease, to cleave factor B to form Ba and Bb. Bb remains associated with C3(H_2O) to form the C3(H_2O)Bb complex. Factor D appears to function as a serine protease in its native state but can cleave factor B only when bound to C3.

C3(H_2O)Bb is an enzymatic complex capable of cleaving native C3. This complex is a fluid-phase C3 convertase. Although it is formed only in small amounts, it can cleave many molecules of C3. Much of the C3b produced in this process is inactivated by hydrolysis, but some attaches covalently to the surface of host cells or pathogens. C3b bound in this way is able to bind factor B, allowing its cleavage by factor D to yield Ba and Bb. The result is the formation of C3bBb, a C3 convertase akin to C4bC2a found in the classical and MBL pathways, with the capability of initiating an amplification cascade.

In light of the nonspecific nature of C3b binding in the AP, it is not surprising that a number of complement regulators exist both in the plasma and on host cell membranes to prevent complement activation on self tissues. Some of these regulatory components are mentioned now for the sake of clarity; more detailed attention is provided later in this chapter (Table 49–1). CR1 and DAF (CD55) compete with factor B for binding to C3b on the cell surface and can displace Bb from a convertase that has already formed.[24] Factor I, a serum protease, in concert with CR1 or MCP (CD46) can prevent convertase formation by converting C3b into its inactive derivative, iC3b.[25] Another complement regulatory protein found in the plasma is FH. FH binds C3b and is able to compete with factor B and displace Bb from the convertase. In addition, FH acts as a cofactor for factor I to convert C3b to iC3b.

Table 49–1 Control Proteins of the Classical and Alternative Pathways

Name	Role in Regulation of Complement Activation
C1 inhibitor (C1INH)	Binds to activated C1r, C1s, removing it from C1q
C4-binding protein (C4BP)	Binds C4b, displacing C2b; cofactor for C4b cleavage by factor I
Complement receptor 1 (CR1)	Binds C4b, displacing C2b, or C3b displacing Bb; cofactor for factor I
Factor H (H)	Binds C3b, displacing Bb; cofactor for factor I
Factor I (I)	Serine protease that cleaves C3b and C4b; aided by factor H, MCP, C4BP, or CR1
Decay-accelerating factor (DAF)	Membrane protein that displaces Bb from C3b and C2b from C4b
Membrane cofactor protein (MCP)	Membrane protein that promotes C3b and C4b inactivation by factor I
CD59	Prevents formation of membrane attack complex on autologous cells; widely expressed on membranes

Pathogen surfaces normally are not afforded the protection offered by these regulators. Persistence of the C3bBb convertase on microbial surfaces may, in fact, be favored by the positive regulator properdin (factor P). Individuals with deficiencies in factor P have a heightened susceptibility to infection with *Neisseria* species.[26] Once formed, the C3bBb convertase rapidly cleaves more C3 to C3b, which can participate in the formation of more molecules of C3bBb convertase. The AP thereby activates an amplification loop that can proceed on the surface of a pathogen but not on a host cell.

Although specific antibody is not required for AP activation, many classes of immunoglobulin can facilitate AP activation.[27] The mechanism by which this occurs remains elusive. However, in contrast to CP activation, which requires Fc, AP activation can occur with F(ab)′2 fragments.

An instructive demonstration for the role of antibody in continuing the AP cascade, with possible ramifications for human disease, comes from a murine model of rheumatoid arthritis. Mice do not spontaneously develop rheumatoid arthritis.[28] However, a murine model has been developed in which expression of antibodies specific for the ubiquitously expressed cytoplasmic protein glucose-6-phosphate can cause joint destruction reminiscent of human rheumatoid arthritis. Interestingly, the disease state, through complement-mediated joint destruction, can occur even if the specific antibodies are of isotypes incapable of fixing complement through the CP. The response may be localized to the joints because of the absence of complement cascade regulators on cartilage.

C3, C5, and the Membrane Attack Complex

The formation of the C3 convertase, C4bC2a (CP and MBL) and C3bBb (AP), is the point at which the three pathways converge (Fig. 49–1). The function of these complexes is to convert C3 to C3a and C3b. C3 is the most abundant complement protein in plasma, occurring at a concentration of 1.2 mg/ml, and up to 1000 molecules of C3b can bind in the vicinity of a single C3 convertase.[29]

The attachment of C3b to either C4bC2a or C3bBb converts this enzyme into a trimeric complex (C5 convertase) capable of binding and cleaving C5 into C5a and C5b. C5b is the initiating component of the membrane attack complex (MAC). The MAC is a multiprotein complex whose components are C5b, C6, C7, C8 and multiple C9s.[30,31] The constituent components of the MAC associate in the numerical order C5b-C6-C7-C8-C9.

The MAC, when viewed by electron microscopy, resem cylinder that possesses a hydrophobic outer face and a hydrop central core. If assembled near a lipid bilayer, such as a cell or bacteri membrane, the MAC can associate with and insert into the lipid bilayer. Such insertion can be thought as "punching holes" into the membrane, allowing for passage of water and small ions into the cell. Osmotic equilibrium is thereby lost, leading to eventual lysis of the targeted cell or bacterium. C5b678 are sufficient to form small pores in the target membrane. The role of C9 appears to be to enlarge the channel, through multiple C9 polymerization, thereby causing more rapid loss of membrane function and lysis. Deficiencies in complement components C5–C9 have been associated with only increased susceptibility to *Neisseria* species–based infections such as gonorrhea and bacterial meningitis. It can be concluded from this observation that the requirement for MAC is limited in host protection.

Complement Receptors and Their Role in Immune Complex Clearance and Activation

As described in the previous section, complement can act by the direct lysis of targeted cells. Another important function of complement in host protection is facilitating the uptake and destruction of pathogens by phagocytic cells. This occurs by the specific recognition of C3b/C4b–coated (opsonized) particles by complement receptors.[32,33]

The best characterized complement receptor for the uptake of C4-coated immune complexes is CR1 (CD35). CR1 binds C4b/C3b–bearing immune complexes. CR1, like most proteins that bind activation products of C4 and C3 molecules, shares a structural motif known as the short consensus repeat. Each short consensus repeat consists of approximately 60 amino acids. CR1 in humans is composed of 30 linked short consensus repeats. CR1 possesses three binding sites for C4b and two for C3b.

CR1 is expressed on a wide variety of cell types in humans, including erythrocytes, macrophages, polymorphonuclear leukocytes, B cells, monocytes, and FDCs. The role of CR1 expression on B cells and FDCs in activating and maintaining the adaptive immune response is detailed below. For now, the focus is on the other cell types that express CR1.

Binding of C3b by CR1 expressed on phagocytic cells is not, in itself, capable of inducing endocytosis. A secondary signal is required to induce phagocytosis. This second signal can be provided by IgG binding to the phagocyte's Fc receptor, by carbohydrates commonly found on bacterial surfaces, or by exposure of the phagocytic cell to the appropriate cytokines. In addition, some phagocytic cells, such as macrophages, are activated by binding of C5a through C5a receptor (CD84; see following section).

The largest pool of CR1-expressing cells is erythrocytes.[34] Erythrocytes bearing opsonized material are removed from the circulation presumably to prevent deposition in tissue sites such as the renal glomerulus. Erythrocytes bearing opsonized material traverse the sinusoids of the liver and spleen, where they come into close contact with fixed phagocytic cells. These phagocytic cells effect the transfer of opsonized material from the erythrocyte onto their own membrane. The transfer is enhanced by cleavage of C4b/C3b to iC4b/iC3b by factor I and complexes taken up by complement receptor of the Ig superfamily (CRIg; see below).

CR2 (CD21) recognizes targets that have been coated with breakdown products of C3b/iC3b/C3dg/C3d. Given its central position in the complement cascade, the presence of C3b is tightly regulated. This regulation is brought about by cleaving C3b into inactive derivatives that cannot participate in forming an active convertase. One of the inactive derivatives of C3b, iC3b, can act as an opsonin in its own right. In addition to iC3b, CR2 binds C3dg and C3d, which are additional breakdown products of C3b. CR2 is the only complement receptor that recognizes C3dg. Likewise, CR3 (CD11b/CD18) binds iC3b and plays a major role in inducing phagocytosis but probably not activation in the absence of a second signal (i.e., Fc receptor or pattern recognition receptor). CR4 (CD11c/CD18) also binds iC3b opsonized particles, resulting in direct endocytosis. Although its role as a phagocytic receptor is not well characterized, CD11c is the major marker for dendritic cells (DCs). It will be important to understand the functional importance of this complement receptor on DC and how it participates in uptake of antigen for presentation to T lymphocytes.

CR2 expressed on B cells augments cognate antibody receptor signaling (see section below). Activation of complement plays a contributing role in producing a strong antibody response. An interesting aside is that CR2 is the cell surface receptor on human B cells that is recognized by the Epstein-Barr virus.[35]

CrIg is a recently described complement receptor that plays an important role in the clearance of C3b opsonized complexes by phagocytic cells of the liver.[36] It is also expressed on subsets of macrophages, but less is known about this role. The recent cocrystallization of C3b and CrIg revealed binding to the C3b β chain, which is in contrast to all other known complement receptors in which binding to the activated C3 occurs via the α chain.

Biologic Activity of C3a, C4a, and C5a

The role of the complement fragments C3a, C4a, and C5a in the immune response is to produce localized inflammation.[37] C3a, C4a, and C5a are anaphylotoxins and are structurally similar to chemokines. When produced in large amounts or injected systemically, they induce a generalized circulatory collapse and shock-like syndrome similar to that seen in a systemic allergic reaction involving IgE antibodies.[38]

Of the three fragments, C5a is the most stable and possesses the best characterized and possibly highest specific biologic activity. All three induce smooth muscle contraction and increased vascular permeability. C5a and C3a also act on endothelial cells lining blood vessels to induce adhesion molecule expression.[39,40] Additionally, C3a and C5a can activate the mast cells that populate submucosal tissues and line vessels throughout the body to release histamine, tumor necrosis factor α, and protease.[41] The changes induced by C3a and C5a recruit antibody, complement, and phagocytic cells to the site of infection, thereby hastening the adaptive immune response. C5a also induces the upregulation of CR1 and CR3 on the surfaces of these cells.

Regulation of Complement Activation

Activation of the complement system must be tightly regulated in order to prevent autologous tissue damage (Table 49–1).[42] Some of the proteins involved in regulating complement action have been described (see Alternative Pathway above). In addition to these regulators, a number of other checkpoints limit the scope and target of complement activation.

As a result of binding to antibody or pathogen, conformational changes to C1q induce the enzymatic activity of C1r and C1s. Both of these enzymes are regulated by the C1 inhibitor (C1-INH). C1-INH is a member of a family of *ser*ine *p*rotease *in*hibitors termed serpins.[43] Serpins provide a bait sequence that mimics the active site of the substrate. When C1r or C1s cleaves this sequence, a new functional site on C1-INH is revealed that covalently binds to C1r or C1s, thereby destroying their proteolytic activity. C1-INH is responsible for preventing fluid-phase activation and degradation of C1 after complement activation has occurred, but it can be overridden by immune complexes.

Although C1 is capable of cleaving multiple C4 molecules, only approximately 10% of the produced C4b clusters about the targeted antigen.[44] The rest is released into the fluid phase. C4b in the fluid phase is rapidly bound by C4 binding protein (C4bp), which is a cofactor for factor I. Factor I cleaves C4b into two fragments, C4c and C4d, which are quickly cleared from the circulation.

In addition to its role in cleaving C4b, factor I is responsible, in combination with specific cofactors, for regulating C3b by cleavage. Factor I in association with FH in the serum or with CR1 and MCP on the cell surface cleaves C3b into iC3b and C3dg. Both of these products are incapable of participating in the formation of the C3 convertase.

CR1 also regulates the complement cascade by promoting the dissociation of C3 convertases (C4bC2b and C3bBb). DAF is involved in regulating the complement cascade in a similar manner. The importance of CR1 or CR1-like molecules in curbing the complement response can be witnessed in a rather unexpected condition. Complement receptor 1–related gene (Crry) is a murine homologue of the human CR1 gene.[45,46] Mice lacking Crry are unable to properly regulate C3. Crry mice spontaneously abort due to C3-dependent injury to the fetus. This presumably is the result of uncontrolled C3 deposition on the placenta. This observation in mice sheds light on the possibility that CR1 plays a role in recurrent fetal loss manifest in patients suffering from antiphospholipid syndrome.

Biologic Consequences of Complement Cascade Deficiencies

The important role of the complement system in preventing disease is witnessed in cases where components of the system are absent either due to random mutation in the human population or by design in gene-targeted "knock-out" mice. Some complement cascade deficiencies have been described. This section focuses on the biologic consequences of deficiencies in complement cascade activation that have profound biologic consequences and completeness, followed by a discussion on deficiencies in complement regulatory proteins.

Homozygous deficiencies in C1q, the most common form of C1 deficiency in humans, is a powerful susceptibility factor for the development of systemic lupus erythematosus (SLE).[47,48] Patients lacking C1q nearly always present with SLE. They have increased susceptibility to viral and bacterial infections, but it is not nearly as pronounced as in C3 deficiency (see below). C1q knock-out mice show increased mortality, with up to 25% of mice having histologic evidence of glomerulonephritis.

C4 in humans is encoded by two separate loci giving rise to two distinct protein products: C4A and C4B.[49] In certain populations, the absence of C4A is associated with greatly elevated risk for development of autoimmune diseases such as SLE or other lupus-like autoimmune disease. Moreover, as with C1q, mice deficient in C4 are predisposed to SLE-like disease.

C2 deficiency appears to be relatively benign.[50] Humans lacking C2 appear to have a normally functioning immune system, although autoimmune disorders and, less commonly, infections are observed with increased frequency.

In light of the central role of C3 in the complement cascade, it is not surprising that C3 deficiency has dire consequences for the host organism. Of all known cases of C3 deficiency among humans, no patients have been reported as disease-free. Infectious complications, predominately pyogenic in nature, occur frequently and recurrently. *Streptococcus pneumoniae* and *Neisseria meningitidis* are the major pathogens reported. In addition, SLE, vasculitic syndromes, and glomerulonephritis have been documented in up to 21% of C3-deficient patients. Mice deficient in C3 show, not unlike humans, greatly increased susceptibility to streptococcal infection and death.[51] The 50% lethal dose (LD_{50}) is 50-fold less for C3-deficient mice than for C3-sufficient controls. This may be due in large part to the inability of mice deficient in C3 to effectively opsonize the bacteria. Moreover, the deficient mice have an impaired humoral response (see section below).

Biologic Consequences of Complement Regulatory Protein Deficiencies

Deficiencies in C1-INH have been observed in the human population.[52] C1-INH deficiency can be inherited as an autosomal dominant trait or can result from autoantibodies that recognize C1-INH, blocking its function.[53] The inherited form of this deficiency is the cause of hereditary angioedema. Patients with hereditary angioedema experience chronic spontaneous complement activation leading to the production of excess cleaved fragments of C4 and C2. The biochemical cause of angioedema in these patients is not definitively elucidated. One line of reasoning points to excess production of C2 kinin and bradykinin. The peptide C2 kinin is a breakdown product of C2a after cleavage of C2. This peptide causes extensive swelling; the most dangerous is local swelling in the trachea, which can lead to suffocation. Bradykinin, which has similar actions to C2 kinin, also is produced in an uncontrolled fashion in this disease as a result of the lack of inhibition of another plasma protease, kallikrein, which is activated by tissue damage and is regulated by C1-INH. Although C1 is unregulated in patients with hereditary angioedema, large-scale cleavage of C3 is prevented by C4 and C2 control mechanisms and by regulation of C3 convertase formation on host cells. Increased risk of infection is not associated with C1-INH deficiency. This disease can be fully corrected by infusion of purified C1-INH.

Acquired C1-INH deficiency may be associated with lymphoproliferative disorders and in most cases represents development of an autoantibody that binds to and neutralizes C1-INH. In two examined cases, autoantibodies abrogate C1-INH activity by preventing formation of the C1s–C1-INH complex. However, once the complex formed, the autoreactive antibodies had no effect on C1-INH function. To date there is no uniform, fully effective therapy for these patients.

The role of factor I in complement cascade regulation can be witnessed in patients who suffer from factor I deficiency.[54] In the presence of a cofactor protein, Factor I cleaves C3b, producing iC3b, the inactive form of C3b. iC3b is incapable of reacting with factor B to form the AP C3 convertase, thereby preventing uncontrolled AP activation. In the absence of factor I, unrestrained C3 consumption occurs secondary to accelerated spontaneous AP turnover. Patients with factor I deficiency suffer from recurrent infections caused by pyogenic organisms, including meningococcal meningitis.

Likewise, mice deficient in the central protein FH exhibit unrestrained C3 activation via AP, leading to near depletion of serum C3. An important outcome of the failure to regulate C3 activation is glomerulonephritis. Strikingly, mice deficient in FH develop a disease resembling the human disorder membrane glomerulonephritis. The phenotype of the mice confirms the general notion that the AP is always "on" and that failure to regulate activated C3 results in consumption of circulating C3 and tissue injury.

The MAC is one mechanism used by the host to rid itself of certain microorganisms. Host cells are protected from MAC-mediated lysis by CD59 (protectin), a membrane-bound protein. CD59 performs its function by inhibiting the binding of C9 to the C5b-C6-C7-C8-C9 complex. CD59 as well as DAF are linked to the cell surface by a phosphoinositol glycolipid (PIG) tail. One of the enzymes involved in the synthesis of PIG tails is encoded on chromosome X. Mutation of this gene leads to a failure to synthesize PIG tails and with it an inability to express CD59 or DAF on the cell surface.[55–57] Lack of CD59 and DAF expression on host cell surfaces is the cause of paroxysmal nocturnal hemoglobinuria. This disease is characterized by episodes of chronic intravascular hemolysis and propensity to thrombosis.

Another example of the importance of FH regulation are reports of genetic association between variant alleles of FH and age-related macular degeneration. More functional studies are required, but it appears that even minor reductions in the efficiency of this important serum regulator lead to dramatic disease susceptibility.

Autoimmunity and Complement Deficiencies

There exists a strong correlative relationship between the lack of certain components of complement system (i.e., C1 and C4) and autoimmune disease, particularly SLE. Two general nonmutually exclusive hypotheses have been put forward to explain the increased incidence of SLE among complement deficient individuals: the clearance hypothesis and the tolerance hypothesis.[58–60] The clearance hypothesis is based on the known role of the CP of complement in binding to foreign antigens and transporting them to the liver and spleen for degradation and removal from the circulation. Thus, defects in clearance of apoptotic cells or debris would lead to inappropriate accumulation of self-antigen and overstimulation of self-reactive lymphocytes.

The tolerance model proposes that innate immunity protects against SLE by delivering lupus autoantigens to sites where immature B lymphocytes are tolerized, thereby eliminating a source of autoreactive antibody molecules. SLE is characterized by high-affinity antibodies specific for autoantigens such as double-stranded DNA (dsDNA), ribonuclear proteins, and histones. Validation of the model comes in part from studies with human B cells demonstrating that self-reactive B cells are eliminated or anergized at two major checkpoints: bone marrow and spleen. Thus, counterselection of potentially pathogenic B cells is an active process and most likely involves components of innate immunity.

The first part of this section familiarized the reader with the general aspects of the complement system. The remainder of this section focuses on the role of the complement system in the initiation and propagation of the adaptive immune response and begins with a description of natural antibody.

Natural Antibody

Natural antibody, in contrast to antibody secreted in response to active immunization, is continuously released, mostly by the B1 subpopulation of lymphocytes. Predominantly IgM but also IgA and IgG3 (in mice), natural antibodies tend to be polyreactive, with low-affinity binding for antigens such as nuclear proteins, DNA, and phosphatidylcholine, which are common structures among both pathogens and host tissue. These antibodies rarely show evidence of somatic mutation. It has been speculated that the variable region genes that predominate among natural antibodies have been selected evolutionarily for their ability to recognize pathogens and act as a rapid response to infection, thereby acting as a stop gap to provide sufficient time for the adaptive immune response to form. Natural antibody mediates its protective effects via the CP of complement.

Certain antibody specificities direct B cells into the B1 subset. An example comes from work using transgenic mice that express an immunoglobulin heavy chain originally derived from a B1 cell. In these mice, the vast majority of observed B cells are phenotypically B1-like.

IgM natural antibody is important in initiating CP leading to enhanced humoral immunity. In addition to its role in protecting against pathogens, natural antibody protects against lupus-like disease based on studies in mice. Thus, like C1q and C4, deficiency in IgM predisposes to an SLE-like phenotype.

Complement Links Innate and Adaptive Immune Responses

One of the critical functions of CP complement is providing a bridge between innate and acquired immune systems. The process is achieved through attachment of complement products to the antigen/pathogen, either directly to the surface or via antibody (see section above). This complement "tag" consists of breakdown products of C3 (i.e.,

C3b, C3dg, and C3d) that facilitate recognition of pathogens by the immune system. The recognition phase is mediated principally through complement receptors CD21 and CD35. This section details complement-dependent mechanisms of immune detection and humoral responses to thymus (T)-dependent antigens.

Soluble Complement Mediators of Antibody Responses

The first clue that complement is important in regulating B lymphocyte responses came from the observation that B lymphocytes bind activated C3 fragments.[61] Soon thereafter, it was noted that mice depleted of serum C3 by treatment with cobra venom factor had diminished responses to T-dependent antigens.[62] The discovery of naturally occurring genetic deficiencies in C3, C4, and C2 in species as diverse as guinea pigs,[63–65] dogs,[66] and humans[67,68] allowed description of impaired antibody responses as well. Because the impaired responsiveness is comparable among animals deficient in CP activators (C4, C2) and C3-deficient or C3-depleted animals, a model emerged suggesting that the effect is mediated through the CP of the complement system. That the impaired responsiveness is comparable among diverse animal species indicated the importance of CP complement in regulating antibody responses to T-dependent antigens.

The advance of gene targeting technology in the murine system led to development of engineered strains devoid of various components of CP complement. C1q-, C4-, and C3-deficient mouse strains generate reduced antibody responses to T-dependent antigens.[69–72] Furthermore, these strains fail to switch immunoglobulin isotypes normally, suggesting that germinal center responses are impaired.[70] Germinal centers are microanatomic structures whose purpose is to provide for increasing affinity of serum antibody for antigens (affinity maturation), isotype switching, and development and differentiation of memory B lymphocytes and plasma cells.[73] Consistent with this theory, immunized complement-deficient mice produce fewer and smaller germinal centers compared with immunized wild-type mice.[70] Importantly, humoral responses in each of the C1q-, C4-, and C3-deficient strains can be rescued by transplantation of wild-type bone marrow.[74–76] Therefore, bone marrow–derived cells can produce sufficient complement to reconstitute antibody responses to T-dependent antigens administered intravenously.

It is suggested that CP potentiates antibody responses through involvement of immune complex formation. The implication is that natural antibodies or specific IgM released early in the response by B cells responding to antigen recognize and bind pathogens, thereby activating the CP. Alternatively, binding of antigen by B cells through the B-cell receptor (BCR) is sufficient to activate CP on the B-cell surface. Several lines of evidence support this model. For example, genetically engineered mice producing only membrane IgM (i.e., with gene-targeted deletion of secretory signals) produce significantly reduced antibody responses to T-dependent antigens.[77] Although immune complex formation likely is important for stimulating antibody responses, it is not necessary. Antigens directly conjugated to C3b or C3d fragments are more potent immunogens compared to unconjugated antigen.[78,79] Furthermore, the magnitude of the immune response is directly influenced by the number of C3d fragments conjugated to the antigen.[78] Therefore, activated products of complement component C3 act as a natural adjuvant in driving efficient antibody responses.

Complement Receptors and Antibody Responses

B Lymphocyte Coreceptors

The effects of complement-coated antigens on antibody responses are mediated primarily through complement receptors CD21 and CD35 (Fig. 49–2). CD21 and CD35 are expressed predominantly on B lymphocytes and FDCs (Fig. 49–3).[80,81] CD35 is also found on polymorphonuclear cells, macrophages, mast cells, and DCs.[80] CD21 and CD35 are encoded for by separate, yet closely linked genes in human.[82] In mice, CD21 and CD35 originate from the same locus (Cr2) and are generated by alternative splicing events at the RNA level.[83,84]

Two novel sets of experiments demonstrated that CD21 and CD35 are important in regulating B-lymphocyte responses to T-dependent antigens. In the first set of experiments, antibodies specific for both CD21 and CD35 or CD35 alone were administered to immunized mice.[85–88] In the second set of experiments, a soluble form of CD21 was administered to immunized mice, thereby competing for C3d-coupled antigen interactions.[89] In both sets of experiments, treatment impaired antibody responses. In the first approach, blocking both CD21 and CD35 was more effective at blocking antibody responses compared to anti-CD35 antibody treatment, suggesting that, although both receptors contribute, CD21 is more important in regulating antibody responses.[85]

Because CD21 and CD35 are found on B lymphocytes and FDCs, two important cell types for humoral responses, two nonmutually exclusive models are proposed for their function. In the first model, CD21 augments antibody responses through activity as a coreceptor on B lymphocytes.[90] The second model proposes that CD21/CD35 on FDCs trap and focus antigen such that B lymphocytes can efficiently cross-link their antigen receptor to become activated.[91] As a coreceptor, engagement of CD21 by complement-coupled antigen on the surface of a B lymphocyte, in combination with membrane immunoglobulin (BCR) cross-linking, would lower the strength of signal through the BCR to activate the cell.[90] Accordingly, naive B lymphocytes bear low-affinity receptors for antigen; therefore, additional signaling by the CD21 coreceptor is required for efficient activation. This was demonstrated in vitro by culturing B lymphocytes with cognate antigen, either uncoupled or coupled to C3d. By measuring Ca^{2+}, it was estimated that 100 to 1000 less C3d-conjugated antigen was required to activate B lymphocytes compared to unconjugated antigen.[78]

The opportunity to test the importance of CD21 and CD35 as B-lymphocyte coreceptors in vivo came from studies using mice with targeted disruption in the Cr2 locus. Importantly, Cr2-deficient mice have impaired humoral responses similar to C1q-, C4- and C3-deficient mice (Fig. 49–3).[92–94] Using embryonic stem cells with a disrupted Cr2 locus, Croix et al.[95] used blastocyst complementation of $Rag2^{-/-}$ mice, such that chimeric mice expressed CD21/CD35 on FDCs but not on B lymphocytes. These chimeric mice displayed impaired antibody responses to the T-dependent antigen NP-KLH compared with controls. Therefore, CD21/CD35 on B lymphocytes is important for normal antibody responses.

Complement's covalent attachment to antigen engages CD21 as a complex with CD19/CD81 and BCR on the cell surface.[90,96,97] Dual binding of CD21/CD19/CD81 with BCR generates a stronger signal compared to BCR engagement alone.[90] If the combined signal is sufficient, the B lymphocyte is activated. If insufficient, then the B lymphocyte likely is eliminated by apoptosis.[98–101] The major ligand-binding receptor within the CD21/CD19/CD81 complex is CD21. CD19 appears more important in initiating a signaling cascade within the cell.[102] CD81 is a tetra-spanning molecule that stabilizes the complex within the membrane. Absence of any of the CD21/CD19/CD81 components adversely affects antibody responses to T-dependent antigens, although the degree of impairment varies.[92,103–105]

Focusing Antigen on Follicular Dendritic Cells

The second role of complement receptors CD21 and CD35 in regulating humoral responses is that they permit FDCs to trap antigen (Fig. 49–4).[91,106] FDCs concentrate in regions of ongoing immune responses, such as germinal centers, and they appear necessary for antibody responses. Germinal centers (see section above) promote somatic hypermutation within immunoglobulin heavy- and light-chain genes, along with isotype switching and production of memory

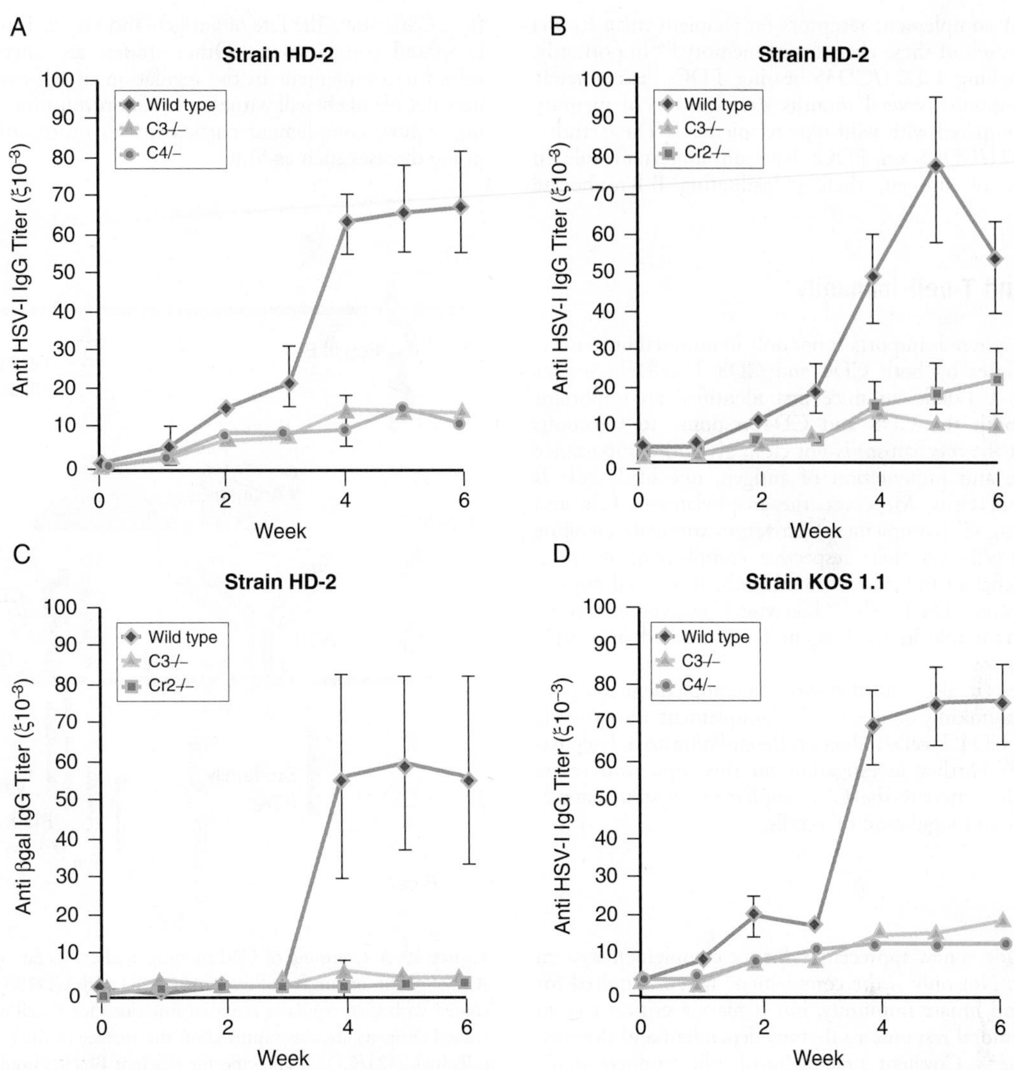

Figure 49–2 Classical pathway complement and complement receptors CD21/CD35 are required for the humoral response to replication-defective HD-2 virus or replication-sufficient KOS1.1 wild-type (WT) virus. Mice were injected at days 0 and 21 with 2×10^6 plaque forming units of replication-defective (**A–C**) or replication-sufficient (**D**) virus, HD-2, and KOS1.1, respectively. Antibody titers were determined by enzyme-linked immunosorbent assay. Mean titer ± SD represents at least five mice analyzed in two separate experiments. **A**, Deficiency in either C3 or C4 results in an impaired secondary humoral response to infectious HSV. **B**, Cr2–/– mice have an impaired secondary response similar to mice deficient in C3. **C**, Humoral response to recombinant virus-expressed heterologous protein (β-galactosidase) is also impaired in mice deficient in C3 or CD21/CD35. **D**, Secondary humoral response to replication-sufficient HSV-1 (strain KOS1.1) depends on complement C3 and C4. *(From Da Costa XJ, Brockman MA, Alicot E, et al: Humoral response to herpes simplex virus is complement-dependent. Proc Natl Acad Sci U S A 96:12708, 1999.)*

B lymphocytes and plasma cells. They can be divided into two regions: dark zone and light zone. To gain entry into the dark zone, B lymphocytes are activated by receiving above threshold signals from the CD21/CD19/CD81 and BCR, in combination with costimulation from helper T lymphocytes.[107] Within the dark zone, activated B lymphocytes divide and mutate their immunoglobulin receptor genes.[108–111] After several rounds of proliferation in the dark zone, B lymphocytes enter the light zone, where they are subjected to selection on antigen deposited on FDCs (i.e., clonal selection).[112,113] The selection of high-affinity B lymphocyte clones into memory B-lymphocyte and plasma cell pools ensures future protection against repeat antigen exposure.

How antigen is retained on FDCs, both for primary B lymphocyte responses and for long-term memory responses, is subject to intense research. However, supporting evidence indicates that complement receptors on FDCs are important in both short- and long-term B-lymphocyte responses. Papamichail et al.[91] demonstrated that retention of antigen–IgG immune complexes on FDCs was reduced upon depletion of C3 using cobra venom factor. Therefore, it appears that immune complex deposition on FDCs is complement dependent. In addition, antibody production in vitro using FDCs demonstrates that antibody production is dependent on CD21/CD35.[114]

Availability of Cr2-deficient mice has shed light on the importance of FDC-derived CD21/CD35 on humoral responses. Because FDCs, the other major cell type expressing CD21/CD35, are radioresistant, it was possible to generate chimeric mice that restricted CD21/CD35 expression to B lymphocytes by bone marrow transplantation. Ahearn et al.[92] made chimeric mice with Cr2-deficient FDCs by transplanting wild-type bone marrow (B-lymphocyte $Cr2^{+/+}$) into lethally irradiated Cr2-deficient recipient mice (FDC-$Cr2^{-/-}$).[115] After secondary challenge with antigen, the chimeric mice failed to sustain high-level antibody production, suggesting that CD21/CD35 on FDCs is important for recall or memory responses.

CD21/CD35 do appear important for persistence of antibody titers, normal frequencies of memory B lymphocytes and plasma cells, and affinity maturation. Adoptively transferring memory B lymphocytes into recipient mice lacking FDC-derived CD21/CD35 demonstrated that complement receptors on recipient mice stroma were required for each of these elements of memory.[116] Importantly, chimeric mice lacking CD21/CD35-bearing FDCs had severely impaired recall responses several months after transfer of memory B lymphocytes compared with wild-type recipients.[116] These studies suggest that CD21/CD35 on FDCs have an important role in long-term storage of antigen, thereby facilitating B-lymphocyte memory.

Complement and T-cell Immunity

The complement system is important not only in humoral immunity; it enhances responses by both CD4 and CD8 T cells.[117] Studies with influenza in C3-deficient mice first identified an important role for C3 in both the CD8 and CD4 response to infectious virus.[118] Although the mechanism is not clear, given the importance of DC in uptake and presentation of antigen, one likely role is C3 opsonization of virus. Moreover, the anaphylatoxins C3a and C5a released during C' (complement) activation stimulate cytokine releases by mast cells via their respective complement receptor. Studies of mice deficient in C3a receptor identified reduced responsiveness of a subset on CD4 T cells.[119] Likewise, C5a receptor appears to play an important role in the lung in T-cell–dependent allergic responses.

T-cell responses are also "tuned down" via complement receptor. Interestingly, cross-linking of the CD46 complement receptor via C3b on activated CD4 T cells induces differentiation to a T-regulatory phenotype.[120] Further investigation on this topic will reveal additional examples whereby the C' (complement) system participates in activation and regulation of T cells.

Conclusion

Over the past decade, a new appreciation for the complement system has come to light. Not only is the complement system required for host protection and innate immunity, but it plays a critical role in "directing" the humoral response to thymus-dependent and thymus-independent antigens. Covalent attachment of split products of C3 (i.e., C3d) alters the fate of antigen and targets it to FDC within the lymphoid compartment. Other studies are uncovering additional roles for complement in the regulation of self-reactive B cells. The next decade likely will witness a similar revolution as our understanding of how complement participates in protection against autoimmune diseases such as SLE.

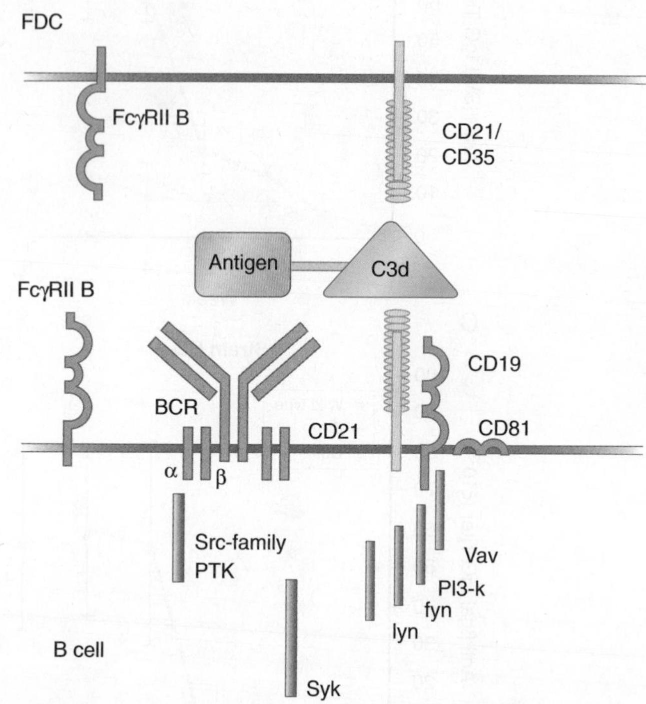

Figure 49–3 Coupling of C3d to antigen alters its fate in B-cell response. **A**, Coligation of the B-cell receptor (BCR) with CD19/CD21 by antigen coated with C3d regulates essential functions for B-cell activation. **B**, C3d-coated antigens are also captured on the surface of the follicular dendritic cells by CD21/CD35, allowing for efficient B-cell stimulation.

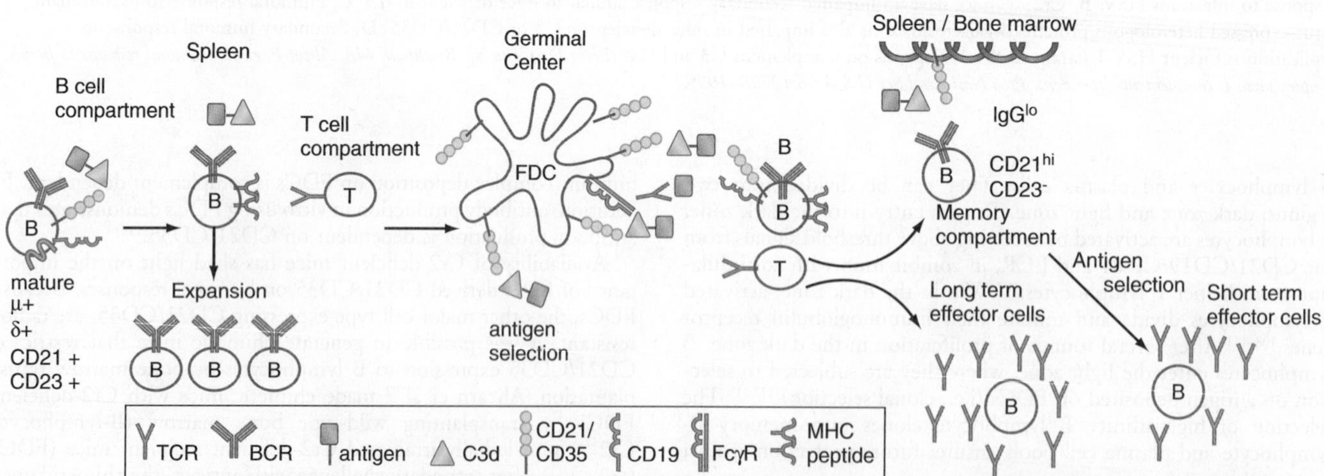

Figure 49–4 Role of complement-tagged antigen in directing B-lymphocyte activation and formation of memory B lymphocytes. Mature B lymphocytes survey secondary lymphoid tissues in search of antigen. Survival of mature B lymphocytes following antigen contact and T-cell help within splenic follicles depends on coreceptor signals through CD21/CD35. Lymphocytes receiving requisite signals expand and continue to differentiate within germinal centers, where CD21/CD35 is again important. B lymphocytes not receiving complement–ligand interactions in germinal centers die. In addition, complement-mediated deposition may localize antigen to follicular dendritic cells (FDCs), thereby providing the substrate for B-lymphocyte selection. Selection and differentiation in germinal centers lead to production of long-lived memory B lymphocytes and effector cells. The lifespan of memory B lymphocytes may also depend on continued interaction of antigen deposited on FDCs with CD21/CD35 in spleen and in bone marrow.

IMMUNOGLOBULINS

Properties and Structure

The mammalian immune system responds to the almost unlimited array of antigens by producing antibodies that react specifically with the molecules that induced their production. During the immune response, the structure of the inducing antigen is imprinted on the immune system, and subsequent challenges with the same or structurally related molecule(s) causes a more rapid rise in antibody levels to much greater concentrations than were achieved after the primary antigenic challenge. Thus, the hallmarks of the humoral immune system include induction, specific protein interaction, and memory.

Antibodies belong to the family of proteins called the *immunoglobulins*. The basic structure of all immunoglobulins consists of a monomer that contains four polypeptide chains: two identical heavy (H) chains and two identical light (L) chains covalently linked by disulfide bonds (Fig. 49–5).[121] A model of the monomeric form of immunoglobulin has been prepared based on x-ray crystallographic data obtained on the IgG myeloma protein Dob (Fig. 49–6).[122] The immunoglobulin monomer consists of a Y- or T-like structure. The size of the arms, called the Fab (fragment-antigen binding) domain of the Y or T, is 80 × 50 × 40 nm, and the size of base, called the Fc (fragment crystallizable) region, is approximately 70 × 45 × 40 nm according to models based on x-ray diffraction data. The immunoglobulin molecule exhibits considerable flexibility. In electron microscopic, low-angle x-ray scattering, transient electric birefringence, and resonance energy transfer studies, the angle between the Fab domains has been observed to vary from 0° to 180°. All antibodies have two identical combining sites for each antigen located at the ends of the Fab domains.

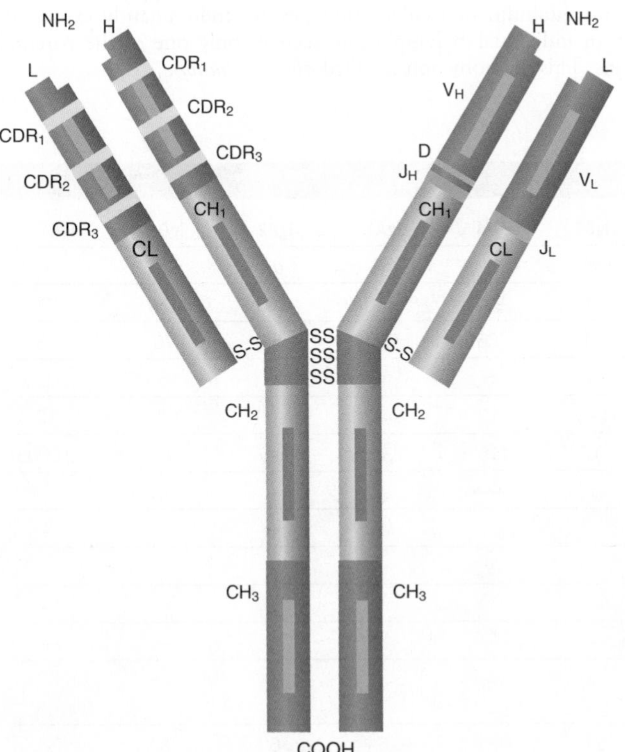

Figure 49–5 Diagrammatic representation of the structural features of an IgG molecule. NH_2 indicates the NH_2-terminus and COOH the C-terminus. V_H, C_{H1}, V_L, and C_L homology domains are shown as boxes. Only the disulfide linkages that join H and L chains are shown. **Left**, Approximate boundaries of the complementarity-determining region (CDR) regions in the V_L and V_H regions. **Right**, Sequences encoded by V_H, D, J_H, V_L, and J_L segments in the V_H and V_L regions.

Fab and Fc represent functional domains in immunoglobulins. They were discovered by performing limited proteolytic digestion of the molecule. Both the H and L chains contribute amino acids that constitute the antigen-binding site in Fab. The Fab will bind to, but will not precipitate, multivalent antigens, in contrast to native IgG. A fragment can be prepared, called $F(ab')_2$, which is devoid of Fc but still precipitates antigen. This form of immunoglobulin consists of two Fabs disulfide bonded at a part of the molecule called the *hinge region*. The hinge region is the part of the immunoglobulin molecule that is responsible for the molecular flexibility exhibited by all immunoglobulins. The other major function of immunoglobulins, binding to specific receptors on cells and certain effector proteins such as protein A and C1q, is associated with binding site(s) also found in Fc.

The chain structure of immunoglobulins explains neither antibody structural diversity nor antibody binding to antigen. The discovery of variable and constant regions of amino acid sequence formed the basis for understanding both phenomena. Thus, in the L chain, the 100 or so amino acids in the amino-terminal half of the protein (variable region [V_L]) vary between antibody molecules, but in the second half (constant region [C_L]) there is virtual complete correspondence in amino acids, position for position, to the carboxy-terminus. The H chains exhibit a similar pattern and can be divided likewise into V_H and C_H1, C_H2, and C_H3. Comparison of the amino acid sequence of many V_Ls has revealed that certain parts of the variable region exhibit excess variability, whereas others are less variable. The former regions are called *hypervariable* or *complementarity-determining regions* (CDRs). The latter framework regions function as a structural scaffold to support the CDRs. Antigen binding is mediated by six CDRs, three in each of the V_H and V_L domains. The combining site for antigen is a trough or cavity composed of parts of the hypervariable regions of both the H and L chains. It is a small region, representing only 25% of the antibody V region. The region that interacts directly with the epitope on the antigen is even smaller and is formed by the association of the CDR regions, each of which consists of approximately 20 amino acids. Thus, the variation in a few amino acids accounts for the specificity and diversity of antibodies with respect to antigen binding.[123]

Immunoglobulins exhibit additional physical heterogeneity, which imparts to each immunoglobulin a special effector function that is reflected in unique biologic properties independent of antigen-binding activity. Heterologous and autologous antisera raised against

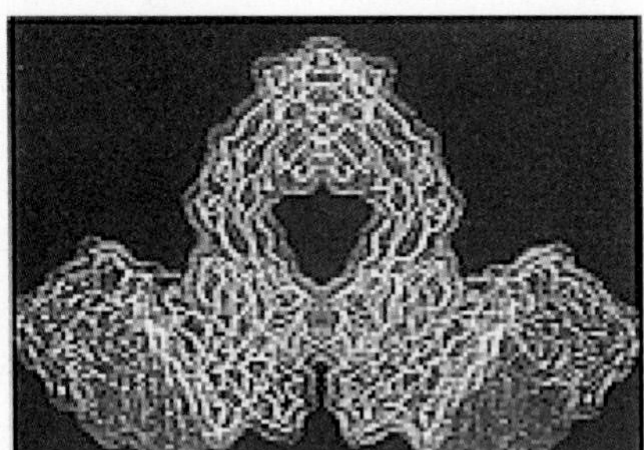

Figure 49–6 α-Carbon backbone and overall surface shape of the intact Dob IgG structure. The antigen-combining sites are located at the ends of the two horizontal Fab arms formed by the association of the light chains (α-carbon backbone as red lines and surface as light blue dots) and heavy chains (α-carbon backbone as yellow lines and surface as blue dots). On the basis of amino acid sequence studies, Dob has a substantial deletion in the hinge region, which probably limits its segmental flexibility. The molecular surface represents the area accessible to a probe sphere the size of a water molecule (1.4-Å radius). In this representation, the surface of the IgG is composed of convex regions, formed by the solvent-accessible van der Waals surface of individual atoms and concave regions. Small gaps and crevices inaccessible to the probe sphere are smoothed over. *(From Getzoff ED, Tamer JA, Lerner RA, et al: The chemistry and mechanism of antibody binding to protein antigens. Adv Immunol 43:1, 1988.)*

immunoglobulins have been used to classify three types of physical heterogeneity. The first kind is based on the antigenic heterogeneity exhibited by immunoglobulin when it is used as an immunogen in other species. This is called *class* or *isotypic variation.* In humans, five isotypes can be distinguished based on unique antigenic (isotypic) determinants found on the H chain. These are designated by capital Roman letters as IgG, IgM, IgA, IgD, and IgE. The H chain of each class is designated by the lower case Greek letter corresponding to the Roman letter of the class. Thus, the H chain for IgG is γ, for IgM is μ, for IgA is α, for IgD is δ, and for IgE is ε. Some of the immunoglobulin classes are composed of polymers of the basic monomer. In humans the two antigenic varieties of the L chain are kappa (κ) and lambda (λ). Each immunoglobulin has two identical L chains; the κ and λ are shared by all classes. The monomeric form of any immunoglobulin is described by its chain structure. The molecular mass of the immunoglobulins can vary from 150 to 1000 kd. This variation is due to polymerization of the basic monomer form. None of the immunoglobulins are polymeric forms of another class. IgG is the most prevalent, constituting 75% of the total immunoglobulin in blood. It is present in normal adults at concentrations of 600 to 1500 mg/dL. IgG is designated γ2κ2 or γ2λ2. It is the only class of immunoglobulin that crosses the placenta (Table 49–2).[124]

The isotype IgM is a pentamer consisting of five monomeric units disulfide linked at the C-terminus of the H chain. Each monomer of IgM is 180 kd due to the presence of an additional C_H domain. The complete protein has a sedimentation coefficient of 19 S, which corresponds to a molecular mass of 850 kd. IgM is designated $(\mu 2\kappa 2)_5$ or $(\mu 2\lambda_2)_5$. IgM also contains a 15-kd protein called the *J chain.* In the current structural model of IgM, the J chain forms a disulfide-bonded clasp at the C-terminus of two H chains (Fig. 49–7).[121]

The structure of the other isotypes of immunoglobulins are summarized as follows. The isotype IgA has a variable number of monomeric units and is designated $(\alpha 2\kappa_2)_n$ or $(\alpha 2\lambda_2)_n$, where n = 2 to 5. Serum IgA constitutes 20% of the total serum immunoglobulin, and 80% of this is monomeric. The remainder exists as polymers, where n = 2 to 5. The other form of IgA is found in external secretions such as saliva, tracheobronchial secretions, colostrum, milk, and genitourinary secretions. Secretory IgA consists of four components: a dimer of two monomeric molecules, a 70-kd secretory component that binds noncovalently to the IgA dimer, and the 15-kd J chain that is believed to form a disulfide-bonded clasp at the C-terminus of the H chains (Fig. 49–7). The isotype IgD has a molecular mass of 180 kd. Its serum concentration is very low, approximately 3 mg/dL. IgD apparently functions as a membrane molecule, being associated on mature but unstimulated B cells in association with IgM. IgE is the homocytotropic or reaginic immunoglobulin and mediates immediate hypersensitivity. It has a molecular mass of 180 kd and, like IgM, has four C domains. The Fc portion of IgE binds strongly to a receptor on mast cells, and this is how this immunoglobulin exerts its particular activity. The overall properties of the immunoglobulins are summarized in Table 49–2.[124,125]

Subclasses of isotypes IgG, IgA, and IgM have been identified. The structural basis for this heterogeneity is antigenic variation (e.g., amino acid sequence differences) in the Fc portion of the H chain of a given class. The subclasses of IgG, called IgG1, IgG2, IgG3, and IgG4, are the best characterized. Each has a slightly different structure, with the most notable difference being the interchain disulfide-bonding pattern (Fig. 49–7 and Table 49–2). IgG1 constitutes 70% of the total IgG and IgG2 20%. IgG3 and IgG4 constitute 8% and 2%, respectively, of the total IgG. The subclasses of IgG exhibit different catabolic rates and bind differentially to cell-associated Fc receptors. IgG2 crosses the placenta slightly more slowly than the other three subclasses. The other known subclasses of immunoglobulin isotypes are associated with IgM (IgM1 and IgM2) and IgA (IgA1 and IgA2). The properties and function of these subclasses are less well known.

The second type of variation is called *allotypic variation.* It is due to genetically controlled antigenic determinants found on both the H and L chains. Although each human has all immunoglobulin isotypes, an individual has only one form of each allotype on his or her immunoglobulin molecules. Allotypes are codominantly expressed, but an individual B lymphocyte secretes only one of the parental forms. This phenomenon is called *allelic exclusion.*

Table 49–2 Properties and Function of Human Immunoglobulins

	IgG1	IgG2	IgG3	IgG4	IgM	IgA1	IgA2	IgD	IgE
H chain	γ1	γ2	γ3	γ4	μ	α1	α2	δ	ε
Molecular weight (kd)	146	146	170	146	970	160	160	194	199
Molecular weight of H chain (kd)	51	51	60	51	65	56	52	70	73
No. of H-chain domains	4	4	4	4	5	4	4	6	5
Carbohydrate (%)	2–3	2–3	2–3	2–3	12	7–11	7–11	9–14	12
Serum concentration (mg/dL)	90	30	10	0.5	15	30	0.5	0.3	0.0005
Classical pathway complement fixation	++	+	+++	+	+++	–	–	–	
Alternative pathway complement activity			–			+	+		–
Placental transfer	+	+	+	+	+				–
Binding to mononuclear cells	+	–	+					–	–
Binding to mast cells and to basophils	–	–	–	–	–			–	+++
Reaction with protein A from *Staphylococcus aureus*	+	+	–	+	–			–	–
Half-life (days)	21	20	7	21	10	6	6	3	2
Distribution (% intravascular)	45	45	45	45	80	42	42	75	50
Fractional catabolic rate (% intravascular pool catabolized/day)	7	7	17	7	9	25	25	37	71
Synthetic rate (mg/kg/day)	33	33	33	33	33	24	24	0.4	0.002

Data primarily from Golub1[24] and Glynn and Steward.[125]

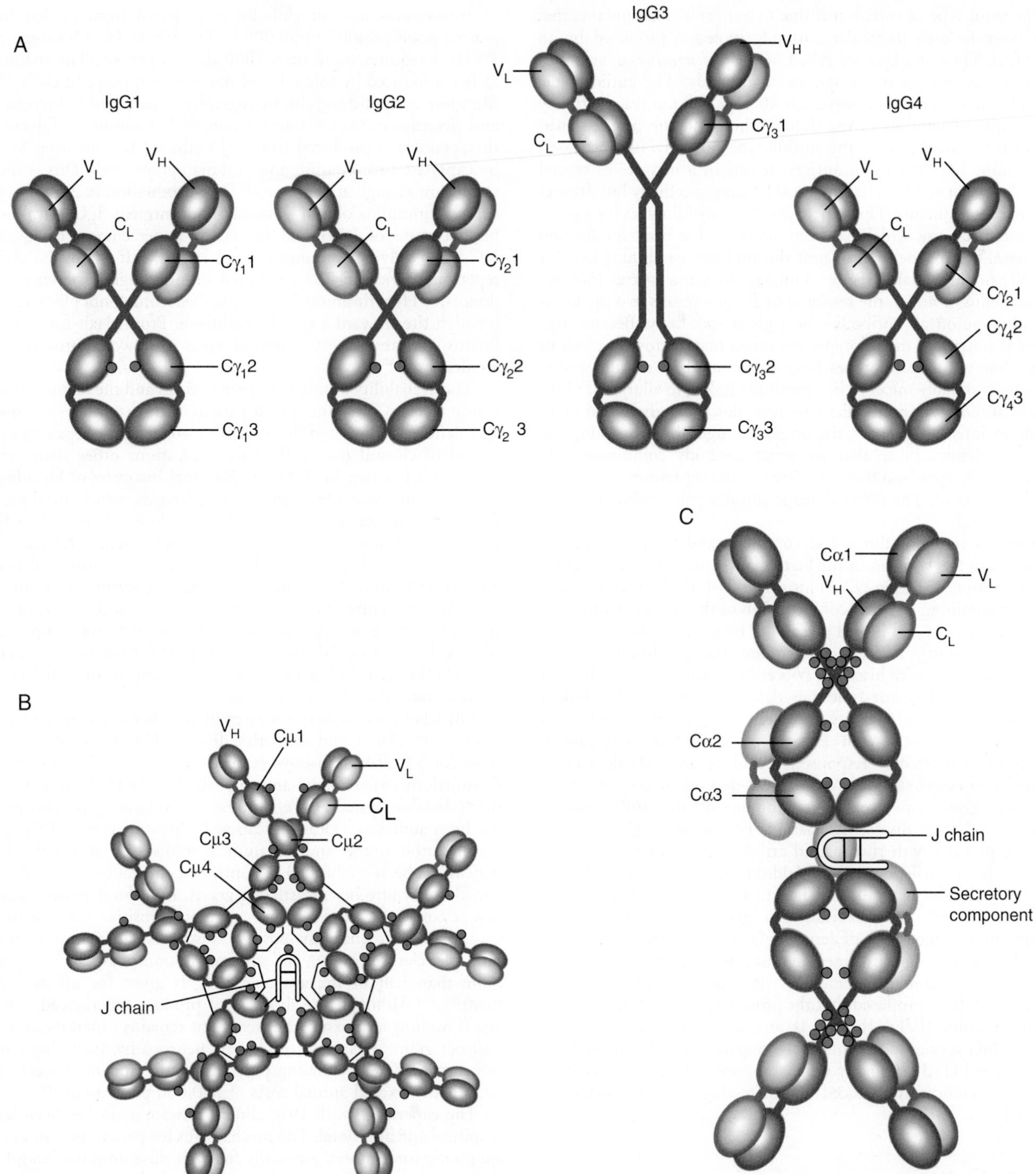

Figure 49–7 **A**, Structure of the four subclasses of human IgG. Constant region domains are indicated by C_nN, where n is the subclass and N is the domain. **B**, Structure of human IgM. The J chain is shown in the model as disulfide linked to two μ-chains. Other models have been proposed. Filled circles indicate carbohydrate. **C**, Structure of human secretory IgA. This model shows the possible arrangement of the two IgA monomers in relation to the secretory component and J chain. As the IgA molecule passes through the epithelial cells, the secretory components are synthesized and attached covalently to the Fc domain of the α-chains that have previously been joined to the J chain with disulfide links. Light chain are shown in pink, heavy chain in red, disulfide bonds as black lines, and carbohydrates as black circles. *(From Turner MW: Mannose-binding lectin: The pluripotent molecule of the innate immune system. Immunol Today 17:532, 1996.)*

The third type of variation is due to antigenic determinants that are unique to each particular antibody molecule produced by an individual. These markers are called *idiotypic determinants,* and they are associated with a single species of antibody. The antiidiotypic antibodies that recognize a particular idiotype will not react with any other immunoglobulins in the donor other than the purified antibody that was used to raise the antiidiotype antibody. In most cases, the immune response to an antigen results in a mixture of several antibodies, each of which has identical binding specificity but distinct idiotypic determinants. Thus, there can be many idiotypes for a given antigenic specificity, which has been interpreted as being a reflection of physical heterogeneity in or near the antibody combining site, for example, in the variable region domains. In some species (notably certain strains of mice), the response to antigen results in a predominant idiotype on all antibodies of a given specificity. Because this quality is inherited, the idiotypes are called major, cross-reactive, or public. Some public idiotypes have been found in certain species (again most notably mice) to be genetically linked to allotypes. Three kinds of antiidiotype antibodies have been described: those that function as an internal image of the original antigen by mimicking the antigen structure, those that recognize antibody combining site-associated idiotypes, and those that are specific for framework-associated determinants. The internal image antiidiotypic antibodies are of clinical interest.

Every immunoglobulin is a glycoprotein, and the critical glycan is attached to the H chain in the Fc domain at the conserved asparagine at position 297 (Asn297). This single, N-linked glycan is essential for maintaining an open conformation of the two H chains. The core structure of the N-linked glycan is a biantennary heptapolysaccharide containing *N*-acetylglucosamine plus additional sugars (fucose, galactose), with bisecting *N*-acetylglucosamine and sialic acid variably present. Effector functions depend on the Asn297-linked glycan and are influenced by its structure.[126] Deglycosylated IgG does not interact effectively with Fcγ receptors (FCγRs) and cannot support in vivo effector responses, including antibody-dependent cell-mediated cytotoxicity or complement-dependent cytotoxicity.[127] Individual glycoforms contribute to modulating inflammatory responses and have disease association. For example, glycosylation differs in patients with rheumatoid arthritis[128] or vasculitis[129] compared to the normal population. Addition of sialic acid to the N-linked glycan reduces binding of IgG to FcγRs and reduces in vivo cytotoxicity. Regulation of sialylation of IgG contributes to the antiinflammatory homeostasis of serum IgG. Upon antigen challenge, reduced sialic acid–IgG can mediate immune clearance and protective immunity through interaction with subclass specific FcγRs. Ravetch et al. have proposed that the protective effect of intravenous immunoglobulin (IVIg) therapy is due to the minor fraction of sialylated IgG species in the total IVIg preparation and that the high doses required (1–3 g/kg body weight) for antiinflammatory activity could be significantly reduced by increasing the percentage of sialylated IgG.[130]

Therapeutic Use

Immunoglobulin G was one of the first plasma proteins prepared in a purified state as a therapeutic drug for treatment of clinical disorders. It remains, along with albumin and alpha-proteinase inhibitor, the most widely used therapeutic plasma derivative, and is currently the major plasma product on the global market. Polyvalent human immunoglobulin preparations have been used to reconstitute humoral immunity in agammaglobulinemic patients for more than three decades. Until 25 years ago, intramuscular treatment was the mode of administration. Intramuscular preparations caused severe adverse reactions when injected intravenously.[131–133] The most serious were anaphylactoid reactions, and were probably complement mediated. Efforts to reduce anticomplementary activity (ACA) and the prekallikrein activator activity (PKA) were initiated in the early 1980s and safer IVIg preparations became available.

Intravenous immunoglobulin is prepared from pooled human plasma pools of 3000 to 50,000 L. The World Health Organization (WHO) requires more than 1000 donors per lot. The majority of IVIg is produced by cold ethanol fractionation procedures,[134,135] with filtration and polishing chromatography steps added to increase yield and decrease pathogen transmission.[136,137] Gamunex (Talecris Biotherapeutics) is produced from cold ethanol fractionation followed by caprylate precipitation and chromatograpy.[136,138] This is the first significant change in commercial IVIg production in 20 years. Intravenous immunoglobulin contains concentrated IgG with normal plasma ratios of IgG1 and IgG2, lower percentages of IgG3 and IgG4, and only trace amounts of IgA and IgM. It retains the antibody repertoire, reflecting the combined immunologic experience of the donors.[139] Hyperimmune IGIV is purified from donor plasma selected for high titer toward a specific pathogen. Prophylaxis for cytomegalovirus and respiratory syncytial virus are two approved clinical applications.[140,141]

The availability of safe IVIg preparations and the fortuitous observation that IgG treatment of a patient with thrombocytopenia and IgG deficiency increased the patient's platelet count began an intense period of clinical use of IVIg for indications other than primary immune deficiency. In 1990, the National Institutes of Health sponsored a Consensus Development Conference, which produced the first consensus statement on IVIg clinical indications.[142] As a result, six disease indications—primary immunodeficiency, Kawasaki syndrome, chronic lymphocytic leukemia, human immunodeficiency virus (HIV) infections during childhood to prevent infections, bone marrow transplantation to prevent graft-versus-host disease or bacterial infections in adults, and idiopathic purpura—were approved by the Food and Drug Administration (FDA) for labeling and marketing. The licensed indications remain unchanged, but off-label uses include more than 100 conditions.[143,144]

Off-label uses include a variety of immune-mediated, presumed immune-mediated, and idiopathic diseases. Consensus recommendations for 53 off-label uses were developed by a University Hospital Consortium Expert Panel and published in 1995.[145] In addition to the indications listed above, chronic demyelinating polyneuropathy has been added as a clear indication for treatment with IVIg. Additional autoimmune and inflammatory diseases in which clinical benefit has been established in controlled clinical trials include Guillain-Barré syndrome, myasthenia gravis, multifocal motor neuropathy, corticosteroid-resistant dermatomyositis, antineutrophil cytoplasmic-autoantibody–positive vasculitis, autoimmune uveitis, multiple sclerosis, cancer, and solid organ transplant.[146–153] Currently, more than half of the available IVIg is given for off-label treatment.[144,154] Although the shortage of product experienced a decade ago is no longer an issue, the treatment remains expensive at $50 to $80 per gram. Treatment of chronic neuropathy, including chronic inflammatory demyelinating polyneuropathy and multifocal motor neuropathy, exceed annual costs of $50,000 per patient.[144]

The experience with IVIg clinical development has been largely empirical and anecdotal. The mechanisms for patient benefit or harm are poorly understood, especially for high-dose immune modulation therapy. Various known and some yet undiscovered functions of immunoglobulins in immune homeostasis may contribute, including modulation of the function and expression of Fc receptors, interaction with complement and cytokine systems, antiidiotypic antibodies, and regulation of T-cell and B-cell function.[155–157]

Many effects of IVIg are explained by mechanisms beyond antigenic recognition of pathogens. Intravenous immunoglobulin preparations contain up to 30% dimers composed of idiotype–antiidiotype antibody pairs. These dimers appear to be very effective as a sink for activated complement and can inhibit complement activation.[158] Benefit for treatment of immune thrombocytopenia purpura seem to be mediated by Fc-receptor blockade of reticuloendothelial cell salvage receptor (FcRn) combined with an antiidiotypic neutralization of antiplatelet antibody that together eliminate antiplatelet antibody from the blood. Other indications of antibody neutralization can be seen in IVIg treatment of myasthenia gravis. The dramatic success of IVIg in treating Kawasaki syndrome may be due to several mechanisms, including antiidiotypic neutralization of antiendothelial antibodies, inhibition of cytokine production and function, and elimination of causative superantigens.[159,160] Intravenous immunoglobulin inhibits B-cell activation and autoantibody production by enhancing $CD8^+$ suppressor T-cell function. Cell-mediated immunity also is affected.[155]

Adverse Events Related to Intravenous Immunoglobulin Infusion

Adverse events associated with IVIg can be characterized as (a) early systemic events, (b) infectious disease transfer, and (c) high-dose treatment related adverse effects.[133]

Early Systemic Events

Common transfusion-related early events are listed in Table 49–3. Most early events are self-limiting and infusion rate dependent. Premedication with steroids, aspirin, or other nonsteroidal antiinflammatory drugs often decreases symptoms. Prophylaxis propanolol can be effective for induced migraine. Aseptic meningitis is a rare early event, is observed 1 to 2 days postinfusion, is unrelated to infusion rate, and can be treated with IV steroids and analgesics.[133,161]

The frequency of reported adverse events varies considerably, ranging from 10% to 85%.[133,142,162–164] There are many reason for this high variability in reporting: (a) differences in product,[137,152,162] (b) infusion rate, (c) dose and frequency of dosing, (d) patient population, and (e) relative experience of patient and physician. Both patients and physicians become steeled to the adverse events, and because incidents are not life threatening and often respond to prophylaxis medication, they are ignored as "normal." Nonetheless, these events are common and affect health and quality of life of patients.[144,162]

Infectious Disease Transfer

A few early preparations of IVIg transmitted hepatitis C virus. Manufacturers have added viral inactivation and partitioning steps, and current licensed products are safe with respect to HIV, hepatitis C virus, hepatitis B virus, and other blood-born pathogens.[165] The industry has responded to the threat of prions with process validation,[163,166] donor screening, donor testing, inventory management (look back), and plasma pool testing.

Table 49–3 Early Systemic Adverse Events Associated with Intravenous Immunoglobulin Infusion

Fever	Rash/urticaria
Chills	Chest tightness
Sore throat	Dyspnea
Face flush	Wheezing
Tachycardia	Low/high blood pressure
Palpitations	Shock
Lumbar pain	Anxiety
Abdominal pain	Nervousness
Nausea	Headache
Vomiting	Migraine
Shaking	Anaphylaxis
Fatigue	Malaise
Myalgia	Leukopenia

High-Dose Treatment-Related Adverse Events

Intravenous immunoglobulin treatment for immune modulation of neurologic diseases requires doses of 1 to 2 kg per kilogram of body weight, or two to five times the dose recommended for replacement therapy. Adverse events with high-dose administration include those listed in Table 49–3 and occasionally thromboembolic events, renal complications, and anemia.[133,164,167–170] Thromboembolic events include deep vein thrombosis, pulmonary embolism, myocardial infarction, and stroke. Thromboembolic events and renal failure seem to be independent of infusion rate. The cause of thromboembolic events is not known. Dalakas[171] has suggested that increased serum viscosity plays a role. Factor XIa has also been identified in IVIg preparations.[172] Factor XIa could directly lead to shortening of coagulation time and risk of thrombosis. Renal complications are rare but result in high morbidity and mortality. Whether IgG, contaminants, or excipients are responsible is not clear. Of the 88 renal adverse events reported to the FDA, 90% were stabilized with sucrose.[133,161] Whether the adverse events observed with IVIg treatment of neurologic diseases are related to a preexisting medical condition or the high doses required for treatment is not clear.

Monoclonal Antibody Therapy

Monoclonal antibody (mAb) technology as described in 1975 by Kohler and Milstein[173] is now well established for the production of diagnostic and therapeutic mAbs. Despite early enthusiasm and much research and development effort, the development of clinical mAb was frustrated for 20 years by reports of severe toxicity and poor clinical efficacy. Only one mAb, OKT3, an anti-CD3, was licensed for clinical use before 1994. Over the last decade the situation has changed. Monoclonal antibody products constitute as much as 25% of new biologicals in clinical development, with a first in humans to regulatory approval success rate of 27%, which compares very favorably to the 11% rate for small-molecule drugs.[174,175] Table 49–4 lists the 18 mAbs that have received FDA approval; 17 are marketed and one has been withdrawn.[176]

The list includes antibodies for diverse clinical conditions, including oncology, chronic inflammatory conditions, solid organ transplantation, infectious disease, and cardiovascular medicine. Approved antibody therapy includes unmodified mAb, radio-immunoconjugates, immuno-drug conjugates, and antibody fragments. More than 150 mAbs are in clinical development, with at least 33 in clinical trials for conditions including colorectal cancer, melanoma, postmenopausal osteoporosis, cutaneous T-cell lymphoma, rheumatoid arthritis, and respiratory syncytial virus infection.[174] Part of the progress is due to the advent of genetic engineering, which has allowed the production of "humanized" mAbs. Human–mouse chimerized Ab with limited mouse determinants or fully human mAb now are produced by DNA technology or with transgenic mice. The humanization of mAbs provides some protection from the patient's immune system, prolonging the circulation half-life from less than 24 hours for murine mAbs in humans and approaching the 21-day half-life of native IgG. Increased circulation time is due in part to the reduction in immune reactivity and subsequent opsonization of mAbs but also because human but not murine IgG is recycled by receptors (FcRn) on human epithelial cells.[177,178]

ReoPro (abciximab) is a chimeric Fab fragment directed to glycoprotein IIb/IIIa and is one of the early successful clinical mAbs (approved for marketing in 1994). ReoPro prevents thrombus formation in patients undergoing procedures such as percutaneous coronary intervention.[179] Another example of a chimeric mAb (IgG1) is Remicade (infliximab), which is an anti–tumor necrosis factor α. Remicade was approved in 1998 for treatment of Crohn disease and in 1999 for treatment of rheumatoid arthritis.[180,181]

Monoclonal antibodies for cancer therapy are divided into two stratagems. "Naked" mAbs target specific tumor-related antigens or

Table 49–4 Monoclonal Antibody Products Approved by the Food and Drug Administration

Product Name, Antibody Name (Company)	Antibody Format	Antigen	K_d (nM)	Proposed Mechanisms of Action	Approved Indications
Orthoclone OKT3, muromonab-CD3 Ortho Biotech Products, LP)	Mouse IgG2a	CD3	0.83	Blocking of function of T-cell expressed CD3; reversal of graft rejection	Prophylaxis of acute kidney transplant rejection
ReoPro, abciximab (Centocor, Inc.)	Chimeric Fab	GpIIb/IIIa and $\alpha_1\beta_3$-integrin	5	Receptor binding and antagonism; inhibition of platelet aggregation	Prevention of platelet-mediated clots in coronary angioplasty
Rituxan, rituximab (Genentech, Inc., and Biogen Idec Inc.); Mab Thera (F. Hoffmann-La Roche Ltd.)	Chimeric IgG1	CD20	8.0	Sensitization of cells to chemotherapy; induction of apoptosis, ADCC and CDC	Non-Hodgkin lymphoma and rheumatoid arthritis
Zenapax, daclizumab (F. Hoffmann-La Roche Ltd.)	Humanized IgG1	CD25	0.3	Receptor binding and antagonism	Prophylaxis of acute kidney transplant rejection
Simulect, basiliximab (Novartis AG)	Chimeric IgG1	CD25	0.1	Receptor binding and antagonism	Prophylaxis of acute kidney transplant rejection
Synagis, palivizumab (MedImmune Inc., and Abbott Laboratories)	Humanized IgG1	RSV gpF	0.96	Binding neutralization of RSV; inhibition of viral fusion and replication	Prophylaxis against RSV infection in children at high risk
Remicade, infliximab (Johnson & Johnson, and Schering-Plough Corporation)	Chimeric IgG1	TNF	0.1	Ligand binding and receptor antagonism	Crohn disease, rheumatoid and psoriatic arthritis, ulcerative colitis, ankylosing spondylitis
Herceptin, trastuzumab (Genentech, Inc., and F. Hoffmann-La Roche Ltd.)	Humanized IgG1	ErbB2	5	Sensitization of cells to chemotherapy; inhibition of angiogenesis and proliferation; induction of ADCC	Metastatic breast cancer that overexpresses ERBB2
Mylotarg, gemtuzumab ozogamicin (Wyeth)	Humanized IgG4, calicheamicin conjugated	CD33	0.08	Induction of double-stranded DNA breaks and cell death (caused by calicheamicin)	Acute myeloid leukemia that expresses CD33
Campath, alemtuzumab (Genzyme Corp. and Schering AG)	Humanized IgG1	CD52	10–32	Induction of ADCC and CDC	B-cell chronic lymphocytic leukemia
Zevalin, ibritumomab tiuxetan (Biogen Idec, Inc.)	Mouse IgG1, Y-labelled	CD20	14–18	Induction of cell death by radiation; induction of apoptosis	Non-Hodgkin lymphoma
Humira, adalimumab (Abbott Laboratories)	Human IgG1	TNF	0.1	Ligand binding and receptor antagonism; induction of CDC	Rheumatoid and psoriatic arthritis
Xolair, omalizumab (Genentech, Inc., and Novartis AG)	Humanized IgG1	IgE	0.17	Ligand binding and receptor antagonism; reduction release of allergic-response mediators from mast cells and basophils	Persistent asthma
Bexxar, I-tositumomab (GlaxoSmithKline)	Mouse IgG2a, I-labelled	CD20	1.4	Induction of cell death by radiation; induction of apoptosis, ADCC, and CDC	Non-Hodgkin lymphoma

Table 49–4 Monoclonal Antibody Products Approved by the Food and Drug Administration—cont'd

Product Name, Antibody Name (Company)	Antibody Format	Antigen	K_d (nM)	Proposed Mechanisms of Action	Approved Indications
Raptiva, efalizumab (Genentech, Inc., and Serono S.A.)	Humanized IgG1	CD11a	3	Receptor binding and antagonism; inhibition of leukocyte adhesion to other cells	Plaque psoriasis
Erbitux, cetuximab (ImClone Systems, Inc., and Bristol-Myers Squibb Company)	Chimeric IgG1	EGFR	0.2	Receptor binding and antagonism; inhibition of cell proliferation; induction of apoptosis; sensitization of cells to chemotherapy and radiotherapy; inhibition of angiogenesis, invasion, and metastasis; induction of ADCC	Metastatic colorectal cancer
Avastin, bevacizumab (Genentech, Inc., and F. Hoffmann-La Roche Ltd.)	Humanized IgG1	VEGF	1.1	Ligand binding and receptor antagonism; inhibition of angiogenesis and metastatic disease progression	Metastatic colorectal cancer, head and neck cancer
Tysabri, natalizumab (Biogen Idec, Inc., and Eland Corporation, PLC)	Humanized IgG4	α_4-Subunit of $\alpha_4\beta_1$-integrin and $\alpha_4\beta_3$-integrin	0.3	Receptor binding and antagonism; inhibition of leukocyte adhesion to their counterreceptors	Multiple sclerosis

Sources include drug prescribing information, company Web sites.[174] Products are listed in order of first regulatory approval, from Orthoclone OKT3 (1986) to Tysabri (2004).

ADCC, antibody-dependent cell-mediated cytotoxicity; CDC, complement-dependent cytotoxicity; EGFR, epidermal growth factor receptor; ErbB2, Her-2/neu, CD340, erythroblastic leukemia viral oncogene homolog 2 neurolglioblastoma derived oncogene homolog (avian); RSV gpF, Human respiratory syncytial virus glycoprotein F; TNF, tumor necrosis factor; VEGF, vascular endothelial growth factor.

cell receptors to recruit the immune system or to modify the growth of tumor cells. Examples of approved naked mAbs are Rituxan (rituximab),[182] an anti-CD20 approved for non-Hodgkin lymphoma, and Herceptin (trastuzumab),[183] an anti-HER2 approved for advanced breast cancer. To date most naked mAb candidates have been disappointing, and the most efficacious are used as adjuvant therapy. The most promising naked mAbs may not directly affect the tumor cell but instead may modify the patient's immune response to the tumor. An example of immune-modulating mAbs in development is anti-CD152,[184] which may modulate the way T cells respond to cancer cells.

The second strategy is to attach or conjugate an antitumor agent to an antitumor mAb. The mAbs deliver the toxic agent to the tumor or tumor cells in an attempt to obliterate the cancer cells. Both radioactive and chemical toxins have been conjugated to a variety of tumor-specific mAbs. Two mAbs that deliver radioactivity directly to the tumor are Zevalin (ibritumomab tiuxetan) and Bexxar (tositumomab), which were approved in 2002 and 2003, respectively, for B-cell non-Hodgkin lymphoma.[185,186] Many immunotoxins have been developed, but without much clinical success. Mylotarg (gemtuzumab ozogamicin), an anti-CD33 mAb, is approved for myelogenous leukemia when chemotherapy is not effective or appropriate.[187]

A listing of approved mAb therapy for cancer can be found online on the American Cancer Society web page (at www.cancer.org) under Monoclonal Antibody Therapy (Passive Immunotherapy). For a review of therapeutic MAbs, see Carter.[176]

SUGGESTED READINGS

Abdul Ajees A, Gunasekaran K, Volanakis JE, Narayana SV, Kotwal GJ, Murthy HM: The structure of complement C3b provides insights into complement activation and regulation. Nature 444:221, 2006.

Ahearn JM, Fischer MB, Croix D, et al: Disruption of the Cr2 locus results in a reduction in B-1a cells and in an impaired B cell response to T-dependent antigen. Immunity 4:251, 1996.

Bayary J, Dasgupta S, Misra N, et al: Intravenous immunoglobulin in autoimmune disorders: An insight into the immunoregulatory mechanisms. Int Immunopharm 6:528, 2006.

Carter RH, Fearon DT: CD19: Lowering the threshold for antigen receptor stimulation of B lymphocytes. Science 256:105, 1992.

Carroll MC: The complement system in regulation of adaptive immunity. Nat Immunol 5:981, 2004.

Dalakas MC: Mechanisms of action of IVIG and therapeutic considerations in the treatment of acute and chronic demyelinating neuropathies. Neurology 59:S13, 2002.

Fischer MB, Goerg S, Shen L, et al: Dependence of germinal center B cells on expression of CD21/CD35 for survival. Science 280:582, 1998.

Helmy KY, Gorgani NN, Kljavin NM, et al: CRIg: A macrophage complement receptor required for phagocytosis of circulating pathogens. Cell 124:915, 2006.

Hopken UE, Lu B, Gerard NP, et al: The C5a chemoattractant receptor mediates mucosal defence to infection. Nature 383:86, 1996.

Jordan SC, Vo AA, Peng A, Toyoda M: Intravenous gammaglobulin (IVIG): A novel approach to improve transplant rates and outcomes in highly HLA-sensitized patients. Am J Transplantation 6:459, 2006.

Kang YS, Do Y, Lee HK, et al: A dominant complement fixation pathway for pneumococcal polysaccharides initiated by SIGN-R1 interacting with C1q. Cell 125:47, 2006.

Kelsoe G: Life and death in germinal centers (redux). Immunity 4:107, 1996.

Kemper C, Chan AC, Green JM, et al: Activation of human CD4+ cells with CD3 and CD46 induces a T-regulatory cell 1 phenotype. Nature 421:388, 2003.

Kopf M, Abel B, Gallimore A, Carroll M, Bachmann MF: Complement component C3 promotes T-cell priming and lung migration to control acute influenza virus infection. Nat Med 8:373, 2002.

Minard S, Papa SM, Campiglio M, Tagliabue E: Biologic and therapeutic role of HER2 in cancer. Oncogene 29:6570, 2003.

Thiel S, Vorup-Jensen T, Stover CM: A second serine protease associated with manna-binding lectin that activates complement. Nature 386:506, 1997.

REFERENCES

For complete list of references log onto www.expertconsult.com

CHAPTER 50

DISORDERS OF PHAGOCYTE FUNCTION AND NUMBER

Mary C. Dinauer and Thomas D. Coates

INTRODUCTION

Phagocytic leukocytes are an essential component of the innate immune system that has evolved to rapidly respond to the presence of invading bacteria, fungi, and parasites. This first line of host defense also includes natural killer lymphocytes, complement, and other plasma proteins. As reviewed in Chapters 10 and 26, phagocytes are responsible for ingesting, killing, and digesting pathogens. Granulocytic phagocytes (neutrophils and eosinophils) circulate in the bloodstream until they sense chemotactic signals from infected tissues, which result in adhesion to the vascular endothelium and subsequent migration into the site of infection. Mononuclear phagocytes (macrophages and their circulating precursor, the monocyte), on the other hand, function primarily as resident cells in a variety of tissues such as lung, liver, peritoneal cavity, and spleen, where they perform a surveillance role and also interact closely with lymphocytes to promote specific immune responses. Microbial killing is accomplished by two types of mechanisms: (a) de novo synthesis of highly toxic and often unstable derivatives of molecular oxygen by an enzyme known as the respiratory burst oxidase and (b) preformed polypeptide "antibiotics" and proteases stored within several types of lysosomal granules that are delivered into phagocytic vacuoles containing the ingested microbes.

This chapter reviews the major congenital and acquired disorders of phagocyte function and number, which from the clinical standpoint largely involve neutrophils. As would be predicted, these disorders are manifested clinically by recurrent bacterial and fungal infections, often with atypical pathogens or unusual presentations. Interestingly, the converse of this is only rarely observed. Most patients with recurrent infections do not have any identifiable abnormality in their phagocytes. There are at least two explanations for the clinical rarity of phagocyte disorders. First, given their critical role in host defense, nature may be quite intolerant of major abnormalities in phagocytes. Prior to the modern antibiotic era, patients afflicted with severe disorders probably did not survive into their childbearing years. Second, there is a remarkable redundancy in the antimicrobial machinery of the phagocytes that permits one system to compensate for a defect in another. For example, the host does not rely on a single chemotactic signal or neutrophil membrane receptor to ensure that phagocytes accumulate at sites of infection. Instead, multiple chemotactic signals and receptors are employed. A similar phenomenon is seen in the reactions that kill microbes as both oxidative and nonoxidative systems are employed.

This chapter is divided into two sections. The first is focused on functional abnormalities and is organized according to the cellular functions outlined above: disorders of the respiratory burst microbicidal pathway, abnormalities of phagocyte adhesion and chemotaxis, and defects in the structure and function of lysosomal granules. The second section outlines the quantitative abnormalities—leukocytosis and leukopenia—with a particular emphasis on neutropenia. The chapter is not meant to be an encyclopedic review of the numerous papers published on phagocyte abnormalities. It is important to note that many of these reports describe marginal in vitro defects, with little evidence that they are responsible for a clinical problem. Many comprehensive reviews offering additional information on phagocyte disorders are available.[1–8]

DISORDERS OF PHAGOCYTE FUNCTION

Inherited and acquired clinical disorders of phagocyte function result from defects in one or more of the major steps leading to microbial killing—adhesion, chemotaxis, ingestion, degranulation, and production of microbicidal oxidants (Fig. 50–1). Patients with inherited disorders typically present in infancy or childhood with recurrent, unusual, or recalcitrant bacterial and fungal infections, and it is usually not difficult to determine that these are outside the range of normal. The presentation of these different inherited disorders can overlap, so that a specific diagnosis cannot be made on clinical grounds alone. Infections commonly seen include those of the skin or mucosa, lung, lymph node, deep tissue abscesses, or childhood periodontitis. These can often have an indolent presentation with only low-grade fevers. Bacterial sepsis is an unusual initial symptom, and usually reflects dissemination from an infected site. Inherited defects in phagocyte function are rare, and represent only approximately 20% of the primary immunodeficiencies.[1] Thus, children with suspected disorders of host defense should be also screened for defects in humoral, cellular, and complement-mediated immunity. An approach to evaluating the patient with significant recurrent infections is shown (Fig. 50–2). If a defect is identified, it is recommended that the patient be referred to a center specialized in care of such patients.

In clinical practice, although nearly all patients with well-characterized phagocyte abnormalities have recurrent or unusual infections, the majority of those individuals with histories of persistent or recurrent infections do not have identifiable phagocyte disorders or other immune defects. In some cases, these reflect another underlying medical condition or nonimmunologic problem related to an anatomic or obstructive defect. This chapter will focus largely on those disorders in which a good correlation exists between the clinical condition and an identifiable defect in phagocyte function.

DISORDERS OF THE RESPIRATORY BURST PATHWAY

Reactive oxygen species generated by the phagocyte respiratory burst are critical for microbial killing. The enzyme responsible for the initial reaction in this pathway is a nicotinamide adenine dinucleotide phosphate (NADPH) oxidase found in plasma and phagolysosomal membranes. Upon activation by inflammatory stimuli, the NADPH oxidase catalyzes the transfer of an electron from NADPH to molecular oxygen, thereby forming superoxide (as the O_2^- ion) (Fig. 50–2, reaction 1).[9–11] This NADPH oxidase, along with the enzymes and reactions that are directly involved in the production or metabolism of O_2^-, constitute the respiratory burst pathway as depicted in Fig. 50–2. Superoxide is the precursor to numerous microbicidal oxidants, including hydrogen peroxide and hypochlorous acid. Five clinically significant defects have been identified in the respiratory burst, involving the following enzymes: NADPH oxidase (reaction 1), leukocyte glucose-6-phosphate dehydrogenase (G6PD) (reaction 8), myeloperoxidase (reaction 4), glutathione reductase, and glutathione synthetase (reaction 9).[2,12–14] These reactions are involved in the production of O_2^- (reactions 8 and 1), in the conversion of O_2^- and hydrogen peroxide to other toxic derivatives (reaction 4), or in the

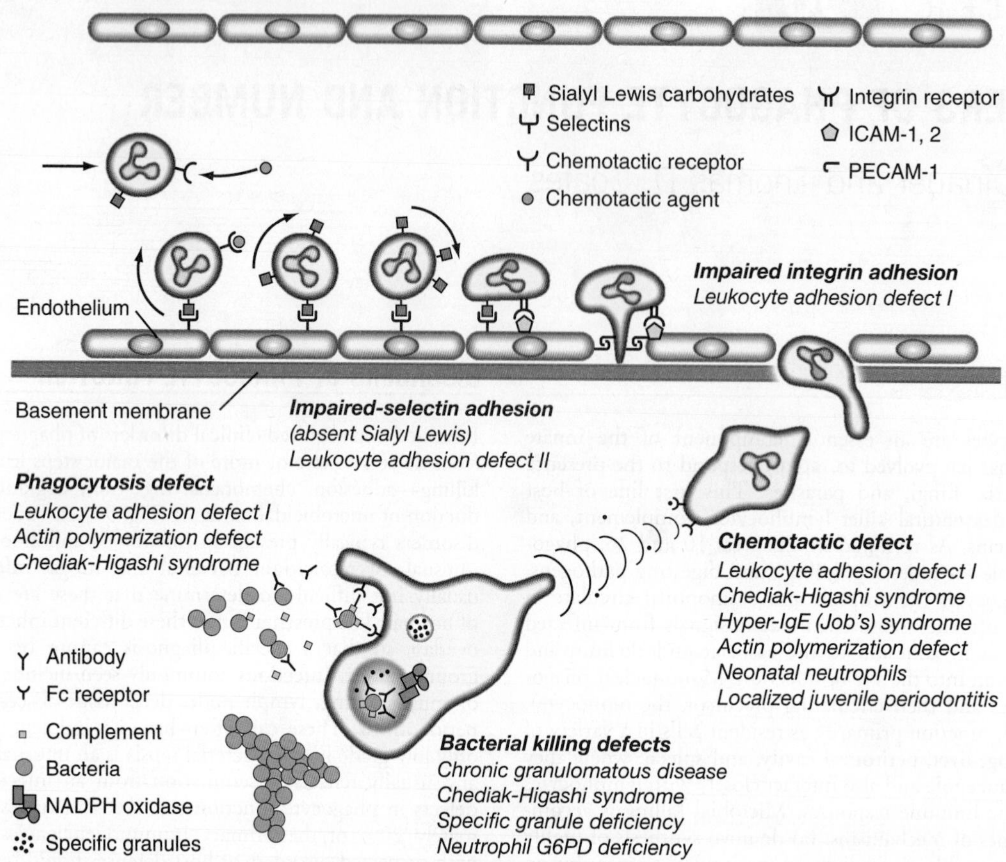

Figure 50–1 Steps in the response of circulating neutrophils to infection or inflammation in tissues. The adhesion molecule E-selectin is upregulated on endothelial cells in response to inflammatory mediators (IL-1, endotoxin, and TNF-α) resulting in the rolling attachment and margination of neutrophils through interactions with sialyl Lewis carbohydrates on its surface. Chemoattractants, such as IL-8, released by endothelial cells cause upregulation of neutrophil β2 integrins, which, in turn, mediate tight adhesion to ICAM-1 and PECAM-1 on endothelial cells. Activated neutrophils can detect as little as a 2% change in the chemoattractant gradient and move toward the site of infection. Neutrophils phagocytose bacteria opsonized by antibody and complement. Both oxidative and nonoxidative antimicrobial mechanisms are then used to kill bacteria. Disorders of phagocyte function associated with each of these steps are listed. *(Modified from Kyono W, Coates TD: A practical approach to neutrophil disorders. Pediatr Clin North Am 49:929, 2002, with permission.)*

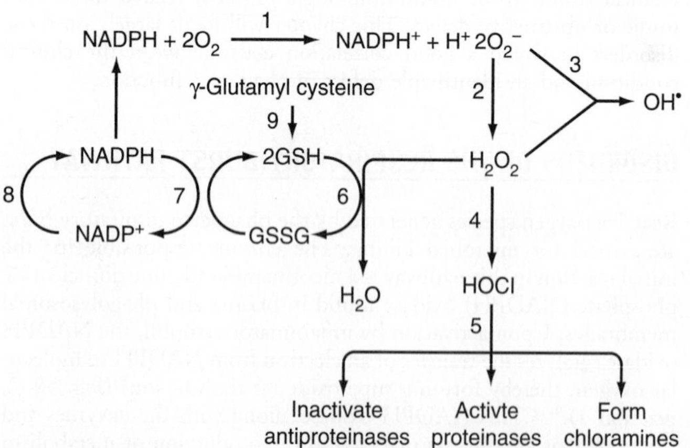

Figure 50–2 Reactions of the respiratory burst pathway. The enzymes responsible for reactions 1 to 9 are as follows: (1) The respiratory burst oxidase (NADPH oxidase); (2) superoxide dismutase or spontaneous; (3) nonenzymatic, Fe^{2+}-catalyzed; (4) myeloperoxidase; (5) spontaneous; (6) glutathione peroxidase; (7) glutathione reductase; (8) glucose-6-phosphate dehydrogenase; (9) glutathione synthetase.

detoxification of excess hydrogen peroxide needed to protect the phagocyte during the respiratory burst (reactions 7 and 9). Of note, homologues to the oxidase NADPH oxidase have recently been discovered in the gut, vascular cells, and other tissues, which may generate oxidants for local host defense or for regulation of other cellular functions.[15,16]

Chronic Granulomatous Disease

Chronic granulomatous disease (CGD) is a genetically heterogeneous group of defects that share in common the failure of neutrophils, monocytes, macrophages, and eosinophils to undergo a respiratory burst and generate O_2^-.[2,9,12,17–20] CGD is relatively rare, having an estimated incidence of between 1/200,000 and 1/250,000 live births based on data from the United States CGD Registry.[17] The absence of respiratory burst-derived oxidants results in recurrent, often life-threatening, bacterial and fungal infections and is also associated with formation of inflammatory granulomas. The disease was first described in 1957 in two independent reports by Good and colleagues[21] and Landing and Shirkey,[22] both of which describe severe recurrent infections in boys associated with visceral granulomas containing pigmented histiocytes. The disease was termed fatal granulomatous disease owing to this distinguishing histologic feature and the grim clinical course in most patients. It was not until the late 1960s and early 1970s that the defect in oxygen consumption and O_2^- production was identified and a convenient diagnostic assay, the nitroblue tetrazolium (NBT) test, was developed.[23,24] In the 1980s, a combination of biochemical and molecular genetic approaches led to the identification of four critical subunits of the NADPH oxidase, and the recognition that mutations in the corresponding genes are responsible for four different genetic subgroups of CGD (Fig. 50–3).[2,9,12,18,25]

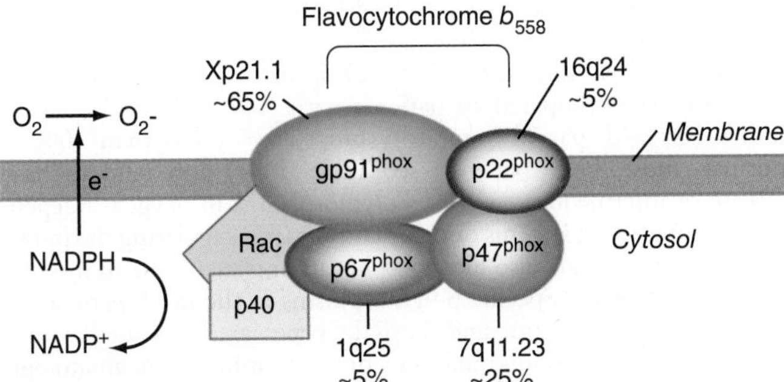

Figure 50–3 NADPH oxidase and molecular genetics of chronic granulomatous disease. Shown is the assembled form of the enzymatically active NADPH oxidase, along with subunits affected in the four different genetic subgroups of chronic granulomatous disease (CGD), the approximate incidence, and the chromosomal location of the corresponding gene. Flavocytochrome b_{558} is the redox center of the enzyme, and is located in plasma, specific granule, and phagolysosomal membranes. This heterodimer is composed of the gp91*phox* and p22*phox* subunits of the NADPH oxidase, which are affected in X-linked and an autosomal recessive form of CGD, respectively. The soluble regulatory proteins p47*phox*, p67*phox*, and p40*phox* are found in the cytosol until phagocyte activation by soluble or particulate inflammatory stimuli, on which they move to the membrane where p47*phox* and p67*phox* bind flavocytochrome b_{558}. Mutations in the genes encoding p47*phox* and p67*phox* account for two autosomal recessive forms of CGD. Another essential regulatory component of the NADPH oxidase is the small GTPase, Rac, which in its active GTP-bound state, becomes membrane-bound and associates with the oxidase. By a mechanism that is not fully understood, binding of these multiple regulatory subunits activates the flavocytochrome to catalyze the transfer of electrons from cytosolic NADPH across the membrane via the FAD and heme redox centers to molecular oxygen, thereby forming superoxide in the extracellular or intraphagosomal compartment. No cases of CGD have been described owing to mutations in p40*phox* or Rac.

Molecular Genetics of Chronic Granulomatous Disease

CGD results from mutations in any of the four genes encoding essential subunits of the NADPH oxidase, which forms the basis of a modern classification scheme (Table 50–1). In turn, the biochemical and genetic analysis of CGD has been instrumental in characterizing this complex enzyme.[2,9,12,18,20] The oxidase subunits are referred to by their apparent molecular mass (kd), and have been given the designation *phox*, for *ph*agocyte *ox*idase. A b-type cytochrome known as flavocytochrome b_{558}, a membrane-bound heterodimer composed of gp91*phox* and p22*phox*, is the redox center of the oxidase. Approximately two-thirds of CGD cases result from defects in the X-linked gene encoding the gp91*phox* subunit of flavocytochrome b_{558},[26–29] which contains both the flavoprotein and heme-binding domains responsible for electron transport. A rare autosomal recessive form of CGD is caused by mutations in the gene encoding p22*phox*,[30] the smaller subunit of flavocytochrome b_{558}, which provides a critical docking site for p47*phox*, a regulatory subunit of the oxidase. The remaining cases of autosomal recessive CGD involve genetic defects in either p47*phox* or p67*phox*, two regulatory proteins that are associated with each other in the cytosol of unstimulated cells but rapidly move to the membrane to activate flavocytochrome b_{558} and superoxide formation when neutrophils are exposed to inflammatory or phagocytic stimuli. Computerized databases for all four genetic subgroups of CGD have been developed that are accessible through the Web site bioinf.uta.fi/idr.[31]

A fifth *phox* protein, p40*phox*, is also associated with p67*phox* and, indirectly, p47*phox*.[32] Although p40*phox* is not essential for enzymatic activity, this subunit is important for high-level superoxide production in response to certain stimuli, including immunoglobulin-opsonized particles and *Staphylococcus aureus*.[33,34] Formation of the active NADPH oxidase complex also involves the activation of the small GTP-binding protein Rac2, which then binds to the plasma membrane and p67*phox*.[35,36] No cases of CGD have been identified resulting from genetic defects in either p40*phox* or Rac2, although a mutation in the latter was found in an infant with recurrent infections and abnormal neutrophil adhesion, motility, and partial NADPH oxidase defects.[37,38]

The gene for gp91*phox*, termed CYBB (MIM306400), spans approximately 30 kb in the Xp21.1 region of the X chromosome and contains 13 exons.[39–41] More than 300 distinct mutations have been identified in the gp91*phox* gene in X-linked CGD, which include deletions, frameshifts, splice site, nonsense, and missense mutations that are distributed throughout the gene (Table 50–2).[18,42,43] Approxi-

Table 50–1 Classification of Chronic Granulomatous Disease

Component Affected	Gene Symbol	Gene Locus	Inheritance	Subtype[a]	NBT Score (% Positive)	O_2^- Production (% Normal)	Flavocytochrome *b* Spectrum (% Normal)	Defect in Cell-Free NADPH Oxidase Assay	Frequency (% of Cases)[b]
gp91*phox*	*CYBB*	Xp21.1	X	X91°	0	0	0	Membrane	68
				X91⁻	80–100 (weak)	3–30	Low	Membrane	5
				X91⁻	5–10	5–10	Low	Membrane	<1
				X91⁺	0	0	N	Membrane	1
p22*phox*	*CYBA*	16p24	AR	A22°	0	0	0	Membrane	4
				A22⁺	0	0	N	Membrane	<1
p47*phox*	*NCF1*	7q11.23	AR	A47°	0	0–1	N	Cytosol	17
p67*phox*	*NCF2*	1q25	AR	A67°	0	0	N	Cytosol	5

X, X-linked inheritance; AR (or A), autosomal recessive inheritance; NBT, nitroblue tetrazolium; N, normal.

[a]In this nomenclature, the first letter represents the mode of inheritance (X-linked [X] or autosomal recessive [A]) and the number indicates the *phox* component that is genetically affected. The superscript symbols indicate whether the level of protein of the affected component is undetectable (°), diminished (–), or normal (+) as measured by immunoblot analysis.

[b]Combined data from 209 kindreds evaluated at the Scripps Research Institute/Stanford University CGD Clinic and a cooperative European study[1] representing 57 kindreds and 63 patients (Modified from Casimir C, Chetty M, Bohler MC, et al: Identification of the defective NADPH-oxidase component in chronic granulomatous disease: A study of 57 European families. Eur J Clin Invest 22:403, 1992; and Curnutte JT: Chronic granulomatous disease: The solving of a clinical riddle at the molecular level. Clin Immunol Immunopathol 67:S2, 1993.).

Table 50–2 Summary of Mutations in the CYBB Gene Encoding gp91*phox* in 261 Kindreds with X-linked Chronic Granulomatous Disease

Type of Mutation	Number of Kindreds	Frequency (%)	Phenotype
Deletions	63	24.2	X91°
Insertions	27	10.3	X91°
Splice-site mutations	42	16.1	X91°
Missense mutations	59	22.6	X91°, X91⁻, X91⁺
Nonsense mutations	70	26.8	X91°

Data are from Roos D, Curnutte J, Hossle JP, et al: X-CGDbase: A database of X-CGD-causing mutations. Immunol Today 17:517, 1996.

mately 10% to 15% of X-linked CGD is caused by new germline mutations. In most X-linked CGD, gp91*phox* is completely absent and there is no measurable cytochrome *b*, NBT reduction, or intact cell superoxide production (the X91° subtype). In about 5% of X-linked cases, gp91*phox* can be present in normal levels but be nonfunctional (X91+), mutated in such a way that gp91*phox* is poorly functional (X91–), or expressed in only a small fraction of phagocytes (X91+).[18,43] The first two "variant" forms of X-linked CGD result from coding sequence mutations whereas the latter are due to mutations in the regulatory portion of the gp91*phox* gene. Some X-linked CGD patients have large deletions that affect not only the gene encoding gp91*phox* but also portions of or all the flanking gene loci for the McLeod hemolytic anemia syndrome (absence of the Kell erythrocyte antigen, Kx), Duchenne muscular dystrophy, and X-linked retinitis pigmentosa.

Autosomal recessive CGD involving p22*phox* occurs in approximately 5% of CGD patients and usually involves the complete absence of cytochrome *b* (A22°). The p22*phox* gene, termed CYBA (MIM 233690), resides at chromosome 16q24 and contains six exons that span 8.5 kb.[30] Mutations in A22 CGD are heterogeneous and range from large interstitial gene deletions to point mutations associated with missense, frameshift, or RNA-splicing defects.[18,44] Because the full expression of flavocytochrome *b* in the membrane requires the production of both subunits, a primary deficiency of either component leads to a secondary loss of the other. Thus, neither subunit can be detected on immunoblot analysis in either X91° or A22° CGD. A single patient with A22⁺ CGD has been described, who has a missense mutation disrupting the binding site for p47*phox*.[45]

Autosomal recessive patients with p47*phox*)-deficient CGD account for approximately one-fourth of cases in the United States and Europe, but only about 7% of cases in Japan.[2,9,25] The gene for p47*phox*, termed NCF1 (MIM 233700), resides on chromosome 7 at q11.23[46] and contains nine exons spanning 18 kb.[47] A limited number of mutations have been identified in the p47*phox* gene. Virtually all patients are either homozygotes or compound heterozygotes for a mutant allele with a GT deletion at the beginning of exon 2 that predicts a premature stop codon and results in absence of the p47*phox* protein.[18,48,49] The high frequency of the p47*phox* GT deletion mutation appears to reflect the existence of at least one closely linked highly conserved p47*phox* pseudogene(s) that contains this GT deletion. This close physical proximity leads to recombination events between the wild-type gene and pseudogene(s).[48]

Finally, a heterogenous group of mutations in the p67*phox* gene are responsible for A67 CGD, a rare autosomal recessive form of CGD accounting for approximately 5% of cases overall.[2,50] This gene, referred to as NCF2 (MIM233710), is located on the long arm of chromosome 1 at position q25[46] and contains 16 exons that span 40 kb.[51] Almost all of the mutations identified to date in A67 CGD lead to absent expression of the p67*phox* protein. However, one A67⁺ patient has been reported in which a nonfunctional form of p67*phox* with an amino acid deletion is expressed, but is unable to translocate to the membrane or bind to Rac.[52]

Despite the fact that more than 90% of patients with CGD have respiratory burst defects that result in undetectable levels of O_2^- production, there is a surprising heterogeneity in the clinical manifestations of the disease.[17,25] At one end of the spectrum are the patients who begin to suffer from severe bacterial and fungal infections during infancy, and who rarely have more than 4 to 12 months between such serious infections. At the other end of the spectrum are patients who are well for many years and then unexpectedly develop a serious infection typical of CGD, such as a staphylococcal hepatic abscess or Aspergillus pneumonia. After their first major infection, some of these patients may be relatively healthy again for another 3 to 10 years before the next severe infection occurs. As a group, patients with X-CGD, A22 CGD, and A67 CGD seem to have a more severe clinical course compared to patients with A47 CGD.[17,25,53] Those individuals with partial respiratory burst activity less than 10% of normal (most X91– patients; see Table 50–1) also tend to have disease of intermediate severity. Polymorphisms in oxygen-independent antimicrobial systems or other components regulating the innate immune response are also likely to play an important role in modifying disease severity. Specific polymorphisms in the myeloperoxidase, mannose-binding lectin, and FcγRIIa genes are associated with a higher risk for granulomatous or autoimmune/rheumatologic complications.[54] Because of this heterogeneity, the diagnosis of CGD should be entertained not only in young children with recurrent severe infections but also in adolescents and young adults who experience exceptionally severe or unusual infections.

Clinical Manifestations

In approximately two-thirds of patients, the first symptoms of CGD appear during the first year of life with the onset of recurrent, purulent bacterial and fungal infections.[17] Table 50–3 summarizes the types of infections and infecting organisms most frequently encountered in CGD. The most common types of infections are those that involve sites in contact with the outside world—consistent with the role of neutrophils as the first line of defense against infection. *S aureus*, enteric gram-negatives, *Serratia marcescens*, *Burkholderia cepacia*, and *Aspergillus* species represent the most frequently encountered pathogens. Although *S aureus* is the most frequently isolated organism overall, the most common causes of death reported in a recent series were pneumonia and/or sepsis due to *Aspergillus* and *B cepacia.*[17]

Most CGD pathogens share the property of being catalase-negative and as such, inadvertently "lend" H_2O_2 secreted from the pathogen to the peroxide-starved CGD phagocyte that in turn uses it (once converted to HOCl by myeloperoxidase; see Fig. 50–2) to kill the microbe. It also appears that at least some of the CGD pathogens are resistant to the nonoxidative killing mechanisms of the phagocyte.[55] It is somewhat surprising how often one fails to identify the infecting organism in CGD—perhaps greater than half the time despite aggressive culturing. In this situation, one treats empirically with the antibiotic that ought to work and if it fails, one then aggressively pursues more invasive diagnostic procedures looking for one (or more) of the less commonly seen microbes such as *Nocardia* species, *Candida*, atypical mycobacteria, and a host of other bacteria and fungi (see Table 50–3). Other unusual organisms that cause infection in CGD include other members of the Burkholderia family,[56,57] including *B. cenocepacia*, *B. gladioli*, and *B. Mallei* (the causative agent in melioidosis, a septic illness common in East Asia) and *Chromobacterium violaceum*, found in brackish fresh water and which can cause a febrile illness with bacteremia in CGD.[58] A previously unknown gram-negative bacteria, *Granulobacter bethesdensis*, was recently identified in a CGD patient with recurrent fevers associated with chronic necrotizing deep lymphatic infection.[59] This organism appears to be a member of the Acetobacteraceae family, which has previously not been linked to invasive human disease.

Pneumonia is the most common type of infection seen in CGD with *S aureus*, *Aspergillus* species, *B cepacia*, and enteric gram negatives as the major pathogens. It is noteworthy that *B cepacia* has

Table 50–3 Infections in Chronic Granulomatous Disease

Infections	% of Infections	Infecting Organisms
Pneumonia	70–80	*Aspergillus, Staphylococcus, B cepacia, Pseudomonas, Nocardia, Mycobacterium* (including atypical), *Serratia, Candida, Klebsiella, Paecilomyces*
Lymphadenitis	50–60	*Staphylococcus, Serratia, Candida, Klebsiella, Nocardia*
Cutaneous infections/impetigo	50–60	*Staphylococcus, Serratia, Aspergillus, Klebsiella, Candida*
Hepatic/perihepatic abscesses	20–30	*Staphylococcus, Serratia, Streptococcus viridans, Nocardia, Aspergillus*
Osteomyelitis	20–30	*Serratia, Aspergillus, Paecilomyces, Staphylococcus, B cepacia, Pseudomonas, Nocardia*
Perirectal abscesses/fistulae	15–30	Enteric gram-negative organisms, *Staphylococcus*
Septicemia	10–20	*B cepacia, Pseudomonas, Salmonella, Staphylococcus, Serratia, Klebsiella*
Urinary tract infections/pyelonephritis	5–15	Enteric gram negatives
Brain abscesses	<5	*Aspergillus, Staphylococcus*
Meningitis	<5	*Candida lusitaniae, Hemophilus influenzae, B cepacia*

The relative frequencies of different types of infections in CGD are estimated from data pooled from several large series of patients in the United States, Europe, and Japan: (a) Mouy R, Fischer A, Vilmer E, Seger R, Griscelli C: Incidence, severity, and prevention of infections in chronic granulomatous disease. J Pediatr 114:555, 1989; (b) Bemiller LS, Roberts DH, Starko KM, Curnutte JT: Safety and effectiveness of long-term interferon gamma therapy in patients with chronic granulomatous disease. Blood Cells Mol Dis 21:239, 1995; (c) Forrest CB, Forehand JR, Axtell RA, Roberts RL, Johnston RB Jr: Clinical features and current management of chronic granulomatous disease. Hematol Oncol Clin North Am 2:253, 1988; (d) Hitzig WH, Seger RA: Chronic granulomatous disease, a heterogeneous syndrome. Hum Genet 64:207, 1983; (e) Tauber AI, Borregaard N, Simons E, Wright J: Chronic granulomatous disease: A syndrome of phagocyte oxidase deficiencies. Medicine (Baltimore) 62:286, 1983; (f) Cohen MS, Isturiz RE, Malech HL, et al: Fungal infection in chronic granulomatous disease. The importance of the phagocyte in defense against fungi. Am J Med 71:59, 1981; (g) Hayakawa H, Kobayashi N, Yata J: Chronic granulomatous disease in Japan: A summary of the clinical features of 84 registered patients. Acta Paediatr Jpn 27:501, 1985; (h) Johnston RB, Newman SL. Chronic granulomatous disease. Pediatr Clin North Am 24:365, 1977. These series encompass approximately 550 patients with CGD after accounting for overlap between reports. Unpublished data from the United States CGD Registry encompassing 368 patients was also used to estimate the relative frequencies of infections and the responsible organisms. The infecting organisms are arranged in approximate order of frequency for each type of infection. Note: *Burkholderia cepacia (B cepacia)* was previously classified as *Pseudomonas cepacia*.

emerged as a particularly lethal organism in CGD.[17,60] This organism often is not covered with the first line of antibiotics used for *S aureus* and most gram negatives, and can quietly proliferate (with persistent fevers) to the point of quick, explosive collapse due to endotoxic shock. Intravenous trimethoprim-sulfamethoxazole has been most effective in treating patients if given before widespread dissemination of the infection. An open lung biopsy is often needed to establish the diagnosis. *Aspergillus* pneumonia is also difficult to treat, but usually responds to 3 to 6 months of daily (then thrice weekly) amphotericin B therapy (with interferon gamma). Surgery has generally not been needed except for biopsy or resection of large cavitary lesions.

Lymphadenitis is the second most common infection and is usually caused by gram negatives, *S aureus*, or *Serratia marcescens*. Incision and drainage should not be delayed if the lesion fails to respond to parenteral antibiotics. Cutaneous abscesses should be similarly managed. Recurrent perinatal impetigo is almost a signature infection in CGD and often requires months of therapy (mostly oral antibiotics) to clear. Hepatic (and perihepatic) abscesses are also common in CGD and are usually, but not always, caused by *S aureus*.[61,62] Most lesions require drainage (needle or surgical) to permit efficient healing to occur. Bone infections, most commonly due to *Serratia* species or *Aspergillus*, are particularly problematic in CGD and arise from either hematogenous or contiguous spread (as often is the case with *Aspergillus* infections in the lung invading ribs, vertebral bodies, or the diaphragm).[17,63] Perirectal abscesses are difficult to treat even with months of therapy and can lead to fistula formations.

Chronic inflammation with granuloma formation is a distinctive hallmark of CGD and contributes to some of its more problematic complications. In some cases, this results from imperfectly controlled infections in which stalemates develop between the pathogen and the patients' leukocytes. These lesions become granulomas as the host employs lymphocytes and activated macrophages to assist in containing the pathogens. However, this complication is not always clearly linked to persistent infection, and in these cases has been speculated to involve a dysregulated inflammatory response and/or inefficient degradation of debris.[64–66] In the absence of oxidant production, excessive production of cytokines and delayed neutrophil apoptosis at inflammatory sites appear to contribute as underlying mechanisms.[66–68]

As a result of persistent inflammatory stimulation, CGD patients can suffer from a variety of more chronic complications (Table 50–4). Lymphadenopathy, hepatosplenomegaly, eczematoid dermatitis and anemia of chronic disease (hemoglobin levels usually 8–10 g/dL) are common manifestations of this process and are most prominent in the first 5 to 10 years of life in CGD. Throughout the body, granuloma formation can lead to dysfunction and obstruction in the esophagus,[69] intestine,[70] and urinary bladder and kidneys.[71–74] In the stomach, the gastric antral narrowing can be severe enough in infants and children to resemble pyloric stenosis. Inflammatory involvement of the gastrointestinal tract can be seen in up to one-third of CGD patients, typically in association with the X-linked form.[75] A chronic ileocolitis resembling Crohn disease occurs in about 10% of patients and can range from mild diarrhea to a debilitating syndrome of bloody diarrhea and malabsorption that can necessitate a colectomy.[17,61,75,76] Other types of chronic inflammation include gingivitis, chorioretinitis, destructive white matter lesions in the brain,[77] and glomerulonephritis.[17,78] Occasional patients may develop either discoid or systemic lupus erythematosus, sarcoidosis, or rheumatoid arthritis.[17,19,79] The underlying mechanisms are poorly defined although recent studies suggest that these manifestations may be in part related to subtle defects in the absence of the NADPH oxidase in memory B cells[80] or T cells.[81]

Carriers of CGD, whether the X-linked form or any one of the autosomal recessive forms, are usually asymptomatic, with two important exceptions. First, about one-fourth of X-linked carriers are at risk of developing mild to moderately severe discoid lupus erythematosus characterized by discoid skin lesions and photosensitivity.[82–84] The onset is usually in the second decade of life. The disease does not progress to systemic lupus nor does one find serologic evidence of even subclinical disease. Severe discoid lupus can be treated with hydroxychloroquine (Plaquenil). Recurrent stomatitis or significant gingivitis, or both, have also been noted in as many as half of X-CGD carriers.[25] A few will also suffer from arthralgias, polyarthritis, and Raynaud phenomenon. The second important complication of the X-linked CGD carrier state is serious infection in those women who

Table 50–4 Chronic Conditions Associated With Chronic Granulomatous Disease

Condition	Relative Frequency (%)
Lymphadenopathy	98
Hypergammaglobulinemia	60–90
Hepatomegaly	50–90
Splenomegaly	60–80
Anemia of chronic disease	Common*
Underweight	70
Chronic diarrhea	20–60
Short stature	50
Gingivitis	50
Dermatitis	35
Hydronephrosis	10–25
Granulomatous ileocolitis	10–15
Gastric antral narrowing	10–15
Ulcerative stomatitis	5–15
Granulomatous cystitis	5–10*
Pulmonary fibrosis	<10*
Esophagitis	<10*
Granulomatous cystitis	<10
Chorioretinitis	<10
Glomerulonephritis	<10
Discoid lupus erythematosus	<10

The relative frequencies of chronic conditions associated with CGD were estimated from the series of reports listed in Table 50–3. In some instances (asterisks), the incidence is estimated from the 50 cases of CGD followed at Scripps Research Institute and Stanford University (unpublished data).

have a usually high degree of inactivation of the normal X chromosome in their myeloid cells. If the circulating neutrophil population is skewed to the point that fewer than 10% to 15% of the cells function, then the carrier has an increased risk of bacterial infections that in some cases have been severe.[85–87] Those with fewer than 5% oxidase positive cells have full-blown CGD.

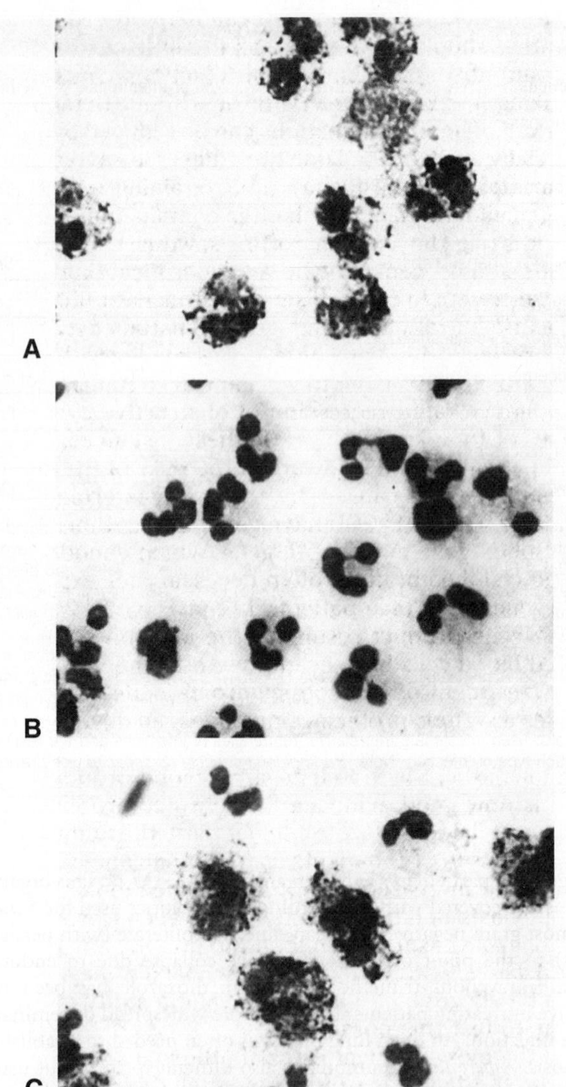

Figure 50–4 Nitroblue tetrazolium (NBT) slide test. Peripheral blood neutrophils and monocytes from a drop of fresh whole blood were made adherent to glass slides and stimulated with phorbol myristate acetate. **A**, Normal neutrophils and monocytes, all of which are NBT-positive. **B**, Neutrophils and monocytes from an X-linked CGD patient, which are all NBT-negative. **C**, A mixture of NBT-positive and NBT-negative neutrophils from the X-linked carrier mother of the patient in part **B**. CGD, chronic granulomatous disease.

Diagnosis

The diagnosis of CGD is usually suggested by the unusual clinical histories outlined above or by a family history of CGD. The nitroblue tetrazolium (NBT) slide test on fresh blood is the classic diagnostic test.[24] A typical result is shown in Fig. 50–4. Figure 50–4A shows the normal positive staining of a group of seven neutrophils and one monocyte. Figure 50–4B shows the complete absence of NBT staining in a patient with X91° CGD, the classic X-linked form of the disease. Figure 50–4C shows the mixed population of NBT-positive and NBT-negative cells observed in that patient's mother, reflecting random X-chromosome inactivation. Because in this test nearly 100% of the normal cells are positive, the carrier state in X-linked CGD can be detected when as few as 5% of the cells are NBT-negative. This test also permits detection of diffuse populations of weakly positive cells such as those seen in X91$^-$ CGD, which are characterized by a partial deficiency of flavocytochrome *b*. Because X-linked CGD can arise by new mutations in the maternal germ line, one does not always see NBT-negative cells in the mother. Flow cytometric assays of oxidase activity, such as those based on the conversion of dihydroxyrhodamine 123 (DHR) to rhodamine 123,[88,89] can also provide both quantitative measurements of oxidant generation and the cell-by-cell distribution of activity. The DHR 123 assay for oxidase activity is now available in many referral centers and through reference laboratories. In addition to X91$^-$ CGD neutrophils, weak staining in the NBT test or a small but measurable level of DHR fluorescence can be seen in A47° cells because of a small amount of residual oxidant production. Regardless of diagnostic assay employed, it is important to have these tests performed on appropriately handled blood samples and by experienced laboratories to avoid inconclusive or false normal results.

Genetic classification is useful primarily for purposes of genetic counseling and prenatal diagnosis. With the exception of classic X-linked disease in a male whose mother is a carrier, determining the specific oxidase gene affected in a given CGD patient (Table 50–1) requires additional laboratory studies. Genetic testing for all four genetic subgroups is now commercially available. Prenatal diagnosis can be performed using fetal DNA from the chorionic villus or amniocytes, or by in utero fetal blood sampling and NBT slide test

Table 50–5 Efficacy of Interferon (IFN)-γ in Preventing Serious Infections in Chronic Granulomatous Disease

	Clinical Study				
Variable	Phase III Placebo[a]	Phase III IFN-γ[a]	Phase IV (U.S.) IFN-γ[b]	Phase IV (Europe) IFN-γ[c]	Phase IV IFN-γ[d]
No. of patients	65	63	30	28	76
Average duration of therapy on study (years)	0	0.83	1.03	2.4	4.3
Patient-years on study	50.9	52.1	31.10	67.2	328
Serious infections per patient-year	1.1	0.38	0.13	0.4	0.30
Number of hospital days per patient-year	28.2	8.6	2.2	15.0	not reported

[a]Results from The International Chronic Granulomatous Disease Cooperative Study Group: A controlled trial of interferon gamma to prevent infection in chronic granulomatous disease. N Engl J Med 324:509, 1991.

[b]Results from Weening RS, Leitz GJ, Seger RA: Recombinant human interferon-gamma in patients with chronic granulomatous disease—European follow up study. Eur J Pediatr 154:295, 1995.

[c]Results from Bemiller LS, Roberts DH, Starko KM, Curnutte JT: Safety and effectiveness of long-term interferon gamma therapy in patients with chronic granulomatous disease. Blood Cells Mol Dis 21:239 , 1995.

[d]Results from Marciano BE, Wesley R, De Carlo ES, et al: Long-term interferon-gamma therapy for patients with chronic granulomatous disease. Clin Infect Dis 39:692, 2004.

analysis of fetal neutrophils.[2,17] Laboratories specializing in neutrophil biochemistry can also perform immunoblot analysis of neutrophil extracts, flavocytochrome *b* spectroscopy, and/or functional analysis of membrane and cytosol fractions in the cell free oxidase assay. In a male with absent flavocytochrome *b* without clear evidence for a maternal carrier, it is necessary to search for the mutation in both the gp91*phox* and p22*phox* genes by DNA sequencing or another method of analysis.

Prognosis and Treatment

The cornerstones of therapy in CGD are currently (a) prevention and early treatment of infections; (b) aggressive use of parenteral antibiotics for most infections; (c) use of prophylactic trimethoprim/sulfamethoxazole (5 mg/kg/day of trimethoprim) or dicloxacillin (25–50 mg/kg/day) for sulfa-allergic patients; (d) prophylactic itraconazole (200 mg daily if 13 years of age or older or if weighing at least 50 kg, or 100 mg daily if less than 13 years of age or weighing less than 50 kg), and (e) use of prophylactic recombinant human gamma-interferon (rIFN-γ) (0.05 mg/m^2 or 0.0015 mg/kg if <0.5 m^2 three times per week). Using these guidelines, the prognosis for patients afflicted with CGD has improved dramatically since the disorder was first described in the 1950s, at which time almost all patients died in childhood.[21,22] In a large study based on data collected by a CGD registry in the United States in the 1990s, the overall mortality was estimated to be 5% per year for X-CGD and 2% per year for autosomal recessive CGD.[17] A more recent single-institution study on seventy-six patients reported an overall mortality rate of 1.5% per year.[90] There is a general consensus that a large majority of newly diagnosed children should survive well into their adult years with aggressive and careful management. As already noted, patients with deficiency of p47*phox* have a tendency for milder disease compared to those with flavocytochrome-negative CGD. On the other hand, there are some patients (usually X-linked) that prove to have more frequent serious infections and/or inflammatory complications, likely due to the effects of modifier genes, who may warrant more aggressive treatment such as bone marrow transplantation (see below).

Several approaches can be used to prevent infections. Patients with CGD should receive all their routine immunizations on schedule (including live virus vaccines), with influenza vaccine administered each year as well. Cuts and skin abrasions should be cleansed promptly with soap and water and a topical antiseptic applied (2% hydrogen peroxide and/or povidone-iodine ointment). Frequent brushing, flossing, and professional cleaning of teeth can help prevent gingivitis. Constipation should be avoided as it can lead to rectal/anal fissures and abscesses. Early anal infections can be treated with soaking in soapy water (with or without Betadine). The frequency of pulmonary infections can be reduced by not using commercially available bedside humidifiers, by avoiding smoking (cigarettes and marijuana), and refraining from handling decaying plant materials, which often contain numerous *Aspergillus* spores (eg, hay, mulch, rotting sawdust).[91]

There is clear evidence that chronic prophylactic trimethoprim/sulfamethoxazole can decrease the number of bacterial infections in CGD patients by more than half without a concomitant increased risk of fungal infection.[92,93] In addition, itraconazole has recently been shown to be an effective agent for prophylaxis for fungal infections in CGD, as studied in a randomized, double-blind, placebo-controlled study.[94] Liver function tests should be monitored on patients receiving itraconazole.

Prophylactic rIFN-γ is another mainstay of current management of CGD. The clinical benefit of rIFN-γ is probably related to generally enhanced phagocyte function and killing by nonoxidative mechanisms, because its use is not accompanied by any measurable improvement in NADPH oxidase activity in the vast majority of CGD patients.[95] In a multicenter trial, patients were randomized in a double-blind fashion to receive either placebo or rIFN-γ (0.05 mg/m^2 three times per week).[96] As summarized in Table 50–5, there was a substantial decrease in the number of serious infections in the rIFN-γ arm. Side effects were observed in some of the patients, but typically restricted mild fever and flu-like symptoms. No additional adverse reactions, including any increased incidence of chronic inflammatory complications, have been noted with more prolonged courses of prophylactic rIFN-γ (more than 10 years) and the patients continue to have a substantial benefit with fivefold fewer serious infections compared to the placebo group in the Phase III study in Table 50–5.[90,97,98] On average, this group of patients is averaging one serious infection per patient every 4 to 5 years.

One of the most frequent errors in the management of CGD patients is the failure to treat potentially serious infections promptly and aggressively with appropriate parenteral antibiotics. Even the best antibiotics can be rendered ineffective if given too late in the course of an infection in CGD. Therefore, early intervention is advisable. Although many of the minor infections and low-grade fevers in CGD patients can be managed on an outpatient basis, episodes of consistently high fever over a 24-hour period or clearly established infections (such as pneumonia or lymphadenitis) should be treated with parenteral antibiotics that cover, at least initially, *S aureus* and enteric gram negatives. Reasonable attempts to define the source of the infection and the responsible microbe should also begin promptly. Monitoring the erythrocyte sedimentation rate (ESR) can be very useful, both as a clue to the presence of a significant infection as well as following the patient's response to therapy. If the patient fails to respond, then more aggressive diagnostic procedures should be instituted (CT, bone, and gallium scans; open biopsies if indicated) and empirical changes in the antibiotics used to broaden coverage to *Pseudomonas cepacia*. If fungus is identified or strongly suspected, amphotericin B has been the drug of choice in the past, although newer azole antifungal agents such as voriconazole are supplanting its use.[99–101] Even with appropriate antibiotics, certain types of infections respond slowly and may require months of therapy, particularly *Aspergillus* infections. In this instance, 4 to 12 months of parenteral antifungal therapy followed by a 1- to 3-year course of daily oral itraconazole has been effective in clearing most infections and preventing their recurrence. Surgical drainage or resection can sometimes play a key role in accelerating healing of certain types of infection such as lymphadenitis, osteomyelitis, and abscesses of visceral organs such as the liver or lung. Finally, granulocyte transfusions may be of benefit in the treatment of stubborn or life-threatening infections.[17,102,103]

Use of corticosteroids should generally be avoided, including extensive topical use, except in cases of severe asthma, esophageal strictures, gastric antral narrowing, granulomatous cystitis, or inflammatory bowel disease. There is clear evidence that corticosteroids are beneficial in these clinical settings as the steroids induce rapid regression of obstructive symptoms at low oral doses (eg, 1 mg/kg/day of prednisone).[75,104] In these cases the physician and patient should be aware of the risks of the additional immunosuppression caused by the corticosteroids.

Rare patients with X91° CGD have genomic deletions that span the gp91^{phox} gene and the Xk gene, which encodes a membrane protein necessary for expression of the Kell genes.[105] Absence of the Xk gene product results in the McLeod syndrome, in which red blood cells have weak Kell antigens and variable acanthocytosis, along with nerve and muscle disorders related to its expression in nonerythroid tissues.[105,106] Transfusion of McLeod syndrome patients poses a serious problem, because they can develop alloantibodies of wide specificity that can preclude any further transfusions except with Kell-negative blood products.

Allogeneic bone marrow transplantation can be used to treat CGD and has been successfully employed.[107–111] However, because of the risks associated with this procedure, marrow transplantation is generally considered only for those patients who have a fully HLA-matched sibling and frequent and severe infections despite aggressive medical management. Reduced-intensity conditioning regimens for allogeneic transplantations have recently been used for bone marrow transplantation in CGD, including several cases with ongoing fungal infections.[108,111,112] Cord blood transplants have also been reported.[113,114] Graft-versus-host disease can be a significant problem for adult patients.[108] Finally, genetic therapies aimed at correcting the defective gene in bone marrow stem cells hold promise for the future, if obstacles can be solved to achieve effective and safe gene delivery with prolonged expression of delivered genes.[19,115,116] Observations on female carriers of X-linked CGD with skewed X-inactivation and preclinical studies in murine CGD models suggest that complete correction of NADPH oxidase activity in 10% of circulating neutrophils will lead to clinically relevant improvements in host defense.[20]

Neutrophil Glucose-6-Phosphate Dehydrogenase Deficiency

NADPH, the primary substrate for the respiratory burst oxidase, is generated by the first two reactions of the hexose monophosphate shunt pathway, which are catalyzed by glucose-6-phosphate dehydrogenase (G6PD) (Fig. 50–2, reaction 8) and 6-phosphogluconate dehydrogenase (6PGD).[14] The leukocyte and erythrocyte G6PD are encoded by the same gene. Thus, a severe deficiency of G6PD in neutrophils can result in a greatly attenuated respiratory burst because of low levels of NADPH. However, the vast majority of individuals with inherited G6PD deficiency do not have problems with a decreased respiratory burst or recurrent infections. A CGD-like syndrome has very rarely been observed in G6PD-deficient patients who have congenital nonspherocytic hemolytic anemia (CNSHA), where hemolysis occurs in the absence of redox stress.[14,117–120] Even in CNSHA, most G6PD mutations cause the enzyme to decay over a period of days and weeks, so that levels in the short-lived neutrophil usually do not become critically low, even in some of the most unstable G6PD variants. A few rare and poorly understood G6PD mutations that cause CNSHA are associated with extremely low (less than 5% of normal) levels of G6PD in the neutrophil, resulting in a deficient respiratory burst and CGD-like symptoms. The combination of chronic, severe hemolytic anemia, recurrent infections, and the laboratory demonstration of extremely low G6PD levels in neutrophils and erythrocytes serves to distinguish this disease from CGD. The treatment for neutrophil G6PD deficiency is the same as for CGD except that the efficacy of rIFN-γ has not been demonstrated in the former. The chronic hemolytic anemia is treated by supportive means, including transfusions.

Disorders of Glutathione Metabolism

As depicted in Fig. 50–2 (reaction 6), the reduced form of glutathione (GSH) serves to protect the neutrophil from the harmful effects of hydrogen peroxide on NADPH oxidase and other neutrophil proteins such as microtubules.[121,122] Adequate intracellular levels of reduced glutathione are maintained by recycling oxidized glutathione (GSSG) to GSH by glutathione reductase (Fig. 50–2, reaction 7) as well as by de novo synthesis of glutathione by glutathione synthetase (Fig. 50–2, reaction 9). Severe deficiencies in either of these enzymes are extremely rare and are apparently inherited in an autosomal recessive manner. In the case of glutathione reductase deficiency, the respiratory burst terminates prematurely, presumably owing to the toxic effects of accumulating hydrogen peroxide on NADPH oxidase.[123] This brief burst of O_2^-, however, appears to be sufficient for adequate microbial killing, because the few patients reported have not had problems with recurrent infections.[124] However, they do have a congenital hemolytic anemia during periods of oxidant stress owing to diminished levels of glutathione reductase in erythrocytes.[124] In glutathione synthetase deficiency, the respiratory burst proceeds normally.[122] Patients have a severe metabolic acidosis as a result of elevated levels of 5-oxoproline, which is the product of the first step in glutathione synthesis and is present in increased levels because of a lack of feedback of GSH on the synthetic pathway. Patients with glutathione synthetase deficiency also have intermittent neutropenia[125] (perhaps caused by the acidosis) as well as oxidant-induced hemolysis.[122] There are mild problems with recurrent infections. Therapy with vitamin E (400 IU/day) has been found to be beneficial in patients with severe glutathione synthetase deficiency suffering from hemolysis and infections.[125]

Myeloperoxidase Deficiency

Myeloperoxidase (MPO) deficiency is the most common inherited disorder of phagocytes, but is almost always asymptomatic.[126,127] MPO is present in azurophilic granules of neutrophils and monocytes, and catalyzes the production of a potent antimicrobial agent, hypochlorous acid (HOCl) from chloride and hydrogen peroxide (Fig. 50–2, reaction 4).[13] HOCl in turn reacts with a variety of primary and secondary amines to form chloramines, some of which can be toxic. Moreover, HOCl is capable of activating latent metalloproteinases (eg, collagenase) and inactivating antiproteinases.

Complete MPO deficiency is seen in approximately 1 in 4000 individuals, and partial deficiency is even more common (1 in 2000 persons).[126,127] The key features of MPO deficiency are summarized in Table 50–6. The disorder is inherited in an autosomal recessive manner. In the few cases reported, several different mutations have been identified, which generally appear to affect the posttranslational processing of a precursor polypeptide for MPO.[126,128,129] Acquired

Table 50–6 Summary of Myeloperoxidase (MPO) Deficiency

Incidence	1 in 2000 (partial deficiency) 1 in 4000 (total deficiency)
Inheritance	Autosomal recessive with variable expression; MPO gene on chromosome 17 at q22–q23
Molecular defect	Defective posttranslational processing of an abnormal MPO precursor polypeptide; eosinophil peroxidase encoded by different gene and levels normal
Pathogenesis	Partial or complete MPO deficiency leads to diminished production of HOCl and HOCl-derived chloramines; MPO products are necessary for rapid killing of microbes (especially *Candida*) but not absolutely required
Clinical manifestations	Usually clinically silent Disseminated candidiasis/fungal disease (rare; usually in conjunction with diabetes mellitus) Acquired deficiency in M2, M3, and M4 acute myeloid leukemias (AMLs) and myelodysplasia
Laboratory evaluation	Deficiency of neutrophil/monocyte peroxidase by histochemical analysis (eosinophil peroxidase normal) Delayed, but eventually normal, killing of bacteria in vitro Failure to kill *Candida albicans* and hyphal forms of *Aspergillus fumigatus* in vitro
Differential diagnosis	Acquired partial MPO deficiency seen in M2, M3, and M4 AML, myelodysplastic syndromes, and Batten disease
Therapy	None in asymptomatic patients Aggressive treatment of fungal infections when they occur Control of blood glucose levels in diabetics
Prognosis	Usually excellent

forms of MPO deficiency are also seen. The gene that encodes for MPO is located on chromosome 17 at q22–q23 near the breakpoint for the 15–17 translocation of promyelocytic leukemia. Subpopulations of MPO-deficient cells can be seen not only in the M3 (promyelocytic) form of acute myeloid leukemia but also in the M2 and M4 forms.[126,114] MPO-deficient cells are also seen in approximately 25% of patients with chronic myeloid leukemia and myelodysplastic syndromes.[130–132]

One of the most curious features of MPO deficiency is the remarkable lack of clinical symptoms in affected persons, given the prediction that severe MPO deficiency would cripple important antimicrobial reactions catalyzed by HOCl. In vitro, an impressive defect in killing *Candida albicans* and hyphal forms of *Aspergillus fumigatus* is observed.[127,133,134] Bacterial killing in vitro is also abnormal in being somewhat slower than normal, but eventually it is complete. MPO-deficient mice also exhibit abnormalities in host defense against Candida and Klebsiella.[135,136] Excessive or unusual infections in MPO-deficient patients, however, are uncommon, except for rare individuals who also suffer from diabetes mellitus.[126,127] In these individuals, disseminated fungal infections (usually candidiasis) are seen.

The discrepancy between the in vitro and in vivo manifestations of MPO deficiency in most patients can be explained in several ways. First, the respiratory burst in MPO-deficient neutrophils is substantially augmented, presumably from the absence of HOCl-mediated toxic effects on the NADPH oxidase.[126] Second, other products of the respiratory burst, together with the oxygen-independent antibacterial proteins, appear to have sufficient potency to compensate for the loss of MPO-dependent reactions. Finally, residual amounts of MPO coupled with the normal levels of eosinophil peroxidase may provide at least some degree of peroxidative activity at the sites of infection.

Treatment is usually not required for MPO deficiency except in those individuals suffering from fungal infections. In these patients aggressive use of antifungal antibiotics is indicated. The prognosis is excellent in the majority of patients with MPO deficiency.

DISORDERS OF PHAGOCYTE ADHESION AND CHEMOTAXIS

Since 1970 numerous investigators have found in vitro chemotactic abnormalities in neutrophils from patients suffering from a wide variety of clinical disorders associated with increased susceptibility to bacterial and fungal infections.[131,132,137–139] In most circumstances the chemotactic abnormality identified was only marginal and not always clearly related to the clinical status of the patient. In other instances, clear and major defects were identified in vitro that correlated with the in vivo propensity for infection. Extensive classification systems have been devised to categorize the numerous acquired defects in chemotaxis,[140] and several reviews are available on this subject.[4,140,141] The problem in many of these reports is that it is unclear whether the infections were caused by the in vitro chemotactic abnormality or by the medical complications of the underlying disorder (eg, acidosis, malnutrition, or exposure to nosocomial infections). A further complicating factor is that there are inherent limitations in the in vitro chemotaxis assay, which is subject to laboratory artifacts both as a result of neutrophil purification procedures as well as the assay itself. Furthermore, the extent to which these in vitro chemotactic assay systems faithfully reflect prevailing in vivo conditions is not known. Our understanding of chemotactic disorders has been hampered by the limitations of these assays, just as the elucidation of respiratory burst defects was obscured when the major available assay was in vitro bacterial killing. In this section the most important and best characterized of the chemotactic disorders, leukocyte adhesion deficiency, will be discussed in detail. A brief discussion of several other clinically significant chemotactic disorders will also be provided.

Leukocyte Adhesion Deficiency Type I

Leukocyte adhesion deficiency type I (LAD I) is a rare autosomal recessive disorder of leukocyte adhesion, chemotaxis, and ingestion of C3bi-opsonized microbes as a result of decreased or absent expression of the leukocyte β_2 integrins (Table 50–7).[142–145] The hallmark of LAD I is the occurrence of repeated, often-severe bacterial and fungal infections without the accumulation of pus despite persistent granulocytosis (Table 50–7). The molecular basis for LAD was first suggested by Crowley and colleagues, who found that neutrophils from a patient with this clinical syndrome lacked a high-molecular-weight membrane glycoprotein.[146] The patient's neutrophils could not be made to adhere to plastic surfaces or to respond to serum-opsonized particles in terms of ingestion and respiratory burst activity.[146] Several other reports quickly followed, which described other patients in whom a similar glycoprotein was missing.[147,148] In 1984, it was found that the missing glycoprotein was actually a group of three closely related glycoproteins with molecular weights ranging from 95 kd (the β2 subunit) to 150 to 180 kd (three distinct α subunits) that form three types of α–β heterodimers.

The molecular basis of LAD I is now known to result from mutations in the gene for the common CD18 β2 subunit for these three leukocyte glycoproteins, now termed β2 integrins, that belong to the integrin superfamily of adhesion molecules.[133,134,149,150] Integrins are noncovalently linked heterodimeric glycoproteins consisting of an α and a β subunit. Within each of the eight known integrin subfamilies the β subunit is identical (and defines the subfamily) whereas the α

Table 50–7 Summary of Leukocyte Adhesion Deficiency Type I (LAD 1)

Incidence	Approximately 60 patients described in literature
Inheritance	Autosomal recessive
Molecular defect	An absent, diminished, or structurally abnormal β subunit (CD18) caused by one of several types of mutations in the β gene; in the absence of a normal β subunit, the three types of α chains in the β_2 integrin subfamily (CD11a, b, c) cannot assemble into normal α-β heterodimers
Pathogenesis	All three β_2 integrins (CD11a/CD18, CD11b/CD18, and CD11c/CD18) are deficient on all leukocytes, causing multiple abnormalities in cell function: adherence, chemotaxis, and C3bi-mediated ingestion/degranulation/respiratory burst
Clinical manifestation	Persistent granulocytosis (neutrophil count of 12,000–100,000/mm^3) Severe or moderate phenotypes depending on severity of deficiency Recurrent pyogenic infections with absent neutrophil infiltration Delayed umbilical cord separation Severe gingivitis/periodontitis
Laboratory evaluation	Flow cytometric measurement of surface CD11b in stimulated neutrophils with monoclonal anti-CD11b
Differential diagnosis	Chronic Granulomatous Disease May be associated with severe neutrophil actin dysfunction
Therapy	Bone marrow transplant in clinically severe patients (CD11b <0.3% of normal) Aggressive use of parenteral antibiotics Possible benefit of prophylactic trimethoprim/sulfamethoxazole
Prognosis	Severe: high incidence of death before 2 years Moderate: Can survive into twenties and thirties but with recurrent infections

subunit varies and confers the functional specificity on the integrin. The molecular defect in LAD involves all members of the β2 integrin subfamily: αL β2 (CD11a/CD18), αm β2 (CD11b/CD18), and αx β2 (CD11c/CD18).[142,143,151] CD11a/CD18 is often referred to as LFA-1 whereas CD11b/CD18 is also called Mac-1, Mo1, or CR3. In the dozens of patients with LAD who have been studied thus far at the molecular level, an absent, diminished, or structurally abnormal β2 subunit (CD18) has been identified.[152] In the absence of a normal β subunit, the three types of α chains in the β2 integrin subfamily cannot assemble into normal α–β heterodimers. Thus, all three β2 integrins are moderately to severely deficient on all leukocytes in LAD.

The β2 integrins serve as receptors for the opsonic complement fragment C3bi, the intercellular adhesion molecules 1 and 2 (ICAM-1 and ICAM-2) that are expressed on endothelial cells and leukocytes, and fibrinogen.[142] The diminished or absent expression of β2 integrins in LAD I leukocytes results in the failure of phagocytes to emigrate from the bloodstream to sites of infection.[153] The early interactions with the endothelium, termed *rolling*, are normal in LAD I, as these are mediated by a different family of adhesion molecules known as selectins.[153] However, β2 integrins are responsible for the subsequent tight binding of neutrophils and monocytes to cytokine-activated endothelium, and this step is therefore severely defective in LAD I. Transendothelial migration is also impaired. A second major functional defect in LAD is the failure of phagocytes to bind C3bi opsonized microbes. Because CD11b/CD18 is the predominant phagocyte receptor for this complement fragment, C3bi-mediated ingestion, degranulation, and respiratory burst activity are severely affected in LAD.[142] Finally, β2 integrin-dependent signals play a key role in activating neutrophils for enhanced migration, phagocytosis of antibody-opsonized microbes, and degranulation.[154,155]

Despite in vitro defects in lymphocyte responses dependent on LFA-1 (CD11a/CD18), patients with LAD I rarely have clinical manifestations related to impaired lymphocyte function.[143,149,151] It is believed that the role CD11a/CD18 plays in lymphoid cell function can be compensated by other adhesion proteins (CD2, CD4, CD8, etc).[142]

Molecular Genetics of Leukocyte Adhesion Deficiency Type I

The fact that LAD I involves a deficiency of all leukocyte β2 integrins focused attention on the common β2 chain (CD18), and mutations in the corresponding gene have been identified in all LAD I patients who have been analyzed at the molecular level to date. Although expression of the leukocyte integrin α subunits is normal in LAD I, these are not transported to the cell surface because the β2 chain is absent or contains mutations that disrupt its structure or its interaction with the α subunit. Mutations in the α subunits have not been found thus far in patients with LAD I. The gene encoding CD18 is located on the long arm of chromosome 21 at position q22.3 (the genes for β2 integrin α subunits are clustered on chromosome 16p11.1-p13).[142,156] The CD18 glycoprotein has a large extracellular domain at the N terminus, a single transmembrane domain, and a 46-residue cytoplasmic tail. As with X-linked CGD, CD18 mutations in LAD I are heterogeneous in nature, family-specific, and can lead to either undetectable or low (9%–20% of normal) levels of α–β dimer expression that correlates with the clinical severity of the disease. More than 30 different mutations have now been characterized in more than 35 patients.[2,133,143,152] These include missense mutations, mRNA splicing defects, small deletions, and a premature termination signal. Many patients are compound heterozygotes, and have two different mutant alleles for CD18. About one-half of patients with LAD I in whom the genetic defect has been identified have point mutations in a stretch of 250 amino acids in the extracellular domain of CD18. This region is highly conserved among all β subunits, and appears to be important for interaction with the α subunit.

Clinical Features

The key features of LAD I are summarized in Table 50–7. The clinical presentation of LAD is heterogeneous and is related to the severity of the deficiency of the β2 integrins. The severe clinical phenotype is associated with less than 0.3% of the normal amount of these glycoproteins on the leukocyte surface, whereas the moderate phenotype has 2.5% to 6% of normal levels.[157] In both the severe and moderate forms of the disease, persistent granulocytosis (neutrophil count of 12,000–100,000/mm^3) is a constant finding, as are recurrent cutaneous abscesses and aggressive periodontitis and/or gingivitis.[143,149,151,158,159] Additional clinical features seen more often in the severe clinical phenotype include delayed umbilical cord separation, omphalitis, perirectal cellulitis, severe ulcerative stomatitis, and bacterial sepsis. A striking finding in LAD I is that abscesses and other sites of infections are devoid of pus despite the marked neutrophilia, because neutrophils are unable to emigrate to tissues. *S aureus* and gram-negative enteric bacteria cause the majority of infections in LAD I. Fungal infections can also occur, in particular from *Candida albicans* and *Aspergillus* species.

Note that infants with delayed separation of the umbilical cord who are healthy and have normal blood counts are very unlikely to have LAD I. Although the mean age of cord separation ranges from 7 to 15 days, 10% of healthy infants can have cord separation at 3 weeks of age or later.[160,161]

Diagnosis

The diagnosis of LAD I is made by flow cytometric measurement of surface CD11b (Mac1) (or the shared CD18 subunit) in unstimulated and stimulated neutrophils using commercially available monoclonal antibodies directed against CD11b or CD18.[142,162] Neutrophils contain an intracellular pool of CD11b/CD18 in their secondary (specific) and tertiary granules, which can be mobilized to the cell surface during stimulation.[142,163] Therefore, the deficiency of CD11b can be more dramatically demonstrated by using stimulated neutrophils. Carriers of LAD I can be identified by this method, because they have been found to express approximately 50% of normal levels of CD11b on the surface of their stimulated neutrophils.[157,163]

Prognosis and Treatment

Treatment for LAD I depends on the clinical severity of the disorder. In those patients with the moderate clinical phenotype, cutaneous and oral infections can be managed as they occur. The use of prophylactic antibiotics such as trimethoprim/sulfamethoxazole appears to be beneficial, as does aggressive prophylactic treatment of periodontal disease. It is important to note that even patients with the moderate phenotype can die of overwhelming infection.[142,157,162] In patients with severe LAD I, aggressive management is indicated because of the high incidence of death before the age of 2 years, and bone marrow transplantation is recommended.[19,109,142,164–167] Graft versus host disease can be problematic.[164,167,168] LAD I should also be amenable to gene replacement therapy in the future, and studies in canine LAD suggest that restoring CD18 expression to even approximately 10% of leukocytes will improve the clinical symptoms.[19,169]

Leukocyte Adhesion Deficiency Types II and III

LAD II is a very rare clinical syndrome closely related to LAD I, but caused by a defect in selectin-mediated adhesion events due to a deficiency in leukocyte sialyl Lewis X ligands. It was first reported by Etzioni and colleagues in two unrelated boys of Moslem Arab origin, and since described in a total of five individuals (four Arab and one Turkish).[170–174] The disease is inherited in an autosomal recessive manner. Patients presented with neutrophilia, recurrent bacterial infections, and periodontitis, similar to LAD I although these symptoms were generally not as severe. In addition, LAD II is associated with dysmorphic features and psychomotor retardation. LAD II neutrophils express normal levels of CD18. A clue as to the molecular cause of LAD II came from the observation that LAD II red cells were Lewis antigen negative and also had the rare Bombay (hh) erythrocyte phenotype, in which red cells express a nonfucosylated variant of the H antigen. These antigenic defects share in common the failure to form certain fucose carbohydrate linkage. The defect in fucose metabolism in LAD II has now been shown to result from mutations in the Golgi GDP-fucose membrane transporter.[172,173] This leads to a generalized loss of expression of fucosylated glycans on the surface of cells, in particular, the sialylated and fucosylated tetrasaccharide, SleX (CD15a), on the neutrophil surface. As a result, LAD II neutrophils are unable to bind to E- and P-selectin receptors on endothelium and therefore have an impairment in the early steps of rolling and loose binding to blood vessel walls prior to tight adhesion and emigration into infected tissues. Fucose supplementation has been partially successful in increasing expression of SLeX and decreasing clinical problems.[175,176]

LAD III has recently been described in a handful of patients with severe, recurrent infections similar to LAD I as well as a bleeding tendency.[177–181] The inheritance appears to be autosomal recessive and is associated with functional defects in the activation of multiple classes of integrins in response to G protein-coupled receptor stimulation. In one patient, activation of the Rap1 GTPase, known to be involved in the regulation of integrin signaling, was defective,[182] and a mouse genetically engineered to lack a blood cell-specific enzyme catalyzing the formation of Rap1 GTP had manifestations similar to LAD III. Because the clinical manifestations are typically severe, early bone marrow transplantation may be indicated for patients with LAD III.[180,181]

Hyperimmunoglobulin E Syndrome

The hyperimmunoglobulin E syndrome (HIES) is a complex disorder characterized by markedly elevated serum IgE levels, serious recurrent staphylococcal infections, chronic dermatitis, and skeletal and dental abnormalities.[183–188] Although not a primary phagocyte defect, neutrophils from patients with this syndrome exhibit a variable and at times profound chemotactic defect.[184,185,189,190] HIES was first described in 1966 and was called Job syndrome, in reference to the biblical description of Job as being afflicted with "sore boils from the soles of his feet unto his crown."[184] The skin abscesses in patients with HIES lack the erythema that is typical of such lesions and are referred to as cold abscesses. The key features of the hyperimmunoglobulin E syndrome are described in Table 50–8.

Although many cases of HIES are sporadic, autosomal dominant inheritance and, rarely, autosomal recessive inheritance are also described.[186,191] HIES has been described in all racial and ethnic groups. The molecular basis for the syndrome is also not known. The

Table 50–8 Summary of Hyper-IgE Syndrome (HIES)

Incidence	More than 200 patients reviewed in the literature
Inheritance	Sporadic is most common; also autosomal dominant with variable penetrance and autosomal recessive forms
Molecular defect	Unknown
Clinical manifestations	Staphylococcal pneumonia Pneumatoceles Fungal superinfection of lung cysts "Cold" cutaneous skin abscesses and furuncles Chronic eczematoid dermatitis Mucocutaneous candidiasis Coarse facies, growth retardation Osteopenia, recurrent fractures Sinusitis, keratoconjunctivitis Scoliosis Hyperextensible joints Delayed shedding of primary teeth Severe viral infections (autosomal recessive) Neurologic problems (autosomal recessive)
Laboratory evaluation	Serum IgE >2500 IU/mL Peripheral blood eosinophilia
Differential diagnosis	Atopic dermatitis Wiskott–Aldrich syndrome, DiGeorge syndrome Hypergammaglobulinemia Chronic granulomatous disease
Therapy	Prophylactic anti-*S aureus* antibiotics Aggressive treatment of acute infections with parenteral antibiotics Surgical drainage of deep infections and resection of lung cysts Monitor for scoliosis, fractures
Prognosis	Generally good if managed aggressively Some patients develop lymphoid malignancies

extremely high serum IgE level is believed to reflect a T-lymphocyte imbalance, leading to abnormal regulation of IgE production as well as decreased production of IFN-γ and tumor necrosis factor.[192,193] Further evidence for a more broad-based immune disorder is the finding that HIES patients mount abnormal antibody responses to vaccines.[194] The recurrent bacterial infections are thought to arise by two mechanisms: (a) excessive production of IgE directed against *S aureus* that occurs at the expense of protective antistaphylococcal IgG[195] and (b) a variable neutrophil chemotactic defect that occurs independently of fluctuations in the serum IgE level.[196,197] The underlying T-cell defect may be responsible for this chemotactic defect, as it may cause the release of chemotactic inhibitors from mononuclear cells. How the immunologic abnormalities relate to the dental and skeletal defects that are the other hallmarks of this disorder (see Table 50–8 and below) is not known.

Clinical Manifestations

The clinical manifestations of HIES are at times dramatic.[186–188] Onset is generally in the first 2 months of life and is manifested by chronic dermatitis. By 5 years of age patients have a history of recurrent skin abscesses, pneumonias, chronic otitis media, and sinusitis. As patients grow older, recurrent staphylococcal pneumonia is a common problem and can be complicated by the formation of pneumatoceles. Septic arthritis, cellulitis, and osteomyelitis are also observed, and are usually caused by *S aureus*, although other bacterial pathogens have also been found. Patients can have chronic mucocutaneous candidiasis and occasionally exhibit keratoconjunctivitis, sometimes complicated by corneal scarring. One feature noted in the majority of patients by the time they reach the teenage years is the presence of coarse facial features (broad nasal bridge, prominent nose). Dental and bone abnormalities are also common features of HIES. Delayed or failure to shed primary teeth occur in the majority. Hyperextensible joints and scoliosis are frequent. Osteopenia of unknown etiology is observed in most patients, and there is an increased risk of fractures to the long bones and vertebral bodies even in the absence of osteopenia.[186]

Diagnosis

The diagnosis of HIES should be entertained in any child or young adult who has the above-described clinical picture or simply a history of recurrent infections. The hallmark laboratory finding is a marked elevation of serum IgE, almost always greater than 2500 IU/mL.[187,188] Levels can be as high as 150,000 IU/mL. Most patients also have peripheral eosinophilia. However, there is no correlation of clinical disease activity with the level of either IgE or peripheral eosinophilia.[3,187,188] Atopic dermatitis is the major differential diagnosis, as comparably high serum levels of IgE can be seen in patients in this disorder, as well as superficial skin infections. The severe and recurrent nature of the staphylococcal furuncles and pneumonias usually seen in HIES can help distinguish these patients from those with atopic dermatitis. Patients with other primary immunodeficiency syndromes may also manifest elevated IgE levels.

Therapy

The therapy for HIES is largely supportive.[187,188] Prophylactic antibiotics (eg, dicloxacillin or trimethoprim/sulfamethoxazole) can be effective in preventing *S aureus* infections. Dermatitis can be treated with topical steroids. Intravenous antibiotics are used for deep-seated infections or for resistant cutaneous infections. Surgical resection of persistent pneumatoceles is sometimes indicated to prevent superinfection by fungal and gram-negative organisms. Plasmapheresis has been reported to be effective in treating patients who have not responded to the above-mentioned therapies. Recombinant IFN-γ has been used with inconsistent results.[188] Recently, either cyclosporin A or intravenous Ig infusions have shown some success in the management of HIES.[188]

Miscellaneous Chemotactic Disorders

It is extremely rare to have primary defects in neutrophil actin polymerization as a cause of abnormal chemotaxis and recurrent infections. In one case, neutrophils had diminished actin polymerization, chemotaxis, and phagocytosis of serum opsonized particles.[198] Family members had decreased CD11b/CD18 expression and a partial decrease in actin polymerization, which suggested that this disorder might be a variant of LAD I; however, no similar cases have otherwise been described. An apparent autosomal recessive disorder of actin polymerization has been described in a male infant of Tongan descent who presented with severe skin infections, recurrent pulmonary infiltrates, thrombocytopenia, and invasive *Candida tropicalis* infection.[199] Neutrophil actin polymerization was markedly abnormal, and associated with increased expression of an actin-binding protein.[200] Finally, a heterozygous point mutation in β-actin affecting binding to actin-regulatory proteins was discovered in a female patient with recurrent infections, photosensitivity, and mental retardation.[201] Neutrophils had a marked impairment in chemotaxis and in the formyl peptide-induced respiratory burst.

A new syndrome of severe neutrophil dysfunction due to a dominant-negative mutation in Rac2, a small GTPase expressed in blood cells that acts in many signal transduction pathways, was recently described in an infant boy born to unrelated parents.[37,38] This baby presented with rapidly progressive and deep-seated soft tissue infections, along with neutrophilia and poor formation of pus but normal expression of β2 integrins and fucosylated proteins. Neutrophils had marked defects in actin polymerization, chemotaxis, degranulation, and the respiratory burst in response to chemoattractants. Neutrophil responses to other agonists were normal, suggesting that the dominant negative Rac2 mutation produces a selective intracellular signaling defect.

Localized juvenile periodontitis (LJP) is a heterogeneous disorder of unknown etiology characterized by chronic and recurrent periodontal infections and severe alveolar bone loss with onset at the time of puberty.[202–205] Nearly three-quarters of patients with LJP have been reported to have defective neutrophil chemotaxis in vitro.[202,206–209] At present it appears that LJP is an acquired disorder in some patients and a genetic disorder in others. It may also be a combination of both in certain patients as they may inherit an unusual sensitivity to the chemotactic inhibitors released by certain periodontal microorganisms. The diagnosis of the disorder is made on the basis of severe periodontal disease and destructive alveolar bone loss involving the first molars and incisors developing during adolescence. It is important to note that many qualitative and quantitative neutrophil disorders are also associated with severe periodontal disease.[210] Therefore, the differential diagnosis should include neutropenia (both chronic and cyclic), LAD, CGD, and Chediak–Higashi syndrome.

One of the most consistently observed chemotactic abnormalities is seen in neonatal neutrophils.[141,211–214] These cells exhibit impaired chemotaxis in vitro in response to a wide variety of chemotactic factors.[143] It appears as though this abnormality is due, at least in part, to defects in cellular adhesion as a result of diminished mobilization of intracellular adhesion-promoting molecules to the cell surface.[211] Defective neutrophil chemotaxis can be seen in normal neonates between birth and 5 days of age. In severely ill infants, the defect may persist for a longer time.

DEFECTS IN THE STRUCTURE AND FUNCTION OF LYSOSOMAL GRANULES

Two major disorders of neutrophil granules have been described: Chediak–Higashi syndrome and specific granule deficiency. A great deal has been learned about the structural and functional abnormalities of neutrophils from patients with these conditions. Although rare, these disorders are also obligatory components in the differential diagnosis for any patient with recurrent bacterial/fungal infections.

Chediak–Higashi Syndrome

The Chediak–Higashi syndrome is a rare autosomal recessive, multisystem disease resulting from widespread defects in granule morphogenesis, with giant lysosomes in leukocytes and other cells throughout the body.[215–221] The disorder is characterized by partial oculocutaneous albinism, frequent (and sometimes fatal) bacterial infections, a mild bleeding diathesis, and peripheral as well as cranial neuropathies associated with defects at the optic chiasm. Those who survive the recurrent infections develop an "accelerated phase" of the disease—a progressive lymphoproliferative syndrome that is eventually fatal owing to a profound pancytopenia that develops.

The most dramatic granule defects are manifested in the various blood cells. Neutrophils contain a highly inhomogeneous population of huge granules derived from coalescence of azurophilic (primary) and specific (secondary) granules.[222–224] The giant granules are often more prominent in the bone marrow than in the peripheral blood,[225] because many of the abnormal myeloid precursors are apparently destroyed before they leave the marrow, resulting in moderate neutropenia with absolute neutrophil counts ranging from 500 to 2000 cells per cubic millimeter. Granules are also markedly deficient in antimicrobial granule enzymes such as cathepsin G and elastase, consistent with a defect in granule morphogenesis.[226] Degranulation is delayed and incomplete in Chediak–Higashi neutrophils, resulting in impaired bacterial killing.[140,216] Chemotaxis is also defective, perhaps related to poor deformability due to the presence of the large granules.[217] Monocytes and macrophages exhibit similar giant cytoplasmic granules, with resultant abnormalities in their phagocytic functions.[216] Giant granules are also seen in lymphocytes and are associated with defects in cytotoxic T lymphocyte and natural-killer cell function.[227–229] Eosinophils contain large granules, the functional significance of which is not known.[230] Platelets in this disorder have a storage pool deficiency of ADP and serotonin, presumably because of the abnormal granule morphogenesis in megakaryocytes, leading to a defect in platelet aggregation.[218,221]

Abnormal giant granules are also present in other cell types. These include melanocytes, which contain abnormal melanosomes that cannot transfer their contents to adjacent keratinocytes, Schwann cells, astrocytes, and certain cells in the liver, spleen, pancreas, gastric mucosa, kidney, adrenal gland, and pituitary gland.[219,221,231]

Molecular Genetics

A gene termed CHS1 or LYST (for its presumed function as a lysosomal trafficking regulatory protein) affected in the majority of Chediak–Higashi syndrome (CHS) cases has recently been identified, and is on the long arm of chromosome 1.[218–220,232,233] The encoded protein is very large (3801 amino acids); its specific function is unknown but recent studies suggest that it may inhibit lysosome fusion with other intracellular membrane vesicles.[234] A variety of frameshift and nonsense mutations that predict synthesis of truncated forms of the protein have been identified in most, but not all, CHS patients studied to date.[218,220,232,233,235] There is no correlation between the length of the truncated CHS1 protein and the severity of the disease. Disorders similar to human CHS have also been described in many mammalian species, including Aleutian mink, *beige* mice, blue foxes, cats, killer whales, and Hereford cattle.[219] Identification of the human CHS1 gene was aided by positional cloning of the mouse *lyst* homolog affected in *beige* mice.[232,236]

Clinical Manifestations

The key features of Chediak–Higashi syndrome are summarized in Table 50–9. The disease usually presents in infancy or early childhood, with infections involving the lungs, skin, and mucous membranes being most commonly encountered.[215] Dental caries and periodontal disease are also common. The most frequent offending organism is *S aureus*.[216] Gram-negative bacteria, *Aspergillus* spp and *Candida* spp also are responsible for many infections. Platelet granule defects result in easy bruising and epistaxis. There is partial oculocutaneous albinism and photosensitivity. Patients can have a white forelock or an ashen or grayish silver sheen to the hair, which can vary from blond to dark brown. In younger patients, there may be a cartwheel distribution of pigment in the iris and an abnormal red reflex. Neurologic manifestations include peripheral or cranial neuropathies, gait abnormalities, muscle weakness, sensory loss, seizures, or spinocerebellar degeneration.[221] Neurologic symptoms worsen with age.

Table 50–9 Summary of Chediak–Higashi Syndrome (CHS)

Incidence	Approximately 200 cases described
Inheritance	Autosomal recessive
Molecular defect	A defect in granule morphogenesis in multiple tissues resulting from mutations in the CHS1 (LYST) gene encoding a lysosomal trafficking regulator protein
Pathogenesis	Giant coalesced azurophil/specific granules in neutrophils resulting in ineffective granulopoiesis and neutropenia, delayed and incomplete degranulation, and defective chemotaxis
Clinical manifestations	Partial oculocutaneous albinism Recurrent severe bacterial infections (usually *S aureus*) Cranial and peripheral neuropathies (muscle weakness, ataxia, sensory loss) Hepatosplenomegaly and complications of pancytopenia in the accelerated phase
Laboratory evaluation	Giant granules in peripheral blood granulocytes and in bone marrow myeloid progenitor cells Widespread lymphohistiocytic infiltrates in accelerated phase
Differential diagnosis	Other genetic forms of partial albinism Giant granules can be seen in acute and chronic myelogenous leukemias
Therapy	Prophylactic trimethoprim/sulfamethoxazole Parenteral antibiotics for acute infections Ascorbic acid (200 mg/day for infants; 6 g/day for adults) Bone marrow transplant at beginning of accelerated phase
Prognosis	Most patients die from infection or complications of the accelerated phase during the first or second decade of life. A few patients have survived into their thirties

Approximately 85% of children surviving into the second decade of life develop an accelerated phase of the disease, with fever, lymphadenopathy, and progressive pancytopenia. A reactive-appearing lymphohistiocytic proliferation occurs in the liver, spleen, lymph nodes, and bone marrow.[215,237,238] Occasionally, younger children with Chediak–Higashi syndrome present in the accelerated phase. The cellular infiltration is not neoplastic by histopathologic criteria, although the prognosis is uniformly fatal unless patients undergo bone marrow transplantation. The accelerated phase resembles the virus-associated hemophagocytic syndrome because the invading histiocytes often exhibit hemophagocytosis.[237] The bone marrow infiltration and progressive hepatosplenomegaly lead to pancytopenia and death due to infection and bleeding. The accelerated phase is thought to be precipitated by Epstein–Barr virus (EBV) infection, and may become fulminant because of a lack of NK cell function.[238,239]

Diagnosis

The diagnosis of Chediak–Higashi syndrome is made on the basis of the giant peroxidase-positive lysosomal granules in the peripheral blood granulocytes or in bone marrow myeloid cells. Identification of large, acid phosphatase-positive lysosomes in amniocytes and chorionic villus cells has been used to diagnose CHS prenatally.[240,241] Other clinical features characteristic of CHS can support the diagnosis, including mild oculocutaneous albinism, silvery hair, and a bleeding diathesis. The accelerated phase of the disease is characterized by diffuse infiltrates of lymphohistiocytic cells seen on biopsy and by pancytopenia.[237] Occasionally, giant granules that resemble those of Chediak–Higashi syndrome can be seen in both acute and chronic myelogenous leukemias.[242]

Therapy

The treatment for the stable phase of Chediak–Higashi syndrome is similar to that for other neutrophil disorders. Prophylactic antibiotics such as trimethoprim/sulfamethoxazole appear to be beneficial. Parenteral antibiotics are indicated for acute infections and responses are often slow. Treatment with high-dose ascorbic acid (200 mg/day for infants, 6 g/day for adults) has been found to improve the clinical status of some patients in the stable phase.[243,244] Although there is some controversy regarding the efficacy of ascorbic acid,[245] given the safety of this medication it seems prudent to administer it to all patients.

The treatment of the accelerated phase is extremely difficult. The lymphohistiocytic infiltrates respond poorly, if at all, to vincristine and corticosteroids.[215,228,237] The only curative therapy appears to be bone marrow transplantation,[246,247] which is ideally performed prior to or at the beginning of the accelerated phase. If transplantation is successful, the accelerated phase of the disease does not recur, and NK cell activity is improved. However, transplantation does not prevent the progressive neuropathy of CHS.

Specific Granule Deficiency

Neutrophil specific granule deficiency (SGD) is an extremely rare congenital disorder characterized by recurrent bacterial and fungal infections, primarily involving the skin, ears, and lungs.[216,248–250] Infections are often indolent and smoldering, and *S aureus*, *Pseudomonas aeruginosa*, enteric gram-negative bacteria, and *C albicans* are the major pathogens. Inheritance appears to be autosomal recessive,[248,251,252] suggesting that it is inherited in an autosomal recessive manner. Neutrophils from patients with SGD have atypical bilobed nuclei, absent specific granules, and multiple deficiencies of secondary and tertiary granule mRNAs and proteins, including lactoferrin, vitamin B_{12}-binding protein and gelatinase B.[248–251] Although azurophil granules in this disorder are present and contain myeloperoxidase and lysozyme, they are markedly deficient in defensins.[226] Monocytes display cell surface and functional defects,[253] eosinophils lack eosinophil-specific granule proteins such as eosinophil cationic protein,[254] and platelets have abnormal α granules,[255] suggesting that the underlying defect may be related to regulation of the synthesis of certain granule and membrane proteins. This defect in synthesis is confined to bone marrow-derived cells, as lactoferrin secretion is normal in the glandular epithelia of SGD patients despite the severe deficiency in the neutrophils.[256]

The recurrent skin and pulmonary infections characteristic of SGD appear to be caused by two fundamental defects in the neutrophils. One defect is the marked deficiency of at least two important microbicidal granule proteins, lactoferrin[251] and defensins.[226] The other defect is a relatively severe chemotactic abnormality presumably caused by the absence of the intracellular pool of leukocyte adhesion molecules that normally reside in the specific granules. As discussed above, these $\beta 2$ integrins play a key role in phagocyte chemotaxis.

The molecular defect responsible for most cases of SGD has recently been shown to involve a myeloid transcription factor known as C/EBPε that regulates expression of certain genes activated during granulocyte differentiation. This came about serendipitously when it was recognized that mice with a targeted deletion in the C/EBPε gene had similar characteristics to SGD patients, including neutrophils with bilobed nuclei, absent secondary granules and impaired chemotaxis, along with increased susceptibility to bacterial infections.[257–259] To date, mutations in the C/EBPε gene have been identified in two SGD patients that encode truncated, nonfunctional proteins.[250,260,261] However, DNA sequencing of the C/EBPε gene of several other SGD patients has not revealed abnormalities, suggesting that SGD is a genetically heterogeneous disorder.[262] The diagnosis of SGD can be readily made by microscopic examination. Wright-stained neutrophils are devoid of specific granules but contain normal numbers of azurophilic granules.[216] Electron microscopy reveals small peroxidase-negative vesicles, which presumably represent empty specific granules.[216] The diagnosis of SGD can also be established by demonstrating a severe deficiency in either lactoferrin or vitamin B_{12}-binding protein. An acquired form of SGD can be seen in burn patients[216] or in individuals with various myeloproliferative disorders.[263] The treatment for SGD is similar to that for other neutrophil disorders. If medical management is aggressive, the prognosis appears quite good, with patients surviving into their adult years.

MISCELLANEOUS INHERITED AND ACQUIRED DISORDERS OF PHAGOCYTE FUNCTION

Defects in phagocyte production of inflammatory cytokines or their intracellular signaling pathways are now being identified, in parallel with our improved understanding of the molecular basis of these important regulatory networks.[264,265] All of these disorders are rare. Inherited defects in macrophage IL-12 production or expression of the IFNγ receptor have been described that present with recurrent and severe atypical mycobacterial infections.[255,256,264,266] Another patient with deficient mononuclear cell production of IL-12 presented with recurrent episodes of pneumococcal pneumonia with the unusual absence of fevers.[267] A variety of genetic defects in a scaffolding protein known as IKK-gamma or NEMO that is important for activation of the NF-κB signaling pathway have been reported in patients with anhydrotic ectodermal dysplasia and immunodeficiency; affected children have recurrent pyogenic infections with a minimal systemic inflammatory response, and can also develop opportunistic infections with atypical mycobacteria or *Pneumocystis carinii*.[265,268–271] Several other kindreds have been described with genetic deficiency of another protein, IRAK-4, important for NF-κB activation by pyogenic bacteria via the Toll-like receptor/Il-I receptor superfamily.[265,271,272] Affected children also had recurrent infections with *S pneumonia* and *S aureus* and a poor inflammatory response but no dysmorphic features or opportunistic infections. A similar patient with endotoxin and IL-1 hyporesponsiveness has also been reported,[273] which may involve a similar genetic defect.

There are a variety of noncongenital defects in phagocyte function that can be associated with an increased risk of bacterial or fungal infection. Several have already been mentioned above, including neonatal neutrophil dysfunction manifested as poor adhesion and chemotaxis. Patients with myelodysplastic syndromes and acute nonlymphoblastic lymphoma can have subpopulations of neutrophils variably defective in adhesion, migration, production of reactive oxidants, and microbicidal activity that can be correlated with an increased risk of infection.[4] Similar defects have been described in diabetes mellitus, Gaucher disease, and renal failure. Severe bacterial infections, surgical trauma, and severe burns can also result in transient depression of a variety of neutrophil functions.[2–4] The underlying mechanism(s) are incompletely defined, and may be related to effects of high levels of inflammatory mediators produced in response to infection or trauma, or to products released by bacteria.

Leukocytosis and Leukopenia

Leukocytosis or leukopenia is defined according to the respective age and population-based means of neutrophils, lymphocytes, monocytes, or eosinophils as the distribution of leukocytes or "differential" undergoes specific developmental changes as well as changes reflecting disease states (Chapter 164). Changes in the number of circulating leukocytes may represent a primary disorder of leukocyte production or reflect a secondary response to some disease process or toxin. This chapter focuses on abnormal elevation or depression of mature neutrophils.

Definitions of Leukocytosis and Neutropenia

Leukocytosis refers to an elevation of the white blood cell count greater than 2 standard deviations above the mean value of circulating white cells. Neutrophilia refers specifically to elevation of the absolute neutrophil count. The latter is calculated by multiplying the percentage of neutrophilic granulocytes by the total white cell count. The usual explanation for leukocytosis is neutrophilia. Abnormal elevations of eosinophils and lymphocytes are considered elsewhere in this text.

Neutrophil counts show considerable variability during the neonatal period with a mean of 11,000/mm^3 and a range of 6000 to 26,000/mm^3. Total white cell counts may be as high as 38,000/mm^3 at 12 hours of age.[274] The white cell count drops after 12 hours, reaching a mean neutrophil count of 5500/mm^3 (1500–10,000) at 1 week. The differential in the first week of life resembles that of the adult, with approximately 60% neutrophils. From 1 week until 5 to 6 years, however, there is a predominance of lymphocytes. Thereafter, neutrophils increase to about 60%. The mean adult total leukocyte count is 7500/mm^3 (4500–11,000) and the mean neutrophil count is 4400/mm^3 (1800–7700).[274] Total neutrophil counts of premature infants are about 30% lower than those of term infants. The sequential changes noted after birth also occur in premature infants but with wider variability.[275]

Neutropenia is defined as a neutrophilic granulocyte count of less than 1500/mm^3. This definition can be used for all ages and races, though, strictly speaking, separate standards should be used for particular groups. For example, newborn infants have elevated granulocyte counts in the first few days of life[274,275] and certain populations of Africans and Yemenite Jews normally have lower granulocyte counts.[276,277]

The absolute neutrophil count (ANC) is calculated by multiplying the total white blood cell count (WBC) by the percentage of bands and mature neutrophils:

$$\text{Absolute neutrophil count} = \text{WBC} \times (\%\ \text{bands} + \%\ \text{mature neutrophils}) \times 0.01$$

Granulocytes less mature than bands are not included in the calculation.

Regulation of Granulocyte Counts

The peripheral neutrophil count reflects the equilibrium between intra and extramedullary compartments. The bone marrow contains a mitotic pool, a maturation pool, and a storage pool. Outside the marrow, there is a circulating pool, a marginated pool of neutrophils adherent to vascular endothelium, and a tissue pool. A complex interplay of factors regulates the production of granulocytes and their movement from one pool to another.[278–282] The clinical assay reporting the number of neutrophils, that is, the white blood cell count (WBC) and the differential, only monitors neutrophils that are in the circulating pool during a brief 3- to 6-hour period of transit from marrow to tissue and thus does not provide definitive information regarding the cause of neutrophilia or neutropenia.

Granulocytes are derived from a common progenitor that also gives rise to erythrocytes, megakaryocytes, eosinophils, basophils and monocytes. The biology of hematopoiesis is quite complex and is regulated by a number of cytokines with overlapping activities. The hematopoietic stem cells normally reside in the bone marrow in a state of quiescence/dormancy. Cytokines that lead to proliferation (or exit from dormancy) of the early progenitor/stem cells are stem cell factor (SCF), thrombopoietin (TPO), FLT3 ligand, interleukin-11 (IL11), granulocyte stimulating factor (G-CSF), and interleukin-6 (IL6). Interleukin-3 (IL3) and GM-CSF act on the later progenitor cells, whereas cytokines supporting differentiation along specific lineages are G-CSF, monocyte colony stimulating factor (M-CSF), and erythropoietin (Epo), leading to granulocytic, monocytic, and erythroid differentiation, respectively.[283–288] Some of these cytokines along with components of complement[289–292] release granulocytes from the marrow storage pool into the circulation. This can result in a two- to threefold increase in the granulocyte count within 4 to 5 hours.[289,293]

It is now clear that neutrophils not only move from the marrow to the circulation, but also reenter the marrow pool from the periphery.[280,294–296] This process involves complex and regulated interactions between hematopoietic growth factors, proinflammatory cytokines, and marrow adhesion receptors. Stromal cell-derived factor-1α (SDF-1α/CXCL12), the ligand for the chemokine receptor, CXCR4, is important in the regulation of B-cell lymphopoiesis and myelopoiesis during embryonic life and of CD34$^+$ cell and lymphocyte trafficking postnatally.[297] This receptor is also responsible for retention of neutrophils in the bone marrow and for homing of peripheral neutrophils back into the marrow.[298] The CXCR4/SDF-1α pathway plays an important role in homing of CD34$^+$ progenitors to the marrow through regulation of α4-integrin and α4-integrin/VCAM-1 engagement, though cooperation of CXCR4 is not an absolute requirement.[280] The bone marrow is important in the release of neutrophils that have reached maturity and in the accelerated release of less mature cells in response to inflammation. However, it also plays an important role in regulating circulating neutrophil counts and in controlling their reentry into the marrow from the periphery. In animal models at least, infused peripheral neutrophils redistribute equally between the marrow and the liver whereas activated neutrophils, such as those found in exudates, home to the liver and marrow-derived neutrophils return primarily to the marrow.[296] This suggests that the marrow recaptures circulating neutrophils and can re-release them. This is supported in humans by the fact that radiolabeled neutrophils infused into humans can be detected in the bone marrow.[299] Retention of neutrophils in the marrow is increased by activation of CXCR4 and blocking neutrophil CXCR4 reduces neutrophil retention and mobilizes neutrophils from the marrow into circulation in animal models[298] and in humans.[300,301] In fact, myelokathexis, a rare congenital disorder where CXCR4 activity is increased, is characterized by neutropenia and marked retention of neutrophils in the marrow, supporting a role for this mechanism in humans.[297,302–304] Similarly, infusion of AMD3100, a CXCR4 antagonist, results in marked increase in the neutrophil count as well as release of CD34+ cells into the periphery.[305,306] Furthermore, inflammatory mediators cause much greater release of neutrophils when CXCR4 is blocked,[298] providing additional support for the role of CXCR4 in regulation of neutrophil counts. Surface expression of CXCR4 on neutrophils decreases with maturation and with activation. This would favor the retention of immature cells in the marrow and cause mature and stimulated neutrophils to remain in the circulation. Although surface levels of CXCR4 are low on freshly isolated human neutrophils, intracellular stores are high, suggesting a high level of spontaneous endocytosis.[307] CXCR4 surface expression increases as neutrophils become senescent, resulting in clearance from circulation and return to the marrow. Furthermore, activation of CXCR4 reduces the chemotactic response of neutrophils to CXCR2 agonists,[307] perhaps explaining the chemotactic defects reported in some patients with myelokathexis.[294,308] The adhesion of hematopoietic cells in the bone marrow is mediated through the interaction of α4β1 integrin (VLA-4) with marrow fibronectin and VCAM-1 in the stroma and is regulated in part by CXCL12/SDF-1α activation of CXCR4.[298,307,309]

During acute inflammation, elevated levels of CXC cytokines stimulate mobilization of neutrophils from the bone marrow and this response is enhanced by inhibition of marrow retention by blockade of CXCR4.[307] It has been suggested that inactivation of SDF-1α by serine proteases such as neutrophil elastase or cathepsin-G released from neutrophils upon activation by cytokines may promote egress by decreasing CXCR4 stimulation.[307,310–312] These studies suggest that the CXCR4/SDF-1α axis is critical in maintenance of neutrophil homeostasis.

More than half of the granulocytes in the peripheral circulation at any given time are attached to the vascular endothelium.[313] These "marginated" neutrophils can be released almost immediately at times of stress, an effect mediated in part by epinephrine.[314] Margination is regulated by specific receptors called selectins that mediate rolling adhesion of leukocytes to the endothelium.[278]

Normally, 1.5×10^9 granulocytes/kg body weight are produced per day, of which approximately 20% are in the myeloid precursor pool, 75% in the marrow storage pool, 3% in the marginated pool, and 2% in the circulating blood.[313,315] Granulocytes spend about 9 days in the marrow, 3 to 6 hours in the blood, and 1 to 4 days in the tissues.[313] Thus, the total granulocyte count as measured from peripheral blood represents a sample of only 2% of the total population.

Movement of neutrophils from one compartment to another as well as changes in production contribute to states of neutrophilia and neutropenia. Thus, neutrophilia can be due to increased production as in infection or myeloproliferative disorders or inhibition of egress from the blood as in certain chemotactic disorders or steroid therapy.[293] Neutropenia may be due to decreased production, to increased margination and egress as in systemic complement activation or burns,[316,317] to destruction as in immune neutropenia, or to increased apoptosis of neutrophils.[318–325]

Practically, evaluation of these processes is limited to examination of the peripheral blood and of the bone marrow. Although sophisticated radiotracer techniques exist, they are not clinically useful. Similarly, clinical tests such as hydrocortisone challenge and epinephrine stimulation, which reflect a releasable marrow storage pool or marginated pool, have limited differentiating power.

Secondary Causes of Neutrophilia

Most leukocytosis occurs as a reaction to some inflammatory process. Infection was documented in 207 of 400 patients (53%) in a prospective study of 400 inpatients with white cell counts greater than 15,000 cells/mm³. Of these 207 patients, 47% had pneumonia, 29% had urinary tract infection, 16% had soft-tissue infection, and 16% had *C difficile* infection. *C difficile* infection was present in 25% of patients with WBC counts greater than 30,000 cells/mm³. Other causes of leukocytosis included physiological stress (38%), medications or drugs (11%), hematologic disease (6%), and necrosis or inflammation (6%).[326]

Leukemoid Reaction

Leukocytosis exceeding 50,000/mm³ is referred to as "leukemoid reaction"[327] and is characterized by a significant increase in early neutrophil precursors in the peripheral blood. The differential count has a marked "left shift," evidenced by presence of myelocyte, metamyelocyte, and band forms. Progranulocytes and myeloblasts may be observed in severe reactions. In contrast to acute leukemia, proliferation and orderly maturation of all normal myeloid elements is observed in the bone marrow and the morphology of the myeloid elements is normal. Presence of the Philadelphia chromosome on karyotypic analysis of the bone marrow distinguishes adult chronic myeloid leukemia from a leukemoid reaction. Leukemoid reactions due to infections may be accompanied by toxic granulation, Doehle bodies, and cytoplasmic vacuoles in the neutrophils.[327]

Newborns have unique responses to stress and infection. The relative number of band forms and less mature granulocyte precursors in the differential of newborn infants has been correlated with sepsis and with depletion of the marrow neutrophil storage pool.[328,329] In the normal infant, the band to neutrophil ratio is less than 0.14 to 0.11 in the first 48 hours, irrespective of birth weight or gestational age.[329] An immature/total neutrophil ratio exceeding 0.8 in the peripheral blood indicates that the marrow reserves are depleted and the risk for death in septic infants is significantly increased.[328] Some infants have extreme responses to stress and as many as 15% of extremely low birth weight infants (<1000 g) presented with leukemoid reactions with no identifiable cause.[330,331] Transient leukemoid reactions have also been seen in phenotypically normal infants who had trisomy 21 limited to their hematopoietic cells.[332,333]

When the marrow is directly invaded by tumor, or in cases of marrow fibrosis or granulomatous reactions, neutrophilia associated with immature granulocytes, nucleated red cells, "stubby elliptocytes,"[334] and teardrop-shaped erythrocytes may be seen, often accompanied by thrombocytosis.[335] Vasculitis and marrow infarction can also cause this picture.[336,337] This is called a leukoerythroblastic response. Essentially, presence of leukoerythroblastosis suggests the presence of an irritative or inflammatory process in the marrow itself. A bone marrow aspirate and biopsy should be performed in these cases to look for granuloma, tumor, or marrow fibrosis. Cultures of the marrow for fungus and tuberculosis[338] should be obtained. Leukoerythroblastic reaction may also be seen during recovery from marrow suppression after chemotherapy. Interestingly, transient erythroblastopenia of childhood has been reported to present with leukoerythroblastosis.[339]

Pelger–Huet Anomaly

Although technically not leukocytosis, the Pelger–Huet anomaly can raise the question of serious infection because of an apparent high band count. The Pelger–Huet anomaly is a benign, dominantly inherited defect of terminal neutrophil differentiation with a frequency at birth of 1:6000. Most of the neutrophils have bilobate nuclei and excessively coarse clumping of nuclear chromatin. The two lobes are joined by a thin, hair-like bridge, which is much thinner than that seen in a normal band. This gives the characteristic "pince-nez" spectacle appearance to the nucleus. Nevertheless, the function of these cells is normal.[340] Interestingly, Pelger–Huet cells can develop multiple lobes during vitamin B_{12} or folate deficiency but return to their bilobate state when the vitamin deficiency is corrected.[341] Colchicine, sulfonamides, ibuprofen, taxoids,[342] and valproate induce the anomaly reversibly.[343–347] This so-called pseudo Pelger cell has also been reported to transiently appear during certain acute infections, acute myelogenous leukemia and in myelofibrosis. In particular, the defect has been associated with cytogenetic abnormalities of chromosome 17 in leukemias.[348–350] Most cases of genetic Pelger–Huet anomaly are due to mutations in the lamin-B receptor, LBR, which is located on chromosome 1q41–43. LBR is a sterol reductase integral to the inner nuclear membrane and targets heterochromatin and lamin to the nuclear membrane.[351–353] Neutrophils of homozygotes have ovoid nuclei with clumped chromatin and varying degrees of developmental delay, epilepsy, and skeletal anomalies.[351,352] Eosinophils and basophils may also be involved. An unusual case of Pelger–Huet anomaly has been reported in association with four generations of one family with late-onset progressive proximal muscular dystrophy.[354] Neutrophilia and a differential "left shift" can be indicative of disease or may be totally benign. An outline of the major primary and acquired causes of neutrophilia is presented in Table 50–10. We have divided the causes of neutrophilia into two groups, those that seem to be due to intrinsic problems with the neutrophil or with the regulation of neutrophil production, and those that are secondary to some other disease process.

Table 50–10 Classification of Neutrophilia

Primary (no other evident associated disease)
Hereditary neutrophilia
Chronic idiopathic neutrophilia
Chronic myelogenous leukemia (CML) and other myeloproliferative diseases
Familial myeloproliferative disease
Congenital anomalies and leukemoid reaction
Leukocyte adhesion factor deficiency (LAD)
Familial cold urticaria and leukocytosis
Secondary
Infection
Stress neutrophilia
Chronic Inflammation
Drug induced
Nonhematologic malignancy
Generalized marrow stimulation as in hemolysis
Asplenia and hyposplenism

Chronic Myelogenous Leukemia

The major differential diagnosis of leukemoid reaction is chronic myelocytic leukemia (CML). This topic is considered in detail in Chapter 69. Leukemoid reactions and CML can be difficult to distinguish. The classic differentiating features are the presence of a low leukocyte alkaline phosphatase (LAP) score and Philadelphia chromosome in CML. The LAP score is also low in familial myeloproliferative disease[355] and paroxysmal nocturnal hemoglobinuria.[356] However, the LAP score can be normal in CML and thus is of little diagnostic value. Juvenile CML (see Chapter 74) can be distinguished from the usual adult form by the ability of circulating stem cells to form monocyte colonies in vitro[357] and the absence of Philadelphia chromosome. Leukocyte counts in CML can be extremely high, occasionally exceeding 500,000/mm^3. Patients with granulocyte counts above 200,000/mm^3 to 300,000/mm^3 require emergent intervention to prevent the vasoocclusive complications of hyperviscosity related to the markedly elevated white blood cells.

Acute Infection

Modest leukocytosis with a left shift is commonly seen in association with many acute bacterial infections. Certain bacterial agents such as *pneumococcus* or *staphylococcus* may cause particularly high leukocyte counts. Leukocytosis is seen in association with acute otitis media, with 9% of patients having greater than 20,000 WBC/mm^3, whereas 27% of culture-proven positive acute otitis media cases have WBC below the mean for age.[358] The predictive value of leukocytosis and increased band forms (WBC >15 × 10^9/L; immature/total >0.2) in detecting bacterial disease was increased from 32% to 71% when associated with depressed fibronectin levels (1 SD < Mean for age). This is of particular interest in view of the role of fibronectin in promoting phagocytosis by PMN and monocytes.[359] The risk of positive blood cultures in children between 3 and 36 months of age with fever >39.5°C (103°F) directly related to white cell count. If the temperature is >39.5°C (103°F) and the WBC is >15,000/mm^3, 16% have a positive culture, whereas 43% of cultures from children with a WBC >30,000/mm^3 are positive. In contrast, only 3.7% of children with counts less than 15,000/mm^3 and none with counts <10,000/mm^3 had positive blood cultures.[360] In hospitalized adults, *C difficile* infection was present in 25% of patients with WBC counts of >30,000 cells/mm^3,[326] and a poor outcome is predicted in elderly inpatients[361] by a WBC >20,000 cells/mm^3. Neutrophilic leukocytosis can also be associated with severe viral disease. Patients with Hantavirus infection, for example, have WBC as high as 65,000/mm^3 (median 26,000/mm^3) with 67% bands (median 27%).[362]

Stress Neutrophilia

Modest elevation in the neutrophil count has been associated with many types of "stress." Neutrophilia can occur within minutes of exercise[363] or stress[364] or epinephrine injection[314] and is presumed to be related to movement of neutrophils from the marginated pool into the circulating pool. The neutrophilia secondary to catecholamine injection has been related to reduced neutrophil adherence to endothelium. The neutrophilia and the adherence-inhibiting ability of plasma can be blocked by pretreatment of the subject with propranolol[365] or by treatment of neutrophils in the in vitro adherence assay system with an antibody to cyclic AMP.[314]

Propanolol does not block exercise-induced neutrophilia, despite measurable increases in plasma epinephrine.[366] The neutrophilia was directly related to the workload and cardiac output during exercise, suggesting a larger role for mechanical- and flow-related effects on dislodgment of the leukocytes sequestered in the lung than for a possible direct effect of catecholamines upon the neutrophils. Other studies show no effect of exercise upon circulating CFU-GM or CFU-GEMM,[363] although it has been suggested that the delayed leukocytosis (up to 235% increase at 5 hours postexercise) may be related to marrow release of leukocytes.[367]

Mild neutrophilia and lymphopenia have been associated with unipolar depression[368] but may be related to the use of antidepressant medications.[369]

Neutrophilia is also seen in the postoperative period. There is a doubling of the leukocyte count approximately 3 hours after surgery. This does not seem to be related to the type of anesthesia.[370,371]

Leukocytosis in the 12,000 to 20,000/mm^3 range has been reported in the postictal state. This can be associated with fever or pulmonary edema and resolves in a few hours to days.[372]

There is an interesting association between leukocyte count and myocardial infarction. Subjects with a leukocyte count greater than 9000 had a 4.5-fold higher incidence of myocardial infarction than those with a leukocyte count less than 6000.[373] It is also not clear whether the leukocyte count is a risk factor or merely an indicator of chronic stress.[374] However, WBC has been shown to be an independent indicator of atherosclerotic cardiovascular disease.[375]

Drug-Induced Neutrophilia

Leukocytosis has been seen in association with a number of drugs and drug reactions. Steroids are well known to induce release of neutrophils from the bone marrow[293] and result in a chronic low-grade neutrophilia. Leukocytosis as high as 200,000/mm^3 in neonates has been associated with maternal steroid administration.[331,376,377] Beta agonists produce an acute neutrophilia by releasing neutrophils from the marginated pool[378] and phenytoin and other anticonvulsants have been associated with leukocytosis.[379–383] Lithium is well-known to produce leukocytosis by increasing production of the colony-stimulating factor and has been used with varying success to treat several neutropenic states.[384] Tetracycline has also been associated with leukemoid reaction with a white cell count greater that 80,000/mm^3.[385] Granulocyte colony stimulating factor is now in common clinical use and can cause significant neutrophilia if its use is not closely monitored.

Nonhematologic Malignancy

Leukocytosis is frequently seen in large-cell lung cancer.[386] Usually, the leukocytosis seen with solid tumors is modest, in the 12,000 to 30,000/mm^3 range,[386–390] although it can be as high as 106,000/mm^3 in the absence of marrow metastasis.[391] Leukemoid reactions have been seen in patients with marrow involvement with tumors from lung, stomach, and breast or with neuroblastoma in children.[391] In some cases, solid tumors of lung, tongue, and kidney have been shown to secrete colony-stimulating activity.[392–394]

Marrow Stimulation

Significant leukocytosis can be seen in states of chronic stimulation of the bone marrow, such as hemolytic anemia or immune thrombocytopenia.[395] For example, patients with sickle cell anemia commonly have leukocyte counts in the 12,000 to 15,000/mm^3 range and have an exaggerated elevation in leukocyte counts with infection. The mechanism of leukocytosis may be related to production of placenta-derived growth factor by erythroid progenitors that stimulates production of inflammatory cytokines by monocytes.[396] This response may be further augmented by functional asplenia seen in sickle cell disease. Likewise, significant rebound leukocytosis can occur in the recovery phase of marrow suppression.[397,398] These reactions can last several weeks. In one instance, there were 90% myeloblasts in the marrow and as many as 20% myeloblasts in the peripheral blood.[399]

Primary Causes of Neutrophilia

Hereditary Neutrophilia

A family of four was described in 1974[400] with leukocyte counts chronically in the 20,000 to 70,000/mm^3 range, splenomegaly and widened diploe of the skull. There was no apparent propensity to bacterial infections. The defect seemed to be dominantly inherited. Subsequent follow-up (W. Herring, personal communication, 1989) revealed that two more children had been born to the same mother and both had chronic leukocytosis. The LAP scores were high in all affected subjects. None of the family members have had any serious medical problems other than a bleeding diathesis related to platelet dysfunction.[400] We have studied one of the members of this family and found normal neutrophil function and normal expression of surface CD18/CD11b (W. Herring, T. D. Coates, unpublished data), indicating that it is not a variant of leukocyte adhesion deficiency. We have seen a second family with this syndrome (D. Powars, personal communication). In this case, the father had marked leukocytosis and splenomegaly and eventually had his spleen removed. His son had similar problems with neutrophil counts at times in the 100,000/mm^3 range and with massive splenomegaly. The neutrophil function and CD18/CD11b expression in the affected father and son were also normal (D. Powars and T. D. Coates, unpublished data).

Chronic Idiopathic Neutrophilia

Chronic leukocytosis can occur in patients who are otherwise well. A series of thirty-four patients with leukocyte counts between 11,000 and 40,000/mm^3 were followed for up to 20 years without occurrence of clinical problems. Bone marrow aspirations were generally normal as were the LAP scores. The remainder of the blood counts were normal, except for occasional thrombocytosis.[401] These data point out that certain normal subjects fall outside of the 95th percentile with respect to WBC. This entity is obviously a diagnosis of exclusion.

Familial Myeloproliferative Disease

A syndrome encompassing growth retardation, hepatosplenomegaly, anemia, and leukocytosis has been described.[355] Some of the affected children died in early life whereas others remained stable or improved. All of the affected subjects had low LAP scores. Several other members of the family in four generations had low LAP scores but no other findings. Chromosomal analysis showed no significant consistent abnormalities and no subject had a Philadelphia chromosome. Other families have been reported with familial occurrence of polycythemia vera, CML, and myelofibrosis.[402–404] Furthermore, there is evidence that some myeloproliferative syndromes associated with monosomy 7 may have familial features.[405,406] Subsequent studies of families with familial myeloproliferative syndromes suggest that there is an inherited predisposition to the acquisition of JAK2 (V617F) mutations that are involved in the final pathway in the development of the myeloproliferative disorder.[407] This acquired mutation is found in some children[408] and in two-thirds of adults with familial myeloproliferative syndrome. Homozygosity is associated with disease progression.[409]

Congenital Anomalies and Leukemoid Reaction

Leukemoid reactions have been associated with amegakaryocytic thrombocytopenia and congenital deformities, such as Tetralogy of Fallot, dextrocardia and absent radii, and rudimentary little toes.[410,411] Transient leukemoid reactions and myelodysplastic syndrome have also been associated with the Noonan Syndrome.[412–414]

Down Syndrome

Infants with Down syndrome may have a transient leukemoid reaction that resembles congenital leukemia.[415] These children can also have an exaggerated leukemoid response to stress.[416] A transient leukemoid reaction has been seen in a phenotypically normal child who expressed trisomy 21 mosaicism in myeloid cells but not in skin fibroblasts. The chromosomal abnormality disappeared after the leukemoid reaction resolved.[333,417] The transient leukemoid reaction in Down syndrome has been associated with several mutations in important regulatory genes, which provide important insights into the control of myelopoiesis.[418,419]

Leukocyte Adhesion Deficiency

Since the 1970s, several patients have been described with persistent leukocytosis, delayed separation of the umbilical cord, recurrent infections, and a stimulus-dependent activation defect of the neutrophil. The laboratory hallmark of these disorders is leukocytosis. White blood cell counts may be only mildly elevated (10,000–12,000/mm^3) but often are in the 18,000/mm^3 to 30,000/mm^3 range and may be as high as 150,000/mm^3 during infection.[420,421] There are no specific morphologic abnormalities seen in the granulocytes. The diagnosis is established by demonstration of marked reduction (<10% of control) or absence in the CR3 receptor (CD11b/CD18) on granulocytes. These patients have severe functional defects as well and are described in detail earlier in this chapter.

Familial Cold Urticaria and Leukocytosis

A very interesting syndrome of leukocytosis, fever, urticaria, rash, and muscle and skin tenderness upon exposure to cold has been reported. This syndrome appears to be dominantly inherited. The onset of symptoms is in infancy and symptoms have been provoked by exposure to cold in the delivery room. Urticaria followed by fever starts about 7 hours after cold exposure. Leukocytosis, sometimes up to 34,000/mm^3, starts approximately 10 hours after cold exposure and begins to subside 12 to 14 hours later.[422,423] In contrast to other causes of urticaria, the skin rash in these patients is characterized histologically by a marked infiltration by neutrophils. The leukocytosis and urticaria were blocked when the patients were infused with endotoxin prior to cold exposure. This has been related to "cold activation of clotting system," as it is associated with a transient decrease in levels of C1 esterase inhibitor.[424,425] The gene has been mapped to a 10-cM region on chromosome 1q44, and the gene (CIAS1) responsible was subsequently identified.[426]

Approach to the Evaluation of Neutrophilia

Laboratory error must always be considered in the differential diagnosis of unexplained, isolated neutrophilia or neutropenia. With current technology, much of the human error has been removed,[427] although some clinicians continue to believe that manual counts are more accurate. Blood counts that do not fit the context of the clinical findings should be repeated before extensive evaluation is undertaken.[428]

Factitious leukocytosis can occur because of blood sampling problems or certain primary disease states. Inadequate anticoagulation of the specimen can result in platelet clumps that are being counted as leukocytes by automated cell counters. The WBC is rarely increased more than 10% and is usually associated with spurious thrombocytopenia.[429,430] In cryoglobulinemia, a temperature-dependent increase in leukocyte and platelet counts occurs at about 30°C and can result in white cell counts as high as 50,000/mm^3 and in a doubling of the platelet count, presumably because of various sizes of precipitated cryoglobulin particles.[431,432] This effect is increased if the sample is allowed to cool to lower temperatures.

The general approach to the evaluation of the patient with neutrophilia will depend on the degree of neutrophilia and the signs and symptoms of the associated diseases. Neutrophilia is most commonly seen secondarily to some acute or chronic inflammatory processes and the diagnosis and treatment are dictated by the nature of the primary illness. In the absence of clear history or physical examination findings, we find the sedimentation rate to be very helpful. An elevated sedimentation rate suggests that a more extensive evaluation for collagen vascular disease or other occult inflammatory disease is warranted whereas a normal value suggests that watchful waiting may be the best course. Examination of the bone marrow is of little help in cases of mild leukocytosis. In leukemoid reactions or leukoerythroblastosis, direct invasion of the marrow and myelodysplasia must be excluded. Bone marrow biopsy, marrow cytogenetics, and fungal, tubercular, and collagen vascular disease evaluation should be assessed. The marrow biopsy may reveal granulomata, which may intensify the search for fungus, or may reveal metastatic tumor that is often missed in marrow aspirate. Marrow cytogenetics may reveal mosaic trisomy 21[332,333] and monosomy 7,[405] Philadelphia chromosome, or other markers of dysplastic states. Much has been written about the leukocyte alkaline phosphatase score, which classically is high in infection and low in CML; however, this test is not diagnostic and is of limited utility.

Many factors contribute to the wide variability in granulocyte counts in normal populations. Particularly in the asymptomatic patient with persistent mild neutrophilia, one must remember that, by definition, the white blood cell count in 2.5% of the normal population must be greater than two standard deviations above the mean. Because regulation of granulocyte production is genetically controlled (W. Herring, personal communication, 1989),[276,277,401] examination of the parents' or siblings' blood counts may be of help in these few cases.

Leukopenia

Neutropenia is usually discovered when a blood cell count is performed as part of an evaluation for fever or as an incidental finding on a blood count done for some unrelated reason. In one study of adults with incidentally discovered neutropenia the causes were chronic idiopathic (34%), exposure to chemical agents (16.5%), infection (9.3%), autoimmune (9.3%), hematologic disorders (9.3%), thyroid disease (8.2%), ethnic neutropenia (7.5%), drug induced (2.1%), and others (4.2%).[433] The biggest concern in the neutropenic patient is the propensity to infection. In this case, the ability to deliver neutrophils to the tissue is the most important parameter, not the absolute neutrophil count.[434]

Table 50–11 Clinically Significant Neutrophil Counts

Absolute Neutrophil Count	Clinical Significance
>1500/mm^3	Normal
1000–1500	No significant propensity to infection. Fevers can be managed as an outpatient.
500–1000	Some propensity to infection. Occasionally fever can be managed as an outpatient.
<500	Significant propensity to infection. Always should be managed as inpatient with parenteral antibiotics. Few clinical signs of infection.

These rules apply strictly for neutropenia with hypoplastic marrow, early myeloid arrests and decreased granulocyte reserve pools. There is more latitude for clinical judgment in neutropenias with normocellular marrow. The only regular exception to these rules is documented chronic benign neutropenia of childhood.

Relation of Absolute Neutrophil Count to Propensity to Infection

Adequacy of the marrow reserve pool of neutrophils is the most important determinant of propensity to infection, and bone marrow aspiration is the single most helpful way to assess neutrophil reserve pool adequacy. When the reserve pool is significantly depleted, the propensity to infection is directly related to the absolute neutrophil count (see Table 50–11). In contrast, there is no good correlation between degree of neutropenia and propensity to infection in patients with good bone marrow reserve. If the marrow cellularity is good and there is no early myeloid arrest, it is unlikely that a patient's propensity to infection is due solely to the neutropenia.

Patients with neutropenia secondary to chemotherapy, marrow failure, or marrow exhaustion are at great risk for overwhelming bacterial infection.[328,329,435] In contrast, children with chronic benign neutropenia of infancy and childhood may have neutrophil counts less than 200/mm^3 for months or years but do not have any serious infectious problems.[435] Similarly, some adults with immune neutropenia may have severe depression of their neutrophil counts and suffer no serious episodes of infection. Changes in the number of circulating leukocytes may represent a primary disorder of leukocyte production or reflect a secondary response to some disease process or toxin. Both of these entities are characterized by neutropenia and cellular marrow. The marrow differential usually shows normal early granulocyte precursors but may have maturation arrest at the metamyelocyte or band stage.

Many patients with chronic neutropenia have normal or increased monocytes. These cells are functioning phagocytes, which may explain the lack of correlation between neutrophil count and propensity to infection in certain patients.[436,437] Tissue delivery of neutrophils in chronic immune-mediated neutropenia has been shown to be greater than in chemotherapy-induced neutropenia of equal degree, suggesting that the peripheral blood count may not accurately reflect neutrophil availability.[434] Although adequacy of the marrow reserve pool of granulocytes is a very important determinant of propensity to infection in neutropenic patients, the clinical setting in which the neutropenia occurs is also of great importance. For example, patients with severe congenital neutropenia have a markedly reduced marrow myeloid reserve but do not develop fulminant sepsis as rapidly as a chemotherapy patient would when mucosal barriers have been broken and both lymphocyte-mediated and phagocytic immunity have been destroyed.[1,438]

The types of infections encountered in neutropenic patients depend on the degree and chronicity of the neutropenia as well as the nature of the associated diseases causing the neutropenia. Patients in good clinical condition with severe neutropenia secondary to decreased production may have prolonged periods without serious infection, although pyogenic infection is inevitable. If the patient is debilitated or receiving suppressive chemotherapy, the frequency of infection is greater. *S aureus*, *P aeruginosa*, *Escherichia coli*, and *Klebsiella* spp are common causes of infection in these patients.[436,437,439] Patients with less severe chronic neutropenia (ANC >300) may have recurrent sinusitis, stomatitis, perirectal infection and gingivitis,[436,437,440] but usually do not become septic.

Patients with significant chronic inability to produce neutrophils almost always have some evidence of gingival disease. However, the converse is not always true, particularly in the case of autoimmune disease. Autoimmune disorders can independently cause neutropenia and oral vasculitis associated with significant oral ulcerations and gingival disease. In this case, the oral lesions may not be secondary to the neutropenia at all. Although it is tempting to attribute the oral symptoms to the neutropenia, they can get worse with administration of G-CSF and resolve with immunosuppressive treatment of the vasculitis, despite persistence of severe neutropenia.

Classification of Neutropenia

It is simplest to classify neutropenia as primary or acquired (Table 50–12). From a mechanistic standpoint, neutropenia can be due to decreased production of neutrophils, shift of granulocytes from the circulating pool to marginated or tissue pools, peripheral destruction, apoptosis,[321,323–325,441,442] or a combination of these causes.[324,325] Regardless, the clinical implications for the patient depend on the effectiveness of delivery of neutrophils to the tissue and the nature of the primary disorder responsible for the neutropenia. These depend on marrow reserve and comorbidities such as collagen vascular disease, T or B cell abnormalities, or cytogenetic abnormalities. We have listed the various neutropenic disorders based on adequacy of the marrow reserve pool and mechanisms in Tables 50–13A and 50–13B.

The laboratory characteristics of many of the neutropenia syndromes overlap; thus, the differential diagnosis can be very difficult. Classification of some of the neutropenia syndromes depends on the clinical course. If there is no family history of neutropenia and the bone marrow is normocellular or hypercellular, there is no certain way to differentiate the various neutropenia syndromes other than to follow the patient clinically. In fact, the syndromes called "chronic benign neutropenia," "chronic idiopathic neutropenia," "chronic benign neutropenia of infancy," and "autoimmune neutropenia" are all very similar, differing only in age of onset, or association with recognizable immune disease. Chronic idiopathic neutropenia (CIN) with mildly hypocellular marrow is associated with mild to moderate neutropenia (1000–1500) and is due to increased apoptosis at the early myeloid progenitor stage.[441] The clinical course is also benign. Differentiating these syndromes is probably not important. It may be better to lump them into a category of "neutropenia with adequate marrow neutrophil reserve" as this better predicts the clinical behavior. The algorithm in Fig. 50–5 outlines an approach to these disorders that is based largely on the patients' symptoms and physical examination (see also Table 50–14).

Table 50–12 Classification of Neutropenia

Acquired neutropenia
Postinfectious
Drug induced
Chronic benign neutropenia
Chronic benign neutropenia of childhood
Autoimmune neutropenia
Isoimmune neonatal neutropenia
Pure white cell aplasia
Neutropenia associated with immunologic abnormalities
Neutropenia and lymphoproliferation of granular lymphocytes
Neutropenia associated with metabolic diseases
Neutropenia due to increased margination
Hypersplenism
Nutritional deficiency
Intrinsic defects
Ethnic neutropenia
Nonimmune chronic idiopathic neutropenia
Severe congenital neutropenia (SCN; Kostmann's syndrome)
Cyclic neutropenia
Myelokathexis (WHIM Syndrome)
Schwachman–Diamond–Oski syndrome
Barth syndrome
Chediak–Higashi syndrome
Griscelli syndrome
Hermansky–Pudlak II
Reticular dysgenesis
Dyskeratosis congenita

Acquired Neutropenia

Many acquired neutropenia have decreased survival of neutrophils in the peripheral circulation. Bone marrow examination reveals normal or increased cellularity with a late maturation arrest, usually at the metamyelocyte or band stage. Elevation of serum lysozyme or lactoferrin helps demonstrate destruction of circulating neutrophils but does not help with clinical management.[316,443] Bone marrow examination is the most helpful test in the evaluation of neutropenia. However, this can be delayed or omitted in the absence of other clinical findings (Fig. 50–5).

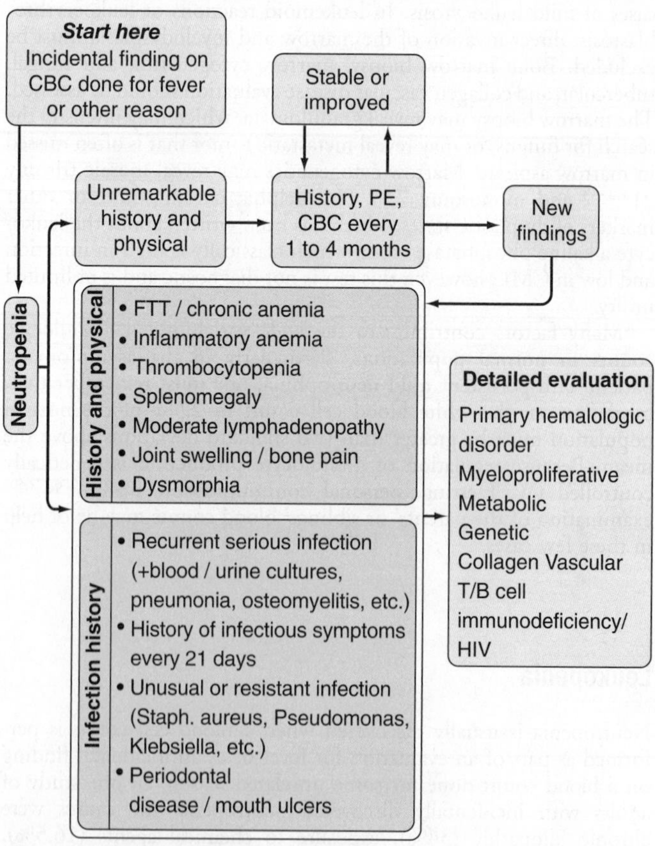

Figure 50–5 Algorithm for evaluation of neutropenia. Patients with neutropenia who are otherwise normal are followed clinically unless one of the noted danger signs or events occurs. Presence of one of the noted physical findings or infectious events should trigger an immediate detailed evaluation as outlined in Table 50–14. CBC, Complete blood count; FTT, failure to thrive; PE, physical examination.

Table 50–13A Neutropenia With Decreased Marrow Reserve

	Disorder	Mechanism	Inheritance/ Frequency	Clinical Characteristics	Diagnosis	Treatment
Primary	Severe congenital neutropenia	Apoptosis of precursor cells; *ELA2* gene mutations	AR, AD, S 1–2/million	Severe neutropenia in newborn; 2% a year progress to MDS or AML	Promyelocyte-myelocyte arrest on BMA, *ELA2* mutation analysis	G-CSF at 6–100 μg/kg/day to maintain ANC 500–1500/mm^3; and keep ESR low
	Shwachman–Diamond syndrome	Abnormal bone marrow stroma; Fas-mediated PMN precursor apoptosis	AR, S Extremely rare	Infections and steatorrhea; exocrine pancreatic deficiency; metaphyseal dysplasia; physical anomalies; 50% survival; 1/3 progress to MDS and AML; ANC <500/mm^3; thrombocytopenia; macrocytic anemia; chemotactic defect	Hypoplastic bone marrow; normal sweat chloride, increased 72-hour fecal fat, short stature. SBDS mutation analysis	G-CSF in selected cases; pancreatic enzyme replacement; CBC 2–3×/year. BMA + cytogenetics if marrow failure develops
	Cyclic neutropenia	Precursor apoptosis; also linked to *ELA2* mutations	AD, S 1–2/million	Regularly recurring fever every 21 days with associated oropharyngeal and skin infections	CBC 2–3 times per week for 8 weeks. Marrow aspirate not helpful. *ELA2* mutation	G-CSF at 2–3 μg/kg qd-qod; G-CSF dosage adjusted to maintain ANC >500/m^3 and keep ESR low
Secondary	Lymphoproliferative disorder of granular lymphocytes	Increased apoptosis due to circulating FAS ligand	Uncommon	Recurrent infection, fever, mouth ulcers, splenomegaly, arthritis. Primarily adults.	Clonal proliferation of granular lymphocytes. CD3$^{+/-}$ and CD8$^+$, or CD16$^+$ or CD56$^+$ or CD57$^+$	Cyclosporin or methotrexate primary treatment. Treat sepsis. Careful use of G-CSF
	Chemotherapy	Direct toxicity to neutrophil precursors	Common	Severity of neutropenia dependent on treatment intensity and cytotoxic agents used; poor marrow reserve = high risk of infection	Appropriate clinical history; BMA done when neutropenia is unusually prolonged or severe	Supportive; prophylactic TMP/SMX at 5 mg/kg divided BID on 3 consecutive days is often used; G-CSF in selected cases
	Drug-induced (nonimmune)	Direct suppression of myelopoiesis	Not uncommon	Medications account for 72% of all cases of neutropenia; mortality rates as high as 12%–25% (chloramphenicol, etc.)	Appropriate clinical history; often empiric discontinuation of drug will assist in diagnosis	Stop unnecessary medications; G-CSF can be used
	Nutritional	Ineffective myelopoiesis	Uncommon	Protein-calorie malnutrition; folate, B_{12}, copper deficiency. Unusual cause of isolated neutropenia	Appropriate clinical history. BMA	Supportive care; correct nutrition/deficiency
	Viral Infection (varicella, EBV, measles, CMV, hepatitis, HIV)	Direct effect; immune-mediated	Uncommon	General—neutropenia can be mild to severe HIV—aspergillosis; pyomyositis		G-CSF sometimes used in severe neutropenia with infection

AML, acute myeloid leukemia; ANC, absolute neutrophil count; BMA, bone marrow aspirate; CBC, complete blood count; CMV, cytomegalovirus; EBV, Epstein–Barr virus; ESR, erythrocyte sedimentation rate; G-CSF, granulocyte colony stimulating factor; MDS, myelodysplasia; TMP/SMX, trimethoprim-sulfamethoxazole.

Postinfectious Neutropenia

Neutropenia can be commonly seen after viral infections, particularly in children. The neutropenia can start within a few days of the onset of infection and last several weeks. Neutrophil counts usually return to normal as the viremia resolves. Viral diseases that have been implicated include varicella, measles, rubella, hepatitis A and B, infectious mononucleosis, influenza, parvovirus, cytomegalovirus,[444–446] and Kawasaki disease. The mechanisms of the neutropenia are multiple and can involve decreased production, redistribution, and destruction of neutrophils.[447–450] In addition, virus-induced antibody can result in protracted immune neutropenia. Parvovirus B19 is commonly associated with transient neutropenia and can cause protracted leukopenia in immunosuppressed patients.[451,452]

Leukopenia is seen in more than 70% of patients with AIDS and can be associated with hypersplenism and with the presence of antineutrophil antibodies[453–455] and disordered T-cell function.[457]

Infection with *S. aureus*, brucellosis, tularemia, rickettsia, mycobacterium tuberculosis, ehrlichiosis, and leishmaniasis[447,458,459] can cause moderate neutropenia. Marked neutropenia can occur in any patient with overwhelming sepsis. This is more likely to occur in debilitated adults or in the newborn. The mechanism is probably due to exhaustion of the marrow reserve pool, and is particularly well documented in newborn sepsis.[328,329,460] Furthermore, systemic activation of complement during sepsis with production of C5a, a neutrophil activator, can result in increased adherence of neutrophils to the vascular endothelium and margination of activated cells, resulting in neutropenia.[461]

Table 50–13B Neutropenia With Normal Marrow Reserve

Neutropenia	Mechanism	Inheritance/ Frequency	Clinical History	Diagnosis	Treatment
Chronic benign neutropenia of infancy and childhood	Anti-PMN antibody most likely	Common	Median age of detection 8 months; 90% detected before 14 months of age; ANC generally <500/mm^3; no significant predisposition to infection	Normal to increased myeloid precursors. See text for details of diagnosis	Supportive, risk of infection is not high; treatment specifically to raise ANC is not indicated
Nonimmune chronic benign neutropenia	Increased apoptosis	Not uncommon	Described mainly in adults. Incidental finding on CBC. Mild neutropenia; ANC >800–1000. No evidence of rheumatic disease	Selective hypoplasia of myeloid series. Serology negative for collagen-vascular disease	Supportive, risk of infection is minimal
Ethnic or benign familial neutropenia	Unknown	Not uncommon AD	Mild neutropenia in the 800–1400 range. No increased infections. American and South African blacks, Yemenite, Black Beduin, and Falasah Jews	Diagnosis of exclusion. Low ANC in family member	None required
Autoimmune neutropenia	Antibody mediated destruction; sequestration can also occur	Not uncommon	Associated with idiopathic thrombocytopenic purpura, immune hemolytic anemia, systemic lupus erythematosus, and Felty syndrome	Increased marrow cellularity and a late maturational arrest. Some have early arrest	Treat primary autoimmune disorder; G-CSF only if marrow reserve decreased
Alloimmune neutropenia	Maternal allo-immunization	Not uncommon	Moderate to severe neutropenia in newborn period; may have increased cutaneous infections	Resolves by 3 to 4 months of age. See Fig. 50–2	G-CSF if appears septic, otherwise supportive care and observation
Drug-induced neutropenia	Antibody or complement mediated	3.4/million	Fever, sore throat, sepsis, stomatitis, pneumonia; 12%–25% mortality; 80% recover	Medication history; BMA when done demonstrates late maturation arrest	Stop unnecessary medications; can observe if normal marrow cellularity and ANC >500/mm^3
Infection-related neutropenia	Virus-induced antibody	Common	Infection specific clinical history. If bacterial sepsis, patient may have decreased marrow reserve.	Parvovirus B19 and HIV screen. See Fig. 50–2	None required to raise ANC unless early arrest
Hypersplenism	Sequestration; possible PMN destruction	Not uncommon	Usually mild neutropenia; associated with a variety of diseases: infection (malaria, TB), neoplasm, collagen-vascular diseases, hemolytic anemia	Clinical examination; blood smear with spherocytes and tailed cells	Treatment of underlying disorder; splenectomy in rare cases (usually done for anemia or thrombocytopenia)

AD, autosomal dominant; AML, acute myelogenous leukemia; ANC, absolute neutrophil count; AR, autosomal recessive; BMA, bone marrow aspirate; G-CSF, granulocyte colony stimulating factor; MDS, myelodysplastic syndrome; S, sporadic; TMP/SMX, trimethoprim-sulfamethoxazole.

Table 50–14 Screening Evaluation for Patients With Symptomatic Isolated Neutropenia

Screening Tests	SCN SDS	CN	LDGL	SLE RA	CVID	ID	MDS	Comments
Bone marrow aspirate/biopsy	↓ PA[1]		↑↓→		↑	↑↓	↓ ABN	Arrows refer to cellularity
Marrow cytogenetics	ABN[3]						ABN	
CBC 2–3 ×/week for 8 weeks	(CY[2])	CY	(CY[2])			(CY[2])		Only done it there is suggestive history
ANA, RF, anti-DNA, immune complexes			+	+				
Quantitative immunoglobulins			↑	↑	↓→	↓		CVID and ID require at least one deficiency
T + B cell quantitation					↓→	→↓		
Clonal granular lymphocytes (FACS)[4] $CD3^{+/-}$ and $CD8^+$ or $CD16^+$ or $CD56^+$ or $CD57^+$			+	±				Cytotoxic clone >5%–20%[5]
HIV screen	Should be done for most cases of neutropenia							

→ normal, ↓ decreased, ↑ increased; ABN, abnormal; CN, cyclic neutropenia; CVID, common variable immunodeficiency; ID, immunodeficiency; LDGL, lymphoproliferative disorder of granular lymphocytes; MDS, myelodysplastic syndrome; PA, progranulocyte arrest; RA, rheumatoid arthritis; SCN, severe congenital neutropenia; SDS, Shwachman–Diamond syndrome; SLE, systemic lupus.

[1]Progranulocyte arrest (PA) is classic for SCN; SDS marrow findings are variable.

[2]Seen rarely with these syndromes.

[3]May show chromosome 7 abnormality in SDS. This is not a diagnostic criteria for SDS.

[4]Double stain CD3 with other markers. A clone with 5% to 20% of lymphocytes is highly suggestive.

[5]Polyclonal patterns may evolve into a monoclonal pattern over 4 to 6 months.

Drug-Induced Neutropenia

Many therapeutic agents cause neutropenia.[462] Common agents associated with neutropenia are listed in Table 50–15.[463] The mechanism can involve direct bone marrow suppression as seen with many antineoplastic agents, antibody and complement-mediated damage to precursor cells,[464,465] or peripheral destruction and clearance of neutrophils.[363,466–468] The rapid increase in our ability to look for genetically determined drug sensitivities will likely increase our understanding of the mechanisms of many episodes of neutropenia previously thought to be idiosyncratic. The relation of clozapine-induced agranulocytosis to TNF and HLA polymorphisms is an excellent example.[458,469]

The most common presenting symptoms are fever, sore throat, pharyngitis, sepsis, stomatitis, or pneumonia.[463] Mortality rates as high as 12% to 25% have been reported, though full recovery can be expected in more than 80% of patients.[463,470] An overall annual risk of agranulocytosis of 3.4 cases per million has been reported in an ambulatory population from Israel, Europe, and northeast United States. Approximately 72% of all cases of agranulocytosis in the United States are attributed to medications, with procainamide, antithyroid drugs, and sulfasalazine being the most commonly implicated.[471] Most episodes of drug-related neutropenia are due to dose-dependent marrow suppression. Phenothiazine, semisynthetic penicillins, nonsteroidal antiinflammatory agents, aminopyrine derivatives, benzodiazepines, barbiturates, gold compounds, sulfonamides and antithyroid medications are the most common causes.[471,472] The cardiac drugs, propanolol (relative risk 2.5), dipyridamole (3.8), digoxin (2.5), and acetyldigoxin (9.9) are significantly associated with agranulocytosis. The excess risk from these drugs ranges from 1 to 3 cases per 10 million persons exposed for up to 1 week.[473] A more extensive list can be seen in Table 50–14.[463] Usually, the neutropenia becomes evident within 1 to 2 weeks of exposure to drug.[472] Recovery typically starts within a few days of stopping the drug and is preceded by the appearance of monocytes and immature neutrophils in the peripheral blood.[467] Changes in the number of circulating leukocytes may represent a primary disorder of leukocyte production or reflect a secondary response to some disease process or toxin. Early recovery occurs more frequently in patients with normal or increased marrow cellularity. In patients with pancytopenia, the median leukocyte recovery time was 14 days for patients with marrow hypoplasia and 10 days for those without marrow hypoplasia.[474] Rebound leukocytosis with marrow and peripheral blasts has been reported, simulating a leukemic state.[398,399]

Although it is always best to stop the drug if neutropenia occurs, clinical circumstances often make it difficult to do so. With certain medications, such as sulfamethoxazole, the neutropenia depends on the dose and duration of therapy. It is often possible to continue the medication with careful observation. Neutropenia secondary to anticonvulsants often places the clinician in the difficult situation of having to balance the risk of neutropenia with losing control of the seizures by stopping the medication. As long as the ANC remains above 500 to 700 cells/mm^3 and there is no infection, it may be safe to continue the medication, albeit with careful follow-up. A bone marrow aspiration can be helpful under these circumstances. A cellular, late-arrested marrow suggests the neutropenia is immune-mediated. In this case, the neutropenia is less likely to be associated with infectious risk.

Chronic Benign Neutropenia

Chronic benign neutropenia is a syndrome occurring in older children and adults. Onset can occur from childhood to late adulthood. The clinical findings and presentation are quite variable.[436,437] Neutrophil counts are commonly between 200 and 500/mm^3 and the bone marrow examination usually reveals normal to increased numbers of myeloid precursors with an arrest at metamyelocyte or band stage. Often, peripheral monocytosis is also present. Hepatosplenomegaly is not seen and no other infectious, inflammatory, or malignant diseases can account for the neutropenia. Frequently, these patients have a benign course despite the degree of neutropenia. They are able to mobilize more neutrophils to the tissue better than patients with acute drug-induced suppression of equal degree.[434] Antineutrophil antibodies, as well as other immunologic abnormalities have been seen in some patients, although these studies are usually normal.[437,475–477] Bone marrow cytogenetic studies are normal.[437,478]

Corticosteroids, splenectomy, and cytotoxic agents have been used successfully to increase neutrophil counts in these patients.[437] A patient with idiopathic neutropenia was effectively treated with human G-CSF.[479] This patient's course was benign for several years until his marrow became hypocellular, whereupon he developed multiple infections. This particular case underscores the relation between marrow reserve and propensity to infection. G-CSF has been shown to decrease the rate of infection in patients with chronic idiopathic neutropenia.[480] Because the clinical course of this disease is usually benign, treatment intended to increase the neutrophil count should be reserved for those patients with significant recurrent infectious complications.[438,458] In such cases, if the patient's marrow is cellular, other causes of immune deficiency should be explored.

Chronic Benign Neutropenia of Infancy and Childhood

Chronic benign neutropenia of infancy and childhood[481–483] is a chronic state of mature neutrophil depletion with a compensatory increase in immature granulocytes in the bone marrow.[483] This interesting subset of chronic benign neutropenia also highlights the relation between marrow reserve pool and propensity to infection. Even though these patients have severe neutropenia, they have no significant propensity to infection. They may have purulent otitis despite a neutrophil count less than 200/mm^3, emphasizing the fact that neutrophils can go to sites of infection, even though they are not seen in the peripheral blood. It is common for these patients to go several months with neutrophil counts less than 200/mm^3 and have no febrile episodes.

The median age of detection is 8 months. Though it can present any time in the first 3 years of life, 90% of patients are detected before 14 months of age. There is a slight female predominance (3 : 2) and no correlation with birth order. Neutrophil counts are usually normal at birth but very low at presentation. There is no family history of neutropenia.[435,481–483] Antineutrophil antibodies have been detected in 98% of patients by both immunofluorescent and agglutination assays.[435,482,484,485] Although the exact mechanism of the neutropenia is unclear, the fact that antineutrophil antibodies are frequently no longer detectable late in the course of the disease[435] and that antiimmune therapy is effective in raising the neutrophil counts[435,486,487] suggests an immune mechanism.[435] In spite of the immune nature of this disorder, measuring antineutrophil antibodies is of little or no practical help in diagnosis or management of the patient. There is a significant false negative rate depending on the type and number of assays used and antibodies can be found in many subjects who are not neutropenic.

Some children and adults with benign neutropenia have mucosal infections in spite of normal marrow reserve. Although the children do not become septic, the ulcers can be very bothersome. These cases are difficult to explain. However, we speculate that an antibody-induced neutrophil functional defect may contribute to the symptoms. Some of these patients have measurable defects in neutrophil movement and have been described as having the so-called lazy leukocyte syndrome.[488,489] Antibodies against functional epitopes have been seen in subjects with benign neutropenia[490] and can induce neutrophil dysfunction.[491,492] Alternatively, the mouth ulcers may be a direct effect of a vasculitis-like syndrome that is also producing the neutropenia.

Table 50–15 Causes of Agranulocytosis/Neutropenia (206 Patients, More Than One Cause Per Patient Possible)[420]

	Agranulocytosis/Neutropenia Probable[h]		Agranulocytosis/Neutropenia Possible[i]			
Drug	***A***	***B***	***A***	***B***	***Total***	***Total Agranulocytosis***
Dipyrone	7	5	4	5	21	17
Mianserin	8	2	2	3	15	13
Salazosulfapyridine (sulfalazine)	6	1	4	2	13	13
Cotrimoxazole	5	1	1	4	11	10
Antiarrhythmic agents[a]	4	1	4	1	10	10
Penicillins[b]	4	1	3	1	9	8
Thiouracil derivatives[c]	4		3	1	8	8
Phenylbutazone	2	2	2	2	8	8
Cimetidine	1	3	4		8	7
Penicillamine	1	2	1	4	8	7
Diclofenac		3	3	1	7	5
Carbamazepine	2	1	4		7	5
ACE inhibitors[d]	2	1	3		6	6
Hydrochlorothiazide with potassium sparing diuretic		3		3	6	6
Indomethacin	1	1		4	6	3
Cephalosporins[e]	1	1	1	2	5	5
Oxyphenbutazone	1		3	1	5	5
Nitrofurantoin	2	1	1	1	5	4
Salicylic acid derivatives		1		4	5	4
Clozapine	2	1	2		5	4
Carbimazole	1		3	1	5	2
Sulfonylurea derivatives[f]		2		2	4	4
Methyldopa	1	1		2	4	4
Thiamazole	2		2		4	4
Nucleosides				4	4	4
Aminoglutethimide	2	1		1	4	4
Ibuprofen		2	1	1	4	4
Pentazocine		1		3	4	3
Levamisole	2		2		4	3
Promethazine	2	2			4	3
Choramphenicol		2		1	3	3
Paracetamol and combination preparations		3			3	3
Perazine		1	1	1	3	3
Mebhydrolin	2	1			3	3
Ranitidine	1			2	3	2
Imipramine	1		2		3	2
Other drugs (all mentioned twice or less)[g]	14	13	10	12	49	42
Total	81	60	66	69	276	241

Agranulocytosis: nadir of neutrophil count ≤0.5 × 109/L . Neutropenia: nadir of neutrophil count >0.5 × 109/L but ≤1.5 × 109/L.

A = causal relation certain or probable: Drug taken within 10 days of onset of neutropenia, recovery when drug stopped, no other likely cause of the agranulocytosis or neutropenia. **B** = causal relationship possible: Same as **A**, but more than one possible cause of neutropenia present.

[a]Procainamide (2), ajmaline (l). tocainide (l), aprindine (5), and amiodarone (l)

[b]Amoxicillin (l), azlocillin (l), benzylpenicillin (3), phenethicillin (l), cloxacillin and penicillin (2)

[c]Methylthiouracil (l) and propylthiouracil (7).

[d]Captopril (5) and enalapril (l).

[e]Cephalexin (l), cephazolin (l), cefuroxime (l), cefotaxime (l), and cephradine (l).

[f]Glibenclamide (l) and tolbutamide (3).

[g]Phenytoin (2), chlorthalidone (2), sulfamethizole (2), norfloxacin (2), naproxen (2), clomipramine (2), Trazodone (2), omeprazole (2), alimemazine (2), pirenzepine. ticlopidine, ibopamine, hydralazine, nifedipine, spironolactone, nalidixic acid, doxycycline, clindamycin, gentamicin, fusidic-acid, dapsone, azapropazone, combination preparations with aminophenazone, respectively, prophenazone, sulindac, piroxicam, pirprofen, niflumic acid, allopurinol, glaphenine, valproate, levodopa with carbidopa, chlorpromazine, haloperidol, zuclopenthixol, zopiclone, cinnarizine, metronidazole, combination preparations with pyrimethamine, and theophylline.

[h]Isolated agranulocytosis or neutropenia: marrow results and complete blood count information available.

[i]Agranulocytosis or neutropenia present but results of hemoglobin, platelet count, or bone marrow aspiration not available.

Autoimmune Neutropenia

Autoimmune neutropenia has been seen as an isolated phenomenon,[466,493] secondary to other known autoimmune diseases,[466,493,494] related to infections,[448] or related to administration of drugs.[466] There is overlap with the chronic benign neutropenia syndromes mentioned previously. The term *autoimmune neutropenia* is probably more appropriately used when there is evidence for other associated immune phenomena. Immunologic mechanisms are found in cases of neutropenia that have been classified as "idiopathic."[435,466,477,480,494] Immune neutropenia can be seen in association with immune thrombocytopenia and immune hemolytic anemia.[466] In the neutropenia associated with Rh hemolytic disease, there is evidence of downregulation in neutrophil production associated with increase in erythropoiesis.[495]

Patients with autoimmune neutropenia have moderate to severe neutropenia, usually accompanied by monocytosis. Marrow cellularity is increased with a late maturation arrest. The propensity to infection is poorly correlated to the degree of neutropenia.[466,494,496] Hepatosplenomegaly has been seen in about half of the patients. The age of presentation is wide, ranging from early childhood to old age.

Neutrophil-specific antibodies to the neutrophil antigens NA1, NA2, ND1, ND2, NB1 as well as to antigens shared by erythrocytes and to HLA antigens have been detected.[485] They are detected by a variety of assays, including leukoagglutination,[485,497] opsonization,[378,494] immunochemical assays,[466] direct antibody binding,[493] complement activation[466,498] and various modifications of these techniques.[499] The antibodies are usually of the IgG and IgM type. Because of the lack of a good, readily available panel of known neutrophil antigens, most assays detect only the presence of neutrophil-associated antibody. Antibodies to CD13 have been detected in some neutropenic patients with cytomegalovirus.[500] Detection of antineutrophil antibodies is rarely helpful in establishing the diagnosis of immune neutropenia. Many people have antineutrophil antibodies and do not have neutropenia. Conversely, a negative assay does not exclude the diagnosis.[466,485] This may be due to antibody specificity for neutrophil progenitors rather than mature neutrophils.[464,465,477] When antineutrophil antibodies have been measured, the degree of neutropenia has been related to the specificity of the antibody as well as the titer.[466,493,494] In addition to neutrophil-associated antibodies, circulating immune complexes have been detected in about one-third of patients with immune neutropenia[494] and in patients with chronic idiopathic neutropenia.[476]

Antineutrophil antibodies of the IgG type have been reported in systemic lupus. These antibodies have been seen both before and after correction of neutropenia by therapy of the lupus.[466,501] Neutropenia in lupus has been attributed to neutrophil-reactive IgG, increased neutrophil apoptosis, and marrow dysfunction.[320,501–504] The mechanism of the increased neutrophil apoptosis seen in lupus may be linked to increased levels of TNF-related apoptosis-inducing ligand (TRAIL) and relative decrease in the TRAIL receptor 3, and anti-apoptotic receptor.[505] Although approximately 50% of patients with lupus are neutropenic, recurrent infection due to neutropenia is rare.[325,501]

Treatment of autoimmune neutropenia depends on the severity of the neutropenia-related symptoms and the nature of the underlying disease. Because many of these patients have a benign course, therapy solely to increase the neutrophil count is not indicated. If the patient has significant neutropenia (ANC <500/mm^3) and recurrent or severe infections, high-dose gamma globulin[486,487,506] or steroids may be used. Splenectomy provides only transient correction of the neutropenia, and results in a subsequent propensity to infection. Other cytotoxic therapy may be considered, particularly in lupus or rheumatoid arthritis.[501,507]

G-CSF has been used successfully in patients with immune neutropenia and may be considered if the patient is having problems with infection.[480] However, G-CSF must be used at the lowest dose needed to raise the neutrophil count in patients with rheumatic disease as it has been associated with flaring of lupus-associated symptoms and general worsening of the patient's condition.[508,509]

Isoimmune Neonatal Neutropenia

Moderate to severe neutropenia can occur in newborn infants secondary to IgG antibodies transferred from mother to infant. The pathogenesis of this disorder is identical to that of Rh hemolytic disease with prenatal sensitization to neutrophil antigens resulting in production of antibodies to FcRγIIIb that then cross the placenta.[458,485,510] The incidence has been estimated at 2 per 1000 live births.[458,510] If the infant is clearly septic or if subsequent episodes of bacterial infection occur, then marrow aspiration should be considered to rule out primary neutropenia. If there is early arrest or storage pool depletion, treatment with granulocyte transfusion or colony-stimulating factor should be considered.

Neutropenia in Infants of Hypertensive Mothers

Neutrophil counts as low as 500/mm^3 have been reported in infants of hypertensive mothers.[511] Forty-nine percent of infants of hypertensive mothers had neutropenia that lasted from 1 hour to 30 days.[512] Neutropenia was more common in infants who had growth retardation or whose mothers had severe hypertension. Thrombocytopenia to 90,000/mm^3 was also seen.[512] The neutropenia seems to be due to marrow suppression and may be associated with a slightly increased incidence of infection.[511–513]

Pure White Cell Aplasia

Pure white cell aplasia (PWCA) is a rare syndrome characterized by severe pyogenic infections and neutropenia. Many (70%) of these patients have an associated thymoma. In some cases, PWCA occurred years after thymoma removal. Bone marrow examination shows almost complete absence of myeloid precursors with normal erythroid precursors and megakaryocytes. This is in contrast to T-gamma neutropenia or Kostmann syndrome, where early myeloid precursors are seen. Marrow inhibitory activity is found in both IgG and IgM fractions of patient's serum and goes away as the marrow recovers.[464,465,514–516] In some cases, the inhibitory activity is in the lymphocyte fractions and not in the serum. PWCA has been associated with ibuprofen therapy. In vitro serum inhibitory activity required the presence of the drug and of complement. The clinical syndrome resolved when ibuprofen was discontinued.[465] PWCA has also been associated with chlorpropamide[517] and certain natural remedies.[518] In cases associated with thymomas, removal of the mass is indicated but may not result in resolution of the neutropenia. Cytoxan, steroids, as well as cyclosporin A have been effective in treatment of PWCA, as has IV IgG.[519,520]

Neutropenia Associated with Immunologic Abnormalities

Neutropenia has been seen in association with a number of immunologic abnormalities. The patients usually present in childhood with frequent bacterial infections, hepatosplenomegaly, and failure to thrive. Some of these children die in the first few years of life. Hypergammaglobulinemia or hypogammaglobulinemia,[521–524] T-cell defects,[525,526] NK cell abnormalities,[475] and autoimmune phenomena[526,527] have been seen. Many of the reported patients had a positive family history of neutropenia.[521–523] Neutropenia is seen in 26% of patients with X-linked agammaglobulinemia and 40% to 50% of patients with X-linked hyper-IgM syndrome and has been associated with decreased marrow production of neutrophils.[524,528] The neutropenia can be chronic, episodic, or cyclic. The most common form of hyper-IgM syndrome is due to mutations in CD40, resulting in marked depression of IgG and IgA with elevation of IgM.[529] Chronic diarrhea, skin rashes, recurrent viral infection may also be seen in these children. The treatment in these disorders depends on the constellation of immunologic abnormalities present. Some of these patients have been treated with bone marrow transplantation.[525]

Neutropenia is also associated with a number of other rare primary immunodeficiency syndromes.[529] Common variable immunodeficiency (CVID) is the most frequent primary immunodeficiency. Its frequency has been estimated at 0.0092 and is associated with certain HLA haplotypes.[530] These patients usually present in the second decade, although they may present in childhood. They have a variety of immunologic abnormalities and usually present with recurrent infection. They are prone to autoimmune disorders, including autoimmune neutropenia.[529] This syndrome should be considered in patients who present as benign neutropenia and subsequently develop significant recurrent infection. In contrast to benign neutropenia, children with global immune defects associated with neutropenia have manifestations of recurrent or unusual infections.

The majority of patients with AIDS have neutropenia as well as anemia. About 30% have thrombocytopenia.[531] Neutropenia has been seen in up to 8% of asymptomatic HIV carriers. The bone marrow is usually hypercellular and has lymphoid aggregates and plasmacytosis. There are commonly dysplastic changes in the granulocytes. The neutropenia is felt to be due to ineffective hematopoiesis. The immunoglobulin fraction of HIV-positive serum inhibits CFU-GM and BFU-E in vitro and thus may contain antibodies to progenitors.

Neutropenia and Lymphoproliferative Disorders of Granular Lymphocytes

A number of somewhat heterogeneous disorders can be grouped under the general name of lymphoproliferative disorders of granular lymphocytes (LDGL) and have been variously called large granular lymphocyte (LGL) leukemia, Felty syndrome, T-gamma lymphocytosis, and T- and natural killer (NK) cell-LGL leukemia.[325,532,533] Approximately 80% of patients with LDGL present with neutropenia during the course of evaluation for recurrent infections.[534] The median age of onset is 55 to 65 years, although it has also been seen in children. There may also be a history of rheumatoid arthritis. Splenomegaly occurs in many of the patients but enlarged liver or lymphadenopathy is not common. The peripheral blood usually, but not always, shows lymphocytosis, with prominent large granular lymphocytes. The bone marrow in these disorders is normocellular to somewhat hypocellular and may have an early myeloid arrest. Most patients follow a benign course for many years. However, some patients die of progressive lymphoproliferation or of sepsis related to neutropenia. Although the course may be relatively protracted and benign, the lymphocytosis does represent a clonal proliferation and is felt by some to be malignant.[527,535]

More than 50% of LDGL patients have other associated disorders such as lupus or rheumatoid arthritis. The most common clinical features are recurrent infection (>50%), splenomegaly (>45%), severe neutropenia (>30%), lymphocytic marrow infiltration (>57%), recurrent infection (>50%), anemia (>45%), positive ANA (>30%), positive rheumatoid factor (>40%), hypergammaglobulinemia (>40%), and immune complexes (>40%).[533] Interestingly, these findings overlap with those of rheumatoid arthritis and Felty syndrome. About one-third of patients with rheumatoid arthritis and neutropenia have LGL proliferation. Felty syndrome (rheumatoid arthritis, splenomegaly, and neutropenia) is associated with decreased granulocyte survival as well as decreased production.[536–538] Infection is the major cause of death in Felty syndrome. Nearly all patients with Felty syndrome are HLA-DR4 positive, whether LGL clones are present or not, whereas patients with LGL proliferation not associated with arthritis have a normal prevalence of HLA-DR4. These findings suggest that rheumatoid arthritis, Felty syndrome, and LDGL may be part of the same general disease process.[539–541]

Lymphoproliferative disorders of granular lymphocytes are associated with a chronic clonal proliferation of $CD3^+$ or $CD3^-$ lymphocytes that are also $CD8^+$, $CD16^+$, $CD56^+$, or $CD57^+$. The disorder was initially associated with lymphocytosis and has been defined as a granular lymphocytosis greater than 2000/μL of more than 6 months' duration.[542] However, it is now recognized that patients can have increased populations of LGL without absolute lymphocytosis. These lymphocytes can be either $CD3^+$ or $CD3^-$, reflecting a T-LGL or NK-LGL phenotype, respectively. Most $CD3^+$ granular lymphocytes (GL) are $CD16^+$. Because the $CD3^+CD16^+$ subset represents less than 5% of lymphocytes in healthy subjects, an increase in this population is very suggestive of LDGL. Approximately 75% to 80% of LDGL patients have $CD3^+CD8^+$ clones and 90% to 100% have $CD57^+$ clones. Approximately 30% have $CD3^-CD16^+CD56^+$ clones. Most cases show a single clone, although polyclonal cases have been seen. In the latter case, repeat study over a 6-month period is recommended to see if a single clone evolves. Although a homogeneous pattern of monoclonal antibody reactivity strongly suggests LDGL, confirmation by studying T-cell receptor rearrangement is optimal.[325,533] Cytotoxic T-cell clones have also been seen in association with other immunologically mediated hematologic disorders including pure red cell aplasia, aplastic anemia,[543] autoimmune hemolytic anemia,[544] post organ transplant,[545] and in other hematologic disorders not associated with neutropenia.[545]

The neutropenia in LDGL has been associated with increase in the rate of apoptosis of granulocytes likely mediated through FAS. In fact, these patients have increased circulating levels of FAS ligand, which drop substantially or disappear after treatment with methotrexate.[323]

Neutropenia and associated infection is the most common reason that LDGL patients require treatment. Methotrexate or cyclosporin A is the treatment of choice for the neutropenia associated with LDGL.[325] In a series of 29 patients, the overall response rate to methotrexate was 85.7% with doses in the 10 mg/M^2 per week range. The overall response rate to cyclosporine A, 1 to 6.7 mg/kg/day, was 78.2%, with a median time to response of about 1 month. The median time to recurrence was 4.5 years. Therapy can be stopped with no recurrence in some patients. Deoxycoformycin and cyclophosphamide have also been used.[546] Improvement in neutropenia and decrease in antineutrophil antibody levels with methotrexate treatment or with cyclosporin A has been reported in patients with Felty syndrome,[507,547] even though the LGL clone persists after treatment.[548] About half of patients do not experience any infections in spite of continued neutropenia.[549]

Treatment with G-CSF has been reported to be successful in management of complications of neutropenia due to Felty syndrome.[549] Although G-CSF can be a useful adjunct to therapy in selected cases, it should always be used with caution as exacerbation of vasculitis has been reported with its use. The dose should start low (3 μg/kg/day) and be increased gradually, usually with concomitant low- to medium-dose prednisone.[325] A high dose of GCSF may be required initially to overcome the effects of the T-cell clone. However, as cyclosporin becomes effective, the dose of GCSF may have to be reduced dramatically to prevent significant neutrophilia.

Neutropenia Associated with Metabolic Diseases

Neutropenia can be associated with ketoacidosis in patients with hyperglycemia, hyperglycinuria, orotic aciduria, and methylmalonic aciduria.[550–553]

Glycogen-storage disease type 1a is due to mutations in glucose-6-phosphatase (GSDase) and type 1b is due to mutation in the glucose-6-phosphate transporter. Both type 1a and 1b are associated with hypoglycemia, dyslipidemia, hyperuricemia, elevated lactic acid, and hepatosplenomegaly. Although not seen with glycogen storage disease type Ia, neutropenia is commonly observed in association with glycogen storage disease type Ib. Recurrent infections are a major source of morbidity in these patients. In particular, gastrointestinal inflammation leads to an inflammatory bowel disease-like picture.[554] The degree of neutropenia is variable but absolute neutrophil counts commonly are less than $500/mm^3$. The bone marrow is normocellular or hypercellular. Variable functional defects have been seen in the neutrophils from these patients, including motility and oxidative metabolism defects.[555–558] The gene for the glucose-6-phosphate transporter that is defective in glycogen storage disease type Ib has been mapped to chromosome 11q23[559,560] and there are now at least sixteen known mutations of the gene encoding glucose-6-phosphate translocase (G6PT1). Some of these mutations abolish transport activity whereas others result in up to 23% residual activity. There seems to be no correlation between the mutation or level of residual enzyme activity and presence or degree of neutropenia. Overall, mutations have been seen in 94% of 284 independent alleles, with the 400X mutation being most common and present in 23.6 of the alleles.[561] Inhibition of G6PT1 found in neutrophil microsomes results in increased apoptosis[562] and is consistent with the finding of apoptosis of circulating neutrophils of patients with GCS1b.[322] Furthermore, transfer of $G6PT^{-/-}$ marrow into to wild type mice produced chimeric ($BM\text{-}Gls\text{-}6\text{-}PT^{-/-}$) mice that have impaired neutrophil function and neutropenia, suggesting that G6PT is necessary for neutrophil function and may play a role in the neutropenia of GSC1b.[563] Patients with glycogen storage disease Ib have been treated with G-CSF and GM-CSF.[554] Two patients with severe Crohn-like symptoms were greatly helped by treatment with GM-CSF.[554,564] Interestingly, both of these patients had hypercellular marrows with no evidence of arrest. Neutrophil counts went up within hours of injection of G-CSF and twice daily dosing was required to maintain granulocyte counts, suggesting a clear role in promoting release of granulocytes from the marrow storage pool.[554]

Neutropenia Due to Increased Margination

Both acute and chronic neutropenia can occur because of complement activation.[443,461,565–568] This mechanism was first recognized in patients undergoing hemodialysis and is associated with pulmonary dysfunction.[566,567] The C5a generated during activation stimulates neutrophils, resulting in increased adherence and aggregation and subsequent entrapment in the pulmonary vasculature.[461,568] Similar activation of complement and neutropenia has been seen with the use of membrane oxygenators.[569] Complement-mediated neutropenia due to shifts in the neutrophil pools has also been seen with burns[316] and transfusion reactions.[443] Because lung dysfunction and pulmonary infiltrates have been seen in some of these processes, the neutrophil has been implicated in the pathophysiology of adult respiratory distress syndrome (ARDS).[316,443,568] However, the occurrence of ARDS and severe neutropenia without neutrophilic infiltration of the lungs suggests that mechanisms other than direct damage to the lungs by neutrophils are possible.[570] Neutropenia may be related to complement-mediated destruction of neutrophils as seen in PNH[571,572] or due to similar destruction of granulocyte precursors.[464,465,498]

Neutropenia Associated with Hypersplenism

Neutropenia can be seen in association with hypersplenism. Usually, the neutropenia is not severe enough to cause symptoms, unless there is an antibody present. Anemia and thrombocytopenia are usually also present. Improvement in the hypersplenism-induced neutropenia in a patient with AIDS was obtained by splenic embolization.[573]

Neutropenia Associated with Nutritional Deficiency

Neutropenia has been seen in association with anemia in nutritional deficiency of vitamin B_{12}, folate, and copper.[574–576] All of these neutropenia syndromes are characterized by ineffective myelopoiesis and megaloblastic changes in the bone marrow. Similar findings have been seen in the inherited deficiency of transcobalamin II.[577] Neutropenia and megaloblastic changes have also been seen in association with sideroblastic anemia in the DIDMOAD syndrome (diabetes insipidus, diabetes mellitus, optic atrophy, deafness). The hematologic abnormalities were responsive to thiamine.[577]

Primary Causes of Neutropenia

There have been significant advances in our understanding of the mechanisms of primary neutropenia that have come in large part from the study of very rare primary neutropenia syndromes or hereditary bone marrow failure states. It is very likely that many of these disorders will eventually be diagnosed by molecular diagnostic approaches in the near future. The primary neutropenia syndromes with known genetic mechanisms are noted in Table 50–16, many of which have commercially available mutational analysis.

Ethnic or Benign Familial Neutropenia

Neutropenia has been seen in several ethnic groups and has been referred to as ethnic, pseudo-, or benign familial neutropenia. The level of neutropenia is usually mild and is not associated with any increased propensity to serious infection. Benign familial neutropenia is characterized by neutrophil counts in the 800 to $1400/mm^3$ range and no propensity to infection.[578] The disorder has dominant inheritance. The bone marrow is normocellular.[579,580] Ethnic neutropenia has been seen in American Blacks,[276] South African Blacks,[276,581] Yemenite Jews,[277,581] Black Beduin, and Falasah Jews.[581] Although this entity is generally benign,[578,580,582] periodontal problems have been described in some of these patients.[583–585]

Nonimmune Chronic Idiopathic Neutropenia

Nonimmune chronic idiopathic neutropenia is described mainly in adults and is characterized by a mild neutropenia below the normal range for a given ethnic population and a benign course. It differs from what we have called chronic benign neutropenia in that the neutropenia is generally milder and marrow shows selective hypoplasia of the granulocyte lineage with increased immature-to-mature cell ratio. The patients are asymptomatic, have no concomitant rheumatic disease or other systemic disease and no detectable antineutrophil antibodies. Although there is no significant splenomegaly, some enlargement can be detected by ultrasound.[586] They have few infections and the outcome of the infections is favorable. There is a female predominance and an HLA class II genetic predisposition.[587–589] We list it separately because the neutropenia is now believed to be secondary to apoptosis of early myeloid precursors at the $CD34^+/CD33^-$ stage. This is associated with increased expression of Fas in $CD34^+/CD33^-$ cells but not in later myeloid cells. Decreased clonogenic potential and increased production of TNF-α, IFN-gamma, and FasL have also been reported in stromal cells from chronic idiopathic neutropenia subjects.[441] There is some evidence that mutations in GFL-1 may be responsible for some cases of nonimmune chronic neutropenia.[590]

Severe Congenital Neutropenia

Severe congenital neutropenia (SCN) was described by Kostmann in 1956.[591] It presents in early infancy with severe, recurrent infections and neutropenia. There is a significant monocytosis associated with the neutropenia, as is also seen in cyclic neutropenia, suggesting a reciprocal relation between these two cell types that are derived from the same progenitor.[592] Most cases of SCN arise sporadically, consistent with the transmission as an often lethal autosomal dominant disorder.[570,592,593] In the original cohort, transmission appeared

Table 50–16 Neutropenia Syndromes With Known Gene Defects
Neutropenia due to genetic mutations

Syndrome	Incidence	Genetics	Gene	Chromosome	% with a mutation	Comments	References[b]
Severe congenital neutropenia[a]	1–2:10⁶	Sporadic AD	ELA2	19p13.3	≈60%	ELA2 mutations more common in severe forms. Progranulocyte arrest in bone marrow. Preleukemic	1, 2
		AR	HAX1	1q	≈10%	"Classic Kostmann syndrome." HAX1 deficiency: Increased threshold for apoptosis. Preleukemic	3
		AD	GFI-1	1p22	<5%	Neutropenia and T/B cell deficiency. Regulates ELA2 leading to increased elastase. Other mutations may give milder phenotypes	4, 5
Cyclic neutropenia*	1–2:10⁶	AD	ELA2	19p13.3	60%–80%	Diagnose by getting a CBC 2 to 3 times/week for 8 weeks with ANC nadir <200/mm³	1, 4
Shwachman–Diamond*	Estimate carrier 1:277, disease 1:76,563	AR	SBDS	7p10–7q11	90%	Neutropenia, short stature, pancreatic dysfunction, may have anemia or thrombocytopenia as well. G-CSF helps, not always needed. Preleukemic	6, 8
Wiskott–Aldrich*	4:10⁶	X	WASP	Xp11.23		Rare cause of SCN. Decreased lymphocyte/NK numbers	6, 26
Myelokathexis (WHIM syndrome)	40 cases	AD	CXCR4	2q21		Hypersegmented PMN, more prominent in BMA. CXCR4 mediates homing of stem cells to marrow and retention of mature neutrophils. G-CSF may help	6, 7
Dyskeratosis congenita*	1:10⁶	X, AD, AR	DKC1 TERC	Xq28 3q21–28	36%	Integument disorder, marrow failure in 80% by third decade, marrow failure can precede skin changes. Disordered telomerase function. Median survival 16 years. Preleukemic	9, 10
Cartilage hair hypoplasia	1:23,000	AR	RMRP	9p13		Impaired cellular immunity, 27% have neutropenia, the marrow shows a myelocyte arrest in some. G-CSF may be of benefit	11, 12
Chédiak–Higashi	1:10⁶	AR	LYST	1q42		Hypopigmentation, large inclusions in myeloid, lymphoid, and other cells. Develop HLH picture that can be fatal	13–15
Griscelli syndrome		AR	Rab27a	15q21		Hypopigmentation of skin and hair, abnormal immune regulation. Develop HLH picture	6, 16
Hermansky–Pudlak II	4 cases	AR	AP3B1	5q14.1		Hypopigmentation, T-cell defects, bleeding, neutropenia	17
P14 deficiency	1 family	AR	P14	1q21		Albinism, neutropenia, cellular marrow with maturation, T- and B-cell defects. Short stature. Reason for neutropenia not clear	18
Cohen syndrome	136 cases	AR	COH1	8q22–q23	94%	Typical facies, developmental delay, retinal dystrophy, intermittent neutropenia with normal marrow	19–23
Barth syndrome*	1:400,000	X	TAZ1	Xq28		3-Methylgluconic aciduria, short stature, myocardiopathy, skeletal myopathy. Severe cardiolipin deficiency; 25% have neutropenia, which may be cyclic	24, 25
Glycogen storage disease 1b*	1:100,000	AR	G6PT1	11q23	97%	IBD like picture, hypoglycemia, hepatosplenomegaly, neutrophil and platelet dysfunction. Hypoglycemia, Responds to G-CSF, marrow hypercellular. Mutations do not correlate with clinical phenotype	4, 30

Table 50–16 Neutropenia Syndromes With Known Gene Defects—cont'd

Syndrome	Incidence	Genetics	Gene	Chromosome	% with a mutation	Comments	References[b]
Hyper-IgM*	1:10^6	X AR	CD40-LG	Xq26–28 12p13	91%	IgG, IgA, IgE deficient. 60% present with neutropenia. Neutropenia is due to immune dysfunction	27–29
Chronic nonimmune neutropenia in adults	1:60 overall in Crete	AD	GFI-1	1p22		One CIN patient identified with this mutation which not the same mutation seen in SCN	5, 31

IBD, inflammatory bowl disease, AP, apoptosis; X, X-linked; AD, autosomal dominant, AR, autosomal recessive; ELA2, Elastase; AP3b1, adapter-related protein 3 beta-1; Rab27a, RAS associated protein 27a; G6PT1, glucose-6-phosphate translocase, TAZ, taffazin; GFI-1, growth factor independent-1;WASP, Wiskott–Aldrich protein; LYST, Lysosomal trafficking regulator; P14, mitogen activated protein kinase binding partner interacting protein; DKC1, Dyskerin-1; TERC, telomerase RNA component; HAX1, HS1 associated protein X1; SBDS, Shwachman–Bodian–Diamond syndrome; RMRP, RNA component of mitochondrial RNA processing endoribonuclease; WHIM, Warts hypogammaglobulinemia immune deficiency myelokathexis.

[a]Mutational analysis available commercially.

[b]*References:* (1) Bellanne-Chantelot C, Clauin S, Leblanc T, et al: Mutations in the ELA2 gene correlate with more severe expression of neutropenia: A study of 81 patients from the French Neutropenia Register. Blood 103:4119, 2004; (2) Horwitz MS, Duan Z, Korkmaz B, Lee HH, Mealiffe ME, Salipante SJ: Neutrophil elastase in cyclic and severe congenital neutropenia. Blood 109:1817, 2007; (3) Klein C, Grudzien M, Appaswamy G, et al: HAX1 deficiency causes autosomal recessive severe congenital neutropenia (Kostmann disease). Nat Genet 39:86, 2007; (4) Welte K, Zeidler C, Dale DC: Severe congenital neutropenia. Semin Hematol 43:189, 2006; (5) Person RE, Li FQ, Duan Z, et al: Mutations in proto-oncogene GFI1 cause human neutropenia and target ELA2. Nat Genet 34:308, 2003; (6) Stein SM, Dale DC: Molecular basis and therapy of disorders associated with chronic neutropenia. Curr Allergy Asthma Rep 3:385, 2003; (7) Kawai T, Choi U, Cardwell L, et al: WHIM syndrome myelokathexis reproduced in the NOD/SCID mouse xenotransplant model engrafted with healthy human stem cells transduced with C-terminus-truncated CXCR4. Blood 109:78, 2007; (8) Shimamura A: Shwachman-Diamond syndrome. Semin Hematol 43:178, 2006; (9) Vulliamy T, Dokal I: Dyskeratosis congenita. Semin Hematol 43:157, 2006; (10) Knight S, Vulliamy T, Copplestone A, Gluckman E, Mason P, Dokal I: Dyskeratosis congenita (DC) registry: Identification of new features of DC. Br J Haematol 103:990, 1998; (11) Ammann RA, Duppenthaler A, Bux J, Aebi C: Granulocyte colony-stimulating factor-responsive chronic neutropenia in cartilage-hair hypoplasia. J Pediatr Hematol Oncol 26:379, 2004; (12) Liu JM, Ellis SR: Ribosomes and marrow failure: Coincidental association or molecular paradigm? Blood 107:4583, 2006; (13) Ward DM, Shiflett SL, Kaplan J: Chediak-Higashi syndrome: A clinical and molecular view of a rare lysosomal storage disorder. Curr Mol Med 2:469, 2002; (14) Introne W, Boissy RE, Gahl WA: Clinical, molecular, and cell biological aspects of Chediak-Higashi syndrome. Mol Genet Metab 68:283, 1999; (15) Dufourcq-Lagelouse R, Lambert N, Duval M, et al: Chediak-Higashi syndrome associated with maternal uniparental isodisomy of chromosome 1. Eur J Hum Genet 7:633, 1999; (16) Gazit R, Aker M, Elboim M, et al: NK cytotoxicity mediated by CD16 but not by NKp30 is functional in Griscelli syndrome. Blood 2007; (17) Enders A, Zieger B, Schwarz K, et al: Lethal hemophagocytic lymphohistiocytosis in Hermansky-Pudlak Syndrome Type II. Blood 2006; (18) Bohn G, Allroth A, Brandes G, et al: A novel human primary immunodeficiency syndrome caused by deficiency of the endosomal adaptor protein p14. Nat Med 13:38, 2007; (19) Kolehmainen J, Black GC, Saarinen A, et al: Cohen syndrome is caused by mutations in a novel gene, COH1, encoding a transmembrane protein with a presumed role in vesicle-mediated sorting and intracellular protein transport. Am J Hum Genet 72:1359, 2003; (20) Kolehmainen J, Wilkinson R, Lehesjoki AE, et al: Delineation of Cohen syndrome following a large-scale genotype-phenotype screen. Am J Hum Genet 75:122, 2004; (21) Chandler KE, Biswas S, Lloyd IC, Parry N, Clayton-Smith J, Black GC: The ophthalmic findings in Cohen syndrome. Br J Ophthalmol 86:1395, 2002; (22) Kivitie-Kallio S, Rajantie J, Juvonen E, Norio R: Granulocytopenia in Cohen syndrome. Br J Haematol 98:308, 1997; (23) Taban M, Memoracion-Peralta DS, Wang H, Al-Gazali LI, Traboulsi EI: Cohen syndrome: Report of nine cases and review of the literature, with emphasis on ophthalmic features. J Aapos 2007; (24) Spencer CT, Bryant RM, Day J, et al: Cardiac and clinical phenotype in Barth syndrome. Pediatrics 118:e337, 2006; (25) Schlame M, Ren M: Barth syndrome, a human disorder of cardiolipin metabolism. FEBS Lett 580:5450, 2006; (26) Ancliff PJ, Blundell MP, Cory GO, et al: Two novel activating mutations in the Wiskott-Aldrich syndrome protein result in congenital neutropenia. Blood 108:2182, 2006; (27) Winkelstein JA, Marino MC, Ochs H, et al: The X-linked hyper-IgM syndrome: Clinical and immunologic features of 79 patients. Medicine (Baltimore) 82:373, 2003; (28) Kitchen BJ, Boxer LA: Large granular lymphocyte leukemia (LGL) in a child with hyper IgM syndrome and autoimmune hemolytic anemia. Pediatr Blood Cancer 2006; (29) Cham B, Bonilla MA, Winkelstein J: Neutropenia associated with primary immunodeficiency syndromes. Semin Hematol 39:107, 2002; (30) Melis D, Fulceri R, Parenti G, et al: Genotype/phenotype correlation in glycogen storage disease type 1b: A multicentre study and review of the literature. Eur J Pediatr 164:501, 2005; (31) Papadaki HA, Palmblad J, Eliopoulos GD: Non-immune chronic idiopathic neutropenia of adult: An overview. Eur J Haematol 67:35, 2001.

to be as a recessive trait.[591,594] Rare cases of X-linked inheritance have also been described that are now recognized as mutations of the Wiskott–Aldrich syndrome gene. The mutations resulting in neutropenia differ from other WASP mutations in that they do not result in complete loss of the WASP protein.[595,596] Bone marrow examination reveals myeloid hypoplasia with an arrest at the promyelocyte stage and ultrastructural examination shows abnormalities in granule production in some patients.[570] Bone marrow culture studies generally show colony growth[478,597] when exogenous colony-stimulating factors are provided.

Mutations in the neutrophil elastase gene (*ELA2*) have been found in patients with SCN.[319,590,598–603] At least 45 different heterozygous constitutional mutations of ELA2 have been seen in patients with SCN, with frequencies ranging from 38%[604] to 78%.[592] ELA2 mutations are also seen in patients with cyclic neutropenia. There are no clear relationships between the specific mutations and the type of neutropenia. There seems to be a set of mutations that are seen in SCN but not in cyclic neutropenia and a group that are seen in both disorders.[592] In addition to direct mutations in *ELA2*, mutations in GFI-1, a transcriptional oncoprotein, have been found in a kindred with SCN. The severity of the neutropenia associated with this dominant mutation was variable within the family. Mutations in GFI-1 cause overexpression of *ELA2*, suggesting that they may be involved in the mechanism of the neutropenia. Interestingly, other mutations in GFI-1 have been seen in patients with chromic nonimmune neutropenia.[590] In contrast to the dominant inheritance of the *ELA2* mutations, the original kindred described by Kostmann seemed to be autosomal recessive in inheritance.[591] Evaluations of patients with recessive inheritance including members of the original kindred revealed mutations in HAX1, which participates in B-cell receptor–mediated signal transduction and may be involved in control of apoptosis.[605] This suggests that HAX1 is responsible for the recessively inherited or "classical" form of Kostmann syndrome. Although there are some theories regarding common pathways in these disorders, there is no clear genetic mechanism for the neutropenia.[592,601] Moreover, although the exact pathways remain unclear, the neutropenia is ultimately due in part to increased apoptosis of marrow myeloid cells.[606]

The G-CSF receptor seemed like a logical choice in the search for the cause of SCN. Although mutations have been found, they are a very rare cause of SCN and can be associated with hyporesponsiveness to G-CSF.[607,608] Mutations in the G-CSF receptor (CSF3R) have been detected in patients who developed leukemia.[609] However, it is not clear how much these contribute to malignant transformation in SCN patients.[602] Such mutations have not been detected at birth but they seem to arise spontaneously, including in SCN subjects who do not have malignancy.[592] This suggests that they are not responsible for the neutropenia and are acquired postnatally.[610] Approximately 78% of SCN patients with evidence of malignant transformation have a CSF3R mutation. However, when patients with CSF3R mutation and no evidence of malignancy were followed, rapid progression to leukemia did not ensue in spite of evidence for highly clonal hematopoiesis.[609]

Approximately 90% of SCN patients respond to G-CSF with increased cell counts or total correction of their neutropenia.[610–614] Treatment may require doses of G-CSF of 5 to 20 μg/kg/day up to as much as 100 μg/kg/day.[610–612,615] Prior to the availability of G-CSF, most of these patients died of infection at an early age. Some patients also develop myelodysplastic syndrome or myeloid leukemia, regardless of their response to treatment. Although there have been some concerns that G-CSF may provoke malignant transformation, there is no clear evidence that this is the case.[612] According to data from the Severe Congenital Neutropenia International Registry (SCNIR), the likelihood of malignant transformation is dependent on responsiveness to G-CSF. Those patients who required more than 8 μg/kg/day and still were not able to maintain an absolute neutrophil count greater than 2188/μL had a cumulative risk for myelodysplasia (MDS) or acute myeloid leukemia (AML) of 40% at 10 years and a 14% risk of death from sepsis. Patients who required less than 8 μg/kg/day and had neutrophil counts more than 2188/μL had a cumulative incidence for MDS/AML of 15% at 10 years and 3% for death from sepsis.[616] In one study, SCN patients could also be classified as high or low risk based on presence of the ELA2 mutation. Presence of this mutation correlated with a younger age at diagnosis (median 2.8 months vs 16.8 months), lower absolute neutrophil counts (0.13 × 109/L vs 0.38 × 109/L), higher monocyte counts (1.33 × 109/L vs 0.96 × 109/L), higher incidence of infection, and a higher incidence of malignant transformation.[604]

More than 90% of patients with this previously fatal disorder respond well to G-CSF. The usual starting dose is 5 μg/kg/day subcutaneously. However, as mentioned earlier, a higher dose is often required. Blood counts in patients with SCN cycle as seen in cyclic neutropenia in response to treatment with GCSF.[603] This can make monitoring of the counts and dose adjustment difficult, especially if the cycle of the neutrophil count is poorly synchronized with the frequency of clinic visits. We find the routine monitoring of the sedimentation rate and C-reactive protein to be useful in following these patients. If the neutrophil counts on average are in an acceptable range, the sedimentation rate and CRP will be in a normal range. Elevation in these parameters or inflammatory anemia should evoke a search for occult infection, particularly in the sinuses and lung. Because the neutrophil counts can vary significantly with administration of the same dose of G-CSF, the G-CSF dose should not be increased on the basis of a single low neutrophil count, especially if the patient is otherwise doing well and the sedimentation rates have been low. The possibility that the neutrophil counts are cycling should be considered before increasing the G-CSF dose. Because of the chance of malignant transformation, progressive anemia, thrombocytopenia, or macrocytosis warrants reexamination of the marrow and evaluation of marrow cytogenetics.

Although G-CSF is the primary treatment for SCN, bone marrow transplantation should be considered, if there is a sibling donor. This is particularly true if the patient is in a high-risk group by virtue of high G-CSF requirement or presence of the ELA2 gene.[604,616] In small uncontrolled series, 9 of 11 patients had a favorable outcome with marrow transplantation.[617] Transplantation is also an important option in SCN patients who develop progressive myelodysplastic changes or frank leukemia, although the outcome is very poor for patients transplanted under these circumstances.[618]

Cyclic Neutropenia

Cyclic neutropenia is a rare, dominantly inherited disorder with variable expression and is characterized by neutropenia that recurs every 14 to 35 days, although more than 90% of the patients exhibit a cycle period of 21 days.[321] Associated recurrent fever, pharyngitis, gingivitis, stomatitis, and bacterial infections are observed in most patients. The severity of the infections parallels the severity of the neutropenia, and can vary from patient to patient. Although the disease tends to be benign, several patients have died of infection.[619] Most of the patients present in the first year of life; however, there is also an adult-onset form. The disorder can persist for many years but tends to decrease in severity with time. Cyclic fever due to cyclic neutropenia must be differentiated from cyclic fevers associated with TNF-receptor mutations or hyper-IgD,[620–623] which are not associated with neutropenia.

Cyclic neutropenia can be cured by bone marrow transplantation in an animal model[619] and has been transferred from an affected human donor to a recipient during bone marrow transplantation.[624] The bone marrow during times of neutropenia is usually hypoplastic with a myelocyte arrest.[619,625,626] At the onset of the neutropenia, postmitotic cells are absent from the marrow but earlier precursors are present. Microscopic studies during all phases of the cycle show cellular blebbing and nuclear condensation, typical of apoptosis. Furthermore, flow cytometric studies show increased numbers of annexin-V labeled myeloid precursors, indicating selective apoptotic death resulting in removal of neutrophil precursors.[627] Consistent with these observations, early mathematical models of hematopoiesis predicted that oscillations would occur if there were an increased rate of irreversible cell loss in the stem cell pool.[606,628–630]

Cyclic neutropenia has been attributed to mutations in the elastase gene (ELA2) on chromosome 19p13.3.[600,601,603,631] The mutations occur in exon 4 or 5 or at the junction of exon 4 and intron 4. Mutations occur in only one allele of the ELA gene, suggesting a gain of function or aberrant function mutation.[321,600,603] Unlike in SCN, presence of the ELA2 mutation does not have a significant effect on disease severity and does not predict a worse outcome.[604] Also, unlike SCD, cyclic neutropenia is not associated with malignant transformation.[616]

The diagnosis of cyclic neutropenia is established by documentation of periodic neutropenia. This requires monitoring of the neutrophil counts at least twice and preferably three times a week for 8 weeks. Bone marrow aspiration is not helpful. The nadir of the neutropenia usually lasts 3 to 5 days and can be missed if the patient is monitored less frequently than two to three times per week. To establish the diagnosis, there must be regular cyclic fluctuations in neutrophil count with a nadir of less than 200/mm^3 at a period of approximately 21 days. Interestingly, patients may report an increased sense of well-being as their counts recover to greater than 500/mm^3.[472] Note that the cycling phenomenon can occur intermittently throughout the course of cyclic neutropenia.[603] It is not uncommon to see patients whose neutrophil counts cycle with nadirs in the 500 to 1000/mm^3 range. These patients usually do not have any symptoms nor do they have the signs of chronic gingival infection characteristic of patients with chronic severe neutropenia. The diagnosis of cyclic neutropenia is reserved for patients with neutrophil counts that periodically fall below 200 to 300/mm^3.

Patients with cyclic neutropenia as defined above almost always have or will soon develop severe dental, gingival, and mucosal infection and therefore should be treated with G-CSF. Most patients respond at doses in the range of 2 to 3 μg/kg every 1 to 2 days and do not usually require the higher doses often needed in SCN.[592] Treatment should also include regular and aggressive dental care. The antibacterial mouthwash chlorhexidine (Peridex), is useful in decreasing gingivitis.[472,611,632] Shwachman syndrome, neutropenia with LDGL, and neutropenia with primary immunodeficiencies can also present with a cyclic pattern.

Myelokathexis

Myelokathexis is a rare syndrome associated with neutropenia and characterized by a cellular marrow with retained mature neutrophils (*kathexis* = retained) and abnormal nuclear morphology of the myeloid series. Since the initial descriptions,[633,634] several patients with the constellation of warts, hypogammaglobulinemia, infections, and myelokathexis have been described,[308,570,635,636] leading to the acronym WHIM syndrome.[637] The inheritance appears to be dominant and considerable heterogeneity in clinical characteristics exists among these patients.[119,297,303,635,637]

Neutrophil counts are in the 100 to 450/mm^3 range. The bone marrow cellularity is usually increased. In some cases, mature neutrophils, some bands, and metamyelocytes have bi- or tetraploid nuclei whereas early precursors are normal. Only rare abnormal neutrophils are found in the peripheral blood.[308,635,636] Myelokathexis is associated with an increased rate of apoptosis and decreased expression of bcl-x pro-survival gene in myeloid precursors, which explains in part the abnormal nuclear morphology.[318,606,638] In addition to neutropenia, these patients also have marked T-cell lymphopenia. The onset of verrucae may not be until the second decade and is absent in some patients, as is the case for hypogammaglobulinemia.[297,303,637,639]

Most of the cases of WHIM syndrome have been linked to autosomal dominant mutations in the CXC chemokine receptor 4 (CXCR4), all of which cause mutations in the carboxy-terminus of CXCR4.[297,304,639] Mutations of CXCR4 in WHIM syndrome cause failure of receptor downregulation and internalization, resulting in prolonged activation.[281,640] Activation of CXCR4 leads to increased retention and homing of neutrophils to bone marrow.[297,298] It is the decreased ability of mutant CXCR4 to downregulate that causes increased retention and apoptosis of neutrophils,[640] likely explaining the neutropenia, hypercellular marrow, and apoptosis seen in patients with myelokathexis.[282,302,318]

Patients with this syndrome respond to treatment with GCSF.[641,642]

Shwachman–Diamond–Oski Syndrome

The combination of neutropenia, metaphyseal dysplasia, and pancreatic insufficiency is known as Shwachman–Diamond–Oski syndrome.[643–646] These patients present in the first 10 years of life with steatorrhea, growth failure, and infections. Severe or fatal infections occur in more than half of the patients whereas many have relatively few problems with infection in spite of the neutropenia.[647] A 72-hour fecal fat measurement is useful to demonstrate fat malabsorption. Although pancreatic insufficiency is detectable by fecal fat determination, trypsin or lipase measurements, some patients have minimal problems with steatorrhea. Half of patients show moderate improvement in fat malabsorption by 5 to 8 years of age.[644] Thus, absence of a clear history of bowel problems does not rule out this diagnosis. Physical examination reveals short stature and a variety of other physical anomalies including strabismus, cleft palate, syndactyly, and microcephaly. Twenty-five percent have metaphyseal dysplasia. The pancreas is normal or enlarged and has a characteristic fatty appearance by magnetic resonance imaging.[648] The liver may be enlarged and liver enzymes may be elevated two- to threefold in patients under 2 to 3 years and normalizes with age.[644,649] Determination of characteristic polymorphisms is now very helpful in making the diagnosis. Note that there is great variability in the clinical phenotype, including absence of neutropenia or fat malabsorption. Thus, DNA analysis has become an essential part of the evaluation.

The neutrophil counts are usually less than 500/mm^3. Thrombocytopenia is present in 24% to 60% of the patients and a mildly megaloblastic, prednisone-responsive anemia is seen in 10% of patients.[643] Pancytopenia develops in 10% to 44% of patients and can progress to full aplastic anemia.[643,644] Although rare, patients can present in the newborn period with severe pancytopenia[650] and diabetes.[651]

The bone marrow is usually hypoplastic but can also be normal. In addition to neutropenia, a neutrophil capping and chemotactic defect is present. A partial chemotactic defect may be seen in the parents,[652] consistent with the presumed recessive inheritance. The reported functional defects have been corrected by injection with thiamine in some patients.[653,654] The mechanism for this response is unknown. Sweat chloride determination is normal.

The disorder has been mapped to the centromeric portion of chromosome 7[655] and has not been associated with mutations in elastase.[603] Detailed studies have identified various mutations in this region of the chromosome that may be related to the pathophysiology of the disorder.[656–659] Between 75% and 90% of patients have mutations in the *SBDS* gene (Shwachman–Bodian–Diamond syndrome), which may regulate ribosomal RNA maturation, that maps to the 7q11 centromeric region of chromosome 7.[649] There seems to be no relation between the polymorphisms seen and the clinical phenotype.[660] Mutational analysis is available commercially from several laboratories and is helpful in establishing the diagnosis as well as for genetic counseling. Most of the mutations found to date result in decreases in production of the SBDS protein.

The most common clonal cytogenetic abnormalities seen with malignant transformation or development of myelodysplasia in SDS are associated with chromosome 7.[661–663] About 44% of mutations are associated with i(7q), and other mutations involving chromosome 7 in combination with i(7q) accounted for another 35%.[649] It is important to note that these chromosomal abnormalities in SDS may be present without development of marrow failure and may be transient,[659,664,665] making it unclear whether patients should be transplanted simply because of presence of a chromosome 7-related clone.[666] In one small prospective study, none of four patients with del(20q) or i(7q) developed marrow failure.[664] The rate of MDS/AML seems to be about the same as for SCN at about 2% per year and does not seem to be related to treatment with G-CSF.[616] The marrow dysfunction and propensity to malignant transformation has been associated with shortened telomere length,[667] increased p53 expression,[657,668] and increased apoptosis of myeloid cells.[664,669]

The steatorrhea responds to pancreatic enzyme replacement and resolves by 5 or 10 years of age in about 50% of the patients, although the pancreatic insufficiency remains.[645] Treatment consists of management of infections and supplementation with pancreatic enzymes. The anemia may respond to treatment with prednisone. However, chronic inflammatory anemia can also occur and warrants a thorough search for the source of chronic inflammation and aggressive treatment. The neutropenia responds to G-CSF and in general the required dose is lower than for SCN.[616] Some patients have neutrophil counts in the 600/mm^3 or higher range and do not have problems with infection. Thus, it is not necessary to treat all patients with G-CSF. However, if the patient develops any serious infection related to the neutropenia or any evidence of chronic infection, G-CSF should be started. Furthermore, patients must be monitored closely for evidence of chronic inflammation, particularly chronic sinopulmonary infection.

The overall expected survival is approximately 50%. As with other constitutional marrow failure syndromes, there is an increased incidence of malignancy. Both lymphocytic and nonlymphocytic leukemias have been seen,[670,671] accounting for some of the mortality associated with this syndrome. Blood counts should be routinely monitored three to four times per year and bone marrow examination and cytogenetics be done in case of any evidence of deterioration of the hematologic status.

Barth Syndrome

Barth syndrome (BTHS) is an X-linked disorder characterized by neutropenia, cardiomyopathy, skeletal myopathy, and growth delay. Cognitive function is usually, but not always, normal. It is caused by mutations in the taffazin (*TAZ*) gene at Xq28 that result in cardiolipin deficiency and abnormal mitochondria. The patients also have 3-methylgluconic aciduria, though this is not specific to BTHS. Clinically, the patients present at an early age with heart failure, arrhythmia, gross motor delay, and may have a positive Gower sign. Half of the patients have height less than the 5th percentile but the BMI and growth velocity seem to be normal. The neutropenia, which may be present at birth, is often cyclic. The clinical findings are quite variable, with about 20% having leukopenia and 25% having neutropenia. There is no correlation between neutropenia and cardiac findings or genotype.[672,673]

Chediak–Higashi Syndrome

The Chediak–Higashi syndrome (CHS) is a rare inherited disorder characterized by oculocutaneous albinism, progressive neurologic impairment, and giant granules in many cells, including neutrophils (see also Table 50–9). The patients also develop severe neutropenia, felt to be due to ineffective granulopoiesis.[674] Chediak–Higashi syndrome results from mutations in the lysosomal trafficking regulator (*LYST*) gene on chromosome 1q42 that code for an adapter protein related to intercellular membrane fusion reactions.[675] The neutropenia and neurologic symptoms are not present at birth, although the abnormal neutrophil granules, diagnostic of the syndrome, are. Patients have defects in neutrophil chemotaxis, natural killer cell activity, T-cell cytotoxicity, and bactericidal function of neutrophils and monocytes.[221,676] Death ensues from a lymphoproliferative syndrome called the "accelerated phase." The accelerated phase of CHS is indistinguishable from hemophagocytic lymphohistiocytosis (HLH). In fact, CHS has been classified as one of the genetic forms of primary HLH.[677] The accelerated phase can be successfully treated using etoposide-containing regimens.[677] However, cure can only be achieved by marrow transplantation.[677,678] Bone marrow transplant is successful in eliminating the immunologic defects with an overall survival of 62%, although only 4 of 11 patients transplanted in accelerated phase survived.[676] Although bone marrow transplant may help the hematologic problems, it does not correct the neurologic abnormalities. In fact, neurologic dysfunction can develop years after successful marrow transplant.[679]

Griscelli Syndrome

Griscelli syndrome is an autosomal recessive disorder characterized by hypopigmentation of the skin and hair and abnormal regulation of the immune system. Neutropenia occurs in association with pancytopenia.[680] In spite of the apparent immunodeficiency, these patients, like CHS patients, develop a progressive HLH syndrome, which is fatal if not treated.[680–682] Mutations in *RAB27A*, *MYO5A*, and *MLPH* have been reported, with Rab27a being associated with immunologic impairment.[681]

Hermansky–Pudlak Syndrome Type II

The seven genetically defined Hermansky–Pudlak syndromes present primarily as bleeding disorders and oculocutaneous albinism. Like Chédiak–Higashi, Griscelli syndrome, and familial hemophagocytic lymphohistiocytosis (HLH), HPS is associated with abnormalities in lysosomal trafficking. All reported cases have nystagmus and bleeding, and some have pulmonary fibrosis. HPSII, like diseases that predispose to HLH, has disordered secretion of lytic granule by cytotoxic T cells and NK cells. The bleeding is due to abnormal platelet granules. HPS-II is consists of oculocutaneous albinism, bleeding, recurrent infection, and neutropenia and is caused by mutations in AP3B1, the cytosolic adaptor protein AP-3, which is involved in lysosomal trafficking. The neutrophil counts are less than 1000/uL and the bone marrow has an early myeloid arrest at the progranulocyte and myelocyte stage, reminiscent of SCN. GCSF is effective in raising the neutrophil counts.[683–685]

Cohen Syndrome

Cohen syndrome is an autosomal recessive condition associated with developmental delay, facial dysmorphism, pigmentary retinopathy, and neutropenia.[686–688] Of the 136 reported cases,[687] 35 are from Finland and are the most clinically homogeneous.[688] The subjects do have oral mucosal infections and can have chronic gingivitis. The neutropenia is isolated, mild to moderate, and intermittent but not cyclic and starts as soon as 2 days of life. The bone marrow cellularity is normal, with no characteristic changes. It is left-shifted in some cases. G-CSF was effective in the patients in whom it was tried.[689]

The disorder is associated with mutations in *COH1* whose function is unknown. It is homologous to the VPS13 protein in yeast, suggesting a role in vesicle-mediated sorting and intracellular protein trafficking.[686,690–692] Ninety-four percent of patients who meet five of eight clinical criteria have mutations in *COH1*.[686]

Reticular Dysgenesis

A syndrome of agranulocytosis, lymphoid hypoplasia, and thymic dysplasia with normal megakaryocyte and erythroid precursors has been called reticular dysgenesis.[693,694] These patients have low IgM and IgA and abnormal T cells.[694] The marrow is hypoplastic, with very few neutrophilic or lymphocytic precursors. The few early myeloid cells present have decreased granule formation.[694] These patients die in infancy. Immediate bone marrow transplantation should be considered.

Dyskeratosis Congenita

Dyskeratosis congenita is an inherited disorder involving abnormalities of integument and usually mild neutropenia,[695] though some patients have pancytopenia.[696,697] Although it is usually X-linked, autosomal dominant, and recessive, inheritance is also seen.[642] It is characterized by nail dystrophy, oral leukoplakia, and reticular pigmentation of the skin. Bone marrow failure develops in more than 80% of cases by the third decade and is the primary cause of death. About 10% of patients develop malignancy and 20% have pulmonary complications that can prove fatal. Now that the genes associated with DC have been identified, it is clear that patients may not present with typical physical findings. In fact, the diagnosis of marrow failure can precede the mucocutaneous manifestations.[698]

The gene for the x-linked form of DC was assigned to band Xq28 and is a mutation in the gene *DKC1* with codes for dyskerin, a protein expressed in all tissues of the body. Mutations in *DKC1* are seen in most x-linked DC patients.[698] Mutations have also been seen in the telomerase RNA component (TERC) as well as telomerase reverse transcriptase (TERT), which are part of the complex that is responsible for maintaining the telomeric ends of chromosomes. These have most commonly been seen in dominant forms of DC. Both DKC1 and TERC are part of the telomerase complex leading in part to the hypothesis that DC is primarily a disorder of telomere maintenance. Interestingly, mutations in TERC and TERT have been reported in other marrow failure syndromes, including aplastic anemia, myelodysplastic syndrome, paroxysmal nocturnal hemoglobinuria, and essential thrombocythemia. Thus, it may be that the pathophysiology of neutropenia and marrow failure in DC is related to stem cell failure due to the role of dyskerin in processing of ribosomal RNA as well as maintenance of the telomere by participation of TERC, TERT, and dyskerin in the telomerase complex.[698,699]

MANAGEMENT OF NEUTROPENIA

The clinical management of neutropenic states depends on the cause and degree of the neutropenia and on associated disease states. The major problem is management of infectious complications. Patients with severe neutropenia and little marrow reserve have acute severe pyogenic infection, whereas patients with hypercellular marrows tend to have chronic infection or no infection problems at all.

The approach is greatly influenced by the clinical context. The clinical approach for patients who are known to be on cytotoxic chemotherapy and present with fever and neutropenia has been well studied and reviewed.[700–702] The approach is largely dictated by the risk level, which is in turn dependent on the intensity of chemotherapy and the nature of the underlying malignancy. In this setting, patients on conventional chemotherapy who are hemodynamically stable and have a predicted short duration of neutropenia may be treated as an outpatient.[700,701,703] However, in the absence of a history of cytotoxic chemotherapy, the situation is less clear. Patients with ANC lower than 500 and fever require prompt evaluation and the rapid initiation of broad-spectrum parenteral antibiotics, regardless of the ultimate cause for the neutropenia. It usually takes days or weeks to establish the specific diagnosis. Until a diagnosis of a benign form of neutropenia is firmly established, the risk associated with not treating a patient with fever and markedly decreased marrow reserve is too grave. Thus, empiric parenteral antibiotic therapy that covers the most common infecting organisms in individuals with severe neutropenia (*S aureus*, *P aeruginosa*, *E coli*, and *Klebsiella* spp) should be started immediately. If the patient is nontoxic, the follow-up is reliable, and the patient has none of the signs of more serious neutropenia syndromes, management can proceed as an outpatient with parenteral ceftriaxone 50 to 75 mg/kg/day. The patient should be seen within 24 hours to follow up on the cultures, to check the patient status, and to give a second dose of antibiotic. This approach can avoid hospitalization in many patients. However, admission is recommended if there is any question that the patient may be toxic. Any possible causative drugs should be stopped and the blood counts followed weekly. As many acquired neutropenia episodes resolve spontaneously, this approach often avoids the need for marrow aspiration and expensive laboratory evaluation.

Table 50–11 gives the relation of the absolute neutrophil count to propensity to infection. These guidelines should be used in patients with chemotherapy-induced neutropenia and in neutropenia associated with granulocyte hypoplasia, such as aplastic anemia, SCN, or familial severe neutropenia. These patients have no marrow reserve and tend to have decreased marrow cellularity with an early myeloid arrest. Because these patients cannot respond to infection, many of the inflammatory signs of infection may be absent. For example, radiographs may not reveal pneumonias or there may be no abdominal tenderness with an early-ruptured viscus. The organisms causing infection come from the gastrointestinal tract or skin and can result in overwhelming sepsis very quickly. Thus, febrile patients with neutropenia related to marrow suppression should be treated immediately with broad-spectrum parenteral antibiotics. Antibiotics should be continued for several days, past the end of fever. If fever and neutropenia persist more than a week, consideration should be given to the empiric use of an antifungal agent. Granulocyte transfusions are effective in certain instances of culture-proven gram-negative sepsis. They should be used in patients with severe neutropenia with culture proven gram-negative sepsis and who have not shown a clinical response to antibiotics within 24 to 48 hours. Enthusiasm for the use of granulocyte transfusion has waned in recent years, in part due to difficulties in procurement and in part due to better antibiotics. There is some recent increase in interest with the availability to increase yields by treating the donor with G-CSF.[704,705] Routine reverse isolation procedures are of no benefit[706,707] and serve to decrease contact with medical personnel. Whereas empiric antibiotics are clearly indicated in case of fever, prophylactic antibiotics should not be routinely used.

Patients with late marrow arrest and normocellular marrow may be able to handle infections reasonably well. Children in whom the diagnosis of chronic benign neutropenia of infancy has been confirmed can be treated like normal children. In older patients with evidence of marrow reserve and a several-month history of severe neutropenia without serious infections, less aggressive therapy may be reasonable as well. When these patients are first encountered, however, they should be treated like other patients with more severe forms of neutropenia.

All patients with chronic neutropenia should receive regular dental care. Chronic gingivitis and recurrent stomatitis can be major sources of morbidity. Antibiotic mouthwash such as Peridex can be very helpful in preventing gingivitis.

Recombinant G-CSF has been effective in correcting neutropenia in cyclic neutropenia and severe congenital neutropenia and is recommended for these patients.[480,611,613,614,632] Bone marrow transplantation has been used successfully in certain cases of severe neutropenia and should be considered if an appropriate donor is available.

MONOCYTOPENIA AND MONOCYTOSIS

Alterations in the number of circulating monocytes are seen in a number of clinical situations (Table 50–17), although generally the disorders are less well defined than those of neutrophils. Production of monocytes is regulated by IL-3 and GM-CSF produced by T-lymphocytes and M-CSF produced by endothelial cells and by monocytes themselves. IL-3 and GM-CSF selectively induce M-CSF production by monocytes, suggesting one mechanism for production of the monocytosis associated with certain chronic infections and enhanced T-lymphocyte activity.[708] Monocytes comprise 1% to 9% of peripheral leukocytes, except during the first 2 weeks of life where the total monocyte count is higher.[709,710]

The blood monocyte and tissue monocyte–macrophages undoubtedly play an important role in defense against bacteria and fungal invasion; however, there is no clear association between circulating numbers of monocytes and propensity to infection as is clearly documented with neutrophils. Decrease in the number of monocytes has been seen with endotoxemia and with glucocorticoid administration.[711] Noncirculating monocytes seem to be relatively resistant to radiation and cytotoxic chemotherapy.[712]

Monocytosis is generally observed in association with chronic inflammatory processes, whether infectious or immune in nature. Monocytosis has been seen with tuberculosis,[713] subacute bacterial endocarditis, syphilis, and fever of unknown origin.[713,714] Collagen vascular diseases such as rheumatoid arthritis, systemic lupus erythematosus, myositis, periarteritis, and temporal arteritis have been associated with monocytosis as well as granulomatous diseases such as sarcoid, regional enteritis, and ulcerative colitis.[713,715]

Monocytosis has been seen with several primary neutropenic syndromes, including cyclic neutropenia, chronic idiopathic neutrope-

Table 50–17 Disorders Associated with Monocytosis

Inflammatory diseases:
Infectious diseases
Tuberculosis
Syphilis
Subacute bacterial endocarditis
Fever of unknown origin
Autoimmune/granulomatous
Systemic lupus erythematosus
Rheumatoid Arthritis
Temporal arteritis
Myositis
Polyarteritis
Ulcerative colitis
Regional enteritis
Sarcoidosis
Malignant disorders:
Preleukemia
Nonlymphocytic leukemia
Histiocytoses
Hodgkin disease
Non-Hodgkin lymphoma
Carcinomas
Miscellaneous:
Chronic neutropenia
Post splenectomy

nia, and Kostmann syndrome.[483,579,591,619] An increase in monocytes usually heralds recovery from agranulocytosis.

Monocytosis is commonly seen in a number of primary hematologic malignancies. Patients with chronic and acute nonlymphocytic leukemias as well as in preleukemic states have increased promonocytes and monocytes.[716–718] In many of these cases, the monocytes may be malignant but are indistinguishable from normal by light microscopy.[718] In addition to leukemia, monocytosis has been seen in both Hodgkin's and non-Hodgkin lymphomas, histiocytoses, as well as nonhematologic malignancies.[719–721] Monocytic leukemoid reactions have been seen in association with corticosteroids in myelodysplastic syndrome.[722]

Acknowledgment

This work was supported by the National Institutes of Health Grants R01HL45635 and PO1HL53586 (MCD) and RO1HL071801 and the Joseph Drown Foundation (TDC).

SUGGESTED READINGS

Berliner N, Horwitz M, Loughran TP Jr: Congenital and acquired neutropenia. Hematology Am Soc Hematol Educ Program 63, 2004.

Dinauer MC: Chronic granulomatous disease and other disorders of phagocyte function. Hematology Am Soc Hematol Educ Program 89, 2005.

Dror Y, Sung L: Update on childhood neutropenia: Molecular and clinical advances. Hematol Oncol Clin North Am 18:1439, 2004x.

Grimbacher B, Holland SM, Puck JM: Hyper-IgE syndromes. Immunol Rev 203:244, 2005.

Holland SM, Gallin JI: Evaluation of the patient with recurrent bacterial infections. Annu Rev Med 49:185, 1998.

Ku CL, Yang K, Bustamante J, et al: Inherited disorders of human Toll-like receptor signaling: Immunological implications. Immunol Rev 203:10, 2005.

Kyono W, Coates TD: A practical approach to neutrophil disorders. Pediatr Clin North Am 49:929, 2002, viii.

Lapidot T, Dar A, Kollet O: How do stem cells find their way home? Blood 106:1901, 2005.

Malech HL, Hickstein DD: Genetics, biology and clinical management of myeloid cell primary immune deficiencies: Chronic granulomatous disease and leukocyte adhesion deficiency. Curr Opin Hematol 14:29, 2007.

Matzner Y: Acquired neutrophil dysfunction and diseases with an inflammatory component. Semin Hematol 34:291, 1997.

Newburger PE: Disorders of neutrophil number and function. Hematology Am Soc Hematol Educ Program 104, 2006.

Palmblad J, Papadaki HA, Eliopoulos G: Acute and chronic neutropenias. What is new? J Intern Med 250:476, 2001.

Rosenberg PS, Alter BP, Bolyard AA, et al: The incidence of leukemia and mortality from sepsis in patients with severe congenital neutropenia receiving long-term G-CSF therapy. Blood 107:4628, 2006.

Ward DM, Shiflett SL, Kaplan J: Chediak-Higashi syndrome: A clinical and molecular view of a rare lysosomal storage disorder. Curr Mol Med 2:469, 2002.

Welte K, Zeidler C, Dale DC: Severe congenital neutropenia. Semin Hematol 43:189, 2006.

REFERENCES

For complete list of references log onto www.expertconsult.com

CHAPTER 51

DISORDERS OF LYMPHOCYTE FUNCTION

David B. Lewis, Kari C. Nadeau, and Aileen C. Cohen

Disorders of lymphocyte function can be categorized as either primary defects or secondary defects, such as those due to malnutrition, human immunodeficiency virus infection, or treatment with immunosuppressive or cytotoxic agents. This chapter emphasizes primary lymphocyte defects (Table 51–1)[1–4] involving the three major lineages of lymphocytes: T cells, B cells, and natural killer (NK) cells. Genetic immunodeficiencies that are mainly associated with the hemophagocytic syndromes (e.g., deficiency of perforin or MUNC 14–3) are discussed in Chapter 52. Immunodeficiency secondary to Epstein–Barr virus (EBV; e.g., X-linked lymphoproliferative syndrome) are discussed in Chapters 54 and 90. The autoimmune lymphoproliferative syndrome secondary to defects in Fas-mediated apoptosis in lymphocytes is discussed in Chapter 90. Treatment of primary immunodeficiency and other inherited disorders by transplantation of hematopoietic cell precursors contained in bone marrow, peripheral blood, or cord blood is discussed in detail in Chapter 100.

Primary immunodeficiencies of lymphocytes arise from abnormalities in development, maturation, or function. They can be divided into those giving rise to immunodeficiency diseases primarily involving antibody production and those characterized by combined defects in both antibody production and T-cell function (see Table 51–1). A few of these disorders, particularly certain forms of severe combined immunodeficiency (SCID), also have NK-cell deficiency as a prominent feature. Excluding selective immunoglobulin (Ig) A deficiency, which affects approximately 1:600 persons, primary immunodeficiency disorders due to inherited gene defects occur in approximately 1:10,000 live births and often but not invariably manifest in the first 6 years of life.[5] The immunodeficiency diseases are characterized by an increased frequency or severity of infections and by infections with unusual, relatively avirulent organisms, such as opportunistic pathogens or attenuated viruses used in vaccination (see box on Evaluation for Suspected Immunodeficiency). Antibody deficiency diseases, which are more common than T-cell disorders, are most frequently characterized by recurrent pyogenic infections, particularly with encapsulated bacteria involving the sinopulmonary tract. T-cell deficiency directly results in difficulty handling intracellular infections with viral and certain fungal (e.g., *Candida, Aspergillus, Pneumocystis*), parasitic (e.g., *Toxoplasma*), and bacterial (e.g., *Mycobacteria, Salmonella, Listeria*) pathogens. T-cell deficiency often includes infections with pyogenic bacteria, secondary to impaired production of opsonizing or neutralizing antibody by B cells from the lack of $CD4^+$ T-cell help as well as invasive infection with aerobic gram-negative bacteria (e.g., *Pseudomonas, Enterobacter*), most likely because of a lack of interleukin (IL)-17–producing helper T (T_H)17 $CD4^+$ cells. Diarrhea and malabsorption often manifest as failure to thrive in early infancy, autoimmune disorders, especially autoimmune cytopenias, and malignancies frequently occur in primary immunodeficiency diseases. The majority of malignancies are observed in patients with ataxia-telangiectasia, Wiskott–Aldrich syndrome (WAS), common variable immunodeficiency (CVID), and the hyper-IgM syndrome.

Immunodeficiency diseases may reflect discrete defects of lymphocyte development along a maturational pathway, as detailed in Chapters 11 and 12 and summarized in Figure 51–1, or in the function and cooperative interaction of mature lymphoid cells with each other, as shown in Figure 51–2 for interactions of T cells and B cells (see Chapter 14), or of T cells with dendritic cells and mononuclear phagocytes, as shown in Fig. 51–2. Primary defects of lymphocyte function usually are inherited, but whether this is true for some disorders, such as CVID, is uncertain in most cases. Autoantibodies can cause acquired immunodeficiency (see IFN-γ/T_H1 Pathway Deficiencies later). The gene defects for many primary immunodeficiencies have been described, often in great molecular detail, and have provided important insights into the immunobiologic role of the affected genes as well as the nature of clinically important genetic mutations in humans.

ANTIBODY DEFICIENCIES

X-Linked Agammaglobulinemia

Etiology and Pathophysiology

Primary immunodeficiencies in which B-cell development is blocked are characterized by early postnatal hypogammaglobulinemia and markedly depressed numbers of peripheral B cells. These disorders have an incidence of approximately 5:1,000,000; approximately 85% of these cases are due to X-linked agammaglobulinemia (XLA).[6] In XLA, mature B cells are absent or markedly decreased in the peripheral blood, plasma cells are absent in lymphoid tissue and bone marrow, and functional antibody is not produced or is present in low amounts.[6–8] Pre-B cells, $CD19^+CD34^-$ cells that express intracytoplasmic IgM heavy chain (Cμ) but not light chain or surface Ig, are present in low to normal numbers or are absent in the bone marrow.[6] When pre-B cells are present in XLA, a smaller proportion is proliferating. In contrast, pro-B cells, defined by a Cμ^-, $CD10^+CD19^+CD34^+$, terminal deoxytransferase-positive (TdT^+) phenotype, are present in normal numbers, suggesting a block at the Cμ^+ pre–B-cell stage of B-cell development (see Fig. 51–2). Rare B cells can be detected in the circulation of patients and, when present, have an immature surface phenotype with a high ratio of surface IgM to IgD and low levels of human leukocyte antigen (HLA) class II surface proteins.[9] Occasionally, circulating mature B cells and serum IgG levels higher than those observed in typical XLA are detected in patients, but deficiency of antibody production usually persists. At least one adult patient with normal levels of IgG but with B-cell lymphopenia and an apparently selective inability to mount antibody responses to unconjugated polysaccharide vaccines has been reported.[10]

The defective gene in XLA is intrinsic to the B cell, maps to Xq21.3-q22, and encodes the B-cell–specific, 77-kd, cytoplasmic Bruton tyrosine kinase (btk), named after the discoverer of human agammaglobulinemia.[6,7,11] This Tec family tyrosine kinase is expressed in all hematopoietic lines except T cells and plasma cells and is involved in signal transduction from surface Ig. More than 600 unique *btk* mutations involving all five domains of the protein have been shown to give rise to XLA,[11] with the kinase domain the most frequent target. In most patients, a direct correlation between clinical phenotype and specific *btk* mutations has not been demonstrated. In fact, phenotypical differences can be observed even among males in a single kindred,[12] indicating the importance of modifying genes or the environment in influencing the immunologic phenotype. The role of btk in signal transduction from a pre–B-cell receptor (pre-

Table 51–1 Primary Lymphocyte Defects

Disorder	Inheritance	Locus	Gene Defect/Pathogenesis	Associated Features
Predominantly Antibody Deficiencies				
X-linked agammaglobulinemia	XL	Xq21.3–22	Defective pre–B-cell maturation secondary to abnormality of Btk, a B-cell–lineage cytoplasm tyrosine kinase	
BLNK deficiency	AR	10q23.2	Lack of the BLNK protein signal transduction molecule compromises B-cell development at the pre–B-cell stage	
Igα (CD79a) deficiency	AR	19q13.2	Defect in Igα, which associates with BCR and pre-BCR, blocks pre–B-cell maturation	
Ig μ heavy-chain deficiency	AR	14q32.3	Mutations of Ig heavy chain gene locus prevents pre-BCR expression and blocks pre–B-cell maturation	
λ5/14.1 deficiency	AR	22q11.21	Absence of λ5/14.1, surrogate light-chain component of the pre-BCR arrests development at pre–B-cell stage	
LRRC8 deficiency	AD, chromosomal translocation	9q34.13	Truncation of C-terminal coding region of LRRC8 gene resulting in a dominant negative impact on B-cell development	Mild facial dysmorphism
κ-chain deficiency	AR	2p11	Point mutation at κ light-chain gene locus	Clinically significant(?)
Hyper-IgM syndrome due to AID (HIGM2) or UNG (HIGM5) defect	AR	12p13 (AID) 12q23–q24.1 (UNG)	B-cell isotype switching defect due to AID or UNG deficiency; decreased IgG and IgA and normal to elevated IgM; T-cell function presumably normal	
Hyper-IgM syndrome due to IKK-γ/NEMO deficiency	XL	Xq28	Defective activation of NF-κB signaling after engagement of CD40 resulting in defective B-cell isotype switching (in most patients); poor innate immune response to gram-positive bacteria due to impaired Toll-like receptor signaling	Hypoplastic/conical teeth, absence of sweat glands, sparse hair
CVID			Defect of B-cell maturation/differentiation, often with defective T-helper function or augmented suppression by T cells; autoimmunity in 10%–15%	
ICOS deficiency	AR	2q33	CVID phenotype: Defect of B-cell maturation/differentiation due to defective costimulation of B cells by T cells	
TACI deficiency	AD or AR	17p11.2	CVID phenotype: Intrinsic defect of B-cell maturation/differentiation	
CD19 deficiency	AR	16p11.2	CVID phenotype: Intrinsic defect of B-cell maturation/differentiation	
Antibody deficiency with normal Ig	?	?	Impaired responses to unconjugated polysaccharide antigens may be prominent; forme fruste of CVID(?)	
IgA deficiency	AR(?)	6p21.3(?)	Failure of deletional isotype switching to and terminal differentiation of IgA-secreting B cells or function may overlap with CVID or TACI deficiency	Autoimmunity, allergy
Selective IgG subclass deficiency	AR(?)	14q32.3(?)	Selective defects of isotype differentiation associated with poor antibody responses to antigens such as polysaccharides, often with IgA deficiency; very rare AR form due to deletion of IgG subclass switch regions	
Hypoimmunoglobulin M syndrome	?	?	Selective decrease in IgM, which usually is depressed but not undetectable; often associated with poor antibody responses to polysaccharide vaccines	
Combined Immunodeficiencies				
SCID				
T⁻B⁺ SCID				
X-linked (γ_c deficiency)	XL	Xq13.1–13.3	Defect of T-cell and NK-cell development secondary to mutation of common γ chain (γ_c) of IL-2, IL-4, IL-7, IL-9, IL-15, and IL-21 receptors	
Jak3 deficiency	AR	19p13.1	Mutations in Jak3, signaling molecule for γ_c; phenotype identical to X-linked SCID phenotype	
IL-7 receptor deficiency	AR	5p13	Defect of T-cell but not NK-cell development due to block in IL-7 and possibly TSLP signaling	
PNP autoimmunity deficiency	AR	14q13.1	Defect of T-cell development and function secondary to toxic metabolites due to deficiency of PNP	Anemia, neurologic symptoms
CD3δ, CD3ε, CD3ζ deficiencies	AR	11q23 (CD3δ and CD3ε), 1q22–q23 (CD3ζ)	Defect in intrathymic signaling via the pre-TCR or TCR resulting in thymocyte maturational arrest	
CD45 deficiency	AR	1q31–32	Defect in intrathymic signaling leads to perturbed thymocyte development and maturational arrest	
WHN/FOXN1 (nude) deficiency	AR	17q11–q12	Defective thymic microenvironment with impaired thymocyte maturation	Alopecia

Table 51–1 Primary Lymphocyte Defects—cont'd

Disorder	Inheritance	Locus	Gene Defect/Pathogenesis	Associated Features
T⁻B⁻ SCID				
RAG1/RAG2 deficiency	AR	11p12–13	Maturation defect of T-cell and B-cell development secondary to absence of antigen receptor gene recombination from mutations of RAG1 or RAG2 recombinase proteins	
Artemis deficiency (includes Athabascan SCID)	AR	10p	Maturation defect of T-cell and B-cell development secondary to absence of Artemis protein required for TCR and Ig antigen receptor gene recombination	Radiation sensitivity
DNA ligase IV deficiency	AR	13q22–q34	Maturation defect of T-cell and B-cell development secondary to absence of DNA repair enzyme required for TCR and Ig gene recombination and lymphocyte survival	Radiation sensitivity, microcephaly
Cernunnos/XLF	AR	2q35	Maturation defect of T-cell and B-cell development secondary to absence of Cernunnos/XLF, which is required for nonhomologous DNA repair during TCR and Ig antigen receptor gene recombination	Radiation sensitivity
ADA deficiency	AR	20q13–ter	Defect of T-cell, B-cell, and NK-cell development secondary to toxic metabolites due to ADA deficiency	Cartilage and neurologic abnormalities in some patients; autoimmunity if partial defect; sensorineural hearing loss
Reticular dysgenesis	AR	?	Stem cell defect affecting maturation of lymphoid and myeloid cells, particularly T cells and neutrophils	Sensorineural hearing loss
T⁺B⁻ SCID				
Omenn syndrome eosinophilia	AR	11p12–13 (RAG1/RAG2), 5p13 (IL-7Rα), 9p21–p12 (RMRP)	Hypomorphic mutations in *RAG1/RAG2*, *IL-7Rα*, or *RMRP* genes resulting in severe but partial block of T-cell and B-cell development with oligoclonal expansion of peripheral T cells with limited TCR repertoire; usually no peripheral B cells but elevated IgE	Erythroderma, hepatosplenomegaly, severe diarrhea, failure to thrive
Other Forms of SCID				
MHC class II deficiency	AR	16p13.1–2 (CIITA), 1q21, (RFX5), 13q (RFXAP)	Mutation of transcription factors (CIITA, RFX5, RFXAP, RFXANK) required for transcription of MHC class II, invariant chain, and HLA-DM molecules	Diarrhea, severe viral infections
ZAP-70 deficiency	AR	2q12	Mutations in ZAP-70 kinase gene required for TCR signaling resulting in decreased intrathymic development of CD8⁺ T cells and peripheral CD4⁺ T cells that are functionally defective	
CD25 (IL-2 receptor α chain) deficiency	AR	10p15–p14	Mutation in IL-2 receptor α gene resulting in abnormal T-cell compartment and defective T-cell activation; possible effect on regulatory CD4⁺ T cells	Lymphadenopathy, hepatosplenomegaly
lck Deficiency	AR	10p15–p14	Mutations in $p56^{lck}$ associated with other T-cell defects	
Orai1 deficiency	AR	12q24	Ion channel defect resulting in decreased generation of an intracellular increase in calcium in T cells after engagement of T-cell receptor	
Hyper-IgM Syndromes with T-cell Immunodeficiency				
X-linked hyper-IgM syndrome (HIGM1; CD40-ligand deficiency)	XL	Xq26–27	Defective B-cell activation and T-cell function due to abnormal CD40-ligand (CD154) expression on activated T cells	Neutropenia, autoimmune cytopenias, rheumatoid arthritis
X-linked hyper-IgM with ectodermal dysplasia	XL	Xq28	Defect in NEMO gene resulting in defective signaling after engagement of CD40	Similar to HIGM1 plus ectodermal dysplasia and NK-cell dysfunction
CD40 Deficiency (HIGM3)	AR	20q12–q13.2	Lack of CD40 blocks CD40-ligand– dependent signaling of B cells, APC-mediated activation of T cells, and mononuclear phagocyte activation by CD40 ligand	Likely similar to CD40 deficiency (HIGM1)
Other Disorders Affecting T-cell Number or Function				
Cartilage-hair hypoplasia syndrome	AR	9p13	Mutation of RMRP gene encoding a nonmessenger RNA resulting in perturbed T-cell development and function; can present as T⁻B⁺ SCID in severe cases	Absence of hair, short-limbed dwarfism

Table 51–1 Primary Lymphocyte Defects—cont'd

Disorder	Inheritance	Locus	Gene Defect/Pathogenesis	Associated Features
Schimke immunoosseous dysplasia	AR	2q34–q36	Mutation of *SMARCAL1*, a gene likely involved in regulating chromatin configuration and gene expression; associated with decreases in peripheral T-cell compartment; thymic hypoplasia(?)	Spondyloepiphyseal dysplasia, focal segmental glomerulosclerosis, thyroid and ocular abnormalities, cerebral ischemia
DiGeorge/velocardial facial syndrome	Most commonly due to haploinsufficiency due to chromosomal deletions	22q11.2 10p14–p13	In 22q11.2 interstitial deletion, haploinsufficiency of *Tbx1* and *CrkL* genes may block development of third and fourth branchial arch derivatives; thymic hypoplasia with normal B-cell and NK-cell compartments; if hypoplasia is severe, can manifest clinically similar to other forms of T^-B^+ SCID syndromes	Abnormal facies, hyperparathyroidism, anomalies of cardiac outflow tract, velopharynx, lower airway, kidney; developmental delay autoimmunity
CD3γ or CD3ε deficiency	AR	11q23	Defective expression of the $\alpha\beta$ TCR–CD3 complex on thymocytes and T cells and abnormal signal transduction capacity; either CD3γ or CD3ε can also present as SCID	
TAP1 and TAP2 deficiencies	AR	6p21.3	Defect in TAP function resulting in decreased MHC class I expression and intrathymic $CD8^+$ T-cell generation	Bronchiectasis (mechanism?)
CD8-α	AR	2p12	Absence of CD8 T cells with increased $CD4^-CD8^-$ T-cell population in periphery	Bronchiectasis (mechanism?)
IFN-γ/T_H1 pathway defects				
IL-12 p40 deficiency	AR	5q31.1–q35	Lack of IL-12 resulting in limited generation of T_H1 cells; IFN-γ responsiveness is normal	
IL-12 receptor β1 deficiency	AR	19p13.1	Lack of IL-12 receptor signaling resulting in limited generation of T_H1 cells; IFN-γ responsiveness is normal	
IFN-γ receptor deficiency	AR or AD	6q23–q24 (IFNGR1) 21q22.1–22.2 (IFNGR2)	Lack of responsiveness to IFN-γ	Can be mimicked by autoantibodies to IFN-γ
STAT1 deficiency	AR or AD	2q32.2–q32.3	Partial form: Blockade of IFN-γ–mediated STAT1 activation; severe form in which STAT1 responses to type I IFN and IFN-γ are ablated	
Other Immunodeficiencies				
Wiskott-Aldrich syndrome	XL	Xp11.22–11.3	Defect of cytoskeletal signaling secondary to *WASP* gene mutation affecting activation of T cells, B cells, and APCs	Thrombocytopenia, small platelets, eczema, malignancies, IgA-mediated autoimmunity
Ataxia-telangiectasia	AR	11q23.1	Disorder of cell-cycle checkpoint pathway and cellular responses to DNA damage secondary to mutation of *ATM* gene	Ataxia, telangiectasia, malignancies, radiation sensitivity
IPEX syndrome	AR	Xp11.23–q13.3	Deficiency of FOXP3 transcription factor resulting in decreased numbers of regulatory $CD25^+CD4^+$ T cells	Autoimmune enteritis, endocrinopathy
STAT5b deficiency	AR	17q11.2	Deficiency of cytokine-and hormone-driven STAT5b signal transduction resulting in T-cell lymphopenia and decreased regulatory $CD25^+CD4^+$ T cells	Laron dwarfism, autoimmune diathesis(?)

AD, autosomal dominant; ADA, adenosine deaminase; AID, activation-induced cytidine deaminase; APC, antigen-presenting cell; AR, autosomal recessive; ATM, ataxia-telangiectasia mutated; BCR, B-cell receptor; BLNK, B-cell linker protein; btk, Bruton tyrosine kinase; CVID, common variable immunodeficiency; HIGM, hyperimmunoglobulin M syndrome; HLA, human leukocyte antigen; ICOS, inducible T-cell costimulator; IFN, interferon; Ig, immunoglobulin; IKK, inhibitor of κB kinase; IL, interleukin; IPEX, immune dysregulation, polyendocrinopathy, enteropathy, and X-linked inheritance; Jak, Janus kinase; LRR8, leucine-rich-repeat-containing 8; MHC, major histocompatibility complex; NEMO, NF-κB essential modulator; NK, natural killer; PNP, purine nucleoside phosphorylase; RAG, recombination-activating gene product; RMRP, RHA component of the RHA-processing endo ribonucleave; SCID, severe combined immunodeficiency; SMARCAL1, SWI/SNF-related, matrix-associated, actin-dependent regulator of chromatin, subfamily A-like protein 1; STAT, signal transducer and activator of transcription; TACI, transmembrane activator and CAML interactor; TAP, transporter associated with antigen processing; TCR, T-cell receptor; TH1, T helper-1; TSLP, thymic stromal lymphopoietin; UNG, uracil N-glycosylase; WASP, Wiskott-Aldrich syndrome protein; WHN, winged-helix nude; XL, X-linked, XLF, XRCC4-like factor.

BCR; IgM heavy chain with surrogate light chain) or other receptors, the substrates phosphorylated by btk, and the mechanism(s) of inhibition of pre–B-cell maturation with *btk* gene defects are only partially understood.[6,7] The btk appears to be involved in activation of phospholipase Cγ, which in turn acts to increase calcium fluxes in B-lineage cells. The btk-dependent activation of phospholipase Cγ involves interaction of btk with the B-cell linker (BLNK) adapter protein.[13] In female carriers of XLA, B cells in which the non-inactivated X chromosome encodes the normal btk allele predominate in the periphery. This is believed to be secondary to decreased proliferation or survival of developing B cells in which the non-inactivated X chromosome expresses the mutant *btk* allele.[14] As in other X-linked disorders, female carriers may have clinically evident agammaglobulinemia due to an extreme proportion of the normal *btk* allele being inactivated, although this is extremely rare in btk deficiency.[15]

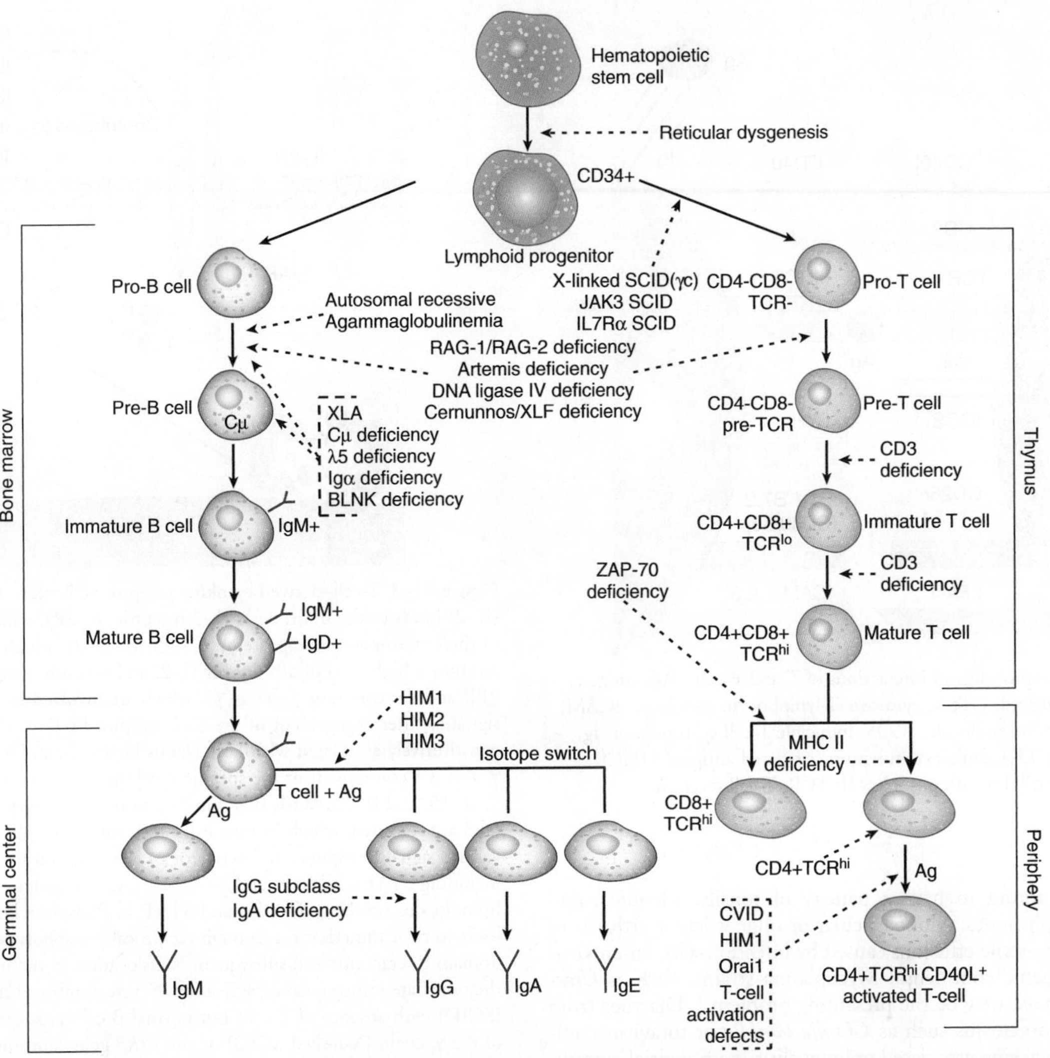

Figure 51–1 Select immunodeficiency diseases associated with maturation of T and B cells. Ag, antigen; Ig, immunoglobulin; BLNK, B-cell linker protein; CD40-L, CD40-ligand; CVID, common variable immunodeficiency; HIGM, hyper-IgM syndrome; ICOS, inducible T-cell co-stimulator; IL-7Rα, interleukin-7 receptor α; JAK, Janus kinase; MHC II, major histocompatibility complex class II; RAG, recombination activating gene; SCID severe combined immunodeficiency; TACI, transmembrane activator and CAML interactor; TCR, T-cell receptor; XLA, X-linked agammaglobulinemia; XLF, XRCC4-like factor.

Non–X-Linked Agammaglobulinemia

Rare disorders of absent B cells and panhypogammaglobulinemia that resemble XLA but are inherited in an autosomal recessive mode have been described. Patients with one form have defects of the μ heavy-chain constant region gene (Cμ deficiency) and defective expression of membrane μ heavy chain. Membrane μ heavy chain is an obligatory component of the pre-BCR and is required for normal B-cell development. Cμ deficiency results in failure of B-cell development at the pro–B-cell to pre–B-cell transition (see Fig. 51–1).[16] Compared with patients with btk deficiencies, persons with genetic defects of the Cμ region tend to have more severe disease, with an earlier clinical presentation and an increased frequency of complications.[17] Defects of other components of the pre-BCR complex, which include a surrogate light chain composed of λ5/14.1 and Vpre-B and the Ig-associated signal-transducing chains Igα (CD79a) and Igβ (CD79b), or of intracellular molecules required for pre-B-cell signaling, also give rise to a clinical picture similar to that of Cμ deficiency. Human mutations have been identified in λ5/14.1,[18] Igα,[19] and the B-cell signaling adaptor molecule BLNK.[20] Another non–X-linked, presumably autosomal recessive form of agammaglobulinemia is characterized by an arrest of B-cell development at the CD10$^+$CD34$^+$ pre–B-cell stage, with complete absence of pre-B cells in the bone marrow and mature B cells in the periphery.[21] The genetic cause is unknown. A single case of agammaglobulinemia in a girl with unusual facial features and a chromosomal translocation that truncates the leucine-rich-repeat-containing 8 (LRRC8) gene product of chromosome 9 has been reported; this condition appears to act in a dominant manner to somehow inhibit B-cell development.[22]

Clinical Manifestations

In affected boys with XLA, recurrent pyogenic infections begin during the latter half of the first year of life as maternal antibody titers wane. The clinical presentation may include chronic or recurrent otitis media, sinusitis, conjunctivitis, pneumonia, or pyoderma.[23,24] Infections occur at more than one anatomic site and usually are caused by pyogenic bacteria such as *Streptococcus pneumoniae*, *Streptococcus pyogenes*, or *Haemophilus influenzae*. There is a striking tendency for boys who present in the first year of life to have a more severe clinical presentation that may include pyoderma gangrenosum, perirectal abscess, cellulitis, or impetigo associated with sepsis due to gram-negative bacteria (e.g., *Pseudomonas*) or *Staphylococcus aureus* and neutropenia.[25,26] On physical examination, patients

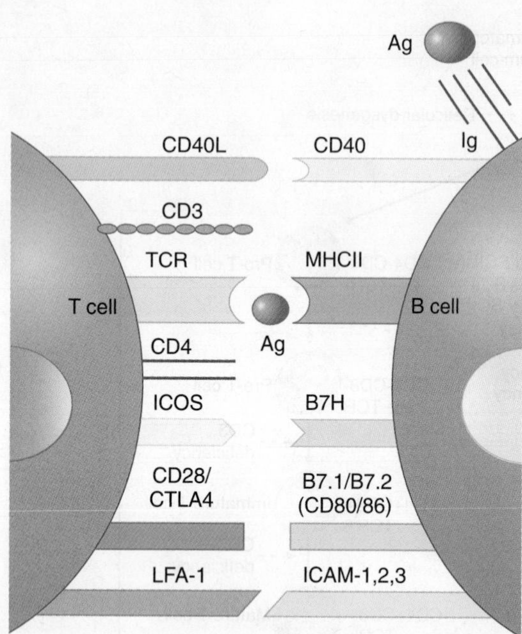

Figure 51–2 Receptor–ligand interactions of T and B cells. Ag, antigen; CD40L, CD40 ligand; CTLA, cytotoxic T-lymphocyte associated; ICAM, intercellular adhesion molecule; ICOS, inducible T-cell costimulator; Ig, immunoglobulin; LFA, leukocyte function-associated antigen; MHCII, major histocompatibility complex class II; TCR, T-cell receptor.

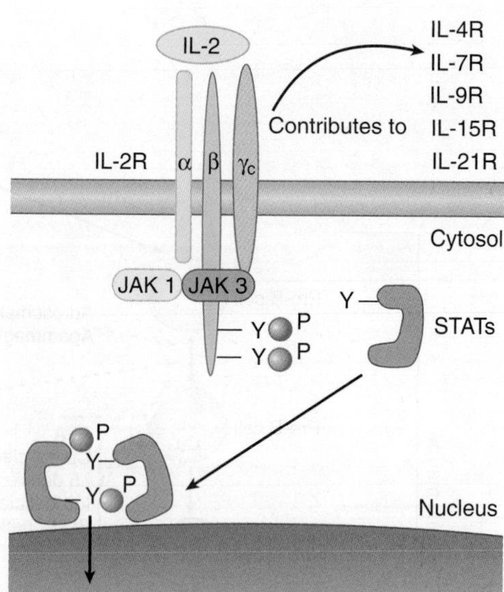

Figure 51–3 T-cell–derived cytokine receptor activation. Interleukin-2 (IL-2) binds to the multimeric IL-2 receptor (IL-2R), which is composed of three transmembrane proteins: CD25 (IL-2Rα), which confers on the receptor a high level of affinity for IL-2, and two other surface chains, IL-2Rβ and the common γ chain (γ_c), which are involved in intracellular signaling after engagement of the IL-2 receptor by IL-2. IL-2Rβ is constitutively associated with Jak1 (Janus kinase 1), and γ_c binds Jak3. The γ_c also is a component of the specific cytokine receptors for IL-4, IL-7, IL-9, IL-15, and IL-21. With IL-2 binding to the IL-2 receptor, Jak1 and Jak3 are activated, which in turn leads to tyrosine (Y) phosphorylation of various signal transducer and activator of transcription (STAT) proteins, including STAT1, STAT3, and STAT5. STAT5 includes two highly homologous proteins, STAT5a and STAT5b. Phosphorylation of STATs leads to their dimerization through reciprocal phosphotyrosine–SH_2 domain interactions and subsequent translocation to the nucleus, where they mediate transcriptional activation. Severe combined immunodeficiency (SCID) with absence of T cells but normal B cells arises from mutation of the γ_c chain (X-linked SCID) or the *JAK3* gene (autosomal recessive SCID) and is due mainly to blockade of IL-7R signaling by developing thymocytes. A SCID-like immunodeficiency also occurs with mutations of CD25. STAT5b deficiency mainly impairs upregulation of CD25 that occurs in response to IL-2 and maintenance of $CD25^+CD4^+$ T cells that express the FOXP3 transcription factor and have regulatory activity (i.e., are capable of inhibiting the function of effector T cells).

with XLA are found to have a paucity of tonsils, adenoids, and peripheral lymph nodes. Monoarticular or oligoarticular arthritis of large joints with sterile effusions caused by infection with enterovirus or a nonpathogenic commensal Mycoplasma strains, such as *Ureaplasma urealyticum*, may be the presenting problem.[27] Diarrhea from infection with organisms such as *Giardia lamblia* or rotavirus commonly occurs. Vaccine-associated poliomyelitis is a potential complication caused by the persistence and mutation of the attenuated live poliovirus vaccine strain into a virulent neurotropic form.[28] Eradication of natural poliovirus infection in most of the world and phasing out of immunization with oral poliovirus vaccine should make this condition mainly an historic medical problem in developed countries. Before diagnosis and institution of therapy with Ig replacement therapy, neutropenia may occur in approximately 25% of affected patients.

Infectious diseases can cause significant morbidity. Chronic infections of the upper and lower respiratory tracts with otitis media, sinusitis, pneumonia, and even bronchiectasis may occur in spite of early institution of Ig replacement therapy.[29] In the past, chronic pulmonary disease was described in almost half of patients with XLA, and hearing loss, resulting from chronic otitis media or meningoencephalitis, occurred in approximately one third of patients.[23] Rarely, sensorineural hearing loss associated with btk deficiency is due to a contiguous gene defect involving deletion of *btk* and an adjacent deafness-dystonia protein gene.[30] Chronic, disseminated enteroviral infection, usually from echovirus, is a potentially fatal complication. It almost always involves the central nervous system (CNS) and may include hepatitis, pneumonia, vasculitis, and a dermatomyositis-like syndrome consisting of rash, brawny edema of the subcutaneous tissues and myositis with muscle weakness.[31–33] In the past, these complications as well as other serious infections accounted for a mortality rate of approximately 15% of patients by age 20 years.[23] In recent times, earlier diagnosis and more effective Ig replacement therapy using the intravenous or subcutaneous route rather than the intramuscular route have decreased the incidence of these complications. However, a recent series found that the majority of patients with XLA were not diagnosed until they had been hospitalized for infection, which suggests there is still room for earlier clinical recognition of the syndrome.[25]

Laboratory Evaluation

Absent antibody responses after immunization or natural antigenic exposure, low levels of serum Ig, and absence or very low levels of peripheral blood B cells are characteristic of the disease (see box on Laboratory Evaluation for Suspected Immunodeficiency). The B cells present usually have an increased surface density of IgM. The IgG level usually is less than 100 mg/dL, and all other Ig isotype levels usually are low or undetectable. However, approximately 10% to 20% of patients may have higher levels of serum Ig and detectable circulating levels of B cells. In rare cases, these can reach normal levels of Ig, although B-cell numbers still are markedly low. Patients with higher Ig levels often present later in life, which may indicate the impact of other modifying genes. T-cell numbers and antigen-specific function are intact, with a tendency for greater T_H1 responses (interferon [IFN]-γ predominant) than T_H2 responses (IL-4, IL-5, and IL-13 predominant).[34] Peripheral neutropenia accompanied by a maturation arrest in the bone marrow is a frequent presenting feature.[26,35] Possible mechanisms of neutropenia include consumption of neutrophils and their immediate precursors after cell activation by endotoxin or other bacteria-derived products during severe bacterial infections. Alternatively, there might be a requirement for btk in stressed myeloid lineage cells. Lymph nodes show an absence of plasma cells, lymphoid follicles, and germinal centers. Definitive diagnosis, prenatal diagnosis, and diagnosis of the carrier state can be performed by genetic analysis. Screening for btk protein expression using either flow cytometry after intracellular staining[36] or Western blotting will rapidly identify most patients with the deficiency, but confirmatory gene sequencing is important, particularly in cases where result of flow cytometry are normal or equivocal and the clinical presentation is strongly suggestive of XLA.

Therapy

Ig replacement therapy is the mainstay of treatment and should be started once the diagnosis is made (see box on Immunoglobulin Replacement Therapy), preferably before repetitive infections have caused irreversible pulmonary damage.[37] Although subcutaneous replacement with Ig can be used to maintain adequate IgG levels in most patients, initial replacement with intravenous immunoglobulin (IVIG) should be used to rapidly achieve normal levels. Maintaining adequate levels of IgG can prevent chronic pulmonary disease and chronic enteroviral meningoencephalitis. Although the latter has been reported even with IVIG therapy, most patients received relatively low doses of Ig compared with current recommendations.[33] The subcutaneous route for rapid Ig administration is an alternative means of antibody replacement,[38] although it requires more frequent dosing than does the intravenous route.

Pyogenic infections should be treated with antibiotics promptly and vigorously to prevent organ damage. Chronic or recurrent infections of the upper and lower respiratory tracts may require the addition of continuous prophylactic antibiotic therapy.

Persistent enteroviral infections have been treated successfully with Ig preparations containing high titers of antibody specific for the infecting enterovirus.[32,39] For treatment of enteroviral meningoencephalitis, these high-titer antibodies specific for the infecting virus may require administration directly into the ventricles of the brain to obtain sufficiently high levels at that site.[40] However, even with this therapeutic approach, infections have not always been cleared.[33] Pleconaril, a drug with activity against enteroviruses, may be useful for this complication in patients with XLA or other primary immunodeficiencies, including hypogammaglobulinemia. However, the development of pleconaril resistance has been reported in this setting.[41] Single positron emission computed tomographic scanning may be a useful noninvasive method for following patients with chronic enteroviral meningitis.[42]

Common Variable Immunodeficiency

Etiology and Pathophysiology

CVID is the most common symptomatic primary antibody deficiency syndrome. It includes a group of heterogeneous disorders associated with recurrent infections, poor antibody responses, and hypogammaglobulinemia.[43,44] Both genders are affected. Onset often is insidious and usually occurs during the second or third decade of life. In approximately 10% to 20% of cases, the disorder is familial, with predominance of an autosomal dominant over an autosomal recessive inheritance pattern.[45] Offspring and first-degree relatives may have selective IgA deficiencies or autoimmune diseases, such as systemic lupus erythematosus (SLE), hemolytic anemia, or immune thrombocytopenic purpura.[45–47] In some instances, SLE may evolve into CVID.[48] Viral infections, including congenital rubella and EBV, have been suspected in the etiology of CVID. In contrast, human immunodeficiency virus and hepatitis virus infections have been reported to restore IgG and antibody production in some patients.[49,50]

Evaluation for Suspected Immunodeficiency

Laboratory studies should be used to confirm a diagnosis of an immunodeficiency disease after a thorough history and physical examination have been performed to exclude a localized anatomic or physiologic defect that may predispose to recurrent infections. An immunodeficiency should be suspected with the occurrence of infections of unusual frequency, location, type, or severity. Recurrent infections may occur at multiple sites, and infections may be caused by unusual or opportunistic organisms, such as *Pneumocystis, Candida, Mycobacterium avium, Pseudomonas, Serratia,* or Cytomegalovirus (CMV). Often the patient lacks a history of exposure. Excessive severity or complications of infections and poor response to treatment are common. With immunodeficiency diseases, organisms may disseminate more widely, multiply in greater numbers, or remain alive in phagocytes. Patients with immunodeficiency diseases often fail to recover to normal health between infections and may experience weight loss or poor weight gain. Autoimmune diseases may accompany antibody deficiency states and other disorders in which T-cell tolerance is compromised.

Recurrent infections such as otitis media, sinusitis, pneumonia, meningitis, arthritis, and osteomyelitis from encapsulated bacteria (e.g., *S. pneumoniae, H. influenzae* type b, *Neisseria meningitidis, Staphylococcus aureus*) suggest a deficiency of antibody or, less commonly, an abnormality of phagocytes or serum complement. Low numbers or poor function of polymorphonuclear leukocytes also is commonly associated with abscesses and infections with unencapsulated nonpathogenic bacteria that reside in the skin or mucosal surfaces. Recurrent infections from viruses, fungi, or intracellular bacteria, such as *Mycobacteria, Listeria,* or *Salmonella,* suggest a defect in T-cell function. Intracellular bacterial infection also is characteristic of defects in the T_H1 pathway involving the generation of IFN-γ–producing T cells or the responsiveness of cells to IFN-γ. Infection with *Pneumocystis* strongly suggests T-cell deficiency. CD40-ligand deficiency is strongly suggested if T cells are present in normal numbers in a male with documented *Pneumocystis* pneumonia. Combined deficiencies of T-cell and B-cell function are characterized by infections with bacteria or viruses. Recurrent systemic *Neisseria* infections suggest deficiency of a terminal complement component or, in male patients, of properdin, a component of the alternative complement pathway encoded in the X chromosome. Antibody deficiency in young children usually does not predispose the patient to infections until the latter half of the first year of life due to the passive protection provided by maternal antibody. However, T-cell immunity is not transplacentally transmitted and is not present at birth.

Laboratory evaluation initially should be directed to the type of deficiency suspected on the basis of the history and results of physical examination. Studies should begin with less expensive and more readily available tests. Results must be compared with age-related normal values. Examinations of the complete blood count and peripheral blood smear may suggest the diagnosis. In patients with suspected T-cell deficiency, live viral immunization should be withheld. Blood products should be obtained from donors who are CMV-antibody seronegative and should be irradiated before administration to prevent graft-versus-host disease.

Although the exact nature of the defects giving rise to CVID are unknown in approximately 85% of cases, many immunologic abnormalities have been described.[51,52] Most patients with CVID have normal numbers of mature B cells that fail to differentiate into antibody-secreting cells. Failure of in vivo B-cell maturation and differentiation usually is believed to be due, at least in part, to defective interactions between T and B cells and possibly between dendritic cells and T cells or B cells. Intrinsic B-cell defects include a failure to proliferate and to secrete one or more Ig isotypes, most often IgG or IgA, with appropriate stimuli. This failure may be explained in part by the observation that many patients with CVID have markedly decreased circulating levels of $CD27^+$ memory B cells, including those of the IgM^+IgD^+ cell subset that have not undergone isotype switching.[53,54] This unswitched B-cell population is also absent in patients who have undergone splenectomy and may be enriched in B cells originating from the marginal zone of the spleen, which has a natural antibody repertoire for the immune control of encapsulated bacteria.[54] Consistent with this idea, CVID patients who have low levels of $CD27^+IgM^+IgD^+$ memory B cells appear to be at particularly high risk for infections with *S. pneumoniae* and marked impairment of the production of antibodies against the capsules of *S. pneumoniae* after vaccination.[55] CVID patients can be divided into those with detectable numbers of switched memory B cells ($CD27^+IgM^-IgD^-$) and those lacking such cells.[56] The latter group tends to have lower levels of IgG, poorer responses to vaccination with polysaccharides, and higher incidences of autoimmune and granulomatous disease and bronchiectasis.[55,56] Many patients also have a dramatic reduction in the degree to which expressed Ig genes have undergone somatic hypermutation,[57,58] a finding that has been suggested to be a better predictor of severe respiratory tract infection than decreases in peripheral blood memory B-cell numbers.[59] As isotype switching, somatic hypermutation, and memory B-cell generation typically require help from $CD4^+$ T cells, particularly in response to protein antigens, these observations are consistent with a defect in interactions between T cells and B cells. Intrinsic limitations in T-cell function may contribute to CVID immunopathology, as T cells from CVID patients may have abnormalities in signal transduction and the ability to express CD40 ligand and cytokines that are important for B-cell help.[51,60] CVID B cells also may not effectively increase expression of B7–2 (CD86), a molecule that is important in providing costimulation to T cells through engagement of CD28.[61] Several studies have focused on potential intrinsic defects or dysregulation in innate immune mechanisms mediated by antigen-presenting cells (APCs) and B cells that might account for poor specific antibody production. A subset of patients with decreased numbers of peripheral $CD4^+$ T cells and splenomegaly have evidence of persistent activation of mononuclear phagocytes, apparently as a result of chronic production of tumor necrosis factor (TNF)-α.[62] Results have been conflicting as to whether CVID patients have increased or decreased production by APCs of IL-12,[63,64] a potent cytokine for T_H1 differentiation. Defects in the ability of CVID dendritic cells to activate T cells also have been reported,[64,65] although these studies used dendritic cells generated in vitro from monocytes using high doses of cytokines and may not be accurate predictors of the function of circulating and tissue-associated myeloid dendritic cells. CVID B cells and plasmacytoid dendritic cells may be impaired for Toll-like receptor (TLR)-9 signaling.[66] TLR-9–dependent activation of plasmacytoid dendritic cells (i.e., by viral or bacterial DNA) normally results in high levels of production of type I IFN, which is a potent stimulus for B-cell activation that synergizes with B-cell TLR-9 signaling. Thus, it is plausible that defects in both plasmacytoid dendritic cell and B-cell TLR-9 signaling are major mechanisms for limiting antibody responses in CVID.

Monogenetic defects in transmembrane activator and calcium modulator ligand interactor (TACI, TNF receptor superfamily member 13B), inducible costimulatory (ICOS) receptor, or CD19 can present as CVID, particularly in kindreds in which multiple family members are affected (see Table 51–1).[52,67,68] TACI, which binds to the secreted ligands BAFF and APRIL, may be particularly important for isotype switch recombination by B cells. ICOS, which is expressed by activated and memory T cells, appears to provide important B-cell activation and differentiation signals, such as for memory cell generation and isotype switching, by binding to ICOS ligand on B cells. CD19 is a B-cell surface protein that is essential for signal transduction after engagement of surface Ig by antigen; it also is important in memory B-cell generation. These gene defects clearly show that both intrinsic T-cell and B-cell genetic defects can present as CVID in humans.[69] TACI mutations, which usually act in a dominant negative manner, may involve 5% to 10% of patients with CVID.[52,67] TACI defects are also found at an increased rate in relatives of patients with CVID who have IgA deficiency.[52,67] The other monogenetic defects act in an autosomal recessive manner and probably account in aggregate for less than 1% of CVID patients in most countries.

Clinical Manifestations

CVID occurs in both genders, Age at onset varies from early childhood to late adulthood. Recurrent pyogenic infections with otitis media, sinusitis, bronchitis, and pneumonia, often from pneumococci, staphylococci, *H. influenzae*, *Moraxella*, or *Mycoplasma pneumoniae*, are typical.[43] Bronchiectasis is a frequent complication and may be the presenting abnormality. Cor pulmonale and respiratory failure associated with chronic lung disease are common causes of death. Patients who are not receiving adequate Ig replacement are at increased risk for disseminated enteroviral infections, although this complication is less common than in patients with XLA.[33] In contrast to XLA, lymphoid tissue is normal or enlarged as a result of B-cell proliferation and prominent germinal center formation. Nodular lymphoid hyperplasia of the gastrointestinal tract is common. Splenomegaly, secondary to reactive follicular hyperplasia, occurs in approximately 25% of patients and may be associated with neutropenia and thrombocytopenia from hypersplenism and with expansion of B cells that are $CD19^{high}CD21^{low/negative}$.[70] Noncaseating granulomas that resemble those found in sarcoidosis may occur in the spleen, liver, lung, bone, and other tissues. Arthritis and arthralgia are common. Gastrointestinal abnormalities with chronic gastritis and achlorhydria, diarrhea, and a sprue-like syndrome with malabsorption, lactose deficiency, and protein-losing enteropathy may complicate the clinical course.[71] Pernicious anemia develops in some patients because of atrophic gastritis and absence of intrinsic factor due to autoantibodies. Reactivation of varicella-zoster virus and recurrent herpes simplex virus infection can occur, suggesting a diminution of T-cell–specific responses to these viruses.

Autoimmune disorders, including autoimmune hemolytic anemia, thrombocytopenia or neutropenia, rheumatoid arthritis, SLE, chronic active hepatitis, and thyroiditis, are frequently seen (see box on Peripheral Blood Abnormalities in Immunodeficiency).[43,72] There is an overall fivefold increase in the incidence of cancer, with a 51-fold increase in gastric cancer and at least a 30-fold increase in lymphoma.[73–77] This increased incidence of gastric cancer may be related to the high frequency of achlorhydria and atrophic gastritis in patients with CVID.[78] A nonmalignant lymphoproliferative disorder with follicular hyperplasia of lymph nodes or nodular lymphoid hyperplasia of the intestine and splenomegaly also may occur and must be distinguished from a malignancy.[79]

Laboratory Evaluation

Serum Igs, especially IgG and IgA, are moderately to markedly decreased, and antigen-specific antibody responses are impaired. The peripheral blood B-cell number is normal in approximately 75% of patients, but the surface phenotype may be immature, and the cells of some patients fail to differentiate to antibody-secreting cells after appropriate stimuli. Decreased numbers of memory ($CD27^+$) B cells is a frequent finding. Atypical XLA must be excluded when a low number of B cells is detected in a male with a presumed diagnosis of CVID. T-cell numbers may be decreased, and a reversal of the ratio of T_H/cytotoxic ($CD4^+/CD8^+$) T-cell ratio may be noted, usually secondary to an increase in $CD8^+$ T cells. Some patients have an expanded number of activated $CD57^+CD25^+$, $HLA\text{-}DR^+$ circulating $CD8^+$ T cells,[80] which also are commonly found in chronic viral infection. Depressed T-cell function and absent delayed-type hypersensitivity skin test reactivity may occur, especially in patients who are older or have lymphopenia. As described above, in the Etiology and Pathophysiology section, CD40-ligand expression and the elaboration of soluble cytokines by T cells activated in vitro may be decreased. In males with CVID that manifests during childhood, care should be taken to exclude two X-linked genetic disorders, btk deficiency (XLA) and SLAM-associated protein (SAP) deficiency (the cause of X-linked lymphoproliferative syndrome), which in the past have been misdiagnosed as CVID. Mutation of the lck protein tyrosine kinase gene has presented as CVID in one instance.[80a]

Therapy

Ig replacement and aggressive antibiotic therapy are indicated (see box on Immunoglobulin Replacement Therapy).[37] After Ig replacement therapy is instituted, pulmonary radiographic and functional changes may stabilize. Serial pulmonary function tests are important for clinical assessment. However, acute infections still may occur with Ig replacement therapy, necessitating prolonged use of antibiotics to prevent deterioration of lung function. In the face of chronic lung disease and bronchitis, some patients require higher doses of Ig replacement (e.g., 600 mg/kg IV every 3–4 weeks or 150 mg/kg subcutaneously every week) than are commonly used to prevent acute lung exacerbations.[81] Therapy with IL-2 has been used experimentally in a limited number of patients, with some improvement of in vitro T-cell function and the ability to mount antibody responses to a neoantigen.[82] Whether such IL-2 therapy has long-term clinical benefits for patients with CVID is unknown. CVID-related granulomatous disease has been responsive to therapy with glucocorticoids or TNF-α inhibitors in some patients. The addition of hydroxychloroquine, a relatively mild immunosuppressive agent, may reduce the need for glucocorticoid therapy in some cases of lymphoid interstitial pneumonitis associated with CVID.

Selective Immunoglobulin A Deficiency

Etiology and Pathophysiology

Deficiency of serum IgA, defined as serum IgA concentration less than 5 mg/dL, is found in approximately 1:600 persons in Europe and North America but occurs in only 1:18,000 in Japan and 1:4000 in China.[83] Most affected persons are asymptomatic, but some IgA-deficient persons suffer from recurrent sinopulmonary infections, autoimmunity, or allergies.[47,83,84] Autoimmunity or allergies may occur in some patients as a consequence of increased absorption of environmental and dietary antigens into the systemic circulation due to the lack of secretory IgA at mucosal surfaces or, alternatively, reflect a broader underlying immunologic defect with poor regulation of autoantibody production.

IgA deficiency may be primary or secondary. It can occur in a sporadic form or with an autosomal dominant or autosomal recessive pattern of inheritance.[85,86] IgA deficiency or CVID may be found in extended families with evidence of linkage or no linkage to the major histocompatibility complex (MHC) locus. A CVID susceptibility locus, designated *IGAD1*, has been fine mapped to the HLA-DQ/HLA-DR region of chromosome 6.[87] This finding suggests an autoimmune pathogenesis in CVID/IgA deficiency that may involve $CD4^+$ T-lineage cells, as these cells mainly recognize antigenic peptides that are associated with MHC class II molecules.

IgA deficiency can be transitory in children, especially when the serum IgA level is only moderately decreased, but in adults the deficiency usually is permanent.[88,89] Congenital infections with rubella virus, cytomegalovirus (CMV), or *Toxoplasma gondii* and acquired EBV infection have been associated with IgA deficiency. In addition, IgA deficiency may occur after use of drugs such as penicillamine, phenytoin, sodium aurothiomalate, captopril, sulfasalazine, or antimalarial agents.

The susceptibility to infection in IgA deficiency may be secondary not to IgA deficiency per se but to concomitant deficiencies of IgG2 and IgG4 subclasses of Igs,[90–92] although this is a highly controversial issue. In some patients, IgA deficiency is a manifestation of a more widely based immunologic defect with similarities to CVID, which also is, at least in part, an arrest in B-cell differentiation. As noted previously, CVID also occurs in family members and shares MHC haplotypes with IgA deficiency. IgA deficiency may evolve into CVID and is frequently found in ataxia-telangiectasia, which also is associated with IgG subclass deficiency.

IgA deficiency usually is associated with an intact structural IgA heavy-chain gene segment (Cα switch region of the Ig heavy-chain gene). Surface IgA-bearing B cells are present in normal or reduced numbers, and the cells may display an immature phenotype with coexpression of surface IgM in some patients.[93] The primary defect appears to be failure of B cells to differentiate to mature isotype-switched surface IgA-positive B cells and IgA-secreting plasma cells with appropriate stimuli.[83] The basis for the defect is not known.

Clinical Manifestations

The majority of persons with IgA deficiency are healthy, but many have various clinical symptoms. Patients with IgA deficiency who were asymptomatic when young may develop symptoms in later life. The frequencies of upper and lower respiratory tract infections are increased. Infections occur more commonly when IgA levels are low with a deficiency in IgG subclasses and with decreased levels of antipneumococcal polysaccharide antibodies.[83,90–92] Some patients have recurrent bacterial infections with recurrent sinusitis, otitis media, or bronchitis and may develop bronchiectasis. The incidence of autoimmune diseases, especially rheumatoid arthritis and SLE, is increased.[72] Other autoimmune diseases may occur, although autoantibodies may be present without symptoms. Allergic diseases, including rhinitis, urticaria, eczema, and asthma, occur with increased frequency. Gastrointestinal and hepatic complications associated with IgA deficiency include malabsorption, celiac disease, giardiasis, nodular lymphoid hyperplasia, pernicious anemia, atrophic gastritis, primary biliary cirrhosis, and chronic active hepatitis. Gastric and colon carcinomas are found with increased frequency. Production of antibodies to food antigens, such as cow's milk, may cause immune complexes that may be pathogenic.

Laboratory Evaluation

The serum concentration of IgA is less than 5 mg/dL, and the levels of IgG and IgM are normal. Secretory IgA is decreased. Approximately 25% of patients have decreased levels of IgE. Some patients, especially those with recurrent sinopulmonary infections, have a concomitant deficiency of IgG2 and IgG4 subclasses and defective antibody responses to polysaccharides, such as those contained in the 23-valent pneumococcal polysaccharide vaccine. Determination of IgA and IgG levels should be repeated at a later date to determine if the deficiency of IgA is persistent and, if so, whether the immunologic disorder has evolved to resemble CVID. IgA-deficient patients have an increased incidence of autoantibodies directed against nuclear proteins, Igs, thyroglobulin, or adrenal, parietal, smooth muscle, or pancreatic cells, or of antibodies to food antigens, such as cow's milk protein. Serum antibodies to IgA occur in greater than 20% of patients with IgA deficiency, especially if IgA is completely undetectable. However, the presence of these antibodies is not highly predictive of adverse reactions to blood products containing IgA. Exposure to blood products with IgA may, however, induce IgE anti-IgA antibodies that can cause anaphylactic reactions.[94]

Therapy

Treatment should be directed at the associated infections and allergic, autoimmune, and gastrointestinal diseases. Precipitating drugs should be discontinued. Antibiotic therapy is indicated for bacterial infections. If infections are severe or cause significant sequelae, prophylactic antibiotics should be considered. Ig replacement therapy is not usually indicated for IgA deficiency unless a defect in specific antibody production to antigens, such as pneumococcal polysaccharides, is documented. Severe or fatal anaphylactic reactions can occur with intravenous administration of IgA-containing blood products to IgA-deficient patients.[94] This may be caused by anti-IgA antibody of the IgE isotype, which may increase after Ig replacement therapy. Treatment with IVIG preparations containing low levels of IgA may be helpful for IgA-deficient patients for whom IVIG therapy is indicated but who have anaphylactic reactions to IgA-containing products.[95] Blood products should be washed prior to transfusing IgA-deficient individuals or if obtained from IgA-deficient donors, including the recipient, before surgery. Plasma for transfusion also should be collected from IgA-deficient persons. Oral administration of γ-globulin has led to improvement in some patients with chronic diarrhea.

Immunoglobulin Deficiency with Normal or Increased Immunoglobulin M (Hyper-IgM Syndrome)

Etiology and Pathophysiology

The hyper-IgM syndrome is so named because of the frequent and characteristic finding of an elevated level of serum IgM and low levels of other Ig isotypes, particularly IgG.[96,97] Two forms of the disease are inherited in a X-linked manner: hyper-IgM syndrome type 1 (HIGM1), which is due to CD40-ligand deficiency, and X-linked hyper-IgM ectodermal dysplasia (XHM-ED), which is due to deficiency of the NF-κB essential modulator (NEMO) protein. Other forms are inherited in an autosomal recessive manner, including hyper-IgM syndrome type 2 (HIGM2), which is due to deficiency of activation-induced cytidine deaminase (AID), and hyper-IgM syndrome type 3 (HIGM3), which is due to CD40 deficiency.

HIGM1, which maps to Xq26, is due to failure of activated T cells, particularly those of the $CD4^+$ subset, to express functional CD40 ligand (CD154).[98,99] CD40 ligand is a type II transmembrane glycoprotein and a member of the TNF ligand family that binds to CD40 on B cells. The interaction between CD40 ligand on the CD4 T cell and the CD40 molecule on APCs, mononuclear phagocytes, and B cells is essential for many adaptive immune responses, but it is not required for normal T- and B-cell development. Because the number of T and B cells and the absolute lymphocyte count is normal, diagnosis requires assaying for functional CD40-ligand surface expression on activated $CD4^+$ T cells by flow cytometry.[97] The engagement of CD40 by CD40 ligand activates NF-κB–dependent transcription by a kinase complex that includes the inhibitor of κB kinase γ (IKK-γ) protein, also known as NEMO. CD40 engagement by CD40 ligand signals the B cell to proliferate and undergo deletional isotype switching (also referred to as *switch recombination*).[96,98,99] CD40-ligand/CD40 interactions are also required for induction of germinal center formation in lymphoid follicles and generation of memory B cells, which occurs in germinal centers. As a result, the main isotypes expressed on B cells in HIGM1 usually are IgM and IgD. When these B cells are immortalized with EBV, they mainly secrete IgM and not other isotypes. Cross-linking of CD40 on B cells from patients with HIGM1 with anti-CD40 antibody or functional CD40 ligand and stimulation with appropriate cytokines (e.g., IL-4, IL-10) can bypass the defect and activate normal isotype switching and Ig secretion. The engagement of CD40 by CD40 ligand also results in increased expression or upregulation of costimulatory molecules (e.g., B7–1 [CD80] and B7–2 [CD86]) on APCs, such as dendritic cells and mononuclear phagocytes. These costimulatory molecules are required for effective activation of T cells by APCs. CD40 engagement also induces secretion of cytokines, such as IL-12, from APCs, which promotes differentiation of naive $CD4^+$ T cells into T_H1 immune effector ($CD4^+$ T cells that produce high levels of IFN-γ). Defective CD40-ligand expression may lead to impaired generation of memory T cells, including T_H1 cells. CD40-ligand/CD40 interaction is essential for control of certain opportunistic infections, such as *Pneumocystis*. Another frequent abnormality in HIGM1 is neutropenia, whose underlying mechanism is elusive.[26]

XHM-ED, which maps to Xq28, is due to mutations in NEMO that result in a primary immunodeficiency characterized by hypoplasia of hair, teeth, and sweat glands (hypohidrotic ectodermal dysplasia) in combination with some features of the hyper-IgM syndrome. The ectodermal abnormalities observed are due to the NEMO mutation, which compromises signaling through ectodysplasin 1 anhidrotic receptor, which, like CD40, is a member of the TNF receptor superfamily. Susceptibility to infections, particularly encapsulated gram-positive and gram-negative bacteria,[96,98,100,101] is characteristic and appears to mainly reflect limitations in NF-κB–mediated immunity. In contrast to HIGM1, opportunistic infections characteristic of T-cell immunodeficiency are less common in XHM-ED, suggesting substantial signaling via CD40 engagement in the absence of NEMO.

HIGM2 is a form of hyper-IgM syndrome maps to 12p13 and arises from defects in AID.[102] It is inherited in an autosomal recessive manner. AID is a member of the RNA-editing deaminase family that contains proteins able to create new functional products from messenger RNA (mRNA) by base substitution. AID expression is limited to germinal center B cells, suggesting a role of AID in terminal B-cell differentiation. AID is directly involved in the isotype switching process. Because T-cell development and function are unaffected in patients with HIGM2, patients experience increased bacterial infections due to antibody deficiency but are not at increased risk for the opportunistic infections seen in HIGM1 and other T-cell disorders. An autosomal recessive form of hyper-IgM syndrome, also known as HIGM5, results from mutations of the enzyme uracil *N*-glycosylase (UNG).[102,103] It is phenotypically almost indistinguishable from AID deficiency.

An autosomal recessive form of hyper-IgM syndrome, termed HIGM3, due to mutations in CD40 has been described.[104] HIGM3 is similar to HIGM1 (CD40-ligand deficiency), resulting in the combination of increased risk of pyogenic and T-cell deficiency opportunistic infections. This phenotype fits with CD40 being the only major receptor for CD40 ligand.

Clinical Manifestations

HIGM1 and HIGM3 result in severe qualitative defects in B-cell function and recurrent sinopulmonary infections, such as otitis media, upper respiratory tract infections, and pneumonia, with encapsulated bacteria. Rarely, the humoral immunodeficiency results in chronic parvovirus-induced anemia or enteroviral meningoencephalitis. A partial but important qualitative defect in T-cell function has been demonstrated by the extreme susceptibility of these patients during infancy to *Pneumocystis jiroveci* pneumonia. This finding highlights the importance of CD40 ligand produced by $CD4^+$ T cells in the normal control of this fungus, perhaps by activating alveolar macrophages of the lung. Other infections indicative of T-cell immunodeficiency have been reported, including hepatobiliary infection with *Cryptosporidium*, cryptococcal meningitis, disseminated histoplasmosis, oral candidiasis, disseminated toxoplasmosis, severe CMV disease, enteroviral pneumonia, and progressive multifocal leukoencephalopathy due to JC virus.[105] The susceptibility of CD40-ligand or CD40 deficiency also may be due to failure of CD40 ligand on activated T cells to activate CD40-expressing macrophages or to induce dendritic cells to secrete IL-12, which is required for memory T_H1-type immune responses. Diarrhea and sclerosing cholangitis occur secondary to *Cryptosporidium* infection, which is a major risk factor for the development of tumors of the hepatobiliary system.[106] Lymphoid hyperplasia with lymphadenopathy, tonsillar enlargement, and hepatosplenomegaly are common. In contrast, hyper-IgM syndrome due to AID and UNG deficiencies are not associated with increased susceptibility to T-cell opportunistic infections but only pyogenic bacterial infections.

Chronic neutropenia occurs in about half of patients with HIGM1 and usually appears after the first year of life. Although the precise mechanism is unclear, neutropenia appears to arise from defective myeloid differentiation at the promyelocyte or myelocyte stage and probably is not due to autoantibodies. The neutropenia may be cyclic or episodic and associated with infection. Stomatitis and chronic recurrent oral or rectal ulcers may complicate the neutropenia but can occur independently. Autoimmune manifestations include arthritis or arthralgia, nephritis, and hemolytic anemia. Surface IgM-positive non-Hodgkin and Hodgkin lymphomas with gastrointestinal tract involvement may occur.

Laboratory Evaluation

Serum levels of IgM and, at times, IgD are markedly elevated. Other Ig isotypes, particularly IgG and IgA, are present in low levels or are absent. However, the IgM level may be normal at an early age. In one study, only half of the patients with HIGM1 had increased serum IgM levels at the time of diagnosis, and one third of patients failed to develop increased levels of IgM during follow-up.[105] IgM is polyclonal, and antibody responses, when they occur, are restricted to the IgM isotype. Peripheral blood B cells are normal in number and express IgM and IgD, but cells with surface IgG or IgA usually are absent. In vitro stimulation of peripheral blood B cells with anti-CD40 antibody or CD40-ligand–expressing cells in the presence of IL-10 or IL-4 will activate isotype switching and secretion of IgG or IgE, respectively, in HIGM1. Definitive diagnosis of HIGM1 is made by demonstrating lack of surface expression of CD40 ligand on activated T cells and failure of soluble forms of CD40 to bind such cells. Lymph nodes lack secondary follicles within germinal centers and show severe depletion of follicular dendritic cells. Female carriers of HIGM1 can be diagnosed by demonstrating expression of functional CD40 ligand on approximately half of their activated T cells. Rarely, female carriers are symptomatic as a result of excessive expression of the cells bearing the X chromosome encoding the abnormal CD40-ligand allele.[107] CD40 deficiency should be suspected in male or female patients who have the clinical features of HIGM1 but have normal expression of functional CD40 ligand (i.e., able to bind to recombinant CD40). XHM-ED should be suspected in patients with clinical findings similar to HIGM1, particularly with recurrent severe infections with encapsulated bacteria, but that is accompanied by hypoplasia of the hair, teeth, and sweat glands. Patients with normal CD40 and CD40-ligand expression should be examined for mutations in AID and UNG, particularly if no evidence of T-cell opportunistic infections is seen.

Therapy

Hematopoietic cell transplantation (HCT) with hematopoietic precursor cells contained in bone marrow, peripheral blood, or cord blood should be strongly considered because of the high morbidity and mortality rates associated with the HIGM1.[105] Even in cases of preexisting cholangiopathy, a nonmyeloablative approach to HCT has been successful in some patients.[108] With Ig replacement therapy, increased IgM levels fall to normal in about half of patients, presumably as a result of feedback inhibition and prevention of infection. Lymphoid hyperplasia and neutropenia also may be reversed with Ig replacement therapy. The neutropenia may respond to therapy with granulocyte colony-stimulating factor. Prophylaxis against *Pneumocystis* pneumonia should be initiated immediately after diagnosis and maintained indefinitely for all forms of the disorder, except possibly in patients with AID or UNG deficiency. Identification of the genetic causes of hyper-IgM syndrome has improved diagnosis, prenatal detection, and counseling and may allow for development of gene therapy.

Selective Deficiencies of Immunoglobulin G Subclasses and Immunoglobulin Isotypes other than Immunoglobulin A

Patients evaluated for recurrent infections may have selective IgG subclass deficiency, such as abnormally low levels of IgG2 and IgG4 or selectively decreased IgG3 levels. Such subclass deficiencies usually are not associated with structural gene abnormalities of the heavy-chain gene locus, and the mechanism for these decreases is unknown. Caution is indicated in the diagnosis of IgG4 subclass deficiency in young children because this subclass has the most delayed appearance after birth of the four IgG subclasses. As in the case of IgA deficiency, IgG subclass deficiencies may be more common in CVID and certain other primary immunodeficiencies, such as ataxia-telangiectasia. Treatment of these IgG subclass deficiencies with Ig replacement usually is not indicated unless reduced antibody-specific responses to vaccines, such as the 23-valent pneumococcal polysaccharide vaccine, is documented. Rare deletions of the heavy-chain gene involve several or single constant region IgG subclass segments.[109,110] Most patients with these partial deletions usually are healthy, potentially as a result of the increased generation of protective IgG3 antibacterial antibodies.[110]

Selective IgM deficiency is a rare immunodeficiency disorder characterized by a low level of serum IgM and severe or life-threatening recurrent infections.[111] Pneumococcal and meningococcal sepsis or meningitis may occur. IgM antibodies are not produced, and IgG antibody responses usually are decreased, although the IgG level is normal. Defects of T_H and excessive suppressor T-cell activity have been described. Some of these patients subsequently develop a CVID-like syndrome.

Absence of either κ or λ light chains associated with hypogammaglobulinemia or IgA deficiency and recurrent respiratory tract infections, pernicious anemia, diarrhea, or malabsorption have rarely been reported. One individual with κ light-chain deficiency had a point mutation in the Cκ gene segment involving amino acid residues required for formation of intrachain disulfide bonds and protein folding, but no clinical immunodeficiency was apparent.[112]

SEVERE COMBINED IMMUNODEFICIENCIES

Etiology and Pathophysiology

SCID is an inherited severe immunodeficiency of T-cell and B-cell function[113] that occurs in approximately 1 : 50,000 live births. The term *combined* reflects the fact that severe T-cell deficiency usually compromises B-cell function because of a lack of T-cell help, even if B cells are present in normal numbers and have the potential for intrinsically normal function. About 80% of affected patients are boys, and only approximately one third of patients with SCID have a positive family history. SCID may result from single X-linked or autosomal recessive gene defects or, less commonly, from chromosome abnormalities. Peripheral T-cell dysfunction in all forms of SCID is mainly or entirely due to perturbed intrathymic maturation of αβ T cells (i.e., T cells that express αβ T-cell receptors [TCRs]) resulting in thymic hypoplasia.[113]

The most common causes of SCID are defects in expression of cytokine receptors or associated kinases by immature thymocytes. X-linked SCID, which accounts for approximately 45% of SCID cases in most series, is characterized by an absence of mature T and NK cells and normal to increased numbers of peripheral B cells.[113] X-linked SCID is due to abnormalities of the gene encoding the common γ chain (γ_c, or CD132), which is an obligate component of the IL-7 receptor (IL-7R) as well as other cytokine receptors. Deficiencies of other components of IL-7R, such as the IL-7R α chain, or of proteins required for IL-7R signal transduction, such as Janus kinase 3 (Jak3), which is intracellularly associated with the cytoplas-

Immunoglobulin Replacement Therapy

Replacement therapy with Ig is indicated for patients with recurrent infections who have defects in antibody production. Such therapy can be lifesaving and prevent recurrent infections and progressive lung damage. However, the cost of Ig replacement therapy is high, so it should not be used indiscriminately. Antibody titers before and after immunization with protein and polysaccharide antigens should be evaluated to assess the need for replacement therapy whenever possible (see Table 51–1). Usual indications include X-linked agammaglobulinemia, common variable immunodeficiency, severe combined immunodeficiency disease, hyper-IgM syndrome, and Wiskott-Aldrich syndrome.

Replacement therapy should not be given to patients with isolated IgG subclass deficiency or low IgM levels unless they have a documented deficiency of specific antibody production and have not benefited from antibiotic prophylaxis. IgG replacement therapy usually is not indicated for isolated IgA deficiency, but some patients with IgA deficiency and concomitant deficiency of IgG antibody production and severe, recurrent infections have improved with replacement therapy. Patients with IgA deficiency may develop anti-IgA antibodies of the IgE isotype that can cause severe or fatal anaphylactic reactions with intravenous administration of IgA-containing blood products. Ig replacement therapy with Ig preparations containing low levels of IgA that are administered by the intravenous or subcutaneous route has been used successfully in these patients.

Development of safe IVIG formulations allows administration of high doses without the pain, side effects, and tissue loss experienced with intramuscular γ-globulin replacement. Multiple IVIG preparations have been approved by the Food and Drug Administration (FDA). All preparations are safe, contain predominantly IgG1 and IgG2, have approximately comparable and consistent IgG antibody titers, and generally are therapeutically equivalent. The FDA-licensed Ig preparations do not carry a risk of transmitting the human immunodeficiency virus. IVIG formulations in the 10% concentration can be used for subcutaneous administration, and a higher concentration product (16%) has been licensed specifically for subcutaneous administration.

The half-life of administered IgG varies among patients. The optimal amount and frequency of infusion of Ig and the serum level of IgG to be achieved must be individualized to render the patient asymptomatic from recurrent infections. In general, with IV administration a trough serum level that is at least 200 to 400 mg/dL higher than the pretherapy level (or >500 mg/dL) should be attained before the next injection. In cases of severe hypogammaglobulinemia, an initial IgG dose of 400 mg/kg usually is given, followed by a similar dose 3 to 7 days later and then every 3 to 4 weeks thereafter. Trough levels should be checked bimonthly for the first 8 months and then every 6 months thereafter. This dosage regimen will result in a steady-state level after 4 to 8 months, with trough levels greater than 500 mg/dL. In general, an IVIG dose of 100 mg/kg will increase the IgG peak by 200 to 300 mg/dL and trough levels by 100 mg/dL (28 days postinfusion). Higher doses (≥600 mg/kg) of IVIG may be required to prevent infections in some patients and may prove better at preventing acute infections or exacerbations in patients with chronic pulmonary disease. If patients complain of fatigue, upper respiratory infections, or conjunctivitis during the week before the next infusion or if intercurrent infections occur, the frequency of infusion or the dose should be increased to raise the trough serum level to greater than 500 mg/dL. During infections, extra infusions may be required because of increases in the catabolic rate of the passively provided Ig. Home infusion therapy is now being practiced widely.

Subcutaneous infusion of Ig is an alternative to intravenous infusions, with a low frequency of systemic adverse reactions. For example, postinfusion headaches are extremely rare. Moreover, the serum level of IgG varies much less between doses because of slow absorption of the product, avoiding breakthrough infections that can occur as IgG levels decline following IVIG administration. The main disadvantage of the subcutaneous route is that less Ig can be administered in a single dose than can be given by the intravenous route. Typically, patients receive approximately 100 to 150 mg/kg every 7 to 10 days using multiple sites for infusion of each dose. This method can be technically challenging in patients with limited subcutaneous tissue.

Adverse reactions to IVIG administration include flushing, chest tightness, flank or abdominal pain, nausea and vomiting, chills, fever, headache, myalgias, dyspnea, diaphoresis, and hypotension. These reactions usually can be controlled by decreasing the infusion rate. In general, reactions are more common with the first infused dose and in the presence of an intercurrent infection. In these situations, infusions should be slower. Repeated severe reactions that do not respond to a decrease in the rate or volume of the infusion may be averted in some patients by pretreatment 1 hour before IVIG with aspirin, ibuprofen or acetaminophen, antihistamines, or steroids. Aseptic meningitis, usually manifesting as a severe headache, may occur after IVIG infusion but apparently not after subcutaneous administration of Ig. Rarely, anaphylactic reactions to IVIG occur. Anaphylactic reactions require stopping the infusion and immediate administration of epinephrine, steroids, and antihistamines, together with respiratory and circulatory support. Anaphylactic reactions rarely are caused by production of IgE antibodies to IgA in patients with IgA deficiency or those with common variable immunodeficiencies with absent IgA. Anti-IgA antibodies should be quantitated following an anaphylactic reaction. If anti-IgA antibodies are present, IVIG preparations with low levels of IgA should be used and the subcutaneous route strongly considered. Anaphylaxis after Ig administered subcutaneously can occur but is rare.

mic domain of γ_c, also results in SCID. The phenotype is similar to that in γ_c deficiency, except that these types of SCID have an autosomal recessive rather than an X-linked inheritance pattern and NK cells are present in IL-7R α-chain deficiency.[113] CD25 deficiency, which is a component of the high-affinity IL-2 receptor, is another example of a cytokine receptor deficiency resulting in SCID. SCID with an autosomal recessive inheritance pattern also may be due to any of the following conditions:

- Increased thymocyte death from toxic effects of accumulated purine metabolites, as in deficiency of adenosine deaminase (ADA) or purine nucleoside phosphorylase (PNP) (which accounts for approximately 20% of cases of autosomal recessive SCID)
- Defective thymocyte rearrangement of TCR genes, including defects of recombination-activating gene 1 (RAG1) or RAG2 proteins (which accounts for approximately 10% of cases of autosomal recessive SCID), partial RAG deficiency (major cause of Omenn syndrome), and nonhomologous end-joining DNA repair (deficiency of Artemis, Cernunnos-XLF (XRCC4-like factor), and DNA ligase IV)
- Defects in the ability of developing thymocytes to transmit intracellular signals through the αβ TCR–CD3 complex (deficiency of CD3δ, CD3ε, CD3ζ, CD3ζ-associated protein [CD3-zeta-associated protein of 70 kilodaltons (ZAP-70)] kinase, lck tyrosine kinase, and CD45 protein tyrosine phosphatase)
- Failure of development of bone marrow precursors that normally colonize the thymus and give rise to thymocytes (reticular dysgenesis)
- Deficiencies in expression of class II MHC molecules, which are required for intrathymic development (positive selection) of

Laboratory Evaluation for Suspected Immunodeficiency

General
- Complete blood cell count
- Chest radiograph
- Serology, culture, and polymerase chain reaction or antigen detection for human immunodeficiency virus

Antibody Deficiency

Initial
- Quantitative Ig levels: IgG, IgM, IgA, IgE
- Antibody titers before and after immunization: Tetanus toxoid, diphtheria toxoid, *Haemophilus influenzae* type b, pneumococcal capsular polysaccharides
- Isohemagglutinin titer

Later
- Quantitation of B cells
- IgG subclasses
- In vitro Ig isotype switching and synthesis (generally only available as a research test) btk or other suspected gene mutations: DNA sequencing
- T-cell CD40-ligand expression by flow cytometry using monoclonal antibodies or CD40 fusion protein

T-Cell Deficiency

Initial
- Absolute lymphocyte count
- Quantitation of T cells and T-cell subsets
- Lymphocyte proliferative response to mitogens and vaccine antigens (e.g., tetanus)

Later
- Proliferative responses to other antigens and allogeneic cells
- Flow cytometric analyses for intracellular cytokines and MHC/tetramer binding
- Quantitation of enzyme activity: Adenosine deaminase, nucleoside phosphorylase
- Protein and mutation analyses for SCID: γ_c, Jak3, interleukin-7 receptor α chain (IL-7Rα), RAG1, RAG2, ZAP-70, lck, Artemis, DNA ligase IV, Cernunnos/XLF, Orai1, winged helix nude (WHN), CD3γ, CD3δ, CD3ε, CD3ζ, CD25, CD45
- MHC class I and II expression and mutation analysis for RFXANK, RFX5, RFXAP, and CIITA if MHC class II mRNA is low or undetectable
- In vitro T-cell activation studies

Complement Deficiency

Initial
- Total hemolytic complement (determination of 50% hemolyzing dose [CH_{50}])
- Properdin (in males with *Neisseria* infections)

Later
- Quantitation and functional analysis of individual components

Polymorphonuclear Leukocyte and Macrophage Deficiency

Initial
- Polymorphonuclear leukocyte count and morphology
- Howell-Jolly bodies
- IgE level
- Dihydrorhodamine (DHR) flow cytometric respiratory burst assay (preferable to nitroblue tetrazolium [NBT] reduction test)

Later
- Rebuck skin window test
- Assays for chemotaxis, chemokinesis, random migration, phagocytosis, phagocyte killing, oxidative metabolism, enzyme activity
- CD11/CD18 expression
- Spleen/liver scan (^{35}S colloid uptake)

Ig, immunoglobulin; MHC, major histocompatibility complex; SCID, severe combined immunodeficiency.

CD4+ T cells from CD4+CD8+ thymocytes as well as antigen presentation to mature peripheral CD4+ T cells (RFXANK, RFX5, RFXAP, CIITA deficiency)

- Mutations in the sequence for an RNA (RNA polymerase II subunit 5 [RPB5]-mediating protein [RMP]), which is involved in mitochondrial RNA processing
- Abnormalities in calcium channel function due to mutations in Orai1, which affects T-lineage cell signaling
- Mutations in winged helix nude (WHN), a transcription factor important for normal development of the thymic microenvironment necessary or thymocyte differentiation

T−B+ Severe Combined Immunodeficiency

X-Linked Severe Combined Immunodeficiency

X-linked SCID maps to the chromosome Xq13.1 region. It results from abnormalities of the gene encoding γ_c, which is an obligate component of a specific surface receptor for IL-7 as well as the IL-2, IL-4, IL-9, IL-15, and IL-21 receptors (see Fig. 51–3).[114] A lack of functional γ_c interferes with T-cell development in the thymus, mainly because of a lack of IL-7 signaling by thymocytes. B cells are present in the periphery in normal or increased numbers but usually are not functionally competent. The lack of competence probably is due to an intrinsic impairment in B-cell responsiveness to cytokines[115] such as IL-4 and IL-21. In most instances, memory B cells are absent, and the B cells present have an immature phenotype. NK cells are absent because of their impaired development, probably secondary to a lack of IL-15 signaling. Mutations of γ_c that retain some expression of normal protein (e.g., splice-site mutations) suggest that NK-cell development and IL-15 receptor signaling is retained as the amount of cell surface γ_c becomes limiting for T-lineage cell development. In female carriers of X-linked SCID, there is nonrandom inactivation of the X chromosome bearing the X-linked SCID mutation in T cells, mature differentiated B cells, and NK cells. More than 151 different mutations of the human γ_c gene have been identified, with missense mutations of exon 5 among the most common and gene segment deletions the least common.[116] Up to one third of mutations that result in SCID may allow γ_c protein expression on the surface of leukocytes. Milder forms of the disease due to missense mutations that preserve some intracellular signaling have been described.[117] In one extreme example, a missense mutation resulted in clinical SCID with opportunistic infections despite apparently normal peripheral T-cell, NK-cell, and B-cell development.[118] In up to one third of affected children, the disorder arises spontaneously; therefore, a family history is lacking.

Jak3 Deficiency

Jak3 deficiency is another form of B-cell–positive SCID that is clinically indistinguishable from X-linked SCID except for its autosomal recessive inheritance pattern.[113,119,120] Jak3 is a tyrosine kinase that associates with the cytoplasmic domain of γ_c and is activated on cytokine binding at the cell surface.[121] Activated Jak3 tyrosine phosphorylates STAT (signal transducer and activator of transcription) proteins, which then dimerize and translocate to the nucleus to activate gene transcription. The STAT5 proteins STAT5a and STAT5b appear to be critical for the Jak3-dependent effects of IL-7 on thymocyte development. The immunologic phenotype of low T-cell numbers, absence of NK cells, and defective B-cell signaling in Jak3 deficiency is typically identical to that in X-linked SCID.

IL-7 Receptor α-Chain Deficiency

IL-7R α-chain deficiency is another autosomal recessive cause of SCID that is phenotypically similar to γ_c or Jak3 deficiency in that peripheral T cells are markedly decreased and normal numbers of B

Peripheral Blood Abnormalities in Immunodeficiency

Anemia
- Hemolytic: Antibody deficiency (especially CVID); 22q11.2 syndrome
- Hypoplastic: PNP deficiency, thymoma, X-linked lymphoproliferative syndrome
- Megaloblastic: Transcobalamin II deficiency, PNP deficiency, antibody-mediated pernicious anemia associated with APECED, CVID, IgA deficiency, cartilage-hair hypoplasia syndrome
- Blood loss: Wiskott-Aldrich syndrome, malabsorption and diarrhea associated with antibody deficiency

Lymphopenia
- Combined T-cell and B-cell deficiency: SCID due to deficiencies of ADA, RAG1/RAG2, Artemis, Cernunnos-XLF, DNA ligase IV
- T-cell lymphopenia with relatively preserved or increased B-cell numbers: X-linked SCID, Jak3 deficiency, ZAP-70 deficiency (greater decrease in CD8$^+$ relative to CD4$^+$ T cells), MHC class II deficiency, CD25 deficiency, p56^{lck} deficiency (all three disorders with greater decrease in CD4$^+$ relative to CD8$^+$ T cells), PNP deficiency, CD45 deficiency, 22q11.2 deletion syndromes (CD8$^+$ often more depressed than CD4$^+$ T cells), WHN deficiency, cartilage-hair hypoplasia syndrome, reticular dysgenesis

White Blood Cell Deficiency
- Neutropenia: Antibody deficiency (e.g., XLA before IVIG treatment), hyper-IgM syndromes (CD40-ligand and CD40 deficiencies), cartilage-hair hypoplasia syndrome

Neutrophilia
- Qualitative white blood cell disorders (e.g., LAD due to CD18 deficiency)

Eosinophilia
- SCID, GVHD, Omenn syndrome, T-cell deficiency, Wiskott-Aldrich syndrome, ataxia-telangiectasia, chronic granulomatous disease

Monocytosis
- Antibody, T-cell, white blood cell deficiencies, particularly during infections

Thrombocytopenia
- Wiskott-Aldrich syndrome (small platelets), Evans syndrome, autoantibodies as part of B-cell disorders (e.g., CVID), 22q11.2 deletion syndromes

Other
- Howell-Jolly bodies: Splenic absence or dysfunction
- Giant lysosomal cytoplasmic granules: Chédiak-Higashi syndrome

ADA, adenosine deaminase; APECED, autoimmune polyendocrinopathy-candidiasis-ectodermal dystrophy; CVID, common variable immunodeficiency; GVHD, graft-versus-host disease; IgM, immunoglobulin M; IVIG, intravenous immunoglobulin; LAD, leukocyte adhesion deficiency; MHC, major histocompatibility complex; PNP, purine nucleoside phosphorylase; SCID, severe combined immunodeficiency; XLA, X-linked agammaglobulinemia; WHN, winged helix nude.

cells are present.[122] The lack of a functional IL-7R α chain results in a loss of signaling by IL-7 as well as a related cytokine thymic stromal lymphopoietin (TSLP),[123] which, based on murine studies, appears to also play a role in CD4$^+$ T-cell development.[124] Thus, absent or reduced IL-7 and thymic stromal lymphopoietin–mediated signaling both may contribute to T-cell immunodeficiency. In contrast with X-linked SCID or SCID due to Jak3 deficiency, the number of NK cells is normal, indicating that NK-cell development is not IL-7 dependent.[122] Other cytokines, such as IL-15, likely are critical for NK-cell development, accounting for the absence of NK cells in γ_c or Jak3 deficiency.

CD3δ, CD3ε, and CD3ζ deficiency

The CD3 cell surface complex of proteins consists of CD3δ, CD3ε, CD3γ, and CD3ζ. These proteins are associated with and are required for surface expression of and signal transduction function by the αβ TCR or γδ TCR of the mature T cell.[125] The CD3 complex proteins are expressed beginning during early thymocyte development and are involved in the transduction of signals from the pre-TCR that contains a functionally rearranged TCR β protein. Genetic deficiency of either CD3δ[126,127] or CD3ε[127] can result in an autosomal recessive form of T$^-$B$^+$ SCID in which NK cells are also present in normal numbers. In contrast to many forms of SCID, thymic tissue may be radiologically detected in CD3δ deficiency, possibly because thymocytes may develop to a CD4$^+$CD8$^+$ intermediate stage of development. Two cases of CD3ζ deficiency due to a homozygous nonsense mutation were identified as a cause of SCID in which B cells and NK cells were present in normal numbers, but the number and function of T cells were reduced.[128,129] Interestingly, one of these patients had a subpopulation of clonally diverse CD4$^+$ T cells in the circulation in which one of the mutated alleles had undergone reversion to three different missense mutations, allowing increased expression of CD3ζ expression and improved T-cell function.[128] In the absence of such reversion, the phenotype appears to be a T$^-$B$^+$NK$^+$ form of SCID,[129] and murine studies suggest that a lack of CD3ζ results in an intrathymic maturational arrest just after TCR β-gene rearrangement at the CD4$^-$CD8$^-$ stage of thymocyte development.

CD45 Deficiency

An autosomal recessive form of T$^-$B$^+$ SCID also may result from a deficiency of CD45.[130,131] CD45 is a transmembrane protein tyrosine phosphatase that functions to regulate Src family kinases required for TCR and BCR signal transduction. In this form of SCID, αβ T cells, particularly those of the CD4$^+$ T-cell subset, are markedly decreased in number, whereas the percentage of γδ T cells is unaffected. Peripheral blood mononuclear cells have reduced responses to mitogens, consistent with a severe quantitative deficiency of αβ T cells. Although B-cell numbers are normal, serum Ig levels decrease with age, consistent with a chronic lack of CD4$^+$ T-cell help. Diagnosis is made by demonstrating a lack of surface CD45 and confirming that the lack is due to a genetic defect of the CD45 gene.

WHN (FOXN1) Deficiency

Two cases of an autosomal recessive form of T$^-$B$^+$ SCID that likely result from homozygous mutations of the WHN/FOXN1 gene have been reported.[132–134] The human WHN gene encodes a transcription factor that is required for thymic, hair follicle, and nail development and is the ortholog of the murine WHN gene, which is the cause of the mouse nude phenotype. Nude mice lack most peripheral T cells as a result of thymic hypoplasia. WHN mutation is expressed by nonhematopoietic cells, including those of the thymic epithelium, and its mutation results in a perturbed thymic microenvironment for T-cell differentiation. B-cell and NK-cell development and numbers are normal. The two patients that in retrospect were identified as having WHN nonsense mutations presented with generalized alopecia, hypomorphic nails, and severe T-cell lymphopenia. HCT is unlikely to permanently cure the disease given that the genetic defect is located in nonhematopoietic cells. Thymic transplantation might be considered for future cases that are identified.

DiGeorge Syndrome

DiGeorge syndrome (DGS) may result in a T$^-$B$^+$NK$^+$ form SCID in less than 5% of cases [see DiGeorge/Velocardiofacial Anomalies (Third and Fourth Pharyngeal Pouch Syndrome) later]. This severe form of the disorder is referred to as *complete DGS*. Complete DGS may be more common with deletion of the chromosome 10p14–13 region than with interstitial deletions of chromosome 22q11.2, which by far are the more common cause of DGS. Genetic screening for DGS by fluorescent in situ hybridization is advisable in cases of T⁻B⁺NK⁺ SCID because not all of these patients have other nonimmunologic characteristic features of the syndrome, such as cardiac disease or neonatal-onset hypoparathyroidism.[135] This is particularly important because patients with complete DGS may have a more sustained clinical response to thymic transplantation than to conventional HCT. Complete DGS may be associated with a severe dermatitis with T-cell infiltration and lymphadenopathy and high circulating levels of T cells.[136] These circulating T cells result from extreme oligoclonal expansion and lack signal-joint TCR excision circles (TRECS) and surface expression of CD45RA and CD62-L, indicating that they are not naive T cells. These patients have essentially no detectable antigen-specific T-cell immune responses.

T^-B^- Severe Combined Immunodeficiency

Adenosine Deaminase Deficiency and Purine Nucleoside Phosphorylase Deficiency

Approximately 15% of patients with SCID and 30% to 40% of patients with autosomal recessive SCID have deficiencies of ADA, an enzyme of the purine salvage pathway that deaminates adenosine and deoxyadenosine to inosine and deoxyinosine, respectively.[113,137] Although ADA is expressed by all cell types, ADA deficiency is particularly deleterious to the lymphoid system and interferes with lymphoid development in the thymus, which normally contains the highest level of ADA activity in the body. In the absence of ADA, accumulation of adenosine and deoxyadenosine increases the tendency of immature thymocytes to undergo apoptosis. The accumulation of deoxyadenosine triphosphate (dATP) in particular may inhibit survival signals mediated by signaling from the pre-TCR and the αβ TCR of the thymocyte. B-cell and NK-cell numbers are severely depressed in early-onset ADA deficiency manifesting as SCID,[138] and murine experiments indicate that ADA-deficient B cells are intrinsically sensitive to the accumulation of dATP.[139] ADA genetic deficiency may be complete or partial and usually is due to point mutations giving rise to a nonfunctional protein because of alterations in enzyme activity, stability, or structure. Rarer splicing defects and chromosome deletions of the ADA gene have been described. The immunodeficiency is progressive. Age at presentation is variable, depending on the amount of residual normal ADA activity that results from the particular ADA genotype; it can even first manifest in adulthood.[140] In contrast to most other forms of SCID, ADA deficiency may be associated with thymus development and production of Hassall corpuscles. ADA deficiency can rarely present with neonatal cholestatic jaundice or liver failure during infancy.

PNP deficiency is a rare, autosomal recessive disease of the purine metabolic pathway.[141,142] Although PNP deficiency differs from ADA deficiency in that B cells usually are present in normal numbers, it is discussed here with ADA because its pathogenesis and presentation are similar to that of SCID. PNP immunodeficiency is progressive. Symptoms commonly begin in early infancy as part of an SCID syndrome with enhanced susceptibility to opportunistic viral and fungal infections and failure to thrive. Death may result from overwhelming opportunistic infections, such as CMV or varicella-zoster virus.[143] The immunodeficiency is believed to be due to failure of conversion of deoxyguanosine to guanine and its consequent phosphorylation to deoxyguanylic acid (deoxyguanosine monophosphate [dGMP]) in lymphoid tissue. The toxic metabolite deoxyguanosine triphosphate (dGTP) accumulates in cells and inhibits ribonucleotide reductase, which is required for DNA synthesis and normal proliferation of thymocytes. T-cell numbers are markedly decreased. In vitro T-cell responses are abnormal, with absent delayed-type cutaneous hypersensitivity. B-cell numbers typically are normal, and circulating Ig is detectable. However, cases of complete PNP deficiency with severe depression of T cells usually lack an antibody-specific response to T-cell-dependent antigens, such as proteins. In contrast, autoantibodies, including rheumatoid factor, antinuclear antibodies, and antibodies to blood cells, may be produced, and autoimmune hemolytic anemia, immune thrombocytopenic purpura, and SLE may ensue. These autoimmune phenomena are particularly common with partial PNP deficiency, which can present in adulthood. Other possible features include megaloblastic anemia, neurologic abnormalities with spastic paresis of the trunk and extremities, cerebrovascular disease, developmental delay, and mental retardation. Diagnosis is made by assaying PNP activity in erythrocytes, lymphocytes, or fibroblasts and levels of deoxyguanosine and dGTP in blood. A low serum uric acid level is a useful screening assay for this enzyme deficiency. Prenatal diagnosis is feasible. Attempts at enzyme replacement therapy have not altered the clinical course, but improved methods for in vivo delivery are under development and appear promising.[144] HCT currently is the preferred form of therapy.

Lymphocyte Receptor Gene Rearrangement Defects—RAG1 and RAG2

The generation of a diverse repertoire of TCR and antibody requires VDJ recombination of the TCR α-, β-, γ-, and δ-chain genes and the heavy and light (κ and λ) Ig chain genes, respectively. This rearrangement process requires RAG1 and RAG2, which are expressed only by immature T- and B-lineage lymphocytes and act as DNA endonucleases, as well as widely expressed proteins that are involved in the process of nonhomologous end-joining (NHEJ) DNA repair.[145] SCID due to defects in this rearrangement process was first suggested by the finding of aberrant DJH joining in bone marrow pre-B cells from patients with SCID. In this form of the disease, ADA activity is normal, with failure of maturation of T and B cells resulting in lymphopenia and a complete absence of adaptive immune responses. NK cells are present and functional. About half of patients with the autosomal recessive forms of B⁻ADA⁺ SCID have nonsense, missense, or deletion mutations in *RAG1* and/or *RAG2*, resulting in loss of functional VDJ recombinase activity and an inability to generate antigen receptors in both T and B cells.[145,146] Hypomorphic mutations of RAG can result in other immune phenotypes, including a form of SCID in which γδ T cells are present in normal or increased numbers, possibly because of CMV infection,[147] and some specific B-cell immune responses are preserved.[148] Another RAG hypomorphic mutation was identified in a 6-month-old girl who demonstrated normal circulating levels of CD4⁺ and CD8⁺ αβ T cells but absent B cells; however, the CD4⁺ and CD8⁺ T cells were the product of just a few clones, so the patient was severely T-cell immunodeficient.[149]

Omenn Syndrome—Hypomorphic Gene Mutations of RAG and Other Proteins as Causes of Severe Combined Immunodeficiency

Omenn syndrome (originally called reticuloendotheliosis with eosinophilia by its discoverer, Gilbert Omenn) is an autosomal recessive form of SCID that includes scaly erythroderma, generalized lymphadenopathy, hepatosplenomegaly, intractable diarrhea, failure to thrive, eosinophilia, and increased IgE levels. In most cases, IgE levels are elevated despite an absence of peripheral B cells and decreases in other Ig isotypes.[150] This syndrome can result from RAG deficiency due to hypomorphic mutations,[151] but it also has been associated with other genetic causes of SCID, such as mutations of the IL-7Rα chain,[152] Artemis,[153] or the RNA component of the mitochondrial RNA-processing endoribonuclease (RMRP).[154] Omenn syndrome clinically resembles (GVHD) but the T cells infiltrating the skin and organs and in the circulation are autologous, activated (HLA-DR⁺CD45R0⁺CD25⁺), self-reactive cells with a severely restricted αβ TCR repertoire and a skewing toward the production of T_H2 cytokines, such as IL-4 and IL-5. This cytokine profile explains the eosinophilia and increased IgE levels. Normal or increased numbers of peripheral lymphocytes may be observed as a result of the marked peripheral T-cell expansion. The source of the B-lineage cells for production of IgE is unexplained. A study of several Omenn syndrome patients with hypomorphic RAG deficiencies suggests that these patients also have reduced expression of the *AIRE* gene,[155] which is required for expression of a variety of self-antigens in the thymic medulla. This secondary AIRE deficiency may result in impaired negative selection of the small number of thymocytes that are generated in Omenn syndrome, allowing them to enter the periphery and undergo clonal expansion to self-antigens and attack tissues, such as the skin and gut. Failure of these SCID patients to also produce regulatory T cells within the thymus may compound the autoimmune disease. Families in which one offspring had Omenn syndrome and another had typical lymphopenic SCID have been described, suggesting that the presentation may be strongly influenced by modifying genes or possibly by environmental factors, such as infection. Prompt HCT, often with adjunctive immunosuppressive therapy to control the autoimmune disease, is required to correct the syndrome permanently and prevent death. The correct diagnosis is important; Omenn syndrome can be mimicked by other diseases, such as Netherton syndrome (mutation of the *SPINK5* gene), in which neonatal-onset severe erythroderma and elevated IgE levels are common.[156]

Lymphocyte Receptor Gene Rearrangement Defects—DNA Repair Defects

Other patients with ADA$^+$ T$^-$B$^+$NK$^+$ SCID inherited in an autosomal recessive manner may demonstrate impaired VDJ recombination but normal RAG1 and RAG2 activity. This condition results from mutations in proteins involved in the general process of NHEJ DNA repair, including Artemis, which performs nucleolytic processing of the DNA ends generated by the RAG proteins so that they can be properly ligated,[157] and Cernunnos-XLF (XRCC4-like factor)[158] and DNA ligase IV (*LIG4* gene),[159,160] which are involved in the later DNA ligation step.[161] NHEJ is important not only for resolution of RAG-induced breaks in the TCR and Ig genes in developing lymphocytes but in all cell types for repair of double-stranded DNA breaks that can occur from radiation and other noxious stimuli. Therefore, a characteristic feature of SCID patients with Artemis, Cernunnos-XLF, or DNA ligase IV mutations is marked sensitivity to ionizing radiation, a feature that is not observed with RAG deficiencies. T$^-$B$^+$NK$^+$ SCID in Athabascan-speaking Native Americans occurs at a very high incidence (1 : 2000 live births) and is due to the high gene frequency of a particular Artemis mutant allele from a founder effect.[162] NHEJ also appears to be important for central nervous system development, as developmental delay and microcephaly are frequent findings in some of these patients, such as those with DNA ligase IV mutations.[159,160,163]

Reticular Dysgenesis

This rare autosomal recessive form of SCID is characterized by the absence of T cells and granulocytes in the peripheral blood and bone marrow.[164–166] B cells and monocyte numbers are normal in at least some patients.[167] Maturation of both lymphoid and myeloid lineage cells in the bone marrow is defective, and sensorineural deafness is a frequent complication.[168] Megakaryocyte and monocyte lineage development in the bone marrow usually is normal. The genetic cause of reticular dysgenesis is unknown. Overwhelming infections ensue unless the defect is corrected by HCT.[169]

Severe Combined Immunodeficiency with Preservation of αβ T-Cell Populations

A number of T-cell defects that impair T-cell activation through the αβ TCR–CD3 complex, including gene defects of the CD3γ component of the CD3 complex, CD25, the tyrosine kinases ZAP-70 and p56^{lck}, and Orai1, a protein required for generation of activation-induced intracellular calcium signal, can result in a form of immunodeficiency that clinically resembles other forms of SCID, except that substantial numbers of αβ T cells with a diverse αβ TCR repertoire may be preserved.[113] Increased incidences of infections, autoimmune hemolytic anemia, neutropenia or thrombocytopenia, allergies, cancer, and chronic diarrhea are typical.

CD3γ and CD3ε Deficiency

An autosomal recessive clinical SCID syndrome in which T cells are present in substantial numbers can result from CD3γ deficiency.[125] CD3γ, along with CD3δ, CD3ε, and CD3ζ, is a component of the CD3 complex required for intracellular signal transduction after the TCR is engaged by antigen. However, in contrast to complete CD3δ or CD3ε deficiency, in which a T$^-$B$^+$ form of SCID is typical (see section on CD3δ, CD3ε, and CD3γ deficiency, above), CD3γ does not appear to be essential for thymocyte development. CD3γ deficiency allows for generation of substantial numbers of CD4$^+$ and CD8$^+$ T cells. However, the T cells have reduced surface levels of the αβ TCR–CD3 complex and impaired signaling properties, as indicated by decreased in vitro T-cell responses to mitogens and specific protein antigens. B-cell and NK-cell numbers are normal.[170] The clinical phenotype is highly variable even for a particular genotype. For example, family members bearing the same CD3γ mutation as that of a severely affected patient may have only mild evidence of clinical immunodeficiency. A single patient with compound heterozygote CD3ε deficiency who presented with a relatively mild immunodeficiency characterized mainly by sinopulmonary infections with pyogenic bacteria rather than infections characteristic of T-cell immunodeficiency has been identified.[171] This mild phenotype may be possible because one of the CD3ε alleles is hypomorphic as well as the possible impact other modifying genes.

CD25 Deficiency

A truncation mutation of the IL-2 receptor α chain (CD25), which is an obligatory component of high-affinity IL-2 receptors, results in a clinical presentation of SCID. In contrast with most forms of SCID, there is a moderate level of circulating T lymphocytes, with relative preservation of the CD8$^+$ compared with the CD4$^+$ T-cell subset.[172] Thymic development appears to be perturbed, with a failure of thymocytes to express CD1 and downregulate the Bcl-2 antiapoptotic protein.[172] B-cell numbers are normal. Lymphocytic infiltration of multiple tissues, including the lung, liver, gut, and bone, is prominent. The lymphocytic infiltration may be due, at least in part, to decreased activity of regulatory T cells, which require high-affinity IL-2 receptor signaling for their generation and peripheral maintenance and play an important in peripheral control of potentially autoreactive T cells (see Immune Dysregulation, Polyendocrinopathy, Enteropathy, and X-Linked Inheritance Syndrome below).

ZAP-70 and lck Deficiencies

SCID can arise from mutations of two tyrosine kinases: ZAP-70 and lck. Deficiency of ZAP-70, which encodes a non-Src protein tyrosine kinase of the Syk family, is characterized by decreased CD8$^+$ T cells, with normal to increased numbers of CD4$^+$ T cells.[173,174] ZAP-70 kinase associates with the TCR after T-cell activation to transduce signals from the TCR. The paucity of CD8$^+$ T cells is due to failure of maturation and positive selection in the thymus. Although double-positive thymocytes accumulate in the thymus in this disorder, only single-positive CD4$^+$ thymocytes and not CD8$^+$ thymocytes develop and immigrate to the periphery, that is, peripheral CD8$^+$ T cells are absent. The peripheral CD4$^+$ T cells fail to proliferate in response to mitogens or to antigens that activate through the TCR but normally are activated by stimulation with phorbol esters and calcium ionophore, which bypass the requirement for TCR-associated protein tyrosine kinases. Thus, there is a complete lack of a functional T-cell compartment. B cells and NK cells are normal in number and intrinsic function. A single case of SCID due to defective expression of lck, a Src family tyrosine kinase expressed by lymphocytes of T-cell and NK-cell lineages, has been reported.[175] lck Deficiency results in selective CD4$^+$ T-cell lymphopenia, with the predominant CD8$^+$ T-cell population lacking CD28 expression. T cells have reduced responsiveness to mitogenic stimuli and IL-2, which becomes more severe with aging. B-cell and NK-cell numbers are in the low to low–normal range, and hypogammaglobulinemia is present.

CRAC Channel Function Defects

Ca^{2+}-release activated Ca^{2+} (CRAC) channels are a principal pathway for calcium influx into T cells from the extracellular space after engagement of the TCR by antigen. Activation-induced increases in intracellular Ca^{2+} concentration activate the calcium-dependent enzyme calcineurin, which in turn dephosphorylates serine residues of target proteins, including proteins of the nuclear factor of activated T cells (NFAT) transcription factor family. NFAT proteins then translocate from the cytoplasm to the nucleus, where they are involved in transcription of cytokines and CD40 ligand. T cells from two patients with SCID who had a T-cell defect in generating NFAT-binding activity to cytokine gene promoters[176] were shown to have a defect in the Orai1 gene.[177] Orai1 is an essential component of the CRAC channel,[178] which highlights its importance for lymphocyte activation and normal T-cell–mediated host defense.

Major Histocompatibility Complex and CD8α Deficiencies

MHC class II deficiency (also known as *bare lymphocyte syndrome type 2*) is a disorder of autosomal recessive inheritance characterized by failure of expression of MHC or HLA class II surface molecules on B cells, monocytes, activated T cells, dendritic cells, Langerhans cells in the skin, and epithelial cells in the thymus and intestine.[179] The most typical presentation is clinical SCID with a selective decrease in CD4$^+$ T cells but not CD8$^+$ T cells and normal numbers of B cells. The immunodeficiency arises from mutations of regulatory factors essential for MHC class II gene transcription that are not linked to the *MHC* locus. MHC class II recognition is required for the normal positive selection of CD4$^+$ T-lineage cells in the thymus. MHC class II expression by APCs also engages the αβ TCR of peripheral CD4$^+$ T cells to provide survival signals in the context of bound self-peptides and to activate these cells for immune responses in the context of bound foreign peptide antigens. In addition to decreased MHC gene transcription, expression of other genes involved in MHC class II antigen presentation, including invariant chain and HLA-DM molecules, is reduced. There is heterogeneity in the gene defects in MHC class II deficiency, with four distinct genetic complementation groups (A, B, C, and D) of *trans*-activating factors that regulate MHC class II gene expression. In most patients, there are mutations of the multimeric protein *trans*-activating regulatory factor X (RFX) complex, including RFXANK (complementation group B), RFX5 (complementation group C), and RFXAP (complementation group D), which cause a loss of transcription factor activity or binding to the X box segment of 5′ promoter region common to HLA class II genes. This results in complete loss of MHC class II gene transcription. Another form of the disease (complementation group A) is caused by a defect of the MHC class II *trans*-activator (CIITA), a master coactivator that forms a complex with the other transcription factors and is essential for activating RNA polymerase II at the promoter. These four proteins are also required for upregulation of MHC class II transcription by IFN-γ. In MHC class II deficiency, moderate reductions in HLA class I expression is also observed in some patients, but these decreases are relatively modest and of uncertain clinical significance.

Frequent clinical manifestations of MHC class II deficiency include primarily septicemia and recurrent gastrointestinal, upper and lower respiratory, and urinary tract infections. Patients are prone to bacterial, fungal, viral, and protozoal infections that start within the first year of life[180] and usually are progressively severe. Diagnosis is made by demonstrating absence of MHC class II expression on B cells, monocytes, or activated T cells. Few children reach puberty; the majority die between the ages of 6 months and 5 years. Rarely, patients have hypomorphic mutations resulting in a mild clinical course and a delay in diagnosis until adulthood.

MHC class II deficiency contrasts with a human disorder of MHC class I antigen presentation (also referred to as *bare lymphocyte syndrome type 1*). This condition results from mutations of the *TAP1* and *TAP2* genes.[181] TAP1 and TAP2 form the heterodimeric TAP peptide transporter that is required for transport of cytoplasmic peptides into the endoplasmic reticulum for binding to nascent HLA class I molecules. Because peptide is an obligatory component of the stable HLA class I molecules, these peptide-free molecules are degraded and fail to reach the cell surface. TAP deficiency is associated with reduced CD8$^+$ T-cell numbers, which most likely is the result of decreased positive selection of immature double-positive thymocytes for the single-positive CD8$^+$ T-cell lineage. A SCID phenotype has not been reported. More surprising is the apparent lack of severe viral infections in view of the well-documented importance of CD8$^+$ T cells in viral clearance in animal models and immunodeficient patients, such as HCT recipients. Instead, human TAP deficiency is associated with bronchiectasis, suggestive of chronic bacterial lung inflammation, but the precise pathogenesis of this complication is unclear. It is possible that TAP-independent HLA class I-restricted viral antigen recognition and preserved NK-cell activity may provide substantial antiviral host immunity in humans. A single family with homozygous CD8-α gene deficiency in which surface CD8 expression on peripheral T cells is completely absent has been identified.[182] CD8-α deficiency is associated with an increased percentage of CD4$^-$CD8$^-$ T cells expressing αβ TCRs, but whether these cells are MHC class I–restricted cells, as are most conventional CD8$^+$ T cells in normal individuals, is unclear. In this family, the clinical presentation of CD8-α deficiency ranged from asymptomatic to recurrent bronchitis and chronic lung disease, similar to TAP deficiency.

Clinical Manifestations of Severe Combined Immunodeficiency

Infections related to severe T-cell deficiency, which is shared by all forms of SCID, constitute the predominant feature of the disease. Thus, the different forms of SCID in general are clinically indistinguishable.[113] SCID usually manifests in early infancy with recurrent severe infections or persistent infections with low-virulence, opportunistic organisms, such as *Candida* or *Pneumocystis*, giving rise to chronic thrush or interstitial pneumonitis with severe hypoxemia, respectively. Chronic diarrhea and failure to thrive are usual features. Recurrent otitis media, skin infections, and chronic severe viral infections are frequently present. Invasive infections with gram-negative aerobic bacteria, such as *Pseudomonas* and *Enterobacter*, may occur, possibly because of a lack of IL-17–producing CD4$^+$ T cells. Fungal ulcers of the pharynx and nasal mucosa (Noma) are particularly frequent in patients with the Athabascan form of Artemis deficiency.[162] The diagnosis of SCID should be considered a pediatric emergency because correction of the defect becomes more difficult if serious infection ensues before HCT.

In partial ADA deficiency or hypomorphic mutations in other types of SCID that allow some development of the adaptive immune system, onset of symptoms may be delayed until the latter half of the first or second year of life, or even later (3–8 years).[140] With partial ADA deficiency, progression of the deterioration of immunity is slower because of the time required to accumulate the toxic metabolites. About half of children with ADA deficiencies have anomalies involving the ribs (flared costochondral junctions), scapula, or other parts of the skeleton, but these abnormalities are not specific for ADA deficiency. Neurologic and hepatic abnormalities also have been observed with ADA deficiency.

Patients with MHC class II deficiency present in the first year of life with a clinical picture typical of SCID, with recurrent severe bacterial, viral, or fungal infections causing recurrent bronchopulmonary disease, chronic protracted diarrhea, malabsorption, liver disease, or failure to thrive. Death often is caused by severe viral infections, particularly those of the herpesvirus group, that occur in the first years of life.

GVHD may arise from transfusion of unirradiated blood products or from maternal–fetal transfer of T lymphocytes in utero or at delivery. It may be associated with fever, eczematoid rash, diarrhea, hepatosplenomegaly, and eosinophilia and may be difficult to distinguish from Omenn syndrome. Although engraftment with maternal T lymphocytes occurs in up to 40% to 50% of patients with SCID, symptomatic GVHD often does not ensue, probably because maternal T cells represent a limited repertoire and/or may have suboptimal responses to activation.

Infection in SCID prior to HCT can induce hemophagocytosis in which secondary impairment of production of multiple hematopoietic cell lineages, including neutrophils and megakaryocytes, occurs.[183] Thus, in potential cases of reticular dysgenesis, consideration must be given to the possibility of a different etiology of SCID, such as γ_c or PNP deficiency,[183] in which the neutropenia may be secondary to hemophagocytosis. Hemophagocytosis of any etiology frequently is associated with secondary decreases in the numbers of circulating B cells,[184] which can complicate the clinical interpretation of the pattern of lymphocyte subsets in SCID. Rarely, hemophagocytosis can be the result of maternally engrafted T cells rather than severe infection.

Laboratory Evaluation of Severe Combined Immunodeficiency

Diagnosis of SCID should be established at the earliest age possible so that optimal therapy can be offered.[113] The total lymphocyte count may be markedly low for age in the T⁻B⁻ forms of SCID, but normal counts do not exclude the diagnosis. T-cell numbers, especially $CD4^+$ T cells, usually are markedly decreased, and the T cells that are present may display an immature phenotype. If substantial numbers of T cells are present, they may be derived from engraftment of maternal lymphocytes or result from a marked oligoclonal expansion of a small number of the infant's T cells with a limited αβ TCR repertoire. Omenn syndrome due to partial RAG1 or RAG2 deficiency or other genetic etiologies of SCID is a classic example of such an oligoclonal expansion. A typical sign of Omenn syndrome is the absence of peripheral B cells with markedly elevated IgE levels. Marked expansion of γδ T cells with severe αβ T-cell lymphopenia can occur in some cases of hypomorphic RAG deficiency. In addition, some forms of SCID may affect only certain subsets of T cells or have only a modest impact on T-cell numbers while having a more severe effect on T-cell function (see section on Severe Combined Immunodeficiery with Prevervation of αβ T-cell populations). For example, with MHC class II deficiency, there may be an increase in $CD8^+$ T-cell numbers and normal numbers of B cells, which conceals the absence of $CD4^+$ T cells. ZAP-70 deficiency is associated with a normal number of dysfunctional $CD4^+$ T cells with a paucity of $CD8^+$ T cells. In X-linked SCID, Jak3 deficiency, and CD45 deficiency, T cells are markedly depressed; B cells are normal or increased in number, but they fail to mature and function. PNP deficiency tends to selectively decrease T cells but leaves B cells unaffected. Deficiencies of ADA, RAG1, RAG2, Artemis, Cernunnos-XLF, and DNA ligase IV are associated with decreases in T and B cells.

In vitro T-cell responses to mitogens and allogeneic cells are absent or very limited, and responses to antigens, such as cell proliferation of peripheral blood mononuclear cells, are absent in SCID. Cutaneous delayed-type hypersensitivity reactions are absent. Ig levels usually are decreased, and specific antibody responses usually are absent, except in some patients with partial ADA deficiency. NK cells are decreased in γ_c-deficient, Jak3-deficient, and ADA-deficient SCID, although any NK cells found in ADA-deficient SCID may display normal function. The thymus in SCID typically is hypoplastic and fat filled, with markedly reduced thymocyte cellularity. Some mutations may permit sufficient thymic development to allow radiographic detection (e.g., CD3δ deficiency). Hassall corpuscles typically are absent, except with ADA or PNP deficiency.

Special studies that may be necessary for diagnosis include assays of the γ_c chain, Jak3, CD3 complex proteins, CD25, CD45, ADA and PNP enzyme activity, dATP, deoxyadenosine, dGTP, deoxyguanosine, ZAP-70 and lck tyrosine kinases, Orai1, and WHN. Analysis of signal transduction in T cells, αβ TCR repertoire, thymic output based on polymerase chain reaction for signal-joint TCR excision circles, MHC class I and class II MHC surface expression, and evaluation of peripheral T cells for maternal genetic markers (e.g., HLA type) as well as skin biopsies of rashes may be useful for establishing the diagnosis of SCID and GVHD.

For many of these diseases, diagnoses by genetic analysis or immunologic evaluation of fetal blood can be performed. For example, in ADA-deficient SCID, prenatal diagnosis is performed by assaying ADA activity or dATP levels in cultured amniotic cells, fetal blood obtained by fetoscopy, or chorionic villus samples. However, some children have small amounts of residual ADA activity, which may make diagnosis difficult. Prenatal diagnosis of SCID can be performed by molecular approaches once the specific gene defect in family members has been identified. Strategies are being developed for population-wide neonatal screening for SCID using polymerase chain reaction to measure the levels of TRECs in DNA isolated from Guthrie card blood spots.[185]

Therapy for Severe Combined Immunodeficiency

The optimal preparative regimen for HCT is a complex and controversial issue and must consider the risk of peritransplantation complications, including death, with the immunologic outcome (see Chapter 100). Although HCT with omission of such preparation usually results in T-cell engraftment and reconstitution of T-cell immunity in recipients with X-linked SCID, these patients usually do not have engraftment of donor B cells and have poor antibody-specific responses to antigen, requiring chronic Ig replacement. NK-cell engraftment may also not occur.

If the immunodeficiency is not corrected, SCID is invariably fatal. Transplantation of hematopoietic cells from HLA genotypically identical family donors completely restores the immunologic function of patients with various forms of T⁻B⁻ and T⁻B⁺ SCID and also is successful in correcting MHC class II deficiency and PNP deficiency.[113] Pretransplantation preparative cytoablation is not required; mortality with this approach has been minimal. T-cell–depleted haploidentical parental transplantation without cytoablative therapy has been successful in cases where HLA-matched relatives were not available. The frequency of GVHD with this approach has been relatively low, but the procedure may carry the risk of a late decline in T-cell immune function, particularly after the first decade following transplant.[186] However, to the best of our knowledge, no study has directly compared long-term immune reconstitution for different cell lineages with cytoablative versus noncytoablative preparative regimens. HCT using matched unrelated donors from cord blood, peripheral blood, or bone marrow may achieve more complete immune reconstitution of both donor T cells and B cells but also may carry a higher risk of posttransplantation mortality than approaches in which pretransplant cytoablation is avoided.[187] Lymphoid and hematopoietic stem cell engraftment is required to correct SCID from reticular dysgenesis and MHC class II deficiency. The presence of preexisting infection or GVHD hinders the success rate for transplantation. Although in utero transplantation of parenteral CD34+ hematopoietic progenitor cells has corrected X-linked SCID diagnosed in the fetus, HCT performed during the neonatal period appears to provide the best results in terms of outcome and is technically less challenging.

All blood products should be irradiated before transfusion of patients with SCID to prevent GVHD. Ig replacement therapy, nutritional support, and prophylaxis against *Pneumocystis* infection usually are required before HCT. Family members should be immunized with a killed rather than live vaccines (e.g., for influenza) to prevent infection in patients.

In the absence of an HLA-identical bone marrow donor, gene therapy has been used in infants with X-linked SCID or ADA deficiency (see Chapter 109).[188] Gene therapy has involved retroviral transduction of a normal cDNA for γ_c or ADA under the control of constitutive promoters into autologous CD34+ hematopoietic precursor cells that have the gene defect. This is followed by infusion of the transfected cell cultures into SCID patients. The initial results of treatment in 10 patients with γ_c deficiency were promising, with evidence of acquisition of normal T-cell and T-cell–dependent B-cell immunity and transduction of multiple lineages, including hematopoietic stem cells. However, several patients developed γδ T-cell leukemia that was related, at least in part, to retroviral integration of the gene therapy vector into the *LMO2* gene, with subsequent dysregulated LMO2 expression, an event that has been implicated in leukemogenesis. A similar retroviral transduction approach also resulted in substantial reconstitution of immunity in ADA deficiency, which appears to be stable. In contrast, leukemias have not been observed as yet in these ADA-deficient patients, perhaps because of technical differences in the retroviral transduction protocol or transgene (see Chapter 109).

Patients with ADA deficiency may be given ADA enzyme replacement therapy by intramuscular injection of polyethylene glycol (PEG)-modified bovine ADA.[189] Modification of ADA with PEG prolongs the circulating half-life of the enzyme and decreases its immunogenicity. PEG-ADA can improve the immunologic and clinical status of patients with ADA deficiency. The exogenous ADA lowers the level of the toxic metabolites in ADA-deficient lymphocytes by deaminating adenosine and 2′-deoxyadenosine. However, immune reconstitution provided by PEG-ADA can result in antibodies to ADA with a loss of secondary loss of immune function. In the absence of an HLA-identical donor, an HLA-haploidentical or matched-unrelated donor HCT is an alternative to ADA replacement therapy. However, use of PEG-ADA before HCT may restore host immunologic function and predispose to graft rejection. Similarly, ADA activity in the transplanted marrow may stimulate immunologic function of the recipient's residual T cells, preventing engraftment. This can be avoided by use of pretransplantation cytotoxic agents.

Interferon-γ/T Helper-1 Pathway Deficiencies

Etiology and Pathophysiology

Defects in the T_H1 pathway (Fig. 51–4) result in markedly increased susceptibility to infections with intracellular bacterial organisms, such as *Mycobacteria* and *Salmonella*. Mutations in five different genes (those encoding IL-12p40, IL-12Rβ1, IFN-γR1, IFN-γR2, and STAT1) result in disorders whose common pathogenesis is impaired IFN-γ–mediated immunity.[190] The T_H1 pathway of T-cell differentiation is initiated by APCs producing IL-12 in response to certain microbial and inflammatory stimuli. IL-12 is a heterodimer composed of p40 and p35 subunits. IL-23 is a close relative of IL-12. It consists of the IL-12 p40 subunit in association with a novel p19 subunit that is homologous to p35. IL-23 may be particularly important in the generation or maintenance of CD4 T cells that produce IL-17 (T_H17 cells), which have a role in host defense distinct from that of T_H1 cells (one at the period control of infections with gram-negative bacteria).[191] IL-12 and IL-23 mediate their effects by binding to specific receptors that are highly expressed by T cells and NK cells. The IL-12 receptor is composed of IL-12Rβ1 and the IL-12Rβ2 subunit. The IL-23 receptor consists of an IL-12Rβ1 subunit that associates with an IL-23R subunit. Many of the effects of IL-12 are mediated by STAT4. In response to IL-12 receptor engagement, STAT4 undergoes tyrosine phosphorylation by Jak2 and Tyk2, homodimerizes, and then moves to the nucleus, where it influences gene expression. IL-12 signaling results in the synthesis and secretion of IFN-γ by T cells and NK cells and in other effects, such as enhanced lymphocyte proliferation and induction of an antiapoptotic state. The IFN-γ receptor consists of two surface proteins, IFN-γR1 and IFN-γR2, both of which are required for receptor function. IFN-γ receptor signaling activates Jak2, resulting in translocation of STAT1 homodimers to the nucleus, where they increase transcription of IFN-γ response genes. STAT1 also is a component of a heterotrimeric complex consisting of STAT1/STAT2/IRF9 that mediates signaling by the type I IFN receptor, which specifically binds IFN-α or IFN-β proteins. In addition to these genetic deficiencies, the acquisition of autoantibodies against IFN-γ may mimic the phenotype due to genetic defects of the IFN-γ receptor.[192–194]

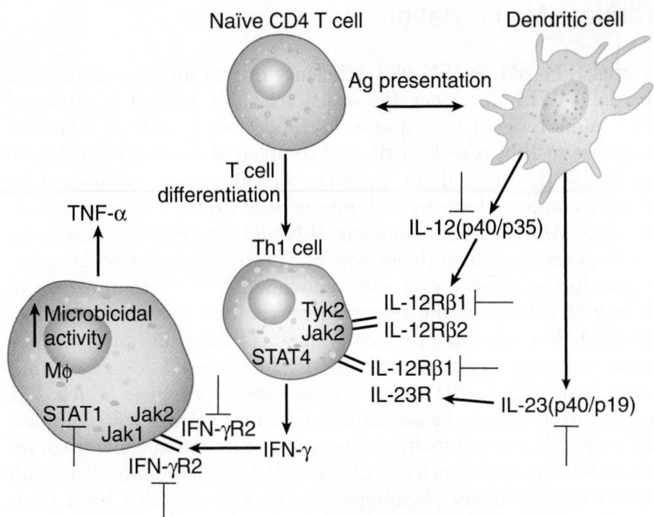

Figure 51–4 Interferon-γ/T helper-1 cell subset 1 (T_H1) pathway deficiencies. T_H1 differentiation is initiated when dendritic cells or mononuclear phagocytes are activated by foreign antigen (Ag) to produce interleukin-12 (IL-12), a heterodimer composed of p40 and p35 subunits. IL-23 is composed of the IL-12 p40 subunit and a unique p19 subunit. IL-12 and IL-23 bind to their specific receptors, IL-12Rβ1 and IL-12Rβ2 and IL-12Rβ1 and IL-23R subunits, respectively, on activated T cells and natural killer cells. IL-23 is less potent than IL-12 at T_H1 differentiation and, although not indicated in the figure, may be an important cytokine for the generation and/or maintenance of CD4 T cells that produce IL-17 (T_H17 cells). IL-12 binding to its receptor activates the Jak/STAT4 pathway of signal transduction and the release of the signature T_H1 cytokine interferon-γ (IFN-γ). IL-23 binding to its receptor may preferentially activate STAT3 than STAT4, accounting for its different effect from IL-12 on CD4 T-cell differentiation. The IFN-γ receptor (IFN-γR) consists of IFN-γR1 and IFN-γR2 subunits and is widely expressed. Upon IFN-γ binding to IFN-γ receptors to cells, such as macrophages, and natural killer cells, Jak1 and Jak2 are activated and phosphorylate STAT1, leading to induction of many proteins that enhance microbicidal activity, including the production of tumor necrosis factor α (TNF-α). Abnormalities in the T_H1 pathway result from mutations in five distinct genes that encode IL-12p40, IL-12Rβ1, IFN-γR1, IFN-γR2, and STAT1. Blocks in these genes are indicated in the figure (by ⊥ in various orientations). Spontaneously arising autoantibodies to IFN-γ that interfere with its biologic activity have been described. Jak, Janus kinase; STAT, signal transducer and activator of transcription.

Clinical Manifestations

Partial IFN-γR1 or IFN-γR2 deficiency due to missense mutations, partial STAT1 deficiency (in which a STAT1 protein is expressed that cannot signal in response to IFN-γ but is able to signal in response to IFN-α or IFN-β), and complete deficiency of IL-12p40 or IL-12Rβ1 all result in a similar clinical picture, manifested by usually curable infections with intracellular bacterial infections, particularly *Mycobacteria*. Complete IFN-γR1 or IFN-γR2 deficiency predisposes the patient to overwhelming intracellular bacterial infections during infancy and early childhood.[190,195,196] In the case of IFN-γR2 deficiency, the severe phenotype can result from gain of glycosylation mutants in which amino acid substitutions from missense mutations create de novo glycosylation sites.[196] A partial dominant form of IFN-γR1 deficiency has been reported in which T_H1 immunity appears to be less impaired than for persons with complete IFN-γR deficiency but with greater vulnerability to infection than for those with partial deficiencies.[197] The IFN-γR1 mutant allele with this partial dominant phenotype encodes a protein that has a truncated cytoplasmic domain and is defective in signaling. This truncation also removes a domain involved in receptor recycling from the cell surface, resulting in accumulation of abnormally high levels of the mutant IFN-γR1 on the cell surface. Because IFN-γ receptors require two normal IFN-R1 molecules for normal function, only a small number of surface IFN-γ receptors in patients with this partial dominant mutation effectively signal.[197] Complete STAT1 deficiency is similar to complete IFN-γR deficiencies, except that patients also are highly susceptible to viral pathogens, such as herpes simplex virus,[198] as a result of the absence of type I IFN receptor signaling.

Patients with complete or partial IFN-γR deficiency usually have disseminated infections caused by bacille Calmette-Guérin (BCG) vaccine and environmental nontuberculous *Mycobacteria*, including organisms not usually pathogenic in an immunocompetent host, such as *Mycobacterium smegmatis*. Infected tissue lacks well-defined granulomas, demonstrating the importance of the T_H1 pathway in this form of tissue reaction. Disseminated infections with *Salmonella* are seen in approximately 50% of patients, and *Listeria* infection occurs occasionally. Severe oral or respiratory tract infections with CMV, herpes simplex virus, varicella-zoster virus, respiratory syncytial virus, and parainfluenza virus may occur. In some of these patients, prior lung infection with *Mycobacteria* may contribute to the severity of viral infections. Patients with partial dominant IFN-γR1 deficiency appear to be particularly prone to develop mycobacterial osteomyelitis.[190,197] Deficiency of IL-12p40 or IL-12Rβ1 predisposes affected patients to intracellular bacterial infections that are similar to those seen with the IFN-γR deficiencies but often are less severe. Extraintestinal infections with nontyphoidal *Salmonella* is much more frequent than mycobacterial infections in IL-12p40 or IL-12Rβ1 deficiency.[199] This striking vulnerability to *Salmonella* infection may reflect a greater role of IL-23 as well as IL-12 in the control of these pathogens.

Several cases of adults with an acquired T_H1 immunodeficiency due to autoantibodies to IFN-γ have been reported. Most patients presented with persistent infection with atypical *Mycobacteria* of low virulence and did not have underlying diseases that would predispose to production of autoantibodies, such as frank SLE or CVID.[191–193] In one series, all six reported cases were Asian women.[193] Both IgG and IgM antibodies have been isolated with anti–IFN-γ activity.[193] The mechanism underlying the production of IFN-γ autoantibodies is unknown.

Laboratory Evaluation

Most patients with complete IFN-γR deficiency will not express the receptor on the surface of mononuclear phagocytes and do not secrete TNF-α in response to IFN-γ. Cells from patients with partial IFN-γR deficiencies may respond weakly to IFN-γ, and deficient responses may be overcome with increasing doses of IFN-γ. The partial dominant phenotype of IFN-γR1 deficiency is distinguished from other forms of the deficiency by increased rather than decreased expression on the cell surface, as the mutation impairs receptor internalization after ligand binding. As with other primary immunodeficiencies, gene sequencing, guided by functional or biochemical assays, often is essential for a definitive diagnosis. An accurate molecular diagnosis is crucial to determine the optimal treatment strategy for individual patients and family members. A useful set of screening assays for these deficiencies evaluates IFN-γ responsiveness by determining the ability of IFN-γ to induce TNF-α production by lipopolysaccharide-primed peripheral blood mononuclear cells IL-12 production; the ability of lipopolysaccharide (LPS) to induce IL-12p70 secretion by IFN-γ primed peripheral blood mononuclear cells; and IL-12 responsiveness by the ability of IL-12 and IL-23 to induce IFN-γ by peripheral blood mononuclear cells (T cells are the main producers in this assay), screening for high circulating levels if IFN-γ may also help identify IFN-γ receptor defects.[200]

Therapy

Treatment of all IFN-γ pathway deficiencies requires prompt administration of antimicrobials to treat infection. Mycobacterial infections in patients with complete IFN receptor deficiency or complete STAT1 deficiency should be treated aggressively with at least four different drugs. Surgery to remove a refractory infectious site may be effective. For patients with complete IFN-γR deficiency, prophylactic administration of antibiotics is recommended. Because of the poor outcomes in these patients, definitive correction of the defect by HCT is the treatment of choice. For patients with the partial dominant form of IFN-γ deficiency, prophylactic antibiotics may be useful, but HCT is not indicated. Patients with partial IFN-γR deficiency or partial dominant deficiency of STAT1, in which type I IFN receptor signaling (mediated by binding of IFN-α or IFN-β) is preserved, have good outcomes; therefore, neither prophylactic antibiotic therapy nor HCT is indicated. Patients with IL-12p40 deficiency and IL-12Rβ1 deficiency also appear to have generally good outcomes, and recalcitrant infections in these individuals often are responsive to IFN-γ treatment.

Wiskott-Aldrich Syndrome

Etiology and Pathophysiology

WAS is an X-linked recessive syndrome characterized by the triad of eczema, thrombocytopenia, and immunodeficiency.[201] Lymphoid as well as other hematopoietic cell types, such as APCs, are affected. The Wiskott-Aldrich gene maps to chromosome position Xp11.22–11.3 and encodes a 502-amino-acid protein termed WASP (WAS protein).[202] More than 160 different *WASP* mutations spanning all 12 exons of the gene have been identified. WASP couples TCR engagement with transcriptional activation and actin polymerization.[201] Defects in signal transduction and actin polymerization of APCs and B cells may contribute to the immunodeficiency.

Abnormal thrombocytopoiesis makes a major contribution to thrombocytopenia. This may be explained by a tyrosine kinase signaling pathway that signals through WASP and controls the assembly of actin, which is essential for megakaryocyte differentiation. Increased platelet destruction due to an intrinsic platelet defect also contributes to thrombocytopenia. Mean platelet volume is reduced, but there is a broad overlap with the normal range. The platelets in WAS express decreased surface glycoproteins IIb, IIIa, and IV and display defective thrombin-induced expression of CD62P (P-selectin) and CD63 and a decreased actin content. After splenectomy, the platelet count usually increases, and the mean distribution of the platelet volume returns to normal, indicating that platelet circulation through the splenic microarchitecture leads to reduced platelet size. Platelet-associated IgG frequently is present but disappears after splenectomy.

Female carriers are asymptomatic because of selection against cells that have the X chromosome carrying the mutant *WASP* gene as their active X chromosome. Nonrandom X chromosome inactivation patterns are observed in obligate carriers in T and B cells, monocytes, polymorphonuclear leukocytes, and platelets but not in fibroblasts. However, affected carriers with symptomatic WAS most likely due to skewed X chromosome activation have been discovered. Hereditary X-linked thrombocytopenia is characterized by thrombocytopenia and small platelets, similar to findings in WAS, without the immunodeficiency or eczema. This disorder is an allelic variant of WAS arising from mutations of the *WASP* gene that often result from missense or splice-site mutations that permit residual detectable WASP expression by cells rather than null mutations, such as frameshifts, deletions, and insertions, which usually ablate all protein expression.[203]

Clinical Manifestations

The initial manifestations usually are petechiae or bleeding in the skin, mouth, nose, or gastrointestinal or urinary tract, or from the umbilical cord, beginning in the first several months of life. Thrombocytopenia is present at birth. A life-threatening bleeding episode (gastrointestinal, intracranial, or severe oral) occurs before a diagnosis is made in up to one third of patients. Early in life, an eczematoid rash usually appears, although it can be quite subtle in some patients. Typically, the rash is prominent in the antecubital and popliteal fossae and tends to become petechial. At the time of diagnosis, only approximately 25% of patients with WAS have the classic triad of thrombocytopenia, eczema, and recurrent otitis media. Infections with bacteria cause recurrent otitis media with chronic purulent drainage and perforated tympanic membranes, recurrent pneumonia, sinusitis, and bacteremia. Viral infections may include recurrent and severe disease due to herpes simplex virus or varicella-zoster virus. Patients lacking all cellular WASP expression may be at particular risk for more severe opportunistic infections, such as *Pneumocystis* pneumonia or invasive fungal infections.[203] The thrombocytopenia and bleeding tendency often are worsened with infection. Autoimmune disorders develop in up to 40% of patients and include arthritis, vasculitis, uveitis, inflammatory bowel disease, and autoimmune hemolytic anemia. Certain instances of autoimmune disease, such as that involving the gastrointestinal tract and kidney, appear to be due to IgA deposition.

The median survival time in untreated WAS patients is 6.5 years. The cause of death is infection, usually from pneumonia or sepsis, in 59% of patients, bleeding in 27%, and malignancy in 5%. The risk of malignancy in patients with WAS is 100-fold higher than normal. A high incidence of lymphoreticular tumors that initially manifest at extranodal sites, especially non-Hodgkin lymphomas with B-cell immunoblastic sarcomas, is observed in patients who survive to later childhood.

Laboratory Evaluation

Immune abnormalities in WAS include a reduced antibody response to unconjugated polysaccharide antigens (severely depressed), protein antigens (moderately depressed), low serum IgM levels, and often elevated serum IgA and IgE levels.[201,203] Moderate T-cell lymphopenia, particularly of $CD8^+$ T cells, is observed in some cases, and T-cell function in vitro usually is depressed after stimulation with allogeneic cells or CD3 monoclonal antibody. The capacity of T cells activated in vitro to differentiate into effector cells producing IFN-γ is impaired.[204] The platelet count is decreased, ranging from $5000/mm^3$ to $100,000/mm^3$, and the platelet size is characteristically small, a feature that is highly specific for WAS or X-linked thrombocytopenia. The platelet count may vary considerably in an individual patient, with a decrease occurring with acute infections, such as with viruses. The number and morphology of megakaryocytes in the bone marrow are normal. The bleeding time is more prolonged than predicted from the platelet count, indicating platelet dysfunction. Rare cases of constitutively activating *WASP* mutations resulting in severe congenital neutropenia have been reported.[205] The carrier state can be diagnosed by demonstrating nonrandom X-chromosome inactivation patterns in leukocytes, although this technique has largely been supplanted by molecular diagnosis. Prenatal diagnosis can be made by detecting polymorphisms flanking the *WASP* gene or its mutations and by decreased fetal platelet count and size. The diagnosis after birth is suggested by the distinct clinical features of the syndrome and can be screened for by flow cytometry following cellular permeabilization and intracellular staining for WASP protein. Confirmation of the diagnosis requires molecular analysis of the *WASP* gene sequence. Determination of WASP expression by cells using Western blotting may be particular helpful in determining prognosis,[203] with detectable protein associated with a milder clinical course.

Therapy

Ig replacement therapy is indicated to decrease the risk of infections. This modality also may decrease the severity of autoimmune disease. HCT can correct all of the defects of this otherwise fatal disorder, including the susceptibility to malignancy and autoimmune disease.[206] Successful engraftment requires preparative ablation or cytoreduction of the recipient's bone marrow. The success rate with HLA-identical HCT is high. Matched unrelated donor HCT for WAS has resulted in some success, especially when performed at an early age. Unfortunately, the success rate of haploidentical parental HCT has been disappointing, and outcomes include a relatively high incidence of severe viral infections, lymphomas, EBV-induced B-cell lymphoproliferative disease, or chronic GVHD in the posttransplantation period.

Splenectomy combined with regularly administered prophylactic antibiotics has been used to manage some patients with severe bleeding problems who could not undergo transplantation.[207] Splenectomy increases the platelet count and decreases the bleeding tendency, but it also may increase the susceptibility to overwhelming sepsis, even with use of prophylactic antibiotics. A majority of splenectomized patients have a sustained increase of platelet counts by at least $20,000/mm^3$, and over half of these patients have a sustained increase by at least $100,000/mm^3$. Recurrences of thrombocytopenia with an acute immune thrombocytopenic purpura–like episode can occur after splenectomy; therapy with corticosteroids and IVIG may be useful in such cases.

Ataxia-Telangiectasia

Etiology and Pathophysiology

Ataxia-telangiectasia is an autosomal recessive disorder caused by mutations of the ataxia-telangiectasia mutated (*ATM*) gene. The disease is characterized by progressive cerebellar ataxia, telangiectasia, recurrent sinopulmonary infections, combined immunodeficiency, increased incidence of malignancies, and premature aging.[208] The frequency of ataxia-telangiectasia is estimated to be between 1 : 40,000 to 1 : 100,000 live births. The *ATM* gene encodes a 350-kd protein kinase with a phosphatidylinositol-3-kinase domain involved in multiple signaling pathways of cellular responses to DNA damage and in control of the cell cycle and DNA replication, recombination, and repair.[208,209] Mutations have included nonsense, splice-site variants, small insertions or deletions causing frameshifts with premature stop codons, missense mutations, and, rarely, large genomic deletions.[210] Ataxia-telangiectasia cells display chromosomal instability and hypersensitivity to agents that cause DNA strand breaks, including γ-rays and x-rays, ionizing radiation, and radiomimetic chemicals such as bleomycin. Ataxia-telangiectasia cells have an increased number of spontaneous and radiation-induced chromosome breaks, which are not rejoined as efficiently as in normal cells. Cells of heterozygous carriers have a sensitivity that is intermediate between those of cells from normal persons and homozygotes. These carriers may be at increased risk for cancer compared to the general population.

Ataxia-telangiectasia cells do not reduce their rate of DNA synthesis after irradiation, as do normal cells, because of dysfunction or absence of the ATM protein. In normal cells, irradiation-induced double-strand breaks in DNA lead to an arrest at the G_1–S transition, S, or G_2–M transition phase of the cell cycle. These cell-cycle checkpoints ensure that damaged DNA is not replicated and cell division does not occur until DNA strand breaks have been repaired. The ataxia-telangiectasia gene product functions in several irradiation-induced signal transduction pathways that recognize DNA damage and transduce a signal from damaged DNA to arrest the cell cycle and repair damaged DNA.[209,210]

The ATM protein is also required for maintaining immature B cells and thymocytes undergoing VDJ recombination from dividing during this process, which also requires double-stranded breaks, in this case by the endonuclease activity of the RAG genes acting on the Ig and TCR gene loci. Failure to prevent cell cycle entry in these developing lymphocytes in ataxia-telangiectasia accounts for the high frequency of lymphocytes with chromosome translocations and aberrant interlocus TCR and Ig gene rearrangements,[211] which also is important in the genesis of lymphoid tumors.[212] Aberrant TCR gene rearrangement may contribute to the relatively low number of peripheral αβ T cells, although these numbers usually are not severely depressed. This is paralleled by thymic hypoplasia and a lack of Hassall corpuscles. Isotype switching by ataxia-telangiectasia B cells may be impaired by a similar mechanism. Double-stranded DNA breaks in the Ig heavy chain switch region are part of normal isotype switching, and failure of the ATM protein to prevent entry of these B cells into the cell cycle may perturb this process.[209] Ataxia-telangiectasia may result in a persistence expression of proteins characteristic of early development, including elevated levels of serum α-fetoprotein and carcinoembryonic antigen. Ovarian agenesis and hypogonadism are frequent. In the absence of cell cycle arrest with *ATM* gene dysfunction, even low levels of DNA damage in ataxia-telangiectasia cells may activate an apoptotic cell death in various tissues, which in normal cells would be activated only by irreparable DNA damage. The increased apoptosis may explain organ atrophy in ataxia-telangiectasia.

Clinical Manifestations

The most common initial presentation of ataxia-telangiectasia is a progressive cerebellar ataxia that typically has onset in the second year of life.[208] Other neurologic symptoms occurring later are choreoathetosis, nystagmus, strabismus, dysarthric speech, and decreased deep tendon reflexes. Telangiectasias appear later in childhood and are most prominent on the bulbar conjunctivae, exposed areas of the skin, external ear, eyelids, face, flexor folds of the neck, extremities, and dorsa of the hands and feet. Recurrent sinopulmonary infections occur in a majority of patients and may become chronic, resulting in bronchiectasis and respiratory insufficiency. The overall risk of cancer is 60 to 180 times normal, with development of malignancies in up to 10% of patients.[73–75,208,213] Black patients with ataxia-telangiectasia have even higher risks of malignancy, especially lymphomas and leukemia. Most neoplasms occur before age 15 years, with a predominance of non-Hodgkin lymphomas having histologic subtypes that are observed with chromosome 14 translocations, Hodgkin lymphoma (mostly of the lymphocytic depletion type), T-cell leukemia, and epithelial carcinomas. Heterozygotes for the *ATM* gene have an approximately threefold to fourfold increased risk of malignancy. It is suggested that heterozygous females, who have an approximately fivefold increased risk of breast cancer, account for up to 8% of all patients with breast cancer in the United States. Caution must be exercised in the treatment of neoplasms because of the increased sensitivity of patients with ataxia-telangiectasia to radiation therapy. Endocrinologic abnormalities occur commonly and include delayed somatic growth, insulin resistance, delayed development of secondary sexual characteristics in females (secondary to absent or hypoplastic ovaries), hirsutism in females, and hypogonadism in males. Premature aging of the skin and diffuse graying of the hair usually occur. Venoocclusive disease of the liver has occurred in association with ataxia-telangiectasia.

Laboratory Evaluation

Absence or deficiency of serum and secretory IgA and of serum IgE are found in approximately 75% of patients. This finding may reflect impaired isotype switch recombination. Low levels of IgG2 and IgG4 and decreased antibody responses to immunization, particularly to purified polysaccharides, also are found. Anergy to delayed-type hypersensitivity skin testing, decreased T-cell numbers, and abnormal in vitro lymphocyte proliferative have been reported. In the mouse knockout model of ATM, thymocyte differentiation is perturbed because of frequent biallelic disruption of the TCRα gene locus. Production of T_H1 and T_H2 cytokines by T cells from patients with ataxia-telangiectasia after polyclonal stimulation in vitro is normal,[214] consistent with the relative rarity of infections characteristic of T_H1 deficiency (e.g., infection with *Mycobacteria*, *Salmonella*, and *Listeria*), in this disorder. Serum levels of α-fetoprotein are increased in greater than 95% of patients, and levels of carcinoembryonic antigen may be elevated. Nonrandom chromosome breaks and chromosome 14 translocations are frequently detected. Early diagnosis can be facilitated by demonstrating the radiosensitivity of EBV-transformed B-cell lines.[215] Genetic confirmation of the diagnosis is difficult because of the large size of the *ATM* gene (66 exons) and the diverse mutations that have been reported. Specialized assays, such as DOVAM-S (detection of virtually all mutations-SSCP),[216] may help with genetic confirmation.

Therapy

There is no established therapy for halting the disease. For ataxia-telangiectasia due to single nucleotide changes resulting in premature stop codons, treatment consisting of in vitro incubation of cells with aminoglycosides may allow increased read-through and expression of full-length protein.[217] Whether aminoglycoside treatment of patients with these mutations has clinical benefits is unclear. Antibiotics are indicated for recurrent pulmonary infections, and IVIG replacement therapy may be indicated. Exposure to excessive sunlight should be minimized to prevent skin changes. Treatment of malignancies in patients with ataxia-telangiectasia may require use of lower doses of radiotherapy and chemotherapy. Radiologic investigations using ionizing radiation, such as computed tomography scans, should be minimized whenever possible in favor of other modalities.

Digeorge/Velocardiofacial Anomalies (Third and Fourth Pharyngeal Pouch Syndrome)

Etiology and Pathophysiology

The DiGeorge or velocardiofacial syndromes most frequently result from a monosomic deletion of genes contained in the chromosome 22q11.2 region.[218] The 22q11.2 interstitial deletions of one chromosome may occur at a frequency of 1 : 3000 live births, with approximately 90% of cases due to deletion of a three-megabase segment flanked by low-copy repetitive sequences.[219] Most cases are sporadic, but the deletion can be either maternally or paternally inherited. In rare cases, a phenotypically similar syndrome results from monosomy for the chromosome 10p13 region. However, this is a relatively rare disorder and is not discussed further here.

This hemizygous genetic defect results in abnormal development of tissues derived from the third and fourth pharyngeal pouches. These pouch derivatives normally develop during the fourth to seventh weeks of fetal development and contribute to thymus, parathyroid glands, and conotruncal components of the heart, ear, and facial structures.[218,220] Possible clinical consequences of the 22q11.2

deletion include severe congenital heart disease, abnormal facies, thymic hypoplasia, cleft palate, and hypocalcemia. Haploinsufficiency for the *TBX1* gene, possibly in combination with other genes, such as *CrkL*, which is involved in intracellular signal transduction, as part of the 22q11.2 deletion may affect the migration of cephalic neural crest mesenchymal cells into the pharyngeal pouches, thereby disrupting tissue differentiation.[221] Haploinsufficiency of *TBX1* and *CrkL* appears to increase local retinoic acid signaling. It is intriguing that the DiGeorge anomaly also may arise from an environmental insult, including retinoid exposure as well as maternal alcoholism and diabetes. The observation that monozygotic twins with the 22q11.2 deletion can have markedly different phenotypes suggests that environmental or postzygotic events have important influences on the clinical expression of the syndrome.[222,223]

The thymus may be completely absent in the most severe form of this developmental field defect. However, more frequently the thymus is small, hypoplastic, and ectopic in location as a result of the lack of descent into the mediastinum. Most patients have a relatively clinically mild partial T-cell deficiency (i.e., without frank opportunistic infections), with decreased numbers of $CD4^+$ and $CD8^+$ αβ T cells that may improve with time. The $CD8^+$ T-cell compartment tends to be more affected than the number of $CD4^+$ T cells.[224] Rarely, complete thymic aplasia results in profound T-cell deficiency accompanied by a marked susceptibility to infections with intracellular pathogens typical of SCID. These severe cases usually do not improve with time.

Clinical Manifestations

A broad and variable spectrum of malformations is possible.[218,225] Affected infants often present with hypocalcemic tetany in the newborn period. Cardiac malformations include interrupted, right-sided, or double aortic arch; truncus arteriosus; pulmonary atresia; aberrant subclavian artery; ventricular septal defect; tetralogy of Fallot; and patent ductus arteriosus. These defects may give rise to cyanosis and cardiac murmurs. Type B interrupted aortic arch or truncus arteriosus are particularly suggestive of the diagnosis. Facial dysmorphic features include hypertelorism, antimongoloid slant of the eyes, midline facial clefts, micrognathia, shortened philtrum of the lip, cleft palate, choanal atresia, low-set posteriorly rotated ears, and notched ear pinnae. If the T-cell deficiency is severe, which occurs in less than 5% of patients, the infant may present with a SCID-type syndrome, with development of chronic or recurrent rhinitis, pneumonia, candidal infections, diarrhea, and failure to thrive. Moderate–to-severe developmental delays, renal anomalies, and dysphagia are common, and hearing loss may be present. Autoimmune disease, including autoantibody-mediated cytopenias, thyroid disease, and juvenile rheumatoid arthritis, are present in approximately 10% of patients with 22q11.2 hemizygous deletions.[218]

Laboratory Evaluation

In the approximately 70% of patients with thymic hypoplasia, total numbers of T cells are low, and B-cell numbers may be normal or increased, resulting in a normal total lymphocyte count. In vitro T-cell responses to nonspecific mitogens or allogeneic lymphocytes may range from normal to absent but in general are directly related to the numbers of T cells present. T-cell signal transduction through the TCR and the TCR repertoire appear to be normal in most patients.[226] Thus, most studies suggest that T-cell deficiency of the DiGeorge or velocardiofacial syndrome is mainly a quantitative rather than a qualitative disorder. The increased incidence of autoimmunity indicates that the 22q11.2 hemizygosity may have a relatively greater impact on mechanisms involved with tolerance, such as the production of regulatory T cells.[227] Unless the T-cell defect is severe, Ig levels of IgG, IgA, and IgM are normal or sometimes increased. Selective IgA deficiency may occur at an increased incidence compared with the general population.[228] Patients with partial T-cell immunodeficiency typically have normal specific antibody responses to T-dependent antigens.[229] A subset of patients with an increased susceptibility to sinopulmonary infections also may demonstrate a decreased antibody response to T-independent antigens, such as polysaccharide antigens.[230] Infants with $CD4^+$ T-cell counts less than 400/μL and decreased in vitro T-cell responses to mitogens are likely to be highly susceptible to infections and to have a persistent immunodeficiency. Profound T-cell deficiency is accompanied by defective antibody responses due to a lack of $CD4^+$ T-cell help. Decreased serum calcium, increased phosphorus, and decreased parathyroid hormone levels are typical with parathyroid hypoplasia. Cytogenetic studies with fluorescent in situ hybridization are used to identify chromosome 22q11.2 abnormalities in the patient and the parents.

Therapy

Hypocalcemia should be treated with intravenous calcium replacement, but the condition may prove difficult to control. Long-term treatment with oral calcium replacement, vitamin D, and a low-phosphate formula usually is required. Cardiac abnormalities, which may be severe, must be evaluated completely. Therapy usually is not required for partial T-cell deficiency because of frequent spontaneous improvement in T-cell function with increasing age and the usually mild clinical phenotype. For patients who present early life with severe, persistent T-cell deficiency and marked susceptibility to infections and failure to thrive, transplantation therapy is indicated because improvement from the immunodeficient state is much less likely. Treatment using transplantation of the thymus of fetal or postnatal origin has been successful.[231] Some severe cases of immunodeficiency also have received HCT,[232,233] but the durability of immune reconstitution after HCT is not known. Blood products from CMV-negative donors should be used and should be irradiated before administration to prevent GVHD. Antibiotic prophylaxis to prevent *Pneumocystis* pneumonia also is indicated in the face of severe T-cell deficiency. Prenatal diagnosis is possible and may be indicated if molecular evaluation is informative in a parent of an affected child.

Cartilage-Hair Hypoplasia Syndrome

Etiology and Pathophysiology

Cartilage-hair hypoplasia syndrome is a rare disorder of autosomal recessive inheritance that includes short stature due to metaphyseal chondrodysplasia, thin and sparse scalp and eyebrow hair, and immunodeficiency. This disorder is particularly common in Finland and among the Amish in the United States. The gene for cartilage-hair hypoplasia, *RMRP*, was identified by positional cloning and encodes an untranslated 267-basepair RNA that is part of a ribonucleoprotein complex.[234] This complex may be involved in multiple cellular processes, including nuclear and mitochondrial functions. Based on studies in yeast,[235] it is believed to include a role in normal cell cycle progression. Presumably, certain cell types, such as chondrocytes and lymphocytes, are more dependent on the function of RMRP-containing ribonucleoprotein than others. The immunodeficiency of cartilage-hair hypoplasia syndrome usually involves decreased numbers of $CD4^+$ and $CD8^+$ T cells, with relative sparing of B-cell numbers. The gene defect may result in thymic hypoplasia, perhaps by resulting in increased apoptosis, which has been documented for peripheral T cells.[236] Although B cells are present in normal numbers, IgA and IgG subclass deficiency is common, as is macrocytic anemia and neutropenia.

Clinical Manifestations

Although the best characterized immune defects of patients with cartilage-hair hypoplasia involve T cells and neutropenia, recurrent sinopulmonary infections are the most frequent problems.[237] In cases with severe T-cell deficiency, the presentation may be similar to that in T⁻B⁺ SCID, with characteristic opportunistic infections, such as *Pneumocystis* pneumonia. The chondrodysplastic skeletal manifestations are invariably part of the syndrome and can be present in the absence of immunodeficiency. In addition to skeletal, hair, and immunologic defects, the syndrome may include many other manifestations, such as hypoplastic anemia, ligamentous laxity, increased risk for malignancy (especially for non-Hodgkin lymphoma), Hirschsprung disease, and impaired spermatogenesis.

Laboratory Evaluation

Patients with cartilage-hair hypoplasia syndrome typically have modest T lymphopenia, predominantly of $CD4^+$ T cells, neutropenia, and hypoplastic anemia. Proliferation of peripheral blood mononuclear cells to mitogens may be reduced, and this effect probably is a result of a combination of $CD4^+$ T-cell lymphopenia as well as intrinsic defects in T-cell proliferation, such as reduced production of IL-2 and increased apoptotic tendency. Diagnosis requires identification of mutations in the *RMRP* gene. Insertional mutations involving the 5′ flanking region have been described, and the region encoding RMRP also displays a number of single-nucleotide polymorphisms, both of which can make the proper genetic diagnosis challenging.

Therapy

IVIG replacement therapy may be helpful in cases of recurrent sinopulmonary infections, particularly if specific defects in antibody production are documented. Prophylaxis for *Pneumocystis* infection with trimethoprim-sulfamethoxazole (TMP-SMX) is indicated in patients in whom $CD4^+$ T-cell numbers are substantially depressed. Treatment with IL-2 may improve T-cell function in vitro, but the clinical significance is less clear. In patients with severe infections whose immunodeficiency mimics T^-B^+ SCID or Omenn syndrome, prompt HCT is indicated. HCT also corrects neutropenia and the predilection to develop lymphoma but not other features of the disorder.

Schimke Immunoosseous Dysplasia

Etiology and Pathophysiology

Schimke immunoosseous dysplasia is a very rare autosomal recessive disorder due to mutations in the SWI/SNF2-related matrix-associated, actin-dependent regulator of chromatin subfamily A-like 1 (SMARCAL1) gene.[238] SMARCAL1 appears to regulate gene expression by its impact on the configuration of DNA, but why SMARCAL1 deficiency has particularly deleterious effects on certain organs is unclear. Characteristic pathology includes spondyloepiphyseal dysplasia with short stature and unusual facies, focal glomerulosclerosis, cerebral ischemia, thyroid dysfunction, and T-cell lymphopenia.[239] Whether the T-cell lymphopenia is mainly due to thymic hypoplasia or decrease survival of peripheral T cells is unclear. T-cell proliferative responses to cytokines, such as IL-2, are reduced.

Clinical Manifestations

Patients are at increased risk for opportunistic infections characteristic of T-cell immunodeficiency, such as *Pneumocystis* pneumonia, particularly if they are also receiving immunosuppressive drugs. Anemia, neutropenia, thrombocytopenia, and pancytopenia are frequent. Progressive renal failure and hypothyroidism are common.

Laboratory Evaluation

Patients with Schimke immunoosseous dysplasia frequently have decreased numbers of both $CD4^+$ and $CD8^+$ T cells, poor responses, even with addition of IL-2, to mitogenic stimuli, and reduced responses to delayed-type hypersensitivity skin tests. Ig levels may be reduced. Specific diagnosis can be made by evaluating the *SMARCAL1* gene for mutations.

Therapy

HCT has been reported to improve the outcome of T-cell immunodeficiency and bone marrow abnormalities, suggesting that these abnormalities are due to an effect that is cell autonomous for hematopoietic cells.[240] Renal transplantation has been performed for treatment of chronic renal failure, although these patients are at relatively high risk for opportunistic infection because of chronic lymphopenia.

Immune Dysregulation, Polyendocrinopathy, Enteropathy, and X-Linked Inheritance Syndrome

Etiology and Pathophysiology

The immune dysregulation, polyendocrinopathy, enteropathy, and X-linked inheritance (IPEX) syndrome is a rare primary immunodeficiency syndrome in which profound early autoimmune disease involving the gut and endocrine tissues is characteristic.[241,242] IPEX is the first example in humans of a single-gene deficiency that results in a selective defect of regulatory T cells rather effector T cells. The syndrome maps to the chromosome Xq11.23-Xq13.3 region and is caused by defects in the gene encoding Forkhead P3 (FOXP3), a member of the Forkhead protein family of transcription factors. FOXP3 is expressed by $CD4^+$ T cells, with particularly high levels contained in the $CD4^+CD25^+$ subset of T cells, which include cells with potent regulatory (immunosuppressive) function. Based on studies in mice lacking FOXP3, this transcription factor appears to be required for the generation and survival of regulatory $CD4^+$ T cells. Intrathymic generation of $FOXP3^+$ regulatory $CD4^+$ T cells is well characterized. More controversial is the importance of the generation of regulatory $CD4^+$ T cells from nonregulatory $CD4^+$ T cells in the periphery. Transfection of FOX3P into naive murine $CD4^+$ T cells confers a regulatory phenotype, suggesting that this transcription factor acts as the key factor for regulatory $CD4^+$ T-cell function, perhaps by inhibiting effector function genes, such as those encoding cytokines. Adoptive transfer studies in mice indicate that $CD4^+CD25^+$ T cells potently suppress immune responses that otherwise may lead to autoimmune disease. For example, these regulatory $CD4^+$ T-cell populations are critical in preventing autoimmune gastrointestinal disease from endogenous bacterial flora.

Clinical Manifestations

An enteropathy present in all patients results in watery or mucoid/bloody diarrhea.[241,242] Small-bowel biopsies may reveal villus atrophy and mucosal erosions with lymphocytic infiltration of the lamina propria or submucosa. The most frequently observed endocrinopathies include insulin-dependent diabetes mellitus and Hashimoto-type thyroiditis, often accompanied by lymphocytic infiltration of these organs. Skin involvement most commonly consists of eczema but can include erythroderma, exfoliative dermatitis, and pemphigoid nodularis. Virtually all children manifest severe failure to thrive, which is due to the enteritis as well as other features of the chronic illness, such as diabetes. Autoimmune hemolytic anemia, immune thrombocytopenic purpura, or both are frequent. Lymphadenopathy, hepatosplenomegaly, arthritis, and glomerulonephritis have been reported less frequently. Viral infections or immunizations may trigger severe clinical symptoms, most likely as a result of T-cell activation. Female carriers with one affected allele are healthy despite the random occurrence of X-inactivation.

Laboratory Evaluation

Absolute lymphocyte and T- and B-cell numbers usually are normal, although increases in $CD4^+$ T cells have been reported. In patients with FOXP3 null mutations, flow cytometry can be used to detect a lack of FOXP3 protein expression after intracellular staining of $CD4^+$ T cells with FOXP3 monoclonal antibodies. The development of better markers for regulatory T-cell populations in humans, which would be expected to be markedly decreased or absent in these patients, should improve laboratory diagnosis in the future. Responses to in vitro lymphocyte stimulation to mitogens or antigens have ranged from normal to slightly decreased. These and other immune abnormalities often are difficult to interpret because most patients require immunosuppression to control enteritis. Increased responses, with enhanced IL-2 production, have been observed only infrequently. Complement and serum levels of total IgM, IgG, and IgA usually are normal. Total IgE levels may be elevated. Specific antibody responses may be decreased, but this is variable. Even within a single family, only some affected members may have decreased antibody responses to protein or unconjugated polysaccharide antigens. Antiislet cell, anti-GAD65, antinuclear antibodies, and other autoantibodies may occur in addition to those reactive with red blood cells and platelets.

Therapy

Immunosuppression with cyclosporine A or FK506, often combined with glucocorticoids, has been the mainstay of therapy but usually is not able to control autoimmune symptoms for prolonged periods. HCT is curative and demonstrates that the genetic defect is caused by autonomous effects on hematopoietic cells. In one patient, beneficial effects included resolution of insulin-dependent diabetes mellitus, which started with the conditioning regimen; partial donor chimerism was sufficient for control of autoimmunity.[243] Based on the handful of patients who have undergone transplantation, the mortality rate associated with this procedure may be relatively high. With the identification of the FOXP3 genetic defect, it now is possible to identify female carriers as well as perform prenatal diagnoses in affected families.

STAT5b Deficiency

Two patients with Laron dwarfism resistant to human growth hormone therapy and lymphopenia have been identified as homozygous defects in the STAT5b gene.[244,245] Both patients had moderate CD4 and CD8 T-cell lymphopenia, most likely reflecting a role for STAT5b in conjunction with STAT5a in signal transduction by T-cell growth-promoting cytokines, such as IL-7 and thymic stromal lymphopoietin. However, peripheral T-cell function appears to be relatively normal. In contrast, the T cells of these patients have substantial defects in expression of CD25 in response to IL-2 and in the generation of regulatory $CD4^+$ T cells that express FOXP3. Hypergammaglobulinemia and idiopathic lymphoid interstitial pneumonia also occurred in one of the patients, consistent with an autoimmune diathesis secondary to decreased regulatory T cells. Opportunistic infections have been observed only in conjunction with immunosuppressive therapy.

SUGGESTED READINGS

Bayry J, Hermine O, Webster DA, et al: Common variable immunodeficiency: The immune system in chaos. Trends Mol Med 11:370, 2005.

Castigli E, Geha R: Molecular basis of common variable immunodeficiency. J Allergy Clin Immunol 114:740, 2006.

Cerundolo V, de la Salle H: Description of HLA class I- and CD8-deficient patients: Insights into the function of cytotoxic T lymphocytes and NK cells in host defense. Semin Immunol 18:330, 2006.

Conley ME, Broides A, Hernandez-Trujillo V, et al: Genetic analysis of patients with defects in early B-cell development. Immunol Rev 203:216, 2005.

Durandy A, Revy P, Imai K, Fischer A: Hyper-immunoglobulin M syndromes caused by intrinsic B-lymphocyte defects. Immunol Rev 203:67, 2005.

Kovanen PE, Leonard WJ: Cytokines and immunodeficiency diseases: Critical roles of the gamma(c)-dependent cytokines interleukins 2, 4, 7, 15, and 21, and their signaling pathways. Immunol Rev 202:67, 2004.

Lawrence T, Puel A, Reichenbach J, et al: Autosomal-dominant primary immunodeficiencies. Curr Opin Hematol 12:22, 2004.

Lindvall JM, Blomberg KEM, Valiaho J, et al: Bruton's tyrosine kinase: Cell biology, sequence conservation, mutation spectrum, siRNA modifications, and expression profiling. Immunol Rev 203:200, 2005.

Markert ML, Boeck A, Hale LP, et al: Transplantation of thymus tissue in complete DiGeorge syndrome. N Engl J Med 341:1180, 1999.

Minegishi Y, Rohrer J, Coustan-Smith E, et al: An essential role for BLNK in human B cell development. Science 286:1954, 1999.

Notorangelo L, Casanova J-L, Conley ME, et al: Primary immunodeficiency diseases: An update from the International Union of Immunological Societies Primary Immunodeficiency Diseases Classification Committee Meeting in Budapest, 2005. J Allergy Clin Immunol 117:883, 2005.

Notorangelo LD, Gambineri El, Badolato R: Immunodeficiencies with autoimmune consequences. Adv Immunol 89:321, 2006.

Ochs HD, Ziegler SF, Togerson TR: FOXP3 acts as a rheostat of the immune response. Immunol Rev 203:153 2005.

Orange JS, Hossny EM, Weiler CR, et al: Use of intravenous immunoglobulin in human disease: A review of evidence by members of the Primary Immunodeficiency Committee of the American Academy of Allergy, Asthma, and Immunology. J Allergy Clin Immunol 117:S525, 2006.

Pesu M, Candotti F, Husa M, et al: Jak3, severe combined immunodeficiency, and a new class of immunosuppressive drugs. Immunol Rev 203:127, 2005.

Ridanpaa M, van Eenennaam H, Pelin K, et al: Mutations in the RNA component of RNase MRP cause a pleiotropic human disease, cartilage-hair hypoplasia. Cell 104:195, 2001.

Saler U, Grimbacher B: Common variable immunodeficiency: The power of co-stimulation. Semin Immunol 18:337, 2006.

Sekiguchi JM, Ferguson DO: DNA double-strand break repair: A relentless hunt uncovers new prey. Cell 124:260, 2006.

Winkelstein JA, Marino MC, Lederman HM, et al: X-linked agammaglobulinemia: Report of a United States registry of 201 patients. Medicine (Baltimore) 85:193, 2006.

Xu Y: DNA damage: A trigger of innate immunity but a requirement for adaptive immune homeostasis. Nat Rev Immunol 6:261, 2006.

REFERENCES

For complete list of references log onto www.expertconsult.com

CHAPTER 52

HISTIOCYTIC DISORDERS

Jeffrey M. Lipton and Robert J. Arceci

The histiocytic disorders comprise a broad grouping of hematologic diseases united by the observation that a dendritic cell or monocyte/macrophage appears to be the principal pathologic protagonist. The ubiquitous nature of these histiocytes, their varied metabolic capabilities and lineage plasticity, their role as regulators of hematopoiesis, their prominence in immune and inflammatory responses, and the uncertainty regarding dendritic cell and monocyte/macrophage ontogeny all have contributed to the confusion regarding the nosology of these disorders. To help clarify the nomenclature, Favara et al.[1] refer to "histiocytes" as ". . . a group of immune cells . . . that include macrophages and dendritic cells." Thus, the term *histiocyte* is ". . . analogous to 'lymphocyte' in that both denote groups of immune cells that are phenotypically and functionally diverse." Based upon this definition, a classification system derived from information on cell lineage and biologic behavior has been developed[1] and has replaced earlier classification systems.[2] In so doing, the World Health Organization's Committee on Histiocytic/Reticulum Cell Proliferations and the Reclassification Working Group of the Histiocyte Society have created a paradigm for continued reassessment of the classification of these disorders as new laboratory and clinical data come to light.

Currently, two broad categories of disease, "disorders of varied biological behavior" and "malignant disorders," are each subdivided into dendritic (antigen-presenting) cell or macrophage/monocyte (antigen-processing cell) related disorders. Other disorders in which histiocytes are implicated include ". . . storage diseases, hyperlipidemic xanthomas, well-defined chronic infections such as tuberculosis and leprosy and granulomatous reactions to foreign materials, are excluded."[1]

This chapter focuses on Langerhans cell histiocytosis (LCH), previously known as histiocytosis X, as the primary dendritic cell-related disorder.[3,4] Juvenile xanthogranulomatosis disease and related disorders, such as Erdheim-Chester disease, derived from dermal dendrocytes, are briefly considered. Macrophage-related histiocytoses include primary or secondary hemophagocytic lymphohistiocytosis (HLH), previously referred to as familial erythrophagocytic lymphohistiocytosis, and infection-associated hemophagocytic lymphohistiocytosis or malignancy-associated hemophagocytic lymphohistiocytosis, in addition to sinus histiocytosis with massive lymphadenopathy, also referred to as Rosai-Dorfman disease. Malignant histiocytic disorders (which include malignant proliferations of the monocyte/macrophage lineage), such as acute monocytic leukemia (FAB-M5), acute myelomonocytic leukemia (FAB-M4), chronic myelomonocytic leukemia, macrophage-related histiocytic sarcoma, and dendritic cell-related neoplasms, are more appropriately discussed in Chapters 59, 62, and 74. Table 52–1 lists a currently accepted classification of the histiocytic syndromes.

DENDRITIC CELL DISORDERS

Langerhans Cell Histiocytosis

Etiology and Epidemiology

The etiology of LCH remains unclear, although arguments and data support both neoplastic and primary immune dysfunction etiologies. Spontaneous remissions have been reported occasionally in patients with LCH, even with multiple sites of involvement.[5,6] In addition, variable morbidity and mortality have been reported in untreated patients with LCH, depending on the extent of disease. Pathologically, the lesions of LCH are characterized by a mixed cellular infiltrate. The hallmark is proliferation and accumulation of immature Langerhans cells, which do not show the cellular atypia characteristic of most malignancies. Using flow cytometry, most investigators have found no evidence of DNA aneuploidy.[7–9]

Studies by Willman et al.[10,11] and Yu et al.[12] demonstrated that LCH is characterized by clonal proliferation of $CD1a^+$ cells, based on differences in repetitive sequences between paternal and maternal X chromosomes. Clonality was observed in both localized and multisystem LCH.[10,13] The identification of clonality does not, however, necessarily indicate malignancy. However, additional data now have demonstrated specific chromosomal regions in lesional cells that display loss of heterozygosity and microsatellite instability.[14,15] In addition, a chromosome t(7;12) translocation has been reported in a single case.[16] Telomere shortening, found in many pre-neoplastic and neoplastic disorders, has also been reported.[16a,16b] A significant concordance of LCH has been observed in twins.[17] Furthermore, aberrant expression of proteins that both promote and block cell cycle progression has been reported in LCH.[18–21] The lesional Langerhans cell is also characterized by its immunophenotypic and functional immature phenotype that can be matured in vitro after exposure to CD40 ligand.[22] No abnormalities inherent to other cells that characterized LCH lesions have been observed.

These data demonstrate that LCH is a clonal proliferative disorder of immature Langerhans cells with variable clinical behavior. Therefore, it is possible that certain forms of LCH that show spontaneous remission represent a disorder similar to that observed in infants with Down syndrome and transient myeloproliferative disease. While the great majority of these cases spontaneously remit, approximately 20% may progress to acute megakaryoblastic leukemia. Interestingly, both transient myeloproliferative disease and acute megakaryoblastic leukemia in patients with Down syndrome are characterized by mutations in the *GATA1* gene, which may contribute to abnormal expansion of megakaryoblasts, facilitating the chance of a subsequent genetic event leading to acute megakaryoblastic leukemia. More data, particularly information documenting specific genetic mutations, may help clarify the etiology and nature of LCH. Although one could conclude that understanding the true etiology of LCH is only an academic issue, this determination has immense implications on the development of future approaches to treatment.[23–27]

Historically, the classic LCH syndromes comprise monostotic i.e. solitary, or multifocal eosinophilic granuloma localized lesion(s) confined to bone[28,29]; Hand-Schüller-Christian disease, which is characterized by protracted multisite and multisystem involvement with the classic but relatively rare triad of skull defects, diabetes insipidus, and exophthalmos[30–33]; and Abt-Letterer-Siwe disease, which is characterized by extensive involvement of the skin, liver, lungs, bone marrow, lymph nodes, spleen, and other organs.[34,35] The prevalence of these disorders has been estimated to be approximately 1 : 50,000, with an incidence of approximately 5 to 10 cases per million per year in children younger than 15 years.[36] An approximately 2 : 1 male predominance has been reported.[37–41] Although infants and children are predominantly affected, adults with LCH, including the elderly,[27,42] have been described; however, well-defined incidence figures have not been reported for adults.

Biologic Characteristics

In order to understand the histiocytic disorders, particularly LCH, it is important to review monocyte/macrophage and dendritic cell differentiation, which is characterized by the developmental sequence shown in Fig. 52–1.[43–48] In the bone marrow, this process begins with the pluripotent hematopoietic stem cell, which may give rise either to a lymphoid progenitor capable of T- or B-lymphocyte lineage commitment or to a multipotent myeloid progenitor capable of differentiation to the erythroid, megakaryocytic, eosinophil, basophil/mast cell, or granulocyte/macrophage cell line. The granulocyte and macrophage share a progenitor, the colony-forming unit granulocyte-macrophage (CFU-GM). CFU-GM, which is capable of granulocyte or monocyte differentiation, gives rise to the monocyte/macrophage progenitor (colony-forming unit-macrophage [CFU-M]). CFU-M gives rise to the monoblast, then to the bone marrow promonocyte (the first morphologically identifiable macrophage precursor), and finally to the monocyte, a process that takes approximately 6 days.[49] The promonocyte ranges from 10 to 18 μm in diameter and has a well-developed Golgi apparatus as well as peroxidase-positive granules. The typical monocyte has a folded nucleus, lightly basophilic cytoplasm, and faint azurophilic granules.

Table 52–1 Classification of Histiocytic Disorders

Disorders of varied biologic behavior
Dendritic cell-related
Langerhans cell histiocytosis
Secondary dendritic cell processes
Juvenile xanthogranuloma and related disorders
Solitary histiocytomas of various dendritic cell phenotypes
Macrophage-related
Hemophagocytic syndromes
Primary hemophagocytic lymphohistiocytosis
Secondary hemophagocytic syndromes
Infection-associated
Malignancy-associated
Other
Rosai-Dorfman disease (sinus histiocytosis with massive lymphadenopathy)
Solitary histiocytoma with macrophage phenotype
Malignant disorders[a]
Monocyte-related
Leukemias (FAB and revised FAB classifications)
Monocytic leukemia M5A and B
Acute myelomonocytic leukemia M4
Chronic myelomonocytic leukemia
Dendritic cell–related histiocyte sarcoma (localized or disseminated)
Macrophage-related histiocytic sarcoma (localized or disseminated)

[a]Data from Favara BE, Feller AC, Pauli M, et al: Contemporary classification of histiocytic disorders. The WHO Committee on Histiocytic/Reticulum Cell Proliferations. Reclassification Working Group of the Histiocyte Society. Med Pediatr Oncol 29:157, 1997.

Bone marrow monocytes enter the circulation and can migrate into tissues where they transform into tissue-specific macrophages under the influence of the local environment and become the cells of the mononuclear phagocyte system.[49] Dendritic cells likewise have their origin in the bone marrow[50] and can be cultured from progenitors residing in both the bone marrow and peripheral blood.[45] A $CD34^+$ progenitor can, in single cell culture, give rise to either dendritic cells or macrophages, confirming that dendritic cells and macrophages share a progenitor. Proliferative precursors of the dendritic cell enter the circulation from the bone marrow in a fashion similar to the monocyte. They then enter the tissues[51,52] in which proliferation and differentiation lead to functional, antigen-presenting dendritic cells. The morphology of the dendritic cell may vary depending upon its functional (veiled vs dendritic) state. The dendritic cell is a large cell, essentially devoid of phagolysosomes and other cytoplasmic organelles, with multiple cytoplasmic extensions. The cytoplasm of this mobile cell is rich with mitochondria. The nucleus is eccentric with small nucleoli. Langerhans cells are characterized by Birbeck granules, which appear ultrastructurally as "tennis-racquet shaped pentalaminar structures."[43]

Functionally the mononuclear phagocyte system, also known as the reticuloendothelial system, consists of a multitude of ordinary tissue histiocytes (fixed macrophages) that provide host defense by

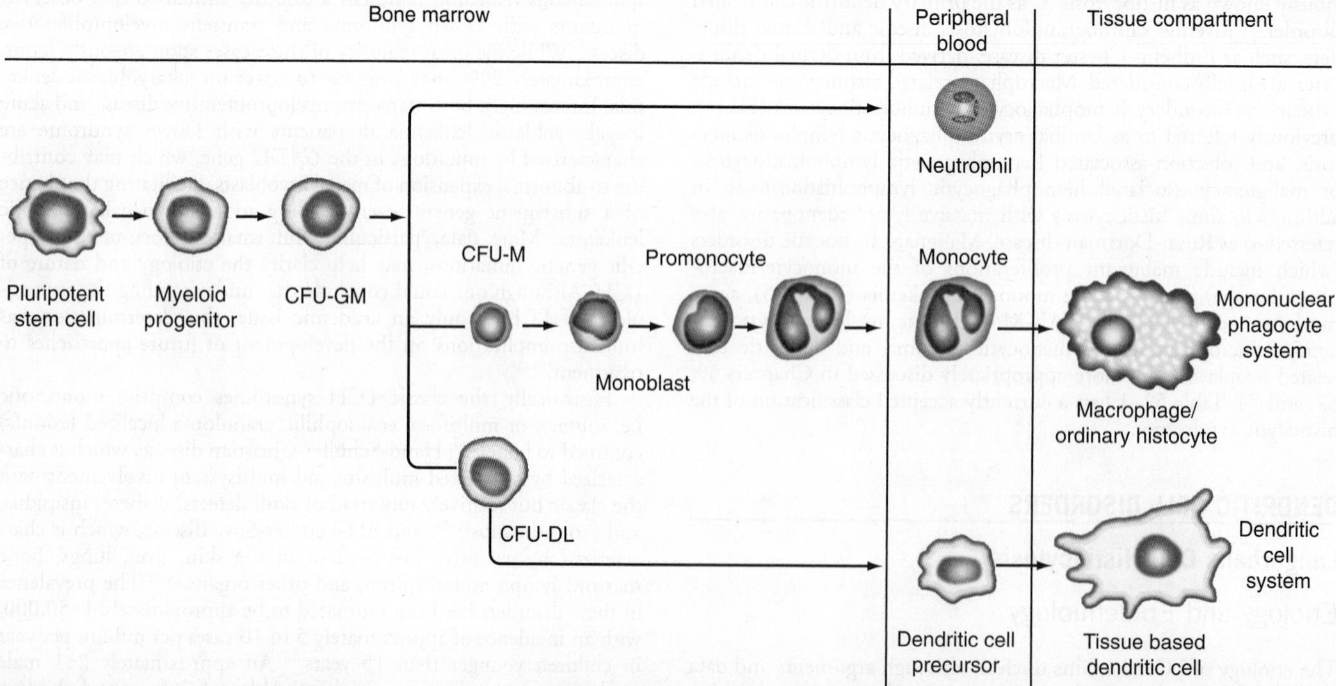

Figure 52–1 Development of cells of the monocyte/macrophage lineage. CFU-DL, colony-forming unit dendritic Langerhans cell; CFU-GM, colony-forming unit granulocyte-macrophage; CFU-M, colony-forming unit macrophage.

Table 52–2 Types of Dendritic Cells

Cell Type	Location	Function
Peripheral blood dendritic cell	Peripheral blood	Migratory
Langerhans cell[a]	Skin, epidermis, cervix, vagina, stomach, esophagus	Antigen uptake and processing transport to lymph nodes
		Antigen transfer
Veiled cells[a]	Afferent lymphatics	Antigen transfer
Interdigitating dendritic cell	Lymph node paracortex (T area), periarteriolar lymphatic sheath of the spleen	Antigen presentation for T cells
Thymic dendritic cell[a]	Thymic medulla	Induction of immune tolerance
Interstitial dendritic cell	Parenchymal organs (excluding brain and central cornea)	Antigen uptake/processing?
Indeterminate cells of the skin (dermal dendrocytes)	Dermis	Antigen presentation
Follicular dendritic cell[b]	Germinal center of lymph nodes	Antigen presentation in B cells and maintenance of long-term immunologic memory

[a]Contains Birbeck granules.
[b]Derived from the lymphoid lineage.
Data from Wright-Browne V, McClain KL, Talpaz M, Ordonez N, Estrov Z: Physiology and pathophysiology of dendritic cells. Hum Pathol 28:563, 1997.

disposing of senescent or damaged blood cells, ingesting invading organisms, processing antigens for the immune system, and stimulating the inflammatory process through production of cytokines,[44,49,53,54] such as interleukin (IL)-1 and tumor necrosis factor (TNF), which activate T lymphocytes as well as other macrophages. Tissue-specific cells of the mononuclear phagocyte system include splenic sinusoidal macrophages, hepatic Kupffer cells,[55] pulmonary alveolar macrophages,[56] bone osteoclasts,[57] pleural, peritoneal, and synovial macrophages, and microglial cells of the brain.[58,59]

Ordinary tissue histiocytes have strong IgG Fc receptors, whereas tissue-based dendritic cells, which comprise the dendritic cell system, have less phagocytic capacity, peroxidase, esterase, or Fc receptor expression, but they are potent antigen-presenting cells.[43,60] Found in virtually all tissues,[43] the Langerhans cell is the major immunologic cellular component of the integument and mucosa. Normal Langerhans cells reside within the epidermis, regional lymph nodes, thymic epithelium, and bronchial mucosa.[61] Functionally, cells of the dendritic cell system process antigen then migrate to lymphoid organs, where they participate as effector cells stimulating primary T-cell responses, thus generating a cellular and, indirectly, a humoral immune response.[43] The types of dendritic cells are summarized in Table 52–2. As with the cells of the mononuclear phagocyte system, dendritic cells are capable of elaborating a wide array of cytokines, including IL-1 and TNF.[62]

Hematopoietic differentiation is regulated by a family of glycoproteins termed colony-stimulating factors and interleukins (see Chapter 16). A large family of these growth factors has been purified, cloned, and functionally characterized. Colony-stimulating factor granulocyte-macrophage (CSF-GM), IL-3 or multi-CSF, CSF-M, and CSF-G[63,64] exert a major influence on monocyte/macrophage and dendritic cell differentiation.[65–67] CSF-GM and IL-3 have a broader range of activity, influencing differentiation of primitive as well as committed progenitors.[68,69] In addition, CSF-GM increases functional activity of mature granulocytes, eosinophils, and monocytes.[70–72] CSF-M and CSF-G are more restricted in their activity and modulate monocyte/macrophage and granulocyte differentiation and function.[73] Early work implicated T cells as a source of stimulating activity.[74] Since then, the monocyte/macrophage, the fibroblast, and other cells have also been shown to be involved in factor production.[75–77] The production of these factors by cells outside the bone marrow supports the finding that some factors have the dual functions of stimulating marrow progenitor differentiation and proliferation and enhancing the activity of mature myeloid cells.[78]

Dendritic cells can be generated from progenitors in vitro using CSF-GM plus IL-4 or TNF.[51] CSF-GM appears to serve as a survival rather than a differentiation factor, whereas TNF induces maturation of these cells.[79,80] Thus, a complex regulatory network with activation by a wide variety of stimuli controls the proliferation and function of macrophages and dendritic cells along with other inflammation-associated cells. The ability of dendritic cells and macrophages to produce cytokines and activate T lymphocytes and other inflammatory cells likely contributes to the varied and sometimes protean clinical manifestations encountered in the histiocytic disorders. In particular, since Nezelof et al.[81] first concluded that histiocytosis X was characterized by proliferation of Langerhans cells, a better understanding of the pathobiology of what is now called LCH has resulted from more focused investigations.

Clinical Manifestations

The signs and symptoms of LCH vary considerably depending on which organs are infiltrated by the Langerhans cells and accompanying immunoreactive cells. Bone, skin, teeth, gingival tissue, ear, endocrine organs, lung, liver, spleen, lymph nodes, and bone marrow all can become involved and exhibit dysfunction secondary to cellular infiltration.[82] Although patients rarely fall into discrete categories defined by the classic designations of eosinophilic granuloma, Hand-Schüller-Christian disease, and Abt-Letterer-Siwe disease, this nomenclature remains valuable if only to catalog the clinical manifestations of LCH and preserve the important historic perspective of these disorders.

Solitary or multifocal eosinophilic granuloma is found predominantly in older children and young adults, usually within the first three decades of life. The incidence peaks between 5 and 10 years of age.[83] Solitary or multifocal eosinophilic granuloma represents approximately 60% to 80% of all instances of LCH.[83] Patients with systemic involvement frequently have similar bone lesions in addition to other manifestations of disease.[82] Patients often cannot bear weight and have tender swelling due to tissue infiltrates overlying the bone lesions.[82,84] Radiographically, the lesions are sharply marginated, round or oval, and usually have a beveled edge that gives the appearance of depth.[82]

Hand-Schüller-Christian disease (multisystem disease) is most commonly described in younger children aged 2 to 5 years. It represents 15% to 40% of these patients, although this type of involvement can be observed in patients of all ages.[26] Signs and symptoms include bony defects, with exophthalmos due to tumor mass in the orbital cavity being characteristic. This condition usually occurs from involvement of the roof and lateral wall of the orbital bones (although skeletal involvement is not necessary).[85] In addition, teeth are often lost due to gum infiltration and/or mandibular involvement (Fig.

52–2). The most frequent sites of skeletal involvement include the flat bones of the skull, ribs, pelvis, and scapula. There may be extensive involvement of the skull, with irregularly shaped, lucent lesions giving rise to the so-called geographic skull.[86] Long bones and lumbosacral vertebrae, usually the anterior portion of the vertebral body, are involved less frequently. In one series, the majority of children with vertebral involvement had only a single affected vertebra, but nine of the 15 patients had other skeletal lesions. Two patients had visceral involvement.[87] In long bones, growth of lesions in the medullary cavity leads to pressure that may result in erosion through the cortex, stimulating the formation of periosteal new bone accompanied by soft-tissue extension.[88] Differential diagnosis includes Ewing and osteogenic sarcoma, bone lymphoma, benign bone tumor and cyst, and infection. Involvement of the wrists, hands, knees, feet, or cervical vertebrae is less common.[82] Orbital involvement may result in vision loss or strabismus due to optic nerve or orbital muscle involvement, respectively. Oral involvement commonly affects the gums and/or palate. Erosion of the lamina dura gives rise to the characteristic "floating tooth" seen on dental radiographs.[89] The entire mandible may be involved (Fig. 52–2), with loss of bone leading to diminished height of the mandibular rami. Erosion of gingival tissue causes premature eruption, decay, and tooth loss.[90] Parents of affected children, particularly infants, frequently report precocious eruption of teeth, when, in fact, the gums are receding leading to exposure of immature dentition. Chronic otitis media, due to involvement of the mastoid and petrous portion of the temporal bone, and otitis externa are not uncommon.

Figure 52–2 Computed tomographic scan of a destructive Langerhans cell histiocytosis mandibular lesion in a child.

Diabetes insipidus (DI) affects 5% to 40% of patients with LCH, depending upon the report.[91–94] Most instances of DI occur in children who present with systemic disease and involvement of the orbit and skull.[95] Fewer than one third of children who ultimately develop DI have polydipsia and polyuria as presenting symptoms of LCH.[95,96] Most children present within 4 years of diagnosis. DI is due to infiltration by Langerhans cells and macrophages into the hypothalamus with or without involvement of the posterior pituitary gland (Fig. 52–3).[97] DI may occur at any time during the course of LCH.[96,98,99] Patients should be instructed to report signs of DI as soon as they develop because dehydration and electrolyte imbalance may be quite serious. In addition, definitive documentation of DI with measurement of serum and urine electrolytes and osmolality before and after a several-hour water deprivation period should be performed. Vasopressin levels can be measured to document a deficiency. Infants who are being tested should be carefully monitored in the clinic or hospital setting to ensure that they do not become severely dehydrated. Once the definitive studies are obtained, a test dose of desmopressin acetate (DDAVP) can be used to determine whether the concentration of urine is increased. Treatment of new-onset DI is controversial.

Short stature has been found in up to 40% of children with systemic LCH.[94,97,100] Chronic illness and steroid therapy play an important role in this phenomenon. However, short stature also may be a consequence of anterior pituitary involvement and growth hormone deficiency,[94,97,100] which can occur in at least half of patients with initial anterior pituitary dysfunction. Other endocrine manifestations include hyperprolactinemia and hypogonadism due to hypothalamic infiltration.[101,102] Pancreatic and thyroid involvement have been reported.[101–103]

Gastrointestinal tract disease has been identified.[104–106] In one retrospective series, only 2% of 348 children had biopsy-proven gastrointestinal involvement.[107] However, in the prospective DAL HX-83 trial, 13% of 78 patients had digestive tract symptoms.[108]

Abt-Letterer-Siwe disease is the rarest (10% of cases) and most severe form of LCH.[83] Typically, patients are younger than 2 years and present with a scaly seborrheic, eczematoid, sometimes purpuric rash involving the scalp, ear canals, abdomen, and intertriginous areas of the neck and face (Fig. 52–4). The diagnosis of LCH in neonates often is delayed beyond the neonatal period and may be unpredictable in terms of outcome when skin only is involved. However, when multisystem disease is evident, outcome is significantly worse.[109] The rash may be maculopapular or nodulopapular. Ulceration may result, especially in intertriginous areas. Ulcerated and denuded skin may serve as a portal of entry for microorganisms, leading to sepsis. Draining ears, lymphadenopathy, hepatosplenomegaly, and, in severe cases, hepatic dysfunction with hypoproteinemia and diminished synthesis of clotting factors can occur. Anorexia, irritability, failure to thrive, and significant pulmonary symptoms, such as cough, tachypnea, and pneumothorax, may occur. One of the most significant areas of

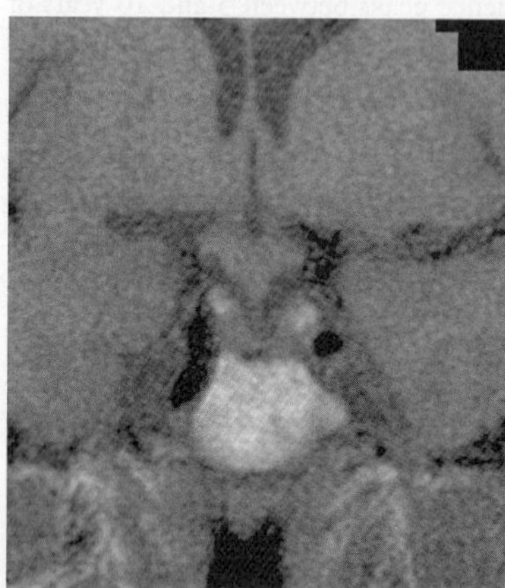

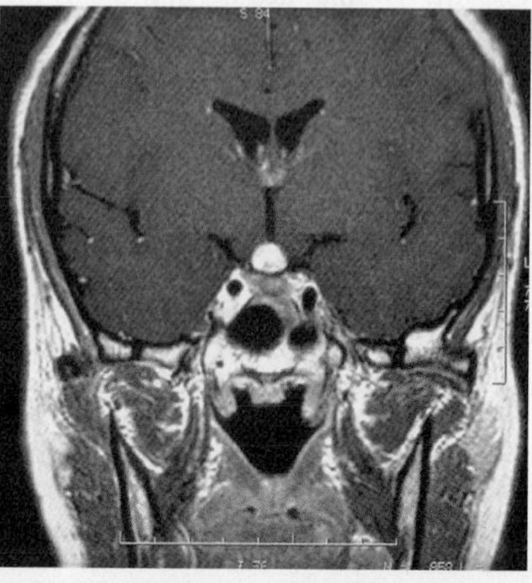

Figure 52–3 Magnetic resonance imaging contrast coronal views showing two patients with diabetes insipidus and pituitary involvement due to Langerhans cell histiocytosis.

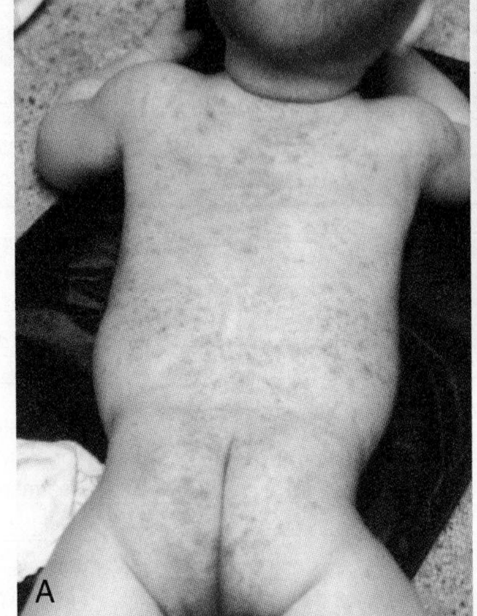

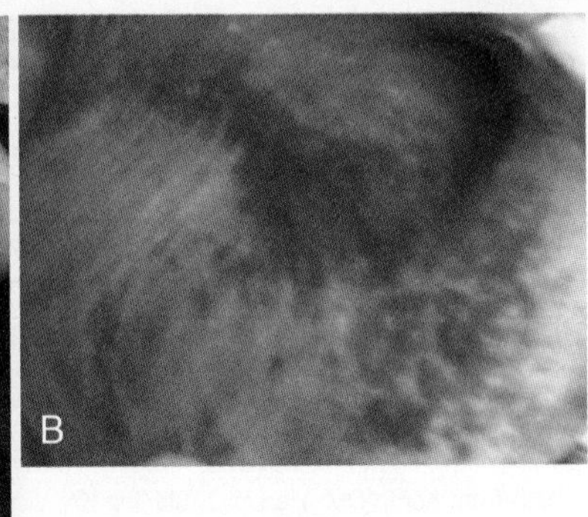

Figure 52–4 Skin involvement in Langerhans cell histiocytosis. **Left**, Diffuse maculopapular rash. **Right**, Hemorrhagic scalp rash.

involvement is the hematopoietic system, with the potential for pancytopenia. The pathophysiology of hematopoietic dysfunction can be hypersplenism as well as direct involvement by Langerhans cells and/or reactive macrophages. Thrombocytopenia frequently portends a fatal outcome.[37]

A severe manifestation of LCH is nonhypothalamic–pituitary involvement of the central nervous system (CNS).[110,111] Bernert et al.[112] reviewed the course of 38 children with LCH and CNS involvement. The majority of patients with CNS involvement had associated skull, orbit, or mastoid disease. Magnetic resonance imaging with contrast is the best method for identifying lesions of the CNS. As expected, the hypothalamic–pituitary region, characterized by DI, was the most common site of involvement, followed by the cerebellum, pons, and cerebral hemispheres. Lesions of the basal ganglia, spinal cord, and optic nerves also were seen. Involvement of the CNS was frequently observed years after the initial diagnosis. Extraaxial lesions of the dura, meninges, or choroid plexus can be treated effectively with surgery, radiotherapy, or systemic treatment. However, infiltrative and atrophic lesions of the cerebellum or pons frequently result in severe, even fatal, sequelae and have been characterized as primarily neurodegenerative.[98] Rare biopsy material of such involvement has shown a primarily inflammatory, lymphocyte infiltrate associated with gliosis, demyelination, and neuronal death.[113] The etiology of this neurodegenerative process is unknown but is believed to be an immune-mediated paraneoplastic response.[26,110,113,114]

LCH can have a strictly nodal presentation, not to be confused with sinus histiocytosis with massive lymphadenopathy, also known as Rosai-Dorfman disease. This presentation is characterized by significant enlargement of multiple lymph node groups, with little or no other signs of disease. Isolated pulmonary involvement usually is seen in young adults in their third or fourth decade of life and occasionally in adolescents. It may follow a severe and often chronic debilitating course; patients may present with pneuomothorax.[115] Cigarette smoking has been strongly implicated in primary pulmonary histiocytosis.[115] In contrast, pulmonary involvement in younger patients with systemic disease frequently is mild, although fulminant pulmonary disease may occur in this age group.[116,117] Findings on chest radiograph vary, from a diffuse infiltrate consistent with bilateral interstitial pneumonia to a "honeycomb lung" appearance (Fig. 52–5).[117,118] Cutaneous disease with no evidence of dissemination has been described in children and adults.[119] Rarely, patients present with deep subcutaneous skin nodules only (formerly described as Hashimoto–Pritzker syndrome).[120]

With such a vast spectrum of disease, adherence to strict labels such as eosinophilic granuloma, Hand–Schüller–Christian disease, or Abt–Letterer–Siwe disease cannot adequately describe a particular patient. Thus, the development of a classification scheme predictive of prognosis becomes particularly useful.

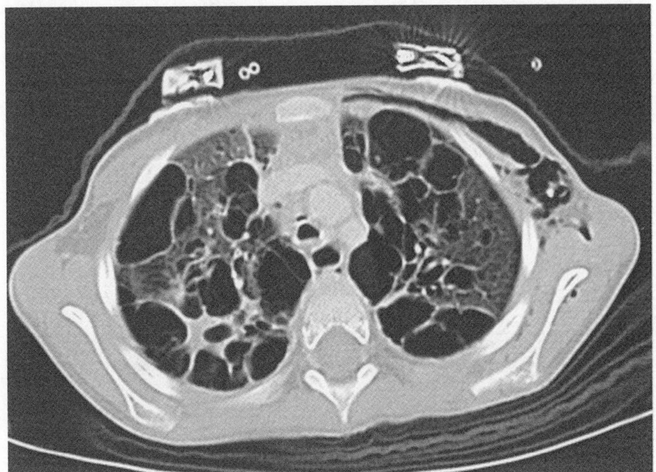

Figure 52–5 Computed tomographic scan of the lungs showing cystic changes associated with Langerhans cell histiocytosis. (*Courtesy Dr. Melanie Committo.*)

Natural History and Prognosis

As originally proposed by Lahey,[121] the prognosis for patients with LCH depend on three factors: age at onset, number of organs involved, and degree of dysfunction of specific organs (Tables 52–3 and 52–4). An adolescent or adult who presents with solitary bone eosinophilic granuloma has the best prognosis, and an infant with multiple affected organs has the worst prognosis.[37–40,121,122] Prognosis-based classification allows one to discard the labels of eosinophilic granuloma, Hand–Schüller–Christian disease, Abt-Letterer-Siwe disease, and other presentations to group patients according to optimizing treatments. One system grouped patients according to age at onset, disease site and severity. Specifically, patients older than 2 years had a good prognosis, whereas patients younger than 2 years did more poorly.[121] Involvement of fewer than four organ systems was a relatively good prognostic sign, whereas involvement of four or more organ systems predicted a less favorable outcome. Dysfunction of three specific organ systems (hepatic, pulmonary, and hematopoietic)

Table 52–3 Survival Experience by Age and Organ Dysfunction

	Patients	Deaths	Median Survival (months)	*P* value (Survival)
Age at Diagnosis				
<2 years	95	35	74+	0.002
≥2 year	56	9	147	
Organ Dysfunction				
Present	59	27	43	0.002
Absent	92	17	145	

Data from Komp DM, Herson J, Starling KA, Vietti TJ, Hvizdala E: A staging system for histiocytosis X. A Southwest Oncology Group Study. Cancer 47:798, 1981.

Table 52–4 Organ System Involvement as a Prognostic Indicator[a]

Organ Systems Involved	Patients	Response to Therapy (CR + PR)[a]	Dead
1–2	13	8	0
3–4	20	15	4
5–6	22	12	9
7+	18	7	11

[a]Complete response (CR) plus partial (PR) response.
Data from Lahey E: Histiocytosis X—An analysis of prognostic factors. J Pediatr 87:184, 1975.

Table 52–5 Grouping System for Langerhans Cell Histiocytosis

Factor	Points
Age	
≥2 years	0
<2 years	1
Extent of Disease	
<4 organs	0
≥4 organs	1
Dysfunction[a]	**(1, 2, or 3; see below)**
No	0
Yes	1
Group	**Total Points[b]**
0	Monostotic eosinophilic granuloma
I	0
II	1
III	2
IV	3

[a]Dysfunction includes the following:
1. Hepatic dysfunction: one or more of the following—hypoproteinemia (total protein <5.5 mg/dL or albumin <2.5 mg/dL), hyperbilirubinemia (>1.5 mg/dL), edema, ascites
2. Pulmonary dysfunction: one or more of the following—tachypnea, dyspnea, cyanosis, cough, pneumothorax, pleural effusion
3. Hematopoietic dysfunction: one or more of the following—anemia in the absence of iron deficiency or significant infection (<10 g/dL hemoglobin), leukopenia (<4000/mL), thrombocytopenia (<100,000/mL)

[b]By arbitrarily assigning either 0 or 1 point for the absence or presence of one of the three important prognostic variables, a number of total points is obtained and a patient is assigned a group.

Modified from Osband ME, Lipton JM, Lavin P, et al: Histiocytosis-X. N Engl J Med 304:146, 1981.

Table 52–6. Risk Groups According to the Histiocyte Society LCH-III Trial

Group 1—Multisystem "Risk" Patients

Multisystem patients with involvement of one or more "risk" organs (i.e., hematopoietic system, liver, spleen, or lungs). Patients with single-system lung involvement are not eligible for randomization.

Treatment includes vinblastine plus steroids, with randomization to receive intermediate-dose methotrexate during first course of therapy followed by lower-dose maintenance methotrexate versus no methotrexate. Duration of therapy is 12 months.

Group 2—Multisystem "Low Risk" Patients

Multisystem patients with multiple organs involved but without involvement of "risk" organs.

Treatment includes vinblastine plus steroids, with randomization to receive 6 versus 12 months of therapy.

Group 3—Single-System "Multifocal Bone Disease" and Localized "Special Site" Involvement

Patients with multifocal bone disease (i.e., lesions in two or more different bones). Patients with localized special site involvement, such as "CNS-RISK" lesions with intracranial soft-tissue extension or vertebral lesions with intraspinal soft-tissue extension.

Treatment includes 6 months of vinblastine plus steroid therapy.

CNS, central nervous system; LCH, Langerhans cell histiocytosis.

was an extremely important adverse predictor of outcome (Table 52–5).[121] In a review covering a 25-year experience at a single institution, seven of 28 patients with multisystem disease died; among these patients, five of 14 had single and nine of 14 had multiple disease recurrences.[123] When LCH presents after age 65 years, regardless of site and extent of disease, the prognosis often is poor.[124]

Organ dysfunction must be distinguished from involvement (e.g., hypoproteinemia hyperbilirubinemia vs hepatomegaly), because involvement alone is not as adverse a prognostic sign as is dysfunction. Such a classification is a reliable prognostic tool and helps to indicate which patients may benefit most from systemic therapy. A review of 62 patients aged birth to 14 years (median age 18 months) confirmed these observations, stressing the importance of the two factors age and localized disease. All but one of the 15 patients who died were younger than 2 years at diagnosis. With regard to local involvement, the presence of skeletal involvement was a good prognostic sign, and skin involvement that was localized to the scalp predicted a considerably better outcome than generalized cutaneous involvement.[125]

The international Histiocyte Society initiated clinical trials that identified the response after the initial 6 weeks of therapy with weekly vinblastine and daily prednisolone as the single most important factor in predicting outcome, especially mortality.[126] Of the approximately 79% of patients who responded to initial therapy, 94% were alive at 5 years, whereas only 11% of the 14% of nonresponders survived. These important data suggest that alternative therapies should be tested early during the course of therapy for patients with poor early responses.[126] From these clinical trials, a staging system has been developed for the LCH-III trial (Table 52–6).

Pathologic Diagnosis

The typical histologic appearance of LCH varies with the age of the lesion examined (Fig. 52–6). The Langerhans cell is the prominent diagnostic feature in the histology of LCH.[127,128] Early lesions often are locally destructive, with proliferation and accumulation of phenotypically and functionally immature Langerhans cells.[61,124] Mitoses usually are not present in great numbers but when found are of no known prognostic significance.[129] Multinucleated giant cells are

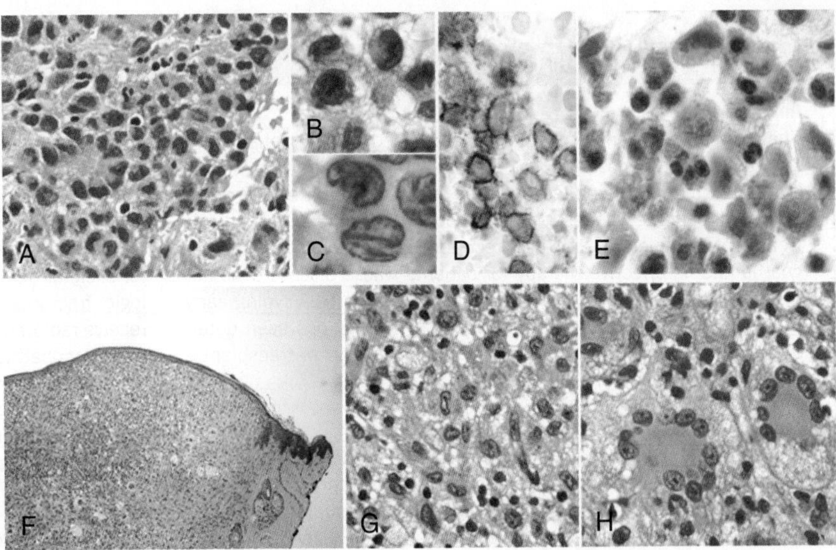

Figure 52–6 **A-E**, Langerhans cell histiocytosis. (**A**, **B**) Biopsy sample shows sheets of histiocytes with abundant pink cytoplasm and folded nuclei with prominent nuclear grooves. **C**, Cell with a central longitudinal nuclear groove gives the cell a coffee-bean appearance. **D**, Immunohistochemical stain for CD1A shows the histiocytic cells are positive. **E.** Some cases of Langerhans histiocytosis are associated with prominent eosinophilia. Another term for such cases is *eosinophilic granuloma*. **F–H**, Juvenile histiocytosis. Histologic features of juvenile xanthogranuloma vary. **F**, In this case, low-power magnification shows a dome-shaped lesion with an attenuated epidermis. **G**, At higher power, the bulk of the lesion is composed of a proliferation of histiocytes with abundant pink cytoplasm. Sometimes these histiocytes show more vacuolization or xanthomatization. **H**, Scattered Touton-type giant cells are present.

Table 52–7 Surface markers of Langerhans Cells, Activated Langerhans Cells, and Langerhans Cell Histiocytosis Langerhans Cells

Marker	LC	LC	Activated LCH LC
Surface ATPase	+	+	+
MHC II	+	+	+
MHC I	+	+	+
Fc IgG receptor	+	+	+
Fc IgE receptor	+	+	?
C3bi receptor	+	+	+
CD1a and CD1c	+	+	+
CD4	±	+	+
CD45	+	+	+
CD14	+	+	?
CDw29	+	+	?
IL-2R	–	+	+
CD80, CD86	–	+ (Cultured)	?
CD11b and CD11c	+	+	+
S100	+	+	+
PLAP	–	+ (Transient)	+
PNA	–	–	+
IFN-γR	–	–	+

IFN-γR, interferonγ receptor; IL-2R, interleukin-2 receptor; LC, Langerhans cell; LCH, Langerhans cell histiocytosis; MHC, major histocompatibility complex. Data from Chu T, Jaffe R: The normal Langerhans cell and the LCH cell. Br J Cancer Suppl 23:S4, 1994.

often present.[130] Other inflammatory cells, such as granulocytes, eosinophils, macrophages and lymphocytes, are present. Giant cells and macrophages may be phagocytic[129] and, over time, may accumulate cholesterol. As lesions mature or show signs of regression, fewer Langerhans cells are present and development of fibrotic reaction is less.

Pathologically, a "presumptive diagnosis" of LCH can be made on the basis of a biopsy demonstrating the characteristic histopathology.[124,127,129,131,132] The Langerhans cell is 15 to 25 μm in diameter, with a ". . . central to slightly eccentric ovoid to uniform-shaped nucleus with a delicate chromatin network and inconspicuous nucleoli. An indentation or groove across the face of the nucleus is a feature of many cells."[132] Additional diagnostic criteria beyond standard histopathology, such as immunochemical staining with ATPase, S100 protein, α-mannosidase, peanut lectin, vimentin, and other markers,[129,133,134] are necessary for a "diagnosis." An extensive immunophenotype of normal and LCH Langerhans cells has been reviewed (Table 52–7).[43] A "definitive diagnosis" of LCH relies upon the immunohistochemical identification of the presence of Langerhans cells by cell surface CD1a or by the presence of Birbeck granules by electron microscopy.[81] Thus, pathologic criteria for the diagnosis of LCH have been established and were formalized by the Histiocyte Society in 1987.[135] With the availability of antibodies to CD1a for use in routinely processed paraffin-embedded specimens, electron microscopy is rarely needed.

Differential diagnosis of LCH is limited and depends on the clinical presentation. It includes immunodeficiency syndromes with graft-versus-host disease, viral infection, infiltrative malignant disease such as leukemia, lymphoma or metastatic solid tumor, reticuloendothelial storage disease, congenital infection, benign and malignant bone tumor and cyst, and papular xanthoma.

Careful evaluation of biopsy material generally results in a diagnosis. However, one of the historic dilemmas in the evaluation of LCH is that the histopathology of lesions from patients with single-site eosinophilic granuloma is similar, if not identical, to that of multisystem disease.[82,131] This is consistent with the finding that tissue in lesions from patients with localized or systemic disease cannot be distinguished on the basis of clonality.[10,11,13] As expected on the basis of these observations, efforts to distinguish "favorable" from "unfavorable" histology[136] have not been shown to be prognostically useful.[137] Although patients are grouped in large part based upon their extent of disease, untreated patients generally do not progress to a higher stage.[82] Within a few months after presentation, it will become apparent that the lesions seen initially are limited to the skeleton or were the "heralding lesion(s)" of diffuse systemic involvement. When cutaneous involvement is the only obvious presenting sign, several months may be required to determine the ultimate extent of disease.[6,82,109]

These observations enforce the need for a complete clinical and laboratory evaluation with proper imaging studies once a definitive diagnosis of LCH is made. In general, baseline evaluation of a newly diagnosed patient requires a reasonable search for all sites of disease. The laboratory and imaging evaluation must be guided by a complete history and thorough physical examination, including a dental examination. All patients should be evaluated with a complete blood count, chemistries including liver function tests, coagulation workup, urine osmolality, chest radiograph, and complete skeletal survey. In a series of children with LCH for whom both radiographic and radionucleo-

Therapy for Langerhans Cell Histiocytosis

Approach

The optimal management, yet to be determined, for the patient with LCH balances the most effective therapy with the desire to minimize both short-term and long-term disease-related morbidities. Currently almost all patients who respond to therapy will be able to discontinue treatment completely, although recurrences are common. Another goal is finding effective therapy for patients whose disease does not respond to therapy. These patients should undergo HLA typing early after diagnosis and their initial response to therapy has been determined, and they should be considered for bone marrow transplantation or other experimental therapies.

Prognostic Grouping

When patients are grouped using three prognostic variables (age, extent of disease, and presence of organ dysfunction(, the prognosis and extent of treatment can be evaluated. The grouping or staging of patients currently is best evaluated according to the Histiocyte Society LCH-III clinical trial, which stratifies treatment arms based on measurement of the initial extent and sites of disease (Table 52–6).

Supportive Care

Severely ill patients are hospitalized. They are given antibiotic, ventilatory, nutritional (including hyperalimentation), blood product, skin care, physical therapy, and medical and nursing support as required in addition to definitive treatment. Scrupulous hygiene is helpful in limiting auditory canal, cutaneous, and dental lesions. Débridement, and even resection of severely affected gingival tissue, is used to limit oral involvement. The seborrhea-like dermatitis of the scalp may improve with use of a selenium- or phenolic-based shampoo twice per week. Topical steroids occasionally are effective but should be used sparingly and only for short-term control of small affected areas. Topical tacrolimus also can be considered. DI may occur at any time during the course of LCH. Patients should be instructed to report signs of DI as soon as they develop because dehydration and electrolyte imbalance may be quite serious. The results of hypothalamic and pituitary radiotherapy instituted early in the course of DI have been poor, and use of this modality is not recommended. Some evidence indicates that a short course of systemic chemotherapy given early after onset of DI may be helpful in reversing the signs and symptoms of DI.

Local Therapy (Surgery and Radiotherapy)

After complete evaluation, patients with disease involving a single bone and (in some cases) patients with disease involving multiple lesions and multiple bones are managed with local therapy. This involves surgical curettage for patients whose lesions are in easily accessible, noncritical locations. Complete "cancer operation" resections usually are not indicated. Surgical restraint must be exercised to avoid drastic cosmetic and orthopedic deformities and loss of function. Local soft-tissue disease (e.g., scalp, thymus, lymph nodes) generally recurs despite surgery; thus, systemic treatment or low-dose radiation in emergent situations is recommended for these types of lesions. Localized radiotherapy (usually 600–1200 cGy) in 200-cGy fractions, utilizing only megavoltage equipment, is currently used. Older patients may require slightly higher doses (1500–2000 cGy), although this idea has not been definitively studied. Patients at risk for skeletal deformity, visual loss secondary to exophthalmos, pathologic fractures, vertebral collapse, and spinal cord injury should receive radiotherapy. Patients suffering from severe pain or symptomatic adenopathy, even when multiple lesions exist, may also warrant low-dose radiotherapy to affected areas if systemic therapy is not rapidly effective. Lesions in poorly accessible sites, such as the orbit, or lesions recurring after curettage also should be irradiated if chemotherapy is not rapidly effective.

Chemotherapy

If symptomatic lesions or failure to thrive is evident, treatment should be pursued. The LCH-III international clinical trial is pursuing risk-stratified therapy depending on the extent and sites of disease involvement as well as the response to initial therapy (Table 52–5). Experimental modalities, such as bone marrow transplantation, are being pursued at specialized centers for group IV patients who are nonresponsive to conventional chemotherapy.

The persistent philosophy for treatment of LCH has been use of an appropriate amount of the least toxic therapy to effectively treat the disease. In patients with potentially morbid or life-threatening disease at presentation or in those who develop morbid or life-threatening disease during the course of treatment, alternative therapy, including bone marrow transplantation, should be implemented. This approach emphasizes the need for treatment protocols based upon careful prognosis-based risk stratification. Whether more intense up-front therapy in lower-risk patients with systemic disease can reduce disease sequelae such as DI, CNS degeneration, sclerosing cholangitis, or disease recurrence and whether a reduction in these problems outweighs the risk of more intense therapy is under evaluation. Patients with this rare disease are best served by treatment according to collaborative protocols such as those of the Histiocyte Society. *Pneumocystis carinii* and fungal prophylaxis in patients for whom long-term immunosuppressive therapy is anticipated should be used.

Long-Term Followup

All patients with LCH should undergo long-term followup. In addition to late malignancies, patients should be monitored for signs of long-term disabilities, including cosmetic and functional orthopedic and cutaneous deformities that may lead to loss of function and severe emotional disorders, loss of permanent dentition, endocrinologic disorders and growth failure, hearing impairment, CNS abnormalities, psychosocial problems, sclerosing cholangitis, pulmonary fibrosis, and cor pulmonale. Patients with chronic disabilities, such as sequelae of LCH, should be followed by appropriate subspecialists.

tide skeletal evaluations were performed, radiologic evaluation detected virtually all significant skeletal lesions.[138] Other tests such as panoramic dental radiographs, pulmonary function tests, imaging of the brain and middle ear, and bone marrow aspirates/biopsies and biopsies of other tissue should be performed based on the findings of initial evaluation. However, an increasing awareness of CNS involvement in LCH has led some clinicians and investigators to obtain magnetic resonance imaging scan with contrast of the brain to evaluate radiographically evident but clinically silent disease or to serve as a baseline comparison for future studies.

Therapy

A generally accepted standard for initial treatment of patients with LCH is use of an appropriate amount of the least toxic therapy to treat the disease (see box on Therapy for Langerhans Cell Histiocytosis). In patients with potentially morbid or life-threatening disease at presentation or in those who develop morbid or life-threatening disease during the course of treatment, alternative and sometimes more aggressive treatment should be implemented. This approach emphasizes the need for treatment protocols based upon careful prog-

Table 52–8 Treatment[a] Versus No Treatment[b]

Patients	Treatment	Dead	Alive	Mean Age (months)
27	No	27	0	10.5
64	Yes	40	24	15.0

[a]Variable chemotherapy (steroids, antimetabolites, and alkylating agents).
[b]Supportive care.
Data from Lahey ME: Prognosis in reticuloendotheliosis in children. J Pediatr Hematol Oncol 60:664, 1962.

nosis-based risk stratification. Whether more intense up-front therapy in lower-risk patients with systemic disease can reduce disease sequelae such as diabetes insipidus, CNS degeneration, sclerosing cholangitis, or disease recurrence and whether a reduction in these problems outweighs the risk of more intense therapy is under evaluation.

For the majority of patients with localized or limited systemic disease, the goal of therapy should be minimizing loss of function and preventing cosmetic deformity. Severely ill patients often are hospitalized and given intensive supportive care in addition to definitive treatment. Scrupulous hygiene plays an important role in limiting auditory canal, cutaneous, and dental lesions. Débridement, and even resection of severely affected gingival tissue, is sometimes used to limit oral involvement. Seborrhea-like dermatitis of the scalp may improve with use of a selenium- or phenol-based shampoo. Topical steroids can be effective, but prolonged exposure or use on the face should be avoided. Topical tacrolimus (FK506) has become available and can be used for skin involvement. Topical nitrogen mustard has been used for problematic focal skin lesions.[139] In patients with particularly refractory and extensive skin involvement, Psaraler Ultraviolet-A (PUVA) can be effective.[140–142] These topical therapies have not been studied in clinical trials.

Surgery and Radiotherapy

Patients with disease involving a single bone usually can be managed with local therapy. This most often involves surgical curettage for patients whose lesions are in easily accessible, noncritical locations. Complete "cancer operation"' resections are not considered necessary and should be avoided in order to reduce cosmetic or orthopedic deformities as well as loss of function. Local soft-tissue disease (e.g., scalp, thymus, lymph nodes) generally recurs despite surgery; thus, additional treatment usually is required. Because of concerns about the development of secondary malignancies, systemic therapy usually is favored over radiation. However, local radiotherapy is indicated under certain circumstances, for example, when patients are at risk for visual or hearing loss, skeletal deformity, spinal cord injury, or severe pain when systemic therapy is not rapidly effective. Localized radiotherapy (usually 600–1500 cGy) in 200-cGy fractions is currently recommended.[143,144] Lesions in poorly accessible sites, such as the orbit or lesions recurring after curettage, can be effectively treated with radiotherapy. A review of 40 patients who received radiotherapy between 1970 and 1984 indicated that patients with unifocal disease have a higher rate of response for individual lesions than do patients with multifocal disease (two or more soft-tissue sites).[145] In this review, the complete plus partial response rate for bone lesions was 100%, with 35 patients evaluated and 24 complete responses. Soft-tissue lesions adjacent to involved bone healed better than did isolated soft-tissue lesions. No patients responded to irradiation applied for liver, spleen, or lung lesions, and none of eight patients with DI responded.[145] The results of hypothalamic and pituitary radiotherapy instituted early in the course of DI have been poor overall, but with anecdotal successes; use of this modality is not recommended.[91,100,109–111] Use of chemotherapy has been reported in anecdotal cases.[146]

Table 52–9 Comparison of Selected Chemotherapy Trials for Langerhans Cell Histiocytosis

Drug(s)[a]	Study Group		Patients	Response (CR + PR)[b]
Single Agent				
VCR	SWCCG	1972	6	50
VBL	SWCCG	1972	20	55
VBL	CCSG	1975	18	56
VBL	Mayo	1980	18	77
CTX	SWCCG	1972	22	63
PCB	SWOG	1974	10	50
CMB	SWOG	1980	32	56
CMB	CCSG	1980	26	27
VP-16	Italy	1988	18	83
VP-16	AIEOP (Italy)	1993	17	88
ADM	AIEOP (Italy)	1993	7	71
VBL	AIEOP (Italy)	1993	54	85
Combination Therapy				
MTX + PRED	ALGB	1974	17	53
VCR + PRED	ALGB	1974	11	64
VBL + PRED	CCSG	1975	18	67
6-MP + PRED	CCSG	1975	25	48
CTX + VCR + PRED + PCB	SWOG	1977	21	38
CTX + VBL + PRED	SWOG	1977	25	25 < 1 year
MTX + CMB + VBL + PRED	Mexico	1988	68	75
VBL + PRED + VP-16	DAL HX-83	1994	Gr A 27	89
			Gr B 57	91
			Gr C 21	67
VBL/PRED	LCH-I	1994	74	58
VP-16/PRED	LCH-I	1994	69	65 ($P = 0.38$)

[a]Pre-1972: Anecdotal responses reported with antibiotics, corticosteroids, vincristine, vinblastine, methotrexate, cyclophosphamide, nitrogen mustard, 6-mercaptopurine, daunorubicin.
[b]CR, complete response; PR, partial response in which >50% of lesions resolve.
ADM, Adriamycin (doxorubicin); CMB, chlorambucil; CTX, cyclophosphamide; 6-MP, 6-mercaptopurine; MTX, methotrexate; PRED, prednisone; PCB, procarbazine; VBL, vinblastine; VCR, vincristine; VP-16, etoposide.
Data from references 93, 108, 148–150, 152–156, 159, 322, 323.

Chemotherapy

Historically, drugs used in therapy for classic malignant diseases have been used systemically for treatment of LCH. Nitrogen mustard, vincristine, vinblastine, cyclophosphamide, procarbazine, chlorambucil, etoposide, methotrexate, corticosteroids and 6-mercaptopurine have been used, alone or in combination, with variable success. Response to chemotherapy varies from 25% to 90%. Lahey[37] showed that treatment improves survival in patients younger than 2 years (Table 52–8). Table 52–9 summarizes selected and mostly early single-arm chemotherapeutic trials.[147–156]

A reasonable therapeutic approach to systemic therapy is to observe patients with limited disease who respond to local (i.e., surgery, radiation) or nonsystemic (i.e., topical steroids) therapy and look for signs of continuing disease resolution. If symptomatic lesions or evidence of progressive disease is seen, systemic treatment should be pursued. Patients in groups II and III with multisystem or systemic disease usually will benefit from chemotherapy, although significant numbers of patients with systemic disease and risk-organ involvement still show poor responses and mortality. Because of the rarity of LCH and the large number of therapeutic questions for which answers must be sought, all patients with disseminated disease should be placed in well-designed studies whenever possible. Based on data from several small studies demonstrating the efficacy of etoposide in previously untreated patients[155,157] and those with resistant disease,[158] in 1991 the Histiocyte Society sponsored its first international randomized study, LCH-I, for patients younger than 18 years. The purpose of the study was to compare the efficacy of vinblastine to that of etoposide in patients with previously untreated multisystem or disseminated LCH.[159] Treatment in each arm consisted of a single pulse of high-dose methylprednisolone for "induction" followed by weekly vinblastine (6 mg/m^2 intravenous bolus) versus every-3-week etoposide (150 mg/m^2 intravenous over 2 hours per day for 3 days). The total treatment period was 24 weeks. LCH-I showed that the rapidity of the initial response correlated with prognosis and that patients with a poor initial response to either arm tended not to benefit from crossover to the alternative arm.[126,159,160] No difference in outcome measures with use of vinblastine compared to etoposide was observed.

Comparison of the results from the DAL HX-83/90 study to those of the LCH-I trial suggested that the more aggressive DAL HX-83/90 might be responsible for a lower recurrence rate and a lower incidence of diabetes insipidus.[161] Therefore, the subsequent LCH-II trial was designed to test this suggestion in a randomized fashion for high-risk patients with multisystem disease. The LCH-II trial used part of the framework of the DAL HX-83 study,[160] in which all patients receive a 6-week "induction" with prednisone, vinblastine, and etoposide. The subsequent treatment period for 1 year and consisted of only oral 6-mercaptopurine, vinblastine, and prednisone (treatment a) or 6-mercaptopurine, vinblastine, and prednisone plus either etoposide (treatment b) or etoposide and methotrexate (treatment c) for patients with multifocal bone involvement (treatment a), soft-tissue involvement without organ dysfunction (treatment b), and organ dysfunction (treatment c), respectively.[160] In the LCH-II trial, patients were stratified into "low risk" (patients older than 2 years with no involvement of the hematopoietic system, liver, lungs, or spleen) or "at risk" (patients younger than 2 years with involvement of the hematopoietic system, liver, lungs, or spleen). Patients with multisystem disease in the "low-risk" group received initial treatment consisting of a 6-week course of prednisone and weekly vinblastine, followed by continuation treatment with oral 6-mercaptopurine, prednisone pulses, and weekly vinblastine for 24 weeks. Patients in the "at-risk" group were randomized to the low-risk treatment arm versus that same treatment but with the addition of etoposide to both initial and continuation treatment. Results from the LCH-II trial show no significant advantage to adding etoposide in terms of survival or frequency of disease recurrence in the overall patient group. However, patients with risk organ involvement had a between 5 years survival when treated with the more intensive Arm B.[160,106a,162] In an attempt to improve the response rate and possibly reduce the frequency of recurring disease, the LCH-III trial currently is addressing whether the initial response rate is improved by the addition of intermediate-dose methotrexate to prednisone and vinblastine and whether overall outcome is improved using 6 or 12 months of continuation therapy.

Alternative treatment has not been standardized for patients with recurrent and/or refractory disease. Patients with recurrent disease (i.e., disease that reappears after a period of remission) often respond well to the drugs with which they initially were treated. A variety of experimental modalities, such as hemibody irradiation,[163] thymic hormone therapy,[164,165] and α-interferon[166] have been explored for treatment of advanced or refractory disease, but these approaches have been largely abandoned. A number of chemotherapeutic approaches have had limited success and require evaluation in prospective studies.[167–169] Alternatively, several studies, including an international phase II trial, have demonstrated significant activity of 2-chlorodeoxyadenosine (2-CdA) against recurrent and refractory LCH.[106,146,169–181] In addition, the combination of 2-CdA and high-dose cytarabine has been used in refractory patients.[106,182] An anecdotal experience using TNF-inhibitors has been reported,[183] as has pamidronate for bone lesions.[184–187] Thalidomide has shown activity in treating skin disease.[188–191] Bone marrow transplantation for high-risk or refractory patients warrants further evaluation in the context of a controlled clinical trial.[192–198]

Table 52–10 Late Malignancy After Treatment of Langerhans Cell Histiocytosis

Patients	Treatment	Malignancy	Interval Between Histiocytosis and Malignancy (years)
1	CMB	Hepatocellular carcinoma	14
2	CMB + RT	Thyroid carcinoma	16
3	CMB (CT) + RT	Acute leukemia	2
4	CMB, NM (CT) + RT	Acute leukemia	6.5
5	CMB, NM (CT) + RT	Acute leukemia	5
6	RT	Thyroid carcinoma	28

CMB, chlorambucil; CT, combination therapy; NM, nitrogen mustard; RT, radiotherapy.

Data from Greenberger JS, Crocker AC, Vawter G, Jaffe N, Cassady JR: Results of treatment of 127 patients with systemic histiocytosis. Medicine (Baltimore) 60:311, 1981.

Long-Term Follow-up

A retrospective analysis by Willis et al.[123] of 71 patients from a single institution followed for a median of 8.1 years from diagnosis revealed the presence of significant late sequelae in 64% of patients followed for more than 3 years despite a relatively good survival rate of 88%, 88%, and 77% at 5, 15, and 20 years, respectively. Skeletal defects were found in 42%, dental problems in 30%, DI in 25%, growth failure in 20%, sex hormone deficiency in 16%, hypothyroidism in 14%, hearing loss in 16%, and CNS dysfunction in 14%. These data emphasize the importance of appropriate therapeutic choices, as sequelae such as bone malformations, including scoliosis, appeared to be a consequence of treatment with radiation. Although Gadner et al.[108,160] found a lower incidence of DI and fewer recurrences in their study that used aggressive initial chemotherapy, including etoposide and methotrexate, for patients with multifocal bone and disseminated disease, the study by Willis et al. included 28 patients with multisystem disease, many of whom received aggressive chemotherapy and still had recurrences and late sequelae.[108,123]

This risk of malignancy in patients with LCH undergoing radiation and chemotherapy is well documented. In the study by Willis et al.,[123] three of 51 patients followed beyond 3 years developed a malignancy. All three patients were younger than 3 years at the time of diagnosis. Two tumors were in a radiation field, but one was a leukemia in a patient treated with an etoposide-containing chemotherapy regimen. Of 127 patients with LCH reported by Greenberger et al.,[40] 84 received chemotherapy, and six developed late malignancies (Table 52–10). Two patients who received radiotherapy developed an in-field tumor, and one of these patients received no chemotherapy. Late malignancy developed in five of 54 patients who received chlorambucil as a single agent or in combination with other chemotherapeutic agents. Two of 29 patients received nitrogen mustard as part of combination therapy, including chlorambucil, vincristine, procarbazine, and prednisone. The risk of malignancy is similar to that reported after chlorambucil given for treatment of polycythemia vera. Thus, judicious use of radiotherapy, avoidance of potentially carcinogenic chemotherapeutic agents, and good supportive care are recommended. Although patients with LCH could have an inherently increased risk of malignancy,[199] the experience cited strongly suggests an excess of malignancy was associated with chlorambucil use. Leukemia in LCH patients treated with etoposide as a single agent[156,200,201] and in combination with other agents[202,203] has been reported. Because etoposide was not shown to be any more effective than vinblastine in both the LCH-I and LCH-II trials for patients without risk organ involvement, there does not appear to be reason to include this leukemogenic agent in the treatment of these patients with newly diagnosed LCH.

Another serious late effect of LCH is sclerosing cholangitis, which may lead to secondary biliary cirrhosis and liver failure.[204–213] The only successful treatment of sclerosing cholangitis has been liver transplantation. Another late complication of LCH is pulmonary cyst formation, fibrosis, and chronic pneumothoraces.[92,214–218] No effective treatment is available, and progression to cor pulmonale and respiratory failure are not uncommon.[219,220] Lung transplantation has been used for treatment of such patients.[221–224] Thus, all patients with LCH require long-term followup. In addition to late malignancies, patients should be monitored for signs of long-term disabilities, including cosmetic, orthopedic, and cutaneous deformities that may lead to loss of function and emotional disorders, loss of permanent dentition, endocrinologic disorders and growth failure, hearing impairment, CNS abnormalities and neurocognitive function, sclerosing cholangitis with biliary cirrhosis, and pulmonary fibrosis and cor pulmonale. More effective treatments that reduce the incidence of these sequelae are needed.

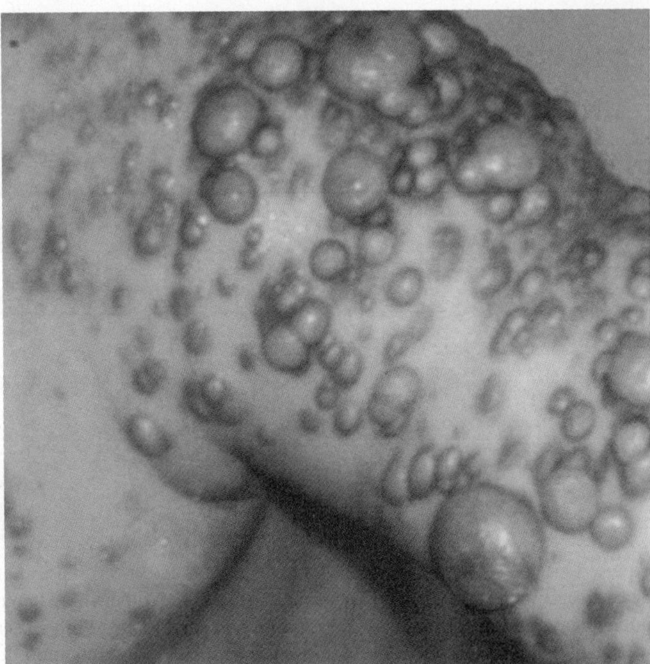

Figure 52–7 Extensive juvenile xanthogranulomatous disease in an infant.

Juvenile Xanthogranulomatous Disease and Erdheim-Chester Disease

Juvenile xanthogranulomatous disease (JXG) is particularly common in infants and young children. The cell of origin and classification of the type of disease represented by JXG have been debated for more than 50 years, but current information demonstrates several important insights. The immunophenotype of JXG cells shows that they are positive in expression for CD14, CD68, CD163, factor XIIIa, and often fascin.[225] The cells usually are negative for CD1a, S100, and the plasmacytoid monocyte antigen CD123. These data support that JXG lesions originate from dermal dendrocytes.[226,227]

JXG most commonly presents as a single skin lesion in infants and young children (see Fig. 52–6). The lesions are nodular and usually yellowish to reddish purple. Lesions may vary significantly in size and number but often are several millimeters to 1 cm in size and solitary. However, in some patients, the lesions become widespread and quite disfiguring (Fig. 52–7). Furthermore, JXG may become systemic, involving multiple organs including the liver, lungs, heart, and CNS. CNS involvement can present with seizures, hemiplegia, and increased intracranial pressure.[228]

Cutaneous JXG lesions usually resolve over several months and require no treatment.[229,230] Benign cephalic histiocytosis is a closely related disorder that presents during infancy. It is characterized by multiple, small reddish-brown, palpable macular lesions primarily involving the head and upper extremities.[231–235] This disorder usually slowly regresses spontaneously over several weeks to months. With both JXG and benign cephalic histiocytosis, residual pigmented regions may persist even after lesions have regressed. In patients in whom JXG becomes systemic and involves multiple organs, systemic chemotherapy similar to that for patients with LCH has been used. In patients who do not respond to initial treatment with vinblastine and steroids, use of other agents, such as methotrexate, steroids, and 2-CdA, has led to responses according to anecdotal reports.[236]

Erdheim-Chester disease is seen most commonly in patients 50 years or older. It usually presents with xanthoma-like skin nodules and bilateral lower limb bone pain. Patients with more disseminated disease may have cardiopulmonary insufficiency, renal failure due to characteristic perinephric constrictive changes, and CNS involvement manifested by ataxia, diabetes insipidus, and altered mental status.[237–240] Periorbital involvement with exophthalmos and impingement on the optic nerves.[225] The disease may be progressive and fatal. Successful effective treatment has been limited, although responses have been observed with steroids, vinblastine plus steroids, methotrexate, 2-CdA, bisphosphonates, and interferon-α.[241–247] Autologous hematopoietic bone marrow transplantation has been reported.[248]

HEMOPHAGOCYTIC SYNDROMES

Hemophagocytic Lymphohistiocytosis

Familial HLH was formerly known as familial erythrophagocytic lymphohistiocytosis. Familial HLH usually is a rapidly fatal, inherited disorder characterized by either persistent or intermittent fevers with hepatosplenomegaly (often presenting initially as isolated splenomegaly), thrombocytopenia and anemia, pancytopenia, coagulation abnormalities with hypofibrinogenemia, and hepatic dysfunction.[249–253] The Histiocyte Society has developed five "diagnostic criteria" for HLH, specifying the clinical criteria of (a) fever and (b) splenomegaly in the presence of the laboratory criteria of (c) cytopenias involving at least two lineages accompanied by (d) hypofibrinogenemia and/or hypertriglyceridemia and (e) hemophagocytosis, in the absence of malignancy, in the bone marrow, spleen, or lymph nodes.[249–253] In addition, three additional criteria have been included: (f) low or absent natural killer (NK) lymphocyte activity, (g) hyperferritinemia, and (h) high levels of soluble IL-2 receptor.[254] Five of the eight criteria must be fulfilled unless a patient has a molecular diagnosis consistent with HLH.

Most affected children are infants (age 2 weeks to 7 years), and two thirds of affected children present within the first 3 months of life.[251,255] Patients usually present with pallor, irritability, anorexia, diarrhea, and failure to thrive. Occasionally, a nonspecific, maculopapular skin rash is seen. Pulmonary effusions are present in one third of patients. The clinical course usually is progressive, resulting in death within approximately 6 weeks without effective treatment.[251,256,257] Most patients die of sepsis, bleeding, or a lymphohistiocytic-mediated meningitis accompanied by refractory seizures. Approximately 75% of patients have CNS involvement at diagnosis.[255] Disease essentially confined to the CNS, leading to seizures, has been reported.[255,258,259] There is no gender predilection, and the presence of the disorder in siblings and in cousins as well as the presence of parental consanguinity supports an autosomal recessive mode of inheritance.

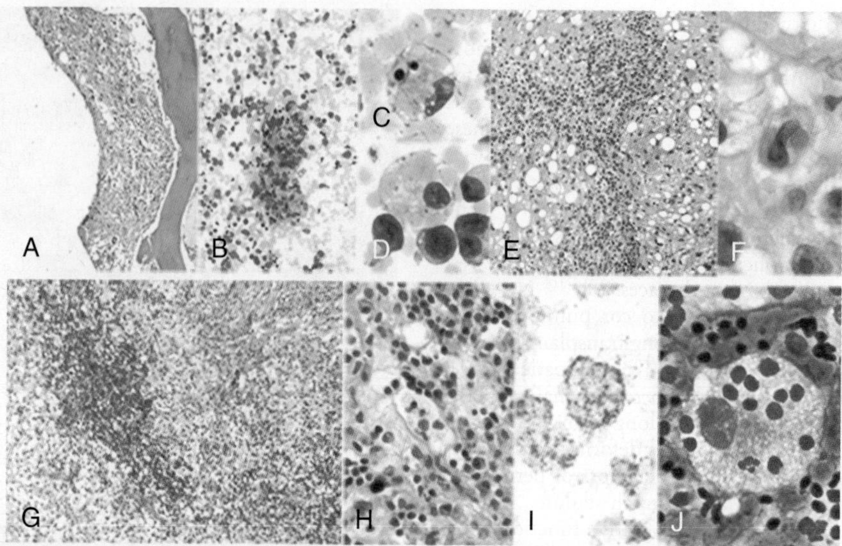

Figure 52–8 A–F, Familial hemophagocytic lymphohistiocytosis. Illustrations from a 3-month-old girl who presented with diarrhea, pancytopenia, hepatomegaly, and liver failure. bone marrow (**A, B**) showed left-shifted granulopoiesis and increased histiocytes, which at high power (**C, D**) were undergoing prominent phagocytosis of erythrocytes, platelets, and other cells. Liver biopsy sample (**E**) showed a lymphohistiocytic infiltrate also associated with hemophagocytosis (**F**). The patient was shown to harbor a mutation of the perforin gene in exon 2. **G–J**, Sinus histiocytosis with massive lymphadenopathy (Rosai-Dorfman disease). Low-power magnification of the biopsy sample (**G**) shows a mottled appearance of the lesion due to dark areas containing small lymphocytes and lighter areas containing histiocytes. At higher magnification (**H**), the histiocytes have abundant pale cytoplasm with scattered cells within. This is emperipolesis, or a process of cells traveling through the cytoplasm but not becoming phagocytized or degraded. Note plasma cells in the background. The emperipolesis can be better visualized with a CD68 stain for histiocytes (**I**). This process delineates the cell boundary and the cells within the histiocyte cytoplasm. The emperipolesis can also be seen on a Wright-stained touch preparation (**J**).

Pathology of the liver shows focal fatty changes, necrosis, and infiltration by lymphocytes and histiocytes. The infiltrate is periportal but can extend into adjacent lobules. Typical hemophagocytosis may be evident only at presentation in as few as one third of patients with verified HLH.[251,260] Thus, convincing evidence of hemophagocytosis should be pursued with serial bone marrow examinations when there is clinical suspicion of HLH. The spleen demonstrates similar focal necrosis along with lymphohistiocytic infiltrates associated with hemophagocytosis. Involvement of the thymus and lymph nodes is similar; however, lymph nodes show significant lymphocytic depletion later in the course of disease. Hemophagocytosis may be present. The lungs are infiltrated with lymphocytes and histiocytes, again with some hemophagocytosis. The bone marrow usually is hyperplastic, with increased numbers of hemophagocytic histiocytes (Fig. 52–8).[260,261] The cellular infiltrate lacks features of malignant cells. The characteristic pathology and clinical presentation clearly distinguishes HLH from LCH and other histiocytic disorders.

Advances in immunology and molecular biology have allowed clinicians to increasingly refine the diagnostic category of HLH. Initial clinical observations had permitted a somewhat crude distinction of the familial syndrome known as familial erythrophagocytic lymphohistiocytosis from viral-associated or infection-associated hemophagocytic syndrome or malignancy-associated HLH.[262–264] In addition, rheumatologists and immunologists have been able to identify a clinically similar "macrophage activation syndrome" in a subset of patients with juvenile rheumatoid arthritis or certain immunodeficiency states.[265]

Aricò et al.[266] have proposed a "diagnostic algorithm" incorporating the current understanding of HLH. The path to a correct diagnosis begins with a patient who meets the described diagnostic criteria. A search for infectious agents, such as Epstein-Barr virus, cytomegalovirus, parvovirus B19, and a number of bacteria, fungi, mycobacteria, and parasites, should be undertaken. A detailed history, physical examination, and laboratory screening usually eliminates from consideration the macrophage activation syndrome associated with juvenile rheumatoid arthritis. Hypoparathyroidism, thymic dysfunction, and orofacial and cardiac anomalies resulting from abnormal development of the third and forth pharyngeal pouches characterize DiGeorge syndrome, which can be associated with secondary HLH.[266,267] The presence of hyperammonemia is characteristic of the metabolic disorder lysinuric protein intolerance that may result in an immunodeficiency state and HLH.[268]

Other rare immunodeficiency syndromes in addition to DiGeorge syndrome and lysinuric protein intolerance can be associated with HLH. The accelerated phase of Chédiak-Higashi and Griscelli syndromes are indistinguishable from other forms of HLH.[266,269–272] Both syndromes are characterized by albinism. Classic granules found in the neutrophils of patients with Chédiak-Higashi syndrome and melanin inclusions in the hair of patients with Griscelli syndrome support the diagnosis. The presence of mutations in *LYST*[273] or *RAB27A*,[270] respectively, confirms the diagnosis.

In males, a diagnosis of X-linked lymphoproliferative disease should be ruled out. In this disorder, a mutation in the *SH2D1A* gene leads to an inhibitory mutation in the lymphocyte 2B4 receptor, resulting in the inability of NK cells to kill cells infected with Epstein–Barr virus.[274–278] This, in turn, results in the sustained proliferation of ineffective cytolytic effector cells and the syndrome of HLH.[279]

Familial HLH is an autosomal recessive disorder whose underlying pathophysiology is impaired NK and cytotoxic T-lymphocyte activity.[257,269] In 1999, the two chromosomal loci 9q21.3–22 and 10q21–22 were linked to the disease, defining HLH type 1 and type 2, respectively.[280–282] Shortly thereafter, mutations in the gene on chromosome 10q22, coding for perforin (PRF1), were identified.[283–285] Perforin functions by creating holes in target cell membrane that in turn allow for entry of granzymes that initiate apoptotic cell death. The pathways leading to perforin synthesis, subcellular compartmentalization, and directional targeting and release of cytolytic granules all represent potential points that could be mutated and contribute to different genetic causes of inherited HLH syndromes. An example of this is the description of mutations in the *Munc13–4* gene, located at chromosome 17q25, which is essential for cytolytic granule fusion.[286] Inactivating mutations in this gene now have been shown to cause familial HLH, termed *FHL3* subtype.[286] Similarly, mutations in syntaxin, another product involved in assembly and trans-port of cytolytic granules in lymphocytes, have been linked to HLH.[287,288]

In the absence of perforin activity, the resulting inability to kill infected target cells results in sustained NK and cytolytic T-lymphocyte activity. This, in turn, results in overexpression of inflammatory cytokines (soluble IL-2 receptor, IL-6, TNF-α, IL10, and IL-12), leading to excessive macrophage activation, dissemination, and organ infiltration along with the signs, symptoms, and laboratory abnormalities that characterize HLH.[256,269,289]

Impaired NK cell activity and number are important keys to the diagnosis. The absence of intracytoplasmic perforin can be used as a reliable marker in the 20% to 40% of patients with familial HLH type 2 (NLH1) associated with the 10q21–22 locus and perforin gene mutations.[266,290,291] The remaining familial cases may be recognized by impaired NK cell function not associated with the absence of perforin expression. HLH type 1 linked to the 9q21.3 locus represents approximately 10% of the cases.[266] However, a substantial proportion of familial cases of HLH remains genetically uncategorized. Patients with absent perforin expression should undergo PRF1, MUNC 13–4, and syntaxin mutation analysis. In the absence of a positive mutation analysis, reevaluation of NK function after successful treatment should be undertaken.

Etoposide has induced clinical remissions accompanied by resolution of clinical, hematologic, and biochemical abnormalities.[292] Although all patients relapse with familial disease, etoposide, usually in combination with prednisone and intrathecal methotrexate,[255] has resulted in complete to very good responses in patients with familial HLH and has been used prior to more definitive therapy with bone marrow transplantation in patients with this otherwise lethal disorder.[293,294] Thus, based on our understanding of the pathophysiology of these disorders, the initial strategy for HLH therapy consists of initial use of etoposide, dexamethasone, and cyclosporine A according the International HLH-2004 clinical trial.[254] Even when an associated infection or malignancy can be identified and treated, therapy directed toward the HLH also may be necessary. Patients with known familial disease or severe or persistent acquired disease should go on to hematopoietic stem cell transplantation (see Chapters 59, 62, and 74). The 3-year actuarial survival using this approach in patients with familial HLH has been reported as 51% ± 20%.[254,256,295]

Sinus Histiocytosis With Massive Lymphadenopathy

First described in 1969, sinus histiocytosis with massive lymphadenopathy, or Rosai-Dorfman disease, is clinically characterized as a benign, frequently chronic, painless massive lymphadenopathy usually involving cervical lymph nodes and, less frequently axillary, hilar, peritracheal, and inguinal nodes.[296] Extranodal disease is present in approximately 28% of patients.[297–299] The upper respiratory mucosa is involved in 20% of patients,[300] bone in 25%,[301,302] and orbit or eyelid in 10%.[303,304] Occasionally there is involvement of skin,[305] CNS, lung, liver, and kidney.[306–308] Ocular manifestations, such as uveitis, have been observed.[309]

Although sinus histiocytosis with massive lymphadenopathy is a histologically reactive and molecularly polyclonal disorder,[310] significant morbidity and death have been associated with massive tissue invasion of the liver, kidney, lung, brain, and other critical structures.[306,311] In these instances, the disease may have a rapid downhill course. Respiratory distress due to tracheal obstruction[312] as well as paraplegia secondary to epidural involvement have been described.[313] Death from sinus histiocytosis with massive lymphadenopathy has occurred as a consequence of severe hemolytic anemia.[311]

Eighty percent of patients are diagnosed in the first or second decade of life; however, the disorder also can affect the elderly.[314] Typically, patients are of African descent.[315] Males and females are equally affected. The incidence of sinus histiocytosis with massive lymphadenopathy is greatest in Africa and the West Indies.[315]

Laboratory evaluation frequently reveals an elevated erythrocyte sedimentation rate, moderate polyclonal hypergammaglobulinemia, anemia, and granulocytosis.[305,312] Involved lymph nodes (see Fig. 52–8) show marked sinusoidal dilation with proliferation of foamy histiocytes within the sinuses. Eosinophils usually are low in number, but plasma cells are abundant.[296,297,300,301] A characteristic finding, referred to as emperipolesis, demonstrates lymphocytes surrounded by the membranes of histiocytes as observed best by electron microscopy.[312] The proliferating histiocytes share properties of macrophages and interdigitating cells. These large pale cells show variable expression of S100. They can be distinguished from Langerhans cells found in the lymph nodes of patients with classic LCH by the absence of Birbeck granules, the presence of α_1-antichymotrypsin, and the absence of CD1a expression.[312]

The etiology of Rosai-Dorfman disease is unknown, but disordered immune regulation has been proposed as a significant contributor. It was originally thought that Rosai-Dorfman disease represented an unusual response to a *Klebsiella* antigen or Epstein-Barr virus,[314] but this has not been confirmed.[305] There has also been an association of the disease with herpesvirus 6.[316] Although patients frequently are febrile, infectious agents are not commonly implicated, and the fever is presumed to be a manifestation of systemic disease.

Disease manifestations can subside over several months to years. Of 215 cases in a patient registry, 21% had complete resolution of disease. However, 14 patients died. Five died of "immunologic" causes, such as severe hemolysis, three died of infections and six probably died as a direct consequence of disease infiltration.[317] As the disease resolves, extranodal disease regresses prior to nodal disease. Corticosteroids, vinblastine, and low-dose cyclophosphamide are sometimes effective; however, the results with these agents have been inconsistent.[297,313,318,319] Thalidomide has been used in some cases, with anecdotal responses.[320] Similarly, 2-CdA has been reported to have activity in Rosai–Dorfman disease.[321] Attempts at treatment should be reserved for special circumstances, such as tracheal or epidural compression or invasion of other vital structures, as well as for significant cosmetic disfigurement. Local excision may be useful in selected patients.[301]

SUGGESTED READINGS

Arceci RJ, Longley BJ, Emanuel PD: Atypical cellular disorders. Hematology (Am Soc Hematol Educ Program). 297, 2002.

Arico M, Girschikofsky M, Genereau T, et al: Langerhans cell histiocytosis in adults. Report from the International Registry of the Histiocyte Society. Eur J Cancer 39:2341, 2003.

Arico M, Allen M, Brusa S, et al: Haemophagocytic lymphohistiocytosis: Proposal of a diagnostic algorithm based on perforin expression. Br J Haematol 119:180, 2002.

Arico M, Danesino C, Pende D, Moretta L: Pathogenesis of haemophagocytic lymphohistiocytosis. Br J Haematol 114:761, 2001.

Bechan GI, Egeler RM, Arceci RJ: Biology of Langerhans cells and Langerhans cell histiocytosis. Int Rev Cytol 254:1, 2006.

Ericson KG, Fadeel B, Andersson M, et al: Sequence analysis of the granulysin and granzyme B genes in familial hemophagocytic lymphohistiocytosis. Hum Genet 112:98, 2003.

Favara BE, Feller AC, Pauli M, et al: Contemporary classification of histiocytic disorders. The WHO Committee On Histiocytic/Reticulum Cell Proliferations. Reclassification Working Group of the Histiocyte Society. Med Pediatr Oncol 29:157, 1997.

Feldmann J, Callebaut I, Raposo G, et al: Munc13-4, is essential for cytolytic granules fusion and is mutated in a form of familial hemophagocytic lymphohistiocytosis (FHL3). Cell 115:461, 2003.

Feldmann J, Le Deist F, Ouachee-Chardin M, et al: Functional consequences of perforin gene mutations in 22, patients with familial haemophagocytic lymphohistiocytosis. Br J Haematol 117:965, 2002.

Gadner H, Grois N, Arico M, et al: A randomized trial of treatment for multisystem Langerhans' cell histiocytosis. J Pediatr 138:728, 2001.

Goransdotter Ericson K, Fadeel B, Nilsson-Ardnor S, et al: Spectrum of perforin gene mutations in familial hemophagocytic lymphohistiocytosis. Am J Hum Genet 68:590, 2001.

Grois N, Prayer D, Prosch H, Lassmann H: Neuropathology of CNS disease in Langerhans cell histiocytosis. Brain 128:829, 2005.

Henter JI, Karlen J, Calming U, Bernstrand C, Andersson U, Fadeel B: Successful treatment of Langerhans'-cell histiocytosis with etanercept. N Engl J Med 345:1577, 2001.

Henter JI, Arico M, Elinder G, Imashuku S, Janka G: Familial hemophagocytic lymphohistiocytosis. Primary hemophagocytic lymphohistiocytosis. Hematol Oncol Clin North Am 12:417, 1998.

Henter JI, Horne A, Arico M, et al: HLH-2004: Diagnostic and therapeutic guidelines for hemophagocytic lymphohistiocytosis. Pediatr Blood Cancer 48:124, 2007.

Henter JI, Samuelsson-Horne A, Arico M, et al: Treatment of hemophagocytic lymphohistiocytosis with HLH-94, immunochemotherapy and bone marrow transplantation. Blood 100:2367, 2002.

Rodriguez-Galindo C, Helton KJ, Sanchez ND, Rieman M, Jeng M, Wang W: Extranodal Rosai-Dorfman disease in children. J Pediatr Hematol Oncol 26:19, 2004.

Stepp SE, Dufourcq-Lagelouse R, Le Deist F, et al: Perforin gene defects in familial hemophagocytic lymphohistiocytosis. Science 286:1957, 1999.

Weitzman S, Jaffe R: Uncommon histiocytic disorders: The non-Langerhans cell histiocytoses. Pediatr Blood Cancer 45:256, 2005.

Willman CL, Busque L, Griffith BB, et al: Langerhans'-cell histiocytosis (histiocytosis X)—A clonal proliferative disease. N Engl J Med 331:154, 1994.

Willman CL, McClain KL: An update on clonality, cytokines, and viral etiology in Langerhans cell histiocytosis. Hematol Oncol Clin North Am 12:407, 1998.

Yu RC, Chu C, Buluwela L, Chu AC: Clonal proliferation of Langerhans cells in Langerhans cell histiocytosis. Lancet 343:767, 1994.

REFERENCES

For complete list of references log onto www.expertconsult.com

CHAPTER 53

LYSOSOMAL STORAGE DISEASES: PERSPECTIVES AND PRINCIPLES

Gregory A. Grabowski and Nancy D. Leslie

THE CONCEPT OF THE LYSOSOME

The lysosome was first described by deDuve as an acid phosphatase-containing, unit membrane-bound organelle within the cytoplasm of eukaryotic cells.[1] As their name implies, lysosomes participate in the lysis or breakdown of cellular material, functioning as a digestive tract within the cell. An array of more than 50 hydrolytic enzymes is contained within the organelles to prevent autodigestion of cellular contents. Since the original description, the role of the lysosome has expanded to that of a dynamic and heterogeneous subcellular organelle with functions tailored to specific cell types and tissues. For example, the specialized lysosomes of neutrophils and osteoclasts extrude hydrolytic enzymes into the extracellular microenvironment, providing a critical component of host defense and bone remodeling, respectively.

The concepts of lysosomes as hydrolytic sacs and the need for specific targeting of enzymes to the lysosome have provided a fertile milieu for research during the past three decades. deDuve was the first to delineate engorged lysosomes in patients with α-glucosidase deficiency (Pompe disease)[2] and, in concert with Van Hoof, in patients with other lysosomal storage diseases.[3] The initial descriptions of lysosomal storage diseases focused on a pathophysiologic view relating morbidity and cellular dysfunction to architectural distortion produced by lysosomal storage. More recently, a more active role for the accumulating catabolic intermediates (eg, lysosphingolipids) has been suggested because of their toxic effects on cells.[4] Further investigation of lysosomal function and derangements has delineated additional categories of disease, including defects of lysosomal membrane proteins, transport, and defects of enzyme processing and uptake.

An important element in understanding the biology and pathobiology of the lysosome is the concept of receptor-mediated endocytosis. The Goldstein and Brown model of receptor-mediated endocytosis for the low-density lipoprotein (LDL) particle[5] and its general implications for the uptake and targeting of proteins to cells were expanded by Neufeld[6] and others. Fratantoni described the phenomenon of cross-correction of lysosomal storage diseases during coculture of skin fibroblasts from patients with two different types of mucopolysaccharidoses (MPSs).[6] Specific "corrective factors" secreted by one MPS cell type could be internalized by the other cell type,[6] resulting in depletion of accumulated substrate. These corrective factors were later identified as enzymes, reinforcing the notion that a single lysosomal hydrolase usually is defective in each MPS variant. However, cross-correction requires the secretion of a functional enzyme containing a signal for receptor-mediated endocytosis by other cells. This signaling system, subsequently characterized by the groups of Sly,[7] Kornfeld,[8,9] von Figura,[10] and others, involves modification of the secreted enzyme to include a mannose-6-phosphate (M6P) recognition signal and its interaction with a specific receptor, allowing reuptake of the tagged enzyme back into the cell or similarly equipped neighbors. This ligand-mediated targeting system is central to selective sorting of most soluble lysosomal proteins within many cells,[9] and to their uptake into cells and delivery to the lysosome. By comparison, membrane-bound lysosomal proteins use different, incompletely defined, amino acid-based targeting systems.[11] These concepts of storage, cross-correction, and targeting have provided the foundation for the development of therapeutic interventions for lysosomal storage diseases, including enzyme reconstitution by transplanted tissue or direct replacement. Both approaches may stabilize or reverse the pathophysiologic process in select lysosomal storage diseases. These findings imply a dynamic and interactive communication of the lysosome with intra- and extracellular compartments. Comprehensive reviews of individual lysosomal diseases are presented in Tables 53–1 and 53–2.

PHYSIOLOGY OF LYSOSOMES

Lysosomal biogenesis is a continuous process that requires synthesis of lysosomal hydrolases, membrane constitutive proteins and membranes, as well as establishment of the acidic milieu required for hydrolytic function. Unlike mitochondria, lysosomes do not contain DNA and therefore cannot self-replicate. Thus, biogenesis includes the fusion of vesicles from the *trans*-Golgi network (TGN) with late endosomes (multivesicular bodies [MVBs]) (Fig. 53–1).[12,13] The TGN vesicles contain lysosomal hydrolases. The maturation of TGN vesicular bodies to lysosomes and of endosomes from early to late compartments accompanies progressive intravesicular acidification. A gradient is established, so that early endosomes have an internal pH of approximately 6.0 to 6.2, whereas late endosomes and lysosomes have pH values of approximately 5.5 to 6.0 and less than 5, respectively. This acidification is needed for the pH-dependent dissociation of receptors and ligands (eg, the M6P receptor and M6P-containing oligosaccharides) and the optimal functioning of lysosomal hydrolases.[14] Dissociation occurs in a virtual compartment termed CURL (*c*ompartment of *u*ncoupling of *r*eceptors and *l*igands). Formation and segregation of lysosomes with their constitutive integral and associated membrane proteins are less well understood.[15] These proteins are essential for lysosomal integrity and function. In particular, the lysosomal membrane contains a proton pump needed for developing and maintaining the acidic internal environment required for lysosomal hydrolase function. The signals for the fusion of TGN vesicles with endosomal vesicles (PL-EN) require the interaction of several membrane components, the sorting of proteins destined for the lysosome, the loss of the M6P receptors, the recycling of these receptors to the *mid*- (*medial*-) Golgi bodies and plasma membrane,[14] and segregation of endosomal membrane and contents. Consequently, the view of the lysosome as an end-stage compartment has been replaced by one of a dynamic communicating organelle with continuously changing contents that, at least in part, exchanges material with other lysosomes in the cell. This leads to a lysosomal compartment that is composed of heterogeneous populations of similar organelles whose individual contents differ greatly in time and space.

Posttranslational modifications of lysosomal hydrolases are important both for specific sorting and targeting of enzymes and for their enzymatic activity. Lysosomal enzymes are glycoproteins that are synthesized on ribosomes of the rough endoplasmic reticulum (ER). As with all secretory proteins, lysosomal hydrolases are synthesized with an amino-terminal (N-terminal) hydrophobic leader or signal peptide that is required for penetration through the ER membrane and into the lumen of the ER. During penetration through the ER membrane, the lysosomal proteins are cotranslationally glycosylated on select N-glycosylation consensus sequences (asparagine–X–serine or -threonine). This occurs by the en bloc transfer of a core mannosyl

Table 53–1 Select Lysosomal Storage Diseases (See Box on Perspective on Diagnosis of Lysosomal Storage Diseases)

Disease*	Common Name	Enzyme Defect	Major Organs Involved; Phenotype Variation	Stored Substrate(s)
MUCOPOLYSACCHARIDOSES (MPSs)[137]				
MPS IH	Hurler syndrome	α-L-Iduronidase	Liver, spleen, brain, heart, cornea, bone; mild and severe variants	Dermatan and heparan sulfate
MPS II	Hunter syndrome	Iduronidate sulfatase	Liver, spleen, brain, heart, bone	Dermatan and heparan sulfate
MPS III[138,139]	Sanfilippo syndrome type A	Heparan *N*-sulfatase	Brain, liver, spleen, heart, bone	Heparan sulfate
	Sanfilippo syndrome type B	*N*-Acetyl-glucosaminidase	Brain, liver, spleen, heart, bone	Heparan sulfate
MPS IV[138]	Morquio syndrome type A	*N*-Acetyl-galactosamine 6-sulfatase	Bone, cornea	Keratan sulfate, chondroitin 6-sulfate
	Morquio syndrome type B	β-Galactosidase	Bone, cornea	Keratan sulfate
MPS VI	Maroteaux–Lamy syndrome	*N*-Acetyl-galactosamine 4-sulfatase	Bone, cornea, liver, spleen, heart; moderate and severe variants	Dermatan sulfate
MPS VII	Sly syndrome	β-Glucuronidase	Brain, liver, spleen, bone, coronary arteries	Dermatan sulfate, heparan sulfate, chondroitin 4- and 6-sulfate
GLYCOPROTEINOSES[56]				
Mannosidosis		Lysosomal α-mannosidase	Brain, liver, spleen and bone; several variants	α-Mannose-rich oligosaccharides
Fucosidosis		Glycoprotein α-fucosidase	Brain, liver, spleen, heart, skin; several variants	Fucose-containing oligosaccharides
Aspartylglucosaminuria[140]		Aspartyl-glucosaminidase	Brain, liver, spleen, bone, heart	Aspartylglucosamine-containing peptides
Sialidosis		Glycoprotein α-neuraminidase	Brain, liver, spleen, bone, retina; several variants	Sialylated glycopeptides
Galactosialidosis[141]		Protector protein-combined α-neuraminidase/β-galactosidase deficiency	Brain, liver, spleen, bone; several variants	Ganglioside G_{M1} and sialylated glycopepetides
Mucolipidosis II[142]	I-Cell disease	*N*-Acetylglucosamine-1-phosphotransferase	Brain, bone, connective tissue	Glycoproteins, glycolipids
Mucolipidosis III[142]	Pseudo-Hurler (syndrome) polydystrophy	*N*-Acetylglucosamine-1-phosphotransferase	Brain, bone, connective tissue	Glycoproteins, glycolipids
SPHINGOLIPIDOSES				
Gaucher disease[52]	Gaucher disease Type 1 (nonneuronopathic)	Acid β-glucosidase; glucocerebrosidase	Liver, spleen, bone, bone marrow; highly variable phenotype	Glucosylceramide
	Gaucher disease type 2 (acute neuronopathic)	Acid β-glucosidase; glucocerebrosidase	Brain, brainstem, liver, spleen, bone marrow, lungs	Glucosylceramide; glucosylsphingosine
	Gaucher disease type 3 (subacute neuronopathic)	Acid β-glucosidase; glucocerebrosidase	Brain, liver, spleen, bone marrow, lungs; variable phenotype	Glucosylceramide; glucosylsphingosine
Metachromatic leukodystrophy (MLD)[143]	Infantile MLD	Arylsulfatase A	Brain, peripheral nerves	Sulfatide
	Juvenile MLD	Arylsulfatase A	Brain, peripheral nerves	Sulfatide
	Adult MLD	Arylsulfatase A	Brain, peripheral nerves	Sulfatide
		Saposin B deficiency	Brain, peripheral nerves normal	Sulfatide
	Pseudo deficiency	Partial arylsulfatase A deficiency		None
Fabry disease[35,144]		α-Galactosidase A	Kidney, vascular endothelial system, heart, CNS vessels	Globotriaosylceramide
Schindler disease[145]		β-*N*-acetyl-galactosami dase	Brain; probably several variants	*N*-Acetylgalactose linked oligosaccharides; ? other
Krabbe disease[146]		Galactocerebrosidase	Brain	Galactocerebroside
Niemann–Pick disease[147,148]	Niemann–Pick disease type A (infantile)	Sphingomyelinase	Brain, liver, spleen, lungs	Sphingomyelin
Multiple sulfatase deficiency[61]		Cysteine modification enzyme	Brain, liver, spleen, bone	Sulfatide, dermatan, and heparan sulfate
GANGLIOSIDOSES				
G_{M2} gangliosidoses[68]	Infantile Tay–Sachs disease (TSD)	β-Hexosaminidase A (α-chain)	Brain	Ganglioside G_{M2}
	Juvenile TSD	β-Hexosaminidase A (α-chain)	Brain	Ganglioside G_{M2}
	Adult TSD	β-Hexosaminidase A (α-chain)	Brain	Ganglioside G_{M2}
	Activator deficiency	G_{M2}-activator	Brain	Ganglioside G_{M2}
	Sandhoff disease	β-Hexosaminidase B, A (β-chain)	Brain, liver, spleen, bone	Ganglioside G_{M2}, globoside

Table 53–1 Select Lysosomal Storage Diseases (See Box on Perspective on Diagnosis of Lysosomal Storage Diseases)—cont'd

Disease*	Common Name	Enzyme Defect	Major Organs Involved; Phenotype Variation	Stored Substrate(s)
G_{M1} gangliosidoses[55]	Landing disease	α-Galactosidase	Brain, liver, spleen, bone	Ganglioside G_{M1}, keratan sulfate
NEUTRAL LIPID STORAGE DISEASES				
Wolman disease[36]		Lysosomal acid lipase	Liver, spleen, adrenal glands, bone marrow	Cholesteryl esters, triglycerides
Cholesterol ester storage disease (CESD)[36]		Lysosomal acid lipase	Liver, spleen, blood vessels	Cholesteryl esters
Farber disease[149]		Ceramidase	Brain, joints, tendons, skin, liver	Ceramide

CNS, central nervous system.
*Reference numbers refer to major reviews.

Table 53–2 Non-Hydrolase-Mediated Lysosomal Diseases

Protein	Function	Mouse Model[150]	Human Disease	Pathology
LAMP-1	Not defined			
LAMP-2	Lysosomal biogenesis, chaperone-mediated autophagy[152]	Vacuoles in liver, pancreas, muscle, heart[153]	Danon disease[151]	Cardiomyopathy, skeletal myopathy
LIMP-2	Endosomal transport, lysosomal biogenesis	Demyelinating neuropathy, deafness, ureteropelvic junction obstruction[154]	Not defined	
Cystinosis	Lysosomal cystine transport	Cystine storage in eye and bone, but NO renal disease[155]	Cystinosis	Cystine storage in renal tubules and cornea
Sialin[156]	Free sialic acid transport		Salla disease, infantile sialic acid storage disease	
Mucolipin-1[157]	Calcium-permeable channel, abnormal sorting of lysosomal proteins		Mucolipidosis IV	Mental retardation, cloudy corneas
Cathepsin K[158]	Osteoclast degradation of bone protein matrix (collagen)		Pyknodystostosis	Skeletal dysplasia
Niemann–Pick type C[73]	Lysosomal accumulation of cholesterol	Yes	Niemann–Pick disease type C	Neurodegeneration, liver disease
Tripeptidyl peptidase I[159]	Protein trafficking/degradation		Late infantile neuronal ceroid lipofucsinosis (LINCL)	Neurodegeneration, seizures, visual and motor disturbances

LAMP, lysosomal-associated membrane protein; LIMP, lysosomal-integral membrane protein.

Perspective on Diagnosis of Lysosomal Storage Diseases

The increasing elucidation of the molecular lesions underlying the lysosomal storage diseases has provided insight into the great heterogeneity within each of these diseases. In addition, the proliferation of tests for the specific genetic lesions has led many practitioners to substitute molecular testing for enzyme-based diagnosis. The great specificity of molecular testing is its downfall, whereas the more generic nature of enzyme testing is a major strength. For any of the disease categories listed in Table 53–1, the diagnosis is established by detection of the specific enzyme defect. In experienced laboratories, many of these activities are accurately determined and will establish the specific diagnosis. Once the diagnosis is established, additional molecular testing can provide supplementary information and, in some cases, prognostic insight. In some lysosomal diseases, the frequency of pseudodeficiency alleles mandates the use of molecular testing, and other adjunct investigations (eg, sulfatide loading studies in metachromatic leukodystrophy) are necessary to fully establish a phenotype and prognosis, particularly in presymptomatic siblings or in prenatal testing. As the therapeutic armamentarium expands, there will be a push to establish diagnoses earlier, perhaps before the onset of clinical symptoms. Population-based screening for lysosomal storage disorders is more complicated than newborn screening for small metabolites, but a number of analytic techniques are being explored. Regardless of the method and timing of ascertainment, every effort should be made to thoroughly and completely characterize these patients at the clinical, biochemical, and molecular levels. Periodic detailed neurologic and physical assessments by imaging and clinical examinations are indicated in all patients to evaluate the effects of intervention or relationship of specific mutations to phenotype. As clinical trials for therapeutic approaches to an increasing number of conditions evolve, it is expected that surrogate markers for disease control will be developed and validated. These markers are likely to add to the armamentarium of modalities for the management of lysosomal disease. The development of registries for several of these conditions will foster the collection of valuable data as new approaches become available.[17]

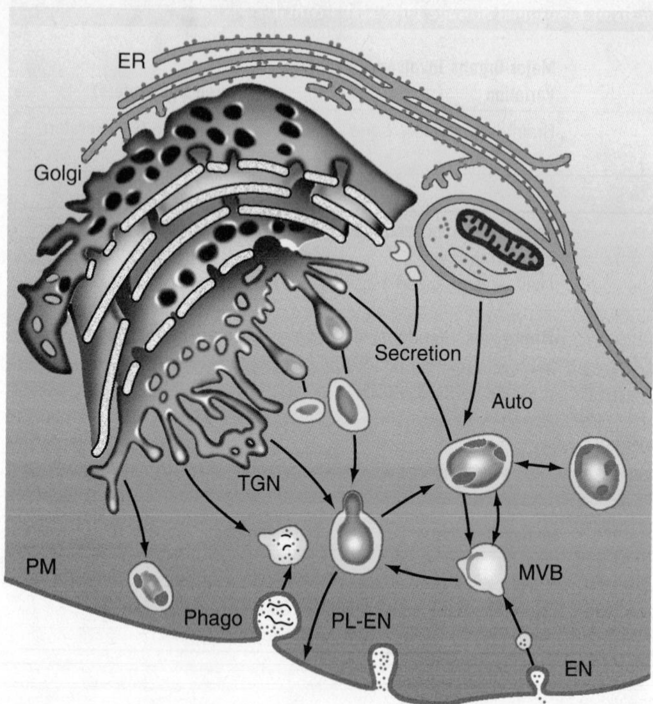

Figure 53–1 Schematic diagram of lysosomal development from the endoplasmic reticulum (ER), through the Golgi apparatus (GOLGI), and the endosomal compartments (EN). EN is shown to develop from the plasma membrane (PM) coated pits. The EN and TGN pathways converge in vesicles containing material from newly synthesized lysosomal proteins, and ER and/or MVB (multivesicular body) contents. Between the MVB, PL-EN, and return to the PM exists the CURL, a virtual compartment for the uncoupling of receptors and ligands. The various EN and lysosomal compartments are distinguished by the progressive acidification of the vesicles from early to late endosomes and the loss of the mannose-6-phosphate (M6P) receptors in the CURL. The MVB is an ultrastructural compartment that contains internal small vesicles derived from the PM. Vesicles that bud from the TGN fuse with late EN or MVB to form the lysosomal compartment. M6P receptors are recycled to the PM and to the mid-Golgi. Secretion indicates a direct route from the TGN to EN for delivery outside of the cell. Auto and Phago refer to autophagy and phagocytosis, respectively, by which internal and external materials are delivered to preexisting lysosomes. *Larger arrows* indicate a major common pathway through the maturing lysosomes. The *double-headed arrows* depict a necessary interaction between various types of lysosomes to account for the major similarities of lysosomes in cells. Lysosomes are inherently heterogeneous. This indicates a dynamic compartment that communicates, probably bidirectionally, with other components of the endosomal/lysosomal system. In addition to what is shown, vesicular transport is needed between the ER and GOLGI.

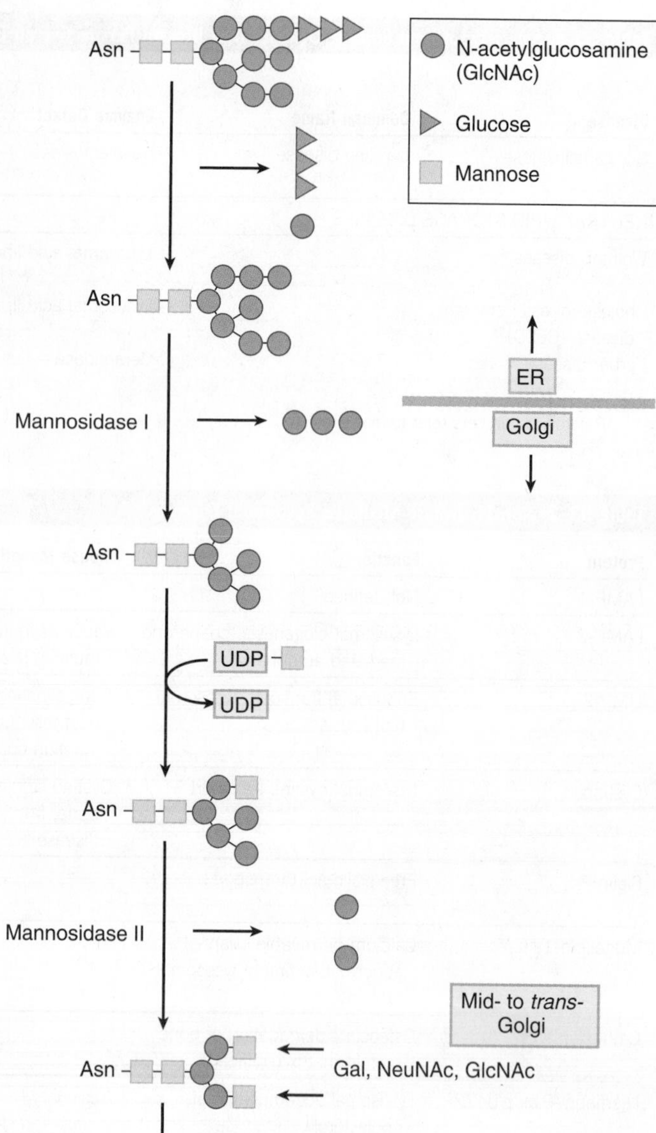

Figure 53–2 Compartmentalized N-linked oligosaccharide modifications of lysosomal proteins. Attachment of the core mannosyl-glucose to select Asn-X-Ser/Thr consensus sequences occurs cotranslationally in the endoplasmic reticulum (ER) lumen through en bloc transfer of the illustrated core oligosaccharide structure from a dolichophosphate. Initial removal of terminal glucosyl residues and a mannosyl residue are removed before exit from the ER to the Golgi. Additional α-mannosyl residues are removed by specific mannosidases in the *cis*-Golgi to a pentamannosyl core. *N*-acetyl-glucosamine-1-phosphate is transferred by glucoaminylphosphotransferases for the creation of a mannose-6-phosphate (M6P). In the *medial-* (*mid-*) and *trans*-Golgi, β-galactosyl and sialyl (NeuNAc) residues are added by transferases localized to those compartments. The final oligosaccharide structures can contain mostly mannose (high mannose), short mannose cores, *N*-acetyl-glucosamines, β-galactosyl and sialyl residues on the core structure (complex), or several combinations of these on different branches of the structure.

oligosaccharide chain from a long-chain lipid phosphate, terminal dolichophosphate (Fig. 53–2). It is unclear how N-glycosylation sequences are selected for occupancy,[16] except that asparagine–proline–serine or–threonine sites are not used and the surrounding protein sequences appear important for transfer of the dolichophosphate oligosaccharide.

Following complete synthesis and glycosylation, the lysosomal enzymes may undergo additional proteolytic processing or assembly and are incorporated into transport vesicles for delivery to and further processing in the *cis*-Golgi apparatus. At this stage, all proteins destined for the lysosomes contain only branched mannosyl chains that terminate with short-chain α-glucosyl moieties. Most enzymes destined for the lysosome acquire complex oligosaccharide modifications during transport through the Golgi apparatus (see Fig. 53–2). A series of glycosylhydrolases and glycosyltransferases within specific regions of the *cis*-, *mid*-, or *trans*-Golgi participate in these sequential modifications. In the *cis*-Golgi network, α-glucosidases and α-mannosidases remove terminal glucose and mannose residues to produce mannose-terminated core oligosaccharides. For each branch point of the mannosyl chain, there are specific α-mannosidases for cleavage.

Following mannosyl trimming, additional sugars including β-*N*-acetylglucosamine and β-galactoside are added to the short mannosyl core by the *mid*-Golgi system. The addition of terminal sialic acid

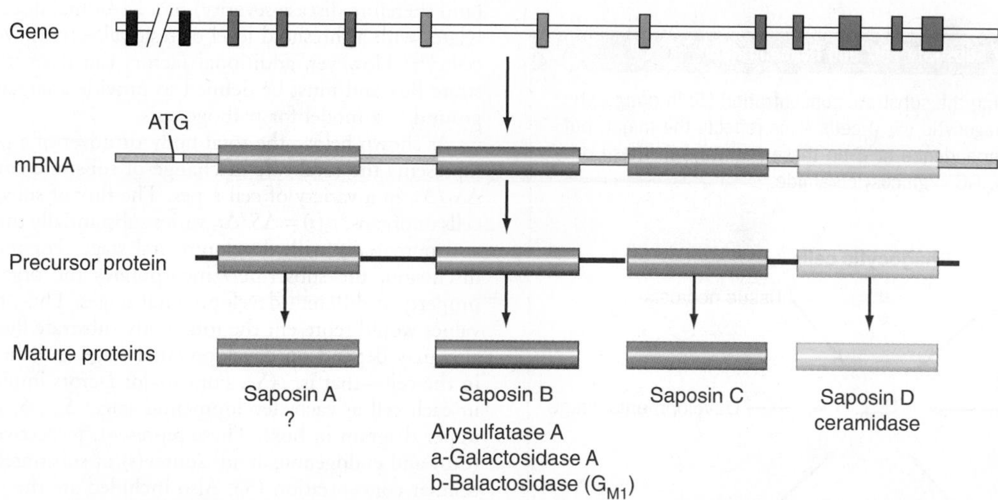

Figure 53–3 Diagram of the processing of prosaposin from the chromosomal gene to messenger RNA (mRNA) to mature saposin proteins that interact with lysosomal enzymes. The chromosomal gene is more than 30 kb in length; the first intron is longer than 20 kb and is located on chromosome 10p. Introns are shown as the *white rectangles*, and exons are filled and matched to the domains for each saposin. The mRNA contains four highly homologous, but not identical, domains that code for the saposins A, B, C, and D. The mature mRNA encodes the saposins and intersaposin peptide links in the same reading frame. The intersaposin peptides are removed by proteolysis. The individual saposins are produced by proteolytic cleavage mostly within the lysosomes, where they interact with their respective lysosomal hydrolases.

residues occurs in the *trans*-Golgi. Each of these sugars is added by glycosyl transferases that have been retained in their respective Golgi compartments by specific signals. Thus, the carbohydrate composition of the lysosomal proteins is indicative of its passage through regions of the Golgi during the synthetic process. Before, or coincident with, ER or *cis*-Golgi modifications is the attachment of an *N*-acetylglucosamine-1-phosphate to the sixth position on mannosyl residues of the mannosyl core oligosaccharide. This modification can be uni- or multivalent and is selective for various branches of the oligosaccharides on a specific lysosomal protein. An *N*-acetylglucosylaminyl-1-phosphotransferase[8,10] is essential for this process, and its deficiency leads to a severe condition, I-cell disease, in which many soluble lysosomal enzymes are lost by default secretion out of the cell.[8]

Shortly after the attachment of the phospho-sugar group, a specific hydrolase cleaves the protecting *N*-acetylglucosamine from the phosphate to expose the M6P residue, the targeting signal for soluble lysosomal proteins. These modification processes culminate in most lysosomal enzymes having several oligosaccharide chains with nonidentical antennerary modifications. As a result, the lysosomal enzymes can have portions of the attached oligosaccharide tree having only mannose residues (high-mannose modification), mannosyl-, *N*-acetyl-glucosylaminyl-, β-galactosyl-, and sialyl-containing oligosaccharides (mixed type modification), or only terminal sialyl acid residues (complex-type modification).[18,19] Of importance, many soluble enzymes employ ill-defined M6P-independent intracellular trafficking signals alone or in combination with the M6P system.

Defective M6P targeting of soluble lysosomal proteins, as occurs in I-cell disease, has no effect on the integrity of the lysosome per se or its membrane. Lysosomal integral or associated membrane proteins (LIMPs or LAMPs) are sorted to the lysosomal membrane or to the interior of the lysosome through M6P-independent trafficking systems. Signals for such trafficking have been identified as strategically located tyrosine residues near the carboxyl-terminal (C-terminal) end of some LIMPs and LAMPs.[15] Additional signals are required for targeting of other lysosomal membrane components. Of importance, for the diseases involving LIMPs and LAMPs, cross-correction of cocultured cells would not occur; this has significance in considering therapeutic strategies of such diseases.

In addition to glycosylation, some lysosomal proteins require proteolytic clipping, phosphorylation, or macromolecular assembly for the development of full function within the lysosomal environment. Proteolytic processing can occur at the N or C termini or by clipping of single-peptide precursors into mature subunits or active peptides. For example, prosaposin is cleaved into four biologically active saposins—A, B, C, and D—that are functional in the lysosomal compartment (Fig. 53–3).[20–22] A "protector protein" precursor is involved in galactosialidosis and is clipped from its zymogen form into two disulfide-linked subunits within the Golgi apparatus before its achieving proteolytic activity.[22,23] Some proteins also may acquire phosphorylation of serines or threonines or sulfation of tyrosines. Macromolecular assembly is required for several heteromeric lysosomal proteins. The association of the β-hexosaminidase α- and β-chains in the mid-Golgi is necessary for synthesis of active hexosaminidase A (α- and β-heteromers) or hexosaminidase B (β-homomers). Macroassembly of the β-galactosidase/neuraminidase/protector protein complex probably occurs within the Golgi apparatus coincident with other processing required for the assembly of the active catalytic complex.[23]

Although the control of tissue expression of many lysosomal proteins has not been characterized, tissue- and cell-specific expression have been described for prosaposin and lysosomal acid lipase[24,25] and probably exist for other lysosomal proteins. These expression patterns may have importance in explaining the variability of the phenotypes of these diseases. Most tissues contain similar lysosomal hydrolases for degradation of macromolecules, such as mucopolysaccharides, glycoproteins, and glycosphingolipids, because these are essential to cell function. Thus, excessive lysosomal storage can be demonstrated in most tissues using histological or biochemical tools. However, concordant levels of lysosomal hydrolase activities are not found in all tissues. The specialized lysosomes of neutrophils contain myeloperoxidases that are not in fibroblast lysosomes.[26] This variation may play an important role in diagnostic assays, because some of the lysosomal proteins are found at measurable levels in plasma, but others require isolation of circulating leukocytes. The activity of α-L-iduronidase, the enzyme deficient in MPS I, is easily detected in amniocytes and placental tissue, but is nearly absent in early chorionic villi. Acid β-glucosidase (deficient in Gaucher disease) is present at nearly 10-fold lower levels in myeloid-derived cells compared with fibroblastic cells.[27]

A formal explanation for variability in both expression and cellular dysfunction is proposed in the Conzelmann and Sandhoff threshold hypothesis for the development of manifestations of specific lysosomal hydrolase deficiency diseases.[28,29] This working hypothesis

Factors Influencing Substrate Flux and Concentration

Factors influencing the substrate concentration (S) in phagocytic (S_{exo}) and nonphagocytic (S_{end}) cells. This reflects the major, but not exclusive, dependence of S on these pathways in these different cell types. GC = glucosylceramide.

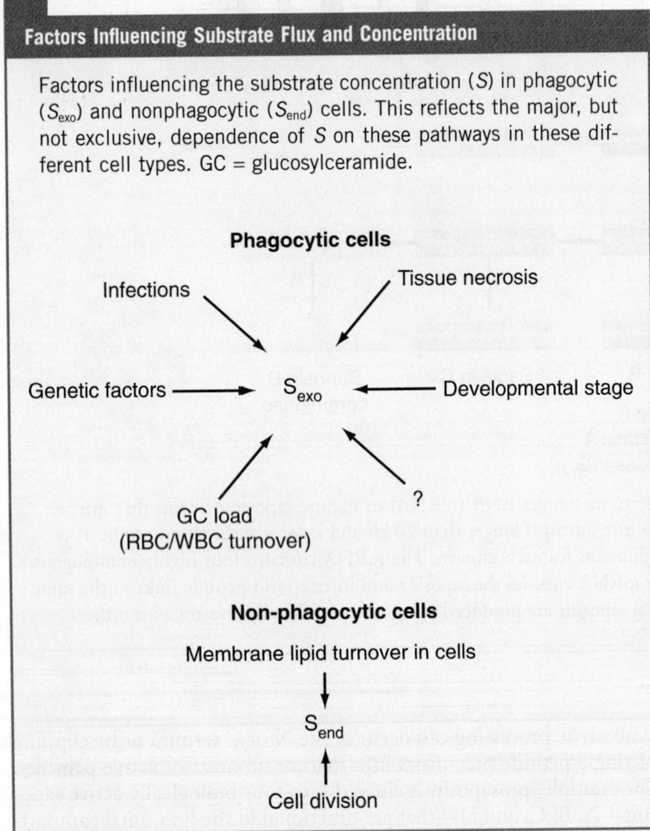

implies that a set level of residual enzymatic activity, or substrate flux, is necessary to prevent lysosomal disease manifestations. Below this threshold, disease manifestations (in tissues or specific cell type) will be expressed, whereas above this threshold, there will be no phenotype. This formalizes the commonsense notion that less enzyme activity leads to more severe disease and that more enzyme activity results in less severe or delayed disease manifestations. The hypothesis also implies that each tissue or cellular type may require specific levels of activity. The therapeutic importance of threshold is clear, because the existence of attenuated disease variants demonstrate that 1% to 10% of normal lysosomal enzyme levels may be sufficient to correct metabolism in many tissues and prevent, reverse, or significantly delay localized disease manifestations. Similarly, very small incremental changes in enzyme activity or substrate flux could have profound effects on disease development and severity. However, expansion of this hypothesis also incorporates the caveat that threshold levels may vary during development. Failure to meet critical thresholds during these stages may result in irreversible changes not amenable to later therapeutic interventions. For example, after progression to a pathologic stage, dysostosis multiplex of bones, cardiac valvular involvement, or neurodegeneration in the MPSs may not be reversed by bone marrow transplantation (BMT) or enzyme replacement therapies.

The threshold hypothesis leads directly to a model for the pathogenesis of lysosomal disease phenotypes; that is, necessary and sufficient conditions can be identified for the occurrence of the disease state. The presence of deleterious mutations that lead to the deficiency of specific proteins is a necessary prelude to the phenotype. However, the relationships of the residual mutant activity to the level of substrate flux through the lysosome, to the temporal and spatial metabolic needs of a particular tissue, and to the phenotype, are poorly understood. Conzelmann and Sandhoff studied ganglioside G_{M2} and sulfatide degradation in fibroblasts from patients with Tay–Sachs disease and metachromatic leukodystrophy (MLD), respectively. Their data support the contention that the age at onset (and therefore disease severity) of a lysosomal disease phenotype correlates with a threshold level of residual activity within lysosomes of cells.[28,29] However, additional factors can dramatically impact substrate flux and must be defined to provide a larger conceptual background as a model for pathogenesis.

As shown below, the total body turnover of a particular substrate represents the total rate of change of substrate concentrations, $v_T = \Delta S_T/\Delta t$, in a variety of cell types. The flux of substrate in individual cells or organs, $v_i(t) = \Delta S_i/\Delta t$, varies substantially throughout the body and potentially with developmental stage. For the purposes of this discussion, the subscript i incorporates the organ- or cell-specific property at different developmental stages. Thus, the sum of all $v_i(t)$ values would represent the total body substrate flux. The quantity v_T also may depend on developmental stage and the level of substrate in the cell—that is, $v(S_i)$. Four major factors impinge on S_i attained in each cell at each developmental stage: S_{exo}, S_{end}, L_{ex}, and L_{en} (see upper diagram in box). These represent, respectively, the exogenous (exo) and endogenous (end) source(s) of substrate(s) that alter intracellular concentration (S_i). Also included are the pathways that lead to decreases in substrate levels (L) through excretion/secretion (ex) and enzymatic degradation (en) to end products within the lysosome. L_{en} represents decreases in substrate concentration due to the residual activity. Although such an equation is a heuristic device, it provides a means of examining, both qualitatively and quantitatively, each of the factors that influences intracellular substrate concentration. This could provide an overall conceptual framework for the dissection of the various phenotypes in lysosomal storage disease and potential targets for therapeutic intervention that may have the greatest impact on the phenotype.

$$v_T = \partial S_T/\partial t = \Sigma \partial S_i/\partial t = \Sigma[v_{xi}(S_i) + v_{ni}(S_i) + v_{Li}(S_i) + v_{eni}(S_i)]$$

The equation calculates the flux (v_T) of substrate (S_i) through various cell types. The sum of various rates of substrate change in n tissues ($\Delta S_i/\Delta t$) equals the total flux of substrate ($\Delta S_T/\Delta t$) through the body of an affected person. The term $v(S_i)$ represents the developmental stage-specific rate of substrate concentration changes in a particular cell type and its potential dependence on the concentration of substrate (S_i) in that tissue. The subscripts of v represent substrates from various sources (ie, x_i = exogenous, phagocytosis, n_i = endogenous sources from catabolism of more complex macromolecules, L_i = losses due to excretion/secretion, en_i = decreases due to enzymatic degradation).

As shown in the box on Factors Influencing Substrate Flux and Concentration (see diagram), the level of S_{exo} is influenced by genetic factors, that is, genetic determinants of cellular turnover or substrate delivery; by exogenous (environmental) agents that lead to increased substrate availability; and by the developmental stage, which could include increased cellular and substrate turnovers. This last aspect may be of importance for changes in the progression of various lysosomal diseases with age. Thus, different developmental stage-specific genes and substrate turnovers could affect an age-dependent threshold for the balance of $v_{in} \rightarrow v_{out}$. It is implicit in this discussion that disease progression is likely to be nonuniform, and exacerbations and remissions of symptoms may occur depending on exogenous factors and other genetic factors. Also, the balance of v_{Sex} and v_{Send} between cells and organs may differ substantially. This will depend greatly on the pathophysiology of various organs. Gaucher disease is a prime example. In many visceral tissues (hepatocytes, skin cells, lymphoid cells), v_{Sexo} for glucosylceramide is much less than v_{Sen}. The v_{Sen} value probably is very low, because even in the most severe variants, storage of glucosylceramide cannot be detected ultrastructurally in such cells. In comparison, in phagocytic cells of the viscera, $v_{Sexo} >> v_{Send}$. This implies that phagocytic cells will have a much greater variation in degree of involvement because of the inherent greater dependence on the exogenous supply of substrate (ie, greater variation in S_{exo} and v_{xi}) (see upper diagram in the box). In contrast, involved central nervous system (CNS) cells are dependent primarily on the S_{exo} for glucosylceramide and other substrates that accumulate in the brain. The contribution of S_{exo} is small. Detailed histologic examination of brains from patients with Gaucher disease type 2 consistently shows significant regional variations in neuronal loss, neuronophagia, and gliosis. There is a rostral-to-caudal gradient of involvement, with greatest severity in the basal ganglia and the dentate nucleus.[30,31] Thus, in Gaucher disease, not only are the pathophysiologic findings in the viscera and the brain fundamentally different, but also within the CNS there are regional variations. The greater dependence of the visceral pathology on S_{ex} implies a potentially greater number of steps that could be altered to influence the rate and degree of disease progression.

These considerations indicate that a necessary condition for the development of disease is the *relative* enzymatic deficiency within the lysosome—that is, is there sufficient hydrolytic power in the lysosome to cleave the substrate presented at any given time? The enzyme deficiency reduces the ability of cells and, therefore, the individual, to adapt to changes in v_T. Thus, the variation in v_T, either endogenous or exogenous, determines to a great extent the eventual phenotypical severity. Because v_T can vary, the progressivity of the specific disease manifestations may be variable at different stages of the disease. The most maladaptive mutations (eg, a homozygous null mutation) frequently may be associated with the most severe phenotypes, but modifier factors (genes) could alter disease severity. The converse also applies. Currently, little is understood about the essential factors that influence substrate flux in the tissues of patients with lysosomal storage diseases.

Definition of these thresholds of activity also may provide clues to dose–response relationships for treatment of various storage diseases and the evaluation of exogenous enzyme replacement therapy. Once delivered to the tissue and cellular sites of pathology, exogenous enzymes will have finite life spans. Assuming appropriate stoichiometric relationships for components required for intracellular activity, the initially high hydrolytic rates will decrease to background levels over several half-lives of the supplied enzyme. Thus, large amounts of enzyme, potentially several-fold above threshold levels, may be needed to eliminate the extreme excess tissue burden of the substrate. Normal metabolism could then be maintained with pulses or intermittent dosing of lesser amounts of enzyme or other therapeutic agents, presumably at levels slightly above the disease threshold, because only catabolism of new substrate would be required.[29] This pulse model of therapy assumes that small amounts of reaccumulating substrates are not irreversibly toxic. Otherwise, a continuous supply of enzyme would be required to avoid such toxic effects. This model also assumes metabolic interaction between lysosomal compartments in cells and that the exogenous enzyme is delivered to the cells that are causal to the disease manifestations.

PATHOPHYSIOLOGY OF LYSOSOMAL STORAGE DISEASES

A majority of lysosomal enzyme deficiencies result from point mutations or genetic rearrangements at loci encoding a single protein required for the activity of the lysosomal hydrolase (see Table 53–1). Defects in lysosomal membrane proteins, transporters, and other nonhydrolytic enzymes also have been described (see Table 53–2), resulting in abnormalities in macromolecular association or trafficking (see later). The final common pathway for lysosomal storage diseases is the accumulation of macromolecules within tissues and cells that synthesize or ingest particular substrates or toxic metabolites in substantial amounts. For many lysosomal storage diseases, the clinical manifestations derive from the accumulation of substrates that are endogenously synthesized within particular tissue sites of pathology. The degree of involvement of any particular organ or organ system reflects the rate of endogenous synthesis or degradation, or both, of those specific compounds in particular tissues. The stored substrates are macromolecules—mucopolysaccharides, glycoproteins, or glycosphingolipids—that require degradation through a pathway with the sequential removal of single components of the substrate molecules at each step in a catabolic cascade (Fig. 53–4). Most of the enzymes are exo-hydrolases. Table 53–1 lists select lysosomal storage diseases categorized according to substrate groups and indicates some of the

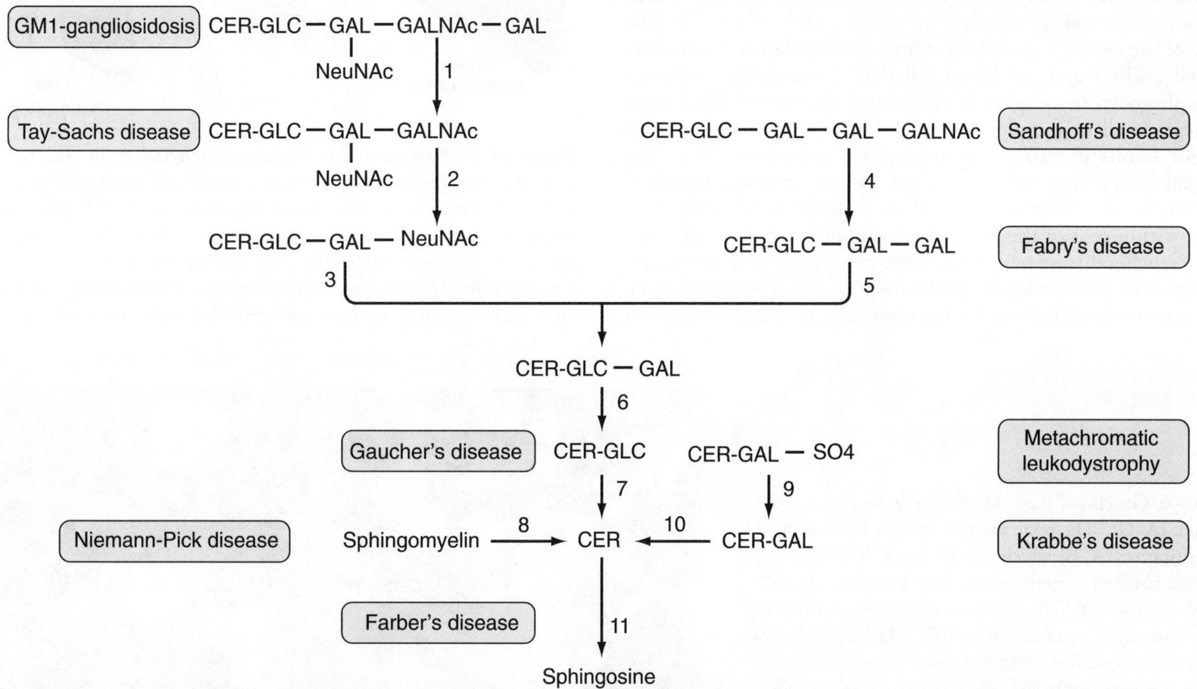

Figure 53–4 Pathway of glycosphingolipid degradation and the diseases that result from specific enzyme deficiencies. The numbers refer to the following lysosomal hydrolases: 1, β-galactosidase; 2, β-hexosaminidase A; 3, ganglioside neuraminidase; 4, β-hexosaminidase B; 5, α-galactosidase A; 6, β-galactosidase for lactosylceramide; 7, acid β-glucosidase (glucocerebrosidase); 8, sphingomyelinase; 9, arylsulfatase A; 10, β-galactocerebrosidase; 11, ceramidase. The deficiency of each of the respective enzymes leads to the accumulations of the substrate preceding the hydrolytic step. Diseases due to the deficiencies of either enzyme 3 or 6.

tissues involved by the various diseases. Specific organ systems are involved by particular diseases to a greater or lesser extent, reflecting the balance of endogenous and exogenous substrate presentations (see above). For example, in Hurler syndrome (comprising mucopolysaccharidoses IA), dermatan and heparan sulfate accumulate in connective tissue leading to joint contractures and abnormal skin consistency. Tissue-specific pathology also is present in several other diseases. Galactocerebroside is found in the greatest concentrations within the myelin sheaths of the CNS and peripheral nervous system (PNS). Although the deficiency of galactocerebrosidase in Krabbe disease occurs in all tissues, the synthesis of galactocerebroside is much greater in CNS and PNS.[32,33] Consequently, the manifestations of the disease are localized to the nervous system. Similarly in Tay–Sachs disease (TSD) or Sandhoff disease, the deficiencies of β-hexosaminidase A or of β-hexosaminidase A and B, respectively, result either in primarily CNS disease or in combined CNS and visceral diseases due to the different accumulated substrates.[34] β-Hexosaminidase A cleaves the specific substrate ganglioside G_{M2}, whereas β-hexosaminidase B cleaves primarily sialylgangliosides and globosides. Ganglioside G_{M2} is synthesized in large amounts only in brain or other nervous tissues, and globoside is synthesized primarily in visceral tissues.

Additional mechanisms, other than endogenous substrate synthesis, must be involved in pathologic substrate deposition in Fabry disease, Gaucher disease, and cholesterol ester storage disease (CESD). Fabry disease (α-galactosidase A deficiency)[35] and CESD (lysosomal acid lipase deficiency)[36] result from an inability to catabolize globotriaosylceramide and cholesterol esters, respectively. Both of these compounds are carried in the plasma associated with LDL particles. These LDL particles are internalized through receptor-mediated endocytosis and presented to the lysosome for degradation. In these two disorders, the major respective pathophysiologic features, endothelial cell and macrophage involvement, are due to the LDL uptake of these substrates and the inability to degrade them within the lysosomes. Endogenous synthesis of globotriaosylceramide and of cholesterol esters is relatively low within most tissues. Most accumulated substrate is derived from distant sources (ie, hepatocytes). The visceral manifestations of Gaucher disease (acid β-glucosidase deficiency) derive from the storage of glucosylceramide, primarily in cells of monocyte-macrophage origin (Figs. 53–5 and 53–6).[37] The vast majority of the viscerally stored substrate probably derives from white blood cell (WBC) and red blood cell (RBC) membrane turnovers through phagocytosis of aging blood-formed elements.[38] The inability to degrade all of the glucosylceramide from the membranes of these cells results in storage in macrophage lysosomes. Thus, the major pathophysiology of the visceral disease involves imported glycosphingolipid substrate rather than endogenously synthesized substrate within cells of the monocyte-macrophage system. By comparison, Gaucher disease type 2 is a severe neurodegenerative disorder of infancy. The visceromegaly, particularly of the spleen and liver, and bone marrow infiltration by Gaucher cells in this disease result from a defect in the phagocytic pathway. However, the severe neurodegenerative disease appears to be related to the presence of toxic by-products derived from degradation of endogenously synthesized glucosylceramide within CNS neurons of affected patients. These endogenous toxic metabolites and the importation into the brain of glucosylceramide from peripheral sources conjointly contribute to severe neurodegenerative disease. The contribution of transported and imported substrates to the pathophysiology of other diseases (ie, metachromatic leukodystrophy, the mucopolysaccharidoses, and the glycoproteinoses) is not fully understood and certainly would have an impact on therapeutic approaches. Thus, several mechanisms—thresholds of enzyme activity, tissue or developmental specificity, substrate localization, and substrate importation—play roles in the pathophysiology of specific lysosomal storage diseases. The relative importance of each process varies among diseases and may explain differential organ involvement within a specific disease category.

The direct distortion of the lysosomal architecture (ie, engorgement of lysosomes) probably has significant pathologic consequences, but the pharmacologic effects of the accumulated substrates or by-products are increasingly recognized as major components of the disease pathophysiology.[4,39] In the glycosphingolipidoses, the toxic metabolites of these complex lipids derive from their incomplete or improper degradation in the lysosome. The deacylated analogs of

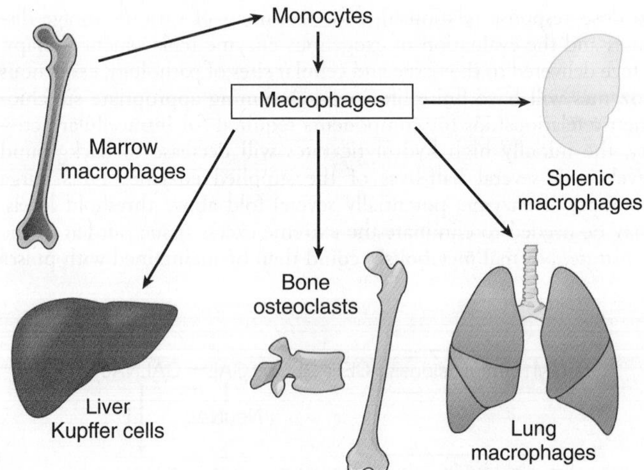

Figure 53–5 Diagram of the cellular pathophysiology of Gaucher disease. Monocytes are produced in the bone marrow and mature to macrophages in the marrow or in specific sites of distribution as liver Kupffer cells, bone osteoclasts, and lung and tissue macrophages. Once resident, they accumulate glucosylceramide by phagocytosis and become end-stage Gaucher cells. The resultant tissue fibrosis, ischemia, osteoporosis, and other pathologic features have not been adequately explained.

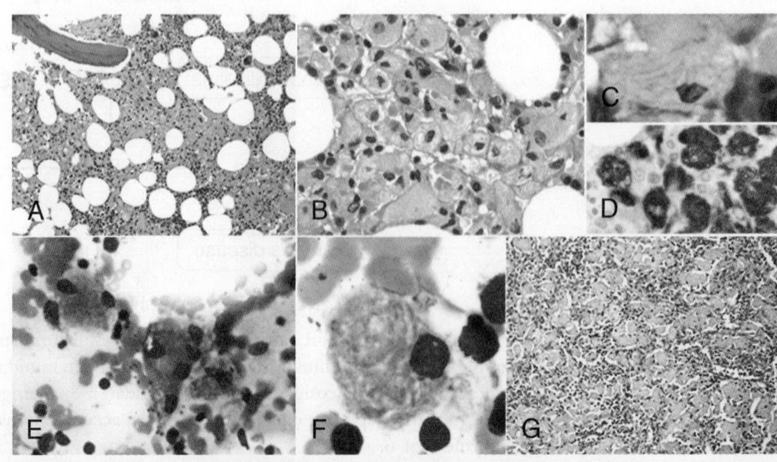

Figure 53–6 Gaucher disease: bone marrow biopsy, aspirate, and spleen: (**A–G**). The bone marrow space is filled with plump histiocytes (**A, B**) which at high power (**C**) show cytoplasmic fibrillary material producing striations. The cells are CD68 positive (**D**). The aspirated material shows clusters of similar histiocytes or macrophages (**E**), which at high power (**F**) illustrate the so-called crumpled tissue paper effect in the cytoplasm (Gaucher cell). The spleen, from a separate case (**G**), has pale clusters of similar histiocytes.

glycosphingolipids are known as sphingoid bases. These compounds are potent inhibitors of a variety of cellular enzymes including protein kinase C isozymes and other membrane proteins.[39,40] Sphingoid bases (lyso-glycosphingolipids) accumulate in Tay–Sachs disease, Sandhoff disease,[41] Krabbe disease,[42] and Gaucher disease type 2 and type 3.[43] The toxicity of sphingoid bases is the most clear-cut in Krabbe disease and Gaucher disease type 2. The excessive accumulation of galactosylsphingosine and glucosylsphingosine in these diseases, respectively, leads to the destruction of neurons within the brains of affected persons. Consequently, the CNS disease manifestations probably are the results of neuronal loss and death rather than the storage of galactosyl- or glucosylceramide per se. In Gaucher disease type 1, small amounts of glucosylsphingosine are known to accumulate in visceral organs and may be related directly or indirectly through cytokines[44,45] to the fibrosis in liver, spleen, and bone marrow of affected patients.[46] The increase in cytokines could provide a unifying pathophysiologic basis (ie, cell death and scarring) for the manifestations of Gaucher disease. In Tay–Sachs disease, ganglioside G_{M2} and lyso-ganglioside G_{M2} accumulate.[41] The formation of meganeurites in TSD indicates that at least one of these stored substrates may alter the growth and development of neurons, as well as accumulating in lysosomes.[47]

In some categories of lysosomal diseases, characteristic pathologic patterns are present. In MPSs I, II, and VI, a pattern of bone abnormalities known as *dysostosis multiplex* is observed, as well as short stature and degenerative joint disease. In cultured articular chondrocytes from rats and cats with MPS VI, increased nitric oxide release and tumor necrosis factor-α (TNF-α) secretion were observed; this phenomenon could be reproduced by exposing normal cells to dermatan sulfate, suggesting that the increased chondrocyte death observed in affected animals might be due to metabolite exposure or inflammatory cytokines.[48] Decreased formation of insoluble elastin can be demonstrated in both Hurler fibroblasts and those from certain forms of MPS IVb, suggesting mechanisms for coronary artery disease or joint disease in some of these conditions.[49] The enormous variation in clinical manifestations in each of these lysosomal storage diseases is of major clinical relevance. Each disease has very severe, rapidly progressive variants, and more attenuated variants that are late in onset, mildly symptomatic, and, in some cases, nearly normal phenotypes.[50,51]

MOLECULAR GENETIC MECHANISMS OF LYSOSOMAL STORAGE DISEASES

The molecular mechanisms that result in the lysosomal storage diseases are as varied as the diseases. The following mechanisms have been identified:

- Deficiency of a single hydrolase, predisposing to multiple phenotypes
- Deficiencies of multiple lysosomal proteins mediated by a single gene defect
- Specific in vivo substrate accumulation with intact in vitro hydrolase activity
- Absence of functional lysosomal hydrolysis with intact hydrolase activities
- Lysosomal membrane transporters of specific metabolites

Single Gene, Multiple Phenotypes

The vast majority of the lysosomal storage diseases result from mutations at single loci that involve a single gene product and are either point mutations or deletions/insertions in genes encoding subunits of particular proteins. Missense or nonsense mutations result in the production of proteins with abnormal catalytic function, stability, or processing. For many of these mutations, an abnormal protein with low enzyme activity is synthesized. For example, numerous mutations have been described at the respective loci for Gaucher disease, Fabry disease, or Tay–Sachs disease. These mutations have differential effects on enzyme stability, catalytic activity, and effector interactions (reviewed by Beutler et al[52]). Because Gaucher and Tay–Sachs diseases are found at high frequencies in the Ashkenazi Jewish population, a few common mutations would be expected as a result of either founder effect or selective pressures. The phenotypical variation in these two diseases represents a continuum of degrees of involvement or age at onset of symptoms. For Gaucher disease, this continuum extends to the asymptomatic population. Approximately 50% of affected Ashkenazi Jews with the *N370S/N370S* genotype are minimally symptomatic and never come to medical attention.[53,54]

By comparison, two completely different disease phenotypes appear to result from the same enzymatic deficiency due to mutations at the β-galactosidase locus: the G_{M1} gangliosidoses and Morquio syndrome type B (MPS IVB). In the former, ganglioside G_{M1} accumulates preferentially in the CNS and mucopolysaccharide metabolites in the visceral organs.[55] In Morquio syndrome type B, keratan sulfate accumulates in visceral organs, leading to skeletal dysplasia and abnormal connective tissue properties (eg, hypermobility). The CNS is not directly involved. These very different phenotypes result from mutations in structural loci for β-galactosidase, affecting different protein domains of β-galactosidase.[55,56] Thus, mutations in single lysosomal polypeptides can result in multiple disease variants that differ in molecular etiology. The severe infantile variant (G_{M2} gangliosidosis) can be associated with a protein that poorly interacts with its protector protein (see later) and is rapidly degraded. The later-onset variant has a protein peptide that can be improperly targeted, with little enzyme routed to the lysosome. The MPS IVB protein binds to protector protein, is properly routed to the lysosome, but exhibits little catalytic activity toward keratan sulfate.[57]

Single Gene, Multiple Enzymes

Several lysosomal hydrolases are multimeric or occur as multienzyme complexes. A mutation in a component of the multienzyme structure or a common subunit could result in selective deficiencies of individual enzyme components or in all of the components of the complex, respectively. Tay–Sachs disease and Sandhoff disease are typical examples of heteromeric proteins in which distinct phenotypes result from mutations in different subunits. β-Hexosaminidase A is composed of α- and β-chains, whereas β-hexosaminidase B is composed of only β-chains. Mutations at the α-chain locus result in Tay–Sachs disease (β-hexosaminidase A deficiency), whereas those in the β-chain result in Sandhoff disease (β-hexosaminidase A and B deficiencies).[58] Because the substrates for β-hexosaminidase B occur in the viscera and those for β-hexosaminidase A, that is, ganglioside G_{M2}, occur predominantly in the CNS, Sandhoff disease has manifestations in the CNS and in the viscera. The β-galactosidase–neuraminidase–protector protein complex is more complicated. Isolated deficiencies of each of these enzymatic components have been described.[55,59] Neuraminidase deficiency results in sialidosis, a glycoprotein storage disease, and protector protein defects result in deficiencies of both β-galactosidase and neuraminidase. The so-called protector protein is a protease that attaches to the neuraminidase–β-galactosidase complex at some time during synthesis and "protects" this complex from inactivation or degradation.[23] Thus, point mutations in the protector protein can lead to galactosialidosis, a triple enzymatic deficiency producing variable phenotypical effects.[60]

A unique and important example of a mutation in a nonlysosomal enzyme causing multiple enzyme deficiencies is multiple sulfatase deficiency (MSD). In this disease, hydrolysis of sulfated mucopolysaccharides and glycolipids is impaired, and a phenotype is produced that resembles a composite of metachromatic leukodystrophy (arylsulfatase A deficiency), MPS II (iduronate sulfatase deficiency), and ichthyosis (microsomal steroid sulfatase deficiency). Because the structural genes for the sulfatases are not involved, a co- or posttranslational modification defect common to cellular sulfatases was suspected. By direct analyses of cellular sulfatases, von Figura and coworkers showed that active sulfatases require a specific posttranslational modification of a conserved cysteine. An enzyme is required to modify this cysteine to 2-amino-3-oxo-propionic acid that acts as a carrier of the sulfite group at the active site of sulfatases. MSD cells are deficient in this posttranslational process.[61,62]

Normal In Vitro/Deficient In Vivo Substrate Cleavage

Mutations in protein activators or cofactors necessary for the catalytic activities of a variety of glycosphingolipid hydrolases result in diseases that are phenocopies of particular enzyme deficiencies. For glycosphingolipid hydrolysis, five such protein activators have been described. Four of these, termed saposins A, B, C, and D, are encoded by a single locus on chromosome 10 (see Fig. 53–3). The G_{M2} activator required for catabolism of ganglioside G_{M2} by β-hexosaminidase A is encoded by a locus on chromosome 5.[63] The hallmark of the saposin deficiencies is the accumulation of specific lipid substrates for a suspected deficient enzyme activity but normal in vitro activity of the associated enzyme. Gaucher-like diseases due to deficiencies of saposin C and prosaposin have been described.[64,65] Metachromatic leukodystrophy-like diseases result from saposin B deficiency,[66,67] and Tay–Sachs-like diseases are due to G_{M2} activator deficiencies.[68] Of these saposin deficiencies, the defects in the prosaposin locus are particularly interesting. Each of the saposins A, B, C, and D participates in the hydrolysis of a variety of glycosphingolipids (see Fig. 53–4). These saposins are believed to participate in specific interactions with the cognate enzyme in glycosphingolipid catalysis,[69] in ganglioside transport,[70] and in substrate presentation. As expected, the deficiency of prosaposin leads to a complex disorder mimicking the deficiency of several glycosphingolipid hydrolases.[71] Of importance, the in vitro activities of the corresponding enzymes are nearly normal in tissues from patients with the saposin defects. It is anticipated that several other activator or cofactor molecules, required for the assistance in hydrolysis of complex macromolecules, will be discovered in the future.

Intracellular Deficiencies/Extracellular Excess

I-cell disease exemplifies the impact on lysosomal enzymes of mutations at loci for nonlysosomal proteins. The enzyme, *N*-acetylglucosamine-1-phosphotransferase is required for the attachment to many lysosomal proteins of the M6P ligand-sorting signal.[8,10] Mutations at the loci for subunits encoding this enzyme result in the absence of the M6P ligand and the secretion into the media of most soluble lysosomal enzyme proteins. The lysosomes are nearly devoid of M6P receptor-targeted enzymes. Consequently, the phenotypes resemble a mixture of various mucopolysaccharide, glycoprotein, and glycosphingolipid degradation defects due to the loss of many enzymes and proteins involved in the respective catabolic pathways. Because some of the membrane-bound proteins of the lysosome are targeted through M6P-independent pathways, they are retained within the lysosomes. Their catalytic activity may be affected, however, by the loss of activator proteins and other lysosomal components, which require the M6P receptor-mediated sorting.

Lysosomal Membrane Transporters of Specific Metabolites

For recycling and use, metabolic products of the hydrolytic reactions within the lysosomes require movement out of the lysosome and into the cytoplasm. The defective transport of such metabolites has been discovered to lead to specific disease phenotypes. Of importance to the hematologist is Niemann–Pick disease type C1 (NPC). This disease is associated with a specific defect in the transport of free cholesterol across the lysosomal membrane and into the cytosol. The deficiency of this transporter leads to the accumulation of free cholesterol within the lysosomes in visceral tissues, lack of negative feedback of cholesterol synthesis within cells, and accumulation of sphingolipids, particularly within the brain and macrophages. The connection of this accumulation and CNS deterioration requires elucidation. Histologically, the bone marrow and other tissues contain numerous macrophage storage cells and "sea-blue histiocytes." The molecular description of NPC indicates that additional lipid storage diseases may be associated with transport deficiencies that will require characterization in the future.[72,73]

GENOTYPE–PHENOTYPE CORRELATIONS

Implicit in the threshold hypothesis is a relationship between the level of enzymatic activity in cells and the phenotype expressed in the tissues. Consequently, for lysosomal storage diseases and other inherited defects, investigators have attempted to relate genetic mutations to phenotypical manifestations. For three lysosomal storage diseases, good, albeit imperfect, correlations have been obtained: metachromatic leukodystrophy (MLD), Tay–Sachs disease, and Gaucher disease. In each of these disorders, major variants include rapid-onset to slowly progressive-onset types. In MLD, combinations of two mutant arylsulfatase A alleles account for a majority of infantile, juvenile, and adult-onset variants of this disease.[74–76] The presence of two copies of a null allele (splicing defect in intron 2) results in a severe infantile disease. By comparison, homozygotes for a P426L substitution develop an adult-onset disease. The combination of a null and P426L mutant alleles can lead to a juvenile-onset variant. These results correlate well with the measured in situ lysosomal cleavage of exogenously supplied sulfatide substrate.[8] It is noteworthy that a very common "pseudodeficiency allele" at the arylsulfatase A locus results in deficient activity toward artificial substrates as measured in vitro, whereas the in vivo flux of sulfatide is low-normal in these cells. This mutant allele contains an altered polyadenylation signal in the 3′ untranslated region leading to inefficient polyadenylation and a decrease in available messenger RNA (mRNA) for protein synthesis. In combination with the glycosylation or null alleles for MLD, persons with a pseudodeficiency allele appear to be deficient for arylsulfatase A activity and would be expected to develop MLD symptoms, but they are asymptomatic. Because this pseudoallele is present in 10% to 15% of the population, it is important to exclude its presence in suspected MLD families, particularly before the institution of therapies.[74] Disease-causing mutations can occur on the background of the pseudodeficiency allele. Thus, the detection of the pseudodeficiency mutation does not exclude a disease mutation on the same allele. In situ measurement of sulfatide cleavage is required to ensure proper diagnosis, and interpretation can be difficult.[77] The pseudodeficiency alleles for β-hexosaminidase A[78] and α-L-iduronidase[79] raise similar concerns.

In Tay–Sachs disease combinations of null and missense mutations produce varying levels of β-hexosaminidase A deficiency that lead to clinical forms with differing rates of progression. The most common allele in the Ashkenazi Jewish population is a 4–base–pair insertion that results in the production of a nonfunctional mRNA—that is, a null allele resulting in the total lack of α-chains for β-hexosaminidase A synthesis. By comparison, the missense mutation leading to a glycine 269 to serine (G269S) substitution produces residual β-hexosaminidase A activity and a more slowly progressive disease. The onset of neurodegeneration and dementia occurs between adolescence and adulthood.[80] As in MLD, the combinations of null mutations with those that lead to partially functional enzymes lead to the different ages at disease onset. In these disease variants, neuronopathic manifestations are progressive, and the rate of deterioration correlates inversely with the in situ level of enzyme activity from 0% to 5% of normal.

By comparison, all Gaucher disease types are associated with residual enzymatic activity within cells. Although good correlations have not been obtained between the level of in vitro enzymatic activity of acid β-glucosidase and the disease phenotype, improved correlations have been found when in situ lysosomal glucosylceramide cleavage is estimated.[81] Within this more physiologic environment, lower levels of residual activity were found in the more severe type 2 and type 3 variants than in the type 1 nonneuronopathic variants. Unlike in the Tay–Sachs and MLD variants, the genotype-phenotype correlations in Gaucher disease relate to the presence or absence of neuronopathic disease, not the delayed onset of CNS involvement (reviewed by Agmon and colleagues[81]).

Gaucher disease is the prototype for lysosomal storage diseases in which several thresholds of substrate flux are apparent. The first threshold is for the preservation of normal glucosylceramide metabolism. This threshold (approximately 50% of normal) is apparent in carriers, because they do not develop disease manifestations or have Gaucher cells in their tissues. The next level is that in affected homozygotes who are enzyme deficient (levels <20% of normal) and are relatively mild to asymptomatic. These patients have enzyme deficiency and Gaucher cells in their bone marrow, but minimal to no disease involvement. The next threshold is for children, adolescents, or young adults with significant to severe visceral manifestations and shortened life spans. Within this group of persons with type 1 disease, the presence of the N370S and other disease alleles modifies the disease expression. Although the degree of involvement is highly variable, it is less severe in homozygotes for N370S, some of whom are asymptomatic. Indeed, approximately 50% of N370S homozygotes in the Ashkenazi Jewish population are minimally symptomatic to asymptomatic.[53] By comparison, the N370S/null allele genotype usually leads to a very severe, but nonneuronopathic, disease course. The next threshold is for the development of neuronopathic disease. Within this group are patients with type 2 and type 3 disease; type 3 patients have later onset of neuronopathic manifestations. Among type 3 variants there is significant heterogeneity, with two different subtypes of neuronopathic disease designated 3a and 3b.[82] From studies of in situ glucosylceramide metabolism, as well as genotype analyses among homozygotes for the L444P mutation, the type 3 patients appear to have significantly greater flux of glucosylceramide through their fibroblasts than that in type 2 patients. The most severely affected type 2 patients may have one L444P mutation and an additional allele that is null, or two null alleles. The latter leads to an early lethal phenotype termed the collodion variant. These thresholds are relative, because even in normal persons, the massive substrate load presented by acute myelogenous leukemia (ie, leukocyte membranes) leads to the presence in bone marrow of Gaucher-type cells in patients with completely normal enzymatic activity. Thus, not unexpectedly, other factors or genes can modify the disease expression, even in patients with the same genotype. These factors or genes have yet to be identified, and the role of ethnic or racial background on disease expression requires definition.

From a practical view, the level of residual enzymatic activity could determine the eventual need for enzyme or gene therapy. In patients with substantial amounts of residual enzymatic activity, such as symptomatic N370S homozygotes, less total enzyme may be needed than in patients who have the genotype N370S/null or other severely compromised alleles. The former patients can supply significant amounts of endogenous enzymatic activity for the cleavage of glucosylceramide and may have lesser needs for exogenous enzyme. For other lysosomal diseases, calculations based on in situ activity of enzymes indicate that very small differences in the quantity of enzyme in cells have major impacts on the phenotype.[29,83] Exogenously supplied enzyme might also influence the onset of specific organ, tissue, or cellular disease manifestations. The findings in Tay–Sachs disease, MLD, and Gaucher disease variants anticipate those in other lysosomal storage diseases. Clearly, mutation analysis for the defective gene alone will not provide an accurate prognosis. Considerable intrafamilial variations exist among affected members with these diseases. This variability makes it difficult to counsel and prognosticate from historic family data.

THERAPEUTIC APPROACHES AND IMPLICATIONS

The threshold hypothesis implies that small amounts of enzymatic activity may be sufficient for prevention of various disease manifestations in the lysosomal diseases. During the past 2 decades, two major approaches have been exploited to reach these thresholds and correct the underlying metabolic defects: (a) direct enzyme therapy in which a specific, pure, lysosomal enzyme that is missing is delivered and (b) transplantation of normal organs or cells to supply the missing normal enzyme. For the latter strategy, bone marrow, liver, spleen, or skin cells, natural or gene enhanced, could act as metabolic or enzyme pumps for delivery of enzyme to the plasma for uptake at distant sites, to contiguous host cells, or for direct replacement and correction of specific cell types. Both of these approaches require receptor-mediated endocytosis effected through specific recognition in the target sites of pathology. This approach implies the need to correct only specific cell types, such as those using the specific receptor system or derived from bone marrow precursor cells. The normal enzyme could be supplied to deficient cells through partially corrected cell populations (chimerism) or by the administered enzyme. This therapeutic strategy applies to enzymes that are soluble or can be solubilized into plasma or interstitial spaces. For membrane-bound proteins, cell–cell contact (ie, metabolic cooperation) may be required for the direct transfer of the enzyme with subsequent targeting to the lysosome. This mechanism may constrain delivery of the enzyme only to cells in direct proximity to the nondeficient cell and could lead to nonuniform correction. In diseases in which the target sites of pathology may be distant from the sites of synthesis of a membrane-bound protein, delivery of enzymes through a secretory pathway will not work, and alternative strategies will be required for delivery of enzyme. Thus, the approach with enzyme therapy or cellular transplantation strategies is disease dependent and requires knowledge of enzyme distribution and intra- and intercellular transport.

Substantial amounts of accumulated substrates in various tissues may be of exogenous origin—that is, transported from distant sites and deposited in lysosomes within particular sites of pathology. Consequently, depletion of the plasma pool of these accumulating substrates may lead to a reequilibration of previously stored material from tissue sources into the plasma. Although this mechanism is hypothetic for most diseases, in Fabry disease, previously stored substrate can be mobilized from tissue storage sites. Such a depletion mechanism has obvious therapeutic implications and implies an interaction of several organs and cell types in phenotypical development. In the neuronopathic Gaucher disease phenotypes, some accumulating substrate in adventitial layers of CNS blood vessels is derived from visceral sources.[83] Depletion of substrate from these visceral sources might lead to a modified progression of the phenotype, depending on the impact of this pathologic process on CNS function. This depletion approach has not been exploited in many of the lysosomal storage diseases, because little is known about glycosphingolipid, mucopolysaccharide, and glycopeptide systemic trafficking. If such depletion and reequilibration can occur, the delivery of particular enzymes for specific diseases to the target sites of pathology may not be essential, and transport of soluble disease metabolites from tissues might prove efficacious alone or in combination with enzyme reconstitution.

The implications for genetic therapeutic approaches to the treatment of lysosomal storage diseases are clear. If the deficient enzyme must be delivered directly to the target site of pathology, transplantation of the appropriate stem cell containing the appropriate genes is attainable in select visceral tissues. The macrophages/monocytes of liver, spleen, bone marrow, lungs and other reticuloendothelial tissues can be replaced with normal cells using BMT. Thus, irrespective of the complex practical and theoretical issues surrounding gene therapy approaches, gene transfer into bone marrow progenitor stem cells of the affected persons should prove efficacious. Of note, metabolites might not reequilibrate out of brain rapidly enough to prevent the manifestations of the disease in the CNS. In that case, the enzyme or cells would need to be delivered to the CNS or areas that are pathologically involved. The delivery of macromolecules, cells, and recombinant viruses to the brain has proved to be difficult and continues as a significant barrier to the development of gene delivery for neurologic diseases, as it has been for their enzyme therapy.

Animal models of human lysosomal storage diseases are essential to the continuing development of therapies and pathophysiology studies. Although numerous naturally occurring models have been identified in mice, rats, dogs, cats, cattle, and other species, targeted gene disruption techniques provide for the generation of null and missense mutations in any desired gene, particularly in mice. Although critical to applied and basic advancements, caution is needed in extrapolating data from such mice directly to humans. There are several examples of knockout mice[84] that have either no disease or lethal phenotypes and for which phenotypes do not correspond well to those in the humans. For the lysosomal storage diseases, the generated phenotypes have been similar to those in humans when similar mutations are compared, such as with Gaucher disease, Tay–Sachs disease, and Niemann–Pick disease type A. The presence or absence of alternative metabolic pathways in different species, however, can have a major impact on the phenotype or the efficacy of a therapeutic intervention.

RESULTS AND LESSONS FROM THERAPY

The principal objective of therapy is to reconstitute a balance between substrate accumulation and degradation, with the therapeutic set point below the threshold of pathology for all involved tissues. The accumulated experience of 20 years has focused on BMT for a number of disorders and enzyme replacement therapy (ERT) for Gaucher disease. In recent years, additional ERTs have become available (Fabry disease and MPS I) and therapeutic augmentation through substrate deprivation or enzyme enhancement has been explored in animal models and clinical trials (Table 53–3). These experiences are critically important to the development of future strategies for lysosomal storage disease. Based on the pluripotency of bone marrow stem cells, most transplantation studies have focused on these cells. The isolation and characterization of stem cells from other organs, including neuronal stem cells, have been encouraging and may provide pluripotent sources of enzyme in the future. The expanding plasticity of such stem cells or bone marrow mesenchymal stem cells[85,86] suggests an expanded potential for multicell reconstitution, particularly neurons. As indicated in Table 53–1, various lysosomal storage diseases have preferential sites of pathology. However, all cells in the body are involved with the enzyme deficiency and most tissues can manifest symptoms and signs of these diseases. For BMT or other organ transplantations to be effective, the cells containing enzymes must be able to catabolize the supplied substrate. This ultimately depends on the mass of cells transplanted because each cell can synthesize only limited amounts of enzyme for supply to the body. Such considerations are particularly relevant for organs such as the kidney or liver, where the donor cells do not migrate from the organ.

Transplantation Approaches

Most lysosomal storage diseases are pleiotropic, and solid organ transplantation is rarely effective as a sole strategy, although kidney or liver transplantation may be necessary to replace a failing organ. Because all cells are enzyme deficient, and most tissues have some evidence of disturbed function from this deficiency (see Table 53–1), BMT has been widely applied as a therapeutic approach, with a variety of outcomes. For any transplantation therapy to be effective, the cells containing the enzymes must be able to catabolize accumulated and newly supplied substrate. This ultimately depends on the mass of cells engrafted, because each cell can synthesize only limited quantities of enzyme.

Animal and human studies identified a critical limitation to BMT, that of engrafting sufficient bone marrow-derived cells into brain substance. Insufficient data are available from autopsy or clinical material of humans who have undergone BMT to show conclusively the extent of biochemical or clinical improvement in the CNS; thus, data obtained from animal models are important in the design of therapies.

The MPS I dog results from a point mutation in the α-L-iduronidase gene leading to a truncated protein.[87] The visceral phenotype is similar to the moderately severe MPS IHS in humans, although the CNS storage resembles the more severe MPS IH. BMT from unaffected litter mates leads to functional and pathologic improvements in bony deformities, cardiac abnormalities, corneal

Table 53–3 Therapy for Lysosomal Diseases*

Disease	Transplantation	ERT†	Substrate Deprivation†	Gene Therapy	Adjunctive Therapy
Gaucher disease	BMT	Yes[108]	Yes[160]	Mice[161,162]	Alendronate disodium in adults[163]
Fabry disease	Kidney	Yes[104]	Mice[123]	Mice[164]	
MPS I	BMT	Yes[103]			
MPS II		Yes[98]			
MPS VI	BMT	Yes[99]		Mice	
GSD II		Yes[100]			
Niemann–Pick disease type B	BMT	Yes			
Krabbe disease	Stem cell			Mice[165]	
Tay-Sachs/Sandhoff disease	Mice[166]		Investigational	Mice[167]	
MPS VII	BMT: mice	Mice		Mice	
LINCL				Mice	
Wolman disease/CESD	Yes	Mice[168]	HMG CoA reductase inhibitors: mice[170]	Mice[169]	
Niemann–Pick disease type C				Mice[171]	Cholesterol mobilization: mice[172]

BMT, bone marrow transplantation; CESD, cholesterol ester storage disease; ERT, enzyme replacement therapy; GSD, glycogen storage disease; HMG CoA, 3-hydroxy-3-methylglutaryl coenzyme A; LINCL, late infantile neuronal lipid fuscinosis; MPS, mucopolysaccharidosis.

*If therapeutic modality is reported only in animals, then species and reference are given.

†"Investigational" indicates that clinical trials are under way in humans.

clouding, and hepatosplenomegaly of affected dogs.[88] The host hepatocytes were cleared of storage material, consistent with uptake of α-L-iduronidase from donor Kupffer cells. Vertebral and joint pathologies continue to progress, although at slower rates than in untransplanted affected dogs. The CNS effects were difficult to evaluate functionally, but lysosomal distention was decreased in glial cells, and there were various improvements in neurons.

The efficacies of BMT, enzyme infusions, and gene therapy have been compared in the MPS VII mouse, a naturally occurring strain with a single base deletion in exon 10 of the *gus* gene encoding β-glucuronidase.[89] BMT using marrow from syngeneic unaffected mice transplanted into irradiated MPS VII-affected mice increased life span and cleared storage material from liver, spleen, kidney, and cornea. Early BMT resulted in greater improvement in the skeleton and in auditory function, but neurologic and behavioral improvements were not demonstrated. The pre-BMT irradiation regimen was shown to directly affect CNS development in young mice, producing CNS dysplasia in these animals. In comparison, infusion of recombinant β-glucuronidase had no effect on the cornea and limited ability to slow the skeletal disease when initiated at 6 weeks of age. The combination of neonatal enzyme infusion, followed by later BMT, showed synergistic effects even though brain enzyme levels were restored to only 0.75% of normal, compared with 20% in the spleen of treated mice. Clearly, poor entry of enzyme into the brain, either by infusion or BMT, is a barrier. More recent attempts to treat the brain of these mice with gene therapy have used a lentivirus vector. Such experiments were successful in reducing storage within the CNS, accompanied by evidence of improvement in cognitive function.[90] The results indicate that reconstitution toward normal substrate flux may require very small amounts of enzyme. However, the threshold amount probably will prove to be disease and tissue dependent.

Conclusive outcomes of BMT in human lysosomal storage disease accrue only over many years. For many conditions, only limited numbers of patients have undergone transplantation, and rigorous long-term evaluation and appropriate natural history controls have been difficult to compile. For MPS I, however, greater than 800 patients have undergone transplantation procedures, and considerable data are available on these patients, both in the United States[91] and in Europe.[92] Durable engraftment of MPS I (severe phenotype) results in prolonged life, improved cardiorespiratory disease, dramatic reduction in hepatosplenomegaly, and, if transplantation is performed early, some protection of the brain. Skeletal disease remains a considerable problem, resulting in significant functional disability and sometimes death (Fig. 53–7). The neurocognitive outcomes in these patients depend on the age at transplantation and the pretransplantation developmental quotient (DQ). The trajectory of development does improve, even with BMT from unrelated donors, but the absolute mean developmental index decreases in 50%. The residual impairment appears to be multifactorial.

In assessing the comparative therapeutic effects in animals and humans, the effects of different genotypes at the disease-producing locus may be considerably greater in humans, in whom the genetic background variation is large compared with that in inbred animals. Nevertheless, responses to transplantation vary within and between disease types. The effects of cytoreductive therapy and graft-versus-host disease, and their interactions with the underlying disease, make the analysis of effectiveness even more complicated in humans, in whom controlled trials are difficult. Also, the therapeutic goals should be carefully delineated. In humans, the natural evolution of tissue lesions in many of the lysosomal storage diseases and, particularly in the brain and bones, are poorly documented. However, with time, these lesions probably become irreversible in a tissue-dependent manner, and a window of opportunity may exist for achieving reversal of disease manifestations in each disease. Once this disease-specific developmental threshold is passed, the damage to the brain or other organs may progress in spite of therapy. Progressive CNS involvement in Krabbe disease (human and murine) and Sanfilippo syndrome, and the worsening skeletal disease of MPS IH following BMT support this notion. In addition, the various levels of reconstitution

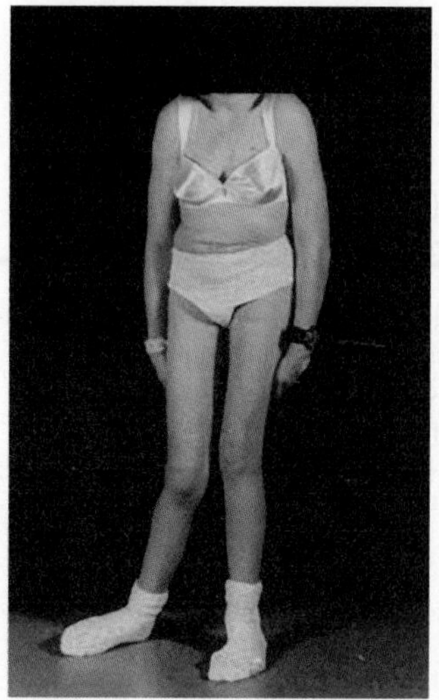

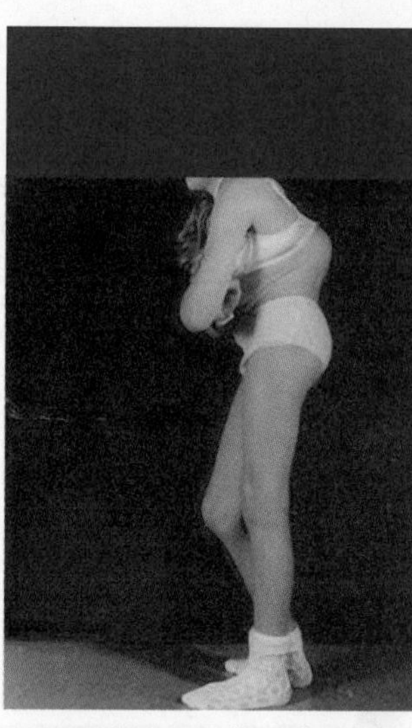

Figure 53–7 Skeletal deformities in a patient with mucopolysaccharidosis (MPS) IH more than a decade after bone marrow transplantation. Central nervous system function was nearly normal, but the axial skeletal disease continued to progress. Additional deformities of the long bones also were present but did not constitute the typical dysostosis multiplex of MPS IH. *(Courtesy of J. E. Wraith.)*

of metabolic flux in each tissue may lead to differing results in patients. For example, variable reconstitution in the CNS following BMT may convert infantile to juvenile MLD—that is, from an earlier-onset, severe abnormality to a later-onset progressive disease. BMT will have its greatest potential beneficial effects in diseases that are pathophysiologically derived from a single cell line that can be replaced by BMT. Gaucher disease is the prime example in which BMT "cures" the visceral lesions if instituted before irreversible damage in liver, spleen, lung, or bone marrow.[93–95] The visceral components of this disease derive from monocyte/macrophage-lineage cells. Clearly, BMT effects on the resolution and/or progression of signs and symptoms have been disease variant and stage-specific. BMT is probably not warranted in patients with severe irreversible pathology. Careful baseline evaluation, selection, and follow-up evaluation of patients will be required to assess the therapeutic impact of BMT in the individual lysosomal storage diseases.

The results of transplantation of other organs in these diseases including the liver, kidney, and spleen have been limited. In those diseases that result from soluble enzyme defects, hepatic, splenic or other solid organ transplantation may be beneficial if sufficient amounts of enzyme can be synthesized and secreted for delivery to distant sources. In comparison, diseases such as Gaucher disease where the enzyme is not normally secreted, transplantation of liver into such patients has resulted in the reaccumulation of Gaucher cells and redevelopment of pathology in transplanted livers.[96] These results indicate that hepatic transplantation alone is insufficient for preventing redevelopment of symptoms in such severely involved patients. Blood chimerism may develop following hepatic transplantation, because the donor liver may supply small amounts of enzyme and bone marrow-derived cells to recipient organs. In the absence of concomitant enzyme replacement therapy, patients receiving hepatic transplantation and small amounts of donor bone marrow may become chimeric and develop two populations of bone marrow-derived cells in their bodies: those that are normal and those that are not. At a low level of chimerism, the storage cells would be expected to accumulate in tissues and, in the absence of cross-correction, eventually result in recurrence of disease manifestations. Greater degrees of monocyte/macrophage chimerism could lead to improvement if the normal cells can prevent accumulation of end-stage Gaucher cells in tissues.[97]

Enzyme Therapy Approaches

Enzyme replacement therapy (ERT) has been available for treatment of Gaucher disease for more than a decade, and has been recently approved for treatment of Fabry disease, MPS I,[50] MPS II,[98] MPS VI,[99] and GSD II[100] (see box Management of Gaucher Disease) Clinical trials are ongoing for Niemann–Pick disease type B. Animal model studies have been published for some of these conditions, as well as for several additional diseases of human relevance.[84,101] With rare exceptions, enzymes for replacement therapy are produced by recombinant methods of gene amplification, resulting in enhanced production of the desired protein product. In most human clinical trials or treatment protocols, the enzymes have been infused intravenously every 1 to 2 weeks.

A significant concern in enzyme therapy is the development of antibodies to the exogenous enzyme. This has been assessed in both animal and human studies. MPS I dogs given recombinant canine or human α-L-iduronidase developed antibodies. Similarly, in dogs implanted with retrovirally transduced myoblasts expressing canine α-L-iduronidase, anti-iduronidase antibodies were produced, with eventual loss of the transduced cells in these animals.[102] In clinical trials of ERT for MPS I,[103] MPS II,[98] MPS VI,[99] Fabry disease,[104] and GSD II,[100] most patients developed antibodies and many developed infusion-associated reactions. It would be expected that the presence or absence of endogenous enzyme protein would alter the cadence and clinical significance of antibody development. These difficulties cannot be ascribed only to the presence or absence of endogenous enzyme protein, however, because 15% of treated Gaucher disease patients develop antibodies to administered enzyme, and all have

Management of Gaucher Disease

The clinical management and enzyme replacement/replenishment therapy (ERT) for Gaucher disease type 1 are complicated by the marked variation in phenotype and in the rates of disease progression. In addition, significant ethnic variation exists in disease severity, and the involved organ systems involved and their progression rates. Much of the literature has focused on the description of the disease in the Ashkenazi Jewish population that is skewed to the adult population of less severely involved patients with slower progression rates.[1,2] Recent studies have clearly shown that within other ethnic groups, and even within the Ashkenazi Jewish population, subsets of affected patients exist with more progressive and severe disease even within specific genotypes.[3] Homozygosity for a common mutation, termed N370S, in the Ashkenazi population can be associated with minimal symptomatology in many patients (approximately 50%). However, a significant number (approximately 30%) of children (<20 years) with this genotype have severe progressive disease.[4] Lacking genetic or validated biomarkers to provide prediction for eventual outcome or track disease progression also complicates treatment programs.

Comprehensive treatment plans are significantly influenced by the clinical context of individual patients. Recently, therapeutic goals or guidelines and timelines to the achievement of therapeutic effects have been developed and can be used to provide a background of therapeutic assessments.[5,6] Increases in hemoglobin and platelet levels, and splenic and liver volumes within the first 6 to 24 months of ERT provide instructive approaches to facilitate dosing and/or goal achievement. However, until recently, dose response characteristics have been lacking for ERT. An extensive analysis using statistical methods (propensity scoring) to diminish significant phenotypic variations show significant incremental dose responses between 15 U (0.375 mg) and 60 U (1.5 mg/kg) [Cerezyme™, imiglucerase, Genzyme Corp., Cambridge, MA] every 2 weeks for the above clinical parameters, as well as bone mineral density.[7,8] In these matched populations over a period of approximately 8 years, greater rates and total responses to enzyme therapy were found at the higher doses. These dose responses can provide guidance for physicians to the attainment of therapeutic goals and the relevant timelines. Such data also provide guidance for dose adjustments in patients who have inadequate responses to initiating doses. For example, in patients with severe thrombocytopenia and very enlarged spleens with extensive bone marrow infiltration and significant losses of bone mineral density, higher doses of enzyme could be chosen to initiate therapy to alleviate potential devastating consequences of severe involvement. On the other hand, adults who have slowly progressing disease over a decade or more, whose platelet counts have slowly decreased, and whose bone mineral density is slowing decreasing may do well on lower doses of enzyme. Either case requires careful follow-up monitoring of responses to ERT. For example, in the high-dose case with severe thrombocytopenia, a patient may be monitored very intensively for platelet values and other parameters to ensure that responses are adequate to avoid complications. Similarly, a patient with very large liver and spleen and mechanical interference with eating or breathing should be monitored carefully to ensure that adequate doses are given. For the patients with less severe involvement on the lower-dose ERT, good responses to therapy after 6 or 8 months might suggest dosage adjustments are not needed. These judgments can be conducted in conjunction with physicians with extensive experience in the management of many patients with Gaucher disease, because hard-and-fast rules cannot be made for each patient.

Some general recommendations can be made on the basis of specific judgments of the physician and the individual patient. Adults with more slowly progressing disease without major complications of Gaucher disease, for example, severe hepatic or splenic involvement or rapidly progressing bone disease, usually are instituted on approximately 30 U/kg every 2 weeks and therapeutic response monitored initially at 6 months. During that period of time, if the therapeutic goals are met, judgments can be made as to whether or not dosage should be decreased, and whether the goals are maintained on that new dose. This author rarely uses less than 20 U/kg every 2 weeks. This is based on clinical observations of a significant number of patients redeveloping progressive disease and/or symptomatology on lower doses. However, lower doses could be appropriate in certain adult patients. In children, the disease is generally more rapidly progressing with more severe involvement (eg, larger livers, spleens and degrees of anemia and thrombocytopenia),[2,4] a higher dose (60 U/kg every 2 weeks) is used to initiate therapy. Also, the clinical impression that bony disease progresses more rapidly during puberty gives impetus to using higher doses in children until the skeleton has matured. This author adjusts to lower doses once puberty has been completed and a mature skeleton has developed, if other parameters have responded well. The objective is to facilitate entrance of children into adult life with adequate bone structure and as normal other parameters to support a normal adult life.

Approximately 13% of patients (close to 500/4000) receiving ERT for Gaucher disease type 1 develop antibodies to the drug; approximately 50% of these develop adverse infusion-related events within 6 to 12 months of initiation.[9] The majority of these antibodies and adverse events disappear within 24 months of regular ERT and create no major problems. Infusion-related adverse events are usually managed with NSAID and/or antihistamines. Rare (3 or 4) patients have developed neutralizing antibodies that inactivate the enzyme with consequent redevelopment of disease signs. These patients have been tolerized by using high dose (120–240 U/kg every 2 weeks) enzyme therapy in combination with cytotoxic drugs although rigorous evaluation and development of protocols has not been undertaken.[10] In addition, IgE mediated anaphylaxis has resulted from ERT in one

Management of Gaucher Disease—cont'd

or two cases. These patients would be candidates for alternative forms of therapy, such as substrate reduction or bone marrow transplantation.

Because of the expense of therapy, the use of this resource to move children and adults to more normal lives can be accomplished within the framework of the therapeutic guidelines and goals. The next series of studies should evaluate the effect of enzyme dose on the achievement of therapeutic goals using a consensus severity score to match patients.

REFERENCES

1. Zimran A, Kay A, Gelbart T, et al: Gaucher disease. Clinical, laboratory, radiologic, and genetic features of 53 patients. Medicine 71:337, 1992.
2. Grabowski GA, Kolodny EH, Weinreb NJ, et al: Gaucher disease: Phenotypic and genetic variation. In Scriver C, Beaudet A, Sly W, Valle D (eds.): The Metabolic and Molecular Bases of Inherited Diseases. New York, McGraw-Hill, 2006. genetics.accessmedicine.com.
3. Sobreira E, Pires RF, Cizmarik M, Grabowski GA: Phenotypic and genotypic heterogeneity in Gaucher disease type 1: A comparison between Brazil and the rest-of-the-world. Mol Genet Metab 90:81, 2007.
4. Kaplan P, Andersson HC, Kacena KA, Yee JD: The clinical and demographic characteristics of nonneuronopathic Gaucher disease in 887 children at diagnosis. Arch Pediatr Adolesc Med 160:603, 2006.
5. Weinreb N, Charrow J, Andersson HC, et al: Effectiveness of enzyme replacement therapy in 1028 patients with type 1 Gaucher disease after 2 to 5 years of treatment: A report from the Gaucher registry. Am J Med 113:112, 2002.
6. Pastores GM, Weinreb NJ, Aerts H, et al: Therapeutic goals in the treatment of Gaucher disease. Semin Hematol 41:4, 2004.
7. Wenstrup RJ, Kacena KA, Kaplan P, et al: Effect of enzyme replacement therapy with imiglucerase on BMD in type 1 Gaucher disease. J Bone Miner Res 22:119, 2007.
8. Grabowski GA, Charrow J, Hollak CEM, et al: Analysis of Enzyme Replacement Therapy Dose-Response Relationships in Patients With Type 1 Gaucher Disease. New Orleans, LA: American Society of Human Genetics, 2006.
9. Richards S, Olson TA, McPherson JM: Antibody response in patients with Gaucher disease after repeated infusion with macrophage-targeted glucocerebrosidase. Blood 82:1402, 1993.
10. Zhao H, Bailey LA, Grabowski GA: Enzyme therapy of gaucher disease: Clinical and biochemical changes during production of and tolerization for neutralizing antibodies. Blood Cells Mol Dis 30:90, 2003.

residual enzyme activity. Similarly, antibodies developed in cross-reacting immunologic material-positive (CRIM$^+$) patients with Pompe disease who were infused with recombinant human acid α-glucosidase as well as in patients with MPS HS and IS treated with α-L-iduronidase. These antibodies can lead to direct neutralizing effects[105] and, potentially, to misdirection or redistribution of enzyme to "nontherapeutic" sites.[106] From a clinical standpoint, antibody therapies appear manageable in terms of both efficacy and infusion safety, but must remain under scrutiny as ERT for other lysosomal storage diseases becomes a reality.

Enzyme therapy has been studied extensively in human Gaucher disease for more than a decade.[107,108] This therapy exploits the receptor for α-mannosyl-terminated oligosaccharides on the surface of cells of monocyte/macrophage origin. The membrane-bound human acid β-glucosidase is extracted from media of overexpressing Chinese hamster ovary cells, purified to homogeneity, treated with exoglycosidases to expose α-mannosyl groups, and intravenously administered to affected patients. Several independent studies have demonstrated the usefulness of this approach, and many patients have demonstrated excellent responses.[108–113] The population of reported patients is varied, and insight can be gained into responses for individual patients during treatment. Response to therapy varies significantly, but by 1 year of enzyme therapy, responses can include (a) an approximately 20% to 30% decrease in liver volume if the liver is initially enlarged, (b) an approximately 30% to 50% decrease in splenic volume, (c) an increase in hemoglobin level by 1.5 g/dL if the patient initially is anemic, with approximately 33% to 50% of such patients achieving normal hemoglobin levels, and (d) an increase in platelet counts. In many patients with massive or heavily scarred spleens, thrombocytopenia may persist for several years. For liver and splenic volume decreases and hemoglobin increases, approximately 50% of patients met or exceeded these responses by 1 year. Patients on higher doses have somewhat better responses in terms of decreased splenic volume than those on smaller doses, but dose–response relationships are highly individualized. Patients with massive splenic enlargement (>20-fold greater) in general have poor hematologic responses until the splenic volume decreases by 50% to 70%. This correlation suggests that there may be a threshold size of spleen for adequate hematologic response as a result of intrasplenic hemolysis and platelet consumption. The variation in response to enzyme therapy is great among patients and at different times during therapy in one patient. Consequently, continued follow-up and monitoring are required to evaluate responses and to initiate treatment changes. Guidelines for monitoring therapy are available.[114]

Hepatic and splenic changes are more rapid than those in the bone and lungs. One cannot exclude the possibility of a different dose-response threshold for each tissue. This is particularly concerning in light of the inability to discern bone or pulmonary changes during a period of rapid dose reduction while hematologic, hepatic, and splenic improvement rates are maintained. Data on the tissue, cellular, and subcellular distribution, or on the half-lives of the administered enzyme, are scarce. Evidence obtained in mice suggests that the enzyme has relatively low uptake by monocyte/macrophage cells,[115] with very different and distinct uptake and survival patterns in the bone marrow, liver, and lung.[111,116] Also, the cellular distribution of exogenous enzyme in affected patients is unknown, but the slowness of response to enzyme suggests that the pre-Gaucher cell compartment may be the major target for enzyme uptake. These "corrected cells" would then ingest Gaucher cells and degrade the contained glucosylceramide. Such a mechanism has implications for enzyme therapy of other lysosomal diseases.

In view of the high cost of enzyme therapy with all current infusion protocols, the timing of the initiation of therapy must be carefully evaluated. Highly symptomatic patients should begin therapy immediately. In addition, other patients with major hematologic and visceral involvement should receive high priority for therapy. Although bone disease appears to be the slowest to respond,[117] patients with substantial bone involvement are candidates for treatment to recover bone integrity and to prevent irreversibility of some bone damage. (see box Management of Bone Crises in Gaucher Disease). A more difficult decision must be made in presymptomatic patients whose susceptibility to major disease manifestations can be anticipated by genotype analysis.[53] Clearly, the issue of the timing and use of an apparently universally effective therapy must be carefully considered and evaluated as a potential preventive intervention. The major inhibition to the use of BMT for Gaucher disease is the risk of the procedure compared with that associated with enzyme therapy, for which the major barrier is cost. If the risk of BMT could

Management of Bone Crises in Gaucher Disease

Bone crises are the most devastating and frightening clinical complications of Gaucher disease type 1. Although the etiology and exact pathogenesis of the bone crisis are not well delineated, the final common pathway appears to be bone infarction. Such infarction leads to localized intramedullary edema and swelling with increased pressure, and occasionally localized erythema and swelling. These crises are exceedingly painful, can be incapacitating, and necessitate the use of narcotic analgesics or even general anesthesia to alleviate the pain. The caricature of the clinical bone crises is a localized episode that begins with an undefined period of a dull aching pain in a specific bone region with increasing pain to excruciating levels over a period of 3 to 4 days. The excruciating pain plateaus for 4 to 7 days with a subsequent period of gradual resolution that can extend from weeks to a month or more. The bone crisis can occur in any bone and in any region of a bone, but most commonly presents as AVN of the head and/or neck of the femur. The shaft of the femur, the head of the humeri, vertebral bodies and the ischial tuberosities of the pelvis can be involved. The immediate consequences of a bone crises, other than pain, are relatively minor. On x-ray or MRI, little evidence is present for structural change in the bone, that is, lytic lesions at the site of infarction. However, a technicium sulfur colloid or pyrophosphate nuclear scans will show a localized area absent blood flow in the acute painful phase. Over a period of several weeks to months, the involved area may develop lytic lesions evident on plain radiographs. That can heal to become normal bone or remain as isolated lytic lesions. Involvement of the heads of the femurs and humeri, or the infarction of vertebral bodies, can lead to functional impairment, need for joint replacement, and/or chronic degenerative disease. Less intense bone crisis episodes probably occur frequently in some patients with intermittent bone pain, but these are difficult to document.

The accompanying localized swelling, pain, and elevation of sedimentation rate, leukocytosis, and fever can simulate an osteomyelitis. Osteomyelitis needs to be excluded, because its occurrence can be life threatening and can be caused by difficult-to-treat organisms within the bone marrow.

Approximately 10% of patients with Gaucher disease experience at least one bone crisis during their disease course.[1] They are more common in children than adults, although the hip involvement with AVN is relatively more common in adults. Recurrent infarctions and/or structural alterations can lead to destructive secondary bony lesions collapse of the hip and the need for hip replacement. Treatment of the acute episode includes the exclusion of osteomyelitis and analgesic treatment as needed. Hyperbaric oxygen and corticosteroids have been tried with variable success.[2] On a short-term basis, high-dose corticosteroids may be beneficial, after osteomyelitis has been excluded, and do not pose any significant threat or complication risk to the patient. Data are lacking on the use of hyperbaric oxygen. Core decompression to alleviate the secondary edema, and reestablish more normal blood flow to the bone marrow, may be an alternative for some patients. Although not critically evaluated, this approach has been accomplished on numerous occasions to alleviate pain and higher intramedullary pressures. Core decompression must be done early in the crisis course and under completely sterile conditions, preferably in an operating room, to avoid secondary contamination and the development of osteomyelitis. The results of early intervention with core decompression suggest utility in selected patients.

An evaluation of bone pain and bone crises in patients who had follow-up for ERT showed that bone crises diminished dramatically within the first year of enzyme therapy.[3] Bone pain also decreased significantly, but a residual level of bone pain could not be alleviated by ERT. This is probably secondary to complications of irreversible bone disease rather than Gaucher disease itself. Thus, ERT has been shown to have significant effects on bone mineral density[4] and on the alleviation and prevention of bone crises.[3] ERT has no role in the acute management of bone crises but rather a preventive role.

REFERENCES

1. Grabowski GA, Kolodny EH, Weinreb NJ, et al: Gaucher disease: Phenotypic and genetic variation. In Scriver C, Beaudet A, Sly W, Valle D (eds.): The Metabolic and Molecular Bases of Inherited Diseases. New York, McGraw-Hill, 2006. genetics.accessmedicine.com.
2. Cohen IJ, Kornreich L, Mekhmandarov S, Katz K, Zaizov R: Effective treatment of painful bone crises in type I Gaucher's disease with high dose prednisolone. ArchDisChild 75:218, 1996.
3. Charrow J, Dulisse B, Grabowski GA, Weinreb NJ: The effect of enzyme replacement therapy on bone crisis and bone pain in patients with type 1 Gaucher disease. Clin Genet 71:205, 2007.
4. Wenstrup RJ, Kacena KA, Kaplan P, et al: Effect of enzyme replacement therapy with imiglucerase on BMD in type 1 Gaucher disease. J Bone Miner Res 22:119, 2007.

be decreased dramatically, possibly through autologous BMT of corrected cells, this may become the treatment of choice.

Several difficult issues need to be resolved to promote optimal use of therapeutic strategies in the lysosomal storage diseases. There is extensive interpatient variability in dose response. What are the determinants of this variability? Will the effects of more easily accessed tissues be preferentially evaluated rather than those in more difficult, potentially more relevant, tissues? Will certain tissues require specific doses of enzyme that will determine overall efficacy of therapy? Is there a concomitant diminution in the need for intense therapy for continued improvement as the tissues are healed? Is there a role for combined BMT/ERT, for example, in MPS I? Most important, what is the window of opportunity for effective therapy? Is it more efficacious to prevent the disease manifestations than to attempt to return a very sick person, with potentially irreversible tissue damage, to health? This issue is particularly relevant for those disorders that involve the CNS.

CNS disease represents a substantial challenge to effective therapy. Although BMT remains the recommended therapy for severe (neuropathic) MPS I, the window of opportunity for clinically significant effects on cognitive function is relatively short. For early-onset neurodegenerative diseases, including Krabbe and Tay–Sachs diseases, even stem cell transplantation in the first weeks of life may not produce the desired level of CNS protection. Enzyme therapy for MPS III is feasible, but as demonstrated in mouse models, little of conventionally infused enzyme penetrates the blood–brain barrier.[118] Clearly, different approaches must be taken in significant CNS disease. Animal experiments have demonstrated expression of TPP-I (the defective protein in late-infantile neuronal ceroid lipofuscinosis [LINCL]) after direct injection of adenovirus vectors in mouse brain.[119] Using a cell-based approach to treat murine Niemann–Pick disease, Jin and colleagues demonstrated prolonged cell survival and a protective effect on Purkinje cells, but limited spread of the effect beyond the injection site.[120]

Substrate Deprivation

Substrate deprivation approaches have demonstrated a potentially more viable approach to CNS disease compared with current technically limited approaches to enzyme-, cell-, or gene-based therapy. The theoretical basis for this approach is the "supply side" of the threshold hypothesis, limiting inflow rather than enhancing outflow. Proof of principle was provided in animal experiments in which Sandhoff mice were crossed with a knockout line lacking the ability to synthesize ganglioside G_{M2} de novo.[121] These animals demonstrated significant delays in onset of neurologic symptoms and prolonged life span compared with controls, although little effect was seen in animals with heterozygote levels of G_{M2} synthesis. Further pharmacologic attempts at synthetic inhibition have shown efficacy in Sandhoff[122] and Fabry mice,[123] and human trials for late-onset Tay–Sachs disease are in the planning stages. The results in human trials of Gaucher disease showed minor effects, with significant adverse event profiles.[124] The appeal of substrate inhibition, beyond its potential ability to affect the CNS, is that these drugs tend to be small molecules that can be administered orally and may have a therapeutic effect on more than one disease, a significant factor in these orphan conditions. However, the generalized effect has drawbacks, including side effects due to the more general pharmacologic activity and distribution.

Gene Transfer

Lysosomal diseases that can be treated successfully by BMT should be amenable to permanent correction by gene therapy using hematopoietic stem cells carrying a copy of the normal gene. Following autologous transplantation with these corrected cells, somatic genetic reconstitution could be achieved by the repopulation of tissues with monocyte/macrophage-derived cells. For diseases due to defects of soluble enzymes, only a portion of stem cells would need to be corrected, because the corrected cells could supply enzymes to other tissues. For diseases that result from membrane-bound enzymes, such as Gaucher disease, all or most of the cells would need to be corrected, unless the transduced cells exhibited a selective advantage. For either of these types of enzyme defects, the amount of enzyme supplied to tissues directly or via cellular replacement would be mass dependent, and insufficient amounts of enzyme or cells would lead to the redevelopment or delay of onset of symptoms and signs. Also, stem cells that produce active lysosomal enzymes do not have any obvious proliferative advantage over those that do not. Thus, therapeutic effects would be expected only if the patient's untransformed cells were ablated by chemotherapy or irradiation. Rational strategy for the treatment of these diseases would include marrow ablation followed by autologous transplantation with transformed hematopoietic stem cells. Considerable effort has been expended to develop the required efficient gene transfer technology and hematopoietic stem cell culture systems. Significant long-term expression of transgene has been accomplished for several of these enzymes.[125–128] Protocols for somatic gene therapy of lysosomal diseases will continue to be evaluated during the next several years.

Gene therapy studies in animal analogs have attempted to exploit targeted enzyme delivery and cell transplantation strategies. The objective of the former is to implant a continuous source of enzyme for delivery to distant sites. The latter approach attempts to replace the primary cells of pathologic involvement with gene-corrected cells. The major motivation for cellular replacement approaches in gene therapy is to avoid the real and potential immunologic barriers to tissue transplantation using allogeneic transplants of corrected cells. Overexpression of β-glucuronidase or α-L-iduronidase from retrovirally transduced fibroblasts, implanted as neo-organs, results in secretion of sufficient enzyme for detection in distant organs. The levels achieved in these enzyme-deficient organs are modest, up to 2% of control levels in liver, compared with those achieved with enzyme infusion or BMT, approximately 5% to 18%.[129] Immunohistochemical studies show detectability of the secreted enzyme only in periadventitial macrophages in the brain and not in brain substance, even though in vitro studies showed enzyme uptake into neuronal and glial cells. Many enzyme deficiency states are being approached similarly. The use of neuronal stem cell transplantation appears to have promise for neuronopathic diseases. Ideally, these cells would be pluripotent neuronal cells that when transplanted into neonatal or adult mice would migrate to specific brain regions and differentiate into appropriate neurons. These cells, allogeneic or "immunotolerized," could then replace diseased neurons or supply enzymes to neighboring diseased cells for metabolic correction. Initial animal studies are promising, but clinical trials are in the future. The recent development of leukemia in SCID patients who received corrected autologous stem cells has raised significant safety concerns.[130]

Pharmacologic Chaperone Approaches

In theory, point mutations lead to expression of mutant proteins with altered stability, folding, targeting, or catalytic activity. Those in the first three groups can accumulate the mutant proteins in prelysosomal compartments, including the endoplasmic reticulum or Golgi (*cis*, mid or *trans*). These accumulations can evoke a cellular response, particularly the ER stress response, endoplasmic reticulum-associated degradation response, or unfolded protein response.[131] If sufficiently severe, these responses promote cellular apoptosis and inflammatory responses that can propagate disease manifestations. Use of chemicals that can promote more appropriate folding and/or stability have been termed pharmacologic chaperones.[132–135] For the lysosomal storage diseases, the counterintuitive use of potent competitive, active site-directed inhibitors has been proposed as potential chaperones to direct the refolding and, potentially, retargeting of mutant lysosomal enzymes to enhance their delivery and targeting to the lysosomes, as well as their stability within the lysosomes (Fan). Several studies in tissue culture[134,135] have indicated that such compounds can lead to enhanced mutant enzyme refolding, activity, and/or stability of selected Gaucher disease enzymes. Intravenous galactose in high doses was used in one Fabry disease cardiac variant patient to alter the mutant α-galactosidase A with some clinical effect.[136] To date, additional in vivo studies in animal models or humans are needed to assess the clinical effectiveness of this interesting and promising approach across a broad spectrum of mutations that produce enzymes with partial activity.

SUGGESTED READINGS

Boelens JJ: Trends in haematopoietic cell transplantation for inborn errors of metabolism. J Inherit Metab Dis 29:413, 2006.

Bonifacino JS, Traub LM: Signals for sorting of transmembrane proteins to endosomes and lysosomes. Annu Rev Biochem 72:395, 2003.

Charrow J et al: The Gaucher registry: Demographics and disease characteristics of 1698 patients with Gaucher disease. Arch Intern Med 160(18):2835, 2000.

Desnick RJ et al: Fabry disease, an under-recognized multisystemic disorder: Expert recommendations for diagnosis, management, and enzyme replacement therapy. Ann Intern Med 138(4):338, 2003.

Enquist IB et al: Effective cell and gene therapy in a murine model of Gaucher disease. Proc Natl Acad Sci U S A 103(37):13819, 2006.

Grabowski GA, Hopkin RJ: Enzyme therapy for lysosomal storage disease: Principles, practice, and prospects. Annu Rev Genomics Hum Genet 4:403, 2003.

Hopkin RJ, Bissler J, Grabowski GA: Comparative evaluation of alpha-galactosidase A infusions for treatment of Fabry disease. Genet Med 5(3):144, 2003.

Kakkis ED et al: Enzyme-replacement therapy in mucopolysaccharidosis I. N Engl J Med 344(3):182, 2001.

Kornfeld S, Mellman I: The biogenesis of lysosomes. Annu Rev Cell Biol 5:483, 1989.

Sidransky E: Gaucher disease: Complexity in a "simple" disorder. Mol Genet Metab 83(1–2):6, 2004.

Zhao H, Grabowski GA: Gaucher disease: Perspectives on a prototype lysosomal disease. Cell Mol Life Sci 59(4):694, 2002.

REFERENCES

For complete list of references log onto www.expertconsult.com

CHAPTER 54

INFECTIOUS MONONUCLEOSIS AND OTHER EPSTEIN–BARR VIRUS-ASSOCIATED DISEASES

Stephen Gottschalk, Cliona M. Rooney, and Helen E. Heslop

INTRODUCTION

The initial clinical descriptions of primary Epstein–Barr virus (EBV) infections are credited to Filatov and Pfeiffer at the end of the 19th century. Pfeiffer coined the term *glandular fever*, which described an illness consisting of fever, malaise, sore throat, and lymphadenopathy.[1] In 1920, Sprunt and Evans introduced the term *infectious mononucleosis* (IM) describing a series of patients with fatigue, fever, lymphadenopathy, and prominent mononuclear lymphocytosis (Fig. 54–1).[2] Serologic diagnosis of IM became available in the 1930s with the heterophile agglutination test developed by Paul and Bunnel and later modified by Davidson.[3,4]

The identification of EBV as the causative agent of IM was impeded for many years by the inability to transmit the disease to animals or to grow the virus ex vivo. In 1958 Burkitt described a lymphoma in African children and investigators suspected an infectious etiology because the lymphoma's geographic distribution pattern coincided with the African mosquito belt.[5] In 1964 Epstein, Achong, and Barr described herpesvirus-like particles in tumor biopsies from Burkitt lymphoma patients.[6,7] Werner and Gertrude Henle developed an indirect immunofluorescent antibody assay to this new virus, now called Epstein–Barr virus, and showed that Burkitt lymphoma patients as well as 90% of American adults had antibodies against EBV.[8] In 1965 the Henles documented seroconversion to EBV of an individual who presented with clinical symptoms of IM.[9] This initial observation was corroborated by larger studies confirming the association of EBV and IM.

Since then EBV has been linked to a heterogeneous group of diseases.[10–12] EBV was the first human virus implicated in oncogenesis and the biology of the virus has been studied extensively on a cellular and molecular level.[7,12,13] Because primary EBV infection is a self-limiting disease in almost all individuals, therapeutic strategies have focused on the treatment of rare, potentially fatal EBV-associated diseases. Over the last decade, successful immunotherapeutic approaches have been developed for EBV-associated lymphoproliferative disease using either monoclonal antibodies or the adoptive transfer of EBV-specific T cells.[14,15]

BIOLOGY OF EPSTEIN–BARR VIRUS

EBV belongs to the family of herpesviruses, which has almost 100 members.[16] Membership is based on the architecture of the viron that is 120 to 300 nm in size and contains (a) a core of linear, double-stranded DNA, (b) an icosadeltahedral capsid with 162 capsomers, (c) an amorphous material between the capsid and envelope designated tegument, and (d) an envelope containing viral glycoproteins. Besides EBV, designated human herpesvirus 4, seven other herpesviruses have been isolated from humans: herpes simplex viruses 1 and 2, cytomegalovirus, varicella-zoster virus, human herpesvirus 6, human herpesvirus 7, and the Kaposi's sarcoma-associated herpesvirus (KSHV, human herpesvirus 8). Herpesviruses are further divided into subfamilies to reflect evolutionary relatedness and similar biological properties. EBV and KSHV belong to the human gamma herpesvirus subgroup and have a limited tissue tropism to B and T lymphocytes and certain types of epithelial cells.

Several variants of EBV have been identified by genomic polymorphisms. Initially, two EBV types were distinguished by sequence changes in EBV nuclear antigens 2 and 3 (EBNA-2 and -3). However, using polymorphisms in the latent membrane protein 1 (LMP-1) further subtypes have been described.[17] EBV strains vary by geography and have not been linked to a particular EBV-associated disease.

EBV-ASSOCIATED CLINICAL SYNDROMES

- Infectious mononucleosis[36]
- Chronic active EBV infection[60,164]
- Hemophagocytic lymphohistiocytosis[165]
- X-linked lymphoproliferative disease[78]
- Oral hairy leukoplakia[83]

PRIMARY EBV INFECTION

Primary EBV infection usually occurs through the oropharynx, where mucosal epithelial cells and/or B cells become productively infected (see Fig. 54–1).[18] Infection of B cells by EBV is initiated by binding of the dominant viral glycoprotein gp350/220 to CD21, the C3d complement receptor, and subsequent cell entry is mediated by a complex of three viral glycoproteins, gH, gL, and gp42. Gp42 binds to HLA class II, which functions as a coreceptor, and gH is most likely involved in virus–cell fusion.[19] The entry of EBV into epithelial cells may occur through multiple mechanisms because the majority of epithelial cells are CD21 negative.[20–22] After viral entry, the capsid is dissolved and the EBV genome is transported into the nucleus, where it circularizes. Infection of epithelial cells results in lytic or

EBV-ASSOCIATED MALIGNANCIES[119]

Malignancy	EBV Frequency
Hodgkin disease[166]	~40%
Non-Hodgkin Lymphomas	
Burkitt Lymphoma[167]	20%–95%
Diffuse large B-cell lymphoma and CD30+ Ki-1+ anaplastic large cell lymphoma[124,126]	10%–35%
Lymphatoid granulomatosis[168]	80%–95%
T cell-rich B-cell lymphoma[125]	20%
Angioimmunoblastic lymphoma[169]	>80%
T-cell, NK-cell, and T/NK-cell lymphomas[132,170]	30%–90%
Nasopharyngeal carcinoma[154]	>95%
Gastric adenocarcinoma[171]	5%–10%
Pyothorax-associated lymphoma[172]	>95%
Leiomyosarcoma in immunocompromised patients[173]	>95%

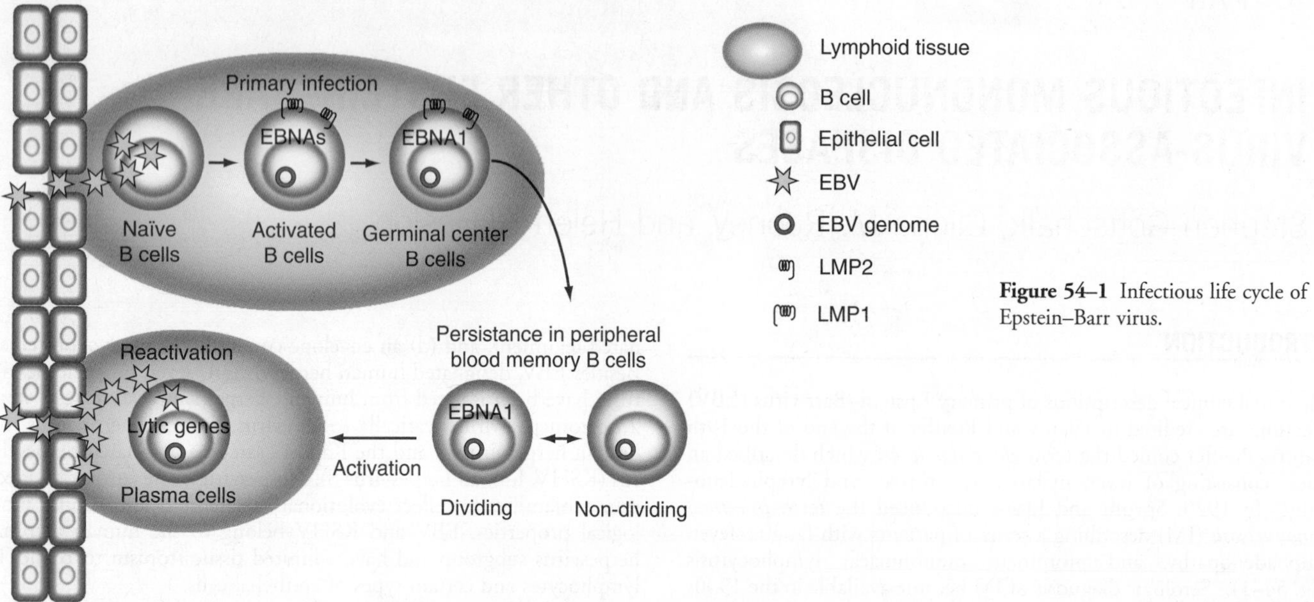

Figure 54–1 Infectious life cycle of Epstein–Barr virus.

abortive infection, and whereas B-cell infection results predominantly in latency, the lytic infection also occurs resulting in the release of infectious virus into the saliva and other secretions. During primary infection, EBV establishes lifelong latency in B cells and it is estimated that 1 to 50 cells per 1×10^6 B cells in the peripheral circulation are infected with EBV. The number of latently infected B cells within a person remains stable over years; however, intermittent reactivation of EBV in B cells into the lytic cycle at mucosal sites is probably responsible for the observed shedding of infectious virus into the saliva of asymptomatic carriers (Fig. 54–1).[12]

Although EBV can infect any B cell and express the full spectrum of latency proteins, extensive studies by the group of Thorley-Lawson have suggested that only infection of naïve B cells results in persistent infection (Fig. 54–1).[23,24] EBV infection pushes the naïve B cell into a memory state independent of an antigen-dependent germinal center reaction by upregulation of cytosine deaminase, which induces both class switching and somatic hypermutation. The former also requires the expression of EBV-encoded LMP1, a constitutively activated CD40 molecule, or CD40 ligation, most likely provided by germinal center Th3 cells that can provide T-cell help for B-cell differentiation by provision of CD40 ligand, IL-4, and IL-10 while preventing antigen-dependent effector T cell-mediated B-cell elimination by expression of TGF-β.[25] This reaction occurs within the lymph node and also involves downregulation of latency proteins and expression of latency type II. On exit from the lymph node, expression of latency proteins is completely inhibited. In this way infected B cells can evade immune elimination. By contrast, primarily infected memory B cells enter and remain in latency type III and are rapidly eliminated by effector T cells and therefore do not contribute to virus persistence.

LATENT EBV INFECTION

During latent infection, EBV persists episomally in resting memory B cells. Initially it was thought that EBNA-1 and LMP-2 is expressed in memory B cells; however more recent studies indicate that the majority of infected cells do not express viral proteins and that of the almost 100 viral proteins, only EBNA-1 is expressed during memory B cell division (see Fig. 54–1).[24,26] This extremely limited expression of viral proteins allows EBV to persist long term despite a robust cellular EBV-specific immune response.

Three other distinct types of EBV latency have been characterized in a heterogeneous group of malignancies (Fig. 54–2).[10–12] Latency type III, which can be readily produced by infecting B cells in vitro

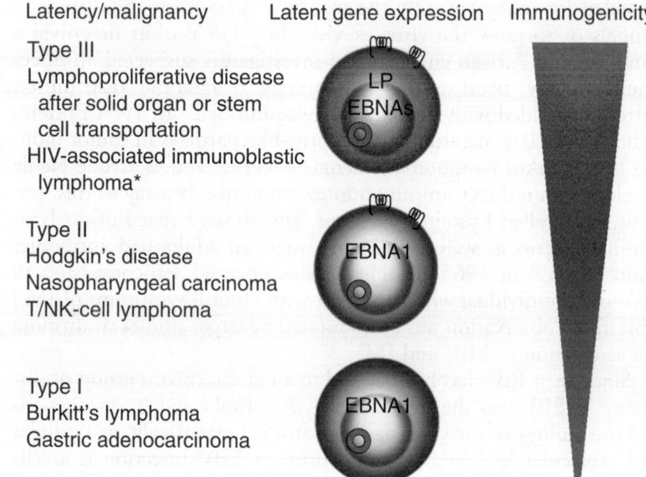

Figure 54–2 Epstein–Barr virus (EBV) latent gene expression and immunogenicity of common EBV-associated malignancies. EBNA: Epstein-Barr nuclear antigen, LP: leader protein. For explanation of symbols, see Fig. 54–1. *Not all lymphomas are latency type III.

with EBV, is expressed in lymphoblastoid cell lines (LCL). These cells express the entire array of nine EBV latency proteins: EBNAs-1, 2, 3A, 3B, 3C, EBNA leader protein (LP), and the two viral membrane proteins LMP-1 and LMP-2. This pattern of EBV gene expression characterizes the EBV-associated lymphoproliferative diseases (EBV-LPD) that occur in individuals severely immunocompromised by solid organ or hematopoietic stem cell transplantation, congenital immunodeficiency, or human immunodeficiency virus (HIV) infection. Latency type II is the hallmark of EBV-positive Hodgkin disease and non-Hodgkin lymphomas (NHL), and nasopharyngeal carcinomas.[11,12] EBV proteins expressed in these malignancies are EBNA-1, LMP-1 and LMP-2. In latency type I, found in EBV-positive Burkitt lymphoma and gastric adenocarcinomas, only EBNA-1 is expressed. However variants in which all EBNAs are expressed in the absence of LMP1 have also been desribed.[27]

The EBV proteins expressed during type III latency are involved in the transformation and growth of EBV-infected B cells. EBNA-1 binds to the origin of replication of the latent viral genome and is

Table 54–1 Frequently Determined EBV-Specific Antibodies

Antibody Specificity	Positive in IM (%)	Time of Appearance in IM	Persistence	Comments
Viral capsid antigen				
VCA-IgM	100	At clinical presentation	4–8 weeks	Highly sensitive and specific; of major diagnostic utility
VCA-IgG	100	At clinical presentation	Lifelong	Useful for documentation of past EBV infection
Early antigen				
Anti-D	70	Peaks 3–4 weeks after onset	3–6 months	Correlates with disease severity; seen in NPC patients
Anti-R	Low	2 weeks to several months after onset	2 months to >3 years	Occasionally seen with unusually severe cases; seen in African Burkitt lymphoma patients
EBNA	100	3–4 weeks after onset	Lifelong	Presence excludes primary EBV infection

EBNA, EBV nuclear antigen; EBV, Epstein–Barr virus; IM, infectious mononucleosis; NPC, nasopharyngeal carcinoma; VCA, viral capsid antigen.
Adapted from Schooley RT: Epstein–Barr virus (infectious mononucleosis). In Mandell GL, Bennett JE, Dolin R (eds.): Principles and Practice of Infectious Diseases. Philadelphia, Churchill Livingstone, 2000, p 1599.

responsible for the maintenance of the EBV episome in host B cells.[28] EBNA-2 upregulates the expression of the viral proteins LMP-1 and LMP-2 and cellular proteins that contribute to transformation. EBNAs-3A and -3C are essential for EBV-induced B-cell transformation, and although EBNA-3B is not essential for transformation it is highly conserved and therefore must provide a survival function in vivo.[29] EBNA-LP cooperates with EBNA-2 in the induction of viral and cellular genes. LMP-1, a viral oncogene, behaves like a constitutively activated CD40 molecule and is essential for EBV mediated B-cell transformation.[30] LMP-2 mimics an activated B-cell receptor (BCR) allowing for long-term B-cell survival in the absence of antigen. In addition it prevents the reactivation of EBV into the lytic phase of infection.[31]

In addition to EBV proteins, small nonpolyadenylated viral RNAs termed EBERs 1 and 2 and the BamHI-A rightward transcripts (BARTS) are expressed in all forms of latency. In addition, the expression of at least 17 distinct EBV-derived microRNAs has been reported.[32] The EBERs are the most abundant viral RNAs in latently infected cells. They enhance the oncogenic phenotype of EBV-transformed cells but are nonessential for EBV-mediated transformation.[33,34] The expression pattern of the microRNAs depends on the latency type and it is therefore likely that they play an important role during the life cycle of the virus.[32,35]

IMMUNE RESPONSE TO EBV

Healthy individuals mount vigorous humoral and cellular immune responses to primary EBV infection.[12,36] Although antibodies to the viral membrane proteins neutralize virus infectivity, the cellular immune response is essential for controlling virus-infected cells during both lytic and latent phases.

Humoral Immune Responses

Heterophile Antibodies

Heterophile antibodies, originally described by Paul and Bunnell, are present in 90%–95% of EBV infections at some point during the illness. However, in infants and children under the age of 4 with primary EBV infection, heterophile antibody responses are often not detected. Heterophile antibodies are IgM antibodies, which agglutinate erythrocytes from different species including bovine, camel, horse, goat, and sheep. EBV-induced heterophile antibodies have no reactivity against guinea pig kidney cells in contrast to naturally occurring antibodies (Forssmann antibodies) or antibodies present in patients with serum sickness and other conditions.

In addition to heterophile antibodies, cold agglutinins directed preferentially against the anti-I antigen on red cell membranes are frequently detected in the sera of IM patients; however, hemolytic anemia is rare. Other antibodies including anti-I, anti-N, Donath–Landsteiner antibodies, platelet antibodies and anti–smooth muscle antibodies have been described.

EBV-Specific Antibodies

EBV-specific antibody responses are detected with immunofluorescence assays developed in the first decades of EBV research. EBV antibodies are directed against (a) EBNA, (b) early antigen (EA), (c) the membrane antigen (MA) expressed on the surface of cells late in the lytic cycle, and (d) the viral capsid antigen (VCA) expressed within cells late in the lytic cycle.[37] Each antigen is a composite of several distinct viral proteins and attempts have been made to replace the above-mentioned assays with tests using specific viral proteins; however, no single test has attracted widespread use.

VCA-IgM and -IgG antibodies are usually present at the onset of clinical symptoms because of the prolonged viral incubation period (Table 54–1). VCA-IgM antibodies are a good marker for an acute infection because they rapidly disappear within 4 to 8 weeks. VCA-IgG antibodies persist for life and are commonly used to document prior EBV infection. IgG antibodies against EA are present at the onset of the clinical illness in approximately 70% of patients. EA antibodies are divided into methanol-sensitive (anti-D) and methanol-resistant (anti-R) antibodies, and the majority of EA antibodies detected are anti-D antibodies. The presence of anti-D antibodies is consistent with recent infection, because titers disappear after recovery. IgG antibodies to EBNA appear late in the course of almost all cases of EBV infection and persist throughout life and the presence early in a suspected case of primary EBV infection excludes the diagnosis. Aberrations in this pattern of serum reactivity are observed in many EBV-associated diseases and will be discussed under the specific disease sections. For example, the absence of EBNA antibodies despite previous EBV infection is one of the serologic markers suggestive for chronic active EBV infection (see section Chronic Active EBV Infection).

Cellular Immune Responses

In normal individuals primary EBV infection often results in a massive expansion of activated, antigen-specific T cells.[38–40] Using tetramer technology to enumerate antigen-specific T cells, it has been documented that the CD8 positive T-cell response may be dominated by T cells specific for a limited number of epitopes, as seen with T-cell responses against other herpesviruses.[40] T cells specific for epitopes derived from immediate early and several early EBV proteins of the lytic cycle are dominant during the acute phase of IM, and long-term persistence of EBV-specific, CD8-positive T cells has been documented after primary EBV infection.[12] As many as 5.5% of the circulating CD8-positive T cells in a healthy virus carrier may be positive for a single EBV epitope, illustrating how persistent EBV infection can influence the composition of the host's T-cell pool.[41] Besides EBV-specific CD8-positive T cells, EBV-specific CD4-positive T cells play an important role in the control of EBV infections, and EBNA-1-specific CD4-positive T cells have been implicated in the control of newly infected B cells.[42] As for CD8-positive T-cell responses there is a marked hierarchy of immunodominance, with the majority of CD4-positive T cells' responses directed against EBNA-1 and to a lesser extent against EBNA-3C.[43,44]

EBV VACCINE DEVELOPMENT

At present there is only limited experience with human EBV vaccines.[12,45] In one study, nine seronegative children in Southern China were vaccinated with a recombinant vaccinia virus expressing the major EBV viral glycoprotein gp350.[46] All nine patients developed neutralizing antibodies and six patients remained EBV-negative over a 16-month period in contrast to none of the 10 controls. Another vaccine trial with a gp350 subunit vaccine has been completed but efficacy data are not yet available.[12] Although potentially ideal for preventing EBV-associated malignancies, vaccines providing life-long immunity against primary EBV infection may not be feasible because the type of immunity required to avoid repeated infection through mucosal surfaces is not clearly defined. Moreover, a recent study suggests that the natural immune response to EBV is not sufficient to protect healthy EBV-positive individuals from repeated infections with different EBV strains.[47]

Vaccine strategies for the immunotherapy of EBV-associated malignancies should seek to elicit or boost the EBV-specific cellular immune response against EBV latency.[48] Individuals likely to benefit from this approach are EBV-seronegative patients scheduled to undergo solid organ transplantation or patients who have an EBV-associated malignancy with a low tumor burden or are in remission. In a recent study to evaluate the latter strategy, sixteen nasopharyngeal carcinoma (NPC) patients with local recurrence or distant metastasis after conventional therapies received injections of dendritic cells pulsed with peptides derived from LMP2, one of the EBV proteins expressed in NPC. Peptide-specific T-cell responses were elicited or boosted in nine patients and a partial tumor reduction was observed in two patients.[49] In another trial, EBV-seronegative, HLA-B8 positive individuals were vaccinated with an MHC class I-restricted EBV peptide epitope derived from EBV latent viral protein EBNA-3A; the peptide vaccine was well tolerated but immunologic and virologic studies are pending.[45]

In the past, EBV vaccine development was impeded by the lack of a suitable animal model. Most vaccination studies so far have been done in cottontop tamarins, a species of New World monkeys that develop B cell lymphomas after intraperitoneal injection of EBV.[50] This model lacks key features of human EBV disease such as oral transmission and long-term viral persistence, which are considered to be important for vaccine development. Since 1997 a rhesus monkey model for acute and persistent EBV infection is available that takes advantage of the rhesus lymphocryptovirus, which belongs to the same herpes virus subgroup as EBV.[51] This animal model reproduces the salient features of human EBV infection, such as oral transmission, lymphadenopathy, atypical lymphocytosis, serologic responses to EBV proteins, and viral latency in B cells. In the future, this model has the potential to become a useful platform to test different vaccination strategies.

INFECTIOUS MONONUCLEOSIS

Epidemiology

EBV infections occur worldwide and in most populations 90% to 95% of adults have antibodies against EBV. Depending on geographic and socioeconomic factors, there is a wide variation in the age of primary EBV infections. Early, asymptomatic primary EBV infection occurs in individuals from lower socioeconomic groups and in third world countries. In higher socioeconomic groups in industrialized countries, the age of primary infection is often delayed until the second decade of life and clinically apparent IM is more prevalent.

Humans are the only source of EBV. EBV is present in the saliva of IM patients. A majority of EBV-positive adults shed virus into their saliva and this percentage is increased in immunocompromised patients such as solid organ transplant recipients. EBV is viable outside the body for 2 weeks at 4°C but is susceptible to drying; the virus has not been recovered from environmental sources, suggesting that close contact is needed for viral spread. The incubation period of IM is estimated to be 30 to 50 days.

Table 54–2 Clinical Manifestations of Infectious Mononucleosis

Manifestation	Percentage (Range)
Symptoms	
Sore throat	82 (70–88)
Malaise	57 (43–76)
Headache	51 (37–55)
Anorexia	21 (10–27)
Myalgias	20 (12–22)
Chills	16 (9–18)
Abdominal discomfort	9 (2–14)
Signs	
Lymphadenopathy	94 (93–100)
Pharyngitis	84 (69–91)
Fever	76 (63–100)
Splenomegaly	52 (50–63))
Hepatomegaly	12 (6–14)
Palatal enanthem	11 (5–13)
Rash	10 (0–15)
Jaundice	9 (4–10)

Adapted from Schooley RT: Epstein–Barr virus (infectious mononucleosis). In Mandell GL, Bennett JE, Dolin R (eds.): Principles and Practice of Infectious Diseases. Philadelphia, Churchill Livingstone, 2000, p 1599.

Clinical Manifestations

Primary EBV infection in infants and young children either is asymptomatic or accompanied by mild, nonspecific symptoms and signs such as fever, upper respiratory tract infection, pharyngitis with or without tonsillitis, and cervical lymphadenopathy. In contrast, approximately 50% of adolescents and young adults present with the clinical picture of IM. Frequently, a prodrome consisting of fatigue, malaise and low-grade fever is present for 1 to 2 weeks. Prominent pharyngitis with exudative tonsillitis is often the cardinal sign of IM; other signs and symptoms are listed in Table 54–2.[36,52] The adenopathy in IM most commonly affects the posterior cervical lymph nodes although diffuse adenopathy can occur. The enlarged lymph nodes are not fixed, may be tender to palpation, and lack overlying skin erythema. Hepatomegaly is uncommon; however splenomegaly develops in more than 50% of patients and is more prominent in the second to fourth week of the illness. Skin manifestations include a faint, morbilliform rash reminiscent of rubella and less commonly erythema multiforme and erythema nodosum. Most patients with primary EBV infection have symptoms for 2 to 4 weeks and recover without significant complication s or sequelae.

Complications of Primary EBV Infections

The incidence of complications associated with primary EBV infection is low, although any organ system can be affected.[53]

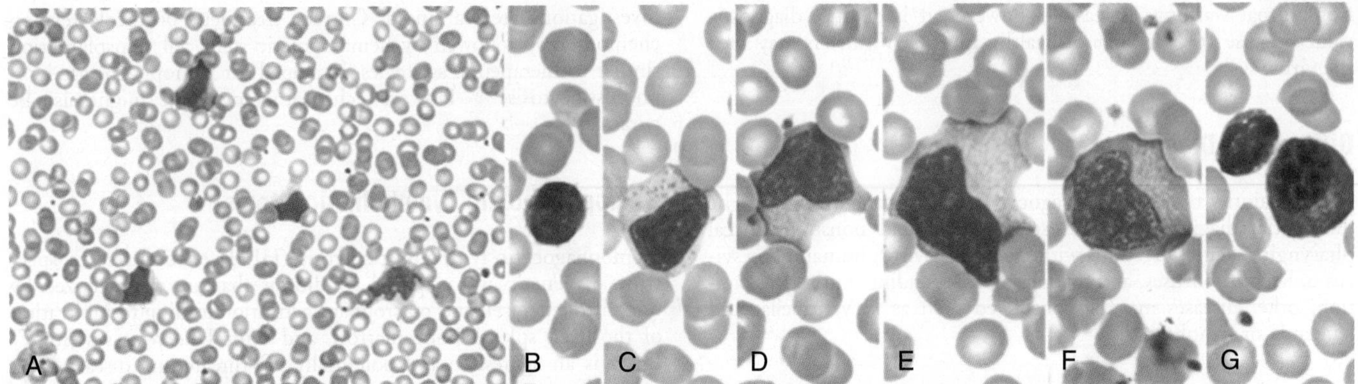

Figure 54–3 Peripheral blood smear in infectious mononucleosis (**A–G**). Low power (**A**) shows moderately high white blood cell count and high number of reactive, or "atypical" lymphocytes. Higher power (**B–G**) illustrates spectrum of lymphoid morphology, including small resting lymphocyte (**B**) for comparison, large granular lymphocyte (**C**), atypical forms (**D**, **E**, **F**), also referred to as "reactive" lymphs, and circulating plasma cell (**G**).

Hematologic Complications

Patients with IM may present with a wide range of hematologic findings besides the atypical lymphocytosis (Fig. 54–3). These include anemia, neutropenia, thrombocytopenia, and rare cases of aplastic anemia.[54]

Anemia

Autoimmune hemolytic anemia occurs in approximately 3% of patients with IM. It presents in the first 2 weeks of the illness, and the majority of patients recover within 1 to 2 months. Patients usually have a positive direct Coombs test. Most common anti-I antibodies are present; however anti-I, anti-N and Donath-Landsteiner antibodies have also been reported. In addition to hemolysis, IM-associated anemia can be caused by erythroblastopenia.

Neutropenia

Mild, self-limiting neutropenia is a common finding during the first 4 weeks of the disease. However severe neutropenia associated with fatal bacterial infections has been reported.

Thrombocytopenia

Mild thrombocytopenia (50,000–150,000/mm^3) is a common finding in patients with IM. It usually occurs within the first 2 weeks of presentation and resolves within 2 months. Severe thrombocytopenia with overt bleeding is rare; however, death from intracranial hemorrhage has been described. The etiology of the thrombocytopenia is not completely resolved, and a variety of explanations have been suggested. Because bone marrow examination shows normal or increased numbers of megakaryocytes, peripheral platelet destruction is most likely due to the presence of antiplatelet antibodies or platelet pooling and destruction within an enlarged spleen.

Splenic Rupture

Splenic rupture occurs predominately in males with an incidence of 1/1000 to 1/3000. The incidence of rupture is highest in the second and third week of illness and can be the first sign of IM. Clinical symptoms include abdominal pain or pain referred to either shoulder. Because abdominal pain is an unusual symptom of uncomplicated IM, a splenic rupture should be strongly considered in IM cases whenever abdominal pain is reported. Although a life-threatening complication, with current management the mortality rate is very low.[55]

Neurologic

Neurologic complications develop usually during the first 2 weeks of IM and can be the only manifestation of IM. EBV infection can cause a wide spectrum of neurologic diseases; including encephalitis, meningitis, Guillain–Barre syndrome, acute transverse myelitis, and peripheral neuritis. Patients with neurologic complications have an excellent outcome, with most patients having a complete recovery.

Other Organs

Although symptomatic heart disease with IM is uncommon, in one cohort of patients, unspecific ST- and T-wave abnormalities were found in 6% of patients. Renal involvement manifested as microscopic hematuria and proteinuria is seen in 10% to 15% of patients; however significant renal dysfunction is rare. Airway compromise due to hypertrophy of the adenoids and tonsils or mucosal inflammation and edema is uncommon but potentially fatal.

Diagnosis

Atypical lymphocytosis is the cardinal hematologic finding in IM (see Fig. 54–3).[54] It develops during the first week of the illness and peaks between the second and third week. Atypical lymphocytes represent 60% to 70% of the total white cell count, which ranges between 12,000/mm^3 and 18,000/mm^3. In general, the atypical lymphocytes are large and vary in size. Nuclei are large and eccentrically placed; the cytoplasm is basophilic and vacuoles are often present. The variable morphologic pattern of atypical lymphocytes in IM distinguishes them from the monotonous appearance of immature leukemic blasts. Atypical lymphocytosis is not pathognomonic for IM and is associated with other diseases like acute viral hepatitis, cytomegalovirus infections, mumps, toxoplasmosis, rubella, roseola, and drug reactions.

The diagnosis of EBV infection depends on serologic testing.[56] Tests for heterophile antibodies, including the monospot test and slide agglutination tests, are routinely available. The results of these tests are often negative in children less than 4 years of age, but they identify 90% of cases in older children and adults. Of the available EBV-specific serologic tests, VCA-IgM antibodies are most commonly determined to diagnose primary EBV infection in heterophile-negative IM cases; determining antibodies against EA may also be helpful (Table 54–1). VCA-IgG antibodies are positive during an acute infections as well as the convalescent period. The presence of anti-EBNA antibodies excludes an acute infection.[37] Isolation of EBV from throat washings is feasible; however, it is of little diagnostic value because 10% to 20% of healthy adult EBV carriers may shed the virus.

Differential Diagnosis

In the majority of cases, the diagnosis of IM is straightforward. The differential diagnosis includes streptococcal and nonstreptococcal pharyngitis, acute infections with cytomegalovirus, human herpesvirus 6, hepatitis viruses, and toxoplasma. Depending on the presentation, other diseases may be considered such as HIV, rubella, and leukemia or lymphoma.

Treatment

Supportive therapy should include rest and analgesia in the acute stage of IM. Contact sports should be avoided until the patient has fully recovered and the spleen is no longer palpable. The use of corticosteroids is not indicated for uncomplicated IM; however, a trial of corticosteroids is warranted in patients with marked tonsillar inflammation and hypertrophy resulting in impending airway obstruction.[57] Although acyclovir reduces EBV shedding into oral secretions, treatment of IM with acyclovir has resulted in no clinical benefit.[58,59]

OTHER EBV-ASSOCIATED DISEASES

Most individuals recover from the acute phase of primary EBV infection with no long-term sequelae. In a minority of patients, a chronic disease follows the acute phase of IM. Mild/moderate chronic active EBV infections (CAEBV) present with fever, malaise, arthralgia, myalgia, and lymphadenopathy.[60] To establish the diagnosis of CAEBV, patients must have (a) signs and symptoms for at least 6 months and (b) an abnormal EBV serology with high antibody titers of VCA-IgG and EA-IgG and little or no antibodies against EBNA. Affected individuals may also have measurable EA-messenger-RNA or EBV-DNA in the peripheral blood, serum, or affected tissues. The life-threatening form of CAEBV is characterized by high fevers, hepatosplenomegaly, and extensive lymphadenopathy, followed by hepatic, cardiac, or pulmonary dysfunction.[61] These patients have very high EBV-VCA titers and EBV-DNA levels in their peripheral blood. Although EBV usually resides in B cells, in severe CAEBV either T cells or natural killer (NK) cells are infected, predisposing to lethal T-cell or NK-cell lymphomas.[62,63] Severe, often fatal CAEBV is more common in Japan, whereas mild/moderate CAEBV is more common in the western hemisphere. These patients do not have mutations in the SH2D1A gene (see section X-Linked Lymphoproliferative Disease) and the etiology of CAEBV remains poorly understood.[64] No effective therapy is available; however, sporadic clinical improvements of mild/moderate CAEBV have been reported after infusion of interleukin 2, high-dose immunoglobulin, antiviral drugs, anti–tumor necrosis factor (TNF)-α antibodies or steroids. We have infused autologous EBV-specific CTL in five patients with mild or moderate CAEBV, because of the successful use of donor-derived EBV-specific CTL for the prophylaxis and therapy of EBV-associated lymphoproliferative disease after hematopoietic stem cell transplantation (see section Lymphoproliferative Disease). Infusion of EBV-specific CTL resulted in resolution of fatigue, malaise, fever, lymphadenopathy and splenomegaly. Four of five patients had responses lasting from 6 to 36 months of follow-up, with 1 patient having recurrence of fatigue and myalgia 12 months after CTL therapy.[65] These results suggest that the infusion of EBV-specific CTL may play a role in the treatment of mild or moderate CAEBV; however, larger number of patients need to be treated with longer follow-up. For severe CAEBV in which EBV resides in the T- or NK-cell compartment, the use of EBV-specific CTL has been investigated anecdotally without encouraging results; nevertheless, further investigations are warranted. Current treatment protocols rely on chemotherapy followed by hematopoietic stem cell transplantation similar to therapeutic strategies developed for hemophagocytic lymphohistiocytosis.[66,67] However, chemotherapy alone might also be curative.[68]

Hemophagocytic Lymphohistiocytosis

Hemophagocytic lymphohistiocytosis (HLH) encompasses a spectrum of genetic and acquired conditions that are characterized by uncontrolled T-cell and macrophage activation leading to infiltration of the liver, spleen, bone marrow, and central nervous system.[69,70] HLH is an aggressive and potentially life-threatening disease most often affecting infants from birth to 18 months of age, but cases of older children and adults have been reported. Familial HLH is a heterogeneous genetic disorder and in the majority of patients the genetic defect is not yet defined. Twenty to 40% of familial HLH cases are caused by mutations in the perforin gene.[71] Ten percent of cases are linked to chromosome 9q21.3-q22, and in addition male patients with HLH have been described who harbor germline mutations in SH2D1A, the gene responsible for X-linked lymphoproliferative disease.[72] Secondary HLH is caused by a variety of infectious agents, including viruses like EBV, CMV, and Parvovirus B19, bacteria, fungi, and parasites. EBV-associated HLH (EBV-HLH) is more commonly seen in the Japanese and Chinese population and is not associated with perforin or SH2D1A gene mutations.[73] In EBV-HLH CD8-positive T cells are infected with EBV in contrast to CAEBV, where CD4-positive T cells or NK cells are infected.[74]

Because there is no definitive diagnostic test for HLH, the International Histiocyte Society has developed criteria for establishing the diagnosis. The patient must have (a) fever, (b) cytopenia (two of three lineages), (c) splenomegaly, (d) hypertriglyceridemia and/or hypofibrinogemia, and (e) hemophagocytosis. Without aggressive therapy, familial HLH is uniformly fatal and high mortality rates have also been reported for secondary HLH. Curative treatment relies on hematopoietic stem cell transplantation.[75,76] The current treatment protocol of the International Histiocyte Society results in a 3-year survival rate of 62%. It consists of initial therapy with decadron, cyclosporine A, etoposide (VP16), and in selected patients intrathecal methotrexate; once the disease is in remission a hematopoietic stem cell transplantation from matched related and unrelated donors is performed.[75]

X-Linked Lymphoproliferative Disease

Mutations or deletions in the SH2D1A (src homology 2 domain protein 1A) result in X-linked lymphoproliferative disease (XLP; Duncan disease), an immunodeficiency characterized by fatal IM, agammaglobulinemia, or B-cell lymphoma.[77,78] SH2D1A interacts with SLAM (signaling lymphocyte activation molecule), which plays a central role in the stimulation of B and T cells. SH2D1A controls several distinct key T-cell signaling pathways, and mutant SH2D1A does not bind SLAM, suggesting that it is a natural SLAM inhibitor. Following infection with EBV, XLP patients mount a vigorous, uncontrolled polyclonal expansion of T and B cells. Infiltrating T cells cause extensive tissue destruction of the liver and bone marrow, resulting in death in 50% of XLP patients during primary EBV infection. Approximately 30% of patients have acquired hypogammaglobulinemia and 25% of patients develop malignant B-cell lymphomas that are often extranodal, involving the intestinal ileocecal region. It is important to realize that some patients with SH2D1A mutations may only present with hypogammaglobulinemia mimicking common variable immunodeficiency and a diagnosis of XLP should be considered when more than one male patient with hypogammaglobulinemia is encountered in the same family.[79] Currently, the only curative therapy for XLP is hematopoietic stem cell transplantation.[80–82]

Oral Hairy Leukoplakia

Oral hairy leukoplakia (OHL) develops frequently, although not exclusively, in HIV-positive patients.[83] It is a nonmalignant hyperplasia of epithelial cells and most patients present with white, corrugated lesions on the tongue. OHL besides IM is the only EBV-associated disease in which active viral replication is apparent and multiple strains are often present within the same lesion. Inhibiting EBV replication in vivo with antivirals such as valacyclovir results in resolution of OHL. However, after valacyclovir treatment, EBV replication recurs in normal tongue epithelial cells, indicating that productive EBV replication is necessary but not sufficient to induce OHL.[84]

EBV-Associated Malignancies

Over the past decades, EBV has been associated with a heterogeneous group of malignancies. Although there is strong circumstantial evidence linking EBV to these malignancies, the potential causative relationship between EBV and these tumors remains to be firmly established. The following section focuses on EBV-associated lymphoproliferative disease, Hodgkin disease, NHL including Burkitt lymphoma, and nasopharyngeal carcinoma. All EBV-associated malignancies are associated with viral latency, and spontaneous viral replication occurs at a very low frequency. Because antiviral agents, like acyclovir, only prevent viral replication and do not affect latency, these agents are of limited therapeutic value.[85]

Lymphoproliferative Disease

EBV-LPD develops in patients with congenital or acquired immunodeficiencies, including severe combined immunodeficiency, XLP, HIV infection, and immunosuppression in recipients of solid organ transplants (SOT) or hematopoietic stem cell (HSC) transplants.[86,87] Besides EBV and a dysfunctional cellular immune system, genetic alterations in B cells have also been implicated in the pathogenesis of PTLD, especially in SOT recipients, including microsatellite instability, DNA hypermethylation, aberrant somatic hypermutation and mutations in specific genes such as MYCC, BCL-6, N-ras, and p53.[88] Most cases of EBV-LPD are lymphomas of B-cell origin, histologic high-grade NHL of the immunoblastic or undifferentiated large cell type that respond poorly to cytotoxic therapy.[89] In the setting of solid organ transplantation, the reported incidence of EBV-LPD ranges from 1% to 25%, with the highest risk in seronegative recipients, patients receiving intensive immunosuppressive therapy, and patients receiving grafts with a high lymphoid content.[90] After HSC transplantation, the incidence of EBV-LPD varies with the transplant regimen and may be as high as 25%. Risk factors for the development of EBV-LPD include the use of stem cells from an HLA-mismatched family member or closely HLA-matched unrelated donor, T-cell depletion of the donor cells, intensive immunosuppression, and an underlying diagnosis of primary immunodeficiency.[91] The incidence is much lower when methods that also deplete B cells are employed.[92] The onset of EBV-LPD seems to be preceded by a large increase in virus load as well as the proliferation of EBV-infected B cells. Frequent monitoring of the EBV-DNA load in peripheral blood is a valuable diagnostic test for early detection of EBV-LPD after HSC or solid organ transplantation. The threshold level of EBV-DNA suggestive of impending EBV-LPD varies according to the PCR method of quantifying viral DNA.[93–95] However, it should be emphasized that not all patients with high EBV-DNA levels, especially those with a solid organ transplant, develop EBV-LPD. Several distinct patterns of EBV latent gene expression have been identified in the memory B cells of high-load EBV carriers, with type III latency conferring the highest risk for EBV-LPD development.[96] Besides EBV-DNA levels, determining the frequency of EBV-specific T cells or the functionality of T cells in patients with high EBV-DNA load might also assist in identifying patients who are at increased risk for developing EBV-LPD.[97,98] In addition, host factors like polymorphisms in the promoter regions of cytokines have been implicated in increasing the risk of developing EBV-LPD.[99] Thus, an elevated EBV-DNA load can lead to early diagnosis of EBV-LPD, with consequent reductions in mortality and treatment-related morbidity, although additional results such as clinical signs and symptoms as well as radiographic findings must be taken into account before therapy is initiated.

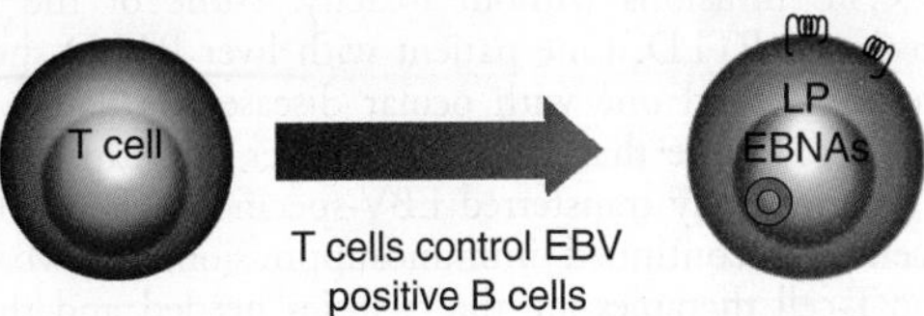

Figure 54–4 Treatment strategies for Epstein–Barr virus-associated lymphoproliferative diseases (EBV-LPD). For explanation of symbols see Fig. 54–1.

Treatment of Lymphoproliferative Disease

A variety of treatment approaches have been explored for EBV-LPD (Fig. 54–4).[86,100] These include (a) conventional chemotherapy, (b) reduction or withdrawal of immunosuppression, (c) adoptive transfer of T cells or EBV-specific cytotoxic T cells (CTL), and (d) infusion of monoclonal antibodies. Other potential strategies include the use hydroxyurea to eradicate EBV episomes or inducing the lytic cycle of EBV so that the lymphoma cells become sensitive to ganciclovir.[101–103] In solid organ transplant recipients, simple withdrawal of immune suppression can result in the regression of localized EBV-LPD by allowing recovery of the suppressed cellular immune system.[104] This approach is limited by the risk of graft rejection, nor is it useful post-HSC transplant because of the profound immunosuppression and the risk of inducing graft-versus-host disease (GVHD). Donor T-cell infusions have been used successfully to treat EBV-LPD post-HSC transplantation but carry the inherent risk of GVHD.[105] One strategy to prevent GHVD after T-cell infusion is the administration of donor-derived ex vivo expanded polyclonal EBV-specific CTL.[106,107] To determine whether adoptive transfer of donor-derived EBV-specific CTL is effective prophylaxis for EBV-LPD, EBV-specific CTL lines were infused into 56 recipients of HSC transplant.[106,108] Infused CTL induced no GVHD, survived long-term, and reconstituted immunity against EBV, and no infused patient developed EBV-LPD compared with an incidence of 11.5% in a comparable untreated control group. Immunotherapy with EBV-specific CTL was also used to treat six HSC transplant recipients who developed overt lymphoma. Five of these patients responded well with complete regression of bulky tumors, although infused CTL caused inflammation at the tumor site. One of the responders had central nervous system (CNS) PTLD, indicating that EBV-specific CTL can cross the blood–brain barrier to eradicate CNS lesions.[102] One patient died of progressive disease, a failure attributed to a deletion in the EBV protein EBNA-3B in the tumor virus causing resistance to killing by the infused CTL.[109]

In solid organ transplant recipients who develop EBV-LPD, donor-derived T cells are of limited value, because the tumor almost always arises in recipient B cells and donor T cells are unlikely to survive in the recipient's hematopoietic system.[110] Initial studies using autologous or partly HLA-matched EBV-specific CTL for the treatment or prevention of EBV-LPD after SOT have shown promising results but need further investigation.[111–113] In our study, twelve SOT recipients at high risk for EBV-LPD, or with active disease, received autologous CTL infusions without toxicity. None of the treated patients developed PTLD. One patient with liver PTLD showed a complete response, and one with ocular disease has had a partial response stable for more than 1 year. However, the expansion and persistence of adoptively transferred EBV-specific CTL was limited in the presence of continued immunosuppression. Drawbacks of EBV-specific T-cell therapies are the facilities needed and the time required (3–4 months) for CTL production. Thus, reliable predictive parameters are needed to select patients who are at high risk for developing EBV-LPD allowing the early initiation of CTL lines.

In addition to cellular immunotherapy, monoclonal antibodies have been used for the treatment of EBV-LPD. Of 58 patients treated with CD21 and CD24 murine monoclonal antibodies in an European multicenter study, 35 (61%) entered complete remission, but these antibodies are no longer available.[114] Rituximab, a humanized CD20 monoclonal antibody, has been used successfully for the treatment of EBV-LPD as for other NHLs.[14,15,115] In a multicenter retrospective analysis of 32 patients with EBV-LPD developing after solid organ or HSC transplantation, rituximab was well tolerated and the overall response rate was 69%, with 20 complete responses and 2 partial responses.[14] These findings have been recently confirmed in a prospective, multicenter Phase II study for SOT patients with biopsy-proven PTLD.[15] Forty-three patients were treated with four weekly infusions of 375 mg/m^2 rituximab. At day 80, 86% of patients were alive and the response rate was 44.2%, including 12 complete responses/complete responses unconfirmed. The overall survival rate was 67% at 1 year. Other centers have reported similar results, with response rates ranging from 20% to 100%.[116,117] Besides B-cell antibodies, interleukin 6 monoclonal antibodies have been used successfully to treat EBV-LPD after solid organ transplantation.[118] Despite these promising results, the overall efficacy of monoclonal antibodies in the treatment of EBV-LPD after solid organ transplantation remains difficult to assess, because the majority of studies lacked controls and were confounded by other therapeutic interventions. As with T-cell therapies for EBV-LPD, the success of monoclonal antibodies will most likely depend on early diagnosis and intervention. Currently, the use of Rituximab seems to be a reasonable alternative in clinical situations where patients present with bulky disease, or EBV-specific CTL are not available.

EBV-Positive Hodgkin Disease and Non-Hodgkin Lymphomas

EBV is associated with Hodgkin disease as well as non-Hodgkin lymphomas (NHLs) in immunocompetent patients.[119,120] All EBV lymphomas are associated with the virus latent cycle (see Fig. 54–2). The majority of EBV-associated lymphomas in immunocompetent patients are latency type II and express EBNA-1, LMP-1 and LMP-2 except for Burkitt lymphoma, which is latency type I and only expresses EBNA-1.

Hodgkin Disease

Hodgkin disease is a malignant neoplasm of lymphoreticular cell origin and 40–50% of cases in immunocompetent individuals are associated with expression of EBV derived antigens in malignant Reed-Sternberg (H-RS) cells and their variants (see Fig. 54–5A,B).[121,122] EBV positive Hodgkin disease is more commonly seen in young children and in less developed countries. EBV association with Hodgkin disease differs by histologic subtype, being highest with the mixed-cellularity subtype. Evidence linking EBV to the pathogenesis of Hodgkin disease include the findings that (a) every H-RS cell in a EBV-positive tumor mass carries the virus and (b) the EBV genome is clonal, indicating that the malignant H-RS cells originated from a single EBV-infected cell. In addition LMP-1, one of the EBV proteins expressed in H-RS cells, activates the transcription factor NF-κB, which is thought to a play an important role in the pathogenesis of Hodgkin disease. EBV-positive HD patients also differ in their antibody response to the major EBV-associated antigens in comparison to healthy controls. The overall outcome of EBV-positive and EBV-negative Hodgkin disease is similar; with combination chemotherapy and radiation, the prognosis is excellent for low-stage disease and overall survival rate for advanced-stage disease are between 65% and 80%. Depending on age and histologic subtype, the presence of EBV might be associated with better survival.[123]

Non-Hodgkin Lymphomas

NHLs expressing type II latency include large B-cell lymphoma, CD30$^+$ Ki-1$^+$ anaplastic large cell lymphoma (ALCL) of B-cell type, T cell-rich B-cell NHLs and lymphatoid granulomatosis. The association of these lymphomas with EBV varies, ranging from 10% to 95%.[124–126]

EBV-associated NK/T-cell lymphomas include extranodal NK/T-cell lymphoma (nasal type), angioimmunoblastic lymphoma, and large granular lymphocyte (LGL) leukemia/lymphoma (NK- or T-cell type).[127,128] Between 30% and 100% of these lymphomas are EBV-positive, expressing a type II latency pattern. In addition, severe chronic active EBV (SCAEBV) infection of NK/T-cell type has been associated with fulminant forms of lymphoma, which are >95% positive for EBV.[62,129] The overall outcome of EBV-associated NHL depends on histologic subtype and risk factors present at diagnosis, but most are high-grade malignancies with an unfavorable prognosis using current treatment modalities.[125,130–132]

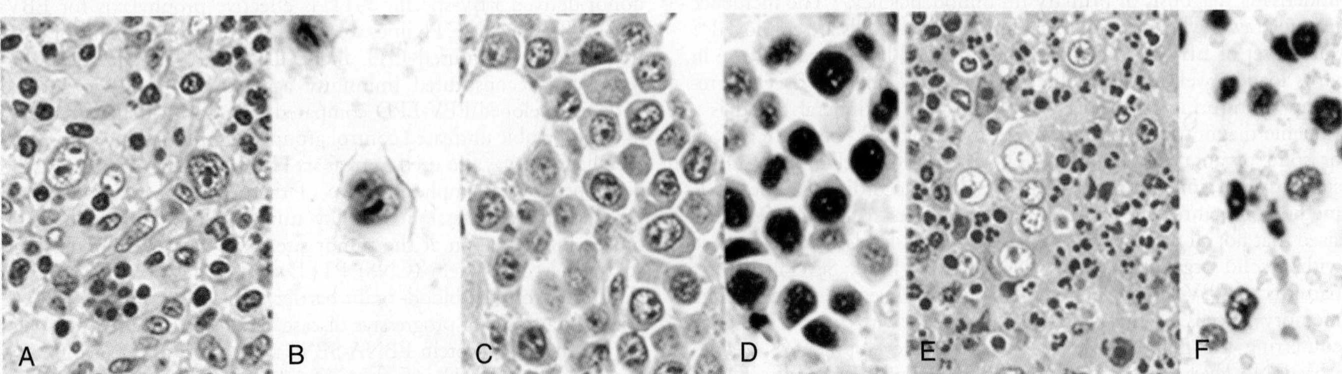

Figure 54–5 Examples of Epstein–Barr virus (EBV)-positive malignancies: Hodgkin lymphoma, nasopharyngeal carcinoma, and large B-cell lymphoma (**A–F**). Hodgkin lymphoma (**A**) and EBV-positive Reed–Sternberg cells (**B**). Large B-cell lymphoma (plasmablastic type) in an HIV+ patient (**C**), diffusely EBV-positive (**D**). Nasopharyngeal carcinoma (**E**), EBV-positive (**F**). (Note: all EBV studies are in situ hybridizations for EBV mRNA, EBER).

Adoptive Immunotherapy for EBV-Positive Hodgkin Disease and Non-Hodgkin Lymphomas in Immunocompetent Individuals

In contrast to EBV-LPD only a limited number of EBV-derived antigens, EBNA-1, LMP-1, and LMP-2, are present in EBV-positive Hodgkin disease and NHL. Nevertheless, EBV-specific CTL have been used to treat 20 patients with EBV-positive Hodgkin disease.[133–135] CTL localized to tumor sites, persisted for prolonged periods of time, and produced resolution of B symptoms. After CTL infusion, five patients were in complete remission at up to 40 months, two of whom had measurable disease at the time of CTL infusion. One additional patient had a partial response, and five had stable disease.[134] Although these results are encouraging, the antitumor activity of infused CTL was lower than in HSCT recipients treated for EBV-LPD. This lack of efficacy could be due in part to immunosuppressive factors secreted by H-RS cells or may simply be quantitative in that the method used for EBV-specific CTL generation produces CTL lines that are dominated by clones reactive to viral proteins not expressed in Hodgkin disease. To improve CTL efficacy, methods to expand CTL specific for the EBV proteins LMP1 and LMP2 expressed in Hodgkin disease and to genetically modify the expanded CTL to render them resistant against inhibitory cytokines have been developed.[48,136–139] The safety and efficacy of LMP2-specific CTL have been evaluated in patients with EBV-positive Hodgkin disease and EBV latency type II NHL.[140] So far 14 patients have been infused and we have observed an increase in the frequency of infused CTL in 8 of 10 evaluable patients. In addition, LMP2-specific CTLs were detected at tumor sites. Of six patients with detectable disease at the time of CTL infusion, five had clinical responses. These results indicate that LMP2-specific CTLs are safe, accumulate at tumor sites, and have antitumor activity.

EBV-Associated Non-Hodgkin Lymphoma in HIV Patients

Patients infected with HIV are at high risk to develop NHL. The incidence increases with age and the male-to-female ratio is approximately 2 : 1. Depending on certain histologic features, the EBV association ranges from 30% in systemic HIV-related Burkitt lymphoma (HIV-BL) to 70% to 80% in HIV-related immunoblastic lymphoma (HIV-IBL), and virtually all cases of primary central nervous system lymphoma (PCNSL) are EBV positive.[141–143] In biopsies of EBV-associated HIV-NHL, there is considerable variation in the number of EBV-positive cells, and the pattern of EBV latent gene expression varies among tumor types as in immunocompetent individuals (see Fig. 54–5C,D) . In HIV-infected patients, the development of EBV-associated HIV-NHL is preceded by a loss of functional EBV-specific CTL, suggesting that strategies to boost the endogenous EBV-specific T-cell response might prevent lymphomas.[144,145] Restoring CD4-positive T-cell counts in HIV patients with highly active retroviral therapy (HAART) has decreased the incidence of PCNSL and HIV-NHL.[146,147] The clinical experience with T-cell therapy for EBV-associated HIV-NHL is limited.

Burkitt Lymphoma

Burkitt lymphoma (BL) is a high-grade malignant small noncleaved B-cell lymphoma.[131] Histology usually reveals a "starry-sky" pattern resulting from numerous benign macrophages that have ingested apoptotic tumor cells. Although almost all endemic BLs in equatorial Africa are associated with EBV, the virus has been implicated less often in sporadic cases and in the United States only 20% of BL are EBV positive. In developing countries, an intermediate type of BL has been described, both in its clinical presentation and association with EBV, which varies from 25% to 80%. As with NPC and Hodgkin disease, there is strong circumstantial evidence linking EBV to BL. The EBV genome is clonal as in other EBV-associated maligancies.[148] The majority of BLs carry a translocation between the long arm of chromosome 8, the site of the MYCC oncogene (8q24), and the Ig heavy chain region on chromosome 14, t(8;14).[133] Although the t(8;14) translocation is seen in endemic as well as sporadic BLs, the exact location of the chromosomal breakpoints on chromosome 8 and 14 differ.[149] Other chromosomal translocations seen in BLs are between MYCC and the κ-light chain locus on chromosome 2, t(2;8), or the λ-light chain locus on chromosome 22, t(8;22).

Current treatment strategies rely on intensive chemotherapy, and overall survival depends on extent of disease at presentation, being 90% to 100% for local and 60% to 70% for advanced disease. The prospect for the development of an EBV-specific immunotherapy for BLs is problematic because lymphoma cells evade the immune system by downregulating the expression of EBV latency antigens, cell adhesion molecules, and MHC class I molecules. EBNA-1, the only EBV protein expressed in BL, autoregulates its own translation and inhibits HLA class I presentation because of an internal glycine-alanine repeat region.[150,151] However, the characterization of EBNA-1-specific CD4-positive T cells as well as rare CD8-positive T cells that can recognize BL through EBNA-1 has provided impetus to explore the role of CD4-positive T cells in the control and therapy of BL.[42–44,152] In addition, EBNA-1-specific CD4-positive T cells had potent antitumor activity in a murine model of Burkitt lymphoma.[153]

Nasopharyngeal Carcinoma

Nasopharyngeal carcinoma (NPC) arises from the epithelial cells of the nasopharynx. The WHO classifies NPC into keratinizing squamous cell carcinoma (type 1), nonkeratinizing carcinoma (type 2), and undifferentiated carcinoma (type 3, most common). Type 2 and 3 carcinomas are associated with EBV (see Fig. 54–5E,F); however, environmental and genetic factors play an important role in oncogenesis, because the incidence of NPC varies 50- to 100-fold from Southern China to western countries.[11,154] EBV was initially linked to NPC by the observation that patients had elevated levels of VCA-IgG, VCA-IgA, and EA-IgG antibodies. Further studies showed that EBV-DNA is present in every tumor cell of type 2 and 3 carcinomas with remarkable consistency. As in Hodgkin disease, the EBV episome in an individual tumor is clonal.[155]

EBV antibody responses have been used to follow tumor burden in NPC patients; in addition, VCA-IgA antibodies and antibodies against EBV DNAse are predictive for NPC in high-risk populations.[156] More recently, detection of EBV-DNA in serum by different PCR methods has shown to be useful for the diagnosis, prognosis, and monitoring of NPC patients.[157] Most NPC patients are treated with radiation. Other modalities such as surgery, chemotherapy, and combined approaches may be appropriate in selected circumstances and a detailed discussion is beyond the scope of this chapter. In NPC, as for EBV-positive lymphomas, only a limited number of EBV latent antigens are expressed. A therapeutic vaccine study targeting LMP2 has been conducted and the results of this trial were discussed in the section EBV Vaccine Development. Three groups of investigators have reported on the use of autologous EBV-specific CTL for the adoptive immunotherapy of patients with recurrent/refractory NPC.[158–161] In one study, four NPC patients with advanced disease were infused and an increase in EBV-specific CTL precursor frequency was observed as well as a reduction in plasma EBV-DNA levels. No decrease in tumor size was observed; however, all patients had a large tumor burden.[158] In the second study, 10 patients were treated with EBV-specific CTL and in 6 of 10 patients, control of disease progression was achieved.[160] We have evaluated the use of EBV-specific CTL in patients with refractory or high-risk NPC in two Phase I clinical studies.[159,161] In the first clinical study, EBV-specific CTL was given alone and in the second clinical trial patients received a monoclonal antibody prior to CTL infusion to enhance T-cell expansion in vivo. Patients with EBV-positive NPC were eligible if they had recurrent, locally advanced-stage disease or metastatic disease. To date, 21 patients have received CTL and completed their evaluation. Six patients were in remission at the time of EBV-specific CTL infusion and remain in remission 6 to 50 months post-CTL infusion. In the 15 NPC patients with active disease, we have observed responses in 10 of 15 patients; 4 patients are in complete remission 12 to 42 months after CTL infusion. Of the other 11 patients, 4 had stable disease (2–32 months), 1 had a partial response (12 months), and 6 had progressive disease. As for the adoptive immunotherapy for EBV-positive Hodgkin disease and NHL, current efforts are focused in increasing the frequency of LMP1- and LMP2-specific T cells in the CTL product and rendering T cells resistant to inhibitory factors secreted by NPCs such a Fas ligand.[162,163]

SUMMARY

Since its discovery in 1964, EBV has been linked to a heterogeneous group of diseases. EBV was the first human virus implicated in oncogenesis and the biology of the virus has been studied extensively on a cellular and molecular level. Over the last decade, successful immunotherapeutic approaches have been developed for EBV-associated lymphoproliferative disease using either monoclonal antibodies or the adoptive transfer of EBV-specific T cells. Further insights into the function of EBV proteins and host–virus interactions hold the promise of improving the outcome of patients with EBV-associated diseases in the future.

SUGGESTED READINGS

Bollard CM, Aguilar L, Straathof KC, et al: Cytotoxic T lymphocyte therapy for Epstein-Barr virus+ Hodgkin's disease. J Exp Med 200:1623, 2004.

Cohen JI: Epstein-Barr virus infection. N Engl J Med 343:481, 2000.

Gottschalk S, Rooney CM, Heslop HE: Post-transplant lymphoproliferative disorders. Annu Rev Med 56:29, 2005.

Heslop HE: Biology and treatment of Epstein-Barr virus-associated non-Hodgkin lymphomas. Hematology (Am Soc Hematol Educ Program) 260, 2005.

Heslop HE, Ng CYC, Li C, et al: Long-term restoration of immunity against Epstein-Barr virus infection by adoptive transfer of gene-modified virus-specific T lymphocytes. Nat Med 2:551, 1996.

Loren AW, Porter DL, Stadtmauer EA, et al: Post-transplant lymphoproliferative disorder: A review. Bone Marrow Transplant 31:145, 2003.

Schooley RT: Epstein-Barr virus (infectious mononucleosis). In Mandell GL, Bennett JE, Dolin R (eds.): Principle and Practice of Infectious Diseases. Philadelphia, Churchill Livingstone, 2000, p 1599.

Thorley-Lawson DA, Gross A: Persistence of the Epstein-Barr virus and the origins of associated lymphomas. N Engl J Med 350:1328, 2004.

Weinstock DM, Ambrossi GG, Brennan C, et al: Preemptive diagnosis and treatment of Epstein-Barr virus-associated post transplant lymphoproliferative disorder after hematopoietic stem cell transplant: an approach in development. Bone Marrow Transplant 37:539, 2006.

Williams H, Crawford DH: Epstein-Barr virus: The impact of scientific advances on clinical practice. Blood 107:862, 2006.

Young LS, Rickinson AB: Epstein-Barr virus: 40 years on. Nat Rev Cancer 4:757, 2004.

REFERENCES

For complete list of references log onto www.expertconsult.com

PART VI

Hematologic Malignancies

CHAPTER 55

CONVENTIONAL AND MOLECULAR CYTOGENETIC BASIS OF HEMATOLOGIC MALIGNANCIES

Vesna Najfeld

Over the past 35 years, cytogenetic analysis of malignant hematologic disorders has been one of the most rapidly growing areas in hematology. Chromosome studies and karyotype information provide both biologic and significant clinical value. Refinements in cell culture methods and the application of chromosome banding techniques have advanced our understanding of disease-specific abnormalities, and molecular cytogenetic methods now have made possible the identification of genes involved at translocation breakpoints in specific chromosomal rearrangements. These advances in molecular cytogenetic methods permit mapping of structural rearrangements even within a single gene[1,2] and fundamentally contribute to current knowledge of the biology of leukemia. This evolution in our understanding of cell biology has resulted in new terminology (Table 55–1). Application of conventional and molecular cytogenetic methods has identified 264 gene fusions involving 238 different genes in almost 35,000 reported patients with hematologic malignancies. This represents 75% of all gene fusions currently known in human neoplasia.[3] Application of these methods has played a pivotal role in the diagnosis, treatment, and prognosis of malignant hematologic diseases. This chapter discusses specific cytogenetic events and delineates molecular phenotypes that are important to understand the molecular pathogenesis of hematologic malignancies. Several genetic testing algorithms are suggested for clinical application of chromosome and fluorescence *in situ* hybridization (FISH) studies. The remarkable hypothesis put forward by Boveri[4] at the turn of the twentieth century, namely, that an abnormal chromosome pattern is intimately associated with the malignant phenotype of the tumor cell, has proved correct for many malignant disorders in general and for leukemia specifically. Knowledge of the molecular cytogenetic phenotype of hematologic malignancies has led to innovative and specifically tailored treatments. The first example of such gene-targeted therapy has already been successfully applied to chronic myelogenous leukemia (CML).[5,6]

METHODS

Cytogenetic Analysis

Cells arrested in metaphase are obtained by exposing marrow cells sequentially to mitotic inhibitors, hypotonic KCl, and fixative. Chromosomes obtained from leukemic marrow then are subjected to the most widely used banding method, trypsin-Giemsa banding (Fig. 55–1). The criteria used to define clonal abnormalities are listed in Table 55–1 and described in the International System for Human Cytogenetic Nomenclature.[7]

Fluorescence *In Situ* Hybridization

FISH is a molecular method that allows detection of the number, size, and location of DNA and RNA segments within individual cells in a tissue sample. It is based on the ability of single-stranded DNA to anneal to complementary DNA. In hematologic disorders, the target DNA is the marrow or peripheral blood nuclear DNA of interphase cells or the DNA of metaphase chromosomes that is fixed on a microscope slide. Other biologic material that may be involved in the leukemic process, such as spleen cells, ascites, and spinal fluid, are particularly useful for FISH studies. In lymphoma, the target DNA is a lymph node, and FISH studies are performed on touch preparation, frozen sections, or paraffin-embedded tissue.

Figure 55–2 shows four general types of FISH probes that are used alone or in combination to determine both numerical and structural rearrangements: (a) centromere enumeration probes, as the name implies, are used most frequently in interphase nuclei for detection of numerical chromosome anomalies, (b) whole chromosome painting probes are used only on the metaphase cells and are very useful in delineating complex rearrangements or the origin of marker chromosome, (c) subtelomeric probes, and (d) unique gene loci probes applied to both interphase and metaphase cells in single, dual, triple, or multiple colors to determine specific chromosomal rearrangements, deletions, or amplifications.

Four different FISH probe strategies are used in probe design for detection of chromosomal translocations in hematologic malignancies (Fig. 55–3): (a) conventional strategy, (b) extrasensitive strategy, (c) dual-fusion strategy, and (d) breakapart strategy. The first application of FISH technology for detection of chromosomal translocation in hematologic malignancy was in 1990, when the *BCR-ABL* hybrid gene was identified using two-color FISH in interphase cells as well as in metaphase marrow-derived CML cells.[8] In the standard strategy for interphase evaluation of chromosomal translocation, a DNA probe comprising sequences mapped proximally to the breakpoint in one of the chromosomes involved in reciprocal translocations is combined with a differentially labeled DNA probe that includes sequences mapped distantly to the breakpoint in the other chromosome. Positive nuclei for the translocation display one dual-color fusion signal, representing one of the derivative chromosomes generated by the translocation, and two single-color signals, one for each of the normal alleles. This standard FISH strategy has been used for detection of translocations in hematologic disorders at diagnosis.

For detection of residual disease, the conventional strategy lacks specificity because cells with random spatial colocalization of normal signals with different colors, found at a frequency from 1% to 10% of scored nuclei, are seen as false positive. To minimize this problem, an extrasensitive method was developed in which a probe for one abnormal chromosome is designed to generate an extra, smaller signal in positive nuclei. Hybridization with this strategy results in abnormal cells showing colocalization of two signals in dual colors, additional two signals in one single color and one signal in another single color. Application of the extrasensitive probe can discriminate between *BCR-ABL* fusion-positive blast crisis of CML and de novo acute lymphoblastic leukemia (ALL).

A dual-fusion strategy was developed not only to minimize false-positive results but also to detect additional deletions at the translocation breakpoints. The dual-color/dual-fusion strategy includes a probe set with DNA sequences that encompasses proximally and distally the translocation breakpoints on both chromosomes involved in translocation. The sequences for each chromosome are labeled with a specific color, and the translocation generates fused signals in both derivative chromosomes. Positive nuclei exhibit two copies of fusion signals and one copy of each of the single signals representing the normal alleles. If a third color is added for detection of particular sequences, such as deletion of chromosome 9 at the site of the Philadelphia (Ph) translocation (Figs. 55–8, *C,* and 55–12*),* the

Table 55–1 Glossary of Cytogenetic and Fluorescence *In Situ* Hybridization Terminology

Term	Definition
Aneuploidy	Abnormal chromosome number, either gain or loss
Balanced translocation	Exchange of chromosomal material that creates no extra or missing DNA
Banding	Set of dark and pale segments along the length of chromosomes, resulting from treatment with enzyme prior to staining Each chromosome is identified by its unique set of bands
Breakpoint	Specific site on a chromosome containing a break in the DNA that is involved in chromosomal structural rearrangement, such as translocation or deletion
Centromere	Constriction on the chromosome at the spindle site attachment During cell mitosis two copies of the DNA in each chromosome are separated by shortening of the spindle fibers attached to opposite sides of the dividing cell Position of the centromere determines whether the chromosome is metacentric (X shaped, e.g., 1, 3, 19, 20), submetacentric (centromere positioned more toward the short arms, e.g., 2, 4, 5, 6–12, 16–18, X), or acrocentric (inverted V shaped, e.g., 13–15, 21, 22, Y)
Centromere enumeration probe (CEP)	Highly repetitive α (or β) satellite DNA, located in the heterochromatin of the centromeric area of chromosomes CEP targets repetitive α (or β) sequences and produces bright compact signals; particularly useful for detection of numerical loss or gain of chromosomes
CGH	Comparative genomic hybridization, molecular cytogenetic technique that provides a copy-number karyotype at the chromosome and band level Array CGH is a higher-level CGH technology that provides gene copy information Variety of arrays include disease specialized, chromosome arm specific, and others.
Chromosomal rearrangement	Aberration in which chromosomes are broken and rejoined
Clonal abnormality	In cytogenetic analysis, two cells showing the same additional or structural abnormality or three cells with loss of the same chromosome In FISH analysis, any abnormality present after the probe has been validated and normal reference range established, above the normal reference range
Deletion	Segment of chromosome that is missing (terminal) or segment of chromosome missing between two breakpoints (interstitial)
DNA sequence	Order of nucleotides in a DNA segment, usually displayed from the 5′-triphosphate (5′ end) to the 3′-hydroxyl (3′ end) nucleotides
Enhancer	DNA sequence that increases the rate of transcription
Exon	Portion of gene that encodes protein
Fiber FISH	Application of FISH technology to extended DNA or free DNA fibers
FISH	Fluorescence *in situ* hybridization, a method for detection of the number and location of DNA sequences (genes) in tissue section or cell population
Fluorochrome	Fluorescence molecule that, when conjugated to a molecule, binds to a hapten to facilitate detection of the chromosomal probe By definition, a fluorochrome is a molecule that will become excited by the light of one wavelength
Gene construct	Recombinant DNA containing a gene of interest surrounded by sequences engineered to promote a measure of its expression
Gene map	Order of genes within a chromosome or entire genome
Genotype	Genetic constitution, usually with reference to particular alleles at a locus
Haploid	Half of a normal complement (i.e., 23 chromosomes)
Haploinsufficiency	Deletion or inactivation of one allele to produce disease due to inadequate activity of the remaining allele
Hybrid gene	Fusion of two different genes as a result of a structural chromosomal rearrangement that functions as one transcriptional unit
Hybridization	Method for rejoining (reannealing) complementary DNA or RNA strands
Hyperdiploid	Additional chromosomes (e.g., 47 or 48 chromosomes)
Hypermetaphase FISH	Application of FISH to accumulated large number of metaphase cells
Hypodiploid	Loss of chromosomes (e.g., 45 or 44 chromosomes)
I-FISH	Interphase fluorescence *in situ* hybridization, application of FISH to nondividing (resting) cells
Interphase	Stage of mitosis in which the cell is not dividing
Inversion	Structural chromosomal rearrangement as a result of two breaks occurring in the same chromosome Paracentric inversion refers to both breaks occurring on the same side of the centromere Pericentric inversion refers to breaks occurring on the opposite side of the centromere
Isochromosome	Structural chromosomal rearrangement that consists of doubling of one of the two chromosome arms (connected by the centromere) and loss of the other arm

Table 55–1 Glossary of Cytogenetic and Fluorescence *In Situ* Hybridization Terminology—cont'd

Karyotype	Arrangement of metaphase chromosomes from a particular cell according to size and banding so that the largest chromosome is placed first and the smallest one last (see Fig. 55–1)
kb (kilobase)	Unit of DNA/RNA length = 1000 base pairs of DNA
Locus	Unique location of a gene on a chromosome
Locus (sequence)-specific probe (LSI)	Probe targeted to unique sequence region of the chromosome Useful for localization of genes on normal chromosomes (gene mapping) and for detection of gene amplification, deletion, inversion, or translocation
Marker chromosome	Chromosome whose morphology cannot be identified using banding method Marker chromosomes are frequent in hematologic neoplasms
M-FISH	Multicolor FISH karyotyping, which allows identification of 24 different human chromosomes (22 autosomes, and the X and Y chromosomes) (see text for details)
Oncogene	Locus that is activated in association with tumor growth One abnormal allele is sufficient to cause tumor formation or cancer
PCR	Polymerase chain reaction, by which individual gene segments are amplified through sequential cycles of polymerization, heat denaturation, and reannealing
Pseudodiploid	Diploid number of chromosomes (46) accompanied by structural rearrangement
Recurrent abnormality	Structural or numerical abnormality observed in multiple patients with the same or similar disease Recurrent chromosome abnormalities in hematologic neoplasms have prognostic significance
Telomeric probe	Used to detect repeated DNA sequences present at the end of the chromosome, which is called the telomere Telomeric DNA contains 10–15 kb of TTAGGG repeats Adjacent to the telomere is a region called the proximal subtelomeric region, and centromeric to it is a unique chromosome telomeric region Chromosome-specific telomeric probes are useful for detection of cryptic translocations involving ends of chromosomes
Translocation	Structural chromosome abnormality resulting from a break in at least two chromosomes with an exchange of material In reciprocal or balanced translocation, no loss of chromosomal material occurs In unbalanced translocation, loss of chromosomal DNA occurs
Tumor suppressor gene	Locus that prevents tumor growth when at least one allele is functional Loss of both alleles, first through constitutional and then through somatic mutation, is associated with tumor formation or cancer
Whole chromosome painting probe (WCP)	Spans the entire length of chromosomal DNA sequences and, as the name implies, targets the entire length of DNA sequences Useful for identification of complex or cryptic structural rearrangements as well as for identification of marker chromosomes
	Nomenclature
p	= Short arm
q	= Long arm
+	When placed before the chromosome, denotes a gain of a whole chromosome (e.g., +8)
–	When placed before the chromosome, indicates a loss of a whole chromosome (e.g., –7); in rare situations, when placed after the chromosome, as in 5q–, indicates loss of a part of the long arms of chromosome 5
t	translocation
del	deletion
der	derivative
inv	inversion
i	isochromosome
mar	marker chromosome
con	connected
nuc ish	nuclear *in situ* hybridization
nuc ish 21q22(D21S65X2)	two copies of D21S65 DNA segment on chromosome 21
nuc ish 9q34(ABLx2),22q11.2(BCRx2) (ABL con BCRx1)	two ABL and two BCR loci, but one of each locus is juxtaposed on one chromosome as a result of t(9;22)

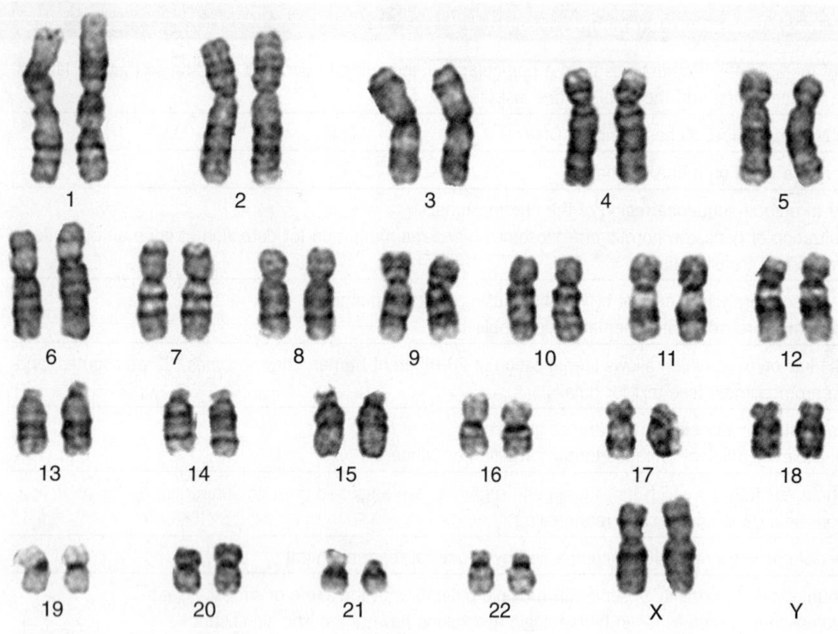

Figure 55–1 Normal arrangements of chromosomes in a karyotype from a bone marrow metaphase cell showing a slightly fuzzy morphology compared to a normal karyotype obtained from phytohaemagglutinin-stimulated peripheral blood cells.

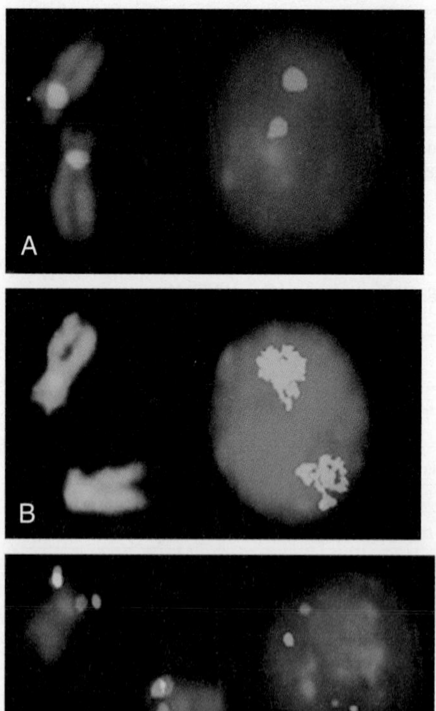

Figure 55–2 Types of chromosomal probes (see text for details). **A,** Pair of chromosome 12 (left) and interphase cell (right) after FISH study with centromere enumeration probe (CEP) showing two hybridization signals (red) in the centromeric area of chromosome and two tight signals in interphase cell consistent with disomy (normal copy number). CEP probes are most useful for detection of numerical abnormalities. **B,** Hybridization with whole chromosome 8 painting probe showing the hybridization signal (green) along the length of the entire chromosome 8 (left) and hybridization domains in interphase cell (right). Whole chromosome painting probes are useful for identifying unknown chromosomes in metaphase cells. **C,** Target of locus-specific indicators (LSI) are specific gene sequences such as *P53* seen after hybridization as two small signals (red) on chromosome 17, band p13. The main application of LSI probes are gene mapping, numerical enumeration in interphase cells, and detection of translocations. Telomeric probe, shown in green for the short arms of chromosome 17, are repetitive probes and are useful for detection of cryptic translocations involving ends of chromosomes. Chromosomes and nuclei are counterstained with DAPI (blue).

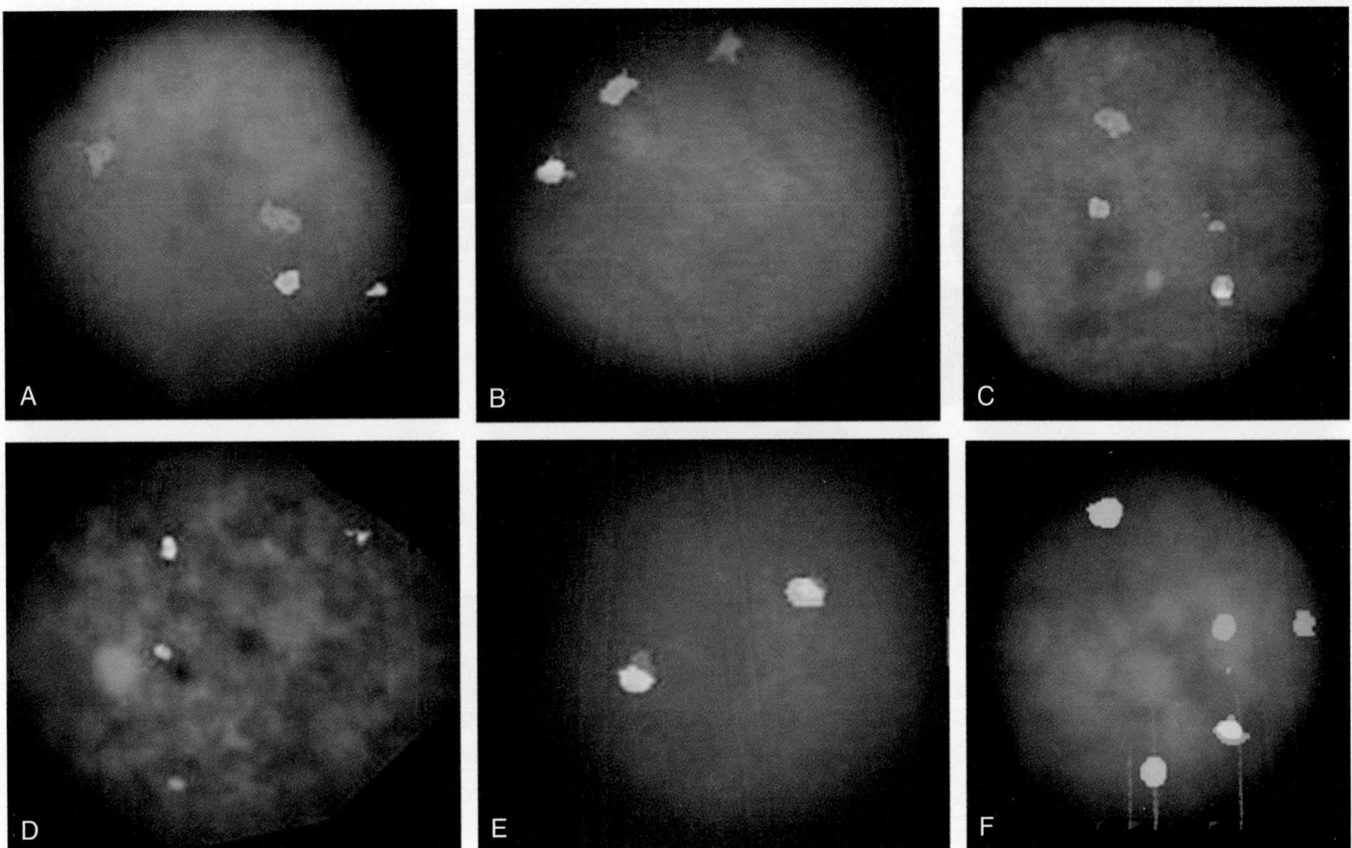

Figure 55–3 Four different probe strategies for detection of chromosomal translocations (see text for details). **A,** Normal cell after *in situ* hybridization with *BCR* (green) and *ABL* (red) showing a normal distribution of two red and two green single signals. **B,** Conventional fusion strategy after *in situ* hybridization shows one fusion (yellow) signal representing derivative chromosome generated by the translocation and one single-color signal, red and green for normal homologues in positive nuclei. **C,** An extrasensitive fusion approach generates an extra small (red) signal as well as a fusion signal (yellow) and one signal in single color (green and red) on normal homologues. **D,** Dual-fusion strategy generates two fusion signals (yellow) on two derivative chromosomes and one single-color signal on each of two normal chromosomes. **E,** "Breakapart" approach in a normal cell appears as two fusion signals (yellow). In this strategy, the 3′ end and the 5′ part of the gene are labeled in two colors. **F,** When the rearrangement occurs, the normal chromosome shows colocalization of red and green (yellow) as a result of the proximity of the sequences on the chromosome, whereas abnormal derivative chromosomes each have one single red and single green signal, indicating that the rearrangement occurred between the two ends of the gene separating the green and red signals on two different chromosomes. The third-color probe (blue) can be used as an internal control (usually CEP probe) to determine the disomic number of chromosomes.

lack of one copy of the third color is consistent with sequence deletion at the site of the translocation of one derivative chromosome. Dual-color/dual-fusion probes are very useful in differentiating various leukemia and lymphoma-associated translocations.

Multiple translocation partners are well known for genes commonly associated with leukemias such as *MLL*, retinoic acid receptor α *(RARA),* and the lymphoma gene *ALK,* and the fourth FISH strategy with "breakapart" probes was developed to address this issue. The breakapart probe includes DNA sequences mapped proximally and distally to the breakpoint within a critical gene (the 3′ end and the 5′ end) labeled with two different fluorochromes. The fused fluorescence signals represent a normal gene, whereas nuclei with rearrangements within the target gene show one single-color signal and one for each derivative chromosome, regardless of which chromosome is the partner in translocation.

One of the most significant advances in diagnostic leukemia cytogenetics has been the application of interphase FISH. *Interphase cytogenetics* is the term used to describe detection of chromosomal abnormalities in nondividing, interphase nuclei (Fig. 55–4).[9] Six aspects of interphase FISH are particularly useful. (a) Interphase cytogenetics allows screening of a large number of cells. This permits investigation of hematologic malignancies with a low mitotic yield, such as chronic lymphocytic leukemia (CLL) or multiple myeloma (MM). (b) Interphase cytogenetics permits detection of chromosomal rearrangements in peripheral blood samples, thus obviating the need for marrow aspiration. For instance, in CML, which rarely yields a large number of dividing cells in peripheral blood, conventional cytogenetics usually is uninformative. However, detection of *BCR-ABL,* a molecular equivalent of the Ph, in peripheral blood using interphase FISH provides reliable, fast, quantitative results (see Chronic Myelogenous Leukemia below). (c) Interphase FISH offers a quantitative assay for monitoring disease progression or detection of minimal residual disease after ablative chemotherapy or hematopoietic cell transplantation (HCT). (d) Use of specific probe sets allows detection of specific disease-associated abnormalities such as t(8;21), which denotes the M2 subtype of acute myeloid leukemia (AML), or t(15;17), which is associated with acute promyelocytic leukemia, in a very short time period, allowing for timely and appropriate therapy. (e) Abnormalities can be detected accurately in archival specimens kept up to 15 years. (f) Simultaneous use of interphase FISH and immunophenotyping is a powerful tool for investigation of lineage involvement in diseases such as myelodysplasia and to determine which cell population carries the specific chromosome abnormality. FISH nomenclature is described in the International System for Human Cytogenetic Nomenclature.[7]

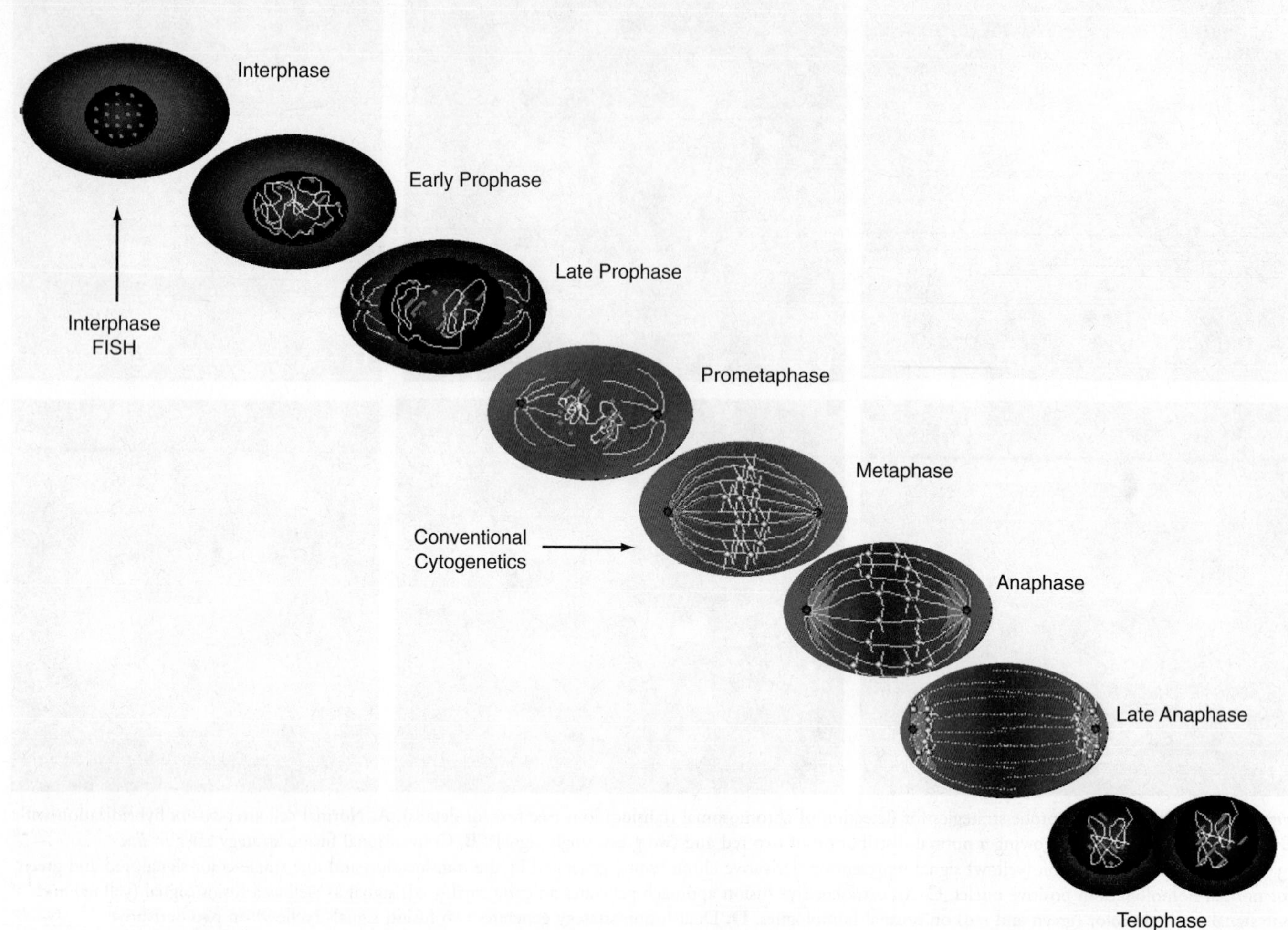

Figure 55–4 Schematic representation of cell division. Most clinical FISH studies are performed on nondividing interphase cells, whereas conventional cytogenetics is performed at the metaphase stage of cell division. *(Courtesy Dr. Ari Melnik, Mount Sinai Medical Center New York.)*

Higher resolution of chromosomal abnormalities can be achieved when fluorescently labeled probes are hybridized to extended DNA or free chromatin (chromatin strands released from their chromosomal scaffold) or free DNA fibers. This approach is termed *fiber FISH* (Fig. 55–5, top). The hybridized signals have the appearance of a "string of pearls" along the fiber rather than tight fluorescing spots observed in interphase cells. Although at the present time fiber FISH has limited clinical applicability because it requires special techniques of target DNA preparation on a glass slide, it has been successfully applied in basic studies, such as mapping chromosomal breakpoints of the *cyclin D* gene in mantle cell lymphoma and for detailed mapping of the breakpoint site region in the *BCL2* gene involved in follicular lymphoma.[10,11]

Multicolor karyotyping permits examination of the entire genome in a single analysis (Fig. 55–6). In 1996 it became possible to identify 24 different human chromosomes (12 autosomes and the X and the Y sex chromosomes), each with a unique color, with the help of fluorochrome-specific optical filters. This method is called *multicolor FISH* (M-FISH).[12] When interferometer-based spectral imaging is used, the method is called *spectral karyotyping*.[13] The starting point in both methodologies is the use of whole chromosome painting probes for each chromosome. Thus, each chromosome is labeled with a different combination of fluorescence dyes. The fluorochrome colors are not distinct enough for the unaided human eye to distinguish the combination with which the chromosome is labeled. In M-FISH, images are sequentially obtained using five different fluorochrome-specific optical filters. A computer program combines the data and displays each chromosome as if it were stained with a distinct color. Spectral karyotyping is based on the use of an interferometer (used by astronomers to measure the light spectra of distant stars) to determine the full spectrum of light emitted by each stained chromosome. A computer program then displays all the chromosomes simultaneously, each with its own unique color. These methods are applied with increasing frequency to resolve complex karyotypes, to detect cryptic translocations in patients with normal karyotype, and to define karyotypes with deletions.[14–17] Their clinical use may be limited because the cost of equipment and probes is beyond what can be afforded by most clinical laboratories. The M-FISH technology cannot be used to discriminate structural intrachromosomal rearrangements such as duplications, deletions, and inversions.

Another powerful method used for identifying locations of chromosomal gains, losses, deletions, or amplifications, without prior knowledge of the chromosomal target that may be altered, is *comparative genomic hybridization* (CGH). Briefly, isolated DNA from leukemic marrow or tumor tissue is labeled with a one-color fluorochrome (e.g., red), whereas DNA isolated from normal control tissue is labeled with a different color (e.g., green). These differently labeled DNAs are hybridized against each other in a competitive hybridization reaction onto normal metaphase spreads. Computer-assisted image analysis detects colors generated after hybridization, which indicate equal hybridization, relative excess, or deficiency of the target DNA (relative to control). The ratio of color intensity provides a "copy-number" karyotype. CGH has been successfully applied to

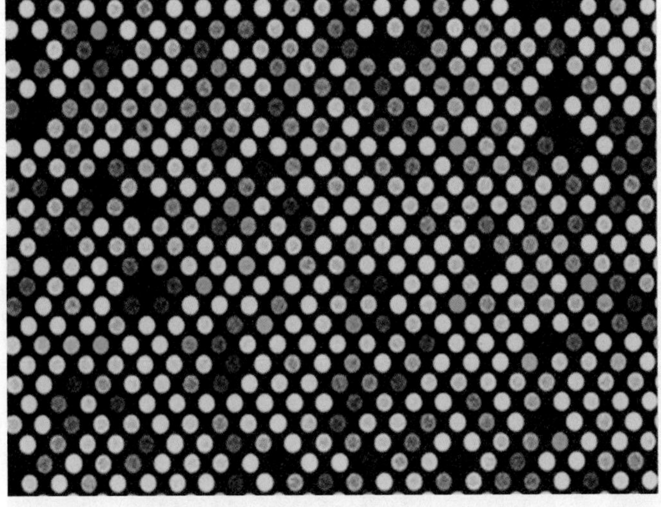

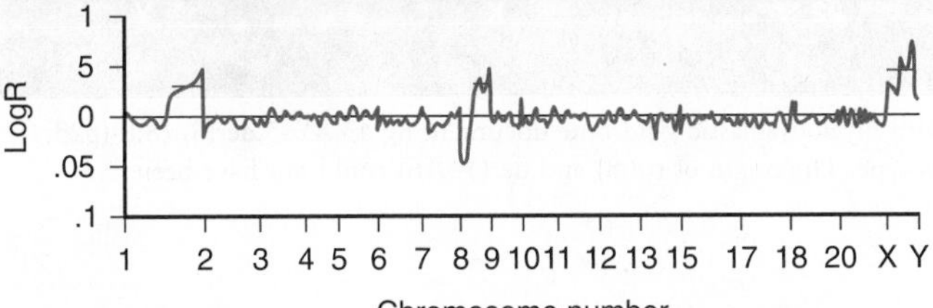

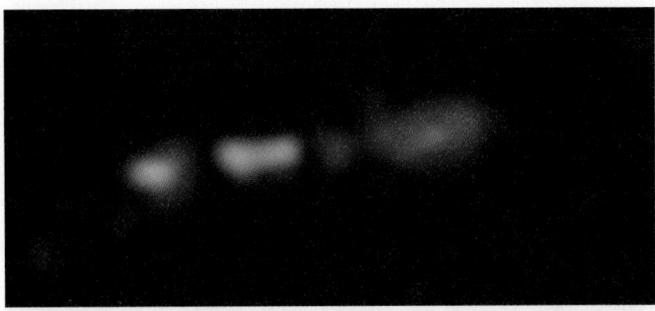

Figure 55–5 Top panels, Application of higher-resolution FISH, fiber FISH, to extended DNA fibers. The hybridization signals have the appearance of a "string of pearls" along the fiber rather than tight fluorescing spots observed in interphase nuclei. **Bottom panel,** Portion of array CGH image. The tumor or normal cell fragmented DNA sample was labeled with Cy5 or CY3, respectively. Yellow spot indicates the intensity signal of the genomic element on that spot in the tumor equals that of the normal cell reference. Red or green spot indicates intensity of the tumor and is greater or less than the reference, suggesting copy-number change for the genomic element on that spot. Graph underneath is the copy-number change profile. Y-axis is the log2 ratio of the intensity of each gene in the order of its position on the genome in tumor sample versus that of normal liver sample. Gained or lost regions are marked by red or green line, respectively. Gains of 1q and 8q and loss of 8p were observed in this tumor. *(Courtesy Dr. D. Weijia Zhang, Mount Sinai School of Medicine, New York, NY. In: Molecular Genetic Pathology. eds. Liang Cheng and David Y. Zhang Humana Press, Totowa, NJ, 2008.)*

many leukemias, but its clinical use remains limited because it cannot detect balanced translocations, which are the hallmark of many hematologic malignancies.[18,19] Nevertheless, CGH is the first efficient approach to scanning the entire genome for variations in DNA copy number.[20,21]

A newly emerging investigational method is a "microchip array" in which labeled DNA or RNA from the sample of interest is hybridized with defined target sequences immobilized on a solid support. The advantage of this method is the ability to screen genes that are amplified or deleted from the genome on a very large scale or, in the case of RNA, to learn whether such genes are expressed at a particular stage of disease. The first example of successful RNA application of the microchip array technique was the differentiation of AML from ALL based solely on gene expression.[22] As shown in Fig. 55–5 (bottom panels), in the "array CGH" procedure, large-insert genomic clones, oligonucleotides, or single nucleotide polymorphisms (SNPs) have replaced metaphase chromosomes used in the regular CGH.[23,24] Array CGH is a higher-resolution CGH technology and provides diagnostic information for diseases associated with DNA dosage. It also can be used to discover previously unexpected sites of gene dosage associated with specific hematologic malignancy type.[25–28] The concept of obtaining gene copy number from multiple genome locations in a single measurement has been used to characterize numerous hematologic malignancies in the last 3 to 4 years, and its clinical usefulness is demonstrated throughout this chapter.

These modern cytogenetics methods have increased the resolution at which chromosomal rearrangements can be identified. Whereas in conventional cytogenetics the target is the whole chromosomes in the metaphase spreads at a resolution of approximately 5 Mb, molecular cytogenetics methods may use analysis of interphase nuclei at a resolution of 50 kb to 2 Mb or fiber FISH analysis of chromatin strands at a resolution of 5 kb to 500 kb. Moreover, the current resolution of array CGH is restricted only by clone size and by the density of clones on the array, some of which may contain resolution at the level of a single nucleotide.

Conventional cytogenetics and FISH methodologies are complementary. Each has its own advantages and limitations in investigating genome rearrangements of malignant cells. Although conventional cytogenetics is the comprehensive study of all chromosomes, it requires a large number of dividing cells, which, in some diseases, such as myelofibrosis, is difficult to obtain. Furthermore, many small deletions or structural rearrangements are beyond the microscopic level of detection. FISH can be used in conjunction with conventional cytogenetics in both interphase and metaphase cells. It is a more sensitive method and can detect rearrangements smaller than 1 kb. The main disadvantage of interphase FISH is that it cannot be used unless a known abnormality is suspected. When the abnormality is known, interphase FISH can pinpoint the clonal aberration at the single-cell level in a very short period of time. Other investigative FISH methods provide further refinement.

Clonal Origin of Leukemia

The question of whether cell proliferation is monoclonal or polyclonal is fundamental to understanding the underlying etiology of hematologic malignancies. Markers of clonality are used to determine the origin of disease, to differentiate malignant from nonmalignant populations, to establish hematopoietic hierarchy, clonal evolution, and clonal remission, and to delineate steps involved in multistep pathogenesis.

The clonal origin of leukemias and lymphomas can be assessed by either intrinsic or extrinsic cellular markers. Intrinsic cellular markers are specific for a cell population, arising either during normal differentiation or as a part of disease process. For instance, cell surface-associated immunoglobulin (Ig) markers such as the λ or κ light chain or idiotypes and T-cell receptors (TCRs) can be useful for evaluating lymphoid diseases.[29,30] Application of Ig markers demonstrated for the first time that MM has a clonal development.[31] Somatic cytogenetic alterations are useful intrinsic markers for identifying abnormal clones and following disease progression. Thus, the observation of identical chromosome anomalies in different cells of the same tumor is evidence of clonality. Since the discovery of the Philadelphia chromosome (Ph) in 1960, it is well established that nonrandom, recurrent chromosomal abnormalities characterize many hematopoietic malignancies.[32] The finding of the Ph in different CML-derived hematopoietic cell lineages led to the hypothesis that CML might originate in a single precursor cell and may have a clonal development.[33,34] Moreover, the presence of additional recurrent chromosomal abnormalities in the Ph positive clone, such as trisomy 8, duplication of the

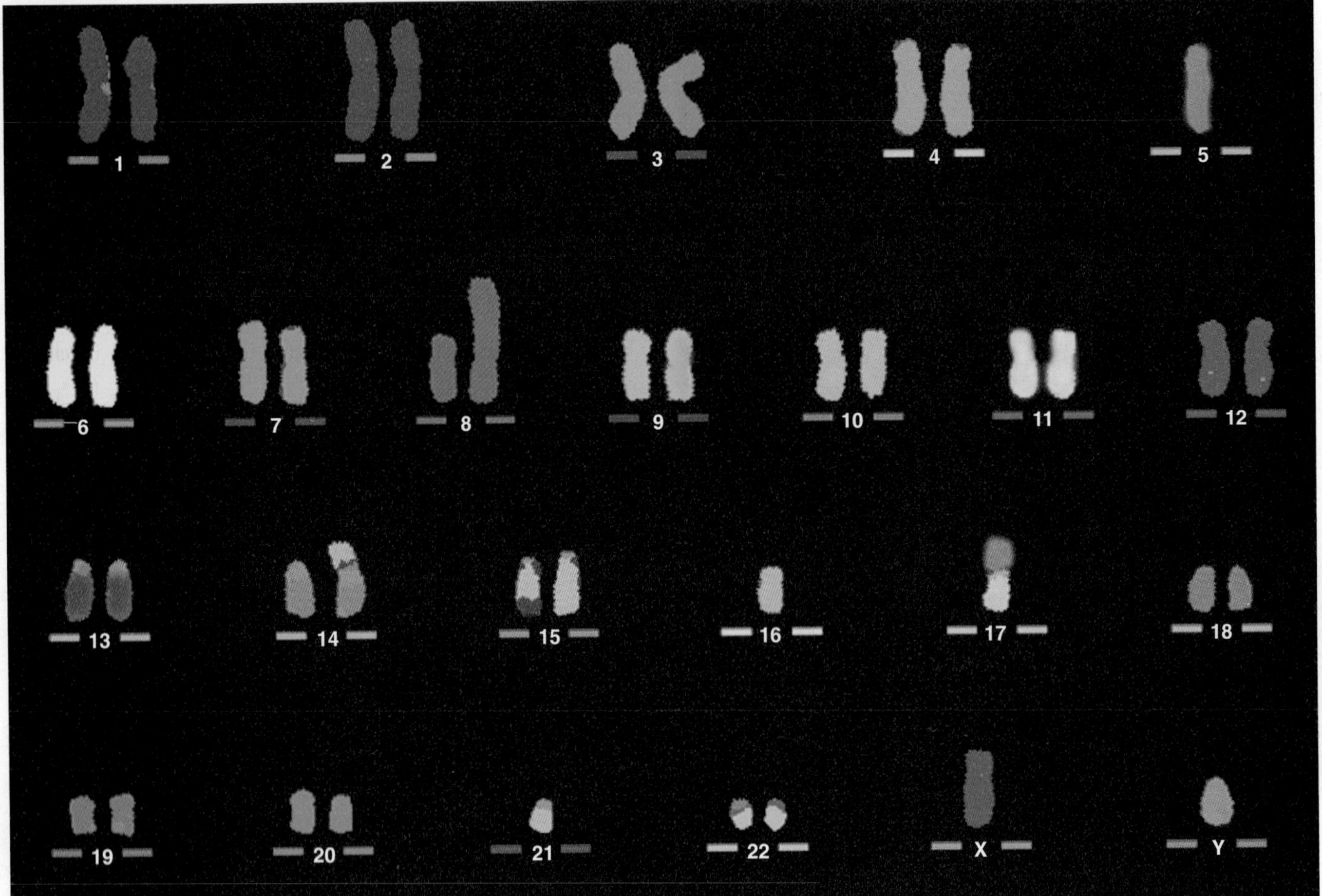

Figure 55–6 Multicolor metaphase FISH of a bone marrow cell from a patient with myelodysplastic syndrome documenting 43,XY,-5,der(8)t(8;8)(p23;q11.2),der(14;16)(p12;p11.1), inv(15)(q21;q24),der(17)t(5;17)(p13;p13),-21 karyotype. The origin of t(8;8) and der(14;16) could not have been determined by conventional cytogenetic study alone.

Ph, or trisomy 19, not only indicates the clinical worsening of the disease and the occurrence of the accelerated phase or blast crisis, but it demonstrate the subclonal evolution of the Ph positive clone. Currently, disease-associated somatic genomic mutation, such as rearrangements of *MLL, AML1, TEL/ETV6, PML-RARA*, and many others, can be identified by polymerase chain reaction (PCR)-based assays or by FISH assay and may serve, with or without conventional cytogenetics, as intrinsic marker of disease processes.

On the other hand, extrinsic marker systems use cellular mosaicism that is completely independent of the disease being studied and is not restricted to the cell lineages. Individuals with Turner or Klinefelter syndrome are mosaic for XX or XY and X cells or XXY and XY cells, respectively. The mosaicism created by X-chromosome inactivation in females is much more widely applicable and has provided fundamental insights into the pathogenesis of hematologic malignancies.[35] Original studies with X-linked glucose-6-phospate dehydrogenase (G6PD) as a marker of clonality was based on the Lyon hypothesis that, early in embryogenesis, one X chromosome in females is inactivated in somatic cells, and the activation status is stably transmitted to daughter cells during mitosis (Fig. 55–7).[36] The choice of maternal versus paternal X-chromosome inactivation is random; however, once it occurs it is maintained in all daughter cells.[37] Random X inactivation occurs by embryonic day 6.5 around the start of gastrulation and results in a mosaic pattern that characterizes adult females.[38–40] Therefore, an adult female is a mosaic for two cell populations, one expressing genes from an active X chromosome and the other expressing genes from the inactive X chromosome. Incidentally, mammalian X-chromosome inactivation is a mechanism that equalizes the dosage of X-linked genes between sexes.[36] Although the exact mechanism of X-chromosome inactivation remains to be elucidated, the process of X inactivation starts with methylation of CpG islands.[41–43] The inactivation process is believed to occur before differentiation of embryonic stem cell into various cell lineages. Hematopoietic cells do not originate from a single embryonic stem cell but from several progenitors, thereby allowing for mosaic expression from both X chromosomes.[43,44]

The observation that human females are heterozygous for the *G6PD* variant A and A⁻ and that two mosaic cell populations may be distinguishable by electrophoretic mobility was first published by Davidson et al.[45] in 1963. The X-inactivation *G6PD* mosaic system was first applied to the study of clonality in human tumors in 1964 by Gartler and Linden.[46] They studied uterine leiomyomas and recognized that the presence of normal cells might mask the ability to detect individual clonal uterine leiomymas.[47] In females who are heterozygous for the *G6PD* polymorphism and have malignant hematologic disorder such as CML, the finding of a single *G6PD* type in marrow or blood cells and both the A and B type *G6PD* in normal tissue control demonstrated that CML has a clonal origin and provided evidence that the malignant transformation occurred in the stem cell common to most cell lineages.[33,34] Additional studies with heterozygous *G6PD* females who had CML demonstrated that some CML-derived B lymphocytes had a single *G6PD* type, but these clonal cells were Ph negative; thus, leukemic transformation predates development of the chromosomal abnormality. This observation provided evidence that CML has a multistep pathogenesis.[34,48,49] Application of *G6PD* studies to hematologic malignancies demonstrated clonal and stem cell origin for AML, ALL, Ph negative chronic myeloproliferative disorder (MPD), myelodysplastic syndrome (MDS), and

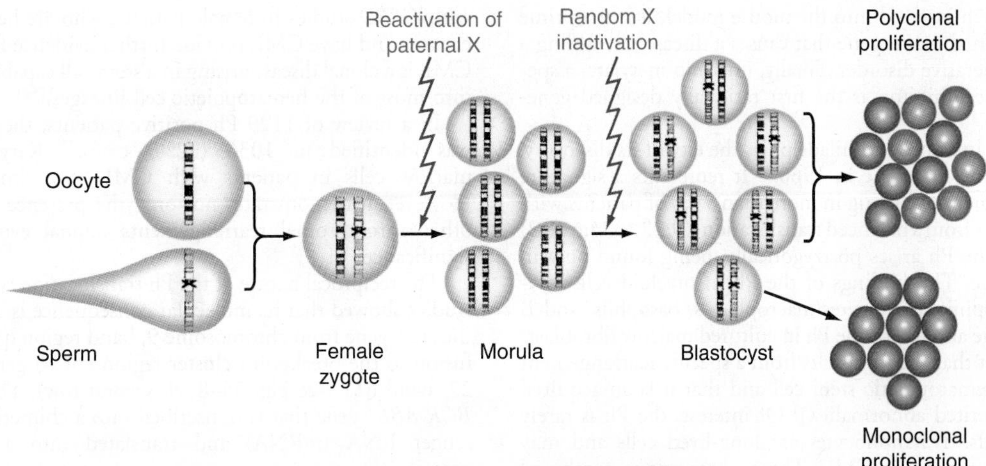

Figure 55–7 X-chromosome–linked enzyme glucose-6-phosphate dehydrogenase (G6PD) as a marker to investigate clonal development of human hematopoietic disorders. Early in embryogenesis, regions of all but one X chromosome are inactivated in each cell containing two or more X chromosomes. The choice of maternal versus paternal X chromosome for inactivation is random. Once the inactivation occurs, it is fixed and is stably transmitted to daughter cells during mitosis (Lyon hypothesis). Females who are heterozygous for the common B type and the less frequent A type, G6PD (localized on Xq27), are mosaic. This cellular mosaicism is used to study monoclonal versus polyclonal cell proliferation and development of malignant hematopoietic diseases. *(Courtesy Dr. W Raskind, University of Washington, Seattle, WA. From Zucker-Franlin D, Grossi CE [eds.]: Atlas of Blood Cells, 3rd ed. Edi-Ermes, Milan 2003.)*

CLL.[50–56] In some patients with AML, *G6PD* studies demonstrated a single enzyme phenotype without the presence of the diagnostic cytogenetic abnormality at the time of hematologic remission, indicating a clonal remission and a possibility of clonal preleukemic phase of AML. This observation provided evidence that, like in CML, a stepwise evolution occurs in AML.[57,58] In MDS, the *G6PD assay* demonstrated that lymphoid cells are part of the MDS clone.[55] Particularly informative were patients with myelofibrosis whose marrow cells had trisomy 8. In sharp contrast, cultured marrow fibroblasts had disomy 8 and expressed both B and A *G6PD* types in equal amounts as control skin fibroblasts, whereas marrow-derived granulocytes, erythrocytes, and platelets expressed only type A enzyme. This indicated that marrow fibroblasts were not clonal and were not part of the disease process.[59] *G6PD* studies were particularly useful in the investigations of red blood cells and platelets in hematologic malignancies because these cells cannot be studied by cytogenetics or DNA analysis because they do not have nuclei. Although it is now a "common knowledge" that hematological malignancies have a clonal development, it is greatly due to what is now known as classic Fialkow's work, whose profound insight contributed towards the current concepts and understanding.

Despite the importance of the *G6PD* approach, it is limited by the rarity of females who are heterozygous for the *G6PD* isoenzyme. An alternative and more extensive *DNA-based X-chromosome clonal assay* uses common polymorphic markers that are caused by changes in DNA methylation patterns that accompany inactivation of the X chromosome. These X-linked loci, such as phosphoglycerine kinase, hypoxanthine phosphoribosyltransferase, *DXS25* (M27β), and human androgen receptor (HUMARA), have been extensively used in assessment of clonality, and now it is possible to identify clonal cell populations in virtually all females.[60–66] DNA-based marker systems rely on a sequence polymorphism that has adjacent differences in methylation on the active and inactive X chromosomes.[60] The inactive X chromosome is more highly methylated than its active homologue, but this is only true for certain regions of genes as 10% to 20% of X-linked genes escape inactivation and can be found both in clusters and in isolation.[67–69] The most widely used *HUMARA assay* appears to maintain the stringent methylation differences. The number of CAG tandem repeats differentiates the maternal from the paternal X chromosome.[65,67]

The DNA-based X-chromosome clonal assay is limited to females younger than 60 years because they usually have 1 : 1 distribution of two mosaic cell population. A ratio greater than 3 : 1 is found in women older than 60 years, probably as a result of stem cell kinetics influenced by X-linked genetic factors.[70] When the ratio of two cell populations is greater than 3 : 1, this phenomenon is called a *skewed X-inactivation pattern.* With the HUMARA assay, acquired unequal or skewed X-chromosome inactivation (excessive lyonization) is found in 35% to 40% of women older than 60 years. Thus, X-chromosome–based clonality studies must incorporate age-matched controls.[70,71] Despite the enormous contribution of clonality assays to the understanding of disease processes, they usually are performed in research investigations and rarely are used as diagnostic tools.

Table 55–2 History of Discovery of Philadelphia Chromosome and BCR-ABL Fusion

1960	Philadelphia chromosome (Ph) is identified
1973	Ph is t(9;22)(q34;q11.2)
1983	*ABL* is translocated from chromosome 9 to chromosome 22
1984	*BCR* is localized to 22q11
1987	Ph′ is BCR-ABL fusion

CHRONIC MYELOPROLIFERATIVE DISORDERS

The World Health Organization (WHO) classification characterizes myeloproliferative disorders (MPDs) as having clonal and effective hematopoiesis.[72] CML has a unique place among hematologic malignancies and is described separate from other Ph negative MPDs.

Chronic Myelogenous Leukemia

The knowledge about CML accumulated during the last 46 years serves as an example of molecular medicine (Table 55–2). The Ph chromosome is the first example of a specific chromosome abnormality associated with malignant disease. *ABL1* and *BCR* genes are the first oncogenes localized at the site of chromosomal breakpoints in t(9;22)(q34;q11). The *BCR-ABL1* fusion is the first example of a "hybrid" gene leading to the production of dysregulated tyrosine kinase protein. When inserted into the mouse model, it is the prime example of a human aberrant gene that causes a disease resembling a human myeloproliferative disorder. Finally, imatinib mesylate, a specific tyrosine kinase inhibitor, is the first rationally designed gene-targeted therapy.[5,6,73]

The Ph, named in honor of Philadelphia, the city of its discovery, was described for the first time in 1960.[32] It represents a signature genomic rearrangement occurring in more than 95% of patients with CML. The Ph results from a balanced translocation t(9;22)(q34;q11.2) (Fig. 55–8, *A*).[74] The Ph arises postzygotically, being found only in hematopoietic tissue. The findings of the Ph in myeloid cells, erythroid cells, eosinophils, monocytes/macrophages, basophils, and B lymphocytes and the absence of the Ph in cultured marrow fibroblasts support the concept that the Ph results from a specific rearrangement in a multipotent hematopoietic stem cell and that it is an acquired rather than an inherited abnormality.[49] Of interest, the Ph is rarely identified in T cells. T lymphocytes are long-lived cells and may antedate the development of CML. These observations combined with *G6PD* studies in female patients who are heterozygous for this enzyme and have CML provide further evidence for the concept that CML is a clonal disease arising in a stem cell capable of differentiation into most of the hematopoietic cell lineages.[75,76]

In a review of 1129 Ph positive patients, the 9;22 translocation was identified in 1036 (92%) cases.[77] Karyotype analysis of marrow cells in patients with CML is a time-consuming task. However, it demonstrates not only the presence of the Ph but also other chromosomal rearrangements (clonal evolution) of clinical significance.[78]

The reciprocal nature of the Ph translocation was confirmed when studies showed that its molecular consequence is the translocation of the *ABL* gene from chromosome 9, band region q34, and subsequent fusion to the breakpoint cluster region (*BCR*) gene on chromosome 22, band q11 (see Fig. 55–8, *A*, second row). This creates a hybrid *BCR-ABL1* gene that is transcribed into a chimeric *BCR-ABL1* messenger RNA (mRNA) and translated into a specific chimeric protein.[79,80]

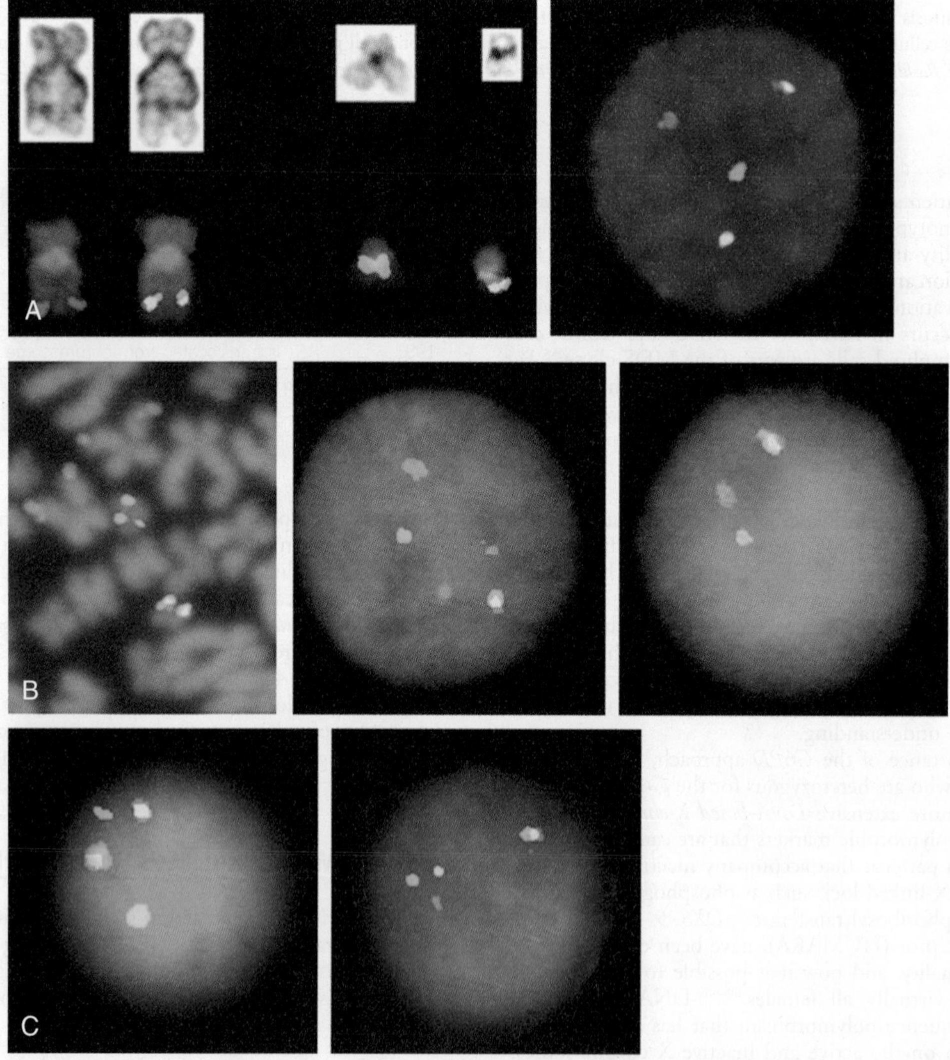

Figure 55–8 Identification of the Philadelphia (Ph) chromosome. **A,** Conventional cytogenetics (left) shows t(9;22)(q34;q11.2), and metaphase FISH with dual-color/dual-fusion *BCR-ABL* probe (underneath) shows two fusion signals (yellow) on abnormal chromosomes 9 and 22, one red single signal on normal homologue 9 and one single green signal on normal chromosome 22. Right, Nucleus after hybridization with dual-color/dual-fusion probe indicating two fusion signals. **B,** Metaphase cell (left) and interphase cell (middle) after hybridization with BCR-ABL extrasensitive probe indicating a fusion signal (yellow) on the Ph chromosome, *BCR* (green) on normal chromosome 22, *ABL* (red) signals on normal chromosome 9, and part of *ABL* on der(9) to reduce the number of false-positive cells. The interphase nuclei on the right is hybridized with a single-fusion BCR-ABL probe showing one fusion signal (yellow) and one single red and green signal on normal homologues. **C,** Two interphase nuclei after hybridization with triple-color BCR-ABL-ASS probe in which *ASS* is aqua. The left nuclei indicate a *BCR-ABL* fusion and disomy for *ASS*. The right nucleus shows deletion for *ASS* locus, consistent with deletion of der(9) (see Fig. 55–11).

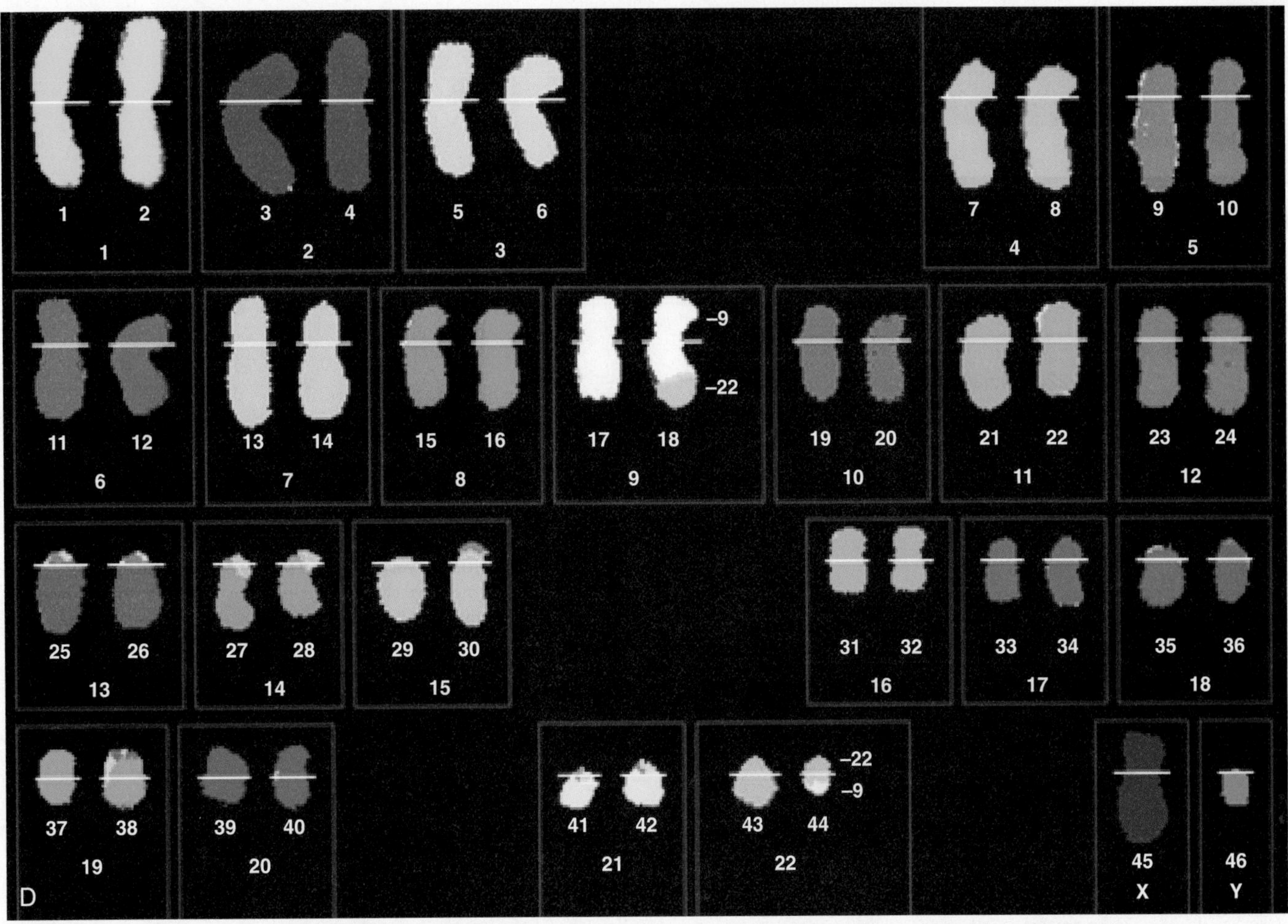

Figure 55–8, cont'd D, In multicolor FISH, identification of t(9;22) is indicated as an exchange of white and pink colors. *(M-FISH courtesy Dr. D. Zimonjic, NCI, NIH, Bethesda, MD. Adapted from Zucker-Franlin D, Grossi CE [eds.]: Atlas of Blood Cells, 3rd ed. Edi-Ermes, Milan 2003.)*

Three major breakpoint locations along the *BCR* gene on chromosome 22 result in three chimeric proteins. They include P210$^{BCR\text{-}ABL1}$, P190$^{BCR\text{-}ABL1}$, and P230$^{BCR\text{-}ABL1}$ and are associated with three distinct types of leukemia. P210$^{BCR\text{-}ABL}$ is found in the majority of patients with classic Ph positive, *BCR-ABL1* fusion-positive CML and approximately 30% of patients with Ph positive ALL. Expression of P190$^{BCR\text{-}ABL1}$ is seen in 20% to 30% of adult and 80% of children with ALL, in rare CML patients, and in the majority of patients with rare Ph positive AML, whereas expression of P230$^{BCR\text{-}ABL1}$ is associated with indolent chronic neutrophilic leukemia variant.[79–83]

The *BCR-ABL1* fusion is demonstrated in both standard and variant translocations, in cases where chromosome 9 involvement is cytogenetically not detectable, and when a masked Ph is present. In the majority of patients, the fusion of *ABL1* and *BCR* takes place on chromosome 22 (Fig. 55–9). However, a small group of patients are described in whom the *BCR* gene is translocated to chromosome 9, and the fusion of two genes is localized to 9q34.[84–86] The prognosis of these patients may be poorer, but at this time the number of reports is too small for a definitive conclusion. The *BCR-ABL1* fusion transcript is present in neutrophils, monocytes, eosinophils, erythrocytes, B cells, rarely in T cells, and in CD34$^+$ cells and is associated with increased proliferation of CD34$^+$ myeloid progenitor cells but not of other more mature myeloid precursors. These observations are consistent with previous Ph and *G6PD* studies and confirm that CML originates in a multipotent stem cell capable of differentiating to all hematopoietic cell lineages with the exception of T cells.[75,87,88] B-lymphoid differentiation and *G6PD* studies in CML provide evidence for the existence of clonal *BCR-ABL1* fusion-negative and Ph negative stage. The formation of *BCR-ABL1* and Ph occurs in the already abnormal and genetically unstable clone of pluripotent hematopoietic cells.[76,89] Thus, it is the preexisting genetic instability that predisposes to formation of *BCR-ABL1* and Ph. Once Ph formation occurs, it has a further selective growth advantage over normal cells, in the multistep pathogenesis, resulting in overwhelming *BCR-ABL1 positive*, Ph positive marrow cells at the time of diagnosis of CML.

In the 5% of patients with CML who are Ph negative by cytogenetic studies, like Ph positive patients, clonal and stem cell origin can be demonstrated, and molecular analysis reveals *BCR-ABL* fusion in approximately 2% to 3% of these patients (Fig. 55–10).[90,91] In the majority of Ph negative patients, an *ABL* insertion from chromosome 9 to 22q11.2 results in a BCR-*ABL1* fusion product without reciprocal translocation of sequences from chromosome 22 to chromosome 9. Approximately 2% of patients truly are Ph negative, *BCR-ABL* fusion negative. They may not have CML but rather another myeloproliferative disorder such as chronic myelomonocytic leukemia or refractory anemia with excess blasts.

The concept that the *BCR-ABL* fusion plays a central role in the pathogenesis of CML is strongly supported by two lines of evidence: (a) retroviral transduction experiments in which P210$^{BCR\text{-}ABL1}$ is expressed in murine marrow cells, resulting in a myeloproliferative disorder resembling CML; and (b) imatinib, a tyrosine kinase inhibitor, selectively inhibits the *BCR-ABL* fusion protein in mice and specifically inhibits the growth of human Ph positive cells in vitro and in vivo.[5,6,92,93] Although considered necessary, *BCR-ABL* may not be initial or sufficient to cause malignant transformation in CML.[49,89]

Genomic PCR and *Southern blot analysis* can determine the exact breakpoints of DNA fusion products. *Reverse transcriptase PCR* (RT-PCR) and *Northern blot analysis* allows detection of *BCR-ABL* tran-

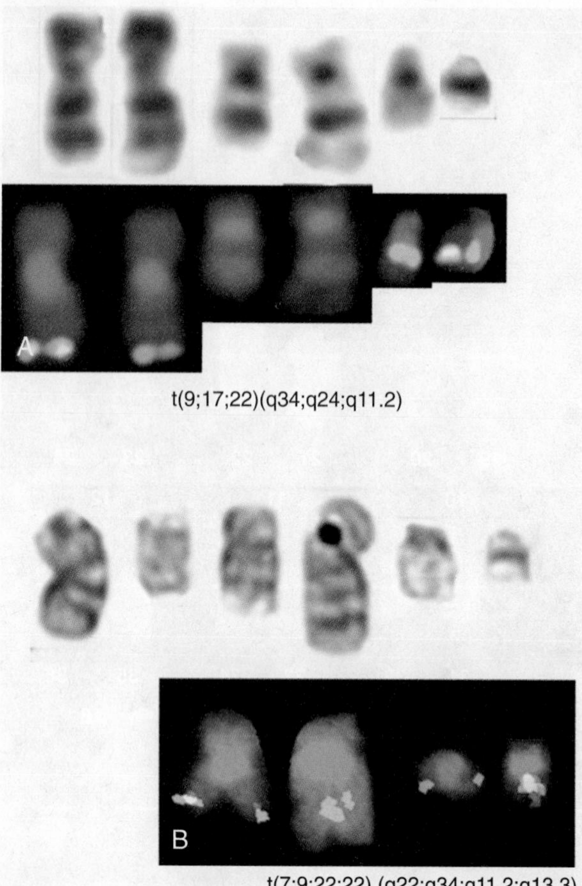

Figure 55–9 Identification of *BCR-ABL* fusion in patients with complex karyotypes. Partial karyotype from a patient with chronic myelogenous leukemia showing t(9;17;22) **(A)** and from a patient showing a four-way translocation with t(7;9;22;22) karyotype **(B)** indicating the *BCR-ABL* fusion is on the Philadelphia chromosome even in complex chromosomal translocations.

scripts at the RNA level. The P210$^{BCR\text{-}ABL1}$ protein can be demonstrated using antibodies against *BCR* and *ABL1* regions by *immunoprecipitation* or in *Western blot analysis.* Current FISH studies for detection of *BCR-ABL1* fusion at diagnosis uses a dual-color *BCR-ABL* ES probe or *BCR-ABL1* dual-fusion probe (Fig. 55–8, *A* and *B,* and Fig. 55–11). A triple-color *BCR-ABL1*-ASS probe is used for detection of deletions on both chromosomes 9 and 22. Approximately 12% to 15% of patients with CML have large deletions adjacent to the Ph translocation breakpoint on the derivative 9 chromosome, and initial reports demonstrated inferior survival in these patients (see Fig. 55–8, *C*).[94,95] Subsequent quantitative PCR and FISH studies demonstrated that deletions are heterogeneous and may involve both chromosomes 9 and 22 (majority of cases), only chromosome 9 (8% of patients with deletions; Fig. 55–12), or only chromosome 22 (4% of cases with deletions). They are associated with adverse prognosis, inferior survival, and higher probability of relapse after hematopoietic cell transplantation.[96,97] A multivariate analysis of 339 patients, with a median observation of 7 years, confirms that deletions on 9q alone, spanning the *ABL1-BCR* breakpoint, are significant independent predictors of adverse prognosis.[98]

At diagnosis of CML, conventional cytogenetics remains a gold standard because the chromosome analysis will identify not only the t(9;22) but also other chromosomal abnormalities that may indicate accelerated or blast phase of the disease or clonal proliferation of Ph negative cells.[99,100] The current international recommendation is that FISH studies should be performed at diagnosis in conjunction with conventional cytogenetics to determine deletion status on der(9q) and to identify patients who are *BCR-ABL1*$^+$ but have the Ph negative karyotype.[101]

Figure 55–10 Partial karyotype from a patient with Philadelphia chromosome (Ph) negative chronic myelogenous leukemia (top) showing normal chromosomes 9 and 22. Two pairs of chromosomes 9 and 22 after hybridization with dual color (middle) and triple color (bottom) demonstrating *BCR-ABL* fusion on the Ph chromosome without apparent t(9;22). Tricolor strategy showed *ABL* and *ASS* in close proximity and appearing as fusion on normal 9 (bottom left chromosome) and *BCR-ABL-ASS* fusion (white) on normal 22.

Imatinib mesylate has revolutionized therapy for CML and, for many patients, has transformed a deadly disease into a chronic disorder that is compatible with normal life.[102] The standard method for monitoring a patient's response to therapy is conventional cytogenetic analysis of cells obtained from marrow aspirate. In the phase III International Randomized Study of Interferon versus STI571 (IRIS), 89% of patients had Ph negative marrow aspirates as determined by conventional cytogenetics at 5 years.[6] However, conventional cytogenetics has limited sensitivity. The degree of tumor load reduction is determined to be an important prognostic factor for patients with CML on therapy. CML patients without discernible Ph detected by conventional cytogenetics analysis may still harbor up to 10^{10} leukemic cells.[103]

Hypermetaphase FISH has greater sensitivity compared to conventional cytogenetics and may detect 31% of *BCR-ABL1*$^+$ metaphase cells in patients who are Ph negative as assessed by conventional cytogenetics.[104] Interphase FISH does not depend on the cycling status of cells, and use of double-fusion probes has reduced false-positive results to approximately 1%. However, if peripheral blood cells rather than marrow aspirate cells are used to monitor residual disease, the high percentage of *BCR-ABL1 fusion*-negative lymphoid cells may underrepresent actual residual tumor load. In most direct comparison studies, interphase FISH of peripheral blood compared to conventional cytogenetics of marrow in patients who are treated with interferon or imatinib showed good correlations ($r = 0.91–0.97$).[105,106] *Real-time quantitative PCR* (RQ-PCR) is by far the most sensitive method. It provides an accurate measure of the total leukemia cell mass and the degree to which *BCR-ABL1* transcripts are reduced by therapy, and it correlates with progression-free survival.[101,107]

The goal of therapy in CML is to achieve a molecular response as measured by the reduction or elimination of *BCR-ABL1* transcripts. In IRIS, at 5-year followup, complete cytogenetic response combined with major molecular response at 12 months is associated with a 97% progression-free survival rate. This compares with an 89% progression-free survival for those with complete cytogenetic response but without major molecular response.[6,108] Current international recommendations for optimal molecular monitoring of patients receiving imatinib treatment includes an RQ-PCR assay expressing the *BCR-ABL1* transcript levels on an internationally agreed scale.[101,109] These

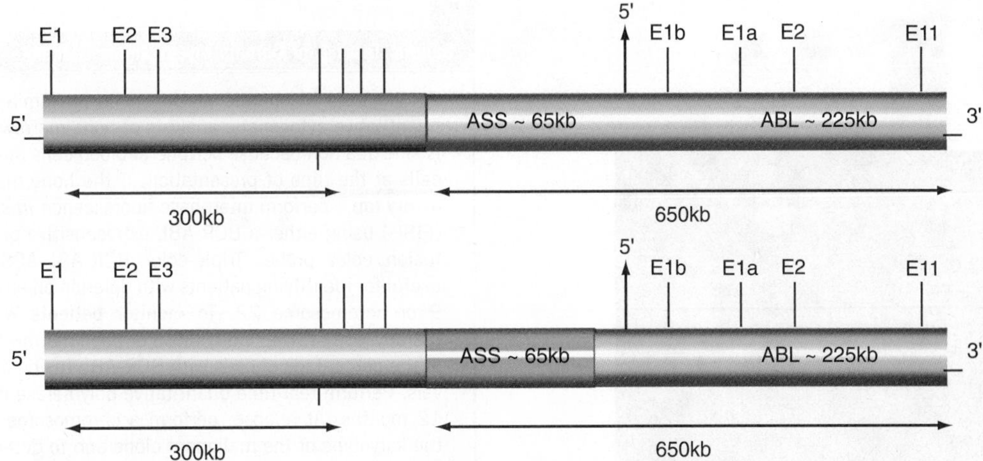

Figure 55–11 Schematic representation of the most frequently used BCR-ABL probes. Dual-color/single-fusion extrasensitive probe strategy, as indicated in text, uses a 650-kb probe in which two loci, *ABL* and *ASS,* both are labeled in red. *BCR-ABL* fusion-positive nuclei show three red signals: one small red signals on der(9), one red signal on normal homologue 9, and a third red signal in fusion with *BCR.* When a triple-color probe is applied, the *ASS* locus usually is labeled in aqua and the *BCR-ABL* fusion-positive cells show two aqua signals, unless there is deletion of der(9). The most useful application of triple-color probe is documentation of deletion of derivative chromosome 9.

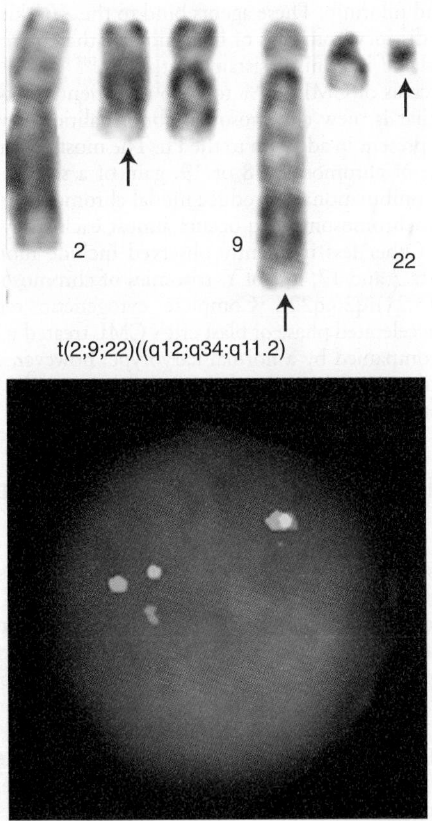

Figure 55–12 Application of triple-color *BCR-ABL-ASS* probe to cells from a patient with chronic myelogenous leukemia and t(2;9;22) karyotype (top). Interphase cell (bottom) shows *BCR-ABL* fusion signal (yellow) on the Philadelphia chromosome and one *ASS* (aqua) signal indicating loss of DNA sequences from derivative chromosome 9 as a result of this complex translocation.

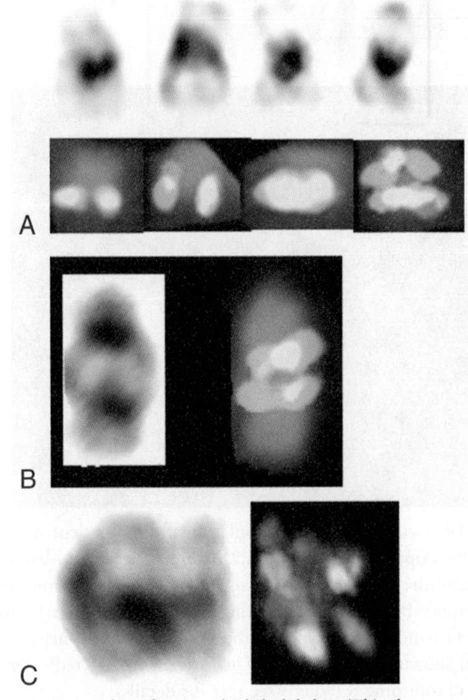

Figure 55–13 Examples of unusual Philadelphia (Ph) chromosomes associated with imatinib resistance and blast crisis of chronic myelogenous leukemia. **A,** Amplification of the Ph chromosome (top row) and the *BCR-ABL* fusion in a patient treated for 3 months with imatinib. The patient developed five copies of the Ph chromosome and 5 copes of the *BCR-ABL* fusion (yellow). B) G banding of dicentric Ph chromosome (left) dic der(22)t(9;22)(q34;q11.2) and after FISH studies (right) showing two copies of *BCR-ABL* fusion. C) G-banding of isoderivative Ph, ider(22)t(9;2 2)(q34;q11.2) (left) and after FISH studies showing two copies of *BCR-ABL* fusion (yellow) on the end of both arms.

recommendations are provisional and may require revision as new evidence emerges. It should be noted, however, that use of highly sensitive PCR-based technologies for detection of minimal residual disease is being questioned because of detection of *BCR-ABL1* transcripts in peripheral blood from normal subjects.[110,111] This finding raises the question of whether cure should be defined on a functional rather than a very sensitive molecular basis.[112]

The two major obstacles to successful imatinib-based therapies for patients with Ph positive, *BCR-ABL1* fusion-positive CML are the persistence of *BCR-ABL* fusion-positive cells and relapse of the disease due to emergence of resistance to imatinib.[108] Acquired resistance to imatinib treatment is manifested in two ways: amplification of *BCR-ABL1* fusion product (Fig. 55–13) and mutations in the ABL kinase

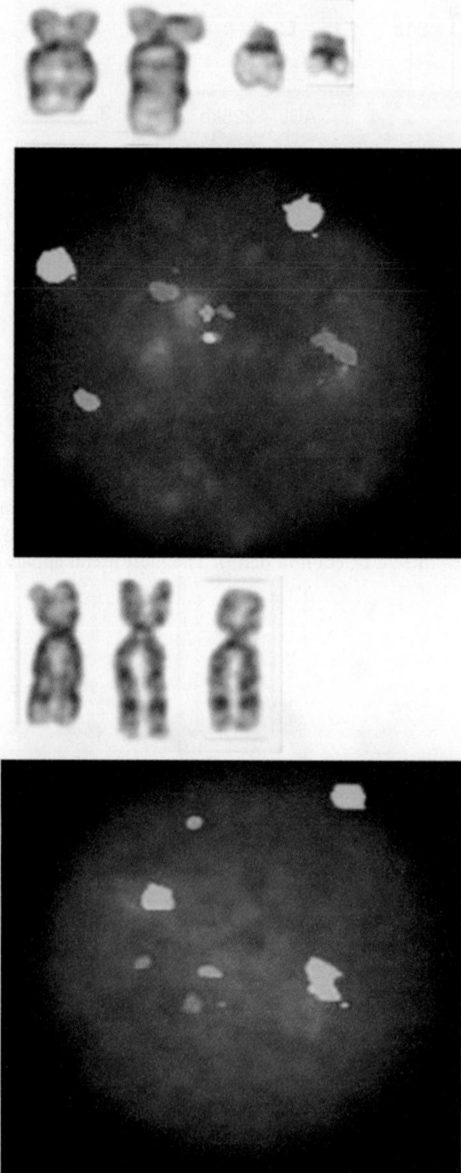

Figure 55–14 Two different cell populations from a patient treated with imatinib. One population shows t(9;22) (top row, partial G-banded karyotype) and the *BCR-ABL* fusion signal (yellow, second row) as well as disomy 8 (aqua). In contrast, the second population shows trisomy 8 (third row, partial G-banded karyotype) in the *BCR-ABL* fusion-negative cells (fourth row) showing disomy for the *BCR (green), ABL* (red) as well as trisomy for chromsome 8 (aqua) (see text for details).

domain. Currently 40 different ABL1 kinase domain mutations have been described.[112]

Between 5% and 8% of patients undergoing treatment with imatinib will develop chromosomal abnormalities such as trisomy 8, monosomy 7, del(20q), and other anomalies in *BCR-ABL1* fusion-negative cells.[113,114] Imatinib may induce chromosomal abnormalities in *BCR-ABL1*⁻ cells. Alternatively, imatinib may uncover chromosomal abnormalities present prior to therapy after significant reduction of overlying Ph positive cells (Fig. 55–14). Presence of +8 and other chromosomal anomalies in Ph negative cells in patients treated with imatinib suggests that CML has a multistep pathogenesis and that clonal Ph negative cells precede development of the Ph positive clone (Fig. 55–15).[114] This important observation about the pathogenesis of CML demonstrates the power of conventional cytogenetics, even in the era of molecular assays, and should be used at least annually while patients are undergoing imatinib treatment.

Genetic Testing for Chronic Myelogenous Leukemia

At diagnosis of chronic myelogenous leukemia (CML), perform quantitative cytogenetic analysis of bone marrow aspirate, which is sine qua non because peripheral blood cells rarely contain blast cells at the time of presentation. If the bone marrow aspirate is a "dry tap," perform interphase fluorescence *in situ* hybridization (FISH) using either a BCR-ABL extrasensitive or BCR-ABL dual-fusion color probe. Triple-color BCR-ABL-ASS is particularly useful for identifying patients with deletion on either chromosome 9 or chromosome 22. To monitor patients with CML during therapy, use FISH to study blood or bone marrow to track changes in the percentage of cells with BCR-ABL fusion at 3-month intervals. Perform real-time quantitative polymerase chain reaction at 12 months. At relapse, perform a chromosome study to assess the karyotype of the malignant clone and to determine whether a new chromosomally abnormal clone has developed or a new subclone in the Philadelphia chromosome (Ph) positive clone.

CML patients who cannot tolerate or are resistant to imatinib may benefit from the second generation of tyrosine kinase inhibitors, such dasatinib and nilotinib. These agents bind to the *ABL* kinase domain in a matter distinct from that of imatinib and thereby retain activity against nearly all imatinib resistant mutations.[108,115]

In blast crisis of CML, 80% to 85% of patients show karyotypic evolution, that is, new chromosomal abnormalities in very distinct patterns are present in addition to the Ph. The most common changes include gain of chromosome 8 or 19, gain of a second Ph, i(17q), alone or in combination, to produce modal chromosome numbers of 47 to 50. Isochromosome 17q occurs almost exclusively in myeloid blast crisis. Other less frequently observed include monosomies of chromosomes 7 and 17, loss of Y, trisomies of chromosomes 17 and 21, and t(3;21)(q26;q22). Complete cytogenetic remission for patients in accelerated phase or blast crisis CML treated with imatinib is rarely accompanied by a normal karyotype; however, 6% to 17% of these patients may have some cytogenetic response[108] (see box on Genetic Testing for Chronic Myelogenous leukemia).

Ph-Negative Chronic Myeloproliferative Disorders

Ph negative MPDs are disorders arising in a single clone of multipotent precursor cells in which one or all myeloid lineages are abnormally amplified. Classic and more frequently encountered Ph negative MPDs include polycythemia vera (PV), primary myelofibrosis (PMF), and essential thrombocytopenia (ET). Less frequently encountered are neutrophilic leukemia, hypereosinophilic syndrome/chronic eosinophilic leukemia, systemic mast cell proliferations, atypical CML, and unclassifiable myeloproliferative disorders. Classic Ph negative MPDs exhibit overlapping clinical and cytogenetic features and have a variable tendency to evolve into acute leukemias. Their clonal origin and multistep pathogenesis are established with use of X-chromosome–based clonality assay demonstrating a single *G6PD* phenotype in all hematopoietic cell lineages with the exception of T lymphocytes.[52–55,59,116] These disorders are also characterized by the recently discovered somatic point mutation within the Janus kinase 2 *(JAK2)* gene. The substitution from guanine to thymine results in an amino acid change from valine (V) to phenylalanine (F) at position 617 in the JH2 domain, constitutively activating *JAK2*.[117–120] Up to 97% of PV patients are positive for the *JAK2* 617V > F mutation, as are approximately 50% of ET and PMF patients.[121] The observation that *JAK2* V617F mutation is present in all hematopoietic lineages, including T and B lymphocytes, suggests clonal development of Ph negative MPDs.[122]

Despite technologic advances, cytogenetic analysis of marrow cells from patients with Ph negative MPD remains a laborious and

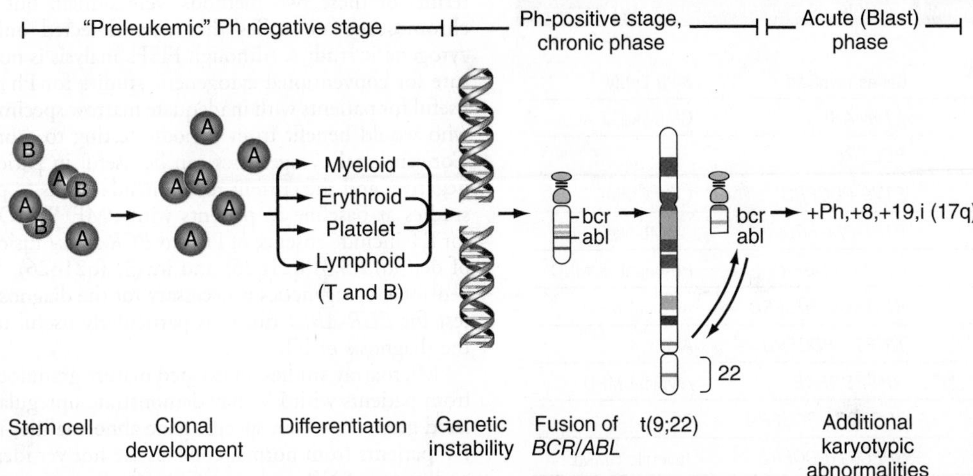

Figure 55–15 Hypothetical model of multistep pathogenesis of Philadelphia chromosome (Ph) positive chronic myelogenous leukemia. The first detectable event is a clonal proliferation of cells that are capable of differentiating to all hematopoietic lineages. These cells are genetically unstable and give rise to *BCR-ABL* fusion and the Ph chromosome. The blast crisis is characterized by nonrandom abnormalities occurring in a genetically unstable Ph positive clone. At least six events can be delineated. *(From Raskind.[35])*

time-consuming technology. Between 5% and 20% of marrow specimens may have a low mitotic yield or are otherwise uninformative due to a "dry tap." This is a particularly important problem in patients with myelofibrosis. The unifying concept of genetic instability in Ph negative MPD is a loss or a gain of genetic material. However, rare recurrent balanced translocations have been identified in MPDs (Table 55–3). In patients with these diseases, marrow cytogenetic studies should be performed because an abnormal MPD clone in the marrow may be present at a very low frequency and not in peripheral blood granulocytes. For example, del(20q)-bearing cells in some patients represent a subclone that is retained only in marrow and is not present in clonal peripheral blood granulocytes,[122] suggesting that examination of blood granulocytes is not a reliable surrogate for marrow cells in detecting karyotype abnormalities of myeloid cells using conventional cytogenetics methods.

At diagnosis, conventional cytogenetic examination of marrow cells reveals chromosome abnormalities in 20% to 25% of PV cases, 45% to 50% of PMF cases, and 8% of ET cases. In the case of PV, detection of the five most common chromosomal abnormalities may be increased to 29% in marrow cells and to 23% in peripheral blood granulocytes when more sensitive FISH methods are used.[123,124] Similar chromosomal abnormalities are found in all classic Ph negative MPDs; however, their frequencies differ in each of these disorders (Fig. 55–16). PV is more likely to exhibit +9/+9p and/or del(20q), whereas PMF is more likely to exhibit del(13q) and/or 12q abnormalities (Fig. 55–17).[125–127] Additionally, these rearrangements are observed in other myeloid neoplasms, such as MDS,[128] atypical Ph negative MPD,[129] and AML.[130]

Trisomy of chromosome 9 and gain of the short arms of chromosome 9 are most frequently observed in PV.[123] Different chromosomal rearrangements may contribute to trisomy, tetrasomy, or amplification of 9p (Fig. 55–18). Unbalanced der(9)t(1;9) resulting in trisomy of both 1q and 9p appears to be the most frequent and relatively specific abnormality observed in PV.[131–133] The prognostic clinical value of +9/+9p is not known, but it appears to occur exclusively in patients positive for the *JAK2* 617V > F mutation.[134,135] Duplication, triplication, or amplification of the mutated *JAK2* allele on the 9p24.1 chromosomal region as a result of +9/+9p may be associated with an increased level of constitutive signaling.[117] Loss of 9p heterozygosity as a result of uniparental disomy has been detected in 30% of PV patients.[136] Interestingly, the *JAK2* gene has been reported to be fused with three different genes, *TEL/ETV6*,[137] *BCR*,[138] and *PCM1*,[139] in atypical MPDs and lymphoid neoplasms. All of these fusion genes have *JAK2* rearrangements of either the JH1 or JH2 domain that produce a phenotype similar to the *JAK2* 617V > F mutation.

Deletion of the long arms of chromosome 20 is a recurrent nonrandom clonal chromosomal abnormality in Ph negative MPDs; it is found in MDS and rarely in AML.[123,140–142] Heterogeneity of this abnormality is suggested by the observation that two minimally deleted regions characterize different disorders. A 2.7-Mb region spanning D20S108 (proximal) and D20S481 (distal) is identified in Ph negative MPD, whereas a 2.6-Mb region spanning R52161 (proximal) and WI-12515 (distal) region is found in other myeloid malignancies.[143] A common overlapping region is 1.6 kb and as such may constitute the major mechanism for loss of heterozygosity. In myeloproliferative disorders, the sole del(20q) does not appear to adversely affect survival.[144–146] Interphase FISH greatly enhances detection of del(20q).[145] Its use is important because the abnormality, at least in PV, may be dormant for many years before del(20q) cells gain proliferative advantage.[123] Molecular cytogenetics using M-FISH, CGH, and genomewide screening failed to detect cryptic or occult 20q aberrations within the 20q11.2/q13.1 region in patients with PV and normal karyotype.[147] Deletion 20q is identified primarily in patients positive for the *JAK2* 167V > F mutation, but rare PV and ET patients with del(20q) are negative for the *JAK2* V167V > F mutation.[131,134,148]

Gain of chromosome 8 is a nonrandom recurrent abnormality not only in Ph negative MPD. It also is one of the three most frequent abnormalities in MDS and is present in 10% of patients with malignant hematopoietic disorders of both myeloid and lymphoid lineages. The prognostic significance in PV is unknown. Some patients with PV have trisomy 8 for more than 20 years.[149] The simultaneous presence of both +8 and +9 is observed in 3% to 4% of PV cases. It is rarely seen in any other hematologic malignancies.

The unbalanced translocation resulting in trisomy 1q is demonstrated in 11% of PV patients, 22% of PMF patients, and 14% of ET patients. It is the third most frequent abnormality in PV (Fig. 55–19).[131] Moreover, 70% of patients with PMF following PV show trisomy 1q as a result of unbalanced translocations. In all cases, a common trisomic region spanning 1q21q22 to 1q32 is present. PMF following PV is considered cytogenetically different from both PMF and PV.[150]

Deletions of the long arms of chromosome 13 are more frequent in PMF (25%–30% of abnormal karyotypes) than in PV (9%–13%) but also are found as recurrent abnormalities in MDS and lymphoid malignancies (different breakpoints).[126] Fine FISH mapping has defined commonly deleted region to 13q13.3–q14.3 encompassing

Table 55–3 Chromosomal Translocations in Ph-Negative MPD[a]

Chromosomal Abnormality	Genes Involved	MPD Entity
t(9;12)(q34;p13)	*ETV6-ABL*	CML-like, T-ALL
5q33	*PDGFRB*	
t(5;12)(q33;p13)	*ETV6-PDGFRB*	CEL, CMML
t(5;7)(q33;q11)	*HIP1-PDGFRB*	CMML-like
t(5;10)(q33;q21)	*CCDC6-PDGFRB*	Ph-negative MPD
t(5;14)(q33;q32)	*KIA1509-PDGFRB*	Atypical MPD
t(5;14)(q33;q32)	*TRIP11-PDGFRB*	AML
t(5;14)(q33;q22)	*NIN-PDGFRB*	Atypical MPD
t(5;15)((q33;q15)	*TP53BP1-PDGFRB*	CEL
t(5;17)(q33;p11)	*SPECC1-PDGFRB*	Juvenile CMML
t(5;17)(q33;p13)	*RABEP1-PDGFRB*	CMML
8p11	*FGFR1*	CMML
t(8;13)(p11;q12)	*ZNF198-FGFR1*	MPD syndrome, leukemia, lymphoma
t(7;8)((q32;p11)	*TRIM24-FGFR1*	MPD syndrome
t(6;8)((q27;p11)	*FGFR1OP-FGFR1*	Stem cell MPD
ins(12;8)(p11;p11p22)	*FGFR1OP2-FGFR1*	MPD syndrome
t(8;17)(p11;q11)	*MYO18A-FGFR1*	MPD syndrome
t(8;22)(p11;q11.2)	*BCR-FGFR1*	Lymphoproliferative disorder
4q12	*PDGFRA*	
del(4)(q12q12)	*FIP1L1-PDGFRA*	CEL
t(4;22)(q12;q11.2)	*BCR-FGFR1*	Atypical CML
4q12	*KIT*	SM
9p24	*JAK2*	
t(9;22)(p24;q11.2)	*BCR-JAK2*	CML-like
t(9;12)(p24;p13)	*JAK2-ETV6*	CML-like
der(9)t(9;12)(p24;q13)	*JAK-NF-E2*	MDS
t(8;9)(p22;p24)	PCM1-JAK2	CMPD, AL,
der(9;18)t(p13;p11)	Not reported	PV, PV→MF
der(9;18)(p10;q10)	Not reported	PV, PV→MF, ET→ AML
der(9)t(1;9)(q12;q12)	Not reported	PV, MF
der(1;7)(q10;p10)	Not reported	ET
t(12)(q21 or q21)	Not reported	MF

AL, acute leukemia; ALL, acute lymphoblastic leukemia; AML, acute myelogenous leukemia; CEL, chronic myeloproliferative disorder ; CML, chronic myelogenous leukemia; CMML, chronic myelomonocytic leukemia; CMPD, chronic eosinophilic leukemia; ET, essential thrombocytopenia; MDS, myelodysplastic syndrome; MF, myelofibrosis; MPD, myoproliferative disorder; T-ALL, T-cell acute lymphoblastic leukemia.

[a]Modified from reference 167.

RB1, D13S319, and *D13S25* loci. Cryptic 13q deletions do occur but are rare and easily identified with FISH in both marrow and peripheral blood. Most patients with del(13q) are negative for the *JAK2* 617V > F mutation.[134,148]

To compare the efficacy of chromosome studies and FISH, blood and marrow from 42 patients who had myelofibrosis were studied using both methods.[151] The FISH method used probes to detect common anomalies of chromosomes 5, 7, 8, 11, 13, 20, and 21. The results of these two methods were similar, but some patients had chromosome anomalies that were detected only by conventional cytogenetic studies. Although FISH analysis is not generally a substitute for conventional cytogenetic studies for Ph negative MPD, it is useful for patients with inadequate marrow specimens and for patients who would benefit from periodic testing to monitor disease status. Conventional cytogenetics can be useful in patients who are *JAK2*-negative, and the current recommendation is to perform cytogenetic studies at baseline in patients with PMF. WHO diagnostic criteria for ET include absence of Ph and *BCR-ABL1* fusion as well as absence of del(5q),t(3;3)(q21q26) and inv(3) (q21q26). Consequently, conventional cytogenetics is necessary for the diagnosis of ET.[152] A FISH test for *BCR-ABL1* fusion is particularly useful to rule out CML in the diagnosis of ET.

Microarray studies on isolated mature granulocytes or CD34+ cells from patients with PV may demonstrate upregulated and downregulated genes; however, specific gene abnormalities that can distinguish PV patients from normal controls are not yet identified. In contrast, preliminary SNP studies of CD34+ cells from nine patients with PV positive for the *JAK2* V617F mutation confirm previous cytogenetic observations that amplification of 9p in a region harboring the *JAK2* locus along with 17q12.3 region are the most common genomic gains. More specifically, 21 genes in recurrently amplified chromosomal regions have significantly elevated expression levels, including *NFIB* on 9p24, and seven genes in recurrently deleted regions have significantly depressed expression level, including *TOPI* on 20q12.[153]

Molecular detection of the *JAK2* 617V > F mutation in patients with clonal hematopoiesis is diagnostic for Ph negative MPD but does not differentiate among PV, ET, PMF, and rare cases of AML and MDS. No doubt the *JAK2* 617V > F somatic mutation is the major genetic contributor to the Ph negative MPD phenotype. However, in this rapidly evolving field, currently six lines of evidence indicate that the *JAK2* 617V > F somatic mutation is neither an initiating event nor the only genetic event resulting in the Ph negative phenotype. (a) From 3% to 7% of patients are negative for the *JAK2* 617V > F mutation, and approximately 50% of PMF and ET patients do not harbor the mutation. (b) Other novel *JAK2* mutations are described in 5% to 15% of Ph negative, *JAK2* V617F-negative MPD patients. One such mutation in *JAK2* exon 12 results in a myeloproliferative phenotype when transfected in a murine model. The *JAK2T7875N* activating mutation results in MPD with features of megakaryoblastic leukemia. The *JAK2ΔIREED* mutation, which involves a five-amino-acid deletion within the JH2 pseudokinase domain, is detected in B-cell precursor ALL, indicating that other *JAK2* mutations may contribute to the lymphoid leukemic phenotype.[154–157] (c) Chromosomal translocations that fuse *JAK2* to another protein are also capable of inducing both myeloproliferative and lymphoid disease. (d) Wild-type *JAK2* is identified in EPO-independent erythroid colonies in a proportion of PV patients with clonal hematopoiesis.[116] (e) Transformation of MPD to AML occurs in *JAK2* V617F-negative clones from patients with *JAK2* 617V > F-positive disease.[158] (f) Recurrent chromosomal abnormalities such as del(20q), trisomy 8, and 12q translocations are detected in a number of patients with PV, ET, and PMF who have *JAK2* 617V > F-negative disease (Fig. 55–20).[148,159]

Rare recurrent balanced abnormalities in atypical Ph negative MPD generally involve the *PDGFRB* gene found at 5q33, *FGFR1* gene on 8p11 (these disorders are referred to as myeloproliferative syndrome or stem cell leukemia syndrome), and *PDGFRA* gene on 4q12. The best described are t(5;12)(q33;p13) resulting in *ETV6-PDGFRB* fusion protein[160] and t(8;13)(p11;q12) resulting in the *ZNF198-FGFR1* fusion gene.[161]

The most frequent recurrent abnormality is the cryptic deletion on 4q12 as a result of *FIP1L1-PDGFRA* fusion gene reported to occur at frequencies ranging from 3% to 56% in patients with chronic eosinophilic leukemia/hypereosinophilic syndrome.[162] The disparity in frequencies reflects differing levels of stringency criteria in the diagnosis of disorders with hypereosinophilia as well as different methodology used for detection of *FIP1L1-PDGFRA* fusion. The

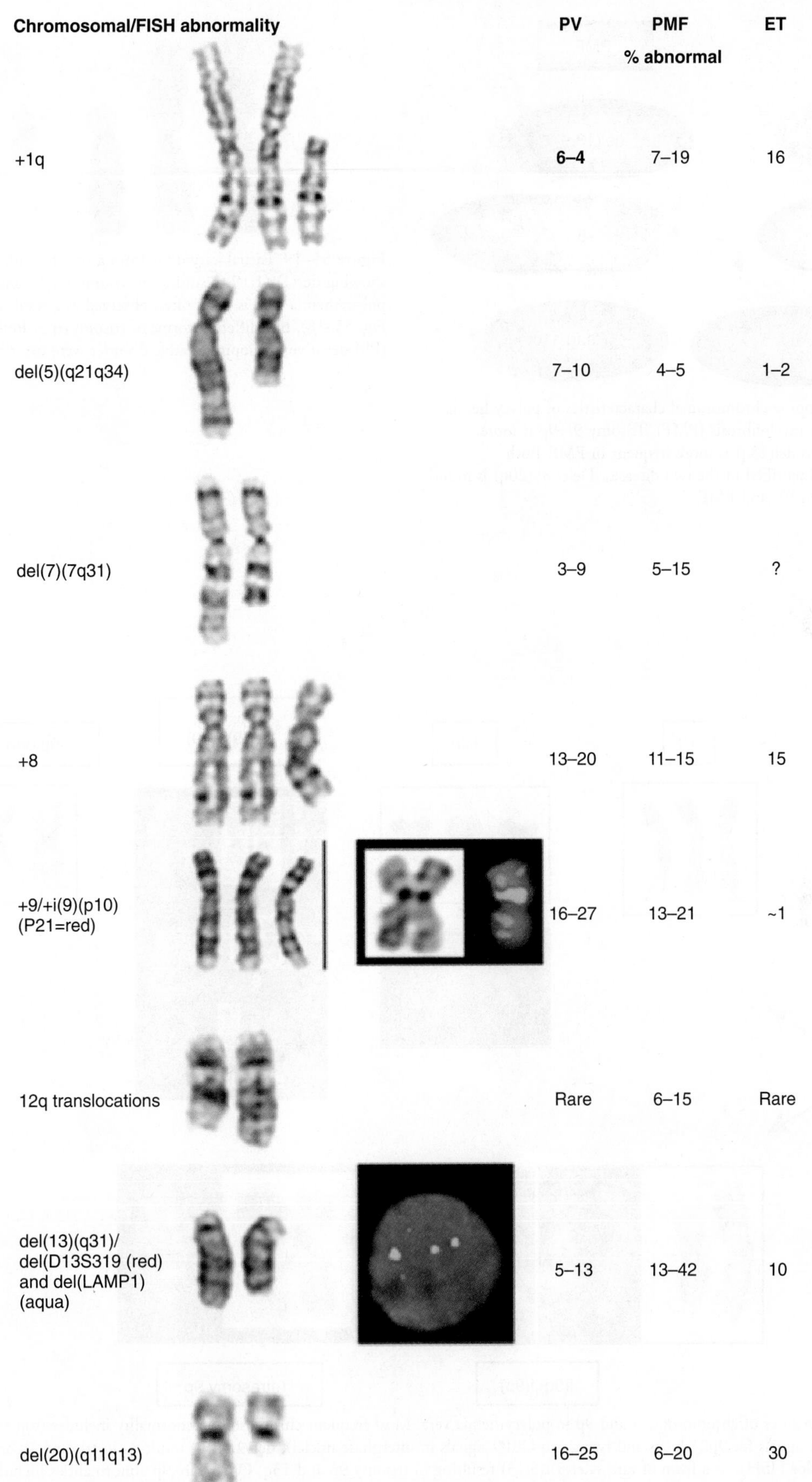

Chromosomal/FISH abnormality
PV
PMF
ET
% abnormal
+1q
6–4
7–19
16
del(5)(q21q34)
7–10
4–5
1–2
del(7)(7q31)
3–9
5–15
?
+8
13–20
11–15
15
+9/+i(9)(p10)
(P21=red)
16–27
13–21
~1
12q translocations
Rare
6–15
Rare
del(13)(q31)/
del(D13S319 (red)
and del(LAMP1)
(aqua)
5–13
13–42
10
del(20)(q11q13)
16–25
6–20
30

Figure 55–16 Most common recurrent chromosomal abnormalities and their approximate frequencies in three classic Philadelphia chromosome (Ph) negative myeloproliferative disorders: polycythemia vera, primary myelofibrosis, and essential thrombocythemia. *(From Silver RT, Tefferi A [eds.]: Myeloproliferative Disorders. Informa, New York, London 2007.)*

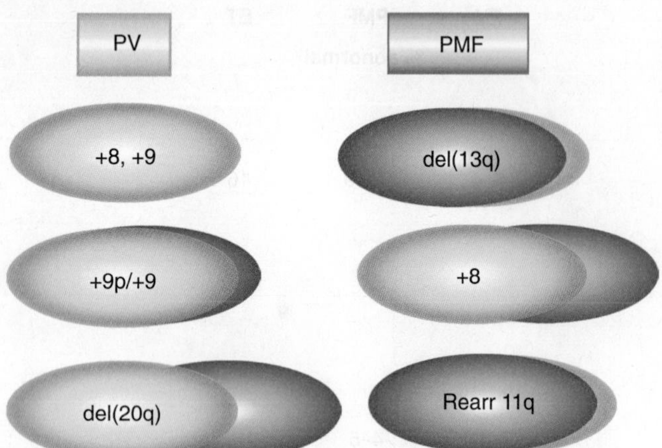

Figure 55–17 Overlapping chromosomal characteristics of polycythemia vera (PV) and primary myelofibrosis (PMF). Trisomy 9/+9p is more frequent in PV, whereas del(13q) is more frequent in PMF. Both abnormalities may be identified in the two diseases. Deletion(20q) is found at similar frequencies in PV and PMF.

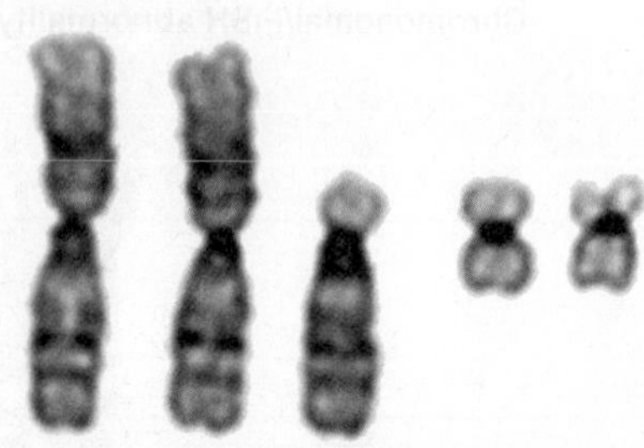

Figure 55–19 Partial karyotype from a patient with primary myelofibrosis showing der(1)t(1;19) resulting in trisomy for 1q and 19p. Trisomy 1q in polycythemia vera is most often observed as a result of der(9)t(1;9) (see Fig. 55–18), but different forms of trisomy1q in Philadelphia chromosome (Ph) negative myeloproliferative disorder were described.

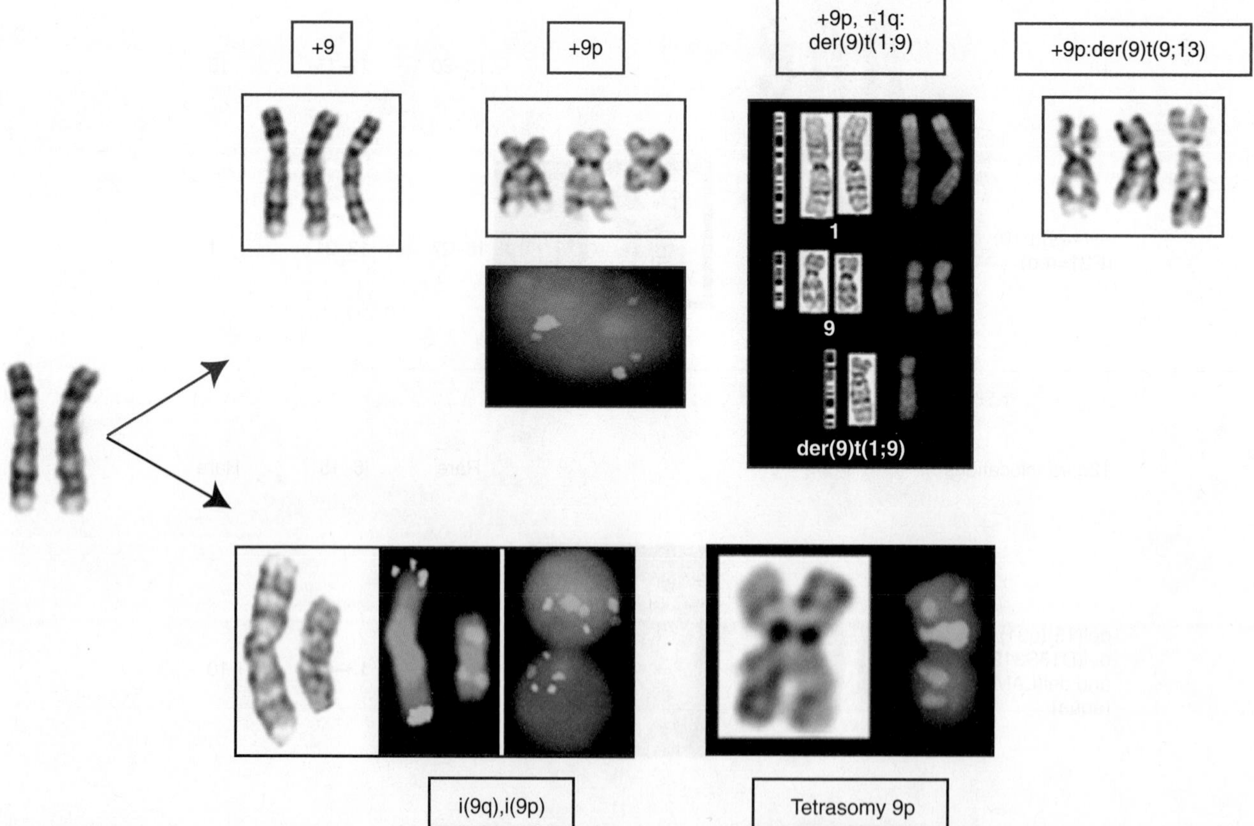

Figure 55–18 Abnormalities of chromosome 9 and 9p in polycythemia vera. Most frequent chromosome abnormality includes (top row) trisomy 9, isolated +9p (three red signals for 9p21 locus and two green CEP9 signals in interphase nuclei), der(9)t(1;9) resulting in trisomy 1q and 9p (documented by original Rx multicolor FISH), or a form of rare +der(9)t(9;13) resulting in trisomy 9p and 13q. Other rare 9p abnormalities include isochromosome (9q) and i(9p) (bottom row), G banding (left), and after FISH study (middle and right), indicating two *ASS* loci on both arms of i(9q) and two 9p21 loci on both i(9p) formation. Interphase FISH shows normal disomy for all tested loci. Isochromosome 9p in a patient with two normal chromosome 9 indicating tetrasomy 9p (G banding) and after dual-color FISH study showing two copes of 9p21 (red) on both arms and one copy of CEP9 (green) consistent with isochromosome 9p. *(Modified from V. Najfeld. In: Molecular Genetic Pathology. eds. Liang Cheng and David Y. Zhang Humana Press, Totowa, NJ, 2008.)*

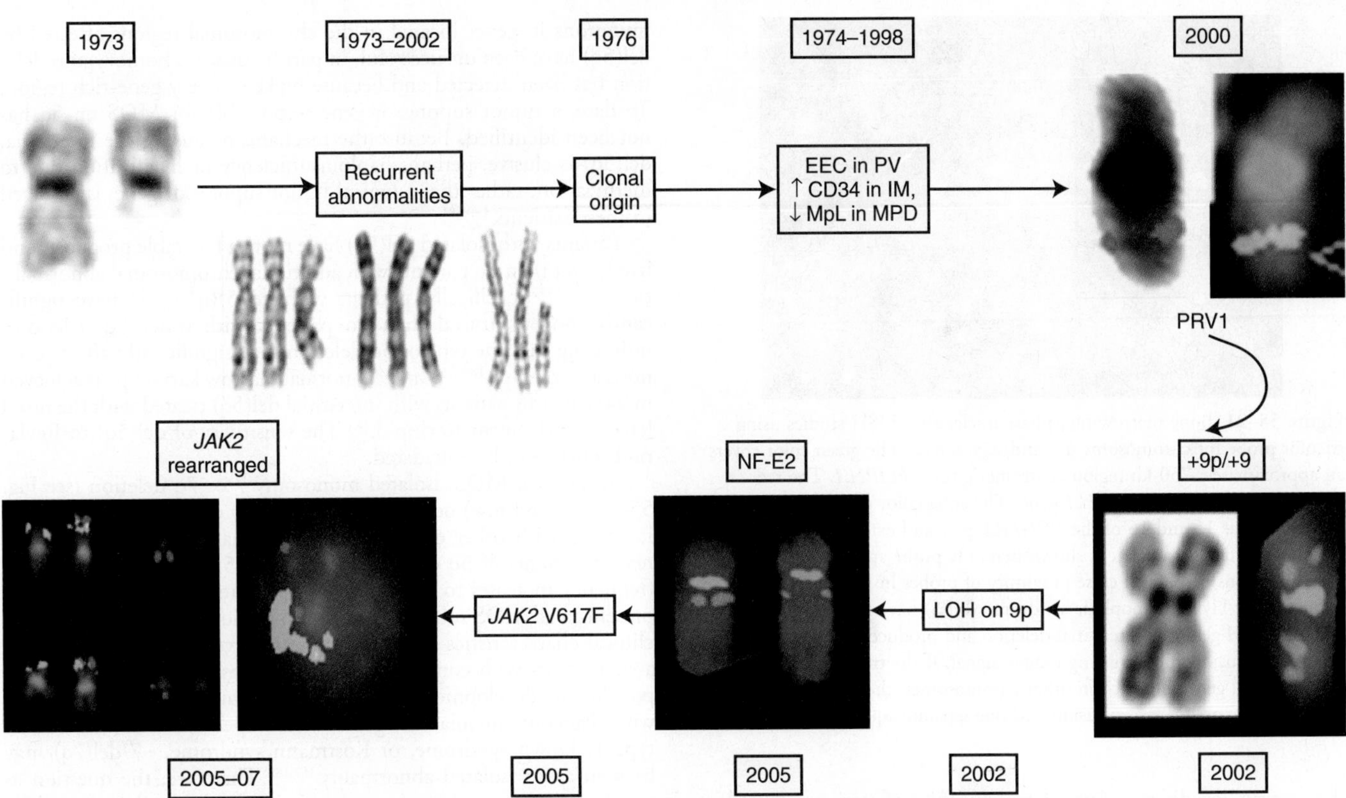

Figure 55–20 Chromosomal and molecular journey of Philadelphia chromosome (Ph) negative myeloproliferative disorder. In 1973, application of G banding to metaphase cells from patients with polycythemia vera resulted in identification of del(20q). During the next 20 years, other recurrent chromosomal abnormalities, such as +8, +9, and +1q, were identified using conventional cytogenetics. In 1973, *G6PD* isoenzyme studies demonstrated clonal origin of polycythemia vera. A number of biologic markers were identified between 1978 and 1998. Observation of increased *PRV1* constitutive activity in patients with myeloproliferative disorder represented the first step in molecular understanding and was followed by FISH findings that +9p is the most frequent abnormality. In the same year, Loss of hetezozygosity (LOH) on 9p was established for approximately 30% of polycythemia vera patients. Two years later, the role of the *NF-E2* gene on 12q was identified through array studies. In the spring of 2005, four papers demonstrated *JAK2* V617F point mutation in the majority of patients with polycythemia vera and in approximately 50% of patients with primary myelofibrosis and essential thrombocytopenia. In the period from 2005 to 2007, other *JAK2* molecular rearrangements, such as amplification and translocations, were documented, as were other point mutations. The exact molecular pathogenesis in Ph negative myeloproliferative disorder awaits elucidation.

most recent investigation of 376 patients with persistent unexplained hypereosinophilia revealed an 11% incidence of *FIP1L1-PDGFRA* fusion detected using highly sensitive RQ-PCR.[163] Patients with *FIP1L1-PDGFRA* fusion are characterized by male predominance, marrow fibrosis, increased number of mast cells, elevated serum tryptase levels, and favorable response to low doses of imatinib.[164–166] Most of these patients have a normal karyotype because a cryptic deletion of *CHIC2* locus on 4q12 is only 800 kb in size, but a more sensitive FISH technology and RQ-PCR will detect the majority of cases with this deletion at diagnosis. Moreover, the most recent commercially available tricolor FISH probe will detect not only deletion 4q12 as a result of *FIP1L1-PDGFRA* but will a rare *BCR-PDGFRA* fusion resulting from the t(4;22)(q12;q11.2) rearrangement (Fig. 55–21). Serial monitoring with RQ-PCR demonstrates exquisite sensitivity of *FIP1L1-PDGFRA*–positive patients to low-dose imatinib treatment.[163]

Conventional and molecular cytogenetic findings in atypical Ph negative MPDs as well as the presence of the *JAK2* 617V > F mutation in typical Ph negative MPDs provide support that abnormalities in tyrosine kinase genes are central to the molecular pathogenesis of these disorders[167] (see box on Genetic Testing for Ph-Negative Myeloproliferative Disease).

Genetic Testing for Ph-Negative Myeloproliferative D

At diagnosis, perform *JAK2* V617F real-time allele-specific polymerase chain reaction as well as cytogenetic analysis of marrow aspirate. Unstimulated peripheral blood can be used instead of marrow aspirate for patients with primary myelofibrosis. Perform fluorescence *in situ* hybridization (FISH) studies with BCR-ABL for patients with essential thrombocytopenia. FISH studies also can be performed when cytogenetics is uninformative for detection of most frequent abnormalities: +9, +9p,+8,del(13)(q14), and del(20)(q11q13). The panel of five probes includes CEP9, P21 at 9p21, CEP8, RB1, and D20S108. To monitor patients after therapy, use FISH study to detect diagnostic abnormality. At diagnosis and to monitor patients with hypereosinophilic syndrome, perform FISH using triple-color *FIP1L1* probe.

MYELODYSPLASTIC SYNDROMES

The MDSs are a clinically heterogeneous group of hematologic disorders with differing biology and clinical manifestations.[168] They have in common a clonal origin, dysplastic cellular morphology, abnormalities of cellular maturation, increased propensity to develop acute leukemia (20%–40%), and multistep pathogenesis.[55,169] Cytogenetic studies are important for patients with these disorders because the results can provide both diagnostic and prognostic information.[170–174] A chromosomally abnormal clone can be detected in 40% to 60% of patients with de novo MDS and in approximately 90% of patients with therapy-related MDS.[128,170] There appears to be a correlation between the frequency of chromosomal abnormalities and

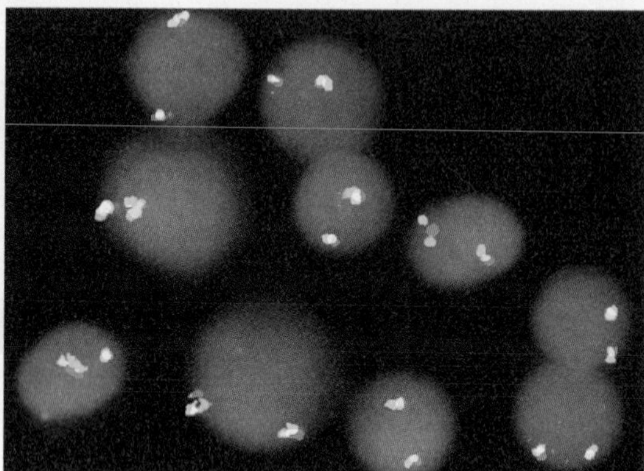

Figure 55–21 Bone marrow interphase nuclei after FISH studies using tricolor probe for chromosome 4, band region q12. The green color covers an approximately 750-kb region centromeric from *FLIP1L1*. The red probe is telomeric of the *FIP1L1* gene. The aqua color probe begins between exons 15 and 16 of the *PDGFRA* gene and extends toward the 4q telomere. In normal nuclei, as shown here, the probe appears as two tricolor fusions because of close proximity of probes in interphase DNA. Patients with Hypereosinophilie syndrome (HES) have fusion of *FIP1L1* and *PDGFRA* genes by interstitial deletion and produce one signal with green–aqua fusion and a missing orange signal. If the translocation involves the *PDGFRA* gene with loci on other chromosomes, the expected signal pattern is one orange–green fusion and one separate aqua signal.

the severity of disease. Approximately 35% of patients with less aggressive MDS, such as refractory anemia and refractory anemia with ring sideroblasts, have clonal chromosomal rearrangements, whereas approximately 60% to 70% of patients with refractory anemia with excess blasts in transformation have such chromosomal abnormalities. A single or complex chromosomal abnormality may be present initially, and evolutionary change may occur during the course of the disease. Even at diagnosis of MDS, complex genomic lesions involving five or more different chromosomes are not unusual. Despite heterogeneity of chromosomal defects (gain, loss, deletion, amplification, rare balanced translocations, transcriptional silencing via methylation or point mutation), the unifying concept of genetic instability in MDS is hemizygosity of specific genes or chromosomal regions. The most common chromosome anomalies in MDS involve del(5q)/−5, del(7q)/−7, trisomy 8, del(11)(q23),del(12p), +13/del(13q), t(11q23), del(12p), del(17p), del(20)(q11q13), +21, and idic(X)(q13) (Fig. 55–22).[72,128,173]

The clinical relevance and the power of conventional cytogenetics in MDS were recognized by the WHO classification for hematologic malignancies, which accepted a strong association between del(5)(q13q33) and 5q− syndrome, and idic(X)(q13) and refractory anemia with ring sideroblasts. The 5q− syndrome is a unique subtype of International Prognostic Scoring System low-risk MDS with a favorable prognosis, lack of other cytogenetic abnormalities, low rate of leukemic transformation, and more common occurrence in elderly females (Fig. 55–23).[174,175]

Among patients who do not have 5q− syndrome (with or without other chromosome abnormalities), interstitial deletions of the long arms of chromosome 5 occur in 10% to 15% and are among the most frequent chromosomal abnormalities in MDS (see Fig. 55–22, first row).[176,177] The finding of del(5q) in $CD34^+CD38^-$ cell indicates its occurrence in a stem cell capable of differentiating into myeloid and lymphoid cell lineages and represents an early event in the pathogenesis of MDS.[178] Data on 1432 patients with del(5q) show a great heterogeneity in breakpoints. FISH methods delineated the commonly deleted segment, currently estimated to be 1.5 Mb in size, on 5q31.1.[176–179,184] The clustering of genes responsible for growth and differentiation of hematopoietic cells and the recurrent nature of −5/del(5q) in MDS caused many investigators to speculate that a tumor suppressor gene(s) is located in the 5q31 or 5q22–23 band region. Despite numerous research efforts for more than 20 years, mutations in genes located in the chromosomal regions affected by del(5q) have been unsuccessful, in part because no homozygous deletion has been detected and because 5q31 is a very gene-rich region. To date, a tumor suppressor gene responsible for MDS on 5q has not been identified. Because the mechanism causing the interstitial del(5q) is elusive, perhaps haploinsufficiency or inactivation due to methylation, rather that a typical tumor suppressor gene, is involved in these patients.[180,181]

Patients with isolated del(5q) have more a favorable prognosis and live longer than do patients with additional chromosomal abnormalities.[177,182,183] Specifically, patients with del(5)(q13q31) have significantly longer survival than do patients with other 5q deletions, indicating that the type of 5q deletion may significantly affect prognosis and therapy.[183–184] Indeed, normal marrow karyotype is achieved in 44% of 148 patients with interstitial del(5q) treated with the novel lenalidomide agent Revlimid.[185] The sensitivity of del(5q) to Revlamid remains to be elucidated.

In de novo MDS, isolated monosomy 7 or 7q deletion (see Fig. 55–22, second row) occurs with a frequency of 1%. However, when it occurs with other chromosomal abnormalities, most commonly rearrangements of 3q or del(12p) (see Fig. 55–22, eighth row), the frequency increases to 5% to 10% of patients.[128,186] Monosomy 7 is present in all MDS subtypes and is seen predominantly in males with clinical characteristics similar to those of juvenile CMML. In pediatric patients with constitutional disorders associated with a predisposition to development of myeloid leukemia, such as individuals with Fanconi anemia, congenital neutropenia, neurofibromatosis type 1, Down syndrome, or Kostmann syndrome, −7/del(7q) may be seen as an isolated abnormality.[187,188] Therefore, the question as to whether these patients have genetic imprinting and preferentially lose chromosome 7 from one parent is relevant to understanding the origin of the genetic abnormality. Evidence unequivocally shows that preferential parental origin of the missing chromosome 7 is not present because approximately half of patients have loss of either the maternal or paternal homologue, excluding the genomic imprinting phenomenon as a cause for monosomy 7.[189] Embryonic origin of partial chromosome 7 deletion in monozygotic twins with juvenile chronic myelomonocytic leukemia has been reported.[190]

The presence of monosomy 7 or deletion 7q is associated with poor clinical outcome in MDS (Fig. 55–23). Allele typing studies implicated three regions in patients with deletion 7q that are most frequently deleted: 7q22, 7q31.1, and 7q31.3. Cytogenetic results indicated that retention of 7q31 band may be associated with longer survival (Fig. 55–24).[191] Consequently, there is speculation that a putative myeloid suppressor gene(s) is located in the regions that are frequently deleted. Because prototypic tumor suppressor genes have not been identified in patients with 7q deletions, an alternative explanation may be haploinsufficiency whereby the level of protein is critical, or a complex of two cooperating proteins is affected as a result of inactivation due to methylation.

Trisomy 8 (see Fig. 55–22, third row) is the third most frequent chromosomal abnormality in MDS. As a sole abnormality, it is found in 11% of patients with MDS and overall is found in 17%.[192] There is a significantly higher incidence of males with trisomy 8 than in females. Trisomy 8 is present in all age groups of patients with MDS. Although trisomy 8 is detected in $CD34^+CD38^-Thy\text{-}1^+$ hematopoietic stem cell of patients with MDS, a sizable fraction of stem cells is disomic but functionally abnormal, suggesting that trisomy 8 is a secondary event in MDS pathogenesis.[193] These findings provide evidence for a multistep pathogenesis of MDS, whereby gain of chromosome 8 is not an early event in stepwise evolution. Although trisomy 8 carries an intermediate risk when detected at diagnosis, findings suggest that MDS patients treated with the hypomethylating agent 5-azycytidine have a significantly better survival than patients with other chromosomal abnormalities.[194,195]

Deletions of 17p are seen in 3% to 4% of MDS and AML patients. These patients often display several other chromosomal rearrangements, including monosomy 17, isochromosome 17q, and unbalanced translocations between chromosome 17 and another chromosome. Approximately 30% of these deletions are therapy

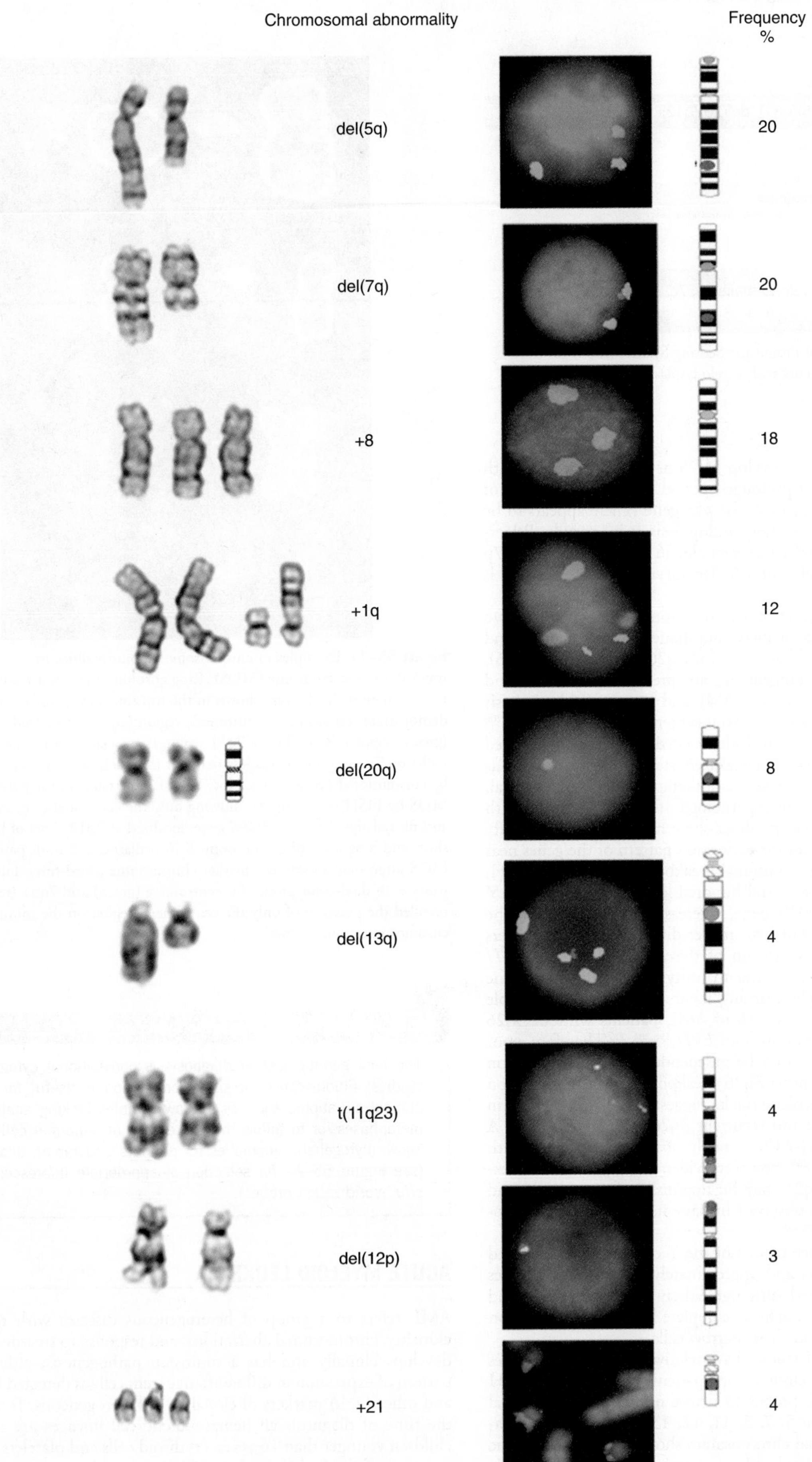

Figure 55–22 Most frequent nonrandom chromosomal abnormalities and their frequencies in myelodysplastic syndrome. G banding of chromosomal abnormalities (left) and their detection in interphase cells (middle). Schematic representation of chromosomes and probe locations for detection of recurrent abnormalities (right).

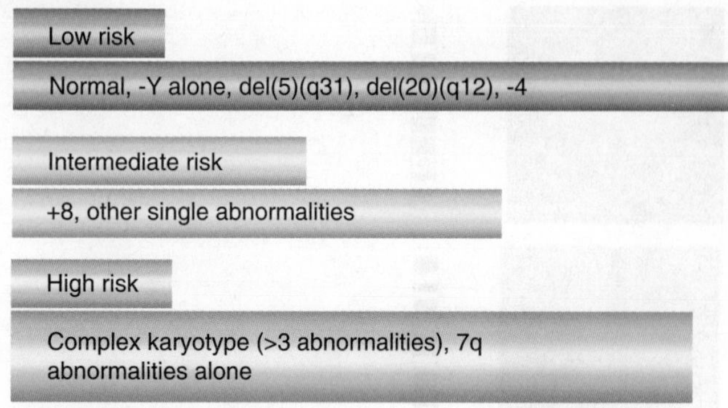

Low risk
Normal, -Y alone, del(5)(q31), del(20)(q12), -4
Intermediate risk
+8, other single abnormalities
High risk
Complex karyotype (>3 abnormalities), 7q abnormalities alone

Figure 55–23 International Prognostic Scoring System (IPSS) for evaluating prognosis in patients with myelodysplastic syndromes.

related. Most patients who develop MDS or AML are treated with hydroxyurea, usually for a prolonged period of time. The extent of 17p deletion in all cases involves the *p53* gene. There appears to be a close correlation between dysgranulopoiesis (e.g., pseudo–Pelger-Huet hypolobulation) and small vacuoles in neutrophils with 17p abnormalities and *p53* deletion. Median survival of these patients is poor.[196,197]

The most frequent rearrangement of chromosome 3 involves two bands on chromosome 3, namely, simultaneously band 3q21 and 3q26, which produces either t(3;3)(q21;q26) or inv(3)(q21q26). These chromosomal rearrangements are present in de novo and therapy-related MDS as well as in AML and megakaryoblastic crisis of CML. The incidence of 3q rearrangements is 2% to 5%.[198–200] Characteristic clinical features include elevated platelet count, marked hyperplasia with dysplasia of megakaryocytes, and poor prognosis with minimal or no response to chemotherapy and a short survival. In addition to similar clinicopathologic features, patients with 3q21q26 chromosomal abnormalities share molecular heterogeneity in both the breakpoints and the expression pattern of the genes near these breakpoints. The chromosomal breakpoints, defined by FISH, in 3q26 are scattered over several hundred kilobases in either the 5′ or the 3′ region of the *EVI1* gene, whereas the breakpoints in the 3q21 region are restricted to two smaller different genomic clusters approximately 100 kb downstream of the *RPN1* gene.[201–203] *EVI1* overexpression is observed in the majority of patients, but some patients with the 3q21q26 rearrangement do not have detectable *EVI1* expression, and at least 9% of AML patients without 3q26 abnormalities show overexpression of *EVI1*.[198,204–206] Therefore, poor prognosis in these patients may be independent of *EVI1* expression despite the fact that extensive 3q26 breakpoint FISH mapping on both metaphases and interphase nuclei suggests *EVI1* involvement in numerous novel sporadic and recurrent 3q26 rearrangements.[207] A fusion transcript of *RPN1-EVI1* is rarely observed in patients with 3q21q26 rearrangements.[208] However, evidence suggests that overexpression of *GATA2* at 3q21 may be responsible for erythroid and megakaryocytic dysplasia observed in patients with 3q21q26 chromosomal abnormalities.[198,203]

The clinical significance of loss of the Y chromosome, observed in 10% of MDS patients and approximately 7% of elderly males without MDS, is undefined, although elderly males with MDS and loss of Y chromosome who achieve complete hematologic remission show the Y chromosome in their marrow cells.

Cytogenetic and FISH studies have relatively similar sensitivities in detecting an abnormal clone among patients with MDS. A FISH test for MDS should use probes to detect numeric and structural anomalies of chromosome 5, 7, 8, 11, 12, 13, and 20.[209–211] Occasional patients with normal chromosomes show an occult neoplastic clone by FISH. On the other hand, some patients exhibit a neoplastic clone by conventional cytogenetic studies that is not detected by FISH (see box on Genetic Testing for Myelodysplastic Syndrome and Fig. 55–22, column 4).

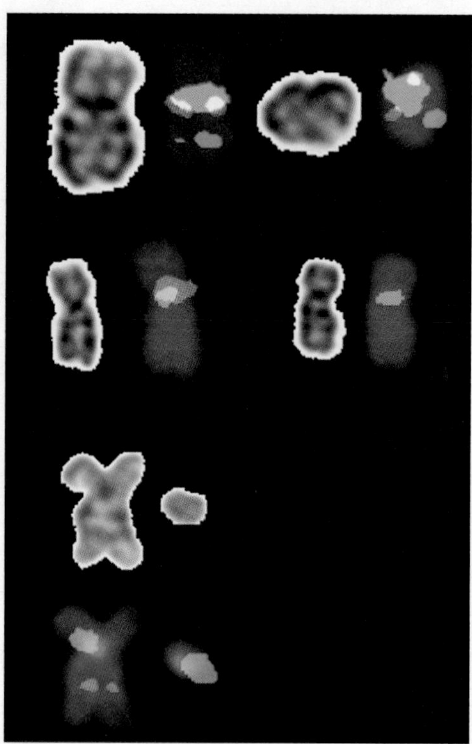

Figure 55–24 Examples of chromosome 7 abnormalities in myelodysplastic syndrome (MDS). Ring chromosome 7 is a recurrent but rare formation. In the case shown in the top row, FISH study (right) demonstrates retention of centromeric region (aqua), 7p12 (red), and 7q31 (green) regions. Retention of 7q31 region is associated with longer survival. Deletion 7p (second row) is less frequent than del(7q) and may be missed by conventional cytogenetics. Note loss of 7p12 band in the patient with MDS by FISH study (right), showing only the centromeric (green) signal and no red signal for the *EGFR* gene, localized at 7p12. Loss of both the short and long arms of chromosome 7 in pediatric and adult patients with MDS often may appear as a marker chromosome (third row), but FISH study with dual-color probes for centromere (green) and 7q31 (red) revealed the presence of only the centromeric region on the minute chromosome (fourth row).

Genetic Testing for Myelodysplastic Syndrome Disorder

The best genetic test at diagnosis is conventional cytogenetic studies. Fluorescence *in situ* hybridization is useful for some clinical situations, such as marrow samples lacking analyzable metaphases, or to follow the percentage of abnormal cells with known cytogenetic anomalies for patients undergoing treatment (see Figure 55–22 for selection of appropriate fluorescence *in situ* hybridization probes).

ACUTE MYELOID LEUKEMIA

AML refers to a group of heterogeneous diseases with respect to clonality, chromosomal aberrations, and response to treatment. AML develops clonally and has a multistep pathogenesis, although the pattern of expression in differentiative stem cell (as detected by *G6PD* and other DNA markers of clonality) is heterogeneous. In adults, at the time of diagnosis all hematopoietic cell lineages are clonal. In children younger than 16 years, erythroid cells and platelets often are not part of the leukemic clone.[50,62] Based on karyotype status, two major groups of AML can be discriminated: (a) those with an abnormal karyotype, which accounts for approximately 52% of patients and (b) those that demonstrate a normal karyotype by conventional cytogenetics, which accounts for 48% of AML patients.[212] Among patients with an abnormal karyotype, 25% have balanced translocations [t(8;21),t(15;17),inv(16)], and 27% showed unbalanced abnormalities [−5/del(5q), −7/del(7q) or complex karyotype]. Within the normal cytogenetic category, 45% to 63% have *NPM* mutations (localized on chromosome 5, band q35), 23% to 33% show *FLT3* (localized on chromosome 13, band q12), 5% to 30% have *MLL* tandem duplications (localized on chromosome 11, band q23), and 8% and 19% have C/EBP α mutations (localized on chromosome 19, band q13.1).[213] The prognosis of patients with normal karyotype in the presence of each of these mutations is different (Table 55–4). Patients with *NPM* mutation alone have a favorable prognosis, with 60% of patients living longer than 11 years.[213,214] In contrast, the presence of *FLT3* and *MLL* mutations is associated with adverse prognosis, and coexistence of *FLT3* and *NPM* does not improve the prognosis. In childhood AML with normal cytogenetics, *NPM* mutations are relatively uncommon, occurring at frequency of 8%.[215] Gene expression profiling as a diagnostic or prognostic indicator in patients with AML and a normal karyotype has limited or moderate accuracy, which probably reflects the molecular heterogeneity of this AML subtype.[216,217]

The pretreatment karyotype in AML constitutes an independently prognostic determinant for attainment of complete remission and risk of relapse and survival.[218] Four broad cytogenetic risk categories of AML are applied in clinical practice: favorable, intermediate, unfavorable, and unknown (Fig. 55–25 and Table 55–5).[219,220] It is

Table 55–4 Gene Mutations in Patients with Acute Myelogenous Leukemia and Normal Karyotype

Gene Mutation	Frequency (%)	Prognosis
NPM	45–63	Favorable
FLT3	23–33	Adverse
MLL	5–30	Adverse
C/EBP	8–19	Favorable

Table 55–5 Cytogenetic Risk Categories in Acute Myelogenous Leukemia

Category	Abnormality
Favorable	t(8;21),[a] t(15;17), inv(16) with or without other abnormalities
Intermediate	Normal, +6, +8, +21, +22 −Y, del(9q)
Unfavorable	−5/del(5q), −7/Del(7q), abn(3q) t(9;22),t(6;9), abn(11q), 20q or 21q, abn(17p), complex karyotype

[a]Without deletion 9q or complex karyotype.

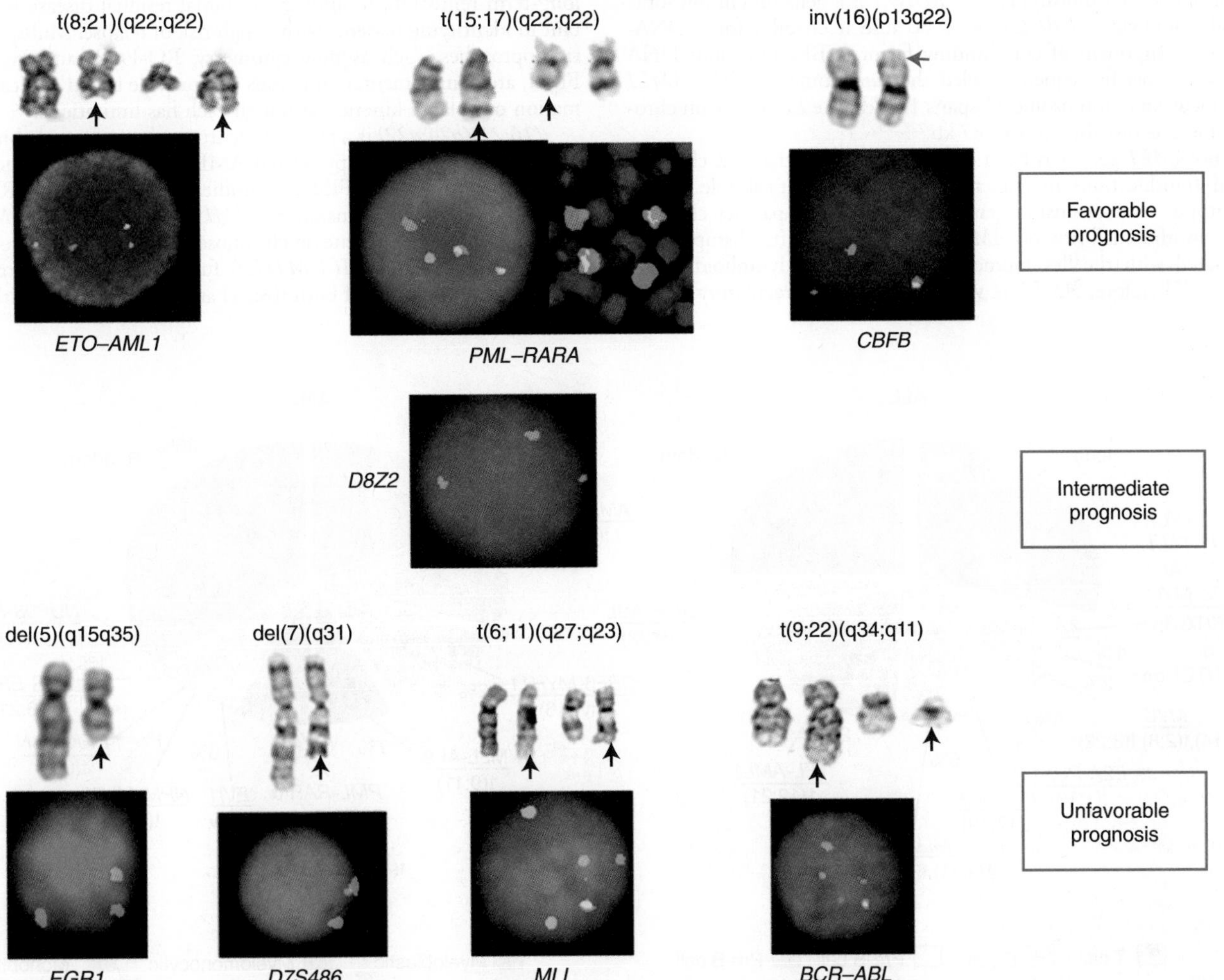

Figure 55–25 Prognostic cytogenetic risk categories in acute myeloid leukemia. Favorable prognosis includes t(8;21) and *ETO-AML1* fusion, t(15;17) and *PML-RARA* fusion, and inv(16) and rearrangements of *CBFB* on 16q22. Trisomy 8 is associated with intermediate prognosis. Unfavorable cytogenetic risk categories include monosomy 5/del(5q), −7/del(7q), and translocations of 11q23 and *MLL,* represented here by t(6;11), and the Philadelphia chromosome.

important to perform appropriate cytogenetic and FISH studies to establish the correct cytogenetic risk category. Patients displaying normal karyotype are in the intermediate prognostic category because their survival probabilities usually are lower than those with t(8;21), inv(16), t(16;16), or t(15;17).[221,222]

Tables 55–6 and 55–7 list show 166 recurrent chromosomal translocations in leukemia, including AML (Fig. 55–26, right). Because of their specific association with distinct subtypes of leukemia, some AML-specific translocations have been incorporated in the WHO classification as the criteria for subclassification of AML, including t(8;21), t(15;17), inv(16), and 11q23 rearrangements, regardless of the morphology or percent blast cells.[72]

The t(8;21)(q22;q22), described for the first time in 1973 and associated with the M2 subtype, may be present alone, although 30% to 35% of patients also display loss of Y chromosomes in males and loss of X chromosome in females (see Fig. 55–25, top left).[223] Another 20% of patients with t(8;21) show deletion of 9q12–23, including a commonly deleted segment that spans 7 to 8 Mb. Trisomies for chromosomes 4 and 8 together with t(8;21) are observed in 6% to 10% of patients. At the time of diagnosis, t(8;21) is present in 10% to 15% of adult patients with de novo AML and up to 40% in the M2 subtype of the French-American-British classification.[224] Virtually all patients with t(8;21) achieve complete remission. Additional cytogenetic abnormalities, irrespective of their nature or complexity, do not have a deleterious effect on remission, relative risk, and overall survival. The t(8;21) interrupts two genes—*RUNX1 (AML1, CBFA2)* on chromosome 21, band q22, and *ETO (e*ight, *t*wenty-*o*ne gene; also called *MTG8*-myeloid translocated gene) on chromosome 8, band q22—and joins them to form a new chimeric gene on the abnormal der[8] chromosome.[225,226] *RUNX1* is a gene on chromosome 21, also known as *CBFA2/AML1* because it encodes for a DNA-binding component of core-binding factor (CBF) and binds DNA through a specific sequence called the *runt* domain.[227] The *AML1* gene locus on chromosome 21 spans 120 kb; the *ETO* gene on chromosome 8 is distributed over 87 kb.[228,229]

The *AML1* gene has been identified in more than 32 chromosomal translocations in leukemia and plays a critical role during hematopoiesis. The fusion gene is located on the partner chromosome in the majority of *AML1* translocations. Its disruption is associated with the development of myeloid and lymphoid leukemias.[230] Therefore, *AML1* is viewed as a master regulatory switch that controls development of a definitive hematopoietic lineage. Moreover, the *AML1* transcription factor is critical for proliferation and differentiation of hematopoietic stem cells. Haploinsufficiency of *AML1* has been linked to a propensity to develop AML, and biallelic nonsense mutations in the *AML1* gene have been identified in most immature AMLs of the FAB M0 subtype.[231] The ETO protein belongs to the ETO family of proteins involved in protein–protein interactions but not in protein–DNA interactions.[232]

In the hybrid ETO-AML1 protein, the C-terminus of AML1 is replaced by the entire ETO protein. A main functional characteristic of ETO-AML1 chimeric protein is its ability to bind DNA containing AML1 binding sites and thereby exert a dominant negative inhibition of the endogenous AML1 protein.[233] The exact function of the ETO-AML1 fusion protein in the onset and progression of AML is not fully understood; however, accumulating evidence indicates that even a point mutation in the AML1 protein, responsible for assembling and organizing the machinery for hematopoietic gene expression at multiple sites in target genes, results in a block of differentiation of myeloid progenitors to granulocytes.[234] Most recent evidence indicates that *AML1/RUNX1* mutations are present in 46% of AML patients with the M0 subtype and in 80% of AML patients with trisomy 13.[235] As mentioned earlier, *FLT3* is localized on chromosome 13, and quantitation of *FLT3* transcript levels is associated with a fivefold increase in patients with *AML1/RUNX1* mutations and trisomy 13 compared to patients without trisomy 13. The exact cooperation of *FLT3* and *AML1/RUNX1* in leukemogenesis remains unknown. Multiple copies of *ETO-AML1* fusion have been demonstrated (Fig. 55–27).

Although 60% to 70% patients with t(8;21) achieve complete and long-term remission, monitoring minimal residual disease is important in identifying patients with a high risk of relapse. Multiparametric approaches, such as flow cytometry, RQ-PCR, and interphase FISH, are complementary methods and provide useful clinical information on relapse kinetics, although each has limitations.[236]

t(16;21)(q24;q22) is a rare but recurrent chromosomal abnormality associated with therapy-related AML or MDS. It was identified for the first time with FISH.[237] Studies using FISH and RT-PCR methods demonstrate fusion of *AML1* on 21q22 and *MTG16* (*m*yeloid *t*ranslocation *g*ene on chromosome 16) on chromosome 16, which produces an *AML1-MTG16* fusion gene on chromosome 16.[238] The breakpoints of both t(8;21) and t(16;21) occur within the

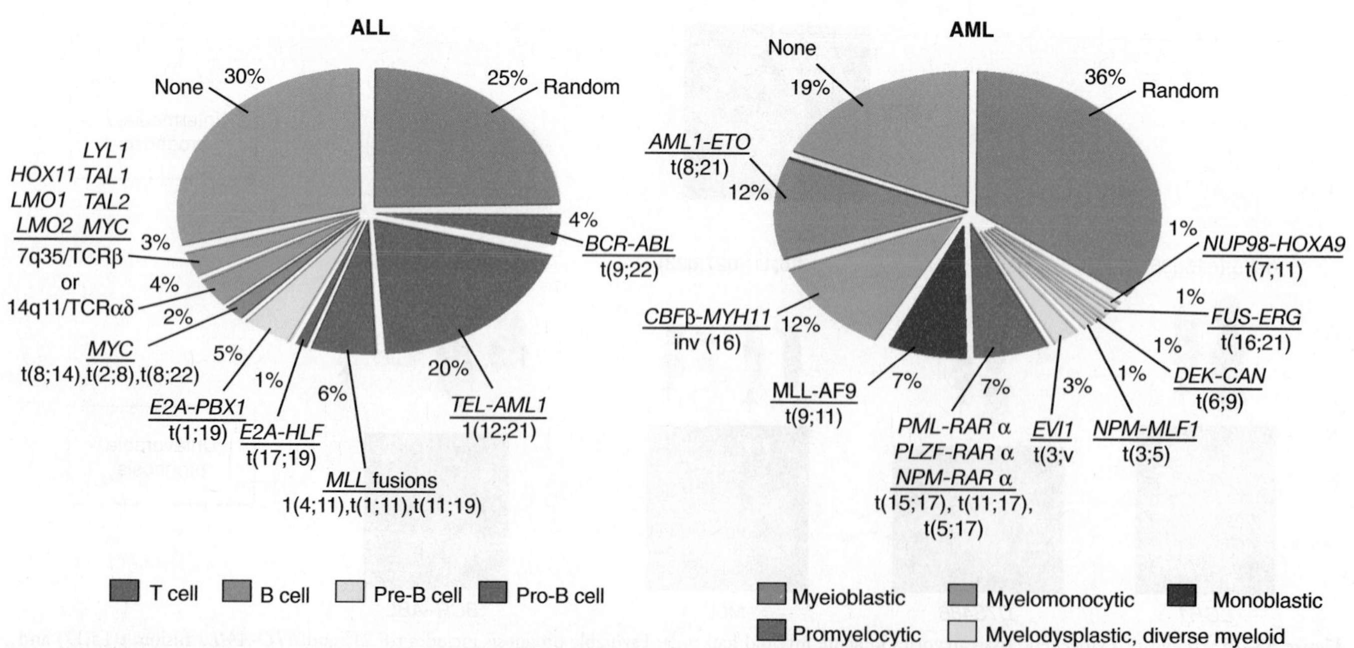

Figure 55–26 Distribution and frequency of chromosomal translocations and associated fusion transcripts in acute lymphoblastic leukemia and acute myeloid leukemia.

Table 55–6 Recurring Chromosome Translocations in Leukemia and the Genes Involved

Translocations	Genes Involved	Associated Diseases
(1) *CBF (AML1/CBFA* and *CBFB)* and *TEL/ETV6*-Associated Translocations/Inversions		
t(X;21)(p22;q22)	*PRDX4-AML1*	AML
t(3;21)(q26;q22)	*EVI1-MDS1-EAP-AML1*	t-AML/CML-ACC/BC
t(8;21)(q22;q22)	*ETO-AML1*	AML
t(8;21)(q23q22)	*FOG2-AML1*	MDS
t(8;21)(q24q22)	*TRPS1-AML1*	ALL/AML
t(16;21)(q24;q22)	*MTG16-AML1*	t-AML
t(19;21)(q13;q22)	*AMP19-AML1*	t-AML
t(12;21)(p12;22)	*ETV6-AML1*	ALL
t(21;21)(q11;q22)	*UPS25-AML1*	MDS
inv(16)/t(16;16)(p13;q22)	*MYH11-CBFB*	AML-M4
t(1;12)(p36;p13)	*MDS2-ETV6*	CML/MDS
t(1;12)(q21;p13)	*ARNT-ETV6*	AML
t(1;12)(q25;p13)	*ARG-ETV6*	AML
t(3;12)(q26;p13)	*MDS1-EV1-ETV6*	MPD
t(4;12)(p11;p13)	*BTL-TV6*	AML
t(5;12)(pq31;p13)	*ACS2-ETV6*	AML
t(5;12)(q33;p13)	*PDGFRB-ETV6*	CMML
t(6;12)(q23;p13)	*STL-ETV6*	ALL
t(7;12)(q36;p13)	*HLXB9-ETV6*	AML
t(9;12)(p24;p13)	*JAK2/-ETV6*	ALL, aCML
t(9;12)(q22;p13)	*SYK-ETV6*	MDS
t(9;12)(p34;p13)	*ABL-ETV6*	CMML
t(12;13)(p13;q12)	*ETV6-CSX2*	AML
t(12;13)(p13;q14)	*ETV6-TTL*	ALL
t(12;15)(p13;q25)	*ETV6-NTRK3*	AML
t(12;17)(p13;p12)	*ETV6-PER1*	AML
t(12;21)(p13;q11)	*ETV6-MN1*	AML
t(12;16)(p13;p11)	*CHOP-TLS/FUS*	AML
t(16;21)(p11;q22)	*TLS-FUS/-RG*	AML, MDS
(2) *RARA*-Associated Translocations		
t(15;17)(q22;21)	*PML-RARA*	APL
t(5;17)(q32;q21)	*NPM-RARA*	APL
t(11;17)(q23;q21)	*PLZF-RARA*	APL
t(11;17)(q13;q21)	*NuMA-RARA*	APL
der(17)	*STAT5-RARA*	AML
t(3;5)(q25;q35)	*MLF1-NPM*	AML/MDS
(3) *E2A*-Associated Translocations		
t(1;19)(q23;p13)	*PBX1-E2A*	B-ALL
t(17;19)(q23;p13)	*HLF-E2A*	B-ALL
(4) Tyrosine Kinase-Associated Translocations		
del(4)(q12q12)	*FIP1L1-PDGFRA*	HES
t(4;22)(q12;q11)	*PDGFRA-BCR*	
t(1;5)(q23;q33)	*Myomegalin-PDGFRB*	MPD
t(5;7)(q33;q11.2)	*PDGFRB-HIP1*	CMML
t(5:10)(q33;q21)	*PDGFRB-H4*	MPD
t(5;12)(q33;p13)	*PDGFRB-ETV6*	CMML, CEL
t(5;14)(q33;q32)	*PDGFRB/-AV14*	AML
t(5;14)(q33;q24)	*PDGFRB/-IN*	MPD
t(5;15)(q33;q15)	*PDGFRB/-P53BP1*	MPD
t(5;17)(q33;p13)	*PDGFRB-RABEPI*	CMML
t(5;17)(q33;p11.2)	*PDGFRB-HCMOGT*	JMML
t(q;22)(p24;q11.2)	*BCR-JAK2*	CML-
t(q;12)(p24;q13)	*JAK2-ETV6*	CML-
t(8;9)(p22;p24)	*PCMI-JAK2*	MPD, AL
(5) *NUP98/NUP214* Associated Translocations		
t(1;11)(q23;p15)	*PMX1/NUP98*	AML
t(2;11)(q31;p15)	*HOXD13/NUP98*	t-AML
t(4;11)(q21;p15)	*RAP1GDS1/NUP98*	T-ALL
t(5;11)(q35;p15)	*NSD/NUP98*	AML
t(7:11)(p15;p15)	*HOXA9/NUP98*	AML
t(9;11)(p22;p15)	*LEDGF/NUP98*	AML

Table 55–6 Recurring Chromosome Translocations in Leukemia and the Genes Involved—cont'd

Translocations	Genes Involved	Associated Diseases
inv(11)(p15q22)	*NUP98/DDX10*	t-AML
t(11;20)(p23;q34)	*NUP98/TOP1*	t-MDS
t(6;9)(p23;q34)	*DEK/NUP214(CAN)*	AML
Normal Karyotype	*SET/NUP214(CAN)*	AML
(6) *FGFR1*-Associated Translocations		
t(8;13)(p11;q12)	*ZNF198-FGFR1*	CMML, MPD
t(7;8)(q32;P11)	*TRIM24-FGFR1*	
t(6;8)(q27;P11)	*FGFR1OP-FGFR1*	
ins(12;8)(p11;p11p22)	*FGFR1OP2-FGFR1*	
t(8;17)(p11;q11)	*MYO18A-FGFR1*	
t(8;22)(p11;q11,2)	*BCR-FGFR1*	

AL, acute leukemia; ALL, acute lymphoblastic leukemia; AML, acute myelogenous leukemia; APL, acute promyelocytic leukemia; B-ALL, B-cell acute lymphoblastic leukemia; CEL, chronic eosinophilic leukemiac; CML, chronic myelogenous leukemia; CMML, chronic myelomonocytic leukemia; HES, Hypereosinophilic syndrome; JMML, juvenile myelomonocytic leukemiac; MDS, myelodysplastic syndrome; MPD, myoproliferative disorder; T-ALL, T-cell acute lymphoblastic leukemia; t-AML, therapy-related; t-MDS, therapy-related.

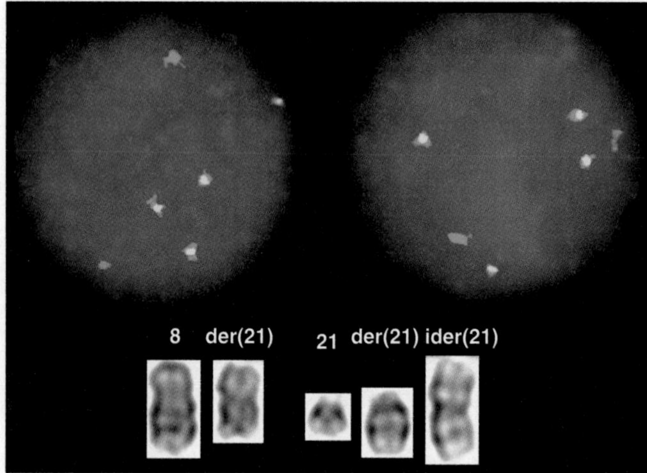

Figure 55–27 Four copies of *ETO-AML1 (RUNX)* fusion (yellow) shown in two interphase cells (top) from a patient with acute myeloid leukemia and t(8;21) (bottom) karyotype as well as ider(21). This formation is equivalent to the Philadelphia chromosome (Ph) duplication in the blast crisis of chronic myelogenous leukemia because of duplication of der(21) without accompanying t(8;21).

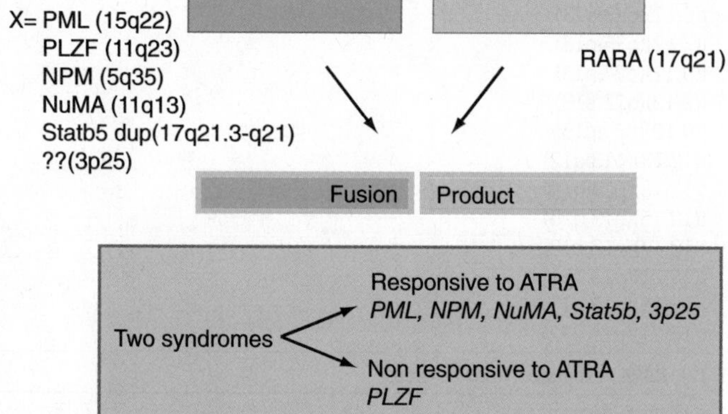

Figure 55–28 Molecular cytogenetic defects in acute promyelocytic leukemia are responsible for different response to all-*trans* retinoic acid differentiation therapy. Patients with t(11;17)(q23(q22) and *PLZF-RARA* fusion do not respond to all-*trans* retinoic acid differentiation therapy, whereas patients with classic t(15;17) and other four cytogenetic variants have exquisite sensitivity to differentiate in response to all-*trans* retinoic acid. *(Modified from V. Najfeld. In: Molecular Genetic Pathology. eds. Liang Cheng and David Y. Zhang Humana Press, Totowa, NJ, 2008.)*

same intron of the *AML1* gene. *AML1-MTG16* gene fusion results in the production of a protein that is very similar to the *AML1-ETO* (*AML1-MTG8*) protein in t(8;21).

(16;21)(p11;q22) is a rare chromosomal rearrangement associated with M1-M2 AML.[239] A proportion of patients may have additional abnormalities. This translocation fuses the *TLS/FUS* gene on chromosome 16, band p11, to the *ERG* gene on chromosome 22, band q22.[240] The *ERG* gene is a member of the ETS family of transcription factors and is a sequence-specific transcriptional activator. The presence of a fusion transcript is detected by RT-PCR, at the time of diagnosis, at relapse, and during remission. These observations are consistent with the impression that patients with t(16;21) have a poor prognosis and may benefit from early detection of this chimeric gene in order to determine the need for more aggressive therapy.

t(15;17)(q22;q21), recognized for the first time in 1977,[241] involves the *PML* (promyelocytic leukemia) gene on chromosome 15, band q22, and *RARA* on chromosome 17, band q21. This abnormality constitutes the genetic basis for approximately 97% of all cases of acute promyelocytic leukemia (see Fig. 55–25, middle panels).[242–245] The remaining 3% of cases include four rare variant translocations: t(11;17)(q23;q21),[246,247] t(11;17)(q13;q21),[248] t(5;17)(q35;q21),[249] and dup(17)(q21.3–q21).[250] Therefore, acute promyelocytic leukemia is associated with several different genetic rearrangements fusing the *RARA* gene with different partner gene in each case.[251–253] Variant *RARA* fusion partners include *PLZF* (promyelocytic leukemia zinc finger) gene on 11q23, *NPM* (nucleophosmin) gene on 5q35, *NuMA* (nuclear matrix-associated) gene on 11q13, and *STATb5* gene on 17q11. Based on these genomic rearrangements, a FISH assay, using a breakapart probe strategy with dual-color *RARA,* can identify two different clinical syndromes. These syndromes occur in patients who are not responsive to all-*trans* retinoic acid (ATRA) therapy and carry the *RARA-PLZF* fusion gene and in patients whose promyelocytes have exquisite sensitivity to differentiate in response to ATRA treatment and have one of the other three *RARA* fusion rearrangements (Fig. 55–28).[254–257] FISH study also identifies patients with cryptic translocations[258] and unusual chromosomal variants (Fig. 55–29). It is important to recognize patients who will or will not respond to ATRA so that appropriate therapy can be administered.

Acute promyelocytic leukemia is a disease characterized by accumulation of blasts blocked at the promyelocytic stage of granulocytic differentiation. Investigators have capitalized on this unique feature by designing highly effective therapy that blocks differentiation.[256,259]

Our current understanding of the molecular pathogenesis of acute promyelocytic leukemia is that *PML-RARA* behaves as a potent

Table 55–7 MLL Translocations and Rearrangements[a]

Cytogenetic Abnormality	Breakpoint	Partner Gene	HUGO Name	Leukemia Type
Characterized on Molecular Level				
t(1;11)(p32;q23)	1p32	*AF1P*	*EPS15*	ALL, AML, CML
t(1;11)(q21;q23)	1q21	*AF1Q*	*MLLT11*	AML
t(2;11)(q11.2–q12;q23)	2q11.2–q12	*LAF4*	*AFF3*	ALL
t(2;11)(q37;q23)	2q37	*SEPT2*	*SEPT2*	t-AML
t(3;11)(p21;q23)	3p21	*AF3P21*	*NCKIPSD*	t-AML
t(3;11)(p21.3;q23)	3p21.3	*DCP1A*	*DCP1A*	ALL
t(3;11)(q21.3;q23)	3q21.3	*SELB*	*EEFSEC*	ALL
t(3;11)(q24;q23)	3q24	*GMPS*	*GMPS*	t-AML
t(3;11)(q27–q28;q23)	3q27–q28	*LPP*	*LPP*	t-AML
t(4;11)(p12;q23)	4p12	*FRYL*	*FRYL*	t-ALL
t(4;11)(q21.1;q23)	4q21.1	*FLJ10849*	*SEPT11*	CML
t(4;11)(q21;q23)	4q21	*AF4*	*AFF1*	ALL, t-ALL, (AML)
t(4;11)(q35.1;q23)	4q35.1	*ARGBP2*	*SORBS2*	AML
Complex chromosomal abnormalities	5q12.3	*AF5-α*	*CENPK*	AML
ins(5;11)(q31;q13q23)	5q31	*AF5Q31*	*AFF4*	ALL
t(5;11)(q31;q23)	5q31	*GRAF*	*ARHGAP26*	JMML
t(6;11)(q12–13;q23)	6q12–q13	*SMAP1*	*SMAP1*	AML
t(6;11)(q21;q23)	6q21	*AF6Q21*	*FOXO3*	t-AML
t(6;11)(q27;q23)	6q27	*AF6*	*MLLT4*	AML, t-AML, ALL
t(7;11)(p22.1;q23)	7p22.1	*KIAA1856*	*KIAA1856*	ALL
t(9;11)(p22;q23)	9p22	*AF9*	*MLLT3*	AML, t-AML, (ALL)
t(9;11)(q33.1–q33.3;q23);	9q33.1–q33.3	*AF9Q34*	*DAB2IP*	AML
ins(11;9)(q23;q34)inv(11)(q13)(q23)	9q34	*FBP17*	*FNBP1*	AML
t(9;11)(q31–q34;q23)	9q31–34	*LAMC3*	*LAMC3*	AML
t(10;11)(p11.2;q23)	10p11.2	*ABI-1*	*ABI1*	AML
ins(10;11)(p12;q23q13)	10p12	*AF10*	*MLLT10*	AML, t-AML, (ALL)
t(10;11)(q21;q23)	10q21	*TET1, LCX*	*CXXC6*	AML
t(11;11)(q13.4;q23)	11q13.4	*ARHGEF17*	*ARHGEF17*	AML
t(11;11)(q13.4q23)	11q13.4	*DKFZP586P0123*	*DKFZP586P0123*	AML
inv(11)(q14q23)	11q14	*CALM*	*PICALM*	AML
inv(11)(q21q23)	11q21	*MAML2*	*MAML2*	t-T-ALL
t(11;15)(q23q;q21)inv(11)(q23q23)	11q23	*UBE4A*	*UBE4A*	MDS
del(11)(q23q23.3)	11q23.3	*LARG*	*ARHGEF12*	AML
del(11)(q23q23.3)	11q23.3	*CBL*	*CBL*	AML
del(11)(q23q23.3)	11q23.3	*BCL9L*	*BCL9L*	ALL
del(11))(q23q24.2)	11q24.2	*TIRAP*	*TIRAP*	AML
del(11))(q23q24.2)	11q24.2	*DCPS*	*DCPS*	AML
t(11;12)(q23;q13.2)	12q13.2	*CIP29*	*CIP29*	AML
t(11;14)(q23.3;q23.3)	14q23.3	*GPHN*	*GPHN*	AML, t-AML
t(11;14)(q32.33;q23.3)	14q32.33	*KIAA0284*	*KIAA0284*	AML
t(11;15)(q23;q14)	15q14	*AF15Q14*	*CASC5*	AML, ALL
t(11;15)(q23;q14)	15q14	*MPFYVE*	*ZFYVE19*	AML
t(11;16)(q23;p13.3)	16p13.3	*CBP*	*CREBBP*	t-MDS, t-AML, t-ALL, t-CML
t(11;17)(q23;p13.1)	17p13.1	*GAS7*	*GAS7*	t-AML
ins(11;17)(q23;q21)	17q21	*ACACA*	*ACACA*	AML
t(11;17)(q23;q21)	17q21	*AF17*	*MLLT6*	AML
t(11;17)(q23;q11–q21.3)	17q11–q21.3	*LASP1*	*LASP1*	AML
t(11;17)(q23;q25)	17q25	*AF17Q25*	*SEPT9*	t-AML, AML
t(11;19)q23;p13.1)	19p13.1	*ELL*	*ELL*	AML, t-AML
t(11;19)q23;p13)	19p13.3	*EEN*	*SH3GL1*	AML
t(11;19)(q23;p13.3)	19p13.3	*ENL*	*MLLT1*	ALL, AML, t-AL
t(11;19)q23;p13.3)	19p13.3	*ACER1*	*ASAH3*	ALL
t(11;19)q23;p13.3-p13.2)	19p13.3-p13.2	*MYO1F*	*MYO1F*	AML
t(11;19)q23;q13)	19q13	*ACTN4*	*ACTN4*	ALL
t(11;20)q23;q11)	20q11	*MAPRE1*	*MAPRE1*	ALL
t(11;22)(q23;q11.21)	22q11.21	*CDCREL*	*SEPT5*	AML, T-ALL
t(11;22)(q23;q13.2)	22q13.2	*P300*	*EP300*	t-AML
t(X;11)(q13.1;q23)	Xq13.1	*AFX*	*FOXO4*	ALL, AML
ins(X;11)(q24;q23)	Xq24	*SEPTIN6*	*SEPT6*	AML
ins(11;X)(q23q28q13.1)	Xq28	*FLNA*	*FLNA*	AML
No Partner Gene Directly Fused to *MLL* Gene				
t(1;11)(p13.1;q23)	1p13.1			
t(9;11)(p13.3;q23)	9p13.3			
t(11;19)q23;p13)	19p13.3			
t(11;21)(q23;q11.21)	21q22			

Table 55–7 MLL Translocations and Rearrangements[a]—cont'd

Cytogenetic Abnormality	Breakpoint	Partner Gene	HUGO Name	Leukemia Type
Not Characterized at Molecular Level				
t(1;11)(p36;q23)				
t(1;11)(q31;q23)				
t(1;11)(q32;q23)				
t(2;11)(p21;q23)				
t(2;11)(q37;q23)				
t(3;11)(p13;q23)				
t(4;11)(p11;q23)				
t(6;11)(q13;q23)				
t(7;11)(p15;q23)				
t(7;11)(q22;q23)				
t(7;11)(q32;q23)				
t(8;11)(q11;q23)				
t(8;11)(q21;q23)				
t(8;11)(q24;q23)				
t(9;11)(p11;q23)				
t(9;11)(q33;q23)				
t(10;11)(q25;q23)				
t(11;11)(q11;q23)				
t(11;11)(q13;q23)				
t(11;11)(q21;q23)				
t(11;12)(q23;p13)				
t(11;12)(q23;q13)				
t(11;12)(q23;q24)				
t(4;13;11)(q21;q34;q23)				
t(11;14)(q23;q11)				
t(11;14)(q23;q32)				
t(11;15)q23;q15)				
t(11;17)(q23;q11)				
t(11;17)(q23;q23)				
t(11;18)(q23;q12)				
t(11;18)(q23;q23)				
t(11;20)(q23;q13)				
t(11;21)(q23;q11)				
t(Y;11)(p11;q23)				
t(X;11)(q22;q23)				

ALL, acute lymphoblastic leukemia; AML, acute myelogenous leukemia; ML, chronic myelogenous leukemia; CMML, chronic myelomonocytic leukemia; JMML, juvenile myelomonocytic leukemia; t-AL, therapy-related acute; t-ALL, therapy-related ALL; t-AML, therapy-related AML; t-CML, therapy-related CML; t-MDS, therapy-related MDS; t-T-ALL, therapy-related T-cell ALL.

[a]Courtesy C. Meyer and R. Marschalek, Diagnostic Center of Acute Leukemia, Institute of Pharmaceutical Biology, JWG University of Frankfurt, Germany, on November 17, 2007.

transcriptional repressor and that supraphysiologic doses of retinoic acid can overcome this repression. In the presence of retinoic acid, *PML-RARA* behaves as a transcriptional activator.[260] In patients with variant *PLZF-RARA,* an additional corepressor complex binding site is present, and histone deacetylase inhibitors are used to restore sensitivity to retinoic acid.[257]

Accurate identification of the acute promyelocytic leukemia-associated genomic lesion at diagnosis is important because acute promyelocytic leukemia is a medical emergency that frequently presents with abrupt onset, high risk of early death (10%–20%), and potential for high cure rate (>80%) if appropriate treatment, based on genetic profile, is initiated. Initial workup may include conventional karyotyping, FISH studies, RT-PCR, and anti-PML antibodies.[261] Longitudinal monitoring of disease with RQ-PCR is currently recommended in order to provide early intervention should relapse occur.

In patients with 16q22 abnormalities such as inv(16)(p13;q22) and t(16;16)(p13;q22), the marrow contains an increased percentage of abnormal eosinophils. Combined May-Grünwald-Giemsa staining with FISH demonstrates that the abnormal eosinophils have inv(16) and, therefore, are part of the leukemic clone.[262,263] Trisomy 22 is a frequent accompanying abnormality.[264] Both inv(16) (see Fig. 55–25, top, right) and t(16;16) (Fig. 55–30) are abnormalities of the core-binding factor β *(CBFB)* gene at 16q22 and are associated with M4Eo subtype according to the French-American-British classification of AML. Both rearrangements result in fusion of *CBFB* and *MYH11* (myosin heavy chain) gene on 16p13. The exact role of the resulting hybrid protein, CBFB-SMMHC (smooth muscle myosin heavy chain) is unknown, but it probably is involved in impaired hematopoietic differentiation. Both t(8;21) and inv(16) rearrangements result in abnormal repression of CBF target genes. Both translocations have favorable prognosis, but they exhibit different leukemic morphologies.[265–269]

Approximately 4% of patients with *CBFB-MYH11* rearrangement do not have a cytogenetically detectable inv(16) or t(16;16). Cytogenetic detection of inv(16) may be difficult, and interphase FISH with dual-color *CBFB* probe at diagnosis is a crucial genetic test. Detection of *CBFB-MYH11* fusion by either RT-PCR or FISH is found in patients without eosinophilia[270]; therefore, *CBFB* testing should be included in the standard testing panel for genomic rearrangement in AML. The presence of additional abnormalities, such as trisomy 8, does not adversely affect clinical outcome. The *CBFB-MYH11* chimeric fusion is detected in utero with approximately 10 years of

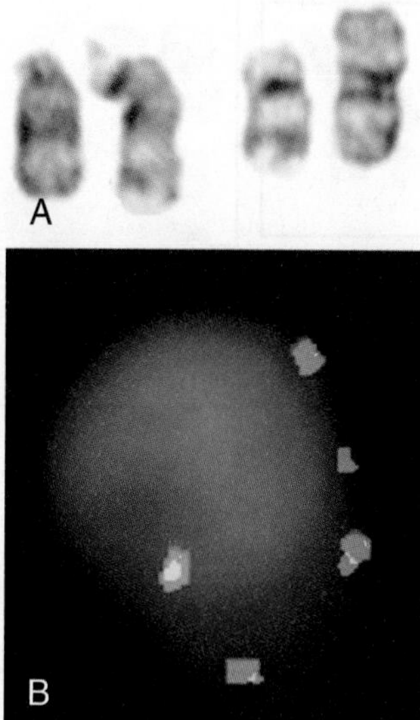

Figure 55–29 Partial karyotype from a patient with acute promyelocytic leukemia showing ider(17)t(15;17)(q22;q21) (top). The karyotype shows isochromosome for the long arms of chromosome 17 and deletion of the short arms. FISH studies revealed three copies of *PML-RARA* fusion in bone marrow nucleus (bottom), confirming that the first event in the pathogenesis was *PML-RARA* fusion, and the subsequent event was a structural rearrangement of isochromosome. *(From V. Najfeld. In: Molecular Genetic Pathology. eds. Liang Cheng and David Y. Zhang Humana Press, a part of Springer Science, Totowa, NJ, 2008.)*

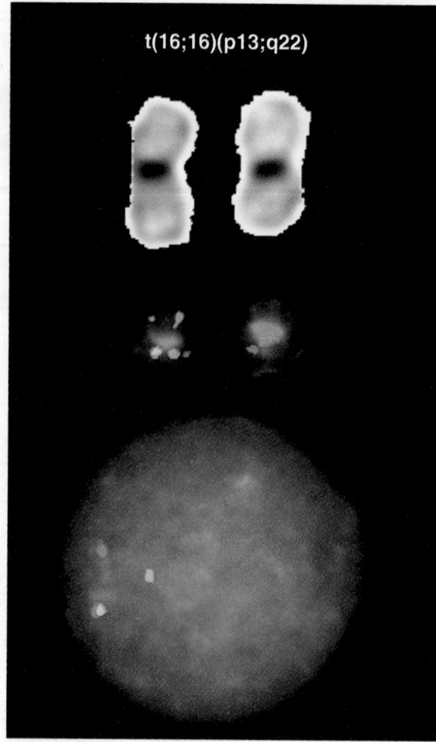

Figure 55–30 Partial G-banded karyotype from a patient with M4 acute myeloid leukemia showing t(16;16) (top), after FISH study using a "breakapart" *CBFB* probe (at 16q22) demonstrating that the 5′ end (red) of the gene remains on 16q of one chromosome 16, whereas the 3′ end (green) translocated to the short arms of the other chromosome 16. Separation of 5′ and 3′ ends as single signals is indicated in the bone marrow nucleus (bottom).

postnatal latency before development of childhood leukemia.[269] This observation suggests that formation of *CBFB-MYH11* is not enough to cause leukemia and that subsequent genetic events must occur before clinically recognizable leukemia is identified.

Less than 1% of patients with AML have Ph (see Fig. 55–25, bottom left). In rare patients with AML, late appearance of Ph either as a sole abnormality or in a clone showing t(8;21) is taken as evidence that Ph in these patients is a secondary event. The late-appearing Ph in AML is characterized by P190$^{BCR\text{-}ABL1}$ protein.[271,272]

The coexistence of Ph and inv(16) is a rare but recurrent finding in both CML and AML. In CML the fusion transcript is P210$^{BCR\text{-}ABL1}$, whereas in AML the fusion transcript is P190$^{BCR\text{-}ABL1}$. The presence of both Ph and inv(16) in AML seems to have a favorable prognosis, whereas in CML the coexistence of *BCR-ABL* and *CBFB-MYH11* suggests rapid transformation to blast crisis.[273]

The *MLL (myeloid lymphoid lineage,* also called "mixed-lineage leukemia," also referred to as *ALL1* or *HRX)* gene, at 11q23 is responsible for 95% of all 11q23 translocations, including AML and ALL (Fig. 55–31 and Table 55–7). Approximately 20% of all translocations in human neoplasia involve the *MLL* gene.[274] The *MLL* abnormalities are found in approximately 15% of patients with AML and ALL. To date, 88 partner genes participate in *MLL* translocations, and 51 of these are characterized at the molecular level.[274–276] The most common translocations involving the *MLL* gene in AML (Table 55–7) are t(9;11)(p23;q23) (Fig. 55–31, *M)* resulting in *MLL-AF9* fusion and t(11;19)(q23;p13.1) (Fig. 55–31, *L)* producing the *MLL-ELL* fusion. A partial tandem duplication of the amino-terminus region of the *MLL* gene is associated in patients with or without trisomy 11 (Fig. 55–31, *B, C, F,* and *G).*[277] The *MLL* gene is encoded by 37 exons. 11q23 translocations cluster within an 8.3-kb region that encompasses exons 8 to 14 of *MLL* and fuses the N-terminal portion of *MLL,* which contains the AT hook and methyltransferase domains, to numerous different proteins. In infant and in therapy-related AML, the *MLL* genomic breakpoints cluster in the 3′ end, near exon 12. In childhood and adult de novo AML, the breakpoints usually occur in the 5′ end, between exons 9 and 10.[278–280] AML patients with *MLL* rearrangements have a poor prognosis despite treatment with aggressive multiagent chemotherapy.[218,281] Identical *MLL* rearrangements have been detected in three pairs of infant monozygotic twins, raising the possibility of in utero *MLL* rearrangements.[282]

Until recently the contribution of various *MLL* fusion partners to transformation was not known. The partner genes in the translocations did not appear to have any unifying characteristics that would clarify their role in leukemogenesis. However, two observations suggest that *MLL* fusion partners are not randomly chosen. First, a precise localization of genomic *MLL* breakpoints in 414 samples with *MLL* rearrangements, using a novel long-distance inverse PCR method, shows that the most frequent translocation fusion partners *(AF4, AF9, ENL, AF10)* belong to the same nuclear protein network involved in histone methylation.[274] Second, observation indicates that several chromatin structural elements, such as topoisomerase II cleavage sites, DNase I hypersensitive sites, and other chromatin sites, are associated with *MLL* rearrangements observed in infant and therapy-related AML.[283] These characteristics of *MLL* suggest that specific chromatin sites are functionally selected in *MLL* rearrangements rather than being randomly chosen.[274]

t(6;9)(p23;q34) is a rare cytogenetic abnormality, described for the first time in 1976 and subsequently reported in 1986 to be associated with AML and marrow basophilia.[284,285] Basophilic leukemia now is recognized by the WHO classification as a separate entity. In addition to t(6;9) other chromosomal abnormalities such as t(8;21)(q22;q22), del(12)(p11–13), t(X;6),(p11;q23), and t(2;6)(q23;p22) may be found in basophilic leukemia.[286] As a result of t(6;9), the 3′ part of the *CAN (NUP214,* nuclear pore complex protein 214 kd) gene located on chromosome 9, band q34, is fused to the 5′ part of the *DEK* gene located on chromosome 6, band p23. The resulting *DEK-CAN/NUP214* fusion gene is a derivative of chromosome 6.[287] The translocation breakpoints occur in a single intron of 8 kb in the *CAN* gene and in a single intron of 12 kb in

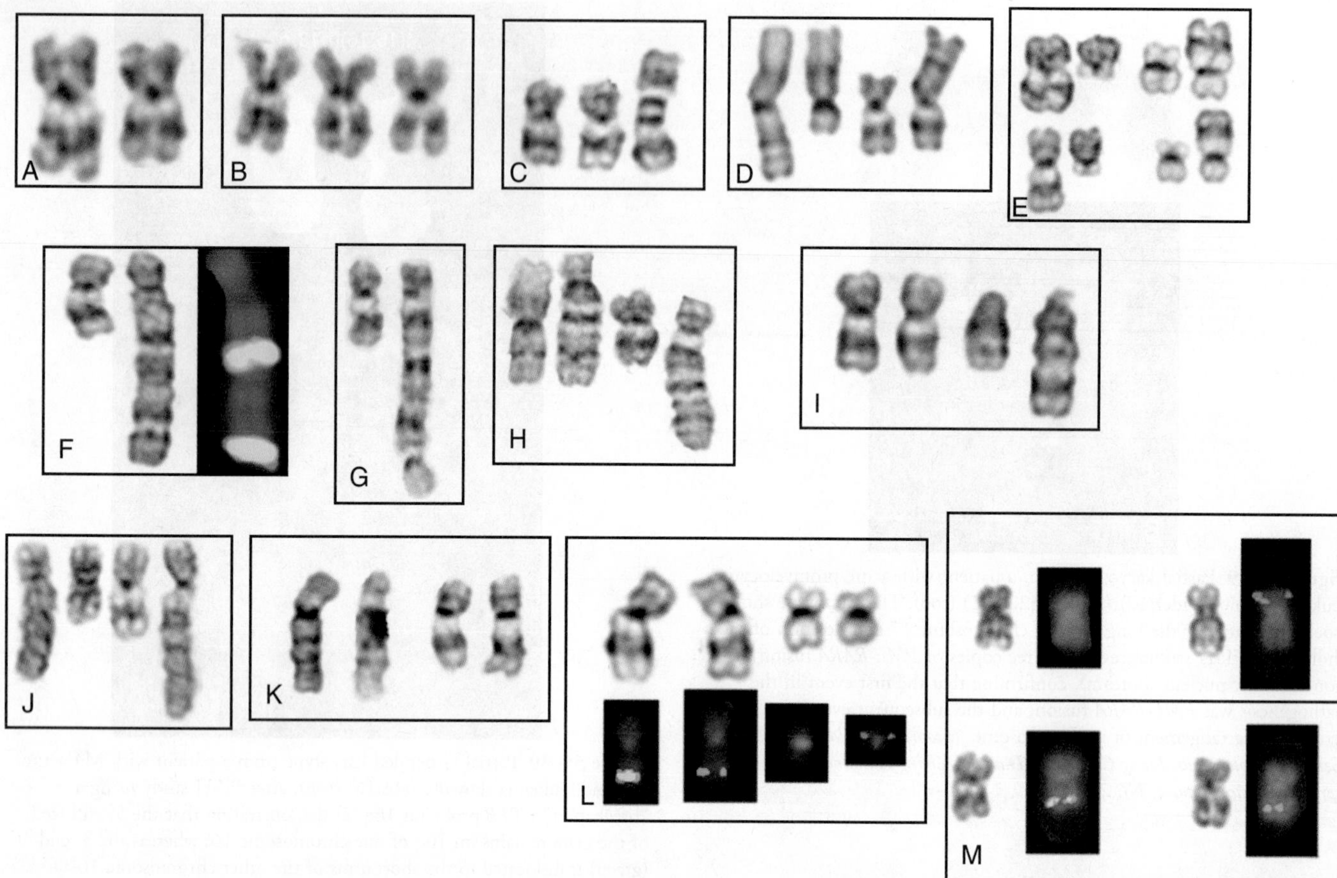

Figure 55–31 Examples of chromosome 11 abnormalities. **A,** Deletion of chromosome 11 at band q23. **B,** Gain (trisomy) of chromosome 11. **C,** Gain of isodicentric, idic(q11) in myelodysplastic syndrome (MDS). **D,** Balanced t(1;11)(q13;p15) in MDS. **E,** t(11;19)(q13;p13) in a pediatric patient with acute myeloid leukemia. **F,** Duplication of the long arms of chromosome 11 and FISH image of *MLL* duplication. **G,** Duplication (11;22) in the form of dicder(11;22)dup(11)(q13q14)t(11;22)(q23;p11) in a patient with MDS. **H,** der(11)dic(1;11)(q12;q23) in a patient with myelofibrosis transforming to acute myeloid leukemia. **I,** der(14)t(11;14)(q23;q23) resulting in trisomy for part of the long arms of chromosome 11. **J,** t(4;11)((q23;q23) in pediatric acute lymphoblastic leukemia. **K,** t(6;11)(q27;q23) in pediatric acute lymphoblastic leukemia. **L,** t(11;19)(q23;p13) in pediatric acute lymphoblastic leukemia and after FISH study showing separation of MLL breakapart probe where the 5′ end of the *MLL* (green) remains on der(11) and the 3′ end (red) is translocated to 19p. **M,** t(9;11)(p22;q23) in pediatric acute myeloid leukemia and after metaphase FISH study (right) showing the 3′ end of the *MLL* (red) is translocated to 9p but the 5′ end (green) remains on der(11).

the *DEK* gene. As a result, the presence of the *DEK-CAN* fusion can be identified in blood or marrow cells by Southern blot analysis and PCR methods. Dual-color commercial FISH probes currently are not available for this translocation.

The nuclear pore complex is a massive structure that extends across the nuclear envelope, forming a gateway that regulates the flow of macromolecules between the nucleus and the cytoplasm. *NUP214* may serve as a docking site in the receptor-mediated import of substrates across the nuclear pore complex and plays a role in nuclear protein import, mRNA export, and cell cycle progression. The hybrid protein contains almost the entire DEK protein fused to the C-terminal two-thirds of the CAN protein. The role of DEK-CAN/NUP214 hybrid protein in leukemogenesis awaits elucidation.

The M7 or megakaryocytic subtype of AML is a clonal disease arising in a multipotent stem cell capable of differentiating along the megakaryocytic and granulocytic pathway. This acute leukemia subtype has a variety of genetic and morphologic characteristics.[288] The M7 subtype has an estimated frequency of 3% to 14% of all AML and is more frequent in children than in adults. In adults, megakaryocytic leukemia is frequently observed as a secondary leukemia after chemotherapy or leukemic transformation of several chronic MPDs, including CML. Approximately 65% of acute megakaryocytic leukemia is associated with myelofibrosis. No specific chromosomal abnormality is associated with the adult form of megakaryocytic leukemia. Approximately 50% of M7 AML patients have chromosomal abnormalities at diagnosis. Observed diverse abnormalities include 3q21–3q26 rearrangements, partial or total deletion of chromosomes 5 and 7, gain of chromosomes 8 and 19, and t(9;22). In multivariate analysis, M7 diagnosis in adults is an independent adverse prognostic factor for overall survival.[289,290]

Three manifestations of childhood megakaryocytic leukemia are observed. First is the t(1;22)(p13;q13) with constitutional trisomy 21 associated with *GATA1* mutation.[291] Children with constitutional trisomy 21 have 10- to 20-fold increased risk for developing leukemia. The incidence of developing M7 leukemia is up to 500 times higher in children with constitutional trisomy 21 than in children without it.[292] However, children with constitutional +21 and megakaryocytic leukemia have a more favorable prognosis compared to patients without constitutional +21. Somatic mutation of transcription factor *GATA1* in these patients leads to exclusive expression of a truncated form of *GATA1.* The second form of childhood acute megakaryocytic leukemia involves t(1;22)(p13;q13) encoding *OTT-MAL* (*RBM15-MKL1*) fusion protein in infants without constitutional trisomy 21 (Fig. 55–32). It is found in 22% of all patients with infantile M7 and 33% of all patients with FAB-M7.[293,294] Detection of t(1;22) is diagnostic. Adults with t(1;22)(p13;q13) encoding the *OTT-MAL* fusion transcript are not reported to date. Third, approximately 19% of infants with constitutional trisomy 21 (or mosaic +21C) and transient myeloproliferative disorder subsequently develop M7 leukemia at a mean age of 20 months.[292] With development of leukemia, these children acquire diverse chromosomal abnormalities, most notably tetrasomy 21 and trisomy 8. The t(1;22)

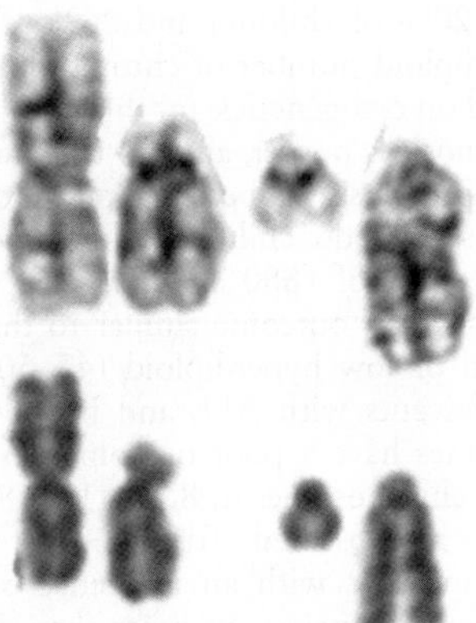

Figure 55–32 Partial bone marrow karyotype from two metaphase cells from a 4-week-old baby with M7 megakaryocytic leukemia showing a diagnostic t(1;22)(p13;q13) abnormality.

rearrangement has been observed in a set of monozygotic twins, suggesting an in utero origin in some cases.

Preliminary results using gene expression profiling are providing the first insight into the molecular pathogenesis of M7 leukemia in children with and without constitutional trisomy 21. These two groups of patients have distinct molecular phenotypes, with increased expression of chromosome 21 genes in patients with constitutional +21 compared to M7 leukemia patients without constitutional +21. The *AML1* (*RUNX1*) gene, localized on chromosome 21 and essential for normal megakaryopoiesis, is expressed at lower levels in children with constitutional +21 and M7 leukemia, indicating a mechanism that may contribute to a block in differentiation in megakaryocytic leukemia.[295]

Approximately 15% to 20% of patients with AML show a numerical gain or loss of a single chromosome as the sole primary karyotypic abnormality. Each of the autosomes and sex chromosomes contributes to the numerical changes. The most common trisomies in decreasing order of frequency are gain of chromosome 8, 22, 13, 21, and 11. The gain of chromosome 8, the most frequent abnormality seen in AML, is found as a sole abnormality in 6.3% and overall in 16%.[192] The incidence of +8 detected by FISH is reported to vary between 19% and 25%. The prognosis of AML with +8 depends on whether +8 occurs as an isolated abnormality or accompanies other cytogenetic aberrations. In the latter situations, +8 does not appear to adversely affect the favorable outcome of patients with t(15;17), inv(16)t(16;16), and t(8;21). In contrast, patients with +8 and a complex karyotype and/or an unfavorable aberration such as del(5q) or −7 usually have very poor outcome. Isolated +8 has been considered to be associated with either intermediate or unfavorable prognosis.[218]

Whether PCR-based molecular screening, conventional cytogenetics, or both, should be used at diagnosis of AML is an important question with major consequences for treatment strategy, monitoring therapy, and overall genetic risk assessment. A prospective comparison study demonstrated approximately 20% discrepancy between broad molecular screening using a multiplex RT-PCR system and cytogenetic testing. This discrepancy has the potential to influence treatment strategies.[296] Cryptic translocations detected as submicroscopic genetic lesions detected by RT-PCR may have no influence on prognosis or treatment strategy. In contrast, cytogenetic results influence treatment decisions by conferring unfavorable risk assignment on patients with negative broad molecular screening. These methodologies provide complementary genetic information for diagnosis, treatment, and followup.

Cytogenetic studies are valuable in assessing the effectiveness of therapy (see box on Genetic Testing for Acute Myeloid Leukemia and Fig. 55–25). In most patients with AML, a clonal cell population cannot be detected during remission. However, in some cases hematopoiesis remains clonal, with normal karyotype showing only a single *G6PD* enzyme type, hence the fourth aspect of AML heterogeneity.[35,57–58] When disease relapses, cells with the original chromosome anomalies are observed. If an appropriate FISH or RT-PCR test is available, these are the genetic tests of choice for predicting relapse because these methods are less expensive and more sensitive than chromosome studies.

Genetic Testing for Acute Myeloid Leukemia

At diagnosis, conventional cytogenetic studies should be performed. In addition, fluorescence *in situ* hybridization and molecular genetic tests are available to detect many classic chromosome anomalies that may be cryptic by conventional cytogenetics. The panel of chromosomal probes for acute myeloid leukemia at diagnosis includes *ETO-AML*, *PML-RARA*, *CBFB*, *BCR-ABL*, *MLL*, and for +8. These tests are performed at diagnosis to establish a benchmark for the percentage of neoplastic cells and are used in followup studies to help assess the effectiveness of therapy.

The biology of AML changes with age. The spectrum of cytogenetic abnormalities in the elderly includes a higher percentage of patients with abnormalities involving −5/del(5q), −7/del(7q), and 17p and a lower incidence of translocations associated with favorable prognosis and treatment outcome.[297] In addition, multidrug resistance is demonstrated in 57% of patients older than 75 years but in 33% of AML patients younger than 56 years. The different biology of AML in older patients may be a consequence of the age of hematopoietic stem cells, shortened telomere length (associated with older cells), and presence of fewer normal stem cells to compete with malignant clones and repopulate marrow following chemotherapy. Therapy-related AML and therapy-related MDS are distinctive clinical syndromes occurring as late complications after high-dose chemotherapy, radiation therapy, and autologous HCT.[298,299] In the best studied series of 306 patients with therapy-related leukemias, normal karyotype is observed in 8% and abnormal karyotype is detected in 92%.[300] From the cytogenetic point of view, two different categories of therapy-related AML and therapy-related MDS can be distinguished. The first is found in patients exposed to alkylating agents who developed therapy-related approximately 5 years after therapy. These leukemias are associated with the presence of monosomy 5/del(5q) or monosomy 7/del(7q). Many of these patients initially develop myelodysplastic features before transforming into a frank AML. Recurrent abnormalities of chromosomes 5, 7, or both account for 70% of all abnormalities observed in therapy-related leukemia.[301] These patients have a poor response to therapy and poor overall survival. A second group of patients develop therapy-related AML without prior MDS. Leukemia cells in these patients often exhibit 11q23 (3%) and 21q22 (3%) balanced rearrangements, attributed to late effects of topoisomerase II inhibitors combined with alkylating agents and radiation.[302] The leukemia may develop within a few months to 3 years after therapy. Polysomy (tetrasomy, pentasomy, hexasomy) of chromosome 8 defines a clinicocytogenetic entity associated with therapy-related myeloid malignancies and poor overall survival[303] (see box on Genetic Testing for Therapy-Related Neoplasms).

ACUTE LYMPHOBLASTIC LEUKEMIA

ALL is a clonally derived disease involving progenitor cells with differentiation expression detected only in the lymphoid lineage.[51] ALL accounts for at least 85% of acute leukemias in children and 20% of acute leukemias in adults.[218] Most published series of patients with acute ALL indicate that more than 85% have an abnormal clone by conventional cytogenetic studies (see Fig. 55–26, left). Genomic rearrangements detected with intensive interphase FISH screening are found in up to 91% of cases.[304] Today cytogenetic analyses combined with FISH and/or RT-PCR investigations are mandatory in most ALL treatment trials, and genetic findings play a pivotal role in proper risk stratification and treatment options.

Pretreatment cytogenetics is an independent prognostic factor in children and adults presenting with ALL and is important in determining risk categories. As shown in Fig. 55–33 and Table 55–8, the risk categories in children include (a) low risk: [hyperdiploidy (trisomies for chromosomes 4, 10, and 17) and t(12;21)/*TEL-AML1*]; (b) high risk: t(1;19)/*E2X-PBX1;* and (c) very high risk: t(9;22)/*BCR-ABL* and 11q23/*MLL* rearrangements.[311] In adults the low-risk category includes high hyperdiploidy and del(9p), whereas the high-risk category includes hypodiploidy/near triploidy, t(9;22)(q34;q11), t(4;11)(q21;q23), t(8;14)(q24;q32), and complex karyotype (five or more chromosomal abnormalities).[305,306]

Genetic Testing for Therapy-Related Neoplasms

The best genetic test for therapy-related myelodysplastic syndrome or acute myeloid leukemia is a conventional cytogenetic study. Fluorescence *in situ* hybridization studies with probes for loci on chromosomes 5 and 7, *MLL,* and *AML1* should be performed if therapy-related leukemia is suspected. This approach is useful for t(8;21), t(9;22), t(11;var), t(15;17), inv(16), −5/5q, −7/7q−, rearrangements of *ETV6* on 12p, and some others.

Approximately 20% of children and 26% of adults with B-cell ALL have a hyperdiploid number of chromosomes. Two groups are distinguished based on cytogenetics: (a) those with 51 to 55 chromosomes, whose prognosis is poorer, and (b) those with 56 to 67 chromosomes, whose prognosis is better. Both groups have a more favorable prognosis than do children with hypodiploidy or near-haploid ALL. In a study of 1880 children with ALL, patients with 45 chromosomes have an outcome similar to that of ALL patients with pseudodiploid or low hyperdiploid (47–50 chromosomes).[307] Children and adolescents with ALL and hypodiploidy with fewer than 44 chromosomes have a poor outcome despite contemporary therapy.[308] Gain of chromosomes 4, 8, 10, 17, 18, and 21 as well as other chromosomes are observed. Trisomy 21 is the most common numerical change in ALL, with an incidence of 1% to 2%.[309,310] Pretreatment cytogenetic analysis of more than 5400 children with ALL unequivocally shows that simultaneous trisomies for chromosomes 4, 10, and 17 are associated with long-term event-free survival (see Fig. 55–33, *D).*[311] In contrast to children who have a favorable prognosis when a hyperdiploid karyotype is present, such a favorable constellation has not been found in adult ALL. The reason may be that adult patients often have poor-risk chromosomal translocations, such as the Ph, which confer a poor outcome irrespective of otherwise good-risk ploidy groups. Modal chromosome numbers of 45 or less are rare (specifically, the near-haploid numbers of 24–36), but they do occur in less than 1% of cases and confer a poor prognosis. Similarly, ALL in adults presenting with low hyperdiploid/near-triploidy is associated with poor outcome.[306] Loss of chromosome 7

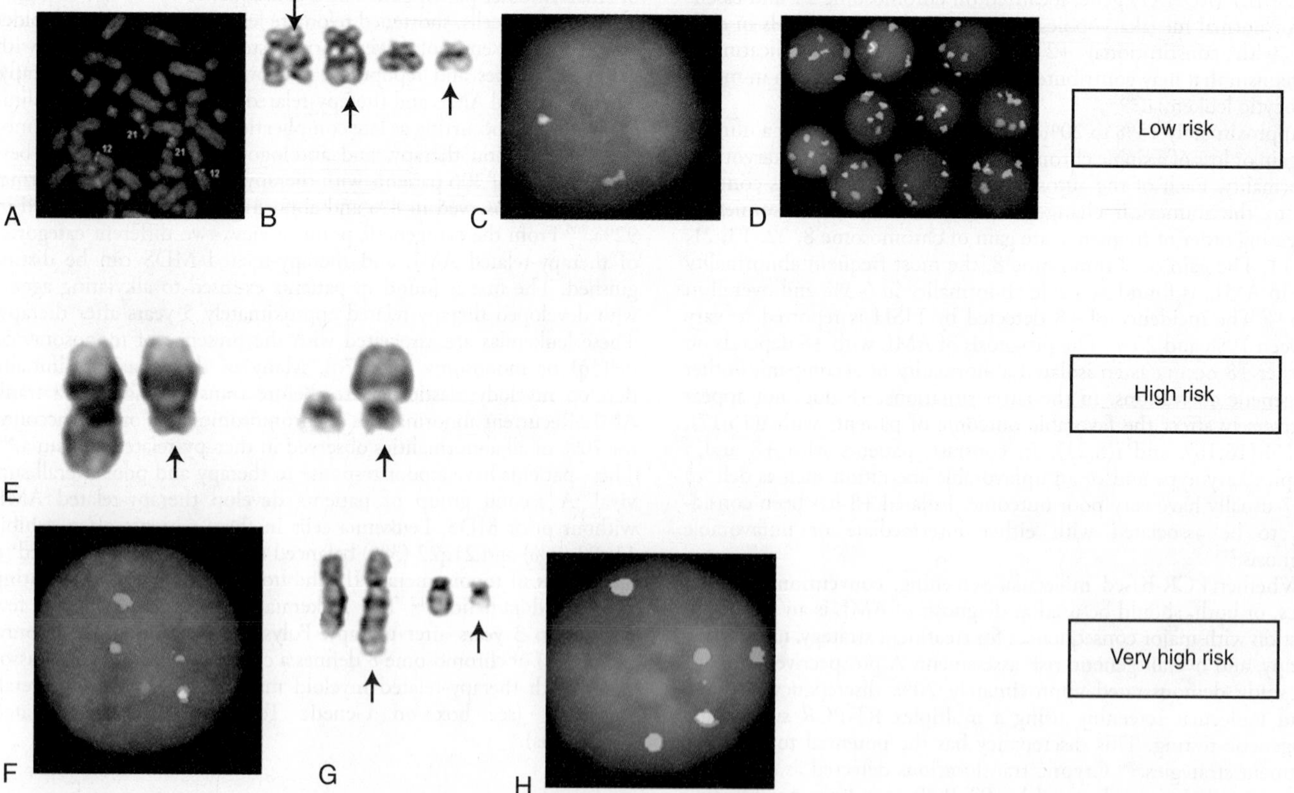

Figure 55–33 Prognostic cytogenetic categories in acute lymphoblastic leukemia. **A,** Localization of *TEL/ETV6* and *AML1* fluorescence probes to chromosomes from a normal bone marrow metaphase cell. *TEL/ETV6* is on 12p13 (green) and *AML1* is on 21q (red). **B,** Partial karyotype showing t(12;21)(p13;q22) *(arrows).* The *short arrow* at 12p indicates a possible *TEL* deletion from normal chromosome 12. **C,** FISH study showing loss of *TEL* (green) from normal 12 homologue in interphase nucleus, a frequent subclonal evolution in patients with t(12;21). **D,** Hyperdiploidy, specifically trisomies for chromosomes 4 (green), 10 (red), and 17 (aqua), is associated with low-risk cytogenetic category (see text for details) and is present in disomy in interphase cells (top left). **E,** Partial G-banded karyotype showing t(1;19)(q23;p13.3), which occurs in approximately 6% of patients with B-cell precursor childhood acute lymphoblastic leukemia. **F,** FISH hybridization to bone marrow nucleus showing *BCR-ABL* fusion (yellow). **G,** as a consequence of t(9;22), occurring in 5% of children and 20% to 25% of adults with acute lymphoblastic leukemia. **H,** Interphase nucleus after FISH study with tricolor probe. Dual-color/breakapart *MLL* shows separation of the 3′ end and the 5′ end as a result of 11q23 rearrangement. CEP11 (aqua) indicates disomy for chromosome 11, used as internal control. *MLL* rearrangements in acute lymphoblastic leukemia are associated with unfavorable prognosis.

Table 55–8 Frequencies of Cytogenetic Aberrations in Adult and Childhood ALL and Their Prognostic Relevance

		Adults		Children	
Cytogenetic Abnormality	**Genes Involved**	***Frequency (%)***	***Prognosis***	***Frequency (%)***	***Prognosis***
Normal karyotype	NA	15–36	Intermediate–good	31–40	Intermediate—good
High hyperdiploidy (>55)	NA	2–11	Good	23–26	Good
Low hyperdiploidy (>50)	NA	10–15	Poor	10–11	Intermediate
Near haploidy (<35)	NA	Rare	NA	1–4	Poor
Pseudodiploidy	NA	31–50	Poor	18–26	Intermediate
Hypodiploidy (35–44)	NA	4–9	Poor	6	Poor–intermediate
t(9;22)(q34;q11.2)	*BCR-ABL*	11–29	Poor	2–6	Poor
t(4;11)(q21;q23)	*MLL- MLL T2*	3–7	Poor	2	Poor
t(1;19)(q23;p13.3)	*TCF3-PBX1*	2–3	Poor	4–5	Poor
t(12;21)(p12;q22)	*TEL/ETV6-AML1*	0–3	Not known	20–25	Good
Abnormal 9p	*P16 (CDKN2A, MTS1)*	6–30	Intermediate-	7–11	Adverse
Abnormal 12p	*TEL (ETV6)/ETV1*	4–6	Favorable–unfavorable	7–9	Not prognostic
del(6q)	Not known	3–6	Not prognostic	6–9	Not prognostic
del(7p)/del(7q)/–7	Not known	6–11	Not prognostic	4	Adverse
del(5q)	Not known	<2	Not prognostic	1	Adverse
Trisomy 8	NA	10–12	Poor	2	Not known
14q11	*TCR-α*	5–7 (26% in T-ALL)	Excellent	3–4 (17%–22% in T-ALL)	Not prognostic
t(10;14)(q24;q11)	*TRD-TLX1*	2–3	Excellent	Not known	NA

ALL, acute lymphoblastic leukemia; T-ALL, T-cell acute lymphoblastic leukemia.

is frequent in adult ALL. The majority of these patients also have t(9;22).

In childhood ALL, t(12;21), was first reported in 1994 as a fortuitous FISH finding.[312] This translocation is difficult to detect by conventional cytogenetics because the translocated portions of 12p13 and 21q22 have virtually identical G-banding patterns. In contrast, the *ETV6-AML1* (*ETV6-AML1*) fusion product of t(12;21) is detected using PCR or FISH in 17% to 41% of pediatric patients with ALL (see Fig. 55–33, *A–C*).[313] The *ETV6-AML1* fusion, found almost exclusively in children 1 to 15 years old with B-precursor ALL, represents the most frequent molecular rearrangement in childhood cancer. Children with the *ETV6-AML1* fusion gene have significantly lower rates of relapse compared with *ETV6-AML1*–negative patients.[314–316] *ETV6-AML1*–positive B-precursor ALL is characterized by a long duration of first remission and excellent cure rates. Prospective analysis demonstrates that the survival rate in t(12;21)-positive patients is significantly better when compared with negative cases; however, this abnormality in multivariate analysis is not found to be an independent predictor of outcome.[317] The *ETV6-AML1* fusion is rare in adult ALL. t(12;21)(p13;q22) fuses the helix-loop-helix domain of the *ETV6* gene, located on chromosome 12, band p13, to the DNA-binding and transactivation domain of the *AML1* gene, located on 21q22. FISH studies allow visualization of the fusion gene on 21q22. Fusion with *ETV6* converts *AML1* from an activator to a repressor of transcription. The *ETV6-AML1* fusion is frequently accompanied by the loss of the other normal unrearranged *TEL/ETV1* allele. This deletion probably represents a subclonal evolution.[318,319] *ETV6-AML1* has been detected in utero, probably in a committed B-cell progenitor, and is present in normal cord blood and peripheral blood samples at frequencies 100-fold greater than the risk of corresponding leukemia. The current view of development of *ETV6-AML1*–positive leukemia is that these early events are followed by a long "preleukemic" phase followed by loss of the normal *ETV6* homologue, which appears to be an important event in the multistep pathogenesis of this leukemia.[320–322] Currently, of the 397 children with *ETV6-AML1*–positive leukemia reported, approximately 60% harbor additional karyotypic abnormalities that contribute to the pseudodiploid or near-diploid karyotype in these cases. The most common secondary change, which occurs in approximately 50% of cases with additional abnormalities, is trisomy 21.[323]

A rare group of patients with B-precursor ALL has no fusion of *TEL* and *AML1*. Instead, marrow cells from these patients show three to 15 copies of the q22 band of chromosome 21, including the *AML1* locus. Amplification of the 21q22 band of chromosome 21 is a clonal marker of the leukemic cells (Fig. 55–34).[324] Following this initial observation, the British Childhood Leukemia Working Party prospectively screened 1630 patients with childhood ALL and identified 28 children with intrachromosomal amplification of chromosome 21 (iAMP21) (Fig. 55–34, *A*).[325] Children with iAMP21 have a common or pre–B-cell immunophenotype, median age of 9 years, and significantly inferior event-free and overall survival at 5 years compared with children exhibiting other cytogenetic subgroups. Even children with Ph positive ALL, known for its poor prognosis, have a better 5-year event-free survival compared to children with iAMP21. These children have a threefold increased risk for relapse and are twice as likely to die than their counterparts without iAMP21.

ETV6 or *TEL* (for *t*ranslocation, ETS, *l*eukemia") transcription factor gene, most frequently found in translocations, was first identified as a part of a *TEL*–platelet-derived growth factor receptor β fusion (*TEL-PDGFRB)* created by t(5;12)(q33;p13) in chronic myelomonocytic leukemia.[326] It was detected using FISH because, as mentioned earlier, of difficulties in detecting cytogenetic rearrangements at the 12p13 site. As a result of this translocation, the helix-loop-helix domain of *TEL/ETV6* is fused in frame to the *PDGFRB* transmembrane and tyrosine kinase domain. Fusion of *TEL/ETV6* to a tyrosine kinase also occurs as a result of t(9;12)(q34;p13), leading

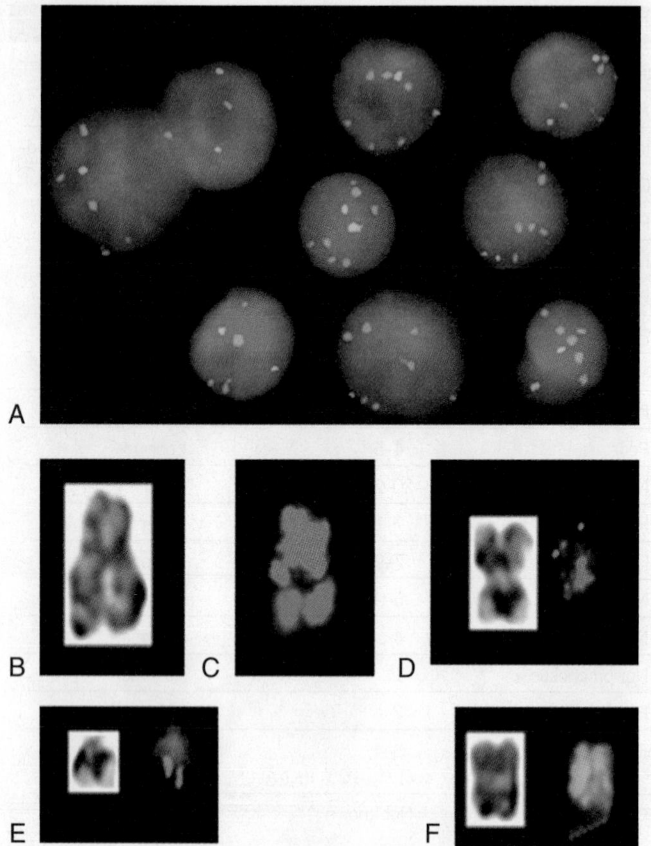

Figure 55–34 Detection of *AML1* and 21q22 amplification. **A,** Intrachromosomal amplification of *AML1* (red) (*TEL* [green], present in disomy) in a pediatric patient with pre–B-cell acute lymphoblastic leukemia. This finding is associated with poor prognosis. **(B)** G banding of der(18) chromosome and after FISH study **(C)** with WCP 18 (green) and LSI 21q22.13 (red) documenting der(18)t(18;21) and amplification of 21q22 region in a patient with myelodysplastic syndrome/acute myeloid leukemia. **D,** Amplification of 21q22 region in myelodysplastic syndrome may be present in another formation: der(21) (G banding, left). FISH study shows amplification of 21q22.13 locus (red) and identified der(21) as t(5;21) with 5p15.2 probe (green). **E,** Localization of 21q22.13 LSI probe on normal chromosome 21. **F,** Homogeneous staining region (hsr)(21), G banding (left), and after FISH study (right) with locus-specific probe for 21q22.13 (red) consistent with 21q22.13 band amplification in a patient with myelodysplastic syndrome.

to the *ABL-TEL* fusion that has been observed in patients with ALL, AML, and atypical CML.[327,328] More than 22 partner genes are known to participate in fusions with *ETV6/TEL*, primarily in ALL and less frequently in myeloid malignancies.

Other rearrangements involving 12p include deletions, duplications, and translocations and are observed most often as part of a complex karyotype, frequently associated with chromosome 5 and/or 7 abnormalities. Deletion of 12p13 is much more frequent in children than in adults with ALL and is observed in patients with myeloid disorders, specifically in adults with MDS.[329] Two other genes residing on 12p also are rearranged: *CCND2* is frequently amplified and *CDKN1B* is commonly often deleted.

Approximately 5% of children and 20% to 25% of adults with ALL have Ph, making it the most common structural rearrangement in adult ALL (see Fig. 55–33, *F* and *G*). The breakpoint on Ph is more centromeric than in CML (see Chronic Myelogenous Leukemia above). It includes the 5′ breakpoint on chromosome 22, distal to the first exon (falling between exon e1 and e2) of the *BCR* gene resulting in the P190$^{BCR\text{-}ABL1}$ variant, providing a diagnostic distinction between lymphoid blast crisis of CML and de novo ALL.[83,330,331]

Ph positive ALL is characterized by the smallest *BCR*-ABL1 (P190) protein containing less BCR than the P210 and P230 fusion proteins. Among Ph positive patients with ALL, approximately 58% to 70% of adults and 80% of children have this genomic breakpoint variant. Up to 19% of Ph positive ALL patients may express both the P190 and the P210 *BCR-ABL1* fusions.[332] A number of earlier studies indicated that the P190 type of the *BCR-ABL1* breakpoint is associated with a more aggressive form of disease, with higher tyrosine kinase transforming ability than the P210 protein associated with CML.[333] Ph positive ALL was classified as a *stem cell* disorder because of the presence of the BCR-ABL transcript in both the myeloid and lymphoid lineages.[334] More recent reports suggest that the presence of the P190 protein does not confer a poorer prognosis.[306,323,333]

The *BCR-ABL1* fusion variants are easily detectable by FISH testing using the extrasensitive probe strategy, and *BCR-ABL1*$^+$ leukemia can be identified in up to 10% of Ph negative cases. Moreover, FISH testing will identify *ABL* rearrangements in *BCR-ABL1* fusion-negative ALL patients.[335] The role of imatinib used alone or in combination with conventional chemotherapy in elderly patients with de novo Ph positive ALL is being studied.[336] Initial gene expression profiling failed to identify specific genes associated with differences in overall survival of adult patients with P190$^+$ or P210$^+$ ALL.[337]

Reactivation of BCR-ABL kinase activity is most commonly associated with the emergence of point mutation in the *ABL* kinase domain implicated in resistance to imatinib treatment (see Chronic Myelogenous Leukemia above). Retrospective analysis reveals that 40% of newly diagnosed and imatinib-naive Ph positive ALL patients have kinase domain mutations, and 83% to 90% have identical mutation at relapse or at the time of hematologic or cytogenetic resistance to imatinib.[338,339] The frequency of the mutant allele is always below the level of detectability by direct cDNA sequencing method at diagnosis, and use of more sensitive methods, such as denaturing high-performance liquid chromatography, is recommended.

More than 60% of adult patients with Ph positive ALL show additional chromosomal abnormalities in the Ph positive clone. Most frequent are gain of Ph, monosomy 7, +8, +X, del(9p) as well as high triploidy.[306,340] The additional chromosomal abnormality has no effect on survival of Ph positive patients.

t(1;19)(q23;p13.3) occurs in 5% to 6% of patients with B-cell precursor childhood ALL. However, among patients with a pre-B (cytoplasmic immunoglobulin positive) immunophenotype, t(1;19) is found in approximately 25%. t(1;19) occurs in 2% to 3% of adults (see Fig. 55–33, *E*).[341–344] Cytogenetically, two forms of t(1;19) can be identified: 25% of cases have a balanced reciprocal t(1;19), whereas 75% of cases have a more common rearrangement of unbalanced der(19)t(1;19)(q23;p13.3).[345] The unbalanced der(19)t(1;19) arises from the initial trisomy of chromosome 1 followed by the t(1;19) translocation, with subsequent loss of the derivative chromosome 1.[346] More than 95% of t(1;19) is associated with the *E2A* (*TCF3*)-*PBX1* fusion gene. The *E2A* gene (originally identified by binding of E2A proteins to the kE2DNA sequence motif contained in the Ig κ light-chain enhancer) on chromosome 19, band p13.3, is fused to the *PBX1* (homeobox) gene on chromosome 1, band q23.[342–343,347] Approximately 1% of pediatric B-ALL patients have a variant t(17;19)(q21–q22;p13) translocation resulting in two different genomic rearrangements. The first is the fusion between the *HLF* gene (breakpoint in intron 3) on chromosome 17 and the *E2A* gene (within intron 13) on chromosome 19, associated with disseminated intravascular coagulation. The second is the breakpoint in intron 12 of *E2A* and intron 3 of *HLF* associated with hypercalcemia.[348] In contrast to *ETV6-AML1* rearrangements, which have a prenatal origin, current evidence suggests a postnatal etiology for t(1;19) translocations.[349]

Currently, it is thought that an unbalanced der(19) in pediatric patients with ALL is associated with significantly improved outcome compared to patients with balanced t(1;19), which remains an adverse prognostic factor.[344] In adults the prognostic relevance of t(1;19) is unclear, and both favorable and unfavorable outcomes have been reported.[350,351] In contrast, a variant t(17;19) rearrangement is associated with poor prognosis.[352] Both t(1;19) and t(17;19) are easily identifiable by conventional cytogenetics, FISH, and RT-PCR, and the latter two methodologies are particularly useful in posttreatment specimens that are cytogenetically normal.[353,354]

In ALL, the most frequent MLL translocations include t(4;11) (see Fig. 55–31, J) leading to MLL-AF4 fusion and t(11;19)(q23;p13.3) (Fig. 55–31, L) resulting in MLL-ENL fusion. These abnormalities are present in more than 80% of infant leukemia and 10% of childhood and adult leukemia.[274–276] MLL rearrangements are associated with poor outcome in both children and adults (see Acute Myelogenous Leukemia above and T-Cell Lymphoproliferative Diseases below).[306] t(4;11) is one of the most common 11q23 abnormalities, occurring in 2% of children and approximately two thirds of adults with *MLL*-associated translocations.

t(8;14)(q24;q32) is seen in fewer than 5% of all ALL patients (children and adults). Variant translocations t(8;22)(q24;q11) and t(2;8)(p12;q24) are seen in less than 1% of children and adults. These patients have CD10+, CD19+, CD20+, surface IgM+ immunophenotype and extremely poor prognosis. The same translocation is found in Burkitt lymphoma, and both entities likely represent the same disease with different manifestations. It has been reported that the majority of adult patients with t(8;14) die within 1 year of diagnosis.[306]

Approximately 2% of children and 8% of adult pre–B-cell precursor ALL show recurrent *IGH* translocations usually identified by FISH as t(8;14)(q11;q32), t(14;19)(q32;q13), inv(14) (q11q32/ t(14;14)(q11;q32), and t(14;20)(q32;q13).[355] These five recurrent *IGH* translocations have in common deregulated expression of unmutated *CEBP* genes (CCAAT enhancer-binding protein transcription factors), and approximately 1% of all B-cell precursor ALL are characterized by novel *CEBP-IGH* fusions.

Abnormalities of the short arms of chromosome 9 (p21–22) occur at a frequency of 7% to 13%. In adults the presence of del(9p) appears to be associated with improved outcome, whereas in children will ALL del(9p) is associated with poor outcome (Fig. 55–35).[306] The most frequent abnormalities are co–deletions of two genes, $p15^{INK4B}$ and $p16^{INK4A}$, as well as the interferon α and β genes found in many, but not all, cases. Among the structural rearrangements involving the short arms of chromosome 9, t/dic(9;12)(p11–12;p11–13) is a rare recurrent abnormality associated with L1 morphology (FAB classification), pre–B-cell phenotype, and excellent prognosis.

Other chromosomal abnormalities detected in nonrandom fashion in adult ALL include deletions, both terminal and interstitial, of the long arm of chromosome 6, and isochromosomes of 7q, 9q, 17q, and 21q. Adult patients with ALL showing t(9;22), t(4;11), t(8;14), −7, +8 chromosomal aberrations have a poorer prognosis and significantly lower probability of long-term complete remission and survival than do patients with a normal karyotype or patients with other chromosomal rearrangements.

Gene expression profiling in childhood ALL suggests that ALL segregates according to cell lineage and primary genomic defects.[356] However, some clues about the genes that participate in drug resistance and influence treatment are provided by a comparison between gene expression profiling and response to therapy. In this study of 187 children with ALL, 14 functionally related genes with roles in

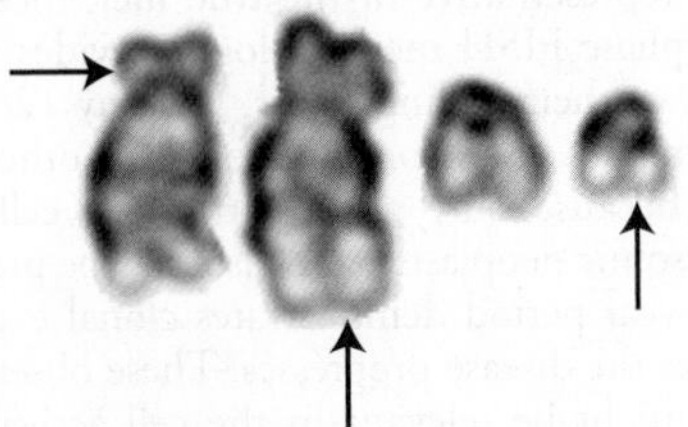

Figure 55–35 t(9;22)(q34;q11) *(arrows)* in a patient with acute lymphoblastic leukemia. Note the first chromosome 9 has deletion of the short arms, a frequent finding in both adult and pediatric acute lymphoblastic leukemia patients.

regulation of cell proliferation were independently associated with risk of relapse.[357]

Epidemiologic and twin studies indicate a multistep pathogenesis of B-cell ALL in infants and children, with initial leukemogenic event(s) occurring in utero and subsequent genomic changes occurring postnatally.[358,359] Twin studies provide insight into the pathogenesis of pediatric leukemia because most common chromosomal translocations and their resultant gene fusions could be traced by molecular analysis of neonatal blood spots or Guthrie cards. If a unique gene fusion sequence is present in at least one cell per 30,000 in peripheral blood, it will be detected by sensitive PCR-based assay. The first in utero origin was demonstrated for *MLL* rearrangements in three children with ALL,[360] and the first demonstration that monozygotic twins shared the identical *TEL-AML1* fusion was demonstrated in a pair of twins diagnosed at age 3 with B-precursor ALL.[361] The concordance rate of twins who share monochorionic placenta and develop leukemia probably is 100%, whereas older twin children have a discordant rate of 90%, indicating that they need additional postnatal leukemic events.[359] The frequency of in utero origin of B-cell precursor ALL in non–twin children as measured by clonal *IGH* rearrangements is reported to be 71%,[362] supporting the notion that, in the majority of infants older than 1 year, development of ALL occurs in fetal hematopoiesis. Subsequent physiologic postnatal switch may eliminate these abnormal clones in the vast majority of the cases; however, a small number of children have "preleukemic" clone for some variable time, with later emergence of leukemia[360] (see box on Genetic Testing for Acute Lymphoblastic Leukemia).

B-CELL CHRONIC LYMPHOCYTIC LEUKEMIA

CLL is a clonal disease arising in a progenitor cell after the B-cell pathway has diverged from the myeloid and T-cell pathways.[56] Approximately 40% to 50% of patients have clonal abnormalities identified by conventional cytogenetics.[363,364] This may be an underestimate because chromosomal changes may occur in one or more cell subsets of the malignant clone. Classic cytogenetic analysis of B-CLL has remained difficult because of the low mitotic yield of neoplastic B cells despite the use of B-cell mitogens, such as 12-*O*-tetradecanoylphorbol-13-cetate (TPA) and stimulation with CD40 ligand and interleukin 4. Molecular cytogenetics, such as interphase FISH, CGH, and array CGH, have raised the detection rate to 80% to 90%.[365] Analysis of clinically relevant chromosomal loci, combined with immunophenotyping, mutation analysis of the immunoglobulin heavy-chain variable region (IgV_H), and *ZAP*-70 overexpression, are of prognostic importance even though oncogenic events that lead to the origin of B-CLL remain unknown (see box on Genetic Testing for B-Cell Chronic Lymphocytic Leukemia, Fig. 55–37, and Table 55–9). Although microarray and high-density SNP array studies have not identified genes involved in the pathogenesis of CLL, they clarify

Genetic Testing for Acute Lymphoblastic Leukemia

At diagnosis, conventional cytogenetic studies should be performed, especially for pediatric patients in whom solely numerical anomalies occur in 25%. Fluorescence *in situ* hybridization (FISH) and molecular genetic methods are valuable to detect certain cryptic chromosome anomalies, such as *TEL/AML1* fusion associated with t(12;21)(p12;q22). The panel of FISH probe at the diagnosis of pediatric acute lymphoblastic leukemia includes *TEL(ETV6)-AML1, MLL, BCR-ABL, P21* at 9p, and centromeric probes for chromosomes 4, 10, and 17. In adults, the role of hyperdiploidy as it relates to prognosis is uncertain, therefore thus FISH testing with centromeric probes is not useful. Establishing benchmarks with FISH and/or molecular testing is crucial for followup of patients during and after therapy.

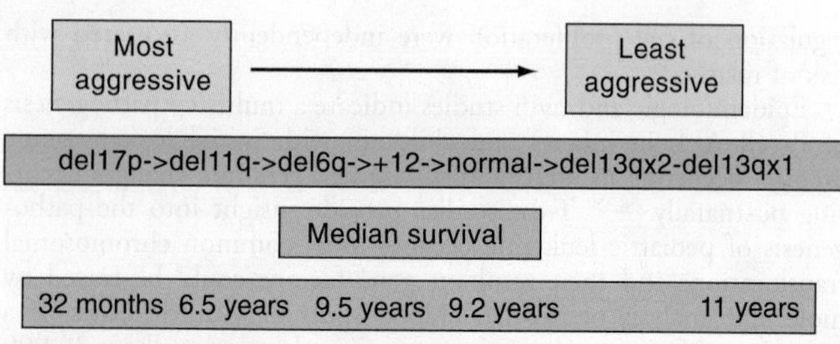

Figure 55–36 Survival of patients with specific genomic defects in chronic lymphocytic leukemia.

Genetic Testing for B-Cell Chronic Lymphocytic Leukemia

Interphase fluorescence *in situ* hybridization (FISH) is used in lieu of chromosome studies because FISH detection of abnormalities in chronic lymphocytic leukemia correlates with clinical risk groups and prognosis. FISH studies should be performed on blood for detection of trisomy 12, deletions of 11q22.3, 13q14.3, and P53 loci, as well as rearrangement of 14q32.3, *IGH* locus. The FISH test can distinguish between patients with B-cell chronic lymphocytic leukemia and those with the leukemic phase of certain lymphomas, such as mantle cell lymphoma and follicular lymphoma.

Table 55–9 Recurrent Chromosomal Translocations in B-Cell Lymphoproliferative Disorders

Translocations	Genes Involved	Associated Diseases
(1) Immunoglobulin (*IG*)-Related Translocations		
t(2;8)(p12;q32)	*IGK-cMYC*	ALL (Burkitt)
t(4;14)(p16.3;q32.3)	*FGFR3-IqH*	Multiple myeloma
t(5;14)(q31;q32)	*IL3-IGH*	B-CLL
t(7;14)(q21;q32)	*IGH/-DK6*	B-CLL
t(8;14)(q24;q32)	*IGH/-cMYC*	ALL (Burkitt)
t(8;22)(q24;q11)	*IGL-CMYC*	ALL (Burkitt)
t(11;14)(q13;q32.3)	*CCND1-IGH*	Multiple myeloma
t(14;16)(q32.3;q23)	*IGH-MAF*	Multiple myeloma
t(14;19)(q32;p13)	*IGH-BCL-3*	B-CLL
(2) Lymphoma-Associated Translocations		
t(11;14)(q13;q32.3)	*CCNDI-IGH*	Mantle cell
t(14;18)(q32.3;q21)	*IGH-BCL2*	Follicular
t(3;14)(q27;q32)	*BCL6-IGH*	Follicular
t(11;18)(q21;q21)	*API2-MALTI*	MALT
t(14;18)(q32.3;q21)	*IGM-MALT*	MALT
t(1;14)(p22;q32.3)	*BCL10-IGH*	MALT
3q27 rearrangements	*BCL 6*	Diffuse large B cell
t(14;15)(q32.3;q11–13)	*IGH-BCL8*	Diffuse large B cell
t(3;14)(p14;q32.3)	*FOXPIF-IGH*	MALT
t(9;14)(p13;q32.3)	*PAX5-IGH*	LPL

ALL, acute lymphoblastic leukemia; B-CLL, B-cell chronic lymphocytic leukemia; LPL, lymphoplasmacytoid lymphoma; MALT, mucosa-associated lymphoid tissue.

that CLL, despite its heterogeneous nature, is one disease entity with a common genetic phenotype resembling memory B lymphocytes.[366,367] Genetic testing is strongly recommended for all CLL patients, particularly in the context of novel therapeutic trials for CLL.[368]

Chromosome abnormalities detected by FISH are of prognostic significance.[365] Four genomic aberrations, as well as normal findings, are independent predictors of disease progression and survival. Genomic aberrations of prognostic significance include 17p deletion, 11q deletion, trisomy 12, and 13q deletion. Survival in these groups was 32, 79, 114, and 133 months, respectively, and the treatment-free interval was 8, 12, 33, and 92 months, respectively (Fig. 55–36). Survival of patients with a normal karyotype was 111 months, and the treatment-free interval was 49 months. Comparison of known prognostic features of B-CLL with interphase FISH results indicate that FISH-detected anomalies are frequent in B-CLL cases, even in Rai stages 0 to 1, but are more frequent among patients with progressive disease (88%) than in patients with stable disease (66%). Two risk groups are recognized: (a) low risk includes patients with normal karyotype or isolated del(13q), and (b) high risk includes patients with del(11q) and del(17p). Patients with +12 are high risk, but in contrast to del(11q) and del(17p), they respond to fludarabine-based therapies (Fig. 55–37).[369] Comparison of a quantitative PCR method with FISH for assessment of the four most frequent aneuploidies revealed a tight correlation in 103 of 110 patients examined, with FISH being more sensitive in detecting subclonal genetic evolution.[370]

The frequency of abnormalities of chromosome 13 in CLL detected by conventional cytogenetics is 10% to 15%.[371] However, with the application of FISH, smaller or larger deletions of band q14.3 are detected in up to 60% of patients over time.[372,373] When multiple DNA probes are used, D13S319 and D13S25 DNA markers are deleted more frequently in B-CLL than is *RB1*. Molecular analyses has detected deletions of 13q in cells that are cytogenetically normal as well as abnormal. Homozygous deletion of D13S25 and/or D13S319 DNA segments from the 13q14.3 band region is a rare but consistent finding in a subset of patients with B-cell CLL. The 13q14.3 deleted segment contains micro-RNA (miRNA) genes. Micro-RNA is made normally by cells, including B lymphocytes, and regulates the function of many genes. Preliminary findings demonstrate that all patients with homozygous 13q deletion have dramatic miRNA15a downregulation, whereas patients with hemizygous 13q deletion are indistinguishable from controls, providing the first molecular clues for the genetic basis and pathogenesis of CLL.[374,375] Trisomy 12 or 13q rearrangements are found separately in a substantial proportion of patients with CLL. They coexist in only 2% to 5% of patients, suggesting that each change may have a distinct pathogenetic route. The presence of del(13q) as the sole abnormality in CLL is associated with the most favorable prognosis, with a median survival of 11 years.

Among the first-degree relatives of patients with familial CLL, population studies demonstrate a sevenfold increased risk for developing CLL and a twofold increased risk for developing lymphoproliferative disorders, indicating genetic predisposition. More than 80 families with aggregation of CLL are reported. Linkage studies suggest a region of interest in band q22.1 of chromosome 13 (marker D13S156). Fine FISH mapping of six CLL-prone families (63 individuals) reveals deletion of 13q14 in 85% of patients with familial CLL, and four CLL families shared a 3.6-Mb minimal region in 13q21.33–q22.2. This region included 12 candidate genes, but thus far no mutations as determined using direct DNA sequence analysis are identified in patients with familial CLL.[376–379]

Trisomy 12 was the first reported recurrent abnormality in CLL. It is detected by classic cytogenetics in 7% to 15% of all cases. FISH assessment detects +12 in 15% to 20% of patients with CLL.[380] FISH studies are more representative of the true incidence of trisomy 12 because the interphase FISH methodology provides information on cells independent of their cycling status. Trisomy 12 may be present as the sole abnormality or in combination with other chromosomal rearrangements. Because only a proportion of cells are trisomic, normal cells or disomic neoplastic cells also may be present. Followup analysis over a 4-year period demonstrates clonal expansion of cells with trisomy 12 as the disease progresses. These observations suggest that trisomy 12 might be relevant in the cell activation process in CLL. The observation that trisomy 12 is documented in B cells and is absent from T lymphocytes and $CD34^+$ cells in the majority of patients is consistent with the original hypothesis that CLL has a clonal origin and that trisomy 12 arises in a progenitor cell already

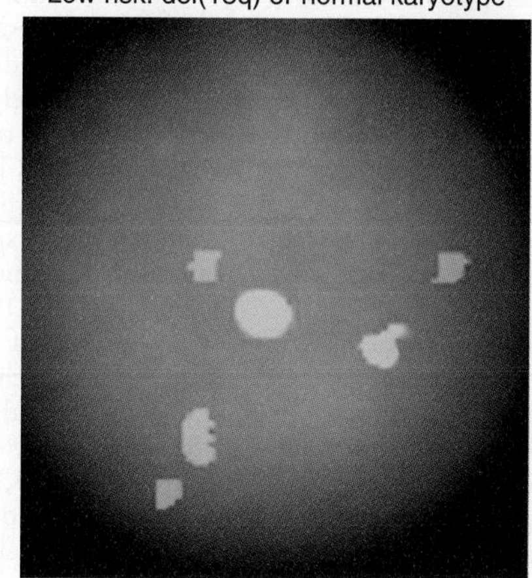

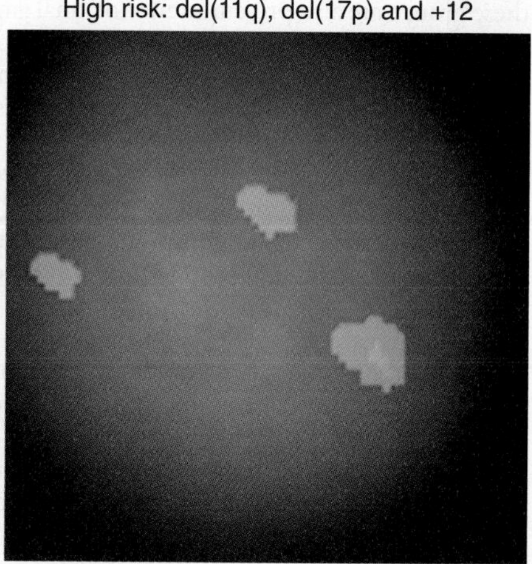

Figure 55–37 Panel of chromosomal probes used for detection of genomic defects in chronic lymphocytic leukemia. They include 13q14.3 (red), 13q34 (aqua), and CEP12 (all present in disomy; left) and 11q22.3 (*ATM,* green) and 17p13.1 (*P53;* red, right). Note only one copy of the *ATM* gene (green, right) consistent with deletion of sequences from the 11q22.3 band region, which is associated with unfavorable prognosis.

committed to the B-cell pathway.[381] Routine FISH genetic testing identifies patients with trisomy 12 because it uses the probe that is hybridized only to the centromeric area of chromosome 12. More sophisticated molecular cytogenetic methods may be useful. High expression of the *CLLU1* gene on 12q22 has been discovered in CLL samples from patients with or without trisomy 12. Overexpression of *CLLU1* in CLL patients without IgV_H hypermutation combined with restricted and CLL-unique expression pattern suggest that *CLLU1* is among the first disease-specific genes identified in CLL.[382]

The frequency of deletions of the long arm of chromosome 11 in CLL as detected by conventional cytogenetics is reported to be 5% to 8%. An interphase FISH study identified a clinical subset of B-cell CLL defined by deletion of 11q22.3–23.1 in 7% to 10% of these cases. FISH characterization of aberrations involved in 11q21–q23 demonstrate a minimal consensus deletion segment of 2 to 3 Mb, containing a number of genes including *ATM* at 11q22.3 (see Fig. 55–37, right). Up to 12% of patients have simultaneous deletions of *ATM* and *MLL* at 11q23. The *ATM* gene is responsible for ataxia-telangiectasia and functions as a cell-cycle checkpoint regulator. Somatic disruptions of both alleles of the *ATM* gene by deletion or point mutation are detected in approximately 34% of cases. This finding strongly suggests the pathogenic role of ATM in some patients with B-CLL.[383] A study revealed discontinuous deletions at 11q23.1–q23.3, indicating that genes in this region may have pathogenic significance because they constitute independent targets for amplification or deletion in cases of B-CLL. Patients with 11q deletion exhibit extensive lymphadenopathy, more rapid disease progression, a shorter treatment-free interval, inferior molecular remission, and reduced overall survival.[384]

Structural aberrations of chromosome 17 are observed in 4% of cytogenetically evaluable B-CLL cases. This abnormality frequently affects the short arm of chromosome 17, the site of the *P53* tumor suppressor gene. Monoallelic deletions of *P53,* detected by FISH, are present in 7% to 20% of patients and represent the strongest predictor of survival in B-cell CLL. The median survival time of these patients is only 32 months.[365] B-CLL in patients with deletion of the *P53* gene is associated with refractory advanced disease, resistance to treatment, and shorter survival. A comprehensive assessment of genetic and molecular features predicting outcome in previously untreated CLL patients receiving either fludarabine or fludarabine plus cyclophosphamide identified del(17)(p13) along with del(11q), but not IgV_H, CD38 expression, or ZAP-70 status, as significant risk factors for early relapse.[384]

Because the leukemic phase of certain lymphomas can clinically mimic B-CLL, FISH testing for translocation using an *IgH* probe is important. Fewer than 5% of patients with CLL/prolymphocytic leukemia morphology have t(11;14)(q13;q32), and these conditions usually transform into prolymphocytic leukemia. Moreover, *IGH* testing in CLL is important for detecting patients with recurrent del(14)(q24.1) associated with unmutated IgV_H status (66%) and trisomy 12 (47%).[385]

Current work provides solid evidence that chromosomal translocations detected by conventional cytogenetics independently predict treatment failure, treatment-free survival, and overall survival in untreated and cladribine-treated B-cell CLL patients.[386,387] When CLL-derived metaphase cells are obtained with systematic stimulation using B-cell mitogens and activators, balanced and unbalanced translocations are seen in 34% to 42% of patients. In multivariate analysis, unbalanced translocations are independently associated with risk of treatment failure. Because del(13q) usually is cryptic by conventional cytogenetics but easily detected with FISH studies,[388] both conventional cytogenetics and interphase FISH should be performed at baseline in patients with advanced CLL.

The validity of hierarchical interphase FISH categories at diagnosis in predicting overall survival of CLL patients is confirmed by long-term followup studies. Interphase FISH testing can identify approximately 27% of patients with clonal chromosomal evolution occurring after 5 or more years of followup, with approximately two third of patients acquiring del(13q) and del(17p).[389] These observations have important clinical implications for management of patients with highest-risk early-stage CLL.

MULTIPLE MYELOMA

MM is a malignancy of terminally differentiated B cells. These plasma cells have a very low proliferative rate, a characteristic that has limited its application in cytogenetic studies. Conventional karyotyping reveals chromosome abnormalities in 25% to 30% of newly diagnosed patients, especially in cases with exceptionally high plasma cell proliferative rates.[390] Karyotypes obtained from these cells usually are complex and exhibit more than 20 aberrations in approximately about 10% of cases.[391]

When reassessed by FISH, CGH, and multicolor karyotyping using a large panel of centromere-specific and translocation-specific probes, interphase plasma cell nuclei revealed chromosomal aneuploidy in almost all patients with MM or monoclonal gammopathy of unknown significance.[392–399] Even during complete clinical remission, 12% to 71% of cells still show a numerical gain or loss of chromosomes 3, 7, 8, 9, 11, 13 15, 21, and X.[400]

Analysis of numerical abnormalities reveals two broad groups of MM patients: hyperdiploid and nonhyperdiploid. Hyperdiploid MM is associated with trisomies of chromosomes 3, 5, 7, 9, 11, 15, 19, and 21 and fewer *IGH* translocations. Nonhyperdiploid MM is characterized by a high frequency of *IGH* translocations (>85%). Both these groups are also present in monoclonal gammopathy of unknown significance, suggesting that they occur early in the evolution of disease.[397–399,401] The prognostic relevance of numerical abnormalities is difficult to ascertain because other adverse genetic changes frequently are present in the same clone. Even with the application of gene expression profiling, MM-specific oncogenes associated with hyperdiploidy have not been identified.[402–404] However, in such a genetically heterogeneous group, it is anticipated that molecular techniques such as array CGH may provide more precise and predictive tools.

An IGH rearrangement on 14q32.3 is found in most patients with MM. The rearrangement consists of complex and heterogeneous translocations with the breakpoint involving either the switch region of *IGH* or the V, D, or J gene (see Table 55–9). The primary translocations are due to somatic hypermutation or errors in the VDJ portion of the switch region recombination. The translocations include a promiscuous array of at least 20 nonrandom chromosomal partners and the characterization of these translocations have led to the identification of critical deregulated oncogenes (e.g., *BCL2*, cyclin D). In each translocation, a potent enhancer is juxtaposed to deregulated oncogenes. The most frequent *IGH* translocations include t(4;14)(p16.3;q32.3), t(11;14)(q13;q32.3), and t(14;16)(q32.3;q23) (Fig. 55–38).

Patients with a recurrent *CCND1-IGH* have an overexpression of cyclin D1. In contrast to mantle cell lymphoma, breakpoints on 11q13 in MM are not clustered but are scattered over a relatively large genomic region. Therefore, the *CCND1-IGH* commercial probe for MM involves another gene, *MYEOV*, that is distinct from the *CCND1-IGH* probe used for detection of t(11;14) in mantle cell lymphoma (Fig. 55–39, bottom left). In contrast to other abnormalities involving the *IGH* locus, clonal t(11;14) MM cells tend to be diploid. There appears to be an association of the t(11;14) with oligosecretory or light chain only, CD20 expression, and lymphoplasmacytic morphology.[397,405–407]

Approximately 15% of patients have a recurrent t(4;14)(p16.3;q32.3) abnormality. This cytogenetic abnormality is associated with IgA subtype, λ light chain, immature plasma cell morphology, and poor response to therapy. This abnormality is cytogenetically cryptic and is detected by FISH and other molecular cytogenetic methods.[397,398,407–410] Two genes on chromosome 4p16.3 and the *IGH* switch region on 14q32.3 are involved. The fibroblast growth factor receptor 3 gene *(FGFR3)* is detected on der(14), where it is overexpressed along with a fusion of the multiple myeloma set domain *(MMSET)* gene, located on 4p16.3.[410] This is the first example of a translocation that simultaneously deregulates two genes with oncogenic potential, the *FGFR3* gene detected on der(14) and the *MMSET* gene detected on der(4). *FGFR3* is 50 to 100 kb telomeric to *MMSET*. Loss of *FGFR3* on der(14) is detected in approximately 20% of cases.[411] A significant proportion of these patients display del(13q) in the same clone and are hypodiploid.

Genetic lesion	Frequency (%)
del(13)(q14.3)	10-20
t(11;14)(q13; q32.3)	15-30
t(14;16)(q32.3; q23)	2-8
t(4;14)(p16.3; q32.3)	15
del(17)(p13.1)	10

Figure 55–38 Most frequent structural chromosomal rearrangements in multiple myeloma and their frequencies.

Translocation (14;16)(q32.3;q23) had never been cytogenetically detected because of the telomeric positions of both loci. However, with FISH studies the incidence of t(14;16) has been estimated to be approximately 2% to 8%.[412] In this translocation, the *MAF* protooncogene is translocated from its normal position on 16q23 to chromosome 14, band q32.3, and is overexpressed. Rare variants t(14;20) and t(8;20) are included in this group because they share a similar gene expression signature and clinical outcome.[413,414] The clinical outcome of patients with t(14;16) is significantly shorter compared to a t(14;16)-negative cohort.[415]

Deletion of either band q14 or q14.3 *(RB1,* DNA marker *D13S319)* on chromosome 13 is detected in 10% to 20% of patients by conventional cytogenetics and in 50% by FISH (see Fig. 55–39, top right).[390,416,417] Microarray CGH data of the critical region on chromosome 13 is consistent with previous findings. Loss of the entire chromosome 13 (82%) is more frequent than is deletion of the long arms of chromosome 13.[418,419] The most commonly deleted region has not been delineated. The median percentage of plasma cells carrying del(13q), identified by FISH, ranges from 75% and 90%.[398,418,420,421] Deletion of 13q is associated with specific clinicopathologic features, including a higher frequency of λ-type MM, high plasma cell labeling index, female predominance, and inferior survival after standard chemotherapy.

Numerous studies have demonstrated that del(13q) represents an adverse prognostic marker in MM. However, molecular cytogenetics analyses revealed that del(13q) is present in 90% of patients showing t(4;14) or t(14;16); therefore, the apparent adverse impact of del(13q) may not be the only genomic defect influencing unfavorable prognosis in these patients.[422–424]

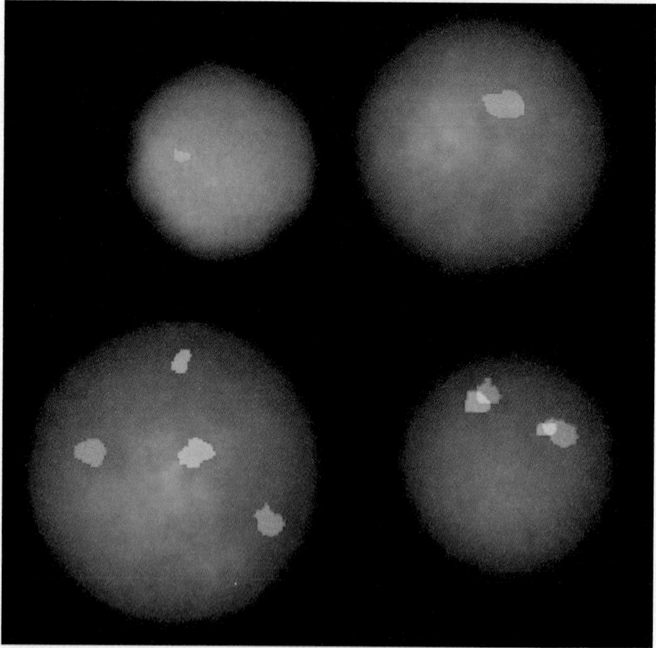

Figure 55–39 Composite image of marrow nuclei from a patient with multiple myeloma after hybridization with five probes. The following probes are the most frequently used for detection of genomic structural rearrangements in clinical testing of multiple myeloma. Left top cell has 17p13.1 deletion (one red signal). Right top nucleus also shows a single red signal after hybridization with D13S319 probe, consistent with deletion of 13q14.3 locus. The patient had codeletion of both loci, which is associated with unfavorable prognosis. Bottom left cell shows two green and two red signals after FISH study with *CCND1* and *IGH,* indicating disomy for both probes and lack of *CCND1-IGH* fusion. Also shown are confirmatory results (bottom right) obtained after application of breakapart *IGH* probe showing lack of separation of green and red signals, consistent with intact *IGH* gene.

The adverse prognostic impact of del(13q) detected by conventional cytogenetics versus interphase FISH remains controversial. Comparative analyses using conventional cytogenetics and metaphase and interphase FISH studies demonstrate different survival depending on whether del(13q) abnormality is detected by metaphase or only in interphase nuclei, or by both.[390,425]

Deletion of *P53* at 17p13.1, which occurs in 10% of patients, is a powerful independent predictor of shortened survival in MM and is associated with stage III disease, clonal evolution, drug resistance, and genetic instability (see Fig. 55–39, top left). This deletion is not found in patients with other high-risk groups such at t(4;14), or t(14;16), and it appears mutually exclusive.[409] Patients characterized by *P53* deletion have significantly shorter overall survival irrespective of therapy administered.[406,426,427]

The gain of 1q21 locus is identified in 45% of cases of monoclonal gammopathy of unknown significance, 43% of newly diagnosed MM, and 72% of relapsed MM and represents one of the most frequent recurrent chromosomal abnormalities in MM.[428] Gain of 1q can be detected cytogenetically as isochromosome, duplications, or jumping translocations or detected with a 1q21-specific FISH probe.[429,430] Among 479 patients with newly diagnosed MM, 43% with amplq21 also have either a hypodiploid and hyperdiploid karyotype, del(13q) by FISH, immunoglobulin A predominance, and poor prognosis compared to patients lacking amp1q21.[428]

The molecular basis of MM is slowly emerging, but the precise role of oncogenes is not yet defined. In order to address this issue and to understand the molecular basis of aneuploidy, work has evaluated the role of centrosome amplification in plasma cell neoplasm. Preliminary evidence indicates that centrosome amplification is common in all stages of plasma cell neoplasm, including monoclonal gammopathy of unknown significance, and probably is integral to disease pathogenesis and genomic instability of MM.[431] The recently described gene Dickkopf-1 *(DKK1)* may be associated with the presence of lytic bone lesions in patients with MM.[432,433]

Molecular abnormalities such as *CCND1-IGH, IGH-MAF,* and *FGHR3-IGH* are found in approximately 40% of patients presenting with MM. In the remaining 60% of cases, chromosomal translocations cannot be identified, but hyperdiploidy is present. These presenting features are followed by further karyotypic instability and often include deletions/monosomy of chromosome 13 or chromosome 17, band region p13.1 (P53). Amplification of 1q21 represents a late event in this multistep process and is associated with a malignant phenotype. From a practical point of view (see box on Genetic Testing in Multiple Myeloma and Fig. 55–39), recommended basic genetic testing for newly diagnosed MM patients must include FISH testing for *CCND1-IGH,* deletions of *P53* and 13q13.4 loci, and rearrangements of *IGH.* Conventional cytogenetics can be performed to detect del(13q) in dividing metaphase cells as an indicator of a highly proliferating tumor. If progression of MM is suspected, FISH testing for amplification of 1q21 is recommended.

LYMPHOMA

Non-Hodgkin lymphoma (NHL) comprises a heterogenous group of disorders characterized by localized proliferation of lymphocytes. Analogous to other hematopoietic disorders, the pathogenesis of these malignancies is attributable to a multistep process involving progressive and clonal accumulation of genetic lesions. The majority of NHLs are of B-cell origin and involve translocations of immunoglobulin loci (see Table 55–9). *IGH* translocations usually are detected by cytogenetics, often in conjunction with FISH probes that span the *IGH* loci[434] and/or PCR-based technologies. These molecular abnormalities exhibit enormous complexity with multiple and complex translocations, deletions, and amplifications within one clone. The WHO recognizes that genetic anomalies represent one of the most reliable criteria for classification of malignant lymphomas. The most common associations between chromosome anomalies and specific lymphomas include t(14;18)(q32;q21) and follicular lymphoma; t(8;14)(q24;q32) and Burkitt lymphoma; t(11;14)(q13;q32) and mantle cell lymphoma; and t(11;18)(q21;q21) and mucosa-associated lymphoid tissue (MALT) lymphoma (see box on Genetic Testing for Non-Hodgkin Lymphoma and Fig. 55–40). However, identification of a specific translocation is not diagnostic of a specific lymphoma subtype. Chromosome studies are difficult and expensive for the study of lymphomas. Thus, many investigators use FISH and/or molecular genetic methods to study touch preparations or paraffin-embedded lymphoid tissue to detect important genetic anomalies in lymphomas.[435–437]

Approximately 85% to 90% of patients with follicular lymphoma and some patients with large cell lymphoma exhibit t(14;18)(q32.3;q21.3), which results in fusion of *BCL2* on 18q21 and *IGH* on 14q32 and represents one of the most common abnormality in NHL (see Fig. 55–40, *D*). Although the exact underlying mechanism is not known, t(14;18) results from a mistake of VDJ recombination and juxtaposes the *BCL2* oncogene with the nonexpressed *IGH* allele.[437] As a consequence, the *BCL2* gene comes under the control of *IGH* enhancer, causing dysregulated expression of *BCL2* protein, one of the proteins involved in regulation of apoptosis. The breakpoints within *BCL2* occur mostly within the 3′ region of the gene, whereas the breakpoints in *IGH* fall within the D_H and J_H regions. Although 75% of breakpoints are clustered within a remarkably narrow region of 15 to 20 bp at the 3′ end of the *BCL2* gene, they are frequently missed by standard PCR.[438] With regular and fiber FISH methods using *BCL2* breakpoint flanking probes, individual 5′ and 3′ breakpoints can be detected. *BCL2* rearrangements are detected with immunohistochemical staining for BCL2 protein.[11] With disease progression, 100% of patients have *BCL2* overexpression. Variant translocations, such as t(2;18)(p12;q21) and t(18;22)((q21;q11) involving the *IGK* or *IGL* gene, respectively, rather than *IGH,* also show overexpression of *BCL2.*[439]

Numerous secondary chromosomal abnormalities are identified by conventional cytogenetics, and at least five recurrent anomalies, each occurring in at least 20% of follicular lymphomas, may distinguish two subgroups of follicular lymphoma patients. Patients with t(14;18) showing additional trisomy for chromosome 2, 7, or 8 are associated with more favorable course of disease compared to patients with additional del(1p), del(1q), del(6q), der(18), del(22q), or gain

Genetic Testing for Multiple Myeloma

Chromosome studies of isolated plasma cells from the marrow are very useful at diagnosis. Perform interphase fluorescence *in situ* hybridization and molecular genetic studies for detection of *CCND1-IGH* [t(11;14)], del(13)(q14.3)/D13S319, del(17)(p13.1)/P53, and *IGH*/14q32.3. If *IGH* rearrangements are detected using a breakapart *IGH* locus, refine the partner and use the following set of probes: *MAF-IGH* for detection of t(14;16) and *FGFR3-IGH* for detection of t(4;14).

Genetic Testing for Non-Hodgkin Lymphoma

Fluorescence *in situ* hybridization (FISH) testing can be performed on touch preparations, paraffin-embedded tissue, or bone marrow cells if bone marrow is involved. Peripheral blood cells are not appropriate for genetic testing of non-Hodgkin lymphoma. Bone marrow cytogenetics at diagnosis is not useful but may be important for staging in some cases. Figure 55–40 lists the most useful FISH probes for detection of genomic defects in non-Hodgkin lymphoma. They include *CCND1-IGH, IGH-BCL2, MYC-IGH, BCL6, MYC* breakapart for detection of Burkitt variant not associated with t(8;14), and *MALT1* breakapart for detection of t(11;18). For patients with suspected anaplastic large cell lymphoma, *ALK* breakapart probe should be informative.

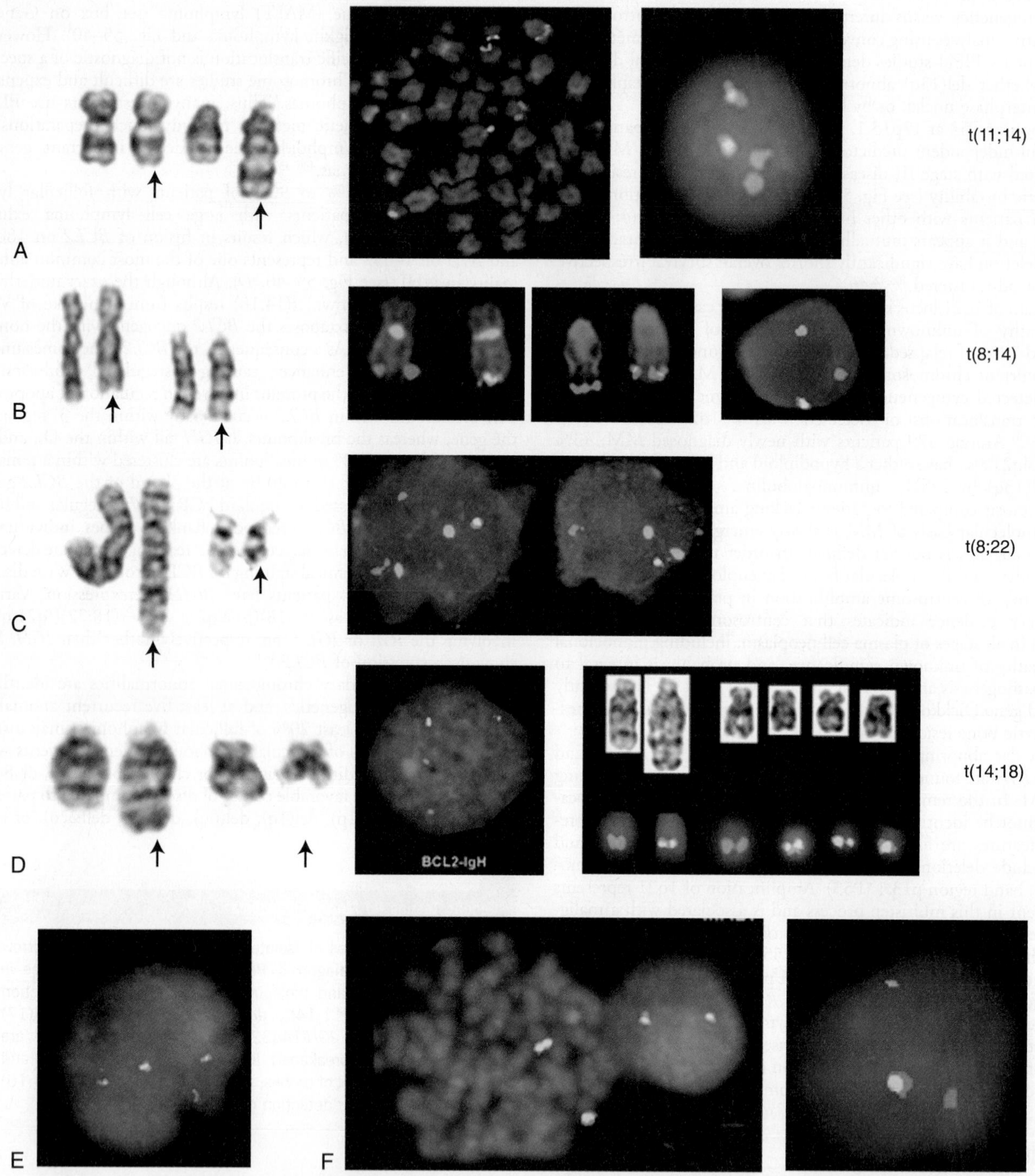

Figure 55–40 Most frequent chromosomal abnormalities in non-Hodgkin lymphoma. **A,** Partial G-banded karyotype of t(11;14)(q13;q32.3) (left), resulting in *CCND1-IGH* fusion (yellow) on metaphase (middle) and in interphase cell (right) present in the majority of patients with mantle cell lymphoma. **B,** Partial G-banded karyotype of t(8;14)(q24;q32.3) (left) resulting in *MYC-IGH* fusion [yellow on der(8) on isolated chromosomes]. Application of *MYC* breakapart probe shows separation of red and green signals consistent with MYC rearrangement. Approximately 80% of Burkitt lymphomas are characterized by t(8;14); **C,** Partial G-banded karyotype of t(8;22)(q24;q11), a variant of Burkitt lymphoma (left). Two interphase lymph node cells after hybridization with *MYC* breakapart probe and CEP8 (aqua). Separation of green and red signals is consistent with *MYC* relocation from 8q24 to 22q11: **D,** Partial G-banded karyotype of t(14;18)(q32.3;q21.3) (left) resulting in *IGH-BCL* fusion (two yellow signals, middle). A composite image on the right shows both a partial karyotype and FISH study of triplicated der(18)t(14;18) and three copies of *IGH-BCL2* fusion (yellow) as well as normal chromosome 14 and 18. Multiple copies of abnormal der(18) chromosome is associated with progressive disease similar to a duplication of the Philadelphia chromosome in the blast crisis of chronic myelogenous leukemia. **E,** Lymph node cell from a patient with diffuse large B-cell lymphoma (DLBCL) showing four copies of *BCL6* (breakapart probe). *BCL6* is localized at 3q27 and is numerically or structurally rearranged in 35% of DLBCL. **F,** Bone marrow metaphase and interphase cell hybridized with breakapart *MALT1* gene at 18q21 (left) indicating two fusion (yellow) signals when *MALT1* gene is intact. In contrast, rearrangement of the *MALT1* gene in MALT lymphoma usually is the consequence of t(11;18)(q21;q21.1)m as shown in the cell (right) with clear separation of the 3′ end (green) and the 5′ end (red).

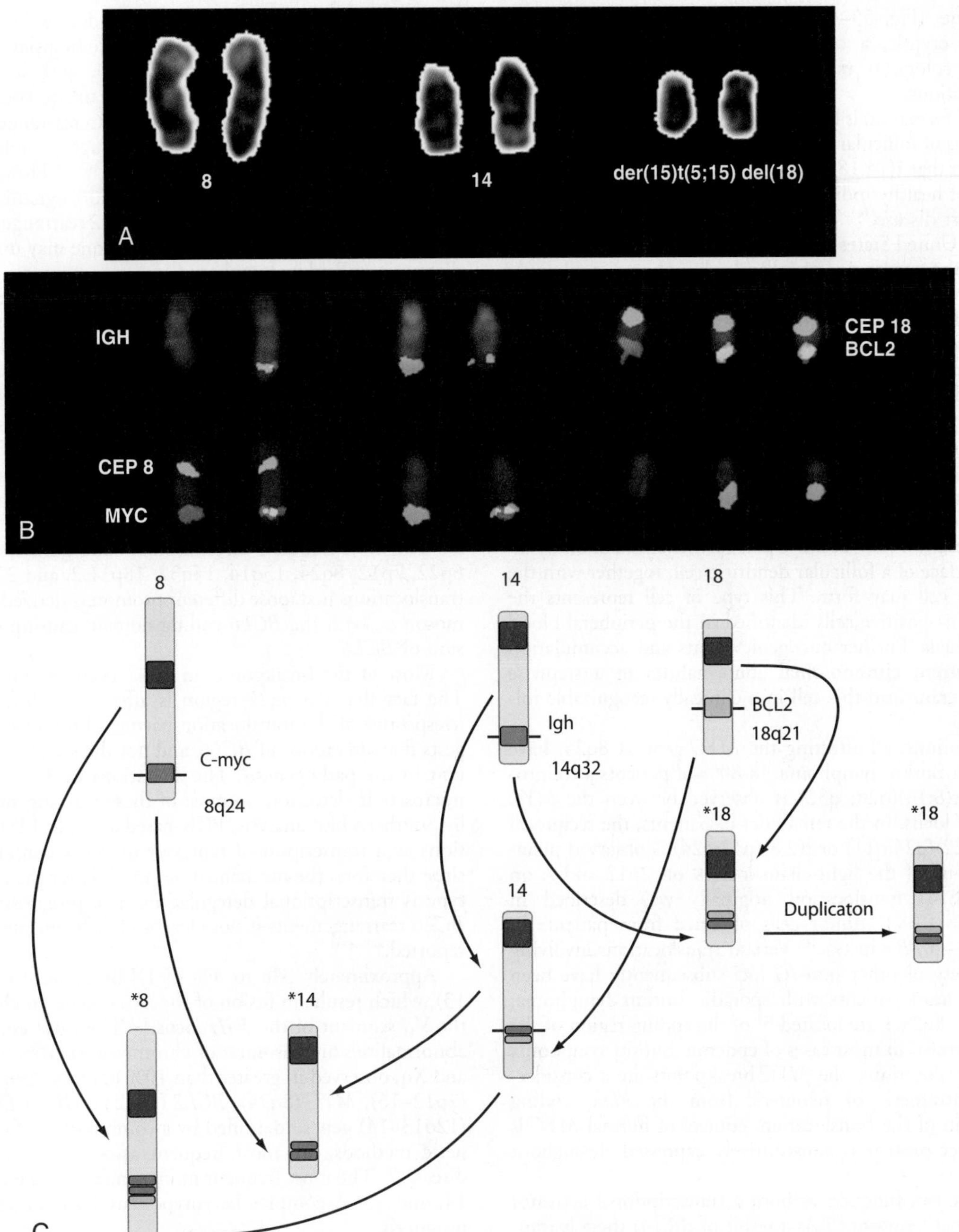

Figure 55–41 Identification of simultaneous *BCL2* and *MYC* rearrangements in high-grade B-cell lymphoma leukemia (see text for details). Partial G-banded karyotype (top) of chromosomes 8 and 14 and what is initially identified as der(15)t(5;15) and der(18). Partial karyotype of the same chromosomes after FISH study (bottom) with probes for *IGH* (green), CEP8 (aqua), and *MYC* (red) indicating *IGH-MYC* fusions (yellow) on both chromosomes 8 and 14. Sequential hybridization with CEP18 (aqua), *BCL2* (red), and *IGH* (green) also revealed *IGH-BCL2* fusion (yellow) on both der(15) and der(18), indicating that der(15) actually is a duplication of rearranged chromosome 18. **C,** Schematic representation of genomic events leading to duplication 18. Rearrangements of both *MYC* and *BCL2* show a complex molecular array.

of chromosome 12 and X, which is associated with inferior outcome. Unfavorable outcome of patients with loss of X chromosome is confirmed by CGH, and del(6)(q25–q27) is identified as the strongest predictor of poor prognosis and shorter survival time. Rearrangements of chromosome 1, such as del(1)(p32–36), +¹(p11–q44), and unbalanced translocations of der(1)(1;1)(p36;q11–23) regions are among the most frequent secondary chromosomal abnormalities in follicular lymphoma.[440–443] Progression of follicular lymphoma to diffuse large cell B-cell lymphoma occurs in 60% to 80% and is accompanied by accumulation of secondary abnormalities, of which homozygous del(9p) might be associated with histologic progression.[444]

The combination of *BCL-2* and *MYC* rearrangements resulting from t(8;14)(q24;q32) and t(14;18)(q32;q21) or variants in the same karyotype is characteristic of high-grade B-cell lymphoma/leukemia, which occurs in fewer than 2% of patients and is associated with aggressive histology and poor prognosis.[445,446] In these cases, a translocation within a single *IGH* allele separates the 3′ from the 5′ *IGH* enhancer element, with relocation of the *BCL2* 5′ *IGH* enhancer fusion to the der(8) and translocation of *MYC* adjacent to the 3′ *IGH* enhancer element that is retained on the der(14). The ISCN cytogenetic description der(8)t(8;14)(q24;q32) t(14;18)(q32;q21), der(14)t(8;14)(q24;q32), der(18)t(14;18)(q32;q21) does not reflect the complexity of the underlying molecular rearrangements (Fig. 55–41A–C). Because one of the translocation may be cryptic, a combination of three FISH probes, labeled in three colors, is especially useful in identifying these complex translocations.

The *IGH-BCL* formation is believed to represent a very early event in the pathogenesis of follicular lymphoma. This notion is supported by the observation that t(14;18) is also found in peripheral blood in more than 50% of healthy individuals and may persist for at least 3 years without overt disease.[447–450] Because the incidence of follicular lymphoma in the United States is approximately one case per 24,000 persons per year, the occurrence of follicular lymphoma is relatively rare.[451] Gene expression profiling shows a distinct pattern associated with an indolent form of disease (median survival 11.1 years) and a more aggressive form (median survival 3.9 years), indicating that these different conditions may represent distinct stages in the evolution of follicular lymphoma.[452] These and other observations point to an immune response that may regulate the pace of the malignant process and may restrain the proliferation of t(14;18)-positive B cells in healthy individuals.[450,451] The molecular pathogenesis of follicular lymphoma may include formation of t(14;18) in a naive B cell. If stimulated by an exogenous agent such as a virus or autoantigen, a germinal center reaction may occur. Upon further stimulation by an antigen on the surface of a follicular dendritic cell, together with the T-cell, a memory cell may form. This type of cell represents the majority of t(14;18)-positive cells identified in the peripheral blood of normal individuals. Further oncogenic events and accumulation of different, recurrent chromosomal abnormalities in a stepwise pathogenesis may transform this cell into clinically recognizable follicular lymphoma.

Three translocations, all affecting the *MYC* gene at 8q24, have been recognized in Burkitt lymphoma. In 80% of patients a reciprocal translocation t(8;14)(q24; q32) is observed between the *MYC* gene and the *IGH* locus. In the remainder of patients, the reciprocal translocation t(8;22)(q24;q11) or t(2;8)(p12;q24) is observed juxtaposing MYC to one of the light-chain loci (κ on 2p12 and λ on 22q11). The t(8;14) translocation originally was described in Epstein-Barr virus (EBV)+ tumor cells obtained from patients in Africa (see Fig. 55–40, *B* and *C*).[453] Variant translocations involving MYC with a variety of other non-*IG* loci subsequently have been reported.[454,455] In most patients with sporadic Burkitt lymphoma, the breakpoints on 8q24.1 are located 5′ of the coding region of the *MYC* gene. In contrast, in most cases of endemic Burkitt lymphoma and in variant translocations, the *MYC* breakpoints are a considerable distance centromeric or telomeric from the *MYC* coding exons.[456] As a result of the translocation, control of normal *MYC* is lost, and the intact protein is constitutively expressed throughout the cell cycle.

The *MYC* gene can function as both a transcriptional activator and a transcriptional repressor.[457] As a result of t(8;14) there is transcription of a truncated MYC protein, whereas in t(2;8) and t(8;22) the rearrangement of the *MYC* gene can occur within sequences downstream of the transcribed region. The exact molecular mechanism by which the rearranged *MYC* is activated is not fully elucidated, but its activation constitutes an important step in malignant transformation. An increased level of *MYC* constitutive synthesis in leukemic disorders is found not only as a result of translocation but also as a result of *MYC* mutations and amplification. Approximately 65% of Burkitt lymphomas demonstrate *MYC* point mutations. Overexpression of *MYC* is linked to amplification of *MYC* genes reported in plasma cell leukemia, AML, CML, and T-cell lymphoma.

The most common secondary change associated with t(8;14) is duplication of the long arms of chromosome 1, and these rearrangements are associated with disease progression.[458,459] A common duplicated region of 93 kb at 1q21.2 is defined by FISH studies.[460] This section of chromosome contains at least three putative oncogenes, including the *OTUD7B* gene. This gene encodes a cytoplasmic protein and functions as a negative regulator of the nuclear factor (NF)-κB transcription factor, known to be implicated as a critical pathogenic factor in lymphoma.[461]

Rearrangements of *MYC* now can be detected in nondividing cells as well as paraffin-embedded lymph node biopsies using a very sensitive interphase FISH assay for t(8;14), with less than 2% false-positive results. Genomic profiling study unequivocally demonstrated that the majority of patients with *MYC* rearrangements should be classified as Burkitt lymphoma even though pathologists called some of the cases diffuse large cell lymphoma.[462,463] However, these studies also indicate that rare cases with the Burkitt signature gene expression lack *MYC* rearrangements and have *BCL2* rearrangements, suggesting that in rare cases *MYC* rearrangement alone may not be sufficient for diagnosis of Burkitt lymphoma.

According to the WHO classification, a Burkitt-like lymphoma is a separate entity characterized by one of the Burkitt lymphoma translocations. However, many such cases fail to show Burkitt lymphoma translocations but do exhibit increased *MYC* expression.[464]

Approximately 35% of patients with diffuse large B-cell lymphoma (DLBCL) and approximately 5% to 10% of patients with follicular lymphoma have rearrangements in the *BCL6* gene normally residing at 3q27. Translocation of 3q27 is the third most frequent translocation in NHL, and at least 33 different partners have been described as participating in these rearrangements (see Fig. 55–40, *E*). The most frequent chromosomal band partners are 2p13, 4p13, 6p22, 7p12, 8q24, 13q14, 14q32, 18p11.2, and 22q11.[465–467] These translocations juxtapose different promoters derived from other chromosomes, with the *BCL6* coding domain causing persistent expression of *BCL6*.

Most of the breakpoints in 3q27 occur within a 10-kb region. The fact that the 3q27 region is affected in different lymphomas, irrespective of the translocation partner chromosomes, strongly suggests that alterations of *BCL6*, and not the reciprocal loci, are important in the pathogenesis. The alterations in 3q27 are too small for microscopic detection, so most of these rearrangements are detected by Southern blot analysis, PCR-based assay, or FISH.[468] *BCL6* functions as a transcriptional repressor of genes containing its binding sites; therefore, the mechanism responsible for the malignant phenotype is transcriptional deregulation. The prognostic significance of *BCL6* rearrangements is not clear, and different outcomes have been reported.[469–471]

Approximately 3% to 4% of DLBCLs have t(14;15)(q32;q11-13), which results in fusion of the *BCL8* gene on chromosome 15 to the V_H segment of the *IGH* locus.[472] The most common secondary abnormalities are trisomies of chromosomes 3, 5, 7q, 11, 12p, 18q, and Xq, observed in greater than 10% of cases. Amplification of *REL* (2p12–16), *MYC* (8q24), *BCL2* (18q21), *GLI*, *CDK4*, and *MDM2* (12q13–14) genes, identified by a combination of molecular cytogenetic methods, are most frequent associated with advanced stage disease.[473] The most frequent monosomies include chromosomes 13, 14, and 15. A complex karyotype may have an adverse impact on prognosis.

Modern molecular cytogenetic methods such as CGH identify three major subgroups in DCLBC. Patients with activated B-cell-like DLBCL (ABC-DCLBC) exhibit frequent trisomy 3, gains of 3q and 18q21–23, and loss of the 6q21–23 region. Patients with germinal center B-like (GCB) DLBCL have frequent gains of the 12q12 chromosomal region. Patients with primary mediastinal lymphoma (PMBCL) has gains of 2p14-p16 and 9p21-pter.[474] Apparently, only gains in several regions of chromosome 3 are significantly associated with inferior survival. Moreover, genomic gains involving the 3p11-p12 region have an independent prognostic power for survival based on previously defined optimal gene expression-based models.[474,475]

All patients with mantle cell lymphoma exhibit the t(11;14)(q13;q32) abnormality by FISH.[476,477] t(11;14)(q13;q32) is also found in a variety of other B-cell malignancies, including MM, splenic lymphoma with villous lymphocytes, and B-cell prolymphocytic leukemia. Most breakpoints on chromosome 11, band q13, are dispersed over a region approximately 130 kb centromeric to the *cyclin D1 (CCND1)* gene. At the molecular level, the *BCL1* locus *(CCND1)* on chromosome 11q13 is juxtaposed to an enhancer sequence within the immunoglobulin heavy-chain gene *(IGH)* on 14q32, leading to overexpression of the *cyclin D* gene, which is not expressed in normal B and T cells or in other malignant lymphomas. The consequence of this translocation is overexpression of *cyclin D1*, a gene involved in cell cycle control.

Each method for detection of t(11;14), including cytogenetics, Southern blot, and PCR-based analyses, has limitations. Cytogenetics is hampered by a low mitotic index of neoplastic B cells. Southern blot and PCR-based analyses for 11q13 rearrangements are positive in only 50% to 60% of patients with mantle cell lymphoma because the breakpoints within 11q13 are scattered along a 130-kb distance. In practical terms, dual-color FISH has proved to be the most sensitive assay for detection of *IGH-CCND1* fusion, which is found in 100% of cases.[478,479] Furthermore, the *CCND1* fusion rearrangement can be detected in formalin-fixed, paraffin-embedded samples, making this method rapid, reliable, independent of cell cycle, and applicable to all cases of mantle cell lymphoma (see Fig. 55–40, *A*).[480]

Gene expression studies have identified a subset of patients with D1-negative mantle cell lymphoma, so called because of the lack *cyclin D1* expression and t(11;14).[481,482] However, both cyclin D1-positive and cyclin D1-negative patients have the same secondary genomic alterations when assessed with conventional cytogenetics, CGH, and array-based CGH.[479,483] These secondary chromosomal alterations include gains of 3q, 8q, and 15q and losses of 1p, 8p23-pter, 9p21-pter,11q21–23, and 13q. Some of the genes residing in these chromosomal regions are dysregulated and involved in cell proliferation, DNA repair mechanism of chromosome stability, and cellular homeostasis and apoptosis mechanisms. Unlike other lymphomas, in mantle cell lymphoma DNA amplifications of several chromosomal regions appear to be associated with a blastoid variant.[484] Loss of 9p21-pter, inactivation of P53, gain of 3q, and high *cyclin D* expression are reported molecular and cytogenetic markers of shorter survival and a more aggressive clinical evolution. The prognostic value of 3q27-qer gains and loss of 9q21–32 region are determined to be independent of the gene expression-based signature.[483] Extra copies of 3q are prognostic in patients with low proliferation, whereas loss of 9q has improved clinical value in subgroup of patients with high proliferation.

Marginal zone lymphoma and MALT lymphoma are considered the third most frequent NHL subtype. According to the WHO classification, they are subdivided into splenic marginal zone lymphoma, nodal marginal zone lymphoma, and MALT lymphoma. An etiologic link between low-grade gastric MALT lymphoma and the lymphoid reaction associated with *Helicobacter pylori* infection is well established.[485] Growing evidence suggests that chronic antigenic stimulation in autoimmune diseases, such as Hashimoto thyroiditis, contribute to an increased risk of developing MALT lymphoma.[486]

The most frequent and specific aberration occurring in MALT lymphomas is t(11;18)(q21;q21.1).[487] Although it has been described in other B-cell lymphomas, t(11;18) in MALT lymphoma usually is the only genetic lesion and does not show additional chromosomal anomalies.[488] It is the only recurrent translocation that does not involve *IG* genes even though it presents as a B-cell lymphoma. As a consequence of t(11;18), *API2* gene on chromosome 11, band q21, which encodes an inhibitor of apoptosis (also known as *IAP2, HIAP1,* and *MIHC),* and a novel gene *MALT1* on chromosome 18, band q21, characterized by several Ig-like C2-type domains, are often rearranged.[489] The resultant chimeric transcript consists of 5′-*API2* and 3′-MAT located on der(18). More than 90% of breakpoints in the *API2* locus occur in intron 7, whereas the breakpoints within *MALT1* are variable and occur in four different introns.[490] The *API2-MALT1* fusion is easily identified using a dual-color *API2-MALT1* FISH probe or the "breakapart" strategy of dual-color *MALT1* probe on lymph node biopsies (see Fig. 55–40, *F*). However, detection of deletions and duplications occurring at high frequencies in both the *API2* and *MALT1* genomic sequences requires more precise molecular cytogenetic methods.

t(1;14)(p22;q32) and its variant t(1;2)(p22;p12) occur in less than 5% of MALT lymphomas, typically display other chromosomal abnormalities, and are associated with an advanced stage of disease at diagnosis (reviewed in[491] and references within). This translocation relocates the entire *BCL10* gene from 1p22 to chromosome 14, bringing it under the control of an *IGH* enhancer. Currently, a specific probe for detecting *BCL10-IGH* fusion is not available, but *IGH* dual-color "breakapart" FISH strategy may determine *IGH* rearrangements without identifying the partner chromosome. The t(3;14)(p13;q32) abnormality, which results in fusion of the *FOXP1F* gene on chromosome 3 to *IGH,* is a rare rearrangement that causes *FOXP1F* overexpression. Its significance in lymphoma remains unknown. t(14;18)(q32;q21), which occurs in 2% to 18% of all MALT lymphomas, results in fusion of *IGH-MALT*.[491,492] The 18q21 breakpoint involving the *MALT1* gene is 5 Mb centromeric from the *BCL2* breakpoint on chromosome 18 associated with follicular lymphoma. In contrast to *API2-MALT1*$^+$ cases, patients with *IGH-MALT1* fusion have disease outside the gastrointestinal tract, presenting usually with ocular, skin, liver, or salivary gland tumors.[493] FISH studies are useful for detecting the *IGH-MALT* fusion in paraffin-embedded lymph node biopsies. Although a unifying concept linking MALT-associated translocations to the pathogenesis of MALT lymphoma is not available, compelling evidence links these translocations to constitutive activation of the NF-κB pathway.[461,491]

Lymphoplasmacytoid lymphoma (LPL) is a small lymphocytic lymphoma with plasmacytoid differentiation (CD5$^-$CD10$^-$) characterized by t(9;14)(p13;q32) in approximately 50% of cases.[494] As a result of this translocation, the paired homeobox 5 gene *(PAX5)* on 9p13 moves to the *IGH* locus on der(14), causing dysregulation of *PAX5*. Molecular characterization of t(9;14) revealed that the coding region of the *PAX5* gene remains intact in some patients. In those individuals, t(9;14) should be considered a regulatory mutation in which the *PAX5* gene is brought under the control of the *IGH* locus. In other cases, molecular studies of t(9;14) reveal that the breakpoint occurs upstream of the *PAX5* promoter, leading to insertion of the *IGH* enhancer upstream of the *PAX 5* gene.

Waldenström macroglobulinemia is a plasma cell dyscrasia characterized by a CD138,CD19 phenotype, with a lympho/plasmacytic clonal expansion in the marrow. The biologic nature is different from lymphoplasmacytoid lymphoma because patients do not display t(9;14)(p13;q32). Recurrent chromosomal abnormalities include deletion of the long arms of chromosome 6 in 55% of cases by cytogenetics[495] and in 21% of cases by FISH.[496] Trisomy 4 is present in approximately 20% of cases.[497] In contrast to other B-cell disorders, abnormalities of *IGH* at 14q32 as measured by FISH and Southern blot are rarely identified in Waldenström macroglobulinemia.

Not much progress has been made in delineating recurrent chromosomal abnormalities in Hodgkin lymphoma (HL). Less than 1% of the cells in HL are Reed-Sternberg cells, of B-cell origin, and the paucity of dividing tumor cells for karyotype analysis has represented a major obstacle for conventional cytogenetics. In one study, simultaneous fluorescence, immunophenotyping, and interphase FISH (FICTION) demonstrated numerical aberrations of CD30$^+$ cells in all HL patients.[498] The most specific chromosomal abnormalities in HL are hyperdiploidy/tetraploidy with tremendous variations in chromosome number, indicating heterogeneity from patient to patient. Even with use of nine different centromeric probes, no specific numerical chromosomal abnormality has been identified. Deletions of 1p, 4q, 6q, and 7q are recurrent, and *JAK2,* located on 9p21, frequently is amplified in patients with HL.[499] Another gene, *c-REL,* on chromosome 2, band region p14-p15, is amplified in 50% of patients.[500] Interestingly, *c-REL* is under the influence of NF-κB transcription factor, and constitutive NF-κB activation is a critical prerequisite for HL/Reed-Steinberg cell survival and proliferation.[461] Thus, it appears that the unifying concept and the hallmark of HL is also constitutive NF-κB activation.

T-Cell Lymphoproliferative Diseases

This is a diverse group of hematologic disorders. The group includes T-cell ALL, T-cell CLL/promyelocytic leukemia as well as several

Table 55–10 Frequent Translocations and Mutations in T-Cell ALL[a]

Translocations	Genes Involved	Children	Frequency (%)	Adults
TCR-Associated Translocations				
t(7;10)(q34;q24) and	*TCRB-TLX1 (HOX11)*	7		31
t(10;14)(q24;q11)	*TCRA-TLX1*			
t(5;14)(q35;q32) (cryptic)	*TLX3 (HOX11L2)*	20		13
inv(7)(p15q34), t(7;7)	*HOXA cluster*		5	
t(1;14)(p32;q11) and t(1;7)(p32;q34)	*TCRA-TAL1*		3	
t(7;9)(q34;q32)	*TCRB-TAL2*		<1	
t(7;19)(q34;p13)	*TCRB-LYL1*		<1	
t(9;14)(p21;q11)	*TCRA_TAL1*		<1	
t(14;21)(q11.2;q22)	*TCRA-HLHB1*		<1	
t(11;14)(p15;q11)	*TCRA-LMO1*		2	
t(11;14)(p13;q11) and	*TCRA-LMO2*		3	
t(7;11)(q35;p13)	*TCRB-LMO1*			
t(1;7)(p32;q34)	*LCK*		<1	
t(7;9)(q34;34.3)	*NOTCH1*		<1	
t(7;12)(q34;p13) and t(12;14)(p13;q11)	*CCND2*		<1	
Formation of Fusion Genes				
1p32 deletion (cryptic)	*SIL-TALI*	9–30		Decreases with age
t(10;11)(p13;q14) (often cryptic)	*CALM-AF10*		10	
t(11;19)(q23;p13)	*MLL*		8	
t(6;11)(q27;q23)	*MLL-AF6*			
t(10;11)(p13;q23)	*MLL/AF10*			
t(X;11)(p13;q23)	*MLL-AFX1*			
t(4;11)(q21;q23)	*MLL-AF4*			
t(9;9)(q34;q34) (episomal or hsr)	*NUP214-ABL1*		<6	
t(9;14)(q34;q32) (cryptic)	*DML1-ABL1*		<1	
t(9;12)(q34;p13)	*ETV6(TEL)-ABL1*		<1	
t(9;12)(p24;p13)	*ETV6(TEL)-JAK2*		<1	
t(9;22)(q34;q11)	*BCR-ABL1*		<1	
t(4;11)(q21;p15)	*NUP98-RAP1GDS1*		<1	
t(10;11)(q25;p15)	*NUP98-ADD3*		<1	
(Cryptic) Deletions				
9p21 (homozygous/hemizygous)	*P16*		65/15	
del (6q)	Unknown		20–30	
Mutations				
NOTCH1	*NOTCH1*		56	
FLT3 ITD and m835	*FLT3*		5	
N-RAS	*N-RAS*	<10		?

ALL, acute lymphoblastic leukemia; TCR, T-cell receptor.
[a]Modified from.[509]

Table 55–11 Frequency of TCR Rearrangements Using Conventional Cytogenetics Versus FISH*

Locus	Conventional Cytogenetics (%)	FISH (%)	
		Total Karyotype	*Abnormal Karyotype*
TCR-αδ	9.5	17.4	24.7
TCR-β	3.1	19	26.9
TCR-γ	0	0	0

FISH, fluorescence *in situ* hybridization; TCR, T-cell receptor.
*Modified from reference 513.

indolent or small T-cell disorders, large granular lymphocyte leukemia, natural killer leukemia/lymphoma, and anaplastic large cell lymphoma (ALCL)

T-cell ALL represents 15% of childhood ALL cases and 25% of adult ALL cases.[501] Table 55–10 lists recurrent cytogenetic and molecular genomic changes associated with T-cell ALL. Immunophenotypic and gene expression analyses are consistent with genetic heterogeneity in T-cell ALL, reflecting, to some degree, distinct stages of T-cell maturation arrest.

One of the common themes in T-lymphoid malignancies is the juxtaposition of T-cell receptor gene *(TCR)* enhancer element adjacent to a variety of transcription factors located at or near breakpoints on the partner chromosome. The chromosomal bands most frequently involved are 14q11, where *TCRA* and *TCRD* are located; 7q35, the site of *TCRB*; and 7p15, the site of the *TCRG*. TCR translocations are found in approximately 35% of T-cell ALL cases

(Table 55–11).[502,503] The rearrangements of *TCRB* and *TCRG* are relatively rare, whereas 14q11 rearrangements involving both *TCRA* and *TCRD* are frequent in T-lymphoid neoplasms.

In children, the overall frequency of T-cell ALL translocations is 40% to 50%, and several molecular/cytogenetic abnormalities have prognostic relevance. *TAL1* rearrangements include t(1;14)(p32;q11), t(1;7)(p32;q35), and rare t(1;3)(p32;p21) and t(1;5)(p32;q31). Generally, *TAL1* rearrangements are submicroscopic and best identified with FISH. They are observed in approximately 3% of patients with T-cell ALL and are more frequent in pediatric than in adult ALL. In children, rearrangements involving *TAL1* gene occur at a frequency of 20% and tend to be associated with better outcome.[504] *TAL2,* residing at 9q32, is detected in rare t(7;9)(q34;q32) as a result of juxtaposition of *TAL2* to *TCRB.*[505] *LYL1,* originally described as a fusion partner of TCRB in rare (7;19)(q34;p13), is associated with poor prognosis.[506] Rearrangements of *HOX11L2,* which include cryptic t(5;14)(q35;q32), t(5;7)(q35;q21), and other variants, occur at a frequency of 24% in children and represent a predictor of poor outcome, irrespective of treatment strategies.[504,506] Similarly, the presence of t(10;11)(p13;q14), which results in the *CALM-AF10* fusion gene and occurs at a frequency of 2% to 5% in children, may be associated with poor outcome.[504,507] Abnormalities of *HOX11* are more common in adults (31%) than in children (7%) and are associated with t(10;14)(q34;q24) and t(7;10)(q34;q24). According to the French collaborative study, t(10;14) is the most frequent chromosomal translocation in patients with T-cell ALL. It is associated with excellent outcome in both children and adults.[504,508] In t(10;14) the homeobox-contain gene *HOX11 (TCL3)* is fused with *TCRD.* The coding regions of *HOX11* are not disturbed by the translocation. In the variant translocation t(7;10)(q35;q24), *HOX11* is juxtaposed to *TCRB,* which results in overexpression of normal *HOX11* mRNA by bringing *HOX11* under the influence of *TCR* promoter sequences.

MLL rearrangements are present in 8% of T-cell ALL cases. The most frequent *MLL* translocation partners in T-cell ALL include *ENL,* which results from t(11;19)(q23;p13.3) and is associated with better prognosis than are other fusion partners.[305] Gene expression profiling data characterized T-cell ALL with *MLL* rearrangements as a distinct molecular subtype with specific molecular signature.[506,509] Homeobox genes, regulators of embryonic development, are known targets of *MLL* and are overexpressed in patients with T-cell ALL and *MLL* rearrangements.[510]

Deregulation of *NOTCH,* tyrosine kinase genes *(ABL1, JAK2),* and *LIM* domain genes *(LMO1, LMO2)* also is common in T-cell ALL. NOTCH has been discovered to be a fusion partner of *TCRB* in t(7;9)(q34;q34.3). These mutations are present in 56% of T-cell ALL cases.[511]

The *LIM* family of genes is found at the breakpoint of rare but consistent chromosomal translocations in T-cell ALL. *LMO1,* located at 11p15, is involved in t(11;14)(p15;q11). *LMO2,* located at 11p13, is involved in t(11;14)(p13;q11) and t(7;11)(q35;p13). As an oncogenic transcription regulator, *LMO2* overexpression in erythroid and T cells leads to differentiation arrest, which is a prerequisite for development of T-cell malignancies.

The *C-MYB* gene, localized on chromosome 6, band q23.3, in normal cells, is rearranged in rare T-cell ALL subtype observed in young patients (median 2.2 years). Two types of recurrent *C-MYB* genomic alterations are found in T-cell ALL: (a) a reciprocal t(6;7)(q23;q34) that results in juxtaposition of *C-MYB* near to *TCRB* regulatory sequences on chromosome 7; and (b) short genomic tandem duplication, identified using genomewide copy-number analysis.[512] Both rearrangements are cytogenetically cryptic. The breakpoints in t(6;7) are subtelomeric and usually missed. The translocation was discovered using a locus-specific FISH probe for C-MYC. The tandem *MYB* duplication is cryptic using both conventional cytogenetics and locus-specific FISH. It is mapped using high-density oligonucleotide array CGH. Discovery of *MYB* highlights the strength of high-density array CGH in identifying cryptic copy-number abnormalities associated with leukemia.

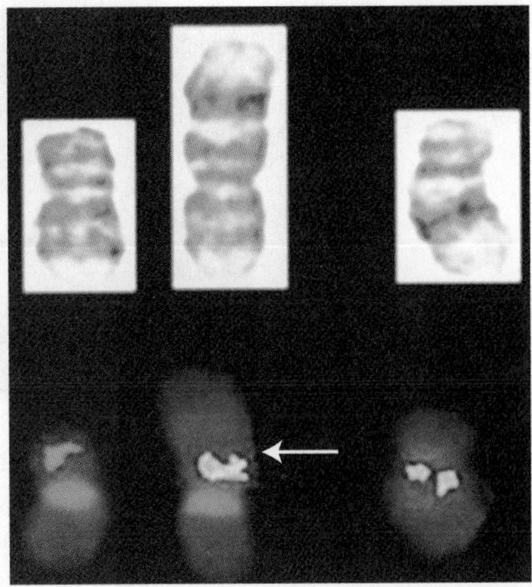

Figure 55–42 Partial karyotype of t(9;12)(p24;q23) (top) and after FISH study (bottom) with *JAK2* (red) and *TEL/ETV6* (green) showing *JAK2-TEL* fusion (yellow) at 9p24.

Although only 1% of Ph positive ALL consist of patients with T-cell ALL, the *ABL1* gene, which is involved in *BCR-ABL1* fusion-positive B-cell ALL and CML, is also involved in fusion with *NUP21,* creating *NUP214-ABL1* chimeric gene, which is identified in up to 6% of T-cell ALL cases.[513] Additionally, this fusion gene is found amplified only in T-cell ALL. When identified with FISH using *ABL1* probe, it appears as an amplified episome between the chromosomes in metaphase cells. RT-PCR also can be used for its detection.[514,515] In rare cases of T-cell ALL, *JAK2* has been identified as a partner chromosome with *ETV6* in t(9;12)(p24;q13) (Fig. 55–42), one of the three JAK2 fusion transcripts seen in hematologic malignancies (see Ph-Negative Myoproliferative Disorders above and Table 55–3).

Numerical changes are rare except for tetraploidy, which occurs in less than 5% of cases and is of unknown prognostic significance. In contrast, cryptic cytogenetic abnormalities revealed by FISH are frequent in ALL. They include deletion of 9p21 *(INK4/ARF)* and 1p32 regions. Deletion of 6q is less common, and the region 6q16 appears to be the common deletion band region.

In contrast to childhood B-cell ALL, the majority of childhood T-cell ALL cases develop after birth. In utero origin of this leukemia is rare. Dramatic treatment advances has been achieved in children with T-cell ALL in the last 4 decades.[516] Initial results with gene expression profiling to determine specific molecular prognostic markers for children with T-cell ALL who may benefit from more intense therapy identified that expression of three genes, *CFLAR, NOTCH2,* and *BTG 3,* at the time of diagnosis may accurately predict disease outcome. All three genes are involved in regulation of apoptosis and cellular proliferation.[517] Expression of *NOTCH2,* but not of the other two gene abnormalities, is implicated in T-cell ALL. Genomewide expression profiling at the time of diagnosis likely can identify novel molecular markers that may be used to predict the clinical outcome of patients.

T-cell CLL and *prolymphocytic leukemia* are characterized by T-cell leukemia 1 gene *(TCL1)* rearrangements. They include inv(14)(q11q32.1), t(14;14)(q11;q32.1), and t(7;14)(q35;q32.1). In patients showing these karyotypic changes, *TCL1* is found to be dysregulated.[518]

Adult T-cell leukemia/lymphoma is associated with human T-cell lymphotropic virus type 1. The most frequent genetic lesions include altered expression of *CDKN2* (cyclin-dependent kinase inhibitor) gene on 9p21 (15%–20%) and loss of heterozygosity at 6q15–q21. The most frequent chromosomal gains are 3p, 7q, and 14q and loss of 6q and 13q. Translocations involving 14q32 or 14q11 are frequently observed. Patients with more chromosomal gains than losses show significantly shorter survival.[519]

Natural killer lymphoma/leukemia, a group of highly aggressive hematolymphoid malignancies of natural killer cell lineage, exhibit

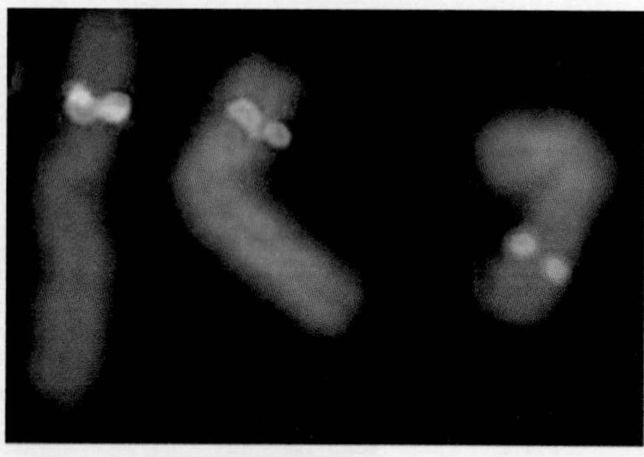
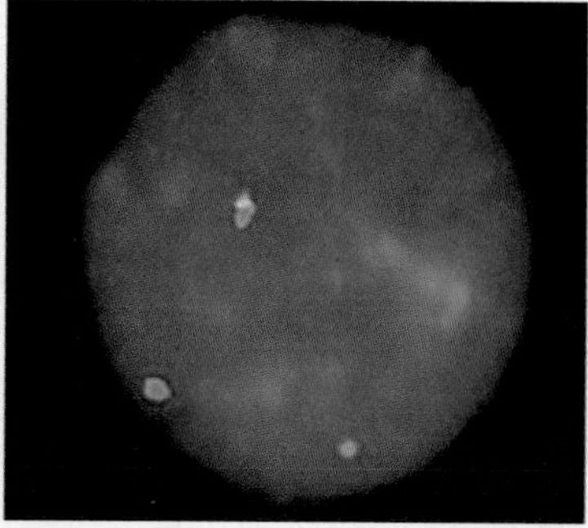

Figure 55–43 FISH study with breakapart *ALK* gene at 2p23 in a patient with anaplastic large cell lymphoma. Partial karyotype shows a normal chromosome 2 (left) with yellow signal, as the 3′ end and the 5′ end of *ALK* gene are in close proximity on chromosome 2. The other chromosome 2 homologue (middle) has only a single green signal (5′ end) as a result of t(2;5)(p23;q35), the most frequent translocation in anaplastic large cell lymphoma. The 3′ end (red) of the *ALK* gene is translocated to 5q35. Abnormal *ALK* gene is also shown in interphase cell (right).

chromosomal rearrangements in greater than 80% by conventional karyotyping. The most frequent abnormalities include del(6)(q21–23) and gain of the X chromosome. FISH, CGH, and spectral karyotyping confirmed the presence of del(6) in $CD3^-CD56^+$ tumor cells.[520] Other less common but recurrent karyotypic changes include isochromosome 1q, 6p, and 17q as well as del(11q), 13q, and 17p and trisomy 8.

Angioimmunoblastic T-cell lymphoma and *unspecified peripheral T-cell lymphoma* are the most frequent nodal T-cell lymphomas. Losses of 5q/10q/12q, identified by CGH, characterize a subtype of peripheral T-cell lymphoma associated with a better prognosis. Gain of 11q13 may represent a primary change in angioimmunoblastic T-cell lymphoma. In general, chromosomal imbalances are more common in unspecified peripheral T-cell lymphoma than in angioimmunoblastic T-cell lymphoma. Both disorders may share similar genomic imbalances.[521,522]

The molecular basis of *ALCL* is the result of t(2;5)(p23;q35), which fuses part of the nucleophosmin gene *(NPM)* on 5q35 with part of the anaplastic lymphoma kinase *(ALK)* receptor tyrosine kinase gene on 2p23 to produce a chimeric *NPM-ALK* gene.[523] This encodes a chimeric NPM-ALK protein that has a constitutively activated kinase. ALK is thought to play a direct role in the malignant transformation of lymphoid cells, probably by aberrant phosphorylation of intracytoplasmic substrates because accumulation of the ALK protein is observed only in cytoplasm. The WHO classification of lymphoid tumors considers ALCL as a distinct clinical entity, with t(2;5) detected by cytogenetics in 60% to 85% of patients. The *NPM-ALK* fusion is identified by FISH (Fig. 55–43) and by RT-PCR assay in 88% of pediatric patients and 60% of adult patients.[524] The other cases of ALCL have variant translocations. They include rearrangements of the 2p23 region: t(1;2)(q25;p23), t(2;5)(q37;q31), t(2;19)(p23;p13), and inv(2)(p23q35), all associated with *ALK* gene expression. They also include rearrangements of the 5q35 region: t(1;5)(q32;q35), t(3;5)(q12 ;q35), and t(3;5)(q25;q34–35).[525] Detection of *ALK* rearrangements by FISH corresponds to a cytoplasmic staining pattern associated with translocations other than t(2;5).

As a result of these variant rearrangements, three new fusion genes have been identified. *ATTIC-ALK* is a fusion gene resulting from inv(2)(p23q35). This translocation fuses *ALK* and 5-aminoimidazole-4-carboxamide ribonucleotide formyltransferase/IMP cyclohydrolase *(ATIC).* This molecular variant is detected by RT-PCR and is the most common *ALK* variant. *TFG-ALK* is a consequence of t(2;3)(p23;q21), which fuses *TRK*-fused gene *(TFG)* with *ALK* at the same breakpoint as found in t(2;5). In t(1;2)(q25;p23), the *TPM3* gene on chromosome 1, which encodes nonmuscular tropomyosin, is fused to *ALK,* producing the *TPM3-ALK* fusion gene.

Prognosis of patients with t(2;5) or variant translocations is excellent but is clearly different from *ALK*-negative ALCL. The true nature of *ALK*-negative ALCL remains obscure. Gene expression profiling showed that ALK^+ ALCL and ALK^- ALCL have different gene expression profiles, indicating that different, as yet unknown, oncogenic mechanisms may be associated with each type.[526] Interestingly, C/EBPβ transcription factor, which is implicated in leukemogenesis of AML, is constitutively active and overexpressed in patients with ALK^+ ALCL but not in ALK^- patients or other lymphomas.[527] C/EBPβ expression is transcriptionally induced through the kinase activity of *NPM-ALK,* which provides insight into the molecular pathogenesis of ALK^+ ALCL.

A variety of genomic rearrangements are seen in the T lymphocytes of patients with *mycosis fungoides* and *Sézary syndrome.* However, specific cytogenetic abnormalities are not associated with these disorders. Most frequent abnormalities involve loss of chromosome 10, deletion of 1p, isochromosome 17q, additions of 17p and 19p, and translocations involving 1p, 10q, and 14q. Both CGH and M-FISH identify chromosome 10, region 10q22–26, as the most frequent abnormality in these disorders.[528,529]

Posttransplant lymphoproliferative disorder (PTLD) is a morphologically diverse group of lymphoid disorders that occurs in immunosuppressed organ transplant recipients. Chromosomal abnormalities are detected in 51% to 72% of B-cell diseases and in almost all T-cell proliferations as measured by CGH, FISH, and conventional karyotyping. Although a variety of recurrent genomic imbalances is observed, the unfavorable prognostic effect on survival is observed in two main WHO morphologic groups, monomorphic PTLD (M-PTLD) and polymorphic PTLD (P-PTLD), and can be correlated with the grafted organ.[530,531] Generally three groups of nonrandom abnormalities are of importance. The pathogenetic role of abnormalities known to be involved in lymphomas, such as 8q24 and *MYC,* 17p13 and *P53,* and 18q21 associated with *BCL2* and *MALT1,* and those associated with large genomic imbalances, such as 2p24–25, 9q22–34, 12q22–24, and 14q32, await elucidation. Trisomy for chromosomes 9 and 11 appears to be associated with EBV^+ PTLD and prolonged survival. In contrast, PTLD patients showing MYC rearrangements are associated with Burkitt lymphoma and an aggressive clinical course. PTLD associated with T cells develops late after transplantation. These disorders are EBV^- and have poor outcome and short survival.

ALLOGENEIC HEMATOPOIETIC CELL TRANSPLANTATION

Molecular and cytogenetic analyses can be used to characterize the origin of engrafted cells and the development and evolution of recurrent malignancies after allogeneic HCT. Newly developed hematopoietic cells that emerge after allogeneic HCT may be of host, donor, or both origins. Genetic studies of posttransplant hematopoiesis are called *chimerism* analysis. This term was introduced into medicine by Anderson et al.[532] in 1951 to indicate an organism whose cells are derived from two or more distinct zygote lineages.[533] Chimerism should be distinguished from mosaicism, which is characterized by two or more different cell populations originating from one zygote. Monitoring chimerism in recipients of allogeneic HCT is essential to identify early engraftment, monitor residual disease in leukemia patients, predict relapse, and optimize posttransplantation therapy in case of graft failure.

Historically, karyotype analysis was used to evaluate engraftment after sex-mismatched allogeneic HCT. Polymorphism of chromosomes 1, 9, and 16 as well as satellite polymorphism of chromosomes 13, 14, 15, 21, and 22 were used to differentiate donor from recipient cells in sex-matched allogeneic HCT. Karyotype analysis not only could identify chimerism also but recurrence of hematologic malignancies. However, it is time-consuming process and has low sensitivity (5%). In the past 2 decades, many methods for detection of chimerism have been developed. All follow the basic principle of using the differences in polymorphic genetic markers to distinguish donor from patient hematopoiesis. These methods, such as restriction fragment length polymorphism, red cell phenotyping, and interphase FISH, do not offer the possibility to study all patients. The most widely used technique is PCR for variable number of tandem repeats/short tandem repeats (VNTR/STR-PCR). This technique has a moderate sensitivity of 3% to 5%, and the quantitation of donor and recipient cells may be cumbersome. The method that allows study of chimerism in all patients involves fluorescence labeling of the primers and resolution of PCR products with capillary electrophoresis. It provides high quantitative accuracy with 1% to 5% sensitivity. Real-time PCR or RQ-PCR for analysis of the *SRY* gene on the Y chromosome allows identification of male cells in the background of 100,000 female cells, providing a high sensitivity for mixed chimerism. However, this approach is limited to the 50% of patients who receive sex-mismatched transplants. Nevertheless, it remains the most sensitive and fastest method for chimerism analysis, providing reliable quantitative results within 2 hours.[534]

Detection of SNPs by chimerism analysis (SNP-PCR) is highly sensitive. In one study using 11 different SNP loci, SNP-PCR analysis identified independent predictors of relapse after HCT.[535] The two most commonly used methods for detection of chimerism after HCT are fluorescence-based PCR amplification of short tandem repeats (STR-PCR) and interphase FISH (Fig. 55–44). Both methods have high quantitation accuracy and reproducibility The sensitivity of both methods approaches 1%; however, STR-PCR is sex independent and can be applied to all patients.[536,537] FISH analysis, on the other hand, permits simultaneous evaluation of chimerism and residual disease in the same cell when high sensitivity is not a requirement. FISH analysis for diagnostic genomic abnormalities in conjunction with conventional cytogenetics remains useful and reliable in determining the presence of residual disease.

Leukemia relapse occurring in donor cells after allogeneic HCT is a rare complication reported in 0.12% to 5% of cases.[538] It was first described in 1971, and more than 50 cases have been reported.[538,539] Careful genetic analysis of relapse cells is essential. VNTR, restriction fragment length polymorphism, or FISH XY analysis alone may not definitively assign the origin of the leukemic clone because genomic deletions or amplifications of chromosomal segments may occur during the transplantation or disease process.[540] The increased use of unrelated cord blood as a source of stem cells for allogeneic HCT raises the concern that hematopoietic progenitors containing preleukemic clonal molecular rearrangements may be inadvertently transplanted.[541] Systematic screening of unselected cord blood samples revealed putative preleukemic rearrangements such as *ETV6-AML1* and *AML1-ETO*. Specific mechanisms that result in development of donor cell leukemia are unknown. A common cytogenetic abnormality has not been recognized, and almost half of cases are associated with a normal karyotype.[538] Nevertheless, these patients must be carefully evaluated using an array of molecular methods for determination of leukemia in donor cells (see box on Genetic Testing for Hematopoietic Cell Transplantation).

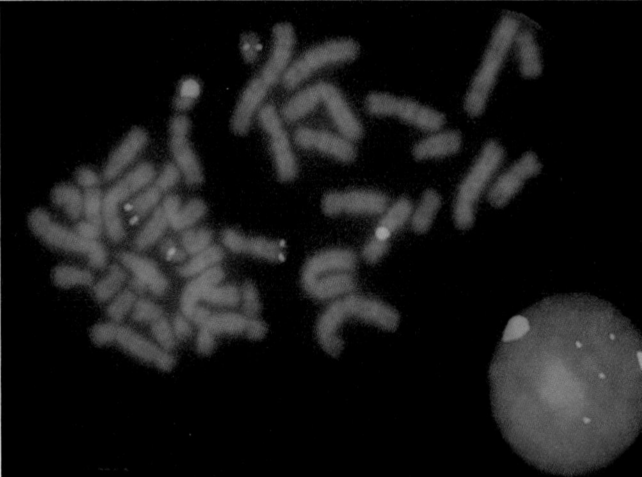

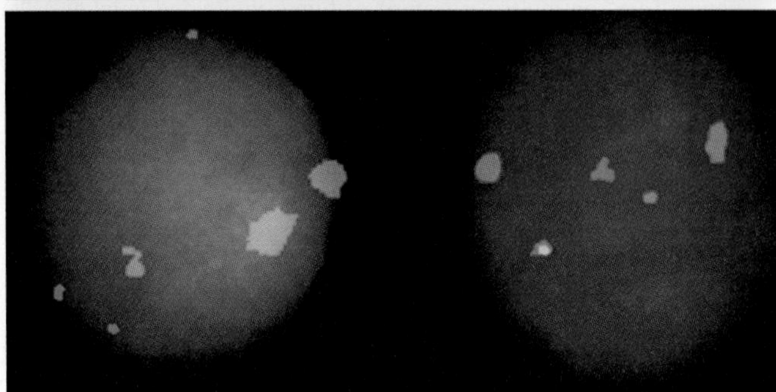

Figure 55–44 Detection of engraftment and residual disease with FISH in sex-mismatched hematopoietic cell transplantation. Metaphase and nondividing cell (blue) after DAPI counterstaining, hybridized with X (large red) and Y (large green) for detection of engraftment and with *ABL* (small red) and *BCR* (small green) for detection of residual chronic myelogenous leukemia (top panel) left nucleus (bottom panel) is showing a donor male (XY) cell origin and lack of *BCR-ABL* fusion. In contrast, a host female (XX), BCR-ABL fusion (yellow)-positive cell is shown on the right. Combination of XY FISH probes with diagnostic genomic markers is a powerful and fast FISH method for simultaneous detection of chimerism and minimal residual disease.

Genetic Testing for Hematopoietic Cell Transplantation

Testing consists of either variable number of tandem repeats/short tandem repeats polymerase chain reaction (PCR) for detection of engraftment in patients with sex-matched hematopoietic cell transplantation (HCT) or single nucleotide polymorphism PCR, which has a high sensitivity. In sex-mismatched HCT, both interphase fluorescence *in situ* hybridization (FISH) with XY probes and real-time quantitative PCR for analysis of *SRY* gene on the Y chromosome can be used for detection of engraftment. Detection of both engraftment and minimal residual disease is best accomplished by FISH simultaneously using probes for XY and the probe for diagnostic genetic defect, such as XY and BCR-ABL.

FUTURE DIRECTIONS

The question of how initial genetic damage in hematopoietic stem cell disorders causes a cascade of other genetic events leading to development of malignancy is unresolved for many diseases. However, major advances have been made, and molecular unraveling of the Philadelphia chromosome led to the rationally designed imatinib treatment that transformed CML from a fatal disease into a chronic disorder compatible with normal life in many patients. Molecular diversity is currently the genetic hallmark of many leukemias, even within a single disease entity such as AML or T-cell ALL. We are at the threshold of understanding other genetic events and common genetic pathways. Such an understanding is crucial to designing molecular interventions for specific abnormalities of genetic pathways underlying hematologic malignancies.

SUGGESTED READINGS

Baccarani M, Saglio G, Goldman J, et al: Evolving concepts in the management of chronic myeloid leukemia: Recommendations from an expert panel on behalf of the European LeukemiaNet. Blood 108:1809, 2006.

Bernasconi P, Boni M, Cavigliano PM, et al: Clinical relevance of cytogenetics in myelodysplastic syndromes. Ann N Y Acad Sci 1089:395, 2006.

Busque L, Gilliland DG: Clonal evolution in acute myeloid leukemia. Blood 82:337, 1993.

Daley GQ, Van Eitan RA, Baltimore D: Induction of chronic myelogenous leukemia in mice by the $P210^{BCR\text{-}ABL}$ gene of the Philadelphia chromosome. Science 247:824, 1990.

Dave SS, Wright G, Tan B, et al: Prediction of survival in follicular lymphoma based on molecular features of tumor-infiltrating immune cells. N Engl J Med 351:2159, 2004.

De Keersmaecker K, Cools J: Chronic myeloproliferative disorders: A tyrosine kinase tale. Leukemia 20:200, 2006.

Druker BJ, Guilhot F, O'Brien SG, et al: Five year follow-up of patients receiving imatinib for chronic myeloid leukemia. N Engl J Med 355:2408, 2006.

Fialkow PJ, Martin PJ, Najfeld V, et al: Evidence for multistep pathogenesis of chronic myelogenous leukemia. Blood 58:158, 1981.

Flynn CM, Kaufman DS: Donor cell leukemia: Insight into cancer stem cells and stem cell niche. Blood 109:2688, 2007.

Graux C, Cools J, Michaux L, et al: Cytogenetics and molecular genetics of T-cell acute lymphoblastic leukemia: From thymocytes to lymphoblast. Leukemia 20:1496, 2006.

Greaves MF, Maia AT, Wiemels JL, Ford AM: Leukemia in twins: Lessons in natural history. Blood 102:2321, 2003.

Grever MR, Lucas DM, Dewald GW, et al: Comprehensive assessment of genetic and molecular features predicting outcome in patients with chronic lymphocytic leukemias: Results from the US Intergroup Phase III Trial E2997. J Clin Oncol 25:799, 2007.

Hiddemann W, Spiekermann K, Buske C, et al: Towards a pathogenesis-oriented therapy of acute myeloid leukemia. Crit Rev Oncol Hematol 56:235, 2005.

James C, Ugo V, Le Couedic JP, et al: A unique clonal JAK2 mutation leading to constitutive signaling causes polycythemia vera. Nature 434:1144, 2005.

Jovanovic JV, Score J, Waghorn K, et al: Low-dose imatinib mesylate leads to rapid induction of major molecular responses and achievement of complete molecular remission in *FIP1L1-PDGFRA* positive chronic eosinophilic leukemia. Blood 109:4635, 2007.

Kurzrock R, Kantarjian HM, Druer BJ, Talpaz M: Philadelphia chromosome-positive leukemias: From basic mechanisms to molecular therapeutics. Ann Intern Med 138:819, 2003.

List AF, Kurtin S, Rose DJ, et al: Efficacy of lenalidomide in myelodysplastic syndrome. Proc Natl Acad Sci U S A 352:549, 2005.

Melnick A, Licht JD: Deconstructing a disease: RARa, its fusion partners, and their roles in pathogenesis of acute promyelocytic leukemia. Blood 93:3167, 1999.

Meyer-Monard S, Parlier V, Passweg J, et al: Combination of broad molecular screening and cytogenetic analysis for genetic risk assignment and diagnosis in patients with acute leukemia. Leukemia 20:247, 2006.

Milligan DW, Grimwade D, Cullis JO, et al: Guidelines on the management of acute myeloid leukemia in adults. Br J Haematol 135:450, 2006.

Moorman AV, Harrison CJ, Buck GAN, et al: Karyotype is an independent factor in adult acute lymphoblastic leukemia (ALL): Analysis of cytogenetic data from patients treated on the Medical Research Council (MRC) UKALLXII/Eastern Cooperative Oncology Group (ECOG) 2993 trial. Blood 109:3189, 2007.

Mufti GJ: Pathobiology, classification and diagnosis of myelodysplastic syndrome. Best Pract Res Clin Haematol 17:543, 2004.

Najfeld V, Montella L, Scalise A, et al: Exploring polycythemia vera with fluorescence *in situ* hybridization: Additional cryptic 9p is the most frequent abnormality detected. Br J Haematol 119:558, 2002.

Pinkel D, Alberson DG: Array comparative genomic hybridization and its application to cancer. Nat Genet Suppl 37:S11, 2005.

Raskind WH, Steinmann L, Najfeld V: Clonal development of myeloproliferative disorders: Clues to hematopoietic differentiation and multistep pathogenesis of cancer. Leukemia 12:108, 1998.

Shaughnessy JD, Haessler J, van Rhee F, et al: Testing standard and genetic parameters in 220 patients with multiple myeloma with complete data set: Superiority of molecular genetics. Br J Haematol 137:530, 2007

REFERENCES

For complete list of references log onto www.expertconsult.com

CHAPTER 56

PHARMACOLOGY AND MOLECULAR MECHANISMS OF ANTINEOPLASTIC AGENTS FOR HEMATOLOGIC MALIGNANCIES

Stanton L. Gerson, Kapil N. Bhalla, Steven Grant, Kavita Natarajan, Richard J. Creger, and David DeRemer

Treatment of hematologic malignancies has undergone a continuing scientific revolution in the past 5 years as new targets identified through studies of the molecular and cell biology of these malignancies have spawned the discovery of mechanistic-based therapeutics. A surprising number of these have progressed from discovery, validation, animal modeling, and successful clinical testing. In addition, there has been a broadening of the spectrum of agents to include small molecules, peptides, antibodies, radiolabeled molecules, and complex delivery systems. This updated chapter provides information on all new therapeutic agents available for the treatment of hematologic malignancies. It reviews the "classic" agents as well as the new, targeted agents. Both cytotoxic and growth-inhibitory agents are covered; however, the use of therapeutic antibodies is reviewed within the disease chapters.

CELL KINETICS, THE CELL CYCLE, AND TUMOR GROWTH

Hematologic malignant cells proliferate more than their normal counterparts. The cell cycle consists of a series of stages through which normal and neoplastic cells proceed during the course of cellular replication (shown schematically in Fig. 56–1). It is divided into G_1 (pre-DNA synthetic phase), S phase (in which DNA replication takes place), G_2 (post-DNA synthetic phase), and mitosis (M), during which chromosomal division and segregation occurs.[1] In addition, nonproliferating, resting cells are said to reside in G_0, a phase that may theoretically last for an indefinite period. Such cells remain in G_0 until they are induced to enter the cell cycle (at G_1) by specific triggers, for example, hematopoietic growth factors. The *growth fraction* of a tumor represents the percentage of cycling cells relative to the total cell population and is given by the formula $[G_1 + S + G_2 + M]/[G_0 + G_1 + S + G_2 + M]$. The *noncycling fraction* is given by the formula $[G_0]/[G_1 + S + G_2 + M]$. Growth fractions of various neoplasms range from less than 10% in the case of certain slowly growing solid tumors to more than 90% in the case of certain hematologic malignancies (eg, Burkitt lymphoma). The *generation* time represents the time required for a cell to proceed through a single cell cycle (generally 24–36 hours for hematopoietic tissues). Surprisingly, in the case of AML, the generation time of leukemic blasts is not significantly shorter than that of normal hematopoietic progenitors, and may in fact be longer. The proliferative advantage of malignant hematopoietic cells (and of many nonhematopoietic tumors) stems, at least in part, from the fact that a higher percentage of cells are in cycle at any one point in time (ie, the growth fraction is higher). The *doubling time* represents the period required for a tumor to double in mass and is, in general, inversely related to the tumor's growth fraction. Tumor-doubling times range from greater than 120 days in the case of some solid tumors (eg, lung and colon) to less than 2 weeks (in the case of some leukemias and lymphomas). Tumor-doubling times are influenced by multiple other factors, including the rate of spontaneous cell death (or apoptosis) and the availability of appropriate nutrients. The importance of these considerations stems from the fact that tumors with high growth fractions and short doubling times tend to be more sensitive to chemotherapy than slowly growing neoplasms with low growth fractions and long doubling times. It is unlikely to be a coincidence that many advanced neoplasms that are potentially curable by chemotherapy (eg, hematologic malignancies such as leukemia, lymphoma, and testicular cancer) fall into the former group; conversely, most incurable advanced malignancies (eg, non-small-cell lung cancer, colon cancer) fall into the latter.

The transition of neoplastic cells through the cell cycle, as in the case of their normal counterparts, is governed by a complex network of proteins consisting of cyclins, cyclin-dependent kinases (CDKs), and CDK inhibitors.[2] The progression through S phase is regulated primarily by CDK2 in association with cyclins A and E; the progression through G_2M is regulated by CDK1 ($p34^{cdc2}$) and cyclin A and cyclin B; and progression through G_1 involves CDKs 4 to 6 in conjunction with cyclin D. CDK inhibitors fall into two major categories: The low-molecular-weight inhibitors (pINK14, 15, 16, 17, and 18), which primarily inhibit cyclin D (and to some extent, CDK2) complexes, and the higher-molecular-weight inhibitors, p21, p27, and p57, which are more universal in their actions and inhibit most or all CDKs.[3] Signals for progression of cells through G_1S are clearly essential for maintenance of the neoplastic phenotype. In the commonly accepted model of G_1S progression, inactivation of the retinoblastoma protein (PRB) is required. In quiescent cells, PRB is in an active dephosphorylated state and bound to the transcription factor E2F. Phosphorylation of PRB by CDK4 and CDK6 and CDK2 leads to release of E2F, which is then free to activate diverse genes essential for S-phase progression, such as *MYC* (also known as c-Myc), *TYMS* (thymidylate synthetase), and *DHFR* (dihydrofolate reductase). Conversely, induction of CDK inhibitors (eg, by TGFB [formerly known as TGFB] or differentiation-inducing agents) results in inactivation of CDK4 and CDK6 and CDK2, dephosphorylation of PRB, inactivation of E2F, and inhibition of the progression through S phase. Aberrant expression of cyclins and CDK inhibitors is commonly encountered in human malignancies, including those of hematopoietic origin, and it has been postulated that the resultant cell-cycle dysregulation contributes to the neoplastic phenotype.

In addition to cellular growth control, cell-cycle proteins are intimately involved in the regulation of programmed cell death (apoptosis) and checkpoint control mechanisms.[4] Consequently, cell-cycle regulatory proteins can exert a major influence on the response of neoplastic cells to various cytotoxic agents. For example, when cells undergo DNA damage, they may arrest in G_2M or G_1, during which repair occurs, or if the damage is too severe, the cells undergo apoptosis. In particular, the tumor suppressor gene *TP53* and its downstream inducible target p21 have been implicated in the G_1 arrest process following genotoxic insult.[5] During the last several years, it has been shown that dysregulation of various cell-cycle regulatory proteins can have a major impact on the sensitivity of neoplastic cells to various chemotherapeutic agents. Loss of the *TP53* gene renders cells resistant to diverse chemotherapeutic agents, presumably by preventing cells from undergoing repair in G_1 and thereby inhibiting the cell death processes and allowing DNA damage to accumulate, culminating in cellular transformation. Conversely, transfection of

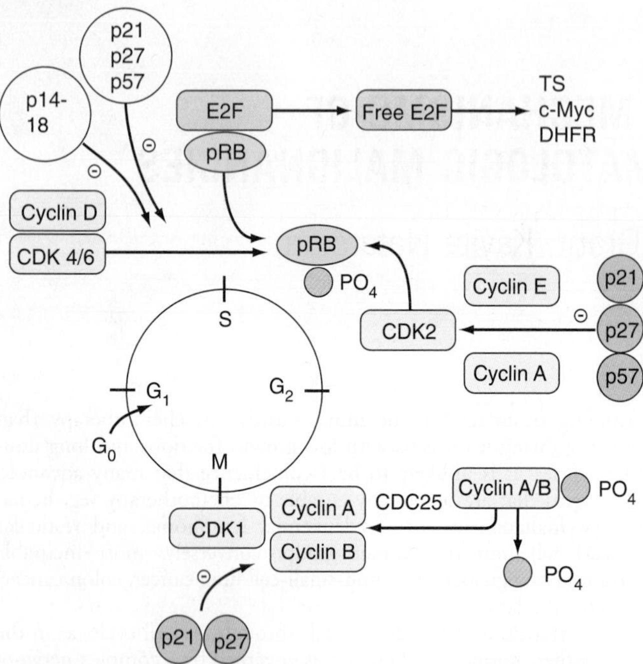

Figure 56–1 Progression through the cell cycle is controlled through complex interactions between cyclins, cyclin-dependent kinases (CDKs), and CDK inhibitors. Progression across the G_1S interface and through S phase involves the E2F transcription factor, which activates numerous enzymes (eg, thymidylate synthase, dihydrofolate reductase) required for DNA replication. The retinoblastoma protein (pRb) in its dephosphorylated state binds to and inactivates E2F in conjunction with DP proteins, thereby inhibiting S-phase progression. Conversely, phosphorylation of pRb antagonizes binding to E2F, allowing S-phase events to proceed. Phosphorylation of pRb results from activation of (1) cyclin-dependent kinase-2 (CDK2):cyclin A/E and (2) CDK4/6:cyclin D complexes. The former complexes are inhibited by the CDKIs p21, p27 (and p57), whereas the latter are inhibited by the low-molecular-weight CDK inhibitors (p14-18), but also by p21 and p27. The complex formed by CDK1 ($p34^{cdc2}$) and cyclins A and B regulates G_2M progression and is inhibited by the "universal" CDK inhibitor, p21. Moreover, its phosphorylation status, which plays a major role in determining activity, is regulated by the phosphatase cdc25. Proteins such as pRb, E2F, p21, and p27 can influence the response of cells to chemotherapeutic agents by controlling cell-cycle progression, and possibly via cell cycle-unrelated actions.

P53-negative cells with wild-type P53 restores responsiveness to most drugs.[6] Dysregulation of the CDK inhibitors p21 (a downstream target of P53) and p27 increases the sensitivity of neoplastic cells to various cytotoxic agents, possibly by uncoupling S-phase progression and mitosis.[7,8] In this model, loss of CDK inhibitor p21 or p27 prevents cells that have sustained DNA damage from arresting in G_1 and allows them to progress inappropriately through S and ultimately G_2M, eventually leading to cell death. Mutations in the E2F protein have been shown to lengthen S phase and increase the sensitivity of malignant cells to S phase-specific agents.[9] Furthermore, cells lacking functional PRB have been shown to be significantly less sensitive to the actions of antimetabolites, including methotrexate.[10] Aside from regulating cell-cycle status and the susceptibility of neoplastic cells to cell-cycle-specific agents, cell-cycle regulatory proteins can actively contribute to the cell death response.

The growth of tumors is best described by Gompertz's law, rather than classic exponential kinetics. For neoplasms that grow exponentially, the tumor growth rate remains constant as the number of cells increases. However, in the in vivo setting, the growth of tumors is limited by various factors such as vascular supply, nutritional requirements, and possibly physical restraints. Consequently, the rate of tumor growth declines as the number of cells increases. To the extent that tumor-doubling times are inversely correlated with drug responsiveness, large, late-stage tumors would be predicted to be less susceptible to cytotoxic drugs than their earlier, higher growth fraction counterparts. It is important to note that most chemotherapeutic drugs kill by *first-order kinetics*. This indicates that a given drug dose kills a constant fraction, rather than number, of tumor cells. The implication of this phenomenon is that it requires the same drug dose to reduce the number of tumor cells from 10^4 to 10^1 cells as it does to reduce the tumor burden from 10^{10} to 10^7 cells.

Recent emphasis on leukemic and lymphoma stem cells has raised a new cellular target for therapeutics and the analysis of available agents provides another level of analysis of efficacy both in clinical and preclinical settings. This progress remains premature and at the moment, the value of targeting leukemia, lymphoma, and myeloma stem cells either in clinical trial design or therapeutic development are not clear. However, for noncurative diseases, a focus on this cell subpopulation may lead to curative therapies. Regardless of targeted therapies, the ability to identify and track such cells will improve appreciation of minimal residual disease and the need for more focused therapies. One factor in common for most malignant stem cells is the overexpression of the ABC transporters. ATP binding cassette transporters (ABC transporters) are often highly expressed in early hematopoietic stem cells and other tissue stem cells that are CD44 positive. Inhibition of these transporters would seem a logical approach to therapeutically targeting leukemic stem cells. Progress in this area will be discussed in the section on MRP and the ABC transporters.

Cytotoxic agents may be divided into several categories with respect to their effects on the cell cycle or the cell-cycle specificity of their actions, or both.

1. *Non-cycle-active drugs* kill both cycling and noncycling cells in all phases of the cell cycle. Examples include steroids and antitumor antibiotics (except bleomycin).
2. *Cycle-active, non-phase-specific drugs* are more active against cycling cells and can kill cells in each phase of the cell cycle. However, such cells may preferentially kill cells in a particular phase of the cell cycle. Examples include alkylating agents, cisplatin, and 5-fluorouracil.
3. *Cycle-active, phase-specific drugs* primarily kill cells in a specific phase of the cell cycle. Examples include most antimetabolites, which are active against cells engaged in DNA synthesis (S-phase cells), and microtubule-active drugs (eg, vinca alkaloids, taxanes), which kill cells in G_2M.

An example of a cytokinetically rational approach to chemotherapy involves the combination of a non-cycle-active agent (eg, daunorubicin) with a cycle- and phase-specific agent (eg, cytosine arabinoside [ara-C], fludarabine, decitabine, clofarabine and nelarabine). From a theoretical standpoint, administration of a non-cycle-active agent may reduce tumor mass, leading in turn to an increase in the growth fraction via recruitment of cells into cycle. Such cells would then be more susceptible to a cycle- and phase-specific agent, particularly one administered over a prolonged interval. In the case of hematopoietic malignancies, attempts have been made to recruit neoplastic cells into the more susceptible S phase of the cell cycle through the use of *hematopoietic growth factors*. The success of such a strategy may be limited by several factors, including the inability of growth factors to increase the S-phase fraction significantly, the lack of selectivity of this strategy, and the theoretical possibility that growth factors may protect neoplastic cells from apoptosis.

Unfortunately, cytokinetic differences between normal and neoplastic tissues have been difficult to identify and exploit. Both normal hematopoietic stem cells and hematologic malignancy stem cells also share a low proportion of cells in cell cycle of G1. However, prolonged dosage schedules can provoke these malignant cells into cell cycle and may explain the efficacy of these approaches. Consequently, rapidly dividing normal tissues such as gastrointestinal epithelium and normal hematopoietic progenitors tend to be very sensitive to most chemotherapeutic agents. As a result, mucositis and myelosuppression represent frequent dose-limiting toxicities for many cytotoxic drugs.

TUMOR CELL HETEROGENEITY OF HEMATOLOGIC MALIGNANCIES

Whereas hematopoietic malignancies are of *clonal* origin (ie, they are derived from a single transformed cell), individual neoplastic cells from a patient's malignancy exhibit a great deal of phenotypic diversity and secondary mutations that affect proliferation, drug sensitivity, and resistance. Although this diversity arises from progeny of clonal populations, and subsets of stem cells have been identified, in animal models it has been shown that the clones themselves can give rise to frequent progeny that can transmit clonal malignancy in transplantation settings, suggesting that at least in these settings, rarefied stem cells are not required to transmit the malignant phenotype. Perhaps these cells even have conflicting phenotypes to the more common malignant cell. For instance, perhaps leukemia stem cells are more quiescent, have higher levels of protective proteins such as efflux pumps for drugs and higher levels of DNA repair proteins or antiapoptosis proteins than the more abundant cell making up the circulating population of cells. Tumor cell heterogeneity arises as a consequence of spontaneous mutational events, changes in gene promoter methylation, impact of abnormal expression of transcription factors, lymphoid reactivity, and cytokine responsiveness. In fact, these can be reinforced if they provide a survival, tissue homing, or proliferative advantage for the affected cells and their progeny.[11] For example, a mutation or change in expression that renders a hematopoietic cell clone autonomous or growth factor-independent would be expected to render such cells less susceptible to adverse environmental conditions, for example, growth factor withdrawal. Similarly, one would also predict that a genetic change facilitating cell-cycle entry or disruption of cellular maturation would ultimately lead to overgrowth of affected clones. For obvious reasons, mutations that interfere with drug metabolism or the cell death pathway itself would provide a net survival advantage, particularly under the selection pressure of cytotoxic drug treatment.

Malignant myeloid and lymphoid cells have many reasons to have increased mutations rates. Genomic instability can arise from dysregulation of the cell cycle, disruption of replication, loss of DNA repair enzymes such as mismatch repair, which gives rise to microsatellite instability and loss of checkpoint regulation. These processes give rise to intraclonal emergent point mutations, translocations, and intragenic loss that not only result in the malignant transformation but also to disruption of genomic stability and selection in favor of proliferative and apoptosis resistance subclones.

Common mechanisms may be involved in events associated with malignant transformation and the development of mutations that result in tumor heterogeneity. For example, the cell-cycle checkpoint and tumor suppressor gene, *TP53*, is induced during DNA damage, leading to G_1 arrest and, if the damage is too severe to repair, cell death by apoptosis. The presumed goal of this process is to eliminate cells that develop deleterious mutations as a result of damage to the genome. Loss of *TP53* may not only increase cellular survival by inhibiting the cell death process, but may also promote the transmission of mutations in cells that would otherwise be deleted. In this manner, a defect of the cell death pathway can have multiple consequences: (a) selection of cells exhibiting a growth advantage over their normal counterparts, (b) development of drug resistance, and (c) promotion of mutations that result in either (a) or (b) as well as neoplastic cell heterogeneity.

A model for understanding the relationship between tumor growth rate, the occurrence of spontaneous mutations, and the development of drug resistance was first described by Goldie and Coldman, and is referred to as the Goldie and Coldman hypothesis.[12] In this model, the size of a tumor depends on a complex interaction between tumor growth rate and cell loss, the latter stemming from the status of the cell death process, exhaustion of available nutrients, and outstripping of the blood supply. As tumors increase in size, the cell death rate tends to increase. The heterogeneous nature of such mutations makes it likely that multiple mechanisms of resistance will develop as well. From an operational standpoint, this model has clear implications for the rational design of therapeutic strategies and provides a basis for early and intensive therapy, as proposed by Hyrniuk and Bush.[13] The successful implementation of this strategy is exemplified by the administration of dose-intensive multidrug regimens (ie, the Stanford 5 regimen in Hodgkin disease, in non-Hodgkin lymphoma [NHL]), and combinations of cytotoxic and immune therapies, such as CHOP-rituximab, which are potentially curative when given early in the course of the disease. Other examples include combined use of multitargeted agents such as lenesolid and bortezomib for myeloma, fludarabine and rituximab for chronic lymphocytic leukemia, or maneuvers to overcome resistance of pretreated disease outside of cell-based therapies. However, as predicted by the model, administration of these or other intensive regimens in patients with relapsed or late-stage disease generally fail because of a generalized resistance of tumor cells to all classes of chemotherapeutic agents.

DEVELOPMENT OF CHEMOTHERAPEUTIC AGENTS

The modern quest for anticancer agents for hematologic malignancies began with the nitrogen mustard class of compounds developed from the chemical warfare agent sulfur gas used in World War I. Since that time, the National Cancer Institute and the pharmaceutical industry have developed complex techniques for drug development, screening, and evaluation.[14] Initial screening consisted of toxicity assessment against murine tumor cell lines.[15] Current screening is directed toward numerous cell targets including receptor and downstream signaling kinases, inducers of cell death pathways including those at the cell surface, mitochondrial DNA and nuclear DNA, DNA processing and repair proteins including topoisomerases and telomerase and histone deacetylase inhibitors, cell-cycle proteins, agents that block protein processing and degradation, and the mitosis and spindle machinery. Killing cells remains the backbone of chemotherapeutic approaches to human malignancies, although a number of differentiating agents, kinase inhibitors, and cytostatic agents have now entered the chemotherapy armamentarium. In addition, agents that target tumor angiogenesis have impressive efficacy. Although cytotoxic alkylating agents cause myelosuppression, newer agents cause more systemic side effects.[16] Secondary leukemias induced by hematopoietic progenitor cell damage occur with the older alkylating agents,[17] topoisomerase inhibitors,[18,19] and combination chemotherapy and radiation[20] but are not seen with the newer classes of compounds. The emphasis on targeted therapeutics in current drug development is focused in two areas: Newly recognized fusion or mutant specific to the malignant cell, such as bcr-abl in CML and the activated JAK2V617F mutation present in myeloproliferative disorders, and fundamental antiapoptotic pathways such as bcl-2.

Screening for Antitumor Activity Among Chemotherapeutic Agents

Current approaches to the discovery of new agents to treat hematologic malignancies relies on the large National Cancer Institute (NCI) Division of Cancer Treatment initative to maintain a large cell bank of malignancies for drug testing. NCI has evaluated more than 60,000 compounds for cytotoxic and growth inhibitory activity using a standard human tumor cell line screen[21,22] that includes K562, MOLT-4, and HL-60.[23] Routine exposure of such tumor cell lines to drug dilutions at 10^{-4} to 10^{-8} molar concentrations are performed with a 48-hour drug incubation followed by a monitoring of the tumor cell growth rate.[22] Following an initial in vitro screen, human tumor cell activity is evaluated using a series of athymic mouse xenograft studies targeting tumors from tissues that show promise in in vitro assays.[24] Drugs with promising efficacy and novel mechanisms of action then go on to formulation and toxicology testing and ultimately are developed for phase I clinical testing[22,25] through the NCI Cancer Therapy Evaluation Program. Weinstein and colleagues[22] used the database to identify clustered cytotoxic activity among agents based on similar cytotoxicity profiles against the 60-cell panel. Among many observed clustered responses, agents with clustered activity against p53 wild-type or mutant cells, multiple drug resistance (MDR-1), gene-expressing cells, and agents that cause G_1 checkpoint arrest have been identified. With this information, a better understanding of mechanisms of drug action and disease-specific responses can be proposed.

More recently, these and other cell lines are being used, along with cell line banks of human hematologic malignancies for high throughput screening efforts that are especially useful for noncytotoxic screens that result in evaluation of agents that affect gene expression, differentiation, migration, and other cell-based assays. In addition, drug discoveries that start as a survey of specific pathway inhibition, such as signaling kinsases (bcr-abl, JAK2, PDGF, kit, and FLT3) and src kinases, represent new approaches validated by the discovery of therapeutic agents such as imatinib and related agents, dasatinib and AMN107.

Human tumor xenografts have been used as a requisite screen in preclinical testing of new chemotherapeutic agents. For leukemia and lymphoma cell lines, increase in life span is used as an end point measured at the percent increased life span (ILS), ((T − C/C) × 100), where T is the life span after drug treatment and C untreated.[26] The best predictive mouse systems are primary malignancies grown in immunodeficient mice and mice with specific chromosomal translocations and oncogenes that mimic human disease. In mice with severe combined immune deficiency (SCID), the RPMI 8226 human myeloma cell line and the multidrug-resistant subline, 8226-C1N, inoculated intraperitoneally led to a lifespan that was numbered in days and the tumor cells in vivo were completely resistant to treatment with doxorubicin.[27] Zhang and colleagues[28] established a human acute promyelocytic leukemia ascites model in the SCID mice and found responses to all-transretinoic acid. Other investigators have used the SCID leukemia model to test antisense oligonucleotide strategies[29] for such tumor-specific genes as *BCR-ABL*[30] in CML. Use of primary and serially passaged human leukemias and myelomas in the SCID model have facilitated drug screening. In both instances, infusion of antisense constructs increased the ILS significantly and led to clinical studies with these agents. Others have used the SCID model for B-cell lymphomas to study chemotherapy or lymphotoxins.[31] Although these models have not entered the NCI drug screen, they represent significant systems to test new agents, in particular novel gene therapy and immunotoxin approaches.

Phase I Clinical Trial Design

New anticancer agents are assessed through a series of clinical trials termed *phase I*, *phase II*, and *phase III* (Table 56–1). The purpose of phase I clinical trials is to establish the safe and optimal biochemically active dose of the compound in question with acceptable toxicity that can be used in disease-targeted phase II testing. During phase I development, pharmacokinetics and pharmacodynamic measures are studied in detail so that appreciable information can be forthcoming from the very first set of patients targeted for treatment and to allow confirmation of these observations in larger phase II disease-focused trials. Dose schedule and route of administration are key considerations in early phase I development. Numerous considerations have guided dose escalation strategies that accompany phase I trial development. The starting dose is typically approximately 10% of the lethal dose (LD)10 in animals adjusted for species dose-equivalency. In classic phase I development, a modified Fibonacci dose schedule is used.[32] Groups of three patients are treated at each of the following doses until the maximum tolerated dose is observed: 1N (the starting dose), 2N, 5N, 7N, 9N, 12N, 16N. Typically, the maximum tolerated dose is defined as the maximum tolerated dose not causing irreversible toxicity of any type and causing less than grade 4 toxicity in any organ. For some myeloablative strategies used in high-dose therapy, grade 4 myelosuppression, mucositis, and diarrhea are acceptable, but only with careful consideration of supportive care including the use of hematopoietic growth factors, antidiarrheal agents, narcotics, and IV alimentation to manage patients through severe mucositis. Typically, if one dose-limiting toxicity is observed, the patient cohort is expanded to six patients; and if two patients develop dose-limiting toxicity, typically defined as grade 4 toxicity except as previously noted, then further entry at this dose is not pursued and the next lower dose level is used to establish the maximum tolerated dose with a total of six patients accrued at that dose level.

Table 56–1 Clinical Trial Design

Phase I
Evaluate safety by dose escalation, multiple dose schedules. Establish maximum tolerated dose and dose-limiting toxicity. Consider use of hematopoietic support if myelosuppression is dose limiting.
Phase II
Establish response (complete, partial, objective) in specific diseases.
Phase III
Compare new treatment with established regimen for the disease in randomized trials.

Alternative strategies of drug escalation have included the use of toxicity grades to enhance dose escalation in early drug development; that is, if no toxicity is observed, fewer patients may be accrued to each dose.[33–35] Using the modified Fibonacci scheme, one patient is entered at each dose level until grade 2 toxicity is observed, at which point cohorts of three patients are entered at each level. Early in drug development, level skipping may take place if no toxicity is observed. The overall impact of this is to reduce the number of patients treated at suboptimal doses of therapy and to enhance the ultimate number of patients evaluated at biologically active doses.

With the rapid development of new anticancer agents in preclinical and early clinical testing, emphasis has shifted toward mechanism-based targeted therapeutics. These phase I trials evaluate both toxicity and "drug-effect" end points.

Phase II Drug Development

Phase II drug development utilizes the established phase I dose to define therapeutic efficacy, typically in a two-stage design. If an expectant response rate in excess of 20% is deemed clinically significant, 15 patients are accrued, and if two or more responses are seen, accrual is continued to a total of 26 patients to establish the definite response rate.[36] At this point, combination therapies are instituted in an effort to optimize therapeutic efficacy. For instance, topotecan was found in phase I testing to have efficacy against refractory leukemias leading to combinations of topotecan with ara-C and other agents.[37–39] Likewise, fludarabine was initially evaluated as a single agent for activity against low-grade lymphomas and acute and chronic leukemias, and is now used in combination with ara-C for the treatment of acute lymphocytic leukemia and with chlorambucil for the treatment of chronic lymphocytic leukemias (CLLs).[40–42] In the past, strategies for combination chemotherapeutic agents have included the use of non-cross-resistant agents with nonoverlapping toxicities. However, more recently, mechanism-based therapeutics has become the focus of drug development. For instance, with the combination of fludarabine and cisplatin, fludarabine may inhibit nucleotide excision repair and enhance persistence of cisplatin-induced DNA adducts, resulting in increased antitumor efficacy in CLL.[43] Likewise,

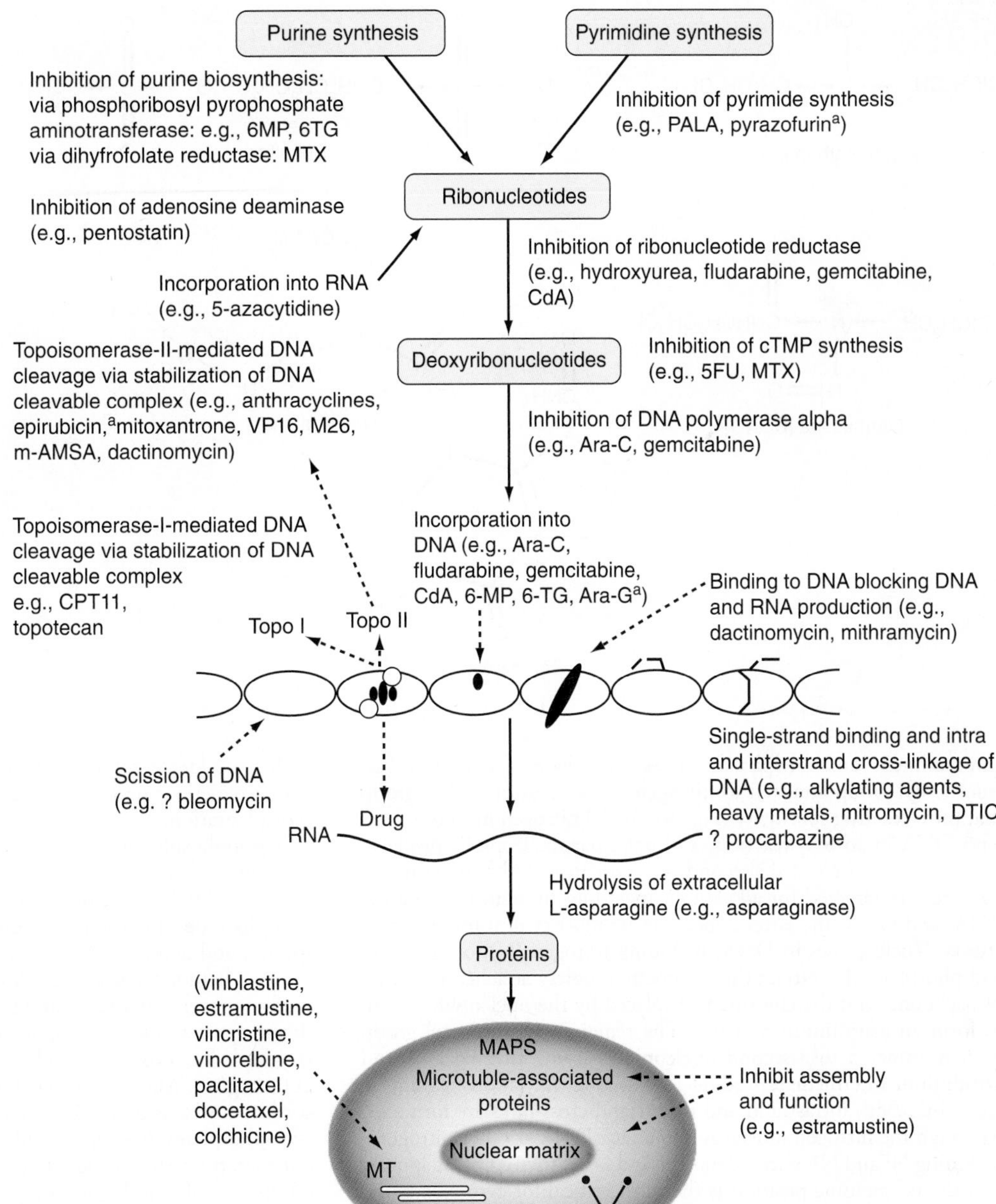

Figure 56–2 Overview of sites and mechanisms of action of the most useful chemotherapeutic agents.

combining a receptor kinase inhibitor with a cell-cycle inhibitor may potentiate efficacy in leukemias.

Most phase III trials randomize between an established standard therapy and a new therapy that has appeared promising in the phase II setting. These studies are usually multiinstitutional and many involve large national and international cooperative groups. The end point of these studies is disease response, survival, and patient tolerance. Linking multiple centers removes the vagaries of reports from single centers, which remain the focus of phase II trials. Phase III trials are important for positive and negative results.

PHARMACOLOGY OF CHEMOTHERAPEUTIC AGENTS

As noted earlier, although cytotoxic anticancer agents may be divided into several categories based on the cell-cycle specificity of their action, in keeping with traditional classification they are more appropriately divided into alkylating agents, antimicrotubule agents, antimetabolites, inhibitors of topoisomerases, platinum analogs, and miscellaneous agents. The pharmacology and cellular mechanisms of action of these agents are schematically presented in Fig. 56–2. Targeted therapeutics such as imatinib and bortezomib are discussed in later sections.

Alkylating Agents

Drug treatment for cancer began with the use of the mustard class of alkylating agents, initially mechlorethamine (nitrogen mustard), which entered into clinical use in the mid-1940s.[44] Alkylating agents are used in many regimens but are rapidly being supplanted by newer classes of agents.

Nitrogen Mustard

The nitrogen mustard class includes mechlorethamine, cyclophosphamide, 4-hydroperoxy cyclophosphamide, ifosfamide,

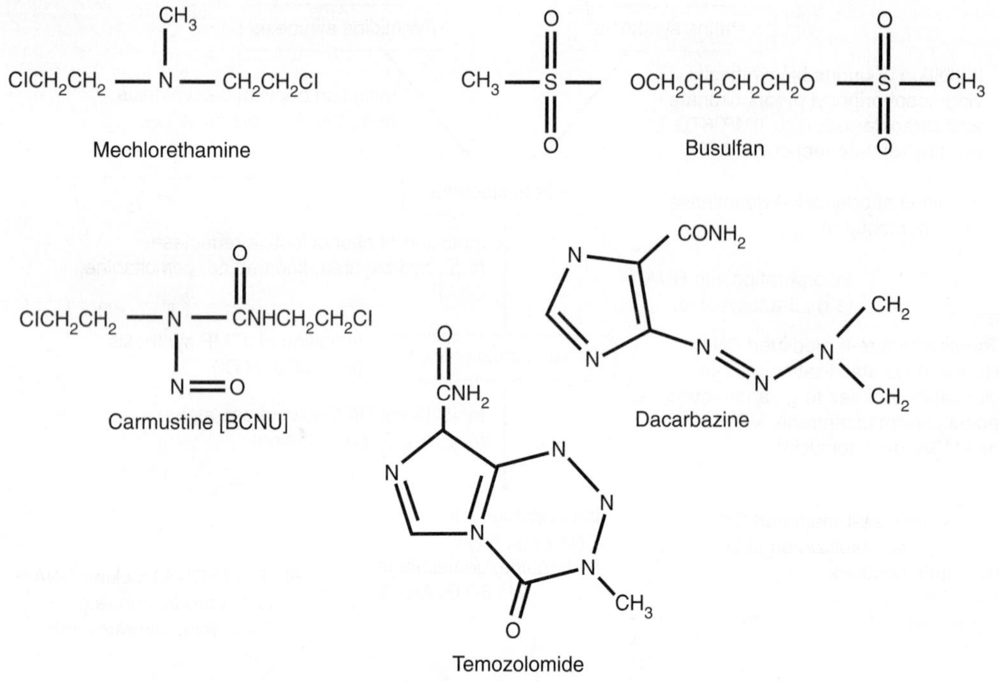

Mechlorethamine

Busulfan

Carmustine [BCNU]

Dacarbazine

Temozolomide

Figure 56–3 Structure of common alkylating agents.

chlorambucil, and melphalan. These all share a common bis-chloroethyl group attached to nitrogen and a substituted "R" group that provides drug specificity (Fig. 56–3). All nitrogen mustards react with DNA in an SN_2 reaction, a bimolecular nucleophilic displacement reaction, also called a second-order reaction.[45] Although numerous sites are targeted for alkylation, including protein, membranes, RNA, and DNA, the latter appears to be most critical for cytotoxic effects. Nucleophiles in DNA, including nitrogen (N), oxygen (O), and phosphate (P), attract the chloroethyl moiety attached to the R-N backbone, and the chlorine is displaced by the nucleophilic atom to form an aziridinium moiety.[46] The remaining chloroethyl group is then attracted to a second nucleophilic atom, forming a second aziridinium intermediate leading to a second alkylation, forming a cross-link. Both intrastrand and interstrand cross-links are formed.[47] Although the nitrogen mustards also attack DNA at other nitrogens, including N^1 and N^3 of the adenosine and N^3 of thymidine, it appears that the N^7 guanine position is the most critical for cytotoxic cross-link formation.[48] Clinical use of mechlorethamine has largely fallen out of favor since the MOPP regimen (mechlorethamine, vincristine [Oncovin], procarbazine, prednisone) has been replaced by ABVD (doxorubicin [Adriamycin], bleomycin, vinblastine, dacarbazine) in Hodgkin disease.[48] Local use of mechlorethamine occurs in a dermatologic suspension for the treatment of cutaneous T-cell lymphomas.[49]

Cyclophosphamide is a nitrogen mustard with a ringed structure off the end-chloroethyl backbone that decreases spontaneous decomposition (see Fig. 56–3). Enzymatic activation is required through multifunction P450 enzymes in the liver. Phenobarbital and corticosteroids may alter activation. Bioavailability of cyclophosphamide orally and intravenously is quite similar, although most use of the drug is by bolus IV injection. Cyclophosphamide is detoxified through oxidation to 4-keto-cyclophosphamide and carboxyphosphamide by aldehyde dehydrogenase.[45] Cyclophosphamide is used in doses as little as 50 to 100 mg/day orally, and in bolus doses of 400 to 700 mg/m^2 for solid tumors and 750 mg/m^2 in combination with doxorubicin and vincristine and prednisone as part of the CHOP regimen for NHLs.[50] It is also used at doses of up to 60 mg/kg daily for 4 days in autologous and allogeneic bone marrow transplantation protocols.[51–53] Cyclophosphamide is used in numerous protocols for NHLs and high-dose therapy regimens designed to eradicate tumor and bone marrow in patients with lymphomas and leukemias, and those undergoing bone marrow transplantation. It is commonly used with granulocyte colony-stimulating factor (G-CSF) for mobilizing hematopoietic stem cells to be collected before autologous transplantation.

Cyclophosphamide is metabolically activated by cytochrome P450 mixed function oxidases in the liver to 4-hydroxycyclophosphamide.[54] 4-Hydroxycyclophosphamide is further converted to aldophosphamide and then to phosphoramide mustard, the alkylated species, and acrolein. Acrolein is a highly reactive aldehyde and the cause of hemorrhagic cystitis. Mercaptoethane sulfonate (mesna)[55] is used to prevent recurrence and to provide prophylaxis against hemorrhagic cystitis due to cyclophosphamide and ifosfamide and is now standard for doses of cyclophosphamide and ifosfamide above 1000 mg/m^2. Mesna is given in divided doses every 4 hours or as a continuous infusion for 18 to 24 hours in a dose equivalent to either cyclophosphamide or ifosfamide.[55] Other than hemorrhagic cystitis, bone marrow suppression is dose limiting and can be rescued by reinfusion of autologous or allogeneic hematopoietic progenitor cells.[56,57] Other toxicities observed include alopecia and cardiac toxicity,[58] which is unusual and most often seen after high-dose therapy.

4-Hydroperoxycyclophosphamide is a chemically stable form of the reactive intermediate of cyclophosphamide, 4-hydroxycyclophosphamide, is more toxic to committed hematopoietic progenitors such as colony-forming unit–granulocyte/macrophage (CFU-GM), burst-forming unit–erythroid (BFU-E), and colony-forming unit–erythroid (CFU-E), but spares early progenitors, presumably on the basis of their expression of the detoxifying enzyme aldehyde dehydrogenase, which is quite high in early progenitor populations.[58,59]

Melphalan, or phenylalanine mustard, has an amino acid side chain that alters its cellular uptake and stabilizes its structure, allowing oral administration (see Fig. 56–3). It is available in both oral and IV dosing and has a similar intracellular pathway to DNA cross-linking as cyclophosphamide and the other nitrogen mustards. Melphalan uptake into cells is by means of a neutral amino acid transporter.[60,61] Its rate of cross-link formation is much slower than that of mechlorethamine, presumably because of delayed metabolism. Orally, melphalan is used predominantly in the treatment of multiple myeloma and intravenously in high-dose regimens for multiple myeloma.[60]

Chlorambucil has been used for more than 40 years for the treatment of chronic lymphocytic leukemia[62] but is being replaced by fludarabine and rituximab. Chlorambucil is the phenylbutyric acid derivative of nitrogen mustard and is very stable, entering the cell by diffusion rather than by a specific uptake mechanism. It is typically administered orally on a daily basis or intermittently. It appears to have greater bioavailability than melphalan and a more consistent half-life of approximately 2 hours.

Busulfan is an alkylsulfonate, unique among alkylating agents because of two sulfur groups and the lack of a chloroethyl moiety (see Fig. 56–3). Busulfan, like the nitrogen mustards, reacts predominantly at the N^7 position of guanine and produces an N^7–N^7 biguanyl DNA cross-link, although the precise nature of this cross-link appears different than that of the nitrogen mustards.[63] This may explain the different clinical utility of busulfan than the nitrogen mustards. The pharmacokinetics of busulfan is important for its use in high-dose therapy for ablation of the bone marrow in patients undergoing autologous transplantation for acute leukemia or allogeneic transplantation. Busulfan clearance does not appear to be accurately predicted by creatinine clearance. Because the incidence of venoocclusive disease is lower in patients receiving high-dose busulfan with predosing pharmacokinetics performed, this is now recommended in high-dose regimens, the target being an AUC of 800 to 1200 ng h/mL.[64,65] Busulfan is a potent stem cell toxin, killing both early and late hematopoietic progenitor cells and damaging the bone marrow stroma.[66,67] Other toxicities of busulfan include nausea and vomiting, and pulmonary interstitial and intraalveolar edema, leading to fibrosis.[68,69] The pulmonary fibrosis is distinct from the interstitial pneumonitis, which accompanies allogeneic bone marrow transplantation and is not related to cytomegalovirus or other viral infections.

Nitrosoureas

There are four chloroethyl nitrosoureas and one methyl nitrosourea in clinical use. The chloroethyl nitrosoureas were derived from methyl nitrosourea by Montgomery.[70] These agents are different from the nitrogen mustards in that they alkylate through an SN^1 reaction, forming a highly reactive intermediate in the presence of N, O, and P nucleophiles in DNA. The commonly used clinical agent is (2-chloroethyl)-*N*-nitrosourea (BCNU).[71,72] *N*-[(4-amino-2-methyl-5-pyrimidinyl) methyl]-*N*-(2-chloroethyl)-*N*-nitrosourea (ACNU) is commonly used in Japan.[73] A third agent, *N*-(2-chloroethyl)-*N*-cyclohexyl-*N*-nitrosourea (CCNU), is used predominantly as an oral nitrosourea in children with brain tumors.[74] All of these compounds have high hydrophobicity, actively penetrating the blood–brain barrier.

The DNA alkylation sites[75,76] include N^7 and O^6 of guanine. Chloroethylation at the O^6 position of guanine appears critical to cytotoxicity. DNA cross-linking by chloroethyl nitrosoureas include at 1-(3-cytosinyl), 2-(1-guanyl) ethane, and 1-2-bis(7-guanyl) ethane.[72,74] The former appears to be responsible for much of the cytotoxicity observed with the chloroethyl nitrosoureas. It is formed after alkylation at the O^6 position of guanine. This adduct undergoes intramolecular rearrangement to a circular intermediate, N^1. O^6 ethanoguanine is formed, which can then rearrange by attack at the opposite hydrogen-bonded base N^3 of cystine forming the interstrand cross-link.[77] This is a unique DNA cross-link and is poorly recognized by DNA repair processes, leading to marked cytotoxic potency of this cross-link.

The pharmacokinetics of the chloroethyl nitrosoureas has been evaluated in both conventional and high-dose schedules. A very short half-life has been detected, which is quite variable, but an association between the AUC of BCNU and pulmonary toxicity has been observed.[78,79] BCNU is predominantly used for high-dose treatment of recurrent lymphomas.[80,81] In both settings, it is an effective form of therapy with sustained complete remission rates of approximately 40% to 60%. Doses of between 600 and 1000 mg/m^2 have been safely administered. The chloroethyl nitrosoureas cause profound and cumulative bone marrow suppression at conventional doses of 120 to 150 mg/m^2, limiting treatment to three to five cycles at 6-week intervals.[78,82–84]

Complications of high-dose BCNU therapy include pulmonary toxicity and renal toxicity at doses higher than 600 mg/m^2. Pulmonary toxicity, as evidenced by a decrease in the DL_{CO}, occurs in up to 40% of patients and is symptomatic in 10% to 15% of patients.[78–80] It can be managed with steroids during the inflammatory but not fibrotic phase and is lethal in some cases.[80,85] Fibrosis is associated with an early interstitial infiltrate followed by evidence of hyaline membrane formation and replacement of the chronic inflammatory cells by fibrosis over a 4- to 6-week period.[86] Renal dysfunction associated by nitrosourea therapy occurs less frequently than severe cumulative myelosuppression and pulmonary fibrosis and is typically seen at doses above 1000 mg/m^2. Interstitial nephritis with glomerulosclerosis, interstitial fibrosis, and dropout of tubules have been reported[87,88] with BCNU or CCNU.

Methylating Agents

Four methylating chemotherapeutic agents are available for clinical use. These include procarbazine, dacarbazine (DTIC), streptozotocin, and temozolomide. Procarbazine and DTIC are triazines.[89] Streptozotocin is a monofunctional methyl nitrosourea derivative with an attached sugar moiety,[15,90] and temozolomide is an imidazotetrazine synthesized in England in the 1960s, reaching clinical trials in the late 1980s.[91] All react with DNA by undergoing SN^1 reactions forming a methyldiazonium ion, resulting in methylation of N^7 guanine, O^6 guanine, O^4 and O^2 thymine, and N^3 adenine.[92–94] None form DNA cross-links. However, all induce high levels of DNA methylation. N^7 methylguanine is unstable, leading to ring opening and both spontaneous and enzymatically mediated depurination. Repair proceeds through the base excision repair system.[95,96] Recognition by the *N*-methylpurine glycosylase results in removal of the adducted base with formation of an abasic site that is recognized by the apurinic (AP) endonuclease, which then cleaves the backbone at the apurinic site. Subsequently, the free 5′ sugar is released by DNA lyase with repair initiated by beta polymerase and DNA ligase.[95] Base excision repair effectively removes N^7 methylguanine and N^3 methyladenine and restores DNA to normal. These lesions appear to contribute little to cytotoxicity and appear to be up to 500-fold less potent as cytotoxic adducts than O^6 methylguanine.[94]

O^6 methylguanine mispairs with thymine during DNA synthesis, resulting in a lesion recognized by the mismatch repair system.[94,97] This system consists of two sets of enzyme homologs of mismatch repair in prokaryotes, mutS and mutL.[97] Mispair recognition proteins are MSH6, MSH3 and MSH2, homologs of the mutS system in bacteria. MSH2 and MSH3 form a stable heterodimer with MSH6.[97] Recognition of the mispair recruits additional proteins to the complex, including MLH1 and PMS1/PMS2, which are homologs of mutL in bacteria. These proteins initiate exonuclease cleavage of a long patch in the newly synthesized strand of DNA. This is then repaired by polymerases delta and epsilon. Unfortunately, if the O^6 methylguanine adduct is not removed before repair synthesis, a thymine is again inserted opposite the O^6 methylguanine and the repair process begins again, resulting in an aberrant episode of repair and multiple single-strand breaks.[94,97–100] Cell protection from methylating agents arises either by removal of O^6 methylguanine (vide infra) or inactivation of the mismatch repair system.[94] Cells expressing high levels of the DNA repair protein for O^6 methylguanine, O^6 alkylguanine DNA alkyltransferase are approximately 10-fold more resistant to methylating agents than alkyltransferase-negative cells.[94,101] Mismatch repair-mediated single-strand patches promote chromosomal aberrations, homologous and nonhomologous recombination, and induction of apoptosis in a p53-dependent and p53-independent manner.[102] Absence of one or more protein components of mismatch repair, leading to the phenotype of replication error repair (RER), is commonly observed in hereditary colon cancer as well as endometrial cancer, gastric cancer,[97,102] and approximately 15% of lymphomas.[103,104] Cells lacking mismatch repair are up to 100-fold more resistant to methylating agents than cells with mismatch repair, regardless of alkyltransferase activity.[94] Acquisition of mismatch repair defects is associated with acquired resistance to methylating agents and cisplatin, which is also recognized by this protein complex.[94,97–100]

Procarbazine was originally synthesized as a monoamine oxidase inhibitor but has been used since the 1950s for the treatment of Hodgkin and NHLs, as well as in combination therapies for gliomas.[105–108] Recent use has been superseded by newer agents. Patients receiving procarbazine form O^6 methylguanine DNA adducts with depletion of the alkyltransferase enzyme, a suicide protein that removes the methyl group in irreversible stoichiometric reaction.[109] Chromosomal breaks, single-strand breaks, and chromosomal aberrations and sister chromosome exchanges observed after procarbazine treatment support its association with treatment-related myelodysplasia and leukemia.[110,111]

DTIC is metabolically activated by cytochrome P450 microsomal oxidoreductases, ultimately leading to formation of the methyldiazonium ion and DNA methylation.[92] DTIC is used in combination with doxorubicin, vinblastine, and bleomycin (ABVD) in Hodgkin disease[43] and is also used in metastatic malignant melanoma in combination with BCNU, cisplatin, and tamoxifen.[112] Activation of DTIC requires hydroxylation of one terminal methyl group caused by demethylation forming 5(3-methyltriazeno)-imidazole-4-carboxamide (MTIC), with spontaneous decomposition to the methyldiazonium ion, which alkylates the DNA, as noted earlier.[113–115] Like procarbazine, DTIC has been shown to form N^7 methylguanine and O^6 methylguanine DNA adducts in human peripheral blood lymphocytes and to deplete alkyltransferase through repair of O^6 methylguanine DNA adducts. A correlation has been found between tumor response and formation of O^6 methylguanine DNA adducts,[116] indicating the importance of this lesion in clinical antitumor effects. Maximum tolerated doses of DTIC are approximately 1000 mg/m^2, with myelosuppression and gastrointestinal toxicity (including severe watery diarrhea) as the most common side effects.[117,118]

Temozolomide represents an imidazotetrazinone.[91,119,120] It differs from DTIC in that it is chemically degraded to the monomethyl triazine, MTIC, at neutral pH and does not require P450 enzymatic demethylation.[121] Compared with DTIC in phase I and phase II trials, temozolomide has much more consistent pharmacokinetic parameters, including peak serum concentrations, volume of distribution and clearance, and conversion to MTIC.[91,119,120] Clinical studies found considerable activity in acute leukemias. Dose-limiting toxicity was thrombocytopenia and, less frequently, neutropenia, with maximum tolerated doses of 1000 mg/m^2 given over 5 days on a daily or twice daily regimen.[91,119,120] Nausea and vomiting were the other common side effects, easily controlled with antiemetics. Formation of O^6 methylguanine has been documented in clinical trials with temozolomide with much more rapid depletion of the alkyltransferase, suggesting that temozolomide may be more effective than the other methylating agents according to its ability to form higher levels of toxic O^6 methylguanine DNA adducts. Early-phase clinical trials using temozolomide in patients older than 60 years with acute myeloid leukemias indicated that the drug is well tolerated and has a modest response rate.[122] A second study has shown that combination therapy including temozolomide, which may induce neoantigens, is also effective.[123] The investigational alkylating agent cloretazine is also in phase II trials in acute leukemia.[124]

Alkylating Agent-Induced Leukemias

Alkylating agents induce dose-limiting myelosuppression, and thus it is not surprising that these agents also cause sublethal DNA damage to hematopoietic progenitors, causing mutational events leading to both myelodysplastic syndromes and malignant transformation to preleukemic and leukemic states. A concern has been the use of hematopoietic growth factors after exposure to alkylating agents. There is evidence of increased cytotoxicity to hematopoietic progenitors during simultaneous exposure to these agents and growth factors.[75] Treatment-related acute myeloid leukemia (T-AML) accounts for approximately 15% of all adult AML. Approximately 50% of T-AML patients have a preleukemic phase as compared with only 10% of patients with de novo AML.[35] Complete remission rates are 15% to 30% in patients with T-AML,[125] and remission duration is a mean of 2 months. Chromosomal abnormalities are common in T-AML, with more than 90% of cases expressing a chromosomal rearrangement, loss, or addition.[20]

Historically, patients with Hodgkin disease treated with mechlorethamine and procarbazine in the MOPP regimen or with CCNU are at highest risk if exposed to radiation as well as an alkylating agent combination.[76] Patients with polycythemia vera treated with chlorambucil are at much higher risk than patients treated with phlebotomy alone, which can contribute to a shift in treatment strategy.[126] Patients with myeloma and ovarian cancer have developed T-AML, especially following prolonged exposure to alkylating agents.[127] The recent introduction of temozolomide for the treatment of glioblastoma multiforme is of concern given its use as a 5 day per month or daily regimen for an extended period of time. There have been a number of reports of secondary leukemia in this patient population indicating that the mutagenic effect of temozolomide seen preclinically will need to be monitored in treated patients.[128,129] Patients treated with alkylating agents for benign diseases such as nephritis, lupus, psoriasis, rheumatoid arthritis,[130] and Wegener granulomatosis[131] also have an increased risk of T-AML. The mean latency between exposure and T-AML from alkylating agents is 4 to 5 years,[17,20,126,127,132] in contrast to T-AML from etoposide, which has a latency as short as 1 year.[133] The cumulative risk for developing T-AML is between 10% and 17% at 4 to 6 years for myeloma treated with melphalan, and between 2% and 10% at 7 to 10 years in patients with Hodgkin disease.[76] More recently, alkylating agent-associated T-AML has been recognized in patients with breast[134,135] and colon[136] cancer. A series of nonrandom chromosomal aberrations associated with T-AML have been identified.[132] Loss or deletion of all or part of the long arm [q] of chromosomes 5 or 7[127] are common, as are trisomy chromosome 8, and deletions of the short arm of chromosomes 12 and 17, and 21.[20]

Antimicrotubule Agents

The antimicrotubule drugs include vinca alkaloids (eg, vincristine, vinblastine, and vinorelbine), taxanes (eg, paclitaxel and docetaxel), and a unique synthetic compound (estramustine).

The vinca alkaloids are naturally occurring (vincristine and vinblastine) or semisynthetic (vinorelbine) nitrogenous bases derived from the pink periwinkle plant, *Catharanthus roseus*.[137] Paclitaxel was originally isolated from the bark of the Pacific yew, *Taxus brevifolia*.[138] Paclitaxel can also be isolated from other members of the *Taxus* genus and from a fungal endophyte that grows on the Pacific yew.[139] Docetaxel is derived semisynthetically from 10-deacetyl-baccatin III, which is obtained from the needles of the European yew, *Taxus baccata*.[140]

Vincristine and vinblastine bind to the protein tubulin at a site distinct from that of the taxanes and, at low concentrations, inhibit microtubule dynamics. At higher concentrations, these vinca alkaloids disrupt microtubules and mitotic spindle, resulting in cell-cycle mitotic arrest and apoptosis of cells (see Fig. 56–3). In contrast, after binding to a-tubulin, taxanes kinetically stabilize microtubule dynamics at their plus ends, as well as shift the equilibrium toward tubulin polymerization into micrutubule bundles. This also causes mitotic arrest and apoptosis of cells.[141] The mitotic arrest caused by antimicrotubule drugs is associated with phosphorylation of the BCL2 protein and increased intracellular levels of the BCL2-associated X protein (BAX), which promote apoptosis.[141]

These agents are used in the management of lymphomas and leukemias and continue to be used in the mainstay of clinical chemotherapeutic regimens. Because of their mechanism of action, they are best used in combinations where potentiation of efficacy with other classes of agents such as antimetabolites and DNA-damaging agents provide better therapeutic responses and well-tolerated treatments, particularly in the relapsed setting. A recent phase II study combining fludarabine with paclitaxel achieved a 60% overall response rate with 32% complete remissions in 28 patients with relapsed non-Hodgkin lymphoma with moderate toxicity other than a high incidence of neutropenia and fever, and a prolonged complete remission (CR) duration of 32 months.[142]

Antimetabolites

The antimetabolites consist of low-molecular-weight compounds that interfere with micromolecular synthesis. As a group, they may be contrasted with agents such as the anthracycline antibiotics, which interfere with macromolecular synthesis. The nucleoside analogs exhibit structural similarities to naturally occurring nucleosides and are incorporated into either DNA or RNA with lethal consequences. Alternatively, they block key enzymes in de novo purine or pyrimidine biosynthesis. The antimetabolites in use in hematologic disorders can be divided into the following broad categories:

1. Inhibitors of de novo purine or pyrimidine synthesis (eg, hydroxyurea)
2. Folic acid analogs (eg, methotrexate)
3. Pyrimidine analogs (eg, ara-C, 5-azacytidine, gemcitabine)
4. Purine analogs (eg, 6-thioguanine, 6-mercaptopurine, fludarabine, chlorodeoxyadenosine, deoxycoformycin, clofarabine, nelarabine).

These categories are not mutually exclusive; for example, some nucleoside analogs (eg, ara-C and 6-thioguanine) also inhibit enzymes involved in DNA or deoxyribonucleotide biosynthesis. As noted previously, the antimetabolites are predominantly cycle-active agents and in most cases are phase-specific, being primarily active against cells in S phase. Because the growth fraction of hematologic malignancies tends to be higher than that of nonhematologic malignancies, antimetabolites are particularly useful in the former disorders. In contrast to alkylating agents, antimetabolites have limited carcinogenic and leukemogenic potential. The fluorinated pyrimidines (eg, 5-fluorouracil) are generally not employed in hematologic disorders and will not be discussed here.

Clofarabine (2-chloro-2′-arabino-flouro-2′-deoxyadenosine) is a purine analog with demonstrated activity in relapsed acute leukemias. To be active, it requires cellular uptake, conversion to the triphosphate nucleotide. It then decreases ribonucleotide reductase, alters nucleotide precursors, inhibits and reduces the function of antiapoptotic proteins such as Bcl-X(L), Mcl-1, and Bax with dephosphorylation of akt,[143] and causes inhibition of DNA synthesis. It appears more active against B-cell than T-cell malignancies but also has activities in AML and MDS.[144] Reversible liver toxicity and myelosuppression can be dose limiting.

Nelarabine (9-beta-D-arabinofuranosylguanine) is the most recently FDA-approved purine analog for the treatment of refractory T-cell leukemias and lymphomas. It preferentially accumulates in T-cells and is incorporated into DNA, causing chain termination and inhibiting DNA synthesis. The FDA approved the drug after analyzing the results of two phase II clinical trials, one in pediatric T-cell acute lymphoblastic leukemia (ALL) and the other in adults with T-cell lymphoblastic lymphoma. In both cases patients had relapsed after at least two induction regimens. Because complete remissions were seen in 13% of the 39 pediatric patients and in 18% of the 28 adult patients, the FDA granted approval.[145] Neurologic toxicity is dose limiting. Good response rates including complete remissions have been seen in refractory T-cell leukemias.[145–148]

Inhibitors of DNA Topoisomerase I and II

The inhibitors of DNA topoisomerases I and II are some of the most commonly used antineoplastic agents in the treatment of hematologic malignancies, and include such drugs as doxorubicin, daunorubicin, mitoxantrone, etoposide, and topotecan. Before describing the specific inhibitors, a brief review of the drug targets (topoisomerase enzymes) will be presented (Table 56–2).

DNA Topoisomerase I

Topoisomerase I is a ubiquitous enzyme whose function in vivo is to relieve the torsional strain in DNA, specifically, to remove positive supercoils generated in front of the replication fork and to relieve negative supercoils occurring downstream of RNA polymerase during transcription.[149–151] Topoisomerase I is catalytically active as a 100-kd monomer and is concentrated in nucleoli, although lower amounts are found in a diffuse nuclear distribution. The gene for this enzyme is located on human chromosome 20q12-13.2. Topoisomerase I does not require adenosine 5′-triphosphate (ATP) for catalytic activity. It binds double-strand DNA over 15 to 25 bp (with a preference for supercoiled or bent DNA), followed by cleavage of one DNA strand and forming a transient covalent phosphotyrosyl bond at the 3′-end of DNA. DNA torsional strain is then relieved by a

Table 56–2 Characteristics of Mammalian DNA Topoisomerases

	Topo I	Topo IIα	Topo IIβ
Size of monomer	100 kd	170 kd	180 kd
mRNA	4.2 kb	6.2 kb	6.5 kb
Chromosome	20q12-13.2	17q21-22	3p24
DNA cleavage	Single-strand breaks	Double-strand breaks	Double-strand
Covalent intermediate	$3'PO_4$-Tyr^{723}	$5'PO_4$-Tyr^{804}	$5'PO_4$-Tyr^{821}
ATP requirement	No	Yes	Yes
Nuclear location	Nucleoli, diffuse	Nuclear matrix and scaffold, nucleoli	Nucleoli Nuclear matrix
Cell-cycle dependence	None	Yes, maximum in G_2/M	None
Nuclear localization signal	NH_2-end	COOH-end	COOH-end
Phosphorylation	By CK II and PKC (increases activity)	By CK II, PKC, p34^{cdc2}, MAP kinase	Increases mass to 190 kd
Role	In replication, transcription, and recombination	In replication, transcription, chromosome condensation/segregation, and recombination	rRNA transcription
Inhibitors	Camptothecins	(see Table 56–3)	

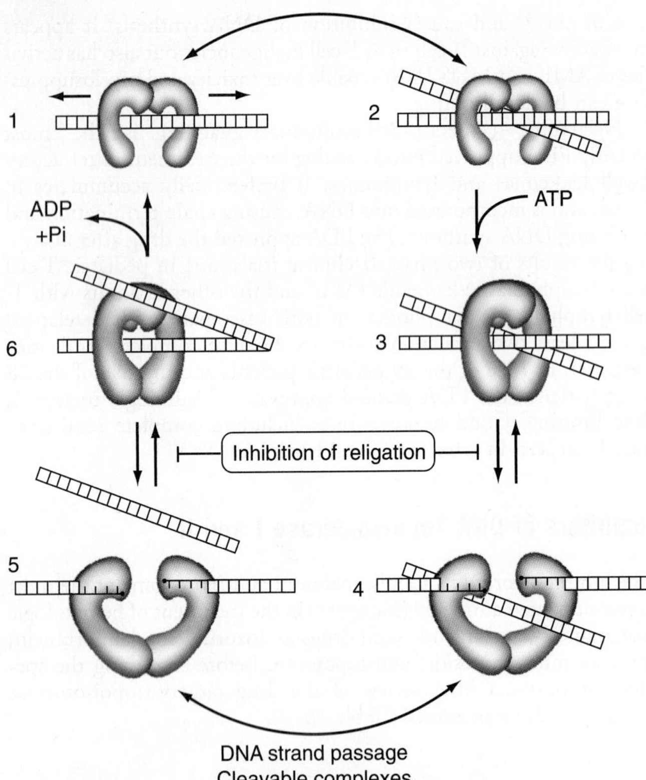

Figure 56–4 DNA topoisomerase II catalytic cycle. (1) Noncovalent binding of DNA by the topoisomerase II homodimer. (2) DNA recognition and preferential binding to crossovers by topoisomerase II. (3) Binding of ATP promotes the formation of a topologic complex. (4) DNA cleavage with covalent linkage of each topoisomerase II monomer to the 5′-DNA terminus of the break. (5) Poststrand passage cleavable complex. (6) Religation of the cleaved DNA is followed by ATP hydrolysis and enzyme turnover. DNA topoisomerase II inhibitors generally increase cleavable complexes by inhibiting the religation activity. *(Adapted from Pommier et al.[171])*

"controlled rotation" mechanism (see Fig. 56–1) subsequent to which the cleaved DNA is religated. The three-dimensional crystal structure of human topoisomerase I, both in covalent and noncovalent complexes with DNA, has defined the structural elements of the enzyme that contacts DNA.[85,86] The association between topoisomerase I and the −3′ end of cleaved DNA has been termed the *cleavable complex*, and it is this complex that is stabilized by topoisomerase I inhibitors.

DNA Topoisomerase II

Two isoforms of human topoisomerase II (alpha and beta) exist. They act as homodimers to cleave double-strand DNA and they require ATP for full activity.[149,151–153] Their role in vivo is to relieve torsional strain in DNA, and their cellular distribution is determined by nuclear localization signals contained in the C-terminal domain.[154,155] These isoforms are distinct in that they have different-size monomers (see Table 56–2), their genes are on separate chromosomes, their nuclear distribution is different, and only the α-isoform shows cell-cycle variations in amount and activity (with maximal activity in G_2/M). The mechanism of action of topoisomerase II involves several steps (Fig. 56–4): DNA recognition and binding (curved and supercoiled DNA, as well as DNA crossovers, are preferred); the sequential cleavage of the two strands of DNA with covalent attachment of a monomer to each 5′-end of the cleaved DNA; passage of another DNA duplex through the break site (eg, to relieve DNA torsional strain or decatenate daughter chromosomes at the end of replication); religation of the cleaved DNA; and ATP hydrolysis-dependent enzyme turnover. The binding of ATP by topoisomerase II is required for the strand passage reaction. Again, the association between topoisomerase II monomers and the 5′ end of the cleaved DNA has been termed the *cleavable complex*, the stabilization of which generally correlates with the cytotoxic activity of specific topoisomerase II inhibitors.

Because topoisomerase I and II inhibitors convert their respective enzymes into DNA-damaging agents, it is usually true that the more enzyme target a cell contains (provided it is in the nucleus), the more cytotoxic the specific inhibitor is. An exception to this generalization is found in CLL cells, which have abundant topoisomerase I, yet are not very sensitive to topoisomerase I inhibitors. This is because topoisomerase I inhibitors are S phase specific and CLL cells have very few cells in S phase. Finally, in addition to topoisomerase I and II, a mammalian DNA topoisomerase III has recently been described and found to be essential for early embryogenesis in the mouse.[156] In addition to the presumed lethality of a homozygous deletion of the topoisomerase II gene, topoisomerases I and III appear to be essential for cell growth and division in mammals.[157,158] The specific role of topoisomerase III in humans is not known at present.

9 7 10 A B C N O 11 12 N D E O CH_3CH_2 OH O

	C-10	C-9	C-7
Camptothecin	H	H	H
Topotecan	OH	$(CH_3)_2NCH_2$	H
9-Aminocamptothecin	H	NH_2	H
SN-38	OH	H	CH_3CH_2
CPT-11	N N–C(=O)–O	H	CH_3CH_2

Figure 56–5 Structure of camptothecin analogs.

DNA Topoisomerase I Inhibitors

Camptothecin is a plant alkaloid first identified in 1966 from the tree *Camptotheca acuminata.* Early clinical studies with camptothecin were stopped primarily because of hemorrhagic cystitis, resulting from conversion of the sodium salt form given to the active lactone form owing to the acidic pH in the bladder. Renewed interest in camptothecin occurred in 1985 when topoisomerase I was identified as the target of this drug,[158] and as new more water-soluble analogs became available. At present, there are two topoisomerase I inhibitors approved by the FDA as second-line agents for the treatment of ovarian carcinoma and colorectal cancer; these are topotecan and irinotecan (CPT-11), respectively. Other analogs, including 9-aminocamptothecin, are currently in clinical trials (Fig. 56–5). With respect to hematologic malignancies, topotecan has been shown to be active in the treatment of myelodysplastic syndromes[159] and inactive in the treatment of CLL.[39] Responses to topotecan have also been seen in refractory multiple myeloma[160] and in refractory acute leukemia.[161,162]

There are several recent reviews of topoisomerase I inhibitors and the clinical trials using these agents.[163–166] The lactone forms of topotecan and SN-38 (the active form of CPT-11 generated in vivo by the action of a carboxylesterase) are as much as 1000-fold more active

Table 56–3 Mechanism(s) of Action of Antineoplastic Agents That Are Primarily Topoisomerase II Inhibitors

Drug	Topo II Inhibition Poison	DNA Suppressor	Free Radical Intercalation	Formation
Epipodophyllotoxins VP-16 VM-26	+++	–	–	+
Anthracyclines Doxorubicin Daunorubicin Idarubicin Epirubicin	++	++	++	+
Anthracenedione Mitoxantrone	++	++	++	+
Acridine m-AMSA	+++	+	+	–
Catalytic inhibitors Aclarubicin	–	+++	+	–
Others (merbarone, fostriecin, bis-2,6-dioxopiperazines)	–	+++	–	–

inhibitors of DNA topoisomerase I than are their carboxylate forms. The lactone form predominates at an acidic pH. Topoisomerase I inhibitors stabilize the DNA–enzyme cleavable complex and thus inhibit DNA religation, but it is the production of DNA double-strand breaks that result from a collision of the DNA replication fork with the ternary drug–enzyme–DNA complex that is the lethal event (see Fig. 56–4).[167–169] Topoisomerase I inhibitors are considered S phase-specific agents because they require ongoing DNA synthesis to exert their cytotoxic effect.

DNA Topoisomerase II Inhibitors

Inhibitors of DNA topoisomerase II are some of the most commonly used agents in the treatment of hematopoietic malignancies, and their biochemical and pharmacologic properties have recently been reviewed by several investigators.[170–173] There now exist three general types of topoisomerase II inhibitors (Table 56–3). The first are the topoisomerase II *poisons*, typified by etoposide, whose activity results in the stabilization of cleavable complexes. The second group are the *catalytic inhibitors*, represented by aclarubicin, merbarone, and the bis-2,6-dioxopiperazine derivatives (ICRF-193, ICRF-159, ICRF-187); these are drugs that, except for aclarubicin, do not bind DNA and do not stabilize cleavable complexes but rather interfere with some aspect of topoisomerase II catalytic activity (eg, ICRF-187 inhibits topoisomerase II adenosine triphosphatase [ATPase] activity). The final class includes drugs that can inhibit both DNA topoisomerases I and II, and are represented by intoplicine[174] and saintopin.[175]

DNA topoisomerase II poisons, the most frequently used drugs in the clinical setting (see Fig. 56–5 for structures) are most likely cytotoxic because they trap DNA topoisomerase II complexes on nascent DNA in the nuclear matrix.[176,177] Recent evidence suggests that the topoisomerase II poison-stabilized enzyme–DNA complex acts as a replication fork barrier and leads to the generation of irreversible DNA damage and cell death in proliferating cells,[178] whereas other experiments in yeast show that although DNA synthesis is a major determinant for cell killing by topoisomerase I inhibitors, topoisomerase II poisons may be cytotoxic during other phases of the cell cycle as well.[179,180]

Drug Resistance to Topoisomerase Inhibitors

Essentially all of the topoisomerase II poisons (see Tables 56–2 and 56–3) are substrates for the drug efflux pump p-glycoprotein (PGP), and many are substrates for multidrug resistance protein (MRP) and lung resistance-related protein. In addition, several point mutations and gene deletions have been defined in the gene for topoisomerase II resulting in the production of an enzyme with altered catalytic and/or cleavage activity.[181,182] The third mechanism is a decrease in expression of the enzyme such that there is less target for the inhibitor to "convert" to a DNA-damaging agent. This can result from a proliferation-dependent or cell cycle-dependent decrease in topoisomerase II,[183] from a specific attenuation of topoisomerase II,[184,185] or from an intrinsic absence of topoisomerase II (identified in some acute and chronic leukemias). The fourth resistance mechanism involves alterations in the subcellular distribution of the enzyme. Truncation of the COOH-end of topoisomerase II has resulted in the cytoplasmic distribution of enzyme caused by a loss of nuclear localization signals, so that the enzyme cannot interact with DNA in the presence of an inhibitor and the cell is resistant.[186–188] However, mutations in the gene for topoisomerase II do not appear to be a common clinical event, as only a single patient with AML has been found to have a point mutation. CLL cells are resistant to topoisomerase II inhibitors because they express very low levels of the protein.

Platinum Analogs

During a study of the effects of electric current on growing bacteria, the antibacterial and, later, the antitumor activities of the platinum compounds were fortuitously discovered. The antitumor agent, cisplatin, and its cis-carboxylester analog, carboplatin, are heavy metal platinum complexes. Both are activated by displacement of their ligands (cisplatin : chloride and carboplatin : carboxylester) by water to form positively charged aquated platinum complexes. This allows platinum to stably bind DNA, RNA, proteins, or other critical biomacromolecules (see Fig. 56–2). With DNA, platinum complexes form covalent links to the N^7 position of guanine and adenine. The N^7 adducts at d(GpG) or d(ApG) result in intrastrand or interstrand DNA cross-links that bend the DNA helix and inhibit DNA synthesis. The cytotoxicity of platinum analogs correlates with the total platinum binding to DNA, as well as with the intrastrand or interstrand cross-links. This results in DNA damage, which triggers apoptosis of sensitive cells.

Cisplatin and carboplatin are used in the treatment of refractory lymphomas as part of high-dose and intensification therapy.

Miscellaneous Agents

Among the agents included in this category, only plicamycin, bleomycin, procarbazine, L-asparaginase, gallium nitrate, and glucocorticoids are of current interest to the hematologist; these are discussed in Appendix 56–6.

Targeted Agents

Imatinib Mesylate and Other Kinase Inhibitors

Imatinib mesylate (formerly GCP57148; Gleevec; STI571) is a phenylaminopyrimidine that was developed as an inhibitor of the BCR-ABL tyrosine kinase, which is expressed in the cells of most patients with CML.[189] The role of the BCR-ABL kinase in the pathogenesis of CML and its use in CML treatment are discussed in detail in Chapter 69, and will not be dealt with in depth here.

Imatinib mesylate represents the prototypical molecularly targeted agent in that it is directed specifically against the BCR-ABL kinase, which is selectively expressed in CML but not normal cells.[190] Imatinib mesylate is not absolutely specific for the BCR-ABL kinase, inasmuch as it also inhibits other kinases, including KIT (formerly designated c-KIT), PDGF, and TEL-ARG.[191] Radiographic crystallographic studies revealed that imatinib mesylate binds to the ATP-binding site of the kinase and stabilizes it in an inactive form. The 50% inhibitory concentration (IC_{50}) of imatinib mesylate for BCR-ABL is in the submicromolar range, and substantially lower than the supramicromolar levels achievable in the plasma of patients receiving the drug by the oral route.

Exposure of BCR-ABL$^+$ leukemic cells to imatinib mesylate not only blocks their proliferation but also induces apoptosis.[192] Such a finding suggests that these cells have become "addicted" to constitutive activation of BCR-ABL for their survival. This is believed to be secondary to activation of a large number of downstream BCR-ABL survival pathways, including those related to STAT5A (previously designated STAT5), MEK/ERK, NF-kB (nuclear factor-κB), AKT, and BCL2L1 (also known as Bcl-xL), among others.[193,194] In addition to promoting survival in BCR-ABL$^+$ cells, activation of these pathways also confers resistance to conventional cytotoxic drugs.[195]

Despite the success of imatinib mesylate in the treatment of chronic phase CML and, to a lesser extent, accelerated or blast phase CML, the preexistence or development of resistance represents a major therapeutic challenge. This success is further tempered by the emergence of mutations within the abl kinase rendering cells resistant to Inhibition, and intolerance due to skin rash, diarrhea, heart failure. In many patients with bcr-abl + ALL, abl kinase mutations are present at the time of diagnosis and emerge with imatinib treatment.[196] Resistance to imatinib can take multiple forms, including the development of standard multidrug resistance mechanisms (eg, PGP-related), *BCR-ABL* gene amplification, increased levels of the BCR-ABL protein, and perhaps most commonly, mutations in the BCR-ABL kinase domain (eg, $_{thr}315_{ile}$), which alter the conformation of the kinase domain and inhibit imatinib mesylate binding.[197–199] A recent study of 171 patients failing imatinib identified 62 patients with mutations in 23 amino acids, most commonly the phosphate-binding loop in the abl kinase gene.[200] In addition, mutations distant to the kinase domain can occur that also have the net effect of antagonizing BCR-ABL binding.[201] Very recently, a new form of imatinib resistance has been described characterized by loss of the BCR-ABL kinase and a reciprocal upregulation of the SRC kinases LYN and HCK.[202] A recent study in an experimental model of Ph-positive CML has shown that targeting multiple kinases improves therapeutic outcome.[203]

One logical approach to enhancing imatinib mesylate activity or overcoming resistance, or both, is to combine it with more conventional cytotoxic agents including ara-C, interferon, and others.[204,205] Clinical trials based on this strategy are currently underway. An alternative approach is to combine imatinib mesylate with other novel agents that interrupt various survival signaling or cell-cycle regulatory pathways. In this regard, potentiation of imatinib mesylate activity in BCR-ABL$^+$ cells has been reported when combined with MEK inhibitors,[206] the CDK inhibitor Flavopiridol,[207] histone deacetylase inhibitors (eg, suberoylanilide hydroxamic acid [SAHA]),[208,209] farnesyl transferase inhibitors,[210] arsenic trioxide,[211] and the FRAP1 inhibitor rapamycin.[212] Clinical trials involving regimens combining imatinib mesylate with Flavopiridol, farnesyl transferase inhibitors, 17-allylaminodemethoxy geldanamycin (17-AAG), arsenic trioxide, and FRAP1 inhibitors are currently underway. Finally, an alternative approach to circumvent imatinib mesylate resistance involves the use of non-cross-resistant agents such as the tyrphostin adaphostin,[213,214] or the SRC tyrosine kinase inhibitor (PD 173955).[215] Another approach is combining an mTor inhibitor, rapamycin, or the novel RAD001 agent, which in preclinical models improves the efficacy of imatinib.[216]

Dasatinib is the second abl kinase inhibitor approved for the treatment of CML. Dasatinib is an oral abl, kit, and src kinase inhibitor that induces responses in most patients who are treated in the chronic and accelerated phase of CML.[217,218] As a multikinase inhibitor, it can be expected to have a higher response rate and perhaps to have broader toxicity profile. However, it is well tolerated, with some patients experiencing pulmonary edema, pleural effusions, skin rashes, and neutropenia. Few patients are removed from treatment for these reasons. There is a high response rate in patients with wild-type sequences of bcr-abl and also in patients with imatinib resistance mutations in the abl protein.[219] Resistance to dasatinib has been observed most likely as a result of mutations at positions 315 or 317 of the abl kinase.[220] Other agents such as nilotinib, AMN 107, are also kinase inhibitors in clinical trials for imatinib-intolerant or imatinib-resistant settings. AMN107 is a much more potent abl-kinase inhibitor and is well tolerated in early trials. As a more potent agent, it will be of interest to define whether it has a better tolerance and efficacy profile compared to imatinib.[221]

Hypomethylating Agents

Promoter methylation within CpG islands regulates gene expression in all cells. Disruption of normal gene expression profiles accompanies the malignant transformation, giving rise to complex patterns of gene expression. As a consequence, promoters of many genes have an altered pattern of methylation resulting in either gene activation or gene repression. The link between these concepts and the interest in agents that alter promoter methylation began with the realization that azacytidine, an agent used sparingly for myeloid leukemias, had efficacy when given at low doses either intravenously or subcutaneously for extended periods of time and that in these cases, altered gene expression accompanied responses. Both azacytidine and 5-aza-2′-deoxycytidine (decitabine) act by irreversible inhibition of the DNA methyltransferases responsible for methylation of the cytidine in CpG islands[222] and are thus S phase-specific agents. Wijermans et al first described that a related compound, 5-aza-2′-deoxycytidine, was effective when given as a continuous infusion to elderly patients with high-risk MDS, with a 54% response rate.[223] The mechanism of action included both direct change in promoter methylation[222,224] and independent changes, with up to 70% genomewide demethylation, suggesting either that genes with altered expression either up- or downregulated a second set of genes through altered pathways such as induction of WAFp21, p15, and p16 or in a more direct fashion through altered transcription factor expression.[225–227] More recent studies have identified activity of these agents in both acute and chronic myeloid leukemias.[228–230] Most often, partial responses or short-lived complete responses are seen in AML with complete responses more common in MDS. Recent studies also describe a number of extended therapy regimens. Kantarjian et al reported a comparison of 20 mg/m^2 decitabine intravenously for 5 days with 20 mg/m^2 subcutaneously daily for 5 days and 10 mg/m^2 intravenously for 10 days. The 5-day IV dose schedule was judged superior on the basis of clinical outcome with 39% complete remissions, a higher proportion of reactivation of p15 and induced hypomethylation as well as clinical tolerance.[231]

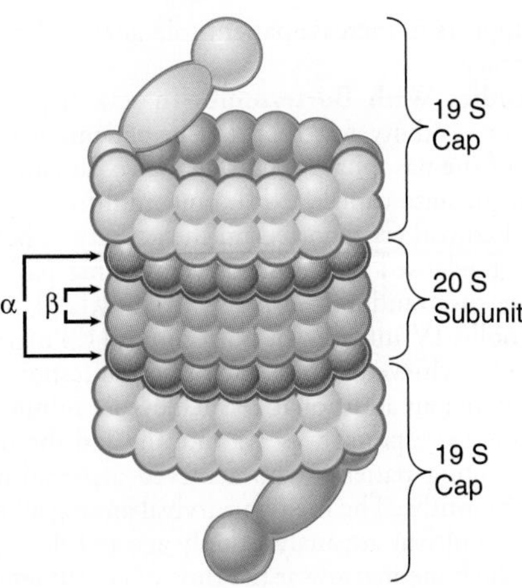

Figure 56–6 26S Proteasome.

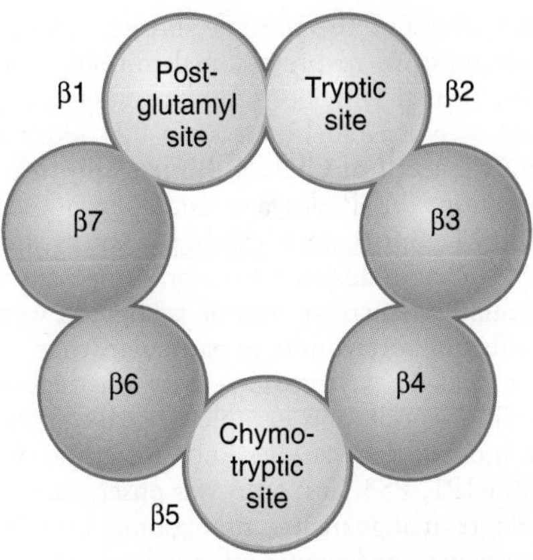

Figure 56–7 Cross section of beta ring of the 20S of the 26S proteasome.

Ubiquitin–Proteasome Inhibitors

The 26S proteasome is the central proteolytic machinery of the highly conserved ubiquitin proteasome system. In eukaryotic cells, whereas the lysosomal pathway degrades extracellular proteins imported into the cell through endocytosis or pinocytosis, the proteasome controls the degradation of intracellular proteins. Numerous studies have demonstrated that the ubiquitin–proteasome system controls basic cellular functions such as cell-cycle progression, signal transduction, and programmed cell death. Hence the interest in therapeutic interventions that manipulate proteasomal activity and potentially restore cellular homeostasis into transformed cells.

Ubiquitin is a highly conserved 76-amino-acid polypeptide that is expressed in all eukaryotic cells.[232] Under the sequential action of E1 (ubiquitin-activating enzyme), E2 (ubiquitin-conjugating enzyme), and E3 (ubiquitin ligase), ubiquitin is activated and covalently conjugated to potential proteasome substrates via an isopeptide bond between the C-terminal glycine residue of ubiquitin and the ε-amino group of internal lysine residues in target proteins.[232] The same set of enzymes also catalyzes the formation of the isopeptide bond between G76 and the lysine residue (K48) of previously conjugated ubiquitin, leading to formation of a polyubiquitin chain. Polyubiquitinated substrates are usually targeted for proteasomal degradation.[232–235]

The 26S proteasome is a large (2000-kd) threonine protease present in the nucleus and cytoplasm of all eukaryotic cells.[236,237] This ATP-dependent, multicatalytic protease eliminates damaged or misfolded proteins and regulates cyclins and cyclin-dependent kinase inhibitor cell-cycle regulatory proteins as well as other proteins that govern the transcription factor activation, apoptosis, and cell trafficking. Its structure consists of two parts: The 20S core and the 19S cap regulatory particle (Fig. 56–6). The 19S cap is involved in the recognition, binding, and unfolding of ubiquitinated proteins, and in the regulation of the opening of the 20S core.[238,239] The 20S core is a cylinder composed of four stacked heptameric rings, each containing seven different α or β subunits (α7β7β7α7) (Figs. 56–6 and 56–7). Three different active sites are located inside the cylindrical core within the β-subunit rings. At least three distinct proteolytic activities are associated with the proteasome: Chymotryptic, tryptic, and peptidylglutamyl.[236,240–242] Following release from the substrate, the polyubiquitin chain is hydrolyzed into single ubiquitin moieties whereas tagged proteins are degraded to small peptides. Both the assembly of the 26S proteasome and the degradation of protein substrates are ATP dependent.[239,240]

Transformed cells are much more sensitive to blockade of the proteasome than are normal cells; the exact mechanism of this selective susceptibility is not fully understood. Early studies revealed that proteasomes are abnormally highly expressed in rapidly growing metazoan embryonic and human neoplastic cells, but not in their well-differentiated and normally growing cells. The selectivity of proteasome inhibitors is not solely dependent on proliferative status, as both transformed and normal fibroblasts have similar growth rates although proteasome inhibitors are selectively toxic to SV-40-transformed cells.[243] Cyclins A, B, D and E, cyclin-dependent kinase inhibitors (p21, p27), inhibitory proteins (I-κB), oncogenes (*FOS*, *MYC*), and tumor suppressors (eg, cyclin B1, p21WAF1/CIP1, p27, p53) are known substrates for the ubiquitin–proteasome pathway. The specificity of the ubiquitin proteasome is such that the degradation of individual substrates can be upregulated without affecting the proteolysis of others. Different classes of proteasome inhibitors have been described thus far and include peptide aldehydes (MG132, PSI, LLnV, ALLN, CEP1612, Z-LLF), streptomyces metabolite (lactacystin), dipeptidyl boronic acid bortezomib, vinyl sulfone tripeptides (NLVS), and natural products like Epoxomycin.[244,245]

Proteosome Targeted Agents (Bortezomib)

Bortezomib (pyrazylcarbonyl-Phe-Leu-boronate), the first in this class of agents to enter clinical trials, is a dipeptidyl boronic acid that is a specific and selective inhibitor of the 26S proteasome. The Boron atom interacts reversibly with the catalytic threonine residue of the proteasome, primarily inhibiting its chymotrypsin-like activity.[244] The inhibition of the ubiquitin–proteasome pathway with bortezomib was demonstrated to arrest the growth of malignant cells (breast, colon, prostate tumor cell lines, Burkitt lymphoma, adult T-cell leukemia, Lewis lung carcinoma, CLL, and myeloma cell lines) and sensitize them to chemotherapeutic agents (5-fluorouracil, cisplatin, taxol, doxorubicin, CPT-11, and gemcitabine). Bortezomib mediates these effects through multiple mechanisms by regulating the expression of proteins involved in cell-cycle progression ($P21^{cip1}$, $P27^{Kip1}$), oncogenesis (P53, I-κB), apoptosis (BCL2, BIRC2, BIRC3, BIRC4, BAX), and more recently DNA repair (DNA-PKcs, ATM).[245–247] Loss of I-κB destabilizes NF-κB, reducing expression of a critical plasma cell cytokine stimulatory molecule, IL-6. The process of cell death appears to be p53-independent and to result in mitotic catastrophy although classical caspase 8-dependent apoptosis pathway has also been implicated.[248] A recent study found a strong correlation between immunoglobulin production and apoptotic sensitivity to bortezomib, suggesting that the active requirement for protein folding in the endoplasmic reticulum provides a direct target and explains sensitivity to proteasome inhibition. It also suggests a selective mechanism that could explain the emergence of less differentiated myeloma cells with decreased immunoglobulin production during treatment.[249,250] These processes also increase oxidative stress and contribute to apoptotic signaling, explaining the sensitivity of myeloma plasma cells to proteasome inhibition.[251]

Preclinical Studies With Bortezomib. Screening of the National Cancer Institute (NCI) tumor cell lines revealed that bortezomib is active against a broad range of tumor types. The average growth inhibition of 50% (GI_{50}) value for bortezomib across the entire NCI cell panel (60 human derived cell lines) was 7 nM.[244] Among solid tumor cell lines, those of the prostate, breast, colon, and pancreas were exquisitely sensitive to proteasomal inhibition. PC-3 prostate carcinoma cells, treated with bortezomib, underwent growth arrest in G2-M phase with a parallel increase in P21 levels and decreased activity but not the levels of CDK-4. Bortezomib treatment also led to caspase activation, PARP cleavage, and apoptotic cell death with an IC_{50} of 20 nM. Bortezomib exhibited synergistic effect when combined in SN-38 and radiation in colon tumor cells and in mouse xenografts. Similarly, pancreatic tumor xenografts were sensitive to the cytotoxic effect of bortezomib, in particular when combined with gemcitabine or CPT-11. Cytotoxic activity was reported as well in Lewis lung carcinoma cells and nasopharyngeal squamous cell carcinoma cells. In most of these studies, increase in the cellular levels of P21WAF1, P27KIP1, P53, and I-κB was observed.[252–256]

In hematologic malignancies, proteasome inhibitors exhibited cytotoxic activity in a wide range of cell lines, including multiple myeloma, U937 human monoblast leukemia, HL-60 promyelocytic leukemia, Jurkat T-cell leukemia, K562 CML, Ramos Burkitt lymphoma, and primary B-cell CLL.[246,257–259] In multiple myeloma cells, bortezomib induced p53 and MDM2 protein expression, induced phosphorylation (Ser15) of p53 protein, and activated JUN NH2-terminal kinase (JNK), which in turn activated caspase 8 and caspase 3. Bortezomib was also shown to activate the intrinsic (mitochondria/cytochrome C/caspase 9) and extrinsic (JNK/death receptor-activated caspase 8) apoptotic pathways of the myeloma cells. Bortezomib blocked TNF-induced NF-κB activation through inhibition of IκB degradation. TNF-induced intracellular adhesion molecule (ICAM)-1 expression on RPMI8226 and MM.1S cells was also inhibited. The unfolded protein response not only is increased in plasma cells producing large quantities of immunoglobulin but also induces a stress apoptosis response.[260] Bortezomib also induces osteoblast activity through the Runx2/Cbfa2 pathway.[261] Furthermore, bortezomib inhibits RANKL-induced osteoclastogenesis through inhibition of P38 kinase.[262] Increased osteoblast activity should help restore the clinical osteoporosis with or without the use of bisphosphonates. Moreover, it prevented the adherence of myeloma cells to bone marrow stromal cells and the NF-κB-dependent production of IL-6. Importantly, bortezomib demonstrated synergistic activity with dexamethasone, thalidomide, melphalan, and doxorubicin, and did not appear to be a substrate for multidrug-resistance transporters.[263–266] However, as shown by Hideshima and colleagues, NF-κB blockade could not account for all of the antimyeloma activity of bortezomib, and clearly other mechanisms contribute to its antineoplastic effects.[266–268] Finally, IC_{50} concentration of bortezomib in myeloma cells had no effect on peripheral blood mononuclear cells from healthy volunteers and did not affect cultured bone marrow stromal cells. This did not preclude the clinical observation of myelosuppression during treatment with bortezomib as a single agent.

Pharmacology of Bortezomib. Bortezomib is primarily metabolized through cytochrome P450 (CYP) and not via phase II pathways, for example, glucuronidation and sulfation. In vitro studies indicated that the primary metabolic pathway is deboronation mediated by CYP3A4. Bortezomib was also metabolized by CYP2D6, but the rate of metabolism was slower than that observed with CYP3A4. Deboronated metabolites have been shown to be inactive in the 20S proteasome assay. Bortezomib rapidly exits the plasma compartment with more than 90% cleared within 15 minutes of IV administration. In whole-body autoradiography of [^{14}C] boretezomib-treated rats, the central nervous system, testes, and eyes appeared to be protected from bortezomib. Bortezomib specifically and selectively inhibits proteasome function by binding tightly ($K_i > 0.6$ nM) and reversibly to the enzyme's chymotrypsin-like site.[242,269] In ex vivo 20S proteasome activity bioassays, proteasome was inhibited within 1 hour of bortezomib administration, and baseline proteasome activity was restored within 48 to 72 hours. Intermittent but high inhibition (>70%) of proteasome activity was better tolerated than sustained inhibition.[270,271] Thus, a twice-weekly clinical dosing regimen is better tolerated. Nonetheless, this dose schedule is often associated with significant myelosuppression and onset of peripheral neuropathy. Reducing the dose schedule to a weekly regimen ameliorates these toxicities and appears to increase patient tolerance without jeopardizing clinical efficacy.

Clinical Studies With Bortezomib. In several phase I clinical studies, antitumor activity was reported in patients with squamous cell carcinoma of the nasopharynx, bronchoalveolar carcinoma, renal cell carcinoma, prostate cancer, NHL, and multiple myeloma.[271,272] Richardson and coworkers reported on the activity of bortezomib in the treatment of relapsed and refractory myeloma patients.[273] In a large multicenter nonrandomized phase II study, 202 patients were treated with a bolus IV infusion of bortezomib (1.3 mg/m^2). Of the 202 patients, 27% achieved a complete or partial response as defined by the Blade criteria; an additional 7% achieved a minimal response. The median time to response was 1.3 months and the median time to progression among patients who achieved a partial or complete response was 13 months. The median survival among all patients was 16 months. In a multivariate analysis, only age and the percentage of plasma cells in the bone marrow at the time of enrollment predicated response to bortezomib. A recent study further defines the safety of using bortezomib in older patients with myeloma.[274] The most common grade 3 to 4 adverse events were thrombocytopenia (31%), fatigue (12%), neuropathy (12%), and neutropenia (14%).[273] The thrombocytopenia, although significant with a mean drop of more than 60%, was rapidly reversible and associated with shorter platelet survival rather than a direct toxic effect on megakaryocytes.[275] The randomized phase III clinical trial compared bortezomib with dexamethasone and concluded that there was a significant advantage for bortezomib-treated patients.[276] A response rate of 38% was seen with a greater than a median 6-month time to progression. A second trial added dexamethasone after two cycles of bortezomib with an overall response rate of 88%.[277] Additional clinical trials have shown the efficacy of bortezomib in multiple myeloma in combination with other cytotoxic agents, including dexamethasone, melphalan, liposomal doxorubicin, lenalidomide, and thalidomide. A recent study showed a significantly prolonged time to disease progression in patients with myeloma who had undergone at least one prior treatment regimen of bortezomib plus liposomal doxorubicin (Doxil) compared to bortezomib alone.[278] The combination of melphalan and bortezomib is well tolerated, with an overall response rate of 68% in pretreated patients.[279] Combining bortezomib, thalidomide, and dexamethasone is also well tolerated, with an overall response rate of 53% in pretreated patients.[280] These combinations are also being explored in other hematologic malignancies (CLL, mantle cell lymphoma, and indolent NHL). In relapsed mantle cell lymphoma, an overall response rate of 33% was noted with a mean time to progression of 9 months.[281]

Newer Proteasome Inhibitors

The success of bortezomib in multiple myeloma and mantle cell lymphoma has stimulated interest in newer-generation proteasome inhibitors such as NPI-0052[282] and PR-171.[283] For example, PR-171 is an irreversible inhibitor of the proteasome and can be administered on a daily × 5 day schedule, potentially yielding more sustained plasma concentrations of the drug. Efforts to define the activity of these second-generation proteasome inhibitors in multiple myeloma and non-Hodgkin lymphoma are currently planned or underway.

Immunomodulatory Agents

Thalidomide and Lenalidomide

These related compounds provide effective therapy for multiple myeloma. They have complex mechanisms of action. Further details on their therapeutic impact are found in the chapter on multiple myeloma.

Thalidomide has been in clinical use for more than 50 years and has well documented and sometimes serious side effects of severe birth defects, somnolence, an axonal length-dependent peripheral neuropathy,[284] orthostatic hypotension, neutropenia, bradycardia and occasional heart block, and increased HIV load in HIV-positive patients. Thrombosis risk is elevated in patients on either agent, giving rise to the recommended use of an anticoagulant regimen such as low-molecular-weight heparin or coumadin.[285] It is an oral immunomodulatory agent. Experimental studies have identified that thalidomide reduces expression of the cellular inhibitor of apoptosis protein and potentiates proapoptotic processes such as TRAIL/po2L.[286] Thalidomide also reduces NF-κB and I-κB expression, thereby reducing IL-6 expression.[287] In addition, thalidomide decreases VEGF and reduces angiogenesis and vessel density in the marrow of patients with multiple myeloma.[288] The lack of a simple mechanism of action has been confusing in the clinical setting because it is unclear which if any biomarker is an appropriate correlate of clinical success or toxicity. Nonetheless, efficacy is certainly seen clinically and validated in SCID models of human myeloma.[289] Recent data point to its clinical efficacy in solid tumors and myelodysplastic syndrome.

Lenalidomide was identified as an analog of thalidomide with more potent immunomodulatory functions but less side effects, and it has emerged as a more potent agent.[290,291] Both have similar anti-angiogenic properties, block IL-6 production, and reduce NF-κB and I-κB levels. Lenalidomide also induces caspase 8-mediated apoptosis, and mitochondrial-mediated cell death. In addition, lenalidomide induces T-cell activation and NK activity, providing some measure of anticancer immune response.[290] It leads to similar and dose-dependent peripheral neuropathy as thalidomide and more significant marrow suppression, both of which are dose limiting. It is also associated with a significant increased risk of thrombosis, leading to recommendations for the use of anticoagulation in this population. Hypersensitivity rash occurs in up to 10% of patients.[292,293] However, a variety of dose schedules provide a flexible therapeutic approach and a high response rate in relapsed settings with an overall response rate of 25% and median overall survival of 28 months.[294] Excellent results with 31 of 34 patients achieving an objective response combining lenalidomide 25 mg/m^2 for 21 days and dexamethasone 40 mg daily for 4 days on days 1, 9, 17, of the 28-day cycle.[295] Ongoing studies are evaluating combination therapy with Doxil,[296] bortezomib, and melphalan.[297] Both thalidomide and lenalidomide are under evaluation for the treatment of primary amyloidosis, MDS, chronic lymphocytic leukemia, and solid tumors. In amyloidosis, the combination of lenalidomide and dexamethasone resulted in a well-tolerated regimen with an overall response rate of 67%, including complete hematologic remissions.[298] Lenalidomide has been approved by the FDA for the treatment of 5q minus myelodysplastic syndrome based on studies indicating more than a 40% response rate owing to the rate of transfusion independence that occurred in this group of patients.[299] In a randomized trial of patients with relapsed or refractory multiple myeloma comparing dexamethasone and lenalidomide to dexamethasone alone, a much higher and sustained response rate of 58% was observed. Effective dose ranges appear to be 5 to 25 mg daily for 21 days on a 4-week cycle, with a range of patient tolerance and adverse reactions that in large part are dose dependent.

TARGETING APOPTOSIS SIGNALING IN HEMATOLOGIC MALIGNANCIES

In humans, the processes of cell division and cell death are tightly coupled so that no net increase in cell numbers occurs. Alterations in the expression or function of the genes that control cell division and cell death can upset this delicate balance, and are hallmarks of cancer, contributing to expansion of neoplastic cells. Although conventional anticancer drugs either cause cell-cycle perturbation or DNA damage, they do not directly interact with the intracellular machinery for apoptosis. Tumor selectivity of such agents is largely caused by the increased sensitivity to apoptosis of tumor cells following DNA damage or cell-cycle perturbation. Novel therapeutic agents or strategies that target critical regulators or effectors of apoptosis are under development and clinical testing, and these agents or strategies have the potential to exert selective cytotoxicity against cancer cells.

Caspases are the "executioners" for apoptosis. These are proteases that exist as inactive zymogens and are activated by proteolytic cleavage of their proforms in response to a variety of death stimuli (explained in the next section). This processing occurs at conserved aspartic acid residues, thus generating the enzymatically active caspases.[300] Caspase activation is organized as a cascade, with upstream initiator and downstream effector caspases.[300] Upstream initiator caspases contain large prodomains that interact with specific proteins involved in triggering the cascade. The downstream caspases, which function as the ultimate effectors of apoptosis, possess small prodomains and are activated predominantly by proteolytic cleavage by upstream caspases. The irreversible cleavage of specific protein death substrates by the downstream effector caspases directly or indirectly accounts for the biochemical and morphologic changes that are recognized as apoptosis.

At least three pathways of caspase activation leading to apoptosis have been elucidated (Fig. 56–8): (a) the receptor-initiated apoptosis pathway, where the TNF family of cytokine receptors activate initiator caspases such as caspase 8; (b) the mitochondria-initiated apoptosis pathway, where cytochrome C and other pro-death effectors are released from mitochondria into cytosol that results in activation of caspase 9; and (c) a pathway of caspase activation, which involves a serine protease, granzyme B, that directly cleaves and activates several caspases, including procaspase 3.

Proapoptotic Targets of Anticancer Agents

Most cancer cells have active antiapoptotic pathways that prevent cell death in response to growth, checkpoint, DNA damage, and metabolic stimuli. A number of current anticancer agents in development target these pathways and are designed to be effective alone or in combination with other agents that disrupt the cell cycle, DNA synthesis, invoke DNA damage, etc.

Death Receptor-Initiated Apoptotic Signaling

Several TNF family receptors are known to transduce signals that result in apoptosis. These include TNFRSF1A (also known as CD120a and previously designated TNFR1), TNFRSF6 (also known as CD95, APO-1, or FAS), TNFRSF25 (also designated TRAMP and known as DR3 or APO3), TNFRSF10A (also known as DR4 or TRAIL-R1), and TNFRSF10B (also known as DR5 or TRAIL-R2). These receptors, also called death receptors, are characterized by the presence of a death domain within their cytoplasmic region, and have been shown to trigger apoptosis upon binding to their cognate ligands or specific agonist antibody.[301] The activating ligands for these death receptors are structurally related molecules that also belong to the TNF gene superfamily such as TNFSF6 (also known as Fas ligand), TNF, and TRAIL.

Ligation of death receptors produces receptor trimerization and formation of death-inducing signaling complex (DISC). This is composed of TNFRSF6, FADD (Fas [TNFRSF6]-associated via death domain), and procaspase 8, an apical signaling complex that mediates receptor-induced apoptosis. FADD binds directly to FasR, TNFRSF10A or TNFRSF10B, and indirectly to TNFRSF1A via TRADD (TNFRSF1A-associated via death domain protein). FADD is essential for cell death signaling from all three receptors. FADD interacts through its C-terminal death domain to cross-link TNFRSF6, TNFRSF10A, or TNFRSF10B receptors and recruits procaspase 8 and procaspase 10, or TRADD, through its N-terminal death effector domain to the DISC (Fig. 56–8). Oligomerization of caspase 8 within the DISC results in a high local concentration of the zymogen. The induced proximity under these crowded conditions generates low levels of intrinsic proteolytic activity of caspase 8, enough to allow the various proenzyme molecules to mutually cleave each other.[302] Processing of caspase 8 removes the DED-

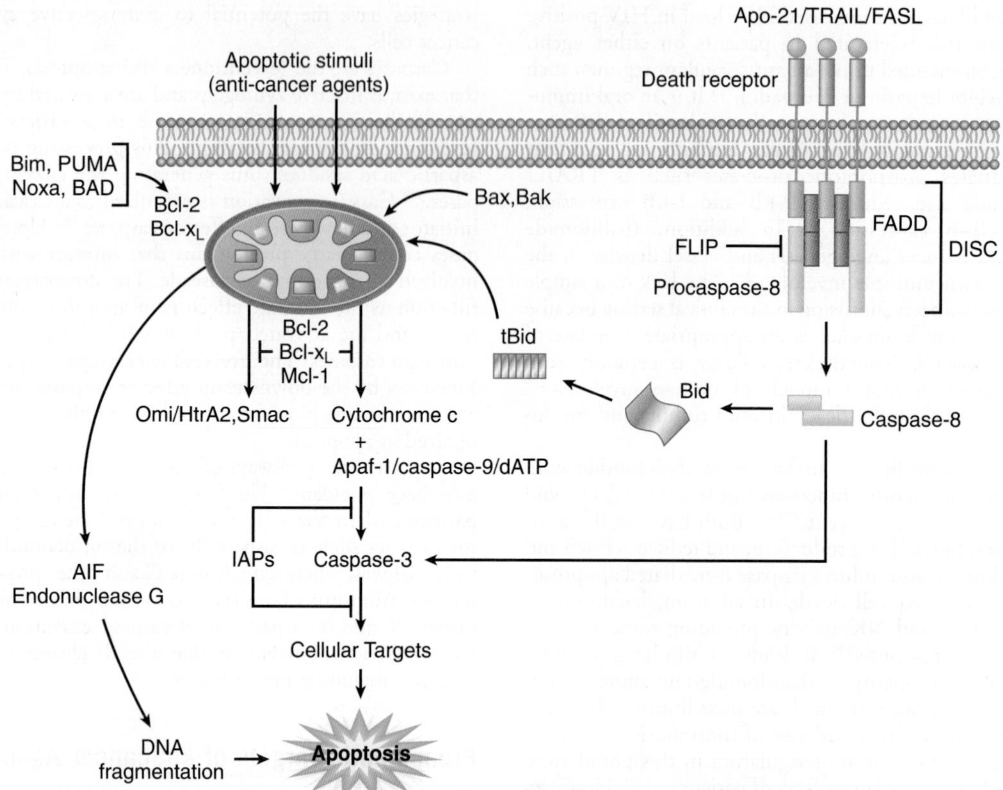

Figure 56–8 Schematic representation of apoptotic pathways.

containing prodomain, thus releasing the activated protease into the cytosol, where it can cleave and activate other downstream procaspases. In certain types of cells (type I), enough caspase 8 is activated by the activation of the death receptor to cause apoptosis. In other cell types, such as hepatocytes (type II), a high level of caspase 8 activation is not achieved and the apoptotic signal is amplified by the mitochondrial pathway.[303] The active caspase 8 cleaves the cytosolic p22Bid into a BH3-only domain containing, proapoptotic, truncated p15 tBid fragment, which translocates to the mitochondria and triggers the release of cyt c into the cytosol.[304] Recently, cleavage by caspase 8 has been shown to cause exposure of a glycine residue on p15Bid that is myristoylated, thereby targeting p15 Bid to the mitochondria.[305] Thus, N-myristoylation acts as an activating switch that enhances tBid-induced release of cyt c and apoptosis. The ability to cleave Bid may not be limited to caspase 8. Other caspases, such as caspase 3, as well another proteases, such as Granzyme B and lysosomal proteases, have been shown to activate Bid.[304] This indicates that Bid probably serves to amplify the caspase cascade rather than to initiate it (Fig. 56–8).

The Fas ligation has also been shown to initiate an alternative pathway to apoptosis, involving activation of c-Jun N-terminal kinase/stress-activated protein kinase (JNK/SAPK).[306,307] After ligation, Fas recruits an adaptor protein called Daxx that interacts with the apoptosis signal-regulating kinase 1 (ASK1), activating the transcription factors AP-1 and ATF-2. Once activated, ASK-1 launches a phosphorylation cascade that culminates in the activation of c-Jun N-terminal kinase (JNK).[308] Activated JNK phosphorylates substrates such as c-Jun, p53, and a pro-death Bcl-2 member Bim.[309] This, in turn, has been shown to trigger the mitochondrial or death-receptor-initiated apoptotic signaling.[310]

Mitochondria-Initiated Apoptotic Signaling

Mitochondria sequester a potent cocktail of proapoptotic proteins. These proteins promote apoptosis either by activating caspases, for example, by cyt c, or by inducing DNA fragmentation, for example, by endonuclease G or apoptosis-inducing factor (AIF), or by neutralizing cytosolic inhibitors of apoptosis or IAPs, for example, by SMAC or Omi/HtrA2.[311,312] On induction of apoptosis, unlike other pro-apoptotic proteins, mitochondrial AIF translocates to the nucleus to induce DNA fragmentation and apoptosis. Cyt c is a well-known component of the mitochondria electron transfer chain. Cyt c is released from the mitochondria during apoptosis. After release into the cytosol, cyt c binds to Apaf-1 (Apoptosis activating factor), a cytosolic adapter protein that contains a caspase recruitment domain (CARD), a nucleotide-binding domain, and multiple WD-40 repeats. Binding of cyt c to Apaf-1 increases its affinity for dATP or ATP by approximately 10-fold. It also triggers the oligomerization of Apaf-1 into a multimeric Apaf-1/cyt c complex, also called the apoptosome. This exposes the CARD domain of Apaf-1, which recruits several molecules of procaspase 9, inducing their autoactivation. Only the caspase 9 bound to the apoptosome is able to efficiently cleave and activate downstream executioner caspase, caspase 3.

Smac/DIABLO is a 25-kd mitochondrial protein that is released from mitochondria into the cytosol during apoptosis.[313] Smac contains mitochondria-targeting sequence at its N-terminus. This sequence is removed on import into the mitochondria, generating the mature Smac protein. In the mitochondria-initiated and common effector pathways of apoptosis, the processing and proteolytic activity of caspase 9 followed by caspases 3 and 7 are inhibited by the IAP (inhibitor of apoptosis) family of proteins.[314] IAP family members include XIAP, cIAP1, cIAP2, and survivin. All IAPs contain at least one BIR domain, although some contain three. Another region, the RING domain, has ubiquitin ligase activity and promotes the self-degradation of IAPs through the proteasomes in response to some apoptotic stimuli.[315] Furthermore, during Fas death receptor-mediated apoptosis, XIAP is cleaved by activated caspase 3 into the amino-terminal BIR1 and 2 and BIR3-RING finger fragments.[313] BIR3 domain binds and sequesters the monomeric and inactive caspase 9, thereby inhibiting its activation.[316] Overexpression of XIAP inhibits anticancer drug (including Ara-C)-induced caspase activity and apoptosis.[317] In contrast, downregulation of XIAP sensitizes cancer cells to apoptosis induced by chemotherapeutic drugs.[318] The antiapoptotic activity of NF-κB has also been shown to be mediated by the induction of IAPs.[319] The first four amino acids of the mature Smac, Ala-Val-Pro-Ile (AVPI) binds to the BIR (baculovirus repeat) domain of IAP (inhibitor of apoptosis protein) proteins.[320] The four amino acids (AVPI) of Smac that bind to the BIR3 domain of XIAP are similar to the XIAP-binding sequence of active caspase 9. In addition, Smac has also been shown to form a stable complex with the BIR2 domain of XIAP. Smac binds to the linker-BIR2 domain and presumably disrupts its inhibition of the active caspase 3 and caspase 7 by steric hindrance. On induction of apoptosis, another mitochondrial protein, Omi/HtrA2 (a serine protease), is released from the mitochondria and can induce caspase-independent cell death.[321] Additionally, like Smac, the mature Omi protein contains a conserved IAP-binding motif (AVPS) at its N-terminus. Omi complexes with XIAP at high stoichiometry and promotes apoptosis by neutralizing the caspase-inhibitory effect of XIAP. Recently, Omi has also been shown to process XIAP and promote its proteasomal degradation.[322]

The Bcl-2 family of proteins is divided into three subfamilies.[323] Members of the subfamily that includes Bcl-2, Bcl-x_L, and Mcl-1 inhibit apoptosis (Fig. 56–8). The Bax subfamily members that promote apoptosis including Bax and Bak share with Bcl-2 three of the four Bcl-2 homology domains, BH1 to BH3.[324] A C-terminus hydrophobic tail is responsible for the localization of these proteins to the outer membranes of the mitochondria and endoplasmic reticulum. The third BH3-only subfamily of proteins that includes Bid, Bim, and Bad also promotes apoptosis by binding and inactivating pro-survival Bcl-2 family members.[325,326] The prosurvival Bcl-2 family members, to a variable degree, are bound to the membranes of the mitochondria, endoplasmic reticulum (ER), and the nuclear envelope. Recent studies have shown that, in the event of an apoptotic stimulus, BH3-only proteins require Bax and Bak to trigger mitochondrial apoptotic signaling.[324–326] For example, the exposed BH3 domain of tBid oligomerizes with Bak and Bax, causing their mitochondrial membrane insertion and cyt c release. In response to apoptotic stimuli, Bax and Bak undergo conformational change and form membrane-associated homooligomers, disrupting the outer membrane of the mitochondria and ER and releasing the pro-death molecules into the cytosol. Besides tBid, Humanin peptide has been shown to activate Bax. Bcl-2 can block these events involving Bax activation by titrating tBid or Bim and/or heterodimerization with Bax and preventing mitochondrial permeabilization.[327]

Induction of $P53^{wt}$ in cells triggers apoptosis by transcriptional activation of pro-death effectors, including Bax, Noxa, Puma, Apaf-1 and DR5 and by transcriptional repression of Bcl-2 and IAPs. P53-dependent apoptosis has also been shown to occur in the absence of any gene transcription or translation.[328] In response to apoptotic stimulus such as irradiation, p53 translocates to the mitochondria, where it directly induces permeabilization of the outer membrane by forming complexes with the protective Bcl-2, resulting in the release of cyt c into the cytosol.[329] The E2F transcription factor, normally restrained by the Rb tumor suppressor to inhibit cell proliferation, has been shown to induce apoptosis though p53-dependent and p53-independent mechanisms.[330] These mechanisms include transcriptional activation of ARF (the alternate reading frame product of the INK4a/ARF tumor suppressor locus) or p73 (a member of the p53 family), repression of Mcl-1, and inducing the levels of caspase proenzymes.[331,332]

Selective Antitumor Agents or Strategies

BCL2 Family of Proteins as Targets for Anticancer Drug Design

The antiapoptotic protein BCL2 was originally identified through involvement in the t(14;18) chromosomal translocation found in human follicular lymphoma.[333] Since this elucidation, overexpression of BCL2 has been shown in both hematologic and solid malignancies and mediates resistance to traditional chemotherapeutic agents, radiation, and other antitumor treatments (Table 56–4).[334]

Table 56–4 Effectors of Apoptosis Pathways as Targets for Cancer Therapy

Receptor-Mediated Pathway	Mitochondrial Pathway Targets or Agents
At the death receptors:	Antisense oligos to BCL2 (Genasense)
TNFSF10	BH3 mimetic (peptides)
Anti-DR5 and anti-DR4 Antibodies	BCL2/BCL2L1 small molecule Antagonists
CDDO	Tea polyphenols

Bcl-2 Antisense

Initial efforts to construct antisense deoxyoligonucleotides (ASODN) evolved from Reed.[334] Liposomal antisense Bcl-2 oligonucleotide (Bcl-ASODN) has been shown to cause apoptosis in many types of cancer and leukemia. Bcl-2-ASODN also sensitized tumor cells in vitro and in vivo to chemotherapeutic drugs.[335,336] Thus far the most promising agent to target Bcl-2 is Genasense (oblimersan sodium; G3139), an 18-mer phosphorothioate oligodeoxynucleotide antisense compound. Clinical studies suggest safety and efficacy in solid and hematologic malignancies. In a recent phase III trial, 241 patients were randomly assigned to receive oblimersan 3 mg/kg/day as a 7-day continuous infusion in addition to fludarabine/cyclophosphamide versus fludarabine/cyclophosphamide. This study met its primary objective by demonstrating a significantly superior complete remission or nodular partial remission (CR/nPR) (17% vs 7%; $P = 0.025$); however, no significant differences in overall response rates as well as time to progression were found.[337] Similar results of another phase III study were reported when the addition of oblimersan to high-dose dexamethasone did not improve overall survival or time to progression in myeloma patients.[338]

BH3 Peptide/Mimetics or Bcl-2/Bcl-xL Small-Molecule Antagonists

Another strategy to create Bcl-2 inhibitors has focused on developing small molecules that mimic the action of the endogenous Bcl-2-binding death agonists. Compounds that mimic the BH3-only class of death agonists such as Bad inhibit the survival proteins Bcl-2 and Bcl-x_L but do not appear to have independent proapoptotic activity. Degterev et al identified two classes of novel small molecule cell-permeable inhibitors of the Bcl-x_L-BH3 domain (BH3I). Their studies demonstrated that BH3Is induce apoptosis by preventing BH3 domain-mediated interaction between proapoptotic and antiapoptotic members of Bcl-2 family.[339] Two natural products have been suggested to antagonize the antiapoptotic function of Bcl-2 or Bcl-x_L. Tetrocarcin A was reported to inhibit mitochondrial functions of Bcl-2 and suppress its antiapoptotic activity.[340] In another report, Antimycin-A was shown to mimic activity of BH3 peptides and selectively induce apoptosis in cell lines overexpressing Bcl-x_L.[341] Certain green tea catechins and black tea theaflavins were identified as potent inhibitors (K_i in the nanomolar range) of the antiapoptotic Bcl-2 family of proteins.[342] On the basis of the high-resolution three-dimensional structure of the target receptor, small organic molecules that bind to this interface have been designed. One of the newly designed BH3 mimetics, ABT-737, binds to Bcl-2, Bcl-xL, and Bcl-w with high affinity ($K_i < 1$ nM) but not to Mcl-1.[343] Preclinical data demonstrate cytotoxic activity in B lymphoid tumor cell lines, human follicular lymphoma, myeloma, and CLL as well as synergism with other chemotherapy agents.[343,344] Also, ABT-737 effectively kills

AML blast, progenitor, and stem cells without disturbing normal hematopoietic cell development.[345] Obatoclax (GX15-070) has demonstrated binding to multiple antiapoptotic Bcl-2 members including Mcl-1.[346] As a single agent, GX15-070, induces cytotoxic responses against patient-derived myeloma cells. Combination studies with melphalan, dexamethasone, and bortezomib have also shown promise in myeloma and mantle cell lymphoma cell lines.[346,347]

Apo-2L/TRAIL

Although TRAIL is a member of the TNF family, differences exist between TRAIL and other major death ligands, including TNF-α and FasL. Unlike Fas, whose expression is limited to certain tissues, TRAIL receptors are widely expressed. In a study by LeBlanc and Ashkenazi, soluble TRAIL induced apoptosis in a variety of leukemia and solid tumor cell types.[302] In contrast, normal tissues including prostate, colon, fibroblasts, and smooth muscle cells were unaffected by exposure to TRAIL; however, TNF or FasL induced fulminant liver damage. Also, in vivo studies indicate that TRAIL interacts synergistically with both chemotherapy and radiation, as well as inducing apoptosis regardless of p53 status.[302]

Clinical Studies

In two phase I clinical studies, PRO1762 (rhApo2L) demonstrated antitumor activity in both solid and hematologic malignancies. Patients received PRO1762 for 5 consecutive days every 3 weeks up to 8 cycles at doses of 0.5 to 15 mg/kg. Following 586 administered doses, no dose-limiting toxicities or clearly attributable toxicities have been noted. In 32 of 51 patients, posttreatment tumor assessment was reported to show 17 (53%) with stable disease and 13 (41%) with progression. Maximum concentrations (C_{max}) achieved at doses greater than 4 mg/kg were equivalent or greater to preclinical models. Hepatic metastases did not appear to influence pharmacokinetics. Enrollment continues for further dose optimization.[348,349]

Anti-DR5 or Anti-DR Receptor Antibodies

Evidence suggests that decoy receptors TRAIL-3 and TRAIL-4 interfere with TRAIL-induced apoptosis, leading to proliferation and survival signals.[350] Therefore, specific targeting of DR4 and DR5 with a specific agonistic antibody may have an advantage as a result of selective binding and activation of death receptors without interaction of decoy receptors. Three fully human monoclonal antibodies are under development: HGS-ETR1 (mapatumumab; anti-DR4), HGS-ETR2 (anti-DR5), and HGS-TR2J (anti-DR5).[351]

Clinical Studies

In one phase II study, 40 patients with relapsed or refractory NHL received HGS-ETR1 divided into two treatment groups: 3 mg/kg every 21 days (8 patients) or 10 mg/kg (32 patients) every 21 days for 6 cycles.[352] All three patients with follicular lymphoma had a clinical response (1 CR, 2 PR). Additionally, 12 of 40 patients (30%) had stable disease, whereas the remainder had progressive disease at the time of first evaluation. Patients tolerated therapy well with no reported discontinuations due to drug toxicity. Results of two phase I studies administering HGS-ETR2 in solid malignancies have been presented, HGS-TR2J is currently being evaluated in phase I trials.

Neutralization of IAPs by Smac Mimics

The N-terminal tetra- or heptapeptide in Smac reverses inhibition of caspase 9 by XIAP. It also promotes the proteolytic activation of procaspase 3 and the enzymatic activity of mature caspase 3.[353] Consistent with this, human acute leukemia cells show that the ectopic overexpression of the full-length Smac or treatment with N-terminus Smac tetrapeptide enhances Apo-2L/TRAIL-induced effector caspase activity and apoptosis.[354] A recent report demonstrated that Bax-dependent release of Smac, not cyt c from mitochondria, mediates the mitochondrial involvement in Apo-2L/TRAIL-induced apoptosis.[355] These findings suggest that the cytosolic Smac or its N-terminus peptide may bypass Bcl-2 or Bcl-x_L inhibition and promote caspase 3 activation by Apo-2L/TRAIL. Low-molecular-weight Smac mimetic compounds with high affinity for the BIR3 domain of IAPs have been developed.[284,356] In human myeloma xenograft models, a novel Smac mimetic, LBW242, inhibits tumor growth even in the presence of myeloma growth factors such as IL-6 and IGF-1.[357] Like Smac, Omi (through its N-terminal AVPS motif) binds and neutralizes XIAP, thereby potentiating the caspase-dependent pathway of apoptosis. Omi has also been shown to induce cell death via its serine protease activity, independent of caspases Apaf-1 or IAPs.[322] Hence, treatment with Omi peptide may be effective against tumors in which Apaf-1 is not expressed because of promoter-based hypermethylation and gene silencing. A second- generation ASODN (AEG35156/GEM460) against XIAP has demonstrated significant antitumor activity and is currently in phase I studies in combination with cytarabine/idarubicin in the treatment of leukemia.[358]

Survivin

Survivin is a 16-kd protein that contains a single BIR domain, followed by a C-terminal, long α-helical region that is required for its binding to the microtubules in the mitotic spindle. Survivin is phosphorylated on Thr34 by CDK1-cyclin B1, and survivin levels and activity increase during G_2/M phase in a cell-cycle-dependent manner. Overexpression of survivin inhibits caspase activity and apoptosis induced by Fas, Bax, and anticancer drugs.[359] Overexpression of survivin has been shown in various cancers and is not expressed in normal terminally differentiated tissue. Survivin expression has also been correlated with poor clinical outcome in AML and other cancers.[360] These observations have made survivin an attractive target for new therapies. The first targeted antagonist of survivin was an ASODN reported in 1999.[361] Preclinical data of ASODN (LY2181308) has demonstrated caspase 3-dependent apoptosis, cell-cycle arrest at G2/M, and sensitization to chemotherapy-induced apoptosis.[361–363] Owing to these encouraging results, phase I clinical studies have been started for LY2181308. In addition to ASODN, other therapeutic strategies that target survivin include gene therapy, siRNA, hammerhead ribozymes, gene therapy, and immunotherapy.[364]

Cyclin-Dependent Kinase Inhibitors as Therapeutic Targets

Orderly progression through the cell cycle is regulated by the coordinate expression of a variety of genes and proteins. In a commonly accepted model of cell-cycle regulation, the decision of a cell to progress through the cell cycle is determined by the activity of cyclins, levels of which fluctuate throughout the cell-cycle traverse, cyclin-dependent kinases (eg, CDKs 1-9), and several endogenous small molecule CDK inhibitors (eg, $p21^{CIP1}$, $p27^{KIP1}$, and $p57^{KIP2}$) (see Fig. 56–1). In general, CDK1, in association with cyclins A and B, is involved in G_2M progression, whereas CDK2, CDK4, and CDK6, in association with A, D, and E, are involved in G_1S progression.[365] Activation of CDKs results in phosphorylation of the retinoblastoma protein (PRB), which leads to its dissociation from the E2F transcription factor. Once freed, E2F triggers the transcription of diverse genes involved in cell-cycle progression (thymidylate synthase and dihydrofolate reductase, among numerous others).[366] Endogenous small-molecule inhibitors such as $P21^{CIP1}$ and $P27^{KIP1}$ bind stoichiometrically to CDKs and inhibit their activity.[367] Activity of CDKs can also be regulated through inhibitory phosphorylations of these proteins (eg, on threonine 14 or tyrosine 15 residues) or, conversely, activating phosphorylations on threonine 160 or 161 (mediated by CDK5 or cyclin-dependent activating kinase [CAK]). Interference with the activation of CDKs results in dephosphorylation of PRB, leading in turn to binding and inactivation of E2F and inhibition of cell-cycle progression.

Cell-cycle dysregulation is a cardinal characteristic of cancer in general,[368] and hematopoietic malignancies in particular. A classic example of this phenomenon is the regular association of increased expression of cyclin D_1 in mantle cell lymphoma.[369] Regulation of the cell cycle has been found to be closely related to apoptosis. Disruption of the cell-cycle traverse has been shown to be a potent cell death stimulus in a wide variety of neoplastic cell types, including those of hematopoietic origin. A corollary of this observation is that agents that interfere with the cell cycle, in addition to blocking cell-cycle progression, can be potent inducers of programmed cell death. For these reasons, inhibitors of the cell cycle have become logical targets for therapeutic intervention in hematologic and other malignancies. Cell-cycle inhibitors can be subdivided into several categories. For example, they can act directly, as in the case of CDK inhibitors, or indirectly, as in the case of histone deacetylase inhibitors, compounds that block cell-cycle progression by inducing endogenous cell-cycle inhibitors such as $P21.^{CIP1}$ The latter agents are discussed later in this chapter. CDK inhibitors can also be classified as specific (ie, directed against a particular CDK, such as CDK2) or those that nonspecifically inhibit most CDKs (eg, flavopiridol). The development of cell-cycle inhibitors has primarily focused on CDK inhibitors, several of which have entered clinical trials in humans, including those involving hematopoietic malignancies. A brief summary of the status of CDK inhibitors, with an emphasis on hematologic malignancies, follows.

Flavopiridol

Flavopiridol (L86-8275) is a semisynthetic flavonoid derived from the Indian plant *rohitukine.* It was the first CDK inhibitor to enter clinical trials in humans.[370] Flavopiridol binds to the ATP-binding site of CDKs, resulting in reversible, competitive enzyme inhibition at concentrations of less than 100 nM. As noted earlier, flavopiridol is a relatively nonspecific CDK inhibitor and inhibits all CDKs, although it is less effective against CDK7. Flavopiridol induces G_1S or G_2M arrest, presumably a consequence of inhibition of CDK1 and CDK2.[371] flavopiridol may also act to block cell-cycle progression by downregulating cyclin D_1 levels or by inhibiting the CDK-activating complex (CDK7), or both.

In addition to blocking cell-cycle progression, flavopiridol has been shown to be a potent inducer of apoptosis in malignant hematopoietic cells (eg, acute and chronic leukemia) at low concentrations (eg, u100 nM).[372] Moreover, flavopiridol has shown activity against a variety of multiple myeloma cell types in vitro.

Recently, the proapoptotic actions of flavopiridol have been attributed to its capacity to inhibit the positive transcription elongation factor-β (PTEF-β), cyclin T/CDK9 complex by inhibiting phosphorylation of the carboxy-terminal domain of RNA polymerase II.[373] This leads to downregulation of several antiapoptotic proteins, including BIRC4, $P_{21}{}^{CIP1}$, and, in the case of multiple myeloma cells, Mcl-1.[374] flavopiridol has also recently been shown to block the antiapoptotic actions of the IAP family member survivin.[375]

In clinical studies, flavopiridol was initially administered as a 72-hour continuous infusion every 2 weeks, with a maximally tolerated dose of 40 mg/m^2. Steady-state plasma levels in excess of those necessary to inhibit CDKs and induce apoptosis in leukemia cells (eg, 350 nM) were achieved.[376] Dose-limiting toxicities were fatigue, diarrhea, nausea, and myelosuppression. However, the occurrence of thromboembolic phenomena and the general lack of single-agent activity have limited enthusiasm for administering flavopiridol by this schedule. More recently, flavopiridol has been administered as a daily IV bolus for 1, 3, or 5 days every 3 weeks with manageable toxicity, and other schedules are being examined,[377] including a hybrid schedule with half the dose administered as an IV bolus and the other half as a more prolonged infusion. When administered as a daily bolus infusion for 3 days every 3 weeks, flavopiridol exhibited modest activity in patients with mantle-cell lymphoma.[378] Very recently, a novel pharmacologically directed schedule of flavopiridol has been developed in which half of the dose (eg, 30 mg/m^2) is administered as a 30-minute bolus loading infusion and 30 mg/m^2 as a 4-hour infusion.[379] In a phase I study, objective response rates of 45% were obtained with this schedule in patients with progressive CLL, including some with high-risk disease. Because of the rapidity of response, particularly in patients with high white blood cell counts, aggressive measures designed to avoid tumor lysis syndrome (eg, hydration, alkalinization of the urine, administration of rasburicase) is advisable. Efforts are now underway to employ this novel flavopiridol schedule in combination with other agents, and in other hematologic malignancies.

Because of limited single-agent activity, combination regimens involving flavopiridol are being explored in hematologic malignancies. On the basis of preclinical evidence of synergism with the antimetabolite ara-C, a regimen combining flavopiridol on a daily IV bolus schedule followed by high-dose ara-C has been initiated in patients with acute leukemia and has shown some activity.[380] In a successive phase II study, flavopiridol was administered as a 1-hour bolus infusion of 50 mg/m^2 daily × 3 days prior to administration of high-dose ara-C (day 6) and mitoxantrone (day 9). Complete response rates of more than 50% were obtained in patients with high-risk AML.[381] More recently, evidence of synergism between flavopiridol and other signal transduction modulators has become the focus of considerable attention. For example, the observation that flavopiridol interacts synergistically with imatinib mesylate in CML cells, including some that are imatinib mesylate resistant,[207] has prompted the initiation of a phase I trial of flavopiridol and imatinib mesylate in patients with progressive BCR-ABL$^+$ hematologic malignancies. Evidence that flavopiridol interacts synergistically with histone deacetylase and proteasome inhibitors in human leukemia cells has appeared,[382,383] and clinical trials combining flavopiridol with the histone deacetylase inhibitor vorinostat or the proteasome inhibitor bortezomib in patients with refractory AML/MDS and multiple myeloma/indolent non-Hodgkin lymphoma are currently underway.

UCN-01

UCN-01 (7-hydroxystaurosporine) was originally developed as a selective PKC inhibitor but was subsequently shown to exert multiple other activities that may be more closely related to its antiproliferative and lethal effects. For example, UCN-01 broadly inhibits CDKs at submicromolar concentrations and arrests cells in G_1S.[384] Recently, UCN-01 has been shown to be a potent inhibitor of the CHEK1 (also known as CHK1) kinase at low (eg, <100 nM) concentrations[385] and as a result an abrogator of both the G_2M and G_1S checkpoints.[163,386] By inhibiting CHEK1, UCN-01 blocks phosphorylation of the cd25C phosphatase, thereby sparing it from proteasomal degradation. This leads in turn to activation of p34cdc2 as a consequence of inhibition of an inhibitory phosphorylation on tyrosine 15.[387] More recently, UCN-01 has been found to be an inhibitor of the PDK1 and AKT kinases,[388] important components of a pathway that exerts multiple antiapoptotic functions.

In preclinical studies, UCN-01 has been shown to induce apoptosis in both myeloid and lymphoid leukemia cells through a process associated with activation of CDK1 and CDK2. In addition, UCN-01 interacts synergistically with various DNA-damaging agents in both hematopoietic and nonhematopoietic cells. For example, antileukemic synergism between UCN-01 and ara-C or fludarabine has been observed in several human leukemia cell lines.[367–369] An interesting recent development is the finding that exposure of human hematopoietic cells to UCN-01 results in activation of the MEK1/2/ERK1/2 pathway, and that inhibition of this process (eg, by pharmacologic MEK inhibitors) results in a dramatic increase in apoptosis. For example, highly synergistic interactions between the MEK inhibitor

PD184352 (CI-1040) and UCN-01 have been observed in human leukemic and myeloma cells.[389,390] Antileukemic synergism between UCN-01 and the HSPCA (also known as Hsp90) antagonist 17-AAG has also been reported.[391]

Initial clinical trials of UCN-01 involved a 72-hour continuous infusion schedule every 2 weeks. Dose-limiting toxicities included nausea, vomiting, hypotension, hyperglycemia, and pulmonary toxicity. The recommended phase II dose was 37 to 42 mg/m²/day for this schedule.[392] Unexpectedly, UCN-01 was found to have an extremely long half-life owing to prolonged binding to plasma 1 acidic glycoprotein. Nevertheless, free UCN-01 levels were achievable that exceeded those necessary to inhibit CHEK1 (eg, 75–100 nM). Subsequently, the regimen was modified so that following the first dose, subsequent doses were administered for 36 rather than 72 hours. To date, single-agent UCN-01 has shown some activity in patients with NHL.[393] More recently, a 3-hour infusional schedule has shown promise in maintaining high plasma levels of free UCN-01.[394]

In view of evidence of synergism between UCN-01 and DNA-damaging agents, several combination regimens are currently undergoing evaluation in patients with hematologic malignancies. A phase I trial of UCN-01 and ara-C was initiated in patients with refractory acute leukemia but was placed on hold secondary to the occurrence of cardiovascular toxicity. Trials combining UCN-01 with either gemcitabine or fludarabine are currently ongoing in patients with lymphoid malignancies (eg, CLL and NHL). Based in part on preclinical evidence of synergism,[395] a trial of UCN-01 and perifosine in patients with refractory leukemia has been initiated. Finally, newer Chk1 inhibitors (eg, AZD7762) with potentially superior pharmacokinetic characteristics than UCN-01 have recently entered the clinic.

CYC202

Roscovitine is a purine analog CDK inhibitor that is primarily active against CDK1, CDK2, and CDK5.[396] CYC202 is the R-enantiomer of roscovitine. In preclinical studies, CYC202 was found to induce cell-cycle arrest (in G1) and apoptosis in several tumor types. It also displayed significant activity in a human colorectal carcinoma xenograft model.[397] In malignant hematopoietic cells (ie, multiple myeloma), CYC202 lethality has been closely correlated with Mcl-1 downregulation via a transcriptional mechanism.[398]

Phase I trials of CYC202 have recently been initiated in humans. Two schedules have been examined: (a) daily by mouth for 7 days, repeating every 21 days, and (b) twice daily for 5 days, repeating every 21 days, with the duration of administration increasing in the second phase of the trial. Toxicities for both schedules include nausea, vomiting, skin rashes, and hypokalemia. Maximum tolerated doses have not yet been reached.[399,400] Very recently, a schedule of CYC202 twice daily × 7 days every 21 days has been shown to be tolerable.[401]

Currently, little information is available at either the preclinical or clinical level concerning the activity of CYC202 in hematologic malignancies. However, given the susceptibility of malignant hematopoietic cells to CDK inhibitor-mediated apoptosis, a possible role for CYC202 in malignant hematopoietic disorders warrants further investigation.

BMS 387032

BMS 387032 is a small-molecule CDK inhibitor discovered through high-throughput screening that is primarily active against CDK2.[402] In preclinical studies, BMS 387032 has shown potent antiproliferative activity against ovarian and breast cancer cells in vitro.[403] As is the case with other CDK inhibitors, BMS 387032 induces cell-cycle arrest, PRB dephosphorylation, and, under some circumstances, apoptosis. One issue that will have to be addressed in the case of BMS 387032 is the implications of findings suggesting that at least in some tumor cell lines, CDK2 may be dispensable for cell-cycle progression.[404]

Several phase I trials of BMS 387032 have been initiated. BMS 387032 has been administered as either a 24-hour or 1-hour infusion every 3 weeks.[405,406] Dose levels of 4 to 59 mg/m² have proved to be tolerable; the maximum tolerated dose for either of these schedules has not been reached. Toxicities have been mild and include rash, nausea and vomiting, diarrhea, and fatigue. A limited number of responses have been noted in patients with solid tumors, and combination trials are planned for the future.

As in the case of CYC202, the activity of BMS 387032 in hematologic malignancies has not yet been established. Nevertheless, based on the theoretical considerations cited earlier, BMS 387032 deserves evaluation in these disorders.

Farnesyltransferase Inhibitors

RAS proteins represent low-molecular-weight proteins that bind GTP and are located at the cell membrane. They are critically involved in the regulation of signal transduction pathways implicated in the control of cell proliferation, differentiation, and survival.[407] One of the key effectors of RAS proteins is the serine-threonine kinase RAF1, which is recruited to the cell membrane by activated RAS, and in turn activates the survival/proliferation-associated kinases MEK1/2 (mitogen-activated kinase 1/2) and ERK (extracellular signal-regulating kinase).[408] RAS is also involved in regulation of the AKT pathway, which exerts multiple antiapoptotic functions.[409]

There are four separate RAS proteins: H-RAS, N-RAS, K-RAS4A, and K-RAS4B. Of these, H-RAS mutations are most commonly encountered in hematopoietic malignancies (ie, myeloid leukemia).[409] Because of the frequency of RAS mutations in human neoplasia and the importance of RAS downstream targets (eg, RAF1/MEK/ERK and AKT) in the survival of neoplastic cells, the RAS pathway has become a logical target for therapeutic intervention.

To function, Ras must be localized to the cell membrane. This in turn requires posttranslational modifications of the RAS protein, most notably farnesylation. This primarily involves addition of a 15-carbon isoprenoid farnesol to the C terminus of RAS following recognition of a CAAX motif. This process is catalyzed by the enzyme farnesyl transferase. Inhibitors of farnesyl transferase (FTIs) thus block RAS farnesylation, preventing the protein from associating with the plasma membrane and subsequently participating in downstream signaling events.[410]

Initial preclinical studies suggested that FTIs inhibited the proliferation and survival of several tumors driven by RAS mutations. However, it soon became clear that tumors with H-RAS mutations were more sensitive to FTIs than those with N-Ras or K-RAS mutations.[375] Furthermore, the antiproliferative effects of FTIs did not always correlate well with their effects on RAS farnesylation or the presence of Ras mutations. Two possible explanations may account for these findings. First, alternative prenylation events, for example, geranyl-geranylation of the RAS protein may also promote its membrane localization, particularly in cells bearing N-RAS or K-RAS mutations, and could theoretically confer resistance to FTI lethality. Second, several other non-RAS candidate proteins have been identified in which interference with farnesylation might contribute to FTI-associated lethality. These include small GTPases (eg, RHO family members) and a variety of nuclear proteins (eg, CENP-E and CENP-F).[411]

To date, four FTIs have undergone extensive clinical evaluation: R115777, BMS-214662, L-778, 123, and SCH 66336.

R115777

R115777 (Zarnestra) is an orally active FTI that has undergone extensive evaluation in patients with solid tumors and hematologic malignancies. In patients with hematologic malignancies, the generally accepted dose and schedule is 600 mg/m² orally twice daily for

21 days repeated at monthly intervals or for 28 days repeated at 6-week intervals. Dose-limiting toxicities include myelosuppression, nausea, vomiting, diarrhea, rash, neurotoxicity, and fatigue. In a series of phase I and II studies, promising activity has been observed in patients with AML, ALL, CML, and myelodysplastic syndrome. For example, in one study, 6 of 22 patients with CML achieved complete or partial responses, and 2 of 8 patients with myelofibrosis achieved objective responses.[412] In a phase I trial of R115777 in patients with refractory or high-risk acute leukemia, an overall response rate of 29% was achieved.[413] Responses in patients with multiple myeloma have also been seen but have been modest.[414] Interestingly, blasts obtained from a number of leukemic patients who responded did not exhibit RAS mutations, suggesting that the lethal effects of R115777 may proceed, at least in part, through RAS-independent pathways.[414] On the basis of these promising initial results, several combination regimens involving R115777 in patients with hematologic malignancies are under development.

SCH 66336

SCH 66336 (lonafarib) is an orally active tricyclic FTI that inhibits farnesyltransferase at concentrations in the low nM range. In preclinical studies, it has demonstrated significant activity against a variety of solid tumor types, particularly those driven by H-RAS.[415] However, it has also shown preclinical activity in CML and ALL model systems.[416,417] Several phase I trials of SCH 66336 have been carried out in patients with solid tumor and hematologic malignancies. The maximally tolerated dose appears to be 200 to 300 mg/m^2 twice daily with nausea, vomiting, diarrhea, fatigue, and renal dysfunction representing the dose-limiting toxicities. Clinical responses were observed in 6 of 16 patients with CML, advanced myelodysplastic syndrome, CMML, AML, and ALL.[418] In phase II studies involving a schedule of 200 mg/m^2 twice daily, responses were observed in patients with MDS and high-risk AML.[419]

One particularly exciting development is the discovery that SCH 66336 interacts synergistically with the BCR/ABL kinase inhibitor imatinib mesylate to induce apoptosis in BCR/ABL$^+$ cells.[210] On the basis of such findings, a clinical trial has been initiated in which SCH 66336 is combined with imatinib mesylate in patients with progressive BCR/ABL$^+$ hematologic malignancies.

BMS-214662

BMS-214662 is a parenterally administered FTI that demonstrated impressive preclinical activity against a panel of solid tumor cell types, particularly those bearing H-RAS mutations.[420] In studies involving hematologic malignancies, the maximally tolerated dose was 118 mg/m^2 administered weekly.[421] Dose-limiting toxicities are similar to those of other FTIs. In one trial, reduction in the percentage of bone marrow blasts to less than 5% was observed in 18% of patients.[422] Interestingly, as in the case of R115777, responses have been noted in patients whose cells lacked RAS mutations.

Inhibitors of the RAF1/MEK/ERK Pathway

The MAPK (mitogen-activated protein kinase) pathways consist of three parallel serine-threonine kinase modules that are intimately involved in the control of cell survival, proliferation, and differentiation. Two of these, JUN N-terminal kinase (JNK) and p38 MAPK, are activated in response to environmental stresses including DNA damage and osmotic stress, whereas p42/44 MAPK (also known as ERK; extracellular signal-regulating kinase) is primarily induced by growth factors and other mitogenic stimuli.[423] Although exceptions exist, JNK and p38 MAPK primarily exert proapoptotic functions, whereas ERK activation is generally associated with cell survival.[424] The only well-defined activator of ERK is the serine-threonine kinase MEK1/2 (mitogen-activated protein kinase kinase 1/2), whereas numerous ERK targets have been identified, including ELK-1, CREB, BCL2, Bad, FRAP1 (also known as mTOR), and caspase 9 among numerous others. The activating effects of MEK1/2 on ERK are opposed by phosphatases that dephosphorylate and inactivate the enzyme (eg, MAP kinase phosphatase 1/2 [MKP1/2]).[425]

The major activator of MEK1/2 is the serine-threonine kinase RAF, of which three forms exist: RAF1, B-RAF, and A-RAF. RAF can be activated by Ras (discussed earlier) as well as through various RAS-independent pathways, including PKC, KSR, as well as the SRC and JAK family of kinases among others.[426] The activation of RAF involves several processes, including recruitment to the plasma membrane, phosphorylation on serine and threonine residues, and dimerization. Interference with any of these processes can lead to inhibition of Raf activation as well as downstream targets.

Dysregulation of the RAF/MEK/ERK pathway has been observed in most hematopoietic malignancies, including acute leukemia, CLL, multiple myeloma, and lymphomas.[408,427] Consequently, there has been considerable interest in the development of pharmacologic inhibitors of the RAF/MEK/ERK pathway in these disorders. In addition to their potential intrinsic activity against malignant hematopoietic cells, there is evidence that such agents might also enhance the activity of conventional cytotoxic drugs.

Raf Inhibitors

Initial approaches to RAF inhibition focused on efforts to destabilize the protein. For example, geldanamycin and the related compound 17-AAG act as inhibitors of HSPCA, a chaperone protein necessary for Raf processing and stabilization. Interference with HSPCA results in destabilization and proteasomal degradation of RAF as well as numerous other proteins, including AKT.[428] Interestingly, mutant kinases appear to be particularly sensitive to 17-AAG-mediated degradation. For example, 17-AAG has been shown to be a highly effective inducer of BCR/ABL degradation and of induction of apoptosis in BCR/ABL$^+$ leukemic cells.[429] There have also been suggestions that 17-AAG-mediated Raf downregulation may contribute to lethality in such cells.[430] Based on these and other data, clinical trials combining 17-AAG and imatinib have been initiated in patients with refractory/progressive CML and related malignancies.

Oxime derivatives KF25706 and KF58333 also disrupt the RAF pathway through a mechanism similar to that of 17-AAG and geldanamycin, that is, destabilization of the RAF protein.[431] More recently, however, a Raf kinase inhibitor, BAY43-9006 (sorafenib), has been developed and has entered phase I and II clinical trials in humans.[432–434] Whether this compound, which has recently been approved for the treatment of renal cell carcinoma, acts primarily or solely as an RAF inhibitor is unclear, and its activity has been ascribed to "off-target actions," including inhibition of VEGF. In preclinical studies, induction of leukemic cell death by sorafenib has been shown to stem from inhibition of translation and downregulation of the short-lived antiapoptotic protein Mcl-1[435] and induction of endoplasmic reticulum stress.[436] Whether sorafenib will display significant activity in hematopoietic malignancies, either alone or in combination with other agents, remains to be determined. Phase II trials of sorafenib in chronic and acute leukemias, and in non-Hodgkin lymphoma are currently underway.

MEK1/2 Inhibitors

Several MEK1/2 inhibitors have been evaluated and have now entered clinical trials. The first of the MEK1/2 inhibitors to be developed was PD98059, a compound that binds to MEK1 and blocks its phosphorylation. PD98059 does not compete with ATP for binding to the enzyme. In preclinical studies, PD98059 has been shown to inhibit the proliferation of and induce apoptosis in leukemia and other malignant hematopoietic cell types.[437] Another MEK inhibitor is U0126, a compound whose mode of action appears to be similar to that of PD98059.[409,438]

Because these agents exhibit limited solubility, attempts have been made to develop alternative MEK1/2 inhibitors suitable for in vivo administration. One such agent, PD184352, has shown activity against human colon cancer cells in a murine xenograft model.[439] Phase I trials of PD184352 (designated CI-1040) have been initiated. However, CI-1040 has now been supplanted by other non-ATP competitive MEK1/2 inhibitors with superior pharmacokinetic characteristics, including PD325901 and AZD6244.[440] AZD6244 has recently shown activity in a multiple myeloma xenograft model.[441]

In addition to exerting antiproliferative effects toward human leukemia cells, MEK inhibitors also increase the lethality of conventional cytotoxic agents (eg, ara-C), resulting in synergistic interactions.[442] One particularly interesting finding is that MEK1/2 inhibitors appear to be very effective in enhancing the antileukemic potential of several novel molecularly targeted agents. For example, PD184352 has been shown to interact synergistically with imatinib in BCR/ABL$^+$ cells, including those resistant to imatinib as a result of increased BCR/ABL expression.[206] Similar findings have recently been observed in the case of the second-generation Bcr/Abl kinase inhibitor dasatinib.[437] In addition, as noted earlier, synergistic interactions between PD184352 and UCN-01 have been reported in human leukemia and myeloma cells,[383,390] and MEK1/2 inhibitors have been found to potentiate the antileukemic activity of small-molecule Bcl-2 antagonists.[437] Collectively, these findings raise the possibility that the ultimate role of MEK1/2 inhibitors in hematologic malignancies may be to enhance the activity of other targeted agents.

PI3K/AKT Inhibitors

The phosphoinositide-3 kinase (PI3K) /AKT (PKB) pathway is involved in the regulation of diverse cellular functions including cell growth, protein synthesis, cell-cycle regulation, glucose metabolism, and motility. PI3K catalyzes the conversion of phosphatidylinositol diphosphate to phosphatidylinositol triphosphate, which activates, through PDK1, the phosphorylation and activation of AKT.[443] The dual-specific phosphatase PTEN opposes the actions of PI3K, and is mutated in many cancers.[444] Activation of AKT signals to multiple downstream targets, generally resulting in prosurvival actions. Targets of AKT involve proteins involved in cell survival (eg, Bad, procaspase 9, CREB, forkhead transcription factors [FHKR], IB), cell-cycle regulation (p21^{CIP1}, p27^{KIP1}, cyclin D_1), glycogen synthesis (GSK3), and protein synthesis (FRAP1, p70^{S6K}).[445] Because of the frequency of PTEN mutations in transformed cells and the dependence of numerous cancers on an intact PI3K/AKT pathway for survival, the PI3K/AKT cascade has become an attractive target for therapeutic intervention.

There is evidence that dysregulation of the PI3K/AKT pathway is a key proliferative pathway in hematopoietic malignancies. For example, the fusion protein nucleophosmin/anaplastic large cell lymphoma (NP-ALK) constitutively activates the PI3K/AKT cascade and has been shown to play a functional role in NP-ALK-related transformation.[446] In addition, inhibitors of PI3K have been shown to be potent inducers of apoptosis in human leukemia and other malignant hematopoietic cells.

PI3K Inhibitors

The most widely used pharmacologic inhibitors of PI3K are the fungal metabolite wortmannin and the flavonoid derivative LY294002.[447] Both inhibit the ATP-binding site of PI3K and interfere with its activity at submicromolar concentrations. These agents are not completely specific for PI3K, however, and variably inhibit other kinases, for example, DNA-PK. Although these agents have shown in vitro and in vivo activity in preclinical model systems, including leukemia, poor pharmacokinetic properties and a relative lack of selectivity have limited their therapeutic potential. However, derivatives of these compounds are currently under development and may eventually prove to be of use in hematopoietic malignancies. For example, PI3K inhibitors such as PX-866 are either in or will shortly enter clinical trials.[448]

AKT Inhibitors

The approach to inhibition of the AKT pathway has focused on agents that act either directly or indirectly. The latter type of agent is exemplified by HSPCA antagonists such as 17-AAG, which disrupts HSPCA chaperone function and results in the degradation of client proteins. For example, downregulation/inactivation of AKT has been implicated in the lethal actions of 17-AAG in human breast cancer cells.[449] It has also been shown to be involved, at least in part, in the lethality of 17-AAG toward human leukemia cells.[430] Because HSPCA antagonists such as 17-AAG are so pleiotropic in their actions, it seems very likely that downregulation of proteins other than AKT (eg, RAF1, BCR/ABL) are involved in antileukemic actions.

The search for specific inhibitors of AKT as chemotherapeutic agents remains the subject of great interest. Although AKT kinase inhibitors have been described,[413] their activity in hematologic malignancies remains to be determined. Several newer agents have been described that appear to act by disrupting the membrane translocation of AKT, and in so doing, preventing its activation. Such agents include perifosine, an alkyl-lysophospholipid,[450] which has entered clinical trials in humans. In addition, novel phosphatidylinositol derivatives have been described that interfere with the activation of AKT, presumably through disruption of its membrane translocation.[451] In preclinical models, perifosine has shown promise in multiple myeloma.[452] The potential of these agents may lie not only in their intrinsic antitumor activity, but possibly as potentiators of cytotoxic drug action.

FRAP1 Inhibitors

FRAP1 (also known as mTOR; mammalian target of rapamycin) is a large (280-kd) serine-threonine kinase that belongs to the family of PI3K-related kinases.[453] A FRAP1-dependent, amino acid or growth factor-signaling pathway controls the initiation of protein translation in mammalian cells.[453,454] It is well recognized that growth factor signaling initiated through the receptor tyrosine kinases (RTKs) or due to the activity of cytosolic tyrosine kinases (TKs), such as BCR-ABL, results in the activation of the PI3K/AKT signaling.[455,456] AKT has been shown to phosphorylate and inactivate TSC2 (tuberous sclerosis 2; also known as tuberin), thereby disrupting its interaction with TSC1 (or hamartin) (Fig. 56–9).[457] Inhibition of TSC1-TSC2 complex de-represses RHEB, which is a small G protein that activates FRAP1.[458] When RHEB is in an active GTP-bound state, its localization to the membrane stimulates FRAP1-mediated phosphorylation of the downstream eukaryotic initiation factor 4E (eIF4E) binding protein 1 (4E-BP) and ribosomal protein S6 kinase 1 (S6K1) (1,2) (see Fig. 56–9). However, the association of FRAP1 with the 150-kd Raptor (regulatory associated protein of FRAP1) is necessary for the phosphorylation of 4E-BP and S6K1.[459,460] Both 4E-BP and S6K1 are involved in the initiation of cap-dependent mRNA translation. At their 5′ termini, the cellular mRNAs contain a cap structure (m7GpppN, where N is any nucleotide), which promotes the binding of the ribosome to the AUG initiation codon of the mRNA.[454] This function of the cap is mediated by the trimeric complex eIF4F that has three subunits, including eIF4A (with cofactor 4B), eIF4G, and eIF4E, which together help unwind the inhibitory secondary structure in the 5′ untranslated region (5′UTR) of the mRNAs.[454] The hypophosphorylated 4E-BP binds tightly to and inhibits 4E, resulting in the inhibition of 4E-dependent translation of cap-containing mRNA. In contrast, FRAP1-mediated phosphorylation of 4E-BP causes its dissociation from 4E, enabling the latter to participate in the cap-dependent translation of mRNAs. FRAP1-mediated phosphorylation and activation of S6K1 results in the

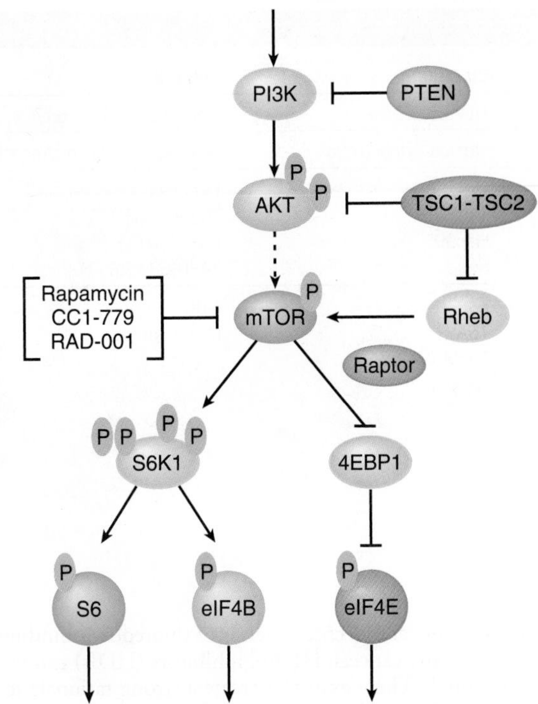

Figure 56–9 Rapamycin or its analogs inhibit mTOR and the downstream phosphorylation of S6K1 and 4EBP1, thereby attenuating the translation initiation of mRNAs with highly structured 5′UTR. Activation of the receptor (FLT-3) or cytosolic tyrosine kinase (eg, Bcr-Abl) can lead to increased activity of PI3K/AKT. Although it can directly phosphorylate mTOR, AKT activity inhibits the TSC1–TSC2 complex, thereby derepressing Rheb and activating mTOR. The phosphorylation and activation of S6K1, and phosphorylation and inactivation of 4E-BP through Raptor, results in the phosphorylation of S6, eIF4B, and eIF4E, which are involved in the cap-dependent translation of mRNAs with highly structured 5′URT.

phosphorylation of the ribosomal S6 protein and eIF4B (see Fig. 56–9).[454] AKT has also been shown to directly activate S6K1.[461] S6K1 activity is involved in regulating the translation of a group of mRNAs that have highly structured 5′UTR, including those mRNAs that have a 5′TOP (terminal oligopyrimidines, a stretch of 4–14 pyrimidines).[454] The presence of highly structured 5′UTR, including a 5′TOP, dictates a stringent translation regulation.[453,454] Therefore, it is clear that the increased activity of PI3K/AKT, either due to the upstream signaling through receptor or cytosolic TKs or the loss of the tumor suppressor phosphatase gene *PTEN*, results in the phosphorylation and activation of FRAP1 signaling.[462,463] This, through S6K1 and 4E-BP phosphorylation, enhances the translation of mRNAs with structured 5′UTR (eg, MYC and cyclin D_1) or 5′TOP (eg, ribosomal elongation factor 1a and poly [A] binding protein).[451,455]

Rapamycin is a lipophilic macrolide fungicide that binds intracellularly to a small ubiquitous protein termed FKBP12 (FK506-binding protein, molecular mass of 12 kd).[453,459,463] Rapamycin is known to possess antimicrobial, immunosuppressant, and antitumor activity.[463] Rapamycin-FKBP12 complex binds and inhibits FRAP1 and its downstream signaling through S6K1 and 4EBP.[453,459,463,464] Rapamycin has been shown to inhibit growth and induce apoptosis of cancer, leukemia, and lymphoma cells owing to its inhibitory effect on FRAP1 signaling and the downstream inhibition of the translation of mRNAs with a 5′TOP or complex secondary structure in their 5′UTRs, which are involved in cell proliferation.[464–467] It also blocks T-cell activation and has been proposed as an agent for the treatment of graft-versus-host disease. However, rapamycin has poor aqueous solubility and chemical stability, which has hampered its clinical development as an anticancer agent.[464] Recently, more soluble ester analogs of rapamycin, for example, CCI-779 (Wyeth Ayerst, PA) and RAD001 (Novartis Pharma, Basel, Switzerland), have been developed. Preclinical studies have shown that similar to rapamycin, these agents also inhibit phosphorylation of S6K1 and 4E-BP, resulting in cell-cycle G_1 phase arrest of a variety of cancer and leukemia cell types.[468,469] This is also associated with attenuation of cyclin D1 levels or upregulation of p27 and inhibition of cyclin A-dependent kinase activity.[470,471]

CCI-779 and RAD001 have been evaluated in phase I studies in patients with solid tumors.[464,472] The main toxicities have been skin rash, thrombocytopenia, and reversible deterioration in the liver function. Although partial responses have been observed in patients with renal and non-small-cell cancers, minor responses have been observed in NHLs. These studies suggest that the optimal therapeutic dose of CCI-779 may be lower than the maximal tolerated dose.[464] In a pharmacodynamic study in patients with renal cancer, inhibition of S6K1 activity in the peripheral blood mononuclear cells could be correlated with time to disease progression.[473] Phase I and II studies of these promising agents in the hematologic malignancies have not been carried out. In these studies, the dose selection could be guided by the pharmacodynamic end points in peripheral blood mononuclear cells. It is clearly important to investigate the clinical antitumor activity of FRAP1 inhibitors in hematologic malignancies that are dependent on FRAP1 signaling and/or its downstream effectors, including S6K1, MYC (eg, Burkitt lymphoma), and cyclin D (eg, mantle-cell lymphoma), for their growth and survival.[474,475] This may be due to upregulation of PI3K/AKT activity, as seen in malignancies with the loss of PTEN (eg, multiple myeloma) or due to increased activity of the upstream tyrosine kinase (eg, BCR-ABL, KIT, and FLT3).[455,475,476] There may also be merit in investigating whether cotreatment with FRAP1 inhibitors would enhance the activity of conventional cytotoxic agents. These studies will define the future role of FRAP1 inhibitors against hematologic malignancies.

Histone Deacetylase Inhibitors

Histone acetyl transferases control gene expression through the modification of chromatin structure through acetylation of chromatin-bound histones. Regulation of acetylation is through histone deacetylation. Without the ability to fine-tune histone binding to chromatin regions, gene expression is perturbed. Inhibition of this process by a group of agents termed histone deacetylation inhibitors alters gene expression in both normal and malignant cells. Often the result is differentiation of malignant cells or induction of apoptosis.

Posttranslational Histone and Nonhistone Protein Modifications and Gene Transcription

Nucleosomes are regularly repeating, structural units of chromatin, which are essential in packaging eukaryotic DNA. Each unit is composed of 146 base pairs of DNA tightly wrapped around a core histone octamer.[477] Each histone octamer consists of 2 units each of histones H2A, H2B, H3 and H4 and each nucleosome in turn is connected to its neighbor by a short segment of linker DNA, approximately 10 to 80 base pairs in length. Histone H1 binds and stabilizes linker DNA.[478] Each core histone has an amino (N) terminal tail, which is lysine rich and positively charged. Specific amino acid residues at the N-terminal undergo a variety of enzymatic posttranslational modifications.[479] Modifications can also occur within the globular domain of histones that make extensive contacts with DNA.[480] Histone code is the name given to the combination of several biochemical modifications affecting different histone residues that specify chromatin function. However, it has been suggested that

Table 56–5 Human Histone Deacetylases

Characteristics	Class I	Class IIa	Class IIb	Class III
Members	HDAC1, 2, 3, 8, 11	HDAC4, 5, 7, 9	HDAC6, 10	SIRT1, 2, 3, 4, 5, 6, 7
Localization	Nuclear	Nucleo-cytoplasmic	Nucleo-cytoplasmic	Nuclear/cytoplasmic/mitochondrial
Substrates	Histones p53 (HDAC1) NF-κB (HDAC3)	Histones Hsp90	Histone Tubulin Hsp90?	Histones Tubulin (SIRT2) p53 (SIRT1) TAF(I)68 (SIRT1)
Binding site inhibitors	Zn^{++} TSA SAHA/LAQ824 Depsipeptide Trapoxin Butyrate VPA	Zn^{++} TSA SAHA/LAQ824 Trapoxin Butyrate VPA	Zn^{++} TSA SAHA/LAQ824 Tubacin	NAD^+ Nicotinamide

various postsynthesis histone modifications be considered an epigenomic alphabet. Each modification is a letter and the combination of modifications at a specified genomic region is a word that may have different functional meanings depending on the context.[480]

Histone acetyl transferases (HATs) and histone deacetylases (HDACs) are two classes of enzymes that mediate the acetylation and deacetylation, respectively, at evolutionarily conserved N-terminal lysine residues.[481] Acetylated histones are negatively charged and do not bind as tightly to negatively charged DNA, thereby facilitating gene transcription. In contrast, deacetylated histones bind closely to DNA, preventing transcription.[482] Acetylation status of chromatin and hence gene transcription is dictated by balanced activity of HATs and HDACs. Acetylation of core histone bases has also been implicated in chromatin assembly, DNA repair, and replication timing of specific genomic regions.[483–485] Cross talk also exists between acetylation and ubiquitination. HDACs, thus, can decrease the half-life of substrates by exposing the lysine residue for ubiquitination.[486–489] Other crucial functions affected by the delicate balance between HATs and HDACs include activation of the apoptotic program via interaction between Ku70 and BAX, protein localization (nuclear vs cytoplasm) and DNA binding of transcription factors like p53, E2F1, GATA1, RelA, YY1 and hormone receptors.[480,490,491] There is a growing list of nonhistone proteins, whose function is modulated by HATs/HDACs. These include HIF-1α, β-catenin, α-tubulin, Ku70, importin-α 7, cortactin, and most recently heat shock protein (hsp) 90.[492–501] HATs and HDACs can be classified into subfamilies according to the presence of highly conserved structural motifs. Please refer to Table 56–5 for details.

Aberrant Histone Acetyl Transferase and Histone Deacetylase Activity in Hematologic Malignancies

Aberrant activity of HATs and HDACs resulting in aberrant gene transcription is a hallmark of many cancers, including many hematologic malignancies.[490,502] Several chromosomal translocations in leukemia that produce chimeric fusion oncoproteins have been shown to recruit HDACs to promoters, repress genes involved in cell-cycle growth inhibition and differentiation. For example, PML-RARα in acute promyelocytic leukemia (APL) and AML1-ETO generated by t(8;21) translocation in AML recruit HDACs to their target genes, resulting in chromatin modification and repression of genes, leading to blocked differentiation and inhibition of apoptosis.[502] HDACs have also been found in complexes with proteins that regulate cell-cycle checkpoints such as Rb and its family members.[490,502] Resistance to chemotherapy can occur because of increased levels of thioredoxin, a thiol reductase, and decreased levels of thioredoxin-binding protein (TBP-2) in many cancers; HDAC inhibitors (HDIs) can reverse this phenomenon.[503] These examples create a strong rationale to develop inhibitors of HDAC activity that would correct transcriptional deregulation of genes involved in cell-cycle regulation and apoptosis.

Mechanisms of Anticancer Activity of Histone Deacetylase Inhibitors

Treatment with HDIs modulates expression of 2% to 10% of a selective subset of genes in various cell types with as many genes upregulated as are downregulated.[504–507] Normal cells are more resistant than cancer cells to the effects of HDIs.[508] HDI-induced cell cycle arrest and apoptosis is usually correlated with upregulation of p21, p27, and p16 and attenuation of cyclin A and D levels leading to decreased activity of CDK4 and CDK2.[209,497,509] Induction of GADD45α and β and upregulation of TGF-β, which inhibits c-Myc, may also contribute to the cell-cycle arrest in G1 or G2.[497,510,511] Promoter regions of p21 and the telomerase catalytic unit TERT have been shown to contain SP1 sites that bind HDAC-recruiting transcription complexes.[497] HDIs also activate the mitochondrial apoptotic pathway by transcriptional activation of apoptotic proteins like TBP2, Bad, Bim, Bid, BAK, Bax, caspases 3 and 9, and repression of antiapoptotic proteins like thioredoxin, bcl-2, XIAP and Mcl-1.[512,513] HDIs have also been shown to upregulate Fas and the Apo-2L/TRAIL receptors DR4 and DR5, downregulate c-FLIP, and enhance Apo-2L/TRAIL-induced DISC and apoptosis.[514–517]

Treatment with HDI alone or in combination with other agents like ATRA has been shown to overcome the inhibition of differentiation due to chimeric fusion oncoproteins such as PML-RARα. PLZF-RARα, or AML-ETO.[502,510,518,519] HDIs have also been shown to induce the expression of gelsolin, an actin-binding protein involved in morphologic and cytostructural changes associated with differentiation.[519,520]

Several HDIs were shown to induce acetylation of hsp90 and inhibit its chaperone association with important prosurvival client proteins such as AKT and c-Raf.[209,497,501] This directs these client proteins to polyubiquitylation and proteasomal degradation, thus contributing to the lowering of the threshold for apoptosis in cancer cells. Inhibition of HDAC6 results in marked accumulation of ubiquitinated proteins (inhibition of the aggresome), via acetylation of α-tubulin, which in turn results in increased cellular stress and cytotoxicity.[521]

There is evidence to suggest that treatment with HDIs leads to tumor regression not only by directly inhibiting cell-cycle progression

Table 56–6 Histone Deacetylase Inhibitors

Name	Type of Compound	Cell Culture (Activity)	Animal Tumor Models	Clinical Trial
Butyrates	Short-chain fatty acids	Yes (uM)	Yes	Phase I/II
Valproic acid	Short-chain fatty acid	Yes	Yes	Phase I/II
Trichostatin A	Hydroxamic acid	Yes (nM)	Yes	—
Pyroxamide	Hydroxamic acid derivative	Yes (nM)	Yes	Phase I
Oxamflatin	Hydroxamic acid derivative	Yes (uM)	Yes	—
Suberoylanilide hydroxamic acid (SAHA)	Hydroxamic acid derivative	Yes (nM)	Yes	Phase I/II
TPX-HA analog (CHAP)	Hydroxamic acid derivative	Yes (nM)	Yes	—
LAQ824	Hydroxamic acid derivative	Yes (nM)	Yes	Phase I
MS-275	Benzamide derivative	Yes (uM)	Yes	—
CI-994 (N-acetyl dinaline)	Benzamide derivative	Yes	Yes	Phase I
Depsipeptide (FR901228, FK-228)	Cyclic tetrapeptides	Yes (nM)	Yes	Phase I/II
Trapoxin	Cyclic tetrapeptides	Yes (nM)	—	—
Apicidin	Cyclic tetrapeptides	Yes (nM)	Yes	—

Activity reported as "Yes" indicates that the compound has been shown to inhibit HDAC activity, that is, growth of transformed cells in culture and in vivo tumor growth in animal studies. (—) indicates no data reported. CI-994 is reported to inhibit histone deacetylation but does not directly inhibit HDAC.

and apoptosis, but also indirectly by exerting antiangiogenic and immune modulatory effects via downregulation of HIF-1α and VEGF.[497,502,522] HDIs also affect cancer cell migration, invasion, and metastasis by altering expression of extracellular matrix proteins and metastasis genes in favor of reduced cell invasion.[513]

Classes of Histone Deacetylase Inhibitors

Several structurally diverse classes of naturally occurring and synthetic compounds have been investigated for their ability to inhibit HDAC activity (Table 56–6).[523] These include short-chain fatty acids (eg, valproic acid), hydroxamic acid derivatives (eg, vorinostat), synthetic benzamides (eg, MS-275), and cyclic tetrapeptides (eg, romidepsin). The various classes of HDIs studied so far are listed in Table 56–6 and described below.

Short Chain Fatty Acids

Sodium butyrate (SB), a well-studied member of this class of compounds, induces in vitro growth arrest and differentiation of human leukemia cells at millimolar concentrations.[524] Its clinical development has been hampered by its short half-life and difficulty in achieving millimolar levels in vivo. Phenylbutyrate, another derivative of butyric acid, is able to induce in vitro growth arrest and differentiation of leukemia cells at clinically achievable submillimolar concentrations.[525,526] Importantly, at these levels, phenylbutyrate is able to synergize with retinoids in inducing cell cycle arrest and differentiation of myeloid leukemia cells.[527] Valproic acid (VPA), a well-tolerated antiepileptic, was shown to be effective as an HDI at levels ranging between 0.5 and 2.5 mM.[510]

Two phase I trials have looked at phenylbutyrate in patients with AML and MDS. No responses were noted in either study, with neurotoxicity being the dose-limiting toxicity. Several studies have employed valproic acid as monotherapy or in combination with other agents in hematologic malignancies.[511,528] As monotherapy in MDS, response rates have been as high as 16% using the IWG criteria. Responses have been higher in low-risk MDS groups and low-risk karyotypes. Neurotoxicity has been the major side effect. Other side effects of VPA include thrombocytopenia, weight gain, asthenia, and rarely hepatic failure and pancreatitis.[529]

However, in general, because they possess short side chains, this class of HDIs are unable to make significant contact with the catalytic pocket of HDACs, and this may account for the low potency of these compounds.[502]

Vorinostat and Other Hydroxamic Acid Derivatives

Members of this class are some of the most potent HDIs.[504] They contain a functional group that interacts with the critical zinc atom at the base of the catalytic pocket of the class I and II HDACs.[490,502] These HDIs also possess a hydrophobic cap and an aliphatic side chain that interacts with the edge and fits into the hydrophobic catalytic pocket, respectively, of the HDACs. Members of this class inhibit both class I and II HDACs.[490,523] Vorinostat (SAHA, Zolinza) is a second-generation polar-planar compound that induces in vitro growth arrest, differentiation, and/or apoptosis of a variety of cancer, leukemia, and multiple myeloma cell types.[490,504] In phase I studies, vorinostat was administered intravenously to patients with solid tumors or hematologic malignancies daily × 3 or daily × 5 for up to 3 weeks.[530] The maximum tolerated dose of vorinostat in patients with hematologic malignancies was 300 mg/m^2 daily × 5 for 3 weeks; thrombocytopenia and leukopenia were the notable toxicities. Responses were seen in patients with lymphoma and bladder cancer. Thirty-nine patients with advanced hematologic malignancies were enrolled in a trial composed of 2 cohorts looking at IV and oral (PO) formulations of vorinostat.[531] The median age of patients in the IV cohort was lower than that in the oral cohort. Up to 70% of patients had diffuse large B-cell lymphoma. Median number of prior treatments was seven and five in the IV and PO cohorts respectively. A substantial number of patients had undergone a prior stem-cell transplant. Most patients tolerated vorinostat well. Major adverse events of the oral formulation included fatigue, diarrhea, anorexia, and dehydration, whereas myelosuppression and thrombocytopenia were more prominent with the IV formulation. The mechanism of thrombocytopenia is unlike conventional chemotherapy; the drug appears to impair megakaryocytic differentiation. In the IV cohort, three patients with Hodgkin Disease (HD) had a benefit, whereas in the PO cohort, three heavily pretreated patients with diffuse large B-cell lymphoma and one patient with cutaneous T-cell lymphoma (CTCL) and one with HD each experienced a clinical benefit.[531]

A phase II trial, evaluated vorinostat in thirty-three heavily pretreated patients with CTCL[532] enrolled in three different dose groups. Dosing schedules were either 400 mg PO daily, 300 mg daily × 3 days followed by 4 days' rest or 300 mg twice a day for 14 days followed by 7 days' rest. Intent-to-treat analysis revealed a response rate of 24.2%; there were no CRs; eight patients achieved PR, including four with Sezary syndrome. Additional patients had minor responses and disease stabilization; a substantial number had relief from pruritis. Median time to response, duration of response, and time to progression were 11.9, 15.1, and 30.2 weeks respectively.[532] Vorinostat was approved by the FDA for patients with refractory CTCL at a dose of 400 mg daily, which had the most favorable safety profile in the above study.

Several other hydroxamic acid-based hybrid polar HDIs have been developed and tested both in vitro and in vivo tumor models and in clinical trials.[490,523] LBH 589 and LAQ824 are novel cinnamic hydroxamic acid analogs. LBH589 induces apoptosis in a dose-dependent manner on human CML blast crisis K562 cells and acute leukemia MV4-11 cells with the activating length mutation of FLT-3.[533] Exposure to LBH 589 is associated with hyperacetylation of H3, H4, Hsp 90, increase in p21, and induction of cell-cycle G1 phase accumulation.

Fifteen patients with a median age of 63 years and refractory AML, ALL, or MDS received IV LBH 589 in a phase I trial at the following dose levels (mg/m^2): 4.8, 7.2, 9.0, 11.5, and 14.0.[534] Grade III QTc prolongation was observed in four patients at the 14.0 mg/m^2 level and in one patient at the 11.5 mg/m^2 level. QTc prolongation was asymptomatic and reversible on drug discontinuation. Other toxicities included nausea, diarrhea, vomiting, hypokalemia, and thrombocytopenia. Eight of 11 patients with peripheral blasts had transient reductions in blast counts, which increase shortly after drug discontinuation.[534] LBH589 has shown to be highly effective in CTCL. In a recent abstract, at an MTD of 20 mg M, W, F, two patients achieved CR, four attained PR, and one patient had SD for an overall response rate of 60%.[535]

Synthetic Benzamide Derivatives

Although structurally diverse, these compounds contain a benzamide moiety.[523] Two important members of this class of HDIs are MS-275 and CI-994.[536] MS-275 exerts antiproliferative effects at micromolar levels against pancreas, breast, colorectal, lung, and ovarian cancer cell types.[537] It has been shown to induce TGF-β receptor, which may enhance the antitumor effects of TGF-β.[538] DLT was reached with the starting dose of 2 mg/m^2 daily × 28 days in a 42-day cycle.[539] Pharmacokinetic data revealed a 30- to 50-fold longer half-life in humans than that predicted from animal models. Twenty-eight patients were subsequently treated on a q14 day schedule with no complete or partial responses noted. Fifteen patients had stable disease. Toxicities common to HDAC inhibitors like nausea, vomiting, and fatigue were noted; no symptomatic cardiac toxicity was noted. Hypoalbuminemia, thought to be due to decreased production and lymphopenia were noted. Three episodes of herpes simplex virus stomatitis were noted in patients who received more than one course; one patient with CTCL experienced herpes zoster recurrence.[539] A recent phase I trial of MS-275 in patients with advanced leukemias reported an MTD of 8 mg/m^2 weekly for 4 weeks every 6 weeks.[540] Dose-limiting toxicities included neurotoxicity and infections. No CR or PR was noted by standard criteria. Another compound, CI-994, also has broad antitumor activity against murine and human xenograft models, and is undergoing clinical evaluation in phase I and II trials.[541]

Cyclic Tetrapeptides

The main members of this class of agents are depsipeptide (Romidepsin, FK228, FR901228)) and apicidin.[522,542] Depsipeptide is a potent HDI that exerts in vitro antitumor effects at nanomolar levels against several cancer cell types. It also induces apoptosis of human acute leukemia and CLL cells.[543] Additionally, depsipeptide was shown to exert antiangiogenic effect by modulating the expression of genes involved in angiogenesis.[544] A phase I study of depsipeptide in patients with CLL and AML at a dose of 13 mg/m^2 IV on days 1, 8, and 15 of a 4-week cycle showed antitumor activity in several patients, though no CRs or PRs were observed.[545] Response was greater in patients with CLL than AML. There were no life-threatening toxicities, but constitutional symptoms characteristic of HDAC inhibition were observed in the majority of patients. This fact brings forth an important aspect of putting patients on chronic therapy with HDAC inhibitors, that is, managing chronic toxicity. Another important clinical aspect is the sequence of use of HDAC inhibitors. Depsipeptide was shown to upregulate MDR1 and induce doxorubicin resistance when used with ATRA in APL cells.[546] However, prior treatment with doxorubicin followed by ATRA/depsipeptide resulted in increased cell death.[546] A phase I study of apicidin is another cyclic tetrapeptide that has been shown to exert antiproliferative effects against several human cancer cell types associated with upregulation of p21$^{CIP1/WAF1}$ and gelsolin.[542]

Combinations of Histone Deacetylase Inhibitors With Other Agents

Histone Deacetylase Inhibitors With Conventional Cytotoxic Agents

Because treatment with HDI lowers the threshold for apoptosis by multiple mechanisms, it would be expected to enhance the apoptotic effects due to conventional chemotherapeutic agents, which generally trigger apoptosis by perturbing the cell cycle and/or inducing DNA damage. Combination of HDI and conventional chemotherapy has resulted in enhanced cytotoxicity in a variety of solid tumor cell lines.[547,548] SB was shown to induce the topoisomerase α expression and sensitize human leukemia cells to etoposide.[549] Cotreatment with phenylbutyrate increases the activity of conventional chemotherapeutic agents such as cytarabine, etoposide, and topotecan against non-Hodgkin lymphoma, CLL, and multiple myeloma cells.[550] Recently, the combination of vorinostat and valproic acid was studied in MOLT4 and HL60 cell lines.[547] It was hypothesized that exposure of cells to the idarubicin prior to HDI would result in disruption of matrix attachment complexes, thereby facilitating HDI access to polynucleosomes, which are involved in temporal control of gene expression. The combination resulted in increased cell loss, but the sequence of drug exposure on cells did not appear to play a role.

Histone Deacetylase Inhibitors With DNA Hypomethylating Agents

DNA methyltransferase (DNMT) induces transcriptional silencing by promoting cytosine hypermethylation of CpG islands in the promoter regions of genes.[551] Aberrant methylation is now well known to silence the expression of tumor suppressor genes (TSGs). The silenced TSGs can be reexpressed by treatment with demethylating agents, for example, 5′-azacytidine and 5′-aza-2′-deoxycytidine (DAC or decitabine), which inhibit DNMT by inducing a stable complex formation between the enzyme and DAC-substituted DNA.[551,552] DNMT and a group of methyl cytosine-binding proteins, for example, MECP2, can also recruit and direct HDACs to the chromatin associated with silenced genes.[552] DNA methylation is a dominant gene-silencing process, and methylated genes show resistance to reexpression by treatment with HDIs alone.[553,554] However, a combined treatment with a DNMT inhibitor and an HDI such as TSA or depsipeptide has been shown to synergistically derepress silenced TSGs such as p16 and p15, resulting in increased growth inhibition and apoptosis of tumor cells.[545–556] Additionally, in the multiple myeloma U266 cells, combined treatment with phenylbutyrate and DAC restored the expression of p16 and induced apoptosis.[557]

In one of the first clinical studies done to verify the above concept, patients with AML or MDS were treated with SQ Aza-CR for 5, 10, or 14 days followed by a 7-day IV infusion of phenylbutyrate.[558] Treatment cycles were repeated every 28 days unless toxicities supervened. Thirty-two of thirty-six screened patients were enrolled. Of the 29 evaluable patients, 11 responded. There were four CRs and one PR, with three patients having a complete cytogenetic response.

Injection site reactions with azacitidine and neurotoxicity with phenylbutyrate were seen that reversed on drug discontinuation. Bisulfite sequencing of the p15 promoter in bone marrow DNA during the first treatment cycle showed heterogenous allelic demethylation in three responding patients.[558] This denoted ongoing demethylation in responding patients versus no demethylation in nonresponders. Six responders with pretreatment methylation of p15 or CDH-1 promoters showed evidence of demethylation during the first treatment cycle.

Issa et al conducted a phase I/II study of decitabine in combination with valproic acid in patients with previously treated and untreated AML.[559] A total of 54 patients received decitabine at a dose of 15 mg/m^2 IV × 10 days. Valproic acid was administered at escalating doses PO for 10 days. A response rate of 22% was noted including 19% CRs and 3% CRs with incomplete platelet recovery. Of 10 older patients with AML, 4 patients had a CR and 1 patient achieved a PR. Induction mortality in this group was 2%. A major cytogenetic response was noted in six of eight responders. Duration of remission was 7.2 months, with an overall survival of 15.3 months in responders. Studies are underway to determine optimal dosing of these novel agents, best sequence of combination treatments, and combination with more potent HDIs like LBH.[560]

Histone Deacetylase Inhibitors With Other Differentiation-Inducing Agents

HDIs have also been tested in combination with ATRA against APL cells expressing PML-RARα or PLZF-RARα. Enhanced differentiation and significant apoptosis due to the combination has been reported.[518] TSA combined with ATRA is especially effective against ATRA-resistant PLZF-RARα-containing APL cells.[518] Similarly, phenylbutyrate was shown to reverse ATRA resistance in a patient with APL.[490] Primary leukemia blasts also demonstrate differentiation following combined treatment with ATRA and TSA or VPA.[519] The combination was noted to induce RARα-targeted genes, suggesting that in AML cells HDIs release a block to RARα-mediated gene expression involved in differentiation.

Valproic acid with ATRA either as upfront therapy or ATRA added to VPA in nonresponding patients was looked at in 58 older patients with AML who were deemed unfit for conventional chemotherapy.[528] The RR was 5% by the IWG criteria for AML but 16% if IWG criteria for MDS was used. A smaller Italian trial looked at sequential valproic acid followed by ATRA in a similar patient population as the aforementioned trial. ATRA was added when adequate concentration of VPA was achieved. Six of 11 evaluable patients had a hematologic improvement. Neurotoxicity was the major adverse event in the trial.[561]

Histone Deacetylase Inhibitors With Cell Cycle and Cell-Signaling Modulators

Both vorinostat and SB have also been combined with the cell cycle-dependent kinase (CDK) inhibitor flavopiridol. The combination of HDI and flavopiridol dramatically increased apoptosis of cultured and primary AML cells, resulting in a synergistic cytotoxic response.[382,562] Because treatment with flavopiridol also transcriptionally downregulates several antiapoptotic gene expressions, this may be responsible for the synergistic effect observed with the combination. Recent studies have shown that treatment with vorinostat or LAQ824 attenuates the mRNA level of *bcr-abl* and promotes polyubiquitylation and proteasomal degradation of Bcr-Abl.[209,563] In addition, a combined treatment with LAQ824 and Bcr-Abl tyrosine kinase inhibitor imatinib or PD180970 was shown to induce apoptosis of imatinib-sensitive or imatinib-refractory CML cells.[563] Similarly, the combination of vorinostat and dasatinib on cultured human, primary CML or murine pro-B BaF 3 cells, expressing unmutated or mutated form of bcr-abl showed enhanced apoptosis.[562] The more potent TKI, AMN107, has also been studied with the HDI, LBH589, in cells with ectopic expression of *bcr-abl* and mutated clones (T315I, E255K) that are imatinib resistant.[564] Taken together, these preclinical findings support the rationale to study the safety and efficacy of the combinations of these HDIs with specific inhibitors of progrowth and survival signaling triggered by oncoprotein tyrosine kinases.

Histone Deacetylase Inhibitors With Other Novel Agents

On the basis of the ability of HDIs such as vorinostat to lower the threshold for apoptotic signaling initiated both by the extrinsic and mitochondrial pathways of apoptosis, the activity of these agents in combination with Apo-2L/TRAIL has been preclinically tested against human leukemia cells. Cotreatment with vorinostat or LAQ824 significantly enhanced APO-2L/TRAIL-induced apoptosis of cultured and primary acute leukemia cells.[514] A similar effect was also seen for vorinostat plus APO-2/TRAIL in multiple myeloma cells.[565]

Recently, the combined effects of HDIs such as SB or vorinostat with the hsp-90 antagonist, 17-AAG were determined in human leukemia cells.[566] The combination was highly synergistic in inducing the mitochondrial pathway of apoptosis. The synergistic effect of the combination was associated with downregulation of Raf-1 and phospho-AKT, as well as inactivation of MEK and ERK1/2. More recently, the combination of the potent HDI LBH589 and 17-AAG was studied in CML blast crisis K562 cells and AML MV4-11 cells with the FLT-3 mutation.[533] 17-AAG induced polyubiquitylation and proteasomal degradation of FLT-3 and bcr-abl by reducing their chaperone association with hsp90. The combination resulted in increased apoptosis of primary imatinib-resistant cells, cells carrying the T315I mutation, and AML cells with the FT-3 mutation. In a separate study, coadministration of minimally toxic concentrations of the proteasome inhibitor bortezomib with either SB or vorinostat resulted in marked increase in caspase activation and apoptosis of Bcr-Abl-positive leukemia cells sensitive or resistant to imatinib.[567] Synergistic cytotoxicity was also noted with LBH589 in combination with bortezomib against MM cells sensitive and resistant to dexamethasone as well as primary patient MM cells. Another novel strategy was explored in a study combining the HDI NVP-LAQ284 with the VEGFR TKI, PTK787/ZK222584.[568] The combination resulted in significant inhibition of prostate and breast tumor growth in vivo. NVP-LAQ824 was shown to downregulate angiogenesis-related genes like HIF-1α, VEGF, Ang-2/tie-2, and survivin. The combination was thought to be more effective because of actions on independent, parallel pathways as well as vertical inhibition of the VEGF pathway.[568] Taken together, these findings suggest that combined hsp90/histone deacetylase, proteasome/histone deacetylase, or histone deacetylase/VEGF inhibition may be a promising strategy against leukemia or other hematologic malignancies where these agents have individually shown promising activity.

Heat Shock Protein Inhibitors

The "heat shock response" was first described by Ferruccio Ritossa in 1962. He made the crucial observation that certain regions of the chromosomes of the fruit fly *Drosophila* puffed out in response to a sudden increase in temperature.[569,570] The gene products encoded on these chromosomes were later termed heat-shock proteins (HSPs). Contrary to most cellular proteins, HSP production increases several-folds in response to environmental stresses, including heat shock, nutrient deprivation, oxidative stresses, heavy metals, and alcohol exposure. They form multimolecular complexes with variable cellular proteins, regulating their correct folding, repair, degradation, and function; hence, the HSPs' more accurate designation is "molecular chaperones."[571,572] A number of multigene families of HSPs exist and their individual products vary in cellular expression, function, and localization. They are classified according to their molecular weight, for example, HSP90, HSP70, and HSP27. Exceptions to this rule are the chaperones identified as glucose-regulated proteins (GRP94 and GRP75).[573] Heat shock proteins (HSPs, also designated as molecular chaperones) are highly conserved proteins that form multimolecular complexes that regulate the functional activity of client proteins that mediate numerous signal transduction pathways. A number of multigene families of HSPs exist and their individual products vary in cellular expression, function, and localization.[571,572] They are classified according to their molecular weight, for example, HSP90, HSP70, and HSP27. HSP90 has received considerable attention as a target for cancer therapy.[573]

HSP90 regulates the function and stability of many key signaling proteins that help cancer cells to escape the inherent toxicity of their environment, to evade the effects of chemotherapy, and to protect themselves from the results of their own genetic instability.[573,574] In humans, HSP90 consists of four genes, cytosolic HSP90α and HSP90β, GRP94, and HSP75/tumor necrosis factor-associated protein 1 (TRAP1).[575] The monomer HSP90 consists of conserved 25-kd N-terminal and 55-kd C-terminal domains. The N-terminus contains a highly conserved ATP-binding domain. Dimerization of these nucleotide-binding domains is essential for ATP binding and hydrolysis.[576] Phosphorylation leads HSP90 to interact with cochaperones such as HSP70 and p23 to form heteroprotein complexes which is essential for various protein functions. Such proteins include several transcription factors (eg, steroid hormone receptor, retinoid receptors, and hypoxia inducible factor HIF-1α), serine/threonine and tyrosine kinases (eg, c-SRC/v-SRC, RAF-1, ERB2, EGFR, MEK, CDK4, AKT, BCR-ABL, LCK, FAK, c-MET), and other proteins with various functions (eg, mutant p53, catalytic subunit of telomerase hTERT, TNFR1, and RB).[577] HSP90 inhibition leads to misfolded client proteins that are involved in malignancy to be polyubiquitinated and degraded by proteosomes.[578] Significant interest in HSP90 inhibition has led to the following compounds.

Benzoquinone Ansamycins (Herbamycin A, Geldanamycin, 17-AAG)

The first class of HSP90 inhibitors to be discovered was the benzoquinone ansamycins, which include herbamycin A and geldanamycin. These natural products were first isolated from the actinomycete broths in the 1970s.[579] Hemamycin A was later shown to reverse the malignant phenotype of *v-Src* transformed fibroblasts, with potent antitumor activity in vitro and in vivo animal models. The effects of this drug on other tyrosine kinases, including $p210^{bcr\text{-}abl}$, were also described, leading to the frequent use of herbimycin A as a general tyrosine kinase inhibitor. However, Whitesell and colleagues later identified HSP90 as the prominent benzoquinone ansamycin-binding protein, and they described the ability of these drugs to disrupt the complex between v-Src and HSP90, resulting in destabilization of v-Src protein and its eventual loss from treated cells.[580] Subsequent immunoprecipitation and x-ray crystallography studies showed that geldanamycin competes at the ATP-binding site and inhibits the intrinsic ATPase activity of HSP90, preventing the formation of mature multimeric HSP90 complexes capable of chaperoning client proteins (Fig. 56–10).[576,581] As a result, the client proteins are ubiquitinated and targeted for proteasomal degradation. Although clearly active in human tumor xenograft models, preclinical evaluation of geldanamycin demonstrated significant hepatotoxicity at therapeutic drug levels.[582] Screening for geldanamycin analogs resulted in the discovery of 17-allylamino-17-demethoxygeldanamycin (17-AAG), a semisynthetic geldanamycin derivative in which an allyl amino group replaces the methoxy in the 17 position (Fig. 56–10). 17-AAG has a significantly improved toxicity profile but like geldanamycin retains the ability to inhibit HSP90.[583] In addition, 17-AAG has been shown to have greater affinity for binding to HSP90 from cancer versus normal host cells.[584]

Preclinical Studies of 17-AAG′: 17-AAG exhibited significant antiproliferative and cytotoxic effects against a wide panel of transformed cell lines, inhibiting pathways that regulate cell-cycle progression, apoptosis, invasion, and angiogenesis. In the NCI in vitro cancer screen, the mean GI_{50} for 17-AAG was 0.19 μM, with greater

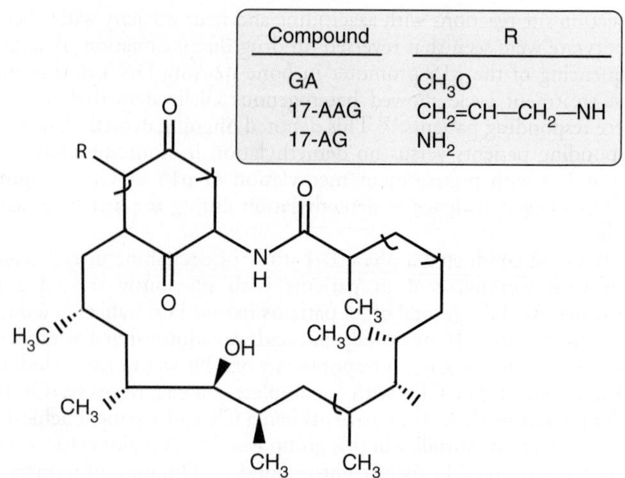

Figure 56–10 Chemical structure of geldanamycin (GA), 17-allylamin-17-demethoxygeldanamycin (17-AAG), and 17-amino-geldanamycin (17-AG).

than average sensitivity in melanoma, leukemia, non-small-cell lung, ovarian, breast, prostate, and renal cancer panels.[585]

Benzoquinone ansamycins have been reported to induce G1 as well as G2/M block. In a panel of breast cancer cell lines, 17-AAG and geldanamycin caused a G1 arrest.[586,587] This G1 block resulted from downregulation of signaling pathways controlling cyclin D or CDK4/cyclin D1 activity, in particular depletion of tyrosine kinases (ERBB2, EGF receptor), degradation of c-RAF-1 with reduced phosphorylation of extracellular signal-regulated kinase (ERK). A G2/M block has been reported in RB-deficient cells treated with 17-AAG; however, the requirement for RB deficiency appears to be cell dependent. A number of G2 checkpoint kinases such as WEE1 and MYT1 have also been identified as HSP90 client proteins.[588]

HSP90 plays a crucial role in regulating apoptosis. 17-AAG induced cytosolic accumulation of cytochrome C and cleavage and activation of caspases 9 and 3, triggering apoptosis in HL-60/Bcr-Abl with ectopic expression of p185-Bcr-Abl and K562 with endogenous p210-Bcr-Abl cells. 17-AAG treatment led to proteasomal degradation of Bcr-Abl in these cells along with AKT depletion.[589] However, high ectopic expression of HSP70 inhibits 17-AAG-induced Bax conformation change, mitochondrial localization, and apoptosis.[560] This is important due to 17-AAG and other analogs of geldanamycin (17-DMAG and IPI504) or radicicol induce HSP70 levels.[590,591] Therefore, strategies leading to abrogation of HSP70 induction would further antileukemic effects of HSP90 inhibitors.

In addition to their modulation of the cell cycle and programmed cell death, geldanamycin and 17-AAG have been implicated in the regulation of invasion, metastasis, and angiogenesis. 17-AAG treatment of H322 and H358 cells enhanced E-cadherin expression and inhibited secretion of MMP-9 and VEGF. Geldanamycins have also been shown to inhibit the HGF/SF-MET signaling pathway, resulting in decreased cell motility and invasion of c-MET transformed cells.[592] HSP90 inhibitors also significantly reduce VEGF secretion by decreasing HIF1α expression as well as inducing degradation of all three VEGF receptors.[593,594]

Combination studies incorporating 17-AAG have shown promise. In lung and colorectal cell lines, combinations of 17-AAG with cisplatin, doxorubicin, or paclitaxel have been synergistic or additive.[595,596] In addition, 17-AAG has shown synergy with novel agents, including imatinib, bortezomib, ERK inhibitors, and SAHA.[533,597–599] Combined treatment of LBH589, a histone deacetylase inhibitor, with 17-AAG exerted synergistic effects in AML and CML cells with decreased Bcr-Abl, p-AKT, AKT, and p-STAT5 levels.[533]

Metabolism of 17-AAG: In human and murine microsome assays, three metabolites of 17-AAG were identified: 17-aminogeldanamycin (17-AG), a diol, and an epoxide.[600] The 17-AAG diol is the major metabolite in human hepatic microsomes, followed by 17-AG. Cytochrome P450 (3A4) was identified as the enzyme responsible for 17-AAG metabolism. Acrolein, a known nephrotoxin, is a by-product of 17-AG. Also, the 17-AG metabolite has shown biological activity equivalent to that of the parent compound. The quinone-metabolizing enzyme DT-diaphorase has been shown to alter 17-AAG's antitumor properties. A positive correlation between DT-diaphorase expression levels and growth inhibition by 17-AAG has been established.[585] Transfection of an active DT-diaphorase gene NQO1 into a human carcinoma cell line increased 17-AAG's growth-inhibitory activity 32-fold. Polymorphisms of the NQO1 gene, which is found in 5% to 20% of the population, as well acting as a substrate for p-glycoprotein efflux pump may limit 17-AAG's clinical efficacy.

Clinical Investigation With 17-AAG: Several phase I trials in adult patients have investigated different scheduling regimens of 17-AAG.[601–605] Administration of 17-AAG on daily × 3 schedule or daily × 5 schedule has been associated with dose-limiting toxicities, namely, hepatotoxicity, diarrhea, and thrombocytopenia at substantially lower doses (40–56 mg/m^2).[603,605] Grade III GI toxicities including nausea, vomiting, and diarrhea are associated with the formulation of 17-AAG, which contains 4% DMSO. No objective clinical responses were reported on the daily × 5 or weekly schedule; however, in xenograft models the effects of 17-AAG on HSP90 client proteins lasted up to 72 hours, suggesting that twice-weekly dosing might be more effective. Thus, additional trials have evaluated twice weekly and weekly × 3 every 4 week schedules. A recent study recommended phase II doses of 175 to 200 mg/m^2 given twice weekly. This schedule was associated with a persistent increase of HSP70; however, no consistent changes in PBMC phosphorylated Akt, HSP90, or Raf-1 during treatment.[604] Combination phase I studies of 17-AAG with docetaxel, irinotecan, imatinib, trastuzumab, and bortezomib, are currently ongoing.

Clinical Investigation With Tanespimycin (KOS-95): Tanespimycin (KOS-953) or (17-AAG in Cremophor) has demonstrated major responses and stable disease in relapsed and refractory multiple myeloma. In a multicenter phase I study, the combination of tanespimycin and bortezomib demonstrated antitumor activity in myeloma patients.[606] Patients received a 1-hour infusion of tanespimycin on days 1, 4, 8, 11, and 21 following bortezomib. The group receiving 1.3 mg/m^2 bortezomib + 340 mg/m^2 tanespimycin is being expanded following 1/10 patients experiencing a DLT (myalgias/cramps). Grade III to IV toxicities include anemia, back pain, and thrombocytopenia, all of which are reversible. HSP70 induction was observed in PBMCs prior to day 11. A phase II study of this combination in refractory myeloma is planned.

Clinical Investigation With IPI-504: Because 17-AAG suffers from poor aqueous solubility and must be administered with DMSO or newer Cremophor formulations, synthesis of HSP90 inhibitors with more favorable pharmaceutical properties is needed. IPI-504, the highly soluble hydroquinone hydrochloride derivative of 17-AAG, has been shown to be 4000-fold more soluble than 17-AAG.[607] In preclinical studies, single agent IPI-504 as well as in combination with bortezomib has shown antitumor effects in xenograft models of multiple myeloma.[608] Also, treatment with IPI-504 resulted in BCR-ABL protein degradation, decreased numbers of leukemia stem cells, and prolonged survival of leukemic mice bearing the T315I mutation.[609] A phase I study has been initiated in relapsed myeloma patients. IPI-504 is administered over 30 minutes on days 1, 4, 8, and 11 every 21 days. Thus far, 15 patients have been treated, with doses ranging from 90 to 300 mg/m^2, no dose-limiting toxicities have been observed to date.[610]

Clinical Investigation With Alvespimycin (KOS-1022): Alvespimycin (KOS-1022) is a second-generation HSP90 inhibitor that has begun phase I trials in IV and oral schedules.[611] Escalating doses of alvespimycin were given intravenously over 1 hour twice weekly every 3 weeks. Alvespimycin demonstrated antileukemic activity with tolerable toxicity at 24 mg/m^2 twice weekly. In 23 patients with AML, 3 patients experienced complete response and 1 patient demonstrated stable disease while on study × 9 cycles. Clinical trials of alvespimycin in combination with trastuzumab in solid malignancies are also ongoing.

17-DMAG: The water-soluble stable geldanamycin derivative, 17-(dimethylaminothylamino)-17-demethoxygeldanamycin (17-DMAG), has demonstrated more potent in vitro and in vivo antitumor activity than 17-AAG.[612] In addition, 17-DMAG offers three potential advantages over 17-AAG: (a) aqueous solubility eliminates formulation problems associated with 17-AAG, (b) 17-DMAG undergoes limited metabolism, and (3) it has higher oral bioavailability.[613] Phase I studies evaluating 17-DMAG have been recently initiated.

Other HSP90 Inhibitors

In addition to benzoquinone ansamycins and the semisynthetic analog 17-AAG, several other compounds were found to bind HSP90 and disrupt its chaperone function.

Radicicol: Radicicol, a macrocyclic antibiotic isolated from *Monosporum bonorden*, binds the N-terminal domain of HSP90 competing with its natural ligand, ATP.[614] Although a more potent inhibitor of HSP90 ATPase compared to geldanamycin, radicicol lacks antitumoral activity in vivo owing to its unstable chemical nature. Oxime-derivative compounds, which retain the HSP90 inhibitory activity and have a more stable chemical structure, were developed.

Novobiocin: Novobiocin, a coumarin antibiotic, binds the C-terminus domain of HSP90, as opposed to N-terminus binding with geldanamycin and radicicol.[615] However it was shown to retain inhibitory activity against HSP90 and degrade its client-signaling proteins. Thus, it appears that N- and C-terminal domains are both essential for HSP90 chaperone functions.

Bryostatin 1: Bryostatin 1 (NSC339555) is a macrocyclic lactone isolated from the marine bryozoan *Bugula neritina*. It originally attracted attention in view of its activity against a wide variety of tumor types in an NCI screen. In hematopoietic cells, bryostatin 1 displays the unique capacity to inhibit the growth of human leukemia cells[616] while stimulating the growth of their normal counterparts.[617]

Bryostatin 1 has been shown to act like the phorbol ester phorbol myristate acetate (PMA) in that it binds to and activates the serine-threonine kinase protein kinase C.[618] However, in contrast to PMA, it is a weak inducer of leukemic cell maturation[619] and in fact blocks PMA-mediated differentiation.[620] This may reflect the ability of bryostatin 1, on chronic administration, to downregulate PKC activity.[621]

In preclinical studies, bryostatin 1 has shown activity against continuously cultured and primary human leukemia and lymphoma cells when administered at nanomolar concentrations.[622,623] In addition, bryostatin lowers the threshold for leukemic and lymphoma cell apoptosis in response to conventional cytotoxic agents. The latter include ara-C, fludarabine, vincristine, paclitaxel, and chlorodeoxyadenosine.[624–628] It is postulated, although not definitively established, that such actions may reflect bryostatin 1-mediated downregulation of PKC, which exerts antiapoptotic actions.[629] More recently, bryostatin 1 has been shown to interact synergistically with more novel agents, including flavopiridol, through a process that may involve induction of TNF.[630] In clinical studies, bryostatin 1 has been administered according to several schedules, including a 1-hour infusion, a 24-hour infusion, and a split day 1 and 4 course weekly × 3 every 4 weeks[631,632] or a 24-hour infusion weekly for 8 weeks.[633] More recently, bryostatin 1 has been administered as a 72-hour continuous infusion every 2 weeks.[634] The maximally tolerated doses for the former schedules are 40 to 50 μg/m^2 and 120 μg/m^2 (40 μg/m^2/day for 3 days) for the latter.[631–633] Dose-limiting toxicity consists of myalgias, which are cumulative and which do not respond well to standard analgesic therapy. Other toxicities include fatigue, hepatotoxicity, nausea and vomiting, and phlebitis.

Bryostatin 1 as a single agent has shown some although limited activity. For example, when administered as a 120-hour continuous infusion every 2 weeks at a dose of 120 μg/m², 3 of 25 patients with CLL or NHL achieved a CR or objective PR.[633] On the other hand, out of nine patients with multiple myeloma, none responded to this bryostatin 1 dose and schedule.[635]

Results have been somewhat more promising when bryostatin 1 was combined with established cytotoxic drugs. For example, administration of bryostatin 1 as a 24-hour infusion (50 μg/m²) immediately before and after a split course of high-dose ara-C resulted in 4 CRs in 23 patients with highly refractory disease.[636] Administration of escalating doses of bryostatin 1 as a 1-hour infusion immediately before or after a 5-day course of fludarabine (doses of 16–25 mg/m²/day) resulted in 17 of 53 objective responses, including six in patients who had progressed on fludarabine previously.[637] Neither sequence was clearly superior to the other. Finally, in a phase I study, patients with B-cell malignancies were treated with a 24-hour continuous infusion of bryostatin 1 followed by a bolus injection of vincristine every 2 weeks. The maximally tolerated dose of bryostatin 1 was 50 μg/m².[638] Of the 24 evaluable patients, 5 patients had durable CRs or PRs, and an additional 5 patients had stable disease. Collectively, these findings suggest that bryostatin 1 may have a role in hematologic malignancies when combined with established cytotoxic agents.

DRUG RESISTANCE TO CHEMOTHERAPEUTIC AGENTS/MULTIDRUG RESISTANCE

Although many hematologic malignancies develop resistance to a specific class of chemotherapeutic agents, especially to targeted therapeutics, through the development of kinase region point mutations, emergence of resistance to multiple cytotoxic chemotherapeutic agents is also common among hematologic malignancies. Etiology of resistance includes specific drug resistance mechanisms, overexpression of the ABC transports such as MDR-1 for drug efflux, and overexpression of antiapoptotic proteins. The Goldie–Coldman hypothesis predicts that drug-resistant tumor cell clones survive because of a favorable spontaneous mutation, which occurs in approximately one in a million cells. Because 1 g of tumor contains 1×10^9 cells, it becomes obvious that high tumor burden states have a tremendous number of mutations, which can contribute to drug resistance. This is the rationale for using combination chemotherapy at specific dose intervals to maximize dose intensity.

Drug resistance mechanisms have been discovered and subsequently defined at the molecular level by investigators working in vitro with tumor cell lines selected in the presence of specific antitumor agents, by analysis of primary samples of untreated and treated hematologic malignancies, and through screening of tumor banks. Classes of resistance include acquired protein deficiency, loss of sensitivity to apoptotic signals, and age-related defects in the cellular pathways that normally lead to apoptosis.

P-Glycoprotein (ABC-B1 transporter)

Structure and Function

The ABC superfamily of membrane transporters mediates the cross membrane flux of xenobiotics, naturally occurring toxic compounds, drugs, peptides, and ions. ABC stands for ATP-binding cassette transporter family. They have profound impact on homeostasis and are critically important to proliferation and differentiation signals in normal progenitor cells. They also mediate drug sensitivity.[639] The terminology remains challenging because many earlier works referred to PGP and MRP, whereas the more recent consensus on the ABC superfamily has created a more simple approach going forward. PGP (ABC B1 transporter) has been the subject of intense biochemical and clinical studies since it was first discovered in drug-resistant cell lines more than 20 years ago.[640] The biochemistry of PGP has been reviewed in detail by several investigators.[641–643] This phosphorylated glycoprotein has a molecular mass of approximately 170 kd and is localized to the plasma membrane where it functions as a drug efflux pump (see Table 56–7). The ATP-dependent extrusion of antineoplastic agents confers a relative level of resistance to the cell that overexpresses PGP. Recently, the family of drug-transporting proteins has been more carefully characterized, leading to the use of the terms ATP-binding cassette transporters.[644] The observation of double minute chromosomes and homogeneously staining regions in several MDR cell lines suggested that gene amplification is involved in PGP-mediated MDR. The human *MDR1* gene, which codes for PGP and is involved in antitumor drug resistance,[645,646] and the human *MDR2* gene (the product of which is expressed by hepatocytes) are located very near each other on human chromosome 7q21.1. The human *MDR1* gene has 28 exons and codes for a protein of 1280 amino acids. The PGP molecule has two homologous halves, each with a hydrophobic region containing six transmembrane domains and a hydrophilic region containing an ATP-binding site. The N-linked glycosylation occurs on the extracellular side (Fig. 56–11). PGP is a member of the ABC superfamily, which includes, among more than a hundred others, the multidrug resistance-associated protein (MRP); the pf*mdr* pump in *Plasmodium falciparum*, which results in chloroquine resistance; STE6, the transporter of the "a" peptide mating factor in yeast; the cystic fibrosis transmembrane conductance regulator (CFTR); and the TAP-1 and TAP-2 proteins that transport antigenic peptides for association with class I molecules and surface antigen presentation.[642,643] MRP has been demonstrated in several MDR mammalian cell lines and in human tumors (see below), whereas a recent study[647] in human tumor cell lines has shown TAP overexpression associated with MRP as well as drug resistance resulting from transfection of the *TAP* genes.

PGP has a broad specificity for hydrophobic compounds and can both reduce the influx of drugs into the cytosol and increase efflux from the cytosol. To accomplish the former, this "hydrophobic vacuum cleaner" must detect drugs and expel them while they are still in the plasma membrane. Drugs are thought to be effluxed from the cytosol through a single barrel of the PGP transporter, although an exact mechanism has been lacking. A recent study has utilized electron microscopy to generate an initial structure of PGP to 2.5-nm resolution.[648] The structure was further refined by three-dimensional reconstructions from single particle image analysis of detergent-solubilized PGP and by Fourier projection maps of small crystalline arrays of PGP. This demonstrates that PGP is monomeric, with the shape of a cylinder 10 nm in diameter with a maximum height (in the plane of the membrane) of 8 nm (Fig. 56–11). Approximately one-half of the PGP molecule is within the membrane, as the lipid bilayer is approximately 4 nm in depth. When viewed from the extracellular surface of the membrane, PGP is pteroidal with a large central pore 5 nm in diameter. This large aqueous chamber in the membrane that is open to the extracellular space is closed on the cytoplasmic side presumably by the two 3-nM intracellular lobes (putative nucleotide-binding domains) and the hydrophilic cytoplasmic loops between the transmembrane domains. Thus, this large pore has a "gate" on the cytoplasmic side of the membrane that can regulate the transport of different-sized substrates.

Substrates of PGP include (see Table 56–7)[642,647] anthracyclines (doxorubicin, daunorubicin, epirubicin, and idarubicin); anthracenediones (mitoxantrone); aminoacridines (*m*-AMSA); taxanes (taxol and taxotere); epipodophyllotoxins (VP-16 and VM-26); *Vinca* alkaloids (vincristine, vinblastine, and vinorelbine); bortezomib.[649] and actinomycin D. Mitomycin C and one of the topoisomerase I inhibitors (topotecan) are both weak substrates for PGP. Several drugs reverse the resistance mediated by PGP overexpression and sensitize cells to the cytotoxic effects of antineoplastic agents. These drugs compete with antitumor agents for efflux from the cell, effectively increasing the intracellular concentration of the cytotoxic drug, and include Immunosuppressants (cyclosporin A, FK 506, rapamycin, PSC 833), calcium-channel blockers (verapamil, nifedipine), antiarrhythmics (quinidine), and other miscellaneous agents.[642,643,650,651] Several of these MDR-modulating agents have been used in clinical trials in an effort to sensitize resistant tumor cells (see below).

Table 56–7 Characteristics of Three Mechanisms of Multidrug Resistance That Result From Overexpression of P-Glycoprotein (PGP), Multidrug Resistance-Associated Protein (MRP), or Lung Resistance-Related Protein (LRP)

	PGP	MRP	LRP
Gene on chromosome	7q21.1	16p13.1	16p11.2
Protein			
Molecular mass	170 kd	190 kd	110 kd
Cellular location	Plasma membrane	Plasma membrane	Cytoplasm >> nuclear membrane
Function	Efflux pump, chloride channel	Drug transporter	Major vault protein (nucleocytoplasmic transport?)
Energy source	ATP	ATP	
Post-translational modifications	N-glycosylation, phosphorylation	N-glycosylation, phosphorylation	*No* N- or O-glycosylation
Analogs	Member ABC superfamily	Member ABC super-family; GS-X pump, MOAT, LTC_4 transport	
Drug resistance phenotype			
Antitumor agents	Act-D, AMSA, dauno, dox, epi, ida, mito-C (low), mtz, nav, tax, txtr, tpt (low), vbl, vcr, VM-26, VP-16	Act-D, chlor, CDDP-GSH, dauno, dox, epi, mel, tax (low), vbl (low), vcr, VM-26, VP-16	Carbo, CDDP, dox, mel, vcr, VP-16
Other drugs	Colch, rhod	As, Cd, colch (low), GSH conjugates, GSSG, LT_4, Sb	
Reversing agents	CSA, FK506, nifed, PSC833, quin, rap, verap	CSA, gnstn, indo, nicard, prbn, PSC833, verap, VX-710	
Normal hematopoietic tissues with increased expression	NK (CD56+) T cells, suppressor T cells (CD8+), B cells, CD34+ stem cells	PBMNs (esp. T cells), rbc membranes; liver and spleen low level	Macrophages
Prognostic significance	AML, MM, NHL	AML (inv 16)	AML, ALL

ABC, ATP-binding cassette; act-D, actinomycin D; As, arsenicals; carbo, carboplatin; Cd, cadmium; CDDP-GSH; cisplatin glutathione conjugate; chlor, chlorambucil; colch, colchicine; CSA, cyclosporin A; dauno, daunomycin; dox, doxorubicin; epi, epirubicin; gnstn, genistein; GS-X, glutathione conjugate; GSSG, oxidized glutathione; ida, idarubicin; indo, indomethacin; LTC_4, cysteinyl leukotriene; mel, melphalan; mito-C, mitomycin C; mtz, mitoxantrone; MOAT, multispecific organic anion transporter; NK, natural killer; nav, navelbine; nicard, nicardipine; nifed, nifedipine; prbn, probenecid; quin, quinidine; rap, rapamycin; rhod, rhodamine; Sb, antimonials; tax, taxol; txtr, taxotere; tpt, topotecan; vbl, vinblastine; vcr, vincristine; verap, verapamil; VM-26, teniposide; VP-16, etoposide.

Methods of Detection

Several monoclonal antibodies that recognize PGP and are commercially available for routine analyses have been described.[642,643,652] Monoclonal antibodies C219[653] and JSB-1[654] recognize internal epitopes of PGP, whereas antibodies MRK16[655] and UIC2[656] detect external antigens and are more suited for FACS analysis.

P-Glycoprotein Expression in Normal Human Tissue

High levels of expression of *MDR1*/PGP have been found in the epithelia of several human tissues with excretory function, suggesting that PGP is normally involved in transporting both exogenous toxic compounds and endogenous metabolites.[642] These tissues include the adrenal cortex, renal proximal tubule epithelium, biliary hepatocytes, small and large intestinal mucosa, pancreas, and endothelial cells of the brain and testis. Normal human hematopoietic tissues with high levels of *MDR1*/PGP include $CD34^+$ progenitor cells, $CD56^+$ (NK) cells, and $CD8^+$ (T-suppressor) cells.[657,658] Lower levels of expression have also been observed in $CD4^+$ (T-helper) cells, $CD19^+$ B cells, and $CD14^+$ cells (monocytes).

P-Glycoprotein Expression in Human Malignancies

Increased expression of PGP has been observed in several human tumors, especially those malignancies that arise in tissues that normally have high levels of PGP expression. A recent analysis of 61 human tumor cell lines (from leukemia, CNS tumors, melanoma, breast cancer, ovarian cancer, colon cancer, lung cancer, and kidney cancer), which were not selected for resistance to antitumor agents, demonstrated coexpression of two or three of the MDR proteins (PGP, LRP, or MRP) in 64% of the cell lines.[659] PGP and LRP were overexpressed in 3% of the tumors; MRP and LRP in 43%; and PGP, LRP, and MRP in 18%. The cell lines with the highest levels of drug resistance were found to overexpress all three proteins. Whether this is true in primary human tumors awaits further investigations.

Acute Myeloid Leukemia

An earlier meta-analysis of studies that examined the expression of *MDR1*/PGP in blasts of patients with AML[660] found that 40% (105/261 patients) who were PGP positive achieved a CR, whereas 81% (192/238) PGP-negative patients obtained a CR. An analysis of 96 untreated patients with AML showed that PGP expression predicted induction failure ($P < 0.0001$) and decreased overall survival ($P < 0.001$), as did unfavorable cytogenetics.[661] PGP expression was not detected in patients with favorable cytogenetic abnormalities [t(15;17), inv(16), t(8;21)], was found in 29% of those samples with a normal karyotype, and expressed in 62% of patients with an unfavorable cytogenetic abnormality. PGP was also detected in 63% of those with secondary AML, compared with 25% of those with de novo disease.[662] PGP analysis with the MRK16 antibody in 211 elderly patients (older than 55 years) with untreated AML once again showed that PGP expression is significantly associated with a decreased CR rate and resistant disease.[663] Patients in this report with de novo PGP-negative AML with favorable cytogenetics have a CR rate of 81%, compared with 12% for those with secondary AML, which is PGP-positive and has unfavorable cytogenetics. Recent clinical trials using the PGP substrate PSC833 acting as a competitive inhibitor have not shown the dramatic benefit expected, especially in older patients with acute leukemias.[664,665]

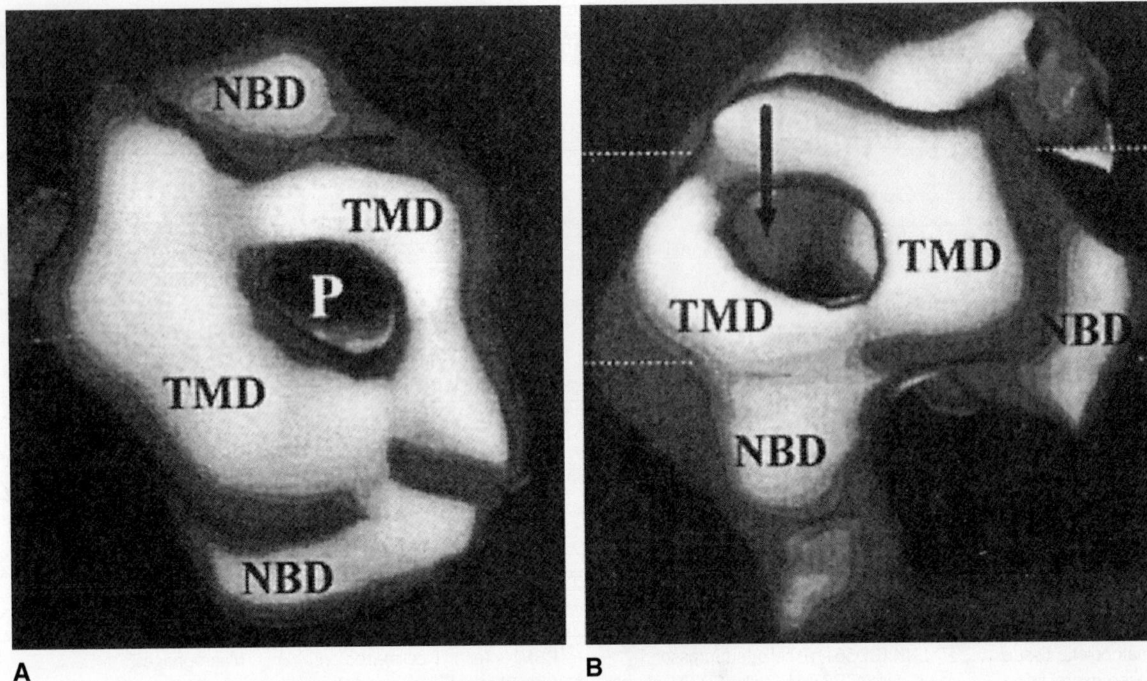

Figure 56–11 Structure of P-glycoprotein determined by electron microscopy; a computer graphic representation of the three-dimensional reconstruction is shown as a shaded surface representation of the structure. The straight arrow shows the putative ATP-binding domains. P represents the aqueous pore open at the extracellular face of the membrane. TMD, two thumbs, each of which probably corresponds to one of the two transmembrane domains. NBD, 3-nm lobes projecting from the structure at the cytoplasmic face of the membrane, probably corresponding to the two nucleotide-binding domains. **A,** View perpendicular to the extracellular surface of the lipid bilayer; **B,** side view of P-glycoprotein in which the approximate position of the lipid bilayer is indicated by the two horizontal dashed lines. Arrow, asymmetric opening providing access from the lipid phase to the aqueous core of the protein. *(Reproduced with permission from Rosenberg MF, Callaghan R, Ford RC, Higgins CF: Structure of the multidrug resistance P-glycoprotein to 2.5 nm resolution determined by electron microscopy and image analysis. J Biol Chem 272:10685, 1997.)*

Impact of P-Glycoprotein in Other Hematologic Malignancies

The role of PGP in the drug resistance of NHL, myeloma, and ALL is ill-defined.[666–669] CLL is another chronic leukemia where few PGP-related antineoplastic agents are used. However, a single study has shown a correlation between *MDR1* expression and survival, in which the 10 B-CLL patients who were *MDR1* positive had a median survival of 19 months compared with 46 months for the 17 patients who were *MDR1* negative ($P < 0.01$). Nonetheless, a recent study identified bortezomib as a substrate for PGP raising the possibility that myeloma PGP levels affect clinical response.[649] There have not been recent studies of the role of PGP in drug resistance in non-Hodgkin lymphoma in the past 5 years.

Clinical Studies With Modulators of P-Glycoprotein

The clinical trials that have employed various modulators of PGP have been reviewed by several investigators.[650,651,670] An early study in VAD-refractory multiple myeloma resulted in short-lived partial responses to VAD plus racemic verapamil in 5 of 22 patients.[671,672] Four of the five responders overexpressed PGP; however, cardiac side effects precluded further dose escalation of IV *R,S*-verapamil. Continuous IV infusion of cyclosporin A (CSA) with VAD in VAD-resistant myeloma patients resulted in 7 of 15 responses, which were more common in those who overexpressed PGP.[673] A randomized SWOG phase III study of VAD and oral verapamil in 120 patients with refractory myeloma demonstrated a 41% and 36% response in the VAD and VAD/verapamil arms, respectively, with median survivals of 10 and 13 months.[674] Continuous-infusion CSA has been dose-escalated in combination with daunorubicin and ara-C.[675] A transient hyperbilirubinemia was seen in 62% of the patients; these same patients had increased serum daunorubicin levels and a higher response rate. A complete response was seen in 26 of 42 patients; however, the MDR phenotype was not found to influence the response. A study of PSC833 in patients with acute leukemia treated with cytarabine, daunorubicin, and etoposide showed a modest benefit in patients under 45,[664] raising the potential of developing an effective strategy in patients more than 60 years of age in whom PGP expression in leukemic cells is more common.

Multidrug Resistance-Associated Protein (ABC G2 Transporter)

Structure and Function

The multidrug resistance-associated protein (MRP) was first described in 1992 in the doxorubicin selected small-cell lung cancer cell line,[676] and its biochemical characteristics and biologic properties have been reviewed.[677] It has now been classified within the larger context of ABC transporters, termed ABC G2 transporter.[644] Because much of the literature use the MRP nomenclature, we refer to this herein except for the studies using the ABC terminology. This N-glycosylated plasma membrane phosphoprotein has a molecular mass of 190 kd (1531 amino acids) and is a member of the ABC transporter superfamily (see Table 56–7 and Fig. 56–12). This transporter has 18 transmembrane domains (12 in the amino end and 6 in the carboxyl end) and is coded on human chromosome 16p13.1.

The overexpression of MRP has been shown in vitro to result in different levels of drug resistance to several classes of antineoplastic agents,[677–681] represented by actinomycin D, chlorambucil, melphalan, CDDP, daunomycin, doxorubicin, epirubicin, VM-26, VP-16, and vincristine. Low levels of resistance have also been reported to taxol, vinblastine, and colchicine. In addition to antitumoral agents, MRP (and its isoforms) are capable of transporting heavy metals

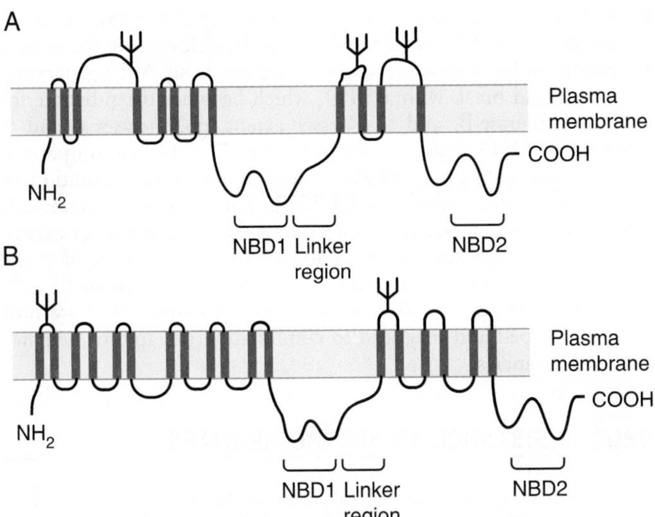

Figure 56–12 Models of multidrug resistance protein (MRP) membrane topology. MRP possesses features common to all members of the ATP-binding cassette transporter superfamily, in that each half of the protein is predicted to consist of several transmembrane domains followed by a cytosolic nucleotide-binding domain (MBD). The first model (**A**) is based on computer-assisted hydropathy analyses of the human MRP amino acid sequence and predicts that MRP is composed of 12 transmembrane domains (*solid bars*), eight of which are within the NH-2 proximal half of the protein. The second model (**B**), based on a comparison of human and murine MRP with other ATP-binding cassette transporters, suggests that there are up to four additional transmembrane domains in the NH2-proximal half of the protein. *(Adapted from Loe DW, Deley RG, Cole SPC: Biology of the multidrug resistance-associated protein, MRP. Eur J Cancer 32A:945, 1996.)*

(arsenicals, cadmium, and antimonials) as well as glutathione conjugates and cysteinyl leukotriene. Compounds reported to modulate MRP-mediated drug resistance in vitro include the calcium channel blocker verapamil, nocardipine, the protein kinase C inhibitor GF109203X, the cyclosporin analog PSC 833, the tyrosine kinase inhibitor genistein, the gyrase-inhibiting antibiotic difloxacin, and amiodarone.[677] More recently, VX-710, a nonmacrocyclic ligand of the FK506-binding protein FKBP12 and a potent modulator of PGP-mediated MDR, has been found to restore sensitivity of MRP-expressing HL60/ADR cells to the cytotoxic action of doxorubicin, VP-16, and vincristine.[682] The NSAID indomethacin has also been shown to significantly increase the sensitivity of HL60/ADR cells to doxorubicin and vincristine and may be a specific inhibitor of MRP.[683]

MRP Expression in Hematologic Malignancies

The expression of MRP mRNA (measured by an RNase protection assay) and/or the level of MRP protein (by immunohistochemistry) has been assessed in 148 patients with hematopoietic malignancies.[684–686] MRP mRNA expression was found to be significantly increased in 84% of patients with CLL and in 30% of those with AML. The vast majority of patients with ALL, CML, multiple myeloma, hairy cell leukemia, and NHL were found to have low levels of MRP mRNA expression in the malignant cells. MRP protein was assayed using monoclonal antibody MRPr1, and the results generally followed those of the message with increased expression in most patients with CLL. A study of 40 patients with refractory lymphoma and 16 with newly diagnosed lymphoma suggests a limited role for MRP mRNA expression in drug resistance in NHL, as 15 paired samples in the refractory group showed no difference in MRP expression pre- and post-EPOCH treatment.[687] In addition, the untreated patients had MRP mRNA levels that were no different from the pre- or post-EPOCH patient levels. A study of 49 patients with AML and 29 with ALL demonstrated significantly higher expression of MRP in ALL ($P < 0.007$) and in secondary AML ($P < 0.016$), but not in de novo AML.[688] Although there was initial enthusiasm for the likely association between the biology of hematologic malignancies, expression of MRP, and clinical response to therapeutic agents, there has been loss of interest in modulating expression of MRP or in developing targeted agents that block its function. For instance, between 2003 and 2007 there are few publications providing evidence of therapeutic impact of MRP expression or its modulation on the treatment of hematologic malignancies. One study provided an update on the expression of MRP in hematologic malignancies.[689] A second identified a new MRP inhibitor in preclinical models that could have therapeutic impact.[690] This group used a drug targeting the peripheral benzodiazepine receptor (pBR) ligand, PK11195. This molecule promotes mitochondrial apoptosis and blocks P-glycoprotein (PGP)- and ABC transporter-mediated drug efflux and potentiates apoptosis in malignant cells. MRP mRNA expression was found to be significantly ($P < 0.05$) elevated at second and later relapses (but not before treatment or at first relapse) in a group of 60 patients (52 children and 8 adults) with ALL.[691] Finally, 14 patients with relapsed AML were found to have a twofold increase in blast MRP mRNA relative to 29 patients with newly diagnosed AML ($P < 0.01$).[692] Paired blast samples (obtained at diagnosis and at relapse) from 13 AML and 4 ALL patients showed a twofold increase in 80% of the patients at relapse, suggesting that the expression of the MRP transporter at relapse may be involved in drug resistance.

The larger family of transporters, the ABC group including ABC G2 and ABC B1, are overexpressed in leukemic cells and in many malignant stem cells.[693] In fact in addition to CD44, high levels of ABC transporters assist in the characterization and isolation of the transplantable subpopulation of malignant stem cells. Brendel and coworkers found that both imatinib and nilotinib used to block the abl kinase in CML were effective blocking the ABC transporter in CML cells.[694] This suggested both that these agents might function in part by blocking expression of an important leukemic stem cell protein and that they would potentiate CML cells to other agents transported by the ABC system.

DNA Repair Pathway Mechanisms of Drug Resistance

O^6-Alkylguanine-DNA Alkyltransferase (MGMT)

As noted previously, the nitrosoureas and methylating agents are cytotoxic in large part due to formation of DNA adducts at the O^6 position of guanine.[695] The most efficient means of protection from the cytotoxicity of adducts at the O^6 position of guanine is rapid repair by the O^6-alkylguanine-DNA alkyltransferase (AGT or MGMT).[695] This protein serves as the stoichiometric acceptor protein for O^6-alkylguanine DNA monoadducts, transferring the alkyl group from DNA to the active site of the protein, inactivating the protein, and restoring DNA to normal.[695,696] However, the N^1G-N^3C DNA cross-link that follows chloroethylation is not a substrate for AGT. There is a striking correlation between drug resistance and alkyltransferase activity.[109,697] Of interest, high levels of AGT are found in many leukemias,[698] whereas low AGT is observed in normal human CD34 cells,[122] perhaps explaining why nitrosoureas are not used in leukemia management and why nitrosoureas are effective myeloablative agents used in high-dose chemotherapy regimens. Recently, a novel inhibitor of AGT, O^6-benzylguanine (BG) has been used to sensitize human tumors to BCNU.[697,699,700] Recent studies indicate activity of the combination of BG and BCNU in myeloma and in cutaneous lymphomas.[701] Therapeutic benefit from the methylating and alkylating agent cloretazine appears to be related to lower levels of AGT.[124] Likewise, temozolomide has some therapeutic efficacy in leukemia in a manner inversely related to AGT levels in the tumor cells.[122]

Mismatch Repair

The spectrum of drug resistance and sensitivity to methylating agents does not end with AGT. Recent evidence suggests that methylating agent-induced cell death involves an aborted effort at mismatch repair. Karran and others, in mammalian systems, have shown that the replicative DNA polymerase and the repair polymerase pauses at O^6-mG and preferentially inserts a thymine (T) at the site.[98,702] The O^6-mG:T base pair is recognized by the mismatch repair (MMR) system, which initiates base excision repair (BER, see below). In human cells, the MMR complex consists of at least 6 proteins involved in the recognition and repair of mismatch lesions: HMLH1, hMSH2, hMSH3, hPMS1, hPMS2, and GTBP (GT-binding protein, also called MSH6), all of which appear to be homologs of MMR proteins found in *E Coli* and in yeast.[97,703,704] Following binding recognition, an endonuclease removes a patch of approximately 100 to 1000 bp containing the T mismatch, DNA polymerase δ or γ fills in the patch, with reinsertion of a T opposite the O^6-mG and a DNA ligase closes the strand break.[97] Because the O^6-mG:T is re-formed, cytotoxicity ensues as a result of repetitive efforts at DNA repair and induction of both chromosomal breakage, rearrangements, energy depletion, and apoptosis.[705] Drug resistance based on mutation or loss of expression of an MMR protein, owing to mutation within one of the gene coding regions, or promoter methylation leading to loss of gene expression, has been noted in solid tumors and in leukemias and lymphomas. The mutator phenotype was originally described in cells with acquired resistance to methylnitrosourea, methylmethanesulfonate or *N*-methyl-*N*-nitroso-*N*-nitrosoguanidine, which were tolerant to G→A point mutations according to the inability to repair O^6-mG[601] and are cross-resistant to 6-thioguanine (6-TG) used in childhood leukemia maintenance regimens, which forms the 6-TG:T mismatch.[98,99]

MMR Mutations and Methylating Agent Resistance

Mismatch repair defects in humans were initially described in hereditary nonpolyposis colon cancer, or HNPCC, which comprises approximately 15% of all colon cancer,[97,104,704] lymphomas, and relapsing acute leukemias.[682] The genetic defect results in a high rate of spontaneous mutations within microsatellite DNA, resulting in the replication error (RER) phenotype arising as the expansion or contraction of mono-, di-, or trinucleotide repeats within the microsatellites.[97] Tumor cells defective in MMR are remarkably resistant to temozolomide regardless of AGT activity or its inhibition by BG, confirming the importance of MMR in sensitivity to methylating agents.[94] Of interest, MMR mutant cells are also two- to threefold resistant to cisplatin,[706] perhaps because the cisplatin DNA adduct is bound by the MMR complex, slowing its recognition and repair by the nucleotide repair pathway and increasing its cytotoxicity.[707] Such MMR-deficient cells also exhibit microsatellite instability, a measure of genomic instability and the propensity to develop further mutations during therapy leading to subclones of resistant cells. Loss of PMS2 has been identified in a family of childhood lymphomas.[708] Microsatellite instability is seen in acute leukemias and in T-cell leukemias,[709,710] suggesting both that these malignancies have lost MMR function and that they are more prone to drug resistance and acquisition of additional mutations that give rise to further drug resistance. Evidence of microsatellite instability and loss of MMR is much more common in treatment-related leukemias,[711] again providing a mechanism of drug resistance.

Base Excision Repair

Methylating agents such as procarbazine and temozolomide form large numbers of N^3-A and N^7-G adducts in addition to O^6-mG (with TMZ, the relative amounts are 72 N^7mG: 8 O^6mG: 5 N^3mA). Thus, under normal circumstances, cells process many more N^7mG and N^3mA lesions than O^6mG lesions, even though the latter appears much more cytotoxic, except in MMR defective cells. Repair of N^3-A and N^7-G adducts through BER is efficient and normally leads to cell survival rather than cell death. Adducts are recognized by the methylpurine glycosylase (MPG) with removal of the base, generating an abasic (or AP) site. The AP site is then cleaved by the class II hydrolytic endonuclease (or apurinic endonuclease, APE) generating a single strand break with a $5'PO_4$ which becomes the substrate for DNA polymerase-β, and to a lesser extent, polymerases δ and γ, followed by DNA ligase (reviewed by Sancar[95]). Other compounds induce nucleotide pool imbalance leading to misincorporation of bases that become substrates for BER. These compounds include folate antagonists such as Methotrexate, 5-FU, and to a lesser extent, nucleoside analogs such as fludarabine. Misincorporation of uracil after 5-FU inhibition of thymidilate synthase also leads to BER.[712] Compounds to disrupt BER, such as methoxyamine,[713,714] are now being developed and may lead to combination therapy for hematologic malignancies.

DRUG RESISTANCE TO ANTIMETABOLITES

Although overlap exists, antimetabolites can be classified into nucleoside analogs that are incorporated into RNA and/or DNA and agents that inhibit de novo purine and pyrimidine biosynthetic pathways. Mechanisms of resistance to these agents fall into several broad categories. For example, many antimetabolites are prodrugs in that they must be converted intracellularly into active nucleotide forms in order to exert their cytotoxic actions. Consequently, events that interfere with cellular accumulation of drug and/or nucleotide formation will reduce activity. Examples include decreased transport of methotrexate or decreased nucleotide formation of Ara-C and 6-thioguanine by reductions in activity of deoxycytidine kinase or HGPRT, respectively. Alternatively, enhanced drug catabolism reduces cytotoxicity. Examples include the deamination of Ara-C (to inactive Ara-U) by cytidine deaminase or catabolism of 6-TG by thiopurine methyltransferase. A third mechanism of resistance stems from the presence of increased intracellular levels of a competing metabolite (eg, dCTP in the case of Ara-C, or hypoxanthine or guanine in the case of 6-TG). Fourth, alterations in the level of activity of a target enzyme or the presence of a mutant form that is less inhibitable will also confer resistance. Examples include increased activity or a mutant form of DHFR (in the case of methotrexate), an altered DNA polymerase α (in the case of Ara-C), or increased activity of ribonucleotide reductase (through overexpression of either subunit). Finally, cytokinetic factors represent a common theme in the case of most (but not all) antimetabolites in that a reduction in the S-phase fraction generally leads to reduced drug sensitivity. Note that these resistance mechanisms are agent specific and are distinct from the more general modes of resistance (eg, increased expression of BCL2) associated with defects in the distal cell death pathway.

FUTURE THERAPEUTIC IMPLICATIONS OF CANCER BIOLOGY

Future treatment strategies against hematologic malignancies are likely to be directed against those cellular targets that are responsible for the altered biology and transformed phenotype of cancer versus normal cells. This altered biology results from the accumulation of genetic mutations and alterations secondary to the unique genomic instability of cancer cells. Major development is taking place targeting protein kinases, translocation fusion proteins, promoter demethylation and histone deacetylation, immunomodulator proteins such as lenazolid, and inhibitors of cytokines such as IL-6 that are overexpressed in hematologic malignancies. As noted above, defects in the DNA repair pathway and in cell-cycle checkpoints that cause inappropriate progression through the cell cycle facilitate the genomic instability of cancer cells. These too are critical to transformation, and agents that overcome these abnormalities are important targets for drug development.

Because dysregulated cell-cycle progression is a common feature of neoplastic cells, several strategies are being developed and tested to exploit this as a therapeutic target. These strategies include the use of drugs that inhibit the function of the mitotic kinase $p34^{cdc-2}$ (CDK1), for example, flavopiridol or inhibitors of the dual-specific phosphatase cdc25, which dephosphorylates and activates $p34^{cdc-2}$. Flavopiridol also inhibits CDK2 and CDK4 by binding to the hydrophobic, adenine binding pocket of the ATP site of these G_1-S kinases, thereby inducing G_1 arrest. An additional strategy is to inhibit mitogenic signaling mediated by oncogene products such as activated Ras, Raf, and Bcr-Abl. Antisense oligonucleotides to RAF, BCR-ABL, MYB, RAS, and BCL2 are being tested for their antitumoral effects alone or in combination with other cytotoxic drugs. Inhibitors of Ras farnesylation exert their antitumoral effects by, as yet, unclear mechanisms.

The relentless growth of tumors and leukemia requires the delivery of nutrients and growth factors through new blood microvessels (angiogenesis). Inhibitors of angiogenesis have an exciting potential in cancer and leukemia therapy. Bevacizumab (anti-VEGF) is approved for solid tumors and is being evaluated in hematologic malignancies. These agents target the vascular endothelial growth factors (eg, VEGF, bFGF, and PDGF) or their receptor-mediated signaling (eg, SU 5416).

SUGGESTED READINGS

Brandwein JM, Yang L, Schimmer AD, et al: A phase II study of temozolomide therapy for poor-risk patients aged > or = 60 years with acute myeloid leukemia: Low levels of MGMT predict for response. Leukemia 21:821, 2007.

Caporaso P, Turriziani M, Venditti A, et al: Novel role of triazenes in haematological malignancies: Pilot study of Temozolomide, Lomeguatrib and IL-2 in the chemo-immunotherapy of acute leukaemia. DNA Repair (Amst) 6:1179, 2007.

Chauhan D, Neri P, Velankar M, et al: Targeting mitochondrial factor Smac/DIABLO as therapy for multiple myeloma (MM). Blood 109:1220, 2007.

DeAngelo DJ, Yu D, Johnson JL, et al: Nelarabine induces complete remissions in adults with relapsed or refractory T-lineage acute lymphoblastic leukemia or lymphoblastic lymphoma: Cancer and Leukemia Group B study 19801. Blood 109:5136, 2007.

Demo SD, Kirk CJ, Aujay MA, et al: Antitumor activity of PR-171, a novel irreversible inhibitor of the proteasome. Cancer Res 67:6383, 2007.

Ghoshal K, Bai S: DNA methyltransferases as targets for cancer therapy. Drugs Today (Barc) 43:395, 2007.

Guilhot F, Apperley J, Kim DW, et al: Dasatinib induces significant hematologic and cytogenetic responses in patients with imatinib-resistant or -intolerant chronic myeloid leukemia in accelerated phase. Blood 109:4143, 2007.

Giuliani N, Morandi F, Tagliaferri S, et al: The proteasome inhibitor bortezomib affects osteoblast differentiation in vitro and in vivo in multiple myeloma patients. Blood 110:334, 2007.

Kantarjian H, Oki Y, Garcia-Manero G, et al: Results of a randomized study of 3 schedules of low-dose decitabine in higher-risk myelodysplastic syndrome and chronic myelomonocytic leukemia. Blood 109:52, 2007.

Manochakian R, Miller KC, Chanan-Khan AA: Bortezomib in combination with pegylated liposomal doxorubicin for the treatment of multiple myeloma. Clin Lymphoma Myeloma 7:266, 2007.

Meister S, Schubert U, Neubert K, et al: Extensive immunoglobulin production sensitizes myeloma cells for proteasome inhibition. Cancer Res 67:1783, 2007.

O'Brien S, Moore JO, Boyd TE, et al: Randomized phase III trial of fludarabine plus cyclophosphamide with or without oblimersen sodium (Bcl-2 antisense) in patients with relapsed or refractory chronic lymphocytic leukemia. J Clin Oncol, 25:1114, 2007.

Perez-Galan P, Roue G, Villamor N, et al: The BH3-mimetic GX15-070 synergizes with bortezomib in mantle cell lymphoma by enhancing noxa-mediated activation of Bak. Blood, 109:4441, 2007.

Pfeifer H, Wassmann B, Pavlova A, et al: Kinase domain mutations of BCR-ABL frequently precede imatinib-based therapy and give rise to relapse in patients with de novo Philadelphia-positive acute lymphoblastic leukemia (Ph+ ALL). Blood 110:727, 2007.

Richardson PG, Sonneveld P, Schuster MW, et al: Safety and efficacy of bortezomib in high-risk and elderly patients with relapsed multiple myeloma. Br J Haematol 137:429, 2007.

Sanchorawala V, Wright DG, Rosenzweig M, et al: Lenalidomide and dexamethasone in the treatment of AL amyloidosis: Results of a phase 2 trial. Blood 109:492, 2007.

Soverini S, Colarossi S, Gnani A, et al: Resistance to dasatinib in Philadelphia-positive leukemia patients and the presence or the selection of mutations at residues 315 and 317 in the BCR-ABL kinase domain. Haematologica 92:401, 2007.

Strauss SJ, Higginbottom K, Juliger S, et al: The proteasome inhibitor bortezomib acts independently of p53 and induces cell death via apoptosis and mitotic catastrophe in B-cell lymphoma cell lines. Cancer Res 67:2783, 2007.

Trudel S, Stewart AK, Li Z, et al: The Bcl-2 family protein inhibitor, ABT-737, has substantial antimyeloma activity and shows synergistic effect with dexamethasone and melphalan. Clin Cancer Res 13:621, 2007.

Trudel S, Li ZH, Rauw J, et al: Pre-clinical studies of the pan-Bcl inhibitor obatoclax (GX015-070) in multiple myeloma. Blood, 2007.

von Metzler I, Krebbel H, Hecht M, et al: Bortezomib inhibits human osteoclastogenesis. Leukemia 21:2025, 2007.

White DJ, Paul N, Macdonald DA, et al: Addition of lenalidomide to melphalan in the treatment of newly diagnosed multiple myeloma: The National Cancer Institute of Canada Clinical Trials Group MY.11 trial. Curr Oncol 14:61, 2007.

Yan L, Bulgar A, Miao Y, et al: Combined treatment with temozolomide and methoxyamine: Blocking apurininc/pyrimidinic site repair coupled with targeting topoisomerase IIalpha. Clin Cancer Res 13:1532, 2007.

Zheng LM, Li Z, Liu L, et al: Anti-tumor efficacy of Cloretazine (VNP40101M) alone and in combination with fludarabine in murine tumor and human xenograft tumor models. Cancer Chemother Pharmacol 60:45, 2007.

REFERENCES

For complete list of references log onto www.expertconsult.com

APPENDIX 56–1

CLINICAL PHARMACOLOGY OF ALKYLATING AGENTS

MECHLORETHAMINE (Mustargen)

Chemistry: Mechlorethamine, also called nitrogen mustard, is a water-soluble and alcohol-soluble analog of sulfur mustard gas. It is a bifunctional chloroethylating agent that alkylates DNA, RNA, and protein.

Absorption, Fate, and Excretion: The parent compound is highly reactive and has a biologic half-life of approximately 15 minutes. The principal route of degradation is spontaneous hydrolysis, but some enzymatic demethylation also occurs.

Preparation and Administration: Mechlorethamine is supplied in vials of 10 mg with 100 mg of sodium chloride, and is reconstituted with 10 mL sterile water to yield a 1-mg/mL solution, ideally prepared immediately before use. However, the manufacturer considers the drug expired 1 hour after reconstitution. The drug is injected over a few minutes through a tubing as a freely running IV infusion. For topical application (eg, in mycosis fungoides), 10 mg of drug is dissolved in 60 mL of tap water. Alternatively, a 10 mg% ointment has been used by dissolving the drug in 95% ethyl alcohol and petrolatum (Aquaphor). Mechlorethamine is a powerful vesicant. In the event of extravasation, vigorous irrigation followed by 0.25% sodium thiosulfate injection at the site of extravasation should be attempted. Ice packs may be placed for 6 to 12 hours to minimize the local reaction.

Toxic Effects: Myelosuppression is the dose-limiting systemic side effect. This worsens with each additive cycle. Severe nausea and vomiting, infertility, alopecia, and pain at the site of injection, which can sometimes spread to involve the venous system (tracking), are also common. Occasionally, a macular papular rash is observed, but this does not appear to be allergic in nature and does not contraindicate continuation of therapy. Infertility is common, but may be reversible. Infrequent adverse effects include alopecia, anorexia, weakness, and diarrhea. The drug has also been shown to induce chromosomal abnormalities and may contribute to the development of secondary leukemias, as seen in patients treated with this agent as part of the MOPP regimen.

Potential Drug Interactions: None has been reported.

Therapeutic Indications in Hematology: Mechlorethamine is incorporated in many chemotherapy combinations used in the treatment of Hodgkin disease (MOPP [mechlorethamine, vincristine, procarbazine, prednisone] and MOPP/ABV [Adriamycin, bleomycin, and vinblastine] hybrid) and in some NHLs (prednisone, etoposide, methotrexate, doxorubicin [Adriamycin], cyclophosphamide, Leucovorin [PROMACE]/MOPP). However, its use has largely been supplanted by other agents.

CYCLOPHOSPHAMIDE (CYTOXAN)

Chemistry: Cyclophosphamide is a cyclic phosphamide ester of mechlorethamine. Once metabolically activated, it alkylates DNA, forming cross-links.

Absorption, Fate, and Excretion: The drug is relatively well absorbed orally, with approximately 75% oral bioavailability. The parent compound is not active. The drug is metabolized by the hepatic CYP system, which ultimately generates at least two active compounds: Phosphoramide mustard and acrolein. The latter appears to be responsible for cyclophosphamide's bladder toxicities. The plasma half-life of cyclophosphamide varies from 4 to 6.5 hours. Approximately 15% of the drug is excreted unchanged in the urine. Dose reduction should be considered in patients with severe renal failure.

Preparation and Administration: Cyclophosphamide is supplied as 25- and 50-mg tablets and as a powder for parenteral administration in 100-, 200-, and 500-mg and 1- and 2-g vials. It is dissolved by adding 5 mL of preservative-free sterile water for every 100 mg of drug. Cyclophosphamide is chemically stable for 24 hours at room temperature and for 6 days if refrigerated.

Toxic Effects: Marrow suppression is the major side effect. The myeloid series is primarily affected, although thrombocytopenia also occurs at high doses and alopecia is common. Nausea and vomiting can be severe and are usually delayed, occurring 6 to 8 hours after administration. Hemorrhagic cystitis occurs in 10% of patients receiving nontransplant doses and is apparently due to the formation of the urotoxin acrolein. Because of this potential side effect, patients should be well hydrated. Mesna disulfide (sodium 2-mercaptoethanesulfonate disulfide) has also been used on a weight equivalent basis to ameliorate cyclophosphamide-induced bladder toxicity. Other potential toxic effects include stomatitis, skin and nail hyperpigmentation, interstitial pulmonary fibrosis, and the syndrome of inappropriate secretion of antidiuretic hormone. Rare episodes of acute congestive heart failure have been reported. After bone marrow transplant doses, hemorrhagic cystitis is common and cardiac toxicity (cardiomyopathy) may be seen. Late sequelae include bladder fibrosis (more common with daily [oral] therapy), bladder cancer, leukemogenesis, and infertility.

Potential Drug Interactions: Corticosteroids may increase P450 enzyme-induced metabolism and is often avoided in high-dose therapy. When combined with doxorubicin, it may increase cardiac toxicity. This may be prevented by amifostine. In animal studies, conflicting results were reported when the P450 enzyme inducer, phenobarbital, was given with cyclophosphamide. Most investigators, however, have observed a reduction in the amounts of active metabolites. Conversely, when cimetidine (but not ranitidine) was administered in leukemia-bearing mice before treatment with cyclophosphamide, a significant prolongation of their survival and higher plasma concentrations of alkylating metabolites were observed. Although one should remain alert for these potential drug interactions, none has been demonstrated in humans. Cyclophosphamide reduces serum pseudocholinesterase levels, which may prolong the neuromuscular blocking effects if given simultaneously. Caution must be exercised when administering high doses of these two drugs to critically ill patients. Life-threatening hyponatremia may develop when used in conjunction with indomethacin, although the precise incidence is unknown.

Therapeutic Indications in Hematology: Cyclophosphamide is a key drug in the treatment of lymphomas and myeloma. It is incorporated in many chemotherapy regimens, including CHOP, MACOP-B, PROMACE/CYTABOM, CVP, and VMCP (see chapter for details). In addition, cyclophosphamide is the drug most commonly used in preparatory regimens for bone marrow transplantation. It is also used in solid tumors and as an immunosuppressant in nonmalignant conditions such as glomerulonephritis and systemic lupus erythematosus.

IFOSFAMIDE (IFEX)

Chemistry: Ifosfamide is an oxazaphosphine nitrogen mustard that differs from cyclophosphamide by the placement of chloroethyl groups.

Absorption, Fate, and Excretion: As in the case of cyclophosphamide, the parent compound is inactive and is metabolized by the cytochrome P450 system in the liver. The metabolism of ifosfamide is influenced by the dose and schedule of administration. When administered as a single bolus, 60% is eliminated into the urine, 53% as unchanged inactive drug. When administered daily for 5 consecutive days, 56% is excreted into the urine, 15% as the inactive parent compound. The half-life is 7 hours when administered daily for 5 consecutive days, and 15 hours when given as a single bolus dose. There is poor penetration across the blood–brain barrier. Its longer half-life and slower metabolic activation allows higher doses to be given.

Preparation and Administration: The drug is provided in 1-g vials and should be reconstituted in sterile water or bacteriostatic water to a final concentration of 50 mg/mL. Ifosfamide can be diluted further in 5% dextrose, normal saline, or Ringer's solution for injection to achieve concentrations of between 0.6 and 20 mg/mL. The solution should be infused over 30 minutes. To prevent hemorrhagic cystitis, patients must receive mesna disulfide for protection against urotoxicity and must be kept well hydrated (2 L/day). Mesna is a thiol compound that is rapidly oxidized to dimesna in vivo. Mesna and dimesna are filtered by the glomeruli, reabsorbed in the proximal tubule, and finally secreted back into the tubular lumen of the kidney. In the tubules, approximately one-third of the filtered dimesna is readily converted back to mesna. The free sulfhydryl group of this compound reacts with the urotoxic metabolite acrolein produced by both ifosfamide and cyclophosphamide (see Fig. 55–6). This reaction creates a nontoxic acrolein-mesna thioether that is safely eliminated in the urine. Mesna has also been shown to inhibit the degradation of ifosfamide or cyclophosphamide to acrolein.

Mesna has been given in combination with ifosfamide in different doses and schedules. One recommended schedule employs IV bolus injection in a dosage equal to 20% of the ifosfamide dose (on a milligram-to-milligram basis) at the time of ifosfamide administration and 4 and 8 hours after each dose of ifosfamide. Mesna has also been given by continuous infusion with excellent results. The two agents may be mixed together in the same IV solution; however, mesna is not compatible with cisplatin.

Toxic Effects: With the use of mesna to protect against urotoxicity, myelosuppression—especially leukopenia and, to a lesser extent, thrombocytopenia—is the dose-limiting side effect. Renal tubular acidosis can occur. Central nervous system effects, observed in approximately 10% of patients treated, include somnolence, confusion, depressive psychosis, and hallucinations. Less commonly, dizziness, disorientation, and cranial nerve dysfunction occur. Nausea and vomiting are common. Low serum albumin and elevated serum creatinine may enhance central nervous system toxicity. As with cyclophosphamide, such side effects as alopecia, leukemogenesis, and infertility also occur. Cardiac toxicity is rare.

Potential Drug Interactions: Because ifosfamide is also metabolized by the P450 system, physicians should remain alert for the same type of potential drug interactions that have been reported with cyclophosphamide. A recent report advises close monitoring of warfarin anticoagulant control in patients receiving ifosfamide/mesna.

Therapeutic Indications in Hematology: Ifosfamide was recently approved for treatment of patients with refractory testicular cancer. In hematologic malignancies, its major indication is in the treatment of refractory lymphomas.

MELPHALAN (Melphalan)

Chemistry: Melphalan is synthesized from nitrogen mustard and phenylalanine. It is a bifunctional chloroethylating agent that forms DNA cross-links.

Absorption, Fate, and Excretion: The oral bioavailability of melphalan is quite variable, 20% to 50% of the drug being excreted in the stool. Some patients show virtually no oral absorption. This fact is particularly pertinent in the treatment of myeloma patients, in whom a lack of response to melphalan may be due simply to poor oral absorption. Melphalan has a half-life of approximately 90 minutes. It is extensively metabolized, with only approximately 10% to 15% of an administered dose excreted unchanged in the urine.

Preparation and Administration: Melphalan is commercially available in 2-mg tablets and in IV formulation for high-dose therapy.

Toxic Effects: The dose-limiting toxicity is myelosuppression, manifested by leukopenia and thrombocytopenia and generally occurring 2 to 3 weeks after therapy. Recovery may take 6 weeks, however, in patients who have been heavily pretreated with chemotherapy drugs or radiotherapy, or both. Nausea, vomiting, and alopecia are uncommon side effects and are usually mild. Occasionally, amenorrhea and azoospermia, pulmonary fibrosis, dermatitis, and secondary malignancies (eg, leukemia) occur, especially in patients receiving the drug over the long term. At cumulative doses of less than 600 mg, the incidence of second hematologic malignancy is probably less than 2% but may be greater than 15% at higher doses. Higher doses used in transplant patients result in gastrointestinal toxicity that is dose limiting. At these doses, the syndrome of inappropriate secretion of antidiuretic hormone, pneumonitis, and hepatic venoocclusive disease have been observed.

Potential Drug Interactions: Administration of high-dose IV melphalan with cyclosporine increases the risk of cyclosporine nephrotoxicity.

Therapeutic Indications: The major use of melphalan is for the treatment of multiple myeloma, either as a single agent or in combination with other alkylating agents and prednisone (eg, the MP and VMCP regimens). The IV formulation has been approved for isolated limb perfusion in melanoma. It is used in high-dose protocols for myeloma and solid tumors at doses of 140 to 200 mg/m^2.

CHLORAMBUCIL (Chlorambucil)

Chemistry: Chlorambucil is an aromatic derivative of mechlorethamine.

Absorption, Fate, and Excretion: Chlorambucil is well absorbed after oral administration. It is extensively metabolized in the liver to its major metabolite, phenylacetic acid mustard (PAAM), which also has bifunctional alkylating activity. The half-lives of chlorambucil and PAAM are 1.5 and 2.5 hours, respectively; less than 1% of either chlorambucil or PAAM is excreted in the urine.

Preparation and Administration: Chlorambucil is commercially available as 2-mg tablets.

Toxic Effects: Treatment is usually well tolerated, with myelosuppression the dose-limiting toxic effect. Patients on a daily oral schedule should have biweekly complete blood counts (CBCs). Nausea and vomiting are uncommon, but mild alopecia and skin rashes occasionally occur. As with the other alkylating agents, azoospermia (especially above cumulative dose of 400 mg), amenorrhea, and secondary leukemia are potential risks of prolonged therapy. Rare cases of pulmonary fibrosis have also been reported.

Potential Drug Interactions: None has been reported.

Therapeutic Indications in Hematology: The major uses are in the treatment of Waldenström macroglobulinemia, low-grade lymphomas, CLL, and Hodgkin disease. Except for CLL, chlorambucil has been supplanted by newer agents.

BUSULFAN (Myleran)

Chemistry: Busulfan is an alkylsulfonate bifunctional alkylating agent not chemically related to mechlorethamine. It forms DNA intrastrand and interstrand cross-links.

Absorption, Fate, and Excretion: Busulfan is well absorbed after oral administration. When given by the IV route, greater than 90% is cleared from the plasma after 3 minutes. The drug is extensively metabolized to inactive compounds that are excreted renally. The major metabolite is methane sulfonic acid, although more than 10 other not fully identified metabolites exist. Virtually no intact busulfan is found in the urine. The biologic half-life of busulfan is approximately 2.5 hours.

Preparation and Administration: The drug is commercially available as 2-mg tablets.

Toxic Effects: Although at low doses the major effect of busulfan is on the granulocytic series, at high doses all three hematologic series are affected. As compared with the other alkylating agents, its nadir of myelosuppression may be relatively late, in a range of 11 to 30 days. Hematologic recovery is also prolonged and may take approximately 54 days. A relatively common side effect is an Addisonian-like syndrome characterized by skin hyperpigmentation and weakness, but without abnormalities in adrenal function. Cumulative pulmonary toxicity has been well described and consists of a mixed alveolar and interstitial pneumonitis. As with the other alkylating agents, infertility and leukemogenesis can occur. Nausea and vomiting are rare. At high doses it is associated with hepatic venoocclusive disease in up to 19% of patients. Seizures may also occur and are controlled by diphenylhydration.

Potential Drug Interactions: A metabolic interaction may take place between busulfan and various anticonvulsant medications; however, further description of the specific effects are awaited.

Therapeutic Indications in Hematology: Busulfan is used mainly in the treatment of CML. More recently, high-dose busulfan has been incorporated into preparatory regimens for bone marrow transplantation. Blood level monitoring with adjustment for higher close levels improved therapeutic outcome and reduced toxicity.

CARMUSTINE (BCNU)

Chemistry: Carmustine, also called BCNU (1,3[bis]-2-chloroethyl-nitrosourea), decomposes spontaneously into a chloroethyl hydroxide that can alkylate the DNA, and into an isocyanide molecule, which may produce carbamylation of proteins. Cytotoxicity is due to DNA cross-links.

Absorption, Fate, and Excretion: Intravenously administered carmustine is rapidly metabolized, with a half-life of 70 minutes. Approximately 30% to 80% of metabolites are eliminated in the urine within 24 hours. The drug or its metabolites, or both, readily cross the blood–brain barrier, resulting in cerebrospinal fluid concentrations within the range of 15% to 70% of plasma levels. Peak serum levels vary widely in patients treated at 200 to 600 mg IMF.

Preparation and Administration: Carmustine is commercially available in 100-mg vials as a white lyophilized powder. The drug is reconstituted with 3 mL of absolute alcohol provided by the manufacturer and 27 mL of sterile water, and can be further diluted with normal saline or 5% dextrose in water. It should be used immediately after reconstitution and can be infused over 1 to 2 hours.

Carmustine is chemically stable for 3 hours at room temperature and for 24 hours when refrigerated.

Toxic Effects: Myelosuppression is the dose-limiting toxic effect and tends to increase with successive cycles of therapy. Leukopenia and thrombocytopenia are characteristically delayed and reach their maximum between the 3rd and 6th weeks after drug administration. Nausea and vomiting can be severe. Abnormal liver function tests may be found, but the abnormalities are usually mild and reversible. Two rare but serious toxic effects include cumulative pulmonary/interstitial pneumonitis progressing to fibrosis and progressive renal damage, which are dose related. Secondary leukemias can also occur 5 to 10 years after treatment. Patients who receive greater than 1100 mg/m^2 are at increased risk of pulmonary fibrosis. Carmustine is not a vesicant, but rapid infusion often produces a burning sensation at the injection site.

Potential Drug Interactions: Cimetidine may enhance the myelosuppressive effect of carmustine. Carmustine may decrease the pharmacologic effects of phenytoin. In rats with intracerebrally implanted tumors, pretreatment with phenobarbital eliminated the antitumor activity of carmustine. The reduction in carmustine antitumor activity correlated with increased carmustine metabolism, which is apparently the result of hepatic microsomal enzyme induction.

Therapeutic Indications in Hematology: Carmustine in combination with other cytotoxic agents may be used in the initial treatment of Hodgkin disease (BCVPP regimen) and multiple myeloma (VBAP regimen). In high-dose therapy, it appears in BEP, for relapsed lymphomas.

LOMUSTINE (CCNU)

Chemistry: Lomustine, also called CCNU, is a nitrosourea derivative with choloroethyl and cyclohexyl side chains.

Absorption, Fate, and Excretion: The drug is rapidly absorbed from the gastrointestinal tract and is rapidly and completely metabolized. Its active metabolites have prolonged plasma half-lives, within a range of 16 to 48 hours. Approximately 50% of an administered dose is detectable (as metabolites) in the urine within 24 hours, and 75% is detectable within 4 days. Active metabolites cross the blood–brain barrier and can be detected in significant concentrations in the cerebrospinal fluid.

Preparation and Administration: The drug is commercially available in 10-, 40-, and 100-mg capsules.

Toxic Effects: The toxicity profile of lomustine is similar to that of carmustine. Because lomustine can produce vomiting, and the drug is given orally, special attention should be directed to emesis control. If the patient vomits soon after ingestion, the vomitus should be inspected for the presence of intact capsules. The drug should be given again if capsules are identified with certainty. Secondary leukemias are reported 3 to 10 years after use.

Potential Drug Interactions: These are similar to those of carmustine.

Therapeutic Indications in Hematology: Lomustine is occasionally used as second-line treatment for patients with Hodgkin disease and NHL, and for childhood gliomas.

STREPTOZOCIN (Zanosar)

Chemistry: Streptozocin is a naturally occurring nitrosourea derived from *Streptomyces acromogenes*. The drug is a glucosamine-1-methyl-nitrosourea, which, unlike the other nitrosoureas, methylates DNA and is cytotoxic owing to induced mismatch repair.

Absorption, Fate, and Excretion: After IV administration, the drug is rapidly metabolized, with no intact drug detectable in the plasma after 3 hours. Its half-life is 40 hours. Within the first 24 hours after administration, approximately 10% of the parent compound is excreted in the urine.

Preparation and Administration: The drug is commercially available in 1-g vials and is reconstituted with either 9.5 mL of normal saline or 5% dextrose in water for injection to form a 100-mg/mL solution. IV infusion of the drug over 30 to 45 minutes usually prevents discomfort at the injection site. Patients should be kept well hydrated to preclude renal tubular toxicity.

Toxic Effects: Although nausea and vomiting have been considered by some investigators to be the limiting toxic effects, in most phase I trials nephrotoxicity was the principal dose-limiting effect. Nausea and vomiting are severe and require aggressive antiemetic support. Streptozocin may also aggravate duodenal ulcers. Renal toxicity frequently occurs and includes mild proteinuria, glycosuria, hypophosphatemia, renal tubular acidosis, and occasionally irreversible azotemia. Although the myelosuppressive effect of streptozocin is mild, it can potentiate the bone marrow suppression of other cytotoxic drugs. Slight increases in hepatic enzymes can also occur. Occasionally, patients (primarily those with insulinomas) may experience transient alterations in glucose metabolism.

Potential Drug Interactions: Streptozocin can potentiate the hyperglycemic effect of glucocorticosteroids. Phenytoin therapy decreases the cytotoxic effect of streptozocin on the pancreatic b cells, leading to potential interference with its therapeutic effect in patients with pancreatic islet cell tumors. Streptozocin is a potent renal toxin, and every effort should be made to avoid concomitant administration of other nephrotoxins.

Therapeutic Indications in Hematology: Streptozocin has been used in the initial treatment of Hodgkin disease and, less commonly, in NHLs.

DACARBAZINE (DTIC)

Chemistry: Dacarbazine is also called DTIC [5-(3,3-dimethyl-1-triazeno)imidazole-4-carboxamide]. After undergoing metabolic activation by microsomal enzymes in the liver, it acts primarily as an alkylating agent.

Absorption, Fate, and Excretion: After IV administration, the drug is extensively metabolized. Activated DTIC has an elimination half-life of 5 to 7 hours. Approximately 40% to 50% of the parent drug is found in the urine within the first 24 hours after administration.

Preparation and Administration: DTIC is commercially available in 100- and 200-mg vials, which must be protected from light and stored at a temperature of 2°C to 8°C. The drug is reconstituted with normal saline or sterile water to produce a 10-mg/mL solution. It can be administered as a slow IV push or by infusion over 15 to 30 minutes.

Toxic Effects: Myelosuppression, primarily represented by leukopenia, is the dose-limiting toxic effect. Use of the drug leads to considerable problems with emesis and requires aggressive antiemetic support. A flu-like syndrome consisting of fever, malaise, and myalgias may occur. Direct sunlight during the first 2 days after drug administration may result in facial flushing, facial paresthesias, and light-headedness. Hepatotoxicity and diarrhea have also been reported. Pain along the injection site can occur if the drug is rapidly infused, but can usually be lessened by prolonging the infusion rate. Secondary leukemias are reported between 3 and 10 years after use.

Potential Drug Interactions: DTIC activation may be enhanced by phenytoin or phenobarbital although the clinical significance of this potential interaction remains uncertain. There may be a potential (as yet poorly characterized) drug interaction with levodopa, whereby the response to levodopa is diminished.

Therapeutic Indications in Hematology: DTIC is used primarily in the treatment of Hodgkin disease as part of the ABVD (doxorubicin [Adriamycin], bleomycin, vinblastine, and DTIC) regimen and for melanoma.

PROCARBAZINE

Chemistry and Mechanism of Action: Procarbazine is a substituted hydrazine derivative with a chemical structure similar to that of the monoamine oxidase inhibitors (MAOIs). Accordingly, procarbazine exhibits weak MAOI effects. Procarbazine itself is inert and must undergo metabolic activation to generate cytotoxic reactants, the mode of action of which is not clear. They may inhibit transmethylation of methyl groups of methionine into tRNA or may also directly damage DNA. Hydrogen peroxide, formed during the autooxidation of procarbazine, may attack protein sulfhydryl groups contained in residual proteins tightly bound to DNA.

Absorption, Fate, and Excretion: Procarbazine is rapidly and completely absorbed by the oral route, with peak plasma levels occurring within 60 minutes. It penetrates well into the cerebrospinal fluid. The drug is readily metabolized in the liver and has a plasma half-life of 10 minutes after IV injection. The major sites of elimination are the kidneys, where approximately 70% of the drug is excreted as *N*-isopropylterephthalamic acid and less than 5% is excreted unchanged.

Preparation and Administration: Procarbazine is commercially available as 50-mg capsules.

Toxic Effects: The usual dose-limiting toxic effect is myelosuppression. Occasionally nausea and vomiting may be dose limiting, although tolerance to those effects may develop during continued administration. Other less common side effects include paresthesias, headache, dizziness, depression, apprehension, insomnia, nightmares, hallucinations, drowsiness, ataxia, foot drop, decreased reflexes, tremors, coma, confusion, convulsions, skin rash, alopecia, myalgia, and arthralgia. Procarbazine may possibly be leukemogenic.

Potential Drug Interactions: Combination chemotherapy that includes procarbazine may result in a decrease in digoxin plasma levels. Because procarbazine is a weak MAOI, hypertensive reactions could theoretically occur following concurrent ingestion of sympathomimetics, levodopa, tricyclic antidepressants, or foods with high tyramine content (eg, dark beer, yogurt, cheeses, and red wines). However, such reactions have not been reported. Concomitant use of narcotics or other strong sedatives may result in exaggerated depressant effects, leading to coma and possibly death. Procarbazine also interacts with alcohol, causing a disulfiram-like reaction.

Therapeutic Indications in Hematology: Procarbazine is often used in combination with other cytotoxic agents in the treatment of

Hodgkin disease (MOPP and MOPP derivatives) and to a lesser extent in the treatment of NHLs (PROMACE-MOPP).

TEMOZOLOMIDE

Chemistry and Mechanism of Action: Temozolomide is not active but undergoes rapid nonenzymatic conversion at physiologic pH to the reactive compound monomethyl 5-triazino imidazole carboxamide (MTIC) which is also the active methyl group-donating metabolite of dacarbazine. Unlike dacarbazine, formation of MTIC from temozolomide does not required metabolic activation (liver) and thus, there is much more consistent conversion from temozolomide to the methyl donating MTIC. The cytotoxicity of MTIC is thought to be primarily due to alkylation of DNA. Alkylation (methylation) occurs mainly at the O6 and N7 positions of guanine. Cytotoxicity results from processing of these lesions by methylguanine methyltransferase, mismatch repair, and base excision repair.

Absorption, Fate, and Excretion: Temozolomide is rapidly and completely absorbed after oral administration; peak plasma concentrations occur in 1 hour. Food reduces the rate and extent of temozolomide absorption.

Temozolomide exhibits a mean elimination half-life of 1.8 hours and exhibits linear kinetics over the therapeutic dosing range. Temozolomide is spontaneously hydrolyzed at physiologic pH to the active species, 3-methyl-(triazen-1-yl)imidazole-4-carboxamide (MTIC) and to temozolomide acid metabolite. MTIC is further hydrolyzed to 5-amino-imidazole-4-carboxamide (AIC) which is known to be an intermediate in purine and nucleic acid biosynthesis and to methylhydrazine, which is believed to be the active alkylating species. Approximately 38% of the administered temozolomide total radioactive dose is recovered over 7 days; 37.7% in urine and 0.8% in feces. The majority of the recovery of radioactivity in urine is as unchanged temozolomide (5.6%), AIC (12%), temozolomide acid metabolite (2.3%), and unidentified polar metabolite(s) (17%). Overall clearance of temozolomide is approximately 5.5 L/hour/minute.

Preparation and Administration: Temozolomide is given orally with each capsule containing either 5, 20, 100, 140, 180, or 250 mg of temozolomide. The inactive ingredients for TEMODAR capsules are lactose anhydrous, colloidal silicon dioxide, sodium starch glycolate, tartaric acid, and stearic acid.

Toxic Effects: Bone marrow depression, including neutropenia, lymphopenia, anemia, and thrombocytopenia, occurs frequently with Temozolomide. Mild transaminase elevations of up to 40% of patients and hyperbilirubinemia of up to 19% are seen, mild to moderate headache is among the most commonly reported adverse effects along with moderate nausea and vomiting although this may be secondary to the use of antiemetics.

Drug Interactions: None described.

Therapeutic Indications in Hematology: Temozolomide may have some activity in both acute myelogenous leukemia and acute lymphocytic leukemia, but the correct dose is presently unknown. Temozolomide has no activity in Non-Hodgkin lymphoma.

APPENDIX 56–2

CLINICAL PHARMACOLOGY OF ANTIMICROTUBULE AGENTS

VINCRISTINE (Oncovin) AND VINBLASTINE (Velban)

Chemistry and Mechanism of Action: Both vincristine and vinblastine are asymmetric dimeric compounds that bind to the protein tubulin at a site distinct from that for the taxanes. At low concentrations, vincristine and vinblastine inhibit microtubule dynamics. At higher concentrations, they disrupt microtubules that constitute the mitotic spindle, resulting in metaphase arrest. They are relatively M phase specific. Owing to their lipophilicity, vinca alkaloids are rapidly taken into cells and achieve several-hundred-fold higher intracellular than extracellular concentrations. Overexpression of the multidrug resistance transporters PGP or MRP can reduce the intracellular accumulation, whereas alterations in the α or β tubulins can affect drug–target interaction for vinca alkaloids.

Absorption, Fate, and Excretion: After IV injection, both drugs are rapidly distributed to the body tissues, especially the red blood cells and platelets. Their elimination follows a triphasic pattern. The elimination half-lives are as follows: α, less than 5 minutes; β, 50 to 155 minutes; and γ, 20 to 85 hours. Both vinca alkaloids are primarily eliminated through the liver into the bile and feces, making patients with obstructive liver disease more susceptible to toxic effects. A 50% reduction in the dose is recommended for serum bilirubin concentrations of 1.5 to 3.5 mg/dL. Dose modification for renal dysfunction is not indicated. After brief IV bolus administration, peak plasma vincristine concentrations of 100 to 400 mM are achieved, which decline to less than 10 mM in 2 to 4 hours. Continuous infusion doses of 1.0 mg/m^2/day produce vincristine plasma concentrations ranging from 1 to 10 nM.

Preparation and Administration: Vincristine is commercially available in 1-, 2-, and 5-mg vials. Each milliliter contains 1 mg vincristine sulfate, 100 mg mannitol, 1.3 mg methylparaben, and 0.2 mg propylparaben. Vincristine is a powerful vesicant that should be administered only intravenously into a freely running infusion of normal saline or dextrose solution. If the drug is given by continuous infusion, it must be infused through a central IV line. In case of extravasation, infusion should be discontinued and any residual drug aspirated through the line. The manufacturer also recommends infiltrating the area with 1 to 2 mL of hyaluronidase, 150 U/mL, and then applying warm compresses for 72 hours to facilitate dispersion of the drug. Vinblastine is commercially available as a lyophilized powder and a 1-mg/mL solution in 10-mg vials. The lyophilized drug is reconstituted by adding sodium chloride for injection (which may be preserved with either phenol or benzyl alcohol) to the 10-mg vial. Administration of vinblastine should follow the same guidelines described for vincristine.

Toxic Effects: Vincristine's dose-limiting toxic effect is neurotoxicity, which appears to be related to its relative polarity. Peripheral neurotoxicity usually manifests as sensory impairment, decreased deep tendon reflexes, and paresthesias. Less commonly, severe painful dysesthesias, ataxia, foot drop, and cranial nerve palsy (eg, affecting the extraocular and laryngeal muscles) can occur. Autonomic neurotoxicities include constipation, abdominal cramps, and ileus, which may be prevented by use of mild laxatives. Alopecia occurs frequently, but myelosuppressive effects are minimal. Rare side effects include inappropriate secretion of antidiuretic hormone and ischemic cardiac toxicity. Vinblastine's dose-limiting toxic effect is myelosuppression, with leukopenia more pronounced than thrombocytopenia. Anemia is uncommon. Neurotoxicity can also occur but is significantly less common than with vincristine. Vinblastine is also a vesicant.

Potential Drug Interactions: Both vinca alkaloids have been reported to increase the accumulation of methotrexate and etoposide in tumor cells. Acute shortness of breath and bronchospasm can occur when vincristine or vinblastine is given in conjunction with mitomycin C. Because asparaginase may impair the hepatic clearance of vincristine, it is preferable to administer the vincristine 12 to 24 hours before the L-asparaginase. Vincristine may decrease the absorption and plasma levels of orally administered drugs such as digoxin. Dilantin may increase the cytotoxicity of vincristine in multidrug-resistant tumor cells; however, this remains to be demonstrated in the clinic. When concurrently administered, erythromycin may increase the toxicity of vinca alkaloids, especially vinblastine.

Therapeutic Indications in Hematology: The vinca alkaloids are among the most important drugs in the treatment of hematologic malignancies. They have a broad spectrum of activity and are often incorporated into many chemotherapy regimens used in the treatment of ALL, Hodgkin disease, NHLs, CLL, and multiple myeloma.

VINORELBINE (Navelbine)

Chemistry and Mechanism of Action: Vinorelbine is a semisynthetic derivative of vinblastine (5′ -nor-hydrovinblastine) with an eight-member catharanthine ring. Similar to other vinca alkaloids, it also binds to tubulin, inhibits microtubule assembly, and produces a mitotic arrest of cells. This occurs at concentrations that relatively spare axonal microtubules, which may reduce neurotoxicity.

Absorption, Fate, and Excretion: Short (6–10 minutes) IV infusions of 30 mg/m^2 produce peak plasma concentrations approximately 1.0 μg/mL with a triphase decay. Rapid α (<5 minutes) and β (49–168 minutes) half-lives result in a rapid decline in the plasma concentration in the first hour posttreatment, followed by a prolonged terminal half-life of 18 to 49 hours, reflecting slow efflux from the peripheral compartment. The volume of distribution at steady state is 20 to 75.6 L/kg. The drug is extensively bound to platelets, lymphocytes, and plasma proteins. The major site of metabolism is the liver, with 33% to 80% of the drug excretion in feces and approximately 20% in urine.

Preparation and Administration: Vinorelbine is available for injection in single use as 10 mg/mL in 1- or 5-mL vials without preservatives. The calculated dose is diluted to 1.5 to 3.5 mg/mL for a slow injection (6–10 minutes) by a syringe with 5% dextrose or 0.9% saline, or between 0.5 or 2.0 mg/mL in an IV bag. Because vinorelbine is a strong vesicant, it should be administered through a freely flowing IV access avoiding all extravasation.

Toxic Effects: Vinorelbine shares many of the principal toxicities of vinblastine. Myelosuppression is dose limiting but not cumulative, with nadirs occurring 7 to 10 days after administration.

Anemia and thrombocytopenia occur infrequently. Because of lower affinity for axonal versus spindle microtubules, neurotoxicity is less prominent with vinorelbine. Mild to moderate peripheral neuropathy and constipation occurs in approximately 30% of patients, and the incidence of neuropathy increases with the duration of treatment. Mild to moderate nausea and vomiting is seen in 33% of patients. Stomatitis and diarrhea are less frequent. Transient elevations of transaminases have been reported. Among the miscellaneous side effects noted are chest pain with or without electrocardiographic changes (6%—most with underlying cardiac disease), as well as bronchospasm and dyspnea (5%). Alopecia is seen in 10% of patients.

Therapeutic Indications in Hematology: Objective responses have been observed in approximately 33% of patients with Hodgkin disease or NHLs.

PACLITAXEL (Taxol) AND DOCETAXEL (Taxotere)

Chemistry and Mechanism of Action: Both paclitaxel and docetaxel are complex diterpene alkaloid esters consisting of a taxane system linked to an oxetane ring and a C-13 side chain that is necessary for their cytotoxic effects in mammalian cells. After binding to the N-terminal 31 amino acids of the β-tubulin subunit in the tubulin oligomers or polymers, these taxanes kinetically stabilize microtubule dynamics at plus ends. They also decrease the lag time and shift the equilibrium toward tubulin polymerization into microtubule bundles. The disequilibrium of tubulin-microtubule polymerization results in mitotic arrest and apoptosis of cells. Taxane-induced mitotic arrest is associated with phosphorylation of BCL2 protein and increased intracellular levels of free BAX protein, which promote apoptosis. As compared with paclitaxel, docetaxel demonstrates 1.9-fold greater affinity for tubulin-binding sites and greater potency in mediating BCL2 phosphorylation.

Absorption, Fate, and Excretion: Taxanes generally are administered by IV infusion lasting over 3, 24, or 96 hours (paclitaxel) or 1 hour (docetaxel). Depending on the dose and schedule, peak plasma concentrations of paclitaxel range between 0.05 and 15.0 mM. Its steady-state volume of distribution ranges between 48 and 182 L/m^2, with rapid uptake in almost all tissues except the central nervous system and 98% plasma protein binding. Plasma decay for paclitaxel is biphasic, with α and β half-lives of 0.34 and 5.8 hours, respectively. Saturable distribution and elimination appear to be responsible for paclitaxel's nonlinear pharmacokinetics. This means that paclitaxel dose escalation in shorter schedules may result in disproportionate increases in area under the concentration–time curve and peak plasma concentration. It is metabolized to 6 hydroxy paclitaxel by the CYP3A isoform of the PU_{50} mixed-function oxidases in the hepatic microsomes. Total fecal and urinary excretion of paclitaxel and its metabolites is approximately 70% and 10%, respectively. Although dose modification is not necessary for renal insufficiency, a 50% reduction in dose is recommended even for moderate hyperbilirubinemia or significant elevations in hepatocellular enzymes. When administered as a 1-hour IV infusion, docetaxel has linear pharmacokinetics that fit a three-compartment model. Similar to paclitaxel, docetaxel also has a high clearance rate (0.36 L/h), steady-state volume of distribution (67.3 L/m^2), and terminal half-life of 12 hours. Docetaxel also has high protein binding (97%) and extensive tissue distribution. The drug or its metabolites also have high fecal (80%) and low urinary elimination (5%). Metabolism of docetaxel also primarily occurs in hepatic microsomal P450 mixed-function oxidases, CYP3A, CYP2B, and CYP1A.

Preparation and Administration: Paclitaxel is available as a 30 mg/5 mL single-dose vial in polyoxyethylated castor oil (Cremophor EL) 50% and dehydrated alcohol, USP 50%. The contents of the vial must be diluted before use. Docetaxel for injection is available as a concentrate in polysorbate 80 in two vial contents (23.6 mg/0.59 mL or 94.4 mg/2.36 mL), along with the appropriate diluent (1.83 or 7.33 mL) in separate vials. Adding diluent that is 13% (w/w) ethanol in water for injection to the concentrate produces a final premix concentration of 10 mg docetaxel/mL. The required amount of premix is transferred by a calibrated syringe into 0.9% saline or 5% dextrose to produce a final concentration of 0.3 or 0.9 mg/mL. The IV infusion is administered over 1 hour.

Toxic Effects: Hypersensitivity reaction (HSR) was noted in up to 30% of patients in the early phase I studies. HSR occurs early in the first or second infusion and may be caused by vehicle Cremophor EL or paclitaxel itself. HSR consists of dyspnea, bronchospasm, urticaria, and hypotension. Most HSRs regress completely after stopping the infusion and treatment with antihistamines, fluids, and vasopressors. Prolonged infusions (>3 hours) and premedication (dexamethasone 20 mg orally, 12 and 6 hours before treatment, diphenhydramine 50 mg, and ranitidine 150 mg IV 30 minutes before treatment) have reduced the incidence of major HSRs to less than 3%. Patients with a history of HSR may be rechallenged with paclitaxel at a markedly slower infusion rate, 20 mg dexamethasone IV every 6 hours for 4 doses prior to treatment. Although not formulated in Cremophor EL, HSRs can occur in up to 25% of patients receiving docetaxel. Most HSRs are minor, consisting of flushing, chest tightness, and low back pain. Premedication with dexamethasone 8 mg orally twice daily for 3 days, starting a day before treatment with docetaxel, considerably reduces the incidence of HSRs and fluid retention. Neutropenia is the main toxicity of paclitaxel and docetaxel, but it is not cumulative. With higher doses of paclitaxel (250 mg/m^2 over 24 hours), this can be ameliorated with subsequent administration of G-CSF. Severe thrombocytopenia and anemia are rare. Symmetric, distal, peripheral sensory neuropathy is usually seen with higher doses or multiple doses of paclitaxel. This often limits chronic use of paclitaxel. Diffuse areflexia and neuronopathy are less commonly seen. Higher doses can also cause motor and autonomic neuropathy as well as myalgias, especially in patients with preexisting neuropathy or when paclitaxel is used with cisplatin. Severe peripheral neuropathy or myalgias are less common after repetitive docetaxel at 100 mg/m^2. Cardiac rhythm abnormalities, especially brady arrhythmias and (rarely) heart blocks, have been reported secondary to paclitaxel treatment. A direct causal link between paclitaxel and myocardial ischemic episodes and tachyarrhythmias has not been established. Although noted, a direct link has also not been established between the occurrence of cardiac conductance abnormalities or ischemia and docetaxel treatment. Nausea, vomiting, diarrhea, and stomatitis are uncommon and generally mild to moderate. Alopecia is universal with both drugs. Skin toxicity is more severe and common with docetaxel. It is characterized by an erythematous pruritic maculopapular rash affecting forearms and hands. Onychodystrophy with discoloration, ridging, and brittleness of fingernails also occurs. Docetaxel can cause cumulative fluid retention resulting in peripheral edema, third-space fluid collection, and weight gain, which usually resolves slowly after stopping docetaxel. Concurrent treatment with dexamethasone, as noted earlier, delays the onset and decreases the incidence of these side effects.

Potential Drug Interaction: When paclitaxel infusion (24 hours) is administered following cisplatin, there is a 33% reduction in the clearance rate of paclitaxel. This produces suboptimal antitumor cytotoxicity and more profound neutropenia. Hence, the sequence of paclitaxel followed by cisplatin is commonly recommended. The use of carboplatin following paclitaxel has been reported to cause less thrombocytopenia than carboplatin alone. Mucositis is more pronounced when paclitaxel is used before doxorubicin, a sequence that reduces the clearance of doxorubicin. Hematologic toxicity is more prominent with the sequence of cyclophosphamide followed by paclitaxel, as compared with the reverse sequence of administration. Anticonvulsants such as phenytoin and phenobarbital induce the metabolism of paclitaxel and docetaxel by the P450 mixed-function oxidases. Conversely, in vitro studies have shown that inhibitors of the P450 system can interfere with the metabolism of both drugs. These inhibitors include erythromycin, testosterone, ketoconazole, and fluconazole.

Therapeutic Indications in Hematology: Both paclitaxel and docetaxel have significant activity against previously treated patients with NHLs. Paclitaxel is also very active against HIV-associated Kaposi's sarcoma.

APPENDIX **56–3**

CLINICAL PHARMACOLOGY OF ANTIMETABOLITES

CYTOSINE ARABINOSIDE

Chemistry and Mechanism of Action: Cytosine arabinoside (1′-β-D-arabinofuranosylcytosine; ara-C) is a nucleoside analog that differs from its naturally occurring counterpart (2′-deoxycytidine) by virtue of the presence of a hydryoxyl group in the 2′-β configuration. The altered reactivity of the resulting arabinosyl sugar moiety confers on ara-C its cytotoxic activity. Ara-C enters the cell by a facilitated nucleoside diffusion mechanism, and is converted to its nucleoside monophosphate form, ara-CMP, by the pyrimidine salvage pathway enzyme, deoxycytidine kinase. This represents the rate-limiting step in ra-C metabolism. Ara-C may also be catabolized intracellularly to an inactive form, ara-U, by the enzyme cytidine deaminase. Ara-C is ultimately converted to its lethal triphosphate derivative, ara-CTP, by a mono- and di-phosphate kinase. Ara-CTP is an inhibitor of DNA polymerases α, β, and γ, and is also incorporated into replicating DNA strands, leading to inhibition of chain initiation and elongation, and premature chain termination. The extent of incorporation of ara-C into DNA closely correlates with lethality in leukemic cells. Although ara-C is generally thought of as a prototypical S phase-specific agent, its ability to interfere with DNA repair polymerases (eg, β and γ) as well as lipid biosynthetic enzymes may account for lethal effects in noncycling cells.

Absorption, Fate, and Excretion: Following IV administration, ara-C is rapidly deaminated to an inactive form, ara-U, by cytidine deaminase. This enzyme is present in the plasma, liver, and kidney, but is present at very low levels in the CNS. The initial plasma half-life of ara-C has been estimated to be 10 to 12 minutes. Approximately 90% of the administered ara-C dose is excreted by the kidney as ara-U or other inactive metabolites. The terminal half-life of ara-C is approximately 2 to 3 hours. CNS ara-C levels following a 2-hour infusion approximate 50% of plasma concentrations. Steady-state plasma concentrations following standard-dose therapy (eg, 100–200 mg/m^2/day as a continuous infusion) approximate between 10^{-7} and 10^{-6} M. When ara-C is given as a high-dose bolus infusion (eg, 1–3 g/m^2 over 1–3 hours), plasma levels as high as 100 μM can be achieved.

Preparation and Administration: Ara-C is provided as a sterile, lyophilized powder for reconstitution in vials containing 100 mg, 200 mg, 1 g, or 2 g of material. The powder is reconstituted with sterile bacteriostatic water for injection with benzyl alcohol (0.945%) added as a preservative. When reconstituted in this way, solutions are stable for up to 48 hours under controlled temperatures (eg, between 15°C and 30°C or 60°–86°F). Material reconstituted without preservative should be used immediately. For intrathecal injection, ara-C should be reconstituted in a diluent that does not contain preservative, for example, preservative-free 0.9% sodium chloride, USP, and used immediately.

Toxic Effects: Ara-C is primarily toxic to rapidly dividing tissues; consequently, myelosuppression and gastrointestinal toxicity represent the major side effects of this agent. Patients receiving ara-C regularly experience leukopenia, anemia, and thrombocytopenia, with nadirs appearing 7 to 14 days after drug administration. Gastrointestinal toxicity includes nausea and vomiting, abdominal pain, mucositis, and a chemical hepatitis characterized by elevation of liver function enzymes. The latter is generally reversible. Patients receiving ara-C as a high-dose infusion (eg, 1–3 g/m^2 repeated every 12 hours for a total of 6–12 doses) experience standard toxicities and several unique ones. These include alopecia, an exfoliative dermatitis, a chemical conjunctivitis (generally ameliorated by the prophylactic administration of a steroid or saline ophthalmic solution), a respiratory distress-like syndrome (characterized by the appearance of rales, an abnormal radiogram, and pulmonary insufficiency), and cerebellar toxicity. The latter, which is characterized by nystagmus, ataxia, and other cerebellar signs, may be irreversible, and its appearance mandates discontinuation of therapy. Intrathecal administration of ara-C has been rarely associated with toxicities described below for methotrexate.

Potential Drug Interactions: None has been reported.

Therapeutic Indications in Hematology: Ara-C represents a mainstay in the treatment of AML (eg, as part of the "7 and 3" regimen in which it is given in conjunction with daunorubicin).

It is also incorporated into some induction regimens for ALL.

High-dose ara-C (HIDAC), either alone or in combination with anthracycline antibiotics, is frequently employed in the treatment of refractory or relapsed AML or ALL. HIDAC has also been used in some salvage regimens for NHL (eg, ESHAP). Chronic low-dose ara-C has been used in the treatment of patients with the myelodysplastic syndrome.

METHOTREXATE

Chemistry and Mechanism of Action: Methotrexate (*N*-4-[[(2,4-diamino-6-pteridinyl)methyl]methylamino]benzoyl]-L-glutamic acid) represents a member of a class of compounds referred to as antifolates. Methotrexate is a potent inhibitor of dihydrofolate reductase, an enzyme responsible for the reduction of dihydrofolates to tetrahydrofolates. The latter are required in 1-carbon transfer reactions involved in de novo purine and pyrimidine biosynthesis, including conversion of deoxyuridylate (dUMP) to thymidylate (dTMP) by thymidylate synthase. As in the case of most antimetabolites, methotrexate is primarily active against S-phase cells. Methotrexate is transported across cell membranes by an energy-dependent, temperature-sensitive, concentrative process involving folate-binding proteins, after which it is polyglutamylated by the enzyme folylpolyglutamyl synthetase. Polyglutamylation of methotrexate enhances its intracellular retention and in some studies has been shown to correlate with the sensitivity of leukemic cells to this agent. The mechanism by which methotrexate kills cells may stem from interference with DNA synthesis (leading to a "thymine-less death") secondary to DHFR inhibition; disruption of purine biosynthesis; or a combination of these actions. The lethal actions of methotrexate may be reversed by reduced folates such as 5-formyltetrahydrofolate (leucovorin). The possibility that tumor cells may exhibit impaired transport of such reduced folates serves as the basis for strategies involving administration of high-dose methotrexate in conjunction with leucovorin rescue.

Absorption, Fate, and Excretion: In adults, oral absorption is dose dependent, with mean bioavailability approximating 60% at doses ≤30 mg/m^2. At higher doses (eg, ≥80 mg/m^2), bioavailability is less. Peak plasma concentrations occur 1 to 2 hours following oral administration. Methotrexate bioavailability approximates 100% for parenteral routes of administration; with these routes, peak plasma methotrexate levels are achieved within 30 to 60 minutes after administration. For each route, the steady-state volume of distribution ranges from 40% to 80% of body weight. Methotrexate tends to accumulate in third-space fluids (eg, ascites or pleural effusions) and can result in prolonged release and accompanying toxicity. Consequently, it is generally not advisable for patients with fluid accumulations to receive methotrexate. Methotrexate competes with reduced folates for transport across cell membranes; however, at high doses (eg, ≥100 mg/m^2), passive diffusion is the primary mechanism through which intracellular accumulation occurs. Methotrexate is approximately 50% protein bound, and does not penetrate the CNS barrier when administered orally or parenterally at conventional doses. However, when given by the intrathecal route, high CNS levels are achieved. Administration of high-dose methotrexate with leucovorin rescue can also result in therapeutic CNS levels.

The primary route of excretion is renal, with 80% to 90% of the drug appearing unchanged in the urine within 24 hours following IV administration. The terminal half-life of methotrexate is 4 to 10 hours for patients receiving low-dose therapy and 8 to 15 hours for those receiving high-dose therapy. Because of the primary renal rate of excretion and the possibility of nephrotoxicity, methotrexate should be withheld or administered at reduced doses in patients with impaired renal function. Patients receiving high-dose methotrexate therapy should be hydrated and their urine alkalinized before administration to reduce the risks of toxicity.

Preparation and Administration: Methotrexate is available in multiple formulations: (a) tablets, containing 2.5 mg methotrexate and inactive ingredients (lactose, magnesium stearate, and pregelatinized starch; (b) methotrexate sodium injection, available in vials of 25, 50, and 250 mg, containing benzyl alcohol as a preservative, sodium chloride, and water for injection. Preservative-containing solutions should not be used for intrathecal or high-dose administration; (c) methotrexate sodium injection without preservative, which can be used for intravenous, intraarteriolar, intrathecal, and high-dose administration; (d) lyophilized powder, which is provided in 20-mg vials, and is reconstituted with preservative-free sodium chloride or 5% dextrose in water to a final concentration not exceeding 25 mg/mL.

For intrathecal administration, solutions of 1 to 1.5 mg/mL should be prepared using preservative-free 0.9% sodium chloride as the diluent. For high-dose therapy, leucovorin rescue is required to prevent significant toxicity. Leucovorin is administered 12 to 24 hours after the methotrexate at a dose of between 15 and 25 mg intravenously, intramuscularly, or orally every 6 hours until the methotrexate dose declines to levels of less than 5×10^{-7} M.

For patients receiving intermediate or high-dose methotrexate (eg, ≥500 mg/m^2), serum methotrexate and creatinine levels should be monitored at 24-hour intervals. If, after 48 hours, serum methotrexate levels are greater than 5×10^{-7} M but less than 1×10^{-6} M, leucovorin is continued at a dose of 25 mg/m^2 every 6 hours for 8 doses until methotrexate levels decline to below 5×10^{-7} M. If levels are greater than 1×10^{-6} M but less than 2×10^{-6} M at 48 hours, the dose of leucovorin is increased to 100 mg/m^2 every 6 hours × 8 doses. For methotrexate levels $\geq 2 \times 10^{-6}$ M at 48 hours, the dose of leucovorin is 200 mg/m^2 every 6 hours × 8 doses.

Toxic Effects: Methotrexate primarily exhibits its toxic effects toward proliferating tissues. Consequently, dose-limiting toxicities include bone marrow suppression (leukopenia, thrombocytopenia, anemia), mucositis, and diarrhea. High-dose therapy is occasionally accompanied by transient elevations in liver function tests, whereas chronic low-dose therapy is more often associated with hepatic fibrosis. Standard-dose therapy is rarely associated with nephrotoxicity, but acute renal failure can be seen with high-dose therapy secondary deposition of 7-*OH*-methotrexate in the renal tubules. The risk of methotrexate nephrotoxicity is significantly reduced by insuring adequate hydration and alkalinization of the urine. Other reported toxicities include a maculopapular rash, and an idiosyncratic pulmonary toxicity characterized by cough, fever, dyspnea, hypoxia, and interstitial infiltrates.

A necrotizing leukoencephalopathy has been reported in patients receiving methotrexate who have had prior cranial irradiation. Intrathecal methotrexate has been associated with several toxicities, including (a) chemical arachnoiditis; (b) motor paralysis accompanied by cranial nerve dysfunction, seizures, and coma; and (c) chronic demyelinating syndrome. Each of these may be exacerbated by prior craniospinal irradiation.

Potential Drug Interactions: Methotrexate exhibits many potential drug interactions that are related to plasma protein binding. For example, many compounds are known to displace methotrexate from serum albumin, potentially increasing its bioavailability. These agents include sulfonamides, salicylates, tetracyclines, chloramphenicol, and phenytoin. However, the clinical implications of such interactions are not clear. Nonsteroidal antiinflammatory drugs should not be administered in conjunction with methotrexate when the latter is given at intermediate or high doses, owing to the potential for elevation and prolongation of methotrexate plasma concentrations. Penicillins can reduce renal clearance of methotrexate and should be used with caution in this setting. Probenecid may also reduce renal transport of methotrexate. Administration of methotrexate can also reduce the clearance of theophyllines, and concomitant use of these agents requires careful monitoring. Increases in methotrexate toxicity have been observed in some patients receiving trimethoprim/sulfamethoxazole, possibly as a consequence of enhanced antifolate effects. Administration of folates in vitamin preparations may reduce the efficacy of methotrexate by bypassing DHFR inhibition. Methotrexate may increase the toxicity (and potentially the activity) of various antineoplastic agents in a schedule-dependent manner (eg, when given before 5-FU).

Therapeutic Indications in Hematology: Methotrexate is widely employed in the treatment of ALL, particularly in the maintenance phase. Methotrexate is frequently administered intrathecally in patients with CNS leukemia, and prophylactically in certain patients with ALL. It also represents a component of various multidrug regimens used in the treatment of NHL (eg, M-BACOD, PROMACE-CYTABOM).

HYDROXYUREA

Chemistry and Mechanism of Action: Hydroxyurea is an inhibitor of the ribonucleotide reductase system that catalyzes the rate-limiting step in the de novo biosynthesis of purine and pyrimidine deoxyribonucleotides, that is, the conversion of ribonucleotide diphosphates to their deoxyribonucleoside diphosphate derivatives. Ribonucleotide reductase consists of two subunits: a binding and allosteric effector component and an iron-binding catalytic component. Hydroxyurea binds to and inactivates the catalytic subunit of the enzyme. Like most antimetabolites, hydroxyurea is an S phase-specific agent, and blocks cells in the G_1S phase of the cell cycle. Exposure of cells to hydroxyurea leads to a depletion of deoxyribonucleotide triphosphate (dNTP) pools, the extent of which correlates with DNA synthesis inhibition and cell death. Two consequences of hydroxyurea administration include potentiation of the metabolism/cytotoxicity of nucleoside analogs (eg, ara-C) as a result of dNTP pool depletion and elimination of amplified genes present extrasomally in double minute chromosomes.

Absorption, Fate, and Excretion: Hydroxyurea is generally administered orally, although IV regimens are currently being investigated. The drug is readily absorbed from the gastrointestinal tract, with peak plasma levels as high as 2.0 mM occurring approximately 2 hours after oral administration. Serum concentrations decline to undetectable levels after 24 hours. The drug is primarily excreted via the renal route, with 75% to 80% of the drug appearing in the urine 12 hours later. The drug penetrates the CSF, although it has not been established that therapeutic levels are achieved following standard oral administration.

Preparation and Administration: Hydroxyurea is provided as 500-mg capsules. The drug is stored at room temperature in tightly capped containers and protected from heat.

Toxic Effects: The most common adverse reactions include myelosuppression (leukopenia, thrombocytopenia, anemia), gastrointestinal symptoms (eg, nausea and vomiting, stomatitis, anorexia, appetite disturbances), and dermatologic toxicity, such as rashes, skin ulcerations, and facial erythema. Rarer toxicities, generally seen at high doses, include neurologic disturbances, such as drowsiness, dizziness, headache, and convulsions, altered renal function, and alopecia. The mutagenic potential of hydroxyurea is unknown, and the drug should be avoided when possible in pregnant women.

Potential Drug Interactions: As noted earlier, hydroxyurea may increase the toxicity of certain nucleoside analogs. Hydroxyurea may also serve as a radiosensitizing agent; consequently, patients receiving concurrent radiation therapy may experience enhanced toxicity.

Therapeutic Indications in Hematology: Hydroxyurea has become, along with interferon-α, the mainstay of therapy in patients with chronic or accelerated phase CML. It is currently recommended for initial therapy of CML over busulfan and may prolong the chronic phase of this disease compared with the latter agent. Hydroxyurea has also been successfully used in the treatment of other myeloproliferative disorders, including myeloid metaplasia and myelofibrosis, polycythemia vera, and essential thrombocytosis. Its leukemogenic potential is uncertain, however, and it should be used with caution, particularly in younger patients. Hydroxyurea has also been shown to reduce the incidence of painful crises in individuals with sickle cell anemia in a subset of patients, a phenomenon that may result from increases in red blood cell fetal hemoglobin levels.

FLUDARABINE

Chemistry and Mechanism of Action: Fludarabine phosphate is a fluorinated derivative of the nucleotide analog 9′-β-D-arabinofuranosyladenine (ara-A) that is resistant to deamination by the degradative enzyme cytidine deaminase. It is converted intracellularly to its triphosphate derivative, which inhibits ribonucleotide reductase, as well as DNA polymerase α and DNA primase. Fluoro-ara-ATP is also incorporated into DNA, a process that appears to be essential for the induction of apoptosis in leukemic cells. Fludarabine is toxic to S-phase cells, but its ability to interfere with DNA repair may contribute to lethality in their noncycling counterparts.

Absorption, Fate, and Excretion: Following IV injection, fludarabine phosphate is rapidly deaminated (ie, within minutes) in the plasma to its nucleoside derivative, 2′-fluoro-ara-A, which is then converted intracellularly to its nucleotide form, 2′-fluoro-ara-AMP by the pyrimidine salvage pathway enzyme, deoxycytidine kinase. The half-life of 2′-fluoro-ara-A is approximately 10 hours; the primary mode of elimination is renal, with 25% of the total dose appearing in the urine as unchanged 2-fluoro-ara-A. Total body clearance of fludarabine is inversely correlated with serum creatinine.

Preparation and Administration: Fludarabine is supplied as a sterile powder in 50-mg vials containing 50 mg of mannitol and sodium hydroxide to adjust the pH to 7.7. Material is reconstituted in 2 mL of sterile water to yield a 25 mg/mL solution for injection. The material may be stored at 4°C (40°F); because the reconstituted solution contains no antimicrobial preservative, drug should be administered within 8 hours of formulation.

Toxic Effects: The most common dose-limiting toxicity is myelosuppression (neutropenia, thrombocytopenia, and anemia). Other toxicities include fever, chills, infection, nausea, and vomiting. Rarer toxicities include malaise, fatigue, anorexia, and weakness. Patients with CLL receiving fludarabine have experienced serious opportunistic infections and tumor lysis syndrome. The most serious toxicity of fludarabine when administered at high doses (>40 mg/m²/day for 5 days) is irreversible neurotoxicity, including cortical blindness, necrotizing leukoencephalopathy, and death. This phenomenon has rarely if ever been seen in patients receiving conventional doses (eg, 25 mg/m²/day for 5 days). Rare reports of interstitial pneumonitis have appeared.

Potential Drug Interactions: Fludarabine has been shown to potentiate the intracellular metabolism and activity of ara-C, although the toxicity of this combination may also be enhanced. No other interactions have been reported.

Therapeutic Indications in Hematology: Fludarabine has shown marked activity in both untreated CLL and in disease refractory to standard alkylating agent therapy. Fludarabine has also shown activity as a single agent, and particularly in combination with others (eg, mitoxantrone, cytoxan) in indolent NHL.

2′-CHLORODEOXYADENOSINE

Chemistry and Mechanism of Action: 2′-Chlorodeoxyadenosine (CdA; cladribine) is a derivative of deoxyadenosine that differs from its parent compound by the presence of a chlorine moiety at the 2′-position of the purine ring. It is transported intracellularly by facilitated nucleoside diffusion and phosphorylated by the pyrimidine salvage pathway enzyme deoxycytidine kinase. CdA is relatively resistant to deamination by cytidine deaminase. CdA is readily converted to its triphosphate derivative, 2′-chlorodeoxyadenosine-5′-triphosphate, particularly in cells of lymphoid origin, and is incorporated into tumor cell DNA by DNA polymerase α. CdATP is also an effective inhibitor of ribonucleotide reductase, which may contribute to lethal effects. CdA induces cell death (apoptosis) in both cycling and noncycling cells, possibly by promoting DNA fragmentation and by depleting cells of ATP or NAD, or both.

Absorption, Fate, and Excretion: Relatively little pharmacokinetic information concerning CdA is available. The drug is most commonly administered as a 7-day continuous infusion or as a 2-hour infusion over 5 days. Bioavailability of CdA following subcutaneous administration approximates that of the IV route, but is less than that after oral administration. Renal excretion appears to be the major route of elimination. When given as a 2-hour infusion, CdA has a relatively long terminal half-life (eg, approximately 6 hours), and plasma concentrations following such a schedule may approximate those associated with the continuous infusion. CSF levels are approximately 25% of plasma concentrations.

Preparation and Administration: For daily infusions, CdA is diluted under sterile conditions in bags containing 500 mL of 0.9% sodium chloride injection, USP. The use of 5% dextrose solutions is not recommended because of enhanced degradation of the drug. For preparation of longer infusions (eg, 7 days) the use of bacteriostatic sodium chloride injection, USP, is recommended. Once prepared, solutions of CdA should be refrigerated at a temperature between 4°C (40°F) and 8°C (47°F) for no more than 8 hours prior to administration.

Toxic Effects: The major toxicity of CdA is myelosuppression, which is primarily observed following intermittent rather than continuous infusion. Other toxicities include fever, generally beginning several days after initiation of therapy, and increased susceptibility to opportunistic infections. Rare side effects include nausea and hepatic and renal toxicity.

Potential Drug Interactions: None has been reported.

Therapeutic Indications in Hematology: CdA has shown significant activity in CLL and hairy cell leukemia. However, response rates in the former disorder appear to be somewhat less than those obtained with fludarabine; moreover, patients who have progressed on fludarabine therapy infrequently respond to CdA. Other diseases in which CdA has shown activity include NHL and Waldenström macroglobulinemia.

2′-DEOXYCOFORMYCIN (Pentostatin; DCF)

Chemistry and Mechanism of Action: 2′-Deoxycoformycin is an adenosine analog that is a highly effective inhibitor of the purine biosynthetic enzyme adenosine deaminase (ADA). It is transported across cell membranes by facilitated nucleoside diffusion, where it binds tightly to ADA. Inhibition of ADA results in accumulation of deoxyadenosine metabolites, most notably dATP. dATP exerts its toxic effects through inhibition of ribonucleotide reductase and induction of global imbalances in deoxyribonucleotide triphosphate pools. These result in interference with DNA synthesis and repair. 2′-Deoxycoformycin is particularly toxic to certain lymphoid cells with low levels of ADA activity. It is also toxic to both cycling and resting cells; the mechanism underlying its cytotoxicity toward quiescent cells is unknown.

Absorption, Fate, and Excretion: After IV injection of 2′-deoxycoformycin, the plasma clearance follows a biphasic pattern, with a terminal elimination half-life of 3 to 15 hours. Protein binding is limited. The drug is only partially metabolized, with approximately 60% to 80% of the drug appearing unchanged in the urine after 24 hours. The total body clearance of 2′-deoxycoformycin correlates well with creatinine clearance. Patients with impaired renal function may require reductions in the 2′-deoxycoformycin dose.

Preparation and Administration: 2′-Deoxycoformycin is unstable when reconstituted in solutions of pH less than 5.0. Consequently, it is customarily reconstituted in normal saline. 2′- Deoxycoformycin is provided in vials containing 10 mg of drug, 50 mg of mannitol, and sodium hydroxide to adjust the pH to <7.0. It is administered as an IV infusion over 20 to 30 minutes. Hydration is recommended before and after 2′-deoxycoformycin administration.

Toxic Effects: The major toxicities of 2′-deoxycoformycin include myelosuppression, nausea and vomiting, immunosuppression, acute renal failure, keratoconjunctivitis, fever, and elevations of liver function enzymes. At high doses, neurologic toxicity, including somnolence, seizures, and coma have been reported, although these are seen infrequently in patients receiving standard dose therapy. When administered at such doses (eg, 4 mg/m^2 biweekly), side effects are relatively minor.

Potential Drug Interactions: 2′-Deoxycoformycin may augment the toxicity of ara-A (vidarabine) as a consequence of inhibition of ADA.

Therapeutic Indications in Hematology: 2′-Deoxycoformycin is primarily used in the treatment of hairy cell leukemia, where response rates of up to 90% have been reported, even in patients refractory to other therapy, including α interferon. Activity has also been reported in other lymphoid malignancies, such as T-cell lymphoma, CLL, prolymphocytic leukemia, and Waldenström macroglobulinemia, although its precise role in the treatment of these disorders remains to be fully evaluated.

6-THIOGUANINE

Chemistry and Mechanism of Action: Thioguanine (6-TG) is a guanine analog in which the 6′-hydroxyl group is replaced by a sulfhydryl group. It interferes with de novo purine biosynthesis at multiple levels. Following transport across the cell membrane by facilitated diffusion, 6-TG competes with hypoxanthine and guanine for phosphorylation by hypoxanthine-guanine phosphoribosyltransferase (HGPRT) and is converted to its nucleotide form, 6-thioguanylic acid (TGMP), which accumulates within cells. TGMP inhibits several purine biosynthetic enzymes, including glutamine-5-phosphoribosylpyrophosphate aminotransferase and IMP dehydrogenase. 6-TG nucleotides are also incorporated in DNA and RNA, where they function as fraudulent bases. It is presently unknown which of these actions (interference with purine interconversions, blockade of de novo purine biosynthesis, or nucleic acid incorporation) is primarily responsible for 6-TG cytotoxicity, although DNA incorporation appears to play a significant role. 6-TG is considered to be an S phase-specific agent.

Absorption, Fate, and Excretion: Following oral administration, the bioavailability of 6-TG is variable, ranging from 14% to 46% of the administered dose (mean = 30%). Peak plasma levels are achieved 8 hours after administration and decline slowly thereafter. The average plasma disappearance of 6-TG is approximately 80 minutes, with a range of 25 to 240 minutes. Relatively little unchanged material appears in the urine; the major excreted product is the methylated derivative 2-amino-6-methyl thiopurine. CNS penetrance after parenteral administration is minimal.

Preparation and Administration: 6-TG is available in tablet form for oral administration. Each tablet contains 40 mg of 6-TG and inactive ingredients including gum acacia, lactose, magnesium stearate, potato starch, and stearic acid. IV preparations are available only in experimental settings.

Toxic Effects: The major dose-limiting toxicity of 6-TG is myelosuppression. Other less common toxicities include gastrointestinal disturbances (nausea and vomiting, anorexia, diarrhea), jaundice, and elevated liver function tests.

Potential Drug Interactions: In contrast to 6-MP, the metabolism of 6-TG is not modified by allopurinol, and consequently dose adjustments do not have to be made when these agents are administered concurrently.

Therapeutic Indications in Hematology: The primary indication for 6-TG is in the treatment of AML, generally in conjunction with other agents (eg, daunorubicin and ara-C). However, it has not been firmly established that addition of 6-TG to such regimens improves therapeutic efficacy. 6-TG also has activity in CML, although it has been supplanted by other agents (eg, hydroxyurea, interferon α) in this disorder.

6-MERCAPTOPURINE

Chemistry and Mechanism of Action: 6-Mercaptopurine (1,7-dihydro-6*H*-purine 6-thione monohydrate; 6-MP; purinethol) is an analog of the purine bases adenine and hypoxanthine. It is both an antineoplastic and immunosuppressive agent. Like 6-TG, 6-MP and its metabolites act at multiple levels to interfere with purine biosynthesis and interconversions. It competes with hypoxanthine and guanine for HGPRTase, and, following conversion to thioinosinic acid (TIMP), blocks conversion of IMP to xanthylic acid and IMP to AMP. Both TIMP and another metabolite, 6-methylthioinosinate (MTIMP) inhibit glutamine-5-phosphoribosylpyrophosphate aminotransferase. 6-MP is also incorporated into RNA and DNA, thereby functioning as a fraudulent base. It is unknown which of these actions is primarily responsible for the lethal actions of 6-MP, although available evidence points to DNA incorporation as a prime determinant of cytotoxicity.

Fate, Absorption, and Excretion: Following oral administration, the bioavailability of 6-MP is highly variable, presumably due to interpatient differences in gastrointestinal absorption, which averages 50% of the administered dose. Extensive catabolism by hepatic xanthine oxidase also contributes to drug elimination. Approximately 50% of the administered 6-MP or its metabolites are recovered in the urine. The volume of distribution generally exceeds the total body water. Following IV administration, the plasma disappearance half-life was 47 minutes in adults. Plasma protein binding is modest (approximately 19%), and CNS penetrance is minimal.

Preparation and Administration: 6-MP is supplied as tablets for oral administration. Each tablet contains 50 mg of 6-MP and the inactive ingredients corn and potato starch, lactose, magnesium stearate, and stearic acid. An IV preparation containing 500 mg of 6-MP per vial is available for investigational use.

Toxic Effects: The major dose-limiting toxicity of 6-MP is myelosuppression. This is dose-related, and is manifested by leukopenia, thrombocytopenia, and anemia. The hematologic effects of 6-MP may be delayed, so it is important to withdraw the medication temporarily at the first sign of unusual hematologic toxicity. Individuals with an inherited disorder of thiopurine methyltransferase deficiency may be particularly susceptible to 6-MP-mediated hematopoietic suppression. Other toxicities include hepatotoxicity (elevated liver function tests, cholestasis, hepatic necrosis, ascites), nausea, vomiting, mucositis, fever, rash, and diarrhea. The hepatotoxicity, which occurs in 10% to 40% of patients, requires close monitoring, and discontinuation of therapy until recovery occurs. Patients receiving 6-MP uniformly experience immunosuppression.

Potential Drug Interactions: Allopurinol, an inhibitor of xanthine oxidase, significantly reduces the catabolism of 6-MP when the latter is given orally, leading to major increases in plasma concentrations. Allopurinol does not alter the pharmacokinetics of IV 6-MP, presumably because the absence of first-pass metabolism of 6-MP when administered by this route. When administered in conjunction with allopurinol, the dose of 6-MP should be reduced by one-third to one-fourth. Increased toxicity has been reported in patients receiving concurrent 6-MP and trimethoprim-sulfamethoxazole. 6-MP may also modify the effects of warfarin.

Therapeutic Indications in Hematology: The major use for 6-MP is in the maintenance phase of treatment for ALL. 6-MP has also been used in the treatment of patients with ITP or autoimmune hemolytic anemia refractory to all other forms of therapy.

5-AZACYTIDINE

Chemistry and Mechanism of Action: 5′-Azacytidine is an analog of the nucleoside cytidine, differing from the parent compound by virtue of the presence of nitrogen at the 5′ position of the heterocyclic ring. 5′-Azacytidine is transported across the cell membrane by facilitated nucleoside diffusion and is converted to its nucleotide monophosphate form, 5′-aza-CMP, by the pyrimidine salvage pathway enzyme uridine-cytidine kinase. 5′-Azacytidine is also a substrate for the degradative enzyme cytidine deaminase. It is ultimately converted to its lethal derivative, 5′-aza-CTP, which is incorporated into RNA, and to a lesser extent, DNA. The lethal actions of 5′-azacytidine are believed to result from its ability to interfere with protein synthesis through disruption of RNA processing. The chemical instability of the 5′-azacytidine ring structure is also felt to contribute to the cytotoxicity of this compound.

Absorption, Fate, and Excretion: The drug distributes into a volume corresponding to the total body water after IV administration, and is also well absorbed following subcutaneous injection.

It is extensively deaminated in the plasma and liver and displays minimal plasma binding. Peak plasma concentrations following IV injection approximate 1.0 mM. The initial half-life of 5′-azacytidine (and/or its metabolites) is approximately 4 hours, although the drug is rapidly converted to various derivatives within minutes of administration. There is minimal CSF penetrance.

Preparation and Administration: 5′-Azacytidine is an investigational agent provided by the National Cancer Institute as a group C drug for patients with refractory AML. It is supplied in 100-mg vials and is reconstituted in 19.9 mL of sterile water for injection. When further diluted to a concentration of 0.2 to 2 mg/mL in normal saline, 5% dextrose in water, or lactated Ringer's solution, 10% of the drug undergoes decomposition within 3 hours. Consequently, the drug should be administered immediately after reconstitution and not stored. When administered as a continuous infusion, fresh solutions should be prepared every 3 to 4 hours.

Toxic Effects: The major toxicity of 5′-azacytidine has been leukopenia and, to a lesser extent, thrombocytopenia. Nausea and vomiting, often refractory to standard antiemetic therapy, have also been encountered, most frequently in patients receiving bolus infusions. Gastrointestinal toxicity is ameliorated by administering 5-azacytidine as a continuous infusion. Other potential side effects include diarrhea, fever, hepatotoxicity (most frequently in patients with preexisting hepatic disease), neuromuscular toxicity, rash, and hypotension.

Drug Interactions: None has been reported.

Therapeutic Indications in Hematology: 5′-Azacytidine is primarily used in the treatment of refractory AML, with response rates ranging from 17% to 30% when used as a single agent. 5′-Azacytidine has also yielded clinical responses in a subset of patients with the myelodysplastic syndrome when administered as a low-dose continuous infusion. In early trials, low-dose 5′-azacytidine has increased fetal hemoglobin levels in some patients with sickle cell anemia and thalassemia; however, its mutagenic potential has limited the use of this agent in nonmalignant conditions.

GEMCITABINE

Chemistry and Mechanism of Action: Gemcitabine (2′,2′-difluorocytidine monohydrochloride) is a nucleoside analog that differs from 2′-deoxycytidine by virtue of the presence of fluorine atoms in the 2′α and 2′β positions of the cytidine ring. It is transported across the cell membrane by facilitated nucleoside diffusion, phosphorylated by deoxycytidine kinase, and ultimately converted to its lethal metabolites, dFdCDP and dFdCTP. The diphosphate form (dFdCDP) inhibits ribonucleotide reductase, leading to disruption of dNTP pools, and resultant interference with DNA synthesis and repair. The triphosphate form (dFdCTP) competes with dCTP for incorporation into DNA. Reductions in dCTP pools (secondary to ribonucleotide reductase inhibition) result in self-potentiation of gemcitabine action. Incorporation of gemcitabine into DNA in S phase inhibits elongation of the replicating strand, leading to DNA chain termination. The lethal actions of gemcitabine in leukemia cells have been related to the induction of apoptosis, and are not restricted to cells actively engaged in DNA synthesis. Gemcitabine has been shown to be considerably more potent in inducing apoptosis in cultured human leukemia cells than ara-C.

Absorption, Fate, and Excretion: In studies involving intravenously administered labeled gemcitabine, up to 98% of the drug was recovered in the urine after 1 week. The excreted dose was composed of a minor fraction (gemcitabine; <10%) and inactive metabolites (eg, 2′-deoxy-2′,2′-difluorouridine). Plasma protein binding was minimal. In studies involving both short and long gemcitabine infusions, the pharmacokinetics were found to be linear and best described by a two-compartment model. Plasma half-life and clearance are influenced both by age and gender. For short infusions, half-lives varied from 32 to 94 minutes; for longer infusions, half-lives varied from 245 to 638 minutes. Volume of distribution was approximately 50 L/m^2 for short infusions and 370 L/m^2 for long infusions.

Preparation and Administration: Vials of gemcitabine contain 200 mg or 1 g of the HCL derivative formulated with mannitol (200 mg or 1 g) and sodium acetate (12.5 mg or 62.5 mg) as a sterile lyophilized powder. HCL or NaOH have been used for pH adjustment.

Toxic Effects: The major dose-limiting toxicity of gemcitabine is myelosuppression, although anemia and thrombocytopenia have also been encountered. Other toxicities include nausea and vomiting, transient elevations in liver function tests, mild hematuria, proteinuria (and in rare cases, HUS), fever, rash, dyspnea, edema, and a flu-like syndrome. Other infrequent toxicities included alopecia, parasthesias, and bronchospasm.

Potential Interactions: Gemcitabine may function as a radiosensitizing agent, and can increase the toxicity of ionizing radiation. No other interactions are known.

Indications in Hematology: The primary indication for gemcitabine is in the treatment of patients with pancreatic carcinoma. However, as an experimental agent, gemcitabine is being evaluated for the treatment of ALL and CLL.

NELARABINE

Arabinofuranosylguanine (Ara-G)

Chemistry and Mechanism of Action: Nelarabine is a pro-drug of the deoxyguanosine analog 9′-β-D-arabinofuranosylguanine also known as ara-G. Accumulation of a metabolite ara-GTP in leukemic blasts allows for incorporation into deoxyribonucleic acid (DNA), leading to inhibition of DNA synthesis and cell death.

Absorption, Fate, and Excretion: Nelarabine is demethylated by adenosine deaminase (ADA) to ara-G, then mono-phosphorylated by deoxyguanosine kinase and deoxycytidine kinase, and subsequently converted to the active 5′-triphosphate, ara-GTP. Nelarabine is only available in an IV formulation. Nelarabine and ara-G are both partially eliminated by the kidneys. Approximately 5% to 10% of nelarabine is excreted by the kidney compared to 20% to 30% of ara G. Nelarabine exhibits a half-life of 30 minutes and ara G, the active metabolite, has a half-life of 3 hours.

Preparation and Administration: Nelarabine for injection is supplied as a clear, colorless, sterile solution in glass vials. Each vial contains 250 mg of nelarabine (5 mg nelarabine per mL) and sodium chloride (4.5 mg/mL) in 50 mL water for injection, USP. Nelarabine is not diluted prior to administration. The dose is transferred into polyvinylchloride (PVC) infusion bags or glass containers and administered as a two-hour infusion in adult patients or as a one-hour infusion in pediatric patients.

Toxic Effects: Bone marrow suppression encompassing all cell lines causing anemia, leucopenia, thrombocytopenia, and neutropenia occurs in all patients. Neurologic complications of nelarabine including asthenia, altered mental states including severe somnolence, central nervous system effects including convulsions, and peripheral neuropathy ranging from numbness and paresthesias to motor weakness and paralysis. Demyelinating disease of the central nervous system may occur when combining nelarabine with other drugs that may have central nervous system toxicity. Nausea and vomiting are seen and antiemetics are necessary.

Drug Interactions: Pentostatin has been shown to be a strong inhibitor of adenosine deaminase (ADA) in vitro. Concurrent administration of nelarabine and pentostatin may result in reduced ADA-dependent conversion of nelarabine to its active moiety, thereby potentially decreasing nelarabine efficacy and/or altering nelarabine adverse event profile. Therefore, concomitant administration of nelarabine and pentostatin is not recommended.

Therapeutic Indications in Hematology: Nelarabine is effective in T-cell acute lymphoblastic leukemia, T-cell lymphoma, and T-cell lymphoblastic lymphoma. The dose in adults of nelarabine is 1500 mg/m^2 administered intravenously over 2 hours on days 1, 3, and 5 repeated every 21 days. The pediatric dose of nelarabine is 650 mg/m^2 administered intravenously over 1 hour daily for 5 consecutive days repeated every 21 days. The proper number of cycles for adult or pediatric patients has not been determined.

CLOFARABINE

Chemistry and Mechanism of Action: Clofarabine is a purine nucleoside antimetabolite formulated in unbuffered normal saline with a pH range of 4.5 to 7.5. It inhibits DNA synthesis by decreasing cellular deoxynucleotide triphosphate pools by inhibiting ribonucleotide reductase, terminating DNA chain elongation and inhibiting repair through incorporation into the DNA chain by competitive inhibition of DNA polymerases.

Absorption, Fate, and Excretion: Clofarabine is 47% bound to plasma proteins, primarily albumin. Clofarabine is phosphorylated intracellularly to the cytotoxic active form (clofarabine triphosphate) by deoxycytidine kinase. The terminal half-life is estimated to be 5.2 hours with the metabolite clofarabine triphosphate, yielding a half-life greater than 24 hours, and 49% to 60% of the dose is excreted in the urine unchanged. Systemic clearance and volume of distribution at steady state were estimated to be 28.8 L/hour/m^2 and 172 L/m^2, respectively.

Preparation and Administration: Clofarabine is supplied in a 20-mL, single-use vial that contains 20 mg clofarabine in 20 mL unbuffered normal saline at a concentration of 1 mg/mL. Clofarabine should be filtered through a sterile 0.2 μm syringe filter and diluted with 5% dextrose injection, USP, or 0.9% sodium chloride injection, USP, prior to IV infusion to a final concentration between 0.15 mg/mL and 0.4 mg/mL.

Toxic Effects: Bone marrow suppression encompassing all cell lines causing anemia, leucopenia, thrombocytopenia and neutropenia occurs in all patients. A capillary leak syndrome also known as systemic inflammatory response syndrome (SIRS) thought related to cytokine release leading to respiratory distress, hypotension, pleural effusions, pericardial effusions, and multiorgan failure may occur in a small number of patients. Elevations of liver transaminases are seen and are transient (typically, less than 2 weeks' duration) and occurred within 1 week of clofarabine initiation. Elevations in bilirubin may also occur.

Drug Interactions: None described.

Therapeutic indications in Hematology: Clofarabine is effective in treating acute lymphocytic leukemia. The recommended pediatric dose is 52 mg/m^2 administered by IV infusion over 2 hours daily for 5 consecutive days. Treatment cycles are repeated following recovery or return to baseline organ function, approximately every 2 to 6 weeks. Clofarabine has been used in adults at a dose of 40 mg/m^2 administered by IV infusion over 2 hours daily for 5 consecutive days. Clofarabine has also been used in combination with cytarabine. As this drug is excreted to a major extent by the kidneys extreme caution should be used in patients with renal dysfunction.

APPENDIX **56–4**

TOPOISOMERASE I INHIBITORS AND TOPOISOMERASE II INHIBITORS

TOPOISOMERASE II INHIBITORS

Etoposide (Vepesid), Etoposide Phosphate (Etopophos), Teniposide (Vumon)

Chemistry and Mechanism of Action: Etoposide (VP-16), etoposide phosphate, and teniposide (VM-26) are semisynthetic derivatives of epipodophyllotoxin. The mechanism of action of these drugs appears to be related to their ability to stabilize a topoisomerase II–DNA cleavable complex, which acts as a replication fork barrier and leads to the generation of irreversible DNA damage and cell death in proliferating cells.

Absorption, Fate, and Excretion: *Etoposide* has an oral bioavailability of 25% to 75%. Its terminal half-life is 6 to 8 hours, with approximately 30% to 40% excreted in the urine, two-thirds as unchanged drug. There is no accumulation with consecutive daily administration, but cytotoxicity has strict schedule dependency. Clinical studies suggest that in patients with a plasma creatinine level greater than 130 mol/L, the etoposide dose should be reduced by more than 25%.

Etoposide phosphate is rapidly and completely converted in vivo to VP-16 by the activity of phosphatase, and has been shown to have the same pharmacokinetics as VP-16. Because of its increased water solubility, etoposide phosphate can be given intravenously in much less volume. In addition, the metabolic acidosis and hypotension seen with the infusion of VP-16 are not seen with this prodrug.

Teniposide has a multiphasic pattern of clearance from plasma with a terminal half-life of 9.5 to 21 hours. Unlike those of etoposide, metabolites of teniposide account for greater than 80% of the drug excreted in the urine. Like etoposide, there is significant interpatient and intrapatient variation in clinical pharmacokinetics. There are currently no formal recommendations for dose modification in patients with renal insufficiency.

Preparation and Administration: *Etoposide* is commercially available as 50-mg capsules and in vials of 50 and 100 mg at a concentration of 20 mg/mL. When the drug is diluted with normal saline or 5% dextrose in water to a concentration of 0.2 or 0.4 mg/mL, it is stable for 96 or 48 hours, respectively. Etoposide must be administered slowly over more than 30 minutes to prevent hypotension.

Etoposide phosphate is available commercially as single-dose vials containing etoposide phosphate equivalent to 100 mg of etoposide. When it is diluted with water, 5% dextrose, or normal saline to a concentration of 10 to 20 mg/mL, it can be administered without dilution over 5 to 10 minutes. When reconstituted, etoposide phosphate is stable for 24 hours at room temperature or under refrigeration.

Teniposide is supplied in 50-mg vials for IV use only. The IV solution may be taken orally but is unpalatable. Currently, no oral preparation is available in the market; however, for investigational purposes each 50-mg vial may be dissolved in 50 to 100 mL of syrup or juice. To achieve optimal absorption, a single oral dose of 60 mg/m^2, which may be repeated at 6-hour intervals, is advised. As with etoposide, rapid infusion can produce hypotension.

Toxic Side Effects: Myelosuppression, especially leukopenia, is the dose-limiting toxic effect of *etoposide* and *teniposide*. Nausea and vomiting are usually mild and easily prevented with antiemetics. Rapid infusion of etoposide (<30 minutes) may cause hypotension. Anaphylactoid reactions (eg, bronchospasm) occur in less than 2% of patients and may be related to the cremaphor vehicle. Alopecia occurs in approximately 20% of patients treated with etoposide. This side effect is more common with teniposide. When the drug is given in bone marrow transplantation doses, mucositis and diarrhea are prominent and may be dose limiting.

Potential Drug Interactions: Theoretically, any drug that increases the S-phase fraction will increase the cytotoxicity of epipodophyllotoxins and other topoisomerase inhibitors. Conversely, drugs that inhibit DNA synthesis antagonize the effect of *etoposide* and *teniposide* (eg, 5-fluoro-2′-deoxyuridine given before etoposide in some human cancer cell lines decreases the cytotoxicity of the latter). More recent in vitro data suggest that synergistic cytotoxic effects are seen when VP-16 is given after a topoisomerase I inhibitor, which appears to upregulate the amount of topoisomerase II enzyme. Antagonistic effects have been reported when a topoisomerase II inhibitor is given before a topoisomerase I inhibitor. In hematology, etoposide and teniposide may inhibit the intracellular ara-CTP formation leading to reduced ara-C cytotoxicity. Potentiation of teniposide activity has been seen with methotrexate and dipyridamoles. There is at least a twofold increase in the clearance of teniposide with concomitant administration of phenobarbital or phenytoin. Cyclosporine and other PGP antagonists (PSC 833) potentiate the cytotoxic effects of etoposide.

Therapeutic Indications: *Etoposide* is employed in the treatment of NHLs and as a second-line treatment for Hodgkin disease. It is also incorporated in the preparatory regimens for bone marrow transplantation of refractory lymphomas (CBV) and acute leukemia. *Teniposide* has been approved as a front-line agent with combination chemotherapy for childhood ALL. Combination chemotherapy with teniposide has been used successfully in some cases of refractory adult ALL and acute monocytic leukemia, but duration of remission is not significantly different from that with other standard salvage regimens. In NHL, teniposide has shown comparable activity to vincristine. *Etoposide phosphate* has been given in both standard-dose and high-dose (as a single agent) chemotherapy regimens and appears to have the same pharmacokinetics and antitumor activity as VP-16.

Daunorubicin

Chemistry and Mechanism of Action: Daunorubicin is an anthracycline that inhibits DNA topoisomerase II, acting as a poison at lower concentrations and a suppressor of cleavable complex formation at higher doses. Daunorubicin is also a DNA intercalator and generates reactive oxygen intermediates.

Absorption, Fate, and Excretion: After IV injection, daunorubicin undergoes rapid tissue uptake and concentration. It is rapidly metabolized in the liver, where approximately 25% of the drug concentrates and has a half-life of 20 to 50 hours. The principal metabolite is daunorubicinol, which also displays antineoplastic activity. Biliary excretion accounts for approximately 75% of the drug and metabolite elimination. Patients with significant hepatic dysfunction should receive an attenuated dose of daunorubicin.

Preparation and Administration: Daunorubicin is supplied with 100 mg of mannitol in 20-mg vials, from which it is reconstituted with 4 mL of sterile water for injection. The vial should be protected from sunlight. Daunorubicin is a powerful vesicant that should be administered into the tubing of a freely flowing IV infusion of either 5% dextrose in water or normal saline. In the event of extravasation, as much infiltrated drug as possible should be aspirated from the tissue, and cold compresses should be maintained on the site for several hours. Despite these measures, skin grafting may be necessary. Daunorubicin is not physically compatible with heparin, and the two drugs should not be coadministered in the same IV tubing. The patient should be informed that daunorubicin may impart a red color to the urine for up to 72 hours after administration.

Toxic Effects: Myelosuppression, predominantly leukopenia, is the dose-limiting toxic effect. Mucositis, nausea and vomiting, and alopecia are common. Facial flushing, conjunctivitis, and lacrimation may occur in rare cases. Erythematous streaking near the site of injection occurs as a benign local allergic reaction and should not be confused with extravasation. The drug can produce a severe local reaction (eg, pneumonitis, esophagitis) in previously irradiated areas, even when both therapies are not administered concomitantly (radiation recall). Cardiac toxicity is a unique characteristic of the anthracycline antibiotics and can be acute or chronic. In the acute form, abnormal ECG changes such as ST-T wave elevation and arrhythmias may be seen. Transient reduction in the ejection fraction can also occur acutely and is often associated with pericarditis (pericarditis-myocarditis syndrome). The chronic form of anthracycline cardiac toxicity is related to the cumulative dose. The dose limit of doxorubicin is generally considered to be 450 to 500 mg/m^2, where the risk of clinical cardiotoxicity is between 1% and 10%. The corresponding cumulative dose limit for daunorubicin is 900 to 1000 mg/m^2. The cardiac toxicity is clinically characterized by congestive heart failure, usually refractory to medical therapy. Cardiac irradiation or the administration of cyclophosphamide may increase the risk of cardiotoxicity. The cardiotoxic effects appear to be related to the formation of free radicals and not to the inhibition of DNA topoisomerase II. The cardioprotective agent dexrazoxane (Zinecard) is now available and recommended to be started at a doxorubicin cumulative dose greater than 350 mg/m^2.

Potential Drug Interactions: Daunorubicin is not physically compatible with heparin or dexamethasone. The drug interactions described for doxorubicin (description follows) probably occur with daunorubicin as well.

Therapeutic Indications in Hematology: Daunorubicin is used in combination with other drugs in the treatment of AML and ALL.

Doxorubicin (Adriamycin)

Chemistry and Mechanism of Action: Doxorubicin is also an anthracycline glycoside antibiotic. It differs from daunorubicin at C-8, where a hydroxyacetyl group replaces an acetyl group. Because of this, doxorubicin is also called hydroxyl daunorubicin. Its mechanisms of action also involve stabilizing DNA–topoisomerase II complexes, DNA intercalation, and free radical formation.

Absorption, Fate, and Excretion: Doxorubicin has a triphasic plasma clearance with a half-life of approximately 30 hours. The drug is extensively metabolized in the liver to yield an active metabolite (doxorubicinol) and a number of inactive metabolites (aglycones). Within 7 days, more than 50% of an injected dose is excreted in the bile, but only 5% to 10% of the drug is excreted in the urine. Penetration into the cerebrospinal fluid is poor.

Preparation and Administration: Doxorubicin is commercially available in vials of 10, 20, 50, 150, and 200 mg. The lyophilized powder is reconstituted with either normal saline or sterile water for injection to yield a 2 mg/mL solution. The reconstituted solution must be protected from sunlight. The drug should be injected slowly into the tubing of a freely running IV infusion of normal saline or 5% dextrose in water. Erythematous streaking along the vein is often an indication that the administration rate is too rapid. The drug is a powerful vesicant, and in case of extravasation the measures described for daunorubicin should be followed.

Toxic Effects: The toxic effects are similar to those of daunorubicin. It is important to emphasize that weekly low-dose regimens or administration by continuous infusion can decrease the risk of cardiotoxicity with doxorubicin.

Potential Drug Interactions: When used in combination with other drugs as treatment for leukemia or lymphoma, doxorubicin may decrease the oral bioavailability of digoxin. It is not physically compatible with heparin or 5-fluorouracil. Barbiturates may increase the plasma clearance of doxorubicin and decrease its cytotoxic effect. Doxorubicin is compatible with vincristine, and the two drugs can be administered together in the same IV solution.

Therapeutic Indications in Hematology: Doxorubicin is one of the most important drugs in the treatment of hematologic malignancies. It is used in the treatment of Hodgkin disease (ABVD regimen), NHLs (CHOP, MACOP-B), and multiple myeloma (VBAP, VAD).

Idarubicin (Idamycin)

Chemistry and Mechanism of Action: Idarubicin, also called 4′-demethoxydaunorubicin (4-DMDR), is an analog of daunorubicin in which the methoxy group from the aglycone has been replaced with hydrogen. Idarubicin is also a topoisomerase II inhibitor and generates free radicals.

Absorption, Fate, and Excretion: The elimination half-life of the parent compound is 11.3 hours and that of the primary metabolite, 13-epirubicinol, is 40 to 60 hours. The major metabolite is as active as idarubicin. The oral bioavailability of this drug is approximately 30%; 80% of the drug is excreted in the urine as 13-epirubicinol.

Preparation and Administration: Idarubicin is supplied in 5- and 10-mg vials from which it is reconstituted with sterile water or normal saline to obtain a 1 mg/mL solution. The drug should be infused from 10 to 15 minutes through the tubing of a freely running IV infusion. Extravasation precautions should be instituted during administration. The oral formulation remains investigational.

Toxic Effects: The side effects of idarubicin are similar to those of daunorubicin and doxorubicin but are of lesser intensity at equal myelosuppressive doses.

Potential Drug Interactions: None has been reported.

Therapeutic Indications in Hematology: Idarubicin in combination with ara-C is equivalent, if not superior, to combination chemotherapy with daunorubicin in the treatment of adult AML and myelodysplastic syndromes. Idarubicin has been approved for use in combination therapy for adult AML.

Mitoxantrone (Novantrone)

Chemistry and Mechanism of Action: Mitoxantrone is a synthetic anthracenedione. Its mechanism of action appears to involve primarily the inhibition of DNA topoisomerase II. Its reduced potential for free radical formation may explain the decreased cardiotoxicity of this drug.

Absorption, Fate, and Excretion: Mitoxantrone is excreted via the renal and hepatobiliary systems, but the hepatobiliary elimination accounts for approximately 30% of active drug elimination and appears to be of greater importance. The half-life is quite variable, with a range of 23 to 42 hours. Patients with severe hepatic dysfunction have been shown to eliminate the drug more slowly.

Preparation and Administration: Mitoxantrone is commercially available as a 2 mg/mL solution in 10-mL, 12.5-mL, and 15-mL vials (20, 25, and 30 mg per vial, respectively). The drug is further diluted in normal saline or 5% dextrose in water for injection and is administered for approximately 15 to 30 minutes into the tubing of a freely running IV infusion. As with the anthracyclines, erythema or streaking along the vein of infusion indicates that the drug is being infused too rapidly. Although mitoxantrone is not a vesicant, there have been rare reports of tissue necrosis following extravasation.

Toxic Effects: Myelosuppression, principally leukopenia, is the dose-limiting toxic effect. Thrombocytopenia is relatively mild. Nausea, vomiting, and alopecia are usually mild and occur in less than 30% of patients treated. Rarely, mucositis and elevation of liver enzymes occur. The drug imparts a blue color to the urine of patients treated. One of the primary advantages of mitoxantrone, in comparison with doxorubicin, is its reduced incidence of cardiac toxicity. Occasionally patients will develop congestive heart failure after treatment with mitoxantrone in the absence of prior anthracycline exposure, although the incidence appears to be less than 5%.

Potential Drug Interactions: None has been reported.

Therapeutic Indications in Hematology: Mitoxantrone is approved for induction therapy of AML in adults.

Amsacrine

Chemistry and Mechanism of Action: Amsacrine, or 4′-(9-acridinylamino) methanesulfon-*m*-anisidide (AMSA) is a synthetic aminoacridine derivative. Amsacrine is a DNA intercalator and also inhibits the activity of DNA topoisomerase II.

Absorption, Fate, and Excretion: When given intravenously, this drug has an initial half-life of 30 minutes and a terminal half-life of 7.9 hours. It is 50% protein bound after 2 hours. It is metabolized by conjugation with glutathione, and approximately 50% of the drug is eliminated in the bile. The remainder of the drug is eliminated via the urinary route as metabolites and parent drug.

Preparation and Administration: Amsacrine is an investigational agent supplied by the National Cancer Institute as a group C drug. It is provided in a dual pack containing two sterile liquids that must be combined before use. One vial contains 1.5 mL of 50 mg/mL of AMSA in anhydrous *N,N*-dimethylactamide and the other contains 13.5 mL of 0.0353 mL lactic acid diluent. When these are combined, the resulting orange-red solution contains 5 mg/mL of AMSA. Because of the *N,N*-dimethylactamide solvent, plastic syringes should not be used with the undiluted AMSA solution.

Toxic Effects: The dose-limiting toxic effect is myelosuppression, predominantly affecting granulocytes. Alopecia is common, and nausea, vomiting, and mucositis can occur. Cardiotoxicity, manifested as a decrease in ejection fraction, acute arrhythmias, or ECG changes was reported in 2.3% of 3200 patients, but most of these patients had been heavily pretreated with anthracyclines. Hypokalemia seems to enhance amsacrine cardiotoxicity and if present should be corrected prior to administration of the drug.

Potential Drug Interactions: The reconstituted solution is physically incompatible with chloride-containing solutions.

Therapeutic Indications in Hematology: Amsacrine is a group C investigational drug approved for the treatment of refractory AML, although it is being evaluated in combination with other cytotoxic agents in the initial treatment of this disease. As a group C drug, amsacrine must be administered as a single agent.

TOPOISOMERASE I INHIBITORS

Topotecan (Hycamtin)

Chemistry and Mechanism of Action: Topotecan is a semisynthetic derivative of camptothecin that stabilizes a complex between DNA topoisomerase I and DNA. The cytotoxic effect of this drug is believed to result from the collision of DNA replication forks with a ternary complex of topoisomerase I, DNA, and topotecan. The resulting double-strand DNA breaks are lethal. The lactone form of topotecan, which predominates at an acidic pH, is a much more potent inhibitor of DNA topoisomerase I.

Absorption, Fate, and Excretion: At neutral or physiologic pH, the carboxylate form of topotecan is favored, and at a pH less than 7, the lactone form is favored. Topotecan has been given as a bolus or by continuous infusion. In less than 1 hour after infusion, most of the circulating drug in the plasma is in the carboxylate form as a result of the physiologic pH. The terminal half-life of the lactone form of this S phase-specific agent is 2.6 hours, whereas the terminal half-life of the total drug is 3.3 hours. In an IV dose, 36% is excreted unchanged in the urine, and there is a 1.5-fold concentration of the drug in bile. CSF levels of topotecan lactone reach approximately 32% of plasma levels. Dose adjustment is required for a creatinine clearance less than 60 mL/min, but no adjustment is necessary for a bilirubin up to 10 mg/dL.

Preparation and Administration: Topotecan is commercially available as 4-mg vials that are reconstituted with 4 mL of sterile water. This solution can be further diluted in normal saline or 5% dextrose in water and should be used immediately.

Toxic Effects: The dose-limiting toxicity for topotecan for all schedules is neutropenia. Thrombocytopenia and anemia are less common, although there is an increase in thrombocytopenia with continuous infusion schedules. Other less common and mild toxicities include nausea, vomiting, diarrhea, fever, fatigue, alopecia, skin rash, and increased liver function tests. Mucositis has been seen with prolonged infusion schedules over 5 days or when topotecan is given in higher doses.

Potential Drug Interactions: In vitro data suggest that there may be some synergism if a topoisomerase I inhibitor is given before a topoisomerase II inhibitor. In vitro data also suggest that synergism may be seen if a topoisomerase I inhibitor (topotecan) is given after an alkylating agent, suggesting that topoisomerase I may be involved in the repair of alkylator-induced DNA damage.

Therapeutic Indications in Hematology: Phase II studies suggest that topotecan has activity in myelodysplastic syndromes, AML, and multiple myeloma.

Irinotecan (Camptosar or CPT-11)

Chemistry and Mechanism of Action: CPT-11 is a prodrug that has a bulky piperidino side chain at C-10 that is cleaved in vivo by a carboxylesterase-converting enzyme to generate SN-38. SN-38 is approximately 1000-fold more potent a topoisomerase I inhibitor than CPT-11. The lactone forms of both SN-38 and CPT-11 are more potent inhibitors of topoisomerase I than the carboxylate forms, which is felt to be the mechanism of action of these drugs as described for topotecan.

Absorption, Fate, and Excretion: The terminal half-life of the lactone form of CPT-11 is 7 hours and that of the total drug, 10.5 hours. The terminal half-life of SN-38 lactone is 8.7 hours and that of the total drug, 14.7 hours. Of a dose of irinotecan, 22% is excreted unchanged in the urine. SN-38 is excreted into the bile and can undergo glucuronidation. The plasma protein binding of CPT-11 is reported to be between 30% and 68%, whereas that of SN-38 is 95%.

Preparation and Administration: Irinotecan is available as a 100-mg single-dose vial with 20 mg/mL irinotecan. This preparation also contains 45 mg of sorbitol per mL and 0.9 mg lactic acid per mL with the pH adjusted to 3.5. This solution can be diluted with 5% dextrose in water (preferred) or in normal saline to a final concentration of 0.1 to 1.2 mg/mL. The solution is stable for up to 24 hours at room temperature or 48 hours when refrigerated. The dose should be modified for severe diarrhea.

Toxic Effects: The major toxic effect of irinotecan is diarrhea. This can be early-onset diarrhea, occurring within hours of administration, or during the infusion, which can be associated with cramping, vomiting, flushing, and diaphoresis. These side effects are due to the cholinergic effects of CPT-11 and can be managed with atropine. Severe later-onset diarrhea can be treated with high-dose loperamide, which has been found to decrease the incidence of grade 4 diarrhea from 20% to 2%. Diarrhea has been found to be the dose-limiting toxicity when irinotecan is given on a weekly schedule, and neutropenia is the dose-limiting toxicity when the drug is given every 3 weeks. Also seen are alopecia, nausea, vomiting, mucositis, fatigue, increased liver function tests, and rare cases of pulmonary toxicity.

Potential Drug Interactions: As described for topotecan, in vitro data suggest some synergism when topoisomerase I inhibitors precede topoisomerase II inhibitors or follow alkylating agent administration.

Therapeutic Indications in Hematology: Phase I and phase II studies have shown responses in refractory leukemia and lymphoma.

APPENDIX 56–5

CLINICAL PHARMACOLOGY OF PLATINUM ANALOGS

CISPLATIN (Platinol)

Chemistry and Mechanism of Action: Cisplatin [cisdiaminedichloroplatinum(II)] is an inorganic heavy metal complex. This complex can have *cis*- and *trans*-isomers; the *cis*-isomer is the active antitumor drug. In the relatively higher chloride concentrations of plasma, cisplatin is uncharged in the dichloroform and passes through plasma membranes. Intracellularly, the low chloride concentrations allow the displacement of the chloride ligands by water to form the positively charged aquated complex. This forms covalent cross-links between two nucleophilic atoms of macromolecules such as the N^7 positions of guanine and adenine in DNA. The cytotoxicity of cisplatin correlates closely with total platinum binding to DNA, to interstrand cross-links, and to the formation of intrastrand bidentate N^7 adducts at d(GpG) and d(ApG), resulting in intrastrand cross-links that bend the DNA helix and inhibit DNA synthesis. Cisplatin damage to DNA induces apoptosis of sensitive cells.

Absorption, Fate, and Excretion: Following its IV injection, the drug concentrates in the liver, kidneys, and bowel. Plasma levels of cisplatin decay in a biphasic manner, with an initial half-life of 25 to 49 minutes and a terminal half-life of 58 to 73 hours. Although 15% of the administered cisplatin is excreted unchanged in the urine, up to 90% of the administered dose of the drug can be recovered from the urine.

Preparation and Administration: Cisplatin is commercially available as a lyophilized powder, supplied in 10- and 50-mg vials also containing mannitol, sodium chloride, and hydrochloric acid, and as an aqueous solution in 50- and 100-mg vials. Reconstitution of the powder for injection is achieved by adding sterile water to make a 1 mg/mL solution. The reconstituted solution should be further diluted in normal saline (usually 500 mL to 1 L) and administered over 1 to 3 hours. To prevent nephrotoxic effects, 25 to 50 g of mannitol is often added to the saline solution, and patients are aggressively hydrated before and after cisplatin infusion. Magnesium sulfate (12–24 mEq) is commonly added to the saline solution to preclude the development of hypomagnesemia.

Toxic Effects: Nephrotoxicity is the dose-limiting toxic effect. Cisplatin produces a dose-dependent impairment of renal tubular function, manifested by an increase in serum creatinine as well as potassium and magnesium wasting. The renal dysfunction is usually reversible, but repeated treatments may produce a cumulative and permanent mild-to-moderate impairment of renal function. Administration of other nephrotoxic agents such as aminoglycosides, even between courses, can potentiate its toxicity. Nausea and vomiting are usually severe and require the use of aggressive antiemetic support. When doses greater than 70 mg/m^2 are used, it is also important to protect against delayed nausea and vomiting by administering antiemetic agents (eg, prochlorperazine plus dexamethasone) for 3 days after therapy. Myelosuppression is usually mild. High-frequency hearing loss, tinnitus, and frank deafness may occur. Peripheral neurotoxicity, characterized by paresthesias or sensory loss in a glove-and-stocking distribution or as muscular weakness, is relatively common in patients who receive total cumulative doses of greater than 500 mg/m^2. The peripheral neuropathy may take many months to resolve, if it does at all. Vestibular toxicity and anaphylactic reactions may occur rarely.

Potential Drug Interactions: Aminoglycosides and amphotericin may enhance cisplatin nephrotoxicity. Caution should be exercised when cisplatin is administered with bleomycin and methotrexate, as cisplatin-induced renal damage may delay the excretion and thus increase the toxicity of these agents.

Therapeutic Indications in Hematology: Cisplatin is used in the treatment of refractory lymphomas, usually in combination with ara-C and high-dose dexamethasone.

CARBOPLATIN (Paraplatin)

Chemistry and Mechanism of Action: Carboplatin is a second-generation platinum (II) complex. Its mechanism of action is very similar to that of cisplatin. However, the carboxyl ester groups in this platinum complex are less easily displaced and less chemically reactive. The peak levels of DNA cross-linking also occur 6 to 12 hours later for carboplatin than for cisplatin.

Absorption, Fate, and Excretion: Carboplatin is primarily eliminated through the kidneys. Its elimination is slower than cisplatin with a terminal half-life between 2 and 6 hours. After IV injection, approximately 60% of the total drug is excreted within 24 hours.

Preparation and Administration: Carboplatin is commercially available as a lyophilized powder in 50- and 150-mg vials containing carboplatin and mannitol. It is reconstituted with sterile water to a final concentration of 10 mg/mL. For injection, further dilution with 5% dextrose and water or normal saline to a concentration of 0.5 or 2 mg/mL, it is stable for 8 hours at room temperature. Carboplatin is often administered by IV injection over 15 to 30 minutes. Patients with reduced renal function (creatinine clearance of <60 mL/min) should have the dose of carboplatin decreased according to the formula described by Egorin et al:

For previously untreated patients:

Dosage (mg/m^2) =
(0.091) (creatinine clearance / body surface area) ×
[pretreatment platelet count –
platelet nadir desired / pretreatment platelet count × 100]
+ 86

For heavily pretreated patients:

Dosage (mg/m^2) =
(0.091) (creatinine clearance / body surface area) ×
[(pretreatment platelet count –
platelet nadir desired / pretreatment platelet count × 100) – 17]
+ 86

A formula developed by Calvert and colleagues also takes into account the patient's pretreatment renal function, as follows:

Dose (mg) =
target AUC (mg/mL × min) H [GFR (mL/min)
+ 25]

where the dose in mg (not mg/m² body surface area) equals target AUC (area under the plasma clearance curve) × GFR (glomerular filtration rate) + 25

In previously untreated adults, the AUC can be estimated at 7 when carboplatin is used alone, and 4.5 when used in combination. If AUC is set lower, less toxicity is expected.

Toxic Effects: The dose-limiting toxic effect is myelosuppression, thrombocytopenia being more significant than leukopenia. Carboplatin leads to less emesis than cisplatin. Although nausea and vomiting are common, they can be easily controlled with antiemetics. At high doses such as those used for bone marrow transplantation, hepatotoxicity, renal dysfunction, and moderate to severe cytotoxicity can occur.

Potential Drug Interactions: None has been reported.

Clinical Indications in Hematology: Carboplatin has been recently approved for the treatment of ovarian cancer. It is also used to treat small cell lung, testicular, head-and-neck, and genitourinary cancers. High-dose carboplatin is presently under evaluation in acute leukemias and lymphomas.

APPENDIX 56–6

CLINICAL PHARMACOLOGY OF MISCELLANEOUS AGENTS

ARSENIC TRIOXIDE

Chemistry and Mechanism of Action: The mechanism of action of arsenic trioxide is not completely understood. Arsenic trioxide causes morphologic changes and DNA fragmentation characteristic of apoptosis in NB4 human promyelocytic leukemia cells in vitro possibly mediated by activation of cysteine-proteases (caspases). Arsenic trioxide also causes damage or degradation of the fusion protein PML/RAR-alpha.

Absorption, Fate, and Excretion: The metabolism of arsenic trioxide involves reduction of pentavalent arsenic to trivalent arsenic by arsenate reductase and methylation of trivalent arsenic to monomethylarsinic acid and monomethylarsinic acid to dimethylarsinic acid by methyltransferases. The main site of methylation reactions appears to be the liver. The pharmacokinetics of trivalent arsenic, the active species, have not been characterized.

Preparation and Administration: Arsenic trioxide is available in 10-mL, single-use ampules containing 10 mg of arsenic trioxide.

It is formulated as a sterile, nonpyrogenic, clear solution of arsenic trioxide in water for injection using sodium hydroxide and dilute hydrochloric acid to adjust to pH 8. TRISENOX should be diluted with 100 to 250 mL 5% dextrose injection, USP, or 0.9% sodium chloride injection, USP, arsenic trioxide should be administered intravenously over 1 to 2 hours. The infusion duration may be extended up to 4 hours if acute vasomotor reactions are observed. A central venous catheter is not required.

Toxic Effects: Arsenic trioxide has electrocardiographic abnormalities including QT interval prolongation, T-wave flattening, and atrioventricular block. Nonspecific edema and weight gain have been reported. Dry skin, pruritis, and rashes have occurred relatively frequently. Anemia, thrombocytopenia, and neutropenia are also observed.

Drug Interactions: Arsenic trioxide can cause QT interval prolongation and complete atrioventricular block. QT prolongation can lead to a torsade de pointes-type ventricular arrhythmia. The risk of torsade de pointes is related to the extent of QT prolongation, and concomitant administration of QT-prolonging drugs may exacerbate this phenomenon.

Therapeutic Indications in Hematology: Arsenic trioxide is effective in newly diagnosed acute promyelocytic leukemia, FAB M3.

Moreover, in patients who are refractory to or have relapsed from retinoid and anthracycline chemotherapy, arsenic trioxide has some activity as a single agent for relapsed or refractory multiple myeloma. Arsenic trioxide produced hematologic improvement in a subset of patients with myelodysplastic syndrome.

BORTEZOMIB (VELCADE)

Molecular Formula: $C_{19}H_{25}BN_4O$ molecular weight 384.24 g/mol Bortezomib (*N*-pyrazinecarbonyl-L-phenylalanine-L-Leucine boronic acid).

Absorption, Fate, and Excretion: Following IV administration of 1.3 mg/m^2 dose, the median estimated maximum plasma concentration of bortezomib was 509 ng/mL (range = 109–1300 ng/mL). The mean elimination half-life of bortezomib after first dose ranged from 9 to 15 hours at doses ranging from 1.45 to 2.00 mg/m^2 in patients with advanced malignancies. In vitro studies with human liver microsomes and human cDNA-expressed cytochrome P450 isozymes indicate that bortezomib is primarily oxidatively metabolized via cytochrome P450 enzymes, 3A4, 2D6, 2C19, 2C9, and 1A2. The major metabolic pathway is deboronation to form two deboronated metabolites that subsequently undergo hydroxylation to several inactive metabolites.

Preparation and Administration: Bortezomib for injection is supplied as a lyophilized powder for reconstitution. Each sterile single-use vial contains 3.5 mg of bortezomib and 35 mg of mannitol USP. Each vial is reconstituted with 3.5 mL normal (0.9%) saline such that the reconstituted solution contains bortezomib at a concentration of 1 mg/mL. The pH of the reconstituted solution is between 5 and 6. The drug is given without any further dilution as an IV bolus over 3 to 5 seconds. Intact vials of lyophilized bortezomib for injection are stored in a refrigerator at 2°C to 8°C (35°F to 47°F) and protected from light. Stability studies are ongoing to monitor each clinical lot. Product should be administered immediately after reconstitution. The solution as reconstituted is stable for 43 hours at room temperature. Bortezomib is administered as an IV bolus (over 3–5 seconds) twice weekly for 2 weeks followed by a 1-week rest period.

Toxic Effects: The most commonly reported adverse events were asthenic conditions (including fatigue, malaise, and weakness; 65%), nausea (64%), diarrhea (51%), decreased appetite (including anorexia; 43%), constipation (43%), thrombocytopenia (43%), peripheral neuropathy (including peripheral sensory neuropathy and peripheral neuropathy aggravated; 37%), pyrexia (36%), vomiting (36%), and anemia (32%). Fourteen percent of patients experienced at least one episode of grade 4 toxicity, with the most common being thrombocytopenia (3%) and neutropenia (3%).

Potential Drug Interactions: No formal drug interaction studies have been conducted with bortezomib. In vitro studies with human liver microsomes indicate that bortezomib is a substrate of cytochrome P450 3A4, 2D6, 2C19, 2C9, and 1A2. Bortezomib may inhibit 2C19 activity (IC_{50} = 18 μM, 6.9 μg/mL) and increase exposure to drugs that are substrates for this enzyme. Patients who are concomitantly receiving bortezomib and drugs that are inhibitors or inducers of cytochrome P450 3A4 should be closely monitored for either toxicities or reduced efficacy. Patients on oral antidiabetic agents receiving bortezomib treatment may experience hypo- or hyperglycemia and require close monitoring of their blood glucose levels and adjustment of the dose of their antidiabetic medication. Finally, patients should be cautioned about the use of concomitant medications that may be associated with peripheral neuropathy (such as amiodarone, antivirals, isoniazid, nitrofurantoin, or statins), or with a decrease in blood pressure.

Therapeutic Indications in Hematology: Bortezomib is FDA approved for the treatment of multiple myeloma patients who have received at least two prior therapies and have demonstrated disease progression on the last therapy.

DASATINIB

Chemistry and Mechanism of Action: Dasatinib is an orally active tyrosine kinase inhibitor against BCR-ABL, SRC family, c-KIT, EPHA2, and PDGFR-beta. The primary mechanism of resistance to dasatinib is the T315I mutant clone.

Absorption, Fate, and Excretion: Dasatinib is orally absorbed and extensively metabolized in human liver microsomes, primarily by cytochrome P450 CYP3A4 to an active metabolite. CYP3A4 is the primary enzyme responsible for the formation of the active metabolite. Flavin-containing monooxygenase 3 (FMO-3) and uridine diphosphateglucuronosyltransferase (UGT) enzymes are also involved in the formation of dasatinib metabolites. In human liver microsomes, dasatinib was a weak time-dependent inhibitor of CYP3A4. The exposure of the active metabolite, which is equipotent to dasatinib, represents approximately 5% of the dasatinib AUC.

Preparation and Administration: Dasatinab is an oral agent usually taken twice daily without regard to meals.

Toxic Effects: Treatment with dasatinib is associated with severe thrombocytopenia, neutropenia, and anemia and platelet dysfunction. Also seen is fluid retention, including pleural and pericardial effusion, pulmonary edema, severe ascites, and generalized edema. Prolonged QT interval has been observed as well as extensive skin rashes.

Drug Interactions: Dasatinib is a CYP3A4 substrate. Administering with drugs that are CYP3A4 inhibitors may cause increased dasatinib plasma concentrations and subsequent increase in toxicities. Drugs that induce CYP3A4 activity may decrease dasatinib plasma concentrations and decrease its effectiveness. The solubility of dasatinib is pH dependent. Simultaneous administration of SPRYCEL with antacids should be avoided and there should be 2 hours' separation in the administration of dasatinib and antacids. Long-term suppression of gastric acid secretion by H2 blockers or proton pump may reduce dasatinib exposure and antacids are preferred. Dasatinib is a time-dependent inhibitor of CYP3A4; therefore, CYP3A4 substrates may have their plasma concentration altered by dasatinib.

Therapeutic Indications in Hematology: Treatment with dasatinib results in hematologic and cytogenetic responses in patients with lymphoid blast crisis (LBC), Philadelphia chromosome-positive (Ph+), chronic myeloid leukemia (CML), and Ph+ acute lymphoid leukemia (ALL), as initial treatment and in disease resistant or intolerant to imatinib.

PLICAMYCIN

Chemistry and Mechanism of Action: Plicamycin, also called mithramycin, forms complexes with DNA and inhibits DNA-directed synthesis of RNA. Plicamycin also inhibits the effect of parathyrin on osteoclasts. The hypocalcemic effect is independent of the antitumor effect.

Absorption, Fate, and Excretion: The pharmacology of plicamycin has been poorly described. Within 15 hours of IV administration, 40% is excreted in the urine. The elimination half-life has been estimated to be approximately 2 hours.

Preparation and Administration: Plicamycin is commercially available as a lyophilized powder in 2.5-mg vials, from which it is reconstituted with 4.9 mL of sterile water for injection. This dose should be further diluted in 1 L of 5% dextrose in water or normal saline and infused over 4 to 6 hours.

Toxic Effects: When plicamycin is employed as an antitumor agent, its most common side effects include myelosuppression, elevated liver enzymes, increased serum creatinine and proteinuria, and coagulopathy due to decreased clotting factors II, V, VII, and X. The drug also causes nausea and vomiting, diarrhea, stomatitis, headache, and irritability. Cutaneous toxicity may occur in up to one-third of patients, manifested by progressive blushing of the face and thickening and coarsening of the skinfolds. The drug can produce severe local irritation if extravasation occurs.

Potential Drug Interactions: None has been reported.

Therapeutic Indications in Hematology: Plicamycin is primarily used to treat hypercalcemia of malignancy. Claims of antitumor activity in the blast phase of CML have been made but have not been confirmed.

BLEOMYCIN

Chemistry and Mechanism of Action: Bleomycin is a glycopeptide. Its antitumor effect correlates with its ability to cause scission of both double- and single-stranded DNA via activated oxygen formed by the iron–bleomycin complex. Bleomycin also affects DNA repair by inhibiting DNA ligase.

Absorption, Fate, and Excretion: Bleomycin is rapidly distributed throughout the body and concentrates in the skin, lung, kidney, peritoneum, and lymph nodes. Its plasma half-life is 2 to 4 hours. Within 24 hours of injection, approximately 50% of an administered dose is excreted unchanged in the urine. Bleomycin elimination correlates well with creatinine clearance; accordingly, patients with renal failure should receive a reduced dose. In the tissues, bleomycin is inactivated by bleomycin hydrolase. Tissues lacking this enzyme, such as lung and skin, are more susceptible to the drug's toxic effects.

Preparation and Administration: Bleomycin is commercially available in vials containing 15 U (approximately equivalent to 15 mg), from which it is reconstituted for injection with 3 to 5 mL of sterile water, normal saline, 5% dextrose in water, or bacteriostatic water. For IV infusion, the reconstituted solution can be further diluted with either normal saline or 5% dextrose in water and administered over 5 minutes. Bleomycin can also be administered by the subcutaneous, intravenous, intramuscular, intracavitary, and intraarterial routes. Because patients with lymphomas are at an increased risk of anaphylactoid reactions, which may not occur until 12 hours after administration, the first 2 doses should be intramuscular "test doses"' of 1 to 2 mg. If no reactions occur, full doses may be given.

Toxic Effects: The most serious toxic effect is interstitial pneumonitis, which is dose related and occurs in approximately 10% of patients treated with cumulative doses of greater than 350 to 400 U. The interstitial pneumonitis may evolve into life-threatening pulmonary fibrosis. Pulmonary toxicity is more common in patients older than 70 years, in those receiving a total dose of greater than 400 U, and in those who received prior radiotherapy to the lung. It is important to emphasize, however, that the pulmonary toxicity is unpredictable; it has been reported in patients who had none of these risk factors and has occurred in a patient after administration of only 20 U. Some reports suggest that an increased concentration of inspired oxygen acts synergistically with bleomycin to produce pulmonary fibrosis. During critical illness and perioperatively, therefore, an attempt should be made to maintain the inspired oxygen concentration at 21%. The early phases of the pulmonary toxicity are clinically manifested by dyspnea and fine rales. Although corticosteroids are often employed in this setting, it is not clear that they are of benefit.

Mucocutaneous toxicity occurs in 50% of patients treated and is manifested by hyperpigmentation, pruritic erythema, mucositis, desquamation of the plantar surface skin of the hands and/or feet, ridging of the nails, and alopecia. The mucositis can be severe and is the acute dose-limiting toxic effect. Febrile reactions, which occur a few hours after bleomycin administration and may last 4 to 12 hours, are also common. Fever becomes less frequent with continued use of the drug and can usually be prevented by concurrent administration of glucocorticosteroids (eg, 100 mg of hydrocortisone). Bleomycin has virtually no myelosuppressive effect. Anaphylactoid reactions are observed in approximately 1% (up to 8% in some series) of patients with lymphomas treated with bleomycin.

Potential Drug Interaction: Bleomycin, administered with other drugs for the treatment of lymphorrhea, can decrease the oral bioavailability of digoxin and the pharmacologic effect of phenytoin and certain anesthetic drugs.

Therapeutic Indications in Hematology: Bleomycin is often incorporated in the chemotherapy regimens of Hodgkin disease (ABVD and MOPP-ABV hybrid regimens) and NHLs (MACOP-B, PROMACE-CYTABOM, M-BACOD, and CHOP-Bleo).

ASPARAGINASE

Chemistry and Mechanism of Action: Asparaginase contains the high-molecular-weight enzyme L-asparaginase amidohydrolase, type EC-2, derived from *Escherichia coli*. Asparaginase hydrolyzes serum asparagine to nonfunctional aspartic acid and ammonia, depriving tumor cells of a required amino acid; thus, tumor cell proliferation is blocked by the interruption of asparagine-dependent protein synthesis. The drug appears to be most active in the G_1 phase.

Absorption, Fate, and Excretion: Asparaginase is not absorbed orally. Its plasma half-life varies from 8 to 30 hours and is not influenced by dosage, age, sex, surface area, or renal or hepatic function.

Preparation and Administration: Asparaginase is commercially available in vials containing 10,000 IU of asparaginase in 80 mg of mannitol. For IV use, the drug should be reconstituted with 5 mL of either sterile water or sodium chloride for injection and injected in the tubing of a freely running infusion of either normal saline or 5% dextrose in water over 30 minutes. For intramuscular or subcutaneous use, each vial should be reconstituted with 2 mL of sodium chloride for injection to obtain a 5000-U/mL solution. For dosages that exceed 2 mL, use of two injection sites is recommended. For both IV and intramuscular administration, the drug must be used within 8 hours of reconstitution, and only if it is clear. Because of the possibility of hypersensitivity reactions (particularly in patients with lymphomas), an intradermal skin test is recommended before initial administration of asparaginase or when 1 week has elapsed between doses. For this test, 2 IU should be injected intradermally and observed for a wheal or erythema for 1 hour. A negative skin test, however, does not preclude possible development of a hypersensitivity reaction. It is recommended that oxygen, epinephrine, and corticosteroids be available at the bedside during administration of the drug. For allergic patients, the *E coli* form of asparaginase should be replaced by the asparaginase derived from *Erwinia carotovora*, provided by the National Cancer Institute as an investigational group C agent.

Toxic Effects: The toxicity of asparaginase is reported to be greater in adults than in children. Anorexia, nausea, or vomiting occurs in approximately one-third of patients. Most of the other side effects can be divided into two main groups, those related to hypersensitivity reactions to the foreign protein and those resulting from decreased protein synthesis. The hypersensitivity reaction is characterized by urticaria, laryngeal edema, bronchospasm, or hypotension and may occur with the initial dose of the drug, even if the skin test is negative. More commonly, however, allergic phenomena are observed after multiple courses of treatment. Adverse effects related to the inhibition of protein synthesis include hypoalbuminemia and decreases in serum fibrinogen, prothrombin, antithrombin III, and other coagulation factors, which may lead to both clotting and hemorrhagic complications; decreased serum insulin with hyperglycemia; and decreased serum lipoproteins. In ≤25% of patients, cerebral dysfunction, characterized by confusion, stupor, and frank coma, can occur. Although the neurotoxic effects resemble those of ammonia toxicity, they are apparently due to low concentrations of either L-asparagine or L-glutamine in the brain. Acute pancreatitis, which may progress to severe hemorrhagic pancreatitis, may occur in 15% of patients. Elevation of liver enzymes and serum bilirubin is almost universal and is histologically represented by fatty metamorphosis. Liver toxicity, although usually not clinically significant, has resulted in occasional fatalities. Asparaginase can occasionally produce renal functional impairment with oliguric renal failure.

Potential Drug Interactions: When asparaginase is administered immediately before or concurrent with methotrexate, it decreases the cytotoxic effect of the latter. When administered to patients with acute leukemia 9 to 10 days before or shortly after methotrexate, however, asparaginase appears to enhance the cytotoxic effect of methotrexate. Concurrent administration of asparaginase with vincristine may increase vincristine's neurotoxic effects, but this effect appears to be less pronounced when asparaginase is given after vincristine. The effects of asparaginase on liver function may potentially interfere with the activation or metabolism of other cytotoxic agents.

Therapeutic Indications in Hematology: Asparaginase is used in combination therapy for remission induction of patients with ALL.

GALLIUM NITRATE

Chemistry and Mechanism of Action: Gallium nitrate is a group IIA metal salt, of which the mechanism of action is not completely understood. Its selective cytotoxic effects in humans are probably related to its predominant concentration in certain malignant tumors. Gallium nitrate binds to intracellular calcium and magnesium sites. Transferrin binding appears to be necessary to produce the cytotoxic effect.

Absorption, Fate, and Metabolism: Gallium nitrate is primarily eliminated by renal excretion and follows a biphasic pharmacokinetic pattern. The reported half-life is within a range of 6 to 36 hours.

Preparation and Administration: Gallium nitrate is an investigational agent supplied as a 25 mg/mL solution in 20-mL vials (500 mg per vial), which also contain trisodium citrate and sodium hydroxide to adjust the pH. Gallium nitrate can be administered by slow IV infusion, although in the treatment of hypercalcemia it is usually given by continuous infusion for 5 to 7 days.

Toxic Effects: When gallium nitrate is given as a single bolus injection, the dose-limiting toxicity is renal impairment. The renal toxicity is significantly minimized when the drug is given by continuous infusion. Other toxic effects include mild myelosuppression, hypocalcemia (when not desired), nausea, vomiting, diarrhea, and mucositis. Rarely, gallium nitrate can produce neurotoxic effects such as hearing loss, visual disturbances, paresthesias, and mental status changes.

Potential Drug Interactions: None has been reported.

Clinical Indications in Hematology: Gallium nitrate has shown promising results in the treatment of hypercalcemia associated with malignancy, in prevention of bone loss in patients with multiple myeloma, and in the treatment of refractory lymphomas.

GLUCOCORTICOIDS

Chemistry and Mechanism of Action: Glucocorticoids are synthetic compounds derived from the natural adrenal hormone, cortisol. Glucocorticoids mediate their biologic actions predominantly by binding to their cytosolic receptor, which then translocates to the nucleus. There, as a homodimer, it binds to specific DNA sequences located in the regulatory regions of a number of genes. Gene transcription can be upregulated or downregulated by glucocorticoids. They can also inhibit binding of the AP-1 transcription factor to its DNA consensus sequence site. Lymphocytes treated with glucocorticoids undergo apoptosis mediated by glucocorticoid receptors. An early cytostatic phase is marked by growth inhibition and cessation of proliferation due to inhibition of cellular uptake of glucose, amino acids, and nucleosides as well as inhibition of macromolecular synthesis. This is followed by a cytolytic phase characterized by chromatin condensation and internucleosomal DNA cleavage.

Absorption, Fate, and Excretion: Many synthetic glucocorticoids are available, the three most commonly used in hematology being prednisone, dexamethasone, and methylprednisolone. The glucocorticoids are well absorbed orally and are primarily metabolized in the liver. Unlike the other two glucocorticoids, the activity of prednisone is dependent on hepatic conversion to the 11-hydroxy form (prednisolone). The biologic half-lives of prednisone and methylprednisolone are approximately 12 to 36 hours, whereas dexamethasone has a biologic half-life of 36 to 72 hours. Plasma half-lives for all three drugs are within the range of 3 to 4 hours. Compared with cortisol, the relative antiinflammatory potencies of dexamethasone, methylprednisolone, and prednisone are 25, 5, and 4, respectively, for equivalent doses.

Preparation and Administration: Prednisone is available only for oral administration, whereas methylprednisolone and dexamethasone are available in oral and parenteral dosage forms.

Toxic Effects: When glucocorticoids are used for less than 14 days, as is often done when they are employed in combination with other cytotoxic agents, the most common side effects include euphoria, insomnia, psychosis, hyperglycemia, hypokalemia, increased appetite, metabolic alkalosis, proximal muscular weakness, and fluid retention with edema formation and hypertension. When used on a chronic basis, glucocorticoids also may induce a "Cushingoid" appearance, easy bruisability, peptic ulcers, osteoporosis, subcapsular cataracts, and increased susceptibility to infections related to impaired cellular immunity. Because of this, H_2 blockers, antifungal agents (eg, ketoconazole), and/or sulfamethoxazole trimethoprim have been employed in certain glucocorticoid chemotherapy combinations.

Potential Drug Interactions: Glucocorticoids interact with a variety of drugs, including barbiturates, oral contraceptives, erythromycin, hydantoins, rifampin, isoniazid, and salicylates. Given the wide range of doses of glucocorticoids used, however, these interactions are of no major clinical relevance.

Clinical Indications in Hematology: Glucocorticoids have direct anticancer activity in many hematologic malignancies, including ALL, CLL, Hodgkin disease, NHLs, and plasma cell neoplasms. Because of their efficacy and toxic profiles, which do not overlap with the toxic effects of the other cytotoxic agents, glucocorticoids are employed in many chemotherapy regimens. In addition, they are useful in the management of hypercalcemia secondary to myeloma and lymphomas and are of paramount importance in the treatment of autoimmune hematologic disorders.

BRYOSTATIN

Chemistry and Mechanism of Action: Bryostatin is a macrocyclic lactone that activates protein kinase C by causing translocation of the enzyme from the cytoplasmic to the membrane-associated active fraction during short-term exposure and protein kinase C membrane depletion and inactivation at long-term exposure.

Absorption, Fate, and Excretion: There is no reliable assay for determining the fate of bryostatin in humans.

Preparation and Administration: Bryostatin is supplied and prepared as a two-part formulation. Vial one contains 0.1 mg of lyophilized bryostatin as a white powder and is combined with 1 mL of a PET diluent (60% polyethylene glycol 400, 30% dehydrated ethyl alcohol, and 10% polysorbate 80). This solution must be further diluted with 9 mL of 0.9% sodium chloride injection and yields a 10-µg/mL solution of bryostatin. Polyvinyl chloride (PVC) bags should not be used, as there may be leaching of a plasticizer and some limited adsorption. The drug may be further diluted with 0.9% sodium chloride, or dextrose 5% in water, to a concentration of 0.15 µg/mL to 0.75 µg/mL in a glass or polyolefin container. Non-PVC tubing is recommended.

Toxic Effects: Dose-limiting myalgias, eye pain, and photophobia are frequently seen. Phlebitis is common with peripheral administration. Fatigue, headache, nausea and vomiting, along with diarrhea, are also seen. Thrombocytopenia, neutropenia, and anemia occur, although infrequently.

Drug Interactions: No known reports.

Therapeutic Indications in Hematology: Bryostatin has activity against myeloid leukemia, CLL, NHL, and multiple myeloma. Enhanced tumor effect has occurred with the combination of bryostatin with vincristine, cisplatin, and cytarabine.

FLAVOPIRIDOL

Chemistry and Mechanism of Action: Flavopiridol is a semisynthetic flavone and selective inhibitor of CDKs 1, 2, 4-7, PKC, PKA, and PDGF causing cell-cycle arrest. It also may inhibit CDK9/TEFb, which causes downregulation of Mcl-1, BIRC4, cyclin D1, and p21CIP1.

Absorption, Fate, and Excretion: Flavopiridol is 94% protein bound and is metabolized by the UDP glucuronyltransferase isoenzymes. Its half-life varies with infusion duration and ranges from 3.5 hours (1-hour infusion) to 27 hours (72-hour infusion).

Preparation and Administration: Flavopiridol is supplied as a 10 mg/mL yellow-greenish solution in a 5-mL vial. Contents may be diluted in either 5% dextrose injection or 0.9% sodium chloride injection to achieve a final concentration of 0.09 to 1 mg/mL. If the drug is administered through peripheral IV access, a concentration of less than 0.5 mg/mL is thought to decrease thrombotic complications. Flavopiridol has been administered as a 1-, 24-, and 72-hour infusion.

Toxic Effects: Grade 4 neutropenia and grade 3 lymphocytopenia occur and are more common with shorter durations of infusion. Thrombocytopenia is seen infrequently. Secretory diarrhea is a dose-limiting toxicity and may last for up to 3 days. Orthostatic hypotension is a frequently seen occurrence. Thrombosis with the 72-hour infusion duration was far more common than in the shorter infusion durations. A fatigue rate approaching 75% has been reported. Other toxicities include pleuritic chest pain, hyperbilirubinemia, and nausea.

Potential Drug Interactions: Paclitaxel in combination with flavopiridol has been associated with severe dose-limiting neutropenia.

Therapeutic Indications in Hematology: Flavopiridol's place in therapy is still being assessed. It has activity and use in hematologic malignancies including mantle cell lymphoma, leukemias, and multiple myeloma. It may cause potential solid tumors in combination with other agents.

TANESPIMYCIN (17-AAG, GELDANAMYCIN, NSC 330507)

Chemistry: Tanespimycin is a water soluble, benzoquinone ansamycin antibiotic that binds to heat shock protein 90.

Fate, Absorption, and Excretion: Tanespimycin has a mean terminal half-life of 2.3 hours and is primarily metabolized by liver microsimal enzymes, specifically CYP3A4. One metabolite, 17-AG is known to be active and has a mean terminal half-life of 4.6 hours. Peak plasma concentrations of 17-AAG and 17-AG occur at 30 and 60 minutes, respectively. 10.6% of 17-AAG and 7.8% of 17-AG is recovered in the urine over a 72-hour period.

Preparation and Administration: Tanespimycin is available as a single use amber vial containing 50 mg of Tanespiycin in 2 mL of dimethylsulfoxide. Prior to administration, the Tanespimycin concentrate must be completely thawed at room temperature (over approximately 1 hour). Incomplete thawing affects the concentration of the drug due to changes in volume. Tanespimycin concentrate must be diluted to 1 mg/mL by withdrawing 2 mL and adding it to 48 mL of EPL diluent 2% egg phospholipids with 5% dextrose in water. A clear solution should be obtained with gentle mixing. Shaking should be avoided to prevent foaming. No further dilution is required and the final solution should be dispensed in a glass bottle. A 0.45 micron filter may be used, but is not required. The infusion should be completed within 8 hours of mixing. Intact vials of Tanespimycin should be stored in the freezer (−10 to −20°C). EPL diluent should be stored in the refrigerator (2 to 8°C) and not frozen. Administration is by intravenous infusion.

Toxicity: Anemia, diarrhea, nausea, vomiting, fatigue, transaminitis, and muscle pain.

Drug Interactions: Tanespimycin is metabolized by CYP3A4. Agents that alter CYP3A4 activity may affect drug levels and metabolism although this has not been shown to affect clinical use.

Therapeutic Uses: Lymphoma and leukemia, in clinical trials.

IMATINIB (GLEEVEC)

Chemistry and Mechanism of Action: Imatinib, a phenylaminopyrinadine derivative, is a selective protein tyrosine kinase inhibitor effecting BCR-ABL tyrosine kinase. This enzyme is found commonly in CML and in some clones of ALL. Imatinib also inhibits the kinases for PDGF, SCF, and KIT.

Absorption, Fate, and Excretion: Imatinib is well absorbed and achieves peak levels within 2 to 4 hours and follows linear pharmacokinetics at the standard doses. The cytochrome P450 is the major route of metabolism with CYP3A4 being the primary pathway. An *N*-desmethyl piperazine is the main metabolite and is active. Pediatric patients follow the same pharmacokinetics as in adults.

Preparation and Administration: Imatinib is available in a film-coated tablet. In its pure form, it is a white to brownish to yellowish powder and is soluble in aqueous buffers of less than 5.5.

Toxic Effects: Gastrointestinal effects are common and include nausea and diarrhea. Muscle cramps are seen in one-third of all patients receiving imatinib. Myelosuppression reflected as thrombocytopenia, anemia, and neutropenia occurs, with thrombocytopenia and neutropenia seen more frequently in patients in accelerated phase or blast crisis. Fluid retention is dose related and is exhibited as edema and weight gain, but pleural and pericardiac effusions are also seen. Fatigue and headache, although low grade, occur in 25% of patients.

Potential Drug Interactions: Drugs that inhibit CYP3A4 may increase imatinib plasma concentrations; these include ketoconazole, itraconazole, erythromycin, and clarithromycin. CY3A4 inducers that may decrease plasma concentration of CY3A4 are dexamethasone, rifampin, phenytoin, and carbamazepine. Imatinib increases concentrations of simvastatin, cyclosporine, and warfarin, along with other medications that are metabolized by CYP3A4.

Therapeutic Indications in Hematology: Imatinib is considered first-line therapy in Philadelphia-positive CML and has activity in accelerated or blast-phase CML. Some effect has been shown in ALL as well as hypereosinophilic syndrome and polycythemia vera.

TOPOTECAN (HYCAMTIN)

Chemistry and Mechanism of Action: Topotecan is a semisynthetic derivative of camptothecin that stabilizes a complex between DNA topoisomerase I and DNA. The cytotoxic effect of this drug is believed to result from the collision of DNA replication forks with a ternary complex of topoisomerase I, DNA, and topotecan. The resulting double-strand DNA breaks are lethal. The lactone form of topotecan, which predominates at an acidic pH, is a much more potent inhibitor of DNA topoisomerase I.

Absorption, Fate, and Excretion: At neutral or physiologic pH, the carboxylate form of topotecan is favored, and at a pH less than 7 the lactone form is favored. Topotecan has been given as a bolus or by continuous infusion. In less than 1 hour after infusion, most of the circulating drug in the plasma is in the carboxylate form because of the physiologic pH. The terminal half-life of the lactone form of this S phase-specific agent is 2.6 hours, and the terminal half-life of the total drug is 3.3 hours. Thirty-six percent of an IV dose is excreted unchanged in the urine, and there is a 1.5-fold concentration of the drug in bile. CSF levels of topotecan lactone reach approximately 32% of plasma levels. Dose adjustment is required for a creatinine clearance less than 60 mL/min, but no adjustment is necessary for a bilirubin up to 10 mg/dL.

Preparation and Administration: Topotecan is commercially available as 4-mg vials that are reconstituted with 4 mL of sterile water. This solution can be further diluted in normal saline or 5% dextrose in water and should be used immediately.

Toxic Effects: The dose-limiting toxicity for topotecan for all schedules is neutropenia. Thrombocytopenia and anemia are less common, although there is an increase in thrombocytopenia with continuous infusion schedules. Other less common and mild toxicities include nausea, vomiting, diarrhea, fever, fatigue, alopecia, skin rash, and increased liver function tests. Mucositis has been seen with prolonged infusion schedules over 5 days or when topotecan is given in higher doses.

Potential Drug Interactions: In vitro data suggest that there may be some synergism if a topoisomerase I inhibitor is given before a topoisomerase II inhibitor. In vitro data also suggest that synergism may be seen if a topoisomerase I inhibitor (topotecan) is given after an alkylating agent, suggesting that topoisomerase I may be involved in the repair of alkylator-induced DNA damage.

Therapeutic Indications in Hematology: Topotecan has activity in myelodysplastic syndromes, AML, CML, and multiple myeloma.

VORINOSTAT (ZOLINZA)

Chemistry and Mechanism of Action: Vorinostat is a histone deacetylase (HDAC) inhibitor. It inhibits HDAC 1, HDAC2, HDAC3 and HDAC6 at nanomolar concentrations. Inhibition prevents removal of the acetyl groups from lysine residues in target histones and transcription factors. Loss of deacetylase function results in persistence of acetyl groups on histones, resulting in larger segments of open chromatin and a general increase in gene expression. Often this promotes differentiation and cell cycle arrest with apoptosis. The number of genes affected continues to grow so that the impact of vorinostat is complex.

Absorption, Fate, and Excretion: Reported pharmacokinetics after a 400-mg oral administration are an AUC of 5.5 micromolar-hours, a C_{max} of 1.2 micromolar, and T_{max} of 2 to 10 hours. Fatty meals decrease rate of absorption but increase in overall drug levels. There is no recommended dosing relative to meals. Vorinostat is heavily plasma protein absorbed. It undergoes glucuronidation hydrolysis and later beta oxidation to inactive metabolites. Little is excreted unchanged.

Preparation and Administration: Oral dosing of 400 mg is standard, with food. If side effects are noted, reduce the dose to 300 mg. There is no approved pediatric dosing.

Toxic Effects: Many side effects are noted. Common are fatigue, thrombocytopenia, muscle spasms and anorexia. Serious reported adverse effects in clinical trails included pulmonary embolism, in 4.7% and anemia in 2.3%.

Potential Drug Interactions: Vorinnostat can prolong coumadin effect, raising the INR. It can also induce glucose intolerance.

Therapeutic Indications in Hematology: Vorinostat is approved for cutaneous manifestations of cutaneous T-cell lymphoma who have become refractory to standard treatments. It is being tested in other disorders such as myeloma and leukemias to determine whether it works through the histone deacetylases and/or through altered expression of numerous proteins.

CHAPTER 57

RADIATION THERAPY IN THE TREATMENT OF HEMATOLOGIC MALIGNANCIES

Andrea K. Ng and Peter M. Mauch

HISTORICAL BACKGROUND

In 1895, x-rays were first described by German physicist Wilhelm Conrad Roentgen. Shortly after, in 1898 Antoine Henri Becquerel discovered radioactivity, and in the same year the Curies isolated radium. The therapeutic potential of x-rays was first demonstrated in 1897, when German surgeon Wilhelm Alexander Freund showed the disappearance of a hairy mole after x-ray treatments. In the early part of the century, radiation therapy consisted of primitive equipment, crude dosimetry, and little knowledge of normal tissue or tumor radiation biology. Although initial tumor shrinkage was achieved, the superficial characteristics of radiation therapy deposited high doses in the skin and subcutaneous tissues, causing skin burns and ulceration, and underdosed deeper tumor tissues, resulting in suboptimal long-term control. By 1930, the development of reliable orthovoltage machines enabled treatment of deeper tumors. The concept of fractionated radiation therapy was also developed in the 1930s. However, even with the more penetrating beams, adequate treatment of tumors deep in the abdomen or chest frequently was associated with complications to the skin, muscles, heart, or bowel. Modern high-energy megavoltage equipment became available in the 1950s with cobalt-60 (^{60}Co). The linear accelerator, designed from microwave technology developed for radar in World War II, was first used in the United States by Kaplan and his group at Stanford University in the late 1950s.

Many of the principles and early techniques of radiation therapy for hematologic malignancies came from pioneering work in Hodgkin lymphoma. Vera Peters, in 1950, was the first physician to present definitive evidence that radiation therapy was a curative modality for early-stage Hodgkin lymphoma.[1] She did this by identifying patients with limited-stage disease who were cured with high-dose, fractionated radiation therapy. Patients received 1800 to 5000 Roentgen to areas of involvement, with the highest dose given to patients with early-stage disease. She reported 5- and 10-year survival rates of 88% and 79%, respectively, for patients with stage I Hodgkin lymphoma, rates that were notably high for a disease in which virtually no one survived 10 years. The early success of radiation therapy in the treatment of lymphoma and Hodgkin lymphoma provided encouragement for treatment of other tumors. These developments in radiation therapy are detailed in the next sections.

RADIATION PHYSICS

Types of Radiation

Electromagnetic Radiation

The ionizing radiation (photons) used in clinical treatment is part of the electromagnetic spectrum.[2] The energy of x-rays, described in terms of electron volts (eV), chosen for therapy is such that they eject an electron from the target tissue, thus the term *ionizing radiation*. High-energy radiation is produced by linear accelerators from radioactive decay. The photons produced from radioactive decay are called gamma rays. They are identical to the x-rays produced by linear accelerators. Radioactive isotopes can be produced that emit gamma rays at sufficient energy and dose rates to be used in clinical external-beam therapy. The most common isotope for external-beam irradiation is ^{60}Co (half-life 5.26 years). This isotope was in use before the availability of linear accelerators. The decay of ^{60}Co to nickel produces two gamma rays of energy that are 1.17 and 1.33 MeV. Linear accelerators generate photon beams by bombarding a target with electrons. Higher-energy and thus more penetrating x-rays can be produced. Furthermore, linear accelerators have a smaller source and as a result, can produce a much sharper beam edge compared with the cobalt machine.

Particle Radiation

High-energy electrons are one of the most frequently used particle radiation in cancer treatment. They can be produced directly from a linear accelerator with the proper extraction technique. The typical energy range for electrons is 6 to 20 MeV, which allows treatment of superficial tumors up to a depth of 5 cm, with a characteristic sharp drop in dose beyond the prescribed depth.

Neutrons, protons, helium, carbon ions, and pi-mesons are other particles used for experimental radiation therapy.[3] Because of their mass and charge, these particles can be sharply localized in tissue (Bragg peak). They are, therefore, useful for precise localization, usually of relatively small lesions. However, their use is limited and are available only in a few centers in the country.

Radiation Treatment Planning and Delivery

Radiation treatment requires a precise knowledge of normal anatomy and a detailed knowledge of growth patterns of tumors. Patient treatment plans are developed at a simulator before commencement of radiation therapy. The conventional simulator contains a diagnostic x-ray tube, usually with fluoroscopic capabilities, but otherwise it has geometry similar to that of the treatment unit. Bony landmarks, or other anatomical structures visible fluoroscopically, are typically used to guide treatment field design. Three-dimensional conformal radiation therapy (3D CRT), which provide a 3D model of the patient's anatomy and tumor, allows more accurate tumor targeting while sparing neighboring critical normal organs.[4–7] Beams' eye view display is used to select optimal beam directions and design beam apertures. Intensity-modulated radiation therapy (IMRT) is increasingly adopted in a number of disease sites.[8,9] This technique is based on the use of optimized nonuniform radiation beam intensities incident on the patient, allowing dose "sculpting" and dose "painting," and has the potential to further improve the therapeutic ratio and reduce radiation toxicity. Despite the relatively low doses used in the treatment of hematologic malignancies, there may be a role for IMRT in specific clinical scenarios in which limitation of dose to surrounding normal structures is critical.[10–12] Other innovative treatment delivery systems that not only optimize dose distribution but also take into account organ motion by integrating onboard imaging systems are becoming increasingly more available.[13]

The introduction of whole-body positron emission tomography (PET) scanning using ^{18}F-fluorodeoxyglucose has a major impact on initial cancer staging and assessing response to therapy. The accuracy of tumor targeting could be improved by incorporating PET scan information into the radiation treatment plan. The fusion of PET data with computed tomography (CT) simulation information allows simultaneous outlining of the treatment volumes with higher anatomic accuracy.[14] New-generation simulators are designed to include both x-ray–based CT and PET and will simplify multiple-source data acquisition. Future application of this new technology may include establishing the optimal radiation dose based on the level of residual metabolic activity.

RADIATION BIOLOGY

Four R's of Radiation Biology

The laboratory and clinical findings of classic radiation biology have been defined in terms of the four R's of repair, redistribution, repopulation, and reoxygenation.[15]

Repair

Two basic types of repair have been defined operationally: sublethal damage repair and potentially lethal damage repair. A radiation cell survival curve is characterized by a shoulder region and a terminal exponential portion (Fig. 57–1). In the shoulder region, a minimum number of targets must be hit before cell death occurs. This is defined as sublethal injury. Sublethal damage repair refers to the repair that occurs within the shoulder region, with the reappearance of another shoulder during that time. Potentially lethal damage repair refers to the increase in survival over time after a single treatment. If the cells remain in situ for a number of hours posttreatment, the proportion of surviving cells will increase. It is likely that similar biochemical mechanisms are involved to some extent for both, although the importance to clinical outcome of each of these repair processes is not completely understood.[16,17]

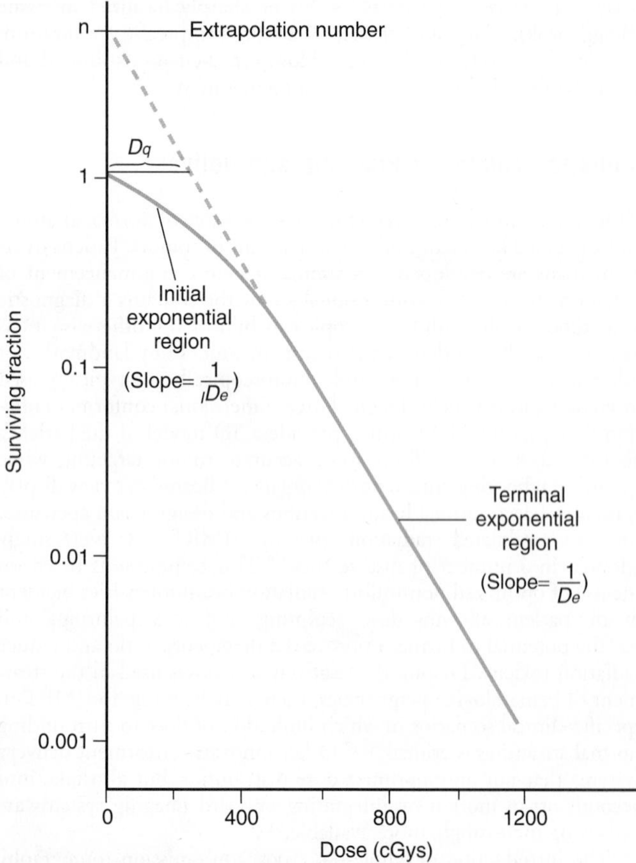

Figure 57–1 Cell survival curve. (*Adapted from Withers HR: Biologic basis of radiation therapy. In: Perez CA, Brady LW (eds.): Principles and Practice of Radiation Oncology, 2nd ed. Philadelphia, JB Lippincott, 1992, p 72*).

Redistribution

Redistribution refers to the synchronization of the cell cycle that occurs after a single dose of radiation. Cells have decreasing radiosensitivity as from M/G2 to G1, to early S to late S phase. The relative radioresistance of S phase has prompted the combined use of radiation with S-phase–specific drugs. An example is the delivery of radiation therapy concurrently with cycle active agents such as 5-FU in gastrointestinal malignancies.

Repopulation

Tumors and normal tissues repopulate during a course of irradiation. Normal tissue repopulation is observable with the healing of mucosal and skin reactions that takes place despite continuing radiation. The repopulation of tumors has been inferred from split-course radiation regimens in which there are a few weeks of no treatment between treatment segments. In settings in which the total dose is the same, local control is worse for split-course than for continuous treatment.

Reoxygenation

Hypoxic cells are relatively radioresistant. For the same portion of cell killing, hypoxic cells require 2 to 3 times the dose as the same cells treated in normoxic conditions.[18] It would be expected that the proportion of hypoxic cells would increase rapidly after a few treatments as the more sensitive oxygenated cells are killed. In general, however, this is not the case. A process called reoxygenation takes place that maintains the proportion of hypoxic cells at a relatively constant number. The exact mechanism of reoxygenation is not known, but likely involves shifts in blood flow. Without reoxygenation, radiation therapy probably would not cure many solid tumors.

Fractionation and Dose

The standard fractionation scheme for radiation therapy is 180 to 200 cGy per day, 5 days per week. The total dose depends on the clinical setting and type of tumor. The approximate dose needed for a probability of more than 95% local control for indolent non-Hodgkin lymphoma is 3600 to 4000 cGy, and 4000 to 5000 cGy for more aggressive histologies. Accelerated fractionation refers to keeping the same total dose, but decreases the time over which it is given. Such a regimen might be used for a rapidly growing or chemotherapy-refractory tumor. Hyperfractionation uses a small single dose given two to three times per day such that the total time is approximately the same as with standard fractionation, but the total dose must be higher to obtain the same effect. The lower dose per fraction spares late-responding tissues relative to tumor. Accelerated hyperfractionation is a hybrid regimen of delivering small doses two to three times per day over a shortened time period. In considering the total dose received by a patient, it is imperative to consider the dose per fraction, the number of doses per week, the total dose, the total treatment time, and when considering retreatment, the time elapsed since completion of the previous course of therapy. In the palliative setting, hypofractionation (high dose per fraction), such as 3000 cGy in 10 fractions, is useful for more aggressive histology. For lymphoma of indolent histology, a good response and effective palliation can be achieved with doses as low as 400 cGy in two fractions.[19,20]

Clinical Radiation Tolerance

The extent and frequency of injury to normal tissues depend on both radiation dose and volume treated. The risk can be enhanced by surgery and chemotherapy. Precise organ tolerances are not known, but estimates can be derived from published case reports and small series.

Central Nervous System

Brain tolerance is approximately 5500 to 6000 cGy in small fractions, but small volumes can tolerate higher doses. Radiation myelitis can occur at doses in excess of 5000 cGy. The combined use of certain cytotoxic agents may increase the risk of spinal cord injury. The peripheral nervous system has a higher tolerance, and is uncommon unless fields have been overlapped.

Heart

Radiation injury to the heart may involve a number of different cardiac tissues. Cardiac injury is rare unless the entire heart is treated to more than 3000 cGy. Anthracycline enhances the risk of myocardial injury, and the total cardiac dose is limited to 1500 cGy in patients who received anthracycline-containing chemotherapy. A more detailed discussion of late cardiac and pulmonary injury is presented in the section on Hodgkin lymphoma.

Lung

Fractionated doses as low as 2000 cGy or single doses as low as 800 cGy can cause radiation pneumonitis. Acute radiation pneumonitis can occur up to 6 months after treatment and is characterized by dry cough, dyspnea and low-grade fever, and radiographic changes within the radiation fields. Long-term fibrosis and loss of pulmonary function depends on the presence of underlying lung pathology, and the use of chemotherapeutic agents, in particular bleomycin, may lower the threshold of clinical radiation lung injury.[21,22] Using 3D radiation planning, dose-volume histograms of the lungs can be generated. In a typical mantle field, 25% to 30% of lungs may receive up to 2000 cGy, but most patients remain asymptomatic in this dose range.

Kidney

A portion of the kidney that receives a total dose in excess of 2000 cGy will permanently lose function. The development of late hypertension or renal failure depends on the volume of kidney irradiated. Even if a portion of one kidney is treated to a high dose, it is rare to see any clinical signs or symptoms. If cisplatin is administered after kidney irradiation, the toxicity of platinum may be increased.

Liver

The irradiation of a large segment of liver to a dose in excess of 3000 cGy produces a clinical syndrome of hepatomegaly, ascites, and elevated liver function tests. Radiation injury is similar to that of venoocclusive disease, a syndrome that occurs with the high-dose alkylating agent regimens used in some stem cell transplantation programs. If not fatal, radiation hepatopathy completely resolves.

Gastrointestinal Tract

The gastrointestinal tract is modestly sensitive to irradiation, with small-bowel tolerance lower than that of esophagus or large bowel. During radiation therapy, patients receiving large abdominal or pelvic fields get some degree of bowel irritation. Permanent gastrointestinal injury occurs at doses above 4500 cGy, and may require surgical excision of the damaged bowel segment, but this should done only after a trial of conservative management.

Other Organs

Virtually all organs are susceptible to injury. The following are the lower limits for a permanent injury for some other organs: bone marrow stroma, 4000 cGy; spleen with functional asplenia, 4000 cGy; ovary, 2000 cGy; skin, 5500 cGy; salivary and endocrine glands, 4500 cGy; bladder, 6000 cGy; peripheral nerve, bone, and muscle, 6000 cGy; oral cavity mucosa, 6000 cGy. Acute reactions (eg, bowel, skin, mucus, hair, blood count depression) occur 2 to 3 weeks after the start of treatment. These systems may recover despite an early decrease in function and the continuation of therapy. Conservative management helps a patient get through treatment with a minimum of treatment breaks. As a rule, the presence or extent of an acute reaction does not predict the likelihood of a late reaction. A major concern after treatment with radiation or chemotherapy is the development of secondary malignancies. The risk is especially well documented in long-term survivors of Hodgkin lymphoma, which is discussed in more detail in the chapter on Hodgkin lymphoma.

SPECIFIC USES OF RADIATION THERAPY FOR TREATMENT OF HEMATOLOGIC AND LYMPHOID MALIGNANCY

Early-Stage Hodgkin Lymphoma

Historically, radiation therapy alone has been the mainstay of treatment in patients with early-stage Hodgkin lymphoma, with disease control rates of 80% to 85%. With the development of less toxic and better tolerated chemotherapy regimens, combined modality therapy is currently the standard treatment for early-stage Hodgkin lymphoma. The major advantages of this approach are that it obviates the need to perform staging laparotomy, allows treatment with smaller radiation fields, and randomized trials have shown it to be associated with greater freedom from treatment failure. Radiation therapy-related issues include the optimal radiation field size and dose in the setting of combined modality therapy (Table 57–1).

Three randomized trials have been conducted comparing involved-field versus extended-field radiation therapy after chemotherapy in early-stage Hodgkin lymphoma.[23–25] The median follow-up time ranged from 39 to 116 months, and all three trials showed no significant difference in failure-free survival between the treatments arms. The Italian trial and the German Hodgkin's Lymphoma Study Group (GHSG) HD8 trial results suggested that the use of a more limited radiation field was associated with a lower risk of second malignancy, although longer follow-up time is needed to confirm the findings.[24,25] In addition to reducing radiation field size in combined modality therapy, lower radiation doses are also being studied as part of the treatment reduction effort in early-stage Hodgkin lymphoma. The European Organisation for Research and Treatment of Cancer (EORTC) H9F trial is a three-arm trial in which all patients receive six cycles of epirubicin, bleomycin, vinblastine, and prednisone (EBVP II).[26] After a complete response, patients were randomized to receive no further treatment, 36 Gy, or 20 Gy of involved-field irradiation. Patients with a partial response all received 36 Gy of involved-field irradiation with or without a 4 Gy boost. No difference in 4-year event-free survival was detected between 20 Gy and 36 Gy doses, although the no radiation therapy arm was closed early owing to a higher than expected relapse rate. The GHSG HD10 and HD11 trials on low-risk and high-risk early-stage patients, respectively, showed no differences between 20 Gy and 30 Gy of involved-field radiation therapy.[27] These results are only available in abstract form with a short follow-up, and additional time is needed to establish the safety of 20 Gy of radiation treatment.

Investigators have also explored the omission of radiation therapy in patients with early-stage Hodgkin lymphoma through randomized trials.[26,28–32] However, five of six available randomized trials that included early-stage Hodgkin lymphoma patients have shown a significantly inferior disease-free survival with chemotherapy alone, with two of the trials closing the chemotherapy-alone arm early owing to a high relapse rate.[26,28–30,32] Treatment with chemotherapy alone in this population is therefore not recommended as standard therapy at this time.

Table 57–1 Trials on Optimal Radiation Dose and Field Size for Early-Stage Hodgkin's Disease

Trial	Prognostic Group	Treatment Arms
GHSG HD 10	Favorable	ABVD × 2 vs ABVD × 4 → 20 Gy IFRT vs. ABVD × 2 vs ABVD × 4 → 30 Gy IFRT
EORTC H9F	Favorable	EBVP II × 6 → 20 Gy IFRT vs. EBVP II × 6 → 30 Gy IFRT vs. EBVP II alone
GHSG HD 11	Unfavorable	ABVD × 4 vs. BEACOPP × 4 → 20 Gy IFRT vs. ABVD × 4 vs. BEACOPP × 4 → 30 Gy IFRT
EORTC H8U	Unfavorable	MOPP/ABV × 4 vs. MOPP/ABV × 6 → IFRT vs. MOPP/ABV × 4 → STNI
GHSG HD 8	Unfavorable	COPP/ABVD × 2 → IFRT vs. COPP/ABVD × 2 → STNI

ABVD: adriamycin, bleomycin, vinblastine, and dacarbazine; BEACOPP: bleomycin, etoposide, adriamycin, cyclophosphamide, vincristine, procarbazine, and prednisone; COPP: cyclophosphamide, vincristine, procarbazine, and prednisone; EBVP: epirubicin, bleomycin, vinblastine, and prednisone; IFRT: involved-field radiation therapy; MOPP: mechlorethamine, oncovin, procarbazine, and prednisone; STNI: subtotal nodal irradiation.

Early-Stage Non-Hodgkin Lymphoma

Non-Hodgkin lymphoma is a heterogeneous disease. The two most common histologic subtypes are diffuse large B-cell lymphoma and follicular lymphoma, accounting for three-quarters of all cases of non-Hodgkin lymphoma.[33,34] Radiation therapy plays an important role in both of these subtypes of non-Hodgkin lymphoma in patients with limited-stage disease. Another subtype of non-Hodgkin lymphoma in which the role of radiation therapy is increasingly recognized is marginal zone lymphoma or mucosa-associated lymphoid tumor (MALT).[35]

Stage I–II Diffuse Large B-Cell Lymphoma

Historically, patients with localized diffuse large cell lymphoma, many of whom were staged surgically, were treated with radiation therapy alone, with a cure rate of less than 50%.[36] Since 1980, doxorubicin-based combination chemotherapy regimen with or without radiation therapy became the treatment of choice, yielding significantly improved relapse-free survival and overall survival rates.[37–40]

To date, there have been four randomized trials that compared chemotherapy alone with combined chemotherapy and radiation therapy in patients with stage I–II aggressive lymphoma.[41–44] Although these four trials appeared to address a similar question in a group of patients with localized disease, each of these trials differ in patient characteristics, study design, and number of cycles or type of chemotherapy in the treatment arms (Table 57–2).

The Southwest Oncology Group (SWOG) 8637 trial compared eight cycles of CHOP (Cytoxan [cyclophosphamide], hydroxydaunorubicin [Adriamycin], Oncovin [vincristine], and prednisone/prednisolone) alone versus three cycles of CHOP followed by radiation therapy.[41] Despite a progression-free and overall survival benefit with combined modality therapy initially, updated results showed no difference between the two arms because of late relapses in the abbreviated chemotherapy and radiation therapy arm.[45] The Groupe

Table 57–2 Recent Randomized Trials Comparing Chemotherapy Alone and Chemotherapy Followed by Radiation Therapy in Localized Diffuse Large B-Cell Lymphoma

ECOG	Stage I (bulky or EN only); Stage II (bulky and nonbulky)	215	12 y	CHOP × 8 → IFRT 40 Gy	6-y DFS: 69% 6-y FFS: 70% 6-y OS: 79%	
				CHOP × 8	6-y DFS: 53% 6-y FFS: 53% 6-y OS: 67%	(p = 0.05) (p = 0.05) (p = 0.23)
SWOG 8736*	Stage I or IE (bulky and nonbulky) Stage II or IIE (nonbulky only)	401	4.4 y	CHOP × 3 → IFRT 40–55 Gy	5-y PFS: 77% 5-y OS: 92%	
				CHOP × 8	5-y PFS: 64% 5-y OS: 72%	(p = 0.03) (p = 0.02)
LNH-93–4	Age > 60 (9% bulky; 57% EN)	576	7 y	CHOP × 4 → IFRT 40 Gy	EFS: 61% OS: 72%	
				CHOP × 4	EFS: 64% OS: 68%	(p = 0.6) (p = 0.5)
LNH-93–1	Age < 60 (10% bulky, 50% EN)	647	7.7 y	ACVBP → MTX, Ifosfamide, VP16, ara-C	EFS: 82% OS: 90%	
				CHOP × 3 → IFRT 30–40 Gy	EFS: 74% OS: 81%	(p < 0.001) (p = 0.001)

ACVBP, doxorubicin, cyclophosphamide, vindesine, bleomycin, and prednisone; CHOP, Cytoxan (cyclophosphamide), hydroxyldaunorubicin (Adriamycin), Oncovin (vincristine), and prednisone/prednisolone; DFS, disease-free survival; ECOG, Eastern Coast Oncology Group; EN, extranodal; EFS, event-free survival; FFS, failure-free survival; IFRT: involved-field radiation therapy; SWOG, Southwest Oncology Group; See Table 57–1 for explanation of abbreviations used.

*Updated in abstract form: at median f/u of 8.4 y, FFS curves overlap at 7 y, and OS curves overlap at 9 y.

d'Etude des Lymphomes de l'Adulte (GELA) 93–1 trial (age < 60) showed a significant event-free and overall survival with doxorubicin, cyclophosphamide, vindesine, bleomycin, and prednisone (ACVBP) (which has a theoretical dose intensity of at least 150% of that of three cycles of CHOP) compared with three cycles of CHOP followed by radiation therapy.[43] Rather than showing that there is no role for radiation therapy in localized diffuse large cell lymphoma, the results of these two trials essentially showed that radiation therapy cannot replace inferior and inadequate chemotherapy.

Both the Eastern Coast Oncology Group (ECOG) trial and the GELA LNH 93–1 trial employed the same chemotherapy on both comparison arms and were therefore appropriately designed to test the role of consolidative radiation therapy.[42,44] The ECOG trial used eight cycles of CHOP, and randomization to radiation therapy or no further therapy was only for patients who had a complete response to the chemotherapy.[42] Patients on the GELA 93–1 trial (age > 60) were randomized upfront to four cycles of CHOP alone versus four cycles of CHOP followed by radiation therapy.[44] In the ECOG trial, despite some slight arm imbalance with more bulky disease in the combined modality therapy arm and the somewhat suboptimal adherence to the assigned treatments, there was a significant disease-free survival benefit favoring the addition of radiation therapy. There was a 12% gain in overall survival at 6 years with the addition of radiation therapy, although it was not statistically significant as this trial was only powered to detect a 20% difference in disease-free survival. The GELA 93–1 trial showed no event-free or survival benefit with the addition of radiation therapy after four cycles of CHOP. In this trial the addition of radiation therapy reduced isolated relapse at initial sites from 13% to 5%. The benefit of improved local control with the addition of radiation therapy will translate into a disease-free and overall survival improvement only with effective systemic therapy that allows the eradication of occult distant disease. To meaningfully clarify the role of radiation therapy in localized aggressive lymphoma, the most informative trial will be one that employs CHOP and rituximab, which is considered the current standard systemic therapy for diffuse large B-cell lymphoma.[46–48]

Stage I–II Follicular Lymphoma

A number of studies have shown that radiation therapy alone can result in long-term cure in 30% to 40% of patients with stage I–II follicular grade I–II lymphoma. Large series reporting results of treatment for limited-stage follicular lymphoma are shown in Table 57–3.[49–58] The median radiation doses vary from 30 to 40 Gy in eight of the nine series, with the two largest series reporting a median dose of 35 Gy.[49,50] Infield recurrences range from 0% to 11%, with higher percentages occurring in patients with bulky disease or who receive a radiation dose of less than 30 Gy.[55,57] A variety of field sizes have been used ranging from involved fields to total nodal irradiation. There were no differences in survival by field size utilized. Freedom from recurrence was better in the Stanford University study with total nodal irradiation[51] and in the Royal Marsden Hospital study with larger field sizes.[56] The most common fields used were involved or regional fields (including the immediate adjacent prophylactic nodal sites). The use of smaller (involved or regional) fields preserves the ability to effectively treat patients who have later recurrence with the same histology or who transform to a higher grade histology. More than half the patients with early-stage disease will eventually develop recurrent disease and increasingly, there will be new and more effective approaches for these patients.

Stage I–II Mucosa-Associated Lymphoid Tumor Lymphoma

The indolent extranodal marginal zone or MALT lymphomas most commonly involve the gastrointestinal tract, salivary glands, breast, thyroid, orbit, conjunctiva, skin, and lungs.[59–64] As this subtype of lymphoma tends to remain localized for long periods of time, local treatment (surgery or local/regional irradiation) is very effective at long-term control of disease and provides the opportunity for cure. In particular, low doses of radiation therapy (30 Gy) to involved

Table 57–3 Large Series (>50 Patients) on Radiation Therapy for Localized Follicular Lymphoma

Institution	No.	Median f/u (y)	Median RT dose (Gy)	RT field	Infield relapses	10-y FFTF (%)	10-y OS (%)
PMH*,†	573	10.6	35	IF	NR	48	>60
BNLI*	208	NR	35	NR	NR	47	64
Stanford*,†	177	7.7	35–50	IF/RF/ER (77%) TLI (23%)	13.8%	44	64
Harvard†	106	12	36.7	IF (60%) RF (36%) EF (4%)			
Foundation Bergonie†	103	8.3	35–40	IF (54%) RF (46%)	NR	49	56
Edinburg	64	5	30–40	Nr	Nonbulky: 0% at 30–40 Gy Unk/bulky: 9% at 30–40 Gy, 11% at 40 Gy	49	78
U. Florida†	72	8.5	NR	IF (53%) EF (43%) TNI (4%)	<30 Gy: 10% >30 Gy: 0%	46	59
NCI†	54	9	36	IF (38%) EF (48%) TLI/TBI (14%)	2%	48	69
Royal Marsden	58	NR	40	IF (52%) EF (48%)	9%	43	79

EF, extended field; FFTF, freedom from treatment failure; IF, involved-field; NCI; National Cancer Institute; NR, not reported; OS, overall survival; PMH, Princess Margaret Hospital; RF, regional field; TBI, total body irradiation; TLI, total lymphoid irradiation; TNI, total nodal irradiation.

*Included patients with follicular grade 3.

†Included patients who received chemotherapy.

nodal regions or extranodal sites almost always will control sites of disease. These doses are somewhat lower than used for patients with localized follicular grade I–II disease. Three recent retrospective studies provide dose control data for this type of lymphoma. Schechter and colleagues first reported in a small series of 17 patients with gastric MALT that low doses of radiation (median 30 Gy, range 28.5–43.5 Gy) were associated with a 100% probability of local control.[59] Tsang and colleagues reported local control data in 70 patients with stage I (62) and stage II (8) MALT presenting in the stomach and other sites treated to a median dose of 30 Gy (range 17.5–35 Gy).[65] The most common doses used were 25 Gy (mostly orbit presentations) and 30 Gy. The overall local control rate was 97%. Of the two local recurrences, one occurred after 17.5 Gy and the other after 30 Gy. The 5-year disease-free and overall survival rates were 76% and 96%, respectively. In a report by Hitchcock and colleagues, 66 patients with stage I–IV marginal zone lymphoma were evaluated.[66] The median radiation dose was 33.5 Gy. All 35 stage I–II patients who received radiation therapy as initial treatment achieved local control. Among stage I–II patients the 5-year progression-free and overall survival rates were 75% and 93%, respectively. The available data support the use of 30 Gy, which results in a local control rate of nearly 100%. Although there is limited data with lower doses such as 25 Gy, there is a suggestion that local control rates are high with this dose as well. This should allow for modification of dose in settings where normal tissue risks are somewhat higher (orbit, salivary glands).

1. Preferred Treatment for Early-Stage Diffuse Large B-Cell Lymphoma Treated with Combined Modality Therapy

Use of involved fields

After a complete remission after six to eight cycles of CHOP or CHOP-R: 36 Gy if initial bulky disease; 30 Gy for the remainder of patients.

After three to four cycles of CHOP or CHOP-R: 35 to 40 Gy

After a partial remission: 40 Gy

2. Preferred Treatment for Early-Stage Follicular Grade 1 and 2 Lymphoma

Use of involved or regional fields

Carefully planned radiation therapy to limited fields with modest doses can significantly reduce the risk of significant damage to the marrow reserve, the risk of developing a treatment related malignancy, and the risk of long-term toxicity to other normal tissues such as the salivary glands, lungs, heart, kidneys and bowel.

The recommended dose is 30 to 36 Gy with a boost to areas of initial involvement to 36 to 40 Gy. Bulky disease should be treated to the upper end of the range; 30 to 36 Gy should suffice for smaller disease.

3. Preferred Treatment for Early-Stage Mucosa-Associated Lymphoid Tumor or Extranodal Marginal Zone Lymphoma

Use of radiation therapy alone to involved nodal regions or extranodal sites

Doses of 30 Gy result in a near 100% local control rate. Although there are limited data with lower doses such as 25 Gy (except for orbital MALT), local control rates can be high with this dose as well. This should allow for modification of dose in settings where normal tissue risks are somewhat higher (orbit, salivary glands).

Although there are high complete response rates with chemotherapy for marginal zone lymphoma, there is little evidence that it is curative. Therefore, outside of clinical trials, chemotherapy should be reserved for patients with stage III–IV disease. Asymptomatic individuals with generalized disease may be considered for observation, similar to patients with generalized follicular lymphoma.

Leukemia and Myeloma

The primary treatment for the leukemias and multiple myeloma is systemic therapy. The overall management of these disease entities is described elsewhere in this book. The role of radiation therapy in the management of these patients is complex and depends on the overall treatment plan. Therefore, only a few of the principles of radiation therapy are included here.

Acute Lymphoblastic Leukemia and Lymphoma

The predominant role for radiation therapy in the management of acute lymphoblastic leukemia (ALL) is for central nervous system (CNS) prophylaxis given the pattern of relapse. For childhood ALL, there is increasing movement away from using cranial irradiation because of concerns of delayed neurocognitive dysfunction and growth compromise.[67,68] However, recent data suggest that CNS-directed chemotherapy, even in the absence of cranial irradiation, is associated with attentional dysfunction in survivors of childhood ALL.[69,70] Adult ALL is much less common and is associated with a far worse prognosis, and long-term sequelae from the radiation treatment is less of an issue. Prophylactic cranial irradiation dose of 1800 cGy is recommended in these patients as part of CNS prophylaxis. Radiation therapy is occasionally used for palliation or for salvage for CNS or testicular relapse. In these cases, doses of 2400 to 3000 cGy are recommended.

Solitary Plasmacytomas and Multiple Myeloma

Solitary plasmacytomas may occur in bone or in soft tissue. Radiation therapy produces long-term local control of more than 80%.[71] Traditionally, doses of 4000 to 5500 cGy have been used, although a recent multiinstitutional study of 258 cases of solitary plasmacytoma failed to show a dose-response beyond 3000 cGy.[72]

Radiation therapy is often used as palliation for patients with bony lesions from multiple myelomas. A typical palliative regimen might be 3000 cGy over 2 weeks. The dose and fractionation must be tailored to the clinical setting. A patient with newly diagnosed multiple myeloma who is expected to live many years should be treated with a higher total dose and a lower dose per fraction. In patients presenting with cord compression, longer-course radiation therapy had been shown to be associated with significantly better functional outcome.[73]

COMMONLY USED RADIATION TREATMENT FIELDS IN HEMATOLOGIC MALIGNANCIES

The radiation field designs frequently employed in lymphoma therapy include:

1. Mantle field: This treatment field and its variations are the most commonly used treatment field in patients with supradiaphragmatic Hodgkin lymphoma. It includes the submental, cervical, supra- and infraclavicular, axillary, hilar and mediastinal lymph nodes (Fig. 57–2). The dose inhomogeneity in a mantle field is a result of variation in separation of a patient's upper body, and the irregularly contoured lung blocks that affect the scatter doses to different areas within the field.[74,75] For instance, the dose to the cervical and axillary regions tends to be higher because of decreased patient thickness in the soft tissue of the neck and axilla, whereas the dose toward the inferior border of the mantle field tends to be lower, because of the thicker separation in that region of the body as well as loss of scatter doses due to the adjacent lung blocks.[76] Some of the techniques that are employed to minimize dose inhomogeneity include the use of an extended source-to-node distance of 110 cm or greater, and by the use of higher-

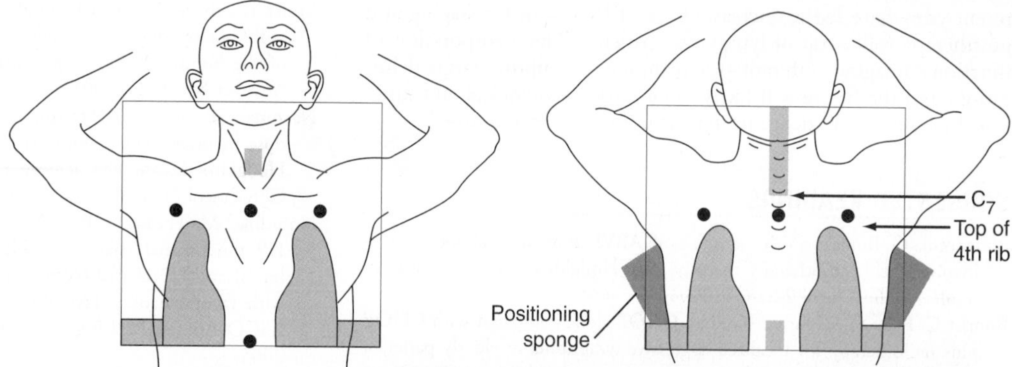

Figure 57–2 A typical mantle irradiation field.

energy megavoltage machines. However, the energy used is limited by the need to ensure adequate doses to superficial nodes, which can fall within the "build-up" regions of the radiation beams, and be potentially underdosed if energy higher than 6 MV is used.

2. Mantle and paraaortic (MPA) ± splenic field: Also known as subtotal nodal or lymphoid irradiation, it treats the paraaortic lymph nodes in addition to the mantle field. The spleen is included in the treatment field in patients who do not undergo surgical staging and splenectomy.
3. Total nodal irradiation (TNI) or total lymphoid irradiation: This encompasses most of the lymphoid tissue, with the addition of a pelvic field to the mantle and paraaortic field. However, other nodal groups, such as the brachial, epitrochlear, popliteal, sacral, and mesenteric nodes are not specifically included in the total nodal irradiation field. MPA radiation therapy and TNI are used less frequently today because of the widespread use of chemotherapy.
4. Inverted-Y field: This is used in patients presenting with infradiaphragmatic lymphoma, and includes treatment to the paraaortic and pelvic lymph nodes.
5. Involved-field radiation: By definition, this includes at least the entire contiguous lymph node group, but may also contain the next echelon of nodes. For example, in a patient presenting with an enlarged cervical lymph node, an involved field treatment would include the entire ipsilateral cervical chain and the supraclavicular region, as these nodes are considered one region (Fig. 57–3). In a patient with mediastinal involvement, the field would include the mediastinal, hilar, subcarinal and medial supraclavicular nodes. Although the hilar nodes are scored separately traditionally, the hilar and subcarinal nodes are included in the mediastinal field (Fig. 57–4). In addition, the medial supraclavicular nodes are included in order to cover the upper mediastinum (top of T1). The current definition of involved-field irradiation with detailed description of specific examples were recently summarized by Yahalom et al.[77]

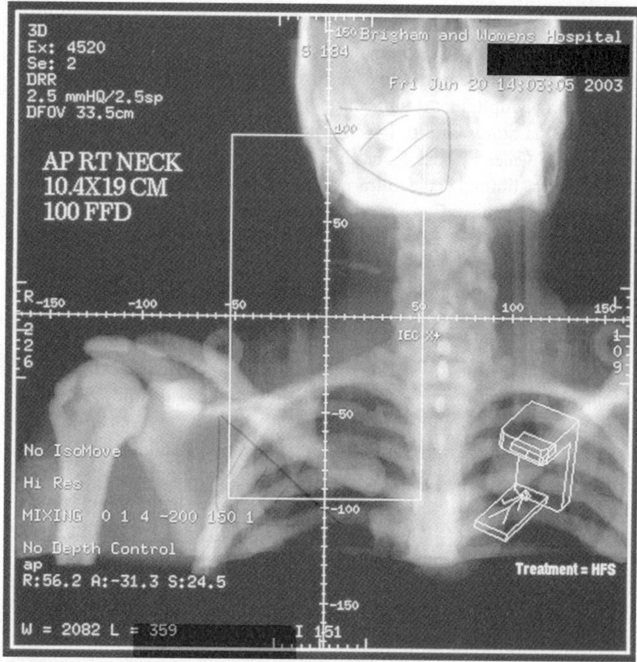

Figure 57–3. Involved field to the cervical and supraclavicular nodal chain in a patient with cervical node involvement only.

FUTURE DEVELOPMENTS

Over the last several decades, tremendous advances have been made in the field of radiation oncology. Modern radiation biology has evolved from initial in vivo cell survival essays for tumor and normal tissues to detailed knowledge of the cellular, molecular, and genetic effects of radiation. Exciting research efforts have been made and clinical applications are ongoing in areas including hypoxia,[78] hyperthermia,[79] radiation sensitizers/protectors,[80,81] and radiolabeled monoclonal antibodies.[82,83] Treatment planning and delivery have also made significant progress in recent years. Three-dimensional conformal treatment planning, including IMRT, has greatly improved tumor targeting while sparing normal tissues. However, careful consideration needs to be given for its use in the lymphoma population, which typically includes younger patients, as the improved dose conformation comes at the expense of low doses spread through a larger volume of normal tissues.[11] Advances in functional imaging in

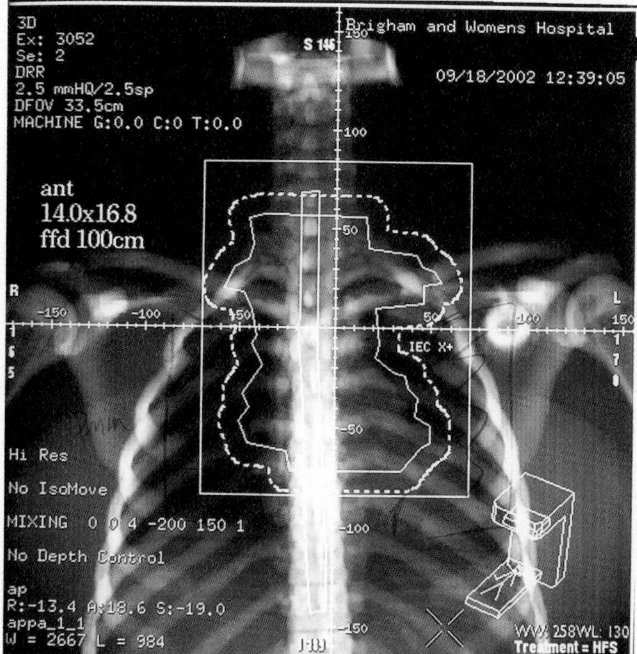

Figure 57–4 Involved field to the mediastinum.

recent years have led to increasing use of PET scan for staging and posttherapy follow-up of lymphoma patients. The incorporation of functional imaging with radiation planning can improve target delineation, and the future will likely involve use of biological and functional parameters in determining the optimal radiation dose.[84]

SUGGESTED READINGS

Bonadonna G, Bonfante V, Viviani S, et al: ABVD plus subtotal nodal versus involved-field radiotherapy in early-stage Hodgkin's disease: Long-term results. J Clin Oncol 22:2835, 2004.

Bonnet C, Fillet G, Mounier N, et al: CHOP alone compared with CHOP plus radiotherapy for localized aggressive lymphoma in elderly patients: A study by the Groupe d'Etude des Lymphomes de l'Adulte. J Clin Oncol 25:787, 2007.

Engert A, Schiller P, Josting A, et al: Involved-field radiotherapy is equally effective and less toxic compared with extended-field radiotherapy after four cycles of chemotherapy in patients with early-stage unfavorable Hodgkin's lymphoma: Results of the HD8 trial of the German Hodgkin's Lymphoma Study Group. J Clin Oncol 21:3601, 2003.

Horning SJ, Weller E, Kim K, et al: Chemotherapy with or without radiotherapy in limited-stage diffuse aggressive non-Hodgkin's lymphoma: Eastern Cooperative Oncology Group study 1484. J Clin Oncol 22:3032, 2004.

Laskar S, Gupta T, Vimal S, et al: Consolidation radiation after complete remission in Hodgkin's disease following six cycles of doxorubicin, bleomycin, vinblastine, and dacarbazine chemotherapy: Is there a need? J Clin Oncol 22:62, 2004.

Mac Manus M, Hoppe R: Is radiotherapy curative for stage I and II low-grade follicular lymphoma? Results of a long-term follow-up study of patients treated at Stanford University. J Clin Oncol 14:282, 1996.

Meyer RM, Gospodarowicz MK, Connors JM, et al: Randomized comparison of ABVD chemotherapy with a strategy that includes radiation therapy in patients with limited-stage Hodgkin's lymphoma: National Cancer Institute of Canada Clinical Trials Group and the Eastern Cooperative Oncology Group. J Clin Oncol 23:4634, 2005.

Miller TP, Dahlberg S, Cassady JR, et al: Chemotherapy alone compared with chemotherapy plus radiotherapy for localized intermediate- and high-grade non-Hodgkin's lymphoma. N Engl J Med 339:21, 1998.

Miller T, Leblanc M, Spier C, et al: CHOP alone compared to CHOP plus radiotherapy for early stage aggressive non-Hodgkin's lymphomas: Update of the Southwest Oncology Group (SWOG) Randomized Trial. ASH Abstract No. 3024, 2001.

Nachman JB, Sposto R, Herzog P, et al: Randomized comparison of low-dose involved-field radiotherapy and no radiotherapy for children with Hodgkin's disease who achieve a complete response to chemotherapy. J Clin Oncol 20:3765, 2002.

Noordijk EM, Thomas J, Fermé C, et al: First results of the EORTC-GELA H9 randomized trials: The H9-F trial (comparing 3 radiation dose levels) and H9-U trial (comparing 3 chemotherapy schemes) in patients with favorable or unfavorable early stage Hodgkin's lymphoma (HL). ASCO Annual Meeting Proceedings 23(No 16S, June 1 Suppl):6505, 2005.

Reyes F, Lepage E, Munck J, et al: Chemotherapy alone with the ACVBP regimen is superior to three cycles of CHOP plus radiotherapy for treatment of low risk localized aggressive lymphoma: The LNH 93–1 GELA study. ASCO Abstract No. 2394, 2003.

Schechter NR, Yahalom J: Low-grade MALT lymphoma of the stomach: A review of treatment options. Int J Radiat Oncol Biol Phys 46:1093, 2000.

Shenkier TN, Voss N, Fairey R, et al: Brief chemotherapy and involved-region irradiation for limited-stage diffuse large-cell lymphoma: An 18-year experience from the British Columbia Cancer Agency. J Clin Oncol 20:197, 2002.

Straus DJ, Portlock CS, Qin J, et al: Results of a prospective randomized clinical trial of doxorubicin, bleomycin, vinblastine and dacarbazine (ABVD) followed by radiation therapy (RT) vs. ABVD alone for stages I, II and IIIA non bulky Hodgkin's disease. Blood (First Edition Paper prepublished online:10.1182), 2004.

Tsang RW, Gospodarowicz MK, Pintilie M, et al: Stage I and II MALT lymphoma: Results of treatment with radiotherapy. Int J Radiat Oncol Biol Phys 50:1258, 2001.

Yahalom J, Mauch P: The involved field is back: Issues in delineating the radiation field in Hodgkin's disease. Ann Oncol 13(Suppl 1):79, 2002.

REFERENCES

For complete list of references log onto www.expertconsult.com

CHAPTER 58

CLINICAL USE OF HEMATOPOIETIC GROWTH FACTORS

Jacob M. Rowe and Irit Avivi

INTRODUCTION

Hematopoietic growth factors are glycoproteins that can be produced by recombinant DNA technology. They have many potential clinical uses in patients with both malignant and nonmalignant hematologic disorders.

The development of in vitro marrow clonogenic culture systems led to the discovery of a family of interacting hematopoietic growth factors which have been demonstrated to have critical physiologic roles for controlling hematopoiesis in vivo (Table 58–1). Of the many hematopoietic growth factors that have been cloned, to date only erythropoietin (EPO), granulocyte colony-stimulating factor (G-CSF), and granulocyte-macrophage colony-stimulating factor (GM-CSF) have seen widespread clinical use.

Other growth factors evaluated for clinical use, for example, interleukin 2 (IL-2), IL-3, IL-11, macrophage colony-stimulating factor (M-CSF), stem cell factor (SCF), IL-6 and IL-1, were generally found to be too toxic for extended clinical use.

ERYTHROPOIETIC GROWTH FACTORS

Recombinant human erythropoietin (rHuEPO) is a purified glycoprotein that stimulates erythroid blood cell development.[2,3] It is produced from mammalian cells into which the gene coding for human erythropoietin has been inserted, and is indistinguishable from human erythropoietin by biologic activity and immunologic reactivity.[2] Endogenous erythropoietin is the only hematopoietic growth factor that behaves like a hormone. Produced mostly in the kidneys,[4–6] but also in the liver,[7] and several other tissues (eg, neuronal and glial cells of the central nervous system, retina, bone marrow macrophages),[8,9] erythropoietin interacts with the erythroid progenitor cells in the bone marrow to promote their proliferation and maintain their viability (Table 58–1).[3,10] Production of erythropoietin in humans is regulated by tissue oxygenation such that hypoxia or anemia stimulates erythropoietin production whereas erythrocytosis suppresses it.[11,12] Hypoxic stimulation results in the production of hypoxia inducible factor (HIF-1), the major factor responsible for transcriptional activation of erythropoietin production (see Chapter 68). Through the interaction of EPO with receptor-bearing cells within the bone marrow, physiological oxygen demands are translated into increased red cell production. In general, plasma erythropoietin concentrations reflect erythropoietin production and can be used to define deficient states in which anemia may be amenable to correction by administration of recombinant EPO (Table 58–2).

Subtypes of Recombinant Human Erythropoietin (rHuEPO) in Clinical Use

Recombinant human erythropoietin introduced into the clinical setting almost 2 decades ago, binds to the dimerized EPO receptor on the surface of the erythroid progenitor cells, inducing a conformational change in the receptor, resulting in the stimulation of several intracellular pathways, for example, JAK-2 kinase on the STAT-5 molecule, responsible for proliferation and inhibition of apoptosis of erythroid progenitor cells. Both epoetin alfa and beta were shown to be highly effective in patients with cancer-associated anemia and anemia caused by renal dysfunction, providing an increase in hemoglobin (HB) level, decrease in red blood cell transfusion requirements, and improvement in quality of life. Both products (epoetin alfa and beta), administered three times weekly, have the same sequence of amino acids but differ in their branching and carbohydrate attachment. Longer-acting versions of rHuEPO (darbepoetin alfa, pegylated-epoietin beta) permit less frequent injections, without adversely affecting treatment efficacy.[13]

Darbepoetin alfa administered once weekly, at a dose of 2.25 μg/kg for 12 weeks has been approved for the treatment of cancer and kidney failure-related anemia.[14,15] General recommendations on the use of rHuEPO are presented in the box below.

General Recommendations for Therapy With rHUEPO

1. The cause of anemia must be clearly established prior to initiation of recombinant erythropoietin (rHuEPO). Even if EPO deficiency has been demonstrated, other factors such as iron deficiency, B_{12}, or folate deficiency must be corrected.
2. In general, rHuEPO therapy should only be given in those conditions where data from clinical trials (preferably Phase III) have demonstrated its efficacy.
3. Recombinant erythropoietin should only be given to patients who have a symptomatic anemia (Hb 9–11 g/dL) or are transfusion-dependent (Hb <9 g/dL). This category also includes patients who are candidates for blood transfusions.
4. In general, begin with a dose at the lower level known to be effective. Escalate after 1 month if this has been inadequate.
5. The target hemoglobin is not always a "normal hemoglobin." A hemoglobin level of 11 g/dL appears to be optimal for patients receiving rHuEPO for chronic renal failure, improving quality of life with a relatively low incidence of serious complications. The targeted hemoglobin level for patients with cancer-associated anemia is considered to be 12 to 13 g/dL (according to the EORTC 2006 guidelines), although large phase III studies are absent.
6. Once-weekly administration of rHuEPO (or even longer—darbepoetin) may replace the more frequent administration of rHuEPO.
7. A longer-acting "EPO," administered every 3 to 4 weeks, has been recently confirmed in phase III clinical trials to be safe and effective and might substitute the current rHuEPO derivatives.

Table 58–1 Biologic Activities of the Hematopoietic Growth Factors

Factor	Bioactivities
Erythropoietic factors	
EPO	• EPO and EPO receptors are mainly expressed by the kidney, but also by the liver, neurons, astrocyte, brain endothelial cells, microglia, retina, and trophoblasts • Stimulates clonal growth of CFU-E and a subset of BFU-E • Suppresses apoptosis in erythroid progenitor cells • Induces release of reticulocytes from marrow • Induces globin synthesis in erythroid precursor cells • Stimulates murine megakaryocyte colony growth and terminal maturation in vitro but not in vivo
Granulopoietic factors	
GM-CSF G-CSF	• Stimulates multilineage hematopoietic progenitor cells • Stimulates BFU-E growth • Stimulates granulocyte, macrophage, and eosinophil colony growth • Stimulates functional activity of eosinophils, neutrophils, monocytes, and macrophages • Induces IL-1 gene expression in neutrophils and peripheral blood mononuclear leukocytes • Costimulates T-cell proliferation with IL-2 • Induces or coinduces TNF-α gene expression with IFN-γ in monocytes. • Stimulates proliferation of myeloid leukemic cells • Stimulate growth of certain nonhematopoietic cancer cells in vitro • Induces migration and proliferation of vascular endothelial cells in vitro • Stimulate growth of progenitor cells committed to the neutrophil lineage • Stimulates neutrophil maturation of certain leukemic cells • Activates phagocytic function of mature neutrophils • Stimulates quiescent pluripotent hematopoietic progenitor cells to enter G_1-S phase • Stimulates mobilization of stem cells and progenitors from hematopoietic niches into peripheral blood • Maintenance of steady-state neutrophil numbers
Megakaryocytopoietic factors	
TPO IL-11	• Stimulates in vitro growth of CFU-Mk, megakaryocytes, and platelets • Stimulates clonal growth of individual $CD34^+CD38^-$ cells • Synergizes with SF, IL-3, and FL • In single $CD34^+CD38^+$ cells, TPO synergizes with SF and IL-3 but not Flt3 ligand; no increase in colony growth or colony size is seen when TPO is added to multicytokine combinations • Increases megakaryocyte ploidy in vitro and in vivo • Enhances the proliferation and differentiation of yolk-sac erythroid lineage precursors • Stimulates production of PDGF, platelet factor 4 and β-thromboglobulin from megakaryocytes • Supports continuous growth of cytokine-dependent human leukemic cell lines • Stimulates adhesion of hematopoietic progenitor cells to fibronectin by activation of VLA-4 and VLA-5 • No direct effect on platelet aggregation but primes the response to ADP, epinephrine, and thrombin; also increases platelet release of ATP and thromboxane B_2 production and platelet expression of CD62 (P-selectin) • Stimulates proliferation of c-mpl-positive AML blasts • Stimulates $CD4^+$ T cell-dependent proliferation of antigen-specific plaque-forming B cells • Shortens the duration of G_0 of primitive hematopoietic progenitor cells • Acts synergistically with IL-3 or SF to stimulate the clonal growth of erythroid (BFU-E and CFU-E) and primitive megakaryocytic (BFU-Mk) progenitors • Increases the ploidy of cultured megakaryocytes • Increases peripheral platelet and neutrophil counts

AML, acute myeloid leukemia; BFU, burst-forming unit; CFU, colony-forming unit; EPO, erythropoietin; G-CSF, granulocyte colony-stimulating factor; GM-CSF, granulocyte–macrophage colony-stimulating factor; TPO, thrombopoietin.

From Bagby GC Jr, Heinrich MC: Growth factors, cytokines, and the control of hematopoiesis. In Hoffman R, Benz EJ Jr, Shattil SJ, et al (eds.): Hematology: Basic Principles and Practice, 3rd ed. Churchill Livingstone, 2000, p 156.

Table 58–2 Clinical Use of Recombinant Erythropoietin

Absolute Recommendation	Often Useful	Possibly Useful
1. Anemia of chronic renal failure 2. Anemia associated with cancer in patients receiving chemotherapy/radiotherapy with Hb level less than 11 g/dL, if symptomatic 3. Anemia of chronic disease, including with symptomatic anemia due to cancer, not receiving chemotherapy 4. Low-risk myelodysplasia	1. Anemia of multiple myeloma 2. Myelodysplasia 3. Anemia of HIV infection	1. Perisurgical (alone or followed by preoperative autologous blood donation) 2. Post allogeneic bone marrow transplantation 3. Anemia of prematurity

rHuEPO in Patients with Renal Failure

As one would expect, nonfunctioning kidneys fail to produce rHuEPO in the quantity sufficient to support red blood cell production.[16,17] The use of rHuEPO over the past 2 decades represents one of the most important advances in the management of patients with advanced renal disease with or without dialysis.[18–21] Not only has this resulted in freedom from transfusion dependency and elimination of many of the associated risks,[18] but it has also led to a significant improvement in quality of life for these patients.[22,23] More than 95% of hemodialysis patients respond to rHuEPO and are able to achieve a hematocrit level of 33% to 36% within 3 months of the initiation of such therapy.[18] Although rHuEPO is not dialyzable, it is commonly administered intravenously (70 U/kg per week) or subcutaneously (lower dose) at the end of each dialysis.[14–26] Practically, treatment dosage is scheduled according to the severity of anemia and response to therapy. The variability in the required rHuEPO dose is related to the enormous variation in the steady-state plasma rHuEPO level at any given level of anemia.

Initially, based on theoretical considerations, there was serious concern that rHuEPO treatment might accelerate the progression of renal failure and thus rHuEPO was often withheld from predialysis patients with renal failure. The results of several prospective studies have been published and it is now standard practice to offer rHuEPO to all patients with chronic renal failure if they have significant anemia and are symptomatic.[18] Patients failing to respond to the subcutaneous rHuEPO at the initial dose of 70 U/kg/week are recommended to be considered for dose escalation. Recent prospective randomized trials suggest that the targeted HB level should be around 10.5 to 11.5 g/dL,[20,21] providing a significant reduction in RBC transfusion requirements, without "paying the price" of increased serious adverse events such as hypertension, myocardial infarction, stroke, congestive heart failure associated with a higher HB level of 13 g/dL or more.[21] Furthermore, neither improvement in quality of life[21] nor preservation of cardiovascular function (eg, cardiac hypertrophy) were better in patients attaining a higher HB level.[20,21] Raised HB levels may increase blood viscosity, enhancing the risk for thrombosis. Furthermore, the altered shape of red cells and their decreased deformability may also contribute to the higher viscosity reported in patients with kidney dysfunction.

During treatment with rHuEPO it is essential to maintain adequate iron stores. Hemodialysis patients often receive iron therapy intravenously, as recommended by the National Kidney Foundation[26,27]; however, the use of an oral iron preparation is perfectly acceptable. Inadequate iron store is the commonest cause of a poor response to rHuEPO. Other, less common causes of a poor response to rHuEPO are inadequate folic acid stores, intercurrent infections, or excessive splenic hemolysis.

Cancer Patients Receiving Chemotherapy

Anemia is a frequent finding in patients with cancer and should be carefully assessed. Additional causes of anemia, iron deficiency, active bleeding, nutritional deficiencies, or hemolysis should be corrected before initiating rHuEPO therapy. rHuEPO therapy should be considered in patients with cancer-related anemia treated with chemotherapy/radiotherapy, presenting with HB levels lower than 9 g/dL, providing a significant reduction in RBC transfusion requirements and improvement in quality of life.[28–32] The use of rHuEPO for patients with less severe anemia (between 9 and 11 g/dL) should be determined by individual clinical circumstances, whereas it is unclear whether an increase in hemoglobin above 12 to 13 g/dL is of clinical benefit.[32] Once this level is achieved, maintenance doses should be titrated individually.[32] Recent data suggest that rHuEPO is likely to be also beneficial in patients with cancer-related anemia not receiving chemotherapy.[32]

Current guidelines recommend an administration of subcutaneous rHuEPO thrice weekly (150 U/kg) or once-weekly darbepoetin for at least 3 to 4 weeks (see box). Response is expected in less than 8 weeks of therapy; escalation in rHuEPO dosage may be considered on an individual basis in patients who fail to respond to initial dose and should be gradually titrated once the hemoglobin level reaches 12 g/dL.[32] The role of iron supplements remains debated. The recently reported EORTC guidelines have failed to find convincing evidence for increased erythropoietic response with the addition of oral iron supplements, but reported some evidence for improved responses with the addition of intravenous iron.[32] However, the doses and schedules for intravenous iron supplements are not well defined yet.[32] Nevertheless, for the majority of ambulatory patients receiving rHuEPO, in whom intravenous iron supplementation is impractical, the use of oral iron supplementation continues to be acceptable.

The risk of both thromboembolic events and hypertension are slightly elevated in patients treated with rHuEPO with chemotherapy-induced anemia, but there are no data for increased risk for patients with pure red cell aplasia.[32]

It is still uncertain if rHuEPO treatment has any significant impact on tumor progression and long-term outcome.[32] The rHuEPO receptor is expressed by several cancer cell lines[33] (eg, breast carcinoma, gastric cancers, tumors of the female reproductive system, and CNS), raising the theoretical possibility of rHuEPO inducing tumor growth, by inhibiting tumor cell apoptosis through several intracellular signaling pathways (eg, JAK-STAT),[34] and by improving oxygenation of tumor cells. In contrast, improvement in tumor oxygenation may increase the effectiveness of radiotherapy and chemotherapy agents (dependent on oxygen tension in the tumor microenvironment) or shut down the hypoxia-inducible factor 1-alpha–vascular endothelial growth factor angiogenesis pathway that promotes tumor growth and metastasis, thereby increasing response to therapy and tumor regression.[35]

However, these in vitro effects, and possible competing interactions, have not been demonstrated in human cancer in vivo. Furthermore, the different rHuEPO subtypes, rHuEPO alpha, beta, or darbepoetin, as well as differing doses targeted to achieve different HB levels might have different effects on the growth of different tumor subtypes.[35]

Despite possible theoretical considerations, the available data do not clearly support a clinical concern for tumor progression with the use of rHuEPO.[32] The cumulative data confirm its ability to reduce transfusion requirement and to improve quality of life. rHuEPO is thus currently recommended for use in cancer patients receiving chemotherapy.[28–32,36]

Anemia Due to Malignant Disease

Myelodysplastic Syndrome

Myelodysplastic syndromes (MDSs) comprise a heterogeneous group of clonal myeloid stem cell disorders characterized by peripheral cytopenias and dysplasia of bone marrow progenitor cells. MDS occurs primarily among older adults with a median age between 65 and 70. The most important clinical problems arise from chronic anemia (80%) and from red cell transfusion-induced iron overload, bleeding due to low platelet counts, and infections as a consequence of neutropenia. A significant number of patients succumb to these complications of cytopenia prior to the onset of overt acute myeloid leukemia. Younger adults are often considered for an allogeneic stem cell transplantation, whereas older adults are mainly treated supportively with growth factors, for example, rHuEPO with or without G-CSF, and blood transfusions in the absence of an effective curative therapy apart from allogeneic transplantation.

A double-blind prospective randomized trial, comparing rHuEPO versus placebo, showed a significantly increased response rate in MDS patients treated with rHuEPO (14/37 vs 4/38, $P = 0.007$),[37] most noticeable in patients with refractory anemia (RA). However, there were no statistical differences in response rate among patients with refractory anemia with ring sideroblasts (RARS) or refractory anemia with excess of blasts (RAEB). A baseline rHuEPO level above

Recommendations for the Use of Recombinant Human Erythropoietin (rHUEPO) in Patients With Cancer

1. The two major goals of erythropoietic protein therapy are improvement of quality of life and prevention of transfusions.
2. The use of rHuEPO is recommended as a treatment option for patients with chemotherapy-associated anemia and a hemoglobin concentration that has declined to a level less than or equal to 10 g/dL. Red blood cell transfusion is also an option depending on the severity of anemia or clinical circumstances.
3. For patients with less severe chemotherapy-associated anemia (those with hemoglobin concentration below 12 g/dL but who have never fallen below 10 g/dL), the decision whether to use epoetin immediately or to wait until hemoglobin levels fall closer to 10 g/dL should be determined by clinical circumstances. Red blood cell transfusion is also a therapeutic option when warranted by severe clinical conditions.
4. Although there is no absolute evidence of an increased response to erythropoietic proteins with the addition of oral iron supplementation, this modality is commonly used in ambulatory patients in an attempt to enhance the erythropoietic effect. Intravenous iron supplement has been convincingly demonstrated to improve response to rHuEPO.
5. There are no predictive factors of response to erythropoietic proteins that can be routinely used in clinical practice if functional iron deficiency or vitamin deficiency is ruled out; a low serum EPO level (in particular in hematologic malignancies) is the only verified predictive factor of some importance. Values must be interpreted relative to the degree of anemia present. Further studies are needed to define the value of hepcidin, c-reactive protein, and others.
6. Patients with cancer-related anemia not receiving chemotherapy might be considered for rHuEPO. The recommended starting dose for subcutaneous rHuEPO is 150 U/kg thrice weekly for a minimum of 4 weeks, with individualized consideration given for dose escalation to 300 U/kg thrice weekly for an additional 4 to 8 weeks in those who do not respond to the initial dose. An alternative weekly dosing regimen (40,000 U/week), based on common clinical practice, can be considered. Dose escalation of weekly regimens should be under similar circumstances to thrice-weekly regimens.
7. Continuing rHuEPO treatment beyond 6 to 8 weeks in the absence of response (e.g., less than 1–2 g/dL rise in hemoglobin), assuming appropriate dose increase, has been attempted in nonresponders but does not appear to be beneficial. Patients who do not respond should be investigated for underlying tumor progression or iron deficiency. As with other failed individual therapeutic trials, consideration should be given to discontinuing the medication.
8. Hemoglobin levels can be raised to (or near) a concentration of 12 g/dL, at which time the dosage of rHuEPO should be titrated to maintain that level or restarted when the level falls to near 10 g/dL. Insufficient evidence to date supports the "normalization" of hemoglobin levels to above 12 g/dL.
9. There is evidence from one well-designed, placebo-controlled randomized trial that supports the use of rHuEPO in patients with anemia associated with low-risk myelodysplasia. Treatment with rHuEPO for myeloma, non-Hodgkin lymphoma, or chronic lymphocytic leukemia patients experiencing chemotherapy-associated anemia should follow the recommendations outlined above.

*Not included into the EORTC guidelines yet, but proven by several large studies.

Portions reproduced with permission from Rizzo JD, Somerfield MR, Hagerty KL, et al: Use of epoetin and darbepoetin in patients with cancer: 2007 American Society of Hematology/American Society of Clinical Oncology clinical practice guideline update. Blood 111:25–41, 2008.

Portions reproduced with permission from Bokemeyer C, Aapro MS, Courdi A, et al: EORTC guidelines for the use of erythropoietic proteins in anaemic patients with cancer: 2006 update. Eur J Cancer 43:258, 2007.

Suggested Management of Anemic Patient With Myelodysplastic Syndrome (MDS)

There is no role for prophylactic therapy using recombinant EPO (rHuEPO), with or without G-CSF, among MDS patients who do not have symptomatic anemia.

For patients who are symptomatic and/or transfusion-dependent, the baseline EPO levels should be obtained.

Patients who have an EPO level less than 200 mU/L should be started on EPO at a dose of 150 U/kg daily, subcutaneously, or high dose darbepoetin.

Recent data support this approach even with an EPO level less than 500 mU/L.

If the response has not been inadequate, then G-CSF at the dose 1 μg/kg/day subcutaneously should be considered.

If there is no response to this combination after 4 to 6 weeks, the dose of rHuEPO may be escalated to 300 U/kg/day.

If no response is demonstrated after 2 months, then EPO should be discontinued. There is no point in attempting this therapy again at a future point.

Patients who have responded to any dose of rHuEPO, or to a combination of EPO and G-CSF, should be maintained on this dose for 3 months.

If the hemoglobin is maintained on this dose, then a judicious attempt at gradual reduction of the rHuEPO dose may be attempted.

Most responses to erythropoietin, with or without G-CSF, are not maintained for more than 12 months.

Most patients with an endogenous level of erythropoietin more than 500 mU/L will not respond to rHuEPO, with or without G-CSF. However, because there is a small subgroup of patients who respond to rHuEPO, it is reasonable to begin with a trial of rHuEPO with G-CSF for 3 months. Among this group, rHuEPO should be offered to patients who are transfusion-dependent and symptomatic.

If no response is seen, then the therapy with these growth factors should be discontinued.

200 mU/L is predictive of a nonresponse.[37] Based on these data, rHuEPO is currently recommended for low-risk MDS patients with endogenous rHuEPO levels below 200 mU/L.[38]

Recent phase II studies reported a high response rate to high-dose darbepoetin in low-risk MDS patients (35%–55% major responses),[39,40] higher than reported with EPO-alpha (10%–20%), almost comparable with that observed with an rHuEPO–G-SCF combination (39%–60%).[41]

Of interest, synergy between granulocyte colony-stimulating factor (G-CSF) and rHuEPO has been demonstrated for the production of normal as well as MDS erythroid precursors.[42] A concurrent administration of rHuEPO and G-CSF appeared to produce a high erythroid response rate (39%), with durable responses being documented in low-risk patients. rHuEPO–G-CSF therapy was not shown to increase the risk for transformation to AML compared with that observed in historical controls treated conservatively, without rHuEPO or G-CSF.[41]

In a randomized trial, the combination of rHuEPO and G-CSF administered sequentially was shown to produce a higher erythroid response rate (38%) than the regimen of rHuEPO alone.[42] It has also been shown that patients responding to rHuEPO and G-CSF tend to have a significantly lower serum rHuEPO level (<500 mU/L).[43] However, these criteria are not exclusive and patients with higher rHuEPO levels are also known to respond.

Myeloma, Lymphoma, and Chronic Lymphocytic Leukemia

There are currently several, however small, randomized trials that examined the value of rHuEPO in myeloma, chronic lymphocytic leukemia (CLL) and non-Hodgkin lymphoma (NHL) patients, irrespective of the chemotherapy that was given.[44–50] Two of these studies included myeloma patients only[44,47] and another study reported on aggressive lymphoma patients, whereas the rest of the recruited patients had various lymphoproliferative disorders including myeloma. The combination of heterogeneous groups of patients and different parameters assessed for evaluation of response, make interpretation of these studies somewhat difficult. However, the fact that each of these trials reported a significant reduction in RBC transfusion requirements and an improvement in quality of life in patients receiving rHuEPO suggests that rHuEPO is valuable and beneficial in these clinical situations.

One of the major concerns nowadays is the potential risk of developing thromboembolic (TE) events in myeloma patients treated concurrently with rHuEPO and thalidomide. rHuEPO has been recently reported to be an independent risk factor for venous thromboembolism in patients with various types of cancers.[51] Thalidomide, especially when given in combination with chemotherapy and steroids, is associated with a high risk of thrombosis (20%–40%). Therefore, the coadministration of rHuEPO and thalidomide-containing regimens may potentially increase the risk for TE significantly. However, the current data related to this subject is limited[52] and further studies are warranted to clarify this issue.

Anemia of Prematurity

Anemia of prematurity, although multifactorial in origin, is characterized by inappropriately low rHuEPO levels. It usually responds to rHuEPO at a dose of 250 to 400 U/kg subcutaneously three times a week.[53,54] However, both retrospective and prospective randomized trials have failed to detect a significant clinical benefit for rHuEPO treatment compared with placebo; although rHuEPO did facilitate a reticulocyte recovery, there was no significant reduction in transfusion requirements despite early treatment with rHuEPO and iron supplements.[54–57] Furthermore, early administration of rHuEPO has been recently suggested to increase the risk of premature retinopathy (ROP).[56]

A recent randomized trial suggested the addition of B_{12} supplementation to a combination of folic acid, intravenous iron, and rHuEPO results in a higher HB level as compared to an identical combination without B_{12}; however, there was no difference in RBC transfusion requirements.[58]

In contrast, there are a few prospective randomized trials that reported a significant reduction in transfusion requirements in very-low-birth-weight infants in stable condition.[59] These differences may arise from patient selection such as the clinical condition of the patient, patient weight, as well as differences in rHuEPO dosage and iron supplementation.

It seems likely that rHuEPO is of value in treating the anemia of prematurity; however, more studies are needed to determine the clinical parameters that are associated with response. Nevertheless, with no convincing evidence of the clinical benefit of such therapy and in consideration of accumulating data regarding potential contribution of rHuEPO to the development of ROP, early administration of rHuEPO is currently not recommended outside of clinical studies.

Autologous Blood Donation

The use of rHuEPO to prime patients for autologous red blood cell donation has been perceived as a major step toward reducing the risks associated with blood transfusions.

Administration of rHuEPO preoperatively has been demonstrated to promote an increase in the number of autologous units collected.[60–64] Furthermore, patients having an autologous RBC donation supported by rHuEPO required a lower number of allogeneic RBC transfusions as compared with those undergoing an autologous RBC donation without rHuEPO support ($P < 0.005$).[64]

Another strategy is to administer rHuEPO 14 to 17 days prior to operation without performing an autologous RBC donation (possible/feasible in patients whose baseline level is relatively low), aiming to increase the preoperative HB level and thereby reduce the number of allogeneic RBC required.[65,66] A recent prospective study comparing this strategy with autologous blood donation without rHuEPO supports showed no significant difference in the incidence of allogeneic transfusions between the two groups.[67]

It appears that preoperative treatment with rHuEPO provides an effective method for autologous blood donation as well as achieving a reduction in the postoperative transfusion requirements.[65,66] However, owing to its high cost, a relatively low number of red blood cell transfusions routinely required following the majority of operations and the absolute reduction in RBC number required (often one unit only), rHuEPO support with or without RBC donation has failed to become common practice. This strategy is usually reserved for patients with rare blood types or those known to be at a high risk for a significant bleeding following surgery.

Stem Cell Transplantation

Serum rHuEPO levels following high-dose chemotherapy initially increase[68] but gradually decline with red cell engraftment.[69] Therefore, early use of rHuEPO following transplant, when erythroid precursors are depleted and endogenous rHuEPO level is relatively high, is unlikely to be of value.[70–74] In contrast, rHuEPO applied following engraftment might be much more effective. Recent publications suggest that rHuEPO therapy is highly effective following conventional allogeneic stem cell transplantation[75] but to a lesser extent following a reduced-intensity allogeneic stem cell transplantation (RIC).[76] rHuEPO therapy is most effective following a conventional allograft when administered between days 35 and 100 post transplant,[75] whereas the maximal effect following RIC appears much earlier.[76,77] The lower number of RBC transfusions required following an RIC along with the high cost of rHuEPO suggests that rHuEPO therapy should be more often considered as a therapeutic option in the conventional myeloablative allograft setting and to a lesser extent with reduced-intensity conditioning.

A reduction in RBC transfusion requirements has been reported when rHuEPO was started on day 30 post transplant following autologous stem cell transplantation.[78,79] Alternatively, rHuEPO administered prior to high-dose therapy has also been suggested to significantly reduce the number of RBC transfusions required following transplant.[80]

Despite these encouraging results, rHuEPO is rarely used in patients undergoing high dose chemotherapy and autologous stem cell transplantation, mostly because of the rapid erythropoietic reconstitution achieved nowadays with peripheral blood stem cell transplantations along with the high cost of rHuEPO.

rHuEPO in the Critically Ill Patient

Critically ill patients have inappropriately low rHuEPO levels, contributing to their anemia. Several studies conducted to assess the potential benefits of exogenous rHuEPO supplementation showed a significant reduction in the number of red blood cell transfusions required, but with no effects on outcome in terms of ICU infection rates or mortality.[81,82] Larger prospective studies, aiming to assess the impact of rHuEPO dosing and iron supplements[83] on patient outcome and define subgroups of critically ill patients in whom rHuEPO might also improve overall survival are warranted.

rHuEPO Therapy in Patients with AIDS

In patients with human immunodeficiency virus (HIV), anemia is the most common hematologic abnormality. In general, as HIV disease progresses, the prevalence and severity of anemia increases. Anemia has been shown to be a significant predictor of progression to the acquired immunodeficiency syndrome and is independently associated with a reduced quality of life and increased risk of death.

Anemia can be caused by several mechanisms, including medication, dietary deficiencies, infections, neoplasms, and blood loss. Management of anemia includes correction of the underlying causes, blood transfusion, and erythropoietin therapy. However, blood transfusions and iron supplementation may activate HIV expression. rHuEPO is an effective means of improving hemoglobin levels and reducing transfusion requirements, especially in patients who have relatively low (<500 mU/L) endogenous erythropoietin levels.[84]

Resolution of HIV-related anemia has been shown to improve the quality of life,[85] physical functioning, and energy and lessen fatigue in individuals with HIV.[86,87] The use of highly active antiretroviral therapy has also been associated with a significant increase in hemoglobin concentrations and a decrease in the prevalence of anemia.[88]

Novel Strategies for Stimulating Erythropoiesis and Potential New Treatments for Anemia

Continuous Erythropoietic Receptor Activator

Continuous erythropoietic receptor activator is an "extremely long-acting EPO" with a half-life of 130 hours, which can therefore be delivered every 3 to 4 weeks. Having successfully completed a phase III trial of its clinical development,[89] continuous erythropoietic receptor activator is the next erythropoietic agent that is likely to be officially approved for treatment of renal failure-associated anemia.[90] Patients with renal insufficiency, particularly those receiving dialysis, as well as patients receiving chemotherapy every 3 weeks for different types of cancers, might benefit from having less frequent rHuEPO injections.[91]

Erythropoietin-Mimetic Peptides (Hematide)

Hematide is a synthetic, dimeric peptidic erythropoiesis-stimulating agent covalently linked to polyethylene glycol developed for the treatment of anemia associated with renal failure and cancer. Having a unique amino acid sequence, unrelated to that of recombinant erythropoietin, Hematide is unlikely to induce a cross-reactive immunologic response against endogenous erythropoietin, resulting in a pure red cell aplasia.

Hematide binds and activates the human rHuEPO receptor, stimulating the proliferation and differentiation of human red cell precursors in vitro. Recent studies confirmed its safety and potential efficacy in healthy volunteers[92] resulting in a dose-dependent increase in both reticulocyte and HB levels. These encouraging results support the design of phase II studies in patients with anemia related to cancer and chronic kidney dysfunction.[93]

Other Strategies for Stimulating Erythropoiesis

Hemopoietic Cell Phosphatase Inhibitors

Hemopoietic cell phosphatase is an intracellular enzyme that negatively regulates the JAK-STAT signaling. Inhibition of hemopoietic cell phosphatase, therefore, enhances erythropoiesis,[94] providing another mechanism for inducing erythropoiesis.

Hypoxia-inducible factor stabilizers

Oxygen-dependent regulation of endogenous rHuEPO production is mediated by hypoxia-inducible factor (HIF), an alpha, beta transcription factor. HIF beta is constantly expressed, whereas HIF alpha concentrations are dependent on oxygen levels. Under normal oxygen level, both the amount of HIF alpha and its ability to stimulate EPO gene transcription are inhibited by oxygen-dependent hydroxylation. Inhibition of these hydroxylation reactions stabilizes HIF, mimicking hypoxia, thereby inducing erythropoiesis. Recently, an orally active hydroxylase inhibitor was reported to induce rHuEPO production and stimulate rHuEPO in normal volunteers[95] and patients with renal failure not yet on dialysis.[96]

rHuEPO Potential Uses Outside Erythropoiesis

As previously mentioned, rHuEPO was traditionally thought to be an erythroid-specific hormone; however, messenger RNA for rHuEPO and its receptor are detected in neuronal and glial cells of the central nervous system and in the retina. rHuEPO was found to protect neurons from harmful stimuli[97] and to induce neuronal proliferation following injury.[98] Preclinical studies showed that rHuEPO is able to cross the blood–brain barrier and decrease infarct size in experimental stroke animal model.[99–101] This potential advantage was also suggested by a single clinical trial[102] demonstrating a tendency for a reduction in neurologic impairment. Results from ongoing studies, assessing the impact of rHuEPO with or without G-CSF (and other GF), should be awaited before introducing GF as a common therapeutic strategy for stroke.[103]

MYELOID GROWTH FACTORS

Myeloid growth factors, mainly G-CSF and GM-CSF, have multiple potential roles in the therapy of patients with hematologic malignancies. Guidelines for their use have been published by the American Society of Clinical Oncology in 1996[104] and have been updated on several occasions.[105,106] Similar guidelines have also been published by the National Comprehensive Cancer Network.[107] The following are the areas with the greatest clinical experience:

Table 58–3 Controlled Trials of Growth Factors After Induction Therapy in Acute Myeloid Leukemia

Study	N	Reduction in days to ANC 1000/μL	Documented Reduced Morbidity	Leukemia Stimulation
GM-CSF (sargramostim)				
Büchner[112]	86	6–9*	+	No
Rowe[113]	117	6*	+	No
GM-CSF (molgrastim)				
Stone[114]	379	2*	+	No
Zittoun[115]	53	–		Yes
Löwenberg[116]	316	5*		No
Witz[117]	209	6*		No
Löfgren[118]	110	8*		No
G-CSF (lenograstim)				
Dombret[119]	173	6*	+	No
Link[120]	187	6*		No
Goldstone[121]	803	5*		No
Amadori[122]	722	5*		No
G-CSF (filgrastim)				
Ohno[123]	67	12*	+	No
Ohno[124]	58	6*	+	No
Heil[125]	521	5*	+	No
Godwin[126]	234	3–4*	+	No
Usuki[127]	270	6*		No
Lehrnbecher[128]	317	5*		No
Estey[129]	197	13*		No

ANC, absolute neutrophil count; G-CSF, granulocyte colony-stimulating factor; GM-CSF, granulocyte-macrophage colony-stimulating factor.
*$P \leq 0.05$.

Potential Uses of Growth Factors in Acute Myeloid Leukemia

- Reducing period of neutropenia
- Recruitment of cells into S-phase of the cell cycle (priming)
- Enhancement of antimicrobial function
- Induction of differentiation of leukemic cells
- Direct antileukemic effects
- Interruption of autocrine-paracrine loops
- Stem cell protection

1. Acute myelogenous leukemia
2. Acute lymphocytic leukemia
3. Stem cell transplantation
4. Myelodysplasia
5. Chemotherapy-induced neutropenia
6. Aplastic anemia

Acute Myeloid Leukemia

Multiple potential uses exist for the administration of colony-stimulating factors in the treatment of acute myeloid leukemia (AML). Because of the potential for cytokine stimulation of acute leukemia cells,[108–111] there was initially great hesitation for conducting clinical trials with colony-stimulating factors in acute leukemia patients. These early reports demonstrated unequivocally the potential for augmenting leukemia blast cell proliferation by GM-CSF, G-CSF, and IL-3. Much of the early work highlighting this concern used experiments demonstrating blast cell proliferation and leukemia progenitor cell differentiation in culture systems containing these growth factors. It is not surprising, therefore, that when clinical trials finally did get underway they were conducted in older patients where the risk of death from marrow aplasia was great enough to outweigh the potential risk of stimulating leukemia cells.

Reducing Period of Neutropenia

Over the past 15 years, 18 major controlled trials of growth factors used after induction therapy in AML have been reported (Table 58–3).* Studies have been grouped according to the product used. Most importantly, the concern for safety has been laid to rest. Apart from one very small study, the preponderance of the data from all of these clinical trials shows that the administration of growth factors at any time after induction therapy for acute leukemia is safe. This safety has been demonstrated not only by the published results of the effects on the success of induction therapy, but also follow-up of these studies have failed to show any increase in the relapse rate among patients who went into complete remission with growth factors when compared with patients who did not receive growth factors.[131] All of these studies, with the exception of one small trial, demonstrated a significant reduction in the time required to reach an absolute neutrophil count of 500/μL or 1,000/μL. Several studies reported varying degrees of reduction in morbidity, and one study showed a significant reduction in mortality.[112,118,122,123,125–127] Despite these 16 well-controlled clinical investigations including more than 4500 patients, controversy still abounds over the use of growth factors in AML. The results obtained are not consistent, and the conclusions of the various authors differ. A meta-analysis cannot be performed because of differences in the design and conduct of these clinical trials. Particularly important may be differences in patient age, induction regimen, disease state, and stage of the disease. Also important is the timing of the growth factor administration, particularly in relation to the documentation of marrow hypoplasia. Differences in study product may exist, even among different preparations of the same cytokine. Finally, the statistical endpoints used in these studies need to be considered carefully. Some of the studies were designed and sized to show differences in hematopoietic recovery, for example, but not to show differences in complete response rate or survival. It is also possible that at least in some of the studies, patient selection may have

*References 72, 112–119, 121, 123–127, 130.

Table 58–4 Clinical Results of Induction Chemotherapy With Cost From Cooperative Group Studies of Cytokine vs Placebo

Clinical Study	Growth Factor	Patients	Reduction in Neutropenia (Days)	Percent of Documented Infections CSF vs Control	Days of Hospitalization	Incremental Cost of CSF Use	Correlative Cost Analysis Study
Pui et al., CCG[134]	G-CSF	148	7	12 vs 27*	6 vs 10*	+$152	Pui et al., 1997[134]
Laver et al., POG[135]	G-CSF	88	Same	NA	9 vs 9	+$2497	Laver et al., 1998[135]
Heil et al., International AML study[125]	G-CSF	521	5	37 vs 36	20 vs 25*	–$2230	Bennett et al., 1999[136]
Godwin et al., SWOG[126]	G-CSF	211	3	163 vs 141	29 vs 29	+$120	Bennett et al., 2001[137]
Rowe et al., ECOG[113]	GM-CSF Yeast	117	4	52 vs 70 10 vs 36* Grade 4,5	36 vs 38	–$2310	Bennett et al., 1999[136]
Löwenberg et al.,** Hovon, EORTC[116]	GM-CSF *Escherichia coli*	316	5*	NA	Same	+$6317	Uyl-de-Groot, 1997[138]

*$P < 0.01$.
**Not placebo-controlled.

Variability in the Design and Conduct of Clinical Studies of Cytokines in Acute Myeloid Leukemia

- Patient age
- Induction regimen used
- Disease state
- Timing of growth factor administration
- Documentation of marrow hypoplasia
- Differences in study product
- Statistical endpoints
- Patient selection

affected interpretation of the data. Thus, it is simply impossible to compare published results.

Among studies investigating the use of growth factors during consolidation therapy, very few have shown benefit. Because patient numbers in these trials were small and because the studies were not sized to show differences in neutrophil recovery during consolidation, failure to demonstrate such a difference does not imply that cytokines do not work when administered during consolidation therapy. In fact, the largest trial of growth factors in AML,[125] which had an adequate sample size to assess reduction in neutropenia, demonstrated a statistically significant shortening of neutropenia among patients receiving growth factors during consolidation. Similar results were also reported by the Cancer and Leukemia Group B when cytokines were given after consolidation therapy with diaziquone and mitoxantrone[132] and in a report of the GOELAM study.[133]

Over the past 4 years, several studies have evaluated the cost-effectiveness of cytokine therapy when used during induction therapy. Table 58–4 outlines these clinical studies and their correlative cost analyses. Most studies in adults demonstrated a cost-benefit for growth factors although a cost-effectiveness study using the more toxic *Escherichia coli*–derived GM-CSF was an exception.[138] Thus, one of the major considerations for withholding the use of cytokines in AML may no longer be compelling.

There are few areas in clinical medicine where so many prospective clinical trials have been carried out to answer a single question, yet at the end the data remain equivocal. Although the major reason for the reluctance to initiate clinical trials of cytokines in the AML was a concern for safety, it can now be stated unequivocally that this concern was unwarranted. With the apparent benefit of cytokine therapy reported in so many studies and the uniform finding of an improved neutrophil recovery time, it is not clear why there is a continued hesitation to use cytokines in AML patients. The probability of infection and the risk of increased morbidity and mortality correlate directly with severity of neutropenia, although these observations may at times not be easy to demonstrate objectively. It is therefore difficult not to acknowledge the benefit of cytokine therapy to a patient undergoing induction therapy because its use is associated with an improved neutrophil recovery time of approximately 1 week. A sense of well-being among patients (and physicians) was achieved after appreciating that neutrophil recovery will be hastened and cannot be ignored and, therefore, it seems that cytokines (GM-CSF or G-CSF) should be administered to all patients undergoing induction therapy for AML who are at high risk for therapy-related morbidity and mortality. The earlier published data were analyzed on the basis of an expectation of major differences in response rate or survival. This is clearly not the issue or the reason for the use of growth factors. Rather, cytokines need to be considered as important supportive care measures, much like, for example, central venous catheters. These indwelling catheters are not cost-effective and they increase rather than decrease infections; nevertheless, virtually all physicians use them for the comfort and well-being of the patients. These same considerations might be employed as a rationale for the use of cytokines in this setting.

Enhancement of Antimicrobial Function

Considerable speculation in preclinical investigations has focused on the potential for enhancing antimicrobial therapy with cytokines. In vitro, GM-CSF increases phagocytic and fungicidal activity of neutrophils against *Candida albicans* and *Torulopsis glabrata*.[139,140] Similarly, in vitro exposure of peripheral blood mononuclear cells to GM-CSF increases phagocytosis of *Cryptococcus neoformans*, and exposure of monocytes to GM-CSF results in increased killing of *C Albicans* and *Aspergillus fumigatus*.[141] The mechanism of increased activity against *Candida* and *Aspergillus* appears to be unrelated to increased phagocytosis; rather, it is due to increased oxidative metabolism and production of toxic superoxide anions by monocytes.[141]

Clinical data that support the use of cytokines in fungal infections have been limited to several early phase I and II trials. A hint of effectiveness was suggested by an Eastern Cooperative Oncology Group phase III study of cytokines in the AML.[113] In this study, 20 of 117 patients had unequivocally documented fungal infections and the overall mortality in the GM-CSF group was 13% compared with 75% in the placebo group (Table 58–5).[142] Most of these patients, as expected, had *Aspergillus* or *Candida* infections and there was no difference in the fungal prophylaxis administered to the two groups. Basically, most patients receiving GM-CSF survived their fungal infections, whereas most of those receiving placebo died. Clearly, caution is mandatory when dealing with relatively small numbers, but these data are intriguing. It is not known whether these results are due to direct stimulation of monocyte activity by GM-CSF or to earlier neutrophil recovery, as initially hypothesized during the design of the study.

Recruitment of Cells Into S-Phase of the Cell Cycle (Priming)

Over the past decade, several groups have attempted to determine whether hematopoietic growth factors can be used to prime leukemic blasts by increasing the proportion in the active phase of the cell cycle, thereby theoretically increasing their susceptibility to S-phase-active agents such as cytosine arabinoside. In vitro studies have shown that growth factors such GM-CSF, G-CSF, stem cell factor (c-kit ligand), and interleukin-3 (IL-3) can increase the fraction of leukemic blasts in the S-phase. The effect that in vivo priming might have on leukemic blasts in their ultimate response to chemotherapy is unclear, despite a multitude of phase II and phase III studies. Detailed analysis of these studies shows that the clinical data remain conflicting and confusing. It is important to understand that in vitro data must be cautiously interpreted when they are described without concurrent controls. The finding of an increased number of blasts or recruitment into the S-phase of the cell cycle following the administration of a cytokine must be compared carefully with control patients, because untreated patients with AML often change their cell-cycle kinetics and increase their blast cell counts. Table 58–6 outlines the 15 controlled studies that have evaluated the role of cytokines as priming agents for AML.* This clearly shows the enormous variability in patient selection, cytokine used, type of therapy administered, and, of course, the results. Despite the vast number of clinical trials examining the use of cytokines as priming agents for AML, the results remain confusing. Only one study demonstrated stimulation of leukemia and a lower response rate among patients receiving priming therapy with *E coli*-derived GM-CSF[130] but considerable caution is needed when interpreting this study—it was not prospectively controlled and the control group consisted of a historical cohort of patients treated on several different studies. It is of interest that in the two studies that have demonstrated a statistically significant clinical benefit for priming with cytokines, this benefit was confined to disease-free survival and there was no effect on the initial response rate.[117,148] In one of the studies this benefit was limited to patients with intermediate cytogenetic abnormalities.[148] To confuse the issue further, a more recent study reported an improved initial response rate after priming with G-CSF.[122]

*References 115–118, 122, 124, 129, 130, 143–149.

Table 58–5 Incidence of Infection With Granulocyte-Macrophage Colony-Stimulating Factor vs Placebo

	GM-CSF ($n = 52$)	Placebo ($n = 47$)	*P*
Therapy-related mortality	3/52 (6%)	7/47 (15%)	0.18
Infection			
• Grade 3, 4, 5	27/52 (52%)	33/47 (70%)	0.068
• Grade 4, 5	5/52 (10%)	17/47 (36%)	0.002
Pneumonia			
• Death/grade 3, 4	2/14 (14%)	7/13 (54%)	0.046
Fungal infection			
• Death/grade 3, 4	1/8 (13%)	9/12 (75%)	0.02

From Rowe JM, Rubin A, Mazza JJ, et al: Incidence of infections in adult patients (>55 years) with acute myeloid leukemia treated with yeast-derived GM-CSF (sargramostim): Results of a double blind prospective study by the Eastern Cooperative Oncology Group. In Hiddeman W, Büchner T, Worrman B (eds.): Acute Leukemias, V: Experimental Approaches and Management of Refractory Diseases. Berlin-Heidelberg, Springer-Verlag, 1996, p 178.

Table 58–6 Controlled Trials of Growth Factors on Priming Therapy in Acute Myeloid Leukemia

Study	Patients, *N*	Growth Factor	Administration, D	Leukemia Stimulation	Cytokine vs Control CR, %	Cytokine vs Control, Disease-Free Survival
Büchner[143]	75	GM-CSF (yeast) vs control	−2	No	81/84	63/52
Rowe[144]	245	GM-CSF (yeast) vs placebo	−2	No	38/40	Same
Estey[130]	232	GM-CSF (*Escherichia coli*) vs control	−8	Yes	48/65*	Worse w/GM
Zittoun[115]	51	GM-CSF (*E coli*) vs control	−1	No	72/77	Same
Heil[145]	80	GM-CSF (*E coli*) vs placebo	−2	No	81/79	Same
Witz[117]	229	GM-CSF (*E coli*) vs placebo	+1	No	62/61	44/19* 24 months
Peterson[146]	174	GM-CSF (*E coli*) vs placebo	−5	No	56/55	Same
Löwenberg[116]	316	GM-CSF (*E coli*) vs control	−1	No	Same	Same
Thomas[147]	192	GM-CSF (*E coli*) vs placebo	−2	No	65/59	Same
Löfgren[118]	110	GM-CSF (*E coli*) vs placebo	−1	No	56/58	Same
Ohno[124]	58	G-CSF vs placebo	−2	No	50/37	Same
Estey[129]	197	G-CSF vs control	−1	No	63/53	Same
Löwenberg[148]	640	G-CSF vs control	−1	No	79/83	42/33* 48 months
Büchner[149]	895	G-CSF vs control	−2	No	**N/A	Same
Amadori[122]	722	G-CSF vs control	+1	No	58/48*	Same

N/A, not available.
*$P \le 0.05$.
From Rowe JM, Liesveld JL: Commentary review. Hematopoietic growth factors in acute leukemia. Leukemia 11:328,1997 (updated).

Thus, the body of evidence has established the safety of cytokines when used as priming agents, and the results of one study should not negate this overall conclusion. In contrast to the established role of growth factors following induction therapy to ameliorate morbidity, no clear role of hematopoietic growth factors as priming agents as yet has been defined, and the use of cytokines as priming agents in AML cannot be recommended outside of well-designed clinical studies.

Growth Factors for Acute Myelogenous Leukemia (AML)

Data from a multitude of prospective clinical trials have demonstrated that growth factors are safe when given at any time during induction therapy for AML.

Growth factors given after induction therapy shorten the period of neutropenia by anywhere from 2 to 7 days.

Six of the 16 major randomized studies have shown a significant reduction in morbidity if growth factors are administered during induction.

No major study has shown a detrimental effect from growth factors.

Studies of cost-effectiveness, although limited in scope, have also, in most instances, demonstrated a benefit for growth factors.

Although glycosylation may confer important biological properties, both the glycosylated and nonglycosylated G-CSF preparations and GM-CSF seem to be equally efficacious in reducing the period of neutropenia. However, nonglycosylated *Escherichia coli*-derived GM-CSF is more toxic than all other growth factors for AML and should not be used.

GM-CSF has a potential advantage when neutropenia is accompanied by fungal infection, and consideration should be given to the preferential use of GM-CSF in such instances.

The data suggest that the best time to administer growth factors is after marrow aplasia has been demonstrated on day 10 to 14 of bone marrow. Thus, growth factors are recommended, as a supportive care measure, both following induction and consolidation therapy for AML.

In contrast to the role of growth factors following induction therapy to ameliorate morbidity, no clear role for growth factors as priming agent has yet been defined and the use of cytokines for priming cannot be recommended outside of a well-designed clinical trials.

Acute Lymphocytic Leukemia

The use of growth factors for patients with acute lymphocytic leukemia (ALL) has largely bypassed the controversy that was described in AML patients. The data suggest that the use of cytokines in ALL, either during induction[151–153] or in subsequent intensification therapy,[134,154,155] reduces the period of neutropenia, and in several prospective, randomized studies affects the morbidity and even mortality (Table 58–7). Thus, it has become fairly established to recommend the use of growth factors, G-CSF or GM-CSF, at every stage of the comprehensive therapy for ALL patients where profound life-threatening neutropenia is expected as part of the therapeutic course.

Stem Cell Transplantation

There are three major uses of growth factors in patients undergoing bone marrow transplantation: enhancement of neutrophil recovery, prevention or therapy of graft failure, and mobilization of stem cells.

Enhancement of Neutrophil Recovery

Over the past 15 years it has been unequivocally established that growth factors given after the infusion of autologous or allogeneic bone marrow grafts significantly shorten the period of neutropenia and reduce the duration of hospital stay (Table 58–8). Various randomized studies show significant reduction in duration of neutropenia of anywhere from 4 to 7 days with a similar shortening in the length of the overall hospital stay.[159,162–168] There are differences in Table 58–8 between the recovery after GM-CSF and G-CSF that do not reflect differences in study product; rather, they reflect evolving clinical practice. Most of the early studies with GM-CSF were conducted using bone marrow as the source of stem cells, whereas most of the published randomized studies with G-CSF used mobilized peripheral blood stem cells. Although not shown in Table 58–8, the available data with growth factor administration after allogeneic bone marrow transplantation—based on several phase II and phase III studies—confirm that in this setting there is also a more rapid neutrophil recovery and reduced hospital stay.[169,170]

In general, the efficacy of enhanced neutrophil recovery is similar whether glycosylated or nonglycosylated G-CSF is used (lenograstim or filgrastim) or glycosylated GM-CSF (sargramostim). The nonglycosylated GM-CSF (molgramostim) is more toxic and should probably not be used. During the last decade there have been multiple

Table 58–7 Growth Factors in Acute Lymphoblastic Leukemia

Study	*N* G-CSF vs Control	Days to ANC >500 or 1000/μL G-CSF vs Control	Incidence of Infections G-CSF vs Control	Early Death G-CSF vs Control	Leukemia Stimulation
Kantarjan[156] Hist*	14/14	4/18	14%/28%	0%/14%	No
Ottman[151] Rand**	37/39	8/12.5	43%/56%	3%/6%	No
Geissler[152] Rand**	25/26	16/26	40%/77%	4%/9%	No
Larson[153] rand, placebo***	102/96	6/22	Same	5%/11%	No

*Historical controls.
**Randomized.
***Randomized, placebo-controlled.
From Hoelzer D: Acute lymphocytic leukemia. Education book of the Sixth Congress of the European Hematology Association. Frankfurt, Germany, June 22nd, 2001, p 17.

Table 58–8 Randomized Trials of Growth Factors Following Autologous Bone Marrow Transplantation

GM-CSF	Days to ANC >500 or 1000/μL Cytokine or Placebo		Days of Hospitalization Cytokine vs Placebo	
Nemunaitis[158]	19	26	27	33
Rabinowe[159]	14	21	23	28
Advani[160]	12	16	27	27
Gulati[161]	16	27	32	40.5
Greenberg[162]	18	27	29	32
Legros[163]	NS		NS	
G-CSF				
Spitzer[164]	10	16	19	21
Klumpp[165]	10.5	16	18	24
Linch[166]	9	12	13	16
McQuaker[167]	10	14	13	16

trials attempting to use other cytokines post-stem cell transplantation. These involved predominantly the combination of GM- and G-CSF therapy, concurrently or sequentially, or combinations involving interleukin 3. Although various combinations of IL-3 with GM- or G-CSF appeared to promote accelerated hematopoietic recovery, the toxicity of IL-3 does not seem to warrant routine use of IL-3 alone, in combination, or as a hybrid (PIXY 321), in routine clinical practice. In any event, the evolving clinical practice of mobilized peripheral blood stem cell grafts has made use of growth factors following autologous transplantation less of a critical issue.

Graft Failure

Graft failure, as well as poor graft function leading to prolonged cytopenias, increases the risks of bone marrow transplantation and affects patient survival. Graft failure, either primary or secondary, was more common during the early days of bone marrow transplantation where the constitution of cells in the graft was somewhat empiric. With current technologies and measurement of precise numbers of CD34-positive cells in the graft, graft failure is far less common. Nevertheless, a small proportion of patients undergoing allogeneic transplantation or, less commonly, autologous transplantation fail to engraft. Studies with GM-CSF have shown that growth factors significantly reduce the rate of graft failure, primary or secondary,[168] and that sequential administration of different growth factors, that is, GM-CSF followed by G-CSF, offered no advantage over GM-CSF alone in accelerating hematopoiesis or preventing lethal complications in patients with poor graft function after transplantation.

Because of the potential for enhancing antimicrobial function with GM-CSF, it is not known whether the routine use of small doses of GM-CSF post bone marrow transplantation is indicated. On the basis of theoretic considerations, in situations where the neutrophils have recovered but the patient remains infected and severely immune-compromised, due to graft-versus-host-disease or the therapy thereof, the use of GM-CSF may help prevent, or be an adjunct to the treatment of, fungal or other opportunistic infection. However, there are no prospective studies to date confirming such a benefit.

Mobilization of Peripheral Blood Progenitor Cells

For the successful mobilization of progenitor cells of peripheral blood for clinical use, several approaches have been used:

1. Collecting cells during the recovery following intensive myelosuppressive chemotherapy;
2. Following the administration of growth factors, G-CSF or GM-CSF; and
3. Using the combination of hematopoietic growth factors and myelosuppressive chemotherapy.

General Guidelines for Mobilization of Peripheral Blood Stem Cells (PBSC)

- Both G-CSF and GM-CSF mobilize PBSC.
- There is a dose response effect for both G-CSF and GM-CSF in PBSC mobilization.
- Combinations of cytokines and chemotherapy mobilize more PBSC than cytokines alone.
- Patients who have received no or minimal prior chemotherapy have a greater than 90% likelihood of achieving an adequate collection of PBSC with cytokine/chemotherapy combinations.
- Patients who have received more than 6 months of alkylating agent therapy, fludarabine or radiation therapy have only a 70% chance of obtaining adequate number of PBSC ($>1.5 \times 10^6$ CD34 cells/kg) using standard technique.
- For heavily pretreated patients, in whom there is a significant risk of nonmobilization using standard techniques, use of an early-acting cytokine such as stem cell factor (SCF) or flt3 ligand (Flt3 L) together with a late-acting cytokine (G-CSF or GM-CSF) is likely to significantly enhance the rate of PBSC mobilization and enable the transplant to take place.

Reproduced with permission from Stiff PJ: Peripheral blood stem cell mobilization: Contemporary issues and early studies using Flt3 ligand. In Rowe JM, Lazarus HM, Carella AM (eds.): Handbook of Bone Marrow Transplantation. London, Martin Dunitz, 2000, p 22.

In practice, progenitor cell grafts are most efficiently collected following the administration of the combination of chemotherapy and growth factors although there is a significant proportion of patients in whom an adequate number of progenitor cells can be collected following the use of growth factors alone. Current understanding of peripheral blood stem cell mobilization is outline in the box below.[171–174]

Although the rate of engraftment using mobilized peripheral blood stem cells is more rapid than following the use of immobilized bone marrow stem cells,[175–178] the published data suggest that there is no fundamental difference in the rate of engraftment between mobilized peripheral blood stem cells or mobilized cells obtained from the bone marrow. In practice, mobilization of peripheral blood stem cells has become commonplace and is easily performed in the outpatient settings. The vast majority of autologous transplants are performed in this manner and an increasing number of allogeneic stem cell transplants are performed using this approach. Some countries prohibit the use of growth factors to healthy children who act as donors; however, the evolving data suggest that the risks, if any, are minimal.

Recently there have been several reports on the efficacious use of a single dose of pegfilgrastim as an alternative to daily injections of cytokines for mobilization.[179,180] This may ease the burden on patients but more mature data are awaited before this becomes standard of care for mobilization.

Myelodysplasia

The administration of the myeloid growth factors, GM-CSF and G-CSF, have also been reported to be occasionally beneficial in increasing the neutrophil count and function in patients with myelodysplasia.[181–185] The initial concerns about the safety of using growth factors known to stimulate leukemic blast cell proliferation have been previously discussed. Clinical data, however, perhaps surprisingly, have demonstrated that stimulation of leukemia does not appear to be of major concern in patients with myelodysplasia.[186] Most studies have not shown an uncontrolled proliferation of leukemic blasts or significant negative effects on survival beyond the expected rate of transformation to frank AML associated with GM-CSF or G-CSF administration. Although most studies have shown a small, but often significant, effect on neutrophil production, the biological significance of this is not always clear as the clinical response of a patient has often not been described in detail.

MDS is a disease of older adults, and conventional therapy is usually unsatisfactory. There is evidence that more than 90% of patients have an increase in their neutrophil count in response to cytokines.

It appears that GM-CSF and G-CSF have the capacity to effect a modest increase in mature myeloid elements. The clinical effects of these cytokines are clearly limited, but in a palliative clinical setting they may be important adjuncts to the supportive care of patients with MDS.

Chemotherapy-Induced Neutropenia

The routine use of growth factors for the primary prophylaxis of neutropenia following chemotherapy for solid tumors or lymphoma is not supported by prospective data.[105–107] Several randomized studies using GM-CSF or G-CSF have been conducted to evaluate the role of primary prophylaxis in patients with lymphoma undergoing induction chemotherapy.[187–189] None of these studies showed a clear benefit in terms of tumor response or survival, although meta-analyses did report a reduction in the incidence of neutropenia and infections.[190,191] The original guidelines published by the American Society of Clinical Oncology suggested that cytokines should only be offered when a therapeutic regimen has an expected rate of febrile neutropenia of at least 40%.[104,105] A subsequent recent update has modified this to an expected rate of febrile neutropenia of at least 20%.[106] A similar recommendation appears in the published guidelines of the National Comprehensive Cancer Network.[107]

Once a patient has developed febrile neutropenia following a course of chemotherapy, it is common practice to administer growth factors in future cycles as secondary prophylaxis. There are clear advantages in maintaining dose intensity and, thus, although convincing prospective data are lacking, such a practice seems reasonable. Growth factors are also used routinely as an adjunct to the therapy of febrile neutropenia following chemotherapy for patients with solid tumors or lymphomas. In most cases, no more than a few days of growth factor administration are required.

An alternative to the administration of daily growth factor has been development of pegfilgrastim, which is a pegylated recombinant G-CSF designed specifically for sustained duration of action and requiring only a single injection per each cycle of chemotherapy.[192,193] Administration of pegfilgrastim as opposed to daily growth factor injections reduces the burden on the patients and may affect the quality of life and compliance of the patient. Typically, pegfilgrastim produces a rapid rise in the absolute neutrophil count with a more sustained duration of response than achieved with daily courses of growth factor.[194] Randomized studies have established the efficacy and safety of pegfilgrastim in chemotherapy-induced neutropenia following treatment of breast cancer,[195] lung cancer,[196] lymphoma,[197] and Hodgkin lymphoma.[198]

Aplastic Anemia

Although often used empirically, there are scanty data supporting the use of myeloid growth factors in acquired aplastic anemia. Nonrandomized data suggest that the degree of response to cytokines is likely to be most pronounced in the less severe forms of aplastic anemia—when its use is less critically needed.[199] There are some data that cytokines may be useful as an adjunct to the therapy of severe bacterial or fungal infections, although they do not appear to be of benefit as prophylaxis for infections in patients with acquired aplastic anemia.[200]

A lingering concern in the use of cytokines for patients with acquired aplastic anemia has been the potential role of cytokines in promoting the development of MDS and AML. The initial concern was first reported from Japan in 1997[201] demonstrating an incidence of more than 40% of MDS in children with acquired aplastic anemia receiving cytokines. Although these data could not be confirmed in a subsequent Italian study,[202] the issue remains unresolved. A recent survey performed by the European Group for Blood and Marrow Transplantation included 840 patients. Among the 43% of patients who received first-line therapy with cytokines, the incidence of MDS/AML was 10.9% compared with 5.8% among patients who did not receive cytokines with their primary therapy.[203] At this time, the retrospective nature of this analysis of registry data does not permit a definitive conclusion on this issue.

In contrast to acquired aplastic anemia there are considerable data supporting the use of myeloid growth factors in patients with congenital aplastic anemias, including Kostmann syndrome, Fanconi anemia, Pearson syndrome, and Shwachman–Diamond syndrome.[199]

Although the outlook for those patients has improved dramatically following the use of myeloid growth,[204] the Severe Chronic Neutropenia International Registry has reported on the increased risk of MDS or AML developing in those patients receiving cytokines.[205] The precise relationship between the duration or dose of cytokine therapy and the risk of development of MDS/AML has not been established.[206]

The recent report from the Severe Chronic Neutropenia International Registry documented a cumulative incidence after 10 years of 21% of patients developing MDS or AML after therapy with G-CSF and 8% of patients having mortality due to sepsis. However, in less responsive patients with congenital neutropenia, who required higher doses of G-CSF (greater than 8 μg/kg/day), 40% developed MDS or AML and 14% died from sepsis, as compared with 11% and 4%, respectively, for the more responsive patients who also received lower doses of G-CSF.[207]

THROMBOPOIETIC GROWTH FACTOR

Thrombopoietin (TPO) is a naturally occurring glycosylated peptide that stimulates the differentiation of bone marrow stem cells into megakaryocyte progenitor cells, induces the expression of megakaryocyte differentiation markers, promotes megakaryocyte proliferation and polyploidization and, ultimately, increases the number of platelets in the circulation.[9,208–212] It also primes platelets to aggregate in response to otherwise subthreshold levels of thrombin, collagen, or diphosphate. In addition to stimulating megakaryocyte production, TPO is essential for the survival and expansion of hematopoietic stem cells.

Two recombinant thrombopoietins have been extensively studied and demonstrated some clinical activity. One is the full thrombopoietin molecule[213] and the other is a truncated form of the protein produced in *Escherichia coli* and modified with polyethylene glycol to provide stability in vivo.[213,214] The latter agent is known as megakaryocyte growth and development factor (MGDF).[213]

Early clinical trials of these two forms of the recombinant protein—the full-length molecule, recombinant human thrombopoietin, rHuTPO, and the truncated molecule, MGDF—have demonstrated a dose-dependent increase in circulating platelet counts when given to healthy donors.[215,216] Administration of both agents after chemotherapy has enhanced platelet recovery, reducing the degree of thrombocytopenia after moderately myelosuppressive regimens.[217–219] Their use following more intensified chemotherapy regimens (induction for acute leukemia, high-dose therapy for transplantation), given in multiple doses, has generally failed to reduce the severity of thrombocytopenia or the need for platelet transfusion.[218,219] TPO can also increase the number of hematopoietic stem cells mobilized with G-CSF[220] and improve the amount of platelets derived from plateletpheresis, if administered pre-pheresis to platelet donors.[213,221,222]

An emerging potential indication for TPO is idiopathic thrombocytopenic purpura. Despite the abundant number of megakaryocytes observed in patient bone marrow, endogenous levels of TPO in these patients are low and the response rate to the thrombopoietin receptor agonist AMG531 (a peptide mimetic TPO), in patients with refractory idiopathic thrombocytopenic purpura, is around 60% to 80%.[223]

Unfortunately, administration of MGDF to healthy donors was reported to be unsafe, inducing the development of severe thrombocytopenia is some of the healthy donors receiving TPO. Antibodies produced by the donors against unrecognized epitopes on the MGDF-truncated product cross-reacted against endogenous TPO, resulting in thrombocytopenia. This side effect led to the abandonment of the use of MGDF and encouraged investigators to currently search for peptide and nonpeptide mimetics that bind and stimulate the thrombopoietin receptor on hematopoietic cells.

IL-3, IL-6, and IL-11 are potent stimulators of platelet production. However, IL-3 and IL-6 are too toxic for routine clinical use. On the other hand, the use of IL-11 is far less toxic and, in fact, has been approved by the FDA for the prevention of chemotherapy-induced thrombocytopenia.[224] IL-11 is a thrombopoietic growth factor directly stimulating the proliferation of the hematopoietic stem cells and megakaryocyte progenitor cells and induces megakaryocyte maturation resulting in increased platelet production.[224]

On the basis of two randomized double-blind placebo-controlled trials,[225,226] the current indication for IL-11 is for the prevention of severe thrombocytopenia and the reduction of platelet transfusions following myelosuppressive chemotherapy in patients with non-myeloid malignancies who are at high risk for developing severe thrombocytopenia.[227] However, despite some encouraging reports, suggesting IL-11 to be able to reduce platelet transfusion requirements,[227] its use has been modest owing to side effects, including edema, dyspnea, pleural effusions, and in some patients, atrial arrhythmias, papilledema, and periosteal bone formation.[227,228]

At the current time there are insufficient data to support the use of IL-11 following intensive chemotherapy for AML or bone marrow transplantation.[229,230] Several prospective randomized trials, though small, have compared IL-11 with placebo, following high-dose chemotherapy and autologous stem cell transplantation. There was a tendency for reduction in platelet transfusion requirements in the IL-11 group; however, the median time to platelet transfusion independence was similar.[230]

Although these thrombopoietic growth factors are of great potential theoretic value, a clinical role similar to the myeloid growth factors or erythropoietin has not been established for them.

SUGGESTED READINGS

Bokemeyer C, Aapro MS, Courdi A, et al: EORTC guidelines for the use of erythropoietic proteins in anaemic patients with cancer: 2006 update. Eur J Cancer 43:258, 2007.

Bussel JB, Kuter DJ, George JN, et al: AMG 531, a thrombopoiesis-stimulating protein, for chronic ITP. N Engl J Med 355:1672, 2006.

Dale DC, Cottle TE, Fier CJ, et al: Severe chronic neutropenia: Treatment and follow-up of patients in the Severe Chronic Neutropenia International Registry. Am J Hematol 72:82, 2003.

Jadersten M, Montgomery SM, Dybedal I, et al: Long-term outcome of treatment of anemia in MDS with erythropoietin and G-CSF. Blood 106:803, 2005.

Kaushansky K: Lineage-specific hematopoietic growth factors. N Engl J Med 354:2034, 2006.

Littlewood TJ, Bajetta E, Nortier JW, et al: Epoetin Alfa Study Group. Effects of epoetin alfa on hematologic parameters and quality of life in cancer patients receiving nonplatinum chemotherapy: Results of a randomized, double-blind, placebo-controlled trial. J Clin Oncol 19:2865, 2001.

Lowenberg B, van Putten W, Theobald M, et al: Effect of priming with granulocyte colony-stimulating factor on the outcome of chemotherapy for acute myeloid leukemia. N Engl J Med 349:743, 2003.

Lyman GH: Guidelines of the National Comprehensive Cancer Network on the use of myeloid growth factors with cancer chemotherapy: A review of the evidence. J Natl Compr Cancer Netw 3:557, 2005.

Mannone L, Gardin C, Quarre MC, et al: High-dose darbepoetin alpha in the treatment of anaemia of lower risk myelodysplastic syndrome results of a phase II study. Br J Haematol 133:513, 2006.

Nosari A, Cairoli R, Ciapanna D, et al: Efficacy of single dose pegfilgrastim in enhancing the mobilization of CD34+ peripheral blood stem cells in aggressive lymphoma patients treated with cisplatin-atracytin-containing regimens. Bone Marrow Transplant 38:413, 2006.

Osterborg A, Brandberg Y, Molostova V, et al: Randomized, double-blind, placebo-controlled trial of recombinant human erythropoietin, epoetin Beta, in hematologic malignancies. J Clin Oncol 20:2486, 2002.

Rosenberg PS, Alter BP, Bolyard AA, et al: The incidence of leukemia and mortality from sepsis in patients with severe congenital neutropenia receiving long-term G-CSF therapy. Blood 107:4628, 2006.

Smith TJ, Khatcheressian J, Lyman GH, et al: 2006 update of recommendations for the use of white blood cell growth factors: An evidence-based clinical practice guideline. J Clin Oncol 24:3187, 2006.

Socie G, Mary JY, Schrezenmeier H, et al: Granulocyte-stimulating factor and severe aplastic anemia: A survey by the European Group for Blood and Marrow Transplantation (EBMT). Blood 109:2794, 2007.

Straus DJ, Testa MA, Sarokhan BJ, et al: Quality-of-life and health benefits of early treatment of mild anemia: A randomized trial of epoetin alfa in patients receiving chemotherapy for hematologic malignancies. Cancer 107:1909, 2006.

REFERENCES

For complete list of references log onto www.expertconsult.com

CHAPTER 59

PATHOBIOLOGY OF ACUTE MYELOID LEUKEMIA

Gerlinde Wernig and D. Gary Gilliland

INTRODUCTION

Acute myeloid leukemia (AML) is a complex disease with considerable phenotypic and genotypic heterogeneity. There are more than 100 recurring cytogenetic abnormalities observed in AML and numerous point mutations. AML is challenging from a clinical perspective as well as from a genetic perspective. Most adults who develop AML will die of their disease or complications related to therapy. Furthermore, patients with AML are still treated with the same empirically derived cytotoxic chemotherapy today, comprising anthracycline and cytosine arabinoside, as was used two decades ago. There is clearly a compelling need to develop more effective and less toxic therapies for this disease.

How can we approach the development of molecularly targeted therapies against the backdrop of almost overwhelming genetic diversity? First, because there are a limited number of AML phenotypes, many of the observed mutations and gene rearrangements associated with AML must target similar transcriptional and/or signal transduction targets. Second, there are several mutations that occur at relatively high frequencies, such as FLT3 mutations, that are attractive targets for therapeutic intervention. This chapter provides a general overview of our current understanding of the genetics of AML and the therapeutic implications.

ETIOLOGY

Most cases of AML are sporadic, characterized by acquisition of somatic mutations in hematopoietic progenitors that confer a proliferative and/or survival advantage, impair hematopoietic differentiation, and confer properties of limitless self-renewal. It is usually not possible to identify a cause for development of AML, either as an inherited predisposition to disease or as a consequence of environmental exposure. However, analysis of rare heritable cases of AML and of cases related to exposure to environmental agents including chemotherapy and ionizing radiation have provided valuable clues to the etiology of AML.

Environmental Exposures

Exposure to a variety of environmental agents has been implicated in the pathogenesis of AML. Ionizing radiation and alkylating agents induce DNA, usually by inducing double-strand breaks that may result in point mutations, genomic deletions, or the chromosomal translocations associated with hematopoietic stem cell transformation.[1] For example, an increased incidence of AML has been noted in survivors of atomic bomb explosions, with a risk that is proportional to the degree of radiation exposure.

Chemical exposure to organic solvents such as benzene and occupational exposure to petroleum products have been associated with a higher risk of developing AML[1]; however, case–control studies of leukemia have demonstrated only a slight increase in risk of disease for persons with occupational or chemical exposures. Except for special groups exposed to high levels of benzene or radiation, the reported risks associated with occupational and chemical exposure have generally been less than twofold, making these exposures of questionable pathogenetic significance in a disease with a yearly incidence on the order of 1/100,000. The presence of RAS mutations in patients with AML has been associated with specific occupational exposure to chemicals, suggesting that these exposures may induce genetic damage that may culminate in acute leukemia.[2]

Therapy-Related Leukemia

Ionizing radiation used in the treatment of malignancies such as Hodgkin lymphoma has also been linked to the development of AML, although the risk appears to be quite low when radiation alone is used as treatment, and is related to the age of the patient and doses of more than 2000 cGy.[3] Whether irradiation adds to the risk of therapy-related AML associated with chemotherapy remains controversial. Although some studies suggest that the risk of development of AML is significantly increased when the two modalities are combined, other studies have demonstrated that the combination of high-dose radiation therapy confined to small volumes and chemotherapy did not significantly increase the leukemogenic risk.

The development of AML after chemotherapy administered for a variety of other malignancies, ranging from Hodgkin lymphoma to breast cancer, is a devastating complication of curative treatment strategies.[3] Leukemia develops after a latency period of varying length, which suggests that the initial mutations resulting in clonal hematopoiesis may occur without any obvious hematologic change (no dysplasia or cytopenia). The subsequent acquisition of a variety of additional genetic lesions may be essential for the development of a preleukemia (myelodysplasia) or overt leukemia. Clonal chromosomal abnormalities have been reported in the majority of cases of therapy-related AML. The most frequently reported abnormalities involve complete loss or interstitial deletions of the long arm of chromosome 5 or 7 (or both). Typically these leukemias develop after alkylating agent-induced damage a median of 3 to 5 years after therapy for the primary malignancy and are associated with an antecedent myelodysplastic disorder.[4] A second group of therapy-related leukemias is associated with rearrangements of the MLL gene in chromosome band 11q23.[5] 11q23-associated AML often develops after treatment with drugs that target DNA-topoisomerase II (eg, epipodophyllotoxins, anthracyclines), with a very short latency of 12 to 18 months after treatment, and is not typically associated with an antecedent myelodysplastic syndrome.[6] Of concern are recent reports of the development of myelodysplastic syndrome and AML after dose-intensive therapy with (and without) autologous stem cell and hematopoietic growth factor support for the treatment of Hodgkin and non-Hodgkin lymphoma and breast cancer.[7,8] The identification of an increasing incidence of therapy-related AML consequent on attempts to improve cure rates for other malignancies emphasizes the importance of understanding the underlying pathogenetic mechanisms.

The genetic damage induced by chemotherapeutic agents can result in clonal proliferation, which may be an essential early step in leukemogenesis, occurring before the development of clinical abnormalities. Clonal hematopoiesis has been demonstrated in clinically asymptomatic patients who received prior cytotoxic chemotherapy for a variety of non-Hodgkin lymphomas.[9] Recently it has also been shown that sequential X-linked clonality assays may help predict subsequent evolution to frank myelodysplasia or AML.[10,11] The specific genetic events induced by chemotherapeutic agents remain unknown; nevertheless, the resultant clonal proliferation and observed cytogenetic abnormalities provide a valuable model for multistep leukemogenesis.

Antecedent Hematologic Disorders That Predispose to Leukemia

Several hematologic disorders increase the risk of development of acute myeloid leukemia. Patients with myelodysplastic syndrome have a relatively high risk of progression to AML of approximately 30% over the lifetime of the affected individual. The risk is lower among patients with myeloproliferative diseases such polycythemia vera, essential thrombocythemia, and myeloid metaplasia with myelofibrosis. Paroxysmal nocturnal hemaglobinuria patients also have a low, but increased, risk for development of leukemia.

Inherited Predisposition to Leukemia

Familial leukemia may occur in the context of a clinical syndrome in which it is one component of the overall disease, or as an isolated leukemia-predisposition trait that is not specifically associated with comorbid conditions.[12] Syndromes associated with an increased risk of leukemia include a rare constitutional trisomy 8 syndrome associated with a characteristic facial and skeletal muscle dysmorphism and an increased risk of hematologic disorders, including aplastic anemia, myelodysplasia, and acute and chronic myeloid leukemia[13]; and Down syndrome, trisomy 21, in which there is a 10- to 18-fold increased risk for leukemia. In individuals with Down syndrome who are less than 3 years old, the leukemia is most frequently AML, of the FAB M7 subtype; after age 3, the development of ALL is more common. Analysis of atypical Down karyotypes in individuals who have progressed to AML has suggested that the 21q22.3 locus that includes the AML1 gene may be important. In has also recently been demonstrated that patients with Down syndrome who develop AML may have acquired loss-of-function mutations involving the hematopoietic transcription factor GATA-1.[14]

Defective DNA repair syndromes are also associated with a high incidence of hematologic malignancies, including AML. These heritable disorders include Bloom syndrome, in which AML, ALL, lymphoma, or other malignancies occur in approximately 25% of affected individuals[15]; Fanconi anemia, in which approximately 50% of patients develop AML or myelodysplasia by the age of 40[16]; neurofibromatosis that results from loss-of-function mutations in the neurofibromin (NF-1) tumor suppressor gene on chromosome 17q11.2 and is associated with the development of juvenile CML, ALL, lymphomas, and a disproportionately high rate of myelodysplastic syndrome evolving into AML in young patients[17]; Li-Fraumeni syndrome, an autosomal dominant disorder caused by mutations of the p53 tumor suppressor genes and is associated with the development of multiple tumor types including leukemia[12]; and Wiskott–Aldrich syndrome, an X-linked immunodeficiency syndrome caused by mutations in the WASP gene and is associated with the occasional development of lymphomas, AML, and ALL.[18] Other syndromes associated with a high risk of developing AML include Kostmann infantile genetic agranulocytosis, an autosomal recessive disorder that has been associated with mutations in the G-CSF receptor on chromosome 1p35-p34.3,[19,20] and the Blackfan–Diamond syndrome, consisting of congenital hypoplastic anemia and growth retardation.[21]

There have also been reported cases of familial leukemias not associated with any defined syndrome. For example, several families have an autosomal recessive pattern of inheritance of childhood-onset myelodysplasia associated with monosomy 7 and evolution to AML.[22] Autosomal dominant patterns of inheritance of leukemia have also been reported, with a variety of morphologic and cytogenetic subtypes.[12,23] These include the familial platelet disorder with propensity to develop AML (FPD/AML syndrome) that is due to inherited loss-of-function mutations in AML1.[24,25]

Although the environmental and hereditary conditions described above serve as excellent models for obtaining insights into the molecular pathogenesis of AML, it must be emphasized that the vast majority of patients with de novo AML show no evidence of any of these risk factors, and the etiologic factors contributing to the development of AML in the majority of affected individuals is poorly understood.

THE LEUKEMIC STEM CELL

What is the target cell for transformation in leukemia? It has recently been appreciated that the hierarchical organization of normal hematopoiesis that includes a small fraction of stem cells with self-renewal capacity, and larger numbers of committed progenitors that lack these properties, also applies to leukemia, and in all likelihood to other cancers.[26,27] That is, only a small fraction of leukemic blasts that are observed clinically have the capacity to self-renew. These observations are important because they suggest that this small subpopulation may be the most important to target therapeutically and also may be the most appropriate cell type in which to monitor response to therapy.

Several lines of evidence indicate that leukemic cells with self-renewal properties, or "leukemic stem cells," exist among the $CD34^+/CD38^-$ population in humans. Perhaps the most compelling evidence in support of the $CD34^+/CD38^-$ (multipotent) stem cell as the target for leukemic transformation in AML comes from recent studies in which purified AML subpopulations were transplanted into mice with severe combined immunodeficiency disease (SCID).[28] These experiments defined a SCID mouse leukemia-initiating cell (SL-IC) in the bone marrow of patients with AML. SL-ICs comprise approximately 1 in 105 AML cells and can repopulate immune-deficient mice with leukemic cells that are phenotypically identical to those of the AML patient from which they were derived.[28] In several AML patient samples studied, the SL-ICs resided in the most primitive compartment of cells—those that are $CD34^+/CD38^-$. $CD34^+/CD38^-$ cells purified from normal marrow give rise to mixed-lineage granulocytic–erythroid–megakaryocytic colonies in culture and can repopulate immune-deficient mice with normal cells. These experiments indicate that the SL-ICs share an immunophenotype expressed by normal multilineage stem cells and that the target for leukemic transformation may reside in this primitive pluripotent population of cells rather than in a lineage-restricted cell.

Using nonobese diabetic mice with SCID (NOD–SCID), a modified SCID mouse,[29] it has been shown recently that in AML patient samples, the SL-ICs reside only in the $CD34^+/CD38^-$ fraction and not in the $CD34^+/CD38^+$ fraction.[26] The SL-IC phenotype was consistent regardless of the FAB subtype (M1, M2, M4, M5), lineage markers, or percentage of leukemic blast cells expressing the CD34 antigen. The SL-ICs also demonstrated self-renewal capacity, a requirement for maintenance of the leukemic clone, assessed by their ability to be serially transplanted into secondary recipient mice. The uniformity of the leukemic stem cell phenotype, together with the observation that normal stem cell repopulating cells are also found in the $CD34^+/CD38^-$ fraction, has suggested the hypothesis that the leukemia-initiating transformation- and progression-associated genetic events always occur in primitive cells and not in committed progenitors.

However, recent data shed interesting new light on these observations. Expression of certain leukemia oncogenes in committed hematopoietic progenitors that are destined to apoptotic cell death can confer properties of self-renewal to these cells. For example, transduction of the MLL–ENL fusion gene into purified common myeloid progenitors (CMP) or granulocyte–monocyte progenitors (GMP) that lack the potential for self-renewal confers properties of leukemia stem cells. These include the ability to serially replate in methylcellulose cultures, and to engender an AML phenotype that can be

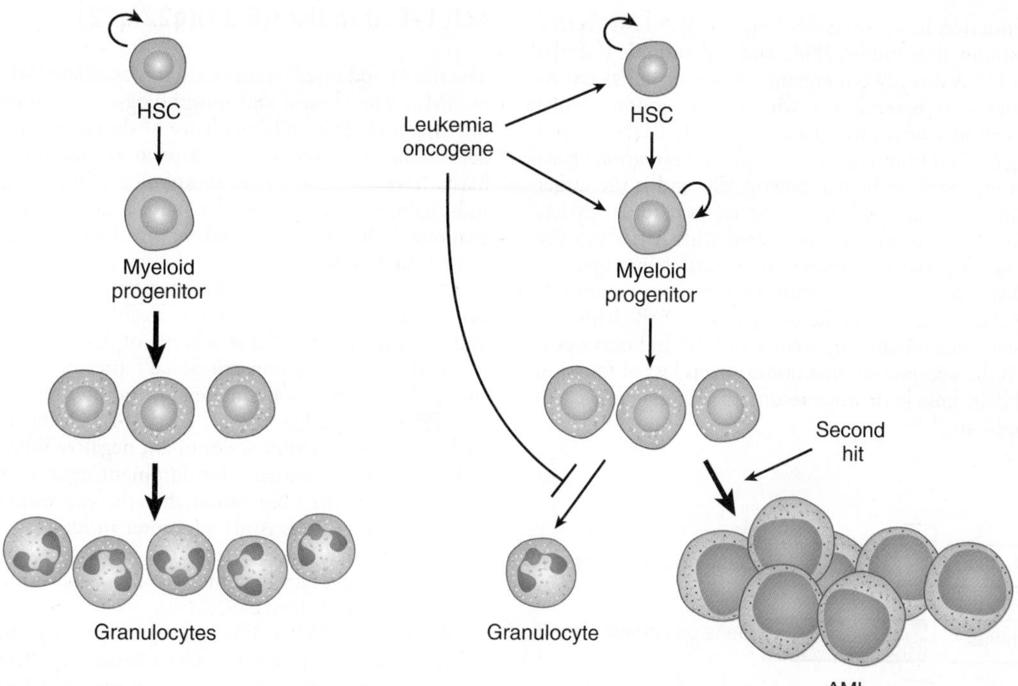

Figure 59–1 The leukemic stem cell. It has been hypothesized that there is a hierarchical development in leukemic cells as in normal hematopoietic cells in which only a small population of early hematopoietic progenitors have self-renewal capacity, as depicted on the left panel. Data derived from injection of human leukemic cells into NOD–SCID mice indicate that among leukemic populations, there is also only a small fraction of cells that have self-renewal capacity, and these have been termed leukemia stem cells (*left panel*). It has recently been shown in murine model systems that expression of certain leukemia oncogenes, such as MLL–ENL, can convert a hematopoietic stem cell that has intrinsic self-renewal capacity, or even a committed hematopoietic progenitor that has no capacity for self-renewal, into a cell that has properties of a leukemic stem cell. Subsequent mutations in this population, such as FLT3 mutations, would confer additional proliferative and survival advantage to these cells. These data indicate that although leukemia-associated mutations may occur in the self-renewing hematopoietic stem cell, they may also occur in committed progenitors and activate transcriptional programs that confer properties of self-renewal (*right panel*).

serially transplanted into secondary recipient mice.[30] The leukemias are immunophenotypically identical, regardless of whether the starting cell population is HSC, CMP, or GMP. These data suggest that certain leukemia oncogenes, such as the MLL–ENL fusion gene, can commandeer programs of self-renewal in committed progenitors and enforce phenotypic expression of markers associated with the hematopoietic stem cell (Fig. 59–1). There are several caveats, including the possibility that retroviral transduction contributes to the phenotype as a consequence of insertional mutagenesis and that this is a mouse model system, and mice may be different from humans in this regard. Nonetheless, these findings provide strategies for understanding the programs that control self-renewal. These may not only be valid targets for therapeutic intervention but may provide insights into approaches to confer properties of self-renewal to adult somatic cells for therapeutic benefit, such as tissue regeneration.

GENE REARRANGEMENTS AND MUTATIONS IN ACUTE MYELOID LEUKEMIA

Most cases of AML can be attributed to acquired somatic mutations that occur in hematopoietic progenitors. Many AML disease alleles were identified by molecular cloning of recurring chromosomal translocations that often pinpoint the genomic location of leukemogenic fusion genes. As detailed in the following sections, examples include fusions involving core binding factor, retinoic acid receptor-alpha, HOX family members, the MLL gene, and transcriptional coactivators such as CBP, MOZ, and TIF2. More recently, it has been appreciated that point mutations also contribute to a significant proportion of cases, including activating mutations in receptor tyrosine kinases such as FLT3 and KIT, and in RAS family members. In addition, loss of function point mutations have been identified in hematopoietic transcription factors such as AML1 (RUNX1), C/EBPalpha, and GATA-1. Most recently, mutations that result in aberrant localization of the nucleophosphim (NPM) have been identified and causally implicated in the pathogenesis of AML—in fact these appear to be the most frequent genetic alterations in AML and are associated with a favorable prognosis.

Chromosomal Translocations

Chromosome translocations result in aberrant expression of an otherwise normal gene because of juxtaposition to active promoter/enhance elements, or can result in expression of fusion genes (Fig. 59–2).[31] In AML, the majority of chromosome translocations result in the generation of chimeric fusion genes (Table 59–1). As detailed in the next section, characterization of the genes involved in these translocations has provided important insights into pathobiology of AML, and has also identified a spectrum of genes that are important in normal hematopoietic development. There are more than one hundred recurring chromosomal translocations observed in hematological malignancies, but many fewer clinical phenotypes. This observation suggests that despite genomic diversity of translocations, some of the resultant fusion genes must target similar signal transduction and/or transcriptional pathways in leukemia.

Core Binding Factor

More than a dozen different chromosomal translocations in AML target Core Binding Factor (CBF). The members of the CBF group function as heterodimeric complexes to regulate diverse target genes involved in differentiation in many tissues (Fig. 59–3).[32] CBF factors consist of an α-subunit that binds DNA, and a β-subunit (CBFβ) that does not bind DNA directly but enhances transcriptional activation of target genes as a heterodimer with the α-subunit. Three α-subunits have been identified, designated RUNX1, RUNX2, and RUNX3 according to their homology to *Drosophila melanogaster* runt gene.[33] RUNX1 is expressed in hematopoietic cells and is the target of translocations in AML, and will herein be referred to as AML1, based on its cloning as a fusion gene associated with AML and the t(8;21). CBF is an important regulator of normal hematopoietic development, and transactivates a spectrum of genes that are important for both myeloid and lymphoid development.[32] Perhaps the most convincing evidence for the importance of CBF in hematopoietic development is the observation that homozygous loss of function of AML1 or CBFβ in knockout mice results in a complete lack of definitive hematopoiesis.[34–36]

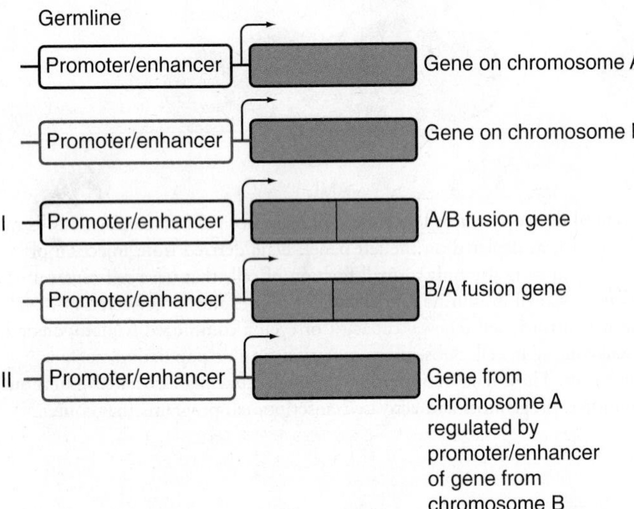

Figure 59–2 Molecular consequences of chromosome translocations. In (I), the chromosomal breakpoints occur within the transcription units, leading to the formation of chimeric genes and thus to the expression of fusion proteins. In (II), an intact transcription unit is juxtaposed to regulatory elements from a gene on another chromosome, resulting in aberrant expression of an otherwise normal gene.

AML1–ETO in the t(8;21)(q22;q22)

The t(8;21)(q22;q22) translocation is associated with the M2 subtype of AML. The clinical and morphologic correlations of this subtype of AML include a high incidence of development of extramedullary collections of leukemic blasts known as granulocytic sarcomas. The blasts have a characteristic morphology, including prominent Auer rods, salmon-colored granules, and large cytoplasmic granules and vacuoles. When the characteristic histologic appearance of these cells is identified in AML blasts that do not contain a t(8;21), the AML1–ETO fusion can often be identified by PCR, indicating that formation of the molecular fusion is responsible for the specific morphologic and clinical features of this subtype of AML.[37]

AML1–ETO is a transcriptional repressor that aberrantly recruits the nuclear corepressor complex, including histone deacetylase (HD) to CBF sites (see Fig. 59–3). AML1–ETO and other CBF fusions each appear to function as dominant negative inhibitors of the native CBF. Convincing evidence for dominant negative activity of AML1–ETO includes the observation that the expression of AML1–ETO from the endogenous Aml1 promoter in knockin mice results in an embryonic lethal phenotype that is identical to the $Aml1^{-/-}$ phenotype, despite the fact that there is a residual normal allele of Aml1 present in these animals.[38,39]

Because the AML1–ETO knockin has an embryonic lethal phenotype, it was not possible to characterize the effects of expression in adult hematopoietic cells. To circumvent embryonic lethality, a conditional allele was generated that allowed for normal development, followed by expression in the hematopoietic compartment. Expression of AML1–ETO appears to confer a subtle proliferative or survival advantage, in that these cells increase with time in the bone marrow. In addition, AML1–ETO appears to confer certain properties of self-renewal, such as the ability to serially replate in methylcellulose cultures. However, these animals do not develop AML unless chemical mutagens such as ethyl-nitrososurea are used, indicating that AML1–ETO expression alone is not sufficient to cause AML.[40]

CBFβ–MYH11 in the inv(16)(p13q22) and the t(16;16)(p13;q22)

The inv(16)(p13q22) and the t(16;16)(p13;q22) are observed primarily in the M4Eo subtype of AML. These patients, similar to those

Table 59–1 Correlation Between Morphologic Subtypes of Acute Myeloid Leukemia (AML) and Recurring Chromosomal Translocation

FAB Subtype	Cytogenetic Aberration	Molecular Aberration
M0, M1, and ALL	t(10:11)	*CALM-AF10*
M1	Trisomy 11	Partial duplication of *MLL*
M2	t(8;21)	*AML1-ETO*
M3	t(15;17), t(11;17), t(5;17)	*PML-RARα, PLZF-RARα, NPM-RARα*
M4eo	inv(16)	*CBFβ-MYH11*
M4 with erythrophagocytosis	t(8;16)	*MOZ-CBP*
M5	11q23 translocations	*MLL* fused to one of its partner genes
M6	t(3;5)	*NPM-MLF1*
M1, M2, M4, and MDS	t(6;9), t(9;9)	*DEK-CAN, SET-CAN*
Multiple FAB subtypes, MDS, and CML	t(16;21)	*TLS/FUS-ERG*
M2, M4, CML	t(7;11)	*NUP98-HOXA9*
MDS, de novo/T-AML	inv(11)	*NUP98-DDX10*
MDS, T-AML, CML	t(3;21)	*AML 1-EAP/MDS1/EVI1*

ALL, acute lymphocytic leukemia; CML, chronic myelomonocytic leukemia; FAB, French-American-British (Cooperative Group); T-AML, T-cell acute myeloid leukemia.

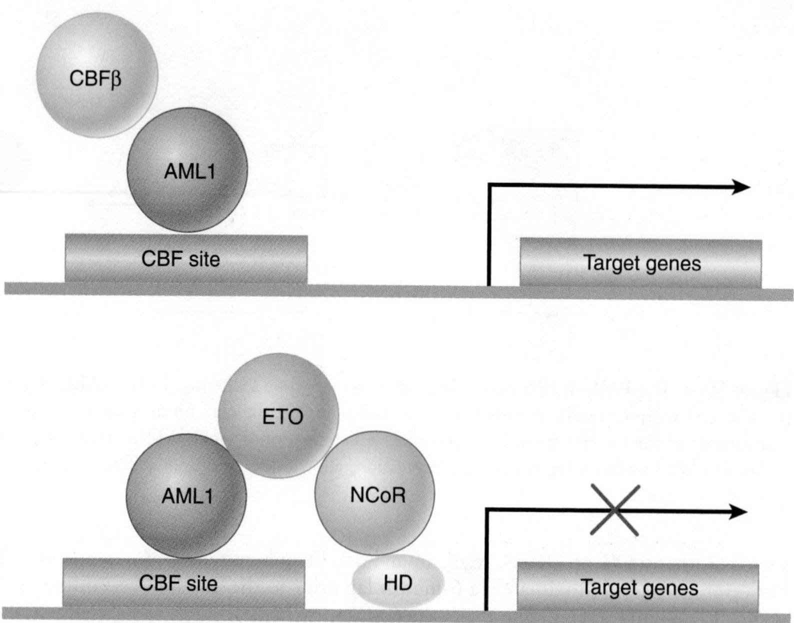

Figure 59–3 Core binding factor (CBF) and leukemia. Core binding factor is a heterodimeric transcription factor containing an AML1 and a CBFβ subunit. AML1 directly contacts DNA, and its transactivation potential is enhanced by binding to CBFβ, which does not contact DNA. Core binding factor fusions, including AML1–ETO (as depicted), CBFβ–MYH11, and TEL–AML1 act as dominant negative inhibitors of CBF through aberrant recruitment of the nuclear corepressor complex, including histone deacetylase. Histone deacetylase inhibitors are currently being explored as therapeutic agents for acute myeloid leukemia (AML) in clinical trials.

with the t(8;21), have a relatively good prognosis and a high likelihood of responding to regimens that include high-dose cytosine arabinoside.[41] The β-subunit of CBF, located at 16q22, is disrupted as a result of either this chromosomal inversion or a translocation leading to the formation of a fusion transcript with the gene for smooth muscle myosin heavy chain, MYH11, located at 16p13.[42] The CBFβ–MYH11 chimeric protein contains nearly all of CBFβ, including the heterodimerization domain for AML1, fused to the C-terminal sequences of MYH11, including its coiled-coil dimerization motif. The chimeric CBFβ–MYH11 protein thus retains its ability to bind to AML1 and is also capable of forming high-molecular-weight multimers through the coiled-coil domain of MYH11. Like AML1–ETO, the CBFβ–MYH11 fusion is a dominant negative inhibitor of transactivation mediated by CBF.[32]

Further support for the hypothesis that the CBFβ–MYH11 fusion is a dominant negative inhibitor of CBF includes the observation that mice that express the CBFβ–MYH11 allele from the endogenous promoter have a similar phenotype to that observed with the AML1–ETO fusion.[35] These mice exhibit phenotype nearly identical to either the $Aml1^{-/-}$ or $Cbf\beta^{-/-}$ mice, with midgestation embryonic lethality, absence of fetal liver hematopoiesis, and central nervous system hemorrhage. The chimeric mice generated from embryonic stem cells containing CBFβ–MYH11 do not develop leukemia unless chemical mutagens are employed.[43] Thus, like AML1–ETO, expression of CBFβ–MYH11 is not sufficient to cause AML.

Translocations Involving the Retinoic Acid Receptor-α Locus

One of the remarkable successes in molecularly targeted therapy of AML over the past decade has been the use of all-trans-retinoic acid (ATRA) to induce complete responses in patients with acute promyelocytic leukemia (APL). This empiric observation fueled efforts to clone the t(15;17)(q22;q22) breakpoint, with a focus on the retinoic acid receptor alpha locus on 17q22. The consequence of the translocation is fusion of the retinoic acid receptor α (RARα) gene on chromosome 17 to a novel partner on chromosome 15, PML (promyelocytic leukemia).[42–44] Two reciprocal fusion RNA species are produced as a consequence of the translocation, RARα–PML and PML–RARα. The PML–RARα fusion protein contains the zinc finger of PML fused to the DNA- and protein-binding domains of RARα. Several other chromosomal translocations associated with an APL phenotype have been cloned and characterized. Each of these targets the RARα locus, with fusion to various partners that include PLZF and NPM. The best studied of these is the PLZF–RARα fusion that also aberrantly recruits the nuclear corepressor complex. However, in contrast with the PML–RARα fusion, ATRA is not able to relieve corepression mediated by the PLZF–RARα fusion, and thus is not effective in patients that harbor the t(11;17) associated with this fusion gene.[44]

The PML–RARα and PLZF–RARα fusion proteins are dominant negative inhibitors of retinoid induced transactivation (Fig. 59–4).[45] In addition to interfering with normal RARα interacting proteins, such as RXRα, the PML–RARα fusion also interferes with the function of the native PML protein, which is thought to function as a tumor suppressor gene on the basis of analysis of mice that are deficient in Pml.[46] The PML protein is a component of a novel nuclear structure referred to by several names, including PML oncogenic domains, nuclear bodies, or nuclear domain 10.[47,48] This nuclear structure was initially discovered by immunohistochemical analysis of the targets of autoantibodies obtained from patients with primary biliary cirrhosis. The Sp100 protein was the first component of this structure to be identified. Type I and II interferons induce the expression of both PML and Sp100. Infection of cells with adenovirus or herpesvirus leads to the delocalization of Sp100 and PML. In APL cells, the integrity of the nuclear body is disrupted and a microspeckled distribution of PML–RARα is observed. Treatment of APL cells with ATRA causes the nuclear bodies to regenerate, with proper relocalization of PML. Recently, arsenic trioxide has also been found to target PML and PML–RARα to nuclear bodies and to induce degradation of these proteins.[49] Thus, the restoration of nuclear body structures by either ATRA or arsenic trioxide correlates with the ability of these agents to induce remission of APL.

The dominant interfering activities of the PML–RARα fusion protein results in a phenotypic block in differentiation at the promyelocyte stage of development. The clinical response of these patients to ATRA, as discussed in more detail below, is explained by the ability of this retinoid to bind to the PML–RARα fusion protein and reverse repression of target genes required for normal hematopoietic development. The ability of the PML–RARα fusion protein to repress transcription is due in part to the aberrant recruitment of the nuclear corepressor complex, including histone deacetylase,[50–52] suggesting that pharmacologic agents that inhibit histone deacetylases may be useful in the therapy of APL.[53–55]

Murine models of APL, like those for CBF mutations associated with leukemia, indicate that multiple mutations are required for the APL phenotype. Expression of PML–RARα in transgenic mice from promoters that direct expression to the promyelocyte compartment,

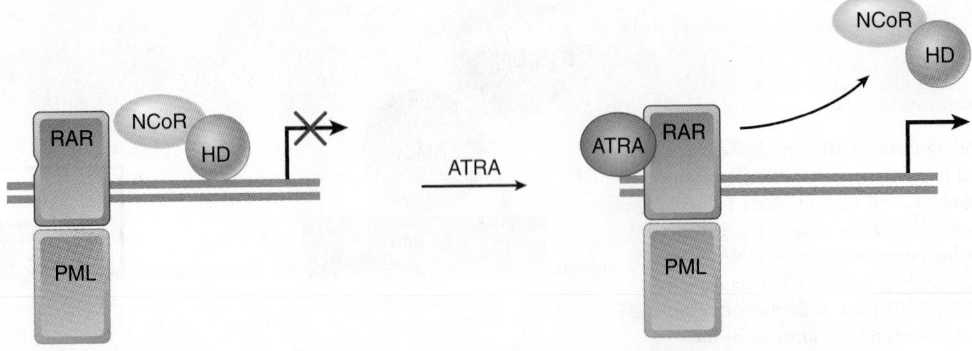

Figure 59–4 The PML–RARα fusion in acute promyelocytic leukemia. PML–RARα is a dominant negative inhibitor of transactivation mediated by retinoic acid receptor family members such as RXRα. As for the core binding factor fusions, dominant negative inhibition can be attributed to aberrant recruitment of the nuclear corepressor complex. All-trans-retinoic acid (ATRA) induces complete remission in the majority of cases of acute promyelocytic leukemia (APL) by inducing release of corepression, allowing for terminal differentiation and apoptosis of leukemic cells.

such as cathepsin G or MRP8, result in an APL-like phenotype.[56–58] However, there is approximately a 6-month lag prior to the development of leukemia, incomplete penetrance of approximately 15% to 30%, and acquired karyotypic abnormalities, all suggesting that second mutations are required for induction of leukemia. Coexpression of both the PML–RARα and RARα–PML under the cathepsin G promoter results in increased penetrance, but prolonged latency and acquisition of cytogenetic abnormalities, still supporting the need to additional mutation.[59] In at least some cases, activating mutations in FLT3, as discussed below, may be the additional mutation required. ATRA is efficacious in these animals, and the model has allowed for preclinical testing of novel agents currently in clinical trials, such as arsenic trioxide.[60]

MLL Gene Rearrangements in Leukemia

Translocations involving chromosome band 11q23 occur frequently in both AML and ALL and have several unique features in comparison with other subtypes of leukemia. There are at least 30 different partner chromosomes involved in recurring reciprocal 11q23 translocations.[5] This exceeds the number of known translocations affecting the immunoglobulin loci, suggesting that the 11q23 breakpoint region may contain genomically unstable sequences that lead to chromosomal recombination events. Translocations involving 11q23 are the single most common cytogenetic abnormality in infants with acute leukemia, regardless of phenotype, occurring in approximately 70% to 80% of these cases. 11q23 translocations are also observed frequently in therapy-related leukemias in patients who have previously been treated with chemotherapy drugs that inhibit topoisomerase II, especially the epipodophyllotoxins.

The chromosomal partners in 11q23 translocations are usually lineage specific. In AML, the t(9;11)(p22;q23), the t(11;19)(q23;p13.1), and the t(6;11)(q27;q23) are the most common, and in ALL, the t(4;11)(q21;q23) and the t(11;19)(q23;p13.3) predominate. The MLL gene was isolated from the 11q23 breakpoint by several groups and is referred to by other names, including HRX, ALL-1, and Htrx.[61–64] 11q23 translocations have been observed in several FAB subtypes but occur most commonly in the M4 myelomonocytic and M5 monoblastic leukemias. Myeloid leukemias with 11q23 translocations often coexpress lymphoid markers, whereas 11q23 lymphoid leukemias often express myeloid or monocytoid markers in addition to B-cell markers. These observations suggest that rearrangement of MLL may affect a pluripotent stem cell or, alternatively, that disruption of MLL may affect a common differentiation pathway shared by lymphoid and myeloid progenitor cells.

MLL encodes a large protein, with a predicted molecular weight of 430 kd, that contains two regions of extensive homology to the Drosophila trithorax gene.[65] The regions that are conserved with trithorax include a series of Cys4–His–Cys3 zinc fingers in the middle portion of the protein that have been referred to as PHD or LAP domains.[66,67] The C terminus of MLL contains a conserved motif, named the SET domain, because it is present in several proteins, including Su(var)3–9, enhancer of zeste, and trithorax.[68] At the N terminus of MLL, there are three AT-hook motifs similar to those present in the HMG-I(Y) proteins that bind to AT-rich sequences in the minor groove of DNA. There is also a region of homology to mammalian DNA methyltransferases. Neither the AT hooks nor the DNA methyltransferase domain is present in trithorax. The MLL protein also contains transcriptional activation and repression domains. In Drosophila, trithorax is essential to maintain the proper expression of homeotic genes but not to initiate their expression. Targeted disruption of Mll in mice causes lethality at embryonic day 10.5.[69] Mll heterozygous mice also exhibited a phenotype with growth retardation, bidirectional homeotic transformations of the axial skeleton, and sternal malformations. In the Mll homozygous deficient mice, expression of Hoxa-7 and Hoxc-9 was abolished, whereas in Mll heterozygous mice, the anterior boundaries of expression of these genes were shifted posteriorly. These findings indicate that MLL is a positive regulator of Hox gene expression.

A broad spectrum of MLL partner genes have been cloned at 11q23 partner chromosomal breakpoints. These include AF4 in the t(4;11)(q21;q23), ENL in the t(11;19)(q23;p13.3), ELL in the t(11;19)(q23;p13.1), AF9 in the t(9;11)(p22;q23), AF6 in the t(6;11)(q27;q23), AF1p in the t(1;11)(p32;q23), AF1q in the t(1;11)(q21;q23), AF-X in the t(X;11)(q13;q23), AF10 in the t(10;11)(p12;q23), AF17 in the t(11;17)(q23;q21), EEN in the t(11;19)(q23;p13), and CBP in the t(11;16)(q23;p13.3). Two MLL partner genes are involved in other chromosome translocations as well. For example, AF10 is fused to the CALM gene in the t(10;11)(p13;q14), and CBP fuses to the MOZ gene in the t(8;16)(p11;p13). The functions of most MLL partner genes are not yet known. Although no consistent homologies or motifs among the partner gene sequences have been identified that might explain how their fusion to MLL results in leukemia, certain partner genes have similar features (Fig. 59–5). For example, ENL and AF9 contain transcriptional activation domains and share extensive homology at their C termini. AF10 and AF17 contain leucine zipper and zinc finger motifs and also share extensive homology with each other. In addition, AFX and AF6q21 contain forkhead domains and also share other regions of homology. Three MLL partner genes have well-characterized functions. ELL has been shown to function as an RNA polymerase II transcriptional elongation factor. It serves to increase the catalytic rate of RNA polymerase II by suppressing transient pausing by the polymerase along the DNA template. CBP and p300 are transcriptional coactivators that mediate interactions between multiple transcription factors and the basal transcriptional machinery. The pattern of protein–protein interactions of MLL partner genes may provide insight into the nature of the aberrant functions of MLL fusion proteins in leukemia.

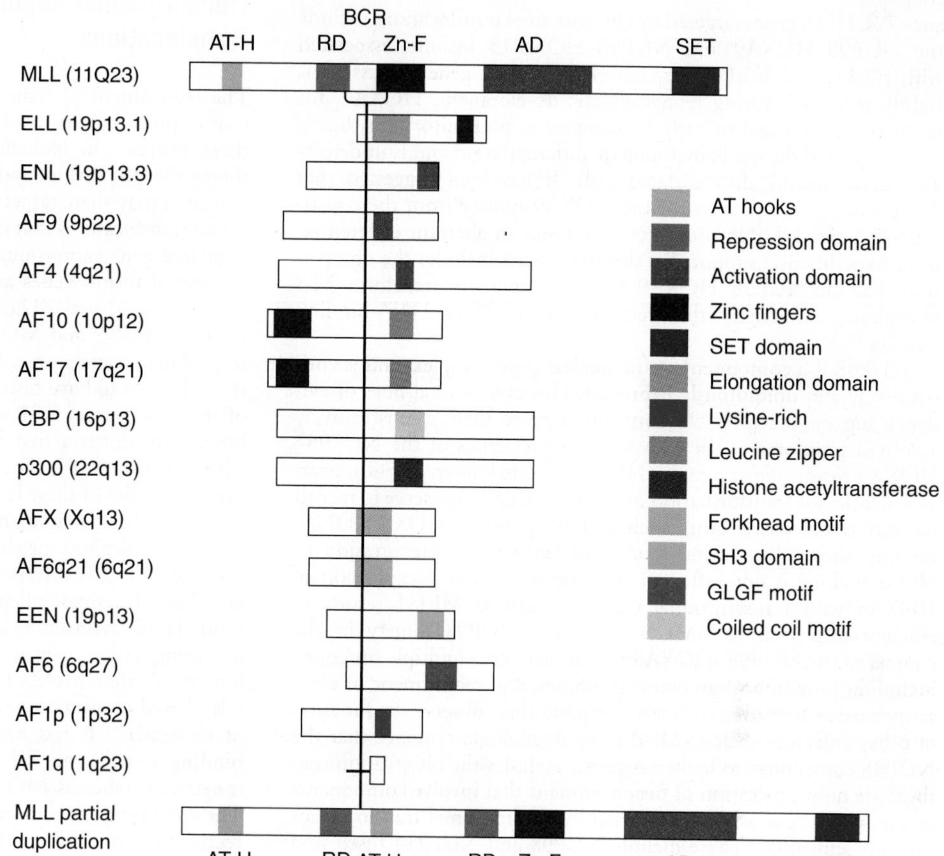

Figure 59–5 Motifs in MLL partner genes. The partner genes can be grouped into several classes that share common motifs. AT-H, AT hooks; RD, repression domain; Zn-F, zinc fingers; AD, activating domain.

In a subset of patients with AML and either trisomy 11 or a normal karyotype, a unique pattern of rearrangement of the MLL gene has been observed. As in the translocations that affect MLL, a fusion occurs involving one of the exons in its breakpoint cluster region. However, rather than fusing to a partner gene, the fusion is to 5′ sequences from MLL itself.[70,71] For example, the structure of the partial duplication might contain MLL exons 1 to 7 fused to exon 2 through the 3′ end of the gene. The largest duplication identified contains exons 2 to 9, and the smallest, exons 4 to 6. The region of the duplication contains the AT hooks, methyltransferase, and repression domains of MLL. In several cases, the 5′ and 3′ genomic breaks within MLL occur at similar points within Alu repetitive sequences, suggesting that partial duplications may be generated as a result of homologous recombination. In contrast to the reciprocal translocations involving MLL, the partial duplications of MLL appear to occur primarily in older patients and are infrequent in childhood and therapy-related leukemias. The morphology of the leukemias also differs in that the partial duplication patients usually are classified as FAB-M1 or -M2, rather than the M4 or M5 typically observed in cases with MLL translocations. These findings suggest that the critical transforming event may be related to rearrangement of MLL itself, as opposed to contributions from the respective fusion partners.

In support of this hypothesis, it has been reported that the MLL gene product is a propeptide that is cleaved by a novel protease, taspase 1. There appears to be aberrant regulation of HOX gene expression by noncleaved MLL, and it has been suggested that the MLL fusion genes and the MLL partial tandem duplications are surrogates for the noncleaved MLL protein.[72] This is an attractive hypothesis, in that it explains the remarkable lack of similarity between the multitude of MLL fusion partners in structure and function, and suggests that a cardinal transforming event that is related to dysregulated HOX gene expression, with MLL fusion proteins as noncleavable surrogates of the native MLL.[72,73] The fusion partners might then contribute to lineage specificity or other phenotypic aspects of transformation related to MLL gene rearrangements.

The t(4;11)(q21;q23) may also be observed in AML, particularly in infants and children.[74] This translocation was originally described in association with ALL, but later studies documented the myeloid or hybrid nature of blasts in some of the patients. New insights into pathogenesis of infant acute leukemia associated with the t(4;11) MLL–AF4 fusion have been gained from analysis of global patterns of gene expression.[74] These analyses indicate that infant leukemia with the MLL–AF4 fusion represents a distinct subclass of leukemia that can be readily delineated from AML or ALL by gene expression profiles. These data, and the target genes that are overexpressed in infant leukemia with the MLL–AF4 fusion such as FLT3, suggest novel approaches to therapy of this subtype of leukemia.

Two different strategies have been used to generate mouse models of 11q23 leukemias. To create an Mll–AF9 knockin mouse, the AF9 cDNA was targeted into the murine Mll genomic locus by homologous recombination in embryonic stem cells.[75] The chimeric mice generated from these embryonic stem cells all developed AML within 6 to 9 months. Chimeric mice that expressed only the N-terminal sequences of Mll did not develop leukemia. In addition, retroviral transduction of bone marrow has been used to express another 11q23 fusion gene, MLL–ENL, in hematopoietic cells.[76] In serial replating assays on methylcellulose, the MLL–ENL-transduced cells could be immortalized, whereas constructs containing either N-terminal MLL, ENL alone, or vector controls could not maintain proliferative capacity beyond three passages. After transplantation of MLL–ENL-transduced bone marrow, syngeneic recipient mice developed AML.

Homeotic Genes in Acute Myeloid Leukemia: HOX and CDX Family Members

Regulation of expression of the large family of HOX paralogs is important in patterning in vertebrate development, and also plays a critical role in normal hematopoietic development (reviewed in reference 77). HOX genes targeted by chromosomal translocations include the NUP98–HOXA9 and NUP98–HOXD13 fusions, associated with t(7;11) and t(2;11), respectively.[78,79] HOX gene expression is tightly regulated during hematopoietic development. HOXA9, for example, is expressed in early hematopoietic progenitor cells, but is downregulated during hematopoietic differentiation and is undetectable in terminally differentiated cells. It has been suggested that unregulated overexpression of the HOXA9 moiety from the constitutively active NUP98 promoter may result in aberrant differentiation. Experimental support for this hypothesis includes the observation that the NUP98–HOXA9 fusion protein can transform 3T3 fibroblasts, an activity that requires the HOXA9 DNA-binding domain.[80]

NUP98 is a component of the nuclear pore complex, and is constitutively and ubiquitously expressed. However, several lines of evidence suggest that NUP98 contributes more than a constitutively activated promoter to the transforming properties of the NUP98–HOXA9 fusion. For example, NUP98 motifs known as FG repeats are essential for transformation in fibroblasts, and may serve to recruit transcriptional coactivators such as CBP/p300 to HOXA9 DNA-binding sites.[80] In murine models of leukemia, overexpression of HOXA9 alone is not sufficient to cause AML, but coexpression of HOXA9 with transcriptional cofactors such as MEIS1 results in efficient induction of AML.[81] Thus, the NUP98 moiety in the context of the NUP98–HOXA9 fusion may serve multiple functions including provision of an active promoter, and recruitment of transcriptional coactivators such as CBP/p300 that subserve the function of other cofactors such as MEIS1. Epidemiologic evidence that the NUP98 contributes to leukemogenesis includes the observation that there are now a spectrum of fusion proteins that involve components of the nuclear pore that are targeted by chromosomal translocations in acute leukemias. These include NUP98 and NUP214 fused to a diverse group if partners include HOX family members, HOXA9 and HOXD13; and the DDX10, PMX1, and DEK genes, respectively.

It has been hypothesized that dysregulated HOX gene expression may be important in leukemias that do not directly target HOX family members. Several proteins that are upstream of HOX expression have been implicated in AML as fusion genes associated with AML. The most frequent of these are MLL gene rearrangements (see Fig. 59–5). As described above, more than 40 chromosomal translocations target MLL and result in fusions of MLL with a broad spectrum of partners. However, a common biological feature of all of these may be the ability to dysregulate HOX gene expression during hematopoietic development in that HOX genes have been shown to be direct targets of various MLL fusions.[82]

In addition, t(12;13) associated with AML results in the expression of high levels of CDX2 from the TEL locus.[83,84] CDX2 is a homeotic protein that regulates expression of HOX family members in the colonic epithelium. As in hematopoietic development, HOX gene expression is highest in colonic stem cells in the colonic crypts, and is downregulated with maturation to epithelial cells. It is thus plausible that high levels of expression of CDX2 dysregulate HOX expression in hematopoietic progenitors and result in leukemia. Evidence to support this includes the ability of CDX2 to induce leukemia in murine retroviral transduction models.[84] Although CDX2 is not normally expressed in hematopoietic cells, a family member, CDX4, has recently been cloned and appears to play a similar role in hematopoietic development as CDX2 does in the gut. Of note, CDX4 in hematopoietic cells appears to either be downstream or epistatic with MLL in the regulation of HOX gene expression.[85]

Taken together, these data indicate that the NUP98–HOXA9 fusion transforms hematopoietic progenitors in part through dysregulated overexpression of HOX family members, and by transactivation mediated through the NUP98 transactivation domain that recruits CBP. Recent evidence indicates, however, that like the other gene rearrangements involving hematopoietic transcription factors, expression of NUP98–HOXA9 alone is not sufficient to cause leukemia. In murine bone marrow transplant models, NUP98–HOXA9 induces AML only after markedly prolonged latencies indicative of a requirement for second mutation.[86]

Transcriptional Regulatory Proteins in Chromosomal Translocations

The recruitment of transcriptional coactivators and corepressors by transcription factors involved in leukemia suggests a critical role for these proteins in leukemogenesis. In keeping with the recurring theme that the diverse and numerous chromosomal translocations in leukemia may share targets and functional activity, there are chromosomal translocations that involve proteins that modulate and facilitate regulated gene expression.

Several fusion genes associated with leukemia involve transcriptional coactivators. These include the MLL–CBP, MLL–p300, MOZ–CBP,[87–89] and MOZ–TIF2[90,91] fusions that incorporate transcriptional coactivators CBP, p300, and TIF2. Although TIF2 itself is not known to have histone acetylase transferase activity, a hallmark of the coactivators CBP and p300, it has a well-characterized CBP interaction domain that may serve to recruit CBP into a complex with MOZ or TIF2. The transcriptional activation and transformation properties of these large fusion proteins are not well understood. One hypothesis is that the fusions have dominant negative activity for CBP and p300, or that the translocation leads to simple loss of function of CBP expressed from one allele. In support of this hypothesis, loss of a single allele of CBP or p300 in the human Rubenstein–Taybi syndrome increases predisposition to malignancies, including colon cancer. However, recent data also support the hypothesis that MOZ–TIF2 may represent a gain of function for CBP based on mutational analysis in cell culture and murine models of leukemia.[92] It has been demonstrated that MOZ nucleosome-binding activity and TIF2–CBP interactions are required for leukemogenesis, whereas MOZ histone acetyl transferase activity is not. These data suggest that the leukemogenicity of the fusion is based on recruitment of CBP to MOZ nucleosome-binding sites.[92]

The t(1;22) Translocation Associated With Infant Acute Megakaryoblastic Leukemia

Megakaryoblastic leukemias have proven challenging to study. Until recently little was understood about the molecular pathobiology of these diseases, in part due to the challenges of collecting clinical material for analysis in the context of severe bone marrow fibrosis. GATA-1 truncation mutations had been demonstrated in Down syndrome-associated AMKL, but these hypomorphic alleles are not observed in sporadic cases of AMKL.[93] However, new insights into non-Down syndrome AMKL have been obtained through the cloning of the t(1;22) that is associated with the majority of non-Down infant AMKL.[94,95] The consequence of t(1;22) in infant AMKL is expression of an aberrant OTT1–MAL fusion protein in the hematopoietic compartment. OTT1 (RBM15) contains three amino-terminal RNA recognition motifs, as well as motifs conserved in evolution through Drosophila, including a Spen paralog and an ortholog C terminal. Ott1 deletion in mice has identified multiple roles in hematopoietic development including effects on megakaryocyte growth.[96] The MAL (MKL1) gene is ubiquitously expressed and has functional motifs that include a coiled-coil dimerization motif and a proline-rich transcriptional activation domain. MLK1 is a Rho–GTPase-regulated cofactor for serum response factor.[97] Although these genes have certain functions that might be ascribed to leukemogenesis, the role of the fusion gene and its respective wildtype counterpart alleles in the development of leukemia is not known.

POINT MUTATIONS IN ACUTE MYELOID LEUKEMIA

Activating Mutations in RAS Family Members

Oncogenic RAS mutations are associated with AML and myelodysplastic syndrome (MDS), typically at codons 12, 13, or 61 or N- or K-RAS. The reported incidence varies widely between studies from 25% to 44% (reviewed in reference 98). One carefully conducted

Figure 59–6 Activating mutations in FLT3 and KIT in AML. Approximately 20% to 25% of cases of AML have internal tandem duplication (ITD) mutations that occur in the juxtamembrane (JM) domain of FLT3, and may range in size from a few to more than 50 amino acids. The ITD disrupts an autoinhibitory structure in the JM domain and results in constitutive kinase activation in the absence of ligand. These mutations confer a proliferative and survival advantage to leukemic cells. Activation loop mutations occur in FLT3 and in KIT at a frequency of approximately 5% each, and also result in constitutive activation of these receptor tyrosine kinases.

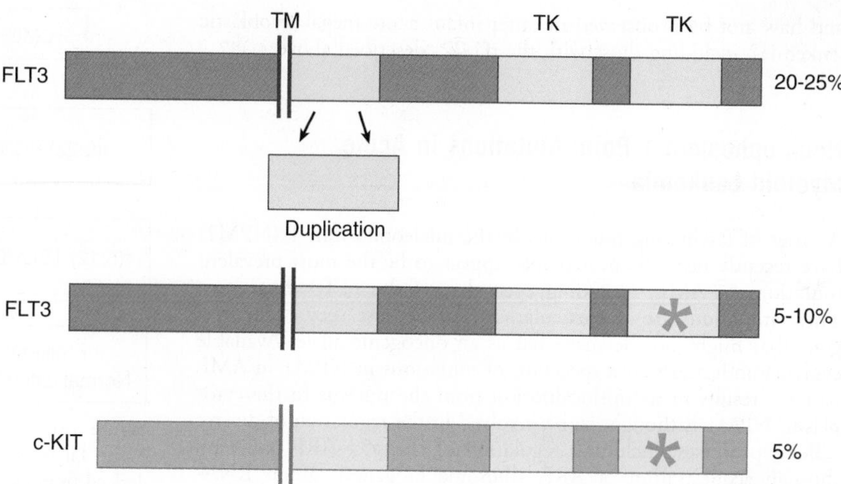

cooperative group trial in which mutant RAS alleles were assessed by direct sequencing reported an 18% incidence of N- or K-RAS mutations, and that RAS mutations conferred a poor prognosis.[99] Considerable effort has been devoted to develop small molecule inhibitors of RAS activation, with a focus on prenylation inhibitors including farnesyl transferase and geranyl-geranylation inhibitors that preclude appropriate targeting of activated RAS to the plasma membrane.[100,101] Prenyltransferases have activity in AML, though responses do not correlate with the presence of activating mutations in RAS, [100,101] or even with inhibition of the target farnesyl transferase itself. There are several possible interpretations of these observations, including the possibility that RAS is activated by mechanisms other than intrinsic point mutations (such as constitutively activated tyrosine kinases like FLT3), or that other proteins that are targets of prenylation are important in leukemia pathogenesis, or that farnesyl transferase inhibitors target an as yet unidentified target.

Mutations That Constitutively Activate Receptor Tyrosine Kinases

Acquired activation loop and juxtamembrane mutations that result in constitutive activation of FLT3 and c-KIT have been identified in a significant proportion of AML cases. These findings may have important therapeutic implications with the recent demonstration of the efficacy of molecular targeting of the ABL kinase in BCR- and ABL-positive CML and CML blast crisis with imatinib (Gleevec).[102,103] FLT3 is the most commonly mutated gene in human AML, occurring in approximately 30% to 35% of cases of AML.[104,105] In 20% to 25% of cases, there are internal tandem duplications (ITDs) of the juxtamembrane domain that result in constitutive activation of FLT3 (Fig. 59–6). The ITDs may range in size from a few to more than 50 amino acids and are always in frame. Because of the extensive variability in size and exact position of the repeats within the juxtamembrane domain, it has been hypothesized that these are loss-of-function domains that impair an autoinhibitory domain, resulting in constitutive kinase activation in the absence of ligand. In support of this hypothesis, the crystallographic structure of FLT3 demonstrates a 7-amino acid extension of the juxtamembrane domain that intercalates into the catalytic domain, thereby precluding kinase activation.[106] It is likely that ITD mutations in this region would disrupt structure of the autoinhibitory domain resulting in kinase activation. In an additional 5% to 10% of cases there are so-called activating loop mutations that occur near position D835 in the tyrosine kinase.[107,108] Several large studies have confirmed the frequency of these mutations in both adult and pediatric AML populations, and that mutations in FLT3 appear to confer a poor prognosis.[109–111]

FLT3 mutations may occur in conjunction with known gene rearrangements such as AML1–ETO, PML–RARα, CBFβ–MYH11, or MLL. Analogous activating loop mutations at position D816 have also been reported in C-KIT in approximately 5% of cases of acute myeloid leukemia. These data suggest that constitutive activation of tyrosine kinases may play an important role in the pathogenesis of acute leukemia as well as in chronic myeloid leukemia. FLT3, KIT, and RAS mutations, as discussed below, form a complementation group in that these rarely overlap in the same patient, and each results in constitutive activation of signal transduction pathways in leukemic cells. However, they collectively account for only approximately 50% of cases, suggesting that other mutations that activate signal transduction pathways may be present in the remainder of cases of AML.

Loss-of-Function Point Mutations in AML1, C/EBPα, and GATA-1

As described above, AML1 is a frequent target of translocations in human leukemias. In addition to frequent involvement of AML1 as a consequence of chromosomal translocations, it has recently been determined that loss-of-function mutations in AML1 are responsible for the inherited leukemia syndrome FPD/AML (familial platelet disorder with propensity to develop acute myelogenous leukemia.[24,25] In addition, approximately 3% to 5% of sporadic cases of AML harbor loss-of-function mutations in AML1,[25,112] with a higher frequency in M0 AML (25%) and in AML or MDS with trisomy 21.

C/EBPα is a hematopoietic transcription factor that is required for normal myeloid lineage development. Because many translocations associated with acute myeloid leukemia phenotypes result in loss of function of hematopoietic transcription factors, it has been hypothesized that C/EBPα may also be a target for loss-of-function mutations in human leukemia. In fact, it has recently been reported that point mutations that result in expression of a mutant C/EBPα protein has dominant negative activity for wildtype C/EBPα in a fraction of M2 AML cases.[113] Thus, these mutations would be predicted to impair hematopoietic differentiation. Recent data indicate that C/EBPα mutations confer a favorable prognosis.[114]

GATA-1 mutations are associated with a subset of acute megakaryoblastic leukemias (FAB M7), in particular leukemias arising in patients with Down syndrome (constitutional trisomy 21). These mutations appear to result in loss of function or dysregulation of GATA-1 and are thought to contribute to leukemogenesis.[14] The mechanism through which hypomorphic alleles of GATA-1 contribute to leukemogenesis in the context of +21 is not known. GATA-1 mutations thus far have only been associated with Down syndrome, and have not been observed in other infant acute megakaryoblastic leukemias, including those with the t(1;22) described above.

Nucleophosmin 1 Point Mutations in Acute Myeloid Leukemia

A series of fascinating mutations in the nucleophosmin 1 (NPM1) have recently been discovered that appear to be the most prevalent mutations in AML, exceeding even that of the FLT3 mutations. These mutations are of particular interest because they occur in a gene that might not be suspected as an oncogenic allele. Available evidence indicates that a spectrum of mutations in NPM1 in AML patients results in its mislocalization from the nucleus to the cytoplasm. NPM1 is thought to be involved in the regulation of diverse cellular processes, including regulation of the p53–ARF pathways through sequestration of ARF, ribosome biogenesis as an RNA-binding protein, and duplication of centrosomes during mitosis. NPM1 had been previously identified in acute leukemias as a translocation fusion partner with RAR and MLF as well as with ALK in anaplastic large-cell lymphoma. However, recent data indicate that NPM1 mutations occur in 25% to 30% of adult AML. These cases of AML have acquired somatic mutations in exon 12 that engender a novel nuclear export motif, resulting in constitutive cytoplasmic localization that is readily apparent by cellular fluorescence in situ hybridization.[115] The mechanism by which mutated NPM1 causes leukemia is not fully understood, although cytoplasmic localization of NPM1 is thought to be intrinsic to its transforming potential.[116] NPM1 mutations are found more frequently in normal karyotype AML, accounting for approximately 50% to 60% of cases. Furthermore, these NPM1 mutant cases are more likely to have concurrent FLT3–ITD mutations as well, in consonance with multihit pathogenesis of AML (discussed below). Among AML patients with normal cytogenetics, the presence of cytoplasmic NPM1 in the absence of the FLT3–ITD is associated with a more favorable prognosis.[116]

LOSS OF GENETIC MATERIAL IN ACUTE MYELOID LEUKEMIA: THE MODEST ROLE OF TUMOR SUPPRESSOR GENES

In contrast with solid tumors, mutations resulting in the loss of function of tumor suppressor genes are relatively uncommon in leukemia. However, several of the known tumor suppressor genes have been well characterized in myeloid leukemias, such as the association of p53 mutations with progression to blast crisis in CML.[117–119] In AML, p53 mutations occur less frequently. Only approximately 7% of cases have known p53 mutations at the time of diagnosis. The incidence of p53 abnormalities may be slightly higher in patients with AML evolving from a prior myelodysplastic syndrome and in cases with 11q23 translocations.[119,120] The p16INK4 gene is another critical cell-cycle regulatory gene that has been shown to be inactivated by a variety of mechanisms in a number of tumors, including frequent deletion in ALL but only very rarely in AML.[121] As noted above, patients with neurofibromatosis and mutations of the NF1 tumor suppressor gene have a high rate of developing neoplasms, including progression of myelodysplastic syndrome to AML, although these might be most appropriately viewed as mutations that result in activation of signal transduction pathways, and are thus more analogous to oncogenic RAS or tyrosine kinase mutations.[17,122] The Wilms tumor suppressor gene, WT1, has been found to be overexpressed in the leukemic blasts of approximately 75% of cases of newly diagnosed AML.[123,124] The WT1 gene, located in the 11p13 region, encodes a transcription factor normally expressed in a time- and tissue-dependent manner, mainly in the kidneys and gonads,[125,126] although it is also expressed in normal $CD34^+/CD38^-$ hematopoietic progenitor cells.[127] In AML, high WT1 levels at diagnosis correlate with lower remission rates and higher overall survival rates.[123,124]

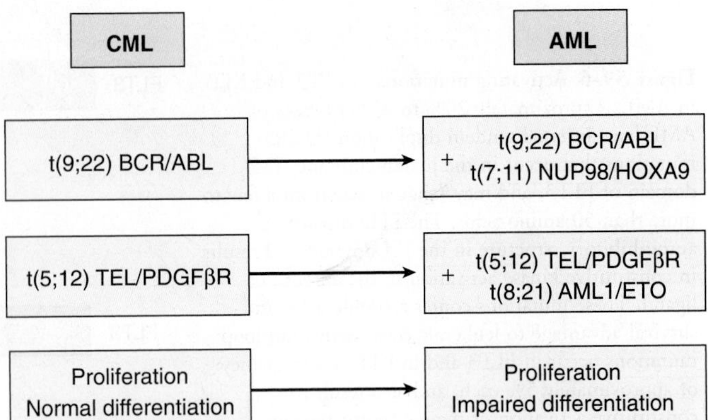

Figure 59–7 Disease progression in CML: Multistep pathogenesis of AML. There are clues to multistep pathogenesis of AML that can be derived from analysis of informative cases of disease progression in CML. Some cases of BCR–ABL positive CML, for example, progress to AML (CML blast crisis) with acquisition of a t(7;11) that results in expression of the NUP98–HOXA9 fusion. Similarly, progression of chronic myelomonocytic leukemia associated with the TEL–PDGFβR fusion may be associated with acquisition of the t(8;21) translocation associated with expression of the AML1–ETO fusion. These data suggest a model of AML in which there are cooperating mutations that confer a proliferative and survival advantage without affecting differentiation, such as BCR–ABL or TEL–PDGFβR; and those that contribute to impaired hematopoietic differentiation such as the AML1–ETO or NUP98–HOXA9 fusions.

A Role for Haploinsufficiency in Pathogenesis of Myelodysplastic Syndrome and Acute Myeloid Leukemia

Certain genetic alterations that result in loss of genetic material are specific to AML. These include loss of the long arms of chromosomes 5, 7, and 20, which occurs commonly in therapy-related AML and AML associated with prior myelodysplastic syndrome, and is associated with a poor prognosis.[3,4,128] These deletion events are discussed in detail elsewhere in this textbook. Despite decades of intensive effort, and the availability of the complete human genome sequence, classical tumor suppressor genes have not been identified in these intervals. Although it is possible that genes will be identified whose homozygous loss of function contributes to the leukemic phenotype, it seems increasingly likely that haploid dosage of one or more genes may be the critical genetic lesion. In support of this hypothesis, several genes, such as p27Kip1, have tumor suppressor activity at haploid gene dosage,[129] and haploinsufficiency of the hematopoietic transcription factor AML1 has been implicated in a familial leukemia syndrome.[24]

COOPERATING MUTATIONS: MULTISTEP PATHOGENESIS OF ACUTE MYELOID LEUKEMIA

More than one mutation is necessary for the development of acute myeloid leukemia. For example, there is evidence for acquisition of additional cytogenetic abnormalities with disease progression from CML to AML (ie, CML blast crisis). Disease progression in BCR- or ABL-positive CML include acquisition of t(3;21) AML1–EVI1, t(8;21) AML1–ETO, or t(7;11) NUP98–HOXA9 gene rearrangements (Fig. 59–7). Progression of chronic myelomonocytic leukemia to AML in a patient with the TEL–PDGFβR gene rearrangement was associated with acquisition of a t(8;21) AML1–ETO gene rearrangement.[130] Furthermore, expression of the AML1–ETO or CBFβ–MYH11 fusion proteins in murine models is not sufficient

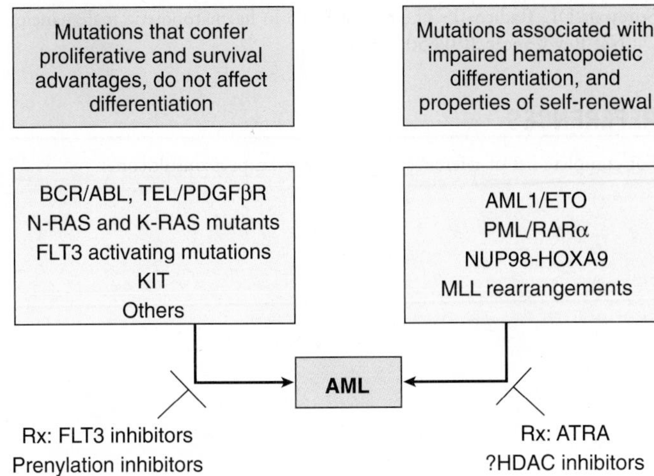

Figure 59–8 A model for cooperating mutations in AML. There are two broad complementation groups in AML. One group, characterized by activating mutations in signal transduction pathways, included oncogenic RAS, FLT3, or KIT mutations. These can be considered as complementation groups because they do not occur together in the same patient with leukemia, and thereby may subserve redundant functions that confer proliferative and survival advantage to hematopoietic progenitors. A second complementation group, exemplified by core binding factor fusions, or RARα fusions, are associated with impaired hematopoietic differentiation and may confer certain properties of self-renewal. These are also mutually exclusive in leukemias, indicating that they may also subserve an overlapping function in AML. When expressed together, components of these two complementation groups result in a phenotype of AML characterized by enhanced proliferative and survival advantage of leukemic blasts, impaired differentiation, and limitless self-renewal capacity.

to cause AML.[40,43] Chemical mutagens must be utilized in these contexts to generate second mutations that cause the AML phenotype. Lastly, transgenic mice that express the PML–RARα fusion protein develop AML only after a long latency of 3 to 6 months, with incomplete penetrance, indicating a need for a second mutation.[56–58]

The genetic epidemiology of AML provides important clues to the nature of the collaborating mutations (Fig. 59–8). There is one broad complementation group in AML that is composed of mutations that activate signal transduction pathways. These include activating mutations in FLT3, RAS, and KIT, and more rarely the BCR–ABL and TEL–PDGFβR fusion associated with disease progression in CML. These can be viewed as a complementation group because although they are collectively present in approximately 50% of cases of AML, they rarely if ever occur together in the same patient.

A second complementation group, typified by translocations involving hematopoietic transcription factors, includes AML1–ETO, CBFβ–SMMHC, PML–RARα, NUP98–HOXA9, MLL gene rearrangements and MOZ–TIF2. These mutations form a complementation group in that they are never observed together in the same leukemia. In general, this second class of mutations impairs hematopoietic differentiation and may confer properties of self-renewal to the leukemic stem cell, but is not sufficient to cause leukemia when expressed alone (see above). However, one mutation from each of these complementation groups is often coexistent in the same leukemia. For example, activating mutations in FLT3 and RAS have been observed in association with virtually all of the fusion genes in the second class described above.[131]

There is also support for the hypothesis of collaborating classes of leukemia oncogenes derived from analysis of genotypes of CML patients who progress to AML (also called CML blast crisis). Some cases of BCR- and ABL-positive CML progress to AML associated with acquisition of the t(7;11) translocation associated with expression of the NUP98–HOXA9 fusion gene discussed above. As another example, TEL–PDGFβR-positive chronic myelomonocytic leukemia may progress to AML associated with acquisition of the t(8;21) translocation associated with expression of the AML1–ETO fusion. These cases of disease progressions from CML to AML suggest the hypothesis that constitutively activated tyrosine kinases cooperate with mutations in hematopoietic transcription factors to cause the AML phenotype.

These findings suggest a hypothesis for pathogenesis of AML in which there are at least two broad classes of cooperating mutations.[131] One class, exemplified by activating mutations in FLT3 or RAS, confer proliferative and/or survival advantage to hematopoietic progenitors but do not affect differentiation. These mutations do not confer self-renewal capacity as assessed in part by the ability to serially replate in culture, or to serially transplant disease in murine models.[132,133] A second class of mutations, exemplified by AML1–ETO, CBFβ–SMMHC, PML–RARα, NUP98–HOXA9, MLL gene rearrangements, and MOZ–TIF2 serve primarily to impair hematopoietic differentiation and confer properties of self-renewal. Together these cooperating mutations induce the AML phenotype characterized by enhanced proliferative and survival advantage, impaired differentiation, and limitless self-renewal capacity. There is experimental evidence to support this model of cooperativity in murine models between BCR–ABL and NUP98–HOXA9,[86] TEL–PDGFβR and AML1–ETO,[134] and FLT3–ITD and PML–RARα.[135] These findings have important therapeutic implications, in that it may be possible to target both classes of mutations. For example, in acute promyelocytic leukemia with activating mutations in FLT3, it may be possible to target FLT3 with small-molecule inhibitors, and PML–RARα with ATRA (see Chapter 60, Fig. 60–2).[136] However, it is important to note that AML, as for other cancers, is likely the cause of multiple mutations. Although this "two-hit" paradigm provides a rationale for targeted therapeutic approaches to treatment of AML, it is likely that additional alleles are required for development of AML—and that these must be identified and studied in detail with attention to novel potential therapies.

SUGGESTED READINGS

Chan IT et al: Conditional expression of oncogenic K-ras from its endogenous promoter induces a myeloproliferative disease. J Clin Invest 113(4):528, 2004.

Cozzio A et al: Similar MLL-associated leukemias arising from self-renewing stem cells and short-lived myeloid progenitors. Genes Dev 17(24):3029, 2003.

Davidson AJ et al: cdx4 mutants fail to specify blood progenitors and can be rescued by multiple hox genes. Nature 425(6955):300, 2003.

Deguchi K et al: MOZ-TIF2-induced acute myeloid leukemia requires the MOZ nucleosome binding motif and TIF2-mediated recruitment of CBP. Cancer Cell 3(3):259, 2003.

Falini B et al: Acute myeloid leukemia carrying cytoplasmic/mutated nucleophosmin (NPMc+ AML): Biologic and clinical features. Blood 109:874, 2007.

Falini B et al: Cytoplasmic nucleophosmin in acute myelogenous leukemia with a normal karyotype. N Engl J Med 352:254, 2005.

Gilliland DG: FLT3-activating mutations in acute promyelocytic leukaemia: A rationale for risk-adapted therapy with FLT3 inhibitors. Best Pract Res Clin Haematol 16(3):409, 2003.

Griffith J et al: The structural basis for autoinhibition of FLT3 by the juxtamembrane domain. Mol Cell 13(2):169, 2004.

Grisolano JL et al: An activated receptor tyrosine kinase, TEL/PDGFbetaR, cooperates with AML1/ETO to induce acute myeloid leukemia in mice. Proc Natl Acad Sci USA 100(16):9506, 2003.

Hsieh JJ et al: Proteolytic cleavage of MLL generates a complex of N- and C-terminal fragments that confers protein stability and subnuclear localization. Mol Cell Biol 23(1):186, 2003.

Miralles F et al: Actin dynamics control SRF activity by regulation of its coactivator MAL. Cell 113:329, 2003.
Raffel GD et al: Ott1(Rbm15) has pleiotropic roles in hematopoietic development. Proc Natl Acad Sci USA 104:6001, 2007.
Rawat VP et al: Ectopic expression of the homeobox gene Cdx2 is the transforming event in a mouse model of t(12;13)(p13;q12) acute myeloid leukemia. Proc Natl Acad Sci USA 101(3):817, 2004.
Stirewalt DL, Radich JP: The role of FLT3 in haematopoietic malignancies. Nat Rev Cancer 3(9):650, 2003.

REFERENCES

For complete list of references log onto www.expertconsult.com

CHAPTER 60

CLINICAL MANIFESTATIONS OF ACUTE MYELOID LEUKEMIA

Kenneth B. Miller and German Pihan

Acute myeloid leukemia (AML) is not a single disease but a heterogeneous group of neoplastic disorders characterized by the proliferation and accumulation of immature hematopoietic cells in the bone marrow and blood. These malignant cells gradually replace and inhibit the growth and maturation of normal erythroid, myeloid, and megakaryocytic precursors.

The clinical evaluation and prognosis of patients with AML has changed dramatically over the last decade. The initial evaluation of a patient with acute leukemia should be directed at defining the factors that are important in assessing the long-term prognosis and planning treatment. Molecular, cytogenetic, and immunologic studies have contributed to our understanding of the pathogenesis and prognosis of the AMLs. The initial evaluation should address the patient's history of possible exposure to known or suspected environmental or occupational leukemogenic agents. A personal or family history of prior illnesses that predisposes the patient to development of AML is important in planning treatment. The new classification system for AML attempts to incorporate in the final diagnosis the patient's prior exposures to leukemogenic agents with the morphology and the molecular and cytogenetic markers.

HISTORY

In 1827 Velpeau reported the first accurate description of a case of leukemia. The patient was a 63-year-old florist who developed an illness characterized by fever, weakness, urinary stones, and massive hepatosplenomegaly. Velpeau reported that the blood of this patient was "like gruel." He speculated that the appearance of the blood was due to white corpuscles and that the unique appearance was not the result of an infection.

In 1845 Bennett, a brilliant and controversial pathologist from Edinburgh, reported a series of patients who died with enlarged spleens and changes in the "color and consistency of their blood."[1] Although he found no infectious etiology for the peculiar appearance of the blood, he attributed these changes to the presence of "purulent material" in the blood and introduced the term *leucocythemia*. Virchow, the noted German pathologist, reported a similar case. Virchow commented on the reversal of the normal ratio of pigmented red to colorless white cells in his patient but did not attribute these changes to an infection. Unsure of the etiology of his finding, he was content to simply describe his observations and used the descriptive name "white blood" and named the disorder *leukemia*, derived from the Greek meaning "white blood."[2]

In 1877 Ehrlich developed aniline-based stains for use on air-dried films of blood and described the appearance of normal and abnormal white blood cells (WBCs). In 1889 Ebstein introduced the term *acute leukemia* to describe a rapidly fatal illness that failed to respond to available therapy.[3] In 1869 Neumann first suggested that the WBCs were made in the bone marrow and not the spleen and proposed term the *myeloid*, meaning marrow-derived. In 1879 Mosler described the aspiration of bone marrow as a means to diagnose leukemia.[4] In 1900 Naegeli described the myeloblast and divided the leukemias into either myelocytic or lymphocytic.[5]

The development of cytogenetic, immunologic, molecular, and biochemical markers has helped to further define the lineage of the leukemic cell and to classify the leukemias. Effective therapy and advances in supportive care have changed the approach to the patient with AML from a disease that was uniformly and rapidly fatal to one that responds to chemotherapy and is potentially curable. The new classification of AML now attempts to incorporate clinically and biologically important disease characteristics to better define prognosis and plan treatment of this heterogeneous group of disorders.

ETIOLOGY

Approximately 8000 new cases of AML occur per year, and the incidence has remained stable over the last decade. AML represent approximately 1.2% of all cancer deaths in the United States.[6,7] AML is a disease of adults. The median age at diagnosis is 65 years, and the incidence increases with age (Fig. 60–1). AML represents approximately 90% of all acute leukemias in adults but accounts for only 13% of leukemia cases in children younger than 10 years. In children younger than 15 years, acute lymphoblastic leukemia (ALL) is approximately five times more common than AML.[8] The incidence of AML rises rapidly after age 50 years. The age-specific incidence is 3.5 : 100,000, 15 : 100,000, and 22 : 100,000 in individuals 50, 70, and 80 years, respectively. The incidence of secondary AML (therapy-related AML [t-AML]) appears to be increasing, currently accounting for 10% to 20% of all cases of AML in adults.[9] Drugs, genetic factors, and environmental and occupational exposures are implicated as possible leukemogenic agents in both children and adults (Table 60–1).[8–10] Leukemogenesis is a multistep process that requires the susceptibility of a hematopoietic progenitor cells to inductive agents at multiple stages. The different subtypes of AML may have distinct causal mechanisms, suggesting a functional link between a particular molecular abnormality or mutation and the causal agent.[11] No one factor has been shown to cause leukemia in all individuals exposed.

Evidence supporting a genetic predisposition for leukemia has come from epidemiologic and family studies.[12] The highest incidences of AML in adults are found in North America, western Europe, and Oceania; the lowest incidences are found in Asia and Latin America.[13,14] Acute promyelocytic leukemia (APL) is more common among populations of Latino or Hispanic background.[15,16] Moreover, APL in patients originating in Latin America and southern Europe is associated with an increased frequency of the breakpoint in the promyelocytic leukemia gene *(PML)* at intron 6 representing the breakpoint cluster region 1 (BCR1). This higher rate of BCR1 APL subtype in Latin Americans is, in part, genetically determined and may be related to the American Indian forebears who immigrated to the Americas from eastern Asia approximately 12,000 years ago.[15,17] Individuals with APL have a significant greater body mass index than do patients with other types of AML.[18] This observation may be explained by the involvement of the retinoic acid receptor α *(RARA)* gene in the regulation of both hematopoiesis and adipogenesis. APL presenting as a secondary or treatment-related leukemia also has unique clinical and epidemiologic features. The secondary APLs are more often associated with a prior exposure to an anthracycline, and the breakpoint in the *PML* gene is different from de novo APL.[19] The highest incidence of secondary APL was in women with breast or ovarian cancer. Patients with breast cancer may have an increased risk for APL that is further increased by administration of anthracycline chemotherapy.[20]

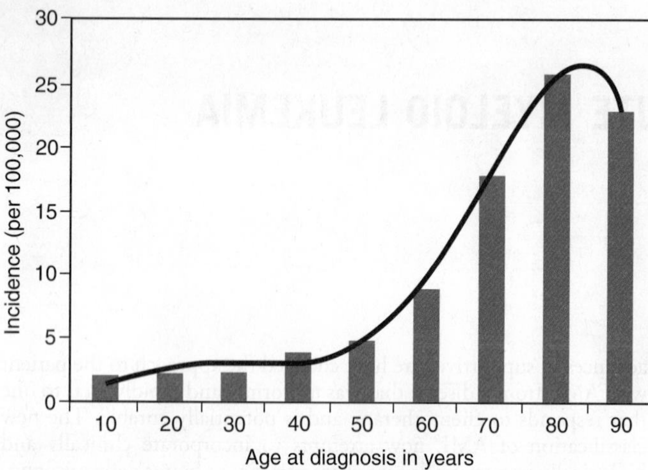

Figure 60–1 Age-specific incidence of acute myeloid leukemia in the United States.

Table 60–1. Risk Factors for Development of Acute Myeloid Leukemia

Genetic Disorders
Down syndrome
Bloom syndrome
Klinefelter syndrome
Patau syndrome
Ataxia-telangiectasia
Neurofibromatosis
Shwachman syndrome
Kostmann syndrome
Fanconi anemia
Li-Fraumeni syndrome
von Recklinghausen disease
Congenital neurofibromatosis
Familial platelet disorder syndrome
Acquired Disorders
Myeloproliferative disorders
Myelodysplastic syndromes
Aplastic anemia
Paroxysmal nocturnal hemoglobinuria
Multiple myeloma
Nonseminomatous mediastinal germ cell tumors
Physical and Chemical Exposure
Benzene
Cigarettes
Embalming fluid (ethylene oxide)
Thorotrast
Radiation (therapeutic and nontherapeutic)
Chemotherapy

Genetic Factors

Multiple cases of both acute lymphoblastic leukemia (ALL) and AML occurring within the same family have been reported.[21,22] The concordance of each of the leukemia subtypes in families is more common than would be expected based on chance alone.[22] Reports of familial leukemia suggest that highly penetrant mutations in leukemia-susceptible genes could be a common mechanism of inherited AML.[23,24]

For all types of AML, a threefold increase in leukemia incidence is observed among first-degree relatives of patients with acute leukemia.[25] Monozygotic twins have an increased concordance for childhood leukemia. If one twin develops leukemia before age 6 years, the second twin has up to 25% risk of developing leukemia.[26] The clinical presentation of AML in monozygotic twins is atypical. The leukemia usually occurs before age 2 years; it occurs in both twins in close succession, typically in the same year; and it is of the same morphologic and cytogenetic subtype.[27] These results suggest a single cell origin of the AML occurring simultaneously in both twins or more likely a single leukemogenic event occurring in utero affecting both twins as a result of shared placental fetal circulation.[22,28,29] No similar excess of leukemia has been observed in nonidentical twins. Moreover, adult twin studies do not demonstrate such a high concordance for acute leukemia.[30]

The existence of a genetic predisposition to development of AML is suggested by the increased leukemia incidence associated with a number of congenital disorders. In Down syndrome (DS; trisomy 21), the incidence of acute leukemia before age 4 to 5 years is 150 times that of the general population, and the incidence of megakaryoblastic leukemia is 500 times higher than expected.[31–33] Moreover, families with a DS child may have be an increased incidence of acute leukemias in the genetically normal parents and siblings.[25,34,35] These reports of familial clustering of DS and leukemia have led to speculations that an inherited mutation in a group of mutator genes subsequently could induce karyotype instability that results in an increased risk for developing leukemia.[36] The AML in DS, classified as myeloid leukemia of Down syndrome (ML-DS), is associated with mutations in exon 2 of the transcription factor GATA1, which is acquired in utero.[37] The GATA1 mutation appears to be unique to DS and is detectable in virtually all cases of ML-DS.

The risk of childhood AML appears to increase with increasing maternal age.[38–40] The risk of childhood leukemia also is higher in children born to mothers who smoke and higher in children of women with a history of multiple miscarriages.[41] Moreover, in a case-control study, paternal preconception smoking was associated with an increased incidence of AML in the children.[42] Mothers of children with AML diagnosed before age 2 age had a fivefold increase in previous fetal loss and a 12-fold increase in two or more fetal losses.[24]

Disorders associated with chromosomal instability and increased chromosome breakage, including Fanconi anemia, ataxia telangiectasia, Bloom syndrome, and Kostmann syndrome, are associated with an increased incidence of AML.[43–45] The genetic disorders presumably give rise to a cellular environment that results in chromosomal instability, hypersensitivity to DNA damage, and increased susceptibility to mutations.[43] von Recklinghausen disease (congenital neurofibromatosis) is associated with an increased incidence of childhood AML.[44] Klinefelter syndrome (XXY) and Patau syndrome (trisomy 13) have been associated with an increased incidence of AML.[41]

Family studies suggest that the increased incidence of AML is part of a multistep process originating in leukemia-susceptible genes.[46,47] The initial molecular events leading to AML may not be localized to the cytogenetic deletions and translocations noted in the leukemic cell but rather predispose the cell to acquire the observed secondary mutations and cytogenetic translocations.[23] Hematopoietic transcription factors are frequent targets for leukemia-associated gene rearrangements.[48] The *AML1* (acute myeloid leukemia 1) gene, located on chromosome 21q22, is also called *RUNX1* (Runt-related protein 1) or *CBFA* (core-binding factor-α). RUNX1 is a highly conserved transcription factor that is critical for normal hematopoiesis. Mutations in the gene encoding AML1/RUNX1 have been in identified in families with an autosomal dominant syndrome called *familial platelet disorder*, members of which have a propensity to develop familial platelet disorder AML.[40] Mutations in the *AML1* gene may result in defective DNA binding, which leads to secondary karyotypic abnormalities that result in the development of AML. Although *AML1* mutations are present in the germline of these families, affected individuals do not develop AML until later in life. Mutations of *CEBPA*, the gene that encodes the granulocytic differentiation factor CCAAT/enhancer binding protein (C/EBP) α, has been shown to be the primary events in some forms of familial leukemia.[47] The factors responsible for the additional mutations necessary for the development of AML are not known.

Exposure History

Exposure to ionizing radiation and a number of chemicals has been linked to the development of acute leukemia. The evidence linking radiation exposure and leukemia comes in part from the long-term followup of survivors of the atomic bomb explosions in Hiroshima and Nagasaki.[49–52] The latency time from exposure to the development of leukemia was between 5 and 21 years, and the risk was related to age at the time of exposure and to radiation dose.[51] The development of leukemia was predictable and dose related. In Hiroshima, individuals had a 30-fold increased incidence of both AML and chronic myelogenous leukemia (CML). The highest rates were observed in persons younger than 10 years or older than 50 years at the time of exposure. In Nagasaki, where victims were exposed to a higher amount of gamma radiation, the incidence of AML was even greater.[53]

Exposure to even moderate doses of radiation is associated with an increased risk for developing AML. Workers at radium plants and military personnel exposed to ionizing radiation during nuclear test explosions have a higher than expected incidence of AML.[54,55] Patients who received low doses of radiation for treatment of benign disorders, such as ankylosing spondylitis,[56,57] menorrhagia,[58] tinea capitis,[59] benign thymic enlargement,[59] and rheumatoid arthritis,[60] develop AML at a greater than expected rate. Exposure to thorotrast, a colloidal suspension of thorium dioxide used widely in the 1940s as a radiographic contrast medium, has been associated with an increased risk of AML, specifically the acute erythroleukemia subtype.[61] The principal thorium isotope is ^{232}Th, which on decay exposes the individual to chronic low-dose α particles. The thorotrast-associated leukemia occurred 10 to 30 years after exposure. The genetic events resulting in the increased incidence of AML in individuals exposed to low doses of radiation are unclear but may be related to somatic point mutations of the *AML1* gene.[62]

Exposure to extremely-low-frequency electromagnetic fields generated by high-voltage power lines has been reported to be associated with an increased incidence of acute leukemia, but this association remains controversial and unproven.[63] It is unclear from the reported cohort and case-control studies whether exposure to electromagnetic radiation generated from wiring and power lines is physiologically, clinically, or epidemiologically important.[64,65]

Chronic exposure to a number of chemicals has been associated with the development of acute leukemia. Benzene is the best studied and has been the most widely used chemical leukemogenic agent.[66–69] Leather and rubber industry workers chronically exposed to benzene and benzene derivatives have a significantly increased incidence of AML.[70] Case-control studies have found that truck drivers, filling station attendants, workers in petroleum and gas plants, and painters have an increased incidence of AML, which perhaps is related to their chronic exposure to benzene and other hydrocarbons.[71–74] Persons exposed to embalming fluid, ethylene oxides, and herbicides may be at increased risk for acute leukemia.[75] Workers exposed to organic solvents used in the processing of medical radiographs and the manufacturing of electrical wiring may have an increased incidence of AML.[76] The interpretation of many of these case–control studies has been challenged, and the overall risk of leukemia for individuals exposed remains controversial. Cigarette smokers and individuals chronically exposed to cigarette smoke appear to be at increased risk for developing AML.[77,78] Heavy cigarette smoking is associated with the development of clonal, nonrandom, cytogenetic abnormalities.[79] Cigarette smoke contains measurable quantities of benzene, and metabolites of benzene are found in the urine of chronic cigarette smokers.[80,81]

Therapy-Related Acute Myeloid Leukemia

An increased incidence of acute leukemia has been reported in patients who received chemotherapy for a number of malignant and nonmalignant disorders (Table 60–2). Most commonly these secondary t-AMLs occur after administration of either alkylating agents or topoisomerase II inhibitors.[9,82] Estimating the risk of developing AML after chemotherapy is confounded by the frequent use of combination therapy; an increased risk of leukemia may be part of the natural history of various treated disorders. The combination of chemotherapy and radiation therapy further increases the risk of developing leukemia.[9,83]

Table 60–2 Drugs Associated with Increased Risks of Myelodysplastic Syndrome and Acute Myeloid Leukemia

Alkylating Agents	
Mechlorethamine	Cyclophosphamide
Ifosfamide	Busulfan
Melphalan	Chlorambucil
Carmustine	Lomustine
Cisplatin	Carboplatin
Topoisomerase II Inhibitors	
Etoposide	Teniposide
Doxorubicin	Daunorubicin
4-Epidoxorubicin	Mitoxantrone
Other Agents	
Procarbazine	Hydroxyurea[a]
Fludarabine[a]	Paclitaxel[a]
Docetaxel[a]	Irinotecan[a]
Methoxypsoralen[a]	Chloroquine[a]
Chloramphenicol[a]	Topotecan[a]

[a]Association is unclear and based on a limited number of case reports.

The t-AMLs are associated with clonal cytogenetic abnormalities, a defined clinical course, and a poor response to standard treatments. The risk of developing t-AML is proportional to the age of the patient, the cumulative dose of the administered alkylating agent, and the underlying disease. In Hodgkin lymphoma, the cumulative risk of developing AML after treatment with alkylating agents increases steadily 1 year after start of treatment and reaches a peak of 13% at 7 years.[84,85] The incidence of AML in patients treated with the mechlorethamine-Oncovin [vincristine]-procarbazine-prednisone (MOPP) regimen containing the alkylating agent mechlorethamine is 3%, 4%, and 7% at 3, 5, and 7 years, respectively. This is in contrast to a less than 1% incidence of AML in patients treated with a regimen that does not include alkylating agents or with radiation therapy alone. AML occurs after autologous bone marrow and stem cell transplants. The actuarial risk for secondary AML after chemoradiation therapy and autologous transplantation for Hodgkin lymphomas is between 6.8% and 18% at 10 years after transplant and is determined in part by the type and intensity of the pretransplant chemotherapy with alkylating agents.[86–88] Patients older than 40 years at the time of transplant who received prior radiation therapy or four or more chemotherapy regimens and required more than 5 days of apheresis to harvest sufficient cells and receive total body irradiation as part of the preparative regimen were at highest risk for developing AML.[89,90]

An increased incidence of leukemia has been reported in patients receiving alkylating agents for malignant and nonmalignant disorders.[91,92] Therapy-related leukemias now represent between 10% and 20% of all cases of AML. The t-AMLs are clinically and prognostically different from AML that occurs de novo. The t-AMLs are divided into two distinct types based on the type of agents administered.[19,83,93] The *alkylating agent–associated t-AMLs* usually are preceded by a variable period of myelodysplasia characterized by anemia, neutropenia, or thrombocytopenia. Clonal, nonrandom, cytogenetic abnormalities involving chromosomes 7, 5, and 8 in addition to other complex abnormalities occur in 50% to 90% of patients.[94] This pattern reflects the multistep process of alkylating agent–induced leukemia, which likely involves DNA damage-induced genomic instability and mitotic recombination with gain of oncogenes and loss of tumor suppressor genes.[94] These t-AMLs are associated with an overall poor prognosis.

A clinically and cytogenetically distinct group of secondary leukemias has been reported in individuals who have received a topoisomerase II inhibitor.[95,96] This group includes the epipodophyllotoxins etoposide and teniposide and the anthracyclines daunomycin, mitoxantrone, and doxorubicin. The topoisomerase II inhibitors cause DNA damage via the intranuclear enzyme topoisomerase II. In contrast to alkylating agent–related AML, the *topoisomerase II–related t-AMLs* typically lack a preceding myelodysplastic phase and are characterized by a shorter latency of onset, generally less than 2 to 3 years.[97–99] These topoisomerase II–related t-AMLs are associated with chromosomal rearrangement involving chromosomes 3, 11, and 21 and characterized by a balanced translocation involving bands 11q23. They typically lack numerical chromosome abnormalities or complex karyotypes, a feature that may reflect the mechanism of topoisomerase II–induced genetic damage, which includes DNA cleavage at hotspots follow by illegitimate recombination.[100–102] The mixed lineage or myeloid–lymphoid leukemia *(MLL)* gene located on chromosome 11 band q23 is the most frequent site of the leukemogenic translocation induced by topoisomerase II inhibitors.[94] The treatment outcome for these patients is much worse than for patients with de novo AML having similar clinical and cytogenetic abnormalities. Secondary acute promyelocytic leukemia (t-APL) usually is associated with exposure to an anthracycline (mitoxantrone) and less often VP-16.[18] Unlike other t-AMLs, t-APL does not have a different prognosis from the de novo APL.[18]

In patients treated with adjuvant chemotherapy for breast cancer, the risk of developing AML/myelodysplastic syndrome (MDS) is related to the dose of both epirubicin (a topoisomerase II inhibitor) and cyclophosphamide (Cytoxan). The incidence of AML/MDS was 0.37% compared with 4.97% for the low and high doses of epirubicin and cyclophosphamide, respectively. Moreover, the risk for secondary AML/MDS may be more closely related with the dose intensity of the treatment than with the cumulative dose and may be independently correlated with the granulocyte colony stimulating factor (G-CSF) dose used.[103] The association between use of G-CSF and development of AML/MDS remains controversial. In a retrospective analysis, use of G-CSF after immunosuppressive therapy for severe aplastic anemia was associated with an increased incidence of AML/MDS: 10.9% versus 5.8% in patients who did or did not receive G-CSF, respectively.[104] A similar increased risk of AML/MDS after immunosuppressive therapy was noted in patients treated with G-CSF for severe congenital neutropenia.[105] The role of colony-stimulating factors in the development of MDS/AML in high-risk patients is unclear and may be confounded by other factors such as age and prior treatments.[106]

In children with ALL, the incidence of t-AML after exposure to one of the epipodophyllotoxins is approximately 5%.[98] However, in children with a T-cell ALL who received a topoisomerase II inhibitor, the incidence of t-AML is 19%. Cytogenetic studies suggest that the second leukemogenic event occurs in a normal hematopoietic progenitor and not in the initial ALL leukemic cell. The outcome for these children treated with standard cytotoxic chemotherapy is poor. Cases of t-AML with inv[16] or t(8;21) occurring after therapy with a topoisomerase II inhibitor have been reported.[107,108] These leukemias are associated with rearrangements of the CBF genes *AML1/CBFA* at 21q22 and *CBFB* at 16q22.[107,108] As with other secondary leukemias, a genetic predisposition for AML has been proposed.[109] Individual differences in DNA stability and repair as well as variations in metabolism of chemotherapy may be important contributing factors. Polymorphism of the glutathione transferase gene *GSTP1* and the NAD(P)H:quinone oxidoreductase NQ01 is overrepresented in some patients with t-AML.[109,110]

Drugs other than the cytotoxic agents reported to be associated with development of acute leukemia include chloramphenicol,[111] phenylbutazone,[112] chloroquine,[113] and methoxypsoralen.[114] The strength of these associations remains unclear.

Certain acquired diseases are associated with transformation to AML. Patients with one of the myeloproliferative disorders, including polycythemia vera, essential thrombocythemia, chronic idiopathic myeloid metaplasia, and myelofibrosis, have an increased incidence of leukemic transformation. In patients with polycythemia vera, the incidence of AML is only approximately 1% for those treated only with periodic phlebotomies.[115] However, addition of chemotherapy or radiation therapy significantly increases the incidence of AML.[92,116–118] The incidence of AML appears to be related to the intensity and duration of the alkylating agent therapy. The relative risk for AML was 4 to 10 times greater for patients treated with daily continuous alkylating agents versus administration of intermittent pulse treatment.[116] Aplastic anemia is associated with late development of acute leukemia.[119] In patients with aplastic anemia treated successfully with antithymocyte globulin, 26% developed AML or one of the MDSs after 8 years. The risk for AML appears higher in patients with aplastic anemia occurring after irradiation or chemical exposure.[120] AML occurs in patients with paroxysmal nocturnal hemoglobinuria and appears to involve the same clone from which the abnormal erythrocytes are derived.[121] Multiple myeloma is associated with the development of AML.[122] The association between AML, multiple myeloma, and administration of multiple alkylating drugs is well documented, but AML can occur in patients with myeloma who have not received prior chemotherapy or radiation therapy.[123]

Primary nonseminomatous mediastinal germ cell tumors are associated with development of the acute megakaryocytic subtype of AML.[124] The secondary leukemias may be associated with the primary germ cell tumor and not result from the chemotherapy administered.[125] A number of AML subtypes are characterized by mutations that confer a proliferative or survival advantage to hematopoietic progenitors without altering differentiation. Mutations of members of the *RAS*, *FLT-3*, *KIT*, and other hematopoietic signaling molecules may play an important role in the proliferation and response to treatment. These factors must work in concert with additional acquired genetic lesions to affect both differentiation and proliferations resulting in AML. FLT-3 is a receptor tyrosine kinase and is important in hematopoietic stem cell survival and proliferation.[126] FLT-3 is mutated in approximately 25% to 30% of AMLs either by internal tandem duplications (ITDs) of the juxtamembrane domain or by point mutations of the kinase domain. It is one of the most frequent somatic alterations in AML. Both types of mutations activate FLT-3. Mutations in FLT-3 are associated with a poor prognosis. AML with *FLT-3*/ITD mutation is associated with a very poor prognosis that is independent of other prognostic factors.[127] However, the prognosis is partly dependent on the ratio of mutant to wild-type *FLT-3* as well as the size of the ITD. Larger ITDs appear to have a poorer prognosis.[128]

CLINICAL MANIFESTATIONS

The presenting signs and symptoms of AML are nonspecific and are related to decreased production of normal hematopoietic cells and invasion of other organs by the leukemic cells. Patients usually complain of a brief viral-like illness characterized by fatigue and malaise or may present with a progressive skin infection after a minor abrasion. Although anorexia is common, weight loss is unusual, generally reflecting the acute onset of the disease. Diffuse bone tenderness involving the long bones, ribs, and sternum is the initial clinical manifestation in 25% of patients. Joint pain and swelling, localized to large joints, may antedate other symptoms by weeks. The bone pain, which can be severe, is caused by expansion of the intramedullary space or direct involvement of the periosteum by the leukemic cells.

Findings on physical examination relate to the interference with normal hematopoiesis by the leukemic cells. Typically, in AML all three cell lines are affected. Anemia results in pallor and cardiovascular symptoms. Thrombocytopenia produces hemostatic defects, which result in petechiae and ecchymosis. Oozing from the gums, epistaxis, and excess bleeding after dental procedures or minor trauma are common initial manifestations. Petechiae are most prominent in the lower extremities and may appear suddenly after minor physical

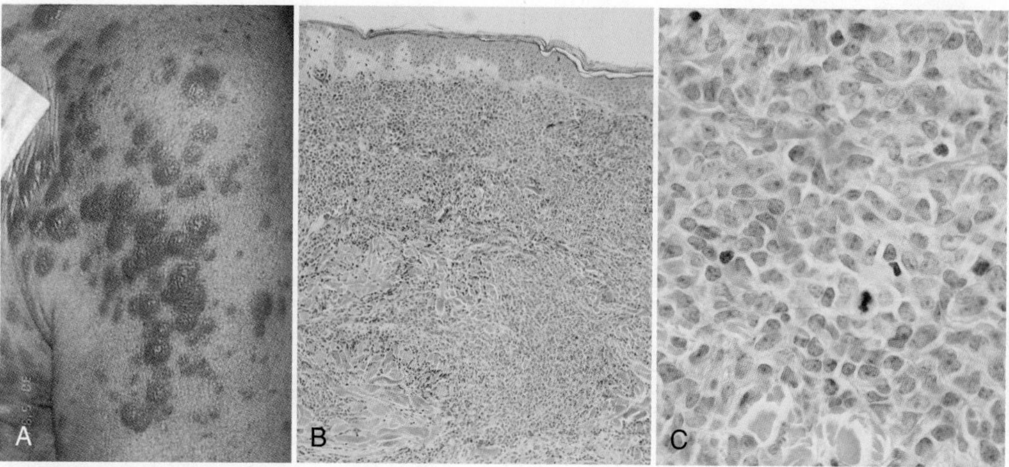

Figure 60–2 A, Leukemia cutis in a patient with monoblastic leukemia. **B,** TK, Tyrosime Kinase.

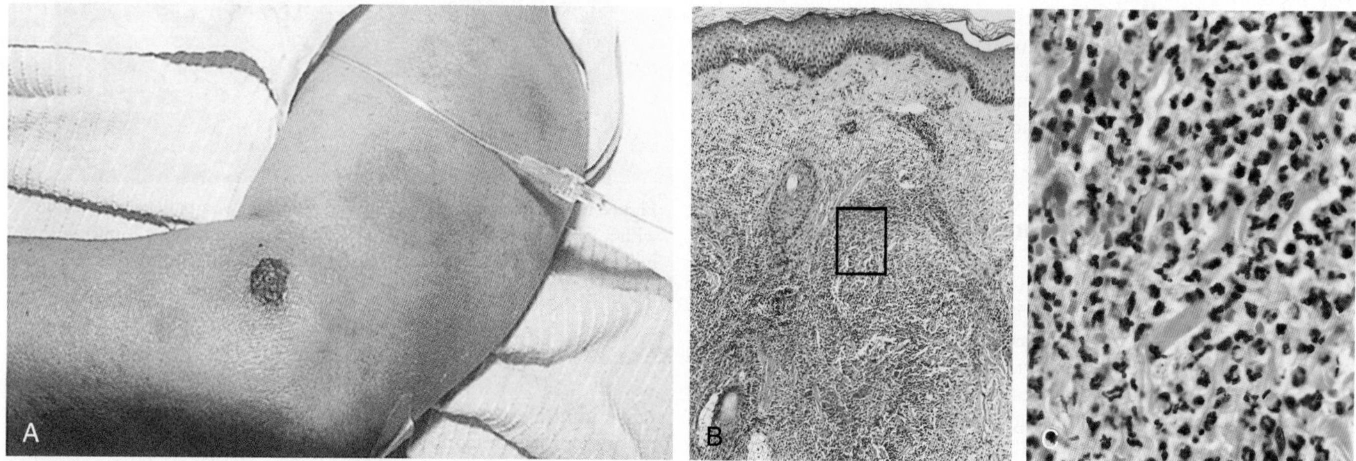

Figure 60–3 A, Sweet syndrome in a patient with acute myeloid leukemia. Tender, pseudovesicular, erythematous plaques are a characteristic feature of this syndrome. (From Cohen PR: Acral erythema: A clinical review. Cutis 51:175, 1993, with permission.) **B,** Histologic features of an early skin lesion in Sweet syndrome at low magnification (40×). **C,** Histologic features of an early skin lesion in Sweet syndrome at high magnification (600×, hematoxylin and eosin stain).

activity. Splenomegaly occurs in up to 50% of patients with AML, but the splenic enlargement usually is modest and rarely extends more than 5 cm below the left costal margin. A very large spleen suggests that the leukemia has evolved from an preexisting chronic myeloproliferative disorder. Lymphadenopathy is rare in AML, in contrast to ALL, in which lymphadenopathy may be a prominent presenting finding. Involvement of the thymus or hilar nodes is very uncommon in AML. Skin involvement (leukemia cutis) occurs in approximately 10% of patients and usually presents as violaceous, raised, nontender plaques or nodules, which on biopsy are found to be infiltrated with myeloblasts (Fig. 60–1). Diffuse involvement of the skin may be seen. Biopsy may reveal prominent diffuse infiltrate involving the deep dermal surface but preservation of the superficial dermis (Fig. 60–2). Skin involvement is more common with the monocytic leukemic subtypes.[129] Sweet syndrome (acute neutrophilic dermatosis) is a cutaneous paraneoplastic syndrome that is associated with AML and other hematologic disorders.[130] It is characterized by fever and tender red plaques and nodules usually on the extremities. Sweet syndrome may precede the diagnosis of AML by several months (Fig. 60–3). Sweet syndrome is more common in the monocytic leukemias. The histologic finding in Sweet syndrome consists of a dense infiltrate primarily composed of mature neutrophils located predominantly in the mid and upper dermis.[131] Sweet syndrome may be associated with leukemia cutis. Skin lesions reveal the presence of leukemia cutis, with abnormal mature neutrophils and blast forms.[132] The pathogenesis of Sweet syndrome in AML is unknown. It has been postulated that leukemia-related growth factors (interleukin [IL]-1, IL-6, or G-CSF) directly or indirectly stimulate epidermal or dermal cells, which inducing the local accumulation of neutrophils. In some patients the neutrophils appear to be clonal and are derived from the leukemic cell, possibly as a result of chemotherapy-induced differentiation.[133] Sweet syndrome may occur in patients with normal, low, or elevated white blood counts. Similar lesions have been noted in patients with inflammatory diseases and associated with use of G-CSF.[133] Systemic steroids are the treatment of choice for leukemia associated Sweet syndrome and usually result in prompt improvement and resolution of the clinical symptoms and lesions.[134]

Myeloid granulocytic sarcomas (chloromas) are collections of blasts in extramedullary sites, which may present as isolated subcutaneous masses and may be confused with a primary or metastatic carcinoma.[135,136] The term *chloromas* is derived from the greenish appearance on sectioning, which is secondary to the presence of myeloperoxidase (MPO) granules in the myeloblasts. Myeloid sarcomas may precede the development of AML and are more common in the undifferentiated and minimally differentiated AML subtypes.[137] The presence of extramedullary leukemia is associated with a generally poorer response to treatment and shorter overall survival.[138] However, the presence of extramedullary disease may be a biologic marker for other adverse prognostic factors and therefore not an independent predictor of response.[139] Gingival hyperplasia caused by

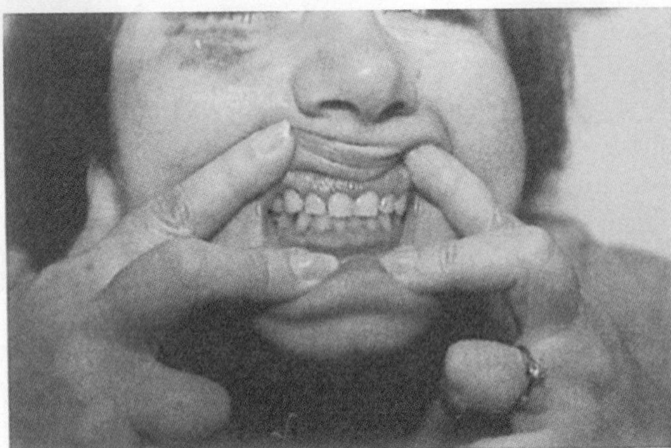

Figure 60–4 Gingival infiltration in a patient with myelomonocytic leukemia.

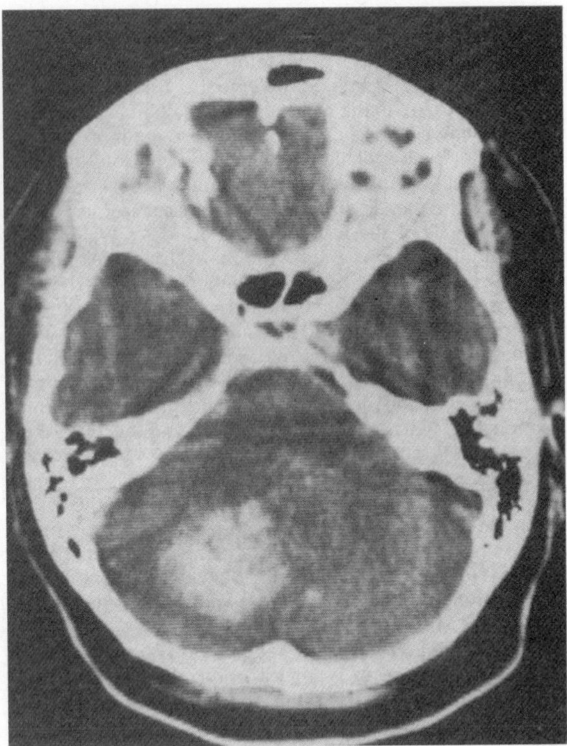

Figure 60–5 Head computed tomographic scan of a patient presenting with a white blood cell count of 100,000/mm³ and massive intracranial hemorrhage secondary to leukostasis.

leukemic infiltration is more frequent in the monocytic leukemias (Fig. 60–4) but may occur in all the leukemic subtypes. The patient initially may present to a dentist complaining of painful gums, rapidly progressive gingival disease, and gum bleeding after dental brushing.

Central and Peripheral Nervous System Manifestations

Central nervous system (CNS) involvement in AML is an uncommon presenting finding. From 5% to 7% of all patients have asymptomatic CNS involvement as determined by positive cerebrospinal fluid cytology.[140] Magnetic resonance imaging is the imaging study of choice to detect meningeal involvement in suspected cases of CNS leukemia.[141] The finding of asymptomatic CNS disease does not alone appear to predict a poor prognosis.[142] Patients at highest risk for developing CNS leukemia include those with a high circulating blast count, elevated lactate dehydrogenase activity, and one of the monocytic leukemic subtypes.[143,144] Of note is the very high frequency of CNS involvement, up to 35%, in AML with increased eosinophils [M4Eo variant in the French-American-British (FAB) classification; AML with abnormal bone marrow eosinophils and inv[16] (p13;q22) in the World Health Organization (WHO) classification], which is associated with inversion of chromosome 16. Leptomeningeal leukemia and intracerebral myeloid sarcomas occur frequently in this otherwise prognostically favorable subtype.[145] Unless signs of overt CNS involvement requiring therapy is evident, it is preferable to defer a lumbar puncture until the peripheral blasts have been cleared with chemotherapy in order to prevent accidental contamination of the spinal fluid with leukemic cells.[89,146] AML may recur in the CNS without evidence of systemic disease. Effective treatment of the CNS disease with either intrathecal chemotherapy and/or radiation therapy does not appear to prevent the subsequent development of recurrence in the bone marrow. Recurrence in the CNS has been associated with an overall poor prognosis.[147]

The majority of patients with leukemic involvement of the CNS are asymptomatic; however, some patients present with meningeal signs and symptoms associated with increased intracranial pressure. In these patients a lumbar puncture is required and typically reveals an elevated opening pressure with increased protein level and low glucose concentration in the cerebrospinal fluid. The cell count may be low; therefore, a cytocentrifuge preparation of the cerebrospinal fluid is required to detect the presence of leukemic cells. Cranial nerve palsies secondary to leukemic infiltration of the nerve sheath occur but are rare in AML. The fifth and seventh cranial nerves are most frequently involved.[148–150] Patients may present with sudden onset of facial muscle weakness, which rapidly progresses to paralysis. Optic nerve infiltration can result in papilledema, eye pain, blurred vision, or sudden onset of unilateral blindness. Retinopathy can occur and result in progressive impairment of vision.[149] Cranial nerve involvement can occur in the absence of overt CNS disease, and in these cases the cerebrospinal fluid may be negative for leukemic cells.[150] Magnetic resonance imaging of the affected nerve root may demonstrate thickening of the nerve sheath, which is suggestive of leukemic involvement. The affected cranial nerve roots should be irradiated as soon as possible after onset of symptoms to prevent permanent loss of function.[149] Patients presenting with neurologic findings and greater than 50,000/μL circulating leukemic cells are at high risk for a major CNS event and require emergency intervention to rapidly lower the blast count. The high number of circulating blasts increases the blood viscosity and is associated with small-vessel leukoblastic emboli, resulting in leukostasis in the cerebral vessels.[151] The leukemic blasts can infiltrate the arteriolar endothelial walls and cause secondary hemorrhage. Suspected or developing CNS leukostasis requires emergency efforts to rapidly lower the blast count and maintain the platelet count greater than 25,000/μL.[151–153] The combination of hyperleukocytosis and thrombocytopenia is associated with an increased risk for CNS hemorrhage.[152] Patients may complain of diffuse headaches and fatigue, which rapidly progress to confusion and coma. Leukostatic hemorrhage clinically resembles a major cerebrovascular accident (Fig. 60–5). Adhesion and aggregation of leukemic cells as well as local anatomic factors appear to play a role in development of CNS leukostasis.[153] Leukostasis is more intensive in the white matter and leptomeninges, with involvement of medium-sized vessels. The risk of CNS leukostasis rapidly increases when the blast count (blasts plus promyelocytes) is greater than 50,000/μL.[154] Patients with hyperleukocytosis generally should not receive red cells in order to avoid a further increase in blood viscosity. Despite most efforts to rapidly lower the white blood count and the blood viscosity, the prognosis for patients with CNS leukostasis remains very poor.[153]

Metabolic and Electrolyte Abnormalities

Metabolic and electrolyte derangements are common in patients with AML due to either leukemic organ infiltration or the effects of the cytotoxic chemotherapy and concomitant medications.[155] Hyperuricemia is the most frequent leukemia-related biochemical abnormality. It results from increased turnover of the proliferating leukemic clone and subsequent purine catabolism. Hyperuricemia and hyperuricuria can develop before therapy is started. Typically, however, the uric acid level rises rapidly once therapy is initiated as a result of release of intracellular nucleic acids by lysis of large numbers of cells. Urate crystals can precipitate in the renal tubules and ureters, causing acute renal failure. To prevent the development of urate nephropathy, all patients should receive intravenous hydration and should be started on allopurinol before chemotherapy is started. Allopurinol, by inhibiting xanthine oxidase, causes an increase in urine xanthine levels and can produce xanthine crystalluria. Xanthine nephrolithiasis and xanthine nephropathy resulting in acute renal failure, which is a rare complication associated with administration of allopurinol and chemotherapy-induced tumor lysis.[156] It is important to maintain adequate hydration as well as to administer allopurinol before and during induction chemotherapy. Alternatively, rasburicase, an analogue of urate oxidase that converts uric acid to allantois, which is five times more soluble than uric acid, is given intravenously and is not associated with elevated xanthine levels.[157] Rarely, leukemic cells produce an obstructive uropathy as a result of direct infiltration of the prostate gland.[158] Direct bilateral cortical, medullary, and interstitial kidney involvement with myeloblasts may rarely result in renal failure.[159,160] However, in AML, in contrast to ALL, kidney infiltration with blasts is uncommon.

Hypokalemia is a common finding in patients with AML.[155,161] The hypokalemia, which can be profound and require large doses of intravenous potassium, is most pronounced in the myelomonocytic and monocytic leukemias.[162] Ineffective myelopoiesis or destruction of the leukemic cells with therapy causes release of large amounts of lysozyme from the leukemic blasts. This enzyme is toxic to renal tubular cells, resulting in proximal renal tubular dysfunction and leading to renal potassium wasting. In most cases, however, lysozyme-induced tubular damage is not the sole mechanism of the hypokalemia.[163] Attempts to directly correlate elevated serum and urinary lysozyme levels with the leukemic subtype and the development of hypokalemia and the renal tubular defect have produced conflicting results.[164,165] Hypokalemia also may be induced by potassium entry into the metabolically active leukemic cell, which has higher sodium/potassium adenosine triphosphatase activity.[161] Leukemic cells can synthesize other factors, such as renin-like activity that may contribute to the development hypokalemia.[166] Renal potassium wasting with inappropriate kaliuresis is associated with hypomagnesemia.[155] Antibiotics and chemotherapy-induced nephropathy, diarrhea and vomiting contribute to the development of hypomagnesemia and hypokalemia during and prior to induction therapy. Hyperkalemia is a rare finding in patients with AML unless renal failure or a tumor lysis syndrome develops. Pseudohyperkalemia may occur in patients with hyperleukocytosis due to lysis of the leukemic cells and release of intracellular K^+ in collection vials in the laboratory.[167]

Hypercalcemia has been reported in association with AML.[168] The mechanism is unclear but may be related to the release of parathyroid hormone (PTH) or PTH-like fragments produced by leukemic cells.[169] The hypercalcemia may be caused by direct bone involvement or stimulation of osteoclasts and the development of lytic bone lesions.[170,171] In these instances, the blood calcium level parallels the activity of disease. Hypocalcemia presumably as a result of release by leukemic cells of factors that result in accelerated bone formation has been reported. The hypocalcemia is associated with hypoalbuminemia in many patients. The most common cause of the hypocalcemia is the coexisting hypomagnesemia, which impairs release of PTH and induces resistance to PTH.[155] The hypocalcemia can be profound, and patients can present with tetany and potentially fatal cardiac arrhythmias. The hyperphosphatemia and hyperphosphaturia associated with underlying renal insufficiency also can contribute to the hypocalcemia.

Rapid lysis of leukemic cells can acutely precipitate a number of serious metabolic problems due to release of intracellular phosphate, potassium, and urate. Tumor lysis syndrome is characterized by rapid development of hyperuricemia, hyperkalemia, hyperphosphatemia, and hypocalcemia.[172,173] The consequences of tumor lysis syndrome are directly related to metabolic abnormalities: hyperuricemia produces urate nephropathy and acute renal failure; hyperkalemia is associated with potentially lethal cardiac arrhythmias; and hyperphosphatemia causes reciprocal depression of serum calcium level and progressive renal insufficiency, with further reduction of excretion of potassium and phosphate. Hypocalcemia, a result of hyperphosphatemia, can cause tetany, cardiac arrhythmias, and muscle cramps. The tumor lysis syndrome is rare in patients with AML. Tumor lysis is more common in patients who present with an elevated WBC count and elevated serum creatinine, uric acid, and lactate dehydrogenase (LDH) levels.[174,175] It is important to recognize patients at risk for this syndrome and to address and correct metabolic and electrolyte abnormalities before starting therapy. Allopurinol and intravenous hydration should be started before beginning chemotherapy. Renal function can rapidly deteriorate, and patients should be monitored daily to correct developing electrolyte abnormalities. Dialysis may be required and should be considered early in the course to prevent the complications of rapidly rising serum potassium, phosphate, and uric acid levels.[176] In the majority of patients, recovery of renal function after tumor lysis occurs early, and most patients can be supported through the relatively brief period of renal insufficiency.[177] Even with careful attention to electrolyte levels and use of intensive hydration, patients still may develop tumor lysis syndrome and acute renal failure. In the majority of patients with AML, development of renal insufficiency is associated with acute tubular necrosis, sepsis, and use of nephrotoxic drugs.[177] Use of nephrotoxic antibiotics and other medications is a frequent contributing factor to the development of renal failure during induction therapy.

Lactic acidosis has been associated with AML.[178] The etiology of this metabolic acidosis is unclear but may be the result of anaerobic glycolysis by the leukemia cells. When lactic acidosis occurs, it usually is associated with a very high or rapidly rising blast count, extramedullary disease, and leukostasis. The lactic acidosis parallels disease activity in these cases and improves with treatment of the leukemia.[179]

A spuriously low serum glucose level, potassium level, and arterial oxygen saturation can occur in the presence of high numbers of circulating blasts.[180] These spuriously low values reflect use by the leukemic blasts of glucose, potassium, and oxygen and typically reflect a delay in processing of the test sample. A spurious elevation of blood potassium levels may occur with hyperleukocytosis as a result of release of potassium from leukocytes undergoing lysis during clotting or as a result of prolonged storage of the sample before analysis.[167] If a spuriously elevated potassium or low glucose level is suspected, serum electrolyte studies should be repeated with an anticoagulated blood sample that is rapidly analyzed to prevent in vitro lysis of leukemic blasts.[161,180,181]

Specific Organ Involvement

Cardiorespiratory symptoms are common findings at presentation and during therapy in patients with acute leukemia. In the first week after treatment is started, infection and pulmonary hemorrhage associated with diffuse alveolar damage and/or infection contributed to the majority of early deaths in AML.[182,183] Pneumonia is the most common pulmonary problem. At presentation or early in the treatment course, gram-positive and gram-negative bacteria are the major pathogens. Patients who are neutropenic have an increased risk for pulmonary infection with fungi or other opportunistic organisms. Pulmonary leukostasis is a serious potential problem in patients who present with a blast count greater than 50,000/μL.[153,184] In this setting, leukocyte thrombi and plugging of pulmonary microvascular

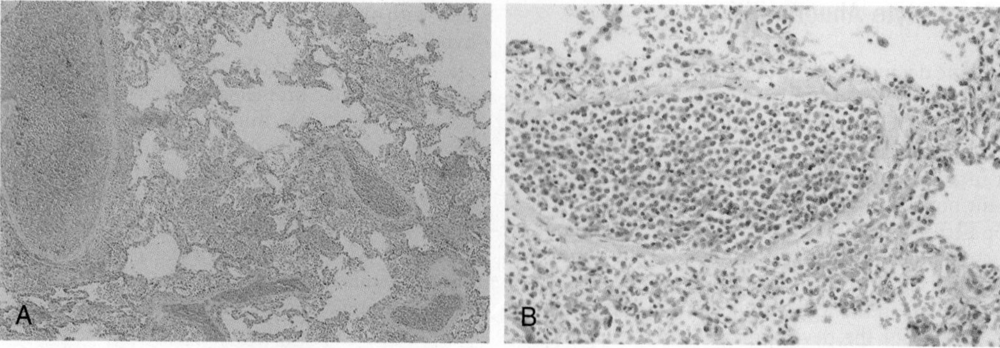

Figure 60–6 A, Pulmonary leukostasis with diffuse involvement of small and large vessels. **B,** Pulmonary leukostasis with involvement of a small pulmonary vessel. The vessel is occluded by aggregates of monoblasts.

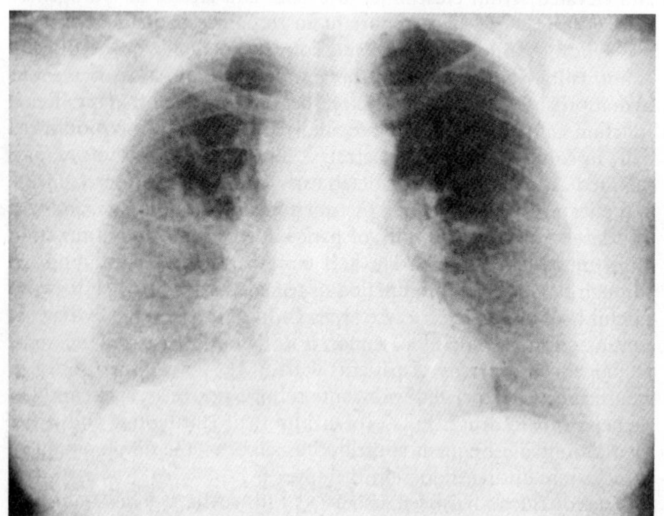

Figure 60–7 Chest radiograph showing pulmonary leukostasis in a patient with monoblastic leukemia and a white blood cell count of 150,000/mm^3.

channels lead to vascular rupture and infiltration of the lung parenchyma (Fig. 60–6). Leukemia-associated acute respiratory failure may be due to pulmonary hemorrhage or to direct damage of the pulmonary endothelium from the lysed leukemic blasts.[185] Patients may note sudden onset of shortness of breath and progressive dyspnea. On physical examination they are tachypneic, with diffuse bilateral rales. Chest radiograph usually shows a diffuse interstitial infiltrate (Fig. 60–7). Fever is common. Hypercapnia, hypoxemia, and progressive respiratory acidosis are signs of a very poor prognosis.[186] Pulmonary leukostasis and the hyperleukocytosis syndrome are more common in patients with one of the monocytic subtypes and the microgranular variant of APL.[153] Hyperleukocytosis, defined as a blast count greater than 50,000/µL, increases the risk of fatal pulmonary and CNS leukostasis and should be considered a medical emergency. Measures to prevent or treat suspected pulmonary leukostasis should be directed at rapidly lowering the WBC count, correct any underlying coagulopathy, and avoiding measures that increase the blood viscosity.[187,188] Emergency treatment should include use of hydroxyurea and platelet transfusions to maintain the platelet count greater than 20,000/µL.[188] Transfusion of packed red cells should be avoided unless necessary for the clinical condition of the patient because a low hemoglobin level is a major determinant for preventing leukostasis in hyperleukocytosis.[153,187] Leukapheresis should be performed to rapidly lower the blast count in patients who present with greater than 50,000/µL myeloblasts or when early signs of leukostasis are present.[189]

The mechanism of hyperleukocytosis syndrome is not clear. Leukostasis is the clinical manifestation of hyperleukocytosis and results in microcirculatory dysfunction and sludging of leukemic cells in the capillary vessel. The interaction of intercellular adhesion molecule 1 (ICAM-1) and lymphocyte function-associated antigen 1 (LFA-1) appears to play a critical role in the adhesion and migration of AML and is responsible for the vascular disruption and distribution of blast cells.[190] The vascular disruption and bleeding in leukostasis appear to be result from interaction of the leukemic cell and the vascular endothelial surface. The interaction of the leukemic cell and the vascular endothelial appears to be critical in causing leukostasis. The absolute white blood count may be less important for the development of leukostasis than the presence of adhesion molecules displayed by the leukemic cell and their chemotactic response to local cytokines in the vascular microenvironment. Dexamethasone in vitro inhibits upregulation of adhesion molecules such a L-selectin and IL-8 receptor on myeloid leukemic cells and may have a role in treating the leukostasis.[153] Pulmonary hemorrhage and leukostasis may mimic the signs and symptoms of a bacterial or fungal pneumonia. Pulmonary hemorrhage may be diffuse, involving both lungs, or localized to a single segment or lobe. Patients typically complain of sudden onset of shortness of breath. Hemoptysis may occur, and hypoxemia and hypercapnia are common. Hyperleukocytosis can be associated with a spurious hypoxemia because of the metabolic requirements of the high blast count.[191] The prognosis for patients who develop pulmonary leukostasis is very poor, even with the rapid lowering of WBC count and initiation of chemotherapy. The presentation may be similar to other forms of noncardiogenic pulmonary edema that can occur during treatment of AML.[192] Physical examination may reveal few objective pulmonary findings, although chest radiograph typically reveals an interstitial pattern in the area of the hemorrhage.

Cardiovascular abnormalities usually result from derangements in metabolic, electrolyte, and pulmonary function. Leukemic infiltration of the heart or great vessels is rare, but leukemic involvement of the conduction system, pericardium, and myocardium as well as involvement of the arterial endothelial wall with monoblasts and subsequent formation and rupture of an aortic aneurysm have been reported.[193] Chemotherapy-related toxicities produce the majority of cardiovascular problems in patients with AML. The cardiotoxicity of the anthracyclines is dose related, and these agents act synergistically with other cardiotoxic agents. Left and right ventricular ejection fractions should be measured in all patients who have received a known cardiotoxic drug or who have a history of cardiac disease before they are given an anthracycline. Anthracycline cardiotoxicity is a multifactorial process and is related to oxidative stress and myocyte induction of apoptosis. Whether the therapeutic effects of the anthracyclines are different from the cardiotoxicity is unclear.[194] An echocardiogram may be more helpful in assessing wall-motion abnormalities. However, a pretherapy "baseline" ejection fraction or echocardiogram is not warranted for all patients before starting induction therapy. Unless the patient has known or suspected cardiac disease that would alter the chemotherapy regimen, treatment need not be delayed pending the result of ejection fraction. Patients who develop progressive cardiorespiratory failure and require intubation and respiratory support continue to have a grave prognosis.[195]

Gastrointestinal abnormalities are frequent in AML patients. Dysphagia is common and usually results from oral or pharyngeal infections, mucosal involvement with leukemia, or chemotherapy-induced mucositis. Oral candidiasis is a common presenting finding and may involve the tongue and/or the soft or hard palate. Esophageal candidiasis can produce substernal pain and a midepigastric "burning" sensation. Dysphagia is common with oral and esophageal candidiasis. The clinical appearance of oral and esophageal candidiasis may be deceptive, and mixed fungal and viral infections are common.[196] Leukemic involvement of the gingiva can occur in any of the AML subtypes. Gingival hypertrophy is most frequent in the well-differentiated monocytic types. Gastrointestinal involvement with AML is rare, but granulocytic sarcomas (chloromas) can form in the esophagus or small intestine and lead to obstructive symptoms.[197,198]

The anal and perirectal areas are important potential sources of infection in neutropenic patients. Patients initially may complain only of pain on defecation and diffuse anal tenderness without signs of infection or cellulitis. Perirectal abscesses usually are due to gram-negative bacteria and in the setting of granulocytopenia can rapidly progress to perirectal cellulitis and septicemia. Although routine digital rectal examinations are generally avoided in patients who are granulocytopenic, the perirectal area can be examined when a local infection is suspected.

Patients should be instructed on the importance of perirectal hygiene. Constipation should be avoided to prevent small mucosal tears. Agents that cause diarrhea should be carefully monitored, and use of harsh laxatives or agents that cause prolonged diarrhea should be avoided. Use of contrast agents that are cathartics must be critically evaluated before their routine use in patients with AML. The perirectal and oral areas are two important portals for infection.

Use of more intensive chemotherapy regimens and broad-spectrum antibiotics has resulted in an increased incidence of gastrointestinal complications.[199] Typhlitis, derived from the Greek word meaning *cecum*, is a fulminant necrotizing colitis related to granulocytopenia and cytotoxic therapy. It occurs in up to 10% of patients with leukemia who are undergoing intensive therapy.[200] Patients present with sudden onset of abdominal pain, fever, and a distended and tense abdomen. Bowel sounds are decreased, and abdominal radiographs are nonspecific, usually revealing an incomplete small bowel obstruction, a questionable right lower quadrant mass, pneumatosis, or no appreciable abnormality. Computed tomographic scanning frequently shows an edematous right colon with spiculation of the pericolic fat and subcutaneous edema. The clinical presentation frequently mimics that of acute appendicitis. The diagnosis of typhlitis usually is made based on clinical findings. Computed tomographic scan may be helpful in differentiating appendicitis from other causes of abdominal pain and fever.[201] The pathogenesis of neutropenic colitis is multifactorial and related to the chemotherapy administered and local mucosal damage. The cecum is the most common site because of limited vasculature and distensibility. The factors implicated in the pathogenesis of neutropenic colitis include a direct toxic effect of chemotherapy, local bacterial invasion, intramural hemorrhage, and leukemic infiltration of the bowel wall.[199] Treatment of typhlitis is controversial, and for many patients the prognosis is poor. Medical management includes bowel rest, broad-spectrum antibiotics directed at bowel pathogens including anaerobes and fungi, intravenous fluid replacement, total parenteral nutrition, and transfusion support.[202] Surgical intervention, usually a hemicolectomy, should be reserved for patients with localizing peritoneal signs suggesting an abscess or clear evidence of bowel perforation, as well as for those who do not respond to medical therapy. Patients who are neutropenic and thrombocytopenic can tolerate an exploratory laparotomy, but their postoperative course is more complicated.[203] The morbidity and mortality of surgery must be carefully weighed against the risk of medical therapy and support therapy in the individual patient. A majority of patients with typhlitis can be managed medically with intensive supportive therapy and antibiotics; only a minority of patients require surgical intervention.[199]

DIAGNOSIS

General Approach to Diagnosis of Acute Myeloid Leukemia

Advances in the understanding of the molecular and genetics of myeloid stem cell disorders have helped in defining clinically and biologically important subtypes of AML.[204–208] This expanding spectrum of AMLs coupled with efforts to institute risk-adapted therapy for these disorders[209,210] requires a comprehensive, yet algorithmic, approach to the diagnosis and classification of AML (see box on Stepwise Algorithm for Diagnosis and Classification of Acute Myelogenous Leukemia Using Cytomorphology, Cytochemistry, Immunophenotyping, Cytogenetics, and Molecular Cytogenetics).[211,212] Collection of adequate samples for cytomorphologic, immunophenotypic, cytogenetic, and molecular studies as well as timely exchange of information among the clinician, pathologist, and cytogeneticist are necessary for the diagnosis and classification of AML.

In many cases diagnosis is possible based on examination of the peripheral blood smear. However, a bone marrow aspirate should be performed to confirm the leukemia subtype and obtain marrow for cytogenetic and immunophenotypic studies. Air-dried marrow smears freshly prepared at the bedside from the aspirated marrow are stained with Wright-Giemsa or May-Grünwald-Giemsa to allow for detailed study of qualitative cytomorphology. Although a core biopsy is not required to make the diagnosis of acute leukemia,[213] a bone marrow core biopsy and touch preparation should be performed on all patients because the aspirate and core biopsy assess different aspects of normal and neoplastic hematopoiesis. A biopsy is particularly important when the marrow cannot be aspirated ("dry tap"). Under these circumstances, the marrow imprints or touch preparations may prove useful for determining cell lineage and performing cytochemical staining. The bone marrow biopsy is routinely stained with hematoxylin-eosin and/or Giemsa stain; it also can be stained by immunohistochemical methods if needed.

Immunophenotyping is best accomplished by multiparameter flow cytometry on aspirated marrow. When an aspirate cannot be obtained, flow cytometric studies can be performed with cells dissociated from a core biopsy.[214] Cytogenetic studies are important prognostic indicators and should be performed on all patients at the time of initial bone marrow biopsy. Samples for cytogenetics must be collected in heparin tubes because ethylenediaminetetraacetic acid (EDTA) interferes with cell growth. Conversely, samples for cytomorphology should be collected in EDTA tubes because heparin interferes with metachromatic stains. Cell suspensions from marrow collected in EDTA should be cryopreserved for possible molecular studies.[213] Cytogenetic, molecular, cytochemical, and immunophenotypic studies are important in diagnosing AML and defining major subtypes of AML in the FAB and WHO classifications. Cytogenetic analysis is performed on Giemsa-banded karyotypes and requires viable dividing cells. Cytogenetic analysis for a complete karyotype can take up to 2 weeks. The introduction and widespread use of fluorescent in situ hybridization (FISH) on interphase nuclei, although not supplanting standard cytogenetics, can provide additional information and is rapidly becoming more available.[215,216] Unlike cytogenetics, FISH analysis requires the clinician to direct the cytogeneticist to search for specific abnormalities. For instance, in suspected cases of APL, FISH analysis of interphase nuclei can rapidly detect the 15:17 translocation. FISH studies do not require dividing cells and therefore can be performed on peripheral blood samples. Test results are generally available in 24 to 72 hours. FISH analysis also can identify cryptic, structural, and numerical abnormalities that can be missed by conventional cytogenetic studies.[217] FISH analysis can help increase the yield of conventional cytogenetic analysis and is a useful adjunct to conventional cytogenetics.

Gene expression profiling using microarray technology to generate gene expression profiles in AML is an area of active research.[218,219] The amplification and hybridization of small amounts of RNA allow for gene expression profiling in AML and have identified potentially important differences in subtypes and biology not defined by traditional morphology or cytogenetics. Microarrays may be able to replace some existing genetic tests as well as add a new method for evaluating genomic abnormalities in AML. Newer high-content "tiled arrays" or single nucleotide polymorphism arrays can successfully identify common and specific somatic DNA lesions in AML as well as pinpoint small deletions or amplifications of chromosome segments. Global profiling of CpG methylation and chromatin posttranslational modification (chromatin code) are capable of uncovering epigenetic changes in AML.[220,221] Combined, these technologies promise to define and map relevant genomic lesions, transcriptional signatures, and epigenetic changes that currently are not defined by traditional morphology or cytogenetics.[208]

Morphology in Diagnosis of Acute Myeloid Leukemia

Microscopic examination of a properly prepared and stained bone marrow or peripheral blood smear remains the cornerstone of AML diagnosis. Morphologic findings can direct the appropriate selection of additional diagnostic tests. The bone marrow aspirate should be evaluated for cellularity, number and morphology of megakaryocytes, myeloid/erythroid ratio (M:E), cellular maturation, and presence of dysplasia or asynchronous maturation. The blast percentage should be determined on a 500-cell differential of the bone marrow aspirate. The original FAB classification recognized three types of myeloblasts: I, II, and III (Table 60–3).[222] Type I blasts lack granules, have fine chromatin, a high nucleocytoplasmic ratio, and prominent nucleoli, and lack Auer rods. Type II blasts have a slightly more basophilic cytoplasm with few azurophilic granules (up to 20) and nuclear features similar to type I blasts except for a lower nucleocytoplasmic ratio. Type III blasts have a variable number of granules (>20) and basophilic cytoplasm with numerous azurophilic granules. The differences in blast types are determined by nuclear features and cytoplasm granules. Importantly, blasts lack a visible Golgi zone.[223] Myeloid precursors are classified as promyelocytes when they have moderately basophilic cytoplasm with numerous azurophilic granules and eccentric nuclei, largely resulting from an incipient Golgi apparatus. It is the absence of Golgi apparatus and not the paucity of granules that is the common cytologic denominator of myeloblasts. For diagnostic purposes, only type I and type II blasts should be reflected in the marrow cell differential count. Pre–B-cell ALL and some forms of natural killer cell leukemia may contain azurophilic cytoplasmic granules resembling those of myeloblasts. Subtle morphologic differences may not be sufficient to make the distinction, and immunophenotyping is necessary to confirm the lineage. Iron stores should be assessed with Prussian blue stain and the presence or absence of ringed sideroblasts specifically noted. Evaluation of the cellularity of a bone marrow aspirate is a qualitative assessment and may reflect the number of spicules obtained, slide preparation technique, and volume of diluting blood. Despite these limitations, the cellularity of a bone marrow aspirate should be noted. Marrow aspirate cellularity is grouped into five broad categories ranging from 0

Table 60–3 Type Blasts in Acute Myeloid Leukemia

Myeloblast	Features
Type I	Agranular basophilic cytoplasm, nucleus with fine chromatin, high nuclear/cytoplasmic ratio, two to four distinct nucleoli
Type II	Granulated basophilic cytoplasm with few (≤20) azurophilic granules, nuclear features similar to those of type I blasts but lower nuclear-to-cytoplasmic ratio
Type III	Heavily granulated basophilic cytoplasm with numerous (>20) azurophilic granules, nuclear features similar to those of type I blasts

Stepwise Algorithm for Diagnosis and Classification of Acute Myelogenous Leukemia Using Cytomorphology, Cytochemistry, Immunophenotyping, Cytogenetics, and Molecular Cytogenetics

The criteria are based on Wright-Giemsa–stained blood and marrow smears and biopsy. The percentage of blast cells separates acute myeloid leukemia (AML) from myelodysplastic syndrome (MDS). The World Health Organization (WHO) classification defines AML as greater than 20% blasts in the marrow or blood. The next step is to define the blast population by immunophenotyping and/or immunohistochemistry. The initial evaluation separates AML from ALL. A history of exposure to prior cytoxic chemotherapy or agents associated with AML defines the leukemia as *therapy-related acute myeloid leukemia* (t-AML). The WHO recognizes the unique clinical and biologic features of the therapy-related leukemias (t-AML). This subtype results from prior exposure to cytotoxic chemotherapy and/or radiation therapy. A majority of patients will have clonal cytogenetic abnormalities and now account for more than 40% of all patients with AML. The WHO recognizes two types of t-AML based on the type of prior exposure or treatment: alkylating agent–related AML and topoisomerase II inhibitor–related AML. The WHO classification defines major subgroups of AML that manifest recurring cytogenetic abnormalities. As a group, these AMLs have chromosomal translocations that result in the production of chimeric proteins, which are pivotal in the leukemogenic process. The genetic abnormalities define a specific biology, clinical course, and prognosis and therefore are important to classify them separately. In this group of patients, the diagnosis is defined by the cytogenetic abnormality independent of the percentage of blasts. There are four recurrent translocations in this group. The diagnosis is defined by the cytogenetic abnormalities and is not dependent on the number of blasts: (a) AML with t(8;21)(q22;q22), (AML1/ETO) (RUNX/CBFA2T1); (b) AML with abnormal bone marrow eosinophils and inv^{16}(p13;q22) or t(16;16)(p13;q22), (CBFB/MYH11); (c) acute promyelocytic leukemia: AML with t(15;17)(q22;q21)(PML/RARA) or t(11;17)(q23;q12) (PLZF/RARA) or t(5;17)(q23;q12)(NPM/RARA), or t(11;17)(q13;q12) (NuMA/RARA); and (d) AML with 11q23 (MLL) abnormalities. If multilineage dysplasia is present, then the leukemia is classified as *acute leukemia with multilineage dysplasia.*

AML with multilineage dysplasia is characterized by the presence of 20% or more blasts in the marrow and dysplasia in at least 50% of the cells of at least two of the three main hemopoietic lines. The leukemia may occur de novo or after a preceding myelodysplastic, myeloproliferative, or overlap myelodysplastic/myeloproliferative syndrome unrelated to prior exposure to chemotherapy. If such a syndrome preceded the development of acute leukemia, the AML is best designated as AML "evolving from a myelodysplastic syndrome." When a leukemia fails to satisfy the cytogenetic, morphologic, or clinical criteria for the newly defined subgroups, it is classified as AML not otherwise categorized. The *not otherwise categorized* designation essentially applies the original FAB classification with some modifications, namely, acute promyelocytic leukemia (M3) is no longer included; a pure erythroleukemia has been distinguished from erythroleukemia, acute erythroid/myeloid type; and acute basophilic leukemia (very rare) has been added, as is a rare entity termed acute panmyelosis with myelofibrosis and the solid tumor myeloid sarcoma.

CD, cluster designation; MPO, myeloperoxidase; NEC, nonerythroid cells; NSE, nonspecific esterase; PAS, periodic acid–Schiff; SBB, Sudan black B; TdT, terminal deoxynucleotidyl transferase; TNC, total nucleated cells.

Stepwise Algorithm for Diagnosis and Classification of Acute Myelogenous Leukemia Using Cytomorphology, Cytochemistry, Immunophenotyping, Cytogenetics, and Molecular Cytogenetics—cont'd

1. Morphology
WG. PB, TP
HE: BMbx

≥ 20% blasts in the bone marrow or peripheral blood

Yes

Acute leukemia

No

Dysmyelopoiesis present

Yes

Work up MDS

No

Other

2. Immunophenotype
Multicolor flow cytometry
(immunohistochemistry)

Lymphoid lineage-specific (LS) markers only

Precursor-B or -T cell leukemia/lymphoma

Myeloid and lymphoid LS markers on same blasts population

Acute biphemotypic leukemia

Myeloid and lymphoid LS markers on separate blasts population

Acute bilineal leukemia

Myeloid LA markers only

Acute myeloid leukemia

Neither

Acute undifferentiated leukemia

Previous exposure to leukemogenic therapy

Yes

AML therapy-related

No

3. Cytogenetics
FISH, MplxRT-PCR
karyotype

WHO-defines recurrent genetic abnormalities

Multilineage dysplasia

No

AML not otherwise categorized

Yes

AML with multilineage dysplasia

AML with recurrent genetic abnormalities

AML with CBFα fusion proteins
t(8;21)(q22;q22) *AML1/ETO*
(RUNX1/CBFA2T1)

AML with CBFβ fusion proteins
inv(16)(p13;q22) *CBFβ/MYH11*
t(16;16)(p13;q22) *CBFβ/MYH11*

AML with RARα fusion proteins
t(15;17)(q22;q12) *PML/RARa*;
t(11;17)(q23;Q12) *PLZF/RARa*
t(11;17)(q13;q12) *NuMA/RARa*;
t(5;17)(q35;q12) *NPM/RARa*

AML with MLL fusion proteins
t(9;11)(q34;q23)MLL/DAB21p;
t(10;11) (p12;q23) MLL/MLLT10;
t(11;19)(q23;p13.1) MLL/ELL;
t(11;19)(q23;p13.1) MLL/ELL;
t(11;19)(q23;p;13.3) MLL/MLLT1)
t(6;11)(q21;q23) MLL/FOXO3A

Acute myeloid leukemia minimally differentiated

Acute myeloid leukemia with maturation

Acute myeloid leukemia without maturation

Acute myeloid leukemia

Acute monoblastic and monocytic leukemia

Acute erythroleukemia and pure eryhroid leukemia

Acute megakaryoblastic leukemia

Acute basophilic leukemia

Acute panmyelosis with myelofibrosis

Myeloid sarcoma

to +4 (aplastic, hypocellular, normal cellular, hypercellular, and intensely hypercellular).

The initial bone marrow in AML typically is hypercellular, with absent or decreased megakaryocytes. However, elderly patients or those with secondary or treatment-related AML may have a normal cellular or hypocellular bone marrow aspirate.[224] Dysplastic myeloid and erythroid maturation may be noted. Myeloid precursors may be morphologically bizarre with asynchronous granulation. The prognostic significance of dysplasia by itself in de novo AML is controversial.[225,226] In addition, prominent dysplasia may suggest prior exposure to hematotoxins or may suggest that the patient's leukemia evolved from a prior MDS or is secondary to prior cytotoxic chemotherapy. Therefore, the presence or absence of dysplasia must be considered in the context of other defined prognostic indicators.[227]

Auer rods (or bodies), which are reddish rod-like filaments of aggregated primary granules, may be present in leukemic cells. These bodies (or rods), first described by Joseph Auer, are derived from incorporation of primary azurophilic granules into autophagic vacuoles. The term *phi body* has also been used to describe small spindle-shaped bodies not easily visualized by Giemsa stains. Phi bodies are best visualized by peroxidase reaction and may constitute a precursor of Auer rods. Cells containing multiple Auer bodies, sometimes referred to as *faggot cells* (from the term meaning "bundle of sticks"), are typical but not restricted to APL. They are faintly birefringent in polarized light. Ultrastructurally they have a defined three-dimensional crystal structure with a characteristic periodicity of 6 to 13 nm, which is different for each of the leukemic subtypes.[228] Auer rods are found in approximately 30% to 50% of newly diagnosed patients with AML and in a greater proportion (60%–70%) with use of cytochemical stains.[229] The myeloblasts in AML with (t8;21)(q22;q22) characteristically have thin and elongated Auer rods, which is a useful feature for recognizing this generally favorable subtype. The remission rate and duration of remission may be higher in patients whose leukemic cells demonstrate Auer rods.[230]

Hematoxylin-eosin stain of the bone marrow biopsy sample of undifferentiated immature AMLs typically exhibits a blue (basophilic) color due to close apposition of blasts with scant cytoplasm and basophilic stained nuclei. In contrast, biopsy samples of the more differentiated AMLs typically show a pale to orange (amphophilic to acidophilic) tinge due to the presence of blasts with more abundant cytoplasm. Monoblasts and promonocytes usually exhibit folded/convoluted nuclei and may contain prominent acidophilic nucleoli. Occasionally the marrow is hypocellular or contains clusters of blasts amidst more maturing myeloid progeny. Some of these cases may represent a diagnostic challenge. In cases with extensive fibrosis, as in some forms of megakaryoblastic leukemia and AML developing in the background of a chronic myeloproliferative disorder, the combination of morphology and immunocytochemistry on the core biopsy may be the only way to establish the diagnosis.

Cytochemistry in Diagnosis of Acute Myeloid Leukemia

Myeloid cells exhibit characteristic staining profiles for esterase, MPO, and periodic acid–Schiff (PAS) reagent (Table 60–4 and Fig. 60–8).[231] MPO and the specific esterase chloroacetate esterase (CAE) are markers for granulocytic differentiation, whereas the "nonspecific" esterases stain monocytic precursors. MPO is one of the most specific markers for the granulocytic lineage and is present in both primary and secondary granules. MPO is positive in myeloblasts, and activity increases as myeloblasts mature into promyelocytes. Auer rods are intensely positive for MPO, as are granules of eosinophils. Lymphoblasts and megakaryoblasts are MPO negative. Sudan black B (SBB) has a reactivity profile similar to that of MPO but is less specific for the myeloid lineage, occasionally staining diffusely the cytoplasm of lymphoblasts. MPO reactivity in 3% or more blasts is the criterion for classifying a leukemia as AML. MPO is negative in AML with minimal differentiation, acute monoblastic leukemia, and acute megakaryoblastic leukemia, which does contain platelet peroxidase but is demonstrable only by electron microscopy. PAS is positive in differentiated granulocytes and megakaryocytes, variably stains monocytes, and is negative in normal erythroid precursors. It weakly

Table 60–4 Cytochemical Stains Used for Diagnosis and Classification of Acute Leukemia

Cytochemical Stain	Specificity
Myeloperoxidase (MPO)	Stains primary and secondary granules of cells of myeloid/neutrophil lineage, eosinophil granules (granules appear solid), granules of monocytes, Auer rods Granules of normal mature basophils do not stain
Sudan black B (SBB)	Stains primary and secondary granules of cells of myeloid/ neutrophil lineage similar to MPO Eosinophil granules, granules of monocytes, Auer rods are positive Basophil granules usually are negative but sometimes show metachromatic staining (red/purple)
Naphthol AS-D chloracetate esterase ("specific" esterase)	Stains neutrophil and mast cell granules Auer rods usually are negative except in acute myeloid leukemia associated with granules), some T and B lymphocytes Abnormal eosinophils are positive
α-Naphthyl acetate esterase ("nonspecific" esterase)	Monocytes and macrophages, megakaryocytes, platelets, most T lymphocytes, some T lymphoblasts (focal)
α-Naphthyl butyrate esterase ("nonspecific" esterase)	Monocytes and macrophages Variable staining of T lymphocytes
Periodic acid–Schiff (PAS)	Neutrophil lineage (granular, increasing with maturation), leukemic promyelocytes (diffuse cytoplasmic), eosinophil cytoplasm but not granules, basophil cytoplasm (blocks), monocytes (diffuse plus granules), megakaryocytes, platelets (diffuse plus granules), erythroblasts positive in block-like pattern Negative in normal erythroid precursors
Acid phosphatase	Neutrophils, most T lymphocytes, T lymphoblasts (focal) Variable staining of eosinophils, monocytes, platelets Strong staining of macrophages, plasma cells, megakaryocytes, some leukemic megakaryoblasts
Toluidine blue	Metachromatic granules in basophils, mast cells
Perls stain, Prussian blue stain	Hemosiderin, and iron in erythroblasts, macrophages occasionally, plasma cells

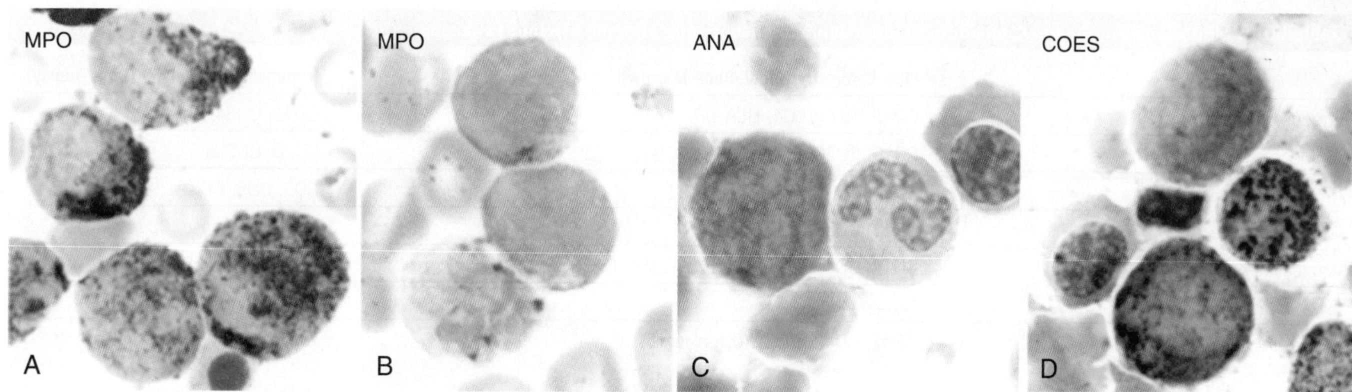

Figure 60–8 Cytochemistries: myeloperoxidase (MPO), α-naphthyl acetate esterase (ANA), and combined esterase (COES) reactions. The MPO reaction is easily performed, can be done in less than a few minutes, and provides important initial information about the lineage of the blasts, particularly in cases where morphology is difficult. In many laboratories the MPO reaction is routinely performed for all new acute leukemias. The MPO reaction should be interpreted in the blastic population and expressed as a percent of blasts that are positive. **A,** Positive MPO reaction is strong. **B,** Reaction is weak and seen in only some blasts. A counterstain would have obscured the weak reaction product. A weak MPO reaction is not uncommon in cases of acute myeloid leukemia associated with myelodysplasia (as in **B**). The neutrophils in such cases are only weakly positive (bottom cell, **B**). The ANA-reaction is a nonspecific esterase reaction positive in most monocytic cells (**C,** orange–brown cell on left compared to negative neutrophil, and erythroid cell, middle and right). The ANA reaction is interpreted as positive cells as a percent of nonerythroid elements. A significant monocytic component usually is defined as 20% or greater of the nonerythroid elements and usually is required to make a diagnosis of acute myelomonocytic leukemia. Of note, in some cases of acute myeloid leukemia with inv[16] (i.e., acute myelomonocytic leukemia with abnormal eosinophils), the monocytes are ANA negative. A COES reaction uses another nonspecific esterase reaction for monocytes, α-naphthyl butyrate esterase (ANB) together with the specific esterase chloroacetate esterase (CAE) for granulocytes. The combination allows simultaneous evaluation of granulocytes (blue reaction product) and monocytes (orange–brown reaction product). **D,** Acute myelomonocytic leukemia. Monocyte (top), granulocyte (right), and myelomonocytic hybrid cell that exhibits both orange–brown and blue reaction products (bottom).

stains the cytoplasm of the majority of AML blasts in a diffuse pattern. It is most useful in the diagnosis of pure erythroid leukemia, where it intensely stains the cytoplasm of erythroblasts in a "block positivity pattern," a finding that is very useful in recognizing this form of erythroid leukemia.

Multiparametric Immunophenotyping in Diagnosis of Acute Myeloid Leukemia

The availability of well-characterized antibodies classified under the uniform terminology of *clusters of differentiation* (CD) has expanded the application of flow cytometry and made phenotyping of AML more precise, reproducible, and comprehensive. Immunophenotyping now is routinely used to distinguish AML from ALL and for lineage assignment. Individual cells can be stained with multiple antibodies directly labeled with various fluorophores. Several "gating" strategies specifically identify blast cells by combining side (orthogonal) scatter and CD45 staining (Fig. 60–9).[232] This strategy identifies blasts by cytoplasm complexity (granularity) on the side scatter channel Y-axis and "brightness" of staining with CD45 on the X-axis, creating specific zones or "gates" of the most common morphologic variants of AML blasts. This strategy permits the gating of even a small group of blasts in a background of numerous more mature cells. Immunophenotyping has been most useful in distinguishing between AML and lymphoid leukemias and in defining hybrid or biphenotypic leukemias (Table 60–5). Certain immunophenotypic profiles are strongly suggestive of the underlying cytogenetic abnormality (Table 60–6). The expression of a number of antibodies correlates relatively well with morphologic classification. Expression of CD34 and CD117 is common in undifferentiated or minimally differentiated AML, whereas strong expression of CD33 and loss of HLA-DR are characteristic of APL. However, the overall expression of surface antigens on myeloblasts does not entirely agree with either morphology or cytochemical staining.[233,234] Use of multiple monoclonal antibodies has identified certain phenotypic groups that may be clinically important, such as the association of AML with t(8;21) with the B-cell surface antigen CD19 and CD79a.[235] The majority of myeloid

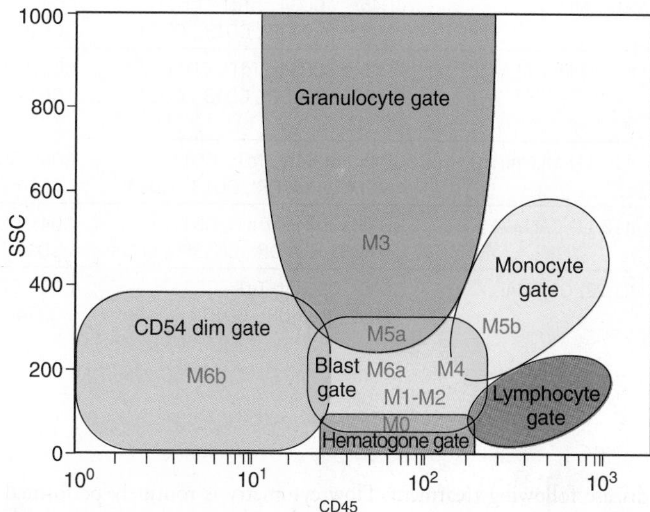

Figure 60–9 Side scatter versus CD45 flow cytometry ploy with approximate areas of "gates" where myeloblasts of the FAB acute myeloid leukemia subtypes usually are positioned. Gates are named according to the predominant normal peripheral blood cell population that normally inhabits them. Side scatter is a measure of "cytoplasm granularity," and CD45 represents the log of the intensity of staining with a common leukocyte antigen antibody.

blast cells express differentiation markers asynchronously, and the unusual coexpression of differentiation antigens is common. Myeloblasts also frequently express lymphoid associated antigens, most frequently CD2, CD7, and CD19.[236,237] CD19 is present in up to 34% of newly diagnosed AMLs.[236] The prognostic significance of this phenotypic heterogeneity is unclear, but it is not associated with a uniformly adverse prognosis. Use of immunophenotyping is particularly important for identification of AML with minimal differentiation, erythroid leukemias, and megakaryoblastic leukemia.[238] Immunophenotyping may be helpful for detecting minimal residual

Table 60–5 Monoclonal Antibodies Commonly Used for Immunophenotyping of Acute Myeloid Leukemia

	Flow Cytometry (Blood/Bone Marrow)	Immunohistochemistry (Core Biopsy)
Precursor antigen	CD45, TdT, CD34, HLA-DR	CD34, CD34, TdT
B lineage	CD19, CD20, CD22, CD79a, CD10	CD20, CD79a
T lineage	CD2, CD3, CD5, CD7	CD3, CD5, CD7
Myeloid lineage	CD13, CD33, CD117, CD15	Myeloperoxidase, CD117, CD15
Monocytic-monocytic	CD14, CD4, CD11b, CD11c, CD64, CD36	Lysozyme, CD68
Erythroid	Glycophorin A	Glycophorin A, hemoglobin A
Megakaryocytic	CD41, CD42, CD61 (cytoplasmic)	von Willebrand factor, factor VIII

Table 60–6 Genotypic/Phenotypic Correlation in Molecularly Defined Acute Myeloid Leukemia

t(8;21) RUNX/CBFA2T1	CD45^{+Dm}, CD34^{+Br}, TdT^{-}, CD117^{+}, MPO^{+Br}, HLA-DR^{+}, CD13^{+Br}, CD33^{+Br}	CD4$^{+/-}$, CD11b^{+}, CD11c, CD18$^{+/-}$, CD15^{+Br}, CD14^{-}, CD64$^{+/-}$, CD65, NG2^{-}	CD19^{+}, CD10^{-}, CD2^{-}, CD7^{-}, CD56$^{+/-}$, CD41^{-}, CD61^{-}
inv(16) CBFB/SMMHC	CD45^{+Dm}, CD34^{+Nn}, TdT^{-}, CD117^{+}, MPO^{-}, HLA-DR^{+}, CD13^{-}, CD33^{-}, CD4$^{-/+}$	CD11b$^{-/+}$, CD11c, CD18$^{+/-}$, CD15^{+Br}, CD14$^{-/+}$, CD64$^{+/-}$, CD65, NG2^{+}, CD19^{+}	CD10^{-}, CD2^{-}, CD7^{-}, CD56^{-}, CD41^{-}, CD61^{-}
t(15;17) PML/RARA	CD45^{+Int}, CD34^{-}, TdT^{-}, CD117$^{+/-}$, MPO^{+Br}, HLA-DR^{-}, CD13^{+Br}, CD33^{+Br}	CD4^{-}, CD11b^{-}, CD18$^{+/-}$, CD15^{-}, CD14^{-}, CD64^{-}, CD65, NG2^{-}, CD19^{-}, CD10^{-}	CD2$^{-/+}$, CD7^{-}, CD56$^{-/+}$, CD41^{-}, CD61^{-}
t(11) MLL	CD45^{+Dm}, CD34$^{-/+}$, TdT^{-}, CD117$^{+/-}$, MPO^{-}, HLA-DR^{+}, CD13^{-}, CD33^{+}	CD4$^{+/-}$, CD11b^{+}, CD11c, CD18$^{+/-}$, CD15$^{+/-}$, CD14$^{+/-}$, CD64$^{+/-}$, CD65, NG2^{+}	CD19$^{-/+}$, CD10^{-}, CD2^{-}, CD7^{-}, CD56$^{+/-}$, CD41^{-}, CD61^{-}
t(4;11) MLL/AF4	CD45^{+Dm}, CD34^{-}, TdT^{+}, CD117^{-}, MPO^{-}, HLA-DR^{+}, CD13^{-}, CD33^{-}, CD4$^{-/+}$	CD11b$^{-/+}$, CD11c, CD18$^{+/-}$, CD15^{+Dm}, CD14$^{-/+}$, CD64$^{+/-}$, CD65, NG2^{+}	CD19+, CD10^{-}, CD2^{-}, CD7^{-}, CD56^{-}, CD41^{-}, CD61^{-}
t(10;11) MLL/AF10	CD45^{+}, CD34^{+Br}, TdT^{-}, CD117^{+}, MPO^{+Br}, HLA-DR^{+}, CD13^{-}, CD33^{+}	CD4^{+}, CD11b^{-}, CD11c, CD18^{-}, CD15^{-}, CD14^{-}, CD64^{-}, CD65^{+}, NG2^{-}	CD19^{-}, CD10^{-}, CD2^{-}, CD7^{-}, CD56$^{+/-}$, CD41^{-}, CD61^{-}
t(10;11) CALM/AF10	CD45^{+}, CD34^{+Br}, TdT^{-}, CD117^{+}, MPO^{+Br}, HLA-DR^{+}, CD13^{+Dm}, CD33^{-}	CD4^{-}, CD11b^{-}, CD11c, CD18^{-}, CD15^{-}, CD14^{-}, CD64^{-}, CD65^{-}, NG2^{-}	CD19^{-}, CD10^{-}, CD2^{-}, CD7^{-}, CD56$^{+/-}$, CD41^{-}, CD61^{-}
t(1;22) OTT/MAL	CD45^{+}, CD34$^{-/+}$, TdT^{-}, CD117^{-}, MPO^{-}, HLA-DR^{+}, CD13$^{-/+}$, CD33$^{-/+}$	CD4^{-}, CD11b^{-}, CD11c, CD18^{-}, CD15^{-}, CD14^{-}, CD64^{-}, CD65^{-}, NG2^{-}	CD19^{-}, CD10^{-}, CD2^{-}, CD7^{-}, CD56$^{+/-}$, CD41^{+}, CD61^{+}

disease following treatment. Flow cytometry is routinely performed at the time of diagnosis; however, it should not replace standard differential cell counting to diagnosis leukemia and evaluate response to treatment.[213]

Classification of Acute Myeloid Leukemia

The classification and diagnosis of AML (Table 60–7) has evolved from the primarily morphologic and cytochemical system proposed by the FAB Cooperative Group in 1976[222,223,239] to the current WHO classification, which explicitly includes clinical information, cytogenetics, and/or molecular abnormalities (Table 60–8). The FAB classification attempted to define relatively homogeneous morphologic categories. The FAB classified the acute leukemias according to the resemblance of the predominant leukemic cell type to a normal differentiating hematopoietic precursor cell.[240] The FAB group divided the myeloid leukemias into eight broad categories based on morphology, cytochemical staining, and immunologic phenotype of the predominant cell type, based on a Wright-Giemsa–stained blood and marrow smear or biopsy. In an attempt to incorporate relevant cytogenetic and clinical features into the classification of AML, the WHO developed a new classification of AML. The WHO-proposed classification retains much of the content of the FAB classification but defines unique clinical and biologically important subgroups by incorporating cytogenetics, adding the morphologic finding of multilineage dysplasia, and incorporating certain clinical data into the definition of four unique subgroups (Table 60–8).[241,242] The WHO classification also attempts to formally address the relationship of AML to MDS and the importance of multilineage dysplasia.[240,242] A fundamental change introduced by the WHO classification reduces the defining blast threshold for the diagnosis of AML from 30% blasts to 20% blasts in the marrow or blood. This new defining threshold eliminates the FAB-MDS subtype refractory anemia with excess blasts in transformation (RAEB-T). In addition, cases with certain recurring cytogenetic abnormalities are defined as AML regardless of the percent blasts in the blood or bone marrow. The WHO classification defines four major subgroups of AML that manifest recurring cytogenetic abnormalities. When a leukemic cell fails to satisfy the cytogenetic, morphologic, or clinical criteria for the newly defined subgroups, it is classified as AML not otherwise categorized. The *not otherwise categorized* designation essentially applies the

Table 60–7 Summary of Diagnostic Features of AML in the FAB Classification

FAB Subtype (%)	Diagnostic Features
AML-M0 (3%–5%)	≥30% blasts; >3% blasts reactive to MPO, SBB, or NSE; immunophenotyping CD33+, CD13+, may be CD34+, TdT+
AML-M1 (15%–20%)	≥30% blasts; ≥3% blasts reactive to MPO or SBB; <10% of marrow nucleated cells are promyelocytes or more mature neutrophils
AML-M2 (25%–30%)	≥30% blasts; ≥3% blasts reactive for MPO or SBB; ≥10% of marrow nucleated cells are promyelocytes or more mature neutrophils; t(8:21) chromosome abnormality
AML-M3 (10%–15%)	≥30% blasts and abnormal promyelocytes; intense MPO and SBB reactivity; promyelocytes and blasts with multiple Auer rods (faggot cells); t(15:17) cytogenetic abnormality
AML-M4 (20%–30%)	≥30% myeloblasts, monoblasts, and promonocytes; ≥20% monocytic cells in marrow; ≤5 × 10^9/L monocytic cells in blood: ≥20% neutrophils and precursors in marrow; monocytic cells reactive for NSE; abnormal eosinophils in M4 with associated inv(16) chromosome abnormality
AML-M5a (2%–7%)	≥80% monocytic cells; monoblasts ≥80% of monocytic cells; monoblasts and promonocytes NSE positive; monoblasts usually MPO and SBB negative
AML-M5b (2%–5%)	≥80% monocytic cells; monoblasts ≥80% of monocytic cells; promonocytes predominate; monoblasts and promonocytes NSE positive; promonocytes may have scattered MPO- and SBB-positive granules
AML-M6 (3%–5%)	≥50% erythroid precursors: ≥30% of nonerythroid precursors are myeloblasts; Auer rods may be present in myeloblasts; dysplastic erythroid precursors frequently are PAS positive
AML-M7 (3%–5%)	≥30% blasts; ≥50% cells megakaryoblasts by morphology or electron microscopy; immunophenotyping CD41+, CD61+

AML, acute myeloid leukemia; CD, cluster designation; FAB, French-American-British; MPO, myeloperoxidase; NSE, nonspecific esterase; PAS, periodic acid–Schiff; SBB, Sudan black B; TdT, terminal deoxynucleotidyl transferase. (Percent of all AML)

original FAB classification with some modifications, namely, APL (M3 and M3 variant) is no longer included as a separate subtype but is placed with the group AML with recurrent genetic abnormalities, which is defined by cytogenetics and not morphology, percent blasts, or immunophenotyping. Pure erythroleukemia has been distinguished from erythroleukemia, acute erythroid/myeloid type; acute basophilic leukemia (very rare) has been added, as is a rare entity termed *acute panmyelosis with myelofibrosis* and the solid tumor myeloid sarcoma. The WHO classification now is widely accepted by most cooperative groups and is replacing the FAB classification of AML. It is expected that the WHO classification will continue to evolve as new biologic markers become available. The new WHO classification requires greater interexchange among the pathologist, clinician, and cytogeneticist for the diagnosis and classification of AML.

When evaluating a patient with acute leukemia, the most important initial morphologic distinction is between AML and ALL or one of the MDSs. The prognosis and therapeutic strategies remain very different for patients with these disorders. In most cases the morphologic, cytochemical, and immunophenotyping analyses will define the appropriate lineage and diagnosis. The MDSs are most frequently confused with acute erythroid leukemia or hypoplastic AML.[243] In cases where nucleated erythroid cells constitute greater than 50% of all bone marrow nucleated marrow cells, the diagnosis may be difficult. In these cases, if the combined number of blasts, type I, and II is less than 20% of the nonerythroid elements (excluding lymphocytes and plasma cells), the case is classified as MDS. If the nucleated red cells comprise less than 50% of bone marrow cells, the percent of blasts is calculated as the percent of all nucleated cells (excluding lymphocytes and plasma cells). In many cases, the difference between an MDS and AML is a difficult diagnostic problem. The AMLs with no or minimal differentiation, the monoblastic leukemias without differentiation, and some of the acute megakaryocytic leukemias (AMKLs) can be difficult to differentiate from ALL by morphology or cytochemical stain alone. In these instances, immunophenotypic studies with lineage-specific monoclonal antibodies are critical.

Subtypes of Acute Myeloid Leukemia According to World Health Organization Classification (see Table 60–7)

The WHO classification explicitly defines AML subtypes with recurrent genetic abnormalities. As a group, these AMLs are relatively common and have chromosomal translocations that result in the production of chimeric proteins, which are pivotal in the leukemogenic process. These genetic abnormalities define a specific biology, clinical course, and prognosis, so classifying them separately is important. In this group of cases, the diagnosis is defined by the cytogenetic abnormalities and is not dependent on the number of blasts in either the bone marrow or blood.

Acute Myeloid Leukemia with Recurrent Genetic Abnormalities

The WHO incorporates a new approach to AML with this subclassification of AML. As a group, AMLs with recurrent genetic abnormalities are frequent and exhibit characteristic morphologic, immunophenotypic, genetic, and clinical features. Their clinical course is well defined, and their prognosis, except for those with involvement of the *MLL* gene, is generally favorable.[207,244] This subtype includes patients with AML associated with abnormalities of the CBFs. The CBFs are a group of heterodimeric transcriptional factors essential for normal hematopoiesis. The CBF-associated AMLs include the leukemias with t(8;21) and inv[16]. The chimeric CBFs resulting from these genomic rearrangements interfere with the normal CBF transcriptional complex, leading to transcriptional repression of CBF-responsive genes and inhibition of normal myeloid differentiation.[125] CBF leukemias generally occur in younger patients (median age 39 years), with a slight male predominance. They respond to standard induction therapy.[245] The complete remission (CR) rate is 87% with both t(8;21) and inv[16], and the CBF-associated AMLs have a generally favorable prognosis. However, as with the other AML subtypes, other prognostic factors affect the response to treatment and overall survival. Older age, presence of blasts with additional complex cytogenetic abnormalities, and presence of *KIT* mutations are associated with a worse prognosis.[246] Patients who present with a higher blast count at diagnosis have a shorter overall survival and a poor response to treatment. In this subtype, the overall survival was improved for younger patients who received a more intensive treatment regimen that contained either high doses of cytarabine or a stem cell transplant.[247,248]

Table 60–8 Relationship between the WHO and the FAB classifications of Acute Myeloid Leukemia
World Health Organization (WHO) Classifications of Acute Myeloid Leukemia

WHO subtype	FAB subtype equivalent	WHO to FAB
Acute myeloid leukemia with recurrent genetic abnormalities		
- Acute myeloid leukemia with CBFα fusions – t(8;21)		M2
- Acute myeloid leukemia with CBFβ fusions – inv(16)		M4eo
- Acute myeloid leukemia with RARα fusions – t(15;17)		M3, M3v
- Acute myeloid leukemia with 11q23 translocations – MLL		M5a, M1, M0
Acute myeloid leukemia with multilineage dysplasia		
Acute myeloid leukemia, therapy related		M5, M1, M2, M0
Acute myeloid leukemia not otherwise categorized		
- Acute myeloblastic leukemia, minimally differentiated	Acute myeloblastic leukemia, minimally differentiated (M0)	M0
- Acute myeloblastic leukemia, without maturation	Acute myeloblastic leukemia, without maturation (M1)	M1
- Acute myeloblastic leukemia, with maturation	Acute myeloblastic leukemia, with maturation (M2)	M2
	Acute promyelocytic leukemia, hypergranular (M3)	M3
	Acute promyelocytic leukemia, hypogranular (M3v)	M3v
- Acute myelomonocytic leukemia	Acute myelomonocytic leukemia (M4)	M4
	Acute myelomonocytic leukemia, with eosinophilia	M4eo
- Acute monoblastic leukemia and monocytic leukemia	Acute monoblastic leukemia (M5a)	M5a
	Acute promonocytic Leukemia (M5b)	M5b
- Acute erythroleukemia (erythromyeloid)	Acute Erythroleukemia (M6a)	M6a
- Pure erythroid Leukemia	Acute Erythroleukemia (M6b)	M6b
- Acute Megakaryoblastic leukemia	Acute Megakaryoblastic leukemia (M7)	M7
- Acute basophilic leukemia		-
- Acute panmyelosis with myelofibrosis		M7
- Myeloid sarcoma		-
Acute myeloid leukemia of ambiguous lineage		
- Unfifferentiated acute leukemia		
- Bilineal acute leukemia		
- Biphenotypic acute leukemia		

Acute Myeloid Leukemia with t(8;21)(q22;q22), (AML1/ETO) (RUNX/CBFA2T1) (Core-Binding Factor Acute Myeloid Leukemia) (Fig. 60–10) (8;21) (10%–30% of Acute Myeloid Leukemia; M2 by FAB Classification)

AML with t(8;21)(q22;q22) is one of the most common subtypes of AML.[249–251] It occurs most frequently in younger adults and less frequently in elderly patients. Most cases are de novo AML, but the frequency is also increased after administration of topoisomerase II inhibitors.[252] Extramedullary disease and splenomegaly are noted in 20% and 25% of patients, respectively.[227] Patients with t(8;21)(q22;q22) generally respond to standard remission induction standard chemotherapy and have a favorable prognosis.[248] Morphologically the blasts demonstrate evidence of maturation to and beyond the promyelocyte. The blasts may exhibit nuclear clefting with large ill-defined nucleoli. Auer rods are common and typically are thin and elongated. Most of the cells have a basophilic cytoplasm with small azurophilic granules. In a minority of cases, blasts, promyelocytes, and myelocytes exhibit prominent basophilic granules (pseudo–Chédiak-Higashi granules). Increased marrow eosinophils and/or basophils are not infrequent, but monocytes and promonocytes are generally not increased. Prominent dysplastic features in the neutrophils are common. Dysplastic erythroid or megakaryocytic precursors are rare. The neutrophilic dysplastic features are not associated with a poorer response to therapy or change in the otherwise favorable prognosis of this subtype. Myeloblasts are strongly positive for MPO and SBB, often with a "clumpy" cytoplasmic pattern. CAE is positive as well, reflecting maturation beyond myeloblasts.

Immunophenotype. Blasts in most cases of AML with t(8;21)(q22;q22) exhibit characteristic immunophenotype. Blasts express the stem cell markers CD34 and CD117 and the myeloid markers CD13 and CD33. Blasts are HLA-DR$^+$ and CD11b$^-$ and CD15$^-$, although the latter two are also strongly expressed by the maturing neutrophilic component. CD14 and CD64, two monocytic markers, usually are negative. The blasts characteristically coexpress lymphoid markers including CD19, occasionally CD56, but only rarely CD2 or CD7.

Cytogenetics and Genetics. In the majority of cases, t(8;21)(q22;q22) is present on standard GTG-banded karyotypes. In a minority of patients, t(8;21)(q22;q22) is not detectable by conventional cytogenetics. These patients harbor either complex karyotypes or cryptic translocations that can be detected by FISH analysis using RUNX and CBFA2T1 nucleic acid probes. Frequent secondary cytogenetic abnormalities in t(8;21) AML are loss of a sex chromosome, loss of part or all of chromosome 9q, trisomy 8, and trisomy 4.[245,247,253] These additional cytogenetic abnormalities, when adjusted for age and white blood count, are not associated with a worse prognosis.[245,247] However, the presence of additional complex cytogenetic abnormalities is associated with poorer overall survival.[245,247]

Acute Myeloid Leukemia with Abnormal Bone Marrow Eosinophils and inv^{16} (p13;q22) or t(16;16)(p13;q22), (CBFB/MYH11) (Fig. 60–11) (5%–10% of AMLs; M4Eo by FAB Classification)

AML with inv^{16} has differentiating characteristics of both neutrophils and monocytes. A distinguishing morphologic feature is the presence of abnormal eosinophil precursors in the bone marrow. Patients with *CBFB/MYH11* fusion genes often present with a high WBC count (range 30,000–100,000/μL) and hepatosplenomegaly.[254] Extramedullary disease, gingival hypertrophy, leukemia cutis, and meningeal leukemia are more common in this subtype than in the less well-differentiated myeloid leukemias. Extramedullary disease (myeloid sarcomas) may be present at the time of diagnosis or may be the

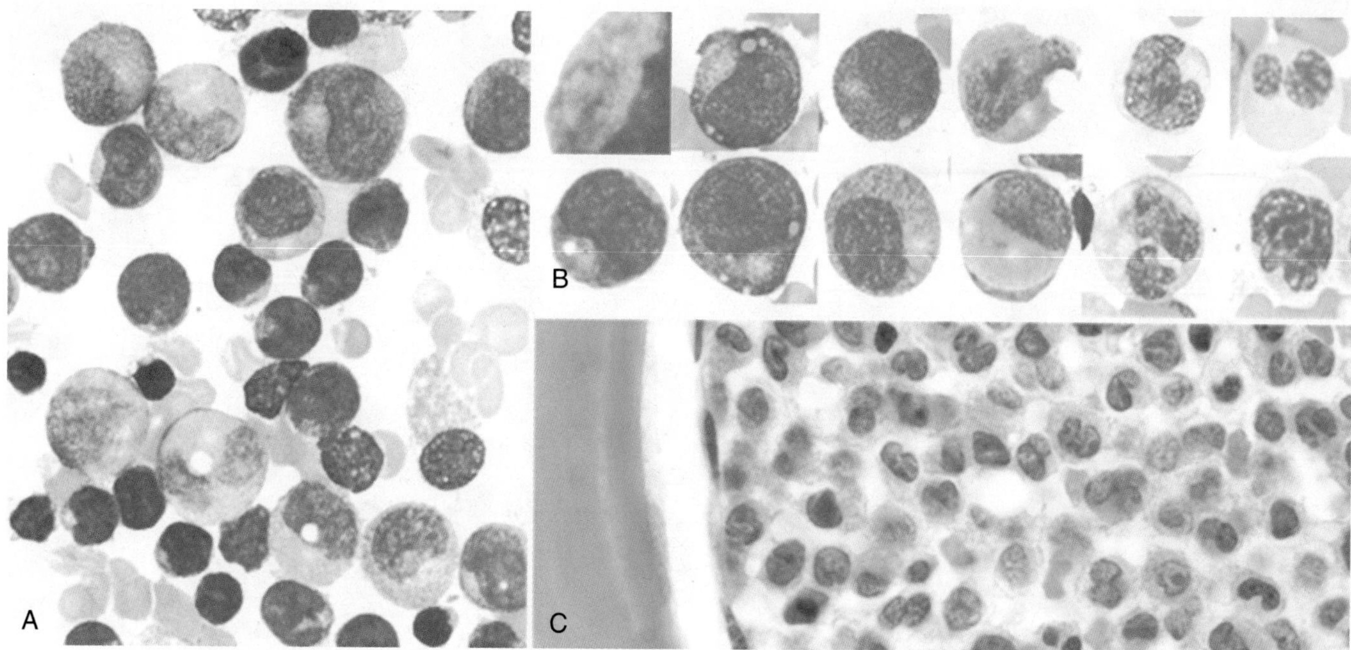

Figure 60–10 Acute myeloid leukemia with t(8;21)(q22;q22), *(AML/ETO)*. **A,** Low-power, Wright-stained bone marrow aspirate smear showing increased blasts associated with differentiating myeloid cells. **B,** Details illustrating some of the features associated with the leukemia. They include blasts with long thin Auer rods (top left), immature cells with abnormal eosinophilic globules (top and bottom, second from left), abnormal salmon-colored granulation in the maturing cells, sometimes associated with a basophilic periphery (top and bottom, fourth from left), and slightly abnormal features in the mature neutrophils (far right). Pseudo–Chédiak-Higashi granules were not seen in this case. **C,** Biopsy shows the significant degree of maturation that is sometimes seen. In some cases the blast count is less than 20%, but the diagnosis of acute myeloid leukemia still can be made with the cytogenetic finding of t(8;21).

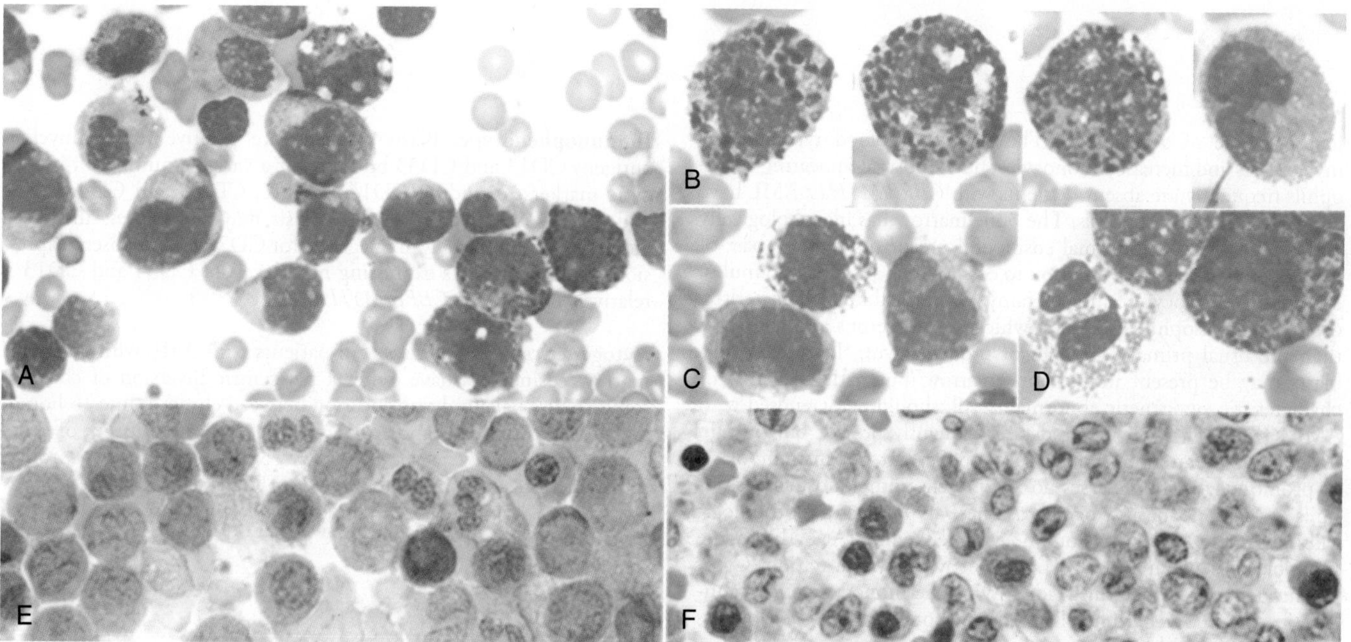

Figure 60–11 Acute myeloid leukemia with abnormal bone marrow eosinophils and inv(16)(p13;q22) or t(16;16)(p13;q22), *(CBFB/MYH11)*. **A,** Low-power, Wright-stained bone marrow aspirate showing blasts, monocytic cells, granulocytic cells, and abnormal eosinophils. **B,** Features of the abnormal eosinophils in three abnormal eosinophils (left three cells). Note the abnormal basophilic granules in the eosinophilic myelocytes. These granules are large, tend to cluster or coalesce, and are interspersed among the large eosinophilic granules, which are more difficult to see. As the eosinophils mature, the abnormal basophilic granules are less prominent and sometimes disappear (far right). A common misconception is that the basophilic granules are the granules of basophils and that the abnormal eosinophils are "hybrid cells." This is not true. **C,** Basophil in the same case (top cell) shown for comparison. **D,** Some cells from a case of reactive eosinophilia also shown for comparison. Immature eosinophils (cell to the right) have primary blue granules. However, they usually are less prominent and less atypical than the basophilic granules of the abnormal eosinophils. Of note, the monocytes in cases of acute myeloid leukemia with inv(16) or t(16;16) sometimes are ANA-reaction negative. **E,** ANA reaction. **F,** Abnormal eosinophils cannot be recognized in hematoxylin and eosin-stained sections of the biopsy sample.

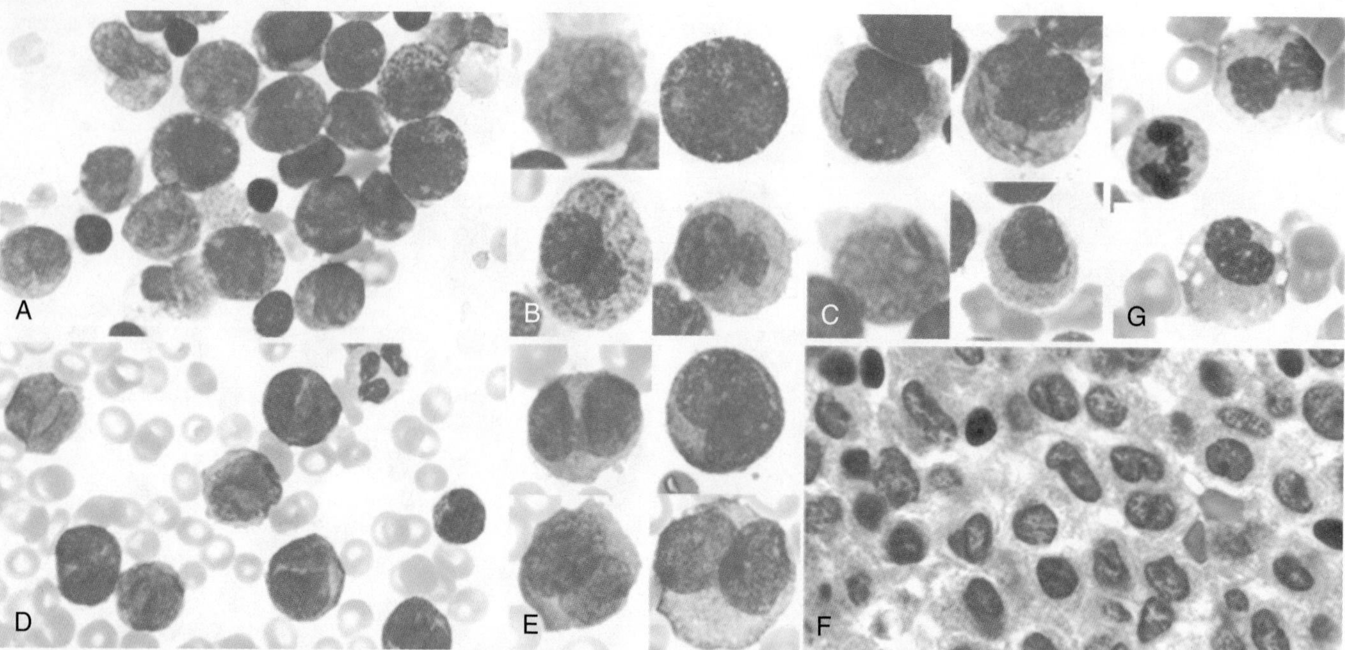

Figure 60–12 Acute promyelocytic leukemia (APL), acute myeloid leukemia with t(15;17)(q22;q21) *(PML/RARA)*. **A–C,** APL. **D, E,** Hypogranular or microgranular subtype. **F,** Bone marrow biopsy. **G,** APL cells maturing after all-*trans* retinoic acid (ATRA) therapy. In the typical granular type of APL **(A)**, the abnormal promyelocytes can exhibit variable morphologic features. Even within the same case, the granules can range from coarse, dark, and dense to fine and dust-like **(B)**. The nuclei in the abnormal promyelocytes frequently exhibit a bilobed, dumbbell, or reniform shape. This is a diagnostically important feature, which can be difficult to recognize beneath the granules **(B)**. Auer rods can be single, multiple, coalesced into Auer bodies, or even present in maturing cells **(C)**. The microgranular type usually presents with an elevated white blood cell count **(D)**. Although granules cannot be readily appreciated at the light microscope **(E)**, granules can be demonstrated by electron microscopy. The abnormal nuclear shapes (bilobed, dumbbell, and reniform) can be easily appreciated **(E)**. Bone core biopsy typically reveals sheets of cells with abundant granular cytoplasm. After ATRA therapy, the abnormal promyelocytes mature to abnormal neutrophils (**G**, top and bottom right, vs normal neutrophil, left). These can be seen for weeks after therapy and do not signify a failed response to the differentiating agent.

first evidence of a relapse.[254] The peripheral blood typically has myeloblasts and increased monocytes, but abnormal-appearing eosinophils frequently are absent. Patients with *CBFB/MYH11* AML have a favorable overall prognosis. The bone marrow has morphologically and cytochemically abnormal eosinophil precursors that are part of the leukemic clone.[255] In addition to eosinophilic secondary granules, eosinophil myelocytes and metamyelocytes exhibit characteristic cytoplasmic basophilic granules, which are numerous and are larger than the usual primary granules of promyelocytes. Less than 20% blasts may be present in the bone marrow, but patients with this characteristic cytogenetic abnormality still should be diagnosed with AML *CBFB/MYH11*. Auer rods are frequently present but only in myeloblasts or rarely in mature neutrophils, but not in monoblasts or promonocytes. Some cases do not present with abnormal eosinophils in the bone marrow or blood. These atypical cases morphologically resemble acute myelomonocytic leukemia (AMML), acute monoblastic leukemia, or AML with or without maturation. Cytochemical stains are helpful in identifying the monocytic and granulocytic cells in the peripheral blood and bone marrow. Myeloblasts typically stain with MPO and SBB. CAE is present in the more mature granulocyte precursors and, unlike in normal eosinophils, is present in abnormal eosinophils. Monoblasts usually are negative or only weakly positive for nonspecific esterases. Serum and urinary lysozyme levels, reflecting the monocytic component, frequently are elevated. The eosinophilic secondary granules stain positive with SBB, CAE, and nonspecific esterases, which is typical of granulocytic but not eosinophilic precursors. The hybrid morphologic and histochemical features of monocytes, eosinophils, and granulocytes in these cells result from abnormal differentiation of a primitive uncommitted leukemic cell.

Immunophenotype. Blasts typically are positive for panmyeloid antigens CD13 and CD33 but also for a variable number of monocytic markers, including CD14, CD11c, CD64, and CD4. CD34 and CD117 usually are positive. Blasts may also express the T-cell antigen CD2 but usually are negative for CD7. Dim or absent expression of CD33 in cells expressing high levels of CD34 and CD13 is relatively specific for *CBFB/MYH11* AML.[256–258]

Cytogenetics and Genetics. All patients with AML with abnormal marrow eosinophils have either a pericentric inversion of chromosome 16 or a balanced translocation between chromosome 16 homologues that transpose bands p13 and q22, leading to fusion of genes *CBFB* and *MYH11*.[254,259] The most common secondary chromosomal abnormalities in the typical *CBFB/MYH11 AML* are trisomy 22, trisomy 8, and 7q−. *KIT* mutations occur in up to one third of AML with *CBFB/MYH11* and are associated with a shorter disease-free response.[260,261]

Acute Promyelocytic Leukemia: Acute Myeloid Leukemia with t(15;17)(q22;q21) (PML/RARA) or t(11;17)(q23;q12) (PLZF/RARA) or t(5;17)(q23;q12) (NPM/RARA), or t(11;17)(q13;q12) (NuMA/RARA) (Fig. 60–12) (5%–10% of Acute Myeloid Leukemia; FAB M3, M3v by FAB Classification)

APL is characterized by distinctive morphology, younger patient age at presentation, associated coagulopathy, and unique response to treatment with all-*trans* retinoic acid (ATRA). In APL, t(15;17)(q22;q21) results in fusion of the *RARA* gene on chromosome 17 with the *PML* gene on chromosome 15. RARA is a member of the nuclear steroid hormone receptor family and is important in the regulation of cellular differentiation. Normally, RARA heterodimers bind to promoter retinoic acid response elements (RARE) and recruit chromatin repressors, shutting down transcription. Upon binding to retinoic acid, RARA releases repressors and recruits transcriptional activators, reestablishing gene expression. PML/RARA retains RARE binding function and binds chromatin repressor more strongly.[262] Treatment of patients with APL with ATRA results in differentiation of leukemic cells, with approximately 70% to 85% of patients attaining CR.[263] APL has two morphologic variants: a "typical" or hypergranular variant found in 75% of cases and a less frequent microgranular (hypogranular) variant.[264] These two variants differ in clinical presentation, prognosis, and morphologic features.[263,265–269] The typical APL is hypergranular. Patients present with a low WBC count (3000–15,000/μL); a majority present with WBC count less than 5000/μL. Patients with microgranular APL typically present with a higher WBC count (range 50,000–200,000/μL). Leukostasis and fatal CNS or pulmonary hemorrhage are more common in patients with the microgranular variant.[270] The clinical features of APL depend to some extent on the type of fusion transcript resulting from the translocation.[271] APL with PLZF/RARA: t(11;17) or NPM/RARA: t(5;17) usually present with leukocytosis, which can be as high as that seen in the microgranular variant. APL with PLZF/RARA is resistant to therapy with ATRA as well as with arsenic trioxide.[272,273]

Patients with APL often present with thrombocytopenia, prolongation of prothrombin time and partial thromboplastin time, increased levels of fibrin degradation products, and hypofibrinogenemia. The coagulation disorder in APL results from at least three distinct mechanisms: disseminated intravascular coagulation, fibrinolysis, and proteolysis.[272] Disseminated intravascular coagulation is attributed to the spontaneous or chemotherapy-associated release of a tissue factor with procoagulant activity present in the granules of the leukemic promyelocytes. However, the bleeding disorder, cannot always be related solely to disseminated intravascular coagulation. Many patients have signs of primary fibrinolysis. The promyelocytic leukemic cell has both strong procoagulant activity on its cell membrane and proteolytic activity in the cytoplasmic granules, a combination that is unique to the leukemic promyelocyte and may explain the severe coagulopathy seen in some patients. Enhanced fibrinolysis is suggested by the increase in fibrin/fibrinogen degradation products, reduced α_2-antiplasmin levels, and normal antithrombin III and protein C levels present in all patients at diagnosis and up to initiation of therapy. Plasma from patients with APL has a plasminogen activator of tissue origin. APL cell express high levels of annexin II on their cell surface.[274] Annexin II is a fibrinolytic protein that increases the efficiency of plasmin formation.

Proteolysis is due to release from the leukemic cells of lysosomal neutrophilic enzymes, human leukocyte elastase, cathepsin G, and proteinase 3, all of which can cleave fibrinogen.[275] Leukemic promyelocytes also express high levels of tissue factor, a membrane glycoprotein that functions as a receptor for factor VII and as a site of activation of factor VII to VIIa. Tissue factor is an initiator of coagulation in normal tissues and may be a cellular activator of the coagulation system in malignant diseases.[276] The coagulopathy is present at diagnosis in 80% to 90% of cases and is exacerbated by cytotoxic chemotherapy. Treatment of bleeding disorders in patients with APL is controversial. Supportive therapy with fresh frozen plasma, fibrinogen, and platelets should be given until the coagulopathy resolves.[263] Use of ATRA with or without chemotherapy has changed the prognosis, course, and management of APL. The bleeding and clotting problems generally respond promptly to treatment with retinoic acid.

The microgranular variant occurs in approximately 20% of cases. It typically presents with a very elevated WBC count (frequently >100,000/μL), and the cells have minimal rather than excessive cytoplasmic granulation.[264] Patients have the typical t(15;17) of the "standard" hypergranular promyelocytic leukemia. The microgranular form can be confused morphologically with a monocytic leukemia. A minority of patients with the microgranular variant present with hyperbasophilic cytoplasm and cytoplasmic projections that may resemble megakaryoblasts. In the microgranular variant, the appearance of blasts in the peripheral blood and bone marrow may be very different.

The promyelocytes of hypergranular APL are larger than normal promyelocytes, and the nucleus varies from folded to reniform to bilobed. Granules may be so numerous that they obscure the nuclear outline. Auer rods may be so numerous as to form Auer bundles *(faggot cells)*.[222,277] Promyelocytes are strongly positive for SBB, MPO, and CAE.[277] Patients with the microgranular variant of APL present with abnormal promyelocytes devoid of normal primary azurophilic granules, and Auer rods are rare.[278] The cytoplasm may appear transparent and devoid of granules, or they may appear dusty, sometimes with large clusters of dust-like granules polarized within the cytoplasm. Electron microscopic studies demonstrate that the promyelocytes of microgranular APL have numerous granules smaller than 250 nm, which is below the limit of resolution of ordinary light microscopy.[279] The nucleus is irregular, folded or bilobed with delicate chromatin and inconspicuous nucleoli. As in the hypergranular form, the abnormal promyelocytes of microgranular APL are strongly reactive for MPO and CAE. The morphologic features of APL with the variant translocations may differ from those of typical APL.[280] For instance, APL with NPM/RARA generally lacks Auer rods, whereas APL with PLZF/RARA exhibit round nuclei, more condensed chromatin, and abundant cytoplasm that is less basophilic, suggesting that cells are arrested at the promyelocyte/myelocyte stage rather than the promyelocyte stage, as is typical of APL.[280] Additionally, Pelger-Huet–like cells are frequent in PLZF/RARAAPL.[280]

Immunophenotype. Both hypergranular and microgranular APL with PML/RARA fusion have characteristic immunophenotypes.[281,282] Cells strongly express CD33, lack or weakly express HLA-DR, are CD34⁻, and frequently coexpress CD2 and CD9. The cells can express variable amounts of CD13, whereas more mature myeloid and monocytic markers, such as CD11b, CD14, and CD15, are expressed weakly or not at all.[281,282] The phenotype of the microgranular variant of APL is similar to that of the hypergranular form but may be $CD34^+$ and $CD2^+$ and express greater amounts of CD45.[283,284] CD56 expression is both variants correlates with lower CR rate and shorter overall survival.[280,285,286]

Cytogenetics and Genetics. t(15;17)(q22;q21) is present in 85% of APLs patients with PML/RARA. The remainder of cases have a cryptic PML/RARA (4%), have complex translocations masking t(15;17) (2%), or are cytogenetic failures.[287,288] FISH is useful for demonstrating cryptic or complex translocations. t(15;17) can rarely not be detected by FISH because of small insertion events that may be missed by large locus-specific FISH probes.[289] PML/RARA–negative APLs result from t(11;17)(q23;q12) due to PLZF/RARA fusion (0.8%), t(5;17)(q23;q12) leading to NPM/RARA fusion (0.2%), or t(11;17)(q13;q12) resulting in NuMA/RARA fusion (<0.1%). RARA fusions not involving PML account for only 2% of all cases of APL.[288] Secondary chromosome abnormalities present at diagnosis do not confer a poor prognosis.[290,291]

Acute Myeloid Leukemia with 11q23 (Mixed Lineage Leukemia) Abnormalities (Fig. 60–13) (5%–10% of Acute Myeloid Leukemias; FAB M5 by FAB Classification)

Acute leukemias with abnormalities of the *MLL* gene (also known as HRX or ALL-1) are clinically and biologically heterogeneous. MLL leukemias include AMLs, ALLs, and leukemias of ambiguous phenotype.[292–294] Although the majority of AMLs with *MLL* abnormalities are therapy-related leukemias and are associated with prior exposure to topoisomerase II inhibitors, a subgroup of de novo AMLs presents with the *MLL* abnormality.[295] In infants with AML it is the most

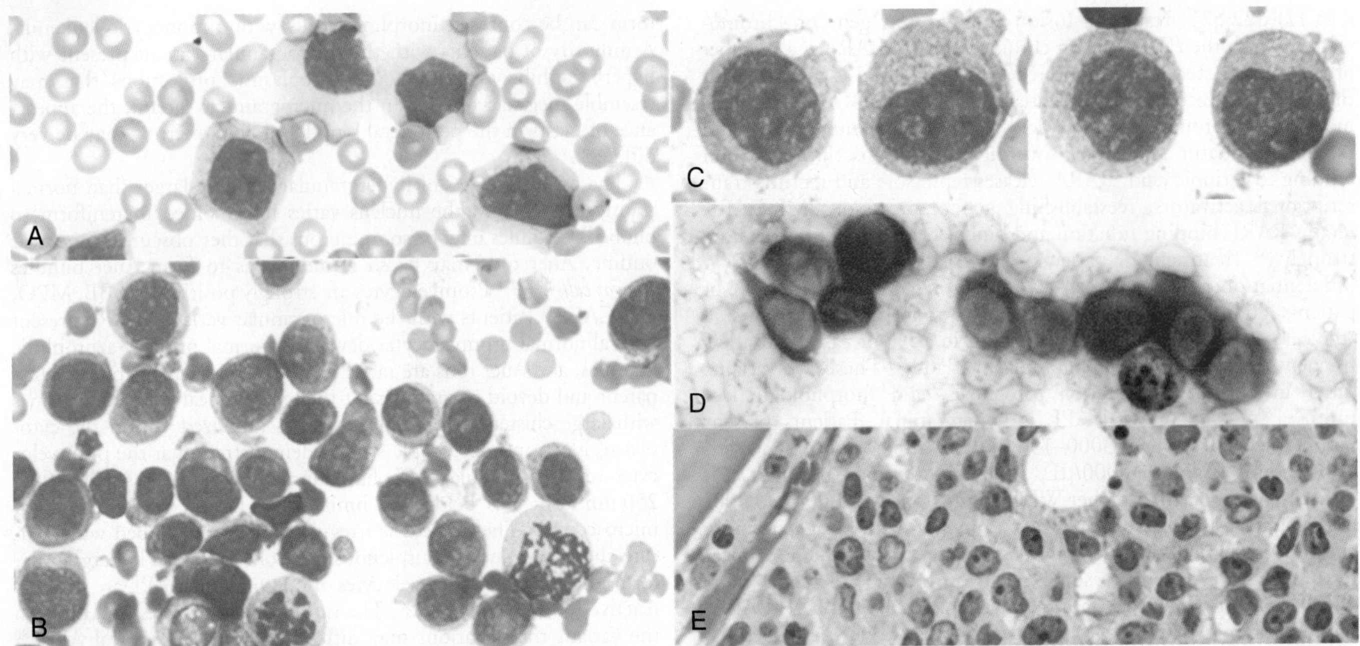

Figure 60–13 Acute monoblastic leukemia with t(9;11)((q31;q23), (*MLL* rearrangement). Case of acute monoblastic leukemia with t(9;11). **A,** Cases typically present with high counts due to circulating monoblasts. **B,** Bone marrow aspirate is packed with monoblasts and shows few granulocytic elements. **D,** Absence of a granulocytic component can be illustrated with the combined esterase reaction. Most cells show the α-naphthyl butyrate reaction product (orange–brown). Only rare granulocytes show the blue reaction product from the chloroacetate esterase reaction. **E,** The biopsy sample usually is packed with sheets of monoblasts with fine nuclear chromatin and abundant pink cytoplasm.

common cytogenetic abnormality, whether lymphoid, myeloid, or biphenotypic.[296–299] De novo AMLs involving the *MLL* gene present with high blood and marrow blast counts as well as higher platelet counts than typically seen in t-AML.[295] Hepatosplenomegaly and extramedullary disease are common. Patients with de novo AMLs with *MLL* translocations appear to have a better overall survival than those with t-AML/t-MDS, whether treated with conventional chemotherapy or marrow transplantation.[295] In infants, however, AML with *MLL* translocations is associated with a high blast count at presentation, hepatosplenomegaly, CNS involvement, and overall poor prognosis.[299] The blasts in de novo AML with *MLL* abnormalities resemble monoblasts. They are large and contain abundant cytoplasm that varies from pale to basophilic. Although primary granules often are present, they usually are small and inconspicuous. A minority of cases have blasts that resemble those of AML with or without maturation.

Immunophenotype. No immunophenotypic features are specific for AML with *MLL* translocation. Noninfant MLL leukemia with monoblastic morphology lacks CD34 and expresses markers of the monocytic lineage, including CD4, CD11b, CD11c, and CD36 but not CD14 or CD56. De novo AML with partial tandem duplication usually is CD11c+.[300]

Cytogenetics and Genetics. The most common abnormalities of the *MLL* gene in de novo AML with karyotypic abnormalities of 11q23 are the reciprocal translocations t(9;11)(q34;q23), t(10;11)(p12;q23), t(11;19)(q23;p13.1), and t(11;19)(q23;p13.3) and in infants t(9;11)(q34;q23) and t(10;11)(p12;q23).[99,293,295,301–303] Additional 51 *MLL* partner genes have been characterized.[292]

Acute Myeloid Leukemias with "Disease-Defining Genetic Abnormalities" Not Included in the Current World Health Organization Classification

Not included in the current WHO classification are a number of other AMLs with recurrent genetic abnormalities. These abnormalities include translocations involving the genes *FGFR1*, *NUP98*, *MYST3 (MOZ)*, and *EVI1* and AML with t(6;9)(p23;q34), t(8;16) associated with hemophagocytosis. Leukemias with normal karyotypes and gene mutations, such as *NPM1*, *CEBPA*, and *RUNX (CBFA)*, currently are not addressed in the WHO classification (Table 60–9).

Acute Leukemia with Multilineage Dysplasia (Fig. 60–14)

AML with multilineage dysplasia is characterized by the presence of 20% or more blasts in the marrow and dysplasia in at least 50% of the cells belonging to at least two hematopoietic cell lines. This leukemia may occur de novo or after a preceding myelodysplastic/myeloproliferative or overlap myelodysplastic/myeloproliferative syndrome. The leukemia that occurs with a documented preceding MDS is best designated AML "evolving from a myelodysplastic syndrome." This type of AML occurs primarily in older individuals and often presents with pancytopenia. The incidence of this form of leukemia increases with age and shares cytogenetic, clinical, and biologic features with MDS. The prognosis with current AML therapy is very poor. MDS-related AMLs appear to differ biologically from de novo leukemias. The WHO emphasizes the background multilineage dysplasia and a documented history of MDS.

Morphology. Dysgranulopoiesis is characterized by neutrophils with hypogranular cytoplasm, hyposegmented nuclei (pseudo–Pelger-Huet anomaly), or multisegmented nuclei. Dyserythropoiesis is characterized by megaloblastic nuclei, with nuclear-to-cytoplasm asynchrony, nuclear fragments, or bizarre nuclei. Dysmegakaryopoiesis includes micromegakaryocytes and mononuclear or large multilobed megakaryocytes. The bone marrow may be hypocellular, normal cellular, or hypercellular.

Immunophenotype. Myeloblasts express lymphoid and/or myeloid markers. The blasts usually express CD34 and coexpress the myeloid markers CD13 and CD33 and the lymphoid marker CD7 or CD56.

Table 60–9 Genetically Defined Leukemias Not Included in the World Health Organization Classification

CURRENT AND PROPOSED MOLECULARLY DEFINED AML TYPES

AML type[1]	HUGO[2] Gene Name	Karyotype[3]	Genotype[4]	Morphology/immunophenotype/clinical features[5]
Core binding factor (CBF) AML group	*RUNX1*	t(8;21)(q22;q22)	*RUNX1-RUNX1T1* fusion gene	AML with differentiation; coarse 1° granules, dysgranulopoiesis; favorable prognosis
•[6]	•	t(3;21)(q26;q22)	*RUNX1-EVI1* fusion gene	MDS > AML; acute megakaryoblastic leukemia; dysmyelopoiesis, ↓ platelets
•	•	t(1;21)(q36;q22)	*RUNX1-PRDM16* fusion gene	MDS > AML with minimal differentiation; AML w/o diff and AML differentiation
•	•	Normal	Acquired *RUNX1* point mutations	Up to 30% of AML with minimal differentiation; some AMKL; ~20% with FLT3 mutations
•	•	Normal	Germline monoalleic *RUNX1* point mutations	Familial platelet disorder with predisposition for acute myelogenous leukemia (FPD/AML).
•	*CBFB*	inv(16)(p13q22) t(16;16)(p13;q22)	*CBFB-MYH11* fusion gene	Acute myelomonocytic leukemia with abnormal eosinophils; extramedullary involvement (CNS, skin, spleen, liver); favorable prognosis
Retinoic acid receptor alpha (RARA) AML group	*RARA*	t(15;17)(q22;q12)	*PML-RARA* fusion gene	APL hypergranular (Auer rods, faggot cells) and microgranular variant (invisible granules); coagulopathy; ATRA sensitive; favorable prognosis
•	•	t(11;17)(q23;q12)	*PLZF-RARA* fusion gene	APL hypergranular with frequent mononuclear Pelger-Huet cells and absent binucleate promyelocytes; coagulopathy; ATRA resistent
•	•	t(11;17)(q13;q12)	*NuMA-RARA* fusion gene	APL hypergranular with bilobed and faggot cells; coagulopathy; ATRA sensitive
•	•	t(5;17)(q35;q12)	*NPM1-RARA* fusion gene	APL hypergranular with bilobed cells but absent Auer rods; coagulopathy; ATRA sensitive
MLL (mixed linage leukemia gene) AML group[7]	*MLL*	t(9;11)(p22;q23)	*MLL-MLLT3* fusion gene	De novo or therapy related (topo II inhibitors only) acute monoblastic/monocytic leukemia; CD34-; CD117-; poor prognosis
•	•	t(6;11)(q27;q23)	*MLL-MLLT4* fusion gene	•
•	•	t(10;11)(p12;q23)	*MLL-MLLT10* fusion gene	•
•	•	t(11;19)(q23;p13.1)	*MLL-ELL* fusion gene	•
EVI1 AML group	*PRMD3 (EVI1)*	inv(3)(q21q26) t(3;3)(q21;q26)	*EVI1::RPN1; RPN1_E::EVI1* enhancer effect	AML with multilineage dysplasia; therapy related AML ↑ platelet; trilineage dysplasia; prominent dysmegakaryopoiesis; poor prognosis
•	•	t(3;12)(q26;p13)	*ETV6-EVI1* fusion gene	•
•	*PRDM16 (MEL1)*	t(1;3)(p36;q21)	*RPN1_E::MEL1* enhancer effect	•
MYST AML group	*MYST3 (MOZ)*	t(8;16)(p11;p13)	*MYST3-CREBBP* fusion gene	De novo and therapy related acute monoblastic/monocytic or myelomonocytic leukemia; Erythrophagocytosis MPO+ NSE+ CD34– CD117– CD56+; poor prognosis
•	•	t(8;22)(p11;q13)	*MYST3-EP300* fusion gene	•
•	•	inv(8)(p11;q13)	*MYST3-NCOA2* fusion gene	•
•	*MYST4 (MORF)*	t(10;16)(q22;p13)	*MYST4-CREBBP* fusion gene	•
EMS (8p12 stem-cell myeloliferative syndrome) AML group	*FGFR1*	t(8;13)(p11;q12),	*ZNF198-FGFR1* fusion gene	Rapidly progressive yeloproliferative disorder, ↑ eos, enlarged LN, spleen; Nodal pre-T, pre- B ALL culminating in AML; poor prognosis
•	•	t(8;9)(p11;q33)	*CEP110-FGFR1* fusion gene	•
•	•	t(6;8)(q27;p11)	*FGFR10P(FOP)-FGFR1* fusion	•
•	•	t(8;17)(p11;q23)	*MYO18A-FGFR1* fusion gene	•
•	•	ins(12;8)(p11;p11p22)	*FGFROP2-FGFR1* fusion gene	•
Nucleophosmin (NPM1) AML	*NPM1*	Normal	*NPM* insertion mutations	40% of AML with normal karyotype; CD34-: good prognosis if FLT3 wild type, poor prognosis in FLT3 with ITD mutations
•	•	t(3;5)(q25;q34)	*NPM-MLF1* gene fusion	MDS>AML CMPD>AML; poor progmosis
HOX AML group[8]	*HOXA*	t(7;11)(p15;p15)	*NUP98-HOXA9* gene fusion	De novo AML; sometimes aCML>>AML; older age
•	*HOXA9*	•	*NUP98-HOXA* gene fusion	De novo AML with maturation; older age
•	*HOXC11*	•	*NUP98-HOXC11* gene fusion	•
•	*HOXC13*	t(2;11)(q31;p15)	*NUP98-HOXC13* gene fusion	•
•	*HOXD13*	t(11;12)(p15;q13)	*NUP98-HOXD13* gene fusion	De novo AMML; older age
•	*NSD1*	del(5q)	*NUP98-NSD1* gene fusion	De novo AML with maturation; younger age
MKL1 AML	*MKL1*	t(1;22)(p13;q13)	*RBM15-MKL1* gene fusion	Infant AMKL (60–80% of non-Down syndrome AMKL <6mo); organomegaly, thrombocytopenia, micromegakaryoctes, myelofirosis
PICALM AML	*PICALM*	t(10;11)(p13;q14–21)	*PICALM-AF10* gene fusion	AML; also T-ALL
DEK-SET AML	*DEK*	t(6;9)(p23;q34)	*DEK-NUP214* gene fusion	MDS>AML with maturation or AMML; Basophilia
•	*SET*	t(9;9)(q34;q34)	*SET-NUP214* gene fusion	•
FUS/TLS-ERG AML	*FUS ERG*	t(16;21)(p11;q22)	*FUS-ERG* gene fusion	Children and young adults; variable morphoogy; erythrophagocytosis; poor prognosis
CEBP AML	*CEBP*	Normal	CEBP point mutations	Accounts for 15% of AML without differentiation
GATA1 AML	*GATA1*	Constitutional +21	GATA1 point mutations	Transient myeloproliferative disorder of the newborn (TMD) > AMKL; Down syndrome pts

1, grouped by gene defect thought to have a dominant and/or early effect in defining the biological and clinical characteristics of acute myelod leukemia (driver mutations); mutations in the genes NRAS and FLT3 are not included as they are acquired during clonal evolution, occur over a wide spectrum of leukemia types and do not define specific groups of AML; 2, Human Genome Organization accepted gene nomenclature/gene symbol; 3, common but not exclusively associated cytogenetic changes; 4, disease-defining molecular event; 5, salient morphologic, immunophenotypic and/or clinical features, not all listed; 6, of the more than fifty translocation partners of the MLL gene, only those most commonly associated with AML are listed; 7, the symbol indicates features similar to those described immediately above; 8, designated HOX AML group since the HOX gene, and not the NUP98 gene, appears to be responsible for leukemogenesis. APL, acute promyelocytic; AMML, acute myelomonocytic; AMKL, acute megakaryoblastic leukemia; MDS, myelodysplastic syndrome.

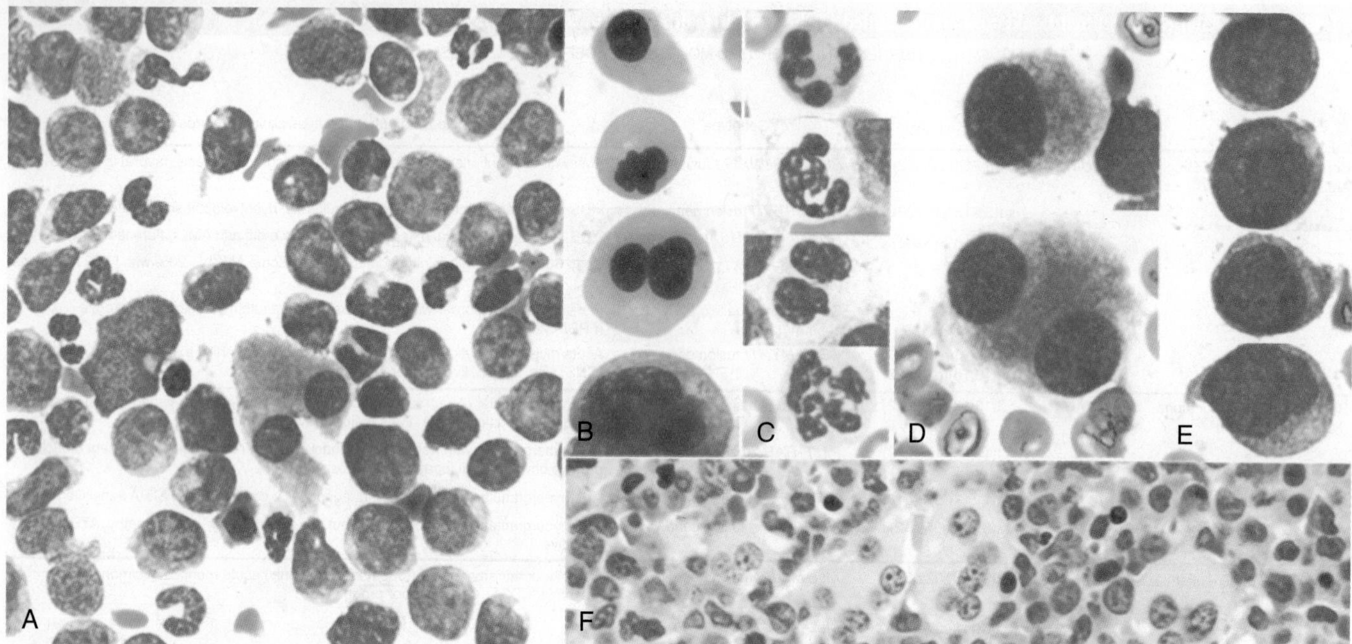

Figure 60–14 Acute myeloid leukemia with multilineage dysplasia. **A,** Bone marrow aspirate shows increased blasts and maturing cells with dysplastic features. **B–D,** Details of the dysplasia. **B,** Maturing erythroid elements exhibit megaloblastoid change and bizarre nuclear abnormalities. **C,** Dysplastic granulocytes (bottom three) are compared to a rare normal granulocyte (top). The dysplastic forms have pale cytoplasm and abnormal nuclear shapes with hypolobation, hypersegmentation, and prominent nuclear excrescences. **D,** Dysplastic micromegakaryocytes have single or double small nuclei but mature cytoplasm with platelet material within. **E,** Increased blasts. **F,** Dysplasia is difficult to appreciate on a biopsied section. This is true except for the megakaryocytes. Dysplastic megakaryocytes can be recognized on the biopsy sample by their abnormally small nuclei, which sometimes are multiple and widely spaced.

Cytogenetics and Genetics. AML-MLD typically exhibits gains and losses of entire or large segments of chromosomes found in MDS. Gains or losses of chromosomes are most common and include −5, −7/del(7q), +8, +9, +11, del(11q), del(12p), del(17p), −18, +19, del(20q), +21. Most of these partial or complete chromosome abnormalities are the same as those that characterize the alkylating agent–associated myelodysplastic syndrome (t-MDS) and secondary acute leukemia (t-AML).

Acute Myeloid Leukemia and Myelodysplastic Syndromes, Therapy-Related (30%–40% of Acute Myeloid Leukemias: M0 by FAB Classification)

The WHO recognizes the unique clinical and biologic features of the therapy-related leukemias (t-AML). This subtype results from prior exposure to cytotoxic chemotherapy and/or radiation therapy. A majority of patients have clonal cytogenetic abnormalities.[304] Secondary leukemias now account for approximately 40% of all AMLs.[305] The WHO recognizes two types of t-AML based on the type of prior exposure or treatment. Alkylating agent–related AML and topoisomerase II inhibitor–related AML have different clinical patterns and cytogenetic abnormalities (Table 60–10).

Alkylating Agent–Related Acute Myeloid Leukemia and Myelodysplastic Syndrome

Alkylating agent/radiation–related disorders occur 5 to 7 years after exposure and are generally preceded by a progressive MDS. The risk for developing AML is partly related to the total cumulative dose of the alkylating agent and the patient's age at the time of treatment.[305] A majority of patients present with dysplasia in two or more lines and are diagnosed with the MDS subtype refractory cytopenia with multilineage dysplasia. The majority of patients are older and respond poorly to chemotherapy. Expression of multidrug resistance glycoprotein 1 (MDR-1) is increased, and many cases are refractory to standard induction chemotherapy.[306]

Table 60–10 Secondary AML (Therapy-Related AML)

	Topoisomerase II Inhibitor	Alkylator
Latency	18–36 months	60–84 months
Morphology	Monocytic	Undifferentiated
Cytogenetics	11q23	Monosomy 7, 5q−, 7q−, trisomy 8
FAB type	M2, M3, M4	M0, M1
Prognosis	Variable–poor	Poor
Prior MDS	No	Yes

AML, acute myeloid leukemia; FAB, French-American-British; MDS, myelodysplastic syndrome

Morphology. The dysplastic changes usually are apparent on peripheral blood smear and include trilineage dysplasia with basophilic stippled red cells and prominent red cell shape abnormalities. Hypogranulated neutrophils with nuclear hypolobulation are common. Ringed sideroblasts are found in the majority of cases. The bone marrow usually is hypercellular for the patient's age. Bone marrow fibrosis occurs in approximately 15% of cases and results in teardrop-shaped red cells in the peripheral smear. Most patients present with a variable period of MDS, but some patients present with overt AML. Morphologically most of the cases correspond to acute leukemia with minimal maturation; however, the morphology may not be lineage specific.

Immunophenotype. The blasts usually express CD34 and myeloid markers, including CD13 and CD33. Aberrant expression of lymphoid markers, including CD56 and CD7, is common.

Cytogenetics and Genetics. More than 90% of patients have a clonal cytogenetic abnormality.[304] Abnormalities involving loss or part of chromosomes 5 and/or 7 are most common. Deletions consisting of loss of all or part of the long arm of chromosomes 5 and/or 7 (5q−, 7q−) in addition to multiple complex chromosome abnormalities are common. As in the other subtypes of AML, the finding of complex cytogenetic abnormalities is associated with a poor response to chemotherapy and short overall survival.

Topoisomerase II Inhibitor–Related Acute Myeloid Leukemia

Topoisomerase II AML occurs in individuals all ages, has a short latency period, and is not generally preceded by an MDS or a period of pancytopenia. The time from exposure to the development of AML usually is 18 to 36 months. The most common drugs include the epipodophyllotoxins etoposide and teniposide and the anthracyclines doxorubicin and mitoxantrone. Morphologically most of the AMLs have a monocytic component, either acute monoblastic or acute myelomonocytic leukemia. APL and CBFB AMLs have been reported after administration of topoisomerase II inhibitors.

The most frequent cytogenetic finding is a balanced cytogenetic translocation involving 11q23 (*MLL* gene),[99] with the translocations t(9;11), t(11;19), and t(6;11) being the most common. Translocations involving 21q22 are the second most common.[307] The prognosis is variable and depends, in part, on the partner chromosome.

Acute Myeloid Leukemia Not Otherwise Categorized (Fig. 60–15)

AMLs that are not defined by previously noted criteria are subclassified into AML not otherwise categorized. The subclassification is similar to the FAB criteria and attempts to define the cell lineage using morphologic, immunophenotypic, and cytochemical criteria (see Table 60–8). The WHO not otherwise categorized criteria subdivide the myeloid leukemias according to their predominant cell type. Some cases of AML cannot be classified according to the WHO criteria. These unclassifiable cases are more frequent among patients with secondary leukemia and represent approximately 2% to 5% of all cases. The WHO includes the subclassification acute leukemia of ambiguous lineage to define a group of AML with blasts of indeterminate lineage. This group includes the hybrid or biphenotypic leukemias that cannot be classified on the basis of morphology or cytochemistry alone. The division between each of the myeloblast subtypes is somewhat arbitrary, and there is a spectrum of myeloid differentiation. The criteria are based on findings in the bone marrow aspirate and blood smear. The WHO does acknowledge that the biopsy is necessary for assessment of cellularity and for diagnosis of leukemias associated with fibrosis.

Acute Myeloblastic Leukemia, Minimally Differentiated (3%–5% of Acute Myeloid Leukemias; FAB M0 by FAB Classification)

Minimally differentiated AML (AML-MD) is a subtype of AML without morphologic or cytochemical evidence of myeloid differentiation. Myeloid differentiation can be ascertained only by immunophenotyping or, if necessary, by immunohistochemistry or ultrastructural cytochemistry.[308,309] AML-MD is more frequent in patients 60 to 80 years of age.[238] An elevated WBC count and extensive replacement of the bone marrow are common presenting findings.[238,310] The blast morphology is variable in this group but relatively homogeneous within each case.[309] The blasts have a pale basophilic to clear agranular cytoplasm without Auer rods. The nuclei chromatin texture usually is fine with prominent nucleoli. Multilineage dysplasia with prominent cytoplasmic budding is commpon.[309,310] Cytochemical stains reveal that less than 3% of the blast cells are MPO positive. Morphologically, the blasts may resemble megakaryoblasts or undifferentiated monoblasts or lymphoblasts. The majority of the cells express CD34, HLA-DR, CD13, and CD33. Coexpression of the lymphoid marker CD7 and TdT, a marker of immaturity, is present in more than one third of cases.[309,310] T- and B-cell lineage-specific markers are absent.[309]

AML-MD has no unique cytogenetic abnormality. The most common abnormalities are complex karyotypes, including abnormalities of chromosomes 7 and 8 and trisomy 13. A proportion of AML-MD with normal karyotype carries mutations of AML1 (RUNXS1) and/or FLT-3.[312] These findings suggest that AML-MD is composed of a group of disorders that represent an early stage of myeloid maturation that share a common morphologic phenotype but differ biologically and genetically. AML-MD is associated with a generally poor prognosis.[262,311]

Acute Myeloblastic Leukemia Without Maturation (10%–20% of Acute Myeloid Leukemias: FAB M1, M2 by FAB Classification)

AML without maturation is defined by ≥90% myeloblasts without evidence of maturation. The myeloid lineage is confirmed by greater than 3% of blasts staining with MPO or SBB. The bone marrow usually is hypercellular. The myeloblasts are poorly differentiated and contain rare azurophilic granules and occasional Auer rods. Nuclei are round or oval with fine chromatin and often, conspicuous nucleoli. There are less than 3% promyelocytes and less than 10% maturing granulocytes or monocytes. A distinctive but rare variant of leukemia with "cup-like" nuclei and fine azurophilic granules is classified in this morphologic category.[265,313] This variant can be easily confused both morphologically and immunophenotypically with the hypogranular variant of APL but has a normal karyotype.

Blast cells frequently express CD34, CD117, D13, and CD33. The mature monocyte markers CD14 and CD11b are rarely expressed, and, unlike AML-MD, the blasts rarely express TdT. Lymphoid lineage-specific markers are generally absent. Unlike AML-MD, more than half of the AMLs without maturation have a normal karyotype, and only 20% have complex karyotypes.[302] The prognosis is variable and depends on the prognostic variable of the specific case. Patients who present with hyperleukocytosis have a poor prognosis.

Acute Myeloblastic Leukemia with Maturation (25%–35% of Acute Myeloid Leukemias; FAB M2 by FAB Classification)

AML with maturation is defined by the presence of maturation to and beyond the promyelocyte stage (≥10%). Monocytes account for ≥20% of marrow or peripheral blood cells. This AML subtype is the largest group of morphologically defined AMLs.[302] This subtype is clinically heterogenous; 25% of patients younger than 25 years and 40% are older than 60 years. Hepatosplenomegaly and lymphadenopathy can be prominent presenting findings. Leukocytosis is present in half of patients, but leukopenia occurs in 25%.[314] Disseminated intravascular coagulation is present in up to 20% of patients. The percent of myeloblasts varies widely, but more mature neutrophils are always present and exhibit dysplastic features, including nuclear hyposegmentation (pseudo–Pelger-Huet anomaly) or hypersegmentation. Auer rods are present in 60% to 70% of cases. Azurophilic granules nearly always are present and range from few to many. Type II blasts may predominate in the bone marrow. Eosinophil precursors are increased but do not have the cytologic abnormalities characteristic of the eosinophils in AMML with inv[16]. Increased basophils or mast cells may be noted and is associated with recurrent cytogenetic abnormalities, including t(6;9)(q22;q22) and translocations or deletions at 12p11–13. Rare cases present with erythrophagocytosis and are associated with t(8;16). The myeloblasts express the myeloid associated antigens CD13, CD33, and CD15. CD34, HLA-DR, and CD117 are variably expressed but less often than the immature AML subtypes. Up to 50% of cases have normal karyotypes, and

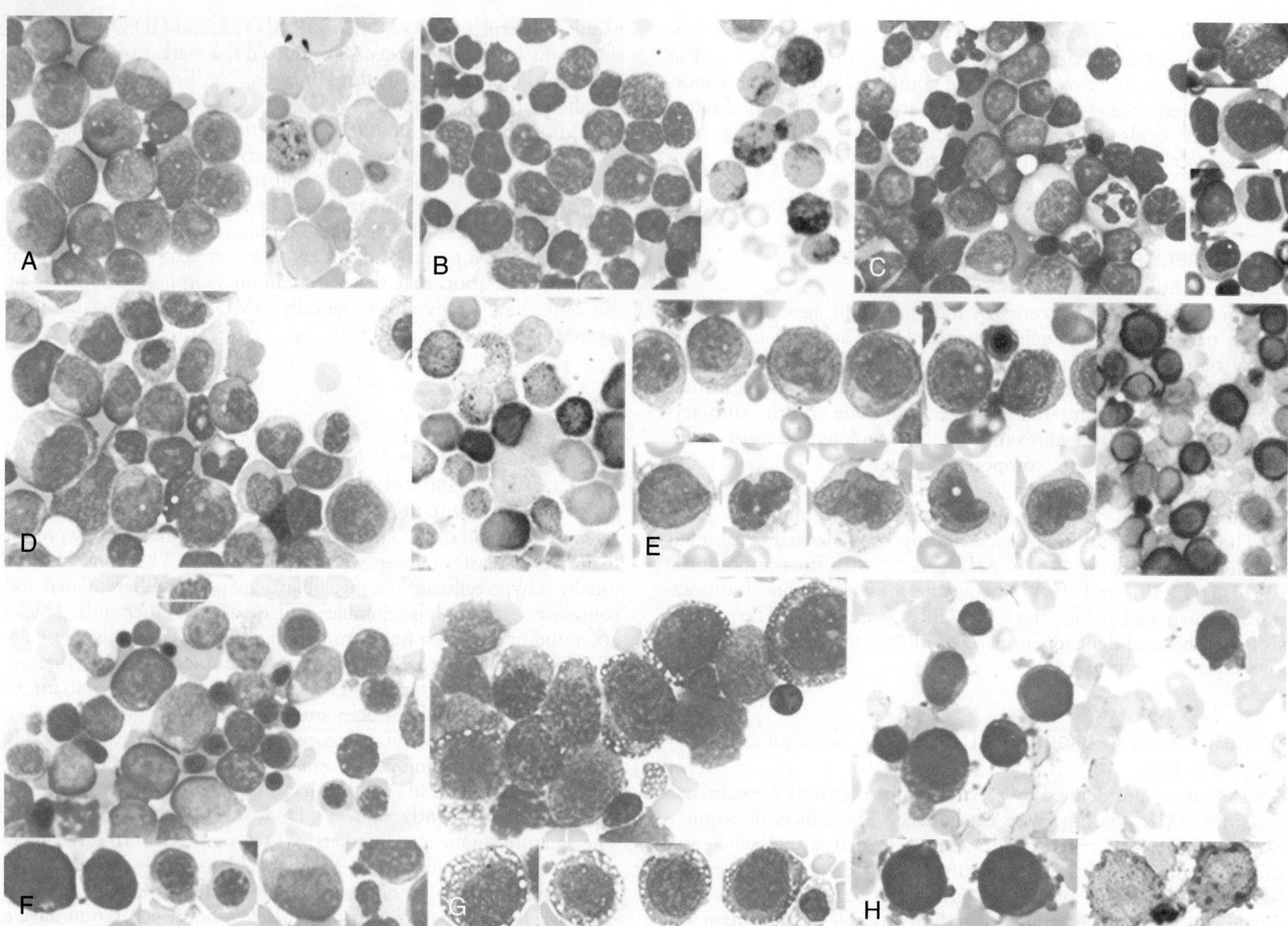

Figure 60–15 Acute myeloid leukemia not otherwise categorized (AML NOC). **A,** AML with minimal differentiation. Sheets of blasts are seen on the aspirate, and the myeloperoxidase reaction (right) is negative in the blasts. The rare positive neutrophil is useful as an internal control. To diagnose AML, flow immunophenotyping of the blasts must demonstrate myeloid markers. In this case, the blasts were CD13, CD33, and CD117 positive but negative for lymphoid markers. **B,** AML without maturation. Sheets of blasts are present, with fewer than 10% maturing granulocytes. The myeloperoxidase reaction (right) is positive in the blasts. **C,** AML with maturation. The aspirate (detail right) shows blasts, maturing granulocytes, and less than 20% monocytes. **E,** Acute myelomonocytic leukemia (AMML). The aspirate shows increased blasts, monocytes, and granulocytic maturation. The monocytic component may be difficult to see on Wright-stained aspirate smear but is obvious on the combined esterase reaction (**D,** right). The monocytes are butyrate esterase reaction positive (orange–brown), and the granulocytic cells are chloroacetate esterase reaction positive (blue). **E,** Acute monoblastic and acute monocytic leukemia. Cells from an acute monoblastic leukemia are illustrated in the top row and those from an acute monocytic leukemia are in the bottom row. Note the absence of differentiation above and differentiation to monocytes in the form of nuclear folding, cytoplasmic vacuolization, and faint granulation below. The combined esterase reaction for either type will show almost all monocytic cells with few granulocytes (right). **F,** Acute erythroleukemia, erythroid/myeloid type. Note that maturing erythroid precursors account for greater than 50% of cells, and that myeloblasts are increased in the nonerythroid component. **G,** Pure erythroleukemia. In contrast to the erythroid/myeloid type, pure erythroleukemia shows greater than 80% erythroid precursors, many of which are abnormal pronormoblasts with prominent vacuolization. **H,** Acute megakaryoblastic leukemia. Megakaryoblasts can sometimes resemble lymphoblasts, with dense nuclear chromatin and scant cytoplasm (top, center). Sometimes megakaryoblasts have cytoplasmic pseudopods or projections (bottom left). Flow cytometric analysis can be used to demonstrate a megakaryocytic origin of the cells, or immunocytochemistry can be used. In this case, the cells were positive for CD41 (bottom, right).

approximately 20% have complex karyotypes that are similar to those of more immature AMLs. Trisomy 8, monosomy 7, and del(5q) are the most common single chromosome abnormalities.[315] The prognosis of this subtype is variable. Cases with t(6;9)(p23;q34) and deletions of 12p have an overall poor prognosis.

Acute Myelomonocytic Leukemia (15%–20% of Acute Myeloid Leukemias; FAB M4 by FAB Classification)

AMML is characterized by differentiating neutrophilic and monocytic precursors. AMML is defined by the presence of ≥20% blasts, with both monocytic and granulocytic lineages each composing at least ≥20% of precursors. Anemia, thrombocytopenia, and leukocytosis (>90%) are typical. Serum and urinary lysozyme levels, which reflect the monocytic component, frequently are elevated.[302,315] Patients often present with extramedullary disease, gingival hypertrophy, leukemia cutis, and meningeal leukemia. Although this subtype occurs in individuals of all ages, it is more common in older patients (median >50 years). Some patients have a preceding history of chronic myelomonocytic leukemia. Morphologically there is a mixed population of myeloblasts, monoblasts, and more mature neutrophils, and monocyte precursors typically are present. Monoblasts are larger than myeloblasts and contain more abundant cytoplasm and a prominent centrally placed nucleolus. Some cells have morphologic features intermediate between myeloblasts and monoblasts. Auer rods are present in the majority of cases. Cytochemical stains are helpful in identifying the monocytes in the peripheral blood and bone marrow. The bone marrow typically stains with the cytochemical markers for both neutrophilic and monocytic precursors, and the leukemic blasts stain positive with MPO, SBB, and CAE as well as the nonspecific butyrate esterase. The blasts cells usually express the myeloid antigens CD13 and CD33 and monocytic markers including CD14, CD4, CD11b, CD64, CD36, and lysozyme. A subset of undifferentiated blasts may express CD34, HLA-DR, and panmyeloid markers. AMML is genetically heterogeneous. This subtype has no defining cytogenetic abnormalities. The prognosis is variable in this group and dependent on other prognostic variables.

Acute Monoblastic Leukemia and Acute Monocytic Leukemia (2%–9% of Acute Myeloid Leukemias; FAB M5a, M5b by FAB classification)

In the WHO classification, acute monocytic and acute monoblastic leukemias are defined by the presence of greater than 80% cells of the monocytic lineage in the marrow, including monoblasts, promonocytes, and monocytes. A minor neutrophil component, not exceeding 20%, also may be present. This subtype of AML is more common in younger patients (median age 49 years).[302] A majority of patients present with an elevated WBC count, and up to 30% of patients present with WBC count greater than 100,000/μL and symptoms of hyperleukocytosis. CNS involvement occurs in up to 22% of patients.[316] Extramedullary disease involving the liver, spleen, and lymph nodes is more common in the monocytic leukemias than in other AMLs, occurring in up to 54% of patients.[317] Gingival hyperplasia and skin involvement are frequent features of the monocytic leukemias and in many patients may be the presenting findings. The WHO classification does not make a distinction between undifferentiated monoblastic leukemia and more mature monocyte leukemia. However, there are meaningful clinical differences between the two monocytic leukemias.[318] Patients with the monoblastic variant are younger, present with a higher blast count, and have an overall poorer prognosis.[317] The difference in prognosis may be due to the high prevalence of unfavorable cytogenetics within the monoblastic (FAB-M5a) leukemia group. The blasts in the monoblastic form usually are large and contain abundant pale to basophilic cytoplasm, which may contain vacuoles or form prominent pseudopods. Auer rods are absent. Finely textured, dispersed azurophilic granules often are present. In the more mature monocytic variant, the predominant cell type is the promonocyte, which has a characteristic oval or lobulated nucleolus with dispersed chromatin. Nucleoli are present but generally are not as prominent as in the monoblastic form. Monoblasts are variably NSE positive and MPO and SSB negative. Promonocytes are NSE positive and often weakly positive for MPO. Up to 20% of monoblastic/monocytic leukemias may lack NSE reactivity. The acute monoblastic and monocytic leukemias stain with more than one of the monocytic markers, including CD11b, CD11c, and CD64. The exception is CD14, which often is absent, particularly in the monoblastic form. The blasts are generally CD34⁻. The blasts variably express myeloid antigens, including CD13, CD33, CD117, HLA-DR, and CD45, and lysozyme is positive. CD15 often is positive in the monocytic form but negative in the monoblastic form.

There is no characteristic cytogenetic finding. A majority of patients have a normal karyotype.[302] Trisomy 8 is present in as many of 6% of monoblastic cases and 23% of monocytic cases.[302] The monoblastic leukemias frequently have abnormalities of 11q23 but include subtype AML with recurrent genetic abnormalities.

The prognosis of the monocytic leukemias is generally poor. The prognosis reflects the poor prognostic features common in this subtype, including high blast count, extramedullary disease, and older age.

Acute Erythroid Leukemia (3%–6% of Acute Myeloid Leukemias; FAB M6 by FAB Classification)

The WHO classification of AML recognizes two forms of acute erythroid leukemia: acute erythroleukemia (erythroid/myeloid) and a pure erythroid leukemia. In the acute erythroleukemia (erythroid/myeloid), progenitors are committed to both the myeloid and erythroid lineages, whereas in the pure erythroid leukemia, progenitors are committed exclusively to the erythroid lineage. Erythroleukemia (erythroid/myeloid) is defined by the presence of more that 50% erythroblasts, usually at all stages of maturation, *and* more than 20% myeloblasts in the nonerythroid marrow cells. Pure erythroid leukemia, on the other hand, is defined by the presence of greater than 80% erythroid precursors among marrow cells, without evidence of a myeloblastic component.[319] Pure erythroid leukemia is extremely rare, can occur at any age, and usually does not evolve from a preceding MDS. Erythroleukemia (erythroid/myeloid) presents with a low WBC count, anemia, and thrombocytopenia. In the erythroleukemia (erythroid/myeloid), dysplastic erythropoiesis is prominent. The erythroid precursors are megaloblastic with prominent multinucleated forms. Nuclear-to-cytoplasm dyssynchrony, that is, immaturity of the nucleus for comparable cytoplasmic hemoglobinization, is common. Myeloblasts range from immature agranular myeloblasts to myeloblasts with prominent azurophilic granules with Auer rods. In the pure erythroid leukemia, early erythroblasts are highly dysplastic and contain round nuclei with immature chromatin and large blotchy nucleoli. The cytoplasm is abundant and deeply basophilic and often contains numerous vacuoles that may coalesce into large tubular structures. Maturation into intermediate and late erythroblasts often is impaired. Some cases of pure erythroid leukemia may demonstrate minimal morphologic erythroid differentiation and are difficult to differentiate from an undifferentiated leukemia or ALL. Staining the biopsy for hemoglobin A is helpful in differentiating erythroid precursors from myeloblast or lymphoblasts. Erythroid leukemias are MPO and SBB negative. NSE may be weakly reactive. PAS always is positive, with clear differences between the two subtypes, a feature that may help in their recognition and differentiation. PAS stain in the erythroleukemia (erythroid/myeloid) leukemia stain the cytoplasm with a diffuse or punctate pattern. In contrast, in the pure erythroid leukemia the PAS staining is coarse and in a block pattern ("block positivity"). Ring sideroblasts are common in the erythroleukemia (erythroid/myeloid), particularly when it has evolved from a prior MDS. The immunophenotyping reflects the dual population of blasts in the erythroleukemia (erythroid/myeloid) leukemia. Myeloblasts express myeloid markers CD13, CD33 and/or CD117, CD34, and HLA-DR are variably expressed. The erythroid blasts typically express high levels of CD71 (transferrin receptor), glycophorin A, and CD36. In contrast, the erythroblasts of the pure erythroleukemia subtype are rarely glycophorin⁺ or strongly CD71⁺. CD36, Gero antibody against the Gerbich blood group, usually is positive. CD36 is not specific for erythroid precursors and can be expressed on monocytes and megakaryocytes. In the pure erythroid leukemia, mature erythroid precursors are absent, and less than 3% of the blasts are MPO positive. Auer rods are usually not present. The proerythroblasts usually are positive for glycophorins A and B, antigens of the AB blood group system, which are strongly expressed on erythroblasts, and fetal erythrocytes. In rare cases, dysplastic differentiating erythroblasts account for more than 90% of marrow cells without an increase in myeloblasts. Patients with erythroleukemia (erythroid/myeloid) tend to be older at diagnosis (mean age >50 years) and frequently present with rheumatic and immunologic findings. One third of patients complain of diffuse joint pain and/or abdominal, back, and chest pain.[320] Many patients have a positive rheumatoid factor, increased polyclonal immunoglobulins, positive antinuclear antibody test, and positive Coombs test.[321] The erythroleukemias, which frequently are preceded by an MDS, represent 10% to 20% of secondary leukemias and 3% to 5% of all de novo AML cases.[320] Hepatomegaly and splenomegaly can be prominent but occur in less than 25% of patients. The red cells may demonstrate other prominent abnormalities, including basophilic stippling, abnormal red blood cell shape, and rare circulating undifferentiated blast forms.

Patients with this subtype generally respond poorly to therapy, with a short remission duration.[320] The response to treatment may reflect the increased incidence of secondary leukemias and patients with a prior MDS having this subtype.

Acute Megakaryoblastic Leukemia (3%–10% of Acute Myeloid Leukemias; FAB M7 by FAB Classification)

AMKL is characterized by greater than 50% marrow megarkaryoblasts.[322,323] The WHO recognizes the controversy regarding the relationship between acute panmyelosis with myelofibrosis and acute megakaryoblastic leukemia with fibrosis and defines a separate subtype: acute panmyelosis with myelofibrosis.[324] In the majority of cases, the predominant cell is the megakaryoblast and therefore should be subtyped as a megakaryoblastic leukemia (AMKL). Patients with a prior myeloproliferative disorder, myelofibrosis, or CML have a higher incidence of AMKL. AMKL is a common form of childhood leukemia that occurs in 7% to 10% of cases and is associated with a poor prognosis.[325] AMKL in adults occurs in an older population (median age 56 years). A majority of patients have an antecedent hematologic disorder or MDS. AMKL is associated with a lower WBC count at presentation, lower percent of bone marrow blasts, and fibrosis. The presenting WBC count usually is low (<5000/μL), and the platelet count is normal or increased in more than one third of cases (range 5000–2,292,000/μL). Hepatosplenomegaly is common in children but rare in adults unless there is a preceding myeloproliferative disorder. Children with DS have a higher incidence of AMKL that may be related to mutations of the hematopoietic transcription factor gene GATA1.[326] The *GATA1* gene located on the X chromosome is essential for normal erythroid and megakaryocytic differentiation. Somatic mutations in exon 2 of GATA1 are detected exclusively in trisomy 21–associated AMKL but not in non–DS AMKL.[327]

Megakaryoblasts are morphologically heterogeneous and vary from small round cells, resembling ALL or an undifferentiated AML, to large atypical megakaryocytes with or without cytoplasmic granules. Binuclear or multinuclear blasts with deeply basophilic cytoplasm, cytoplasmic projections, and vacuoles are common. Undifferentiated blasts may be surrounded by shed platelets and recognizable micromegakaryocytes. Megakaryocytic fragments are seen In the peripheral blood, as are large atypical cells with prominent cytoplasmic blebs representing megakaryoblasts. The bone marrow typically cannot be aspirated (dry tap), so biopsy is essential to make the diagnosis. The bone biopsy shows increased reticulin and fibrosis, the latter a result of stimulation of normal fibroblasts in the bone marrow by local secretion of platelet-derived growth factor by the leukemic megakaryoblasts.[244]

Megakaryoblasts are SBB and MPO negative, and the PAS reaction is often, but not universally, positive. In many cases the megakaryoblastic features of the blasts are not recognized by light or electron microscopy, so use of monoclonal antibodies specific for platelet glycoproteins is necessary to define this subtype. Immunophenotyping with monoclonal antibodies to platelet glycoproteins CD41 (glycoprotein IIb/IIIa) and/or CD61 (glycoprotein IIa), CD41, or factor VIII-related antigens may be needed to identify the megakaryoblasts.[269] The CD61 antibody reacts poorly in B5 fixed tissues. Moreover, von Willebrand factor (vWF) expression frequently is decreased in cases of AMKL with poorly differentiated blasts. α Granules store vWF, and their synthesis is decreased in immature megakaryocytes. CD42b is a better marker for detecting megakaryoblasts.[328] The ultrastructural platelet peroxidase reaction is technically difficult to perform and has been largely replaced by immunologic techniques. When flow cytometry is used to determine surface antigen profiles of leukemic cells, membrane staining must be demonstrated to distinguish adherent platelets that may cause false-positive results with antibodies to platelet glycoproteins.[329] Cytospin immunofluorescence techniques are needed to distinguish adherent platelets from true-positive cytoplasmic and membrane staining. Myeloid markers including CD13 and CD33 may be positive, but CD34, HLA-DR, and CD45 are negative. The platelet-associated antigen is variably expressed, and its presence is a marker for better prognosis and drug sensitivity in AMKL.[330] Cytogenetic abnormalities of chromosomes 3 and 21 have been associated with the AMKL subtype.[329] The clinical and hematologic features of the AMKL subtype are varied and reflect the evolution of AMKL from a prior myeloproliferative disorder. The clinical course is highly variable and atypical for an acute leukemia.[331] Some patients whose disease has evolved from a preexisting myeloproliferative disorder have a slowly progressive indolent disease that extends over a number of months to years. The response to conventional induction chemotherapy is generally poor, with a lower complete response rate and a shorter overall surival.[14,323,332] CR frequently is associated with reversal of the bone marrow fibrosis.

Variant: Acute Myeloid Leukemia/Transient Myeloproliferative Disorder in Down Syndrome

Patients with DS have an increased incidence of AMKL.[332] In some of patients the AMKL appears to originate in an early progenitor cell and expresses markers of mixed lineages; these patients may have a better prognosis. The WHO acknowledges that patients with DS are predisposed to developing a related transient myeloproliferative disorder (TMD). At least 10% of infants with DS develop a TMD, a disease in which megakaryoblasts accumulate in the liver, bone marrow, and blood. In most cases the TMD requires no treatment and goes into a spontaneous remission.[333] However, within 3 years of development of TMD, 30% of DS infants develop AMKL.

The TMD usually presents in the neonatal period with marked leukocytosis. Greater than 30% blast forms are present in the blood or bone marrow. The blasts in TMD are morphologically and phenotypically indistinguishable from AMKL blasts. The later appearance of AMKL in infants with TMD appears to be derived from the original TMD clone.[333]

Acute Panmyelosis with Myelofibrosis (Fig. 60–16) (<1% of Acute Myeloid Leukemias; M7 by FAB Classification)

Acute panmyelosis and myelofibrosis (APMF) is a rare form of AML. The WHO defines APMF as an entity distinct from acute megakaryoblastic leukemia. However, the clinical and hematopathologic finding partially overlap. APMF is primarily a disease of adults, but it can occur at any age. The disease can occur de novo or as a secondary AML in patients who have received prior alkylating agent chemotherapy.

Patients present with pancytopenia, lack of splenomegaly, bone marrow fibrosis, and normal erythroid maturation.[215] The disorder previously has been called acute myelofibrosis or acute myelosclerosis. The median age at presentation is greater than 70 years (i.e., 72 years; range 2–84 years). The common presenting symptoms are pancytopenia, fatigue, spontaneous bruising, and fevers. Red cell morphology reveals macrocytic red cells with teardrop forms. Neutrophils are dysplastic, with hypogranulation and pseudo–Pelger-Huet anomaly. Platelets frequently are abnormal, with hypogranular, hypergranular, and giant forms in the blood. Megakaryocytic fragments and platelet clumps are rare. Circulating blasts are rare and undifferentiated. The bone marrow cannot be aspirated in all cases (dry tap). The marrow biopsy is variably hypercellular with dysplastic atypical megakaryocytes. Usually a polymorphic cellular background is seen and includes erythroblasts, dysplastic megakaryocytes, and maturing myeloid precursors with foci of immature cells scatted throughout. The overall blast count may be difficult to estimate, but myeloblasts do not represent the majority of marrow cells. The WHO does not require precise determination of the number of blast forms for the diagnosis. The dysplastic megakaryocytes are a prominent feature, with nonlobulated nuclei and dispersed chromatin. The cytoplasm is uniformly eosinophilic. Distinguishing APMF from AMKL, chronic idiopathic myelofibrosis, and AML with fibrosis can be difficult. The lack of prominent splenomegaly helps to distinguishing APMF from

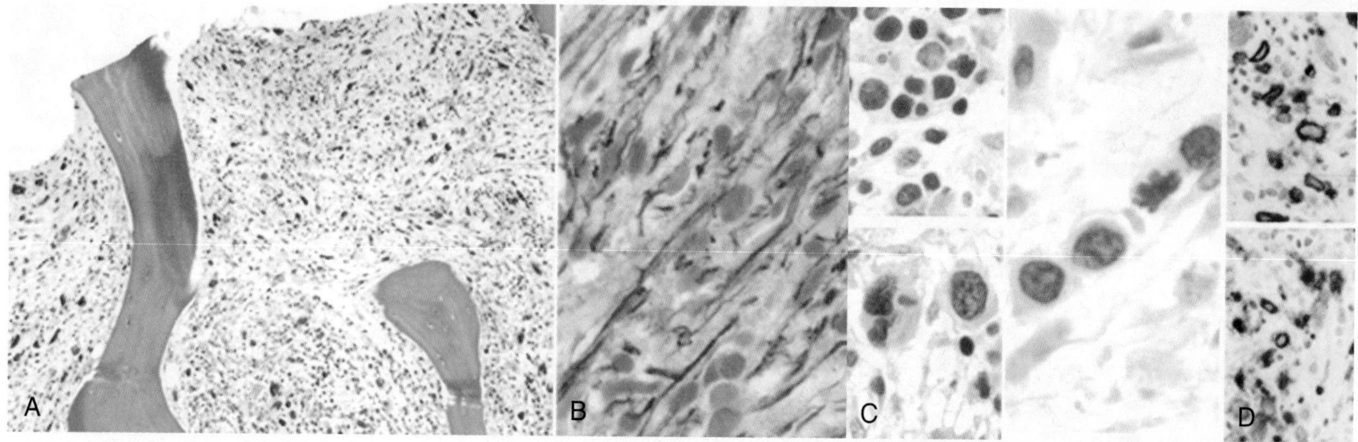

Figure 60–16 Acute panmyelosis with myelofibrosis. **A,** Bone marrow biopsy shows a loosely packed marrow with a swirling appearance to the cellular elements due to underlying fibrosis. B, The latter is illustrated on the reticulin stain. **C,** Proliferations of erythroid cells (top left), megakaryocytes (bottom left), and immature cells within the fibrotic areas (right). **D,** Immunohistochemical staining shows increased megakaryocytes (top, CD61) and increased blasts (bottom, CD34).

one of the myeloproliferative disorders. Moreover, the megakaryocytes in chronic idiopathic myelofibrosis have markedly convoluted nuclei with condensed chromatin.

Immunotyping reveals that the majority of the blasts are CD34$^+$. A variable proportion expresses MPO.[328] A majority of blasts express early myeloid or precursor antigens, including CD34, CD33, and CD117. Megakaryoblasts may be rare, in contrast to AMKL, in which megakaryoblasts are numerous.

Cytogenetics may be difficult to obtain due to the lack of circulating blasts and fibrotic bone marrow. The majority of patients reported have abnormalities of chromosome 5, 7, or 8 [del(5q), del(7q), trisomy 8]. The cytogenetics are consistent with a malignant myeloid disorder similar to MDS or MDS-related AML. APMF may represent a multilineage disease characterized by a heterogeneous blast population with secondary fibrosis.[334] The prognosis for patients with APMF is generally very poor, with a rapid progressive course.

Acute Basophilic Leukemia (<1% of Acute Myeloid Leukemias)

Acute basophilic leukemia (ABL) is a rare form of AML characterized by basophilic blasts. The FAB classification does not include this subtype, and cases usually were included in the M2 or M4 category.[335] Although ABL has been recognized for years, there were no specific guidelines for its diagnosis.[336] Many cases of ABL resemble the blast transformation of CML or AML with basophilia.[337] CML in the accelerated and blast transformation is characterized by an increase in circulating mature basophils. ABL has a high incidence of cutaneous involvement, organomegaly, and lytic bone lesions caused by hyperhistaminemia. The blasts are medium size, with a high nuclear-to-cytoplasmic ratio, round or bilobed nucleus with dispersed chromatin, and one to three prominent nuclei. The cytoplasm is moderately basophilic and contains a variable number of coarse basophilic granules. The blasts can be identified by either light microscopy or ultrastructure as deriving from the basophilic lineage. The peripheral smear usually shows both blast cells and maturing basophils that may be hypogranular. Mature differentiated circulating basophils are only moderately increased. The blasts are MPO and PAS negative by light microscopy but are generally positive with electron microscopy, which is a diagnostic feature of ABL.[336] Electron microscopy reveals numerous electron-dense granules containing varying intramembranous scrolls and the lamellae feature of immature mast cells. The most characteristic cytochemical feature is that the granules have metachromatic features with toluidine blue. Bone marrow biopsy reveals diffuse replacement with medium-sized blasts. Basophils may be increased in the bone marrow. In cases with mast cell differentiation, the mast cells are generally located close to the bone trabeculae and have an oval nucleus with elongated cytoplasm.

Immunophenotyping reveals the blasts are CD33$^+$, CD13$^+$, CD34$^+$, and variably HLA-DR$^+$. The blasts usually do not express lymphoid markers but may be CD9$^+$; some cases are TdT$^+$. Cytogenetics are helpful for excluding a missed CML, Philadelphia chromosome–positive t(9;22)(q34;q11). Chromosomal abnormalities include del(5q), monosomy 7, and del6(q22)t(6;9).[338] ABL is very rare, and information concerning prognosis or response to treatment is limited. The cases reported have had a poor prognosis.[336]

Myeloid Sarcoma (Fig. 60–17)

Myeloid sarcomas, also known as *granulocytic sarcomas* or *chloromas*, are an extramedullary tumor of immature myeloid cells. Myeloid sarcomas can occur concomitantly with AML or precede the development of systemic disease by months to years.[339] Myeloid sarcomas can occur with CML or other myeloproliferative disorders. When myeloid sarcoma occurs in the setting of MDS or a myeloproliferative disorder, the WHO considers it equivalent to blast transformation. The most common sites for myeloid sarcoma are the skin, subperiosteal bone, lymph nodes, and soft tissues.[339] The interval between the diagnosis of myeloid sarcoma and the development of overt AML can be months to more than 9 years. In some instances, no evidence of subsequent AML was found, but this may reflect the time of the reporting.[339,340] It is assumed that all patients subsequently will manifest findings of AML or systemic blast transformation of an underlying myeloproliferative disorder. The WHO defines three major types of myeloid sarcoma based on the degree of maturation: (a) blastic, composed primarily of myeloblasts and the most common; (b) immature, composed of myeloblasts and promyelocytes; and (c) differentiated, composed of promyelocytes mature neutrophils and the least common.[340] The diagnosis is based on the reactivity of blast cells as determined by cytochemical reactions or by immunophenotyping. Imprints of the mass are useful for cytochemical staining. The blasts have an antigenic profile similar to the underlying disease. MPO, lysozyme, CD43, and CD68 are helpful in identifying the tumor as a myeloid sarcoma.

Myeloid sarcomas are common in AML with t(8;21), are noted in 18% to 24% of cases and in patients with inv[16] (M14Eo).[339] The monoblastic sarcomas may be associated with 11q abnormalities. Myeloid sarcomas have been reported following allogeneic stem cell transplantation and may be the first sign of recurrent disease.[341]

The prognosis is that of the underlying disease. When myeloid sarcoma occurs as an isolated lesion, local radiation therapy may

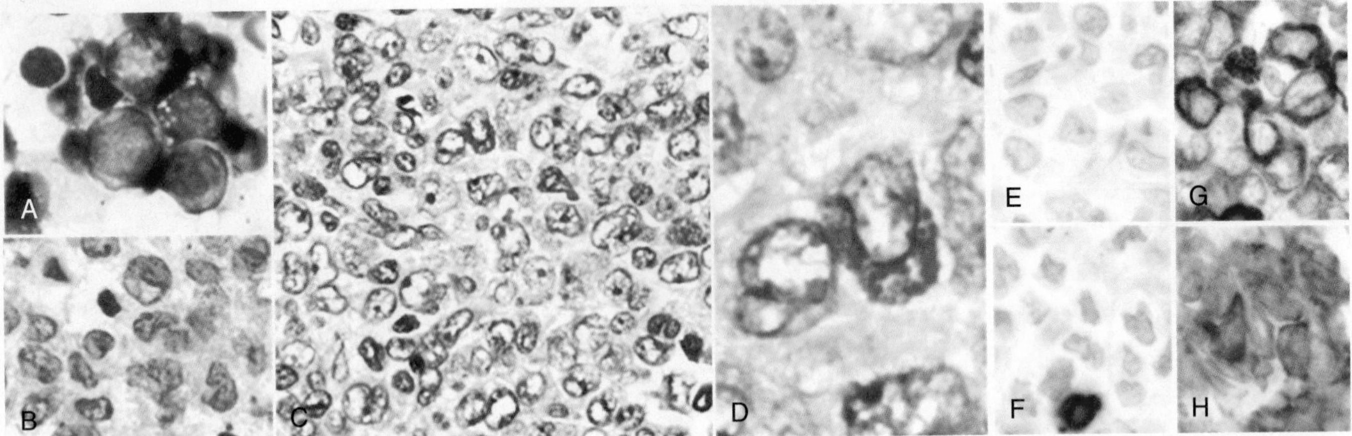

Figure 60–17 Myeloid sarcomas can sometimes present a diagnostic challenge. In this case, touch imprints **(A)** and frozen section preparation **(B)** from a mass lesion in the cecal area from a 44-year-old patient were thought to represent a high-grade lymphoma. However, initial immunohistochemical stains did not support the diagnosis. Closer inspection of the tumor and use of subsequent immunomarkers allowed a diagnosis to be reached. The tumor **(C)** is composed of sheets of noncohesive cells. A diagnostic clue to the origin was the presence of eosinophilic myelocytes **(D)**, which indicates that some tumor cells have the capacity to differentiate to eosinophils. The granules of neutrophilic myelocytes cannot be recognized on tissue section. Immunohistochemical stains showed the cell was CD45+ (not shown), B and T marker negative **(E, F)**, but myeloid marker (myeloperoxidase and CD33) positive **(G, H)**. Cytogenetic analysis showed the case was inv(16)(p13;q22).

result in prolonged responses before systemic disease recurs or progresses. Optimal therapy depends in part on the clinical circumstances, underlying disease, and location of the myeloid sarcoma.

Acute Leukemias of Ambiguous Lineage (<5% of Acute Myeloid Leukemia Syndromes)

The WHO defines acute leukemias of ambiguous lineage as leukemias in which the morphology, cytochemical, and immunophenotyping features cannot classify the leukemia as either myeloid or lymphoid. The classification of AML attempts to assign a specific lineage to each subtype based on morphology, cytogenetics or cytohistochemical staining, and immunophenotyping. In some cases a specific lineage cannot be assigned based on these criteria. In an attempt to explain this phenomenon, a number of different terms have been used, including *lineage infidelity, mixed lineage leukemias, biphenotypic or bilineage leukemias, hybrid or biclonal leukemias*, and *lineage switches*.[236,342,343] This confusing and sometimes arbitrary terminology reflects the heterogeneous nature of these disorders and the lack of specificity of currently available markers.[236] The monoclonal antibodies that are used to characterize lymphoid or myeloid leukemias recognize hematopoietic differentiation antigens. These antigens, which are expressed on a number of epithelial cells and overlapping subsets of hematopoietic cells, have important roles in the biology of normal and malignant hematopoiesis.

The WHO has assigned the term *acute leukemias of ambiguous lineage* to define this population of leukemias. In the present classification, system lineage cannot be assigned in less than 5% of all acute leukemias. Acute bilineage leukemias are defined by detection of dual populations of blasts, with each population expressing markers of a distinct and different lineage. Biphenotypic include leukemias that have a population of myeloid and lymphoid blasts. The leukemic blasts lack markers that are considered lineage specific and may express HLA-DR, CD34, CD38, TdT, and CD7 or demonstrate cytochemical and phenotypic markers of both myeloid and lymphoid precursors. This phenomenon may reflect a fundamental abnormality of gene expression that is specific for the malignant clone.[236,344] The clinical significance of lymphoid antigen expression in myeloid leukemias is unclear. Lymphoid antigens may be positive in up to 48% of myeloid leukemias.[345] The most common lymphoid antigens expressed in myeloid leukemias are CD2 and CD7, which are expressed in 34% and 30% of patients with AML, respectively.[345,346] The leukemic cells may express markers of more than one lineage, reflecting the abnormal maturation of an earlier uncommitted stem cell prior to myeloid lineage commitment. Monoclonal antibodies and molecular probes have shown that leukemic cells can demonstrate characteristics of more than one hematopoietic lineage.[347] These cells may demonstrate Auer rods, stain with peroxidase and/or Sudan black, and react with monoclonal antibodies typical of both myeloid precursors and mature T cells. A number of classification systems have attempted to address the biphenotypic leukemias, but none has been widely accepted.[344] Many cases express myeloid and lymphoid antigens; these cases do not represent evidence of biphenotypia but reflect inappropriate expression of lymphoid antigens on immature myeloblasts. Biphenotypic leukemias express multiple antigens of more than one lineage. The biphenotypic leukemias are recognized as leukemias with true ambiguous lineage.

A majority of bilineage and biphenotypic leukemias present with cytogenetic abnormalities. Rearrangements of the *MLL* gene 11q23 and the Philadelphia chromosome t(9;22) are most common. Other cases can present with complex cytogenetic abnormalities. Moreover, molecular studies have demonstrated that some cases of AML have rearrangement of the Ig heavy-chain gene or T-cell receptor chain genes.[348,349] Bilineage leukemias can be suspected on morphologic grounds when two distinct populations of blast cells are noted. Biclonal leukemias represent approximately 7% of all adult acute leukemias.[345] In these cases, the malignant transformation presumably occurred in a progenitor cell capable of differentiating into separate myeloid and lymphoid progenitors. This is in contrast to mixed lineage or hybrid leukemias, in which the leukemic cell expresses characteristics of more than one lineage.

Lineage switch is the expression of markers of one lineage at diagnosis but markers of a different phenotype or lineage at the time of leukemic relapse.[346] This transformation, which usually occurs after a treatment interval of 1 year, may reflect the selection of a clone from a bilineage leukemia or modulation of antigens expressed on leukemic cells. Clinically the biphenotypic and biclonal leukemias present with the usual findings of AML. However, they may present with features of both myeloid and lymphoid leukemias, including prominent diffuse lymphadenopathy and higher circulating blast and platelet counts. Otherwise, the clinical presentations are indistinguishable from those of the other forms of AML.

Current models of hematopoietic differentiation are based on evidence that normal pluripotential precursors give rise to committed precursors of a single-cell lineage and then undergo a series of discrete developmental steps. The AMLs are believed to arise from a single clone that is arrested at a normal stage of committed differentiation. The currently used classification system is based on the premise that leukemic cells adhere morphologically and immunologically to a single lineage. Cases of biphenotypic leukemias, mixed lineage, or lineage switch leukemias demonstrate the heterogeneity of these neoplastic disorders and support the concept that, in at least some acute leukemias, the transforming event occurs at the level of the pluripotential stem cell.

PREDICTORS OF RESPONSE

Treatment of patients with AML is divided into two phases: induction, and postinduction. The primary objective of induction therapy is induction of CR. CR is conventionally defined morphologically by the presence of less than 5% blasts in the bone marrow together with recovery of peripheral blood counts. The blood should have no circulating blast forms, hematocrit greater than 30 vol%, and platelet count greater than 100,000/μL without transfusion support. The term *complete remission–platelets* is applied to patients who have a platelet count less than 100,000 μL but meet the other criteria of CR. The outcome of induction therapy is dependent on a number variables. Patients must tolerate the side effects of chemotherapy and the prolonged period of neutropenia and thrombocytopenia resulting from the disease and the treatment. True resistant leukemia accounts for less than 20% of all induction failures. The major determinant of the outcome of remission induction therapy is the capacity of the patient to tolerate intensive therapy. A majority of patients who fail to attain CR do so because of the complications of therapy, which include infection and hemorrhage. Therefore, prior medical problems and performance status are important predictors of response. Factors that predispose to serious infections decrease the likelihood of a patient attaining CR. Whether administration of hematopoietic growth factors decreases the incidence of serious infections for all patients receiving induction chemotherapy is unclear. A number of clinical and biologic characteristics have been defined that are important prognostic factors predicting the likelihood that a patient will respond to induction treatment (Table 60–11). Cytogenetics are the most important independent prognostic factor for remission induction and duration.[350] Favorable cytogenetic abnormalities of the CBF, including t(8;21) and inv[16], are associated with a significantly better response and longer remission and survival, whereas abnormalities of chromosomes 5 and 7 and complex cytogenetic abnormalities are associated with a poor response to therapy and shorter overall survival. Other factors that are predictors of remission duration include the presence of extramedullary disease and a high blast count. Patients with the previously noted subtypes of undifferentiated AMKL and t-AMLs are associated with a poorer prognosis.

Age is an important predictor of response to induction therapy. The outcome for younger patients has improved with advances in supportive care and more intensive postremission therapy. However, the outcome for elderly patients continues to be poor (Fig. 60–18). The definition of a "elderly "patient varies among studies and is not uniform across cooperative groups. Generally, patients older than 60 years tolerate intensive treatment poorly and have an increased incidence of unfavorable prognostic variables, including unfavorable cytogenetics and expression of the multidrug resistance gene *MDR*.[351] Older patients with AML have an increased incidence of multilineage dysplasia, suggesting a more primitive stem cell origin or t-AML. Favorable cytogenetics are less common in elderly patients, and the proportion of patients with unfavorable cytogenetics is increased.[352] The combination of age greater than 70 years and poor prognosis cytogenetic was associated with a poor response to intensive chemotherapy and a limited survival benefit.[353,354] Cytotoxic chemotherapy in elderly patients is also associated with higher morbidity and mortality because of the presence of comorbid diseases, poor tolerance of prolonged pancytopenia, and perhaps altered drug metabolism and excretion.[355] Moreover, the majority of reports on treatment of elderly patients reflects selection bias. Most elderly patients do not participate in cooperative trials, and both patient and physician selection bias makes the generalization of findings in reported trials difficult. The true outcome of induction therapy and the survival of most elderly patients with AML are not known. Use of aggressive, intensive, induction therapy is of unclear benefit in elderly patients with AML.[355] Elderly patients with complex karyotype with at least three abnormalities or rare aberrations had a lower CR rate. Moreover, elderly patients with complex karyotype with more than five cytogenetic abnormalities or rare aberrations had a 0% 5-year survival rate.[355] Elderly patients with favorable cytogenetics, including abnormalities of CBF, had a 5-year survival rate of only 19%. The current treatments are of limited benefit in elderly patients with complex or rare cytogenetic abnormalities.[355] The CR rate was independently associated with older age and increasing WBC count. In elderly

Table 60–11 Prognostic Factors in Acute Myeloid Leukemia

Factor	Favorable	Unfavorable
Age	<55 years	>60 years
Leukemia	De novo	Secondary
White blood cell count	<25,000/μL	>100,000/μL
WHO subtype	Core-binding factor AML	AML with multilineage dysplasia, therapy-related-AML Acute megakaryocytic leukemia, acute erythroid leukemia, acute basophilic leukemia
FAB type	M3, M4Eo	M0, M5a, M5b, M6, M7
Cytogenetics	t(15;17), t(8;21), inv(16) Normal cytogenetics	Abnormalities of chromosomes 5 and 7, multiple >3 abnormalities, rare abnormalities 11q23, t(6;9)
Extramedullary disease	Absent	Present
Auer rods	Present	Absent
Phenotype	CD34⁻	CD34⁺ CD56⁺
Other	Nucleophosmin 1 (NPM-1)	High lactate dehydrogenase level, low albumin level KIT mutations FLT-3 internal tandem duplication MDR-1 expression

AML, acute myeloid leukemia; FAB, French-American-British; WHO, World Health Organization.

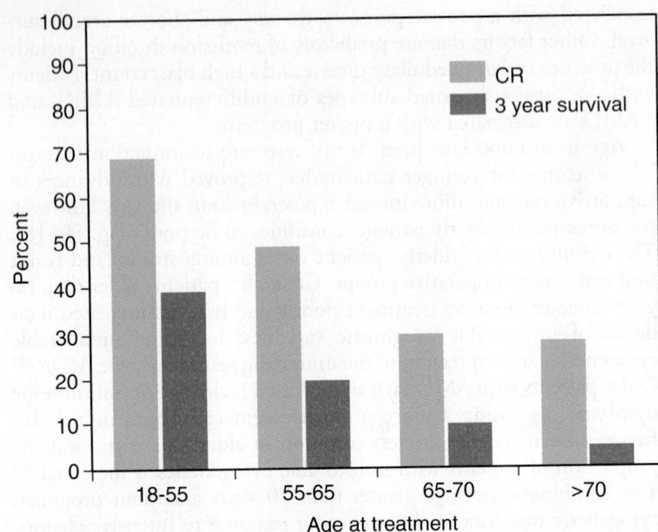

Figure 60–18 Age-associated complete remission and survival in acute myeloid leukemia.

patients older than 60 years, the overall 5-year survival rate was 6% to 7%.[355,356] In elderly or high-risk patients, cytogenetics identify a group of patients who are unlikely to benefit from intensive chemotherapy and should be offered alternative treatments or supportive therapy.[354–356]

Attempts to reduce the toxicity of treatment in elderly patients are controversial. Use of colony-stimulating factors to improve neutrophil recovery and the outcome of treatment in elderly patients with AML remains controversial. Colony-stimulating factors have been shown to reduce the duration of neutropenia in elderly patients undergoing induction chemotherapy, but their overall effect on morbidity or mortality is unclear.[357–360] Less intensive chemotherapy has been administered to elderly patients in an attempt to decrease toxicity, with variable results.[360,361]

Patients with secondary AML or a history of a prior MDS or myeloproliferative disorder respond poorly to standard chemotherapy regimens. Pretreatment serum albumin and serum LDH levels and performance status are important predictors of response.[362] The lower the serum albumin level, the less likely the patient will attain CR and/or tolerate intensive chemotherapy. A poor performance status or elevated serum LDH level is associated with a lower complete response rate and shorter remission duration.[363] A leukemic cell count greater than 20,000/μL is associated with a lower CR rate and shorter duration of remission.[363]

The presence of c-KIT mutations and FLT-3 ITD mutations is associated with a higher relapse rate and decreased overall survival.[354,355] Expression of *MDR* has been implicated as a poor prognostic factor.[351] *MDR-1* encodes an ATP-binding transmembrane protein that extrudes a variety of antineoplastic compounds from the cells, including the anthracyclines. Twenty percent of de novo AML cases and 75% of secondary AML cases express MDR-1. MDR-1 expression is linked to expression of the CD34 antigen. The MDR-1 phenotype identifies a group of high-risk, poor-prognosis leukemias, but its role as an independent prognostic indicator is unclear. Moreover, expression of CD34 on leukemic cells is associated with a poor response to induction chemotherapy, but whether this is an independent predictor of response is unclear.[364] Prospective studies are needed before therapy can be altered based on prognostic factors.

Use of intensive postinduction therapy has resulted in longer remissions and improved overall survival. In most studies, 60% to 70% of patients younger than 60 years will attain CR with induction therapy, but 40% to 70% will relapse in the first 18 to 24 months. The factors that determine remission duration are highly controversial and dependent in part on the type of postinduction chemotherapy used.[365,366] Patients who require two courses of induction chemotherapy to attain CR appear to have shorter remission duration.

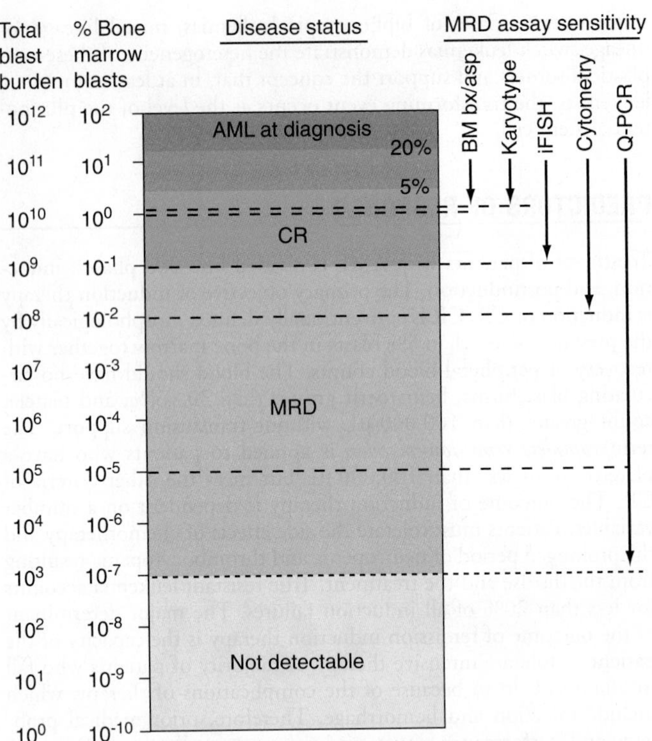

Figure 60–19 Hypothetical disease burden in acute myeloid leukemia (AML; assuming 100% blasts at the time of diagnosis) at different stages of disease evolution and approximate sensitivity levels of the assays used to monitor patients after remission induction. Blasts refer to leukemia blasts only. Segmented and dotted lines depict usual and optimized levels of detection by quantitative polymerase chain reaction (Q-PCR). iFISH and Q-PCR target AML-specific genome changes (translocations, deletions, mutations, etc.). Flow cytometry targets AML-specific aberrant phenotypes. Suitable targets for MRD assessment may not be available in all AML cases. BM bx/asp, combined assessment of marrow biopsy and aspirate smear; CR, complete remission; iFISH, interphase fluorescent in situ hybridization; MRD, minimal residual disease.

tion. The morphologic appearance of the bone marrow biopsy sample at the time of CR may be an important predictor of remission duration. The presence of morphologic dysplasia involving more than one cell line may be associated with shorter remission duration. However, chemotherapy can result in dysplastic features in the bone marrow; therefore, the finding of dysplastic erythroid and myeloid precursors following high-dose induction and consolidation therapy must be interpreted with caution.[225] All these prognostic factors are determined from retrospective studies. None of these variables has been critically analyzed in controlled prospective trials.

Patients in remission for more than 3 years have a markedly increased chance of prolonged survival; 75% to 80% of patients in CR at 3 years will have a prolonged disease-free survival.[367,368] However, patients continue to relapse 3 to 15 years after attaining CR. The biologic factors responsible for these late relapses are unknown and may reflect one or more of the etiologic events in the development of AML.[369]

Minimal Residual Disease Monitoring

Use of modern intensive induction chemotherapy regimens for AML results in CR rates greater than 60% in patients with AML. Intensive regimens lead to a 2- to 3-log decrease in leukemia cells. Accurate monitoring of minimal residual disease at the completion of induction or consolidation therapy may be important in the management of adults with AML. Minimal residual disease can be monitored in a number of ways, and each method has its advantages and disadvantages (Fig. 60–19). Minimal residual disease status, detected by either multiparameter flow cytometry or real-time quantitative polymerase chain reaction (QPCR), at the completion of consolidation therapy is a better predictor of relapse. Detection of abnormal disease-specific phenotypes by multiparameter flow cytometry may be of greater value in the assessment of early clearance of myeloblasts after completion of induction therapy, whereas QPCR, which measures disease-specific genetic changes, may be more informative and a marker of "persistent" minimal residual disease after consolidation therapy. Selection of targets for QPCR also may be important. Future treatments will be directed by prognostic factors and may allow for risk-adjusted induction and consolidations regimens.

SUGGESTED READINGS

Appelbaum FR, Kopecky KJ, Tallman MS, et al: The clinical spectrum of adult acute myeloid leukaemia associated with core binding factor translocations. Br J Haematol 135:165, 2006.

Beaumon M, Sanz M, Carli PM, et al: Therapy-related acute promyelocytic leukemia. A report on 106 cases. J Clin Oncol 21:2123, 2003.

Cheson BD, Bennett JM, Kopecky KJ, et al: Revised recommendations of the international working group for diagnosis, standardization of response criteria, treatment outcomes, and reporting standards for therapeutic trials in acute myeloid leukemia. J Clin Oncol 21:4642, 2003.

Deschler B, Lubbert M: Acute myeloid leukemia: Epidemiology and etiology. Cancer 107:2099, 2006.

Dohner K, Schlenk RF, Habdank M, et al: Mutant nucleophosmin (NPM1) predicts favorable prognosis in younger adults with acute myeloid leukemia and normal cytogenetics: Interaction with other gene mutations. Blood 106:3740, 2005.

Farag SS, Archer KS, Mrozek K, et al: Pretreatment cytogenetics add to other prognostic factors predicting complete remission and long-term outcome in patients 60 years of age or older with acute myeloid leukemia: Results of Cancer and Leukemia Group B 8461. Blood 108:63, 2006.

Frohling S, Schlenk RF, Kayser S, et al: Cytogenetics and age are major determinants of outcome in intensively treated acute myeloid leukemia patients older than 60 years: Results from AMLSG trial AML HD98-B. Blood 108:3280, 2006.

Frohling S, Scholl C, Gilliland DG, Levine RL: Genetics of myeloid malignancies: Pathogenetic and clinical implications. J Clin Oncol 23:6285, 2006.

Greaves MF, Maia AT, Wiemels JL, Ford AM: Leukemia in twins: Lessons in natural history. Blood 102:2321, 2003.

Haferlach T, Kohlmann A, Schnittiger S, Hiddeman W, Kem W, Schoch C: Global approach to the diagnosis of leukemia using gene expression profiling. Blood 106:1189, 2005.

Kalaycio M, Rybicki L, Pohlman B, et al: Risk factors before autologous stem-cell transplantation for lymphoma predict for secondary myelodysplasia and acute myelogenous leukemia. J Clin Oncol 24:3604, 2006.

Pedersen-Bjergaad J: Insights into leukemogenesis from therapy-related leukemia. N Eng J Med 352:1591, 2005.

Smith RE, Bryant J, DeCillis A, Anderson S: Acute myeloid leukemia and myelodysplastic syndrome after doxorubicin-cyclophosphamide adjuvant therapy for operable breast cancer: The National Surgical Adjuvant Breast and Bowel Project. J Clin Oncol 21:1195, 2003.

Smith ML, Cavenagh JD, Lister A, Fitzgibbon J: Mutation of CEBPA in familial acute myeloid leukemia. N Eng J Med 351:2403, 2004.

Vardiman J, Harris NL, Brunning RD: The World Health Organization (WHO) classification of myeloid neoplasms. Blood 100:2292, 2002.

REFERENCES

For complete list of references log onto www.expertconsult.com

CHAPTER 61

THERAPY FOR ACUTE MYELOID LEUKEMIA

Jacob M. Rowe and Martin S. Tallman

Approximately 13,000 patients in the United States are diagnosed annually with acute myeloid leukemia (AML). The median patient age at presentation has been steadily increasing over the past 2 decades and now is approaching 70 years. In an analysis by the Eastern Cooperative Oncology Group (ECOG) of the outcome of approximately 3000 patients with previously untreated AML entered into five consecutive clinical trials, the 5-year overall survival (OS) rate among 2000 patients younger than 55 years improved from 11% in the 1970s to 37% in the 1990s (Figs. 61–1 and 61–2). The overall incidence of AML in the United States is 3.4 patients per 100,000 population; 1.2 patients per 100,000 at age 30 years and more than 20 patients per 100,000 population at 80 years.[1] Considerable progress has been made in the therapy for younger AML patients, yet two thirds of young patients still die of their disease. The treatment of older adults remains entirely unsatisfactory, and greater progress in the treatment of this age group is required.

OBJECTIVES OF TREATMENT AND CRITERIA FOR RESPONSE

The traditional goal of treatment of AML is to produce and maintain a complete remission (CR).Criteria for CR are platelet count higher than 100,000/μL, neutrophil count higher than 1000/μL, and bone marrow specimen with less than 5% blasts.[2] In the 1960s, Freireich et al.[3] demonstrated that patients who achieved CR lived longer than patients who did not. The difference in survival time was entirely attributable to the duration of time spent in CR, suggesting a correlation between achievement of CR and survival time.[3] These findings have been confirmed for patients treated in the 1980s and 1990s. In general, after 3 years have elapsed from the beginning of CR, the probability of recurrence sharply declines, becoming less than 10%. Patients who have been in continuous CR for 3 years can, for operational purposes, be considered potentially cured.[4] Only patients who reach CR are potentially cured. A partial remission, with blood counts as in a CR but with 6% to 25% blasts in the marrow, occurs so infrequently with conventional anti-AML chemotherapy regimens that its effect on survival is difficult to judge.

Other response criteria have been proposed, such as CR with incomplete platelet recovery (CRp).[5] Although they meet other criteria for CR, such patients have platelet counts higher than 30,000 rather than the 100,000/μL standard. CRp is relatively rare after typical therapies. Subsequent survival of patients given such therapies is worse than for patients who meet the criteria for CR.[6] However, the motivation for defining CRp is the advent of newer, targeted therapies. Such therapies may be more likely to produce CRp, and, with such therapies, survival may be independent of the distinction between CR and CRp. The former point remains to be proved, and results with at least one drug, gemtuzumab ozogamicin (Mylotarg), suggest the latter hypothesis is not accurate. A *cytogenetic CR* implies that in patients whose blasts have cytogenetic abnormalities, the abnormalities can no longer be detected on standard analysis after CR is achieved. It appears that cytogenetic CRs last longer than CRs in which an initial abnormality persists[7,8]; however, most CRs also are cytogenetic CRs. A *molecular CR* extends the concept of cytogenetic CR to the molecular level and is especially relevant in acute promyelocytic leukemia (APL). APL constitutes less than 10% of cases of AML, so our focus remains on CR.

Two types of events, sometimes indistinguishable, can interfere with the achievement and maintenance of a CR.[9,10] First, patients can die as a result of therapy administered to produce a CR; therapy-induced death in CR is less common. These events are classified as supportive care failures. Second, and more common, disease can be resistant to therapy. Resistance can manifest as failure to enter CR (i.e., primary refractory AML) but more often manifests as recurrent disease after a transient CR. These two types of resistance correspond to the two principal phases of chemotherapy: remission induction and therapy in remission.

Relapse-free survival, also called *disease-free survival (DFS),* is a better measure of the effectiveness of postremission therapy than remission duration. This is because when analyzing remission duration, patients who die in CR are *censored* at time of death. Such censoring assumes that patients who die in CR have the same underlying risk of relapse (had they lived) as patients who do not die in CR. This assumption has not been proved. In contrast, relapse-free survival counts relapse and death in CR as evidence that a regimen is ineffective.[11]

STANDARD REMISSION INDUCTION THERAPY

Cytosine Arabinoside

Modern remission induction therapy for AML usually consists of a combination of cytosine arabinoside (ara-C) and an anthracycline (see box on Induction Therapy for Adults with AML up to Age 60). Ara-C, an antimetabolite that is an analogue of the normal nucleoside cytidine, is converted to ara-C triphosphate (ara-CTP). Once converted to ara-CTP, ara-C is incorporated into DNA and causes cell death. Mechanisms of cytotoxicity that do not require ara-CTP formation also may exist. When originally used in the 1960s and 1970s,[12] ara-C was administered at daily doses of 100 to 200 mg/m^2 (i.e., standard-dose ara-C) by twice-daily intravenous infusions or by continuous intravenous infusion. The latter approach was used because of the drug's very short half-life (15 minutes). When given by continuous infusion, CR rates were higher when the same total dose of ara-C was given over 5 days rather than 2 days. Despite the pharmacologic rationale previously mentioned, whether administration of ara-C by continuous infusion is preferable to bolus (over 1–3 hours) infusion is unknown. Given at standard doses, the principal adverse affects of ara-C are myelosuppression and, rarely, nausea and vomiting or diarrhea.

Anthracyclines

Anthracyclines include drugs such as daunorubicin, rubidazone, and idarubicin. Anthracyclines, such as the related agents mitoxantrone and etoposide, appear to exert cytotoxicity by stabilizing the normally occurring complex between DNA and the enzyme topoisomerase II. Stabilization of the complex leads to cell death. Daunorubicin, when given at 60 mg/m^2 daily for 3 to 7 days, produces CR rates of 40%, similar to the rates seen with ara-C.[13] Anthracyclines and ara-C have

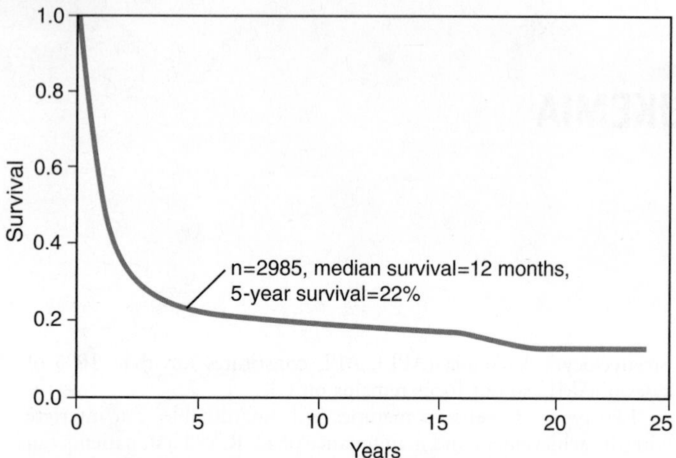

Figure 61–1 Survival of almost 3000 consecutive patients treated with Eastern Cooperative Oncology Group (ECOG) protocols for newly diagnosed acute myeloid leukemia (AML) since 1973. *(Data from Appelbaum FR, Rowe JM, Radich J, et al: Acute myeloid leukemia. Hematology Am Soc Hematol Educ Program 62, 2001:62.)*

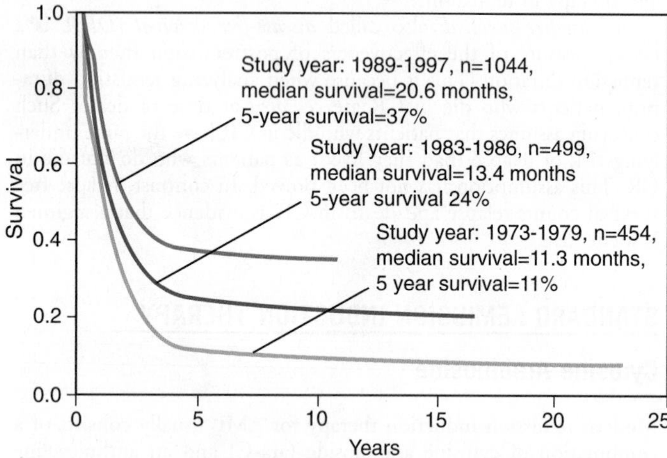

Figure 61–2 Patients ≤ 55 years with newly diagnosed acute myeloid leukemia (AML) treated with Eastern Cooperative Oncology Group (ECOG) protocols since 1973. *(Data from Appelbaum FR, Rowe JM, Radich J, et al: Acute myeloid leukemia. Hematology Am Soc Hematol Educ Program 62, 2001.)*

Induction Therapy for Adults with Acute Myeloid Leukemia Up to Age 60

- Aim of induction therapy is to reduce the number of leukemia cells to levels undetectable by morphology or standard cytogenetics (2–3 log cell kill).
- Once diagnosis is made, treatment should not be delayed.
- Gold standard remains treatment with an anthracycline and cytarabine.
- Daunorubicin 60 mg/m^2 for 3 days with cytarabine 100 mg/m^2 for 7 days (3 + 7) is a standard to which other regimens are compared.
- Multiple clinical trials suggest that daunorubicin 45 mg/m^2 is a suboptimal dose.
- There is no definitive evidence that therapy with another anthracycline or anthracenedione is superior.
- Standard 3 + 7 regimen is effective for all cytogenetic or molecular subtypes.
- Higher doses of anthracyclines (e.g., daunorubicin 90 mg/m^2) are safe, but no definitive data of improved efficacy are available.
- Induction therapy can be safely repeated at day 14 if unequivocal residual leukemia is present in a cellular marrow.
- No convincing data to indicate that addition of 6-thioguanine improves efficacy.
- Increasing the dose of cytarabine from 100 to 200 mg/m^2 does not improve outcome.
- Continuous infusions of cytarabine are preferable to bolus administration.
- Intensifying induction by using higher doses of cytarabine or addition of etoposide does not affect the remission induction rate.
- High doses of cytarabine or addition of etoposide may prolong disease-free survival.
- Administration of cytokines (granulocyte colony-stimulating factor and granulocyte-macrophage colony-stimulating factor) shortens the period of neutropenia by 4 to 7 days and is useful as supportive care strategy during induction.
- Use of cytokines as priming agents remains controversial.
- Preliminary data suggest that addition of gemtuzumab ozogamicin during induction therapy may improve the disease-free survival in patients with favorable- and intermediate-risk cytogenetic abnormalities.

similar toxicities, but anthracyclines are more likely to cause mouth sores. They also produce alopecia and a cardiomyopathy that can be prevented by limiting the total dose administered.[14] Cumulative doses of at least 180 mg/m^2 probably can be safely given to patients younger than 70 years with no prior exposure to anthracyclines. The probability of congestive heart failure in these patients was zero compared with 10% to 20% at the same dose level in patients older than 70 years, with hypertension, or with prior exposure to anthracyclines.

3 + 7 Regimens

Effective induction therapy for patients with AML was introduced more than 3 decades ago and included a combination of 7 days of cytarabine 100 to 200 mg/m^2/daily and 3 days of daunorubicin.[15] The so-called "3 + 7" regimen remains the gold standard against which all new combinations of agents are compared. CR can be achieved in 30% to 40% of adults younger than 60 years using either of these drugs[16,17] alone as compared to approximately 60% to 80% using a combination of an anthracycline and cytarabine. The results of induction therapy are greatly influenced by prognostic factors, most importantly the leukemia cell karyotype at presentation (Tables 61–1 and 61–2).[18] Caution is required when comparing published results for any given subtype of AML with a particular induction regimen. These results may vary among the major cooperative oncology groups due to differing criteria for the establishment of a CR, including the requirement for central pathology review.

Although the most frequently used dose of daunorubicin has been 45 mg/m^2 for 3 days, a careful analysis of the available data suggests that this dose should be modified to a higher dose, nearer to 60 mg/m^2. Multiple randomized studies have compared daunorubicin at a dose of 45 to 50 mg/m^2 with other anthracyclines, including idarubicin,[16,17,19,20] amsacrine,[21] aclarubicin,[22] and mitoxantrone.[23] Each of these studies revealed superiority of these alternative anthracyclines or the anthracenedione mitoxantrone. This improvement was observed through significantly improved CR rate, improved DFS, improved OS, or more rapid response rate as measured by the number of courses required to attain CR (Table 61–3). Furthermore, sequential studies by the Southwest Oncology Group (SWOG) reported a substantially improved CR rate among patients younger than 50 years receiving daunorubicin at a dose of 70 mg/m^2,[24] compared with 45 mg/m^2.[25] Although this was not a randomized comparison, these

Table 61–1 Risk Stratification of Acute Myeloid Leukemia Patients Based on Cytogenetic Analysis

	SWOG Criteria	MRC Criteria: As for SWOG, Except:
Favorable	t(15;17)—with any other abnormality inv(16)/t(16;16)/del(16q)—with any other abnormality t(8;21)—without del(9q) or complex karyotype	t(8;21)—with any other abnormality
Intermediate	+8, −Y, +6, del(12p) normal karyotype	abn11q23 del(9q), del(7q)—without other abnormalities Complex karyotypes (≥3 abnormalities but <5 abnormalities) All abnormalities of unknown prognostic significance
Unfavorable	−5/del(5q), −7/del(7q), t(8;21) with del(9q) or complex karyotype inv(3q), abn11q23, 20q, 21q, del(9q), t(6;9) t(9;22), abn17p, complex karyotypes (≥3 abnormalities)	Complex karyotypes (≥5 abnormalities)
Unknown	All other clonal chromosomal aberrations with <3 abnormalities	

MRC, Medical Research Council; SWOG, Southwest Oncology Group.

Table 61–2 Results of Induction Therapy in Adults with Acute Myeloid Leukemia According to Cytogenetic Prognostic Groups

	Favorable		Intermediate		Unfavorable	
	n	*CR Rate*	*n*	*CR Rate*	*n*	*CR Rate*
MRC[47] (excluding children)	389	90%	853	84%	130	57%
ECOG/SWOG[48]	121	84%	278	76%	184	55%
GOELAM[53]	48	87%	226	76%	36	58%

Results of induction therapy from three cooperative groups. Identical standard induction therapy was used in all cytogenetic subtypes. A remarkable concordance among the three groups is demonstrated, although a rigorous comparison cannot be made due to minor differences among the studies in the classification of the cytogenetic prognostic groups.

MRC, Medical Research Council; ECOG, Eastern Cooperative Oncology Group; SWOG, Southwestern Oncology Group; GOELAM, Groupe Ouest-est Leukemias Aigues Myeloblastiques.

Data from Rowe JM: Current standard therapy of adult acute myeloid leukemia. In Appelbaum FR, Rowe JM, Radich J, Dick JE (eds.): Acute Myeloid Leukemia. Hematology Am Soc Hematol Educ Program 62, 2001.

Table 61–3 Daunorubicin 45–50 mg/m² and Cytarabine Versus Other Combinations in Adults Aged 50–60 Years

Author	Daunorubicin (mg/m²)	Other	CR Rate (%)	*P* Value	Improved Disease-Free Survival[a]	Improved Overall Survival[a]	More Patients in CR After One Course[a]
Randomized Studies							
Vogler[16]	45	Idarubicin 12 mg/m²	58 vs 71	0.03			
Wiernik[17]	45/m2	Idarubicin 13 mg/m²	70 vs 88	0.03		+	
Berman[19]	50	Idarubicin 12 mg/m²	58 vs 80	0.005		+	+
Mandelli[20]	45	Idarubicin 12 mg/m²	Same	—			+
Arlin[23]	45	Mitoxantrone 12 mg/m²	53 vs 63	0.1			+
Hansen[22]	45	Aclarubicin 75 mg/m²	50 vs 64	0.04	+		
Berman[21]	50	Amsacrine 190 mg/m²	54 vs 70	0.03	+		
Sequential Studies							
Hewlett[24] Weick[25]	45	Daunorubicin 70 mg/m²	58 vs 70				
Cassileth[26] Cassileth[27]	60	Idarubicin 12 mg/m²	Same				

[a]$P \leq 0.05$.
CR, complete remission.

data were generated by analyzing sequential studies, performed by the same cooperative group, in which only the dose of daunorubicin varied. Furthermore, sequential studies by ECOG have shown that the CR rate with idarubicin (12 mg/m^2 daily for 3 days) was identical to the historical control among a similar number of patients in the same age who used 60 mg/m^2 daily for 3 days of daunorubicin (Table 61–3).[26,27] Consequently, because of the question of dose equivalence, it is impossible to conclude from any of these studies whether any anthracycline or anthracenedione is superior.

Multiple attempts have been made to intensify induction therapy, but no unequivocal benefit has been demonstrated. Furthermore, reports of improved survival with an intensified induction regimen must be cautiously interpreted because OS might be influenced by the choice of postremission therapy.

Comparisons of dose intensity in AML therapy are fraught with hazards as multiple variables exist among the studies, including patient age and prognostic factors that lead to patient selection.

Although a higher dose of daunorubicin can be safely administered,[28] a direct comparison of 45 mg/m^2 with 90 mg/m^2, together with the identical dose of cytarabine, currently is being studied in a prospective fashion by both ECOG and the Dutch Haemato-Oncology Association (HOVON). DFS of AML patients can be improved by adding etoposide to standard induction therapy.[29,30] However, no data demonstrate that this strategy is superior to that which can be achieved by appropriate intensification therapy during the consolidation phase of AML therapy.

Caution is in order when interpreting what appears to be impressive data obtained by the completion of phase II studies. A study adding high-dose cytarabine directly after a standard 3 + 7 regimen was reported to yield a complete response rate of 89%.[31] However, this study, which was performed in a limited number of institutions, was compared with historical controls and could not be reproduced by several large cooperative group studies.[32]

3 + 7 Variants

Although 6-thioguanine often is included in the 3 + 7 regimen (spurring acronyms such as DAT and TAD), a Cancer and Acute Leukemia Group B (CALGB) study randomizing 427 patients to receive daunorubicin plus ara-C with or without 6-thioguanine found no difference in the CR rate, remission duration, or survival between the regimens.[33] Similarly, although an earlier Australian Leukemia Study Group (ALSG) trial suggested that patients younger than 55 years randomized to receive etoposide in addition to 3 + 7 had longer remissions and survival,[29] subsequent, larger randomized trials by the Medical Research Council (MRC) in Great Britain conducted with patients younger than 55 years[35] and older than 55 years[36] found that replacement of 6-thioguanine in DAT by etoposide had no effect on CR rate, remission duration, or survival. Such discrepancies emphasize the difficulty inherent in generalizing even from randomized trials while suggesting that any advantage gained by combining etoposide with the 3 + 7 regimen is relatively small at best. Although once cited as a possibility, neither the MRC nor ALSG found any benefit for etoposide in patients with French-American-British classification system (FAB) types M4 and M5.

Targeted delivery systems have been introduced for treatment of relapsed patients. Ongoing studies are using such systems as an adjunct to standard induction and consolidation therapy in young adults with AML. Preliminary data from a study conducted by the MRC in Great Britain reported a substantially improved DFS, except in patients with a high-risk karyotypic abnormality, with its use during induction with 3 + 7 of gemtuzumab ozogamicin, which consists of anti-CD33 conjugated to calicheamicin.[37] Additional followup and data from other cooperative groups are awaited before a definitive conclusion can be made on the usefulness of such therapy.

Similarly, new studies are about to be undertaken using targeted chemotherapeutic agents, such as tyrosine kinase inhibitors of the internal tandem duplication of FLT-3, as adjuncts to standard induction therapy. No data are yet available for such agents, which have minimal activity when used as single agents in patients with advanced disease.[38,39]

Causes of Failure

Between 40% and 45% of patients who fail to enter CR with 3 + 7 or the variants described die before response to induction therapy can be assessed; this proportion is heavily dependent on age and pretreatment performance status.[40,41] Death usually results from multiorgan failure, with the lung often the initially affected organ and pneumonia frequently the inciting event. The most commonly identified pathogens are fungi, particularly *Aspergillus* spp., and gram-negative bacilli.[42] Microbiological and autopsy studies essentially never implicate *Pneumocystis carinii* or viruses such as cytomegalovirus,[42] although the same techniques readily identify viral infections in allogeneic stem cell transplant patients or patients with chronic lymphocytic leukemia. In about half of the cases of fatal pneumonia studied at autopsy, no pathogen is identified.[42] Hemorrhagic exudation frequently contributes to pulmonary failure. Despite profound thrombocytopenia due to the disease and its treatment, this process usually is not accompanied by bleeding elsewhere. Central nervous system hemorrhage as a cause of death appears to be decreasing.[41] This suggests that pulmonary hemorrhage is an inflammatory response to underlying infection or to chemotherapy-induced lysis of tumor cells. The latter phenomenon most often occurs in the week after chemotherapy begins and is more likely in patients who present with high white blood cell (WBC) counts (>25,000–50,000/mL), particularly if accompanied by monocytosis.

With the exception of patients older than 75 years or patients of any age with a poor pretreatment performance status, the typical patient whose disease fails to respond to 3 + 7 will survive for at least 4 to 5 weeks, but not in CR due to resistant AML. These patients are divided into those in whom marrow hypoplasia is never observed and those in whom hypoplasia develops but is followed by reappearance of AML rather than achievement of CR. In clinical practice, a bone marrow aspirate usually is obtained 2 to 3 weeks after beginning therapy. A biopsy is needed only if the quality of the aspirate does not permit determination of cellularity. If the marrow continues to show blasts and is cellular, a second course of the same therapy is often given, sometimes at reduced total dose (e.g., 2 + 5 regimen). If the day 14 or 21 marrow is hypoplastic, therapy usually is delayed until it is clear that leukemia has reappeared, at which time the second course begins. A second course of therapy can produce remissions, but they usually are shorter in duration than are remissions produced after one course of therapy,[43] illustrating the connection between results of induction therapy and results of postremission therapy. The initial marrow sample obtained after a period of hypoplasia may demonstrate up to 10% to 20% blasts as a reflection of the regeneration of normal, not "leukemic," marrow, especially if cytokines have been given. In this circumstance, followup (e.g., at 1- to 2-week intervals) marrow samples show a reduction in percentage of blasts concomitant with a rise in the concentrations of neutrophils and platelets. If the patient presented with a cytogenetic abnormality, cytogenetic analysis may predict whether subsequent regeneration will be normal or leukemic.[44] The former possibility is suggested if the cytogenetic abnormality can no longer be detected in the followup marrow. In contrast, a persistent abnormality suggests that regeneration will be leukemic or that, if CR occurs, it will be short lived.

STANDARD POSTREMISSION THERAPY

Three types of postremission therapy can be distinguished. *Maintenance therapy* usually is defined as therapy that is less myelosuppressive than that used to produce remission. This typically is used in patients with APL and often in older patients. Most groups do not routinely use maintenance therapy for young adults with AML. The terms *consolidation therapy* and *intensification therapy* often are interchangeable and refer to an intensive form of postremission therapy that is intensely myelosuppressive and includes drugs similar to those used in induction, often at higher doses.

Alternatively, postremission therapy may comprise an autologous or an allogeneic stem cell transplant, with or without prior standard consolidation therapy.

Alternative Strategies for Postremission Therapy

A variety of approaches to preventing relapse have been explored. Such strategies have included intensive consolidation chemotherapy or high-dose chemotherapy or chemoradiotherapy with either human leukocyte antigen (HLA)-matched sibling allogeneic hematopoietic stem cell transplantation (allo-HSCT) or autologous HSCT, or low-dose maintenance therapy.

Allogeneic Stem Cell Transplantation

Allo-HSCT provides the most potent antileukemic effect of any postremission therapy in AML, as demonstrated by the lowest rates of relapse (see box on Allogeneic Hematopoietic Stem Cell Transplantation for AML). The clinical impact of graft-versus-leukemia effect was convincingly demonstrated by the International Bone Marrow Transplant Registry (IBMTR).[45] The most important limiting factor for allo-HSCT still is the high transplant-related mortality. The mortality from established grade III to IV graft-versus-host disease has not changed significantly over the past 3 decades.

If an HLA-matched sibling donor (MSD) is available, this is the preferred therapy for most patients up to age 55 to 60 years, if they present with an intermediate-risk karyotype, the most common cytogenetic group, composing approximately 50% of all AML patients. Data have shown that this form of therapy provides the best antileukemic effect as judged by the relapse rate.[46–48] Similarly, allo-HSCT is the treatment of choice for patients with a poor-risk cytogenetic abnormality.[49] Although offering allo-HSCT to AML patients with unfavorable cytogenetics has been the standard of care, a paucity of prospective data support this approach. In fact, the MRC AML-10 study reported that among the group with unfavorable cytogenetic abnormality, allo-HSCT did not offer any advantage.[47] In contrast, a U.S. Intergroup study reported a clear advantage for patients undergoing allo-HSCT, resulting in a survival of 44% compared with 15% for patients undergoing chemotherapy.[48] However, these studies are based on small subgroups of fewer than 20 patients, so seemingly conflicting data are not unexpected. In contrast, prospective data from the EORTC/GIMEMA AML-10 trial demonstrated, for the first time in a significant cohort of patients, an unequivocal benefit for allo-HSCT in patients with unfavorable cytogenetic abnormalities (Fig. 61–3).[50]

Patients with favorable-risk cytogenetic findings usually are not offered allo-HSCT during their first CR (Table 61–4). Although the rate of relapse is significantly lower with this mode of therapy, the high transplant-related mortality abrogates the value of allo-HSCT in such patients.

The timing of allo-HSCT following induction has never been prospectively defined. Historically, some form of consolidation therapy was often given prior to allogeneic transplantation.[51,52] Some cooperative groups use an attenuated form of consolidation,[27] generally for logistic reasons such as to establish the availability of a donor and transplant center. Other groups proceed immediately to allo-HSCT if an HLA-matched donor is available.[53] A retrospective analysis from the IBMTR[54] as well as an analysis from the European Group for Bone and Marrow Transplantation (EBMT) registry[55] showed no benefit of administering consolidation therapy prior to allo-HSCT for patients in first CR. This issue remains open because it has never been studied prospectively. Furthermore, the data from the registries are applicable only to patients in first CR. No studies, prospective or retrospective, have addressed the need for consolidation therapy prior to allo-HSCT in patients beyond first CR. More importantly, no

Allogeneic Hematopoietic Stem Cell Transplantation for Acute Myeloid Leukemia

- Provides superior antileukemic therapy.
- Standard of care in first complete remission of young patients with intermediate and unfavorable cytogenetic abnormalities.
- Reduced-intensity conditioning is reserved for older patients or those with comorbidities.
- Emerging data suggest a role for alternative donor stem cell transplants for patients with unfavorable cytogenetics in first complete remission.
- Standard of care for all patients in second remission.
- High rate of relapse in patients in whom transplants are performed while in relapse.
- For relapsed patients who achieve a remission, alternative donor transplants are an acceptable and recommended option.

Table 61–4 Indications for Matched-Sibling Allogeneic HSCT in Acute Myeloid Leukemia

Remission Status	Prognostic Parameters	Decision to Proceed with Allogeneic HSCT
CR1	Favorable cytogenetics Intermediate cytogenetics Unfavorable cytogenetics	No Young; ± poor prognostic factors—Yes Yes
≥CR2	All	Yes
Relapse	If cannot reinduce	Yes

CR, complete remission; HSCT, hematopoietic stem cell transplantation.

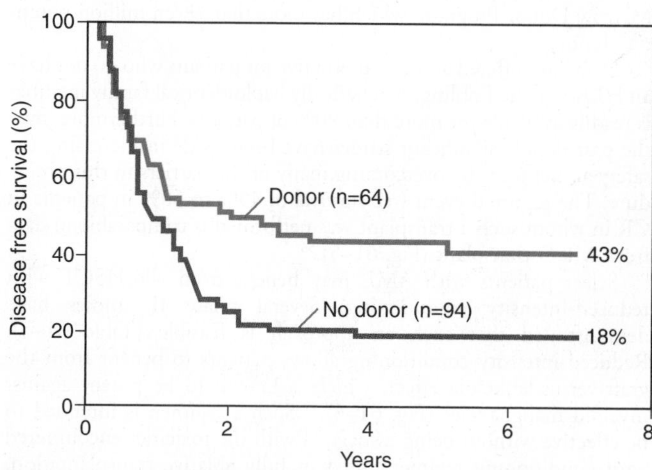

Figure 61–3 Allogeneic versus autologous stem cell transplantation for adults <46 years with acute myeloid leukemia, unfavorable cytogenetics. *(Data from Suciu S, Mandelli F, de Witte T, et al: Allogeneic compared with autologous stem cell transplantation in the treatment of patients younger than 46 years with acute myeloid leukemia (AML) in first complete remission (CR1): An intention-to-treat analysis of the EORTC/GIMEMAAML-10 trial. Blood 102:1232, 2003.[50])*

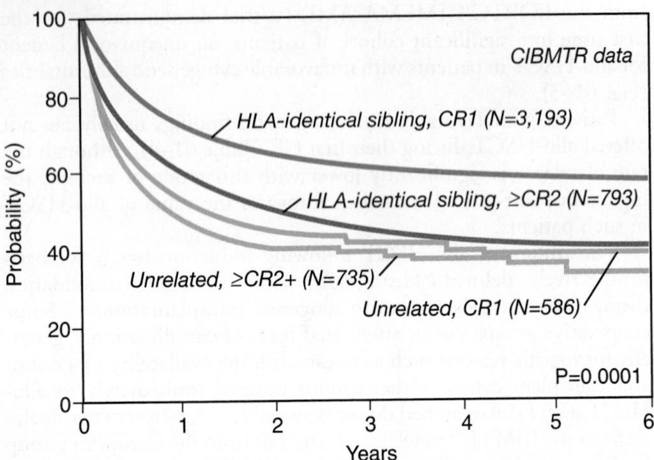

Figure 61–4 Probability of survival after allogeneic transplants for acute myeloid leukemia by donor type and remission status, 1996–2001. *(Data from Loberiza F: Report on state of the art in blood and marrow transplantation. IBMTR/ABMTR Newsletter 10: 20046.[307])*

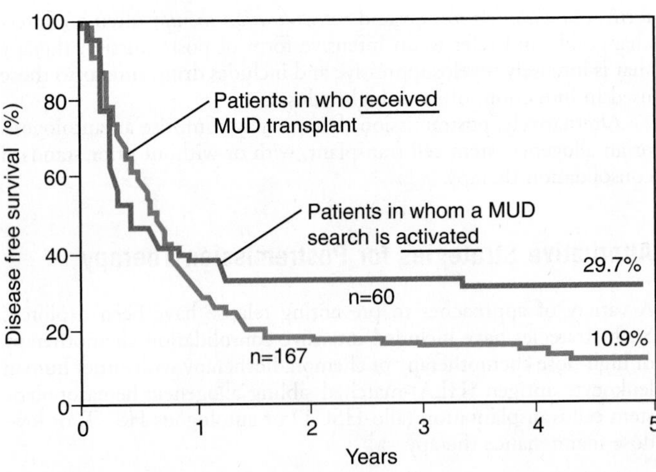

Figure 61–5 Haploidentical stem cell transplantation in acute myeloid leukemia. Results are better in patients in complete remission than in patients who have relapsed. *(Data from Aversa F, Terenzi A, Tabilio A, et al: Full haplotype-mismatched hematopoietic stem-cell transplantation: A phase II study in patients with acute leukemia at high risk of relapse. J Clin Oncol 23:3447, 2005.[56])*

data provide guidance as to when reduced-intensity conditioning should be applied.

Alternative sources of stem cell grafts has vastly increased the available pool of AML patients who can be offered allo-HSCT. The Center for International Blood and Marrow Transplant Research (CIBMTR) has reported data on the outcome of AML patients in first CR and beyond transplant with grafts from a matched unrelated donor (MUD) demonstrating a long-term probability of survival of 35% to 40% (Fig. 61–4). The performance of MUD HSCT has become widespread. Data suggest that the outcome with MUD is approaching that of sibling allo-HSCT from a matched related donor. However, no intention-to-treat analysis of MUD HSCT for AML has been performed. Currently, only a minority of patients for whom MUD HSCT is planned actually undergo such a transplant, because in many instances the disease progresses prior to the availability of a donor. More recently, encouraging results with MUD HSCT has been facilitated by the vast number of potential donors who are available through several worldwide registries, including the National Marrow Donor Program, which has more than seven million potential donors.

Data have offered another alternative for patients who do not have an HLA-matched sibling. A genetically haploidentical family member is readily available for more than 90% of patients. Furthermore, over the past decade significant strides have been made in increasing the safety and efficacy by overcoming many of the barriers to this procedure. The reported event-free survival of 45% to 50% in patients in CR in whom such a transplant was performed is comparable to data from MUD transplant (Fig. 61–5).[56]

Select patients with AML may benefit from allo-HSCT with reduced-intensity conditioning. Several phase II studies have demonstrated that such an approach is feasible (Table 61–5). Reduced-intensity conditioning allows patients to benefit from the graft-versus-leukemia effect, which is known to be potent against myeloid malignancies (Fig. 61–6).[45] Such a regimen is intended to be effective without being associated with the toxicities encountered with conditioning regimens used in fully ablative transplantation. Use of this strategy in AML has never been studied prospectively, but phase II studies have demonstrated that reduced-intensity conditioning transplantation can be performed with modest activity and acceptable toxicity in older adults or in patients with significant comorbidities (Fig. 61–7).[57,57a] Another study of patients older than 40 years who were treated with either reduced-intensity conditioning or a traditional conditioning regimen demonstrated no significant

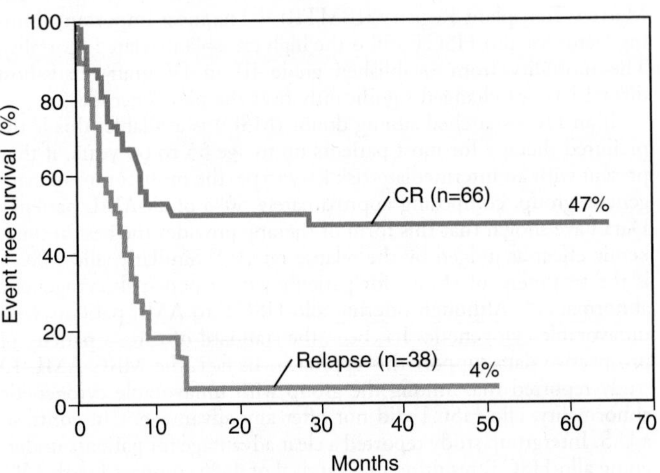

Figure 61–6 Effect of graft-versus-host disease on relapse rate of patients undergoing allogeneic hematopoietic stem cell transplantation. *(Data from Horowitz MM, Gale RP, Sondel PM, et al: Graft-versus-leukemia reactions after bone marrow transplantation. Blood 75:555, 1990.[45])*

Table 61–5 Reduced-Intensity Conditioning for Allogeneic Hematopoietic Stem Cell Transplantation

Study	N	TRM (1 Year)	EFS/PFS/DFS (1–3 Years)
Maris[308]	59	16%	38%
Sayer[309]			
CR/PR	59	12%[a]	40%–50%
No CR	54	30%[a]	15%
Kroger[310]	37	27%	38%
de Lima[311]	94	30%	27%
Martino[312]	37	5%	66%
Ho[313]	62	15%	62%

[a]100 days.
CR, complete remission; DFS, disease-free survival; EFS, event-free survival; PFS, progression-free survival; PR, partial remission, TRM, treatment-related mortality.

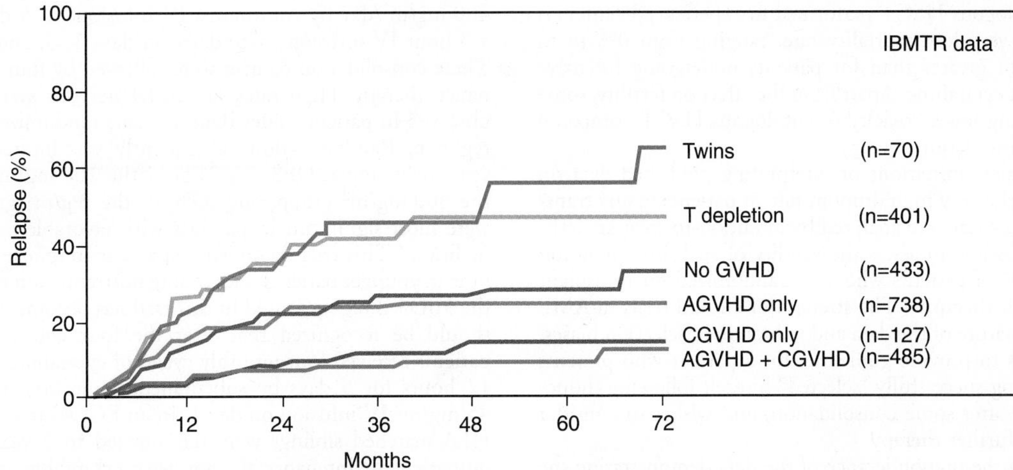

Figure 61–7 Results with reduced-intensity transplant for acute myeloid leukemia. *(Data from Hegenbart U, Niederwieser D, Sandmaier BM, et al: Treatment for acute myelogenous leukemia by low-dose, total-body, irradiation-based conditioning and hematopoietic cell transplantation from related and unrelated donors. J Clin Oncol 24:444, 2006.[57a])*

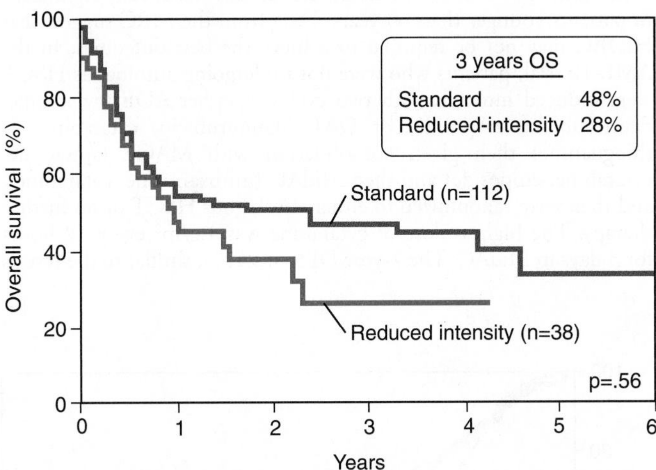

Figure 61–8 Standard versus reduced-intensity conditioning for patients with acute myeloid leukemia. *(Data from Scott BL, Sandmaier BM, Storer B, et al: Myeloablative vs nonmyeloablative allogeneic transplantation for patients with myelodysplastic syndrome or acute myelogenous leukemia with multilineage dysplasia: A retrospective analysis. Leukemia 20:128, 2006.[58])*

difference in patient outcomes between the two different approaches to conditioning (Fig. 61–8).[58]

Patients with unfavorable cytogenetic abnormalities have an extremely poor prognosis without allo-HSCT.[50,52,59] In fact, the data are identical to those of patients with Philadelphia chromosome-positive acute lymphocytic leukemia (ALL) who do not undergo allo-HSCT in first CR. In contrast to such ALL patients, AML patients with unfavorable cytogenetic abnormalities historically have rarely been referred for alternative donor HSCT in first CR. This reluctance likely will be overcome in the near future. A report from the German 01/99 study described a cohort of 250 high-risk patients, followed prospectively, who encountered an unequivocal benefit from allo-HSCT from MUD compared to other forms of postremission therapy.[60,61]

Autologous HSCT

After allo-HSCT, autologous HSCT offers the most potent form of postremission therapy, relying on the antileukemic effect provided by the myeloablative regimen (see box on Autologous Hematopoietic Stem Cell Transplantation for AML). Use of autologous HSCT has generated a fair amount of controversy, in part because of the difficulties in interpreting the historic outcome data and applying them to current day practice. Data are further confounded by the degree and intensity of prior chemotherapy and patient selection. Most of the major prospective studies reported over the past decade have described a lower relapse rate for patients undergoing autologous HSCT in comparison with chemotherapy (Table 61–6). The lower relapse rate following autologous HSCT has also been demonstrated in patients with favorable cytogenetic finding (Table 61–7). Thus, the preponderance of data suggests that autologous HSCT provides a more potent antileukemic efficacy than intensive chemotherapy alone.

In many instances, the overall outcome from these trials does not support a primary role for autologous HSCT, mostly because of the high mortality reported in patients undergoing an autologous HSCT: 18% in the MRC trial and 14% in the U.S. Intergroup study.[27,51] Other studies demonstrated superior DFS, but OS was not significantly improved due to subsequent rescue of patients who had relapsed and entered a second remission.[52,53]

Autologous Hematopoietic Stem Cell Transplantation for Acute Myeloid Leukemia

- Autologous stem cell transplantation provides a more potent antileukemic effect than chemotherapy.
- In most prospective studies of autologous stem cell transplant, high mortality rates are associated with use of bone marrow as the stem cell source.
- Mortality using peripheral blood stem cell grafts is only 1% to 2%.
- Mortality and morbidity are not greater than the rates with standard consolidation therapy using high-dose cytarabine with the exception of impact on fertility.
- Appears to have a role in consolidation for patients with favorable cytogenetic abnormalities and for those with intermediate-risk cytogenetic abnormalities who do not have a human leukocyte antigen-compatible donor.
- Definitive data in patients with unfavorable cytogenetic abnormalities are lacking, but it is reasonable to offer this to patients who are not eligible for some form of allogeneic stem cell transplant.
- Although leukemia cells may be present in the graft, a definitive role for purging grafts harvested during remission has not been demonstrated.

Currently autologous HSCT performed in experienced centers is associated with a very low mortality rate, ranging from 0% to to 2%,[32] which is not greater than for patients undergoing intensive consolidation with cytarabine. Apart from the effect on fertility, some centers are reporting lower toxicity of autologous HSCT compared with intensive consolidation therapy.[62]

One of the major limitations of interpreting published data on transplantation is the very high dropout rate of patients in any transplant group. Because data are analyzed by intention-to-treat analysis, it is virtually impossible to assess the validity of such interpretation when 40% to 50% of patients who were randomized for transplant never received such therapy.[18] The strength of clinical trials in AML is the prospective nature of the data and reduction of selection biases. However, this fails to provide guidelines for a patient who presents to a clinician having successfully "selected" himself following induction, and possibly after some consolidation, and wishes to consider the most suitable further therapy.

Thus, based on the preponderance of the data demonstrating the potent antileukemic activity of autologous transplantation and the low morbidity and minimal mortality associated with this procedure using current technologies, there appears to be a clear role for this technique in patients with a favorable cytogenetic finding and for those with intermediate-risk cytogenetic abnormalities who are not suitable candidates for allo-HSCT. Some investigators have recognized the validity of autologous HSCT in AML but have suggested that it be "reserved" for patients who relapse.[63] Such considerations should be discouraged because of the very poor rate of survival for patients with relapsed AML, irrespective of their prognostic factors, when based on information that may be available at diagnosis.[64]

Intensification Therapy

A variety of studies have suggested that increasing the intensity of postremission therapy prolongs remission duration and improves OS in patients younger than 60 years with AML. Several studies have prospectively evaluated the role of intensive postremission consolidation with high-dose cytarabine (HiDAC). CALGB randomly assigned 596 patients in CR to receive four courses of cytarabine at one of three doses: 100 mg/m²/day by continuous IV infusion for 5 days; 400 mg/m²/day by continuous IV infusion for 5 days; or 3 g/m² as a 3-hour IV infusion twice daily on days 1, 3, and 5 (Fig. 61–9).[65] These consolidation courses were followed by four cycles of maintenance therapy. High rates of central nervous system toxicity were observed in patients older than 60 years randomized to the HiDAC regimen. Randomization subsequently was limited to patients 60 years or younger. DFS was 21% in the 100 mg/m² group, 25% in the 400 mg/m² group, and 39% in the 3 g/m² group. The results were most significant in patients with favorable cytogenetic abnormalities.[66] This trial demonstrated a dose–response effect for cytarabine in younger patients undergoing postremission therapy. Although the HiDAC regimen used in this trial has become widely adopted, it should be recognized that after the four courses of HiDAC, all patients received four monthly cycles of cytarabine 100 mg/m² every 12 hours for 5 days by subcutaneous injection and daunorubicin 45 mg/m² IV infusion on day 1. In an ECOG trial, patients without HLA-matched siblings were randomized to 2 years of continuous outpatient maintenance therapy with cytarabine and 6-thioguanine or a single course of intensive consolidation with cytarabine 3 g/m² IV every 12 hours for 12 doses followed by amsacrine 100 mg/m² per day IV for 3 days. The 4-year event-free survival at 4 years was 27% for the intensive consolidation arm and 16% for the maintenance arm *($P = 0.068$)*.[26] This difference was statistically significant in patients younger than 60 years. Data from the MRC suggest that HiDAC may not be required to achieve the best outcomes. In the AML-10 trial, patients who were not undergoing autologous HSCT were induced into CR with two cycles of either ADE (cytarabine, daunorubicin, etoposide) or DAT (daunorubicin, cytarabine, 6-thioguanine) then given consolidation with MACE (amsacrine, cytarabine, etoposide) and then MidAC (mitoxantrone, cytarabine), and then were randomized to either autologous HSCT or no further therapy. The highest dose of cytarabine was 1 g/m² every 12 hours for 3 days in MidAC. The 7-year DFS was 40%, similar to the results

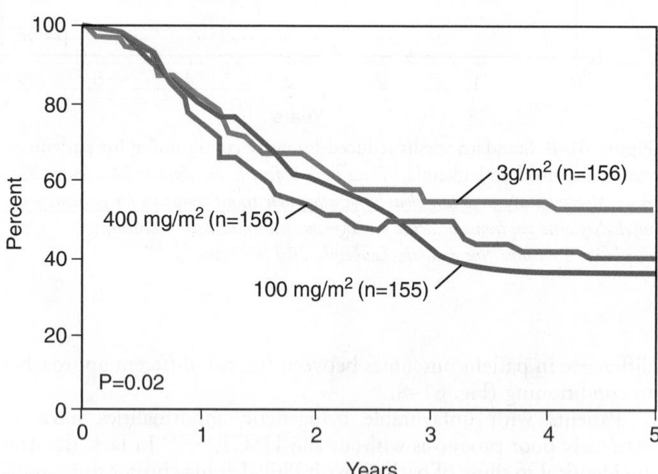

Figure 61–9 Escalating postremission therapy with cytarabine: acute myeloid leukemia < 60 years. *(Data from Mayer RJ, Davis RB, Schiffer CA, et al: For the Cancer and Leukemia Group B: Intensive postremission chemotherapy in adults with acute myeloid leukemia. N Engl J Med 331:896, 1994.[65])*

Table 61–6 Relapse Rate Following Autologous Stem Cell Transplantation and Chemotherapy for Acute Myeloid Leukemia in CR1

	Autologous Transplant	Chemotherapy
GIMEMA[50]	40%	57%
GOELAM[53]	45%	55%
MRC[51a]	35%	53%
ECOG/SWOG[48]	48%	61%

[a]Excluding children.
Adapted from Appelbaum FR, Rowe JM, Radich J, Dick JE: Acute myeloid leukemia. Hematology Am Soc Hematol Educ Program 62, 2001.

Table 61–7 Relapse Rate Following Postremission Therapy for Patients with Acute Myeloid Leukemia in CR1 with Favorable Cytogenetics

	Allogeneic BMT		Autologous BMT		Chemotherapy	
	n	*Relapse Rate*	*n*	*Relapse Rate*	*n*	*Relapse Rate*
MRC[283]	50	8%	50	20%	242	38%
ECOG/SWOG[48]	19	20%	20	17%	22	59%

BMT, bone marrow transplantation.

reported in the CALGB discussed. These data suggest that among patients not receiving HSCT, the critical factor may be administration of intensive chemotherapy rather than the requirement for HiDAC.[67]

The number of courses of HiDAC, or any other form of intensive chemotherapy, required for optimal postremission therapy is uncertain and remains an important question for future large cooperative group studies. The Finnish Leukemia Group randomized patients younger than 65 years in CR after two courses of induction and two courses of HiDAC to four additional HiDAC consolidation courses.[68] No benefit was observed for patients randomized to the longer consolidation program, suggesting early intensive consolidation likely is the most important influence on outcome rather than the number of cycles of intensive chemotherapy. Furthermore, in the U.S. Intergroup trial among patients receiving chemotherapy only, one cycle of HiDAC resulted in a 5-year DFS of 52%.[27] Thus, although two to four cycles of intensive postremission chemotherapy are given commonly to most patients, no prospective data support this strategy.

Data suggest that the outcome of patients with core-binding factor (CBF) AML is very favorable when multiple (3–4) cycles of HiDAC (3 g/m^2 per dose) are administered. Byrd et al.[69] for the CALGB retrospectively reviewed their experience of patients with t(8;21). The 5-year DFS and OS for patients given ≥3 cycles of HiDAC (71% and 76%, respectively) was significantly higher than the rates for patients given one cycle of HiDAC followed by further cycles of chemotherapy without HiDAC (37% and 44%, respectively; $P = 0.03$ and $P = 0.04$, respectively; Fig. 61–10). However, similar favorable outcomes have been reported by the MRC in larger number of patients with regimens lacking HiDAC.

Maintenance Therapy

A prospective randomized trial conducted by the ECOG suggested that maintenance therapy with 6-thioguanine plus cytarabine 60 mg/m^2 once per week for 2 years offered a benefit in remission duration compared to no maintenance treatment (median remission duration 8.1 months vs 4.1 month; $P = 0.003$), although no significant survival difference was identified.[26] Buchner et al.[70] analyzed long-term followup data and observed a benefit to monthly maintenance for 3 years (5-year DFS 23% vs 6%). In an EORTC-HOVON trial, 76 older patients (age ≥61 years) achieving CR were randomized to no further therapy and 75 patients to eight cycles of low-dose cytarabine (10 mg/m^2 subcutaneously) every 12 hours for 12 days every 6 weeks following consolidation with the same agents used during induction.[71] An advantage in DFS was observed among patients receiving maintenance low-dose cytarabine every 6 weeks for 1 year (median DFS 20% vs 7% and 5-year DFS 13% vs 7%; $P = 0.006$). However, OS was not different (5-year OS 18% vs 15%; $P = 0.29$).[71] The AML-9 study conducted by the MRC randomized patients in CR to maintenance treatment for 1 year with eight courses of cytarabine 70 mg/m^2 subcutaneous every 12 hours and 6-thioguanine 100 mg/m^2 orally every 12 hours for 5 days per month followed by four courses of COAP (cyclophosphamide, vincristine, cytarabine, prednisone) or observation. Such therapy delayed, but did not prevent, relapse with no improvement in OS at 5 years. Therefore, contemporary studies using various maintenance regimens consistently show a benefit in DFS, but not OS, resulting from maintenance therapy.

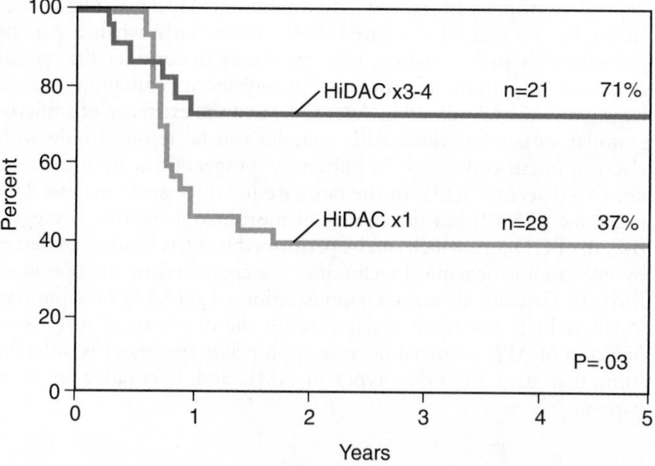

Figure 61–10 t(8,21) Acute myeloid leukemia disease-free survival. Effect of multiple cycles of high-dose cytarabine. *(Data from Byrd JC, Dodge RK, Carroll A, et al: Patients with t(8;21) (q22;q22) and acute myeloid leukemia have superior failure-free and overall survival when repetitive cycles of high-dose cytarabine are administered. J Clin Oncol 17:3767, 1999.[69])*

SPECIFIC AML SUBTYPES

Based on the karyotype status, two major groups of AML can be discriminated: those with an abnormal karyotype, accounting for 52%–60% of patients, and those with a normal karyotype by conventional cytogenetics, composing 40%–48% of AML patients.[47,48,59,72a] Among the patients with an abnormal karyotype, 25% have balanced translocations [t(8;21),t(15;17),inv(16)], and 27% show unbalanced abnormalities [−5/del(5q), −7/del(7q) or complex karyotype]. Within the normal cytogenetic category, 45% to 63% have nucleophosmin (*NPM;* localized on chromosome 5, band q35*)* mutations, 23% to 33% show *FLT-3* (localized on chromosome 13, band q12) length mutations, 5% to 30% have *MLL* (localized on chromosome 11, band q23) tandem duplications, and 8% to 19% have CCAAT enhancer-binding protein (C/EBP; localized on chromosome 19, band q13.1) α mutations.[73a] The prognosis of patients with normal karyotype in the presence of each of these mutations is different. Patients with an *NPM* mutation alone have a favorable prognosis, especially if associated with the absence of *FLT-3* ITD, with 60% of patients living longer than 11 years.[73a,74a] In contrast, the presence of *FLT-3* and *MLL* mutations is associated with an adverse prognosis, and coexistence of *FLT-3* and *NPM* does not contribute toward better prognosis. In contrast to adults, in childhood AML with normal cytogenetics, *NPM* mutations are relatively uncommon, occurring at a frequency of 8%. Gene expression profiling and microRNA expression as diagnostic or prognostic indicators in patients with AML and a normal karyotype have limited or moderate accuracy, probably reflecting the molecular heterogeneity of this AML subtype.[88,88a]

The pretreatment karyotype constitutes an independent prognostic determinant for attainment of CR and risk of relapse and survival.[47,48,59] Four broad cytogenetic risk categories of AML are applied in clinical practice: favorable, intermediate, unfavorable, and unknown (see Table 61–1).[47,48] It is important to perform appropriate cytogenetic and fluorescent in situ hybridization studies to establish the correct cytogenetic risk category. Patients displaying normal karyotype are in the intermediate prognostic category because their survival probabilities usually are lower than those with t(8;21), inv(16)/t(16;16), or t(15;17). Their 5-year survival rate is only about 25%.[47,48,59] The incidence of intermediate- to high-risk AML increases with age (Fig. 61–11).

AML with Intermediate-Risk Cytogenetic Abnormalities

In the United States and Europe, between 40% and 50% of all AML patients have a normal karyotype (Table 61–8).

Patients with a normal karyotype are classified as having intermediate risk; however, unlike patients with favorable or unfavorable cytogenetics, such patients are heterogeneous and do not have a uniform prognosis.

Prognosis of AML patients with normal cytogenetics may be discriminated by the presence of the gene mutations resulting in *FLT-3* internal tandem duplication,[83,84] the partial tandem duplication of

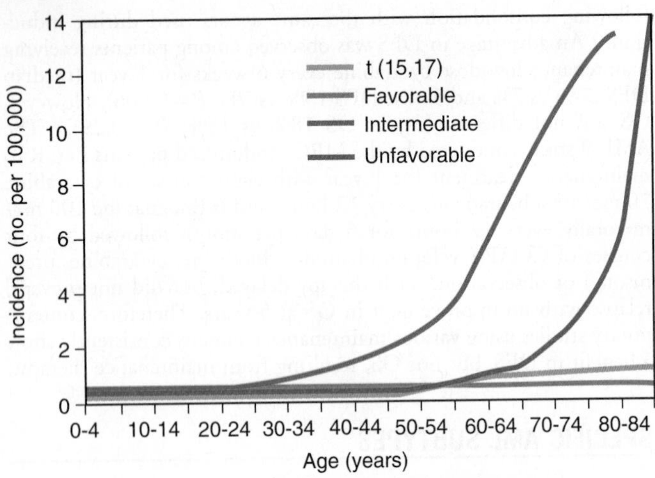

Figure 61–11 Age-specific incidence rates for acute myeloid leukemia by cytogenetic risk groups. *(Data based in part on Mauritzson N, Johansson B, Albin M, et al: Survival time in a population based consecutive series of adult acut myeloid leukemia-the prognostic impact of karyotype during the time period 1976–1993. Leukemia 13:1039, 2000.)*

Table 61–8 Incidence of Intermediate Risk Cytogenetic Abnormalities in Acute Myeloid Leukemia

	Intermediate-Risk Group	Normal Karyotype
ECOG/SWOG	46%	40%
MRC	66%	42%
CALGB	71%	48%
German-Austrian AML Group		45%

Data from Rowe JM: Preface: Significant advances in the biology and therapy of AML over the past four decades. Best Pract Res Clin Haematol 19:259, 2006.

Acute Myeloid Leukemia with Intermediate-Risk Cytogenetic Abnormalities as Determined by Karyotypic Analysis

- Overall incidence increases with age but not to the same degree as acute myeloid leukemia (AML) with unfavorable cytogenetic abnormality.
- Intermediate-risk AML composes 45% to 70% of all AML cases.
- From 40% to 50% of all AML patients have a normal karyotype.
- Patients with a normal karyotype represent a group with diverse prognostic factors; thus, current classification is unsatisfactory.
- Prognostic factors for patients with normal cytogenetics include the following:
  1. Partial tandem duplication of the MLL gene
  2. Presence of the FLT-3 internal tandem duplication
  3. Wilms tumor antigen expression
  4. Multidrug resistance (MDR-1)
  5. Overexpression of other specific genes, such as BAX, BCL-2/BAX, BALC, EVI-1, KIT, ERG
  6. CD56 expression
- Prognostication can also be made by hierarchical cluster analysis using gene expression profiling.
- More favorable prognosis associated with expression of CCAAT enhancer-binding protein α (CEBPA) or nucleophosmin 1 (NPM1).
- Most young patients with intermediate cytogenetic abnormalities should be referred for an allogeneic stem cell transplant if a human leukocyte antigen (HLA)-compatible sibling is available.
- Stem cell transplants from a matched unrelated or haploidentical donor may be reasonable in young fit patients with other demonstrated unfavorable prognostic features.
- Autologous stem cell transplant is a reasonable option for those who do not have an HLA-matched donor.

the *MLL* gene,[85,86] or Wilms tumor gene (WT1) expression.[87] When gene expression profiling is used with application of hierarchical cluster analysis, distinct prognostic groups also can be discriminated among AML patients with a normal karyotype.[88,89] A more favorable prognosis is associated with the presence of gene mutations of NPM1[90] or C/EBP α (CEBPA).[91] The traditional classification of patients with a normal karyotype is rapidly evolving, resulting in a predictive model based on genetic analysis. Thus, young patients with a normal karyotype who have distinct poor prognostic features may be candidates for an alternative donor stem cell transplant if an HLA-matched donor is not readily available. Conversely, it may well be that patients with an intermediate karyotype who have a more favorable prognosis (presence of CEBPA or NPM1) may be offered postremission therapy that does not include allo-HSCT. It is likely that patients with a normal karyotype will be further defined by molecular markers, allowing for more precise prognostic classification over the next few years (see box on AML with Intermediate-Risk Cytogenetic Abnormalities as Determined by Karyotypic Analysis).

AML with Favorable-Risk Cytogenetic Abnormalities

APL is caused by translocations disrupting the retinoic acid receptor α *(RARA)* locus on chromosome 17, resulting in fusion products with other nuclear proteins such as the promyelocytic leukemia (PML) protein, whose gene is located on chromosome 15 in 99% of cases.[92] The PML-RARA fusion protein, acting in a dominant negative manner, causes APL, presumably by recruiting histone deacetylase activity and preventing transcription of genes important in promyelocyte differentiation.[93] Standard cytogenetic analysis demonstrates the 15;17 translocation [t(15;17)] in 95% to 100% of cases. Polymerase chain reaction (PCR) methodology provides a more sensitive means of detecting the PML-RARA rearrangement underlying the t(15;17). Its potential can be used to detect minimal residual APL in patients in CR. APL constitutes less than 10% of unselected cases of AML, and independent risk factors for a diagnosis of APL in a patient with AML are younger age, Hispanic background, and obesity. The chief clinical feature is a bleeding diathesis resulting from plasmin-dependent primary fibrinolysis and disseminated intravascular coagulation. In any case of untreated AML, particularly when a patient presents with such a picture, it is important to consider the typical morphologic pattern (i.e., abnormal promyelocytes containing coarse, large granules and numerous Auer rods) and the existence of a microgranular variant in which APL granules can be resolved only with electron microscopy. More importantly, cytogenetic analysis must be done to detect t(15;17). In the rare case in which such analysis does not show t(15;17) but the clinical or morphologic picture is suggestive, the POD test, which can be performed in a few hours, can detect by immunohistochemical techniques the characteristic disruption of PML in virtually all cases. Demonstration of t(15,17) or a positive POD or PCR test result is requisite for the diagnosis of APL. Recognition of APL is crucial because appropriate treatment is different from that used for other types of AML and is curative in most patients.

Acute Promyelocytic Leukemia

Hillestad[98] is credited with the first description of APL as a distinct clinical entity in 1957. Since then, more has been learned about the pathogenesis and therapy of APL than for any other subtype of AML.

Table 61–9 Distinctive Features of Acute Promyelocytic Leukemia

• 10%–15% of adult acute myeloid leukemia (1200 new patients per year in the United States)
• Leukopenia in 85%
• Coagulopathy (disseminated intravascular coagulopathy, fibrinolysis, proteolysis)
• t(15;17)
• Promyelocytic leukemia-retinoic acid receptor α (PML-RARA) fusion transcript
• Differentiation with all-*trans* retinoic acid
• Apoptosis with arsenic trioxide

Previously, this subtype of AML was highly fatal, primarily because a severe life-threatening bleeding disorder often manifested as intracerebral hemorrhage, which accounted for an induction mortality rate of 20% to 30%.[99] However, since the introduction of all-*trans* retinoic acid (ATRA) therapy in the early 1990s and its administration with anthracycline-based chemotherapy, APL is curable in the majority of patients.

APL is distinguished from other subtypes of AML in several ways, including the peculiar sensitivity of the leukemia cells to anthracyclines,[100] frequent presentation with leukopenia, presence of life-threatening coagulopathy, presence of the PML-RARA fusion transcript, which results from the t(15;17),[101,102] ability of leukemia cells to undergo differentiation with ATRA[103] and apoptosis with arsenic trioxide (ATO),[104] and high cure rate now achieved in the great majority of patients (Table 61–9).[105] Achieving CR without prior marrow aplasia also is unique to APL. This treatment approach has become a paradigm for directing therapy at the specific molecular abnormality and one of the true therapeutic triumphs in the treatment of malignant disease. Current therapy generally consists of three phases: induction, consolidation, and maintenance (see box on How to Treat Acute Promyelocytic Leukemia).

How to Treat Acute Promyelocytic Leukemia

1. Initiate treatment with all-*trans* retinoic acid (ATRA) as soon as the diagnosis is suspected without waiting for genetic confirmation in an effort to decrease the induction mortality most often related to the coagulopathy.
2. If coagulopathy is present, administer frequent platelet transfusions to maintain platelet count greater than 30,000 to 50,000/μL and cryoprecipitate to maintain fibrinogen level greater than 100 to 150 mg/dL. There is no role for routine use of heparin or antifibrinolytic agents.
3. For induction, administer anthracycline-based chemotherapy with ATRA. Give concurrent ATRA and chemotherapy for patients who present with a high white blood cell count greater than 10,000/μL. If a patient is older or unable to tolerate anthracyclines, consider ATRA plus arsenic trioxide.
4. Maintain a high index of suspicion for the retinoic acid syndrome. At the first sign of dyspnea, pleural or pericardial effusions, hypotension, or pulmonary infiltrates, initiate dexamethasone 10 mg twice daily.
5. For consolidation, give anthracycline-based chemotherapy with ATRA (1 week with each cycle) for two to three cycles until molecular remission is achieved.
6. For high-risk patients (presenting white blood cell count 10,000/μL or higher), consider either high-dose anthracyclines, intermediate- or high-dose cytarabine during either induction or consolidation, or administer arsenic trioxide.
7. For maintenance, consider either ATRA or ATRA plus low-dose chemotherapy with 6-mercaptopurine and methotrexate. Studies have suggested that patients in molecular remission may not benefit from maintenance therapy.
8. Patients can be monitored by checking the peripheral blood for promyelocytic leukemia-retinoic acid receptor α (PML-RARA) using reverse transcriptase polymerase chain reaction every 3 to 6 months, probably more frequently for high-risk patients.
9. For relapse, consider arsenic trioxide for two cycles until molecular remission is achieved, followed by high-dose chemotherapy and autologous hematopoietic stem cell transplantation. Consider prophylactic intrathecal chemotherapy for any patient who has relapsed.

Efficacy of ATRA Combined with Anthracycline-Based Chemotherapy for Induction in Patients with APL

Based on in vitro studies documenting differentiation of leukemic promyelocytes in the presence of retinoic acid, phase II clinical trials were initiated that demonstrated the remarkable effectiveness of ATRA initially in patients with relapsed and refractory APL and then in newly diagnosed patients in which the majority of patients achieved CR.[106–111] Subsequently, cooperative oncology groups carried out clinical trials comparing ATRA to conventional chemotherapy.[112–115] In a trial conducted by the North American Intergroup (protocol I0129), 350 patients were randomized to ATRA induction therapy or to conventional induction chemotherapy with daunorubicin and ara-C.[113,115] After two courses of intensive consolidation chemotherapy, patients were randomized to 1-year maintenance with daily oral ATRA or no maintenance. Patients who received ATRA during induction and during maintenance had the best outcome, and approximately 75% of these patients appear cured of their disease. The benefit of ATRA maintenance therapy also was demonstrated in the conventional chemotherapy group (5-year DFS 47% in maintenance group vs 16% in no maintenance group). The European APL group conducted a randomized trial comparing the sequential versus concurrent addition of ATRA to standard induction chemotherapy. They found benefit associated with the concurrent approach due to a decrease in the relapse rate rather than an increase in the CR rate.[114] In phase II studies the Spanish Cooperative Group PETHEMA (LPA96 and LPA99) and the GIMEMA investigated induction therapy with ATRA and idarubicin,[119,120] without cytarabine, prompted by the apparent peculiar sensitivity of leukemic promyelocytes to anthracyclines.[121]

ATRA plus idarubicin appears to be equally effective in inducing remission as was the combination of cytarabine, ATRA, and an anthracycline.[100,109] Furthermore, in the PETHEMA studies, no cytarabine was administered during any phase of treatment. However, in a prospective randomized trial by the European APL group, a higher relapse rate was observed among patients treated with ATRA plus daunorubicin than among patients treated with ATRA plus daunorubicin and cytarabine.[122] Enrollment in the noncytarabine arm was discontinued prematurely. Of the 11 relapses in the noncytarabine arm, nine were hematologic and two were molecular, compared to only one hematologic and one molecular relapse in the cytarabine arm. Possible explanations for the different results observed in the European APL group and PETHEMA studies include differences between idarubicin and daunorubicin, differences in the total cumulative doses of the two anthracyclines, and the fact that ATRA was used during consolidation in PETHEMA but not in the European group study. It appears that if idarubicin is used in the doses reported and perhaps daunorubicin is used in higher doses than previously reported, cytarabine is not needed.

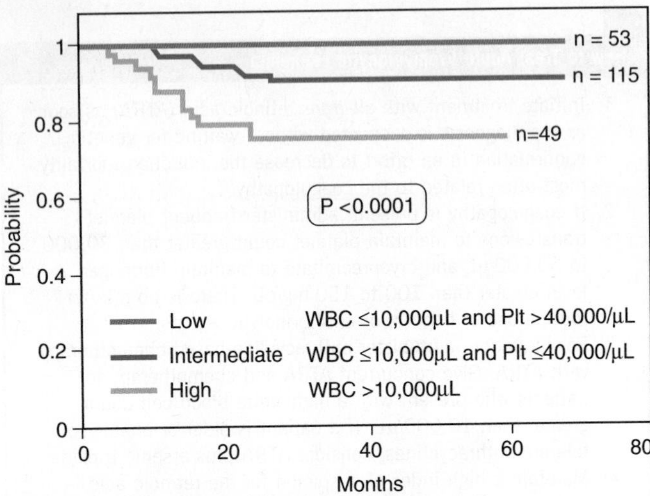

Figure 61–12 GIMEMA and PETHEMA study. Relapse-free survival of patients with acute promyelocytic leukemia by risk group. *(Data from Sanz MA, Lo Coco F, Martin G, et al. Definition of relapse risk and role of nonanthracycline drugs for consolidation in patients with acute promyelocytic leukemia: A joint study of the PETHEMA and GIMEMA cooperative groups. Blood 96:1247, 2000.[116])*

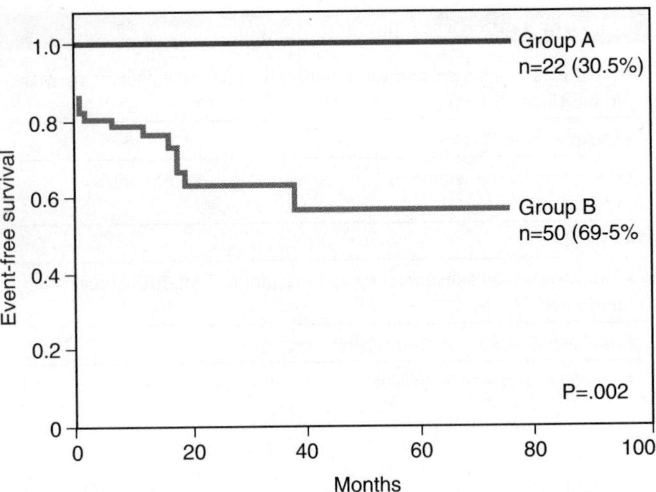

Figure 61–13 Comparison of event-free survival with single-agent arsenic trioxide therapy between good-risk acute promyelocytic leukemia patients (group A: white blood cell count <5000) and the rest (group B). *(Data from Mathews V, George B, Lakshmi KM, et al: Single-agent arsenic trioxide in the treatment of newly diagnosed acute promyelocytic leukemia: Durable remissions with minimal toxicity. Blood 107:2627, 2006.[138])*

The most important factor predicting outcome in APL is the WBC count at initial presentation. The GIMEMA and PETHEMA cooperative groups used both WBC count and platelet count to identify patients at low risk (WBC ≤ 10,000/µL, platelet count >40,000/µL), intermediate risk (WBC ≤ 10,000/µL, platelet count = 40,000/µL), or high risk (WBC > 10,000/µL) for relapse (Fig. 61–12).[116] Advanced age is another important unfavorable prognostic factor.[118] In addition, the FLT-3 internal tandem duplication mutation occurs in approximately 35% of patients with APL and appears to confer an unfavorable prognosis in patients with APL[117,123–126] The presence of the bcr3 isoform of the PML-RARA fusion transcript also has been reported to confer an unfavorable prognosis.[127]

Induction Therapy with ATO in Patients with APL

Excellent results have been observed with ATO as a single agent in patients with relapsed and refractory APL[128–133] In the U.S. multicenter trial of 40 patients with relapsed and refractory APL, all of whom previously exposed to ATRA, 85% of patients achieved CR after induction with ATO.[132] Furthermore, of 29 assessable patients who achieved CR, 86% achieved molecular remission after induction or consolidation with ATO. These data encouraged the studies of ATO as part of initial induction regimen.[134–138]

A number of studies have shown that single-agent ATO is a very effective therapy for patients with newly diagnosed APL (Table 61–10). Investigators in Iran treated patients with only two courses of ATO and found an 86% CR rate and a 92% molecular remission rate.[137] Investigators from India reported an identical CR rate among 72 patients given ATO for induction and up to six courses of ATO for consolidation.[138] In this study, CR rate and 3-year event-free survival, DFS, and OS rates were 80%, 75%, 87%, and 86%, respectively. The molecular remission rate was 76%. Patients with WBC count less than 5000/µL and platelet count greater than 20 × 10,000/µL had 3-year event-free survival, DFS, and OS rates of 100%, whereas patients not in this good-risk group had 3-year event-free survival, DFS, and OS rates of 63%, 80%, and 79% respectively (see Fig. 61–12). Investigators at the Shanghai Institute of Hematology conducted a trial in which 61 patients with newly diagnosed APL were randomized to receive ATRA, ATO, or the combination of ATRA plus ATO (Table 61–11).[136] All patients subsequently received intensive consolidation chemotherapy and maintenance therapy.

Table 61–10 Induction Therapy with Single-Agent Arsenic Trioxide of Untreated Acute Promyelocytic Leukemia Patients

Study	N	CR Rate (%)	PCR Negative (%)	Postremission Therapy
China[134]	124	88	NR	Chemotherapy
Iran[137]	111	86	92	ATO × 1
India[138]	72	86	76	ATO × 6

ATO, arsenic tetroxide; CR, complete remission; PCR, Polymerase chain reaction.

Patients randomized to the combination arm achieved complete hematologic remission in a significantly shorter median time period (25 days) than did those who received ATRA alone (40 days) or ATO alone (35 days). Furthermore, there was a significantly greater reduction in the amount of PML-RARA fusion transcript detected among patients in the combination arm. At median followup of 18 months, there were no relapses among the 20 patients who achieved CR after receiving combination therapy, whereas seven of the 37 patients who achieved CR with monotherapy relapsed.

A single small randomized study suggested that addition of ATRA to ATO in patients with relapsed and refractory APL did not improve outcome compared to ATO therapy alone.[142] However, in patients with untreated APL the combination appears to induce more rapid CR and results in a more profound molecular remission rate in newly diagnosed patients, with apparently no greater toxicity than experienced with each agent alone. Therefore, for patients who cannot be treated with anthracyclines (e.g., older patients, those with abnormal cardiac function) and who have low-risk or intermediate-risk disease, it is reasonable to consider treatment with a combination of ATO plus ATRA, or perhaps ATO alone if the patient has very low-risk disease (WBC < 5,000/µL; Fig. 61–13).

Consolidation Therapy for Patients with APL

The PETHEMA group suggested that addition of ATRA to consolidation chemotherapy may be beneficial for patients with intermediate- and high-risk disease.[120] In the LPA99 study, such patients received ATRA at the standard dosage of 45 mg/m^2/day on days 1 through 15, in combination with three courses of single-agent con-

Table 61–11 Randomized Trial of Arsenic Trioxide and ATRA in Untreated Acute Promyelocytic Leukemia

Induction/Maintenance Therapy	*N*	CR Rate (%)	Time to CR (Days)	↓PML/RARA (fold)	Relapse (%; Median Followup 18 Months)
ATRA	20	95	40 ± 10	6.7	26.3
ATO	20	90	35 ± 3	32	11.1
ATRA + ATO	21	95	25 ± 5	119	0
P value	—	NS	<0.05	<0.01	<0.02[a]

[a]All patients also treated with consolidation chemotherapy and 6-mercaptopurine plus methotrexate as maintenance.
ATO, arsenic tetroxide; ATRA, all-*trans* retinoic acid; CR, complete remission; PML-RARA, promyelocytic leukemia-retinoic acid receptor α.
Data from Shen ZX, Shi ZZ, Fang J et al: All-trans retinoic acid/As2O3 combination yields a high quality remission and survival in newly diagnosed acute promyelocytic leukemia. Proc Natl Acad Sci USA 2004;101:5328–5335.104.[136]

solidation chemotherapy. The impact of adding ATRA during consolidation was difficult to evaluate because patients in these groups also received an increased dose of idarubicin during the first course and 2 consecutive days of idarubicin during the third course, instead of 1 day as in their previous study (LPA96).[119] Nevertheless, the relapse rate was lower and the survival rate was better. However, the impact of both adding ATRA during consolidation and the higher doses of chemotherapy appeared to have less of an influence on patients with high-risk disease.

Therapy for Patients with High-Risk APL

Patients with high-risk APL currently are a major focus of clinical investigations. The 3-year cumulative incidence of relapse for patients with high-risk disease is approximately 21%. Three studies have suggested that administration of intermediate- or high-dose cytarabine to patients at high risk for relapse is beneficial.[122,143,144] The GIMEMA group administered intermediate-dose cytarabine during consolidation to patients with high-risk disease. The first course of consolidation included cytarabine 1 g/m²/day for 4 days plus idarubicin; the second course included mitoxantrone and etoposide; and the third course included idarubicin, cytarabine 150 mg/m² every 8 hours subcutaneously for 5 days, and 6-thioguanine. Patients also received ATRA at conventional doses for 15 days during each consolidation course. After a median followup of 2 years, the cumulative incidence of relapse in high-risk patients was only 2%. The European APL group observed a low relapse rate among patients with WBC count greater than 10,000/μL who received consolidation with cytarabine at a dosage of 1 to 2 g/m² every 12 hours.[122]

In the completed North American Intergroup protocol C9710, patients received conventional ATRA, daunorubicin, and cytarabine induction therapy and then were randomized to receive or not receive two 25-day courses of ATO as an initial consolidation.[127] Patients subsequently received further consolidation with two 3-day courses of daunorubicin with 1 week of ATRA therapy. Preliminary results indicate a very low relapse rate among low- and intermediate-risk patients of 3% and 7%, respectively and a relapse rate of 16% in high-risk patients.[139a]

Maintenance Therapy for Patients with APL

Although the initial randomized trials suggested that maintenance therapy was beneficial, subsequent studies have indicated that maintenance may not be important for APL patients who have achieved a molecular remission after intensive consolidation.[141,147] In a trial conducted by the GIMEMA, between 1993 and 1997, 318 of patients were randomized to one to four maintenance arms: oral 6-mercaptopurine (6-MP) and methotrexate, ATRA alone, ATRA alternating with 6-MP and methotrexate, or no further therapy after consolidation.[147] Beginning in 1998, 268 patients in molecular remission after consolidation were randomized to ATRA alone or ATRA plus 6-MP and methotrexate. A total of 78 PML-RARA–negative patients were randomized to 6-MP plus methotrexate, 83 to ATRA alone, 81 to ATRA plus 6-MP methotrexate, and 76 to no further therapy. No difference in molecular DFS was observed among the randomized arms. A study conducted by the Japanese Adult Leukemia Study Group (APL97), which randomized patients in molecular remission to either six courses of intensive maintenance chemotherapy (no ATRA) or observation after consolidation, also could not demonstrate any benefit of maintenance.[141] These studies suggest that patients who have low- or intermediate-risk disease and who achieve molecular remission after consolidation therapy may not benefit from maintenance therapy. These results have important implications because reports have suggested a small percentage of patients may develop therapy-related secondary myelodysplastic disorders or AML.[139,140]

Treatment of Patients with Relapsed APL

ATO has become the treatment of choice for patients with relapsed or refractory APL. ATO has a greater likelihood of inducing a molecular CR (approximately 50% after a single 25-day course and 80% after two courses) and may be less toxic than chemotherapy (Table 61–12).[150] Once a molecular CR is achieved with ATO, high-dose chemotherapy followed by autologous HSCT should be considered considered.[145,150,152] For the unusual patient who remains molecularly positive following ATO, allo-HSCT appears to be an effective strategy.[146] CD33 is expressed on the surface of APL cells. For patients who experience a molecular relapse, gemtuzumab ozogamicin anti-CD33 antibody linked to calicheamicin is effective therapy.[148] Among 11 evaluated patients treated for molecular relapse with gemtuzumab ozogamicin, nine achieved a molecular remission after two doses, and these remissions were sustained. Although experience is limited, ATO also appears to be an effective approach.[149]

Prophylactic and intrathecal therapy should be considered for patients with bone marrow relapse because of an apparent increased incidence of extramedullary disease at relapse, particularly in the central nervous system.[153,154] Although not clearly beneficial, prophylactic intrathecal therapy also may be useful for patients who present with or who develop leukocytosis during the initial phase of treatment.

CBF Leukemias

CBF AML is associated with a good prognosis. AML with the specific translocation t(8;21) (Table 61–13) is associated with a younger median age at onset than many other subtypes of AML, extramedullary disease, and has a relatively favorable prognosis when treated with intensive consolidation chemotherapy in the absence of extramedullary disease.[151] Chloromas or extramedullary collections of leukemia cells, historically referred to as *granulocytic sarcomas,* may be associated with expression by leukemic blasts of CD56, which is a neural

Table 61–12 Studies with Arsenic Trioxide in Relapsed and Refractory Acute Promyelocytic Leukemia

Patients Achieving Complete After One Course of Arsenic Trioxide Therapy

Study	N	CR Rate (%)	Comments
Zhang[134]	42	22 (52)	73% of the 30 patients with previously untreated achieved CR with As_2O_3
Shen[136]	10	9 (90)	Duration of As_2O_3 treatment needed to obtain CR was between 28 and 44 days (median 38 days)
Niu[131]	47	30 (85.1)	31 patients were treated with As_2O_3 alone: CR rate 83.9% 11 patients with combination of As_2O_3 and chemotherapy; CR rate 81.8% 5 patients with As_2O_3 and ATRA: CR rate 100.0%
Soignet[130]	12	11 (92)	8 of 11 patients in CR also tested negative molecularly by RT-PCR for the PML-RARA transcript
Soignet[132]	40	34 (85)	Using a 10^{-4} sensitivity level, 78% of patients exhibited molecular conversion form positive to negative by RT-PCR for the PML-RARA transcript
Kwong[314]	8	8 (100)	All patients achieved morphologic but not molecular remission after As_2O_3 treatment, but all patients attained molecular remission after subsequent idarubicin treatment

As_2O_3, arsenic tetroxide; ATRA, all-*trans* retinoic acid; CR, complete remission; PML-RARA, promyelocytic leukemia-retinoic acid receptor α; RT-PCR, reverse transcriptase polymerase chain reaction.

Table 61–13 Clinical, Biologic, and Molecular Characteristics of Acute Myeloid Leukemia with t(8;21)

Clinical Features

- Younger median age at onset
- 20% of adult and 40% of pediatric M2
- EMD
- Favorable prognosis

Biologic Features

- Most common cytogenetic abnormality associated with EMD
- EMD may have poor prognosis
- Expression of AML1-ETO fusion protein
- Leukocytosis may have poor prognosis
- Loss of sex chromosome common and may have poor prognosis
- EMD associated with CD56 expression

Molecular Features

- AML1 activates transcription
- ETO binds corepressor–HDAC complex
- HDAC removes hydrophobic acetyl groups from histones, suppressing transcription of AML1 target promoters
- AML1-ETO represses transcription

AML, acute myeloid leukemia; EMD, extramedullary disease; HDAC, High-dose Ara-C.

Table 61–14 Core-Binding Factor Leukemias

Translocation	Genes Involved
t(8;21)	AML1-ETO
t(3;21)	AML1-EAP, MDS1, EVI1
t(12;21)	TEL (ETV6)
inv(16) t(16;16)	CBFβ-MYH11

Current Treatment Recommendations for Adults with Core-Binding Factor Leukemias

- Induction therapy includes an anthracycline and cytarabine.
- Consolidation chemotherapy includes three to four courses of intensive chemotherapy.
- One effective regimen is high-dose cytarabine at a dose of 3 g/m², given twice daily over 1 hour for 4 to 6 days.
- The dose of cytarabine can be reduced to 1.5 g/m² twice daily for older adults ages 55 to 70 years.
- Patients older than 70 years can receive cytarabine at a dose of 1.5 g/m²/day for 6 days.
- There is little role for allogeneic hematopoietic stem cell transplantation in first complete remission given the associated toxicity with the procedure.
- Autologous hematopoietic stem cell transplantation often used as postremission consolidation.
- The presence of extramedullary disease indicates a poorer prognosis and warrants more intensive therapy.

crest adhesion molecule that plays a role in trafficking of leukemic cells.[155,156] Insights into our understanding of the molecular features of leukemogenesis in patients with t(8;21) serve as a foundation for studying both leukemogenesis and chemotherapy resistance (see box on Current Treatment Recommendations for Adults with Core-Binding Factor Leukemias).

Molecular Features of t(8;21) and inv(16) or t(16;16)

The balanced reciprocal translocation between chromosomes 8 and 21 is the most common balanced translocation in de novo AML and is associated with fusion of the AML1 and ETO genes. AML with t(8;21), together with inv(16) or t(16;16), and t(12;21) also are classified as CBF leukemias (Table 61–14). The AML1 gene (also called $CBFA_2$) encodes the DNA-binding component of CBF-β, one subunit of a CBF complex that binds to DNA sequences and activates transcription of a number of genes important in hematopoiesis, including myeloperoxidase, the colony-stimulating factor (CSF)-α receptor, subsets of the T-cell antigen receptor, neutrophil elastase, interleukin-3, and granulocyte-macrophage colony-stimulating factor (GM-CSF), through recruitment of coactivators. Expression of AML1/CBF-β also may contribute to transcriptional repression and plays a major role in control of normal hematopoiesis. The normal function of the ETO gene remains elusive, but the gene is expressed as a nuclear phosphoprotein in brain tissue and in $CD34^+$ hematopoietic progenitor cells. The structure of ETO, as a nuclear zinc-finger-containing protein, implicates its role as a regulator of transcription. ETO can bind nuclear corepressor N-COR and Sin33A, which binds histone deacetylase. These observations suggest that in healthy cells, ETO functions as an adaptor protein within the nuclear corepressor complex to stabilize the interaction of these corepressor proteins. Therefore, the chimeric fusion protein AML1/ETO appears to repress transcription of genes normally activated by AML1/CBF-β. AML1/ETO inhibits CEBPA–dependent activation of the myeloid-specific NP-3 promoter and blocks granulocyte (G)-

Table 61–15 Complete Remission Duration by Cytogenetic Group According to Cytarabine Dose Randomization

Cytogenetic Group	Cytarabine Dose	No. of Patients	Median Time of CR (months)	5-Year CR (%)
Core-binding factor	3 g/m²	18	NR	78
	400 mg/m²	20	NR	57
	100 mg/m²	19	14.3	16
Normal	3 g/m²	45	18.2	40
	400 mg/m²	48	21.4	37
	100 mg/m²	47	12.5	20
Other	3 g/m²	27	13.3	21
	400 mg/m²	31	10.6	13
	100 mg/m²	30	9.6	13

CR, complete remission; NR, No response.

Data from Bloomfield CD, Lawrence D, Byrd JC et al. Frequency of prolonged remission duration after high-dose cytarabine intensification in acute myeloid leukemia varies by cytogenetic subtype. Cancer Res 1998;58:4173–4179.49.

CSF–induced differentiation of myeloid progenitors and thereby contributes to leukemogenesis.[157]

As a result of the 8,21 translocation, AML fuses to ETO, not normally expressed by hematopoietic cells. Patients with CBF leukemias with alteration of either the AML1 or CBF gene, such as patients with AML M4Eo involving either inv(16)(p13;q22) or t(16;16)(p13;q22) and a fusion between MYH11 and CBF-β genes, have demonstrated a more favorable prognosis than patients with either normal or more complex karyotypic abnormalities when given repetitive cycles of intensive consolidation with high doses of cytarabine (Table 61–15).[158–160]

AML with Unfavorable Cytogenetics

Patients with unfavorable cytogenetics constitute approximately 30% of patients with previously untreated de novo AML.[48] The proportion of patients with an unfavorable karyotype increases with age.[161] Patients with unfavorable karyotypes have a poor prognosis. The definition of unfavorable karyotypes as defined by SWOG/ECOG includes −5 or deletion 5q, −7 or deletion 7q, t(6;9), t(9;22), abn3q, 11q, 20q, 17p, or 11q23 abnormalities and patients with complex karyotypes, which include three or more clonal cytogenetic abnormalities (see Table 61–1).[48] Some differences in cytogenetic classifications exist among various cooperative oncology groups. The MRC defines complex karyotype as ≥ 5 clonal abnormalities.[47] In addition, in this classification, del(7q) and del(9q) as well as 11q23 abnormalities are classified as intermediate risk. In the series by the CALGB, the outcome for patients with complex karyotypes as defined by ≥ 3 abnormalities fared slightly better than those with ≥ 5 abnormalities.[59] In the MRC series, the presence of an unfavorable karyotype constituted a heterogeneous group of patients with respect to outcome.[47] For example, patients with −5 had OS of 21% at 5 years compared to patients with a complex karyotype who had OS of only 4% at 5 years. The presence of an additional cytogenetic abnormality, even if complex, does not appear to have an unfavorable influence on outcome among patients with favorable cytogenetics.[59,162,163] Patients with unfavorable cytogenetic abnormalities have a poor probability of continuous complete CR.[47,48] Such patients appear to fare poorly with intensive chemotherapy or with MSD allo-HSCT. However, the U.S. Intergroup trial, the EORTC/GIMEMA AML-10 trial, and one small single institution study suggest that patients with unfavorable cytogenetic abnormalities may benefit from HLA-identical sibling HSCT.[48,50,164] The graft-versus-leukemia effect associated with MUD HSCT may be potent enough to overcome the otherwise poor prognosis associated with unfavorable cytogenetics.[165] Isolated trisomies of chromosomes 8, 11, 13, and 21 also have been shown to have adverse prognostic implications in adults with previously untreated AML.[166,167] However, SWOG found that the outcome of patients with sole trisomy 8 was similar to patients with an abnormal karyotype.[168] Patients with trisomy 8 and an associated favorable cytogenetic abnormality appear to have an outcome similar to that of patients with favorable cytogenetics.[167,168] Therefore, the prognosis of patients with trisomy 8 depends to a large extent on whether this abnormality occurs alone or in association with other cytogenetic abnormalities. The presence of unfavorable cytogenetic abnormalities also has prognostic importance in patients with therapy-related AML.[162,171] Expression of CD56, the neural crest adhesion molecule, has been associated with unfavorable cytogenetics abnormalities.[172]

Table 61–16 Therapy-Related Leukemia Versus De Novo AML by Cytogenetics Analysis

	Favorable	Intermediate	Unfavorable
De Novo AML			
n	363	996	134
3-year relapse risk	32%	47%	78%
3-year survival	68%	46%	17%
Therapy-Related Leukemia			
n	14	76	29
3-year relapse risk	19%	62%	67%
3-year survival	79%	25%	14%

AML, acute myeloid leukemia.

Data from Grimwade D, Walker H, Oliver F et al: The importance of diagnostic cytogenetics on outcome in AML: Analysis of 1,612 patients entered into the MRC AML 10 trial. The Medical Research Council Adult and Children's Leukaemia Working Parties. Blood 92:2322, 1998.

Therapy-Related AML

Therapy-related AML is the most serious long-term complication of therapy for cancer. Almost all malignancies treated with cancer chemotherapy have been associated with development of AML. The optimal therapy for therapy-related leukemia continues to be debated.

The overall incidence of therapy-related leukemia in adults ranges between 5% and 10% of all patients with AML, although differences in the reported incidence likely are affected by the chosen definition of therapy-related leukemia. In essence, the ultimate prognosis of patients with true therapy-related leukemia is dependent on the cytogenetic and molecular prognostic factors at diagnosis, much like de novo AML (Table 61–16).[47] The definition of therapy-related leukemia in published series has been far broader, making comparisons and interpretation of appropriate therapies more difficult. The largest published series of therapy-related myelodysplasia or AML included

Table 61–17 Cytogenetic Abnormalities in 306 Patients with T-MDS/T-AML

Karyotype	No. (%)
Normal karyotype	24 (8)
Clonal abnormalities	282 (92)
Clonal abnormalities of chromosome 5, 7, or both	
(±other abnormalities)	214 (70)
Abnormal chromosome 5[a]	63 (21)
Abnormal chromosome 7[a]	85 (28)
Abnormal chromosomes 5 and 7	66 (22)
Recurring balanced rearrangements	31 (10)
t(11q23)	10 (3.3)
t(21q22)[a]	8 (2.6)
t(15;17)	6 (2.0)
inv(16)[a]	6 (2.0)
t(8;16)	1 (0.3)
Other clonal abnormalities	39 (13)[b]

[a]One patient with an abnormality of chromosome 5 and t(3;21) and one patient with an abnormality of chromosome 7 and inv(16) are listed twice in the table.

[b]Includes eight patients with +8, three patients with −13/del(13q), and one patient each with del(20q), del(11q), +11, +21, or −Y.

T-AML, therapy-related acute myeloid leukemia; T-MDS, therapy-related myelodysplasia.

Data from Smith SM, Le Beau MM, Huo D et al: Clinical-cytogenetic associations in 306 patients with therapy-related myelodysplasia and myeloid leukemia: The University of Chicago series. Blood 102:43, 2003.

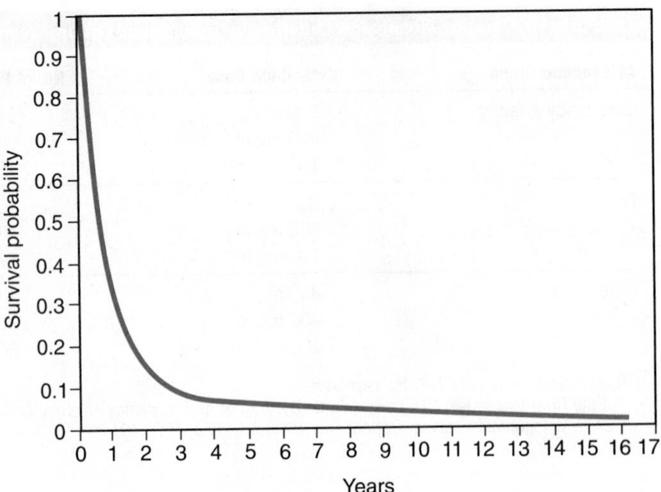

Figure 61–14 Overall survival from diagnosis of therapy-related myelodysplasia/therapy-related acute myeloid leukemia in 306 patients. *(Data from Smith SM, Le Beau MM, Huo D, et al: Clinical-cytogenetic associations in 306 patients with therapy-related myelodysplasia and myeloid leukemia: The University of Chicago series. Blood 102:43, 2003.[173])*

306 patients reported from the University of Chicago.[173] Ninety-two percent of patients had cytogenetic abnormalities, the most frequent being abnormalities of chromosome 5 and 7 (Table 61–17). The OS of such patients remains dismal and is very similar to that of AML patients with unfavorable cytogenetics at presentation (Figs. 61–14 and 61–15). The two types of drugs most commonly associated with therapy-related leukemia are the alkylating agents and topoisomerase II inhibitors. Since the initial report of the association of therapy with melphalan and the development of AML,[174] virtually all the alkylating agents have been implicated (Table 61–18).[175] Similarly, since the earliest report implicating the epipodophyllotoxins in the genesis of leukemia, many other inhibitors of topoisomerase II, such as the anthracyclines, mitoxantrone, and the dioxopiperazine derivatives razoxane and bimolane, all have been associated with development of secondary AML (Table 61–18).

Definition

One of the major obstacles to progress in the treatment of therapy-related leukemia has been the variable definitions, as outlined in Table 61–19. It is clear that in the treatment of any AML, "patient issues" must be considered. Thus, any patient who had a prior malignancy or previously had been exposed to chemotherapy or radiation may have additional comorbidities that may affect the ultimate outcome. However, from a biologic standpoint, it is desirable to define therapy-related leukemia as any AML that has specific cytogenetic or molecular markers, usually associated with a poor prognosis, which define leukemogenesis as a secondary rather than a primary event. In essence, there is little biologic difference between a patient who presents with a true therapy-related leukemia and a patient with de novo AML who presents with unfavorable cytogenetic abnormalities. Although many reports have emphasized the dismal overall prognosis of patients with therapy-related leukemia,[176] the optimal

Table 61–18 Diseases and Drugs with a Reported Risk of Treatment-Related Myelodysplasia or Acute Myeloid Leukemia

Hematologic neoplasias	Alkylating agents
Multiple myeloma	Melphalan
Hodgkin lymphoma	Mechlorethamine
Non-Hodgkin lymphomas	Cyclophosphamide
Polycythemia vera	Busulfan
Essential thrombocythemia	Dihydroxybusulfan
Acute lymphoblastic leukemia	Chlorambucil Carmustine
Solid tumors	Lomustine
Breast cancer	Semustine
Lung cancer	Dacarbazine
Testicular cancer	Cisplatin
Childhood tumors	Carboplatin
Nonmalignant diseases	Topoisomerase II inhibitor
Rheumatoid arthritis	Etoposide
Psoriasis	Teniposide
Wegener granulomatosis	Doxorubicin 4-epi-doxorubicin Daunorubicin Mitoxantrone Razoxane Bimolane

Data from Pedersen-Bjergaard J: Insights into leukemogenesis from therapy-related leukemia. N Engl J Med 352:1591, 2005.

treatment depends on biologic features, with the cytogenetic findings being most important. Patients with therapy-related leukemia who have a more favorable karyotype have a far better outcome than do patients with therapy-related leukemia who have an unfavorable karyotype (Fig. 61–16).[169,171] These data are consistent with older data that confirmed the favorable prognosis for patients with therapy-related leukemia who present with favorable cytogenetic abnormalities, such as t(8;21), inv(16), and t(8;18).[170,177] Whether patients with

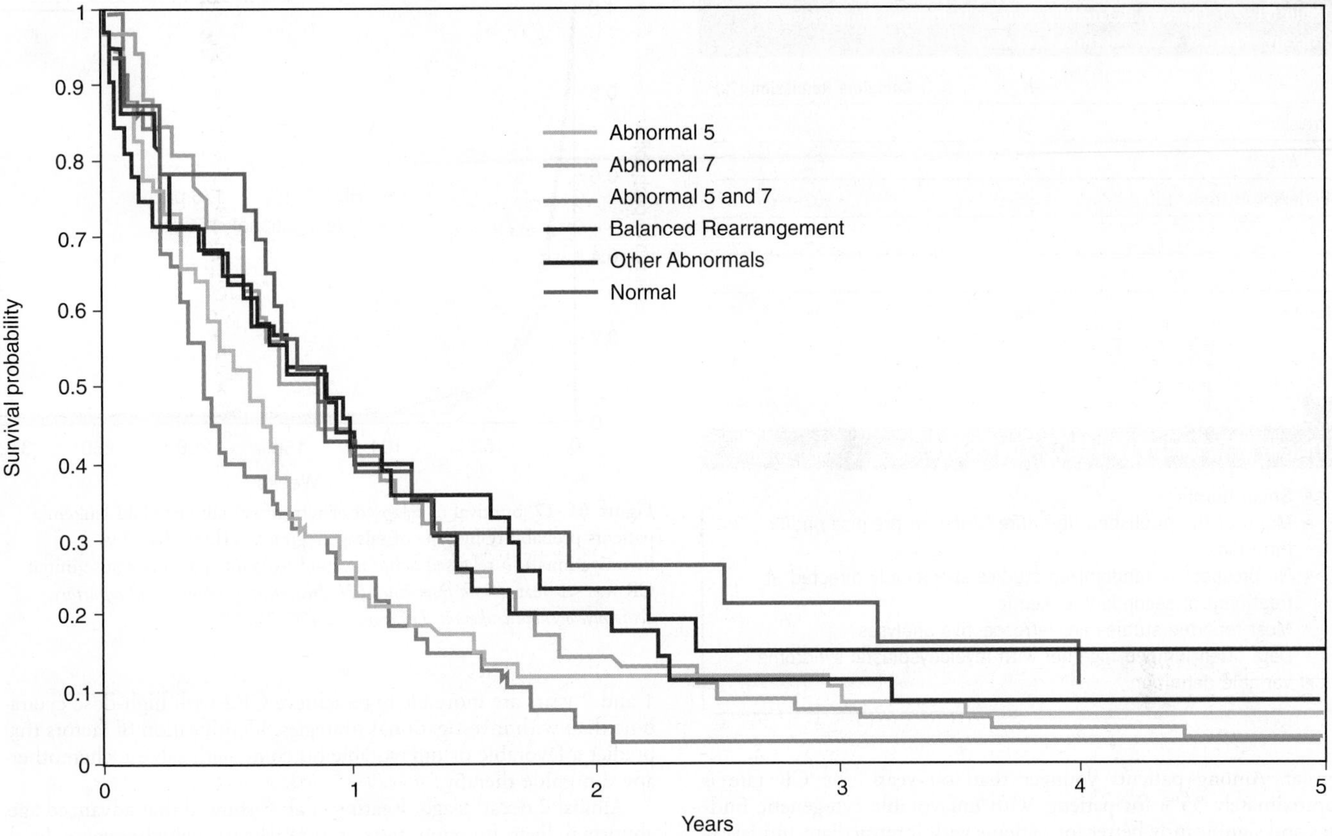

Figure 61–15 Survival of therapy-related myelodysplasia/therapy-related acute myeloid leukemia based on cytogenetic abnormalities. *(Data from Smith SM, Le Beau MM, Huo D, et al: Clinical-cytogenetic associations in 306 patients with therapy-related myelodysplasia and myeloid leukemia: The University of Chicago series. Blood 102:43, 2003.*[173]*)*

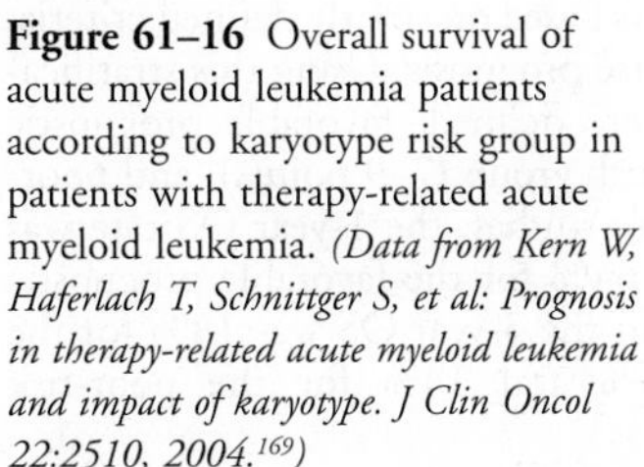

Figure 61–16 Overall survival of acute myeloid leukemia patients according to karyotype risk group in patients with therapy-related acute myeloid leukemia. *(Data from Kern W, Haferlach T, Schnittger S, et al: Prognosis in therapy-related acute myeloid leukemia and impact of karyotype. J Clin Oncol 22:2510, 2004.*[169]*)*

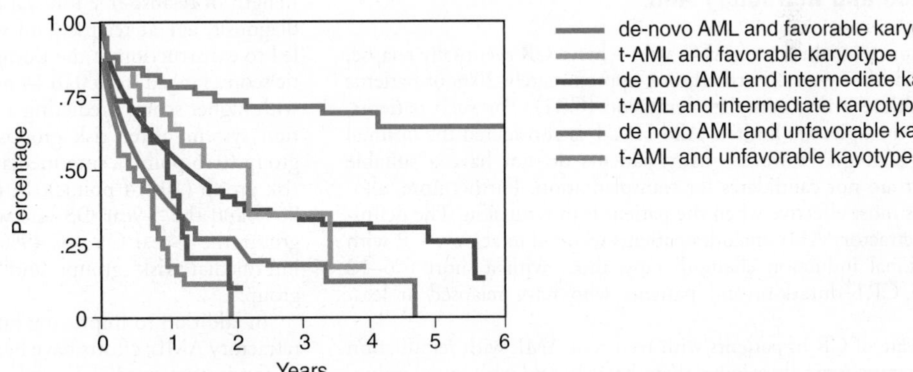

Table 61–19 Therapy-Related Leukemia: Possible Definitions

- Any leukemia with a history of prior malignancy
- Any leukemia with a history of prior exposure to chemotherapy or radiation ("therapy-related leukemia")
- Any MDS with above
- AML that evolved from MDS
- AML or MDS with specific cytogenetic or molecular markers—usually associated with a poor prognosis—that define the leukemogenesis as a secondary rather than a primary event

AML, acute myeloid leukemia; MDS, myelodysplasia.

secondary leukemia have a poor prognosis independent of their cytogenetic findings continues to be debated (see box on Therapy of Secondary Leukemia—The Problem). In 2002 the MRC reported an apparently independent poor prognosis for patients with therapy-related leukemia.[178]

Induction and Postremission Therapy

Multiple induction regimens have been proposed for treatment of therapy-related leukemia (Table 61–20). Not surprisingly, the CR rate is best in the smallest studies and worsens as the studies accrue larger numbers of patients.

No evidence indicates that any form of therapy is more optimal than standard induction therapy using the classic 3 + 7 regimen or

Table 61–20 Therapy-Related Leukemia: Induction Therapy for Therapy-Related Acute Myeloid Leukemia

	N	Complete Remission (%)
Preisler[315]	11	73
De Witte[316]	22	62
Pederson-Bjergaard[317]	36	62
Hoyle[318]	66	36
Kantarjian[319]	72	29
Kantarjian[177]	148	34

Therapy of Secondary Leukemia—The Problem

- Small numbers
- Much of the published literature based on premise and/or intuition
- No prospective randomized studies specifically directed at treatment of secondary leukemia
- Most reported studies are retrospective analyses
- Data often lumped together with myelodysplastic syndrome
- Variable definition

similar. Among patients younger than 60 years, the CR rate is approximately 55% for patients with unfavorable cytogenetic findings and significantly better for patients with intermediate and favorable cytogenetic findings. Thus, the overall direction when treating such a patient should be based on the prognostic indicators and the patient's overall performance status rather than the history.

Relapsed and Refractory AML

The majority of adults with AML who achieve CR eventually relapse, usually within 2 years. Furthermore, approximately 20% of patients never achieve a first complete remission (CR1). For such patients, effective therapies are limited. Allo-HSCT is considered the optimal curative strategy. However, many patients do not have a suitable donor or are not candidates for transplantation. Furthermore, allo-HSCT is most effective when the patient is in remission. The definition of refractory AML includes patients who fail to achieve CR with conventional induction chemotherapy, those with a short (<6–12 months) CR1 duration, and patients who have relapsed at least twice.[179]

The rate of CR in patients with recurrent AML with reinduction chemotherapy typically is lower than that achieved with initial induction therapy, and most patients have a shorter duration of second complete remission (CR2) compared to CR1.[180] If CR2 is achieved, the median duration of remission and DFS are generally short (<12 months). In addition, reinduction therapy often is associated with substantial treatment-related morbidity and mortality. These patients are candidates for clinical trials exploring innovative therapeutic strategies. There is no lack of new agents to explore.

Prognostic Factors in Patients with Relapsed or Refractory AML

With the exception of patients with APL, the prognosis for the majority of adults with relapsed or refractory AML with CR1 duration less than 12 months is poor whether treatment includes conventional cytotoxic chemotherapy such as high-dose cytarabine or investigational agents (Fig. 61–17).[181] Patients whose CR1 duration is between

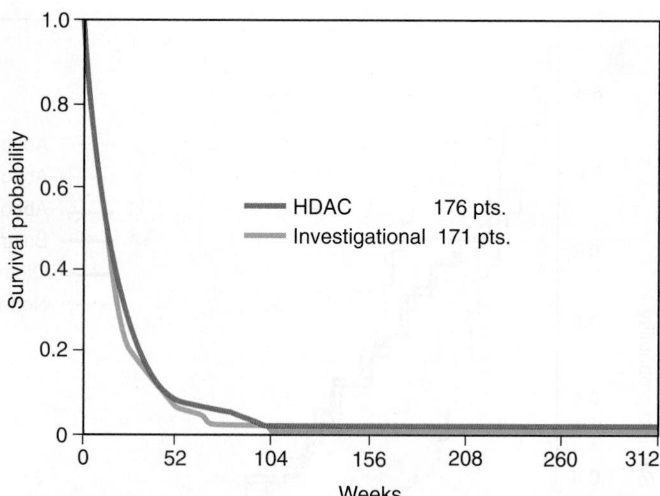

Figure 61–17 Survival of relapsed or refractory acute myeloid leukemia patients probability by type of salvage regimen (HDAC-based vs investigational) in relapsed acute myeloid leukemia patients whose initial CR was <1 year. *(Data from Estey EH: Treatment of relapsed and refractory acute myelogenous leukemia. Leukemia 14:476, 2000.[181])*

1 and 2 years are more likely to achieve CR2 with high-dose cytarabine than with investigational strategies. Identification of factors that predict a favorable or unfavorable outcome with salvage chemotherapy can guide therapy.

Almost 2 decades ago, Keating et al.[182] showed that advanced age, abnormal liver function tests, serum lactate dehydrogenase level, marrow karyotype, proportion of blasts plus promyelocytes, and shorter (<1 year) CR1 duration were significantly associated with response to therapy and survival after salvage chemotherapy. Two studies that reported the outcome of approximately 1200 younger patients with AML in first relapse based on four clinical parameters (length of relapse-free interval after first CR, cytogenetic findings at diagnosis, age at relapse, and whether HSCT had been performed) led to construction of the European Prognostic Index.[183,184] Prognostic scores ranged from 0 to 14 points based on strictly defined criteria, with higher scores predicting a worse prognosis. Using this stratification system, three risk groups were defined: favorable prognostic group (0–6 points), intermediate-risk group (7–9 points), and poor-risk group (10–14 points). In these studies, the 1-year OS rate was 70% and the 5-year OS rate was 64% for the favorable prognostic group, the 1-year OS was 49% and the 3-year OS was 18% for the intermediate-risk group, and 16% and 14% for the poor-risk group.

In addition to improving outcomes in patients with relapsed and refractory AML, efforts have been undertaken to identify quantitative methods that predict for relapse in patients who are in apparent morphologic CR. For example, a persistently abnormal karyotypic abnormality in patients in apparent CR by morphologic criteria predicts for relapse.[185]

Age

The CR rate with conventional cytotoxic salvage chemotherapy of patients who relapse during their first CR is inversely related to age (Table 61–21).[179,182,186–188] In a retrospective study by Rees et al.[188] that included a large number of patients in each age subgroup, the CR2 rate among 375 patients was 33% for younger patients compared to 19% among older patients.

Duration of CR1

The most important predictor of achieving CR2 with salvage chemotherapy appears to be the duration of CR1.[179,188,189–192] Patients with relapsed AML usually are categorized into one of two groups: those

Table 61–21 Impact of Age on Achieving a Second Complete Response Among Patients with Relapsed and Refractory Acute Myeloid Leukemia

	Age <60 Years		Age >60 Years	
Study	***CR2/Total Patients***	***CR2 (%)***	***CR2/Total Patients***	***CR2 (%)***
Rees[188]	124/375	33	21/110	19
Keating[181]	75/208	36	5/35	14
Hiddemann[179]	56/104	54	14/32	44
Kern[187]	67/138	49	21/48	44
Sternberg[186]	10/22	45	19/25	76

CR, complete remission.

Table 61–22 Impact of Duration of Initial Complete on Achieving a Second Complete Response Following Relapse Remission of Acute Myeloid Leukemia

	CR <1 Year		CR >1 Year	
Study	***CR2/Total Patients***	***CR2 (%)***	***CR2/Total Patients***	***CR2 (%)***
Rees[188]	32/251	13	113/234	48
Keating[181]	20/105	19	51/82	62
Hiddemann[179]	40/87	46	29/49	60
Estey[190]	6/24	25	9/10	90
Thalhammer[191]	40/121	33	26/47	55

CR, complete remission.

Table 61–23 Impact of Diagnostic Cytogenetics on Second Complete Response Rate and Survival in Patients with First Relapse Acute Myeloid Leukemia

	Weltermann[196]		Kern[197]		Wheatley[194]
Risk Group	***CR Rate (%)***	***3-Year Survival (%)***	***CR Rate (%)***	***CR Rate (%)***	**5-Year Survival (%)**
Good	88	43	80	90	72
Intermediate	64	18	49	54	43
Poor	36	0	30	45	17

Good risk: Presence of t(15;17), t(8;21) or inv (16).
Intermediate risk: Presence of a normal karyotype or cytogenetic abnormalities not included in favorable or poor-risk groups.
Poor risk: Presence of a complex karyotype or abnormalities of chromosome 3, 5, or 7.
CR, complete remission.

with CR1 greater than 1 year or those with CR1 less than 1 year (Table 61–22).

Cytogenetic Abnormalities

Pretreatment cytogenetic abnormalities have important prognostic implications in patients with relapsed and refractory AML.[193–196] Kantarjian et al.[193] reported that a favorable karyotype was more frequent in patients whose first CR persisted for least 12 months, whereas the opposite was found in patients with an unfavorable karyotype. Other investigators have provided similar observations concerning the prognostic significance of pretreatment cytogenetic findings in patients with relapsed and refractory AML (Table 61–23).[194–196] Kern et al.[195] reported that unfavorable cytogenetic findings were associated with a lower rate of achieving a second CR and were a poor prognostic factor with regard to survival following first relapse. Kern et al.[197] suggested that cytogenetic findings at relapse tend to be predictive of outcome more strongly than cytogenetic finding at diagnosis. However, Estey et al.[198] found that a change in the cytogenetic pattern at first relapse did not influence the prognosis of therapy after first relapse in the majority of patients.

Treatment of Patients with Relapsed or Refractory AML

Conventional Cytotoxic Chemotherapy

Many salvage chemotherapy regimens have been studied in patients with relapsed or refractory AML, with modest success. No standard chemotherapy regimen provides a durable second or greater CR. One of the most active agents is high-dose cytarabine. Doses range from 500 mg/m^2 to 3 g/m^2 every 12 hours for up to 6 days, given either alone or in combination with other active agents including anthracyclines, asparaginase, etoposide, mitoxantrone, or amsacrine.[199–206] In general, CR rates in the range from 30% to 65% have been observed, with associated reinduction mortality rates of 12% to 25%. Whether the higher doses of cytarabine are more effective is not clear.

The German AML Cooperative Group trial compared cytarabine 3 g/m² with 1 g/m² administered twice daily on days 1, 2, 7, and 8 given with mitoxantrone in patients younger than 60 years. No substantial difference in CR rate (approximately 47%) was noted.[187] Therefore, although dose-intense cytarabine is viewed as an essential component of many conventional salvage programs, dose escalation to 3 g/m² may not be justified in many patients given the increased toxicity. It is desirable to select a salvage chemotherapy regimen with minimal toxicity because many suitable patients subsequently are offered HSCT.

Similarly, there is no definitive proof that additional agents given with intermediate- or high-dose ara-C improves OS. A large randomized trial conducted by SWOG did not show a benefit in OS with the addition of mitoxantrone to HiDAC every 12 hours for a total of 6 days.[204] Similarly, in a study of etoposide combined with HiDAC, a CR rate of 45% was observed compared to a CR rate of 40% with HiDAC.[206] Novel regimens with cytotoxic chemotherapy or other agents, including mitoxantrone plus etoposide, or purine analogues, have been explored, but there is no evidence that they represent an improvement over intermediate- or high-dose cytarabine-based regimens.[189,209–213]

Novel Agents Combined with Conventional Cytotoxic Chemotherapy

Several novel therapies have been combined with conventional chemotherapy in an effort to improve outcome (Table 61–24). These include targeted therapies, many of which are small molecules directed toward specific genetic abnormalities. Therapies to promote intracellular drug retention by inhibiting the efflux pump P-glycoprotein, a product of the multidrug resistance (MDR)-1 gene, have a particularly compelling rationale based on in vitro observations. Cyclosporine[208,214] and its analogue PSC-833 have been studied, but their use has not been associated with improved outcomes compared to conventional chemotherapy.[215,216] Other novel inhibitors, such as zosuquidar, which has pharmacokinetic properties such that concomitant chemotherapy need not be reduced as with other MDR inhibitors, also have not been associated with better outcomes.[217] Despite strong preclinical data, trials using MDR inhibitors alone or in combination with chemotherapy and gemtuzumab ozogamicin[218,219] have shown variable and generally disappointing results. A phase III trial conducted by the SWOG demonstrated significant improvement in relapse-free-survival and OS when cyclosporine was combined with daunorubicin and high-dose cytarabine,[208] but these results were not validated by other studies using a similar strategy.[214]

Allogeneic HSCT in Relapsed AML

Allo-HSCT remains the only known curative treatment of relapsed or refractory AML. However, only a minority of patients are candidates for this approach. Gale et al.[220] demonstrated significantly better leukemia-free-survival withMSD HSCT compared to chemotherapy in adults 30 years or younger and CR1 longer than 1 year (41% vs 17%; $P = 0.017$) or adults older than 30 years and CR1 shorter than 1 year (18% vs 7%). Three-year probabilities of treatment-related mortality with chemotherapy and HSCT were 7% versus 56%, respectively. It is reasonable to consider HSCT in early first relapse in young (age <60 years) adults if a suitable MSD is readily available. Clift et al.[221] demonstrated a 5-year DFS of 28% and a cure rate of 25% to 30% among 126 patients transplanted for AML in first untreated relapse. These results are comparable when MSD HSCT is carried out in CR2.[222] Reiffers et al.[223] demonstrated a 3-year DFS of 35% among 459 patients. Moreover, approximately 50% of patients in first relapse successfully achieved CR2, and 15% to 20% died during reinduction chemotherapy.

A routine strategy is reinduction with salvage chemotherapy to achieve CR2 followed by HSCT. There is no standard chemotherapy

Table 61–24 Studies with Novel Cytotoxic Drugs for Treatment of Relapsed/Refractory Acute Myeloid Leukemia

Agent	Class	Mechanism of Action	Comments
Clofarabine	Nucleoside analogue	Inhibits RNR	Phase II trials in combination with Ara-C, particularly in elderly underway[249,250]
Gemtuzumab ozogamicin	Immunoconjugates	Antitumor Antibiotic Calicheamicin	Odds ratio 30% in older adults in late first relapse[252–256]
Troxacitabine	Nucleoside analogue	Inhibits RNR	Odds ratio 18% in refractory acute myeloid leukemia; combination studies show antileukemia activity; causes hand–foot syndrome[250,251]
Cloretazine	Alkylating agent	DNA damage	Phase III trials underway evaluating chemotherapy ± cloretazine[260,261]
FLT-3 inhibitor	Small molecule inhibitor	Inhibits tyrosine kinase	Reduction in blasts in blood and marrow, but rare CR; in phase III trials evaluating chemotherapy ± inhibitor[39]
SU5416	Small molecule inhibitor	Inhibits vascular endothelial growth factor receptor	Modest clinical efficacy as a single agent[263]
Farnesyltransferase	Nonpeptidometric enzyme-specific linked inhibitor	Inhibits farnesyl protein transferase	Modest clinical activity but with few CR[264]; phase III trial in older adults in CR1 or any patient in CR2 after consolidation as maintenance underway
Oblimersen	Antisense	Inhibits bcl-2	Can be combined with chemotherapy[266]
Decitabine	Nucleoside analogue hypomethylating agent	Removes methyl groups from certain genes	Includes CR[267]

Ara-C, cytosine arabinoside; CR, complete remission; RNR, ribonucleotide reductase; FLT-3, fms-like tyrosine kinase 3.

regimen for this clinical setting. The selection of one regimen over the other is often based on CR1 duration and patient age. The FLAG ± idarubicin regimen (fludarabine, ara-C, G-CSF) had been used for cytoreduction, followed by either matched sibling or MUD HSCT, with some success.[224] Promising results have been reported with either autologous HSCT or allo-HSCT using a preparative regimen that includes increased radiation dose delivered by ^{131}I-labeled anti-CD45 antibody.[225,226] The role of autologous HSCT in younger patients with CR1 greater than 1 year is unclear because no randomized trials have compared this approach with MUD HSCT.

Interpretation of data comparing HSCT and chemotherapy as consolidation therapy is difficult. Differing results likely are attributable in part to patient selection and difficulties in defining duration of response in the chemotherapy arms because most patients proceed to other therapies, including HSCT.

Relapse After Transplantation

The best approach for patients relapsing after allo-HSCT is controversial. Without further therapy, their median survival is approximately 3 to 4 months. Options such as immunotherapy, donor lymphocyte infusion (DLI), or a second allo-HSCT after myeloablative conditioning have been studied but have limited effectiveness. Choi et al.[227] treated 16 patients who relapsed after allogeneic HSCT with cytoreductive chemotherapy followed immediately by G-CSF–primed DLI. Ten of the 16 patients achieved CR; four of the patients remained in CR at the time of publication. OS at 2 years was 31%. Duration of CR after HSCT (>6 months or <6 months) was the only significant prognostic factor for OS. All five patients who relapsed after chemotherapy followed by DLI strategy did so in extramedullary sites, as has been observed by other investigators.[228] Response rates to DLI for relapsed AML range from 15% to 30%. However, CR rates are durable only in a minority of patients.[229] Associated toxicities of DLI include acute graft-versus-host disease (>grade II in 30%), with treatment-related mortality rates estimated to be up to 20%. In young patients refractory to DLI or among those with longer CR duration after allo-HSCT, a second allo-HSCT should be considered.[230] However, both relapse and mortality rates associated with second transplants are high (42% and 30%, respectively) in the series from the CIBMTR,[231] and reduced-intensity conditioning transplantation frequently is required. Further investigation and development of new approaches for patients in this clinical setting to maximize the graft-versus-leukemia effect and to minimize graft-versus-host disease and toxicity are underway. Umbilical cord blood stem cells are another source of stem cells for transplantation for patients who lack a suitable MSD or MUD.[232,233] To increase the graft cell dose present in a single umbilical cord unit, double cord unit transplantations have been evaluated, with limited success.[234] None of these transplant approaches from alternative donor stem cell sources can be considered standard of care and remain investigational.

Refractory AML

Allo-HSCT offers the best chance for achieving sustained CR in patients with primary refractory AML. The outcome appears to be better among patients without peripheral blood blasts and with bone marrow containing less than 30% blasts prior to conditioning for transplant.[235] Forman et al.[236] reported a cumulative probability of DFS of 43% at 10 years in 21 young (age <41 years) AML (n = 16) and ALL (n = 5) patients after MSD HSCT. Biggs et al.[237] described 88 AML patients (age <52 years) who were refractory to at least two courses of cytotoxic chemotherapy and subsequently proceeded to MSD HSCT. The 3-year probability of leukemia-free survival in these patients was 21% (14%–31%), with 3-year treatment-related mortality rate of 44%. Cook et al.[238] showed that allo-HSCT can cure a small proportion of patients refractory to induction chemotherapy. On the other hand, relapsed patients who are refractory to reinduction have a dismal prognosis. Nevertheless, it is reasonable to offer some form of allo-HSCT if the patient has not undergone this procedure during CR1.

Similar to MUD HSCT, use of partially mismatched related donors expands the population of patients who potentially can benefit from allo-HSCT for primary refractory AML. This strategy is a reasonable alternative in patients with no MSD available and may result in a similar outcome.[239] In a retrospective trial by Singhal et al.,[240] the outcome of 24 MSD (median age 24 years) and 19 partially HLA-mismatched related donor (PMRD; median age 34 years; P = 0.04) allo-HSCT recipients with primary refractory AML and other hematologic malignancies were compared. All PMRD patients and 90% of the MSD patients achieved CR2. The advantage of PMRD transplantation over MUD HSCT is the rapid availability of the donor, a factor that is of critical importance in patients with refractory progressive acute leukemia. Haploidentical stem cell transplantation is another alternative strategy that has met with considerable success.[56,241,242] The emerging data suggest that this form of transplant may have some efficacy for AML.[213a]

Autologous HSCT

The exact role of autologous HSCT in younger patients with relapsed AML without an HLA matched donor for allo-HSCT is not established. Without randomized studies, the data are unclear and demonstrate variable results. The EBMT registry data show DFS probabilities in the range from 30% to 35% for patients undergoing autologous HSCT in CR2.[243,244] These numbers clearly are better than those reported in prospective nonregistry studies. When compared with chemotherapy, autologous HSCT has not been shown to lead to a statistically significant improved survival for patients in CR2.[245] Moreover, for the majority of AML patients who receive autologous HSCT in CR1 and relapse, a second autologous HSCT rarely is feasible. Data from the EBMT registry show that only 56 (3.5%) of 1579 AML patients who relapsed after an autologous HSCT in CR1 have been treated with a second autologous HSCT.[246]

An analysis by Lazarus et al.[247] for the CBMTR showed superior outcomes with autologous HSCT (n = 668) compared with MUD HSCT (n = 476) in patients in CR1 (n = 692) and patients in CR2 (n = 452). Multiple confounding factors may have accounted for these results, including limitations in defining the degree of match between unrelated donor–recipient pairs, accrual of older patients, and inclusion of patients with adverse cytogenetic findings among patients undergoing MUD HSCT.

Investigational Agents in Relapsed and Refractory AML (Table 61–24)

New Purine Analogues

Clofarabine (2-chloro-2′β-fluoro-deoxy-9-β-D-arabinofuranosyladenine) is a newer second-generation purine adenosine nucleoside analogue with improved toxicity profile.[210] The drug is highly resistant to cleavage by bacterial purine nucleoside phosphorylase and is resistant to deamination by adenosine deaminase. Clofarabine acts by inhibiting ribonucleotide reductase and DNA polymerase, depleting the amount of intracellular dNTPs available for DNA replication, resulting in premature DNA chain termination. In a phase II trial of relapsed and refractory patients with AML and other hematologic malignancies, an overall response rate of 48% was achieved, including a CR rate of 32%.[248] In a subsequent phase I/II trial of relapsed and refractory leukemias, predominantly AML, clofarabine was combined with cytarabine in an effort to modulate cytarabine triphosphate accumulation.[249] The overall response rate was 38%, with a CR rate of 22%. Dose-limiting toxicities include reversible hepatotoxicity and rash but no neurotoxicity.

Several other important cytotoxic agents have been introduced. Phase I/II trials with these novel agents have demonstrated some therapeutic efficacy, and these agents currently are under further investigation in combination regimens (see Table 61–3). Troxacitabine is a novel L-nucleoside analogue with activity in refractory AML both as a single agent activity and combined with other cytotoxic agents.[250,251]

Gemtuzumab Ozogamicin

Gemtuzumab ozogamicin is an immunoconjugate of a humanized anti-CD33 monoclonal antibody chemically linked to the potent cytotoxic antitumor antibiotic calicheamicin.[252] The immunoconjugate is internalized into the leukemia cell expressing CD33, and the calicheamicin is freed intracellularly after the acid environment of the cell results in hydrolysis of the chemical linker.[253] A compilation of three phase II trials showed an overall response rate of approximately 26% (13% CR and 13% CRp among patients in first relapse who had a more favorable prognosis because they had a prolonged CR and did not have therapy-related AML or AML that had evolved from an antecedent hematologic disorder).[254]

These results led to the approval of this drug for use in older adults with AML in first relapse who were not candidates for intensive chemotherapy.[255] In a final analysis of 277 patients in first relapse treated with gemtuzumab ozogamicin, 26% achieved remission (13% CR and 13% CRp), with a median recurrence-free survival of 6.4 months for patients who achieved CR.[256] Data have shown that the results of gemtuzumab ozogamicin as monotherapy correlate with P-glycoprotein–mediated drug efflux.[257] Unique toxicities are hepatic venoocclusive disease and sinusoidal obstructive syndrome, which are rare (<1%), but the incidence is higher among patients who undergo allo-HSCT within 3.5 months of exposure to gemtuzumab ozogamicin.[258,259] Given the limited effectiveness of this agent as monotherapy, phase II studies exploring combinations of gemtuzumab ozogamicin with chemotherapy have been performed, with encouraging results. Therefore, gemtuzumab ozogamicin has been incorporated in ongoing randomized trials of untreated patients with AML evaluating its benefit when combined with induction chemotherapy and as an in vivo purging agent of grafts prior to autologous HSCT. Preliminary data from the MRC study using gemtuzumab ozogamicin in combination with standard induction chemotherapy were most encouraging.[37]

Novel Alkylating Agents

Cloretazine is a sulfonylhydrazine alkylating agent with modest activity in high-risk relapsed AML patients (CR1 duration <6 months) that may prove more effective when combined with other agents.[260,261]

Other Targeted Agents

Many other agents with novel mechanisms of action are being investigated in patients with relapsed or refractory AML (see Table 61–24).[262] They include FLT-3 inhibitors[39]; receptor tyrosine kinase inhibitors such as SU5416[263]; farnesyltransferase inhibitors, which interfere with Ras signaling[264,265]; agents that promote apoptosis, such as the bcl-2 antisense oligonucleotide, which downregulates bcl-2[266]; and methyltransferase inhibitors, such as decitabine, which induce hypomethylation of CpG-containing parts of the genome.[267] FLT-3 inhibitors such as CEP-701 have modest antileukemic activity as single agents, as demonstrated by reductions in peripheral blood and occasionally bone marrow blasts, but few, if any, patients achieve CR. Data suggest that combining these agents with cytotoxic chemotherapy may be useful.[268,269] Studies have explored the FLT-3 inhibitor PKC-412 combined with daunorubicin and ara-C in newly diagnosed patients. Ninety-one percent of patients with FLT-3 mutations achieved CR compared to 53% of patients without FLT-3 mutations. In a trial of CEP-701 (lestaurtinib) restricted to patients in first relapse, greater than 85% inhibition of FLT-3 occurred in 76% of patients. Decitabine is an exciting new hypomethylating agent with activity in patients with AML.[267]

Strategies to Detect Early Relapse in AML

Current remission criteria are inefficient in detecting residual leukemic cells, that is, minimal residual disease (MRD). More sensitive methods, such as cytogenetics, flow cytometry, and reverse transcriptase (RT)-PCR, are not routinely used. These methods, when combined with morphologic criteria for remission, may decrease the relapse rate and provide insight into the clinical efficacy of different therapeutic strategies and might improve overall prognostic stratification in AML patients. Marcucci et al.[276] retrospectively evaluated 118 AML patients with abnormal cytogenetic finding at diagnosis (n = 118). Patients who converted to normal cytogenetic findings at CR1 (NCR1; n = 103) were compared with those with abnormal cytogenetic findings at both diagnosis and CR1 (ACR1; n = 15). ACR1 patients had significantly shorter OS ($P = 0.006$) and DFS ($P = 0.0001$) and higher cumulative incidence of relapse ($P = 0.0001$). In multivariable models, the NCR1 and ACR groups were predictors for OS ($P = 0.03$), DFS ($P = 0.02$), and cumulative incidence of relapse ($P = 0.05$; Fig. 61–18). The relative risk of relapse or death was 2.1 times higher for ACR patients than for NCR patients (95% confidence interval 1.1–3.9). Notably, there was no significant difference in time of attaining CR1 between the NCR and ACR groups. At 3 years, all patients in the ACR1 group had relapsed compared to 61% in the NCR1 group.

The ability of immunophenotyping to identify a leukemia-associated phenotype has significantly increased the sensitivity of MRD detection in patients with AML. Buccisano et al.[270] used this technique to evaluate MRD at the end of induction and following consolidation in a total of 92 patients. The threshold discriminating MRD^- from MRD^+ cases was set at 3.5×10^{-4} residual leukemic cells. The results showed that the MRD status at the end of consolidation was the most significant predictor of outcome, with 5-year actuarial probability of relapse-free survival and OS at 5 years of 71% and 64%, respectively, for MRD^- patients compared to 13% and 16%, respectively, for MRD^+ patients. Interestingly, the majority of patients with MRD^+ status at the end of consolidation relapsed after autologous HSCT.

Controversy exists as to the prognostic significance of FMS-like receptor tyrosine kinase (FLT-3) mutations. Although the exact mechanism by which FLT-3 mutation leads to an increased relapse risk remains to be defined, it appears to relate to an increased proliferative potential caused by a cytokine-independent phenotype rather than resistance to conventional chemotherapy, making it another possible therapeutic target. Del Poeta et al.[271] suggested that the bax/bcl-2 ratio is a predictor of both OS and time to relapse. However, the value of this index in risk-stratifying AML patients remains to be determined. In patients with APL, the more sensitive method of RT-

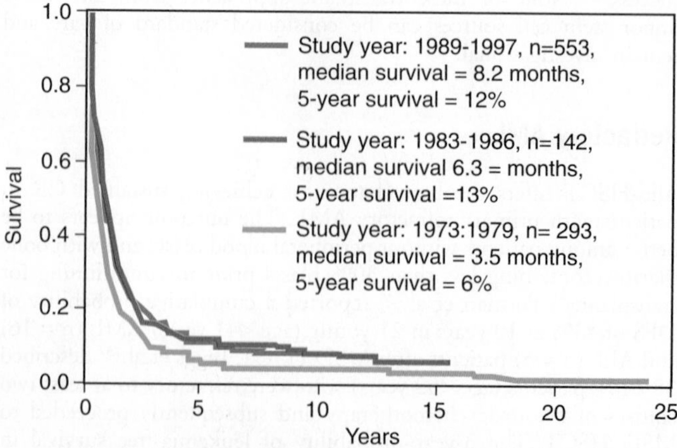

Figure 61–18 Patients older than 55 years with newly diagnosed acute myeloid leukemia treated with Eastern Cooperative Oncology Group (ECOG) protocols since 1973. *(Data from Appelbaum FR, Rowe JM, Radich J, et al: Acute myeloid leukemia. Hematology Am Soc Hematol Educ Program 62, 2001.)*

Table 61–25 Clinical and Biologic Features That Distinguish AML in Older Adults from the More Characteristic AML Occurring in Younger Adults

- More common
- Dismal long-term prognosis
- Published data often misleading
- More unfavorable prognostic factors
- Cytogenetics
- MDR-1
- Morphology
- Often indistinguishable from "classic" secondary leukemia
- Inability to withstand rigors of chemotherapy
- Inadequate postremission therapy

AML, acute myeloid leukemia; MDR, multidrug resistance.
Data from Rowe JM: Treatment of acute myelogenous leukemia in older adults. Leukemia 14:480, 2000.

Table 61–26 CR Rate in Older Adults with Acute Myeloid Leukemia: Treatment in the Modern Era

	N	CR Rate (%)	CR, Unfavorable Rate (%)
MRC AML-11[276]	1314	55	26
CALGB[277]	388	52	
SWOG[278]	328	38	34
German AMLCG[70]	297	60	
ECOG[275]	348	42	30

CR, complete remission.

PCR for detecting PML-RARA transcript, especially when increases in the quantity of transcript are observed serially, correlates with an increased probability of hematologic relapse.[272] Such data are used to identify patients who require early salvage therapy with ATO and subsequent HSCT. All these approaches are of value in detecting patients at high risk for relapse in whom an early therapeutic intervention would be justified.

AML in Elderly Adults

Elderly adults have dismal long-term prognosis that has not improved much over the past 3 decades (see Fig. 61–18). Such patients generally have more unfavorable prognostic factors at presentation, including a high proportion of intermediate-risk and unfavorable-risk cytogenetic findings; high incidence of antecedent hematologic disorders, such as myelodysplasia; high frequency of leukemic cells that express the MDR-1 gene; high incidence of trilineage dysplasia; and increased incidence of the FLT-3 internal tandem duplication. Furthermore, treatment of the elderly with AML Is made more difficult by the inability of the elderly to tolerate intensive chemotherapy. The type of postremission therapy that such patients receive is generally considered suboptimal. In essence, the difficulty of managing AML in older patients is due the suboptimal therapy offered to poor-risk patients (Table 61–25).[273]

Induction Therapy

Older adults who do not have significant comorbidities should be treated with standard induction therapy (see box on How to Treat Older Patients). The mortality from induction therapy is clearly related to the presence and severity of comorbidities.[274] In general, older patients tolerate induction therapy well. Full doses of 3 + 7 induction should be given. Dose attenuation does not shorten the period of aplasia and significantly reduces the likelihood of achieving CR. With such therapy, approximately 50% of patients can achieve CR (Table 61–26), except for older patients who have unfavorable cytogenetics in whom the CR rate is only 25% to 30%.[275–278]

Therapy for Patients Older Than 75 Years

A difficult but common dilemma is the optimal therapy for newly diagnosed AML patients older than 75 years. A strict age cutoff is to be discouraged; the decision should be based on the biologic status of the individual patient. Thus, a fit 75-year-old may tolerate induction therapy well, albeit with a higher mortality than a 30-year-old. The inherent improved quality of life for a patient in CR often will tip the scales in favor of standard induction therapy. The alternative to standard induction therapy usually includes a palliative approach with hydroxyurea, low-dose cytarabine, or similar agents, and supportive care with antibiotics and red cell and platelet transfusions. This therapy should be reserved primarily for patients who are deemed to have an excessive expected mortality from standard induction therapy. Such patients should be encouraged to enter clinical trails using some of the new targeted agents (see previous section Investigational Agents in Relapsed and Refractory AML) that are not severely myelosuppressive.

How to Treat Older Patients

- Older adults represent the greatest challenge in the management of acute myeloid leukemia (AML).
- Older patients represent the majority of AML patients.
- Little progress over the past 3 decades in treatment of AML in the elderly.
- Standard 3 + 7 induction therapy at full dose should be offered if patient has no serious comorbidities.
- Chemotherapy dose attenuation leads to a similar degree of aplasia but with a reduced chance of achieving remission.
- Patients with serious comorbidities should be treated with either hydroxyurea or low-dose cytarabine.
- In the group as a whole, 40% to 50% of patients can achieve a complete remission but only approximately 25% of those with unfavorable karyotypic abnormalities.
- No absolute data that any form of postremission therapy makes a difference.
- Standard of care is some form of postremission therapy.
- An effective regimen is cytarabine 1.5 g/m^2 given twice daily over 1 hour for 12 doses. Patients older than 70 years should receive six doses.
- Probably one cycle of consolidation therapy is appropriate; more is not better.
- Patients with unfavorable cytogenetic abnormalities should not receive standard consolidation therapy.
- Patients should be encouraged to enter studies for targeted therapy or maintenance therapy using low-dose cytarabine.
- Patients who have a histocompatible allogeneic stem cell donor should be encouraged to enter a clinical trial of allogeneic hematopoietic stem cell transplantation using reduced-intensity conditioning.

Postremission Therapy

The selection of postremission therapy for the elderly with AML remains a dilemma. Whether any form of postremission therapy prolongs OS in older patients is unknown. In addition, the regimen and the number of courses of such a regimen have not been established.[279] Several studies have compared the role of intensive consolidation therapy in older adults.[70,276,277,280] Each of these studies demonstrated that further intensification of the dose of chemotherapy after a single course of consolidation was of no value. Thus, for postremission therapy for older adults, the correct approach likely depends on the patient prognostic factors at presentation. Assuming that the patient is fit, it is reasonable to offer one cycle of intensive consolidation therapy. Additional intensive chemotherapy consolidation should be considered investigational. For uncommon older patients who have favorable cytogenetic findings, maximal tolerated chemotherapy should be given, as, occasionally such patients may be cured.[47] At the other end of the spectrum, there probably is no justification to administering standard intensive consolidation therapy to older patients who have unfavorable cytogenetics and have achieved CR. Such patients have a uniformly poor prognosis, irrespective of the therapy offered.[276,283] These patients probably should be offered some form of experimental therapy or entered into a trial of maintenance therapy.[285]

Use of reduced-intensity HSCT[57a,58] has offered new opportunities to therapy for AML in older patients and may increase the number of patients who may achieve long-term DFS. However, prospective data in this regard are limited.

Autologous HSCT is feasible in older patients with a good performance status and offers significant promise. The EORTC-GIMEMA AML-13 study reported a 3-year DFS of 28%and OS of 39% among 35 patients who received an autologous HSCT.[286] More data are required to establish the optimal conditioning regimen as well as the timing of such a procedure.

To decrease morbidity and mortality in older adults, several investigators have explored other approaches to induction and postremission therapy.[287] Use of targeted agents, such as tipifarnib and lestaurtinib, clearly would be attractive due to their reduced toxicity. Data on the use of these agents during induction for previously untreated older patients have been disappointing.[281,284] Nontargeted agents that nevertheless have a significant cytotoxic activity, such as clofarabine,[282] decitabine,[288] ahnd cloretazine,[289] have undergone major trials and clearly hold major promise. Further studies with decitabine are awaited, especially because of the significant promise of this agent during treatment of patients with myelodysplasia.[290,291]

Maintenance Therapy

For patients who are not candidates to receive any form of intensive therapy, several therapeutic options are available. Hydroxyurea is an effective agent used by many. However, a prospective study by the MRC compared hydroxyurea with low-dose cytarabine given at a dose of 20 mg twice daily for 10 days. The study reported a superior outcome for low-dose ara-C therapy, with a greater percentage of patients who could achieve CR: 18% versus only 1% for hydroxyurea.[292] Whether this is due to the mechanism of action of ara-C or to the more profound myelosuppression associated with such therapy, which is not a goal when hydroxyurea is given, is unclear.

SPECIAL CONSIDERATIONS

Hyperleukocytosis and Leukostasis

Significant abnormalities may be observed when the blood count exceeds 100,000/μL. Many of these abnormalities are spurious. False elevations of platelet count arise because blast fragments may be sensed by electronic particle counters as platelets, based on size. This problem can be readily resolved by a manual platelet count or review of the peripheral blood smear. The serum glucose level and partial pressure of oxygen (pO_2) may be depressed due to consumption of glucose and oxygen by blast cells in the in vitro collection system.[293] Immediate placement of sample on ice at the time of collection may prevent these abnormalities. However, many patients with leukocytosis have true hypoxia due to pulmonary shunting and increased arterio-alveolar gradients. Therefore, careful clinical evaluation of an abnormal pO_2 is required. Pseudohyperkalemia can occur.

The hyperleukocytosis syndrome requires urgent reduction of the blast burden, which can be accomplished almost immediately by leukapheresis.[294] Each leukapheresis procedure should lower the blast count by approximately 20%, but the effect is transient and often requires serial procedures until cytoreductive therapy is effective. Although commonly used in practice, one publication reported lack of impact of leukapheresis on mortality and the incidence of intracranial hemorrhage.[295]

Hydroxyurea often is given immediately in doses of 4 to 8 g/day to lower the blast count. By approximately 36 hours a significant reduction in peripheral blast count usually will be accomplished, at which time the dose can be decreased. Historically, radiation therapy was used emergently for central nervous system leukostasis. However, since the advent of leukapheresis, this mode of therapy, although effective, is rarely used.[296,297] Another indication of emergently lowering of blast count in hyperleukocytosis is the potential for tumor lysis syndrome. Leukostasis may occur in patients with hyperleukocytosis, and patients with a rapidly increasing peripheral leukemic cell level (usually >50,000/μL) are at greatest risk.[272] The lungs and central nervous system are the areas most vulnerable to leukostasis because of sludging of blasts in the microvasculature of these organs. True hyperviscosity is uncommon in the hyperleukocytosis syndrome in AML due to the usual presence of concurrent anemia. Thus, the clinical effects of leukostasis are caused primarily by a mechanical obstruction of microvasculature rather than true hyperviscosity.[298]

Therapy of Tumor Lysis Syndrome

The optimal management of the tumor lysis syndrome is prevention. The goals are to reduce the formation of uric acid and to establish brisk urinary flow. The formation of uric acid from purine nucleic acids requires xanthine oxidase.

Allopurinol reversibly inhibits xanthine oxidase, causing a reduction of serum uric acid concentration. Patients who present with markedly elevated serum uric acid level may be candidates for recombinant urate oxidase (rasburicase), which converts uric acid to soluble allantoin.[299] Brisk diuresis is required to prevent renal tubular deposition of calcium phosphate and the metabolic intermediates xanthine and hypoxanthine that accumulate during therapy with allopurinol.

Therapy of Transfusion-Related Graft-Versus-Host Disease

There is no known therapy for this condition. The only effective strategy is prevention. In general, patients who are at risk for this condition must receive only cellular blood products that have undergone γ irradiation in order to interfere with cellular proliferation.[300] Lymphocyte proliferation in vitro assays indicate that an irradiation dose of 2500 cGy should be used. This dose inflicts only a minor degree of damage on other cellular components, such as red blood cells.[301] Blood component irradiation can be provided by most well-equipped and adequately staffed universities as well as community cancer centers.

Other newer methods that inhibit T-cell proliferation and prevent this syndrome, including photochemical therapy, appear to be promising.[302]

Treatment of Toxicity from High-Dose Cytarabine

The unique toxicities related to cytarabine are corneal toxicity and neurotoxicity. Corneal toxicity results from inhibition of corneal DNA synthesis and usually resolves within 1 to 2 weeks of discontinuing cytarabine. Administration of corticosteroid eye drops given 12 hours before initiation of high-dose cytarabine therapy and at the time of each dose may virtually prevent the corneal toxicity.[303]

Primary midline cerebellar toxicity has been recognized as a serious neurologic complication of high-dose cytarabine and is one of the major limiting factors. It occurs most frequently in older patients and those with impaired hepatic and/or renal function. For younger adults, a total cumulative dose of 48 g/m^2 has been associated with an almost 10% incidence of cerebellar toxicity.[304] Older patients can safely receive 1.5 g/m^2 every 12 hours for 12 doses; those older than 70 years can receive six doses safely if they do not have hepatic or renal impairment.[305] In general, neurologic toxicity occurs after high-dose cytarabine is completed and usually resolves, but continuing high-dose cytarabine when cerebellar symptoms or objective findings occur during the course of treatment may lead to irreversible damage unless the treatment is stopped immediately. Although cerebellar dysfunction is the most common neurologic complication with high-dose cytarabine, optic neuropathy, somnolence, hemiparesis, coma, and other complications occasionally have been reported.[306]

SUGGESTED READINGS

Armand P, Kim HT, DeAngelo DJ, et al: Impact of cytogenetics on outcome of de novo and therapy-related AML and MDS after allogeneic transplantation. Biol Blood Marrow Transplant 13:655, 2007.

Burnett AK, Milligan D, Prentice AG, et al: A comparison of low-dose cytarabine and hydroxyurea with or without all-trans retinoic acid for acute myeloid leukemia and high-risk myelodysplastic syndrome in patients not considered fit for intensive treatment. Cancer 109:1114, 2007.

Chang MC, Chen TY, Tang JL, et al: Leukapheresis and cranial irradiation in patients with hyperleukocytic acute myeloid leukemia: No impact on early mortality and intracranial hemorrhage. Am J Hematol 82:976, 2007.

den Boer ML, Pieters R: Microarray-based identification of new targets for specific therapies in pediatric leukemia. Curr Drug Targets 8:761, 2007.

Estey E: Acute myeloid leukemia and myelodysplastic syndromes in older patients. J Clin Oncol 25:1908, 2007.

Estey E: Older adults: Should the paradigm shift from standard therapy? Best Pract Res Clin Haematol 21:61, 2008.

Finke J, Nagler A: Viewpoint: What is the role of allogeneic haematopoietic cell transplantation in the era of reduced-intensity conditioning—Is there still an upper age limit? A focus on myeloid neoplasia. Leukemia 21:1357, 2007.

Gardin C, Turlure P, Fagot T, et al: Postremission treatment of elderly patients with acute myeloid leukemia in first complete remission after intensive induction chemotherapy: Results of the multicenter randomized Acute Leukemia French Association (ALFA) 9803 trial. Blood 109:5129, 2007.

Giles FJ, Borthakur G, Ravandi F, et al: The haematopoietic cell transplantation comorbidity index score is predictive of early death and survival in patients over 60 years of age receiving induction therapy for acute myeloid leukaemia. Br J Haematol 136:624, 2007.

Jaff N, Chelghoum Y, Elhamri M, et al: Trisomy 8 as sole anomaly or with other clonal aberrations in acute myeloid leukemia: Impact on clinical presentation and outcome. Leuk Res 31:67, 2007.

Kantarjian HM, O'Brien S, Huang X, et al: Survival advantage with decitabine versus intensive chemotherapy in patients with higher risk myelodysplastic syndrome: Comparison with historical experience. Cancer 109:1133, 2007.

Krug U, Serve H, Müller-Tidow C, et al: New molecular therapy targets in acute myeloid leukemia. Recent results. Cancer Res 176:243, 2007.

Lancet JE, Gojo I, Gotlib J, et al: A phase 2 study of the farnesyltransferase inhibitor tipifarnib in poor-risk and elderly patients with previously untreated acute myelogenous leukemia. Blood 109:1387, 2007.

Mead AJ, Linch DC, Hills RK, et al: FLT3 tyrosine kinase domain mutations are biologically distinct from and have a significantly more favorable prognosis than FLT3 internal tandem duplications in patients with acute myeloid leukemia. Blood 110:1262, 2007.

Medeiros BC, Landau HJ, Morrow M, et al: The farnesyl transferase inhibitor, tipifarnib, is a potent inhibitor of the MDR1 gene product, P-glycoprotein, and demonstrates significant cytotoxic synergism against human leukemia cell lines. Leukemia 21:739, 2007.

Tallman MS, Dewald GW, Gandham S, et al: Impact of cytogenetics on outcome of matched unrelated donor hematopoietic stem cell transplantation for acute myeloid leukemia in first or second remission. Blood 110:409, 2007.

Thomas X, Suciu S, Rio B, et al: Autologous stem cell transplantation after complete remission and first consolidation in acute myeloid leukemia patients aged 61–70 years: Results of the prospective EORTC-GIMEMA AML-13 study. Haematologica 92:389, 2007.

Walter RB, Gooley TA, van der Velden VH, et al: CD33 expression and P-glycoprotein-mediated drug efflux inversely correlate and predict clinical outcome in patients with acute myeloid leukemia treated with gemtuzumab ozogamicin monotherapy. Blood 109:4168, 2007.

Whitman SP, Ruppert AS, Marcucci G, et al: Long-term disease-free survivors with cytogenetically normal acute myeloid leukemia and MLL partial tandem duplication: A Cancer and Leukemia Group B study. Blood 109:5164, 2007.

REFERENCES

For complete list of references log onto www.expertconsult.com

CHAPTER 62

ACUTE MYELOID LEUKEMIA IN CHILDREN

Michael C. Wei, Gary V. Dahl, and Howard J. Weinstein

BACKGROUND

Acute myeloid leukemias (AMLs) represent a clinically and biologically heterogeneous group of diseases caused by the malignant transformation of a hematopoietic stem cell or myeloid progenitor cell.[1,2] The proliferative advantage of the leukemic stem cell, coupled with impairments in differentiation and inhibition of apoptosis, is thought to arise from acquired genetic alterations that lead to accumulation of immature or blast cells in the bone marrow. The blasts eventually suppress normal hematopoiesis and infiltrate other organs and tissues. Conventionally, the French–American–British (FAB) cooperative group classified AML into eight subtypes (M0–M7) based primarily on blast cell morphology and reactivity with histochemical strains. More recently, the World Health Organization (WHO) developed a new classification system that included cytogenetics and lowered the percentage of blasts in the marrow required to make a diagnosis of AML from 30% to 20%.[3] AML accounts for approximately 20% of acute leukemias in children and 80% of those in adults. The biology of AML, and its response to chemotherapy, is quite similar in children and young adults (age <50 years). One difference is the more frequent extramedullary involvement of AML in infants and young children as compared with adults. In contrast to cure rates for childhood acute lymphoblastic leukemia (ALL), cure rates for AML have improved only modestly over the past two decades.[4,5] Approximately 50% of children treated with chemotherapy alone appear to be cured of their leukemia.[6–9] The outcome is somewhat better for children who, while in their first remission, receive hematopoietic stem cell transplants from histocompatible sibling donors, with an 8-year actuarial survival rate of 60%.[10] However, because there is a greater risk of early mortality and long-term morbidity from bone marrow transplantation (BMT) compared to chemotherapy, allogeneic marrow transplants are now recommended in first remission for high-risk patients only. Greater understanding of the biologic and genetic heterogeneity of AML is leading to better classification schemes, new therapeutic strategies, and risk-adapted therapy.

CLASSIFICATION

Careful examination of both the blood smear and the bone marrow aspirate is required to establish the diagnosis of AML, because approximately 10% of patients with acute leukemia do not have circulating blasts at diagnosis. It is not unusual for the morphology of leukemic cells in the peripheral blood to differ from that of cells in the bone marrow. Various methods are available for characterizing the blast cell population in patients with acute leukemia. These include morphologic interpretation of Wright–Giemsa-stained specimens in conjunction with cytochemistry, chromosome analysis, immunophenotyping, and molecular genetic analysis. Precise diagnosis and classification are essential for successful treatment and biological investigation of the childhood leukemias.[5]

Acute myeloid leukemia has been traditionally classified by the pattern of myeloid lineage differentiation noted in the bone marrow (eg, myeloblastic or granulocytic, monocytic, erythroid, or megakaryocytic lineage). In 1976, the FAB cooperative group proposed a classification system based primarily on morphologic and cytochemical features of the blast cells, with subsequent revisions to include immunophenotypic or electron microscopic confirmation for the M0 and M7 subclasses.[11–13] The FAB group recognizes eight subgroups of AML and also requires a minimum of 30% bone marrow blasts for the diagnosis of AML (Table 62–1). This is an arbitrary cutoff point that is sometimes problematic. The distribution of FAB subtypes in most children is similar to that seen in young adults with AML, except for children younger than 2 years of age, who tend to have M4 or M5.[14] Infants and toddlers with M4- and M5-type disease often present with hyperleukocytosis and extensive extramedullary leukemia, especially leukemia cutis and central nervous system (CNS) disease. The M0 subtype is quite rare in children, and appears to confer a worse prognosis.[15] The M7 subtype is most common in children younger than 3 years of age, especially those with Down syndrome.[16]

The FAB system provides a morphological classification; however, in many cases there is no correlation between morphology and the underlying genetic abnormality. Recently, a new classification for hematopoietic and lymphoid neoplasms was developed by WHO in conjunction with the Society for Hematopathology and the European Association of Hematopathology. The basic principle of the WHO system is that the classification of hematopoietic neoplasms should utilize not only morphologic findings but also all available information including genetic, immunophenotypic, biological, and clinical features to define specific disease entities and provide better correlation with prognosis and underlying biology. The current WHO system classifies AML into four separate groups: recurrent cytogenetic translocations, multilineage dysplasia, therapy-related, and not otherwise categorized (Table 62–2). In the WHO classification, the blast threshold for the diagnosis of AML is reduced from 30% to 20% in the blood or marrow. In addition, patients with the clonal recurring cytogenetic abnormalities t(8;21)(q22;q22), inv(16)(p13;q22) or t(16;16)(p13;q22), and t(15;17)(p22;q12) are classified as having AML regardless of blast percentage.[3,17]

New methods for classifying AML include molecular and biological characterization that may supplant or augment traditional classifications. Gene expression profiling of pediatric AML has identified sets of genes whose expression patterns confer prognostic significance.[18–20] Whether expression-based classifications are better than traditional cytogenetics remains to be determined, although they may certainly be used as an additional diagnostic tool. Another classification schema based on the pattern of intracellular phosphoprotein phosphorylation measured by multiplex flow cytometry has described new subsets of AML.[21]

EPIDEMIOLOGY

Approximately 400 new cases of AML are diagnosed in children each year in the United States.[22] In contrast to the early-age peak (3–4 years) for childhood ALL, the incidence of AML is quite constant from birth throughout the first 10 years, with a slight peak in late adolescence. AML also appears to account for the majority of the very rare instances of congenital leukemia. The predominance of AML in this age group may in part be due to the inclusion of infants with the transient myeloproliferative disorder associated with Down syndrome (see discussion later in this chapter). The incidence and

Table 62–1 FAB Subtypes of Recurring Chromosome Abnormalities and Clinical Features

FAB Subtype	% of Total	Chromosome Abnormality	Clinical or Laboratory Features
M0	2	−5 or del(5), −7 or del(7)	Blasts often express CD34 and terminal deoxynucleotidyl transferase (TdT)
M1	10–18		
M2	27–29	t(8;21)(q22;q22) t(6;9)(p23;q34)	Myeloblastomas (especially orbital)
M3	5–10	t(15;17)(q22;q21)	Disseminated intravascular coagulation
M4eo		inv(16)(p13;q22) or t(16;16)(p13;q22)	CNS leukemia, eosinophilia
M4	16–25	t(9;11)(p22;q23) t(11;19)(q23;p13.1) t(10;11)(p12;q23)	Congenital leukemia and young age (<2 y), extramedullary leukemia (especially leukemia cutis), hyperleukocytosis
M5	13–22	t(9;11)(p22;q23) t(11;19)(q23;p13.1) t(10;11)(p12;q23)	Congenital leukemia and young age (<2 y), extramedullary leukemia (especially leukemia cutis), secondary leukemia after epipodophyllotoxins, hyperleukocytosis
M6	1–3		
M7	4–8	t(1;22)(p13;q13)	Infants <1 y old with t(1;22), myelofibrosis, Down syndrome
All		+8	Prior myelodysplastic syndrome
All		−5 or del(5)(q11-q35)	Older adults, toxic exposure, prior myelodysplastic syndrome
All		−7 or del(7)(q22-q36)	Older adults, toxic exposure, prior myelodysplastic syndrome

subtypes of acute leukemia in children do not have significant geographic variation. In Japan, Shanghai, and among the Maori of New Zealand, however, the rates of AML are the highest. In India and Kuwait, the lowest rates are reported.[23] Patterns of presentation also vary. For example, an unusually high percentage of children diagnosed with AML in Turkey and several African countries present with myeloblastomas or chloromas involving the orbital area.[24] There is no known relationship between race and the incidence of AML, although Hispanics experience the highest rate of leukemia per million population, from 1.3- to 1.7-fold higher than other racial/ethnic groups.

ETIOLOGY

As in other forms of leukemia, the precise cause of AML is unknown. The vast majority of children with AML have no obvious predisposing factors. Known risk factors include several congenital/genetic disorders, ionizing radiation, and certain drug or toxin exposures (Table 62–3).[25–38] For example, occupational exposure to benzene and treatment with alkylating agents or topoisomerase-2 inhibitors (especially the epipodophyllotoxins) are associated with an excess incidence of AML.[37,38] The likelihood of developing secondary AML from epipodophyllotoxin therapy (etoposide or teniposide) appears to be schedule- and cumulative-dose-dependent. Increased risk has been noted with twice-weekly or weekly administration of etoposide/teniposide.[38] In contrast to alkylating agent-induced AML, which generally causes chromosomal loss of 5q or 7q, the secondary leukemias observed after treatment with etoposide or teniposide are usually of the FAB M4 or M5 subtypes, have a shorter latency period (2–4 years), and usually have chromosomal translocations involving band 11q23 (*MLL* gene rearrangement). The *MLL* gene is also rearranged in 60% to 70% of cases of infant acute leukemia,[39,40] and de novo AML, most frequently in the FAB M5 and M4 subtypes (rearranged in 50% of M5 and 20% of M4).[41] In utero exposure to naturally occurring topoisomerase II inhibitors such as dietary flavonoids has been hypothesized to increase the risk of *MLL*-rearranged infant AML.[42,43] Children who were exposed to radiation from the atomic bombs in Japan had an increased incidence of leukemia, but no excess of leukemia was noted in Japanese children who were exposed prenatally to the atomic explosions.[35] Several studies have addressed whether exposure to low-frequency, nonionizing radiation (eg, electromagnetic fields) is leukemogenic.[44] Recent reports did not find an increased risk of acute lymphoblastic leukemia in children exposed to residential magnetic fields.[45,46]

Unusual concordance of AML has been observed in monozygotic twins and in children with certain genetic disorders. The increased concordance of acute leukemia observed in identical twins approaches 100% for infant leukemias, and a risk on the order of 1 in 10 for older twin pairs. These leukemias are the consequence of the transplacental passage of a single leukemic clone rather than a genetic predisposition in most cases.[26,47] Patients with diseases associated with chromosome fragility and impaired DNA repair mechanisms (eg, Fanconi anemia and Bloom syndrome) are predisposed to develop AML.[23] Children with congenital disorders of granulopoiesis and erythropoiesis, such as Kostmann syndrome and Diamond–Blackfan anemia, are also at increased risk for developing AML.[27,28] The cumulative incidence of myelodysplastic syndrome or AML in patients with severe congenital neutropenia receiving long-term G-CSF therapy is 21% after 10 years.[48]

Children with trisomy 21 or Down syndrome have an approximately 10- to 20-fold increased risk for developing acute leukemia compared with children without Down syndrome. Although most leukemia seen in children is lymphoid, in children with Down syndrome, more than 50% of cases are myeloid. From birth through 4 years of age, the incidence of AML (especially FAB M7 or acute megakaryocytic leukemia) is much greater than ALL in children with Down syndrome. In children with Down syndrome, the incidence of acute megakaryoblastic leukemia is up to 500-fold greater than in the general pediatric population. After 5 years of age, the ratio of ALL to AML reverts to that of the general pediatric population.

Some neonates with Down syndrome or trisomy 21 mosaicism may manifest a transient myeloproliferative disorder (TMD). This intriguing syndrome is diagnosed in 10% of neonates with Down

Table 62–2 WHO Classification of Acute Myeloid Leukemia

Acute myeloid leukemia with recurrent genetic abnormalities
Acute myeloid leukemia with t(8;21)(q22;q22), (AML1/ETO)
Acute myeloid leukemia with abnormal bone marrow eosinophils and inv(16)(p13;q22) or t(16;16)(p13;q22), (CBFβ/MYH11)
Acute promyelocytic leukemia with t(15;17)(q22;q12), (PML/RARα) and variants
Acute myeloid leukemia with 11q23 (MLL) abnormalities
Acute myeloid leukemia with multilineage dysplasia
Following MDS or MDS/MPD
Without antecedent MDS or MDS/MPD, but with dysplasia in at least 50% of cells in two or more myeloid lineages
Acute myeloid leukemia and myelodysplastic syndromes, therapy related
Alkylating agent/radiation-related type
Topoisomerase II inhibitor-related type (some may be lymphoid)
Others
Acute myeloid leukemia, not otherwise categorized
Classify as:
Acute myeloid leukemia, minimally differentiated
Acute myeloid leukemia without maturation
Acute myeloid leukemia with maturation
Acute myelomonocytic leukemia
Acute monoblastic/acute monocytic leukemia
Acute erythroid leukemia (erythroid/myeloid and pure erythroleukemia)
Acute megakaryoblastic leukemia
Acute basophilic leukemia
Acute panmyelosis with myelofibrosis
Myeloid sarcoma

Table 62–3 Congenital Disorders or Acquired Factors Predisposing to Acute Myeloid Leukemia

Genetic factors
Down syndrome
Fanconi anemia
Bloom syndrome
Neurofibromatosis type I
Klinefelter syndrome
Turner syndrome
Congenital bone marrow failure syndromes
Kostmann syndrome
Diamond–Blackfan anemia
Drugs
Benzene
Alkylating agents
Epipodophyllotoxins
Ionizing radiation
Myelodysplastic syndromes

syndrome, usually during the first week of life.[32,49] TMD cannot be readily distinguished from congenital AML. The blasts have been shown to be clonal in origin and there is complete clinical and hematologic recovery in approximately 80% of children with TMD within weeks to 3 months without therapy. Infants with TMD or transient leukemia may have very elevated white blood cell counts with circulating blasts (megakaryoblasts or erythroblasts), hepatosplenomegaly, and an increased percentage of blasts in the bone marrow. There is a small subgroup of infants with TMD who die from liver failure and multiorgan system failure. In some of these patients, hepatic fibrosis is associated with megakaryoblast infiltration of the liver. Because the majority of infants with TMD never require any therapy in the first months of life, these neonates should be observed and given supportive care. However, for the small group of infants with liver failure or hydrops fetalis, a course of low-dose cytarabine may be helpful.

Data from retrospective surveys indicate that 30% of infants with TMD eventually develop AML (mostly M7) before 4 years of age.[32] It is not known whether this is a recurrence of the original disease or the appearance of a new disease. Prior to the onset of AML, there is often a several-month prodrome characterized by thrombocytopenia and bone marrow myelofibrosis with dysplastic megakaryocytes. Mutations in the *GATA-1* gene, an erythroid/megakaryocytic transcription factor, are present in the blast cells from infants with TMD as well as patients with Down syndrome and AML (FAB M7).[50,51] An unexpected finding has been the high cure rate of AML in children with Down syndrome, including those who had TMD as neonates.[52–54] This may in part be due to an increased in vitro sensitivity of Down syndrome myeloblasts to chemotherapy, especially cytarabine and daunorubicin. In in vitro studies with cytarabine, there is greater generation of ara-C triphosphate (ara-CTP) compared to myeloblasts from children without Down syndrome.[55–57]

Children with neurofibromatosis 1 (NF1) are at increased risk for developing acute and chronic myeloid leukemias as well as certain benign and malignant tumors that primarily arise in cells derived from the embryonic neural crest.[34] In patients with NF1 and leukemia, loss of both *NF1* alleles in bone marrow blasts has been detected in some patients.[36] These data are consistent with a tumor-suppressor function for the *NF1* gene. Inactivation of *NF1* may contribute to leukemogenesis by aberrantly activating the *RAS* signaling pathway.

PATHOPHYSIOLOGY

Chromosomal Rearrangements

The chromosomal abnormalities detected in blasts from the majority of children with AML are important for diagnostic and prognostic purposes and have been equally important for cloning genes involved in leukemogenesis.[58,59] Common cytogenetic abnormalities observed in patients with AML in relation to the FAB classification are listed in Table 62–1. Monosomies or deletions of chromosomes 5 or 7 and trisomy 8 are not associated with a specific FAB subtype of AML and are most commonly detected in older adults. In contrast, the balanced translocations and inversions are more frequently observed in children and young adults with AML.[58] Younger children have a higher incidence of translocations involving 11q23.[60] Most of the described chromosome changes are not unique to a specific age group, except for the t(l;22)(pl3;ql3) translocation that has been reported only in infants with M7 AML.[61] Fluorescence in situ hybridization can detect cryptic abnormalities that are not evident in banding studies.[62] Many of the genes at the breakpoints of chromosomal translocations have been cloned and proved to be transcription factors involved in normal hematopoiesis and myeloid differentiation.[63,64]

The translocation t(8;21) is the most frequently occurring translocation in AML. Three-way rearrangements may occur, and the t(8;21) is frequently associated with loss of a sex chromosome. The t(8;21) produces a fusion protein involving *AML1* on chromosome 21 and *ETO* on chromosome 8.[65] The *AML1* gene encodes one of the DNA-binding subunits of the core binding factor transcription factor complex. The chimeric fusion protein is thought to function as a transcriptional repressor and recruits corepressors, which interfere with normal *AML1*-dependent transcription, thereby inhibiting differentiation and enhancing self-renewal.[66] The *AML1/ETO* gene has been detected by molecular methods in patients with t(8;21) in long-term complete remission.[67] In patients with t(8;21) AML, qualitative minimal residual disease can be detected during and after chemotherapy. Minimal residual disease quantitation by real-time reverse-transcriptase polymerase chain reaction (RT-PCR) allows for identification of patients with a higher risk of relapse.[68]

Chromosomal abnormalities involving chromosome 16, inv(16)(p13;q22) or t(16;16)(p13;q22), comprise approximately 5% of AML and are associated with a favorable prognosis and characteristic morphology.[69] The morphology is of the FAB M4 subtype, with the distinctive presence of dysplastic eosinophils containing a dense infiltration of large, violet-purple eosinophilic granules. *CBFβ*, encoding the β subunit of core binding factor, is disrupted at the 16q22 breakpoint, and *MYH11*, encoding smooth muscle myosin heavy chain, is disrupted at the 16p13 breakpoint. The resultant fusion product, CBFβ–MYH11, exerts a dominant-negative effect on the core binding factor transcription factor complex, resulting in a block in myeloid differentiation. A high proportion of these leukemias have cooperating mutations thought to lead to increased cell proliferation.[70]

As noted earlier in this chapter, chromosome band 11q23 translocations are commonly seen in infants and toddlers with the M4 and M5 subtypes and secondary leukemias after epipodophyllotoxin therapy. The 11q23 translocation disrupts the *MLL* gene (mixed-lineage leukemia) that encodes a large protein with regions of homology to the Drosophila trithorax protein. In mammals, the wild-type MLL protein functions as a histone methyltransferase involved in maintenance of homeobox (Hox) gene expression and plays a critical role in definitive hematopoiesis.[71] *MLL* oncogenic rearrangements result in aberrant Hox gene expression. The most common chromosome 11 translocations observed in childhood AML are t(9;11)(p21;q23), t(11;19)(q23;p13.1), and t(10;11)(p12;q23), although more than 50 *MLL* translocation partners have been identified.[41,72] *MLL* translocations are found in both ALL and AML, and the precise reasons for development of one or the other is likely related to the cell of origin and the biology of the specific *MLL* translocation.

The translocation t(15;17)(q22:q21) is uniquely associated with both the hypergranular and the hypogranular variants of M3 AML. The cloning of the breakpoint revealed rearrangement of a retinoic acid receptor gene (*RARa*), with fusion to the *PML* gene.[73] The *PML-RARa* hybrid gene is expressed in leukemic cells from most patients with APL, though rarely other fusion partners, such as t(11;17) or t(5;17) have been reported. The fusion protein is an abnormal retinoic acid receptor with decreased sensitivity to retinoic acid, thereby antagonizing normal differentiation. This molecular marker (*PML-RARa* transcript) provides a convenient assay for diagnosing acute promyelocytic leukemia (APL) and determining the presence of minimal residual disease.[74] Before the *RARa* gene was shown to be rearranged in t(15;17), observations were made that M3 AML cells differentiated in response to retinoic acid both in vitro and in vivo (see section on APL).[75] Now it is understood that the mechanism involves driving differentiation by saturating the retinoic acid receptor with pharmacologic levels of retinoic acid.

Cell of Origin and Biological Properties of Leukemia Stem Cells

Cytogenetic studies and assays using X-linked polymorphisms confirmed the clonal nature of AML.[58,76] The chromosomal changes vary but predominantly involve balanced translocations, deletions, or inversions.[58] These cytogenetic findings are restricted to the leukemic cells. The bone marrow karyotype returns to normal when the disease is in complete remission. At relapse, the original clone reappears (plus or minus additional genetic changes), suggesting that the leukemic clone was suppressed, but not eliminated, by treatment.

At what stage of hematopoiesis the initiating leukemogenic event occurs is unknown. There is evidence that the cell of origin in AML is a primitive hematopoietic stem cell (HSC). In several adult patients with AML, a clonal marker has been detected in both erythroid and granulocytic cells, suggesting transformation of a less-committed progenitor (colony-forming unit granulocyte, erythroid, megakaryocyte, macrophage).[77] Studies of human AML leukemic stem cells (LSC) transplanted into immunodeficient mice indicated that the LSC closely resembles primitive HSC immunophenotypically.[1] However, model systems of human AML using AML oncogenes introduced into phenotypically defined populations of mouse bone marrow cells has demonstrated that both primitive HSC and more differentiated granulocyte-macrophage precursors can be transformed and give rise to AML.[78] Thus, more committed progenitors have the potential to be transformed, but whether this occurs in human disease remains uncertain.

As discussed in the section above, many of the oncogenic chromosomal rearrangements in AML give rise to chimeric proteins involving nuclear transcription factors that alter their normal function. These chimeric nuclear oncoproteins are thought to initiate leukemic transformation by impairing the ability of hematopoietic progenitors to differentiate and enhance their self-renewal. Transformation of granulocyte-macrophage precursors with the MLL-AF9 oncogene gives rise to AML leukemic stem cells that share properties with more undifferentiated stem cells, suggesting that the transformative oncogene has reactivated a stem cell program in a committed progenitor cell.[78] In another model of MLL-AF9 leukemia, alteration of a cell-matrix interaction has been implicated in the transformation process, and it is likely that the microenvironmental niche is important in an instructive or supportive role for leukemia-initiating cells.[79]

Although bulk leukemic blasts have limited capacity for self-renewal, leukemia stem cells have the ability to self-renew and generate precursors that give rise to the entire leukemic hierarchy. These LSC cells are thought to be quite rare,[80] but that view is being challenged.[79] Many AML LSC are found in a quiescent state,[81] which may explain why some patients relapse after treatment with agents that target rapidly dividing cells. Identification of LSC and targeting therapy to these cells is a major goal of AML research.

Cooperating Mutations

Some oncogenic AML translocations can be generated in utero, indicating a long latency for the development of disease.[82] Given this latency, additional secondary mutations are thought to be required for an initiated cell to progress to overt leukemia. A cooperativity model of leukemogenesis suggests that there are two types of mutations required, one conferring a proliferative or survival advantage and another that impairs hematopoietic differentiation.[83] Although most chromosomal translocations act to impair differentiation, many cooperating mutations affect cellular proliferation. The most frequent known examples in pediatric AML include *KIT*, *RAS*, and FMS-like tyrosine-kinase 3 (*FLT3*) mutations. A review of 170 pediatric AML samples showed that 40% harbored a mutation in one of these three genes.[84] Mutations in *RAS*, a critical mediator of growth signal transduction mutated in many cancers, were found in 37 of 99 pediatric AML samples.[85] Mutated *RAS* synergizes with nuclear fusion genes to accelerate leukemia latency in mouse models.[86] *FLT3* is a receptor tyrosine kinase important for cell proliferation and differentiation. Mutations including the internal tandem duplication (ITD) or activating loop mutations are thought to lead to constitutive activation of the receptor. *FLT3* ITD overexpression by itself induces a myeloproliferative disease (but not frank AML) in mice[87]; however, *FLT3* ITD increases the penetrance of acute promyelocytic leukemia in a *PML–RAR* model.[88] Somatic *FLT3* mutations are found in 5% to 44% of pediatric AML, and most studies have found a lower frequency than that in adult AML.[19,89–91] Certainly other signaling path-

Table 62–4 Signs and Symptoms at Presentation in Acute Myeloid Leukemia

Sign or Symptom	Percentage of Patients
Fever	34
Pallor	25
Anorexia, weight loss	22
Weakness, fatigue	19
Sore throat	18
Other respiratory symptoms	23
Bleeding	
Cutaneous	18
Mucosal	10
Menorrhagia	5
Bone or joint pain	18
Lymphadenopathy	14
Gastrointestinal symptoms	13
Neurologic signs or symptoms	10
Swollen gingiva	8
Chest pain	6
Recurrent infection	3

Data from Choi S-I, Simone JV: Acute nonlymphocytic leukemia in 171 children. Med Pediatr Oncol 2:119, 1976.

ways beyond *KIT*, *RAS*, and *FLT3* are likely to be affected in AML. Loss of heterozygosity at multiple loci has been observed in AML samples, representing another mechanism whereby cooperating mutations are generated.[92]

CLINICAL FEATURES

History and Physical Exam

The initial signs and symptoms in the majority of children with AML include some degree of pallor, fatigue, skin or mucosal bleeding, or fever or infection that has not responded to appropriate antibiotic therapy (Table 62–4).[93] These signs and symptoms reflect the anemia, thrombocytopenia, and neutropenia secondary to diminished production of normal blood cells due to bone marrow infiltration with leukemic blasts. AML, in contrast to chronic myelogenous leukemia, is rarely diagnosed as an incidental finding on a routine complete blood cell count in an asymptomatic child. Bone pain and arthralgias are less common presenting symptoms in children with AML than those with ALL. Massive hepatosplenomegaly is uncommon except in infants with AML.[94] Ocular pathology includes retinal hemorrhages due to coagulopathy, leukostasis, and leukemic infiltration, which may be asymptomatic.[95,96]

Congenital Leukemia

The clinical manifestations of leukemia diagnosed in the first 4 weeks of life differ in varying degrees from the typical findings in infants older than 6 months of age and older children with AML.[94] Approximately one half of newborns and infants younger than 2 months of age with AML have leukemia cutis.[97] These babies have been described as looking like a "blueberry muffin" (Fig. 62–1). The skin lesions are described in the following sections. It is important to note that these lesions may precede bone marrow manifestations of leukemia. Transient spontaneous remissions of leukemia cutis may occur but are

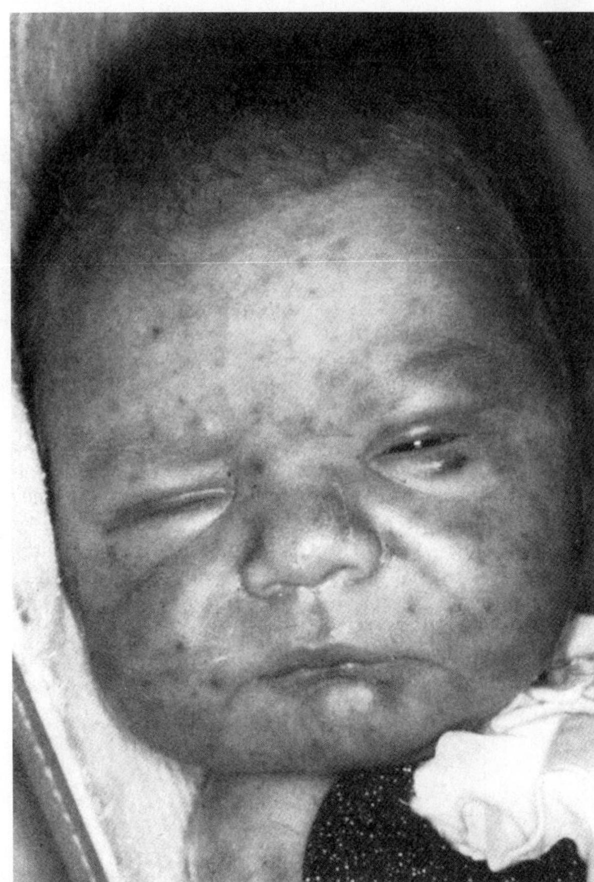

Figure 62–1. Leukemia cutis as commonly seen in congenital leukemia.

usually followed within weeks by their reappearance in association with overt bone marrow involvement.[97] In one review of 117 patients with congenital leukemia, there were six spontaneous remissions.[98] Other signs and symptoms of congenital leukemia include hepatosplenomegaly, lethargy, pallor, and failure to thrive.

Extramedullary Leukemia

The most common sites of extramedullary leukemia in children with AML include skin, gingiva, and CNS and myeloblastomas in the head and neck area (Fig. 62–2). Extramedullary involvement with AML is more common in infants than in older children. In a review of 29 infants with AML at St. Jude Children's Research Hospital, 13 were found to have leukemia cutis and 11 presented with CNS leukemia.[94] The skin lesions are often widespread, range in size from several millimeters to several centimeters, and are palpable as freely mobile, generally painless subcutaneous nodules. The color of the overlying skin may be salmon, red-brown, or bluish to slate gray in color. Testicular involvement is extraordinarily rare in children with AML and, like CNS leukemia, is commonly associated with the M4 and M5 FAB subtypes.

The most common pathologic finding of AML in the CNS is that of meningeal infiltration by blasts, but epidural or brain parenchymal myeloblastomas have also been described. The incidence of meningeal leukemia at diagnosis in children with AML ranges from 5% to 15%,[99–101] but most children are asymptomatic. The diagnosis of CNS leukemia is made by examining a cytocentrifuged specimen of cerebrospinal fluid (CSF) (Fig. 62–3). A currently accepted definition of CNS leukemia is CSF with five or more white blood cells (WBCs) per microliter and definite blasts, cranial nerve palsy, signs of meningeal disease, or a nonhemorrhagic CNS mass or chloroma. If the CSF is contaminated with more than 10 red blood cells per microliter

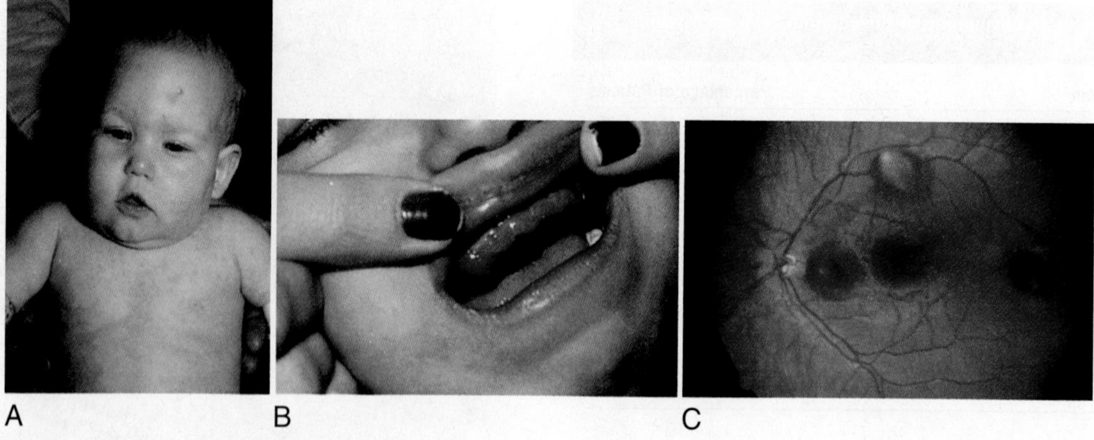

Figure 62–2. **A**, Monoblastic leukemia cutis at diagnosis; lesion on forehead preceded disseminated rash by 6 to 8 weeks. **B**, Gingival infiltration with M5a leukemia in a 21-month-old girl. **C**, Retinal infiltration at presentation of M4 disease in a 5-year-old boy.

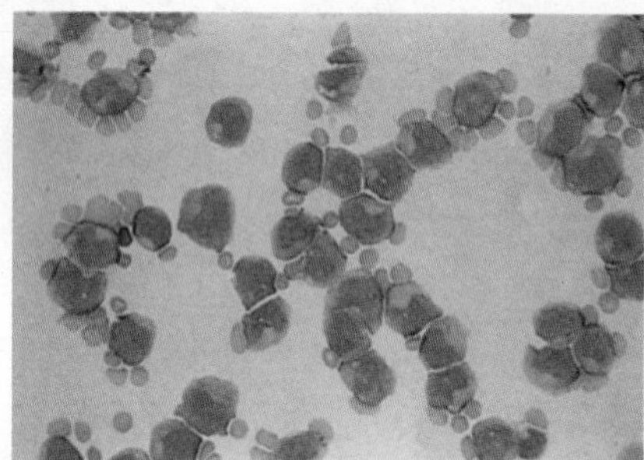

Figure 62–3. Cerebrospinal fluid double-concentrate cytocentrifuge preparation of M5a leukemia cells.

and leukemic blasts, the lumbar puncture is considered traumatic. The rare symptomatic patient with CNS leukemia may have headache, vomiting, papilledema, or a cranial nerve palsy (facial nerve is most common). In contrast, patients with cerebral leukostasis present with seizures, somnolence, or stroke secondary to areas of hemorrhage and infarction in brain tissue.

Fewer than 5% of newly diagnosed patients with AML have myeloblastomas, also known as granulocytic sarcomas or chloromas.[102] These "solid tumors" of myeloid blasts may occur anywhere but are primarily detected in the bones and soft tissues of the head and neck (often orbits), and in intracranial or epidural locations.[102,103] Myeloblastomas may herald overt bone marrow involvement with AML by weeks to months and are associated with FAB M2 and t(8;21) and, in infants, with M4 and M5 subtypes.[14,104]

Laboratory Evaluation

The initial WBC count at presentation in children with AML is variable (1000 → 500,000 μL^{-1}). Approximately 15% to 20% of children have WBC counts higher than 100,000 μL^{-1}.[60,93] Marked leukocytosis is associated with the FAB M4 and M5 subtypes and congenital leukemia, whereas lower leukocyte counts are commonly seen in patients with M3 or APL. The leukocyte differential in most patients includes fewer than 1000 neutrophils per microliter and a variable percentage of blasts. In approximately 10% of patients, no peripheral blasts are detectable.

Most patients with AML have a normocytic anemia, with occasional teardrop forms and nucleated red blood cells noted on the peripheral smear. In one large series of children with AML, initial hemoglobin levels range from 2.7 to 14.3 g/dL (median, 7 g/dL). The rare hemolytic anemia associated with AML is usually microangiopathic, secondary to disseminated intravascular coagulation (DIC).

Approximately 50% of children with AML present with platelet counts of fewer than 50,000 μL^{-1}. Thrombocytopenia is the usual cause of hemorrhage in patients with AML. Bleeding is usually not observed until the platelet count falls below 20,000 μL^{-1} unless there is an associated coagulopathy. The other major cause of bleeding in children with AML is DIC. Patients with APL (FAB M3) are most at risk for DIC, but infants with M4 and M5 types are also at increased risk.[75,105] Prior to the use of all-trans-retinoic acid (ATRA) for patients with APL, prophylactic low-dose heparin and transfusion of fresh frozen plasma and platelets were recommended by several groups of investigators.[106] ATRA appears to downregulate tissue factor expression and thereby reduces the severity and duration of DIC in APL patients. At present, all patients should be carefully followed with serial coagulation studies (partial thromboplastin time, prothrombin time, fibrinogen, and fibrin split products). The optimal management of coagulopathy is controversial. Heparin usage is discouraged now that all patients receive ATRA.

The definitive diagnosis of acute leukemia is made by examination of the bone marrow aspirate.[107] In most patients, the bone marrow is hypercellular, with 30% to 90% blasts. The bone marrow biopsy may be hypocellular, especially in patients with a history of prior MDS, Fanconi anemia, or paroxysmal nocturnal hemoglobinuria. Dysplastic changes have recently been reported in patients with de novo AML and appear to have no prognostic significance. For a diagnosis of hypocellular AML, there need to be less than 20% blasts.

Immunophenotypic Analysis

Normal hematopoietic cells undergo changes in expression of cell surface markers as they mature from stem cells into cells of a committed lineage. Monoclonal antibodies have been developed that react with lineage-specific and stage-specific lymphoid and myeloid activation and differentiation antigens.[108] By using a combination of monoclonal antibodies recognizing B-cell, T-cell, and myeloid antigens, it is possible to confirm the diagnosis of AML and to differentiate AML from ALL if morphology and traditional immunohistochemistry are inconclusive (<15% of cases).

Several unusual immunophenotypes of AML blasts have been described that are FAB subtype-specific and associated with unique chromosomal changes. For example, M2 AML with t(8;21) is characterized by expression of the myeloid and stem cell antigens CD13, CD15, CD34, HLA DR, and expression of the B-cell antigen CD19 and the neural adhesion molecule CD56.[109] In adult AML studies, CD56-positive AML with t(8;21) and t(15;17) translocations was associated with shorter remissions and decreased overall survival.[109,110]

It has been estimated from several studies that 5% to 15% of patients with acute leukemia have morphologic, cytochemical, immunophenotypic, or genetic evidence of more than one hematopoietic lineage. Approximately 10% to 25% of AML patients demonstrate lymphoid antigen expression on myeloid blasts, and similarly 4% to 25% of ALL patients demonstrate expression of at least one myeloid antigen on the blast cell surface.[111–113] The expression of lymphoid antigens in AML lacks prognostic significance.[114] In most instances of hybrid or mixed-lineage acute leukemia, there is coexpression of lymphoid and myeloid markers on the same blast, but in rare cases there have been two distinct populations of blasts.[113] The pathogenesis of these mixed-lineage leukemias remains poorly understood. They may represent a leukemic transformation in a primitive stem cell, or the aberrant expression of a lymphoid gene in a myeloid leukemia. Because few instances of true biphenotypic leukemia have been described, the prognosis is unclear. In a pediatric study, 14 of 16 patients with lymphoid antigen-positive AML expressed a T-cell marker.[113] Interestingly, several of these patients had a poor response to AML induction therapy but subsequently responded to an ALL induction regimen. Despite this, children with AML whose blasts express lymphoid antigens should be treated initially on AML protocols.

Differential Diagnosis

The diagnosis of AML is usually straightforward after an examination of the peripheral blood and bone marrow.[107] Other diagnoses that can sometimes cause diagnostic difficulty include the myeloproliferative disorders (eg, juvenile myelomonocytic leukemia), myelodysplastic (preleukemic) syndromes, and overwhelming bacterial infections that result in leukemoid reactions or neutropenia secondary to a bone marrow maturation arrest in granulocytic precursors. In the last situation, the bone marrow may be confused with APL, but with resolution of the infection, granulocytic maturation ensues. The differential diagnosis of congenital leukemia is somewhat more challenging, in part because of the leukoerythroblastic peripheral blood picture noted in neonates with hypoxia or sepsis. Congenital viral infections, including cytomegalovirus, herpes simplex, human immunodeficiency virus (HIV), and rubella, need to be ruled out as well as the transient myeloproliferative disorder associated with trisomy 21.[115,116]

Prognosis

The prognostic significance of several clinical and biologic features in children with AML is summarized in Table 62–5. In contrast to childhood ALL, very few clinical, laboratory, or treatment-associated factors have been consistently related to prognosis.[117,118] A WBC count greater than 100,000 µL^{-1} at diagnosis, monosomy 7 or 5, del(5q), 3q rearrangements, a complex karyotype, FAB M0 subtype, non-Down syndrome FAB M7, an FLT3 internal tandem duplication, and secondary AML are associated with lower remission rates.[15,91,119–122] Favorable factors for predicting complete remission include FAB M1 with Auer rods, chromosome findings of inv(16) or t(8;21), and the combined use of ATRA and chemotherapy for APL (FAB M3).[120,123,124]

In some studies, the M4 and M5 FAB subtypes, high initial leukocyte count, age younger than 2 years, extramedullary leukemia (other than CNS) at diagnosis, and longer time to enter remission (more than one induction cycle) were found to have an adverse impact on remission duration.[117] In the German BFM studies, two risk groups were identified.[120] The BFM favorable risk group includes children with FAB M1 or M2 with Auer rods, M3 and M4eo, with 5% blasts or less in the bone marrow on day 15 after induction chemotherapy, and Down syndrome. Included in this favorable group are patients with t(8;21) and inv(16). The United Kingdom Medical Research Council trials have separated good-, standard-, or poor-risk groups based on karyotype and response to the first round of induction.[125] The good-risk patients (32%) had karyotypes t(8;21), inv(16), t(15;17), or FAB M3 morphology, and this was irrespective of response to induction course 1. The poor-risk patients (19%) had karyotypes -5, -7, del(5q), abn(3q), and complex karyotype, or more than 15% bone marrow blasts after course 1 but without favorable genetics. The standard-risk patients (49%) included those with neither favorable nor unfavorable cytogenetics and less than 15% bone marrow blasts after course 1. The good-, standard-, and poor-risk patients had overall survival from complete remission at 10 years of 77%, 58%, and 30%, respectively.[125]

Table 62–5 Patient Characteristics Relating to Duration of Remission

Characteristics	Favorable Value
Cytogenetics	t(15;17), t(8;21), inv(16)
Leukocyte count	<100,000 µL^{-1}
Secondary acute myeloid leukemia	Not present
FAB subtype	M1 or M2 with Auer rods, M3 and M4eo
FLT3	Wild-type
Courses to complete remission	1

The presence of acute mixed-lineage or biphenotypic leukemia (AML with lymphoid-associated antigens) does not influence prognosis.[72,112] Age 10 years or more is associated with increased risk of death or recurrence.[126] The role of ethnicity in survival is controversial. Retrospective analysis at St. Jude showed no difference between black and white children in multiple studies.[127] Black children had inferior EFS and OS on recent Children's Cancer Group studies, possibly because of decreased availability of matched bone marrow donors.[128] Several groups of investigators have reported that children with AML and Down syndrome have a very good outcome after treatment with chemotherapy alone.[52,53] Reducing chemotherapy is advisable in Down syndrome AML patients, who appear to be more susceptible to treatment-related mortality, especially in intensive-timed regimens.[53,129,130]

Minimal residual disease (MRD) is being compared to traditional prognostic factors to predict relapse risk. MRD analysis detects leukemic blasts at much higher sensitivity than traditional bone marrow morphological analysis. MRD can be measured with flow immunophenotyping or PCR for specific translocations or genes associated with disease. Assays with RT-PCR for many of the common gene rearrangements in AML are now available for diagnostic purposes and for following minimal residual leukemia.[131] Genetic markers suitable for RT-PCR studies are found in almost 50% of AML patients. Flow immunophenotyping can detect an aberrant leukemic phenotype in more than 85% of AML patients at 0.1% to 0.01% residual cells, and detection of more than 0.1% minimal residual disease after one round of induction or at end of consolidation was associated with a significantly worse risk of early relapse and overall survival.[132–134] Importantly, immunophenotyping detected residual leukemia in 23% of cases in morphological remission. The BFM group, however, has suggested that MRD is not more predictive of relapse than other traditional prognostic factors such as cytogenetics.[135]

Additional mutations or aberrant gene expression beyond the characteristic chromosomal translocation are found in AML that have biologic and prognostic significance. As discussed above, patients who bear a somatic *FLT3* internal tandem duplication produce an abnormal protein with extra amino acids at the juxtamembrane region that confers constitutive activation, and *FLT3* mutant leukemia has poor prognosis regardless of the FAB type (Fig. 62–4).[89–91,136–138] The St. Jude collaborative group now places patients with *FLT3* mutation into a poor-risk category and is evaluating this risk stratification prospectively. A large review of *FLT3* mutation status indicated that mutant *FLT3* by itself is not an

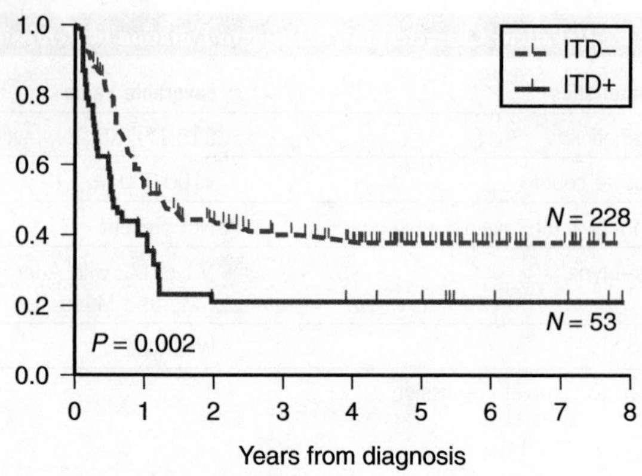

Figure 62–4. Kaplan–Meier estimate of event-free survival (EFS) according to the presence of FLT3/ITD from Pediatric Oncology Group Protocol 9421. Log-rank *P* values are shown.

indication for hematopoietic stem cell transplantation (HSCT) over chemotherapy.[139] The Wilms tumor suppressor gene *WT1* has been found to be overexpressed at diagnosis in 78% of patients in one study; those patients with continued overexpression of *WT1* during therapy had higher risk of relapse and death.[140] However, another study reached the opposite conclusion that *WT1* expression was associated with favorable cytogenetics and better survival.[141] Nucleophosmin is a nucleocytoplasmic shuttling protein that regulates the *P53-ARF* tumor suppressor pathway. Mutations in nucleophosmin have been found that alter its intracellular localization, and mutated nucleophosmin is associated with better response to induction and survival.[142–145] Overall, the use of MRD and specific gene markers to predict patients with higher risk of relapse must be further studied prospectively. Eventually such studies may be used to stratify high-risk patients for more intensive or targeted therapy or HSCT.

THERAPY

The long-term survival (>5 years) rate for children with AML has increased from less than 10% to approximately 50% during the past 30 years.[4,6,9,125,146–148] This improved cure rate has resulted from more effective remission induction chemotherapy and better strategies to prevent relapse. Improvements in supportive care have been equally important, making it safe and feasible to treat patients with myelosuppressive doses of chemotherapy.[149,150] All children with AML should be referred to a pediatric oncology center for treatment and are usually enrolled on a cooperative group clinical trial, such as those of the Children's Oncology Group, Berlin–Frankfurt–Muenster (BFM) Group, and the United Kingdom Medical Research Council, or collaborative institutional protocols.

Supportive Care

Before chemotherapy is started, the infant or child should be stabilized with regard to renal, metabolic, hematologic (anemia, bleeding, DIC, leukostasis), and infectious disease issues. Excellent supportive care to facilitate children surviving therapy without significant morbidity is of paramount importance. A double-lumen indwelling central venous catheter should be placed early in the treatment course. The metabolic derangements associated with leukemic cell death (tumor lysis syndrome) include hyperuricemia, hyperkalemia, hyperphosphatemia, and hypocalcemia.[151] The tumor lysis syndrome is seen more often in children with ALL (especially T cell and mature B cell) than in those with AML. Uric acid nephropathy is avoided by prompt attention to hydration, alkalinization of the urine, and administration of allopurinol. A new agent, recombinant urate oxidase (Rasburicase) converts uric acid to more soluble allantoin and is now used with outstanding efficacy in children expected to have tumor lysis syndrome. Children with AML are at especially increased risk of bacterial and fungal infections during therapy and leukemia-induced neutropenia. The most commonly encountered fungal infections are due to *Candida* and *Aspergillus* species. Given the high risk of fungal disease, it is reasonable to provide antifungal prophylaxis during AML therapy; however, there is no standard antifungal prophylactic regimen. Fluconazole is effective against most *Candida* species, but has no activity against *Aspergillus* species. Current commercially available agents with anti-*Aspergillus* activity that have been used in AML patients include the triazoles (itraconazole, voriconazole, and posaconazole), the echinocandins (caspofungin, micafungin, and anidulafungin), and amphotericin B deoxycholate or the lipid preparations of amphotericin. In patients with AML, septicemia due to α-hemolytic streptococcal organisms is associated with high-dose cytarabine, a component of most AML therapeutic protocols. The α-hemolytic streptococcal infections have a high rate of recurrence and associated toxicities during subsequent episodes of intensive chemotherapy. There is no known prophylactic regimen to prevent this infection. Physicians caring for these children must maintain a high index of suspicion and be prepared to institute appropriate antibiotic coverage in the event of fever or unexplained illness. Prolonged periods of neutropenia have been treated with hematopoietic growth factors (granulocyte- or granulocyte-macrophage colony-stimulating factor) during induction and after cycles of intensification chemotherapy, although not all protocols use them. Blood products should all be leuko-poor and irradiated to prevent transfusion-associated graft-versus-host disease. Platelet transfusions are recommended prophylactically if the platelet count is lower than 10,000 μL^{-1}.

One to 2% of children with AML still die within the first several days to a week after diagnosis. These early deaths usually result from intracranial hemorrhage from either a coagulopathy or CNS leukostasis.[152] If the leukocyte count is greater than 100,000 μL^{-1}, it is important to initiate urgent measures to prevent leukostasis. Leukostasis refers to plugging of blasts in vessels with invasion of vessel walls, leading to hemorrhagic infarction of the brain, lung, or other organs. Children with AML who have leukocyte counts higher than 200,000 μL^{-1} are much more susceptible to leukostasis than patients with ALL and comparable WBC counts.[151] The most clinically relevant target organs for leukostasis are the brain and lung, with signs and symptoms including somnolence, seizures, stroke, tachypnea, and hypoxemia. Treatment should include immediate measures to lower the WBC count, and exchange transfusion or leukapheresis if the patient is symptomatic. Oral hydroxyurea combined with leukapheresis is very effective for rapidly lowering the blast count in patients with AML and preventing the clinical manifestations of leukostasis.[153,154] Although extremely elevated WBC counts and leukostasis are rare in APL, leukapheresis should be avoided in these patients to prevent an exacerbation of DIC.[155]

Remission Induction

Because of the narrow therapeutic index of the active agents in AML, all induction regimens (except for FAB M3) are designed to produce rapid bone marrow hypoplasia, an apparent prerequisite for successful remission induction. A major concern is the appropriateness of current dose adjustments made in chemotherapy protocols for infants less than 1 year of age (generally based on mg/kg arbitrary dose reductions of 25%).[60] The combination of cytarabine (7 days) and daunorubicin (3 days), known as the "7+3" regimen, has been the traditional backbone of induction chemotherapy and results in a complete remission rate of approximately 80%, with a recent survey of protocols showing a range of 70% to 93%.[156] Approximately one-third of these patients require two courses of induction to achieve a remission. Recent protocols using intensified induction by timing or dose intensity have demonstrated improved remission rates, approaching 90%, with superior overall survival.[8,10] The addition of a third agent such as etoposide or thioguanine during induction is now widely used, and a randomization of DAT (daunorubicin, cytarabine, thioguanine) versus ADE (cytarabine, daunorubicin, etoposide) showed no significant differences between the two induction regimens.[8] Although attempts to increase the intensity of induction have not significantly improved complete remission rates, there is evidence that induction intensity improves ultimate outcome. Patients receiving intensified induction have had statistically significant increases in disease-free survival compared with those patients randomized to standard 7+3 induction. These data are consistent with the hypothesis that more effective early leukemic cell kill reduces the likelihood of a subsequent relapse in children and adults with AML.[60] Lower remission rates are seen in patients with secondary AML, a history of a prior myelodysplastic syndrome (MDS), and certain cytogenetic findings (see section on Prognosis). Because of the requisite period of bone marrow hypoplasia and the greater impairment of bone marrow reserve in patients with AML, the remission induction phase of therapy is more toxic than for patients with ALL. Prospectively controlled pediatric and adult cooperative group studies have shown that daunorubicin is preferable to doxorubicin because it is associated with less oral mucositis and gastrointestinal toxicity.[157] The most disturbing gastrointestinal toxicity during induction is an enterocolitis involving the distal ileum, cecum, and proximal colon. This syndrome is referred to as typhlitis or the right lower quadrant syndrome and is noted in approximately 10% of patients.[158] The signs and symptoms of typhlitis develop approximately 10 to 14 days after the start of chemotherapy. Treatment recommendations include bowel rest and double-coverage broad-spectrum antibiotics for gram-negative organisms. Surgery is rarely needed and is reserved for intestinal perforation, abdominal wall fasciitis, or massive bleeding. Several adult and pediatric AML studies have explored the benefits of substituting either mitoxantrone or idarubicin for daunorubicin.[159,160] Mitoxantrone is at least as effective as daunorubicin. Idarubicin is not superior to daunorubicin for remission induction and is associated with more marrow toxicity and greater number of days until neutrophil recovery.

Acute Promyelocytic Leukemia (FAB M3)

In the past, approximately 65% to 75% of patients with M3 AML (also called APL) entered remission after a standard induction with daunorubicin and cytarabine. The remission induction period, however, was associated with significant early mortality secondary to hemorrhagic complications.[161] The use of ATRA alone during induction for patients with acute APL (*PML/RARa*-positive) results in a similar or even higher rate of complete remission with a different toxicity profile and substantially lower mortality rate during induction.[75] The ATRA-induced remissions are associated with differentiation of the blasts/promyelocytes and a peripheral blood leukocytosis during the first two weeks of therapy. European and American clinical trials have established the current standard front-line therapy, which combines ATRA with anthracycline-based chemotherapy for remission induction and consolidation chemotherapy and with ATRA continuing during maintenance, resulting in overall survival higher than 80%.[162,163] Recent results support a potential role for the addition of cytarabine during induction.[164] ATRA is associated with several life-threatening complications, including severe respiratory distress and capillary leak syndrome and pseudotumor cerebri (more common in pediatric patients). The retinoic acid syndrome (respiratory distress and weight gain) has been successfully managed in most patients by temporary cessation of ATRA and administration of dexamethasone. The symptoms of pseudotumor cerebri disappear within days after withdrawal of ATRA, and the drug can usually be safely restarted at a reduced dose.[165,166] This syndrome has also been seen in response to treatment with arsenic trioxide and thus might better be termed the "differentiation syndrome."[167] Patients whose disease is induced into remission with ATRA alone remain PCR-positive for PML/RARa after induction and all eventually relapse if no consolidation chemotherapy is added. The combined use of ATRA and chemotherapy during remission induction followed by consolidation chemotherapy and ATRA maintenance results in an improved disease-free survival rate when compared with the use of ATRA alone either during induction or maintenance.[123] The ability to detect PML/RARa messenger RNA by RT-PCR is a useful method of monitoring the efficacy of therapy. When used at the 10^{-4} sensitivity level, persistent positive RT-PCR findings after the consolidation phase strongly predict hematologic relapse.[74,168] Arsenic trioxide (As_2O_3 or ATO) can be used to achieve remissions in those patients who relapse after ATRA treatment.[169] APL cells express CD33, and gemtuzumab ozogamycin has been used successfully in both untreated and relapsed APL in adults.[170,171]

Central Nervous System Leukemia

There is no evidence that CNS-directed therapy with either intrathecal chemotherapy alone or in combination with cranial irradiation prolongs disease-free survival in children with AML.[5,118,172] Most pediatric AML studies, however, still include intrathecal chemotherapy because isolated CNS relapse occurs in approximately 20% of children with AML who did not receive any CNS-directed therapy.[99,100] Using historical controls, the BFM AML group has made a case for using prophylactic cranial irradiation and tested their hypothesis in a prospectively controlled clinical trial.[173] The current results (including CNS relapse) of recent pediatric AML trials, using intrathecal chemotherapy without CNS irradiation, are similar to those of patients treated on the BFM AML trial that used cranial irradiation for prevention and treatment of CNS involvement.[159] In contrast to ALL, the finding of blasts in the CSF at diagnosis in children with AML does not adversely affect prognosis.[101] An accepted approach for the treatment of CNS leukemia is weekly intrathecal methotrexate or cytarabine until the CSF is clear of blasts. In some protocols, this is followed by CNS irradiation at the end of systemic chemotherapy.[118]

Treatment in Remission

Without further treatment after standard induction chemotherapy, more than 90% of patients relapse within 1 year, and the remainder relapse by 2 years. The intensity and duration of chemotherapy in remission, as well as the role of BMT in first remission, have been areas of active investigation and controversy during the past decades. In the 1970s, pediatric AML studies tested whether modestly myelosuppressive combination chemotherapy given in remission would improve overall survival. These protocols led to a plateau in disease-free survival of 15% to 20% at 5 years.[157,172,174] In an effort to improve upon these disappointing results, other approaches were explored, including early intensification or consolidation chemotherapy and HSCT. Allogeneic HSCT provided an opportunity for delivering very high doses of chemoradiation and possibly stimulating a graft-versus-leukemia effect.[175–177] Although the initial studies were not randomized, the results suggested a benefit for either the intensification of chemotherapy or HSCT early in first remission.[178] Cytarabine, the single most active agent in AML, was the prototype drug for intensification, because laboratory and clinical studies indicated that a log increase in its dose could overcome certain mechanisms of resistance.[179,180] Approximately 40% of patients with AML who are refractory to standard doses of cytarabine achieve a complete remission with high-dose cytarabine.[180] The superiority of high-dose compared to standard-dose cytarabine has also been confirmed in a prospective randomized clinical trial in adults with AML.[181] Most pediatric AML studies that were initiated in the late 1980s included several consolidation cycles of high-dose cytarabine. These protocols resulted in 5-year leukemia-free survival plateaus of 35% to 60%.[182–184] Clinical studies in the most recent decade have evolved and indicate that timed sequential induction[10] and therapies utilizing repeated courses of intensive consolidation[8,159,185] result in 5-year event-free survival rate of 50%. High-dose cytarabine is given in combination with other agents such as mitozantrone, amsacrine, etoposide, or asparaginase, and noncytarabine containing consolidation cycles are used as well. The optimal number of consolidation chemotherapy cycles has not been determined, but is usually three to four cycles. Maintenance chemotherapy with oral thioguanine and standard doses of cytarabine given after consolidation chemotherapy has not been shown to further increase the proportion of patients in long-term remission. Patients who receive maintenance have a poor salvage rate if relapsed because of clinical drug resistance.[185]

Hematopoietic Stem Cell Transplantation in First Remission

Allogeneic HSCT from a histocompatible family donor was first evaluated in children and young adults with AML in first remission in the mid-1970s.[175–178,183] Published data from many pediatric AML bone marrow transplant series show 5-year event-free survival rates ranging from 56% to 74%.[8,159,186–188] Many of the early transplant studies, however, were not prospectively designed, and therefore were biased in their selection criteria, were not controlled for the timing of HSCT in first remission, and excluded patients who were eligible for a transplant but who relapsed before the procedure. In an effort to avoid these and other biases, it was suggested that the outcomes of studies comparing HSCT to chemotherapy be analyzed according to the intention-to-treat analysis, which includes all eligible patients (ie, those having a matched family donor) and not just individuals who actually received the transplant.[183,184] When the data are analyzed in this way, there is still a statistically significant survival advantage for allogeneic HSCT compared with chemotherapy in most studies.

Allogeneic HSCT early in first remission using an HLA-matched related donor results in a significantly better disease-free survival rate as compared with chemotherapy but is limited to approximately 20% of patients with a suitable donor. For those children with AML who have a relatively favorable prognosis after treatment with chemotherapy [eg, t(15;17), t(8;21), inv(16), Down syndrome] or standard risk patients without unfavorable risk factors, it is reasonable to reserve HSCT for early relapse or second remission. In addition, a limited donor pool of histocompatible related individuals, and the acute toxicities (eg, acute graft-versus-host disease, interstitial pneumonia, hepatic veno-occlusive disease) and late effects of HSCT, continue to be major limitations in the more widespread application of this procedure in patients with AML.[189,190] The late effects of HSCT in young children may include growth problems, gonadal toxicity, secondary malignancy, and chronic graft-versus-host disease.[190–193] Because of these issues, many pediatric oncologists are recommending chemotherapy alone, especially for children with a relatively favorable prognosis, and reserving HSCT for those children who have a relapse. In particular, children with promyelocytic leukemia who receive ATRA plus chemotherapy and those with Down syndrome AML are often successfully treated with chemotherapy regimens. Given the current status of biologic characteristics and aggressive chemotherapy regimens, it appears that HSCT should be used in first remission only for children with high-risk features and be reserved for use in second remission or early relapse in all others.[194] Up to 50% to 60% of patients with AML who achieve second remission and receive allogeneic transplantation appear to be long-term leukemia-free survivors.[195] Patients with refractory disease or who relapse after intensive therapy within a year of diagnosis have a very poor prognosis with any form of therapy, including HSCT.

For patients who lack suitable donors (<5 or 6 antigen-matched family member), purged autologous HSCT became an attractive option in first remission, after it was reported to be effective in some patients with AML in second remission (5-year survival rates of 30%–40%).[196] However, the results of three randomized trials in pediatric AML have concluded that autologous HSCT is not superior to intensive chemotherapy in first remission.[10,184,197] Finally, another study indicated that the addition of autologous BMT to four courses of intensive chemotherapy substantially reduces the risk of relapse in patients with AML, leading to an improvement in long-term survival.[198] Because of the good chance of salvage for children who relapse after completion of chemotherapy and the morbidity, mortality, and late effects of autologous BMT, the authors suggest that delay of the autograft until second remission may be appropriate.

The Role of Hematopoietic Stem Cell Transplantation in Pediatric AML

Outcomes in pediatric AML show a benefit for allogeneic transplant in first remission for select patients, but the risk of treatment-related mortality with transplant must be weighed against the improved outcomes with chemotherapy alone because of sequential dose-intensive regimens. The choice of chemotherapy versus hematopoietic stem cell transplantation (HSCT) in first remission therefore depends on prognostic factors and the availability of a suitable donor. The authors recommend matched-related or, if a sibling donor is unavailable, matched-unrelated HSCT for patients with high-risk features, including monosomy 7, *FLT3* internal tandem duplication mutation, and patients with refractory disease after two courses of induction. Allogeneic HSCT in first remission should also be considered for non-Down syndrome patients with FAB M7 morphology given recent reports of poor outcomes with this subtype. Favorable-risk patients (ie, Down syndrome M7, inv(16), t(15;17), t(8;21)) should be treated with chemotherapy alone. All other patients without high-risk features in first remission should be treated with consolidative chemotherapy alone, because multiple studies have shown equivalent outcomes compared to autologous or allogeneic transplant. For these patients without high-risk features, matched-related or matched-unrelated HSCT should be reserved for relapsed disease. An autologous transplant should be considered in second remission when there is no suitable allogeneic donor. Haploidentical transplants are still considered experimental but show promise as an alternative especially with a KIR mismatch.

Management of Relapse

The prognosis for children who do not enter remission with frontline chemotherapy or who suffer an on-therapy relapse is very poor.[199,200] Intensive reinduction therapies and HSCT for second complete remission are associated with significant treatment-related morbidity and mortality. Many different chemotherapy regimens have been evaluated in children and adults with refractory or relapsed AML. Relapse regimens that have been investigated include high-dose cytarabine with L-asparaginase or mitoxantrone, etoposide (VP-16) and amsacrine with or without azacitidine, fludarabine and cytarabine, and 2-chlorodeoxyadenosine (2-CDA). An anti-CD33 monoclonal antibody linked to the chemotherapy agent calicheamicin (gemtuzumab ozogamicin) is an effective agent but is associated with hepatic toxicity (veno-occlusive disease, or sinusoidal obstruction syndrome) in a subset of patients, particularly after HSCT.[201,202] Clofarabine is a nucleoside analog that shows promise in relapsed leukemia as monotherapy or in combination with other agents.[203,204] Other investigational agents include farnesyltransferase inhibitors, inhibitors of the mammalian target of rapamycin, kinase inhibitors, proteasome inhibitors, and epigenetic modifiers.[205]

The best predictor of response to chemotherapy after relapse is the duration of the first remission. Children who relapse within 1 year after achieving remission have a substantially lower likelihood of achieving a second remission when compared with those patients who relapse later.[206–208] The complete remission rate is 30% to 40% for the former group and 60% to 70% for the latter group. Fewer than 20% of the complete responders are projected to remain in remission for more than 2 years, unless they receive an HSCT.[208]

The projected 5-year survival rate after an allogeneic or autologous BMT in second remission is 40% to 60%.[199] Because of the higher rate of relapse after an autologous compared to an allogeneic HSCT, there is a growing experience with matched unrelated donor transplants using bone marrow or cord blood.[209,210] In selected patients (short duration of first remission or early relapse), it is reasonable to undertake an HSCT without an attempt at inducing a second remission. This is feasible only if a transplant option is immediately available and the patient is clinically stable. A second transplant for multiply relapsed AML is feasible.[211]

For relapsed patients without a matched related or unrelated donor, haploidentical transplants have become an option. Outcomes are typically worse compared to matched related transplants.[212] However, mismatch at the KIR locus has been suggested to lead to improved outcomes in haploidentical transplants owing to natural killer (NK) cell alloreactivity.[213,214] A subset of killer immunoglobulin-like receptors (KIR) expressed on NK cells will inhibit NK cell function when engaged by specific major histocompatibility (MHC) class I proteins. In HSCT, NK donor cells are thought to help eliminate recipient leukemia cells if the recipient cells do not express the cognate MHC epitope for the donor's inhibitory KIR. For matched unrelated transplants, the effect of KIR mismatch is not as clear.[214,215]

Approximately 5% of patients who achieve remission develop isolated CNS relapse.[216] Risk factors for CNS relapse include age less than 2 years, hepatosplenomegaly, CNS disease at diagnosis, high WBC, FAB M5 morphology, and chromosome 11 abnormalities. Initial CNS status does not seem to matter.[101] Outcome following CNS relapse following systemic versus local therapy was similar, and thus the rare patients with CNS relapse are typically treated with local therapy alone.[216]

FUTURE DIRECTIONS

The major challenge for the future is to continue improvement on all fronts for the care of patients with AML, including understanding the biology of the leukemic stem cell, disease classification, supportive care, development of more effective therapies, and how to deliver the optimal combination of therapy for an individual patient. Although improved over past rates, the 5-year event-free survival rate is still only approximately 50%, and a substantial portion of children with AML continue to relapse and ultimately die from their disease. The primary cause of relapse is the development of drug resistance. Newer insights into the multiple mechanisms of drug resistance are beginning to be elucidated. Not to be overlooked is the importance of optimizing supportive care, as the treatment-related mortality with AML is still substantial.[152]

In addition to new clinical trials exploring therapy timing and dose issues, investigations are ongoing with new therapeutic agents that interfere with leukemia-related biologic processes. Gemtuzumab ozogamycin is being studied in combination with conventional chemotherapy during induction and consolidation. Lestaurtinib, a small molecule inhibitor of *FLT3*, has selective toxicity against *FLT3* ITD AML cell lines and in mouse models, but cells can develop resistance to *FLT3* inhibition.[217,218] The proteasome regulates the levels of many intracellular proteins, including NF-κB, and proteasome inhibition has been effective in myeloproliferative disorders. Bortezomib is a proteasome inhibitor that has in vitro activity and synergy with chemotherapeutic agents against primary AML cell lines.[219] Regulation of epigenetic modifications with histone deacetylase and DNA methyltransferase inhibitors is also another promising area of research. Intriguing, novel efforts to screen libraries of small molecules based on their effect on gene expression signatures has yielded unexpected compounds active in promoting differentiation of AML.[220,221] Many of these new agents are being tested up-front in high-risk patients in a risk-adapted strategy and in the relapse setting.[222] Eventually, it may be possible to target the genetic lesions of leukemic cells in other AML subtypes, as exemplified by the use of all-trans-retinoic acid in APL or imatinib in chronic myelogenous leukemia. In a completely different approach, the use of NK cells has been studied as a cell-based therapy outside of HSCT. NK cells from haploidentical donors, but mismatched at the KIR locus, can be isolated and infused into recipients and expanded in vivo using a combination of immunosuppressive agents and IL-2 to provide an antileukemia effect.[223]

The improved ability to measure minimal residual disease by PCR, immunophenotyping, or specific genetic alterations, should result in giving therapy when leukemic burden is smaller and selected intensification of therapy in the presence of residual leukemia. Through the development of new agents, improved monitoring, intelligent use of biologic response modifiers, and limiting the use of BMT to high-risk patients, therapy can be closely tailored to improve outcome. For high-risk patients, the increasing availability of alternative sources of hematopoietic stem cells from unrelated bone marrow or cord blood donors will greatly expand the use of hematopoietic stem cell transplantation in all phases of therapy. Strategies based on preclinical models are also being developed that will hopefully achieve a more favorable balance of the graft-versus-host and graft-versus-leukemia reactions.[224]

SUGGESTED READINGS

Arceci RJ, Sande J, Lange B, et al: Safety and efficacy of gemtuzumab ozogamicin in pediatric patients with advanced CD33+ acute myeloid leukemia. Blood 106:1183, 2005.

Baer MR, Stewart CC, Lawrence D, et al: Expression of the neural cell adhesion molecule CD56 is associated with short remission duration and survival in acute myeloid leukemia with t(8;21)(q22;q22). Blood 90:1643, 1997.

Bonnet D, Dick JE: Human acute myeloid leukemia is organized as a hierarchy that originates from a primitive hematopoietic cell. Nat Med 3:730, 1997.

Creutzig U, Reinhardt D, Diekamp S, Dworzak M, Stary J, Zimmermann M: AML patients with Down syndrome have a high cure rate with AML-BFM therapy with reduced dose intensity. Leukemia 19:1355, 2005.

Hasle H, Alonzo TA, Auvrignon A, et al: Monosomy 7 and deletion 7q in children and adolescents with acute myeloid leukemia: An international retrospective study. Blood 2007 [epub online].

Kaspers GJ, Creutzig U: Pediatric acute myeloid leukemia: international progress and future directions. Leukemia 19:2025, 2005.

Massey GV, Zipursky A, Chang MN, et al: A prospective study of the natural history of transient leukemia (TL) in neonates with Down syndrome (DS): Children's Oncology Group (COG) study POG-9481. Blood 107:4606, 2006.

Meshinchi S, Woods WG, Stirewalt DL, et al: Prevalence and prognostic significance of Flt3 internal tandem duplication in pediatric acute myeloid leukemia. Blood 97:89, 2001.

Rao A, Hills RK, Stiller C, et al: Treatment for myeloid leukaemia of Down syndrome: Population-based experience in the UK and results from the Medical Research Council AML 10 and AML 12 trials. Br J Haematol 132:576, 2006.

Ravindranath Y, Yeager AM, Chang MN, et al, for the Pediatric Oncology Group: Autologous bone marrow transplantation versus intensive consolidation chemotherapy for acute myeloid leukemia in childhood. N Engl J Med 334:1428, 1996.

Ross ME, Mahfouz R, Onciu M, et al: Gene expression profiling of pediatric acute myelogenous leukemia. Blood 104:3679, 2004.

Rubnitz JE, Razzouk BI, Lensing S, Pounds S, Pui CH, Ribeiro RC: Prognostic factors and outcome of recurrence in childhood acute myeloid leukemia. Cancer 109:157, 2007.

Sievers EL, Lange BJ, Alonzo TA, et al: Immunophenotypic evidence of leukemia after induction therapy predicts relapse: Results from a prospective Children's Cancer Group study of 252 patients with acute myeloid leukemia. Blood 101:3398, 2003.

Smith BD, Levis M, Beran M, et al: Single-agent CEP-701, a novel FLT3 inhibitor, shows biologic and clinical activity in patients with relapsed or refractory acute myeloid leukemia. Blood 103:3669, 2004.

Tallman MS, Andersen JW, Schiffer CA, et al: All-trans retinoic acid in acute promyelocytic leukemia: Long-term outcome and prognostic factor analysis from the North American Intergroup protocol. Blood 100:4298, 2002.

Webb DK, Harrison G, Stevens RF, Gibson BG, Hann IM, Wheatley K: Relationships between age at diagnosis, clinical features, and outcome of therapy in children treated in the Medical Research Council AML 10 and 12 trials for acute myeloid leukemia. Blood 98:1714, 2001.

Woods WG, Neudorf S, Gold S, et al: A comparison of allogeneic bone marrow transplantation, autologous bone marrow transplantation, and aggressive chemotherapy in children with acute myeloid leukemia in remission. Blood 97:56, 2001.

REFERENCES

For complete list of references log onto www.expertconsult.com

CHAPTER 63

PATHOBIOLOGY OF ACUTE LYMPHOBLASTIC LEUKEMIA

Alejandro Gutierrez, Adolfo Ferrando, and A. Thomas Look

Normal lymphoid precursors undergo somatic recombination at their immunoglobulin (*Ig*) or T cell receptor (*TCR*) gene loci,[1] and the successful completion of V(D)J recombination, with the resultant formation of a functional immunoglobulin or T cell receptor, is required for the survival of lymphocyte precursors. Positive and negative selection steps ensure that only lymphocytes with immunoglobulin or T cell receptors that function appropriately within the context of an individual's immune microenvironment are allowed to proceed through the proliferation and differentiation steps required for the development of mature lymphocytes. This developmental process generates a repertoire of lymphocytes with unique variations in the antigen-recognition portions of the immunoglobulin or T cell-receptor genes, which form the foundation of a fully competent adaptive immune system that can recognize a countless variety of foreign antigens.

The acquisition of somatic genetic alterations involving oncogenes or tumor suppressors can lead to the dysregulated proliferation and clonal expansion of lymphoid precursors that is characteristic of acute lymphoblastic leukemia (ALL). Many genes that are critical to leukemogenesis have been identified through the cloning and characterization of genetic alterations induced by recurrent chromosomal translocations.[2–5] In addition, a number of translocations have prognostic significance and are used in modern ALL treatment protocols to adjust the intensity of therapy. In many cases, the malignant transformation of lymphoid cells is the result of altered expression of transcription factors that play critical roles in normal B- and T-cell development, although it may also involve the aberrant expression of otherwise quiescent genes. More recent evidence has implicated members of signal transduction pathways in leukemogenesis.[6–8] Although the incidence of specific genetic alterations in ALL varies according to patient age, evidence is accumulating that the pathogenesis underlying malignant transformation in similar genetic alterations is similar across age groups.[9,10]

FUTURE DIRECTIONS

The immediate applications of the emerging molecular information include a redefinition of risk classification schemes to emphasize the roles of somatically acquired genetic abnormalities that carry a defined prognosis and likelihood of therapeutic failure. Currently, patients are assigned to treatment according to their initial clinical features and, increasingly, the genetic and biologic properties of their leukemic cells. We are now in a position to view ALL as a group of heterogeneous diseases defined by discrete molecular lesions. As these lesions have been systematically analyzed in larger numbers of patients, it has been possible to devise new classification schemes for ALL that reflect prognosis with exquisite precision. The development of new drugs based on the molecular biology of ALL is clearly a priority for the future, and will likely take the form of compounds developed to specifically interfere with oncoproteins expressed by each patient's leukemic blasts. In addition, the discovery that several kinases play important roles in ALL pathogenesis has provided new opportunities for targeted drug development. The opportunity is now at hand to improve therapy through randomized trials coordinated on a nationwide or even worldwide scale that focus on key subsets of acute leukemia patients whose lymphoblasts harbor specific genetic abnormalities.

CLONAL ORIGIN OF LEUKEMIC LYMPHOID CELLS

Human ALL arises from a single progenitor cell that has acquired somatic genetic changes, which lead to dysregulated proliferation and differentiation arrest. The clonal origin of leukemia was first suggested by the identification of the Philadelphia chromosome in chronic myeloid leukemia.[11] Subsequently, numerous lines of

Clinical Risk Assignment in Childhood Acute Lymphoblastic Leukemia

Risk Group	Features	Recommended Therapy
Low risk	• Simultaneous trisomies of chromosomes 4, 10, and 17 • *TEL–AML1* fusion	Less intensive antimetabolite-based chemotherapy
Intermediate risk	• Standard-risk age/leukocyte count, without other genetic risk features	Intermediate antimetabolite-based chemotherapy
High risk	Presence of any of the following: • Age >10 years • T cell immunophenotype • White blood cell count >50,000 mm^{-3} • CNS leukemia	Intensified multiagent chemotherapy with cranial radiation
Very high risk	• *BCR–ABL* translocation* • *MLL* translocations†,‡ • Hypodiploidy <45 chromosomes • Induction failure or elevated minimal residual disease at the end of induction chemotherapy	Allogeneic bone marrow transplantation in first remission

*Bone marrow transplantation in first remission is clearly beneficial in *BCR–ABL*-positive ALL.

†Current evidence suggests that bone marrow transplantation in first remission may not improve outcomes for children with *MLL*-rearranged ALL.

‡Although *MLL* translocations are almost always associated with very poor outcomes, patients with T-cell ALL who have the t(11;19) MLL–ENL translocation appear to have excellent outcomes with conventional chemotherapy.

evidence have provided additional support for this theory, which is now generally accepted. Uniform structural and numerical chromosomal abnormalities are frequently demonstrated in all leukemic lymphoblasts from an individual patient. Identical rearrangements of *Ig* or *TCR* genes, which are somatic in origin, have been demonstrated in ALL cell populations.[2,12] In addition, identical patterns of X-chromosome inactivation have been demonstrated within all cells of individual patients with ALL by allelic analysis of the glucose-6-phosphate dehydrogenase gene on the X chromosome.[13] As X-inactivation occurs in early embryogenesis, before somatically acquired mutations begin to promote the transformed phenotype, this is particularly strong evidence for the clonal origin of leukemia. In addition, the methylation patterns of restriction-fragment-length polymorphisms in X-linked genes, as detected by Southern blot analysis, have been used to show that even rare ALL cases with two completely different cytogenetic clones probably arise by clonal evolution from a single transformed progenitor.[14]

LINEAGE-SPECIFIC FEATURES OF LEUKEMIC LYMPHOBLASTS

An important advance in the understanding and treatment of ALL was the realization that malignant lymphoblasts share many of the features of normal lymphoid progenitors.[15–17] Thus, ALL cells rearrange their *IG* and *TCR* genes and express components of antigen receptor molecules and other differentiation-linked cell-surface glycoproteins in ways that correspond to features of developing normal B and T lymphocytes. In many cases, leukemic cells appear to represent the clonal expansion of a lymphoid progenitor that has arrested its development at an early stage of B- or T-cell differentiation.[18] Furthermore, research continues with the goal of defining stem cell populations in lymphoblastic leukemia, such as those that have been identified in acute myeloid leukemia.[19] However, with better understanding of the normal patterns of antigen-independent lymphoid cell development, it has become clear that leukemic lymphoblasts can show asynchronous gene expression with subtle variations in phenotype.[20] Hence, it should not be surprising that in some cases of ALL, the blast cell phenotypes differ from those of normal lymphocyte progenitors, which is likely a result of aberrant regulation of gene expression. Still, the general concept that leukemic cells should be classified according to their "normal" developmental stage remains an important one, providing a basis for the study of immunophenotype-specific genetic changes.

B-Cell Acute Lymphoblastic Leukemia

The diagnosis of mature B-cell ALL is based on the detection of surface immunoglobulin on leukemic blasts. This rare phenotype accounts for only 2% to 3% of ALL cases, and the lymphoblasts generally have distinctive morphology, with deeply basophilic cytoplasm containing prominent vacuoles; this morphologic pattern is designated L3 in the French–American–British system.[21–23] Prominent clinical features include concomitant extramedullary lymphomatous masses in the abdomen or head and neck, frequent involvement of the central nervous system and cranial nerves, and tumor lysis syndrome, often complicated by acute renal failure due to uric acid nephropathy.

Acute B-cell leukemia appears to be a disseminated form of Burkitt lymphoma, as these conditions share common cytogenetic, molecular genetic, immunologic, cytologic, and clinical features.[24] Acute B-cell leukemia does not respond well to chemotherapy traditionally used for childhood ALL. However, good outcomes have been obtained with treatments designed for Burkitt lymphoma, which involve relatively brief but intensive regimens that emphasize cyclophosphamide and the rapid rotation of antimetabolites in high dosages.[25–29] Thus, B-cell leukemia is the first form of ALL to be recognized as a distinct clinical entity based on immunophenotypic and cytogenetic features, and the first to be treated by separate protocols designed specifically for the leukemia's unique features.

Pre-B and Early Pre-B Acute Lymphoblastic Leukemia

Approximately 80% of ALL patients have lymphoblasts with phenotypes corresponding to those of B-cell progenitors.[23,30] These cases can be identified on the basis of cell surface expression of CD19 and at least one other recognized B lineage-associated antigen: CD20, CD24, CD22, CD21, or CD79[23,30]; most B-lineage ALL cases also express CD10 (CALLA, or Common ALL Antigen). The lymphoblasts may also express nuclear terminal deoxynucleotidyl transferase (TdT) or CD34. Approximately one-fourth of B-progenitor ALL cases express cytoplasmic Igμ heavy-chain proteins and are designated pre-B cell ALL. Pre-B cases were originally shown to have a worse long-term response to therapy compare to early pre-B cases, an observation that was later attributed to the presence of the t(1;19) translocation that forms the *E2A–PBX1* fusion gene in approximately one-fourth of the pre-B cases.[31] However, with the introduction of more intensive, risk-adjusted treatment regimens, the prognosis for patients with t(1;19)+ ALL has improved significantly.[32,33]

DNA rearrangement of immunoglobulin (*Ig*) genes occurs before heavy-chain gene expression in B-cell development, providing a genetic marker of B-lymphocyte ontogeny. Korsmeyer and coworkers[34,35] pioneered the use of heavy- and light-chain gene rearrangements to support an early B-lineage origin of most ALL blasts. This work was extended to establish synchrony between *Ig* gene rearrangements and the expression of B lineage-restricted cell surface antigens. However, *Ig* heavy-chain gene rearrangements have also been documented in approximately 15% of T-cell ALL cases and a similar percentage of AML cases.[36–38] Thus, caution must be exercised when assigning cell lineage on the basis of studies of *Ig* gene rearrangement.

The identification of specific immunophenotypic, genetic, and clinical features that predict response to therapy in patients with B-lineage ALL, and the incorporation of these predictors into clinical decision making, is now widespread in modern ALL treatment protocols. This ability to predict outcome in these patients has been closely tied to the remarkable improvements in therapy for children with this disease, which 50 years ago was universally fatal. However, many subgroups of pediatric and adult patients face a much poorer prognosis, and much progress remains to be made.

T-Cell Acute Lymphoblastic Leukemia

Leukemias of T-cell precursors can be identified and classified according to the sequence of expression of T cell-associated surface antigens during normal thymocyte ontogeny.[39,40] In this tightly regulated process, the earliest T-cell precursors are characterized by the lack of expression of CD4 and CD8 surface markers. These double-negative (DN) thymocytes express CD7, TdT, and cytoplasmic CD3, and proceed through four different stages of development (DN1 to DN4) defined by the expression of CD44 and CD25. During the DN stages, the TCR-β gene becomes rearranged, driving the production of intermediate single-positive cells (ISPs) with a surface $CD4^+$, $CD8^-$, $sCD3^-$ phenotype. These cells then differentiate into early double-positive ($CD4^+$, $CD8^+$) cells, at which point the *TCR-α* gene rearrangement occurs. Subsequently, these DP progenitors acquire surface CD1 and then differentiate into late cortical thymocytes showing a loss of CD1 and a gain of surface CD3 expression. This thymic T-cell developmental process ends when mature $CD4^+$ or $CD8^+$ single-positive cells are produced,[40,41] although further T cell differentiation occurs in the periphery upon antigen presentation. Numerous investigators, using a battery of monoclonal antibodies specific for T-cell surface glycoproteins, have confirmed the close relationship between the recognizable patterns of surface antigen expression on leukemic T cells and the normal stages of thymocyte development.[42–45]

Lymphoblasts with a T cell phenotype comprise approximately 15% of cases of ALL. These are often associated with distinctive clinical features that include high circulating leukocyte counts, a male predominance, central nervous system involvement, and a radiographically evident thymic mass in many cases at presentation. Historically, patients with T-cell ALL had an adverse prognosis by comparison to patients with B-lineage ALL, but this gap has narrowed with the intensification of therapy for these patients.[46–48] Although several groups have associated the expression of various cell surface antigens in T cell ALL with outcome in retrospective studies,[46,47,49–51] the validation of these markers in prospective studies remains elusive, as does the identification of other clinical or genetic markers of prognosis.[52,53]

The human antigen-specific TCR molecule is a heterodimer composed of disulfide-linked α- and β-polypeptide subunits. Each of these genes undergoes site-specific recombination that generates, at the DNA level, the sequence diversity that allows a wide repertoire of antigen specificity, in a manner analogous to the *Ig* genes. Hence, rearrangement of the *TCR-α/β* genes can be used to establish clonality and lineage derivation within leukemias of T-cell progenitors. Although *TCR-β* genes are generally in a germline configuration in B-lineage leukemic cells, rearrangements at this loci can be seen in approximately 10% of B-cell ALL cases.[54,55] Clonal rearrangements of the *TCR-γ/δ* genes are even less restricted to the T-cell lineage, being observed in a significant number of B-lineage ALL cases.[56,57]

Mixed-Lineage Leukemia

Acute mixed-lineage leukemias are defined by blast cells that coexpress markers of both the lymphoid and myeloid lineages. Two distinct forms of these leukemias are recognized: those with lymphoid morphology that coexpress myeloid-associated antigen[58,59] and those with myeloid morphology and reactivity to myeloperoxidase staining that coexpress cell-surface antigens normally restricted to lymphoid cells. The origin of mixed-lineage leukemias has not been established. One possibility is malignant transformation of pluripotent hematopoietic stem or progenitor cells that retain the ability to differentiate in both the myeloid and lymphoid lineages; another is immortalization of rare progenitor cells that normally coexpress features of both lineages; and a third is aberrant gene expression as a result of specific genetic alterations.[60] There was initially considerable controversy over whether cases of lymphoid leukemia with expression of one or more myeloid cell surface antigens (eg, CD13, CD33, or CD14) had an adverse prognosis. However, most recent data suggest that the coexpression of myeloid antigens in acute lymphoblastic leukemia does not carry an adverse prognosis in the setting of contemporary treatment regiments.[61–63] The expression of lymphoid markers in predominantly myeloid leukemias is relatively rare, and although some studies reported an adverse effect of T-lymphoid markers on outcomes,[64] more recent analyses did not demonstrate a significant prognostic value to lymphoid antigen expression in AML.[65]

GENETIC BASIS OF LYMPHOID LEUKEMIA

Multiple acquired genetic abnormalities are responsible for the aberrant proliferation and differentiation arrest characteristic of ALL. These include chromosomal rearrangements detectable by conventional cytogenetics, as well as lesions that are evident only by molecular analysis. The ability to identify these changes, and the discovery that many of these can be used to predict response to therapy, has led to risk-adapted therapy for ALL. It is worth noting that the vast majority of patients with leukemia have normal constitutional karyotypes, indicating that the genetic abnormalities in ALL lymphoblasts are usually acquired somatically, and thus are restricted to the malignant clone.

Chromosomal translocations are found in 75% of ALL cases (Fig. 63–1).[22,66] They can be broadly classified as recurrent lineage-restricted abnormalities, which account for approximately two-thirds of the translocations in ALL, or as "random" translocations, which have been identified only in single or very small numbers of cases. The characterization of genes that span the breakpoints of recurrent translocations has allowed the identification of genes that play critical roles in leukemogenesis.[3–5]

Central Role of Transcription Factors

Molecular studies on recurrent chromosomal translocations in ALL have demonstrated a central role for the aberrant expression of transcription factors in the pathobiology of leukemia (Table 63–1). The dysregulated expression of these transcription factors, which are often functionally normal, leads to an abnormal proliferation and differentiation arrest of leukemic lymphoid and myeloid progenitors.[3–5] Conserved amino acid sequence motifs within the sequence-specific DNA-binding domains of these nuclear trans-activating proteins allow them to be grouped into families that in many cases, appear to be involved in similar regulatory processes. Thus, the transcription factor genes in Table 63–1 are grouped according to shared structural features of their DNA-binding domains: basic region helix–loop–helix (bHLH), cysteine-rich (LIM), homeodomain (HOX), basic region–leucine zipper (bZIP), zinc-finger, A-T hook minor groove, ETS-like, or runt homology. Another important association is the lineage restriction of transcription factor genes affected by specific chromosomal translocations, suggesting that the proteins they encode disrupt the differentiation of specific lymphoid progenitors. This interpretation implicates a central role for transcription factors in the initiation of leukemia, and suggests that the normal developmental programs of progenitor cells of different lineages are controlled by different regulatory programs.

Rabbitts[67] has aptly described a key group of regulatory transcription factors as the products of "master genes." In his model, the nuclear proteins encoded by these genes act positively to upregulate critical target genes or negatively to interfere with normal regulatory pathways. The net effect is disruption of gene regulatory cascades that control and coordinate the expression of large numbers of proteins required for completion of lymphoid cell differentiation programs. Disruption of transcription factors in leukemic blasts occurs by at least two distinct mechanisms: the dysregulated expression of intact genes and the creation of chimeric transcription factors.

Developmental Biology of Oncogenic Transcription Factors

A surprising connection has emerged from studies of oncogenic transcription factors and the developmental proteins regulating segmentation in *Drosophila*, as the DNA-binding domains of these proteins often show striking homology. The proteins participating in leukemogenesis interfere with a highly regulated network of hematopoietic transcription factors leading to arrested cell development at stages corresponding to those of early lymphoid or myeloid progenitors. Recent evidence implicating the major *HOX* genes in the control of hematopoiesis as well as embryogenesis, together with the established roles of *Drosophila* segmentation genes in controlling *HOM-C* gene expression, suggests that the *HOX* loci may serve as proximal targets of a wide spectrum of hybrid and dysregulated transcription factors in the acute leukemias.[5] In this model, the oncogenic transcription factors inappropriately activate or suppress the expression of *HOX* genes, which in turn regulate gene programs with pleiotropic effects on normal hematopoietic cell development.

The mechanisms that lead to the activation of oncogenic transcription factors in ALL tend to vary according to the ALL subtype. In mature B-cell ALL and in T-cell ALL, genetic lesions that lead to the aberrant expression of structurally intact genes predominate, whereas the chromosomal translocations that often occur in B-precursor ALL generally lead to the formation of chimeric proteins, which are produced as a result of the translocation-induced fusion of the coding sequence of 2 genes.

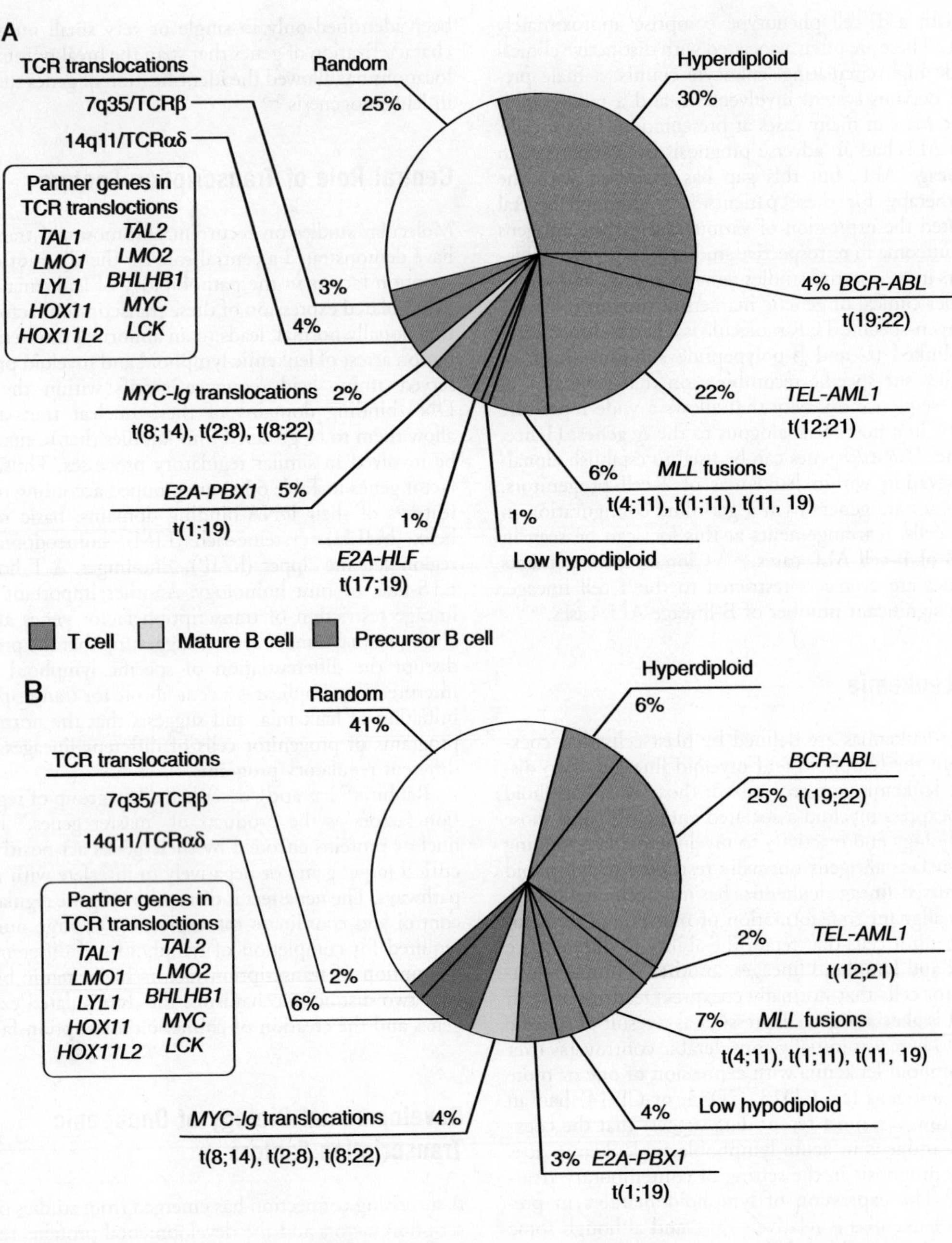

Figure 63–1 Frequency of the major chromosomal translocations in **(A)** pediatric and **(B)** adult ALL. The genes affected by chromosomal translocation are shown in boldface type. TCR translocations in T-ALL can activate a number of different protooncogenes as shown in the insert, including *TAL1, LMO1/2, HOX11, HOX11L2,* and *MYC.*

Dysregulated Expression of Structurally Intact Genes

Activation of MYC in B-Cell Acute Lymphoblastic Leukemia

The vast majority of cases of mature B-cell ALL and Burkitt lymphoma are characterized by a translocation that places one allele of *MYC* from chromosome 8 under the control of the regulatory elements of an *Ig* gene, either the heavy-chain gene on chromosome 14q32 or the κ or λ light-chain genes on chromosomes 2 and 22. This leads to the aberrant expression of *MYC*, a prototypical basic helix–loop–helix oncogenic transcription factor.[68–76] In the predominant t(8;14) translocation, the involved *MYC* locus is translocated into the heavy-chain gene on chromosome 14, adjacent to the coding sequences of the *Ig* constant region.[68–70] The coding sequences of the *Ig* variable region generally are reciprocally translocated to the distal tip of chromosome 8. In variant translocations, the *MYC* gene remains on chromosome 8, and portions of the respective light-chain genes are translocated to that chromosome downstream of the *MYC* locus.[71–75]

Although the *MYC* coding region is not structurally altered by translocation in most cases of B-cell ALL/Burkitt lymphoma, point mutations in the N-terminal phosphorylation domain of *MYC* commonly arise in these tumors at codons 58 or 62.[77–79] These codons are phosphorylation sites involved in the regulation of the activation and degradation of the protein,[80] and these mutations lead not only to the aberrant stabilization of MYC protein[81–83] but also inhibit the ability of MYC to activate the proapoptotic *BIM* gene, although its ability to stimulate proliferation remains intact.[84]

Table 63–1 Transcription Genes Affected by Chromosomal Breakpoints in the Acute Lymphoblastic Leukemias

Family*	Translocation	Affected Gene	Disease
Basic helix–loop–helix (bHLH) proteins	t(8;14)(q24;q32)	*MYC*	Burkitt
	t(2;8)(p12;q24)	*MYC*	lymphoma
	t(8;22)(q24;q11)	*MYC*	and B-cell ALL
	t(8;14)(q24;q11)	*MYC*	T-cell ALL
	t(7;19)(q35;p13)	*LYL1*	T-cell ALL
	t(1;14)(p32;q11)	*TAL1*	T-cell ALL
	t(7;9)(q35;q34)	*TAL2*	T-cell ALL
	t(14;21)(q11.2;q22)	*BHLHB1*	T-cell ALL
Cysteine-rich (LIM) proteins	t(11;14)(p15;q11)	*LMO1*	T-cell ALL
	t(11;14)(p13;q11)	*LMO2*	T-cell ALL
	t(7;11)(q35;p13)	*LMO2*	T-cell ALL
Homeodomain (HOX) proteins	t(10;14)(q24;q11)	*HOX11*	T-cell ALL
	t(7;10)(q35;q24)	*HOX11*	T-cell ALL
	t(5;14)(q35;q32.2)	*HOX11L2*	T-cell ALL
	t(1;19)(q23;p13)	*E2A–PBX1*	Pre-B-cell ALL
Basic-region/leucine-zipper (bZIP) proteins	t(17;19)(q22;p13)	*E2A–HLF*	EPB ALL
A–T hook minor groove binding proteins†	t(4;11)(q21;q23)	*MLL–AF4*	EPB ALL
	t(11;19)(q23;p13.3)	*MLL–ENL*	ALL or AML
ETS-like (TEL, ERG) proteins	t(12;21)(p13;q22)	*TEL–AML1*	ALL
Runt homology (AML1)	t(12;21)(p13;q22)	*TEL–AML1*	ALL

ALL, acute lymphoblastic leukemia; AML, acute myeloid leukemia; EPB, early pre-B.
*Based on the DNA-binding domain.
†Partial list of MLL fusions.

The mechanisms by which *MYC* exerts its potent growth-promoting effects are complex and only partially understood. *MYC* is estimated to regulate the expression of 15% of the genome,[85] and leads to the transcriptional activation of a large number of genes involved in cell division, growth, metabolism, adhesion, and motility,[86] although it also leads to the transcriptional repression of many other genes, such as the cell cycle inhibitors *p27* and *p21*. Many experts currently believe that the potent effects of *MYC* are mediated by relatively subtle effects on a large number of target genes and networks, rather than by large effects on a small number of targets. *MYC* exerts its transcriptional activity via the formation of heterodimers with its DNA-binding partner protein MAX. MYC : MAX heterodimers bind to canonical hexameric E-box DNA sequences (5′-CACGTG-3′) where they activate transcription.[87] MAX can also heterodimerize with other bHLHZip proteins, including MAD,[88] MXI-1 (MAD2),[89] and MNT.[90] Whereas transcriptional activation by MYC : MAX complexes promotes proliferation, binding by MAD : MAX and other MAX heterodimers produces opposite effects; for example, MAD inhibits MYC function both by competing with MYC for binding to MAX and by directly inhibiting transcription.

BHLH, LIM, and HOX Genes in T-Cell Acute Lymphoblastic Leukemia

In leukemias with a T-cell phenotype, chromosomal breakpoints consistently involve the *TCR* enhancer (7q34) or the *TCRα/δ* enhancer (14q11), both of which are highly active in committed T-cell progenitors and can cause dysregulated expression of transcription factor genes located at the breakpoint on the reciprocal chromosome involved in these phenotype-specific rearrangements.[91] The affected transcription factors include (a) genes encoding basic helix–loop–helix (bHLH) family members, such as *TAL1*,[92,93] *TAL2*,[94] *LYL1*,[95] *MYC*,[96–98] and *BHLHB1*[99]; (b) LIM-only domain (*LMO*) genes, such as *LMO1* and *LMO2*[100]; and (c) the orphan homeobox genes *HOX11* and *HOX11L2*.[37,101–106] The observation that T-ALL oncogenes act as master transcriptional regulators during the embryologic development of specific organ systems suggests that their aberrant expression in T-cell precursors may contribute to the onset of leukemia by disrupting the mechanisms that control cell proliferation, differentiation, and survival during the discrete steps of normal T-cell development. Gene expression profiling and mutational analyses have shown that cases of T-ALL can be separated into five subtypes according to the pattern of multistep genetic abnormalities that occur (Fig. 63–2).

The best characterized of the oncogenic transcription factors involved in T-ALL is *TAL1* (also known as *SCL*), which is altered by the t(1;14) or by site-specific deletions in approximately one-fourth of childhood T-ALL cases.[107–112] *TAL1* is aberrantly expressed in the leukemic cells of 60% of children and 45% of adults with T-ALL, and its expression is required for maintenance of the leukemic phenotype in human cell culture studies.[113] TAL1 acts as a master regulatory protein during early hematopoietic development and is required for the generation of all blood cell lineages.[114,115] However, it does not seem to be required for the generation and function of hematopoietic stem cells during adult hematopoiesis.[116] This class II basic helix–loop–helix (bHLH) transcription factor binds to DNA by forming heterodimers with class I bHLH factors such as E2A.[117] Although TAL1 binding to promoter sites that are normally occupied by TAL1, E2A, or HEB can lead to either repression or activation of transcription,[113] TAL1 appears to exert its leukemogenic effects largely via the inhibition of E2A activity.[118] The observation that loss of E2A function induces T-cell leukemias in mice,[119,120] and that the DNA-binding domain of TAL1 is dispensable for transformation in transgenic mouse models,[121] gives additional support to the notion that TAL1-mediated inhibition of E2A plays a central role in its pathogenesis in T-ALL.

The LIM-only domain genes, *LMO1/RBTN1/TTG1* and *LMO2/RBTN2/TTG2*,[100,122,123] encode proteins that possess duplicated cysteine-rich LIM domains involved in protein–protein interactions. LMO2 interacts with TAL1 in erythroid cells and in T-cell leukemias.[124–126] Moreover, homozygous disruption of *LMO2* in mice causes the same phenotype as described above for *TAL1* knockouts, indicating that a multiprotein complex is required for normal hematopoietic development that involves LMO2, TAL1, and other

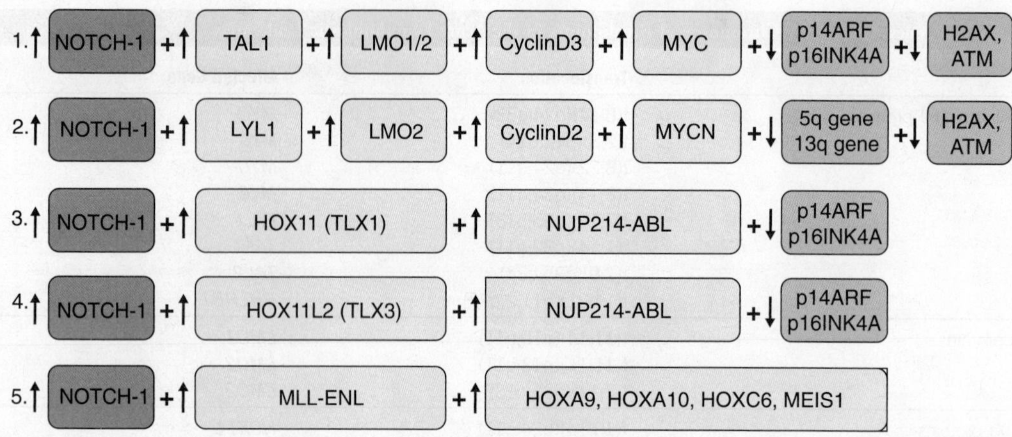

Figure 63–2 Multistep oncogenic pathways in T-cell ALL. Gene expression profiling and mutation analyses have revealed that five different multistep molecular pathways can lead to the malignant transformation of developing thymocytes. *NOTCH1* mutations are seen in samples from all five T-ALL subtypes. *HOX11, HOX11L2,* and *TAL1*-overexpressing cases show high levels of *MYC* expression and share the loss of the tumor suppressor genes *p16/INK4A* and *p14/ARF* on chromosome 9p. *HOX11* and *HOX11L2* are often associated with a novel *NUP214–ABL* episomal fusion gene, which may render these T-ALLs sensitive to imatinib. *LYL1*+ cases show high levels of expression of *N-MYC* and frequently have deletions affecting as yet unidentified loci on chromosomal arms 5q and 13q. Finally, *MLL–ENL*+ cases have a clearly distinct gene expression profile characterized by low expression of *MYC* and other genes involved in cell growth and proliferation, but high expression of *HOXA9, HOXA10,* and *HOXC6* in concert with the HOX gene regulator *MEIS1*. Adapted from Armstrong SA, Look AT: Molecular genetics of acute lymphoblastic leukemia. J Clin Oncol 23:6306, 2005, with permission.

proteins such as GATA1.[127–130] In addition, overexpression of *LMO1* or *LMO2* in thymocytes of transgenic mice leads to T-cell lymphomas, recapitulating human T-cell tumors,[131–135] and accelerates the onset of leukemias in *TAL1* transgenic mice lines.[126]

The homeodomain gene *HOX11*, located on chromosome 10, band 24, is one of the more interesting proteins activated by translocation into the vicinity of the *TCR* loci.[37,102,104–106] *HOX11* is the founding member of a family of *HOX* genes that includes *HOX11L1* and *HOX11L2*[106] and whose family members are characterized by the presence of a threonine in the third helix of the homeodomain, which confers specific DNA-binding properties. *HOX11* was originally isolated from the recurrent t(10;14)(q24;q11) in T-ALL[37,102,104,105] and is aberrantly expressed in 5% of pediatric and up to 30% of adult T-ALL cases.[101,136,137] The relatively low frequency translocations involving the *HOX11* locus on 10q24, 2% to 5% in childhood T-ALL[105] and 14% in adult cases,[138] suggest that alternative mechanisms leading to *HOX11* overexpression account for the activation of this transcription factor oncogene in a significant fraction of T-ALL cases.

Like other *HOX* genes, *HOX11* plays an important role in embryonic development, and functions as a master transcriptional regulator necessary for the genesis of the spleen.[139,140] In the mouse embryo, *Hox11* expression can be detected in the branchial arches, restricted areas of the hindbrain and the splenic primordium,[141,142] where it is required for the survival of early splenic progenitors.[140] The *HOX11* oncogenic transcription factor is associated with T-cell leukemogenesis at the early cortical thymocyte stage and relies on specific homeodomain–DNA interactions for its leukemogenic effects.[143] In addition, *HOX11* also directly interacts with the catalytic subunits of the serine/threonine phosphatases PP2A and PPA, which mediate disruption of the G2/M cell-cycle checkpoint.[144]

A second *HOX11* family member, *HOX11L2*, has also been implicated in the pathogenesis of human T-ALL through characterization of the t(5;14)(q35;q32), a cryptic chromosomal rearrangement detectable only by fluorescence in situ hybridization or by chromosome painting techniques.[103] This translocation leads to the ectopic expression of *HOX11L2*, possibly by bringing it under the influence of regulatory elements in the *CTIP2/BCL11B* gene, which is highly expressed during T-lymphoid differentiation. In contrast to the predominance of *HOX11* expression in adult T-ALL cases, both the t(5;14) and expression of *HOX11L2* can be detected in 20% to 25% of children but in only 5% of adults with T-ALL.[101,137,145–147] The role of HOX11L2 as a master transcriptional regulator upstream of important pathways involved in cell fate determination is supported by its importance during embryonic development.[148] In mice, *Hox11l2* expression is essential for normal development of the ventral medullary respiratory center.[148] Mice deficient in this protein die soon after birth as a result of respiratory failure that resembles congenital central hypoventilation syndrome in humans.

HOX11 and HOX11L2 are closely related in structure, and have a high degree of homology at the amino acid level, especially in the homeobox domain, where their sequences differ by only three amino acids. The high level of structural homology in their DNA-binding domains supports the hypothesis that HOX11 and HOX11L2 may induce T-ALL through regulation of the same transcriptional targets. However, activation of *HOX11* and *HOX11L2* seem to be associated with clinically relevant differences that may result, at least in part, from differences in their mechanisms of action. The expression of HOX11 is associated with a favorable prognosis both in children and in adults.[17,91,136] On the other hand, reports on the prognostic significance of *HOX11L2* expression in T-ALL show conflicting results,[17,145,147,149] and in the absence of more definitive data, it would appear prudent to avoid incorporating *HOX11L2* expression into treatment algorithms.

Recently, the analysis of gene expression profiling using oligonucleotide microarrays has shown that the expression of different transcription factor oncogenes such as *TAL1, LYL1, HOX11* and *HOX11L2* is associated with distinct gene expression profiles. These unique signatures resemble those of thymocytes blocked at discrete stages of T-cell development (Fig. 63–3),[17] and suggest that transcription factor oncogenes contribute to the pathogenesis of T-ALL by interfering with critical regulatory networks that control cell proliferation, survival, and differentiation during T-cell development.[17] On the basis of the patterns of aberrant gene expression, human cases of T-ALL can be classified into five different subtypes (see Fig. 63–2).

HOXA Cluster Translocations in T-Cell Acute Lymphoblastic Leukemia

A recurrent inversion on chromosome 7 that places the *HOXA* cluster in the vicinity of the T cell-receptor beta gene regulatory elements, and that leads to activation of the entire *HOXA* cluster, was recently discovered in approximately 5% of cases of T-ALL.[150,151] Many of these cases also carried cooperating oncogenic lesions consisting of *NOTCH1* gene mutations and deletions of 9p21.[152] This new trans-

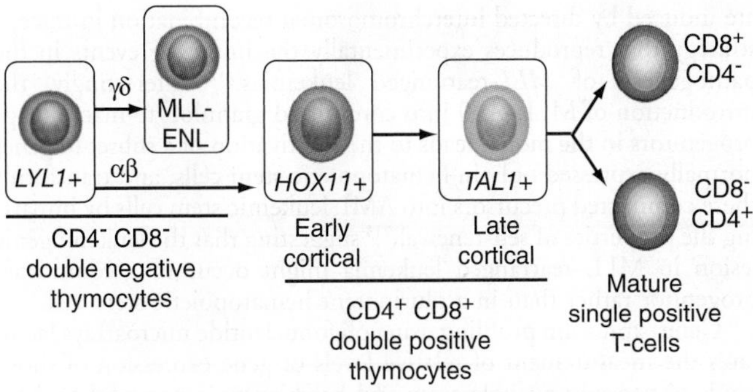

Figure 63–3 Thymocyte development is a tightly regulated process in which progenitor cells undergo sequential stages of differentiation, proliferation, lineage commitment, and selection that result in the production of functionally competent mature T cells. Microarray gene expression profiling shows that T-ALL lymphoblasts expressing high levels of the LYL1 transcription factor oncogene undergo an early arrest at the double-negative thymocyte ($CD4^-$, $CD8^-$) stage of development. In T-ALL cases with aberrant expression of HOX11, the leukemic cells show a developmental arrest at the double-positive ($CD4^+$, $CD8^+$) early cortical stage of thymocyte differentiation, whereas those with aberrant expression of TAL1 are arrested at the double-positive late cortical stage. T-ALL cells with expression of the *MLL–ENL* fusion gene are characterized by an early arrest of differentiation with a gene expression signature that indicates commitment to the gamma-delta lineage. Adapted from Ferrando AA, Neuberg DS, Staunton J, et al: Gene expression signatures define novel oncogenic pathways in T cell acute lymphoblastic leukemia. Cancer Cell 1:75, 2002, and Ferrando AA, Armstrong SA, Newberg DS, et al: Gene expression signatures in MLL-rearranged T-lineage and β-precursor acute leukemia: dominance of HOX dysregulation. Blood 102:262, 2003, with permission.

location that directly activates *HOXA* gene expression provides additional evidence for the role of aberrant *HOXA* activation in leukemogenesis and in the pathogenesis of *MLL-* and *CALM–AF10*-rearranged leukemias.

Other Genes Activated by Translocation

Transcription factors are not the only genes activated by translocation to the sites of the *IG* or *TCR* genes. In cases of B-precursor ALL carrying the t(5;14), for example, the *IL-3* gene is activated by juxtaposition with the *IG* heavy-chain locus.[153,154] Similarly, relocation to the *TCRB* locus activates expression of the *LCK* tyrosine kinase genes in T-ALL cases with the t(1;7).[155–157]

Chimeric Transcription Factor Genes

Formation of chimeric proteins whose functional domains come from two normally separate genes represents a second mechanism of aberrant transcription factor activation, which is more prevalent in B-precursor ALL. These chromosomal translocations result in the production of a chimeric protein by fusing the DNA-binding, dimerization, and trans-activation regions of discrete genes. This process is facilitated by the molecular structure of transcription factors, in which discrete coding regions of each gene encode particular functional domains; this molecular structure likely arose for evolutionary reasons.

E2A–PBX1 Fusion Genes in Pre-B Cell Acute Lymphoblastic Leukemia

A well-known example of a chimeric transcription factor with oncogenic potential is the *E2A–PBX1* rearrangement, which results from the t(1;19)(q23;p13) chromosomal translocation present in approximately 5% of all B-lineage ALLs and in 25% of cases with a pre-B (cytoplasmic immunoglobulin-positive) phenotype.[32,91,158] This translocation fuses the transactivation domain of the *E2A* transcription factor on chromosome 19 to a homeobox gene (*PBX1*) on chromosome 1, leading to the expression of several forms of hybrid E2A–PBX1 oncoproteins.[159–161] *PBX1* is related to the *Drosophila exd* gene, a homeobox gene that plays a role in lymphocyte development.[162,163] The hybrid proteins resulting from the t(1;19) retain the amino-terminal trans-activation domains of E2A (AD1 and AD2), but not the bHLH DNA-binding or protein interaction domain.[160,161,164] The bHLH domain is replaced by the homeobox DNA-binding domain of PBX1, enabling the fusion protein to function as a chimeric transcription factor.[165–167]

The transforming potential of *E2A–PBX1* was first demonstrated by the rapid induction of AML in lethally irradiated mice repopulated with bone marrow stem cells that had been infected with recombinant retroviruses containing *E2A–PBX1* genes.[168] The fusion has also been shown to transform NIH-3T3 fibroblasts and induce T-cell lymphomas in transgenic mice.[169,170] Additional studies have shown that deletion of one of the E2A activation domains diminishes its transforming activity, whereas deletion of the PBX1 homeodomain has no effect.[170,171] However, the homeodomain and flanking sequences are required for interactions with other HOX proteins and for optimal binding of E2A–PBX1 to specific DNA sequences.[172–176] It thus appears that complex interactions between E2A–PBX1 and other HOX proteins target the fusion protein to specific target genes whose activation is critical to lymphoid cell transformation. The presence of the *E2A–PBX1* translocation was originally associated with poor prognosis.[31] However, this translocation no longer imparts an adverse prognosis in the setting of modern risk-adjusted protocols for childhood ALL.[32,177–179]

E2A–HLF Fusion Genes in Early Pre-B Acute Lymphoblastic Leukemia

The t(17;19) is a rare recurrent chromosomal translocation that fuses the amino-terminal transactivation domains of E2A to the C-terminal DNA binding and dimerization domains of HLF,[180,181] which belongs to the PAR subfamily of bZIP transcription factors. Although E2A–HLF can bind DNA either as a homodimer or as a heterodimer with HLF and related proteins, no other PAR proteins are expressed in hematopoietic cells, and the E2A–HLF fusion binds DNA as a homodimer in cells harboring the t(17;19). Like E2A–PBX1, E2A–HLF can transform NIH–3T3 fibroblasts, a process that requires the HLF leucine zipper domain and the E2A transactivation domains.[182] E2A–HLF can also induce lymphoid tumors in transgenic mice.[183]

A major consequence of the activation of E2A–HLF in lymphoid precursors is dysregulation of the mechanisms that control programmed cell death in lymphoid progenitors. Expression of a dominant-negative form of E2A–HLF in t(17;19)-carrying cell lines blocks E2A–HLF function and results in apoptosis.[184] In normal pro-B lymphocytes, expression of E2A–HLF reversed IL-3-dependent and p53-induced apoptosis. HLF is the mammalian homologue of the nematode protein ces-2, which regulates the death of specific nerve cells in *Caenorhabditis elegans*.[184–186] Ces-2 is necessary for the death of the sister cells of a specific pair of serotonergic neurons during worm development. Ces-2 induces apoptosis by inhibiting the expression of *ces-1*, a prosurvival gene that normally inhibits programmed cell death by antagonizing the activity of the proapoptotic factor *egl-1*. This pathway, which is highly conserved through evolution, is disrupted by E2A–HLF fusion. Thus, in contrast to the proapoptotic role of ces-2 in the worm via repression of ces-1, E2A–HLF blocks apoptosis by inducing the expression of *SLUG*, a *ces-1* homologue normally responsible for protecting hematopoietic progenitors from DNA-damage-induced apoptosis.[187–190]

The t(17;19) is seen in less than 1% of ALL cases, typically occurs in adolescents, and is associated with disseminated intravascular coagulation and hypercalcemia at diagnosis. The t(17;19) seems to impart unfavorable prognosis, because each of seven patients whose blasts expressed *E2A–HLF* died of leukemia despite aggressive therapy.[91] It seems likely that resistance to chemotherapy in these cases is mediated by the role of E2A–HLF in driving the expression of *SLUG* and inhibiting apoptosis.[190]

MLL Fusion Genes

Translocations involving chromosome 11 band q23 occur in approximately 80% of infant ALL cases, 5% of AML cases, and 85% of secondary AML cases that occur in patients treated with topoisomerase II inhibitors.[91] The gene bisected by 11q23 translocations is designated *MLL* (also known as *HTRX* or *ALL-1*) and encodes a protein that shares significant sequence homology with trithorax, a *Drosophila* regulator of homeobox gene function during fly embryogenesis.[191–194] Trithorax regulates homeobox genes in the *Antennapedia* and *Bithorax* complexes of the fly and is required for normal head, thorax, and abdomen development.[195] The MLL protein shares three regions of homology with trithorax, including two central zinc-finger domains and a 210-amino acid C-terminal SET domain. Interestingly, a SET domain is also found in the *Drosophila* enhancer of zeste protein that, like trithorax, regulates genes in the *Antennapedia* and *Bithorax* complexes.[196] The *MLL* SET domain contains a histone H3/lysine 4 methyl transferase activity that plays a critical role in the regulation of *HOX* gene expression.[197] Other structural features of *MLL* include three A-T hook domains near the N terminus that are thought to bind the minor groove of DNA in AT-rich regions, and a 47-amino acid region of homology with the noncatalytic domains of human DNA methyltransferase.[198,199] MLL localization and stability depend on proteolytic posttranslational processing by Taspase1, a specialized protease that cleaves the MLL protein into N-terminal and C-terminal fragments that remain associated through intramolecular protein–protein interaction domains.[200–202]

Translocation breakpoints cluster in an 8.5-kilobase region of *MLL* between exons 5 and 11 and fuse the N-terminal region of *MLL*, containing the A-T hook and methyltransferase domains, to a variety of partner proteins. Although the role of each partner protein in leukemogenesis has not been fully determined, it appears that at least some of them may contribute functional domains to the fusion. For example, the t(4;11), t(9;11), and t(11;19)(q23;p13.3) fuse *MLL* to *AF-4*, *AF-9*, and *ENL*, respectively. All three of these partners are small serine- or proline-rich proteins with nuclear localization signals, suggesting that they may function as transcriptional transactivators. An unrelated gene, *ELL*, is fused to *MLL* by the t(11;19)(q23;p13.1).[203,204] *ELL* was also independently isolated as an RNA polymerase II elongation factor.[205] Still other partners seem to have no transcriptional activity but to contribute a dimerization domain to the fusion protein that results in homo-oligomerization of the N-terminal portion of MLL.[206,207]

Homologous recombination techniques have recently been used to create mice lacking one or both copies of *Mll*, the murine homologue of *MLL*. *Mll* heterozygous mice demonstrated the effects of haploinsufficiency, including anemia, thrombocytopenia, and reduced numbers of B lymphocytes. The mice also showed homeotic transformations of the cervical, thoracic, and lumbar regions that reflected shifts in the pattern of *Hox* gene expression, establishing a crucial role for *Mll* in *Hox* gene regulation. These results are consistent with other data suggesting a role for *Hox* genes in normal hematopoiesis. Mice with homozygous inactivation of *Mll* died in utero and lacked *Hox* gene expression, further supporting a key role for *Mll* in *Hox* regulation.

Formal proof that *MLL* fusions play a critical role in the development of leukemias has come from the generation of murine models of *MLL*-induced leukemias. Chimeric mice harboring a *MLL–AF9* fusion gene generated by homologous recombination developed leukemias with a latency of 4 to 12 months.[208] Retroviral transduction of *MLL–ENL*, *MLL–ELL*, and *MLL–CBP* fusion genes in hematopoietic precursors induces transformation upon transplantation into recipient mice.[209–211] Similar results were recently obtained with a model in which chromosomal translocations involving the *Mll* locus are induced by directed interchromosomal recombination in mice, a strategy that reproduces experimentally the initiating events in the pathogenesis of *MLL*-rearranged leukemias.[212] Interestingly, the introduction of MLL–AF9 into committed granulocyte-macrophage progenitors in the mouse leads to the reactivation of a subset of genes normally expressed only in hematopoietic stem cells, and transforms these committed precursors into AML leukemic stem cells by imparting the properties of self-renewal,[213] suggesting that the leukemogenic lesion in MLL–rearranged leukemia might occur in a committed progenitor rather than in a pluripotent hematopoietic stem cell.

Gene expression profiling using oligonucleotide microarrays facilitates the measurement of relative levels of gene expression of thousands of genes in a single assay and has became a powerful tool for the molecular characterization of human malignancies. The analysis of gene expression profiles using DNA arrays in *MLL*-rearranged B-lineage leukemias has shown that these tumors have a characteristic gene expression signature that includes the upregulation of several *HOX* genes and the expression of numerous myeloid markers.[214–216] Both early B- and T-cell ALLs with MLL rearrangements showed a characteristic upregulation of specific *HOX* genes, including *HOXA9*, *HOXA10*, *HOXC6*, and the *HOX* gene regulator *MEIS1*.[214–216] These results, together with the demonstration that HOXA9 plays important roles in the transformation of hematopoietic precursors by MLL fusion oncogenes in murine leukemia models,[217,218] emphasize the central role of *HOX* gene dysregulation in the pathogenesis of *MLL*-rearranged leukemias. In addition, as discussed later in this chapter, overexpression or activating mutations of the *FLT3* receptor tyrosine kinase are frequent in *MLL*-rearranged leukemias,[214,215,219,220] and a model of the multistep pathogenesis of *MLL*-rearranged ALL is depicted in Fig. 63–4.

The presence of MLL rearrangements is associated with dismal outcomes despite aggressive chemotherapy in most cases of ALL.[23,221–223] Additionally, bone marrow transplantation in first remission in these patients is not clearly beneficial, and may actually be associated with a decrease in event-free and overall survival when compared to chemotherapy alone.[223,224] One notable exception is the t(11;19) translocation in T cell ALL in particular. Although this translocation represents a poor prognostic indicator in patients with B-precursor ALL, the largest series published to date demonstrated a surprisingly good outcome in patients with T cell ALL with this translocation.[225]

CALM–AF10 Fusion Gene in T-Cell Acute Lymphoblastic Leukemia

The t(10;11)(p13;q14) detected in approximately 3% to 10% of T-ALL cases and in occasional AML cases results in the fusion of *CALM*, encoding a protein with high homology to the murine clathrin assembly protein ap3, with *AF10*, a gene identified as an MLL partner in the MLL–AF10 fusion resulting from the t(10;11)(p13;q23).[226] Although the mechanism of action of CALM–AF10 remains incompletely understood, the expression of this fusion transcript has been associated with early arrest in T-cell development and to differentiation into the gamma–delta lineage in T-ALL.[227] In addition, recent evidence suggests that aberrant upregulation of HOX gene expression appears to be involved in CALM–AF10-mediated leukemogenesis, at least in acute myeloid leukemia cells that carry this translocation.[228] Interestingly, analysis of a mouse model of CALM–AF10-induced acute myeloid leukemia suggests that the leukemia stem cell in this model has lymphoid characteristics, and cells from human patients with AML can be identified that have similar characteristics to the disease-propagating cell in this animal model.[229]

TEL–AML1 (ETV6–RUNX1) Fusion Gene in Early Pre-B Acute Lymphoblastic Leukemia

Although most t(12;21) translocations cannot be detected by standard cytogenetic analysis, this translocation is detectable by molecular

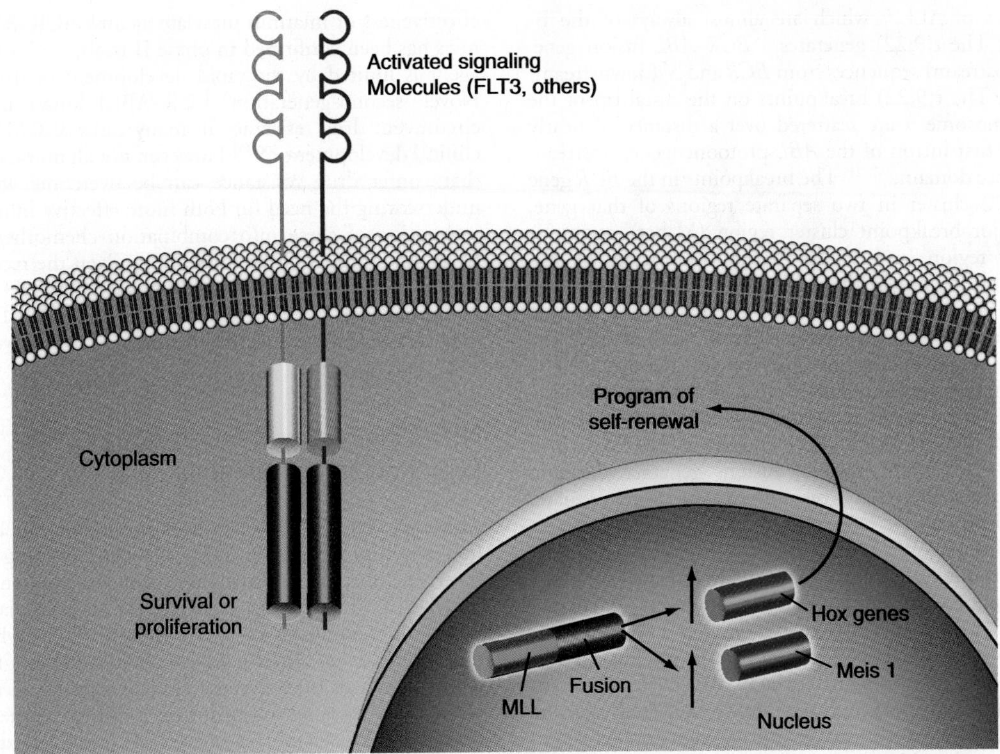

Figure 63–4 Multistep pathogenesis of *MLL*-rearranged ALL. MLL translocations induce self-renewal in hematopoietic progenitors as a first step in leukemogenesis. The presence of FLT3 mutations in *MLL*-rearranged ALLs support activation of FLT3 or other kinases as cooperating events in this disease. Clinical trials designed to assess the efficacy of FLT3 inhibitors in *MLL*-rearranged ALL are being developed. Adapted from Armstrong SA, Look AT: Molecular genetics of acute lymphoblastic leukemia. J Clin Oncol 23:6306, 2005, with permission.

techniques in approximately 25% of childhood B-lineage ALL, which makes this the most common genetic lesion in pediatric ALL.[91] The *TEL–AML1* translocation often arises prenatally and is probably the initiating mutation in ALL, as evidenced by the identification of identical *TEL–AML1* translocations in identical twins with concordant ALL,[230] and in retrospectively analyzed neonatal blood specimens of children diagnosed with ALL.[231] However, *TEL–AML1* is insufficient in causing leukemia, because the incidence of detectable *TEL–AML1* fusions in the blood of normal newborns is approximately 100-fold greater than the incidence of leukemia.[232]

The molecular mechanisms mediating *TEL–AML1*-induced leukemogenesis remain poorly understood. This fusion gene encodes a chimeric protein that contains the helix–loop–helix (HLH) domain of *TEL* fused to nearly all of *AML1* (also known as *RUNX1* or *CBFA2*), including both the transactivation domain and the DNA- and protein-binding Runt homology domain. Both of these genes are found in other leukemia-related translocations, and both are essential for normal hematopoiesis. *TEL* was first identified in the t(5;12) in chronic myelomonocytic leukemia, where it is fused to the platelet-derived growth factor receptor gene (*PDGFRB*), and is also fused to *ABL*, *MN1*, and *EVI1* in AML, and to *JAK2* in T-ALL.[233] The role of TEL in hematopoiesis has been demonstrated with a conditional mouse model in which the absence of TEL in early development leads to the absence of fetal hematopoiesis. Interestingly, the inactivation of TEL in adult mice leads to the selective loss of hematopoietic stem cells from adult bone marrow, whereas hematopoiesis is sustained by committed precursors.[234] Most *TEL–AML1* leukemias show loss of the normal *TEL* allele, suggesting that the leukemogenic effect of *TEL–AML1* may be mediated in part by loss of function of the *TEL* gene.[235–238]

AML1 is the DNA-binding component of the AML1-CBFβ transcription factor complex disrupted by the t(8;21), t(3;21), and inv(16) in AML, making it the most common target of chromosomal translocations in leukemia. AML1 is a transcription factor that has been shown to be required for the expression of several hematopoietic genes involved in myeloid and lymphoid development, including *PU.1* and interleukin 3, although it can also act as a transcriptional repressor in some settings.[239] Homozygous disruption of the murine *AML1* gene or *CBFB* gene results in the lack of definitive hematopoiesis, indicating that genes regulated by AML1 are essential for normal hematopoietic development.[240,241] In addition, rare familial mutations in the *AML1* DNA-binding domain lead to the familial platelet disorder and predisposition to myeloid malignancy syndrome.[242] However, the molecular pathways mediating *TEL–AML1*-induced leukemogenesis remain incompletely understood.

The presence of the *TEL–AML1* translocation is associated with an excellent prognosis, with event-free survival rates of approximately 90% in a variety of studies.[91,243,244] However, *TEL–AML1* may not represent an independent predictor of prognosis when age and white blood cell count at the time of diagnosis are taken into account in multivariate analysis.[244] Nevertheless, this translocation identifies a large subset of children with B-precursor ALL who appear to represent good candidates for less intensive therapy. The *TEL–AML1* translocation is associated with lower expression of the *MDR-1* multidrug resistance gene[245] and of genes involved in purine metabolism,[246] which might account for the particular efficacy of these cases to current combination chemotherapy regimens that rely heavily on methotrexate and mercaptopurine, agents that inhibit de novo purine synthesis.

Tyrosine Kinase Genes

BCR–ABL in B-Precursor Acute Lymphoblastic Leukemia

The 22q- chromosomal marker, often called the Philadelphia (Ph) chromosome, which arises from the t(9;22)(q34;q11), was originally identified in patients with chronic myelogenous leukemia (CML), although it is also found in approximately 4% of childhood cases and

25% of adult cases of ALL,[91] which are almost always of the B-precursor subtype. The t(9;22) generates a *BCR–ABL* fusion gene, consisting of 5′ (upstream) sequences from *BCR* and 3′ (downstream) sequences of *ABL*. The t(9;22) breakpoints on the distal tip of the long arm of chromosome 9 are scattered over a distance of nearly 200 kb within the first intron of the *ABL* protooncogene, upstream of the tyrosine kinase domain.[247–249] The breakpoints in the *BCR* gene on chromosome 22 cluster in two separate regions of that gene, known as the major breakpoint cluster region (M-bcr) or minor breakpoint cluster region (m-bcr). In two-thirds of cases of Ph-positive ALL, the breakpoint in the *BCR* gene occurs in the minor breakpoint cluster region (m-bcr), whereas in all cases of chronic myeloid leukemia and approximately one-third of cases of ALL, the breaks occur in the major breakpoint cluster region (M-bcr).[250] The fusion transcript more commonly present in ALL (m-bcr) encodes a 190-kd protein (p190), whereas the transcripts found in CML and some cases of ALL (M-bcr breakpoint) encodes a 210-kd hybrid protein (p210).[251–253,254] Both types of fusions generate chimeric oncoproteins that are activated as a tyrosine-specific protein kinase, similar to the v-abl protein.[255–257]

The ABL tyrosine kinase is localized both in the nucleus and in the cytoplasm of proliferating cells. It is normally activated by DNA damage downstream of ATM and appears to promote p53-mediated growth arrest.[258–261] Mice deficient in ABL develop a wasting syndrome and die soon after birth.[262,263] In contrast to the nuclear and cytoplasmic distribution of normal ABL, the BCR–ABL fusion oncoprotein has a cytoplasmic location and shows increased tyrosine kinase activity.[264,265] When expressed in murine hematopoietic precursors, both p190 and p210 transform hematopoietic cells in vitro and induce a syndrome similar to CML in mice.[266–269] Transformation by the BCR–ABL oncoprotein involves activation of the RAS/MAPK pathway, PI-3 and JUN kinases, c-CBL and CRKL, JAK-STAT, NFκB, Src, and cyclin D1.[270–277] Among these targets, RAS, JUN-kinase and PI-3 kinase pathways are involved in the induction of cell proliferation.[278] The BCR–ABL oncoprotein affects multiple aspects of cell homeostasis, including apoptosis, differentiation, and cell adhesion. An important cellular effect of BCR–ABL is the induction of cellular resistance to DNA damage agents such as cytostatic drugs and irradiation. After DNA damage, BCR–ABL extends the duration of the G2/M cell cycle checkpoint and facilitates DNA repair. It also upregulates the antiapoptotic *BCLXL* gene, contributing to the suppression of apoptotic cell death.[279]

The factors that determine whether the *BCR–ABL1* translocation leads to B-precursor ALL or CML remain incompletely understood. Clinical observations, mutational studies, and mouse models present a complex picture, and it has been difficult to ascertain whether features of the fusion gene itself, the cell type in which the translocation occurred, or other factors determined whether this translocation led to CML or ALL. However, it has recently been demonstrated that the *BCR–ABL1*-mediated activation of several SRC kinases, including Lyn, Hck, and Fgr, plays crucial roles for the ability of *BCR–ABL1* to induce B-precursor ALL but not CML in the mouse.[280,281]

The presence of the Philadelphia chromosome is associated with an extremely poor prognosis in ALL patients despite treatment on contemporary protocols for high-risk disease.[282–284] Although a relatively small subset of these patients may be cured with the use of standard intensive chemotherapy, particularly those with a low white blood cell count at diagnosis and good initial steroid response,[285–288] bone marrow transplantation in first remission from a matched related donor is clearly beneficial for patients in all risk groups.[286,289,290] In addition, evidence is accumulating that transplantation of Ph-positive ALL using an alternative bone marrow donor is also an advantageous approach.[291,292]

The development of imatinib mesylate (STI-571/Gleevec), a pharmacologic tyrosine kinase inhibitor targeting the BCR–ABL oncoprotein, has opened novel therapeutic opportunities for the management of Ph-positive ALL, especially for patients who are not candidates for bone marrow transplantation. Initial phase I clinical studies with this agent showed marked antileukemic activity in patients with CML[293] or BCR–ABL-positive ALL.[294] Although the effectiveness of imatinib mesylate against BCR–ABL-positive leukemias has been confirmed in phase II trials,[295–297] its utility as a single agent is limited by the rapid development of drug resistance.[298,299] Novel "second-generation" BCR–ABL1 kinase inhibitors that can circumvent drug resistance in many cases of CML are under active clinical development.[300,301] However, not all mutations in *BCR–ABL1* that confer drug resistance can be overcome with newer agents, underscoring the need for both more effective inhibitors and for the integration of these into combination chemotherapy regimens for BCR–ABL-positive leukemias.[302–305] Given the recent recognition of the role of SRC kinases in Ph-positive ALL,[280] the novel kinase inhibitors that are active against both SRC and BCR–ABL kinases may be particularly effective in cases of Ph-positive ALL.[306,307]

NUP214–ABL1 in T-Cell Acute Lymphoblastic Leukemia

Although the *BCR–ABL1* translocation is rare in T-cell ALL, amplified episomes containing *NUP214–ABL1* fusion genes have recently been described in approximately 6% of children and adults with T-cell ALL.[308] These episomes appear to arise via a mechanism in which the genomic region of chromosome 9q34, which contains both the *NUP214* and *ABL1* genes, is circularized in a manner that leads to the fusion of these 2 genes. The breakpoint in the *ABL1* gene in all of these cases occurs in intron 1, which is the same breakpoint observed in Philadelphia-positive CML and B-precursor ALL, whereas the *NUP214* breakpoints are variable. The wild-type NUP214 protein is a component of the nuclear pore complex and may contribute oligomerization motifs to the *NUP214–ABL1* fusion oncogene. The NUP214–ABL1 fusion protein has constitutively activated ABL1 tyrosine kinase activity, which is inhibited by the BCR–ABL kinase inhibitor imatinib.[308] The therapeutic potential of imatinib or second-generation tyrosine kinase inhibitors for NUP214–ABL1-positive T-cell ALL is of considerable interest.

FLT3 in *MLL*-Rearranged Acute Lymphoblastic Leukemia

FLT3 encodes a receptor tyrosine kinase that is highly expressed in early hematopoietic precursors, where it plays important functional roles.[309,310] Multiple studies have shown that activating mutations of *FLT3*, which lead to constitutive receptor tyrosine kinase activity even in the absence of ligand, are common in leukemic myeloblasts in patients with AML, but are rare in adults with ALL.[311–313] However, gene expression studies demonstrated high expression of *FLT3* in most cases of ALL that involve MLL gene rearrangements or hyperdiploidy.[214,215,219] In addition, activating mutations were identified in 18% of infants with *MLL*-rearranged ALL,[220] in 21% to 24% of hyperdiploid ALL cases,[7,220] and in all three cases of the prothymic CD117/KIT$^+$ subtype of T-cell ALL in adults that were examined.[314]

In the absence of FLT3 ligand, wild-type FLT3 receptors are inactive because of autoinhibition mediated by the juxtamembrane domain of the receptor. Upon binding of FLT3 ligand, normal FLT3 receptors homodimerize, become activated by phosphorylation, and lead to the activation of signal transduction pathways that promote proliferation and cell survival.[315] Activating mutations of *FLT3* found in leukemias occur in 2 separate regions of the gene. In-frame tandem duplications in the juxtamembrane domain lead to loss of the autoinhibiton mediated by this domain, with subsequent dimerization and receptor activation in the absence of FLT3 ligand.[316] Alternatively, point mutations or insertions in the second tyrosine kinase domain of the FLT3 receptor lead to autophosphorylation and activation of downstream signaling in the absence of FLT3 ligand.[6,313,317] Small-molecule inhibitors of the FLT3 kinase lead to apoptosis in AML cell lines in vitro, and are currently undergoing phase I and II

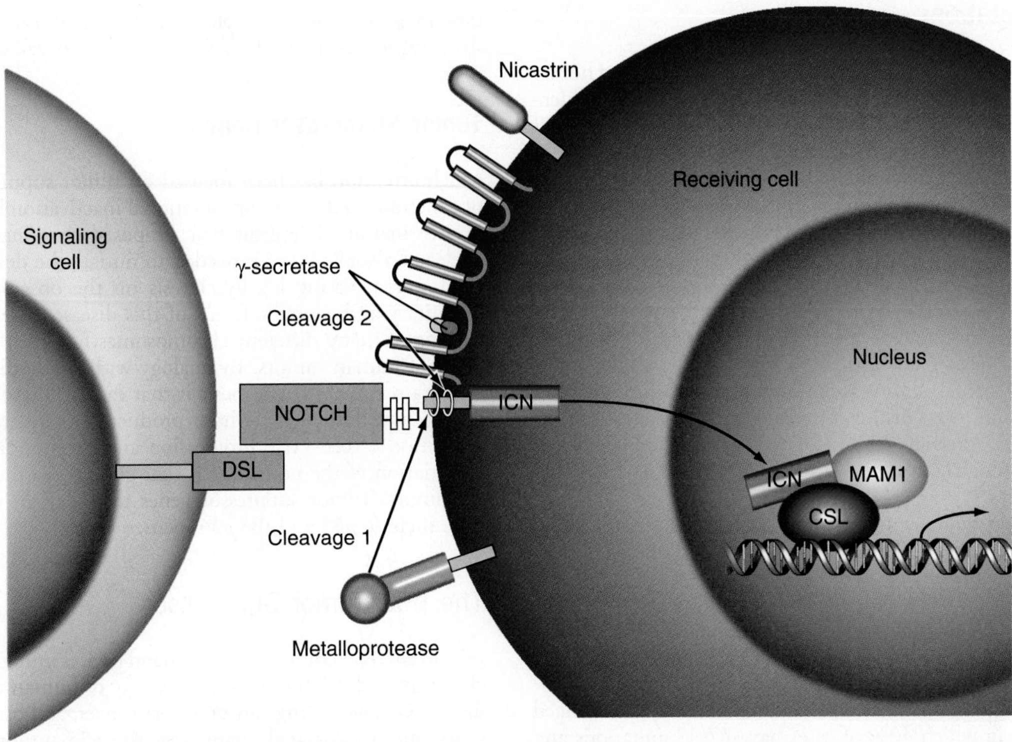

Figure 63–5 Activation of NOTCH signaling via extracellular and intracellular proteolytic cleavage and nuclear translocation of the intracellular NOTCH domain (ICN). Interaction with delta serrate ligand (DSL) stimulates proteolytic cleavage of NOTCH by metalloproteases and γ-secretase. This leads to the release of the intracellular ICN domain, which translocates to the nucleus, where it acts as a transcription factor to regulate gene expression. Adapted from Armstrong SA, Look AT: Molecular genetics of acute lymphoblastic leukemia. J Clin Oncol 23:6306, 2005, with permission.

testing in adults with AML and MDS.[318] These small-molecule inhibitors are also active against *MLL*-rearranged ALL cell lines,[219,319] and hold promise as targeted therapies for cases of ALL that rely on aberrant activation of FLT3.

Mutated Genes

The activation of cellular protooncogenes by point mutation is difficult to detect, because such lesions lack the cytogenetic abnormalities that signal other forms of transforming alterations. Genes of this type must first be identified in experimental systems, so that investigators know in advance the types of activating point mutations that are likely to occur in human tumors. The prototypic genes of this class are *NOTCH1* and members of the RAS family, with mutations that affect defined functional domains of the corresponding proteins.

NOTCH1 in T-Cell Acute Lymphoblastic Leukemia

The *NOTCH1* gene was discovered as a partner gene in a t(7;9) chromosomal translocation that is found in exceedingly rare cases of T-ALL, in which *NOTCH1* is truncated and placed under the control of the T cell-receptor β locus.[320] *NOTCH1* plays several critical roles in promoting T-cell development[40,321–323] and is highly leukemogenic when expressed in murine T-cell precursors.[324] Despite the rarity of translocations involving this gene, a search for activating NOTCH1 mutations demonstrated that these are present in more than 50% of cases of T-ALL, and these occur in all molecular subtypes of T-ALL.[8] NOTCH1 is a transmembrane protein that is proteolytically processed during its transit to the cell surface, where it exists as a heterodimer consisting of extracellular and transmembrane subunits (Fig. 63–5). Upon ligand binding, the transmembrane subunit undergoes additional proteolytic cleavage within the plasma membrane, which leads to the release of its intracellular domain, known as ICN1, into the cytosol. ICN1 subsequently translocates into the nucleus where it is active as a transcription factor. Activating *NOTCH1* mutations in T-ALL can occur as either missense mutations in the heterodimerization domain, which allow constitutive proteolytic activation of the ICN1 domain,[8,325] or as frameshift mutations or stop codons that lead to truncation of the PEST domain,[8,326] which impair the degradation of ICN1. Mutations in both regions are often found on the same allele in cases of T-ALL, and, in experimental systems, mutations in both domains of the same gene indeed are synergistic.[8] Recent work has demonstrated that *MYC* is an important transcriptional target of *NOTCH1*, and it mediates many of the leukemogenic properties of *NOTCH1* in human T-ALL cell lines.[327–329]

The proteolytic activation of the ICN domain of NOTCH1 upon ligand binding is mediated by γ-secretase, and γ-secretase inhibitors have previously been developed because of the role of this enzyme in the pathogenesis of Alzheimer disease. These inhibitors inhibit the growth of many T-ALL cell lines,[8,330] and trials of γ-secretase inhibitors in patients with T-ALL are currently under way.

FBW7 in T-Cell Acute Lymphoblastic Leukemia

FBW7 is an E3 ubiquitin ligase that targets the transcriptionally active intracellular form of NOTCH (ICN) , MYC, and cyclin E for degradation, and this gene is inactivated by mutation or deletion in approximately 10% of T-ALL cases.[331] In T-ALL cell lines, *FBW7* mutation or homozygous deletion leads to resistance to NOTCH pathway inhibition by γ-secretase inhibitor therapy, likely because intracellular NOTCH protein levels remain high in the absence of FBW7-mediated degradation despite inhibition of γ-secretase activity. In addition, tumor-derived FBW7 mutations maintain their ability to bind MYC but do not lead to its degradation, and these may act as dominant negative mutants that protect MYC from degradation.[331]

RAS Gene Mutations

Human tumor DNAs were initially found to contain activated homologues of either *HRAS* or *KRAS*,[332,333] protooncogenes that were identified on the basis of their homology with viral oncogenes. Gene transfer methods identified an additional member of the RAS gene family, called *NRAS*,[334,335] that had not been observed as a component of a transforming retrovirus. Protooncogenes of the RAS family—*HRAS*, *KRAS*, and *NRAS*—encode 21-kd proteins that are associated with the inner surface of the cytoplasmic membrane and are involved in growth factor receptor signaling.[336] The *RAS* protooncogenes are activated to the status of transforming oncogenes by somatic mutations that alter the amino acids specified by codons 12, 13, or 61. Mutated *RAS* genes lose their intrinsic GTPase activity and become insensitive to GAP proteins, thus accumulating in their active, GTP-bound conformation, even in the absence of growth factor binding to surface receptors. Aberrant RAS-mediated signaling contributes to transformation through activation of the PI3K, Raf–MEK–ERK, and RALGDS pathways.[336]

Activated *NRAS* genes appear to be preferentially involved in hematopoietic malignancies. They have been detected in myeloid cell lines,[337,338] in fresh leukemic cell samples from patients with AML or CML,[339–341] and in patients with myelodysplastic syndromes.[342] In acute lymphoblastic leukemia, mutations of codons 12, 13, or 61 of *NRAS* have been found in approximately 10% of patients, whereas *KRAS* mutations have been identified in 5% to 10% of patients.[343,344] RAS mutations are particularly common in cases of *MLL*-rearranged B-precursor ALL, in which 40% of cases have *KRAS* mutations and an additional 10% have *NRAS* mutations.[344] In addition, RAS mutations have also been associated with high hyperdiploidy.[345] The presence of RAS mutations does not appear to have prognostic significance in the setting of contemporary treatment regimens.[343]

Gene Amplification

Gene amplification at the DNA level provides the cell a means to increase expression of critical genes whose products are ordinarily tightly controlled. Clinically important examples of protooncogene amplification have been documented in solid tumors of both adults and children. The *MYCN* gene, for example, is amplified from 10- to 300-fold in tumor cells from approximately one-third of cases of childhood neuroblastoma; such amplification has been linked to an advanced stage of disease and a poor prognosis.[346] However, the cytogenetic hallmarks of gene amplification—double-minute chromatin bodies and homogeneously staining regions—are rarely found in karyotypes of human leukemia cells, making it unlikely that high-level amplification of cellular protooncogenes is widespread in ALL. However, as noted earlier, the *NUP214–ABL1* fusion oncogene is amplified as a small, cytogenetically undetectable episome in T-ALL.

MYB Duplication in T-Cell Acute Lymphoblastic Leukemia

A duplication of the *c-MYB* gene was recently discovered in cases of T-ALL,[347–349] and a chromosomal translocation that juxtaposes *c-MYB* to the T cell-receptor β gene regulatory elements was also identified in a small number of patients.[348] The discovery of this gene duplication involving a small region of the chromosome was made possible by recent technologic advances that now allow the high-resolution detection of small regions of focal amplifications and deletions. The *MYB* transcription factor is the cellular counterpart of the avian *v-MYB* avian myeloblastosis virus, which causes a rapidly fatal monoblastic leukemia in chickens and is essential for normal hematopoiesis, including T-cell development. The *MYB* duplication is mediated by homologous recombination between identical sequence regions that flank the gene,[349] and its expression appears to be important in preventing T lymphoblast differentiation, as knockdown of *MYB* expression in T-ALL cell lines induces T-cell differentiation.[347]

Tumor Suppressor Genes

Much attention has been focused on tumor suppressors, whose loss of function via deletion or mutational inactivation leads to malignant transformation. Knudson first proposed that inactivation of both alleles of a single locus is needed to initiate the development of retinoblastoma, basing his hypothesis on the observed frequencies of hereditary and sporadic forms of this disease. Allelic loss of defined regions of many different chromosomes has been linked to specific types of human tumors. By analogy with the findings in retinoblastoma, a reasonable hypothesis is that each of these regions harbors a tumor suppressor gene whose product is uniquely involved in the inhibition of cell cycle progression and promotion of terminal differentiation of the normal cells that give rise to these different types of tumors. Tumor suppressor genes that play an important role in ALL include *p53* and the *p16* locus.

The p53 Tumor Suppressor

p53, located on chromosome 17, band p13, is mutated or lost through chromosomal deletion in a wide variety of human tumors,[350] including colon cancer, lung cancer, breast cancer, and osteosarcoma. Heritable cancer-associated changes of the *p53* tumor suppressor gene occur in families with Li-Fraumeni syndrome—an unusual aggregation of sarcomas, brain tumors, leukemias, adrenocortical carcinomas, and premenopausal breast cancers.[351–354] *p53* encodes a 53-kd transcription factor that functions as a cell cycle and apoptosis checkpoint regulator.[350,355–359] The p53 protein is induced by DNA damage, blocks cell division at G1 to allow DNA repair, and activates apoptosis in cells that have sustained DNA damage.[360–365] The mechanism of p53 activation is triggered by the loss of activity of MDM2 after DNA damage (via ATM) or oncogenic stress (via p14/ARF). As a negative regulator of p53, MDM2 induces the ubiquitination of p53 and its degradation by the proteasome. Hence, when MDM2 activity is abolished, p53 accumulates and certain cell cycle regulatory genes such as *p21*(*WAF1/CIP1/SDI1/CAP20*) and proapoptotic factor genes such as *BAX*, *PUMA*, and *NOXA* are transcriptionally activated.

p53 is also inactivated in a variety of hematopoietic malignancies, including B-cell ALL and Burkitt lymphoma, but is mutated or deleted in less than 3% of pediatric B-precursor or T-cell ALL cases at diagnosis.[366–368] It thus appears to play a limited role in the etiology of pediatric leukemia. However, *p53* mutations are seen in approximately 25% of relapsed T-cell ALL cases, suggesting a role for *p53* inactivation in the development of resistant disease.[366,367] In addition, *p53* mutations were detected in 3 of 10 ALL patients who failed on induction therapy or suffered early relapse, further supporting a role for *p53* inactivation in disease progression.[369,370]

The Cyclin-Dependent Kinase Inhibitors

The cyclin-dependent kinase inhibitors, which include p15 (INK4B/MTS2), p16 (INK4A/MTS1/CDKN2), p18 (INK4C), p19 (INK4D), p21 (WAF1/CIP1/SDI1/CAP20), p27 (KIP1), and p57 (KIP2), constitute a family of tumor suppressors that negatively regulate the cell cycle by inhibiting cyclin-dependent kinase (CDK) phosphorylation of pRB.[371] The *INK4A* locus, located on the short arm of chromosome band 9q21, contains two different tumor suppressor genes, *p16INK4A* and *p14ARF* (*p19ARF* in mice),[372,373] each with a distinct promoter and first exon but common second and third exons. Despite this close relationship at the genomic level, p16 and p14 have totally unrelated amino acid sequences, as they use different reading frames in their common second and third exons.[374] A third tumor suppressor gene, the cyclin-dependent kinase inhibitor *p15INK4B*, also resides in this region.[375,376] p16INK4A and p15INK4B directly inhibit cyclin D-CDK4/6 complexes and interfere with cell cycle progression. Cyclin D-CDK4/6 complexes promote entry into S phase through phosphorylation of the retinoblastoma protein, PRB, leading to the release of transcription factors, such as E2F, that promote entry into S phase. By contrast, p14ARF lacks a direct effect on the cell cycle machinery, acting instead to stabilize and upregulate p53 through the inhibition of MDM2.[375–379] The role of the *INK4a* locus in tumorigenesis was substantiated when mice with targeted disruption of exon 2 in *p16* developed tumors (primarily lymphomas and fibrosarcomas) whose induction was enhanced by the topical application of carcinogens and ultraviolet light.[380,381] The phenotype of the *p16/p19*$^{-/-}$ mice could be duplicated by selective mutation of the *p19ARF* gene (by targeting the first exon),[372] although mice deficient in *p16INK4A* with intact *p19ARF* also showed increased susceptibility to cancer.[380,381]

The short arm of chromosome 9 is the most frequent target of chromosomal alterations in human cancer. In particular, the human leukemias and lymphomas show a high frequency of 9p21 deletions involving both the *p16INK4A/p14ARF* and the *p15INK4B* loci. Epigenetic silencing of these tumor suppressor genes through hypermethylation of their promoter sequences represents an alternative mechanism of gene inactivation. Although *p16INK4A/p14ARF* and *p15INK4B* are homozygously deleted in 20% to 30% of B-precursor ALL cases and in 70% to 80% of T-cell ALL cases, epigenetic silencing of the p15INK4B promoter has been observed in 44% of primary B-lineage ALLs.[382–394]

The clinical impact of *p15INK4B* and *p16INK4A/p14ARF* deletions in ALL remains controversial.[394] On the one hand, homozygous p16 deletion is related to high-risk features at diagnosis and to an increased risk of relapse and death in childhood ALL,[393,395,396] and on the other, *p15INK4B* and *p16INK4A/p14ARF* deletions were not associated with clinical outcome in a study of adult ALL cases.[397] Interpretation of the clinical significance of the inactivation of these tumor suppressor genes must also take into account alternative mechanisms of gene inactivation, such as aberrant methylation of *p15INK4B* promoter sequences, which has been associated with epigenetic silencing of this locus and a worse outcome in adult ALL cases.[398]

Loss of SMAD3 Protein in T-ALL

Loss of the SMAD3 protein has been described in all 10 cases of T-ALL that were analyzed, although RNA levels of this protein were normal in many of these samples.[399] Both RNA and protein levels of this protein were detectable in normal T cells and in most cases of B-precursor ALL and AML, and the mechanism through which Smad3 protein levels are suppressed whereas RNA levels remain normal in T-ALL is unknown.[399] SMAD3 is one of several of the receptoractivated SMAD proteins that bind to the cell surface receptor for transforming growth factor β (TGF-β) and, upon ligand binding, move to the nucleus, where they regulate transcription.[400] TGF-β signaling leads to tumor-suppressor effects that are mediated at least partly through the transcriptional induction of the cyclin-dependent kinase inhibitors p15INK4b and p21, and by the inhibition of *MYC* expression.[401] However, the specific mechanisms through which SMAD3 mediates the tumor-suppressor effects of TGF-β signaling and through which SMAD3 loss contributes to leukemogenesis remain unknown.

PAX5 and Other B-Cell Developmental Gene Alterations in B-Precursor ALL

A recent high-resolution genome-wide analysis of B-precursor ALL cases using single-nucleotide polymorphism arrays identified copy number alterations in a number of genes that play important roles in B-cell development.[402] Genes involved in B-cell development were found to be altered by deletion, amplification, mutation, or rearrangement in 40% of cases of B-precursor ALL. The most common abnormalities identified were deletions at the *PAX5* locus, and upon further analysis in other cases, other mechanisms that led to inactivation of *PAX5* were identified. These included a number of translocations that led to fusion proteins that maintained the ability to bind to PAX5 transcriptional targets but lost regulatory ability, thus having dominant negative activity, and inactivating point mutations that altered the transcriptional activity of *PAX5*. Deletions were also detected in the *TCF3*, *EBF1*, *LEF1*, *IKZF1*, and *IKZF3* genes, all of which play important roles in B-cell development.

Other Tumor Suppressors

As discussed previously, *FBW7*, which mediates the degradation of the NOTCH and MYC oncoproteins, is mutated in a subset of cases of T-ALL. In addition, the identification of recurring chromosomal deletions in human ALL indicates that other tumor suppressor loci may be involved in this disease. These recurrent deletions, which affect the long arm of chromosome 6, the short arm of chromosome 9, or the short arm of chromosome 12, can be found in leukemic cells from approximately 10% of patients with ALL, making them among the most frequent cytogenetic abnormalities in this disease. Functional deletion can result either from interstitial deletion of the involved chromosome arm or from derivative chromosomes that result from unbalanced chromosomal translocations. For each chromosome, the deleted regions overlap a single target region, which may contain key genes of the tumor suppressor type, whose loss could be an important step in leukemic transformation.

Deletions of the long arm of chromosome 6 are consistently found in approximately 10% of cases of ALL.[403] Interstitial deletions affecting bands 6q15-q24 have been reported most frequently; translocations with breakpoints within this region are also common. Band q21 of chromosome 6 seems to be involved in each of the abnormalities, suggesting that the target gene(s) resides in this region. Deletions of chromosome 6q occur with equal frequency in pro-B, pre-B, and T-cell cases.

Deletions or translocations involving the short arm of chromosome 12 are also found in approximately 10% of ALL cases, with most clustered around band 12p13.[403] These cases generally have a B-precursor phenotype, and the blast cells usually express CD10 and HLA-DR on the cell surface. Abnormalities of the short arm of chromosome 12 are rarely found in T-ALL cases. Translocations involving chromosome 12p13 may be balanced or unbalanced and can involve multiple different donor chromosomes. Molecular studies, however, have revealed that the majority of translocations involving 12p13 are cryptic 12;21 translocations, resulting in the *TEL–AML1* fusion. In the cases with unbalanced translocations, DNA sequences distal to the breakpoint are lost from the affected homologue and subsequently from the leukemic cell genome, so the result is similar to that of interstitial deletion. The frequency of deletions involving the 12p13 region suggests that these lesions primarily inactivate one allele of a tumor suppressor gene in this chromosomal region. Although the *TEL* and *p27KIP1* genes may be targets of deletion in these cases, neither locus is inactivated by point mutations in childhood ALL cases with loss of heterozygosity (LOH) in 12p,[235,404] implicating additional tumor suppressor genes in this region, although *TEL* or *p27KIP1* haploinsufficiency could also contribute to leukemic transformation.[235,404]

Abnormalities of Leukemia Cell Ploidy

Abnormalities of chromosome number, which generally occur in the absence of specific chromosomal translocations, have important prognostic implications in childhood ALL. Found in 25% to 30% of childhood ALL cases, hyperdiploidy greater than 50 chromosomes in the leukemic clone is one of the most powerful means for identifying patients with a very good prognosis.[91,243] In particular, trisomies of chromosomes 4, 10, and 17 impart a particularly good prognosis, and hyperdiploidy in the absence of these trisomies is less of a favorable prognostic factor.[405] As mentioned previously, activating mutations of *FLT3*, a receptor tyrosine kinase, are common in these patients. Patients with hyperdiploidy typically present with favorable prognostic indicators, such as age between 2 and 10 years, a low white blood cell count, and an early pre-B immunophenotype, and can expect cure rates that approach 90%.[406–408] The mechanism accounting for the favorable outcome of patients with hyperdiploid ALL remains elusive, but may reflect an increased sensitivity to antimetabolite therapy[409] and a greater propensity to undergo apoptosis.[410] Conversely, hypodiploidy (< 45 chromosomes) carries an extremely poor prognosis.[411,91,243] Overall, adults with ALL have significantly fewer numeric chromosomal abnormalities than do children; however, abnormalities of ploidy do appear to have prognostic significance in adults also, as one large series demonstrated a favorable prognostic impact of hyperdiploidy, whereas adults with hypodiploidy had extremely poor outcomes.[33]

CHILDHOOD ACUTE LYMPHOBLASTIC LEUKEMIA: A MODEL FOR GENE-BASED RISK ASSESSMENT

Many of the chromosomal and molecular genetic abnormalities in the leukemic blasts of patients with ALL are important predictors of response to currently available chemotherapy. Lymphoblasts from each new case of childhood ALL should be examined for molecular prognostic markers, including leukemia cell ploidy, *MLL* gene rearrangements, and the presence of *BCR–ABL* and *TEL–AML1* fusion transcripts. Additional clinical criteria that have prognostic significance, such as the age of the patient, the peripheral blood white blood cell count at diagnosis, and the presence of central nervous system involvement, are used by modern pediatric ALL treatment regimens to further adjust the intensity of therapy to an individual patient's risk of relapse. In the future, high-density SNP arrays and gene expression arrays may be performed on samples from each patient, to identify genomic alterations and gene expression patterns that have prognostic significance, such as *HOX11* expression in the case of T-ALL.[412] It is worth noting that ALL in patients less than 1 year of age is associated with an extremely poor prognosis secondary to an exceedingly high rate of relapse, and these patients are often treated with unique treatment regimens designed specifically for infant ALL. Finally, response to treatment has independent prognostic significance. Induction failure, defined in pediatric protocols as any morphologic evidence of leukemia at the end of the initial month of induction chemotherapy, represents a very poor prognostic factor and is an indication for bone marrow transplantation once remission is achieved in most centers. In addition, sensitive flow-cytometric and PCR-based methodologies for the detection of minimal residual disease are now available, and the level of minimal residual disease after induction chemotherapy has recently been shown to provide an additional means of identifying patients at low or high risk of relapse.[413,414] With the availability of these prognostic indicators, there remains little justification for uniform treatment of newly diagnosed cases of ALL. Rather, modern trials emphasize risk-based therapy to reduce toxicity in patients likely to become long-term responders, and to intensify therapy for those at high risk of relapse.

A risk classification scheme based on a patient's clinical features and on the genetic features of leukemic blasts has been proposed for patients with B-precursor or T-cell ALL that are 1 year of age or older. Patients with *TEL–AML1* positivity or with simultaneous trisomies of chromosomes 4, 10, and 17 constitute the lower-risk group and are candidates for reduced-intensity treatment regimens. The intermediate-risk group includes patients between the ages of 1 and 9 with standard-risk age and leukocyte count, as defined by the criteria of the National Cancer Institute, and whose leukemic lymphoblasts lack prognostically important genetic features. The high-risk group comprises patients who meet any of the following criteria: age 10 years or older, high leukocyte counts at diagnosis, a T-cell immunophenotype, or a slow early response to therapy. Patients in the very high-risk group, defined by extreme hypodiploidy, *MLL* gene rearrangements, the *BCR–ABL* translocation, or high minimal residual disease at the end of induction chemotherapy are eligible for bone marrow transplantation in first remission. It is worth noting that the evidence supporting a benefit for bone marrow transplantation in first remission is especially strong in the presence of the *BCR–ABL* translocation, although its role in *MLL*-rearranged ALL remains controversial. Among several exceptions to this risk stratification criteria are T-ALL patients with the t(11;19) and expression of *MLL–ENL*, who have a favorable prognosis,[17,415] and infants younger than 1 year of age, in whom separate risk stratification criteria have been devised (reviewed in reference 416). Recent progress in the risk assessment of different subtypes of ALL predicts that gene expression profiling by oligonucleotide microarray analysis[215] will further improve the power of current molecularly based systems of risk classification. The incorporation of highly predictive risk stratification methods into clinical trials, together with the development of novel molecularly tailored therapies, should eliminate the still-significant risk of relapse in patients with newly diagnosed ALL, ensuring permanent cure without the hazard of acute or chronic complications.

SUGGESTED READINGS

Comprehensive Reviews

Look AT: Oncogenic transcription factors in the human acute leukemias. Science 278:1059, 1997.

Armstrong SA, Look AT: Molecular genetics of acute lymphoblastic leukemia. J Clin Oncol 23:6306, 2005.

Specific Genetic Lesions in ALL

Ferrando AA, Neuberg DS, Staunton J, et al: Gene expression signatures define novel oncogenic pathways in T cell acute lymphoblastic leukemia. Cancer Cell 1:75, 2002.

Grabher C, von Boehmer H, Look AT: Notch 1 activation in the molecular pathogenesis of T-cell acute lymphoblastic leukaemia. Nat Rev Cancer 6:347, 2006.

Hsu K, Look AT: Turning on a dimer: New insights into MLL chimeras. Cancer Cell 4:81, 2003.

Krivtsov AV, Twomey D, Feng Z, et al: Transformation from committed progenitor to leukaemia stem cell initiated by MLL-AF9. Nature 442:818, 2006.

O'Neil J, Shank J, Cusson N, et al: TAL1/SCL induces leukemia by inhibiting the transcriptional activity of E47/HEB. Cancer Cell 5:587, 2004.

Sattler M, Griffin JD: Molecular mechanisms of transformation by the BCR-ABL oncogene. Semin Hematol 40:4, 2003.

Weng AP, Ferrando AA, Lee W, et al: Activating mutations of NOTCH1 in human T cell acute lymphoblastic leukemia. Science 306:269, 2004.

Zelent A, Greaves M, Enver T: Role of the TEL-AML1 fusion gene in the molecular pathogenesis of childhood acute lymphoblastic leukaemia. Oncogene 23:4275, 2004.

Clinical Implications of ALL Genetics

Armstrong SA, Kung AL, Mabon ME, et al: Inhibition of FLT3 in MLL. Validation of a therapeutic target identified by gene expression based classification. Cancer Cell 3:173, 2003.

Ferrando AA, Look AT: Clinical implications of recurring chromosomal and associated molecular abnormalities in acute lymphoblastic leukemia. Semin Hematol 37:381, 2000.

Gilliland DG: Molecular genetics of human leukemias: New insights into therapy. Semin Hematol 39:6, 2002.

Pui CH, Evans WE: Treatment of acute lymphoblastic leukemia. N Engl J Med 354:166, 2006.

Schultz KR, Pullen DJ, Sather HN, et al: Risk- and response-based classification of childhood B-precursor acute lymphoblastic leukemia: A combined analysis of prognostic markers from the Pediatric Oncology Group (POG) and Children's Cancer Group (CCG). Blood 109:926, 2007.

Stam RW, den Boer ML, Pieters R: Towards targeted therapy for infant acute lymphoblastic leukaemia. Br J Haematol 132:539, 2006.

Winick NJ, Carroll WL, Hunger SP: Childhood leukemia—new advances and challenges. N Engl J Med 351:601, 2004.

REFERENCES

For complete list of references log onto www.expertconsult.com

CHAPTER 64

CLINICAL MANIFESTATIONS OF ACUTE LYMPHOBLASTIC LEUKEMIA

Karen R. Rabin, Stacey Berg, C. Philip Steuber, and David G. Poplack

BACKGROUND

Before the institution of modern chemotherapy, acute lymphoblastic leukemia (ALL) was a uniformly fatal disease, with most patients surviving only 2 to 3 months. Over the past 40 years, successive studies of improved treatment regimens have been conducted that have not only resulted in improved survival of children with ALL but have also served as a paradigm for the conduct of clinical research in cancer. With current chemotherapy, the majority of children with ALL have prolonged disease-free survival and up to approximately 85% are considered cured.[1]

EPIDEMIOLOGY AND ETIOLOGY

ALL is the most common malignancy of childhood, with about 2400 new cases diagnosed annually in the United States.[2] In the pediatric population, ALL is four times more frequent than acute nonlymphoblastic leukemia (ANLL; or acute myelocytic leukemia [AML]). In contrast, ALL accounts for less than 1% of all adult malignancies, and for less than 20% of the acute leukemias in this population.[3–5] In children, the peak incidence of ALL occurs at approximately 2 to 3 years of age.[2] In adults, the greatest number of cases occur in those older than 65 years.

Children with certain chromosomal abnormalities are at higher risk than the general population for developing leukemia. These include Down syndrome,[6] Bloom's syndrome,[7] Fanconi anemia,[8] ataxia telangiectasia,[9] and neurofibromatosis.[10] In addition, siblings, especially twins, of children with leukemia are at greater risk of developing leukemia, although this risk may be only approximately twice that of the general population.[11] Some cases of childhood ALL may be related to hereditary or acquired mutations in the p53 gene.[12]

Because concordance is only about 25% in monozygotic twins, who share identical genetic makeup, environmental factors clearly also play an important etiologic role. A few environmental exposures have been definitively linked to ALL, including ionizing radiation and certain toxic chemicals and chemotherapeutic agents (although these are far more often associated with development of AML). Most other proposed environmental associations are controversial or relatively modest. Only in a few specific cases have infectious agents been causally linked to ALL: HTLV-1 in adult T-cell ALL/lymphoma, and Epstein–Barr virus (EBV) in mature B-cell ALL/Burkitt lymphoma.

Interestingly, childhood ALL has been shown to originate *in utero* in some cases.[13] Studies of twins concordant for ALL have demonstrated the presence of identical unique gene rearrangements in leukemic cells from both twins, suggesting origin in a single prenatal clone shared via a common blood supply.[14–18] Preleukemic clones have also been detected in archived neonatal blood spots in nontwin cases of ALL.[19] The gene rearrangements detected in these preleukemic clones are presumably the initiating leukemogenic events, but a "second hit" is generally necessary in order for progression to overt leukemia. Greaves has hypothesized that an abnormal immune response to common infections may provide this second hit.[20] A variety of epidemiologic data is consistent with this hypothesis, particularly evidence that early daycare attendance, with its attendant frequent infections, is protective against development of ALL (reviewed in reference 20).

CLASSIFICATION

Morphology

ALL cells are heterogeneous and have been subclassified on the basis of differences in their appearance under the light microscope. The most widely used system, developed by the French-American-British (FAB) Cooperative Working Group divides lymphoblasts into three categories: L1, L2, and L3 (Table 64–1 and Fig. 64–1). The L1 morphology is predominant, occurring in approximately 85% of childhood ALL cases. The L2 subtype represents nearly all the remainder, with the rare L3 subtype constituting only 1% to 2%. Although there is no apparent correlation of the L1 and L2 morphology with particular immunologic cell surface markers, cells of the L3 variety possess cell surface immunoglobulin and other characteristic mature B cell markers, and are identical cytomorphologically to Burkitt lymphoma cells.

Immunophenotype

Immunophenotyping plays a major role in the diagnosis of the acute leukemias. The use of monoclonal antibodies specific for various stages of B-cell, T-cell, and myeloid differentiation enables the clinician to determine more definitively whether a leukemia is lymphoid or myeloid in origin (Table 64–3 and Fig. 64–2). In most cases, immunophenotyping also permits assignment of the relative stage in the process of B- or T-cell differentiation from which the leukemic clone is believed to have arisen or reached a differentiative block. Approximately 80% to 85% of childhood ALL is believed to develop from the monoclonal proliferation of B-cell precursors. In contrast, only approximately 1% to 2% of cases manifest surface immunoglobulin and are classified as mature B-cell ALL. The remainder of cases are of T-cell origin. A variety of classification schemes have been developed that define both B-cell precursor ALL and T-cell ALL according to their degree of differentiation or maturation.

Most cases of ALL express surface antigens and molecular markers that help to identify them as derived from a specific lineage. However, lineage infidelity is not uncommon.[21,22] Lymphoid leukemias may aberrantly express a few myeloid markers, and vice versa, so no single marker can be relied upon consistently across all cases. Accurate classification of lymphoid and myeloid leukemia depends instead on a panel of markers, in conjunction with morphologic and cytogenetic features. Biclonal leukemia, characterized by two separate clones of distinct lineages, is much less common. It occurs in perhaps 1% to 2% of childhood and adult ALL, and generally responds poorly to treatment.[23]

The development of recombinant DNA technology has led to identification of immunoglobulin gene and T-cell receptor (TCR) gene rearrangement in leukemic cells. Although it is possible to relate the patterns of immunoglobulin and TCR gene rearrangement to the stages of development of B-cell precursor and T-cell ALL, respectively, immunoglobulin gene rearrangement is seen in some cases of

PT1: Diagnostic Evaluation of the Patient with Acute Leukemia

The diagnostic evaluation of a patient with acute leukemia is a comprehensive process that includes a detailed history and complete physical examination, morphologic and laboratory assessment of peripheral blood and bone marrow, blood chemistries, comprehensive clotting studies (PT, PTT, thrombin time, and fibrinogen), a lumbar puncture and cerebrospinal fluid (CSF) examination, chest radiograph, and other studies necessary to ensure that the newly diagnosed patient will receive optimal supportive care.

History and Physical Examination

When leukemia is suspected, a detailed history and physical examination should be performed. The history should include the nature of presenting symptoms and their duration, with specific attention to signs and symptoms of anemia, thrombocytopenia and neutropenia. A detailed family history, including the occurrence and nature of any malignancies among family members, should be obtained, as well as any history of environmental exposures (eg, chemicals, radiation). Physical examination should include signs of bone marrow dysfunction like pallor, bleeding (eg, petechiae, and/or purpura) and any evidence of infection. Lymphadenopathy and hepatosplenomegaly should be carefully documented. Generalized lymphadenopathy is more common than regional enlargement in leukemia. In children, palpable small axillary, cervical, and inguinal nodes are common, but enlargement of posterior auricular, epitrochlear, or supraclavicular nodes is abnormal. Careful examination of the optic fundi to rule out evidence of retinal hemorrhages secondary to thrombocytopenia and/or leukemic infiltration is important. The oropharynx should be evaluated, including the gingivae, a common site of hypertrophy in patients with acute myelomonocytic or monocytic leukemia.

Hematologic Evaluation

A complete blood count (CBC) will usually reveal evidence of varying degrees of anemia, thrombocytopenia, and anemia. Isolated thrombocytopenia without any other abnormalities on physical examination or CBC is rare. In most patients, leukemic blasts will be seen on the peripheral blood smear. A bone marrow aspirate prior to the start of therapy is usually required for adequate immunophenotyping and cytogenetic studies, although in patients with very high white blood cell counts consisting almost entirely of blasts, peripheral blood sampling may be adequate. The anterior or posterior iliac crest is the preferred site for marrow aspiration. In cases where aspiration does not yield sufficient material for evaluation, bone marrow biopsy is performed. Bone marrow biopsy also is helpful in assessment of the degree of marrow cellularity. Once the diagnosis of leukemia is confirmed, definitive assignment of the type of leukemia is crucial if appropriate treatment is to be delivered.

Detailed immunophenotyping using a panel of monoclonal antibodies is undertaken in all newly diagnosed cases of acute leukemia. Use of a sufficiently comprehensive monoclonal antibody panel capable of detecting the major lymphoid (both B and T cell), myeloid, and platelet-related antigens enables a definitive lineage assignment to be made in most cases of acute leukemia (Table 64–3). Molecular phenotyping may provide useful information regarding the status of the immunoglobulin or T-cell receptor gene rearrangement in lymphoid leukemic cells. Cytogenetic analysis, including evaluation of both chromosomal number and structure, plays a critical role as discussed below.

Lumbar Puncture

Lumbar puncture (LP) is performed in all newly diagnosed patients because the presence of central nervous system (CNS) leukemia alters treatment. In patients with marked thrombocytopenia, platelet transfusions may be considered prior to performing the LP. The CSF cell count and protein and glucose levels are determined. Examination of a cytocentrifuged specimen of CSF is always performed as this technique increases diagnostic sensitivity.

Other Diagnostic and Laboratory Studies

A chest x-ray is routinely obtained in newly diagnosed patients, particularly prior to administration of sedation or anesthesia. When significant mediastinal enlargement is detected, computed tomography (CT) can help to define its extent more accurately. Patients presenting with significant bone pain often undergo radiologic examination of the involved site. All newly diagnosed patients have a comprehensive battery of blood chemistries performed including uric acid, electrolytes, calcium, phosphorus, blood urea nitrogen, serum creatinine, and liver function tests (including lactate dehydrogenase). In addition, MRI or CT imaging of the brain at diagnosis may be useful, particularly as a baseline for comparison in the event of CNS relapse or toxicity.

Supportive Care

The blood type of all patients is determined and appropriate crossmatching instituted if transfusion is required. Packed red cell transfusions are utilized to maintain an adequate hemoglobin. Platelets are often administered prophylactically to maintain the platelet count at more than 10,000 to 20,000/mm^3. If the patient becomes refractory to random donor platelets, single-donor or HLA-matched platelets may be useful.

All newly diagnosed patients receive vigorous hydration and allopurinol or urate oxidase to prevent uric acid nephropathy and complications from tumor lysis. In patients with extremely high initial white blood cell counts (eg, >100,000/mL) leukapheresis or, in very young patients, exchange transfusion, is sometimes helpful, although its role is controversial, especially in ALL.[124,125]

Newly diagnosed patients who are febrile receive an extensive evaluation to rule out infection. The febrile neutropenic patient is placed on broad-spectrum antibiotic coverage.

The diagnosis of leukemia places extraordinary stress on patient and family alike. Starting at the time of initial diagnosis, careful attention is given to evaluating the psychosocial profile of patient and family so that appropriate psychosocial support for both can be instituted. Optimal psychosocial support requires a concerted, coordinated effort of physician, nurses, social workers, clergy, child life, and other skilled health care personnel.

T-cell ALL and TCR gene rearrangement in some cases of B-cell precursor ALL. Thus molecular phenotyping to assign B- or T-cell lineage is not completely reliable.[3,24]

Cytochemistry

Special histochemical stains once played a primary role in determination of lymphoid versus myeloid lineage (Table 64–2). Since the advent of immunophenotyping, they have been principally helpful in providing supporting information in the relatively small number of cases where immunophenotyping is not diagnostic. The periodic acid–Schiff (PAS) stain is positive in approximately 50% of cases of ALL and often shows a characteristic pattern of block positivity. The PAS reaction may be negative in ALL, however, and has been positive in rare cases of AML, limiting its diagnostic utility. TdT (terminal deoxynucleotidyl transferase) is usually detectable in lymphoblasts of T- and B-cell precursor lineage, but not in mature B-cell ALL or in ANLL. The myeloperoxidase stain detects myeloperoxidase in primary granules and is considered specific for cells of the myeloid lineage. Classically, an acute leukemia in which 3% or more of cells in the bone marrow are myeloperoxidase-positive has been considered

Table 64–1 French–American–British Classification of Acute Lymphoblastic Leukemia

Cytologic Features	L1	L2	L3
Cell size	Small cells predominate	Large, heterogeneous in size	Large and homogeneous
Nuclear chromatin	Homogeneous in any one case	Variable—heterogeneous in any one case	Finely stippled and homogeneous
Nuclear shape	Regular, occasional clefting or indentation	Irregular; clefting and indentation common	Regular—oval to round
Nucleoli	Not visible, or small and inconspicuous	One or more present, often large	Prominent; one or more
Amount of cytoplasm	Scanty	Variable; often moderately abundant	Moderately abundant
Basophilia of cytoplasm	Slight or moderate, rarely intense	Variable; deep in some	Very deep
Cytoplasmic vacuolation	Variable	Variable	Often prominent

Data from Bennett JM, Catovsky D, Daniel MT, et al: French-American-British (FAB) Cooperative Group: The morphological classification of acute lymphoblastic leukaemia—Concordance among observers and clinical correlations. Br J Haematol 47:553, 1981.

Table 64–2 Morphologic, Cytochemical, and Biochemical Characteristics Helpful in Distinguishing Acute Lymphoblastic Leukemia from Acute Myelocytic Leukemia

MORPHOLOGIC FEATURES	ALL	AML
Nuclear/cytoplasmic ratio	High	Low
Nuclear chromatin	Clumped	Spongy
Nucleoli	0–2	2–5
Granules	–	+
Auer rods	–	+/–
Cytoplasm	Blue	Blue-gray
CYTOCHEMICAL REACTION		
Peroxidase	–	+
Sudan Black B	–	+
Periodic Acid–Schiff	+/–	–
Naphthyl AS-D chloroacetate esterase	–	+/–
α-Naphthyl acetate esterase	–	+/–
α-Naphthyl butyrate esterase	–	–
Terminal deoxynucleotidyl transferase	+*	-

Table provides information on characteristics that may be useful in differentiating acute lymphoblastic leukemia (ALL) from acute myelocytic leukemia (AML) (see text for details). Wide variation in morphology is encountered in both disease categories. Diagnostic evaluation should include more refined classification of disease according to FAB subtype.

*Terminal deoxynucleotidyl transferase is usually negative in FAB L3 ALL.

Table 64–3 Monoclonal Antibodies Frequently Used in Immunophenotyping of Acute Leukemia in Children

Cluster of Differentiation (CD) Designation	Cell Lineage
2, 3, 4, 5, 7, 8	T cell
10, 19, 20, 22, 24	Precursor B cell
10, 19, 20, 22, Kappa or Lambda	Mature B cell
11, 13, 14, 15, 33, 34, 41, 42, 117	Myeloid
71 (and other myeloid markers)	Erythroid
42 + 61 (and other myeloid markers)	Megakaryocytic

to be myeloid, although this definition is arbitrary and may cause confusion in cases of mixed-lineage leukemia. The Sudan black stain sometimes has been used as a substitute for myeloperoxidase, but because rare cases of ALL demonstrate Sudan black positivity, the myeloperoxidase stain is preferred. Naphthyl AS-D chloroacetate esterase is an enzyme found in cells of neutrophilic lineage that may help define myeloid disease but is generally considered less sensitive than the myeloperoxidase stain. The α-naphthyl acetate esterase and α-naphthyl butyrate esterase stains are helpful particularly in defining monocytic lineage.

Cytogenetics

As molecular technology has improved, the cytogenetic analysis of ALL, as with other malignancies, has become increasingly important in identifying prognosis and tailoring therapy appropriately. The standard laboratory workup of ALL now includes analysis of both chromosome number and chromosome structure. Chromosome number, or ploidy, can be assessed either by karyotype analysis, or by flow cytometry using a measure called the DNA index (DI), which is the ratio of nuclear fluorescence in leukemic blasts compared to normal diploid cells. Chromosome structure is analyzed by chromosome banding, fluorescence in situ hybridization (FISH), and other molecular cytogenetic techniques, including genomewide techniques such as array comparative genomic hybridization.[25] Further discussion of specific recurrent chromosomal abnormalities and their prognostic significance can be found in the Prognosis section below and in Chapter 63.

Genomewide Expression Patterns

Microarray-based analysis of gene expression patterns is a powerful tool that is starting to be used in the classification of ALL. Microarray studies have both provided biological validation of existing ALL subtypes, and identified new subtypes.[26,27] Another research focus has been identification of sets of genes associated with good and poor prognosis within existing subgroups, such as ALL with MLL rearrangement.[28] Expression array studies also aim to identify highly overexpressed genes that are candidate molecular targets for development of new therapies (eg, FLT3, a receptor tyrosine kinase, in hyperdiploid and MLL-rearranged ALL).[29] Finally, microarray analysis is being used to identify expression patterns that correlate with chemotherapy sensitivity versus resistance.[30]

PATHOPHYSIOLOGY

Leukemia is believed to develop from expansion of a single abnormal lymphoid progenitor cell, which accumulates mutations that allow unregulated proliferation. The pathogenesis of ALL is discussed in further detail in Chapter 63.

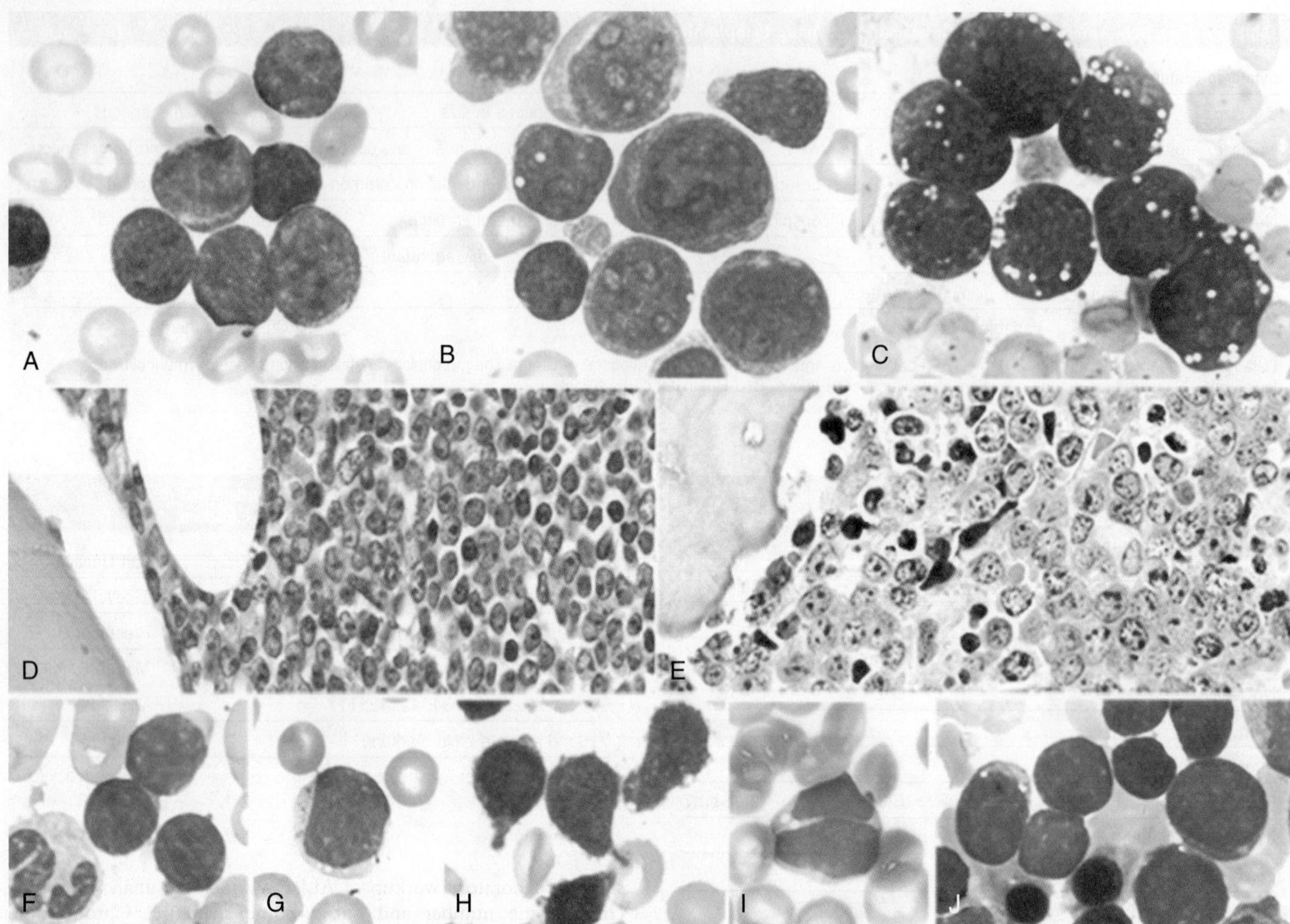

Figure 64–1 Morphologic aspects of acute lymphoblastic leukemia (ALL) (**A–J**). Typical uniform lymphoblasts (**A**) with intermediate-sized nuclei, fine but "smudgy" chromatin, absence of nucleoli, and scant cytoplasm. In the older FAB classification scheme, these would have been considered L1 blasts. Lymphoblasts with more cytologic variation (**B**), including variability in size, number of nucleoli, and amount of cytoplasm. These would have been considered L2 lymphoblasts. Burkitt leukemia/lymphoma cells for comparison (**C**). The cells have intermediate size, more dense chromatin, and deep blue cytoplasm with vacuoles. Histologic features of ALL (**D**) and Burkitt leukemia/lymphoma (**E**) in bone core biopsy. Additional cytologic variants of ALL include a lymphocyte-like variant with small nuclei (**F**), a variant with faint cytoplasmic granules (**G**), and the hand-mirror variant (**H**). The latter might be an artifact of preparation. Lymphoblasts can have deep groves or clefts (**I**). Malignant lymphoblasts must be distinguished from reactive hematogones, or regenerating immature lymphoid cells (**J**).

CLINICAL FEATURES

Patients with ALL present most frequently with signs and symptoms of the uncontrolled growth of leukemic cells in bone marrow, lymphoid organs, and other sites of extramedullary spread. Bone marrow involvement results in varying degrees of anemia, thrombocytopenia, and granulocytopenia that may be manifested by pallor and fatigue, petechiae, purpura or bleeding, fever, and infection. Liver, spleen, and nodal enlargement are present in the majority of patients and are the most common sites of extramedullary disease spread. Hepatosplenomegaly, which occurs in approximately two-thirds of patients, and lymphadenopathy, clinically detectable in over half of presenting cases, are usually asymptomatic. Bone pain, however, is a common presenting feature, particularly in the young child with ALL whose first symptom may be the onset of a limp or refusal to walk.[31] Notably, isolated thrombocytopenia in an otherwise well child with normal white blood cells, red blood cells, and physical examination is very rarely a manifestation of ALL.

Symptoms may be present from a few days to several months before the diagnosis of ALL is made. The nonspecific nature of the signs and symptoms of ALL occasionally leads to delay in diagnosis. In addition, because ALL may imitate a variety of disorders, there may be diagnostic confusion (Table 64–5).[32] For example, arthralgias arising from leukemic infiltration of the joints may be confused with juvenile rheumatoid arthritis or osteomyelitis. In rare cases, ALL has presented with unusual symptoms such as aplastic anemia or hypereosinophilia (Table 64–6).

Extramedullary Spread

ALL frequently involves organs other than bone marrow. Most patients have some extramedullary disease at diagnosis, and extramedullary relapse is a known complication of the disease. The most commonly affected extramedullary sites of disease include the central nervous system, testes, lymph nodes, liver, spleen, and kidney. Of these sites, the central nervous system (CNS) and the testes have the greatest clinical significance. The incidence of occult extramedullary involvement in patients presumed to be in clinical remission is difficult to ascertain, but has been estimated to be as high as 50%, although this is likely treatment-dependent.[33–35] Organ dysfunction due to leukemic involvement is rare, and usually occurs only in patients with progressive, end-stage disease. The occurrence of an extramedullary relapse is most significant because it frequently heralds the development of bone marrow relapse.

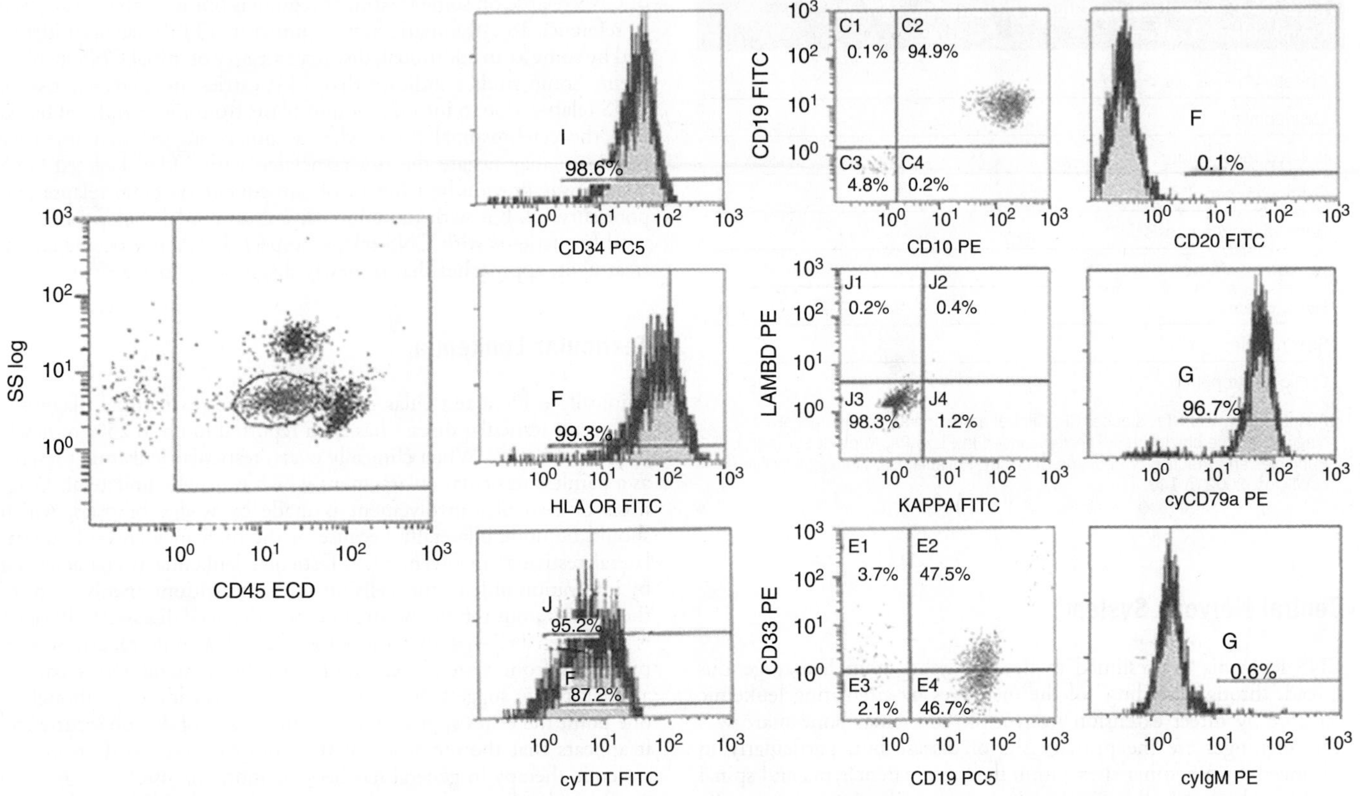

Figure 64–2 Flow data from a typical case of precursor-B acute lymphoblastic leukemia (ALL). The CD45 side-scatter histogram, left shows a distinctive blast population (circled) with weak CD45 reactivity and low side scatter. This is easily distinguished from lymphocytes, monocytes/granulocytes, and nucleated red blood cells. In this case the blasts phenotype was CD34+, HLADR+, TdT+, CD19+, CD10+, CD20−, cyCD79A+, Kappa−, Lambda−, and cyIgM−. There is weak and partial reactivity for a myeloid marker, CD33.

Table 64–4 Uniform Assessment of Risk Factors in Childhood Acute Lymphoblastic Leukemia

Risk Factor	Associated With Better Outcome	Associated With Worse Outcome
Age	1–9 years	≥10 years
WBC	<50,000/μL	≥50,000/μL
DNA index	>1.16	≤1.16
Trisomy 4 and 10	Present	Absent
M1 marrow day 7 or 14	Yes	No
Peripheral blasts at day 8	Absent	Present*
Cytogenetics		t(9;22) t(4;11) t(1;19)
Immunophenotype	B-precursor	T cell*
CNS leukemia	CNS 1	CNS 2* CNS 3

*In some studies.

Adapted from Smith M, Arthur D, Camitta B, et al: Uniform approach to risk classification and treatment assignment for children with acute lymphoblastic leukemia. J Clin Oncol 14:18, 1996.

Table 64–5 Differential Diagnosis of Acute Lymphoblastic Leukemia

INFECTIONS
Viral (eg, EBV, CMV, parvovirus, HIV)
Leukemic reactions secondary to infection
AUTOIMMUNE DISORDERS
Juvenile rheumatoid arthritis
Idiopathic thrombocytopenia purpura
Transient erythroblastopenia of childhood
Systemic lupus erythematosus*
BONE MARROW FAILURE SYNDROMES, CONGENITAL OR ACQUIRED
Megaloblastic anemia
Pure red cell aplasia
Congenital neutropenia
Aplastic anemia
Myelodysplastic syndrome*
Myelofibrosis*
HEMOPHAGOCYTIC LYMPHOHISTIOCYTOSIS
OTHER MALIGNANCIES
Other leukemias
Hodgkin and non-Hodgkin lymphoma
Solid tumors with marrow involvement: neuroblastoma, rhabdomyosarcoma, medulloblastoma, PNET
Multiple myeloma*

*Disorders to be particularly considered in the differential diagnosis of adults.

Table 64–6 Some Unusual Clinical Presentations of Acute Lymphoblastic Leukemia

Aplastic anemia
Eosinophilia
Isolated renal failure
Pulmonary nodules
Bone marrow necrosis
Pericardial effusion
Hypoglycemia
Skin nodules
Cyclic neutropenia

Adapted from Vietti TJ, Steuber CP: Clinical assessment and differential diagnosis of the child with suspected cancer. In Pizzo PA, Poplack DG (eds.): Principles and Practice of Pediatric Oncology. Philadelphia, Lippincott Williams & Wilkins, 2002, p 149.

Central Nervous System

CNS leukemia is presumed to develop either from hematogenous spread, through "seeding" of the meninges by circulating leukemic cells, or by direct extension from involved cranial bone marrow.[36] The meninges are the primary site of disease but, particularly in advanced disease, other sites within the brain parenchyma and spinal cord may be involved.[37] Signs and symptoms, if present, are usually caused by increased intracranial pressure and include headache, nausea and vomiting, lethargy or irritability, papilledema, and nuchal rigidity. Cranial nerves, most commonly the seventh, third, fourth, and sixth, may be involved and may on rare occasions be an isolated site of CNS leukemia at diagnosis or relapse. The hypothalamic-obesity syndrome, in which infiltration of the hypothalamus produces hyperphagia and pathologic weight gain, is a rare complication of CNS leukemia. Because of its varied symptomatology, CNS leukemia must be considered as a possible diagnosis in any patient with ALL who develops neurologic signs and symptoms.

The diagnosis of CNS leukemia is made by evaluation of cerebrospinal fluid (CSF) obtained by lumbar puncture. In symptomatic patients, the opening CSF pressure is usually increased, the CSF cell count is usually elevated, the CSF protein is frequently elevated, and the CSF glucose may or may not be decreased. CSF examination following concentration of cells by cytocentrifugation reveals leukemic lymphoblasts. Because routine CNS surveillance is standard, the diagnosis of CNS leukemia is commonly made in asymptomatic patients. In such cases, the CSF opening pressure, cell count, and protein and glucose levels may all be normal and only examination of a cytocentrifuged CSF specimen may help identify leukemic lymphoblasts.

CNS leukemia is often classified into 3 groups: CNS 1, in which there are less than 5 WBC/μL of CSF and no blasts are seen; CNS 2, in which there are less than 5 WBC/μL of CSF but blasts are present; and CNS 3, in which there are 5 WBC/μL of CSF or more and blasts are present, or cranial nerve palsies are noted. CNS involvement is relatively uncommon at diagnosis, occurring in less than 5% of children and up to 15% of adults.[37] Unless adequate CNS preventive therapy is administered, however, the majority of patients will eventually develop overt CNS disease. Because the blood–brain barrier creates a pharmacologic sanctuary that prevents many systemically administered antileukemic agents from penetrating adequately into the CNS, specific CNS treatment—in the form of intrathecal chemotherapy, high-dose systemic chemotherapy, and/or cranial radiation—is required to prevent the development of CNS leukemia. Patients with CNS 3 status are clearly at increased risk for future CNS relapse and require more intensive CNS-directed therapy, often including cranial radiation. The significance of CNS 2 status, in contrast, has been controversial, with evidence for an increased risk of CNS relapse on some treatment regimens but not others (reviewed in reference 38). Traumatic lumbar puncture (TLP) has been identified by some as an additional, distinct category of initial CNS involvement. Some studies indicate that TLP carries an increased risk of CNS relapse, due to introduction of blasts from the peripheral blood into the cerebrospinal fluid, whereas others suggest that intensive treatment may negate the risk associated with TLP.[38] Isolated CNS relapse was previously a herald of subsequent systemic relapse and poor survival, but with more intensive multimodal therapy, the survival for patients with CNS relapse, especially when it occurs late in treatment, approaches that of newly diagnosed patients.[39,40]

Testicular Leukemia

Clinically evident testicular involvement is rare at initial diagnosis, but occult testicular disease has been reported in up to 25% of newly diagnosed boys.[41] When clinically overt, testicular leukemia presents as a painless testicular enlargement which is usually unilateral. Diagnosis of testicular involvement is made by wedge biopsies, which should be done bilaterally because of the high incidence of contralateral testicular involvement.[42] Testicular leukemia is characterized by infiltration of leukemic cells into the interstitium; involvement of the seminiferous tubules occurs in more advanced disease.[43] Although it had been believed that the testes are a leukemic sanctuary site, protected from systemic chemotherapy by a blood–testes barrier, animal studies suggest this is not the case.[44] In addition, although at one point the testes appeared to be a major site of disease recurrence, it appears that the incidence of this complication has decreased as systemic therapy in general has become more intense.[45]

Testicular disease frequently occurs as an "isolated" clinical relapse in patients in bone marrow remission. The actual incidence of true isolated testicular disease, however, may be less than previously believed. A high percentage of patients with presumed isolated testicular relapse may in fact have occult leukemia present in the bone marrow[46] or other reticuloendothelial organs.[47] The frequent diagnosis of testicular involvement may simply reflect the relative ease with which recurrence can be detected clinically at this anatomic site. In contrast to the case of CNS leukemia, where routine surveillance for occult disease is essential, routine surveillance for occult testicular disease either during therapy or at the end of maintenance therapy is no longer standard. The reason for this is that there is no survival advantage when testicular leukemia is diagnosed at the occult stage rather than at clinical presentation.[48–50]

Lymph Nodes

Nodal involvement is a characteristic feature of ALL and is often responsible for bringing the patient to medical attention. Leukemic involvement usually results in obliteration of the normal microscopic structure of the node. Typically, the lymphadenopathy is generalized and enlarged nodes are painless and freely moveable.

Liver and Spleen

Hepatosplenomegaly is common in newly diagnosed patients with ALL. Pathologically, these organs show diffuse enlargement secondary to infiltration by leukemic lymphoblasts. In the spleen, the normal distinction between red and white pulp is lost. In the liver, leukemic infiltration of the portal areas is common. Even in cases associated with marked hepatomegaly, liver function abnormalities, if present, are usually mild.

Kidneys

Renal enlargement at diagnosis is common and represents diffuse infiltration by leukemic blast cells. Preferential involvement of the cortex occurs. Renal dysfunction due to leukemic cortical infiltration is rare, although many patients, especially those with a high tumor burden, do have renal dysfunction due to uric acid nephropathy.

LABORATORY EVALUATION

Hematologic Findings

Over 90% of patients with ALL have clinically evident hematologic abnormalities at diagnosis. These usually reflect the degree to which normal marrow is replaced with leukemic cells. Anemia, usually normochromic and normocytic and characteristically accompanied by a low reticulocyte count, is present in approximately 80% of cases. In approximately 50% of patients, the initial leukocyte count is elevated; in up to 25% it is greater than 50,000/mL at presentation. Patients with a profoundly elevated leukocyte count at diagnosis (>50,000/mL) have a worse prognosis. Despite the elevation in leukocyte count at diagnosis, however, many patients present with severe neutropenia (<500 granulocytes/mm^3) and are at significant risk of serious infection. Thrombocytopenia is extremely common; over three-fourths of patients present with platelet counts <100,000/mL. Only approximately one-third of patients have a platelet count <50,000/mL at diagnosis. Although petechiae and purpura are present in many patients, severe bleeding is unusual at initial presentation, even when the platelet count is <20,000/mL, unless fever, infection, or an accompanying coagulopathy, such as disseminated intravascular coagulation (DIC), are also present.

Examination of the peripheral blood smear will reveal the presence of leukemic lymphoblasts in most patients at diagnosis. Definitive diagnosis generally requires examination of the bone marrow, which is usually hypercellular and infiltrated with leukemic lymphoblasts. Technically, the presence of greater than 5% leukemic blast cells confirms the diagnosis. Most institutions, however, require at least 25% blast cells before a definitive diagnosis is rendered. More than three-fourths of patients have greater than 50% lymphoblasts in their bone marrow at initial presentation. Occasionally, it is necessary to repeat bone marrow examinations in order to arrive at the definitive diagnosis.

Other Laboratory Studies

At the time of diagnosis, many patients with ALL have elevated serum uric acid levels. The degree of uric acid elevation reflects the extent of tumor burden, higher levels occurring in patients with high initial leukocyte counts and pronounced lymphadenopathy and hepatosplenomegaly. In order to prevent uric acid nephropathy and renal failure, hyperuricemia must be corrected by vigorous use of hydration and administration of either the xanthine oxidase inhibitor allopurinol or urate oxidase (rasburicase), an enzyme that catalyzes the oxidation of uric acid to allantoin.[51]

A variety of metabolic abnormalities, including elevated serum levels of calcium, potassium, and phosphorus, may be observed in the newly diagnosed patient with ALL. These are more frequently encountered in those patients with a high leukocyte count and extensive tumor burden. Hypercalcemia may be due either to extensive infiltration of bone or to the ectopic release of a parathormone-like substance by leukemic lymphoblasts.[52] Hyperphosphatemia may accompany the extensive destruction of tumor cells. It may occur either as a result of ineffective leukopoiesis or as a consequence of chemotherapy-induced tumor lysis.[53] Hyperkalemia also can occur as a result of extensive leukemic cell lysis, although spurious hyperkalemia due to lysis of blasts *in vitro* must be considered when serum potassium levels appear elevated.[54] Lactic acidosis may also be present at diagnosis or relapse.[55]

Other laboratory abnormalities are also occasionally present at diagnosis. Low serum immunoglobulin levels at diagnosis have been reported in up to 30% of children with ALL.[56,57] Significant coagulation abnormalities are not a typical feature of ALL at diagnosis. Although DIC may occur, it is infrequent. Clotting abnormalities are observed, however, in many patients under active treatment with L-asparaginase.[58] Abnormalities in a number of lysosomal enzymes are also evident at diagnosis. Serum lactate dehydrogenase (LDH) is frequently elevated. The degree of elevation appears to correlate with tumor burden.[3,59] In addition, isoenzyme I, an acid hydrolase hexosaminidase, is frequently elevated in B-cell precursor ALL.[60]

Certain radiographic findings can also be strongly suggestive of ALL, including leukemic lines on plain films, and marrow signal abnormalities on MRI.[61]

PROGNOSIS

A number of clinical and laboratory features evident at diagnosis have prognostic value for predicting the remission duration of patients treated for ALL. Some prognostic factors may be related rather than independent. Changes in treatment strategies may result in previously significant risk factors losing their prognostic value. Furthermore, advances in technology, especially in molecular genetics, have led to more precise definition of some risk factors. It seems likely that many clinical features associated with prognosis may be "surrogate markers" for an underlying biologic feature, such as a translocation resulting in abnormal intracellular signal transduction, that actually determines prognosis.

Many clinical features have been related to prognosis. The initial leukocyte count at diagnosis has proven to be an important prognostic factor in virtually all ALL studies. In general, the prognosis is inversely related to the leukocyte count. Those patients with initial leukocyte counts greater than 50,000/mL have a particularly poor prognosis.[62,63] The relationship between white count and prognosis appears to be continuous.

Age at diagnosis also has prognostic importance. Patients who are very young (<1 year) and older patients (>10 years) tend to have a worse prognosis.[64–67] Abnormalities of chromosome band 11q23, such as the t(4;11) translocation, are especially common in the infant age group, and this association may in part be responsible for their poor prognosis.

Immunophenotype also correlates with prognosis.[68–70] ALL patients with either mature B-cell or T-cell immunophenotypes generally have a worse prognosis than patients with B-precursor ALL, although the prognostic influence of T-cell phenotype is less striking after adjusting for its association with high initial leukocyte count. Moreover, on some recent, more intensive treatment protocols, the T-cell phenotype lacks prognostic significance.[71] Highly aggressive treatment also improves the outcome of patients with mature B-cell ALL.[72–74]

The expression of myeloid markers on ALL cells may be associated with a poor prognosis in children with ALL, although this is not apparent in all analyses.[22,75,76] There is also a relationship between morphologic subtype and prognosis. The FAB L3 subtype is associated with mature B-cell ALL and thus conveys a relatively poorer prognosis. In many studies of childhood ALL, the L2 subtype has also been associated with more resistant disease and poorer survival compared to L1.[77,78] However, several studies suggest that L2 morphology does not have prognostic significance independent of other risk factors such as age, sex, and white blood cell count.[79,80] In some studies, low serum immunoglobulins, particularly low IgM levels, have also been associated with poor event-free survival.[56,57,81]

Gender and race may also influence outcome. Female patients have a more favorable prognosis. This appears to be related to the impact of testicular relapse and to the higher incidence of T-cell disease in male patients.[66,82,83] Ethnicity appears to be an important prognostic determinant. African American and Hispanic patients have a lower remission induction rate and a higher likelihood of experiencing bone marrow relapse.[84–86] The reasons for this poor outcome are related in part to the more frequent recurrence of very elevated initial leukocyte counts, mediastinal masses, and L2 morphology in this population.[84,87,88] However, even when these factors are adjusted for, there still appears to be an increased risk of treatment failure for nonwhite patients.[89]

In the past, tumor burden as reflected by hepatomegaly, splenomegaly, massive lymphadenopathy, and/or mediastinal mass demonstrated prognostic significance. However, on multivariate analysis they are closely related to the initial leukocyte count,[90–93] and hence in the current National Cancer Institute classification scheme for ALL, neither organomegaly nor lymphadenopathy is viewed as a primary prognostic factor (Table 64–4).[63]

Advanced molecular diagnosis is providing new insight into prognosis. The association between chromosomal number and prognosis is well characterized. Hyperdiploidy occurs in about 35% of pediatric ALL and is an independent positive prognostic factor, particularly high hyperdiploidy, which has been variously defined in the literature as exceeding a threshold of between 50 and 55.[94–96] More recently, particular trisomies have been identified that appear to be more significant than total chromosome number as predictors of favorable outcome: trisomies 4 and 10,[97] trisomies 10 and 17,[94] and the triple trisomies of 4, 10, and 17.[98]

In contrast, patients with hypodiploidy fare less well.[99] Cases lacking only a single chromosome have similar prognosis to diploid cases, but those with less than 45 chromosomes have a significantly inferior outcome, with the worst outcome in near-haploid cases (24–28 chromosomes).[99,100] Rare cases with near triploidy (68–80 chromosomes) or near tetraploidy (>80 chromosomes) have also been associated with very poor outcome,[101] although a recent large series found a favorable outcome in the B-lineage cases.[102]

Abnormalities in chromosome structure, as well as number, convey important prognostic information. Recent technical advances have led to the identification of previously unappreciated, prognostically significant gene rearrangements. A number of chromosomal translocations are associated with both a high rate of induction failure and early relapse, including the t(8;14) translocation associated with B-cell ALL, the t(9;22) *BCR-ABL* gene rearrangement found in Philadelphia chromosome positive ALL, the t(1;19) *E2A-PBX1* gene rearrangement occurring in B-precursor ALL, and the t(4;11) *MLL* translocation occurring most frequently in infants. In contrast, the t(12;21) translocation, which results in the *TEL-AML1* rearrangement, is present in approximately 25% of cases of B-cell precursor ALL and is associated with improved outcome.[26,103–109] These recurrent genetic lesions are discussed in greater detail in Chapter 63. Identification of the fusion proteins and other functional abnormalities produced by these chromosomal abnormalities may radically change therapy for ALL in the future. Proof of this principle is the remarkable success of imatinib mesylate (Gleevec), a rationally designed inhibitor of the *bcr-abl* fusion tyrosine kinase produced by the t(9;22) translocation.[110]

Perhaps one of the most significant prognostic factors is the response to initial treatment, although strictly speaking it is not a presenting feature of patients with ALL. Nonetheless, patients who fail to achieve complete remission after completing an initial course of induction therapy have markedly reduced remission duration and survival. The rapidity of initial cytoreduction appears to be extremely important. For example, the presence of residual leukemia in the marrow on day 7 or 14 of induction therapy has been associated with shorter event-free survival compared with patients whose marrow shows no evidence of residual disease at that time.[87,90,111,112] In some studies, response to initial therapy has been the overriding prognostic factor regardless of initial disease features.[113,114]

Morphologic examination of the bone marrow is the classic approach to assessing response to treatment, with remission defined as less than 5% blasts. Newer molecular definitions of remission based on minimal residual disease (MRD) detection are far more sensitive in identifying patients at risk of ultimate morphologic relapse. Precisely how and when MRD should be measured in clinical practice remains unresolved, but it is clearly an important disease parameter to follow. MRD can be measured by assessing for the presence of aberrant combinations of immunophenotypic markers by flow cytometry, for clone-specific immunoglobulin or T-cell receptor rearrangements by PCR, or for fusion proteins generated by translocations, also using PCR.[115] Persistent MRD bears adverse prognostic significance at all time points that have been studied, ranging from early induction to 24 months into treatment.[116–120] Conversely, rapid achievement of MRD negativity before the end of induction identifies a favorable prognosis group with a high probability of cure, who might be spared the adverse effects of high-intensity regimens.[121]

CONCLUSION

Current treatment regimens for childhood ALL use prognostic factors to define different risk groups that are subsequently treated according to their relative risk of failure.[122] In turn, improved treatment strategies may reduce the impact on survival of a given prognostic factor. In most centers, patients with poor risk features receive more intensive treatment, while those with good risk features receive treatment designed to be effective yet minimize treatment-related adverse sequelae. The use of different prognostic factors for stratification of risk groups may lead to difficulty in comparing the results of different approaches to therapy. A uniform approach to risk factor assessment based on a combination of clinical and laboratory criteria has recently been developed (Table 64–4),[123] and further characterization of molecular markers of prognosis is a major current research effort. The success of this risk-based strategy and the general principles of treatment in childhood ALL are detailed in Chapter 65.

SUGGESTED READINGS

Cave H, van der Werff ten Bosch J, Suciu S, et al: Clinical significance of minimal residual disease in childhood acute lymphoblastic leukemia. European Organization for Research and Treatment of Cancer—Childhood Leukemia Cooperative Group. N Engl J Med 339(9):591, 1998.

Chessells JM: Pitfalls in the diagnosis of childhood leukaemia. Br J Haematol 114(3):506, 2001.

Greaves M: Infection, immune responses and the aetiology of childhood leukaemia. Nat Rev Cancer 6(3):193, 2006.

Hoelzer D, Gokbuget N, Ottmann O, et al: Acute lymphoblastic leukemia. Hematology Am Soc Hematol Educ Program 2002:162.

Second MIC Cooperative Study Group: Morphologic, immunologic and cytogenetic (MIC) working classification of the acute myeloid leukaemias. Br J Haematol 68(4):487, 1988.

Pui CH: Central nervous system disease in acute lymphoblastic leukemia: Prophylaxis and treatment. Hematology Am Soc Hematol Educ Program 2006:142.

Pui CH, Evans WE: Treatment of acute lymphoblastic leukemia. N Engl J Med 354(2):166, 2006.

Rubnitz J, Downing J, Pui C-H, et al: TEL gene rearrangement in acute lymphoblastic leukemia: A new genetic marker with prognostic significance. J Clin Oncol 15:1150, 1997.

Smith M, Arthur D, Camitta B, et al: Uniform approach to risk classification and treatment assignment for children with acute lymphoblastic leukemia. J Clin Oncol 14(1):18, 1996.

Sutcliffe MJ, Shuster JJ, Sather HN, et al: High concordance from independent studies by the Children's Cancer Group (CCG) and Pediatric Oncology Group (POG) associating favorable prognosis with combined trisomies 4, 10, and 17 in children with NCI Standard-Risk B-precursor Acute Lymphoblastic Leukemia: A Children's Oncology Group (COG) initiative. Leukemia 19(5):734, 2005.

Uckun FM, Sensel MG, Sun L, et al: Biology and treatment of childhood T-lineage acute lymphoblastic leukemia. Blood 91(3):735, 1998.

Weir EG, Cowan K, LeBeau P, Borowitz MJ: A limited antibody panel can distinguish B-precursor acute lymphoblastic leukemia from normal B precursors with four color flow cytometry: Implications for residual disease detection. Leukemia 13(4):558, 1999.

Yeoh EJ, Ross ME, Shurtleff SA, et al: Classification, subtype discovery, and prediction of outcome in pediatric acute lymphoblastic leukemia by gene expression profiling. Cancer Cell 1(2):133, 2002.

REFERENCES

For complete list of references log onto www.expertconsult.com

CHAPTER 65

TREATMENT OF CHILDHOOD ACUTE LYMPHOBLASTIC LEUKEMIA

Sima Jeha and Ching-Hon Pui

INTRODUCTION

Steady progress in the development of treatment strategies for childhood acute lymphoblastic leukemia (ALL) started in the 1950s, when complete remissions were achieved using single chemotherapeutic agents.[1,2] Combining and cycling these agents, with the addition of central nervous system (CNS) prophylaxis, significantly prolonged remissions resulting in cure rates of approximately 50% in the 1970s.[3] Drugs developed over 30 years ago, such as mercaptopurine, methotrexate, vincristine, corticosteroids, anthracyclines, and asparaginase, still constitute the backbone of contemporary ALL protocols resulting in long-term, event-free survival rates exceeding 80%.[4] This progress was accomplished with serial clinical trials using outcome predictors to stratify therapy.[5–12] A uniform risk classification approach based on age and leukocyte count at diagnosis was adapted at a National Cancer Institute-sponsored workshop held in 1993, based on the observation that patients with high presenting leukocyte counts are at greater risk for subsequent relapse than those with lower leukocyte counts at diagnosis, and that children between 1 and 10 years of age have a better outcome than infants, or older patients.[13] This classification proved to be insufficient because up to a third of patients designated as standard-risk may relapse and this criteria cannot be applied to T-cell ALL. With improved understanding of the immunology and molecular pathways involved in ALL, current risk classification typically include age, leukocyte count at diagnosis, blast cell immunophenotype and genotype, as well as early treatment response. The most common form of acute leukemia in children is B-precursor cell, which is frequently associated with extra chromosomes (hyperdiploidy), or expression of *ETV6–CBFA2* (*TEL–AML1*). As discussed in Chapter 63, *E2A–PBX1* and *BCR–ABL* rearrangements are not common in children with ALL, and the *MLL(HRX)* gene rearrangement is predominant in young infants. Hypodiploidy (less than 44 chromosomes per leukemic cell) and rearrangement of *BCR–ABL* or *MLL* are unfavorable prognostic indicators.[14,15] Hyperdiploidy (more than 50 chromosomes) and the *TEL–AML1* gene fusion are associated with favorable outcomes; however, 10% to 15% of these patients relapse despite contemporary therapy. Early response to therapy, as measured by minimal residual disease (MRD) evaluation, has played an increasingly important role in risk stratification of ALL. Accordingly, patients are divided into three risk groups: low-, intermediate-, and high-risk (also referred to as standard-, high-, and very high-risk categories in other risk classification schema). Current childhood ALL therapy emphasizes early and vigorous assessment of the risk of relapse in individual patients, to improve outcome of patients with high-risk leukemia while minimizing long-term sequelae and enhancing the quality of life in patients at low risk of relapse.[4]

PRINCIPLES OF TREATMENT

Accurate assessment of relapse hazard is an integral part of ALL therapy, so that only high-risk patients are treated aggressively, with less toxic therapy reserved for cases at lower risk of failure. The prognostic impact of age and, to a lesser extent, leukocyte count can be explained partly by their association with specific genetic abnormalities. For example, the poor prognosis of infants is associated with *MLL* rearrangement (detected in 70%–80% of patients in this age group), and the overall favorable outcome of patients aged 1 to 9 years is related to the preponderance of cases with hyperdiploidy greater than 50 or *TEL–AML1* fusion.[4,14] As mentioned earlier, primary genetic features do not entirely account for treatment outcome. Although up to 15% of patients with hyperdiploidy greater than 50 or *TEL–AML1* fusion suffer recurrences of their leukemia, a substantial proportion of the patients with the t(9;22) and *BCR–ABL* fusion who are 1 to 9 years old and have low leukocyte counts at diagnosis may be cured with intensive chemotherapy alone.[16] Among patients with *MLL–AF4* fusion, infants and adults have a worse prognosis than children.[17–19] Genetic polymorphisms of drug transporters, receptors, targets, and drug-metabolizing enzymes can influence the efficacy and toxicity of antineoplastic agents.[14] Interindividual variability in the pharmacokinetics and pharmacodynamics of many antileukemic agents might partially explain the heterogeneity in treatment response among patients with specific genetic abnormalities and the difference in outcome by age group. We and others have identified multiple polymorphisms associated with relapse risk, acute toxicity, and late effects.[20–25] Individualizing therapy on the basis of germline genetic status may help optimize treatment (as discussed in Chapter 9). The prime example is the use of polymorphisms of thiopurine methyltransferase, an enzyme that catalyzes the methylation of thiopurines, such as mercaptopurine and thioguanine, to guide treatment.[24] Concomitant administration of drugs that induce cytochrome P450 enzymes (eg, phenobarbital and phenytoin) significantly increases the systemic clearance of several antileukemic agents and may adversely affect treatment outcome. Hence, response to therapy is determined by several factors including the leukemic cell biologic features, the pharmacogenetics of the patient, the treatment regimens administered, and compliance to therapy. Indeed, the degree of reduction of the leukemic cell clone early during remission induction therapy has shown greater prognostic strength than any other individual biological or host-related feature.[26] Assessing MRD by flow-cytometric detection of aberrant immunophenotypes or analysis by polymerase chain reaction of clonal antigen-receptor gene rearrangements provides a level of sensitivity and specificity that cannot be attained by traditional morphological assessment of treatment response.[26] Patients who are in morphological remission but have a postinduction MRD level of 1% or more fare as poorly as those who do not achieve clinical remission by conventional criteria (>5% blasts). Approximately half of all patients show a disease reduction to 10^{-4} or lower after only 2 weeks of remission induction, and they appear to have an exceptionally good treatment outcome. Although MRD positivity is strongly associated with known presenting risk features, it has independent prognostic strength and is increasingly used to intensify ALL therapy in contemporary regimens.

PHASES OF THERAPY

Recognition that ALL is a heterogenous disease and the identification of reliable prognostic factors have led to wide use of risk-directed therapy. With the exception of mature B-cell ALL cases, which are treated with short-term intensive chemotherapy (including high-dose methotrexate, cytarabine, and cyclophosphamide),[27,28] therapy for

Minimal Residual Disease

The rapidity of response to induction therapy is an important independent predictor of outcome. There is strong concordance between the assessment of MRD by flow cytometry and by polymerase chain reaction methods. We monitor MRD using primarily a flow cytometry method, which is simple and rapid, and we reserve polymerase chain reaction methods for the few patients (less than 5%) whose leukemic cells lack a suitable immunophenotype. Approximately half of all patients show a disease reduction to 10^{-4} or lower after only 2 weeks of remission induction, and these patients appear to have an exceptionally good treatment outcome. Persistence of MRD of 10^{-4} or more at 4 months from diagnosis is associated with an especially dismal outcome. The adverse prognosis of high-risk slow early responders can be improved with intensification of induction and consolidation. Standard-risk cases may be spared the increased risk of early morbidity and mortality from intensive induction, provided that they receive postinduction intensification therapy.

Drug Interactions

We have not yet reached a full understanding of the contribution of genetic polymorphisms to interindividual differences in drug effects that allows us to translate this new knowledge into clinical practice. However, by simply avoiding drug interactions, one can prevent increased toxicity or reduced efficacy of chemotherapy. Phenytoin and phenobarbital induce the activity of cytochrome P450 enzymes, significantly increasing the systemic clearance of several antileukemic agents that may adversely affect treatment outcome. We substitute these anticonvulsants with gabapentin in patients receiving antileukemic therapy. On the other hand, azole compounds (eg, fluconazole, itraconazole, ketaconazole) can inhibit cytochrome P450 enzymes and increase the toxicities of various antileukemic agents, especially vincristine.

Dose Schedule

The biologically equivalent doses between the different formulations of corticosteroids, thiopurines, and asparaginase are not known. Trials comparing such agents should be cautiously interpreted taking into account the dose schedule used, and the effect of variability in the pharmacokinetic profile and potency among the agents involved. Simple modification of dose or schedule may result in significant difference in efficacy and toxicity. Also, when comparing regimens containing high-dose intravenous methotrexate, the dose schedule of leucovorin rescue should not be ignored, as it plays a crucial role in modulating the activity and toxicity of methotrexate.

High Risk CNS

Patients with the following characteristics are at increased risk of CNS relapse and require more intense CNS-directed therapy:

1. Patients with high-risk genetic features
2. Large leukemic cell burden
3. T-lineage ALL
4. CNS-3 status (>5 WBC/microliter CSF with presence of lymphoblasts on cytospin)
5. CNS-2 status (<5 WBC/microliter CSF with lymphoblasts)
6. Traumatic CSF with blasts

Consolidation Therapy

The importance of a consolidation phase following remission induction is undisputed, but the treatment regimen and duration varies in the different childhood ALL studies. Commonly used strategies include high-dose methotrexate plus mercaptopurine, frequent pulses of vincristine and corticosteroid plus high-dose asparaginase for 20 to 30 weeks, and reinduction treatment with the same agents given during initial remission induction. Reinduction treatment has become an integral component of contemporary protocols. In one randomized study, double reinduction further improved treatment outcome in patients with intermediate-risk ALL, whereas additional pulses of vincristine and prednisone after a single reinduction course were not beneficial, suggesting that the increased dose intensity of other drugs, such as asparaginase, was responsible for the observed improvement. An "augmented" regimen including Capizzi methotrexate (escalating-dose intravenous methotrexate with no rescue, followed by asparaginase) and additional doses of vincristine and asparaginase during periods of myelosuppression, improved outcome of patients with a slow early response to therapy.

ALL typically consists of a brief remission-induction phase followed by intensification (or consolidation) therapy to eliminate residual disease, and then prolonged continuation treatment to maintain remission. All patients also require treatment directed to the CNS early in the clinical course to prevent relapse due to leukemic cells sequestered in this site.[4]

Contemporary protocols stratify therapy based on risk groups defined by age, leukocyte count, immunophenotype, leukemic genotype, and response to early remission induction therapy.[5–12] The standard or lower risk category includes patients between 1 and 10 years of age with an initial leukocyte count less than $50 \times 10^9\ L^{-1}$, and the remaining patients are considered higher risk. Additional features used by some investigators to stratify patients as lower risk include hyperdiploidy greater than 50 (DNA index > 1.16) and trisomy of chromosomes 4 and 10. Conversely, other characteristics such as T-cell phenotype, adverse cytogenetic translocations [t(9;22) and t(4;11)], overt CNS leukemia at diagnosis, and slow early response to induction chemotherapy have been used to stratify patients as high risk.

Remission Induction

Remission induction therapy aims at eradicating more than 99% of the initial leukemic cell burden and restoring normal hematopoiesis. This treatment phase typically lasts 4 to 6 weeks, and includes the administration of a glucocorticoid (prednisone or dexamethasone), vincristine, and at least a third drug (asparaginase or anthracycline, or both). A two-drug remission induction regimen of weekly vincristine and daily prednisone results in remission in 80% to 90% of children with ALL.[29,30] Addition of a third agent, such as asparaginase or an anthracycline, increases the remission rate to approximately 95%.[31,32] In addition to improving remission rates, intensified induction regimen also prolong remission duration. In a study in which children were randomly assigned to receive identical therapy except for induction drugs, one group received vincristine and prednisone and the other received those two drugs plus an anthracycline.

Although the complete remission rates for both groups exceeded 90%, there was long-term benefit for the more intensively treated group.[32,33] A three-drug induction regimen appears sufficient for most standard-risk cases, provided they receive intensified postremission therapy.[34] The benefit in long-term survival of using 4 or more drugs during induction is widely accepted in higher-risk patients but less clear in lower-risk patients.[35] Among the studies with the best reported outcomes, most rely on at least four drugs for remission induction for all patients, regardless of their risk group status.[5,10,12] Children with high-risk ALL are treated with four or more drugs for remission induction.[4] Addition of a tyrosine kinase inhibitor has greatly improved the remission induction rate, duration of disease-free survival, and quality of life of patients with Philadelphia positive (Ph+) ALL.[36,37]

On the basis of reports of more potent in vitro antileukemic activity and better CNS penetration,[38–41] dexamethasone has replaced prednisone in some induction and many continuation regimens.[12,42–44] However, the biologically equivalent doses between dexamethasone and prednisone are not known, and one study suggested that prednisone can yield results comparable to dexamethasone, provided a higher dose is used (ie, 60 mg/m^2/d).[45] Not surprising, dexamethasone given at higher dose was associated with increased incidence of hyperglycemia, hypertension, myopathy, bony morbidity, severe behavioral changes, and infectious complications.[46] As with glucocorticoids, the pharmacodynamics of asparaginase differ by formulation.[47] The native *Escherichia coli* asparaginase has been the most commonly used preparation. Polyethylene glycol-conjugated asparaginase, a long-acting and less allergenic form, is progressively replacing the native product and is being increasingly administered intravenously instead of intramuscularly.[48] Asparaginase derived from *Erwinia chrysanthemi* has a short half-life and its use is currently limited to patients who are allergic to the *E coli* formulations. The dose schedule for asparaginase should take into account the variability in the pharmacokinetic profile and potency among the different preparations.

The rapidity of response to induction therapy, as measured by clearance of peripheral and bone marrow blasts, is an important predictor of outcome,[4,5] although intensification of postinduction therapy can improve the adverse prognosis of slow early responders.[49] With modern chemotherapy and supportive care, 97% to 99% of children can be expected to attain complete morphological remission (ie, <5% blasts in bone marrow) at the end of remission induction, that is, those who do not have a poor outcome.[50,51] Hence, most investigators offer these patients the option of allogeneic hematopoietic stem cell transplantation at the end of extended induction treatment.[52] We and others have found that patients with 1% blasts identified by MRD studies had an outcome as poor as those with induction failure[53,54] and the patients may also be candidates for allogeneic transplantation.

Consolidation (Intensification)

Following remission induction, consolidation (or intensification) is given to eradicate drug-resistant residual leukemic cells. Therapy is tailored to the leukemia subtype and risk group. Intensifying asparaginase therapy during the early phase of treatment improved results in the Dana Farber Cancer Institute studies.[55] Adding doxorubicin to asparaginase favorably influenced the outcome of high-risk patients, particularly those with T-cell disease.[56,57] Significant improvement was also reported in the outcome of patients receiving early intensification consisting of intermediate-dose or high-dose antimetabolite therapy.[57–60] The optimal dose of methotrexate depends on the leukemic cell genotype and phenotype, as well as host pharmacogenetic and pharmacokinetic parameters. Methotrexate at 2.5 g/m^2 is adequate for most patients with standard-risk B-cell precursor ALL, but a higher dose (5 g/m^2) may benefit those with T-cell or high-risk B-cell precursor ALL.[5] This observation is consistent with the finding that T-lineage blast cells accumulate methotrexate polyglutamates less avidly than do B-lineage blast cells.[61] The increased ability of hyperdiploid ALL blasts cells to accumulate methotrexate polyglutamate could partially explain the excellent outcome of children with hyperdiploidy greater than 50 ALL treated on low-intensity antimetabolites-based regimens.[62–64] The relatively low accumulation of methotrexate polyglutamates in blast cells with either *TEL–AML1* or *E2A–PBX1* fusion suggests that patients with these genotypes may also benefit from an increased dose of methotrexate.[65] Leucovorin rescue is necessary after treatment with high-dose methotrexate; however, overzealous rescue might counteract the antileukemic activity of methotrexate.[66]

Delayed intensification, pioneered by the Berlin–Frankfurt–Münster consortium, consists of using drugs similar to those used in remission induction therapy after 3 months of a less intensive, interim maintenance chemotherapy.[5] The Children's Cancer Group confirmed the efficacy of delayed reinduction therapy in low-risk cases,[67] and showed that double-delayed intensification with a second reinduction at week 32 of treatment improved outcome in patients with intermediate-risk disease.[68] An augmented intensification regimen consisting of the administration of additional doses of vincristine and asparaginase during the myelosuppression period following delayed intensification, and sequential escalating-dose parental methotrexate followed by asparaginase (Capizzi methotrexate), improved the outcome of high-risk patients whose disease had responded slowly to initial multiagent induction therapy.[49]

Continuation (Maintenance)

Continuation or maintenance phase consists of 2 to 2.5 years of low-intensity metronomic chemotherapy designed to eradicate any residual leukemic cell burden. Weekly low-dose methotrexate and daily oral mercaptopurine form the backbone of most continuation regimens. Adjusting chemotherapy doses to maintain neutrophil counts between 0.5 and 1.5×10^9 L^{-1} has been associated with a better clinical outcome.[4,69] Overzealous use of mercaptopurine, to the extent that neutropenia necessitates chemotherapy interruption, reduces overall dose intensity and is counterproductive.[70] It is generally recommended to give mercaptopurine at bedtime to patients with an empty stomach[71] and to avoid taking it together with milk or milk products containing xanthine oxidase, an enzyme that can degrade the drug.[72] Approximately 10% of the population inherit one wild-type gene encoding TMPT and one nonfunctional variant allele, resulting in intermediate enzyme activity, whereas 1 in 300 people inherits two nonfunctional variant alleles and is completely deficient of this inactivating enzyme.[73,74] Patients with heterozygous and especially homozygous deficiency of thiopurine methyltransferase are at high risk of severe myelosuppression. Identification of these patients allows selective reductions in mercaptopurine dosage without modifying the dose of methotrexate.[24,75] Patients with thiopurine methyltransferase deficiency are also at greater risk of developing therapy-related acute myeloid leukemia and radiation-induced brain tumors, in the context of intensive thiopurine therapy.[24,76–78] Conversely, patients with higher levels of enzyme activity might be at a greater risk for relapse as a result of decreased exposure of leukemic cells to active drug metabolites.[5] Substituting thioguanine for mercaptopurine during continuation therapy was associated with a high incidence of profound thrombocytopenia and hepatic veno-occlusive disease.[79–81] Thioguanine use has therefore been limited to short pulses administered during consolidation therapy in some trials, whereas mercaptopurine is selected for prolonged administration.

Many groups add regular pulses of vincristine and corticosteroids to this regimen although the benefit of these pulses in the context of contemporary therapy has not been established.[82] The optimal duration of therapy remains unknown. Attempts to shorten therapy duration from 24 months to 12 or 18 months have resulted in a significant increase in relapses.[83] Many studies extend treatment for boys to 3 years because of their generally poorer outcome compared with girls,[84,85] although the benefit of this approach remains to be demonstrated. Several studies showed no advantage to prolonging treatment beyond 3 years.[86,87]

Central Nervous System-Directed Therapy

The importance of therapy directed to the CNS was first demonstrated by investigators at St. Jude Children's Research Hospital in the 1960s, when the incidence of CNS leukemia as an initial site of relapse became progressively more common as more effective chemotherapeutic regimens resulted in longer duration of hematologic remissions. This was attributed to the CNS's acting as a pharmacologic sanctuary, poorly penetrated by conventional doses of systematically administered chemotherapeutic agents.[88,89] Radiation therapy was the first modality to successfully prevent CNS relapse.[91] The effectiveness of 2400 cGy cranial radiation as preventive therapy was offset by substantial late effects in long-term survivors, including learning disabilities, multiple endocrinopathy, and an increased risk of second malignancies. Subsequent trials demonstrated that, in the context of intensive systemic and intrathecal therapy, cranial irradiation can be reduced[5,92] or even omitted altogether.[5,8,92,93]

Patients with high-risk genetic features, large leukemic cell burden, T-lineage ALL, and leukemic cells in the cerebrospinal fluid (CSF) even from iatrogenic introduction from a traumatic lumbar puncture at diagnosis are at increased risk of CNS relapse and require more intense CNS-directed therapy.[94] Approximately 2% to 3% of patients will present with CNS-3 status (detectable CNS leukemia defined as >5 WBC per microliter CSF with the presence of lymphoblasts on a cytospin preparation) and an additional 5% to 10% with CNS-2 status (<5 WBC per microliter CSF with lymphoblasts) or traumatic lumbar puncture with blasts.[94,95] These patients are at an increased risk of CNS relapse and benefit from more aggressive CNS-directed therapy.[93] Special care is being taken to minimize traumatic lumbar punctures, to deliver intrathecal therapy optimally, and to intensify systemic and intrathecal therapy in high-risk cases.[96] Studies have successfully used triple intrathecal therapy or intrathecal methotrexate alone. A randomized study did not resolve the controversy over the optimal type of intrathecal therapy as the benefit from reduction in CNS relapse was offset by a higher rate of medullary relapse in the patients randomized to receive triple intrathecal therapy with methotrexate, hydrocortisone, and cytarabine.[80] Systematically administered agents, including high-dose methotrexate,[97–99] dexamethasone,[38] and asparaginase,[100] may contribute to the prevention of CNS relapse.

ALLOGENEIC HEMATOPOIETIC STEM-CELL TRANSPLANTATION

Comparisons between allogeneic hematopoietic stem-cell transplantation and intensive chemotherapy have yielded inconsistent results owing to the small numbers of patients studied and differences in case selection criteria.[101,102] Allogeneic transplantation during initial complete remission may improve outcome of children with poor response to initial induction chemotherapy, t(9;22), early hematologic relapse, or T-cell ALL with poor early response or hematologic relapse.[16,37,103] The benefit of allogeneic hematopoietic stem-cell transplantation in infants with t(4;11) ALL remains controversial.[18,104–106] Matched unrelated-donor or cord blood transplantation has yielded outcomes comparable to those obtained with matched related-donor transplantation and should be considered reasonable alternatives if a matched donor is not available.[107,108] Autologous transplantation has failed to improve outcome in ALL.[101] With improving prospects for effective targeted therapy, the need for allogeneic transplantation should be continuously reevaluated.

INFANT ALL

Infant ALL comprises approximately 4% of childhood ALL, and is associated with a high WBC count at presentation, a high frequency of an immature B-cell precursor phenotype characterized by the lack of CD10 expression, and the presence of *MLL* rearrangements.[109,110] Rearrangements of the *MLL* gene on chromosome 11q23 occur in 70% to 80% of infants with ALL, and are mostly associated with the t(4;11) translocation with *MLL–AF4* fusion.[109] Whereas the outcome of the 15% to 20% infants with *MLL* germline ALL is comparable to that of older children with ALL, those with very young age (<6 months), high initial leukocyte count (WBC > 300 × 10^9 L^{-1}), *MLL* rearrangement, and a poor early response to therapy have a dismal prognosis with less than 20% survival rates.[18,104,109,110] As mentioned earlier, the use of hematopoietic stem-cell transplantation in infants is controversial. Two recent publications suggest that the use of hematopoietic stem-cell transplantation contributed to a favorable outcome in infant ALL.[106,107] However, these studies did not have a control arm in which patients only received chemotherapy and the data were not corrected for waiting time to hematopoietic stem-cell transplantation. Moreover, in one of these studies total body irradiation was used and led to substantial late effects in infants.[107] Data from a large retrospective intergroup analysis did not show differences between infant *MLL*-rearranged patients who did or did not receive hematopoietic stem-cell transplantation.[18]

RELAPSE

Most relapses occur during treatment or within the first 2 years after its completion, although relapses have been reported as late as 10 years after an initial ALL diagnosis.[111] The most common site of relapse is the bone marrow. Relapse in extramedullary sites, such as the CNS and testes, has decreased to less than 5% and 2%, respectively.[112] Leukemia relapse occasionally occurs at other sites, including the eye, ovary, uterus, bone, muscle, tonsil, kidney, mediastinum, pleura, and paranasal sinus. Extramedullary relapse in children with ALL frequently presents as an isolated clinical finding. However, in studies that included an MRD assay, many extramedullary recurrences were associated with MRD in the bone marrow.[113] A small fraction of patients experience a recurrence of acute leukemia with an immunophenotype different from that determined at diagnosis. Some of the cases represent relapse of original leukemic clones with a shift in immunophenotype, but others are secondary malignancies caused by the mutagenic effects of leukemia treatment especially from epipodophyllotoxin.[114] Patients with isolated bone marrow relapse generally fare worse than those with combined bone marrow and extramedullary relapse.[113] Factors indicating an especially poor prognosis are a short initial remission and a T-cell immunophenotype. Other adverse factors include t(9;22). The presence of minimal residual disease at the end of second remission induction is also a strong adverse prognostic indicator.[115,116] Salvage regimens are mostly based on different combinations of the same agents used in frontline therapy, and are associated with significant morbidity and dismal long-term survival rates in most cases. Patients with early or multiple relapses and heavy prior chemotherapy exposure have an expected median survival of 9 to 10 weeks even when multiagent chemotherapy is used. Although chemotherapy may secure a prolonged second remission in children with ALL who experience late relapse (defined as more than 6 months after cessation of therapy), allogeneic hematopoietic stem cell transplantation is the treatment of choice for patients who experience hematologic relapse during therapy or shortly thereafter and for those with T-cell ALL. Patients with late-onset isolated CNS relapse who had not received cranial irradiation as initial CNS-directed therapy have a very high remission retrieval rate, with long-term prognosis approaching that of newly diagnosed patients in those who had a long initial remission before the CNS event.[101,117,118]

SUPPORTIVE CARE

Supportive care is especially important during remission induction treatment, when there is an increased risk from cardiovascular, metabolic, and infectious complications. Rapid turnover of leukemia cells before and immediately after the initiation of chemotherapy leads to metabolic disturbances including hyperkalemia, hyperuricemia, hyperphosphatemia, and hypocalcemia.[119] Patients with high levels of uric acid are at risk for the development of acute renal failure secondary to uric acid deposition in the kidneys. All patients require intravenous hydration to prevent or treat hyperuricemia and hyperphosphatemia. Allopurinol, a xanthine oxidase inhibitor, can prevent uric acid formation. Rasburicase, a recombinant urate oxidase that breaks down uric acid to allantoin (a readily excretable metabolite with 5- to 10-fold higher solubility than uric acid), is more effective than allopurinol but is associated with methemoglobinemia or hemolytic anemia in patients with glucose-6-phosphate dehydrogenase deficiency because hydrogen peroxide is a byproduct of the uric acid breakdown.[120] Phosphate binders should also be used to prevent or treat hyperphosphatemia.

Transfusions should be administered slowly in patients with severe anemia to prevent congestive heart failure. In patients with extreme hyperleukocytosis, packed red blood cell transfusion should be delayed until after leukocyte count is decreased by leukapheresis, exchange transfusion, or chemotherapy to prevent complications of leukostasis. We limit the use of leukapheresis to patients presenting with a leukocyte count of 400×10^9 L^{-1} or greater, because they have a high risk of intracranial bleeding, pulmonary complications, and neurologic events as a result of leukostasis.[121] Exchange transfusion is preferred in smaller children. Mechanical reduction of leukocyte count is a short-acting supportive measure and should not delay prompt initiation of chemotherapy. All blood products should be irradiated in patients who are receiving immunosuppressive therapy to prevent graft-versus-host disease.

Patients should avoid foods that may be contaminated with pathogens[122] and reduce salt intake, which could induce hypertension and resultant seizure in patients receiving glucocorticoids during induction.[123] Adolescents, obese individuals, and Down syndrome patients are at increased risk of hyperglycemia and other complications.[124] All febrile patients should be given broad-spectrum intravenous antibiotics until an infectious disease is excluded. Prophylaxis with trimethoprim-sulfamethoxazole successfully prevents *Pneumocystis carinii* pneumonia.[125] Dental evaluation at diagnosis and meticulous oral hygiene during chemotherapy minimizes the oral complications of leukemia and its treatment. Oral candidiasis occurs frequently, especially in young children. Azole compounds (eg, fluconazole, itraconazole, ketaconazole) are frequently used to treat fungal infections. It should be recognized that they can inhibit cytochrome P450 enzymes and increase the toxicities of various antileukemic agents, especially vincristine.[126] Photosensitive skin rash can occur during antimetabolite therapy. The rashes are erythematous, maculopapular, similar to atopic eczema, and most prominent on the face. Children with a history of atopy appear to have a higher incidence of this complication. Topical administration of simple emollients or a weak steroid preparation, and avoidance of external exposure to sunlight should improve the skin condition. Patients with Down syndrome tolerate methotrexate poorly; appropriate dose adjustment is indicated.[127,128] Please refer to Chapters 64, 91, 92, 96, 148, and 152 for more details on supportive measures in children with cancer.

LATE EFFECTS OF TREATMENT

The most problematic late effects of contemporary ALL therapy include neuropsychological impairments, bone morbidity, and obesity.[129–133] Although neuropsychologic deficits are well-recognized side effects of cranial irradiation, intrathecal and systemic chemotherapy (especially methotrexate) can also cause brain atrophy and spinal cord dysfunction.[129,130] Severe CNS toxicity has been attributed to cranial irradiation at doses of 2400 cGy or higher, but lower doses have also been associated with long-term neuropsychological impairments, especially in younger children. Systemic and intrathecal chemotherapy contribute to the development of neurocognitive toxicities.[130] Obesity, most prevalent among female survivors of childhood ALL, may be related to cranial radiation and corticosteroids. Osteopenia, fractures, and osteonecrosis has been observed in up to 30% of survivors of childhood ALL.[131] Osteonecrosis, which can lead to significant pain, loss of function, and total joint replacement, has been reported in approximately 8% of children with ALL, with the highest frequency observed in those diagnosed in adolescence.[132,133] Ovarian and testicular function are relatively unaffected by most antileukemic therapy. Offspring of patients successfully treated for childhood ALL are expected to be normal as general population.[134] Second malignant neoplasms, including malignant gliomas, meningiomas, and AML, occur with increased frequency in patients treated on regimens that included irradiation, epipodophyllotoxins, or alkylating agents.[135–139] Please refer to Chapter 97 on late effects of therapy.

FUTURE DIRECTIONS

The treatment of childhood ALL is based on the concept of tailoring the intensity of therapy to a patient's risk of relapse. As the cure rate approaches 90%, treatment response assessed by MRD measurements of submicroscopic leukemia has emerged as a powerful and independent prognostic indicator for gauging the intensity of therapy. Children at high risk of relapse may now benefit from early intensification of therapy. The next goal is to reduce the intensity of therapy in children at very low risk of relapse, hence avoiding undue toxicity. The successful elimination of preventive cranial irradiation indicates that treatment reduction is feasible if done with caution and appropriate substitution with less toxic alternatives. Gene expression profiling could enhance the accuracy of risk stratification of pediatric ALL. Expanding the application of pharmacogenomics—a science that aims to define the genetic determinants of drug effects—will allow further individualized therapy in the future.[140] Although optimizing the use of old drugs continues through serial studies, new formulations of existing agents are being tested to improve the efficacy and reduce the toxicity of the parent compounds. Such modifications include improving drug transport and delivery, or altering the molecular structure to improve the therapeutic index.[140] Ongoing trials are studying the benefit of the two novel nucleoside analogs, clofarabine and nelarabine, in high risk ALL and T-cell ALL respectively.[140–142] In addition to refining leukemia classification, studies of global gene expression help identify potential molecular targets for therapy. It remains to be determined whether the success in targeting BCR–ABL with tyrosine kinase inhibitors will translate to other pathways, including NOTCH and FLT3. The development of monoclonal antibodies and cellular immunotherapy that exploits the expression of leukemia-associated antigens to stimulate the antitumor activity of cytotoxic T-lymphocytes or natural killer cells offers a new modality of targeted therapies that are under investigation. The challenge is to combine our current knowledge with technology to design effective risk-targeted therapies based on the biological features of leukemic cells, host genetics, and early response to therapy.

SUGGESTED READINGS

Arico M, Valsecchi MG, Camitta B, et al: Outcome of treatment in children with Philadelphia chromosome-positive acute lymphoblastic leukemia. N Engl J Med 342:998, 2000.

Berg SL, Blaney SM, Devidas M, et al: Phase II study of nelarabine (compound 506U78) in children and young adults with refractory T-cell malignancies: A report from the Children's Oncology Group. J Clin Oncol 23:3376, 2005.

Evans WE, Relling MV. Moving towards individualized medicine with pharmacogenomics. Nature 429:464, 2004.

Gaynon PS, Qu RP, Chappell RJ, et al: Survival after relapse in childhoood acute lymphoblastic leukemia: Impact of site and time to first relapse—The Children's Cancer Group experience. Cancer 82:1387, 1998.

Gaynon PS, Trigg ME, Heerema, NA, et al: Children's Cancer Group trials in childhood acute lymphoblastic leukemia: 1983–1995. Leukemia 14:2223, 2000.

Jeha S, Gaynon PS, Razzouk BI, et al: Phase II study of clofarabine in pediatric patients with refractory or relapsed acute lymphoblastic leukemia. J Clin Oncol 24:1917, 2006.

Pui CH, Boyett JM, Rivera GK, et al: Long-term results of Total Therapy studies 11, 12 and 13A for childhood acute lymphoblastic leukemia at St. Jude Children's Research Hospital. Leukemia 14:2286, 2000.

Pui CH, Evans WE: Treatment of acute lymphoblastic leukemia. N Engl J Med 354:166, 2006.

Pui CH, Gaynon PS, Boyett JM, et al: Outcome of treatment in childhood acute lymphoblastic leukemia with rearrangements of the 11q23 chromosomal region. Lancet 359:1909, 2002.

Pui CH, Jeha S. Therapeutic strategies for the treatment of acute lymphoblastic leukemia. Nat Rev Drug Discov 6:149, 2007.

Schrappe M, Reiter A, Zimmermann M, et al: Long-term results of four consecutive trials in childhood ALL performed by the ALL-BFM study group from 1981 to 1995. Berlin-Frankfurt-Munster. Leukemia 14:2205, 2000.

Silverman LB, Declerck L, Gelber RD, et al: Results of Dana-Farber Cancer Institute Consortium protocols for children with newly diagnosed acute lymphoblastic leukemia (1981–1995). Leukemia 14:2247, 2000.

Vora A, Mitchell CD, Lennard L, et al: Toxicity and efficacy of 6-thioguanine versus 6-mercaptopurine in childhood lymphoblastic leukaemia: A randomized trial. Lancet 368:1339, 2006.

REFERENCES

For complete list of references log onto www.expertconsult.com

CHAPTER 66

ACUTE LYMPHOCYTIC LEUKEMIA IN ADULTS

Dieter Hoelzer and Nicola Gökbuget

Acute lymphocytic leukemia (ALL) is a malignant disease characterized by an accumulation of lymphoblasts. In the early 1980s adult ALL was largely an incurable disease with an overall survival (OS) of less than 10%. After pediatric protocols were adopted the OS in adults improved to 30% to 40%. Progress has been made in the tools used to diagnose ALL. In addition, a variety of new drugs for the treatment of ALL are now under evaluation. The prerequisite for comprehensive therapy of ALL, however, requires more than ever standardization and quality control of treatment strategies. Rapid diagnosis and classification is not only important for clinical practice but also helpful in identifying prognostic factors, defining targets for evaluation of minimal residual disease (MRD) and for creation of novel therapeutic agents.

EPIDEMIOLOGY

According the National Cancer Institute, the age-adjusted overall incidence of ALL in the United States was 1.6/100,000 (1.8 in males and 1.4 in females). The incidence is higher in whites compared with blacks. After an initial peak in children younger than 5 years of age (8.3/100,000), the incidence decreases continuously. It increases again above the age of 65 to a second peak in the age group above 85 years (2.0/100,000).[1]

BIOLOGIC AND MOLECULAR ASPECTS

Preferred Approach to Diagnosis

Classification of the phenotype of the blast cells in acute leukemia requires morphologic and cytochemical evaluations, immunophenotyping, cytogenetic analysis, and molecular genetic analysis. Morphology remains the means by which acute leukemia is initially detected and, together with cytochemical reactions, is the major tool in distinguishing between ALL and acute myeloid leukemia (AML) (see Fig. 66–1). For more precise subclassification of ALL into B or T lineages and further subtypes, immunologic techniques must be used to detect lineage-specific antigens as well as surface or intracytoplasmic molecules. These methods also offer the opportunity to identify leukemia-specific surface markers for the detection of minimal residual disease (MRD). Cytogenetic analysis is still part of the diagnostic characterization of ALL, but molecular genetic techniques for identification of particular subsets of ALL (eg, *BCR–ABL*-positive ALL) are of greater importance. Molecular markers, particularly rearrangements of T-cell receptor (TCR) and immunoglobulin heavy chain (IgH) genes, are the most frequently used tools to evaluate MRD.

Morphology

The cytologic features of leukemic blast cells in ALL and their division into L1 to L3 according to the French-American-British (FAB) classification are discussed in Chapter 64. The distribution of L1 and L2 subtypes is of minor relevance for prediction of outcome. The subtype L3, observed in up to 5% of adult ALL patients, should be distinguished because it is indicative of a mature B-cell ALL, which requires different treatment options, but should be confirmed by surface marker analysis. According to the WHO classification ALL is grouped together with lymphoblastic lymphoma as either precursor B-cell or T-cell neoplasm. B-cell ALL is referred to as precursor B-lymphoblastic leukemia/lymphoma. L3-ALL is classified as Burkitt cell leukemia together with Burkitt lymphoma. T-ALL is grouped together with T-cell lymphoblastic lymphoma as precursor T-lymphoblastic lymphoma/leukemia.

Cell Surface Marker Analysis

ALL is divided into subtypes by immunologic criteria based on the presence of specific receptors or antigens on the cell surface of leukemic blast cells. Within the B or T lineage ALLs, the subtypes are defined according to their stage of differentiation. For more details on the immunologic classification of ALL, see Chapters 63 and 64.

The frequency and definition of ALL subtypes in adult and childhood ALLs are outlined in Table 66–1. In the German multicenter trials for childhood ALL (BFM) and adult ALL (GMALL), the phenotypic characteristics of 1756 children and 946 adults with ALL were analyzed prospectively. B-precursor ALL is the most frequent subtype in children and adults (85% and 70%, respectively). T-lineage ALL has a higher incidence in adults (25%). Within the B and T lineages, the more immature subtypes, pro-B ALL and early T ALL, occur more frequently in adults. The European Group for the Immunological Characterization of Acute Leukemia has proposed a unified classification of ALL immunophenotypes.[2] The use of such uniform classifications is of utmost importance to permit results in different trials to be comparable. Immunophenotypes in ALL are often associated with clinical characteristics such as disease manifestations, course of disease, and biologic markers such as cytogenetic and molecular aberrations as illustrated in Table 66–1.

B-Lineage Acute Lymphoblastic Leukemia

Pro-B ALL, also termed *pre-pre-B ALL* or early pre B, lacks B-, T-, and pre-B-cell markers but expresses the human leukocyte antigen (HLA-DR), TdT, and CD19 and has rearranged immunoglobulin genes (Table 66–1). It occurs in approximately 11% of adult and 5% of childhood ALL.

Common ALL is the major immunologic subtype in childhood, as well as in adult ALL. It comprises greater than 50% of cases of adult ALL. Common ALL is characterized by the presence of CD10 (see Table 66–1). Common ALL blast cells do not express markers that characterize relatively mature B cells, such as cytoplasmic immunoglobulins or surface membrane immunoglobulins. The blast cells are positive for CD19 and TdT.

Pre-B ALL is characterized by the expression of cytoplasmic immunoglobulins, which is absent in common ALL, but is identical to common ALL with respect to the expression of all other cell markers (see Table 66–1). Rarely CD10 may be absent in this subtype. Pre-B ALL comprises nearly 10% and 15% of adult and childhood ALL, respectively.

Mature B-cell ALL is found in approximately 4% of adult and 3% of childhood ALL patients. The blast cells express surface antigens of mature B cells, including surface membrane immunoglobulin. CD10

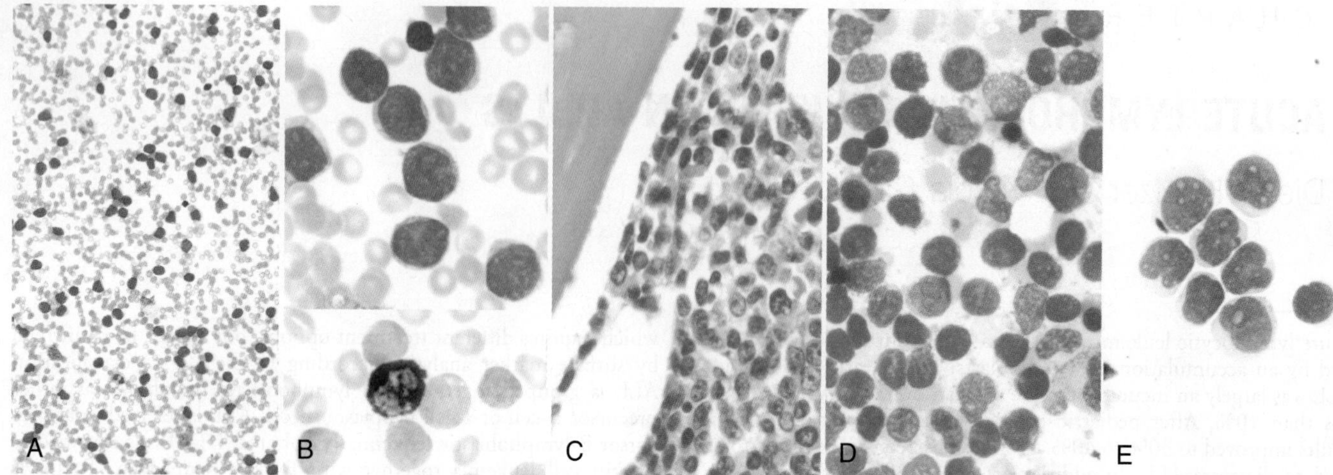

Figure 66–1 Acute lymphoblastic leukemia: peripheral blood, bone marrow biopsy and aspirate, and cerebral spinal fluid (**A–E**). The illustration is from a 37-year-old male who presented with a WBC of 170,000/μL and over 90% blasts with lymphoid morphology (**A** and **B**, top). An initial myeloperoxidase reaction (**B**, bottom) showed the blasts to be negative (positive cell is a segmented neutrophil that serves as an internal control). The bone marrow was packed with blasts as seen on the biopsy and aspirated material (**C** and **D**). The blasts were immunophenotyped by flow cytometry and were shown to be precursor-B lymphoblasts with the following phenotype: $CD34^+$, HLA^-DR^+, TdT^+, $CD19^+$, $CD10^+$, $cyCD79A^+$, $cyIgM^-$, and sIg^-. Cytogenetic studies illustrated the t(9;22), and molecular analysis revealed the p190 *BCR/ABL*. A spinal tap showed a WBC count of 120/μL with an RBC count of 37/μL. The differential showed 80% blasts. The morphology of the blasts on the cytospin of the cerebrospinal fluid (**E**) is somewhat altered by the preparation. Note the absence of significant red blood cells in the specimen. Given the high number of blasts in the peripheral blood, a more traumatic tap would have made it difficult to distinguish between central nervous system disease and contamination of the cerebrospinal fluid specimen by blood.

Table 66–1 Immunologic Subtypes of Acute Lymphocytic Leukemia and Corresponding Cytogenetic/Molecular Markers

Subgroups	Most Important Markers	Incidence in Children (*n* = 1756)*	Incidence in Adults (*n* = 946)*	Cytogenetic/Molecular Marker†
B-Lineage	$HLA\text{-}DR^+$, TdT^+, $CD19^+$ and/or $CD79a^+$ and/or $CD22^+$	85%	72%	
Pro-B (B-I)	$CD10^-$, no other differentiation markers	5%	11%	6% t(4;11)/ALL1-AF4 (70% in pro-B) (20% Flt3 in MLL^+)
Common ALL (B-II)	$CD10^+$	65%	51%	33% t(9;22)/BCR-ABL (30–50% in c/pre-B)
Pre-B (B-III)	cy IgM^+	15%	10%	4% t(1;19)/PBX-E2A
Mature B	cy or s kappa or lambda	3%	4%	5% t(8;14)/c-myc-IgH
T-Lineage	cy or s $CD3^+$, $CD7^+$		26%	
Early T	cy $CD3^+$, $CD7^+$, $CD5^\pm$, $CD2^-$, $sCD3^-$, $CD1a^-$	1%	7%	5% t(10;14)/HOX11-TCR <5% t(11;14)LMO/TCR 2% SIL-TAL1
Cortical (thymic) T	$CD2^+$, $CD5^+$, $CD1a^+$, $sCD3^\pm$		13%	4% NUP213-ABL1 (in T-ALL), 33% HOX11†
Mature T (T-IV)	$CD2^+$, $CD5^+$, $sCD3^+$, $CD1a^-$		7%	5% HOX11L2† (in T-ALL) 50% Notch1† (in T-ALL)

a, and; o or; cy, intracytoplasmic; s, surface.
*According to reference 175.
†According to GMALL data and reference 174.
‡According to experience of the GMALL.
§For newly proposed prognostic factors.

may be present, as well as occasional cytoplasmic immunoglobulins (see Table 66–1).

T-Lineage Acute Lymphoblastic Leukemia

Approximately 25% of adult ALL cases have blast cells with a T-cell phenotype. All cases express the T-cell antigen gp40 (CD7), and they may, according to their degree of T-cell differentiation, express other T-cell antigens (eg, the E rosette receptor [CD2] or the cortical thymocyte antigen T6 [CD1]) (see Table 66–1). A minority of T-cell ALL blast cells may also express CD10 together with T-cell antigens. In most cases of T-cell ALL, one or more of the T-cell receptor genes are rearranged. These properties make it possible to classify T-cell ALLs according to their stage of differentiation.

Early T-precursor ALL (or pre-T ALL) comprises 7% and 1% of adult and childhood ALL, respectively, and shows no further differentiation markers.

Thymic T-ALL (or cortical T-ALL) accounts for 13% of adult ALL and is characterized by CD1a expression. Because this subtype is associated with a better prognosis, its identification is of particular importance.

Mature T-ALL forms 7% of adult ALL and shows expression of surface CD3.

Cytogenetic and Molecular Genetic Analyses

Cytogenetic abnormalities are independent prognostic variables for predicting the outcome of adult ALL.[3] In some cases, cytogenetic or molecular genetic analysis contributes to confirmation of the diagnosis, for example, the correlation between t(8;14) and mature B-ALL. In four multicenter studies, clonal chromosomal aberrations could be detected in approximately 62% to 85% of adult ALL patients[4–7]; 15% to 38% of the cases had normal metaphases. The major cytogenetic abnormalities in ALL are clonal translocations such as t(9;22) (20%–30%), t(4;11) (3%–4%), t(8;14) (5%), t(1;19) (2%–3%), and other structural abnormalities such as 9p- (5%–15%), 6q- (4%–6%) und 12p aberrations (4%–5%). If none of the structural aberrations are present, the abnormalities can be classified according to the modal chromosomal number (<46, 46 with other structural abnormalities, 47–50, or >50).

Molecular analyses, detecting gene rearrangements in ALL by the polymerase chain reaction (PCR), Southern blot analysis, or fluorescent in situ hybridization with chromosome-specific DNA probes, are useful approaches in establishing a more precise diagnosis and in defining the quality of remission, and they may also provide insights into the pathophysiology of the leukemic process (eg, the mechanisms of leukemic cell stimulation by BCR–ABL fusion proteins). The most frequent molecular markers in ALL are BCR–ABL and ALL1–AF4.

The *Ph chromosome t(9;22)(q34q11)* results from a translocation involving the breakpoint cluster region of the *BCR* gene on chromosome 22 and the *ABL* gene on chromosome 9. The *BCR–ABL* gene rearrangement can be demonstrated by molecular techniques. PCR analyses revealed an incidence of 20% to 26% BCR–ABL-positive ALL in adults[8–10] compared with 3% in childhood ALL patients. One-third of adult ALL patients with a Ph chromosome show M (major)-*BCR* rearrangements (resulting in a 210-kd protein), similar to patients with chronic myeloid leukemia (CML), whereas two-thirds have m (minor)-*BCR* rearrangements (resulting in a 190-kd protein). It is noteworthy that *BCR–ABL* is more frequently detected than the corresponding chromosomal abnormality (t[9;22]) because of occasional difficulties in obtaining sufficient material for cytogenetic analysis.

The most frequent form of 11q23 abnormalities in ALL is *t(4;11)(q21;q23).* The involved gene on chromosome 11 is named *MLL* for "mixed-lineage leukemia." Synonyms are *ALL-1, HRX,* and *HTRX1.* The *MLL* gene is fused to a gene located on chromosome 4 that is named *AF-4* (also referred to as *FEL*). The translocation is frequently detected in infant leukemia and in patients with the early pre-B subtype (CD10 negative). The overall incidence in adults is approximately 5%. Typical molecular aberrations in ALL with associated cytogenetic translocations and immunologic subtypes are summarized in Table 66–1.

The role of cytogenetic analysis has to be reevaluated critically. The most frequent cytogenetic aberrations and those with the greatest prognostic impact can also be detected by the corresponding molecular genetic aberrations, such as *BCR–ABL* for t(9;22) and ALL1–AF4 for t(4;11). These techniques are more reliable and have a greater sensitivity, for example, a detection level of 10^{-4} to 10^{-6}. They are, therefore, more useful for initial detection of the aberrations and for follow-up analysis of MRD.

Minimal Residual Disease

Molecular and immunologic techniques have allowed the detection of minimal residual disease (MRD), defined as leukemic cells undetectable by morphologic examination. MRD evaluation is most frequently based on detection of leukemia-specific constellations of surface markers by flow cytometry (FACS), fusion genes related to specific chromosomal translocations (eg, BCR–ABL in t(9;22) by polymerase chain reaction [PCR]) and individual rearrangements of immunoglobulin (IgH, Igκ) and T-cell receptor genes (TCR-β -γ, -δ) by PCR and recently by real-time PCR. These methods reach, in ideal cases, a sensitivity of 10^{-4}, which refers to the detection of 1 malignant cell in 10,000 normal cells. Overall, more than 90% of the ALL patients have at least one target for MRD evaluation.

ETIOLOGY

The cause of ALL remains unknown. However, a number of factors are associated with an increased risk to develop acute leukemia (ALL and AML).[11,12]

Genetic Predisposition

In epidemiologic studies, patients with some rare congenital chromosomal abnormalities have an increased risk for development of acute leukemias, including ALL. In children with leukemia (predominantly AML), there is an 18-fold higher incidence of Down syndrome than would be expected.[13] There is also an increased risk of ALL associated with inherited disorders, such as Klinefelter syndrome, Fanconi anemia, Bloom syndrome, ataxia-telangiectasia, and neurofibromatosis. The impact of genetic predisposition on the pathobiology of ALL may also be inferred from reports of the simultaneous development of ALL in identical twins. Molecular analyses have demonstrated that the disease is not related to genetic predisposition but probably to the exchange of a malignant stem cell between the twins. This was demonstrated for rearrangement of the MILL gene[14] and the TEL–AML1 fusion gene.[15] Particularly in infant leukemias, prenatal molecular aberrations are probably the basis and lead after additional postpartum events to development of leukemia.

Irradiation

The incidence of acute leukemias, mainly AML, but also ALL, was increased almost 20-fold in survivors of the atomic bomb explosions (>1 Gy exposure) in Japan,[16] with a peak incidence occurring 6 to 7 years after the radiation exposure. Induction of leukemia by emissions from nuclear power stations has also been raised as a possible environmental leukemogenic risk; this has never been demonstrated unequivocally. Whether radiation exposure after the Chernobyl accident led to an increased incidence of leukemia is still controversial.

Chemical

The risk for the development of ALL may also be increased after exposure to chemical agents, such as benzene or other agents capable of producing bone marrow aplasia, including chemotherapeutic drugs. Secondary, therapy-related AMLs but also ALLs can occur after exposure to alkylating agents, such as cyclophosphamide, epipodophyllotoxins, topoisomerase II inhibitors, and, rarely, anthracyclines,[17,18] which are used for treatment of other preceding neoplasias.

Viral

There is no direct evidence that a virus causes human ALL. Indirect findings, however, suggest involvement of a virus in the pathogenesis of two lymphoid neoplasias.[19] In the endemic African type of Burkitt lymphoma, the Epstein–Barr virus, a DNA virus of the herpes family, has been implicated as a potential causative agent.[20] The endemic

Table 66–2 Symptoms and Clinical Signs at Diagnosis of 938 Adult Acute Lymphocytic Leukemia Patients

Sign or Symptom	Patients (%)
Symptoms	
Infections/fever	36
Hemorrhages	33
Physical findings	
Lymphadenopathy	57
Splenomegaly	56
Hepatomegaly	47
Mediastinal mass	14
Central nervous system involvement	7
Other organ involvement	9
Pleura	3
Bone	1
Pericardium	1
Retina	1
Skin	<1
Tonsils	<1
Lung	<1
Kidney	<1
Testes	<1

infection with human T-cell leukemia virus I (HTLV-I) in Japan and the Caribbean has been shown to be an etiologic agent for adult T-cell leukemia/lymphoma.[21]

CLINICAL MANIFESTATIONS

Most adult patients initially present with clinical symptoms resulting from bone marrow failure. Physical findings such as pallor, tachycardia, weakness, and fatigue are due to anemia; petechiae or other hemorrhagic manifestations are attributable to thrombocytopenia; infectious complications are due to neutropenia. Clinical signs of leukemia related directly to infiltration of organs with leukemic blasts, such as lymphadenopathy, splenomegaly, and hepatomegaly, are present in most patients but are infrequently the problems for which the patient first seeks medical advice.

Symptoms and clinical manifestations of 938 adult ALL patients, 15 to 65 years of age, entering two consecutive German multicenter trials, are listed in Table 66–2. One-third of the patients had infection or fever at presentation, and one-third presented with hemorrhagic episodes. Weight loss was observed only occasionally. Approximately one-half of the patients presented at diagnosis with lymphadenopathy, splenomegaly, and hepatomegaly, and hilar lymph node enlargement or a thymic mass (detected on chest radiographs or computed tomography scans) in approximately 14% of patients. Most (85%) patients with mediastinal masses had T-cell ALL. Massive thymic enlargement can cause dyspnea, especially when associated with pleural effusions. Although 7% of ALL patients at presentation had CNS involvement (as demonstrated by leukemic blast cells in the cerebrospinal fluid), only 4% of these initially had CNS symptoms, such as headache, vomiting, lethargy, nuchal rigidity, and cranial nerve or peripheral nerve dysfunction.

Virtually any organ can be infiltrated by ALL blast cells, and approximately one-tenth of the patients had such organ involvement (see Table 66–2). Most often a pleural effusion was observed in those patients with mediastinal enlargement and T-cell ALL. Some of those

Table 66–3 Laboratory Findings at Time of Diagnosis of 938 Adult Patients

		Patients (%)
White blood cell count (×10⁶/L)	<5,000	27
	5000–10,000	14
	10,000–50,000	31
	50,000–100,000	12
	>100,000	16
Leukemic blast cells in peripheral blood	Present	92
	Not present	8
Leukemic blast cells in bone marrow	<50%	3
	51%–90%	51
	>90%	46
Bone marrow aspirable		84

Table 66–4 Peripheral Blood Counts at Time of Diagnosis of 938 Adult Acute Lymphocytic Leukemia Patients

		Patients (%)
Neutrophils (×10⁶/L)	<500	23
	500–1000	14
	1000–1500	9
	>1500	54
Platelets (×10⁶/L)	<25,000	30
	25,000–50,000	22
	50,000–150,000	33
	>150,000	15
Hemoglobin (g/dL)	<6	8
	6–8	20
	8–10	27
	10–12	24
	>12	21

patients also had a pericardial effusion. Bone or joint pain was rarely observed as compared with childhood ALL; bone lesions could be found in only 1% of cases. Initial involvement of the testes was very rare (<1%). Leukemic infiltration of the retina, skin, tonsils, lung, or kidney was observed only occasionally, particularly in mature B-cell ALL and to a lesser extent in T-cell ALL, all of them associated with a poorer outcome.

LABORATORY EVALUATION

The peripheral blood cell values at diagnosis of the same cohort of patients are shown in Tables 66–3 through 66–5. The leukocyte count (Table 66–3). was elevated in 59%, 14% had normal counts, and 27% had leukopenia. In 92% of the patients, leukemic blast cells were seen in the blood smear. Thus, "aleukemic" leukemias account for only a small proportion of cases of adult ALL. With automated blood counting, the diagnosis may be missed in patients with normal or decreased white blood cell (WBC) counts and with low or zero blast cells in peripheral blood. For this reason, the need for microscopic examination of blood smears in people suspected of having acute leukemia should be stressed. An elevated blood count ($>100,000 \times 10^6$/L) was observed in 16% of the patients, and, occasionally, WBC counts greater than $500,000 \times 10^6$/L have been observed. In general, a high WBC count is found more frequently in T-cell ALL patients than with B-lineage ALL patients.

Neutrophils (Table 66–4) less than 500×10^6/L were seen in 23% of the patients, and thrombocytopenia, less than $25,000 \times 10^6$/L, in

Table 66–5 Coagulation Parameters at Time of Diagnosis of 938 Adult Acute Lymphocytic Leukemia Patients

		Patients (%)
Fibrinogen (mg/dL)	<100	4
	>100	96
Prothrombin time (%)	<50	7
	50–75	34
	75–100	34
	>100	25
Partial thromboplastin time (sec)	<30	33
	30–40	53
	40–50	11
	>50	3

30% of the patients, corresponding roughly to the symptoms of infection and bleeding present at diagnosis.

Bone marrow aspiration or biopsy is mandatory for a diagnosis of ALL. In less than 15% of patients, the bone marrow cannot be aspirated and a biopsy must be performed. Dry taps are due to densely packed blast cells, fibrosis, or inadequate technique; the first two resolve after therapy. Most patients have greater than 50%, or even greater than 90%, of blast cells in the bone marrow (see Table 66–3). In less than 3% of cases, the blast cells constitute less than 50% of the nucleated marrow cells.

A lumbar puncture should be done to determine whether the CNS is involved. If there is a risk of bleeding due to a very low platelet count or of blast cell contamination due to a high leukemic blast content in the peripheral blood, lumbar puncture should be postponed. When the leukocyte count in the spinal fluid is low, or the morphologic detection of blasts is inconclusive, demonstration of an immunologically defined blast cell population can confirm a diagnosis of CNS involvement.

The most frequent metabolic abnormality is an increased serum uric acid level, which occurs in approximately one-half of the patients; hypercalcemia was rare. Serum lactate dehydrogenase may be elevated as a result of cell destruction in patients with a large tumor mass, particularly in B-cell ALL. Because of liver infiltration some patients may show elevation of liver enzymes. In a small proportion of patients (Table 66–5), the initial fibrinogen level may be less than 100 mg/dL. Disseminated intravascular coagulopathy and other disturbances of coagulation are rarely observed at diagnosis.

DIFFERENTIAL DIAGNOSIS

Difficulty is rarely experienced in establishing the diagnosis of ALL. The differentiation from lymphocytosis, lymphadenopathy, and hepatosplenomegaly due to viral infections and other acute or chronic leukemias can usually be done by lymphocyte surface markers.

Aleukemic pancytopenic ALL patients without blast cells in peripheral blood (less than 10%) must be distinguished from those with aplastic anemia, which may also be a preleukemic syndrome. In contrast to ALL, the bone marrow is hypocellular in aplastic anemia. In rare cases with a limited bone marrow infiltration, an arbitrary distinction between ALL and NHL is usually made according to the degree of infiltration, more or less than 25%.

In approximately 29% of the patients blast cells coexpress myeloid surface markers such as CD13 and CD33 (>20%). Distinct subtypes of ALL are associated with a higher incidence of myeloid marker coexpression, for example, early T-ALL, pro-B-ALL, and Ph/BCR–ABL-positive ALL. These cases of ALL with myeloid marker coexpression must be differentiated from mixed or hybrid leukemias in which blast cells express lymphoid as well as myeloid antigens; they may also be termed *biphenotypic* or *bilineage* leukemias. The European Group for the Immunological Characterization of Acute Leukemia has suggested a score to unequivocally identify this rare subgroup.[2] Biphenotypic leukemias may be allocated to a treatment strategy for either for ALL or for AML and outcome seems to be poor with both approaches.

Occasionally difficulties can occur in distinguishing Ph/BCR–ABL-positive ALL from primary lymphoid blast crisis of CML. Sometimes final diagnosis can be made only after the initiation of treatment. In ALL patients achieving complete clinical remission (CR), the peripheral blood count are normal values, whereas CML cases revert to a chronic phase with a pathologic left shift.

THERAPY

Initial Evaluation and Supportive Therapy

At diagnosis, the evaluation of an adult with ALL should include a history and a careful physical examination. Speed in clinical evaluation and diagnosis is important to initiate supportive measures and to decide on appropriate therapy. Only in a few cases is the leukemic process so far advanced that immediate treatment of leukemia is necessary (eg, in patients with symptoms due to a large mediastinal mass and pleural effusions or to a rapidly progressing B-cell ALL).

A few general measures should be initiated at once. Sufficient fluid intake to guarantee urine production of 100 mL/hour throughout induction therapy should be maintained to reduce the danger of uric acid formation. Parenteral fluid administration may be required when the patient's oral intake is inadequate because of nausea or difficulty in swallowing. Placement of an implantable port system is advantageous when anticipating a long period of induction therapy or when part of the therapy will be carried out on an outpatient basis.

Patients should receive allopurinol to reduce the formation of uric acid and avoid the danger of urate nephropathy. Allopurinol blocks the enzyme xanthine oxidase, which mediates the generation of uric acid from xanthine as a product of purine catabolism. Allopurinol should be given at a dose of 300 mg/day, which may be increased to 600 mg/day if high leukocyte counts or organomegaly persist. The dose of allopurinol has to be reduced when 6-mercaptopurine is given because it potentiates the action of 6-mercaptopurine. Rasburicase is a new recombinant uratoxidase enzyme that catalyses the oxidation of uric acid to allantoin. It has been demonstrated that rasburicase can reduce high uric acid faster and more safely than allopurinol, thereby preventing a tumor lysis syndrome in almost all cases.[22] Therefore it could be an alternative to allopurinol in patients with a high risk of tumor lysis syndrome.

Approximately one-third of adult patients present with infection and bleeding. They are at high risk for infectious and hemorrhagic complications during the induction period because thrombocytopenia and granulocytopenia are aggravated by chemotherapy. In general, platelet transfusions should be given in response to bleeding episodes and to prevent bleeding when platelet counts fall to less than 10,000 μL[10] and to less than 20,000 μL[10] when there is a bleeding tendency or the patient is febrile. HLA-matched platelets are given to patients who become refractory to random donor platelets. The incidence of fatal hemorrhage during induction therapy has been significantly lowered by these measures.

Infection Management

The use of more intense chemotherapeutic regimens has resulted not only in improved response rates of malignancies but also in higher infection-associated morbidity and mortality. Long-term neutropenia is the most important risk factor, but CD4 lymphopenia, antibody deficiency, and immunosuppression in allogeneic stem cell transplantation also lead to severe and lethal infections. Before the 1990s, gram-negative microorganisms were the leading cause of febrile neutropenia, but since then gram-positive bacterial infections caused mostly by staphylococci have increased, frequently correlated to indwelling central venous access. The number of multiresistant bacteria is increasing. Invasive fungal infections are increasing in frequency, particularly mold infections.

ALL patients should receive antibacterial and antifungal prophylaxis depending on the expected duration of neutropenia. In febrile neutropenia, thorough and early diagnostic procedures are necessary. They include physical examination, microbiologic investigations, imaging procedures, and biopsies. Cultures of blood, urine, sputum, and other infected areas are mandatory. Successful treatment of febrile neutropenia is based on immediate empirical administration of broad-spectrum antibiotics.

Hematopoietic Growth Factors

The use of hematopoietic growth factors, such as granulocyte colony-stimulating factor (G-CSF) and granulocyte-macrophage colony-stimulating factor (GM-CSF), is a valuable component of supportive therapy during the treatment of ALL. There is no indication that these CSFs stimulate leukemic cell growth in a clinically significant manner.

Most clinical trials demonstrate that the prophylactic administration of G-CSF significantly accelerates neutrophil recovery[23–28] and several prospective, randomized studies also show that this is associated with a substantially reduced incidence and duration of febrile neutropenia and of severe infections in ALL[24,26,27] and also reduced in mortality during induction.[23,26–28]

The advantage of G-CSF administration was particularly evident in select high-risk patients receiving multiple treatment cycles,[24] whereas clinical effects appeared to be negligible in patients at low risk of infectious complications in one study in childhood ALL.[29] Conversely, the results of the St. Jude trial show that even in cases of acute leukemia with a greater than 40% probability of severe neutropenia, not all patients benefit from G-CSF treatment.[30] A comparison of this study with other trials[26,27] highlights the great importance of CSF scheduling. When CSFs are first given at the end of a 4-week induction chemotherapy regimen, potential benefits are limited.[30] Therefore, it is noteworthy that G-CSF may be given even in conjunction with chemotherapy without aggravating the myelotoxicity of these specific regimens[25–27] and that this scheduling is an important determinant of the clinical efficacy. Alternatively, it was demonstrated that after short consolidation cycles G-CSF application may be postponed from day 12 after high-dose cytarabine/mitoxantrone to day 17 without negative effects on duration of neutropenia.[31] Similar results were reported for consolidation therapy with the Hyper-CVAD regimen.[32] A closer adherence to the dose and schedule of chemotherapeutic regimens should be theoretically possible with the use of G-CSF. So far, no trial has demonstrated a benefit of increased dose intensity made possible by G-CSF application in terms of leukemia-free survival (LFS).

G-CSF is regularly used for mobilization of stem cells in candidates for autologous stem cell transplantation. There are some hints that prophylactic application of G-CSF after intensive chemotherapy cycles or in parallel may reduce the incidence of severe mucositis. Thus, delayed application of G-CSF during induction therapy has led to an increased risk of mucositis.[32]

Chemotherapy

Chemotherapy of ALL is usually divided into several phases, beginning with remission induction. The objective of induction chemotherapy is to achieve complete remission, that is, eradication of leukemia as determined by morphologic criteria and, more recently, also by molecular markers. Although the induction phase is usually well defined, postremission therapy can be subdivided into intensification and maintenance phases. Usually prophylactic CNS treatment is added (Table 66–6).

Remission Induction Therapy

Exact diagnosis and management of initial complications are the prerequisites for successful induction therapy. A cautious cell reduction phase is recommended for patients with a large leukemic cell burden or a high leukocyte count (>25,000 × 10^6/L). Patients with extreme leukocytosis (>100,000 × 10^6/L) have been treated initially with leukapheresis. However, in the majority of patients the cell count can also be reduced with steroids alone or in combination with vincristine or cyclophosphamide.

Standard induction therapy for ALL includes prednisone, vincristine, anthracyclines (mostly daunorubicin), and also L-asparaginase. Other drugs, such as cyclophosphamide, cytarabine (either conventional or high-dose), mercaptopurine, and others, are added in many protocols, sometimes called early intensification. Several new approaches are currently being explored in adult ALL to improve CR rates and thereby remission quality.

Steroids, mostly prednisone and prednisolone, have been administered, although *dexamethasone* (DEXA) has a higher antileukemic activity in vitro and a better penetration to the cerebrospinal fluid.[33] In pediatric trials, the replacement of prednisone by DEXA has led to a decrease of the CNS relapse rate and improved survival.[34] The DEXA schedule has to be designed carefully because continuous application of higher doses may lead to long-term complications[34] and to increased morbidity and mortality due to infections.[35]

Anthracycline dose intensity and schedule may play an important role in induction therapy of ALL.[36] The most frequently used anthracycline is daunorubicin (DNR). Many groups have replaced weekly applications by higher doses of DNR (30–60 mg/m^2 on a 2- to 3-day schedule).[28,37,38] A particularly high CR rate (93%) was reported with intensive anthracycline therapy (270 mg/m^2 for 3 days)[38] from a single-center study, but not confirmed in a larger multicenter trial.[39] Intensive anthracycline therapy may be associated with a higher mortality during the induction phase. Therefore, intensive supportive care and probably the use of growth factors are recommended with these protocols. Overall it remains open whether intensified anthracycline therapy is beneficial—for all subgroups and particularly in terms of achieving a molecular remission.

Asparaginase (A) does not affect the CR rate but improves LFS, and if not used during induction therapy, it is often included as part of the consolidation treatment. The addition of A to conventional induction therapy did not improve the CR rate in one trial in adult ALL. There was, however, a trend toward a higher LFS in patients treated with A.[40] Three different A preparations with significantly different half-lives are available: Native *Escherichia coli* A (1.2 days), *Erwinia* A (0.65 days), and *PEG-L-A* (5.7 days).[41] To reach equal efficacy, the treatment schedule has to be adapted, which is generally daily for *Erwinia*, twice daily for *E coli*, and once weekly for PEG-A. The importance of A pharmacokinetics is illustrated by a randomized trial in childhood ALL, where significantly lower survival rates were achieved with *Erwinia* compared with *E coli* A, both given at the same schedule, which is due to underdosing of *Erwinia*.[42] A randomized trial comparing PEG-A with *E coli* A in childhood ALL showed a higher earlier response rate for the latter but no difference in long-term outcome.[43] Thus, it remains open for debate whether PEG-A is superior to *Erwinia* A or native *E coli* A. During induction, A is often given concurrently to steroids in patients, inducing additional toxicities such as coagulation disorders and hepatic dysfunction, which are not predictable. It may thereby lead to treatment delays and compromise dose intensity in individual patients.

The role of cyclophosphamide (C)—generally administered at the beginning of induction therapy—has been evaluated in several studies. A randomized study by the Italian GIMEMA group comparing a three-drug induction regimen with and without C did not show a difference in terms of CR rate (81% vs 82%).[44] However, in several nonrandomized trials, high CR rates (85%–91%) were achieved with regimens including C pretreatment,[28,45] particularly in adult T-ALL.

High-dose treatment during induction refers particularly to *high-dose cytarabine* (HDAC; 1–3 g/m^2, usually for 12 doses) before

Table 66–6 Overall Treatment Results of Adult Acute Lymphocytic Leukemia

Group	Author	Year	No.	Age	Induction	Consolidation	Maintenance	CR	LFS
GMALL 01[176]	Hoelzer	1993	368	25	V, P, A, D, C, AC, M, MP	V, DX, AD, AC, C, TG	MP, M	74%	35% at 10 years
GMALL 02[176]	Hoelzer	1993	562	28	V, P, A, D, C, AC, M, MP	V, DX, AD, AC, C, TG, VM, AC	MP, M	75%	39% at 7 years
UKALL IX[177]	Durrant	1993	266		V, P, A (MP, M)/D		MP, M, V, P	68%	22% at 8 years
BGMT[119]	Attal	1995	135	31	V, P, A, D;C, AC, MP	HdM, ARC, allo/auto SCT	[Il-2]	93%	44% at 3 years
CALGB 8811[178]	Larson	1995	197	32	V, P, A, D, C	C, MP, AC, V, A, M, AD, DX, TG	MP, M, V, P	85%	30% at 5 years
GIMEMA 0183[179]	Mandelli	1996	358	31	V, P, A, D	V, IdM, IdAC, P, VM, AC	MP, M, V, P[A, AC, VM, IdAC]	79%	25% at 10 years
HOVON[64]	Dekker	1997	130	35	V, P, A, D	HdAC, amsa, MP, VP	-	73%	28% at 5 years
SAKK[65,180]	Wernli	1994, 97	140	31	V, P, D, M, A, HdAC, VP	allo/auto SCT; >50 y: HDC	-	69%	21% at 5 years
UKALL XA[61]	Durrant	1997	618	>15	V, P, D, A	[AC, VP, D, TG]	MP, MTX, V, P	82%	28% at 5 years
PETHEMA[181]	Ribera	1998	108	28	V, P, D, A, C	HdM, V, D, P, A, C, VM, AC	MP, M [VD, P, Mi, A, C, VM, AC]	86%	41% at 4 years
CALGB 9111[28]	Larson	1998	198	35	C, D, V, P, A	C, MP, AC, V, A, MP, M, AD, DX, TG, P	MP, M, V, P	85%	40% at 3 years
LALA-87[89]	Thiebaut	2000	581	33	V, P, D/R, C, [amsa, AC]	D/R, AC, A	MP, M, V, C, P, D/R, DT, BCNU	76%	17% at 5 years
GMALL 05/93[134]	Gökbuget	2001	1163	35	V, P, D, A, C, AC, MP	V, DX, AD, AC, C, TG, VM, AC, HdM, A, C, [HDAC, Mi] ± SCT	MP, M	83%	35% at 5 years
SWEDEN[37]	Hallbook	2002	120	44	HdAC, C, D, V, BM	AM, HdAC, V, BM, C, D, VP +/– SCT	MP, M, D, V, P, AC, TG	86%	36% at 3 years
JALSG-ALL93[54]	Takeuchi	2002	263	31	V, AD, P, A, C	VP, Mi, AC, IdM, A, ACR, P	MP, MTX [V, AD, P, Mi, VP, AC, IdM, A, ACR, AC]	78%	30% at 6 years
UCLA, USA[182]	Linker	2002	84	27	V, P, D, A	HdAC, VP, HdM, MP, D, V, P, A	M, MP	93%	47% at 5 years
GIMEMA 0288[183]	Annino	2002	794	28	V, P, A, D, C, [HDAC, Mi]	V, HDM, HDAC, DX, VM	MP, M, V, [AC, Mi, VM, HDAC, HDM, DX]	82%	29% at 9 years
MRC/ECOG[184]	Rowe	2003	1389	15–60	V, P, D, A, C, AC, MP	HdM, A [AC, VP, V, DX, D, C, TG] ± SCT	MP, M, V, P	91%	41% at 5 years
MD Anderson[123]	Kantarjian	2004	288	40	V, AD, DX, C	HdM, HdAC, P	M, MP, V, P	92%	38% at 5 years
GOELAMS-GOELAL02[91]	Hunault	2004	198	33	P, V, I, A	C, AC, MP, HdM, V, I, C, AC, TG ± SCT	aIFN	86%	41% at 6 years
LALA 94[90]	Thomas	2004	922	33	P, VCR, CP, DNR/IDA	[MI + IdAC] vs [CP/AC/MP] MTX/Asp, CY, AC, V, A, D ± SCT	MP, MTX	84%	36% at 5 years
EORTC ALL-3[94]	Labar	2004	340	33	D, C, V, P	A, C, HdAC, [P, V; AD, BCNU, C, MP, M, AMD] ± SCT	MP, MTX, V	74%	36%*at 6 years
GIMEMA 0496[158]	Mancini	2001	450		P, V, D, A	HDAC, VP, V, D, P, C	MP, MTX	80%	33% at 5 years
Pethema ALL-93[93]	Ribera	2005	222	27	V, D, P, A, C	HdM, HdAC ± SCT	MP, MTX	82%	34% at 5 years

AC, cytosine arabinoside; AD, doxorubicin; BCNU, carmustine; C, cyclophosphamide; CR, cure rate; D, daunorubicin; DT, dactinomycin; DX, dexamethasone; HdAC, high-dose AC; HdM, high-dose M; IdAC, intermediate-dose AC; VM, teniposide; IdM, intermediate-dose M; LFS, leukemia-free survival; M, methotrexate; Mi, mitoxantrone; MP, 6-mercaptopurine; N/M, either/or; P, prednisone; R, rubidazone; TG, thioguanine; V, vincristine; VD, vindesine; VP, etoposide; BM, betamethasone.
*Since 1993, >100 patients, follow-up >3 years.

or after the standard induction therapy. This approach has resulted in a median CR rate of 79%, which is not superior to that obtained with conventional treatment, and it remains uncertain whether and for which subgroups it could be beneficial for LFS.[46] Upfront treatment before conventional chemotherapy yielded higher CR rates[37,47–49] than treatment afterward,[45,50,51] which was, in part, related to a higher induction mortality with the latter approach. Any type of induction therapy with HDAC may lead to an increased incidence of severe neutropenias after subsequent chemotherapy cycles.

With current regimens, the remission rate in ALL is 85% to 90% (see Table 66–6), with low failure rates and a variable early mortality up to 11%. Beyond mortality, even morbidity, for example, due to extended cytopenias, and subsequent infections such as fungal pneumonias may compromise further treatment and dose intensity. Options for increasing the rate of CR are limited in adult ALL. Therefore in the future increased molecular CR rates will be the most important goal. It may be defined as a burden of MRD below the detection limit of 10^{-4} (0.01%); the frequency of molecular CR in adult ALL ranges from 50% for Ph+ ALL treated with imatinib[52] to 60% for standard-risk ALL.[53]

Five percent to 15% of adult ALL patients do not achieve CR after induction therapy, compared with less than 3% of children with ALL, and 5% to 10% of adult ALL patients die during the induction period. Mortality during induction is age dependent, increasing with age from less than 3% in adolescents to 20% in patients greater than 60 years of age. The main cause of death in approximately two-thirds of the patients is infection, often fungal infection. The remaining nonresponders may achieve a partial remission or may be refractory to standard treatment. These patients have an extremely poor prognosis and are, therefore, candidates for new, experimental treatment approaches and are also considered for SCT, even if not in complete remission.

Intensification Therapy

Consolidation therapy refers either to high-dose chemotherapy, to the use of multiple new agents, or to readministration of the induction regimen, also called reinduction. These measures are aimed at eliminating clinically undetectable residual leukemia after induction chemotherapy and thereby preventing relapse, as well as emergence of drug-resistant cells.

Intensive consolidation is standard in the treatment of ALL based on pediatric studies and historic comparisons although randomized trials often failed to demonstrate a benefit of intensification[44,54]; this is probably due to the low number of patients in whom these concepts were evaluated. Consolidation cycles in large studies are very variable and it is impossible to evaluate their individual efficacy (see Table 66–6). Intensification schedules include teniposide, etoposide, amsacrine (*m*-AMSA), mitoxantrone, idarubicin, and HDAC, or intermediate- or high-dose methotrexate (HDM). Allogeneic SCT from sibling or unrelated donors or autologous SCT is now the major approach for intensive postinduction therapy in high-risk patients. Before SCT, a consolidation therapy is usually delivered to achieve a CR with good remission quality. High-dose chemotherapy has been used mainly to overcome drug resistance or to achieve therapeutic drug levels in the cerebrospinal fluid.

High-Dose Cytarabine

Although there is considerable experience with HDAC for the consolidation treatment of ALL,[46] it still remains uncertain what dose is optimal; usually doses ranging from 1 to 3 g/m² every 12 hours for 4 to 5 days are given within several combinations. HDAC has been included in several trials in adult de novo ALL as part of consolidation therapy (see Table 66–6). It seems that specific subgroups of ALL profit from HDAC treatment; thus, encouraging results are achieved for pediatric B-cell ALL. It remains uncertain to what extent HDAC contributes to the effects of HDM in these disease subtypes. Apparently, also for adult pro-B ALL, HDAC is beneficial because cure rates of 50% can be achieved.[55]

An additional argument for the use of HDAC might be its effectiveness in treating CNS leukemia. There is evidence that in ALL and NHL, higher levels of AC triphosphate can be reached with 3 g/m² as compared with the lower dose of 1 g/m² AC; in addition, with the higher dose, the cerebrospinal fluid can be cleared of blast cells.[56]

High-Dose Methotrexate

In general, it seems that intensive application of HDM is beneficial. It has been extensively studied for the treatment of childhood ALL and, to a lesser extent, in adult ALL. HDM appears to be effective in preventing systemic and testicular relapses. However, in adults dosages are probably limited to 1.5 to 2 g/m² if given as a 24-hour infusion. Otherwise toxicities, particularly mucositis, may lead to subsequent treatment delays and decreased compliance. Toxicity, but also efficacy, is reduced with a shortened infusion time, for example, 4 hours.[57] The situation may change when improved prophylaxis of mucositis, for example, with keratinocyte growth factor, becomes available.

The effect of HDM on CNS leukemia may contribute to the favorable results reported with its use. HDM at a dose of 6 g/m² resulted in an 80% CR rate given in children with CNS relapse,[58] indicating that systemic application yields cytotoxic levels in the cerebrospinal fluid. Several studies have investigated the efficacy of HDM as consolidation (Table 66–6). Most favorable results have been achieved in small trials with HDM as part of intensive multidrug consolidation regimens.

Asparaginase

From pediatric ALL trials, there is increasing evidence that intensified application of *Asparaginase* leads to improved overall results.[59,60] In adult ALL this approach appears to be useful particularly in consolidation, where less toxicity can be expected compared to induction.

Reinduction

Pediatric trials and one randomized trial in adults also underline the efficacy of repeated induction also named reinduction or late intensification.[61]

The role of HD anthracyclines and epipodophyllotoxins in consolidation remains open. Overall in adult ALL, stricter adherence to protocols during consolidation with fewer delays, dose reductions, and omission of drugs because of toxicities would be an important contribution to therapeutic progress.

Maintenance Therapy

Maintenance therapy even after intensive induction and consolidation is standard for ALL patients. Some groups even prolong maintenance therapy beyond 2 years of total treatment. MTX preferably given intravenously (IV) and mercaptopurine (MP) given orally are the backbone of maintenance regimens. The potential effects of further intensification cycles for specific subgroups of ALL remains open. It may be useful to aim for leukocyte counts below 3000/μL during maintenance[62] to achieve optimal suppression of residual disease.

Attempts to omit maintenance therapy altogether after induction and consolidation therapy have resulted in inferior results.[63–65] On the other hand the role of periodic cycles of intensive chemotherapy during maintenance remains to be defined.

In a large, multicenter Italian study (GIMEMA 0183), after intensive consolidation treatment, patients were randomly assigned to postconsolidation therapy with conventional maintenance therapy or to additional alternating treatment courses of different intensities.[66] In this report, there was no difference in the survival rate at 10 years between the treatment groups (27% for conventional and 28% for more intensive maintenance), which may suggest that after adequate early consolidation therapy the intensity of the maintenance therapy has no influence on survival. However, only a few patients actually received these regimens as scheduled; adults often show poor compliance to intensive maintenance because of toxicities and moreover social reasons. Therefore maintenance with less intensive cycles with vincristine, for example, and steroids may be more practicable.

Currently, maintenance therapy in adult ALL is being revisited based on the burden of MRD (eg, none for MRD-negative patients), the subtype of ALL, and the use of new therapeutic options (eg, a tyrosine kinase inhibitor for BCR–ABL-positive ALL). It is still open whether and to what extent maintenance therapy is necessary in ALL subgroups.

Prophylaxis of Central Nervous System Leukemia

Central nervous system leukemia occurs in 6% (1%–10%) of patients with adult ALL at diagnosis, with a higher incidence in T-cell ALL (8%) and mature B-cell ALL (13%).[67] Treatment and prophylaxis of CNS leukemia may consist of intrathecal (i.th.) methotrexate alone or in combination with AC or prednisone, similar intraventricular therapy administered by an Ommaya reservoir, cranial irradiation, or systemic treatment with HDAC or HDM.[68]

Adult ALL patients who do not receive specific prophylactic CNS treatment have a CNS relapse rate of 30% (29%–32%),[67] similar to that observed in children without CNS prophylaxis.[69]

With i.th. chemotherapy alone, the rate of isolated and combined CNS relapses can be reduced to 13% (8%–19%). Intermittent treatment during maintenance therapy improves the outcome compared with administration of only a few doses during induction treatment. In most adult ALL trials, additional prophylactic CNS irradiation (24 Gy) has been administered. This combined approach further reduces the CNS relapse rate to 9% (3%–19%). There is some evidence that early irradiation after remission induction is superior to delayed irradiation during consolidation treatment.[70]

In many recent trials, combined treatment approaches have shown greater efficacy. For high-dose chemotherapy together with i.th. therapy, the rate of CNS relapses was 7% (2%–16%); with additional CNS irradiation, the relapse rate was 6% (1%–13%). The efficacy of intensified CNS prophylaxis was also demonstrated in a retrospective analysis from the MD Anderson Cancer Center, where the lowest CNS relapse rate (2%) was achieved in a trial with early high-dose chemotherapy and i.th. therapy for all patients.[71]

Because the risk for CNS relapse is associated with other risk factors, such as T-cell ALL, B-cell ALL, extreme leukocytosis, high leukemia cell proliferation rate, high serum lactate dehydrogenase levels, and extramedullary organ involvement, a risk-adapted CNS prophylaxis has been suggested.[71] This approach, however, compared with childhood ALL, is not widely used in adults. It should be kept in mind that effective CNS prophylaxis not only reduces the risk of isolated CNS relapse but also improves general outcome. Deescalation of CNS prophylaxis should therefore be done carefully. In the future, the use of liposomal cytarabine for i.th. therapy may help reduce the number of i.th. applications and thereby the risk of contamination and improve efficacy with the aim to replace CNS irradiation in defined populations. Due to toxicity risks liposomal cytarabine should not be combined with systemic high-dose therapy.

The risk of CNS relapse can also be affected by skill in the performance of the administration of i.th chemotherapy. Thus, contamination of the CSF with blood at the initial lumbar puncture can be associated with a poor outcome. The Lumbar puncture should be done by experienced physicians; platelet transfusions should be given before in case of low platelet counts; and patients should remain in prone position after i.th. therapy.[72]

Therapy for Relapsed and Resistant Leukemia

Patients who fail to achieve CR or those who relapse subsequently have been treated with a variety of protocols.[73,74] The repetition of regimens, including vincristine, anthracyclines, and steroids, similar to standard induction treatment, have led to CR rates of 61% in earlier studies.[73,74] The use of single-agent HDM, HDAC, and probably the anthracycline derivatives-mitoxantrone and rubidazone have resulted in a second remission in less than or equal to 30% of patients, whereas other agents, such as amsacrine, teniposide, and etoposide are effective in 10% to 15%.of patients.

High-dose AC has been extensively studied in relapsed adult ALL. From several small pilot studies comprising 90 patients in total, the weighted mean CR rate was 37%.[75] Higher CR rates (50%–60%) were achieved with combination regimens that included HDAC and mitoxantrone, amsacrine, or vincristine plus steroids, again with a wide variation that may be attributed to patient selection and nonuniform intensity of pretreatment. Because HDAC is increasingly administered during frontline treatment, its efficacy following relapse may be limited. Therefore, new combinations with idarubicin (46%–64% CR rate)[76–78] or fludarabine (67%–83% CR rate)[79,80] have been evaluated. Median remission duration or survival has been reported by only a few groups, but did not exceed 5 months and 16%, respectively.

HDM followed by rescue with folinic acid combined with asparaginase lead to response rates of 22% to 79% in resistant ALL in early studies.[73] This combination is no longer administered to relapsed patients but is now incorporated in several regimens for patients with de novo ALL.

The most significant predictive factor for treatment response in relapsed patients is the duration of the first remission. Patients with longer previous remission (>18 months) have a higher CR rate and longer remission duration compared to those with a short previous remission (<18 months).[81,82] Therefore decision making concerning therapy should consider the duration of first remission, age, further options (eg, SCT), and other factors as summarized in Table 66–7. In patients with late relapse, a modified induction is often successful whereas in patients with early relapse, during intensive chemotherapy, new, experimental, or more intensive regimens should be considered. Fortunately, at present a variety of new drugs for ALL are being evaluated (reviewed in references 83–85).

For all chemotherapy regimens, the duration of second remission is usually short (<6 months) and the only curative approach for adult patients with relapsed or resistant ALL is SCT. The major aim of relapse treatment is the induction of a second remission with sufficient duration to permit preparation for SCT. Three large study groups have reviewed the outcome of relapsed ALL patients recently. The MRC UK-ALL found in 609 patients with first relapse a 5-year survival rate of 7%. Survival was poor in all subgroups, for example, younger (<20 years) versus older patients (12% vs 3%), short (<2 years) versus longer duration of first remission (11% vs 5%) or immunophenotype. Hundred twenty patients were able to receive an SCT after relapse, with survival rates of 15% for autograft, 16% for unrelated, and 23% for sibling allogeneic SCT after 2 years.[86] Also the French group reported a rate of second remission of 44% in 421 relapsed patients with an LFS of 12% after 4 years. They identified transplantation during second CR and a longer duration of CR (>1 year) as favorable prognostic factors.[87] The German group observed an improvement of outcome for relapsed T-ALL after more frequent application of experimental drugs, including nelarabine and perfor-

Table 66–7 Factors for Decision Making on Therapy of Relapsed Acute Lymphocytic Leukemia Patients

- Duration of first remission: ≥18 months
- Prior therapy (drugs /cycles) not used before
- Available targets
  - Subtype: B-precursor vs T-ALL
  - Antigens: Available monoclonal antibodies
  - Molecular markers: Available kinase inhibitors
- Localization of relapse

Table 66–8 Results of SCT in Adult Acute Lymphocytic Leukemia Patients

Type of SCT	Stage	No.	TRM	Relapse Rate	LFS
Allogeneic					
Family donor	CR1	1100	27%	24%	50%
	≥CR2	1019	29%	48%	34%
	Rel/Refr.	216	47%	75%	18%
Unrelated donor	CR1	318	47%	10%	39%
	≥CR2	231	8%	75%	27%
	Rel/Refr.*	47	64%	31%	5%
Autologous	CR1	1369	5%	51%	42%
	≥CR2	258	18%	70%	24%
Nonmyeloablative	All stages	232	28%	49%	31%

LFS, leukemia-free survival; SCT, stem cell transplantation; TRM, transplant-related mortality.
*One trial.[185]

mance of SCT in up to 70% of the patients achieving a second CR.[88] Thus all attempts—including experimental drugs—should be directed toward obtaining a second remission and proceeding with SCT.

Stem Cell Transplantation

SCT has gained an increasingly important role in the treatment of patients with adult ALL. Although the majority of large prospective studies in adult ALL addressed the issue of indications for SCT in first CR, scheduling and procedures are still not defined satisfactorily. To circumvent the problem with comparability of SCT and chemotherapy, several groups have constructed prospective trials with a "genetic" randomization, offering allogeneic SCT in first CR to all patients with a sibling donor. The study results certainly depend on the "conventional" treatment approach used in the chemotherapy arm. Some groups scheduled autologous SCT only and others a randomized comparison of autologous SCT and chemotherapy.

The most difficult outcome parameter is the OS of the total patient cohort in a prospective trial that answers the question whether an SCT-based treatment concept is able to improve overall outcome. OS of studies with genetic randomization have not documented that transplant is superior to chemotherapy[85]; this may be partly due to the fact that allogeneic SCT was implemented in only 11% to 38% of the patients.[54,89–94] Even if allogeneic SCT yielded favorable results, because of its infrequent implementation the impact on OS is too small.

Allogeneic Stem Cell Transplantation From Sibling Donors

The outcome of allogeneic SCT for patients with ALL depends on the age and remission status of the patient. The best results have been obtained in patients transplanted during the first remission. In a total of 1100 patients collected from published trials, the LFS rate was 50%, albeit with wide variations (21%–66%). The relapse probability (RP) was 24% and the transplant-related mortality rate (TRM) was 27% (Table 66–8). In more recent studies, results are improving, most probably because of a reduction in TRM.[95] According to the data of the International Bone Marrow Transplantation Registry (IBMTR) for HLA-identical sibling SCT between 1996 and 2001, the 3-year probability of survival was 48% for ALL recipients older than 20 years of age who were transplanted during their first remission.[96]

There is evidence that graft-versus-leukemia (GvL) effects are also operational in ALL patients receiving an allograft because several studies have shown that the RP is lower in patients with limited graft-versus-host disease.[97–100] Age is another important prognostic factor for outcome after SCT. The LFS is 62% for patients below and 48% for those above 20 years of age.[96] Nevertheless, age limits for allogeneic matched sibling SCT have been increased continuously up to 50 to 55 years. Experience of transplant centers may also have a role. Specialized centers in the United States report LFSs of 61% to 64% for sibling SCT in ALL in first remission.[101–103]

The LFS rate is 34% after allogeneic SCT in second remission. In advanced ALL (refractory or in relapse), allogeneic SCT results in an 18% long-term survival rate (see Table 66–8). Despite this, SCT is the treatment of choice in patients with relapsed or refractory ALL.

Matched Unrelated Stem Cell Transplantation

SCT using grafts from matched unrelated donors can result in long-term survival of 39% of patients with a lower RP (10%) as compared to allogeneic sibling SCT whereas TRM (47%) is higher. Both facts are probably due to more pronounced GvL and graft-versus-host (GvH) effects. It should be considered, however, that matched unrelated (MUD) series generally include selected high-risk patients, for example, with a high proportion of Ph/BCR–ABL-positive ALL. In the IBMTR registry, for adults older than 20 years, the 3-year probability of survival after MUD SCT in first CR was 42%.[96] In the largest series so far the results of MUD SCT were analyzed retrospectively in adult poor-risk ALL (mainly Ph/BCR–ABL-positive) patients with a median age of 34 years. They were particularly favorable for patients in first CR (42% at 2 years), whereas in second or subsequent CR, the LFS was only 17%.[104] The RP of only 6% for patients in first CR may be due to a more pronounced GvL effect. The high TRM of approximately 40%[104,105] is still the major obstacle to MUD SCT (see Table 66–8). This might be reduced by the use of different, less toxic preparative regimens, including nonmyeloablative SCT, better management of graft-versus-host disease (GvHD), and improved supportive care.

Overall, the results of MUD SCT in ALL are encouraging, particularly considering that these are often patients with advanced stages of disease. There is increasing evidence that results of MUD SCT are approaching those of sibling SCT, particularly if adjusted for bias. MUD SCT is therefore the treatment of choice for high-risk patients in first CR, including Ph/BCR–ABL-positive ALL—and probably also other high-risk patients—if a sibling donor is not available.

In later remission or relapse, MUD SCT may lead to long-term survival of 27% whereas outcome after transplantation in relapse is only 5% (see Table 66–8).

Autologous Stem Cell Transplantation

Another attempt to overcome the limited availability of bone marrow donors is autologous SCT. The results for autologous SCT in first remission are surprisingly good, with an LFS of 42% and a low TRM (see Table 66–8). The major problem is a high RP (51%). Similar results with an LFS rate of 42% in standard-risk ALL (n = 280) and 40% in high-risk ALL (n = 174) have been reported by the European Bone Marrow Transplant Group (EBMT).[106] Favorable results have been achieved in a trial with autologous BMT or PBSC transplantation in adult ALL patients in first CR followed by a 2-year maintenance treatment with 6-mercaptopurine and methotrexate.[107]

The TRM after autologous SCT is very low (3%) and is similar to that of conventional intensification therapy. With the increasing number of MUD transplants being performed and the advantage of GvL effects, the role of autologous SCT is decreasing. However, because of the low TRM, this is still a reasonable approach for elderly patients and probably patients with negative MRD status in autologous bone marrow graft. Several prospective randomized trials in adult ALL showed equal outcomes for chemotherapy consolidation and autologous SCT.

In the second remission, few patients obtain long-term survival with auto SCT (see Table 66–8). It may be considered as interim therapy before an allogeneic SCT if autologous stem cells have been collected during first CR.

Nonmyeloablative Stem Cell Transplantation

Nonmyeloablative SCT or reduced intensity conditioning regimens (NMSCT) is a novel approach that deserves evaluation in ALL and may lead to an extension of indications for allogeneic SCT. In contrast to conventional SCT, which mainly relies on cell kill by high-dose chemotherapy and total body irradiation (TBI), NMSCT uses GvL effects. Immunosuppression (eg, with purine analogs, other cytostatic drugs, or low-dose TBI) is followed by the infusion of stem cells from sibling or MUD donors with adapted immunosuppression to establish host tolerance.[108]

There is, however, the general opinion that GvL effects are less pronounced in ALL as compared to other malignancies. Nevertheless, these effects are present as indicated by lower RR in patients with acute or chronic GvHD,[98–100] lower RR after MUD SCT, induction of remissions by withdrawal of GvHD prophylaxis, or donor lymphocyte infusions (DLIs) in single patients with relapsed ALL.

NMSCT is being increasingly considered as an option for elderly patients with contraindications for conventional SCT. Initial results indicate that in first CR, stable remissions can be achieved in some patients.[109] These studies show an LFS of 31% for patients in all stages, with a 28% TRM and a 49% RR (Table 66–8). According to an EBMT analysis the LFS in 97 adult ALL patients with a median age of 38 years was 37%, with 28% TRM and 49% relapse rate.[110] The LFS was in both studies considerably higher if NMSCT was performed in patients in first remission.[109,110]

Results of Umbilical Cord Blood and Haploidentical Stem Cell Transplantation

The experience with umbilical cord blood (UCB) transplantation in ALL mainly comes from pediatric patients. Registry results of younger adults with acute leukemia indicate, however, that UCB (single or double) can be considered as an alternative donor source—if available.[111]

The experience with haploidentical SCT is restricted mainly to pediatric patients, where it may be considered in patients without a donor and with an urgent need of SCT. In adult patients with acute leukemia, a retrospective analysis indicated that—if feasible—autologous SCT is preferable to haploidentical SCT; despite a higher RR, the overall outcome was slightly superior.[112] According to the available experience, both approaches should be restricted to specialized centers, later stage of disease, and performed as part of a clinical trial.

Comparison of Different Transplantation Procedures and Transplantation Versus Chemotherapy

Allogeneic Sibling and Matched Unrelated Stem Cell Transplantation

Owing to improved supportive care, better donor selection, and extension of indications beyond very high-risk patients, the results of MUD donor SCT are similar to allogeneic sibling SCT. The prospective MRC/ECOG study of SCT showed in 321 patients with allogeneic sibling donor SCT a survival of 55% (standard and high-risk ALL) compared to 46% with MUD donor SCT in 67 patients with very high risk (Ph/BCR–ABL positive) ALL.[92] A study of nine German centers showed in first CR a higher proportion of MUD donor SCT (60% vs 27%) and there was no difference regarding LFS (45% vs 42%).[113] The TRM for allogeneic sibling SCT ranged in prospective trials between 15% and 26%[54,89–94] and reaches 35% in MUD SCT.[92] Several factors such as intensity of therapy before SCT, preparative regimens, immunosuppressive therapy after SCT, and also the experience and conditions at SCT centers may play a role. It can be summarized, however, that MUD SCT is a reasonable option for high-risk patients without a sibling donor.

Donor Versus No Donor Comparisons

This type of comparison represents the intent-to-treat analysis that is an adequate approach only if a significant number of patients actually receive the assigned treatment option. Several trials did not show differences in outcome for patients with (intent to treat: allogeneic sibling SCT) or without donor (intent to treat: randomization of auto SCT and chemotherapy).[54,94,114–116]

The Pethema study for high-risk patients even showed a trend toward an advantage for patients without a donor.[93] In contrast, several other studies demonstrated an advantage of SCT in high-risk patients.[90,91,115]

Recently the large ECOG/MRC group reported their results comparing patients with donor (allogeneic sibling SCT) to those without a donor (randomized comparison of chemotherapy and auto SCT). The special feature of this trial was the use of age (≥35 years) as a prognostic factor. Standard-risk patients were by definition younger than 35 years with a WBC count less than 30000/µL for B-precursor and less than 100,000/µL for T-ALL. Overall, patients with a donor had a superior OS (53%) compared to those without donor (45%) mainly because of a lower RP (29% vs 54%). The difference was particularly evident in standard-risk (62% vs 52% OS) but not in high-risk (41% vs 35%) patients,[117] a finding that is in contrast to all other trials. Because a younger age was the major factor for definition of standard risk, this result can be interpreted in two ways: (a) outcome of SCT is better in younger patients, which is a well-known fact, and (b) the outcome of young standard-risk patients with a donor is not superior to chemotherapy in other trials. A third issue is the fact that the performance of SCT was limited (321 allogeneic sibling SCT of 1508 evaluable patients).[92] The TRM reached 20% even in standard-risk patients. The OS of 39% in this trial was similar to other studies.[118]

Chemotherapy or Allogeneic Sibling Stem Cell Transplantation Versus Autologous Stem Cell Transplantation

In several randomized studies, no significant difference was detected in studies comparing chemotherapy and autologous SCT.[89,90,93,94] In the large randomized ECOG/MRC trial, the outcome of autologous SCT was inferior (33%) compared to chemotherapy (42%) in terms of LFS mainly because of a higher RP.[117] Comparisons of allogeneic and autologous SCT have shown an inferior outcome for autologous SCT. In two trials with an intent-to-treat comparison, the results of autologous SCT were poor (30% and 33%).[91,119]

Preferred Approach to Stem Cell Transplantation

A recently published evidence-based review emphasized that SCT offers an advantage as compared to chemotherapy in high-risk patients and in patients in second remission. The analyses also revealed the lack of prospective, controlled trials for SCT in ALL.[120] This is probably due to the fact that every study design that includes SCT by definition has too many variables, such as donor availability, individual patient condition, and patient wish. Not surprisingly, a meta-analysis of 7 studies[54,90,91,93,94,115,121] showed a broad variation in rates of performance of allogeneic (68%–96%) and autologous (9%–81%) SCT. The meta-analysis showed a correlation of outcome with compliance to allogeneic SCT. Again the OS for SCT was superior

Table 66–9 Indications for Stem Cell Transplantation in the German Multicenter Trials for Adult Acute Lymphocytic Leukemia Patients

	Indication	Priorities*
First remission		
High risk	All patients within 3–4 months from diagnosis	1. Allogeneic sibling† 2. Allogeneic unrelated† 3. Autologous 4. NMSCT
Standard risk	Molecular nonresponders	See above
Relapse, including molecular relapse	All patients in second CR (if necessary in good PR or beginning relapse)	See above (consider cord blood or haploidentical SCT if no donor available)

*Decision depends on age, patient's general condition, and donor availability.
†Matched or one mismatch.

to chemotherapy, with a particular advantage in high-risk patients.[122] Thus the role of allogeneic SCT in standard-risk ALL remains unclear.

In ongoing trials, indications for SCT in first remission are not uniformly defined. The advantages of SCT (short treatment duration, favorable outcome in some trials) must be compared to disadvantages (TRM, late complications, poorer quality of life). The major question is whether all patients with sibling donor should proceed to SCT or only those with specific risk factors.

When considering SCT, one has to balance the expected reduced relapse risk and the increased anticipated mortality. Also, late effects are more pronounced in SCT patients, the quality of life seems to be poorer, and the risk of procedure-related death is 20% to 30%. SCT in first CR from sibling or unrelated donor seems to be justified in subgroups of ALL with OS below 40% with chemotherapy and should probably not be offered to patients with OS after chemotherapy above 50%. These outcomes clearly depend on the different chemotherapy regimens used.

Therefore, in the majority of trials SCT indications are determined by the presence of adverse prognostic factors. The status of MRD is of increasing importance as an indication for the SCT. It remains open to further studies whether SCT is really a favorable option in patients with high MRD and whether patients with high-risk features but negative MRD status are still candidates for SCT. Allogeneic sibling and MUD SCT are considered in a similar way. Although outcome after SCT is better in younger patients, there is a trend to treat adolescents with pediatric-type intensive chemotherapy protocols and to proceed less with transplantation. For older, high-risk patients and those with contraindications, nonmyeloablative SCT is a reasonable alternative, with an expected LFS of 34% in first CR.[110]

There is general agreement that all patients in second or later remission are candidates for SCT. Depending on donor availability and general condition, experimental procedures such as NMSCT, cord blood SCT, and haploidentical SCT may be considered.

Table 66–9 outlines the indications of SCT in the German multicenter study group for adult ALL as an example for a risk-adapted approach.

OUTCOME OF ALL SUBTYPES AND PROGNOSTIC FACTORS

Age is probably the most important prognostic factor for achievement of CR and long-term outcome.[62] Other prognostic factors are of greater importance for duration of remission and survival (Table 66–10). Appreciation of the impact of such risk factors (Table 66–11) on the results in the majority of adult ALL trials have led to the generation of risk-adapted treatment protocols (Table 66–12).

Table 66–10 Outcome of Adult Acute Lymphocytic Leukemia Patients According to Subgroups*

Subgroup	No. of Patients	CR Rate	No. of Patients	LFS
Age				
<30	669	88%	510	42%–60%***
30–59	610	79%	412	33%
≥60	215	58%	141	15%
Subtype				
T-ALL**	976	88%	850	40%–60%***
B-Precursor ALL	2366	82%	2036	40%–60%
Pro-B-ALL	987	75%	107	37%–60%****
Cytogenetics				
Ph/bcr-abl + (without imatinib)	633	72%	633	21%
Ph/bcr-abl + (with imatinib + Chemo)		90%		50%
WBC				
<30,000/μL	698	81%	746	40%
>30,000/μL	387	75%	409	28%
Time to CR				
<4 weeks			1433	44%
>4 weeks			253	36%

CR, complete remission; LFS, leukemia-free survival; MRD, median remission duration.
*Pooled data from published studies.
**Depends on T-ALL subtype.
***Depending on protocal and subtype.
****Including allogeneic SCT.

Table 66–11 Adverse Prognostic Factors for Remission Duration in Adult Acute Lymphocytic Leukemia Patients*

Clinical characteristics	Higher age >50 years, >60 years High WBC >30000/μL in B-lineage
Immunophenotype	Pro-B (B-lineage, CD10⁻), CD10⁻ pre B-ALL Early T (T-lineage, CD1a⁻, sCD3⁻) Mature T (T-lineage, CD1a⁻, sCD3⁺)
Cytogenetics/molecular genetics	t(9;22)/BCR-ABL or t(4;11)/ ALL1-AF4 New molecular markers for T-ALL
Treatment response	Late achievement of CR >3 or 4 weeks MRD positivity

*Adverse prognostic factors as they emerged from the more than 3000 adult ALL patients treated in the GMALL (German Multicenter Studies for Adult ALL) trials. Data from Gökbuget N, Hoelzer D, Arnold R, et al: Treatment of adult ALL according to the protocols of the German Multicenter Study Group for Adult ALL (GMALL). Hemat/Oncol Clin North Am 14:1307, 2000.

Table 66–12 Preferred Approach to the Treatment of Adult Acute Lymphocytic Leukemia Patients

	Low-Risk ALL	High-Risk ALL	Very High-Risk ALL	Mature B-ALL
Definition	B-lineage WBC <30,000/μL Time to CR <4 weeks No Pro-B/ t(4;11) T-lineage Thy ALL Molecular CR	B-lineage WBC >30,000/μL Time to CR >4 weeks Pro-B/ t(4;11) T-lineage Early T, mature T No molecular CR	Ph/BCR-ABL positive	
Multidrug-induction	Yes	Yes	Yes + imatinib	Short intensive cycles including HDM, fractionated C, HDAC and other drugs Rituximab
CNS prophylaxis*	Yes	Yes	Yes	Yes
Consolidation (also other combinations)	Alternating cycles, e.g., HDM, HDAC, Asparaginase reinduction	One cycle	One cycle + imatinib	6 cycles
SCT in CR1	None	Allogeneic SCT (if matched related or unrelated donor) Autologous SCT After additional (if no donor and negative MRD, consolidation)		None
Maintenance	6-MP/M + intensification for 2–2½ years		imatinib	None

AC, cytosine arabinoside; ALL, acute lymphocytic leukemia; CR, complete remission; HDM, high-dose methotrexate; SCT, stem cell transplantation; MRD, minimal residual disease; Thy ALL, thymic ALL.

*Intrathecal therapy with M or triple combination (M, AC, steroid) continued during maintenance therapy; additional CNS irradiation and/or high-dose chemotherapy according to subgroup.

Age

Recent studies have shown that survival of patients with adult ALL decreases continuously with increasing age, from 34% to 57% below 30 years to 15% to 17% above 50 years.[28,44,54,118,123] Some groups used age above 30 to 35 years as an indication for SCT in first CR.[91,93] This is probably counterproductive because the outcome of SCT significantly decreases with age.[117] Increasing attention is being paid to the definition of specific treatment approaches for adult ALL patients at both ends of the age spectrum—adolescents at one and elderly patients on the other.

Table 66–13 Treatment Results in Elderly Acute Lymphocytic Leukemia Patients

Approach	No. of Studies	No. of Patients	CR	ED	OS
Palliative	4	94	43%	24%	7 months
Intensive chemotherapy	11	519	56%	23%	14%
Prospective studies	5	187	58%	16%	22%

CR, complete remission; OS, overall survival.

Elderly Patients

The CR rate is approximately 50% in patients at the age of 50 to 88 years, with a remission duration of 3 to 12 months and a survival rate below 10% (reviewed in references 124 and 125). It is difficult to define an age limit when a change in prognosis occurs. Almost all studies use a cutoff point at the age of 55 to 65 years to determine eligibility for allogeneic HSCT. This age seems to be practical because younger patients are candidates for intensified treatment approaches, such as SCT, whereas for the older group, new strategies need to be explored, carefully weighing the gain in survival against quality of life. Elderly patients at the age of 55 to 65 years or even older who have achieved a CR and are in good clinical condition are potential candidates for autologous SCT or NMSCT.

Several factors such as comorbidity, higher risk of complications, and increased risk of early mortality are associated with the inferior results in elderly patients. The major cause of death is infections. Therefore the increased hematologic toxicity with prolonged severe cytopenias is of particular relevance in elderly patients. Often it cannot be distinguished whether these are due to toxicity or to lack of response. There is the dilemma that on one hand the disease is more resistant in the elderly and on the other hand the tolerability of therapy is lower and there is a higher risk of organ toxicities, for example, of the liver or heart. Altogether, comorbidities and complications lead to treatment delays, omission of single drugs, and prolonged intervals between therapy cycles, which contribute to poorer long-term results. There is also a lower incidence of favorable prognostic subtypes such as T-ALL in the elderly, whereas the incidence of unfavorable subtypes is higher.[126]

Palliative therapy is associated with a short survival (Table 66–13).[124] With the use of intensive chemotherapy protocols developed for younger patients, the CR rate in the elderly was 56%, with 23% early mortality and a median survival of 9 months. It can be assumed that only elderly patients in good general condition were accepted to these trials. Thomas et al showed in three successive treatment periods that the remission rates of elderly patients could be improved by the adoption of specific age-adapted protocols.[127] Fortunately there is a new trend to develop prospective trials for elderly patients to offer a curative option on one hand and to limit toxicity, early mortality, and duration of hospitalization on the other to maintain quality of life. With these approaches, a more favorable remission rate of 58% and survival of 22% have been achieved.[124]

Further improvement of results in the elderly is urgently required. Innovative strategies are based on targeted, subgroup-specific elements with the aim not to increase the typical chemotherapy-associated toxicity. This includes use of the abl-kinase inhibitor imatinib for Ph+ ALL, and antibody therapy for CD20-positive ALL (rituximab). The German study group reported a remission rate of 63% in CD20-positive (Ph/BCR–ABL-negative) elderly patients and a survival of 54% after 1 year with a regimen combining age-adapted chemotherapy and eight doses of rituximab before the chemotherapy cycles.[128] In elderly patients with Ph/BCR–ABL-positive ALL, the remission rate can be improved to above 90% with imatinib monotherapy.

Adolescent Patients

In the recent years the optimal approach to treatment of adolescents has been discussed extensively. Several groups have compared the outcome of adolescents treated with so called "adult" protocols with those treated with "pediatric" protocols. Although entry criteria were quite similar, the outcome was always significantly inferior in those participating in the adult trials (EFS 34%–71%) as compared to the pediatric trials (EFS 64%–80%).[129] The conclusion was that pediatric trials include higher doses of VCR, ASP, and HDMTX and a higher time–dose intensity. However, the poor outcomes associated with adult protocols selected for comparison is probably also due to suboptimal approaches in these specific studies. The GMALL reported a survival of 64% in 417 young adults (15–25 years), with significant differences in outcome for subgroups ranging from 74% for standard risk, 49% for high risk, and 55% for Ph+ ALL.[130] Results are superior to most of those reported from adult protocols in adolescents.

One solution could be the extension of age limits of pediatric protocols to 25, 35, or even higher ages as currently attempted by several US groups. It remains open to question whether a sufficient number of adults will actually be treated in these studies and whether the application of such intensive regimens will be restricted to selected patients and selected, highly experienced pediatric care providers.

The other option, which is currently followed by several adult study groups, is to adopt more successful pediatric treatment elements to their protocols and to aim for a higher time and dose intensity with fewer treatment interruptions and omissions, particularly in adolescents and young adults. Interim results of such studies were reported recently. The CR rates (82%–92%) and EFS (66%–72%)[131–133] are promising but considerable toxicity, for example, neuropathies, and thrombosis was observed, indicating that these protocols may probably not be transferable to all adults.

White Blood Cell Count

An elevated white blood cell count (WBC) at diagnosis (>30,000–50,000/μL) is associated with a higher relapse risk.[28,44,54,89,123] It was even considered as the most deleterious prognostic factor in B-precursor ALL, with an OS of 19%–29%,[118,134] whereas in T-ALL WBC has no significant effect on outcome in a GMALL multivariate analysis.[134] The biological reason for the highly resistant behavior of B-precursor ALL with high WBC is unclear. In the GMALL studies, these patients show a high relapse rate but also seem to have a higher mortality with chemotherapy and SCT.[135] In these patients, evaluation of MRD, use of experimental drugs, and SCT modalities seem to be particularly important.

IMMUNOPHENOTYPE AND CYTOGENETICS

The immunophenotype is an important independent prognostic variable in ALL. In ongoing trials it is used to adjust treatment regimens accordingly (eg, separate regimens for mature B-cell ALL). A further example for clinical application is the identification of patients for antibody therapy (eg, anti-CD20 in CD20-positive B-lineage ALL or B-cell ALL, and anti-CD52 in B- and T-lineage ALL).

T-Lineage Acute Lymphoblastic Leukemia

Results of treatment of T-cell ALL have substantially improved as compared with survival rates of 10% 20 years ago. Many groups have confirmed the superior outcome of T-lineage ALL as compared to B-lineage ALL.[118,134] There is, however, a substantial difference in outcome for the T-ALL subtypes. Thymic T-ALL, which accounts for one-half of the adult T-ALL patients, has a favorable outcome, with CR rates of 85% to 90% and survival rates greater than 50% at 5 years. Early T-ALL and mature T-ALL have poorer outcomes, with CR rates of 70% and LFS rates of approximately 30%.[134] The biologic importance of immunophenotype was underlined by the fact that elevated expression of HOX11, HOX11L2, SIL-TAL1, and CALM-AF10 is associated with subtypes (ie, maturation states) of thymocytes.[136] Other groups observed inferior outcomes for early T-ALL[137,138]; coexpression of CD13, CD33, and/or CD34[137]; HOX11L2- and SIL-TAL-positive T-ALL.[138] The German group reported poor survival associated with overexpression of ERG and BAALC.[139,140] Overexpression of HOX11, which is associated with thymic T-ALL, may confer a favorable prognosis. Notch1-activating mutations with so far unclear prognostic relevance were identified in up to 50% of T-ALL cases.[136] They may be targeted by γ-secretase inhibitors. Five percent of T-ALL show the NUP214-ABL1 aberration, which may identify a target population for imatinib therapy.[141]

The addition of cyclophosphamide and AC to the usual cytostatic drugs for ALL are mainly responsible for the improved outcome in T-ALL. HDM contributed to the improvement of survival in children[142,143] as did HDAC.[144,145] For adults, the benefit of HDM in T-cell ALL has to be confirmed in larger trials. With current treatment regimens, CR rates of more than 80% and an LFS above 50% can be achieved in T-ALL. New treatment approaches in adult T-ALL include purine analogues, such as nelarabine,[132] Forodesine,[146] or antibody therapy (eg, anti-CD52).

B-Lineage ALL

In *common* and *pre-B-ALL*, CR rates in adults have improved to 80% or more, but patients still relapse in most studies over a period of up to 5 to 6 years, and only one-third of these patients survive. With B-precursor ALL, prognostic factors are decisive for outcome; high-risk patients with adverse prognostic features, such as high WBC (>30,000/μL), late achievement of CR (>3–4 weeks), and Ph/BCR–ABL-positive status (see Table 66–11) have a survival rate of 25% or less, whereas standard-risk patients without any of those features have a 5-year survival of greater than 50%.[134]

Philadelphia chromosome/BCR–ABL-positive ALL had until recently been associated with the worst prognosis in children as well as in adults. Outcome is now improved dramatically.

Adults with the subtype *pro-B-ALL* or the *t(4;11)* translocation had a poor prognosis, as do infant ALL patients.[147] With intensive regimens, including HDAC and mitoxantrone as consolidation therapy, the results for adults seem to be improving.[55] Pro-B-ALL patients benefit from allogeneic SCT in first CR with survival rates of 60% in transplanted patients.[148] The adverse impact of the translocation t(4;11) seems to have changed with new treatment modalities.

In mature *B-cell* ALL, CR remission rates were low (40%) a decade ago, and remission duration was short (11 months).[149] A change was brought about by innovative childhood B-cell ALL studies that significantly improved outcome, with CR rates of 80% to 94% and an LFS rate of 63% (weighted mean).[149] The drugs responsible for the improvement were high doses of fractionated cyclophosphamide, HDM (0.5–8 g/m^2), and HDAC in conjunction with the conventional drugs for remission induction in ALL given in short cycles at frequent intervals over a period of 6 months.

The application of these childhood B-cell ALL protocols in original or modified form also brought a substantial improvement in adult patients with B-cell ALL. CR rate reached 75% (62%–83%) and the LFS 55% (20%–71%).[149–151] Adverse-outcome prognostic factors were late CR (more than two cycles of chemotherapy), high WBC (>30 × 10^9/L), and age more than 50 years. B-cell ALL has a higher incidence of CNS involvement at diagnosis and of CNS relapse. Therefore, effective measures against CNS disease, such as HDM and HDAC, as well as i.th. therapy, are important components of treatment regimens. Maintenance treatment has been omitted. Because relapses occur almost exclusively within the first year in childhood, as well as in adult B-cell ALL studies, patients thereafter can be considered to be cured.

Further significant improvement was achieved by the addition of antibody therapy with anti-CD20 (rituximab) because more than 80% of the patients are CD20-positive. With these regimens, survival rates above 70% to 90% can be achieved in adults with mature B-ALL or Burkitt lymphoma.[152,153]

The translocations t(8;14), t(8;2), and t(8;22) or c-myc aberrations are present in most cases of mature B-cell ALL and in Burkitt lymphoma. They may add information in cases with uncertain diagnosis. They have lost their poor prognostic significance, however, because of the improved treatment for patients with B-cell ALL or Burkitt lymphoma.

TREATMENT RESPONSE AND MINIMAL RESIDUAL DISEASE

Besides age, the most relevant prognostic factor in ALL is still the achievement of CR. Further prognostic factors related to treatment response are delayed time to CR or response to prednisone therapy. A more accurate approach to assess individual response is evaluation of MRD[62,154] because this is an independent prognostic factor that reflects primary drug resistance as well as individual completion of therapy and unknown host factors. The methods for detecting the burden of MRD have been described earlier and are summarized in Table 66–14.

Table 66–14 Methods for Detection of Minimal Residual Disease in Acute Lymphocytic Leukemia Patients

Method	Target	Sensitivity	Application B-Lineage ALL	T-Lineage ALL
Flow cytometry	Leukemia-specific immunophenotype	10^{-3}–10^{-4}	~35%	>90%
PCR	Fusion transcripts	10^{-4}–10^{-6}	~30%	~10%
PCR	Ig rearrangements (IgH, IgK)	10^{-4}–10^{-6}	>90%	~20%
PCR	TCR rearrangements (TCR-β, -δ, -γ)	10^{-4}–10^{-6}	~50%	>90%

ALL, acute lymphocytic leukemia; IgH, immunglobulin gene; PCR, polymerase chain reaction; TCR, T-cell receptor gene.

Data from Campana D, Pui C-H: Detection of minimal residual disease in acute leukemia: Methodological advances and clinical significance. Blood 85:1416, 1995; Beishuizen A, van Wering E, Breit TM, et al: Molecular biology of acute lymphoblastic leukemia: Implications for detection of minimal residual disease. In Hiddemann W et al (eds.): Acute leukemias. V. Experimental Approaches and Management of Refractory Disease. Berlin, Springer-Verlag, 1996, p 460.

Identification of High-Risk Patients as Candidates for Stem Cell Transplantation or Experimental Therapy

After start of consolidation a high burden of MRD (>10^{-4}) at any time point is associated with a high relapse risk of 66% to 88%[53] and the predictive value increases at later time points (months 6–9).[155] In the GMALL studies, patients with a high burden of MRD (>10^{-4}) after induction and first consolidation were identified as high risk and were considered candidates for SCT in first CR.[156]

Identification of Low-Risk Patients in Whom Treatment Intensity Reduction May Be Justified

This aim is more difficult to reach. An early and rapid decrease of MRD during induction is associated with a relapse risk of only 8%.[53] However, this course is observed in only 10% of the patients. In the GMALL studies, patients with negative MRD status after induction, which is repeatedly confirmed during the first year and measured with two sensitive markers, are considered as MRD low risk. It remains open whether any treatment reduction is justified in adult AU.

Assessment of Molecular Clinical Remission and Thereby Evaluation of Different Induction Therapies and Detection of Molecular Relapses

These are two important, new items for follow-up analysis in adult ALL. Molecular response provides a more individual impression of the response and is particularly important, because nowadays 85% to 90% of adult ALL patients achieve a cytologic CR. Even in phase II studies, "molecular relapse" is already an inclusion criterion. This makes sense because patients with an increase of MRD burden above 10^{-4} after achievement of a molecular CR are at a high risk for relapse (>80%), and therapeutic action should be taken.[157]

Risk Stratification According to Minimal Residual Disease

The approaches to integrate MRD analysis in prospective risk stratification of adults can be different in terms of (a) the time points sampled, (b) the selection of patients for MRD risk stratification, (c) combination of MRD-based and conventional risk factors, and (d) the MRD-based treatment decisions. It is hardly possible to identify adult low-risk patients in whom reduction of the intensity of therapy would be justified. In the GMALL study, these patients are defined according to very strict criteria to omit maintenance therapy. However, 20% to 30% of these patients relapsed. The major aim in MRD-based studies is therefore to identify patients with high risk of relapse for treatment intensification with SCT. It remains to be demonstrated that this is an effective strategy because patients with high MRD before SCT have an increased risk of relapse and might probably benefit from additional conventional, even experimental, therapy to reduce tumor load. On the other hand, it has to be questioned whether patients who are candidates for SCT based on conventional risk factors including Ph+ ALL should receive allogeneic SCT if they are MRD negative. The best strategy remains unknown.

Evaluation of the burden of MRD has not been without problems. The technical procedure is time-consuming, expensive and requires highly specialized staff. The predictive value depends on the technical quality such as sensitivity, 10^{-4} number of targets (at least two for immunoglobulin or TCR-rearrangements) and on the frequency of evaluations (3-monthly). At least in multicenter studies, these prerequisites can often not be fulfilled. Sensitivity of the evaluation of MRD with the exception of BCR–ABL based analysis is also

Table 66–15 Expression of Surface Antigens on Acute Lymphocytic Leukemia Blast Cells

Subgroup	Antigen	Expression on >20% of LBC*
B-Lineage	CD19	95% precursor
		94% mature
	CD20	41% precursor
		86% mature
	cyCD22	17%
T-lineage	CD25	
	CD7	99%
	CD3	33%
Both	CD52	66%–78%†
	CD33	16%

LBC, lymphatic blast cells; rel, relapsed.
*Data from the GMALL central immunophenotyping, E. Thiel, S. Schwartz, Berlin.
†Data from Faderl S, Kantarjian HM, O'Brien S, et al: A broad exploratory trial of Campath-1H in the treatment of acute leukemias. Blood 96:1397a, 2000.

not sufficient to evaluate the efficacy of consolidation cycles because in most patients MRD is below the detection limit.

DRUG RESISTANCE

MDR-1 function has been associated with a poorer prognosis.[137,158] In vitro sensitivity testing was able to identify patients with resistance to conventional cytostatic drugs that were associated with an inferior prognosis. More recently it was demonstrated that in vitro resistance is associated with distinct gene expression profiles.[159] In vitro resistance testing is also increasingly used for effectivity testing of new cytostatic drugs. In the future, a prediction of response to induction regimens may be possible to adapt therapy to individual susceptibility.

NEW THERAPEUTIC APPROACHES IN ADULT ACUTE LYMPHOBLASTIC LEUKEMIA TREATMENT WITH MONOCLONAL ANTIBODIES

ALL blast cells express a variety of specific antigens such as CD20, CD19, CD22, CD33, and CD52 that may serve as targets for treatment with monoclonal antibodies (MoAb) (Table 66–15). MoAb therapy is an attractive approach because it is targeted, subtype specific, and compared to chemotherapy has different mechanisms of action and side effects. One prerequisite for Ab therapy may be the presence of the target antigen in at least 20% to 30% of the blast cells. Application may be most promising in a stage of low MRD level.[160]

Anti-CD20

Most experience has been had so far with rituximab, which is a chimeric MoAb to CD20 that is expressed on normal and malignant B lymphocytes. It exerts significant antitumor activity and its use has led to an improvement of results in B-cell non-Hodgkin lymphoma (NHL). CD20, defined as expression on more than 20% of the blast cells, is, however, also present on one-third of B-precursor ALL blasts, particularly in elderly patients (40%–50%), and the majority of mature B-ALL blast cells (80%–90%).

The anti-CD20 antibody has been successfully integrated in the therapy of mature B-ALL and Burkitt lymphoma. It is now also being explored in several pilot studies for CD20-positive B-precursor ALL. In a GMALL protocol for elderly patients, rituximab is administered prior to chemotherapy cycles starting during induction for a total of 8 treatments. Also the combination of Hyper-CVAD regimen with rituximab in B-precursor ALL was feasible and a favorable outcome with CD20-positive ALL was reported (reviewed in reference 161).

Anti-CD52

The CD52 antigen is expressed by most lymphatic cells and to a higher degree in T- compared with B-lymphoblasts. CD52 antibodies were first used for ex-vivo T-cell depletion of allogeneic bone marrow grafts to prevent GvHD without further GvHD prophylaxis. The humanized antibody Campath-1H has antitumor activity in CLL, T-PLL, and other T-NHL. Several studies with anti-CD52 therapy in adults with ALL are ongoing, either during relapse or at the time of MRD. The CALGB has integrated anti-CD52 therapy as consolidation in their frontline therapy and demonstrated its feasibility in a dose-finding study. Efficacy data are not available.[162]

Additional MoAbs (B43[anti-CD19]-Genistein, B43[anti-CD19]-PAP, and anti-B4-bR [anti-CD19]) have been investigated in phase I–II pilot trials in ALL. Antibodies developed for other diseases, such as anti-CD22 in lymphoma and anti-CD33 in AML, may be applicable in ALL because these antigens are expressed in 17% and 16% of adult ALL cases, respectively.

Antibody treatment could be administered as single agents or in combination with chemotherapy, for purging, and as posttransplant therapy and may be particularly effective in low burden disease (MRD-positive patients).

IMATINIB IN PH/BCR–ABL-POSITIVE ALL

In Ph/BCR–ABL-positive leukemia, the BCR–ABL fusion gene is causally involved in leukemogenesis and is considered to be essential for leukemic transformation. With a selective inhibitor of the Abl tyrosine kinase (STI571, imatinib), the cellular proliferation of BCR–ABL-positive CML and ALL cells can be inhibited.

Clinical Experience With Imatinib in Advanced Ph-Positive Acute Lymphoblastic Leukemia

In a multicenter phase II study, 56 patients with relapsed or refractory Ph+ ALL received imatinib at an initial daily dose of 400 mg PO, which was later increased to 600 mg; 60% of Ph+ ALL patients achieved a hematologic response. A complete hematologic remission with normalization of peripheral blood (PB) counts (ANC >1.5/nL, platelets >100/nL) was noted in 19% of patients. Rapid blast cell clearance occurred within 1 week of treatment in the majority of patients. It is noteworthy that the PB response did not necessarily correspond with a marrow BM response. Median estimated time to progression for ALL patients was 2.2 months.[163] Despite the rapid development of relapse, which occurs within weeks in many patients, some of these patients went on to SCT.[164] Response to imatinib therapy can be closely monitored by quantitative PCR.

Hematologic toxicity (grades III and IV) was frequent, but was rarely associated with serious infectious or hemorrhagic complications. Nonhematologic toxicity attributed to imatinib consisted primarily of mild to moderate gastrointestinal discomfort, peripheral and facial edema, and muscle cramps, and was readily manageable. No patient discontinued therapy because of nonhematologic adverse events. There were no imatinib-related deaths. Thus imatinib was well tolerated even in heavily pretreated patients.

Imatinib in the Treatment of Ph-Positive Acute Lymphoblastic Leukemia

In *younger patients* imatinib was first administered between chemotherapy cycles. However, with this approach no molecular remissions were achieved. Therefore, studies with parallel application of chemotherapy and imatinib were started, leading to CR rates above 91% to 96% and molecular CR of 38% to 50%.[52,165–167] All studies reported an improved OS of 55% to 65% compared with 15% in studies before the imatinib era. No trial described increased toxicity compared to chemotherapy alone or negative effects on subsequent SCT.

In *older patients* outcomes with de novo Ph+ ALL treatment results have been previously extremely poor, with particularly high induction mortality. Therefore, induction chemotherapy was replaced by single-drug therapy with imatinib. The remission rate was 92% in an Italian trial.[168] The German study group (GMALL) conducted a randomized trial comparing dose-reduced chemotherapy and imatinib monotherapy. After induction, all patients received chemotherapy combined with imatinib. The remission rate for the imatinib arm was 93% as compared to 54% with chemotherapy.[169] The survival was superior to previous trials without imatinib, but in both arms the relapse rate was high and there was no difference in outcome.

At present, combination of chemotherapy and imatinib is the standard for treatment of younger patients with Ph+ ALL. Patients are still referred for SCT in first CR if possible. In elderly patients, imatinib monotherapy for induction seems reasonable—at least if a rapid response is observed. However, it remains unknown whether the high relapse rate may be decreased by a combination of imatinib with mild chemotherapy during induction or by intensification of consolidation. Furthermore, transition to the use of treatment with other tyrosine kinase inhibitors in case of molecular relapse or detection of mutations of BCR/AB2 is important.

Imatinib and Allogeneic Stem Cell Transplantation in Ph-Positive Acute Lymphoblastic Leukemia

It is known that MRD after SCT in Ph+ ALL is associated with a relapse probability exceeding 90%. Starting imatinib in the setting of MRD may decrease this high relapse rate. In a prospective study conducted by the GMALL, 27 Ph+ ALL patients received imatinib upon detection of MRD after SCT. MRD became undetectable in 52% after a median of 1.5 months. Each of these patients remained in remission at least for the duration of imatinib treatment. Failure to achieve MRD negativity shortly after starting imatinib predicted relapse, which occurred in 92% of these patients after a median of 3 months. LFS was 91% after 1 year in the molecular responders compared with 8% in the nonresponders.[170]

It remains unknown whether imatinib should be started in all patients after SCT or only in case of MRD detection. Anyway, continued MRD positivity after 2 to 3 months of imatinib identifies patients who will ultimately experience relapse and in whom additional or alternative antileukemic treatment should be initiated.

Mechanisms of Resistance to Imatinib

MRD detection often leads to early detection of molecular resistance or molecular relapse. Additional treatment can then be initiated before overt relapse occurs. Nowadays, an additional search for mutations of the tyrosine kinase domain of BCR/ABL is required because these mutations can confer resistance to imatinib and partly to the second-generation tyrosine kinase inhibitors Dasatinib and Nilotinib.[171,172] Both drugs have an increased efficacy compared to imatinib and are active in the majority of mutations—with the exception of the T315I mutation. The remission rate achieved with these drugs in patients who fail imatinib is approximately 30%. These second-generation drugs are currently being evaluated in patients who have relapsed, but trials for de novo Ph+ ALL are starting.

New Cytotoxic Drugs

In the past 10 years a variety of new drugs has been developed for use in ALL (reviewed in 83, 84, and 85). Nelarabine is a purine analogue that acts specifically on T lymphoblasts with a remission rate between 30% and 40% in relapsed T-ALL.[132,173] Treatment was generally well tolerated although neurotoxicity occurred in some patients. At present, application in frontline therapy is being evaluated. BCX1777 (Forodesine) is an inhibitor of the enzyme purine nucleoside phosphorylase and thereby acts on the similar system as purine analogues.[146] Clofarabine is a purine analogue without subgroup-specific effects. Other new drugs are liposomal preparations that may improve feasibility of treatment, for example, liposomal vincristine, daunorubicin, or liposomal cytarabine for i.th. application.

Future Risk Stratification and Treatment Concepts for Adult Acute Lymphoblastic Leukemia

The treatment of adult ALL has already become more sophisticated and complicated and will be even more so in the future. Treatment strategies depend on factors unrelated to the disease, such as the availability of a stem cell donor, patient-related factors, disease markers, treatment response, and availability of targeted drugs. Prognostic factors and patient characteristics therefore no longer only serve as the basis for identification of candidates for SCT in first CR but to define individualized treatment approaches, which are discussed in the following examples.

- *Subgroup-adjusted and targeted treatment*: Use of targeted drugs such as tyrosine kinase inhibitors, subgroup-specific purine analogues such as nelarabine, or monoclonal antibodies such as CD20 in mature B-ALL to increase subgroup-specific activity of treatment. These approaches have already led to significant improvement of outcome and will be refined in the future.
- *Age-adapted treatment*: In similar ways to subgroup-adapted treatment, therapies have to be defined for patients at both ends of the age spectrum, that is, for both elderly and adolescent patients. In elderly patients the major focus is on effective targeted therapy with as much quality of life as possible, whereas in adolescents the major aim is to deliver time- and dose-intensive chemotherapy based on pediatric protocols.
- *Individualized treatment*: New methods offer the option to adopt intensity and duration of therapy to individual response as measured by the presence of MRD or to add or omit specific drugs according to the results of an evaluation for drug resistance.
- *New integrated risk classification*: A variety of molecular markers newly detected by microarray analysis have been proposed as prognostic factors.[174] They may possibly be integrated in a conventional risk model that aims to identify patients for SCT in first CR and may rather stimulate analysis of underlying mechanisms, drug targets, or invention of treatment adaptations.
- *Risk-adapted indications for SCT*: Indications for SCT have to be defined carefully, taking into account not only long-term results but also acute and long-term toxicities. At present the majority of study groups stick to risk-adapted indications for SCT.
- *Evaluation of new cytostatic drugs*: Many of these drugs fit in subtype-adjusted, targeted therapies. Taking the number of targets and drugs into account, evidence-based priorities for clinical evaluation in relapsed ALL and for integration in frontline therapy have to be set.

Risk- and subtype-adjusted treatment strategies has led to considerable improvement in the outcome of patients with mature B-ALL, T-ALL, and Ph-positive ALL but to a lesser extent in adult patients with B-precursor ALL. Future strategies will integrate a variety of additional factors, thereby resulting in a more complex, flexible, and patient-specific treatment approach.[85] Besides these sophisticated approaches, a better adherence to protocols, support of patients to improve their compliance, and documentation of compliance would be warranted in adult ALL. Treatment should be done at experienced centers, and closer cooperation between internal medicine and pediatric physicians including cooperative studies would be desirable.

Also, the design of prospective trials will be challenging because they will focus on even smaller subgroups of ALL and phase I studies with new drugs. These trials will only be possible in larger, international study groups that are able to recruit sufficient patient numbers. To enable any intergroup comparison, international efforts similar to that utilized to study childhood ALL are required to define uniform criteria for diagnostic classification, definition of subgroups, and even prognostic factors.

SUGGESTED READINGS

Bruggemann M, Raff T, Flohr T, et al: Clinical significance of minimal residual disease quantification in adult patients with standard-risk acute lymphoblastic leukemia. Blood 107:1116, 2006.

Deangelo DJ, Yu D, Johnson JL, et al: Nelarabine induces complete remissions in adults with relapsed or refractory T-lineage acute lymphoblastic leukemia or lymphoblastic lymphoma: Cancer and Leukemia Group B study 19801. Blood [Epub ahead of print], 2007, Mar 7.

Fielding AK, Richards SM, Chopra R, et al: Outcome of 609 adults after relapse of acute lymphoblastic leukemia (ALL); an MRC UKALL12/ECOG 2993 study. Blood 109:944, 2007.

Gökbuget N, Hoelzer D: Treatment with monoclonal antibodies in acute lymphoblastic leukemia: Current knowledge and future prospects. Ann Hematol 83:201, 2003.

Gökbuget N, Hoelzer D: Treatment of adult acute lymphoblastic leukemia. Hematology Am Soc Hematol Educ Program 133, 2006.

Hahn T, Wall D, Camitta B, et al: The role of cytotoxic therapy with hematopoietic stem cell transplantation in the therapy of acute lymphoblastic leukemia in adults: An evidence-based review. Biol Blood Marrow Transplant 12:1, 2006.

Hoelzer D, Gökbuget N: New approaches in acute lymphoblastic leukemia in adults: Where do we go? Semin Oncol 27:540, 2000.

Kiehl MG, Kraut L, Schwerdtfeger R, et al: Outcome of allogeneic hematopoietic stem-cell transplantation in adult patients with acute lymphoblastic leukemia: No difference in related compared with unrelated transplant in first complete remission. J Clin Oncol 22:2816, 2004.

Mohty M, Labopin M, Boiron J-M, et al: Reduced intensity conditioning (RIC) allogeneic stem cell transplantation (allo-SCT) for patients with acute lymphoblastic leukemia (ALL): A survey from the European Group for Blood and Marrow Transplantation (EBMT) [abstract]. Blood 106:659, 2005.

Moorman AV, Harrison CJ, Buck GA, et al: Karyotype is an independent prognostic factor in adult acute lymphoblastic leukemia (ALL): Analysis of cytogenetic data from patients treated on the Medical Research Council (MRC) UKALLXII/Eastern Cooperative Oncology Group (ECOG) 2993 trial. Blood 109:3189, 2007.

Ottmann OG, Wassmann B, Pfeifer H, et al: Imatinib compared with chemotherapy as front-line treatment of elderly patients with Philadelphia chromosome-positive acute lymphoblastic leukemia (Ph+ ALL). Cancer 109:2068, 2007.

Pui CH: Central nervous system disease in acute lymphoblastic leukemia: Prophylaxis and treatment. Hematology Am Soc Hematol Educ Program 142, 2006.

Raff T, Gökbuget N, Luschen S, et al: Molecular relapse in adult standard risk ALL patients detected by prospective MRD-monitoring during and after maintenance treatment—data from the GMALL 06/99 and 07/03 trials. Blood [Epub ahead of print], 2006, Oct 5.

Rowe J, Buck G, Fielding A, et al: In adults with standard-risk acute lymphoblastic leukemia (ALL) the greatest benefit is achieved from an allogeneic transplant in first complete remission (CR) and an autologous transplant is less effective than conventional consolidation/maintenance chemotherapy: Final results of the International ALL Trial (MRC UKALL XII/ECOG E2993). Blood 108:2, 2006.

Thomas DA, Faderl S, O'Brien S, et al: Chemoimmunotherapy with hyper-CVAD plus rituximab for the treatment of adult Burkitt and Burkitt-type lymphoma or acute lymphoblastic leukemia. Cancer 106:1569, 2006.

Thomas DA, Kantarjian H, Cortes J, et al: Outcome with the hyper-CVAD and imatinib mesylate regimen as frontline therapy for adult Philadelphia (Ph) positive acute lymphocytic leukemia (ALL). Blood 108:284, 2006.

Wassmann B, Pfeifer H, Gökbuget N, et al: Alternating versus concurrent schedules of imatinib and chemotherapy as front-line therapy for Philadelphia-positive acute lymphoblastic leukemia (Ph+ ALL). Blood 108:1469, 2006.

Yanada M, Matsuo K, Suzuki T, Naoe T: Allogeneic hematopoietic stem cell transplantation as part of postremission therapy improves survival for adult patients with high-risk acute lymphoblastic leukemia: A metaanalysis. Cancer 106:1657, 2006.

REFERENCES

For complete list of references log onto www.expertcmsult.com.

CHAPTER 67

MYELODYSPLASTIC SYNDROMES: BIOLOGY AND TREATMENT

Daniel J. DeAngelo and Richard M. Stone

Over the past several decades, many terms have been used to describe the bone marrow failure syndromes, which often terminate in an overt acute leukemia. The terms include refractory anemia (RA), preleukemia, smoldering acute leukemia, oligoblastic leukemia, refractory dysmyelopoietic anemia, and myelodysplastic syndrome.[1–5] Patients typically present with varying degrees of anemia, leukopenia, and thrombocytopenia, rendering many transfusion dependent or susceptible to infection or hemorrhage. The term *myelodysplastic syndrome* (MDS) is the currently accepted norm that is used to describe this clinical entity. MDS may arise either de novo or secondary to ionizing radiation, toxins or chemotherapeutic drug exposure.[6–11] The natural history of these syndromes ranges from an acute precipitous decline over several weeks to a chronic condition that lasts many years. The actual incidence of MDS is unknown. Unfortunately, the incidence rates of MDS were not reported to the National Cancer Institute's Surveillance Epidemiology and End Results (SEER) Program until 2001. Estimates in Europe range from 3 to 20 cases per 100,000, whereas in the United States, greater than 10,000 new cases are diagnosed each year (median age 76 years).[12–14] The incidence in men is significantly higher than in women (4.5 vs 2.7 per 100,000). MDS is rarely seen in patients younger than 50 years but rapidly increases with advancing age and may equal the incidence of acute myelogenous leukemia (AML) by the eighth decade.[15–17] For example, the age-specific incidence rates of MDS are approximately 5 per 100,000 for ages 60 to 69 years but increase to approximately 50 per 100,000 for ages 70 to 79 years.[18]

The various pathologic entities of MDS previously were classified by the French-American-British (FAB) Cooperative Group into five subtypes based on a set of criteria that included bone marrow morphology and the percentage of myeloblasts,[19] with the presence of greater than 30% myeloblasts classified as AML. The FAB classification scheme, based largely on the histologic changes within the bone marrow, has been extremely useful in assessing prognosis in patients with MDS, but the arbitrary division between MDS and AML based on the presence or absence of 30% myeloblasts is biologically inconsistent. In large studies, patients with refractory anemia with excess blasts in transformation (RAEB-T) and AML have similar outcomes. As a result, the World Health Organization (WHO) has adopted the definition of AML in a patient with 20% or greater myeloblasts and have removed the antiquated term RAEB-T.[20]

Most patients with MDS have progressive cytopenias, and a large fraction of patients eventually develop overt AML.[21] Patients with secondary AML from an underlying MDS typically are treated with multiagent chemotherapy in an attempt to delete the leukemic clone.[22] Nevertheless, the same problems exist as with MDS: advanced age, therapy-related toxicity, and resistant disease. Stem cell transplantation (SCT) remains the best chance for cure, but this strategy is not appropriate for the majority of patients due to their advanced age. Treatment of MDS ultimately is intended to extend overall survival by both improving the peripheral blood cytopenias and delaying the leukemic transformation. However, the more immediate goal of therapy is to relieve symptoms and improve the quality of life while minimizing side effects.

BIOLOGY

Pathogenesis

Myelodysplasia is the result of a transformation of a myeloid stem cell. A hematopoietic stem cell is capable of self-renewal and can give rise to more differentiated progeny.[23–26] As the stem cell differentiates it becomes lineage specific. An early pluripotent stem cell can give rise to both lymphoid and myeloid cells. However, the neoplastic transformation of the myeloid stem cell is the initial event that leads to myelodysplasia.[27] MDS rarely transforms into acute lymphocytic leukemia, thus suggesting that the MDS myeloid stem cell has lost its lymphopoietic potential.[28,29] Poorly defined transforming event(s) affects the pluripotent myeloid stem cell in MDS, thus conferring a growth advantage that eventually leads to development of monoclonal hematopoietic progeny. Many genetic mutations regulate this process, and these alterations determine both the biology and clinical aspects of the disease.[30]

The clinical hallmark of patients with myelodysplasia is the development of ineffective hematopoiesis (Fig. 67–1). Interestingly, cellular turnover within the bone marrow often is increased in most patients with myelodysplasia.[31] Cell kinetic studies have revealed a dramatic increase in the rate of cell division. The peripheral cytopenias are thought to be secondary to an increase in apoptosis, or programmed cell death, resulting in a futile increase in cell cycling.[32,33] Impaired cellular function is another important clinical feature of myelodysplasia. Erythroid precursors have a decreased response to erythropoietin (Epo), which may contribute to subsequent anemia.[34] In addition, terminally differentiated cells in MDS have functional defects. Mature granulocytes have decreased myeloperoxidase activity,[35–37] and platelets may have impaired aggregation properties.[38] The oncogenic pathway is not a single-step process. Sequential genetic changes are required to change a transformed myelodysplastic stem cell into a true neoplasm that often leads to development of AML.[39]

MDS is a clonal hematopoietic disorder.[40] Bone marrow cytogenetic analysis has been a great asset in the evaluation of the clonal nature of the MDS stem cell.[41–43] The clonal nature of MDS has been best elucidated by the use of X-inactivation studies.[44,45] These studies use restriction fragment length polymorphism (RFLP) analysis to study the differences between the methylation patterns of inactive versus active X chromosomes. RFLP analysis using the phosphoglycerate kinase and hypoxanthine phosphoribosyltransferase genes as well as the polymorphic genes of glucose-6-phosphate dehydrogenase all have demonstrated clonal hematopoiesis within the granulocyte, monocytic, erythroid, and megakaryocytic lineages in patients with MDS.

Apoptosis

Programmed cell death, referred to as *apoptosis*, is an important and active cellular process that regulates cell and lineage population.[46] The rate of apoptosis is finely regulated by the ratio of proapoptotic pro-

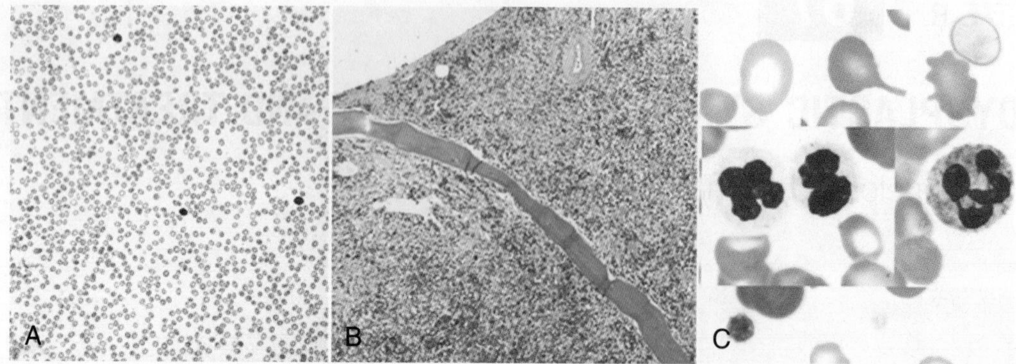

Figure 67–1 Elements of myelodysplastic syndrome. **A–C,** Myelodysplastic syndromes are generally characterized by cytopenias (**A**) due to ineffective hematopoiesis (**B**), which is related to multilineage dysplasia (**C**). **A,** This patient presented with a white blood cell count of 1,500/μL, hemoglobin 8.9 g/dL, and platelet count 47,000/μL. **B,** The bone marrow was hypercellular, indicating ineffective hematopoiesis. **C,** Evidence of trilineage dysplasia was apparent on the peripheral smear. Anisocytosis with macro-ovalocytes and poikilocytosis is seen in the red blood cells (**C, top**). The latter included the somewhat uncommon finding of Cabot ring forms (**right**). A large proportion of the granulocytes were severely hypogranular (**C, middle left**) compared to some normal forms still in the circulation (**right**). Platelets (**C, bottom**) were decreased in number, and many were severely hypogranular (**middle,** barely visible) compared to residual normal platelets (**left**).

teins, such as c-Myc, p53, Bax, and Bad, to the antiapoptotic proteins, which include Bcl-2 and Bcl-X_L.[47–50] Increased apoptosis has been documented within $CD34^+$ bone marrow cells in patients with MDS.[51] This increased apoptosis seems to be highest in patients with RA compared to those with RAEB and may account for the cytopenias that are the hallmark of early-stage MDS.[52–55] For example, the intracellular ratio of c-Myc to Bcl-2 is higher in $CD34^+$ cells in patients with MDS compared to those from normal patients or patients with AML.[56] In addition, an increased level of apoptosis is associated with increased levels of inhibitory cytokines, such as tumor necrosis factor (TNF)-α.[57] TNF-α is increased across all MDS subtypes and may inhibit the development and maturation of the hematopoietic precursors. TNF-α may increase the production and secretion of other proapoptotic cytokines, such as interleukin (IL)-6, transforming growth factor β, interferon γ, and Fas ligand. Use of growth factors, such as erythropoiesis-stimulating agents (ESAs) and granulocyte colony-stimulating factor (G-CSF), has been shown to decrease the rate of apoptosis in some patients.[58–60] These findings suggest that increased levels of apoptosis is associated with early-stage MDS, whereas decreased levels of apoptosis may help propagate the transformation from MDS to AML.[52,54,61–63]

Hematopoiesis

The colony-forming capacities of the pluripotent hematopoietic stem cells and their progeny are low or absent in many patients with MDS.[64] The bone marrow cells as well as peripheral T cells from patients with MDS seem to produce lower levels of granulocyte-macrophage colony-stimulating factor (GM-CSF), IL-3, macrophage colony-stimulating factor (M-CSF), and IL-6. The colony-forming unit granulocyte-macrophage (CFU-GM) is less responsive to both G-CSF and GM-CSF in patients with MDS.[65,66] These findings are more dramatic in patients with RAEB or RAEB-T. In addition, the erythroid progenitor cell, burst-forming unit-erythroid (BFU-E), is less responsive to Epo in vitro.[64] There also seems to be a direct correlation between the size of the BFU-E and the Epo level in patients with MDS. These findings may help explain the peripheral blood cytopenias in patients with MDS and the observation that additional Epo is of limited clinical benefit.

Epigenetic

The term *epigenetics* is the alteration of gene expression without altering the primary DNA sequence.[67–70] These modifications can occur at multiple levels, the most common involving DNA methylation. DNA methylation involves the addition of methyl groups to a cytosine residue.[71–73] Cytosine methylation typically occurs when a cytosine is followed by a guanine in the so-called CpG pair. CpG pairs are underrepresented within the human genome, but when they do occur, they occur clustered in so-called CpG islands. These CpG islands typically are located proximal to gene promoter regions and regulate gene expression.[74,75] For example, methylation of CpG islands is associated with gene silencing. The process of gene silencing may be physiologic in the case of both imprinted genes as well as regulating gene dosage of genes on the X chromosome in females.[67] Tumor suppressor genes are thought to undergo this aberrant gene silencing mechanism, leading to abnormal physiologic consequences.

Epigenetic changes in MDS and AML have become increasingly important. For example, the promoter methylation of the α-catenin gene *CTNNA1* may be an important underlying abnormality involving the loss of chromosome 5.[76] Other examples include promoter methylation of the p15INK4B gene.[72,77,78] This gene often is hypermethylated in patients with therapy-related MDS or therapy-related AML. In addition, methylation changes of this gene are seen more frequently in patients with loss of chromosome 7 and in patients who progress from RA to RAEB.[78]

Genetic Pathways Involved in Disease Progression

The genetic changes that occur in patients who transform from MDS to AML are numerous, complicated, and involve a multistep process characterized by activation of specific oncogenes as well as inactivation of tumor suppressor genes.[39] RAS mutations are frequently identified in patients with hematologic malignancies.[79–81] In patients with MDS, RAS was mutated in as many as one third of the cases, with the highest frequency in patients with chronic myelomonocytic leukemia (CMML).[82] The FMS oncogene encodes for M-CSF and, like RAS, is most preferentially seen in patients with CMML. Mutations involving the p53 tumor suppressor gene on chromosome 17p is rarely identified in patients with MDS, but when seen they often correspond with disease progression and resistance to chemotherapy.[83,84] Although the FMS-like tyrosine receptor III (FLT-3) is the most common single mutated gene in patients with AML, it is mutated in less than 3% of patients with MDS.[85–88]

Most patients develop genetic alterations that include the gain or loss of part or whole chromosomes as well as specific gene mutations and promoter methylation changes.[89] For example, patients with abnormalities involving chromosome 5 and 7 often acquire additional mutations in p53, RAS, or both, followed by promoter methylation changes of p15.[87,90] This process often is involved in patients with therapy-related MDS who previously received alkylating agent therapy and typically occurs 3 to 5 years after chemotherapy exposure.[88]

Genetic mutations that are commonly seen in patients who previously received a topoisomerase II inhibitor, such as the anthracycline doxorubicin, involve the complex acquisition of chromosomal translocations often involving the mixed lineage leukemia (MLL) gene on 11q23.[91–101] More than 30 different translocations have been identified that involve 11q23, and they account for approximately 5% of all translocations that occur in acute leukemia. Reciprocal translocations involving the 11q23 gene have been described in patients with acute lymphoblastic leukemia (ALL), AML, acute biphenotypic leukemia, and MDS. Other chromosomal translocations that are seen less commonly after anthracycline exposure include the AML1 gene on 21q22 often leading to translocation of t(3;21),[91] the core-binding factor β (CBF-β) gene on chromosome 16 leading to inversion of chromosome 16 [inv(16)],[92] and the retinoic acid receptor α (RAR-α) gene on chromosome 17 characterized by translocation t(15;17) and development of acute promyelocytic leukemia.[93–95] In addition, mutations of the NUP98 gene on chromosome 11p15 have been associated with exposure to topoisomerase II inhibitors.[96,97] These cytogenetic changes characterized by specific chromosomal abnormalities, with the notable exception of NUP98 on 11p15, subsequently develop RAS, BRAF, c-KIT, or FLT-3 mutations, followed by changes in the methylation pattern within the p15 promoter.[98,99]

Patients with a normal cytogenetic karyotype or other nonspecific chromosomal abnormalities often evolve from an MDS to an AML phenotype with a different and distinct process. These patients typically develop acquisition of a RAS mutation or another mutation involving a transcription factor,[100] which are known as class II mutations, or mutations involving tyrosine kinases, which are known as class I mutations. Examples of class I mutations include FLT-3, c-KIT, c-FMS, and JAK2.[101,102] Also included are genes further downstream within the RAS-BRAF-MEK-ERK pathway. They include N-RAS, K-RAS, BRAF, and PTPN11. This class of mutations results in the constitutive activation of the cell cycle leading to an increase in cell proliferation. For example, mutations in RAS are commonly seen in monocytic subtypes of AML and in CMML, whereas PTPN11 genes are commonly mutated in juvenile myelomonocytic leukemia.[103,104] The class I mutations are considered "late events" in the pathogenesis of leukemia but are thought to cooperate to a high degree with class II mutations. Examples of class II mutations that can be seen in patients who transform from MDS to AML include CCAAT enhancer-binding protein α (CEBPα), AML1, and rarely internal tandem duplications of MLL (MLL-PTD).[105–107]

As expected, patients with de novo and therapy-related MDS and AML have heterogeneous clinical presentations but often have similar cytogenetic abnormalities.[89,108,109] Although three distinct cytogenetic subgroups can be identified (chromosome 5/7, MLL gene on 11q23, and normal karyotype), many different genetic pathways have been outlined for patients with therapy-related MDS and therapy-related AML. Some of these changes are more consistent with the clinical presentation of MDS (e.g., −5/5q− or −7/7q−), whereas other abnormalities are more often related to the presentation of overt AML [e.g., translocations involving 11q23, inv(16), and t(15;17)]. However, the frequent association of both class I and Class II mutations argues strongly for their cooperative nature in the development of MDS and AML.[110]

DIFFERENTIAL DIAGNOSIS

Before a diagnosis of MDS can be made, it is important to consider alternative diagnoses, especially if the patient is younger than 50 years (Table 67–1). Although most patients with MDS have a normal or hypercellular bone marrow, approximately 10% to 15% of patients have a hypocellular bone marrow that may be difficult to distinguish from aplastic anemia.[111] The presence of a clonal chromosomal abnormality will confirm the diagnosis of MDS.[112] In addition,

Table 67–1 Predisposing Factors and Epidemiologic Associations of Patients with Myelodysplastic Syndrome

Heritable
Constitutional Genetic Disorders
Trisomy 8 mosaicism
Familial monosomy 7
Down syndrome (trisomy 21)
Neurofibromatosis 1
Germ cell tumors [embryonal dysgenesis del(12p)]
Congenital Neutropenia
Kostmann syndrome
Shwachman-Diamond syndrome
DNA Repair Deficiencies
Fanconi anemia
Ataxia-telangiectasia
Bloom syndrome
Xeroderma pigmentosum
Pharmacogenomic polymorphisms (GSTq1-null)
Acquired
Senescence
Mutagen Exposure
Alkylator therapy (chlorambucil, cyclophosphamide, melphalan, N-mustards)
Topoisomerase II inhibitors (anthracyclines)
β Emitters (^{32}P)
Autologous stem cell transplantation
Environmental/occupational (benzene)
Tobacco
Aplastic anemia
Paroxysmal nocturnal hemoglobinuria

patients with aplastic anemia typically have greater TNF receptor expression than do patients with MDS.[113] It is important to rule out the diagnosis of paroxysmal nocturnal hemoglobinuria (PNH).[114] Patients with hypocellular MDS have a clinical presentation similar to patients with aplastic anemia and have a better overall prognosis compared to other patients with MDS, especially patients who respond to immunosuppressive therapy.[115,116]

Similarly, the presence of myelofibrosis may make adequate assessment of the bone marrow aspirate difficult.[117,118] Patients with significant fibrosis within the marrow cavity often have an unaspiratable and/or aspicular aspirate specimen. Therefore, the ability to analyze the bone marrow aspirate for dysplastic features is markedly limited. However, in some patients, the diagnosis of myelodysplasia can be easily made, and the bone marrow biopsy shows an increased number of reticulin fibers.[119] Reticulin stain, typically by silver impregnation, is an important method for identifying underlying marrow fibrosis but should be distinguished from marked collagen fibrosis, which is seen often in patients with chronic idiopathic myelofibrosis (agnogenic myeloid metaplasia with myelofibrosis). Extensive mature collagen fibrosis can be demonstrated by trichrome stain and is extremely uncommon in patients with MDS. Although marrow fibrosis can be seen in all subtypes of MDS, it is more frequent in CMML and therapy-related MDS.[120] Patients with MDS and fibrosis can be distinguished from patients with chronic idiopathic myelofibrosis.[121] The latter entity is associated with marked splenomegaly, an unusual feature in patients with MDS regardless of the degree of marrow fibrosis. The absence of splenomegaly and an unusually rapid progressive clinical course helps distinguish patients between MDS and chronic idiopathic myelofibrosis, which usually is more indolent. Other disorders to consider in cases of extensive fibrosis include chronic myelogenous leukemia (CML), especially accelerated phase disease, and acute megakaryocytic leukemia (FAB-M7).[122]

Variants of CML as well as atypical CML can be difficult to distinguish from CMML.[123] The WHO currently lists CMML in its own category; therefore, it is no longer considered part of the myelodysplastic syndromes.[20] Nevertheless, the differential is important. CML is distinguished by the presence or absence of a BCR-ABL fusion gene.[124] The term *atypical CML* represents a diffuse group of disorders that are BCR negative.[125] Their clinical prognosis is somewhat worse than in patients with BCR-ABL given the inability to target a tyrosine kinase. Patients with atypical CML often have a short overall survival and poor response to therapy. Clinically, they can be distinguished from patients with other forms of MDS by an increase in basophilia and progressive leukocytosis as well as organomegaly, specifically splenomegaly.[126] These patients typically have marked thrombocytopenia and eventually develop marrow failure without transformation to AML. In a review of 76 BCR-negative patients from the MD Anderson Cancer Center, the median overall survival was 24 months, with AML transformation in eight patients. Chromosomal abnormalities were seen in 30% of patients, with trisomy 8 the most common abnormality identified. Patients with atypical CML can be difficult to separate clinically and pathologically from patients with MDS or other myeloproliferative disorders.

Dysplastic hematopoiesis is a common finding accompanying human immunodeficiency virus (HIV) infection.[127,128] An HIV serologic test must be obtained in order to exclude HIV infection, especially in patients with high-risk lifestyles, as well as young patients. The typical bone marrow aspirate and biopsy findings in patients with HIV infection include a hypercellular marrow and evidence of trilineage dysplasia, which is most predominant within the erythroid lineage.[129,130] The erythroid hematopoiesis almost always is megaloblastic, and reticulated fibrosis is often seen in bone marrow biopsies. Most patients have polyclonal plasma cell expansion, and lymphoid aggregates and/or granulomas are often seen. The differential diagnosis of erythrodysplasia in patients with HIV infection includes medications, opportunistic infections, or a direct effect of HIV on the hematopoietic progenitor cells. These findings reaffirm the need for serologic screening for HIV in patients with unexplained cytopenias.

A number of drugs can cause erythrodysplasia and complicate the evaluation and diagnosis of a patient with cytopenias. These medications include valproic acid,[131] mycophenolate mofetil,[132] ganciclovir,[132,133] alemtuzumab,[134] nucleoside analogues such as fludarabine and cytarabine, and the anti-metabolites mercaptopurine and methotrexate. The bone marrow changes associated with these medications include macrocytic anemia, reduced neutrophil lobation, and frank neutropenia and thrombocytopenia. In fact, some patients may have trilineage dysplasia, making an accurate diagnosis difficult.

Nutritional deficiencies must be excluded in any patients in whom the diagnosis of MDS is being entertained. These include vitamin B_{12} and folate deficiency[135] and copper deficiency.[136,137] Copper deficiency in adult patients is rare but can occur after gastrectomy, prolonged parenteral nutrition, or even enteral feeding if copper is not included in the formulation. Rarely, copper deficiency develops after ingestion of large amounts of zinc supplements, as zinc excess results in concomitant copper deficiency. Clinically, patients with copper deficiency present with signs and symptoms of profound anemia. In addition, copper deficiency may cause a variety of neurologic complications, including central nervous system demyelination, peripheral neuropathy, myelopathy, and even optic neuritis. In patients with severe cooper deficiency, hemoglobin levels may fall as low as 3.5 g/dL. The mean corpuscular volume often is normal or slightly increased, and the red cells on the peripheral smear are hypochromic and microcytic. Patients typically present with mild neutropenia with neutrophil counts of 1000/mL. Bone marrow examination will reveal a cellular marrow with early erythroid vacuolization and moderate numbers of ringed sideroblasts.

A number of drugs may induce sideroblastic anemia, including isoniazid[138] and chloramphenicol.[139,140] Cycloserine and pyrazinamide also have been implicated in rare cases. With isoniazid, the anemia is modest, with hematocrits typically in the 26% range, low mean corpuscular volume, and dimorphic red cell morphology. Abundant ringed sideroblasts are present within the bone marrow, and typically the anemia is rapidly reversed with discontinuation of the offending agent. However, administration of large doses of pyridoxine up to 200 mg/day may accelerate reversal of the anemia.

Although chloramphenicol typically produces a ringed sideroblastic anemia, an idiosyncratic marrow failure syndrome associated with chronic administration also can be seen. When this occurs, a prominent feature within the bone marrow is vacuolization, specifically of the early erythroid precursors. Patients often have marked reticulocytopenia and increased serum iron levels. In most cases, the anemia is reversed with discontinuation of the drug; however, some patients may have profound, long-lasting evidence of marrow failure.

Sideroblastic anemia is associated with alcoholism with or without folate and vitamin B_{12} deficiency.[141] As many as one third of patients who are chronic alcoholics may have sideroblastic changes within the bone marrow, including dimorphic erythroid cells. Patients often have a markedly elevated mean corpuscular volume, which is impressively uniform. The ringed sideroblasts often disappear within days to weeks after discontinuation of alcohol intake.[142] However, concurrent vitamin deficiencies and/or liver disease may further affect the peripheral blood cytopenias and, importantly, the recovery phase.

CLINICAL FINDINGS IN PATIENTS WITH MDS

Erythroid Cells

The diagnosis of myelodysplasia in patients with anemia, neutropenia, thrombocytopenia, or a combination thereof depends on the demonstration of dysmorphic features within the bone marrow (Table 67–2 and Fig. 67–2). Both a bone marrow aspirate and a biopsy should be obtained. An aspirate usually can assess cellular morphology and quantitation of myeloblasts, but accurate assessment of bone marrow cellularity and localization of immature precursors

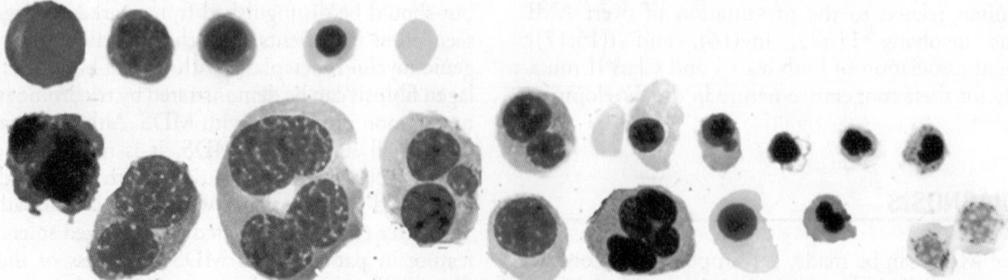

Figure 67–2 Erythroid dysplasia. Examples of dysplastic erythroid precursors (**bottom**) compared to those with normal morphology in the sequence of erythroid maturation (**top**). The dysplastic forms include (**left to right**) abnormal immature forms with multinucleation, maturing forms with multinucleation and nuclear-to-cytoplasmic dyssynchrony, and more mature forms with megaloblastoid change, nuclear budding, cloverleaf forms, cytoplasmic vacuolization, and cytoplasmic stippling. Ringed sideroblasts (**far right**) also are evidence of erythroid dysplasia. Photographs from a patients with refractory cytopenia with multilineage dysplasia and ringed sideroblasts.

Table 67–2 Physical Examination, Medical History, and Laboratory Tests Aiding in Diagnosis of Myelodysplastic Syndrome

Medical History
Duration of symptoms
History of blood disease
History of exposure to occupational toxins or cytotoxic agents
Medication history
Alcohol intake
Comorbid conditions
Physical Examination
Pallor
Petechiae
Purpura
Bruising
Tachypnea
Signs of infection
Splenomegaly
Laboratory Testing
Complete blood count with a manual differential
Reticulocyte count
Vitamin B_{12} and folate levels
Consider methylmalonic acid and red blood cell folate levels
Iron, total iron-binding capacity, and ferritin level
Thyroid-stimulating hormone level
Lactate dehydrogenase
Antinuclear antibody
Coombs test and haptoglobin
Serum erythropoietin level
Human leukocyte antigen (histocompatibility antigens) typing in appropriate patients
Paroxysmal nocturnal hemoglobinuria screen
Bone Marrow Testing
Hematopathology
Percentage of blasts on 200 cell aspirate differential
Presence or absence of Auer rods
Percentage of cellularity of bone marrow biopsy
Iron stain on aspirate (ringed sideroblasts)
Iron stain on biopsy (storage)
Dysplastic features (% and number of dysplastic lineages)
Cytogenetics (karyotype of 20 metaphase cells)
Fluorescent in situ hybridization
Flow cytometry (not useful for quantitation)

require a review of the biopsy sections. Occasionally multiple sampling is required to make a definitive diagnosis because the affected bone marrow is distributed unevenly or the patient develops progressive dysplastic features over time.

Almost all patients with MDS (>90%) present with fatigue and lethargy, which is associated with chronic anemia.[143] The anemia most often is macrocytic, with a significantly reduced reticulocyte index. The most recognized morphologic abnormality of the red blood cells (RBCs) on examination of the peripheral blood smear consists of oval macrocytes; however, in rare cases, teardrop cells or dacrocytes, elliptocytes, and acanthocytes are seen.[144] It remains essential to exclude other causes of macrocytic anemia in this population, including vitamin B_{12} and folate deficiency.[145] The anemia in patients with MDS is a result of ineffective erythropoiesis. Epo levels usually are normal or elevated.[3,146] In addition, most patients have evidence of abnormal iron utilization. Other patients have evidence of increased fetal hemoglobin synthesis,[147] abnormal red cell antigens,[148] increased red cell fragility, and low levels of pyruvate kinase. The latter two abnormalities may result in an abnormal Ham test secondary to increased hemolysis.[149]

It is important to exclude the diagnosis of PNH even in patients without a history of thromboembolic disorders. The most efficient test is the absence of polyinositol glycol-associated antigens by flow cytometric analysis due to the absence of the PIG-A gene. PNH is diagnosed by the absence of CD55 and CD59 on red blood cells, and the absence of CD11b on monocytes.[150,151] Some patients have a small clone of PNH cells, but this finding is of unclear clinical significance.[152,153] Other possible features of MDS include disordered α- and β-globin chain synthesis[154,155] and hemoglobin H inclusions.[156]

Morphologic features within the bone marrow aspirate include megaloblastic erythroid precursors, often with multiple nuclei or asynchronous maturation of the nucleus and cytoplasm. Occasionally, ringed sideroblasts, which are red cell precursors with iron-laden mitochondria, can be identified.[157] Ringed sideroblasts are defined by the presence of at least five Prussian blue-staining iron granules encircling more than one third of the nucleus of an erythroblast. The presence of ringed sideroblasts without morphologic features of dysplasia also can be seen in unrelated congenital and malignant hematologic conditions. RA and refractory cytopenia with multilineage dysplasia (RCMD) typically are differentiated from refractory anemia with ringed sideroblasts (RARS) and refractory cytopenia with multilineage dysplasia and ringed sideroblasts (RCMD-S) by the presence of greater than 15% ringed sideroblasts.[158]

One unusual feature of the FAB classification scheme occurs when greater than 50% of the total cellularity is composed of erythroid precursors.[19] In this case, if greater than 30% of the nonerythroid cells are myeloblasts, a diagnosis of erythroleukemia is made (FAB-M6A). This differs from the pure erythroleukemia described by Deguglielmo (FAB-M6B).

Myeloid Cells

A large proportion of patients, approximately 50%, with MDS either present with neutropenia or develop neutropenia as a result of disease progression.[159] Not only is MDS associated with a quantitative neutrophil defect but also with qualitative defects. Patients with MDS often have a reduced inflammatory response to infections. Patients with MDS have diminished production of many hematopoietic growth factors, and these likely account for the qualitative neutrophil defects and their reduced phagocytic properties. In spite of this, recurrent infections occur in only 10% of patients,[160] but this is the cause of death in approximately one-fifth of the patients with MDS.[161]

The most common infections in patients with MDS are bacterial, usually from the lower respiratory tract, skin, or perineal area. Recurrent infections can occur even in the absence of severe neutropenia, likely from granulocyte functional impairment. In patients with CMML,[162,163] the monocytes are also derived from defective hematopoietic stem cells and similar qualitative defects in terms of cell adhesion and phagocytic and cell killing properties leading to an increased rate of infections.

Abnormalities of the myeloid series range from subtle to rather striking (Fig. 67–3).[19] They include a left shift toward more immature forms, even without an excess of myeloblasts. The myeloid precursors also may show asynchronous maturation of the nucleus and cytoplasm as manifested by a lack of granule formation. The nucleocytoplasmic dyssynchrony is most clearly represented in the early myeloid cells, or *abnormal promyelocytes*. Their granular cytoplasm, reticulated nucleus, and prominent Golgi apparatus characterize these dysplastic promyelocytes. The more mature granulocytes often are hypogranulated and may be hypolobated as well. Granulocytes with a bilobed nuclear structure are referred to as pseudo–Pelger-Huet cells.[164] There is a congenital abnormality in pediatric patients in which all of the neutrophils are bilobed or hyposegmented; this is termed the Pelger-Huet anomaly, which is a benign condition.

The most critical finding in patients with MDS is the presence and quantification of the myeloblasts. The absolute proportion of

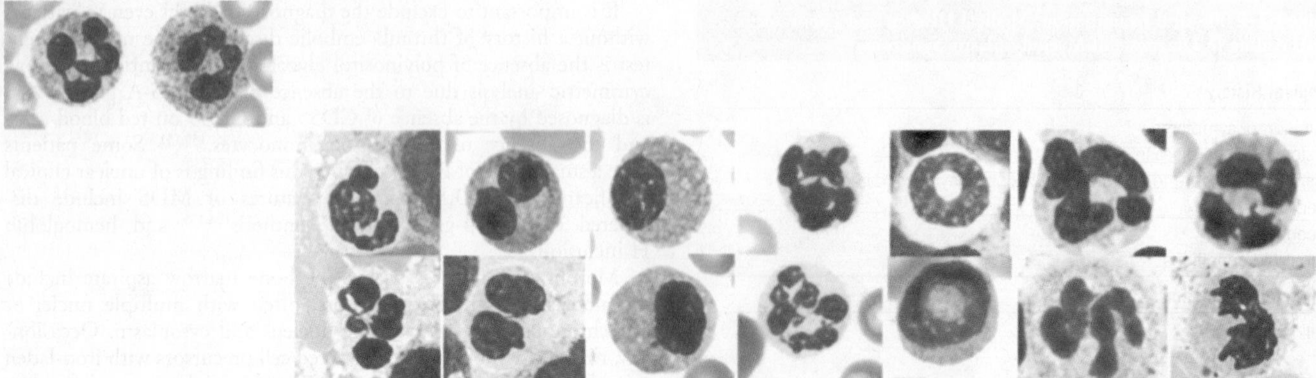

Figure 67–3 Granulocytic dysplasia is most evident in mature neutrophils (**bottom**) and can be contrasted to features of normal forms (**top**), which usually still are present as a subpopulation of the total cells in most cases. Granulocytic dysplasia is characterized by (**left to right**) reduced cytoplasmic granulation, nuclear hypolobation (resulting in the binuclear or single-lobed pseudo–Pelger-Huet forms), hypersegmentation, ringed forms ("rodent cells"), cells with nuclear twinning, and cells with excessive nuclear excrescences. Photographs from a number of cases of refractory cytopenia with multilineage dysplasia and refractory anemia with excess blasts.

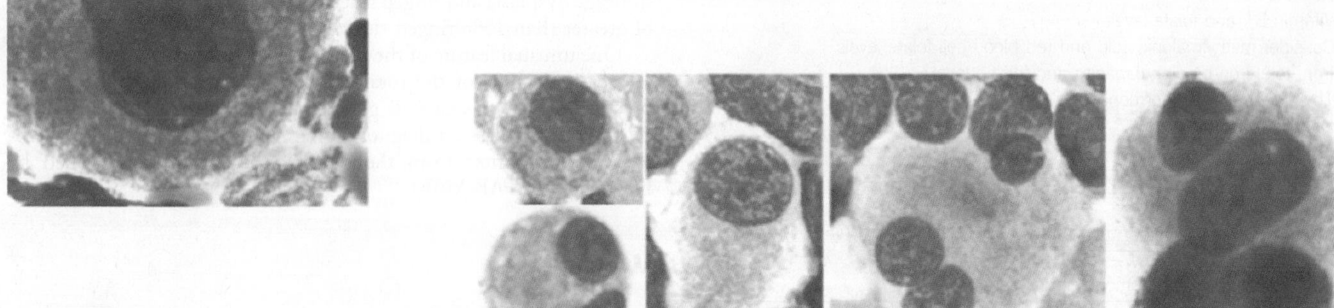

Figure 67–4 Megakaryocytic dysplasia. Dysmegakaryopoiesis is most obvious with the presence of micromegakaryocytes and abnormal larger forms (**bottom, right**). These are compared to a normal megakaryocyte (**top, left**). Micromegakaryocytes have single, two or four small nuclei, which indicate a low ploidy level. Normal low-ploidy megakaryocytes can be seen in the bone marrow, but these are immature forms and do not have mature granular cytoplasm with platelet material, as do the micromegakaryocytes. Larger dysplastic megakaryocytes have multiple, small, widely spaced nuclei. Photographs from a number of cases of refractory anemia with excess blasts and refractory cytopenia with multilineage dysplasia.

myeloblasts reflects the defect in the differentiation capacity of the abnormal hematopoietic stem cell and represents the most important prognostic finding. The diagnosis of AML is established if there are more than 20% myeloblasts based on the WHO classification scheme or greater than 30% based on the older FAB criteria.[19,20] Quantification of myeloblasts should be performed on a cellular and spicular bone marrow aspirate and not by flow cytometric analysis, because the latter can be effected by peripheral blood dilution of the sample.

Megakaryocytes

Thrombocytopenia is present in approximately half of patients with MDS and may represent the only cytopenia in 5% of cases.[165] The finding of thrombocytosis is uncommon and typically associated with either the 5q syndrome[166] or a JAK2 mutation, as is the case in patients with refractory anemia with ringed sideroblasts and thrombocytosis (RARS-T).[167] As in the case with neutrophils, patients with MDS often have both a quantitative as well as a qualitative defect with their platelets.[38] The latter can be identified by careful examination of the peripheral blood smear, on which giant or agranular platelets often are identified. Upon examination of the bone marrow, the megakaryocytes often are small or micromegakaryocytic and contain fewer nuclear lobes (hypolobated) than their normal counterparts (Fig. 67–4).[19,164,168] In patients with the 5q syndrome, the megakaryocytes are nonlobated and mononuclear.[166]

Patients may have disproportionately prolonged bleeding times and abnormalities in platelet aggregation studies.[38,169–171] These may be present even in patients with normal platelet counts. The hallmark is an acquired Glanzmann defect, characterized by abnormal platelet glycoprotein IIb/IIIa. A falling platelet count often is a marker of disease progression. Patients with MDS are at risk for spontaneous bleeding and have increased risk for hemorrhage following surgery and trauma. Again, this is true even in patients without thrombocytopenia.

Autoimmune Manifestations

Immunologic and rheumatologic complications occur frequently in patients with MDS.[172–174] Patients can present with acute episodes of seronegative oligoarthritis or polyarthritis[175,176] as well as symptoms of cutaneous vasculitis, polymyositis, or peripheral neuropathies. Lupus-like symptoms have been reported at the time of the presentation of cytopenias in patients complaining of systemic features of fever, polyarthritis, polychondritis, pleuritis, pericarditis, or even hemolytic anemia. Presentations involving mucocutaneous ulcerations, iritis, polymyositis, peripheral neuropathy, inflammatory bowel disease, and red cell aplasia have been reported in patients with MDS.[177] In addition, cases of relapsing polychondritis, polymyalgia rheumatica,[172,178,179] Raynaud phenomenon, pyoderma gangrenosum, Sjögren syndrome, and glomerulonephritis have been reported, but their association is less clear.[180] Although these paraneoplastic processes may complicate the initial clinical presentation of MDS, they are often responsive to immunosuppressive agents such as corticosteroids.[181]

Dermatologic Manifestations

Cutaneous complications of MDS are rather uncommon.[182] Neutrophilic dermatosis (Sweet syndrome) is one exception. It is characterized by painful plaque-like lesions that often are associated with fever and arthralgias. These lesions can be present on the face, neck, or upper or lower extremities. Sweet syndrome usually responds to corticosteroid or dapsone therapy. It is often present in patients who are transforming to AML. Other dermatologic presentations include monocytic infiltrates, which are more common in patients with CMML[163,183,184]; chloroma or granulocytic sarcoma, which if present would constitute AML; and petechial lesions, which are common in any patient who presents with severe thrombocytopenia.

Findings on Physical Examination

The physical examination of a patient with MDS typically is rather unrevealing (see Table 67–2). Most patients will pallor due to anemia; petechiae is less commonly present as a result of thrombocytopenia.[185] Signs and symptoms of an infectious process, either bacterial or fungal, should be ruled out. Splenomegaly, hepatomegaly, and lymphadenopathy are rather uncommon, except for patients with CMML.[163]

CLASSIFICATION AND PROGNOSIS OF PATIENTS WITH MDS

Classification Systems

The myelodysplastic syndromes are a heterogeneous group of clonal hematologic disorders characterized by persistent peripheral blood cytopenias and proliferation of myeloblastic leukemia cells.[21] Since the early 1980s, several groups have developed classification schemes for patients with MDS that can be used for prediction of survival as well as rate of transformation to overt AML. The FAB consensus conference in 1982 described a classification scheme that includes both acute myelogenous leukemia and myelodysplasia.[19] Five categories of MDS were described based on the bone marrow morphology of bone marrow aspirates, specifically requiring patients to have >10% dysplasia within two or more cell lines. Patients were separated into five groups primarily based on the percentage of myeloblasts within the bone marrow aspirate. These categories are RA, RARS, RAEB, RAEB-T, and CMML (Table 67–3). The diagnosis of acute leukemia required at least 30% myeloblasts within the bone marrow or peripheral blood; patients with 30% or fewer myeloblasts were classified as myelodysplasia.

With the exception of RARS and CMML, the subgroups of MDS are stratified by the percentage of blasts within the peripheral blood or bone marrow. The first two categories, RA and RARS, have fewer than 5% myeloblasts in the bone marrow. Patients with RA and RARS tend to have a longer median overall survival and a lower rate of progression to acute leukemia than patients in the other categories. Patients with RAEB and RAEB-T have between 5% and 20% or between 21% and 30% myeloblasts within the bone marrow, respectively. These patients often have more severe cytopenias, increased risk of progression toward acute leukemia, and shorter overall survival time. Patients with CMML represent a heterogeneous group.[162,163] Some patients have a more MDS-like picture, with significant pancytopenia and trilineage dysplasia within the bone marrow. Other patients have more of a myeloproliferative-like picture, with elevated white blood count, peripheral monocytosis, splenomegaly, and hypermetabolic symptoms. The median survival of patients with MDS-CMML was 23 months versus 15 months for patients with myeloproliferative disorder (MPD)-CMML ($P = 0.31$), and both groups had nearly identical risk of progression to AML.[186,187]

The FAB classification scheme led to marked improvement in the diagnosis of myelodysplasia. It also served as a general prognostic predictor. However, there still exists considerable variation within the groups with respect to overall survival and clinical features. Several prognostic systems have been devised to better predict the outcome of individual patients. For example, prognosis is inversely related to the number of bone marrow myeloblasts, and cytogenetics have an extremely important impact on overall survival.[188] The International Myelodysplastic Syndrome Risk Analysis Workshop (IMRAW) has developed an International Prognostic Scoring System (IPSS) based on an analysis of more than 800 patients (Table 67–4).[189] This analysis revealed that the most important variables for overall prognosis were specific cytogenetic abnormalities, percentage of myeloblasts within the bone marrow, and number of the lineages involved in the cytopenia. Other adverse prognostic features include age greater than 60 years and male sex. Isolated loss of the Y, 5q, or 20q chromosome or the presence of a normal karyotype is associated with a favorable prognosis. Adverse prognostic cytogenetic features included abnormalities of chromosome 7 or complex cytogenetic changes defined as having more than three cytogenetic anomalies. This scoring system divided patients into four categories: low, intermediate-1, intermediate-2 and high-risk groups. The overall median survival for these groups was 5.7, 3.5, 1.2, and 0.4 years, respectively.[189] There are several limitations of using the IPSS for individual patients. First, the IPSS is heavily weighted on the percentage of blasts within the bone marrow aspirate.[190] Second, only a limited number of cytogenetic abnormalities were described within the IPSS, and their prognostic importance is significantly underestimated. Finally, the various cytopenias not only have the same impact on the overall IPSS score, but by themselves they are clinically meaningless.

A significant limitation of the FAB classification scheme derives from the arbitrary boundaries imposed within the continuum of disease categories. Patients with RAEB, RAEB-T, and AML likely represent a similar biologic process. Use of 30% myeloblasts within the bone marrow as the division between myelodysplasia and acute

Table 67–3 French-American-British Classification Criteria

Subtype	Abbreviation	Peripheral Blood	Bone Marrow
Refractory anemia	RA	Blasts <1%	Blasts <5%
Refractory anemia with ringed sideroblasts	RARS	Blasts <1%	Blasts <5%, and >15% ringed sideroblasts
Refractory anemia with excess blasts	RAEB	Blasts <5%	Blasts 5%–20%
Refractory anemia with excess blasts in transformation	RAEB-T	Blasts >5%	Blasts 20%–30% or Auer rods
Chronic myelomonocytic leukemia	CMML	Monocytes >1 × 10^9/L	Any of the above
Acute myelogenous leukemia	AML		Blasts >30%

Description of syndromes from Bennett et al.[19]

Table 67–4 International Prognostic Scoring System for Myelodysplastic Syndrome

Overall Score[a]	Median Survival (Years)	25% AML Evolution (Years)
Low (0)	5.7	9.4
Intermediate-1 (0.5–1.0)	3.5	3.3
Intermediate-2 (1.5–2.0)	1.2	1.1
High (≥2.5)	0.4	0.2

The percent of myeloblasts are scored as follows: <5% = 0; 5%–10% = 0.5: 11%–20% = 1.5: 21%–30% = 2.0.

Cytogenetic features associated with good prognosis are scored as 0 and include normal karyotype, loss of Y, 5q–, or 20q–; those associated with a poor prognosis are scored as 1.0 and include abnormalities of chromosome 7 or three or more cytogenetic changes; all other cytogenetic abnormalities are scored as 0.5 and are of intermediate prognosis.

A score of 0 refers to a patient with either zero or one cell lineage cytopenia, and a score of 0.5 is assigned to two or more lineage cytopenias. Lineage cytopenias are defined as hemoglobin <10 g/dL, absolute neutrophil count <1800/mm³, and platelet count <100,000/mm³.

AML, acute myelogenous leukemia.

[a]The overall score is the sum of the scores from the percent of bone marrow myeloblasts, karyotype, and cytopenias.

Data from Greenberg et al.[189]

Table 67–5 FAB and WHO classifications

FAB	WHO	Dysplasia(s) (>10%)
RA	5q– syndrome	Erythroid lineage only
	RA	Erythroid lineage only
	RCMD	2–3 lineages
	MDS-U	1 lineage only
RARS	RARS	Erythroid lineage only
	RCMD-RS	2–3 lineages
RAEB	RAEB-1	1–3 lineages
	RAEB-2	1–3 lineages
RAEB-T	AML	

The World Health Organization (WHO) has reclassified chronic myelomonocytic leukemia (CMML) within the myeloproliferative disorders (MPD) and RAEB-T to "AML with multilineage dysplasia." AML now is classified as ≥20% myeloblasts.

The following are considered AML regardless of blast percentage: t(8;21)-AML1/ETO, t(15;17)-PML/RARA, inv(16) or t(16;16)-CBFβ/MYH11, 11q23-MLL.

AML, acute myelogenous leukemia; FAB, French-American-British; MDS-U, myelodysplastic syndrome unclassifiable; RA, refractory anemia; RAEB, refractory anemia with excess blasts; RAEB-1, 5%–9% myeloblasts; RAEB-2, 10%–19% myeloblasts; RAEB-T, refractory anemia with excess blasts in transformation; RCMD, refractory cytopenias with multilineage dysplasia; RS, ringed sideroblasts.

From Harris NL, Jaff ES, Drebold J, et al: World Health Organization classification of neoplastic diseases of the hematopoietic and lymphoid tissues: Report of the Clinical Advisory Committee meeting-Airlie House, Virginia, November 1997. J Clin Oncol 17:3835, 1999; and Germing U, Gottermann H, Minning H, et al: Problems in the classification of CMML—Dysplastic versus proliferative type. Leuk Res 22:871, 1998.

leukemia is not biologically consistent and often leads to confusion in the recommendation of treatment options. The European Association of Hematopathologists and the Society for Hematopathology developed a new World Health Organization (WHO) classification scheme.[20] The WHO defines AML as having a myeloblast count of 20% or greater and drops the RAEB-T category (Table 67–5). Inclusion of CMML in MDS under the older FAB classification scheme was problematic, so within the new WHO classification scheme, CMML has been removed from the MDS category and placed within the myeloproliferative disorders (Table 67–6). This change seems more consistent with not only clinical presentation but also with the many treatment choices that are offered to patients with CMML. A new category, refractory cytopenia with multilineage dysplasia (RCMD), also was proposed. This category allows for the classification of patients with morphologic dysplasia within their bone marrow aspirate but who present with isolated neutropenia or thrombocytopenia instead of the typical anemia.

Table 67–6 World Health Organization Criteria for Diagnosis of Chronic Myelomonocytic Leukemia

Peripheral blood monocytosis >1000/mL.
No evidence of Philadelphia chromosome or BCR-ABL gene.
Less than 20% myeloblasts, monoblasts, and promonocytes within the peripheral blood or bone marrow.
Dysplastic changes in one or more myeloid lineages. If myelodysplasia is absent or minimal, the diagnosis of CMML can be made if the above three criteria are met and: Acquired clonal cytogenetic abnormality is present in bone marrow cells, or Persistent monocytosis for >3 months and all other causes of monocytosis have been excluded
CMML-1: Blasts <5% in peripheral blood and <10% in bone marrow
CMML-2: Blasts 5%–19% in peripheral blood or 10%–19% in bone marrow

From Vardiman JW, Harris NL, Brunning RD: The World Health Organization (WHO) classification of the myeloid neoplasms. Blood 100:2292, 2002.

In addition to the number of myeloblasts, the FAB and WHO classification scheme are based on the degree of hematopoietic dysplasia. The FAB classification required patients to have 10% or greater dysplasia in two or more hematopoietic lineages. The WHO modified this requirement, and unilineage erythrodysplasia now is classified as RA or RARS depending on the presence or absence of ringed sideroblasts. Importantly, the dysplasia must have been present for more than 6 months, and no other causes of erythrodysplasia could be present. The WHO introduced a new category of refractory cytopenia with multilineage dysplasia with or without ringed sideroblasts: RCMD and RCMD-S, respectively. Although often subtle, patients with multilineage dysplasia have a significantly poorer overall survival as well as leukemia-free survival compared to patients with unilineage dysplasia.

The WHO classification system has been modified using prognostic scoring variables based on transfusion requirements as well as similar cytogenetic abnormalities within the IPSS.[191] The newer WHO classification-based scoring system (WPSS) is able to stratify patients into five risk groups (Table 67–7). The very-low-risk group has a survival of 11.3 years and 7% risk of transformation into AML at 10 years, whereas the very-high-risk group has a survival of 0.7 years and 50% risk of transformation into AML at 8 months. Although this scoring system has been validated on a separate cohort of patients, use of the WPSS has not gained widespread popularity. What is clear from the WPSS is that the definition of RBC transfusion "dependency" requires further confirmation and prospective large cohort studies.

Other parameters for evaluating the prognosis of MDS have been assessed in a series of scoring systems that follow different clinical and/or cytogenetic features, which include white blood cell count, hemoglobin, platelet count, age, sex, lactate dehydrogenase, and immunophenotyping.[190,192–196] For example, the CD44 antigen, which is a transmembrane glycoprotein, is expressed on bone marrow mononuclear precursor cells as well as peripheral granulocytes and erythrocytes.[193,197] Serum CD44 levels typically are increased in patients with MDS as well as acute myeloid leukemia and acute lymphoblastic leukemia. Increased expression of CD44-6v has been associated with shorter survival in patients with AML. Flow cytometric analysis has been used to evaluate expression of CD44 on early myeloid cells that coexpress CD66. CD66 typically is expressed on monocytes as well as immature myeloid cells. Low CD44 coexpression on CD66 myeloid cells typically is seen in the early stages of MDS as opposed to increased CD44 expression on CD66-weak

Table 67–7 WHO-Based Prognostic Scoring System for Predicting Survival in Patients with Myelodysplastic Syndrome

	Points			
Variables	*0*	*1*	*2*	*3*
WHO subtype	RA, RARS, 5q–	RCMD, RCMD-RS	RAEB-1	RAEB-2
Transfusion requirement	None	Yes[a]	—	—
IPSS cytogenetic risk	Good	Intermediate	Poor	—

[a]Defined as 1 unit of red blood cells every 8 weeks over a 4-month period.
IPSS, International Prognostic Scoring System; RA, refractory anemia; RAEB, refractory anemia with excess blasts; RAEB-1, 5%–9% myeloblasts; RAEB-2, 10%–19% myeloblasts; RCMD, refractory cytopenias with multilineage dysplasia; RS, ringed sideroblasts; WHO, World Health Organization.

WPSS Risk Group	Score
Very low	0
Low	1
Intermediate	2
High	3–4
Very high	5–6

WPSS, World Health Organization Classification-Based Prognostic Scoring System.

Overall Score	Median Survival (Years)	Cumulative Acute Myelogenous Leukemia Evolution at 5 Years
Very low (0)	11.8	0.03
Intermediate (1)	5.5	0.14
Intermediate (2)	4.0	0.33
High (3–4)	2.2	0.54
Very high (5–6)	0.8	0.84

Adapted from Malcovati L, Porta MG, Pascutto C, et al: Prognostic factors and life expectancy in myelodysplastic syndromes classified according to WHO criteria: A basis for clinical decision making. J Clin Oncol 23:7594, 2005.

myeloid cells, which often is seen in the later stages of myelodysplasia, that is, in patients with increased number of blasts. A shift in CD44 expression therefore often has been associated with a trend toward immaturity or increased number of blasts in patients with MDS; therefore, CD44 expression profiling may be useful as a separate prognostic marker for patients with MDS. However, large prospective studies are warranted.

The angiogenic process is extremely important in the growth and metastasis of many solid tumors.[198,199] Its role in hematopoietic malignancies is less well characterized. Both vascular endothelial growth factor and basic fibroblast growth factor are expressed by myeloblasts. Furthermore, analysis of bone marrow samples from patients with untreated AML showed increased microvessel density.[199,200] Vascular endothelial growth factor has been linked to the promotion of atypical localization of immature myeloid precursors, which is a poor prognostic marker in patients with MDS, especially for signaling out those patients who are at highest risk for disease progression.[119,201,202] Furthermore, microvessel density is markedly higher in patients with RAEB-T compared with the other MDS subtypes, suggesting a role between angiogenesis and transformation to acute leukemia in patients with MDS.

RBC Transfusion Dependence

RBC transfusion dependence is associated with a poorer overall survival in patients with MDS. In a retrospective study of 239 patients with low-risk MDS 19% were RBC transfusion dependent and had shorter survival than did patients who had not recently undergone transfusions.[203] A similar retrospective study of 467 patients by Malcovati et al.[191] also demonstrated that RBC transfusion dependency in patients with MDS had a negative impact on both overall survival and leukemia-free survival. The negative effect was dependent on the number of transfusions per month and was an independent prognostic variable regardless of cytogenetic risk assessment.

The etiology for the shorter survival in patients with MDS who are RBC transfusion dependent is unclear. Some patients had secondary hemochromatosis as assayed by increased serum ferritin levels, and some patients developed cardiac dysfunction or arrhythmias.[203] Although iron overload is suggested to be a significant component in the increased mortality of transfusion-dependent patients with MDS, prospective studies are needed to accurately assess the effect of iron chelation on survival and subsequent prognosis in patients with MDS who are RBC transfusion dependent.

CYTOGENETIC AND MOLECULAR ABNORMALITIES

Careful examination of the bone marrow aspirate to detect cytogenetic abnormalities is a critical part in establishing the diagnosis of MDS. Although approximately 60% of patients with MDS have a normal karyotype, the presence of characteristic cytogenetic abnormalities may establish the diagnosis in cases where the dysplastic changes within the bone marrow aspirate are subtle (see Table 67–4).[21] Furthermore, documentation of additional cytogenetic changes may imply an evolving clonal evolution and development of a neoplastic process.

Abnormal karyotypes are identified in about half of all cases of MDS and in more than 80% of therapy-related cases.[6,188] The most common abnormality is trisomy 8. Other common abnormalities include monosomy 5 or 7, loss of the Y chromosome, or deletions involving the long arms of chromosomes 5, 7, 11, 13, and 20. Complex karyotypes, defined as three or more abnormalities, are seen in approximately 15% of cases of MDS and portend an unfavorable prognosis. Chromosomal abnormalities are most often associated with the FAB subtypes RAEB and RAEB-T. The presence of a deletion of the long arm of chromosome 5 (5q–) as the sole abnormality is seen most often in patients with RA[145] ; monosomy 7 is rarely seen in this MDS subgroup. Translocations involving platelet-derived growth factor receptor-β (PDGFR-β) have been identified in 5% to 10% of patients with CMML. The first case was identified in a patient with a translocation involving the transcription factor TEL on chromosome 12,[204] but many other fusion partners have now been described. The TEL–PDGFR-β receptor gene product produces a chronic myeloproliferative disorder in mice and is a potential target for tyrosine receptor kinase inhibition with imatinib therapy.

Therapy-related MDS is associated with specific chromosomal abnormalities.[108] Patients who develop MDS or AML after exposure to alkylator therapy often have either a partial loss or complete monosomy of chromosome 5 or 7.[6,7,109] Patients who were exposed to topoisomerase II inhibitors typically present with a monocytic acute leukemia and not MDS. These patients have a high frequency of chromosomal rearrangements involving the MLL gene on 11q23[91] or less commonly the AML1 gene on 21q21. Other chromosomal abnormalities associated with therapy-related MDS include 3p14-21, 6p21, 12p11-17, and 19p13. Mutations involving p53 on chromosome 17p have been described and are associated with a long latency period between toxin exposure and the diagnosis of MDS or AML.[205,206]

Several diagnostic tests have increased the ability to detect cryptic cytogenetic anomalies. Fluorescent in situ hybridization uses specific DNA probes to identify each chromosome individually.[207] This method can screen hundreds of cells and does not depend on analysis of dividing cells during metaphase. Thus, the sensitivity can be dramatically increased, but use of fluorescent in situ hybridization is limited to detection of standard cytogenetic abnormalities. Polymerase chain reaction analysis can detect specific gene translocations in either the bone marrow or blood. This assay is rapid and can detect abnormalities present in fewer than 1 : 10,000 cells but also is limited to detection of standard cytogenetic abnormalities.

It is important to realize that a normal karyotype does not exclude the diagnosis of MDS. Normal karyotypes are see in about half of all cases of MDS. This is thought to be due to the limitations of standard G banding or the failure of the neoplastic clone to divide in culture. Spectral karyotype analysis or "chromosomal painting" can identify cryptic balanced and unbalanced translocations in most patients with MDS.

Cytogenetic Correlation with Prognosis

One of the limitations with the IPSS is the limited information that was available on cytogenetic data. Cytogenetic analysis since has been performed in more 2000 patients with MDS and was successful in 97% of these patients.[208] Clonal cytogenetic abnormalities were seen in 52.3% of patients. These included numeric as well as structural chromosomal abnormalities. The limitation in terms of prognosis is the varying degree by which patients receive therapy; therefore, the impact of karyotypic abnormalities on the natural history of myelodysplasia was studied in 1286 patients treated with supportive care only (see Table 67–4). Therefore, how overall and leukemia-free survival are affected by therapeutic intervention is unclear.

In patients with a normal karyotype (N = 612), median survival was 53 months. This is compared to an 8.7-month survival for patients with complex abnormalities. The most frequent abnormality involved deletion of chromosome 5q, which occurred in 30% of patients who had a cytogenetic abnormality or 58% of all patients with successful cytogenetic analysis. Isolated deletion of 5q was seen in 14% of patients with clonal abnormalities. Other frequent abnormalities included monosomy 7 or 7q deletion in 21% and trisomy 8 (+8) in 16% of patients with MDS. Less common abnormalities are listed in Table 67–8.

Favorable prognosis measured as a median survival of approximately 3 years was seen in patients with translocations involving chromosome 1q, translocation involving 7q, any chromosome 12 abnormality, translocation involving 17q with a noncomplex karyotype, monosomy 21, trisomy 21, as well as for loss of chromosome X. Median survivals had not been reached for patients with del9q, del12p, and del15q. The favorable survival for these patients was seen only if patients has no additional abnormalities. In addition, 21 other chromosomal aberrations were identified, but their rarity did not allow for prognostic relevance. Therefore, even though numerous cytogenetic abnormalities have been identified, the rarity of a few cytogenetic abnormalities makes prognostic impact limited.

Abnormalities with intermediate prognosis, defined as median survival between 1 and 3 years, was seen in patients with chromosome 3q rearrangements, translocations involving 11q23 as a noncomplex karyotype, and trisomy 19. In addition, regardless of the specific aberrations, an overall correlation was seen between prognosis and extent of abnormalities. Patients with three or more abnormalities had a median survival of 17 months, patients with four to six abnormalities had a median survival of 9 months, and patients with more than six abnormalities had a median survival of only 5 months. This analysis further demonstrates the cytogenetic impact of a complex karyotype on the prognosis of patients with MDS. Cytogenetic analysis remains an important factor in treatment selection as well as monitoring response to therapy. What is unclear from this type of analyses is the impact of pharmacologic therapy on the prognosis of patients with MDS based on their cytogenetic abnormalities.

Table 67–8 Frequency and Median Survival of Cytogenetic Prognostic Subgroups

Anomaly	Frequency (%)	Median Survival (Months)
Good-Prognosis Cytogenetics		
del(9q), NC	0.4	NR
del(15q), NC	0.4	NR
t(15q), NC	0.4	NR
del(12p), NC	0.8	108.0
+21, NC	1.1	100.8
–Y, +1	0.4	84.6
del(5q), isolated	8.2	80.0
+21, or +1	0.8	80.0
del(5q), NC	10.7	77.2
del(20q), isolated	1.9	71.0
del(20q), NC	2.2	71.0
–X, NC	0.5	56.4
No (normal karyotype)	49.5	53.4
del(5q), +1	2.5	47.0
+8, or +1	1.2	44.0
–Y, NC	2.7	39.0
–Y, sole	3.5	36.0
+1/+1q, NC	0.4	34.7
t(1q), NC	0.6	34.7
t(7q), NC	0.6	34.7
t(11q), NC	0.5	32.1
–21, NC	0.5	32.0
Intermediate-Prognosis Cytogenetics		
del(11q), NC	0.9	26.1
+8, NC	5.0	23.0
+8, isolated	3.8	22.0
t(11q23), NC	0.5	20.0
Rea 3q, NC	0.5	19.9
+19, NC	0.4	19.8
del(7q), isolated and NC	0.6	19.0
Any 3 abnormalities	2.8	17.1
del(11q), isolated	0.6	15.9
–7, +1	0.9	14.4
–5, NC	0.4	14.6
–7, sole	2.3	14.0
–7, NC	3.2	14.0
Poor-Prognosis Cytogenetics		
Complex, all	13.4	8.7
t(5q), NC	0.4	4/4
4–6 abnormalities	5.3	9.0
>6 abnormalities	3.9	5.0

NC, noncomplex karyotype (≤3 abnormalities); NR, not reached.

From Haase D, Germing U, Schonz J, et al: New insights into the prognostic impact of the karyotype in MDS and correlation with subtypes: Evidence from a core dataset of 2124 patients. Blood 110:4385, 2007.

CLINICAL SYNDROMES

Patients with MDS often present with symptoms of ineffective hematopoiesis.[209] They usually seek medical attention complaining of recurrent infections, bleeding, easy bruising, progressive fatigue and lethargy, or dyspnea on exertion. Occasionally, patients present without symptoms but with abnormal peripheral counts, such as neutropenia, anemia, thrombocytopenia, or a combination of all three. It is important to realize that bleeding can also occur in nonthrombocytopenic patients due to dysfunctional platelets. Patients will either die of progressive bone marrow failure or progress to overt AML. A subgroup of patients with less than 5% myeloblasts, RA, or RARS may die of nonhematologic causes which typifies this affected elderly patient population. In general patients with MDS have a shorter overall survival than age-matched controls, suggesting that bone marrow failure may be additive to other comorbid diseases.[21]

MDS has been reported to coexist with other hematologic malignancies, the most frequent being multiple myeloma, even in previously untreated patients.[210,211] MDS also has been described in patients with hairy cell leukemia, chronic lymphocytic leukemia,

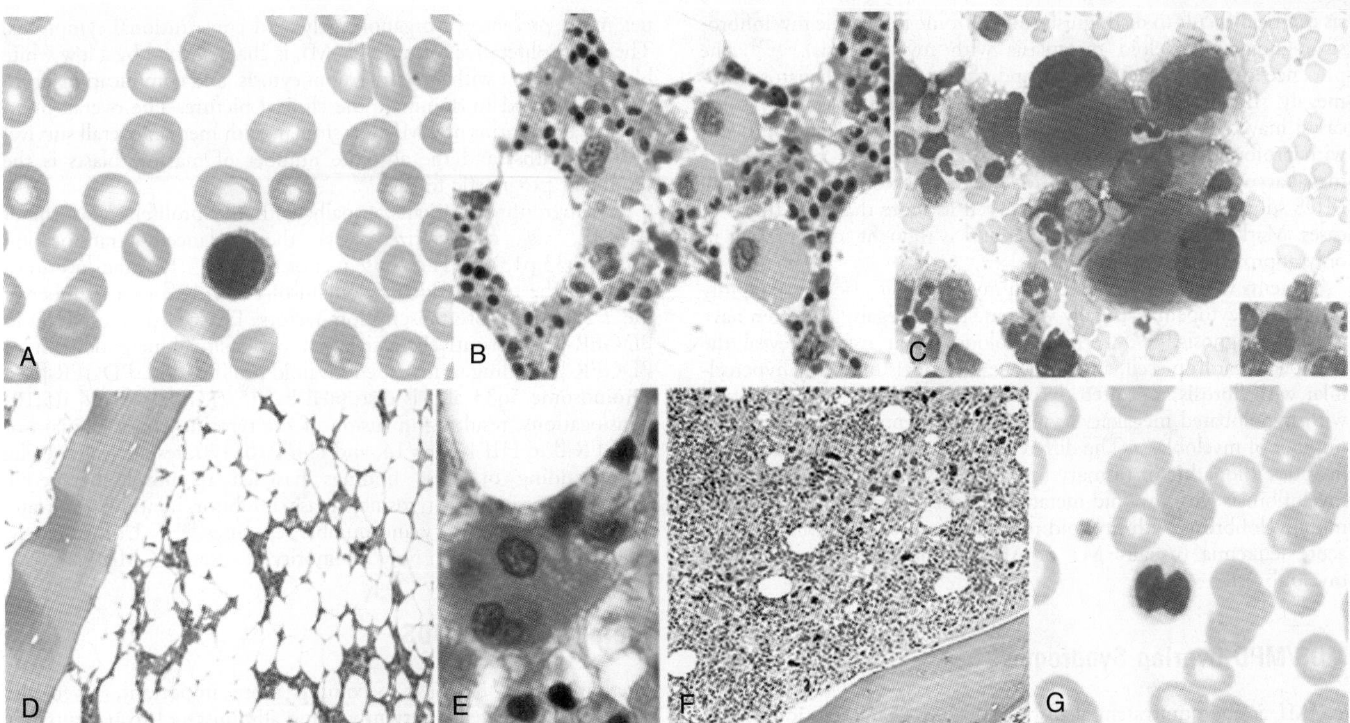

Figure 67–5 Specific syndromes. 5q− syndrome (**A–C**); hypocellular myelodysplastic syndrome (**D, E**), and myelodysplastic syndrome with fibrosis (**F, G**). The 5q− syndrome has specific morphologic correlates. There is a macrocytic anemia (**A**), and a cellular bone marrow characterized by increased small monolobated megakaryocytes (**B, C**). The megakaryocyte nuclei have little segmentation and are fairly round. Although some true micromegakaryocytes may be present (**C, insert,** same magnification), the typical monolobated forms are not as tiny as the micromegakaryocytes. Hypocellular myelodysplastic syndrome (**D, E**) can present a diagnostic problem and differentiation from aplastic anemia. Dysplasia may be difficult to evaluate if the smears are paucicellular. The finding of dysplastic megakaryocytes (note small widely separated nuclei, **E**) on the biopsy sample can be helpful. Myelodysplastic syndrome with fibrosis (**F**) can be difficult to differentiate from myeloproliferative neoplasms. However, the lack of large megakaryocytes, which typically are see in the myeloproliferative diseases, along with presence of dysplasia in the circulating neutrophils (**G**) are useful clues to the correct diagnosis.

non-Hodgkin lymphoma, and large granular lymphocytic leukemia.[212] The association of MDS with these other hematopoietic malignancies suggests a common myeloid/lymphoid stem cell as the transforming cell. However, the association may simply be a statistically random association or be therapy related in some cases. The coexistence of MDS with another hematologic malignancy significantly complicates the treatment options.

5q− Syndrome

Patients with myelodysplasia represent several unique clinical cohorts. Patients with an isolated loss of the short arm of chromosome 5 [del5(q31-q35), or 5q−] are characterized by a prolonged clinical course that progresses to acute leukemia in less than 25% of cases.[213,214] Interestingly, anemia seems to be the principal laboratory abnormality. Neutropenia, if present, typically is mild, and platelet counts often remain elevated. The striking pathologic feature is the presence of mononuclear micromegakaryocytes identified in the bone marrow biopsy (Fig. 67–5, *A–C*).

Women account for a larger proportion of cases, up to 70%.[215,216] Patients with 5q− deletions must be distinguished from patients with additional cytogenetic abnormalities, because these patients often have a more rapid progression to AML. The large arm of chromosome 5 is rich in genes encoding both cytokines and cytokine receptors.[217] Haploinsufficiency of the ribosomal protein encoding RPS14 gene has been shown to cause the phenotypic features of 5q− syndrome.[218] RNA-medicted interference (RNAi) screening technology confirmed the notion that 5q− syndrome is caused by a defect in ribosomal protein RPS14. In addition, a link has been established between acquired 5q− syndrome and congenital bone marrow failure syndromes such as Diamond-Blackfan anemia. Because of the uniqueness of the 5q− syndrome, it often is considered separately from the other myelodysplastic disorders. Patients typically require RBC transfusion as their principal treatment, so careful attention must be paid to management of iron overload. Lenalidomide (Revimid) has been approved for patients with a chromosome 5q abnormality who are transfusion dependent, and its use is discussed in treatment section.[219,220]

Hypocellular MDS

The majority of patients with myelodysplasia have a hypercellular or normocellular bone marrow. A hypocellular bone marrow is found in a minority of patients (<15%) and is referred to as *hypoplastic myelodysplasia* (see Fig. 67–5, *D and E*).[221] In this subgroup of patients, the morphologic features of the bone marrow may be difficult to differentiate from aplastic anemia, and the definitive diagnosis can sometimes be made from cytogenetic analysis. Cytogenetic abnormalities are rarely found in patients with aplastic anemia. The differential diagnosis of patients with a hypoplastic bone marrow includes not only aplastic anemia but also drug toxicity, PNH, and T-cell large granular lymphocytic leukemia.[222,223] These entities usually can be excluded by flow cytometric analysis of the bone marrow aspirate. The natural history of hypoplastic myelodysplasia is similar to that of the standard variants.

MDS with Myelofibrosis

Substantial reticulin fibrosis is rarely found in patients with myelodysplasia (see Fig. 67–5, *F and G*), although there is an increase incidence in patients with CMML. Myelodysplasia with myelofibrosis can be difficult to distinguish from chronic idiopathic myelofibrosis (agnogenic myeloid metaplasia with myelofibrosis).[121,224] The presence of trilineage dysplasia and the absence of hepatosplenomegaly support the diagnosis of myelodysplasia. However, some cases, may reflect an evolving transformation to a leukemic process, with profound bone marrow fibrosis such as is often seen in acute megakaryocytic leukemia (FAB-M7). Myelofibrosis can occur in all MDS subtypes, and mild fibrosis is seen in more than two thirds of cases. Marked fibrosis is much rarer and is thought to be present in only approximately 10% of cases.

Patients who develop MDS with myelofibrosis often have rapidly progressive cytopenias, usually without splenomegaly, and often have a poor prognosis.[117,118] Peripheral blood smear usually reveal the heralded "teardrop" cell, and the bone marrow is markedly hypercellular with fibrosis and often dysplastic megakaryocytic proliferation with hypolobated megakaryocytes; many patients have an increased number of myeloblasts. The differential diagnosis is complicated and includes idiopathic or primary myelofibrosis, postpolycythemia vera myelofibrosis with myeloid metaplasia, post-essential thrombocythemic myelofibrosis with myeloid metaplasia, accelerated phase CML, acute leukemia (usually M7 or AML with dysplasia), and acute myelofibrosis.

MDS/MPD Overlap Syndromes

CMML is the quintessential disorder having characteristic findings of both MDS and MPD (Fig. 67–6, *A*).[158,162,163] Because the majority of patients with CMML have evidence of trilineage dysplasia, the FAB cooperative group categorized CMML as a subtype of MDS. The FAB criteria for diagnosis included a peripheral monocyte count of 1000 per mm^3, less than 5% blasts in the blood, less than 20% blasts in the bone marrow, and absence of Auer rods. The new WHO classification system places CMML with juvenile myelomonocytic leukemia and atypical or BCR-negative CML into the new subgroup MDS/MPD (see Table 67–6).[21]

Many patients with CMML also present with splenomegaly, hepatomegaly, lymphadenopathy, tissue infiltration, or serous effusions.[162,186,187,225] Pleural, pericardial, synovial, and ascitic effusions all have been reported in patients with CMML and are associated with a high circulating monocyte count. Patients with CMML can have vastly different presentations. Certain patients with CMML present with profound cytopenias and marked dysplasia, whereas other patients have a predominately myeloproliferative form. Because of these two rather distinct clinical presentations, some clinicians separate CMML into two separate entities, with the proliferative form characterized by white blood cell WBC count greater than 12,000 per mm^3, presence of organomegaly, and constitutional symptoms. The nonproliferative form of CMML is characterized by a low white blood cell count with a relative monocytosis, and complications from cytopenias tend to dominate the clinical picture. The overall prognosis of both forms of CMML is similar, with median overall survival of 19 months, and the absolute number of marrow blasts is the dominant prognostic feature.[187]

A subgroup of patients, usually with the proliferative form of CMML, is characterized by the balanced translocation t(5;12)(q33;p13).[204] The consequence of the t(5;12) translocationis fusion of the tyrosine kinase domain of PDGFR-β to a member of the *ETS* family of transcription factors TEL. Fusion of TEL to PDGFR-β constitutively activates the tyrosine kinase domain of PDGFR-β, leading to increased myeloid proliferation. PDGFR-β on chromosome 5q33 also is disrupted by t(5;7), t(5;14), and t(5;10) translocations, resulting in fusion of the tyrosine kinase domain of PDGFR-β to HIP1, CEV14, and H4/D10S170, respectively.[226] The understanding of these findings has led to novel therapeutic approaches using the tyrosine kinase inhibitor imatinib mesylate, with remarkable efficacy and durable responses.[183,227] Unfortunately, PDGFR-β is present in only a minority of cases of CMML.

Therapy-Related MDS

Therapy-related MDS is becoming more important, given the increased dose density currently being administered to patients, for example, those with breast carcinoma.[228–231] Furthermore, the use of myeloid growth factors may inadvertently increase this risk.[232] Therapy-related MDS and AML remain one of the most serious long-term complications of current cancer therapy and often are induced by well-defined chemotherapeutic agents and/or radiation. The incidence of secondary or therapy-related MDS is increasing.[228] The term *secondary myelodysplasia* refers to the development of disease following either exposure to environmental or therapeutic toxins or from a previously diagnosed hematopoietic disorder. The term *therapy-related* should be specifically attributed to the presentation of MDS or AML following the use of intensive chemotherapy or radiation therapy.

Many patients with therapy-related MDS/AML have common chromosomal aberrations and/or gene mutations. Most importantly, patients with therapy-related MDS behave in a more aggressive fashion regardless of FAB or WHO classification subtype. Patients with therapy-related MDS are not included in the IPSS schema; therefore, specific prognostic factors are limiting. The risk of secondary MDS is highest in patients who already have been exposed to alkylating agent therapy. The cytogenetic abnormalities of alkylating agent-related therapy-related MDS/AML are quite distinct.[6,10,109]

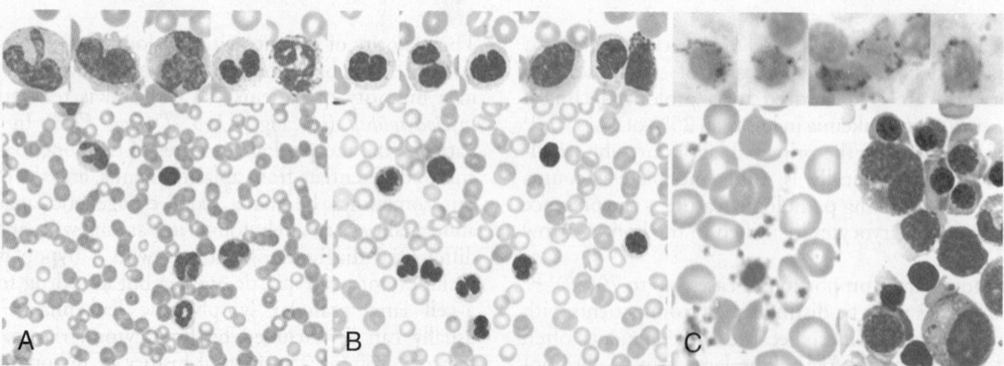

Figure 67–6 Overlap syndromes. Chronic myelomonocytic leukemia (**A**), "atypical chronic myelogenous leukemia" (**B**), and refractory anemia with ringed sideroblasts and thrombocytosis (**C**). In chromic myelomonocytic leukemia there can be granulocytic dysplasia and cytopenias (e.g., anemia, thrombocytopenia), but the characteristic feature is the presence of an absolute monocytosis (**A**). "Atypical chronic myelogenous leukemia" (BCR/ABL-negative) is essentially a "high-count" myelodysplastic syndrome. There typically is severe granulocytic dysplasia. The absence of an absolute monocytosis excludes chronic myelomonocytic leukemia from the diagnosis. The case shown is characterized by numerous pseudo–Pelger-Huet cells, immature hypogranular granulocytic precursors, and some basophils (**B**). The case was shown to be associated with i(17q) as a sole abnormality. Refractory anemia with ringed sideroblasts and thrombocytosis is characterized by anemia and thrombocytosis in the blood (**C, left**), hypercellular marrow with erythroid proliferation (**C, right**), and ringed sideroblasts (**C, top**).

They include either a total loss or a deletion of the long arm of either chromosome 5 or 7. A higher than normal risk for developing therapy-related MDS/AML has been described in long-term survivors of Hodgkin lymphoma, non-Hodgkin lymphoma, multiple myeloma, and gastrointestinal cancers, specifically those treated with semustine (methyl-CCNU).[233–236] The estimated actuarial risk in patients treated for Hodgkin lymphoma is between 6% and 9%. A 17% actuarial risk has been reported in patients treated for multiple myeloma.

The risk of developing MDS following adjuvant treatment of breast cancer, small cell lung cancer, testicular cancer, or ovarian cancer is low but increases with use of regional radiation therapy. Topoisomerase II inhibitors also can induce therapy-related AML[91] but typically involves a balanced translocation of chromosome band 11q23 and less commonly involves 3q26 and 21q22. The topoisomerase II inhibitors include the epipodophyllotoxins and anthracyclines. As opposed to prior exposure from alkylating agents, MDS seldom precedes therapy-related AML caused by the topoisomerase II inhibitors.

Use of adjuvant therapy for treatment of early-stage invasive breast carcinoma has been associated with therapy-related MDS/AML. The incidence of therapy-related MDS/AML after treatment of early-stage breast cancer with mastectomy alone is only 0.27%.[229,237,238] A case-control study of 82,700 women treated for early-stage breast cancer during the 1970s and 1980s reported that the typical cyclophosphamide, methotrexate, and fluorouracil (CMF) regimens with a low cumulative dose of cyclophosphamide is associated with an additional five cases of leukemia for every 10,000 women treated over 10 years.[239] However, with the current use of anthracycline-based adjuvant chemotherapy regimens (cyclophosphamide, epirubicin, fluorouracil [CEF]; or fluorouracil, Adriamycin [doxorubicin], cyclophosphamide [FAC]), the risk of therapy-related MDS/AML has increased compared to the classic CMF regimen. Rates of therapy-related MDS/AML now approach 1.5% after 5 to 10 years of follow-up. There is an even greater risk in women who received radiotherapy.[240,241] In patients who receive four cycles of standard anthracycline and cyclophosphamide therapy (cyclophosphamide 600 mg/m^2 and doxorubicin 60mg/m^2 per cycle), the risk appears quite low. In one study, the incidence of therapy-related MDS/AML in patients who receive four full cycles of cyclophosphamide and anthracycline chemotherapy was only 0.1% with the median followup of 5 years. However, women seem to have a higher risk for therapy-related MDS/AML in the National Surgical Adjuvant Breast and Bowel Project (NSABP) protocols B-22 and B-25, in which a higher dose of cyclophosphamide as well as doxorubicin were used.[237] Of potential importance was the use of G-CSF in these regimens. In one retrospective study of patients with breast cancer, use of G-CSF was associated with doubling of the risk of therapy-related MDS/AML.[232]

A history of autologous bone marrow transplantation has been associated with a substantial risk of developing therapy-related MDS and AML.[240,242–249] The cumulative probability of developing therapy-related MDS/AML after autologous SCT ranges from 4% to 14%, depending on the series. A retrospective study by Friedberg et al.[250] reported a 19.8% actuarial risk of developing MDS by 10 years. All of the 552 patients analyzed in this study were treated with cyclophosphamide and total body irradiation. The patients who developed MDS had on average a lower number of cells reinfused per kilogram at autologous bone marrow transplantation (BMT). The increased incidence of therapy-related MDS/AML has been associated with use of radiation therapy as part of the conditioning regimen, but other risk factors include advanced stage, number and type of prior courses of chemotherapy. and exposure to radiation therapy before transplantation. The prognosis of patients with therapy-related MDS or AML remains extremely poor.

Therapy-related MDS and AML are characterized by three distinct groups of cytogenetic abnormalities.[89,108] The first is an unbalanced aberration along chromosome 5 or 7. Patients typically have loss of the whole chromosome 5 or 7 or loss of various parts, specifically the long arm of chromosome 5 or 7. Another frequently observed abnormality is the gain of a whole chromosome 8 (trisomy 8).[39] Abnormalities of chromosomes 5, 7, and 8 are seen in 15% to 25% of cases in de novo MDS but compose approximately 50% to 70% of cases with therapy-related MDS. Similarly, they occur in 15% to 25% of cases of de novo AML but in 40% to 50% of therapy-related AML. A second cytogenetic subgroup comprises recurrent balance translocations involving the MLL gene on chromosome 11q23.[251,252] Patients with this abnormality typically present with AML without a myelodysplastic prodrome. From 15% to 20% of patients with therapy-related AML have rearrangements of the MLL gene, whereas this abnormality typically is not seen in patients with therapy-related MDS. In fact, the WHO has redefined patients with MLL gene rearrangements or patients with t(8;21) or t(16;16) or inv(16) as having AML regardless of the absolute blast count.[20,158] The final group of patients with therapy-related MDS consists of patients with a normal karyotype or other chromosomal aberrations. This group comprises 50% to 60% of de novo MDS but only 5% to 10% of therapy-related MDS and 10% to 15% of therapy-related AML.

With respect to specific molecular abnormalities, the most common specific gene mutation involves the MLL gene on 11q23, but other abnormalities have been identified, namely, AML1 on 21q22, the RARA locus on chromosome 17q21, and CBFB on chromosome 16q22.[93,94,97,105,107,252–254] Rearrangements of these genes lead to a dominant loss of function of the transcription factor, which results in impairment of differentiation. It is thought that by interfering with myeloid differentiation, leukemia will result. In addition, other abnormalities have been identified, including mutations of the nucleophosmin gene NPM1, which has been designated a class II mutation in leukemogenesis.[255] The critical genetic consequences of unbalanced chromosome aberrations in MDS and AML are unclear. Deletions of chromosome 17p13 or loss of whole chromosome 17 were thought to involve the p53 gene.[206,256–259] In addition, data have suggested that monosomy 5 or loss of the long arm of chromosome 5 is related to haploinsufficiency of the EGR1 gene.[260] However, a study from the Look laboratory at the Dana Farber Cancer Institute has implicated haploinsufficiency and promoter methylation of *CTNNA1*, the gene encoding α-catenin.[76] How either of these genetic defects relates to the haploinsufficiency of the ribosomal protein encoding RPS14 remains unclear.[218]

RARS with Thrombocytosis

Some patients with MDS present with marked thrombocytosis. Most patients have RARS, but with markedly elevated platelet count, and therefore have been reclassified as RARS-T (see Fig. 67–6C).[167,261–264] Bone marrow aspirate and biopsy show features consistent with a myeloproliferative and myelodysplastic overlap syndrome. Importantly, the megakaryocytes resemble those seen in essential thrombocythemia. Patients with RARS-T often have evolved from a low-grade MDS category, such as RA or RARS, but have acquired a JAK2 V617F mutation. This mutation is relatively uncommon in other patients with MDS; therefore, RARS-T represents another JAK2 mutation-associated chronic myeloproliferative disorder.[265–267]

According to the WHO, patients with RARS-T are classified under the provisional MDS/MPD category and listed as unclassifiable.[268] Given the rarity of this syndrome, definitive estimates of overall survival and time to leukemic transformation are unclear. However, a retrospective analysis of 23 patients with RARS-T revealed a 5-year survival of 86% compared to 62% in patients with RARS who did not have a JAK2 V617F mutation.

3q21-q26 Syndrome

Patients with MDS who contain a 3q21-q26 cytogenetic abnormality often have profound trilineage dysplasia, especially of the megakaryocytes.[269] Patients can present with either MDS or AML and typically have a normal or increased platelet count. Cytogenetic analysis at the time of diagnosis often reveals at t(1;3), inv(3), or t(3;3) abnormality. Patients with these cytogenetic abnormalities have an extremely poor response to chemotherapy and, as a result, a poor overall prognosis. The peripheral blood smear often reveals giant platelets or even circulating megakaryocytic fragments. In addition, hypogranular megakaryocytic forms and micromegakaryocytes may be present in the bone marrow aspirate. These morphologic abnormalities involving the megakaryocytes are accompanied clinically with an increased risk of bleeding despite either a normal or increased absolute platelet count. Platelet aggregation studies show decreased platelet aggregation to collagen and epinephrine and may explain the increased risk of bleeding seen in these patients.[38,171]

TREATMENT

General Principles

Treatment of patients with MDS remains challenging for several reasons. First, patients with this disorder are likely to be elderly, so comorbid disease and performance status are critical components in deciding on specific therapy. Second, the disease is heterogeneous, making therapies for one type of MDS less optimal than those for others. Given the lack of precise pathophysiologic understanding of more than a few MDS subtypes, designing truly targeted therapies is impossible. We are left with agents that deal with abnormalities generally thought to play a role in MDS, such as underactive or overactive apoptosis, failure to express silenced genes required for hematopoietic cell differentiation, or overabundant angiogenic signaling. Finally, there is no widely accepted standard of care in that very few, if any, modalities have been definitively proven to change the natural history of this disease. Until recently,[270] response criteria for MDS were not standard, making for difficult interpretation of the multiple phase II trials that included trial-specific response criteria.

The primary goal of most therapeutic strategies in neoplastic diseases is improvement in overall survival. Although this remains the desired result for treatment of patients with MDS, less formidable achievements also might be useful. Such benefits might include delay in time to transformation to leukemia, response rate (rigorously defined), decrease in transfusions, decreased infection, hematologic improvement, and improved quality of life. The only modality historically associated with an appreciable degree of long-term disease-free survival is allogeneic bone marrow transplantation.[270,271] This modality is resource intense, potentially highly toxic, and heretofore available only to a minority of patients with MDS due to age and performance status requirements. On the other hand, analysis of the role of the myriad other valuable medical therapies is complicated (see box on Treatment).

Management Guidelines for a Newly Diagnosed Patient with Myelodysplasia

The only known curative modality for patients with myelodysplastic syndrome (MDS) is stem cell transplantation (SCT). Therefore, all appropriate candidates should be considered for SCT. They include patients younger than 70 years (age 75 years at some centers), with a reasonable performance status and no significant comorbidity. Retrospective data from the International Bone Marrow Transplant Registry suggest that patients with low-risk disease (International Prognostic Scoring System [IPSS] low or intermediate-1) should undergo SCT only at the time of disease progression (see text and Table 67–10). Disease progression includes progressive clinically significant cytopenias such as progressive red blood cell (RBC) and/or platelet transfusion dependency or transformation to a high-risk disease. Transformation to high-risk MDS typically is manifested by an increase in the number of bone marrow blasts but also could represent accumulation of additional cytogenetic abnormalities.

Patients with low-risk disease should be carefully analyzed for the presence of a deletion of the long arm of chromosome 5. Patients with a deletion of 5q or those who have the 5q syndrome should start taking lenalidomide at the time they become RBC transfusion dependent. For patients with hypoplastic MDS who are younger than 6 years, have a low transfusion requirement, and have no increase in marrow myeloblasts, immunosuppressive therapy should be considered with antithymocyte globulin and a calcineurin inhibitor. In all other patients with low-risk MDS, the addition of an erythropoietin-stimulating agent (ESA) should be considered, but only in patients with a serum erythropoietin (Epo) level less that 500 mU/mL. For patients who do not respond to initial ESAs, addition of a myeloid growth factor (granulocyte colony-stimulating factor or granulocyte-macrophage colony-stimulating factor) should be considered. In patients who do not respond or those with an elevated Epo level, aggressive supportive care should continue. The addition of a hypomethylating agent, such as azacytidine or decitabine, may improve the hematologic parameters, but the overall experience of hypomethylating agents in patients with low-risk MDS is limited. The addition of lenalidomide is another option for patients who have isolated anemia, but lenalidomide has no impact on the myeloid or megakaryocytic lineages in patients without the 5q abnormality. Although controversial, iron chelation therapy can be considered for patients with low-risk MDS and a serum ferritin level greater than 1000 mcq/L.

All patients with high-risk MDS classified by an IPSS score of intermediate-2 or higher or patients with more than 10% bone marrow blasts should be seen at a transplant center for consideration of SCT if they are appropriate candidates. For patients who are not eligible for transplantation, a hypomethylating agent should be initiated at the time of presentation. Hypomethylating agents such as azacytidine and decitabine are associated with a small but reproducible complete remission rate, and evidence from Europe has demonstrated that azacytidine may improve median overall survival. In addition, regardless of the IPSS risk category, all patients should be considered for clinical trial participation. Novel strategies hopefully will make an impact not only on patient quality of life but also improve the median survival of patients with MDS.

Role of Iron Chelation in the Management of Patients with Myelodysplasia

The development of secondary hemochromatosis is associated with significant morbidity in chronic hemoglobinopathies such as thalassemia major, Blackfan-Diamond syndrome, and sickle cell anemia. Iron chelation therapy has been shown to improve the outcome in patients with these disorders. However, the same cannot be said for patients with MDS. The majority of patients with MDS become RBC transfusion dependent because since they are exposed to a significant amount of intravenous iron. Each unit of packed RBCs has approximately 200 to 250 mg of elemental iron. More than 75% of patients with MDS who receive chronic RBC transfusions will develop evidence of secondary hemochromatosis documented by a serum ferritin level of 1000 mg/mL or higher. This typically occurs after patients have received a total lifetime of 40 units of packed RBCs. Nevertheless, it remains difficult to document true organ failure as a result of iron overload in most patients with MDS. In patients with MDS, a serum ferritin level of 1000 mg/mL or higher is associated with a reduced median overall survival. What has not been demonstrated in a prospective fashion is whether the addition of iron chelation therapy can improve survival.

Patients with high-risk MDS have a shortened overall survival as a result of progressive cytopenias resulting in infection, bleeding diatheses, or transformation to acute myelogenous leukemia. In these

Role of Iron Chelation in the Management of Patients with Myelodysplasia—cont'd

patients, the role of iron chelation therapy is unlikely to improve the median survival. However, in patients with low-risk MDS, the natural history of the disease is markedly different. Many patients have an indolent course, with a median overall survival greater than 3 years. In addition, use of disease-modifying agents, such as, lenalidomide in patients with the 5q syndrome may alter the natural history of the disease.

Two studies have demonstrated that iron chelation therapy is associated with improved median survival in patients with low-risk MDS. Both studies have limitations. In the Canadian study, which was a retrospective analysis of 178 patients, only 18 patients received iron chelation therapy. The other study from the French MDS group was a nonrandomized prospective analysis of 165 patients of whom 46% received iron chelation therapy. In this latter study, various regimens of iron chelation were used, and but no formal assessment of individual iron stores was made. Thus, the role of iron chelation therapy for patients with MDS is unclear. If it has a role, it should be reserved for patients with low-risk MDS because they are expected to have a prolonged median survival, especially patients who are benefiting from their therapy.

MDS in Young Patients

Although MDS typically occurs in patients older than 60 years (median age 70 years), younger individuals also can be affected. Data on the treatment of young patients with MDS who have an indolent or low-risk presentation are unclear. When the IPSS was developed, few patients were younger than 60 years, but it was clear that young patients within the low and intermediate-1 risk groups had significantly better survival than did older patients within the same IPSS risk group. Because the outcome from SCT is related to patient age, the best approach for young patients with MDS who have a low to intermediate-1 IPSS score remains debated.

Cutler et al. demonstrated a superior outcome when patients in low or intermediate-1 IPSS risk groups were transplanted at the time of disease progression as opposed to the time of their initial diagnosis. Furthermore, data from the German registry revealed that 86% of patients younger than 50 years with low-risk disease were alive at 20 years, and patients with an intermediate-1 IPSS score had a median survival of 176 months. Therefore, patients with low or intermediate-1 risk MDS who are younger than 50 years should be observed, and SCT should be delayed until disease progression. Disease progression includes the development of significant transfusion requirements, progressive cytopenias, or transformation to a higher IPSS subgroup.

Erythropoietin-Stimulating Agents in Patients with MDS

The safety of ESAs, recombinant human erythropoietin (rh-Epo; Epogen or Procrit) and darbepoetin (Aranesp), has come into question, specifically in patients with chemotherapy-induced anemia and chronic renal failure. ESAs can increase hemoglobin and ameliorate the symptoms from anemia that develop in patients with cancer who are undergoing chemotherapy and those with chronic renal failure. However, treatment also increases the risk of thromboembolic complications. Increased risk of tumor recurrences also has been noted.

For patients with chronic renal failure, two trials have demonstrated that patients assigned to a high targeted hemoglobin experience significantly more adverse events, including death, chronic heart failure, myocardial infarction, and stroke than do patients assigned to lower targeted hemoglobin. Use of ESAs for treatment of anemia in patients with MDS has remained a standard approach used by most physicians. Interestingly, most physicians are unaware that this remains an off-label use, as regulatory authorities have not approved ESAs for use in patients with MDS. The efficacy of ESAs in MDS has been difficult to tabulate given the changing definition of response. Now with most authors using the International Working Group (IWG) criteria for response, we have a better appreciation for the low but reproducible responses seen with use of ESAs in patients with MDS. The hemoglobin response from an ESA in patients with MDS ranges from 20% to 40%. It is important to note that a major hemoglobin response includes the development of transfusion independence as well as an increase in hemoglobin of at least 2 g/dL from baseline measurements.

There have been many concerns regarding the safety of ESAs in patients with MDS. Importantly, no significant adverse events, including thromboembolic complications, have been noted in multiple studies. Mounting evidence indicates that a lower baseline serum Epo level is associated with a higher response rate; therefore, all patients should have a baseline Epo level measured before initiation of an ESA (see text and Table 67–9). Patients with a serum Epo level greater than 500 mU/mL have such a low response rate to ESAs that alternative strategies should be considered first. ESA treatment requires a long duration to see maximum benefit, and, because of increased iron utilization, concurrent iron administration may be required to achieve a maximum response. In addition, use of ESAs did not appear to be associated with higher rates of progression to AML. More importantly, it appears that amelioration of chronic anemia in patients with MDS not only may improve their quality of life but also may change the natural history of the disease (see text).

Supportive Care

If there is standard therapy for patients with MDS (other than relatively rare young patients who may be bone marrow transplant candidates), it is supportive care. Supportive care generally consists of administration of blood products and antibiotics when needed. Most also would consider use of iron chelation therapy and hematopoietic growth factors as reasonable supportive care adjuncts.

The development of hematopoietic growth factor therapy held both promise and peril as a therapeutic strategy in the treatment of patients with MDS. Certainly if platelet count, hematocrit, and neutrophil count are low, use of an agent that could stimulate growth of the appropriate precursor cell might prove beneficial in ameliorating symptoms and complications associated with the given cytopenia. On the other hand, it was recognized early on that, in most cases, the pathophysiology of MDS had nothing to do with the failure of growth factor availability. For example, levels of Epo, the renally elaborated protein that regulates red cell production,[272] usually are elevated in anemic patients with MDS[273]; however, the intrinsically diseased bone marrow cannot respond. Moreover, it has been recognized for some time that leukemic cells, the neoplastic counterparts of normal bone marrow stem cells, harbor growth factor receptors and can be induced to proliferate in vitro in response to these agents.[274] As such, it was feared that particularly the myeloid growth factors might be leukemogenic in patients with MDS. Although clinical studies have failed to confirm a major deleterious leukemogenic effect, they also have shown that these treatments do not prevent infection or prolong life expectancy. Nonetheless, when used selectively, hematopoietic growth factors may be useful in the management of certain patients with MDS.

Management of RBC Transfusion Dependence

Because most patients with MDS are anemic, which is a major factor in fatigue and poor quality of life, the issue of primary management of this finding is critical. Transfusion of packed RBCs, generally when the patient is symptomatic or when the hemoglobin falls below 8 to 9 mg/dL, is the usual approach. RBCs should be irradiated to prevent transfusion-associated graft-versus-host disease.[275] Whether routine depletion of white cells to reduce alloimmunization is required is controversial.[276] Despite the caveat about high Epo levels in MDS patients, patients can respond meaningfully to this agent, perhaps because a blunted response curve[277] allows pharmacologic doses of recombinant Epo to stimulate erythropoiesis in MDS. The potential for exogenous Epo to raise the hematocrit, decrease transfusion requirements, and possibly improve the quality of life in patients with MDS spurred the generation of many phase II and III trials with various doses and schedules of Epo. Although the initial trials generally used three times per week dosing (based on the successful use of this drug in patients with renal failure),[278] the impracticability of this approach (based on third-party payment rules requiring patients receive drug administration in a doctor's office) have generated weekly dosing schedules. Moreover, the availability of long-acting Epo[279] has furthered the use of more intermittent schedules.

Selected phase II trials[280–283] using recombinant human erythropoietin (rh-Epo) in patients with MDS report response rates in the 25% range. However, definitions of response are highly variable, most trials were conducted before common use of the International Working Group (IWG) criteria,[270] and the clinical benefit of such responses can be quite heterogeneous. For example, an increase in hemoglobin of 1 to 2 mg/dL could have biologic but very little clinical significance unless the patient becomes transfusion independent. Older patients with MDS who have clinical or subclinical impairment of renal function leading to a relatively lower level of serum Epo for a given degree of anemia might be good candidates for a therapeutic trial with this agent.

Although most patients with MDS have abundant supplies of iron due to prior transfusion or high gut absorption, a small subset of patients may be iron deficient. Therefore, it is important to review iron stores at the time of diagnostic bone marrow examination and, if absent, to provide supplemental iron because Epo responsiveness requires an iron-replete state. Since response to Epo in MDS may be delayed, the drug should be continued for at least 8 weeks before therapeutic failure is declared. Although the drug is well tolerated, keeping severely anemic and/or heavily transfusion-dependent patients on Epo for long periods makes little sense and is costly. Several studies have suggested that adding the myeloid growth factor G-CSF at low doses to erythropoietin can enhance the erythropoietic response.[284–286] Using the combination of Epo plus G-CSF initially or adding G-CSF after the effect of Epo is stable or waning may lead to response rates in the 40% range, which appear to be higher than with Epo alone. Nonetheless, the lack of a true prospective randomized trial of Epo with/without G-CSF has limited the wide acceptance of this strategy.

For patients with low-risk MDS, rh-Epo remains the most commonly used initial therapeutic approach for treatment of patients with MDS who are transfusion dependent to RBCs. In patients with MDS, only 15% to 30% will experience an erythroid response to rh-Epo. There are good predictive features for an observed response. Predictors for response to Epo are unclear. A decision model was developed by Hellstrom-Lindberg[286] (Table 67–9). Patients with MDS who had an Epo level less than 500 mU/mL, low RBC transfusion requirements, and bone marrow blasts less than 10% had a favorable chance of responding to rh-Epo. Interestingly, the presence of a deletion 5q with or without additional cytogenetic abnormalities did not affect the response rate but did shorten the response duration.[287] In addition, patients who do not have RARS[288,289] have a higher and more durable response. The Nordic MDS group suggested that patients with multilineage dysplasia have a poorer response to rh-Epo compared to patients with unilineage erythroid dysplasia (75% vs 9%; $P = 0.003$).[290] However, this has not been uniformly observed. The addition of a granulocyte colony-stimulating factors (G-CSF or GM-CSF) to single-agent rh-Epo can increase response rates by 20% to 40%.[60,284,286,291–293] Darbepoetin, a hypersialated ESA, has a longer half-life than rh-Epo and has yielded similar response rates when administered at intervals of every 1 to 3 weeks.[293] Response durations to either ESA agent range from 1 to 2 years, with longer responses associated with lower blast percentage as well as a low-to-intermediate IPSS score.

Table 67–9 Algorithm for Predicting Response to Erythropoietin and Granulocyte Colony-Stimulating Factor in Lower-Risk Myelodysplastic Syndrome

Parameter	Value of Parameter	Score
Serum erythropoietin	<100 mU/mL	+2
	100–500 mU/mL	+1
	>500 mU/mL	−3
RBC transfusions	<2 units/month	+2
	≥2 units/month	−2

Score	Response
Score >+1	Good response = 74%
Score −1 to +1	Intermediate response = 23%
Score <−1	Poor response = 7%

Response definitions:
Complete = Stable hemoglobin >11.5 g/dL.
Partial = Increase in hemoglobin with >1.5 g/dL or cessation of red blood cell (RBC) transfusion.
Adapted from Hellstrom-Lindberg E, Ahlgren T, Bequin Y, et al: Treatment of anemia in myelodysplastic syndromes with granulocyte colony-stimulating factor plus erythropoietin: Results from a randomized phase II study and long-term follow-up of 71 patients. Blood 92:68, 1998.

Few data regarding the safety of ESA use in patients with MDS are available. Use of ESAs for treatment of chemotherapy-induced anemia and chronic renal insufficiency has been associated with increased morbidity and mortality in many but not all randomized trials. In patients with chronic renal insufficiency, a hemoglobin target of 10 to 12 g/dL was often targeted in a randomized trial in which patients assigned to a targeted hemoglobin of 13.5 g/dL experienced significantly more adverse events, including death, chronic heart failure, myocardial infarction, and stroke compared to patients assigned to a lower targeted hemoglobin.[294] These findings have been supported by a more recent meta-analysis of nine randomized studies comparing different hemoglobin targets suggesting that patients with higher hemoglobin concentration display significantly higher rates of all-cause mortality, including complications from arteriovenous (AV) access thrombosis as well as from poorly controlled hypertension.[295]

As for patients with MDS, amelioration of anemia is thought to improve quality of life, specifically in responding patients. In addition, decreasing the need for transfusion support may have a dramatic impact on RBC supplies as well as decrease the risk of secondary hemochromatosis. More important is the observation that transfusion dependency has a negative impact on the natural history of patients with MDS.[191] A retrospective case-matched study of patients with MDS treated with supportive care compared to rh-Epo demonstrated that patients with a low RBC transfusion requirement (<2 units of RBCs per month) had a significant survival advantage with the addition of rh-Epo (hazard ratio = 0.56; $P = 0.015$).[296] Of major importance is the fact that administration of rh-Epo had no significant adverse effect on leukemic evolution. In fact, there was a suggestion that responding patients had a lower risk of AML progression compared to patients who did not respond. These findings were corroborated by another study of 419 patients with MDS who were treated with an ESA.[287] Patients were compared with case-matched controls with MDS managed by supportive care without use of rh-Epo. Similarly, a survival advantage was observed in the responding patients. Finally, a phase III prospective cooperative group trial also demonstrated a survival advantage in patients with MDS treated with rh-Epo with or without use of the myeloid growth factor G-CSF.[291] This was compared to best supportive care. The median survival in patients responding to treatment was 53 months compared to 23 months in nonresponding patients. These data importantly suggest that decreasing RBC transfusion requirements and resolution of severe anemia in patients with MDS may improve not only overall survival in low-risk patients but also decrease the risk for AML progression.

Management of Neutropenia

Due to the quantitative and qualitative defects in neutrophils, infections are common in patients with MDS and are a source of considerable morbidity and occasional mortality.[21] No data support the routine use of prophylactic granulocyte transfusions or antibiotics in MDS. Once fears about the ability of the myeloid growth factors G-CSF and GM-CSF to stimulate clinically meaningful blast cell proliferation were diminished, studies conducted in the late 1980s and early 1990s documented the efficacy of these agents in routinely increasing the number of normal white blood cells.[297–300] However, the few randomized studies performed did not demonstrate a decrease in the infection rate or an improvement in life expectancy despite achieving blood count improvement.[301] Such a discrepancy may reflect the maturation of dysfunctional or hypofunctional neutrophils that, although increased in number, cannot provide significant host defense benefit. Moreover, the mortality rate from infectious causes in MDS before conversion to AML probably is low. Although selected patients with recurrent suppurative infections might be candidates for myeloid growth factors, these agents should not be routinely used in MDS.

Management of Thrombocytopenia

Patients with MDS, particularly with more advanced subtypes, may have severe chronic thrombocytopenia with associated mucosal bleeding. Thrombocytopenia, defined as platelet count less than 100×10^9/L, occurs in 40% to 65% of patients with MDS. This problem may become life threatening if a significant bleed occurs in the brain or gastrointestinal tract. The reported incidence of hemorrhagic complications ranged from 3% to 53%, and the frequency of death as a result of hemorrhage was 14% to 24% of such cases.[165] Nonetheless, platelet transfusions should be used judiciously in MDS because overuse may result in alloimmunization and failure to respond to subsequent transfusions, even if leuko-poor products are used.[276] As in the case of RBC transfusions, platelets should be irradiated prior to use.[275] Therefore, rather than giving transfusions below a certain threshold, as is routinely done after chemotherapeutic administration,[302] it makes more sense to use clinical bleeding as the trigger. Use of the antifibrinolytic agent ε-aminocaproic acid can be considered for the thrombocytopenic patient who is bleeding but is not responding to transfusional therapy.[303]

Levels of thrombopoietin, the homeostatic hormone responsible for maintaining normal platelet counts, are elevated in thrombocytopenic patients with MDS,[304] making response to pharmacologic doses of the recombinant protein unlikely. However, neither native thrombopoietin nor its pegylated derivative megakaryocyte growth and development factor (MGDF) has been tested in patients with MDS. MGDF underwent limited testing as a supportive agent in patients with AML after induction chemotherapy.[305,306] Not only was MGDF not associated with a decrease in bleeding or need for platelet transfusions in AML, but its development was discontinued due to development of antiplatelet antibodies and thrombocytopenia in normal volunteers. IL-11, a cytokine with pleiotropic effects, is approved for use as a supportive agent for prophylaxis against severe thrombocytopenia after myelointense chemotherapy for solid tumor patients.[307] Limited testing of this agent alone in MDS patients[308] or after myelosuppressive therapy with the antibody–toxin conjugate gemtuzumab ozogamicin demonstrated side effects (e.g., fluid retention) and limited efficacy.

AMG531 (romiplostim) is a thrombopoiesis-stimulating Fc-peptide fusion protein (peptibody) that is being investigated in patients with idiopathic thrombocytopenic purpura.[309] AMG531 binds and activates the thrombopoietin receptor Mpl. Phase II studies have demonstrated durable platelet responses in patients with idiopathic thrombocytopenic purpura and the ability of these patients to subsequently discontinue corticosteroid therapy. AMG531 also is being developed in patients with chemotherapy-induced thrombocytopenia as well as in patients with MDS. A phase I/II study of AMG531 in patients with low-risk MDS who also were thrombocytopenic has been completed. Durable platelet responses were seen in 54% of patients with a decreased need for transfusions and a lower number of severe hemorrhagic events in responding patients.[310] Future studies will further explore the response rates of AMG531 in patients with MDS-related thrombocytopenia as well as patients currently undergoing hypomethylating therapy who develop thrombocytopenia as a complication of therapy.

Eltrombopag (SB-497115) is an oral nonpeptide thrombopoietin receptor agonist that binds to the transmembrane domain of the Mpl receptor, thereby inducing proliferation and differentiation of megakaryocytes.[311] Eltrombopag increased platelet production in patients with thrombocytopenia secondary to hepatitis C virus infection and in adult patients with relapsed or refractory chronic idiopathic thrombocytopenic purpura. Its use in patients with MDS has not been reported.

Management of Iron Overload

In patients with MDS, particularly those with indolent histologic subtypes and/or good prognoses based on the IPSS schema, administration of well over 100 units of packed RBCs is not unusual. The high iron load associated with such transfusion requirements may be harmful to the liver, pancreas, heart, and central nervous system.[312] Chelation therapy with either desferoxamine by continuous subcutaneous administration or the oral agent deferasirox (ICL670) can be administered to such patients, usually after they have received at least 25 to 30 units of blood.[313,314] Side effects of desferoxamine include cataract formation and chronic skin irritation from the subcutaneous injections. Chronic administration of desferoxamine is cumbersome,[315] is not well tolerated, and chelates only approximately 25 mg of iron per day, which compares unfavorably with the 250 mg given in a single unit of blood. Although beneficial in children with thalassemia who receive frequent transfusions,[316] the role of desferoxamine is limited in patients with MDS.

Deferasirox initially is administered at a dose of 20 mg/kg once per day and escalated to 30 or 40 mg/kg/day depending on the response. Typical side effects include development of gastrointestinal toxicity principally manifested as abdominal pain, nausea, vomiting, and diarrhea. Unfortunately, these side effects make dose escalation difficult in some patients. Deferasirox typically is used in patients with low-risk MDS and has been associated with decreases in serum ferritin levels. Prospective randomized trials using this agent in patients with low-risk MDS are warranted before its use can be universally recommended.

The development of secondary iron overload is difficult to define.[209] Secondary iron overload often is defined in patients with serum ferritin level greater than 1000 mg/mL. Patients who have an elevated serum ferritin level greater than 1000 mg/mL have decreased overall survival.[191,317] Whether poorer clinical outcomes are related to increased number of transfusions, a consequence of iron overload, or are due to progressive marrow dysfunction and failure that results in lower hemoglobin levels is unclear. Although these data are provocative, further evaluation and independent validation are needed, especially because few patients live long enough to develop definitive complications of iron overload.

Agents with Limited Efficacy

In the past, virtually every patient with MDS was given pyridoxine (vitamin B_6), probably because of its safety and the fact that rare children with congenital dysmyelopoiesis may respond.[318] However, reports of adults who actually benefit are rare. Androgen therapy, formerly a mainstay in the treatment of patients with bone marrow failure due to aplastic anemia or myelodysplasia, is rarely used today because of the lack of supporting data and its untoward side effects.[319] Danazol is a weak androgen and possibly has immunosuppressive properties. Although danazol therapy occasionally improves anemia and thrombocytopenia,[320] the rarity of such responses and the associated side effects have lead to abandonment of its typical use.

Immunosuppressive Therapy

For many years, patients with MDS were treated with steroids. Response rates in the 20% range were noted, but the increased use of prednisone in patients with myelodysplasia clearly led to more complications than benefit.[321] Nonetheless, several pieces of evidence have caused resurgence in enthusiasm for immunosuppressive therapy for MDS. First, autoimmune phenomena, often polyarthritis,[174] can be associated with MDS. Treatment with steroids in such cases may ameliorate the autoimmune manifestations and improve blood counts.[181] Patients with MDS have aberrant autoimmune hematopoietic inhibitory activity. In a subset of patients, clonal amplification of T lymphocytes has been demonstrated. The implication of this T-cell repertoire is that it suppresses hematopoiesis through a $CD8^+$ cytotoxic T-lymphocyte–mediated pathway.

Hypoplastic MDS bears morphologic similarity to aplastic anemia. Some patients with aplastic anemia who initially respond to immunosuppressive therapy may progress to MDS,[322] which suggests that these two entities share a common pathophysiology, that of T-cell–mediated suppression of a primitive bone marrow stem cell. Indeed, antithymocyte globulin (ATG), the mainstay of nontransplant therapy for aplastic anemia,[323] has a role in certain patients with MDS. A report from the National Cancer Institute suggests that patients with MDS who are young and have low platelet counts may benefit from a trial of ATG, with response rates as high as 50%.[324] The pretreatment variables associated with a higher response to immunosuppressive therapy include younger age (<60 years) and short duration of RBC transfusion dependency (<6 months). Interestingly, findings have shown the presence of a PNH clone or the presence of human leukocyte antigen (HLA) DR15 phenotype is another predictor for response to ATG in MDS.[325] It was originally thought that only those patients with hypoplastic MDS would respond, but now it seems clear that bone marrow hypoplasia is not a requirement for response, that rabbit or horse ATG can be used, and that patients with excess blasts rarely respond.[326]

Although no randomized trials have confirmed a survival benefit in patients treated with immunosuppressive therapy, a comparison of more than 800 patients in the IMRAW managed for prognostic variables showed that immunosuppressive therapy was associated with an improved overall survival (8.1 vs 5.2 years; $P < 0.001$).[116] Immunosuppressive therapy also was associated with a decreased risk of leukemic transformation ($P = 0.001$). The benefit in overall survival due to decreased leukemic transformation was seen in patients with low and intermediate-1 IPSS who were younger than 60 years. In addition, investigators from Prague have shown that approximately 40% of patients with indolent subtype MDS may respond to cyclosporine A.[327] Although a large randomized trial testing the usefulness of ATG in MDS is ongoing, young patients with MDS who do not have excess marrow blasts should be considered for a trial of immunosuppression.

Manipulating the Microenvironment

The pathophysiology of MDS is complex. However, it is increasingly recognized that the bone marrow microenvironment, including endothelial cells, fibroblasts, and other stromal cells, as well as immune effector cells and certain elaborated cytokines may have critical roles in maintenance of the neoplastic MDS clone. For example, microvessel density is increased in the marrows of patients with AML and MDSm[199] and proangiogenic substances such as vascular endothelial growth factor may be required for growth of neoplastic stem cells.[200] Second, at least in the indolent MDS subtypes, peripheral cytopenias in the presence of hypercellular bone marrow have suggested overabundant apoptosis, perhaps due to stromal cell secretion of proapoptotic substances such as TNF.[62] Attempts to modify TNF availability with use of phosphodiesterase inhibitors such as pentoxyphylline in combination with the steroids and ciprofloxacin (pentoxyphylline, ciprofloxacin, and dexamethasone [PCD] therapy)[328] or with the direct anti-TNF molecule etanercept (Enbrel),[329] as used in rheumatoid arthritis,[61] have led to transient and low-level responses in MDS. Amifostine, a thiol-containing compound approved for use as a chemoprotectant and radioprotectant,[330] alone[331] or in combination with PCD,[332] has limited biologic activity, with clinical responses that are too rare to justify the routine use of any of these strategies without an ability to predict which patients will respond.

The proangiogeneic and proapoptotic cytokine milieu of MDS may be counteracted by agents such as thalidomide, which has been effective in treatment of patients with refractory myeloma.[294] Studies suggest that thalidomide can lead to significant improvement in the need for transfusions in approximately 20% of patients with low-grade MDS subtypes.[333,334] However, many in the typical older patient population are poorly tolerant of the constipation, somnolence, and neuropathy typically associated with thalidomide use. The potent and better-tolerated thalidomide analogue lenalidomide (Revimid), which has activity in patients with advanced multiple myeloma,[219,220,335] may well be a real advance in "microenvironment-directed" therapy in MDS. Arsenic trioxide, which is approved for use in relapsed acute promyelocytic leukemia[336] and may modify the cytokine and angiogenic milieu in MDS, has shown only limited clinical activity.[337,338]

Lenalidomide

Lenalidomide is a thalidomide derivative (CC5013) that has more potent inhibition of TNF-α and other inflammatory cytokines compared to the parent compound. In addition, lenalidomide has greater capacity to promote T-cell activation and suppress angiogenesis. Importantly, lenalidomide lacks much of the neurotoxicity of thalidomide but still has myelosuppressive properties. A phase I study (MDS-001) was performed in patients with MDS who had symptomatic anemia and did not respond to treatment with ESAs.[220] Patients received doses of lenalidomide at 25 mg daily, 10 mg daily, or 10 mg daily for 21 days of a 28-day cycle, and 56% of patients experienced a durable erythroid response per the International Working Group (IWG). Twenty of 32 patients who previously were RBC transfusion dependent became independent of transfusion. Importantly, erythroid response rates were dependent on the presence of deletion of chromosome 5q, with 10 of 12 patients responding compared to 57% of patients with a normal karyotype and 12% of patients with abnormal karyotype. For patients with a 5q abnormality, responses were durable, with median duration of major erythroid response exceeding 2 years. The dose-limiting toxicities were different than expected from thalidomide and predominantly included myelosuppression, specifically within the first month of therapy. In fact, grade 3 or greater neutropenia occurred in 58% of patients and grade 3 or greater thrombocytopenia in 50% of patients.

Two multicenter confirmatory trials were performed in patients with MDS and a low or intermediate-1 risk IPSS score. Patients were transfusion dependent and had not responded to an ESA. The MDS-002 study was performed in patients without a 5q abnormality, and lenalidomide was started at a dose of 10 mg daily or 10 mg daily on days 1 to 21 of a 28-day cycle.[339] The overall transfusion response rate was 43,% with 26% of patients achieving transfusion independence. The median duration of response was 41 weeks. Although only a minority of patients had clonal cytogenetic abnormalities 19% experienced a cytogenetic response. The principal toxicity remained myelosuppression, with 30% and 25% of patients developing grade 3 or greater neutropenia and thrombocytopenia, respectively.

A second phase II trial (MDS-003) was performed in transfusion-dependent patients with MDS who contained a deletion of chromosome 5q using a similar dosing regimen as in the MDS-002 study.[219] A total of 148 patients were enrolled, and erythroid responses were seen in 76% of patients, with an amazing 67% of patients achieving a transfusion-independent state. In addition, complete cytogenetic responses were seen in 73% of patients and partial cytogenetic responses in 45% of patients. Development of a cytogenetic response was associated with achievement of transfusion independence. Surprisingly, the presence of additional chromosomal abnormalities was not associated with a decreased erythroid or cytogenetic response rate. Myelosuppression was extremely common in patients with chromosome 5q abnormality, and grade 3 or greater neutropenia or thrombocytopenia was reported in 55% and 44% of patients, respectively. A retrospective analysis suggested that patients who experience a 50% reduction in platelet count or grade 3 myelosuppression during the first 8 weeks of therapy had a higher incidence of response compared to patients who did not suffer myelosuppression. Exogenous use of myeloid growth factors was effective in treatment-related neutropenia.

The long-term outcome of lenalidomide use for treatment of patients with MDS who harbinger a deletion of chromosome 5q has been analyzed.[340,341] The data confirm a long median duration of response of 2.2 years, with some patients responding for more than 5 years. Higher response rates were seen by multivariate analysis for patients with the "actual" 5q syndrome, RBC transfusions of fewer than 4 units per 8 weeks, low-risk IPSS score, and age younger than 70 years. Using Kaplan-Meier estimates, responders had a 10-year overall survival estimate of 78% compared to 4% for patients who failed to respond. Unfortunately, these data are retrospective but nevertheless suggest that lenalidomide may change the natural history of patients with MDS who concurrently have a chromosome 5 abnormality.

Differentiation Therapy

Can the putative block in normal hematopoietic differentiation in patients with MDS be reversed by pharmacologic agents? Many compounds, including the vitamin A analogue retinoic acid,[342] the protein kinase C inhibitors phorbol ester[343] and brysotatin,[344] polar-planar solvents such as phenylbutyrate[345] and hexamethylene bisacetamide,[346] and nucleoside analogues such as low0dose cytarabine (ara-C)[78] can promote maturation of leukemic cells in tissue culture. One of the first clinical efforts with one of these agents suggested that low-dose cytarabine produced responses in patients with MDS without causing aplasia.[347] Initial enthusiasm for low-dose cytarabine in MDS faded because of studies suggesting a low response rate in meta-analysis and that some of the responses really occurred due to hypoplasia, much as would be expected from standard chemotherapy.[348,349] A randomized trial conducted by the Medical Research Council demonstrated a superior overall survival compared to best supportive care in elderly patients with AML or high-risk MDS.[350]

A randomized trial of retinoic acid versus observation, one of the few such efforts in MDS, failed to show any discernible benefit for patients enrolled in the experimental arm.[351] Phase II clinical trials with phenylbutyrate[352] and hexamethylene bisacetamide[353] each produced a few impressive responses, but the low frequency of efficacy and the requirement for cumbersome prolonged infusions prevented major interest. Although not a differentiating agent, melphalan, an orally available alkylating agent, has produced complete remissions in limited testing in patients with MDS.[354]

The mechanism of retinoic acid's differentiation activity in acute promyelocytic leukemia is inhibition of histone deacetylase-mediated transcriptional repression engendered by the PML-RARA fusion protein consequent to the characteristic t(15;17) chromosomal abnormality.[355] Several compounds that, unlike retinoic acid, have direct histone deacetylase inhibitory capability are in development as potential therapeutic agents for MDS. Depsipeptide has undergone phase I testing in patients with AML.[356] The drug appears to be well tolerated and inhibits histone acetylation in vivo. Other histone deacetylase inhibitors, including phenylbutyrate, suberoylanilide hydroxamic acid (Vorinostat), valproic acid, MS-275, LAQ823, LBH589 (panobinostat), and MGCD0103 are undergoing phase I testing in patients with MDS and related disorders.[357,358] Not surprisingly, attempts have already been made to combine DNA hypomethylating agents with histone deacetylase inhibitors in the form of azacytidine plus phenylbutyrate[359] or decitabine plus valproic acid.[360] Such efforts require careful consideration of optimal scheduling and ample ancillary studies to determine if the presumed targets really are affected.

Hypomethylating Agents

Progress in the field of epigenetics,[361] including thoughts concerning promoting expression of transcriptionally silent genes that might be required for the differentiated phenotype, has rekindled interest in the use of small molecules to promote hematopoietic maturation in patients with MDS. Structural barriers to transcription result from either overmethylation of DNA[73] or underacetylation of the histone DNA coat.[362] Cells from patients with MDS typically display overmethylation of genes such as p15INK4B,[363] which argues in favor of the relevance of this mechanism.

The greatest recent therapeutic advance in the management of patients with MDS was highlighted by a phase III trial, albeit with early crossovers permitted, of the putative DNA hypomethylating agent azacytidine given subcutaneously daily for 7 days every 28 days versus observation in patients with MDS conducted by the Cancer and Leukemia Group B.[364] Randomization to azacytidine was associated with a response rate of 60% (mostly hematologic improvement), delay in transformation to AML, and improved quality of life measured by several validated instruments.[365] The benefit of azacytidine was apparent in patients with both high- and low-risk MDS; a trend toward improvement in overall survival in the azacytidine arm did not reach statistical significance. The side-effect profile of the drug included mild nausea and vomiting and transient myelosuppression in some patients. Azacytidine, which now can be given intravenously, is metabolized in vivo to another hypomethylating agent decitabine.

Decitabine (5-aza-2′-deoxycytidine) has significant activity in patients with MDS based on a phase II trial performed in Europe[366] and a low-dose trial performed at the MD Anderson Cancer Center.[164] A phase III trial was performed in 170 patients with IPSS intermediate-1 or higher risk. Patients were randomized to receive either decitabine at a dose of 15 mg/m^2 given intravenously every 8 hours for 3 days or supportive care.[367] The overall response rate in patients treated with decitabine was 17%, including 9% complete remissions. Unfortunately, no effect was observed in terms of overall survival, but in a subgroup analysis, patients with intermediate-2 and high IPSS scores who received decitabine had a longer median time of progression to AML or death compared with patients who received supportive care alone (12.0 months vs 6.8 months; $P = 0.03$). One of the difficult issues with this study is that 43 patients received only two cycles of therapy, yet more than two cycles or 3.3 months of therapy on average was required to demonstrate a clinical response. Both decitabine and azacytidine have been approved by the US Food and Drug Administration and are being tested against supportive care in multiinstitutional prospective phase III trials.

A randomized bayesian phase II trial of patients with MDS was conducted at the MD Anderson Cancer Center. Decitabine was administered in one of three schedules: 10 mg/m^2 intravenously for 10 days, 20 mg/m^2 intravenously for 5 days, or 20 mg/m^2 intravenously for 5 days.[368] All three groups of patients received the same total dose of decitabine, 100 mg/m^2. The 20 mg/m^2 intravenously for 5 days arm was preferentially enrolled, suggesting that this may be the superior regimen. The overall response rate was 48%, with 34% of patients entering a complete remission. Although these results seem to be superior to those achieved using the 3-day regimen, they must be confirmed in a multicenter trial.

Signal Transduction Inhibitors

In MDS subtypes associated with excess blasts, highly analogous to the situation in AML, the underlying biologic problem may include overproliferation and/or lack of apoptosis within the stem cell compartment. Insofar as there are patients with MDS whose disease behaves more like AML, one can think of the same therapies that are in use or in development for the more aggressive neoplasm. Moreover, older adults with AML in particular are generally presumed to have blasts that emanate from a primitive stem cell, much like MDS.[97] As such, remission induction chemotherapy is a variable therapeutic alternative for some patients with MDS.

The constitutively activated tyrosine kinases BCR-ABL in CML[124] and FLT-3 in 30% of cases of AML[102] represent important drug targets. The development of imatinib for treatment of patients with CML[369] has revolutionized the treatment of patients with gastrointestinal stromal cell tumors (GIST) based on the ability of imatinib to inhibit c-KIT,[370] idiopathic hypereosinophilic syndrome (HES) based on its ability to inhibit platelet-derived growth factor receptor α (PDGFR-α).[371] Similarly, the rare patients with the MDS subtype CMML whose cells harbor a cytogenetic abnormality, such as t(5;12), a translocation that activates PDGFR-β,[226,227] also exhibit striking responses to imatinib.[183,227] Therefore, it is important to carefully scrutinize the cytogenetic results in patients with MDS, especially those with CMML, for any translocation involving the long arm of chromosome 5, for the potential of initiating imatinib therapy.

Several drugs that can inhibit the activated version of the FLT-3 tyrosine kinase are in development, particularly for use in AML.[372,373] However, rarely, and again probably more likely in CMML, patients with MDS may have one of two activating FLT-3 mutations, either a so-called *internal tandem duplication*, a copy of between nine and 300 base pairs in the juxtamembrane region, or a mutation in the activation loop, usually a point mutation yielding a D835Y amino acid substitution.[102] As such, a few patients with primary MDS have been treated with PKC412, one of the FLT-3 inhibitors currently in clinical trials, and responses have been noted.[373] Identifying other tyrosine kinases that may be activated in MDS and the drugs that inhibit them could yield future therapeutic advances.

Another cell-signaling therapeutic target in MDS is mutationally activated RAS, a 20-kd guanine nucleotide binding protein.[374] Because a mutation in a RAS family member occurs in approximately 20% to 40% of patients with MDS and most commonly in CMML, drugs that inhibit this enzyme are in development. The so-called *farnesyltransferase inhibitors* were developed because they inhibited an enzyme that catalyzed a key step in the posttranslational modification of RAS, preventing attachment of the farnesyl group required for movement to the cell membrane and enzyme activation.[375] Phase I and II trials with farnesyltransferase inhibitors have been completed in patients with MDS and AML.[376] One of the most important conclusions from these trials, in addition to the presence of only modest clinical activity, was that responses occurred exclusively in patients whose cells did not have RAS mutations, suggesting the likelihood of alternative targets, perhaps farnesylation of some of the many other proteins undergoing this posttranslational modification step, including lamin A or RHOB.[377]

Induction Chemotherapy

Use of cytotoxic chemotherapy for treatment of patients with MDS was generally considered to be an unhelpful strategy based on the typically older age of these patients and their poor tolerance of chemotherapy. Moreover, the proximal nature of the stem cell defect in MDS suggests that patients would be resistant to chemotherapy, based on overexpression of proteins mediating pleiotropic drug resistance,[378] and would have limited normal stem reserve, making them prone to severe myelosuppression. However, Estey et al.[379] demonstrated that patients with MDS can respond as well, or as poorly, to chemotherapy as those with AML, if the key prognostic factors of age and cytogenetic status are controlled for. Complete response rates range from 40% to 50%. Unfortunately, these responses tend to be short lived, even with consolidation chemotherapy, which does support the intrinsic nature of chemotherapy resistance in MDS. Curative intensive consolidation regimens with high-dose ara-C is appropriate only for younger adults with de novo AML in first remission[380] and therefore has no role in the treatment of older patients with MDS, given that older adults with AML do not benefit from such an intensive approach.

The notion that selected patients with MDS might benefit from chemotherapy[379] was altered by the change in the definition of AML and MDS in the new WHO classification system. Patients with 20% or greater blasts, as opposed to 30% in the older FAB system, now are considered to have AML.[20] Second, patients with balanced chromosomal translocations associated with a favorable prognosis, such as inv(16), t(8;21), and t(15;17), are considered to have AML at any level of marrow or peripheral blood leukemic cell involvement.[20] Applying the new definitions of MDS, relatively few patients are obvious chemotherapy candidates.

Induction chemotherapy may be useful in the relatively younger patient with high-risk MDS, defined as greater than 10% blasts in the bone marrow or with serious cytopenias. Such patients can be considered for nonmyeloablative or reduced-intensity conditioning allogeneic transplant.[381] Chemotherapy may be useful as a cytoreductive step prior to a reduced-intensity transplant, but prospective data are lacking. Although regimens containing topotecan alone or with ara-C[382] have activity in patients with MDS, this novel agent is no better than standard anthracycline and ara-C combination regimens[383] and should not be used routinely. Similarly, gemtuzumab ozogamicin, an antibody–toxin conjugate that is associated with a 30% remission rate in relapsed AML,[382] is expensive, myelosuppressive, and not particularly efficacious in patients with MDS.[384]

Stem Cell Transplantation

Recognition that the stem cell defect in MDS is proximal and pervasive suggested that allogeneic transplant would be required to eliminate the malignant clone, thereby making cure a possibility. Numerous studies suggested that up to 60% of selected patients with low-risk MDS and 20% to 40% of patients with high-risk disease can experience long-term disease-free survival after allogeneic transplantation from a matched donor.[270,271,385–387] Albeit in a relatively young and well population, no other modality, including chemotherapy[379] or autologous BMT,[388] is associated with a similarly high success rate. Despite concern that high-dose chemotherapy with autologous marrow or peripheral blood stem cell rescue would be an unworthy approach given that neoplastic stem cells would be difficult to eliminate in MDS and would grow poorly as an autograft, European investigators reported appreciable disease-free survival when this modality is used as consolidation therapy in MDS patients achieving remission with chemotherapy.[388] However,

Table 67–10 Decision Analysis of Allogeneic Bone Marrow Transplantation for Myelodysplastic Syndrome

	Overall Survival (Years)		
International Prognostic Scoring System Category	***Immediate Transplant***	***Transplant in 2 Years***	***Transplant at Progression***
Low	6.51	6.86	7.21
Intermediate-1	4.61	4.47	5.16
Intermediate-2	4.93	3.21	2.84
High	3.20	2.75	2.75

From Cutler CS, Lee SJ, Greenberg P, et al: A decision analysis of allogeneic bone marrow transplantation for the myelodysplastic syndromes: Delayed transplantation for low-risk myelodysplasia is associated with improved outcome. Blood 104:579, 2004.[389]

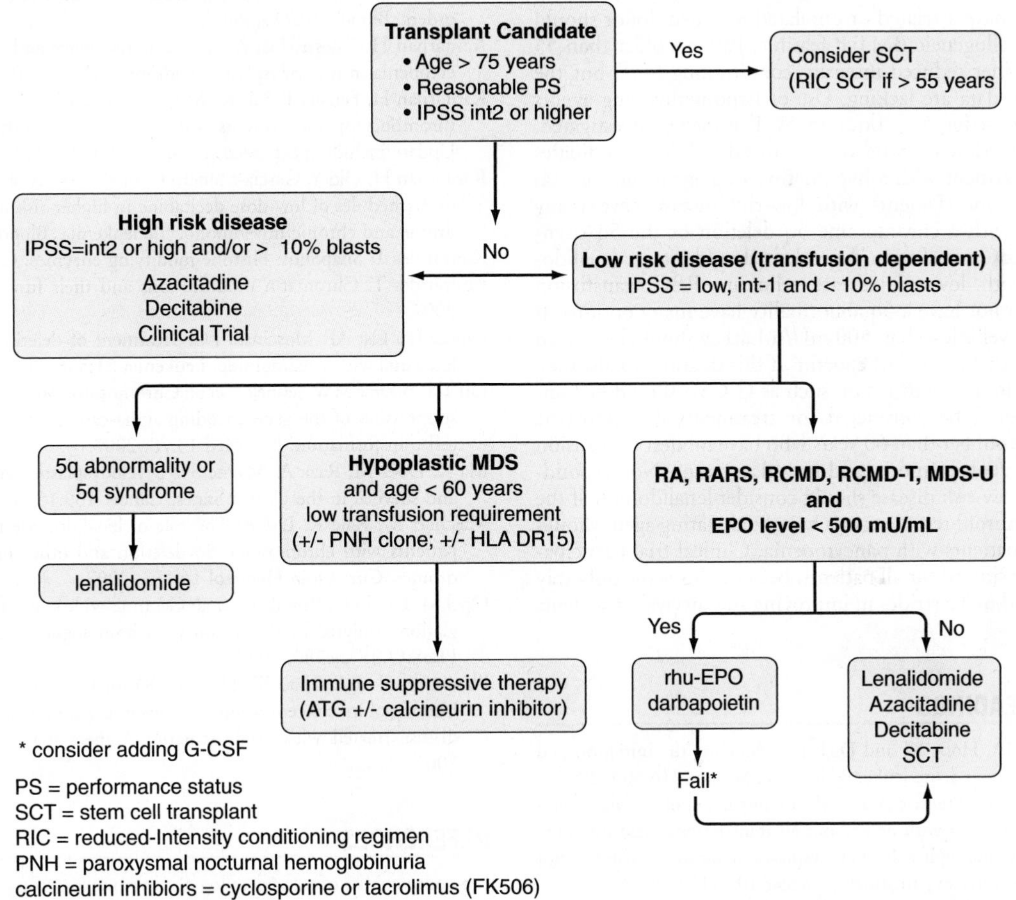

Figure 67–7 Algorithm for management of a patient with myelodysplastic syndrome.

because these patients likely would be more typical of an AML population, autologous BMT still is considered an experimental procedure for MDS.

An important treatment decision concerns the appropriate timing of transplantation, especially in low-risk disease. Upfront SCT potentially can take advantage of a relatively healthier bone marrow, with waiting until disease progression delaying transplant-related morbidity. Cutler et al.[389] analyzed a national database registry of transplant patients with MDS and their outcomes to perform a decision analysis addressing this question. They found that for low and intermediate-1 IPSS groups, delayed SCT was associated with better overall survival (Table 67–10). In contrast, for intermediate-2 and high IPSS groups, SCT at diagnosis maximized overall survival. The analysis focused only on full ablative conditioning regimens. Nevertheless, all patients with MDS who are reasonable transplant candidates based on age and comorbidity should undergo a formal consultation with transplantation specialist.

One clear advantage of allogeneic transplant in MDS, beyond the obvious benefit provided by the proffering of normal stem cells, is the powerful graft-versus-leukemia effect.[383] Evidence that neoplastic MDS cells are targets for killing by the graft emanates from data demonstrating a lower relapse after allogeneic, compared with syngeneic, transplants, the higher relapse rate after T-cell–depleted grafts, and mild graft-versus-host disease.[390] The apparent safety of unrelated matched transplants has improved recently due to the advent and routine use of molecular HLA typing.[391] Although allogeneic transplant seems an attractive option, a major problem remains the mortality associated with regimen-related toxicity and graft-versus-host disease, especially given the older age of the typical MDS patient. Use of nonmyeloablative or reduced-intensity conditioning, seeking to maximize the graft-versus-leukemia to toxicity ratio, is being used with increasing frequency.[381,392,393] Although it appears that reduced-intensity conditioning allogeneic transplantation can be accomplished with an acceptable short-term mortality rate in patients with MDS up to age 70 to 75 years, long-term data on efficacy are lacking.[394–396] Cord blood transplants could extend the availability of allogeneic transplantation to greater numbers of patients with MDS. This technique may prove feasible in older adults, especially if it is associated with an acceptable risk of graft-versus-host disease.[397,398]

CONCLUSION

Despite recent advances in therapy for MDS, the need for improvement is great. Almost all patients with MDS should be referred for a clinical trial. Treatment recommendations involving available approaches and agents can be derived for a given patient, but generally not without prolonged discussion between the physician and the patient and his or her family (Fig. 67–7). All patients younger than 70 years with high-risk disease according to the IPSS (intermediate-2 or high) and who have a related or unrelated matched donor should be considered for allogeneic BMT if feasible. Patients older than 55 years should consider reduced-intensity conditioning SCT, but the long-term efficacy data are lacking. Use of hypomethylating agents as a form of "cytoreduction" prior to SCT is being investigated. Patients with high-risk MDS who are not considered SCT candidates should initiate treatment with a hypomethylating agent such as azacytidine or decitabine. Patients with low-risk disease have many options. Patients with a chromosome 5q deletion or the 5q− syndrome who are RBC transfusion dependent should receive lenalidomide. Patients with low-risk disease who are RBC transfusion dependent and do not have a 5q abnormality have many options. If their serum Epo level is less than 500 mU/mL, they should be started on an ESA, either rh-Epo or darbepoetin. If this treatment fails, then addition of a myeloid growth factor, such as G-CSF, should be considered. ATG should be considered for treatment of hypoplastic MDS in patients younger than 60 years who have modest transfusion requirements, a recent diagnosis, and low blast count. Nonresponding patients with low-risk disease should consider lenalidomide if the goal is only an erythroid response, or a hypomethylating agent should be considered in patients with pancytopenia. Clinical trial participation should be considered for all patients, because this is the only way that we can try and make strides in improving the survival of patients with MDS.

SUGGESTED READINGS

Barabe F, Kennedy JA, Hope KJ and Dick JE: Modeling the initiation and progression of human acute leukemia in mice. Science 316:600, 2007.

Burnett AK, Milligan D, Prentice AG, et al: A comparison of low-dose cytarabine and hydroxyurea with or without all-trans retinoic acid for acute myeloid leukemia and high-risk myelodysplastic syndrome in patients not considered fit for intensive treatment. Cancer 109:1114, 2007.

Bussel JB, Cheng G, Saleh MN, et al: Eltrombopag for the treatment of chronic idiopathic thrombocytopenic purpura. N Engl J Med 357:2237, 2007.

DeAngelo DJ: Role of imatinib-sensitive tyrosine kinase in the pathogenesis of chronic myeloproliferative disorders. Semin Hematol 44:S17, 2007.

Girtovitis FI, Ntaios G, Papadopoulos A, et al: Defective platelet aggregation in myelodysplastic syndromes. Acta Haematol 118:117, 2007.

Haase D, Germing U, Schonz J, et al: New insights into the prognostic impact of the karyotype in MDS and correlation with subtypes: Evidence from a core dataset of 2124 patients. Blood 110:4385, 2007.

Hershman D, Neugut AI, Jacobson JS, et al: Acute myeloid leukemia or myelodysplastic syndrome following use of granulocyte colony-stimulating factors during breast cancer adjuvant chemotherapy. J Natl Cancer Inst 99:196, 2007.

Huff JD, Keung YK, Thakuri M, et al: Copper deficiency causes reversible myelodysplasia. Am J Hematol 82:625, 2007.

Jones PA, Baylin SB: The epigenomics of cancer. Cell 128:683, 2007.

Joslin JM, Fernald AA, Tennant TR, et al: Haploinsufficiency of EGR1, a candidate gene in the del(5q), leads to the development of myeloid disorders. Blood 110:719, 2007.

Kantarjian H, Giles F, List A, et al: The incidence and impact of thrombocytopenia in myelodysplastic syndromes. Cancer 109:1705, 2007.

Kantarjian H, Fenaux P, Sekeres MA, et al: Phase 1/2 study of AMG 531 in thrombocytopenic patients with low-risk myelodysplastic syndrome: Update including extended treatment. Blood 110:250a, 2007.

Kantarjian H, Oki Y, Garcia-Manero G, et al: Results of a randomized study of 3 schedules of low-dose decitabine in higher-risk myelodysplastic syndrome and chronic myelomonocytic leukemia. Blood 109:52, 2007.

Kouzarides T: SnapShot: Histone-modifying enzymes. Cell 131:822, 2007.

Kouzarides T: Chromatin modifications and their function. Cell 128:693, 2007.

Lancet JE, List AF, Moscinski LC: Treatment of deletion 5q acute myeloid leukemia with lenalidomide. Leukemia 21:586, 2007.

Liu TX, Becker MW, Jelinek J, et al: Chromosome 5q deletion and epigenetic suppression of the gene encoding alpha-catenin (CTNNA1) in myeloid cell transformation. Nat Med 13:78, 2007.

Ma X, Does M, Raza A, Mayne ST: Myelodysplastic syndromes: Incidence and survival in the United States. Cancer 109:1536, 2007.

Melchert M, Kale K, List A: The role of lenalidomide in the treatment of patients with chromosome 5q deletion and other myelodysplastic syndromes. Curr Opin Hematol 14:123, 2007.

Opel M, Lando D, Bonilla C, et al: Genome-wide studies of histone demethylation catalysed by the fission yeast homologues of mammalian LSD1. PLoS ONE 2:e386, 2007.

Phrommintikul A, Haas SJ, Elsik M, Krum H, et al: Mortality and target haemoglobin concentrations in anaemic patients with chronic kidney disease treated with erythropoietin: A meta-analysis. Lancet 369:381, 2007.

REFERENCES

For complete list of references log onto www.expertconsult.com

CHAPTER 68

THE POLYCYTHEMIAS

Ronald Hoffman, Mingjiang Xu, Guido Finazzi, and Tiziano Barbui

Under normal conditions, the red blood cell mass in humans is tightly controlled and remains relatively constant in a given individual.[1] The numbers of senescent red cells lost daily are replaced by newly formed ones by a carefully controlled network of growth factors and progenitor cells.[1–4] Erythropoiesis, which leads to a baseline production of red cells, can be augmented by a variety of stimuli that increase the delivery of oxygen to tissues. This delicate balance can be disturbed by various pathologic conditions and can result in either reduced numbers of red cells (anemia) or excessive numbers of red cells (polycythemia).[1–4] Hematocrit values over 52% in males and over 48% in females are abnormal and require further evaluation to determine the nature of a potential polycythemic disorder.[5] These polycythemic states can be caused by various disorders that can be accounted for by many different pathophysiologic mechanisms. Determination of the etiology of an individual's polycythemia is a critical step in defining the patient's appropriate prognosis and treatment plan. Primary polycythemias are the result of innate abnormalities involving hematopoietic progenitors and stem cells that lead to constitutive overproduction of red cells. By contrast, secondary polycythemias are the consequence of external factors such as erythropoietin (EPO), which act on normal progenitors to overproduce red cells.

ERYTHROPOIESIS

Red cell production can be influenced by numerous factors including nutrients, growth factors, numbers and function of marrow progenitor and precursor cells, as well as cellular receptors and transcription factors (see Chapters 21 and 25). The hematopoietic growth factor, EPO, is considered to be the physiologic regulator of the terminal phases of erythropoiesis.[1,2] Alterations in its production are followed by adjustments in the rate of formation of red blood cells.[1,2] In humans, EPO production is controlled by the relative supply of oxygen to the kidney, the major site of EPO.[1–3] In states of severe hypoxia, EPO production can be increased up to 1000-fold.[6] A large body of information is available addressing EPO physiology in patients with erythrocytosis.[1,2,7–12] Following phlebotomy of a healthy person, EPO excretion increases, and an inverse logarithmic relationship between hematocrit and EPO excretion rates is observed.[1] Patients with secondary erythrocytosis due to chronic hypoxia have either normal or increased basal values, but also have increased values following reduction of the hematocrit to normal levels by phlebotomy.[1] By contrast, EPO excretion is invariably subnormal in patients with polycythemia vera (PV), which demonstrates that this disorder is not a result of excessive EPO production.[1,8,12,13]

Different levels of EPO are required at the erythroid precursor and progenitor cell levels.[4] In addition, multipotent myeloid progenitors and primitive erythroid progenitors (burst-forming units–erythroid [BFU-E]), both of which ultimately contribute to erythropoiesis, require additional growth factors such as stem cell factor (SCF), interleukin 3 (IL-3), granulocyte–macrophage-colony stimulating factor (GM-CSF), or thrombopoietin (Tpo) to promote their proliferation and maturation (see Chapter 25).[4,14–16]

ERYTHROPOIETIN, OXYGEN SENSING, AND HYPOXIA-INDUCIBLE FACTOR

Under normal conditions, EPO production is mediated by the decreased oxygen content of hemoglobin within red cells, termed hypoxemia, which leads to decreased oxygen delivery to tissues.[4] Regulation of oxygen homeostasis is critical to survival. The acute reduction of the availability of oxygen leads to the initiation of a cascade of adaptive events occurring at the level of the organism, tissues, cells, and specific genes that sets in place compensatory events to correct the lack of oxygen supply. Low oxygen levels, hypoxia (60 mmHg), in humans result in oxygen-sensing cells within the glomus cells of the carotid body located in the carotid artery undergoing rapid membrane depolarization, leading to the production of action potentials, influx of calcium ions, and release of the neurotransmitter dopamine. These events result in an increase of the lung ventilation rate and restoration of normal oxygen tension to vital organs. Activation of the carotid body results in the sensation of breathlessness experienced by individuals at high altitudes.[17,18] The current candidates for oxygen sensors include the prolyl hydroxylase family of enzymes that require molecular oxygen for activity, the NAD(P)H oxidase family of enzymes that reduce reactive oxygen species and the electron transport systerm.[19] In response to chronic hypoxia, multiple compensatory mechanisms come into play in the kidney, the major site of EPO production.[2,20] Hypoxic stimulation results in production of hypoxia-inducible factor-1 (HIF-1), the major factor responsible for transcriptional activation of the *EPO* gene.[21] Analysis of proteins that bind to the EPO enhancer under hypoxic conditions led to the identification of HIF. The HIF transcriptional system is a master regulator of the hypoxic response controlling a large number of genes in multiple cell types. As key mediators of cellular oxygen maintenance, HIF-1 and HIF-2 facilitate body oxygen delivery and responses to oxygen deprivation by regulating the expression of gene products that are involved in cellular energy metabolism and glucose transport, angiogenesis, erythropoiesis and iron metabolism, pH regulation, apoptosis, cell proliferation, cell–cell and cell–matrix interactions. Classic HIF target genes include phosphoglycerate kinase, glucose transporter-1, vascular endothelial growth factor (VEGF) and EPO. The HIF proteins are members of the Per–ARNT–Sim family of heterodimeric basic helix–loop–helix transcription factors (Fig. 68–1).[22–32]

HIF-1α is continuously synthesized irrespective of oxygen availability. It is barely detectable in normal cells owing to rapid degradation via the ubiquitin proteasome pathway. During hypoxia, the rapid accumulation of HIF-1α is achieved by blocking its degradation, which permits an instantaneous response to hypoxia without activating the transcriptional/translational machinery.[22–32]

HIF-1 is composed of two subunits, HIF-1α and HIF-1β, that form a heterodimer (see Fig. 68–1).[32] In contrast to the constitutively expressed, HIF-1β subunits, HIF-1α is an oxygen-labile protein that becomes stabilized in response to hypoxia.[19] HIF-1α mRNA and protein levels are induced by hypoxia, and HIF-1α protein levels decay rapidly with return to normoxia. The posttranslational

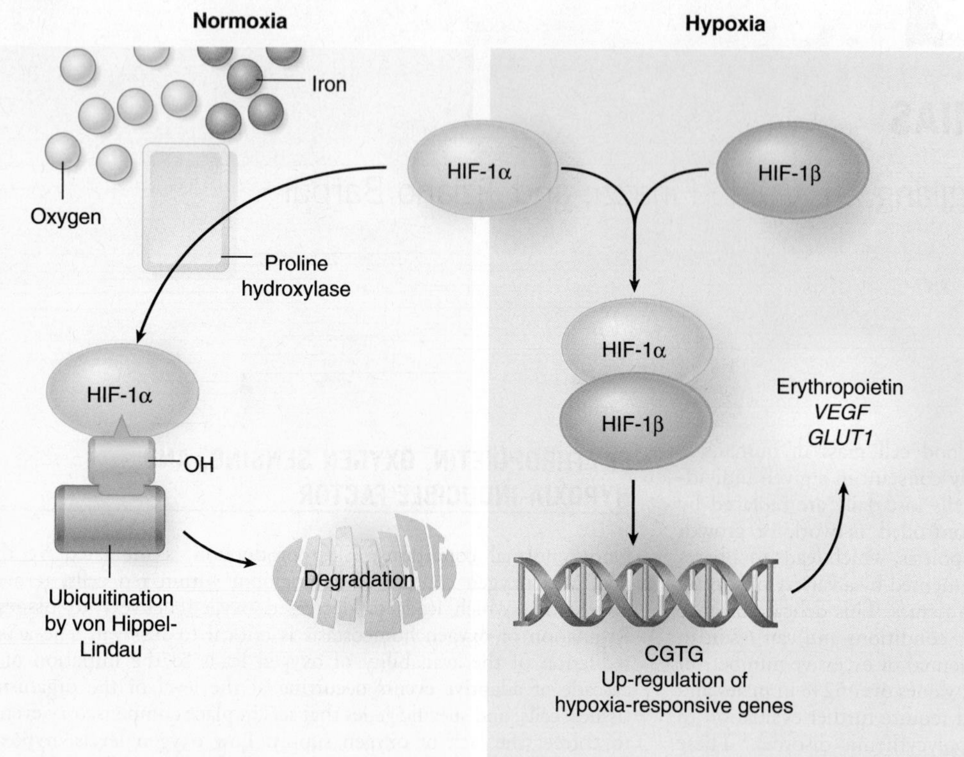

Figure 68–1. Schematic representation of the relationship between hypoxia sensing and erythropoietin production.

regulation of HIF-1α protein accounts for the majority of the regulation of this gene.[17] Normoxia-induced, ubiquitin-mediated degradation of the HIF-1α protein is the major regulator of HIF-1α levels,[33,34] thereby reducing the stimulus for additional EPO production (Fig. 68–1). The targeting and subsequent polyubiquitination of HIF-1α require the von Hippel–Lindau (VHL) protein, oxygen, and three different iron-requiring proline hydroxylase enzymes (Fig. 68–1). VHL protein targets HIF-1α for oxygen-dependent proteolysis[33–41] by a mechanism that involves the interaction of VHL protein with other proteins (Fig. 68–1). Different parts of the HIF-1α chains have different functions. The amino terminus part of HIF-1α is involved in DNA binding and dimerization while the carboxy terminus portion has regulatory functions. One domain at the carboxy terminus influences transcriptional activity without affecting HIF-1α protein levels while the other region termed the oxygen-dependent degradation domain (ODD) affects protein abundance. The ODD is divided into an amino terminus and a carboxy terminus subdomain. The ubiquitin proteasome pathway is responsible for the degradation of HIF-1α chains in the presence of oxygen.[38–41] The VHL protein physically interacts with the ODD of HIF-1α and the VHL protein is part of a multiprotein ubiquitin ligase capable of ubiquitinating HIF-1α subunits and targeting them for destruction by the proteasome. Iron-chelating drugs can also block the interaction of HIF-1α with the VHL protein, suggesting a role for iron in the degradation of HIF-1α.[38–41]

At least three prolyl hydroxylases (PHDs) have been found to hydroxylate HIF at unique proline residues and have been termed PHD-1, PHD-2, and PHD-3.[38–41] Under normoxic conditions, hydroxylation of HIF-1α at these different proline residues is essential for HIF proteolytic degradation by promoting interaction with the VHL tumor-suppressor protein through hydrogen bonding to the hydroxy proline-binding pocket in the VHL-β domain. As oxygen levels decrease, hydroxylation of HIF decreases, and HIF-1α then no longer binds VHL and becomes stabilized. The activity of PHDs depends on the availability of molecular oxygen, which qualifies these enzymes as oxygen sensors. In addition, these dioxygenases require 2-oxoglutarate as a cosubstrate and vitamin C to keep their central nonheme iron in the ferrous state. While PHD-2 appears to be the hydroxylase that is essential for HIF-1α degradation under normoxic conditions, PHD-3 is important for hydroxylation of HIF-1α during reoxygenation. Different effects of individual PHDs on HIF-1α and HIF-2α hydroxylation indicate that the stability of individual HIF-1α subunits and their target gene expression might be affected by tissue- and cell-type differences in PHD expression and activity levels. The activity of PHDs can be modulated by mitochondrial reactive oxygen species implicating mitochondria in oxygen sensing.[22]

Von Hippel–Lindau syndrome is a hereditary cancer syndrome that is associated with exaggerated responses to hypoxia due to post-translational abnormalities in HIF.[42] Von Hippel–Lindau syndrome is characterized by a propensity for developing clear cell renal carcinomas, retinal hemangioblastomas, cerebellar and spinal hemangiomas, pancreatic and renal cysts, islet cell tumors of the pancreas, and pheochromocytomas. The tumors result from somatic mutations that cause a loss of heterozygosity of the *VHL* gene.[42] VHL disease affects approximately 1 in 35,000 individuals and is transmitted in an autosomal dominant manner. Individuals with VHL disease carry one wild-type VHL allele and one inactivated VHL allele. This inactivation can occur by somatic mutation or hypermethylation. Tumor or cyst development is linked to somatic inactivation or loss of the remaining wild-type VHL allele. Approximately 20% to 37% of VHL patients have large or partial germline deletions, 23% to 27% have nonsense or frame-shift mutations, and 30% to 35% have missense mutations. More than 150 different VHL mutations linked to VHL disease have been reported. The tumors linked to VHL inactivation are often highly vascular and can produce angiogenic factors such as VEGF. In addition, renal cell carcinoma, cerebellar hemangioblastomas, and pheochromocytomas have been associated with paraneoplastic erythrocytosis due to overproduction of EPO.[42] Overproduction of HIF-inducible mRNAs is the hallmark of VHL protein defective cells. Genotype–phenotype correlates in VHL disease suggest that VHL has functions independent of HIF regulation that might play a role in tumor formation. VHL protein has other binding partners, including atypical protein kinase C and a family of deubiquitinating enzymes named VHL-interacting deubiquitinating enzymes 1 and 2. In addition, pVHL has been involved in numerous cellular processes, including regulation of extracellular matrix,

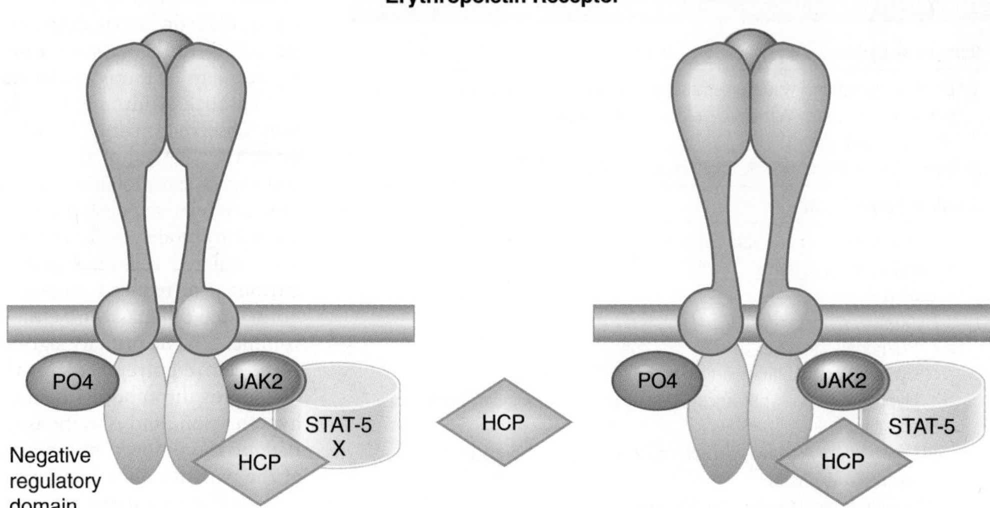

Figure 68–2. Schematic representation of the erythropoietin receptor and the defect in the receptor underlying primary familial and congenital polycythemia. HCP, hematopoietic cell phosphatase.

cytoskeleton stability, cell cycle control, and differentiation.[42] Although VHL disease is not associated with erythrocytosis, Richard and coworkers have recently observed the development of paradoxical polycythemia in three patients with VHL syndrome and central nervous system or retinal hemangioblastomas treated with the VEGF receptor inhibitor SU5416. The cause of these phenomena remains unknown.[43]

THE ERYTHROPOIETIN RECEPTOR

Interaction of EPO with the erythropoietin receptor (EPOR) present on the erythroid progenitor and precursor cells leads to its homodimerization, resulting in (a) stimulation of cell division, (b) differentiation by induction of erythroid-specific gene expression, and (c) prevention of erythroid progenitor and precursor cell apoptosis.[44,45] The cytoplasmic portion of the EPOR contains a positive regulatory domain that interacts with JAK2 (Fig. 68–2).[46,47] Immediately after EPO binding, JAK2 phosphorylates itself, the EPOR, and other proteins such as STAT5. This JAK2/STAT5 signaling plays an essential role in EPO/EPOR-mediated regulation of erythropoiesis.[46]

The C-terminal cytoplasmic portion of the EPOR also possesses a negative regulatory domain.[48] Hematopoietic cell phosphatase (HCP, also known as SHP-1 or PTP N6) interacts with this portion of the EPOR and downregulates signal transduction[48] by promoting dephosphorylation (see Fig. 68–2). Inactivation of the HCP-binding site leads to prolonged phosphorylation of JAK2/STAT5.[48,49] Another negative regulator of erythropoiesis, suppressor of cytokine signaling-3 (SOCS-3), binds to the cytoplasmic portion of the EPOR and suppresses EPO-dependent JAK2/STAT5 signaling.[50] Thus, deletion of the distal C-terminal cytoplasmic portion of the EPOR abolishes negative regulatory elements and results in increased proliferation of erythroid progenitor cells. Mutations in the *EPOR* gene have been observed in some patients with primary familial and congenital polycythemia (PFCP)[51–55] and are occasionally found in erythroleukemia (Fig. 68–2).[56] PV is not caused by mutations in EPOR.[57] Such secondary growth factors as insulin-like growth factor-1 (IGF-1) and the components of the renin–angiotensin system may also influence the production of red cells.

THE RENIN–ANGIOTENSIN SYSTEM AND HEMATOPOIESIS

The renin–angiotensin system (RAS) regulates fluid and electrolyte homeostasis and blood pressure[58–60] and has been hypothesized to also play a role in the regulation of erythropoiesis. The primary function of angiotensin during development is the regulation of tissue growth and differentiation.[58] Angiotensin II (AngII) is a ligand for two distinct receptors, type 1 and type 2 (AT1 and AT2). AT1 appears to play a major role in the regulation of cell proliferation.[59,60]

The RAS was first postulated to influence erythropoiesis in the 1980s after it was discovered that the use of angiotensin-converting enzyme (ACE) inhibitors to treat hypertension could result in anemia.[61] In animals, increased blood levels of renin (a major regulator of AngII synthesis) were found to result in elevated serum EPO levels and erythrocytosis.[62–64] In humans, the infusion of AngII also increases serum EPO levels.[65,66] The pathway underlying AngII-driven EPO secretion is unknown. However, some investigators have suggested that AngII modulates renal EPO production through changes in renal perfusion and sodium reabsorption.[20] This hypothesis is based on the presumption that reduced oxygen pressure in the kidneys triggers HIF-1α to induce release of EPO.[32] AngII also directly stimulates proliferation of hematopoietic progenitors in vitro,[67,68] and inhibition of this effect with ACE inhibitors induces apoptosis of erythroid progenitors in renal transplantation patients.[69] Mice with a knockout of the angiotensin-converting enzyme-1 (ACE-1) develop a normocytic anemia that can be fully reversed by infusion of AngII.[70] ACE-related anemia is most pronounced in patients with renal insufficiency or end-stage renal disease and in patients who have received a renal allograft.[71] The pathogenesis of this anemia is not clear, but reduced levels of circulating EPO are not solely responsible, suggesting that there might be other contributing factors. The AT1 receptor is present on erythroid progenitors, and its ligand, AngII, augments EPO stimulation of erythropoiesis.[72] The involvement of JAK2 kinase in AngII signaling suggests that this signal transduction pathway mediated by EPO and AngII might overlap.[73] Postrenal transplant erythrocytosis likely can be accounted by activation of the renin–angiotensin system.[72]

DEFINITION AND CLASSIFICATION OF POLYCYTHEMIA

The term *polycythemia* is a literal translation from Greek, meaning "too many cells in the blood," and refers to an increase in the red cell mass[12]; it is frequently used interchangeably with the term *erythrocytosis*. Polycythemia may be due to a myriad of causes (Table 68–1).[12,74,75] The polycythemias can be classified as relative and absolute.[12,74,75] Relative polycythemia is a disorder in which the patient characteristically has a modest elevation of the hematocrit level without an elevated red cell mass but rather due to contraction of the plasma volume, whereas the absolute polycythemias are accompanied by an actual increase in the circulating red cell mass.[74,76] Polycythemias can also be classified according to the responsiveness of their erythroid progenitor cells to growth factors or the circulating

Table 68–1 Differential Diagnosis of the Polycythemias

Relative or Spurious Polycythemia
1. Decreased plasma volume—reduced fluid intake, marked loss of body fluids (diaphoresis, vomiting, diarrhea, "third-spacing")
2. Gaisböck syndrome
3. Overfilling of blood in collection vacuum tubes
Absolute Polycythemia
1. Primary congenital and familial polycythemia
2. Secondary polycythemia
Acquired
Hypoxia
Pulmonary disease
Cyanotic congenital heart disease
Hypoventilation syndromes—sleep apnea, Pickwickian syndrome
High altitude
Smokers' polycythemia, carbon monoxide intoxication due to industrial exposure
Postrenal transplantation erythrocytosis
Aberrant erythropoietin production
Tumors—renal cell carcinoma, Wilms tumor, hepatic carcinoma, uterine leiomyomata, virilizing ovarian tumors, vascular cerebellar tumors
Miscellaneous renal and hepatic disorders—solitary renal cysts, polycystic kidney disease, renal artery stenosis hydronephrosis, viral hepatitis
Endocrine disorders—Cushing's syndrome, primary aldosteronism
Androgen use
Erythropoietin use
Congenital
Abnormal high-affinity hemoglobin variants
Biphosphoglycerate deficiency
Congenital methemoglobinemia
Chuvash polycythemia (von Hippel–Lindau mutations)
Prolyl hydroxylase mutations
3. Polycythemia vera

levels of such growth factors. Primary polycythemias are characterized by increased sensitivity of the erythroid progenitors to regulatory growth factors, as a result of acquired somatic or inherited germline mutations expressed by hematopoietic progenitor cells.[77,78] In contrast, secondary polycythemias are characterized by an increase in regulatory growth factors, primarily EPO, and normal responsiveness of their erythroid progenitors to these growth factors.[75,77,78] These conditions can usually be distinguished by in vitro assays of erythroid progenitor cells, quantitation of serum EPO levels, and detection of somatic JAK2 mutations.[79–83]

RELATIVE POLYCYTHEMIA

Individuals with a modestly increased venous hematocrit level that is not accompanied by an increased red cell mass are frequently thought to be polycythemic by imprecise yet widely accepted medical practice. Frequently these individuals are thought to be polycythemic owing to the lack of appreciation by a clinician of what constitutes the upper limit of normal values for a hematocrit (52% in males and 48% in females). Such individuals frequently prove not to have an absolute polycythemia as defined by an actual increase in the measured red cell mass. *Relative* or *spurious polycythemia* is a term used to describe an elevation of the hematocrit level due either to an acute transient state of hemoconcentration associated with intravascular fluid depletion or a chronic sustained relative polycythemia due to contraction of the plasma volume.[74–76]

Transient polycythemias may be a result of acute depletion of the plasma volume from a variety of disorders, including protracted vomiting or diarrhea, plasma loss from external burns, sudden cold exposure or protracted exercise, insensible fluid loss due to fever, sepsis, diabetic ketoacidosis, or acute ethanol intoxication.[74–76] These elevations of hematocrit can be easily corrected by appropriate replacement of intravascular fluids.

Gaisböck syndrome, first described in 1905,[84] is a benign condition observed mainly in obese, hypertensive, middle-aged, male smokers.[73–77] Alcohol, diuretics, obesity, hypoxia, psychological stress, and excess catecholamine secretion have been identified as possible causes of relative polycythemia.[85] Such individuals can have a chronic modest to moderate elevation of the hematocrit level associated with a normal red cell mass and low plasma volume, which has been attributed to reduced venous compliance,[86] or they can have a high normal red cell mass with either a normal or slightly decreased plasma volume.[74,76] The primary significance of the identification of a patient with relative polycythemia is the recognition of the increased risk of developing thrombotic vascular events likely due to excessive smoking, hypertension, and obesity associated with this disease. The optimal therapy is unknown, but treatment is generally directed at correction of the patient's underlying cardiovascular risk factors.

It is also important to emphasize that overfilling of blood collection vacuum tubes can result in pseudopolycythemia, pseudothrombocytopenia, and pseudoleukopenia as a result of inadequate sample mixing.[87] Careful attention to such a seemingly trivial detail can help avoid expensive, unnecessary diagnostic workups.

ABSOLUTE POLYCYTHEMIAS

Primary Familial and Congenital Polycythemia

PFCP is an autosomal dominant disorder.[53–57,89–95] Although PFCP is uncommon, it is more prevalent than polycythemia due to high-oxygen-affinity hemoglobin mutants or a 2,3-biphosphoglycerate deficiency.[92] Unlike patients with PV, patients with PFCP lack splenomegaly and do not progress to acute leukemia. It is not unusual for these patients to present with headaches, which resolve with normalization of the hematocrit level. An increased incidence of cardiovascular events has been reported in affected members.[89] Characteristic laboratory findings are (a) an increased red blood cell mass without increased leukocyte or platelet counts, (b) no activating mutation of JAK2, (c) a normal hemoglobin–oxygen dissociation curve, (d) low serum EPO levels, and (e) in vitro hypersensitivity of erythroid progenitors to EPO.[53–57,79–83,87–94] Even though PFCP is present at birth, many affected patients are incidentally diagnosed later in life following the performance of routine blood counts, or when evaluated in the context of multiple family members having polycythemia. It is of interest that one individual so affected was an accomplished cross-country skier who had won medals at the Olympic games.[88]

To date, 12 mutations of the EPOR associated with PFCP have been described. Nine of the 12 result in truncation of the EPOR cytoplasmic carboxyl terminal (see Fig. 68–2) and are the only mutations convincingly linked with PFCP.[44] Such abnormalities lead to a loss in the negative regulatory domain of the EPOR. Three missense EPOR mutations have also been described, but these have not been linked to PFCP or any other disease phenotype.[56]

The physiologic basis for EPO-mediated activation of erythropoiesis is as follows: EPO activates its receptor by conformational changes of its dimers, leading to initiation of an erythroid-specific cascade of events. The first signal is initiated by the binding of a tyrosine kinase to the EPOR and its phosphorylation and activation of a transcription factor, STAT5, which regulates erythroid-specific genes.[44] This "on" signal is negated by dephosphorylation of the EPOR by HCP, that is, the "off" signal.[53,54] Truncation of the EPOR leads to a loss in the negative regulatory domain of the EPOR, a binding site for HCP, leading to a gain-of-function mutation of the EPOR (see Fig. 68–2). A mouse bearing a normal human EPOR and a mutant, disease-causing human EPOR has been created by flox/cre (gene replacement) technology.[96] This mouse model, with its potential for tissue-specific deletion and augmentation of EPO signaling, should help better understand the role of EPO signaling in other tissues such as the brain and endothelial cells. Recently an alternative explanation for the increased sensitivity of erythroid progenitors to EPO of patients with PFCP has been provided by Meyer and coworkers.[97] These investigators showed that EPOR downregulation provides another mechanism by which EPO desensitization can occur. EPOR downregulation is a complex process that involves EPOR ubiquitination and degradation by proteasomes. This degradation process removes all of the phosphorylated tyrosine residues in the intracellular domain of the receptor, thereby preventing further signal transduction. The remaining part of the EPO–EPOR complex is then internalized and degraded by lysosymes. Meyer and coworkers reported that the E3 ligase B-transducin repeat containing protein-1 (B-Trcp-1) is responsible for EPOR ubiquitination and degradation. Mutations of the B-Trcp abolish EPOR ubiquitination and degradation, making BaF3 cells expressing the EPORs hypersensitive to EPO. Each of the PFCP mutations involving the EPOR results in the loss of the binding site for B-Trcp-1. These findings suggest that the EPO hypersensitivity in PFCP might also be in some cases due to increased EPOR activity occurring as a consequence of diminished ubiquitination and degradation of the EPO–EPOR complex.[97]

The effect of a truncated EPOR is not always predictable. Some patients who inherit an EPOR mutation are not polycythemic.[98] This observation suggests that undefined environmental or genetic factors may mask the development of polycythemia. Also, the heterogeneity of the polycythemic phenotype observed in a PFCP animal model[96] appears to be strain dependent. This indicates that gene modifiers or epigenetic factors may mask the development of the full PFCP phenotype.

Mutations of genes encoding proteins other than the EPOR account for most cases of PFCP. Mutations of the EPOR were found in only 10% to 20% of subjects with PFCP.[45] Additional disease-causing genes and their mutations have yet to be identified.[99]

SECONDARY POLYCYTHEMIAS

Secondary polycythemias can be either congenital or acquired. Conditions leading to hypoxia, such as high altitude, cyanotic heart disease, or chronic lung disease, may result in physiologic polycythemia mediated by increased levels of EPO.[12,75] There are marked variations in EPO levels and the subsequent erythroid response in the face of chronic hypoxia,[78,100–103] suggesting that some of these factors may be genetically determined. The same degree of renal tissue hypoxia may induce substantially different EPO production in response to high altitude.[100–103] It is likely that these individual variations are a function of genetic differences in hypoxia sensing and the hypoxia response pathways; the exact mechanism remains to be clarified. For purposes of simplicity and clinical diagnostic usefulness, the secondary polycythemic disorders are divided into those that are acquired and those that are congenital. It should be kept in mind that this division, although useful for differential diagnosis, is artificial. Patients with inherited germline mutations, for instance, can develop an EPO-secreting pheochromocytoma or renal cell cancer, whereas a patient with PV can smoke and have chronic obstructive pulmonary disease. In other instances, polycythemia due to a germline mutation can be masked by an acquired environmental factor or another gene-modifying mutation.[98]

Acquired Secondary Polycythemias

Polycythemias of Cyanotic Heart Disease and Pulmonary Disease

Patients with cyanotic heart disease and pulmonary disease frequently suffer from arterial hypoxemia leading to increased production of EPO and polycythemia. Excessive EPO production occurs when the Pao_2 is sustained below 67 mmHg as a result of severely impaired pulmonary mechanics.[75] Because patients with severe pulmonary disease and secondary erythrocytosis frequently have elevated plasma volumes, the degree of elevation of the hematocrit level may be modest. Hematocrit levels as high as 65% or rarely 75% have, however, been reported.[75]

Why some patients with pulmonary disease and congenital heart disease develop polycythemia whereas others do not is not clear. Increased oxygen-carrying capacity may improve oxygen delivery; however, it is not obvious at what hematocrit level the resultant elevation in blood viscosity impairs blood flow to the tissues, leading to a reduction in oxygen uptake. In addition, oxygen uptake to the tissues is markedly influenced by whole blood volume. Thus, whereas the optimal hematocrit level for oxygen delivery is about 45% in normovolemic subjects, it rises to over 60% in hypervolemic states,[104,105] likely as a result of engorgement of the vascular bed and a decrease in peripheral resistance. Furthermore, chronic exposure to hypoxia leads to respiratory alkalosis that, in turn, promotes the synthesis of 2,3-bisphosphoglycerate (2,3-BPG), facilitating increased oxygen delivery to tissues.[92]

The practical relevance of an elevated hematocrit level in this clinical situation is whether and at what level it is harmful or beneficial. The seminal studies of Winslow and colleagues have suggested that an extremely elevated hematocrit level might be detrimental to optimal oxygen delivery.[107] They showed that isovolemic hemodilution of the hematocrit in Andean natives led to a general improvement in symptoms, which correlated well with an increased anaerobic threshold and improved mixed venous oxygen saturation during exercise.[107] Although this careful study influenced the understanding of the relationship between an increased hemoglobin concentration and oxygen delivery, it is a single uncontrolled observation and must therefore be interpreted with caution. It is unfortunate that clinical observations regarding the optimal hematocrit level for the treatment of PV have been frequently applied to other polycythemic states. Although it is widely accepted that erythrocytotic pediatric patients with cyanotic heart disease are at an increased risk for developing cerebral vascular accidents, the literature provides conflicting data as relates to the prevalence of such events among adults. Engelfriet et al reported a 10% prevalence of stroke and transient ischemic attacks in a cohort of adult patients with cyanotic heart disease, and Anmash et al reported a 13.6% prevalence of a history of stroke in a similar adult patient population.[105,109] By contrast, Perloff followed a group of 124 patients for over 6.1 years and did not document any strokes.[110]

The major cause of the thrombotic tendency in patients with erythrocytosis and cyanotic congenital heart disease is hyperviscosity due to extreme erythrocytosis and sludging within the microcirculation.[111,112] Iron deficiency occurs in over 30% because of the total depletion of iron stores to support erythropoiesis. Microcytic iron-deficient red cells are less deformable, and therefore further elevate blood viscosity. Evidence of hyperviscosity producing cerebral perfusion abnormalities not resulting from an overt thrombosis may also lead to such symptoms as headache, sluggish mentation, dizziness, blurry vision, muscle weakness, or paresthesias caused by reduced tissue perfusion.

The treatment of hyperviscosity secondary to erythrocytosis in cyanotic heart disease is controversial. Phlebotomy among select patients has been shown to improve cerebral blood flow and neurological symptoms and increase exercise capacity. To date there are no studies that define the optimal target hematocrit level to be achieved with phlebotomy of such a patient.[111,112]

The optimal target hematocrit level is likely to vary for each patient depending on the level of shunting and cardiac output. Phlebotomy based on symptoms may presently be the only practical approach.[111] Phlebotomy must be followed by the infusion of an equal volume of fluids to maintain intravascular volume and blood flow as well as to provide a dilutional effect to reduce the hematocrit level.[111,112] Perloff et al recommended a 1 : 1 replacement with 0.9% normal saline whereas Rosenthal suggested replacing the volume of blood removed with 1 : 1 fresh frozen plasma infused over 30 to 60 minutes. Hydroxyurea therapy has been used occasionally to reduce erythropoiesis in this situation to avoid inducing iron deficiency.[110,113]

The superiority of hydroxyurea therapy versus phlebotomy therapy has not been documented.[111,112]

Large studies of patients with Eisenmenger syndrome[114] and other patients with cyanotic heart disease[114] provide little evidence for the routine use of phlebotomy for the treatment of an asymptomatic patient. These elevations in hematocrit levels cannot, however, be totally ignored. The Framingham Study demonstrated a close correlation between a hematocrit greater than 51% and the risk for stroke.[115] Furthermore, in patients with cyanotic congenital heart disease with hematocrit levels over 80%, cerebral and pulmonary thrombotic events have been shown to correlate with the degree of elevation of the hematocrit level.[110,116] It is unlikely that the degree of hematocrit level elevation is the only factor contributing to this thrombotic tendency. Shibata and colleagues have generated transgenic mice with hematocrit levels greater than 85% due to overexpression of human EPO in an oxygen-independent manner.[117] These animals did not experience thromboembolic complications in any organs at any age. Therefore, factors beyond erythrocytosis likely contribute to the biogenesis of thromboembolism in these mice as well as in humans with polycythemia. The surprising absence of thrombosis in these mice with extreme erythrocytosis has been attributed to poor clot formation due to mechanical interference by the numerous red cells present, reduction in peripheral-blood platelet counts, and reduction of the activity of both the extrinsic and intrinsic coagulation pathways.[117] Similar coagulation abnormalities have been observed in patients with cyanotic congenital heart disease and were believed to be due to hepatic dysfunction from congestive cardiac failure or a chronic disseminated coagulopathy.[118]

Chronic oxygen therapy in patients with severe chronic obstructive pulmonary disease has resulted in relief of hypoxia and a modest reduction in hematocrit levels. Phlebotomy is a more efficient method of reducing the red cell mass.[111,112,119] On the basis of these considerations and the clinical experience with polycythemic conditions of diverse causes, we recommend that only those patients with polycythemia due to cyanotic congenital heart disease or pulmonary disease who develop symptoms that might be attributed to increased whole blood hyperviscosity (difficulty concentrating, headaches, general malaise) undergo a trial of isovolemic phlebotomy. The physician should always be guided by the patient's report of or lack of subjective improvement in well-being immediately following phlebotomy. To avoid problems associated with large-volume phlebotomies, relatively small quantities of blood should be removed repeatedly and colloids or fresh frozen plasma should be infused.[111,112,119]

Obstructive Sleep Apnea-Induced Polycythemia

Obstructive sleep apnea syndrome is characterized by repetitive episodes of partial or complete obstruction of airflow during sleep. Common symptoms include loud snoring and breathing pauses observed by a bed partner, feelings of nonrefreshing sleep, and excess daytime sleeping. Although the evidence is largely anecdotal,[120] secondary polycythemia is a widely recognized complication of long-standing sleep apnea, being found in 5% to 10% of those with nocturnal apnea and hypopnea.[121] Similarly, 25% of those with unexplained polycythemia are subsequently found to have sleep apnea.[122] The mechanism by which sleep apnea causes polycythemia is unclear. McKeon and coworkers found no differences in EPO levels between normoxic and hypoxemic patients referred for suspected sleep apnea.[123] In a later study, Carlson and coworkers also were unable to find any statistically significant differences in EPO levels between sleep apnea patients with and without polycythemia and age- and gender-matched healthy controls.[121] Obstructive sleep apnea is also associated with an increased risk for developing cardiovascular diseases, including systemic hypertension, pulmonary hypertension, cardiac arrhythmias, atherosclerosis, ischemic heart disease, and stroke. Intermittent hypoxia is thought to be a major cause of cardiovascular complications. These patients undergo repeated episodes of hypoxia and normoxia. The hypoxia leads to ischemia and the reoxygenation causes a sudden increase of oxygen. This reoxygenation phase results in the production of reactive oxygen species and the promotion of oxidative stress, leading to an inflammatory response and the development of vascular complications.[124]

Conversely, PV may induce central sleep apnea by decreasing cerebral blood flow to diencephalic respiratory centers, and patients so affected can have complete resolution of their sleep disorder when appropriately phlebotomized.[125]

Pickwickian Syndrome and Polycythemia

Pickwickian syndrome or obesity-hypoventilation syndrome, seen in morbidly obese individuals, is characterized by chronic hypoxemia and hypercapnia due to alveolar hypoventilation, with a resultant increase in EPO production, polycythemia, and cor pulmonale.[75] The three principal causes are the high cost of the work of respiration in morbidly obese individuals, dysfunction of the respiratory centers, and repeated episodes of nocturnal obstructive apnea.[126] Effective treatments include surgically induced weight loss,[127] nasal continuous positive airway pressure ventilation,[128] and the respiratory stimulant medroxyprogesterone acetate.[124]

Polycythemia Due to High Altitude

Polycythemia due to the hypoxic conditions encountered by high-altitude dwellers would appear at first glance to represent a universal adaptive process to altitude. High altitude results in hyperventilation, alkalosis, and shifting of the O_2 dissociation curve to the left, which leads to the impaired release of O_2 from hemoglobin and ultimately tissue hypoxia.[75,130–132] This tissue hypoxia results in markedly increased EPO production, leading to increased plasma iron turnover, reticulocytosis, and a rising hematocrit level. Residents of the Andes Mountains who live 4200 m above sea level frequently have 30% higher hematocrit levels than individuals living at sea level.[75,130–134]

People native to high altitude (highlanders) live in a hypobaric hypoxic environment characterized by a low ambient partial pressure of oxygen. In response to this environment they develop alveolar hypoxia, hypoxemia, and polycythemia.[130–134] Healthy highlanders develop pulmonary hypertension, right ventricular hypertrophy, and an increased amount of smooth muscle cells in the distal pulmonary arterial branches, which leads to increased pulmonary vascular resistance and pulmonary artery pressure as compared to individuals living at sea level. The importance of these structural changes in the pulmonary vasculature in highlanders is confirmed by the slow decline of pulmonary artery pressure, which is normalized after living for 2 years at sea level.[130–134] Despite these adaptive changes, healthy highlanders are able to perform physical activities similar to or often even more strenuous than those living at sea level. In fact, there are differences in ventilation rates between athletes performing at sea level and those at high altitudes.[134] Ventilation rates of athletes increase normally during exercise at sea level, whereas relative hypoventilation occurs in highlanders. This relative hypoventilation is characteristic of Andean natives and has been ascribed to desensitization of the carotid bodies to the hypoxic stimulus.[134] The erythrocytosis observed in individuals who reside at high altitudes for relatively short periods of time (days) can also be attributed in part to excessive water loss and contraction of the plasma volume. Total acclimatization of an individual who moves from sea level to a high altitude may actually require years. Individuals who reside at sea level and are acutely exposed to high altitudes are at increased risks of developing deep venous thrombosis, pulmonary infarction, retinal hemorrhage, and ischemic digits due to increased blood viscosity.[75] High-altitude climbers frequently combat these problems by intravenous administration of isotonic saline, with considerable success.[75]

The chronic responses of various ethnic and racial groups to high altitudes are quite variable. Andean natives, known as the Quechua and Ayamara Indians, experience a gradual increase in their hemoglobin levels with age.[133] In addition, hemoglobin values are almost

10% higher in those living at 5500 m above sea level than in those living at 4355 m above sea level.[133] Curiously, their Tibetan and Ethiopian counterparts living at similar altitudes do not respond to the resultant chronic hypoxia by increasing their hematocrits.[136–140] It has been suggested that high levels of nitrous oxide in the exhaled breath of Tibetans may improve oxygen delivery by inducing vasodilatation and increasing blood flow to tissues, thus making the compensatory increased red cell volume unnecessary.[141] Interestingly, Tibetans and Ethiopians have lived much longer as mountain dwellers than the Quechua or Ayamara Indians, suggesting that extreme elevation of the red cell mass is a maladaptation that Tibetans and Ethiopians have avoided by adopting more physiologic compensatory mechanisms. The molecular basis of these adaptive responses is unknown. Other factors can contribute to the development of erythrocytosis in high-altitude dwellers. Many inhabitants of the mining community of Cerro de Pasco (altitude 4280 m) with excessive erythrocytosis (mean hematocrit 76%, range 66%–91%) have been shown to have toxic serum cobalt levels,[142] suggesting that other EPO-promoting factors such as cobalt might augment the hypoxia-inducing effect on EPO causing the extreme polycythemias.

This individual variability of elevation of serum EPO levels in high-altitude dwellers and the resultant increase in red cell mass appears widespread. For example, acclimatization to moderately high altitudes when combined with low-altitude training (so-called living high, training low) improves sea-level performance in endurance athletes, in part because of the erythropoietic effects of altitude exposure.[102,139,146] This substantial individual variability in response to all forms of altitude training correlates with improved athletic performance and with elevation of EPO levels.[101,143,144] A large component of this individual variability appears to be related to differences in the peak and rate of decay of the increase in EPO in response to altitude exposure.[86] These observations suggest that there are genetically determined variables accounting for individual responses to hypoxia that are different from the EPO-mediated increase of red cell mass.[87] Polymorphisms of candidate genes involved in oxygen sensing and erythropoiesis were examined to detect the genetic variants of response to hypoxia. No evidence of an association between the candidate genes and severe polycythemia were, however, observed.[145]

Chronic mountain sickness (CMS) is a pathological loss of adaptation to altitude by highlanders. CMS is a clinical syndrome that occurs in native or lifelong residents living above 2500 m.[137–140] Anecdotal reports of particularly susceptible families or people to CMS are frequently cited as evidence that certain individuals have an innate susceptibility to develop CMS.[103] It is characterized by excessive erythrocytosis (females, Hb > 19 g/dL; males, Hb > 21 g/dL), severe hypoxemia, and in some cases moderate or severe pulmonary hypertension that may lead to the development of cor pulmonale and congestive heart failure. The clinical picture of CMS gradually disappears after descending to lower altitudes and reappears after returning to high altitude.[75,130–132] The prevalence of CMS is higher in men than women and increases with altitude, aging, associated lung disease, history of smoking, and air pollution. CMS is a public health problem in populations of mountainous regions of the world living above 2500 m.[75,130–132] In China alone, 80 million people live above that altitude, whereas in South America, 35 million people live above 2500 m. CMS is a common problem in these areas. Bolivian investigators have reported a prevalence of CMS in 6% to 8% of males in La Paz (3600 m) and a hospital frequency of 28%.[130–132] Chinese investigators have reported an overall prevalence of 5.6% in Chinese Han immigrants and 1.2% in Tibetan natives living in the Qinghai Tibetan plateau. The major mechanism underlying the development of CMS is relative alveolar hypoventilation.[130–132] Healthy highlanders characteristically hyperventilate. A gradual decline in the rate of alveolar ventilation in these individuals leads to progressive loss of adaptation to chronic hypoxia and the development of CMS.[146] The main components of this syndrome include (a) alveolar hypoventilation leading to relative hypercapnia and increasing hypoxemia; (b) excessive polycythemia leading to increased blood viscosity and expansion of the total lung blood volume; (c) pulmonary hypertension and right ventricular hypertrophy that may evolve to hypoxic cor pulmonale and heart failure; and (d) neuropsychiatric symptoms, including sleep disorders, headache, dizziness, and mental fatigue.[146] Physical examination reveals cyanosis of the nail beds, ears, and lips in contrast to the ruddy color that is characteristic of a healthy highlander. In some cases the face is almost black and the mucosa and conjunctiva are dark red. The fingers are frequently clubbed and auscultation of the heart reveals an increased pulmonary second sound.[130–132,140] The patients are frequently hypertensive and have evidence of heart failure. Chest x-ray and electrocardiographic findings are characteristic of right atrial and right ventricular hypertrophy. The cardiac hemodynamic values of patients with CMS and healthy highlanders and those living at sea level are shown in Table 68–2.[130] Criteria for the diagnosis of CMS have been recently published and are useful in identifying CMS patients as well as monitoring their response to treatment.[131]

The definitive treatment for CMS is descent to lower altitudes or sea level. The degree of polycythemia decreases after a few weeks or months and eventually the hematocrit level returns to sea-level values. Pulmonary hypertension and right ventricular hypertrophy gradually resolve and disappear after 1 to 2 years of living at sea level.[130–132] Phlebotomy or isovolemic hemodilution can reduce the excessive erythrocytosis and hyperviscosity. A variety of drugs has also been evaluated for the treatment of patients with CMS. Ten weeks of the respiratory stimulant medroxyprogesterone acetate at doses of 60 mg/d led to a reduction of the hematocrit level from 60% to 52% and an increase in arterial oxygen saturation from 84% to 90% in 17 highlanders with excess erythrocytes.[147,148] Medroxyprogesterone use however was associated with a loss of libido in males and therefore is infrequently used in this population.[147,148] Therapy with almitrine, a respiratory stimulant, or enalaprial, an ACE inhibitor (10 mg/d for 30 days), has resulted in even more modest reductions of hematocrit levels.[149] Acetazolamide therapy has been evaluated in a small double-blind, placebo-controlled, randomized clinical trial of patients with CMS.[150] Acetazolamide is an inhibitor of carbonic anhydrase and stimulates ventilation by promoting the development of metabolic acidosis. Furthermore, acetazolamide reduces renal EPO production. Patients with CMS were randomized to receive placebo or acetazolamide therapy at a dose of 250 or 500 mg/d for 21 days. Drug therapy at both doses of acetazolamide resulted in reduction of hematocrit levels by 7% ($P < 0.001$) and serum EPO levels by 50% to 67% ($P < 0.1$), with an increase in nocturnal oxygen saturation levels of 5% ($P < 0.01$).[150] According to this small study, 250 mg of acetazolamide daily appears to be an inexpensive, nontoxic, effective therapy for CMS.[150] Whether this conclusion can be validated by larger clinical trials and can be implemented successfully in large populations of patients with CMS has yet to be determined.

Smokers' Polycythemia or Carbon Monoxide-Induced Polycythemia

Smoking is the most common cause of secondary polycythemia.[75,151–154] Those affected have a carboxyhemoglobin-induced increase in red cell mass or decrease in plasma volume,[122–124] either of which is reversible with smoking cessation. Excessive carbon monoxide exposure can also be attributed to exposure to industrial emissions and automobile exhaust.[75] Carbon monoxide binds to hemoglobin with a more than 200 times greater affinity than oxygen, resulting in not only occupation of one of the heme groups of hemoglobin but also an increase in the O_2 affinity by the remaining heme group.[75] Individuals smoking even one pack of cigarettes a day frequently have elevated hematocrit levels.[75] These patients characteristically have normal blood gases and elevation of carboxyhemoglobin levels, resulting in a reduction in $P_{50}O_2$.[75] The elevation of the hematocrit level is reversed with the interruption of the smoking behavior. Increased hematocrit levels have been observed in 3% to 5% of heavy smokers. Although these patients are not immune to thrombotic complications, the number of thromboembolic events is lower than in patients with PV.[153–156] A

Table 68–2 Hemodynamic Values in Chronic Mountain Sickness in Comparison With Healthy Highlanders and Sea Level Subjects

	Sea Level Controls (n = 25; age 17–23 y)	Healthy Highlander Controls (n = 12; Age 19–38 y)	CMS Subjects (n = 10; Age 22–51 y)	P, CMS vs Healthy Highlanders
Hb, g/dL	14.7 ± 0.88	20.1 ± 1.69	24.7 ± 2.36	<0.001
Hct, %	44.1 ± 2.59	59.4 ± 5.4	79.3 ± 4.2	<0.001
Sa_{O_2}, %	95.7 ± 2.07	81.1 ± 4.61	69.6 ± 4.92	<0.001
RAP, mmHg	2.6 ± 1.31	2.9 ± 1.4	3.9 ± 1.8	NS
PPA, mmHg	12 ± 2.2	23 ± 5.1	47 ± 17.7	<0.001
PWP, mmHg	6.2 ± 1.71	6.9 ± 1.4	5.7 ± 2.3	NS
PVR, dynes cm^{-5}	69 ± 25.3	197 ± 57.6	527 ± 218.1	<0.001
CI, L min^{-1} M^{-2}	3.9 ± 0.97	3.8 ± 0.62	4.0 ± 0.93	NS

CI, cardiac index; CMS, PVR, pulmonary vasculan resistance; chronic mountain sickness; Hb, hemoglobin; Hct, hematocrit; NS, nonsignificant; PWP, pulmonary wedge pressure; RAP, right atrial pressure.
Values are mean ± SD.
Data derived from Penaloza D, Arias-Stella J. The heart and pulmonary circulation at high altitudes: Healthy highlanders and chronic mountain sickness. Circulation 115(9):1132, 2007. [review]

retrospective review of patients with either PV or smokers' polycythemia found that 60% of those with PV suffered thromboses, whereas only 41% of those with smokers' polycythemia were so affected (P < 0.05).[154]

Postrenal Transplantation Erythrocytosis

Postrenal transplantation erythrocytosis (PTE) is defined as a persistently elevated hematocrit level greater than 51% after renal transplantation without an elevation of the white blood cell count or platelet count. PTE is a potentially dangerous condition found in approximately 10% to 15% of renal allograft recipients.[156,157] PTE usually develops within 8 to 24 months following a successful renal transplantation and resolves spontaneously within 2 years in about 25% of patients, despite persistently good renal allograft function.[72,158] PTE is more common in males and may recur in the same patient after a second successful renal transplantation.[159] Factors that increase the likelihood of its development are a lack of EPO therapy before transplantation, a history of smoking, diabetes mellitus, transplant-related renal artery stenosis, retention of the native kidney, low serum ferritin levels, and normal or high pretransplantation EPO levels. PTE is also more frequent in patients who do not suffer rejection. At higher hematocrit levels (usually >60%), thrombotic events may complicate the clinical course of patients with PTE.[72,157,159]

Approximately 60% of patients with PTE experience malaise, headache, plethora, lethargy, and dizziness. In addition, from 10% to 20% develop thromboembolic complications involving either arteries or veins. Retention of the native kidney is essential for the development of PTE in most cases. Although the transplanted kidney produces EPO under normal regulatory mechanisms, the native kidney overproduces EPO in spite of the development of erythrocytosis. Frequently the PTE resolves with removal of the native kidney.[72] Plasma EPO levels are higher (10-fold) in patients with PTE as compared to nonerythrocytotic renal transplant recipients. In addition, erythroid progenitor cells isolated from patients with PTE are hypersensitive to EPO.[72]

The molecular basis of PTE remains unclear; AngII is believed, however, to play an important role in its pathogenesis by sustaining the secretion of EPO.[158] There is growing evidence that increased AT1R expression makes erythroid progenitor cells hypersensitive to AngII.[160,161] Furthermore, AngII can modulate release of erythropoietic stimulatory factors including EPO and IGF-1.[55,162] Because men comprise almost all of the transplant recipients who develop PTE, androgens are thought to play a role in the development of the syndrome. Androgens can directly affect erythroid progenitor cells or stimulate EPO production or actually the RAS system.[72] Treatment of patients with PTE includes intermittent phlebotomy or administration of drugs.[72] The ACE inhibitor enalapril suppresses the renin–angiotensin pathway and virtually eliminates the need for therapeutic phlebotomy in these patients.[162] Maximal reduction of hemoglobin levels is evident 6 months after starting therapy with either ACE inhibitor or angiotensin receptor blockers. Some patients are exquisitely sensitive to these medications and may in fact become severely anemic.[163–165] The AT1R antagonist losartan has been shown to be as effective in treating PTE as any ACE inhibitors. Therapy is usually begun at hematocrit levels above 55% with the hope of maintaining hematocrit levels below 50% in order to reduce the risk of thrombosis.[72] Furthermore, the ACE inhibitor fosinopril in an open-label crossover trial with theophylline was shown to produce a dramatic reduction in hematocrits in patients with PTE (51.3%–43.7%, P < 0.005).[166] Low doses of ramipril, another ACE inhibitor, normalized the hematocrit level in 26 of 27 patients with PTE after a mean of 127 days of therapy.[167]

Polycythemia Accompanying Kidney and Liver Diseases and Neoplastic Disorders

Polycythemia has been reported in association with kidney diseases such as renal cell carcinoma, renal artery stenosis, hydronephrosis, Wilms tumor, and polycystic kidney disease.[75] Renal tumors account for approximately one-third of cases of tumor-associated polycythemias. The tumor tissue has been demonstrated to produce excessive amounts of EPO, and the erythrocytosis resolves with surgical resections of the tumor. The mechanisms underlying the activation of EPO gene has been related to somatic mutation of the VHL gene in clear cell renal carcinomas. Wiesener et al reported that clear cell carcinoma associated with erythrocytosis and high serum EPO levels strongly expressed EPO mRNA and HIF-1α and HIF-2α.[168] These abnormalities were related to a point mutation in the VHL gene that impaired the bindings of HIF-1α to VHL leading to its accumulation and increased production of EPO.[168] Polycythemia is also a well-described paraneoplastic manifestation of hepatocellular carcinoma in 2.5% to 10% of patients and is again due to the production of EPO by the tumor.[169,170] Polycythemia in hepatoma patients is strongly related to tumor burden and elevated α-fetoprotein levels.[170,171] Polycythemia has also been associated with cerebellar hemangioblastomas (Fig. 68–3) and very large uterine fibromas.[75,172] In tumor-associated erythrocytosis, EPO production has been shown to be autonomous of hypoxic stimuli.[75]

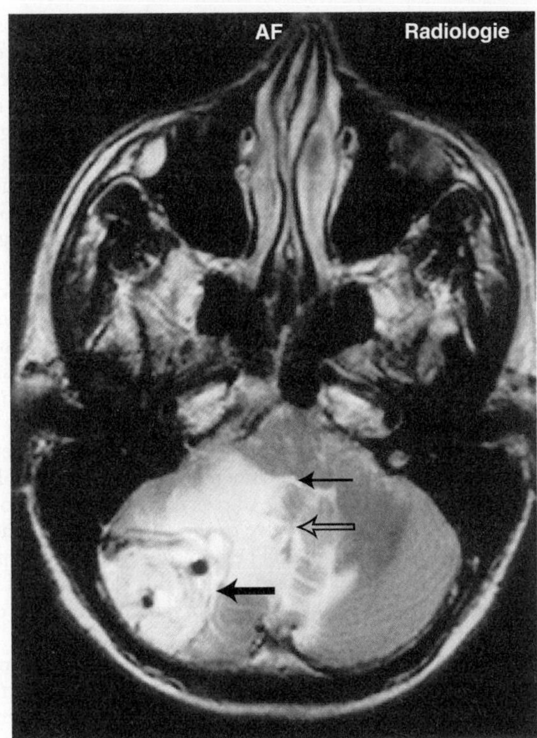

Figure 68–3. This MRI scan discloses a tumor measuring 3 × 4 cm in diameter in the right cerebellar hemisphere (black arrow) with perifocal edema and midline shift (white arrow), resulting in obstruction of the fourth ventricle (thin arrow). (From Kuhne M, Sidler D, Hofer S, Lugli A, Ludwig CH: Challenging manifestations of malignancies. Case 1. Polycythemia and high serum erythropoietin level as a result of hemangioblastoma. J Clin Oncol 22(17):3639, 2004.)

Polycythemia in Endocrine Disorders

Polycythemia is also associated with Cushing syndrome[173] and primary aldosteronism.[174] Secondary polycythemia can also be seen in 24% of older hypogonadal males receiving long-term androgen replacement therapy[175] and a significant number of competitive athletes taking anabolic steroids. For instance, in a small study of professional bodybuilders, 67% of those examined had hematocrit levels above 50%.[176] The effectiveness of drug screening in athletic competitions is demonstrated by the very low rate of positive tests for androgens (<2% of 170,000 tests) on random testing at the Olympic games and other international events.[177] In spite of previous assertions regarding increased EPO excretion following androgen therapy,[178] none of the athletes examined had elevated levels of EPO.[179] Recombinant human EPO has also been abused by athletes competing in endurance sports and can be detected by analyzing the individual's hematocrit level, reticulocyte count, percentage of macrocytic red blood cells, serum EPO level, serum transferrin receptor level, and the electrophoretic mobility of the EPO molecule (recombinant EPO is less negatively charged than endogenous EPO).[143]

Congenital Secondary Polycythemias

High-Oxygen-Affinity Hemoglobins and Biphosphoglycerate Deficiency

There are more than 100 mutations of hemoglobin that lead to increased oxygen affinity, and thus decreased oxygen delivery and compensatory polycythemia (see Chapter 44).[75,180] These mutations involve either the α- or β-chain globin chains. Such polycythemias are usually well tolerated in young patients but may lead to thrombotic complications in older patients.[180] High-oxygen-affinity hemoglobin variants are transmitted as autosomal dominants.[180] Phlebotomy therapy of such patients has been reported to be of no beneficial value, and have been shown to decrease exercise tolerance and anaerobic threshold. The best test to detect a high-oxygen affinity hemoglobin relies on the determination of hemoglobin dissociation kinetics and P_{50} (partial pressure of O_2 at which hemoglobin is 50% oxygenated). If co-oximetry is not available, the P_{50} can be mathematically estimated from a venous blood gas measurement[181] by using the following formula:

$$\text{AS REC } P_{50}\text{std} = \frac{\text{antilog}(\log 1/k)}{n}$$

$$\text{Where } 1/k = \text{Antilog}(n \log Po_{2(7.4)}) \times \frac{100 - So_2}{So_2}$$

A Hill constant (n) for hemoglobin A of 2.7 is used in all calculations. The Po_2 in venous blood measured at 37°C is converted to Po_2 at pH 7.4 with the formula

$$\log Po_{2(7.4)} = \log Po_2 - 0.5(7.40 - \text{pH}),$$

where pH represents the value in the antecubital venous blood. An example of a calculation provided by Lichtman and colleagues[144] follows. The Po_2 = 25 mmHg, So_2 = 44%, Sco = 2.0%, and pH = 7.37.

$$\begin{aligned}\log Po_{2(7.4)} &= \log Po_2 - 0.5(7.40 - \text{pH})\\ &= \log 25 - 0.5(7.40 - 7.37)\\ &= 1.3979 - 0.0150\\ &= 1.3829.\end{aligned}$$

$$1/k = \text{antilog}(2.7 \log Po_{2(7.4)}) \times \frac{100 - So_2}{So_2}$$

$$= \text{antilog}(2.7 \times 1.3829) \times \frac{100 - So_2}{So_2}$$

$$= \text{antilog}(3.7338) \times \frac{100 - 44}{44}$$

$$= 5417.5134 \times 1.2727$$

$$= 6894.8693$$

$$\text{AS REC } P_{50} \text{ std} = \text{antilog} \frac{\log 1/k}{2.7}$$

$$= \text{antilog} \frac{\log 6894.8693}{2.7}$$

$$= \text{antilog}(3.8385/2.7)$$

$$= \text{antilog } 1.4216$$

$$= 26.4$$

A $P_{50}O_2$ below 17 mmHg is indicative of a mutant hemoglobin with high oxygen affinity, whereas a level above 35 is strongly suggestive of a mutant hemoglobin with a low oxygen affinity.[75,181] Hemoglobin electrophoresis is not a reliable screen to rule out hemoglobin mutations as only about one half of these mutants are electrophoretically distinguishable. A hemoglobin electrophoresis will reveal the presence of an abnormal hemoglobin only if the mutation leads to a change in electrical charge. In 30 hemoglobin variants, such a charge differential was not present and more complex studies including isoelectric focusing and high-performance liquid chromatography were required to make the diagnosis.[180]

A rare cause of congenital polycythemia is 2,3-BPG (previously known as 2,3-DPG) deficiency (see Chapter 44). 2,3-BPG is synthesized in red cells and binds to hemoglobin, thereby reducing its affinity for oxygen.[75,106] An absence of 2,3-BPG therefore leads to increased affinity of hemoglobin for oxygen resulting in a lifelong hypoxic stimulus and erythrocytosis.

Congenital methemoglobinemias, whether due to cytochrome b5 reductase mutations or globin mutations, may be associated with mild polycythemia (see Chapter 44). When hemoglobin is oxidized to methemoglobin all of the four subunits of the tetramer may be affected, eliminating the oxygen transport capacity of hemoglobin.[180]

Chuvash Polycythemia

Chuvash polycythemia (CP) is an autosomal recessive disorder associated with germline mutations of VHL and erythrocytosis.[182,183] CP was first described in the mid-1970s and is endemic in the Chuvash population of the Russian republic.[182–187] It has been alleged that there may be thousands of affected individuals among the 1 million Chuvash people.[184–186] The serum EPO concentration in affected individuals is elevated compared with healthy first-degree family members, although some patients may have normal serum EPO levels.[184,185] The erythroid progenitors of patients with CP are also hypersensitive to EPO; thus, CP has characteristics of both primary and secondary polycythemias.[183] A missense mutation in the VHL gene, VHL598C→T mutation, has been identified in CP patients.[186,187] The disorder is characterized by a high hemoglobin level, increased plasma, EPO level, varicose veins, vertebral hemangiomas, low blood pressure, and an elevated concentration of VEGF. The defective VHL gene product is not capable of promoting the ubiquitin-mediated degradation of HIF-1α, thereby leading to increased elaboration of EPO. CP is associated with a high mortality rate due to thrombotic and hemorrhagic vascular complications.[183–187] Cerebral vascular events are especially common causes of death. The median age of death from a cerebral vascular event is 42 years. Estimated survival to age 65 is 29% for individuals with CP and 64% for age-matched community members. There is a perfect genotype–phenotypic correlation, with all patients with CP being homozygotes for the mutation. Interestingly, heterozygous carriers do not develop erythrocytosis but do have lower blood pressures and do not seem to be at increased risk for tumors, which contrasts with patients with VHL syndrome.[187]

Germline mutations of VHL alleles have been reported in several patients with apparent congenital polycythemia that had no evidence of developing a tumor[187–189]; some of these subjects had germline mutations of both VHL alleles. Other subjects with congenital polycythemia of various ethnicities, including Pakistanis, Punjabis, African Americans, and Caucasians, harboring homozygosity for the CP VHL mutation or double heterozygosity for CP and other VHL mutations, have been found.[187–189] The VHL598C→T mutation, has been shown to originate in a single haplotype in the Chuvash patients, as well as in Caucasians, Asian Indians, and one African American individual.[182,187–189] This mutation appears to be the most common genetic defect leading to congenital polycythemia. The mutation originated from a single founder 12,000 to 51,000 years ago.[187] This suggests that such wide dissemination from the original founder may be associated with some survival advantage for heterozygotes carrying this mutation. Such an advantage might be related to a subtle improvement of iron metabolism, erythropoiesis, embryonic development, energy metabolism, or some other yet unknown effect.

Rapidly accumulating data suggest that VHL mutations might be the most common cause of congenital polycythemias, greatly exceeding the number of patients with hemoglobin chain mutations. In point of fact, in one study of over 200 unrelated subjects with apparently congenital polycythemia, none had a 2,3-BPG deficiency, 2 had a globin mutation (Hgb Vanderbilt, and Hemoglobin San Diego), and 12 had EPOR mutations to account for their polycythemia.[183] By contrast, when 50 patients were examined for the VHL mutation, 22 had VHL mutations, most of these being the CP VHL mutation, occurring either homozygously or in combination with another VHL mutation.[187] The failure of patients with CP to develop VHL syndrome tumors is consistent with the concept that deregulation of H1F-1α and VEGF are not sufficient to cause tumors. Recently a cluster of patients with clinical features identical to patients with CP has been documented on the island of Ischia in the Bay of Naples, Italy.[190] All of these patients also had the VHL598C→T mutation. Twelve of the 14 patients were homozygotes and 2 were heterozygotes. The homozygotes have symptoms identical to patients in Chuvashia with this mutation. Unlike heterozygotes in Chuvashia, the two heterozygotes from Ischia developed erythrocytosis associated with high EPO levels, which raises the possibility that genetic alterations of certain components of the oxygen-sensing pathway other than VHL may contribute to the development of erythrocytosis in the Italian patients. The disorder in Ischia has a gene frequency even higher than that in Chuvashia, with 14% of the population estimated to be heterozygotes, which has led Prchal and Gordeuk to suggest that heterozygotes have a survival advantage.[191]

The Chuvash mutation has also been shown to have a profound effect on the cardiopulmonary system. Smith and coworkers have reported that patients with Chuvash polycythemia have significant abnormalities of cardiopulmonary physiology, including elevated basal ventilation rates and increased pulmonary vascular tone, with extremely high ventilatory rates and heightened pulmonary vasoconstriction and heart rates in response to acute hypoxia.[192] These observations indicate that the VHL–HIF pathway might also play a central role in calibrating the pulmonary system to hypoxic challenges. Such undesirable exaggerated hypoxic responses and the resulting elevated pulmonary vascular hypertension may contribute to the morbidity and mortality associated with CP.[192] Increased expression of endothelin 1 has been documented in patients with CP.[193] Endothelin 1 has been associated with the development of hypoxia-related pulmonary hypertension. Endothelin 1 receptor inhibitors might therefore be useful in reversing the associated pulmonary hypertension in these patients. Treatment strategies for patients with CP have included phlebotomy, aspirin, and occasionally chemotherapy. It is unknown whether such therapeutic strategies alter the natural history of this disorder. A variety of HIF-1 inhibitors being currently evaluated for the treatment of tumor patients might potentially also be useful for the treatment of patients with CP.

An additional genetic abnormality of oxygen sensing has been reported that leads to familial polycythemia. A heterozygous C-to-G change at base 950 of the coding sequence of PHD2 (P317R mutation) was detected in all three affected family members with this syndrome. Hydroxylation of HIF-1 by PHD2 facilitates its interaction with VHL, thereby favoring its ubiquitination and degradation by the proteosome.[194] The failure of PHD2 P317R to bind the HIF-1 and HIF-2α and promote HIF hydroxylase activity ultimately leads to increased HIF-l and erythropoietin levels, resulting in the development of erythrocytosis. Mutations involving other PHD isoforms might potentially play a role in the development of erythrocytosis in other cases of familial polycythemia.[40] The PHD2 P317R mutation is inherited as an autosomal dominant trait, in contrast to the Chuvash polycythemia defect, which is an autosomal recessive disorder.[194] Polycythemic patients with PHD2 P317R do not have any evidence of tumors characteristic of the VHL syndrome.[194]

Neonatal Polycythemia

Because of the high oxygen affinity of fetal hemoglobin, many neonates have markedly elevated hematocrit levels. Babies with hematocrit levels over 65% have more neurologic and functional impairments and are more likely to be born to diabetic mothers. Although phlebotomy has been recommended,[195] there is little evidence that it has been beneficial for these babies.

POLYCYTHEMIA VERA

PV is a clonal, chronic, progressive myeloproliferative disorder (MPD) often of insidious onset, characterized by an absolute increase in red cell mass and also usually by leukocytosis, thrombocytosis, and splenomegaly.[4,196,197] PV leads to excessive proliferation of erythroid, myeloid, and megakaryocytic elements within the bone marrow. Vaquez[198] first described this clinical entity in 1892, noting the characteristic physical findings. At the turn of this century, Cabot[199] and Osler[200] independently associated the name PV with this newly described clinical disorder. Limited insight into the pathogenesis of this disorder has been gained. Studies have been performed that demonstrate the hypersensitivity of hematopoietic progenitor cells derived from the malignant clone to a number of regulatory factors.[77,78,201–204]

PV differs from many other hematologic malignancies, in that prolonged survival is enjoyed by most patients if the excessive production of red blood cells and platelets can be controlled.[12,205,206] This prolonged survival, however, is punctuated by the development of other syndromes, such as myelofibrosis and acute leukemia (Fig. 68–4).[12,207,208] Frequently, patients present asymptomatically to a physician only to find that they have splenomegaly, isolated erythrocytosis, or thrombocytosis; left untreated, these patients will become symptomatic, owing to the excessive production of red blood cells or platelets, or both.[5] After a number of years, the erythrocytotic phase of the disease frequently becomes inactive, and the patient may no longer suffer from the sequelae of excessive red cell production. Subsequently, these patients can develop so-called spent-phase or PV related myelofibrosis postpolycythemic myeloid metaplasia (PV related MF), which is frequently indistinguishable from another MPD, primary myelofibrosis (PMF).[207–209] Finally, a significant proportion of these patients will go on to develop acute myeloid leukemia. Only a limited number of patients undergo this orderly transition; many patients can transition from the polycythemic phase directly into an acute leukemia or a myelodysplastic disorder.[12]

The transition from one phase of this MPD to another is not necessarily unidirectional. A number of cases of presumed IM have been described in which chemotherapy treatment has resulted in a striking decrease in marrow fibrosis associated with the development of an elevated red cell mass and a syndrome that was virtually indistinguishable from de novo PV.[209] The constantly changing clinical picture of this malignant hematologic disorder requires careful observation and treatment to deal with the numerous problems that can be encountered.

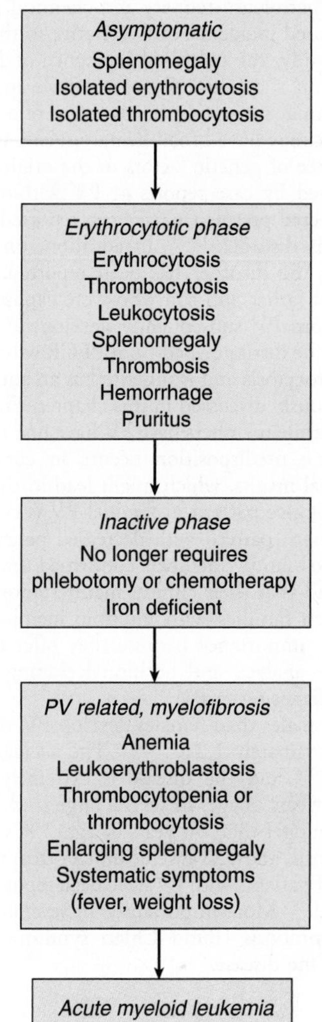

Figure 68–4. Evolution of polycythemia vera.

EPIDEMIOLOGY

PV is the most common primary polycythemia. It has been previously estimated that between 2.3 and 2.8 per 100,000 persons per year are affected.[210–215] Its incidence surpasses that of chronic myeloid leukemia, making it the most common MPD.[214] It is important to emphasize that no or very few population-based estimates of the prevalence of this disorder are presently available. Actual determination of its prevalence is a difficult process because of the need for an extensive diagnostic evaluation to differentiate this disorder from other causes of spurious or absolute erythrocytosis.[205] Ten thousand individuals between 18 and 65 years of age enrolled in the Vicenza Thrombophilia and Atherosclerosis project in Italy were screened for an elevated hematocrit level or platelet count, or both, and followed for 5 years.[5] On the basis of these studies, the prevalence of PV was shown to be 300 cases per 1 million.[5] This higher prevalence data is likely due to the previous inability to identify asymptomatic patients with PV before presentation to a physician. If confirmed, these estimates from Italy are likely conservative, as patients older than 65 years of age were not included in this project. These data indicate that, in fact, PV is not a rare disease but actually a relatively common hematologic malignancy.

The prevalence of PV has been reported by several investigators to be higher among American Jews and lower among African Americans.[210,216–218] The incidence of the disorder is greater among Ashkenazi Jews, who originate from eastern and central Europe, than among Arabs and Sephardic Jews.[218] Interestingly, extremely low occurrence rates have been reported from Japan, where the incidence was found to be 2 cases per 1 million per year.[219] These findings suggest that important environmental or genetic factors might be involved in the biogenesis of this disorder. One notable exception to the low prevalence of PV in Japan has been the higher incidence observed among populations exposed to atomic bomb explosions.[220] The possibility that radiation exposure is an etiologic factor in the generation of PV was also raised by the observation in the United States of four cases of PV 10 to 20 years after a nuclear explosion in which 3000 military observers were exposed.[221]

An epidemiologic investigation that focused on occupational exposure among petroleum refinery and chemical plant workers has revealed an increased incidence of PV relative to the general population.[222] In this study, the increased incidence of PV was linked to similar increases in the frequency of multiple myeloma and non-Hodgkin lymphoma, suggesting involvement of a putative environmental toxin that may have broad hematopoietic toxicity.[222]

The importance of genetic factors in the origin of this disease is further emphasized by case reports of PV within families.[223–232] A greater than expected prevalence has been reported in the parents of patients with this disorder.[223–232] In addition, one family of three sisters all having the disorder has been reported.[228] An additional report describes a father and son who were exposed to organic solvents and in whom PV subsequently developed.[232] These forms of familial PV must be distinguished from PFCP, which is characterized by isolated erythrocytosis and is inherited as an autosomal dominant disorder, as previously discussed in this chapter. The reports of families in which multiple members have PV have first raised the possibility that a genetic predisposition occurs in concert with several additional external insults, which might lead to the development of PV.[231] The inheritance pattern of familial PV is compatible with an autosomal dominant pattern with decreased penetrance.[231] Clinical analyses of affected family members confirmed that they have clonal hematopoiesis and that their clinical manifestations are identical to sporadic PV. Such families with multiple members with PV have been of scientific importance because they offer the possibility for genewide linkage analysis and positional cloning to identify additional genes predisposing to PV.[231]

Slightly more males than females develop PV, the male-to-female ratio being approximately 1.2 : 1.[167–171] The average age at diagnosis is 60 years,[12,210–214] and the disease is extremely rare in patients younger than 30 years of age. In several large studies, 5% of patients with PV were younger than 40 years of age, 1% were younger than 25 years at diagnosis, and 0.1% were younger than 20 years.[12,146,207,230] Small numbers of patients with PV have been reported who presented during childhood.[233] More importantly, in several of these children, hepatic vein thrombosis (Budd–Chiari syndrome) was the initial manifestation of the disease.[234]

BIOLOGICAL AND MOLECULAR ASPECTS

Considerable speculation has centered on the pathobiology of the erythrocytosis that characterizes PV.[235,236] London and colleagues[3] established that the expanded red cell mass of PV was due to a two- to threefold increase in the production of red blood cells by a hyperplastic marrow and was not attributable to prolongation of the red cell life span. Granulocyte and platelet production are also increased in this disorder. This overly exuberant production of all cellular elements of the blood suggests that the basic defect resides at the level of the hematopoietic cellular hierarchy from which each of these cells originates, the pluripotent hematopoietic stem cell.

A variety of studies have documented serum EPO levels in patients with PV, secondary erythrocytosis, and relative polycythemia, and in normal adults.[6–11] Serum EPO levels have been shown to be subnormal in patients with PV, elevated in many but not all cases of secondary erythrocytosis, and normal in patients with relative polycythemia (Fig. 68–5),[6–11] indicating that PV cannot be an abnormality of EPO production.

In 1951, Dameshek[197] postulated that chronic myeloid leukemia, PV, essential thrombocythemia, and IM were related disorders, which he called MPD. He concluded that these disorders resulted from a generalized hyperresponsiveness of marrow cells to myelostimulatory factors and speculated that these disorders were neoplastic in origin.[197]

Since the mid-1970s, much data have accumulated that conclusively demonstrate PV to be the result of a neoplastic proliferation of hematopoietic cells.[78,231,236–242] The cellular origin of the disorder was first established by the analysis of glucose-6-phosphate dehydrogenase (G6PD) isoenzymes in African American women who were heterozygous for this X-linked gene (Fig. 68–6). This approach was based on the random irreversible inactivation of one X chromosome in each female somatic cell during embryogenesis. Inactivation of the same X chromosome occurs in the progeny of these cells.[194] A normal African American female heterozygous for G6PD will therefore have approximately equal populations of marrow cells with a different G6PD isoenzyme.[60] The G6PD isoenzymes can be readily distinguished by electrophoretic methods.[237]

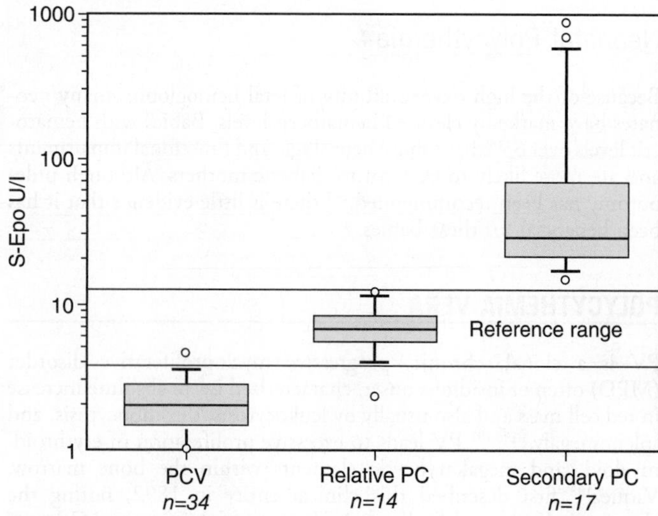

Figure 68–5. Serum erythropoietin levels in polycythemia vera, relative to secondary polycythemia. The middle bar represents the median; the boxes, quartiles, and the end bars, the 95% range. The open circles represent individual values outside the 95% range. (From Birgegaard G, Miller O, Caro J, Erslev A: Serum erythropoietin levels by radioimmunoassay in polycythaemia. Scand J Haematol 29:161, 1982.)

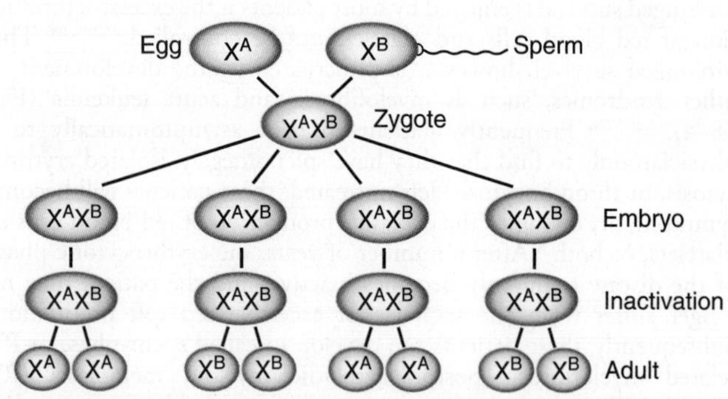

Figure 68–6. Schematic presentation of X chromosome inactivation in an embryo heterozygous at the *G6PD* locus (Gd^b/Gd^a). In this diagram, the maternal X chromosome bears an A gene for G6PD(X^A) and the paternal X chromosome a B gene (X^B). During embryogenesis, one X chromosome in each somatic cell is randomly inactivated, so that half the somatic cells will have an active X^A and the other half an active X^B. Inactivation is fixed for a particular cell and its progeny. All progeny of an active X^A gene will express X^A. Female G6PD heterozygotes are mosaics, with some cells active X^A and others X^B. A tumor with clonal origin will consist entirely of either X^A or X^B cells and therefore will contain only G6PD type A or B but not both. Tumors with multicellular origin will contain X^A and X^B cells and, therefore, both G6PD types. (Adapted from Fialkow PJ: Clonal origin of human tumors. Annu Rev Med 30:135, 1979.)

This approach was exploited in a seminal study by Adamson and coworkers[238] in an effort to determine the cellular origin of PV. They presumed that cells composing a tumor that arises from a single cell in a G6PD heterozygote would express a single isoenzyme type, whereas a neoplasm originating from multiple cells would express both isoenzyme types.[237] These investigators found that circulating

Table 68–3 Relative Amounts of G6PD Isoenzymes in Various Mesenchymal Tissues in Two Patients With Polycythemia Vera

Tissue	%A Case 1	%B Case 2
Skin	55:45	55:45
Lymphocytes	85:15*	55:45
Erythrocytes	100/0	100/0
Granulocytes	100/0	100/0
Platelets	100/0	100/0

*Contaminated with erythrocytes.

Data from Adamson JW, Fialkow PJ, Murphy S, et al: Polycythemia vera stem-cell and probable clonal origin of the disease. N Engl J Med 295:913, 1976.

Table 68–4 G6PD Isoenzyme Analysis of Erythroid Colonies Cloned From Marrow Cells of G6PD Heterozygotes With Polycythemia Vera

Erythropoietin (U/mL)	Patient 1		Patient 2	
	Colonies*	A/B†	Colonies*	A/B†
0	15	19/0	36	27/0
0.25	32	21/1	75	12/0
1.0	47	28/3	115	22/1
5.0	68	26/10	156	44/2
10.0	—	—	161	30/8

*Colonies per 10^5 cells.

†Number of individual colonies analyzed of specific G6PD isoenzyme type per 10^5 cells.

Data from Prchal JF, Adamson JW, Murphy S, et al: Polycythemia vera: The in vitro response of normal and abnormal stem cell lines to erythropoietin. J Clin Invest 61:1044, 1978.

red cells, granulocytes, and platelets obtained from African American females who were G6PD heterozygotes express the same isoenzyme, whereas skin and cultured marrow fibroblasts obtained from these same patients demonstrate both isoenzymes (Table 68–3).[236,238] They concluded that PV represented a clonal proliferation of neoplastic hematopoietic stem cells and was not multicellular in origin or the consequence of excessive proliferation of normal hematopoietic stem cells.[238]

The clonality of blood cell production in PV has subsequently been confirmed using restriction fragment length polymorphisms of the active X chromosome.[240–242] A monoclonal pattern of X chromosome inactivation has been defined in red cells, granulocytes, monocytes, and platelets in females with PV.[78,240–242] Such studies confirm the clonal cellular origin of the disorder.

On the basis of the knowledge that red cell production in PV is not associated with excessive EPO production, several investigators have hypothesized that the erythroid progenitor cell in this disorder is no longer subject to physiologic regulators.[205] With the development of clonal assay systems for hematopoietic progenitor cells, it became possible to analyze the effect of EPO on in vitro colony formation.

Two classes of erythroid progenitor cells, the burst-forming unit–erythroid (BFU-E) and the colony-forming unit–erythroid (CFU-E) present in the marrow and peripheral blood of patients with PV were studied. Prchal and Axelrad[77] first reported that PV bone marrow can form substantial numbers of erythroid colonies in vitro in the absence of exogenous EPO, whereas normal human bone marrow is incapable of forming such colonies without the addition of EPO. These erythroid colonies have been termed *endogenous colonies*.[243,244] When erythroid PV and normal bone marrow were subsequently assayed in the presence of EPO, PV marrow was characterized by a higher cloning efficiency.[78,243–248] Mixed-colony formation has also been shown to be enhanced in PV.[244] Mixed colonies originate from multilineage progenitor cells. Their formation by PV marrow, but not by normal marrow, also occurs in vitro in the absence of exogenous EPO.[244] These observations suggest that the altered response to EPO in PV is characteristic not only of erythroid progenitor cells but of more primitive hematopoietic progenitor cells as well. Cell-cycle analysis of PV hematopoietic progenitor cells revealed another cell progenitor abnormality[245]: A higher proportion of PV progenitor cells were in the synthetic phase of the cell cycle than was observed in normal subjects.[245]

Further insight into the cellular defects in PV was provided by the studies of Prchal and coworkers (Table 68–4).[246] These researchers cloned marrow cells from African American female G6PD heterozygotes with PV in the presence and absence of exogenous EPO and demonstrated that the erythroid colonies that formed in the absence of exogenous EPO contained the same G6PD isoenzyme type as that expressed by peripheral blood elements.[246] Thus, the so-called endogenous erythroid colonies arose from the abnormal clone that was responsible for supplying red cells, granulocytes, and platelets to the peripheral blood. When exogenous EPO was added, increasing numbers of colonies were formed containing cellular elements expressing the other G6PD isoenzymes; presumably, these colonies originated from cells not involved in the malignant process. Similarly, small numbers of granulocyte–macrophage colonies not originating from the PV clone were also observed in these assays. These data collectively indicate the existence of malignant and nonmalignant populations of hematopoietic progenitor cells in PV marrow. The relative frequency of the neoplastic clone in relation to normal progenitor cells was further examined by Adamson and coworkers,[239] who, by monitoring the proportion of neoplastic erythroid clones and their numeric relationship to normal clones over a period of several years, showed disease progression to be associated with a significant decline in the frequency of normal colony-forming cells and increasing preponderance of the neoplastic clone.[239]

The clonal assay systems first used to obtain "endogenous erythroid colonies" contained serum contaminated with trace amounts of EPO.[243] This EPO contamination led to confusion about the responsiveness of the PV cells to the actions of this hormone. Two conflicting hypotheses were entertained: one suggesting that proliferation of abnormal populations of erythroid progenitor cells is completely independent of EPO and the other was consistent with hypersensitivity of polycythemia progenitors to EPO. Using an anti-EPO antiserum to remove trace amounts of EPO present in serum, Zanjani and colleagues[243] concluded that erythroid progenitor cells from PV patients do not proliferate in the absence of EPO but are, in fact, abnormally sensitive to the actions of this hormone. This increased responsiveness allowed these cells to form colonies in the presence of serum containing small amounts of EPO. By constructing EPO dose–response curves from PV marrows and comparing them with those obtained from normal marrow cells, Eaves and Eaves[247] drew similar conclusions. Their studies showed that most PV patients possess two distinct populations of erythroid progenitor cells: a normally EPO-responsive population and a population of cells similar in proliferative and maturational behavior in vitro but requiring little or no EPO.[247] These investigators suggested that because of the exquisite EPO sensitivity of the malignant clone, the proliferation of the normal progenitor cells in vivo was at a disadvantage.[247] The EPO dependence of PV progenitor cells was further demonstrated by Casadevall and coworkers,[248] who used a serum-free culture system, which no longer was contaminated with EPO. They were unable to demonstrate endogenous erythroid colony formation by normal or PV marrow and showed that PV erythroid progenitor cells were exquisitely sensitive to EPO compared with normal progenitors.[248] These data collectively indicated that the abnormality in the erythroid progenitor cell in PV is not only quantitative but also qualitative.

Using semipurified populations of blood and bone marrow BFU-E, a number of investigators have demonstrated that the increased responsiveness of these marrow progenitor populations extends to their responses to SCF, IL-3, GM-CSF, and insulin-like growth factor-1 (IGF-1). These studies also demonstrated that bone marrow fractions enriched for granulocyte–macrophage progenitors as well as megakaryocyte progenitors from the patients had a heightened responsiveness to IL-3 and GM-CSF.[201,202] The dogma that the hyperresponsivity of PV progenitor cells to a variety of growth factors (EPO, IL-3, GM-CSF, steel factor) is the underlying defect that leads to PV has been universally accepted.[237,236]

Many investigators have examined the possibility that the hematopoietic defect in PV could be accounted for by genetic alteration of cytokine receptors expressed by affected hematopoietic cells.[249–252] In PV, the EPOR is structurally similar to the normal EPOR, and mutations in the EPOR do not appear to be directly involved in the pathobiology of PV.[249–252] Furthermore, no significant differences in the number, dissociation constant, or internalization rate of receptors for steel factor have been detected in the erythroid progenitor cells of PV patients.[249]

The receptor for TPO (Mpl) has also been implicated in the biogenesis of PV. Mpl is expressed by the megakaryocytes, platelets, and pluripotent hematopoietic stem cells.[12,253–255] Impaired expression of Mpl in murine knockout models results in a reduction of multipotent and committed hematopoietic progenitors, and TPO increases the proliferation of primitive hematopoietic progenitor cells in vitro.[12,253] The retrovirus, MPLV, which encodes a truncated form of MPL, induces a fatal myeloproliferative disorder in mice.[254,255] Mpl expression has been shown to be abnormal in the megakaryocytes and platelets of patients with PV.[256,257] Two forms of Mpl were detected in PV platelets compared with normal platelets, where a single form is present. The two forms of Mpl in PV have been attributed to an abnormality in posttranslational glycosylation, which has been suggested to be characteristic of PV.[257] The removal of the distal extracellular domain of Mpl in mice results in independent survival of hematopoietic progenitor cells expressing this truncated receptor.[254,255] In PV platelets and megakaryocytes, this extracytoplasmic domain is not detectable by flow cytometry, and total platelet Mpl is reduced, which has recently been shown to be a consequence of JAK2-induced Mpl trafficking.[12,256,257] The abnormal expression of Mpl in PV has been used as a diagnostic tool in distinguishing the etiology of various causes of erythrocytosis. In addition, these data provide the rationale for the belief that abnormal Mpl function may play a fundamental role in the development of PV. Furthermore, the defect in Mpl expression becomes more pronounced with disease progression, suggesting that it may be a useful marker of disease activity.[12,256,257]

Several groups have suggested that the overproduction of red cells in PV is a consequence of progenitor and precursor cell accumulation rather than proliferation.[12,258] This hypothesis was first based on the observation that the antiapoptotic protein BCL-XL was overexpressed in PV progenitor cells, resulting in their resistance to apoptosis in the absence of EPO. This overexpression of such antiapoptotic proteins presumably permits erythroid progenitors to terminally differentiate in the absence of EPO. Additional proof of this pathogenetic mechanism was provided by the demonstration of increased expression of the cyclin-dependent kinase inhibitor INK4α/ARF locus in PV erythroid cells.[259] Furthermore, Pellagatti and colleagues, using cDNA microarray technology to analyze the gene expression profile in PV granulocytes, showed upregulation in PV granulocytes of several protease inhibitors that are known to possess high affinity for proteases that promote neutrophil apoptosis.[260] They have suggested that upregulation of such protease inhibitors might lead to increased survival of neutrophil precursors in PV.

Identification of JAK2V617F Mutation in PV

For more than two decades, a number of research groups have been searching for the genetic defect underlying PV. Most groups predicted that this defect involved the signaling pathways downstream of the EPOR. These pathways include the tyrosine kinase JAK2 and the transcriptional signal transducers and activators of transcription (STAT)3 and STAT5. The initial discovery of a mutation was predicated on a somewhat simplistic yet revealing set of experiments performed by Vainchenker and his colleagues in France and reported in 2005.[79,261] They observed that the inhibition of JAK2 by a small molecule (AG490) or by small interfering RNA (siRNA) reduced erythropoietin-independent colony formation by PV bone marrow mononuclear cells.[261] This observation prompted them to directly sequence JAK2 in the hematopoietic cells of PV and to discover a single recurrent point mutation.[79] A guanine-to-thymine mutation was observed that resulted in a substitution of valine to phenylalanine at codon 617 within the pseudokinase domain (JH2) of JAK2 (*JAK2V617F*) (Fig. 68–7).[79] These findings were quickly confirmed by several different groups.[79–82] Kralovics et al had previously identified a region of loss of heterozygosity (LOH) on chromosome 9p in PV, and identified a 6·2-Mbp region common to all PV patients screened.[262] As this region contained JAK2, with its known role in erythropoiesis, it was screened for mutations and the same JAK2V617F mutation identified.[81] Three other groups targeted JAK2 as part of a global sequencing screen of tyrosine kinases and phosphatases in MPDs.[80,82,263] Analysis of germline DNA demonstrated that *JAK2V617F* is an acquired somatic mutation present exclusively in hematopoietic cells.[79–82,263] All patients with PV have a population of erythroid progenitor cells which are homozygous for the mutation.[268] Using quantitative PCR, patients with a low burden of JAK2V617F in granulocytes have been termed heterozygotes (<50%), while patients with a higher burden of JAK2V617F are termed homozygotes (>50%). A subset of patients with PV are homozygous for *JAK2V617F*, which was demonstrated to be the result of mitotic recombination and duplication of the mutant allele (Fig. 68–8).[81,262] The consequence of this mitotic recombination event has been observed during the clinical course of individual patients leading to JAK2V617F heterozygote patients becoming homozygotes over time.[264] The concept of the conversion of JAK2V617F heterozygosity to homozygosity is further supported by the observation that the median duration of disease at the time of evaluation was 48 months in homozygous PV patients as compared to 23 months in heterozygotes and 15 months in patients with wild-type JAK2.[82] These observations are consistent with a multistep pathogenesis of PV. The multiple steps being the acquisition of JAK2V617F, which results in JAK2V617F heterozygosity, followed by a second step, homologous recombination, that leads to JAK2V617F homozygous progenitor cells and eventually JAK2V617F homozygous granulocytes.[82] It remains unknown at present if a lesion occurring prior to acquisition of the JAK2V617F mutation predisposes an individual to acquire JAK2V617F.

A number of groups have reported the frequency of JAK2V617F in patients with MPDs (Table 68–5).[79–82,265,266] The prevalence of the mutation in PV ranges from 65% to 97%, with an average of 82% in nearly 1000 reported cases. The differences in reported rates of positivity are likely due to at least three causes: first, the stringency of the criteria used to diagnose PV; second, the sensitivity of the method used to detect mutations; and third, the source of DNA (granulocytes, mononuclear cells, or whole blood cells). The majority of studies have used peripheral blood neutrophils as they are derived from the same clonal progenitor that is transformed in PV. Direct sequencing techniques are likely to have a lower sensitivity than techniques that employ PCR amplification of the mutant allele.[267] Approximately 50% to 60% of patients with essential thrombocytosis (ET) and IM are also *JAK2V617F*-positive. ET can be distinguished from PV by cloning erythroid progenitors and analyzing the JAK2V617F status of individual hematopoietic colonies.[268] In the overwhelming majority of cases, PV is characterized by a population of JAK2V617F homozygous colonies with some heterozygous and wild-type colonies. By contrast in ET, there are few homozygous colonies, with the majority being heterozygous or wild-type.[268] The majority of ET and IM patients who are negative for *JAK2V617F* have clonal hematopoiesis,[269] which indicates that these JAK2V617F diseases likely are the consequences of another genetic event. The *JAK2V617F* allele has also been observed in a limited number of

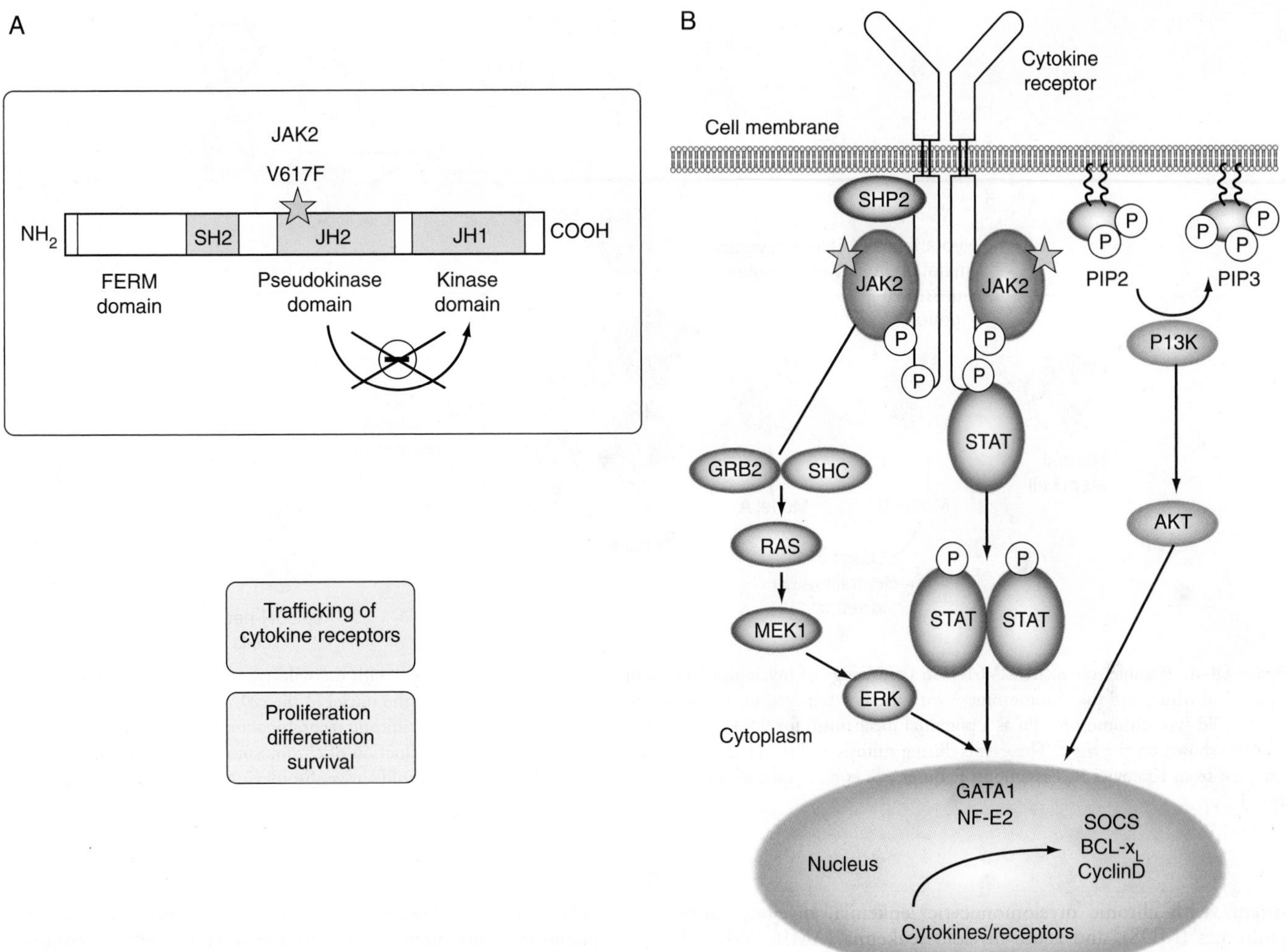

Figure 68–7. JAK2V617F signaling in myeloproliferative disorders. (*a*) Structure of JAK2 V617F: the mutation is located in pseudokinase JAK homology domain 2 (JH2) and disrupts the autoinhibition of this regulatory domain. Consequently, the tyrosine kinase corresponding to the JH1 domain is constitutively activated. (*b*) In the presence of a homodimeric cytokine receptor (eg, EPOR), the two JAK2V617F proteins bound to the intracellular domain of the receptor transphosphorylate its tyrosine residues. In turn, STAT5, PI3K, and RAS signaling pathways are activated, leading to the downstream modulation of transcription and protein levels for cell cycle, proliferation and apoptosis-related factors. P, phosphate; PIP2 and PIP3, phosphatidyl inositol bi- and triphosphate; PVR, pulmonary vascular resistance. (From Delhommeau F et al: Cell Mol Life Sci 63, 2006.)

Table 68–5 Frequency of JAK2V617F Mutations in PV, ET, and IM

	JAK2V617F Detection Method	PV: JAK2V617F (Homozygous)	ET: JAK2V617F (Homozygous)	IM: JAK2V617F (Homozygous)
James et al	Sequencing	89 (30)	43	43
Levine et al	Sequencing	74 (25)	32 (3)	35 (9)
Kralovics et al	Sequencing	65 (27)	23 (3)	57 (22)
Baxter et al	Sequencing	97 (26)	57 (0)	50 (19)
Jones et al	ARMS/pyrosequencing	81 (33)	41 (7)	43 (29)
Levine et al	Allele specific/Taqman	99	72	39

PV, Polycythemia Vera; ET, essential thrombocytosis; and IM, idiopathic myelofibrosis.
Data from Levine RL, Wernig G. Role of JAK-STAT signaling in the pathogenesis of myeloproliferative disorders. Hematology (Am Soc Hematol Educ Program) 233, 2006.

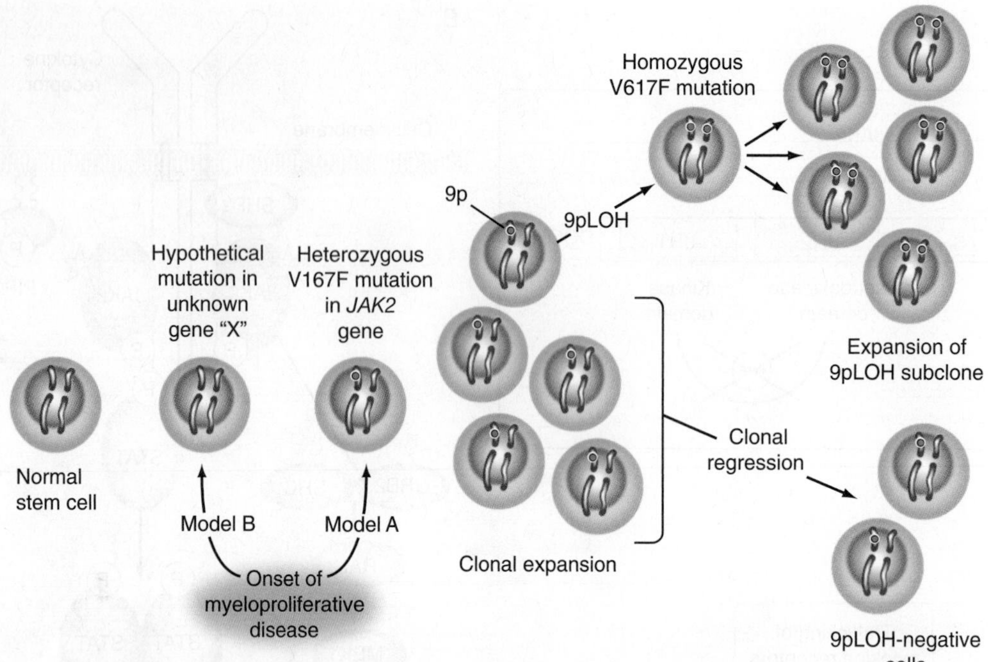

Figure 68–8. Possible role of JAK2V617F in the biology of myeloproliferative disorders. The chromosome 9 with the wild-type *JAK2* sequence (G) is depicted in white, and the chromosome 9 with the GT transversion (T) is shown in red. Circles symbolize the nuclei of the cells. Deletion of the telomeric part of wild-type chromosome 9p as a potential mechanism for 9pLOH is shown on the left. Alternatively, mitotic recombination could also result in 9pLOH, shown on the right. The events during mitosis and the resulting cell progeny after mitotic recombination of chromosome 9p are also shown. (Adapted from Kralovics R, Passamonti F, Buser AS, et al: A gain-of-function mutation of JAK2 in myeloproliferative disorders. N Engl J Med 352:1779, 2005.)

patients with chronic myelomonocytic leukemia, myelodysplastic syndromes (MDS), and acute myeloid leukemia (AML), although most *JAK2V617F* mutations in AML occur in patients with a preceding diagnosis of PV, ET, or IM.[265,266,270] JAK2V617F is an acquired somatic mutation, and does not appear in nonhematopoietic cells and has not been detected in patients with secondary erythrocytosis. Moreover, JAK2V617F has not been observed in lymphoid malignancies although another mutation, *JAK2 L611S*, was identified in one case of pre-B-ALL during a screen for *JAK2* mutations using denaturing high-performance liquid chromatography.[266] Using high-sensitivity allele-specific PCR, JAK2V617F has been detected in small numbers of normal individuals or hospitalized patients who do not have MPD.[271] At this time, it remains unknown whether this observation is a consequence of oversensitivity of the assay utilized or the presence of the mutation in patients with preclinical forms of MPDs. Long-term follow-up of such individuals would be required to determine the clinical significance of such an observation.

The JAK2V617F Mutation Is Present in Hematopoietic Stem Cells in PV

Previous studies had demonstrated that the majority of patients with PV had clonal involvement of multiple lineages, including myeloid, erythroid, and lymphoid cells.[238,240,272,273] These results suggested that PV originates in hematopoietic progenitors with the ability to differentiate into multiple lineages. In addition, loss of heterozygosity at 9p24, now known to correspond to homozygous *JAK2V617F* mutations, can be identified in both myeloid and lymphoid cells in some patients with PV, further suggesting that the underlying mutations occur in progenitor cells with the ability to differentiate into multiple hematopoietic lineages.[262]

The JAK2V617F mutation has been detected in hematopoietic colony-forming cells and more mature progeny, such as neutrophils and platelets.[79–82,274] Jamieson et al have recently isolated, according to phenotypic populations of cells enriched for HSCs, common myeloid progenitors (CMPs), granulocyte–macrophage progenitors (GMPs), and megakaryocytic–erythroid progenitors (MEPs) from patients with PV and analyzed for the presence of the *JAK2V617F* mutation in these progenitor populations.[275] They detected *JAK2V617F* in HSCs, CMPs, GMPs, and MEPs from patients with PV supporting that PV is a disorder that arises in HSCs and involves the myeloid, erythroid, and megakaryocytic lineages.[275] These data are in agreement with a recent report by Ishii et al claiming that *JAK2V617F* can be detected in different hematopoietic lineages in patients with PV,[276] although the mutation could only be detected in lymphoid cells in a minority of patients. Delhommeau et al and Larsen et al have also provided data indicating the JAK2V617F mutation in PV originates in lymphomyeloid progenitor cells.[277,278]

Structural and Functional Aspects of JAK2V617F-Mediated Transformation

The JAK2V617F mutation occurs within the JH2 domain of JAK2, which has significant homology to the kinase domain of JAK2 (JH1) but lacks catalytic activity (see Fig. 68–7). The JH2 domain exerts an inhibitory effect on JAK2 kinase activity and the *V617F* mutation is predicted to disrupt this inhibition.[279] In vitro kinase assays with JAK2V617F and wild-type JAK2 have revealed that JAK2V617F has greatly increased kinase activity, as assessed by autophosphorylation and by substrate phosphorylation.[263] Ectopic expression of JAK2 V617F in either epithelial or hemopoietic cell lines results in autophosphorylation of mutant JAK2, but not the wild-type (WT) JAK2, and activation of downstream signaling events.[79–82,263] BAF3 or FDCP cell lines expressing the EPOR and engineered to stably express JAK2 V617F are largely independent of the addition of exogenous growth factors and are hypersensitive to EPO.[79–82] Lu et al have shown that coexpression of JAK2 V617F and a homodimeric type 1 cytokine receptor (EPOR, TPOR, or G-CSFR) facilitates the transformation of cells to growth-factor independence, suggesting that the mutant JAK2 requires a receptor scaffold in order to be active.[280] This contrasts with the effects of the TEL-JAK2 fusion gene, which can readily transform cells on its own, presumably because of the strong homodimerization effects of the TEL moiety.[281] Ectopic expression of JAK2 V617F can also sensitize cells to the effects of IGF1, a characteristic feature of PV progenitors.[282]

Expression of JAK2V617F in hematopoietic cells activates intracellular signaling pathways downstream of the EPOR including STAT5, STAT3, the MAP kinase pathway, and the PI3K–Akt pathway.[79–82,263] STAT5 is normally phosphorylated by the cytokine receptor–JAK2 complex, and phosphorylated STAT5 then translocates to the nucleus and activates the transcription of target genes. The target genes of STAT5 include Bcl-X_L, an important antiapoptotic protein known to be expressed in increased levels in PV proerythroblasts.[258] The possibility that STAT5-mediated activation of Bcl-X_L is important in the pathogenesis of PV was suggested by a recent report that demonstrated that expression of either constitutively active STAT-5 or Bcl-X_L resulted in spontaneous erythroid colony formation. In addition, cells expressing JAK2V617F display constitutive activation of the MAP kinase pathway (as assessed by phosphorylation of ERK), and of the PI3K pathway (as assessed by phosphorylation of AKT). Furthermore, JAK2 has been shown to play a role in cellular mpl trafficking.[284] The JAK2V617F might also lead to the decreased expression of mpl by platelets observed in PV patients.[284] It is important to note that many other oncogenic tyrosine kinases activate the same signal transduction pathways, and the role and requirement for each of these signaling pathways in the transformation of hematopoietic cells by JAK2V617F remains unknown.

Many PV patients have a low burden of *JAK2V617F* as assessed by DNA sequencing, suggesting that there is either a subpopulation of cells that are homozygous for *JAK2V617F* mixed with wild-type cells or a clonal population of cells with one wild-type copy of *JAK2* and one mutant copy of *JAK2*. In PV, data from clonality/quantitative *JAK2V617F* assessment and from colony assays suggest that most PV patients have a subpopulation of cells homozygous for *JAK2V617F*, whereas in ET clonal progenitor cells are heterozygous for *JAK2V617F*.[268,269] It is therefore important to determine whether the wild-type allele can interfere with the ability of JAK2V617F to constitutively signal in the heterozygous state and whether there is an effect of gene dosage on the activation of signal transduction pathways. Transient coexpression of wild-type JAK2 does not interfere with the ability of JAK2V617F to autophosphorylate, even when wild-type JAK2 is expressed at higher levels than the mutant kinase.[79] This suggests that JAK2V617F kinase activity is unaffected by coexpression of wild-type JAK2. In contrast, when JAK2V617F and wild-type JAK2 were coexpressed in Ba/F3 cells, cytokine-independent growth was attenuated, suggesting in this cellular context that wild-type JAK2 is able to interfere with JAK2V617F-mediated transformation.[79] Suppressors of cytokine signaling (SOCS) proteins bind to the JH1 catalytic loop and target JAK2 for degradation. SOCS1 and SOC3 bind to the catalytic groove belonging to JAK2 and inhibit its catalytic activity. SOCS3 binds to the EPOR and JAK2 to inhibit EPOR signaling. SOCS proteins inhibit JAK2 by functioning as E3 ubiquitin ligases. Hookham and coworkers recently reported that although SOCS1, SOCS2, and SOCS3 inhibit phosphorylation of wild-type JAK2, they are incapable of blocking phosphorylation of JAK2V617F.[285] On the basis of their findings, SOCS3 appears to be unable to inactivate JAK2V617, and SOCS3 itself is not degraded but accumulates and actually promotes the further phosphorylation of JAK2V617F.[285] Such dysregulation likely enhances JAK2V617F-induced cell proliferation and prolongs signaling. These data have been suggested by Hookham to provide an explanation why JAK2V617F hematopoiesis predominates in PV heterozygotes. Low levels of JAK2V617F signaling in JAK2V617F heterozygotes likely induce SOCS3, which would downregulate JAK2 wild-type signaling and enhance signaling by JAK2V617F, permitting the malignant clone to predominate.[285]

Murine Models of JAK2V617F-Mediated Disease

Significant insight regarding the biological consequences of JAK2V617F has been gained by genetic modification of murine bone marrow, allowing them to express JAK2V617F. James et al first reported that the transplantation of marrow cells into lethally irradiated mice that expressed JAK2V617F but not wild-type JAK2 led to the development of marked erythrocytosis and splenomegaly without elevation of granulocyte or platelet counts 28 days after transplantation.[79] This report suggests that JAK2V617F is sufficient for the development of erythrocytosis in PV. Subsequent reports have provided additional insights into the in vivo effects of JAK2V617F.[79,286–289]

Wernig et al have shown that JAK2 V617F expression by marrow cells produces an increased hematocrit and splenomegaly in both C57Bl/6 and Balb/c recipient mice, but marked leukocytosis and bone marrow reticulin fibrosis were only observed in Balb/c mice.[226] Although the bone marrow was characterized by megakaryocyte hyperplasia, recipient mice did not develop thrombocytosis as a result of defects in megakaryocytic maturation and platelet production. These data suggest that there are host modifiers that affect the phenotype induced by JAK2V617F expression. Activation of JAK2 and STAT5 was observed in JAK2V617F-expressing cells but not in cells expressing wild-type JAK2, demonstrating activation of these signal transduction pathways by JAK2V617F in vivo.[286] In addition, erythroid colonies were cloned from marrow cells isolated from mice transduced with JAK2V617F in the absence of EPO and further increased in number in the presence of low levels of EPO. These results suggest that the presence of the JAK2 V617F may be sufficient to induce PV but that the disease phenotype may be affected by other unknown genetic modifiers.

Using a similar approach, Lacout et al also assessed the effects of JAK2V617F on C57Bl/6 mice and followed these mice for 6 months after transplantation.[287] Mice expressing JAK2V617F developed polycythemia and leukocytosis, peaking 3 months after transplant, followed by a progressive reduction in cell counts that was associated with progressive marrow fibrosis and increasing splenomegaly. The degree of bone marrow fibrosis was variable, and interestingly, mice with high-grade fibrosis developed anemia, thrombocytopenia, and neutrophilia consistent with post-PV IM. Again, elevated platelet counts were not observed in mice transduced with JAK2V617F, suggesting that JAK2V617F may not be sufficient for the development of thrombocytosis in patients with PV. One group of secondarily transplanted animals where there was a relatively low level of JAK2 V617F expression was associated with a transient period of thrombocytosis. It has been suggested that this is a situation analogous to that seen in clinical ET where JAK2 V617F homozygosity is rare and may suggest that the lower doses of JAK2V617 lead to thrombocytosis while higher allele frequency results in polycythemia and leukocytosis. These data have also been confirmed by Bumm et al and Zaleskas et al.[288,289]

Data generated from these bone marrow transplant models of JAK2V617F-mediated disease suggest that JAK2V617F is sufficient for the development of PV. Although mice transduced with JAK2V617F display certain features of IM (reticulin fibrosis) and ET (megakaryocytic hyperplasia), the phenotype of these mice more closely resemble that in PV. The dominant erythroid phenotype of JAK2V617F may reflect differences in the pathogenesis of the different MPD. It is possible that PV may result from acquisition and subsequent homozygosity of *JAK2V617F*. Gene dosage or level of expression of JAK2V617F might dictate the phenotype of a particular MPD. This hypothesis is supported by the observation that patients with PV, but not ET, frequently have homozygous *JAK2V617F* mutations and that some patients with ET have monoclonal granulopoiesis even when a minority of cells are *JAK2V617F*-positive.[268] However, the consequences of the expression of JAK2V617F in the heterozygous and homozygous state cannot be assessed using these models, and the genetic basis of the strain-specific differences in phenotype remains unknown. Despite these limitations, these models provide a powerful tool to study a human PV-like illness and provide an in vivo platform for preclinical testing of therapeutic agents that inhibit JAK2V617F.

Other JAK2 Mutations in PV

Other mutations of JAK2 associated with erythrocytosis, however, can also constitutively activate JAK2 kinase activity. Grunebach et al have identified a new mutation in JAK2 that leads to a change of the amino acid aspartate for glutamate at position 620 (JAK2 D620E) in a 27-year-old patient with PV.[290] Scott et al have recently identified four somatic gain-of-function mutations affecting *JAK2* exon 12 in 10 JAK2V617F-negative patients. Those with a *JAK2* exon 12 mutation presented with an isolated erythrocytosis and distinctive bone marrow morphology and had reduced serum EPO levels. Erythroid colonies could be grown from their blood samples in the absence of exogenous EPO.[83] All such erythroid colonies were heterozygous for the mutation, whereas colonies homozygous for the mutation occur in most PV patients with JAK2V617F. BaF3 cells expressing the murine EPOR and also carrying exon 12 mutations can proliferate without added interleukin-3. They also exhibited increased phosphorylation of JAK2 and ERKs, as compared with cells transduced by wild-type JAK2 or V617F JAK2.[83] Three of the exon 12 mutations involved a substitution of leucine for lysine at position 539 of JAK2. This mutation resulted in a myeloproliferative disorder phenotype, including erythrocytosis, in retroviral murine bone marrow transplantation model.[83] *JAK2* exon 12 mutations, therefore, might define a distinctive myeloproliferative syndrome that affects patients who currently carry a diagnosis of idiopathic erythrocytosis. Additional genetic lesions are currently being sought in patients who meet clinical criteria for PV but are JAK2V617F negative.

Familial and Congenital PV—Additional Genetic Events in the Pathogenesis of PV

Despite in vivo data suggesting that *JAK2V617F* might be sufficient for the development of PV, there is evidence that additional genetic events might contribute to the pathogenesis of PV, ET, and/or IM. The fact that the identical *JAK2* mutation is identified in patients with three phenotypically related but clinically distinct MPD suggests that additional genetic and/or epigenetic events likely contribute to the phenotypic divergence of these disorders. Furthermore, Kralovics and coworkers have reported using either restricted fragment length polymorphism analysis or the presence of the cytogenetic abnormality $20q^-$ in patients with MPDs that the percentage of granulocytes and platelets that were JAK2V617F positive was often lower than the percentage of granulocytes belonging to the malignant clone.[291] These findings suggest that the acquisition of JAK2V617F is a relatively late event that is preceded by a genetic event that leads to clonal hematopoiesis. The acquisition of the JAK2V617F apparently occurs in this background of clonal hematopoiesis.

Several investigators have reported families where multiple members have an MPD and have analyzed the JAK2V617F status of family members.[292–295] In a study by Bellane-Chantelot et al, the members of 72 families with multiple members with MPD were analyzed for *JAK2V617F* mutational status.[292] Somatic *JAK2V617F* mutations were identified in some, but not all family members with MPDs. Interestingly, in some families both *JAK2V617F*-positive and *JAK2V617F*-negative members with MPD were observed. A small number of relatives who were JAJ2V617F negative and did not have a diagnosis of PV, ET, or PMF had hematopoietic cells that formed endogenous erythroid colonies in vitro. These results suggest that an as yet unidentified genetic event might contribute to the pathogenesis of PV, ET, and PMF, regardless of *JAK2* mutational status, and that there may be "initiating events" that precede the acquisition of *JAK2V617F* in these disorders. It is anticipated that the recent development of whole genome mapping technologies will permit researchers to identify the disease allele that predisposes these family members to develop an MPD.[292–295]

ETIOLOGY AND PATHOGENESIS

The most frequent cause of mortality in PV patients is vascular thrombosis.[206,207,296,297] This increased thrombotic tendency is believed primarily to be a direct consequence of the expanded red cell mass that characterizes this disorder.[298] However, the thrombotic tendency in PV may be multifactorial in origin, with quantitative defects of platelets and neutrophils contributing to its development.[299–306]

In the European Collaboration on Low-Dose Aspirin in Polycythemia Vera (ECLAP) study,[307] the incidence of cardiovascular complications was higher in patients older than 65 years (5.0% of patients per year; hazard ratio 2.0; confidence interval (CI) 1.22–3.29; $P <$ 0.006) or with a history of thrombosis (4.93% of patients per year; hazard ratio 1.96; 95% CI 1.29–2.97; $P = 0.0017$).[307] Patients both with a history of thrombosis and older than 65 years had the highest risk of developing additional cardiovascular events (10.9% of patients per year; hazard ratio 4.35; 95% CI 2.95–6.41; $P < 0.0001$). These data confirm previous findings that increasing age and history of thrombosis are the two most important prognostic factors for the development of vascular complications.[307]

This information does not negate the increased incidence of thrombotic incidents also observed in younger patients with this disorder.[308] In a series of 58 PV patients younger than 40 years, a disturbingly high incidence of life-threatening thrombotic events was observed. In fact, 7 of the 10 patients in this series who died during the period of observation died from thrombotic events: four from Budd–Chiari syndrome, one from a pulmonary embolism, and two from cerebral thrombosis.[244] Therefore, although a significant factor, preexisting atherosclerotic disease is not the sole etiologic factor in the genesis of thrombosis in PV. Some have suggested an important role for smoking as a secondary factor leading to the increased incidence of thrombotic events in this patient population.[309,310]

The principal hemorrheologic abnormality in PV is an elevated whole blood viscosity.[311–313] The blood viscosity in PV is higher than that of normal controls at all shear rates.[311–313] In a retrospective analysis of the records of 69 PV patients with histories of vascular thrombosis, Pearson and Wetherley-Mein,[298] in a seminal report, demonstrated a strong correlation in univariate analysis between hematocrit level and the development of thrombotic episodes, including many cerebrovascular occlusions (Fig. 68–9). Thomas and coworkers showed that cerebral blood flow is reduced in patients with PV in whom the hematocrit level is 53% to 62%.[298] These abnormalities were observed even in patients with hematocrits at the lower levels of normal, that is, 46% to 52%.[298] Reductions in cerebral blood flow were correctable with phlebotomy. Reduction of the hematocrit by relatively small amounts frequently led to substantial improvements in whole blood viscosity and cerebral blood flow. Some PV patients apparently still maintain a higher than normal whole blood viscosity despite the normalization of the hematocrit, suggesting that an increase in hematocrit may not be the only factor responsible for increased blood viscosity.[312]

A number of possible explanations have been suggested for the observed relationship between hematocrit and the development of thrombotic events in PV patients. Turrito and Weiss[313] presented evidence indicating that platelet adhesion and thrombus formation on the vascular subendothelium are determined in part by the rate at which platelets are transported to the vascular surface. In a polycythemic condition in which increased numbers of red cells are present, a greater number of intercellular collisions between red cells and platelets occur. These collisions could lead to increased platelet movement in a direction perpendicular to blood flow. This facilitation of platelet transport to the vessel wall may be an important factor in the development of thrombosis.[313] An alternative explanation for

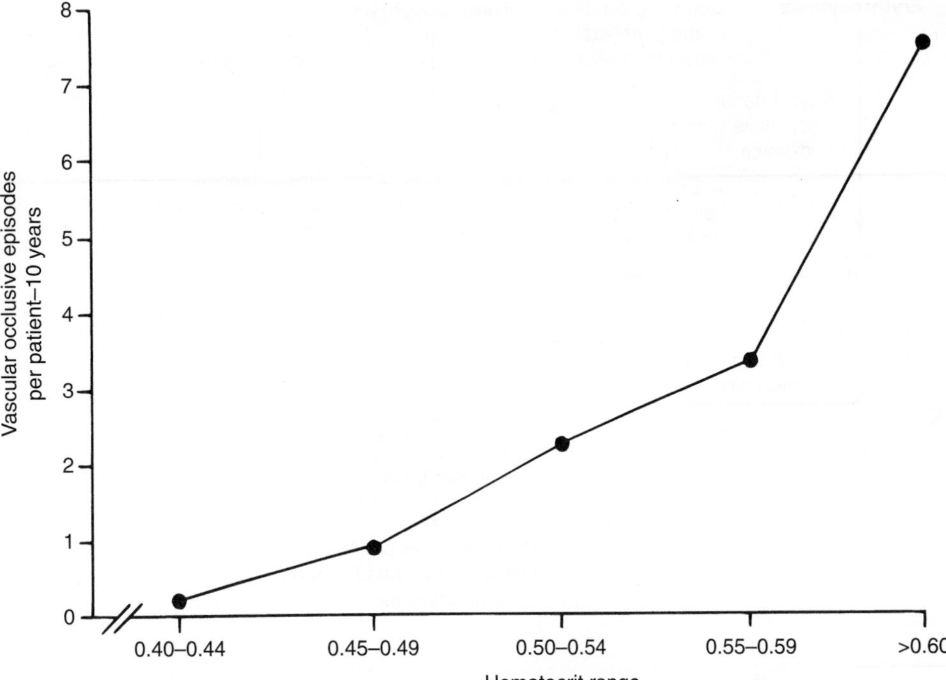

Figure 68–9. Relation of hematocrit to number of vascular occlusive episodes per 10 years in patients with polycythemia vera. (Data from Pearson TC, Wetherley-Mein G: Vascular occlusive episodes and venous haematocrit in primary proliferative polycythemia. Lancet 2:1219, 1978.)

the association between hematocrit level and the risk of thrombosis is based on the knowledge that blood viscosity is particularly sensitive to hematocrit levels.[12,309,310] Increased hematocrits lead to increased blood viscosity, in turn leading to increased peripheral vascular resistance and an actual reduction in blood flow to a variety of organs, predisposing them to the development of thrombosis.[309,310] The issue of hematocrit and thrombosis in PV has been prospectively investigated in a recent analysis of 1638 patients enrolled in the ECLAP study.[314] In this prospective study, in spite of recommendations of maintaining hematocrit levels less than 45%, only 50% of patients achieved this target during the follow-up and 10% had hematocrit levels above 50%.[314] These different hematocrit values were not associated with different thrombotic outcomes as assessed using univariate and multivariable analysis. The clinical significance of this finding appears to be relevant for the construction of future therapeutic guidelines and deserves to be validated in prospective randomized clinical trials. Additional factors have been implicated in the development of thrombosis in PV patients. Almost all patients with PV are iron deficient.[315] Decreased red cell deformability has been said to accompany iron deficiency, leading to increased blood viscosity and a decreased ability of red cells to pass through small-bore polycarbonate filters.[316–320] Such abnormalities have been shown by Tillman and Schröter[320] and Yip and colleagues[252] to be due to increased membrane stiffness rather than to reduced surface–volume ratio, as has been suggested by others. This increased membrane stiffness, however, might be counterbalanced by the effect of a reduced red blood cell size on the adherence of blood platelets to arteriolar subendothelium. Aarts and coworkers[319] have shown that red cell size is a major determinant of platelet adherence, with larger red blood cells leading to increased platelet adherence and smaller red cells to decreased platelet adherence. Whether the increased membrane stiffness associated with iron deficiency is counterbalanced by the decreased platelet adherence associated with smaller red blood cells is yet to be determined.

Studies of patients with hemoglobinopathies due to abnormal oxygen binding who have secondary erythrocytosis provide further support to the belief that hematocrit elevations are not the sole cause of the thrombotic tendency in PV. A survey of patients with these types of hemoglobinopathies has not demonstrated a higher incidence of myocardial ischemia or any other form of thrombosis, even though the red cell mass is frequently as elevated as that in patients with PV.[321] Furthermore, Shibata and colleagues studied the risk of thrombosis in a transgenic mouse model with extreme erythrocytosis due to overexpression of EPO and did not observe an increased incidence of thrombosis.[117]

Thrombocytosis and qualitative platelet abnormalities occur frequently and are likely to be important contributory factors to the development of thrombosis.[206,304,305,322–332] Dawson and Ogston[324] have implicated uncontrolled thrombocytosis as a cause of thrombosis in these patients, but this relation has not been confirmed by Kessler and colleagues[322] or Berk and colleagues.[296] Increased plasma and urinary thromboxane production has been linked to increased platelet activation in these patients.[323] A low-dose aspirin regimen selective for inhibition of platelet cyclooxygenase has been found to suppress increased thromboxane production in vivo and to clinically benefit patients with PV.[302,303,325,326] Furthermore, elevated levels of serum vascular endothelial growth factor and plasma TPO have been observed in PV patients.[301] These growth factors have been shown to lead to platelet activation.[301]

Despite conflicting data, no clear clinical relationship between platelet number or function and the incidence of hemorrhage or thrombosis in PV patients has been delineated.[297,298,314,322–327] An argument in favor of a role of elevated platelet numbers in the genesis of thrombosis in PV and ET is the observation in patients with ET that a reduction of excessive platelet numbers with the use of hydroxyurea is associated with a reduction in the risk of developing thrombotic events.[327] However, this should not be taken as evidence that the reduction in developing additional vascular events was due to platelet count normalization alone; very likely, it may be related to the suppression by hydroxyurea of each of three myeloid lineages. In line with this interpretation are the results of a randomized study performed by the Medical Research Council in the United Kingdom (PT-01) in which patients with ET were randomized to receive either hydroxyurea or anagrelide therapy.[333] This study showed that hydroxyurea therapy rather than anagrelide, a selective platelet number-reducing drug, was associated with a reduction in the number of arterial thrombotic events, especially in JAK2V617F patients.[333] In a recently reported analysis of the ECLAP study, the rate of thrombosis in PV patients during follow-up did not vary according to different platelet numbers.[314] Select patients with PV have, however, been afforded prompt resolution of vascular complications such as erythromelalgia or transient ischemic attacks following institution of platelet antiaggregating agents or cytoreduction.[259,260,262] It is important to emphasize that erythromelalgia does not resolve in PV patients with phlebotomy alone or with anticoagu-

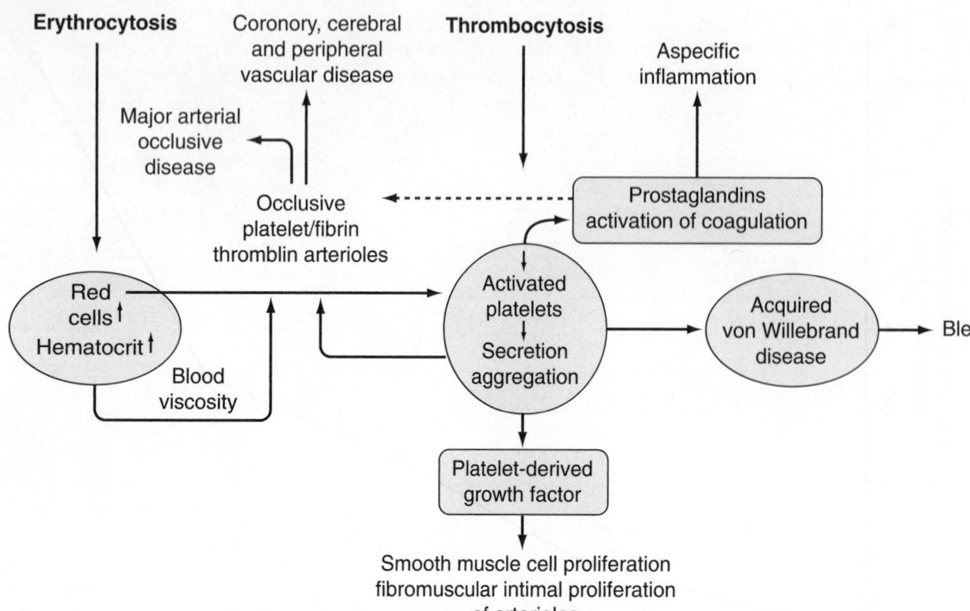

Figure 68–10. Pathophysiology of arteriolar and arterial thrombosis and inflammation, as well as hemorrhage, as a multicellular process in polycythemia vera. (Modified from Michiels JJ, Leenknegt H, Michiels JJ, Budde U: Acquired von Willebrand disease in myeloproliferative disorders. Leuk Lymph 22(Suppl 1):79, 1996.)

lation but requires the use of platelet antiaggregating agents or reduction of platelet numbers.[328] What distinguishes the clinical courses of these patients from those of others is unknown. These reports coupled with the knowledge of abnormal thromboxane metabolism of platelets in PV provide substance to the belief that platelets contribute to the generation of the thrombotic and hemorrhagic tendencies observed in PV (Fig. 68–10).[323–328] Although a number of clinical assessments of platelet function have been used to identify patients who are potentially at a high risk of developing a life-threatening hemorrhagic or thrombotic event, the results of these studies to date have been very disappointing.[323–328] It appears that the etiology of thrombosis and hemorrhage in PV is multifactorial and that the available tools are inadequate to identify those patients at highest risk.[303]

An elevation of white cell number occurs in 50% to 60% of PV patients that may also have a detrimental effect on the rheology of the microcirculation in PV.[299,300,334] A recent analysis of the ECLAP database showed that baseline white blood cell count above 15,000 × 106 L^{-1} was associated with the development of major arterial events, mainly myocardial infarction.[334] Similar results were shown also in two additional studies in patients with ET.[335,336] Activated leukocytes may release proteases and oxygen radicals that alter endothelial cells and platelets so as to favor the development of a prothrombotic state.[299,300] Falanga and coworkers have shown that a series of markers of leukocyte activation, including expression of membrane CD11b and leukocyte alkaline phosphatase antigen, cellular elastase content, plasma elastase levels, and myeloperoxidase levels are elevated in patients with PV.[300] Limited and conflicting data are available as to whether or not there is a correlation between the presence of platelet-leukocyte interactions and thrombotic events. Moreover, the association between these functional abnormalities and the presence of JAK2V617F is unclear.[337] Overall these results would indicate that an increased release of neutrophil proteases may provide a mechanism by which the hemostatic pathway is activated in PV, which ultimately would contribute to the establishment of a prethrombotic state.[300]

PV patients are also at an increased risk of developing life-threatening hemorrhagic complications.[305,329–332] Abnormalities in platelet function and number have been implicated as the cause of this hemorrhagic tendency.[305,306,322–332] Qualitative platelet abnormalities frequently found in these patients include platelet hypofunction as demonstrated by defective in vitro platelet aggregation, acquired storage pool disease, platelet membrane defects, increased platelet reactivity as demonstrated by enhanced platelet aggregation, increased plasma β-thromboglobulin levels, and shortened platelet survival.[323–325,330] With platelet counts greater than 1000 × 10^9 L^{-1}, the development of acquired von Willebrand syndrome has been reported and is associated with life-threatening hemorrhagic episodes.[329,330]

A major cause of morbidity and mortality in PV results from the transition from the polycythemic phase of the disease to PV related MF and to acute leukemia. PPMM is characterized by cytopenias, myelofibrosis, and extramedullary hematopoiesis.[338–340] In a variety of MPDs, the fibroblastic component of the bone marrow has been shown not to be directly involved in the malignant process but to be a reactive event to the neoplastic clone.[341,342] Several investigators have suggested that the release of growth factors, particularly platelet-derived growth factor (PDGF), fibroblast growth factor, and transforming growth factor-β from megakaryocytes or platelets, which are present in abundance in patients with MPDs, might be responsible for this fibroblastic proliferation.[341] Whether the use of any particular therapeutic agents for treatment of PV accelerates the development of PV related MF remains hotly debated. Some have suggested that the use of radioactive phosphorus (^{32}P) favors such a transition, although others have not noted any relation between the treatment modality used and more rapid progression to PV related MF.[271–275] Najean and associates have reported a long-term follow-up of PV patients and noted a high incidence of myelofibrosis in patients treated by phlebotomy alone.[276] In this study, myelofibrosis was rarely observed before the 10th year of follow-up, but occurred in 20% of patients surviving after 15 years and 50% surviving after 20 years.[276] Messinezy and Pearson have reported that of 20 patients known to have survived 15 years with PV, 25% developed myelofibrosis.[277] Surprisingly, in the Italian Natural History Study with a follow-up of 20 years, myelofibrosis was a rare cause of death.[235] After treatment with alkylating agents or irradiation during the proliferative phase, patients with PV related MF have been reported to be more likely to transform to acute leukemia.[166] No randomized studies have been powered to assess the relative risk of malignant transformation in patients given HU. The bulk of evidence does not support a clear leukemogenic role for this drug that is currently considered the standard therapy in high-risk PV patients. Nevertheless, as a cautionary principle, it is wise to consider carefully the use of this agent in very young subjects and in those carrying cytogenetic abnormalities, and to avoid it in pregnant women and in patients previously exposed to radiophosphorus or alkylating agents.[348]

CLINICAL MANIFESTATIONS

The principal clinical manifestations of PV are direct consequences of the excessive proliferation of cellular elements of the various hematopoietic cellular lineages involved in the neoplastic process. With the current widespread use of laboratory screening tests during routine patient examination, increasing numbers of people are being diagnosed with PV before the development of symptoms related to this neoplastic process. Symptomatic patients with PV may present to a physician with a myriad of nonspecific complaints, including headaches, weakness, pruritus, dizziness, excessive sweating, visual disturbances, paresthesias, joint symptoms, epigastric distress, and weight loss.[196,206–208] Thrombosis is a frequent presenting event.[297] In one series, two-thirds of such thrombotic events occurred either at presentation or before diagnosis and the remainder during follow-up.[297] At diagnosis, one-third of patients have already lost 10% of their body weight, presumably secondary to the hypermetabolism associated with this disorder.[206] Arthropathies that are frequently observed in these patients are largely due to the clinical manifestations of gout. The hyperproliferative bone marrow state characteristic of PV and the increased nucleoprotein degradation are contributing factors in the development of hyperuricemia.

The principal findings on physical examination of a patient with PV include ruddy cyanosis, conjunctival plethora, hepatomegaly, splenomegaly, and hypertension.[196,206,208,297]

Untreated patients are at particularly high risk for thrombotic and hemorrhagic events.[285,307,331,332] In several large series of patients with PV, thrombosis was the cause of death in 30% to 40% of patients (Table 68–6).[206–208,285,329–333] Arterial thrombotic events account for two-thirds of such events, with venous thrombotic events representing the remainder. Ischemic stroke, myocardial infarction, and transient ischemic attacks are the most common arterial thrombotic events. Patients may also present with deep venous thrombosis in the lower extremities, pulmonary embolism, or peripheral vascular occlusions.[296–298] It is not unusual for patients with PV to develop thromboses at unusual anatomic sites; in particular, thromboses are relatively frequent in the splenic, hepatic, portal, and mesenteric vessels.[206–208,285,307] A meta-analysis on 120 patients from seven studies indicated that the estimated prevalence of an underlying MPD was 49% for patients with idiopathic hepatic vein thrombosis and 23% for patients with portal vein thrombosis.[350]

Reisner and coworkers have demonstrated by echocardiography that cardiac valvular abnormalities are common in patients with myeloproliferative disorders.[351] In fact, aortic or mitral valve lesions were found in 77% of patients with PV. The most common echocardiography lesion was leaflet thickening, found in 40% of patients, and vegetation, which occurred in 16%. The presence of such lesions was closely associated with the occurrence of arterial or venous thrombosis or embolism. Such vascular abnormalities may account for a significant number of thrombotic events in this patient population.[351]

A particularly serious thrombotic event associated with PV is Budd–Chiari syndrome,[352–359] which results from hepatic venous or inferior vena caval thrombosis and obstruction. These events lead to hepatic venous outflow obstruction, increased hepatic sinusoidal pressure, and portal hypertension. Portal venous perfusion of the liver is frequently reduced, leading to portal venous thrombosis and hypoxic damage of liver parenchymal cells. This cascade of events results in centrilobular hepatic necrosis, centrilobular fibrosis, and nodular regenerative fibrosis, which culminates in the development of cirrhosis of the liver.[356] The cause of Budd–Chiari syndrome can be identified in 75% of cases, including hereditary and acquired prothrombotic disorders; trauma and infection PV account for 10% to 40% of all cases of Budd–Chiari syndrome.[352–359] Paroxysmal nocturnal hemoglobinuria is also a frequent cause of Budd–Chiari syndrome. Because marrow cells from 87% of patients with idiopathic Budd–Chiari syndrome form erythroid colonies in the absence of EPO, such patients are believed to be suffering from a forme fruste of an MPD.[356–358] The identification of these latent MPDs, without elevated blood counts, may be facilitated by screening for the JAK2 mutation. Primignani et al reported that JAK2V617F mutation occurred in 35% of 73 patients with extrahepatic portal vein thrombosis and in 40% of 20 patients with the Budd–Chiari syndrome while Patel and coworkers demonstrated that 58% of patients with idiopathic Budd–Chiari syndrome were JAK2V617F positive.[360] An MPD developed in over 90% of the JAK2V617F-positive patients after a median of 49 months from the diagnosis of Budd–Chiari syndrome.[361] Detection of the JAK2V617F mutation in 38% to 42.8% of patients with splanchnic vein thrombosis and normal/low blood cell counts has been reported.[362] Furthermore, JAK2V617F has been detected in 18% to 37% of patients with portal vein thrombosis.[363,364] The diagnostic value of low serum erythropoietin level in Budd–Chiari syndrome has been questioned since elevated levels have been attributed in JAK2V617F-positive patients to necrotic liver tissue.[365]

There are fulminant, acute, subacute, or chronic forms of Budd–Chiari syndrome.[356] These clinical manifestations are dependent on the extent and rapidity of hepatic vein occlusion and the development of venous collaterals to decompress the venous sinusoids. One should always consider a diagnosis of Budd–Chiari syndrome in any patient with an MPD with ascites, upper abdominal pain, and liver function abnormalities.[344–356] This syndrome is characterized by hepatosplenomegaly, ascites, edema of the peripheral extremities, and distention of superficial abdominal veins due to resultant portal hypertension.[356] Routine biochemical determinations of hepatocellular function and injury are frequently of little diagnostic value in patients with suspected Budd–Chiari syndrome.[356] Doppler ultrasonography is the best tool for screening patients for Budd–Chiari syndrome. This test has a sensitivity and specificity of 85%.[356,359] Characteristic findings include an absence of flow in the hepatic veins or nonvisualization of the hepatic vein. Contrast-enhanced computed tomographic scanning and magnetic resonance imaging are useful in better defining the hepatic venous anatomy.[356,359] Hepatic venous and inferior vena caval catheterization are key diagnostic procedures that indicate the sites of venous obstruction.[356–359] The diagnosis can be definitively made by a spider web pattern on hepatic venography. Transjugular liver biopsy specimens usually reveal intense congestion and cellular atrophy.[356,359]

Table 68–6 Fatal and Nonfatal Thrombotic Events (n = 254) During Follow-Ups in 1213 Patients With Polycythemia Vera

	Type of Complication	
	Nonfatal Event *n* **(%)**	**Fatal Event** *n* **(%)**
Arterial thrombosis	101 (50.5)	44 (81.5)
Myocardial infarction	28 (14.0)	27 (50.0)
Ischemic stroke	19 (9.5)	17 (31.5)
Transient ischemic attack	39 (19.5)	—
Peripheral arterial thrombosis	15 (7.5)	—
Venous thrombosis or embolism	77 (38.5)	10 (18.5)
Deep venous thrombosis	35 (17.5)	—
Superficial thrombophlebitis	37 (18.5)	—
Unknown	5 (2.5)	—
Unknown	22 (11.0)	—
Total	200 (100)	54 (100)

Data from Gruppo Italiano Studio Policitemia: Polycythemia vera: The natural history of 1213 patients followed for 20 years. Ann Intern Med 123:656, 1995.

It has been emphasized that patients with PV can present with portal or hepatic vein thrombosis with normal hemoglobin or hematocrit values. Such patients have leukocytosis, thrombocytosis, or splenomegaly.[355,359] The diagnosis of "inapparent PV" in this patient population can only be made after red cell volume measurements are performed.[355] Screening for the JAK2 mutation should be systematically carried out in such situations, and may substitute for red cell volume measurements.[362] Gastrointestinal bleeding or an increase in plasma volume that is a consequence of splenomegaly often accounts for the normal blood counts in such patients with Budd–Chiari syndrome. The factors operational in the PV patient that lead to the development of hepatic vein thrombosis are believed to be multiple. Splenomegaly causes increased portal blood flow whereas extramedullary hematopoiesis within the hepatic sinusoids frequently obstructs hepatic blood flow.[355] These processes are surely important contributory factors, in addition to the other previously discussed risk factors that lead to the development of thrombosis in this patient population.[355–359]

Neurologic abnormalities occur in almost 60% to 80% of untreated or poorly controlled PV patients and include transient ischemic attacks, cerebral infarction, cerebral hemorrhage, fluctuating dementia, confusional states, and choreic syndromes.[296,298,351,366–372] In addition, complaints of dizziness, paresthesias, visual disturbances, tinnitus, and headaches have been attributed to the increased blood viscosity[296,298,351,366–372] and reduced cerebral blood flow caused by erythrocytosis. The transient neurologic symptoms can also be the consequence of small infarcts in the region of the basal ganglia, which can be detected by computed tomography.[367] These small infarcts are known as lacunae and result from the occlusion of small penetrating arteries, which are particularly susceptible to thrombosis.[367] Cerebrovascular thrombosis occurs more often in PV patients than in the general population.[331,370,366–369] Symptoms due to intermittent carotid or vertebral basilar artery insufficiency (or both) occur so frequently in PV that Millikan and colleagues[369] suggest that every patient with focal cerebrovascular insufficiency should at least have a complete blood count test to rule out an underlying MPD.

Cavernous sinus thrombosis is usually associated with a primary infectious etiology involving a focus in the face, throat, mouth, ear, or sinuses.[371–374] Aseptic cavernous sinus thrombosis is an extremely rare phenomenon that has been reported in patients with PV.[371–379] These patients present with monocular blindness and the characteristic features of ipsilateral cavernous sinus thrombosis, and only retrospectively is the diagnosis of PV made.[374] Therefore, patients found to have this symptom complex who have no known infectious predisposing causes should be carefully evaluated to rule out this diagnosis. The most sensitive diagnostic technique is MRI in combination with magnetic resonance venography. If MRI is not readily available, CT scanning is useful as the initial examination to rule out other acute neurological disorders. In some cases cerebral angiography may be indicated.[375]

Thrombosis of large-caliber arteries is a relatively rare event in PV patients, but there have been case reports of thromboses within the chambers of the heart, leading to refractory congestive heart failure and acute aortic occlusion.[295,296] Such catastrophic thrombotic events in the heart or large vessels would suggest that cardiac catheterization be performed with some caution.[296]

PV frequently manifests with symptoms due to peripheral vascular disease.[254,255,297–299] In these cases, patients may first be seen by surgeons or dermatologists.[298] Intense redness or cyanosis of the digits with or without burning, classic erythromelalgia, digital ischemia with palpable pulses, or thrombophlebitis without other known cause may be the presenting symptoms.[327,380–384]

Erythromelalgia is characterized by burning pain in the digits, an objective sensation of increased temperature, and relief by cooling.[328,380–384] PV is the most common cause of erythromelalgia and is one of the few disorders in which digital ischemia with or without ulceration may exist in the presence of palpable pulses.[384] Other disorders that can lead to this abnormality include embolism, trauma, cutaneous infarction, neuritis, infection, and various types of arteritis.[384] Painful and ulcerating toes and fingers have frequently been observed to be presenting symptoms in patients with PV.[380–384] The likelihood that arterial insufficiency is the cause of such ulceration is quite small in patients who have a palpable dorsalis pedis and posterior tibialis pulses; in this situation, the possibility of an underlying hematologic disorder such as PV should be entertained. Foot pain at rest is a distressing but not widely recognized symptom of PV. In patients with this complaint, peripheral pulses are of normal character and cutaneous circulation appears to be adequate.[328,380–384] The pain is most severe at night, is dull in nature, and occurs primarily in the feet or legs. These symptoms have been shown to be the results of platelet activation and aggregation in vivo, which preferentially occur in arterioles.[261] If untreated, erythromelalgia can progress to ischemic acrocyanosis or gangrene. Phlebotomy alone in PV does not improve erythromelalgia.[328,380–384] These symptoms can be abolished by reducing the platelet counts to normal levels and can be rapidly reversed after the institution of antiplatelet aggregation therapy. Therefore, the cause of erythromelalgia appears to be closely linked to abnormal arachidonic acid metabolism that occurs within platelets in this disorder.[328]

Retrospective reviews have revealed a higher than expected number of patients with PV and pulmonary hypertension.[385–387] Proposed etiologies include direct obstruction of pulmonary arteries by circulating megakaryocytes, extramedullary hematopoiesis in the pulmonary parenchyma, smooth muscle hyperplasia induced by release of platelet-derived growth factor from activated platelets, chronic disseminated intravascular coagulation, and unrecognized recurrent thrombotic events.[387] Endothelin-1 has been associated with development of hypoxia-related pulmonary hypertension and VEGF with protection from this complication. The diagnosis of pulmonary hypertension is made, on average, 9.5 years after the diagnosis of the underlying MPD disorder and is associated with a poor prognosis, with death usually occurring as a result of congestive heart failure or pneumonia.[380] Although anecdotal reports have claimed improvements in patients' pulmonary artery pressure with control of the underlying disease,[386,387] Dingli and coworkers at the Mayo Clinic did not find any change in serial measurements of 11 patients' pulmonary arterial pressures despite good disease control.[386]

As many as 30% to 40% of patients with PV experience some sort of hemorrhagic event,* which can be relatively trivial, such as epistaxis or gingival hemorrhage, or can be life-threatening, such as gastrointestinal hemorrhage or hematomas involving vital organs.[329–331,388] The gastrointestinal tract is a frequent site of hemorrhagic complications, as patients with PV are predisposed to portal vein thrombosis and resultant variceal bleeding and pepticular disease. Gastroduodenal erosions and ulcers and *Helicobacter pylori* infection are all significantly more common in PV patients than in control patients with dyspepsia.[391] This may be due in part to altered mucosal blood flow as a result of increased plasma viscosity or increased histamine release due to peripheral blood basophilia.[391] Cerebral hemorrhage is a common cause of morbidity and mortality.[367] Bleeding events frequently occur with the use of antiinflammatory agents[332]; an association between the hemorrhage and the use of high doses of these platelet-paralyzing drugs has been made in almost one-third of such instances.[389,390] Low-dose aspirin therapy has, however, been recently shown not to lead to an increased incidence of life-threatening hemorrhagic events.[302,303] Spontaneous bleeding in patients with PV is relatively rare,[304,308] although spontaneous retropharyngeal hematomas leading to acute upper-airway obstruction or hematomas in the groin have been reported.[392]

The PV patient who undergoes a surgical procedure is at a very high risk of developing postoperative complications.[393–395] In one series of 62 major operations on 54 patients with PV, postoperative complications occurred in 47% of patients[393]; 52% of complications were due to hemorrhage, 18% to thrombosis, and 14% to hemorrhage and thrombosis.[315] The postoperative mortality rate in this patient population was 18%.[393] In another series of 15 patients, 5

*References 12, 331, 332, 336, and 388–390.

suffered serious complications secondary to thrombosis and hemorrhage.[394,395] A recent study by an Italian group evaluated retrospectively 311 surgical interventions in 105 patients with PV and 150 with ET[394]: 24 arterial or venous thrombosis (7.7%), 23 major hemorrhages (7.3%), and 5 surgery-related deaths (1.6%) were observed within 3 months of the procedure. PV patients with uncontrolled erythrocytosis prior to surgery have been shown to have the highest complication rate. Patients with inadequately controlled disease had a 79% incidence of complications, whereas in those who enjoyed adequate hematologic control before surgery the rate of perioperative and postoperative complications was reduced to 28%.[396] In addition, duration of disease control was an important factor in decreasing surgical risk[393–396]; a prolonged period of effective disease control before surgery reduced the complication rate to 5%.[396] Complication rates following surgery can therefore be dramatically reduced by appropriate therapeutic interventions with normalization of blood counts. The chief deterrent to such an approach has been the failure by physicians to recognize the risk associated with PV in the surgical setting.

Generalized pruritus occurs in approximately 50% of cases of PV.[196,397–400] Water contact, such as during showers or bathing, induces attacks of intolerable pruritus.[398] There appears to be no clear relation between the degree of the pruritus and severity of the disease,[400] and 20% of patients continue to experience itching despite reduction of their red blood cell masses to the normal range.[397–400] Aquagenic pruritus is significantly more common among JAK2V617F homozygous patients than heterozygotes or WT patients.[401,402] The degree of pruritus is so severe in some patients that they are unable to tolerate bathing at all and find it necessary to substitute gentle skin swabbing or to simply not bathe. The etiology of the pruritus in PV remains uncertain. Several groups have attempted to implicate elevated blood and urine histamine levels in its pathobiology.[397,400] Steinman and colleagues[398] have presented data suggesting that water exposure in patients with PV actually leads to elevated histamine levels, which would provide an explanation for the exacerbation of the pruritus frequently observed with water contact. Jackson and associates[399] have been able to establish a strong correlation between skin mast cell numbers and the severity of itching. However, the failure of the pruritus to respond to antihistamine therapy in many patients suggests that abnormally high histamine levels probably do not constitute the sole factor in its development.

Iron deficiency has also been implicated as a factor contributing to pruritus in PV patients who are almost invariably iron deficient.[403] Iron substitution therapy has resulted in symptomatic improvement,[403] but this approach is less than optimal because it frequently results in uncontrollable erythrocytosis.

Several investigators have suggested that patients suffer from serious nonhematologic symptoms secondary to iron deficiency.[404–406] Rector and colleagues[406] evaluated these sequelae in patients with PV who were uniformly iron deficient and followed these patients for more than 25 years. Their data are unique in that they indicate that the quantitative evaluation of symptoms fails to provide convincing evidence that undue fatigue occurs as a result of iron deficiency.[406] In fact, treadmill performances by six patients were equivalent to those observed among normal subjects.[323] None of the patients experienced dysphagia or the esophageal changes associated with chronic iron deficiency.[323] The one symptom that was observed to occur regularly, particularly in women, was picophagia, a pica consisting of compulsive ice eating.[323] This symptom can be resolved with ingestion of extremely small amounts of oral iron.

PV related MF occurs in 5% to 50% of patients with PV.[†] The transition to this stage of the disease occurs, on average, 10 years after the initial diagnosis, but in individual cases it can occur after either shorter or longer intervals. Two extremes of opinion exist on the frequency of this complication. Najean and coworkers have reported that 15 years or more after the initial diagnosis, this complication is a major clinical problem affecting almost 50% of patients.[338] Spivak has, however, questioned the true frequencies of anemia, myelofibrosis, and extramedullary hematopoiesis in the absence of cytotoxic therapy for PV patients.[12] He has suggested that in individuals treated only with phlebotomy PV related MF is a rare event. In the ECLAP study, the development of PV related MF was associated with long duration of disease and was not influenced by patient age or the use of cytoreductive drugs. For patients with disease duration greater than 10 years, hazard ratio was 15.24 (95% CI 4.22–55.06, $P <$ 0.0001).[307] PV related MF is characterized by (a) increasing splenomegaly, (b) teardrop red blood cell morphology, (c) extensive bone marrow fibrosis, (d) a leukoerythroblastic blood picture, and (e) a normal or decreasing red blood cell mass. The patients may be entirely asymptomatic but often complain of fatigue, dizziness, weight loss, and anorexia.[338–390] Splenomegaly can lead to abdominal pain due to repeated splenic infarcts and to early satiety due to mechanical obstruction of the upper gastrointestinal tract.

The anemia that characterizes the spent phase is primarily a result of splenic pooling, ineffective erythropoiesis, and extramedullary production of red blood cells with a shortened red cell survival. Patients positive for JAK2V617F are less likely to require blood transfusion but have a poorer survival.[408] Occasionally, the anemia is exacerbated by a folate or iron deficiency.[309] Before assuming that a patient has entered the spent phase, it is prudent to assess bone marrow iron stores. Replacement therapy with iron may lead to the resurgence of erythropoiesis and prevent the faulty categorization of disease progression.

Bleeding abnormalities due to thrombocytopenia or qualitative platelet abnormalities are especially common during this phase of the disease. Frequent instances of epistaxis or ecchymoses occur,[338–340] and gastrointestinal hemorrhage due to esophageal varices arising from portal hypertension is a recurrent problem.[338–340] The majority of hemorrhagic events are minor in nature. Frequently, patients suffer from generalized wasting characterized by progressive asthenia and weight loss. Severe hyperuricemia, leading to secondary gout or uric acid nephropathy, may also complicate the clinical course.

Patients with PV related MF are at a high risk for the development of acute leukemia.[12,233,340–348,410–422] Of those patients who enter the spent phase of PV, 20% to 50% will eventually undergo leukemic transformation.[339,340] Approximately 70% of patients who enter the spent phase will be dead 3 years after this transition; however, the other 30% of these patients will have much longer survival times averaging 6.5 years.[338–340]

The leukemic transformation of PV has been extensively described.[315,410–424] The possibility that a relation exists between the therapeutic modality used during the erythrocytotic phase and the frequency of development of acute leukemia has been a point of heated discussion.[12,410,411] Some of the controversy surrounding this question was formerly due to a lack of understanding of the basic origins of PV.[12] Clinical hematologists in the 1950s and 1960s frequently thought of PV as a benign hematologic abnormality and believed that therapeutic interventions either with alkylating agents or radiotherapy were solely responsible for the development of acute leukemia. That concept has proved erroneous, and PV, like the other MPDs, has been shown to be a clonal malignant hematologic disorder.[78,336,337] The evolution to acute leukemia can therefore be thought of as a natural consequence of this malignant disorder, which can be accentuated by the therapeutic interventions discussed above.

Further insight into the relation between acute leukemia and PV has been best provided by the results of the PV Study Group (PVSG), which described a randomized trial comparing the use of phlebotomy, chlorambucil, and ^{32}P for the treatment of this disorder.[333] The incidence of acute leukemia was approximately 1.5% in patients treated with phlebotomy alone, 17.5% in patients treated with chlorambucil, and 10.9% in patients treated with ^{32}P after over 15 years of follow-up.[418–421] The incidence of acute leukemia in the patients treated with phlebotomy alone is therefore much higher than that expected in a normal age-matched control group, again indicating that leukemia is a natural evolutionary event in the clinical course of an individual with PV. The incidence of acute leukemia can be

†References 206–208, 307, 338–340, 349, 407, and 408.

increased, however, by institution of therapy with either alkylating agents or ^{32}P.[418–421] The time course for the development of acute leukemia appears to be dependent on the treatment used to control the polycythemia. The development of acute leukemia in patients treated with phlebotomy in the PVSG trial was limited to the first 5 years of treatment, suggesting that the development of acute leukemia is not due solely to the prolongation of survival. In contrast, analysis of the hazard function was virtually flat for patients treated with chlorambucil from years 2 to 7 after randomization; however, the risk for acute leukemia became alarmingly high after 10 years of study, suggesting that the risk of acute leukemia increases with time, even after the drug has been stopped.[412–421] One half of the cases of acute leukemia in the chlorambucil arm occurred in the first 5 years, with the remainder equally split between the second and third 5-year periods. In contrast, 60% of the cases of acute leukemia in the group treated with radioactive phosphorus occurred 6 to 10 years after randomization. Of particular concern is the high incidence of leukemia recently reported in patients who were initially treated with radioactive phosphorous or busulphan and then switched to maintenance therapy with hydroxyurea, previously believed to be a nonleukemogenic agent.[418,419] These findings suggest that a combination of radiotherapy (^{32}P) or an alkylating agent, busulphan, and another chemotherapeutic agent (hydroxyurea) may particularly increase the risk of leukemia.[418,419] In the ECLAP study, independent variables associated with increased risk to transform to AML/MDS were older age, exposure to ^{32}P, busulphan and pipobroman but not hydroxyurea when used alone. The effects of overall disease duration on the development of AML failed to reach statistical significance.[425] Approximately 30% to 50% of patients with PV who develop acute leukemia have previously entered the spent phase.[410–420] In contrast, approximately 50% of patients progress directly from the erythrocytotic phase to acute leukemia.[12] The phenotype of the leukemia cells that characterize the leukemic phase is overwhelmingly myeloid.[419,424] Unusual cases of lymphoblastic transformation of PV have, however, been reported, as have rare cases of biphenotypic leukemias.[423,424] Another adverse effect solely associated with the use of chlorambucil has been the development of large-cell lymphoma in 3.5% of patients.[418–421]

The development of leukemia sometimes can be abrupt, however. In some instances, a preleukemic phase characterized by refractory anemia with excess blasts has been described.[12,421] In fact, one half of such cases of acute leukemia in one series were preceded by a myelodysplastic disorder.[421]

In addition, the incidence of nonhematologic malignancies has been shown to be increased in patients treated with either chlorambucil or radioactive phosphorous but not with phlebotomy therapy.[418–420] The rates of nonhematologic cancers were highest in sites in the skin and gastrointestinal tract. These malignancies are presumed to be treatment related.

A surprising finding that provides some insight into the origins of acute leukemia occurring in PV patients has been provided from studies of the JAk2V617F status of the leukemia blast cells of such patients.[266,426–428] Surprisingly, in only about 50% of these patients, the leukemic cells were JAK2V617F negative even though in excess of 90% of the PV patients and JAK2V617F positive.[428] Furthermore, Theocharides and coworkers showed that 53% of patients with JAK2V617F-positive MPD had JAK2V617F-negative blasts at the time they developed AML. Patients with JAK2V617F-positive MPD who developed JAK2V617F-negative leukemias had a shorter time between the diagnosis of the original MPD and the leukemic transformation (3 + 2 vs 10 + 7 years) than patients with JAK2V617F-positive leukemias.[428] The possible origins of JAK2V617F-negative leukemias from JAK2V617F-positive MPDs are diagrammatically presented in Fig. 68–11.[68] The AML could potentially originate in the normal stem cell pool that persists in MPD patients or it could originate in a malignant clone that has not acquired the JAK2V617F mutation. The other possibility remains that the chronic MPD and the AML represent two subclones originating from a common ancestor, and that the leukemic transformation results in loss of JAK2V617F.

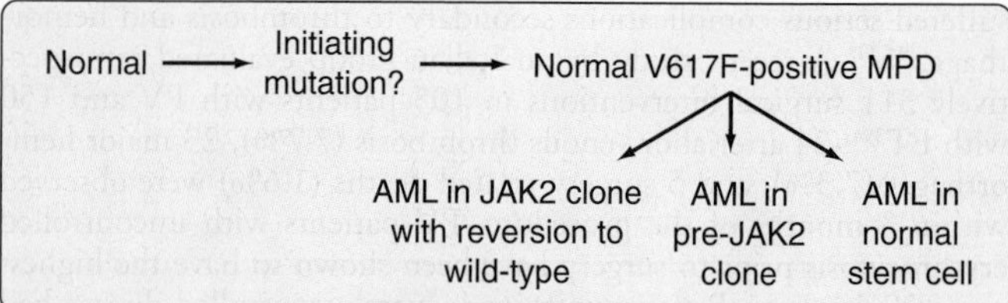

Figure 68–11. Models for the development of JAK2V617F-negative acute myeloid leukemia from JAK2V617F-positive myeloproliferative disorder. Three possible models are shown, in which V617F$^-$ acute myeloid leukemia could develop from (1) a V617F$^+$ cell that subsequently reverts to V617F$^-$; (2) a cell that had some other initiating mutation prior to *JAK2*; or (3) a normal stem cell. (From Campbell PJ, Baxter EJ, Beer PA, et al: Mutation of JAK2 in the myeloproliferative disorders: Timing, clonality studies, cytogenetic associations, and role in leukemic transformation. Blood 108(10):3548, 2006.)

LABORATORY EVALUATION

Laboratory evaluation of the patient with erythrocytosis involves the careful use of a broad range of diagnostic studies. These studies must be employed in a rational manner, or the evaluation can become extremely costly. Because PV is a panmyelosis, the overwhelming number of patients has elevated hematocrits, white blood cell counts, and platelet counts.[196] The diagnosis of PV has been greatly simplified by the discovery of the JAK2V617F mutation, which is present in over 90% of PV patients. Hematocrit values greater than 52% in males and greater than 48% in females are abnormal and require further evaluation.[5] To document the absolute increase in red cell mass, the performance of a blood volume study with direct quantitation of the red cell mass and plasma volume is frequently necessary.[12,429–432] A hematocrit value greater than 60% in men or greater than 55% in women is almost always associated with an absolute erythrocytosis.[12,429–432] In such cases, it is frequently unnecessary to order blood volume studies. In men suspected of polycythemia with a hematocrit level below 60% and women with a hematocrit level below 55%, blood volume measurement if available is suggested to be required for determining whether the elevated hematocrit level is actually due to an expanded red cell mass.[12,429–432] Occasionally, an elevated red cell mass can actually be present in the face of a normal hematocrit. In cases of splenomegaly due to portal hypertension, an expanded plasma volume may mask an elevated red cell mass.[355] In addition, iron deficiency can also lead to a fall in hematocrit in PV, making the diagnosis difficult.[12] PV is associated with a 20% to 30% frequency of gastric ulcers and gastritis, which can be associated with blood loss.[311] In this situation, thrombocytosis may be exacerbated as a consequence of the iron deficiency. Iron supplementation and correction of the bleeding lesion may permit the diagnosis to be established. Administration of iron to such patients must be performed carefully to avoid a rapid increase in red cell mass, which can be associated with a high risk of thrombosis. Lamy and associates have recommended that increased hematocrit and hemoglobin levels do not constitute the only criteria for proceeding with a red cell mass determination to make a diagnosis of PV.[355] They suggest that red cell mass determinations be performed in patients with normal hemoglobin and hematocrit values with portal or hepatic vein thrombosis, splenomegaly, leukocytosis, or thrombocytosis. Performance of JAK2V617F mutational analysis may represent a more direct means of identifying an underlying MPD.[360–365] In such patients, the use of red cell measurements in these settings is intended to aid in the diagnosis of so-called inapparent PV.[12,282,429–432] Indirect calculations of the red cell mass from plasma volume measurements assume a normal body venous hematocrit ratio. Unfortunately, this ratio may be abnormal in patients with spurious PV, and calculations derived from venous-packed red cell volumes may overestimate the red cell mass.[429–432] It is regrettable that red cell mass determinations are no longer available at many institutions.[432] To be assured of the presence of an absolute erythrocytosis in appropriate patients, clinicians should refer individuals to institutions where these analyses are performed. In a world where it is easier to obtain an analysis for a JAK2V617F mutation than a red cell mass, the reality is that the molecular analysis is and will become the more widely used diagnostic tool.

The criteria for establishing a red cell mass has previously been based on values expressed as mL/kg of total body weight. Because adipose tissue is considerably less vascular than lean tissue, it may not contribute equally to the red cell mass.[429–431] Red cell mass measurements, therefore, based solely on body weight can be misleading. Red cell mass measurements more closely correlate with lean body mass than total body weight. Measured red cell mass values in obese subjects are regularly lower when expressed as mL/kg of total body weight than those observed in lean individuals.[429–431] To overcome this difficulty, the International Council for Standardization in Haematology has presented formulas to calculate normal red cell mass values, based on lean body mass, surface area, height, and weight.[429] Implementation of this approach is suggested due to the high incidence of obesity in our society.[429] Modification of the PVSG's criteria for definition of elevation of the red cell mass has been suggested. An elevated red cell mass is now defined as being 25% greater than the mean predicted value of a red cell mass for that individual rather than basing evaluations on the volume per kg of total body weight.[431]

Leukocytosis is present in approximately two-thirds of cases and seems to be proportional to the burden of JAK2V617F.[433] Thrombocytosis is observed in 50% of cases.[196] Abnormalities of red blood cell, white blood cell, and platelet morphology are frequently observed. The morphologic red blood cell changes observed during the erythrocytotic phases are characteristic of iron deficiency and include microcytosis, hypochromia, and frequently polychromatophilia.[12,315] Some anisocytosis and poikilocytosis can be seen as well. Fetal hemoglobin levels and the number of red cells containing fetal hemoglobin, known as F cells, may be increased.[434] The white blood cells are characterized by normal morphology, although the numbers of basophils, eosinophils, and immature myeloid forms can be increased.[196] Platelet morphology is also quite striking in PV. Frequently, megathrombocytes (platelets the sizes of red blood cells) are seen on the peripheral blood smear. Patients frequently have platelet counts of less than 1×10^6 mm^{-3}, but it is not unusual to observe a patient with a platelet count higher than this value. PV related myelofibrosis is characterized by a leukoerythroblastic blood picture, with the appearance in the peripheral blood of dacryocytes or teardrop red blood cells, myelocytes, metamyelocytes, and, rarely, blasts and promyelocytes in addition to nucleated red blood cells in the peripheral blood.[338–340]

Platelet aggregation studies and bleeding times are frequently abnormal in patients with PV, but do not correlate frequently with the risk of bleeding episodes. The most common abnormalities are decreased primary and secondary aggregation to either or both epinephrine and ADP and decreased response to collagen with generally a normal response to arachidonic acid. Abnormal platelet storage pool disease is a characteristic feature and due to abnormal platelet activation.[305,330–332] Prothrombin times (PT) and partial thromboplastin times (aPTT), as well as fibrinogen levels, are usually normal.[435,436] Profound abnormalities of the PT and aPTT are, however, frequently reported. This is largely a laboratory artifact caused by the extreme erythrocytosis, which results in a relatively smaller volume of plasma being present in the whole blood sample. Coagulation assays are performed on blood anticoagulated with sodium citrate, and the citrate concentration in the anticoagulant is calibrated to chelate the plasma calcium and inhibit coagulation reactions. All coagulation assays include the addition of calcium chloride to neutralize the excess citrate and provide free calcium to mediate coagulation reactions. In patients with extreme erythrocytosis, the ratio of citrate in the collection tube to the volume of plasma is too high; therefore, excess citrate is present, and the standard amount of calcium chloride added during the performance of the PT and aPTT is insufficient to neutralize the excessive citrate and the coagulation assays are frequently and factually prolonged. To avoid this problem, the clinician should calculate the relative amount of plasma compared with the normal amount and remove the corresponding volume of sodium citrate from the blood collection tube. Normal values can then be confidently anticipated in patients with erythrocytosis. Tytgat and colleagues[435] have detected a shortened fibrinogen half-life in some PV patients and a significantly increased fractional catabolic rate of the plasma fibrinogen pool per day. Boughton and Dallinger[436] have confirmed these findings. In addition, elevated platelet β-thromboglobulin and plasma β-thromboglobulin levels are observed. The constellation of findings is indicative of increased platelet turnover rates. Furthermore, Falanga and colleagues have shown that prothrombin fragments F1 and 2, thrombin–antithrombin complex, and D dimer levels were elevated in PV patients.[300] These are enzyme–inhibitor complexes or by-products of active thrombosis that serve as a biochemical signature of the hypercoagulable state that characterizes PV.[300]

An acquired von Willebrand syndrome occurs frequently in patients with PV and ET who have extreme elevations of platelet numbers.[329,437,438] This syndrome is characterized by a normal or prolonged bleeding time, a normal factor VIII level and normal von Willebrand factor (vWF) antigen level but abnormal vWF ristocetin cofactor actively associated with a decrease or absence of large vWF multimers.[329,437,438] This acquired defect resembles type II vWF disease. Because the molecular size of vWF is a major determinant of its adhesive function and the larger multimers are most active in achieving hemostasis, the deficiency of large vWF multimers is associated with a bleeding tendency. The decrease in the frequency of large vWF multimers occurs in patients with platelet counts over 1000×10^9 L^{-1}.[329,437,438] This abnormality has been reported not only with patients with severe thrombocytosis due to myeloproliferative disorders but also in patients with reactive thrombocytosis.[329,437,438] An inverse correlation between the proportion of large vWF multimers and platelet numbers has been observed.[263,264,346,347] In addition, normalization of the platelet count is accompanied by restoration of a normal vWF multimer pattern.[329] These findings suggest that thrombocytosis of any etiology may favor the adsorption of larger forms of vWF multimers onto platelet membranes, resulting in their removal from the circulation and subsequent degradation by platelet-associated proteases.[329] Although patients with MPD frequently have bleeding tendencies, this is not the case in secondary thrombocytosis, possibly because of the limited periods of extreme thrombocytosis observed in such patients.[329] Patients with PV with clinical courses punctuated by hemorrhagic events, extreme thrombocytosis, and acquired von Willebrand syndrome should not receive aspirin therapy if they are suffering from a thrombotic episode, but should be phlebotomized and platelet reduction therapy should be initiated.[329] Patients with PV and acquired von Willebrand syndrome suffer from recurrent bleeding from mucous membranes and the digestive tract and easy bruisability. These symptoms frequently resolve with normalization of the platelet count.

Deficiencies of one or more natural anticoagulants as well as the antiphospholid antibody syndrome have been observed in patients with PV and thrombosis.[439–441] These studies indicate that either familial or acquired antithrombin III deficiency, protein C or S deficiency, the factor V Leiden mutation, or the prothrombin G gene mutation may contribute to the hypercoagulable state observed in PV.[439–441] Of note, although hyperhomocyteinemia due to deficiency of cobolamin or folate can be found in 32% to 56% of PV patients, there is no agreement as to its role in the genesis of thrombotic episodes.[442,443] Such inherited disorders associated with the erythrocytosis of PV provide a scenario that frequently favors thrombosis in affected individuals. In attempting to determine if a patient with PV and an active thrombosis suffers from such an inherited predisposition, it is important to be aware that proteins C and S as well as antithrombin III levels can be low in patients with an ongoing acute thrombosis or liver cirrhosis. Normal prothrombin and factor VII levels in such a patient eliminate liver cirrhosis as a cause of the reduction of these circulating anticoagulants in patients with cirrhosis. Individuals with inherited prethrombotic conditions frequently have levels of specific proteins below 10% to 20% of normal during periods of active thrombosis.[439–441]

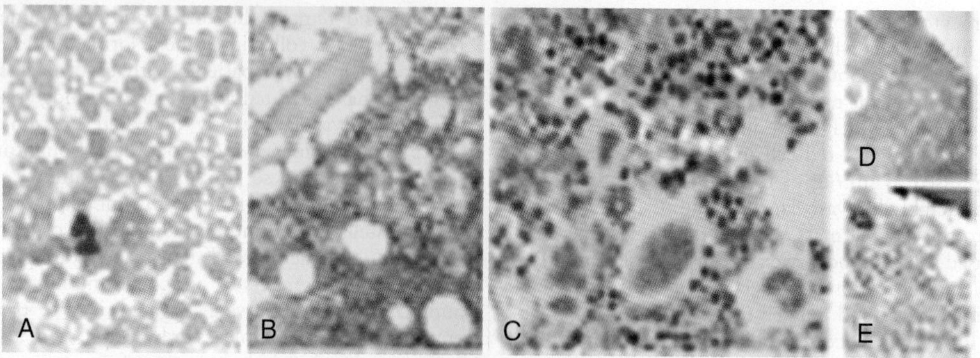

Figure 68–12. Photomicrograph of bone marrow biopsy obtained from a polycythemia vera patient in myelofibrotic phase demonstrating hypercellularity and increased number of megakaryocytes (×160).

The leukocyte alkaline phosphatase activity level is elevated in 70% of patients.[196] Moreover, recent data indicate an increase of neutrophil elastase levels in granulocytes and in plasma that correlates with JAK2 mutational status.[444] Serum B_{12} concentrations have been found to be elevated in 40% of patients, whereas serum B_{12}-binding proteins are elevated in 70% of cases.[196] Hyperuricemia occurs in an overwhelming number of patients, and elevated histamine levels are also frequently observed.[445] Bone marrow aspirates and biopsies obtained at the time of diagnosis of patients with PV are hypercellular and display characteristic erythroid, granulocytic, and megakaryocytic hyperplasia.[310,346,446,447] The cellular elements (Fig. 68–12) are frequently morphologically normal. Iron stores are almost uniformly absent in pretreatment biopsy specimens.[310,346,446,447] Significant increases in bone marrow reticulin may be present in biopsies obtained early in the course but also may develop during the erythrocytotic phase and may be present for long periods before the onset of the myelofibrotic phase.[12,243,275,354,355] It is important to emphasize that individuals may have considerable marrow fibrosis, which occurs as a consequence of the underlying MPD. The presence of such marrow fibrosis should not be considered a harbinger of the development of PV related myelofibrosis. In those patients who enter the spent phase of the disease, a moderate to marked increase in reticulin fiber is observed, either simultaneously with or within 1 year of this clinical transformation.[310,340,343,446,447]

Several investigators have attempted to use bone marrow biopsy morphology as a differential diagnostic tool to differentiate between PV and secondary forms of erythrocytosis. The marked hypercellularity and megakaryocytic hyperplasia that are the hallmarks of myeloproliferative disorders are useful parameters for identifying such individuals (see Fig. 68–12).[310,343,446,447] It is imperative to use the bone marrow biopsy rather than the aspirate specimens for this purpose.[310,343]

The pathologic appearance of the spleen in PV depends on the stage of the disease at which that organ is examined.[448] Spleens from patients in the erythrocytotic phase of the disease are characterized by striking congestion with mature erythrocytes.[448] Small numbers of hematopoietic precursor cells are frequently present. By contrast, spleens examined during the PV-related myelofibrosis phase are characterized by prominent numbers of foci of extramedullary hematopoiesis, with representation of all marrow precursor elements.[448]

The proliferative capacity of PV hematopoietic progenitor cells has been shown to be a useful laboratory adjunctive study.[77,78,449–451] Lemoine and coworkers[449] prospectively used the formation of endogenous erythroid colonies as a diagnostic tool to confirm the diagnosis of PV in the evaluation of a group of patients with isolated erythrocytosis (Table 68–7). In this study, the clinical courses of those patients with marrow cells that formed endogenous colonies were very similar to those of patients who met standard criteria for the diagnosis of PV.[449] Slightly greater than 70% of these patients developed difficulties that eventually required treatment. Conversely, those patients whose marrow cells did not form colonies in the absence of EPO enjoyed benign clinical courses not requiring therapeutic intervention. The usefulness of such assays has also been emphasized by Shih and Lee, who studied patients with idiopathic thrombocytosis who did not meet the diagnostic criteria for PV.[432] Shih and Lee reported that a high proportion of patients with normal or reduced hematocrit levels associated with marked isolated thrombocytosis ($>1 \times 10^6$ mm^{-3}) who had marrow cells that formed endogenous erythroid colonies eventually developed PV within a median period of 24 months.[452] These findings require confirmation because other laboratories have reported endogenous erythroid colonies in 50% of patients with ET.[451,453] It is important to emphasize that although the presence of endogenous colonies in the blood is indicative of PV, the inability to detect these colonies does not entirely eliminate the diagnosis.[12] Assays of bone marrow cells are indicated when endogenous colonies are not detectable in the peripheral blood.[12] Because of the lack of quality assurance in the performance of such clonal erythroid progenitor cell assays in some laboratories, some reservations concerning their widespread use as diagnostic tools have been expressed.[359] The formation of EEC by marrow mononuclear cells can be an important diagnostic tool in those rare patients who are JAK2V617F negative.

Table 68–7 Study of Diagnostic Usefulness of Marrow Erythroid Progenitor Cell Cultures in Patients Suspected of Polycythemia Vera Based on Standard Clinical Criteria

Diagnosis	Standard Criteria*	Endogenous Erythroid Colonies†
Group A‡		
Polycythemia vera	46	43 (93%)
Secondary polycythemia	12	0
Unclassifiable polycythemia	29	18
Total	87	61 (70%)
Group B‡		
Secondary polycythemia	5	0
Unclassifiable polycythemia	16	4 (25%)
Total	21	4 (20%)

‡Group A is defined to include male patients having a red cell mass of >36 mL/kg and female patients with a red cell mass of >32 mL/kg. Group B is defined as male patients having a red cell mass of 30 to 36 mL/kg and female patients with a red cell mass of 25 to 32 mL/kg.

Data from Lemoine F, Najman A, Baillou C, et al: A prospective study of the value of bone marrow erythroid progenitor cultures in polycythemia. Blood 63:996, 1986.

Allele-specific polymerase chain reaction methods can be used to detect the JAK2V617 mutation in approximately 95% of patients with polycythemia vera.[454,455] The very high frequency of JAK2V617F in PV has dramatically improved our ability to diagnose this disease.

Recently Scott et al have identified somatic gain of function mutations affecting JAK2 exon 12 in 10 JAK2V617F negative patients.[83] Each of these patients had isolated erythrocytosis associated with normal neutrophil and platelet counts but low serum EPO levels and the formation of erythroid colonies by peripheral blood mononuclear cells in the absence of EPO in vitro. Bone marrow biopsies from these patients were slightly hypercellular with isolated erythroid hyperplasia.[83] Megakaryocytes were morphologically normal and not clustered. The exon 12 mutations were frequently present at low levels in granulocyte DNA but were readily identifiable in endogenous erythroid colonies generated in vitro. Since granulocyte involvement with JAK2 exon 12 mutations is low, it is important to sequence DNA from bone marrow cells or from endogenous erythroid colonies generated in vitro in order to make this diagnosis.[83] At diagnosis, serum EPO levels in PV are either reduced or at the lower limits of normal. Even following normalization of the hematocrit, the serum EPO level in PV remains low in two thirds of patients.[8–12]

The occurrence of nonrandom cytogenetic abnormalities in PV is not unexpected, as this is a feature of most hematologic malignancies.[456–464] Such abnormalities have been observed, with no single characteristic chromosome abnormality defined; the most frequent abnormalities are the gain of chromosome 9/9p, deletion of chromosome 20q, trisomy 8, deletion of chromosome 13, and gain of the long arm of chromosome 1.[461,462] Interphase fluorescence in situ hybridization (I-FISH) has been used to detect cryptic chromosome 9 rearrangements. FISH uncovered chromosome 9 rearrangements in 53% of patients with abnormal FISH patterns indicating that gain of 9p is the most frequent genomic alteration PV.[370,371] Swolin and coworkers had previously reported that trisomy for 9p was the most frequent finding at initial cytogenetic examination of patients with PV.[456] The association between the trisomy of 9p and PV was one of the keys to the identification of the JAK2V617F mutation.[262] Kralovics and coworkers identified loss of heterozygosity by genomewide screening on the long arm of chromosome 9.[262] Cytogenetic studies of 9p loss of heterozygosity did not indicate any terminal losses or deletions along the entire short arm of chromosome 9, indicating that the loss of heterozygosity was due to mitotic recombination. According to the physical map of the short arm of chromosome 9, 85 genes were present in this arm, one of them being JAK2.[262] Subsequently, the JAK2V617F mutation was identified and homologous recombination was shown to be the event by which PV patients transitioned from being heterozygous to homozygous for JAK2V617F.

At diagnosis, approximately 25% of patients have a recurrent clonal chromosome marker whereas the remainder are cytogenetically normal, as categorized according to the phase of disease (onset, erythrocytotic, or spent phase).[443–464] Certain cytogenetic abnormalities are clearly a result of treatment-induced mutation, associated with the use of ^{32}P or alkylating agents.[461,462] The frequency of detection of cytogenetic abnormalities in PV is a cumulative function, with clonal cytogenetic abnormalities being observed in 8% to 25% at diagnosis, in 35% to 55% following a number of years of treatment, and in greater than 80% in those patients in whom acute leukemia eventually develops.[443–464] Therefore, clonal progression from a normal to abnormal karyotype, especially acquisition of abnormalities involving chromosomes 5 and 7, is an important adverse prognostic parameter.[443–464] It is important to emphasize, however, that patients with del(20q) have been observed without further karyotypic instability for over 10 years.[464] These abnormalities are not predictive of poor outcome unless other chromosome rearrangements or genetic alterations occur. Occasionally, patients lose their cytogenetic abnormality as a result of chemotherapy. This is a very rare event and of unknown clinical significance.[464]

$20q^-$ (q11) has been shown to be the second most common cytogenetic abnormality.[465–469] $20q^-$ is recognized as a genomic constitutive fragile site subject to mutagenic insult in vitro.[470] This cytogenetic defect is not diagnostic of PV. The $20q^-$ (q11) deletion is due to an interstitial deletion.[465–468] To date, an extensive search for a putative tumor suppressor gene at the site of the $20q^-$ deletion that might play a role in the biogenesis of PV has been unrewarding.[465–468]

Serial cytogenetic evaluation of previously karyotypically normal patients indicate that other abnormalities most often acquired with progression of the disease are $13q^-$, $12q^-$, and $1q^-$.[456–462] These particular abnormalities do not necessarily herald transition to acute leukemia, but leukemia or myelofibrosis was observed in 8 of 12 patients with the $1q^-$ abnormality in one study.[461] Deletion of the long arm of chromosome 13 has been observed during the myelofibrotic phase of PV, but this abnormality has been detected also during the erythrocytotic phase. It does not appear, therefore, that a chromosome $13q^-$ abnormality heralds disease transition. PV related myelofibrosis occurring after the use of chemotherapy is often accompanied by additional karyotypic abnormalities, with chromosomes 5 and 7 being the most frequently involved.[458]

One can conclude that chromosome abnormalities such as +8,+9, and $20q^-$ might be related to the biogenesis of the disease rather than to the treatment employed.[462,463] In addition, it appears that, at best, in some patients, an abnormal clone (abnormalities of chromosome 5 or 7) and hypodiploidy develop as a consequence of therapy with chemotherapeutic agents.[456–462] Diez-Martin and colleagues have also suggested that patients with a cytogenetic abnormality at diagnosis have a statistically significantly poorer survival rate than those in whom a normal karyotype is observed.[461] This influence of cytogenetics on prognosis has not been confirmed by others.[459–463]

DIFFERENTIAL DIAGNOSIS OF THE POLYCYTHEMIAS

In most patients, establishing the cause leading to erythrocytosis is not difficult. Initially, it is critical to be certain that one is dealing with a patient with an absolute erythrocytosis. For this purpose, a direct determination of red cell mass is not always necessary.[8–12,429–431] Unfortunately, this test is not presently available at many institutions.[432] Many patients with a raised hematocrit level, however, will require blood volume studies to document an elevated red cell mass.[12,429–431] A hematocrit level greater than 60% on several occasions in men or greater than 55% in women, however, is associated with an elevated red cell mass in virtually every case.[12,429–431] In those situations, it would be reasonable not to proceed with blood volume studies. If the hematocrit is below 60% in men or below 55% in women, blood volume studies are recommended. It has become increasingly apparent that an elevated hematocrit level should not be the only criterion for proceeding with a red cell mass determination.[429] Splenomegaly can lead to an expanded plasma volume, which can mask the diagnosis of polycythemia.[429–431] It is suggested that red cell mass determinations be performed in patients with normal hemoglobin or hematocrit determinations in the context of hepatic or portal vein thrombosis, isolated leukocytosis, or splenomegaly.[355,357] Testing for JAK2V617F can be extremely useful in diagnosing PV and is viewed by some as an alternative to blood volume measurements if they are not available. The presence of splenomegaly is an important finding on clinical examination, and adjunctive laboratory findings include normal arterial oxygen saturation, elevated leukocyte alkaline phosphatase activity, and JAK2V617F assays.[196,78–82] Splenic sizing by ultrasound can be useful in documenting splenic enlargement when the spleen is not palpable by physical examination.[471]

It is initially important to differentiate PV from the large number of other causes of secondary erythrocytosis. Characteristically, the patient with PV will present with erythrocytosis, leukocytosis, and thrombocytosis, and splenomegaly and are positive for JAK2V617F.[78–82] The bone marrow biopsy shows hypercellularity with trilineage hyperplasia. In individuals with less pronounced disease, it is important to determine the SaO_2 using an arterial blood gas, the carboxyhemoglobin level, and the $P_{50}O_2$ in patients with other family members with erythrocytosis to exclude obvious causes of secondary erythrocytosis. Because smokers' polycythemia is the most frequent cause of erythrocytosis, it is wise to measure carboxyhemoglobin levels early on in the investigation. In addition, a PaO_2 greater than 67 mmHg or an O_2 saturation greater than 95%, as quantitated on an arterial blood gas, will be helpful in ruling out hypoxic conditions that lead to erythrocytosis. In patients with intermittent hypoxia, such as sleep apnea syndrome or alveolar hypoventilation due to obesity, such blood gas determinations can be normal. A low $P_{50}O_2$ will be indicative of a hemoglobin mutant with high O_2 affinity leading to tissue hypoxia and erythrocytosis. These patients will often have multiple other family members with erythrocytosis. Tests that can be especially useful for this purpose are the serum EPO level, the ability of bone marrow cells to form erythroid colonies in the absence of exogenous EPO and a JAK2V617F determination.[8–12,78–82,265] Numerous studies have indicated that classification of 90% of patients with erythrocytosis can be achieved by quantitating serum EPO.[8–12] These studies have indicated that patients with PV most frequently exhibit serum EPO levels below the 95% confidence intervals for the range observed in normal controls.[8–12] The subnormal serum EPO levels are maintained even after several phlebotomies have been performed that normalize the serum hemoglobin concentration in PV patients.[8–12]

Spivak has, however, expressed some caution about overreliance on the use of serum EPO levels to define the etiology of erythrocytosis in an individual patient.[12] He has pointed out that although the lowest EPO levels occur in PV, it is not unusual to have a normal EPO level in some patients with hypoxic causes of secondary erythrocytosis unless the hypoxia exists over an extended period of time. Spivak concludes that a normal EPO level cannot be used to exclude a hypoxic cause of erythrocytosis.[12] EPO measurements do, however, remain an important diagnostic tool. Elevation of EPO levels in the face of erythrocytosis are indicative of a hypoxic cause of secondary erythrocytosis, whereas extremely low levels of EPO (<4 mIU/mL) are virtually diagnostic of PV.[8–12] It is the patient with erythrocytosis and a normal EPO level where additional adjunctive diagnostic tests are required to define the cause of erythrocytosis. The availability of newly defined genetic markers such as JAK2V617 or JAK2 exon 12 mutations clearly expedite the diagnosis.[8–12,78–82,265]

Incorporating a mutational screen into the algorithm for investigating a case of suspected polycythemia will help to streamline the diagnosis of PV, although the presence of a JAK2 mutation alone does not distinguish PV from IM or ET. James et al have investigated 88 patients with erythrocytosis, the JAK2 V617F mutation was found in 57 of 61 cases diagnosed as PV and 0 of 11 with idiopathic erythrocytosis.[454] These data and data by others have suggested that mutational analysis can be used to help screen individuals and that this may reduce the need for investigations such as red cell mass determination and bone marrow biopsies. JAK2 analysis has broader applicability than clonality assays, which are restricted to females and are also not evaluable in older women because of the phenomenon of age-related skewing. Of course, it has to be remembered that patients without a JAK2 mutation can still have a primary MPD.

The ability of bone marrow cells to form endogenous erythroid colonies also been used to analyze etiologic factors in the development of Budd–Chiari syndrome.[78,449–453] Valla and associates[357] studied the marrow proliferative capacities of 20 patients with this syndrome and observed endogenous erythroid colony formation in 16 cases. In 2 of these 16 patients, it was quite obvious that an MPD was the underlying etiologic factor in the development of hepatic vein thrombosis. This abnormality in the other 14 patients suggests that the development of Budd–Chiari syndrome may represent, in some cases, a forme fruste of an MPD.[355,357] Furthermore, marrow cells from patients with other MPDs, ET, CML, and IM also frequently form endogenous erythroid colonies. As has been previously discussed, the JAK2V617F mutation can be detected in 20% to 40% of patients with Budd–Chiari syndrome, portal vein thrombosis, or mesenteric vein thrombosis and normal hematological values.[360–365] Clearly, JAK2V617F assays should be performed in such patients to diagnose an early form of an MPD.

Clinical criteria for the diagnosis of PV have been defined by the PVSG and the World Health Organization and have been used successfully to obtain a uniform patient population with PV for evaluation of therapeutic modalities.[12,196,431,472] It is important, however, for the clinician to realize that some patients undoubtedly have a MPD disorder resembling PV but do not fulfill all the diagnostic criteria of the PVSG or the World Health Organization.[12] The criteria for the diagnosis of PV including the use of the JAK2V617 assay have recently been revised by the World Health Organization and are now provided in Table 68–8.[472] These criteria are the consensus of many experts working in this field and represent an advance in this field. There will always be unusual cases with clinical characteristics that cannot be pigeonholed into a particular diagnostic category. If asymptomatic; these patients should be followed carefully until the disorder evolves into a more recognizable entity. This would appear prudent to avoid unnecessary therapeutic interventions. If these patients have serious symptoms, the individual physician must make treatment decisions on the basis of the risk-benefit ratio for that patient.

Table 68–8 Proposed Revised World Health Organization Criteria for Polycythemia Vera

Diagnosis Requires the Presence of Both Major Criteria and One Minor Criterion OR the Presence of the First Major Criterion Together With Two Minor Criteria.

Major Criteria

1. Hemoglobin >18.5 g/dL in men and 16.5 g/dL in women or another evidence of increased red cell volume*
2. Presence of *JAK2*V617F or other functionally similar mutation such as *JAK2* exon 12 mutation

Minor Criteria

1. Bone marrow biopsy showing hypercellularity with trilineage hyperplasia (panmyelosis) with prominent erythroid, granulocytic, and megakaryocytic proliferation
2. Low serum erythropoietin level
3. Endogenous erythroid colony formation *in vitro*

**Hemoglobin or hematocrit >99th percentile of method-specific reference range for age, sex, altitude of residence, or Hemoglobin >17 g/dL in men and 15 g/dL in women if associated with a documented and sustained increase of at least 2 g/dL from an individual's baseline value that cannot be attributed to correction of iron deficiency, or Elevated red cell mass >25% above mean normal predicted value.*

Data from Tefferi et al. Proposals for revision of the World Health Organization diagnostic criteria for polycythemia vera, essential thrombocythemia, and primary myelofibrosis: From an ad hoc international expert panel. Blood 2007, 110:1092–1097.

A particularly difficult dilemma occurs when evaluating patients with isolated pure erythrocytosis.[473–476] These patients have elevated red blood cell masses, normal white blood cell counts, normal platelet counts, no evidence of splenomegaly, and no evidence of any recognizable cause of secondary erythrocytosis. Clearly, some of these patients have JAK2V617F-positive PV or mutations of exon 12 JAK2 leading to isolated erythrocytosis. The familial congenital form of polycythemia due to truncation of the EPOR, characterized by increased sensitivity of erythroid progenitor cells to EPO, can be easily distinguished from PV. These patients frequently present in childhood, and this disorder is characterized by isolated erythrocytosis that is associated with an increased risk of thrombotic events.[88–94] There is a strong family history of polycythemia.[77–83] In contrast to PV, the marrow progenitor cells are hypersensitive to EPO, yet no colonies form in the absence of EPO.[88–94] In addition, patients with other cases of familial polycythemia due to mutations of VHL or PHD should be excluded.[182–190,194]

PV must also be differentiated from the other MPDs, such as CML, ET, and PMF.[477] Such classification has major prognostic implications and influences important therapeutic decisions, including the use of tyrosine kinase inhibitors such as imatinib, dasatinib, or holotinib. With the distinctive cytogenetic abnormalities and molecular genetic abnormalities that are unique to CML (Philadelphia chromosome, *BCR-ABL* gene fusion), these two disorders should not be difficult to differentiate.[196] A less complex test, the leukocyte alkaline phosphatase activity, may also be of assistance. The leukocyte alkaline phosphatase score is elevated in PV but is decreased in patients with CML.[196,309] In addition, the incidence of elevated red cell masses in patients with CML is low.

Patients with PMF can present with abnormalities that are virtually indistinguishable from those of patients with PV related MF.[338–340] Almost 50% of PMF are JAK2V617F positive while over 90% of patients with PPMM are JAK2V617F positive.[78–82] The survival of patients with the latter disorder is much shorter than that of patients with the former condition.[338–340] Some patients with presumed PMF may actually develop PV after the institution of chemotherapy.[209]

A preceding history of PV permits differentiation between these two situations. ET and PV with marked thrombocytosis can easily be confused. When the red blood cell mass is used as a definitive diagnostic test, a distinction between ET and the erythrocytotic phase of PV is usually readily apparent.[457,476] This measurement, however, can be normal or actually low in the patient with PV who is iron deficient because of bleeding or excessive phlebotomy.[12] Campbell and coworkers have recently used sensitive PCR-based methods to assess the JAK2 mutational states in 806 patients with ET.[478] The mutation was present in over 50% of patients with ET. JAK2V617F-positive ET patients were characterized by multiple features that resembled those of patients with PV, including higher Hgb levels, higher white blood cell counts, more prominent marrow erythroid and granulocytic hypoplasia, a higher incidence of venous but not arterial thrombosis, low serum EPO levels, and lower serum ferritin levels.[478] Surprisingly, JAK2V617F-negative patients had higher platelet counts. Furthermore, JAK2V617F-positive ET patients had a higher probability of developing PV with longer follow-up. Acquisition of homozygosity for the JAK2V617 due to homologous recombination is likely the critical event in the development of PV in JAK2V617F ET patients.[81,262] Homozygosity for JAK2V617F occurs in at least 30% of patients with PV, but is extremely rare in ET.[478]

An elevated expression of polycythemia rubra vera 1 (PRV-1) mRNA in granulocytes has been suggested to be diagnostic of PV.[12,78,479–481] PRV-1 is a novel member of the urokinase type plasminogen activator receptor (uPAR) super family.[479] Use of a quantitative reverse transcription–polymerase chain reaction (RT-PCR) assay for the measurement of PRV-1 mRNA expression in PV granulocytes has been useful in distinguishing PV from secondary erythrocytosis.[481] Expression analysis has revealed that PRV-1 is constitutively expressed in the bone marrow of patients with a variety of hematologic disorders and that its usefulness as a diagnostic tool for the MPD is restricted to peripheral blood granulocytes. In PV, PRV-1 is not downregulated in granulocytes within the marrow.[482] Furthermore, the specificity of overexpression of PRV-1 mRNA in granulocytes has been questioned as increased PRV-1 mRNA has also been documented in the granulocytes of patients with ET, idiopathic myelofibrosis, normal patients receiving granulocyte-colony stimulating factor, patients recovering from trauma or surgery, occasional patients with hereditary forms of thrombocythemia due to higher TPO levels, as well as occasional patients with secondary or spurious polycythemia.[483,484] The overexpression of PRV-1 in PV does not involve structural genetic changes.[485] Impaired expression of Mpl by PV platelets has also been examined as a universal marker of PV. Some investigators have reported that this abnormality, however, was observed only in a subset of patients with PV and IM. Both PRV-1 overexpression and impaired expression of Mpl likely represent downstream events of the JAK2V617F mutation.[486]

THERAPY

Dramatic prolongation of survival over that expected from the natural history of patients with untreated PV has been achieved with several therapeutic strategies.[196,207,296,297,302,303] Historic evidence of a median survival period of approximately 18 months of untreated patients from the time of diagnosis is derived from descriptive accounts, but more recent data of the clinical course of untreated patients are not available. It is clear that many patients remain asymptomatic for years before diagnosis.[5] A cumulative median duration of survival for PV patients treated with modern strategies of more than 15 years has been reported.[12,297,302] However, in spite of modern therapies, an excess of mortality in comparison with a matched normal population has been reported.[307] Men have a higher mortality rate than women in each age group of patients with PV.[12,297,302] At present, the therapeutic goals are to reduce the risk of thrombosis by normalizing the hematocrit levels to 45% or lower in males and 42% or lower in females.[12]

A series of studies performed over a 17-year period (1967–1984) by the PVSG has answered several very important questions regarding the efficacy and associated complications of particular therapeutic modalities.[296,418–421] These investigations have aided in the identification of optimal therapy for individual patients, which must be selected on the basis of age and comorbid disease status to minimize treatment-related complications.[12,296,418–421,487]

The first PVSG randomized trial (01 trial) evaluated three treatment strategies: (a) phlebotomy alone, to maintain the hematocrit level at less than 45%; (b) intravenous ^{32}P, 2.3 mCi/m^2 repeated every 12 weeks if needed (maximum 5mCi per dose), supplemented by phlebotomy to maintain the hematocrit level at less than 45%; and (c) myelosuppression with chlorambucil 10 mg per day PO for 6 weeks, then daily on alternate months, with necessary dose reductions

General Principles of Therapy

1. Etiology of erythrocytosis must be correctly categorized to be certain the patient has polycythemia vera (PV). This will avoid inappropriate exposure of patients with nonmalignant disorders to potential leukemogenic agents. To this end, a major contribution will be played by incorporating a JAK2V617F determination in the diagnostic workup, and in this way, early phases of PV can be recognized as well.
2. Therapy should be individualized.
3. Initially, the blood volume should be reduced to normal as rapidly as possible. The speed of phlebotomy will depend on patients' general medical conditions (250–500 mL every other day). Elderly patients with compromised cardiovascular or pulmonary systems should be more carefully phlebotomized (twice a week), or smaller volumes of blood should be removed.
4. Hematocrit levels should be maintained at 42% for females and 45% for males.
5. Excessive doses of chemotherapeutic agents should be avoided. Supplementary phlebotomy rather than potentially toxic doses of chemotherapeutic agents should be used to avoid excessive marrow and systemic toxicity.
6. Hyperuricemia is treated with allopurinol (100–300 mg/d).
7. Pruritus is treated with cyproheptadine 4 to 16 mg/d; if unsuccessful, interferon-α therapy 3.0 × 10^6 units subcutaneously three times a week. A role for serotonin-uptake inhibitors (paroxetine 20 mg/d or fluoxetine 10 mg/d) has been proposed.
8. Elective surgery or dental procedures should be delayed until red cell mass and platelet counts have been normalized for more than 2 months. Aspirin should be withdrawn at least 1 week before surgery. If emergency surgery is contemplated, phlebotomy and cytopheresis should be pursued.
9. Women and men who are contemplating having children should be treated by phlebotomy plus low-dose aspirin therapy (81 mg/d or with interferon-α) to avoid teratogenic effects of chemotherapy. Such avoidance will also prevent deleterious effects on fertility. During pregnancy, therapy is frequently not necessary; if it is, phlebotomy plus low-dose aspirin should be exclusively used. If phlebotomy control is inadequate, treatment with interferon-α should be pursued.

Algorithm for Management of Patients with PV

Low-risk young patients (<60 years) and no prior history of thrombosis, platelet count lower than 1.5×10^6 mm^{-3}

Phlebotomy + low-dose aspirin (81 mg/d) to maintain hematocrit lower than 45% in males and lower than 42% in females. Aspirin should not be used in patients with histories of a hemorrhagic episode or with extreme thrombocytosis (>1.5×10^6 mm^{-3}) or acquired von Willebrand syndrome.

↓

Thrombosis or hemorrhage
Systemic symptoms
Severe pruritus refractory to histamine antagonists
Painful splenomegaly

↓

Pegylated interferon 90 to 180 μg/week or Interferon α (3×10^6 units three times a week; alter dose depending on response and toxicity). Consider the use of pegylated interferon, which can be administered once weekly

↓

If platelet control is inadequate or patient cannot tolerate interferon, one option could be the use of anagrelide. However, the use of this drug is controversial. In this case, supplemental phlebotomy is required to maintain hematocrit lower than 45% in males and lower than 42% in females and the use of hydroxyurea should be considered, especially if patient continues to have thrombotic episodes.

↓

If the patient has increasing splenomegaly, systemic symptoms, or repeated thromboses, in spite of adequate dose of hydroxyurea (2–3 g daily) start busulphan: 4 to 6 mg/d PO for 4 to 8 weeks. It should be mentioned that the sequential use of hydroxyurea and busulphan may be associated with an increased risk of leukemia. Supplemental phlebotomy may be required.

↓

Painful splenomegaly
Splenectomy + continued systemic therapy

↓

High-risk patients (>60 years), previous thrombosis, platelet count higher than 1.5×10^6 mm^{-3}

Phlebotomy to hematocrit of 42% in females and 45% in males

Aspirin (81 mg/d) to be given only in patients with platelet counts lower than 1.5×10^6 mm^{-2}

Myelosuppressive therapy with hydroxyurea 30 mg/kg PO for 1 week

↓

Then 15 to 20 mg/kg

If patient continues to have thrombotic episodes and has extreme thrombocytosis or cannot tolerate hydroxyurea.

Consider pegylated interferon 90 to 180 μg/wk or add busulphan 4–6 mg/d PO for 4 to 8 weeks.

Stop when blood counts are normalized or platelet count is lower than 300,000 mm^{-3}.

Occasional supplemental phlebotomy if hematocrit is greater than 42% in females and greater than 45% in males; when patient relapses (patient is symptomatic), initiate busulphan therapy again at same dose.

↓

If patient is poorly compliant, consider ^{32}P: 2.3 mCi/m^2 IV every 12 weeks as needed (limit 5 mCi per dose).

Increase dose by 25% if no response

Patient age more than 70 years

Phlebotomy + low-dose aspirin + hydroxyurea

↓

No response or poor compliance

Busulphan 4 to 6 mg/d PO for 4 to 8 weeks. Stop when blood counts are normalized or platelet count is lower than 300,000 mm^{-3}.

↓

No response

^{32}P

and supplemental phlebotomy.[418–421] More than 400 patients were randomly assigned to this protocol. Median survival duration from entry into the study until death was 9.1 years for patients treated with chlorambucil, 10.9 years for those treated with ^{32}P, and 12.6 years for the phlebotomy group.[418–421] Long-term survival was inferior for patients treated with chlorambucil when compared with those treated with ^{32}P or phlebotomy.[418–421] An early finding was the appearance during the first 5 years of a significant excess of deaths from acute leukemia in the chlorambucil arm, which reached 17% after 15 years of follow-up.[418–421] As a result, the chlorambucil arm was discontinued, and patients were assigned randomly to one of the other two arms. Even though no statistical difference in overall survival between ^{32}P and phlebotomy alone was apparent through the first 10 years, the morbidity and mortality associated with each type of therapy were attributable to distinctly different causes.[418–421] Thrombosis as a cause of death was much more frequent in the phlebotomy-only group during the first 5 to 7 years of follow-up.[418–421] Analyses of factors associated with thrombosis revealed that the performance of phlebotomy, the rate of phlebotomy, advancing age, and history of previous thrombosis were statistically significant factors predictive of this outcome.[420] In contrast, the use of ^{32}P led to a lower rate of thrombosis during the first 5 years, but the incidences of leukemias, lymphomas, and nonhematologic malignancies increased during the next 5 years to nearly 10%.[417–421] Following a 15-year period of observation, the incidences of leukemia and lymphoma in the chlorambucil group had risen to 17%.[417–421] A statistically significant increase in skin and gastrointestinal cancers occurred in the ^{32}P- and chlorambucil-treated cohorts, compared with the group treated with phlebotomy alone.[417–421]

Given the paradox of equal 10-year survivals but demise due to distinct causes in comparable populations of patients treated by phlebotomy alone or by phlebotomy plus ^{32}P, the PVSG pursued strategies to reduce the thrombotic risk in the phlebotomy-only group. One study attempted reduction of the thrombotic risk by combination antiplatelet therapy. It appeared possible that therapy directed toward altering platelet function might reduce the frequency of thrombosis.[331] Therefore, a randomized trial was performed in which phlebotomy, supplemented with the platelet antiaggregating agents aspirin and dipyridamole, was compared with ^{32}P (PVSG trial 05). The outcome for the group treated with phlebotomy, aspirin, and dipyridamole was disappointingly inferior to the ^{32}P results.[389] In fact, more thromboses occurred in the former than in the latter group, but surprisingly there was also a significantly greater incidence of severe gastrointestinal hemorrhages.[389]

Renewed impetus for the use of nonchemotherapeutic agents for the treatment of PV was provided by an extensive natural history study of 1213 patients reported by the Gruppo Italiano Studio Policitemia.[297] They showed that the age- and gender-standardized mortality rate of patients with PV was 1.7 times greater than the mortality rate of controls in the general Italian population.[297] In addition, four times as many patients who had previously received ^{32}P, alkylating agents, or hydroxyurea died of cancer compared with patients treated with phlebotomy alone.[297] When this group combined the total number of deaths and the number of nonfatal myocardial infarctions and strokes, they found an unsatisfactory risk-benefit profile in patients treated with chemotherapeutic agents and suggested that antithrombotic strategies, such as low-dose aspirin, be carefully evaluated for use in the care of PV patients.[297]

In light of more recent knowledge of the dose requirements for selective antiplatelet therapy with aspirin, it appears that the PVSG study of platelet antiaggregating agents might have failed due to the use of excessive aspirin dosages (900 mg/d). Such aspirin doses appear to diminish vascular endothelial production of the platelet antiaggregatory factor, prostacyclin I_2 (PGI_2).[326,331]

PV platelets are known to have a generalized abnormality of arachidonate metabolism that is characterized by enhanced synthesis of thromboxane A_2, which likely reflects stimuli to platelet activation.[326,331] The exact mechanism responsible for enhanced platelet synthesis of thromboxane A_2 in PV remains unknown and requires further investigation. A low-dose aspirin regimen (50 mg/d for 7–14 days) has been shown to suppress more than 80% of the excretion of the metabolites of thromboxane A_2.[325] A pilot study was performed in which the toxicity of low-dose aspirin therapy in PV patients was evaluated.[325] A very-low-dose aspirin regimen (40 mg/d) was chosen to prevent thrombosis yet minimize the risk of bleeding. After follow-up of the low-dose aspirin treatment group and control group, low-dose therapy was shown not to be associated with an increased incidence of bleeding complications. Aspirin therapy was well tolerated and was associated with complete inhibition of platelet cyclooxygenase activity.[325] A large, randomized, placebo-controlled clinical trial testing the risk–benefit ratio of low-dose aspirin therapy in preventing thrombotic episodes in PV has been recently completed.[302] Treatment with low-dose aspirin (100 mg/d) compared with placebo reduced the risk of the combined endpoint of nonfatal myocardial infarction, nonfatal stroke, pulmonary embolism, major venous thrombosis, or death from cardiovascular courses. Overall mortality and cardiovascular mortality, however, was not reduced significantly by aspirin therapy. Importantly, the incidence of major bleeding episodes was not significantly increased in the aspirin group.[302] It is important to emphasize that patients require aggressive phlebotomy therapy to the appropriate target hematocrit levels as well as the appropriate use of myelosuppressive agents as primary therapy, with the addition of aspirin serving as an adjunct to this strategy. Spivak has questioned the conclusions of this study, as many of the patients had hematocrit levels above the acceptable therapeutic range and were receiving myelosuppressive agents to normalize platelet numbers.[303] However, in the recently reported analysis by ECLAP investigators, multivariate analysis did not show any differences in the rate of thrombosis associated with different hematocrit levels during follow-up. High hematocrit levels were not found to be significant predictors of death, development of thrombotic events, or hematological progression.[314] We can conclude that aspirin therapy appears to be a relatively innocuous therapy but should be avoided in patients with extremely high platelet counts. Surely, in young (<60 years of age), low-risk patients (no prior history of thrombosis, platelet count >1 $\times 10^6$ mm^{-3}), phlebotomy with low-dose aspirin (81 mg/d) therapy is an attractive approach.

It is interesting to compare the results of the PVSG study with those of a randomized trial of ^{32}P versus busulphan for the treatment of PV conducted by the European Organization for Research and Treatment of Cancer (EORTC).[488,489] The two studies were comparable in size, design, and duration of follow-up. In the EORTC trial, induction courses of busulphan 4 to 6 mg/d for 4 to 8 weeks were compared with ^{32}P treatment.[392] Patients treated with busulphan enjoyed a survival advantage over ^{32}P-treated patients.[392,393] This difference was due primarily to a threefold greater incidence of fatal thrombotic events in the ^{32}P group. Interestingly, the incidence of leukemia in both groups was very low (<2%), with an overall malignancy rate of less than 10% (involving mostly solid tumors).[488,489]

It is reasonable to conclude from this trial that busulphan is a myelosuppressive agent with limited leukemogenic potential when used on an intermittent schedule.[488,489] A retrospective study of patients in England treated with phlebotomy and intermittent busulphan supports these same conclusions.[480]

After the disappointing results experienced with the alkylating agent chlorambucil, the PVSG began a nonrandomized phase II investigation of hydroxyurea, an S-phase-specific ribonucleotide reductase inhibitor.[421,490,491] The hope was that this agent would be nonleukemogenic. Of 53 patients with PV treated with hydroxyurea who had never received other forms of myelosuppression, after follow-up for a median period of 8.6 years and a maximum follow-up of 795 weeks, 5.4% developed acute leukemia compared with 1.5% of patients treated with phlebotomy alone on the original PVSG randomized study.[421]

In a comparable trial reported by Sharon and coworkers, 71 patients were treated with hydroxyurea for a mean duration of 7.3 years.[492] Remarkably, the incidence of thrombosis was only 6%, indicating the impressive potential of hydroxyurea to lower the incidence of thrombosis in patients with PV, confirming an observation previously made by Kaplan and colleagues.[491] The incidence of leukemia in the Israeli trial was 5.6%.[492,493] Several other reports are also available reporting the incidence of acute leukemia in PV patients treated with hydroxyurea.[416,490–498] The incidence varies from 10.5% in the 30 patients treated by Weinfeld and associates, to 6.2% in the 65 patients treated by Lovfenberg and colleagues, and 10% in the 150 cases treated by Najean and colleagues.[494,495] Furthermore, in a randomized trial including 296 patients comparing the efficacy of hydroxyurea with piprobroman, an alkylating agent, for the treatment of PV, the incidence of leukemia was similar in both treatment arms. The incidence of PPMM was, however, statistically greater in the patients treated with hydroxyurea.[494] Piprobroman is not available in the United States. In a more recent retrospective series, the incidence of acute leukemia and myelodysplasia in patients with PV treatment hydroxyurea alone was 6.9%.[498] These patients received a greater dose of hydroxyurea than patients who did not develop leukemia. The leukemia associated with hydroxyurea therapy developed over 6.3 years after treatment with hydroxyurea was initiated. In patients treated first with busulphan and then hydroxyurea, the rate of acute leukemia/myelodysplasia was even higher, 13.8%. Finazzi et al examined 22 cases with AML/MDS reported in the ECLAP study that enrolled 1638 patients. AML/MDS were diagnosed after a median of 8.4 years from the diagnosis of PV and variables associated with progression were older age, whereas overall disease duration (more than 10 years) failed to reach statistical significance.[425] Exposure to P32, busulphan, and pipobroman but not hydroxyurea alone had an independent role in producing an excess risk for progression to AML/MDS as compared with treatment with phlebotomy or interferon.[425] However, the documented ability of hydroxyurea to lower the incidence of thrombotic events, even in the face of a possible increasing documentation of its leukemogenic potential, makes this drug a very useful chemotherapeutic agent in older, high-risk patients with disease that cannot be controlled with phlebotomy alone. Excessive myelosuppression, macrocytosis, hypersegmentation of polyps, stomatitis, leg ulcers, creatinine elevations, and jaundice have been attributed to the use of hydroxyurea.[490–498] Aphthous and leg ulcers occur in 20% of patients, usually after 5 years of hydroxyurea maintenance therapy.[490–498] In addition, the use of hydroxyurea requires patient compliance and careful monitoring of blood counts to avoid the sequelae of excessive myelosuppression.

Some clinical investigators have suggested that a program of phlebotomy alone would be the most appropriate for younger patients, who have not experienced a cerebrovascular or cardiovascular event. Strong consideration should be given to the use of phlebotomy therapy in conjunction with low-dose aspirin therapy in addition to the use of such apparently nonleukemogenic drugs as interferon-α in this younger patient population.[12,302,303,497–505]

Anagrelide, a selective inhibitor of platelet production, has been used to treat thrombocytosis in PV patients with thrombotic or hemorrhagic complications.[497] This agent appears to be nonleukemogenic and acts by impairing megakaryocyte maturation.[500,501,505] Its use leads to a selective reduction in platelet numbers, and it has been effective in patients refractory to hydroxyurea and interferon.[497–500,503] This drug does not effectively control the erythrocytosis and leukocytosis or systemic symptoms associated with PV and therefore was suggested to be used as a supplement to phlebotomy therapy.

Pettit and colleagues have reported that anagrelide use in polycythemia resulted in a complete resolution of thrombocytosis as defined as a platelet count of less than 600,000 or a 50% reduction of pretreatment levels in 66% of 113 patients with PV.[503] In nearly all responders, platelet reduction was observed within a week. The time to complete response generally ranged between 17 and 25 days.[503] The dose of anagrelide required to control thrombocytosis remained constant over time in most patients. When anagrelide is discontinued, platelet counts returned to pretreatment levels within 5 to 7 days. The average daily dose required to control thrombocytosis in PV patients was 2.4 mg.[503] After the recent publication of the PT-O1 randomized clinical trial comparing hydroxyurea and anagrelide therapy for ET patients, many physicians are cautious about the use of this drug in preventing vascular events. In fact, major arterial thrombosis was more frequent in the anagrelide arm as compared with the hydroxyurea arm, in spite of a similar normalization of elevated platelet counts.[333] Moreover, the association of anagrelide and low-dose aspirin led to a significant increase of bleeding manifestations. Clinicians presume that the effects of anagrelide observed in ET patients will be relevant to patients with PV. This assumption has not been tested in a randomized clinical trial. Anagrelide should not be used in pregnant patients because it can easily cross the placenta, leading to adverse effects on the platelet count of the fetus.[497]

Approximately 15% to 20% of patients treated with anagrelide discontinued the medication due to nonmyelosuppressive side effects.[497–499,503–505] The spectrum of adverse effects involved neurologic (headaches and dizziness), cardiac (vasodilatation, fluid retention, congestive heart failure, palpitations, and tachycardia), and gastrointestinal (nausea) toxicities. These toxicities reflect the novel mechanism of action of anagrelide as a cyclic nucleotide phosphodiesterase inhibitor. Anagrelide should be used with caution in patients with known or suspected cardiac disease because of its ability to promote fluid retention.[497–499,503] Because many of the patients with PV are elderly, careful attention to fluid status should be maintained to avoid slipping into congestive heart failure following the initiation of anagrelide.

Another potential approach to controlling the erythrocytosis and thrombocytosis in PV involves the use of interferon-α.[506–518] Interferon-α has global effects on hematopoiesis.[518] It inhibits in vitro erythropoiesis and thrombopoiesis and antagonizes the action of PDGF, which likely plays a major role in the pathobiology of myelofibrosis.[518] Silver has suggested that treatment with interferon potentially might alter the natural history of polycythemia by interrupting the development of PPMM and myelofibrosis.[514] Reports of small groups of patients treated with interferon indicate that the erythrocytosis can be controlled in 6 to 12 months, virtually eliminating the need for phlebotomy in approximately 70% of cases.[497,506–513] In addition, interferon is capable of eliminating or reducing the degrees of splenomegaly, leukocytosis, and thrombocytosis in the majority of PV patients.[497,506–513] More importantly, interferon treatment has been shown to be capable of diminishing the severity of pruritus in 80% of patients.[515–517] Occasionally the effect on pruritus can occur in days.[515–517] The mechanism by which interferon eliminates pruritus remains unknown. The usual dose of interferon used to control polycythemia varies between 1.9 to 25 × 10^6 units weekly with a median maintenance dose and 10.5 × 10^6 units weekly administered subcutaneously in divided doses three times a week.[497,506–513] A loss of biologic effect can be attributed to the development of interferon-α-neutralizing antibodies, which may be overcome by retreatment with lymphoblastoid interferon-α N3.[497,506–513] Disease control persists in most patients only as long as interferon-α therapy is continued. Rare patients have, however, enjoyed sustained remissions after discontinuation of interferon.[413,419] Silver updated his experience on the long-term use (median 13 years) of interferon-α in 55 patients with PV.[519] Complete responses, defined by absence of the need to phlebotomize patients to maintain a normal hematocrit level less than 45% and platelet counts below 600,000 μL^{-1}, were reached in the great majority of cases after 1 to 2 years of treatment and the maintenance dose could be decreased in half of the patients. Noteworthy is the absence of thrombohemorrhagic events during this long period of follow-up.[519] Although these results are promising, treatment of larger numbers of patients for longer periods of time is required before the results of long-term interferon therapy in the treatment of PV can be appropriately evaluated. Although one would anticipate that this form of therapy would be nonleukemogenic, insufficient data are available to justify this conclusion. In addition, although interferon-α has a profound effect on PDGF and megakaryocytopoiesis, no data are available to suggest that its use delays or prevents the development of PPMM. Interferon-α has, however, been reported to be capable of suppressing the abnormal clone in PV, similar to its ability to induce cytogenetic remissions in chronic myeloid leukemia.[78,515] In these patients clonal hematopoiesis reverts to a normal polyclonal pattern.[78] Intolerance to therapy with interferon-α leads to drug withdrawal in 14% of patients.[497,505–513] Initially, all patients suffer flu-like symptoms, which are controllable with acetaminophen or aspirin. Such symptoms usually resolve spontaneously after several months of therapy. More serious side effects, including high fevers, severe asthenia, and reversible lower extremity bilateral neuritis, may require cessation of interferon-α therapy. It is anticipated that further evaluation of interferon-α therapy will be pursued in the future. A pegylated form of interferon has been recently used to treat a variety of MPDs with great success.[512] This form of interferon can be administered once weekly and its use is associated with a more favorable toxicity profile.[512] Interestingly, in a multicenter phase II trial of pegylated interferon-α2a in 27 patients, Kiladjian et al reported a decrease in JAK2V617F allele frequency in 24 patients (89%), and in one patient the mutant JAK2 was no longer detectable after 12 months of therapy.[520] Ishii and coworkers have demonstrated the elimination of JAK2V617F-positive cells following pegylated interferon therapy, which was associated with the restoration of polyclonal hematopoiesis.[521] The role of pegylated interferon therapy versus the present standard of care will be defined only after the performance of a randomized phase III trial.

Imatinib mesylate (Gleevec) therapy has also been shown to be effective in reducing phlebotomy requirements, in lowering abnormal platelet counts, and reducing spleen size in PV patients.[522] Imatinib is a potent inhibitor of the BCR–ABL tyrosine kinase and is approved for the treatment of chronic myeloid leukemia. Imatinib also inhibits other tyrosine kinases encoded by protooncogenes such as *KIT* (formerly designated c-kit) and *PDGF-R*.[522] Oehler and colleagues have shown that in vitro Imatinib treatment blocks EPO-independent colony formation by PV marrow cells.[523] The amount of suppression was dose dependent and occurred at drug concentrations that are achieved in patients receiving imatinib therapy for chronic myeloid leukemia PV. Patients undergoing imatinib therapy who achieved a complete hematological remission enjoyed an approximately two- to threefold reduction in the frequency of JAK2V617F.[524]

Symptomatic management of the PV patient may be complicated by the occurrence of intractable pruritus.[196,398–403] Normally, the pruritus occurs on exposure to sudden body cooling, especially after a warm bath[196,398–403] and is experienced by as many as 40% to 60% of patients treated with phlebotomy.[398–403] The frequency of pruritus appears to be somewhat lower in patients treated with myelosuppressive agents.[196] This observation is related to the probable relation between pruritus and degranulation of tissue mast cells and circulating basophils.[397] Some uncontrolled studies have attributed pruritus to hyperhistaminemia or severe iron deficiency, with relief associated with the use of histamine antagonists or ferrous sulfate.[403] Iron replacement is frequently not possible because it can lead to dangerous elevations of the red cell mass. In a number of instances, however, iron replacement has been possible with disease control with interferon-α.[12] The association between pruritus and tissue infiltration by mast cells would appear to explain the response of occasional patients to photochemotherapy with psoralens and ultraviolet irradiation.[522,523] At present, interferon therapy for pruritus appears to be extremely useful.[516] Taylor reported that significant pruritus control occurred in 83% of patients treated with appropriate doses of interferon-α.[394]

This use of interferon-α represents a significant advance in the treatment of a frequently disabling symptom in this patient population. In addition, 80% of patients with pruritus have been reported to respond to paroxetine or fluoxetine, selective serotonin uptake inhibitors.[525–527] Other effective options include psoralen photochemotherapy and narrowband ultraviolet B phototherapy.[528]

Budd–Chiari syndrome is a catastrophic illness that can lead to significant morbidity and mortality in a patient with PV.[352–359] Patients with MPD are at a high risk of developing this syndrome.[196,352–359] Independently, the use of oral contraceptive pills and congenital and acquired thrombophilic factors are involved in its development.[529] A number of cases of hepatic vein thrombosis have been reported in nonpolycythemic women taking oral contraceptives.[356,530] Although no data are available, one must be concerned about the use of oral contraceptives in women with PV.

The optimal approach to the problem of Budd–Chiari syndrome is obviously preventive and involves maintenance of normal blood values in the patient with PV.[356,359,531] Once the Budd–Chiari syndrome develops, the prognosis without treatment is dismal. The goals of therapy are to prevent further propagation of thrombus, relieve the intense hepatic congestion, and manage the severe ascites that often plague these patients.[356,359] If untreated, these patients often have a slowly progressive course, with deterioration and death occurring within 3.5 years.[356] Spontaneous resolution of the hepatic vein occlusion rarely occurs. Diuretics may be of value in the treatment of the ascites but do not affect the long-term outcome.[356] Thrombolytic therapy within 24 hours of onset of diagnosis with urokinase (240,000 units per hour for 2 hours, followed by 60,000 units per hour) or tissue plasminogen activator (0.5–1.0 mg/h) directly infused into the thrombosed hepatic vein for 24 hours results occasionally in success.[356,359] Even if therapy is delayed for 2 to 3 weeks, a favorable outcome can be achieved in some instances with thrombolytic therapy. Such therapy is not innocuous since bleeding can complicate the course of therapy. Angioplasty of localized segments of the hepatic vein can result in the relief of symptoms in the majority of patients but the risk of restenosis is high.[356] Anticoagulant therapy may have a role in the prevention of further clot formation, but there has been no definitive evidence that such therapy promotes resolution of established thromboses.[356]

The clinical deterioration of patients with Budd–Chiari syndrome results from damage to the hepatocytes from necrosis associated with marked elevation in sinusoidal pressure, coupled with ischemia from reduced hepatic arteriole perfusion.[356] The only rational therapeutic intervention therefore involves some sort of portal vein decompression to achieve an effective reduction of sinusoidal pressure.[356,359,531] A variety of surgical procedures resulting in portal-splenic decompression have been shown to be of value in patients with Budd–Chiari syndrome.[356,359] Transjugular intrahepatic portosystemic shunt placement has been used as a bridge to liver transplantation.[356,359,531,532] Surgical portosystemic shunts may reverse hepatic necrosis and prevent cirrhosis.[356] The 5-year survival rate after surgical shunts ranges from 75% to 94%.[356] Liver transplantation is a potential option for treatment of those patients with continued hepatic decompensation.[356,532,533] The indications for liver transplantation are cirrhosis, fulminant hepatic failure, and failure of a portosystemic shunt.[356,359] The overall actuarial survival at 1 year is 76% and was 68% at 10 years.[534] Since PV is a slowly progressive disease, transplantation should not be withheld from these patients.[534] Pretransplant predictors of mortality based on a multivariable analysis were impaired renal function and a history of a shunt.[534] The hematologic consequences of polycythemia must be aggressively treated in the posttransplantation setting, the hepatic vein occlusion may reoccur in the transplanted liver.[356,359,535]

Therapy of cerebral vein thrombosis and sinuses includes anticoagulation with heparin to arrest the thrombotic process and to prevent pulmonary embolism. Low-molecular-weight heparin should be started as soon as the diagnosis is confirmed, even in the presence of hemorrhagic infarcts.[534] After the acute phase, vitamin K antagonists are given for 6 months after a first episode or longer if the MPD disease is not well controlled.[537] There is currently no available evidence from randomized clinical trials regarding the efficacy or safety of thrombolytic therapy.

The performance of any surgical procedures on patients with PV is, as previously discussed, accompanied by excessively high morbidity and mortality.[393–397] Elective surgery should not be contemplated unless the patient's hematologic values have been normalized for several months.[393–397] The longer the hematologic control has been in effect, the lower the incidence of postoperative complications. If emergency surgery is required, the patient should be phlebotomized rapidly until a normal hematocrit is reached, and platelets should be available in case excessive perioperative or postoperative bleeding occurs.[393–397] Following emergency or elective surgery, the patient should be mobilized as soon as possible and strong consideration should be given to anticoagulation with low-molecular-weight heparin, unless the patient has some contraindication. Dental extractions can also result in excessive hemorrhage and should not be performed unless the patient is under strict hematologic control.[393–397]

Perhaps the most difficult and frustrating period encountered during the clinical course of a patient with PV is the development of PV related MF.[339,340] These patients are frequently symptomatic, as a result of the sequelae of anemia, infection, bleeding, and splenic enlargement.[339,340] Because few of these patients have been treated in a uniform, controlled fashion, it is difficult to make strict therapeutic recommendations. In a study by Dingli and coworkers, an unfavorable marrow karyotype (other than 13q$^-$ or 20q$^-$) in patients with PV- and ET-related myelofibrosis was associated with a poor prognosis (median survival of 12 months).[407] Causes of death include transformation into acute myeloid leukemia, sepsis, hemorrhage, thrombotic events, and multiorgan failure.[407]

The anemia that characterizes the spent phase is usually multifactorial in origin. An important factor is splenic pooling of red cells and expansion of the plasma volume, which occurs as a consequence of splenomegaly.[538] It can therefore be useful in these patients to obtain red blood cell mass measurements and to quantitate the degree of anemia directly to detect those patients who have a low hematocrit level but normal red cell mass.[12,409] Folate or iron deficiency may be important in anemic patients and should be corrected.[12] Almost 20% of patients with PV related MF develop overt hemolytic anemia.[338–340] Some of these patients respond to prednisone therapy, but most require splenectomy. By far the most common cause of anemia is ineffective erythropoiesis,[539] and these patients often require transfusion therapy. Androgen therapy (danazol 400–800 mg/d) may be effective in stimulating effective hematopoiesis and diminishing transfusion requirements.[540] Low-dose thalidomide and a short course of prednisone may also be effective in eliminating the red cell transfusion requirement.[541] Iron overload syndrome secondary to ineffective erythropoiesis or transfusion therapy is a dangerous possibility. In this situation, some consideration should be given to chronic oral iron chelation therapy.

The clinical courses of these patients are frequently punctuated by pressure symptoms secondary to splenic enlargement and repeated splenic infarcts.[338–340] Treatment must be directed toward decreasing the expansion of a rapidly enlarging spleen. Small doses of busulphan, hydroxyurea, or melphalan, or occasionally interferon-α therapy, may result in the relief of such symptoms.[338–340,542–544] Radiotherapy in small doses is also sometimes helpful.[541,542] Unfortunately, its effect is frequently transient.[543,545] The chemotherapy or radiation dose must be carefully determined, because overzealous use may lead to granulocytopenia and thrombocytopenia. Often, as a last resort, splenectomy is the only reasonable therapeutic maneuver. This procedure in advanced disease is associated with an operative mortality rate of 25% and should be performed by only the most experienced of surgeons.[545–550] Surgical intervention should not be inappropriately delayed.[546–550] Splenectomy in such patients is frequently complicated by excessive hemorrhage and infected hematomas.[546–550]

Thrombocytopenia may lead to life-threatening hemorrhages in PV related mMF myelofibrosis patients.[338] Its development is due to ineffective thrombopoiesis and platelet sequestration by an enlarged spleen, and patients may rarely respond to splenectomy.[546–550] Bleeding due to qualitative platelet abnormalities has been noted in these patients; when it is severe, platelet transfusions are often required, although because of marked splenomegaly such transfusions frequently do not increase platelet numbers. The clinician therefore must follow the extent of hemorrhage as a means of determining the effectiveness of such transfusions. In patients with refractory bleeding, a trial of epsilon aminocaproic acid or Factor VIIa infusions is suggested.[12] Disseminated intravascular coagulopathy occasionally complicates PV related myelofibrosis and can lead to life-threatening hemorrhage.[546] After careful laboratory documentation, replacement therapy with fresh frozen plasma should be pursued. Some mention should also be made of the use of biologic response modifiers for the treatment of PV related myelofibrosis. A number of investigators have suggested that interferon might be useful in the treatment of PMF and might be successful in reducing spleen size, but in reality responses are rare.[550]

Limited information is available concerning the treatment of those patients who develop acute leukemia following PV.[419,423,424,551–556] The overwhelming majority of such cases involve myeloid leukemias, but a small number of patients have a lymphoblastic phenotype.[419,423,424,551–556] The optimal treatment of such patients is unknown. In the elderly, the choice not to institute chemotherapy is a reasonable option, because results with treatment are so poor.

Rare prolonged remissions of acute leukemia following PV have been reported in the literature.[553] These patients are frequently elderly, and poor results with standard regimens have been reported. Alternative approaches to standard therapy should be entertained in these elderly patients with secondary leukemias. In a recent retrospective analysis on 23 patients with leukemic transformation of PV, the median patient age was 68 and leukemia developed a median of 12.8 years from the diagnosis of PV.[557] Twelve of the 14 patients in which cytogenetic analyses were performed had complex cytogenetic abnormalities associated with high-risk leukemias.[557] Fifteen patients were treated with palliative measures and had a median survival of 2.5 months. Of the eight patients treated with standard induction therapy, one obtained a complete remission and seven died without obtaining a response.[557] The median survival of these chemotherapy-treated patients was 5.6 months. The median survival of the entire cohort of 23 patients was 2.9 months.[559] This poor outcome is likely the result of clinical and biological features of the acute leukemia, advanced patient age, unfavorable cytogenetics, and patient comorbidities associated with advanced age.[557] Allogeneic stem cell transplantation is poorly tolerated in these patients. In Seattle, many of the transplanted patients with acute leukemia that developed following PV or ET died of transplant-related complications.[558] Selected patients are likely to tolerate and to have a favorable outcome with allogeneic stem cell transplantation and reduced intensity condition. Because of these poor outcomes, patients with PV-related acute leukemia should be considered candidates for experimental therapeutic strategies. Arsenic trioxide has recently been shown to induce apoptosis of AML cells and to downregulate activated STAT proteins by targeting JAK2.[559] A trial of low-dose cytosine arabinoside and arsenic trioxide chemotherapy in elderly patients has recently been reported with promising results.[560] Such regimens should be explored in patients with MPD-related acute leukemias.

PV occurs infrequently during the childbearing years.[554–562] When it does, it has been reported to lead to an increased incidence of fetal wastage, with 30% of pregnancies in PV patients terminating in spontaneous abortions.[554–562] In addition, preeclampsia occurs more frequently in these women.[554–562] Pregnancy in PV patients is frequently associated with a gradual normalization of blood values, and it is not unusual for a woman who has required extensive therapy for control of her disease to no longer require phlebotomies during pregnancy.[561–565] Delivery appears not to be complicated by excessive hemorrhage or by an increased risk of venous thrombosis.[561–565]

The normalization of the hematocrit level during pregnancy in PV has been associated with lowering of the red cell mass into the normal range in the few patients in whom these measurements have been performed. Although some degree of hematocrit level normalization can be explained by expansion of the plasma volume or by nutritional deficiencies that occur during pregnancy, it is unlikely that these factors can be solely responsible. It seems more reasonable to assume that the high estrogen levels characteristic of pregnancy suppress erythropoiesis. In the few male patients with PV who have been treated with estrogen, suppression of red cell production has been noted. After termination of the pregnancies, the patients' hematologic values slowly drift back to their previously elevated values in parallel with the return to normal estrogen levels. Because pregnancy is usually associated with spontaneous control of the polycythemic state, no specific therapy is required, except for careful observation. If needed, therapy should be limited to phlebotomy and low-dose aspirin therapy because of the mutagenic effects of chemotherapeutic agents.[240] If this management strategy therapy is unsuccessful, interferon therapy is suggested because it is not known to be leukemogenic or teratogenic and does not cross the placenta.[499] In the puerperium, thromboprophylaxis with 6 weeks of low-molecular-weight heparin therapy is recommended.[562] Aggressive intervention with hematocrit level control and aspirin therapy with low-molecular-weight heparin is associated with a feasible outcare for the pregnancy.[562]

Because PV is ultimately a stem cell disorder, it should be possible to achieve cure with stem cell transplantation.[558,566–568] Thus far, the majority of patients undergoing allogeneic stem cell transplantation have been relatively young (<50 years of age), and have been transplanted either in the "myelofibrotic" or after transformation to acute leukemia.[563–565] In the largest study reported thus far, 36 of 56 patients (64%) with myelofibrosis of various etiologies (including 5 with antecedent PV) are alive for a median of 2.8 years following transplantation.[566] Acute graft-versus-host disease occurred in 68% of patients, and chronic graft-versus-host disease in 59%. Transplantation-related mortality rates were low among patients with marrow fibrosis, but substantial among patients with leukemic transformation, due perhaps to either the biology of the disease itself or to the induction chemotherapy required pretransplantation.[566] Recent promising studies suggest that reduced-intensity conditioning may be better tolerated by older patients who progress to PV related MF before transformation to acute leukemia.[567–569] Transplantation during the polycythemia phase of the disease is rarely appropriate.

Development of JAK2 Inhibitors and Their Implications for the Treatment of PV

The identification of *JAK* mutations in PV has raised the exciting prospect of developing specific JAK2V617F inhibitors to treat PV patients. Given the remarkable clinical success of imatinib therapy for the treatment of *BCR–ABL*-positive CML,[570] *FIP1L1–PDGFR*-positive hypereosinophilic syndrome,[571] and chronic myelomonocytic leukemia associated with *PDGFR*β rearrangements,[572] and the rapid development of second-generation BCR–ABL inhibitors for imatinib-refractory CML,[573,574] the expectations that discovery of *JAK2V617F* will facilitate the development of a molecularly targeted therapy for PV have been heightened.

Although JAK kinase inhibitors with specific activity against JAK2 have been previously identified and characterized,[575] most of these compounds do not have sufficient potency (eg, cellular IC_{50} < 1–2 μM) to be used for preclinical and clinical testing. An enormous amount of effort is currently being expended to identify a specific inhibitor of JAK2V617F. Recently two tyrosine kinase inhibitors currently used clinically, erlotinib[576] and Cephalon-701 (CEP-701),[577] have been identified that inhibit JAK2V617F. Erlotinib (Tarceva) is a kinase inhibitor that inhibits epidermal growth factor receptor-related tyrosine kinase activity. Erlotinib has been used in the treatment of non-small-cell lung cancer and pancreatic cancer associated with mutations of epidermal growth factor receptor.[578] Recently, Li et al have shown that erlotinib also is a potent inhibitor of JAK2V617F activity.[576] In vitro colony assays revealed that erlotinib at micromolar concentrations effectively suppressed the proliferation of PV erythroid progenitor cells while having little effect on normal cells.[576] CEP-701 is an orally active inhibitor of the receptor tyrosine kinase Flt-3 and is currently in phase III clinical trials in patients with AML associated with Flt-3 mutations.[579] Dobrzanski et al recently reported the ability of CEP-701 to inhibit JAK2V617F and to suppress the growth of cells from patients with MPD.[577] A hundred nanomoles of CEP-701 inhibited the growth of over 50% of CD34+ cells isolated from patients with MPD, but did not affect the proliferation of normal cells.[577] Multiple academic groups and pharmaceutical companies are actively working on additional novel JAK2 inhibitors with even more favorable pharmacokinetic and pharmacodynamic properties.

There are several issues that need to be addressed before JAK2 inhibitors can be used for the treatment of chronic MPDs: (a) It has been shown that loss-of-function mutations involving JAK3 and the tyrosine kinase Tyk2 are associated with inherited forms of severe combined immunodeficiency and that JAK3-specific inhibitors are effective immunosuppressive agents.[580] It is, therefore, critical for a candidate JAK2 inhibitor to have minimal inhibitory activity against Tyk2 and JAK3. JAK2 inhibitors with significant inhibitory activity against JAK3 and Tyk2 at pharmacologic doses might suppress cell-mediated immunity, leading to an unacceptable incidence of opportunistic infection. (b) The JAK2 inhibitors should have preferential activity against mutant rather than WT *JAK2* to avoid significant hematological toxicity. Wild-type JAK2 function is indispensable for definitive hematopoiesis, and specifically for erythropoiesis.[581] Thus an agent that inhibits JAK2 might cause dose-dependent cytopenias, particularly anemia. (c) Since the management of many patients with PV with conventional therapies, including venesection, aspirin, and hydroxyurea are associated with a reasonable outcome at relatively modest costs, a cost–benefit analysis of the use of a potentially expensive long-term targeted therapy will be required. (d) The role of JAK2V617F as the initiating event in PV pathophysiology is not as yet clear, and the potential impact of JAK2-directed therapy is uncertain. (e) It has been shown that the blast cells of patients with acute leukemia that develop after an MPD are in about 50% of cases negative for JAK2V617F even if the patient was JAK2V617F positive prior to the malignant transformation.[425–428] It is possible that the use of JAK2V617F inhibitors would promote the proliferation of clones responsible for leukemic transformation by eliminating the JAK2V617F-positive clone. (f) Given the important role of JAK2 signaling in prolactin- and growth hormone-mediated signal transduction, it is possible that endocrine side effects might occur in patients treated with JAK2 inhibitors.[486]

Allele-specific assays such as allele-specific PCR,[82] pyrosequencing,[80] and quantitative real-time PCR[276] can precisely quantitate *JAK2V617F* mutational burden. Such quantitative assessments of *JAK2V617F* mutational burden has clearly been used to demonstrate that the *JAK2V617F* mutant clone persists in PV patients treated with imatinib and interferon-α.[582] Given the need to assess response to therapy with molecular targeted agents, quantitative assays for *JAK2V617F* should be used to follow tumor burden in trials of JAK2 inhibitors. It is imperative that these assays be validated as surrogate assays predictive of long-term survival or reduction of complications associated with PV.

PROGNOSIS

The prognosis of a patient with PV depends on the nature and severity of the complications that occur during the clinical course of that particular patient's disorder.[12,296,297,417–420,531] In addition, an individual patient's prognosis depends on the duration of the erythrocytotic phase or the time for transition to PPMM or acute leukemia.[12,153] Survival is also influenced by whether appropriate treatment is instituted during the erythrocytotic phase of the illness. Patients who have uncontrolled erythrocytosis are at an extremely high risk for the development of thromboses.[12,296,297,417–420,531] The median survival from onset of symptoms may be as short as 1.5 years in untreated patients.[207] Determination of the optimal management of patients with PV has been a difficult task, as the disease, when treated, is associated with a survival period of 10 to 15 years.[12] Studies of new potential therapeutic interventions therefore require prospective studies with prolonged follow-ups before meaningful results can be generated.[302,303]

Table 68–9 Risk Stratification in Polycythemia Vera Based on Thrombotic Risk

Risk Category	Age >60 y or History of Thrombo\sis	Cardiovascular Risk Factors*
Low	No	No
Intermediate	No	Yes
High	Yes	

*Hypertension, hypercholesterolemia, diabetes, smoking (see text). Extreme thrombocytosis (platelet count >1500 × 10^9 L^{-1}) is a risk factor for bleeding. Its role as a risk factor for thrombosis is uncertain. Increasing leukocyte count has been identified as a novel risk factor for thrombosis, but confirmation is required.

Data from Finazzi G, Barbui T: How we treat patients with polycythemia vera. Blood 2007 Jan 30 [Epub ahead of print].

Increasing age and history of vascular events have consistently proven to be independent predictors of developing additional thromboses in patients with PV. In the ECLAP trial, the incidence of cardiovascular complications was higher in patients older than 69, patients with a prior history of thrombosis, and patients with a WBC higher than 15,000 × 109 L^{-1}. Conventional cardiovascular risk factors including hypertension, hyperlipidemia, diabetes, and smoking are assumed to be associated with the same relative risk of developing thrombosis in PV patients as that observed in the general population. Although practicing hematologists are frequently concerned about elevated platelet counts in PV patients, both the PVSG 01 trial and the ECLAP trial failed to show any association between platelet count and thrombotic events, suggesting that therapies in PV targeting reduction of platelet numbers are ill conceived.

These data have led to stratification of therapy in patients with PV based on clearly identifiable risk factors (Table 68–9).[349] The development of acute leukemia was a relatively rare event in PV occurring in 22 of 1638 patients in the ECLAP observational study after a median of 8.4 years from the time of diagnosis.[425] Older age as well as treatment with P32, busulphan, and pipobroman was associated with a four- to eightfold increased risk of developing acute myeloid leukemia of a myelodysplastic syndrome, as compared to patients treated with phlebotomy alone, hydroxyurea, or interferon. For reasons not presently understood, patients presenting with PV and a low blood cholesterol are at an especially high risk for developing acute leukemia.[425]

Recently, the effect of JAK2V617F allele frequency on the prognosis of PV patients has been examined.[401,402] Over 95% of patients with PV are JAK2V617F positive and their mutational load can be determined by allele-specific PCR.[402] Approximately 30% of PV patients have a high JAK2V617F burden (>50%) and the remainder have a lower burden (<50%), with the small numbers being wild-type. Two groups have recently reported that high burdens of JAK2V617F in PV patients is associated with larger splenic volumes, more frequent aquagenic pruritus, and a higher rate of evolution into myelofibrosis.[401,402] A high burden of JAK2V617F, although associated with higher hematocrit levels and white cell counts, were not associated with a higher incidence of thrombosis or a shorter survival.

FUTURE DIRECTIONS

The discovery of JAK2V617F mutations has led to a more comprehensive understanding of the pathophysiology of this clonal neoplastic disorder. The use of JAK2V617F assays as diagnostic tools has dramatically changed the manner in which PV is diagnosed. The use of JAK2V617 and a variety of other biomarkers including PRV-1, cMPL, and cytogenetic abnormalities may prove useful in better identifying patients at risk of developing fatal thrombotic events. Furthermore, JAK2V617F is being pursued as a target for the rational identification of small molecule therapies for the treatment of PV. Furthermore, JAK2V617F allele chimerism is being used as a means of quantitating tumor burden in patients treated with JAK2V617F inhibitors or pegylated forms of interferon-α. The relationship between JAK2V617F burden and disease outcome must be carefully validated before it can be used as a surrogate biomarker for more rapid approval of drug therapies for PV. Randomized clinical trials of such novel agents comparing these outcomes with the standard of care are clearly required in order to be certain that they represent significant advances in the treatment of PV patients.

SUGGESTED READINGS

Bellanne-Chantelot C, Chaumarel I, Labopin M, et al: Genetic and clinical implications of the Val617Phe JAK2 mutation in 72 families with myeloproliferative disorders. Blood 108:346, 2006.

Diller GP, Gatzoulis MA: Pulmonary vascular disease in adults with congenital heart disease. Circulation 115(8):1039, 2007.

Elliott MA, Tefferi A. Thrombosis and haemorrhage in polycythaemia vera and essential thrombocythaemia. Br J Haematol 128(3):275, 2005.

Finazzi G, Barbui T: How we treat patients with polycythemia vera. Blood 109:2446, 2007.

Finazzi G, Caruso V, Marchioli R, et al, and the ECLAP Investigators: Acute leukemia in polycythemia vera: An analysis of 1638 patients enrolled in a prospective observational study. Blood 105(7):2664, 2005.

Gordeuk VR, Stockton DW, Prchal JT: Congenital polycythemias/erythrocytoses. Haematologica 90(1):109, 2005.

James C, Ugo V, Casadevall N, Constantinescu SN, Vainchenker W: A JAK2 mutation in myeloproliferative disorders: Pathogenesis and therapeutic and scientific prospects. Trends Mol Med 11(12):546, 2005.

James C, Ugo V, Le Couedic JP, et al: A unique clonal JAK2 mutation leading to constitutive signalling causes polycythaemia vera. Nature 434:1144, 2005.

Kiladjian JJ, Cassinat B, Turlure P, et al: High molecular response rate of polycythemia vera patients treated with pegylated interferon alpha-2a. Blood 108(6):2037, 2006.

Kim WY, Kaelin WG: Role of VHL gene mutation in human cancer. J Clin Oncol 22(24):4991, 2004.

Kralovics R, Passamonti F, Buser AS, et al: A gain-of-function mutation of JAK2 in myeloproliferative disorders. N Engl J Med 352:1779, 2005.

Marchioli R, Finazzi G, Landolfi R, et al: Vascular and neoplastic risk in a large cohort of patients with polycythemia vera. J Clin Oncol 23(10):2224, 2005.

Mentha G, Giostra E, Majno PE, et al: Liver transplantation for Budd-Chiari syndrome: A European study on 248 patients from 51 centres. J Hepatol 44(3):520, 2006.

Patel RK, Lea NC, Heneghan MA, et al: Prevalence of the activating JAK2 tyrosine kinase mutation V617F in the Budd-Chiari syndrome. Gastroenterology. 130(7):2031, 2006.

Penaloza D, Arias-Stella J: The heart and pulmonary circulation at high altitudes: Healthy highlanders and chronic mountain sickness [review]. Circulation 115(9):1132, 2007.

Perrotta S, Nobili B, Ferraro M, et al: Von Hippel-Lindau-dependent polycythemia is endemic on the island of Ischia: Identification of a novel cluster. Blood 107(2):514, 2006.

Spivak JL: Polycythemia vera: Myths, mechanisms, and management. Blood 100:4272, 2002.

Theocharides A, Boissinot M, Girodon F, et al: Leukemic blasts in transformed JAK2-V617F positive myeloproliferative disorders are frequently negative for the JAK2-V617F mutation. Blood 110:375, 2007.

Vannucchi AM, Antonioli E, Guglielmelli P, et al: Clinical profile of homozygous JAK2V617F mutation in patients with polycythemia vera or essential thrombocythemia. Blood 110:840, 2007.

Wajcman H, Galacteros F: Hemoglobins with high oxygen affinity leading to erythrocytosis. New variants and new concepts. Hemoglobin 29(2):91, 2005.

REFERENCES

For complete list of references log onto www.expertconsult.com

CHAPTER 69

CHRONIC MYELOID LEUKEMIA

Ravi Bhatia and Jerald P. Radich

BACKGROUND

Chronic myeloid leukemia (CML) is a hematopoietic malignancy originating from transformation of a primitive hematopoietic cell. Without treatment, CML progresses from an initial chronic phase (CP) characterized by marrow hyperplasia and increased numbers of circulating differentiated myeloid cells followed by advanced phases of disease (accelerated phase [AP] and blast crisis [BC]) marked by a block in differentiation, an accumulation of blasts, and a depletion of normal hematopoietic cells, especially white blood cells and platelets. CML was the first malignant disease found to be consistently associated with a specific cytogenetic abnormality, the Philadelphia chromosome (Ph), resulting in the formation of the *BCR–ABL* fusion oncogene. Study of *BCR–ABL* has led to sensitive methods to detect residual disease and predict outcome and to "targeted" therapy aimed at inhibiting abnormal tyrosine kinase activity resulting from the *BCR–ABL* fusion oncogene. In addition, CML was one of the first diseases demonstrated to be curable by hematopoietic cell transplantation (HCT). Thus, CML has become the model for "tailored" therapy, where various treatments can be escalated on the basis of molecular response.

ETIOLOGY/EPIDEMIOLOGY/GENETICS

Chronic myelogenous leukemia was recognized as a distinct entity, associated with massive splenomegaly and leukocytosis without other explanations, in the mid-1800s. The modern history of CML was initiated by Nowell and Hungerford in 1960. They used newly developed techniques to detect a small chromosome in metaphase preparations of marrow cells from CML patients.[1] This abnormal chromosome was the first consistent chromosomal abnormality in human malignancies and was termed the Philadelphia chromosome after the city of its discovery. Rowley showed that the Philadelphia chromosome resulted from a translocation between chromosomes 9 and 22 [t(9; 22)(q34;q11)].[2] The genes involved in this translocation were cloned in the 1980s, and the t(9 : 22) translocation was shown to result from the fusion of the BCR (breakpoint cluster region) gene on chromosome 22 to the *ABL* (Abelson leukemia virus) gene on chromosome 9, with formation of the *BCR–ABL* fusion oncogene.[3] This oncogene codes for a constitutively active cytoplasmic tyrosine kinase, which is now believed to be the principal cause of the chronic phase of CML. Until the 1970s, CML was regarded as an incurable and inevitably lethal disorder. It was then recognized that selected patients can be cured, by allogeneic HCT. However, transplantation therapy for CML is limited by donor availability and the risk of life-threatening toxicity. More recently, imatinib mesylate, a tyrosine kinase inhibitor that specifically blocks the enzymatic action of the abnormal tyrosine kinase coded by the fusion oncogene, has resulted in a high rate of remission and improved survival in CML patients.

Chronic myelogenous leukemia is the most common of the myeloproliferative diseases and represents 15% to 20% of all new leukemia cases.[4] The annual incidence of CML is 1 to 1.5 cases per 100,000 population per year. The median age at diagnosis is 67 years and the incidence sharply rises with age. The disease occurs slightly more often in men than in women. Chronic myelogenous leukemia may occur in children but only approximately 10% of cases occur in subjects between 5 and 20 years of age, and represent only 3% of all childhood leukemias. Concordance of disease is not observed between identical twins.[4] Radiation may play a role in some cases, because persons exposed to high-dose irradiation, including survivors of the atomic bomb, have a significantly increased risk of leukemia, and high-dose irradiation of myeloid cell lines in vitro induces the expression of BCR–ABL transcripts indistinguishable from those that characterize CML.[5] The BCR–ABL gene has been reported to be detectable at very low levels in a high proportion of healthy individuals using a very sensitive PCR assay.[6] These findings suggest that fusion genes may develop relatively frequently in hematopoietic cells, but only infrequently lead to development of leukemia. The mechanism by which the Ph chromosome is first formed and the time required for progression to overt disease are unknown.

PATHOPHYSIOLOGY

CML is generally believed to develop from transformation of a primitive hematopoietic stem cell (HSC) by the *BCR–ABL* fusion gene.[7] The progeny of transformed HSC have a proliferative advantage over normal hematopoietic cells, thus allowing the Ph-positive clone gradually to displace residual normal hematopoiesis. The translocation is found in cells of myeloid, erythroid, megakaryocytic and B-lymphoid origin, consistent with a hematopoietic stem cell origin of the disease.[8–10] Hematopoietic expansion in patients with chronic-phase disease primarily involves an increase in myeloid cell mass, which is related to an expansion of mature cells as well as increased numbers of precursor and progenitor cells. In chronic phase, the leukemic cells are minimally invasive and are primarily located in hematopoietic tissues including blood, bone marrow, spleen, and liver. The proliferative advantage of the malignant clone may be related to enhanced responsiveness to hematopoietic growth factors and/or reduced response to inhibitory factors.[11–14] Chronic myelogenous leukemia progenitors also demonstrate defective adhesion to marrow stromal cells and extracellular matrix.[15] Altered microenvironmental interactions may contribute to another feature of CML, which is abnormal progenitor trafficking with increased numbers of circulating progenitors and extramedullary hematopoiesis. Several observations indicate that although the Ph-positive clone displaces normal hematopoiesis, it does not destroy residual normal stem cells. For example, Ph-negative progenitors can be seen after cultures of CML cells in vitro,[16,17] can be selected on the basis of cell surface phenotype,[18] and can be identified in the blood after high-dose chemotherapy.[19] As described later in the Therapy section, treatment with agents such as interferon (IFN) or imatinib mesylate can result in restoration of Ph-negative hematopoiesis in CML patients.

The *BCR–ABL* gene that characterizes CML results from a chromosomal translocation that results in the fusion of the *ABL* gene on chromosome 9 and the *BCR* gene on chromosome 22 (Fig. 69–1). The translocation is related to a break in *ABL* upstream of exon a2, and in the major breakpoint cluster region of the *BCR* gene. This leads to juxtaposition of a 5′ portion of *BCR* and a 3′ portion of *ABL* on a shortened chromosome 22 (the derivative 22q-, or Ph).[3,20–22] The resulting messenger RNA (mRNA) usually contain one of two *BCR–ABL* junctions, designated e13a2 (formerly b2a2) and e14a2 (or b3a2).[23] Both *BCR–ABL* mRNA molecules are translated into a

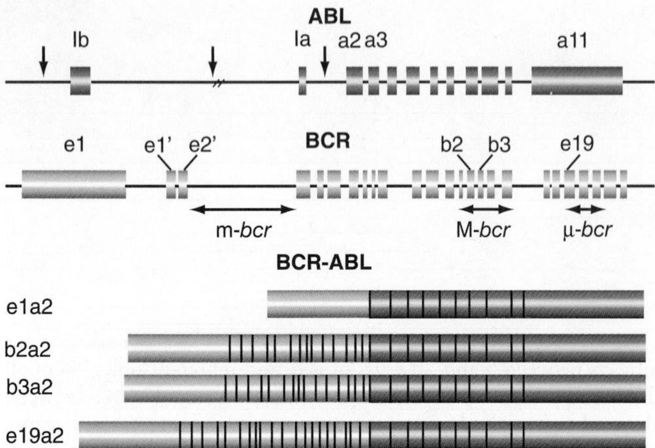

Figure 69–1 Locations of the breakpoints in the *ABL* and *BCR* genes and structure of the chimeric mRNAs derived from the various breaks. (Adapted from Deininger MW, Goldman JM, Melo JV (eds) The Molecular Biology of Chronic Myeloid Leukemia. Blood 96 (10): 3343, 2000.)

210-kd fusion protein, referred to as p210*BCR–ABL*. Rarely, other variant breakpoints and fusions can give rise to full-length, functionally oncogenic *BCR–ABL* proteins, notably p190*BCR–ABL* (associated with an e1a2 mRNA junction) and p230*BCR–ABL* (associated with an e19a2 mRNA junction).[24] Of patients with CML who have a normal-appearing karyotype, one-third have a cytogenetically occult *BCR–ABL* gene, usually located on a normal-appearing chromosome 22 but occasionally on chromosome 9. In the remaining patients with Ph-negative, *BCR–ABL*-negative disease, the molecular basis of leukemia is not known.

Some studies have suggested that pathogenesis of CML may be multistep, with development of clonal hematopoiesis preceding the t(9;22) translocation.[8,25] However there is substantial evidence to suggest that the generation of a classic *BCR–ABL* fusion gene in a hematopoietic stem cell is sufficient to initiate CML. Expression of *BCR–ABL* has been shown to transform mouse fibroblast cell lines, growth factor-dependent hematopoietic cell lines, and primary murine bone marrow cells.[26] Expression of *BCR–ABL* in human $CD34^+$ cells also causes increased proliferation, reduced apoptosis and altered adhesion and migration mimicking alterations seen in progenitor cells from CML patients.[27] Transplantation of murine bone marrow cells made to ectopically express the *BCR–ABL* gene by retroviral transduction induces a myeloproliferative disorder (MPD) that closely resembles human CML with increased numbers of peripheral-blood cells (with a predominance of granulocytes), splenomegaly, and extramedullary hematopoiesis, although the disease is much more fulminant than human CML.[28,29] Initial development of transgenic and knockin mouse models of CML was problematic. It appears to be crucial to express this oncogene in the proper cell type. Expression of BCR–ABL in B-cell lymphocytic and megakaryocytic precursors resulted in the development of B-acute lymphocytic leukemia (B-ALL) and megakaryocytic myeloproliferative syndrome.[30–32] Specific expression of the oncogene in hematopoietic stem cells through a stem cell leukemia (SCL) enhancer to regulate expression induces development of a CML-like disease.[33] Together, these studies indicate that *BCR–ABL* expression alone is sufficient to induce chronic-phase CML-like disease in mice.

The *ABL* gene encodes a nonreceptor tyrosine kinase that is expressed in most tissues (Fig. 69–2). Mice with homozygous disruption of the *ABL* gene demonstrate increased perinatal mortality, lymphopenia, and osteoporosis and are smaller, with abnormal head and eye development.[34] The *BCR* gene also encodes a signaling protein that contains multiple modular domains (Fig. 69–2). Although *BCR*-deficient mice develop normally, their neutrophils produce excess levels of oxygen metabolites following activation.[32,35] The normally regulated tyrosine kinase activity of the *ABL* protein is constitutively activated by the juxtaposition of N-terminal *BCR* sequences. *BCR* acts by promoting protein dimerization, leading to phosphorylation of tyrosine residues in the kinase-activation loops and leading to constitutive activation of kinase activity. The fusion of *BCR* sequences to *ABL* also adds new regulatory domains/motifs to *ABL*, such as the growth factor receptor-bound protein 2 (GRB2) SH2-binding site. The uncontrolled kinase activity of *BCR–ABL* and enhanced interaction with a variety of effector proteins leads to deregulation of cell signaling mechanisms that regulate proliferation. The *ABL* protein is found in both the nucleus and the cytoplasm and shuttles between these two compartments, whereas the *BCR–ABL* is exclusively cytoplasmic and localizes to the cytoskeleton where it appears to contribute to adhesion and migration abnormalities.[36]

The structure of the *BCR–ABL* protein and the biochemical pathways affected have been extensively studied (see Fig. 69–2).[36] However, most such interactions have been studied only in cell lines and conditions of forced overexpression. Their existence in primary leukemia cells and relevance to CML pathogenesis is not certain. The murine transduction–transplantation CML model has been helpful in studying the role of *BCR–ABL* domains and signaling interaction in primary hematopoietic cells. However, the murine CML model is not fully representative of human CML, and the role of different domains in development of disease in CML patients still needs to be confirmed. The *ABL* tyrosine kinase is crucial for oncogenic transformation. Mice that express a form of *BCR–ABL* with a point mutation in the ATP-binding site of *ABL* that inhibits its kinase activity do not develop leukemia. This suggests that the *ABL* kinase activity is essential for *BCR–ABL* leukemogenesis in vivo. The success of kinase inhibitor therapy for CML provides further proof of the importance of kinase activity in maintenance of human disease. Other important domains in *BCR–ABL* have also been shown to regulate the kinase activity of *ABL* or connect to other downstream signaling pathways. The amino-terminal coiled-coil (CC) oligomerization domain of *BCR* is an important activator of *ABL* kinase activity, and also promotes the association of *BCR–ABL* with F-actin fibers.[37,38] Phosphorylation of *BCR* at tyrosine 177 generates a GRB2-binding site, which is important for *RAS* activation. Mutation of the tyrosine-177 residue of *BCR–ABL* to phenylalanine (Y177F) largely abolishes its ability to bind GRB2, without affecting the kinase activity of ABL. The Y177F mutant has a greatly reduced ability to induce MPD in mice.[39] A tyrosine phosphorylation site in the activation loop of the *ABL* kinase domain and the SH2 domain of *ABL* also contribute to *RAS* activation. Mutations in the SH2 domain of *ABL* and a Y1294F point mutation reduce the ability of *BCR–ABL* to induce a CML-like MPD in mice.[40] The carboxy-terminal region of *ABL* is required for the proper function of normal *ABL*. However, deletion of the *ABL* actin-binding domain was reported to not affect the ability of *BCR–ABL* to induce CML-like MPD in mice, suggesting that this domain may be dispensable for *BCR–ABL*-mediated leukemogenesis.[41] Certain *BCR–ABL* domains may have complementary or overlapping functions.

Many signaling proteins become phosphorylated in *BCR–ABL*-expressing cells and/or to interact with *BCR–ABL* through various functional domains. These interactions may in turn activate signaling through mechanisms including *RAS*, *PI3K*, *AKT*, *JNK*, and *SRC* family kinases, protein phosphatase, STATs, nuclear factor-B and *MYC*. *BCR–ABL* also induces expression of cytokines such as interleukin-3 (IL-3), granulocyte colony-stimulating factor (G-CSF), and granulocyte–macrophage colony-stimulating factor (GM-CSF).[36] A CML-like MPD was still induced following expression of *BCR–ABL* in bone marrow cells from *Stat5a*$^{-/-}$*Stat5b*$^{-/-}$, *Cbl*$^{-/-}$, and *Il-3*$^{-/-}$*GM-CSF*$^{-/-}$ mice, indicating that these proteins may not be required for *BCR–ABL*-mediated leukemogenesis.[42,43] *BCR–ABL* expression induced CML-like MPD but failed to induce B-ALL in mice that lacked the *SRC* family kinases LYN, HCK, and FGR, indicating the potential importance of the kinases in lymphoid blast crisis or ALL but not for MPD.[28,44] Disruption of the gene encoding IFN consensus sequence-binding protein (*ICSBP*) results in the development of a CML-like disease in mice. Forced expression of *ICSBP* inhibits *BCR–ABL*-induced CML-like disease.[45] Downregulation of *ICSBP* transcripts was also found in patients with CML, and this reduction

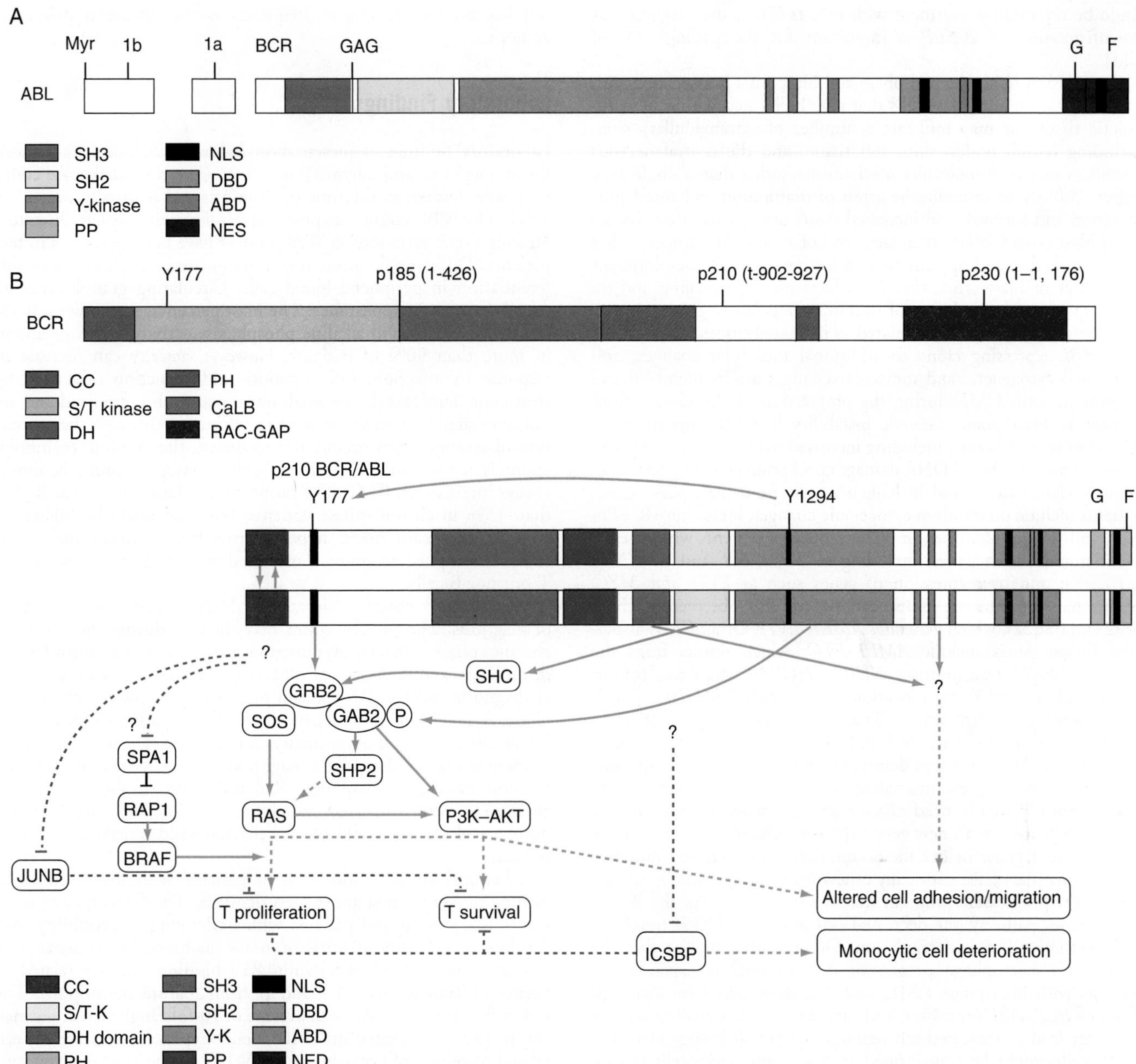

Figure 69–2 **A**, The *ABL* and *BCR* proteins. Several important domains make up the *ABL* and *BCR* proteins. Two isoforms of *ABL* (human types 1a and 1b) are generated by alternative splicing of the first exon, one of them (1b) contains a myristoylation modification site (Myr). The amino-terminal half of ABL contains tandem SRC homology 3 (SH3), SH2, and the tyrosine-kinase (Y-kinase) domains. These domains can assemble into an autoinhibitory structure, in which the SH3 and SH2 domains hold the kinase in the "off" state. In its carboxy-terminal region, *ABL* contains four proline-rich SH3-binding sites (PPs), three nuclear localization signals (NLSs), one nuclear exporting signal (NES), a DNA-binding domain (DBD), and an actin-binding domain (ABD). The actin-binding domain contains binding sites for both monomeric (G) and filamentous (F) forms of actin. The points in ABL that fuses with BCR and GAG (for v-Abl) are indicated. **b |** *BCR* contains a coiled-coil (CC) oligomerization domain, a serine/threonine (S/T) kinase domain, a Dbl/CDC24 guanine-nucleotide exchange factor homology (DH) domain and a pleckstrin homology (PH) domain, a putative calcium-dependent lipid-binding site (CaLB), and an RAC guanosine triphosphatase-activating protein (RAC-GAP) domain. *BCR* also contains binding sites for growth factor receptor-bound protein 2 (GRB2) at tyrosine 177 (Y177), as well as for the GRB10, 14–3-3, and the *ABL* proteins, through its SH2 domain. p185, p210, and p230 indicate the points at which *BCR* most commonly fuses to *ABL*. These forms are associated with acute lymphoblastic leukemia, chronic myelogenous leukemia (CML) and a milder form of CML, respectively. The number of amino acids in each form are indicated in parentheses. **B**, Leukemogenic signaling of BCR–ABL. The BCR–ABL proteins can form dimers or tetramers through their CC domains, and trans-autophosphorylate. Phosphorylation at Y177 generates a high-affinity binding site for growth factor receptor-bound protein 2 (GRB2). GRB2 binds to *BCR–ABL* through its SH2 domain and binds to SOS and GRB2-associated binding protein 2 (GAB2) through its SH3 domains. SOS in turn activates *RAS*. Following phosphorylation (P) by *BCR–ABL*, GAB2 recruits phosphatidylinositol 3-kinase (PI3K) and SHP2 proteins. The SH2 domain of ABL can bind SHC, which following phosphorylation can also recruit GRB2. The *ABL* SH3 domain and the SH3-binding sites in the carboxy-terminal region can bind several proteins that involve regulations of cell adhesion/migration. *BCR–ABL* can promote cell proliferation and survival partly by activating the *RAS, SHP2 and PI3K-AKT* signaling pathways. It can also downregulate transcription of *ICSBP* and *JUNB* and might also inhibit *SIPA1*. Red arrows indicate direct interactions and/or activations. Black arrows indicate negative regulations. Broken arrows indicate multiple steps. (From Ren R: Mechanisms of *BCR–ABL* in the pathogenesis of chronic myelogenous leukaemia. Nat Rev Cancer 5(3):172, 2005.)

could be reversed by treatment with IFN-α. These data suggest that downregulation of *ICSBP* is important for the pathogenesis of CML.

Progression to accelerated phase and blast crisis is associated with increase in immature blast cells that may be located within hematopoietic tissues or may infiltrate a number of extramedullary sites, including lymph nodes, skin, soft tissue, and the central nervous system. A variety of molecular mechanisms, rather than a single gene defect, is likely to underlie the arrest of maturation, enhanced proliferation and survival, and increased tissue invasiveness that characterize blast crisis CML.[46] Increased level of *BCR–ABL* expression is a common feature and appears to be a key factor in the development of features of blast crisis, through effects on cell signaling and on transcription and translation of important regulatory genes. Disease progression is believed to be related to increased susceptibility of the *BCR–ABL*-expressing clone to additional molecular changes, and additional cytogenetic and molecular changes are frequently found in patients with CML during the progression of the disease from chronic to blast phase. Genetic instability in CML appears to be related to several factors, including increased oxidative stress, reduced DNA repair, or reduced DNA damage checkpoint signaling response. Genetic changes observed in leukemic cells from blast-phase CML patients include nonrandom cytogenetic changes, including +8, +Ph, +19, and I(17)q, identified in 60% to 80% of patients with disease; point mutations in genes, including in *TP53*, *RB*, and *CDKN2A* (*p16*^{INK4A}); and overexpression of genes such as *EVI1* and *MYC*. Additional chromosome translocations are also observed, such as t(3;21)(q26;q22), which generates *AML1-EVI1*. Other CML-associated fusion genes include *AML1–ETO*, which results from the t(8;21)(q22;q22) translocation; *NUP98–HOXA9*, which results from the t(7;11)(p15;p15) translocation; and *CBFβ–SMMHC*, which results from inv(16)(p13;q22). These observations suggest that the block in myeloid differentiation in blast crisis may involve cooperation between *BCR–ABL* and defects in hematopoietic transcriptional regulators. Gene expression analyses suggest that the progression of CML from CP to advanced phase may be a two-step rather than a three-step process, with new gene expression changes occurring early in accelerated phase before the accumulation of increased numbers of leukemia blast cells. Especially noteworthy and potentially significant in the progression program were the deregulation of the *WNT*/beta-catenin pathway, the decreased expression of *JUN B* and *FOS*, and alternative kinase deregulation. Other studies suggest that the granulocyte/macrophage progenitor (GMP) pool is expanded in patients with blast-phase CML, and that these cells have increased levels of *BCR–ABL* expression and increased *WNT* signaling activity that may lead to increased self-renewal capacity. It is suggested that GMP cells might be transformed into leukemic stem cells during blast-phase CML, although these findings and the role of *WNT* signaling need to be confirmed.[47,48]

CLINICAL FEATURES

History

Most (>90%) CML patients present in chronic phase (CP). CML is often diagnosed incidentally during routine examination or examination for another illness. Symptoms usually include fatigue, weight loss, bone pain, sweating, and abdominal discomfort and early satiety related to splenomegaly. Symptoms are generally gradual in onset over weeks to months. Uncommon presenting symptoms include those related to leukostasis, acute abdominal pain related to splenic infraction, priapism, and hypermetabolism, hyperuricemia, and gouty arthritis.

Physical Examination

Physical examination may detect pallor and splenomegaly. The incidence of splenomegaly used to be greater than 90% at diagnosis but has been decreasing in frequency as the disease is diagnosed earlier.

Laboratory Findings

Laboratory findings at presentation generally include leukocytosis, thrombocytosis, and anemia (Fig. 69–3). The total leukocyte count is always elevated at the time of diagnosis and is usually over 25 × 10^9/L. The WBC count rises progressively if patients are left untreated. Striking cyclic variations in WBC counts have been described in rare patients. Differential counts reveal granulocytes at all stages of differentiation in peripheral blood cells. Circulating granulocytes are usually normal in appearance. The blast percentage is between 0.5% and 10%. Neutrophil alkaline phosphatase activity is low or absent in more than 90% of patients. However, activity can increase in response to infection, inflammation, and reduction of counts by treatment. Functional abnormalities of neutrophils are mild and are not associated with predisposition to infection. Although the proportion of eosinophils is usually not increased, the absolute eosinophil count is usually increased. The absolute basophil count is almost always increased in CML. The proportion of basophils is usually less than 15% in chronic-phase patients, but may rarely be higher. In contrast to mastocytosis, hyperhistaminemia is uncommon. The absolute lymphocyte count is increased as a result of an increase in T but not B cells.

The platelet count is elevated in 50% of patients at the time of diagnosis. The platelet count may increase during the course of chronic phase. Platelet dysfunction may occur but disorders of thrombosis and hemorrhage are rare. Thrombocytopenia is rare at diagnosis and usually is a sign of progression toward accelerated phase. A deficiency in the second wave of aggregation to epinephrine is the most common abnormality, and is associated with deficiency of adenine nucleotides in the storage pool. The hematocrit is decreased in most patients at diagnosis. Red cells tend to show only mild alterations with increased variability of size and shape. Small numbers of nucleated red blood cells and mild reticulocytosis may be seen.

Chemical abnormalities seen in patients with untreated CML include hyperuricemia and hyperuricosuria. The formation of urate stones is common and patients with underlying susceptibility may develop acute gouty arthritis or urate nephropathy. Patients have increased serum level of Vitamin B12 binding capacity related to release of Transcobalamin I and II from mature neutrophils. The serum B12 level in CML is an average of 10-fold higher than normal. Serum LDH is elevated in CML. Pseudohyperkalemia may be seen related to release of potassium from WBC during clotting. Spurious hypoglycemia or hypoxemia may result from consumption by neutrophils after a sample is drawn.

Examination of the marrow usually reveals a very hypercellular marrow, with 75% to 90% marrow cellularity (see Fig. 69–3B–F). The granulocytic/erythroid ratio is increased to 10 : 1 to 30 : 1, with increased granulopoiesis and reduced erythropoiesis. Eosinophils and basophils may be increased. Blasts usually represent less than 5% of cells. Presence of more than 10% blasts indicates transformation to accelerated phase. Megakaryocytes are typically smaller than usual and may have hypolobated nuclei. Megakaryocyte numbers may be normal or slightly decreased, but 40% to 50% of patients show moderate to extensive proliferation of megakaryocytes. Collagen type III detected by silver staining is typically increased (Fig. 69–3H). Approximately half the patients demonstrate increased reticulin fibrosis which may be associated with increased megakaryocytes in marrow. Increased fibrosis may be associated with larger spleen size, anemia, and increased blasts in blood and marrow. Pseudo-Gaucher cells and sea blue histiocytes, secondary to increased marrow cell turnover, may be seen in 30% of specimens (see H5eC69, Fig. 69–3G). The spleen shows enlargement related to infiltration of the cords of the red pulp with granulocytes at different stages of maturation. The liver may show infiltration with granulocytic cells in the portal areas and hepatic sinusoids.

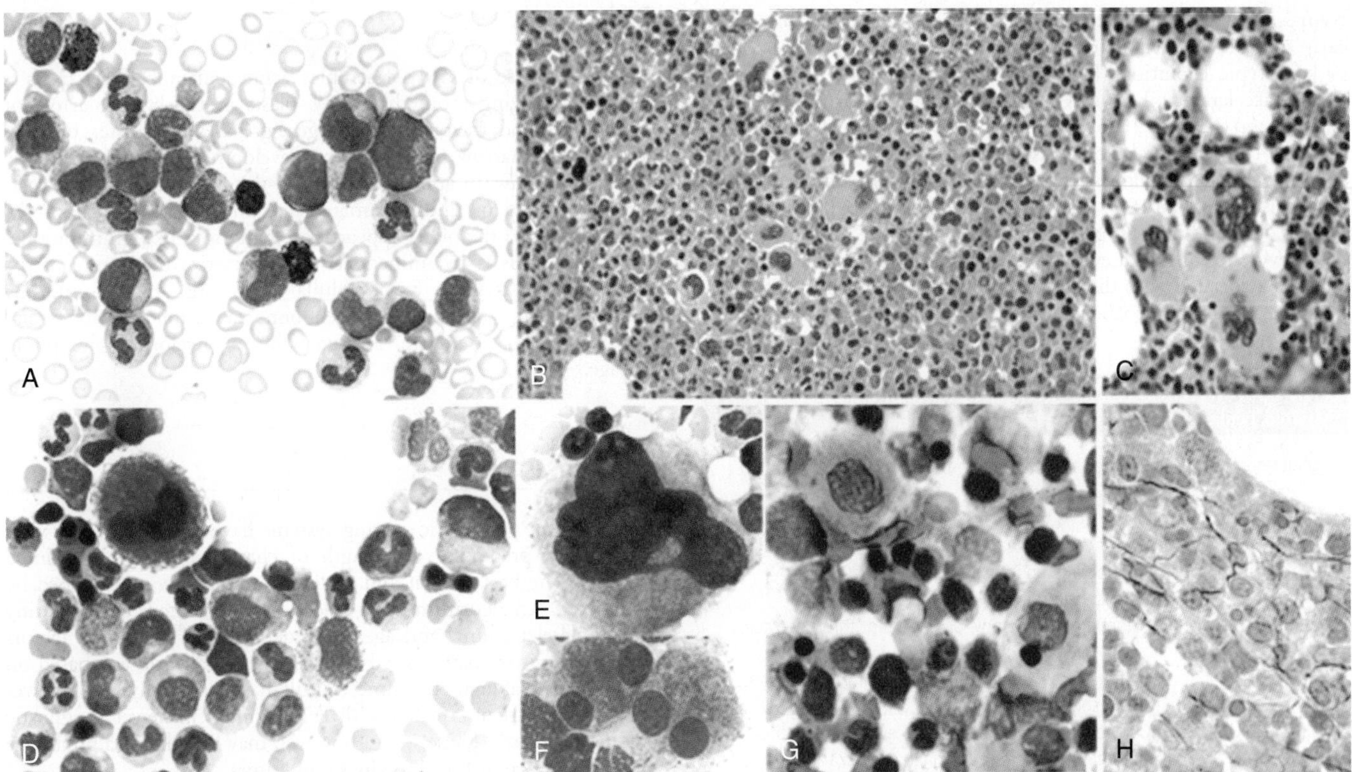

Figure 69–3 Chronic myelogenous leukemia, chronic phase: **A–H**. Peripheral smear (**A**) showing marked leukocytosis due to a granulocytic proliferation of all stages with particularly increased myelocytes and absolute basophilia. Bone core biopsy (**B**) illustrating markedly hypercellular marrow due to granulocytic proliferation and increased small hypolobated megakaryocytes. Compare with large megakaryocytes (**C**) from a myeloproliferative disorder other than CML. Bone marrow aspirate (**D**) showing granulocytic proliferation and small, "dwarf" megakaryocyte, compared with large-sized megakaryocyte (**E**) and micro-megakaryocytes (**F**) typical of MDS. Pseudo-Gaucher cells (**G**) and mild fibrosis (**H**) as seen on reticulin stain.

Cytogenetic examination shows t(9;22)(q34;q11) and Ph chromosome in more than 90% of patients. Additional chromosomal abnormalities besides the Philadelphia chromosome are seen at diagnosis in 20% of patients including –Y and +8, and have not been shown to affect disease course. Variant Ph chromosomes are seen in 5% of patients, with complex rearrangement involving exchange of material with an additional chromosome besides chromosomes 9 and 22. In a small proportion of patients cryptic or complex translocations can be detected by fluorescence in situ hybridization (FISH) or polymerase chain reaction (PCR) assays. The methodology used for identifying *BCR–ABL* transcripts has evolved over the years. Initially it was possible only to identify the presence or absence of *BCR–ABL* transcripts by either single-step amplification or a two-step "nested" amplification with internal primers to increase the sensitivity. Real-time quantitative polymerase chain reaction (RQ-PCR) provides an accurate measure of the total leukemia cell mass, and the degree to which *BCR–ABL* transcripts are reduced by therapy correlates with progression-free survival. A consensus meeting at the National Institutes of Health (NIH) in October 2005 made suggestions for (a) harmonizing the different methodologies for measuring *BCR–ABL* transcripts in patients with CML undergoing treatment and using a conversion factor whereby individual laboratories can express *BCR–ABL* transcript levels on an internationally agreed scale; (b) using serial RQ-PCR results rather than bone marrow cytogenetics or FISH for the *BCR–ABL* gene to monitor individual patients responding to treatment; and (c) detecting and reporting Philadelphia (Ph) chromosome-positive subpopulations bearing *BCR–ABL* kinase domain mutations.

In any new patient whose blood count suggests the diagnosis of a chronic myeloproliferative disorder, the detection of *BCR–ABL* transcripts in a blood specimen is probably the best way to confirm the diagnosis of CML. Current guidelines suggest that circulating *BCR–ABL* transcript numbers be measured, and marrow cytogenetics studied in every new patient with CML before initiation of treatment.[49] Marrow cytogenetics is essential to identify any unusual translocations or additional cytogenetic abnormalities, and RQ-PCR for *BCR–ABL* at diagnosis will identify whether the commonly observed e13a2 (b2a2) or e14a2 (b3a2) transcripts are present, or one of the less common fusion transcripts that are not amplified by the standard primer sets. This can prevent confusion if a patient on therapy has undetectable *BCR–ABL* transcripts because their transcripts were not amplified in the standard assay. If collection of marrow cells is not feasible, FISH on a blood specimen using dual probes for the *BCR* and *ABL* genes is another method of confirming the diagnosis. FISH may also detect cytogenetically "silent" *BCR–ABL* rearrangements and also deletions in the derivative 9q+, which have prognostic significance, and may therefore be performed in conjunction with marrow cytogenetics and RQ-PCR for *BCR–ABL* transcripts.

Natural History

The natural history of CML, determined more than 75 years ago, suggests a median survival from diagnosis of approximately 3 years. Without therapy, CML evolves from a chronic to an accelerated phase (AP) and eventually to blast crisis (BC). In approximately 25% of patients, there is no intervening AP between CP and BC (Table 69–1). Median survival times have been significantly prolonged with therapy (discussed below in the Therapy Section).

Accelerated Phase

In general, accelerated phase is characterized by symptoms of fever, night sweats, weight loss and bone pain, difficulty in controlling counts using conventional therapy, increased numbers of blasts and early myeloid cells in marrow and peripheral blood, and evidence of karyotypic evolution (Fig. 69–4A–C). The WHO classification defines accelerated phase of CML as one or more of the following changes: (a) 10% to 19% myeloblasts in peripheral blood or bone marrow; (b) peripheral blood basophils higher than 20%; (c) persistent thrombocytopenia, less than 100×10^9/L; (d) persistent thrombocytosis, more than 1000×10^9/L unrelated to therapy; (e) increasing WBC count and increasing spleen size unresponsive to therapy; and/or (f) evidence of clonal evolution.[50] The most common cytogenetic changes associated with disease evolution are an additional Ph chromosome, trisomy 8, isochrome I(17q), and trisomy 19.

Table 69–1 WHO Criteria for Accelerated and Blast Phases of Chronic Myeloid Leukemia (CML)

Accelerated phase	Diagnosis can be made if one or more of the following is present: Blasts 10% to 19% of peripheral blood white cells or bone marrow cells Peripheral blood basophils at least 20% Persistent thrombocytopenia (<100 × 10⁹/L) unrelated to therapy, or persistent thrombocytosis (>1000 × 10⁹/L) unresponsive to therapy Increasing spleen size and increasing WBC count unresponsive to therapy Cytogenetic evidence of clonal evolution (ie, the appearance of an additional genetic abnormality that was not present in the initial specimen at the time of diagnosis of chronic-phase CML) Megakaryocytic proliferation in sizable sheets and clusters, associated with marked reticulin or collagen fibrosis, and/or severe granulocytic dysplasia, should be considered as suggestive of CML-AP. (These findings have not yet been analyzed in large clinical studies, however, so it is not clear if they are independent criteria for accelerated phase. They often occur simultaneously with one or more of the other features listed.)
Blast crisis	Diagnosis can be made if one or more of following is present: Blasts 20% or more of peripheral blood white cells or bone marrow cells Extramedullary blast proliferation Large foci or clusters of blasts in bone marrow biopsy

Blast Crisis

The blast phase of CML resembles acute leukemia. Blast crisis is defined as having more than 20% blasts in the bone marrow or peripheral blood, the presence of large aggregates and clusters of blasts in the bone marrow biopsy, or the development of extramedullary blastic infiltrates. In approximately two-thirds of patients, the blasts have a myeloid or undifferentiated-like phenotype whereas in the remaining third the blasts appear more lymphoid-like. Immunophenotypic analysis is recommended to characterize the nature of the blasts (Fig. 69–5A–C). Extramedullary blast crisis most commonly affects the skin, lymph nodes, spleen, bone, or central nervous system, but may occur elsewhere, and may be of myeloid or lymphoid lineage.

PROGNOSIS

A number of prognostic scoring systems have been developed with the goal of predicting the length of chronic phase in individual patients. The best known and widely used index was developed by Sokal et al. An algorithm using spleen size, percentage of circulating blasts, platelet count, and age were identified as prognostic factors for chronic-phase patients.[51] However, the Sokal scale was based on therapies available at that time (busulfan, splenectomy), and newer systems for patients treated with IFN resulted in newer prognostic scoring systems.[52] These scales, however, may have limited predictive value in the age of tyrosine kinase inhibitors.

Approximately 20% of patients with CML have deletions of chromosomal material of varying size on the derivative 9q+.[53] These deletions presumably occur at the same time as the formation of the Philadelphia chromosome, and are thus not considered to be additional clonal changes as would be suggestive of accelerated-phase disease. Patients with der 9q+ have a worse prognosis if they receive IFN therapy; it is unclear whether or not such deletions have a poor prognosis in patients receiving imatinib therapy.[54,55]

THERAPY

Definitions of Response to Treatment

Hematologic, cytogenetic, and molecular response to treatment in CML have been defined (Table 69–2). A complete hematologic remission is defined as the achievement of normal WBC and platelet counts and normal differential, and disappearance of all symptoms

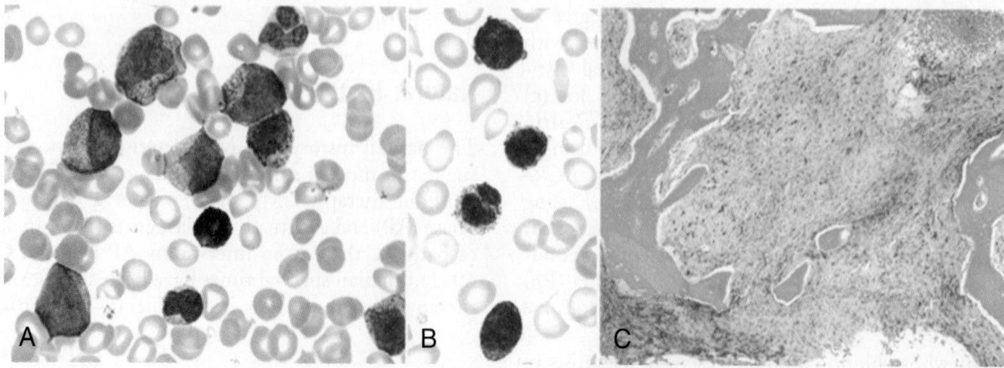

Figure 69–4 Chronic myelogenous leukemia, accelerated phase: **A–C**. Peripheral smear (**A**) showing increased immaturity in a case in which blasts were more than 10% of circulating leukocytes. Peripheral smear (**B**), illustrating increased basophils, in a case in which basophils were more than 20% of circulating leukocytes. Bone core biopsy (**C**) showing increased fibrosis and small dysplastic megakaryocyte. These findings are suggestive of accelerated phase.

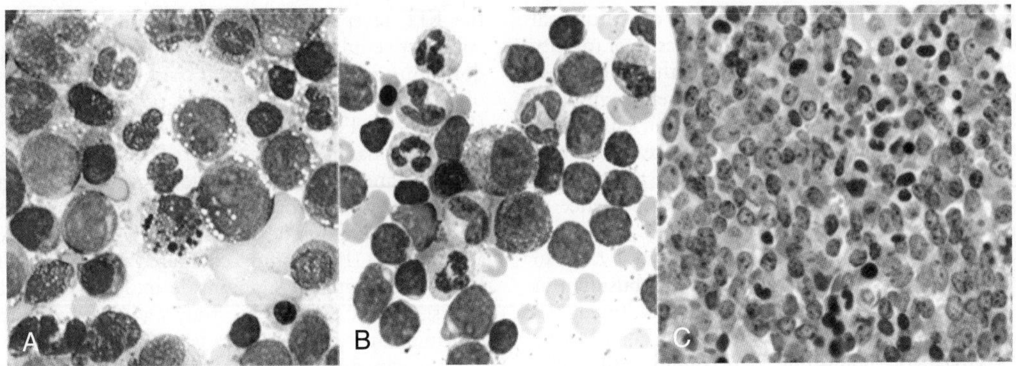

Figure 69–5 Chronic myelogenous leukemia, blast phase: **A–C**. Bone marrow aspirate (**A**) showing myeloid blast phase associated with t(9;22) and inv(16). Note abnormal eosinophil (center). Bone marrow aspirate (**B**) showing lymphoid blast phase in the background of residual CML. Bone core biopsy (**C**) illustrating focal blast phase.

Table 69–2 Response Definition and Monitoring

Hematologic Response	Cytogenetic Response	Molecular Response
Complete: Platelet count <450 × 10^9/L; WBC count <10 × 10^9/L; differential without immature granulocytes and with less than 5% basophils; nonpalpable spleen	Complete: Ph-negative = 0% Major: Ph-positive = 1% to 35% Minor: Ph-positive = 36% to 65% Minimal: Ph-positive = 66% to 95% None: Ph-positive < 95%	Complete: *BCR–ABL* transcripts nonquantifiable and nondetectable Major: *BCR–ABL* transcripts ≤0.10%

To control *BCR–ABL/ABL* gene ratio according to the proposed international scale for measuring molecular response, with a standardized "baseline," as established in the IRIS trial, taken to represent 100% on the international scale and a 3-log reduction from the standardized baseline (MMR) is fixed at 0.10%.

and signs of CML.[49] A partial hematologic response is defined as a decrease in the WBC count to less than 50% of the pretreatment level, or the normalization of the WBC count accompanied by persistent splenomegaly or immature cells in the peripheral blood. A complete cytogenetic response is defined as the absence of Ph-positive metaphases in marrow cells, and partial cytogenetic response as 1% to 34% Ph-positive metaphases. Major cytogenetic remission combines the percentages of complete and partial response. A reduction of *BCR–ABL* mRNA by 3-log or more, compared with a standardized baseline, has been designated a major molecular response (MMR), whereas consistent lack of detection of *BCR–ABL* mRNA is referred to as a complete molecular response (CMR).

Chemotherapy

Busulfan (BU) chemotherapy for CML was introduced in the 1950s. Busulfan was administered in doses of 4 to 6 mg/day and then held when the WBC count fell to 30 × 10^9/L. The drug effect could persist for weeks, and the counts could fall further after therapy was discontinued. Busulfan therapy was associated with serious adverse effects, including prolonged aplasia, pulmonary fibrosis, and a syndrome simulating adrenal insufficiency.

Treatment with hydroxyurea (HU) was started as an alternative to busulfan. Hydroxyurea therapy is usually initiated at doses of 1 to 6 g/day in an attempt to lower counts. Hydroxyurea administered at doses of 1 to 2 g/day is then used to maintain blood counts in the normal range. Hydroxyurea is less toxic than busulfan. Its major adverse effect is reversible marrow suppression. In randomized trials, hydroxyurea was shown to prolong survival of patients with chronic-phase CML when compared to busulfan therapy. Median survival of hydroxyurea-treated patients was 5 years compared with 3.75-year median survival of busulfan-treated patients. Because neither drug results in significant selective suppression of the Ph-positive clone, the aim of therapy with these agents is to control disease and symptoms. Hydroxyurea is now commonly used to achieve control of counts simultaneous with or prior to initiation of treatment with imatinib or other disease-specific therapies.

Several other chemotherapeutic agents can be used to reduce the white cell counts in CML. Low-dose cytosine arabinoside can be used either as an intermittent bolus or as a daily infusion to control disease where hydroxyurea or busulfan are not proving useful. Cytosine arabinoside has also been used in combination with other agents including IFN and imatinib in an attempt to enhance response.

Hyperuricemia and hyperuricosuria are frequently encountered problems in newly diagnosed and relapsed CML patients. Allopurinol, given at a dose of 300 mg daily and adequate hydration should be started prior to initiating treatment. Allopurinol should be discontinued after the WBC count has been controlled.

Interferon

Pioneering observational studies initiated in the 1980s by investigators at the MD Anderson Cancer Center provided evidence for efficacy of IFN in CML and indicated a 70% to 80% probability of complete hematologic remission in selected CML patients.[56–58] Initial research involved the use of human leukocyte IFN, but subsequent clinical studies used recombinant human interferon-α (rIFN-α). Recombinant interferon gamma (rIFN-γ) has been shown to be relatively ineffective for CML. The potential mechanisms by which IFN works in CML are not understood, but may include inhibition of increased proliferation, correction of the adhesion defect of the malignant progenitor in CML, or stimulating an immune response to CML. Rates for complete and partial cytogenetic remissions range from 0% to 38%.[59] Evidence exists for a dose–response relationship, with IFN doses of 4 to 5 million units/m^2/d more likely to achieve remission (and toxicity) than lower doses. Durable remissions are more common in young patients, those treated soon after diagnosis, with less advanced stage disease, and with favorable prognostic stage. Hematologic remissions usually occur within 1 to 3 months after starting IFN. The median time to complete cytogenetic remissions is 9 to 18 months, but may occur after 4 years of therapy. Durable cytogenetic responses, some lasting as long as 10 years, are more common in patients who achieve a complete cytogenetic remission compared with partial cytogenetic remission.

Virtually all patients receiving IFN experience some constitutional adverse effects, and discontinuation of treatment as a result of toxicity is necessary for 4% to 18% of patients compared with 1% of those receiving hydroxyurea. Acute adverse effects are generally mild to moderate and include flu-like symptoms such as fever, chills, and malaise. A constellation of other more severe acute reactions and chronic complications can occur. Overall, the mechanisms underlying the toxic effects are not well understood, but the incidence of adverse effects is usually dose- and duration-dependent.[59]

Randomized studies show an improvement in survival rates in patients receiving IFN compared with patients receiving busulfan or hydroxyurea. The Italian multicenter study randomly assigned 218 patients to receive IFN and 104 patients to receive HU or BU (the control group).[60] Cytogenetic remissions were significantly more common in the IFN group. After a median follow-up of 68 months, the observed 6-year survival rate was 50% for IFN-treated patients and 29% for controls, with median survivals of 72 and 52 months, respectively. The time for progression from chronic phase to accelerated or blast phase was lengthened from 45 months to more than 72 months. In a German multicenter study, 622 patients were randomized to receive IFN, BU, or HU. The 5-year survival rate in the IFN group (59%) exceeded that of the BU group (32%), but was not significantly higher than that of the HU group (44%).[61] Much of the discrepancy between the Italian and German findings can be explained by differences in case mix and treatment regimens. Two other randomized trials also showed benefit for IFN treatment compared with chemotherapy. The UK Medical Research Council randomly assigned 293 patients to receive IFN and 294 patients to receive HU or BU.[62] The 5-year survival rate was 52% for the IFN group and 34% for the control group. A Japanese randomized control trial compared IFN (80 patients) with BU (79 patients).[63] Hematologic and cytogenetic remission rates did not differ significantly. After a median follow-up of 50 months, the predicted 5-year survival rate was 54% for patients receiving IFN and 32% for those receiving BU.

The added value of combining IFN with cytosine arabinoside was shown in a French multicenter trial, wherein 360 patients were randomly assigned to receive IFN combined with cytosine arabinoside (20 mg/M^2/day for 10 days) and 361 patients to receive only IFN.[64] After 3 years, the survival rate was 86% with IFN and cytosine arabinoside and 79% with IFN alone. The rate of hematologic response was higher in the IFN-cytosine arabinoside group than in the IFN group. Major cytogenetic responses were observed 12 months after randomization in 41% patients treated with IFN-cytosine arabinoside and in 24% patients treated with IFN only.

Thus, the accumulated evidence from randomized trials suggests that IFN improves survival in chronic-phase patients with favorable features compared with BU and HU. Meta-analysis suggests that the pooled 5-year survival rate is 57% (50%–59%) for IFN and 42% (29%–44%) for chemotherapy, which results from a delay in the onset of blast crisis.[65] The controlled trials suggest that IFN increases life expectancy by a median of approximately 20 months compared with BU and HU. There is no direct evidence that IFN has a greater impact on survival than HU for patients who are in the later stages of chronic phase or who are sicker (eg, more than 1 year from diagnosis, or more than 10% to 30% blasts in peripheral blood). Adding cytosine arabinoside to IFN appears to add further survival benefit but also increases toxicity. Although IFN clearly is beneficial in patients with CML patients, benefit is limited by low levels of cytogenetic response and considerable toxicity. As discussed below, the use of IFN in the modern treatment of CML patients has been replaced by use of imatinib and other tyrosine kinase inhibitors.

Imatinib Mesylate and Targeted Therapies

Because the tyrosine kinase activity of *BCR–ABL* plays a critical role in cellular transformation, it is an attractive target for inhibition. Imatinib is a small, 2-phenylaminopyrimidine molecule that inhibits the kinase activity of all proteins that contain *ABL*, *ABL*-related gene (ARG) protein, or platelet-derived growth factor receptor, as well as the KIT receptor, at micromole concentrations.[66,67] Imatinib is a competitive inhibitor that acts at the ATP-binding site in the kinase domain to inhibit the normal binding of ATP and blocks the ability of *BCR–ABL* to phosphorylate tyrosine residues on its substrates (Fig. 69–6A–F).

Initial phase 1 and phase 2 trials established that imatinib was well tolerated and induced hematologic as well as cytogenetic response in the majority of chronic-phase CML patients who had failed other treatments.[68] Subsequently the International Randomized Interferon and STI571 (IRIS) study compared imatinib at 400 mg daily with IFN-α plus cytosine arabinoside in 1106 newly diagnosed patients in first chronic phase. This study was closed with the conclusion that imatinib is the initial nontransplant treatment of choice for patients with newly diagnosed chronic-phase CML. This conclusion was based primarily on a higher rate of disease progression in the patient group receiving IFN plus cytosine arabinoside. In the initial report from this study, after a median follow-up of 19 months, the estimated rate of an MCR at 18 months was 87.1% (95% CI, 84.1–90.0) in the imatinib group and 34.7% (95% CI, 29.3–40.0) in the IFN plus cytosine arabinoside group ($P < 0.001$).[69] The estimated rates of CCR were 76.2% (95% CI, 72.5–79.9) and 14.5% (95% CI, 10.5–18.5), respectively ($P < 0.001$). At 18 months, the estimated rate of freedom from progression to accelerated-phase or blast-crisis CML was 96.7% in the imatinib group and 91.5% in the IFN group ($P < 0.001$). Imatinib was better tolerated than combination therapy. In a subsequent 60-month follow-up report for this study, the estimated cumulative incidence rate of CHR, MCR, and CCR for patients on first-line imatinib was 98%, 92%, and 87% at 60 months (Fig. 69–7).[70] Only 7% of patients progressed to advanced phase, and the estimated overall survival was 89%. Crossover between arms was permitted for treatment failure, and 382 (69%) of 553 patients originally allocated to the IFN/cytarabine arm crossed over to the imatinib arm at a median of 60 months from start of treatment. The main reason for crossover from IFN to imatinib was intolerance of treatment, but reasons also included disease progression and failure to achieve hematologic or cytogenetic response.

Pretreatment risk factors have been found to predict the likelihood of achieving and maintaining response to imatinib. At 60 months, the estimated risk of disease progression was significantly higher for patients with a higher pretreatment Sokal score (estimated rates for high-risk, intermediate-risk, and low-risk groups of 17%, 8%, and 3%, respectively; $P = 0.002$). The achievement of certain milestones of response has also been found to predict prognosis. For example, patients who fail to achieve a complete hematologic response by 3 months of treatment, any cytogenetic response by 6 months or a major cytogenetic response by 12 months do poorly in comparison with patients achieving these milestones. Reduction of *BCR–ABL* levels observed with cytogenetic and quantitative PCR monitoring is also predictive of prognosis (Fig. 69–8). A landmark analysis indicated that at 60 months, 97% of the patients (95% CI, 94 to 99) who had achieved CCR at 12 months after the initiation of imatinib treatment ($n = 350$) had not progressed to accelerated phase or blast crisis (Fig. 69–9). For patients who did not have an MCR within 12 months ($n = 73$), the estimate was 81% (95% CI, 70–92; $P < 0.001$). Interestingly, the Sokal score was not predictive of risk of disease progression in patients who had a complete cytogenetic response (95%, 95%, and 99% in the high-risk, intermediate-risk, and low-risk groups, respectively; $P = 0.20$). The molecular responses at 12 and 18 months was predictive of long-term outcome. Patients who had a more than 3-log reduction in *BCR–ABL* transcript numbers at 18 months had 100% progression-free survival at 5 years, whereas patients who had failed to achieve CCR had 83% progression-free survival ($P < 0.001$).

A dose of 400 mg of imatinib daily is currently considered to be the standard dose for initiating therapy in newly diagnosed chronic-phase patients. Nonrandomized studies performed at the MD Anderson Cancer Center suggest that patients receiving initial therapy with 800 mg imatinib daily will achieve CCR more rapidly than patients receiving standard 400-mg daily doses.[71] However, it is not clear that the overall frequency of response will differ between the two groups,

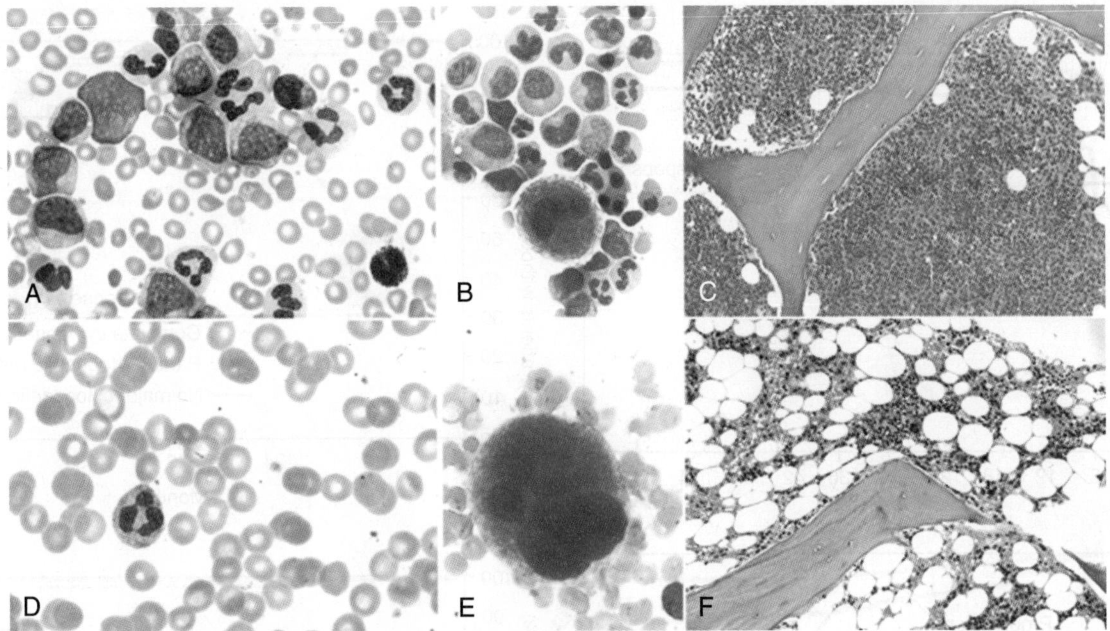

Figure 69–6 Chronic myelogenous leukemia, before and 3 months after imatinib therapy (**A–F**). Chronic-phase CML, as seen in the peripheral blood (**A**), aspirate (**B**), and biopsy (**C**), and after 3 months of imatinib therapy (**D, E, F**). Note normalization of white cell count (**D**), megakaryocyte size (**E**) and marrow cellularity (**F**).

and overall survival and progression-free survival are excellent with standard-dose imatinib (Fig. 69–10). Randomized trails examining the question of optimal imatinib dosing are ongoing.

Results of Treatment of Patients Failing Interferon

In a phase II study, 532 chronic-phase patients who were refractory to or intolerant of IFN-α were treated with imatinib at a dose of 400 mg daily. A CHR was achieved in 95% of patients, MCR in 60% of patients, and CCR in 41% of patients. With a median follow-up of 18 months, the estimated progression-free survival was 89%. Only 2% of patients discontinued therapy because of adverse events. Baseline features that predicted a high rate of MCR included the absence of blasts in the peripheral blood, a hemoglobin level greater than 12 g/dL, less than 5% blasts in the marrow, CML disease duration of less than 1 year, and a prior cytogenetic response to IFN.[72]

Results of Treatment in Accelerated Phase

A phase II study in accelerated-phase patients enrolled 235 patients. Some hematologic response was seen in 82% of patients, with 34% of patients achieving a CHR. A major cytogenetic response occurred in 24% of patients, with 17% complete responses. Estimated 12-month progression-free and overall survival rates were 59% and 74%, respectively.[73]

Results of Treatment in Blast Crisis

A phase II study of 260 myeloid blast crisis patients treated with imatinib showed an overall response rate of 52%, with sustained hematologic responses lasting at least 4 weeks in 31% of patients. Eight percent of patients achieved a complete remission with peripheral blood recovery. Another 4% of patients cleared their marrows to less than 5% blasts but did not meet the criteria for CR because of persistent cytopenias. Eighteen percent of patients either "returned" to chronic phase or had partial responses. Major cytogenetic responses were seen in 16% of patients, with 7% having complete cytogenetic responses. The median survival was 7 months. These results compare favorably with historical controls treated with chemotherapy for myeloid blast crisis in which the median survival is approximately 3 months. In patients with Ph-positive ALL, 29/48 (60%) responded to a single agent, imatinib. However, the duration of response was relatively short, with a median estimated time to disease progression of only 2 months.[74]

Toxicity

Myelosuppression is particularly common in CML patients treated with imatinib and is more common in patients with advanced disease. In the phase III randomized trial of newly diagnosed patients in the chronic phase, grade 3 neutropenia (ANC < 1000/mm^3) was experienced by 11% of patients, grade 4 neutropenia (ANC < 500/mm^3) occurred in 2% of patients, grade 3 thrombocytopenia (platelets <50,000/mm^3) occurred in 6.9% of patients, and grade 4 thrombocytopenia (platelets <10,000/mm^3) occurred in less than 1% of patients. Myelosuppression can occur at any time during imatinib therapy, but it usually begins within the first 2 to 4 weeks of starting therapy for blast crisis, with a slightly later onset in patients in accelerated or chronic phase. Although grade 3 and 4 neutropenia is frequent, particularly in advanced phases, infectious complications are relatively rare, possibly related to the lack of mucous membrane damage in patients on imatinib. Central nervous system and gastrointestinal hemorrhages may occur, most frequently in patients in blast crisis with platelet counts less than 20,000 and with uncontrolled leukemia. The primary goal in treating otherwise healthy patients in chronic phase is to avoid the risk of potentially dangerous neutropenia and platelet transfusion dependence. For patients with blast crisis or high-risk accelerated-phase disease (>15% blasts), a suggested approach is to balance risks and benefits, and support patients with a platelet count under 10,000/mm^3 or under 50,000/mm^3 with clinically evident bleeding with platelet transfusions. In the event of clinically significant bleeding, imatinib should be held immediately, until the bleeding is controlled. In patients whose absolute neutrophil count is less than 500/mm^3, imatinib is continued if the marrow is

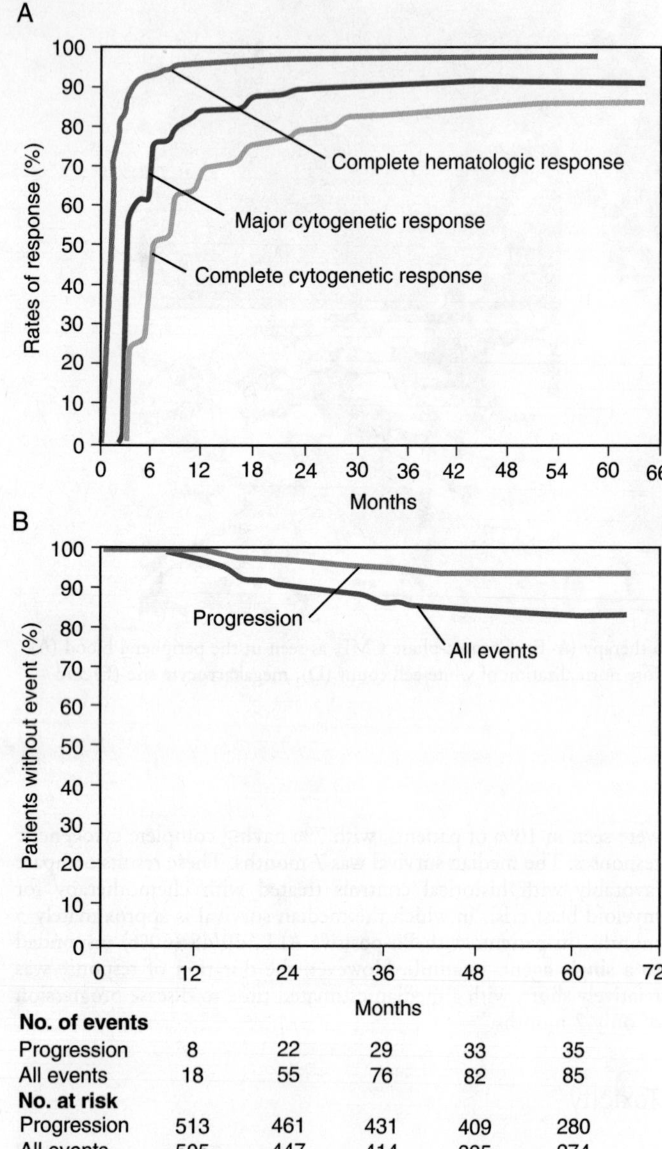

Figure 69–7 Response of newly diagnosed chronic myeloid leukemia (CML) patients to imatinib mesylate based on 5 years' follow-up on the International Randomized Interferon and STI571 (IRIS) study. **A**, Kaplan–Meier estimates of the cumulative best response to initial imatinib therapy. **B**, Kaplan–Meier estimates of the rates of event-free survival and progression to the accelerated phase or blast crisis of CML for patients receiving imatinib. (Data from Druker BJ, Guilhot F, O'Brien SG, et al: Five-year follow-up of patients receiving imatinib for chronic myeloid leukemia. N Engl J Med 355(23):2408, 2006.)

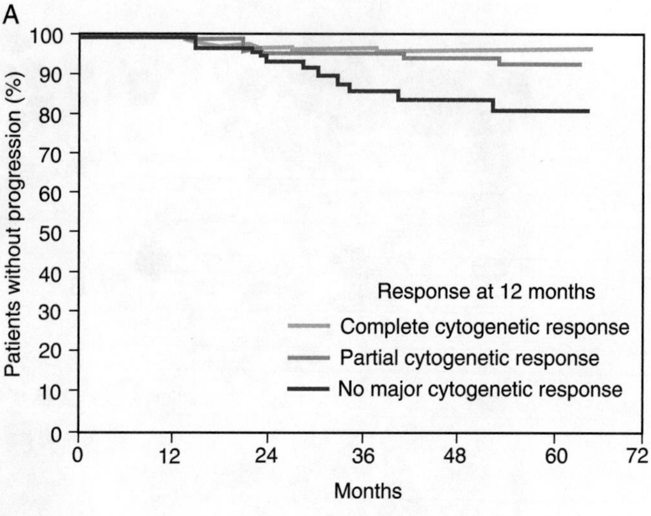

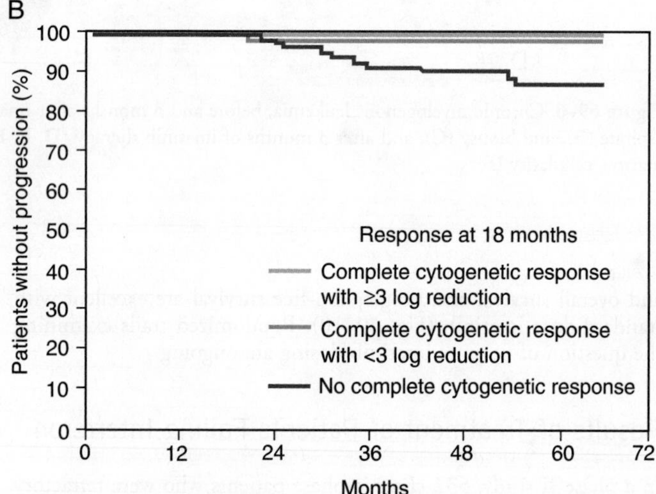

Figure 69–8 Rate of progression to the accelerated phase or blast crisis on the basis of cytogenetic response after 12 months or molecular response after 18 months of imatinib therapy. (Data from Druker BJ, Guilhot F, O'Brien SG, et al: Five-year follow-up of patients receiving imatinib for chronic myeloid leukemia. N Engl J Med 355(23):2408, 2006.)

hypercellular or if there are more than 30% blasts. In cases where the marrow is hypocellular and the ANC is less than 500/mm³ for 2 to 4 weeks, imatinib may be held, the dose reduced or myeloid growth factors can be used.[75] Concurrent administration of growth factors and imatinib is well tolerated and patients have not experienced a greater rate of relapse.[76]

The most common nonhematologic adverse events related to imatinib were nausea, muscle cramps, fluid retention, diarrhea, musculoskeletal pain, fatigue, and skin rashes. Only a minority of patients experienced grade 3 or 4 toxicity, and there was a low rate of discontinuance of therapy because of toxicity of 5%, 3%, and 2% in the phase II studies for blast crisis, accelerated phase, and chronic phase, respectively. The higher rate of severe toxicity in patients with advanced-phase disease may relate to the higher doses administered, or the poorer underlying health of patients. Most adverse effects can be managed successfully with supportive measures. Some toxicities (eg, mild skin rashes, mild elevations of transaminases, bone pain, and arthralgias) may improve spontaneously despite continued therapy at the same dosage.

Imatinib Resistance

Both de novo and acquired resistance have been observed in imatinib-treated CML patients. The two most commonly described mechanisms associated with resistance are point mutations in the *BCR–ABL* gene that prevent imatinib from inhibiting kinase activity and *BCR–ABL* gene amplification. The Sawyers group, in an original study of nine patients who relapsed on imatinib treatment, detected *BCR–ABL* gene amplification in three patients and kinase domain mutations in six.[77] Relapse was associated with reactivation of *BCR–ABL* kinase activity. This group subsequently reported results of sequencing analysis of *BCR–ABL* kinase domain mutations in 32 patients whose disease relapsed after an initial response to imatinib. Twenty-nine of 32 patients had *BCR–ABL* kinase mutations, with 15 different amino acid substitutions affecting 13 residues in the kinase domain.[78] The different mutations conferred varying degrees of

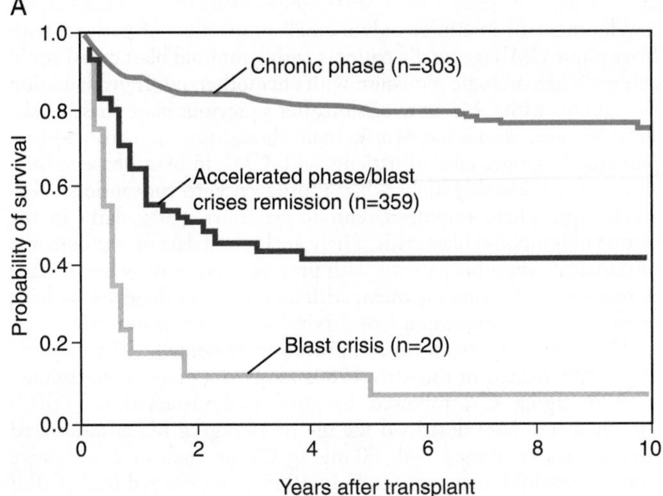

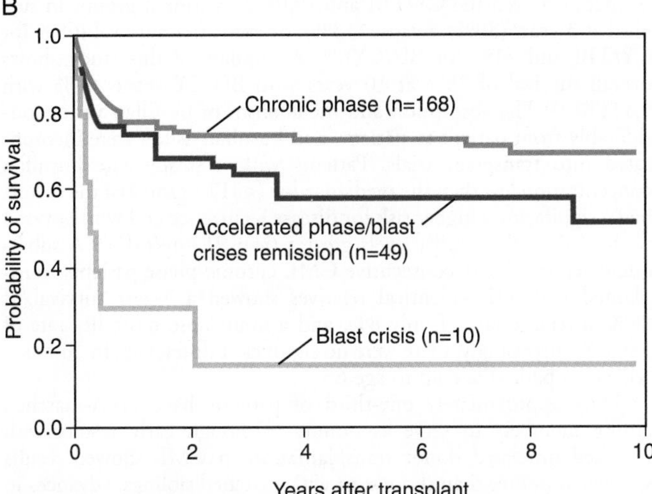

Figure 69–9 Probability of survival following (**A**) related donor transplantation, and (**B**) unrelated donor transplantation for chronic myelogenous leukemia (CML), chronic phase (CP), accelerated phase (AP), and blast crisis (BC), performed after 1992, at the FHCRC, Seattle.

imatinib resistance. In patients with stable chronic-phase disease, detection of mutations correlated with subsequent disease progression. Multiple independent mutant clones were seen in some patients. Subsequent studies have identified mutations in more than 40 different amino acids.[79] Mutations have been found in some patients prior to start of treatment supporting a model in which preexisting *BCR–ABL* mutations that confer imatinib resistance acquire a selective clonal growth advantage during imatinib treatment. There is some evidence that *BCR–ABL*-independent mechanisms may also play a role in imatinib resistance in some patients. Activation of the *SRC* family kinases, *LYN*, has been demonstrated in cell derived from patients with acquired imatinib resistance.[80]

The structure of the *ABL* kinase domain in complex with imatinib has been solved. This information sheds light on the mechanisms by which kinase domain mutations confer drug resistance.[81] Mutations may affect residues that directly contact imatinib such as a mutation resulting in substitution of isoleucine for threonine in the T315 position (T315I). The P-loop of the *ABL* kinase domain undergoes extensive downward displacement upon imatinib binding. Mutations in the P-loop prevent conformational changes required for imatinib binding. Imatinib captures and stabilizes the *ABL* kinase in its inactive conformation, but is sterically excluded from the active conformation. The M351T mutation and mutations in the activation loop result in the kinase remaining in the active conformation rather than the inactive conformation required for imatinib binding.[78]

Because the active conformations of *ABL* and *SRC* bear a high degree of structural similarity, compounds with *SRC* kinase inhibitory activity have been evaluated against native and mutant *BCR–ABL*. BMS-354825 (dasatinib, Sprycel) is a dual *SRC-ABL* kinase inhibitor that exhibits approximately 300-fold higher potency against native *BCR–ABL*.[78] Dasatinib can effectively inhibit most clinically detected *BCR–ABL* kinase domain mutants at low nanomolar concentrations, with the notable exception of T315I. Dasatinib entered clinical trials in late 2003 and has recently been approved by the Federal Drug Administration for the treatment of patients who failed imatinib.[82] Another compound, AMN107 (nilotinib) was generated by rational modification of Imatinib to enhance *BCR–ABL* kinase binding activity. Nilotinib binds *ABL* but with significantly increased avidity and can overcome resistance of most kinase domain mutants, with the exception of T315I. This drug is currently in clinical trials. It is evident however that both agents have significant activity in imatinib-resistant CML. Interestingly, responses occurred in patients with and without *BCR–ABL* kinase domain mutations at trial entry, with the exception of patients with the T315I mutation. Responses in chronic phase and, to a lesser extent, in accelerated phase have been stable. In contrast, many patients with myeloid, and all patients with lymphoid, blast crisis or Ph-positive ALL have relapsed.[83] These data are similar to the results of the initial studies with imatinib and indicate that once the disease has progressed beyond the chronic

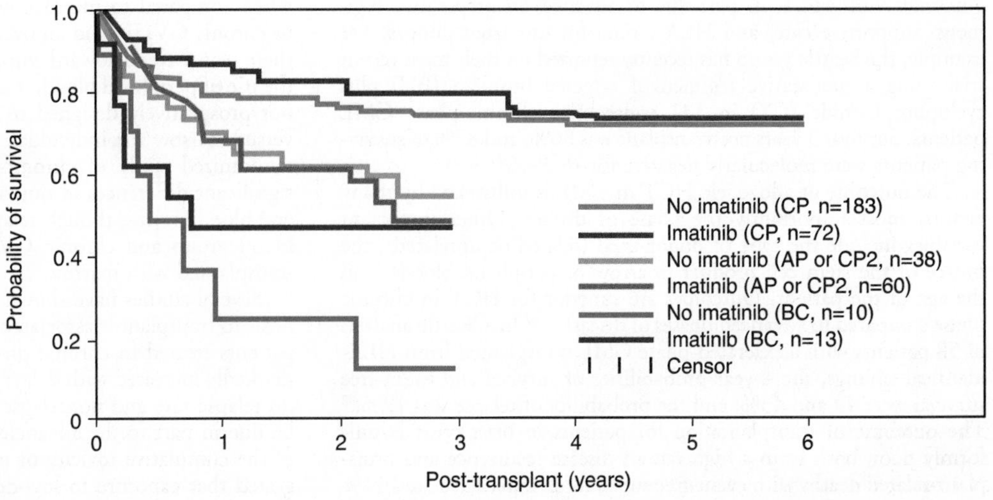

Figure 69–10 Effect of prior treatment with imatinib on overall survival after transplantation. CP2 = a return to chronic phase after treatment for accelerated phase or blast crisis disease. (Data from Oehler VG, Gooley T, Snyder DS, et al: The effects of imatinib mesylate treatment before allogeneic transplantation for chronic myeloid leukemia. Blood 109(4):1782, 2007.)

phase, tyrosine kinase inhibitor-based monotherapy is not sufficient to induce lasting responses.[84]

The fact that the T315I mutant is not responsive to either dasatinib or nilotinib and that this mutant has been detected in some patients with acquired resistance to dasatinib underscores the need to develop a T315I inhibitor. One compound termed VX-680, initially designed as an inhibitor of aurora kinases, is in Phase 1 trials, and several others are in preclinical development.[81,85]

Residual Disease

Currently, the reverse-transcriptase polymerase chain reaction (RT-PCR) is the most sensitive method for detecting low numbers of *BCR–ABL* transcripts in a patient after apparently successful hematopoietic cell transplantation. Most patients who have been treated with imatinib and have responded well continue to demonstrate evidence of residual disease using sensitive PCR assays. Recent updates of clinical trials of imatinib in CP CML patients indicate that an increasing proportion of patients appear to enter a molecular remission over time, including some patients achieving a PCR-undetectable status.[70] However, even patients with negative PCR (so-called complete molecular response) may still have significant numbers of residual malignant cells. Persistence of small populations of leukemia cells raises the concern that they could be a potential source of relapse. It is unclear whether the drug can be stopped in patients with MMR or CMR. Anecdotal observations of patients who discontinued therapy in CCR or CMR for various reasons, indicate that most such individuals experienced disease recurrence.[86–89] Patients who maintain response tend to be individuals who have received imatinib for relapse after allogeneic transplantation or who had been treated with IFN-α before they commenced imatinib.[90,91] Together, these data suggest that imatinib alone may not be capable of eradicating the leukemic cell clone.

Allogeneic Hematopoietic Cell Transplantation

The Seattle team reported initial results of HLA-matched sibling donor hematopoietic cell transplants performed as therapy for 10 CML patients in 1982, and subsequently published a larger study on 167 patients transplanted from matched siblings through 1983.[92,93] Long-term follow-up demonstrates that approximately 40% of patients transplanted in chronic phase nearly 20 years ago are surviving. Hematopoietic cell transplant became the first curative treatment in CML. Data from 4267 recipients of matched-sibling transplants reported to the IBMTR between 1994 and 1999 show a probability of survival of 69% ± 2% for 2876 patients transplanted within the first year from diagnosis, and 57% ± 3% for 1391 patients transplanted more than 1 year from diagnosis.[94] Contemporary results from selected single institutions continue to demonstrate excellent outcomes with HCT, in part due to advances in preparative regimens, supportive care, and HLA typing for unrelated donors. For example, the Seattle group has recently reported on their most recent trial using a preparative regimen of targeted busulfan (BU) plus cyclophosphamide (CY) in 131 consecutive chronic-phase CML patients. Survival 3 years posttransplant was 86%, and 87% of surviving patients were molecularly negative for *BCR–ABL*.[91,95]

The outcome of allogeneic HCT in CML is influenced by many factors, most importantly the phase of disease. Other important variables include the type of donor used (related or unrelated), the source of the stem cell product (marrow or peripheral blood), and the age of the patient. Outcomes are superior for HCT in chronic phase compared to advanced phases of disease.[96,97] In a Seattle analysis of 58 patients with accelerated-phase CML transplanted from HLA-identical siblings, the 4-year probabilities of survival and event-free survival were 49 and 43%, and the probability of relapse was 12%.[98] The outcome of transplantation for patients in blast crisis is uniformly poor, both from a high rate of disease recurrence and transplant-related deaths with event-free survivals of 43%, 18%, and 11% at 100 days, 1 year, and 3 years, respectively.[93,99,100] Prior to the development of imatinib, only a small proportion of patients with blast-phase CML (generally patients with lymphoid blast crisis) could achieve a hematologic remission with chemotherapy. Transplantation for patients with CML in remission after a previous blast phase results in cure rates somewhat worse than those seen in chronic-phase patients. Response rates of patients with CML in blast phase to imatinib are considerably higher than those seen with conventional chemotherapy. These responses tend to be short, particularly in the setting of lymphoid blast crisis. There are limited data on the outcome of transplantation for patients with previous blast crisis who are back in remission following treatment with imatinib, but these few patients seem to have a progression-free survival at 3 years of over 50%.[101]

Preparative regimens have improved incrementally. The majority of patients treated in the early 1980s received a preparative regimen of 120 mg/kg CY, followed by total body irradiation (TBI).[93] Tutschka et al later described the use of 16 mg/kg BU administered over 4 days combined with 60 mg/kg CY on each of 2 successive days, in myeloid malignancies.[102] In 1988 a randomized trial of BU/CY versus CY/12 Gy TBI in myeloid malignancies showed no differences between the CY/TBI and BU/CY treatment groups in survival at 3 years (80%), relapse (13%), or event-free survival (68% for CY/TBI and 71% for BU/CY).[103] An update of this study shows overall survival of 78% at 10 years with BU/CY versus 64% with CY/TBI.[104] The absorption and metabolism of busulfan varies considerably from patient to patient, and busulfan assays were incorporated into transplant trials. Patients with a steady-state busulfan concentration less than the median value (<917 ng/mL) of the cohort had a significantly higher risk for disease recurrence and worse overall survival than those with levels greater than 917 ng/mL.[105] A subsequent report of 131 consecutive CML chronic-phase patients transplanted with HLA-identical relatives showed a 3-year survival of 86%, a relapse rate of only 8%, and a nonrelapse mortality rate of 14%.[106] Surprisingly, there were no significant differences in outcome related to patient age up to age 65.

Only approximately one-third of patients have HLA-matched family members to serve as donors. Although early results with matched unrelated donor transplantation in CML showed results somewhat poorer than those seen with matched siblings, advances in donor selection, GVHD prophylaxis, and supportive care have resulted in continued improvements in outcome.[107–110] Thus, in many institutions results following unrelated transplants are almost equivalent to those seen with matched siblings (with a caveat that unrelated donor transplants have a lower-age patient exclusion), and registry data of multiple centers report 65% survival at 5 years among younger patients transplanted within a year of diagnosis.

Marrow was used as the stem cell source in all initial transplant studies. Two large randomized trials involving a variety of hematologic malignancies have shown that use of filgrastim [granulocyte-colony stimulating factor (G-CSF)] mobilized peripheral blood hematopoietic cells leads to more rapid myeloid and platelet recovery when compared to marrow, with no significant difference in acute or chronic GVHD and an overall survival advantage.[111,112] Although there was a trend toward improved survival in CML patients with the use of peripheral blood, it should be noted that these studies were not prospectively designed to address the role of peripheral blood versus marrow for individual disease states. Lastly, the results of a randomized study of chronic-phase CML showed no statistically significant differences in outcome between the marrow and peripheral blood groups, though relapse rates were lower in the peripheral blood group and chronic GVHD higher compared with patients transplanted with marrow.

Several studies have shown that an increased interval from diagnosis to transplant is associated with a worse transplant outcome, for patients treated in chronic phase.[113,114] No single cause of failure is markedly increased with delay; rather there is a modest effect of delay on relapse rate and nonrelapse mortality. Thus the delay effect may be due in part to the advancing disease over time and/or the effect of the cumulative toxicity of prior therapy. An IBMTR report suggested that exposure to low-dose busulfan led to a worse outcome with subsequent transplantation.[114] Reports have suggested that exposure to IFN might worsen the outcome of unrelated donor transplant, but data on the effect of IFN on matched sibling transplantation were less clear. In a recent German report, the 5-year survival rate from transplant was 46% for the 50 patients who received IFN within the last 90 days before transplant and 71% for the 36 who did not.[115] These observations suggest that IFN should be avoided, if possible, in the months immediately preceding allogeneic hematopoietic cell transplantation.

There have been several studies on the effect of prior imatinib and transplant outcomes. Early reports warned of an increase in regimen-related toxicity and mortality, especially from hepatic causes.[116] Larger studies have failed to show a deleterious effect of pretransplant imatinib.[117,118] A study of only CML patients showed no difference in regimen-related mortality, survival, or relapse between 140 patients who received imatinib versus 200 historical controls.[101] Curiously, in a few studies, chronic GVHD has been significantly less in patients receiving imatinib before transplant. The biology underlying this effect is unknown.

The form of GVHD prophylaxis used in the treatment regimens also influences the outcome of transplantation for CML, especially in chronic phase. Prevention of GHVD by removing T cells from the donor marrow was explored in a number of transplant studies in the 1980s. Although successful in reducing the incidence of GVHD, T-cell depletion in CML was associated with high rates of graft failure and relapse, leading to poorer disease-free and overall survival.[100] These findings illustrated the critical role of the graft versus leukemia (GVL) effect in eradicating CML following allogeneic transplantation. Because of these observations, T-cell depletion was largely abandoned as a method to control GVHD in CML transplants. However, there has been renewed interest in the possibility of preventing GVHD without loss of a GVL effect by combining T-cell depletion with an intensified conditioning regimen and delayed reinfusion of viable donor lymphocytes.[119]

Graft Versus Leukemia Effect in Chronic Myeloid Leukemia

Although evidence for a GVL effect can be found in many settings, nowhere is it as strong as in the setting of allogeneic HCT therapy for CML. Evidence in support of such an effect includes the following[120]: the higher rates of relapse following syngeneic and T cell-depleted transplants compared to unmodified allogeneic transplants[100,121]; the close association between the development of acute and chronic GVHD and freedom from relapse following non–T cell-depleted transplants[122–124]; the high response rate to donor lymphocyte infusions to treat posttransplant relapse (range from 50% to 100%), which is higher than in any other malignancy.[125,126] The markedly increased relapse rates seen with T-cell depletion indicate a role for T cells in GVL. T cell targets might include minor histocompatibility antigens shared by most cells in the body, thus accounting for the association of GVL with GVHD. Alternatively, there may be polymorphic minor histocompatibility antigens, with expression limited to hematopoietic tissue.[127,128] A third possible category of targets for the GVL effect in CML is the overexpression of protein targets in CML cells.[129] Understanding the cells and their targets responsible for the potent GVL effect seen in CML will be critical to the development of more effective, less toxic transplant-based therapies in the future.

Reduced Intensity Conditioning

Investigators have begun to study reduced intensity conditioning (RIC) or nonablative transplant approaches in an attempt to avoid the toxicities of high-dose preparative regimens while retaining the potentially powerful GVL effects. These approaches are of particular relevance for patients with CML because their median age at diagnosis is 67 years. Although the results of these studies are still in the early stages, some of the early observations are intriguing. For example, using a preparative regimen consisting only of 200-cGy TBI, and GVHD prophylaxis using cyclosporine (CSP) and mycophenolate mofetil (MMF), McSweeney et al reported complete molecular responses in five of nine patients transplanted for CML in chronic phase ($n = 6$) or accelerated phase ($n = 3$). The other four patients rejected their grafts. By adding 30 mg/m^2 fludarabine pretransplant, graft rejection has been eliminated as a problem following matched sibling transplantation.[130] Or et al recently reported similar encouraging results using a preparative regimen of fludarabine, low-dose busulfan, and antithymocyte globulin.[131] Thus, nonablative allogeneic hematopoietic cell transplantation may offer a safe and effective way to treat CML in the chronic phase.

Residual Disease Posttransplantation

The detection of *BCR–ABL* transcripts posttransplant is a strong predictor of relapse following transplantation. In a study of 346 patients after transplantation, 40% of patients were positive for *BCR–ABL* residual disease at 3 months posttransplant but this finding was not predictive of outcome, suggesting that eradication of the CML clone posttransplant takes an extended period of time.[132] In contrast, at 6 or 12 months posttransplant, 27% of patients were *BCR–ABL*-positive and at this time the assay was a powerful predictor of outcome, as only 3% of PCR-negative patients eventually relapsed compared with 42% of PCR-positive patients. The predictive power of PCR detection of *BCR–ABL* among longer-term survivors is somewhat weaker. At 18 months posttransplant, 1% of 289 *BCR–ABL*-negative patients subsequently relapsed compared with 14% of 90 *BCR–ABL*-positive patients. The advent of reliable quantitative PCR testing further refined risk prediction of *BCR–ABL* detection. Olavarria et al studied 138 transplant patients at 3 to 5 months posttransplant, and were able to define patients as having a low risk of relapse (16%), an intermediate risk (43%), or a high risk (86%) based on *BCR–ABL* quantification.[133] Further studies have confirmed the importance of quantitative *BCR–ABL* monitoring of minimal residual disease after transplantation for CML, which offers an obvious opportunity for early intervention for patients with residual or recurring disease.[134]

Treatment of Posttransplant Relapse

The pace of disease progression after posttransplant relapse is variable; some patients remain low-level PCR-positive for *BCR–ABL* for years without relapsing and some relapse with low levels of Ph-positive metaphases and remain stable for many years. The EBMT retrospectively studied 130 patients who relapsed after transplant before 1990 and noted that postrelapse survival (without DLI or imatinib therapy) was significantly better for recipients of matched sibling grafts for chronic-phase disease, with a short interval from diagnosis to transplant but a long interval from transplant, with a likelihood of being alive 10 years after posttransplant relapse of 42%.[135,136] An appreciation of the likely tempo of progression is thus important when considering treatment intervention options.

An increasing number of potential interventions are available for relapsing disease. IFN can produce both clinical and cytogenetic remissions in patients who have relapsed after transplantation.[137,138] Results with IFN appear better if treatment is initiated at the time of cytogenetic relapse instead of waiting until hematologic relapse, as IFN induces molecular remissions in some individuals treated early.[95] There are now a large number of studies demonstrating cytogenetic complete response rates of 50% to 100% in patients treated with DLI for clinically relapsed chronic-phase CML.[125] Response rates tend to be higher for patients treated earlier at the time of cytogenetic relapse and lower for patients in accelerated phase. The two major complications of DLI are transient marrow failure and the development of GVHD. Marrow failure only occurs in patients treated in hematologic relapse and likely reflects clearance of host hematopoiesis before donor hematopoiesis recovers, and thus is of particular concern for patients in full-blown hematologic relapse with no evidence of residual donor hematopoiesis.[139] Treatment earlier in the course of relapse can avoid this complication. The overall incidence of GVHD following DLI is approximately 50% in most series. Most early studies of DLI involved a single infusion of a relatively large number of donor T cells. It has since been reported that large numbers of T cells are tolerated with less GVHD if administered in a fractionated fashion rather than as a single bulk dose.[106] A recent report from the EBMT provides further support for starting at lower doses of lymphocytes and escalating dosage as required.[140]

More recently, imatinib mesylate has been shown to be active as posttransplant therapy. In a recent report of 28 patients who were treated with imatinib for posttransplant relapse, an overall response rate of 79% was seen, with CHR seen in 100% of patients in chronic phase, 83% in accelerated phase, and 43% in blast crisis.[72] CCR was seen in 29% of patients. Recurrence of GVHD disease was seen in 18% and granulocytopenia requiring dose adjustments of imatinib developed in 43% of patients. Because imatinib has only recently become available, almost all of the reported cases treated with imatinib for posttransplant relapse had never been treated with the drug previously. However, imatinib appears to be tolerated given early after transplantation to prevent relapse in high-risk Ph+ cases.[141] Twenty-two patients with Ph+ ALL or advanced-phase CML received imatinib at a median of 28 days postengraftment. Seventeen of 19 adults and all 3 children tolerated imatinib at the targeted dose (400 mg/day for adults, 260 mg/m^2/day for children), and 19 completed the planned course of 1 year of imatinib therapy. At a median follow-up of approximately 1½ years, 12 of 15 of the Ph+ ALL and 5 of 7 of the CML patients were in molecular remission.

Autologous Transplantation

The rationale for autologous transplantation in CML has been experimental and clinical evidence for persistence of polyclonal Ph-negative progenitors capable of reconstituting hematopoiesis in CML patients. This is most dramatically demonstrated by the high rate of complete cytogenetic response seen in CML patients treated with imatinib. Furthermore, it has been shown that transplantation of autologous cells may allow restoration of Ph-hematopoiesis.[142–149] Initial studies carried out using unmanipulated autologous marrow or blood cells indicated that autologous transplantation could reestablish CP in patients with advanced disease and induce cytogenetic responses in a small proportion of CML CP patients.[150–155] Subsequent studies indicated that depletion of Ph-positive progenitors by ex vivo graft manipulation was possible and associated with cytogenetic remission posttransplant.[156–159] Another approach to depleting malignant cells from the graft was to treat patients before harvesting marrow or peripheral blood for transplantation, also called in vivo purging.[142,160–173] However, remissions following autologous transplantation were usually of short duration, indicating either ineffective purging or relapse posttransplantation secondary to residual leukemic cells in the patient. In addition, the procedure was often associated with significant toxicity and delayed recovery. Although the compiled results of 200 autologous transplants at eight different centers in Europe and North America indicated a possibility of improved survival,[174,175] it is not possible to make any definite conclusions in the absence of controlled clinical trials. A meta-analysis of six trials in which patients were randomly allocated to receive autologous HCT or an IFN-based regimen did not show an advantage for HCT.[176]

Any trials of autologous HCT now need to be considered in the context of the excellent results of imatinib treatment, and the availability of second-generation kinase inhibitors with significant activity in imatinib-resistant CML patients. Pilot studies to collect PBSC from patients who have received imatinib mesylate and achieved CCR, for use for autologous HCT in case of later progression, have been reported.[177–181] The PBSC collection process is well tolerated and Ph-negative collections are more consistently achieved than with previous strategies. Although the target numbers of CD34$^+$ cells is usually attained, a subset of patients fails to reach this target. Furthermore, many patients mobilize suboptimally and require multiple collections, possibly as a result of the effects of imatinib on normal hematopoiesis and the mobilization process.[67] Collections are usually Ph-negative, but molecular evidence of disease can be found in most patients. Collection of PBSC from patients responsive to imatinib may form the framework of future attempts to perform autologous transplantation in CML; however, additional strategies are required to further deplete cells containing the *BCR–ABL* from PBSC collections as well as improve therapy for residual disease posttransplant.[182] At this point, autologous HCT for CML should probably be limited to investigational clinical trials for patients who fail kinase inhibitor studies therapy and lack allogeneic donors.

CAN TYROSINE KINASE INHIBITOR TREATMENT CURE CHRONIC MYELOID LEUKEMIA?

A fraction of CML patients treated with imatinib may not have detectable levels of the *BCR–ABL* gene even with sensitive PCR assays. This raises the question as to whether patients can actually be cured with tyrosine inhibitor treatment. Patients with negative PCR may still have significant numbers of residual malignant cells. The definition of a "cure" remains controversial. Although cure might theoretically require the total eradication of all leukemia cells, it can be argued that patients may be considered cured if low numbers of leukemia cells persisted but could not reestablish clinical disease. Such a situation may occur in CML post allogeneic transplantation where a graft-versus-leukemia effect may help maintain remission. In AML associated with the t(8;21), many long-term survivors continue to demonstrate molecular evidence of this translocation. On the other hand, late relapses can be observed in patients with childhood ALL more than 10 years after remission, with molecular evidence that the relapse originated from the same clone that caused the disease originally.

Therefore, it is important to consider whether *BCR–ABL*-expressing cells that escape elimination with imatinib include cells with leukemogenic potential. Mathematical modeling of the effect of imatinib on different hematopoietic cell compartments in CML suggests that leukemia stem cells are resistant to elimination by this drug.[89] This is supported by evidence that *BCR–ABL* -positive stem and progenitor cells are retained in patients in CCR on imatinib treatment.[183] In vitro treatment with imatinib and dasatinib effectively inhibits proliferation of CML primitive progenitors but only modestly increases progenitor cell apoptosis.[184–186] Similarly, treatment with imatinib and dasatinib failed to eradicate primitive leukemia cells in a mouse model of CML.[44] These observations suggest that at least short-term treatment with imatinib or dasatinib does not eliminate primitive leukemogenic cells, implying that "cure" of CML is likely to remain elusive with treatment with these agents alone. This is supported by observations of disease recurrence in patients who were *BCR–ABL* negative by PCR and stopped treatment for various reasons.[86–89] Intriguingly, some patients have been reported to have maintained a *BCR–ABL*-negative status for more than 1 year following discontinuation of imatinib treatment, but the long-term durability and frequency of such responses, or factors that predict for such responses, are not clear at present.[86]

The mechanisms underlying "primary resistance" leading to the incomplete elimination of a subset of malignant cells in imatinib-responsive patients are not well understood. Point mutations in the *BCR–ABL* kinase domain and *BCR–ABL* gene amplification are associated with acquired resistance to imatinib and are detectable in patients with a stable CCR.[187] However mutations are not consistently seen, occur in only a small percentage of cells, and do not consistently predict for subsequent relapse. Imatinib resistance could also be related to increased drug efflux and reduced intracellular drug levels in primitive progenitors, which may also express higher levels of *BCR–ABL* than more mature cells.[188] It has been shown that nondividing primitive CML hematopoietic cells are especially insensitive to imatinib-induced apoptosis.[185,189] Microenvironmental interactions through maintenance of dormancy or by inducing antiapoptotic signals may help preserve viability of CML hematopoietic cells treated with imatinib. In the future, a better understanding of the mechanisms underlying persistence of leukemogenic cells may allow development of improved strategies to effect "cures" in CML patients with tyrosine kinase inhibitor treatment.

MANAGEMENT OF THE NEWLY DIAGNOSED CHRONIC MYELOID LEUKEMIA PATIENT IN THE IMATINIB ERA

What should be the initial management for CML patients? After years of clinical research, we know (a) imatinib is remarkably effective for patients treated in chronic phase, as greater than 85% of patients obtain a complete cytogenetic remission (CCyR).[70] In the IRIS trial, approximately 70% of cases remain in CCyR at 5 years of follow-up. Treatment of advanced phase (accelerated or blast disease) is associated with much poorer outcomes[73,74]: (b) allogeneic transplantation is generally associated with 10-year survival rates of 70% or better for younger patients in early chronic phase, but survival likewise falls in accelerated- or blast-phase disease[104]; and (c) relapse occurs for chronic-phase patients treated with imatinib, but outcome can be effectively monitored by sensitive RT-PCR assays.[190]

Imatinib has become the initial treatment of choice for patients with CML. For patients diagnosed in accelerated phase or blast crisis, initial treatment with imatinib results in better responses than seen with other nontransplant therapies, but these responses in general tend to be short-lived, and therefore advanced-phase patients should consider transplantation as soon as possible. For patients diagnosed during chronic phase, imatinib is a reasonable first choice of therapy. Current recommendations from advisory panels, such as the European Leukemia Net and the National Cancer Care Alliance, state that all chronic-phase patients should start on imatinib therapy, but allow for consideration of transplantation based on the patient's age, preference, and response to initial imatinib.

However, there are also questions that make the decision on how early to transplant problematic. For example, given that tyrosine kinase inhibitors such as imatinib do not appear to kill the CML stem cell, is relapse inevitable? Many relapses stemming from *ABL* point mutations act aggressively. Will these patients be especially hard to cure with transplantation? And although short-term tyrosine kinase inhibitor therapy does not seem to adversely affect transplant results, what will happen with long-term exposure to these agents?

For patients with chronic-phase disease, imatinib can be initiated with simultaneous workup of family donors and unrelated donors. Criteria for imatinib failure or suboptimal response are in evolution. Certainly, failure to achieve a complete hematologic response at 3 months of treatment is an indication to switch therapy. At 6 months of therapy, patients should have some cytogenetic response, and by 12 months, patients should achieve a major cytogenetic response, with the elimination of two-thirds of their Ph on cytogenetic exam. By a conservative approach, patients should achieve a complete cytogenetic remission by 18 months of therapy. Patients who relapse after a CCR, especially those with *ABL* point mutations, should consider alternative therapy, including transplant.

SUGGESTED READINGS

Baccarani M, Saglio G, Goldman J, et al: Evolving concepts in the management of chronic myeloid leukemia: Recommendations from an expert panel on behalf of the European LeukemiaNet. Blood 108(6):1809, 2006.
Review and recommendations for disease classification, treatment, and response assessment.

Deininger MW, O'Brien SG, Ford JM, Druker BJ: Practical management of patients with chronic myeloid leukemia receiving imatinib. J Clin Oncol 21(8):1637, 2003.
Practical recommendations for the dosing and management of toxicities in patients treated with imatinib.

Druker BJ, Guilhot F, O'Brien SG, et al: Five-year follow-up of patients receiving imatinib for chronic myeloid leukemia. N Engl J Med 355(23):2408, 2006.
Extended follow-up of landmark study establishing the role of imatinib in the treatment of CML.

Druker B, Tamura S, Buchdunger E, et al: Effects of a selective inhibitor of the Abl tyrosine kinase on the growth of Bcr-Abl positive cells. Nat Med 2(5):561, 1996.
Preclinical studies demonstrating efficacy of imatinib in CML.

Goldman JM, Melo JV: Chronic myeloid leukemia—Advances in biology and new approaches to treatment. N Engl J Med 349(15):1451, 2003.
Comprehensive review of CML pathogenesis and treatment.

Hughes T, Deininger M, Hochhaus A, et al: Monitoring CML patients responding to treatment with tyrosine kinase inhibitors: Review and recommendations for harmonizing current methodology for detecting BCR-ABL transcripts and kinase domain mutations and for expressing results. Blood 108(1):28, 2006.
Report from NIH conference for standardizing methods and criteria for disease monitoring.

Oehler VG, Gooley T, Snyder DS, et al: The effects of imatinib mesylate treatment before allogeneic transplantation for chronic myeloid leukemia. Blood 109(4):1782, 2007.
Analysis of results of transplantation in the context of prior imatinib treatment.

Radich JP, Gooley T, Bensinger W, et al: HLA-matched related hematopoietic cell transplantation for chronic-phase CML using a targeted busulfan and cyclophosphamide preparative regimen. Blood 102(1):31, 2003.
Results of an optimized transplantation regimen for chronic-phase CML.

Ren R: Mechanisms of BCR-ABL in the pathogenesis of chronic myelogenous leukaemia. Nat Rev Cancer 5(3):172, 2005.
Review of BCR-ABL-mediated signaling mechanisms contributing to transformation.

Shah N, Nicoll J, Nagar B, et al: Multiple BCR-ABL kinase domain mutations confer polyclonal resistance to the tyrosine kinase inhibitor imatinib (STI571) in chronic phase and blast crisis chronic myeloid leukemia. Cancer Cell 2(2):117, 2002.
Comprehensive analysis of kinase domain mutations conferring imatinib resistance.

REFERENCES

For complete list of references log onto www.expertconsult.com

CHAPTER 70

PRIMARY MYELOFIBROSIS

Ronald Hoffman, Mingjiang Xu, and Giovanni Barosi

Primary myelofibrosis (PMF) is a chronic, malignant hematologic disorder characterized by splenomegaly, leukoerythroblastosis, teardrop poikilocytosis (ie, dacryocytes), some degree of marrow fibrosis, increased marrow microvessel density, and extramedullary hematopoiesis.[1–12] In PMF, there is a profound hyperplasia of morphologically abnormal megakaryocytes and clonal populations of monocytes that may be responsible for the marrow fibrosis due to the local release of fibrogenic growth factors.[7] This disorder was first described in 1879 by Heuck,[13] who reported the presence of marrow fibrosis and extramedullary hematopoiesis in the liver and spleen of two patients. PMF has also been referred to by a variety of other terms, including agnogenic myeloid metaplasia, myelosclerosis, idiopathic myeloid metaplasia, osteosclerosis and idiopathic myelofibrosis.[1–12] Fibrosis of the bone marrow is not unique to PMF and may accompany many other disorders (Table 70–1).[6,7] The designation PMF rather than idiopathic myelofibrosis was recently chosen by an international group of hematologists and hematopathologists to reflect our greater understanding of the origins of this disorder.[14,15] Furthermore, this same group created the terms post polycythemia vera (PV) myelofibrosis (post-PV MF) and post essential thrombocythemia (ET) myelofibrosis (post-ET MF) to identify myelofibrosis which is preceded by a history of PV or ET.[14,15] In PMF, the marrow fibrosis is believed to occur in response to the progeny of a clonal proliferation of hematopoietic stem cells.[16] This syndrome frequently leads to progressive marrow failure. In 1951, Dameshek[17] included PMF among the myeloproliferative disorders (MPD). This hypothesis was largely based on clinical observations of patients with PV, chronic myeloid leukemia (CML), and ET who developed marrow fibrosis and a clinical picture resembling PMF. Dameshek[17] also noticed that each of these MPDs frequently terminates in a leukemic phase.

EPIDEMIOLOGY

Few epidemiologic studies are available to estimate the incidence of PMF. Since the chronic MPDs have not been considered in the past to be malignancies, case registries have limited data on the incidence of such chronic MPD as PMF. The yearly incidence of PMF in Goteborg, Sweden, during a study period of 1983 to 1992 was calculated to be 0.4 cases per 100,000 persons.[18] Review of previously published reports indicated an annual incidence rate in European, Australian, and North American localities ranging from 0.5 to 1.3 cases per 100,000 persons.[18–23] The annual incidence rate of PMF in Olmstead County, Minnesota, was determined to be 1.33 cases per 100,000 persons, and in southeast England, the annual incidence has recently been reported to be 0.37 per 100,000 persons.[19] In Japan, PMF is considered a rare disorder, with only 84 cases per 100,000 persons determined at autopsy.[24,25] This figure was obtained by monitoring autopsy protocols from all Japanese medical schools, universities, general hospitals, and research institutes over a 10-year period.[24] The incidence of myelofibrosis among survivors who were 10,000 meters or less from the hypocenter of the atomic bomb explosion at Hiroshima was 18 times the incidence reported from the remainder of Japan.[26] These patients became symptomatic an average of 6 years after the bomb blast.[26] Such data indicate a strong link between excessive radiation exposure and development of PMF, which is further substantiated by the high incidence of myelofibrosis in patients who have received the contrast material Thorotrast (which contains 232Th, a radioactive element with a half-life of 1.41×10^{10} years).[27] Thorotrast is taken up and retained indefinitely by cells of the reticuloendothelial system, which results in continuous irradiation of the liver, spleen, lymph nodes, and bone marrow. Chronic exposure to several industrial solvents, including benzene and toluene, has also been associated with development of PMF.[28–31] PMF has been reported as a complication of chronic benzene poisoning since the chemical was first used in the leather and shoe industries during the 1930s and 1940s.[29,31] The average age at diagnosis of PMF is approximately 65 years, and most patients are diagnosed between 50 and 69 years of age.[1–12,23] In several series, men have been affected more frequently than women, but others have failed to confirm this male predominance.[1–12,23] Rarely, PMF has been reported in the pediatric age group.[32,33] In several children, PMF manifested in early childhood, and in one family, twins were affected.[32,33] Evidence of genetic transmission exists: a higher incidence has been reported in Ashkenazi Jews than in Arabs who both live in Northern Israel.[22]

BIOLOGIC AND MOLECULAR ASPECTS

Ward and Block[4] originally proposed that PMF represented a response of an intrinsically normal stem cell to an unidentified stimulus, but Dameshek[17] conjectured that the abnormal fibroblastic proliferation in PMF was not an integral part of the primary disorder. These conflicting hypotheses were first tested in studies using a variety of genetic markers to define the cellular origin of PMF. Jacobson and colleagues[16] demonstrated in an African American female PMF patient who was heterozygous for isoenzymes of glucose-6-phosphate dehydrogenase (G6PD) that circulating hematopoietic cells were derived from a common hematopoietic stem cell and that the bone marrow fibroblasts were nonclonal in origin. Using X chromosome gene probes, Lucas and coworkers[34] confirmed the clonal origin of hematopoiesis in PMF. Using a similar molecular biologic approach, Anger and associates[35] reported that in each of three cases of PMF suitable for clonal analysis, a clear-cut monoclonal X-inactivation pattern was observed. Greenberg and colleagues[36] studied the cytogenetic composition of bone marrow fibroblasts of a PMF patient who had a clonal cytogenetic abnormality in unstimulated peripheral blood cells, which was absent in the marrow fibroblasts. Fully developed fibrosis of the bone marrow in PMF is frequently preceded by a hypercellular phase of variable duration. The diagnosis depends on the demonstration of atypical megakaryocytes and an increased fibrosis within marrow biopsies and the exclusion of other MPDs.[8,37] Kriepe and coworkers[38] used an analysis of X-linked restriction fragment length polymorphisms of blood cells of patients at various stages of PMF to demonstrate clonality of hematopoiesis in advanced stages of PMF and in the prefibrotic phase. An *NRAS* mutation present in the hematopoietic cells of a PMF patient indicated that T and B cells were also involved in the malignant process in some patients, perhaps providing some explanation for the immunologic abnormalities associated with PMF.[39] Similarly, fluorescence in situ hybridization techniques have been used to detect clonal cytogenetic abnormalities in myeloid and in purified B- and T-cell lymphocytes in patients with PMF.[40] These studies indicate that PMF is a clonal hematologic malignancy originating in primitive hematopoietic cells capable of

Table 70–1 Conditions Associated with Myelofibrosis

Nonmalignant Conditions
Infections: tuberculosis, histoplasmosis
Renal osteodystrophy
Vitamin D deficiency
Hypoparathyroidism
Hyperparathyroidism
Gray platelet syndrome
Systemic lupus erythematosus
Scleroderma
Radiation exposure
Osteopetrosis
Paget disease
Benzene exposure
Thorotrast exposure
Gaucher disease
Primary autoimmune myelofibrosis
Malignant Disorders
Primary myelofibrosis
Other chronic myeloproliferative disorders: polycythemia vera, chronic myeloid leukemia, Essential thrombocythemia
Acute myelofibrosis
Acute myeloid leukemia
Acute lymphocytic leukemia
Hairy cell leukemia
Hodgkin lymphoma
Myelodysplasia with myelofibrosis
Multiple myeloma
Systemic mastocytosis
Non-Hodgkin lymphoma
Carcinomas: breast, lung, prostate, stomach

producing lymphoid and myeloid cells and that the marrow fibrosis represents a secondary reaction of marrow stromal cells not involved by the process.[34–41] If marrow fibrosis is truly an epiphenomenon of the neoplastic hematopoietic cell proliferation, it may be expected to disappear if this cell population is eradicated. Reversal of myelofibrosis has been observed after allogeneic stem cell transplantation and infrequently seen after long-term administration of chemotherapy or interferon.[42–44] Such findings indicate that the bone marrow fibrosis in PMF is not irreversible and is clearly a consequence of the neoplastic cellular proliferation.

Erythroid and megakaryocyte colony formation occurs in vitro in the absence of added exogenous cytokines in PMF, a finding common to other MPDs.[45–48] LeBousse-Kerdiles and associates reported that such autonomous colony formation was observed only when the mononuclear cell fractions isolated from peripheral blood of PMF patients were assayed but not when purified CD34+ cells were similarly assayed. These findings indicated that the reported autonomous colony formation in PMF was caused by paracrine stimulation by cytokines secreted in culture by ancillary cell populations.[49] In contrast, Taksin and coworkers[50] provided convincing data indicative of true autonomous megakaryocyte colony formation by PMF progenitor cells. The autonomous megakaryocyte proliferation could not be attributed to a mutation in the cell receptor for thrombopoietin or by autocrine production of thrombopoietin by PMF progenitor cells. To gain insight into the molecular basis for this dysregulation of hematopoietic progenitors, a differential gene expression approach was employed to analyze autonomously proliferating megakaryocytes from PMF patients from their normal counterparts. These studies demonstrated that the gene for the immunophilin, *FKBP59* (also designated *FKBP4*), was overexpressed in 8 of 10 patients with PMF.[51] Their data suggest that FKBP[51] may exert an antiapoptotic effect mediated by inhibition of calcineurin activity.[51] Such a phenomenon may provide a potential biologic basis for increased cell survival signal in hematopoietic cells in PMF that may manifest as autonomous progenitor cell proliferation in vitro. Although a population of autonomous proliferating megakaryocyte progenitor cells may exist, a second and more common population remains dependent on the addition of exogenous growth factors. The hypothesis that marrow fibrosis in PMF is a secondary process has been further explained by the work of Castro-Malaspina and colleagues,[52] Wang,[53] and Hirata and coworkers.[54] These groups found that fibroblasts derived from marrow explants obtained from PMF patients displayed the same physical and proliferative characteristics as normal marrow fibroblasts. PMF and normal marrow fibroblasts exhibited anchorage and serum dependence, contact inhibition of growth, and similar production of hematopoietic colony stimulating activities. These data suggest that marrow fibroblasts and their precursor cells in PMF patients do not differ from those of normal subjects.

Many of the peripheral blood abnormalities associated with PMF may be attributed to the extramedullary hematopoiesis that is characteristic of this disorder. Extramedullary hematopoiesis had previously been attributed to the reactivation of quiescent hematopoietic stem cells, which are retained at sites of prior embryonic hematopoiesis, especially in the spleen.[4] This hypothesis has been questioned, because of the observation that the spleen is not a prominent site of fetal hematopoiesis in humans and by the observation that extramedullary hematopoiesis occurs in a wide variety of sites in PMF that cannot be accounted for by the fetal reversion hypothesis.[55–57] CD34+ cells in PMF exit from the bone marrow; because of abnormal trafficking patterns, they are filtered out by the spleen, accumulate progressively, and continue to proliferate.[56] Ultimately, there is an unequal distribution of CD34+ cells, with a twofold greater number being present in the spleen than the marrow. The myeloid metaplasia of the spleen is characterized by disturbances of splenic architecture, including an increased presence of megakaryocytes and their progenitor cells.[56] Intravascular hematopoiesis within the sinusoids of the bone marrow is a conspicuous finding in PMF.[58] It is likely that this finding is the result of marrow fibrosis distorting the marrow sinuses and allowing entrance of hematopoietic precursors or progenitor or stem cells into the sinusoids and access to the circulation.[58–60] The characteristic changes of the marrow vascular architecture consist of increased quantities of collagen type IV deposits associated with endothelial cell proliferation.[61,62] Moreover, sinusoidal hyperplasia and hypervascularity occur, resulting in increased blood flow.[62] The excessively dilated marrow sinusoids in PMF contain prominent intraluminal foci of hematopoiesis.[62,63] Thiele and associates[61] pursued a morphometric analysis of marrow vascular structures and collagen type IV deposits in PMF. Compared with normal controls and patients with PV, a significant increase in the numbers of marrow sinusoids and subendothelial collagen type IV was observed in cases of PMF.[61] Evolution of the fibroosteosclerotic changes in PMF was accompanied by a striking accumulation of collagen IV and a marked luminal expansion and irregularity. The formation of a network of blood vessels has been shown to be triggered by a broad variety of tumor cells as a consequence of the production and release of angiogenic factors and is therefore not specific to PMF.[63] This increase in marrow vasculature in PMF has been confirmed using immunohistochemical methods and has been shown to correlate with increased spleen size and to be an independent risk factor for overall survival.[64] Vessels from patients with PMF are frequently markedly abnormal and appear as localized vascular nests consisting of numerous short vessels that are highly branched and tortuous.[64,65] Thiele and colleagues[61] hypothesized that the increased marrow microvessel density in PMF was probably mediated by megakaryocyte α-granule constituents. Transforming growth factor β (TGF-β) and vascular endothelial growth factor (VEGF), for instance, has a profound effect on angiogenesis.[65–68] The evolution of the fibroosteosclerotic process in PMF appears to be a coordinated process closely related to the vascular proliferation and also modulated by growth factors present within abnormal megakaryocytes.

Chagraoui and coworkers have reported that the osteosclerosis in mice with MPD due to thrombopoietin overexpression occurs predominantly due to upregulation of osteoprotegerin production by marrow stromal cells.[69] Osteoprotegerin is a secreted molecule that binds to the ligand for the RANK receptor (receptor activator of NF-κB) expressed on osteoblast progenitor cells. The RANK ligand binds to the RANK receptor and promotes osteoblasts differentiation.[70] TGF-β is also a negative regulator of osteoclastogenesis through direct stimulation of transcriptional secretion of osteoprotegerin and downregulation of RANK ligand.[71,72] In patients with PMF, it remains unknown if the degree of osteosclerosis can be corrected with increased levels of osteoprotegerin. By contrast, Garimella and coworkers have also provided evidence that the osteosclerosis observed in GATA1 low mice and myelofibrosis is due to the elaboration of bone morphogenetic proteins by megakaryocytes.[73] Bone morphogenetic proteins cause abnormal stimulation of marrow osteoprogenitor cells resulting in overgrowth of cancellous bone and osteosclerosis.

A number of angiogenic growth factors, including basic fibroblast growth factor (bFGF) and vascular endothelial cell growth factor, have been implicated as causative factors of the increased marrow microvessel density in PMF.[49,66–68] Elevated serum VEGF levels have been reported in PMF, and increased expression of bFGF has been reported in PMF megakaryocytes and platelets.[47,59,60] These angiogenic cytokines are the products of the abnormal megakaryocytes present in PMF marrow and the increased marrow microvessel density observed is ultimately a consequence of a cytokine release characteristic of PMF megakaryocytes. It is yet to be proved that the endothelial cell proliferation in PMF is not part of the malignant clone leading to this disease process. A cell called a *hemangioblast*, which is capable of giving rise to myeloid and endothelial cells, may be the site of the oncogenic event leading to PMF.[75] Groopman[75] first hypothesized that growth factors released from neoplastic hematopoietic cells in PMF were capable of stimulating marrow fibroblast proliferation and suggested that the megakaryocyte was the primary source of such proliferation factors. The role of megakaryocytes in the development of fibrosis in PMF is further supported by the megakaryocytic hyperplasia with dysplastic or necrotic megakaryocytes that characterizes this disorder, by the increased circulating megakaryocytes and megakaryocyte progenitors that are present in PMF, by the association of marrow fibrosis and acute megakaryocytic leukemia, and by the presence of myelofibrosis in gray platelet syndrome, an inherited disorder of platelet α-granules.[76–78] Castro-Malaspina and coworkers[79] subsequently showed that megakaryocyte-enriched marrow cell homogenates and platelet homogenates induced DNA synthesis by human marrow fibroblasts. This group hypothesized that ineffective megakaryocytopoiesis in PMF results in liberation of excessive amounts of such growth factors, leading to marrow fibroblast proliferation and collagen synthesis.[79] Platelet-derived growth factor (PDGF), TGF-β, and epidermal growth factor (EGF), each of which are contained within platelet and megakaryocyte α-granules, stimulate marrow fibroblast proliferation.[81–83] TGF-β enhances type I and type III procollagen and fibronectin synthesis by marrow fibroblasts.[81] Kimura and associates[83,84] presented data to suggest that MPD fibroblasts are more sensitive to human serum mitogens than normal marrow fibroblasts. The PDGF content of platelets from PMF patients is decreased, indicating that a release or leakage of such growth factors by marrow megakaryocytes may occur.[49,85] Their studies indicated that if α-granule constituents were important in the development of marrow fibrosis, their release or leakage would likely occur within the marrow cavity. Such local effects could result in fibrosis without leading to increased concentrations of α-granule constituents in the general circulation. Martyré and colleagues[49,85] further examined the possibility that platelet α-granule constituents may account for marrow fibrosis in PMF. In these studies, PMF platelet PDGF and TGF-β levels were found to be 2.0- to 3.0-fold and 1.5- to 3.0-fold higher, respectively, in PMF than in normal controls, whereas EGF levels in PMF were similar to those of control platelets.[85] The roles of PDGF and TGF-β in the biogenesis of PMF probably are not restricted to promoting fibroblastic proliferation but are also related to the effect of these two growth factors on synthesis, secretion, and degradation of extracellular matrix components.[80,82] Martyré and coworkers[49,85] provided additional data that strengthens the hypothesis that TGF-β plays a pivotal role in the development of progressive fibrosis in PMF. This group documented the increased expression of TGF-β mRNA in peripheral blood mononuclear cells isolated from PMF patients and localized this to peripheral blood megakaryocytes of PMF patients.[85] They have recently reported that the overexpression of PMF megakaryocyte TGF-β is a consequence of NF-κB activation.[86] These data strongly implicate TGF-β as a major player in the biogenesis of fibrosis in PMF.[49,76,85]

TGF-β enhances fibronectin and collagens types I, III, and IV as well as chondroitin or dermatan sulphate and proteoglycan gene expression.[87,88] TGF-β decreases the synthesis of various collagenase-like enzymes that degrade extracellular matrices while at the same time stimulating the synthesis of protease inhibitors such as plasminogen activator inhibitor 1.[89,90] The net effect of these complex interactions is the accumulation of extracellular matrix, which probably contributes to further progression of fibrosis. Additional growth factors probably are involved in the development of progressive fibrosis in PMF. Circulating megakaryocytic cells and platelets from PMF patients have been shown to possess high levels of bFGF.[91] Because bFGF is devoid of a secretion peptide signal, bFGF is not present in media conditioned by megakaryocytic cells from PMF patients.[92] bFGF is a potent angiogenic factor and is a mitogen for human bone marrow stromal cells.[91] Elevated platelet, megakaryocyte, and serum bFGF levels have been reported in PMF patients with progressive fibrosis.[91,93] BFGF may be released or leaked from dysplastic and necrotic PMF megakaryocytes or platelets. These findings suggest that bFGF may also contribute to the progressive fibrosis and pronounced angiogenesis frequently observed in PMF.[91,93]

The roles of the megakaryocytes and platelets in the development of marrow fibrosis were further clarified by the transplantation of marrow cells genetically modified to overexpress thrombopoietin into normal mice.[94,95] These animals possessed increased numbers of platelets and megakaryocytes and developed a syndrome characterized by marrow myelofibrosis, osteosclerosis, extramedullary hematopoiesis, and elevated numbers of circulating hematopoietic precursors within a period of 3 months.[94,95] In these mice, TGF-β and PDGF levels in platelet-poor plasma were elevated twofold to threefold higher than those in normal control mice.[94,95] Retransplantation of these mice with normal marrow cells resulted after 12 to 15 weeks in reduction of platelet and megakaryocyte numbers and reversal of the marrow myelofibrosis and osteosclerosis.[95] These data dramatically demonstrate the roles of megakaryocytes and platelets and their intracellular growth factors in the generation of marrow fibrosis. Remarkably, transgenic mice overexpressing thrombopoietin in the liver but not the marrow have similar degrees of megakaryocytic hyperplasia and thrombocytosis but do not develop marrow fibrosis.[96] The discrepancy between these two animal models emphasizes the unique consequences that marrow thrombopoietin generation may play in the generation of marrow fibrosis. Ozaki and associates[97] reported that thrombopoietin was capable of enhancing the production of megakaryocyte PDGF, PF-4, and TGF-β.

In a number of reports, elevated thrombopoietin levels have been reported in patients with PMF.[98–100] This unanticipated elevation of plasma thrombopoietin levels was not caused by enhanced production of thrombopoietin mRNA by marrow fibroblasts or marrow cells but was probably caused by the reduced expression of the thrombopoietin receptor by the platelets and megakaryocytes of PMF patients, leading to decreased clearance of thrombopoietin.[100,101] Vannucchi and colleagues[102] used another rodent model to determine the relationship between marrow megakaryocytic hyperplasia and marrow fibrosis. They studied mutant mice with reduced expression of the transcription factor GATA1. These mice frequently develop anemia and die during gestation or after birth. The few animals that survive to adulthood recover from the anemia but remain thrombocytopenic throughout life because of a block in megakaryocyte maturation into proplatelets that results in megakaryocyte hyperplasia in the marrow and the spleen and increased production of TGF-β.[103] These animals develop a clinical picture after 15 months that closely resembles PMF, including anemia, teardrop red blood cells, fibrosis of the marrow and spleen, extramedullary hematopoiesis in the liver, and progenitor cell mobilization into the peripheral blood.[102] Unlike PMF in humans, the myelofibrosis in the GATA1 low mice is not the consequence of a clonal disorder and does not progress to acute leukemia. Mutations in the GATA1 functional pathway in human PMF have not been described.[104] However, at the protein level, a large number of the megakaryocytes in the bone marrow of PMF patients are GATA1 negative, suggesting that whatever the genetic defect leading to PMF is, it involves the pathway which affects the posttranscriptional and/or posttranslational regulation of GATA1 in megakaryocytes.[105] Interesting, this study identified that the presence of GATA1 negative megakaryocytes, and not the Jak2V617F mutation, is a marker that distinguishes PMF from other MPDs. Given the central role played by GATA1 in megakaryopoiesis, it is not surprising that megakaryocytes with low GATA1 content are all characterized by common morphological abnormalities. These abnormalities include: lack of proper organization of the α-granules, abnormal P-selectin localization on the demarcation membrane system, increased emperipolesis of neutrophils through the demarcation membrane system and increased levels of para-apoptosis, a TUNEL negative process of cell death mediated by neutrophils and macrophages.[104] It is conceivable that at least some of these megakaryocytes alterations may play a central role in the pathobiology of PMF. The two rodent models of myelofibrosis, GATA1 low mice and mice that overexpress thrombopoietin eventually develop myelofibrosis, but the rate of progression to marrow fibrosis is remarkably different. The thrombopoietin-overexpressing mice develop myelofibrosis in 3 months, whereas the GATA1 animals require 15 months to achieve a similar state. Although both animal models have been shown to have increased levels of the fibrogenic cytokines TGF-β1, PDGF, and VEGF within their femurs compared with normal littermates, the levels of these cytokines in the GATA1 low mice were reduced compared with the animals that overexpressed thrombopoietin.[102,103] The less pronounced elevation in these cytokines probably explains the greater period required to develop marrow fibrosis in the GATA1 low mice.

To further assess directly the role of TGF-β in the development of myelofibrosis, marrow stem cells from homozygous TGF-β1null mice (TGF-$\beta 1^{-/-}$) and wild-type mice were isolated and genetically modified with a retroviral vector encoding the murine thrombopoietin gene and transplanted into lethally irradiated wild-type hosts.[106]

Although thrombopoietin levels and platelet levels were increased in both groups of animals, only animals receiving the wild-type grafts but not the stem grafts from TGF-β1null mice developed myelofibrosis. These studies provide further evidence for the critical role that TGF-β1 plays in the biogenesis of myelofibrosis and provides rationale for the potential use of TGF-β as a drug target in future treatments for this disease. The mechanism by which the pathologic release of growth factors from megakaryocytes occurs in PMF remains unknown. Schmitt and coworkers[107] suggested that megakaryocyte emperipolesis might lead to this liberation of fibrogenic cytokines. *Emperipolesis* is defined as the random entry of hematopoietic cells into the cytoplasm of megakaryocytes. This group documented increased emperipolesis of neutrophils and eosinophils in PMF and the liberation of myeloperoxidase-positive granules by the engulfed neutrophils.[107] They correlated the degree of emperipolesis in PMF marrow biopsies with the degree of marrow fibrosis. They suggested the abnormal P-selectin distribution in megakaryocytes accounted for the selective sequestration of granulocytes by PMF megakaryocytes.[107]

Megakaryocytes are not the only cells capable of releasing cytokines that promote marrow fibrosis. Levels of macrophage colony stimulating factor, a cytokine that regulates macrophage development and proliferation, are elevated in the serum of PMF patients.[108] Monocytes/macrophages from patients with PMF can produce greater quantities of TGF-β and interleukin-1 (IL-1) than normal controls.[109] IL-1 and TGF-β are fibroblast mitogens that induce extracellular matrix protein production. Rameshwar and coworkers[109] showed that monocyte adhesion to extracellular matrix proteins led to the overproduction of IL-1 and TGF-β by PMF monocytes. The monocyte adhesion molecule CD44 appears to be involved in the induction of fibrogenic cytokines by mediating the interaction between monocytes and accumulated extracellular matrix protein deposits.[109] Rameshwar and associates[110] showed that the pro-inflammatory transcriptional factor NF-κB plays a pivotal role in the elaboration of IL-1 and TGF-β in the activation of NF-κB monocytes and that of PMF patients. These investigators suggest that NF-κB stimulates TGF-β production by influencing intracellular IL-1 levels and may serve as another potential therapeutic target for the treatment of PMF. The role of monocytes in the biogenesis of marrow fibrosis was further supported by the report of Frey and colleagues.[111] They showed that although immune-deficient mice that were treated with an adenoviral vector expressing the human thrombopoietin gene developed megakaryocyte hyperplasia, osteomyelofibrosis, and extramedullary hematopoiesis, similarly treated nonobese diabetes (NOD) and severe combined immune deficiency (SCID) mice with similar elevations of thrombopoietin levels did not develop fibrosis of the marrow. NOD/SCID mice possess functionally defective monocytes and macrophages in terms of IL-1β secretion, cytokine receptor expression, and protein kinase C levels. These investigators hypothesized that normal monocytes and macrophages that were present in SCID mice but not NOD/SCID mice were necessary for the development of osteomyelofibrosis.[111] Recently, however, Wagner-Ballon and coworkers have performed similar studies resulting in conflicting data, which suggest that completely functional monocytes are not required to develop myelofibrosis.[112] They showed that thrombopoietin and TGF-β levels in the plasma of NOD/SCID mice engrafted with thrombopoietin overexpressing hematopoietic cells reach levels similar to the levels achieved in immunocompetent mice and that both types of animals develop an MPD characterized by marrow fibrosis. The discrepancies between the studies of Fey et al and Wagner-Ballon et al might be due to the levels of thrombopoietin achieved using two different gene delivery system.[111,112] Frey et al used an adenoviral construct with a human thrombopoietin cDNA, while Wagner-Ballon et al used a retroviral vehicle encoding a murine thrombopoietin DNA to overexpress thrombopoietin in NOD/SCID, SCID, and wild-type mice.[111,112] Wagner-Ballon et al were able to achieve higher levels of thrombopoietin and TGF-β1 than Frey and coworkers.[112] These data lead one to question if monocytes/macrophages play a crucial role in the development of myelofibrosis promoted by thrombopoietin.

Recently, greater insight into the molecular origins of the MPD has been gained following the discovery of a gain of function mutation of an auto-inhibitory domain of the Janus kinase family of protein tyrosine kinases, which is involved in cytokine receptor signaling. The Jak2V617F mutation results from a valine to phenylalanine mutation at amino acid Jak2V617F which leads to ongoing phosphorylation activity which then can bind to a cytokine receptor and promote STAT recruitment.[113,114] This mutation is the likely cause of the hypersensitivity to cytokines that characterizes hematopoietic progenitors from each of the MPD.[113,114] In a mouse marrow transplant model, marrow cells transduced with Jak2V617F results in a clinical phenotype which closely resembles PV including erythrocytosis, extramedullary hematopoiesis, and marrow fibrosis.[115] Although 90% of patients with PV are Jak2V617F positive, approximately 50% of PMF patients harbor this mutation.[14,15,113–116] The Jak2V617F mutation is homozygous in 13% of patients with PMF but 30% of patients with PV.[14,15] Homozygosity has been attributed to homologous recombination. Homozygosity of Jak2V617F in PMF patients is associated with a more frequent occurrence of unfavorable cytogenetic abnormalities.[117] There is conflicting data as to whether the clinical course of patients with Jak2V617F positive and Jak2V617F negative PMF differ.[118,119] Additional somatic mutations have been identified in patients with PMF which likely play a role in the biogenesis of PMF. A mutation in the transmembrane domain of the thrombopoietin receptor (cMPL) has been documented in 9% of patients with Jak2V617F negative PMF (MPLW515L or MPLW515K).[120,121] Pardanani and coworkers have provided data to support the coexistence of MPL515L, MPL515K, and MPL wild-type (WT) alleles in the same patient.[121] Furthermore, 30% of PMF patients with mutations of cMPL also have the Jak2V617F mutation.[121] By studying archival material, the burden of MPL515L and MPK515K and Jak2V617 in PMF patients has been shown to remain constant throughout the clinical course of patients with PMF.[122] In a murine bone marrow transplant assay, expression of MPLW515L but not wild-type MPL resulted in a rapidly progressive, fully penetrable, lethal MPD (18 days) characterized by marked thrombocytosis, leukocytosis, splenomegaly, hepatomegaly, marrow megakaryocytic hyperplasia, and marrow fibrosis, but not erythrocytosis.[120] These data have suggested that the MPL mutation favors the development of thrombocytosis while the Jak2V617F mutation favors the development of erythrocytosis. Guglielmelli and coworkers have recently reported that PMF patients with MPL515L/K mutations as compared with MPL wild-type PMF were older, presented with more severe anemia and were more likely to require transfusional support.[123] Although 50% of patients with PMF have clonal hematopoiesis and lack mutations of either Jak2 or cMPL, they have a similar clinical phenotype to patients with the recently identified somatic mutations.[124] It is, therefore, difficult to attribute to either of these mutations as the sole cause of PMF. It appears, however, that the genetic origins of PMF represent the culmination of multiple genetic and possibly epigenetic events. Additional genetic events which might play a role in this process are being sought by a number of laboratories.[125–127] Comparative genomic hybridization has shown that gains of cytogenetic material occur in over 50% of PMF patients and most commonly involve gains of 9p, 2q, 3p, chromosome 4, 12q, and 13q.[127] Furthermore, Dingli et al have identified an unbalanced translocation between chromosomes 1 and 6 with specific breakpoints (t1,6) that they believe to be highly specific to PMF. These chromosomal sites may harbor additional genes that play a role in the origins of PMF.[125]

Further insight into the phenotypic heterogeneity of Jak2V617F positive and negative MPDs has recently been provided. Teofili and coworkers using immunohistochemical approaches of bone marrow reported that PV is characterized by increased expression of phosphorylated STAT3 and STAT5 protein, whereas PMF is characterized by reduced expression of STAT3 and STAT5.[128] This expression pattern was independent of Jak2V617F status. Such observations suggest that additional or alternative molecular events occur in PMF and PV that might play a role in the development of their distinctive clinical phenotypes.

A number of investigators have shown that myeloid cells (red cells, white cells, and megakaryocytes/platelets) are clonal in this disorder and that they harbor the Jak2V617F or MPL515L/K mutations.[129–131] Furthermore B, T, and natural killer cells isolated from PMF patients have been shown in selected cases to be Jak2V617F or MPL515 L/K positive.[131] These studies indicate that Jak2V617F and MPL mutational events originate in a cell capable of generating both myeloid and lymphoid cells such as the pluripotent hematopoietic stem cell. The ability of primitive human hematopoietic cells to engraft sublethally irradiated immunodeficient mice is the standard surrogate in vivo assay for human hematopoietic stem cells. Xu et al have demonstrated that PMF $CD34^+$ cells are capable of engrafting NOD/SCID mice and generating myeloid and B cells that are clonal, Jak2V617F positive and carry a patient-specific marker chromosomal abnormality.[132] The differentiation program of PMF $CD34^+$ cells following transplant into NOD/SCID mice was also remarkably different from that of normal $CD34^+$ cells, producing greater numbers of $CD34^+$, $CD33^+$, and $CD41^+$ cells but fewer $CD19^+$ cells.[132] This predisposition to produce greater numbers of megakaryocytes was further explored by incubating PMF, PV, and $CD34^+$ cells in vitro in the presence of stem cell factor and thrombopoietin. PMF $CD34^+$ cells displayed a far greater proliferative capacity and produced greater numbers of megakaryocytes which were characterized by a resistance to undergo apoptosis in vitro due to overexpression of the antiapoptotic factor Bcl-XL.[133] The megakaryocyte hyperplasia in PMF, therefore, could be accounted by two factors, an increased ability of $CD34^+$ cells to generate megakaryocytes and the accumulation of megakaryocytes due to Bcl-xL overexpression.[133] Although Bcl-xL overexpression has been linked to Jak2V617F, PMF megakaryocyte Bcl-xL overexpression also occurred to a similar degree in megakaryocytes generated from $CD34^+$ cells isolated from individuals with both Jak2V617F positive and negative disease.[133]

Marrow megakaryocytes PMF have been shown by Ciurea et al to produce greater amounts of TGF-β than MKs generated in vitro from normal volunteers or patients with PV.[133] Komura and coworkers have previously reported that an immunophilin FK506 binding protein 51 (FKB51) is overexpressed in PMF megakaryocytes and that FKB51 overexpression leads to activation of NF-κB in PMF MKs.[86] Cells with activated NF-κB produce greater amounts of TGF-β. This effect of NF-κB is likely indirect since NF-κB cannot directly increase transcription of TGF-β since its promoter does not have NF-κB binding sites. These studies suggest that NF-κB or TGF-β inhibitors might be useful in preventing the progression of marrow fibrosis in PMF.

The number of unilineage and multilineage hematopoietic progenitor cells constitutively mobilized into the blood of PMF patients is dramatically increased.[45–48] The number of CD34+ cells present in the peripheral blood in PMF is 360 times greater than in normal controls and 18 to 30 times higher than in patients with polycythemia vera or essential thrombocythemia.[55] These findings are so striking that some investigators have suggested that the quantitation of CD34+ cells in the peripheral blood might serve as a means of discriminating PMF from other MPDs. A level of 15×10^6/L of $CD34^+$ cells in peripheral blood allows differentiation of PMF from PV and ET.[55] Barosi and coworkers[55] reported that the numbers of circulating $CD34^+$ cells tend to increase as the disease progresses and that there is a close correlation between patients presenting with more than 300×10^6 $CD34^+$ cells/L of peripheral blood and imminent evolution to leukemia. These findings suggest that PMF $CD34^+$ cells trafficking abnormality due to the inability of these cells to be retained within the marrow or their premature release into the peripheral blood.

PMF is characterized not only by the constitutive mobilization of $CD34^+$ hematopoietic cells but also endothelial progenitor cells into the peripheral blood. Endothelial progenitor cell mobilization predominates during the prefibrotic phase of PMF while hematopoietic stem/progenitor cell mobilization occurs characteristically in more clinically advanced phases of the disease.[134,135] This dysregulation of stem cell trafficking likely ultimately leads to the seeding of extramedullary sites with primitive hematopoietic and endothelial cells which results in production of extramedullary hematopoiesis within the liver and spleen as well as a variety of other organs. Several proteolytic pathways have been documented to play a role in cytokine mediated stem cell mobilization. Proteins released by activated neutrophils cleave vascular adhesion molecule-1 (VCAM-1) expressed by stromal cells leading to the disruption of a key adhesive interaction between VCAM-1 and very late antigen-4 (VLA-4) expressed by hematopoietic stem cells and progenitor cells.[136] The interaction between stromal cell-, endothelial cell and osteoblasts derived stromal cell derived factor-1 (SDF-1) and the CXC chemokine receptor-4 (CXCR-4) expressed by hematopoietic stem cells and progenitor cells is also believed to determine patterns of stem cell trafficking. Proteases including neutrophil elastase, soluble matrix metalloproteinase-9 (MMP-9) and cell-bound MMP-9 have been shown to play a role in the constitutive mobilization of $CD34^+$ cells that occurs in PMF patients. The concentrations of soluble VCAM-1, a degradation product of VCAM-1 is elevated in the plasma of PMF patients and these levels correlate with the absolute numbers of $CD34^+$ cells in the peripheral blood. Furthermore, CXCR-4 expression by PMF $CD34^+$ cells is downregulated which may account for altered SDF-1/CXCR-4 interactions participating in $CD34^+$ cell mobilization.[136,137] This down regulation of CXCR4 expression can be reversed in vitro by treatment with chromatin modifying agents which suggest that this event might be due to epigenetic events.[138] Furthermore the expression levels of CXCR4 were significantly lower in patients with a high burden of Jak2V617F (allele frequency 75%) as compared to patients with low burden Jak2V617F, suggesting the dependence of gene expression on the frequency of the mutated allele.[139] Similar degrees of CD34+ cell mobilization are observed in post-ET and post-PV MF as occurs in PMF.[135,136] In PV patients, Passamonti and coworkers have demonstrated a relationship between Jak2V617F gene dosage and the degree of constitutive mobilization of CD34+ cells suggesting that such mobilization may be a consequence of the transition from Jak2V617F heterozygosity to homozygosity which is accompanied by granulocyte activation.[140] Drugs which target the proteases responsible for constitutive CD34+ cell mobilization may present an intriguing strategy to prevent the establishment of or to eliminate extramedullary sites of hematopoiesis in patients with PMF.

ETIOLOGY AND PATHOGENESIS

Exposure of a variety of animal models to chemical agents, industrial solvents, hormones, viruses, immunologic stimuli, and ionizing radiation have led to the development of marrow fibrosis.[3] A model of PMF has been established in the rabbit,[141–147] in which saponin administered intravenously induces extramedullary hematopoiesis and myelofibrosis over a period of weeks.[142] Mice and rats fail to respond to the same doses of saponin.[141] Hoshi and Weiss provided ultrastructural evidence to suggest that saponin causes damage to the endothelium of marrow vascular cells, rendering them incompetent.[141] A series of hemorrhagic events appears to occur, leading to release of normoblasts into the peripheral blood, marrow hypoplasia, fibrosis, and regeneration.[141] This effect is accompanied by the appearance of increased numbers of hematopoietic progenitor cells in the blood and spleen and a simultaneous depletion of such cells in the marrow.[141] Such marrow vascular injury may be a common link leading to the development of myelofibrosis.

Reticulin fibrosis of the marrow represents an exaggeration of the fibrous pattern of normal marrow. In contrast, collagen fibrosis occurs in primary and secondary PMF and results in the disruption and obliteration of the sinusoidal architecture of the bone marrow. The marrow stroma in PMF is composed of an increased deposition of extracellular matrix proteins, including collagen types I, III, V and VI; hyaluronic acid; the noncollagenous glycoproteins; fibronectin; vitronectin; tenascin; and the basement membrane components collagen type IV and laminin.[7] Bone marrow reticulin is composed of types I and III collagen and fibronectin.[144–146] Charron and coworkers[147] documented a progressive increase in marrow collagen content during the course of PMF. The increment in collagen was highest in patients in whom the disease was of longest duration.[147] The degree of collagen fibrosis can be best estimated by silver impregnation or by the use of a trichrome stain of a marrow biopsy specimen.[7] The silver stain stains reticulin, the glycoprotein coating of stromal cells, black (Fig. 70–1), and trichrome stains collagen bluish green. Compared with collagen extracts from normal individuals, PMF extracts showed a moderate increase in neutral soluble collagen and a larger increase in polymeric collagen.[147] Charron and associates[147] also observed changes in the pattern of marrow collagen deposition during the course of PMF. Early in the course, there is a higher percentage of newly synthesized fibers, and later, more polymeric collagen is present, presumably as a result of progressive cross-linking and insolubilization. Charron and colleagues[147] and Gay and coworkers[145] claim that type III collagen preferentially increases in the early stages of the disease but that it is subsequently replaced by type I collagen. The serum level of procollagen N-terminal peptide III (PC III), which is cleared extracellularly during collagen biosynthesis, is increased in most PMF patients.[148] This finding supports the concept that type III collagen synthesis is increased in PMF.[149–151] Some investigators have suggested that PC III levels do not reflect the extent of marrow fibrosis in PMF,[149,150] but PC III elevation in a longitudinal study of patients with PMF was found to be a sensitive marker of disease activity.[151,152] PC III levels were observed to fall in patients responding to chemotherapy and to rise 1 to 2 weeks before elevations in white blood cell and blast cell counts in patients unresponsive to chemotherapy.[152] Bone marrow fibrosis appears to depend on the accumulation of collagen and on the establishment of an equilibrium

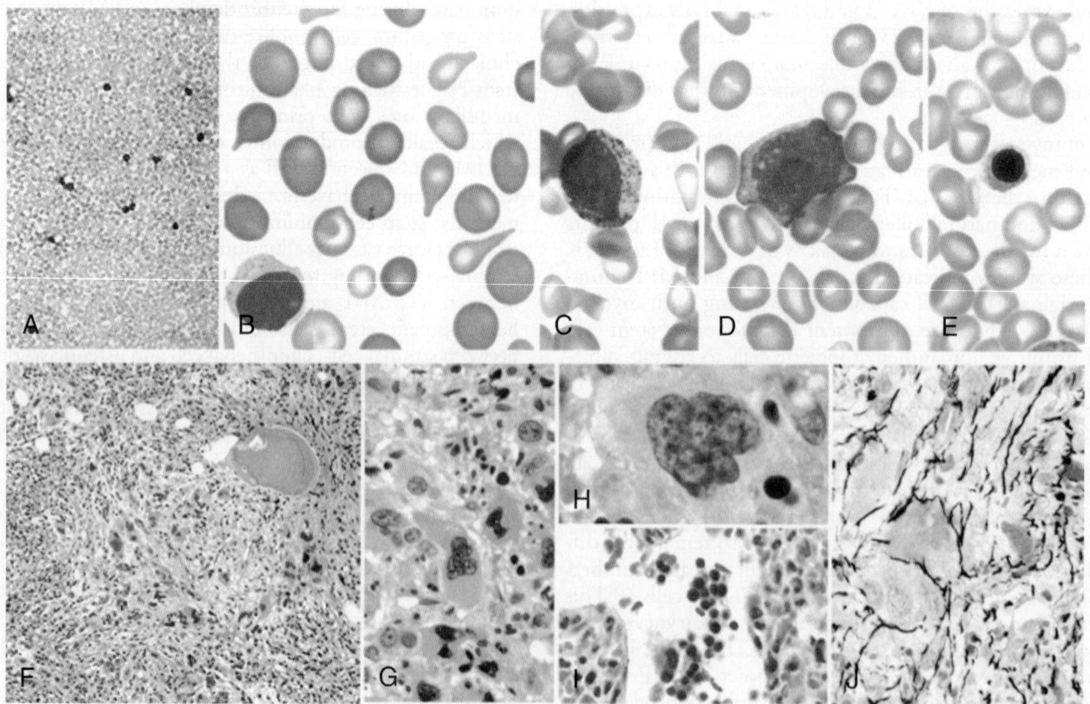

Figure 70–1 PRIMARY MYELOFIBROSIS. Peripheral Blood **A–E**, and Bone Marrow Biopsy **F–J**. The leukocyte count can vary in PMF from leukopenia to marked leukocytosis. In the case illustrated, the count was normal (**A**). However, the smear showed numerous dacryocytes, or teardrop forms (**B**), and a leukoerythroblastic picture (**C, D, E**), ie, the presence leukoblasts, or immature granulocytic precursors (**C**), including blasts (**D**), and circulating nucleated red blood cells or erythroblasts (**E**). The bone marrow biopsy is frequently hypercellular (**F**) and comprised of an atypical megakaryocytic and granulocytic proliferation (**G**), in which some of the megakaryocytes have atypical and pyknotic nuclei. Other megakaryocytes (**H**) are considered to have nuclei that are "cloud-like." The marrow biopsy frequently shows sinusoidal hematopoiesis (**I**) and significant fibrosis as illustrated by a reticulin stain (**J**).

between collagen production and destruction. PC III levels would therefore be expected to reflect collagen synthesis more closely than total marrow collagen content. Extensive deposition of collagen type VI in PMF has been documented.[78] This structural component forms a linkage between individual collagen type I or collagen type III fibers, or both. Advanced marrow fibrosis is associated with increased deposition of fibronectin, tenascin, and vitronectin. In normal bone marrow, collagen type IV and laminin are limited to discontinuous sinusoidal membranes, and myelofibrotic stroma possess continuous sheets of both proteins resulting from increased marrow microvessel density and endothelial cell proliferation. The accumulation of matrix depends on a balance between the synthesis and degradation of matrix components. Extracellular matrix can be degraded by a variety of proteases, including matrix metalloproteinases (MMPs). MMP activity can be inhibited by tissue inhibitors of matrix metalloproteinases (TIMPs). Wang and associates[153] explored whether the marrow fibrosis in MMP could be caused by an imbalance between MMPs and TIMPs. They documented decreased plasma levels of MMP-3 and an elevation of TIMP-1, but normal levels of MMP-1, MMP-2, and MMP-9 in PMF patients and suggested that these enzymes might play a role in the degree of marrow fibrosis of individual patients.[153] Jensen and colleagues[154] reported that plasma levels of soluble plasminogen activator receptor levels were increased in PMF patients. The binding of this single-chain proenzyme of urokinase-type plasminogen activator to its cell bound receptor (CD87) results in the generation of plasmin.[154] Plasmin-mediated activation of MMPs in concert with plasmin can lead to the degradation of a variety of matrix proteins. The elevation of plasma levels of the soluble plasminogen activator receptor is likely an indication of ongoing stromal cell activity and constant tissue remodeling within the marrow of PMF patients.

The kinetics of engraftment of normal stem cells following allogeneic stem cell transplantation in PMF patients and the slow regression of fibrosis after transplant leads one to question if the distorted marrow architecture associated with fibrosis in PMF actually disrupts the functions of the marrow microenvironment.[155–157] In PMF patients, normal stem cells engraft following transplant and hematopoietic cell recovery occurs before the marrow fibrosis has resolved.[155–157] These observations raise some questions concerning the prospects for success with strategies for the treatment of patients with PMF that are directed solely toward reversing the marrow fibrosis rather than eliminating the malignant clone and its progeny. Furthermore in mouse models of myelofibrosis, inhibition of TGF-B1 was capable of preventing the development of marrow fibrosis but did not rescue animals from a fatal MPD.[158]

CLINICAL MANIFESTATIONS

Table 70–2 lists the symptoms and physical findings of patients with PMF at presentation.

Approximately 25% of patients are entirely asymptomatic and come to medical attention because of an enlarged spleen detected during routine physical examination or because of an abnormal blood cell count or peripheral blood smear. The most common symptom in PMF is fatigue, which in the majority of patients affects the quality of daily life and social activities. Fatigue may be the result of anemia, which leads to the associated complaints of weakness, dyspnea on exertion, and palpitations. But when patients were questioned with the aid of specific questionnaires, fatigue was found to be a significant burden even in patients who were not anemic.[159] The presence of anemia, splenomegaly, and other features associated with advanced disease favored the development of higher levels of fatigue. Other nonspecific constitutional symptoms, including fever, night sweats, pruritus, bone pain, and weight loss are present at diagnosis in 20% to 50% of patients with PMF[159] and are more frequent in older patients.[160]

With enlargement of the spleen, various syndromes characterized by abdominal discomfort emerge.[161] Pressure of the spleen on the stomach may lead to delayed gastric emptying and early satiety.[161]

Table 70–2 Summary of Symptoms and Physical Findings of Patients with Primary Myelofibrosis Detected at Diagnosis

	Incidence (%)		
Symptom or Finding	**Varki et al.[5]**	**Silverstein[3]**	**Visani et al[377]**
Asymptomatic	21	30	16
Fatigue	71	58	47
Fever	5	10	5
Weight loss	39	15	7
Night sweats	21	6	NR
Symptoms due to enlarged spleen	11	23	48
Bleeding	20	17	5
Gout/renal stones	13	6	NR
Pallor	NR	60	NR
Petechiae/ecchymoses	20	15	NR
Splenomegaly	89	90	99
Hepatomegaly	64	70	39
Peripheral edema	13	NR	NR
Evidence of portal hypertension	2	6	2
Lymphadenopathy	2	10	1
Jaundice	0	4	NR

NR, not reported.

Patients may merely complain of a dull, heavy sensation in the left upper quadrant. Pain of extreme severity, simulating an acute abdominal emergency, is produced by splenic infarction. Pressure of the spleen on the colon or small bowel may be responsible of severe, disabling diarrhea.

Thrombotic episodes may rarely be the presenting feature of the disease or may occur during its course with a probability of 9.6% at 5 years, a rate higher than in the control general population.[162] Thrombosis may be venous (cerebral venous sinus thrombosis, splanchnic vein thrombosis, deep vein thrombosis, pulmonary thromboembolism) or arterial (stroke, transient ischemic attacks, retinal artery occlusion, myocardial infarction, angina pectoris, and peripheral arterial disease). The cellular phase of PMF with thrombocytosis and presence of cardiovascular risk factors such as hypertension, smoking, hypercholesterolemia, and diabetes are the independent predictors of thrombosis.[162] After splenectomy, the rate of thrombosis increases and is associated with the development of thrombocytosis following the procedure.[162]

Bleeding problems may complicate the clinical course of PMF patients. Bleeding may be trivial, as manifested by petechiae and ecchymoses, or it may be life-threatening as a result of uncontrollable esophageal bleeding.[1–3,7,9] It may result from thrombocytopenia or poor platelet function.[1–3,7,9] Bleeding may be only initially encountered during a surgical procedure such as splenectomy; in this case, the bleeding diathesis may result from inapparent disseminated intravascular coagulopathy (DIC) and has the potential for catastrophic consequences.[6]

Occurrence of isolated sites of ectopic sites of myeloid metaplasia has been reported, particularly in the pulmonary, gastrointestinal, central nervous, and genitourinary systems.[1–3,7,9] Extramedullary hematopoiesis can rarely occur in the skin, manifesting as nontender, occasionally pruritic red, pink, or violaceous plaques, papules, or hemangioma-like nodules. These dermal infiltrates, when biopsied, are composed of combinations of myeloid, erythroid, and megakaryocytic cells.[163–165] Patients with nonsplenic ectopic myeloid metaplasia present with cough and "large lung tumors," headache, or paralysis resulting from "brain tumors or spinal cord tumors," small-bowel obstruction, or intractable ascites from ectopic implants of hematopoietic tissue in the gut or peritoneum.[1–3,7,9,166–170] Myeloid metaplasia of the renal pelvis, ureters, and bladder, and renal parenchymal infiltration have been observed.[170] Expansion of hematopoietic tissue at the urethral meatus may be confused with a urethral carbuncle.[170] Such strategically localized sites of extramedullary hematopoiesis may lead to renal failure or obstruction of both kidneys and bladder dysfunction.[170] Ascites occurring in a patient with PMF may result from peritoneal or mesenteric implants of extramedullary hematopoietic tissue or from portal hypertension.[171,172] If the ascites result from peritoneal implants, the fluid is always exudative and sterile and frequently contains myeloid, erythroid, and megakaryocytic elements.[171,172] Such cytologic studies should routinely be performed on ascitic or pleural fluid obtained from patients with PMF. Unusual sites of extramedullary hematopoiesis have been reported in the gallbladder and lacrimal fossae.[173,174]

Table 70–2 lists the prominent physical findings in patients with PMF.[2,5] Splenomegaly serves as the hallmark of the disease. Its extent may vary, but massive splenomegaly, with the organ occupying the entire left side of the abdomen and extending into the pelvis, may occur in 35% of patients. Hepatomegaly occurs in almost 70% of cases,[1–3,7,9] and lymphadenopathy is observed in 10% to 20%, but the degree of nodal enlargement is frequently only moderate.[2,5] Other important physical findings include pallor, peripheral edema, jaundice, and bony tenderness. Acute monoarticular inflammation caused by secondary gout is seen in 6% of patients.[3]

Portal hypertension may occur and is a result of massive increases in hepatic blood flow and intrahepatic obstruction.[1–3,7,9,161,175,176] Clinical features of portal hypertension, such as ascites or esophageal varices, occur in 9% to 18% of patients with PMF.[161,175,176] Occasionally, cirrhosis or evidence of thrombosis of the portal or hepatic veins has been reported.[171,172] Wanless and coworkers,[175] analyzed a large series of patients with polycythemia vera and PMF at autopsy. In patients with portal hypertension, thrombotic lesions in small- or medium-sized portal veins and in extrahepatic portal veins were observed. Nodular regenerative liver hyperplasia occurred in 14.6% of cases and correlated closely with the presence of portal vein lesions. They concluded that thrombosis is the most likely cause of portal venous obliteration and portal hypertension in PMF and that clinically significant thrombosis confined to small intrahepatic veins or large hepatic veins should be considered in any patient with PMF. In this autopsy series, portal and hepatic venous disease occurred even in the absence of signs of portal hypertension. Such a finding is consistent with subclinical thrombosis with recanalization occurring fairly commonly in this patient group.[175,176]

Rarely, the development of PMF can be preceded by the appearance of multiple cutaneous edematous plaques and nodules characteristic of the Sweet syndrome, a cutaneous process occurring in response to a number of hematologic malignancies.[177] Pyoderma gangrenosum has been reported to be associated with PMF,[178] and atypical pyoderma gangrenosum is reported to be a complication at splenectomy incision.[179]

PMF may be associated with the development of pulmonary hypertension.[180–185] These patients present with progressive dyspnea, signs of biventricular heart failure, and rapidly increasing hepatosplenomegaly. An elevation in pulmonary artery pressure can be documented by transthoracic Doppler echocardiography and right heart catherization.[180,182] Many of these patients succumb to cardiopulmonary complications within 18 months of the documentation of pulmonary artery hypertension.[180–185] The development of pulmonary artery hypertension can be attributed to thromboembolic disease, extramedullary hematopoiesis diffusely involving the lung, or pulmonary fibrosis due to the elaboration of fibrogenic cytokines from dysfunctional circulating megakaryocytes and platelets.[180–185] Marrow fibrosis also occurs in patients with primary pulmonary hypertension and can be associated with anemia and thrombocytopenia. These patients can be distinguished from patients with PMF by their lack of high levels of circulating CD34+ cells, teardrop red cells, hematopoietic cell clonality, and their Jak2V617F negativity.[185]

Nephrotic syndrome associated with PMF has been reported in few cases.[186,187] Renal extramedullary hematopoiesis is a constant finding in these cases, but renal biopsy may reveal also a picture of mesangioproliferative glomerulopathy,[186] or membranous glomerulonephritis.[187] Immunocomplexes deposition with subepithelial electron dense deposits caused by immuno dysfunction of PMF has been proposed as the pathogenetic explanation for this association.[187]

PMF may be associated with a preexisting or simultaneously appearing autoimmune disease, such as systemic lupus erythematosus, scleroderma, primary biliary cirrhosis, ulcerative colitis, polyarteritis nodosa, or juvenile rheumatoid arthritis.[188–191] In addition, autoimmune forms of myelofibrosis have been described distinct from PMF and are most commonly associated with systemic lupus erythematosus. These patients characteristically have cytopenia and marrow fibrosis, but have limited degree of splenomegaly and only mild numbers of teardrop red cell and immature myeloid cells in the peripheral blood. Patients with autoimmune myelofibrosis frequently have a positive direct antiglobulin test and antinuclear antibodies but are Jak2V617F negative.

LABORATORY EVALUATION

Careful examination of the peripheral blood smear (Fig. 70–1) and bone marrow (Fig. 70–1) permits ready diagnosis of PMF. Leukoerythroblastosis with teardrop red cells strongly suggests this diagnosis. The leukoerythroblastic condition is characterized by the presence of nucleated red blood cells and immature myeloid elements in 96% of cases.[1–3,7,9] Megathrombocytes and megakaryocytic fragments are frequent findings. The number of teardrop erythrocytes (ie, dacryocytes) decreases after splenectomy or institution of chemotherapy,[192,193] which has led some to suggest that splenic fibrosis causes the development of these red cell changes.[193,193] In approximately 60% of patients, hemoglobin levels drop to less than 10 g/dL.[1–3,7,9] The degree of anemia is not infrequently difficult to estimate by hemoglobin or hematocrit determinations, because individuals with large spleens often have expanded plasma volumes and apparent anemia, which is largely dilutional in nature. Of the patients with decreased red cell mass, 95% have normochromic normocytic red cell indices.[194] The anemia may be aregenerative or may be caused by ineffective red cell production and shortened red blood cell survival.[195–197] Morphometric analysis of bone marrow biopsies has demonstrated that erythroid hypoplasia is more common than previously appreciated,[198] and ferrokinetic studies have demonstrated that 30% of patients have erythroid failure.[199] Ineffective red cell production in PMF can be demonstrated with ferrokinetic studies by increased plasma iron turnover but decreased incorporation of radioactive iron into circulating red blood cells.[195–197] Ineffective iron incorporation in red blood cells occurs in 90% of patients with PMF.[3] Fifteen percent of patients have major hemolytic episodes during the clinical course of the disease.[3] The cause of the hemolytic anemia is usually multifactorial, with contributions from hypersplenism, a defect in red blood cells resembling paroxysmal nocturnal hemoglobinuria, and antierythrocyte autoantibodies.[1–3,7,9,199]

Hypochromic microcytic anemia resulting from iron deficiency secondary to blood loss may develop in 5% of PMF patients. Blood loss may be caused by leaking esophageal varices, duodenal ulceration, gastritis, or intravascular hemolysis. Occasionally, a patient with PMF may develop an occult malignancy or a site of extramedullary hematopoiesis within the gastrointestinal tract, which may serve as a bleeding source.[161] Unexplained microcytosis (MCV < 80 fL) has been reported as a laboratory feature in PMF and in general not has been shown to have prognostic relevance.[200] Macrocytic anemia may complicate PMF.[201] Folic acid absorption is normal in these patients, and the folic acid deficiency probably results from increased use.[201]

Leukopenia can occur in 13% to 25% of patients, and leukocytosis is seen in one third.[1–3,7,9] Occasional blast cells and granulocytes with the pseudo-Pelger-Huët anomaly are frequent findings.[1-3,7,9] The leukocyte alkaline phosphatase score was studied in 78 patients by Silverstein and Elveback,[202] and was high in 41 patients (>100), normal in 17 patients (30 to 100), and low in 20 patients (<30). In the Mayo Clinic series of 169 patients in the myelofibrotic phase of the disease, platelet counts of less than 100,000/mm^3 were observed in 31% of patients, and platelet counts of more than 800,000/mm^3 were observed in 12%.[3] In the prefibrotic phase of the disease, almost 90% of patients had platelet counts greater than 500,000/mm.[3,37] Defective platelet aggregation is common, and platelets frequently do not respond to collagen or epinephrine.[3] A variety of qualitative platelet anomalies have been documented by abnormal in vitro aggregation patterns.[203,204] In 15% of patients, abnormalities suggestive of ongoing DIC are found, including decreased platelet numbers, decreased levels of factor V and VIII, and increased fibrin-split products.[3] Usually, when DIC occurs in PMF, it produces no symptoms and unfortunately may only become clinically apparent after surgical intervention. Associated liver dysfunction may also be a contributory factor to prolongation of the prothrombin time.

Additional laboratory abnormalities are quite common. In one series, lactic acid levels were elevated in 95% of patients, bilirubin levels in 40%, uric acid in 60%, and alkaline phosphate and serum glutamic oxaloacetic transaminase levels in 50%.[5] Patients with PMF have decreased levels of total cholesterol.[205,206] The ratio of high-density lipoprotein cholesterol to low-density lipoprotein cholesterol is diminished.[205,206]

A variety of immunologic abnormalities have been reported in PMF, including the presence of antinuclear antibodies, elevated rheumatoid factor titers, direct Coombs test positivity, lupus-type circulating anticoagulants, hypocomplementemia, marrow lymphoid nodules, and increased circulating immune complexes.[207-211] In one series of 50 patients with PMF, increased quantities of circulating immune complexes were detected in 39% and found to be associated with increased disease activity as manifested by increased transfusion requirements, bone pain, and fever.[207] Some investigators have suggested that abnormalities of the complement system may be important in the disease progression of PMF,[210] and others have hypothesized that low levels of C3 may predispose these patients to develop serious bacterial infections.[207] A remarkably high incidence of monoclonal gammopathies has been reported in PMF, with such benign gammopathies occurring in 8% to 10% of patients in some series.[212,213] Ten cases of the simultaneous occurrence of a plasma cell dyscrasia and PMF have been reported.[3,212,213]

Successful bone marrow aspiration is unusual, accomplished in only 6 of 48 cases in one series, with the tap completely dry in 50% of cases.[5] A bone marrow biopsy is necessary in all cases for the diagnosis and monitoring of the disease. The amount of residual hematopoietic cellular tissue and the degree of marrow fibrosis are the key elements that should be assessed. Table 70–3 summarizes the appearance of bone marrow biopsies in the series of Varki and associates.[5] Some caution should be taken in using repeated bone marrow biopsy specimens to diagnose PMF. Cases in which a marrow biopsy was performed at the site of a previous bone injury during the healing process frequently results in confusion because of primary callus formation at that site.[214] Most marrow biopsies in PMF are hypercellular and are remarkable for increased numbers of megakaryocytes. Bone marrow fibrosis and osteosclerosis were seen in 67% and 54% of cases, respectively.[5,8] The characteristic morphologic features include patchiness of the hematopoietic cellularity and the reticulin fibrosis, some microscopic fields being cellular and others depleted of hematopoietic cells. The amount of neticulin may vary from field to field. The megakaryocytes are increased in numbers and often are arranged around and within the sinuses and not always clustered in groups. They are large with irregular, roundish, cloud-like nuclei[8] and distended marrow sinusoids frequently containing intravascular hematopoiesis.[8,47,215,216] The marrow biopsies reveal a substantial increase in vascularity. The marrow microvessels are more tortuous and branched than observed in normal controls. The increased microvessel density is correlated with increased VEGF expression by megakaryocytes. A rare histological variant of PMF is the so-called myelofibrosis with fatty bone marrow,[7-9] in which the bone marrow is characterized by myeloid hypoplasia associated with fairly complete fatty substitution, mimicking bone marrow of aplastic anemia. These patients frequently have areas of clusters of densely aggregated hematopoietic elements exhibiting the histopathological characteristics of PMF and large numbers of hematopoietic progenitors circulating in their peripheral blood.[9] This variant of PMF is likely due to the abnormal trafficking of hematopoietic cells from the bone marrow to extramedullary sites. Consistent with the osteosclerosis observed in patients with PMF, increased thickness of some bone units with new lamellae and focal areas of woven bone. There is a net decrease in osteoclast number and conversion of trabecular pillars into plates.[217]

Table 70–3 Bone Marrow Biopsy Findings at Diagnosis of Patients with Primary Myelofibrosis

Finding	Incidence (%)*
Percentage of hematopoietic cells	
0–25	6
26–50	10
51–75	31
76–100	52
Pattern of cellularity	
Diffuse	71
Patchy	29
Megakaryocytes	
Increased	90
Decreased	4
Normal	6
Granulocytes	
Increased	70
Immaturity	8
Percentage of fibrosis/collagen (H&E stain)	
0–10	79
11–25	15
26–50	2
51–100	4
Reticulin fibrosis (Gomori stain)†	
1+	12
2+	21
3+	46
Osteosclerosis	54

*Based on a total of 48 biopsies.
†Based on a scale of 1+ to 4+.
H&E, hematoxylin and eosin.
Adapted from Varki A, Lottenberg R, Griffin R, Reinhard E: The syndrome of idiopathic myelofibrosis: Clinicopathologic review with emphasis on the prognostic variables predicting survival. Medicine (Baltimore) 62:353, 1983.

In Wolf and Neiman's series, morphologic evidence of progression of fibrosis was present in only 1 of 21 cases in which sequential biopsies were obtained.[218] No connection was observed between bone marrow cellularity, fibrosis, and splenic size.[218] In contrast, Lohmann and Beckman[219] observed progressive fibrosis in 18 of 20 patients who did not have maximal myelofibrosis at the time of the initial biopsy.[219] Thiele and colleagues[215] presented data to indicate an early prefibrotic subtype of PMF with no or minimal marrow reticulin and another phase with conspicuous fibrosis and osteosclerotic changes of the marrow. Based on a careful histomorphometric evaluation of the bone marrow they concluded that in a subset of patients there was a progressive fibroosteosclerotic process during the evolution of the disease that was paralleled by an increase in numbers of small megakaryocytes with irregular perimeters and megakaryocytes with naked nuclei.[8,215] The clinical and morphologic findings of patients with the prefibrotic stage of PMF have been further characterized[8,37,220-225] (Tables 70–4 and 70–5). Although a steady progression to marrow fibrosis has been demonstrated in patients with the

Table 70–4 Characteristics of Patients with the Prefibrotic Phase of Primary Myelofibrosis

Characteristics	Patients (%)
Anemia (hemoglobin g/dL £ <12.5 female, <14.0 male)	38
Splenomegaly (≥2 cm below costal margin)	15
Thrombocythemia	
(≥500 × 10^9/L)	88
(≥1000 × 10^9/L)	34
Leukocytosis (≥0 × 10^9/L)	51
Erythroblasts (peripheral blood >1%)	3
Myeloblasts (peripheral blood >0%)	4
Lactate dehydrogenase (>300 U/L)	20
Leukocyte alkaline phosphatase (score >80)	24

Adapted from Thiele J, Kvasnicka HM, Zankovick R, Diehl V: Clinical and morphological criteria for the diagnosis of prefibrotic idiopathic (primary) myelofibrosis. Ann Hematol;80:160,2001.

Table 70–5 Morphologic Findings in Patients with the Prefibrotic Phase of Primary Myelofibrosis

Blood

No or mild leukoerythroblastosis
No or minimal red blood cell poikilocytosis; few or no dacryocytes

Bone marrow

Hypercellularity
Neutrophilic proliferation
Megakaryocytic proliferation and atypia (eg, clustering of megakaryocytes, abnormally lobulated megakaryocytic nuclei, naked megakaryocytic nuclei)
Minimal or absent reticulin fibrosis

Adapted from Thiele J, Pierre R, Imbert M, et al: Chronic idiopathic myelofibrosis. In Jaffe ES, Harris N, Stein H, Vardiman JW (eds): World Health Organization's Tumors of Hematopoietic and Lymphoid Tissues. Washington, DC, IARC Press, 2001, p 35.

prefibrotic phase,[8,37,220–225] fibrosis may remain static or diminish in the more advanced stages of PMF.[225]

Different scoring systems for pathologically grading the marrow cellularity and fibrosis have been employed with the aim of staging and documenting progression of the disease.[222] In a recent European consensus conference, the importance of age-dependent decrease in cellularity was recognized.[226] Grading of myelofibrosis was simplified by using four easily reproducible categories including differentiation between reticulin and collagen. A consensus was reached that the density of fibers must be assessed in relation to the hematopoietic tissue. This feature is especially important in order to avoid a false impression of a reduced fiber content in fatty and/or edematous bone marrow samples after treatment[226] (Table 70–6). Bock and coworkers have shown that progression of marrow fibrosis in PMF is accompanied by expression of subsets of collagenases which is independent of the Jak2V617F status.[227]

Morphologic examination of the spleen reveals foci of extramedullary hematopoiesis in the sinusoids of the red pulp, where megakaryocytes, myeloid elements, and nucleated erythroid elements are seen.[8,175,218,228] Follicular atrophy in the white pulp frequently occurs.[218] The extramedullary hematopoietic cells belonging to each of the myeloid lineages can be distributed in the spleen diffusely or be limited to macronodules. The predominance of immature granulocytic forms is associated with an especially poor prognosis.[8,228]

Table 70–6 Grading of Myelofibrosis according to the European Consensus Criteria

Grading	Description*
MF-0	Scattered linear reticulin with no intersections (cross-overs) corresponding to normal bone marrow
MF-1	Loose network of reticulin with many intersections, especially in perivascular areas
MF-2	Diffuse and dense increase in reticulin with extensive intersections, occasionally with focal bundles of collagen and/or focal osteosclerosis
MF-3	Diffuse and dense increase in reticulin with extensive intersections and coarse bundles of collagen, often associated with osteosclerosis

*The quality of the reticulin stain should be assessed by detection of normal staining in vessel walls as internal control. The degree of myelofibrosis should be assessed by disregarding lymphoid nodules and vessels and disregarding fibers framing adipocytes. Areas of prominent scleredema and/or scarring should be included in the overall grading of myelofibrosis. Fiber density should be assessed in hematopoietic areas.
Data from: Thiele J, Kvasnicka HM, Facchetti F, Franco V, van der Walt J, Orazi A: European consensus on grading bone marrow fibrosis and assessment of cellularity. Haematologica 90:1128, 2005

Pathologic examination of the liver reveals hematopoietic cellular elements within the sinusoids. Sinusoidal dilatation is a common finding, as well as prominent intrahepatocyte and Kupffer cell hemosiderin deposition. A marked increase in the hepatic reticulin network has also been observed.[175]

Approximately 30% to 75% of patients with PMF have karyotypic abnormalities at diagnosis.[229–233] It is important to perform cytogenetic analysis on this patient population to discriminate PMF from CML.[233] Detection of a Philadelphia chromosome or *BCR-ABL* fusion gene indicates that the marrow fibrosis results from CML. In cases that are Philadelphia chromosome negative, it is prudent to perform polymerase chain reaction (PCR) analysis for *BCR-ABL* to exclude the diagnosis of CML. Chromosomal abnormalities in PMF have been reported to involve chromosomes 1, 2, 5 to 13, 15, 17, 18, 20, 21, and the Y chromosome.[125–127,229–233] Reilly and associates[232] reported that three cytogenetic patterns (ie, 13q–, 20q–, and partial trisomy 1q) were seen in 65% of all cases with an abnormal karyotype. In a series from Mayo Clinic,[233] 20q–, 13q–, and trisomy 8 were the most frequent individual abnormalities in PMF, whereas abnormalities of chromosomes 1, 5, 7, and 9 were almost universally associated with coexisting abnormalities.[233] The presence of clones with trisomy 8 or 12p– as well as chromosome 7 deletions have been associated with an adverse prognosis.[233–235] A correlation between the presence of multiple chromosomal deletions and poor survival has been reported.[235] The deletions of chromosome 13 have been shown to include the region of the retinoblastoma gene *(RB1)*, which is a putative tumor suppressor gene.[236] Translocations involving 12q have also been described. Rearrangement of the HMGA2 gene in two PMF patients with 12q aberrations has been described, and overexpression of HMGA2 was observed in these patients as well as in 10 of 10 patients with PMF without 12q abnormalities.[237] Since HMGA2 is known to play a major role in fetal growth and development, HMGA2 activation has been proposed to play an important role in the pathogenesis of PMF.[237] Partial or complete losses of chromosomes, particularly chromosomes 5 and 7, appear to be associated with the use of chemotherapeutic agents for the treatment of PMF.[230–233] An association between erythroid hypoplasia in PMF and a defect on chromosome 11 has been reported.[238] It is not unusual for a leukemic transformation of PMF to be preceded by additional cytogenetic abnormalities, a finding consistent with a multistep process leading to a leukemic transformation.[239] An unbalanced translocation between chromosomes 1 and 6 with specific breakpoints, der(6)t(1;6)(q21–23;p21.3), was described in patients with typical

PMF by Dingli and associates, suggesting that this translocation is a highly specific cytogenetic anomaly for PMF.[125] Since the marrow is almost uniformly unable to be aspirated in PMF, cytogenetic analysis are frequently performed on peripheral blood cells leading to a high proportion of failed studies. Cytogenetic abnormalities can however be detectable by fluorescence in situ hybridization (FISH) on deparaffinized sections of bone marrow biopsy specimens. FISH analysis can also be more sensitive than conventional cytogenetics for detecting specific aberrations such as 20q- and 13q-.[127]

Investigation of PMF by a comparative genomic hybridization technique suggests that genomic aberrations are much more common than has been previously indicated by conventional cytogenetic analysis and occur in the majority of cases.[127] Gains of 9p were the most frequent finding, occurring in 50% of patients, suggesting that genes on 9p may play a crucial role in the pathogenesis of PMF.[185] This observation, together with the observation that loss of heterozygosity at 9p was a frequent stem cell defect in polycythemia vera, served as a foundation for the discovery of normal *V617F* mutation in MPD.[240]

In PMF the proportion of patients with normal V617F mutation in granulocytes has been reported to range from 35% to 95%.[113,114,241,242] The detection rate for Jak2V617F is much higher for patients with post-PV MF (91%) than PMF (45%) or post-ET MF (39%).[119] In PV a high burden of Jak2V617F allele has been associated with an increased rate of evolution to myelofibrosis.[119,243] Such wide differences in the mutational frequencies can be attributed to the different sensitivity of the techniques used to detect the mutation and to differences in the case-mix of the reported series, ie, proportion of idiopathic and secondary PMF cases. Tefferi and coworkers[119] have reported that the Jak2 mutation in PMF is associated with an older patient age at diagnosis and a history of thrombosis or pruritus. The clinical utility of performing normal mutation in patients with PMF is yet to be defined. The quasi-perfect specificity of the mutation for a Philadelphia-negative MPD may be used in the process of diagnosing patients in whom the cause of bone marrow fibrosis cannot be immediately attributed to PMF. Moreover, since the proportion of *Jak2* mutated alleles in granulocytes has been reported to reflect the progression of the disease,[140] this measurement may be also used for monitoring the response to therapeutic agents during cytoreductive therapies.

Gain-of-function mutations of the thrombopoietin receptor, MPLW515L and MPLW515K, are present in patients with PMF at a frequency of approximately 5%, 1% of patients with ET, but not patients with PV.[120,121] MPL mutations may occur concurrently with the normal V617F mutation, suggesting that these alleles may have functional complementation in MPD.[121] In all cases the MPLW515K/L mutant allele is present in excess of the Jak2V617F allele.[120] In contrast to acute myeloid leukemia, mutations in the receptor tyrosine kinases KIT, FMS, FLT3 have not been documented in PMF.[244,245]

The number of circulating cells expressing the CD34 antigen, a phenotypic marker of hematopoietic stem and progenitor cells, in patients with PMF has been reported to be more than 300 times higher than in normal volunteers and 18 to 30 times higher than in patients with PV or ET.[55–57] The clinical utility of the cytofluorimetric measurement of CD34+ cells as a diagnostic marker of PMF is hampered by the fact that a small number of subjects with PMF exhibit a normal number of $CD34^{+}$ cells in the peripheral blood. Arora and coworkers[246] found that 14% of patients with PMF and post-ET and post-PV MF had peripheral blood CD34 positive cell numbers that did not exceed the upper limit of the normal reference range (5×10^6/L). Cases with a very mild disease phenotype, absent or slight reticulin BM fibrosis account for the majority of these patients. CD34+ cell numbers may be otherwise used for monitoring the disease course, and the response to therapies. High values of CD34+ cells (>200 $\times 10^6$/L) indicate an accelerated phase of the disease.[55]

Other biomarkers of a myeloproliferative process, such as decreased expression of the receptor for thrombopoietin (c-MPL) by platelets,[247] or overexpression of the polycythemia rubra vera-1 gene (*PRV-1*),[247–249] have been reported in variable proportions of patients with PMF, but their assessment seems to not have clinical utility in practice.

On radiographic examination, the characteristic features of PMF are a diffuse increase in bone density and increased prominence of the bony trabeculae. This increased bone density may be patchy and can produce a mottled appearance. Such abnormalities have been reported in 25% to 66% of patients with PMF.[3]

Noninvasive imaging of bone marrow is a promising means of evaluating the bone marrow cellularity and distribution in PMF. Magnetic resonance imaging (MRI) can portray the conversion or reconversion of fatty to cellular marrow.[250,251] Fibrotic marrow is easily distinguished from cellular marrow by its strikingly low signal intensity with all pulse signals.[250] Kaplan and colleagues[250] reported that marrow patterns in the proximal femurs of PMF patients correlated with the clinical severity of the disease and that might be useful in staging and evaluating the progression of the disease process.[251] Marrow MRI has been used to differentiate PMF from ET, where the marrow adipose tissue is preserved, while in PMF, the adiposity of the marrow is reduced.[252]

The specificity of ^{18}F-FLT (3′–^{18}F-fluoro-3′-deoxy-L-thymidine) uptake for cycling cells and the high resolution of PET (positron emission tomography) have brought to use ^{18}F-FLT PET to visualize the proliferative activities of bone marrow in PMF.[253] Displacement of tracer uptake in bones of the long extremity, spleen and liver but reduced in the iliac crest and spine was a typical imaging pattern in PMF that might have a diagnostic and staging relevance.[253]

DIFFERENTIAL DIAGNOSIS

A patient with hepatosplenomegaly, peripheral cytopenias, teardrop poikilocytosis, leukoerythroblastosis, and marrow fibrosis probably has PMF, but other disorders may lead to this clinical picture (see Table 70–1 and Fig. 70–2).[9,10] Two sets of criteria for the diagnosis of PMF have been previously created (Tables 70–7 and 70–8).[10,220] The Cologne Criteria are particularly useful because they provide a tool with which to diagnose the prefibrotic phase of the disease.[220]

Table 70–7 The Cologne Criteria for the Diagnosis and Staging of Primary Myelofibrosis

A. No preceding or allied other subtype of myeloproliferative disorders or MDS
B. Splenomegaly (on palpation or >11 cm on ultrasound).
C. Thrombocythemia (platelet count ≥500 $\times 10^9$/L)
D. Anemia (Hb < 12 g/dL)
E. Definite leukoerythroblastic blood picture
F. Histopathology: granulocytic plus megakaryocytic myeloproliferation with large, multilobulated nuclei containing megakaryocytes that show abnormal clustering and definitive maturation defects and
1. No reticulin fibrosis
2. Slight reticulin fibrosis
3. Marked increase (density) in reticulin fibers or collagen fibrosis
4. Osteosclerosis (endophytic bone formation)

Diagnosis and classification of PMF are acceptable if the following combinations are present:

Stage 1 A + B + C + F1 is consistent with a hypercellular (prefibrotic) stage clinically simulating ET.

Stage 2 A + B + C + D + F2 is consistent with early PMF. Stage 3 A + B + D + F3 is consistent with manifest IMF. Stage 4 A + B + D + E + F3 + 4 is consistent with advanced IMF complicated by osteosclerosis (osteomyelosclerosis).

ET, essential thrombocythemia (ET); Hb, hemoglobin; PMF, primary myelofibrosis; MDS, myelodysplastic syndrome

Data from Thiele J, Kvasnicka HM, Diehl V, et al: Clinicopathological diagnosis and differential criteria of thrombocythemias in various myeloproliferative disorders by histopathology, histochemistry and immunostaining by the bone marrow. Leuk Lymphoma 33:207, 1999.

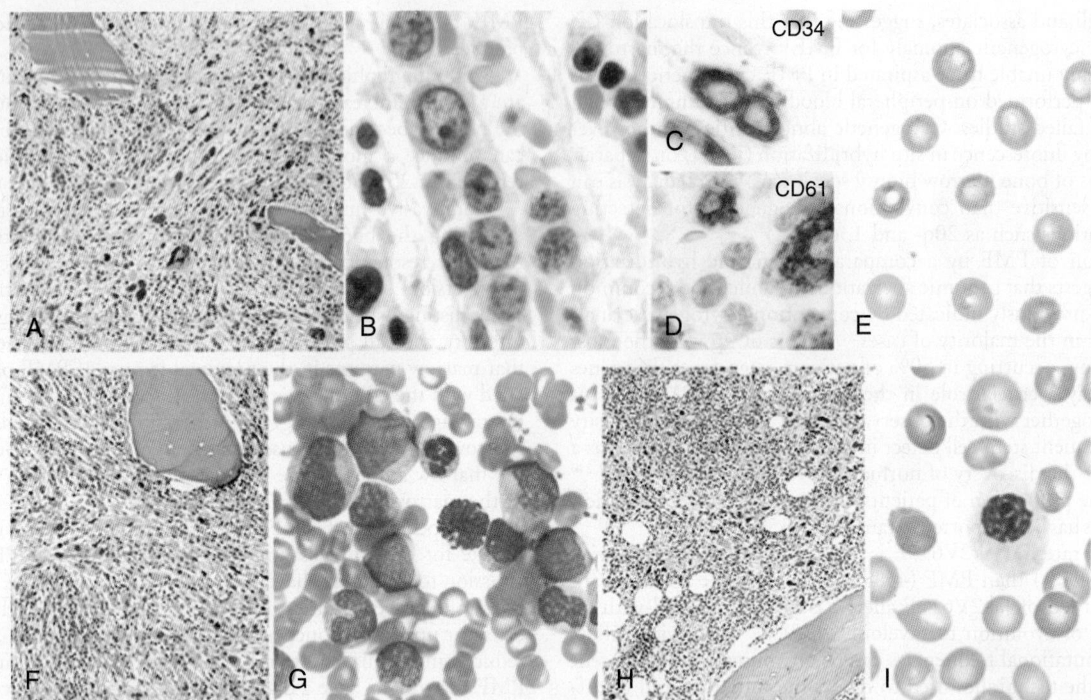

Figure 70–2 DIFFERENTIAL DIAGNOSTIC CONSIDERATIONS IN PMF. Acute panmyelosis with myelofibrosis (APMF) **A-E;** Chronic Myelogenous Leukemia (CML) in advances phase with fibrosis **F,G;** Myelodysplastic Syndrome (MDS) with fibrosis **H, I.** The bone marrow biopsy of APMF, CML in advanced phase with fibrosis, and MDS with fibrosis can all look similar to PMF at low power (**A, F, H**). In APMF the distinction from PMF is made in part by seeing increased immature cells on the biopsy (**B**) interspersed with other hematopoietic precursors. These are usually $CD34^+$ (**C**), but in contrast to acute megakaryoblastic leukemia are usually CD61 negative (**D**). Also the peripheral blood usually shows pancytopenia with neither teardrop red blood cells nor a leukoerythroblastosis (**E**). Although the biopsy of CML presenting in advanced phase can resemble PMF, the peripheral blood usually shows a classic granulocytosis with left shift and basophilia. In the case illustrated, the 30-year-old female patient had a fibrotic bone marrow (**F**), but presented with a WBC of 148K/μL showing a full spectrum of granulocytes, increased blasts (22%) and basophilia. P210 BCR/ABL was demonstrated.

Table 70–8 The Italian Criteria for the Diagnosis of Primary Myelofibrosis

Necessary criteria
A. Diffuse bone marrow fibrosis B. Absence of Philadelphia chromosome or *BCR-ABL* rearrangement in peripheral blood cells
Optional criteria
A. Splenomegaly of any grade B. Anisopoikilocytosis with teardrop erythrocytes C. Presence of circulating immature myeloid cells D. Presence of circulating erythroblasts E. Presence of clusters of megakaryoblasts and anomalous megakaryocytes in bone marrow sections F. Myeloid metaplasia
Diagnosis of PMF is acceptable if the following combinations are present:
• The two necessary criteria plus any other two optional criteria when splenomegaly is present, or • The two necessary criteria plus any other four optional criteria when splenomegaly is absent

Data from Barosi G, Ambrosetti A, Finelli C, et al: The Italian Consensus Conference on Diagnostic Criteria for Myelofibrosis with Myeloid Metaplasia. Br J Haematol 104:730, 1999.

Recently the World Health Organization (WHO) diagnostic criteria were revised, incorporating testing for Jak2V617F and activating MPL mutations (Table 70–9).[14,15] The WHO criteria are based upon the recognition of a prefibrotic form of PMF without reticulin fibrosis and that the primary diagnostic features of PMF are increased megakaryocyte numbers, megakaryocyte morphology and abnormalities of granulocyte mutation.[14,15] Secondary myelofibrosis frequently occurs in patients with lymphoma or metastatic carcinoma of the stomach, prostate, lung, and breast.[6,254–257] The clinician should be extremely careful in making the diagnosis of PMF in a patient who has a previous history of a primary neoplasm. Demonstration of carcinoma cells in the marrow establishes that metastatic carcinoma is the cause of the marrow fibrosis. Careful breast examination and mammography are indicated in all women suspected of having PMF to exclude the possibility of metastatic breast cancer. The finding of blastic or lytic bone lesions in patients with myelofibrosis suggests the presence of an underlying carcinoma. Disseminated tuberculosis and histoplasmosis have been associated with the development of secondary myelofibrosis.[3,258] Caseating or noncaseating granulomas observed on bone marrow biopsy suggest the presence of these infectious disorders. Identification of the causative organisms by culture techniques should be pursued.

A number of other primary hematologic disorders can also be accompanied by marrow fibrosis. The peripheral blood and marrow findings that allow differentiation of these disorders were reviewed by Dickstein and Vardiman (Table 70–9) and can be enhanced by Jak2V617F and MPLW515L/K mutational analysis.[60] A variant myelodysplastic syndrome with myelofibrosis has been described by Pagliuca and coworkers.[259] These patients frequently present with cytopenias and have dysplastic cellular abnormalities indistinguishable from those of other patients with myelodysplasia. Their marrows, however, are characterized by the presence of marrow fibrosis and a striking megakaryocytic hyperplasia, with a predominance of small hypolobulated forms, in some cases surrounding fibrosis. Reticulocytopenia is characteristic of these patients, as are teardrop red blood cells and a clinical picture of leukoerythroblastosis.[259] Unlike patients with PMF, patients with myelodysplasia and marrow fibrosis do not have hepatic or splenic enlargement extending more than 3 cm below the costal margin.[259] The overall survival time of patients with this

Table 70–9 Proposed Revised World Health Organization Criteria for Primary Myelofibrosis

Major criteria

1. Presence of megakaryocyte proliferation and atypia,* usually accompanied by either reticulin and/or collagen fibrosis, or, in the absence of significant reticulin fibrosis, the megakaryocyte changes must be accompanied by an increased bone marrow cellularity characterized by granulocytic proliferation and often decreased erythropoiesis (ie, prefibrotic cellular-phase disease)
2. Not meeting WHO criteria for PV†, CML‡, MDS§, or other myeloid neoplasm
3. Demonstration of *Jak2*617V > F or other clonal marker (eg, *MPL*515W > L/K), or in the absence of a clonal marker, no evidence of bone marrow fibrosis due to underlying inflammatory or other neoplastic diseases¶

Minor criteria

1. Leukoerythroblastosis‖
2. Increase in serum lactate dehydrogenase level‖
3. Anemia‖
4. Palpable splenomegaly‖

Diagnosis requires meeting all 3 major criteria and 2 minor criteria.
*Small to large megakaryocytes with an aberrant nuclear/cytoplasmic ratio and hyperchromatic, bulbous, or irregularly folded nuclei and dense clustering.
†Requires the failure of iron replacement therapy to increase hemoglobin level to the polycythemia vera range in the presence of decreased serum ferritin. Exclusion of polycythemia vera is based on hemoglobin and hematocrit levels. Red cell mass measurement is not required.
‡Requires the absence of *BCR-ABL*.
§Requires the absence of dyserythropoiesis and dysgranulopoiesis.
¶Secondary to infection, autoimmune disorder or other chronic inflammatory condition, hairy cell leukemia or other lymphoid neoplasm, metastatic malignancy, or toxic (chronic) myelopathies. It should be noted that patients with conditions associated with reactive myelofibrosis are not immune to primary myelofibrosis and the diagnosis should be considered in such cases if other criteria are met,
‖Degree of abnormality could be borderline or marked.
Data from Tefferi A, Thiele J, Orazi A, et al: Proposals and rationale for revision of the World Health Organization diagnostic criteria for polycythemia vera, essential thrombocythemia, and primary myelofibrosis: recommendations from an ad hoc international expert panel. Blood 110:1092, 2007.

variant of myelodysplasia has been reported to be 30 months, with death resulting from the effects of cytopenias or transformation to acute leukemia. Two additional studies indicated that the presence of myelofibrosis in patients with myelodysplasia was associated with a particularly short survival time (9.6 months) compared with patients with myelodysplasia without fibrosis (17.4 months).[260,261]

Hairy cell leukemia can also be confused with PMF.[5] In one study, 5 of 61 patients who had originally been diagnosed as having PMF were shown retrospectively to have had hairy cell leukemia.[5] Hairy cell leukemia can present as pancytopenia with splenomegaly and is associated with a dry marrow tap. In one series, marrow reticulin content was increased in 26 of 29 patients with hairy cell leukemia.[262] The presence of hairy mononuclear cells possessing tartrate-resistant acid phosphatase or the appropriate phenotype in the peripheral blood or marrow should facilitate differentiation of PMF from hairy cell leukemia[8] (see Chapter 84). This exercise is important because of the different modalities of treatment that can be successfully employed for hairy cell leukemia.

Marrow fibrosis can occur in patients with other MPDs, especially PV and CML, and less frequently with ET.[263] In CML, progressive marrow fibrosis may herald the onset of accelerated disease or blast crisis. Myelofibrosis in CML occurs in two distinct patterns, one in which patients present with CML and significant associated marrow fibrosis and a second in which the myelofibrosis develops late in the course of the CML.[264] The myelofibrosis in the latter group appears at a mean of 36 months after the diagnosis of CML, is associated with a mean survival time of 4.9 months from the detection of myelofibrosis, and therefore represents an ominous prognostic sign.[264]

Post-PV MF occurs in 5% to 15% of patients with PV.[263] This transition occurs, on average, 10 years after the initial diagnosis of PV is made, but in individual cases, it may appear after shorter or longer intervals.[263] PMF is clinically indistinguishable from post-PV MF except for the previous history of erythrocytosis in the latter group. Of patients with post-PV MF, 25% to 50% will develop leukemia, and 70% will be dead within 3 years of this transition.[263] Post-PV MF represents a transitional myeloproliferative syndrome with relatively grave prognostic implications. Myelofibrosis has also been reported after ET.[223] In a series of 195 patients with ET followed at a single institution, Cervantes and coworkers[223] observed 13 patients who developed myelofibrosis after a median follow-up of 7.2 years. The investigators claimed that these patients did not represent individuals with prefibrotic stages of PMF, but rather evolution of ET. They estimated the probability of developing such a complication to be 3% 5 years after diagnosis, 8% at 10 years, and 15% at 15 years, and considered this evolution to marrow fibrosis a major long-term complication of ET.[223] This evolution of ET was reported not to be associated with or prevented by the use of cytotoxic agents.[223] Thiele and associates,[224] however, suggested that most individuals with a presumptive diagnosis of ET whose disease evolved into post-ET MF suffered from prefibrotic PMF if strict diagnostic criteria were used. They have conjectured that a considerable number of patients who carry a diagnosis of ET already are actually in a prefibrotic phase of PMF.[224] Careful prospective natural history studies using strict histopathologic criteria will be required to resolve this controversy.

Acute panmyelosis with myelofibrosis (APMF) represents a clinical entity distinct from PMF.[265–267] This disorder has been termed also acute myelofibrosis, acute myelosclerosis, acute megakaryocytic myelofibrosis, and acute myelodysplasia with myelofibrosis. APMF is exceedingly rare and corresponds to less than 1% of the cases of acute myeloid leukemias (AML). Patients characteristically present with pancytopenia, fever, absence of clinically significant splenomegaly, minimal or absent teardrop poikilocytosis, and fibrotic bone marrow.[265–267] The bone marrow is characterized by the appearance of immature myeloid cells and the blast cells, which frequently express megakaryocytic phenotypic properties.[265] Survival ranges from 1 to 9 months after diagnosis. Its distinction from PMF is important, because aggressive chemotherapy and possibly stem cell transplantation are the treatments of choice. Even though some authors consider APMF a form of acute megakaryoblastic leukemia,[268] the WHO criteria for diagnosing APMF are somewhat distinct from those for acute megakaryoblastic leukemia (AMKL).[269] The main requirement for the diagnosis of AMKL is a minimum of 20% marrow blasts, a percentage that is significantly higher than observed in APMF. In addition, the blasts in all cases of AMKL stain strongly for CD61 and CD41 and are negative for myeloperoxidase. In contrast, APMF is characterized by a lower percentage of blasts within a polymorphic cellular background, which includes erythroblasts, megakaryocytes, and maturing myeloid elements with variability in their relative proportions from case to case. The blasts in APMF did not express significant reactivity to megakaryocytic phenotypic markers, but are identifiable by their strong reactivity with CD34 and occasional reactivity with myeloperoxidase. These results emphasized the panmyelotic nature of APMF.[265] In PMF, the peculiar cytologic characteristics of the megakaryocytes, which include anisocytosis with a predominance of large size forms arranged into tight cellular clusters, the abnormal chromatin clumping with hyperchromatic nuclei and clumped (cloud shape) nuclear lobulation as well as the characteristic stromal changes that include the presence of intrasinusoidal hematopoiesis allow for a distinction from these more acute disorders.

Pacquette and colleagues[270] reported that up to 12% of patients who present with myelofibrosis might suffer from an underlying autoimmune disorder such as systemic lupus erythematosus. Pullarkat and coworkers[271] suggested that primary autoimmune myelofibrosis (primary AIMF), represent a distinct clinicopathologic syndrome unrelated to other well-defined autoimmune disorders.

They described eight diagnostic criteria for AIMF, including grade 3 or 4 reticulin fibrosis in the marrow, lack of clustered or atypical megakaryocytes, lack of dysplasia or eosinophilia or basophilia, lymphoid infiltration of the marrow, lack of osteosclerosis, absent or mild splenomegaly, presence of autoantibodies, and absence of disorders associated with myelofibrosis. They described seven patients fulfilling most of these criteria, six of whom responded to therapy with steroids.[271] The appearance of the marrow in AIMF is indistinguishable from that of PMF. Autoimmune myelofibrosis occurs predominantly in females with a broad clinical spectrum. Patients may present with myelofibrosis in the setting of established systemic lupus or in patients with minimal manifestations of an autoimmune disorder as in primary AIMF.[269–272] The presence of teardrop erythrocytes or leukoerythroblastosis in a patient with lupus suggests autoimmune myelofibrosis. Such patients universally have a positive antinuclear antibody (ANA) test result or an elevated anti-DNA titer.[269–272] According to these authors, since the physical manifestations of an autoimmune disease may not be evident, all patients with myelofibrosis should have an ANA test to exclude an autoimmune etiology. Moreover, a diagnosis of AIMF is important because the cytopenias and marrow fibrosis in this disorder may partially resolve with steroid or methotrexate therapy.[269–272] However, it must be pointed out that the place of primary AIMF in the classification of fibrotic disorders needs a more precise definition. This is particularly true since in none of the reported cases categorized as primary AIMF was PMF excluded with the use of markers including hematopoietic cell clonality or presence of Jak2V617F or MPLW515L and MPLW515K.

TREATMENT AND COMPLICATIONS

Therapy

The optimal forms of treatment for PMF have not yet been defined, but reports of non-myeloablative allogeneic stem cell transplantation provide hope for cure of a subpopulation of these patients. A conservative approach to management is generally accepted, with observation of asymptomatic patients and therapeutic intervention reserved for patients with symptoms.[7,9,273] An alternative approach proposed by Pegrum and coworkers[274] provides for the institution of single-agent chemotherapy early in the course of the disease. Traditional chemotherapeutic or biologic response modifier regimens used have included busulfan (2–4 mg/day), 6-thioguanine (20–40 mg/day), and a combination of chlorambucil (15 mg/day) and prednisone (30 mg/day), administered intermittently for a course of 3 to 4 weeks with a 2-week rest interval between courses, interferon-α, or low-dose melphalan therapy.[7,9,274–285] Such an approach may be associated with reduction in spleen size, and some investigators have claimed reversal of marrow fibrosis with reduction in the number of teardrop red cells, poikilocytosis, and leukoerythroblastosis.[276–285] Hydroxyurea appears to be a useful agent for the treatment of PMF. Its use has been associated with significantly reduced platelet numbers and a reduction of megakaryocytic abnormalities, as well as a significant reduction of myelofibrosis.[107,280,281] Some investigators have hypothesized that hydroxyurea-induced suppression of megakaryocytopoiesis causes a reduction in the levels of platelet-derived fibrogenic cytokines, resulting in reduced fibroblast proliferation and deposition of reticulin.[280] Manoharan[281] has shown that moderate doses (20–30 mg/kg) of hydroxyurea given twice or three times weekly are effective and safe in PMF patients requiring treatment. Similar reports have appeared after the use of busulfan; Chang and Gross[282] have reported three patients with PMF who responded to daily busulfan therapy with the achievement of hematologic remission and reversal of myelofibrosis. Not only did hematologic parameters, including the hemoglobin and hematocrit levels, improve, but a reduction of the number of teardrop erythrocytes and the degree of leukoerythroblastosis occurred. Most importantly, the quality of life of these individuals improved.[282] Judicious use of busulfan is recommended in this setting, however, because of its potential for producing delayed marrow suppression. Petti and colleagues[284] reported the use of melphalan administered at low doses (2.5 mg given 3 times/week) in 99 evaluable patients with PMF. Melphalan was well tolerated and produced less hematologic toxicity than busulphan. Among 16 patients with severe anemia requiring transfusion therapy, 38% became transfusion independent, and 20% experienced a 50% reduction in their transfusion requirement. Approximately 54% of patients with symptomatic splenomegaly experienced a clinically significant reduction in spleen size.[284] The median duration of the response to melphalan therapy was somewhat longer than 2 years. The disease of more than 20% of the patients receiving melphalan evolved into the leukemic phase. It is impossible to determine whether melphalan therapy played a role in this evolution or if this rate of blastic transformation was a consequence of the advanced stage of the disease at the time of treatment. The use of this agent was associated with acceptable toxicity, with only 13% of patients stopping their therapy because of the development of cytopenias and 17% requiring a dose reduction because of hematologic toxicity.[284] Whether low-dose melphalan therapy is superior to other chemotherapeutic agents or biologic response modifiers and has a significant effect on long-term survival will require further study.

Interferon-α has been suggested as a biologic response modifier that might alter the course of PMF.[285] It can be useful in suppressing thrombocytosis and inhibiting the activity of PDGF, which stimulates the proliferation of fibroblasts. Bourantos and coworkers[286] reported the use of the combination of interferon, granulocyte-macrophage colony-stimulating factor (GM-CSF), and erythropoietin in seven patients with PMF. Each of these patients had an aspirable marrow with megakaryocytic hyperplasia but only mild to moderate deposition of reticulin fibers.[286] Six of seven patients enjoyed marked reductions in spleen size.[286] Each of these patients had an increase of 1 g/dL or more in the hemoglobin concentration. In one patient, the degree of marrow fibrosis was diminished. These investigators suggested that interferon might decrease the rate of fibrosis if administered chronically during the early course of this disease.[286] Tefferi and associates[287] treated 11 patients with PMF with interferon-α (3 million international units given three times each week for the first 3 months). If no unacceptable side effects were experienced, the dose was increased to 15 million international units weekly. Only four patients were able to complete 1 year of therapy; the other seven patients discontinued the drug because of unacceptable toxicity or the development of severe cytopenias. No clinically significant improvement was observed in any of these patients. Interferon therapy did not appear to alter the degree of bone marrow fibrosis, osteosclerosis, or angiogenesis.[287] The clinician probably should expect only modest benefits to be derived from interferon-α therapy for PMF after patients have entered the more advanced phases of the disease. Whether interferon-α may be more effective during the prefibrotic phase of PMF requires careful study in a large randomized trial.

Therapy is indicated for PMF patients with the following conditions: symptoms attributable to anemia, pressure symptoms related to splenomegaly, bleeding problems, or life-threatening thrombocytopenia, significant hyperuricemia bone pain, systemic symptoms (fevers, night sweats and weight loss), and portal hypertension and life-threatening gastrointestinal bleeding.[3,7,11,12,288] Hyperuricemia should be aggressively treated in all patients with PMF. Hydration and chronic administration of allopurinol (300 mg/day) are suggested.[3]

Anemia is a common problem in patients with PMF. It is usually multifactorial in origin; contributing factors are folate deficiency, iron deficiency, ineffective erythropoiesis, erythroid hypoplasia, and hemolysis.[194–196] Patients with documented nutritional deficiencies should receive folate or iron supplementation, or both. Transfusion therapy with packed red blood cells is clearly indicated in patients who are symptomatic from their anemia. Chronic transfusion therapy is frequently required, and the clinician should try to attain a hemoglobin level at which symptoms resolve. Long-term transfusion therapy potentially may lead to the development of iron overload syndrome. Thus, serious consideration should be given to early institution of iron chelation therapy. For a handful of patients, transfusion requirements have been reported to be reduced after desferrioxamine or deferasirox therapy.[289] Since an oral effective iron chelator, deferasirox, is now available; therapy should be initiated early in the course of the disease when repeated cell transfusion therapy is required.[289] The remainder of approaches to the anemic patient deals with therapeutic interventions designed to avoid or diminish the number of transfusions administered.

Low-dose dexamethasone has been reported to be useful in the treatment of patients with transfusion-dependent PMF.[290] Whether these cases represent steroid responses of autoimmune-induced myelofibrosis and not classic PMF remains unknown. Low-dose melphalan therapy has been successfully used to reduce the transfusion requirements of a reasonable number of PMF patients.[284] Corticosteroids (eg, prednisone 1 mg/kg/day taken orally) have also been successfully employed for treatment of the hemolytic anemia associated with PMF.[1–3,7,9,291] Silverstein[3] reported a 2-gram increase in hemoglobin in 29% of men and 52% of women. Folate should be simultaneously administered to all such patients. Bouroncle and Doan[291] reported even more encouraging results with simultaneous administration of busulfan and corticosteroids, with clinical responses lasting 6 to 12 months. After patients have reached a peak response, tapering of prednisone should be initiated to determine an acceptable maintenance dose. The hemolytic process frequently recurs after such tapering. It is important to be aware that the hemolytic anemia in patients with PMF may also be a consequence of a coexisting secondary form of paroxysmal nocturnal hemoglobinuria.[292] In addition, a case of paroxysmal cold hemoglobinuria associated with a Donath-Landsteiner antibody has also been described.[293] Furthermore, patients with PMF who receive multiple transfusions are candidates for developing delayed hemolytic transfusion reactions which occasionally may be severe and persistent.[294] The direct antiglobulin test is usually positive in this setting. It is generally believed that additional transfusions in these patients with delayed hemolytic transfusion reactions should be avoided if possible. Other therapeutic options include steroids, intravenous immunoglobulins, and recombinant human erythropoietin-α (rHuEPO).[294]

Erythroid failure and ineffective erythropoiesis in PMF may respond to anabolic steroids.[1–3,7,9,295–298] Gardner and Nathan[295] have recommended that all patients with PMF and anemia should receive a trial of androgens. A number of preparations have been suggested, including testosterone enanthate (600 mg/week IM), stanozolol (12 mg/day taken orally), nandrolone (3 mg/kg/week IM), fluoxymesterone (10 mg taken orally 3 times daily), and oxymetholone (50 mg taken orally 4 times daily). A good response, as defined by a decrease or total avoidance of transfusion therapy, occurs in about 50% of patients. A course of 3 to 6 months of androgen therapy is indicated to identify responsive patients,[295] but the development of hepatic dysfunction or virilizing side effects may limit long-term androgen administration. Besa and colleagues[298] indicated that patients with associated chromosomal abnormalities were less likely to respond to androgen therapy. Danazol, a synthetic attenuated androgen, has been useful in reducing the requirement for red blood cell transfusion support and correction of thrombocytopenia.[299] Danazol appears to be a potentially effective therapy for PMF, which is mainly characterized by marrow failure.[299] Cervantes and colleagues[300] reported 33 patients with PMF who were either transfusion dependent or had hemoglobin levels below 10 g/dL who received an initial dose of 600 mg/day of danazol. Of the 30 evaluable patients, a favorable response was seen in 11 (37%), with 27% having a complete response. The median time to response was 5 months (range 1–9 months). Variables associated with response were lack of transfusion requirement and higher Hb levels. In 8 out of 30 patients (27%) a moderate increase of liver enzyme levels was reported. It is unknown whether any of the anabolic steroids preparations are superior to the others, or whether they are superior to danazol in improving anemia of PMF.

Early reports of rHuEPO therapy have suggested that rHuEPO alone does not improve the anemia associated with PMF.[301,302] However, the experience with the use of rHuEPO in PMF has been recently reviewed by Cervantes and colleagues in a total of 51 patients,[303] documenting that 28 (55%) of these patients responded to rHuEPO treatment including 16 complete and 12 partial responses. Endogenous serum levels inappropriately low for the degree of anemia is predictive of a favorable response to rHuEPO. Serum Epo levels less than 125 U/L were found to be associated with a favorable response to rHuEPO therapy. Lower number of responders were reported in a small trial, in which only 4 (16%) of 25 patients responded and in which the variables associated with response were favorable cytogenetic abnormalities (13q– or 20q–) and absence of a higher burden of the normal V617F mutation.[304] Responses are also associated with a limited enlargement of the spleen, and a small red cell transfusion requirement.

The use of darbepoetin, a novel hyperglycosylated erythropoiesis-stimulating protein, has been reported in 20 PMF patients.[305] With an initial weekly dose of 150 μg, increased to 300 μg, when no response was observed after 4 to 8 weeks, eight patients (40%) responded to treatment, including six complete and two partial responses, and five maintained their response after a median follow-up of 12 months (range 4–22 months). The median time to response was 2 months. Univariate analysis indicated that older age was the only factor associated with a favorable response to treatment (P = 0.006). None of the patients with elevated serum erythropoietin levels responded. Treatment was usually well tolerated and patients can be successfully switched from rHuEPO to darbepoetin.

Multiple trials have explored the use of thalidomide in the treatment of anemia in PMF, based on this drug's antiangiogenic, immunomodulatory, and antiinflammatory actions.[306–311] A pooled analysis of five small phase II studies published from 2000 to 2002 have indicated that 29% percent of patients with moderate to severe anemia can experience an increase in hemoglobin or reduction/elimination of blood transfusion requirements, with thalidomide therapy at a standard dose of 200 to 800 mg a day.[312] Nevertheless, most of the patients treated with these doses suffered from adverse effects that resulted in an attrition rate of greater than 50% after 3 months. Moreover, increases of white blood cell numbers and/or platelet counts were frequently reported to be associated with such serious adverse events as pericardial effusions secondary to myeloid metaplasia. Using a dose-escalation design and starting with a low dose of thalidomide (50 mg per day), Marchetti and colleagues[313] reported that 31% of patients with transfusion-dependent anemia experienced a response after treatment. Combining low-dose thalidomide (50 mg/day) with prednisone, Mesa and colleagues[314] reported that the regimen was better tolerated and equally or more effective than standard dose treatment.[314] Although the size of the patient population was limited, with this regimen 40% of patients with a red blood cell transfusion requirement became transfusion independent, and 95% of the patients were able to complete the 3-month course of therapy with acceptable toxicity.[314] The median hemoglobin level was reported to increase by 1.8 g/dL after low-dose thalidomide and prednisone therapy. This regimen also had a significant effect on the degree of thrombocytopenia and resulted in a reduction in the degree of splenomegaly in almost 10% of the patients.[314] These responses were frequently maintained after therapy was halted.[315] More recent reports provided further evidence that higher doses of thalidomide were not more effective than lower doses. Abgrall and colleagues[316] reported a prospective phase II B, randomized double-blind multicenter trial comparing therapy with 200 to 400 mg thalidomide with placebo, and documented that in the thalidomide group, in which only 10 of 26 patients completed 6 months of treatment, no difference was observed between the thalidomide and placebo groups as regards improvement of hemoglobin levels or reduction of the number of red blood cell transfusion required.[316] Thomas and coworkers reported the experience with thalidomide therapy in a two-stage phase II dose-escalation trial in 44 patients with advanced PMF.[317] Starting at 200 mg daily and increasing to 800 mg as tolerated, the median tolerated dose was 400 mg for a median duration of 3 months; and 20% of the patients experienced improvement in their degree of anemia (21% became transfusion independent).[317] Recently a more potent thalidomide analog, lenalidomide, has been evaluated in 68 symptomatic patients with PMF at two institutions.[318] Oral lenalidomide was administered at a dose of 10 mg/day if the platelet count was ≥100,000/mm^3 or at a dose of 5 mg/day if the platelet count was <100,000/mm^3 for 3 to 4 months. The overall response rates were 22% for patients with anemia, 33% for patients with splenomegaly and 50% for thrombocytopenia. Several patients normalized their hemoglobin levels or became red blood cell transfusion independent. The most common associated toxicities were grade 3 and 4 neutropenia and thrombocytopenia which occurred in approximately 30% of patients but resolved with discontinuation of therapy. In several patients with del(5)(q31) associated PMF or post-PV MF, lenalidomide therapy was associated with reduction of the numbers of cells with a marker chromosome as assayed by FISH and reduction of the Jak2V617F burden.[319] Lenalidomide therapy in combination with prednisone therapy in PMF is currently being evaluated in a cooperative group setting.

Pressure symptoms caused by splenic enlargement can be treated initially with cytotoxic chemotherapy. Busulfan, chlorambucil and prednisone, 6-thioguanine, radioactive phosphorus, melphalan and hydroxyurea (15–20 mg/kg 3 times each week) have each been used for this purpose.[1–3,9,284] In the Mayo Clinic series, a significant reduction in spleen size with relief of pressure symptoms occurred in 70% of patients receiving chemotherapy.[3] Responses are unfortunately short lived, lasting a median of only 4.5 months.[3] Only 16% of patients with long-term maintenance therapy enjoyed sustained relief of symptoms.[3] Hematologic toxicity often necessitates cessation of therapy.

Splenic irradiation frequently has been used for treatment of the painful, large spleen syndrome.[3,4,320–323] Irradiation in fractions of 0.15 to 1 Gy administered daily or by an intermittent fractionation schedule (ie, 2–3 times/week) to a total dose per treatment course of 2.5 to 6.5 Gy may be effective.[3,4,320–323] Responses are transient, lasting an average of 3.5 months, and hematopoietic toxicity is frequently significant. Wagner and associates[322] recommended simultaneous treatment with splenic irradiation and oral hydroxyurea and have obtained some promising results. Silverstein[3] reported that splenic irradiation was especially useful for treatment of splenic pain of sudden onset and for treatment of ascites due to implants of hematopoietic tissue. Radiation therapy should be considered as a temporary measure to be employed in patients who are too ill to tolerate splenectomy or chemotherapy. In one series, the median duration of response to irradiation was 6 months, and the median survival after irradiation was 20 months.[320] Splenic irradiation is limited by myelosuppression with significant prolonged cytopenias,[320] which is not predictable and is not correlated with the doses of radiation administered. Splenectomy after irradiation can be associated with increased complications, and irradiation should probably be administered only to patients who are not candidates for surgery.[3,7]

Radiotherapy offers a viable treatment option and sometimes may be the therapy of choice for the treatment of symptomatic hepatomegaly, peritoneal and pleural implants or pulmonary infiltration leading to ascites or pleural effusions, and extramedullary hematopoiesis in vital organs leading to organ dysfunction.[324] Because of the inherent sensitivity of myeloid tissue to radiation and profound marrow suppression that may occur after irradiation, therapy is usually initiated at low doses (20–25 cGy/day), with modification of the dose as the clinical situation dictates.[324] An alternative approach using intraperitoneal administration of cytosine arabinoside has been used to treat ascites in PMF.[325] Therapy is initiated at 0.77 mg/kg/day to achieve a concentration of 30 mg per 2 L of peritoneal fluid. The dosage is advanced so that the patient eventually receives 1 g or 13.5 mg/kg/day. Abdominal pain is the most common adverse effect associated with this approach.[325] Low-dose, single-fraction, whole-lung radiotherapy has also been useful in treating pulmonary artery hypertension associated with PMF.[182]

Splenectomy is indicated in patients with hemolysis, thrombocytopenia, painful splenomegaly, recurrent splenic infarction, and portal hypertension refractory to other therapeutic modalities.[3,7] Benbassat and colleagues[326] reviewed the role of splenectomy in PMF by evaluating 321 patients undergoing splenectomy and concluded that this procedure should be considered only in select individuals for specific indications. Splenectomy in patients with PMF is associated with a postoperative morbidity rate of 15% to 30% and a mortality rate of almost 10%. These events largely result from episodes of bleeding, infection, and thrombosis.[326–332] Following splenectomy 77%, 50%, 40%, and 30% of patients, respectively, have been reported to experience long-term improvement in symptomatic splenomegaly, anemia, portal hypertension, and severe thrombocytopenia.[332] Bleeding and thrombotic complications, however, complicated the course of 25% of patients with PMF, and 6.7%% of patients died during the perioperative period.[332] Postoperatively, the major long term complications include leukocytosis, thrombocytosis, and accelerated hepatic enlargement. Such adverse events can frequently be controlled with the immediate institution of hydroxyurea therapy during the postoperative period or if unsuccessful treatment with 2-chlorodeoxyadenosine therapy. The appropriate implementation of splenectomy can result in the improved quality of life of PMF patients who frequently do not have other therapeutic options available. Since splenectomy is associated with significant morbidity and mortality, the physician should only resort to this strategy if thrombocytopenia, anemia or symptomatic splenomegaly is unresponsive to less invasive approaches. Patients should only be considered for this procedure if their performance status allows one to anticipate a favorable surgical outcome with some certainty. Excessive delay of the decision to undergo splenectomy may result in a missed window of opportunity because the patient may become increasingly debilitated, no longer making them a viable surgical candidate. Histopathologic and cytogenetic features of the patient's marrow did not predict the likelihood of response for the cytopenias to splenectomy. Progressive hepatomegaly and marked thrombocytosis occurred, respectively, in 16% and 22% of patients after splenectomy.[332] The latter was associated with increased risk of thrombosis and decreased postoperative survival duration. In this report and several others, an extraordinarily high rate of leukemic transformation was observed after splenectomy.[328–331] Whether this was a function of the absence of the spleen or more likely the consequence of the natural history of the disease is unknown. Barosi and colleagues[331] suggested that splenectomy was an independent risk factor for leukemic transformation, stemming from a disruption of the host-tumor relationship. Porcu and associates,[330] however, argued for the possibility that patients with late-stage PMF who required splenectomy might be undergoing leukemic transformation in areas of splenic extramedullary hematopoiesis without overt marrow transformation. This population may be destined to develop leukemic transformation, and the need for splenectomy may only serve to identify this group of patients before such an event. Ferrokinetic measures of total erythropoiesis and of plasma volume, previously claimed to be useful guides for the choice of splenectomy, have little value for predicting outcome.[333] Compensatory hepatic myeloid metaplasia may accelerate after splenectomy, leading to rapid enlargement of the liver.[7,9,327,334,335] Occasionally, this massive myeloid metaplasia and sinusoidal dilation can result in liver failure and death.[334] This complication can, however, frequently be treated with a variety of agents including low radiation, low-dose melphalan, hydroxyurea, or 2-chlorodeoxyadenosine.[284,336–340] 2-chlorodeoxyadenosine therapy can be a particularly useful agent for patients with increased hepatomegaly, rapidly rising white blast cell counts, a extreme degree of thrombocytosis following splenectomy, or patients with these same clinical features who have not undergone splenectomy.[341] The drug can be administered every four4 weeks according to one of two dosing schedules (0.1 mg/kg/day IV by continuous infusion for 7 days, or 5 mg/m^2/day for 2 hours IV for 5 consecutive days). Responses occur usually by the second cycle and the medium duration of response is 6 months. 2-chlorodeoxyadenosine can be extremely useful in controlling the excessive myeloproliferation in patients awaiting an allogeneic stem cell transplant.

Excessive bleeding in patients with PMF can be a result of thrombocytopenia, qualitative platelet defects, or DIC.[3] Based on his clinical observations, Silverstein and coworkers[3,339] suggested that splenectomy was contraindicated in patients with DIC. Actively bleeding patients with consumption coagulopathy should receive platelet and plasma replacement therapy. Low-dose heparinization has resulted in improvement in some patients.[3] Platelet transfusions are suggested in bleeding patients who are thrombocytopenic or have normal platelet counts but who are known to have qualitative platelet abnormalities. Factor VII infusions should be considered in patients with bleeding refractory to platelet transfusion.

Allogeneic stem cell transplantation is a potentially curative option in patients with PMF who have an appropriate donor available.[155,156,342–351] Successful transplantation is associated with gradual resolution of marrow fibrosis and normalization of hematopoiesis.

Most of the knowledge of allogeneic SCT with conventional conditioning regimens comes from two series of transplants, with more than 50 patients each.[342,343] The first was published by Guardiola and coworkers in 1999, and reported the collected results of European and American transplant centers.[342] The second was published by Deeg and coworkers, and reported the results of the Fred Hutchinson Cancer Center in Seattle.[343] The Seattle experience has been recently updated.[351] In the two cohorts of 55 and 56 PMF patients, the median age of transplanted patients was 42 and 43 years, treatment-related mortality (TRM) was 27% and 33%, and 5-year survival 47% and 58%, respectively. The 5-year probability of treatment failure due to relapse or persistent disease after transplantation was 36% (28% for patients receiving an unmanipulated HLA matched related transplant) in the series of Guardiola and coworkers,[342] whereas in the series of Deeg and colleagues,[343] failure of sustained engraftment was 10.7%, and occurred solely in patients receiving transplants from alternative donors. A hemoglobin level of 10 g/dL or less and osteomyelosclerosis before transplantation adversely affected the outcome. The probability of grade III or IV acute graft-versus-host disease (GVHD) was 33%, with 16 of 45 patients developing extensive chronic GVHD. In a follow-up of the report of Guardiola and colleagues with inclusion of 11 new patients, multivariate analysis demonstrated the influence of age on 5-year survival (14% for patients 45 years or older compared with 62% for those younger than 45 years).[344] In an recent update from the Seattle group, the experience of 95 PMF patients who received busulfan, a total body irradiation conditioning reagent, was provided.[351] The 7-year actual survival was 61%. Although 10% of patients died of recurred a persistent disease and nonrelapse related mortality at 5 years was 34%.[351] An even higher 1-year cumulative nonrelapse mortality of 48% was successively reported from two Canadian centres in 25 patients.[345] Furthermore, Ditschkowski and colleagues[346] reported the experience of the University Hospital of Essen, Germany, in 20 patients. The median age of the patients was 45 years with a range from 23 to 59 years. The estimated TRM was 20%, while overall survival was 38.5%. Three of 20 (15%) died from relapse. By using low hemoglobin level, severe bone marrow fibrosis, and the presence of peripheral blasts prior to allogeneic SCT as predictors for decreased posttransplant survival, the mortality was 33% in the low-risk group and 73% in the high-risk group. Among low-risk patients, the 3-year relapse-free survival was 51%, whereas it was 17% among high-risk patients. From these experiences, myeloablative allo-HSCT in PMF has provided evidence that engraftment can be obtained, and that a complete and durable remission of the disease can be achieved in approximately 50% of patients. However, owing to the poor transplant outcomes in older patients, enrollment to this procedure represents a major therapeutic dilemma in PMF patients who are primarily diagnosed older than 60 years of age.

The advent of nonmyeloablative, reduced-intensity conditioning (RIC) regimens for allogeneic SCT has expanded the use of to procedure to older patients. As a result of diminished transplantation-related toxicity, it has been possible to investigate the usefulness of allo-SCT in patients with PMF previously believed to be unsuitable candidates due to advanced age. The use of RIC regimens were first reported in PMF patients by Devine and colleagues[155] and by Hessling and colleagues,[347] indicating that the use of RIC regimens in older patients with PMF resulted in lower TRM and achievement of histo-hematological responses. The experience from 10 European Centers from the EBMT was successively reported by Hertenstein and coworkers.[348] In 20 patients with a median age at transplantation of 50 years (range 39–65 years) and treated with conditioning regimens containing fludarabine or total body irradiation (TBI) and including antithymocyte globulin (ATG) or antilymphocyte globulin (ALG) in 9 cases, the 1-year TRM was 37% and 1-year overall survival was 54%. Since the cohort of cases included 5 patients who had acute transformation before HSCT, this report should be read with the understanding that a high proportion of high-risk patients are in the study cohort. Indeed, when patients were transplanted before acute transformation, 1-year TRM was 18%.

In recent years, two studies have enrolled over 40 patients in a retrospective registry study, including European and American institutions of the MPD Consortium, Rondelli and coworkers[156] reported 21 patients with a median age of 54 years and a range from 27 to 68 years. All patients had an intermediate or high severity score taking into account hemoglobin and WBC count values. However, no patient had undergone leukemic transformation. Different conditioning regimens, most of whom containing fludarabine, resulted in a TRM of 10% and 2-year overall survival rates of 87%. Eighteen patients were alive 12 to 122 months (median, 31 months) after transplant, and 17 were in remission (1 after a second transplant), with a relapse rate of 14%. Thirty-three percent of the patients developed acute GVHD grades II to IV, and 72% developed chronic GVHD. Posttransplant chimerism analysis showed more than 95% donor cells in 18 patients, and two patients achieved complete donor chimerism after donor lymphocyte infusion (DLI). In a prospective study of 21 patients with a median age of 53 years (range 32–67 years), Kröger and coworkers[349] reported remarkably similar data. The conditioning regimen consisted of busulphan and in vivo T-cell depletion with ATG. TRM was 16% at 1 year. Hematological response was seen in 100%; complete histopathological remission was observed in 75% of the patients, and 25% of the patients showed partial histopathological remission with a continuing decline in the grade of fibrosis. No instance of primary graft failure was observed and only one case of secondary graft failure was documented. After a median follow-up of 22 months (range, 4–59), the 3-year estimated overall and disease-free survival was 84%. These studies, and other successive reports,[350] suggest that RIC regimen followed by related or unrelated allo-HSCT, may reduce TRM and achieve long-term control of the disease in a high proportion of patients. Grafting with an unrelated donor is associated with greater TRM, although not significantly. Although longer-term follow-up data and larger studies are desirable, nonmyeloablative transplantation appears to be a promising therapeutic option in older patients with PMF before leukemic transformation.

Many unresolved issues remain to be clarified concerning the optimal strategy for allo-SCT in PMF. The need for splenectomy prior to allo-SCT remains a major issue. Splenectomy prior to allo-HSCT in PMF results in faster hematopoietic recovery.[342,343] Li and coworkers specifically analyzed the impact of pretransplant splenectomy on posttransplant outcome in 26 patients transplanted for PMF.[352] Posttransplant granulocyte recovery was faster among splenectomized patients: 14 to 51 days (median 18 days) to reach 0.5×10^9/L, compared with 19 to 85 days (median 23) among patients with intact spleen ($P = 0.04$); and the need for both red blood cell and platelet transfusions was greater among patients with intact spleens (mean 9.8 vs 6.1 units for red blood cells, and 21.7 vs 16 units for platelets). The 3-year probability of disease-free survival was 73% for splenectomized patients and 64% for patients without splenectomy; however, this difference was not statistically significant. At this time transplant centers have different policies regarding patients with extensive splenomegaly. The role of splenectomy prior to HSCT should be evaluated in prospective studies. Our initial observations in patients who were prepared with fludarabine and melphalan and then received an allogeneic HSCT, suggest that even severe splenomegaly (>30 cm longitudinal size by CT scan) can be reduced in a relatively short period of time after transplant (Ciurea S, Hoffman R, and Rondelli D, submitted).

The establishment of valid complete remission criteria of PMF after allogeneic SCT remains a major issue because the conventional criteria for response after allo-SCT are often influenced by GVHD, infections, or poor graft function and cannot be used. Conversely, normal blood counts and disappearance of disease-related symptoms do not exclude residual disease. Molecular markers of minimal residual disease monitoring have been evaluated as a biomarker for long-term disease-free survival. A highly sensitive method to monitor and quantify normal V617F positive cells in normal mutation positive patients with PMF after SCT allowed detecting minimal residual disease. This method has proven useful as a parameter for complete remission assessment and as a guide for instituting adoptive immunotherapy.[353] Autologous transplantation has also been investigated based on the premise that bone marrow fibrosis and extramedullary hematopoiesis are related to the bulk of the neoplastic clone, and therefore successful debulking using high-dose chemotherapy may interrupt the disease process and improve the disease manifestations at least until the reestablishment of the abnormal clone in the marrow by the "contaminated" autologous graft is achieved. This hypothesis was tested in a study in 21 patients with PMF.[354] The median patient age was 59 years. The conditioning regimen consisted of oral busulfan (16 mg/kg). The median times to neutrophil and platelet recovery were 21 days and 21 days, respectively. Five patients required backup stem cell infusions because of delayed engraftment. The 2-year actuarial survival rate was 61%. Six patients died of nonrelapse related causes (n = 3) or disease progression (n = 3). Transfusion independence was achieved in 10 of 17 anemic patients, and 4 of 8 patients with platelet counts of less than 100×10^9/L responded with durable counts of more than 100×10^9/L.[354] Although this study clearly demonstrates the feasibility of this procedure, the role of autologous transplantation in PMF remains uncertain.

With increased understanding of the biology of PMF, a number of phase I and II studies have examined more rational therapy for PMF. Imatinib mesylate is a tyrosine kinase inhibitor with specific inhibition of a number of kinases, including BCR-ABL, KIT, and PDGFR.[355] Tefferi and colleagues administered imatinib mesylate at a daily dose of 400 mg to 23 patients with PMF. They reported significant side effects, including neutropenia, musculoskeletal pain, thrombocytosis, edema, diarrhea, and hyperbilirubinemia, but found no significant clinical benefit. Zarnestra, a farnesyl transferase inhibitor interfering with RAS signaling pathways, was evaluated in eight patients with PMF and reported to be effective in the reduction of splenomegaly and attainment of transfusion independence.[356] Etanercept, a soluble tumor necrosis factor (TNF) receptor, has been effectively used to alleviate the constitutional symptoms in a pilot study of 22 patients with PMF.[357] Sixty percent of the patients who were able to be evaluated patients experienced an improvement in their symptoms, and 20% had an objective response with improvement in their cytopenias or splenomegaly.[357]

Small molecule tyrosine kinase receptor inhibitors has been shown to have modest activity in patients with PMF.[358,359] Giles and coworkers administered PTK787/ZK222584 to 20 patients with PMF at dose of 500 or 750 mg twice daily. Twenty percent of patients achieved a response indicating that therapies which target VEGF or its receptor might be active alone or in combination with other chemotherapeutic agents.[359] Several pilot trials of bisphosphonates for bone pain in PMF patients have reported with occasional success.[360] Shi et al recently presented data, which suggest that chromatin modifying agents such as hypomethylating agents and histone deacetylase inhibitors might be candidate agents for the treatment of PMF.[138] Inoue et al have reported the successful treatment of a single patient with PMF with severe anemia and thrombocytopenia with the histone deacetylase inhibitor valproic acid.[361] This class of agents leads to accumulation of acetylated histones which in turn leads to increased gene expression. The therapeutic potential for the use of chromatin modifying agents for the treatment of PMF patients requires careful evaluation.

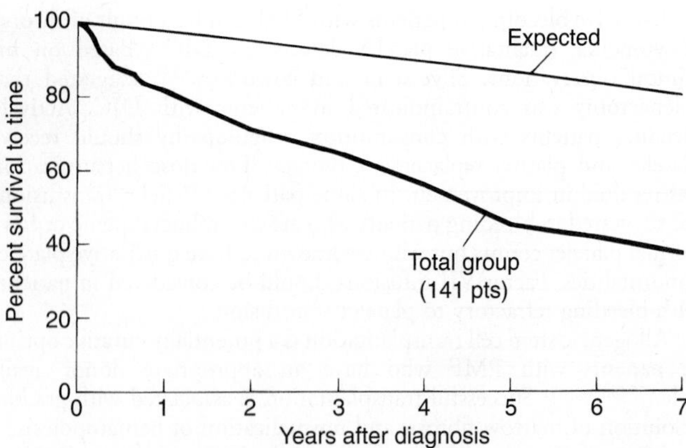

Figure 70–3 Overall survival from time of diagnosis of 141 patients with primary myelofibrosis. *(Data from Silverstein MN: Agnogenic Myeloid Metaplasia. Acton, MA, Publishing Sciences Group, 1975, p 197.)*

PROGNOSIS

The median overall survival period from the time of diagnosis of PMF varies from series to series but is approximately 5 years[1,3,7,9,362] (Fig. 70–3). Individual survival times have been reported to range from 1 year to more than 30 years.[1–8] In one series of 106 cases of PMF, the primary causes of death were determined in 53 cases and included infection (16 cases), leukemic transformation (9 cases), heart failure (9 cases), bleeding (7 cases), hepatic failure due to massive myeloid metaplasia of the liver (5 cases), portal hypertension (4 cases), and renal failure, pulmonary embolism, and post-transplantation GVHD (1 case each).[363] The incidence of acute leukemia as a terminal event ranges from 5% to 22% (Fig. 70–4), depending on the series cited.[1,3,7,9,362–365] Approximately one half of the patients who develop acute leukemia have not received previous treatment with alkylating agents or radiotherapy, suggesting that the evolution into acute leukemia may be part of the natural history of PMF.[362–365] The actuarial cumulative risk of death from leukemic transformation at 1 and 5 years after diagnosis has been reported to be 2% and 16%, respectively.[329,365–368] Immunologic and morphologic characterization of the blast phenotypes comprising these leukemias reveals that a typical myeloid phenotype is most commonly detected; other cell lineages, such as megakaryocytic, erythroid, lymphoid, and even stem cell phenotype, may also be involved, leading to the existence of mixed myeloid and hybrid transformations.[365–375] Megakaryoblastic transformations have been detected in one third of cases in one series, an incidence higher than that found in de novo acute myeloid leukemia.[374] Survival after blast transformation is limited, a phenomenon that is probably a result of patient age and the aggressive biology of these leukemias. In a series of 91 patients the leukemic transformation of PMF was fatal in 98% after a median of 2.6 months.[375] Successful leukemia remission induction therapy in these patients is an extremely rare event.[375] Patients should be sent for transplant prior to leukemic transformation.

Several clinical and biologic parameters that are characteristic of patients at diagnosis have been used to identify subgroups of patients with different outcomes.[9,232,363,369,376–381] Some investigators have suggested that there are two subpopulations of patients in PMF: short-lived and long-lived subpopulations of patients.[363] Such efforts at developing prognostic parameters have met with conflicting results, with the exception that anemia at presentation is consistently associated with short survival.[363] Dupriez and associates[369] developed an extremely simple scoring system, the Lille scoring system, based on two adverse prognostic factors—hemoglobin level less than 10 g/dL and white blood cell count less than 4,000 or more than 30,000/mm^3 and were able to stratify patients into three groups (Table 70–10). The low-risk (0 factors), intermediate-risk (1 factor), and high-risk (2 factors) groups were associated with median survival

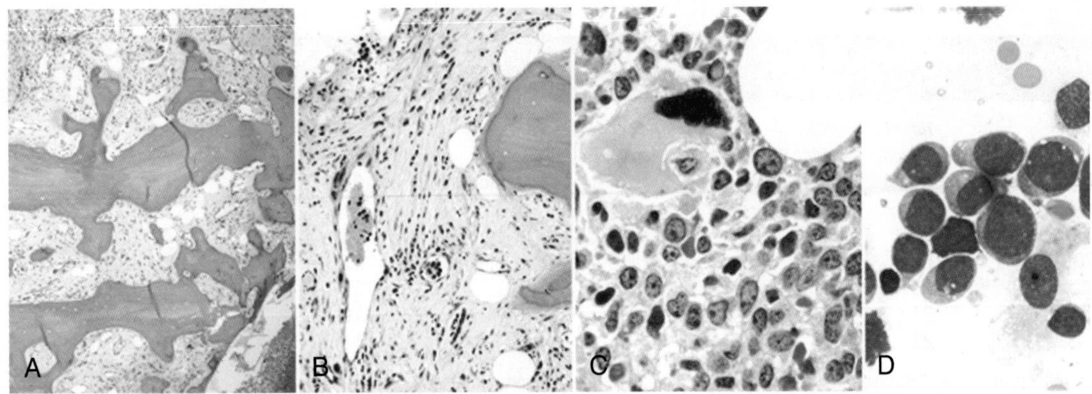

Figure 70–4 DISEASE PROGRESSION IN PRIMARY MYELOFIBROSIS. Marked osteosclerosis **A, B,** and acute leukemia **C, D**. PMF progresses in some patients to severe osteosclerosis in which there is markedly thickened and irregular bone formation (**A**) and a marrow space that is fibrotic and nearly depleted of hematopoietic elements (**B**). A terminal transformation to acute leukemia (**C, D**) occurs in 5% to 22% of cases.

Table 70–10 Distinguishing Features of Myeloid Malignancies Presenting with Marrow Fibrosis

Disorder	Splenomegaly	WBC	Teardrop poikilocytosis	Marrow Fibrosis	% Marrow Blasts	Bilineage or Trilineage Dysplasia	Jak2V617F, MPLW515L/K
MDS with fibrosis	No or mild	Decreased, normal or increased	No or few	+	<20	+	Negative
Acute panmyelosis with myelofibrosis (APMF)	No or mild	Decreased or normal	No	++	<20	+++	Negative
Acute megakaryoblastic leukemia (AMKL)	No or mild	Decreased, normal or increased	No or few	++	>20	++	Negative
PMF	Increased	Decreased, normal or increased	Present	++	<20	+	Positive in 50% of cases
CML, chronic phase	Increased	Increased	No or few	0-+	<20	–	Negative
CML accelerated phase	Increased	Increased	No	0-+	<20	0-+	Negative

CML, chronic myeloid leukemia; MDS, myelodysplastic syndrome; PMF, primary myelofibrosis.
Adapted from: (a) Dickstein JI, Vardiman JW: Issues in the pathology and diagnosis of the chronic myeloproliferative disorders and myelodysplastic disorders. Am J Clin Pathol 99:513, 1993; and (b) Orazi A, O'Malley DP, Jiang J et al: Acute panmyelosis with myelofibrosis: an entity distinct from acute megakaryoblastic leukemia. Mod Pathol 18:603, 2005.

times of 93, 26, and 13 months, respectively.[369] Other scoring systems that use simple clinical hematological parameters have been subsequently proposed. In a large Japanese study of 336 patients,[379] the presence of a hemoglobin level of 10 g/dL or higher, a platelet count of at least 100 × 10^9/L, and less than 3% circulating blasts predicted a median survival of approximately 15 years compared with less than five years in the remaining patients.

In 106 patients with PMF with successful marrow karyotypic analysis, Reilly[232] demonstrated that 35% percent of cases exhibited clonal abnormalities. A Kaplan-Meier analysis defined age ($P < 0.01$), hemoglobin ($P < 0.001$), white blood cell count ($P < 0.06$), platelet count ($P < 0.0001$), and abnormal karyotype ($P < 0.001$) as adverse prognostic parameters.[232] From these results, a prognostic schema was defined (Table 70–11). Median survival times varied from 180 months for the low-risk group (age <68 years, hemoglobin level >10 g/dL, normal karyotype) to 16 months for high-risk group (age >68 years, hemoglobin level ≤10 g/dL, abnormal karyotype).[232] Tefferi and colleagues[215] restricted the negative influence of chromosome changes to the presence of trisomy 8 and deletion of 12p, while deletions of 13q and 20q did not involve a shorter survival.

The impact of cases with a prefibrotic myelofibrosis in staging the disease is difficult to examine since these patients have been rarely considered for inclusion in the published prognostic schemas, thus possibly producing a selection bias against the very early, indolent cases. Kvasnicka and colleagues[380] analyzed a large series of patients, including a high proportion of cases with prefibrotic stage of the disease. Even though the degree of bone marrow fibrosis had prognostic significance after univariate analysis, the authors were able to distinguish three classes of patients on the basis of hemoglobin (Hb) level, white blood cells (WBC), percentage of circulating blasts, and age. What most significantly emerged from this series was the identification of a subset of young patients who were not anemic and who had a normal number of WBC at diagnosis who had a very long duration of disease, ie, median survival of approximately 20 years.

Table 70–11 Lille Scoring System for Predicting Survival in Primary Myelofibrosis

Adverse Prognostic Factors
Hb < 10 g/dL
WBC < 4 or >30 ×10^9/L
The scoring system (number of adverse prognostic factors)

Factor No.	Risk Group	Cases (%)	Median Survival (mo)
0	Low	47	93
1	Intermediate	45	26
2	High	8	13

Adapted from Dupriez B, Morel P, Demory JL, et al: Prognostic factors in agnogenic myeloid metaplasia: A report on 195 cases with new scoring system. Blood 88:1013, 1996.

Results in Fully Myeloablative Regimens and Reduced-Intensity Regimens in Allogeneic Hematopoietic Stem Cell Transplantation for Primary Myelofibrosis

Reference	*No. of Patients*	*Median Age, Years*	*Intermediate/High Risk, Dupriez, %*	*Regimen*	*TRM, %*	*CR, %*	*OS, %*
Guardiola et al 1999, 2000[342,344]	55	42	76	Myeloablative	27	40	14 (>45 years) at 5 years; 62 (<45years) at 5 years
Daly et al 2003[345]	25	48	84	Myeloablative	48	33	41 at 2 years
Deeg et al 2003[343]	56	43	54	Myeloablative	32	53	58 at 3 y
Hertestein et al 2002[348]	20	50	75	RIC	37	60	54 at 1 year
Rondelli et al 2005[156]	21	54	100	RIC	10	76	85 at 2.5 years
Kroger et al 2005[349]	21	53	80	RIC	16	75	84 at 3 years

TRM: transplant-related mortality; CR: complete remission; RIC: reduced-intensity conditioning.

Prognosis in Patients with Primary Myelofibrosis Based on the Presence of Anemia and Cytogenetic Abnormalities

Age (yr)	*Hb (g/dL)*	*Karyotype*	Survival (mo) *(95% CI)**	*(n)†*
<68	≤10	Normal	54 (46–62)	(7)
		Abnormal	22 (14–30)	(7)
	>10	Normal	180 (6–354)	(25)
		Abnormal	72 (32–112)	(11)
>68	≤10	Normal	44 (31–57)	(13)
		Abnormal	16 (5–27)	(14)
	>10	Normal	70 (61–79)	(22)
		Abnormal	78 (26–130)	(7)

*95% confidence interval.
†Number of patients.
Data from: Reilly JT, Snowden JA, Spearing RL, et al: Cytogenetic abnormalities and their prognostic significance in idiopathic myelofibrosis: A study of 106 cases. Br J Haematol 98:96, 1997.

Prognostic scoring systems have been developed for use at the time of referral of a young patient for stem cell transplantation. Cervantes and colleagues documented that in patients younger than 55 years of age, the factors associated with poor prognosis are anemia (Hb value <10 g/dL), constitutional symptoms and presence of blast cells in peripheral blood.[160] Based on the above mentioned three variables, two prognostic groups could be clearly identified among these younger patients: a "low-risk" group, including patients with none or one of the bad prognostic factors, and a "high-risk" group, defined by patients with two or three unfavorable factors. The "low-risk" group encompassed three quarters of the patients overall and median survival approached 15 years, whereas the "high-risk" group included a quarter of the patients, with a median survival of less than three years. In a cohort of 160 patients with PMF younger than 60 years of age and an overall survival of 78 months, Dingli and coworkers[381] identified a hemoglobin level of <10 g/dL, white blood cell count of either <4 or >30 × 10^9/L, platelet count of <100 × 10^9/L, an absolute monocyte count ≥ 1×10^9/L, the presence of constitutional symptoms, and hepatomegaly as independent predictors of inferior survival. By combining four parameters including hemoglobin level of <10 g/dL, white blood cell count of either <4 or >30 × 10^9/L, platelet count of <100 × 10^9/L, an absolute monocyte count at least 1 × 10^9/L, Tefferi et al was able to predict the course of three subpopulations of 334 PMF patients irrespective of age.[382] Almost 47% of patients were in the low-risk group and had a median survival of 134 months; 30% were in an intermediate-risk group and had a median survival of 58 months, and 23% were in the high-risk group with a median survival of 28 months. It is important to note that these laboratory values were obtained at the time of diagnosis or within six months of diagnosis, but prior to therapeutic intervention.[382] Clearly whatever the prognostic scoring system utilized, patients in the high risk group have a grave prognosis and be considered as candidates for stem cell allogeneic transplantation. Patients in a low-risk group should be observed, and patients in an intermediate-risk group should be considered as candidates for experimental therapeutic agents which are increasingly becoming available. If such agents are effective, they might serve as a viable alternative to stem cell transplantation in the future.

The prognosis of post-ET or PV MF has not been as well defined as PMF. Dingli and coworkers have recently reported that Hb levels <10 g/dL, older age and unfavorable cytogenetic abnormalities (clones other than 13q- and 20q- were predictive of a poor survival).[383] Post-ET and PV MF does not appear to be associated with a significantly proorer prognosis than PMF. The median survival for an entire cohort of such patients in one study was 90 months.[383] Patients with unfavorable cytogenetic abnormalities had a median survival approximately only 30 months.[383]

FUTURE DIRECTIONS

A major challenge with PMF remains the definition of the clinical boundaries of the PMF syndrome which will reconcile the disease definition with its clinical features, histological features, and patient prognosis. The scientific community must employ uniformly applicable diagnostic criteria not only for clinical trial enrollment purposes but also for better communication with patients, the development of better prognostic tool for stratification of therapy, and more accurate interpretation of results from molecular testing or targeted therapy. More rationale therapy for PMF should evolve from a better understanding of the basic cellular and molecular biologic abnormalities underlying PMF. Targeting tyrosine-kinases that are specifically activated in PMF, like normal mutated protein, or signalling pathways that are disrupted by disease specific mechanisms, like the TGF-β pathway, may provide promising therapeutic options. Until new drugs are available, allogeneic stem cell transplantation with reduced-intensity conditioning and peripheral blood stem cell grafts remains the only potentially curative therapy available for patients younger than 65 years with a good performance status. Although there is a reluctance to expose such patients to the risks of allogeneic stem cell transplantation, if their underlying disorder is associated with a poor prognosis, this risk appears to be warranted. The decision requires a detailed discussion of the risks and benefits of such a high risk but potentially effective procedure. The establishment of a multi-institutional cooperative group to evaluate therapies and treatment strategies for PMF patients must be a goal for the future. No single institution has sufficient numbers of patients to perform the phase III trials that have been sorely needed in this area. Only with the implementation of a rigorous evaluation of individual therapeutic strategies will we be able to determine the value of a growing number of potentially active agents. Each new therapy must be evaluated using a number of clinical endpoints as well as surrogate biomarkers and the immediate and long-term toxicities associated their use deter-

Approach to Treatment and Complications

When initially encountering a patient with presumed PMF, the physician must be certain that this process is not secondary to carcinoma invading the marrow or involvement of the marrow with lymphoma, an infectious disease such as tuberculosis or an autoimmune process. After a careful history and physical examination, appropriate cultures, chemistries, and radiographic studies should be performed to exclude these secondary forms of myelofibrosis. An ANA screen should be performed on patients with myelofibrosis and signs of immunoreactive process, like fever, high erythrocyte sedimentation rate, arthralgias to avoid missing an immune-mediated myelofibrosis that is treatable with steroids.

The treatment of PMF depends on the major manifestations of the disease in an individual patient. The clinician must consider treatment of anemic patients, patients with symptoms resulting from splenomegaly, those with bleeding abnormalities, those with portal hypertension, and those with ascites, bone pain, or symptoms due to hypermetabolism. Because most patients with the prefibrotic phase of PMF are largely asymptomatic, an approach to the treatment of this newly defined entity remains unknown. Prospective clinical trials will be needed to evaluate treatments to delay or prevent transition to the myelofibrotic phase. Nutritional deficiencies of iron or folate are easily diagnosed and treated. From the analysis of the results of the three most effective drugs in the treatment of the anemia associated with PMF, androgen therapy seems to be the first therapeutic option due to the safety and efficacy of the treatment. Screening for prostate cancer is recommended before using androgen therapy in males.

No evidence exists to determine if any of the anabolic steroids, such as testosterone enanthate, oxymetholone, or danazol are superior. Many centers now prefer danazol because of its better tolerability and absence of virilizing side effects. In the case of a lack of response, thalidomide or rHuEPO should be considered. RHuEPO therapy should be restricted to those patients with serum erythropoietin levels that are inappropriately low in relation to the degree of anemia, especially those without marked anemia and without a high burden of the normal V617F mutation (>50%).

In patients with symptoms resulting from splenomegaly, or with progressing splenomegaly, chemotherapy in the form of hydroxyurea, busulphan, interferon-α, or low-dose melphalan therapy is able to achieve some reduction of spleen size in approximately two thirds of patients; in some cases the response is sustained.

Individuals with acute splenic infarction who do not respond to administration of analgesics may gain pain relief from local irradiation over the spleen at doses of 0.25 to 0.50 Gy/day for 4 to 5 days. Radiotherapy may be also beneficial in those with huge, painful spleens in whom splenectomy is too risky. Patients with symptoms resulting from a profoundly enlarged spleen are best treated with splenectomy. Whenever a patient is considered a candidate for splenectomy, an extensive preoperative evaluation must be pursued. All patients must have an extensive preoperative evaluation of the coagulation system, which should include assays for coagulation factors V and VIII, fibrin-split products, platelet count, and bleeding times. Patients with qualitative platelet abnormalities remain candidates for splenectomy, but successful surgical intervention may require the use of adrenal steroids before surgery and platelet transfusions at the time of surgery. In patients with subclinical DIC, surgery is definitely contraindicated. The operation itself must be considered a major procedure. Morbidity after splenectomy can be minimized by careful selection of patients with respect to cardiac and renal status, improved surgical technique, aggressive blood bank support with platelet transfusions, and early postoperative mobilization of the patient. Only a senior staff surgeon who has performed this type of surgery many times should attempt such an operation. Immunization against pneumococcus, *Haemophilus influenzae* and meningococcal vaccines should be given at least 2 weeks prior to splenectomy. Since thrombocytosis prior to splenectomy is a risk factor for development of thrombosis after surgery, patients at splenectomy should have a platelet counts reduced to 200 $\times$ 10^9/L and, if necessary, this should be achieved with hydroxyurea or short courses of cytosine arabinosine at standard doses (100 mg/day for 5–6 days). Since the occurrence of thrombosis of the portal system is a potentially life-threatening complication after splenectomy in PMF,[384] thrombosis prophylaxis with low-molecular-weight heparins is mandatory. Doppler ultrasonography monitoring of the portal vein system (at least at the first weeks after intervention) is recommended. At the documentation of new thrombosis of the portal system, anticoagulation therapy must be established. Platelet transfusions should be administered to the bleeding patient after splenectomy, even if the platelet count is normal, because PMF is frequently associated with qualitative platelet abnormalities.

Thrombocytopenia and nonapparent DIC may lead to a hemorrhagic diathesis. In patients who have qualitatively abnormal platelet function, platelet transfusions are suggested for serious bleeding or when preparing a patient for surgery. Patients with thrombocytopenia resulting from marrow failure and hypersplenism can often be managed by administering danazol (600 mg/day). For patients with life-threatening thrombocytopenia who do not respond to danazol, splenectomy should be seriously considered.

Portal hypertension in PMF may be caused by increased blood flow from the spleen to the liver (ie, forward-flow portal hypertension) or by an intrahepatic block due to postnecrotic cirrhosis or intrahepatic extramedullary hematopoiesis. Forward-flow portal hypertension is correctable by splenectomy, whereas portal hypertension due to an intrahepatic defect may require a portosystemic shunt procedure. The indications for portosystemic decompression include upper gastrointestinal bleeding and refractory ascites. Some patients can be decompressed with a transjugular intrahepatic portosystemic shunt.[385,386] Limited survival of patients treated medically with variceal bleeding has been observed, but prolonged survival (>3 years) of patients treated surgically has been reported.

Patients with ascites, bone pain, or hypermetabolism present unique problems. If the ascites is caused by portal hypertension, management should be directed at relieving the hypertension. Development of ascites in PMF may also result from seeding of the peritoneal cavity with extramedullary hematopoiesis. In all patients with myelofibrosis who develop ascites, paracentesis should be performed and careful study of the ascitic fluid pursued. If megakaryocytes are found in the samples of ascitic fluid, the ascites probably results from peritoneal implants of myeloid tissue. These implants are treated by intraperitoneal instillation of cytosine arabinoside, initially at a dose of 0.77 mg/kg/day, which can be advanced to 13.5 mg/kg/day, or by abdominal irradiation. Administration of fractionated doses of radiation at 0.25 Gy/day with rotation into the four quadrants of the abdomen is also extremely effective. Radiation therapy to a total dose of 5 to 10 Gy may be very rewarding. Patients with myelofibrosis who develop severe bone pain have an extremely guarded prognosis. Treatment with etidronate at a dose of 6 mg/kg daily on alternating months has resulted in complete recovery from bone symptoms in a few patients.[387] This complication frequently serves as a prodrome of leukemic transformation. In these patients, biopsies at sites of pain may reveal pure populations of leukemic blasts. The pain appears to be the result of invasion of the periosteum by blast cells. Bone pain may also be treated with local irradiation for several days. Symptoms resulting from hypermetabolism, such as weight loss, sweating, and asthenia are not unusual. Such patients may benefit from low-dose hydroxyurea or etanercept. Patients with excessive myeloid proliferation, extensive hepatomegaly or extramedullary hematopoiesis involving the lung may benefit from therapy with 2-chlorodeoxyadenosine.

Approach to Treatment and Complications—cont'd

All patients younger than 65 years with symptomatic PMF should be evaluated for allogeneic stem cell transplantation. Identification of an appropriate donor and rapid referral to an expert stem cell transplantation unit should be expedited. Patients with a poor prognosis (high-risk group) as determined by the Lille scoring system or the system proposed by Dingli should be referred for transplant. If patients enjoy a good performance status, they should be encouraged to consider allogeneic SCT or enter a clinical trial evaluating such procedure. For patients with low-risk disease, allogeneic SCT is not recommended because of the prolonged survival of these patients. Allogeneic transplantation should be considered in intermediate-risk patients. The optimal conditioning regimen for RIC allogeneic SCT for PMF remains unknown. As far as splenectomy before allo-SCT, the recommendation is to consider splenectomy in patients who have significant symptomatic splenomegaly, refractory hemolytic anemia, or complications of portal hypertension refractory to medical management

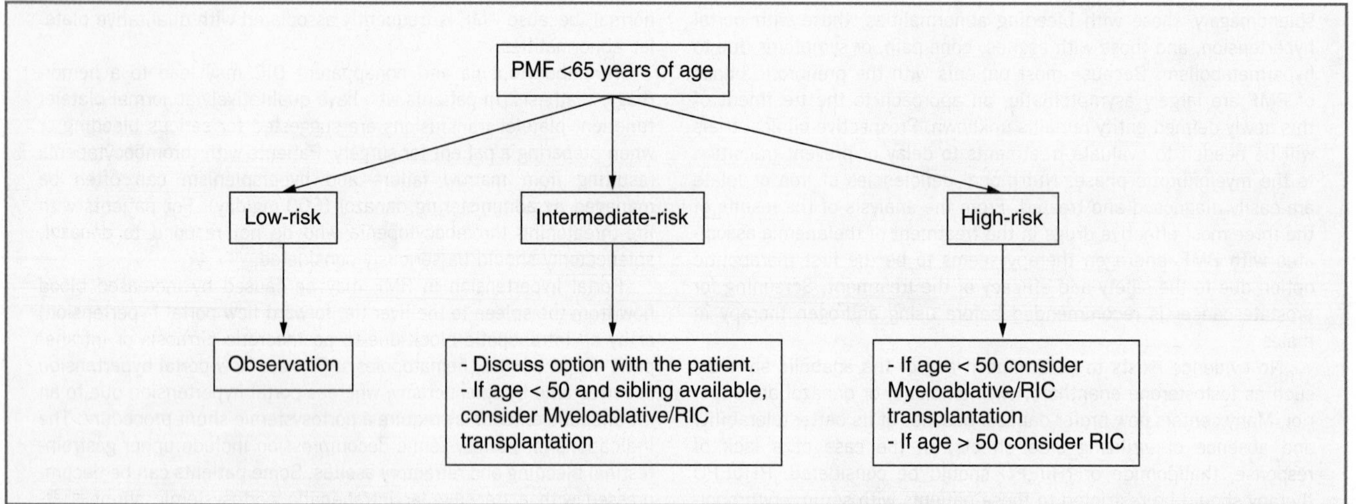

Above, algorithm for selection of PMF patients for allogeneic stem cell transplantation stratified according to clinical characteristics of patients. High-risk patients are those with two of the following abnormalities in the hemopoietic cell lineage: Hb < 10 g/dL, WBC >30 or <4 × 10^9/L and platelet <100 × 10^9/L.[321] Intermediate-risk patients are those with one of these; low-risk patients are those with none of these.

mined. The European Myelofibrosis Network (EUMET) and the International Working Group for Myelofibrosis Research and Treatment (IWG) have independently developed objective criteria by which responses to experimental therapeutic agents might be judged.[388,389] Since it is likely that a large number of such agents will be evaluated in patients with PMF during the next few years, it is recommended that either of these two means of evaluating a response to a therapeutic agent be implemented so that their relative efficacy can be more easily judged.

SELECTED REFERENCES

Barosi G, Hoffman R: Idiopathic myelofibrosis. Semin Hematol 42:248, 2005.

Cervantes F, Alvarez-Larran A, Domingo A, Arellano-Rodrigo E, Montserrat E: Efficacy and tolerability of danazol as a treatment for the anaemia of myelofibrosis with myeloid metaplasia: long-term results in 30 patients. Br J Haematol 129:771, 2005.

Cervantes F, Alvarez-Larran A, Hernandez-Boluda JC, et al: Darbepoetin-alpha for the anaemia of myelofibrosis with myeloid metaplasia. Br J Haematol 134:184, 2006.

Ciurea SO, Merchant D, Mahmud N, et al: Pivotal contributions of megakaryocytes to the biology of idiopathic myelofibrosis. Blood 110:986, 2007.

Dupriez B, Morel P, Demory JL, et al: Prognostic factors in agnogenic myeloid metaplasia: A report on 195 cases with the new scoring system. Blood 88:1013, 1996.

Kerbauy DM, Gooley TA, Sale GE, et al: Hematopoietic cell transplantation as curative therapy for idiopathic myelofibrosis, advanced polycythemia vera, and essential thrombocythemia. Biol Blood Marrow Transplant 13:355, 2007.

Kralovics R, Passamonti F, Buser AS, et al: A gain-of-function mutation of Jak2 in myeloproliferative disorders. N Engl J Med 352:1779, 2005.

Marchetti M, Barosi G, Balestri F, et al: Low-dose thalidomide ameliorates cytopenias and splenomegaly in myelofibrosis with myeloid metaplasia: a phase II trial. J Clin Oncol 22:424, 2004.

Mesa RA, Nagorney DS, Schwager S, Allred J, Tefferi A: Palliative goals, patient selection, and perioperative platelet management: outcomes and lessons from 3 decades of splenectomy for myelofibrosis with myeloid metaplasia at the Mayo Clinic. Cancer 107:361, 2006.

Migliaccio AR, Vannucchi AM, Migliaccio G, Hoffman R: Molecular advances toward the understanding of the pathobiology of idiopathic myelofibrosis. Curr Immunol Rev 2:169, 2006.

Pardanani AD, Levine RL, Lasho T, et al: MPL515 mutations in myeloproliferative and other myeloid disorders: a study of 1182 patients. Blood 108:3472, 2006.

Pikman Y, Lee BH, Mercher T, et al: MPLW515L is a novel somatic activating mutation in myelofibrosis with myeloid metaplasia. PLoS Med 3: e270, 2006.

Reilly JT: Idiopathic myelofibrosis: pathogenesis to treatment. Hematol Oncol 24:56, 2006.

Rondelli D, Barosi G, Bacigalupo A, et al: for Myeloproliferative Diseases Research Consortium: Allogeneic hematopoietic stem-cell transplantation with reduced-intensity conditioning in intermediate- or high-risk patients with myelofibrosis with myeloid metaplasia. Blood 105:4115, 2005.

Strasser-Weippl K, Steurer M, Kees M, et al: Prognostic relevance of cytogenetics determined by fluorescent in situ hybridization in patients having myelofibrosis with myeloid metaplasia. Cancer. 2006;107(12): 2801–2806.

Tefferi A, Cortes J, Verstovsek S, et al: Lenalidomide therapy in myelofibrosis with myeloid metaplasia. Blood 108:1158, 2006.

Tefferi A, Thiele J, Orazi A, et al: Proposals and rationale for revision of the World Health Organization diagnostic criteria for polycythemia vera, essential thrombocythemia, and primary myelofibrosis: recommendations from an ad hoc international expert panel. Blood 110:1092, 2007.

Thiele J, Kvasnicka HM, Facchetti F, Franco V, van der Walt J, Orazi A: European consensus on grading bone marrow fibrosis and assessment of cellularity. Haematologica 90:1128–32, 2005.

Wernig G, Mercher T, Okabe R, Levine RL, Lee BH, Gilliland DG: Expression of Jak2V617F causes a polycythemia vera-like disease with associated myelofibrosis in a murine bone marrow transplant model. Blood 107:4274, 2006.

Xu M, Bruno E, Chao J, et al: The constitutive mobilization of bone marrow-repopulating cells into the peripheral blood in idiopathic myelofibrosis. Blood 105:1699, 2005.

REFERENCES

For complete list of references log onto www.expertconsult.com

CHAPTER 71

ESSENTIAL THROMBOCYTHEMIA

Guido Finazzi, Mingjiang Xu, Tiziano Barbui, and Ronald Hoffman

Essential thrombocythemia (ET) is a chronic myeloproliferative disorder (MPD) characterized by a sustained proliferation of megakaryocytes, which leads to increased numbers of circulating platelets.[1–20] In addition to platelet counts in excess of 450×10^9/L, this disorder typically is characterized by profound marrow megakaryocyte hyperplasia, splenomegaly, and a clinical course punctuated by hemorrhagic or thrombotic episodes or both.[1–20] ET is a clinically heterogeneous disorder with up to two-thirds of patients who meet the criteria for diagnosis being asymptomatic at presentation. ET was first reported in 1934 by Epstein and Goedel,[21] who described a patient with an elevated platelet count who suffered from repeated hemorrhagic episodes.[21] This disease entity has been referred to by a variety of names, including primary thrombocythemia, idiopathic thrombocythemia, primary thrombophilia, and essential thrombocytosis.

Originally, many clinical investigators questioned whether ET represented a distinct clinical entity.[22] However, extensive descriptions of larger series of patients have provided information to dispute this initial skepticism.[1–20] Dameshek[23] in 1951 speculated that ET may represent one of the MPD. Laboratory investigations have confirmed this concept and clearly demonstrated that the disorder is typically a clonal hematologic malignancy.[24–28] Many patients, however, meet the criteria for the diagnosis of ET but have polyclonal hematopoiesis.[11–20,29–31]

In 2005 a breakthrough in our understanding of the pathogenesis and management of ET was made with the discovery of the Jak2V617F mutation in the majority of patients with chronic MPD, especially polycythemia vera (PV).[32–37] This finding has had a major impact on the classification of and diagnostic approaches to these disorders as well as creating drug development strategies based upon molecular pathogenesis.

EPIDEMIOLOGY

The true incidence of ET is unknown because extensive epidemiologic studies are not available. Although many investigators have indicated that this disorder is very rare, information from several institutions suggests that it occurs considerably more frequently than originally believed.[1–20] Following the incorporation of a platelet channel in automated complete blood cell counts, extreme thrombocytosis has been shown to be a relatively common occurrence in a general hospital setting.[38,39] Thus, 94 cases of newly diagnosed ET were identified from 1961 to 1982 at the Saint Louis Hospital in France, whereas 61 patients with this disorder were discovered from 1974 through 1987 at the Medizinische Poliklinik in Munich.[13,14] The incidence of ET has been reported to be approximately 1.5 to 2.4 patients/100,000 population annually.[40–42] Interestingly, a significant increase in the annual incidence rate of ET from 0.69 to 4.35 patients/100,000 inhabitants through the years 1983 to 1999 has been observed in the city of Goteborg, Sweden.[42] This trend was not observed for PV and is most likely due to the more frequent use of automated platelet counters in recent years. These figures are in keeping with the findings of an epidemiological cross-sectional study carried out in the city of Vicenza, Italy reporting a prevalence of ET of 400 per million inhabitants.[43] ET and PV appear to have approximately a 1:1 relative incidence,[42] although this incidence may be influenced by institutional affiliations and geographic differences.

The disorder appears to affect primarily middle-aged people, with an average age at diagnosis of 50 to 60 years.[1–20] In most series, there appears to be no gender predilection; although in several reports, a higher prevalence in females has been noted.[1–20,44,45] This discrepancy might be due to an equal frequency in older patients of both sexes but to a second peak frequency at around 30 years of age for women.[13] This predisposition of young women to develop ET has been reported previously.[45–47]

An abnormality of thrombopoietin production or of the thrombopoietin receptor has been suggested as the basis of inherited disorders leading to thrombocytosis.[48] A Dutch family with 11 family members and a Japanese family with 8 family members were reported with a hereditary form of thrombocytosis that was inherited in an autosomal dominant fashion.[49] The thrombopoietin receptor in the Dutch family was normal, yet there was a G to C transversion in the splice donor site of intron 3 of the thrombopoietin gene.[49] All of the affected members of both the Japanese and Dutch families were shown to have elevated thrombopoietin levels. In each family, a point mutation in the thrombopoietin gene was believed to lead to systemic overproduction of thrombopoietin, leading to a familial form of thrombocytosis.[48,49] The patients with autosomal dominant familial thrombocytosis have a benign course, which is not complicated by thrombotic or hemorrhagic events or transformation to myelofibrosis or acute leukemia. In addition, such patients frequently have lower platelet counts than pediatric patients with ET and a lower incidence of hepatosplenomegaly.[48–52] Recently another form of familial thrombocytosis has been defined. Ding have described a Japanese pedigree of familial thrombocythemia which is inherited as an autosomal dominant.[53] This disorder has been attributed to a dominant-positive activating mutation of the cellular receptor of thrombopoietin (MPL).[53] A unique mutation, serine 505 to asparagine 505 ($MPL^{Ser505Asp}$) has been identified in the transmembrane domain of MPL. These patients all have polyclonal hematopoiesis. Thrombopoietin and MPL mutations do not account for all cases of autosomal dominant familial thrombocythemia-indicating some degree of genetic heterogeneity.[49–53]

Moliterno and coworkers have also described a polymorphism of the thrombopoietin receptor (MPL Baltimore) which is accompanied by thrombocytosis. This polymorphism is due to a single nucleotide substitution that results in a lysine to asparagine (K39N) substitution in the ligand binding domain of MPL.[54] The polymorphism is associated with reduced expression of platelet MPL and the development of thrombocytosis. The polymorphism occurs exclusively in African American and appears to have an autosomal dominant pattern of inheritance with incomplete penetrance. Approximately 7% of African Americans are heterozygous for K39N.[54]

Several cases of ET have been reported in patients in the pediatric age group, but this is an extremely unusual occurrence.[55–63] A review of the literature cannot accurately determine the risk of thrombosis or bleeding of ET in childhood, but the clinical course is not entirely benign. The incidence of ET in childhood has been reported to be approximately 1 per 10^7 population, 60 times lower than that in adults. Approximately 30% of children with this disorder experience thrombotic or hemorrhagic complications at diagnosis or later in their course and 50% have splenomegaly.[61] Interestingly, in a recent study only 20% of pediatric patients with ET, as compared to 45% of adult ET patients, had clonal hematopoiesis, and 20% were Jak2V617F positive as compared to 60% of adult patients.[63]

Several families with multiple members having ET have been described.[64–66] The prevalence of the Jak2V617F mutation in familial cases of MPD has been recently analyzed in 72 families including 174 patients (68 with ET).[67] The Jak2 mutation was found in half of patients with ET, a similar proportion as observed in sporadic, non familial cases. Among 46 families with at least 2 cases of PV, ET, or primary myelofibrosis (PMF) the Jak2 mutation was absent in 6 families, heterogeneously distributed in 18 and present in all patients with MPD in 22. Thus, the Jak2 mutation does not seem to be required for the development of ET or other MPD.

ETIOLOGY

Greater insights into the mechanisms leading to thrombocytosis in ET have been gained. Patients with ET have normal or near-normal platelet survival.[68,69] The thrombocytosis is due to increased platelet production by megakaryocytes. Effective platelet production is increased as much as 10-fold and is associated with an increase in megakaryocyte clustering, volume, nuclear lobe number, and nuclear ploidy.[68,69]

Analysis of circulating blood cells of females with ET who were heterozygotes for isoenzymes of glucose-6-phosphate dehydrogenase has revealed that platelets, erythrocytes, and neutrophils express a single isoenzyme type.[24–28,30,31] In addition, Raskind and colleagues[27] have presented data to indicate that B cells can also be involved in this neoplastic process. Such findings indicate that ET is typically a clonal hematopoietic disorder originating at the level of the pluripotent hematopoietic stem cell. The clonal origin of ET has subsequently been confirmed using restriction fragment-length polymorphisms of X chromosome genes.[28,30,31,70]

Such clonal analyses have revealed that a significant proportion of nonclonally derived leukocytes exist in addition to the clonally derived population of leukocytes in patients with ET.[28,30,70] In one study of 42 patients with ET, 31 patients exhibited clonality of at least one hematopoietic lineage, whereas the remaining 11 patients had polyclonal origin of all lineages studied.[30] The biogenesis of polyclonal ET remains ill defined. It is possible that small numbers of normal hematopoietic stem cells persist to account for this admixture of nonclonal populations. It has been reported by several groups that ET patients with polyclonal hematopoiesis have fewer thrombotic complications.[11,18,29,30,70]

In one patient, Anger and coworkers[70] determined that although the total leukocyte fraction was clonally derived, the T-lymphocyte population was nonclonal in origin. In fact, most studies indicate that T lymphocytes are of polyclonal origin in ET patients.[28] Interestingly, in some patients, monoclonality of hematopoiesis is restricted to platelets, despite the polyclonal origin of the other lineages. Other studies, however, have indicated a common origin of granulocytes, platelets, and B lymphocytes in this disorder.[26] Such studies raise the possibility that the malignant transformation leading to ET occurs at a number of cellular stages along the hematopoietic cellular hierarchy.[56]

The biologic behavior of megakaryocyte progenitor cells present either in the marrow or in the peripheral blood of patients with ET has been extensively studied.[72–85] In each of these studies, the use of serum-containing culture systems has led to the detection of increased numbers of assayable progenitors. These data support the concept that the principal abnormality is an expansion of the progenitor cell pool. In addition, colonies were noted to appear in the absence of exogenous cytokines.[72–85] A second subpopulation of colony-forming unit-megakaryocyte (CFU-MK) assayed from patients with ET was also shown to remain responsive to the addition of cytokines, suggesting the presence of both a MPD clone not requiring exogenous cytokines and a more physiologic clone that does.[72–85]

Several laboratories have demonstrated that megakaryocyte progenitor cells isolated from ET patients are hypersensitive to the action of several cytokines including IL-3, IL-6, and thrombopoietin, but not GM-CSF.[82–85] Investigators have explored the possibility that the defect in ET might actually be due to resistance to inhibitors of megakaryocytopoiesis.[86] Zauli and associates have shown that the ET CFU-MK has a significantly lower sensitivity to the inhibitory effects of low doses of TGF-β and a limited response to the inhibitory effects of high concentrations of autologous platelet lysates.[86] TGF-β was shown to be primarily responsible for the inhibitory activity present in such platelet lysates.[86] Some combination of increased sensitivity to growth factors that promotes platelet production and disrupted sensitivity to negative regulators of thrombopoiesis at the level of the megakaryocyte progenitor cell might account for the thrombocytosis that is characteristic of ET.

Using serum-free cultures, a number of laboratories have reported conflicting data about spontaneous megakaryocyte colony formation by CFU-MK from patients with ET in the absence of the addition of exogenous cytokines.[77–85] Several groups have attempted to use this in vitro characteristic as a diagnostic tool to discriminate ET from reactive thrombocytosis.[84,85] Because there is some degree of spontaneous megakaryocyte colony formation by normal marrow in such serum-free culture systems, these findings remain difficult to interpret.[87] No evidence of an autocrine regulatory defect involving IL-3, IL-6, GM-CSF, or thrombopoietin has been detected to account for the expansion of the megakaryocyte progenitor cell pool in ET.[82,88,89]

Erythroid progenitor cells in ET can also proliferate in response to the small amount of cytokines present in serum alone. Erythroid colony formation in the absence of exogenous erythropoietin is a hallmark of the proliferative defect that characterizes PV.[90] Burst-forming unit-erythroid can be assayed from both marrow and peripheral blood of patients with ET and form erythroid colonies in the absence of exogenous erythropoietin.[91–94] Such an abnormality in these nonpolycythemic patients probably indicates an underlying defect shared by progenitor cells in many MPD.[91–94]

Thrombopoietin is the primary physiologic regulator of megakaryocytopoiesis and platelet production. This growth factor acts by binding to its cell surface receptor, Mpl.[95] The thrombopoietin receptor is expressed by $CD34^+$ hematopoietic progenitor cells, megakaryocytes, and platelets.[95] Normal or slightly elevated thrombopoietin levels have been observed in patients with ET.[96–100] Furthermore, expression of the thrombopoietin receptor and its mRNA have been shown to be dramatically reduced in the platelets of patients with ET.[97–102] Investigators have reported that in PV there is overexpression of the polycythemia rubra vera (PRV-1) gene in leukocytes; however PRV-1 overexpression is found less frequently in patients with ET.[103] Interestingly, decreased Mpl expression and elevated granulocyte PRV-1 expression have been observed in patients with autosomal dominant familial thrombocythemia who carry a mutation in the thrombopoietin gene.[49] These studies question the specificity of c-mpl and PRV-1 expression in identifying patients with MPD.[49]

The Jak2V617F mutation is present in 40% to 60% of patients with ET while gain of function mutations involving the thrombopoietin receptor, MPLW515L and MPL515K are present in approximately 1% of patients with ET.[32–37,104–110] Jak2 is a cytoplasmic tyrosine kinase which plays a key role in mediating intracellular signaling from a variety of growth factors including IL-3, erythropoietin, GM-CSF, G-CSF, and thrombopoietin, Lu et al have shown that coexpression of Jak2V617F with a homodimeric type 1 cytokine receptor (including erythropoietin, thrombopoietin, or G-CSF) is necessary for hormone activation of Jak-STAT signaling pathways and for hematopoietic cell proliferation to become growth factor independent.[111] The Jak2V617F mutation is present in ET patients with both clonal and polyclonal hematopoiesis.[101–110] Patients with clonal hematopoiesis have a higher Jak2V617F mutational burden (26%) than patients with polyclonal hematopoiesis (16%).[112] Gale et al have presented data in ET patients which indicates that the relative size of the Jak2V617F clone is often small and that it remains stable over time in patients with both clonal or polyclonal hematopoiesis.[113] Although an allele burden higher than 50% Jak2V617F indicating the presence of granulocytes homozygous for Jak2V617F has been found in 70% of PV patients, it was observed in only 2% of ET patients.[114] Scott and coworkers examined the Jak2V617F status of hematopoietic colonies cloned from 22 PV patients with either a high or low burden of Jak2V617F.[115] All PV patients had assayable erythropoietic bursts that were homozygous for Jak2V617F and concluded that even in PV patients with low a burden of Jak2V617F that Jak2V617F homozygous progenitors were present.[115] By contrast hematopoietic colonies cloned from ET patients were virtually never Jak2V617F homozygous.[115] The transition from Jak2 heterozygous to homozygous progenitors is a consequence of homologous recombination. These studies suggest that such an event is characteristic of PV, but rarely occurs in ET.[34] If such event occurred in ET, it would likely lead to a transition from an ET phenotype to a PV phenotype.[110] Some investigators, but not all, have reported a higher allelic burden of Jak2V617F in platelets as compared to granulocytes in patients with ET, while the allelic burden in PV and PMF is higher in granulocytes than platelets.[107–110,116–121] Jak2V617F is observed only in platelets in rare patients with ET.[117] Jak2V617F can be detected, not only in granulocytes and platelets of ET patients but also erythroblasts.[122] In PV Jak2V617F produces an increased phosphorylation of signal transducer activator of transcription (STAT).[123] In PV uniformly increased phosphorylated STAT3 and STAT5 expression in bone marrow cells was observed while in ET normal or increased phosphorylated STAT3 but reduced phosphorylated STAT5 has been noted.[123] STAT3 is a pivotal regulator of megakaryocytopoiesis which might provide an explanation for its exclusive upregulation in ET.[123]

The methodology used to detect Jak2V617F influences the proportion of ET patients documented to be positive for the mutation.[124] The frequency of Jak2V617F positive ET tends to be higher if real time PCR is utilized (72%) than if DNA resequencing (23%–32%) or allelic specific PCR (57%) is utilized to detect the mutation.[124] This still leaves a subset (22%) of patients with ET who are Jak2V617F negative, indicating that alternative pathways are likely responsible for the ET phenotype in these patients.[124] Discordance between the percentage of clonal granulocytes and the percent of Jak2V617F positive granulocytes have led some investigators to speculate that the development of a clonal form of ET may precede the acquisition of the Jak2V617F mutation.[112]

The clinical phenotype of patients with Jak2V617F positive and negative ET appears to be different.[107–110,116–121] At diagnosis, patients with the mutation tend to be older and to have a higher hemoglobin level, a higher neutrophil count, but a lower platelet count than patients with Jak2V617F negative ET. Patients with Jak2V617F positive ET, have marrows which are more hypercellular and are characterized by greater degrees of erythroid and granulocytic hyperplasia.[110] Serum erythropoietin levels are lower in Jak2V617F positive patients, and they have lower serum ferritin levels. In addition the rate of thrombosis has been suggested by some, but not all investigators to be higher in Jak2V617F positive ET patients.[110] Furthermore, a greater number of ET patients who have the mutation eventually go on to develop PV.[110] Jak2V617F positive patients have been reported to require smaller doses of hydroxyurea to lower their platelet counts.[110] Campbell and coworkers have hypothesized that since Jak2V617F positive ET shares many phenotypic similarities with PV and that these two disorders should be considered as a continuum rather than being categorized as two separate diseases.[110]

Most clinical sequelae of ET are related to hemorrhagic and thrombotic episodes, which frequently punctuate the clinical course of individual patients.[1–20,125,126] Thrombotic complications occur most frequently in older patients and patients with a previous history of a thrombotic event, whereas hemorrhagic events occur almost exclusively in individuals with extremely high platelet counts (>1000 × 10^9/L).[1–20,127,128] A subset of young patients who are asymptomatic and remarkably free of such complications has also been described.[49,56,128,129] Unfortunately, catastrophic thrombotic complications can be seen in both the young and the elderly.[130,131] The age-related differences in the frequency of these events have been attributed to the coexistence of vascular disease in older patients.[130,132] This hypothesis remains controversial because other studies have described younger patients with a significant incidence of vascular thrombosis, sometimes in usual sites, such as the portal or superior sagittal sinus veins.[13,133] Microvascular thrombosis causing digital or central nervous system ischemia leads to a variety of clinical syndromes closely associated with ET.[9,125–127,130–138]

Past studies have concluded that the degree of elevation of the platelet count in ET is an important determinant of the frequency of thrombotic and hemorrhagic events.[1,4,5] These conclusions were, however, based on observations of a limited number of patients. Many other studies have failed to define a relationship between the frequency of thrombotic complications and platelet numbers.[13,14,137,138]

Some progress has been made in further defining the relationship between platelet numbers and the risks for thrombotic and hemorrhagic events in ET.[125,128,139–142] Cortelazzo has reported in a randomized trial of patients at a high risk of developing a thrombotic event (>60 years of age and/or a previous history of a thrombotic episode) that reduction of platelet numbers was highly effective in preventing additional thrombotic events.[139] Furthermore, Cortelazzo and colleagues have shown that the incidence of thrombotic events was closely correlated with the duration of thrombocytosis.[127] Several groups have now confirmed that the degree and duration of bleeding in this patient population is correlated with the platelet count.[97,134–136] Bleeding events appear to occur exclusively when the platelet counts are excessively high and are reduced in number when the platelet count returns to normal.[96–102,128,140–143] The clinical spectrum of bleeding in ET patients closely resembles that observed in von Willebrand disease.[140–143] Several groups have now shown that high platelet counts (>1000 × 10^9/L) are associated with an acquired form of von Willebrand syndrome and that reduction of platelet numbers is associated with correction of the von Willebrand syndrome like abnormalities and cessation of bleeding episodes.[140–143] The mean platelet count in patients with ET and acquired von Willebrand disease is 2050 ± 1107 × 10^9/L.[144,145] An increase in the number of circulating platelets appears to favor the adsorption of larger von Willebrand multimers onto platelet membranes, resulting in their removal from the circulation and their subsequent degradation.[141,145]

Platelets with patients with ET have been known for a considerable time to be qualitatively abnormal.[4,7,125–128,140,142–145] Although both increased and decreased platelet reactivity has been described, these findings have not been definitively associated with thrombohemorrhagic complications with two noteworthy exceptions; erythromelalgia, where the prompt relief of symptoms by cyclooxygenase inhibitors provides direct evidence that prostaglandins play a role in the development of vascular occlusion, and acquired von Willebrand syndrome, which is a major cause of bleeding in patients with ET.[4,7,126,134–145] Prolongation of the bleeding time has been reported in 7% to 19% of newly diagnosed patients with ET.[128]

A close correlation between prolongation of the bleeding time and the occurrence of hemorrhage in ET patients does not always exist. This is in contrast to correction of the bleeding time in those patients with ET, extreme thrombocytosis, and an acquired von Willebrand syndrome following reduction of platelet numbers to the normal range.[126,142,145] It is important to emphasize that aspirin prolongs the bleeding time of patients with ET to a greater degree than that of normal controls.[128,130,145] Abnormal platelet aggregation has been reported in 35% to 100% of patients with ET.[128] The majority of such studies have used conventional platelet aggregation studies performed on platelet-rich plasma. In one study, the simultaneous measurement of platelet aggregation and ATP dense granule release by whole blood platelet lumi-aggregometry was used to identify ET patients at a risk of developing thrombosis. This observation has not been confirmed and a prospective analysis of larger cohorts of patients is required to confirm the utility of such assays.[146]

Abnormal aggregation studies are not related to prolongation of the bleeding time or to the incidence of episodes of hemorrhage or thrombosis. In ET, platelet aggregation is classically defective in response to epinephrine, adenosine diphosphate (ADP), and collagen, but is usually normal with arachidonic acid and ristocetin.[128,147]

Characteristically, in ET, the first wave of aggregation is diminished and the second wave of aggregation is absent in response to epinephrine.[128,147] Interestingly, preincubation of ET platelets with thrombopoietin corrects, in part, the impaired aggregation in response to epinephrine, ADP, and collagen.[148] Usuki and coworkers have proposed that circulating thrombopoietin levels in this disorder might regulate platelet function and responses to agonists in vivo.[148] An acquired form of platelet storage pool disease occurs frequently in ET. Platelet α-granule content and the release of the content of granules are abnormal resulting in elevated plasma levels of platelet factor-4 and β-thromboglobulin.[128]

Because the content of α-granule constituents has been reported to be normal in ET megakaryocytes, the synthesis of these molecules is not believed to be abnormal, but rather, the release of α-granule constituents is believed to be a consequence of platelet activation.[128] The finding of an acquired storage pool defect again does not correlate with platelet numbers or with the occurrence of clinical symptoms. Numerous individual functional platelet abnormalities have been demonstrated.[149–157] A defect in the metabolism of arachidonic acid by lipoxygenase has been documented, as have decreased numbers of platelet receptors for prostaglandin D_2 and adrenergic receptors for epinephrine.[128,154,155] Platelets from patients with thrombotic episodes have been found to be capable of increased generation of thromboxane B_2 and to have an increased affinity for fibrinogen.[156,158] Elevations in β-thromboglobulin and serum thromboxane B_2 levels in ET patients are suggestive of the presence of enhanced in vivo platelet activation and possibly thrombin generation.[158] These same abnormalities are not detected in patients with secondary thrombocytosis and may provide some explanation for the high incidence of thrombosis associated with ET.

The survival of platelets in ET patients with erythromelalgia and thrombosis has been shown to be reduced to 4.2 ± 0.2 days as compared with normal platelet survival in asymptomatic ET patients (6.6 ± 0.3 days) and patients with reactive thrombocytosis (8.0 ± 0.4 days).[159] Thrombosis in this setting is associated with an increased platelet turnover, which can be quantitated cytometrically by measuring the number of platelets most recently released into the circulation (reticulated platelets).[160] Treatment of erythromelalgia with aspirin increased mean platelet survival from 4.0 ± 0.3 days to 6.9 ± 0.4 days and was associated with a significant elevation of platelet numbers.[143,159] These findings suggest that erythromelalgia results from platelet-mediated thrombosis of the arterial microvasculature of the extremities (Fig. 71–1).[126,143,159] Complete correction of this ischemic circulatory defect is associated with the use of platelet cyclooxygenase inhibitors, such as aspirin and indomethacin.[135] Agents that do not inhibit platelet cyclooxygenase, such as coumadin, sodium salicylate, dipyridamole, sulfinpyrazone, and ticlopidine are not active in the treatment of this disorder. Dazoxiben is capable of inhibiting platelet malondialdehyde and thromboxane B_2 synthesis but does not correct the symptoms of erythromelalgia.[126,143,159] These findings suggest that prostaglandin endoperoxides play a role in the generation of platelet-associated thrombosis in ET (Fig. 71–1).[126]

Abnormalities of platelet membrane constituents have also been demonstrated in ET. Most commonly, decreased concentrations of glycoprotein (GP) Ib and also reduced concentrations of GPIIb and GPIIIa have been reported.[128] A remarkable patient with ET with a prolonged bleeding time was shown to have an acquired deficiency of glycoprotein Ia-IIa, the putative collagen receptor. Collagen-induced platelet aggregation was totally absent.[150] The mechanisms underlying these acquired membrane defects, as well as their clinical significance, remain unclear.

One intriguing explanation for the increased risk of thrombosis in patients with ET has been proposed by Lee and Baglin.[151] These investigators demonstrated that the total amount of thrombin generated on the platelet surfaces of patients with ET was markedly greater than that generated on the platelet surfaces of normal controls or patients with reactive thrombocytosis.[151] The molecular basis of this abnormality has not been defined, but it remains possible that an abnormal membrane structure of ET platelets may account for the enhanced thrombin potential that may lead to a relatively high

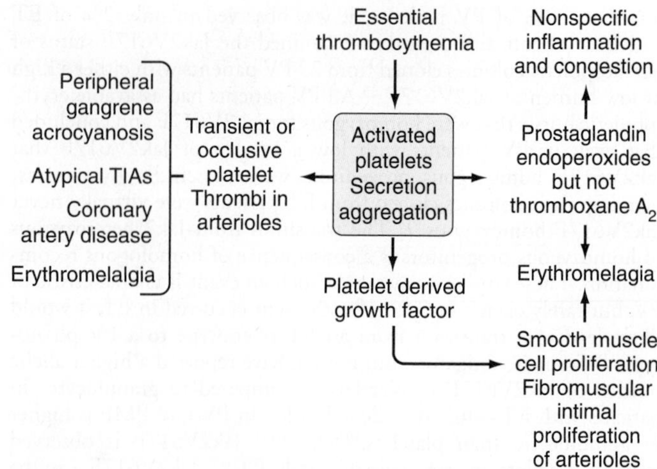

Figure 71–1. Proposed pathophysiologic mechanisms of platelet-mediated inflammatory ischemic atherothrombotic processes in essential thrombocythemia. *Modified from: Michiels JJ, Berneman Z, Van Bockstaele D, van der Planken M, De Raeve H, Schroyens W. Clinical and laboratory features, pathobiology of platelet-mediated thrombosis and bleeding complications, and the molecular etiology of essential thrombocythemia and polycythemia vera: therapeutic implications. Semin Thromb Hemost 32:174, 2006.*

thrombotic risk. Villmow and coworkers have documented increased numbers of platelet microparticles, as well as increased platelet-neutrophil and platelet-monocyte completes, in patients with ET.[161] Platelet microparticles support thrombin generation and leukocyte activation.[161] Increased numbers of platelet microparticles have been associated with the development of vascular thrombosis.[161]

Recently, in vivo leukocyte activation has been shown to occur in ET and to be associated with signs of activation of both the coagulation cascade and endothelial cells. Falanga and associates have speculated that platelet and leukocyte activation may play a role in the generation of the prethrombotic state that characterizes ET.[162–164] Interestingly, the presence of the Jak2 mutation is associated with a greater degree of platelet and leukocyte activation in these patients.[165] Activated neutrophils are able to bind platelets which triggers the expression of tissue factor as well as endothelial cell activation and damage. From a clinical point of view, two recent studies have demonstrated that an increased leukocyte count in patients with ET is an independent risk factor for developing thrombosis and is associated with an inferior survival.[166–168] Therefore, an important role for leukocytes in the pathogenesis of thrombosis in ET is becoming more evident.

CLINICAL MANIFESTATIONS

The presenting symptoms of patients with ET are quite variable. Many patients (12% to 67%) reach medical attention fortuitously, as a result of the extreme degree of thrombocytosis detected when obtaining a routine blood cell count.[1–20] In two series, in fact, 76% to 84% of cases were asymptomatic, and the diagnosis was made incidentally.[127,169] Most patients present with symptoms related to small- or large-vessel thrombosis or minor bleeding.[1–20] In general arterial events predominate over venous events. Presentation with a major bleeding episode is unusual.[170] After thrombocytosis has been detected, 13% to 37% of patients relate symptoms resulting from hemorrhagic events, whereas 22% to 84% of patients report thromboembolic complications.[1–20,127,171] Table 71–1 lists the thrombotic symptoms at diagnosis and subsequently reported from one large series of patients.[127] The thrombotic events primarily involved the microvasculature, with thrombosis of large vessels also occurring. Neurologic complications are common.[1–12,133–136,171–174] Table 71–2 lists representative neurologic complaints,[134] of which headache was

Table 71–1. Thrombotic and Hemorrhagic Events in 100 Patients with ET

Category	No. of Patients	No. of Events (%)	Initial Events	Subsequent Events
No clinically relevant events or asymptomatic	76	—	—	—
Hemorrhage	4	4 (11)	3	1
Gastrointestinal tract bleeding			2	1
Knee hemarthrosis			1	
Thrombosis	20	32 (89)	11	21
Arterial	17	25 (79)	10	15
Distal		7 (27)	2	5
Cerebral		15 (62)	8	7
Cardiac		3 (11)	—	3
Venous	3	7 (21)	1	6
Sup phlebitis		3 (43)	—	3
Iliofemoral DVT		1 (14)	—	1
Splenic mesenteric		2 (29)	—	2*
Cerebral		1 (14)	1	—
Total	100	36 (100)	14	22

*One fatal.

DVT, deep vein thrombosis; Sup phlebitis, superficial leg phlebitis.

Data from Cortelazzo S, Vlero P, Finazzi G, et al: Incidence and risk factors for thrombotic complications in a historical cohort of 100 patients with essential thrombocythemia. J Clin Oncol 8:556, 1990.

Table 71–2. Frequency of Neurologic Complaints Associated with Essential Thrombocythemia

Manifestations	Patients (N)
Headache	13
Paresthesias	10
Posterior cerebral circulatory ischemia	9
Anterior cerebral circulatory ischemia	6
Visual disturbances	6
Epileptic seizures	2
Total number of patients	33

Data from Jabaily J, Iland HJ, Laszlo J, et al: Neurologic manifestations of essential thrombocythemia. Ann Intern Med 99:513, 1983.

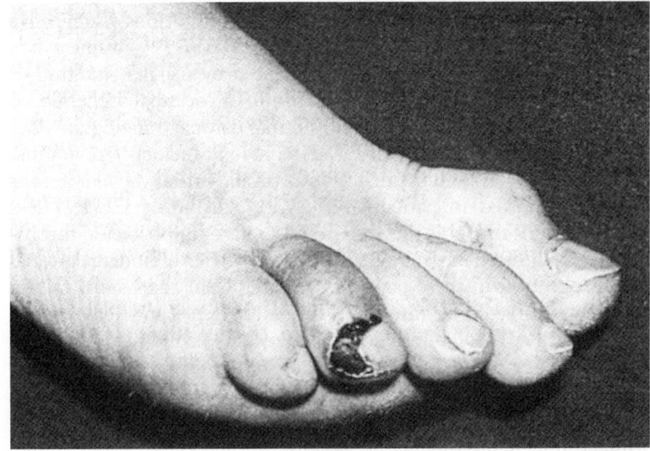

Figure 71–2. Gangrene of the toe in a patient with essential thrombocythemia.

the most common, with paresthesias of the extremities a close second. There was an extremely high incidence of transient ischemic attacks involving both the anterior and posterior cerebral circulation.[172–174] These attacks have a sudden onset, last for a few moments, and are frequently associated with a pulsatile headache.[172–174] The various symptoms occur sequentially rather than simultaneously and can be preceded or followed by erythromelalgia. Transient neurologic symptoms include unsteadiness, dysarthria, dysphoria, motor hemiparesis, scintillating scotomas, amaurosis fugax, vertigo, dizziness, migraine-like symptoms, syncope, and seizures.[172] The syndrome is caused by platelet-mediated ischemia and thrombosis in end-arterial microvasculature. It is not unusual for these symptoms to eventually progress to definitive cerebral infarcts.[173]

Microvascular circulatory insufficiency involving the toes and fingers is frequent.[125–127] Such events can lead to digital pain, enhanced by warmth; distal extremity gangrene (Fig. 71–2), and classic erythromelalgia.[9,125–127,135,136,175,176] The term *erythromelalgia* refers to a syndrome of redness and burning pain in the extremities.[176] Venous thrombosis is not typically observed in these patients. Erythromelalgia, which is characterized by a burning pain and a dusky congestion of swollen extremities, is usually preceded by paresthesias.[96] Cold provides relief to these symptoms, and heat intensifies the symptoms. Patients prefer to wear shoes or slippers without socks and elevate their feet.[126,175] These symptoms may progress in intensity and lead to peeling of the skin in affected appendages or affected toes or fingers, which then may become cold and ischemic with a dark purplish tinge. Erythromelalgia symptoms are asymmetric in the majority of cases.[126] Symptoms related to coronary artery disease or transient ischemic attacks may precede or accompany the onset of erythromelalgia.[126] Occasionally, hemorrhagic episodes may occur in patients experiencing erythromelalgia.[126] Platelet counts in patients with erythromelalgia are frequently below 1000 × 10^9/L, except in those patients with concomitant occurrence of erythromelalgia and hemorrhage.[126,135,136,175] The relief of such pain for several days after a single dose of aspirin is diagnostic of erythromelalgia.[126,135,136] The specific microvascular syndrome of erythromelalgia is readily explained by platelet-mediated arteriolar inflammation and occlusive thrombosis leading to acrocyanosis and even gangrene.[126,135,136] Skin biopsies from affected sites reveal arteriolar lesions without involvement of venules, capillaries, or nerves.[135] The arteriolar endothelial cells are swollen and the vessel walls thickened by cellular swelling and deposition of intracellular material.[135] Compared with atherosclerotic circulatory obstruction, arterial pulses in patients with erythromelalgia remain normal.[135,136]

Although thrombosis of the microvasculature is generally more frequent, thrombosis of large veins and arteries in patients with ET still occurs commonly.[13,14,177] In one series, 51% of patients had symptoms related to large-vessel thrombosis, mostly in the arteries of the legs (30%), the coronary arteries (18%), and the renal arteries (10%).[14] Involvement of the carotid, mesenteric, and subclavian arteries is not unusual. In the same series, 7% of patients suffered from venous thrombosis involving either the splenic vein, hepatic veins, or veins of the legs and pelvis.[14] Unexplained thrombosis of the hepatic veins leads to Budd-Chiari syndrome, whereas thrombosis of the renal vein can result in the development of the nephrotic syndrome.[178–181] Abdominal venous thromboses occur predominantly in young females with ET. Patients with this complication are at a high risk of having a poor survival due to hepatic failure or transformation to myelofibrosis (MF) or acute leukemia.[180] It is worth noting that abdominal venous thrombosis may occur in patients with normal or near-normal blood counts but as an occult MPD. In these cases, an extensive diagnostic work-up, including a bone marrow biopsy and a search for the Jak2V617F mutation, is recommended.[179–181] In one study of 41 patients presenting with the Budd-Chiari syndrome who had a mean hemoglobin concentration (12.4 g/dL, SD 2.8) and a mean platelet count (289 × 10^9/L, SD 192) not previously suggestive of a MPD, 58% were positive for the Jak2V617F.[181] Priapism is a rare complication of ET, presumably caused by platelet sludging in the corpus cavernosum.[172,182] In addition, myocardial ischemia or infarction, or both, associated with normal coronary angiograms has been reported in patients with ET, as has a high incidence of anginal symptoms.[183–185] A high incidence of aortic and mitral valvular lesions has been reported in patients with MPD, including ET.[185] These valvular lesions resemble previous descriptions of nonbacterial thrombotic endocarditis and may be the origin of the peripheral arterial emboli observed in these patients.[185] In addition, acute renal failure has been observed after thrombosis of renal arteries and veins in one patient with ET.[186] Pulmonary hypertension secondary to alveolar capillary plugging by platelets and megakaryocytes has also been reported in patients with ET.[187–189]

Hemorrhagic problems plague many patients with ET;[1–20] the primary site of bleeding is the gastrointestinal tract.[5,125,126,130,142,190] Other sites of bleeding may be the skin, eyes, urinary tract, gums, tooth sockets (following extraction), joints, or brain.[1–20] Bleeding most often is not severe but occasionally may require red cell transfusion support.[1,8,13] The postoperative period appears to be an extremely precarious time, with a high incidence of bleeding episodes following surgical insult,[18,183,191] likely caused by postsurgical thrombocytosis and the development of acquired von Willebrand syndrome. The syndrome of hemorrhagic thrombocythemia is closely correlated with a significant increase of platelet counts in excess of 1000 × 10^9/L and is associated with pseudohyperkalemia.[126]

In one large study, in which 97 ET patients were followed for an average of 7 years, 26 had some type of hemorrhage, mostly of gastrointestinal or mucosal origin, few of which were life threatening; 44 of the 97 patients had some form of thrombosis, mainly in the peripheral arteries. Risk factors for atherosclerotic disease, especially cigarette smoking, increased the risk of thrombosis.[132,192,193] It is important to emphasize that individual patients can suffer from both thrombotic and hemorrhagic episodes and that patients are not necessarily consistent "bleeders" or "clotters."[125,126,130,190]

A controversy revolves around the understanding the risk of thrombohemorrhagic events in asymptomatic patients with ET who are less than 40 years of age.[40,45,47,56,129,194–196] This group represents 25% of the patients studied in a 13-year period at one institution and 34% of those studied at another institution.[56] In one series of 57 such adults with a mean follow-up period of 4.7 years (range from 5 months to 20 years) 43% remained asymptomatic, whereas thrombotic complications developed in another 43%.[56] Hemorrhagic complications occurred in 11% of the patients and 4% suffered a spontaneous abortion (2 of the 16 pregnancies).[56] The thrombotic complications were life-threatening in only 5% of the patients, all of whom recovered. The two deaths that occurred were not attributable to ET.[56] The most common thrombotic complications were migraine headache in 20% of the patients and erythromelalgia in 5% of the patients. None of the hemorrhagic episodes were life threatening.[56] In this series, young patients enjoyed a low incidence of life-threatening complications and a favorable long-term prognosis, findings confirmed by other large series.[56,129,134,194] However, in another study of 44 patients younger than the age of 45, serious thrombotic or hemorrhagic complications occurred in 23% of patients and 4% died as a consequence of thrombotic events.[130] Carobbio and coworkers have shown that an association between leukocytosis and the development of additional thrombotic events was most evident in such untreated low risk ET patients.[166]

In a retrospective study Cortelazzo and colleagues demonstrated that patients older than 60 years of age who had a previous thrombotic event had a major risk of developing additional thrombotic events.[127] By contrast, the incidence of thrombotic and hemorrhagic complications in asymptomatic patients with ET less than 60 years of age who had a platelet count of less than 1500 × 10^9/L has been shown to be comparable with a normal control population.[194] Ruggeri and associates have emphasized the importance of the concurrent absence of both of the formerly mentioned clinical characteristics to define a low-risk profile in young patients with ET.[194] Gender and smoking have been shown to be independent risk factors for developing arterial thrombotic complications in ET. Men have a significantly higher risk of such complications and smoking increases markedly the risk of arterial thrombosis in women but not men.[193] Investigators continue to search for other acquired or congenital defects of hemostatic mechanisms, such as the factor V Leiden mutation, prothrombin G 20210A gene mutation, and so on, to better understand why many patients remain asymptomatic, whereas others experience a serious thrombosis. Screening of patients for such thrombophilic states may identify patients at an even higher risk for both arterial or venous thrombotic events.[11,197]

The identification of the Jak2V617F mutation in about 50% of patients with ET raised the question of whether patients with or without the mutation differ in terms of thrombotic risk.[107–110] In a large study of 806 patients, Campbell and coworkers suggested that the Jak2 mutation was associated with a high risk of developing venous but not arterial thrombotic events.[110] An increased risk of thrombosis in Jak2 mutated patients with ET has also been reported by other investigators.[109,198] However, the rate of vascular complications was reported not to be affected by the presence of the mutation in two other relatively large studies, including 150 and 130 patients, respectively.[108,117] Regardless, it is conceivable that the significantly higher age distribution, hematocrit and leukocyte levels in mutation-positive patients might contribute to the apparent association between Jak2V617F and thrombosis reported in some studies.[108–110,117,198] Vannucchi et al have reported that the rare ET patients with a high Jak2V617F burden are at a particularly higher risk of developing cardiovascular events.[114]

Pregnancy is not contraindicated in patients with ET. The outcome of pregnancy in patients with ET has recently been the subject of intense investigation.[199–209] In a systematic review of the literature, Barbui and coworkers pooled data from 461 pregnancies reported by retrospective and prospective cohort studies.[209] The rate of spontaneous abortions was 44%, which is approximately twofold higher than in the general population. Loss of the fetus late in the pregnancy was also more common in ET than in normals (5%–9.6%

versus 0.5%). Placental infarction was reported in 18 cases: which was often responsible for intrauterine fetal growth retardation (11 cases). Abruptio placenta was reported in 9 cases (3.6%), a rate which is higher than that observed in the general population (1%). Postpartum thrombotic episodes were reported in 13 patients, occurring in 5.2% of the pregnancies.[209] This rate is higher than in the overall population of pregnant women.[210] The average platelet count at the beginning of pregnancy in patients with successful pregnancies was 1,010 × 10⁹/L, and it was 977 × 10⁹/L among those with an unsuccessful outcome; thus, the baseline platelet count was not predictive of pregnancy outcome. ET patients with the Jak2V617F mutation have been reported to be at a higher risk of developing complications with pregnancy.[211] During the second trimester, a spontaneous decline in platelet counts was reported, reaching a nadir of 599 × 10⁹/L.[209] This decrease in platelet counts seems larger than the reduction observed in normal pregnancies, which is attributed to an increase in plasma volume. The mechanism for this reduction in platelet numbers is not known, but could involve placental or fetal production of a factor that downregulates platelet production. In the postpartum period the platelet counts are elevated to their earlier levels and rebound thrombocytosis may occur in some patients. This increases the probability of vascular complications during this period of high thrombotic risk to a level similar to that observed in other conditions of thrombophilia.

In the large majority of cases, the fetal losses in pregnant ET women occur during the first trimester.[201–208] In one series, 65% of the miscarriages occurred in 17% of women.[202] Thus, a previous history of spontaneous abortion may be the greatest risk factor for the development of subsequent spontaneous abortions.[201–208] Excessive bleeding during delivery appeared to be an extremely rare event.[199–209] Maternal complications are rare. Minor thromboses usually occur in the post-partum period, but such major events as deep venous thrombosis, transient ischemic attacks and superior sagittal sinus thrombosis have been reported. Hemorrhage is usually minor and occurs in 4% to 9% of cases. Major hemorrhagic episodes are restricted to patients with acute von Willebrand syndrome.

Physical examination is relatively unremarkable in patients with ET. Most patients are not severely ill at diagnosis, a median Karnofsky score of 90% being reported in one series.[1–20] Splenomegaly is detectable in 40% to 50% of patients, and approximately 20% have hepatomegaly.[1–20] During the course of the disorder, a further increase in the degree of hepatosplenomegaly is reported to not typically occur, but it may be observed.[1–20]

Table 71–3. Laboratory Findings Associated with Essential Thrombocythemia

Findings	Patients N	Patients %
Hemoglobin Level		
>16 g/100 mL	6	6
12–16 g/dL	64	68
<12 g/dL	23	24
Leukocytosis		
<8 × 10⁹/L	23	24
8–12 × 10⁹/L	41	44
12–20 × 10⁹/L	22	22
20–29 × 10⁹/L		8
Platelet Count		
<1 × 10¹²/L	37	38
1–1.5 × 10¹²/L	37	39
>1.5 × 10¹²/L	20	22
Reticulin fibrosis	38/70	54
Normal cytogenetics	49/51	99
Platelet Aggregation		
Normal	4/64	6
Decreased		
After ADP	19/64	30
After collagen	6/64	9
After ADP and collagen	35/64	55

Data from Bellucci S, Janvier M, Tobelem G, et al: Essential thrombocythemias: Clinical, evolutionary and biological data. Cancer 58:2440, 1986.

LABORATORY EVALUATION

The hallmark of ET is a sustained and unexplained elevation of the platelet count (≥450 × 10⁹/L). The level of thrombocytosis required for the diagnosis is arbitrarily determined; the range being 450 to greater than 1000 × 10⁹/L, depending on the series cited (Table 71–3).[1–20,212–214] Table 71–3 lists the laboratory findings reported in one large series of patients with typical ET.[13] Accompanying leukocytosis was a common finding in this series, as in others reported in the literature.[1–20] A leukoerythroblastic blood picture, as well as teardrop-shaped red blood cells are not features of ET.[1–20,212] Mild eosinophilia (>400/mm³) and basophilia (>100/mm³) have been reported in more than one third of patients.[7,8]

The most common morphologic abnormalities are variations in red blood cell size and shape and the presence of megathrombocytes (see Fig. 71–3).[1–20] Enlargement of megakaryocytes with hyperlobulated nuclei and their tendency to cluster in small groups along sinuses are the hallmarks of ET.[212,215] The megakaryocytes are characterized by abundant, mature, cytoplasm and hyperlobulated nuclei with smooth nuclear contours (see Fig. 71–3). Granulopoiesis and erythropoiesis are not remarkable except for increased cell numbers. Reticulin content was increased in 25% of patients, but collagen fibrosis was not evident.[7,12] Significant reticulin fibrosis or any collagen fibrosis argues against a diagnosis of ET.[212] In 70% to 80% of patients, iron stores were present in the marrow, albeit at reduced levels.[213] Almost all patients have normal serum ferritin levels.[215] Cervantes and colleagues[218] have suggested that the absence of iron stores in 30% of patients may merely be an epiphenomenon of a chronic MPD, and not truly reflective of an iron deficiency state. By contrast patients with a prefibrotic form of PMF have marrows with dense clusters of megakaryocytes with maturation defects and bulbous nuclei. Bleeding times are prolonged in 10% to 20% of patients.[13,128] Platelet aggregation studies are frequently abnormal, most often demonstrating impaired aggregation in response to epinephrine, ADP, and collagen but not to arachidonic acid and ristocetin.[128] Spontaneous platelet aggregation has been reported to occur frequently in such patients, but this has not been a universal finding.[128]

Approximately 25% of patients with ET have been reported to have elevated uric acid levels at diagnosis.[10,12,14] The average value of the serum potassium at diagnosis is usually within the normal range, although 23% of patients have been reported to have pseudohyperkalemia and falsely elevated phosphorus concentrations.[219] The laboratory features of acquired von Willebrand syndrome associated with an excessively high platelet count and a bleeding tendency have been previously described in detail.[143] This syndrome in patients with ET is associated almost uniformly with a platelet count greater than 1500 × 10⁹/L, a prolonged bleeding time, a normal factor VIII coagulant activity, and a von Willebrand antigen level but a decreased von Willebrand factor-ristocetin cofactor activity and collagen binding activity, as well as a decrease or absence of large von Willebrand factor multimers simulating a type II von Willebrand disorder.[140–143] The enhanced thrombotic risk of ET patients has been associated with a reduction in the concentration of one of the natural anticoagulants including protein S, antithrombin III protein C, and resistance to activated protein C.[197,220] These studies indicate that such a genetic deficiency of one of the natural anticoagulants might further contribute to the thrombotic tendency of patients with ET. Pseudohypoxemia has also been observed in ET patients with extreme degrees of

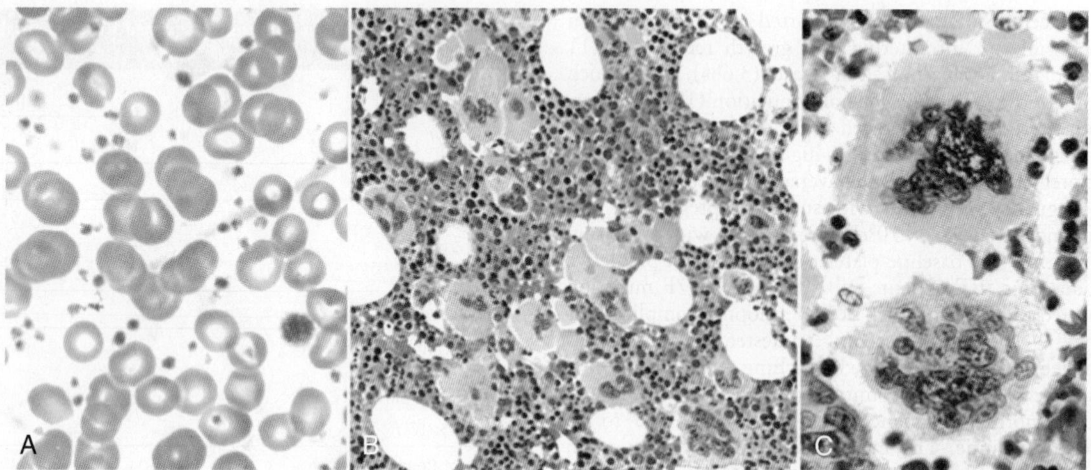

Figure 71–3. Essential thrombocythemia: peripheral blood smear and bone marrow biopsy (**A-C**). The peripheral blood smear in ET shows a marked thrombocytosis with anisocytosis (varying sizes) of the platelets (**A**). The bone marrow (**B**) is hypercellular and exhibits a marked proliferation of large and giant megakaryocytes in loose clusters with other hematopoietic elements in the background. The large megakaryocytes (**C**) tend to be extensively lobulated.

thrombocytosis.[221] The serum B_{12} level can be increased in 25% of cases.[7,12,13]

In ET, marrow karyotypes are characteristically normal.[7–14,222,223] The absence of the Philadelphia chromosome and the BCR/ABL rearrangement excludes the diagnosis of chronic myeloid leukemia (CML).[224–227] The Philadelphia chromosome or the BCR/ABL rearrangement that is seen in patients with CML must be searched for in patients who present with a high platelet count due to the observation that thrombocytosis may be the initial laboratory abnormality in patients with CML.[228] Because the prognosis and management for ET and CML are very different, it is important to rule out chronic myeloid leukemia as the cause of the elevation in platelet numbers. Aneuploidy is seen in the minority of cases. In fact, analysis of 170 cases of ET revealed a definite chromosomal abnormality in only 5.3% of cases. Marker chromosomal abnormalities, such as $1q^+$, $20q^+$, $21q^+$, or $1q^+$, have been reported, but no consistent chromosomal abnormality has been identified.[222,230–233] As has been previously mentioned, approximately 50% of ET patients are Jak2V617F positive with only 4% having a high allele burden.[114] Approximately 1% of patients have the activating MPL mutations.[105]

Table 71–4. Bone Marrow Biopsy Findings in Essential Thrombocythemia

Parameter	Normal	Slightly Increased	Moderately Increased	Markedly Increased
Cellularity	4	7	22	4
Megakaryocyte number	0	3	10	24
Erythroid elements	6	12	15	4
Myeloid elements	7	11	17	2
Reticulin content	29	7	1	0

Data from Iland HJ, Laszlo J, Peterson P, et al: Essential thrombocythemia: Clinical and laboratory characteristics at presentation. Trans Assoc Am Physicians 96:165, 1983.

DIFFERENTIAL DIAGNOSIS

In the pre-Jak2V617F era, the diagnosis of ET was one of exclusion. The discovery of Jak2V617F has provided a definitive diagnostic tool with which to diagnose ET. This mutation, however, can be found only in about half of the patients and the technology required to detect it is based on the polymerase chain reaction (PCR) assays.[234] Hence, it is reasonable to consider Jak2V617F analysis for the evaluation of patients with otherwise unexplained thrombocytosis in order to streamline further investigations. Accordingly, a positive test indicates an underlying MPD. However, further investigations, including a bone marrow biopsy (Table 71–4) and cytogenetic analysis, are still required to differentiate ET from the other chronic MPD as well as from myelodysplastic syndromes presenting with thrombocytosis, such as the 5q− syndrome and refractory anemia with ringed sideroblasts associated with thrombocytosis (RARS-T) (Table 71–5) and prefibrotic forms of PMF.[235–239]

For those patients who present with thrombocytosis and are Jak2 negative, the first step in determining the cause of thrombocytosis is to exclude reactive forms of thrombocytosis. The causes of secondary or reactive forms of thrombocytosis are numerous. In a hospital population, patients with extreme thrombocytosis (>1000 × 10^9/L) are not particularly rare in adult or pediatric patient populations.[38,39,236,240–243] Examination of the blood smear is important to avoid confusion with so-called pseudothrombocytosis. This occurs in a number of conditions in which platelet-sized particles that are red or white cell fragments (CLL, TTP, Hgb-H disease, and microspherocytosis) are erroneously enumerated as platelets by automatic particle counters.[243] Confirmation of increased numbers of platelets by examination of the peripheral smear will avoid misdiagnosis and unnecessary clinical evaluation.

In one series of 280 patients with extreme thrombocytosis encountered over a 5-year period at a university hospital, reactive thrombocytosis accounted for 82% of cases of extreme thrombocytosis, whereas thrombocytosis due to an MPD accounted for only 14% of cases.[241] In fact, of the patients with MPD, ET accounted for only 29% of the cases. Reactive thrombocytosis was more common in all age groups except those in the eighth decade and older. The causes of extreme thrombocytosis outlined in this series are listed in Table 71–5.[241] Importantly, in this series, the mean peak platelet counts for patients with reactive thrombocytosis (1195 × 10^9/L) was significantly lower than those of patients with thrombocytosis secondary to an MPD (1,808 × 10^9/L).[241] This shows, however, that a significant number of patients with reactive thrombocytosis have platelet counts greater than 1000 × 10^9/L and that it is impossible to distinguish between reactive thrombocytosis and thrombocytosis caused by an MPD, based solely on the degree of thrombocytosis.[31,39,236,240–243] Thrombotic and hemorrhagic events infrequently occur in patients with reactive thrombocytosis.[31,39,236,240–243] These findings are in contrast to the enhanced risk of these two complications in patients with ET. This relatively high frequency of extreme thrombocytosis in an acute care hospital emphasizes the need for caution in making a

Table 71–5. Etiologic Conditions Associated with Extreme Thrombocytosis

Condition	Number (%) (N = 280)
Reactive thrombocytosis	231
Infection (%)	72 (31)
Postsplenectomy (or hyposplenism) (%)	43 (19)
Malignancy (%)	33 (14)
Trauma (%)	32 (14)
Inflammation (noninfectious) (%)	21 (9)
Blood loss (%)	13 (6)
Uncertain etiology (%)	9 (4)
Rebound (%)	8 (3)
Myeloproliferative disorders	38
CML (%)	16 (42)
ET (%)	11 (29)
PV (%)	5 (13)
PMF (%)	2 (5)
Unclassified (%)	4 (11)
Uncertain etiology	11

CML, Chronic myeloid leukemia; ET, essential thrombocythemia; PMF, primary myelofibrosis; PV, polycythemia vera.

Data from Buss DH, Cashell AW, O'Conner ML, et al: Occurrence, etiology and clinical significance of extreme thrombocytosis: A study of 280 cases. Am J Med 96:247, 1994, Excerpta Medica, Inc.

diagnosis ET. A number of groups have shown that reactive thrombocytosis may be a consequence of the elaboration of known cytokines in response to the underlying inflammatory or neoplastic disorder.[244–250] Elevated levels of IL-1, IL-6, GM-CSF, G-CSF, and thrombopoietin have been detected in such patient populations and not infrequently in individuals with thrombocytosis caused by an underlying MPD.[97,98,250–252] Elevation of thrombopoietin levels has not only been found in patients with reactive thrombocytosis but also in patients with ET.[98] IL-6-induced thrombocytosis is mediated in part by secondary thrombopoietin production by the liver in inflammatory disorders and malignant diseases.[247,252] Thus, as opposed to the determination of the erythropoietin levels in patients with erythrocytosis being helpful to differentiate primary from secondary causes, the level of thrombopoietin cannot be used to differentiate ET from secondary causes of thrombocytosis.[98] C-reactive protein is an acute phase reactant, the hepatic synthesis of which is mediated by IL-6.[244] C-reactive protein levels are high in patients with high levels of IL-6.[244] In one series, 81% of patients with reactive thrombocytosis had elevated IL-6 or C-reactive protein levels, whereas patients with uncomplicated thrombocytosis secondary to an MPD had undetectable IL-6 levels.[244] Low levels of both IL-6 and C-reactive protein are strongly indicative of the thrombocytosis being the consequence of an underlying MPD.[244]

A number of investigators have constructed lists of diagnostic criteria useful in identifying individuals with ET.[7,13,45,46,253–258] No such list is infallible. Table 71–6 list useful tests in distinguishing reactive thrombocytosis from ET. Table 71–7 outlines the recently updated WHO criteria for the diagnosis of ET which incorporates Jak2V7617F testing.[259] Although useful in diagnosing adults with ET, the utility of these criteria in diagnosing children with ET has recently been questioned.[260] Red cell mass and plasma volume studies are sometimes necessary to differentiate ET from PV. In males with thrombocytosis and a hematocrit of less than 60% or in a female with a hematocrit of less than 55%, it has been suggested that such studies be performed.[261] Hematocrit values greater than these are associated with an elevated red cell mass, and radioisotope studies are unnecessary to document the presence of an elevated red cell mass.[261] Bone marrow karyotypic analysis or studies for the *BCR-ABL* fusion gene are imperative in every patient to exclude the diagnosis of CML[224–227] or to detect another clonal hematological malignancy.[223] This step is necessary because the natural history of these disorders is very different and early therapeutic intervention with specific medical therapy for CML, such as with imatinib, dasatinib, nilotinib, or stem cell

Table 71–6. Clinical and Laboratory Features Helpful in Distinguishing Essential Thrombocythemia from Reactive Thrombocytosis* (revised)

Feature	ET	RT
Chronic platelet increase	+	–
Known causes of RT	–	+
Thrombosis or hemorrhage	+	–
Splenomegaly	+	–
BM reticulin fibrosis	+	–
BM megakaryocyte clusters	+	–
Abnormal cytogenetics	+	–
Increased acute phase reactants	–	+
Spontaneous colony formation†	+	–
Jak2V617F mutation	+	–

*Acute phase reactants include C-reactive protein and fibrinogen.†Erythroid colonies.

BM, bone marrow; ET, essential thrombocythemia; RT, reactive thrombocytosis.

Modified from Tefferi A, Hoagland HC: Issues in the diagnosis and management of primary thrombocythemia. Mayo Clin Proc 69:651, 1994.

Table 71–7. Proposed Revised WHO Criteria for Essential Thrombocythemia (ET)

1. Sustained platelet count ≥450 × 10^9/L*
2. Bone marrow biopsy specimen showing proliferation mainly of the megakaryocytic lineage with increased numbers of enlarged, mature megakaryocytes; no significant increase or left-shift of neutrophil granulopoiesis or erythropoiesis
3. Not meeting WHO criteria for PV†, PMF‡, CML§, MDS¶, or other myeloid neoplasm
4. Demonstration of Jak2V617F or other clonal marker, or in the absence of a clonal marker, no evidence for reactive thrombocytosis

Diagnosis requires meeting all 4 criteria.

During the work-up period.

††Requires the failure of iron replacement therapy to increase hemoglobin level to the PV range in the presence of decreased serum ferritin. Exclusion of PV is based on hemoglobin and hematocrit levels, and red cell mass measurement is not required.

‡Requires the absence of relevant reticulin fibrosis, collagen fibrosis, peripheral blood leukoerythroblastosis, or markedly hypercellular marrow for age accompanied by megakaryocyte morphology that is typical for PMF—small to large with an aberrant nuclear/cytoplasmic ratio and hyperchromatic, bulbous or irregularly folded nuclei and dense clustering.

§Requires the absence of *BCR-ABL*.

¶Requires absence of dyserythropoiesis and dysgranulopoiesis.

‖Causes of reactive thrombocytosis include iron deficiency, splenectomy, surgery, infection, inflammation, connective tissue disease, metastatic cancer, and lymphoproliferative disorders. However, the presence of a condition associated with reactive thrombocytosis does not exclude the possibility of ET if the first three criteria are met.

From: Tefferi A, Thiele J, Orazi A, et al: Proposals and rationale for revision of the World Health Organization diagnostic criteria for polycythemia vera, essential thrombocythemia, and primary myelofibrosis: recommendations from an ad hoc international expert panel. Blood 110:1092, 2007.

transplantation for appropriate patients is potentially curative.[225,262] In one series, six women presented with the clinical picture of ET without anemia, marked splenomegaly, or extreme leukocytosis characteristic of CML.[225] Each of these patients was shown to have a Philadelphia chromosome on karyotypic analysis, and five of the six entered the accelerated phase or blast crisis within 5 to 7 years of diagnosis.[225]

A highly instructive case was reported by Morris and colleagues.[224] The patient was a 23-year-old woman who presented with a syndrome indistinguishable from ET.[224] Although no Philadelphia chromosome was detected, the patient did develop blast crisis after 4 years of follow-up. By Southern blot analysis, she was shown to have the *BCR-ABL* fusion gene, suggesting that she actually suffered from CML and not from ET.[224] This case emphasizes the importance of molecular studies when evaluating patients suspected of having ET.[224]

Occasionally, ET might be distinguished from acquired sideroblastic anemia associated with thrombocytosis, which has been recognized by the WHO classification of hematologic malignancies.[212,263] These patients present with thrombocytosis that is associated with a moderate-to-severe anemia and frequently splenomegaly. Their marrows are characterized by the morphologic features of ET and the presence of more than 15% ringed sideroblasts.[212,263] This entity likely represents a heterogeneous, poorly defined disorder that includes a spectrum of conditions sharing features of MPD and myelodysplastic disorders. Interestingly, most patients (6 of 9 patients) with acquired sideroblastic anemia associated with thrombocytosis (RARS-T) carry the Jak2V617F mutation.[237–239] In addition, ET clearly needs to be distinguished from the prefibrotic phase of PMF.[212] In the prefibrotic phase of PMF, nucleated red blood cells, teardrop-shaped red cells, immature myeloid cells, and megathrombocytes are observed in the peripheral blood.[212,264,265] In the marrow biopsy the megakaryocytes are markedly abnormal, a morphologic finding that is helpful in distinguishing this entity from ET. In prefibrotic PMF, the megakaryocytes often appear in clusters adjacent to the sinusoids; deviations in the nuclear cytoplasmic ratio in the megakaryocytes are observed with abnormal patterns of chromatin clumping and plump cloud like balloon shaped lobulation of the nuclei are observed associated with minimal fibrosis or even absent reticulin fibrosis during this stage of PMF.[212,263,264]

The presence of clonal hematopoiesis, at least in one lineage, quickly establishes the diagnosis of ET.[11,24–31] Unfortunately, techniques to study clonality are currently not widely available and are restricted to the evaluation of females. Such studies may be particularly useful in young females with thrombocytosis, Probes for a variety of genes on the X chromosome can be informative for clonal analysis of blood cell production in greater than 72% of American females.[28,31] In such patients, analysis of restriction fragment length polymorphisms can be used to establish a pattern of clonal hematopoiesis, which is indicative of a hematologic malignancy and establishes the diagnosis of ET in a young female with thrombocytosis who is Jak2V617F negative.[27] Polyclonal hematopoiesis is found in all cases of reactive thrombocytosis. Polyclonal hematopoiesis, however, does not exclude the diagnosis of ET because in several series, almost one third of patients who met the clinical criteria for ET had polyclonal hematopoiesis in all studied lineages.[28–31] The biogenesis of this polyclonal form of ET is poorly understood. Initial studies, however, have suggested that women with polyclonal hematopoiesis my have fewer thrombotic complications than those with clonal hematopoiesis.[29,30] Further follow-up will be required to confirm these observations.

A number of diagnostic tests, including splenic volume estimates using ultrasound evaluations and assays of bone marrow progenitor cells (erythroid or megakaryocyte), have been suggested as useful means of differentiating reactive thrombocytosis from ET.[11,82,85,91,266] Insufficient numbers of patients, as well as a lack of long-term follow-up, make it impossible to assess the clinical value of such tests. Studies such as PRV-1 gene overexpression in leukocytes, or decreased expression of platelet MPL are not useful in aiding clinicians in differentiating ET from other MPDs.[103] As outlined above, the most important step in improving the diagnosis of ET has been the identification of the Jak2V617F mutation in about 50% of patients with ET.[32–37] The current availability of this relatively simple molecular test makes it easier to establish the diagnosis of a ET, although the utility of the test is limited by suboptimal negative predictive value and lack of diagnostic specificity.

As has been previously discussed, the lack of quality control in many laboratories in the performance of clonal assays for hematopoietic progenitor cells is of concern and limits the usefulness of such information gained by their performance.[77–86] The presence of endogenous erythroid colonies or megakaryocyte progenitors with increased sensitivity to hematopoietic growth factors is, however, helpful in distinguishing reactive thrombocytosis from thrombocytosis due to an MPD.[77–82] Such assays are of limited use in distinguishing ET from the other MPD.[82]

At times it is impossible to define the cause of an individual patient's thrombocytosis. In an asymptomatic patient, the resolution of this problem is easy: one should simply provide follow-up and determine whether the degree of thrombocytosis increases. If additional clues to the cause of the thrombocytosis are subsequently revealed, a diagnosis will become apparent. In a patient with thrombohemorrhagic difficulties, one must make a presumptive diagnosis of the cause of the thrombocytosis and then, after weighing the benefits versus the risks of various treatment plans, determine whether reduction of platelet numbers or simple observation is indicated. Some reassurance is provided by the report of Schilling, who followed a large cohort of patients, each with platelet counts of greater than 1000×10^9/L, for 18 months. None of the patients with reactive thrombocytosis developed a cerebrovascular accident, thrombophlebitis, or peripheral arterial thrombosis.[236] These findings are consistent with the conclusions of Buss and coworkers that thrombohemorrhagic complications are rare in patients with secondary thrombocytosis.[138,241]

THERAPY

The challenge in treating patients with ET is to prevent thrombotic and hemorrhagic events without increasing the risk of transformation to post-ET MF and/or acute myeloid leukemia. Both age (>60 years of age) and a history of a previous thrombosis are predictors of a patient developing additional thrombotic events during follow-up (Table 71–8).[267] Other predictors of cardiovascular morbidity include a history of smoking, diabetes mellitus and congestive heart failure.[267] The use of these parameters have allowed investigators to stratify ET patients according to their risk to develop additional thrombotic events (Table 71–9).[267]

The treatment of asymptomatic low risk patients with ET is controversial and remains largely problematic, yet greater insight into the

Table 71–8. Risk Factors for Thrombosis in 100 Patients with Essential Thrombocythemia

Risk Factor	Incidence of Thrombosis (% Pt-Yr)	Relative Risk (95% Confidence Interval)	*P*
Age (years)			
<40	1.7	1.0[a]	
40–60	6.3	3.9 (0.7–21.5)	NS
>60	15.1	10.3 (2.1–51.5)	<0.001
Previous Thrombosis			
No	3.4	1.0[a]	<0.0005
Yes	31.4	13.0 (4.1–1.5)	

NS: not significant.
[a]Reference category.
Data from: Finazzi G, Barbui T. Risk-adapted therapy in essential thrombocythemia and polycythemia vera. Blood Rev 19:243, 2005.

Table 71–9. Risk Stratification in Essential Thrombocythemia Based on Thrombotic Risk

Risk Category	Age >60 Years Or History Of Thrombosis	Cardiovascular Risk Factors
Low	NO	NO
Intermediate	NO	YES
High	YES	

Cardiovascular risk factors: hypertension, hypercholesterolemia, diabetes, smoking, congestive heart failure. Extreme thrombocytosis (platelet count >1500 × 10^9/L) is a risk factor for bleeding. Its role as a risk factor for thrombosis in ET is uncertain.

Data from: Finazzi G, Barbui T. Risk-adapted therapy in essential thrombocythemia and polycythemia vera. Blood Rev 19:243, 2005.

management of such patients has recently been gained.[9–20,46,131,194,209,254] Management of ET patients with life-threatening hemorrhagic or thrombotic episodes is more straightforward. One approach is platelet pheresis in combination with the institution of myelosuppressive therapy.[268–272] Rapid platelet pheresis using continuous or discontinuous flow centrifugation devices has proved effective in preventing additional morbidity in patients with ET in the setting of a potential life-threatening thrombotic event.[268–272] In this situation, immediate physical removal of large numbers of platelets is preferred. Because chemotherapeutic agents generally require 18 to 20 days before platelet counts can be reduced to normal levels, Taft and colleagues[268] have recommended reducing the platelet count to 500,000/mm^3 by each platelet pheresis and suggest that achievement of such a goal requires the passage of two blood volumes over a 3-hour to 4-hour period.

Such a therapeutic approach has been employed to treat acutely ill patients with problems, such as cerebrovascular accidents, myocardial infarction, transient ischemic attacks, or life-threatening gastrointestinal hemorrhage.[268–272] Long-term platelet pheresis has proved an ineffective means of controlling thrombocytosis, presumably because of the rapid rate of production of platelets.[269] Therefore, most clinicians begin by administering a chemotherapeutic agent that has a rapid onset of action, such as hydroxyurea, simultaneously with the institution of platelet pheresis.[271]

In those patients found to have ET and who are clearly symptomatic and fall into the high risk group, little controversy exists as to the need for lowering the platelet number. The large number of thrombotic complications that occur in patients with ET who smoke, points to the urgent need for these patients to stop smoking immediately.[132,193] Most investigators try to normalize the platelet count or to reach a platelet count at which the symptoms of the high-risk patient resolve. Although major bleeding episodes requiring hospitalization are rare, those patients with extreme thrombocytosis (>1500 × 10^9/L), acquired von Willebrand syndrome, and history of hemorrhagic episode are clearly at risk for developing additional bleeding complications.[140–145] These patients require reduction of the increased platelet numbers to the normal range with use of a variety of agents, including hydroxyurea, anagrelide, or interferon-α. According to some authors, such patients should avoid exposure to aspirin, even if they are suffering hemorrhagic complications and thrombotic episodes simultaneously.[140–145] Thrombotic complications are more frequent, especially when thrombocytosis is less marked, and are the major causes of morbidity and mortality. Symptoms of functional ischemia are the most common clinical presentation, although the majority of patients are asymptomatic at diagnosis (Table 71–1).[1–20,47,127] Many investigators have attempted to identify factors associated with an increased risk of thrombotic complications.[1–20,47,127,197,266] Patients older than 60 years of age or with a history of a vascular occlusive episode have a significantly greater risk of developing additional thrombotic episodes.[90] Such patients define a high-risk population who merit therapeutic intervention (Table 71–9).[127] Cortelazzo and associates, in a randomized trial of high-risk patients, reported that cytoreductive therapy with hydroxyurea which reduced the platelet count to 600 × 10^9/L was effective in preventing additional thrombotic episodes in high-risk patients.[139] The use of anagrelide, with good control of the platelet numbers, has also been shown to minimize thrombotic complications.[273] The target platelet count to be achieved with any of these therapeutic interventions to avoid additional thrombotic events has not been well established.

Another situation that requires treatment is discomfort due to erythromelalgia or progression of erythromelalgia to frank gangrene.[126] Such patients respond within days to low-dose aspirin therapy or platelet reduction therapy.[126]

The therapeutic strategy to be employed with asymptomatic patients younger than 60 years of age remains controversial.[10,11,131,194,254] The risk of the development of thrombotic events, the leukemogenic potential of chemotherapeutic agents used to treat thrombocytosis, and the ability of cytoreductive therapy or a platelet antiaggregating therapy to reduce the incidence of thrombotic events must be considered before embarking on treatment of an asymptomatic younger (<60 years) patient with ET.[194] The Italian treatment guidelines do not recommend the use of chemotherapeutic drugs in these patients.[209]

In the past, groups of ET patients have been successfully treated with a variety of chemotherapeutic agents, including busulfan, melphalan, chlorambucil, pipobroman, thiotepa, radioactive phosphorus P^{32}, hydroxyurea, nitrogen mustard, uracil mustard, and CCNU (lomustine).[1–7,38,39,45,46,274–285] Many of these agents have been used to treat a variety of MPD and solid tumors, and their use has been associated with an increased risk of developing leukemia.[46,222,274–285] Very few phase III studies comparing the efficacy of such agents for the treatment of ET in high-risk patients have been completed.[139,286] In a study of a small group of patients, the response to either melphalan or radioactive phosphorus therapy was studied during the first year of therapy.[277] The only conclusion that could be drawn from this study was that the time to response as defined by platelet count reduction was considerably shorter for patients receiving melphalan than for those receiving radioactive phosphorus.[277] Intermittent use of busulfan (4 mg/day, until the platelet count fell to 400,000/mm^3, followed by a series of 2-week courses when the platelet count rose to >400,000/mm^3) has proved to be another relatively nontoxic and effective regimen.[274,283] These conclusions were based on a lengthy examination of the courses of 37 patients.[274,280]

During the 1980s and 1990s, hydroxyurea became the drug of choice for the treatment of ET.[46,99,139,280,285–289] The impetus for this practice was based on the capacity of ^{32}P and alkylating agents such as melphalan and busulfan to induce acute leukemia.[46] The popularity of the ribonucleoside reductase inhibitor, hydroxyurea, for the management of ET was due to the belief in the early 1970s that it was nonleukemogenic.[46,282] Hydroxyurea can be administered at a dose of 15 mg/kg initially, with adjustment of the dose to maintain a platelet count (at the least) below 600 × 10^9/L[46] without inducing significant neutropenia. Once the agent is started, frequent monitoring of blood counts is mandatory to avoid the development of neutropenia, and until the maintenance dose is determined.[139,285] The use of this drug in a high-risk group of patients with reduction of platelet numbers to less than 600 × 10^9/L has resulted in reduction of thrombotic events when compared with a control population.[139] The reduction of platelet numbers to this level did not entirely eliminate the occurrence of additional thrombotic episodes. One center has suggested that platelet reduction to less than 400 × 10^9/L might be needed to minimize the residual risk of thrombosis during therapy.[290] These findings require confirmation in a large, well-controlled randomized clinical trial.

Hydroxyurea use is associated with some toxicity, including dose-related neutropenia, nausea, stomatitis, hair loss, nail discoloration, and lower extremity and oral ulcerations.[284,285,289] Each of these problems resolves with withdrawal of the drug or dose reduction. Hydroxyurea is also not universally successful in controlling the thrombocytosis. Resistance to hydroxyurea has been reported in 11% to 17% of cases.[285] The criteria for defining resistance or intolerance to hydroxyurea have been recently established by an International Working Group.[291] They include: platelet count greater than 600 × 10^9/L after

Table 71–10. Effects of Essential Thrombocythemia Treatment Options on the Development of Acute Leukemia

Category	Myelosuppressive Therapy	No. of Patients	No. Developing Acute Leukemia
A	None	7	1
B	HU only	22	1*
C	AA or P^{32}	34	4*
D	HU followed by AA &/or P^{32}	7	5*
E	AA or P^{32} followed by HU	21	1*
Totals		91	12

*$P < 0.006$ (Fisher exact test) for B, C, E, versus D.
AA, alkylating agent; HU, hydroxyurea.
Data from Murphy S, Peterson P, Iland H, Laszlo J: Experience of the Polycythemia Vera Study Group with essential thrombocythemia: A final report on diagnostic criteria, survival and leukemic transition by treatment. Semin Hematol 34:29, 1997.

three months of at least two g/day of HU (2.5 g/day in patients with a body weight >80 kg); platelet count greater than 400 × 10^9/L and WBC less than 2,500/mm^3 or hemoglobin less than 10 g/dL at any dose of HU; presence of leg ulcers or other unacceptable mucocutaneous manifestations at any dose of HU; HU-related fever. In such situations, hydroxyurea can be substituted for (or combined with) other platelet-lowering agents, such as anagrelide or interferon-α.[291]

The risk of evolving to acute leukemia is extremely low in untreated ET patients.[1–20,44,46,292] Unfortunately, hydroxyurea has not been proved to be entirely nonleukemogenic.[280,285–289,292,293] In fact, some of the strongest evidence for the leukemogenic potential for hydroxyurea has been provided by the PV Study Group, which had previously been an advocate of hydroxyurea therapy for the treatment of ET.[44,46] A cohort of 29 patients with ET were treated with hydroxyurea between 1977 and 1982.[46] These patients met the diagnostic criteria for this disorder as established by this cooperative group.[44,46] Although five patients were lost to follow-up, the median follow-up time for the remaining patients was 7.3 years (Table 71–10). Disturbingly, 6 of the 24 patients developed acute leukemia. One patient developed acute leukemia 2.4 years after treatment, whereas other cases occurred after 6.7 to 9.7 years of follow-up. One of these patients was treated with hydroxyurea alone, whereas five others were switched from hydroxyurea to either P^{32} or an alkylating agent.[46] Another group of 62 patients was treated by this group initially with P^{32} or melphalan. Of these patients, 21 were later switched to hydroxyurea therapy. After the analysis of patients in all of these groups, the predicted probability of developing acute leukemia was determined to be 21.6% at 10 years with the greatest likelihood being between 5 and 10 years after diagnosis.[46] With careful analysis of this data, the subgroup of patients who were initially treated with hydroxyurea, but subsequently switched to an alkylating agent or p^{32} had a high incidence of acute leukemia (Table 71–10).[34,46] By contrast, those patients initially treated with P^{32} or melphalan, whether or not they were eventually treated with hydroxyurea, had a lower incidence of leukemia (Table 71–10).[34,46] More recent, prospective studies both in ET and PV have confirmed that hydroxyurea therapy was associated with a very low incidence of leukemic transformation when used alone (lower than 5%), with long-term follow-up (up to 14 years). However, the leukemic risk increased significantly when the drug was used before or after treatment with alkylating agents, particularly busulphan.[294–296] One can conclude from these studies and those of others that hydroxyurea therapy alone is less leukemogenic than alkylating agents or P^{32} alone but that some enhanced risk for the development of leukemia secondary to its use can not be completely excluded.[44,46,280,284,288,292] In those patients who cannot tolerate hydroxyurea or who cannot be controlled with its continued use, according to the consensus criteria cited above,[291] anagrelide or interferon-a therapy appears to be an alternate choice.[1–20] Recently, data on the use of anagrelide in ET suggest that it is nonleukemogenic when used in patients with ET; however, further follow-up will be required to confirm this initial observation.[297] When considering the risk-benefit ratio, one can conclude that hydroxyurea therapy is first-line therapy for ET patients at a high risk of developing an additional thrombosis, including those older than 60 years of age or with a history of a thrombotic episode or with significant other cardiovascular risk factors.[139,286,298] Such nonleukemogenic drugs as interferon-α, anagrelide, or pegylated interferon, appear to be good choices in symptomatic patients younger than 40 years of age.[209,291–310] A high proportion of the acute myeloid leukemias and myelodysplastic disorders occurring in ET patients treated with hydroxyurea alone have morphologic, cytogenetic, and molecular characteristics of the 17p deletion syndrome.[223,288] These patients are reported to have a typical form of dysgranulopoiesis characterized by hypolobulated polymorphonuclear leukocytes with small vacuoles in polys, and p53 mutations.[284,288]

Interferon-a has been employed to treat the thrombocytosis associated with MPD with increasing frequency since the 1990s.[299–310] Interferon-α acts by directly inhibiting megakaryocyte colony formation and secondarily by inhibiting the expression of thrombopoietic stimulating cytokines, such as GM-CSF, G-CSF, IL-3, and IL-11 and by stimulating the production of negative regulators of megakaryocytopoiesis, such as IL-1ra (receptor agonist) and MIP-1a.[311] Interferon-a ?inhibits thrombopoiesis by suppressing thrombopoietin-induced phosphorylation of the Jak2 substrates, Mpl and STAT5.[244] Furthermore, interferon-α also induces the production of suppressor of cytokine signalling-1 (SOCS-1), which inhibits thrombopoietin-mediated cell proliferation.[312] In a total of 212 patients treated with interferon-α in a total of 11 different clinical trials, a response rate of approximately 90% has been reported.[306] Therapy was administered to outpatients, most frequently at an initial dose of 3 million units daily, and usually produced a rapid decrease in platelets within 2 months.[306] The mean time to complete response with a daily dose of 3 million units daily was about 3 months.[306] Interferon-α was effective in patients who had received other chemotherapeutic agents and in patients resistant to conventional cytotoxic drugs.[299–310] In the majority of patients, the interferon dose required to maintain a normal platelet count during maintenance therapy was lower than the induction dose.[299–310] In one study, 61% of patients required 3 million units 3 times a week, 15% once a week, and 24% daily.[306] In addition, sustained remissions that persisted for 3 to 36 months were achieved with interferon-α therapy in 9% to 16% of patients. Interferon-α is reported to be nonmutagenic and to not cross the placenta, making it a useful drug for the treatment of the symptomatic pregnant patient with ET.[18,209,299–310] Reduction in platelet numbers with interferon results in a marked improvement in clinical symptoms. Toxicity, especially in older patients, the need for parenteral administration, and cost, limit the usefulness of interferon-α.[299–310] Side effects include flu-like symptoms during induction therapy, such as fever, bone and muscle pain, fatigue, lethargy, and depression. Symptoms are frequently controlled with acetaminophen.[299–310] Long-term administration of interferon-α can result in mild weight loss, alopecia, and late development of autoimmune conditions, including thyroiditis leading to hypothyroidism and autoimmune hemolytic anemia.[299–310] Patients may develop neutralizing antibodies to recombinant interferon, leading to a concomitant rise in platelet numbers.[313] In such a situation, use of leukocyte interferon-a results in an excellent response.[313] In one review, it was reported that 25% of 273 patients failed to continue to receive interferon therapy either because of poor compliance or side effects.[307] To gain a more comprehensive evaluation of the clinical usefulness of interferon-α a prospective clinical trial comparing interferon-α with hydroxyurea in patients with ET is required. Until the results of this trial are available, interferon-α or anagrelide should be considered as reasonable alternatives to hydroxyurea in a patient younger than 40 years of age who has suffered a previous thrombotic episode.[1–20,209]

Recently a semisynthetic protein polymer conjugate of interferon-α 2b, pegylated interferon (PEG-IFNa2b), which was anticipated to be superior to unmodified interferon as related to its adverse event profile and efficacy has been used to treat ET.[308–310] This formulation of interferon provides prolonged activity which permits once weekly dosing. Normalization of blood counts occurred after a median time of 2 to 3 months; 12% of patients discontinued therapy because of inability to tolerate the drug, and 17% did not achieve normalization of their platelet counts. The majority of side effects were WHO grade 1 or 2, although some had grade 3 toxicity, primarily fatigue and flu-like symptoms.[310] More importantly, no thromboembolic or hemorrhagic complications occurred during the period of treatment, although 12 thrombotic events occurred in 42 patients (24%) in the 24 months prior to the institution of therapy.[310] This form of interferon, however, appears to lead to a similar frequency and severity of side effects during long term use as experienced with conventional interferons. Interestingly, the use of another pegylated form of interferon (peg-IFNa-2a) in patients with PV was able to decrease the percentage of mutated Jak2 allele in 24 of 27 treated patients from a mean of 49% to a mean of 27%.[314] The use of this form of interferon appeared to be associated with less side effects then standard forms of interferon or peg-IFNa-2b. A less pronounced effect on the Jak2 mutational burden has been reported following the administration of peg-IFNa-2b in patients with ET.[315]

The use of platelet anti-aggregating agents remains an important area of investigation. Patients with ET have an increased predisposition to hemorrhage, which is likely potentiated by the use of drugs that affect platelet function.[1–20,126,141–145,290] Transient ischemic attacks and erythromelalgia associated with ET have been reported to respond rapidly to aspirin alone, to aspirin and dipyridamole in combination, or to indomethacin alone.[135,136] In erythromelalgia, symptoms disappear for 2 to 4 days after administration of a single dose of aspirin.[135] Although these agents surely have a role in the treatment of these specific complications, their use should be pursued with extreme caution because of the increased risk of hemorrhage. Kessler and colleagues have, in fact, determined that 32% of bleeding episodes in patients with extreme thrombocytosis and MPD occurred concurrently with the use of antiinflammatory agents.[137] By contrast, Hehlmann and coworkers[14] have reported the treatment of 46 patients with ET with 250 mg/day of aspirin without any bleeding complications.

Aspirin, particularly in lower doses, 81 to 100 mg/day has been shown to be useful in preventing thrombotic episodes in patients with ET.[290] Risk for bleeding associated with aspirin can be minimized if it is administered solely to patients with platelet counts of less than 1000×10^9/L or the absence of a bleeding history.[290] Van Genderen and associates have retrospectively analyzed a group of 57 patients receiving aspirin alone or in combination with a chemotherapeutic agent (Table 71–11).[290] Their data suggest that low-dose aspirin, 100 to 500 mg/day, is not only effective in the treatment of erythromelalgia and transient ischemic attacks but also reduces the recurrence of other thrombotic events in symptomatic patients.[290] Impressively, in this admittedly small population of high-risk patients with a mean follow-up of only 6.2 years, myelosuppressive therapy, plus low-dose aspirin therapy totally eliminated the incidence of thrombotic complications.[290] These findings are encouraging and are supportive of the judicious use of aspirin in patients with a history of a thrombotic episode. Low-dose aspirin therapy must be restricted to patients with a platelet count of less than 1000×10^9/L. The diagnosis of acquired von Willebrand syndrome should be excluded before aspirin use and considered a contraindication to the use of aspirin.[290] A large, randomized trial evaluating benefit and risk of low-dose aspirin (100 mg daily) has been carried out in 518 patients with PV. Treatment with aspirin, as compared with placebo, reduced the risk of non-fatal major thrombosis and death from cardiovascular causes without increasing significantly the incidence of major bleeding.[316] These results are reassuring in terms of benefit/risk ratio of this drug in MPD but their relevance to patients with ET is uncertain. Statin therapy has been proposed to be a useful means of reducing platelet activation in patients with MPD.[317] This strategy has not been evaluated in clinical trials as yet.

Anagrelide, has been hailed as a non leukemogenic treatment of ET.[1–20,297,318–328] Anagrelide is a member of the imidazo (2,1-b)quinazolin-2-1 series of compounds. When studied in humans, it was noted that anagrelide in small doses produced thrombocytopenia. The drug acts primarily by reducing megakaryocyte size and ploidy and decreasing megakaryocyte proliferation. Anagrelide, therefore, appears to lower platelet counts primarily by interfering with the development of megakaryocytes.[329] A major study of 577 patients treated with anagrelide has confirmed its usefulness.[273,297] Anagrelide in low doses was effective in lowering the platelet count in 93% of patients. Most importantly, it was effective, despite resistance to previous therapy. Resistance to anagrelide therapy has not been documented.[297,318–328] The recommended initial dose is 0.5 mg orally two to four times a day. The dose should be increased by 0.5 mg/week to control thrombocythemia.[318–328] The dose of anagrelide should not exceed 10 mg/day or 2 mg/dose.[318–328] Excessive use will result in predictable thrombocytopenia and increase the likelihood of side effects. The median maintenance dose in patients with ET is 2.0 mg/

Table 71–11. Incidence of Thrombotic and Bleeding Complications in 68 Patients with Essential Thrombocythemia who had Long-Term Follow-up According to Treatment Strategy

Treatment	Duration of Follow-up Events/100 (person-years)	Thrombotic Complications Events (*n*)	Events/100 (person-years)	Bleeding Complications Events (*n*)	(person-years)
Careful observation	127	27	32.3	2	1.6
Low-dose aspirin	139	5	3.6*a*	10	7.2*d*
Cytoreduction	113	10	8.9*b*	2	1.8*e*
χ^2 Low-dose aspirin and cytoreduction	40	0	0*c*	4	10.0*f*
Total	419	42		18	

aP < 0.001 (χ^2 = 17.3, 1df), for comparison with careful observation (thrombosis).
bP = 0.014 (χ^2 = 6.0, 1df), for comparison with careful observation (thrombosis).
cP = 0.003 (χ^2 = 8.6, 1df), for comparison with careful observation (thrombosis).
dP = 0.032 (χ^2 = 4.6, 1df), for comparison with careful observation (bleeding).
eP = 0.92 (χ^2 = 0.01, 1df), for comparison with careful observation (bleeding).
fP = 0.014 (χ^2 = 6.0, 1df), for comparison with careful observation (bleeding).
Data from Van Genderen PJJ, Mulder PGH, Waleboer M, et al: Prevention and treatment of thrombotic complications in essential thrombocythemia: Efficacy and safety of aspirin. Br J Haematol 97:179, 1997.

day administered in divided doses.[322] Data on over 3000 patients with a variety of MPD complicated by extreme thrombocytosis are available.[322] In addition, follow-up of more than 500 patients for more than 5 years had been reported.[297] Anagrelide has been shown to be an effective drug in the treatment of ET resulting in a median time to response of 2.5 to 4 weeks. An effect on platelet numbers is usually noted in 6 to 10 days.[318–328] Anagrelide leads to a reduction in hematocrit in 36% of patients, but it has no effect on white cell numbers.[318–328] In a long-term study of 35 young patients (17–48 years) followed for a median of 10.8 years (range, 7–15.5 years) more than 3 g/dL decrease in hemoglobin level was reported in 8 cases (24%).[330] Most important, the reduction in platelet numbers attributed to anagrelide use has been reported to be associated with a decrease in symptoms attributable to the thrombocythemia.[297] Silverstein reported that anagrelide use in 1700 patients reduced the incidence of thrombohemorrhagic episodes due to thrombocytosis associated with MPD from 0.66 symptoms per patient before therapy to 0.07 symptoms per patient after 28 to 30 months of therapy.[318] However, in the study of Storen and Tefferi, 7 of 35 (20%) young patients given anagrelide for more than 7 years experienced a total of 10 thrombotic episodes, and a similar proportion experienced major hemorrhagic events.[330]

The most common side effects of anagrelide resulted from its vasodilatory and positive inotropic actions. These effects resulted in complaints of headache, dizziness, fluid retention, palpitations and high output cardiac failure.[318–328] The vasodilatory effect leads to reduced renal blood flow resulting in fluid retention. In addition, gastrointestinal complications, such as nausea, abdominal pain, and diarrhea are prominent. These side effects usually develop within 2 weeks of initiation of therapy and frequently diminish in severity or resolve within 2 weeks of continued therapy. Because of its ability to promote fluid retention and the development of tachyarrhythmias, anagrelide therapy should be avoided in patients with cardiac disease and should be administered carefully to elderly patients.[318–332] If congestive heart failure or arrhythmias other than tachycardia develop, anagrelide therapy should be discontinued.[331,332] Jurgens and coworkers have reported that prolonged anagrelide therapy may be associated with a potentially irreversible drug induced cardiomyopathy which is reminiscent of tachycardia induced cardiomyopathy.[331] Dose reduction can be used to lessen the degree of tachycardia or fluid retention. Acetaminophen may be useful for treatment of the headaches. The carrier for the anagrelide is lactose, and Silverstein reported that patients with nausea, diarrhea, and abdominal pain are usually lactase-deficient and that the use of LactAid results in resolution of such symptoms.[321] Although most adverse effects are mild or moderate, in one series therapy was discontinued in 16% of patients because of intolerable side effects—especially headache, nausea, fluid retention, and, rarely, frank congestive heart failure.[318] Anagrelide has no mutagenic activity but its use is not currently advised during pregnancy. Because of its small molecular weight, it is believed to be capable of crossing the placenta and, thus, may lead to fetal thrombocytopenia.[286,297,318–321] Anagrelide does not appear to be leukemogenic because no cases of leukemic transformation have been attributed to its use.[286,297,318] Anagrelide, therefore, appears to be suitable drug for the treatment of young, symptomatic patients with ET and for those who are resistant or refractory to first-line treatment with hydroxyurea.[209,291] Anagrelide has also been successfully used to treat children with ET.[59,319,326]

Hydroxyurea and anagrelide have been compared head-to head in a large randomized trial of 809 high-risk patients with ET, all treated also with low-dose aspirin (75 mg daily).[286] Overall patients randomized to anagrelide (and aspirin) were more likely to reach the composite primary end point of major thrombosis (arterial or venous), major hemorrhage or death from a vascular causes ($P = 0.03$). When individual end points were assessed arterial thrombosis, major hemorrhage and the development of myelofibrosis were all significantly more frequent in patients treated with anagrelide ($P = 0.004$, 0.008, and 0.01 respectively).[286] Anagrelide and aspirin seemed to offer at least partial protection from thrombosis as the prevalence of thrombotic events (8% at 2 years) was significantly less than that observed in the control arm of a previous study (28%).[286] Intriguingly the number of venous thromboses was less frequent in patients treated with anagrelide ($P = 0.006$).[298] Based on this large randomized study hydroxyurea is presently considered first line therapy for patients with high risk ET. Although equivalent control of the platelet count was achieved with both agents, hydroxyurea proved superior, perhaps due to its ability to reduce not only platelet numbers but also leukocyte numbers which have been associated with thrombosis in ET patients. In addition, the combination of anagrelide and low-dose aspirin was associated with a higher incidence of hemorrhagic episodes, indicating that this combination should be avoided.[286]

A continuing clinical controversy revolves around the question of whether any treatment is indicated in patients with ET in whom the platelet count elevation is initially detected fortuitously and who remain largely asymptomatic.[131,194] Such a decision is particularly important because the use of most chemotherapeutic agents is associated with an increased risk of the development of leukemia, and the use of platelet anti-aggregating agents is not without risk.[136,289,290] The need for such treatment can be questioned, because in several studies a relationship between frequency of thrombotic episodes and degree of platelet elevation has not been established.[13,128,138] One should not lapse into a false sense of security in deferring therapy, however, because the course of ET can include infrequent but dangerous thromboembolic complications, and patients may function normally for long periods of time without experiencing a life-threatening event.[1–20] In a retrospective study of 99 consecutive low risk ET patients (age <60 years) who presented with extreme thrombocytosis (platelet count >1000 × 10^9/L) but without a previous history of thrombohemorrhagic complications, the incidence of major thrombosis and hemorrhagic events was shown to be similar during follow up between those who were treated with prophylactic cytoreductive therapy and those who did not receive such therapy.[196] The clinical course of these patients with a median age of 43 years was, however, not benign since 21% experienced a major thrombotic episode, and 7% a major hemorrhage after a medium follow-up of 147 months.[196] If the clinician feels compelled to use some therapeutic intervention in the young, asymptomatic patient, low-dose aspirin (100 mg/day) appears to be effective in the treatment of microvascular complications and its use is associated with limited toxicity.[246] Still, it would seem reasonable to withhold therapy in younger, asymptomatic patients until the development of a clinically significant thrombotic or hemorrhagic event. The older patient (>60 years) with other significant risk factors for cardiovascular complications is probably best served by immediate institution of therapy.[139] In addition, platelet reduction therapy is indicated in a patient with excessive thrombocytosis (platelet count >1500 × 10^9/L) and a documented acquired von Willebrand syndrome.[140–144] Such an individual is at a very high risk of suffering a serious hemorrhagic episode.

The management of a pregnant patient with ET remains problematic.[201–208] The major goal of any therapeutic intervention in a pregnant patient with ET should be the prevention of the vasoocclusive events that lead to placental infarction, intrauterine fetal growth retardation, and, in some cases, fetal death. Patients with Jak2V617F positive ET have a higher risk of developing such complications.[211] In one large series, there was no significant relationship between the fetal outcome and the degree of maternal thrombocytosis or presence of disease complications.[202] In this series, there were no instances of excessive bleeding or other related complications during delivery.[202] This group did not recommend the use of therapeutic platelet pheresis and, in fact, claimed that specific therapy (aspirin, heparin, or platelet pheresis) did not alter the clinical course.[202] However, of the many patients reported in the literature who did not receive any therapy, a significant number experienced either spontaneous abortion or intrauterine deaths.[201–208] Low-dose aspirin (100 mg/day), because of its profound effect on events involving the microcirculation, such as erythromelalgia and transient ischemic events, has been used with increasing frequency in pregnant patients during the first and second trimesters.[201,206–208,290] Low dose aspirin therapy is safe in pregnant women. It is recommended that aspirin be discontinued at least 1 week before delivery to avoid bleeding complications such as an epidural hematoma during delivery or during the postpartum period.[201] Because of the high risk of bleeding in patients with platelet counts greater than 1000×10^9/L with acquired von Willebrand syndrome, aspirin therapy is contraindicated.[139–145] There is limited experience reported in the literature with aspirin therapy alone and although the results are promising, the sample size is too small to confirm a beneficial effect.[201–208] The observed true birth rate, however, was 75% in those receiving aspirin compared with 43% in the group in the literature who received no therapy.[201,209] Aspirin therapy has, however, recently been found to be ineffective in preventing complications in Jak2V617F positive pregnant ET patients.[211] Chemotherapeutic drugs are to be avoided during the period of conception and especially during the first trimester.[201] Both hydroxyurea and busulfan are known teratogens in animal models.[153] In addition, busulfan and hydroxyurea reduce fertility in males.[201] Because the greatest risk of thrombosis is postpartum, thrombosis prophylaxis should be initiated in the form of low molecular weight heparin and low-dose aspirin following delivery unless there is hemorrhage or evidence of bleeding. These measures should be continued for 6 weeks. Mothers receiving interferon, anagrelide or hydroxyurea should refrain from breast feeding.

With the availability of interferon to treat ET, it is difficult to justify the use of chemotherapeutic agents during the time of conception or during the first two trimesters of gestation. Interferon-α therapy is not known to be leukemogenic or teratogenic, and because it does not cross the placenta, its use may be considered during pregnancy.[306] The manufacturers of interferon-α still advise that interferon-α not be used during pregnancy because adverse effects on the fetus cannot be ruled out.[306] The effect of interferon-α on male fertility remains uncertain. Anagrelide therapy should be avoided in the pregnant patient because of its potential to lead to fetal thrombocytopenia.[313–323]

Because none of the strategies described earlier has been tested in large clinical trials, one must develop a therapeutic strategy for an individual pregnant patient.[18] In the patient who has no history of spontaneous abortions and who is totally asymptomatic but is found to be pregnant, no therapy is presently indicated, although low-dose aspirin therapy (100mg/day) can be initiated without appreciable risk and can be continued throughout the pregnancy. Its use should be discontinued 1 week before delivery. Aspirin therapy is contraindicated in patients with platelet counts greater than 1500×10^9/L or patients with acquired von Willebrand syndrome. If a patient is symptomatic from a thrombohemorrhagic episode or if the platelet count is rising to levels above 1500×10^9/L, therapy with a platelet-reducing agent is indicated. Platelet pheresis therapy can be attempted in selected patients but if incomplete control is obtained, interferon-α therapy is, at this point, the best option. Several successful pregnancies have been reported with interferon-α therapy.[201–208] The patient with a history of a previous spontaneous abortion appears to be at a particularly high risk of developing subsequent spontaneous abortions if left untreated.[201–208] At the minimum, low-dose aspirin therapy in this patient population is a reasonable therapeutic approach.

Hormone replacement therapy including oral contraceptives and estrogen replacement hormone therapy remains controversial in patients with ET. Each of these agents in the normal population is associated with an increased incidence of arterial and venous thrombosis. Intuitively it would seem wise to avoid such agents in patients with ET who are already at an increased risk of developing thrombosis. Gangat and coworkers retrospectively reviewed the consequences of such hormonal interventions in 305 women.[333] Oral contraceptive therapy was associated with a high incidence of venous thrombosis occurring within the abdominal cavity, while estrogen replacement hormone therapy in menopausal women did not appear to be associated with an increase incidence of thrombosis.[333] This observation is surprising and might be a consequence of the limited numbers of patients included within this study.

PROGNOSIS

The probability that a patient with ET will survive 10 years ranges from 64% to 80%.[1–20] In a large study from Spain with extensive follow-up, there was no substantial difference between the probability of survival of patients with ET and that of the control population.[334] However, a more recent cohort study of 322 consecutive patients seen at the Mayo Clinic and followed for a median follow-up of 13.6 years showed a different pattern.[167] Survival of patients with ET was similar to that of the control population during the first decade of disease whereas the survival became significantly worse thereafter.[167] Multivariable analysis identified an age at diagnosis of 60 years or older, leukocytosis, tobacco use and diabetes mellitus as independent predictors of poor survival. The risk of developing leukemia or myelofibrosis was low in the first 10 years (1.4% and 3.8%, respectively) but increased substantially in the second (8.1% and 19.9%, respectively) and third (24.0% and 28.9%, respectively) decades of the disease.[167,335] The presence of the Jak2V617F mutation did not influence either survival or the rate of leukemic transformation.[335] The rate of leukemic transformation was however higher in patients with platelet count 1000×10^9/L and abnormal hemoglobin levels.[335]

Table 71–12 presents the outcome and causes of death in one series of 435 patients with ET.[8] Death predominantly resulted from thrombotic complications.[8] Transformation to acute myeloid leukemia has been reported with increasing frequency in patients with ET and is an important cause of mortality.[46,285,289–293] The rate of leukemic transformation ranges from 3% to 10%.[1–20] The phenotype of the blast cell can be either myeloid, myelomonocytic, megakaryocytic, of mixed lineage, or even lymphoblastic.[285,289–293,336–341] A limited number of patients have been reported who have developed acute leukemia and who had not been previously treated with any

Table 71–12. Outcome of Patients with Essential Thrombocythemia

Essential Thrombocythemia (n = 435)†	
Percentage, Incidence per 1000 Person-years (95% Confidence Interval), or Number (%)	
15-year overall survival (%)	73
Incidence	
Thrombosis	11.6 (8.7–15.5)
Leukemia	1.2 (0.5–2.8)
Myelofibrosis	1.6 (0.8–3.4)
Solid tumor	4 (2.5–6.4)
15-year cumulative risk (%)	
Thrombosis	17
Leukemia	2
Myelofibrosis	4
Solid tumor	8
Cause of death	(n = 77)
Thrombosis	20 (26)
Hemorrhage	1 (1)
Leukemia	6 (8)‡
Myelofibrosis	3 (4)
Solid tumor	11 (14)
Not related to ET§	31 (40)
Unknown	5 (7)

†4303 person-years of follow-up.
‡Including leukemia or postmyelofibrotic evolution of ET.
§Includes degenerative diseases of the nervous system, cardiomyopathy, chronic liver diseases, renal failure, and trauma.
Data from: Passamonti F, Rumi E, Pungolino E, et al: Life expectancy and prognostic factors for survival in patients with polycythemia vera and essential thrombocythemia. Am J Med 117:755, 2004.

chemotherapeutic agents.[289–293,335,340] Most investigators have concluded that the transformation of ET into acute leukemia is a rare event that can be accelerated by the administration of chemotherapeutic agents.[1–20]

The development of acute leukemia is associated with a deletion of the short arm of chromosome 17, which is most frequently deleted in hydroxyurea-treated patients, whereas a trisomy of the long-arm of chromosome 1 and monosomy 7q have been observed in patients treated with piprobroman.[289] These cytogenetic abnormalities are believed to be induced by the use of these chemotherapeutic agents.[288] The median survival after the development of myelodysplasia and/or leukemic transformation is 4 months.[335] Acute leukemia, which develops after ET, is frequently refractory to combination chemotherapy, but stem cell transplantation can be curative.[342,343]

Transformation of ET to a clinical stage that resembles PMF has been well documented.[1–20,46,264,265] In fact, 6% of the patients documented unequivocally as having ET by the criteria of the PV Study Group went on to develop myelofibrosis.[46] Three additional patients who met these diagnostic criteria went on to develop PV.[44,46] These studies emphasize the potential of ET to eventually evolve into a clinical picture that resembles one of the other MPD. In a series of 195 patients with ET evolution into myelofibrosis occurred in 13 cases after a mean of 8 years from the time of diagnosis.[265] After 10 years, the actuarial probability of developing myelofibrosis was 8% in one study and 9.7% in another. The development of myelofibrosis was heralded by the appearance of immature myeloid precursors and dacryocytes in the blood smear and increased serum lactate dehydrogenase levels followed by a reduction in platelet numbers and progressive splenomegaly.[265] This does not represent an instance of misdiagnosis but rather the natural evolution of the underlying hematologic malignancy. In addition, some patients, especially women who are iron deficient, may have their erythrocytosis masked and, thus, may truly have PV although, with the finding of an elevated platelet count, a diagnosis of ET may have been made. According to the data mentioned earlier, the risk of patients with ET transforming into acute leukemia is greater than that of normal individuals.[1–20] This is a phenomenon shared with the other MPD. The risk of developing acute leukemia following treatment with hydroxyurea alone increases only slightly (3%–4%), but the sequential use of hydroxyurea with other cytotoxic agents, such as busulfan or pipobroman significantly increases the risk of developing a secondary leukemia.[285,288,289,294,295]

FUTURE DIRECTIONS

ET is a hematological malignancy with its own distinct clinical manifestations and associated complications.[1–20] Better means of identifying patients at risk for developing fatal thrombotic or hemorrhagic complications are necessary to provide the basis with which to develop the optimal care of such patients. The ability to reduce the incidence of thrombohemorrhagic episodes with cytoreductive therapy in high-risk patients is now well established.

Multi-institutional studies comparing the efficacy of such promising agents as interferon-α or pegylated interferon, for the treatment of high-risk patients compared with hydroxyurea are needed. The use of low-dose aspirin therapy to reduce the number of episodes of erythromelalgia and transient ischemic attacks is now well-established.[88] Another pressing question that requires resolution is the degree of platelet reduction that is required for optimal management to be achieved. Whether reduction of platelet numbers below 400×10^9/L rather than using 600×10^9/L as a therapeutic target will further reduce the rate of thrombotic events will require further study.[290]

Finally, the discovery of the Jak2 V617F and MPL mutations have already had a major impact on disease classification during routine clinical practice. Diagnostic strategies have now incorporated screening for the Jak2 and MPL mutations, although their prognostic significance remains to be clearly established. This new understanding of the molecular pathogenesis of MPD lays the foundation for the development of novel targeted therapies. The use of specific Jak2 inhibitors for Ph negative MPD will clearly be the subject of current investigation.

Personal Approach to Therapy of ET

The optimal therapy for patients with ET remains uncertain. Certain concepts, however, apply to all patients. One is that all patients with ET should stop smoking to minimize the risk factors associated with atherosclerotic disease. Indiscriminant use of high doses of nonsteroidal anti-inflammatory drugs, including clopidogrel, should be avoided because this practice can lead to an increased risk of hemorrhage. Use of such agents is particularly frequent in the elderly in whom ET is common.

In a randomized trial of high-risk patients, cytoreductive therapy has been shown to lessen the chance of developing additional thrombotic events. High-risk patients include patients older than 60 years of age and patients with a history of a previous thrombotic episode, including erythromelalgia, transient ischemic attacks, or large vessel thrombosis. At present, no therapy is indicated in asymptomatic patients younger than 60 years of age. If a patient has a platelet count greater than or equal to 1500×10^9/L and acquired von Willebrand syndrome with bleeding symptoms, platelet reduction therapy is indicated to avoid the high risk of hemorrhage. Patients with acquired von Willebrand syndrome should clearly avoid the use of aspirin.

In those patients requiring platelet reduction therapy, the choice between the use of anagrelide, interferon-α, pegylated interferon, or hydroxyurea therapy is based on patient age, ease of administration, and drug-related toxicity. In patients older than 40 years, hydroxyurea therapy is the treatment of choice, whereas in younger patients, we prefer to initiate therapy with interferon-α. If the patient cannot tolerate interferon-α or fails to respond, we feel comfortable treating the symptomatic patient younger than 40 years of age with hydroxyurea. Although we remain concerned about the leukemogenic potential of hydroxyurea, this potential danger is far less than that associated with the use of the alkylating agents or P^{32}.

Those patients who initially receive hydroxyurea and no longer respond to this agent or suffer toxicity and require another agent should not receive long-term P^{32} or an alkylating agent. This sequence of administration is associated with an extremely high risk of leukemic transformation. Those patients who have had a trial of hydroxyurea and require further treatment should receive either anagrelide, interferon-α, ?or pegylated interferon. Doses of each of these agents required for disease control will, of course, be dependent on the target platelet level that one hopes to achieve. Strict control to a platelet count of less than or equal to 400×10^9/L may lead to greater protection from thrombosis than merely reduction to a level of less than or equal to 600×10^9/L., but there are no randomized trials to support this practice. The success in achieving this goal is obviously dependent on the ability of the patient to tolerate the agents used. In the younger patient, if such strict control is not achievable due to poor compliance or toxicity associated with anagrelide or interferon-α therapy, we are satisfied with continuing therapy and maintaining platelet counts of less than or equal to 600×10^9/L. In these patients, the addition of low-dose aspirin (100 mg/day) should be considered; it is less clear to us if those patients who achieve better platelet control with cytoreductive therapy should also be so treated. However, in studies from Europe addressing this question in PV, the approach of combining aspirin with cytoreduction therapy appears to minimize

Personal Approach to Therapy of ET—cont'd

thrombotic complications. The use of anagrelide and aspirin in combination should be avoided due to the high risk of a hemorrhagic episode. In patients who suffer from thrombotic episodes, especially episodes involving the microcirculation or large vessels, we administer low-dose aspirin (100 mg/day). This dose of aspirin does increase the number of bleeding episodes to a modest degree but is effective in the treatment of thrombotic events. This low-dose aspirin therapy is given in addition to an agent, which reduces platelet numbers.

Hydroxyurea can be started at a dose of 1g/day and then adjusted to achieve the target platelet count (<400 × 10^9/L) without developing leukopenia. Anagrelide is initiated at 0.5 mg twice daily and increased by 0.5 mg/day every 5 to 7 days if platelet counts do not begin to drop. The usual dose to achieve platelet number control is 2.0 to 2.5 mg/day. There are patients who do not tolerate either hydroxyurea or anagrelide. In this patient group, interferon-α therapy is initiated at 3 million units 3 times per week subcutaneously or consideration to therapy with a pegylated form of interferon (peg-IFNa-2a) should be given. Another choice is busulfan at 4mg/day for 2-week courses every time the platelet count rises above the normal range. Busulfan therapy is reserved for patients older than 60 years.

In general, we do not routinely treat patients younger than 40 years of age, unless they have already have had a thrombohemorrhagic event or have significant risk factors for atherosclerotic disease. Complications even in young, otherwise healthy, patients with platelet counts greater than 2000 × 10^9/L are unusual. However, these marked elevations of platelet numbers can be anxiety-provoking situations for the patient and the clinician.

In certain situations, in young, low-risk patients, treatment should be instituted. Surgery can increase the risk of thrombosis, and the use of antiinflammatory agents can increase the risk of bleeding postoperatively. Under these circumstances, the platelet count should be lowered to the normal range. In pregnant patients with ET, low-dose aspirin therapy is the first treatment option. If the patient develops symptoms as a result of thrombosis, platelet reduction therapy is necessary and interferon-α therapy is the treatment of choice. Since interferon does not cross the placenta, it likely will not be teratogenic. Both hydroxyurea and busulfan have been successfully used to treat MPD during pregnancy, but they are probably teratogenic if used during the first trimester. If such agents are needed, they should be instituted after the first trimester.

In a patient with ET and a serious acute hemorrhagic event, the site of bleeding should be determined immediately, and any antiplatelet aggregating agents should be stopped. Although the platelet count may be high, these platelets should be considered to be qualitatively abnormal, leading to defective hemostasis. The patient may be suffering from acquired von Willebrand syndrome. In patients with acquired von Willebrand syndrome, DDAVP or factor VIII concentrates containing von Willebrand factor can be used immediately at the same time chemotherapy is being administered. If acquired von Willebrand syndrome is not present, the transfusion of normal platelets is suggested. In those patients with persistent hemorrhage, immediate reduction of the platelet count can be achieved by platelet pheresis. Hydroxyurea at 2 to 4 g/day for 3 to 5 days should be administered immediately, then reduced to 1 g/day. Any patient receiving hydroxyurea should be monitored for the onset of granulocytopenia or thrombocytopenia. Reduction of platelet counts is usually observed within 3 to 5 days of hydroxyurea treatment.

In contrast, patients with acute arterial thrombosis require immediate institution of platelet antiaggregating agents. Aspirin at a dose of 100 mg/day is suggested. Patients with erythromelalgia or transient ischemic attacks will have a rapid cessation of symptoms following the use of low-dose aspirin. In a patient with a life-threatening arterial thrombosis, the platelet count should be lowered with either a combination of apheresis and hydroxyurea or with hydroxyurea alone, depending on the severity of the event. If the arterial thrombosis involves the microcirculation and is not life threatening (transient ischemic attacks or erythromelalgia), immediate low-dose aspirin therapy is indicated and platelet reduction therapy (hydroxyurea, anagrelide, or interferon-α) can be initiated using a standard dose and schedule.

SELECTED REFERENCES

Barbui T, Finazzi G: When and how to treat essential thrombocythemia. N Engl J Med353:85, 2005.

Bellanne-Chantelot C, Chaumarel I, Labopin M, et al: Genetic and clinical implications of the Val617Phe JAK2 mutation in 72 families with myeloproliferative disorders. Blood108:346, 2006.

Campbell PJ, Scott LM, Buck G, et al: United Kingdom Myeloproliferative Disorders Study Group; Medical Research Council Adult Leukaemia Working Party; Australasian Leukaemia and Lymphoma Group. Definition of subtypes of essential thrombocythaemia and relation to polycythaemia vera based on JAK2 V617F mutation status: a prospective study. Lancet 366:1945, 2005.

Carobbio A, Finazzi G, Guerini V, et al: Leukocytosis is a risk factor for thrombosis in essential thrombocythemia: interaction with treatment, standard risk factors, and Jak2 mutation status. Blood 109:2310, 2007.

Chim CS, Kwong YL, Lie AK, et al: Long-term outcome of 231 patients with essential thrombocythemia: prognostic factors for thrombosis, bleeding, myelofibrosis, and leukemia. Arch Intern Med 165:2651, 2005.

Falanga A, Marchetti M, Barbui T, Smith CW: Pathogenesis of thrombosis in essential thrombocythemia and polycythemia vera: the role of neutrophils. Semin Hematol;42:239, 2005.

Finazzi G, Barbui T: Risk-adapted therapy in essential thrombocythemia and polycythemia vera. Blood Rev 19:243, 2005.

Harrison CN: Essential thrombocythaemia: challenges and evidence-based management. Br J Haematol 130:153, 2005.

Harrison CN, Gale RE, Machin SJ, Linch DC: A large proportion of patients with a diagnosis of essential thrombocythemia do not have a clonal disorder and may be at lower risk of thrombotic complications. Blood 93:417, 1999.

Harrison C: Pregnancy and its management in the Philadelphia negative myeloproliferative diseases. Br J Haematol 129:293, 2005.

Harrison CN, Campbell PJ, Buck G, et al: United Kingdom Medical Research Council Primary Thrombocythemia 1 Study. Hydroxyurea compared with anagrelide in high-risk essential thrombocythemia. N Engl J Med 353:33, 2005.

Levine RL, Belisle C, Wadleigh M, et al: X-inactivation-based clonality analysis and quantitative JAK2V617F assessment reveal a strong association between clonality and JAK2V617F in PV but not ET/MMM, and identifies a subset of JAK2V617F-negative ET and MMM patients with clonal hematopoiesis. Blood 107:4139, 2006.

Lippert E, Boissinot M, Kralovics R, et al: The JAK2-V617F mutation is frequently present at diagnosis in patients with essential thrombocythemia and polycythemia vera. Blood 108:1865, 2006.

Michiels JJ, Berneman Z, Van Bockstaele D, van der Planken M, De Raeve H, Schroyens W: Clinical and laboratory features, pathobiology of platelet-mediated thrombosis and bleeding complications, and the molecular etiology of essential thrombocythemia and polycythemia vera: therapeutic implications. Semin Thromb Hemost 32:174, 2006.

Moliterno AR, Williams DM, Gutierrez-Alamillo LI, Salvatori R, Ingersoll RG, Spivak JL: Mpl Baltimore: a thrombopoietin receptor polymorphism associated with thrombocytosis. Proc Natl Acad Sci U S A 101:11444, 2004.

Randi ML, Putti MC, Scapin M, et al: Pediatric patients with essential thrombocythemia are mostly polyclonal and V617FJAK2 negative. Blood 108:3600, 2006.

Scott LM, Scott MA, Campbell PJ, Green AR: Progenitors homozygous for the V617F mutation occur in most patients with polycythemia vera, but not essential thrombocythemia. Blood 108:2435, 2006.

Tefferi A: Essential thrombocythemia: scientific advances and current practice. Curr Opin Hematol 13:93, 2006.

Tefferi A, Thiele J, Orazi A, et al: Proposals and rationale for revision of the World Health Organization diagnostic criteria for polycythemia vera, essential thrombocythemia, and primary myelofibrosis: recommendations from an ad hoc international expert panel. Blood 110:1092, 2007.

Teofili L, Martini M, Cenci T, et al: Different STAT-3 and STAT-5 phosphorylation discriminates among Ph-negative chronic myeloproliferative diseases and is independent of the V617F JAK-2 mutation. Blood 110:354, 2007.

REFERENCES

For complete list of references log onto www.expertconsult.com

CHAPTER 72

EOSINOPHILIA, EOSINOPHIL-ASSOCIATED DISEASES, CHRONIC EOSINOPHIL LEUKEMIA, AND THE HYPEREOSINOPHILIC SYNDROMES

Steven J. Ackerman and Joseph H. Butterfield

HISTORICAL BACKGROUND, ETIOLOGY, AND PATHOPHYSIOLOGY OF HYPEREOSINOPHILIA

In the 100 years following the initial identification of the eosinophilic granulocyte (Fig. 72–1) by Paul Ehrlich in 1879, an extensive list of diseases and conditions characterized by blood or tissue eosinophilia, or both (Table 72–1), was developed. However, the specific functional roles of eosinophils in host defense, allergic reactions and other inflammatory responses, tissue injury, and fibrosis have only begun to be fully delineated and appreciated during the past 25 years. Recent research has now served to characterize the unique cellular characteristics of activated tissue and peripheral blood eosinophils, their preformed granule protein constituents and inducible lipid, oxidative, and cytokine products, focusing on the eosinophil's proinflammatory and cytotoxic potential in the pathogenesis of allergic, parasitic, neoplastic, and a variety of other idiopathic disease processes.[1] Recognition of the eosinophil as a proinflammatory effector cell in bronchial asthma has in part fueled the surge in interest in this granulocyte in asthma and other respiratory diseases,[2] and the prior epidemic of eosinophil myalgia syndrome related to ingestion of tainted L-tryptophan,[3] and recent increase in cases of eosinophilic esophagitis have served to markedly increase public interest and awareness of the eosinophil.

Studies of the biochemistry, biologic activities, and in particular, the localization in tissues of the distinctive enzymatic and nonenzymatic cationic protein constituents of the eosinophil's secondary or specific granule provided the first convincing evidence for the role of this granulocyte in the pathogenesis of inflammation and tissue damage in eosinophil-associated diseases.[1] In addition, identification of eosinophil-specific granule constituents in tissues by a variety of sensitive and specific immunochemical methods provided additional evidence for the participation of this leukocyte in diseases not normally associated with tissue or blood eosinophilia, for example, certain skin diseases.[4] Investigations over the past 10 to 15 years of the biochemistry, functions, and localization in tissues of these unique enzymatic and nonenzymatic cationic proteins have now provided compelling evidence supporting a pathologic effector role for the eosinophil in directly inducing tissue damage.[5] These distinctive cationic granule protein constituents include the two major basic proteins (MBP-1, MBP-2), the eosinophil peroxidase and the ribonucleases eosinophil cationic protein (ECP), and eosinophil-derived neurotoxin (EDN). Eosinophils have also been shown to have the capacity to express a variety of toxic oxidative intermediates,[6] eicosanoid and other lipid mediators of inflammation,[7] and most recently, inflammatory and hematopoietic cytokines that are integral to the normal and pathologic role of this granulocyte in health and disease.[8] This chapter will provide an overview of current knowledge and understanding of the inflammatory and pathologic activities of this granulocyte in human disease, focusing principally on the consequences of hypereosinophilia in the idiopathic hypereosinophilic syndrome (HES).

Patients presenting with hypereosinophilia provide an often daunting diagnostic challenge to physicians who must navigate multiple medical subspecialties in order to wade through the long and diverse list of potential causes (Table 72–1). This process, an often frustrating experience for both physician and patient, may nevertheless result in an indeterminate diagnosis of hypereosinophilia of unknown etiology. The hypereosinophilic syndrome (HES) comprises a group of myeloproliferative disorders of unknown etiology that are marked by sustained overproduction of eosinophils and tissue infiltration. In addition to the striking and sometimes profound eosinophilia associated with the syndrome, idiopathic HES is characterized by a predilection for end-organ damage most commonly involving the heart, with the development of eosinophilic endomyocardial fibrosis and related cardiac pathologies. However, as heart disease can also develop with eosinophilias due to other known etiologies, for example, tropical eosinophilia and certain cancers,[9,10] the cardiac manifestations of idiopathic HES are not unique to this syndrome. The currently defined criteria for HES as originally presented by Chusid and colleagues[11] and which serve to distinguish HES patients from those with identifiable (reactive) causes for their eosinophilia include (a) persistent eosinophilia of greater than 1500 eosinophils/mm^3 for more than 6 months; (b) exclusion of other potential etiologies for the eosinophilia including parasitic, allergic, or other causes; and (c) presumptive signs and symptoms of organ system dysfunction or involvement that appears related to the eosinophilia that is otherwise unexplained in the clinical presentation. Of interest, the more recent identification of subgroups of patients with profound idiopathic eosinophilia characteristic of HES but who do not go on to develop end-organ damage characteristic of HES (eg, patients with episodic angioedema with eosinophilia[12,13]) complicates the diagnosis, treatment, and management of patients with profound eosinophilia of unknown etiology. This chapter provides a review of the distinguishing, as well as more variable, hematologic and clinical features of HES that should assist the physician in separating this syndrome from more common (reactive) eosinophilias of known etiology. This will include a discussion of the current understanding of HES etiology and pathogenesis, as well as therapeutic approaches and strategies for managing this complex syndrome.

EOSINOPHIL MORPHOLOGY

Eosinophils contain three distinct membrane-bound granule populations that are produced during their differentiation from hematopoietic progenitors in the bone marrow (Fig. 72–2). These include (a) round, uniformly electron-dense primary granules, present mainly at the eosinophilic promyelocyte/myelocyte stages; (b) specific or secondary granules, containing an electron-dense crystalloid core surrounded by a less dense granular matrix (>95% of granules in mature eosinophils and the morphologic hallmark of this granulocyte); and (c) less well characterized small granules, which are sites for hydrolytic

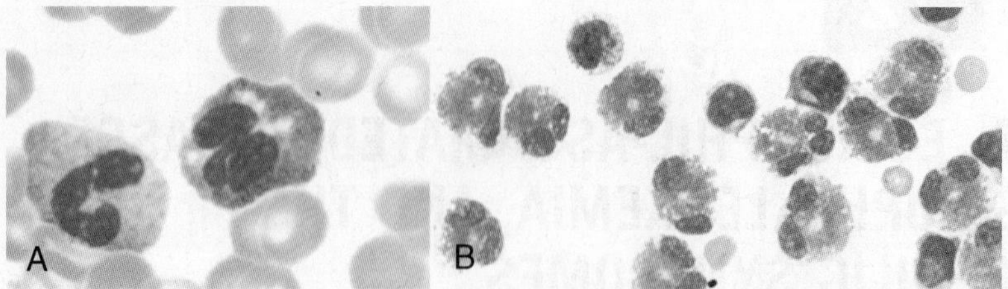

Figure 72–1 Eosinophil and Eosinophilia (**A**, **B**). Eosinophil in a standard peripheral blood smear (**A**) (center) compared to a neutrophilic granulocyte (left). The eosinophil usually has a bilobed nucleus and heavily condensed chromatin usually with two lobes. The granules are considerably larger than those of a neutrophil, and are spherical red-orange and refractile. They fill the cytoplasm and frequently overlie the nucleus. An eosinophilia is illustrated in a CSF specimen (**B**) from a patient with hydrocephalus and a V-P shunt; apparently the eosinophilia is due to an allergic response.

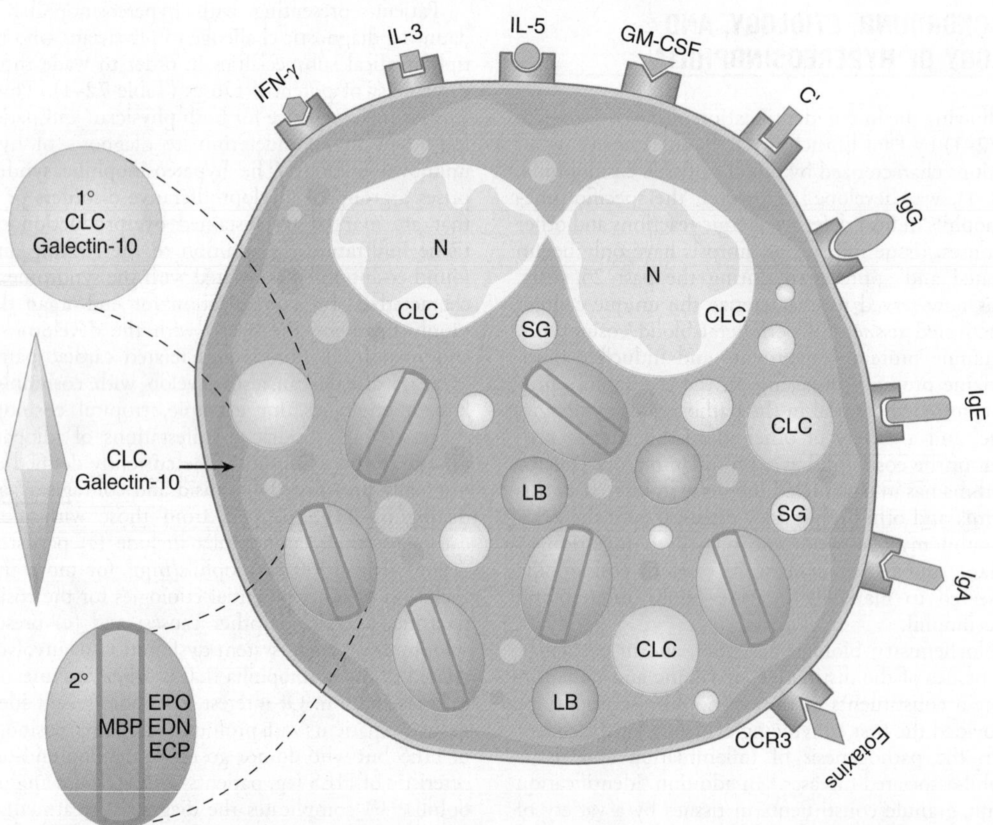

Figure 72–2 Schematic structure of the mature human eosinophil. Primary (1°) and secondary (2°) granules, small granules (SG), and non-membrane-bound lipid bodies (LB) are shown, as are the major cell surface cytokine, chemokine, immunoglobulin, and complement receptors. The subcellular localizations of the eosinophil granule cationic proteins major basic protein (MBP), eosinophil peroxidase (EPO), eosinophil cationic protein (ECP), and eosinophil-derived neurotoxin (EDN) in the secondary granule and the Charcot–Leyden crystal (CLC) protein (galectin-10) in the coreless primary granule, and the nucleus and cytosolic space beneath the plasma membrane are also indicated. (Redrawn from Gleich GJ, Adolphson CR, Leiferman KM: The biology of the eosinophilic leukocyte. Annu Rev Med 44:85, 1993.)

enzymes such as acid phosphatase and arylsulfatase, may contain catalase, and may be functionally analogous to lysosomes and peroxisomes of other cells. The large specific granule is the major repository for the eosinophil's cytotoxic and proinflammatory cationic proteins, which also confer the unique and characteristic tinctorial (eosinophilic) properties of this cell as originally identified by Paul Erlich in 1879. Eosinophils also contain lipid bodies, non-membrane-bound lipid-rich organelles often confused with granules and present in many types of leukocytes and other cells.[7] Normal blood eosinophils contain greater numbers of lipid bodies than do neutrophils, and the numbers of lipid bodies increase during eosinophil activation in vitro and engagement in inflammatory reactions in vivo.[14] Although the functions of lipid bodies are incompletely understood, they incorporate fatty acids such as arachidonate and likely serve as intracellular depots for its storage and metabolism, as suggested by the lipid body localization of all the principal eosinophil eicosanoiden-forming enzymes including 5-lipoxygenase, leukotriene C4 synthase, and cyclooxygenase.[15] As reviewed in detail elsewhere,[16] these four organelles, along with vesiculotubular structures and small vesicles involved in transport and secretion in the activated cell, serve as the major subcellular sites for the eosinophils' armamentarium of preformed cytotoxic and inflammatory mediators.

Table 72–1 Diseases, Syndromes, and Conditions Commonly Associated With Peripheral Blood Eosinophilia and/or Tissue Eosinophilia

Infectious Agents	
	Parasitic
	Tropical eosinophilia
	Visceral larval migrans (VLM, Toxocariasis)
	Helminth infections
	Filariasis (*Wuchereria bancrofti, Brugia malayi*)
	Onchocerciasis
	Schistosomiasis
	Fascioliasis
	Paragonimiasis
	Strongyloidiasis
	Trichinosis
	Hookworm
	Ascariasis
	Echinococcosis/hydatid disease
	Nonparasitic
	Coccidioidomycosis
	Chlamydial pneumonia of infancy
	Scarlet fever and pneumococcal pneumonia (convalescent phase)
	Cat scratch disease
	Cryptococcosis (CSF eosinophilia) in HIV
Allergic Diseases	
	Asthma (atopic and intrinsic, nasal polyps, aspirin intolerance syndromes)
	Bronchopulmonary aspergillosis
	Allergic rhinitis
	Urticarias (acute allergic and chronic idiopathic)
	Atopic dermatitis
	Acute drug (hypersensitivity) reactions (interstitial nephritis, cholestatic hepatitis, exfoliative dermatitis)
Respiratory Tract Disorders	
	Hypersensitivity pneumonitis (rare)
	Allergic bronchopulmonary aspergillosis
	Eosinophilic pneumonia
	Transient pulmonary infiltrates (Löeffler syndrome)
	Prolonged pulmonary infiltrates with eosinophilia (PIE syndromes)
	Tropical pulmonary eosinophilia (TPE)
	Bronchiectasis
	Cystic fibrosis
Endocrinologic Disorders	
	Addison disease
Gastrointestinal Diseases	
	Inflammatory bowel disease (IBD)
	Eosinophilic gastroenteritis, eosinophilic esophagitis (EE)
	Allergic gastroenteritis (young children)
	Celiac disease (when associated with EE)
Toxic Reactions to Ingested Agents	
	Eosinophil myalgia syndrome (L-tryptophan)
	Toxic oil syndrome
Reactions to Cytokine Therapies	
	IL-2 and IL-2 plus lymphokine activated killer (LAK) cells
	GM-CSF for chemotherapy-induced neutropenia
Cutaneous Disorders	
	Atopic dermatitis
	Immunologic skin diseases
	Scabies
	Eosinophilic cellulitis (Wells syndrome)
	Episodic angioedema with eosinophilia
	Chronic idiopathic urticaria
	Bullous pemphigoid
	Herpes gestationis
Immunodeficiency Syndromes	
	Wiskott–Aldrich syndrome
	Selective IgA deficiency with atopy
	Hyper-IgE recurrent infection syndrome (Job syndrome)
	Swiss-type and sex-linked combined immunodeficiency
	Nezelof syndrome
	Graft-versus-host-disease (GVHD)
Connective Tissue Diseases	
	Vasculitis/Collagen Vascular Disorders
	Hypersensitivity vasculitis
	Allergic granulomatosis with angiitis (Churg–Strauss syndrome)
	Serum sickness
	Eosinophilic fasciitis
	Sjögren syndrome
	Rheumatoid arthritis (severe)
Neoplastic and Myeloproliferative Diseases and Syndromes	
	Neoplastic
	Ovarian carcinoma
	Solid tumors (mucin secreting, epithelial cell origin)
	Eosinophil leukemia
	Idiopathic hypereosinophilic syndrome (HES)
	Systemic mastocytosis
	Lymphomas (T cell, Hodgkin)
	Chronic myelogenous leukemia, acute myelogenous leukemia, MDS (myelodysplastic syndrome)
	T-cell lymphocytic leukemia
	Myelomonocytic leukemia with bone marrow eosinophilia (M4Eo, inversion 16)
	Angioimmunoblastic lymphadenopathy
	Angioblastic lymphoid hyperplasia (Kimura disease)
Rare Causes	
	Chronic active hepatitis
	Chronic dialysis
	Acute pancreatitis
	Postirradiation
	Hypopituitarism

Modified and updated from Mahanty S, Nutman, TB: Eosinophilia and eosinophil-related disorders. In Middleton EJ, Reed CE, Ellis EF, et al (eds.): Allergy: Principles and Practice, 4th ed. St. Louis, Mosby-Year Book, 1993, p 1077.

EOSINOPHIL DEVELOPMENT, RECRUITMENT, AND ACTIVATION

Eosinophilopoiesis

Eosinophils are derived in the bone marrow from $CD34^+$ multipotential myeloid progenitors in response to a number of T cell-derived eosinophilopoietic cytokines and growth factors including IL-3, GM-CSF, and IL-5. These cytokines affect the eosinophil lineage at three different levels, including the (a) commitment, proliferation, and differentiation of hematopoietic progenitors in the bone marrow; (b) priming and activation in the blood and tissues for enhanced functional activities; and (c) recruitment and tissue localization (discussed later). Although activated T cells are likely the primary source for IL-3, IL-5, and GM-CSF pertinent to eosinophil differentiation and the development of reactive eosinophilia in disease, other cell types including mast cells, macrophages, natural killer cells, endothelial cells, and stromal cells such as fibroblasts are also producers of GM-CSF. IL-5, produced primarily by activated T_{H2} type helper T cells[17] and mast cells,[8,18] stimulates the proliferation and differentiation of murine activated B cells and regulates the production of eosinophils in vitro and in vivo.[19–21] Both IL-3 and GM-CSF have activities on other hematopoietic lineages, whereas IL-5 is more eosinophil-specific and plays a crucial role in regulating the terminal differentiation and postmitotic activation of eosinophils.[22] IL-5 is therefore a late-acting cytokine that demonstrates maximum activity on an eosinophil progenitor pool that is first expanded by the earlier-acting, multipotential cytokines such as IL-3 or GM-CSF.[22] Although IL-3 and GM-CSF participate in the proliferation and commitment of progenitors to the eosinophil lineage, IL-5 is both necessary and sufficient for eosinophil development to proceed in vivo.[22,23] In humans, IL-5 does not appear to have any effect on B cells or other lymphoid lineages, and its activity, high-affinity receptor, and functions are restricted to eosinophils and hematopoietically related basophils.[22] The expression of the high-affinity receptor for IL-5 is an important prerequisite and very early lineage-specific event in the hematopoietic program for these granuloctyes. Overexpression of IL-5 is observed in many eosinophil-associated diseases[24–26] and IL-5 transgenic mice develop profound eosinophilia,[27,28] indicating that IL-5 plays important roles in promoting the production and function of eosinophils in vivo. These general observations have recently been confirmed and expanded in studies of IL-5 deficient (gene knockout) mice,[29,30] which produce basal levels of normal eosinophils in the bone marrow, but do not develop blood and tissue eosinophilia, airway hyperreactivity, or lung damage in the murine ovalbumin allergic asthma model,[30] nor eosinophilic responses to helminth parasites.[29] For these reasons, IL-5 and its receptor may be excellent targets for therapeutic intervention in eosinophil-associated inflammatory diseases.

Mobilization and Migration of Eosinophils to Sites of Inflammation

In the normal individual, eosinophils produced in the bone marrow reside only briefly in the peripheral circulation in transit to extravascular sites. They tend to localize preferentially in certain tissues and organs exposed to the external environment, principally in the submucous membrane and loose connective tissue of skin, gastrointestinal tract, genital tract, and the lungs.[31] In contrast, the acute and chronic inflammatory recruitment of eosinophils into tissues occurs primarily in response to the early- and late-phase components of immediate hypersensitivity reactions, but also in association with a number of other immunologically mediated reactions, diseases, and idiopathic syndromes to be outlined or discussed in detail later. In addition, diurnal variations in the eosinophil intravascular compartment are well documented, with minimum numbers of blood eosinophils early in the morning and highest numbers late at night, mirroring circadian rhythms in circulating adrenal corticosteroids. Likewise, diurnal variations have also been documented to occur in the mobilization, recruitment, and activation state of eosinophils in tissues, for example, in diseases such as nocturnal asthma.[32,33]

Although eosinophils may represent only part of an inflammatory infiltrate composed of neutrophils, monocytes, and/or lymphocytes, the mechanisms by which they are selectively recruited in large numbers in certain reactions are currently under investigation.[34] The mobilization of eosinophils, as for other leukocytes, from the vasculature involves their rolling and adherence to vascular endothelium via L-selectin, followed by interactions with intercellular adhesion molecule-1 (ICAM-1) through CD18/CD11a,b-dependent mechanisms, and migration in response to specific cytokines or chemoattractants. Adherence via CD18-independent mechanisms involves binding to cytokine-activated endothelial cells utilizing either E-selectin, also known as endothelial leukocyte adhesion molecule-1 (ELAM) or vascular cell adhesion molecule-1 (VCAM). Selective recruitment of eosinophils likely involves adhesion to VCAM via the β_1 integrin very late activation antigen-4 (VLA-4), which is expressed by eosinophils but not by neutrophils.[35] Because no single chemotactic agent identified thus far is uniquely specific for eosinophils, selective eosinophil recruitment likely involves the complex interaction of multiple adhesion pathways and chemotactic gradients. The inflammatory mediators identified to function as potent eosinophil chemoattractants include the complement fragment C5a and platelet activating factor (PAF), along with a number of the eosinophil-active cytokines, including IL-3, IL-5, and GM-CSF, which also prime eosinophils for enhanced migratory responses to agents such as PAF, fMLP, LTB_4, and IL-8. Other potent eosinophil chemoattractants identified thus far are active in the 10^{-12} to 10^{-11} M range, are approximately 1000-fold more active than PAF and C5a, and include both IL-2 and the $CD8^+$ T cell-derived lymphocyte chemoattractant factor (LCF) that utilizes CD4 expressed on the activated eosinophil as its receptor.[36] The chemokine RANTES, which is chemotactic for certain T-cell subsets and monocytes, but not for neutrophils, is likewise a potent stimulus for eosinophil migration[37]; its production by the $CD4^+$ T-cell component of cutaneous and pulmonary allergen-induced late-phase reactions may contribute to the eosinophil infiltration characteristic of these responses. The most potent and eosinophil-selective chemoattractants identified to date are the family of eotaxins (eotaxin-1, 2, 3), chemokines that bind and signal through the CCR3 receptor expressed on eosinophils.[38–41] Recent studies have characterized the selective signals that regulate eosinophil accumulation in tissues in eosinophil-associated diseases. Two interrelated mechanisms for the tissue accumulation of eosinophils have recently been identified and shown to be linked to eosinophil-associated pathophysiology.[42] Interleukin-5 was shown to play a critical role in expanding and terminally differentiating eosinophil progenitor pools in the bone marrow in response to allergenic or other stimuli in peripheral tissues. T_{H2} T cell-derived cytokines such as IL-4 and IL-13 operate within tissues to regulate the transmigration of eosinophils from the vascular bed, a process that exclusively promotes tissue accumulation of eosinophils over other leukocytes, probably by activating eosinophil-specific adhesion pathways on endothelial cells and by regulating the production of IL-5 and eotaxin expression in the target tissue compartment. IL-5 and eotaxin likely cooperate locally to selectively and synergistically promote eosinophilia, the former working both systemically and within tissues to promote the local eosinophil chemotactic signals provided by the latter. The regulation of IL-5 and eotaxin levels within tissues by cytokines that include IL-4 and IL-13, allows T_{H2} cells to coordinate both tissue and peripheral blood eosinophilia. These observations highlight the importance of targeting both IL-5 and eotaxin/CCR3 signaling systems to block eosinophil-associated inflammation and tissue pathology.[42–45]

Eosinophil Activation in Disease: Eosinophil Heterogeneity

Eosinophils secrete their preformed granule constituents and newly synthesized lipid, and cytokine and peptide mediators of inflammation on stimulation (Fig. 72–3). It has become increasingly clear that peripheral blood eosinophils from patients with eosinophilia and eosinophils from the inflammatory tissue microenvironment are heterogeneous with regard to their capacity for stimulation and secretion of the described mediators. Eosinophils from blood and tissues of patients with eosinophilia differ from their normal counterparts by a variety of morphologic, biochemical, and functional characteristics,[46] some of which appear to be linked to a significant decrease in cell density as measured by separation over density gradients of cell separation media such as Percoll. A distinction is now made between the populations of "normodense" (normal density) and "hypodense" (light density) eosinophil phenotypes isolated from the peripheral blood and tissues. The blood of normal individuals contains less than 10% of eosinophils with densities less than 1.082 g/mL, whereas patients with eosinophilia can have markedly increased numbers of the hypodense cells.[25,47,48] Hypodense eosinophils possess a variety of properties consistent with their being primed, activated in vivo, or both, by analogy with classic macrophage activation. On a morphologic level, activated hypodense eosinophils show increased vacuolization, decreased granule size (and content of granule cationic proteins

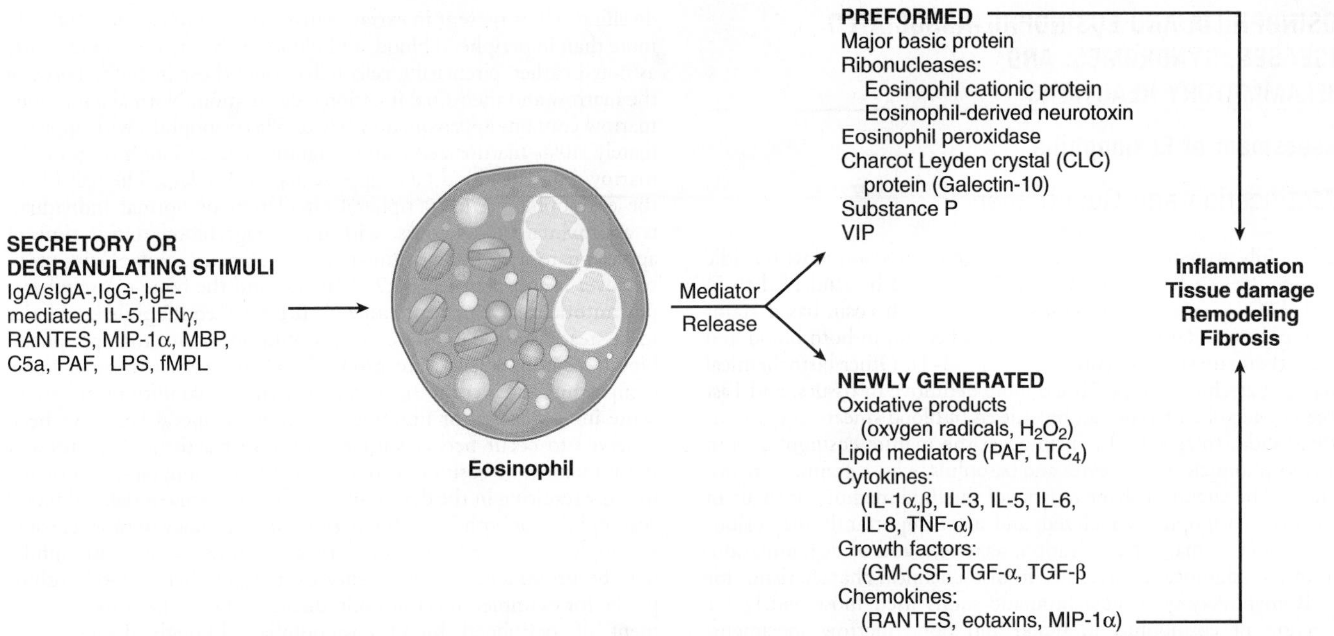

SECRETORY OR DEGRANULATING STIMULI
IgA/sIgA-,IgG-,IgE-mediated, IL-5, IFNγ, RANTES, MIP-1α, MBP, C5a, PAF, LPS, fMPL

Eosinophil

Mediator Release

PREFORMED
Major basic protein
Ribonucleases:
Eosinophil cationic protein
Eosinophil-derived neurotoxin
Eosinophil peroxidase
Charcot Leyden crystal (CLC) protein (Galectin-10)
Substance P
VIP

NEWLY GENERATED
Oxidative products
(oxygen radicals, H_2O_2)
Lipid mediators (PAF, LTC_4)
Cytokines:
(IL-1α,β, IL-3, IL-5, IL-6, IL-8, TNF-α)
Growth factors:
(GM-CSF, TGF-α, TGF-β
Chemokines:
(RANTES, eotaxins, MIP-1α)

Inflammation
Tissue damage
Remodeling
Fibrosis

Figure 72–3 Eosinophil secretory/degranulating stimuli and eosinophil-derived inflammatory mediators. The listed factors have been shown to stimulate the secretion of inflammatory mediators from the eosinophil. These mediators may be either preformed, such as the eosinophil granule-derived cationic proteins, or newly generated mediators such as oxidative products, lipid mediators (eg, LTC_4), inflammatory or hematopoietic cytokines, chemokines, and growth factors. Release of these mediators leads to tissue inflammation, damage, remodeling, and fibrosis. (Redrawn from Furuta GT, Ackerman SJ, Wershil BK: The role of the eosinophil in gastrointestinal diseases. Curr Opin Gastroenterol 11:541, 1995.)

such as MBP[48]), and increased numbers of cytoplasmic lipid bodies.[15] The numbers of surface receptors for a variety of eosinophil-active agonists, including complement cleavage fragments of C3 (CR1 and CR3), immunoglobulins (IgE, IgA), cytokines, and PAF, are increased on hypodense eosinophils from eosinophilic patients, as are a variety of membrane surface antigens such as CD4.[36] Functionally, hypodense eosinophils show increased metabolic activity, oxygen consumption, and generation of superoxide anion as well as an increased capacity for the synthesis and secretion of LTC_4 and certain cytokines, enhanced chemotaxis, and augmented cytotoxicity for antibody-coated targets.

The mechanism by which eosinophils develop the morphologic, biochemical, and functional characteristics of activated cells in vivo has been largely defined through the in vitro analysis of factors capable of prolonging eosinophil survival and inducing the development of the hypodense phenotype. Culture of normal peripheral blood eosinophils with growth factors (GM-CSF), hematopoietic cytokines (IL-3, IL-5), and interferons (IFN-α and IFN-γ), either alone or in coculture with endothelial cells or fibroblasts, induces the development of the hypodense activated phenotype characteristic of eosinophils isolated from patients with hypereosinophilic disorders. In addition, the eosinophilopoietic cytokines (IL-3, IL-5, and GM-CSF) also prolong the survival of mature normodense and hypodense eosinophils in vitro (and possibly in vivo in the tissue microenvironment), likely through the prevention of programmed cell death (apoptosis).[49,50] Of interest, culture of eosinophils with the previously mentioned factors in vitro does not precisely recapitulate all the functional characteristics of the in vivo activated, tissue-derived cell, suggesting a requirement for additional, as yet undefined, factors that may include interaction of adhesion receptors with their ligands during eosinophil recruitment and migration into the tissue or stromal cell-derived factors.

The diagnostic and therapeutic significance of eosinophil heterogeneity has not been fully evaluated. Although the percentage of hypodense eosinophils in the blood may correlate with the degree of peripheral blood eosinophilia,[47] precise relationships between the percentage of hypodense eosinophils and the clinical status of an eosinophilic disorder have not been clearly defined. Rough correlations have been reported between disease severity and numbers of hypodense eosinophils in circulation for particular hypersensitivity disorders such as allergic asthma and allergic rhinitis. However, there is a significant overlap in the percentage of hypodense peripheral blood eosinophils in hypereosinophilic disorders of greatly varying severity, such as bronchial asthma, the hypereosinophilic syndrome, and certain helminth infections. As eosinophils reside primarily in the tissue microenvironment for the majority of their lifespan, it is not surprising that their heterogeneity in the peripheral circulation is at best a crude reflection of disease severity. In vitro models of eosinophil heterogeneity suggest a number of pathways for the development of eosinophil subpopulations, including acute exposure to mediators generated in immediate-type hypersensitivity reactions (eg, PAF, eosinophil-active cytokines such as GM-CSF, IL-3, IL-5, IFN, or TNF) or more chronic exposure to eosinophil-active cytokines in combination with as yet undefined factors in the tissue microenvironment as discussed earlier. Regardless of the specific mechanisms or mediators involved in eosinophil priming or activation, the development of eosinophil heterogeneity as a reflection of the functional, proinflammatory capacity of the cell in vivo suggests the possibility that these processes could be manipulated in a therapeutic manner. For example, in disorders such as HES where excessive levels of IL-5 have been demonstrated in the peripheral circulation (see below),[24] therapies aimed at modulating IL-5 levels to normalize the eosinophil phenotype and attenuate the eosinophilia may be appropriate. One such example has been the use of cyclosporin A to produce a clinical remission in a patient with steroid-resistant HES in which cyclosporin A was shown in vitro to inhibit IL-5 production from T-cell clones derived from the patient.[51] In contrast, because eosinophil infiltration of certain types of malignancies, including colon cancers or lung adenocarcinomas, may be associated with improved prognosis,[52,53] it may be advantageous to induce the development of tissue eosinophilia and enhanced cytotoxicity as demonstrated in response to local production of IL-4.[54] Studies suggest novel roles for the eosinophil in tumor immune surveillance and antitumor effector cell responses in animal models.[55]

EOSINOPHILIA AND EOSINOPHIL-ASSOCIATED DISEASES, SYNDROMES, AND INFLAMMATORY REACTIONS

Assessment of Eosinophilia

Identification and Quantitation

Eosinophils, so named for their unique granular staining with acidic fluorone dyes such as eosin, were first identified by Paul Ehrlich in 1879. Subsequently, histochemical staining with eosin-based stains became the standard for eosinophil identification in both blood and tissues (hematoxylin and eosin) (see Fig. 72–1). Other histochemical dyes such as chromotrope 2R are more definitive in tissues, and Fast Green or Luxol Fast Blue can be utilized in blood smears or cytocentrifuge slides to specifically distinguish the mature eosinophil from polymorphonuclear leukocytes and basophils, whose granules are not stained. The chemical characteristics of the fluid medium or tissue in which the eosinophil is analyzed, and most importantly the eosinophil's degree of maturity, activation, secretion, and/or degranulation, can induce significant variability in histochemical characteristics for the Romanovsky-type metachromatic stains used most widely for detection of eosinophils in blood and bone marrow specimens. For example, eosinophils in urine, as found in eosinophilic cystitis or interstitial nephritis, are best detected by Hansel stain.[56] As a result, it is now appreciated that the definitive identification of the eosinophil's participation in a particular inflammatory response or disease may require immunochemical localization using specific monoclonal or polyclonal antibodies to eosinophil-specific granule proteins such as MBP, eosinophil peroxidase, or ECP, all of which have been used to identify eosinophil infiltration and secretion or degranulation in tissues where they have been missed by more classic histochemical techniques.[4,57] For peripheral blood, absolute eosinophil counts done manually or using automated counting systems provide a much more reliable estimation of eosinophil numbers than does microscopic differential counting of blood smears combined with total leukocyte counts, especially in situations where there is an absolute leukocytosis or leukopenia for another lymphoid or myeloid lineage. Circulating eosinophils are generally present in low numbers in normal healthy individuals with consensus absolute counts ranging from 35 to 350 eosinophils/mm^3 (mean 125 for adults; 225 for children under 12 years). The broad range of variability in normal blood eosinophil levels reflects the multiple sources of both subtle and more obvious physiologic effects due to diurnal variation in endogenous glucocorticoid levels (discussed earlier), degree of atopy in the general population, and other factors that can include exercise, emotional stress, and hormonal influences of the menstrual cycle.

Clinical Assessment of Eosinophilia: Peripheral Blood Versus Tissue Eosinophils

The low numbers of eosinophils in the blood compared to neutrophils and lymphocytes, coupled with their principal localization in tissues, makes accurate quantitation and interpretation of blood eosinophil counts more difficult than that of other cellular elements. As noted earlier, cell differential counts of 100 to 200 are fraught with the problems inherent in sampling error when eosinophils constitute less than 3% to 5% of total peripheral blood leukocytes. Further, automated cell counters may not accurately enumerate eosinophils unless they are present in sufficiently high numbers, and can miss eosinophil peroxidase-deficient cells. A manual differential or absolute cell count should be performed if low-to-moderate eosinophilia is suspected in the clinical evaluation of a patient. The number of circulating eosinophils in the blood reflects a complex interplay of factors, including rates of development and transit from the bone marrow, margination, and subsequent emigration into tissues through postcapillary venules. Because the eosinophil is primarily a tissue dwelling cell, is present in extravascular sites at levels several 100-fold more than in peripheral blood, and blood levels may vary significantly as noted earlier, circulating cells reflect only those in traffic between the marrow and their final functional destination. Normal adult bone marrow contains approximately 3% to 5% eosinophils, with approximately 40% mature cells, and migration of eosinophils from the marrow into the blood takes approximately 3.5 days. The half-life of the eosinophil in the peripheral circulation of normal individuals is approximately 18 hours, with an average blood transit time of approximately 26 hours, similar to that of neutrophils. Daily mean turnover is approximately 0.2×10^9/kg, and the bone marrow has a postmitotic reserve of approximately 0.1×10^9 eosinophils/kg. Under ideal steady-state conditions, one would anticipate that peripheral blood eosinophil levels are proportional to levels in normal tissue compartments. In contrast, under the dynamic conditions of certain acute inflammatory or immune responses, temporal lags have been observed to occur between infiltration into reactive tissue sites and the induction of eosinophil development and emigration from the marrow resulting in the development of eosinopenia or delayed blood eosinophilia, or both.[58–60] Moreover, in the pathology of more chronic eosinophil-associated inflammatory conditions, tissue eosinophilia may be prominent in the absence of any peripheral blood eosinophilia, for example, in certain skin diseases.[4] Thus, the clinical assessment of peripheral blood eosinophilia, although diagnostically important, must be interpreted with these caveats in mind.

The list of diseases, syndromes, and inflammatory processes associated with peripheral blood (>300 eosinophils/mm^3) or tissue eosinophilia, or both, is quite extensive (see Table 72–1). Of course, the most common associations are infections with parasitic helminths and allergic diseases and their related inflammatory reactions. Effective clinical assessment of patients with eosinophilia requires a careful and detailed history, including travel information; where the patient has lived; drug use, including intravenous drugs, L-tryptophan, vitamin supplements, and other over-the-counter nonprescription medications; diet; and allergic symptomatology. In addition, the systemic nature of many of the nonallergic/noninfectious conditions involving eosinophilia dictates that a careful history of fever, weight loss, myalgias, arthralgias, rashes, lymphadenopathy, and so on should be obtained as well. Symptomatic or asymptomatic eosinophilia in patients taking drugs associated with known eosinophil responses and eosinophil-related drug reactions strongly dictates that their use be discontinued and that follow-up evaluation confirms that the eosinophilia and related symptoms have resolved. Patients with eosinophilia who have resided in or visited areas endemic for helminth or other parasites should be examined for intestinal and blood-borne infections, with additional serologic evaluation as necessary to identify the causative agent. Once the more common and obvious causes of eosinophilia have been excluded, that is, drug reactions, parasitic infections, and various allergic conditions, the differential diagnosis of eosinophilia becomes more difficult because of the complexity and number of potential organ systems and conditions involved (see Table 72–1).

Monitoring of Eosinophil Activity

An appreciation of the importance of both numbers of tissue eosinophils and their functional status, as well as differences in functional status between circulating eosinophils and those that have been recruited into and exposed to cytokines and other factors in the tissue microenvironment, has resulted in the development and more routine use of methods to monitor eosinophil activity in situ. Tissue biopsies have become more routinely employed for both the clinical and experimental evaluation of eosinophil function in diseases involving the skin,[4,58,61] lungs,[33,62,63] lymph nodes,[64] heart,[65] and other tissues, greatly contributing to the current understanding of the eosinophil's proinflammatory role in disease pathogenesis. The difficulties, tediousness, and sampling errors inherent in accurately quantitating the numbers of eosinophils, let alone their functional status in tissue biopsy specimens, even using antibodies that recognize specific cell surface activation markers or secretion products and modern morphometric techniques, makes routine clinical evaluation of tissue eosinophils by these methods somewhat impractical. Alternatives such as analysis of tissue secretions from affected organs, for example, bronchoalveolar lavage of the lung, have been used with great success in the clinical and experimental evaluation of eosinophil function in diseases such as asthma.[32,66,67] In addition to the more routine histochemical identification and enumeration of eosinophils, and immunochemical localization of secreted eosinophil granule cationic proteins in tissue biopsies, two additional methods have been extensively used to monitor eosinophil activation, secretion, and involvement in disease pathogenesis. These include the identification of activated eosinophils by staining with a monoclonal anti-ECP antibody EG2 that recognizes a secreted, deglycosylated form of the protein,[68–70] and measurement of the eosinophil granule cationic proteins such as MBP, ECP, and EDN by radioimmunoassay[71–73] in various body fluids including serum, plasma, urine, sputum, nasal lavage, and BAL fluid.[74] Under controlled sampling conditions, measurements of these eosinophil granule products have served as excellent indicators of eosinophil secretory activity in vivo and eosinophil involvement in a variety of allergic, parasitic, and certain inflammatory and skin diseases not normally associated with blood or tissue eosinophilia. Examples include assays of MBP and ECP in bronchoalveolar lavage[75] and nasal lavage[76] in asthma and allergic rhinitis,[74] in serum and plasma in lymphatic filariasis,[58,77] and in skin diseases such as chronic idiopathic urticaria.[78] Such measurements likely reflect in vivo secretion in tissues or secretory activity of eosinophils in the fluid sampled,[74] or both, and have provided compelling evidence for relationships between eosinophil secretory activity and disease severity.[75,79,80]

IDIOPATHIC HYPEREOSINOPHILIC SYNDROME

The hypereosinophilic syndrome (HES) comprises a group of myeloproliferative disorders of unknown etiology that are marked by a sustained overproduction of eosinophils. In addition to the striking and sometimes profound eosinophilia associated with the syndrome, HES is characterized by a predilection for end-organ damage, most commonly involving the heart, with the development of eosinophilic endomyocardial fibrosis and related cardiac pathologies. The currently defined criteria for HES as originally presented by Chusid et al[11] are listed in Table 72–2 and include (a) persistent eosinophilia of greater than 1500 eosinophils/mm^3 for more than 6 months; (b) exclusion of other potential etiologies for the eosinophilia including parasitic, allergic, or other causes; and (c) signs and symptoms of organ system dysfunction or involvement that appears related to the eosinophilia or is of unknown cause in the clinical presentation. Total leukocyte counts are often less than 25,000/mm^3 with 30% to 70% eosinophils. However, extremely high leukocyte counts (>90,000/mm^3) may be associated with poor prognosis in some patients. These three primary features of the syndrome, including sustained eosinophilia of unknown etiology or disease association, along with evidence of organ involvement (see Table 72–2), comprise the defining characteristics of HES. The clinical features of patients diagnosed with HES, as summarized by Spry[81] and most recently reviewed by Weller and Bubley,[82] Brito-Babapulle,[83] and one of us,[84] are shown in Table 72–3 as well as their frequency at presentation. The most commonly encountered features in approximately 50% to 75% of patients studied in detail to date[85–87] include the cardiovascular manifestations, especially endomyocardial disease (discussed later) and its associated thromboembolic complications, the major causes of morbidity (and mortality) in the HES.

Table 72–2 Criteria for the Diagnosis of the Idiopathic Hypereosinophilic Syndrome

Eosinophils >1500/mm^3 for at least 6 months
Reactive causes of eosinophilia excluded
Known eosinophilic disease entities excluded
Evidence of eosinophilic end-organ damage
Clonal eosinophilic disorders excluded
Factors Favoring a Diagnosis of HES
Elevated serum immunoglobulins
Elevated levels of tumor necrosis factor or interleukins (IL-5)
Elevated serum IgE levels
Good therapeutic response to corticosteroids

*Reproduced with permission from Brito-Babapulle, F: Clonal eosinophilic disorders and the hypereosinophilic syndrome. Blood Rev 11:129, 1997.

DIFFERENTIAL DIAGNOSIS OF HYPEREOSINOPHILIC SYNDROME

As shown in Table 72–1, a large number of diseases have been identified that are associated with reactive, secondary eosinophilia and hypereosinophilia. Their clinical presentations vary significantly and must be clearly distinguished from HES. In particular, there are a number of eosinophilic diseases and syndromes of questionable or unknown etiology that must be differentiated from HES according to both clinical and pathologic parameters. The pathology of a number of these eosinophilic syndromes is generally restricted to specific organs; for example, eosinophilic gastroenteritis and eosinophilic pneumonia lack the multiplicity of end-organ damage generally seen in HES, and for this reason they can usually be distin-

Table 72–3 Major Organ Involvement and Prominent Clinical Features of Patients With the Hypereosinophilic Syndrome*

Primary Organ Involvement†
Hematologic[100§]
Cardiovascular[58]
Cutaneous[56]
Neurologic[54]
Pulmonary[49]
Splenic[43]
Hepatic[30]
Ocular[23]
Gastrointestinal[23]
Clinical Manifestations‡
Eosinophilic endomyocardial disease
Skin lesions (eg, angioedema, urticaria)
Anorexia and weight loss
Thromboembolic disease
Lymph node and/or spleen enlargement
Ophthalmological complications
Fever, excessive sweating
Gastrointestinal involvement, including diarrhea
Central nervous system disease
Pulmonary involvement
Psychiatric disturbances
Myalgia
Arrhythmias
Renal impairment
Splenic infarction
Diarrhea alone
Arthralgia
Pericarditis

*In order of frequency.

†Average percentage of 105 patients from American, French, and English studies combined.

‡Reproduced from Table 1 of Weller PF, Bubley GJ: The idiopathic hypereosinophilic syndrome. Blood 83:2759, 1994.

§Reproduced from Spry CJ: The hypereosinophilic syndrome: Clinical features, laboratory findings and treatment. Allergy 37:539, 1982.

guished from HES. In many of these disorders such as eosinophilic gastroenteritis, eosinophilic esophagitis, and eosinophilic cystitis, localized tissue eosinophilia may not be accompanied by eosinophilia in the peripheral blood. For reasons that remain unclear, these syndromes lack the propensity to evolve toward secondary eosinophil-mediated cardiac disease. Because some patients with HES exhibit evidence of vasculitic disease, and the major eosinophil-associated vasculitis is the Churg–Strauss syndrome, this syndrome likewise needs to be ruled out. The Churg–Strauss syndrome is characterized by a history of blood eosinophilia greater than 10%, asthma, pulmonary infiltrates (nonfixed), abnormalities in the paranasal sinuses, mononeuropathy or polyneuropathy, and extravascular eosinophilic infiltrates in biopsied blood vessels.[88] Necrotizing vasculitis of small arteries and veins and extravascular granulomas are characteristic findings in biopsies from most, but not all Churg–Strauss patients.[89,90] Asthma, peak eosinophil counts of greater than 1500/mm^3, and systemic vasculitis involving two or more extrapulmonary organs are generally the identifying characteristics of these patients.[90] Although neurologic, pulmonary, and possibly paranasal findings may accompany HES,[85] asthma is characteristically absent.[91] Nevertheless, it may be difficult to make a clear-cut distinction between HES and Churg–Strauss syndrome in some patients, especially as responses to high-dose corticosteroids would be identical for both at the outset.

Eosinophilic syndromes with cutaneous involvement can generally be distinguished from HES by the histopathology of biopsied skin lesions. These syndromes include Kimura's disease (angiolymphoid hyperplasia with eosinophilia), Wells syndrome (eosinophilic cellulitis), eosinophilic fasciitis, and eosinophilic pustular folliculitis. The syndrome of episodic angioedema with eosinophilia, characterized by a clinical course of periodic recurring episodes of angioedema, urticaria, fever, and marked blood eosinophilia, is not associated with end-organ cardiac damage and has thus been distinguished from HES.[12,13] The eosinophil myalgia syndrome, induced by ingestion of tainted L-tryptophan, is relegated to mainly historic interest, since there have not been any new cases following removal of the "tainted" L-tryptophan from the market.

A differential diagnosis of HES requires the exclusion of all identifiable eosinophilias of reactive, secondary etiologies (see Tables 72–1 and 72–4). These especially include eosinophilias due to parasitic infections caused predominantly by helminthic parasites, but also by two enteric protozoans, *Dientamoeba fragilis* and *Isospora belli*. In adults, filarial infections and strongyloidiasis are most likely to elicit pronounced and prolonged eosinophilias, in contrast to *Trichinella spiralis* infections, which cause an acute eosinophilia that does not persist without reinfection.[92] Infections with *Strongyloides stercoralis*, which have the capacity to induce marked hypereosinophilia that mimics HES,[85,93] are particularly important to exclude, especially because HES has been misdiagnosed in patients with unsuspected strongyloidiasis, and treatment of these patients with immunosuppressive glucocorticoids can lead to disseminated, often fatal disease.[94] Serial stool examinations and, in particular, assays for *Strongyloides* infection should be performed, e.g. strongyloides agar plate culture, since serologic ELISA assays may cross-react with other helminth infections such as Filariasis, Ascaris lumbricoides and Schistosomiasis. Parasitic helminth infections not amenable to or detectable by routine stool examinations, including tissue or blood-dwelling helminths causing filariasis, trichinosis, or visceral larval migrans[95] (*Toxocara canis* infections in children), should be evaluated by diagnostic examinations of blood, tissue biopsies, or specific serologic tests (ELISAs) that are now available.

Table 72–4 Causes of "Reactive" Eosinophilias

Allergic/Hypersensitivity Diseases	Asthma, rhinitis, drug reactions, allergic bronchopulmonary aspergillosis, allergic gastroenteritis
Infections	Parasitic Strongyloidiasis, *Toxocara canis, Trichinella spiralis*, visceral larva migrans, filariasis, Schistosomiasis, *Ancylostoma duodenale, Fasciola hepatica, Echinococcus, Toxoplasma*, other parasitic diseases Bacterial/Mycobacterial (mainly pulmonary TB) Fungal (Coccidioidomycosis, *Cryptococcus*) Viral (HIV, HSV, HTLV-II) Rickettsial
Connective Tissue Diseases	Churg–Strauss syndrome, Wegener's granulomatosis, rheumatoid arthritis, polyarteritis nodosa, systemic lupus erythematosus, scleroderma, eosinophilic fasciitis/myositis
Pulmonary Diseases	Bronchiectasis, cystic fibrosis, Löffler syndrome, eosinophilic granuloma of the lung
Cardiac Diseases	Tropical endocardial fibrosis, eosinophilic endomyocardial fibrosis or myocarditis
Skin Diseases	Atopic dermatitis, urticaria, eczema, bullous pemphigoid, dermatitis herpetiformis, episodic angioedema with eosinophilia (Gleich syndrome)
Gastrointestinal Diseases	Eosinophilic gastroenteritis, eosinophilic esophagitis (EE), celiac disease (in association with EE)
Malignancies	Hodgkin and non-Hodgkin lymphomas, acute lymphoblastic leukemia, Langerhans cell histiocytosis, angiolymphoid hyperplasia with eosinophilia (Kimura disease), angioimmunoblastic lymphadenopathy, solid tumors (eg, renal, lung, breast, vascular neoplasms, female genital tract cancers)
Immune System Diseases/Abnormalities	Wiskott–Aldrich syndrome, hyper-IgE (Job's) syndrome, hyper-IgM syndrome, IgA deficiency
Metabolic Abnormalities	Adrenal insufficiency
Other	IL-2 therapy, l-tryptophan ingestion (eosinophil myalgia syndrome), toxic oil syndrome, renal graft rejection

Reproduced with permission from Gotlib J, Cools J, Malone JM, et al: The FIP1L1-PDGFRα fusion tyrosine kinase in hypereosinophilic syndrome and chronic eosinophilic leukemia: Implications for diagnosis, classification, and management. Blood 103:2879, 2004.

CLINICAL MANIFESTATIONS OF HYPEREOSINOPHILIC SYNDROME

Hematologic Findings

The definitive hematologic manifestation of HES is sustained eosinophilia of 30% to 70%, with total leukocyte counts ranging from 10,000/mm^3 to 30,000/mm^3 (see Fig. 72–4). However, extremely high leukocyte counts of greater than 90,000/mm^3 are not uncommon in some patients with HES, but are often associated with a poorer prognosis.[96] Blood smears from patients with HES generally show more or less normal, mature eosinophil morphology, including typical bilobed nuclei and granule-rich cytoplasm. However, eosinophilic myeloid precursors may also be noted, though less commonly, and eosinophils may also exhibit morphologic abnormalities including nuclear hypersegmentation, decreased size and/or numbers of secondary granules, and cytoplasmic vacuolization when viewed at the light microscope level.[11,97] The presence of myeloblasts and/or

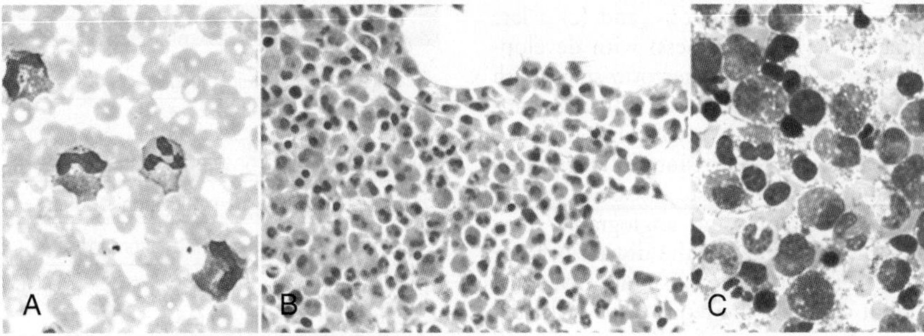

Figure 72–4 Hypereosinophilic Syndrome (**A–C**). The illustration is from the case of a 38-year-old woman who was found to have a marked eosinophilia when she presented with headaches, nausea and vomiting. The WBC was 16,900/uL, with 36% eosinophils (A). The bone marrow was hypercellular and showed sheets of eosinophils (B). On the aspirated material (C) eosinophils and eosinophilic precursors accounted for more than 70% of the cells. The patient had no obvious infectious process and no allergies. There was no malignancy associated with eosinophilia such as T-cell lymphoma, Hodgkin lymphoma, or other myeloid disease. Peripheral blood lymphocyte phenotyping showed no abnormal T-cell subset. Cytogenetic analysis showed a normal female karyocyte, and FISH analysis for del 4q12 showed no deletion of *CHIC2*.

Table 72–5 Clonal Disorders With Peripheral Blood Hypereosinophilia

CEL	Chronic eosinophilic leukemia
AEL	Acute eosinophilic leukemia
CML	Chronic myelogenous leukemia
PRV	Polycythemia rubra vera
ET	Essential thrombocythemia
AML	Acute myeloid leukemia
MDS	Myelodysplastic syndrome
MPD	Myeloproliferative disorder
SM	Systemic mastocytosis
TLL	T-cell lymphocytic leukemia

Reproduced and modified with permission from Brito-Babapulle, F: Clonal eosinophilic disorders and the hypereosinophilic syndrome. Blood Rev 11:129, 1997.

dysplastic findings in the peripheral blood may suggest an alternative, clonal etiology such as AML or a myelodysplastic syndrome (Table 72–5).[83] Ultrastructurally, HES eosinophils may show a selective loss of secondary granule components (crystalloid MBP-containing core or granular matrix, or both), decreased numbers and/or size of granules, and increased numbers of cytoplasmic lipid bodies and tubulovesicular structures of unknown function.[14,48,98,99]

In addition to their hypereosinophilia, patients with HES may also present with an absolute neutrophilia, further contributing to their overall increased leukocyte counts. This may include band forms, less mature precursors, and alterations in neutrophil nuclear segmentation and cytoplasmic granules.[100] Basophilia, when seen in some HES patients, is usually minimal. Levels of leukocyte alkaline phosphatase may be abnormally elevated or decreased in HES patients,[11] and vitamin B_{12} and B_{12}-binding proteins in serum can be normal or elevated.[101,102] In the NIH series, platelet counts were found to be decreased or increased in 31% and 16% of patients, respectively.[100] Approximately 50% of HES patients may be anemic, with nucleated erythrocytes being present in the peripheral blood. The bone marrow in these patients is hypercellular with significant increases in the percentage of eosinophils (generally from 25% to 75% of marrow elements), with a clear left shift in eosinophil maturation.[100] Myeloblasts are generally normal in number, and myelofibrosis is rare, being observed in only a minority of patients in the NIH series.[100] Splenomegaly has been reported in approximately 43% of HES patients (see Table 72–3). Hypersplenism in these individuals may contribute to the development of both thrombocytopenia and anemia. Splenic pain induced by capsular distention or infarction is a frequent complication of splenic involvement in these individuals.[103] The progressive leukocytosis with hypereosinophilia in these patients, along with the hypercellular bone marrow and lack of increased numbers of myeloblasts, can make it difficult to distinguish HES from other myeloproliferative syndromes.

Cardiovascular Findings

The cardiac manifestations of HES can be frequent and considerable (approximately 50%–60% of patients) (see Table 72–3). Prior to the advent of early diagnosis, improved management, and newer therapies, cardiac disease was the leading cause of morbidity and mortality in HES patients. The cardiac and thromboembolic manifestations of HES are likely eosinophil-mediated. However, the risks of developing cardiac disease are not necessarily related to the extent or duration of the eosinophilia,[104,105] as patients who ultimately develop cardiac involvement are more likely to be males with an HLA-Bw44 phenotype, develop splenomegaly and thrombocytopenia, have elevated vitamin B_{12} levels, and have abnormal hypogranular and vacuolated blood eosinophils and circulating early myeloid progenitors.[104] In contrast, those HES patients who do not develop heart disease tend to be females with angioedema, hypergammaglobulinemia, and increased serum IgE levels and immune complexes.[104] The cardiac damage seen in HES, progressing from early necrotic changes through thrombosis and fibrosis, is identical to that seen in patients with hypereosinophilias of diverse etiologies. These include tropical eosinophilias caused by loiasis or other filarial infections and parasitic infections such as trichinosis and visceral larval migrans,[106] drug reactions or administration of GM-CSF,[107] and eosinophilias of neoplastic origin including eosinophil leukemia, various carcinomas,[108] and Hodgkin or non-Hodgkin lymphomas.[109] Because identical forms of cardiac pathology can develop in patients with hypereosinophilias of diverse etiologies, and some patients never go on to develop cardiac involvement, the pathogenesis of eosinophil-associated cardiac disease likely involves both eosinophils and as yet undefined factors required for the recruitment, activation, and secretion of these eosinophilic constituents in the heart and associated cardiovascular tissues.

Eosinophilic endomyocardial fibrosis, as first described by Löffler,[110] is pathologically similar to that of tropical endomyocardial fibrosis,[111,112] save for the frequent absence of eosinophilia in the latter disorder.[110] However, the general absence of hypereosinophilia in patients with tropical endomyocardial fibrosis is thought to be a function of the late stage of helminthic disease in which the heart disease develops. The histopathology of cardiac involvement in HES is well characterized and can evolve through three sequentially defined stages for which eosinophils and secretion of eosinophil-derived mediators may be directly involved in the pathogenesis. These include (a) an initial acute necrotic stage of short duration (5 weeks) involving active endomyocarditis, (b) a later thrombotic stage (10 months) with mural thrombus formation over endocardial lesions, and (c) a late fibrotic stage (after approximately 2 years of illness) with development of endomyocardial fibrosis.[113] The early necrotic stage with damage to the endocardium, involves marked eosinophil and lymphocyte infiltration of the myocardium with myocardial necrosis, formation of eosinophilic microabscesses, and eosinophil degranulation. However, this early necrotic stage of cardiac disease is usually not recognized clinically. Echocardiography and angiography may fail to detect abnormalities in this early stage of the disease because ventricular thickening has not yet occurred, and endomyocardial biopsies, generally from the right ventricle, are required to make the diagnosis of cardiac involvement.[86] Treatment of HES patients with corticosteroids during this acute necrotic stage may avert or control the subsequent development of myocardial fibrosis. However, patients often present at the later stages of the cardiac involvement. In the second stage, thrombi form over the damaged endocardium in either of the ventricles or the atrium, generally with sparing of the aortic and pulmonary valves.[114] Progressive scarring at sites of mural thrombus formation ultimately leads to the late fibrotic stage, with endomyocardial fibrosis resulting in a restrictive cardiomyopathy and mitral or tricuspid valve regurgitation, or both. The more common clinical manifestations in the later progressive stages of endomyocardial fibrosis include dyspnea, chest pain, signs of left or right ventricular congestive heart failure, or both, murmurs from mitral valve regurgitation, cardiomegaly, and T-wave inversions.[114] Most patients who progress to this stage of HES cardiomyopathy will benefit from standard medical therapies for congestive heart failure, or mitral valve replacement where hemodynamically indicated. Two-dimensional echocardiography is the most sensitive method for detecting cardiac abnormalities in these patients, with visualization of mural thrombi and the various manifestations of fibrosis, including thickening of the mitral valve and its supporting structures. Approximately 80% of HES patients in the NIH series had echocardiographic abnormalities, with thickening of the left ventricular free wall the most common finding (68% of patients).[114] Cardiac catheterization may also be useful for demonstrating elevated right and left ventricular end diastolic pressures, and angiography may be used to visualize valvular incompetence. Although electrocardiographic changes in these patients are common, they are not specific to HES. Recently, intractable coronary artery spasm has been reported as the sole cardiovascular manifestation of HES.[115]

Histopathologic evaluation of the heart of HES patients generally shows four dominant features: (a) endocardial fibrosis and thickening, including involvement of mitral valve and supporting structures; (b) mural thrombus and granulation tissue on the endocardium with extensive infiltration by eosinophils; (c) thrombotic and fibrotic involvement of small intramural coronary vessels, including inflammatory cells and eosinophils; and (d) eosinophilic infiltration of the endocardium and, in some cases, of the myocardium. In a multicenter study of biopsy and postmortem specimens of cardiac tissue from HES patients at various stages of eosinophilic endomyocardial disease, activated eosinophils (identified by staining with the EG2 anti-ECP monoclonal antibody) and marked intracardiac extracellular deposition of eosinophil granule cationic proteins, including MBP, ECP, and EDN/EPX in the early necrotic and later thrombotic lesions, were identified mainly in areas of acute tissue damage on and beneath the endocardium, myocardial necrosis, and in the walls of small vessels.[65] The presence of activated eosinophils and toxic granule proteins in the early lesions of this disease suggests an active role for eosinophils and their products in inducing endocardial damage and myofibrillar injury, although the mechanisms involved in eosinophil recruitment into the heart have yet to be identified. In vitro studies have shown that secretion products of activated eosinophils can damage rat heart cell plasma membranes.[116] In addition, eosinophil peroxidase in the presence of hydrogen peroxide and bromide or thiocyanate ion can induce damage to the endothelium of the working isolated rat heart,[117] and eosinophil granule proteins can impair thrombomodulin activity,[118] findings that support a role for these eosinophil products in the development of endocardial injury and subsequent thrombotic events in the HES.[119] The in vitro findings that eosinophil secretion products such as EDN can induce fibroblast proliferation,[120] that ECP alters fibroblast proteoglycan synthesis,[121] and that MBP can augment IL-1 or TGF-β-induced production of inflammatory cytokines (IL-6 and IL-11) by fibroblasts,[122] further implicates the eosinophil in the development of endocardial fibrosis in later stages of the disease.

Table 72–6 Diagnosis of Chronic Eosinophilic Leukemia

Mature eosinophils in blood
Establish clonality
No dysplastic morphological features
Absence of *BCR-ABL*-positive cells
Absence of clonal lymphoproliferation
Presence of the *FIP1L1-PDGFRα* gene fusion (interstitial deletion of *CHIC2* on chromosome 4q12) **OR**
Elevated levels of serum tryptase (a surrogate marker for the *FIP1L1-PDGFRα* gene fusion)
Presence of the *ETV6-PDGRFβ* gene fusion (in patients with chronic myeloproliferative diseases with eosinophilia)

Reproduced and updated with permission from Brito-Babapulle, F: Clonal eosinophilic disorders and the hypereosinophilic syndrome. Blood Rev 11:129, 1997.

OTHER MAJOR CLINICAL MANIFESTATIONS OF HYPEREOSINOPHILIC SYNDROME

Pulmonary Findings

The overall pulmonary involvement reported for HES patients is approximately 50% (Table 72–6), with the most common respiratory problem being a chronic and persistent, usually nonproductive cough. Although the physiologic basis for pulmonary involvement in HES is not known, it may be secondary to aspects of congestive heart failure or numerous other factors, including infiltration and sequestration of eosinophils in lung tissues or pulmonary emboli originating from ventricular thrombi. Of note, although bronchospasm has been noted in some series of patients,[123] asthma is apparently quite rare in HES.[124] Transudative pleural effusions are the most common abnormality in patients with frank congestive heart failure.[11] In contrast to chronic eosinophilic pneumonia,[125] the pulmonary infiltrates seen in 14% to 28% of HES patients[11,122] were either diffuse or focal, without any preference for particular regions of the lung. Pulmonary infiltrates in HES may or may not clear with prednisone treatment, and pulmonary fibrosis can develop in patients with endomyocardial fibrosis.[85]

Neurologic Manifestations

As noted in Table 72–5, neurologic involvement is quite frequent in HES (approximately 50% of patients), encompassing three different complications.[126] The first type of neurologic involvement is caused by thromboemboli, which may originate from intracardiac thrombi in the left ventricle. These thromboembolic episodes may occur even before overt cardiac disease is visible by echocardiography. Patients with thrombotic complications may experience embolic strokes or transient ischemic episodes that may be multiple and recurrent, and these episodes may occur even though the patient is adequately anticoagulated with coumadin and antiplatelet agents.[86,126] The second type of neurologic manifestation involves primary diffuse central nervous system (CNS) dysfunction of unknown etiology. HES patients may variably exhibit changes in behavior, confusion, ataxia, and loss of memory.[126] The third neurologic dysfunction noted in HES is the development of peripheral neuropathies, which can occur in approximately 50% of HES patients exhibiting neurologic involvement.[126] These include symmetric or asymmetric sensory polyneuropathies, including sensory deficits, painful parathesias, or mixed sensory and motor defects.[126–128] These neuropathies may improve with steroid administration or other treatments, may be stable or continue to progress despite therapy, or may improve or resolve with time. The histopathology of the involved nerves usually shows varying degrees of axonal loss, without evidence of vasculitis or direct or peripheral eosinophil infiltration.[126–128] The presence in eosinophils of two granule cationic proteins, eosinophil-derived neurotoxin (EDN)[129] and eosinophil cationic protein,[130] both equally potent in inducing a neurotoxic and paralytic syndrome known as the Gordon Phenomenon[129,131] when injected experimentally (intrathecally) into rabbits,[132] has led to speculation that these proteins might be responsible for inducing the various neuropathies commonly seen in HES. The histopathology of the cerebrocerebellar dysfunction in the brains of experimental rabbits undergoing the Gordon Phenomenon includes a spongiform degeneration of white matter and loss of Purkinje cells,[131] changes not comparable to the peripheral axonal nerve damage seen in HES. Both EDN and ECP, related approximately 16-kd cationic proteins with 70% amino acid sequence homology,[133,134] are members of the ribonuclease gene family and possess potent ribonuclease activity and cellular toxicities in vitro.[134] However, there is no direct evidence that these ribonucleases and cellular toxins have the capacity to mediate the types of neurologic damage seen in HES, nor have these proteins been visualized by immunochemical means at sites of HES neuropathology. Marked elevations in CSF levels of IL-5, MBP, and EDN have been documented in two children with raccoon roundworm infections, progressive neurologic deterioration, and deep white matter changes on magnetic resonance images of the brain. This was the first report of MBP and EDN measurements in the CSF associated with human disease.[137] Thus, the pathogenesis of the encephelopathic, CNS, and peripheral manifestations of HES-associated neuropathy remain speculative.

Cutaneous Manifestations

For reasons that remain unclear, the skin is frequently involved in HES pathology, with cutaneous manifestations present in greater than 50% of patients in most series (see Table 72–6).[11,85,135] The skin lesions associated with HES most commonly fall into three categories: (a) angioedematous and urticarial; (b) erythematous, pruritic papules, and nodules; and (c) mucosal ulcerations. As noted earlier, patients with angioedema and urticaria are more likely to have a benign disease course that is responsive to corticosteroids, without the development of cardiac or neuropathic complications.[85,103] A subgroup of HES patients with cyclic angioedema and eosinophilia are now considered to have a syndrome (episodic angioedema with eosinophilia) that is distinct from classic HES.[13] These patients have a disorder with recurrent attacks of angioedema, urticaria, fever, and bodyweight gain that can be quite pronounced. These clinical manifestations are associated with marked leukocytosis and eosinophilia during the episodes. In HES patients who develop papular or nodular lesions, these usually improve concomitantly with positive responses to systemic therapy.[136] Dermal biopsies in these patients generally show mixed cellular infiltrates including eosinophils, without signs of vasculitis.[136] Perivascular eosinophilic infiltrates are also found in these lesions.[136] The aquagenic erythematous pruritic eruptions and indurated papules and nodules in some HES patients have been found to respond to psoralen and ultraviolet light A therapy (PUVA),[138,139] and in some patients, this treatment has interestingly been accompanied by a return of eosinophil counts to normal.[137] PUVA therapy may also be effective for the cutaneous manifestations of HES associated with HIV infection (exfoliative erythroderma, linear flagellate plaques).[140] HES-associated pruritus and nodular lesions have also been controlled with the addition of Dapsone (75–150 mg/day) to prednisone.[141] Oral sodium cromoglycate (cromolyn sodium) given before meals has also been reported to be efficacious,[142] though neither of these agents had any effect on peripheral eosinophilia. Severe and sometimes incapacitating mucocutaneous ulcerations may be a prodrome to HES and indicate a subset of HES patients with a poor prognosis.[141,142] They can occur at multiple sites, including the mouth, nose, pharynx, penis, esophagus, stomach, and anus,[143,144] and lesions can flare up independent of other clinical manifestations of HES. Biopsies of the ulcerative lesions usually show mixed cellular infiltrates, without a predominance of eosinophils or any evidence of vasculitis or microthrombi.[143] These ulcers have generally been resistant to treatment with topical or systemic corticosteroids, colchicine and hydroxyurea, but have recently been shown to respond remarkably well to IFN-α with complete and durable remissions.[145,146]

Eosinophils are present in many skin diseases and, in certain conditions, may constitute part of the diagnostic histology of the lesion.[147] Although eosinophils in general may not appear prominent in many cutaneous diseases, there is now ample evidence to suggest that they may nevertheless participate in the pathogenesis of cutaneous inflammation[4,148] and contribute to edematous reactions in atopic dermatitis,[61] syndromes associated with acute[149,150] and chronic urticarias,[78] IgE-mediated late-phase reactions,[151] chronic dermatitis associated with parasitic infections such as onchocerciasis,[58] episodic angioedema with eosinophilia,[13] eosinophilic cellulitis,[151] and skin lesions associated with rIL-2 administration for advanced malignancies.[152] Indirect evidence includes the ability of the eosinophil to elaborate its granule cationic proteins, some of which are capable of inducing release of vasoactive amines from basophils and mast cells and inducing cutaneous wheal-and-flare reactions following direct injection into human skin,[148] and production of lipid mediators such as LTC_4 and PAF, both potent inducers of vasopermeability in vivo. In addition, levels of eosinophil-active IL-5 are elevated in the syndromes of episodic angioedema with eosinophilia,[12] eosinophil-associated toxicity due to IL-2 administration,[153] and in the acute inflammatory response (Mazzotti reaction) in human patients with onchocerciasis treated with diethylcarbamazine.[154]

By far, the most direct evidence to date for eosinophil participation in the etiology of the skin diseases listed earlier has been the immunochemical detection, generally by immunofluorescent staining of skin biopsies, of prominent extracellular deposits of eosinophil granule cationic proteins such as MBP, ECP, or EDN, but not neutrophil products (neutrophil elastase) in affected but not unaffected skin, and in the absence of prominent numbers of intact eosinophils in lesional infiltrates. One example is the IgE-mediated late-phase reaction that follows the wheal-and-flare response characteristic of type I, IgE-mediated hypersensitivity. This classic late-phase reaction characterized clinically by erythema, edema, pruritus, and tenderness peaking 6 to 12 hours after intradermal antigen or anti-IgE challenge, involves infiltration by mononuclear cells, neutrophils, basophils, and eosinophils presumably in response to mast cell degranulation, along with extensive extracellular deposition of eosinophil (MBP) and neutrophil (elastase) granule products.[151] The secretion and extracellular deposition of eosinophil granule constituents, shown to possess potent cytotoxic and proinflammatory activities in edematous and eczematous lesions, clearly suggests that eosinophils may contribute to the pathogenesis of both acute and chronic skin diseases, including the cutaneous lesions associated with HES.[155] However, studies elucidating the mechanisms that regulate eosinophil recruitment, activation, and secretion in the skin are still needed to more clearly understand the dynamics of eosinophil participation in these cutaneous disorders and to identify potential therapeutic approaches to selectively block their influx and function.

ETIOLOGY OF HYPEREOSINOPHILIC SYNDROME

Hypereosinophilic Syndrome Versus Eosinophil Leukemia

The hypereosinophilic syndrome has historically been confused with chronic eosinophil leukemia (CEL), especially because distinguishing between malignant versus nonmalignant causes of hypereosinophilia

Table 72–7 Published Reports of Imatinib Use in Hypereosinophilic Syndrome, Chronic Eosinophil Leukemia, and Systemic Mastocytosis With Eosinophilia

Author (Year)[Reference]	No. Patients Treated With Imatinib	Disease	Response*	Comments
Schaller and Burkland† (2001)[159]	1	HES	CR	Initial report; rapid hematologic remission on imatinib 100 mg/day
Gleich et al† (2002)[163]	5	HES	4 CR	IL-5 levels were normal in responders
Ault et al† (2002)[166]	1	HES	CR	Resolution of 70% eosinophilia in 18 days on imatinib 100 mg/day
Pardanani et al† (2003)[160,166]	7	HES,	3 CR	IL-5 levels were elevated in responders
		Eos-CMD	1 PR	
Cortes et al† (2003)[164]	9	HES	4 CR	3 responses at imatinib 100 mg/day; 1 response at 400 mg/day
Cools et al (2003)[165]	11	HES/CEL	9 CR	*FIP1L1-PDGFRα* fusion present in 5/9 responders
Klion et al (2004)[161]	7	HES-MPD	7 CR	Molecular remission in 5 of 6 patients tested for *FIP1L1-PDGFRα* after 1–12 months of imatinib
Klion et al (2003)[162]	6	HES-MPD	6 CR	Serum tryptase is a surrogate marker for the *FIP1L1-PDGFRα* fusion and imatinib responsiveness; an HES subtype with mast cell dysplasia distinct from SM with eosinophilia
Pardanani et al (2003)[268]	6	SM with eosinophilia	3 CR	Responders had *FIP1L1-PDGFRα* fusion and no *D816V KIT* mutation

CR, complete hematologic remission; Eos-CMD, eosinophilia-associated chronic myeloproliferative disorder; HES-MPD, myeloproliferative variant of HES; PR, partial hematologic remission; SM, systemic mastocytosis.

*Refer to individual studies for their specific response criteria.

†*FIP1L1-PDGFRα* fusion was not assessed in these studies.

Reproduced and updated with permission from Gotlib J, Cools J, Malone JM, et al: The FIP1L1-PDGFRα fusion tyrosine kinase in hypereosinophilic syndrome and chronic eosinophilic leukemia: Implications for diagnosis, classification, and management. Blood 103:2879, 2004.

can be quite difficult.[83] Truly malignant acute eosinophil leukemias have several distinguishing characteristics such as a marked increase in the numbers of immature blood and/or bone marrow eosinophils, greater than 10% blast forms in the bone marrow, tissue infiltration with immature eosinophilic cells, and a clinical course and findings that tend to resemble other acute leukemias, including anemia, thrombocytopenia, and increased susceptibility to infections.[57] However, because the cardiac and neurologic manifestations of HES can also develop in chronic eosinophil leukemia, they cannot be used as distinguishing clinical features.

In contrast, CNS infiltration by eosinophils and the tendency to produce bone myeloblastomas are features more frequently associated with acute eosinophil leukemia.[57] Chromosomal abnormalities may occur with both HES and chronic eosinophil leukemia, but eosinophil leukemia is more frequently associated with chromosomal anomalies characteristic of other acute nonlymphocytic leukemias including 8:21 and 10p+11q− translocations, and trisomy-1. In addition, eosinophil leukemia has been reported as a variant of the M4Eo phenotype of acute myelomonocytic leukemia with eosinophilia, now linked to inversion 16 chromosomal abnormalities.[156–158]

Molecular explanations for the development and pathogenesis of HES and CEL have been elusive, and clinical differentiation between these indolent and often aggressive hypereosinophilias has been difficult at best. However, recent reports indicating that some patients with HES or CEL respond effectively to imatinib mesylate (Gleevec) with complete hematologic and cytogenetic remissions (Table 72–7),[159–166] and at fourfold lower doses in most patients than typically employed to treat chronic myelogenous leukemia (CML) (100 mg/day vs 400 mg/day),[159,163,164,166] suggested that these *BCR-ABL*-negative patients might possess abnormal gene fusions or activating mutations that generate novel tyrosine kinase targets of imatinib. These findings sparked a "reverse" bedside-to-bench translational research effort by several research laboratories to rapidly identify the constitutively active tyrosine kinase targets of imatinib in these HES patients. Possible targets included the known activated kinases such as ABL, platelet-derived growth factor receptor (PDGFR), or c-KIT, all of which have been shown to be inhibited by imatinib mesylate. These efforts rapidly bore fruit with the successful identification of an activated tyrosine kinase gene fusion on chromosome 4q12, which is produced by a novel interstitial chromosomal deletion of the *CHIC2* domain, fusing an uncharacterized human gene known as FIP1-like-1 (*FIP1L1*) to the platelet-derived growth factor receptor-α gene (*PDGFRα*).[163] These findings have significantly changed the current paradigm for the diagnosis and therapeutic options available for patients with HES and CEL (see Table 72–8),[167] with significant implications for the reclassification and management strategies for these hypereosinophilias.[167] Of importance, not all HES and CEL patients respond to imatinib,[163] and the majority of patients who do respond with hematologic remissions have been male and not female.[159–166] (There is apparently only a single report thus far of a female HES patient being imatinib responsive. One of us (JHB) has now treated two female patients who are responsive to Gleevec.) Importantly, approximately 40% of the patients who do respond to imatinib lack the *FIP1L1-PDGFRα* gene fusion,[165,167] suggesting genetic heterogeneity in HES/CEL and the likely presence of other novel fusion genes (eg, with *ABL*, *ARG*, *PDGFRα*, *PDGFRβ*, or *KIT*) or gene mutations thereof, that generate imatinib-sensitive constitutively active tyrosine kinases. As for CML patients with the *BCR-ABL* fusion, HES/CEL patients with the *FIP1L1-PDGFRα* fusion may relapse during imatinib therapy through the acquisition of a resistance mutation (T674I) in the PDGFRα ATP-binding region at the same position as the T315I mutation in *BCR-ABL* known to confer imatinib resistance.[168–170] Of note, a recent study by Cools and colleagues[171] has demonstrated in a murine bone marrow transplant model the efficacy of PKC412, an alternative inhibitor of PDGFRα, as a potentially effective treatment for FIP1L1-PDGFRα-induced disease and imatinib-induced resistance due to the T674I mutation.[171]

Diagnosis and Treatment of Hypereosinophilias

The mechanism of action by which the *FIP1L1-PDGFRα* gene fusion leads to the proliferation and differentiation of the eosinophil lineage over other myeloid lineages in these patients is unclear and under investigation in a number of laboratories. Initial investigations suggest that STAT5 may be one of the downstream targets of FIP1L1-PDFGRα tyrosine kinase activity. Studies have demonstrated that retroviral transduction-mediated overexpression of STAT5a in umbilical cord blood-derived CD34+ human stem/progenitor cells selectively amplifies their commitment, proliferation, and terminal differentiation to the eosinophil lineage in vitro in the presence of IL-5,[172] and that STAT5 activation by tyrosine kinases such as BCR-ABL can contribute to the transformation of leukemic cells.[173] Of interest, it was recently shown in a murine transgenic model that the FIP1L1-PDGFRA fusion gene itself is not sufficient to induce an HES/CEL-like disease independently, but requires a second event, that is, overexpression of IL-5.[174] For a comprehensive discussion of the implications of these breakthrough findings, the new screening and therapeutic options for HES, CEL, and related hypereosinophilias (eg, systemic mastocytosis with eosinophilia), and the reclassification of some forms of classic HES to CEL based on identification of the *FIP1L1-PDGFRα* gene fusion and imatinib responsiveness, the reader is directed to the recent review published by Gotlib and colleagues.[167]

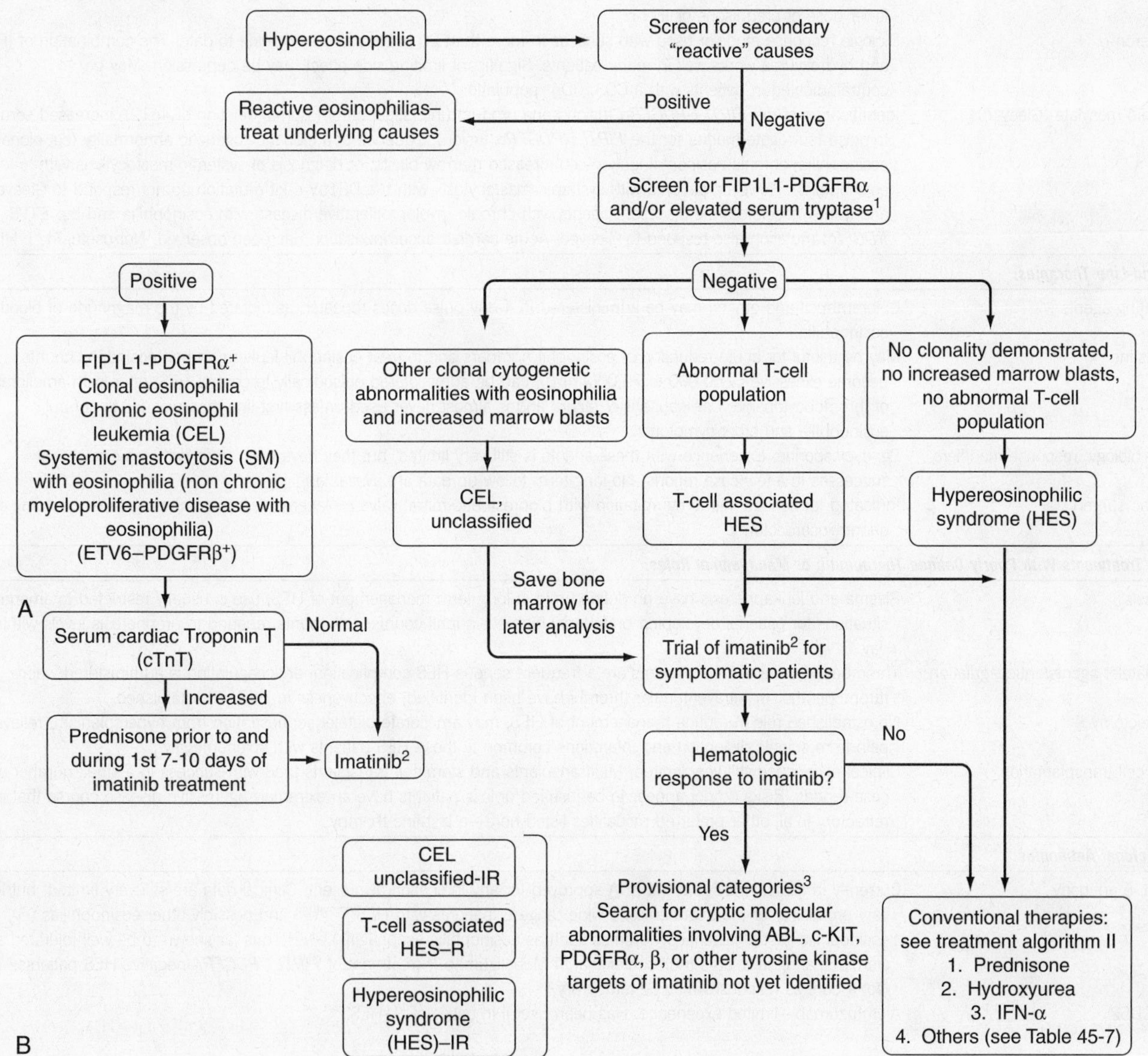

[1] Screen for increased serum tryptase as a surrogate marker if the FIP1L1-PDGFRα test is not available

[2] Assay for increases in cardiac troponin T (cTnT) for the first 7-10 days of imatinib treatment; if elevated, add treatment with prednisone for 7-10 days until serum troponin T levels are normal.

[3] Proposed re-classification of eosinophilic disorders: FIPIL1-PDGFRα-positive chronic eosinophilic leukemia (F-P+CEL); chronic eosinophilic leukemia, unclassified; hypereosinophilic syndrome (HES); T-cell associated HES Provisional categories based on imatinib treatment; CEL, unclassified-imatinib responsive (IR); HES–IR T-cell associated HES-IR.

Table 72–8 Therapeutic Options for the Hypereosinophilic Syndrome

Therapy	Indications
None	If no evidence of organ involvement and eosinophil counts <2000/mm³ (ie, those patients with eosinophilia, but without any other defining features of HES), patients should be monitored closely and periodically without treatment, for at least 6 months and possibly indefinitely. Hold off therapy as long as the eosinophil counts are stable, echocardiograms are normal, and there are no new clinical signs or symptoms of end organ damage. Reinvestigation of the etiology of the eosinophilia is warranted and recommended every 3 months to reconfirm a diagnosis of HES.
First-Line Therapies:	
Prednisone	First-line agent for those with organ involvement; if effective in suppressing peripheral blood eosinophilia, dose (= 7.5 mg/day) may be tapered or changed to every other day, but check eosinophil counts on both the on and off days; response to prednisone is associated with a better patient prognosis. "Pulse" IV with methylprednisolone (1 g/day for 3–5 days) useful for reversing CNS deterioration.
Hydroxyurea	Used in those patients with organ involvement and eosinophilia unresponsive to corticosteroids; anemia, thrombocytopenia, or both, is very common with chronic therapy. Anemia is sometimes responsive to erythropoietin. Not useful as a single agent, but in combination with prednisone or IFN-α, or Gleevec allowing improved response and lower dose of prednisone or IFN-α.
Interferon-α	Biologic response modifier used with success in more than 20 publications worldwide to date. The combination of IFN-α and hydroxyurea works well in many patients. Significant limiting side effect may be depression. May be contraindicated in patients with a $CD3^-/CD4^+$ population[7]
Imatinib mesylate (Gleevec)	Identification of the *FIP1L1-PDGFRα* fusion gene product (interstitial chromosomal deletion of 4q12), increased serum tryptase (surrogate marker for the *FIP1L1-PDGFRα* fusion), evidence of a clonal cytogenetic abnormality (eg, clonal eosinophilia, chronic eosinophil leukemia, increased marrow blasts, or diagnosis of systemic mastocytosis with eosinophilia). However, patients with systemic mastocytosis with the D816V c-kit mutation do not respond to Gleevec, and it may accelerate the disease. Patients with chronic myeloproliferative disease with eosinophilia and the *ETV6-PDGFRβ* mutation also respond to Gleevec. Acute cardiac decompensation has been observed. Not useful in "L-HES."
Second-Line Therapies:	
Alkylating agents	Chlorambucil and others; may be administered in 4-day pulse doses repeated as dictated by the magnitude of blood eosinophilia.
Vincristine	May be useful for acute reduction of eosinophil numbers and to treat eosinophil leukemia when eosinophil counts become excessive (= 50,000 to 75,000/mm³); can be administered episodically to control HES, often with amelioration of thrombocytopenia. Can cause liver failure and is almost never used unless first-line therapies fail to control eosinophilia and other symptoms.
Other biologic response modifiers	Eg, cyclosporine. Experience with these agents is still very limited, but they have been used with some apparent successes in a few case reports. No long-term follow-up data are available.
Cardiac surgery	Indicated for serious mitral regurgitation with bioprosthetic mitral valve replacement; less commonly, thrombectomy or endomyocardectomy.
Other Treatments With Poorly Defined Therapeutic or Management Roles:	
Pheresis	Plasma and leukapheresis have no defined role in long-term management of HES; use is usually restricted to emergency situations for patients developing profoundly high eosinophil counts; cell counts rebound to prepheresis levels within 1 day.
Antiplatelet agents/anticoagulation	Thrombotic/thromboembolic events are a frequent serious HES complication; anticoagulation is administered where thromboemboli or intraventricular thrombi have been identified; effectiveness in HES not established.
Splenectomy	No established role in routine management of HES; may ameliorate platelet sequestration from hypersplenism; relieve pain from splenic distention and infarctions common to those HES patients with splenomegaly.
Stem cell transplantation	Clinical experience still very limited. Minitransplants and stem cell transplants tried with success in a small number of case reports. Risks do not appear to be justified unless patients have an extremely aggressive disease course that is refractory to all other preferred modalities listed here—a last-line therapy.
Monoclonal Antibodies:	
Anti-IL-5 antibody	Currently in clinical trials, but not FDA approved for any indication at present. Clinical data are still very limited, but look very promising for the treatment of a wide range of patients with HES[218,228–231] and possibly other eosinophilias (eg, eosinophilic gastrointestinal syndromes such as eosinophilic esophagitis).[228,234] Thus far shown to be well-tolerated and steroid sparing in a large multicenter trial of Mepolizumab™ treatment of *FIP1L1-PDGFRA*-negative HES patients.[228–234] Not a cure as responses may be temporary.[232]
Anti-CD52	Alemtuzumab—limited experience. Has been useful in cases of "L-HES."[9]

Lymphomas and Hypereosinophilia

A number of lymphomas may be associated with the development of eosinophilia, including Hodgkin lymphoma,[175] T-cell lymphoblastic lymphoma,[176] and adult T-cell leukemia/lymphoma,[177] but the eosinophilia is generally much more modest than that seen in HES. In contrast, there are several reports of patients presenting with classic clinical and hematologic features of HES who have gone on to develop acute lymphoblastic leukemias[178–181] or T-cell lymphomas.[182–185] In a number of T-cell lymphoma cases, the accompanying eosinophilias were shown to be associated with the production of eosinophilopoietic cytokines (GM-CSF, IL-3, or IL-5) by the lymphomas themselves.[186,187]

PATHOGENESIS OF EOSINOPHIL-ASSOCIATED END-ORGAN DAMAGE IN HYPEREOSINOPHILIC SYNDROME

According to the current understanding of eosinophil function and hypereosinophilic conditions, sustained eosinophilia, regardless of origin (whether reactive, clonal, or idiopathic), has the capacity to lead to end-organ damage. The multiple manifestations of such eosinophil-associated end-organ damage are considerable (see Table 72–6), and their identification and management have been discussed in many reports and reviews.[57,82,84,92,124,188] However, not all cases of sustained hypereosinophilia necessarily lead to end-organ damage. For example, patients with syndromes such as eosinophilic pneumonia and episodic angioedema with eosinophilia[13] characteristically fail to develop the cardiac damage characteristic of HES patients. Experimentally, IL-5 transgenic mice, which develop extremely high numbers of peripheral blood eosinophils, do not develop significant end-organ damage, suggesting that other factors in addition to IL-5 are likely necessary for eosinophil recruitment to the tissue, eosinophil activation, and tissue damage.[26,27] Other factors may be necessary to induce eosinophilic end-organ damage, such as secretion of eosinophil-active inflammatory or hematopoietic cytokines (eg, GM-CSF), genetic predisposition, clonal T-cell dysfunction, development of a T_{H2} instead of T_{H1} T-cell profile, or in situ production of cytokines that block eosinophil apoptosis and enhance eosinophil survival and activation. Because of rather limited experience, it is not currently known whether true myeloproliferative eosinophilic disorders of clonal origin have the capacity to lead to end-organ damage. Of note, HES patients in the National Institutes of Health (NIH) series who ultimately developed cardiac disease exhibited features suggestive of a diagnosis of myeloproliferative disease, including splenomegaly, thrombocytopenia, anemia, elevated B_{12} levels, cytogenetic abnormalities, and circulating myeloid precursors and myeloid dysplasia.[82,85] As noted earlier, the eosinophil expresses a number of granule cationic protein mediators capable of inducing thrombotic events,[189] endothelial and endocardial damage,[65] and neurotoxicity (the ribonucleases EDN and ECP).[133,134] Eosinophil granule MBP and ECP are potent cellular toxins capable of damaging normal host cells and tissues in a manner reminiscent of end-organ damage associated with tissue eosinophilia.[1,190] In addition, the eosinophil has the capacity to undergo a potent respiratory burst on activation, generating reactive oxidative species that can directly, or in association with eosinophil peroxidase, induce oxidant-mediated tissue damage.[117,119,191] However, the mechanisms by which eosinophils induce thrombosis and the thromboembolic events associated with hypereosinophilic diseases, such as idiopathic HES, remain unclear, especially because most investigators have failed to identify consistent systemic alterations in coagulation and fibrinolytic pathways in these patients.[85,86] However, studies by Slungaard and colleagues suggest that eosinophil granule cationic proteins have the capacity to alter thrombomodulin activity, suggesting one possible mechanism for thromboembolism in hypereosinophilic heart disease.[118]

THERAPY AND PROGNOSIS FOR HYPEREOSINOPHILIC SYNDROME

The earlier literature on HES is filled with reports of poor to dismal patient prognosis. For example, a 1975 review by Chusid and colleagues of 57 published cases indicated an average survival time of 9 months, with a 3-year survival of only 12%.[11] The high morbidity and mortality reported in these reviews of prior decades likely reflect the fact that most HES patients tended to present late with more advanced disease, in particular, significant cardiovascular problems. Deaths in these patients were generally the result of congestive heart failure and secondary complications of endomyocardial disease, including bacterial endocarditis, progressive valvular incompetence, and the thromboembolic sequelae of the syndrome.[57,124] However, earlier diagnosis of HES, along with improved clinical and echocardiographic methods for monitoring, and use of cardiac medications and cardiothoracic surgical procedures not previously available, has resulted in more successful prevention and management of cardiac disease in these patients, considerably improving clinical outcome and survival. A report in 1989 of 40 HES patients in France reported 80% survival after 5 years and 42% survival at 10 and 15 years.[123] Thus, for many patients, prevention and management of HES end-organ damage, in particular the cardiac sequelae, result in prolonged survival over decades.[82,124] Current previously unavailable supportive therapies for managing the cardiovascular complications of HES, along with therapies aimed at controlling the eosinophilia to prevent end-organ damage in the first place, are the mainstay of HES treatment regimens (Table 72–8).[82] Treatment should focus on controlling end-organ damage, not just on suppressing or eradicating the eosinophilia, especially as the severity of cardiovascular complications of HES do not necessarily correlate with the duration or level of eosinophilia.[104,105] Although more aggressive treatment (eg, cytotoxic chemotherapy or bone marrow transplant) may be indicated and necessary in selected patients, the current goal is chronic maintenance therapy. In a 1992 review of HES, Spry[124] points out that overaggressive cytotoxic therapy for some HES patients may be more deleterious than the HES itself, with the risk of marrow aplasia.[11] Current diagnostic and therapeutic options for the treatment and management of HES are listed in Table 72–4, the box on Diagnosis and Treatment of Hypereosinophilias, and the box on Treatment Strategies for *FIP1L1-PDGFRα*-negative Eosinophilias, and are described in greater detail later. Recent experience with the use of biologic response modifiers, in particular interferon-α, show considerable promise for durable remissions of eosinophilia and clinical signs and symptoms, particularly in patients with resistant disease, but also in HES patients, in general, as a first line-therapeutic option.[84]

INITIAL THERAPEUTIC OPTIONS

Patients meeting the diagnostic criteria for HES (see Table 72–2) or CEL (Tables 72–9 and 72–10) should be managed according to the newest strategies as defined in the two algorithms shown for hypereosinophilias (see box on Diagnosis and Treatment of Hypereosinophilias, and box on Treatment Strategies for *FIP1L1-PDGFRα*-negative Eosinophilias, as adapted and modified from the original algorithm of Schooley and colleagues[192] and recently updated for this chapter based on Gotlib et al[167] with permission). Patients without any overt evidence of organ dysfunction or severe symptoms and with eosinophilia counts less than 1500 to 2000 eosinophils/mm^3 can be monitored closely and periodically without treatment for at least 6 months and possibly indefinitely, so long as their complete blood counts are stable, their echocardiograms normal, and there are no new clinical signs or symptoms of end organ involvement. Periodic reinvestigations of the etiology of the eosinophilia are highly appropriate and recommended every 3 to 6 months to reconfirm the diagnosis of HES. Of note, patients with eosinophilias routinely greater than 2000 eosinophils/mm^3 that meet the previously defined criteria for HES should be treated, regardless of the absence of clinical signs and symptoms of end organ involvement, see box on Diagnosis of Hypereosinophilic Syndrome (HES). Patients with negative clinical evaluations for secondary, reactive causes of their eosinophilia (Table 72–4) should subsequently undergo testing for the *FIP1L1-PDGFRα* fusion gene product, or if this test is unavailable, for elevated serum tryptase as a surrogate marker. Those positive for the fusion or with elevated serum tryptase, or both, can be classified as having one of the *FIP1L1-PDGFRα*-positive clonal eosinophilias (eg, CEL or systemic mastocystosis [SM] with eosinophilia). A negative test for the gene fusion or normal serum tryptase level would classify the patient into one of the three diagnostic categories based on additional laboratory criteria: CEL, unclassified, T cell-associated hypereosinophilic syndrome (HES), or classic HES. A trial of imatinib mesylate is recommended for *FIP1L1-PDGFRα*-positive CEL or SM patients with eosinophilia; there is still some debate whether the latter *FIP1L1-PDGFRA+* patients represent HES with increased bone marrow mast

Table 72–9 End-Organ Damage Produced by Hypereosinophilia

Organ/System	
Cardiac	**Pulmonary**
Constrictive pericarditis[233]	Pulmonary infiltrates[250,251]
Endomyocardial fibrosis[107,234,237]	Fibrosis[85]
Myocarditis[224]	Pleural effusions[252]
Intramural thrombi[235–242]	Pulmonary emboli[252]
Valve regurgitation[240]	**Ocular**
Cardiomyopathy[243]	Microthrombi[253]
Coronary Artery Spasm[115]	Vasculitis[241]
Neurologic	Retinal arteritis[254–257]
Thromboemboli[244]	**Joints**
Peripheral neuropathy[244]	Arthralgia[257]
Central nervous system/dysfunction[245,246]	Effusions[258]
Epilepsy[245]	Polyarthritis[259]
Dementia[245]	Raynaud phenomenon[260,261]
Eosinophilic meningitis[246]	Digital necrosis[262]
Dermatologic	**Gastrointestinal**
Angioedema[247]	Ascites[263]
Urticaria[141]	Diarrhea[86]
Papulonodular lesions[141]	Gastritis[264]
Mucosal ulcers[143]	Colitis[225,265]
Vesicobullous lesions[248]	Pancreatitis[266]
Microthrombi[249]	Cholangitis[267]
	Budd–Chiari syndrome[267]

*Reproduced from Brito-Babapulle, F: Clonal eosinophilic disorders and the hypereosinophilic syndrome. Blood Rev 11:129, 1997.

Table 72–10 Major Factors Supporting a Diagnosis of Clonality in Hypereosinophilia

- Cytogenetic abnormalities
- FISH for FIP1L1-PDGFRA mutations in eosinophils
- G6PD alloenzymes in heterozygote females
- Cultured eosinophil colonies with abnormal cytogenetics
- Grade III bone marrow fibrosis
- Trilineage blood or bone marrow myelodysplasia
- Abnormal localization of immature precursors (ALIP)
- Activating mutations in the *K ras* oncogene
- Abnormal nucleotide content of eosinophils
- Clonal T-cell proliferation or T-cell receptor gene rearrangement
- Clinical response to a trial of imatinib mesylate (Gleevec)
- Elevated levels of serum tryptase (surrogate marker for *FIP1L1-PDGFRα* gene)
- Wilms' Tumor gene expression (WTI)[269]

Minor Factors Supporting a Diagnosis of Clonality

- Increased serum cobalamin (vitamin B_{12}) and unsaturated B_{12} binding capacity (UBBC)
- Hepatomegaly/splenomegaly
- Normal levels of interleukins and immunoglobulins
- Low neutrophil alkaline phosphatase
- Markedly abnormal eosinophil morphology
- Anemia or thrombocytopenia
- Poor therapeutic response to steroid

Factors of Uncertain Significance

- Apoptosis on blood film examination
- Thrombotic events
- Eosinophilic end organ damage

Reproduced and updated with permission from Brito-Babapulle, F: Clonal eosinophilic disorders and the hypereosinophilic syndrome. Blood Rev 11:129, 1997.

cells or SM with eosinophilia.[193,194] For *FIP1L1-PDGFRα*-negative patients, conventional therapies, or possibly a short trial of imatinib mesylate, is suggested for symptomatic patients. *FIP1L1-PDGFRα*-negative patients who have hematologic remissions with imatinib may be provisionally categorized as imatinib responsive (IR), warranting investigation of potential alternative constitutively active tyrosine kinase targets of the drug. The indication for aggressive initial treatment is evidence of progressive organ involvement or symptoms, or both. In asymptomatic eosinophilic patients with no evidence of end-organ involvement, specific therapy need not be administered immediately if eosinophil counts remain less than 1500 to 2000/μL. However, careful and frequent (3–6 month intervals) clinical and echocardiographic follow-ups should be done to evaluate such patients for the onset of cardiac involvement, which may nevertheless develop insidiously despite blood eosinophil counts less than approximately 2000/μL. It may be valuable in such patients to evaluate the effect of a short course of prednisone (60 mg/day or 1 mg/kg/day) to determine whether their eosinophilia will be responsive to corticosteroid suppression, should organ involvement ultimately develop.

Chemotherapeutic Agents

A trial of imatinib mesylate (Gleevec; initially 100 mg/day) is recommended for *FIP1L1-PDGFRα*-positive CEL or SM patients with eosinophilia (Table 72–7). For *FIP1L1-PDGFRα*-negative patients, conventional therapies, or possibly a short trial of imatinib mesylate (100 mg/day) is suggested for symptomatic patients. *FIP1L1-PDGFRα*-negative patients who have hematologic remissions with imatinib may be provisionally categorized as IR as indicated in the box on Diagnosis and Treatment of Hypereosinophilias, warranting further investigation of potential alternative constitutively active tyrosine kinase targets of the drug.[167] In *FIP1L1-PDGRFα*-negative patients who fail a short trial of imatinib and have evidence of end-organ involvement and steroid-resistant eosinophilia, the decision

Treatment Strategies for *FIP1LI-PDGFRα*-Negative Eosinophilias (Classical Hes, T Cell-Associated Hes, and Unclassified Chronic Eosinophil Leukemia)

Several prognostic features mentioned earlier may predict a good response to corticosteroid therapy, including the presence of angioedema and urticaria, elevated serum IgE levels, and a rapid drop in eosinophil counts in response to the initiation of corticosteroids, since eosinophils have surface receptors for glucocorticoids. Initial therapy in patients presenting with evidence of end organ involvement is with prednisone (1 mg/kg/day or 60 mg/day in adults). If an adequate suppression of blood eosinophil counts is obtained, then doses may be slowly tapered and ultimately switched to alternate day therapy (1 mg/kg/day). However, eosinophil counts should be monitored between doses on the "off" days to confirm that eosinophil counts remain level and adequately controlled. In the NIH series, 38% of patients responded well and 31% partially to prednisone treatment.[100,103,114] Patients less likely to respond favorably to prednisone included those with the poor prognostic signs of splenomegaly, cardiac dysfunction, and neurologic symptoms at the time of presentation. The mechanisms of steroid-refractory eosinophilia in HES have not been defined.

Diagnosis of Hypereosinophilic Syndrome*

Patients presenting with eosinophilia of unknown etiology should undergo a thorough clinical and laboratory evaluation consisting of the following:

- Complete/detailed history and physical examination
- Complete blood count with total eosinophil count and review of peripheral blood smear
- Hepatic and renal function tests, urine analysis
- Serologic assays: erythrocyte sedimentation rate, rheumatoid factor, human immunodeficiency virus (HIV)
- Serum tryptase level
- Quantitation of total IgE level
- Stool for ova, parasites ×3, duodenal aspirate
- Serologic assays for *Strongyloides*, *Trichinella*, *Toxocara*, *E Histolytica*, and *Echinococcus*, *Filariasis*, *Schistosomiasis*
- Bone marrow aspirate and biopsy (with cytogenetics)

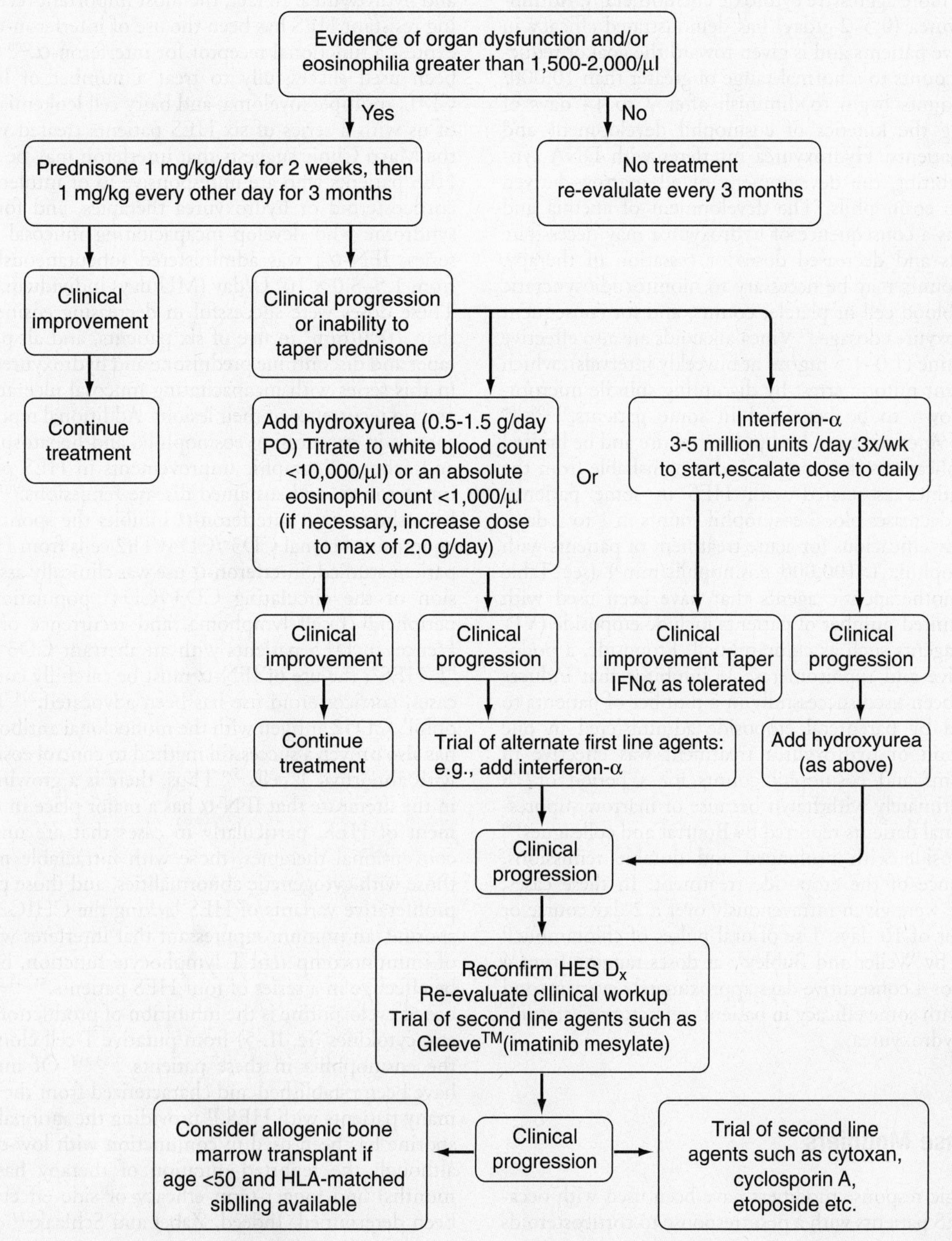

Treatment Strategies for FIP1LI-PDGFRα-Negative Eosinophilias (Classical Hes, T Cell-Associated Hes, and Unclassified Chronic Eosinophil Leukemia)—cont'd

- Chest radiograph, computed tomographic scan of chest, abdomen, and pelvis
- Electrocardiogram and echocardiogram
- Patients meeting diagnostic criteria for HES/CEL:

1. persistent eosinophilia of >1500 eosinophils/mm³ for more than 6 months
2. exclusion of other potential "reactive" etiologies for the eosinophilia including parasitic, allergic, or other causes, and
3. presumptive signs and symptoms of organ system dysfunction or involvement that appears related to the eosinophilia or is of unknown cause in the clinical presentation.

Patients with negative clinical evaluations for secondary, reactive causes of their eosinophilia should subsequently undergo testing for the *FIP1L1-PDGFRα* fusion gene product, or if this test is unavailable, use elevated serum tryptase levels as a surrogate marker. Those positive for the fusion or with elevated serum tryptase, or both, can be classified as having one of the *FIP1L1-PDGFRα*-positive clonal eosinophilias (eg, CEL or SM with eosinophilia). A negative test for the gene fusion or normal serum tryptase level would classify the patient into one of the three diagnostic categories based on additional laboratory criteria: CEL, unclassified, T cell-associated HES, or classic HES. A trial of imatinib mesylate is recommended for *FIP1L1-PDGFRα*-positive CEL or SM patients with eosinophilia (now abbreviated as SM-CEL or HES-MPD).

*Reproduced, modified, and updated from Schenkein and Wolff[220] and Gotlib et al[167] with permission.

may be made to use more aggressive cytotoxic chemotherapy. Administration of hydroxyurea (0.5–2 g/day) has demonstrated efficacy in steroid-nonresponsive patients and is given toward the goal of reducing total leukocyte counts to a normal range of greater than 10,000/mm³. Eosinophil counts begin to diminish after 7 to 14 days of treatment, reflecting the kinetics of eosinophil development and turnover in these patients. Hydroxyurea interferes with DNA synthesis, thereby inhibiting the development of all marrow-derived cells, in addition to eosinophils. The development of anemia and thrombocytopenia as a consequence of hydroxyurea may necessitate red cell transfusions and decreased doses or cessation of therapy. Weekly leukocyte counts may be necessary to monitor idiosyncratic fluctuations in red blood cell or platelet counts, and for consequent adjustment of hydroxyurea dosage.[82] Vinca alkaloids are also effective in HES, and vincristine (1.0–1.5 mg/m² at biweekly intervals), which produces a permanent mitotic arrest by disrupting spindle microtubules, has been shown to be beneficial in some patients.[81,195–198] However, the use of vincristine can lead to liver failure and be limited by neurologic complications that may be indistinguishable from the peripheral neuropathies associated with HES in some patients. Because vincristine decreases blood eosinophil counts in 1 to 3 days, it may be particularly efficacious for acute treatment of patients with marked hypereosinophilia (>100,000 eosinophils/mm³) (see Table 72–8). Other chemotherapeutic agents that have been used with some success in a limited number of patients include etoposide (VP-16) and alkylating agents such as chlorambucil. Etoposide, a podophyllotoxin derivative and topoisomerase II inhibitor that induces DNA damage, has been used successfully in a number of patients to date. Oral followed by parenteral etoposide administered in one patient after cessation of hydroxyurea treatment was effective in controlling symptoms and eosinophil counts for a period of 18 months, but was ultimately withdrawn because of marrow suppression.[193] Two additional patients reported by Bourrat and colleagues[199] responded to etoposide with prolonged and durable remissions, despite discontinuance of the etoposide treatment. In these cases, doses of 300 mg/m² were given intravenously over a 2-day course or 200 mg/m² on 7 out of 10 days. Use of oral pulses of chlorambucil have been reported by Weller and Bubley[82] at doses ranging from 4 to 10 mg/m² daily for 4 consecutive days approximately every second month for 2 years with some efficacy in patients refractory to steroids and intolerant to hydroxyurea.

Biologic Response Modifiers

A number of biologic response modifiers have been used with occasional success in HES patients with a poor response to corticosteroids and hydroxyurea. In fact, the most important recent advance in treating resistant HES has been the use of interferon-α,[84] and eosinophils express a functional receptor for interferon-α.[200–206] Interferon-α has been used successfully to treat a number of leukemias including CML, multiple myeloma, and hairy cell leukemia. Experience by one of us with a series of six HES patients treated with interferon-α at the Mayo Clinic suggests that interferon may be a valuable agent for HES patients who are unresponsive to or intolerant of conventional corticosteroid or hydroxyurea therapies, and for patients with this syndrome who develop incapacitating mucosal ulcers.[143,144] In this series, IFN-α_{2b} was administered subcutaneously at doses ranging from 1.5–8.0 × 10^6 U/day (MU/day) individualized for each patient. These doses were successful in decreasing eosinophil counts to less than 1000/mm³ in five of six patients, and all patients were able to taper and discontinue prednisone and hydroxyurea.[145,146] Two patients in this series with incapacitating mucosal ulcerations had resolution and no recurrence of their lesions. Additional reports indicate variable success in suppressing eosinophilia and hepatosplenomegaly, clinical and echocardiographic improvements in HES patients treated with interferon-α, and sustained disease remissions.[201–206] In vitro studies have shown that interferon-α inhibits the spontaneous high rate of apoptosis of clonal $CD3^-/CD4^+$ Th2 cells from HES patients. In one patient studied, interferon-α use was clinically associated with expansion of the circulating $CD3^-/CD4^+$ population, development of peripheral T-cell lymphoma, and recurrence of hypereosinophilia. Hence, in HES patients with an aberrant $CD3^-/CD4^+$ population, "L-HES", the use of IFN-α must be carefully considered.[207] In these cases, corticosteroid use has been advocated.[208] Targeting the eosinophil's CD52 antigen with the monoclonal antibody alemtuzumab™ has also proven a successful method to control eosinophilia in patients with abnormal T cells.[209] Thus, there is a growing body of evidence in the literature that IFN-α has a major place in the long-term treatment of HES, particularly in cases that are unresponsive to more conventional therapies, those with intractable mucosal ulcerations, those with cytogenetic abnormalities, and those presenting as myeloproliferative variants of HES lacking the CHIC2 deletion.[210] Cyclosporine, an immunosuppressant that interferes with multiple aspects of immunocompetent T lymphocyte function, has been reported to be effective in a series of four HES patients.[51,211,212] The rationale for use of cyclosporine is the inhibition of production of eosinophilopoietic cytokines (ie, IL-5) from putative T-cell clones thought to drive the eosinophilia in these patients.[51,83,211] Of interest, T-cell clones have been established and characterized from the peripheral blood of many patients with HES,[51] providing the rationale for its use. Cyclosporine has been used in conjunction with low-dose corticosteriods, although the reported duration of therapy has been limited (10 months) and longer-term efficacy or side effects in HES have not been determined. Indeed, Zabel and Schlaak[212] demonstrated corticosteroid-sparing effects and durable control of eosinophilia using 4 mg/kg cyclosporine in a series of three HES patients.

Pheresis

As noted in Table 72–8, plasma and leukapheresis have no defined role in the long-term management of HES. The use of leukapheresis has generally been restricted to emergency situations for patients developing profoundly high eosinophil counts. However, cell counts rebound rapidly to pretreatment levels within 1 day of the procedure.[213,214] Even multiple repeated sessions of leukapheresis are usually not sufficient to induce more than a transient decrease in blood eosinophil levels.[213–216] Five repeated plasma and leukapheresis sessions over a period of 2 weeks for a single patient was reported to significantly decrease blood eosinophilia; however, continued sessions in this patient were insufficient by themselves to lower blood eosinophil counts to acceptable levels.[206] The mechanism by which plasmapheresis transiently decreases eosinophil levels is entirely speculative but has been suggested to involve a temporary removal or decrease in the levels of circulating eosinophilopoietic factors.[213,216]

Anticoagulation and Antiplatelet Agents

Because thrombotic and thromboembolic events are frequently serious complications of HES, anticoagulants have often been used, especially in those patients with clear evidence of thromboemboli, neurologic symptoms, and cardiac involvement. Commonly used agents include warfarin, antiplatelet agents, or heparin. However, the efficacy of anticoagulation or antiplatelet agents has not been clearly established in HES disease, and many patients treated with these agents have continued to have thrombotic events, despite their adequate use.[86,124]

Splenectomy

As previously noted, splenomegaly has been reported in approximately 43% of HES patients, and hypersplenism in these individuals may contribute to both thrombocytopenia, anemia, and splenic infarction. Splenic pain induced by capsular distention or infarction is a known complication of HES.[103] In HES, splenectomy has the capacity to ameliorate platelet sequestration from hypersplenism and to relieve the pain associated with splenic distention and infarction.

Stem Cell Transplantation

There is still very limited experience reported with stem cell transplantation for the treatment of HES.[217–221] However, recent reports of stem cell transplantation for refractory HES include two successes with patients apparently in complete remission[219,221] and a third with a course complicated by the development of graft-versus-host-disease (GVHD) requiring cyclosporin-A therapy.[217] In a fourth report, the patient relapsed 40 months after transplantation, but survived for more than 44 months.[220] In a case reported in 1988, an HES patient who received an allogeneic transplant recovered hematologically, but subsequently died within 3 months from a diffuse cytomegalovirus (CMV) infection, thus preventing adequate evaluation of the procedure.[218] Only in HES cases with an extremely aggressive course unresponsive to standard therapies, or in young patients with a refractory course of disease and clinical features suggestive of a myeloproliferative disorder (eg, chromosomal abnormalities) should allogeneic stem cell transplantation be considered a treatment option at this time. Without greater understanding of the underlying mechanisms responsible for the overproduction of eosinophils and the aggressive development of end-organ damage in some of these patients, the risks associated with stem cell transplantation may outweigh its more routine use in treatment of this disorder.

Cardiac Surgery

Treatment of the cardiovascular sequelae of HES continues to be a therapeutic challenge.[57] Surgical intervention in eosinophilic heart disease does not appear to carry any risk of disease recurrence at the operative sites. For patients who develop significant compromise of valvular function, endomyocardial thrombosis, or fibrosis, cardiac surgery has the capacity to provide substantial clinical and quality-of-life improvements.[57] Mitral valve[222] and/or tricuspid valve repair or replacements[223] have been reported in more than 50 eosinophilic patients.[57] Endomyocardectomy and thrombectomy, as performed for advanced stage Löeffler's endomyocardial fibrosis, has also been used effectively in some HES patients[86,224] and ventricular decortication may be performed in combination with valve replacement. For mitral valve replacements, mechanical valves have proven problematic because of recurring thrombotic episodes despite adequate anticoagulation,[224–226] suggesting the use of porcine valves whenever possible.[82,227] HES patients who have received valve replacements have generally experienced long-term improvement in cardiac function,[82] provided the eosinophilia remains controlled.

Ineffective Agents in Hypereosinophilic Syndrome

Agents that have proved either not very useful or totally ineffective in the treatment of HES include antihistamines, anabolic steroids, methotrexate and busulfan (alone or in combination), azathioprine, and cyclophosphamide.

SUMMARY AND CONCLUSIONS

The heterogeneity of HES, ranging from patients with clear features of myeloproliferative disorders, including cytogenetic abnormalities, to patients with more benign clinical courses, such as episodic angioedema with eosinophilia, suggests that multiple disease processes are likely at play. Current research aimed at defining the cause of HES and mechanisms regulating the development of eosinophil-mediated end-organ damage in eosinophil-associated diseases in general, should ultimately lead to more selective and improved therapies. The therapeutic targets for these efforts are likely to include (a) IL-5 and its high affinity receptor; (b) underlying T-cell clones (either immunocompetent or occult T-lymphoid malignancies) that elaborate eosinophilopoietins such as IL-5 or GM-CSF, tissue or organ-specific dysfunctional elaboration of eosinophil-active chemoattractant factors such as eosinophil-selective chemokines (the eotaxins); (c) vascular endothelial adhesion molecules (VCAM/VLA-4); and (d) undefined mechanisms that induce the overproduction of eosinophils and/or serve to recruit and activate eosinophils selectively in certain tissues and organs. The essential absence of end-organ damage in some syndromes of hypereosinophilia contrasts starkly with the morbidity (and mortality) associated with the development of endomyocardial fibrosis in HES and certain other eosinophilias. Because HES patients are clearly a heterogeneous group, clinical management based on current knowledge must be specifically tailored to the individual,[84,167] with the overall goal of controlling the eosinophilia and, in particular, the eosinophil-mediated end-organ damage. In the past 30 years, the clinical and surgical management of patients with idiopathic hypereosinophilias and HES has evolved significantly. Current treatment options permit the control or eradication of eosinophilia and end-organ damage in most HES patients. The recent report of the efficacy of imatinib mesylate in approximately 50% of patients with HES has led to the identification of the *FIP1L1-PDGFRα* gene fusion that encodes a pathogenetically relevant and constitutively active tyrosine kinase. This seminal finding will ultimately lead to a reclassification of hypereosinophilias into several well-defined clinical entities and should stimulate new research that may ultimately translate into improved clinical characterization and therapeutic options. For patients with imatinib-resistant forms of CEL, or with classic HES that does not respond to conventional therapies such as glucocorticoids, hydroxyurea, and IFN-α, treatment options such as stem cell transplantation may hold promise for durable disease remissions. Importantly, treatment with IFN-α should be considered as an initial first-line option for the management of imatinib nonresponsive HES, either alone or in combination with other therapies.[84] Finally, humanized anti-IL-5 antibody (mepolizumab) is currently in clinical trials, but is not FDA approved. The clinical data with this agent, though still preliminary, looks highly promising for the treatment of a wide range of patients with *FIP1L1-PDGFRA*-negative HES[228–232] and possibly other eosinophilias, for example, eosinophilic gastrointestinal syndromes such as eosinophilic esophagitis.[233,219]

Future research on HES and CEL will likely focus on the molecular basis of imatinib responsiveness in both *FIP1L1-PDGFRα*-positive and -negative patients, addressing specifically how the constitutively activated FIP1L1-PDGFRα or other fusion- or mutant-activated kinases selectively lead to chronic hypereosinophilia and end-organ damage. Studies of the effects of imatinib on the proliferation and terminal differentiation of bone marrow-derived eosinophil progenitors, and the survival and intracellular signaling pathways in eosinophils from imatinib-responsive patients may be particularly revealing in terms of the downstream targets of these novel kinases.

Acknowledgments

The authors greatly acknowledge and appreciate discussions and critical input and advice from Dr. Amy Klion and Dr. Gary Gilliland in the development of the new algorithms for the evaluation and therapeutic options now available for patients with hypereosinophilias, specifically in terms of reviewing the treatment options for patients shown to be *FIP1L1-PDGFRα*-positive versus negative, or to have elevated serum tryptase levels as a surrogate marker for the *FIP1L1-PDGFRα* gene fusion. Dr. Ackerman is supported in part by grants from the National Institute of Allergy and Infectious Diseases, NIH (AI25230 and AI33043).

SUGGESTED READINGS

Ackerman SJ, Bochner BS. Mechanisms of eosinophilia in the pathogenesis of hypereosinophilic disorders. Immunol Allergy Clin North Am. 27:357, 2007.

Butterfield JH, Sharkey SW: Control of hypereosinophilic syndrome-associated recalcitrant artery spasm by combined treatment with prednisone, imatinib mesylate and hydroxyurea. Exp Clin Cardiol 11:25, 2006.

Garrett JK, Jameson SC, Thomson B, et al: Anti-interleukin-5 (mepolizumab) therapy for hypereosinophilic syndromes. J Allergy Clin Immunol 113:115, 2004.

Gleich GJ, Schwartz LB, Busse WW, Huss-Marp J, Walsh SR: Baseline demographics and disease characteristics of patients with hypereosinophilic syndrome in a placebo-controlled trial evaluating the steroid-sparing effects of the anti-IL-5 monoclonal antibody, mepolizumab. Blood (ASH Annual Meeting Abstracts) 108:4899, 2006.

Gotlib J: KIT mutations in mastocytosis and their potential as therapeutic targets. Immunol Allergy Clin North Am 26:575, 2006.

Gotlib J, Cools J, Malone JM, et al: The FIP1L1-PDGFR{alpha} fusion tyrosine kinase in hypereosinophilic syndrome and chronic eosinophilic leukemia: Implications for diagnosis, classification, and management. Blood 103:2879, 2004.

Klion AD. Approach to the therapy of hypereosinophilic syndromes. Immunol Allergy Clin North Am 27:551, 2007.

Klion AD, ed. Hypereosinophilic Syndromes. Immunol Allergy Clin North Am Vol. 27. Amsterdam: Elsevier, Inc.; pp. 333–570, 2007.

Klion AD, Bochner BS, Gleich GJ, et al: Approaches to the treatment of hypereosinophilic syndromes: A workshop summary report. J Allergy Clin Immunol 117:1292, 2006.

Klion AD, Robyn J, Akin C, et al: Molecular remission and reversal of myelofibrosis in response to imatinib mesylate treatment in patients with the myeloproliferative variant of hypereosinophilic syndrome. Blood 103:473, 2004.

Klion AD, Law MA, Noel P, et al: Safety and efficacy of the monoclonal anti-interleukin 5 antibody, SCH55700, in the treatment of patients with the hypereosinophilic syndrome. Blood 103:2939, 2004.

Pitini V, Teti D, Arrigo C, Righi M: Alemtuzumab therapy for refractory idiopathic hypereosinophilic syndrome with abnormal T cells: A case report. Br J Haematol 127:477, 2004.

Rothenberg ME, Klion AD, Roufosse FE, et al: Treatment of patients with the hypereosinophilic syndrome with mepolizumab. N Engl J Med 358:1215, 2008.

Simon HU, Cools J. Novel approaches to therapy of hypereosinophilic syndromes. Immunol Allergy Clin North Am 27:519, 2007.

Stein ML, Collins MH, Villanueva JM, et al: Anti-IL-5 (mepolizumab) therapy for eosinophilic esophagitis. J Allergy Clin Immunol 118:1312, 2006.

Yamada Y, Rothenberg ME, Lee AW, et al: The FIP1L1-PDGFRA fusion gene cooperates with IL-5 to induce murine hypereosinophilic syndrome (HES)/chronic eosinophilic leukemia (CEL)-like disease. Blood 107:4071, 2006.

REFERENCES

For complete list of references log onto www.expertconsult.com

CHAPTER 73

MAST CELLS AND SYSTEMIC MASTOCYTOSIS

Animesh Pardanani and Ayalew Tefferi

MAST CELLS

Discovery

The discovery of mast cells is credited to Paul Ehrlich,[1] who first described a subgroup of connective tissue cells ("Mastzellen") localized to a great extent around blood vessels; these cells were thought to be morphologically larger than white blood cells and to contain "protoplasmic deposits" (granules) that display a characteristic reactivity toward aniline dyes. In his thesis, Ehrlich stressed that the identification of mast cells was to be based primarily on the specific histochemical reaction that rendered the cell granules metachromatic, and not simply on the microscopic appearance of these cells. Several years later, Ehrlich discovered the presumed nontissue counterpart of mast cells[3,4]; this basophilic granulocyte was identified in the peripheral blood of patients with myeloid leukemia, which suggested that the particular cell (blood mast cell, basophil, or mast leukocyte) had its origin in the bone marrow with subsequent residence in the peripheral blood as do other leukocytes.

Origin

Although the origin of mast cells remained obscure for many years, it is now accepted that these cells originate from CD34+/c-Kit+/CD13+ pluripotent hematopoietic cells in the bone marrow.[5–8] Mast cells are released into the circulation in the immature state and undergo terminal maturation/differentiation after migration into tissues, where they ultimately reside. In early studies, mouse models were used to investigate the origin and development of mast cells: (a) C57BL/6-bg^j/bg^j, beige Chediak–Higashi syndrome mice. In this model, the giant mast cell granules were used a morphological marker for donor-derived cells.[9] Here, cells from the bone marrow, peripheral blood, liver, thymus, or lymph nodes of beige mice were transplanted into irradiated, congenic C57BL/6 +/+ mice, or alternatively, the beige mouse was parabiosed with a congenic +/+ mouse, (b) dominant white spotting (*W*)- or Steel (*Sl*)-locus mutant mice (vide infra) that are profoundly deficient in mast cells. Kitamura initially demonstrated that the mast cell content in skin and other organs in the adult *W/W^v* mouse could be restored to normal levels after transplantation of bone marrow cells from congenic +/+ mice.[10]

The relationship between human mast cells and cells belonging to other leukocyte lineages remains unclear. Although mast cells share several features with basophils, namely presence of cytoplasmic basophilic granules, expression of high-affinity IgE receptors (FcεRI), and release of histamine upon stimulation, the two cell types are considered to be distinct. Unlike mast cells, basophils circulate in the blood as mature cells and are thought to be incapable of proliferation; that is, basophils undergo apoptosis after their recruitment and activation in the tissues.[11] Studies of developmental pathways in murine hematopoiesis have not been conclusive as to how mast cell-committed progenitors are generated; that is, whether there is a shared bipotent progenitor for mast cell and basophilic lineages or whether mast cells are derived directly from multipotent progenitor cells.[12–14] Molecular studies in patients with mastocytosis however reveal that the pathogenetically relevant mutation Kit Asp816Val (D816V) is found primarily in mast cells and not basophils, thus suggesting that the two cells do not arise from a common progenitor cell.[15] Furthermore, it has been proposed that mast cells and basophils, both of which are metachromatic staining cells, can be distinguished on the basis of cellular immunophenotype,[16–18] gene expression profile,[19] or growth factor responsiveness.[18] With regards to the latter, interleukin-3 (IL-3) and to some extent IL-5 has been shown to promote the growth and differentiation of basophils but not mast cells in humans.[20–22] In contrast, the primary cytokine for mast cell growth and differentiation is the stem cell factor (SCF)/c-Kit ligand.[23–27] Mast cells resemble monocytes, including their responsiveness to IL-4, the expression of mast cell tryptase in human monocytic cell lines, and the ability of murine mast cells to adopt monocytic features in culture.[28,29]

Growth, Proliferation, Survival

The interaction between SCF and its cognate receptor c-Kit (Kit) plays a key role in regulating mast cell growth and differentiation. Kit is expressed on hematopoietic progenitors and is downregulated upon their differentiation into mature cells of all lineages, except mast cells, which retain high levels of cell surface Kit expression.[30] Insight into the biologic function of Kit and SCF came from observations in mice carrying specific mutations at the dominant white spotting (*W*)[31–38] or Steel (*Sl*) loci, respectively (reviewed in 39, 40). A double gene dose of mutant alleles at either locus produces common pleiotropic effects, including a profound decrease in mast cell number, coat color abnormalities/white-spotting (piebaldism), macrocytic anemia, reduced fertility, and abnormalities in intestinal pacemaker activity. Despite the shared phenotype between *W*- and *Sl*-mutant mice, the mechanism underlying the defect in hematopoiesis is quite different. In *W/W^v* mice, for instance, transplantation of bone marrow cells from congenic +/+ mice corrected both the anemia and mast cell deficiency, which indicated that the defect was an intrinsic stem cell disorder.[10,41–44] Many independent mutations of the *W* locus have been described; the alleles are semidominant and vary in their phenotypic effect on hematopoiesis, pigmentation, and fertility in the homozygous and heterozygous state.[45] In contrast, the defect is cell-extrinsic in *Sl/Sl^d* mice; when skin from either *W/W^v* or *Sl/Sl^d* mice was grafted onto the back of congenic +/+ mice, mast cells were found to populate the grafted skin from *W/W^v* mice but not in skin from *Sl/Sl^d* mice.[9,46] Furthermore, the hematologic defects in *Sl/Sl^d* mice were not corrected by transplantation of bone marrow cells from a congenic +/+ host[46] indicating that the disorder is microenvironmental in nature.

Activation and Function

Mast cells are ubiquitous and are found in virtually all tissues, but are most numerous at anatomic sites that are in contact with the environment, such as the mucosa of airways and gut, as well as in the skin. Although mast cells have been long identified as key cellular mediators of the allergic inflammatory response,[47–51] they have myriad other physiologic functions, including a key role in innate immunity.[52–55] The study of mast cell function in humans has been difficult for several reasons. First, these cells are relatively inaccessible; in general, primary culture of mast cells (including those derived from cord blood or peripheral blood-derived progenitor cells) is cumbersome, the yield of cells is quite limited, and it is presently unclear whether fully mature mast cells can be obtained by this approach.[26,56–61] Second, there appears to be significant variation in the functional properties of mast cells depending upon the anatomic location from which they are isolated (eg, skin versus intestinal mucosa).[62–64] Third, mast cells display considerable phenotypic plasticity, with many autocrine, paracrine, or systemic factors influencing various aspects of cell phenotype.[65] Consequently, investigators have often relied on transformed mast cell leukemia cell lines (eg, HMC-1, LAD-1, LAD-2),[66,67] or murine animal models for experimental studies of mast cell function.[52,54] Mouse strains that exhibit a profound mast cell deficiency include (a) *c-kit/W* mutant mice (eg, W/W^v mice; vide infra) also display non-mast cell phenotypic abnormalities including sterility, which entails complex breeding strategies, and (b) W^{sh}/W^{sh} mice, which carry an inversion mutation upstream of the *c-kit* coding region, display abnormal pigmentation and reduced mast cell number but have relatively preserved hematopoiesis and fertility.[68–72] The aforementioned mice can be selectively reconstituted with mast cells by systemic (intravenous) or local (eg, intradermal, intraperitoneal) transfer; this adoptive transfer of genetically compatible, in vitro cultured mast cells (eg, from bone marrow cells) provides a useful model (ie, "mast cell knockin mice") for the study of mast cell function in vivo.[73–75] It remains unclear however whether observations from cell line or mouse experiments can be extrapolated to humans, given that neoplastic transformation significantly alters normal cellular function and given the marked interspecies differences in mast cell biology. Mast cells undergo activation, classically following cross-linking of FcεRI-bound IgE by multivalent allergens in sensitized individuals. The tissue mast cell burden is dynamic and has been noted to increase in chronic allergic inflammatory states.[76] Non-IgE triggers for mast cell mediator release include anaphylatoxins of the complement system (C3a and C5a), neuropeptides (eg, vasoactive intestinal peptide, somatostatin, substance P), lipopolysaccharides, chemokines (eg, CCL3, / MIP1α), and Toll-like receptors (reviewed in 52, 53, 55). Other non-IgE triggers for mast cell activation include specific cytokines, such as SCF, and to some extent IL-4 (in cooperation with SCF) as well as IL-3. Upon activation by either IgE-dependent or IgE-independent mechanisms, three classes of mediators are released: (a) preformed mediators that are stored in cytoplasmic granules (eg, amines, proteases, proteoglycans); (b) lipid mediators synthesized de novo (eg, leukotrienes, prostaglandins); and (c) growth factors, cytokines, and chemokines.[11,48,77–86] Mast cells are primed for multiple cycles of degranulation-mediator release, and display distinct patterns of mediator release depending upon the strength and type of stimulus that is provided.[52,87–89] Mast cells display a wide spectrum of "activation levels" in vivo; however, the mechanisms regulating the secretory phenotype of mast cells in a given individual are not completely understood (reviewed in 52). The key mast cell mediators include (a) vasoactive amines, particularly histamine; (b) several distinct tryptases (α, β, and δ) that comprise the principal protein component of mast cells; (c) anionic proteoglycans (eg, heparin, chondroitin sulphate) that confer metachromasia upon staining with toluidine blue; (d) various lipid mediators; these arachidonic acid-derived eicosanoids, which include leukotriene C_4, leukotriene B_4, and prostaglandin D_2, mediate vasodilation, vasopermeability, smooth muscle constriction, mucus secretion, as well as other proinflammatory processes; (e) other proteases (eg, chymase, carboxypeptidase A); and (f) specific cytokines. The secreted cytokines, which recruit and activate specific cells, include IL-3 (basophils), IL-5 (eosinophils), tumor necrosis factor-α/IL-8 (neutrophils), and IL-4/IL-13 (T and B lymphocytes). Mast cells mediate not only early-phase (eg, anaphylaxis, acute asthma) but also late-phase allergic responses, as well as non-type I hypersensitivity reactions through the aforementioned mediators.[90] Furthermore, mast cells mediate upregulation of T_H2-responses and allergen-specific IgE biosynthesis, which contribute to host defenses against parasitic infections.[91,92] Mast cells have also been implicated in other nonallergic diseases, including viral and bacterial infections,[93–95] autoimmune disorders,[96–98] as well as in angiogenesis related to cancer,[99] although its role(s) in these conditions has not yet been precisely delineated.

Role of Kit and Stem Cell Factor in Mast Cell Biology

c-Kit is the cellular homolog of the *v-Kit* oncogene of the Hardy–Zuckerman 4 feline sarcoma virus[100] and encodes for Kit, which belongs to the type III subfamily of receptor tyrosine kinases. Members of this receptor tyrosine kinase subfamily share both sequence similarity and a common overall structure, with an extracellular domain containing 5 immunoglobulin-like motifs that binds SCF, a short transmembrane (TM) domain that anchors Kit to the cell membrane, a cytoplasmic tyrosine kinase (TK) domain that is split by an insert sequence into ATP-binding and phosphotransferase regions, and a juxtamembrane (JM) domain that lies between the TM and TK domains.[101–103] After *c-Kit* was found to be located on human chromosome 4,[101,104] in a region (4q11-q12) homologous to a region of mouse chromosome 5, that includes the *W* gene locus, further studies sought to examine whether the *W* locus was linked to murine *c-Kit*. Using interspecific backcross analysis, it was determined that the two were tightly linked,[105] and *c-Kit* was subsequently found to be disrupted in two spontaneous mutant *W* alleles, W^x, and W,[44] confirming that Kit was encoded by the *W* locus.[106] Specific mutations at the *W* locus, such as *W* (78, amino acid TM/JM deletion), W^{37} (JM missense mutation), or W^v, W,[41] and W^{42} (TK missense mutations) result in a loss-of-function phenotype and point to the critical role of individual domains/regions in Kit function[38,106–114] (reviewed in 115). The common phenotypic denominator of mutations at the *W* locus is reduced Kit tyrosine kinase activity, whether by expression of decreased number of Kit receptors with normal kinase activity (W,[44] W,[57] and W^x alleles), or expression of normal numbers of kinase-defective Kit (W,[37] W,[42] W,[41] W^v, W^{55} alleles) (reviewed in 115).

SCF was initially isolated from medium conditioned by Buffalo rat liver cells, and exhibited ex vivo growth factor activity toward primitive hematopoietic progenitors as well as mast cells.[27] The subsequent purification, cloning, and mapping of SCF revealed it to be syntenic with the *Sl* locus on mouse chromosome 10, and SCF sequences were found to be deleted in a number of mutant *Sl* alleles such as Sl^d and Sl^{12H}.[116–118] SCF was shown to be a ligand for Kit by cross-linking of ^{125}I-labeled SCF to Kit-expressing cells[119] and the administration of recombinant SCF in vivo rescued both the macrocytic anemia and the mast cell deficiency exhibited by Sl/Sl^d mice.[118] The Steel–Dickie (Sl^d) mutation is a 4.0-kb deletion within the gene SCF, which renders Sl^d only capable of encoding a soluble truncated growth factor that lacks both transmembrane and cytoplasmic domains.[120,121] SCF is synthesized by a variety of mesenchymal cells, including fibroblasts, that express the cytokine as a transmembrane protein that may be proteolytically cleaved to generate a soluble form; two distinct isoforms with differential susceptibility to proteolysis are synthesized.[122] Soluble SCF exists as a homodimer in plasma and can crosslink two Kit receptors on the cell surface, thereby leading to activation of Kit, as well as downstream signal transduction.[123] SCF promotes mast cell development, survival of mature mast cells, as well as adhesion of mast cells to extracellular matrix proteins. SCF also regulates mediator release from human mast cells, potentially by both IgE-dependent and IgE-independent mechanisms.

Mastocytosis

Mast cell disease/mastocytosis is characterized by the abnormal growth and accumulation of morphologically and immunophenotypically abnormal mast cells in one or more organs in the body. In contrast to normal mast cells, its neoplastic counterparts are more variable in appearance, ranging from round to fusiform variants, with long, polar cytoplasmic processes; they additionally display cytoplasmic hypogranularity with uneven distribution of fine granules, as well as atypical nuclei with monocytoid appearance.[124–126] Immunophenotypic evaluation of mast cells reveals virtually invariable expression of aberrant markers in mastocytosis patients.[127–129]

Pathogenesis

Current evidence points to an important role for gain-of-function mutations in *c-Kit*, particularly Kit D816V, in the pathogenesis of mastocytosis. The issue as to whether additional genetic hits are necessary for neoplastic transformation of mast cells, and for full expression of the mastocytosis phenotype, remains to be determined. Other specific mutations, such as *FIP1L1-PDGFRA* and Kit F522C, although rare, exhibit specific genotype–phenotype associations in mastocytosis patients and hence deserve specific mention in this section.

Kit D816V

Furitsu et al showed that Kit expressed on HMC-1 cells, an immature mast cell line established from a patient with mast cell leukemia,[66] was constitutively phosphorylated and activated in the absence of SCF.[130] Sequencing of *c-kit* in these cells revealed two point mutations, one in the juxtamembrane (V560G) and the other in the tyrosine kinase (D816V) domain. Two rodent cell lines, P815 (mouse mastocytoma) and RBL-2H3 (rat mast cell leukemia), were subsequently found to carry mutations corresponding to human D816V (ie, D814Y and D817Y, respectively).[131,132] These mutations, in human, mouse, and rat Kit, were shown to be constitutively activating when expressed in the human embryonic kidney cell line 293T.[130–132] Soon after this report, Nagata et al published the first report of the Kit D816V mutation in human mastocytosis.[133] Since then, other Kit mutations, either involving D816 or an adjacent amino acid residue (eg, D816Y,[134–136] D816F,[134] D816H,[137] I817V or VI815–816,[138] and D820G[139]) or involving other domains (extracellular,[140] transmembrane,[141,142] or juxtamembrane[143,144]) have also been identified in mastocytosis. The juxtamembrane mutations include V560G, K509I, and V559A; some are rare alleles detected in germline DNA in cohorts with familial mastocytosis.[145] Interestingly, several kindreds with combined familial gastrointestinal stromal tumors and mastocytosis, both of which are associated with gain-of-function Kit mutations, have also now been described.[140,143]

Although activating Kit mutations are clearly associated with human mastocytosis, they do not occur universally,[146] and the question as to whether individual mutations are necessary and sufficient to cause mast cell transformation remains currently unsettled. Introduction of human Kit D816V (or its murine homologs) into IL-3-dependent cell lines, either Ba/F3 (pro-B-lymphocyte), IC-2 (mast cell) or FDC-P1 (myeloid), results in their cytokine-independent growth.[147–149] Furthermore, subcutaneous injection of mutant Kit V559G- or Kit D814V-bearing Ba/F3 cells into nude mice produced large mastocytomas and all the mice subsequently died of mast cell leukemia.[148] These experiments do not, however, provide direct confirmation of the neoplastic transformation potential of activating Kit mutations since the IL-3-dependent cell lines are immortalized and have acquired a priori the capacity to self-renew by unknown events. Kitayama and colleagues introduced activated Kit (V559G or D814V) by retroviral infection into murine bone marrow cells and injected these cells into mast cell-deficient irradiated *W/W*^{v} mice.[150] In vitro colony assays revealed that Kit D814V, and to some extent Kit V559G, stimulated cytokine-independent growth of both mast cell and non-mast cell myeloid colonies. Furthermore, a proportion of the transplanted mice developed acute leukemia, likely of B-lymphoid origin; in addition, a subset of transgenic mice expressing Kit D814V developed acute leukemia/lymphoma of immature B-cell origin at 10 to 80 weeks of age. In another study, human Kit D816V was introduced into murine fetal liver cells, with induction of megakaryocytic differentiation, in the absence of cytokines.[151] In the presence of SCF, Kit D816V-expressing cells showed increased mast cell differentiation, as did Kit-wild type (WT)-expressing cells. The Kit D816V-expressing cells however were not transformed, as assessed by colony assays, regardless of the absence or presence of SCF. Furthermore, introduction of Kit D816V induces myelomastocytic differentiation and cluster formation of Ba/F3 cells but does not enhance their growth.[152] Thus, there is conflicting experimental data from mouse studies as to whether activating Kit mutations are sufficient to cause oncogenic transformation. Similarly, Kit D816V mutation alone may not be sufficient to cause oncogenic transformation in humans. This is consistent with the observation that most mastocytosis patients harboring this mutation have indolent disease. In addition, B cells and monocytes carrying mutated *c-kit* display a nonmalignant behavior, despite being derived from the same precursor that gives rise to lesional mast cells in mastocytosis patients.[153] Thus, it is possible that Kit D816V may affect the differentiation and apoptosis potential of human mast cells rather than providing a potent proliferative signal. In support of this theory, human bone marrow mast cells harboring Kit D816V but not normal mast cells have been shown to survive in a medium devoid of SCF.[154] Moreover, enhanced expression of the antiapoptotic protein Bcl-xL was found in lesional mast cells in patient bone marrow biopsies.[155] It is also possible that Kit D816V affects mast cell function; for instance, Taylor and colleagues showed that hematopoietic progenitors and mast cells carrying Kit D816V migrate to SCF more vigorously.[156] Thus, Kit D816V as a single hit may explain the pathology and clinical course of indolent mastocytosis but not of aggressive mastocytosis or mast cell leukemia.

FIP1L1-PDGFRA

Systemic mastocytosis patients frequently exhibit eosinophilia (SM-eo),[157–160] and in at least some cases the eosinophils can be shown to be derived from the neoplastic clone.[161] A subset of cases with eosinophilia harbor the *FIP1L1-PDGFRA* oncogene, which results from an interstitial deletion in chromosome 4q12—leading to constitutively active platelet-derived growth factor receptor A (PDGFRA) tyrosine kinase activity—that is uniquely sensitive to inhibition by imatinib mesylate.[162] In these patients, *FIP1L1-PDGFRA* involves mast cells and eosinophils in addition to lymphocytes, thus pointing to its origin in a multipotent hematopoietic progenitor cell.[163] The bone marrow mast cell infiltration pattern is unusual as compared to the typical mastocytosis patient harboring Kit D816V, in that the mast cells are diffusely distributed, with fewer pathognomonic mast cell clusters.[164,165] The patients harboring *FIP1L1-PDGFRA* are probably best classified as having chronic eosinophilic leukemia (CEL), although, since in at least some cases, they fulfill criteria for both systemic mastocytosis and CEL, their classification as systemic mastocytosis, subtype SM-CEL, may be appropriate.[166,167] Gain-of-function Kit[168] and PDGFRA[169] mutations have also been identified in gastrointestinal stromal cell tumors, where they have a pathogenetic role. Intriguingly, in both gastrointestinal stromal cell tumors and mastocytosis patients, KIT and PDGFRA mutations appear to be alternative and mutually exclusive genetic events.

Other Mutations/Polymorphisms

Presence of Kit D816V alone does not explain the remarkable clinical heterogeneity of human mastocytosis. Kit mutations are not consistently detected in some patients, such as those with childhood-onset cutaneous mastocytosis. Also, other mutations, polymorphisms, and/or karyotypic abnormalities have been detected in mastocytosis (summarized in 146), which likely influence the disease phenotype whether or not these lesions coexist with Kit D816V. Intriguingly, loss-of-function mutations have also been detected in mastocytosis; the dominant-negative Kit E839K mutation, [170] as well as the IL-4 receptor alpha chain polymorphism, Q576R, that is thought to limit mast cell growth and differentiation,[171] are both associated with relatively limited forms of mastocytosis.

Classification

The classification of mastocytosis has evolved over the years; the first recognition of cutaneous mast cell disease came from Unna's recognition in 1887 that urticaria pigmentosa (UP) lesions were histologically composed of mast cell infiltrates.[172] Although the systemic nature of mastocytosis had been alluded to by Sézary and others in the early 1900s,[173,174] systemic mast cell infiltrates were histologically demonstrated by Ellis only in 1949.[175] Subsequently, a dichotomous view prevailed, wherein benign mastocytosis was separated from malignant mastocytosis, based on the presence or not of UP, organomegaly, particular cytologic and cytochemical features of bone marrow mast cells, as well as the clinical course.[176–179] Following this, based on the recognition that not all patients classified as having benign mastocytosis have a favorable outcome, and that malignant mastocytosis was composed of relatively distinct clinicopathologic entities, updated classifications generally with four or five broad mastocytosis subgroups were proposed.[159,180] More recently, updated diagnostic criteria and an updated consensus classification for mastocytosis was proposed and adopted by the World Health Organization (WHO) in 2001.[181,182] This classification incorporates recent advances in our understanding of mastocytosis, including the role of *c-kit* mutations, aberrant expression of cell surface immunophenotypic markers on neoplastic mast cells, as well as the role of mast cell mediators as surrogate measures of mast cell number and/or function. The current WHO classification classifies mastocytosis into seven variants (Table 73–1):[182] cutaneous mastocytosis (CM), indolent systemic mastocytosis (ISM), systemic mastocytosis with an associated clonal hematological non-mast cell disorder (SM-AHNMD), aggressive systemic mastocytosis (ASM), mast cell leukemia (MCL), mast cell sarcoma, and extracutaneous mastocytoma. In addition, two relatively rare variants of mastocytosis with characteristic clinicopathologic features have also been described: well-differentiated systemic mastocytosis (WDSM) and systemic mastocytosis without skin involvement associated with recurrent anaphylaxis (SM-ana).[138] The WHO classification of mastocytosis mandates a number of staging investigations to define the exact subtype of disease.[182] Identification of B findings (Table 73–2) alone such as more than 30% mast cells in the bone marrow or serum tryptase greater than 200 ng/mL are indicative of a high systemic mast cell burden (ie, smoldering SM), whereas the additional presence of C findings (Table 73–3) such as cytopenias, pathologic fractures, hypersplenism, and so on, indicate impaired organ function directly attributable to mast cell infiltration and are diagnostic for presence of aggressive disease (ie, ASM).

Table 73–1 World Health Organization Variants of Mastocytosis[182]

1. Cutaneous mastocytosis (CM): a. Maculopapular CM b. Diffuse CM c. Mastocytoma of skin
2. Indolent systemic mastocytosis (ISM): a. Smoldering systemic mastocytosis (SSM) b. Isolated bone marrow mastocytosis
3. Systemic mastocytosis with an associated clonal hematological non-mast cell lineage disease (SM-AHNMD): a. SM-MDS b. SM-MPD c. SM-CEL d. SM-CMML e. SM-NHL
4. Aggressive systemic mastocytosis (ASM) With eosinophilia (SM-eo)
5. Mast cell leukemia (MCL) Aleukemic MCL
6. Mast cell sarcoma
7. Extracutaneous mastocytoma

CEL, chronic eosinophilic leukemia; CMML, chronic myelomonocytic leukemia; MDS, myelodysplastic syndrome; MPD, myeloproliferative disorder; NHL, non-Hodgkin lymphoma.

Clinical Features

Mast cell disease has a varied clinical presentation with symptoms that may be broadly grouped as follows:

Skin Rash

There are three major forms of cutaneous mastocytosis recognized by the WHO.[182] The commonest is urticaria pigmentosa (also referred to as maculopapular cutaneous mastocytosis [MPCM]), the others being diffuse cutaneous mastocytosis and solitary mastocytoma of the skin. The skin lesions are typically yellow tan to reddish brown macules, and may less frequently present as nodules or plaques (Fig. 73–1). The lesions generally involve the extremities, trunk, and abdomen, but spare sun-exposed areas, including the palms, soles, and scalp. The lesions commonly exhibit an urticarial response to mechanical stimulation such as stroking or scratching (Darier's sign or dermographic urticaria).[183,184] Biopsies of UP/MPCM lesions demonstrate multi-focal MC aggregates mainly around blood vessels and around skin appendages in the papillary dermis.[184,185] An increase in dermal MC, in the absence of typical UP lesions, is not considered diagnostic of CM, given the relatively nonspecific nature of such a finding.[186–189] Children account for nearly two-thirds of all reported cases of cutaneous mastocytosis, with a majority of cases arising before the age of 2 years.[190–192] In contrast, most adult MCD patients with UP/MPCM have systemic disease (often indolent) at presentation that is most commonly revealed by a bone marrow biopsy done as part of the diagnostic workup.[193]

Table 73–2 B Findings: Indication of High Mast Cell Burden[304]

1. Infiltration grade (mast cells) is greater than 30% in bone marrow in histology and serum total tryptase levels greater than 200 ng/mL
2. Hypercellular marrow with loss of fat cells, discrete signs of dysmyelopoiesis without substantial cytopenias, or WHO criteria for an MDS or MPD
3. Organomegaly: palpable hepatomegaly, splenomegaly, or lymphadenopathy (on CT or ultrasound) greater than 2 cm without impaired organ function

MDS, myelodysplastic syndrome; MPD, myeloproliferative disorder; WHO, World Health Organization.

Table 73–3 C Findings: Indication of Impaired Organ Function Attributable to Mast Cell Infiltration[182]

1. Cytopenia(s): Absolute neutrophil count $<1000/\mu L$, or hemoglobin <10 g/dL, or platelets $<100,000/\mu L$
2. Hepatomegaly with ascites and impaired liver function
3. Palpable splenomegaly with hypersplenism
4. Malabsorption with hypoalbuminemia and weight loss
5. Skeletal lesions: large-sized osteolysis or severe osteoporosis causing pathologic fractures
6. Life-threatening organopathy in other organ systems that definitively is caused by an infiltration of the tissue by neoplastic mast cells

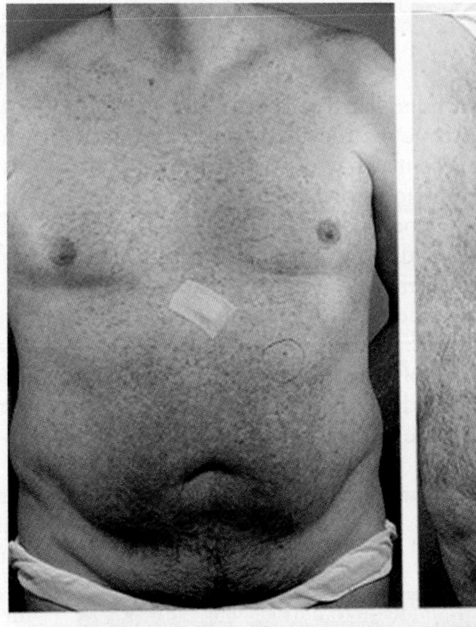
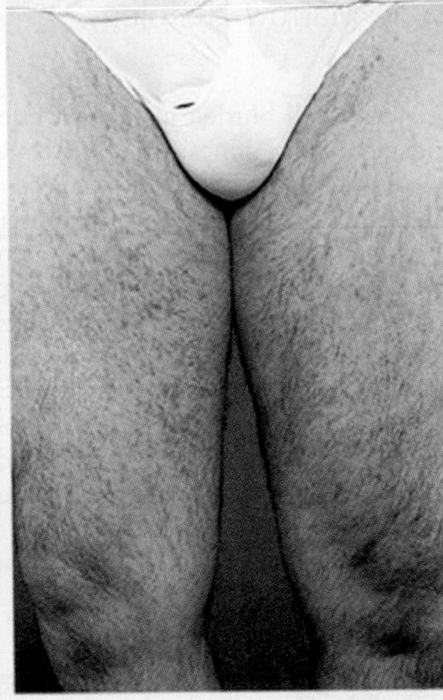

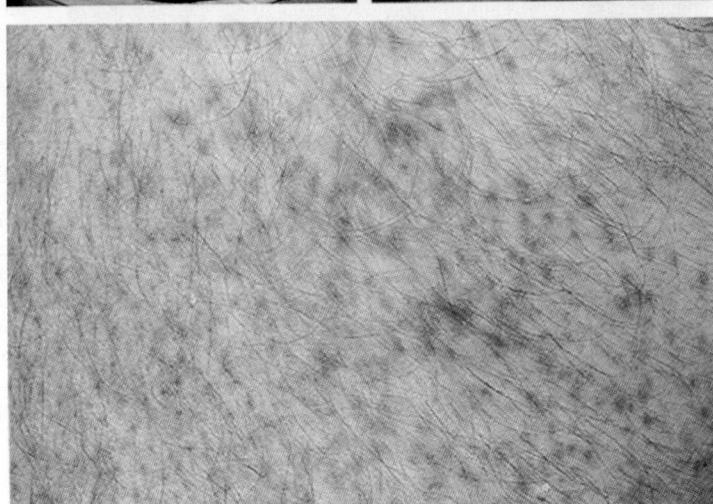

Figure 73–1 Urticaria pigmentosa lesions in a patient with cutaneous mastocytosis.

Symptoms Related to Mast Cell Degranulation

Most adult patients in this category have a low systemic mast cell burden, commonly exhibit CM lesions, and generally have indolent disease. Presenting symptoms include pruritus, urticaria, angioedema, flushing, bronchoconstriction, neuropsychiatric manifestations, and hypotension.[194] Gastrointestinal features such as nausea, vomiting, abdominal pain, diarrhea, and malabsorption may be prominent in some patients. Histamine receptor stimulation increases gastric acid production, which may cause peptic ulcer disease with potential morbidity from a bleeding peptic ulcer and/or perforation.[195,196] Presyncope, episodic vascular collapse, and sudden death represent the more dramatic clinical presentations of mast cell mediator release.[197]

Musculoskeletal Symptoms

Patients may have indolent or aggressive disease and present with poorly localized bone pain, diffuse osteoporosis or osteopenia, myalgias, arthralgias, pathological fractures, skeletal deformities, and/or compression radiculopathies. In the absence of typical cutaneous lesions (UP/MPCM) or mast cell mediator release symptoms, the diagnosis of systemic mastocytosis may prove challenging and diagnosis is frequently delayed in this setting. Systemic mastocytosis in this setting must be distinguished from other disorders including osteoporosis, metastatic cancer, Paget disease, and multiple myeloma.

Symptoms Related to Organomegaly/Organopathy

Systemic mastocytosis patients in this category are generally older, without CM lesions, frequently exhibit organomegaly and mast cell atypia (ie, high-grade morphology), and commonly experience an aggressive disease course.[125,198,199] Organ infiltration by neoplastic mast cells may lead to hepatomegaly (with or without liver dysfunction and ascites), splenomegaly (with or without hypersplenism), lymphadenopathy, large osteolytic lesions with or without pathologic fractures, and malabsorption with hypoalbuminemia and weight loss. Extensive marrow involvement may result in anemia and eventually to pancytopenia.

Diagnosis

The diagnosis of systemic mastocytosis is based on identification of abnormal mast cells by morphological, immunophenotypic, and/or genetic (molecular) criteria in various organs. The WHO criteria for systemic mastocytosis are shown in Table 73–4.[182]

Bone Marrow Histology

The mast cell burden in normal bone marrow is very low (<0.1%) and increases significantly in systemic mastocytosis patients.[200] Consequently, the diagnosis of systemic mastocytosis is most frequently established by histologic and immunohistochemical examination of bone marrow aspirate and biopsy specimens. The bone marrow is virtually always involved in adults and shows characteristic histologic features; in contrast, histological criteria for non-bone marrow organ involvement have not been clearly defined and, consequently, have not been widely accepted to date. Furthermore, a bone marrow examination allows determination of whether an associated clonal non-mast cell lineage hematological disorder is present. The pathognomonic lesion, which represents the WHO major diagnostic criterion, is presence of multifocal, dense mast cell aggregates, frequently in perivascular and/or paratrabecular locations (Fig. 73–2). These aggregates may be relatively monomorphic, composed mainly of fusiform mast cells, or may be polymorphic, with mast cells admixed with lymphocytes, eosinophils, neutrophils, histiocytes, endothelial cells, and fibroblasts.[180] Eosinophils are most commonly observed at the periphery of mast cell aggregates (often focally), but increased numbers of eosinophils may also be seen in areas not involved by mast cells.[125] Although irregular trabecular thickening is commonly noted, particularly when mast cell aggregates abut the trabeculae, other cases may be characterized by a marked thinning of bone marrow trabeculae and osteopenia. Mast cell infiltrates are commonly associated with a dense network of reticulin fibers; in cases with diffuse marrow infiltration by monomorphous, spindled mast cells that resemble fibroblasts, a diagnosis of primary myelofibrosis may be erroneously made, especially when accompanied with a decrease in normal hematopoietic elements.

Table 73–4 World Health Organization Criteria for Diagnosis of Systemic Mastocytosis[182]

MAJOR
Multifocal dense infiltrates of mast cells in bone marrow or other extracutaneous organ sections (>15 mast cells aggregating)
MINOR
a. ≥25% mast cells in tissue sections or bone marrow aspirate smears that are spindle shaped or have atypical morphology
b. C-kit point mutation at codon 816V
c. Expression of CD2 and/or CD25 by mast cells
d. Baseline serum tryptase persistently >20 ng/mL (not valid in presence of another non-mast cell clonal disorder)
Major plus one minor *or* three minor criteria are needed to diagnose systemic mastocytosis

Three distinct patterns of bone marrow mast cell infiltration have been described in systemic mastocytosis.[124,125] The commonest, Type I pattern, is frequently associated with urticaria pigmentosa and indolent disease; the mast cells are focally increased (generally 10%–30% of marrow cellularity), with normal distribution of fat and other hematopoietic elements in the uninvolved marrow space. A spectrum of atypical morphological features including cell spindling, cytoplasmic hypogranulation or uneven granule distribution, cytoplasmic processes, and nuclear abnormalities are seen in mast cells from these patients; much less commonly, the mast cells may be relatively normal appearing.[126,159,176,200,201] In contrast, Type II pattern consists of a significant increase in granulopoiesis in areas not involved by mast cells, as may be seen in ASM patients; some of these cases meet WHO criteria for diagnosis of a clonal non-mast cell lineage hematologic disorder associated with mastocytosis (SM-AHNMD) (see Fig. 73–3). The latter (ie, SM-AHNMD) is the second most common mastocytosis category (more frequent than ASM) and may account for up to a third of systemic mastocytosis patients.[176,178,179,202,203] The coexistence of these two entities (ie, mastocytosis and non-mast cell neoplasm) likely reflects their origin in a common multipotent hematopoietic progenitor cell, although in rare cases the two may develop

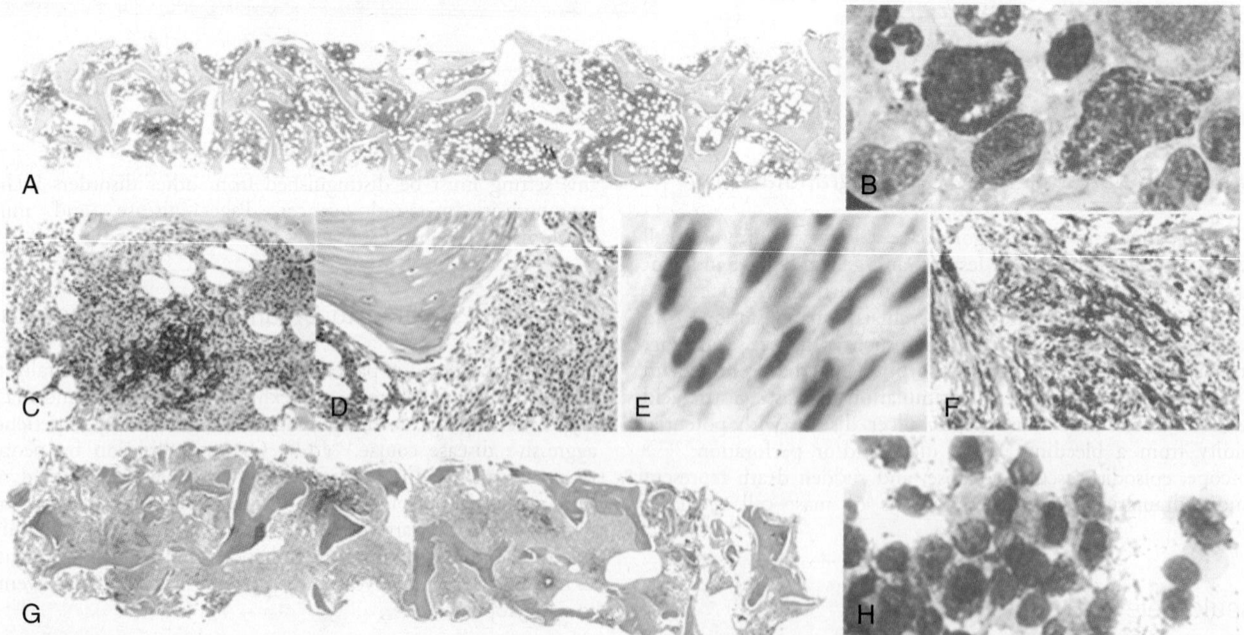

Figure 73–2 Systemic mastocytosis (**A–H**). Bone marrow biopsy (**A**) shows multiple small foci of involvement by systemic mast cell disease. The aspirate (**B**) contained only scattered mast cells. The involved areas include nodules of mast cells (**C**, and far left bottom in **A**) with central accumulations of lymphocytes resulting in the so-called bull's eye pattern, and paratrabecular foci (**D**, and far right bottom in **A**), along thickened bone. The latter can easily mimic lymphoma in the bone marrow, which can also exhibit a paratrabecular pattern of infiltration. High power of the mast cell involvement (**E**) illustrates the typical fusiform or spindle appearance of the mast cells. A mast cell tryptase immunohistochemical stain (**F**) is quite useful diagnostically. CD117 and CD25 were also positive. A second case (**G**) illustrates extensive involvement by an aggressive systemic mastocytosis. Note the extensive replacement of the marrow space and the marked osteosclerosis. Numerous mast cells are seen on the aspirate (**H**).

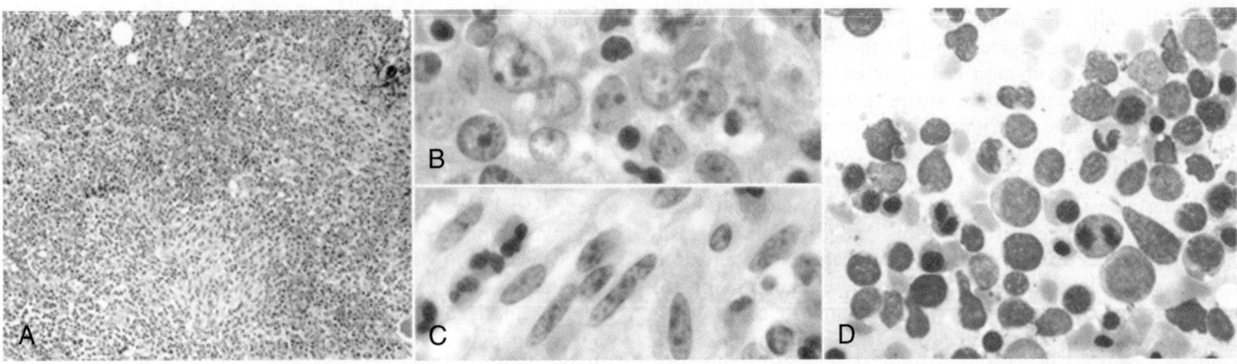

Figure 73–3 Systemic mastocytosis with an associated clonal hematological non-mast cell disorder (**A–D**). Low power of a bone marrow (**A**) from a 57-year-old female with systemic mastocytosis associated with acute myeloid leukemia. A focus of mast cells is present (**A**, bottom center) in the hypercellular marrow. High powers of same area (**B**) demonstrate increased immature cells including blasts, and the mast cell focus (**C**) composed of fusiform mast cells associated with eosinophils. The mast cells were shown to be mast cell tryptase-positive, CD25^{+} and CD117^{+}. The marrow aspirate (**D**) illustrates increased myeloblasts associated with multilineage dysplasia.

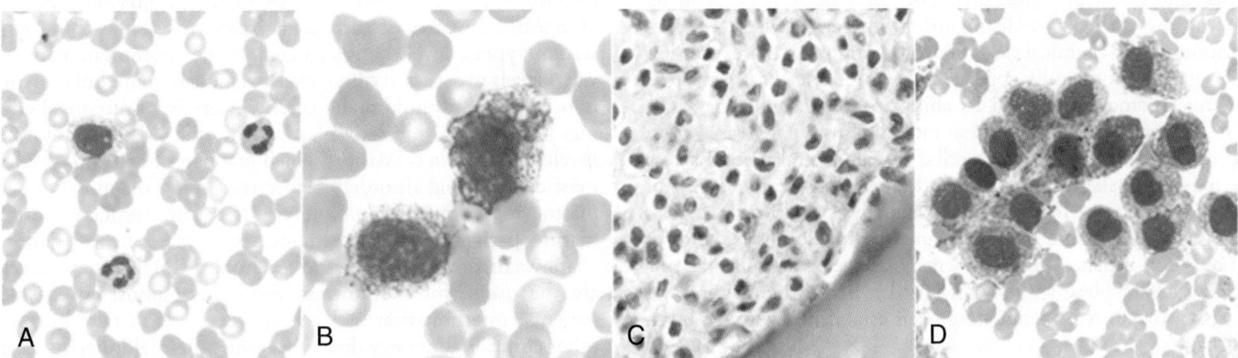

Figure 73–4 Mast cell leukemia (**A–D**). Low power of peripheral blood (**A**) showing 2 granulocytes and a single immature mast cell with sparse metachromatic granules. Two additional circulating mast cells are also illustrated (**B**). The marrow biopsy was packed with mast cells (**C**). Note the cells are held apart from one another due to their abundant cytoplasm. A similar pattern of infiltration is seen in hairy cell leukemia and in acute promyelocytic leukemia. The aspirate (**D**) shows sheets of immature and hypogranular mast cells.

independently.[202,204] The diagnosis of SM-AHNMD is established by WHO criteria, for both the mastocytosis and non-mast cell neoplasm components.[205] In most SM-AHNMD cases, a diagnosis of mastocytosis is made incidentally, usually after an examination of bone marrow for evaluation of the non-mast cell hematologic disorder.[202,203] In such cases, it is difficult to ascertain if mastocytosis existed prior to the onset of the non-mast cell disorder, although some patients provide historical clues (time of onset of UP lesions and/or symptoms of mast cell degranulation) in this regard. In most cases, the non-mast cell neoplasm tends to clinically overshadow the mastocytosis component, thereby reflecting its more aggressive biological nature. The most frequent non-mast cell disorders associated with mastocytosis are the chronic myeloproliferative disorders (except bcr-abl-positive CML), AML, and MDS.[126,179,203] The recognition that chronic myelomonocytic leukemia (CMML), a hybrid myeloproliferative–myelodysplastic disorder, is commonly associated with mastocytosis supports the contention that dysmyelopoiesis is a prominent feature of systemic mastocytosis.[202,204,206,207] In some cases, the bone marrow mast cell involvement may be obscured by the non-mast cell neoplasm if only conventional stains are employed (vide infra).[202] In this regard, mast cell infiltrates are more easily identified within sheets of monotonous blasts in AML than within the polymorphic infiltrates seen in myeloproliferative or myelodysplastic disorders. Patient characteristics that are associated with Type II pattern include older age, absence of UP lesions, organomegaly, anemia, eosinophilia, greater than 10% morphologically atypical mast cells in the bone marrow, elevated serum tryptase level, and a rapid clinical course.[158–160,176,180,200,208] Type III pattern is characterized by diffuse marrow infiltration with atypical mast cells of high-grade morphology, frequently with circulating mast cells; mast cell leukemia (MCL) (see Fig. 74–4) is characterized by increased numbers of mast cells in bone marrow (>20% in aspirate smear) and peripheral blood (>10%), with associated bone marrow failure manifested as peripheral cytopenias. The mast cells are immature, sometimes blastic, and often have sparse metachromatic granules, and hence may be missed on routine staining unless tryptase[200,201] and/or immunophenotyping studies are performed.[209,210] Rare aleukemic variants of mast cell leukemia have also been described.[210] Rarely, patients may present with increased numbers of metachromatically granulated, primitive, blast-like cells. In such cases, differentiating mast cell leukemia from tryptase- and/or kit D816V-positive acute myeloid leukemia (AML),[211,212] acute basophilic leukemia,[213] and myelomastocytic overlap syndrome[214] is a diagnostic challenge, in the absence of well-defined criteria. The aforementioned histologic patterns appear to be relevant for prognosis; in one study, mastocytosis patients with a Type I pattern (ISM) had an actuarial 5-year survival rate of 75%, as compared to 17% and 0% for patients with Type II (ASM or SM-AHNMD) and Type III (MCL) patterns, respectively.[208] Although mast cell cytologic atypia (large, irregularly shaped nuclei, increased mitotic activity, decreased numbers of metachromatic granules, etc) has been historically proposed by some authors as a criterion for aggressive mastocytosis,[199,215–217] such proposals have not been broadly accepted or implemented in routine practice.

In general, mast cells may not be readily recognized by standard dyes such as Giemsa, toluidine blue, or naphthol AS-D chloroacetate esterase (Leder stain), particularly when associated with significant hypogranulation or with abnormal nuclear morphology, and may be confused with a variety of other cells that include fibroblasts, histiocytes, hairy cells, and monocytes, particularly in polymorphic bone marrow mast cell aggregates.[180,218] Furthermore, the metachromatic staining properties of mast cells may be significantly diminished or lost with conventional tissue processing, particularly decalcification with acidic solutions that is necessary for sectioning of paraffin-embedded bone marrow tissue.[218] Among the immunohistochemical markers, staining for tryptase is considered the most sensitive, being able to detect even small-sized mast cell infiltrates (ie, composed of 10–15 cells) (Fig. 73–2).[219,220] Given that virtually all mast cells, irrespective of their stage of maturation, activation status, or tissue of localization express tryptase, staining for this marker detects even those infiltrates that are primarily composed of immature, poorly granulated mast cells.[209] Tryptase immunostaining is particularly useful for the diffuse pattern of mast cell infiltration, particularly when the cells are loosely distributed, in contrast to discrete mast cell aggregates.[219] It must be emphasized that neither tryptase nor other immunohistochemical markers such as chymase, Kit/CD117, or CD68 can distinguish between normal and neoplastic mast cells.[221] Also, abnormal basophils seen in some cases of acute and chronic basophilic leukemia, as well as in chronic myeloid leukemia, and blasts in some AML cases may be tryptase positive, and may prove difficult to distinguish from mast cells.[202] In contrast, immunohistochemical detection of aberrant CD25 expression on bone marrow mast cells appears to be a reliable diagnostic tool in systemic mastocytosis, given its ability to detect abnormal mast cells in all mastocytosis subtypes, including the rare cases with loosely scattered, interstitial mast cells.[209] A unilateral bone marrow biopsy may not be sufficient to exclude low levels (early stages) of mast cell involvement. In a retrospective analysis of 23 mastocytosis patients who underwent bilateral bone marrow biopsies, 4 cases (17%) only had unilateral involvement.[222] Three of the four patients had low serum tryptase levels (<25 ng/mL), hence the diagnosis of systemic mastocytosis may not have been established without bilateral biopsies.

Mast Cell Immunophenotyping

As mentioned previously, the qualitative and semiquantitative profiling of cell surface antigens by multiparametric flow cytometry can be extremely useful in distinguishing normal bone marrow mast cells from their pathologic counterparts in systemic mastocytosis (reviewed by Escribano et al).[223] Normal mast cells typically express KIT/CD117 and Fc RI, and their typical profile is CD117^{++}/Fc RI^{+}/CD34^{-}/CD38^{-}/CD33^{+}/CD45^{+}/CD11c^{+}/CD71^{+}. These cells do not express certain myeloid markers (CD14 and CD15), or lymphoid lineage markers, except CD22.[224] Neoplastic mast cells typically express CD25 and/or CD2, and the abnormal expression of at least one of these two antigens counts as a minor criterion toward the diagnosis of systemic mastocytosis per the WHO system.[182] In general, the detection of CD25 on mast cells, by either flow cytometry or immunohistochemistry, appears to be the more reliable marker (relative to CD2), although some authors have noted significant variation in the percentage of CD2-positive cases by flow cytometry depending upon the specific antibody–fluorochrome conjugate used.[223] Consistent with flow cytometry data,[129] it has been reported that screening for CD2 expression by immunohistochemistry may have relatively low diagnostic value because a significant proportion of cases stain negative, and CD2 expression on bone marrow mast cells is generally weak in the cases that are positive.[209,220,221] Interval monitoring of CD25 expression on bone marrow mast cells may represent one approach for assessing presence of residual disease in patients undergoing mast cell-cytoreductive therapy, generally for the aggressive mastocytosis subtypes.[129,225,226] Other aberrant immunophenotypic features of neoplastic mast cells include abnormally high expression of complement related markers such as CD11c,[227] CD35,[228] CD59,[228] and CD88,[228] as well as increased expression of the CD69 early-activation antigen,[229] and the CD63 lysosomal-associated protein.[230]

Serum Tryptase Measurement

The measurement of tryptase (a mast cell enzyme with trypsin-like enzymatic activity) levels in biological fluids (serum) has proven to be a useful disease-related marker in systemic mastocytosis, and is included as a minor criterion for diagnosing the condition according to WHO guidelines, provided that certain conditions are satisfied.[182,231] There are two major forms of mast cell tryptase–alpha (subtypes alpha 1 and 2) and beta (subtypes beta 1, 2, and 3) (reviewed by Schwartz).[232] Mature beta 2 tryptase is stored in mast cell secretory granules as an enzymatically active tetramer complexed with proteoglycans and is released only during granule exocytosis, thereby largely reflecting mast cell activation. In contrast, the precursor forms of both alpha and beta tryptase are constitutively secreted by mast cells,[233] and the combined total serum levels (including precursor and mature tryptase forms) are thought to correlate with systemic mast cell number, albeit with effects related to tryptase haplotype and gender.[234] The commercially available fluoroimmunoenzymatic assay (Pharmacia, Uppsala, Sweden) measures total tryptase levels; in healthy individuals, levels range from 1 to 15 ng/mL, whereas in most patients with systemic mastocytosis, total serum tryptase levels exceed 20 ng/mL. In cases of suspected mastocytosis, it is important that serum tryptase levels be interpreted in the appropriate context. Elevated levels of serum tryptase have been documented in patients with non-mast cell myeloid malignancies, including acute myeloid leukemia (AML),[211,235] myelodysplastic syndrome (MDS),[236] and chronic myeloid leukemia (CML),[237] which mandates exclusion of such non-mast cell myeloid disorders before reaching a diagnosis of systemic mastocytosis. Furthermore, levels of serum tryptase, particularly mature β-tryptase, can be frequently elevated in association with anaphylaxis or a severe allergic reaction.[231] Total tryptase levels may also be useful for monitoring treatment response in mastocytosis patients; interpretation of levels however has to take into account other clinical/laboratory data, given the potential inherent variability of tryptase levels, as well as other possible confounding effects, such as administration of radiocontrast agents or narcotics, that may lead to mast cell degranulation.

Molecular Studies

In mastocytosis patients molecular studies are important from the diagnostic standpoint and, increasingly, from the therapeutic standpoint as well. Recent studies underscore the high prevalence of the Kit D816V gain-of-function mutation in mastocytosis patients, with high correlation between mutation detection and the proportion of lesional/clonal cells in the sample, as well as the sensitivity of the screening method employed (reviewed by Akin).[145] Accordingly, the likelihood of mutation detection in peripheral blood mononuclear cells in a case of indolent mastocytosis (with low probability of circulating clonal cells), using a low-sensitivity screening test (eg. DNA sequencing), is quite low. Sensitivity of detection may be enhanced by enriching lesional mast cells or other clonal cell populations (eg. neutrophils or eosinophils) by laser capture microdissection, or magnetic bead- or flow cytometry-based cell sorting, respectively.[161,206,238] Furthermore, use of higher-sensitivity methods including allele-specific PCR,[239] or PCR with peptide nucleic acid (PNA) probes to clamp the wild-type allele combined with mutant allele detection with hybridization probes dramatically enhance the probability of mutation detection in bulk cells (sensitivity = 10^{-3}).[136,138] Using the latter method, the D816V mutation was detected in virtually all patients with indolent (ISM) or aggressive (ASM) systemic mastocytosis (93%), but less frequently in patients with well-differentiated systemic mastocytosis (WDSM; vide infra) (29%) in a recent study.[138] Here, Kit mutations other than D816V (eg, I817V, VI815–816) were rarely detected (<3%). Notably, most poor prognosis mastocytosis patients harbored Kit D816V in two or more bone marrow myeloid cell populations (81%), in contrast to indolent mastocytosis cases (27%).

WDSM may represent a distinct, albeit genetically heterogenous, subtype of systemic mastocytosis.[138] A subset of WDSM cases carry the F522C germline mutation located in the Kit transmembrane domain.[142] In contrast to other systemic mastocytosis subtypes, mast cells in WDSM do not (aberrantly) express either CD2 or CD25 antigens and are mature in appearance.

The *FIP1L1-PDGFRA* mutation can be detected by either fluorescence in situ hybridization (FISH) or PCR-based assays.[165,240] Some investigators have suggested that PCR (particularly nested PCR) is a more reliable screening test for *FIP1L1-PDGFRA* (relative to FISH) in primary eosinophilia, given the low sensitivity of FISH in some cases.[240] Limitations of PCR-based assays include the possibility of an unusual *FIP1L1-PDGFRA* transcript, given the heterogeneity of breakpoints with the *FIP1L1* locus and other mechanisms (eg, cryptic splice sites), which may lead to a false-negative test result. Finally, although real-time quantitative PCR assays for monitoring *FIP1L1-PDGFRA* transcript levels have been described, its precise utility in assessing either depth of response with therapy (ie, detection of minimal residual disease) or for molecular relapse remains unclear at this time.

Treatment

Adults with systemic mastocytosis generally seek treatment for one or more of the following disease manifestations: skin rash (eg, UP), symptoms of mast cell degranulation, and/or symptoms related to skeletal involvement or organomegaly/organopathy from mast cell infiltration. Although the treatment of systemic mastocytosis has hitherto been empirically derived, recent advances in our understanding of the molecular pathogenesis of this condition allows for the identification of specific disease subtypes that are uniquely sensitive (or resistant) to specific therapies. Consequently, in this era of increasingly wider access to molecular testing, it is important that mastocytosis patients be molecularly profiled for presence or absence of relevant pathogenetic mutations, to enable optimal therapeutic decisions for a given individual. The relative rarity of mastocytosis, its biologic heterogeneity, and (historically) the lack of simple, widely agreed upon treatment response criteria, have hitherto served as barriers to development of evidence-based therapies for this disorder. Although the therapy of systemic mastocytosis patients has to be individualized, an algorithm illustrating our general treatment approach to these patients is presented in the box below. Investigational therapies for systemic mastocytosis are discussed in the next section. We refer the reader to specialized dermatology texts for the treatment of cutaneous mastocytosis.

Treatment of Mast Cell Degranulation Symptoms

Although mast cell cytoreductive agents (eg, interferon, chemotherapy) can often effectively ameliorate symptoms of mast cell degranulation, these agents may have significant adverse effects; hence, the initial approach to these patients emphasizes measures to prevent mast cell degranulation, as well as use of medications for symptom relief. In all cases, avoidance of triggers for mast cell degranulation (eg, animal venoms, extremes of temperature, mechanical irritation, alcohol, emotional and physical stress) remains the cornerstone of therapy. Some patients cannot tolerate certain drugs or chemicals such as opioid analgesics, alcohol, aspirin/other nonsteroidal anti-inflammatory medications, contrast dyes; the patient history often provides useful clues in this regard. Furthermore, appropriate precautionary measures during anesthesia and surgery are recommended in these patients.[241–244]

Noncytoreductive therapy of mast cell degranulation symptoms includes the use of oral H-1 (eg, hydroxyzine, diphenhydramine, fexofenadine, cetirizine, cyproheptadine, chlorpheniramine) and H-2 (eg, ranitidine, famotidine) antihistaminics for pruritis and peptic ulcer symptoms, respectively, and orally administered cromolyn sodium for nausea, abdominal pain, and diarrhea. Use of the latter is supported by Level I evidence.[187,245] Cromolyn sodium was found in a double-blind crossover study to be therapeutically equivalent to a combination of cimetidine and chlorpheniramine for the treatment of mastocytosis-related symptoms.[246] Corticosteroids are occasionally used for treating recurrent hypotensive episodes, ascites, and diarrhea with malabsorption. Patients with a propensity toward vasodilatory shock ought to wear a medical alert bracelet and carry an Epi-Pen injector for self administration of subcutaneous epinephrine.[247] In the rare case of a patient with severe and/or recurrent life-threatening degranulation-related events that are refractory to the aforementioned agents, cautious consideration may be given to the use of cytostatic or cytoreductive agents; one must keep in mind however the potential adverse effects, including potentially mutagenic effects, of such agents and use them only after a full discussion of potential risks and benefits of such treatment with the patient.

Treatment of Organomegaly/Organopathy Symptoms

Cytoreductive therapy, especially chemotherapy, is generally reserved for patients with progressive symptomatic disease, and organopathy (C findings) that is directly related tissue mast cell infiltration. In certain patients, however, it can be difficult to distinguish whether the organopathy relates to mast cell infiltration or whether it represents an immunological response to the disease or an associated non-mast cell neoplasm (SM-AHNMD). Currently employed first- and second-line therapeutic agents include the following.

Interferon-Alpha (IFN-α)

Interferon-alpha (IFN-α) is often considered the first-line therapy for progressive symptomatic disease, including in the presence of a concurrent non-mast cell myeloproliferative disorder (eg, CMML).[248] IFN-α is generally started at the dose of 1 million units (MU) subcutaneously three times per week, followed by gradual escalation to 3 to 5 MU three to five times per week, if tolerated. IFN-α (with or without concomitant corticosteroids for synergistic effect) has been reported to improve symptoms of mast cell degranulation,[249] decrease bone marrow mast cell infiltration,[250–255] and ameliorate mastocytosis-related ascites/hepatosplenomegaly,[250,251,256] cytopenias,[257] skin findings,[248,252,258] and osteoporosis.[253,254,259,260] Response rates to IFN-α therapy have been difficult to estimate, given the heterogeneous presentation of patients with mastocytosis, use of variable treatment dosages, generally short follow-up, and use of nonuniform treatment response criteria in published studies. The optimal dose and duration of IFN-α therapy for systemic mastocytosis remain uncertain. In a prospective multicenter study, all four patients receiving the highest IFN-α dose (ie, >3 MU/m²/day) responded to treatment.[249] The time to best response may be up to 12 months or longer[257] and delayed responses to therapy have been described.[261] A significant proportion of patients may experience clinical and/or biochemical relapse within several months of IFN-α treatment being discontinued, outlining the largely cytostatic effect of IFN-α on neoplastic mast cells.[249,251] IFN-α is associated with a variable, but significant, incidence (up to 50%) of dose-limiting toxicity, including flu-like symptoms, bone pain, fever, worsening cytopenias (particularly in patients with baseline organomegaly/cytopenias), depression, and hypothyroidism.[249,251] Anaphylaxis, as a response to IFN-α injections, has been described.[262] Consequently, the dropout rate with IFN-α treatment due to adverse events is not trivial and whether the addition of corticosteroids to IFN-α improves either treatment tolerance or efficacy remains to be proven in a randomized setting.[257]

2-Chlorodeoxyadenosine/Cladribine

Single-agent 2-chlorodeoxyadenosine/Cladribine (2-CdA) has therapeutic activity in systemic mastocytosis in IFN-α refractory/intolerant patients; variable treatment schedules have been employed in this setting.[263–267] In a prospective multicenter pilot study of 10 patients, 2-CdA (0.1–0.13 mg/kg by a 2-hr IV infusion on days 1 through 5

Investigational Therapies

Tyrosine Kinase Inhibitors

PKC412 is an *n*-benzoyl-staurosporine, with inhibitory activity against protein kinase C (PKC), Flt3 (FMS-like tyrosine kinase), Kit, vascular endothelial growth factor receptor-2 (VEGFR-2), PDGFR, and fibroblast growth factor receptor (FGFR) tyrosine kinases.[283,284] PKC412 potently inhibits growth of cell lines harboring Kit D816V,[285,286] and early data suggest activity in patients with advanced systemic mastocytosis[287,288]; preliminary data from the latter Phase II study indicated that six of nine patients responded to PKC412 therapy. PKC412 has limited efficacy as a single agent for treatment of AML[289] but may be active against constitutively activated ZNF198-FGFR1 for the treatment of 8p11 myeloproliferative syndrome (EMS).[290]

Dasatinib (BMS354825) is an orally bioavailable thiazolecarboxamide that is structurally unrelated to imatinib. It is a dual Src/Abl kinase inhibitor that is more potent than imatinib, and demonstrates inhibitory activity against a number of Bcr-Abl mutations linked to imatinib resistance in CML, but not T315I.[291] Dasatinib inhibits cell lines harboring Kit WT or Kit D816V at nanomolar concentrations.[292,293] In contrast to imatinib, dasatinib binds to the Abl and Kit ATP-binding sites irrespective of the activation-loop conformation.[294,295] Preliminary data indicates modest activity in systemic mastocytosis; in one report, although 30% had symptomatic benefit, only 2 of 24 patients achieved significant mast cell cytoreduction (both patients were Kit D816V-negative and achieved complete remission).[296]

Nilotinib (AMN107) is a small-molecule kinase inhibitor with activity against a number of Bcr-Abl mutations linked to imatinib resistance in CML, but not T315I.[297] Nilotinib also has in vitro inhibitory activity against cell lines harboring Kit WT or Kit V560G (juxtamembrane mutant) but has limited activity against Kit D816V (IC_{50} in micromolar range).[285,298] These data suggest that nilotinib may be a less than ideal candidate for treatment of systemic mastocytosis, where a majority of the patients carry the Kit D816V mutation.[285] Data pertaining to clinical activity of AMN107 in mastocytosis patients is not yet available.

MLN518 is a quinazoline-based tyrosine kinase inhibitor, which inhibits cell lines harboring Kit D816V as well as juxtamembrane mutant-Kit, thus making it a promising candidate for mastocytosis treatment.[299]

AP23464/AP23848 are ATP-based inhibitors that have low-nanomolar inhibitory activity against Kit D816V.[300] Interestingly, cell lines harboring Kit WT or juxtamembrane mutant-Kit were less sensitive to inhibition, relative to Kit D816V, suggesting a therapeutic window wherein clones carrying the latter mutation could be selectively suppressed/eliminated in mastocytosis patients without disrupting normal hematopoiesis.

EXEL-0862 is a novel tyrosine kinase inhibitor that has been shown to have greater inhibitory activity against the HMC 1.2 cell line that harbors both Kit D816V and Kit V560G, as compared to HMC 1.1 that harbors the juxtamembrane Kit V560G mutation alone.[301] Thus, EXEL-0862 is a promising candidate for the treatment of mastocytosis and other malignancies harboring active site Kit mutations.

Nontyrosine Kinase Inhibitors

17-AAG (17-(Allylamino)-17-demethoxygeldanamycin) is a geldanamycin derivative that binds to heat shock protein 90 (hsp90), thus enhancing the proteasomal degradation of several hsp90 client kinases, including mutant Kit. In one report, a dose-dependent decrease in phosphorylation of Kit, Akt, and STAT3 was observed in both HMC 1.1 and HMC 1.2 cells.[302] Furthermore, 17-AAG inhibited patient-derived neoplastic mast cells ex vivo, relative to mononuclear cells. 17-AAG is currently in phase II clinical trials for the treatment of mastocytosis.

IMD-0354 is an NF-κB inhibitor, which potently suppresses growth of HMC 1.2 cells that harbor both Kit D816V and Kit V560G mutations, and may have promise for treating mastocytosis patients.[303]

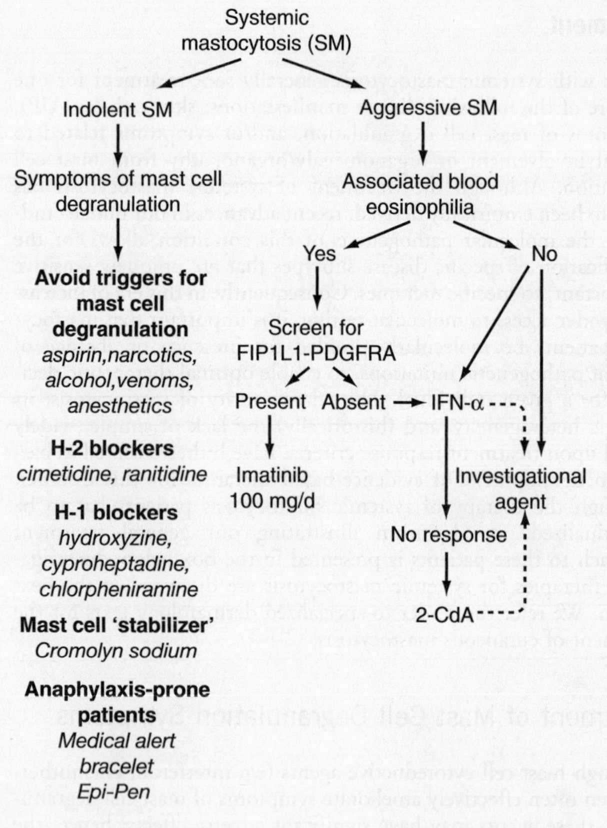

every 4–8 weeks for 6 cycles) was found to be therapeutically active in all mastocytosis subsets.[267] Although all patients had a clinical response, and bone marrow mast cell cytoreduction was also noted in 9 of 10 patients, no complete remissions were observed. Also, in a preliminary report of 33 SM patients treated with 2-CdA (0.15 mg/kg by a 2-hr IV infusion or subcutaneously for 5 days every 4–12 weeks for 1 to 6 cycles), major, partial, or no responses were seen in 24, 2, and 7 patients, respectively.[268] Myelosuppression was the major adverse effect seen in approximately a third of cases in each study. Although single-agent 2-CdA has activity in the treatment of systemic mastocytosis, there is relatively limited experience with its use in this setting; additional data are awaited to clarify the optimal dose/schedule of administration, response rates in specific mastocytosis subtypes, and durability of treatment responses. Given the potential for prolonged bone marrow aplasia and lymphopenia and associated risk of opportunistic infections, its use is probably best restricted to select cases with IFN-α refractory disease, after careful consideration of the risk-to-benefit ratio as well as other available therapies for every patient.

Imatinib Mesylate (Gleevec™)

Imatinib mesylate (Gleevec™) is an orally bioavailable small-molecule inhibitor of Kit, Abl, Arg, and PDGFR tyrosine kinases. The identification of gain-of-function mutations involving *Kit* and *PDGFRA* genes (known imatinib targets) in the pathogenesis of systemic mastocytosis has obvious therapeutic implications in this regard. Consistent with predictions from in vitro data,[154,269] the limited clinical experience to date suggests that the vast majority of mastocytosis patients (who harbor Kit D816V) are likely to be refractory to imatinib therapy.[270,271] In contrast, clinically meaningful responses have been observed for the rare patients with Kit juxtamembrane mutations (eg, F522C, K509I), suggesting that this subgroup of patients has imatinib-responsive disease.[142,144] Furthermore, patients with bone marrow involvement by abnormal mast cells who harbor *FIP1L1-PDGFRA* also uniformly achieve complete clinical, histologic, and molecular/cytogenetic responses with low-dose imatinib therapy, in the absence of mutations that confer imatinib resistance (*PDGFRA*T764I), which may be acquired with clonal evolution (reviewed by Pardanani).[164,165,272–274] Lastly, imatinib is predicted to be effective in systemic mastocytosis with specific mutations such as V560G[275] and del419,[140] although clinical proof of this supposition is lacking to date. The remarkable efficacy of imatinib in treating mastocytosis patients harboring specific mutations provides proof-of-principle for development molecularly targeted therapies for this disease, as well as a treatment-relevant molecular classification. It is currently recommended that patients with primary eosinophilia, particularly in the presence of increased bone marrow mast cells or increased serum tryptase level (ie, SM-CEL), be screened for the presence of *FIP1L1-PDGFRA* by either fluorescence in situ hybridization (FISH) or reverse transcriptase–polymerase chain reaction (RT-PCR). Imatinib mesylate, generally at the 100 mg daily dose level, is considered to be first-line therapy for this group of patients.[276–278] Initiation of imatinib therapy in patients with clonal eosinophilia harboring *FIP1L1-PDGFRA* can rarely lead to cardiogenic shock resulting from rapid onset of eosinophil lysis/degranulation in the endomyocardium.[279,280] Consequently, consideration may be given to starting imatinib concurrently with corticosteroids, particularly in the presence of either an abnormal echocardiogram or an elevated serum troponin level prior to treatment. In contrast to *FIP1L1-PDGFRA*, early data suggest that imatinib is not therapeutically beneficial for patients carrying Kit D816V, who make up the majority of systemic mastocytosis patients.[164,165,271,281] This mutation maps to the Kit enzymatic site and disrupts the imatinib-binding site.[282] For patients harboring D816V or those without detectable imatinib-sensitive mutations, IFN-α may represent an attractive initial treatment option. Although a modest clinical benefit may be observed with imatinib at 400 mg daily in some patients without either Kit D816V or *FIP1L1-PDGFRA*,[281] the use of imatinib in this setting is considered investigational.

FUTURE DIRECTIONS

The approach to a patient with systemic mastocytosis continues to be challenging, with many unanswered questions relating to aspects of (a) diagnosis, (b) pathogenesis, (c) clinical presentation, and (d) treatment of this heterogeneous disorder.

- At the diagnostic interface, a uniform approach to molecular testing is lacking at present; consensus is needed regarding the specific molecular assay(s) as well as biological material(s) that are considered optimal for mutation analysis in mastocytosis patients.
- At present, it is unclear why some mastocytosis patients develop a concurrent non-mast cell hematologic neoplasm (eg, CMML)—do these emerge from the same clone? Are there specific mutations that cooperate with Kit D816V in this regard?
- Questions pertaining to the diverse clinical presentation of mastocytosis patients also remain largely unanswered—for instance, are specific symptoms related to particular mast cell mediators? What determines whether skin rash versus bone disease (or other feature) will be the dominant clinical presentation for a given patient?
- Finally, there is an urgent need for studies of small molecule inhibitors/other novel therapies targeting Kit D816 in mastocytosis patients; given the relative rarity of mastocytosis, this will most effectively be accomplished in the setting of cooperative, multiinstitutional clinical trials.

SUGGESTED READINGS

Akin C: Molecular diagnosis of mast cell disorders: A paper from the 2005 William Beaumont Hospital Symposium on Molecular Pathology. J Mol Diagn 8(4):412, 2006.

Bischoff SC: Role of mast cells in allergic and non-allergic immune responses: Comparison of human and murine data. Nat Rev Immunol 7(2):93, 2007.

Escribano L, Garcia Montero AC, Nunez R, et al: Flow cytometric analysis of normal and neoplastic mast cells: Role in diagnosis and follow-up of mast cell disease. Immunol Allergy Clin North Am 26(3):535, 2006.

Garcia-Montero AC, Jara-Acevedo M, Teodosio C, et al: KIT mutation in mast cells and other bone marrow haematopoietic cell lineages in systemic mast cell disorders. A prospective study of the Spanish Network on Mastocytosis (REMA) in a series of 113 patients. Blood 108(7):2366–72, 2006.

Gleixner KV, Mayerhofer M, Aichberger KJ, et al: PKC412 inhibits in vitro growth of neoplastic human mast cells expressing the D816V-mutated variant of KIT: Comparison with AMN107, imatinib, and cladribine (2CdA) and evaluation of cooperative drug effects. Blood 107(2):752, 2006.

Gotlib J, George TI, Linder A, et al: Phase II trial of the tyrosine kinase inhibitor PKC412 in advanced systemic mastocytosis: Preliminary results. Blood (ASH Annual Meeting Abstracts) 108:Abstract 3609, 2006.

Grimbaldeston MA, Metz M, Yu M, et al: Effector and potential immunoregulatory roles of mast cells in IgE-associated acquired immune responses. Curr Opin Immunol 18(6):751, 2006.

Jovanovic JV, Score J, Waghorn K, et al: Low-dose imatinib mesylate leads to rapid induction of major molecular responses and achievement of complete molecular remission in FIP1L1-PDGFRA positive chronic eosinophilic leukemia. Blood, 2007. doi:10.1182/blood-2006-10-050054.

Pan J, Quintas-Cardama A, Kantarjian HM, et al: EXEL-0862, a novel tyrosine kinase inhibitor, induces apoptosis in vitro and ex vivo in human mast cells expressing the KIT D816V mutation. Blood 109(1):315, 2007.

Pardanani A, Ketterling RP, Li CY, et al: FIP1L1-PDGFRA in eosinophilic disorders: Prevalence in routine clinical practice, long-term experience with imatinib therapy, and a critical review of the literature. Leuk Res 30(8):965, 2006.

Robyn J, Lemery S, McCoy JP, et al: Multilineage involvement of the fusion gene in patients with FIP1L1/PDGFRA-positive hypereosinophilic syndrome. Br J Haematol 132(3):286, 2006.

Schittenhelm MM, Shiraga S, Schroeder A, et al: Dasatinib (BMS-354825), a dual SRC/ABL kinase inhibitor, inhibits the kinase activity of wild-type, juxtamembrane, and activation loop mutant KIT isoforms associated with human malignancies. Cancer Res 66(1):473, 2006.

Schwartz LB: Diagnostic value of tryptase in anaphylaxis and mastocytosis. Immunol Allergy Clin North Am 26(3):451, 2006.

Sellge G, Bischoff SC: Isolation, culture, and characterization of intestinal mast cells. Methods Mol Biol 315:123, 2006.

Shah NP, Lee FY, Luo R, et al: Dasatinib (BMS-354825) inhibits KITD816V, an imatinib-resistant activating mutation that triggers neoplastic growth in the majority of patients with systemic mastocytosis. Blood 108(1):286–91, 2006.

Tokarski JS, Newitt JA, Chang CY, et al: The structure of dasatinib (BMS-354825) bound to activated ABL kinase domain elucidates its inhibitory activity against imatinib-resistant ABL mutants. Cancer Res 66(11):5790, 2006.

Valent P: Diagnostic evaluation and classification of mastocytosis. Immunol Allergy Clin North Am 26(3):515, 2006.

Valent P, Akin C, Metcalfe DD: FIP1L1/PDGFRA is a molecular marker of chronic eosinophilic leukaemia but not for systemic mastocytosis. Eur J Clin Invest 37(2):153, 2007.

Verstovsek S, Kantarjian H, Cortes J, et al: Dasatinib (Sprycel) therapy for patients with systemic mastocytosis. Blood (ASH Annual Meeting Abstracts) 108:Abstract 3627, 2006.

Verstovsek S, Akin C, Manshouri T, et al: Effects of AMN107, a novel aminopyrimidine tyrosine kinase inhibitor, on human mast cells bearing wild-type or mutated codon 816 c-kit. Leuk Res 30(11):1365, 2006.

Zhang LY, Smith ML, Schultheis B, et al: A novel K509I mutation of KIT identified in familial mastocytosis-in vitro and in vivo responsiveness to imatinib therapy. Leuk Res 30(4):373, 2006.

REFERENCES

For complete list of references log onto www.expertconsult.com

CHAPTER 74

MYELODYSPLASTIC AND MYELOPROLIFERATIVE SYNDROMES IN CHILDREN

Franklin O. Smith and Mignon L. Loh

INTRODUCTION

The myelodysplastic (MDS) and myeloproliferative syndromes (MPS) are a heterogeneous group of clonal stem cell disorders that result in ineffective hematopoiesis and an increased risk of developing acute myeloid leukemia (AML). In MDS, ineffective hematopoiesis results in progressive cytopenias whereas, in MPS, at least initially, ineffective hematopoiesis leads to excessive proliferation characterized by increased peripheral blood counts. MDS and MPS are rare in children, with the vast majority of cases diagnosed in older adults. Chronic myelogenous leukemia (CML), characterized by the Philadelphia chromosome (*bcr/abl*-positive) is seen in both children and adults, whereas other forms of MPS (polycythemia vera [PV], essential thrombocythemia [ET], primary myelofibrosis [PMF], chronic neutrophilic leukemia [CNL], chronic eosinophilic leukemia [CEL], chronic basophilic leukemia [CBL], chronic myelomonocytic leukemia [CMML], systemic mastocytosis [SM], and stem cell leukemia-lymphoma syndrome [SCLL]) are exceedingly rare in children. Readers interested in CML and disorders that are predominantly found in adults are referred to in chapters 67, 69, and 70. In contrast, two of these MPS disorders are uniquely pediatric: juvenile myelomonocytic leukemia (JMML) and Down syndrome-associated transient myeloproliferative disorder (TMD).

MYELODYSPLASTIC SYNDROMES

The myelodysplastic syndromes are a heterogeneous group of disorders characterized by ineffective hematopoiesis, impaired maturation of hematopoietic cells, progressive cytopenias, and dysplastic changes in the bone marrow.

Epidemiology

MDS is a common malignancy of adults with an incidence of 50 cases per million in people over the age of 60 years.[1] In contrast, MDS accounts for only 3% to 7% of all hematologic malignancies in children, with an unknown true incidence. Several population-based studies have been performed with reported incidences of 4.0 cases per million in Denmark,[2] 3.1 per million in British Columbia,[3] and 1.35 per million in the United Kingdom.[4] The median age of presentation is 6.8 years with an equal sex distribution.[4–6]

Pathobiology

As in adults, MDS in children can be considered as de novo or secondary. In adults, two predominant patterns of primary, de novo MDSs have been observed. In the first of these patterns, the disease is indolent in nature, is characterized by prolonged survival, little accumulated genetic damage, and a low probability of progression to AML. This group of diseases is best exemplified by the 5q− syndrome, an entity not seen in children. Far more common in adults is a disease characterized by the accumulation of genetic damage, progression to marrow failure, and a high probability of developing AML. This form of the disease is characterized as a mutator phenotype.[7] The primary myelodysplastic syndromes seen in children appear to share this mutator phenotype.

As in adults, secondary MDS in children can also arise as sequelae from exposure to chemotherapy and radiation; however MDS in children may also result from constitutional marrow failure syndromes including Fanconi anemia, congenital neutropenia (Kostmann syndrome), Shwachman syndrome, and Diamond–Blackfan anemia.

Ongoing studies are now defining the molecular pathogenesis and interrelationship between MDS, MPS, and AML.[8–10] Accumulating data suggest that aberrant signal transduction resulting from acquired somatic mutations encoding proteins leading to hyperactivation of the Ras pathway may stimulate proliferation without concomitant differentiation.[9] This has been clearly demonstrated in CML (BCR-ABL).[11,12] A number of other putative pathogenetic mutations have been identified in other myeloproliferative disorders, including *JAK*2V617F in PV, ET, and PMF[13]; *KIT*D816V in SM[14]; *FIPL1-PDGFRA* in CEL-SM[15]; *ZNF198-FGFR1* in SCLL[16]; *RAS/NF1/PTPN11* mutations in JMML[17–19]; and *GATA1* mutations in TMD (Fig. 74–1).[20]

AML is the result of cooperating mutations in genes that confer a proliferative and survival advantage without effecting differentiation (eg, activating mutations in receptor tyrosine kinases [FLT3, c-kit]) and genes that impair differentiation and apoptosis (eg, loss of function mutations in transcription factors [CBF, AML/ETO]) (Fig. 74–2). This multistep model for the pathogenesis of AML is supported by murine models,[21,22] the analysis of leukemia in twins,[23–26] and the analysis of patients with familial platelet disorder with a propensity to develop AML (FDP/AML syndrome).[27]

Classification

Until recently, MDS in children has been poorly defined, characterized, classified, and reported. In fact, MDS was not included in the International Classification of Childhood Cancer until 2005.[28] Also contributing to this lack of information was the use of classification and prognostic systems designed for adults that have had limited applicability to children. A number of classification systems for children and adults have now been proposed. The most commonly used system is the French–American–British (FAB) system originally proposed in 1982.[29] This classification system recognized five forms of MDS in adults: refractory anemia (RA), refractory anemia with ringed sideroblasts (RARS), refractory anemia with excess of blasts (RAEB), refractory anemia with excess of blasts in transformation (RAEB-T) and chronic myelomonocytic leukemia (CMML). Using this system, RAEB, and RAEB-T were commonly reported in children, whereas RA and RARS were thought to be rare in children. However, a recent population-based study in the United Kingdom showed 25% of childhood MDS cases to be RA or RARS[4] suggesting inaccurate diagnosis, or reporting of these subtypes in other pediatric studies. CMML has only rarely been reported in children.

Additional subtypes of MDS are now recognized that do not fit well into the FAB system, including hypoplastic MDS, therapy-related MDS, refractory cytopenias with trilineage dysplasia, MDS associated with myelofibrosis, and MDS associated with inherited disorders (congenital neutropenias, Shwachman syndrome, Fanconi

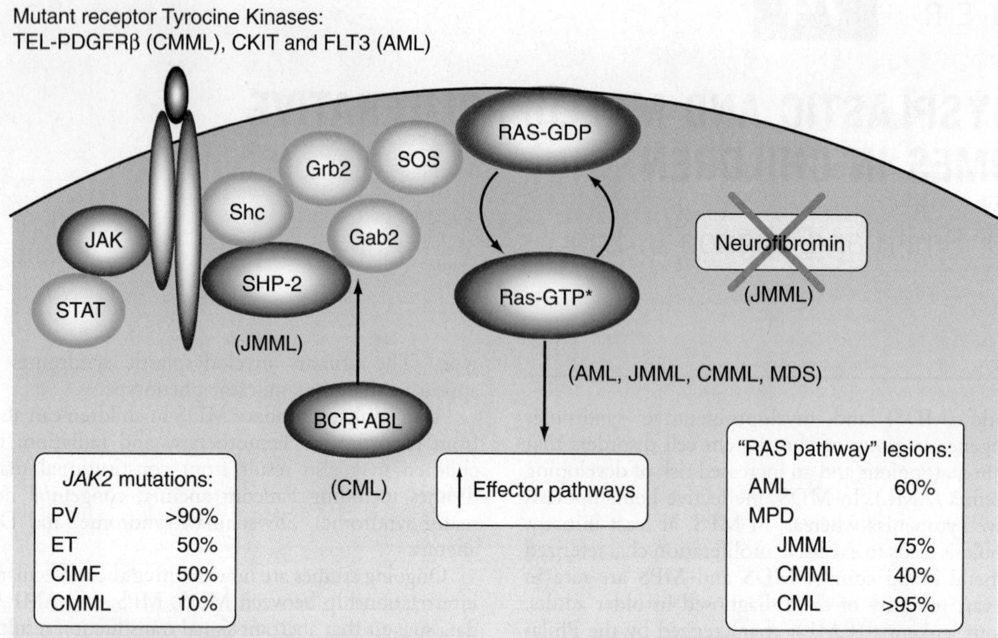

Figure 74–1 Overview of Ras signaling with molecules harboring mutations in patients with myeloid malignancies. AML, acute myeloid leukemia; CML, chronic myelogenous leukemia; CMML, chronic myelomonocytic leukemia; GDP, guanosine diphosphate; GTP, guanosine triphosphate; JMML, juvenile myelomonocytic leukemia; MPD, myeloproliferative disorder.

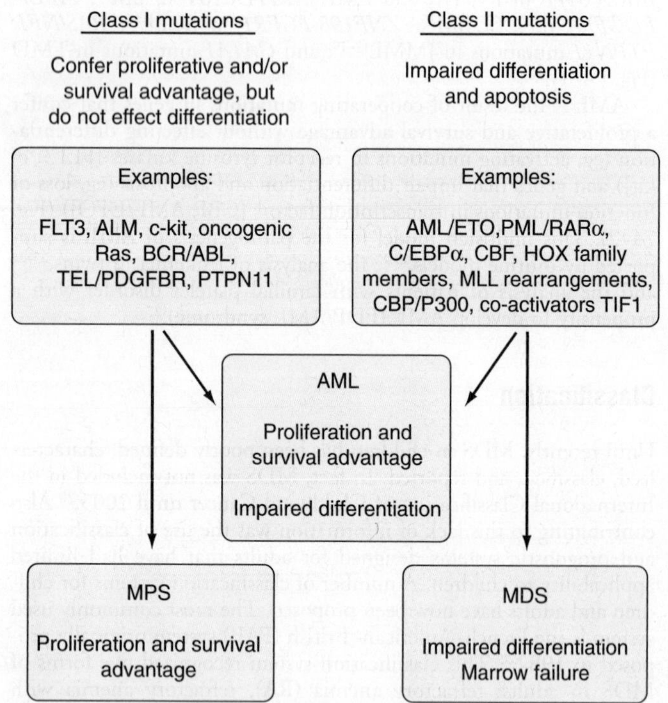

Figure 74–2 Cooperating mutations in AML, MPS, and MDS.

Table 74–1 Proposed Pediatric Myelodysplastic Syndrome Classification

I. Combined Myeloproliferative/Myelodysplastic Diseases
Juvenile myelomonocytic leukemia
Chronic myelomonocytic leukemia
BCR/ABC negative chronic myeloid leukemia
II. Down syndrome Disease
Transient myeloproliferative disease
Myelodysplasia syndrome/acute myeloid leukemia
III. Myelodysplastic syndrome
Refractory cytopenias with multilineage dysplasia (RCMD)
RCMD-EB

anemia), Down syndrome, and neurofibromatosis type 1, and mitochondrial cytopathies.[30,31] Therefore, the World Health Organization (WHO) recently proposed changes to the FAB criteria to account for many of these subtypes.[32] Other significant changes included elimination of the RAEB-T subtype with reclassification of MDS with greater than 20% blasts as AML and reassignment of CMML and JMML to a new category of MDS/MPS.

Despite these improvements to the FAB system found in the WHO classification, there are still a number of limitations for children. Therefore, several pediatric-based classification systems for MDS and MPS have been proposed. Among these is a system to parallel the WHO classification (Table 74–1).[33] In this system, there are three major subtypes. The first category includes myeloproliferative disorders of childhood, including JMML, CMML, and Ph–CML. The second category includes patients with Down syndrome with associated TMD or myeloid leukemia. The third category focuses specifically on MDS and consists of refractory cytopenias (RC) (defined as <5% marrow blasts and <2% peripheral blasts), RAEB with 5% to 19% marrow blasts and 2% to 19% peripheral blasts and RAEB-T, defined as 20% to 29% peripheral blood or bone marrow blasts.

A second system based on category, cytology, and cytogenetics (CCC) allows for classification of individual patients into a very large number of categories.[34] The clinical utility of this system is unclear. However, a recent comparison of these two pediatric systems with the adult WHO and FAB systems suggested that both were superior for children than the corresponding adult classification system.[35]

Taken together, it may be useful to think about childhood MDS as primary or secondary, with secondary MDS arising either from a known congenital bone marrow failure syndrome or prior acquired aplastic anemia, or as a complication from prior chemotherapy or radiation therapy. A diagnosis of primary MDS would then apply to all other cases.

Clinical Manifestations

Signs and symptoms of MDS are nonspecific and are usually attributable to pancytopenia (fever, infections, pallor, fatigue, bruising, and petechiae). Lymphadenopathy, hepatomegaly, and splenomegaly are uncommon presenting signs in children with MDS.

Laboratory Manifestations

Commonly accepted minimal diagnostic criteria for pediatric MDS would include the absence of common de novo AML karyotypic abnormalities and at least two of the following: (a) sustained, unexplained anemia; neutropenia or thrombocytopenia; dysplastic morphology in the erythroid; granulocytic or megakaryocytic lineages (at least bilineage); (b) an acquired, sustained clonal cytogenetic abnormality and 5% or more blasts in the marrow.[7,33] Almost half of all children with MDS in a series reported by Kardos et al presented with refractory cytopenia, most notably neutropenia and thrombocytopenia.[36]

Morphologically, the bone marrow may be hypocellular, normocellular, or hypercellular. A diagnosis of MDS is made based on the presence of dysplastic changes in at least two cell lineages. The dysplastic changes in the granulocytes (hypogranulation, nuclear hyposegmentation, megaloblastoid maturation, and a left shift with an increased number of myeloblasts), megakaryocytes (micromegakaryocytes, abnormal megakaryocyte nuclei), monocytes (increase in marrow monocytes, abnormal granulation with persistence of azurophilic granules, hemophagocytosis, abnormal nuclei, and giant forms), and/or erythroid lineages (megaloblastoid maturation, nuclear budding and multinucleated forms, and ringed sideroblasts) can be multiple and varied. Similar dysplastic changes can occur in the peripheral blood for each of these lineages. Although dysplastic changes in the marrow are a common feature of MDS, it is important to remember that dysplasia, unto itself, is not diagnostic of MDS because dysplastic features are associated with other conditions and can be found in normal marrow donors.[37]

Although flow cytometric analysis can serve to quantitate the number of blasts based on aberrant cell surface antigen expression and detect populations of PNH-like CD91^{+} cells,[38] flow cytometric findings analysis is not generally diagnostic of MDS.

Cytogenetic abnormalities are seen in approximately half of children diagnosed with de novo MDS. Karyotypic abnormalities most commonly seen are −7, 7q−, and +8. Abnormalities in chromosomes 6, 9, 11, 12, and 13 are rare in children. Specific abnormalities seen in adults, including −5, 5q−, and −Y are very rarely seen in children. Finally, chromosome abnormalities commonly found in de novo AML including t(8;21), t(15;17) t(9;11), t(16;16), t(11;19), t(11;17), t(8;16), and inv[16] are not commonly seen in MDS.

Differential Diagnosis

Although the history, physical examination, evaluation of the bone marrow and peripheral blood, and cytogenetic analysis will often make the diagnosis of MDS, other diseases should be considered. Congenital disorders such as Down syndrome, Fanconi anemia, Shwachman syndrome, Diamond–Blackfan anemia, congenital dyserythropoietic anemias, and hereditary sideroblastic anemia should be considered. Hypoplastic MDS can be difficult to distinguish from severe aplastic anemia and may require prospective monitoring and serial bone marrow examinations. The differential should also include AML with a low blast count, mitochondrial cytopathies such as Pearson syndrome, and myeloproliferative disorders. Specifically, PNH, while rare in children, should be considered. Deficiencies of vitamin B_{12} and folate can cause megaloblastic changes that resemble the dysplastic changes seen in MDS. Other nutritional deficiencies, including iron, thiamine, riboflavin, and pyridoxine should be considered. Infections due to human immunodeficiency virus, parvovirus, Epstein–Barr virus, cytomegalovirus, and human herpes virus 6 can cause changes that resemble MDS. Finally, the differential should include toxins (insecticides, chemotherapy agents, and arsenic) as well as cytokine exposure and radiation. In cases where the diagnosis is unclear, serial bone marrow examinations may serve as a useful aid.

Therapy

Although MDS is a heterogeneous, clonal disease of hematopoietic stem cells that can manifest different clinical courses, it is not readily curable by conventional chemotherapy and requires allogeneic hematopoietic stem cell transplantation (SCT) for cure in most cases. Some children with RA and refractory cytopenias with multilineage dysplasia (RCMD) who do not have life-threatening neutropenia and who do not require transfusions may only require close observation (see Red Box). Although children with this disease may eventually develop progressive disease requiring SCT, they may have long periods when minimal treatment is required.[36] The use of AML-like chemotherapy for patients with refractory cytopenias with multilineage dysplasia with excess blasts (RCMD-EB) is controversial but may serve to "de-bulk" patients with a high percentage of blasts prior to SCT.[6,39,40] However, this potential benefit may be offset by toxicities associated with AML-like chemotherapy. Finally, patients with RAEB-T, which is now defined as AML, or t-MDS, should be treated like AML.

A multitude of agents have been studied for the treatment of MDS in adults, but only rarely in children. These include low-dose chemotherapy (cytosine arabinoside, melphalan, hydroxyurea, etoposide, topotecan, 6-mercaptopurine, and busulfan), hormones (glucocorticoids and androgens), differentiating agents (13-*cis*-retinoic acid, all-*trans* retinoic acid), hematopoietic growth factors (granulocyte-macrophage colony-forming factor [GM-CSF], granulocyte colony-forming factor [G-CSF] and erythropoietin), demethylating agents (decitabine, 5-azacytidine), proteosome inhibitors, antiangiogenic agents, amifostine, and arsenic.[41–61] Although the potential to better control MDS in adults with azacitidine, decitabine, and arsenic is exciting, there is currently no safety or efficacy data to support the use of these agents in children with MDS.

Most children with MDS will require allogeneic SCT for curative therapy. Although children have been included in published SCT studies for MDS that are largely focused on adult patients, there are

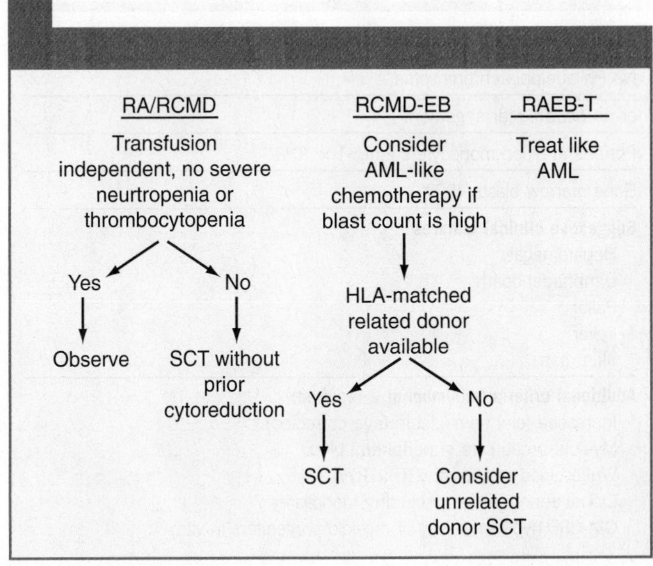

several studies focusing specifically on children.[62–65] Taken together, these studies suggest a probability of disease-free survival in about 50% of patients undergoing HLA-matched related donor SCT.

Prognosis

Although a number of methods have been developed to predict the outcome of adults with MDS, the system now most commonly used in adults is the International Prognostic Scoring System.[66] This system uses percentage marrow blasts, karyotype, and number of cytopenias to assign a score that is then used to predict outcome. Although it is an effective tool for adults, its value for children is very limited.[67]

Secondary Myelodysplastic Syndrome

Secondary MDS can develop in both children and adults after exposure to chemotherapy and radiation. Alkylating agents used to treat Hodgkin disease, non-Hodgkin lymphoma and Ewing sarcoma are particularly concerning in children.[68–80] Interestingly, there is also evidence to suggest that the cardioprotectant, dexrazoxane, a topoisomerase II inhibitor with a mechanism of action that is different from etoposide and doxorubicin, may have increased the incidence of secondary MDS and AML in children treated for Hodgkin disease.[81]

Treatment options for children with secondary MDS are limited. Although AML-like chemotherapy can induce a period of remission and reduction in marrow blasts, it is not curative. Allogeneic SCT has curative potential, but outcomes remain poor, with only 20% to 30% of children surviving.[79,82,83]

MYELOPROLIFERATIVE SYNDROMES

Juvenile Myelomonocytic Leukemia

Juvenile myelomonocytic leukemia (JMML) is a uniquely pediatric clonal disorder of the hematopoietic stem cell. It is among the most common form of MPS in childhood. There is now international agreement on the diagnostic criteria[84] (Table 74–2) with recent progress toward defining common response criteria.

Table 74–2 Diagnostic criteria for juvenile myelomonocytic leukemia[84]

Required laboratory criteria (all three required)
No Philadelphia chromosome
or no *bcr/abl* rearrangement
Peripheral blood monocyte count >1 × 10⁹/L
Bone marrow blasts <20%
Suggestive clinical features
Hepatomegaly
Lymphadenopathy
Pallor
Fever
Skin rash
Additional criteria (minimum of 2 required)
Increased fetal hemoglobin (age corrected)
Myeloid precursors in peripheral blood
White blood cell count >10 × 10⁹/L
Clonal abnormalities, including monosomy 7
GM-CSF hypersensitivity of myeloid progenitors in vitro

Epidemiology

The incidence of JMML has been estimated as 0.69 to 0.9 per million,[4,85] although its true incidence is currently not known. There is a male predominance with a median age of diagnosis of 1.8 years.

Pathobiology

Early clonality studies suggested that JMML arose at the level of at least an immature myeloid precursor cell.[84,86–90] More recent data suggest that JMML may arise in a pluripotent stem cell with involvement of the myeloid, erythroid, and megakaryocyte lineages as well as B lymphocytes and T lymphocytes.[84,91–93]

Several potential causative mutations in JMML cells have been identified, including loss of heterozygosity of *NF1*,[94] activating *RAS* mutations,[95–97] and mutations in the *PTPN11* gene (Fig. 74–1).[17,98] The identification of potential molecular mechanisms involved in the pathogenesis of JMML has been facilitated by two human diseases (neurofibromatosis type 1 (*NF1*) and Noonan syndrome [*PTPN11*]). Approximately 10% to 15% of patients with JMML have clinically evident neurofibromatosis type I,[84,94,99–101] and children with NF1 have a 500-fold increase in clonal malignant myeloid diseases, including JMML. The observation that individuals with NF1 are predisposed to JMML, the high incidence of *RAS* mutations in human cancers, and the identification of neurofibromin as a negative regulator that functions as a GTPase-activating protein that inactivates *Ras* from its active GTP-bound state[84,102–104] led to the hypothesis that *NF1* might function as a tumor suppressor gene in myeloid malignancies. Indeed, the demonstration of loss of heterozygosity of the wild-type *NF1* allele in the leukemic cells from children with NF and JMML supported this hypothesis. Subsequent studies clearly demonstrating homozygous inactivation of the NF1 allele (one allele with LOH, the other allele rendered nonfunctional by a constitutionally inherited mutation) in the leukemic cells from these children as well as demonstration of the accumulation of activated Ras proteins in these cells provided formal proof that NF1 functions as a tumor suppressor gene.[18,101,105,106] Finally, accurate murine models of JMML have been engineered by several groups in which either the *NF1* gene has been homozygously deleted or a *Kras(G12D)* allele has been conditionally activated.[96,97,107,108]

Abnormalities in *NF1* are also detectable in an additional small percentage of JMML patients who do not have clinical manifestations of neurofibromatosis.[84,105] Point mutations with a loss of *NF1* tumor suppressor function is demonstrated in approximately 15% of patients with JMML. This finding is mutually exclusive of *RAS* mutations that occur in another 25% of patients, suggesting that both *NF1* and *RAS* mutations are sufficient to initiate JMML.[84,95,105,109,110] The *RAS* family of proteins are of significance in JMML in that they are involved in signaling pathways for GM-CSF.[84,92,111,112] This deregulation in signaling results in GM-CSF hypersensitivity in in vitro dose–response assays.[113] However, JMML cells do not show selective hypersensitivity to G-CSF or IL-3 despite similar signaling components to those of GM-CSF.[113] Therefore, *NF1* may act as a tumor suppressor gene in immature hematopoietic cells by negatively regulating *Ras*.[84,94,101]

In 2001, Tartaglia et al reported that constitutional mutations in PTPN11 were causative of 50% of cases of Noonan Syndrome (NS).[114] NS is a common congenital disorder, with both acquired and sporadic forms. Patients affected by NS have cardiac defects (pulmonic stenosis of hypertrophic cardiomyopathy), variable levels of developmental delay, skeletal defects, and bleeding diatheses. Some children develop a JMML-like MPS in infancy that generally spontaneously recovers, although rare patients progress to frank JMML. Based on the knowledge that *PTPN11* encodes SHP-2, a nonreceptor protein tyrosine phosphatase that relays signals from activated growth factors to Ras, it was logical to hypothesize that somatic mutations in *PTPN11* might exist in the remaining cases of de novo JMML patients who did not have either clinical NF1 or harbor a RAS mutation. Indeed, 35% of patients with JMML were discovered to have mutations in *PTPN11*, in residues that altered the interaction between the N-SH2 and C-SH2 domains, leading to constitutive activity of the phosphatase.[17,98]

Taken together, these data suggest that deregulated Ras/MAPK signaling is a common feature of JMML. The genetic spectrum of *NF1*, *PTPN1,1* and *RAS* (most commonly *N-RAS* and *K-RAS*) mutations in JMML appear to be largely mutually exclusive,[84,105,109] again supporting the hypothesis that these lesions are functionally redundant and that their common biochemical output is hyperactivation of the Ras/MAP kinase pathway.

The molecular abnormalities occurring in the remaining 25% of patients have yet to be determined, but the evidence is overwhelming that the functional consequence of the as yet unidentified lesion will result in hyperactivation of the Ras/MAPK pathway.

Clinical Manifestations

Children with JMML present with signs and symptoms attributable to a heavy cell burden of organ-infiltrating cells that results in hepatosplenomegaly, lymphadenopathy, and skin rash. As a result of its association with neurofibromatosis, patients may also have café-au-lait spots. Death is usually the result of organ dysfunction due to infiltrating cells, infection, or bleeding. Approximately 10% to 20% of children will progress to a blast-like phase consistent with AML.

Laboratory Manifestations

Laboratory abnormalities may include an elevated white blood cell count with an absolute monocytosis, anemia, and thrombocytopenia (see Fig. 74–3). Monocytes, either circulating in the peripheral blood or in the bone marrow frequently appear dysplastic. The peripheral smear often shows leukoerythroblastic changes and there are often circulating nucleated red blood cells. Fifty percent of patients may also present with elevated fetal hemoglobin levels and hypergammaglobulinemia. International criteria mandate that the bone marrow has fewer than 20% blast cells at diagnosis. Other findings typical in the bone marrow include micro-megakaryocytes.

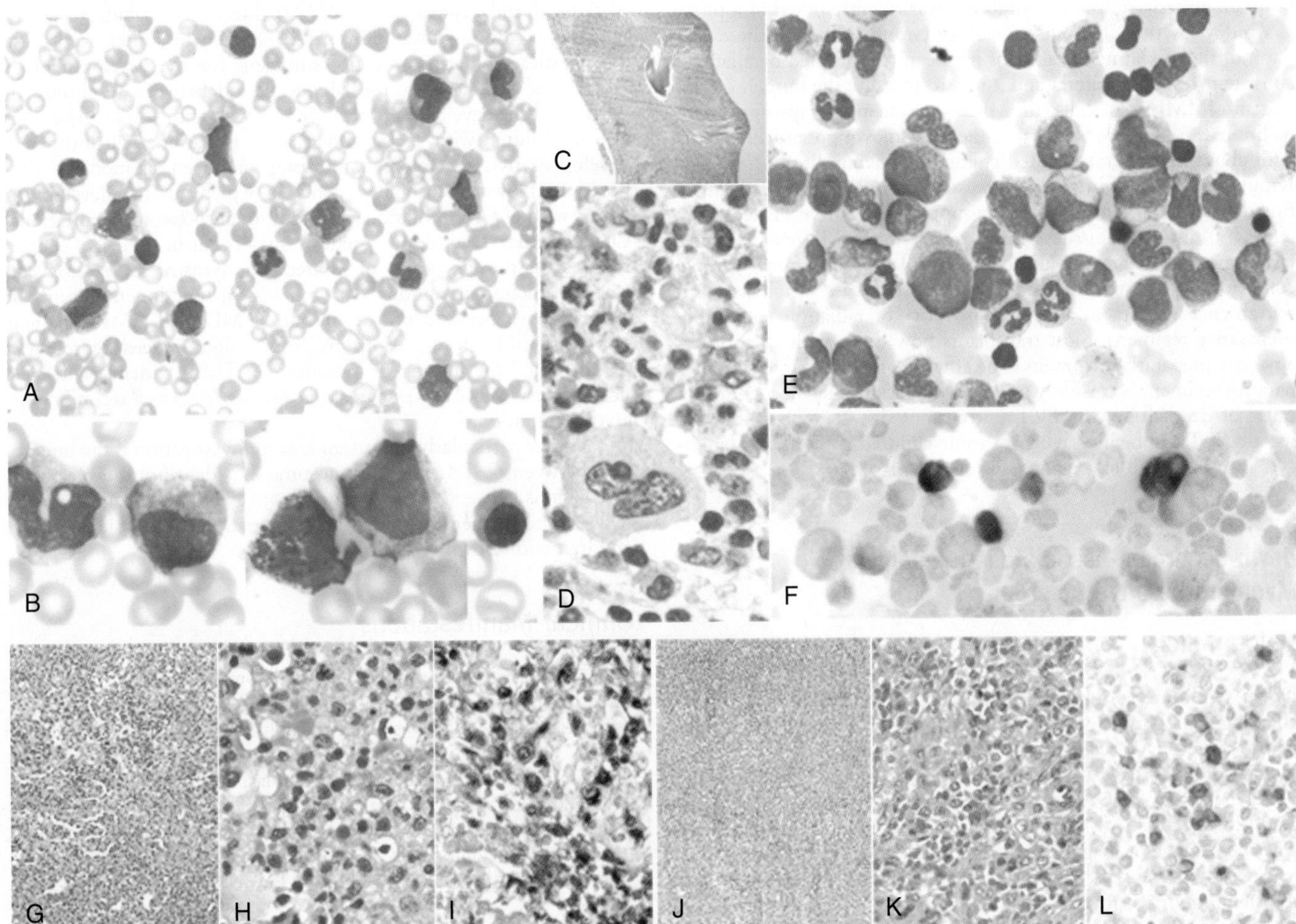

Figure 74–3 Juvenile myelomonocytic leukemia: Blood, bone marrow, lung, and spleen (**A–L**). The illustrations are from the case of a 3-year-old boy who was diagnosed with neurofibromatosis at birth. At 1 year of age, he presented with leukocytosis (58 K/μL) and splenomegaly. The peripheral blood (**A, B**) showed left-shifted granulocytes and increased monocytes (16%). A bone marrow biopsy (**C, D**) was hypercellular as a result of increased granulocytic and monocytic cells that could also be appreciated on the aspirate (**E**). Blasts accounted for only 4% of the marrow elements. A combined esterase reaction (**F**) illustrated the increased monocytes (alpha naphthol butyrate esterase reaction-positive; orange/brown) in the background of granulocytes (chloroacetate esterase reaction-positive; blue). Cytogenetic analysis revealed monosomy 7. At age 2, he presented with respiratory distress and a lung biopsy (**G, H**) demonstrated a monocyte infiltrate (lysozyme stain, **I**) consistent with involvement by JMML. This is not uncommon in such patients. At age 3, his blast count began to rise, and he underwent a splenectomy (**J, K**; lysozyme stain, **L**) followed by a successful stem cell transplant.

Differential Diagnosis

Making a diagnosis of JMML is not always easy, as its clinical and laboratory presenting features can also be associated with other disorders, including other forms of MPS, infections (Epstein–Barr virus, cytomegalovirus, human herpes 6 virus, histoplasmosis, mycobacterium, and toxoplasmosis), Class I Langerhans cell histiocytosis, hemophagocytic lymphohistiocytosis (HLH), Fanconi anemia, Kostmann syndrome, Shwachman syndrome, and Down syndrome.

Therapy

Children with JMML can have a variable course, with rare patients having a spontaneous remission and long-term survival without treatment whereas others have a rapidly fatal course despite aggressive treatment.[115,116] Age, platelet count, and hemoglobin F level have been used to predict the clinical course of patients not undergoing SCT,[100] but biologic features that can reliably predict an individual patient's clinical courses are not currently known. Currently, the most adverse prognostic factor for outcome is age at diagnosis.[117]

A wide variety of agents have been used to treat children with JMML, including AML-like chemotherapy,[40,100,118–122] low-dose chemotherapy,[123,124] interferon-alpha,[125] and 13-*cis*-retinoic acid.[103] Tipifarnib, a farnesyl transferase inhibitor, was recently tested in a phase II window by the Children's Oncology Group. Although the evaluation of these treatment regimens has been complicated by a lack of consistent response criteria and assays to measure the burden of clonogenic JMML stem cells, the efficacy of chemotherapy appears to be limited. Allogeneic SCT offers the only known potential for cure, with about half of transplanted children surviving disease-free.[117,126] Rapid withdrawal of immunosuppression appears to be important in this disease, as mounting evidence supports a graft-versus-leukemia effect.[127] A number of issues related to SCT for JMML remain uncertain. Among these are the value of pretransplant splenectomy, optimal conditioning regimen and graft-versus-host disease prophylaxis. In the absence of data to suggest superiority of radiation containing preparative regimens, most transplants now occur with chemotherapy-only preparative regimens. The efficacy of reduced intensity preparative regimens is currently under investigation. The most common cause of death following SCT is recurrent disease. The efficacy of second SCT can be life-saving for some children.[128,129] Donor leukocyte infusions (DLIs) are not often successful.[130]

Down Syndrome-Associated Transient Myeloproliferative Disorder

Epidemiology

Down syndrome is one of the most common congenital disorders, affecting approximately 1 in every 800 to 1000 live births. It has been demonstrated in a recent population-based study that children with Down syndrome have a 10- to 20-fold overall increased risk of developing leukemia,[131] a 150-fold increased risk of developing AML, and a 500-fold increased risk of acute megakaryocytic leukemia (AMKL). The median age of diagnosis of AMKL in Down syndrome patients is 2 years.[132] Transient myeloproliferative disorder, also known as transient abnormal myelopoiesis and transient leukemia, is thought to occur in at least 10% of children with Down syndrome, although it has been suggested that when cases of TMD that develop and resolve in utero or result in death prior to delivery are taken into account, the incidence may be as high as 20%.[133] Currently it is estimated that approximately 20% to 30% of children with TMD will subsequently develop AMKL, usually by 3 years of age. The probability of progression to leukemia will be further defined in a recently completed Children's Oncology Group study that prospectively follows a cohort of children with TMD.

Pathobiology

The molecular pathogenesis of TMD and AMKL in children with Down syndrome is now providing valuable insights into myeloid leukemogenesis.[20] Recent studies have shown that virtually all patients with TMD and most patients with AMKL harbor mutations in the hematopoietic transcription factor *GATA1*.[134–138] *GATA1* is a double zinc finger DNA-binding transcription factor expressed primarily in hematopoietic cells. It is required for the development of red blood cells, megakaryocytes, mast cells, and eosinophils. A number of different mutations in *GATA1* have been identified, including insertions, deletions, missense mutations, nonsense mutations, and slice site mutations. All of these mutations lead to a block in the expression of the full-length 50-kd isoform of *GATA1* but allow for the expression of a smaller, 40-kd isoform (*GATA1s*).[139] This smaller isoform lacks the N-terminal transactivation domain but retains both zinc fingers involved in DNA binding as well as interactions with its cofactor, Friend of *GATA1* (FOG1).[134] Recent studies have shown that mutations that alter *GATA1–FOG1* binding in the N-terminal zinc finger or result in the expression of the *GATA1s* isoform uncouple megakaryocyte growth and differentiation.[140–142] Similar studies in cell lines derived from Down syndrome children with AMKL have demonstrated that expression of *GATA1* led to erythroid differentiation whereas expression of *GATA1s* did not alter the characteristics of the cell line.[138] Taken together, current data suggests that the loss of *GATA1* and expression of *GATA1s* directly contribute to leukemogenesis. Although mutations in *GATA1* may be sufficient to cause TMD, these mutations are not sufficient for the development of AMKL, as evidenced by the latency period between resolution of TMD and the development of AMKL as well as the observation that not all children with TMD and *GATA1* mutations will ultimately develop AMKL. Therefore, a multistep pathogenesis model is proposed in Down syndrome patients in which AMKL develops in clones with *GATA1* mutations and additional cooperating mutations. One potential "second hit" mutation may occur in the *JAK3* gene, a member of the Jak family of nonreceptor tyrosine kinases. Several gain-of-function mutations[143,144] and loss-of-function mutations in *JAK3*[145] have been identified in both TMD and AMKL patient samples. Although mutations in *JAK3* might indeed represent a "second hit," the finding of mutations in TMD patients who have not progressed to AMKL may argue against *JAK3* as a second cooperating mutation.

Another particularly important area of investigation is the interaction between *GATA1* and chromosome 21. Identification of critical interactions between *GATA1* and relevant genes on chromosome 21 will serve to further inform us about the pathogenesis of leukemia in children with Down syndrome.

Clinical Manifestations

Down syndrome patients typically will present with TMD within three months after birth, although TMD can be manifest at birth. Some of these children present with hydrops fetalis secondary to anemia and cardiac dysfunction. Although some patients may be asymptomatic, others can have myeloblast infiltration of the heart, liver, and spleen that can result in hepatosplenomegaly; hepatic fibrosis; pleural, pericardial, and peritoneal effusions; and disseminated intravascular coagulopathy. In some cases, organ dysfunction can be severe, with failure of the liver, heart, kidneys, and lungs.

Laboratory Manifestations

The complete blood count in infants with TMD typically demonstrates an elevated white blood cell count with myeloblasts present. The percentage of circulating myeloblasts exceeds the percentage of bone marrow myeloblasts. Rarely a neonate without stigmata of Down syndrome will present with similar features—in these cases workup for either Trisomy 21 mosaicism or a *PTPN11* mutation should be pursued. Flow cytometric analysis of the myeloblasts from TMD patients and AMKL associated with Down syndrome show many similarities between these disorders as well as patterns of cell surface antigen expression that is distinct from other types of AML in children.[146] Specifically, all TMD and AMKL blasts express CD45, CD38, and CD33 whereas the majority of cases express CD36 and CD34. CD41 and CD61 also are expressed, consistent with megakaryocyte differentiation. CD14 and CD64 are usually negative. Most cases have aberrant expression of CD7, a T-lineage antigen.

Therapy

The treatment of infants with TMD is generally supportive. Patients without significant organ dysfunction can be followed closely without medical intervention. In infants with significant organ impairment, a number of therapeutic approaches aimed at reducing the burden of myeloblasts are routinely employed, including exchange transfusion, leukophoresis, and chemotherapy. According to reports using cytosine arabinoside in Down syndrome children with AMKL,[147,148] cytosine arabinoside is the chemotherapeutic agent now most commonly used in infants with TMD. The efficacy of very low doses of cytosine arabinoside is being tested in prospective clinical trials. Several additional questions related to the treatment of infants with TMD are also the subject of ongoing clinical trials. Among these is the identification of high-, intermediate-, and low-risk populations with treatment stratified on the basis of risk group and a determination of whether treatment with very low dose cytosine arabinoside will prevent progression of TMD to AMKL and hepatic fibrosis.

Prognosis

Recent data from the Children's Oncology Group reporting the results of the POG 9481 prospective clinical trial offer insights into the natural history of TMD and the identification of prognostic factors.[149] This study followed 48 children with TMD. Eighty-nine percent of infants achieved a spontaneous remission, 74% had a normalization of peripheral blood counts and 64% maintained a clinical remission. Seventeen percent of infants had an early death. Factors associated with early death included a high white blood cell count ($P < 0.001$), increased bilirubin and liver function test values ($P < 0.005$), and a failure to normalize blood counts ($P = 0.001$). Nineteen percent of patients had a progression to AMKL at a median of 20 months. The greatest risk factor for progression to leukemia was the presence of karyotypic abnormalities in addition to trisomy 21 in blasts cells.

OTHER DISORDERS

Essential Thrombocythemia

Essential thrombocythemia has an estimated incidence of 1 to 1.25 cases per million in adults but is rarely diagnosed in children, with an estimated incidence of 0.09 cases per million.[150–154] Recent investigations in children and adults suggests that ET is a heterogeneous disease. Recently, mutations in JAK2 have been reported in patients as well as overexpression of polycythemia rubra vera-1 *(PRV-1) RNA*. It has been proposed that ET consists of several subtypes, with some children and adults having monoclonal disease, whereas in others the disease is polyclonal. Further investigation into the mutational status of V617F*JAK2* also demonstrates mutation-positive and mutation-negative patients.[151,155] Studies suggest that a similar proportion of children and adults display PRV-1 RNA overexpression, V617F*JAK2* mutations, and monoclonal disease.[156]

Patients with ET have thrombocythemia with an increased number of megakaryocytes in the marrow. Platelet clumps on peripheral blood smears are common. Some patients have a concomitant increase in the number of peripheral blood granulocytes. The differential diagnosis includes familial ET (characterized by the dominant-positive activating mutation of *c-mpl*), other forms of MPS, and increased platelets as a reactive process.

Although the clinical course may be uncomplicated, patients can develop thromboembolic complications, including deep-vein thrombosis, transient cerebral ischemia, and peripheral vascular ischemia. The clinical course for children is typically benign, with fewer thrombotic episodes.[156,157] Adult patients have a median survival of at least 10 years, with most deaths due to thrombosis.[158,159] Progression to AML has been reported in adult patients, usually those with a prior exposure to chemotherapy agents.

Asymptomatic children do not require treatment. A number of treatment approaches aimed at controlling thrombocytosis have been attempted for symptomatic patients, including hydroxyurea, interferon-alpha, and anagrelide.[160–162] The successful use of allogeneic bone marrow transplantation has been reported for a small number of adult patients with ET.[163,164] Newer Jak2 inhibitors for those patients harboring *JAK2* mutations are in the early phases of clinical development.

Idiopathic Myelofibrosis

Idiopathic myelofibrosis (IM) is rarely diagnosed in children[165] and should be differentiated from AMKL, metastatic neoplasms, and connective tissue, metabolic, and bone diseases. It is characterized by marrow fibrosis, megakaryocytes with bizarre morphology, splenomegaly, anemia, and extramedullary hematopoiesis. IM is a clonal disorder of unknown pathogenesis but with approximately half of adult patients having mutations in V617F*JAK2*.[166] Recent studies have suggested that angiogenic cytokines produced by megakaryocytes and monocytes and their receptors (platelet-derived growth factor receptors [PDGF-R], vascular endothelial growth factor receptor-2 [VEGF-R2] and fibroblast growth factor [FGF] receptor) may be involved in the pathogenesis of the myelofibrosis.[167]

Numerous treatment approaches have been attempted with variable degrees of success. These include splenectomy, splenic radiation, transfusions, androgens, corticosteroids, hydroxyurea, and interferon-alpha.[168–170] More recently, based on preliminary studies about the potential role of angiogenic cytokines and their receptors, new approaches have been tested, including the tyrosine kinase inhibitor imatinib[171,172] and the antiangiogenic agent thalidomide.[173,174] Finally, allogeneic transplantation has been used successfully, with resolution of marrow fibrosis in donor-engrafted patients.[164,175,176] The survival in children is unknown with a median survival in adults of 4 years.

Polycythemia Vera

Polycythemia vera (PV) has an incidence of 3 cases per 100,000 in adults, but is very rarely seen in children with less than 0.1% of PV patients diagnosed prior to 20 years of age.[177] Polycythemia in children is far more often the result of congenital or acquired causes of an increased red cell mass. These would include primary familial polycythemia (characterized by specific mutations in the thrombopoietic gene (TPO), TPO receptor or erythropoietic receptor gene) and secondary polycythemias due to abnormal hemoglobins, cardiac and pulmonary disease, excessive erythropoietin, and a relative polycythemia that is the result of decreased plasma volume.

Polycythemia vera in children and adults is associated with clonal hematopoiesis,[178] V617F*JAK2* mutations,[156,179–183] overexpression of PVR-1 RNA,[184,185] and endogenous erythroid colony (EEC) growth.[186,187] However, in contrast to adults, children with PV are less likely to have V617F*JAK2* mutations and EEC growth.[156] Thus, although these biomarkers are useful diagnostic tools in adults, thereby necessitating a revision to the World health Organization's diagnostic criteria,[188] they may not be as helpful in the diagnosis of PV in children. Although the pathogenesis is currently unclear, patients also have abnormalities in tissue factor, endogenous anticoagulants mechanisms, hyperhomocysteinemia, and acquired von Willebrand syndrome.

Children with PV may present with signs and symptoms associated with an increased red cell mass such as headache, dizziness, fatigue, pruritis, night sweats, and a ruddy complexion. Hepatosplenomegaly may be present. As a result of hyperviscosity of the blood, elevated platelet counts, and coagulation abnormalities, patients can develop thromboses and central nervous system ischemia, although the incidence of thrombotic events may be lower than that reported in adults.[156]

Many different agents have been used to treat PV, including chlorambucil,[189] melphalan,[190] 6-thioguanine,[191] uracil mustard,[192] busulfan,[193] carboquone,[194] anagrelide,[195] imatinib,[196] hydroxyurea,[197] radioactive phosphorous,[198] and interferon.[199] A total of seven randomized clinical trials have been conducted in adults using some of these agents.[200] Despite these efforts, the best approach to patients with PV remains unclear. Therefore, the British Committee for Standards in Hematology recently formulated recommendations for the initial management of PV.[201] Recommendations include phlebotomy to maintain a hematocrit level less than 45, aspirin unless contraindicated, and cytoreduction if there is poor tolerance to phlebotomy, symptomatic or progressive splenomegaly, evidence of disease progression, or thrombocytosis. For patients less than 40 years of age, interferon was the recommendation for first-line cytoreduction with hydroxyurea and anagrelide as second-line. Finally, allogeneic transplantation has been successfully used to treat a limited number of adult patients.[163,164,202,203] Allogeneic transplantation is considered only for patients with significant thrombotic disease or progression to AML.

FUTURE DIRECTIONS

Although a clearer understanding of the biologic mechanisms underlying MDS in children is slow in coming, dramatic progress has been made in our understanding of the biologic mechanisms for TMD, JMML, PV, ET, and IM. There exists a potential for targeted therapeutics for these disorders.

However, progress for both MDS and MPS in children will require international cooperation. The rarity of these disorders and limitations in resources for pediatric cooperative cancer groups make clinical trials within each individual cooperative group increasingly difficult.

SUGGESTED READINGS

Bhatia S, Krailo MD, Chen Z, et al: Therapy-related myelodysplasia and acute myeloid leukemia after Ewing sarcoma and primitive neuroectodermal tumor of bone: A report from the Children's Oncology Group. Blood 109(1):46, 2007.

Crispino JD: GATA1 mutations in Down syndrome: Implications for biology and diagnosis of children with transient myeloproliferative disorder and acute megakaryoblastic leukemia. Pediatr Blood Cancer 44(1):40, 2005.

Greenberg P, Cox C, LeBeau MM, et al: International scoring system for evaluating prognosis in myelodysplastic syndromes [see comments] [published erratum appears in Blood 1998 Feb 1;91(3):1100]. Blood 89(6):2079, 1997.

Hasle H: Myelodysplastic and myeloproliferative disorders in children. Curr Opin Pediatr 19(1):1, 2007.

Hasle H, Baumann I, Bergstrasser E, et al: The International Prognostic Scoring System (IPSS) for childhood myelodysplastic syndrome (MDS) and juvenile myelomonocytic leukemia (JMML). Leukemia 18(12):2008, 2004.

Hasle H, Niemeyer CM, Chessells JM, et al: A pediatric approach to the WHO classification of myelodysplastic and myeloproliferative diseases. Leukemia 17(2):277, 2003.

Locatelli F, Nollke P, Zecca M, et al: Hematopoietic stem cell transplantation (HSCT) in children with juvenile myelomonocytic leukemia (JMML): Results of the EWOG-MDS/Etrial BMT. Blood 105(1):410, 2005.

Loh M, Shannon K: The role of neurofibromatosis type 1 in myeloid malignancies. American Society of Clinical Oncology Education Book Alexandia, VA, 2007, p. 663.

Loh ML, Vattikuti S, Schubbert S, et al: Mutations in PTPN11 implicate the SHP-2 phosphatase in leukemogenesis. Blood 103(6):2325, 2004.

Luna-Fineman S, Shannon KM, Atwater SK, et al: Myelodysplastic and myeloproliferative disorders of childhood: A study of 167 patients. Blood 93(2):459, 1999.

Occhipinti E, Correa H, Yu L, Craver R: Comparison of two new classifications for pediatric myelodysplastic and myeloproliferative disorders. Pediatr Blood Cancer 44(3):240, 2005.

Shannon KM, O'Connell P, Martin GA, et al: Loss of the normal NF1 allele from the bone marrow of children with type 1 neurofibromatosis and malignant myeloid disorders [see comments]. N Engl J Med 330(9):597, 1994.

Tefferi A, Gilliland DG: Oncogenes in myeloproliferative disorders. Cell Cycle 6(5):550, 2007.

Tefferi A, Gilliland DG: Classification of chronic myeloid disorders: From Dameshek towards a semi-molecular system. Best Pract Res Clin Haematol 19(3):365, 2006.

Tefferi A, Thiele J, Orazi A, et al: Proposals and rationale for revision of the World Health Organization diagnostic criteria for polycythemia vera, essential thrombocythemia, and primary myelofibrosis: Recommendations from an ad hoc international expert panel. Blood 110:1092, 2007.

Webb DK, Passmore SJ, Hann IM, Harrison G, Wheatley K, Chessells JM: Results of treatment of children with refractory anaemia with excess blasts (RAEB) and RAEB in transformation (RAEBt) in Great Britain 1990–99. Br J Haematol 117(1):33, 2002.

Woods WG, Barnard DR, Alonzo TA, et al: Prospective study of 90 children requiring treatment for juvenile myelomonocytic leukemia or myelodysplastic syndrome: A report from the Children's Cancer Group. J Clin Oncol 20(2):434, 2002.

REFERENCES

For complete list of references log onto www.expertconsult.com

CHAPTER 75

PATHOBIOLOGY OF NON-HODGKIN LYMPHOMA

Georg Lenz and Louis M. Staudt

INTRODUCTION

The molecular pathogenesis of non-Hodgkin lymphoma (NHL) has been unraveled over the past two decades, owing to advances in molecular biology and genomics. As with other types of cancer, NHLs arise by a multistep accumulation of genetic aberrations that confer a selective growth advantage on the malignant clone. Recurrent translocations involving the immunoglobulin heavy chain (IgH) locus are often crucial first steps in lymphomagenesis. These translocations juxtapose the potent IgH transcriptional enhancers with various oncogenes that control cell proliferation, survival, and differentiation, leading to their overexpression and/or misexpression. These translocation events alone are insufficient for full malignant transformation, as evidenced by studies of mice engineered to overexpress these oncogenes. Recent efforts have uncovered many additional molecular aberrations that cooperate to produce lymphomas, as detailed below.

Although histologic examination of NHLs has revealed multiple NHL subtypes, the era of genomics has revealed new subtypes that are histologically indistinguishable but yet have distinct molecular etiologies and clinical behaviors. These insights have been achieved using DNA microarrays, which provide a genomewide profile of mRNA expression levels in a cancer sample. The gene expression profile of a tumor sample enables the precise measurement of various biological features of the tumor such as its proliferation rate, the activity of survival pathways, and the nature of nonmalignant tumor-infiltrating cells. By analyzing gene expression profiles and clinical data in concert, molecular models of survival can be constructed that reveal those aspects of tumor biology that are clinically relevant.

This chapter summarizes current concepts about the molecular pathogenesis of the common NHL subtypes. Particular attention is paid to the molecular diagnosis of lymphomas by gene expression profiling, which has led to new pathogenetic pathways and targets for therapeutic attack.

DIFFUSE LARGE B-CELL LYMPHOMA

DLBCL Subgroups Defined by Gene Expression Profiling

Diffuse large B-cell lymphoma (DLBCL) is the most common type of NHL, accounting for 30% to 40% of lymphoma cases in adults.[1] DLBCL has a variable clinical course, with only 40% to 50% of patients cured using anthracycline-based chemotherapy, suggesting that DLBCL is a heterogeneous diagnostic category.[2] This concept was supported by gene expression profiling studies that have distinguished three molecular subgroups of DLBCL, termed germinal center B-cell–like (GCB) DLBCL, activated B-cell–like (ABC) DLBCL, and primary mediastinal B-cell lymphoma (PMBL) (Figs. 75–1 and 75–2).[3–7] These three subgroups differ by the expression of thousands of genes and by this measure are as molecularly distinct as acute myelogenous leukemia and acute lymphoblastic leukemia. The gene expression profiles of these subgroups suggest that they arise from B-cells at different stages of differentiation and use separate oncogenic pathways.[8] Moreover, the DLBCL subgroups differ in clinical presentation and have significantly different survival rates following chemotherapy. Taken together, these observations have led to the view that the DLBCL subgroups represent distinct disease entities that are histologically indistinguishable.

By gene expression profiling, the GCB DLBCL subtype appears to derive from B cells at the germinal center stage of differentiation.[3,4,9] The unique biology of the germinal center reaction requires B cells to proliferate rapidly, mutate their immunoglobulin receptors, undergo positive selection for the ability to bind antigen at high affinity, and be eliminated by apoptosis if they fail to do so. This unique biological repertoire is associated with a broad gene expression signature that distinguishes normal germinal center B cells from other mature B-cell subsets. GCB DLBCLs express most, but not all, of the germinal center B-cell signature genes.[3,4,9] Moreover, GCB DLBCLs frequently have ongoing somatic hypermutation of their immunoglobulin genes within the malignant clone.[10] This specialized mutational mechanism is mediated by AID, an enzyme that is expressed at higher levels in normal germinal center B cells than at other stages of differentiation.[11]

Another gene characteristically expressed in GCB DLBCL is BCL-6, which encodes a key transcription factor that is required for the differentiation of mature B cells into germinal center B cells during an immune response.[12–14] BCL-6 is highly expressed in normal germinal center B cells but is silenced during plasmacytic differentiation.[15] BCL-6 functions as a transcriptional repressor and the target genes that it represses fall into distinct functional categories. Notably, BCL-6 represses *PRDM1*,[16,17] which encodes Blimp-1, a transcriptional repressor that is both necessary and sufficient for plasmacytic differentiation.[18,19] Blimp-1 promotes terminal plasmacytic differentiation by directly or indirectly extinguishing the expression of most mature B-cell differentiation genes as well as *c-myc* and other proliferation-associated genes.[20] BCL-6 also represses a set of genes that are induced when B cells are activated through the B-cell receptor or through CD40, suggesting that BCL-6 may modulate the response of normal germinal center B cells and GCB DLBCLs to antigen and T cells.[16,21,22] A third group of BCL-6 targets are negative regulators of cell cycle progression, including p21 and p27kip1, suggesting that BCL-6 licenses germinal center B cells and GCB DLBCLs for limitless cell cycle progression.[16,23] Finally, BCL-6 blocks the DNA damage response by repressing p53 and perhaps other DNA damage signaling molecules.[24] This function of BCL-6 may allow germinal center B cells and GCB DLBCLs to tolerate the double-stranded breaks that are induced by the enzyme AID, the effector of immunoglobulin somatic hypermutation and class switch recombination.[11] It is likely that BCL-6 expression imparts on GCB DLBCLs several biological attributes of normal germinal center B cells, including unfettered replicative potential and insensitivity to DNA damage.

ABC DLBCL may derive from B cells that are trapped between the germinal center B-cell and plasma-cell stages of differentiation.[4,5] This notion is based on the observation that ABC DLBCLs have downregulated most germinal center B-cell signature genes, including *BCL-6*, and express many genes that are characteristic of plasma cells. In particular, ABC DLBCLs express a key regulator of the secretory phenotype of plasma cells, *XBP-1*, as well as many of its downstream target genes.[5,25] Notably, inactivating mutations, deletions, and rearrangements of *PRDM1* and consequent loss of Blimp-1 expression are present in roughly one quarter of ABC DLBCLs but not in GCB DLBCLs.[26,27]

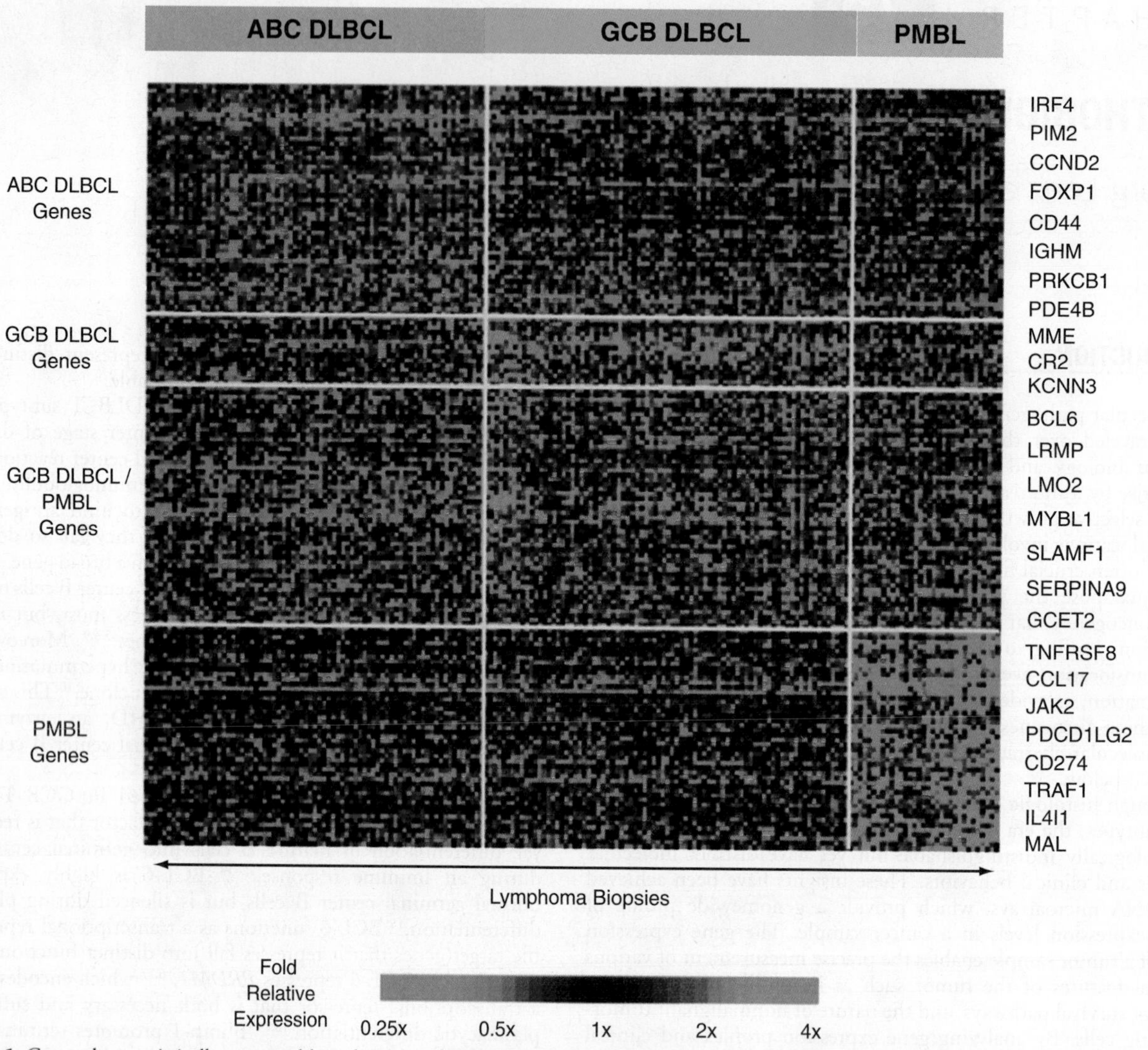

Figure 75–1 Genes characteristically expressed by subgroups of DLBCL: Activated B-cell–like (ABC) DLBCL, germinal center B-cell–like (GCB) DLBCL, and primary mediastinal B-cell lymphoma (PMBL). Each column represents gene expression data from a single DLBCL biopsy sample and each row represents expression of a single gene. Relative gene expression is indicated according to the color scale shown.

Moreover, BCL-6 translocations and genomic alterations in *PRDM1* have not been detected in the same ABC DLBCL cases.[27] Furthermore, BCL-6 translocations are more than twice as common in ABC DLBCL than in GCB DLBCL.[28] These observations support the hypothesis that ABC DLBCLs arise as a result of a block in B-cell differentiation, mediated either by Blimp-1 genomic aberrations or by translocation of BCL-6 and consequent repression of Blimp-1 expression. As further evidence of a post–germinal center origin, ABC DLBCLs carry a high load of mutations in their immunoglobulin genes but rarely have ongoing immunoglobulin gene mutation.[10]

Another characteristic feature of the ABC DLBCLs is the constitutive activation of the nuclear factor-κB (NF-κB) pathway, which suppresses apoptosis.[29] NF-κB signaling is mediated by a family of heterodimeric transcription factors that contribute to a wide range of cellular activation responses (reviewed in 30–32). Several of these factors are kept inactive in the cytoplasm by binding to inhibitory proteins of the IκB family. Stimulation though various receptors activates IκB kinase beta (IKKβ), which phosphorylates the IκBs, leading to translocation of NF-κB factors to the nucleus, where they transactivate their target genes. ABC DLBCLs, but not GCB DLBCLs, are characterized by high expression of NF-κB target genes.[29] ABC DLBCL cell lines have constitutive activation of the NF-κB pathway owing to constitutive activity of IKKβ. Inhibition of NF-κB using a dominant active form of IκBα or a dominant negative form of IKKβ is toxic to ABC DLBCL but not GCB DLBCL cell lines.[29] Moreover, small-molecule inhibitors of IKKβ are selectively toxic to ABC DLBCL cell lines, confirming that ABC DLBCLs are "addicted" to the antiapoptotic effects of NF-κB.[33]

Many upstream signaling pathways can activate NF-κB, generally in a transient fashion.[30–32] Insight into the upstream pathways causing constitutive NF-κB activity in ABC DLBCLs was provided by a genetic screen in DLBCL cell lines using a library of small hairpin RNAs (shRNAs), that mediate RNA interference.[34] shRNAs targeting *CARD11*, *MALT1*, and *BCL10* were all found to be toxic to ABC DLBCL but not GCB DLBCL cell lines. In normal B and T cells, CARD11, MALT1, and BCL10 form an oligomeric signaling complex (the CBM complex) following antigenic stimulation that leads to IKKβ activation.[35] CBM complex formation in normal lymphocytes is transient whereas in ABC DLBCLs it is constitutively engaged to activate IKKβ. The molecular aberrations leading to constitutive formation of the CBM complex in ABC DLBCLs are currently unknown.

PMBL, the third subgroup of DLBCL, was initially defined by clinical criteria.[36] In contrast to other forms of DLBCL that mainly affect patients older than 60 years of age,[37] PMBL typically occurs in young patients, often female, with a median age of only 30 to 35 years. In the majority of patients, the mediastinum is the only site of lymphoma manifestation.[38,39] On pathologic examination, a thymic remnant often can be found associated with the tumor mass, suggesting that PMBL arises from a rare B-cell subpopulation residing in

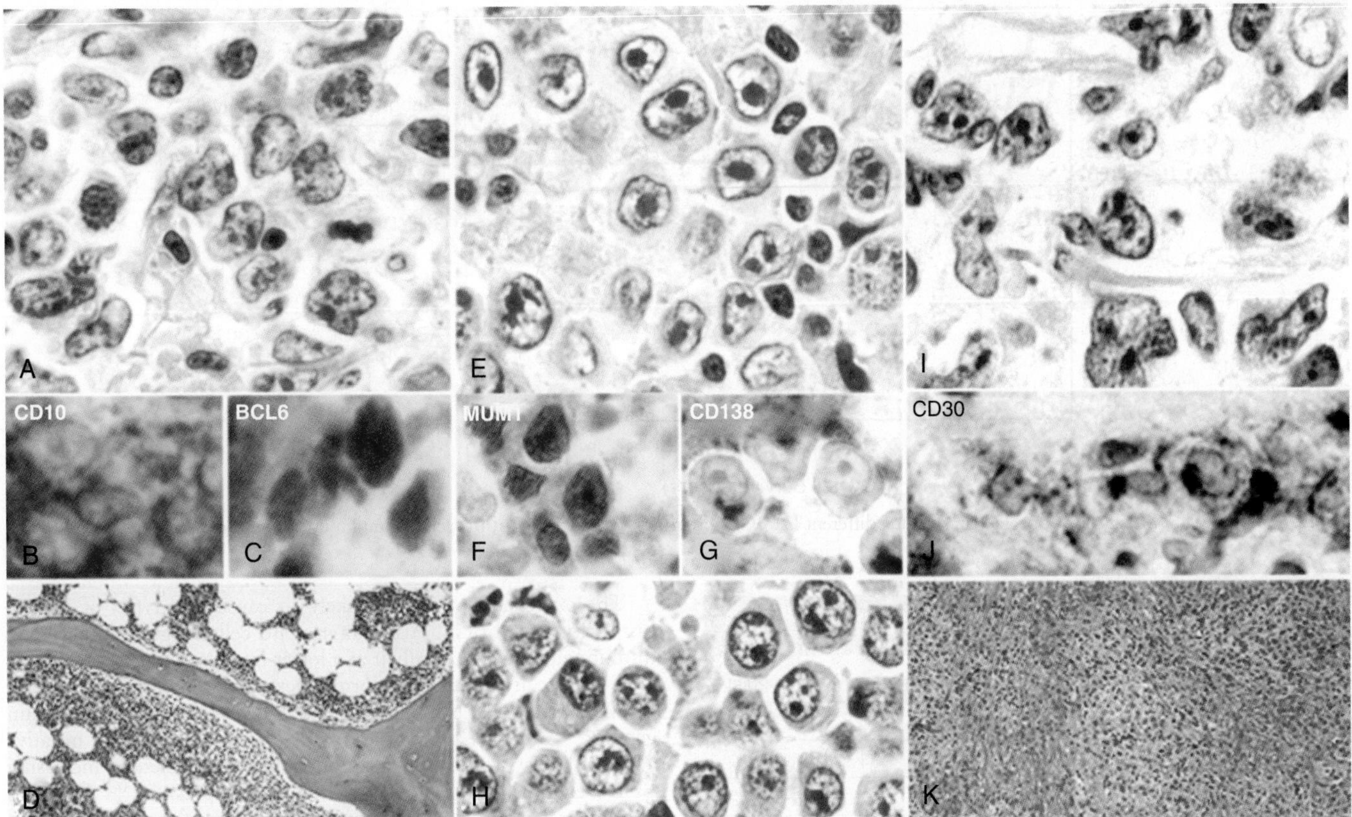

Figure 75–2 Three types of large B-cell lymphoma: germinal center B-cell–like, activated B-cell–type, and primary mediastinal B-cell–type (**A–L**). Germinal center B-cell–like, or germinal center-derived large B cell lymphomas usually have a centroblastic morphology (**A**), are CD20⁺, and express the germinal center markers CD10 (**B**) and BCL6 (**C**). In this case, the patient's staging bone marrow (**D**) showed paratrabecular involvement by small cleaved cells (centrocytes), indicating that the large B-cell lymphoma likely arose from a lower-grade follicular lymphoma. Activated B-cell like large B-cell lymphoma can sometime have an immunoblastic morphology (**E**), and can typically express MUM1 (**F**) and CD138 (**G**). These post–germinal center cell-type of lymphomas can also have a plasmablastic morphology (**H**), as sometimes seen in HIV-related cases. Primary mediastinal large B-cell lymphomas are frequently composed of multilobated centroblasts (**I**). They are typically CD45⁺, CD20⁺, and usually CD30⁺ (**J**), but CD15-negative. Surface immunoglobulin may be negative on such cases. PMBL is commonly associated with fibrosis, which is present in broad bands (**K**) or surrounding individual cells (as in **I**).

the thymus.[40] By gene expression, PMBL can be reliably diagnosed by virtue of a characteristic gene expression signature that distinguishes it from GCB DLBCL and ABC DLBCL.[6,7] PMBLs express some genes in common with GCB DLBCLs, including *BCL-6*, but do not express the ABC DLBCL signature genes and, particularly, do not express genes associated with plasmacytic differentiation.[6] Importantly, PMBL cannot be diagnosed reliably on clinical grounds alone; roughly one-quarter of the cases diagnosed as PMBL by clinical criteria were not PMBL by gene expression, and were instead other types of DLBCL that happened to have prominent mediastinal involvement.[6]

Gene expression profiling revealed an unexpected molecular relationship between PMBL and nodular sclerosis Hodgkin lymphoma.[6,7] More than one-third of genes that distinguish PMBL from the other DLBCL subgroups were also highly expressed in Hodgkin lymphoma cell lines, and many were expressed in the malignant Reed-Sternberg cells of Hodgkin lymphoma.[6] Among those genes are known markers for PMBL (IL4I1, Mal) and Hodgkin lymphoma (CD30).[40,41] In addition, both PMBL and Hodgkin lymphoma express targets of the NF-κB pathway.[6,7,42,43] A PMBL cell line[33,44] and several Hodgkin lymphoma cell lines[42,43] depend on constitutive activity of the NF-κB pathway for survival. The molecular mechanisms of constitutive NF-κB activity in PMBL are unknown, but the CARD11/MALT1/BCL10 pathway is not involved.[44]

The molecular relationship between PMBL and Hodgkin lymphoma extends the previous observation that these two lymphoma entities share several clinical and pathologic features.[45] Both entities often affect young patients, especially women, who present with a mediastinal tumor that has prominent sclerosis. In addition, rare patients with Hodgkin lymphoma who have a complete response to therapy may nonetheless relapse with PMBL. Histologically, a set of "grey zone" lymphomas have been recognized that have features of both PMBL and Hodgkin lymphoma. These considerations suggest that both PMBL and Hodgkin lymphoma originate from the same rare B-cell population in the thymus, which shares some molecular features with these malignancies such as expression of Mal.[40] Despite their similarities, PMBL and Hodgkin lymphoma are readily distinguished histologically and by gene expression, and thus must differ in detail in their oncogenic mechanisms.[6]

Genetic Aberrations in DLBCL Subgroups

The three gene expression subgroups of DLBCL exhibit striking differences in the frequency of genomic abnormalities, supporting the hypothesis that they represent distinct diseases that use different oncogenic mechanisms (Table 75–1). Two common recurrent genetic aberrations in DLBCL are the t(14; 18) translocation involving the *BCL-2* gene and amplification of the *c-rel* locus on chromosome 2p. The t(14;18) translocation is present in almost half of GCB DLBCLs but never in ABC DLBCLs.[4] Likewise, c-rel amplification occurs in one sixth of GCB DLBCLs but is absent in ABC DLBCLs.[4]

In contrast, roughly one-quarter of ABC DLBCLs have trisomy 3 or gain and amplification of chromosome arm 3q, abnormalities

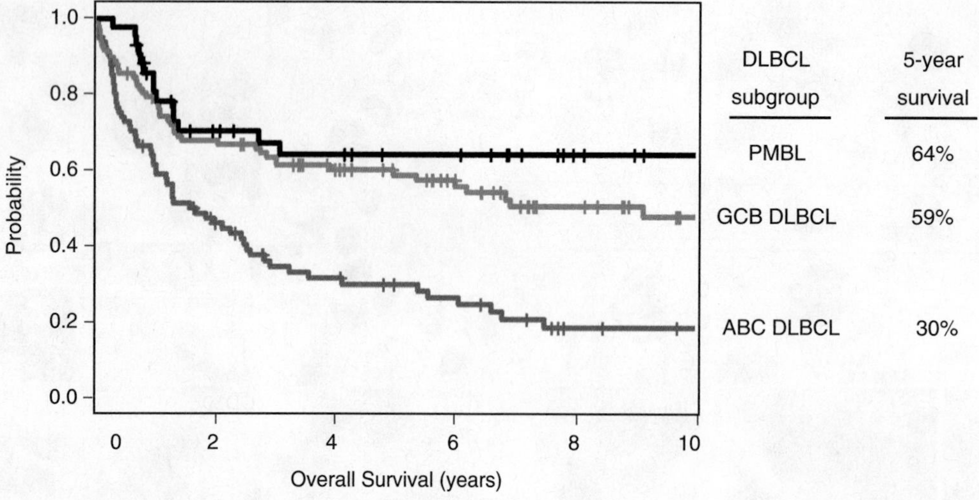

Figure 75–3 Kaplan–Meier plot of overall survival for different DLBCL subgroups treated with anthracycline-containing chemotherapeutic regimens.

Table 75–1 Frequency of Recurrent Genetic Aberrations in DLBCL Subtypes

	GCB DLBCL	ABC DLBCL	PMBL
BCL2 translocation, t(14;18)	45%	0	18%
BCL2 amplification, 18q21	10%	34%	16%
REL amplification, 2p13	16%	0	25%
Gain or amplification of 3q	0	26%	5%
Gain or amplification of 9p24	0	6%	43%
PRDM1 mutation/deletion (Blimp-1)	0	24%	n.d.
BCL6 translocation	11%	29%	23%

Compiled from References 4, 6, 26–28, 46, 77. n.d.: not determined.

that never occur in GCB DLBCLs.[46] Trisomy 3 is also a recurrent feature of MALT lymphomas, raising the possibility that ABC DLBCL might derive from this lymphoma type.[47] However, ABC DLBCLs do not harbor the t(11;18) translocation,[34] a recurrent and characteristic feature of MALT lymphoma, suggesting that trisomy 3 may have a separate selective advantage in both MALT lymphoma and ABC DLBCL. Interestingly, the presence of these chromosome 3 abnormalities in ABC DLBCL is associated with low expression of the "lymph node" signature, which reflects a nonmalignant host response to DLBCL[46] (see below). ABC DLBCLs also have frequent amplifications of a region on chromosome 18q21 containing the *BCL2* and *MALT1* genes, events that are uncommon in other DLBCL subgroups.

PMBLs frequently have gains or high-level amplifications of chromosome band 9p24,[48] events that occur rarely in ABC DLBCL and never in GCB DLBCL.[6,46] This abnormality is also recurrent in Hodgkin lymphoma,[49] in keeping with the clinical and molecular similarities between PMBL and Hodgkin lymphoma. These amplicons include the *JAK2* gene,[6,50] which encodes a key tyrosine kinase that regulates cytokine signaling through STAT family transcriptional factors. A role for cytokine signaling in both PMBL and Hodgkin lymphoma is further supported by recurrent inactivation of *SOCS1*, a negative regulator of cytokine signaling.[51–54] In addition, the PMBL amplicon encodes PD-L1 and PD-L2, which are ligands for the PD receptor on T cells that are highly expressed in PMBL.[6] Engagement of the PD receptor by its ligands generally inhibits signaling through the T-cell receptor, raising the possibility that the chromosomal amplification of these genes modulates the interaction between the PMBL cells and surrounding T cells in the thymus.[6]

The expression of AID is likely to cause two types of genetic instability in DLBCL. AID can mutate cellular genes other than immunoglobulin genes, albeit at a lower frequency. For example, the BCL-6 gene is mutated in normal germinal center B cells and in NHLs at a rate that is roughly 100-fold lower than immunoglobulin genes.[55,56] Some BCL-6 mutations in DLBCL occur in a negative autoregulatory site in the first noncoding exon, thereby increasing BCL-6 expression by relieving BCL-6 of self-repression.[57,58] DLBCLs accumulate AID-dependent somatic mutations in many other cellular genes, including several oncogenes such as *MYC* and *PIM1*.[59] These mutations are generally within 1 to 2 kilobases of the start of transcription, so for some genes, the mutations can alter protein function.

A second form of AID-dependent genetic alteration is aberrant immunoglobulin class switch recombination.[60] In addition to its role in somatic hypermutation, AID catalyzes the deletional joining of immunoglobulin switch regions, thereby effecting a change in immunoglobulin heavy chain isotype.[11] In aberrant class switch recombination, AID-induced breaks in the immunoglobulin switch regions are substrates for joining reactions with other double-stranded breaks in the genome, leading to so-called switch chromosomal translocations. This process is distinctly more common in ABC DLBCL than in other forms of DLBCL or in MALT lymphoma.[60] In addition to switch translocations, ABC DLBCLs have frequent internal deletions, mutations, and duplications with the switch N and switch γ regions, and these are ongoing processes within the malignant clone.[60] Moreover, ABC DLBCLs have a significantly lower frequency of legitimate class switch recombination. Of note, AID is one of the few germinal center B-cell–restricted genes that is expressed at higher levels in ABC DLBCL than in GCB DLBCL.[5,60,61] Because ABC DLBCLs are impaired in normal immunoglobulin class switching, their high AID activity may increase double-stranded breaks in the IgH locus and eventually culminate in translocations.

Clinical Differences in DLBCL Subgroups

Overall survival rates following anthracycline-based chemotherapy differ among the three molecular subgroups of DLBCL. In an initial cohort of patients studied by gene expression profiling, GCB DLBCL and PMBL had relatively favorable 5-year overall survival rates of 64% and 59%, respectively, whereas ABC DLBCL had only a 30% 5-year survival rate (Fig. 75–3).[4,6] The superior survival of patients with GCB DLBCL was subsequently confirmed in two other large cohorts studied by gene expression.[62–64] An immunohistochemical method has been developed that roughly mirrors the GCB DLBCL/ABC DLBCL distinction.[65] This approach divides DLBCLs into a GC phenotype (roughly equivalent to GCB DLBCL) and a non-GC

Table 75–2 International Prognostic Index Table

	Score = 0	Score = 1
Age	<60	>60
ECOG performance status	≤1	>1
Ann Arbor stage	≤2	>2
LDH	<Upper limit of normal	>Upper limit of normal
Extranodal sites	≤1	>1

phenotype (including ABC DLBCLs and other unclassified DLBCLs). In multiple DLBCL cohorts treated with CHOP chemotherapy, this method confirmed that GC cases had a better overall survival rate than non-GC cases.[65–72]

The prognostic value of the DLBCL subgroup distinction is statistically independent of the features included in the International Prognostic Index (IPI),[73] (Table 75–2) demonstrating that this distinction is not merely a surrogate of known clinical prognostic attributes.[3,4] Nonetheless, there are significant differences in the frequency of individual components of the IPI (Table 75–2) in the different DLBCL subtypes. A significantly higher proportion of ABC DLBCL patients are older than 60 years of age and more patients in this cohort have a poor performance status (ECOG > 2). In contrast, PMBL patients are younger, with a median age of 33, and have more frequent extranodal involvement.[4,6] The pattern of extranodal involvement also differs: PMBL frequently involves various thoracic structures, often by direct extension, whereas ABC DLBCL and GCB DLBCL most commonly involve the gastrointestinal tract, bone marrow, liver, and muscle.[6]

Recently, standard therapy for DLBCL has changed to include the anti-CD20 monoclonal antibody rituximab; in patients older than 60 years of age, overall survival in DLBCL is improved by approximately 10% to 15% with the CHOP-Rituximab (CHOP-R) regimen compared to CHOP alone.[74] Immunohistochemical studies using antibodies to BCL-2 and BCL-6 have suggested that biological subgroups of DLBCL may respond preferentially to the addition of rituximab. The expression of BCL-2 protein is an adverse prognostic factor with CHOP chemotherapy but not with CHOP-R.[75] DLBCLs express BCL-2 protein by two distinct mechanisms. Among GCB DLBCLs, those with the t(14;18) translocation express BCL-2 whereas the others do not.[4,76] In ABC DLBCL, many tumors express BCL-2, not by translocation but by transcriptional activation and, in some cases, amplification of the BCL-2 locus on chromosome 18.[46,65] However, a minority of ABC DLBCLs do not express BCL-2 protein, and these have a more favorable prognosis with CHOP chemotherapy.[77] For BCL-6, tumors that lack expression are associated with poor survival with CHOP chemotherapy, but not with CHOP-R.[78] Whole-genome gene expression profiling of tumors in the context of CHOP-R treatment will be needed to fully understand which DLBCL patients are benefiting most from rituximab and which patients are yet to be cured by the current standard of care.

PREDICTION OF SURVIVAL FOLLOWING CHEMOTHERAPY BY GENE EXPRESSION

Other gene expression profiling studies have taken a "supervised" approach to correlate gene expression patterns with the clinical outcome.[4,80] In this approach, statistical methods are used to identify genes whose expression patterns across a series of cancer specimens are associated with favorable or inferior survival. Often, these survival-associated genes can be classified into gene expression signatures, which are sets of coordinately expressed genes that reflect a particular biological phenotype such as cell lineage, stage of differentiation, or activity of an intracellular signaling cascade.[81] In one study of DLBCL, the majority of survival-associated genes could be assigned to one of four gene expression signatures, termed "germinal center B cell," "MHC Class II," "lymph node," and "proliferation."[4] The germinal center B cell, MHC Class II, and lymph node signatures were associated with favorable outcome whereas the proliferation signature was associated with poor survival.

The germinal center B-cell signature consists of genes characteristically expressed in normal germinal center B cells; this signature is another way of identifying the prognostic difference between GCB DLBCL and ABC DLBCL. In a supervised survival analysis of an independent DLBCL cohort,[80] two genes that were strongly associated with inferior prognosis encode protein kinase C β1 and phosphodiesterase 4b, both of which are more highly expressed in ABC DLBCL than in GCB DLBCL.[5,82]

Three other signatures are cross-cutting in that they are variably expressed within GCB DLBCL, ABC DLBCL, and PMBL. The MHC class II signature includes genes encoding the various MHC class II proteins and invariant chain, all of which are involved in antigen processing during an immune response.[4] Immunohistochemical stains showed that the variation of expression of this signature was due to differences in MHC class II protein expression in the malignant tumor cells, not in the nonmalignant bystander cells.[83,84] In addition, tumors with low expression of the MHC class II signature were found to have fewer infiltrating $CD8^+$ cytotoxic T cells.[83] Plausibly, therefore, the inferior prognosis of tumors with decreased expression of the MHC class II signature may reflect an inadequate host immune response.

The third gene expression signature associated with favorable outcome was dubbed the lymph node signature because it reflects the infiltration of nonmalignant cells into the tumor in lymph node biopsies.[4] This signature includes various genes encoding extracellular matrix components as well as genes expressed in macrophages. Histologically, this signature reflects a sclerotic reaction that is a feature of certain DLBCLs. High expression of the lymph node signature is more common in GCB DLBCL and PMBL than in ABC DLBCL but is a variable feature within each subgroup. The reason why this signature confers a favorable prognosis is unclear, but one hypothesis suggests that this signature indicates a dependence of the malignant cell upon the lymph node's microenvironment. This dependence may limit the ability of the malignant cell to establish itself in extranodal environments. Interestingly, certain chromosomal abnormalities in DLBCLs were associated with either low expression or high expression of the lymph node signature, suggesting the nature of the malignant cell may dictate its mode of interaction with its microenvironment. Specifically, gain or amplification of chromosome arm 3q, which occurs exclusively in ABC DLBCLs, was associated with low expression of the lymph node signature whereas gain of chromosome band Xp21 was associated with high expression of the lymph node signature.[46]

The majority of genes associated with poor overall survival in DLBCL belong to the proliferation gene expression signature,[4] called so because these genes are more highly expressed in dividing cells than in quiescent cells.[81] Although the proliferation signature was a variable feature of each DLBCL subgroup, it was most highly expressed in ABC DLBCLs, on average.[4] The particular proliferation genes that predict survival in DLBCL are a specific subset of the proliferation genetic program, specifically the transcriptional network regulated by c-myc.[4,8] Interestingly, c-myc and its target genes are more highly expressed on average in ABC DLBCL than in the other DLBCL subtypes.[85] One of the primary cellular phenotypes controlled by c-myc is cell growth, which specifically refers to an increase in cell size.[86] In this regard, it is notable that ABC DLBCLs frequently have an "immunoblastic" morphology,[4] a cellular phenotype that could be a consequence of c-myc activity.

A multivariate model of survival in DLBCL was constructed from these four gene expression signatures.[4] For every biopsy, a "survival predictor score" was calculated as a weighted average of the four signatures in the biopsy. After ranking according to these scores, DLBCL patients were divided into four equal quartile groups that had 5-year

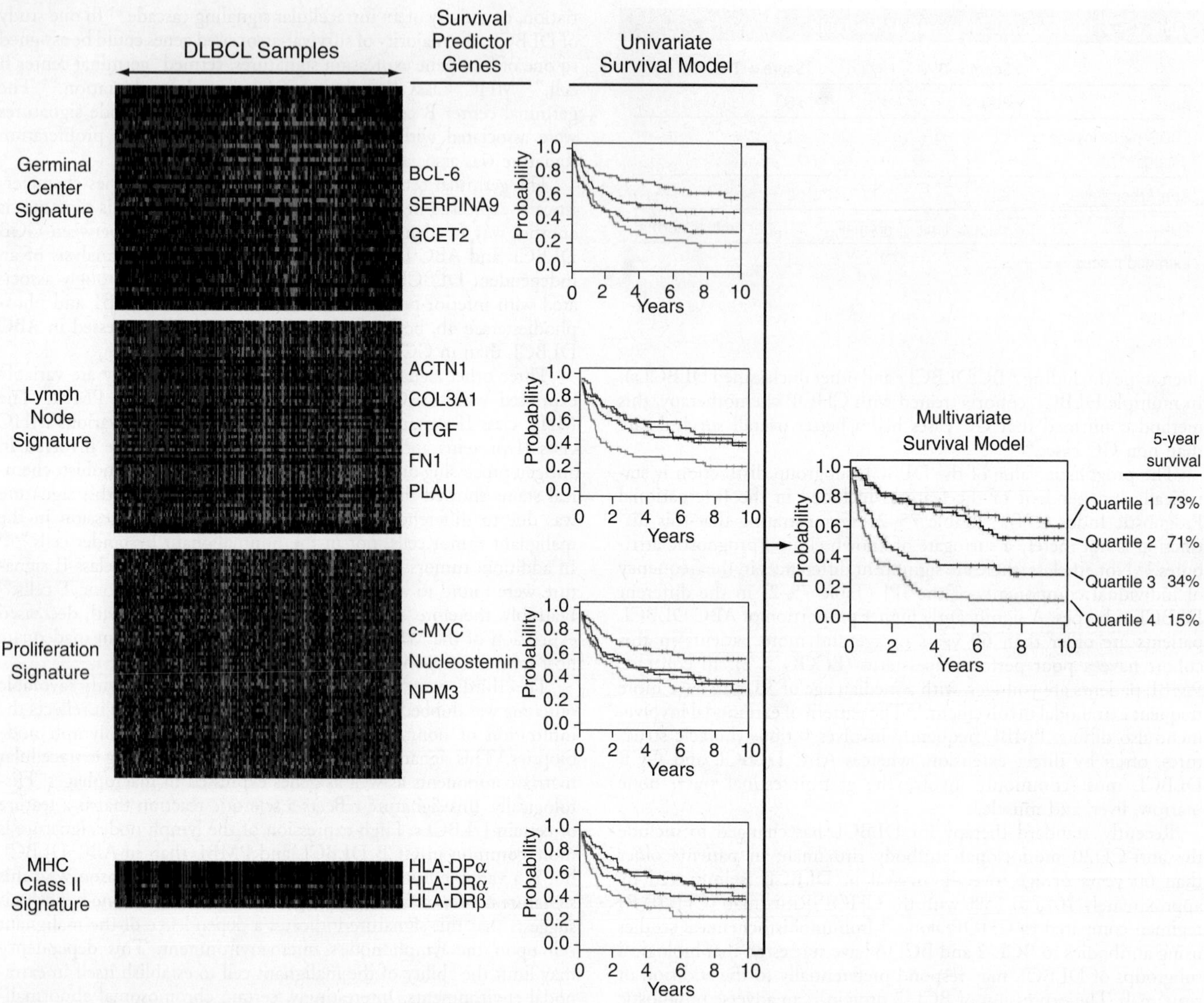

Figure 75–4 Gene-expression–based model of survival following chemotherapy for DLBCL. The left panel shows the expression of the four gene expression signatures used to create the survival model in DLBCL. Expression of the germinal center, lymph node, and MHC class II signatures is associated with favorable prognosis, whereas expression of the proliferation signature is associated with inferior survival. Representative genes from each signature used to create the survival model are shown. For each signature, patients were divided into four equal quartiles based on the expression of the signature in their biopsy samples. The four Kaplan–Meier plots in the middle depict the survival of patients in each signature quartile. These four signatures were combined into a multivariate model of survival and patients were divided into four quartile groups based on this model. The Kaplan–Meier plot at the right depicts the survival of each quartile group of the multivariate model.

survival rates of 73%, 71%, 34%, and 15% (Fig. 75–4).[4] This gene-expression–based predictor was statistically independent of the clinical variables in the IPI (Table 75–2), suggesting that it reflects meaningful aspects of DLBCL biology that alter the response to therapy.

CONCLUSIONS

DLBCL is a heterogeneous diagnostic category consisting of at least three different molecular subtypes. Like subtypes of acute leukemia, these DLBCL subtypes differ with respect to the expression of thousands of genes, in part because they derive from different stages of B-cell differentiation. Perhaps as a consequence of this varied origin, they use different oncogenic pathways and harbor specific chromosomal abnormalities. These attributes, along with their clinical differences, support the view that the DLBCL subtypes are distinct disease entities. These three DLBCL subgroups account for roughly 82% of the cases, demonstrating that additional, less common subtypes of DLBCL remain to be discovered. Layered on top of this subtype distinction is the variable expression of other signatures that reflect biological attributes of the tumors that have prognostic import.

Burkitt Lymphoma

Burkitt lymphoma (BL) (see Fig. 75–5) is a highly aggressive NHL that is often characterized by extranodal involvement or leukemic presentation.[87] BL often arises in adolescents or young adults[88] and is curable in a high fraction of cases by intensive multiagent chemotherapy.[89–91] Three different forms of BL can be distinguished: sporadic BL, endemic BL (occurring mainly in equatorial Africa), and immunodeficiency-associated BL.

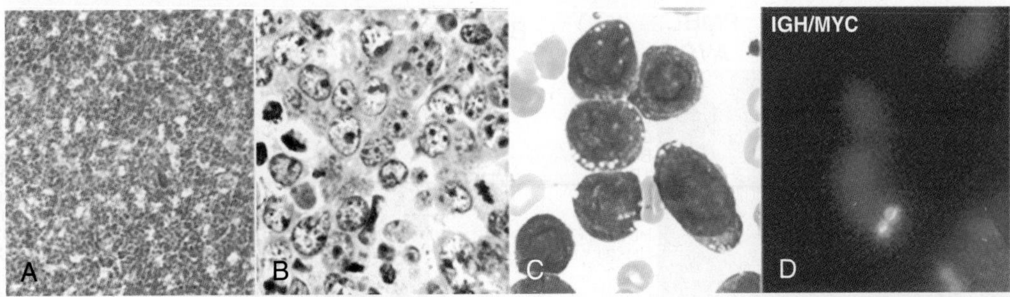

Figure 75–5 Burkitt Lymphoma (**A–D**). A case of Burkitt lymphoma illustrated at low power (**A**), showing the "starry sky" appearance. This is due to the dense proliferating cells producing the dark sky, and the scattered lighter-staining tingible body macrophages (stars) phagocytizing dying cells. Higher magnification (**B**) illustrating the syncytia of intermediate-sized cells with coarse chromatin and multiple nucleoli. Note the tingible body macrophage with abundant light cytoplasm and ingested debris (center bottom). Burkitt cells as seen on a Wright-stained bone marrow aspirate (**C**) in a patient with Burkitt leukemia. Notice deep blue cytoplasm with numerous vacuoles. Fluorescence in situ hybridization (FISH) with probes to MYC and IgH (**D**) illustrate the IgH/MYC fusion (courtesy of Dr. Yanming Zhang, University of Chicago).

Chromosomal Translocations Involving *c-myc*

BL is characterized by chromosomal translocations that dysregulate the expression of the protooncogene *MYC*, encoding the transcription factor c-myc, located on chromosome band 8q24.[92–94] Approximately 80% of cases harbor a t(8; 14) (q24; q32) that juxtaposes *MYC* with IgH enhancer elements, whereas in the remaining cases, *MYC* is translocated to the Igμ or Igκ locus.[95,96] The position of the chromosomal breakpoints in *MYC* and in the Ig genes are widely dispersed.[97] In endemic BL, cases with a t(8; 14) often show breakpoints on chromosome 8 more than 100 kb 5′ of *MYC* whereas the breakpoints on chromosome 14 can be mapped in the Ig joining regions (J_H). The involvement of the J_H regions indicates a role for the Rag1 and Rag2 recombinases that are active during early B-cell development.[98] By contrast, in sporadic BL and immunodeficiency-associated BL, the chromosome 8 breakpoints occur between *MYC* exons 1 and 2 or within a few kilobase 5′ of *MYC*, and the chromosome 14 breakpoints often involve the Ig switch regions.[95,99] It highly likely, therefore, that the AID recombinase that is central to Ig class switching plays an important role in these *MYC* translocations, as illustrated by the ability of AID to direct IgH-*MYC* translocations in mouse B cells.[100] These observations suggest that sporadic BL arises from earlier stages of B-cell differentiation than endemic or immunodeficiency-associated BL.

c-myc is a multipotent transcription factor that may regulate as many as 15% of all genes.[86] Consequently, c-myc plays an important role in many fundamental cellular responses, including cell proliferation, cell growth, protein synthesis, metabolism, differentiation, and apoptosis. The transcription of *MYC* itself is tightly regulated in normal cells, by virtue of a complicated promoter that has built-in autoregulation.[101] Translocations in BL that juxtapose *MYC* with the powerful immunoglobulin enhancers presumably upset this regulatory balance, thereby altering the expression of c-myc target genes in ways that are not fully understood.

Gene Expression Profiling

The importance of constitutive c-myc expression to the biology of BL was confirmed by gene expression profiling experiments comparing sporadic BL with DLBCL.[9] A gene expression signature of *MYC* target genes is more highly expressed in BL than in DLBCL (Fig. 75–6). These signature genes are expressed highly in a subset of DLBCLs bearing the t(8;14) translocation, but BLs have yet higher expression of this signature.[9]

The distinction between BL and DLBCL does not just rely upon *MYC* and its target genes. BL is also characterized by high expression of a subset of the genes that are characteristic of normal germinal center B cells, consistent with an origin of BL from this stage of B-cell differentiation (Fig. 75–6).[9] This "BL-high" subset of the germinal center B-cell signature (eg, *CD10* and *GCET2*) is expressed at much lower levels in GCB DLBCL, even though this lymphoma subtype also originates from germinal center B cells. Conversely, a "BL-low" subset of germinal center B-cell genes (eg, *LMO2*, *CD80*, *CD86*) is more highly expressed in GCB DLBCL than BL. Yet other germinal center B-cell signature genes are expressed equivalently in BL and DLBCL (eg, *BCL6*, *PAG*). One explanation for these observations could be that BL and GCB DLBCL derive from different germinal center B-cell subpopulations. Alternatively, differences in the oncogenic mechanisms of BL and GCB DLBCL may affect the germinal center B-cell gene expression program.

A gene expression signature that is expressed at exceedingly low levels in BL compared to DLBCL is the NF-κB signature.[9] Normal germinal center B cells have very low expression of NF-κB target genes, which may facilitate the apoptosis that is a prerequisite for the antigen-based selection for high-affinity B-cell receptors that occurs in the germinal center.[81,102] BLs inherit this low NF-κB phenotype from their normal counterparts, which may account for the high rate of spontaneous apoptosis in BLs and their characteristic "starry sky" histology.

Finally, in comparison to DLBCL, BL is characterized by low expression of all MHC class I genes.[9] BLs are characterized by a notable lack of immune cell infiltration, which may be due to their inability to effectively present antigens via the MHC class I pathway.

The gene expression differences between BL and DLBCL were used to fashion a molecular diagnosis of BL.[9] In BL cases in which there was no diagnostic disagreement among pathologists, the molecular predictor of BL had 100% accuracy. However, for a number of cases, an original diagnosis of BL was revised to be DLBCL based on the best available pathologic techniques. For some of these cases, the gene-expression–based diagnosis nevertheless declared the sample BL. Treatment of these patients with CHOP chemotherapy was unsuccessful, bolstering the view that they were indeed BL. Overall, one-sixth of the cases that were BL according to gene expression were misdiagnosed as DLBCL by the expert panel of pathologists using the current gold standard diagnostic techniques. Similar results were obtained by another large gene expression profiling study of BL and DLBCL.[63] An incorrect diagnosis of DLBCL in these cases would lead to the use of CHOP chemotherapy, which is incapable of curing BL. Therefore, a gene expression-based diagnosis of BL has the potential to significantly improve the choice of treatment for patients with these aggressive lymphomas.

Additional Genetic Aberrations

Epstein–Barr virus (EBV) infection is detectable in virtually all cases of endemic BL and in 20% to 40% of sporadic and immunodefi-

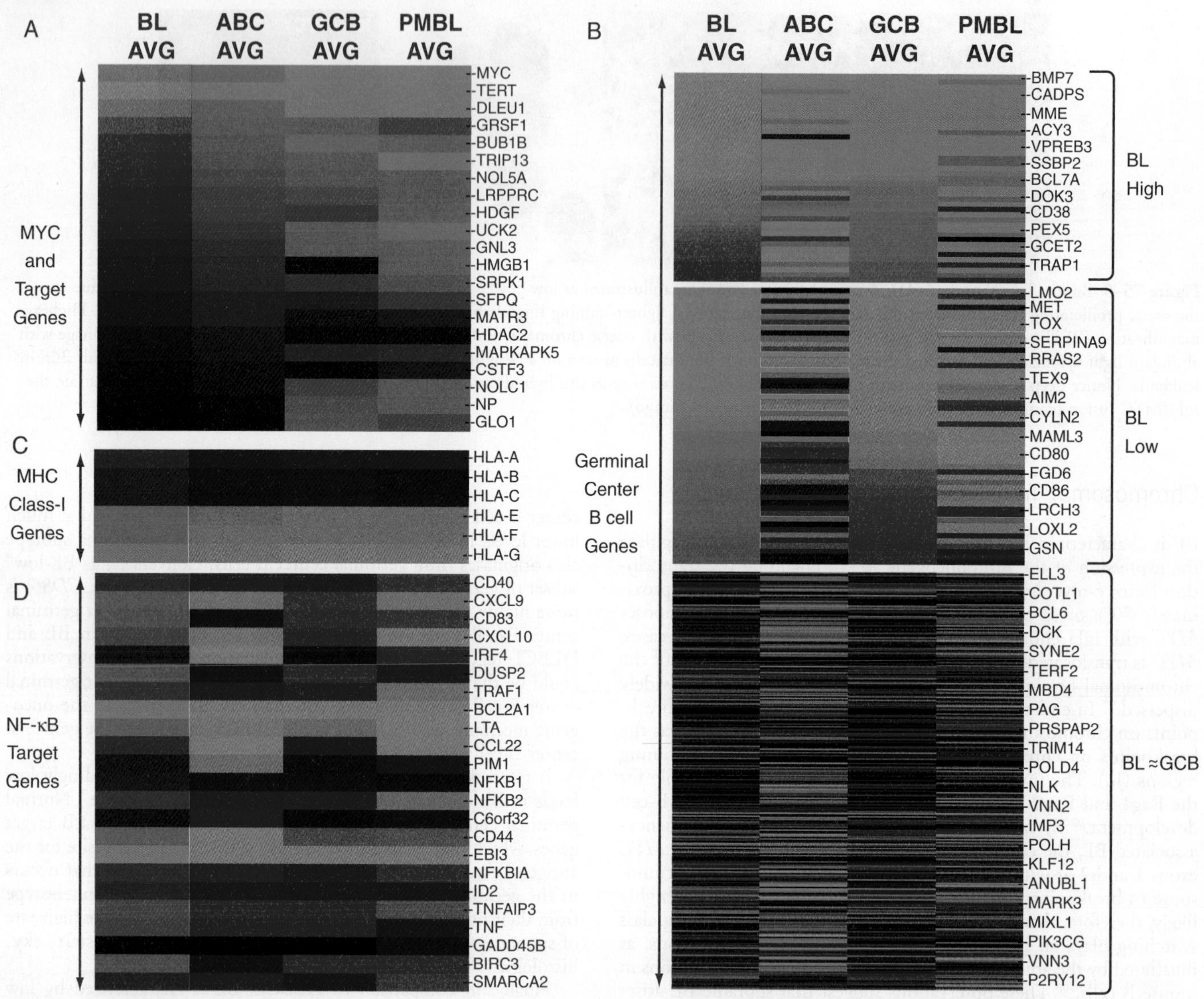

Figure 75–6 Relative expression of genes that distinguish Burkitt lymphoma (BL) from subgroups of DLBCL (ABC DLBCL, GCB DLBCL, and PMBL) is categorized into gene-expression signatures: c-myc and its target genes (**A**); genes that are expressed in normal germinal-center B cells (**B**) and are expressed more highly (BL-high), less highly (BL-low), or equivalently (BL≈GCB) in BL than in GCB DLBCL; MHC class I genes (**C**); and genes targeted by the NF-κB signaling pathway (**D**). Germinal-center B-cell signature genes are those that were overexpressed in normal germinal-center B cells, compared to blood B cells. The "BL-high" genes were expressed at levels twice as high in BL as in GCB DLBCL ($P < 0.001$). The "BL-low" genes were expressed at levels twice as high in GCB DLBCL as in BL ($P < 0.001$). The expression levels of the "BL≈GCB" genes did not differ significantly between the two lymphoma subtypes.

ciency BL.[103–106] This epidemiologic data is compelling evidence for a role of EBV in BL pathogenesis, but no satisfactory molecular mechanism has been elucidated.[107] An additional recurrent genetic event in BL is mutation or deletion of the *p53* tumor suppressor gene, present in approximately 30% of cases.[108]

Like normal germinal center B cells, most cases of BL do not express BCL-2. However, a minority of cases have a t(14;18) translocation or express BCL-2 by an unknown transcriptional mechanism, and these cases have a poor clinical outcome.[109] Interestingly, these BL cases were enriched in the set of cases that were misdiagnosed by pathologists as DLBCL, suggesting that the BCL-2 translocation may define a biologically and clinically distinct subtype of BL.[9]

Follicular Lymphoma

Follicular lymphoma (FL) is the most frequent low-grade NHL and accounts for approximately 20% of all NHL cases (see Fig. 75–7).[1] FL has a variable clinical course with a median overall survival of 8 to 10 years, with 10% to 15% of patients surviving more than 15 years. Conversely, 10% to 15% of patients have a rapidly progressive disease, often associated with transformation to DLBCL and poor prognosis.[110,111]

Chromosomal Translocation Involving *BCL2*

In approximately 90% of FL cases, a t(14; 18)(q32; q21) translocation juxtaposes the *BCL2* gene and the IgH locus,[112,113] thereby deregulating the key antiapoptotic protein BCL-2.[114,115] Less commonly, *BCL2* is deregulated by translocation to the Igκ and Igλloci. Normal germinal center B cells have essentially no BCL-2 expression[116,117] and have a high rate of apoptosis that they require for efficient selection of B cells with high affinity for antigen. The forced expression of BCL-2 due to the t(14;18) allows a B cell to escape this physiological cell death, a first step toward malignancy. A minority of FL cases do not express BCL-2 protein and lack *BCL2* transloca-

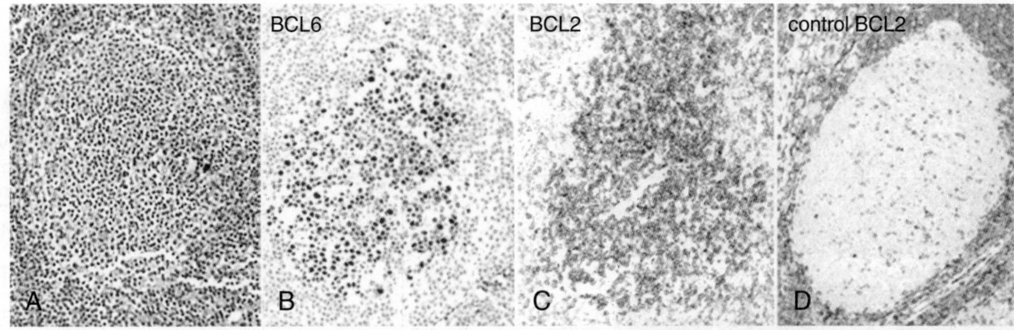

Figure 75–7 Follicular lymphoma (**A–D**). Details from a case of follicular lymphoma, grade 1 of 3 associated with t(14;18)(q32;q21). Malignant follicle (**A**), with immunohistochemical stains for the germinal center marker, BCL6 (**B**), and for BCL2 (**C**). Note the overexpression of BCL2 when compared to a reactive follicle (**D**).

tions[118]; alternative antiapoptotic mechanisms in these cases remain to be elucidated. Interestingly, a subset of FLs lacking BCL-2 expression harbor a BCL-6 translocation, which is otherwise rare in FL.[119]

The t(14; 18), the initiating event in FL, is apparently mediated by the RAG recombinase proteins, which cleave at J segments in the IgH locus and at an unusual non-B-form DNA structure in BCL2.[120] Expression of the RAG proteins is confined to early stages of B-cell differentiation, suggesting that the t(14; 18) occurs in the bone marrow. Interestingly, healthy individuals harbor the t(14;18) in their normal blood B cells.[121–123] These B cells have a surface phenotype and molecular features of memory B cells, suggesting that they have traversed the germinal center and could conceivably be precursors to FL.[124] Indeed, a type of in situ FL has been described in which a t(14;18)-positive B-cell follicle is identified in an otherwise normal lymph node biopsy—some of these cases progress to FL but others remain benign for many years.[125]

The t(14;18)-positive B cells of normal individuals have Ig switch recombination events on the t(14;18) allele, consistent with the activity of the AID recombinase and a germinal center derivation.[124] Nonetheless, the surface expression of IgM and IgD is invariably maintained on these cells, as is also the case in FL. These results suggest that stimulation of the B cells through their IgM/IgD antigen receptors plays a role in the derivation of both the benign t(14;18) B cells and FLs. Analysis of Ig V region sequences in FL is consistent with an antigen-driven selection of high-affinity variable region mutations.[126] Additionally, in most FL cases, somatic mutation creates new sites for N-linked glycosylation in the immunoglobulin variable regions.[127] This process is also observed in DLBCL, but only in those cases with a GCB phenotype harboring the t(14;18).[128] The meaning of these findings is a matter of conjecture but it is possible that sugar addition to the surface immunoglobulin receptor might allow the malignant B cell to participate in pathogenic interactions with lectin-like molecules in the germinal center microenvironment.

Gene Expression Profiling

Like GCB DLBCL, FL is characterized by expression of the germinal center B-cell signature, indicating its close relationship to this stage of B-cell differentiation.[3] Accordingly, FLs have ongoing mutation of their immunoglobulin genes, a hallmark of the germinal center stage of differentiation.[129] Nonetheless, FL and GCB DLBCL are relatively easy to distinguish by gene expression profiling.[3]

The length of survival following diagnosis of follicular lymphoma is highly variable, with some patients living for more than 20 years and others succumbing to the disease in a few years. Gene expression profiles of tumor biopsies at the time of diagnosis can be used to predict the length of survival. In a gene expression profiling study of 191 patients with FL, genes that were associated with longer and shorter overall survival were identified and organized into gene expression signatures by hierarchical clustering.[130] This analysis revealed two signatures associated with overall survival, both of which consist of genes known to be expressed in normal immune cells. One signature, termed "immune-response 1" was associated with favorable overall survival whereas the other signature, termed "immune-response 2," was associated with inferior survival. These two signatures were combined into a statistical model that produced a "survival predictor score" for each patient. After ranking according to these scores, the patients were divided into four equal quartiles that had remarkable differences in median overall survival (Fig. 75–8). Three-quarters of the patients had a very indolent disease, with a median survival of 11.7 years, but one-quarter had an aggressive disease and a median survival of only 3.9 years.

Biologically, the immune-response 1 signature reflects a mixture of immune cells that is enriched for T cells, because many genes in this signature are T-cell–restricted in expression (eg, *CD7*, *CD8B1*, *ITK*). However, this signature is not merely a reflection of the total number of infiltrating T cells in a sample because the expression of pan T-cell gene expression signature was not associated with survival. This implies the presence of specialized T-cell subsets in these tumors and/or the admixture of other immune cells. By contrast, the genes in "immune-response 2" signature reflect an immune infiltrate that is relatively devoid of T cells and enriched for macrophages and/or dendritic cells, as judged by expression of *TLR5*, *FCGR1A*, or *LGMN* and other genes characteristic of these cell types.

Recent studies evaluating immune subsets in FL by immunochemical means support the prognostic value of the immune-response 1 and immune-response 2 signatures. In two studies, a higher tumor CD8 T-cell number was associated with favorable survival,[131,132] consistent with the fact that the CD8 T-cell–restricted gene *CD8B1* is a component of the immune-response 1 signature.[130] Other studies have found associations between higher tumor CD4 cells with favorable survival.[133] Conversely, adverse overall survival has been associated with a high content of CD68-positive or STAT1-positive macrophages.[134,135]

Two general hypotheses that are not mutually exclusive could account the prognostic import of the immune response signatures.[8,130] In an immune-response hypothesis, the reason why the immune-response 1 signature is favorable is that it reflects an active antitumor immune response, dominated by T cells. In a "microenvironment addiction" hypothesis, the immune-response 1 signature represents a quasi-normal germinal center reaction in which the FL cells depend on trophic signals from the immune cells in the microenvironment. Tumors with the immune-response 2 signature may have developed ways to survive independently from the germinal center microenvironment, allowing them to spread more widely and rapidly. It is also certainly possible that genetic differences in the malignant cells, not readily detectable by gene expression, might evoke different immune response signatures.

Clearly, current data provide only a glimmer of the complexity of immune reactions in FL, but the nature of the immune cells could logically have an impact on response to immune modulatory thera-

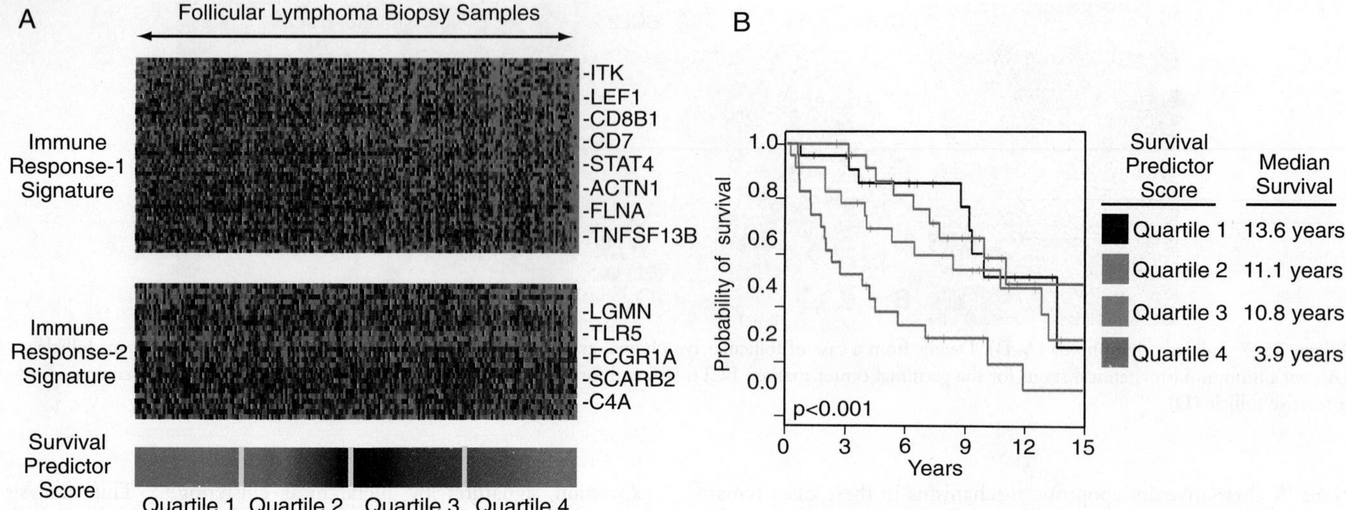

Figure 75–8 **A**, Two sets of coordinately expressed genes, termed the immune response-1 and immune response-2 signatures, are associated with survival in follicular lymphoma. The expression pattern of each gene in these two signatures is shown for follicular lymphoma biopsy samples. Expression of the immune response-1 signature is associated with favorable survival following diagnosis and expression of the immune response-2 signature is associated with adverse survival. These signatures are combined into a multivariate model of survival that generates a survival predictor score for each patient. Patients are ranked according to this survival predictor and divided into four equal quartiles as shown. **B**, Kaplan–Meier plot of overall survival of patients in the four quartiles of the survival predictor.

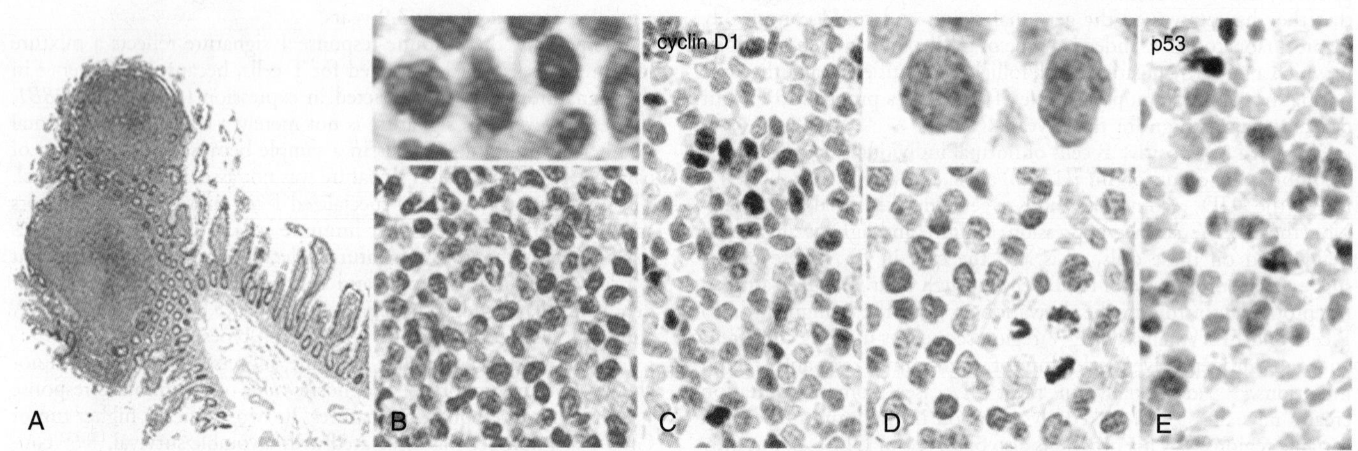

Figure 75–9 Mantle cell lymphoma (**A–E**). A case of mantle cell lymphoma presenting as lymphomatoid polyposis (**A**). The lymphoma cells are small to intermediate in size and have irregular nuclear contours and condensed nuclear chromatin (**B** and detail). The cells were CD19+, monoclonal B cells with lambda light chain restriction, coexpression of CD5, FMC-7, and lack of CD23. The cells showed cyclin D1 expression by immunohistochemical staining (**C**). The t(11;14)(q13;q32) was detected by conventional cytogenetic analysis. In comparison, the blastoid variant of mantle cell lymphoma (**D**) has larger cells with a high mitotic rate and fine chromatin. These cases frequently overexpress p53 (**E**) and are associated with a complex karyotype, including t(11;14).

pies such as idiotype vaccines or rituximab. Response to rituximab could be influenced by the nature and abundance of Fc-receptor bearing immune cells in the tumors because genetic polymorphisms that alter Fc-receptor binding of Rituximab are associated with response to this treatment.[136]

Additional Genetic Aberrations

The t(14;18) is not sufficient to induce lymphoma development in mouse models, suggesting that additional oncogenic hits are required to generate frank FL.[137] Thus far, however, these additional oncogenic mechanisms remain poorly understood. Other genes commonly involved in lymphomagenesis, such as *p53* or *c-myc*, are not frequently altered in FL. By classical cytogenetics, deletions on chromosomes 1 and 6 as well as gains on chromosomes 7, 12, and X are detectable in 20% to 30% of FL samples.[138–140]

During histologic transformation of FL into DLBCL, various genetic aberrations have been defined, including *p53* mutations and inactivation of *p16*.[141,142] By gene expression profiling, transformation appears to occur by two distinct mechanisms, one in which the DLBCL is distinctly more proliferative than the antecedent FL and another in which there is no change in proliferation.[143,144] Of note, *p53* mutation and *p16* inactivation are confined to cases in which transformation is accompanied by increased proliferation.[143]

Mantle Cell Lymphoma (MCL)

With a median age of 65 years at diagnosis, mantle cell lymphoma (MCL) is a disorder of the elderly, with males accounting for roughly 90% of cases.[36,145] Although MCL accounts for only 5% to 10% of all lymphoma diagnoses, it contributes disproportionately to lymphoma deaths because of its often aggressive clinical course and lack of curative therapy; median survival with MCL is only 3 years.[146] Histologically, two forms of MCL can be distinguished, one with "classic" morphology and the other with a "blastoid" morphology that is associated with a worse prognosis (see Fig. 75–9).[145,147,148] As detailed below, these histologic variants correspond to different rates of tumor cell proliferation. MCL is derived in the vast majority of cases from a naive pre–germinal center B cell because its rearranged immunoglobulin genes are unmutated. However, some cases with mutated immunoglobulin loci have recently been described that seem to have a more indolent clinical course.[149]

Deregulation of Cyclin D1 by Chromosomal Translocation

The genetic hallmark of MCL is the chromosomal translocation t(11; 14) (q13; q32) that juxtaposes the *CCND1* gene to the IgH locus, leading to overexpression of the cell cycle regulator cyclin D1. The three D-type cyclins (D1, D2, and D3) play an important role in cellular proliferation by propelling cells from G_1 to S phase of the cell cycle. Each forms heterodimers with the cyclin-dependent kinases CDK4 and CDK6, thus forming active kinase complexes.[150] These complexes inactivate the tumor suppressor retinoblastoma protein (RB) by phosphorylation, thereby inhibiting its activity as a molecular brake on G1- to S-phase progression.[145,151] Of equal importance, cyclin D-CDK4/6 complexes bind stoichiometrically to p27kip1, an inhibitor of cyclin E-CDK2 complexes. This sequestration of p27kip1 allows the cyclin E-CDK2 complexes to drive entry into S phase. Cyclin D1 is not expressed at appreciable levels in normal B cells and thus the t(11;14) significantly alters cell cycle regulation in MCLs.

Gene Expression Profiling

An extensive gene expression signature distinguishes MCL from other forms of NHL, which undoubtedly imparts a unique biology on this malignancy (Fig. 75–10).[152] Interestingly, rare NHL cases have this characteristic signature but lack both the t(11;14) translocation expression and cyclin D1 expression.[153] Instead, these cases express either cyclin D2 or D3 and, in some cases, bear a translocation involving the cyclin D2 gene.[154] These findings emphasize the primacy of D-type cyclins in the pathogenesis of MCL. Another important gene expressed at high levels in most MCLs is *BCL2*. Although MCLs lack *BCL2* translocations, they express *BCL2* mRNA and protein at levels that equal or surpass those in t(14;18) GCB DLBCL. Such high expression of this antiapoptotic gene may confer sensitivity to BCL-2-targeted therapies.[155,156]

Gene expression profiling can also be used to predict the length of survival following diagnosis of MCL.[152] A proliferation signature that reflects tumor cell proliferation rate is a strong predictor of overall survival, with high expression of the signature associated with shorter survival. This signature includes genes involved in cell cycle control, DNA synthesis, DNA repair, and other cellular processes that need to be upregulated to enable cellular proliferation to proceed. The average expression of the proliferation signature can be used to calculate a survival predictor score for each patient with MCL. In a study of 91 MCL patients, patients were ranked according to these scores and divided into four equal quartile groups, with median

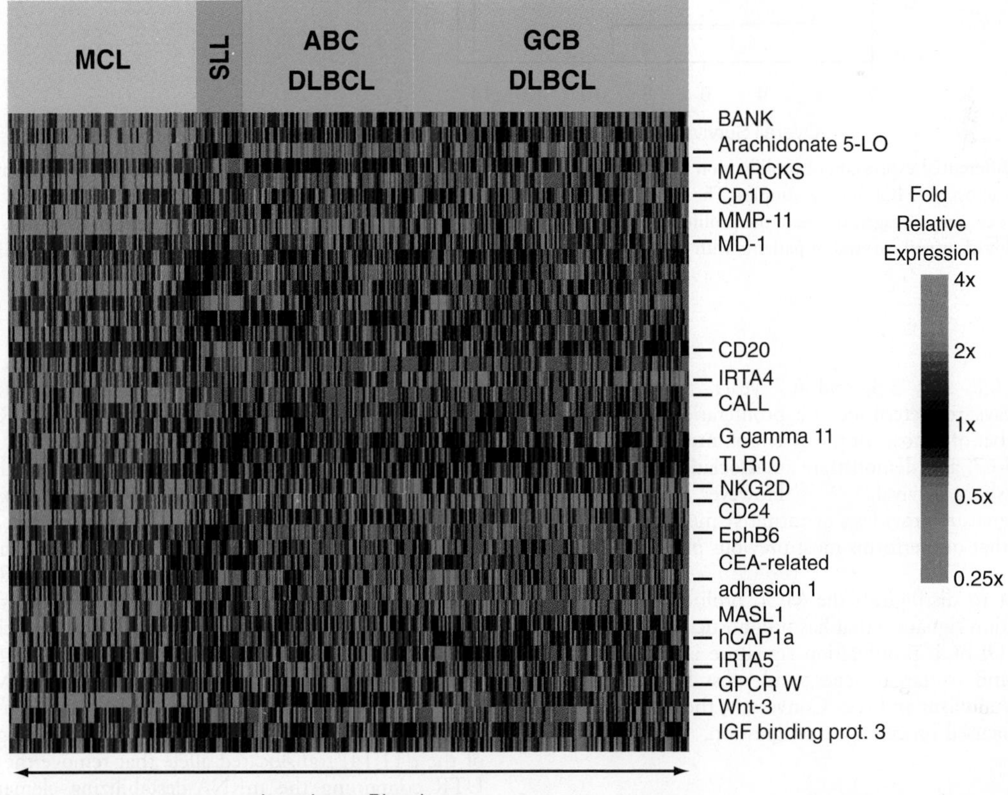

Figure 75–10 Hierarchical clustering of expression measurements from 42 Mantle cell lymphoma (MCL) signature genes that are more highly expressed in MCL samples compared to SLL, ABC DLBCL, and GCB DLBCL samples. Each column represents a single lymphoma specimen, and each row represents expression of a single gene. Red squares indicate increased expression and green squares indicate decreased expression relative to the median expression level according to the color scale shown.

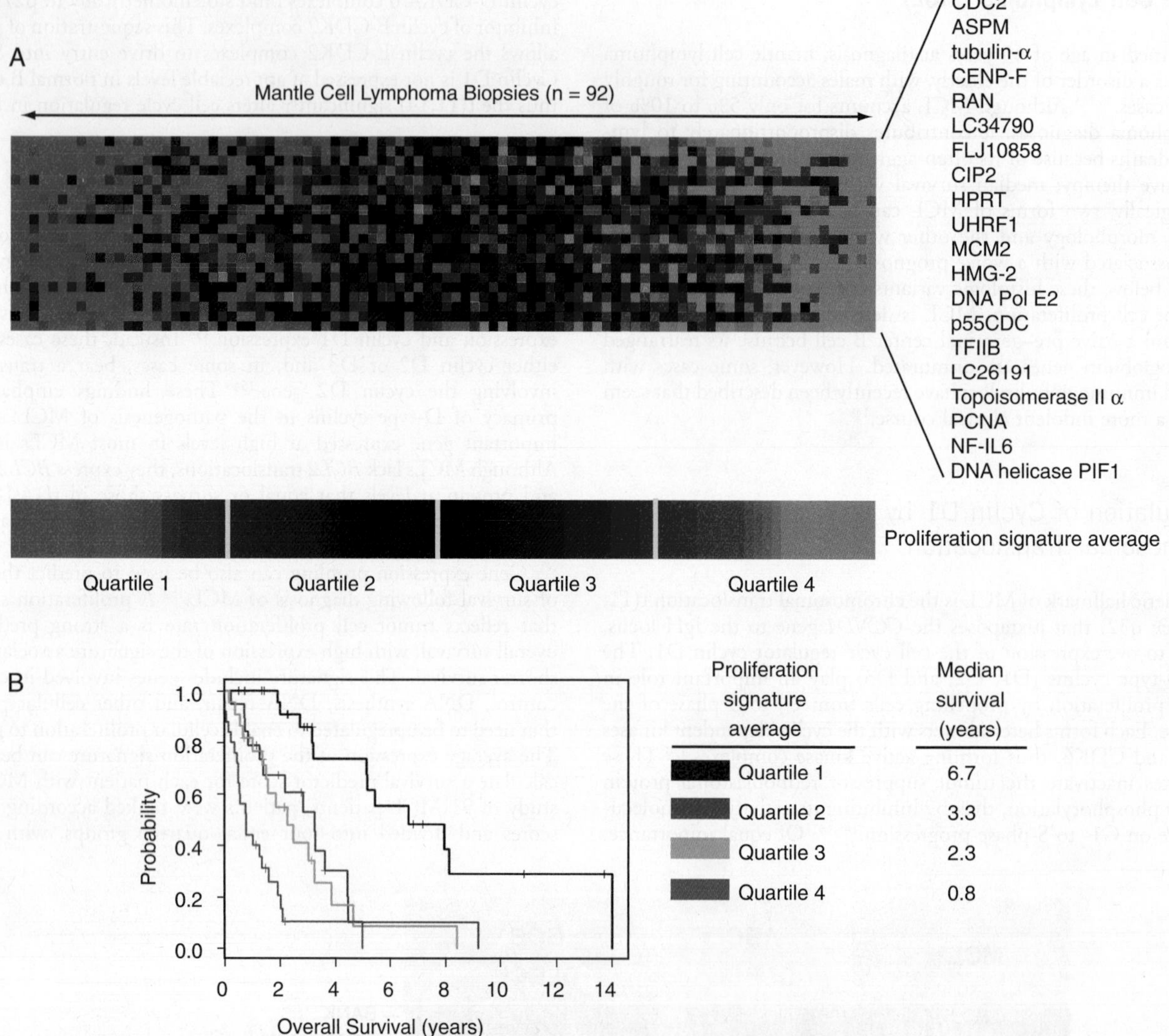

Figure 75–11 **A**, Differential expression of proliferation signature genes in samples from MCL. The expression patterns of 20 genes from the proliferation signature are shown across 92 MCL biopsy samples. The expression of each of these genes was found to be associated with short survival. The expression levels of these 20 genes were averaged to create the proliferation signature average, which was divided into four quartile groups as shown. **B**, Kaplan–Meier plot of overall survival of patients with MCL, divided into four quartile groups according to the expression of the proliferation signature in their tumors.

survival rates of 0.8, 2.3, 3.3, and 6.7 years, respectively (Fig. 75–11). Other ways to determine the proliferation rate, such as counting the number of mitoses or the extent of immunohistochemical staining for Ki-67, also demonstrate an association between high proliferation and short survival.[147,157–159] However, the proliferation gene expression signature provides a quantitative measurement of the proliferation rate that outperforms most previous prognostic tests in MCL.

It is important to distinguish the MCL proliferation signature from the proliferation signature that has prognostic value in DLBCL (see above). The DLBCL proliferation signature is primarily composed of c-myc and its target genes, and most likely reflects an increase in cell metabolism and size. Conversely, the MCL proliferation signature is focused on cell cycle progression.

Additional Genetic Abnormalities

Many recurrent genetic alterations in MCL target the G1–S phase of the cell cycle, and their combined action is reflected in the proliferation signature.[152] One of the most illustrative examples involves Cyclin D1 itself. Though most MCLs bear a t(11;14) translocation that deregulates *Cyclin D1*, levels of *Cyclin D1* mRNA differ significantly among MCL tumors. Elevated *Cyclin D1* mRNA levels are associated with both higher expression of the proliferation signature and shorter overall survival.[152] MCL tumors may express a full-length 4.5-kb mRNA isoform, termed Cyclin D1a, but also may express shorter isoforms in some cases.[160,161] Whereas the longer isoform includes an extended 3′ untranslated region (UTR) that harbors an mRNA-destabilizing element, the shorter isoforms lack the mRNA-destabilizing element and essentially only include the coding region.[161–164] Consequently, the short *Cyclin D1* mRNA isoforms are more stable and accumulate to higher levels. In MCL cases with a high proliferation rate, the short Cyclin D1 isoforms are frequently expressed.[152,164] Many of these cases have discrete genomic deletions of the t(11;14) translocated allele that remove the portion of the 3′ UTR containing the mRNA-destabilizing element.[160,161,164] Other tumors have somatically acquired point mutations that create new polyadenylation and cleavage site in the 3′ UTR of *Cyclin D1* just downstream of the coding region.[164] These events are functionally equivalent to genomic deletions in the 3′ UTR because they give rise to short mRNAs lacking the mRNA destabilizing element. Given the central role of Cyclin D1 in the G1–S phase transition of the cell cycle, it is likely that the higher expression of Cyclin D1 caused by these somatic genetic aberrations contributes directly to higher tumor proliferation.

A second common genetic alteration in MCL affecting the G1–S transition is homozygous deletion of the *INK4A-ARF* locus on chromosome band 9p21.[165,166] This locus encodes two important tumor suppressors, p16(INK4a) and p14(ARF), that share amino-terminal sequences but are unrelated in structure in their carboxy-terminal regions. p16(INK4a) prevents CDK4/6 from interacting with the D-type cyclins, resulting in a block in the cell cycle at the G1–S phase boundary.[150,167] Loss of p16(INK4a) is associated with higher expression of the proliferation signature and shorter survival.[152] MCL tumors that are highly proliferative can also have amplification and/or overexpression of *BMI1*, which encodes a chromatin repressor that can silence the *INK4A-ARF* locus.[152,168] Moreover, *CDK4* can be amplified and overexpressed in some proliferative MCLs.[169] Finally, the *RB* gene, which encodes a critical regulator of the G1–S phase transition, is mutated and inactivated in rare MCL cases with a high proliferation rate.[170]

These findings suggest that MCL tumor proliferation rate is a biological integrator of multiple oncogenic events that separately affect the G1–S phase transition.[152] Indeed, a quantitative model of the MCL proliferation rate (as measured by the proliferation signature) can be constructed using *Cyclin D1* mRNA levels and p16(INK4a) loss as variables.[152] This model suggests that these oncogenic abnormalities quantitatively alter the levels of Cyclin D1-CDK4/6, thereby causing p27kip1 to be neutralized to a varying degree in different MCL tumors. This in turn frees Cyclin E/CDK2 from p27kip1-mediated inhibition, favoring entry into S phase. In this view, the probability of progression from G1 to S phase is regulated in cycling cells as a continuous variable, not in a binary on–off fashion. In keeping with this model, essentially all of the p27kip1 in MCL tumors is physically associated with Cyclin D1 complexes.[171]

MCLs invariably delete or inactivate both p16(INK4a) and p14(ARF), unlike some other cancers that only mutate p16(INK4a), highlighting the potential role of p14(ARF) in MCL pathogenesis. p14(ARF) blocks MDM2-mediated ubiquitination of p53, leading to p53 stabilization. In addition, p14(ARF) blocks proliferation in ways that are not yet understood.[172,173] Thus, p14(ARF) could play an important role in the MCL pathogenesis in addition to p16(INK4a).

p53 mutations are associated with poor prognosis in MCL and are also associated with higher tumor proliferation.[174–177] The rationale for the specific genetic selection of p53 mutations in the more proliferative MCLs is not clear but may relate to the role that p53 plays in cellular senescence.[178,179] Senescence is a process triggered by a variety of oncogenes that limits proliferation. Of note, p16(INK4a) is also an important mediator of senescence.

Another frequently observed genetic abnormality in MCL is mutation or loss of the *ATM* gene, which is detected in 40% to 75% of MCL cases.[152,177,180,181] ATM plays a central role in the cellular response to DNA damage and ATM inactivation is associated with a high frequency of chromosomal aberrations, suggesting that these mutations, at least in part, might be responsible for chromosomal instability of MCL. *ATM* mutations are not associated with the proliferation status of MCL tumors, and are not associated with differences in the overall survival. Given their high frequency in MCL, *ATM* mutations are most likely early genetic events in MCL pathogenesis. The role of *ATM* inactivation in MCL is likely to be unrelated to p53 because *ATM* mutations are not associated with higher MCL proliferation rate, unlike p53 inactivation.

The therapy of MCL remains problematic, but recently a rapamycin analogue has shown clinical activity as a single agent, suggesting a role for the mTOR pathway in this lymphoma type.[182] The protein kinase mTOR lies downstream of signaling by PI-3 kinase and AKT kinase, and controls cellular utilization of nutrients.[183] Phosphorylation and activation of AKT is present in the majority of proliferative MCLs.[184] Furthermore, *PTEN*, a lipid phosphatase that controls PI-3 kinase activation, is recurrently mutated, deleted, or silenced in MCL.[184] Therefore, the activity of rapamycin analogues in MCL may be based on the underlying genetic abnormalities in the PTEN-PI3 kinase-AKT-mTOR pathway.

PERSPECTIVES

This chapter is not meant to exhaustively describe known biological mechanisms in lymphomas but rather emphasize biological themes pertinent to multiple lymphoma subtypes:

1. Quantitative molecular analysis of tumor specimens provides a molecular diagnosis that can define biologically distinct subgroups and reveal the differential engagement of oncogenic pathways. Certain diagnostic distinctions, such as between BL and DLBCL, cannot be made reliably by conventional pathologic methods but are readily distinguished by gene expression profiling. In DLBCL, gene expression profiling has revealed at least three diseases that arise from different stages of normal B-cell development and require distinct genetic aberrations to become malignant. Other diagnostic categories, like MCL, appear to represent single diseases. Nonetheless, gene expression profiling has uncovered signatures of biological pathways that account for differences in survival among patients with the same diagnosis. The logical conclusion from these observations is that quantitative technologies such as gene expression profiling have the potential to greatly enhance the diagnosis and treatment of lymphoma patients. Incorporation of these technologies into clinical trials should help elucidate the molecular differences between responders and nonresponders.
2. Lymphomas interact critically with their microenvironment. In both DLBCL and FL, gene expression signatures of nonmalignant cells in tumor biopsies are strong predictors of survival. These clinical correlations suggest that lymphomas vary in the manner and extent to which they interact with immune cells and stromal cells in their microenvironment. Furthermore, many lymphoma types may depend upon stimulation by either self or foreign antigens. In certain notable cases, such as in marginal zone lymphomas, eradication of the foreign antigen can cure the malignancy.[185–187] In the future, it will be important to model these cell–cell interactions in vitro and in mouse models because this may yield new perspectives on how to interfere with lymphoma biology therapeutically.
3. Pathway-targeted agents hold great promise for the treatment of lymphoma. Inhibitors of the NF-κB pathway may prove active in ABC DLBCL, PMBL, HL (Hodgkin lymphoma), MALT lymphoma, and T cell lymphomas.[30] Inhibitors of B-cell receptor signaling may be toxic for lymphoma types that are stimulated by antigens in their microenvironment, potentially including FL. Such inhibitors may target a wider range of lymphomas given the dependence of normal B cells on tonic B-cell receptor signaling.[188] BCL-2 inhibitors are exciting new agents for those lymphomas with high expression of BCL-2, including t(14;18)-positive GCB DLBCL, ABC DLBCL, MCL, and small lymphocytic lymphoma.

Given the rapid progress that has been made toward a molecular understanding of lymphoma pathogenesis, it seems likely that rational and patient-specific treatments of lymphoma will become a clinical reality.

SUGGESTED READINGS

Adams JM, Cory S: The Bcl-2 apoptotic switch in cancer development and therapy. Oncogene 26:1324, 2007.

Dave SS, Fu K, Wright GW, et al: Molecular diagnosis of Burkitt's lymphoma. N Engl J Med 354:2431, 2006.

Davies AJ, Rosenwald A, Wright G, et al: Transformation of follicular lymphoma to diffuse large B-cell lymphoma proceeds by distinct oncogenic mechanisms. Br J Haematol 136:286, 2007.

Hacker H, Karin M: Regulation and function of IKK and IKK-related kinases. Sci STKE 2006:re13, 2006.

Iqbal J, Greiner TC, Patel K, et al: Distinctive patterns of BCL6 molecular alterations and their functional consequences in different subgroups of diffuse large B-cell lymphoma. Leukemia 11:2332, 2007.

Jost PJ, Ruland J: Aberrant NF-κB signaling in lymphoma: Mechanisms, consequences and therapeutic implications. Blood 109(7):2700, 2007.

Lenz G, Nagel I, Siebert R, et al: Aberrant immunoglobulin class switch recombination and switch translocations in activated B cell-like diffuse large B cell lymphoma. J Exp Med 204:633, 2007.

Ngo VN, Davis RE, Lamy L, et al: A loss-of-function RNA interference screen for molecular targets in cancer. Nature 441:106, 2006.

Nyman H, Adde M, Karjalainen-Lindsberg ML, et al: Prognostic impact of immunohistochemically-defined germinal centre phenotype in diffuse large B-cell lymphoma patients treated with immunochemotherapy. Blood 109(11):4930, 2007.

Pasqualucci L, Compagno M, Houldsworth J, et al: Inactivation of the PRDM1/BLIMP1 gene in diffuse large B cell lymphoma. J Exp Med 203:311, 2006.

Pinyol M, Bea S, Pla L, et al: Inactivation of RB1 in mantle cell lymphoma detected by nonsense-mediated mRNA decay pathway inhibition and microarray analysis. Blood 109(12):5422, 2007.

Sagaert X, de Paepe P, Libbrecht L, et al: Forkhead box protein P1 expression in mucosa-associated lymphoid tissue lymphomas predicts poor prognosis and transformation to diffuse large B-cell lymphoma. J Clin Oncol 24:2490, 2006.

Schulze-Luehrmann J, Ghosh S: Antigen-receptor signaling to nuclear factor kappa B. Immunity 25:701, 2006.

Rawlings DJ, Sommer K, Moreno-Garcia ME: The CARMA1 signalosome links the signalling machinery of adaptive and innate immunity in lymphocytes. Nat Rev Immunol 6:799, 2006.

Tam W, Gomez M, Chadburn A, et al: Mutational analysis of PRDM1 indicates a tumor-suppressor role in diffuse large B-cell lymphomas. Blood 107:4090, 2006.

Wahlin BE, Sander B, Christensson B, et al: CD8+ T-cell content in diagnostic lymph nodes measured by flow cytometry is a predictor of survival in follicular lymphoma. Clin Cancer Res 13:388, 2007.

Wiestner A, Tehrani M, Chiorazzi M, et al: Point mutations and genomic deletions in Cyclin D1 create stable truncated mRNAs that are associated with increased proliferation rate and shorter survival. Blood 109(11):4599, 2007.

REFERENCES

For complete list of references log onto www.expertconsult.com

CHAPTER 76

PATHOBIOLOGY OF HODGKIN LYMPHOMA

Stefano A. Pileri, Brunangelo Falini, Claudio Agostinelli, and Harald Stein

INTRODUCTION

Hodgkin disease is a lymphoid tumor that represents approximately 1% of all de novo neoplasms occurring every year worldwide. Its diagnosis is based on the identification of characteristic multinucleated giant cells within an inflammatory milieu. These cells—termed Reed-Sternberg (RS) or diagnostic cells—correspond to the body of the tumor: they measure 20 to 60 μm in diameter and display a large rim of cytoplasm and at least two nuclei with acidophilic or amphophilic nucleoli, covering more than 50% of the nuclear area (Fig. 76–1). The population of cells within the tumor also includes a variable number of mononuclear elements—Hodgkin (H) cells—showing similar cytological features to RS cells and neoplastic cell variants, each in relation to a specific subtype of Hodgkin disease. Molecular studies have recently shown that in most if not all cases, RS cells, Hodgkin cells, and cell variants actually belong to the same clonal population, which is derived from peripheral B and T lymphocytes in approximately 98% and 2% of cases respectively.[1–10] Accordingly, Hodgkin disease has been included among malignant lymphomas and the term *Hodgkin lymphoma* (HL) has come into use.[6,11,12]

Although regarded as diagnostic, Hodgkin and RS (H&RS) cells are not exclusive of HL, because similar elements may be observed in reactive lesions (such as infectious mononucleosis), B- and T-cell lymphomas, carcinomas, melanomas, or sarcomas.[13] Thus, the presence of an appropriate cellular background—along with the results of immunophenotyping—is basic for the diagnosis. The reactive milieu—which can even represent 99% of the whole examined population—consists of small lymphocytes, histiocytes, epithelioid histiocytes, neutrophils, eosinophils, plasma cells, fibroblasts, and vessels in different proportions depending on the histological subtype of HL. It is sustained by autocrine and/or paracrine production of cytokines including IL-1, -2, -5, -6, -7, -8, -9, -10, -13, TNF-α, GM-CSF, M-CSF, TGF-β, bFGF, VEGF, MCP-1, MIP-1α, MIP-1β, IP10, MIG, TARC, CD70, CD80, and CD86.[14–23] In addition, various numbers of H&RS cells may express cytokine receptors, such as CD30, CD40, IL-2R (CD25/CD122), IL-3R (CD123), IL-6R (CD126), IL-7R (CD127), IL-13R (CD213), TNF-R (CD120), TGF-βR (CD105/endoglin), M-CSF-R (CD115), SCF-R (CD117/c-kit receptor), and FasL (CD178)[14,15,19,20,24–26]; chemokine receptors and their ligands (eg, CXCR6, CCR10, CXCL 16, and CCL28)[27]; and receptor tyrosine kineses (see PDGFRα, DDR2, EPHB1, RON, TRKA, and TRKB).[28] The release of these molecules is also responsible for the characteristics of the nonneoplastic component[29,30] and most of the symptoms recorded in HL patients as well as for the growth and immunosurveillance escape of neoplastic cells. It has also been proposed that hepatocyte growth factor (HGF) and its receptor (c-MET) might constitute an additional signaling pathway between RSC and the reactive cellular background, affecting adhesion, proliferation, and survival of H&RS cells.[31]

HISTOPATHOLOGIC CLASSIFICATION

In 1832, Sir Thomas Hodgkin provided the first description of the process in a paper entitled "On Some Morbid Appearances of the Absorbent Glands and Spleen."[32] In 1898 and 1902, Carl Sternberg and Dorothy Reed independently described the typical "diagnostic" cells.[33,34] In 1944, Jackson and Parker proposed the first comprehensive classification of the tumor (Table 76–1).[35] This classification, however, was subsequently found to be clinically irrelevant, because most patients belonged to the granulomatous subtype and the response to therapy greatly differed from case to case.

In 1956, Smetana and Cohen identified a histopathologic variant of granulomatous Hodgkin disease, provided with a better prognosis and characterized by sclerotic changes[36]: this variant was termed "nodular sclerosis Hodgkin disease" in the classification proposed by Lukes, Butler, and Hicks in 1964 (Table 76–1).[37] The latter classification, simplified at the Rye Conference in 1965, (Table 76–1) was routinely used for some decades, because of the high inter- and intrapersonal reproducibility and satisfying clinicopathologic correlations.[38]

In 1994, in the light of morphologic, phenotypic, genotypic, and clinical findings, HL was listed in the Revised European-American Lymphoma (REAL) classification[39] and subdivided into two main types: lymphocyte-predominant (LP-HL) and classical HL. The latter further included the following subtypes: (a) nodular sclerosis classical HL, (b) mixed cellularity classical HL, (c) lymphocyte depletion classical HL, and (d) lymphocyte-rich classical HL (Table 76–1). In 2001, this approach was adopted by the World Health Organization (WHO) (Table 76–1), which promoted lymphocyte-rich classical HL from provisional entity to accepted entity.[40] On this occasion, the concept of lymphocyte-rich classical HL has been expanded by including a nodular form of the process, as proposed by the European Lymphoma Task Force.[41]

It is worthy of note that HL subtyping should be performed only in lymph node biopsies at the onset of the disease: in fact, chemo- and/or radiotherapy actually modify the histopathologic picture by inducing a lymphocyte-depleted pattern.

LYMPHOCYTE-PREDOMINANT HODGKIN LYMPHOMA

LP-HL represents 4% to 5% of all HL cases[42] and significantly differs from the classical type in terms of morphology, phenotype, genotype, and clinical behavior (Table 76–2). The only feature shared by LP-HL and classical HL is the low amount of neoplastic cells. For a long time, following the Rye Conference, the tumor was also called "nodular paragranuloma," a designation adopted by the Kiel Group[43] based on the term *paragranuloma* introduced much earlier by Jackson and Parker.[35] This designation intended to underline the differences existing between this type of HL and the remaining ones.

Clinicopathologic Findings

LP-HL displays features that are not generally encountered in classical HL and make its behavior closer to that of "indolent" B-cell lymphomas.[44] First of all, it has a unimodal age distribution, with a single peak in the fourth decade, which contrasts with the two peaks usually observed in classical HL.[44] The disease most often affects a single node rather than groups of nodes. Bone-marrow involvement is only occasionally found during staging procedures in patients whose disease appears to be limited to a single node[44]: this pattern of spread differs from the orderly progression classically seen in classical

Lymphocyte-Predominant Hodgkin Lymphoma

Growth pattern:
Nodular (80% of cases)
Diffuse (20% of cases)
Characteristics of neoplastic cells:
Lymphohistiocytic/popcorn cells scattered, but easily found
Hodgkin and Reed–Sternberg cells rare
B-cell phenotype (CD20$^+$, CD79a$^+$, J-chain$^{+/-}$)
CD45$^+$
EMA$^{+/-}$
CD30$^-$
CD15$^-$
LSP1$^-$
TARC$^-$
IgD$^+$/CD38$^+$/IgM$^-$/CD27$^-$ in 27% of cases (corresponding to a subgroup of young male patients presenting with laterocervical lymphadenopathy)
Signaling molecule expression: Fyn$^+$, Syk$^+$, BLNK$^+$, PLC-gamma2$^+$
Transcription factor expression: BASP$^+$, Bcl-6$^+$, Oct-2$^+$, PU.1$^+$, BOB.1$^+$
Follicular dendritic cell meshwork in the nodular form
IgV$_H$ gene status: clonal rearrangements with somatic mutations (ongoing in approximately 50% of cases)
Aberrant somatic hypermutations of PIM1, PAX5, RhoH/TTF, or c-MYC gene in 80% of cases (two or more genes mutated in 50% of cases)
Recurrent genomic imbalances
No correlation with Epstein–Barr virus infection
Normal counterpart: germinal center cell
Reactive milieu:
Small B-lymphocytes in the nodular form
CD57$^+$ T-cell rosettes around neoplastic cells in the nodular form
T lymphocytes predominant in the diffuse form
Possible association with diffuse large B-cell lymphoma
Differential diagnosis with T cell-rich B-cell lymphoma and lymphocyte-rich classical Hodgkin lymphoma.

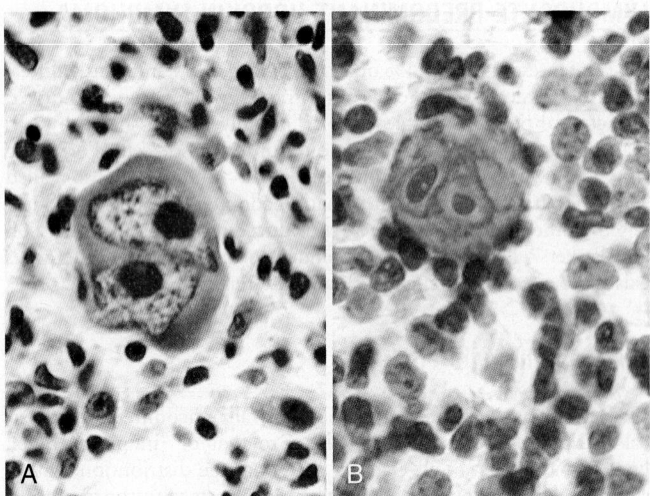

Figure 76–1 A characteristic diagnostic Reed–Sternberg cell (**A**) measuring up to 60 μm shows prominent inclusion-like nucleoli (hematoxylin and eosin, ×800). Another Reed–Sternberg cell (**B**) strongly expressing CD30 is contained within an inflammatory milieu (APAAP technique, Gill hematoxylin counterstain, ×500).

Table 76–1 Approaches Used to Classify Hodgkin Lymphoma

Jackson and Parker Classification (1944)
1. Paragranuloma 2. Granuloma 3. Sarcoma
Lukes and Butler Classification (1964)
1. Lymphocytic and/or histiocytic, nodular 2. Lymphocytic and/or histiocytic, diffuse 3. Nodular sclerosis 4. Mixed cellularity 5. Diffuse fibrosis 6. Reticular
Rye Conference Classification (1965)
1. Lymphocyte predominance 2. Nodular sclerosis 3. Mixed cellularity 4. Lymphocytic depletion
REAL/WHO Classification (1994/2001)
1. Lymphocyte predominance, nodular or diffuse 2. Classical Hodgkin lymphoma: - Lymphocyte-rich classical HL* - Nodular sclerosis (grades 1 and 2) - Mixed cellularity - Lymphocyte depletion

*This form—regarded as a provisional entity in the REAL Classification—includes a nodular (common) and a diffuse (rare) form in the WHO scheme.

HL.[45] Involvement of the thymus is uncommon, unlike the other types of HL.[44] The tumor has a very indolent course with prolonged disease-free intervals, despite a high rate of late relapses, which usually respond well to therapy.[44,46] The benign nature of these relapses and the incidence of delayed treatment-related toxicity have raised questions about the need for an aggressive upfront approach and prompt to the search for novel targeted therapies.[47] At times, LP-HL can be associated with diffuse large B-cell lymphoma: most authors think that the latter behaves more favorably than de novo forms, although conflicting data have been reported.[44,48,49] All these findings per se justify a distinction between LD-HL and classical HL, a concept that is further supported by morphologic and phenotypic data (see also the following morphologic findings and phenotypic findings sections).

Morphologic Findings

In most instances, the growth is—at least in part—nodular (Fig. 76–2).[39,40,44] The detection of a diffuse variant of the process is rare and usually corresponds to the histological progression of a nodular form.[39,40,45,50] Interestingly, Fan et al have proposed a subclassification of LP-HL, based on the prevalent growth pattern: classic nodular, serpiginous or interconnected nodular, nodular with prominent extranodular neoplastic cells, nodular with T cell-rich background, diffuse with T cell-rich background, and diffuse with B cell-rich background.[51] The neoplastic population consists of large elements, called L&H (lymphohistiocytic) or "popcorn" cells.[39,40,44] Although commonly used in the literature, the term L&H is actually incorrect in the light of the definitely proven lymphoid origin of the tumoral elements.[2–7] L&H/popcorn cells show nuclei resembling those of centroblasts, with polylobated profile, finely dispersed chromatin and small nucleoli, that are more often adjacent to the nuclear membrane (Fig. 76–3).[39,40,44] Their cytoplasmic rim is narrow and moderately basophilic at Giemsa staining. Occasionally, neoplastic elements display the features of H&RS cells and/or of lacunar cells of nodular sclerosis classical HL and are associated with minimal sclerosis[39,40,44]:

Table 76–2 Differential Diagnoses Between T Cell-Rich Large B-Cell Lymphoma, Lymphocyte Predominant Hodgkin Lymphoma, and Classical Hodgkin Lymphoma

Diagnostic criteria	TCRBCL	LP-HL Nodular/diffuse	CHL
Neoplastic component			
Cell distribution	Dispersed	Within the nodules (n)	Dispersed
L&H/L&H-like cells	–/+	+	–
RS/RS-like cells	–/+	Rare	+
CD45 expression	+	+	–
CD30 expression	–*	–*	+
CD15 expression	–	–	+/–
CD79a expression	+/–	+	Rare
CD20 expression	+**	+**	–/+
BOB.1 expression	+	+	Rare
Oct-2 expression	+***	+***	–*
PU.1 expression	–	+	–*
LSP1 expression	+	–	+
IgD expression	–	–/+	–
CD3 expression	–	–	Rare
EMA expression	+/–	+/–	Rare
J-Chain expression	+/–	+/–	–
TARC expression	–	–	+
EBV	–	–	+/– or –/+
Ig gene rearrangement	+	+	+#
CGH: number of genomic imbalances	4.7	10.8	NE
CGH: distribution of genomic imbalances	1–5	6–22	NE
Reactive component in each case			
T lymphocytes	Numerous	Moderate (n)	Variable
T cells with irregular nuclei	Numerous	Absent	Variable
Bcl-6+/CD57+ rosettes	Absent	Numerous (n)	Absent
TIA-1+ cells	Numerous	Rare (n)	Numerous
CD20+ small lymphocytes	Some	Numerous (n)	Some
Histiocytes	Variable	Some	Variable
FDC	Absent	Present (n)	Variable
Clinical findings			
Stage	III/IV	I/II	I/III
B symptoms	+/–	–	–/+
Bone-marrow involvement	+/–	–	–
Orderly progression in the spread	–	–	+
Aggressiveness	High	Low	Variable

CGH, comparative genomic hybridization; CHL, classical Hodgkin lymphoma; EBV, Epstein–Barr virus; EMA, epithelial membrane antigen; FDC, follicular dendritic cells; LP-HL, lymphocyte predominant Hodgkin lymphoma; TCRBCL, T cell-rich large B-cell lymphoma.

Note: +, 70% to 100% of cases positive; +/–, 40% to 70% of cases positive; –/+, 10% to 40% of cases positive. Rare, 1% to 10% of cases positive; –, all cases usually negative; NE, not evaluated. n, nodular form of LP-HL.

*Weakly positive in some instances.

**Negative in rare instances.

***Usually overexpressed.

#In 1% to 2% of the cases TCR gene rearrangement.

under these circumstances, immunophenotyping plays a fundamental role for the differential diagnosis between LP-HL and lymphocyte-rich classical HL (see Table 76–2). The reactive milieu consists of small lymphocytes with some plasma cells and epithelioid elements, which at times become so numerous as to mimic a histiocyte-rich large B-cell lymphoma (see also the following differential diagnosis section).[52]

As mentioned before, sometimes diffuse large B-cell lymphoma can be concurrently or subsequently detected in patients with nodular LP-HL: when occurring in the same lymph node, the large B-cell component often surrounds LP-HL nodules.[44,53–56]

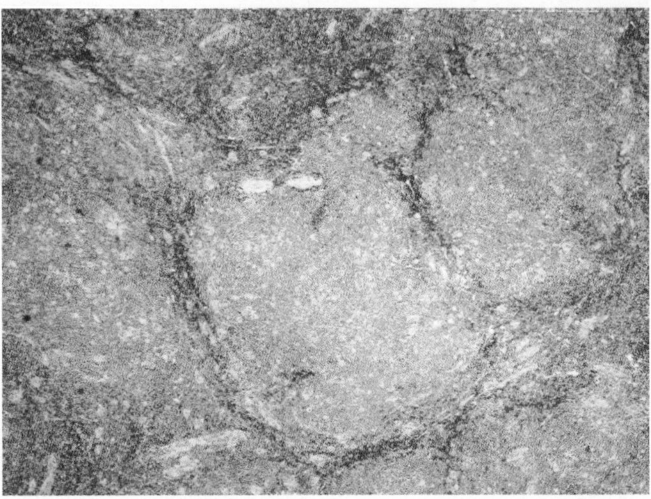

Figure 76–2 Nodular lymphocyte predominant–Hodgkin lymphoma: at panoramic view, the tumor appears as nodular densely packed cellular areas mostly consisting of small lymphocytes (Giemsa, ×40).

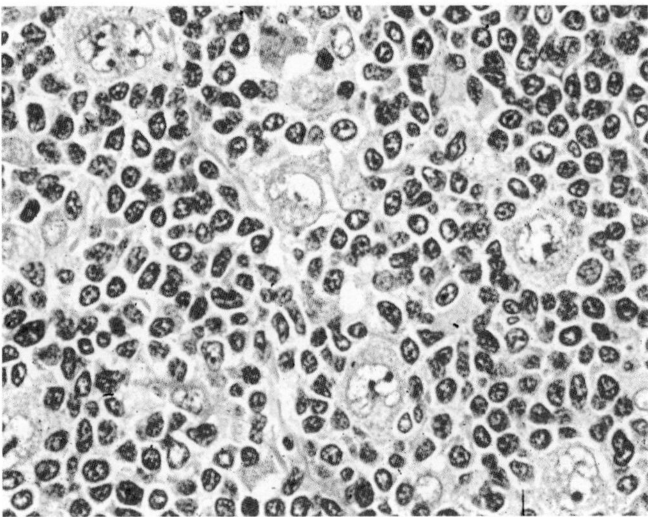

Figure 76–3 Nodular lymphocyte predominant–Hodgkin lymphoma: at closer examination, lymphohistiocytic/popcorn cells are situated among small lymphocytes (Giemsa, ×400).

PROGRESSIVELY TRANSFORMED GERMINAL CENTERS

Progressively transformed germinal centers, first described by Lennert in 1978,[57] represent a peculiar form of follicular hyperplasia, which can be confused with LP-HL.

Progressively transformed germinal centers occur in children and young adults, who have a slightly higher risk of developing LP-HL than the average population. In particular, progressively transformed germinal centers can precede, concur with, or follow LP-HL.[43,44]

On morphologic grounds, progressively transformed germinal centers are 2 to 3 times larger than reactive follicles and predominantly consist of small lymphocytes—mainly mantle cells—intermingled with some centroblasts and follicular dendritic cells (Fig. 76–4). Progressively transformed germinal centers can be differentiated from LP-HL because of the lack of L&H/popcorn elements and their cytologic composition. The latter correspond to a mixture of B (CD20+) and T (CD3+) lymphocytes, histiocytes, and follicular dendritic cells, which overall produce a "moth-eaten" appearance.[57,58]

Molecular studies highlight that progressively transformed germinal centers carry somatic hypermutation, clonal expansion, and antigen selection as classical germinal centers; however, no clonal

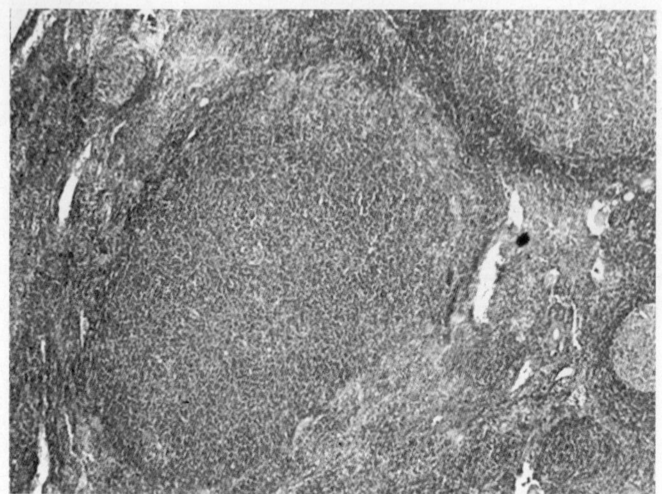

Figure 76–4 Progressively transformed germinal center: at low power, it resembles the nodules of lymphocyte predominant–Hodgkin lymphoma (Giemsa, 40×).

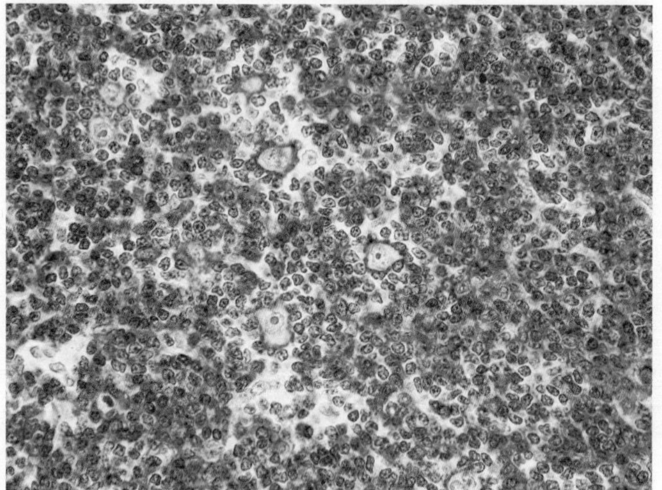

Figure 76–5 Nodular lymphocyte predominant–Hodgkin lymphoma: lymphohistiocytic/popcorn cells and most small lymphocytes within a nodule express CD20 (APAAP technique, Gill hematoxylin counterstain, ×200).

expansion across the borders of individual PTGC is found in contrast to the monoclonal pattern of nodular LP-HL.[59]

Phenotypic Findings

Neoplastic cells—that are primarily cycling as determined by the Ki-67 staining—display a distinct profile, which differs from that of classical HL.[6,39–41,44,60–66] In particular, LP-HL cells are CD45^{+}, CD20^{+}, CD79a^{+}, Bcl-6 protein^{+}, PU.1$^{+/-}$, Oct-2^{+}, BOB.1^{+}, J-chain$^{+/-}$, epithelial membrane antigen (EMA)$^{+/-\text{or}-/+}$, CD3^{-}, CD10^{-}, LSP1^{-}, and CD15^{-} (Figs. 76–5, 76–6, 76–7, and 76–8). Interestingly, CD20 may be lost following rituximab therapy.[67] Expression of Bcl-2 and CD30 is unusual and—when detected—definitely weak.[60,68] Notably, a certain number of extrafollicular reactive blasts (smaller than L&H/popcorn cells) are marked by the anti-CD30 antibodies: in the past, they have been misinterpreted as malignant elements.[41] Recently, Prakash et al have reported that in 27% of LP-HL cases, neoplastic cells express IgD and CD38 in the absence of IgM and CD27.[69] These cases seem to correspond to a distinctive subset of patients with a younger median age (21 vs 44 years), striking male predominance

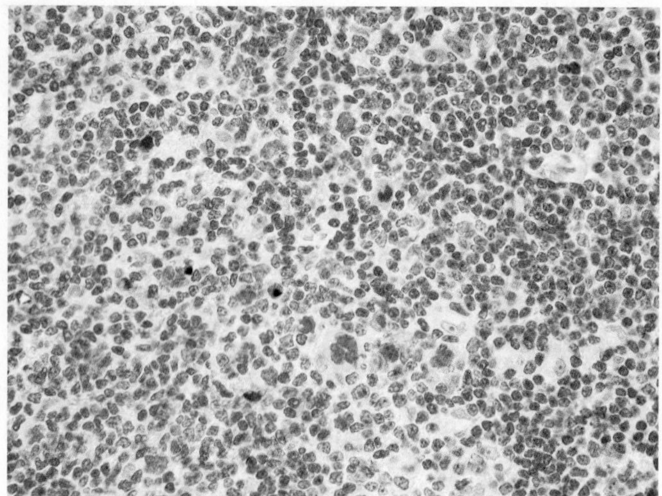

Figure 76–6 Nodular lymphocyte predominant–Hodgkin lymphoma: lymphohistiocytic/popcorn cells carry the Bcl-6 protein (APAAP technique, Gill hematoxylin counterstain, ×200).

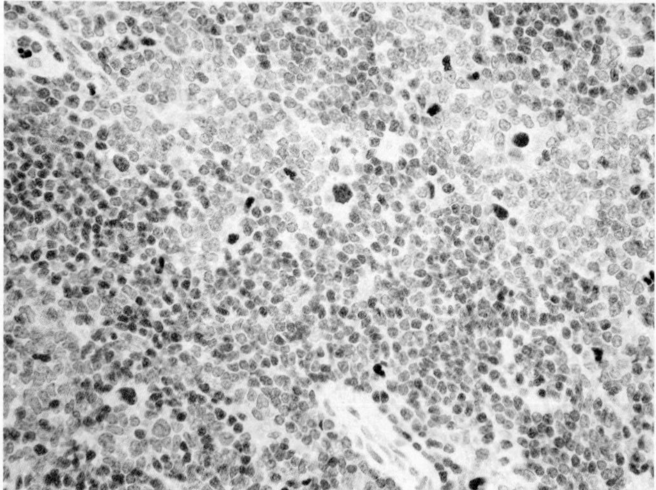

Figure 76–7 Nodular lymphocyte predominant–Hodgkin lymphoma: positivity of neoplastic elements at the determination of the PU.1 transcription factor (Envision^{+} Method, Gill hematoxylin counterstain, ×200).

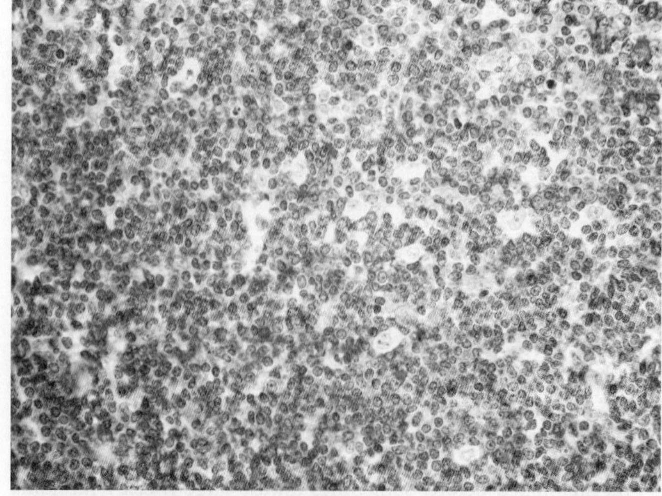

Figure 76–8 Nodular lymphocyte predominant–Hodgkin lymphoma: neoplastic cells are LSP1 negative conversely to the surrounding small lymphocytes (APAAP technique; Gill hematoxylin counterstain, ×200).

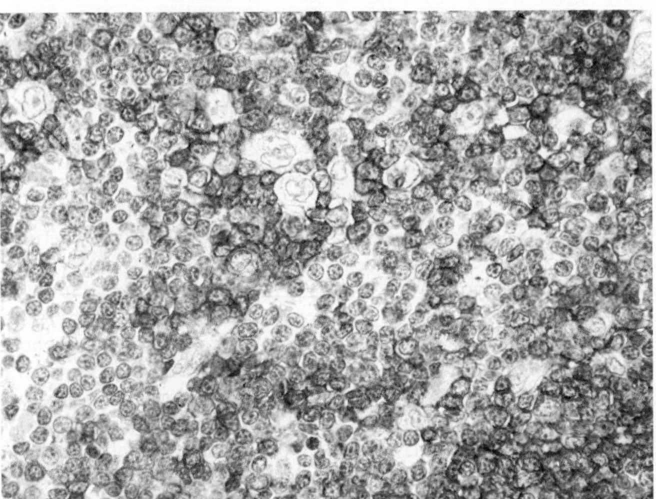

Figure 76–9 Nodular lymphocyte predominant–Hodgkin lymphoma: lymphohistiocytic/popcorn cells are surrounded by rosettes of CD57$^+$ T lymphocytes (APAAP technique, Gill hematoxylin counterstain, ×300).

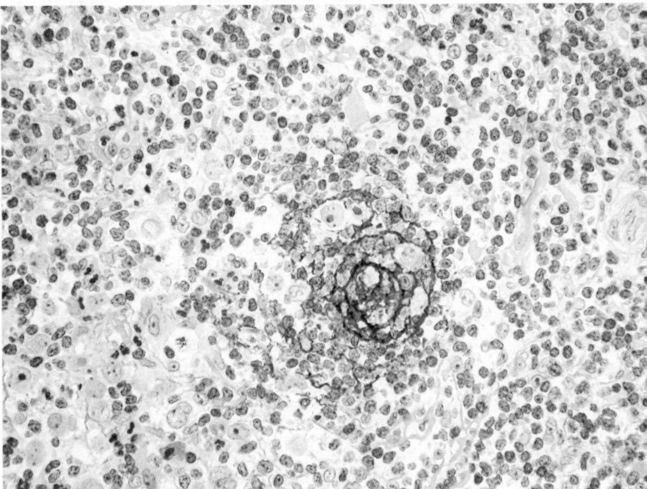

Figure 76–10 Nodular LP–Hodgkin lymphoma: delicate meshwork of CD21$^+$ follicular dendritic cells (APAAP technique, Gill hematoxylin counterstain, ×300).

(32 : 1 vs 1.5 : 1), and more frequent cervical lymph node involvement (56% vs 18.2%).[69]

Phenotypic analysis shows a series of findings that have pathobiological implications. These data support the derivation of L&H/popcorn cells from germinal-center B elements because of

1. their positivity for Bcl-6 protein, CD40, and CD86[60,70–75];
2. their close contact with rosettes of CD4$^+$/CD57$^+$ T-lymphocytes (ie, the same T-cell component found in normal germinal centers and PTGC) (Fig. 76–9)[75]; and
3. their relationship with a meshwork of FDCs (CD21$^+$/CD35$^+$), at least in the nodular form of the disease (Fig. 76–10).[76]

Second, it underlines that LP-HL is not affected by an almost complete silencing of the B-cell program, in contrast to classical HL. This is supported not only by the above-mentioned positivities for CD20, CD79a, J-chain, and transcription factors, but also by the regular detection of intracellular signaling molecules (ie, Fyn, Syk, BLNK, and PLC-gamma2) that are usually abrogated in classical HL.[77]

In the nodular form, the small lymphocyte component mainly consists of B-cell elements.[39,40,44] The progression to a diffuse form, however, is characterized by an increase in the number of T lymphocytes that can finally predominate over B cells. Some recent reports have highlighted that T lymphocytes can coexpress CD4 and CD8.[78] This finding is in keeping with the concept that a proportion of tumor-associated reactive T cells bear an activation profile.[79]

Genotypic Findings

Further evidence of the derivation of the tumor from germinal-center B cells has been provided by recent molecular studies, based on single-cell polymerase chain reaction (PCR).[1–7] These studies have shown that popcorn cells in any given case represent a monoclonal population derived from germinal-center B cells, because of the consistent occurrence of monoclonal Ig gene rearrangements and the high load of somatic hypermutations within variable-region genes. Ongoing mutations are detected in about half LP-HL cases: this finding—not observed in classical HL—identifies mutating germinal-center cells as the precursors of the neoplastic elements.[2,5] The pattern of mutation within these gene segments suggests that tumoral cells, their precursors, or both have been selected for expression of functional antigen receptors.[2,5]

A clonal relationship between the neoplastic cells of nodular LP-HL and concurrent diffuse large B-cell lymphoma was proven by Ohno and coworkers through selective microdissection of immunostained tissue sections and sequence analysis of the immunoglobulin heavy chain gene (IgH) complementary determining region (CDR) III in two cases.[56] This leads to the possible genetic similarities between LP-HL and DLBCL recently suggested by two studies.[80,81] Of these, the former shows that—besides Ig genes—the somatic hypermutation process aberrantly involves four targets (PIM1, PAX5, RhoH/TTF, c-MYC) previously identified in DLBCL.[80] The latter demonstrates recurrent rearrangement of the BCL-6 gene in 48% of LP-HL cases that involve Ig and non-Ig loci similar to those found in DLBCL.[81]

Comparative genomic hybridization studies reveal recurrent genomic imbalances in LP-HL. In particular, gain of 1, 2q, 3, 4q, 5q, 6, 8q, 11q, 12 q, and X and loss of chromosome 17 have been recorded in 36.8% to 68.4% of 19 cases analyzed by Franke and coworkers.[82]

Finally, in situ hybridization studies with EBER1/2 probes, as well as conventional Southern blot, PCR, and immunohistochemistry for the latent membrane protein-1 (LMP-1) show that the L&H/popcorn cells of LP-HD have so far never been found to be infected by Epstein–Barr virus (EBV), conversely to the neoplastic component of classical HL.[83,84] Isolated small lymphocytes belonging to the reactive background carry EBV infection in 25% of cases.[41]

Differential Diagnosis

The distinction between LP-HL, classical HL, and T-cell/histiocyte-rich large B-cell lymphoma is sometimes blurred.[41,52,76,85–88] This is not surprising if one considers that (a) LP-HL and lymphocyte-rich classical HL were in the past lumped under the generic label "lymphocyte-predominant Hodgkin disease"[41] and (b) LP-HL and T cell-rich B-cell lymphoma might share a common histogenesis.[86,87] The difficulties encountered in this field are clearly underlined by the recent proposal of three subtypes of T cell-rich B-cell lymphoma (L&H-like, centroblastic/immunoblastic-like, and RS-like) based on the morphologic and phenotypic characteristics of the neoplastic cells in individual cases.[87] Table 76–2 summarizes the main criteria to be applied to this critical differential diagnosis,[41,66,69,85,88–94] which is of paramount importance because of the dramatic differences in terms of clinical aggressiveness and therapeutic approach among the above-mentioned tumors.[95,96]

CLASSICAL HODGKIN LYMPHOMA

Classical Hodgkin lymphoma represents approximately 95% of all HL cases and shows a typical bimodal age distribution with a peak at approximately 20 years of age and a second peak in late life.[39] It is characterized by a series of clinical, morphologic, phenotypic and genotypic features, which are integrated by specific findings in the four subtypes of the process (nodular sclerosis, mixed cellularity, lymphocyte depletion, and lymphocyte-rich). Classical HL recognizes peripheral B-cell derivation in approximately 98% of cases, the remaining ones originating from peripheral T lymphocytes.[7,8]

Clinicopathologic Findings

Patients with classical HL most often present with lateral-cervical lymph node enlargement whereas peripheral extranodal involvement is definitely rare. Approximately 50% of patients are staged I or II. A mediastinal mass is observed in most nodular sclerosis classical HL cases, at times showing the characteristics of "bulky" disease. Systemic symptoms—fever, night sweats, and body weight loss—are detected in approximately 25% of patients. Conversely to what was reported in the past, the histological subtype is not regarded as a major prognostic indicator.

Morphologic Findings

In classical HL, typical RS cells (Fig. 76–1) can be easily found: their number (from few to many) differs from case to case. They may be associated with peculiar cell variants and an inflammatory background related to the histological subtype. The lymph node structure is largely effaced, although remnants of normal follicles can be detected in some cases. The type of structural alteration is indeed characteristic in nodular sclerosis classical HL.

Phenotypic Findings

In 1982, Schwab et al described a new monoclonal antibody, termed Ki-1, which seemed to specifically identify H&RS cells and a small subset of normal lymphocytes with a perifollicular location. However, with wide use, this antibody was shown not to be specific for H&RS cells, as originally thought, but to react with a variety of lymphoid tumors, including a previously unrecognized category, anaplastic large-cell lymphoma.[97–99] Following the evaluation of Ki-1, other reagents with similar characteristics have been developed[13,100] that were assessed at the III Workshop on Leukocyte Differentiation Antigens (Oxford, 1986) to form the 30th cluster of monoclonal antibodies (CD30). The target recognized by these antibodies is a glycoprotein of 120 kd, expressed by lymphoid elements following activation and formed by three distinct domains (intracytoplasmic, transmembranic, and external).[13] It is encoded by a gene located at 1p36, whose activity is modulated by the number of ATCC-repeats in the 5′ region of the promoter, and represents a member of the receptor superfamily of tumor necrosis factor (TNF).[101,102] Recently, CD30 overexpression has been reported to induce constitutive

Classical Hodgkin Lymphoma

Histotypes:
Nodular sclerosis classical Hodgkin lymphoma (grades I and II, cellular phase, syncytial)
Mixed-cellularity classical Hodgkin lymphoma (interfollicular, epithelioid cell-rich)
Lymphocyte-depleted classical Hodgkin lymphoma (fibrotic, sarcomatous)
Lymphocyte-rich classical Hodgkin lymphoma (nodular, diffuse)
Characteristics of neoplastic cells:
Typical Hodgkin and Reed–Sternberg cells easily found (predominant in the lymphocyte-depleted sarcomatous histotype)
"Lacunar" cell variants in the nodular sclerosis histotype
Mummified (apoptotic) cells possibly found
Null phenotype in most instances (CD20$^-$; CD79a$^-$; J-chain$^-$; T-cell markers$^-$)
B-cell phenotype (CD20$^+$ and more rarely CD79a) in 20% to 25% of cases
T-cell phenotype in 1% to 2% of cases
Cytoplasmic and surface immunoglobulins$^-$
CD45$^-$
EMA$^-$
CD30$^+$
CD15$^{+/-}$
LSP1$^+$
TARC$^+$
AFT3$^+$
HGAL$^{+/-}$
ALK protein$^-$
Signaling molecules expression: Fyn$^{+/-}$, Lyn$^-$, Syk$^-$, BLNK$^-$, PLC-gamma2$^-$
Transcription factor expression: BASP$^+$, IRF4$^+$, T-bet$^+$, Bcl-6$^-$, Oct-2$^-$, PU.1$^-$, BOB.1$^{-/+}$
Follicular dendritic cell meshwork partly preserved in the "follicular form" of the nodular sclerosis histotype (cellular phase)
IgV_H gene status: clonal rearrangements with somatic mutations (not ongoing), crippling in 25% of cases
Aberrant somatic hypermutations of PIM1, PAX5, RhoH/TTF or c-MYC gene in 55% of cases (2 or more genes mutated in 30% of cases)
TCR clonal rearrangements in approximately 1% of cases
Constitutive NF-κB activation
Defective cytokinesis
Recurrent chromosomal aberrations involving 2p, 4p, 8q, 9p, 12p, 14q, and 16q
Correlation with Epstein–Barr virus (EBV) infection in 20% to 40% and 50% to 75% of nodular sclerosis and mixed-cellularity cases, respectively; latency II EBV infection pattern (LMP-1$^+$, EBER1/2$^+$, EBNA2$^-$)
Normal counterpart: post–germinal-center cell?
Reactive milieu:
Small B and T lymphocytes in the lymphocyte-rich histotype
Organized fibrotic bands originating from the lymph node capsule (regularly thickened) and circumscribing nodules with variable reactive cell component in the nodular sclerosing histotype
A mixture of small lymphocytes (predominantly T), plasma cells, neutrophils, eosinophils, and histiocytes in the mixed cellularity histotype
Abundant and randomly distributed collagen fibers in the fibrotic variant of the lymphocyte-depleted histotype
A few lymphocytes in the sarcomatous variant of the lymphocyte-depleted histotype
Possible association with non-Hodgkin lymphoma (B-CCL, follicular lymphoma, extranodal marginal zone lymphoma, diffuse large B-cell lymphoma, Burkitt lymphoma, peripheral T-cell lymphoma, anaplastic large-cell lymphoma)
Differential diagnosis with anaplastic large-cell lymphoma, peripheral T-cell lymphoma, diffuse large B-cell lymphoma (including T cell-rich B-cell lymphoma and primary mediastinal large B-cell lymphoma), fibrosarcoma, malignant fibrous histiocytoma, and undifferentiated nasopharyngeal carcinoma
Possible pathologic unfavorable prognostic indicators: lymphocyte depletion; nodular sclerosis grade II; expression/overexpression of one or more of the following molecules: Bcl-2, Bax, Bcl-X_L, p53, p21, MMP-2, PCNA, and Ki-67; low and high infiltration of FOXP3$^+$ and TIA-1$^+$ cells, respectively; genes related to microenvironment, cell growth/apoptosis, and regulation of mitosis (surrogated by the following molecules: ALDH1A1, STAT1, SH2D1A, TOP2A, RRM2, PCNA, MAD2L1, and CDC2)

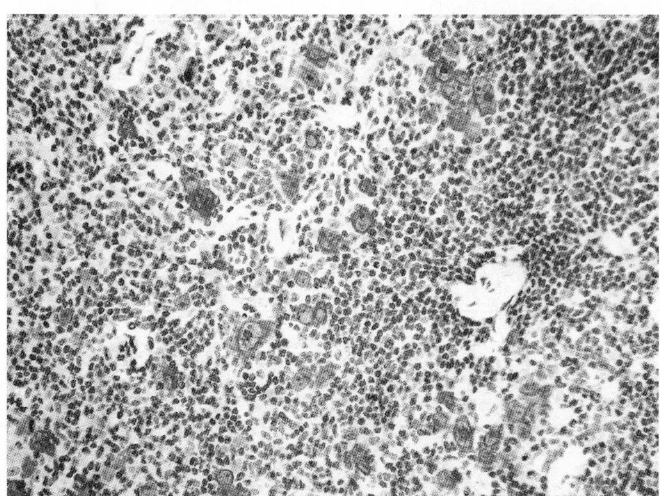

Figure 76–11 Classical Hodgkin lymphoma: Hodgkin and Reed–Sternberg cells express CD30 both at the cytoplasmic membrane level and in the Golgi area (dot-like positivity) (APAAP technique, Gill hematoxylin counterstain, ×250).

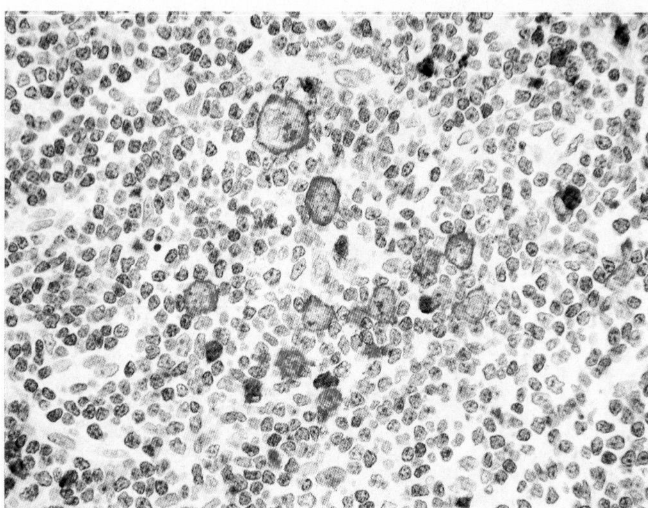

Figure 76–12 Classical Hodgkin lymphoma: neoplastic cells display CD15 membrane-bound and dot-like positivities (APAAP technique, Gill hematoxylin counterstain, ×300).

nuclear factor kappaB (NF-κB) activation (see below).[102] As expected, the CD30 ligand (CD30L) belongs to a group of molecules with homology to TNF: within the classical HL context, it seems to be mostly expressed by tissue mast cells.[103] The external domain of CD30 is cleaved by a metalloproteinase.[13] The levels of soluble CD30 have been reported to correlate with the size and extent of the tumor at presentation, thus representing a new possible prognostic indicator, independent of age, race, symptoms, and bulky disease.[104] The CD30 molecule has also been proposed as a possible therapeutic target for specific antibodies conjugated with plant toxins or iodine-131 for classical HL for therapeutic purposes: such antibodies have produced promising results in cases refractory to conventional therapies, although severe hematotoxicity has been recorded.[105–112]

Following immunohistochemical analysis both of paraffin and frozen sections, CD30 antibody staining results in different patterns: membrane-bound, dot-like in the Golgi area (corresponding to the accumulation of the 90-kd proteic precursor), and diffuse Fig. 76–11). The first two patterns are exclusive of lymphoid elements with the exception of embryonic carcinoma,[13,113,114] whereas the third one can occur in a variety of malignant tumors other than lymphomas, including pancreatic cancer, nasopharyngeal undifferentiated carcinoma, mesothelioma, and malignant melanoma.[100,114] Therefore, the immunophenotypic diagnosis of HL should always be based on the application of a panel of antibodies, including anticytokeratins, melanoma-associated antigens, CEA, and PLAP.[13] Expression of the CD30 molecule by H&RS cells is observed in more than 98% of classical HLs, although the intensity of the immunostaining can vary from case to case and even within the same case. The antigen is sensitive to fixation (especially prolonged fixation in formalin or fixation in B5): thus very efficient antigen retrieval techniques are required to achieve reliable results.[115]

CD15 is another valuable marker for H&RS cells (Fig. 76–12), which is detected in approximately 80% of cases of classical HL.[98,116] CD15 is characteristic, but not specific for H&RS cells, because it can de detected—rarely—in B- and T-cell lymphomas as well as in nonlymphoid tumors.[98,116–119] Among the antibodies available, the MMA seems to be superior for the diagnosis of classical Hodgkin lymphoma.[120]

H&RS cells usually do not express CD45 and epithelial membrane antigen (EMA), whereas B- and T-cell markers are observed in a proportion of cases.[121–130] In particular, CD20 (Fig. 76–13) is observed in 20% to 30% of examples of classical HL—usually EBV—and CD79a even more rarely.[123,126–128] Positivity for one or more T-cell markers is detected in a minority of H&RS cells (Fig. 76–14).[129,130] Under these circumstances, single-cell PCR studies

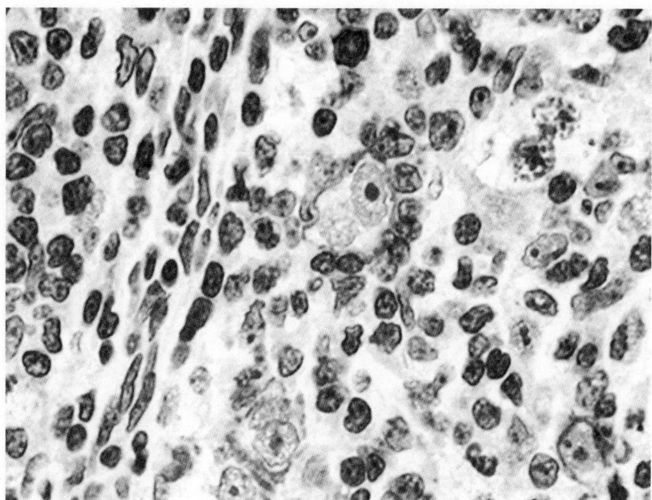

Figure 76–13 Classical Hodgkin lymphoma: Hodgkin and Reed–Sternberg elements show variable degrees of CD20 positivity (APAAP technique, Gill hematoxylin counterstain, ×500).

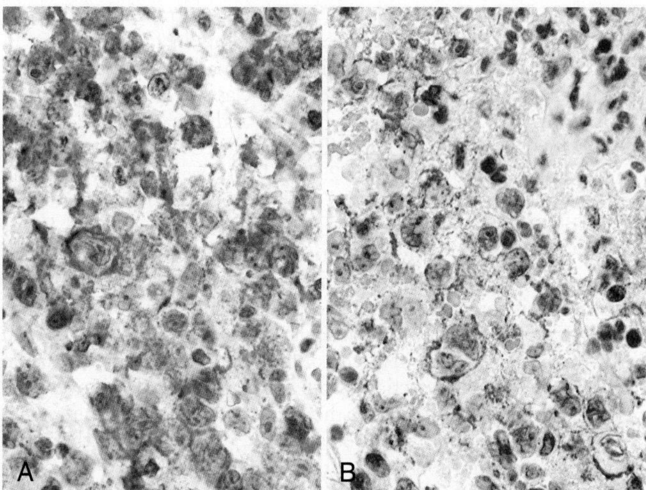

Figure 76–14 Classical Hodgkin lymphoma, sarcomatous lymphocyte-depleted type: Hodgkin and Reed–Sternberg elements express CD3 (a) and CD2 (b) (APAAP technique, Gill hematoxylin counterstain, ×300).

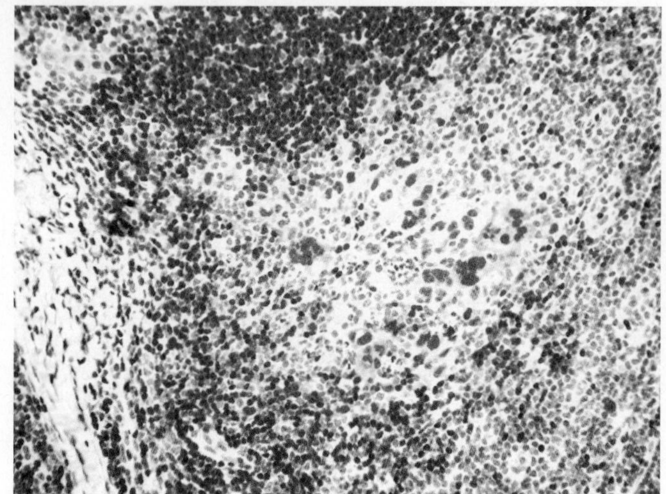

Figure 76–15 Classical Hodgkin lymphoma: neoplastic cells reveal a strong–moderate positivity for B-cell specific activator protein (BSAP); small B lymphocytes stain more intensively (APAAP technique, Gill hematoxylin counterstain, ×250).

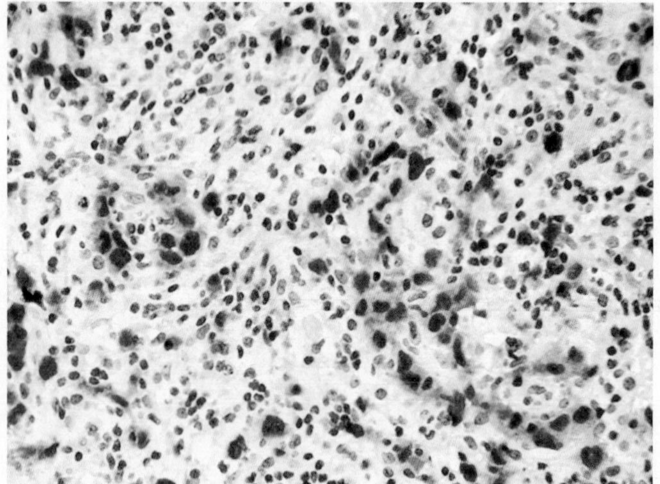

Figure 76–16 Classical Hodgkin lymphoma: Hodgkin and Reed–Sternberg cells express IRF4 (APAAP technique, Gill hematoxylin counterstain, ×250).

have so far shown T-cell receptor (TCR) gene rearrangement in only a few instances, clonal Ig gene rearrangements in fact occurring in most cases of classical HL cases with T-cell marker expression.[8,131,132] In contrast to LP-HL, the elements of classical HL are generally negative for the Bcl-6 molecule.[70,133] In addition, they are usually positive for LSP1, HGAL, PAX5/BSAP, and MUM1/IRF4 and more often negative for BOB.1, Oct-2, and PU1 (see also the following genotypic findings section) (Figs. 76–15, 76–16, 76–17 and 76–18).[7,8,61–65,70,133–136] With the exception of one case report,[132] BSAP has been found to effectively discriminate between classical HL and anaplastic large-cell lymphoma in large series of cases (for further details on this topic, see Table 76–3 and the Nodular Sclerosis Classical HL section).[137,138] In particular, this molecule is expressed throughout all the steps of B-cell differentiation, with the exclusion of plasma cells.[70] Its detection strongly favors classical HL over anaplastic large-cell lymphoma, in the light of the fact that the former recognizes B-cell origin in 98% of cases,[1–8,39,40] whereas the latter indicates—by definition—a T- or null-cell derivation.[39,40] The anaplastic (large cell) lymphoma kinase (ALK) represents another important tool for the differential diagnosis between classical HL and anaplastic large-cell lymphoma. It is expressed in 60% to 80% of cases of anaplastic large-cell lymphomas,[139–145] whereas it has not been

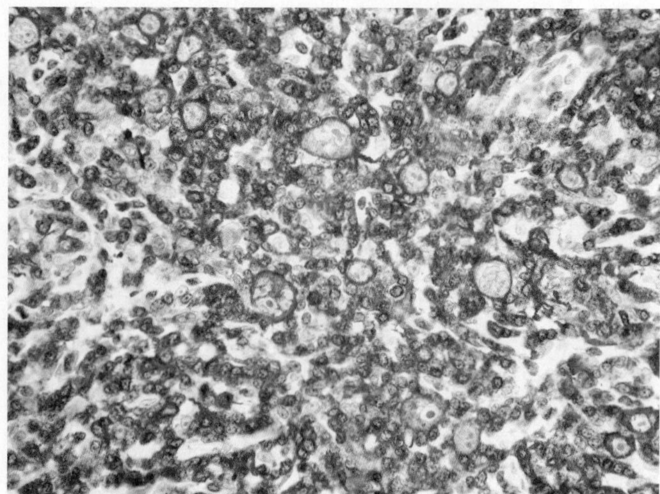

Figure 76–17 Classical Hodgkin lymphoma: neoplastic cells and reactive small lymphocytes strongly express LSP1 (APAAP technique, Gill hematoxylin counterstain, ×300).

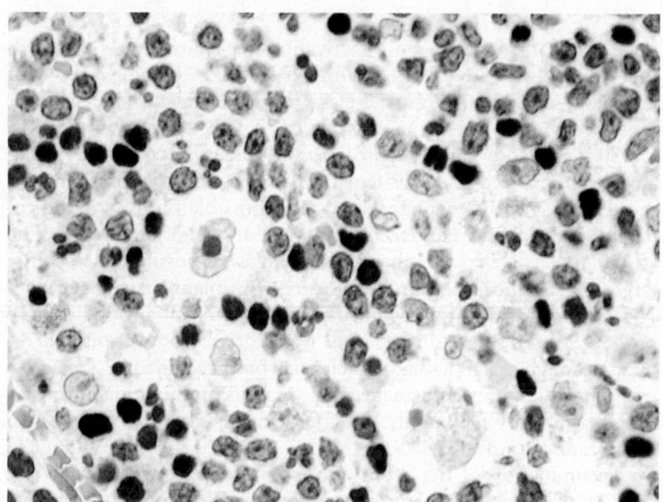

Figure 76–18 Classical Hodgkin lymphoma: Hodgkin and Reed–Sternberg cells lack the Oct-2 transcription factor; the surrounding positive small B lymphocytes represent the internal control (APAAP technique, Gill hematoxylin counterstain, ×500).

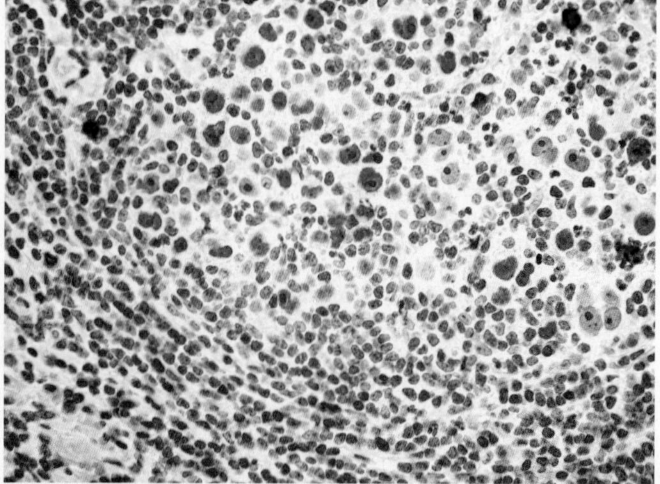

Figure 76–19 Classical Hodgkin lymphoma: neoplastic cells show p53 overexpression (APAAP technique, Gill hematoxylin counterstain, ×300).

Table 76–3 Differential Diagnosis Between Anaplastic Large-Cell Lymphoma Hodgkin-Like and Classical Hodgkin Lymphoma

	ALCL-HL	HL
Morphologic characteristics		
Neoplastic component	Usually cohesive	Usually dispersed
Reactive component	Often minor	Usually prevalent
Reed-Sternberg cells	May be present	Always present
Intrasinusoidal diffusion	Typical	Exceptional
Molecular characteristics		
CD30 expression	+	+*
CD45 expression	+/–	–
CD15 expression	–/+	+/–
EMA expression	+/–	–/+
CBF.78 positivity	+ (80–90%)	–/+ (rare cells)
BHN.9 positivity	+ (60%)**	– (5%)
TARC expression	+	–
TRAF1 expression	Rare	+
T-bet	Rare	+
CD3 expression	–/+***	Rare
B-cell marker expression	–	–/+
BSAP expression	–	+
T-rosettes	–	+/–
p53 expression	–/+	+
EBV positivity	–	+ or +/–
Clonal TCR gene rearrangement	+	–
Clonal Ig gene rearrangement	–	+
ALK protein expression	+#	–

ALCL-HL, Anaplastic large-cell lymphoma–Hodgkin lymphoma; ALK, anaplastic lymphoma kinase; EBV, Epstein–Barr virus; EMA, epithelial membrane antigen; BSAP, B-cell–specific activator protein; TARC, thymus and activation-regulated chemokine; TRAF1, tumour necrosis factor receptor–associated factor 1.

Note: +: 70% to 100% of cases positive. +/–: 40% to 70% of cases positive. /+: 10% to 40% of cases positive. Rare: 1% to 10% of cases positive. –: all cases usually negative.

*The intensity of immunostaining may vary within the same case.

**Results can vary depending on the fixative used.

***Membrane-bound and/or dot-like positivity.

#Some cases showing morphology and phenotypic profile consistent with ALCL-HL (including BSAP negativity) can lack t(2;5)/ALK protein expression: these cases need further studies to assess their definitive inclusion among anaplastic large cell lymphomas.

observed in classical HL,[146–150] with the exception of two controversial studies.[151,152] In anaplastic large-cell lymphoma, ALK overexpression is due to the synthesis of a chimeric protein caused by the occurrence of t(2;5)(2p23;5q35) or more rarely of a variant translocation, which leads to the formation of a hybrid construct between the ALK gene domain encoding for the transmembranic portion of the kinase and the promoter of another gene.[144,145,147,153,154] The latter is represented by nucleophosmin (NPM) in the classical t(2;5).[144,145,147,153] Finally, T-bet, TRAF1, and TARC are additional markers useful for the distinction between classical HL (mostly positive) and anaplastic large-cell lymphoma or diffuse large B-cell lymphoma (usually negative),[91,155,156] whereas clusterin and fascin are unreliable tools.[157,158]

It has been suggested that phenotypic findings might be of prognostic significance. In particular, the value of the following parameters was assessed in a retrospective analysis based on 1751 HL cases: CD30 expression, CD15 positivity, CD20 staining, age, sex, histotype, stage, B symptoms, Hb level, and ESR.[159] CD15-negative cases were characterized by a higher incidence of relapse ($P = 0.0022$) and a shorter survival rate ($P = 0.0035$), independently of the remaining prognostic indicators.[159] Two recent studies, one of which was based on the tissue microarray technology, have further documented that CD20 expression is prognostically relevant in cases treated between 1974 and 1980 but not in patients who received current therapeutic approaches.[127,128] Chemoresistance and tendency to relapses seem to be also influenced by the expression of molecules that determine cell proliferation, such as Bcl-2, Bax, Bcl-X_L, p53, p21, MMP-2, PCNA, and MIB-1 (Fig. 76–19).[160–164] On the whole, tumors with H&RS cells showing expression or overexpression of one or more of these molecules tend to have a poor response to treatment and/or short survival. Very recently, gene expression profiling studies (see also the following genotypic findings section) have identified eight candidate molecules (ALDH1A1, STAT1, SH2D1A, TOP2A, RRM2, PCNA, MAD2L1, and CDC) as surrogates of therapeutically relevant abnormalities related to microenvironment, cell growth/apoptosis, and regulation of mitosis.[165] In line with this, low and high infiltration of FOXP3$^+$ and TIA-1$^+$ reactive T cells respectively have been found to correlate with an unfavorable clinical course.[166]

Genotypic Findings

The origin of RS cells of Hodgkin disease has long been a mystery.[167] As previously discussed in the LP-HL section, micromanipulation of single RS cells isolated from tissue sections and PCR analysis of the cells for rearranged Ig genes have shown that the vast majority of both LP-HL and classical HL cases are of B-cell origin.[1–7] Conversely to that seen in LP-HL, ongoing mutations are not detected in classical HL,[7] including the lymphocyte-rich type.[168] This suggests that classical HL originates from a late germinal-center or post–germinal-center B cell possibly corresponding to "asteroid" cells of thymic medulla or interfollicular dendritic B cells of the lymph node.[169]

To explain the lack of Ig synthesis, emphasis was initially given to the occurrence of mutations resulting in stop codons within originally functional rearrangements of the variable region of the immunoglobulin heavy chain (IgV_H) gene.[5] Such mutations are expected to occur in IgV_H genes of germinal-center B cells, but under physiologic conditions "crippled" germinal-center cells (incapable of functional antibody expression) rapidly undergo apoptosis. RS cells might carry additional crippling mutations contributing to Ig gene silencing, which are not easily detectable, such as replacement mutations interfering with antigen binding or heavy- and light-chain pairing.[5] Marafioti et al, however, showed that crippling mutations were absent from 75% of classical HL cases, thus indicating that they cannot be responsible for the general absence of the Ig transcripts.[7] The latter event was then related to the downregulation of the transcription factors BOB.1, Oct-2 and PU.1.[62–65] Nevertheless, this finding, although characteristic of HL, was not observed in normal B-cell subsets and B-cell non-Hodgkin lymphomas[170] and cannot per se be responsible for the abrogated Ig synthesis. In fact, not sustained by genomic imbalances or gene rearrangements,[171] it likely represents only an epiphenomenon within the context of a much more complex process that leads to silencing of the B-cell program.[172,173] As mentioned in the previous section, clonal TCR gene rearrangements have been documented in rare cases.[8,131,132]

The BCL-6 gene has been found to carry somatic mutations only in the classical HL cases of B-cell derivation: these are represented by irrelevant somatic base substitutions without consequences for Bcl-6 protein expression and classical HL pathogenesis.[174] In contrast to LP-HL, no BCL-6 gene rearrangements have so far been detected in classical HL, thus further supporting the concept that the neoplastic cells of classical HL and LP-HL correspond to different steps of B-cell maturation.[175] Recently, Liso et al have shown that the at least PIM1, PAX5, RhoH/TTF, or c-MYC genes might be involved by an aberrant somatic hypermutation process in 55% of classical HL cases, two or more being mutated in 30% of patients.[80] Such rates are indeed lower than those recorded in LPHL (80% and 50%, respectively).[80]

During the last few years, "gene expression profiling" studies have been carried out mostly using classical HL-derived cell lines.[165,176–182] These studies—whose results might be in the future modified by the analysis of micro-dissected primary H&RS cells—[183] have shown that HL cell lines carry the gene profile of a germinal-center B lymphocyte that resists apoptosis through CD40 signaling and NF-κB activation (see also the following Cell kinetics section).[176] In particular, 45 genes have been recognized whose expression seem to be regulated by NF-κB: seventeen of them are novel NF-κB target genes.[179] The NF-κB-dependent gene profile is composed of chemokines, cytokines, receptors, apoptotic regulators, intracellular signaling molecules, and transcription factors, the majority of which maintain a marker-like expression in H&RS cells. For instance, the downregulation of the intracellular signaling genes Lyn, Syk, BLNK, and PLC-gamma2 has been validated by the lack of the corresponding products at the immunohistochemical level.[77] Using chromatin immunoprecipitation, it has been found that NF-κB is recruited directly to the promoters of several target genes, including the signal transducer and activator of transcription (STAT)5a, interleukin-13, and CC chemokine receptor 7. Intriguingly, NF-κB upregulates STAT5a expression and signaling pathways in H&RS cells, and promotes its persistent activation, as also supported by the detection of the corresponding product in most tumor cells of classical HL. The gene profile thus underscores a central role of NF-κB in the pathogenesis of HL and potentially of other tumors with constitutive NF-κB activation.[179] Other studies have suggested the possible (positive or negative) prognostic impact of the deregulation of genes related to the tumor microenvironment, cell growth/apoptosis, and regulation of mitosis.[165,177] Further studies have focused on the different patterns of gene dysregulation occurring in anaplastic large-cell lymphoma and classical HL.[178,181] A recently published report has provided evidence that the HL cell lines L428, HDLM2, KMH2, and L1236 cluster as a distinct entity, irrespective of their B- or T-cell derivation, and their gene expression resembles that of EBV-transformed B cells and cell lines derived from diffuse large B-cell lymphoma with features of in vitro-activated B cells.[182] Twenty-seven genes, most of which were previously unknown to be expressed in H&RS cells, were reported to be aberrantly expressed, including the transcription factors GATA-3, ABF1, EAR3, and Nrf3. In addition, the gene encoding for the nonreceptor tyrosine kinase FER has been found to be upregulated: this might contribute the constitutive activation of STAT-3.[182] The results of this study might shed new light on the pathogenesis of classical HL and allow the identification of new targets for both diagnostic and therapeutic purposes.[182] Finally, Schweing and coworkers have reported that H&RS cells of classical HL show loss of the B-cell lineage-specific gene expression program, a finding that might explain the lack of characteristic surface markers and Ig as well as of the transcription factors required for their expression, such as Oct-2, BOB.1, and PU.1.[182] Some explanations of this phenomenon have been provided, ranging from downregulation of a few master transcription factors due to hypermethylation[172] to overexpression of the helix-loop-helix proteins ABF-1 and Id2 that antagonize the function of the B cell determining transcription factor E2A.[173]

Several cytogenetic abnormalities have been detected in classical HL, although they may vary from case to case with frequent intraclonal variability, thus suggesting chromosomal instability.[184] Some tumors show 14q alterations, as seen in B-cell lymphomas, but without occurrence of t(14;18), others 2p, 4p, 9p, 8q, 12p, and 16q abnormalities.[184–187] In particular, aberrations of chromosomes 2p and 9p might involve the REL and JAK2 oncogene loci.[187] FISH studies have recently shown recurrent chromosomal breakpoints affecting Ig loci in H&RS cells,[188] whereas CESH has suggested that classical HL can be distinguished from all NHLs, including ALCL-like HL by unsupervised hierarchical cluster analysis.[189]

Cell Kinetics

It is well known that the antibodies raised against the nuclear associated antigens Ki-67 and PCNA (Fig. 76–20) react with the vast majority of H&RS cells, thus indicating that they have entered the cell cycle.[190,191] However, in spite of the Ki-67 and PCNA marking, tumoral cells do not rapidly overwhelm the reactive component.[190,191] A possible explanation for this phenomenon was provided by Leoncini and coworkers, who postulated that H&RS cells have a defective cytokinesis that prevents both their progression in the cell cycle and their entrance into an apoptotic pathway.[192,193] This assumption has recently found support in a series of studies, part of which was based on the application of tissue microarray technology.[164,194,195] They have shown that H&RS cells carry multiple alterations in different pathways and checkpoints, including G1/S and G2/M transition and apoptosis. Relevant findings are the overexpression of cyclins A, B1, D3 and E, CDK2, CDK6, STAT1, STAT3, Hdm2, p16, p23, Rb, Bcl-2, Bcl-X_L, surviving, and NF-κB proteins (Figs. 76–21 and 76–22).[164,194–196] Garcia et al have reported that the overexpression of some of these markers affects survival.[164] In the past, special emphasis was given to the frequent p53 positivity of H&RS cells,[160] which, however, does not correspond to mutations of exons 4 to 8 of the gene.[197] P53 accumulation in the nuclei of neoplastic elements might else be the result of elevated MDM2 protein levels and/or p14(ARF)/Hdm2 nucleolar complexes resulting in stabilization of p53 protein.[198,199] Additional mechanisms influencing proliferation and apoptosis in classical HL cells can be the expression of Notch1, Jagged1, c-FLIP, caspase 3, CCR7, and TRAF proteins.[200–204] The over-expression of CCR7 and TRAF proteins is related to constitutive NF-κB activity, which is characteristic of H&RS cells and causes protection from apoptosis.[205] Studies have recently suggested that the persistent activation of NF-κB in H&RS cells is probably due to defects of members of the I-κB family that are the natural inhibitors of NF-κB[206–208] or by the aberrant activation of I-κB kinase.[209] Additional factors contributing to this activation can be constitutive acti-

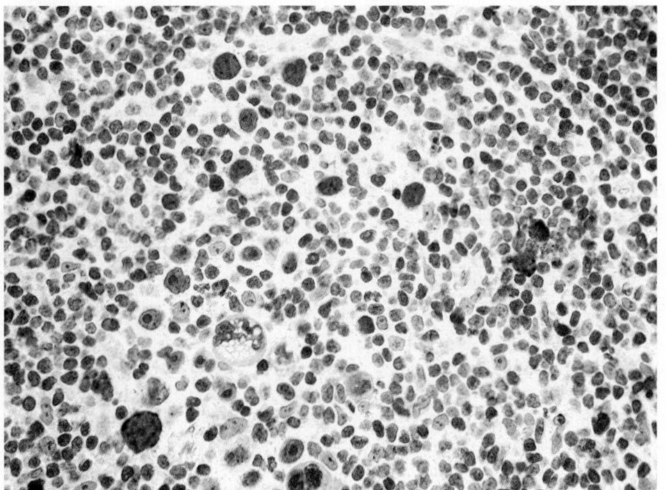

Figure 76–20 Classical Hodgkin lymphoma: most neoplastic cells express the Ki-67 molecule as shown by the Mib-1 monoclonal antibody; some small lymphocytes are also cycling (APAAP technique; Gill hematoxylin counterstain; ×300).

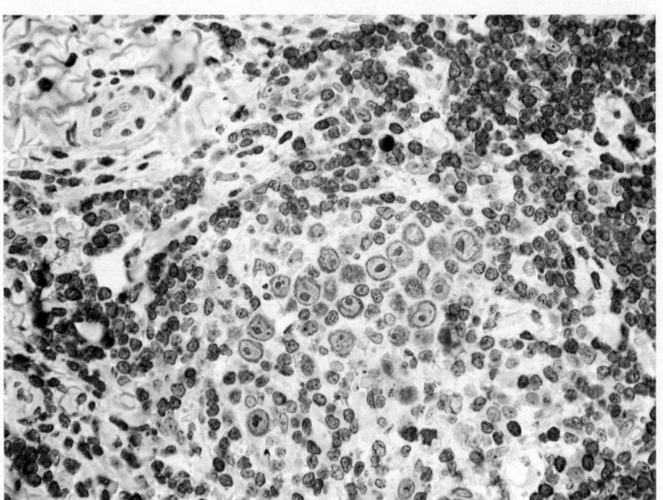

Figure 76–21 Classical Hodgkin lymphoma: Hodgkin and Reed–Sternberg display a strong–moderate Bcl-2 positivity (APAAP technique, Gill hematoxylin counterstain, ×300).

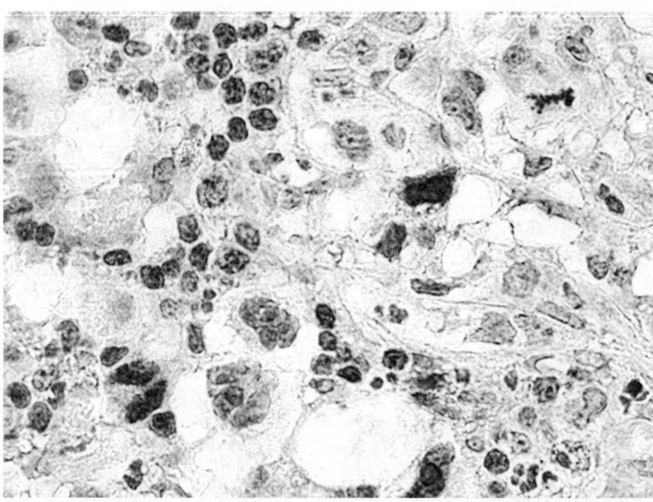

Figure 76–22 Classical Hodgkin lymphoma: cyclin E positivity of tumoral elements (Envision+ Method, Gill hematoxylin counterstain, ×500).

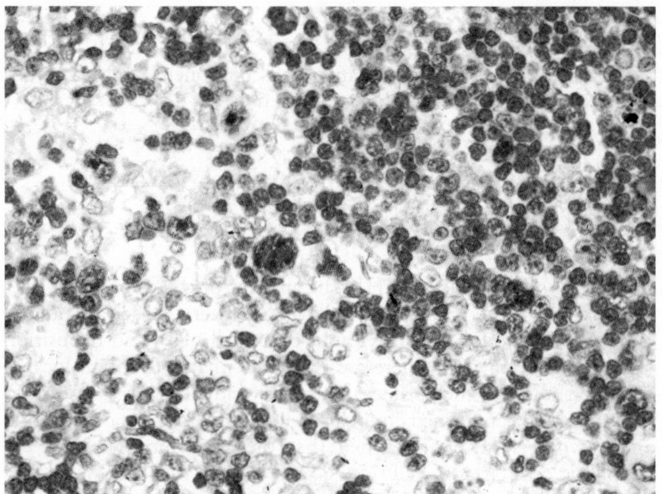

Figure 76–23 Classical Hodgkin lymphoma: positivity of Hodgkin and Reed–Sternberg cells for Epstein–Barr virus at in situ hybridization with EBER1/2 probes (APAAP technique, Gill hematoxylin counterstain, ×400).

vated AP-1 and CD30 and LMP-1 overexpression.[210–212] As mentioned above, NF-κB activity maintains high expression of a gene network, which plays a basic role in H&RS cell survival.[179,213]

EPSTEIN–BARR VIRUS INFECTION

Epstein–Barr virus (EBV) studies reveal viral integration in the genome in classical HL cells in a variable percentage of patients (20%–80%). In particular, in Western countries 20% to 40% of cases of nodular sclerosis and lymphocyte-depleted cases and 50% to 75% of the mixed-cellularity cases are associated with expression of LMP-1 and/or EBER-1/2 (Fig. 76–23) but not EBNA2, thus showing a pattern characteristic of latency type II EBV infection.[214,215] Interestingly enough, these percentages can remarkably vary according to the geographic area examined, as shown by Leoncini and coworkers, who found significant differences in the EBV incidence between classical HL patients from Kenya and Italy (92% vs 48%).[216] In addition, Takeuchi et al have observed that the EBV-positivity rate has significantly decreased among Japanese patients with nodular sclerosis classical HL during the period 1955 to 1999.[217] The type of EBV strain also varies between different geographic areas: in developed countries strain 1 prevails, in developing countries strain 2.[218] HL that is positive for EBV at diagnosis is usually also positive at relapse with persistence of the same EBV strain.[219] The exact role of EBV in the pathogenesis of HIV classical HL (transforming agent as suggested by LMP-1 expression or cofactor for the maintenance of malignant growth?) is still open to question.[84] Niedobitek and coworkers have recently shown that EBV-infected H&RS cells strongly express EBI3: this molecule, which corresponds to an EBV-induced cytokine homologous to the IL-12 p40 subunit, might heterodimerize with IL-12 p35, thus inhibiting the development of a Th1 immune response directed against both the tumor and virus.[220] No convincing data have so far been provided concerning the prognostic impact of EBV-infection in classical HL cases.[221,222] Finally, Huang et al have found amplifiable hCMV DNA in 11/33 EBV-negative classical HL cases recorded in a cohort of Chinese patients; based on this observation, these authors speculate that hCMV infection might play a role in the pathogenesis of HL, particularly in EBV-negative cases.[223]

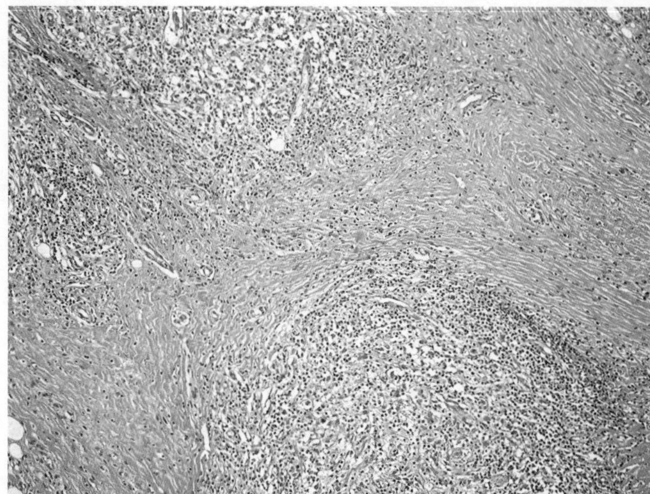

Figure 76–24 Nodular sclerosing classical Hodgkin lymphoma: the lymph node structure is largely effaced because of a nodular growth; the nodule is surrounded by thick collagen bands originating from the capsule (hematoxylin and eosin, ×40).

NODULAR SCLEROSIS

Morphologic Findings

Nodular sclerosis represents the most frequent subtype of classical HL in Italy and the United States, where it corresponds to 75% to 80% of all HL cases; the incidence of the process, however, significantly varies among different geographic areas.[224,225] As stated by Lukes et al in 1966, the tumor is characterized by sclerosis, lacunar cells, and a nodular pattern.[37]

Sclerosis

Fibrotic phenomena do always occur in nodular sclerosis classical HL: they more often correspond to the formation of broad collagen bands, which originate from a regularly thickened lymph node capsule (Fig. 76–24) and subdivide the lymphoid parenchyma into large nodules, at times visible at gross examination. Fibrotic tissue displays a typical birefractive green color with the use of polarized light microscopy, a finding not observed in lymphocyte-depleted classical HL.

Lacunar Cells

Lacunar cells represent the cell variant characteristic of nodular sclerosis classical HL. Lukes et al originally described lacunar cells as large elements with polylobated nuclei, small- to medium-sized

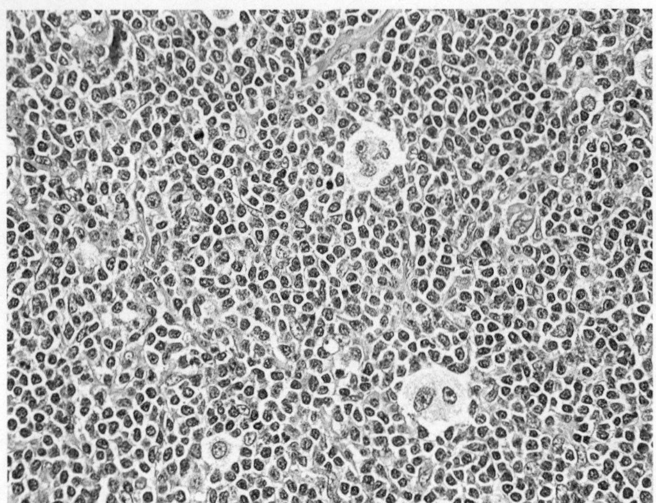

Figure 76–25 Nodular sclerosing classical Hodgkin lymphoma: scattered lacunar cells are detected within a nodule (hematoxylin and eosin, ×300).

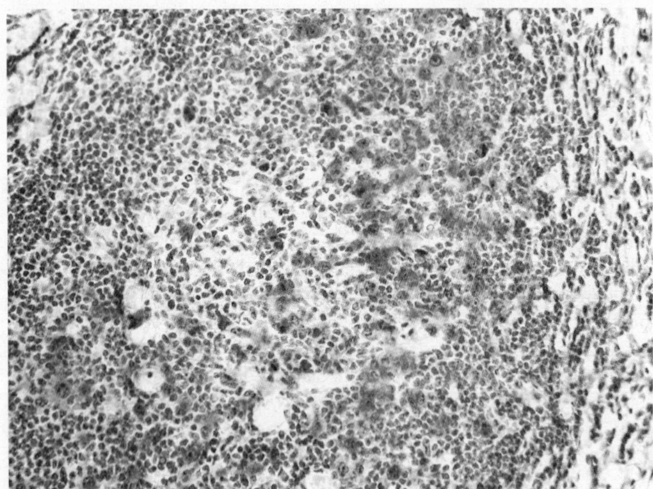

Figure 76–26 Nodular sclerosing classical Hodgkin lymphoma, cellular phase: CD30+ lymphomatous elements display a nodular aggregation without the overt deposition of collagen bands (APAAP technique, Gill hematoxylin counterstain, ×200).

nucleoli and a wide rim of clear or slightly acidophilic cytoplasm, very sensitive to formalin fixation (Fig. 76–25).[37] The latter in fact causes perinuclear condensation of the cytoplasm, which remains connected to the cell membrane via some narrow filaments, limiting empty "lacunar" cytoplasmic spaces. Lacunar cells display a much higher degree of pleomorphism than originally thought. They may be uninucleated, multinucleated, and/or show huge nucleoli, which traits are indeed similar to those of typical RS cells. This morphologic variability seems to depend on the characteristics of the inflammatory component present.[226] Although lacunar cells are easily found, H&RS cells are rare; it should be emphasized that some neoplastic elements appear "mummified" because of apoptotic changes.

Nodular Pattern

The nodules—which should be detected in at least part of the lymph node involved—can contain foci of necrosis and actually show a great

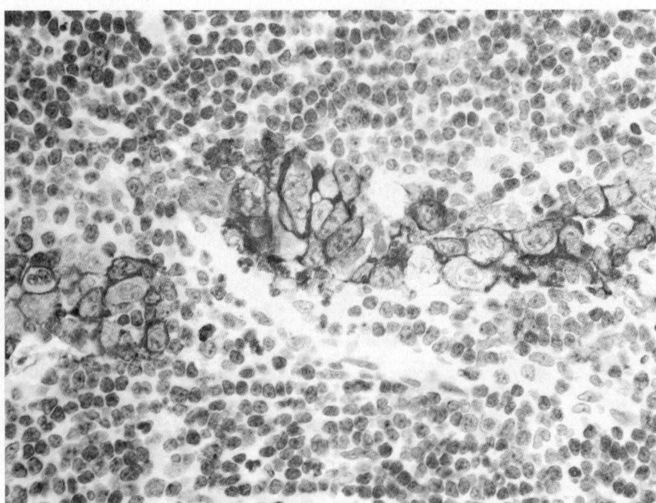

Figure 76–27 Nodular sclerosing classical Hodgkin lymphoma, syncytial variant: CD30+ neoplastic cells show a cohesive growth (APAAP technique, Gill hematoxylin counterstain, ×400).

variability in terms of inflammatory cell component (from lymphocyte predominance to lymphocyte depletion).

Nodular Sclerosis Classical Hodgkin Lymphoma: Cellular Phase

In nodular sclerosis classical HL, the amount of collagen fibres varies remarkably. In the so-called cellular phase, there is a clear-cut tendency to nodule formation without overt collagen band deposition (Fig. 76–26). However, there are typical lacunar cells, often located at the periphery of the nodules or around residual follicles. The latter situation has been termed "follicular Hodgkin lymphoma" by Kansal and coworkers, who underlined that the antigenic profile of the neoplastic cells ($CD30^+$, $CD15^+$, $CD20^{-/+}$, $CD79a^{rare}$) allows its easy distinction from nodular LP-HL.[227] The reactive component mainly consists of small lymphocytes with the phenotype of mantle B cells ($CD20^+$, $CD79a^+$, $CD5^+$, IgM^+, IgD^+, $CD3^-$).[228] The secretion of cytokines by neoplastic cells is currently thought to be the cause of progressive attraction of T lymphocytes, histiocytes, plasma cells, and eosinophils, which give rise to nodules replacing the preexisting follicles and producing the typical pattern of nodular sclerosis classical HL. Within the nodules, there are numerous follicular dendritic cells that seem to represent a favorable prognostic indicator.[229]

Nodular Sclerosis Classical Hodgkin Lymphoma: Syncytial

The term *syncytial* nodular sclerosis Hodgkin disease was coined by Butler in 1983 and then reproposed by Strickler in 1986.[230] This variant is thought to represent 16% of all the nodular sclerosis classical HL cases[231] and to be associated with a more aggressive clinical course,[230] because of the occurrence of mediastinal bulky disease and stage III/IV in 88% of the patients. This variant is characterized by large sheets of neoplastic cells (partly with a lacunar appearance), which may undergo central necrosis (Fig. 76–27).[230] In the past, similar cases have been diagnosed as non-Hodgkin lymphoma, metastatic melanoma, carcinoma or sarcoma, thymic carcinoma, or germ cell tumor. The differential diagnosis requires the application of an adequate panel of antibodies, which allow the identification of the characteristic phenotype: $CD3^-$, $CD15^+$,

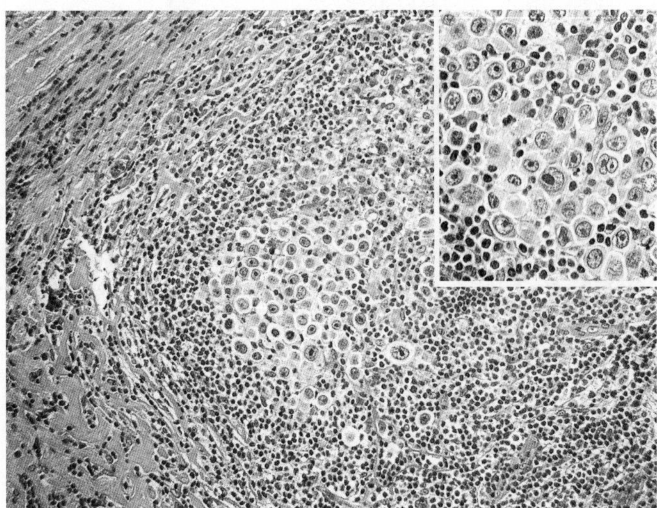

Figure 76–28 Nodular sclerosing classical Hodgkin lymphoma, grade II: mostly mononuclear neoplastic cells cover more than 25% of the examined area (hematoxylin and eosin, ×200); inset: cytologic details at higher magnification (hematoxylin and eosin, ×300).

CD20$^{-/+}$, CD30^{+}, CD45^{-}, CD79a^{-}, cytokeratins^{-}, PLAP^{-}, protein S-100^{-}, HMB.45 melanoma-associated antigen^{-}, EMA^{-}, and ALK protein^{-}.

Histologic Grading of Nodular Sclerosis Classical Hodgkin Lymphoma

The British National Lymphoma Investigation (BNLI) Group has repeatedly proposed to subclassify nodular sclerosis classical HL into two grades: grade II tumors seem to represent 15% to 25% of all nodular sclerosis cases and which have a more aggressive clinical course,[232,233] a finding not confirmed by all studies.[234,235] In the recently developed WHO scheme, the BNLI grading system has been maintained in order to test its real prognostic value in a larger series.[40] It is based on the degree of cellularity of the nodules, the amount of sclerosis and the number and atypia of neoplastic cells. The term *grade II* is applied to cases showing one of the three following patterns:

1. more than 25% of the nodules have a cellular composition consistent with the pleomorphic or reticular subtype of lymphocyte-depleted HL (Fig. 76–28);
2. more than 80% of the nodules display a fibrotic or fibrohistiocytic composition; and
3. more than 25% of the nodules contain numerous large bizarre or anaplastic cells, in the absence of any depletion of the reactive small lymphoid component.

Very recently, the German Hodgkin Lymphoma Study Group has proposed a new grading system based on three criteria: eosinophilia, lymphocyte depletion, and atypia of H&RS cells.[236] In particular, these findings seem to represent useful prognostic indicators in intermediate and advanced stages.[236]

Differential Diagnosis

Anaplastic Large-Cell Lymphoma

The boundaries between classical HL and anaplastic large-cell lymphoma are not always easily defined: in the past this had led to the creation of the category of anaplastic large-cell lymphoma–Hodgkin like, which in approximately 85% of cases presents with a mediastinal mass and stage II disease.[237,238] On practical grounds, this distinction is relevant, because anaplastic large-cell lymphoma can be cured in 80% of cases by the administration of third-generation chemotherapy regimens, whereas HL usually requires different therapeutical approaches.[237] The problems in differential diagnosis are essentially due to the fact that anaplastic large-cell lymphoma–Hodgkin like shares with nodular sclerosis classical HL architectural and cytologic features, including fibrotic reaction and nodule formation. In the authors' experience, the diagnosis of anaplastic large-cell lymphoma–Hodgkin like should be considered only in those cases that display nodules almost exclusively consisting of basophilic blasts with a minimal reactive cell component and phenomena of intrasinusoidal spread.[238] When these morphologic criteria are applied, most of the cases in the past diagnosed as anaplastic large-cell lymphoma–Hodgkin like would be now reclassified as nodular sclerosis classical HL (grade II or syncytial) and might tentatively be termed "anaplastic large cell lymphoma–like Hodgkin disease."[142] By applying more restrictive diagnostic criteria, rare examples of anaplastic large-cell lymphoma–Hodgkin like do still exist.[239] Immunohistochemical and molecular biological analyses are helpful in distinguishing between HL and anaplastic large-cell lymphoma, as shown in Table 76–3. In problematic cases the expression of CD15, possibly in conjunction with positivity for B-cell markers (with special reference to BSAP),[239] and the lack of TCR gene rearrangements and ALK protein favor HL, whereas negativity for CD15, the expression of T-cell markers and/or ALK protein, and the presence of clonal TCR gene rearrangements or an NPM/ALK hybrid gene support the diagnosis of anaplastic large-cell lymphoma; cases that cannot be resolved by the use of the combination of morphology, phenotype, and molecular data should be regarded as "unclassifiable" and submitted to a second biopsy or a treatment equally effective for anaplastic large-cell lymphoma and classical HL.[6]

Primary Mediastinal (Thymic) Large B-Cell Lymphoma

Primary mediastinal large B-cell lymphoma (PMBL) is a distinct clinicopathologic entity, which represents approximately 2.4% of all malignant lymphomas[240] and more often affects young females.[6,39,241,242] The presence of a certain amount of T lymphocytes, eosinophils, and RS-like elements, along with sclerosis, possible nodularity, and frequent CD30 expression by neoplastic cells[243] may suggest classical HL. In most instances, the two processes can be distinguished by the fact that PMBL expresses B-cell markers (CD19; CD20; CD22; CD79a), Bcl-6, Oct-2, BOB.1, PU.1, and the MAL protein (in 70%–75% of cases) and is CD15 negative.[243,244] Nonetheless, similarities between PMBL and classical HL have been observed. For instance, PMBL lacks both Ig mRNA and protein expression, in spite of functional Ig gene rearrangements and intact transcriptional machinery.[243] This concept has been further strengthened by two independent gene expression profiling studies that have shown that the molecular signature of PMBL differs from that of other diffuse large B-cell lymphomas and shares several features of classical HL,[245,246] including the constitutive NF-κB activity that promotes cell survival and favor antiapoptotic TNF-α signaling.[247] Thus, a grey zone between PMBL and classical HL has been proposed that can explain transitional features between NSHL and PMBL.[248,249] Whether the two tumors represent the extremes of the same disease or the ends of a spectrum of biologically related diseases remains uncertain. A recent study has, for instance, shown that the signaling molecules Syk, BLNK, and PCL-gamma2 characteristically silenced in classical HL are regularly expressed in PMBL: a finding that is characteristic to diffuse large B-cell lymphoma rather than to HL.[250]

Undifferentiated Nasopharyngeal Carcinoma

Undifferentiated nasopharyngeal carcinoma occurs in young patients and is associated with involvement of laterocervical nodes, which is

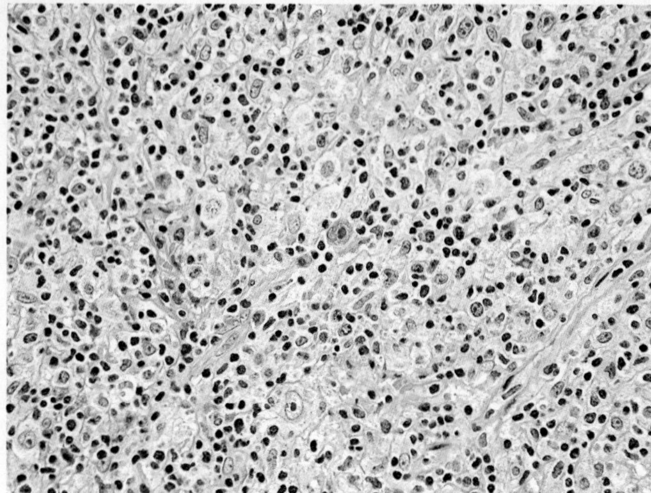

Figure 76–29 Mixed-cellularity classical Hodgkin lymphoma: Hodgkin and Reed–Sternberg cells are seen within a cellular milieu consisting of small lymphocytes, some plasma cells, histiocytes, and granulocytes (hematoxylin and eosin, ×250).

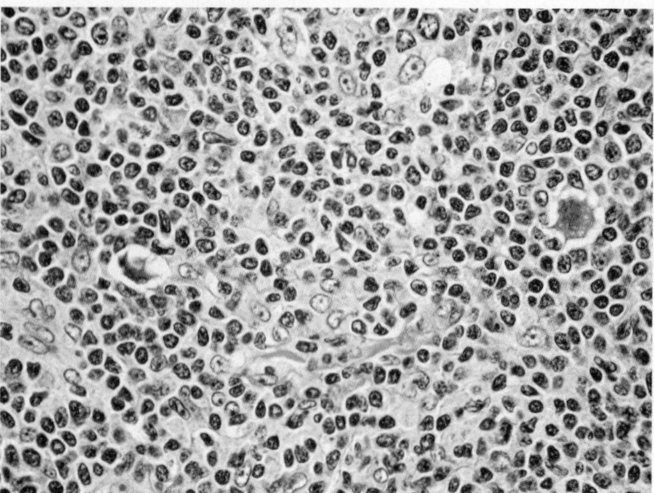

Figure 76–30 Mixed-cellularity classical Hodgkin lymphoma: two mummified (apoptotic) neoplastic cells (hematoxylin and eosin, ×350).

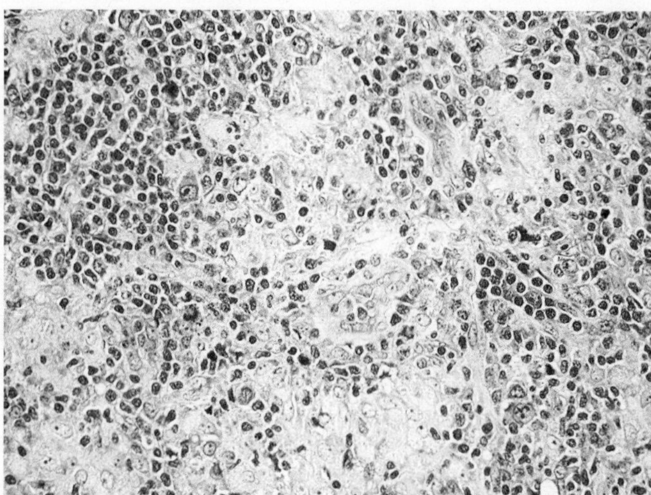

Figure 76–31 Mixed-cellularity classical Hodgkin lymphoma with a high content of reactive epithelioid cells (Giemsa, ×250).

the usual site of diagnostic biopsy. On morphologic grounds, neoplastic cells can resemble H&RS cells and produce a nodular growth with sclerosis, plasmacytosis, and eosinophilia. Because the primary tumor may remain occult, morphologic features can contribute to a misdiagnosis of nodular sclerosis classical HL.[251,253] Immunohistochemistry, however, allows the easy distinction between undifferentiated nasopharyngeal carcinoma and classical HL by showing positivity of the neoplastic cells for cytokeratins, EMA, and LMP-1. The latter is due to regular EBV integration, as shown by in situ hybridization with EBER1/2 probes and PCR techniques.

MIXED-CELLULARITY HODGKIN LYMPHOMA

Mixed-cellularity HL was originally described by Lukes et al as intermediate between LP and lymphocyte-depleted Hodgkin disease.[37] Later on, Lukes included in this category all the cases that according to his criteria remained unclassified, transforming it into a "basket."[253]

Approximately 15% to 25% of HL cases belong to the mixed-cellularity classical HL group.[39,40] The histological picture is characterized by a diffuse growth with frequent paracortical location.[39,40] Involvement of the capsule and necrosis are rare. The term *mixed-cellularity classical HL* reflects the cellular composition of the reactive milieu that consists of plasma cells, epithelioid histiocytes, eosinophils, and T lymphocytes (CD3$^+$, CD57$^-$) forming rosettes around neoplastic elements.[39,40] The latter correspond to H&RS cells that are rather numerous and easy to find, without lacunar or popcorn variants (Fig. 76–29).[39,40] Some neoplastic elements, as in the nodular sclerosis subtype, appear "mummified" because of apoptotic changes (Fig. 76–30).

Morphologic Variants of Mixed Cellularity

Interfollicular Variant

The interfollicular variant is rarely observed and likely represents partial lymph node involvement by classical HL. It is characterized by the occurrence of rather numerous H&RS cells around reactive follicles, which display germinal centers either in the second phase of development[254] or in regressive transformation. The latter usually resemble the germinal centers seen in hyaline-vascular Castleman disease and are probably related to the release of cytokines, such as IL-6, by H&RS cells.[255] This unusual variant of mixed-cellularity classical HL should be taken into consideration to avoid possible confusion with follicular hyperplasia or Castleman disease.

Epithelioid Cell-Rich Variant

It is relatively frequent and shows prominent epithelioid cell reaction with granulomata formation and occasional Langerhans cells (Fig. 76–31). Within this context, typical H&RS cells are always detected, at times following a laborious search. The epithelioid cell-rich variant of mixed-cellularity classical HL should be differentiated from the so-called Lennert lymphoma because of the different therapeutic approaches applied to the two tumors.

Differential Diagnosis

Lennert Lymphoma

Lennert lymphoma is a peripheral T-cell lymphoma characterized by a high content of epithelioid elements and some blasts resembling RS cells.[39] By no means, part of the cases in the past diagnosed as atypical Hodgkin disease do actually correspond to peripheral T-cell

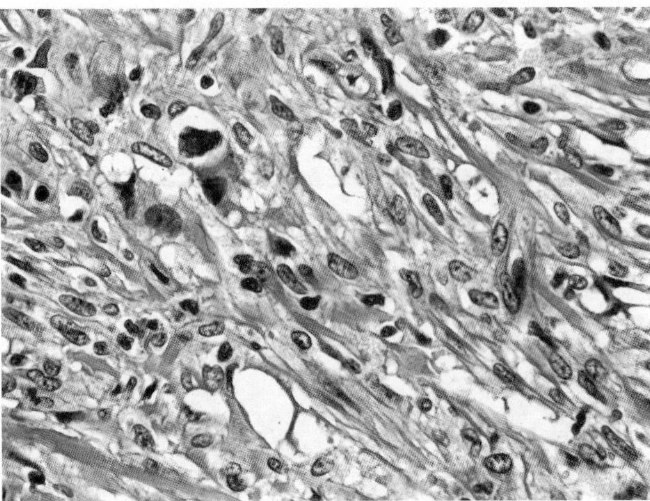

Figure 76–32 Lymphocyte-depleted classical Hodgkin lymphoma, fibrotic variant: rare neoplastic cells are present within a fibrotic matrix; some histiocytes and scanty lymphocytes are seen (hematoxylin and eosin, ×450).

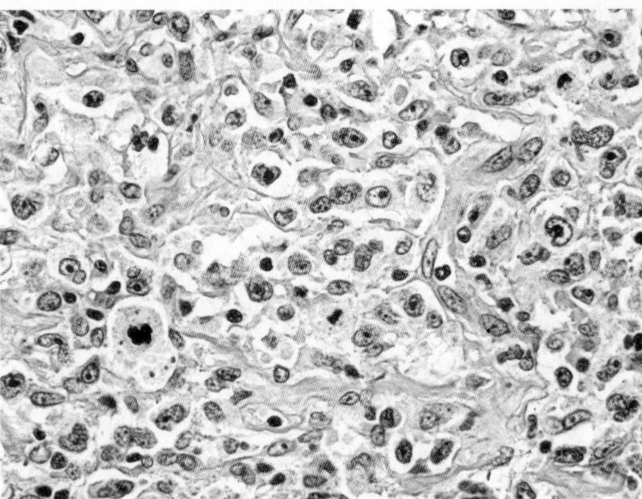

Figure 76–33 Lymphocyte-depleted classical Hodgkin lymphoma, sarcomatous variant: Hodgkin and Reed–Sternberg cells predominate; small lymphocytes are indeed rare (hematoxylin and eosin, ×400).

lymphomas with a high content of epithelioid elements.[226] The following features are of paramount importance for the recognition of Lennert lymphoma: (a) the marked irregularity of the nuclear profiles of the lymphoid component, as opposed to the regular nuclear outline of reactive lymphocytes in HL[256]; (b) the phenotypic profile of the atypical population, which in turn is $CD3^+$, $CD45^+$, $CD30^{occasionally+}$, and $CD15^-$, although some cases can partially lack T-cell markers[117,257]; and (c) higher mitotic index.[258]

T Cell/Histiocyte-Rich Large B-Cell Lymphoma

T cell-rich large B-cell lymphoma, first described in 1984,[259] is an aggressive tumor, usually presenting as stage III–IV disease with splenomegaly, bone-marrow involvement, and mesenteric lymphadenopathy, that is, findings that are rarely observed at the onset of HL.[260–263] The main differences between classical HL and T cell/histiocyte-rich large B-cell lymphoma are summarized in Table 76–2.[52,76,85–87,89,91,92,261–263]

LYMPHOCYTE-DEPLETED HODGKIN LYMPHOMA

Lymphocyte-depleted HL is indeed rare, accounting for approximately 1% of HL cases, and is associated with the worst clinical behavior and prognosis. In most instances, patients present with III–IV disease and display B symptoms and bone marrow involvement.[264] Histopathologically, it is characterized by the paucity of the lymphoid component, absolute or relative abundance of RS cells, and variable fibrotic reaction. According to Lukes et al, two subtypes of lymphocyte-depleted classical HL can be distinguished: fibrotic and reticular/sarcomatous.[37]

Fibrotic Variant

The fibrotic variant is characterized by complete effacement of the nodal structure with possible capsule preservation and has (Fig. 76–32) the following distinctive features:

a) low cellular density with fairly small, although variable amounts of lymphocytes;
b) prominent diffuse reticulin fibre formation, which is not organized in birefringent collagen bands,[253] but includes single neoplastic elements and is associated with deposition of amorphous material (procollagen) around sinusoids;
c) the high variability in the number of H&RS cells, whose detection requires at times a long and laborious search.

At low power, the histopathological picture can resemble the depletion phase of HIV-lymphadenopathy: therefore, careful node examination is required to make a firm diagnosis.[265]

Reticular or Sarcomatous Variant

The reticular or sarcomatous variant is characterized by the huge amount of H&RS cells, some of which appear "mummified" (Fig. 76–33). There is diffuse effacement of the normal lymph node structure; small lymphocytes, plasma cells, histiocytes, and granulocytes are scanty; foci of necrosis are usually found, their extent varying from case to case.

Differential Diagnosis

Thanks to the extensive application of immunohistochemistry and molecular biology techniques, it is now evident that most of the cases diagnosed in the seventies and early eighties as sarcomatous lymphocyte-depleted classical HL are in fact examples of anaplastic large-cell lymphoma,[266] peripheral T-cell lymphoma,[267] primary mediastinal large B-cell lymphoma,[268] or syncytial variant of nodular sclerosis classical HL. In the authors' experience, the differential diagnosis should also include some nonlymphoid tumors, such as inflammatory fibrosarcoma,[269] Langerhans cell sarcoma, inflammatory and giant cell malignant fibrous histiocytoma,[270] lymphocyte-rich well-differentiated liposarcoma,[271] and undifferentiated nasopharyngeal carcinoma. Under these circumstances, immunophenotyping is essential for a correct diagnosis.

LYMPHOCYTE-RICH CLASSICAL HODGKIN LYMPHOMA

Several reports suggest the existence of HL cases with a lymphocyte-predominant background, but differing from the prototypic description of LP-HL due to the presence of some eosinophils, sclerosis, typical H&RS cells, or aberrant phenotypic features (eg, the expression of CD30 and CD15).[43,74,224,272,273] In 1994, the REAL Classifica-

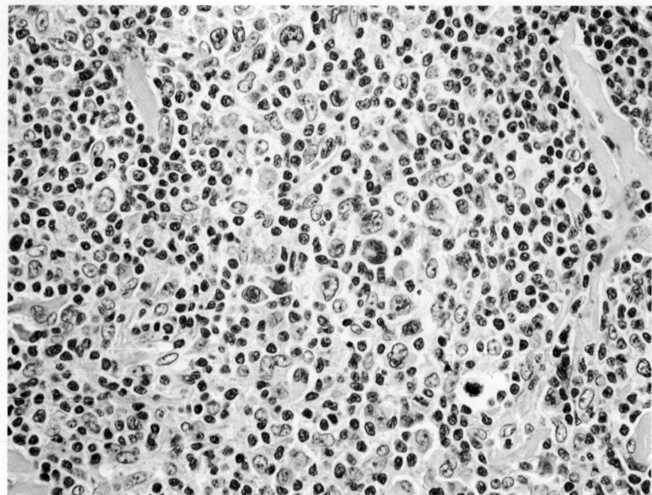

Figure 76–34 Lymphocyte-rich classical Hodgkin lymphoma: mononuclear and diagnostic neoplastic elements are situated within a cellular milieu mostly consisting of small lymphocytes (hematoxylin and eosin, ×300).

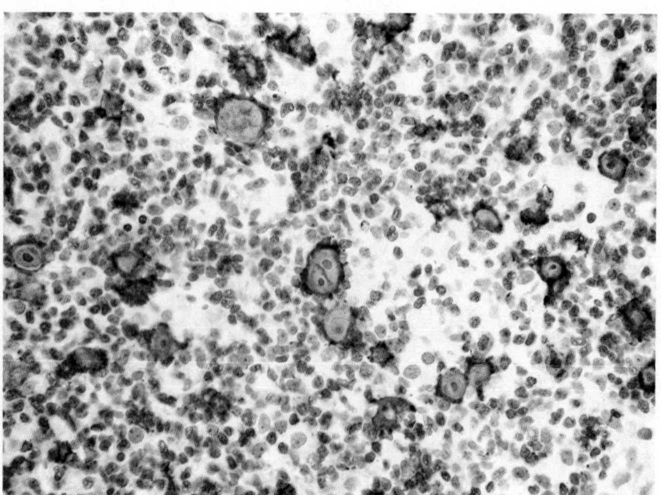

Figure 76–35 Lymphocyte-rich classical Hodgkin lymphoma: neoplastic cells express CD30 (APAAP technique; Gill hematoxylin counterstain; ×350).

tion included a provisional entity called "lymphocyte-rich classical Hodgkin disease," which was thought to have a diffuse growth pattern in most instances.[39] Following two workshops held by the European Association for Hematopathology in 1994 and the European Lymphoma Task Force in 1995, the concept of lymphocyte-rich classical HL was definitely accepted and further expanded by the recognition of two subtypes of the tumor, nodular and diffuse, which should be differentiated from LP-HL and T cell-rich B-cell lymphoma (Table 76–2).[41,88,260,274]

Morphologically,[40] most lymphocyte-rich classical HL cases have a vague nodularity, admixed histiocytes and absent neutrophils and eosinophils, thus closely resembling nodular LP-HL, particularly at low power. Furthermore, a proportion of the neoplastic cells can exhibit features of L&H/popcorn elements. In contrast to LP-HL, however, many lymphomatous cells have the cytomorphologic features of classical H&RS cells, and the nodular structures frequently contain small germinal centers (Fig. 76–34). Focal sclerosis can sometimes be seen.

On phenotypic grounds,[40] the neoplastic cells usually express CD30 and CD15 (Fig. 76–35). Expression of CD20 and CD79a are found in 32.5% and 8.7% of cases, respectively, figures that are much lower than those observed in LP-HL. Approximately 50% of the examples of lymphocyte-rich classical HL harbor EBV-positive H&RS cells. The reactive component consists of abundant mantle B cells with surface IgD and IgM expression and variable amounts of $CD3^+$ T lymphocytes, which produce rosettes around neoplastic elements but seldom express CD57. CD21 immunostaining reveals a loose, ill-defined meshwork of follicular dendritic cells, which becomes much denser and sharper as compared to the small residual germinal centers, when present.

The clinical characteristics of this variant of classical HL, which accounts for approximately 6% of all HL cases,[50,159] has been the object of several studies, including those promoted by the International Project on LP-Hodgkin Disease and the German Hodgkin Lymphoma Study Group.[50,159] These studies have shown that the patients with lymphocyte-rich classical HL differ from those with nodular sclerosis or mixed-cellularity classical HL, because they are usually older than 50 and have a higher incidence of stages I–II and subdiaphragmatic location. On the other hand, they rarely have bulky disease, B symptoms, and mediastinal or extranodal involvement. The clinical profile of lymphocyte-rich classical HL is thus closer to that of LP-HL, although it is associated with a lower frequency of stage II and more common splenic infiltration. By comparison with other types of classical HL, lymphocyte-rich classical HL is associated with more frequent late relapses, which have a low aggressive behavior pattern.

Owing to its peculiar clinicopathologic features, lymphocyte-rich classical HL has been accepted as a distinct entity in the WHO Classification.[40]

UNCLASSIFIABLE HODGKIN LYMPHOMA

In cases with partial lymph node involvement, with small amounts of tissue available for examination or with extranodal location, the classification of HL can be difficult or even impossible. In the past, these problem cases were usually included in the MC subtype. Because it is important to follow the criteria for distinguishing the subtypes of HL as fashion for the purposes of prospective clinicopathologic studies, both the REAL Classification and WHO schema list cases with ambiguous features or insufficient biopsy material as HL unclassified.

EXTRANODAL INVOLVEMENT BY HODGKIN LYMPHOMA

Although the onset is typically nodal, HL can secondarily affect extranodal organs. The criteria for the diagnosis of HL at extranodal sites vary significantly depending on the clinical history and kind of tissue involved. In fact, in needle biopsies taken from the bone marrow (Fig. 76–36) and liver during staging procedures, the diagnosis of HL can confidently be made according to "minimal criteria," that is, by the detection of HC in the appropriate cellular milieu.[256] By contrast, the diagnosis of HL at other extranodal sites requires the recognition of typical "diagnostic" cells and appropriate phenotypic markers, especially in patients without a previous history of HL.

THERAPY-RELATED HISTOLOGIC CHANGES

Relapses of HL at previously treated sites may have morphologic features that completely differ from those recorded at the time of presentation. Under these circumstances, the histologic picture is characterized by numerous atypical H cells, rare RS cells, and severe lymphocyte depletion, which can make the distinction from diffuse large B-cell lymphoma difficult.[226,275]

In patients with bulky disease, a residual mass is often detected following chemo- and radiotherapy, placing into question the efficacy of the administered therapy. In the authors' experience, histological examination of the residual mass frequently shows a fibrotic reaction with sclero-jaline changes and epithelioid cell palisades around necrotic foci, but no active tumor.

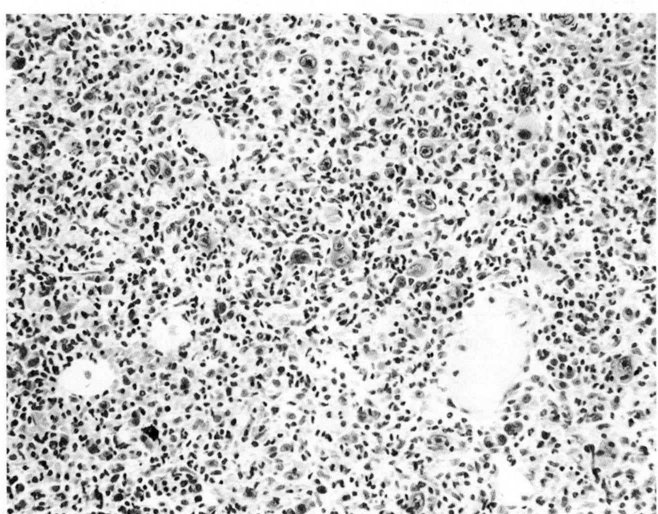

Figure 76–36 Bone-marrow involvement in classical Hodgkin lymphoma: Hodgkin and Reed–Sternberg cells are seen in an inflammatory cellular background that produces a certain fibrotic reaction (hematoxylin and eosin, ×250).

Chemo- and radiotherapy can produce toxic damages in organs not primarily involved by the process, such as postradiation interstitial pneumonitis, thyroid fibrosis, cardiomyopathies, or bone-marrow aplasia. In addition, patients treated for HL have an increased risk of developing acute leukemias, malignant lymphomas, and more rarely nonlymphoid tumors. This concept especially applies to individuals who have received MOPP chemotherapy.[226] On the whole, autopsies performed in subjects with a previous history of HL often show that the cause of death was a therapy-related complication without detectable residual disease.[226]

RELATIONSHIPS BETWEEN HODGKIN LYMPHOMA AND IMMUNODEFICIENCY DISORDERS

Patients with HIV are more at risk than the normal population to develop HL, especially the lymphocyte-depleted or mixed-cellularity types.[276] The tumor frequently presents with extensive subdiaphragmatic and extranodal involvement, a mediastinal mass rarely being detected.[277] Involvement of the liver, bone marrow, skin, or lung may occur in the absence of splenic and regional or mediastinal node involvement. On the whole, HL in HIV patients behaves differently than individuals without HIV, having more extensive dissemination,[226] a more aggressive clinical course and a worse prognosis.[278] On molecular grounds, neoplastic elements in HIV$^+$ HL are more often CD20$^+$ and Bcl-6$^-$/CD138$^+$. The latter finding differs from that usually observed in HIV$^-$ LP-HL (regularly Bcl-6$^+$/CD138$^-$) and classical HL (which displays a mixture of Bcl-6$^-$/CD138$^+$ and Bcl-6$^+$/CD138$^-$ RSC).[279] In addition, most if not all HIV$^+$ HL cases are positive for EBV, as shown by LMP-1 expression and in situ hybridization studies. This observation suggests an active role for EBV in the process of lymphomagenesis in HIV$^+$ HL[267] also in the light of the well-known LMP-1-transforming ability.[280] In particular, in 89% of HIV$^+$ cases (vs 32% of the seronegative ones) the LMP-1 gene has a 30-bp deletion, which allows LMP-1 prolonged half-life and accumulation in the infected cells.[280,281]

Classical HL can occur also in immunosuppressed patients following bone-marrow or solid organ transplantation. In this setting, a HL-like posttransplant lymphoproliferative disorder (PTLD) had also been reported. It remains controversial whether it is truly a form of HL or should be more appropriately classified as a form of B-cell PTLD.[282]

ASSOCIATION OF HODGKIN LYMPHOMA WITH NON-HODGKIN LYMPHOMA

The occurrence of HL and a synchronous or metachronous form of non-Hodgkin lymphoma (NHL) in the same patient is rare. The most frequent combination of the two is a diffuse large B-cell lymphoma that develops following LP-HL.[4,44,48,53–56] However, also classical HL has been reported in conjunction with different types of NHL, including follicular lymphoma, marginal zone lymphoma, diffuse large B-cell lymphoma, B-cell chronic lymphocytic leukemia, anaplastic large-cell lymphoma, Burkitt lymphoma, MALT lymphoma, and peripheral T-cell lymphoma.[283–296]

There are three possible explanations for the occurrence of this association: (a) both neoplasms arise coincidentally from two unrelated lymphoid elements; (b) the HL progresses from a previous NHL lymphoma; and (c) both lymphomas are derived from a common precursor cell. In the past, no reliable answer could be given to these challenging questions. In the last few years, the introduction of single-cell PCR has allowed the molecular analysis of some cases showing simultaneous or subsequent occurrence of HL and NHL. Past reports suggested a direct progression from NHL to HL (either classical or lymphocyte predominant).[53–56,290] Recent studies, however, have revealed that in most instances NHL cells and H&RS cells display the same monoclonal Ig gene rearrangements, as well as the presence of somatic mutations, thus supporting the concept that the two tumors stem from a common precursor cell (ie, a mature germinal-center B cell).[4,292–295]

SUGGESTED READINGS

Falini B: Anaplastic large cell lymphoma: Pathological, molecular and clinical features. Br J Haematol 114:741, 2001.

Falini B, Fizzotti M, Pucciarini A, et al: A monoclonal antibody (MUM1p) detects expression of the MUM1/IRF4 protein in a subset of germinal center B cells, plasma cells, and activated T cells. Blood 95:2084, 2000

Falini B, Pileri S, Pizzolo G, et al: CD30 (Ki-1) molecule: A new cytokine receptor of tumor necrosis factor superfamily as a tool for diagnosis and immunotherapy. Blood 85:1, 1995.

Fan Z, Natkuman Y, Bair E, Tibshirani R, Warnke R: Characterization of variant patterns of nodular LP-Hodgkin lymphoma with immunohistologic and clinical correlations. Am J Surg Pathol 27:1346, 2003.

Hummel M, Marafioti T, Stein H: Immunoglobulin V genes in Reed-Sternberg cells. N Engl J Med 334:405, 1999.

Küppers R, Klein U, Schwering I, et al: Identification of Hodgkin and Reed-Sternberg cell-specific genes by gene expression profiling. J Clin Invest 111:529, 2003.

Liso A, Capello D, Marafioti T, et al: Aberrant somatic hypermutation in tumor cells of nodular-lymphocyte-predominant and classic Hodgkin lymphoma. Blood 108:1013, 2006.

Marafioti T, Hummel M, Anagnostopoulos I, et al: Origin of nodular LP-Hodgkin's disease from a clonal expansion of highly mutated germinal center B cells. N Engl J Med 337:453, 1997.

Marafioti T, Pozzobon M, Hansmann ML, Delsol G, Pileri SA, Mason DY: Expression of intracellular signalin molecules in classical and lymphocyte predominance Hodgkin disease. Blood 103:188, 2004.

Rudiger T, Gascoyne RD, Jaffe ES, et al: Workshop on the relationship between nodular LP-Hodgkin's lymphoma and T-cell rich/histiocyte rich B-cell lymphoma. Ann Oncol 13(Suppl 1):44, 2002.

Sánchez-Aguilera A, Montalbán C, de la Cueva P, et al: Tumor microenvironment and mitotic checkpoint are key factors in the outcome of classic Hodgkin lymphoma. Blood 108:662, 2006.

Seitz V, Hummel M, Marafioti T, Anagnostopoulos I, Assaf C, Stein H: Detection of clonal T-cell receptor gamma-chain gene-rearrangements in Reed-Sternberg cells of classic Hodgkin's disease. Blood 95:3020, 2000.

Stein H, Delsol G, Pileri S, et al: Hodgkin's lymphoma. In Jaffe ES, Harris NL, Stein H, Vardiman JW (eds.): Tumours of Haematopoietic and Lymphoid Tissues. Lyon, IARCPress, 2001, p 237.

Stein H, Herbst H, Anagnostopoulos I, Niedobitek G, Dallenbach F, Kratzsch HC: The nature of Hodgkin and Reed-Sternberg cells, their association with EBV, and their relationship to anaplastic large-cell lymphoma. Ann Oncol 2:33, 1991.

Stein H, Marafioti T, Foss H-D, et al: Downregulation of BOB.1/OBF.1 and Oct2 in classical Hodgkin's disease but not in LP-Hodgkin's disease correlates with immunoglobulin transcription. Blood 97:496, 2001.

Torlakovic E, Tierens A, Dang HD, Delabie J: The transcription factor PU.1, necessary for B-cell development is expressed in lymphocyte predominance, but not classical Hodgkin's disease. Am J Pathol 159:1807, 2001.

Torlakovic E, Torlakovic G, Nguyen PL, Brunning RD, Delabie J: The value of anti-pax-5 immunostaining in routinely fixed and paraffin-embedded sections: A novel pan pre-B and B-cell marker. Am J Surg Pathol 26:1343, 2002.

Traverse-Glehen A, Pittaluga S, Gaulard P, et al: Mediastinal grey zone lymphoma: The missing link between classic Hodgkin's lymphoma and mediastinal large B-cell lymphoma. Am J Surg Pathol 29:1411, 2005.

Tzankov A, Zimpfer A, Pehrs AC, et al: Expression of B-cell markers in classical Hodgkin lymphoma: A tissue microarray analysis of 330 cases. Mod Pathol 16:1141, 2003.

Tzankov A, Zimpfer A, Went P, et al: Aberrant expression of cell cycle regulators in Hodgkin and Reed-Sternberg cells of classical Hodgkin's lymphoma. Mod Pathol 18:90, 2005.

REFERENCES

For complete list of references log onto www.expertconsult.com

CHAPTER 77

HODGKIN LYMPHOMA: CLINICAL MANIFESTATIONS, STAGING, AND THERAPY

Volker Diehl, Beate Klimm, and Daniel Re

BACKGROUND

In his historic paper entitled "On Some Morbid Appearances of the Exorbant Glands and Spleen," Thomas Hodgkin,[1] in 1832, presented the clinical history and postmortem findings of the massive enlargement of lymph nodes and spleens of seven patients.[2] Hodgkin assumed that these pathologic findings more resembled an autonomous lymphatic process that started in the lymph nodes located along the major vessels in the neck, chest, or abdomen than an inflammatory condition or an infectious disease such as syphilis or tuberculosis.

As late as 1865, Sir Samuel Wilks for the first time linked Thomas Hodgkin's name to the disease that he described as "Cases of the Enlargement of the Lymphatic Glands and Spleen (or Hodgkin's Disease)."[3] He was also the first to describe Hodgkin Lymphoma (HL)-associated B symptoms such as anemia, weight loss, and fever. In 1878, Greenfield was the first to publish drawings of the pathognomonic giant cells, which later were named after Carl Sternberg (1898) and Dorothy Reed (1902), who contributed the first definitive microscopic descriptions of HL.[4,5]

Because HL was frequently clinically associated with tuberculosis, for a long time it was considered to be a peculiar form of a granulomatous disease such as tuberculosis. Despite the very strong evidence for the malignant nature of HL over the past century, it has been only recently shown that Hodgkin and Reed-Sternberg (HRS) cells are definitely clonally expanding, preapoptotic, germinal center-derived B lymphocytes that resemble true malignant cells.[6]

The management of HL has undergone a paradigm shift as a result of the availability of effective drug regimens capable of inducing high remission rates, the use of combined chemoradiotherapy with involved field irradiation in patients with early-stage disease, the introduction of effective salvage chemotherapy for relapsed HL with peripheral blood stem cell transplantation (PBSCT), and a more sensitive realization of the magnitude of late-treatment mortality. Future developments will be based on a better understanding of biological prognostic factors and the implementation of PET imaging to allow a more individualized treatment approach.

ETIOLOGY, EPIDEMIOLOGY, AND GENETICS

Incidence and Age of Onset

HL is an uncommon disorder with an annual incidence of 2 or 3 cases per 100,000 persons in Europe and the United States.[7] In industrialized countries, the onset of HL has a bimodal distribution, with a first peak occurring in the third decade and a second peak occurring after the age of 50 years. Because of more refined molecular, cytologic, and immunohistologic techniques offering sensitive discrimination between HL subtypes and non-Hodgkin lymphomas (NHLs), the second peak seems to have disappeared, mainly because the lymphocyte-depleted subtype of HL was recognized more frequently as large B-cell lymphomas.[8] Slightly more men than women (1.4 : 1) develop this malignancy. Among the group of young adults, the most common subtype is nodular sclerosing HL (NSHL), which occurs at a higher frequency (2 : 1) than the mixed-cellularity subtype of HL (MCHL). The frequency of MCHL increases with age, whereas incidence of the NSHL subtypes reaches a plateau in the group of young adults older than 30 years. According to the World Health Organization (WHO) classification, the subtypes of lymphocyte rich-classic HL (LRCHL), nodular lymphocyte-predominant HL (LPHL), and lymphocyte-depleted HL (LDHL) are less commonly diagnosed, with a frequency of 3% to 5% (LPHL and LRCHL) and less than 1% (LDHL) in Western countries.[9,10] There is a great difference in incidence of this disease between developing and industrialized countries. In developing countries, the disorder occurs predominantly during childhood, and its incidence decreases with age, whereas in industrialized countries, young children are much less commonly diagnosed with HL compared with adolescents or young adults. In industrialized countries, there are associations for early birth order, low number of siblings and playmates, high level of maternal education, single-family dwellings during childhood, and occurrence of HL in younger patients.[11,12]

Similar characteristics had also been observed in the epidemiology of poliovirus infection. These similarities suggested that HL might represent the rare consequence of an infection with a common agent that led to HL after a prolonged delay.[13] Several factors point in the direction of an infectious or at least inflammatory pathogenesis of HL: clinical symptoms of fever, night sweats, and weight loss, and the laboratory findings of elevated erythrocyte sedimentation rate (ESR) or increased serum concentrations of inflammatory cytokines such as interleukin-1 (IL-1), IL-2, IL-5, IL-6, IL-10, tumor necrosis factor (TNF), and growth factors such as granulocyte colony-stimulating factor (G-CSF) and granulocyte-macrophage colony-stimulating factor (GM-CSF).[14]

Role of Epstein-Barr Virus in the Pathogenesis of Hodgkin Lymphoma

Several studies have suggested that the Epstein-Barr virus (EBV) might be a transforming agent in HL. Mueller and colleagues[15] analyzed EBV titers in predisease sera and found enhanced EBV activation before the onset of HL. Patients with a history of EBV-related infectious mononucleosis have a twofold to threefold increased risk for development of HL. Another study confirmed that patients with a serologically diagnosed infectious mononucleosis had a fourfold increased relative risk of EBV-positive but not EBV-negative Hodgkin lymphoma.[16] The estimated median incubation time from mononucleosis to EBV-positive Hodgkin lymphoma was 4.1 years making a causal association between infectious mononucleosis-related EBV infection and the EBV-positive subgroup of Hodgkin lymphomas likely in young adults.

To substantiate the role of EBV in HL, a number of researchers investigated EBV in HRS cells using novel molecular techniques and found that EBV DNA is present in the tumor cells of HL patients more frequently in developing than in industrialized countries. In Western countries, about 50% of all cases of classic HL are EBV positive (ie, carry the virus within the tumor cells), with 15% to 30% of NSHL cases being positive and up to 70% of mixed-cellularity subtypes (MCHL) harboring EBV DNA.[17] For comparison, 90% or more of HRS cells are positive for EBV in developing countries.[18] EBV positivity in underprivileged patients and children from industrialized countries shares the frequency of that observed in developing countries.[19] It was also shown that impaired immune status may contribute to the development of EBV-positive cHL in older patients.[20]

HRS cells in EBV-positive patients show an expression pattern of EBV-encoded genes resembling that found in endemic nasopharyngeal carcinoma or in a subset of T-cell lymphomas, called *type 2 latency*. This pattern includes expression of the EBV latent genes *LMP1, LMP2A*, and *EBNA1*. Recently it was shown by three independent studies that EBV can rescue BCR deficient germinal center B-cells from apoptosis adding evidence that EBV plays a role in malignant transformation in HL.[21–23]

Because EBV is present in only half the tumor cells of patients with HL in the Western world, investigators were prompted to search for other viruses involved in the pathogenesis of HL. Although measles virus has been discussed to be associated with HL,[24] the role of other viruses than EBV for the pathogenesis of HL remains uncertain. More specifically, despite initial reports that SV40 virus is present in a variety of lymphomas including HL,[25] polyomaviruses were not detected in HL samples in follow-up studies.[26]

Taken together, these data suggest that EBV is involved in the transformation process in EBV-positive HL cases. In EBV-negative cases, a "hit and run" mechanism was hypothesized, but evidence of EBV as a transforming agent in negative cases is scant.[27]

Inheritance Pattern

In general, a family history of hematopoietic malignancy is associated with an approximately twofold increased risk of HL.[28] More specifically, the risks of family members of patients affected by HL for developing the same disease are three to nine times those of the expected values. These observations led to the hypothesis that at least a portion of cases occurs as an inherited disorder.[29] Mack and colleagues found that of 179 monozygotic twin pairs with HL; both twins in 10 pairs developed HL, strongly supporting the idea of a genetic component in a subset of HL.[30] Recent linkage studies associated family or personal history of autoimmune or chronic inflammatory disease to the development of HL suggesting that characteristics of the immune system might be important for the development of HL.[31,32] Another analysis of the Swedish Cancer Registry found HL fourth in a list of cancers with high familial clustering (52 first-degree relatives, 8766 HL cases), just behind cancers affecting the eye or testis.[33] However, familial HL is estimated to constitute only a minority of cases. No consistent mechanism of inheritance has been identified, and evidence for a genetic translocation unique to all cases of familial HL is lacking.

Hodgkin and Reed-Sternberg Cells and Their Origins

The affected tissue in HL is characterized by a heterogeneous infiltrate with typical mononucleated and multinucleated giant cells in an inflammatory background composed of stroma, lymphocytes, histiocytes, eosinophils, and monocytes (see Chapter 76). In classic HL, the giant cells are called *Hodgkin* and *Reed-Sternberg* (HRS) cells, and in LPHL, they are called *lymphocytic* and *histiocytic* (L&H) cells. Typically, HRS cells represent only 0.1% to 1% of the affected tissue.

Because immunophenotyping did not lead to the identification of the origin of the HRS cells, molecular approaches were used to resolve this issue. Küppers[34] was the first to show that HRS cells harbor somatically mutated clonal rearranged immunoglobulin (Ig) heavy chain genes by using single-cell polymerase chain reaction (PCR) methods on primary HRS cells.

From these results, it was concluded that HRS cells were derived from germinal center B cells. Amplification of identically rearranged and mutated Ig genes from different HRS cells showed they were clonal in origin—a key criterion of malignancy. HRS cells expand clonally within one affected lymph node, clonally disseminate in advanced-stage disease, and recur even after clinical complete remission. Some studies indicate that in a small subset of HL, the HRS cells are probably of T-cell origin.[35,36] HRS cells are derived from germinal center or post-germinal center B cells in most cases. In contrast, lymphocytic and histiocytic cells in LPHL harbor ongoing mutations in their rearranged Ig genes and therefore seem to be malignant B cells at a different stage of maturation.[37]

Malignant Transformation of Hodgkin and Reed-Sternberg Cells

Despite significant progress in understanding the cellular origin of HRS cells, little is known about the mechanisms responsible for the initial transformation event. EBV has been identified as a virus with potential involvement in the transformation of a subpopulation of HL cases. Constitutive activation of nuclear factor-kappa B (NF-κB) seems to be a central mechanism that results in the exit of cells from the hostile environment of the germinal center and contributes to their proliferation and resistance to apoptosis.

Infected HRS cells express the EBV-encoded latent genes *LMP1, LMP2*, and *EBNA1*. Products of the latent genes have transforming capacity. *LMP1*, for instance, can transform primary B cells by mimicking the function of constitutively active CD40, a transmembrane receptor molecule of the TNF receptor family. Physiologically, CD40 ligation results in activation of a signaling cascade terminating in activation of the transcription factor NF-kB. NF-kB itself initiates transcription of proinflammatory and antiapoptotic genes. Constitutively, activation of NF-kB has been demonstrated to be a characteristic feature of HRS cells.[38] Abrogation of constitutive NF-kB activation results in massive, spontaneous apoptosis of HRS cells by downregulation of an antiapoptotic signaling network, thereby providing evidence for its central role in the transformation and acquisition of the apoptosis-resistant phenotype.[39]

SUMMARY OF MECHANISMS UNDERLYING MALIGNANT TRANSFORMATION

Although much has been learned about the derivation of the HRS cells, little is known about the basic mechanisms underlying malignant transformation of HL. The HRS cells in HL are derived from preapoptotic germinal center B cells in most cases, but in some cases, they are of T-cell origin. The expression of EBV latent genes in EBV-positive cases (50%) may play a role in cellular transformation by upregulating the transcription factor NF-kB. The events underlying the transformation process in the EBV-negative cases, however, are still not understood. Several studies have focused on the apoptosis-resistant phenotype of HRS cells, and some data suggest that constitutively expressed Flice-inhibitory protein (FLIP), a protein that inhibits FAS-mediated apoptosis, contributes to apoptosis resistance in HL.[40] Genetic instability is a typical feature of HRS cells, and studies point to distinct genetic imbalances rather than subtle genetic alterations such as point mutations or microsatellite instability.[41] Besides NF-kB, other transcription factors are deregulated in HRS cells contributing to the lost B cell identity of malignant cells in HL.[42,43] The discovery that the HRS cells themselves contribute to the ineffective immune response by expressing immunosuppressive cytokines or by expressing chemokines that predominantly attract Th2 lymphocytes that are incapable of cell killing has widened our understanding of the environmental crosstalk of these peculiar cells.[44]

DIAGNOSIS AND STAGING

From the beginning, it was postulated that HL spread from one lymph node area by contiguity to adjacent lymph node chains. Only in the middle of the 20th century was this knowledge used by investigators such as Peters, Kaplan, Tubiana, and Musshoff for the development of strategies for the treatment of this disorder.[45–47]

The applicability of new radiologic techniques and the information derived from routine exploratory staging laparotomies have provided important insights into the presentation and evolution of HL.[47,48] Although there is strong evidence that HL starts in a single group of lymph nodes and then spreads by the lymphatic route, there is mounting evidence that the gradually more aggressive tumor cells tend to disseminate through the bloodstream rather early and disseminate to organs such as bone marrow, liver, and lung. For the initial diagnosis of HL, an excisional biopsy of a suspicious lymph node should be performed. Assessment of the bone marrow is important for staging and for an evaluation of the normal bone marrow cells before therapy. Bone marrow involvement occurs rarely both in early stage disease (<1%) and in advanced stage disease (<5%).

The extent of HL can be classified using the four-stage Ann Arbor classification. The absence (A) or presence (B) of systemic symptoms (eg, fever, night sweats, and weight loss) further characterizes the severity of disease. The Cotswolds classification is a modification of the Ann Arbor classification using information from staging and treatment gathered over the past 20 years. This classification was proposed in 1989 during a meeting held in the Cotswolds, England.[49] Information about prognostic factors such as size of the mediastinal mass, presence of bulky nodal disease, and the extent of subdiaphragmatic disease is included in this classification (Table 77–1).

The staging procedures recommended for determining the extent of disease have become less invasive in recent years. Staging laparotomy and splenectomy are used only in patients with limited, often infradiaphragmatic or occult disease, for which ultrasound- or computed tomography (CT)-guided fine-needle biopsy is impossible or not informative. CT of the neck, chest, abdomen, and pelvis is routinely performed in the diagnostic evaluation of a patient with HL.

Table 77–1. Cotswolds Staging Classification

Classification	Description
Stage I	Involvement of a single lymph node region or lymphoid structure (eg, spleen, thymus, Waldeyer ring) or involvement of a single extralymphatic site (IE)
Stage II	Involvement of two or more lymph node regions on the same side of the diaphragm (hilar nodes, when involved on both sides, constitute stage II disease); localized contiguous involvement of only one extranodal organ or site and lymph node regions on the same side of the diaphragm (IIE). The number of anatomic regions involved should be indicated by a subscript (eg, II3)
III1	With or without involvement of splenic, hilar, celiac, or portal nodes
III2	With involvement of paraaortic, iliac, and mesenteric nodes
Stage IV	Diffuse or disseminated involvement of one or more extranodal organs or tissues, with or without associated lymph node involvement
	Designations applicable to any disease stage
A	No symptoms
B	Fever (temperature, >38°C [100.4°F]), drenching night sweats, unexplained loss of >10% of body weight within the preceding 6 months
X	Bulky disease (a widening of the mediastinum by more than one-third of the presence of a nodal mass with a maximal dimension greater than 10 cm)
E	Involvement of a single extranodal site that is contiguous or proximal to the known nodal site

Two-thirds of patients with newly diagnosed HL have radiographic evidence of intrathoracic involvement. A *large mediastinal mass* has been arbitrarily defined as a mass in which the ratio is greater than one third for the largest transverse diameter of the mediastinal mass over the transverse diameter of the thorax at the diaphragm on a standing posteroanterior chest radiograph.[49] Alternatively, others have defined extensive mediastinal disease as greater than 35% of the thoracic diameter at T5–6, or wider than 5 to 10 cm. Patients with large mediastinal masses are at increased risk for relapsing in nodal and extranodal sites above the diaphragm after radiation therapy alone.[50,51]

Gallium 67 scintigraphy was used in evaluating the mediastinum or in the evaluation of residual masses in HL patients after treatment but has been replaced by ^{18}F-fluorodeoxyglucose (FDG) positron emission tomography (PET). According to the international harmonization project,[51a] FDG-PET can be used to improve staging techniques at initial diagnosis by detecting lesions not detected by CT; to assess tumor response while on treatment; and to evaluate residual tumor masses at the end of treatment, allowing discrimination between active lymphoma and fibronecrotic tissue.

When using PET in addition to conventional imaging techniques for the initial workup of patients, approximately 10% of HL patients are up-staged and another 10% down-staged[52] but it remains unclear, whether patients would benefit from a subsequent change of the treatment plan. Therefore the value of PET for initial staging of HL patients is limited. When assessing early tumor response rates in HL patients already after one to three cycles of chemotherapy. Hutching and Gallamini[52,53] found a significant correlation between the PET results and the clinical outcome of the patient in terms of progression free survival (PFS) and overall survival (OS).[52] Results are comparable with other published data[54] but patient numbers are small. Whether such an early PET response will be useful to tailor therapies more individually in the future needs to be clarified by prospective trials such as the HD18 trial of the GHSG and future trials of the EORTC.

If PET is used at the end of treatment, it shows an excellent negative predictive value between 91% and 95% in several monocentric studies.[55,56] In contrast, the positive predictive value of PET is around 50%. Based on this data the ongoing HD15 trial evaluates the prognostic value of PET in patients with residual lesions ≥ 2.5 cm at the end of chemotherapy. Only patients with a positive PET scan receive additional radiotherapy in this ongoing trial. Appropriate staging procedures for the initial workup of HL are summarized in the box on Recommended Staging Procedures for HL.

CLINICAL FEATURES

History

Patients with NSHL or MCHL have a central pattern of lymph node involvement (eg, cervical, mediastinal, paraaortic). In 70% to 80% of patients with the subtypes of classic HL, primary lymphadenopathy occurs in the left cervical or supraclavicular region or in the mediastinum. NSHL patients more often have a supradiaphragmatic onset of disease. MCHL patients present with smaller disseminated nodes and predominantly subdiaphragmatic nodes or organ involvement. In contrast, certain nodal chains (eg, mesenteric, hypogastric, presacral, popliteal) are seldom involved. Patients with LPHL always present initially with involved peripheral nodes in the cervical, submandibular, axillary, or inguinal region (in approximately 75% of cases of stage IA disease). B symptoms and involvement of the spleen or other organs rarely occur. The incidence of subclinical node involvement in patients with negative radiographic staging ranges from 6% to 35%. The spleen is involved more frequently in patients with adenopathy below the diaphragm, systemic symptoms, and MCHL histology. Involvement of the liver in untreated patients is rare and almost always occurs with concomitant splenic involvement. Infiltration of the bone marrow at diagnosis is rare, usually focal, and

Recommended Staging Procedures for Hodgkin Lymphoma

The following staging procedures are recommended for the initial workup of Hodgkin lymphoma:

1. Adequate surgical biopsy reviewed by an experienced hematopathologist
2. Core-needle biopsy of bone marrow from the posterior iliac crest; needle or surgical biopsy of any suspicious extranodal (eg, hepatic, osseous, pulmonary, cutaneous) lesions; and cytologic examination of any effusion
3. Detailed history, with attention to the presence or absence of systemic symptoms, and a careful physical examination, emphasizing node chains, size of the liver and spleen, and inspection of Waldeyer ring
4. Routine laboratory tests: complete blood cell count, erythrocyte sedimentation rate, and liver function tests
5. Chest radiographs (posteroanterior and lateral) with measurement of the mass-to-thoracic ratio
6. Neck, chest and abdominal CT
7. 18-FDG PET scan

almost always associated with extensive disease, systemic symptoms, and unfavorable histology.

Bulky lymph node involvement or a contiguous collection of smaller lymph nodes (>10 cm in diameter) may result in regional complications such as vascular, tracheal, bronchial, or gastrointestinal compression or obstruction. Invasion of adjacent anatomic regions such as the lung, pericardium, pleura, chest wall, or bone can occur in patients with HL histology, more with the NSHL subtype. Effusions of the pericardium, pleural cavity, or peritoneal cavity often are associated with extranodal involvement and invasive growth into neighboring structures. Despite a large mediastinal mass, superior vena cava syndrome is seldom observed; if it occurs, it is often associated with venous thrombosis.

The recommended staging procedures have become less invasive in recent years. Staging laparotomy (with splenectomy, needle and wedge biopsy of the liver, and biopsies of para-aortic, mesenteric, portal, and splenic hilar lymph nodes) is necessary only rarely in cases of early-stage HL for which use of limited radiation therapy alone depends on pathologic staging.

Compared with the NHLs, bulky infradiaphragmatic lesions with obstructive symptoms are rare in HL. The spleen is involved in about 30% to 35% of patients at diagnosis, less frequently with NSHL histology, and only rarely in patients with LPHL. Spleen involvement is often subclinical and hard to diagnose with modern imaging techniques. Tumor involvement is not necessarily associated with splenic enlargement; a small spleen can have diffuse HL involvement. Details of organ extranodal involvement (so called E-lesions) are given in Table 77–2.

Hematopoietic spread to organs is mainly seen in the lung, liver, bone marrow, and bone, and it must be distinguished from disease invasion into adjacent organs by extranodal tumor that penetrates the capsule of a lymph node. Skin involvement is seen very rarely and can appear as small, opaque, or red papules or as ulcerating lesions. Involvement of the central nervous system can occur by extension from nodes within the paraaortic region through the intervertebral foramina, manifesting as neurologic symptoms and pain.[57] Similarly, primary involvement of the intestinal wall never occurs, but secondary invasion of the gut from adjacent mesenteric lymph nodes can be seen. Bone marrow infiltration is usually focal and, in most cases, is associated with extensive disease, including systemic symptoms and hematopoietic insufficiency.

A considerable number of undiagnosed patients with HL present with systemic symptoms before the discovery of enlarged lymph nodes. Typical symptoms include fever, drenching night sweats, and weight loss (ie, B symptoms). The characteristic HL-associated fever

Table 77–2. Sites of Disease Involvement in Untreated Patients with Hodgkin Lymphoma

Anatomic Site	Involvement (%)
Waldeyer ring	1–2
Cervical nodes	60–70
Axillary nodes	30–35
Mediastinum	50–60
Hilar nodes	15–35
Paraaortic nodes	30–40
Iliac nodes	15–20
Mesenteric nodes	1–4
Inguinal nodes	8–15
Spleen	30–35
Liver	2–6
Bone marrow	1–4
Total extranodal	10–15

Adapted from Gupta RK, Gospodarowicz MK, Lister TA: Clinical evaluation and staging of Hodgkin's disease. In Mauch PM, Armitage JO, Diehl V, et al (eds): Hodgkin's Disease. Philadelphia, Lippincott Williams & Wilkins, 1999.

(ie, Pel-Ebstein type) occurs intermittently and recurs at variable intervals over several days or weeks. Fever and drenching night sweats are identified in 25% of all patients at the time of initial presentation, increasing to 50% of patients with more advanced disease. Other nonspecific symptoms include pruritus, fatigue, and the development of pain shortly after drinking alcohol. This pain is usually transient at the site of nodal involvement and may be severe. Pruritus, although not a defined B symptom, may be an important systemic symptom of disease, although it affects less than 20% of patients. It often occurs months or even a year before the diagnosis of HL.[58] The underlying pathophysiologic mechanisms leading to pruritus are unknown, but possible causes include an intrinsic production of cytokines such as growth factors by the HRS cells and an autoimmune reaction in which a number of cytokines are activated by tumor lysis.

Is Laparotomy Necessary for Staging?

Staging laparotomy is rarely used in patients with limited, infradiaphragmatic or occult disease when ultrasound- or CT-guided fine-needle biopsy is not feasible or the results would not be representative. With the greater use of reproducible and clinically relevant prognostic factors and imaging techniques to stage patients, most centers and treatment groups determine treatment strategy based on the risk of primary progressive or relapsing disease, applying reduced doses of radiotherapy or chemotherapy in a combined-therapeutic approach.

CHOICE OF TREATMENT

Prognostic Factors and Treatment Groups

Prognostic factors define the likely outcome of the disease of an individual patient at diagnosis allowing selection of appropriate treatment strategies. Despite an enormous effort to define clinically relevant and generally acceptable prognostic factors, there are still two major methods for dividing HL patients according to a risk- or prognosis-adapted therapeutic approach: stage and systemic symptoms. A third factor meets general trans-Atlantic acceptance: massive local tumor burden (ie, bulky disease >10 cm in diameter). Prognostic factors are rarely the subject of specific clinical studies but are recognized and evaluated using data from large cohorts of uniformly

Table 77–3 Definition of Treatment Groups According to the EORTC/GELA and GHSG

Treatment Group	EORTC/GELA	GHSG	NCIC/ECOG
Early-stage favorable	CS I-II without risk factors (supradiaphragmatic)	CS I-II without risk factors	Standard risk group: favorable CS I-II (without risk factors)
Early-stage unfavorable (intermediate)	CS I-II with ≥1 risk factors (supradiaphragmatic)	CS I, CSIIA ≥ 1 risk factors; CS IIB with C/D but without A/B	Standard risk group: unfavorable CS I-II (at least one risk factor)
Advanced stage	CS III-IV	CS IIB with A/B; CS III-IV	High risk group: CS I or II with bulky disease; intraabdominal disease; CS III,IV
Risk factors (RF)	A large mediastinal mass B age ≥50 years C elevated ESR* D ≥4 involved regions	A large mediastinal mass B extranodal disease C elevated ESR* D ≥3 involved areas	A ≥ 40 years B not NLPHL or NS histology C ESR ≥ 50 mm/h D ≥ 4 involved nodal regions

*erythrocyte sedimentation rate (≥50 mm/h without or ≥30 mm/h with B-symptoms).

ECOG, Eastern Cooperative Oncology Group; EORTC, European Organization for Research and treatment of Cancer; GELA, Groupe d'Etude des Lymphomes de l'Adulte; GHSG, German Hodgkin Study Group; NCIC, National Cancer Institute of Canada.

treated, well-documented, and reliably followed patients, usually from large clinical trials.[59,60]

In the United States, most centers still treat HL patients according to the traditional separation of *early stages* (I-II, A and B), representing about 45% of newly diagnosed patients, and *advanced stages* (III-IV, A and B or any stage with bulky disease >10 cm in diameter), representing about 55% of newly diagnosed patients. Patients with early-stage disease are treated with radiotherapy alone or, in most centers or trials, with combined-modality strategies. Patients with advanced-stage disease (IIIB or IV) are assigned to intensive chemotherapy protocols, sometimes followed by adjuvant radiotherapy.

The European Organization for Research and Treatment of Cancer (EORTC) identified in the H1 and H2 trials additional prognostic factors that are now used to assign clinical stage I or II patients to a more unfavorable-prognosis group. The EORTC has, since 1982, defined clinical stage I or II (supradiaphragmatic only) patients as having an *early unfavorable prognosis* HL if any of the following factors is present: age older than 50 years, asymptomatic with an ESR higher than 50, B symptoms with an ESR higher than 30, and a large mediastinal mass. In previous trials, stage II disease with MCHL or LDHL histology and number of involved regions had also been counted as adverse factors.[61]

The German Hodgkin Study Group (GHSG) has, since 1988, assigned clinical stage I or II patients to an *intermediate group* (Table 77–3) if they had any of the following adverse factors: large mediastinal mass (>1/3 of maximum thoracic diameter), three or more involved lymphatic regions (which is not equivalent to lymphatic areas), elevated ESR, and localized extranodal infiltration.[62] Because of the rarity of splenectomy, massive splenic involvement was seldom reported and was abandoned for the current generation of trials. It can be difficult to distinguish consistently between E-lesions and stage IV disease, and various assessments of the prognostic value of this feature have been obtained by different investigators. In 1980, Stanford University began to provide combined-modality treatment for clinical stage I or II patients with large mediastinal masses or multiple E-lesions.

Until recently, the following general treatment strategies have been employed in the United States and in Europe:

1. Early stages, favorable: irradiation alone (extended field)
2. Early stages, unfavorable (intermediate): moderate amount of chemotherapy (typically four cycles) plus irradiation
3. Advanced stages: extensive chemotherapy (typically eight cycles) with or without consolidation (usually local) irradiation

Most centers and groups both in the United States and in Europe tended to favor combined-modality treatment, even for early stage favorable-prognosis patients. Such treatment includes chemotherapy and reduced irradiation therapy. More recently, chemotherapy alone is tested in early stage disease while chemotherapy alone can already be considered standard treatment for patients with advanced stage HL and a complete response after chemotherapy. These typical strategies and the investigation of alternatives are reported in the following sections.

An attempt has also been made to identify very good risk and very poor risk subgroups. The EORTC has investigated the use of localized radiotherapy in a "very favorable subgroup" of early-stage patients. Inclusion criteria were stage IA disease for female patients younger than 40 years and NSHL or LPHL histology without an elevated ESR or large mediastinal mass. However, the failure rate was 29% at six-year follow-up,[63] and this policy was abandoned. Similarly, advanced-stage patients at particularly high risk for failure for intensified therapy were treated with early high-dose chemotherapy (HDCT) with autologous stem cell transplantation (ASCT).[64] As neither the definition of the prognostic groups nor the choice of treatment is uniform, no conclusive data about this early intensification is available.

Despite the different mode of action of chemotherapy compared with radiotherapy, similar prognostic factors have emerged from analyses of cohorts treated with irradiation and with combined-modality therapy. The usefulness of the factors previously listed for radiation-treated patients has been reliably confirmed in cohorts who also received chemotherapy[65,66] in early or in advanced stages of disease. This similarity of prognostic effects is supported by the observation from a meta-analysis of irradiation versus combined-modality treatment in patients with early-stage disease that the difference in failure-free survival between these two treatment strategies was essentially constant across different prognostic groups.[67]

The EORTC includes in its advanced-stage cohorts stage III and IV patients only, without regard to other factors, as did the US National Cancer Institute and several US cooperative groups. Certain other trial groups also include stage I-II patients in the advanced-stage group, if they have B symptoms or bulky disease.[68] The GHSG includes both stage III-IV patients and patients with stage IIB disease and a large mediastinal mass or E-lesions in the advanced-stage cohort. The gradual shift towards more intensive therapy is thus based on the incorporation of prognostic factors into treatment algorithms.

Prognostic Factors for Advanced-Stage Hodgkin Lymphoma

International consensus about uniform treatment strategies and longer and better controlled follow-up periods with a greater fre-

Table 77–4. Final Cox Regression Model of the International Prognostic Score

Prognostic Factor	Log Hazard Ratio	Relative Risk	*P Value*
Serum albumin <4 g/dL	0.40 + 0.10	1.49	<0.001
Hemoglobin <10.5 g/dL	0.30 + 0.11	1.35	0.006
Male gender	0.30 + 0.09	1.35	0.001
Stage IV disease	0.23 + 0.09	1.26	0.011
Age ≥45 years	0.33 + 0.10	1.39	0.001
White blood cell (WBC) count ≥15,000/mm³	0.34 + 0.11	1.41	0.001
Lymphocyte count <600/mm³ or <8% of WBC count	0.31 + 0.10	1.38	0.002

quency of treatment failure events have permitted more conclusive and generally applicable prognostic factor analyses for the advanced-stage disease compared with early-stage disease. The International Prognostic Factor Project produced an International Prognostic Score (IPS),[66] which is not necessarily completely comprehensive, but is widely accepted (Table 77–4).

All of the factors in Table 77–4 were shown to be highly significant in a multivariate analysis of data from 5141 patients treated in 25 centers, and their prognostic power was confirmed in an independent sample. Serum albumin and hemoglobin levels, male gender, and age of 45 years or older are also prognostic factors for early-stage patients. All seven factors were associated with similar relative risks of between 1.26 and 1.49. It was recommended that these factors be combined into a single score by counting the number of adverse factors and giving an integer prognostic score between 0 and 7. However, even patients with five or more factors (7% of cases) had a 5-year failure-free rate of more than 40%. The best failure-free rate was close to 80% for patients with at most one adverse factor (29% of cases), suggesting that a group of advanced-stage patients with a relatively favorable prognosis could be recognized (1618 patients included in the final analysis for freedom from treatment failure according to whether the prognostic score was 0 to 2 or 3 or higher).

A number of other factors have been shown to correlate with prognosis in advanced stages, but their independent importance has not been proved because of conflicting results or lack of validation in a large independent data set. These include pathologic grade in nodular sclerosis HL, the amount of tissue eosinophilia, inguinal involvement, serum lactic dehydrogenase concentration, and β 2-microglobulin level.

Prognostic factors may subsequently be used to for treatment intensification or for treatment reduction. Concerning intensification, various investigators have treated a poor-prognosis subset of advanced-stage patients who had attained a remission by conventional chemotherapy, with HDCT accompanied by hematologic stem cell support.[64] Proctor and coworkers[69] constructed a continuous numeric index for this purpose as a weighted sum of the variables, including age, stage, lymphocyte count, hemoglobin level, and the presence of bulky disease, and included patients with an index greater than 0.5 in the poor-prognosis subset. Federico and colleagues[70] included patients with two or more factors (high lactate dehydrogenase levels, very large mediastinal mass, two or more extranodal sites, inguinal involvement, low hematocrit, and bone marrow involvement) in a high-dose chemotherapy/autologous stem cell transplantation arm after four cycles of ABVD and compared it to eight cycles of ABVD. At 5 years, FFTF rates were in favor of conventional therapy (82% vs. 88%), and OS was 88% in both arms. Relapse rates were slightly higher in the transplantation arm although this was not statistically significant. This observation indicates that the early high-dose intensification is unlikely to result in clinically relevant long-term survival benefit compared with conventional treatment.

In conclusion, the three-level scheme of division into early favorable, early unfavorable (intermediate), and advanced-stage cases remains a suitable instrument to tailor risk-adapted therapy according to our current knowledge. Because clinical and biologic factors do not discriminate the 10% to 15% of advanced-stage patients who will progress or experience an early relapse (<12 months), biologic molecular parameters are urgently needed to save most patients from overtreatment or allow even more intensive treatment for the 10% to 15% of patients resistant to the best modern treatment modalities. There is hope that current approaches using on-treatment imaging techniques such as PET, gene expression profiles of primary tumor material,[71] individual drug metabolism[72] or cytokine profiles of serum samples will detect patterns that can identify poor prognosis patients.

EARLY-STAGE HODGKIN LYMPHOMA

Early-Stage Favorable Disease

The treatment of early-stage HL is changing. In the 1990s, extended field irradiation was considered standard treatment. However, because of recognition of the high relapse rate and the fatal long-term effects, the use of extended field radiotherapy is being abandoned by most study groups. Instead, for favorable-prognosis early-stage disease, limited amounts of chemotherapy for the control of occult lesions is routinely combined with involved field irradiation and there is even evidence, that chemotherapy alone might be sufficient to control disease.

Extended field radiotherapy alone produces complete remissions in 90% to 98% of patients with early-stage favorable HL.[73,74] Unfortunately, 30% to 40% of those patients will relapse, but salvage chemotherapy or combined-modality treatment yields remissions in most of these cases. Taken together, approximately 75% to 85% of patients with early-stage, favorable-prognosis disease who receive extended field radiotherapy as first-line treatment are alive after 10 years.[75,76]

Increasing concern about the long-term consequences of treatment prompted many investigators to reexamine the aggressive approaches developed for early-stage favorable disease in the 1970s and 1980s. Several follow-up studies reported an increased risk of secondary cancer for long-surviving patients. Cumulative risks varied between 17.6% at 15 years,[77] and 26.3% at 30 years for children treated under the age of 16 years.[78] Follow-up evaluation of more than 12,000 patients by the International Database on HL similarly revealed a cumulative incidence rate of 11.2% at 15 years.[79] In the latter study, less than 10% of patients with secondary neoplasias had received chemotherapy alone, whereas most patients were treated with radiotherapy alone or radiotherapy in combination with chemotherapy. Among the high incidence of cancer, breast cancer in young women treated with mantle field irradiation between the age of 15 and 25 years is of a special concern, as the relative risk of breast cancer was elevated by 56-fold in women treated under the age of 19.[80] It was also discussed in that context, that chemotherapy-dependent hormonal factors also play an important role in the pathogenesis of breast cancer.[81]

Considering the impact of chemotherapy in addition to radiotherapy, there is conflicting data. One study pointed out that the occurrence of second malignancies is increased in patients treated with both chemotherapy and radiotherapy when compared to patients treated with irradiation alone.[82] In contrast to that trial, a recent meta-analysis[83] compared data from randomized trials testing radiation therapy versus combined modality treatment (3343 patients), chemotherapy versus combined modality treatment (2861 patients), radiation therapy versus chemotherapy or involved-field versus extended-field radiation therapy (3221 patients) for untreated HL came to different results. It was concluded that administration of chemotherapy in addition to radiation therapy as initial therapy for HL decreases overall risk for second malignancies by reducing relapse and need for salvage therapy. Administration of radiation therapy additional to chemotherapy marginally increased overall risk for second tumors in advanced stages. Breast cancer risk was substantially higher after EF-RT. It has to be pointed out that caution is needed in applying findings of these two trials to current therapies as treatment strategies, drugs and radiation techniques changed considerably over the years.

Besides the occurrence of second cancers, treatment results are challenged by the development of long-term toxicities such as pulmonary dysfunction[84] or heart failure.[85] In a retrospective study analyzing 415 patients that received radiation including the heart or carotid or subclavian arteries, the rates of clinically significant valvular dysfunction (6.2% at 22 years), and coronary artery disease (10.4% at 9 years) were higher than expected.[86]

Many of the ongoing and recently completed studies were developed in an attempt to reduce the long-term complications of treatment without increasing mortality from HL. These include studies that evaluate reduction of radiation dose or field size or even the omission of radiotherapy and evaluate combined-modality treatment in an attempt to identify the optimal chemotherapy regimen, the optimal number of cycles of chemotherapy, and to determine the optimal radiation volume and dose when combined with chemotherapy.

Radiation Dose

Based on a Kaplan meta-analysis showing a continuous reduction in recurrence rates up to doses of 40 Gy, extended field radiotherapy was usually administered to a total dose of 40 Gy as a sole treatment modality.[87] However, subsequent dose-response analyses indicated a plateau in cure rates starting around 30 Gy.[88]

The GHSG thus planned a multicenter, randomized, controlled trial (HD4) to test whether subclinical disease can be adequately controlled by a total radiation dose of 30 Gy (extended field). In this multicenter trial, 376 pathologically staged patients with stage I or II disease without adverse risk factors (eg, large mediastinal mass, E-lesions, massive splenic disease, elevated ESR, ≥3 tumor-involved areas) were recruited.[89] Patients were randomly assigned to receive 40 Gy of extended field radiotherapy (arm A) or 30 Gy of extended field radiotherapy followed by an additional 10 Gy to involved lymph node regions (arm B). Complete remission was attained in 98% of patients in each arm. With a median follow-up of 86 months, the 7-year relapse-free survival rates (78% for arm A and 84% for arm B) and overall survival rates (91% for arm A and 96% for arm B) did not differ significantly. In conclusion, subclinical involvement of HL is sufficiently treated with 30 Gy of radiotherapy alone. However, the relapse-free survival rate in this favorable subgroup of patients treated with radiotherapy alone is unsatisfactory.

Combined-Modality Treatment with Extended Field Irradiation versus Extended Field Radiotherapy Alone

To reduce the high relapse rates observed with radiotherapy alone, combined-modality therapies were introduced and compared with radiotherapy alone in patients with early-stage, favorable-prognosis HL. The HD7 trial (1994–1998) of the GHSG randomized 650 favorable-prognosis clinical stage IA-IIB patients to subtotal nodal and splenic irradiation alone or to two courses of ABVD and extended field radiation therapy.[90] The final analysis after a median follow-up of 87 months showed an advantage in freedom from treatment failure in the patients receiving ABVD (88%) compared with those treated with irradiation alone (67%, $P < 0.0001$). Probably due to effective salvage therapy, overall survival (94% and 92%) did not differ between the two treatment arms.[91]

Results of an American Intergroup phase III trial (#9133) have been published comparing three cycles of doxorubicin and vinblastine (AV) plus subtotal lymphoid irradiation with subtotal lymphoid irradiation alone in clinical stage IA-IIA patients with supradiaphragmatic disease that did not undergo staging laparotomy.[92] The trial had to be closed at the second interim analysis because of a marked superior failure-free survival rate for patients on the combined-modality arm (94% versus 81%, respectively, at a median follow-up of 3.3 years). Nevertheless, the two previously described studies used EF radiotherapy and did not address the issue of whether radiation therapy could be reduced safely when coadministering chemotherapy.

Combined-Modality Treatment with Involved Field Radiotherapy versus Extended Field Radiotherapy Alone

Randomized trials of combined-modality therapy have been based on the premise that this approach results in a very high freedom from recurrence rate and that this high degree of efficacy can even be maintained when using less toxic chemotherapy and radiation therapy regimens. In the EORTC H7F trial (333 favorable patients), six cycles of the EBVP regimen (ie, epirubicin, bleomycin, vinblastine, and prednisone, with one dose per cycle) plus involved field irradiation were compared with mantle and para-aortic-splenic nodal irradiation (STNI) for favorable-prognosis clinical stage IA-IIA patients. At 10 years, the event-free survival rate was significantly better for patients on the combined chemotherapy and radiation therapy arm compared with those receiving radiation therapy alone (88% versus 78%, $P = 0.01$), with similar survival rates (92%) (Table 77–5).[93] As the H7U trial showed that EBVP is less efficient than a hybrid of MOPP (mechlorethamine, vincristine [Oncovin], procarbazine, and prednisone) and ABVD,[93] the latter regimen was used in subsequent studies.

The EORTC H8F trial (1993–1998) testing three cycles of MOPP/ABV and involved field irradiation against mantle and para-aortic-splenic irradiation for favorable-prognosis clinical stage IA-IIA patients was activated in 1993 (n = 543 patients). This trial asked the question whether three cycles of standard chemotherapy are sufficient to control subclinical HL. Because relapse-free survival differed significantly between the two groups (98% versus 74%; $P < 0.001$), it was concluded that combined-modality treatment was the new gold standard of therapy (see Table 77–5).[94] Taken together, these EORTC trials were the first to demonstrate, that STNI could be safely replaced by a combined modality regimen, as smaller radiotherapy (IF) in combination with chemotherapy was shown to be superior to STNI.

Compared with the 12-week Stanford V regimen given to patients with poor-prognosis HL, patients with favorable-prognosis clinical stage IA-IIA disease received a modified eight-week Stanford V regimen that included involved field irradiation to sites of initial disease involvement. This regimen provides information about the ability of brief but intense chemotherapy to control HL beyond the initially involved sites in favorable-prognosis clinical stage I-II patients.[95]

With the objective of reducing acute toxicity and chronic morbidity, Horning and colleagues developed a presumably less toxic chemotherapy regimen of vinblastine, methotrexate, and bleomycin (VBM), which was tested in a randomized trial of pathologic stage IA-IIB and pathologic stage IIIA patients.[96] The trial compared subtotal nodal/total nodal irradiation with involved field irradiation (44 Gy) followed by VBM. The freedom from disease progression at 9 years favored involved field irradiation and VBM (98%) over subtotal nodal/total nodal irradiation alone (78%) ($P = 0.01$). No differences were seen in overall survival ($P = 0.09$) (see Table 77–5).[97] The British National Lymphoma Investigation (BNLI) has confirmed the efficacy of VBM with involved field irradiation, but in their experience, this approach produced unacceptable pulmonary and hematologic toxicity.[98]

Table 77–5. Favorable Prognosis Stage I-II Hodgkin Lymphoma: Studies Analyzing the Radiation Fields and Doses and the Optimal Chemotherapy

Trial	Treatment Regimens	No. of Patients	Outcomes	
			FFTF	*SV (7 yr)*
GHSG HD7[91]	A. EF RT 30 Gy (IF 40 Gy) B. 2 ABVD + EF RT 30 Gy (IF 40 Gy)	311 316	67% 88% (*P* < 0.0001, NS)	92% 94%
SWOG #9133[64]	A. 3 (doxorubicin + vinblastine) + STLI (S) (36–40 Gy) B. STLI (S) (36–40 Gy)	165 161	*FFTF* 94% 81% (*P* < 0.001, NS)	*SV (3 yr)* 98% 96%
			EFS	*SV (10 yr)*
EORTC/GELA H7F[93]	A. 6 EBVP + IF RT (36 Gy) B. STLI (S)	168 165	88% 78% (*P* = 0.0113, NS)	92% 92%
			RFS	*SV (10 yr)*
EORTC/GELA H8F[94]	A. 3 MOPP/ABV + IF RT (36 Gy) B. STLI (S)	271 272	98% 74% (*P* < .001)	97% 92%
Stanford V (favorable CS IA-IIA HL)[95]	Stanford V for 8 weeks + modified IF RT (30 Gy)	65	FFTF (3y) = 95%; SV (3y) = 97%	
			EFS	*SV (4 yr)*
EORTC H9F[94]	A: 6 EBVP + IF RT (36 Gy) B: 6 EBVP + IF RT (20 Gy) C: 6 EBVP (no RT)	239 209 130	88% 85% 69% (*P* < 0.001, *P* < 0.241)	98% 100% 98%
GHSG HD10	A. 2 ABVD + IF RT (30 Gy) B. 2 ABVD + IF RT (20 Gy) C. 4 ABVD + IF RT (30 Gy) D. 4 ABVD + IF RT (20 Gy)	1370 in all arms FFTF (2 vs 4 cycles, 53 mo)	OS (2 vs 4 cycles, 53 mo) 96% vs 97% 91% vs 92%	
GHSG HD13	2 ABVD + 30 Gy IF RT 2 ABV + 30 Gy IF RT 2 AVD + 30 Gy IF RT 2 AV + 30 Gy IF RT	open	Open	

ABVD regimen, doxorubicin, vinblastine, bleomycin, and dacarbazine; CS, clinical stage; EF, extended field; EORTC, European Organization for Research and Treatment of Cancer; EBVP regimen, epirubicin, bleomycin, vinblastine, and prednisone; GELA, Groupe d'Etude des Lymphomes de l'Adulte; FFTF, freedom from treatment failure; FU, follow-up; GHSG, German Hodgkin's Lymphoma Study Group; HL, Hodgkin's disease; IF, involved field; LP, lymphocyte-predominance histology; MOPP regimen, mechlorethamine, vincristine (Oncovin), procarbazine, and prednisone; NS, not significant; OS, overall survival; RFS, relapse-free survival; RT, radiation therapy; Stanford V regimen, mechlorethamine, doxorubicin, vinblastine, prednisone, vincristine, bleomycin, and VP-16; STLI (S), subtotal lymph node irradiation (splenic irradiation); SV, survival; SWOG, Southwestern Oncology Group.

Involved Field Radiation Dose in Combined-Modality Treatment

Two trials enrolling patients with early stage favorable HL are evaluating radiation dose to involved sites after chemotherapy (see Table 77–5). In the multicenter international HD10 trial of the GHSG, 1370 patients were randomized to two or four cycles of ABVD followed by 20 or 30 Gy of involved field radiation therapy. This trial will help to determine the optimal number of cycles of ABVD needed to control occult HL in the abdomen and to prevent recurrence of HL in apparently uninvolved sites. The fourth interim analysis in August 2006 showed no significant differences in overall survival and FFTF between two and four cycles of ABVD (96% and 97% for OS; 91% and 92% for FFTF, respectively) after a median observation time of 53 months.[99] This trial also showed that 20 Gy of involved field radiotherapy is sufficient to control early stage disease.

The HD13 study of the GHSG is designed to determine whether the rather toxic components of the ABVD regimen of bleomycin (lung) and dacarbazine (gastrointestinal) can safely be eliminated in combined-modality treatment schedules. The data safety monitoring committee closed the AV and the ABV arm in 2005 and 2006 due to a fourfold increase in HL related events compared with ABVD alone. ABVD and AVD recruitment will continue probably until 2008.

Another two trials tested chemotherapy-only approaches for early stage patients. The EORTC/GELA H9F trial (n = 783) is evaluating doses of 36 Gy, 20 Gy, or no radiation to involved sites in patients who have achieved complete remission after six cycles of EBVP II (n = 591). The final analysis with arm comparison showed higher relapse rates than expected in the chemotherapy-only arm, which had to be closed early. The event-free survival at 4 years was 88%, 85% and 69% for 36 Gy, 20 Gy and no radiation therapy, respectively ($P <$ 0.001) showing that IF could not be skipped when combined with a mild chemotherapy regimen.[63] Although data are not yet mature, it was postulated that 20 Gy are equally efficient than 36 Gy in these patients.

More recently, Meyer et al published a trial conducted by the National Cancer Institute of Canada Clinical Trials Group and the Eastern Cooperative Group.[100] Patients with stage I-IIA were allocated to a favorable and an unfavorable cohort (inclusion criteria: age

>40 years, erythrocyte sedimentation rate >50 mm/h, mixed cellularity or lymphocyte-depleted histology, and >4 sites of involvement) before random assignment to ABVD as single modality or a radiotherapy containing combined modality treatment. Patients in the chemotherapy-only group received up to six cycles of ABVD. Patients in the radiotherapy group were treated with STNI only or two cycles of ABVD and STNI, if allocated to the favorable or the unfavorable cohort, respectively. There was a statistically significant difference in terms of freedom from progression (FFP) in favor of the radiation-containing regimen (93% vs. 87%) but rates for event-free and overall survival did not reach statistical significance at a median follow-up time of 4.2 years. It might be speculated that the reduced FFP rate for the chemotherapy only arm will be outweighed by a reduced rate of long-term toxicities and secondary malignancies, which needs to be confirmed in a longer follow-up.

Recommendations and Future Directions for Favorable-Stage I-II Hodgkin Lymphoma

Current clinical trials are evaluating the use of alternative chemotherapy combinations, shortened courses of chemotherapy, chemotherapy with smaller radiation fields or lower radiation doses, and chemotherapy without radiation therapy. Fortunately, death from HL of patients with favorable-prognosis, early-stage disease is unusual and overall survival is not a useful parameter to evaluate midterm results in early-stage HL. Current trials should be judged by freedom from first recurrence rates and acute morbidity. On the basis of the available data, it can be concluded that patients with early-stage favorable HL benefit from a short course of ABVD chemotherapy in combination with involved field radiotherapy. Although there is some evidence that radiotherapy might not be necessary for those patients that achieve a complete remission (CR) after two courses of ABVD chemotherapy, it is still advisable to treat all patients with early-stage favorable HL with a combined modality regimen as follow-up of these patients is still too short. Ongoing studies using PET after two courses of ABVD and giving IF-RT only to PET positive patients will demonstrate whether consolidative RT is necessary after achieving a CR after two ABVD.

Early-stage Unfavorable Hodgkin Lymphoma

It is generally accepted that early-stage, unfavorable-prognosis HL patients (see Table 77–3) qualify for combined chemotherapy and radiotherapy. However, the prognostic impact of a single risk factor, the optimal chemotherapy regimen, the number of chemotherapy cycles, the field sizes, and the dosage of radiation within these fields are subjects of debate.

Trials to Identify the Best Chemotherapy Regimen

The first combined-modality trial to test MOPP versus ABVD in patients with unfavorable-prognosis, early-stage disease was the Milan study conducted between 1974 and 1982. Using split-course treatment (ie, 3 cycles of chemotherapy followed by subtotal nodal irradiation), this study did not show a significant difference in freedom from progression between the two treatment groups.[101] However, in the EORTC H6U trial (1982–1988) comparing split-course MOPP and ABVD, the 10-year survival rate was equivalent in both arms, but the freedom from treatment failure rate was significantly higher with ABVD than with MOPP.[102] In the EORTC H7U trial (n = 389), the event-free survival rate was 68% for the EBVP regimen plus involved field irradiation, compared with 88% (P = 0.001) for MOPP/ABV plus involved field irradiation leading to 10-year OS rates of 79% and 87%, respectively (P = 0.0175) (Table 77–6).[93]

The Grupo Argentino de Tratamiento de la Leucemia Aguda (GATLA) trial and the EORTC H7U trial studied modified nonalkylating agent regimens versus standard alkylating agent regimens in patients with unfavorable-prognosis, early-stage disease. All patients received combined radiation therapy and chemotherapy. In the GATLA trial, the event-free survival rate was 66% with the AOPE regimen (ie, doxorubicin, vincristine, prednisone, and etoposide) and 85% (P = 0.009) with the CVPP regimen (ie, cyclophosphamide, vinblastine, procarbazine, and prednisone).[103] In the EORTC H7U and the GATLA trials, the arms using modified chemotherapy were associated with significantly higher recurrence rates. Compared with the effect on favorable-prognosis stage I-II HL, less toxic and less intense chemotherapy regimens in combined-modality therapy regimens do not appear to be equally effective in patients with unfavorable-prognosis disease (see Table 77–6).

Chemotherapy modalities using reduced numbers of cycles of chemotherapy or modified chemotherapy regimens have been also tested in nonrandomized trials.[104,105] Another nonrandomized trial tested the efficacy of the 12-week Stanford V regimen (ie, nitrogen mustard, doxorubicin, vincristine, vinblastine, etoposide, bleomycin, and prednisone plus 36 Gy of involved field irradiation). In that study, 142 patients with stage III-IV disease or locally extensive mediastinal stage I-II HL were enrolled to receive this brief and dose-intense combined-modality regimen.[106] At 5.4 years, the rate of freedom from progression was 89%, and the overall survival rate was 96%. The estimated rates of 5-year freedom from progression for stage I-II and stage III-IV patients were 96.7% ± 6.5% and 84.7% ± 7.4%, respectively. Freedom from progression and overall survival also depended significantly on the IPS (0 to 2 compared with >3). Progressive disease was not observed during treatment. The investigators stressed the fact that there were no treatment-related deaths, no secondary leukemia, and no myelodysplasia and that 42 pregnancies occurred after competition of treatment. The E2496 Intergroup trial which was closed in 2006 is evaluating the benefits and late complications of the Stanford V protocol comparing it with ABVD chemotherapy.

Based mainly on trial results from advanced HL, ABVD has also become the standard regimen for clinical stage I-II patients. ABVD is thus compared in the already mentioned E2496 trial and in three other trials with more intense regimens. The EORTC H9U and the GHSG HD11 trials compared four cycles of ABVD with four cycles of BEACOPP-baseline (ie, bleomycin, etoposide, doxorubicin (Adriamycin), cyclophosphamide, vincristine (Oncovin), procarbazine, and prednisone), and involved field radiotherapy is limited to a dose of 20 or 30 Gy, respectively. The fifth interim analysis of the HD11 trial was presented at the end of 2005.[107] After a median observation time of 3 years, FFTF was 87% and OS was 96%. For both FFTF and OS, there was no significant difference neither between ABVD (FFTF 87% and OS 97%) and BEACOPP (FFTF 88% and OS 96%) nor between 30 Gy (FFTF 90% and OS 97%) and 20 Gy IF-RT (FFTF 87% and OS 97%). The relatively low FFTF rate led the GHSG to investigate the efficacy of two cycles of BEACOPP escalated followed by two cycles of ABVD within the ongoing HD14 trial.

Radiation Field and Dose

In preceding studies, the GHSG randomized responding patients with early-stage, unfavorable-prognosis disease to 40 Gy of extended field irradiation or 20 Gy of extended field irradiation plus 20 Gy of involved field radiotherapy (HD1 trial), with no outcome difference. In the follow-up trial (HD5), patients received 30 Gy of extended field irradiation plus 10 Gy to sites of bulky disease.[108] These trials demonstrated that radiation dose in the extended field can safely be reduced to at least 30 Gy (with 10 Gy delivered to bulky tumors) when given after two cycles of alternating ABVD and COPP (ie, cyclophosphamide, vincristine [Oncovin], procarbazine, and prednisone). Similarly, other groups have aimed at improving combined-modality treatment for HL patients with early-stage, unfavorable-prognosis disease. The cooperative study reported by Zittoun and coworkers[109] compared six cycles of MOPP sandwiched

Table 77–6. Unfavorable-Prognosis Stage I-II Hodgkin Lymphoma: Studies Analyzing the Appropriate Radiation Volume and Dosage and the Most Effective Chemotherapy

Trial	Treatment Regimens	No. of Patients	Outcomes	
			FFP (5 yr)	
Istituto Nazionale Tumori, Milan (1974–1982)[70]	A: 3 MOPP + STLI/TLI + 3 MOPP	33	66%	
	B: 3 ABVD + STLI/TLI + 3 ABVD	36	72% ($P = 0.2$)	
			FFTF	*SV (10 yr)*
EORTC H6U (1982–1988)[71]	A: 3 MOPP + mantle + 3 MOPP	165	68%	87%
	B: 3 ABVD + mantle + 3 ABVD	151	90% ($P < 0.0001$, $P = 0.52$)	87%
			EFS	*SV (6 yr)*
EORTC H7U (1988–1992)[72,93]	A: 6 EBVP + IF RT (36 Gy)	183	68%	79%
	B: 6 MOPP/ABV + IF RT	182	88% ($P < 0.001$, $P = 0.0175$)	87%
			EFS	*SV (5 yr)*
GATLA (1986–1992)[73]	A: 3 CVPP + IF RT (30 Gy) + 3 CVPP	92	85%	95%
	B. 3 AOPE + IF RT (30 Gy) + 3 AOPE	84	66% ($P = 0.009$, $P = 0.16$)	87%
			DFS	*SV (6 yr)*
French Cooperation (1976–1981)[109]	A: 3 MOPP + IF RT (40 Gy) +3 MOPP	82	87%	92%
	B: 3 MOPP + EF RT (40 Gy) +3 MOPP	91	93% (NS, NS)	91%
			FFP	*SV (12 yr)*
Istituto Nazionale Tumori, Milan (1990–1997)[110]	A: 4 ABVD + STNI	65	93%	96%
	B: 4 ABVD + IF RT	68	94% (NS, NS)	94%
			FFTF	*SV (5 yr)*
GHSG HD8 (1993–1998)[111]	A: 4 COPP/ABVD + EF RT (30 Gy) + bulk (10 Gy)	532	86%	91%
	B: 4 COPP/ABVD + IF RT (30 Gy) + bulk (10Gy)	532	84% (NS, NS)	92%
			EFS	*SV (10 yr)*
EORTC/GELA H8U (1993–1998)[94]	A: 6 MOPP/ABV + IF RT (36 Gy)	335	84%	88%
	B: 4 MOPP/ABV + IF RT (36 Gy)	333	88%	85%
	C: 4 MOPP/ABV + STLI	327	87% (NS, NS)	84%
			FFTF	*SV (3 yr)*
GHSG HD11 (1998–2002)	A: 4 ABVD + IF RT (30 Gy)	327	87%	96% for ABVD
	B: 4 ABVD + IF RT (20 Gy)	325	88%	96% for BEACOPP
	C: 4 BEACOPP + IF RT (30 Gy)	319	87%	97% for 20 Gy
	D: 4 BEACOPP + IF RT (20 Gy)	329	90% (all arm comparisons NS)	97% for 30 Gy

Table 77–6. Unfavorable-Prognosis Stage I-II Hodgkin Lymphoma: Studies Analyzing the Appropriate Radiation Volume and Dosage and the Most Effective Chemotherapy—cont'd

Trial	Treatment Regimens	No. of Patients	Outcomes	
			FFTF	*SV (4 yr)*
EORTC H9U (1998–2002)[112]	A: 6 ABVD + IF RT (30 Gy) B: 4 ABVD + IF RT C: 4 BEACOPP + IF RT	277 276 255	94% 89% 91% (NS, NS)	96% 95% 93%
GHSG HD14 (2003-)	A: 4 ABVD + IF RT (30 Gy) B: 2 BEACOPP escalated + 2 ABVD + IF RT (30 Gy)	open	Open	

ABVD regimen, doxorubicin, vinblastine, bleomycin, and dacarbazine; AOPE regimen, doxorubicin, vincristine, prednisone, and etoposide; BEACOPP regimen, bleomycin, etoposide, doxorubicin (Adriamycin), cyclophosphamide, vincristine, procarbazine, and prednisone; COPP regimen, cyclophosphamide, vincristine, procarbazine, and prednisone; CS, clinical stage; CVPP regimen, cyclophosphamide, vinblastine, procarbazine, and prednisone; DFS, disease-free survival; EBVP regimen, epirubicin, bleomycin, vinblastine, and prednisone; EF, extended field; EFS, event-free survival; EORTC, European Organization for Research and Treatment of Cancer; FFP, freedom from progression; FFTF, freedom from treatment failure; GATLA, Grupo Argentino de Tratamiento de la Leucemia Aguda; GELA, Groupe d'Etude des Lymphomes de l'Adulte; GHSG, German Hodgkin's Lymphoma Study Group; IF involved field; MOPP regimen, mechlorethamine, vincristine (Oncovin), procarbazine, and prednisone; NS, not significant; RFS, relapse-free survival; RT, radiation therapy; Stanford V regimen, mechlorethamine, doxorubicin, vinblastine, prednisone, vincristine, bleomycin, and VP-16; STLI, subtotal lymph node irradiation; SV, survival.

around 40 Gy of radiotherapy applied by an involved field or extended field technique (see Table 77–6). In a total of 173 patients evaluated, there was no difference in terms of disease-free survival (87% versus 93%) and overall survival (92% versus 91%).

An Italian study headed by the Milan group[110] (see Table 77–6) entered patients in a randomized study comparing STNI with involved field irradiation after four cycles of ABVD. With a median follow-up of 12 years, treatment outcomes were very similar in both arms (freedom from progression rates of 94% and 93%; survival rates of 96% and 94%, respectively). In their H8U trial, the EORTC compared six cycles of MOPP/ABV plus 36 Gy of involved field irradiation, four cycles MOPP/ABV plus 36 Gy of involved field irradiation, and four cycles of MOPP/ABV plus STLI. There were no differences among the three arms in terms of response rates, failure-free survival, and overall survival, although the median follow-up was still rather short (4 years).[94]

The question of whether radiation fields can be reduced to the involved sites after adequate chemotherapy was answered by the HD8 trial of the GHSG (see Table 77–6).[111] This trial compared 30 Gy of extended field irradiation plus 10 Gy to sites of bulky disease (>5 cm in diameter) with 30 Gy of involved field radiotherapy plus 10 Gy to bulky disease sites after two alternating cycles of COPP/ABVD. Between 1993 and 1998, 1204 patients were randomized. The median observation time was 54 months. The overall survival rate for all eligible patients was 91%, and the freedom from treatment failure rate was 83%. Comparisons of both arms showed similar rates for freedom from treatment failure (86% and 84%) and overall survival at 5 years (91% and 92%). There were also no significant differences between the two arms in terms of complete remission, progressive disease, relapse, death, and secondary neoplasias. In contrast, acute side effects, including leukopenia, thrombocytopenia, nausea, and gastrointestinal and pharyngeal toxicity, occurred more frequently in the extended field arm. This study defines a new standard of treatment for patients with early-stage, unfavorable-prognosis HL consisting of four cycles of effective chemotherapy followed by involved field radiotherapy. The shortcoming of this study is that about 5% of patients with intermediate-stage disease will suffer from progressive disease while on ABVD-like chemotherapy and another 15% will relapse within the next 5 years.

Two large randomized trials are evaluating whether four cycles of combination therapy are equally effective as six cycles in combination with radiotherapy. The EORTC H8U study randomized patients to involved field or STLI irradiation and four or six cycles of MOPP/ABV; at a follow-up neither relapse-free survival nor overall survival differed significantly among the three groups (see Table 77–6).[94] The EORTC H9U trial randomized patients to four or six cycles of ABVD or four cycles of BEACOPP followed by irradiation. According to a recent interim analysis, similar FFTF rates are observed in patients treated with 4 or 6 cycles of ABVD, while BEACOPP basis did not add any benefit but appeared to be more toxic.[112]

Besides the HL6 trial of the National Cancer Institute of Canada reported above,[100] there is only one more prospective trial comparing chemotherapy alone to a combined-modality therapy in unfavorable-prognosis stage I-II HL. The GATLA trial randomized 104 patients with unfavorable disease to six cycles of CVPP alone or six cycles of CVPP sandwiched around involved field irradiation (30 Gy). The 7-year survival rates were 66% and 84%, and the freedom from relapse rates were 34% and 77% ($P < 0.001$), both favoring combined-modality treatment.[113] This trial, however, may not be relevant in view of the fact that there is international agreement that C-MOPP (ie, cyclophosphamide, vincristine [Oncovin], procarbazine, and prednisone; also called COPP regimen) or derivatives are no longer the treatment of choice for any stage of HL.

Summary and Treatment Recommendations

The outcome of treatment for patients with unfavorable-prognosis stage I-II HL has improved dramatically in the past three decades. This mainly results from the use of combined-modality therapy, because radiation therapy alone or chemotherapy alone historically was associated with recurrence rates of approximately 50%. Four cycles of ABVD chemotherapy followed by 30 Gy of involved field radiotherapy is a new standard for patients with unfavorable-prognosis early-stage HL. Nevertheless, this standard is challenged by more intense regimens such as Stanford V and BEACOPP escalated as 5% of the patients progress and another 15% experience a relapse within 5 years when treated with conventional ABVD and radiotherapy. Most clinical trials are exploring new combinations of more effective chemotherapy and reduced radiation doses to determine optimal treatment, with the aim of decreasing late morbidity and mortality while maintaining a high probability of freedom from first recurrence. Whether four to six cycles of chemotherapy without irradiation can produce long-lasting remissions has to be awaited.

ADVANCED-STAGE HODGKIN LYMPHOMA

Treatment Strategies

MOPP: Pioneer Combination Therapy

Up to the middle of the 20th century, patients with advanced stages of HL were incurable. With the advent of more effective drugs used early in childhood leukemia, de Vita and colleagues at the NCI were the pioneers who paved the road for the incredible success of modern chemotherapy in oncology by achieving a 50% cure rate for advanced-stage HL patients with the drug combination MOPP.

The MOPP regimen was administered with each of the four drugs given at full dose over 2 weeks, with a complete remission rate of 81%. These excellent results were confirmed at other centers with complete remission rates of 73% to 81%, long-term freedom from progression rates of 36% to 52%, and long-term overall survival rates of 50% to 64%.[114–116]

Despite the promising initial results with MOPP therapy, many investigators used alternative regimens to improve the efficacy or reduce toxicities. The omission of single drugs, such as the alkylating agents nitrogen mustard or procarbazine, from the MOPP regimen was shown by the Cancer and Acute Leukemia Group B (CALGB) to be associated with inferior complete remission rates.[117] The *four-drug principle* therefore was considered as the standard at that time, with which any other drug combination had to be compared.

A five-drug regimen developed by the ECOG containing carmustine, cyclophosphamide, vinblastine, procarbazine, and prednisone (BCVPP) was compared with MOPP[118] and showed a significantly higher freedom from progression rate (50% versus 33%) and overall survival rate (83% vs 75%) at 5 years. However, a rather heterogeneous selection of patients made the interpretation of these results rather difficult.

In the United Kingdom, the ChlVPP regimen (ie, chlorambucil, vinblastine, procarbazine, and prednisolone) demonstrated similar efficacy with less acute toxicity compared with MOPP, although no randomized comparison was performed. The BNLI performed a randomized trial to compare LOPP (ie, lomustine, vincristine [Oncovin], procarbazine, and prednisone) with MOPP. No significant differences were observed in complete remission or overall survival rates.[119]

In summary, the described efforts to improve the efficacy and reduce the toxicity of the original MOPP regimen did not result in higher cure rates but possibly resulted in acute gastrointestinal and neurologic toxicities.

ABVD: Second Combination Regimen

Despite great accomplishments with MOPP and MOPP-like regimens, there were major drawbacks. Between 15% and 30% of the patients did not obtain a complete remission, and only about 50% of patients could be cured. The use of MOPP was associated with significant acute toxicity and with an increased risk of sterility and acute leukemia because of the use of alkylating agents.

In 1975, Bonadonna and colleagues[120] introduced the ABVD regimen (ie, doxorubicin (Adriamycin), bleomycin, vinblastine, and dacarbazine) in an attempt to develop a treatment for patients who had failed MOPP therapy. Vinblastine had demonstrated high activity as a single agent and lacked cross-resistance with vincristine. Doxorubicin and bleomycin were very active drugs and produced objective responses in about 50% of patients. Dacarbazine was added because it was active as a single agent and showed synergism with doxorubicin.

The Milan group started to compare MOPP and ABVD, using three cycles of each drug combination, followed by extended field irradiation and three additional cycles of the same chemotherapy regimen. The comparison demonstrated a significant superiority for ABVD, with freedom from progression rates of 63% for MOPP compared with 81% for ABVD.[121] Because both regimens were highly active and had no overlapping toxicities, it was therefore appropriate to test MOPP and ABVD in various combinations to further increase cure rates.

The Milan group randomized patients with stage IV disease to MOPP or MOPP/ABVD for up to 12 cycles.[114] The results were significantly superior for the alternating program, with a statistically significant difference in freedom from progression at 8 years (36% for MOPP versus 65% for MOPP/ABVD, $P < 0.005$). Subsequently, three large cooperative trial groups (ECOG, CALGB, and EORTC) confirmed these results and demonstrated superior results with the combination of MOPP/ABVD over MOPP or a MOPP-like regimen. ECOG compared the MOPP derivative BCVPP with MOPP followed by ABVD. Rates for complete remission and overall survival were superior with the MOPP/ABVD combination.

Results of prospective multicenter trials using the traditional standard regimens of MOPP, ABVD, or alternating, sequential, or hybrid combinations of these two very effective, non–cross-resistant drug regimens (mostly supplemented with radiotherapy) have shown complete remission rates of up to 80% to 90%. However, the failure-free survival and overall survival rates at 5 years were only 65% to 70% and 75% to 85%, respectively. The pivotal CALGB trial of treatment for advanced HL, which compared MOPP, ABVD and alternating MOPP/ABVD without additive radiotherapy, revealed equal therapeutic results for ABVD and MOPP/ABVD as far as progression-free survival and overall survival rates were concerned.[122] Both regimens were superior to MOPP. ABVD had less germ cell and hematopoietic stem cell toxicities.[123] Long-term (>15 years) follow-up of this study demonstrated a 45% to 50% progression-free survival rate and a 65% overall survival rate for ABVD and MOPP/ABVD.[124]

Hybrid Regimens

Goldie and Coldman[125] related drug sensitivity of tumors to their spontaneous mutation rate. The model formed the basis of hybrid schemes that were tested by several groups for the treatment of advanced-stage HL. Investigators in Vancouver and Milan independently designed two hybrids of MOPP and ABVD to test the Goldie-Coldman hypothesis prospectively.

The National Cancer Institute of Canada compared the MOPP-ABV hybrid with alternating MOPP/ABVD in patients with stage IIIB-IV HL. At 5 years, there was no significant difference in the overall survival rates between the two arms, but the hybrid regimen was associated with greater hematologic and nonhematologic toxicities.[126]

The Milan group compared their MOPP/ABV hybrid with alternating MOPP/ABVD. Freedom from progression and overall survival rates at 10 years revealed no significant difference between the hybrid and alternating chemotherapy arms.[68]

In the HD5 and the HD6 trial, the GHSG compared a new hybrid scheme of COPP/ABV/IMEP (which included iphosphamide, methotrexate, and etoposide) with their standard COPP/ABVD. Complete remission rates, freedom from treatment failure, and overall survival rates showed no statistically significant difference between the two treatment arms.[127]

The Goldie-Coldman hypothesis could not be confirmed in advanced-stage HL, although this might be attributed to the fact that the optimal hybrid regimen has not been identified. Subsequently, large multicenter trials were started in the United States and Europe to compare the MOPP/ABV hybrid with alternating MOPP/ABVD and sequential MOPP/ABVD. These multicenter trials demonstrated that the MOPP/ABV hybrid was equally effective as alternating MOPP/ABVD but more effective than sequential MOPP/ABVD.[128,129]

As a conclusion to the sequence of these comparative trials, Duggan and associates[130] addressed the important question of whether the inclusion of MOPP in the conventional setting and scheduling adds therapeutic benefit to ABVD or merely enhances toxicity. The investigators presented a carefully designed, randomized US intergroup trial in which they compared ABVD with the MOPP/ABV hybrid in 856 adult patients with stage IIIA, IIIB, or IV HL or following relapse after radiotherapy. Therapy was given for 8 to 10 monthly cycles; radiotherapy and the use of prophylactic hematopoietic growth factors were not permitted. There was no statistical difference observed between the ABVD and the MOPP/ABV arms as far as failure-free survival and overall survival were concerned. After a median observation time of 5 years, the failure-free survival rate after ABVD was 63%, and after MOPP/ABV, it was 66%. The rate of overall survival was 82% after ABVD and 81% after MOPP/ABVD. However, significantly greater toxicity was seen during therapy and after completion of treatment in the MOPP/ABV group, especially concerning objectively measurable parameters, such as hematologic and pulmonary toxicities, and subjective features such as the well-being of patients because of anorexia, fatigue, and hypotension. The total number of treatment-related deaths was 25 for MOPP/ABV and 15 for ABVD, which was not significantly different. Fifty-six of 96 total deaths in the ABVD arm and 49 of 94 deaths in the MOPP/ABV arm were caused by progressive HL, accounting for more than 50% of the total deaths in each arm. After a median follow-up of 6 years, 46 second malignancies have been reported, 18 for ABVD and 28 for MOPP/ABV, with 11 cases of acute myeloid leukemia or myelodysplastic syndrome (AML/MDS) in the MOPP/ABV arm and 2 cases in the ABVD arm. Both patients with leukemia in the ABVD arm received alkylating agents as rescue treatment.

ABVD alone is equally effective as the MOPP/ABV hybrid but less toxic, and all combinations are more effective than MOPP alone. ABVD alone has the advantage of less acute toxicity, especially an absence of sterility, and few or no patients developed secondary AML/MDS. One concern is the cardiotoxicity due to doxorubicin and pulmonary side effects due to bleomycin with the application of six to eight courses of ABVD and even more with consolidation radiotherapy. However, it is internationally accepted that ABVD should be the standard regimen against which all experimental drug combinations should be tested.

Treatment Duration

Many groups have compared different lengths of treatment and numbers of cycles.[122] As a result of these experiences, 8 to 12 cycles of chemotherapy have been given in the phase III trials. From these studies, although the optimal duration or total dose of drugs is not known precisely, it becomes evident that at least six, but maximally eight, cycles of an anthracycline-containing drug combination appear to be sufficient.

Newer Chemotherapy Regimens

The proved comparable efficacy of ABVD and combinations containing alkylating agents in recent trials indicate that cure of advanced-stage HL patients is possible without alkylating agents. However, the pulmonary toxicity of bleomycin, which is especially pronounced in children and in combination with mediastinal irradiation, remains a major issue with the continued use of ABVD. A number of drugs showing significant responses in relapsed HL have become candidates for use in first-line therapy. The topoisomerase inhibitor etoposide has been of special interest to several groups because a 20% to 60% response rate in refractory HL has been reported with single-agent use.[131] Based on these considerations, several etoposide-containing drug regimens have been developed.

Stanford V is a seven-drug regimen, including doxorubicin, vinblastine, mustard, bleomycin, vincristine, etoposide, and prednisone (Table 77–7).[132] The program was applied weekly over a total of 12 weeks. Sophisticated consolidation radiotherapy to sites of initial bulky disease was employed. In a phase II trial, 126 patients had been recruited. The estimated 5-year freedom from progression rate was 89%, and the overall survival rate was 96% at a median observation time of 4.5 years. In this single-center study, results were as expected,[106] however, they were not reproducible and were clearly inferior in a randomized comparison with ABVD and MOPPEBVCAD,[133] which in parts may be explained by the use of smaller consolidating radiotherapy fields in the randomized setting. Reduced long-term toxicities with preserved fertility were major goals and could be achieved in men and women. An intergroup trial of Stanford V versus ABVD has been initiated in select patients with low-risk advanced HL.

The Manchester group developed an abbreviated, 11-week chemotherapy program of VAPEC-B (ie, vincristine, doxorubicin, prednisone, etoposide, cyclophosphamide, and bleomycin) (see Table 77–7). In a randomized trial, VAPEC-B was compared with the hybrid ChlVPP/EVA, with radiotherapy applied to previous sites of bulky disease or residual disease in both arms.[134] This study was stopped after 26 months because of a threefold increase in the rate of progression after VAPEC-B. The final analysis of this important trial[135] (Table 77–8) described 282 untreated patients with stage I-II disease (plus mediastinal bulky lymphadenopathy or B symptoms, or both) and clinical stage III-IV disease at three UK centers and one Italian center who received 6 monthly cycles of ChlVPP/EVA hybrid or 11 weekly cycles of VAPEC-B. Radiotherapy was given to sites of bulky disease (>10 cm in diameter) or residual disease. After a median follow-up time of 4.9 years, freedom from progression, event-free survival, and overall survival rates were significantly better with ChlVPP/EVA than with VAPEC-B (freedom from progression: 82% versus 62%; event-free survival: 78% versus 58%; overall survival: 89% versus 79%). The superiority of ChlVPP/EVA was seen especially in the high-risk group (IPS > 2 risk factors, bulky disease); for the group with fewer risk factors, results were comparable.

Table 77–7 shows the doses and scheduling of combination-chemotherapy regimens used most frequently within and outside clinical trials for advanced-stage HL. Caution should be exercised when comparing results of different trials, because the amount of consolidation radiation therapy varies widely and can influence the outcome significantly. Large prospective, randomized trials provide the only reliable comparison between regimens. The results of such trials are summarized in Table 77–8.

Dose Density and Dose Intensity

Experiences with treating several tumors in animal models have demonstrated a clear relationship between chemotherapy dose and tumor response. Retrospective analyses of drug delivery with MOPP chemotherapy showed that patients with HL who received less than the intended doses had inferior outcomes.[136] Such dose-response relationships also were observed independently with mustard, procarbazine, and vincristine.

Until recently, no prospective, randomized trials that analyzed the role of dose intensity in the treatment of advanced-stage HL had been conducted. There are two principal ways to test the effect of dose intensity on treatment outcome. Doses of cytotoxic drugs can be intensified by increasing individual drug dose or by shortening the interval between treatments, or both. Gerhartz and associates[137] compared COPP/ABVD with a dose and time-escalated COPP/ABVD regimen administered with GM-CSF support. The delivered dose intensity in the dose-intensified arm was 1.22, compared with 0.92 in the standard arm (1.0 = standard intended dose). The analysis revealed a higher complete remission rate in the intensified arm, but definitive results have not been reported.

In 1992, the GHSG initiated a series of clinical trials to address the role of dose intensity in advanced HL in a comprehensive way. Starting with a mathematical model of tumor growth and chemotherapy effects, the data from 705 patients with advanced-stage disease who were treated in previous GHSG studies were reassessed in this model.[138] The investigators predicted that moderate dose escalation would increase tumor control by 10% to 15% at 5 years. The BEACOPP regimen (ie, bleomycin, etoposide, doxorubicin, cyclophosphamide, vincristine, procarbazine, and prednisone) was devised and used as a standard combination-chemotherapy regimen (see Table 77–7).[139] After establishing excellent tolerability and efficacy in a pilot trial, a second regimen of escalated BEACOPP was developed in which the doxorubicin dose was increased to a fixed level and doses of cyclophosphamide and etoposide were increased in a stepwise fashion with G-CSF support.[140] Maximum tolerated doses were determined in a multicenter pilot study to be 190% of the standard dose for cyclophosphamide and 200% for etoposide.

The GHSG then designed a three-arm study, the HD9 trial, comparing COPP/ABVD, standard BEACOPP, and BEACOPP-escalated in patients with advanced HL (see Table 77–8).[141] Radiotherapy was administered to bulky disease at diagnosis or for residual disease after eight cycles of chemotherapy. About two thirds of

Table 77–7. Combination Chemotherapy Regimens Previously or Currently Used in Advanced-Stage Hodgkin Lymphoma

Drug Regimen	Dose (mg/m²)	Route	Schedule (days)	Cycle Length
MOPP				21 days
Mechlorethamine	6	IV	1, 8	
Oncovin (vincristine)	1.4*	IV	1, 8	
Procarbazine	100	PO	1–14	
Prednisone	40	PO	1–14	
ABVD				28 days
Adriamycin (doxorubicin)	25	IV	1, 15	
Bleomycin	10	IV	1, 15	
Vinblastine	6	IV	1, 15	
Dacarbazine	375	IV	1, 15	
COPP				28 days
Cyclophosphamide	650	IV	1, 8	
Oncovin (vincristine)	1.4*	IV	1, 8	
Procarbazine	100	PO	1–14	
Prednisone	40	PO	1–14	
Stanford V				12 weeks
Mechlorethamine	6	IV	Wk 3, 5, 9	
Adriamycin (doxorubicin)	25	IV	Wk 3, 5, 9, 11	
Vinblastine	6	IV	Wk 3, 5, 9, 11	
Vincristine	1.4*	IV	Wk 2, 4, 6, 8, 10, 12	
Bleomycin	5	IV	Wk 2, 4, 6, 8, 10, 12	
Etoposide	60 ´ 2	IV	Wk 3, 7, 11	
Prednisone	40	PO	Wk 1–10 qod	
G-CSF		SQ	Dose reduction or delay	
VAPEC-B				11 weeks
Vincristine	1.4*	IV	Wk 2, 4, 6, 8, 10	
Adriamycin (doxorubicin)	35	IV	Wk 1, 3, 5, 7, 9, 11	
Prednisolone	50	PO	Wk 1–6	
Etoposide	75–100 ´ 5	PO	Wk 3, 7, 11	
Cyclophosphamide	350	IV	Wk 1, 5, 9	
Bleomycin	10	IV	Wk 2, 4, 6, 8, 10	
ChlVPP/EVA				21 days
Chlorambucil	6	PO	1–7	
Vinblastine	6	IV	1	
Procarbazine	80	PO	1–7	
Prednisolone	50 total	PO	1–7	
Etoposide	100	IV	8	
Vincristine	2 total	IV	8	
Adriamycin (doxorubicin)	30	IV	8	
BEACOPP (baseline)				21 days
Bleomycin	10	IV	8	
Etoposide	100	IV	1–3	
Adriamycin (doxorubicin)	25	IV	1	
Cyclophosphamide	650	IV	1	
Oncovin (vincristine)	1.4*	IV	8	
Procarbazine	100	PO	1–7	
Prednisone	40	PO	1–14	
BEACOPP (escalated)				21 days
Bleomycin	10	IV	8	
Etoposide	200	IV	1–3	
Adriamycin (doxorubicin)	35	IV	1	
Cyclophosphamide	1250	IV	1	
Oncovin (vincristine)	1.4*	IV	8	
Procarbazine	100	PO	1–7	
Prednisone	40	PO	1–14	
G-CSF		SQ	8+	
BEACOPP-14				14 days
Bleomycin	10	IV	8	
Etoposide	100	IV	1–3	
Adriamycin (doxorubicin)	25	IV	1	
Cyclophosphamide	650	IV	1	
Oncovin (vincristine)	1.4*	IV	8	
Procarbazine	100	PO	1–7	
Prednisone	40	PO	1–7	
G-CSF		SQ	8–13	

* Vincristine dose capped at 2 mg.
G-CSF, granulocyte colony-stimulating factor.

Table 77–8. Selected Trials for Advanced Hodgkin Lymphoma

Trial	Therapy regimen	# Pts.	Outcome	Reference
Stanford	Stanford V (12 weeks) (+ RT to initial mediastinal bulk+hilar+supracl. nodes)	108	95% (OS) 83% (FFP) [CS III/IV; 12 years]	106 and Blood 2004;308a
Intergroup Italy	A. ABVD (6 cycles) B. Stanford V (12 weeks) C. MEC hybrid (6 courses) (+ RT initial bulk/ residual mass)	98 89 88	83% (FFS); 86% (FFP); 90% (OS) 67% (FFS); 76% (FFP); 83% (OS) 85% (FFS); 93% (FFP); 90% (OS) [5 years]	133
Intergroup GB & Italy	A. ChlVPP/EVA hybrid (6 cycles) B. VAPEC-B (11 weeks) (+/-RT initial bulk/ residual mass)	144 138	 82% (FFP); 78% (EFS); 89% (OS) 62% (FFP); 58% (EFS); 79% (OS) [5 years]	135
GHSG HD9	A. COPP/ABVD (4 cycles) B. BEACOPP baseline (8 cycles) C. BEACOPP escalated (8 cycles)	260 469 466	67% (FFTF); 79% (OS) 75% (FFTF) 84% (OS) 84% (FFTF) 90% (OS) [7 years]	150
GHSG HD12	A. 8 BEA esc. B. 8 BEA esc. C. 4 BEA esc. + 4 BEA baseline D. 4 BEA esc. + 4 BEA baseline (A.+C.: +RT bulk/residual mass)	348 345 351 352	4th interim analysis [2 years] all pts: 88% (FFTF); 94% (OS)	150
GHSG HD15	A. 8 BEA esc. B. 6 BEA esc. C. 8 BEA-14 (+RT to PET+ residual mass ≥2.5 cm)		Ongoing Trial	
Intergroup #20012 EORTC	8 x ABVD 4 BEA esc. +4 BEA baseline		Ongoing Trial	

ECOG, Eastern Cooperative Oncology Group; EF/IF-RT, extended/involved-field radiotherapy; EFS, event-free survival; EORTC, European Organization for Research and Treatment of Cancer; FFP, freedom from progression; FFS, failure free survival; FFTF, freedom from treatment failure; GELA, Groupe d'Etude des Lymphomes de l'Adulte; GHSG, German Hodgkin Lymphoma Study Group; OS, overall survival; RFS, relapse free survival; STNI, subtotal nodal irradiation; SWOG, Southwest Oncology Group.

patients received consolidation radiotherapy. In September 1996, at the time of a planned interim analysis, the COPP/ABVD arm of this trial was closed to accrual because of superior outcomes in the combined BEACOPP arms. In the final analysis in June 2001, 1201 patients were evaluated. Superiority over the COPP/ABVD arm for freedom from treatment failure was observed, with 87% for BEACOPP-escalated, 76% for BEACOPP-baseline, and 69% for COPP/ABVD after a median of 5 years, a highly significant result. A major difference was observed in the rate of primary progressive disease during initial therapy, which was significantly lower with BEACOPP-escalated (2%) than with BEACOPP-baseline (8%) or COPP/ABVD (10%) ($P < 0.001$).

The overall survival rates were 83% for COPP/ABVD, 88% for BEACOPP-baseline, and 91% for BEACOPP-escalated. The survival differences were highly significant ($P < 0.002$), and the survival difference between the COPP/ABVD and BEACOPP-escalated regimens reached an impressive degree of significance ($P < 0.002$).

As expected, BEACOPP-escalated was associated with a greater degree of hematologic toxicity, including the need for a greater number of red blood cell and platelet transfusions. Second malignancies, including AML possibly related to etoposide, were reported: with BEACOPP-escalated, 9 cases of AML/MDS; with BEACOPP-baseline, 4 cases of AML/MDS; and with COPP/ABVD, 1 case of AML/MDS. However, the total rate of secondary neoplasias was highest in the COPP/ABVD arm, with 4.2% compared with 3.4% in the BEACOPP-escalated arm. The death rate at 5 years, including all acute and late causes of deaths, was 18.8% (49 of 260 patients) for the COPP/ABVD arm, 13% (61 of 469 patients) for BECOPP-baseline, and 8.6% (40 of 460 patients) for BEACOPP-escalated.

Dosage, dose intensity, and total dose are decisive factors when comparing similar drug regimens. It is difficult to predict the relative efficacy of regimens that use different drugs. As mentioned above, Hasenclever[138] proposed a theoretical framework as a first step to accomplish that task. Different drug doses in a regimen are assumed to be roughly additive in an efficacy scale when appropriately weighted. If the drug weights are known, a total chemotherapy dose can be derived. This total dose must be further corrected for different treatment durations, assuming a typical regrowth kinetic for each lymphoma entity. The resulting quantity, the effective dose, is a reasonable first-order predictor of relative treatment efficacy. Hasenclever derived drug weight estimates from a model based meta-analysis of all randomized chemotherapy comparing trials of treatment for HL and provided an estimate of the slope of the effective dose-cure rate relationship.

Applying the effective dose model and using the weights estimated from trials up to 1998, MOPP/ABVD, MOPP/ABV, and BEACOPP-baseline were predicted not to be notably different from ABVD in cure rates (all within ±5%) because their effective doses are similar. However, Stanford V was predicted to be of reduced efficacy when given with less additional radiotherapy. This prediction was confirmed by an Italian study.[133]

High-Dose Chemotherapy in Combination with Stem Cell Support as Induction Therapy

The effective dose model predicted that early HDCT with ASCT would not be a promising option to improve the outcome as first-line therapy for advanced-stage HL. The reason is that the total dose in such high-dose therapy is roughly equivalent to two or three conventional cycles of standard chemotherapy, and the effective doses are not sufficiently different. This was confirmed by three trials comparing HDCT and ASCT with conventional chemotherapy (see Table 77–8).[70,142,143]

These three groups tried to improve the outcome of patients at very high risk for treatment failure by using a high-dose regimen such as BEAM (ie, CCNU, etoposide, cytosine arabinoside, and melphalan) or high doses of etoposide and melphalan as first-line therapy after three or four cycles of conventional chemotherapy. Proctor[143] used a numeric prognostic index in a defined population of advanced-stage HL patients to identify a group with a poor prognosis. Of 930 registered patients, he identified 179 (19%) in the poor-prognosis category. There was no difference between the two treatment arms, with one group treated with three cycles of PVACEBOP (ie, prednisolone, vinblastine, doxorubicin, chlorambucil, etoposide, bleomycin, vincristine, and procarbazine) plus high-dose etoposide and melphalan and another group treated with five courses of PVACEBOP. Ninety-three percent of the patients after three courses reached a complete remission; after a median observation time of six years, the high-dose arm had a time to treatment failure rate of 79%, and the conventional arm had a time to treatment failure rate of 85%.

A second French and Italian study[142] defined high-risk HL patients as having a mediastinal mass ratio greater than 45%, more than five involved nodal areas (INAs), or clinical stage IV with more than two contiguous visceral sites, alone or in combination. Sixty patients received four courses of ABVD plus BEAM plus stem cell support (Table 77–8). In the other arm, 53 patients received three monthly courses of intensive chemotherapy with VABEM (ie, vindesine by continuous infusion on days 1 through 5, doxorubicin [Adriamycin], BCNU, etoposide, and prednisolone). Patients in partial or complete remission in both arms received involved field irradiation (20 Gy) plus 20 Gy to INAs. Complete remission rates were 90% for the high-dose arm and 84.9% for the intensive-chemotherapy arm. Rates for freedom from progression at 4 years were 75.3% for the high-dose arm and 81.4% for the comparison arm.

In the third study, Federico and colleagues[70] randomized 160 patients with poor-prognosis, advanced-stage HL who had experienced a good partial response after four courses of ABVD to four additional cycles of ABVD (arm A) or to HDCT plus ASCT (arm B) (see Table 77–8). No additional irradiation was administered. The complete remission rate in arm A was 91%, in arm B 89%. After a median follow-up of 50 months, the event-free survival rate was 85% for arm A and 83% for arm B. Overall survival rates for the two arms were not different. In conclusion, these studies did not show any benefit for late intensification during first-line therapy when ABVD or an equally effective regimen was used.

The 14-Day Variant of the BEACOPP-21 Regimen: the BEACOPP-14

Increased dose intensity can be achieved by two means: increasing the dosage in the same timeframe or shortening the intervals between the treatment courses and shortening the time scale in which drugs are applied. The experiences with the highly effective but toxic BEACOPP-escalated regimen (given in 21-day intervals) led the GHSG to consider a BEACOPP variant, in which the drug dosage and time architecture were altered according to the effective dose model of Hasenclever, with the hope of accomplishing the same efficacy but with a reduced toxicity, especially the rate of AML/MDS development.[144]

The result was the construction of a time-intensified BEACOPP-baseline regimen, which was given in 14-day intervals and administered with G-CSF support for advanced-stage HL (BEACOPP-14) (see Table 77–7). In a multicenter pilot study with 32 centers, the GHSG tested the feasibility, toxicity, and efficacy of the regimen in 99 patients in stage IIB with large mediastinal masses or extranodal disease (23%) or stage III-IV disease (77%) from July 1997 until March 2000. The final analysis with 94 evaluable patients was performed in August 2002 (see Table 77–8).

Ninety-one percent of the 94 patients received eight cycles of therapy; 77% were given within 16 days, and 94% were given within 22 days. Seventy percent of the patients received consolidation radiotherapy. Seven patients with initial bulky disease were not irradiated. Eighty-eight (94%) achieved a complete remission, and only four patients had progressive disease. With a median follow-up of 34 months, five patients relapsed, only one developed a high-grade NHL, and three patients died, one of toxicity and two of progressive disease. The estimated rate for freedom from treatment failure was 90%, and the overall survival rate was 97% at a median of 34 months of observation time.

Acute hematotoxicity was moderate, ranging between that of the escalated and the baseline BEACOPP-21 regimen, with 75% of patients experiencing WHO grade 3 or 4 leukopenia. Twenty-three percent of patients experienced thrombocytopenia, and 65% had anemia, in a few cases necessitating the use of erythropoietin or blood transfusions. Treatment results with the BEACOPP-14 baseline regimen are promising and may help to treat advanced-stage HL patients more effectively and safely.

Role of Radiotherapy in Advanced-stage Hodgkin Lymphoma

Several reports have indicated that patients treated with chemotherapy alone failed to respond or progressed, primarily in previously involved nodal sites. However, the benefits of consolidation radiotherapy must be balanced with the risk for serious side effects, particularly a second malignancy in the irradiated field.

Several phase III trials investigated the role of consolidation radiotherapy after primary chemotherapy with divergent results. After MOP-BAP (ie, mechlorethamine, vincristine [Oncovin], procarbazine, bleomycin, doxorubicin [Adriamycin], and prednisone) chemotherapy, 80% of relapses were detected in initially involved sites; 61% of patients who achieved complete remission were randomized to low-dose involved field radiotherapy or no further treatment in this SWOG study. In this trial, no significant differences in remission duration or overall survival were detected.[145]

The GHSG analyzed the role of low-dose (20 Gy) involved field radiotherapy versus two cycles of additional consolidation chemotherapy in 288 patients in complete remission after initial chemotherapy with COPP/ABVD. There were no significant differences in freedom from progression or overall survival rates between the two treatment arms.[146]

To overcome the insufficient power of randomized studies with too few patients to detect a relevant difference, Loeffler and colleagues[147] performed a meta-analysis of 14 studies involving more than 1700 patients. Two study designs were compared; in the *additional design*, irradiation was added to the same chemotherapy regimen, and in the *parallel design*, more cycles of chemotherapy were substituted for irradiation. In the additional design, radiotherapy reduced the hazard rate by about 40%. The benefit of irradiation was most pronounced among patients with mediastinal involvement and provided no reduction in relapse among patients with stage IV disease. There was no survival benefit detected for radiotherapy in any subgroup analyzed. In the parallel design, there was no significant difference in disease-free survival. However, overall survival was significantly higher among patients treated with chemotherapy alone. In the combined-modality group, there were more deaths from causes other than HL, including leukemia.

An important issue is determining the added efficacy of radiotherapy as adjuvant treatment to modern anthracycline-containing chemotherapy and the added late toxicity of this combined-modality treatment. Prospective, randomized trials, such as the comparison of MOPP-ABV hybrid plus consolidation radiotherapy by the EORTC, are needed to address these questions (Table 77–8).[148] In this trial, patients in complete remission after MOPP/ABV received two further chemotherapy cycles followed by randomization to involved field radiotherapy or observation. This important study recruited patients for more than 10 years and completed the accrual with 700 patients in 2001. A first detailed analysis showed that involved field irradiation did not improve relapse-free survival or overall survival in patients who already achieved a complete remission with MOPP/ABV. Remarkably, those who reached a partial remission and were treated with additional involved field irradiation had comparable overall outcomes compared with those who reached a complete remission. The added late toxicity associated with irradiation was not evaluated in this report because of the short observation time.[149]

A similar approach with a potentially more active chemotherapy regimen, BEACOPP, was performed by the GHSG (HD12 study) (Table 77–8). In this trial, patients were randomized to eight cycles of BEACOPP-escalated or four cycles of BEACOPP-escalated plus four cycles of BEACOPP-baseline. Subsequently, patients were randomized to receive radiotherapy to initial sites of bulky and residual disease or to no further treatment. The fourth interim analysis of HD12 in 2004 with a median follow-up of 30 months showed a FFTF rate of 88% and an OS rate of 94% for the total cohort with a similar toxicity profile as described in the HD9 trial but a reduced number of AML/MDS cases (0.8%). Although there was no difference between the treatment arms with or without radiotherapy, 18% of patients with large residual tumors received consolidating radiotherapy in the non-RT arms.[150]

In the still recruiting HD15 trial, the GHSG is comparing treatment of advanced-stage HL with eight cycles of BEACOPP-escalated with six courses of BEACOPP-escalated plus eight courses of BEACOPP-14 (see Table 77–8). In this trial, radiation therapy is administered only to PET-positive residual tumors.

OUTCOMES

The progress of clinical research in the treatment of HL in the past 40 years is reflected in tumor-free survival rates at 10 years of between 80% and 90% for nearly all stages (see Fig. 77–1). These gains have led to the question of how much overtreatment and how much long-term negative side effects should be allowed to justify such high success rates at the beginning of the course of treatment. We offer some possible solutions to this dilemma:

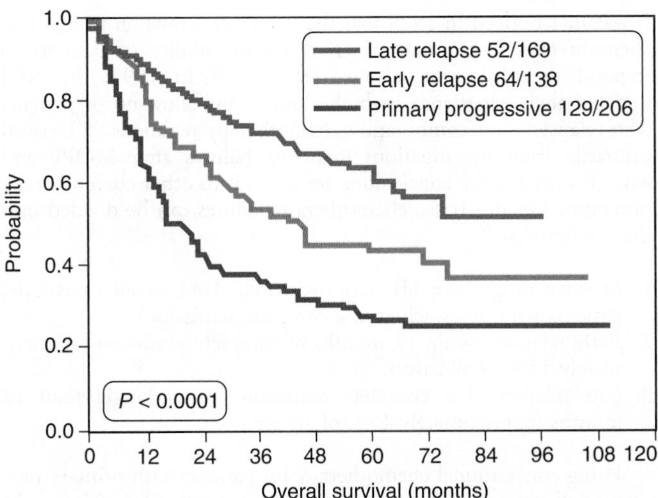

Figure 77–1. Overall survival rates of patients with primary progressive, early relapse, and late relapse of Hodgkin lymphoma after first-line polychemotherapy (German Hodgkin's Lymphoma Study Group, n = 513; total n = 3809). *(Data from Josting A, Rueffer U, Franklin J, et al: Prognostic factors and treatment outcome in primary progressive Hodgkin's lymphoma-a report from the German Hodgkin's Lymphoma Study Group (GHSG). Blood 96:1280, 2000, and from Josting A, Franklin J, May M, et al: New prognostic score based on treatment outcome of patients with relapsed Hodgkin's lymphoma registered in the database of the German Hodgkin's lymphoma study group. J Clin Oncol 20:221, 2002.)*

1. Give six to eight cycles of ABVD to low-risk patients (IPS = 0 to 2) and rescue the 10% to 15% of patients with relapsing or progressive disease with more aggressive salvage strategies, such as HDCT with stem cell rescue. The downside of this approach is high degrees of toxicity for relapsing patients, including secondary leukemias. BEACOPP-escalated is significantly superior to COPP/ABVD in terms of primary progression (2% versus 12%) and freedom from treatment failure (91% versus 72%). The GHSG uses BEACOPP-escalated in all patients independently of risk factors.
2. Give a more intensive initial regimen for patients at higher risk for failure (IPS > 3), such as BEACOPP-escalated with a 10% to 20% higher freedom from progression and an overall survival benefit of about 8% over ABVD or C-MOPP/ABVD at 5 years, accepting the higher initial burden of acute toxicity and higher rate of AML/MDS due to the more aggressive induction treatment.

These strategies are created at the time when an international prospective trial is being conducted under the leadership of the EORTC and with participation of most large cooperative study groups in Europe, Canada, and Australia (EORTC trial #20012).

Table 77–9 demonstrates the risk of early progression, treatment failure rate, and overall survival rates at 5 years when patients are stratified based on IPS scores of 0 to 2 and 3 to 7, as well as treatment with COPP/ABVD (as effective as ABVD), BEACOPP-baseline, and BEACOPP-escalated (see Table 77–8).

Table 77–9. Early Progression Rates and 5-Year Kaplan-Meier Freedom from Treatment Failure Rates According to Treatment Arm and Prognostic Subgroup

International Prognostic Score*	COPP/ABVD	BEACOPP Baseline	BEACOPP Escalated
Early Progression (%)			
0–2	12% (7%–18%)	8% (5%–13%)	2% (0.5%–4%)
3–7	12% (6%–22%)	8% (4%–13%)	2% (0.5%–7%)
5-Year FFTF (%)			
0–2	72% (64%–80%)	77% (71%–83%)	91% (88%–5%)
3–7	66% (55%–77%)	71% (64%–79%)	82% (75%–89%)
5-Year OS (%)			
0–2	86% (83%–89%)	93% (91%–95%)	94% (92%–96%)
3–7	79% (74%–84%)	82% (79%–85%)	86% (83%–89%)

*The International Prognostic Factor Project produced an international prognostic score (IPS): 0–2, 49% of all patients; 3–7, 30% of all patients, the rest were not evaluable for IPS.
ABVD regimen, doxorubicin, vinblastine, bleomycin, and dacarbazine; BEACOPP (baseline) regimen, bleomycin, etoposide, Adriamycin (doxorubicin), cyclophosphamide, Oncovin (vincristine), procarbazine, and prednisone; BEACOPP (escalated) regimen, bleomycin, etoposide, Adriamycin (doxorubicin), cyclophosphamide, Oncovin (vincristine), procarbazine, prednisone, and granulocyte colony-stimulating factor; COPP regimen, cyclophosphamide, vincristine, procarbazine, and prednisone; FFTF, freedom from treatment failure; OS, overall survival.

The question concerning consolidation irradiation to sites of bulky or residual disease after intensive chemotherapy will be answered by the final analysis of the results of the described trials (see Table 77–8) (see also box on Primary Treatment of Hodgkin Lymphoma Outside of Clinical Trials.)

PRIMARY PROGRESSIVE AND RELAPSED HODGKIN LYMPHOMA

Depending on stage and risk factor profile, up to 95% of patients with HL after initial presentation achieve complete remission after standard treatment. Depending on their initial treatment, patients who relapse have different treatment options, including radiotherapy for localized disease in previously nonirradiated areas, conventional salvage chemotherapy, or HDCT followed by ASCT. Conventional chemotherapy is the treatment of choice for patients relapsing after initial radiotherapy for early-stage HL. The survival of these patients is at least equal compared with patients with advanced-stage disease initially treated with chemotherapy.[151] In contrast, patients with relapsed HL after primary chemotherapy generally have a poorer prognosis. The therapeutic options include salvage radiotherapy, salvage chemotherapy, and HDCT with ASCT.

Newer approaches such as sequential HDCT, tandem HDCT, allogeneic SCT, or nonmyeloablative conditioning with allogeneic blood stem cell transplantation (ie, mini-transplantation) have been investigated in cases of relapsed HL.[152–154] Because more aggressive approaches are associated with increased toxicity, an accurate pretreatment prognostic assessment of patients is required to help select the most appropriate therapeutic regimen.

Prognostic Factors for Patients Relapsing After Primary Radiotherapy

Primary radiation therapy is now less often used in the treatment of localized HL. It has been replaced by combined-modality therapy, in which various numbers of cycles of combined chemotherapy are given before low-dose radiotherapy, which is limited to the involved field rather than the extensive radiation therapy used in the past. Combined-modality therapy has reduced the relapse rate to less than 20% for patients presenting with clinical stage I-IIA disease. In the future, chemotherapy alone may replace combined-modality treatment. This is the subject of a number of prospective, controlled trials.

The relapse rate after primary radiation therapy is 30% to 35% and most relapses occur within 3 years of the completion of radiotherapy, although late relapses after 4 years have occurred in 5% to 7% of patients. This small fraction of late disease recurrence is noteworthy because this is generally a more favorable prognostic group when treated with systemic therapy. Their overall survival rate is not different from that of patients who never relapse.[76,155,156]

Most patients who relapse after radiotherapy are treated with systemic combination chemotherapy, often with the inclusion of involved-field radiotherapy if a nodal site was previously unirradiated. The long-term survival of patients varies significantly according to the pattern of relapse. Three major prognostic factors for response to second-line therapy include age (>40 or 50 years), stage at relapse, and the type of therapy used for the treatment of relapse (ie, chemotherapy alone or chemotherapy and radiation). In some series, mixed cellularity or lymphoid-depleted histology were also adverse prognostic factors.

The salvage rate of relapsing patients is likely to get better than the current 60% range with the potential for earlier diagnosis with more sensitive diagnostic techniques such as PET. For those who fail conventional-dose salvage chemotherapy, high-dose therapy can still result in long-term disease-free survival for an additional 30% to 50% of patients.

Recommendations for the Primary Treatment of Hodgkin Lymphoma Outside of Clinical Trials

Group	Stage	Recommendation
Early stages (favorable)	CS I-II A/B, no RFs*	2 cycles ABVD; 6 cycles EBVP; *or* VBM ± IF RT, (20–30Gy)
Early stages (unfavorable, intermediate)	CS I-II A/B + RFs	4–6 cycles ABVD; BEACOPP-baseline, Stanford V; *or* MOPP/ABV ± IF RT, 20–30Gy
Advanced stages	CS IIB + RFs, CS III A/B, CS IV A/B	6–8 cycles ABVD; MOPP/ABV; ChlVPP/EVA; BEACOPP-escalated *or* BEACOPP-14 ± RT, 20–30 Gy for residual tumor (PET positive) and/or bulk disease

*See Table 77–3 for risk factors (RFs)

ABVD regimen, doxorubicin, vinblastine, bleomycin, and dacarbazine; BEACOPP-baseline regimen, bleomycin, etoposide, doxorubicin (Adriamycin), cyclophosphamide, vincristine (Oncovin), procarbazine, and prednisone; BEACOPP-escalated regimen, bleomycin, etoposide, doxorubicin (Adriamycin), cyclophosphamide, vincristine (Oncovin), procarbazine, prednisone, and G-CSF; BEACOPP-14 regimen, bleomycin, etoposide, doxorubicin (Adriamycin), cyclophosphamide, vincristine (Oncovin), procarbazine, prednisone, and G-CSF; ChlVPP/EVA regimen, chlorambucil, vinblastine, procarbazine, prednisolone, etoposide, vincristine, Adriamycin (doxorubicin); CS, clinical stage; EBVP regimen, epirubicin, bleomycin, vinblastine, and prednisone; IF, involved field; MOPP regimen, mechlorethamine, vincristine (Oncovin), procarbazine, and prednisone; PET, positron emission tomography; RT, radiation therapy; Stanford V regimen, nitrogen mustard, doxorubicin, vinblastine, bleomycin, vincristine, etoposide, and prednisone; VBM regimen, vinblastine, methotrexate, and bleomycin

Prognostic Factors for Patients Relapsing After Primary Chemotherapy

It was first noticed in 1979 that the length of remission to first-line chemotherapy had a marked effect on the ability of patients to respond to subsequent salvage treatment.[157] In 1992, the NCI updated their experience with the long-term follow-up of patients who relapsed after combination-chemotherapy regimens.[158] Derived primarily from investigations involving failures after MOPP and MOPP variants, the conclusions are relevant to other chemotherapy programs. On this basis, chemotherapy failures can be divided into three subgroups:

1. Primary progressive HL (approximately 10% of all cases); (ie, patients who never achieved a complete remission)
2. Early relapses within 12 months of complete remission (approximately 15% of all cases)
3. Late relapses after complete remission lasting longer than 12 months (approximately 15% of all cases)

Using conventional chemotherapy for patients with primary progressive disease, virtually no patient survives more than 8 years. In contrast, the projected 20-year survival rate for patients with early relapse or late relapse was 11% and 22%, respectively.

Prognostic Factors for Patients with Primary Progressive Hodgkin Lymphoma

Patients with primary progressive disease, defined as progression during induction treatment or within 90 days after the end of

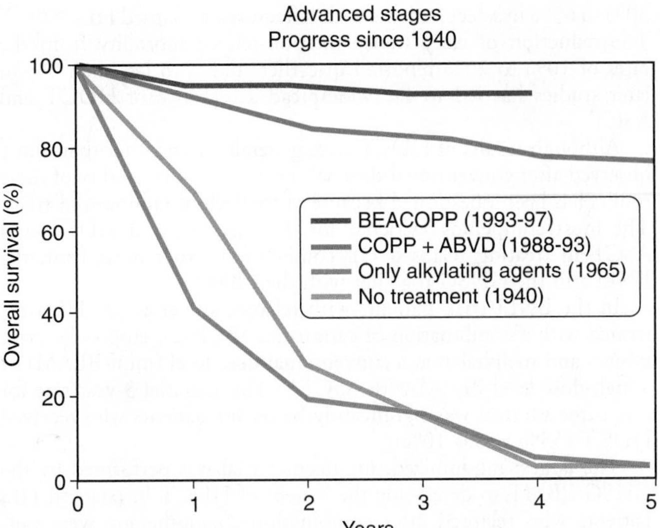

Figure 77–2. Progress made in the treatment of advanced stage Hodgkin lymphoma during the last 40 years. *(modified from: DeVita VT Jr.: The consequences of the chemotherapy of Hodgkin's disease: The 10th David A. Karnofsky Memorial Lecture. Cancer 47:1, 1981; including data from GHSG trials.)*

treatment, have a particularly poor prognosis. Treatment of patients with primary progressive HL has consisted of salvage chemotherapy, radiotherapy, and HDCT with ASCT. Conventional salvage regimens have led to disappointing results for most patients. Response to salvage treatment is low, and the duration of response is often short. The 8-year overall survival rate is between 0% and 8%. The rate of freedom from treatment failure in second remission is 0% at 4 to 8 years in the small series reported.[158,159] Extensive disease often limits the use of radiotherapy.

The GHSG retrospectively analyzed 206 patients with prior disease to determine the outcome after salvage therapy and identified prognostic factors (Fig. 77–2).[160] Rates for the 5-year freedom from second failure and overall survival for all patients were 17% and 26%, respectively. As reported from a number of transplantation centers, the 5-year freedom from second failure and overall survival rates for patients treated with HDCT were 42% and 48%, respectively, but only 33% of all patients were able to receive HDCT.

A high proportion of those rapidly succumb to progressive disease. Life-threatening severe toxicity on institution of salvage treatment occurred in 11% of patients. Insufficient stem cell harvests, poor performance status, and older age also contributed to an ineligibility to participate in HDCT. In a multivariate analysis, Karnofsky performance score at the time to progression ($P < 0.0001$), age ($P = 0.019$), and attainment of a temporary remission to first-line chemotherapy ($P = 0.0003$) were significant prognostic factors for survival. Patients with none of these risk factors had a 5-year overall survival rate of 55%, compared with an overall survival rate of 0% for patients with all three of these unfavorable prognostic factors.

HDCT is an effective treatment for a proportion of patients with primary progressive HL. Because of the poor outcomes of HL patients with progressive disease, future trials must aim at identifying patients at very high risk for induction failure and modifying primary treatment in this group to avoid progressive disease.

Prognostic Factors for Early and Late Relapsed Hodgkin Lymphoma

The overall prognosis is worse for patients relapsing after first-line chemotherapy when treated with conventional chemotherapy. HDCT followed by ASCT is the treatment of choice for patients with relapsed HL after first-line combination chemotherapy. Two randomized studies performed by the BNLI and the GHSG/European Bone Marrow Transplant Registry (EBMT) (HLR1) have shown improved outcome for patients with relapsed HL treated with HDCT.[161,162] Although the results reported with HDCT in patients with late relapse have been superior to those reported in most series of conventional chemotherapy, the use of HDCT in late relapses has remained an area of controversy. Patients with a late relapse have satisfactory second complete remission rates when treated with conventional chemotherapy, with an overall survival rate between 40% and 55%.

However, the HDR1 trial of the GHSG showed improved freedom from treatment failure after HDCT compared with conventional chemotherapy in patients with late relapse. HDCT should be considered as standard treatment for all patients with previous chemotherapy, including those with late relapse. Although these results indicate the superiority of HDCT compared with conventional chemotherapy in patients with relapsed HL, a proportion of patients with early relapse will develop recurrent disease after HDCT. However, a considerable number of good-risk patients may be overtreated with the use of HDCT. An effective assessment of prognostic factors available at the time of relapse is required to guide the physician in selecting the most appropriate therapeutic regimen and to evaluate new experimental approaches in very poor-risk relapses.

Many prognostic factors have been described for patients relapsing after first-line chemotherapy. These include age, gender, histology, relapse sites, stage at relapse, B symptoms, performance status, and extranodal relapse. The impact of these variables is difficult to assess because of a variety of confounding factors, including small numbers of patients, and inclusion of primary progressive HL. Multivariate analyses were not performed systematically.

Lohri and colleagues[163] observed favorable outcomes for patients with favorable risk factors such as an initial stage of less than stage IV at diagnosis, an absence of B symptoms at relapse, and an initial remission duration of more than 12 months. The 5-year failure-free survival rate was 82% for patients lacking all three parameters (n = 22) and 17% for those with one or more risk factors (n = 49). Fermé and coworkers[164] analyzed 100 patients with relapsed or refractory HL who were treated with salvage therapy before high-dose therapy. By univariate analysis, patients with long initial remissions (>12 months), untreated relapses, and a good performance status enjoyed improved overall survival. Reece and associates[165] reported an analysis of 58 patients treated with HDCT and ASCT at the same institution. Four prognostic subgroups were identified according to the presence of the following parameters at relapse: B symptoms, extranodal disease, initial remission duration of less than 12 months, and no risk factors. Patients with no risk factors had a 3-year progression-free survival of 100%, compared with 81% in patients with one factor, 40% in those with two factors, and 0% in patients with all three adverse risk factors.

Brice and colleagues[166] performed one of the largest studies evaluating prognostic factors in relapsed HL. One hundred eighty-seven patients who relapsed after a first complete remission were included. At first relapse, 44% of patients received conventional treatment (chemotherapy or radiotherapy, or both), and 56% received HDCT followed by ASCT. Two prognostic factors were identified by multivariate analysis as correlating with freedom from second failure and overall survival. These factors were the initial duration of first remission (ie, <12 months or >12 months; $P < 0.0001$) and stage at relapse (I-II versus III-IV; $P = 0.0013$). Freedom from second failure rates were 62% and 32%, respectively, and overall survival rates were 44% and 87% according to the presence of 0 or 2 parameters, respectively.

The GHSG performed a retrospective analysis that included a much larger number of relapsed patients (n = 422) than previously reported. The analysis of various prognostic parameters suggests that the prognosis of a patient with relapsed HL can be estimated according to several factors. The most relevant factors were combined into a prognostic score. This score was calculated on the basis of duration

Table 77–10. Prognostic Scores for Patients with Relapsed Hodgkin Lymphoma

Prognostic Factor	4-Year Overall Survival Rates
Duration of first remission	
Early relapse	47%
Late relapse	73%
Stage at relapse	
Stage III/IV	46%
Stage I/II	77%
Hemoglobin level (anemia) at relapse	
F < 10.5; M < 12.0 [g/dL]	40%
F ≥ 10.5; M ≥ 12.0 [g/dL]	72%

From Josting A, Franklin J, May M, et al: New prognostic score based on treatment outcome of patients with relapsed Hodgkin's lymphoma registered in the database of the German Hodgkin's Lymphoma Study Group. J Clin Oncol 20:221, 2002.

of first remission, stage at relapse, and presence of anemia at relapse. Early recurrence within 3 to 12 months after the completion of primary treatment, relapse with stage III or IV disease, and hemoglobin levels at relapse (<10.5 g/dL for female patients, <12 g/dL for male patients) were counted in a score with possible values of 0, 1, 2, and 3 in order of worsening prognosis (Table 77–10).[167] This prognostic score allows the examiner to distinguish patients with different rates of freedom from second failure and overall survival. The actuarial 4-year rates for freedom from second failure and overall survival for patients relapsing after chemotherapy with three unfavorable factors were 17% and 27%, respectively. In contrast, patients with none of the unfavorable factors had rates of freedom from second failure and overall survival at 4 years of 48% and 83%, respectively. The prognostic score could also predict the major candidate groups for dose intensification: patients relapsing after radiotherapy and patients relapsing after chemotherapy who were treated with conventional therapies or with HDCT followed by ASCT.

Treatment of Primary Progressive and Relapsed Hodgkin Lymphoma

Patients who relapse after achieving an initial complete remission can achieve a second complete remission with salvage treatment, including radiotherapy for localized relapse in previously nonirradiated areas, conventional salvage chemotherapy, or HDCT with ASCT. Salvage radiotherapy alone offers an effective treatment option for a selected subset of patients with relapsed HL. This applies to patients with localized relapses in previously non irradiated areas. In a retrospective analysis from the GHSG database including 624 relapsed or refractory HL patients, 100 patients were eligible to receive salvage radiotherapy alone: the 5-year freedom from second failure (FF2F) and OS rates were 28% and 51%, respectively. Prognostic factors for OS were B-symptoms, stage at relapse, performance status and duration of first remission in limited stage relapses.[168] The survival of patients treated with conventional chemotherapy after relapse of irradiated early-stage disease is at least equal to that of patients with advanced-stage disease initially treated with chemotherapy. Rates of overall survival and disease-free survival range from 57% to 71%.[169,170] Patients who relapse after radiation therapy alone for localized HL have satisfactory results with combination chemotherapy and are not considered candidates for HDCT and ASCT.

The optimal treatment for recurrence after primary chemotherapy is less clear. Different modalities such as salvage radiotherapy, conventional chemotherapy, second-line chemotherapy and HDCT with ASCT or allo-SCT are being employed. HDCT followed by ASCT has been shown to produce long-term disease-free survival rates of 30% to 65% in select patients with refractory or relapsed HL.[154,171–174] The reduction of early transplantation-related mortality from the rates of 10% to 25% reported in earlier studies to less than 5% in later studies has led to the widespread acceptance of HDCT and ASCT.

Although results of HDCT have generally been better than those observed after conventional-dose salvage therapy, the validity of these results has been questioned because of the lack of randomized trials. The most compelling evidence for the superiority of HDCT and ASCT in treating relapsed HL comes from two reports from the BNLI and the GHSG together with the EBMT.

In the BNLI trial, patients with relapsed or refractory HL were treated with a combination of carmustine (BCNU), etoposide, cytarabine, and melphalan at a conventional-dose level (mini-BEAM) or a high-dose level BEAM with ASCT.[161] The actuarial 3-year rate for event-free survival was significantly better for patients who received HDCT (53% versus 10%).

The largest randomized, multicenter trial was performed by the GHSG/EBMT to determine the benefit of HDCT in relapsed HL. Patients who relapsed after combination chemotherapy were randomly assigned to four cycles of DexaBEAM (ie, dexamethasone, BCNU, etoposide, cytosine arabinoside, and melphalan) or two cycles of DexaBEAM followed by HDCT (BEAM) and ABMT/PBSCT. The final analysis of 144 evaluable patients revealed that for 117 patients with partial or complete remissions after two cycles of chemotherapy, the freedom from treatment failure rate for the HDCT group was 55%, compared with 34% for the patients receiving an additional two cycles of standard chemotherapy. Overall survival was not significantly different.[175]

Sequential High-Dose Chemotherapy

Sequential HDCT has increasingly been employed in the treatment of solid tumors and hematologic and lymphoproliferative disorders. Initial results from phases I and II studies indicate that this kind of therapy offers safe and effective treatment.[176–179] In accordance with the Norton-Simon hypothesis,[180] after initial cytoreduction, non–cross-resistant agents are administered at short intervals. In general, the transplantation of PBSCs and the use of growth factors allow the application of the most effective drugs at the highest possible doses at intervals of 1 to 3 weeks. Sequential HDCT enables the highest possible dosing over a minimum period (ie, dose intensification).

In 1997, a multicenter phase II trial with a high-dose sequential chemotherapy program and a final myeloablative course was started to evaluate the feasibility and efficacy of this novel regimen in patients with relapsed HL.[181] Patients between the ages of 18 and 60 years with histologically proved relapsed or primary progressive HL in second relapse with no prior HDCT and an ECOG performance status 0 to 1 were eligible for this study.

The treatment program consisted of two cycles of dexamethasone, cytosine arabinoside, and cisplatin (DHAP regimen) in the first phase to reduce tumor burden before HDCT. Patients with partial or complete remissions after two cycles of DHAP received sequential HDCT consisting of cyclophosphamide (4 g/m^2 given IV), methotrexate (8 g/m^2 given IV), vincristine (1.4 mg/m^2 given IV), and etoposide (2 g/m^2 given IV). The final myeloablative course was BEAM followed by PBSCT with at least 2×10^6 CD34$^+$ cells/kg.

At the last interim analysis, 102 patients were available for the final evaluation. At the end of treatment, 10 patients had experienced multiple relapses, 17 patients had progressive disease, 30 patients experienced early relapses, and 45 patients experienced late relapses. After a median of 30 months of follow-up (range, 3 to 61 months), results were as follows. The response rate after DHAP was 87% (23% complete remissions, 64% partial remissions), and the response rate at final evaluation was 77% (68% complete remissions, 9% partial remissions). Toxicity was tolerable, with no treatment-related deaths. Rates of freedom from treatment failure and overall survival rates for patients with early relapse were, respectively, 64% and 87% for early relapse, 68% and 81% for late relapse, 30% and 58% for patients with progressive disease, and 55% and 88% for patients with multiple relapses. This three-phase treatment regimen appears to be well tolerated and feasible in patients with relapsed and primary progressive HL. The preliminary data suggest high efficacy of treatment for relapsed HL patients, warranting further randomized studies.

In January 2001, the GHSG, EORTC, and EBMT started a prospective, randomized study to compare the effectiveness of a standard HDCT (BEAM) with a sequential HDCT after initial cytoreduction with two cycles DHAP. Patients with histologically confirmed early or late relapsed HL and patients in second relapse with no prior HDCT fulfilling the entry criteria receive two cycles of DHAP followed by G-CSF. Patients achieving no change, partial remission, or complete remission after DHAP are centrally randomized to receive BEAM followed by PBSCT (ie, arm A of the study) or high-dose cyclophosphamide plus G-CSF followed by high-dose methotrexate plus vincristine, followed by high-dose etoposide plus G-CSF and a final myeloablative course with BEAM (ie, arm B of the study).[182] The results of this study are eagerly awaited.

Allogeneic Transplantation after Reduced Conditioning in Hodgkin Lymphoma

Allogeneic bone marrow transplantation (allo-BMT) has clear advantages compared with ASCT. Donor marrow cells uninvolved by malignancy are used avoiding the risk of infusing occult lymphoma cells, which may contribute to relapse in patients who undergo autologous transplantation. Donor lymphoid cells can potentially mediate a graft-versus-lymphoma effect.

Generally, the constraints of donor availability and age have limited broader application of allo-BMT in HL. Moreover, allo-BMT is associated with a high treatment-related mortality rate of up to 75% for patients with induction failure, which casts doubt on the feasibility of this approach in HL patients.[183–186] In most cases, allogeneic transplantation from HLA-identical siblings is not recommended for patients with HL. The reduced relapse-rate associated with a potential graft-versus-tumor effect is offset by lethal graft-versus-host toxicity. Nevertheless, patients with induction failure and relapsed patients with additional risk factors also have a poor prognosis after HDCT and ASCT. The role of allo-BMT should be further evaluated in these patients, taking advantage of newer developments such as non-myeloablative conditioning regimens and allo-PBSCT.

To circumvent the problems inherent to the toxicity and treatment-related mortality associated with allografting, the possibility to achieve engraftment of allogeneic stem cells after immunosuppressive therapy combined with myelosuppressive but nonmyeloablative therapy has been assessed. Several groups have updated their experiences with non-myeloablative conditioning regimens.[152,187,188]

As discussed in a recently published article, TRM might be significantly reduced by employing reduced-intensity conditioning (RIC).[189] Furthermore, another recent study using RIC in 49 HL patients indicates the potential for durable responses in patients who have previously had substantial treatment for Hodgkin lymphoma. The low non–relapse-related mortality suggests that allo transplants should be considered earlier in the course of the disease.[190]

Allogeneic SCT following RIC might thus become an appropriate strategy in selected subgroups of young poor-risk patients, eg for those failing autologous transplantation, or patients with early relapse and further risk factors who are chemotherapy sensitive.[191] However to date, the number of patients treated is small, requiring further clinical studies and information in order to define clear indications.

The EBMT together with the Grupo Espanol de Linfomas-Transplante Autologo de Medula Osea (GEL/TAMO) and the GHSG activated a multicenter phase II study to evaluate the treatment-related mortality of patients with primary progressive or relapsed HL (ie, early relapse, multiple relapses, and relapse after ASCT). Patients with an HLA-compatible sibling donor or an HLA-matched unrelated donor are initially treated with one or two cycles of DHAP or other salvage protocols to reduce tumor burden before allo-PBSCT. PBSCs are collected after G-CSF priming of the donor and reinfused after conditioning with fludarabine and melphalan.

SPECIAL CONSIDERATIONS

Lymphocyte-Predominant Hodgkin Lymphoma

The clinical relevance of the Revised European-American Lymphoma (REAL) and WHO classifications, particularly the distinction between LPHL and LRCHL, has been clarified by the international retrospective study of the European Task Force on Lymphoma (ETFL).[192]

Clinical Features

LPHL patients show a similar age distribution to patients with MCHL but are somewhat older on average than patients with NSHL. Approximately 75% of patients are male, which is similar to the profile for MCHL and different from NSHL (only 50%). Fifty-three percent of LPHL patients had stage I disease, and only 6% had stage IV disease. Thus, the proportion of patients with early-stage disease is consistently high compared with classic HL. B symptoms were present in only 10% of cases, far less than in classic HL. LPHL seems to predominantly manifest in lymph nodes in the peripheral upper neck and inguinal node sites and to occur relatively seldom in central sites such as lymph nodes in the mediastinum and upper abdomen.[193]

Treatment

There are reports that certain LPHL patients do well without any therapy beyond excision. LPHL cases appear to relapse just as frequently as other subtypes, but the relapse is less aggressive, resulting in frequent multiple relapses and reasonable survival rates.[192] More recently, the GHSG published data on 131 patients with LPHL stage IA demonstrating no statistical significance in terms of remission induction between IF-RT, EF-RT and combined modality treatment. Patients with early unfavorable or advanced-stage LPHL (20% to 25%) should be treated similarly to patients with classical HL because of worse FFTF and OS rates compared to those with stage IA.[194]

In the case of relapse, the monoclonal CD20 antibody rituximab might be an optional treatment. Two phase 2 trials showed promising results with overall response rates of 86%[195] and 100%.[196] In a follow-up of the GHSG trial, the median time to progression was 33 months while the median OS was not reached yet. Due to these promising results in relapsed patients, the GHSG will start a trial for patients with stage IA LPHL using rituximab as a first-line monotherapy.

Transformation to Non-Hodgkin Lymphoma

In an analysis from the International Database on Hodgkin's Disease,[77] LPDH was associated with a significantly higher risk for developing secondary NHL, by a factor of 1.8, compared with NSHL and MCHL. Several smaller LPHL studies report secondary NHL, occurring at a rate of 2% to 3% on average. Miettinen[197] reported four secondary NHLs among 31 cases of untreated LPHL, suggesting that some, if not all such NHLs develop independently of treatment.

Hodgkin Lymphoma in the Elderly Patient

Clinical experience and data from large prospective trials demonstrate that patients older than 60 years experience more relapses and suffer more treatment-related toxicity than younger patients. From population-based clinical trials, it is known that about 10% to 15% of all patients with HL are older than 60 years.[198,199]

The patient's physical and mental condition, disease history, and the presence of concurrent disorders influence the treatment strategy. Age in general is not a contraindication to aggressive treatment but significantly fewer elderly patients received the intended full chemotherapy dose (75% versus 91%). The survival analysis of one large retrospective trial of the GHSG showed a significantly poorer treatment outcome for elderly patients in terms of 5-year OS (65% v 90%) and FFTF (60% v 80%).[199] Nevertheless, biologically young patients in good physical and mental condition should be treated in a stage-adapted manner, analogous to conventional treatment protocols for patients younger than 60 years. In this subgroup, complete remission, relapse-free survival, and overall survival rates appear to be as good as in younger cohorts.[200] Combined-modality treatment with a conservative combination-chemotherapy regimen and limited radiation fields is considered the standard therapy for favorable- and unfavorable-prognosis, early-stage HL. In advanced stage disease, six to eight cycles of ABVD combination represents a safe regimen for older patients, while more aggressive regimens causing severe hematologic toxicity should be avoided. For instance, the escalated BEACOPP-21 regimen, which has proved especially effective in advanced-stage HL patients under the age of 60 years, appeared to be too toxic for patients older than 60 years.[201] Close monitoring of toxicity (eg, electrocardiogram, echocardiography, pulmonary function tests) and response to treatment are important to modify treatment at any time.

Treatment for patients with impairment of lung, liver, heart, or kidney should be individually adapted. Depending on preexisting impairment of organ function, single drugs with organ-specific toxicities (eg, bleomycin, doxorubicin) may be omitted from the chemotherapy regimen, replaced, or modified in dose. Involved field radiotherapy, or the use of less aggressive drugs such as gemcitabine and Navelbine with or without dexamethasone are possible treatment alternatives. Of note, a concomitant application of bleomycin and gemcitabine should be avoided due a high incidence of pulmonary toxicity in one trial.[202] The GHSG is currently conducting a trial for elderly patients over the age of 60 years introducing gemcitabine as first-line therapy for patients with intermediate- or advanced-stage HL. Patients are treated with six to eight cycles of PVAG (prednisone, vinblastine, doxorubicin, and gemcitabine). They are additionally irradiated (36 Gy) in case of residual lymph nodes at the end of chemotherapy.

Hodgkin Lymphoma During Pregnancy

HL is the fourth most common cancer occurring during pregnancy.[203] One case of HL has been reported per 1000 to 6000 deliveries. Several studies have shown that pregnancy is not associated with a worse clinical course and that the 20-year survival rate of pregnant women with HL is not different from that of nonpregnant women.[204]

The clinical presentation of HL is not influenced by pregnancy. However, there are significant limitations on the ability of the clinician to stage and treat the pregnant patient. CT should be avoided because it exposes the fetus to ionizing radiation. Ultrasound is helpful for assessing the fetal status and detecting tumor lesions in the abdomen of the mother. Magnetic resonance imaging can complete the radiologic staging because it appears not to be associated with risk to the fetus. Decisions about the need for a chest radiograph should be made on the basis of clinical examination.

If HL is diagnosed in the first trimester, most experts agree that a therapeutic abortion should be encouraged. If the mother wishes to continue her pregnancy, treatment should be deferred until the second trimester, if possible, because therapeutic options are limited during the first trimester. If therapy is urgently indicated and the mother does not want an abortion, supradiaphragmatic irradiation with a dose of less than 10 Gy or vinblastine chemotherapy for more advanced disease may be considered.

In the second or third trimester, patients with stage I-II disease may be closely observed, and treatment can be postponed until an early delivery is achieved, usually between gestational weeks 32 and 34. If there is any sign of accelerated disease progression, especially supradiaphragmatic lymphadenopathy, radiotherapy alone is recommended. Most studies recommend doses of 10 to 36 Gy delivered as mantle field or involved field irradiation with abdominal shielding. At this time of fetal development, the risk of adverse sequelae for the child from supradiaphragmatic irradiation is low. In patients with infradiaphragmatic lymphadenopathy or advanced disease, combination chemotherapy is the treatment of choice. Because most chemotherapeutic agents freely cross the placenta and enter the fetal circulation, the patient and the fetus should be closely monitored. Chemotherapy administered in the second and third trimesters may increase the risk of intrauterine growth retardation, microcephaly, and mental retardation.[205] Application of cytotoxic drugs shortly before birth may be particularly hazardous because the placenta is also the primary means of drug elimination, and metabolism and excretion are delayed in the neonate. The current concept is that antimetabolites, especially methotrexate, carry a high risk of teratogenesis, whereas doxorubicin, bleomycin, etoposide, and the vinca alkaloids appear acceptable. The ABVD regimen may be used when chemotherapy is indicated beyond the first trimester. Because chemotherapeutic agents accumulate in the milk, mothers are best advised not to breastfeed during treatment.

Hodgkin Lymphoma in HIV-Positive Patients

Epidemiology and Clinical Presentation

HL is the most common non–AIDS-defining tumor diagnosed in HIV-infected patients. Some reports claim that HIV-associated HL only occurs in patients with high CD4 lymphocyte counts.[206] This goes along well with the observation that at the onset, most HL patients have a perturbed but not depressed immune response and with the fact that HL seldom or never occurs as a consequence of intrinsic or iatrogenic immunosuppression. The impact of HAART on the epidemiology of HL remains unclear.[207]

There are hints that EBV may play a definitive role in the pathogenesis of HIV-associated HL. EBV is found in HRS cells in 80% to 100% of tumors from HIV-infected patients.[208] Tumor cells of most cases of HIV-associated HL express EBV-encoded latent membrane protein 1 (LMP1).[209]

The clinical characteristics differ strikingly from those of HIV-negative HL patients. HL in HIV-infected patients is characterized by the predominance of unfavorable histologic subtypes, mainly mixed cellularity.[210] NSHL occurred less frequently (0% to 40%). The lymphocyte-predominant subtype is rare; in contrast, more than 20% of all cases were classified as lymphocyte depletion.[211]

At the time of diagnosis, 70% to 90% of all patients with HIV-associated HL present with advanced disease. Extranodal involvement is common (60%). The most common sites of involvement include bone marrow, liver, and spleen. In HIV-infected patients, noncontiguous spread of lymphoma can be observed, such as liver involvement without splenic disease or lung involvement without mediastinal adenopathy. Bone marrow involvement occurs in 40% to 50% of patients and may be the first indicator of the presence of HL in almost 20% of cases.[212] HL tends to develop as an early manifestation of HIV infection, at a time when the CD4 cell count is still in a higher range and most patients initially present with persistent generalized lymphadenopathy. Physicians should consider HIV-associated HL in the differential diagnosis of lymphadenopathy in HIV-infected patients.

Treatment

Because of the underlying immune deficiency caused by HIV, treatment of HIV-associated HL is a major problem and may worsen the status of the patient and increase the risk of opportunistic infections by inducing further immunosuppression. Most patients have been treated with combination-chemotherapy regimens such as MOPP and ABVD as they suffer from advanced stage HL. According to one trial, survival of patients with HIV-associated HL is short, with response rates far less than that of HIV-negative patients with HL.[213] There are reports on the use of reduced-intensity regimens such as epirubicin, bleomycin, and vinblastine (EBV) in combination with antiretroviral therapy (in the pre-HAART era), resulting in better responses and fewer opportunistic infections. Overall survival, however, was not significantly improved.[214] Response rates and overall survival could be improved by full-dose regimens such as EBVP[215] or ABVD[216] in combination with antiretroviral therapy with prophylaxis of the most common opportunistic infections, such as *Pneumocystis carinii*, and the use of G-CSF. Treatment with BEACOPP baseline showed promising results regarding complete remission, toxicity, and median survival while it is discouraged from treating HIV positive patients with the dose intense BEACOPP escalated regimen.[217] Hoffmann and colleagues who analyzed 57 patients with HIV-HL found that the only factors independently associated with overall survival were response to highly active antiretroviral therapy (HAART), complete remission after chemotherapy, and age below 45 years. This resulted in a median survival time of 18.6 months for patients without HAART response, whereas the median survival time for patients with HAART response was not reached (89% OS at 24 months).[218]

In summary, treatment of HIV-associated HL is a great challenge for the specialist in infectious diseases and the hematologist, who should closely cooperate in this demanding task. The combination of not too aggressive but still effective chemotherapy and more effective HAART, prophylaxis of opportunistic infections, and the use of hematopoietic growth factors will probably improve survival of more patients with HIV-associated HL.

SEQUELAE OF TREATMENT

Long-Term Complications of Treatment

Because most HL patients can be cured with modern treatment modalities and can have a life expectancy equivalent to age-matched healthy individuals, it is of utmost importance in the formulation of the treatment strategy to take into account the acute treatment-related toxicities and the long-term side effects of chemotherapy and radiotherapy. In a study analyzing 1261 young HL patients treated before 1987, the relative risk of death from all causes other than HL was 6.8 times that of the general population, and still amounted to 5.1 after more than 30 years.[219] This rate of complications counterbalanced the initial success rates for high numbers of tumor-free survivors and resulted in a late decline of the survival curves due to deaths that were consequences of treatment and not caused by the primary disease.

Modern combined-modality treatment strategies with reduced radiation fields and doses and declining intensities of induction chemotherapy regimens probably will diminish the high rate of late complications. Long-term complications of upper diaphragmatic irradiation include lung, heart, and thyroid dysfunction and secondary cancers of the breast and lung (Table 77–11).

Table 77–11. Long-Term Toxicities after Curative Treatment for Hodgkin Lymphoma

Minor Toxicities
Endocrine dysfunctions (eg, hypothyroidism, hypomenorrhea, amenorrhea, decreased libido)
Long-term immunosuppression
Viral infections (eg, herpes simplex, varicella-zoster, papillomaviruses)
Serious Toxicities
Lung fibrosis from radiation therapy plus bleomycin
Myocardial damage from anthracyclines and radiation therapy
Sterility in men and women
Growth abnormalities in children and adolescents
Opportunistic infections
Psychological problems
Psychosocial disturbances
Fatigue
Potentially Fatal Toxicities
Acute myeloid leukemia, myelodysplastic syndrome
Non-Hodgkin lymphomas
Solid tumors (eg, lung, breast, and colon cancers, sarcomas)
Overwhelming bacterial sepsis after splenectomy or splenic irradiation

Pulmonary Complications

Radiation pneumonitis typically occurs 1 to 6 months after completion of mantle radiation therapy. The overall incidence of symptomatic pneumonitis is less than 5% after mantle field irradiation; patients with large mediastinal adenopathy or combined chemotherapy and radiation therapy have a twofold to threefold greater risk (10% to 15%) of developing this complication.[220] A mild nonproductive cough, low-grade fever, and dyspnea on exertion characterize symptomatic radiation pneumonitis. Radiographically, pneumonitis is characterized by the formation of infiltrates confined to the original radiation fields. Infection rather than pneumonitis is more likely if the infiltrates extend into areas of the lung initially protected from radiation. Severe pneumonitis may require treatment with steroids.

Cardiac Complications

Chemotherapy and radiotherapy have overlapping toxic effects on the heart. Modern treatment strategies avoid large radiation fields and doses and excessive doses of cytotoxic drugs such as bleomycin (eg, alveolitis, pneumonitis, lung fibrosis) and anthracyclines such as doxorubicin (eg, myocarditis, myocardial necrosis and fibrosis, arrhythmias, myocardial infarction, pericarditis, coronary syndrome). These sequelae have become less common but still affect 2% to 5% of patients.[220,221] It was found in a retrospective study analyzing 415 patients who received radiation including the heart or carotid or subclavian arteries, that the rates of clinically significant valvular dysfunction (6.2% at 22 years), especially aortic stenosis, and coronary artery disease (10.4% at 9 years) are higher than expected.[86]

The risk of chronic cardiomyopathy appears to increase as the cumulative dose of doxorubicin exceeds 400 to 450 mg/m^2. It is still unknown whether there is an increased risk of cardiomyopathy at lower cumulative does in patients treated with mediastinal irradiation before or after chemotherapy. Careful cardiac evaluation of patients treated with combined radiation therapy and chemotherapy is recommended because mediastinal irradiation may predispose to accelerated coronary arteriosclerosis, especially when increased doses of anthracyclines are administered.

Secondary Neoplasia

The steady but continuing late decline of the historic survival curves in the second half of the 20th century was mainly attributed to the increasing number of secondary tumors.[219] The increasing radiotherapy associated incidence of secondary malignancies is potentiated by the administration of potentially carcinogenic drugs such as nitrogen mustard, procarbazine, and cyclophosphamide.

The highest incidence of acute leukemia usually spikes within the first 10 years after initial treatment and is reported to range from 2% to 6%.[222–224] The incidence and outcome of secondary acute myeloid leukemia (AML) and myelodysplastic syndrome (MDS) was also assessed retrospectively in 5,411 patients with HL treated within GHSG studies (1981 and 1998). After a median observation time of 55 months, incidence of secondary AML/MDS was 1%. Most patients were treated with (COPP)/ABVD or similar combinations (n = 30) or with BEACOPP (n = 11). After 24 months of observation, no difference in freedom from treatment failure and overall survival (2% and 8%, respectively) was observed in patients who developed AML or MDS.[224]

The classic form of a treatment-related leukemia is characterized by a relatively long latency period of 3 to 5 years, a preceding myelodysplastic phase, trilineage bone marrow dysplasia, and abnormalities of chromosome 5 and/or 7. Topoisomerase II inhibitors, primarily the epipodophyllotoxins but also anthracyclines when given in combination with alkylating agents, have been implicated in the development of a clinically and cytogenetically distinct form of secondary AML in adult and pediatric patients.[225]

The histologic pattern of NHLs occurring after HL include intermediate-grade or high-grade histology and are similar to lymphomas seen in patients with immunodeficiency diseases or under chronic immunosuppression after organ transplantation or because of autoimmune disorders. These lymphomas have a cumulative risk of 1.2% to 2.1% at 15 years.[226,227]

The incidence of solid tumors in treated HL patients increases with time and does not reach a plateau, even in the second decade after treatment. The causative role of radiotherapy and chemotherapy is debated, but most epidemiologists tend to place greatest blame on the intensive irradiation with large fields and doses higher than 40 Gy. The major risks appear to be lung cancer (mostly in smokers) and breast cancer among women who were irradiated at a young age during the developmental phase of the breast.[228] A recent study of the GHSG with a median follow-up of 72 months, showed that the cumulative risk of a second malignancy is 2% (relative risk for lung cancer, colorectal cancer and breast cancer is 3.8, 3.2, and 1.9, respectively). This figure is expected to increase over time due to the rather short median observation time and slow progression of solid malignancies.[229] Other cancers include sarcomas, melanomas, connective tissue and bone tumors, and salivary, stomach, and skin cancers.[227,230]

A case-control study[231] from a collaborative group of population-based registries and cancer centers that maintains data on 25,665 cases of HL showed that HL patients treated with chemotherapy alone had about twice the risk of developing lung cancer as those treated by radiotherapy alone or with both modalities. Most of these reports may no longer be relevant because of changes in combination-chemotherapy regimens and reduced-intensity irradiation programs.

Gonadal Dysfunction

Loss of libido, sexual discomfort, impotence, and sterility are major problems for young, sexually active HL patients. Because the mean age of the more than 10,000 patients accrued over the past 25 years in the GHSG is 28 years, treatment-related disturbances of sexual function affect approximately 80% of all treated patients and influence the quality of their lives tremendously.

In men, C-MOPP or C-MOPP-like chemotherapy induces azoospermia in 50% to 100% of male patients. This finding is associated with germinal hyperplasia and increased follicle-stimulating hormone levels, with normal levels of luteinizing hormone and testosterone. Only 10% to 20% of male patients will eventually show recovery of spermatogenesis after a long interval. After MOPP alternating with ABVD, the incidence of permanent azoospermia is about 50%. Results of a current analysis show azoospermia in 64%, dyspermia in 30% and normospermia in 6% of men after HL treatment. Azoospermia is more frequent after BEACOPP compared with COPP/ABVD (85% v 63%, $P = 0.029$). A correlation between abnormal FSH level after treatment and azoospermia has been documented. Of note, when ABVD is administered, azoospermia is observed only in a few patients.[232,233] As already reported before,[234] most HL patients (70%–80%) have inadequate semen quality already prior to treatment.[235] Sperm banking before HL treatment has become standard.

In an analysis which included 405 women, menstruation before the beginning of therapy was mostly (90%) regular. After a median follow-up of 3.2 years, 51% of the women receiving 8 cycles of dose-escalated BEACOPP had continuous amenorrhoea. Amenorrhea was significantly more frequent after dose-escalated BEACOPP compared to ABVD, COPP/ABVD or standard BEACOPP ($P = 0.0066$). Amenorrhea after therapy was most pronounced in women with advanced-stage HL ($P < 0.0001$), in those older than 30 years at treatment ($P = 0.0065$), and in women who did not take oral contraceptives during chemotherapy ($P = 0.0002$).[236]

The preservation of fertility in women is complicated. Methods consist of embryo cryopreservation and cryopreservation of oocytes, requiring 10 to 14 days of ovarian stimulation. Live births after cryopreservation of ovarian tissue and orthotopic transplantation have been reported.[237,238] The protection of fertility with the application of GnRH analogues or oral contraceptives during chemotherapy in women has been reported in single case studies and is currently been tested in a randomized clinical trial of the GHSG. There is still no standard cotreatment for the reduction of ovarian failure in young women during treatment for malignant diseases.

Other Complications

Abnormalities of endocrine function often are not detected or are neglected, but they can be very disturbing to patients. Hypothyroidism is a common event, occurring in about 30% of patients after mantle field irradiation, and typically is detected by an elevated level of thyroid-stimulating hormone. Hormone replacement therapy is required. Herpes zoster infection is another complication, occurring in one third of patients of patients treated with radiation therapy or chemotherapy alone, but the incidence appears higher after combined-modality treatment. Early treatment with antiviral agents may limit the intensity and duration of the infection. Acute, transient radiation myelopathy or Lhermitte sign (ie, paresthesias down the dorsal portion of the extremities after neck flexion) occurs in about 10% to 15% of patients after intensive irradiation, but it is seen rarely with reduced radiation doses and fields. This particular complication typically occurs 6 weeks to 3 months after radiotherapy, and its course is self-limited, persisting for weeks to months. Xerostomia is a temporary complication of mantle irradiation; saliva production returns to normal usually within 6 months of treatment. However, xerostomia may be prolonged in older patients, especially after irradiation of the Waldeyer ring. Fluoride supplementation and careful dental care can minimize the risks of developing radiation-related dental caries. Postsplenectomy sepsis can occur, particularly in children,[239] but the risk can be minimized by immunization with pneumococcal vaccine. Vaccines also have been developed against *Haemophilus* and *Neisseria*, the other microorganisms associated with a small but definite risk of developing overwhelming postsplenectomy sepsis.

Quality of Life

Because 80% to 90% of patients with HL can be cured of their disease, it is of great importance for health providers to know that patients are alive and what that their lives are like. Clinicians should aim at assessing the quantity and quality of life of patients.

A review of the pediatric oncology literature by Bradlyn and colleagues[240] demonstrated that only 3% of all randomized clinical trials reported quality of life data. Primarily retrospective analyses of the quality of life of long-term survivors of HL have been performed.[241,242] These analyses showed that a substantial subgroup of patients still suffers serious side effects of the disease and its treatment many years after therapy. To obtain more complete data, quality of life investigations should be a mandatory component of the clinical trial design and part of the inclusion criteria.[243] Several studies including a quality of life approach have highlighted the difficulties that survivors may experience even long after completion of treatment, including symptoms such as general fatigue, poor health, and social problems.

FUTURE DIRECTIONS IN HODGKIN LYMPHOMA

Generally accessible and innovative experimental therapeutic strategies for HL patients in relapse or with proved or suspected residual disease are being evaluated. Such approaches include immunotherapy with antibody-based regimens for specific targeting of malignant cells and with cellular vaccines. The combination of experimental strategies with chemotherapy seems to offer promise.

Native Monoclonal Antibodies

The CD20 antigen is expressed on all malignant cells in nodular LPHL, and thus may prove to be a good target for treatment with the anti-CD20 antibody rituximab. Two phase 2 trials showed promising results with overall response rates of 86% and 100%.[195,196] In a follow-up study of the GHSG trial, the median time to progression was 33 months while the median OS was not reached yet.[244] Due to these promising results in relapsed patients, the GHSG will start a trial for patients with stage IA LPHL using rituximab as a first-line monotherapy. It has been concluded that rituximab provides safe and effective treatment in a subgroup of patients with CD20$^+$ HL.

Very recently, it was proposed to use anti-CD20 antibodies independently of CD20 expression on the malignant cells with the ultimate aim to target nonmalignant bystander cells and the micorenvironment.[245] In one phase II trial including advanced stage patients (n = 72), the addition of rituximab to ABVD chemotherapy showed overall survival of 100% at a 32 months follow-up. Clinical studies testing this hypothesis have to be performed to add evidence to this experimental approach.

Anti-CD30 antibodies are directed against the mostly H-RS-specific CD30 antigen. Currently, there are two anti-CD30 antibodies under clinical investigation: the humanized chimeric antibody SGN-30 and the fully human antibody MDX-060. Although SGN-30 showed promising activity against CD30-positive H-RS-cells in preclinical tests,[246] Bartlett et al[247] demonstrated only a modest antitumor activity in a first phase 1 clinical trial in 2 of 13 patients without serious side effects. The following phase I/II trial included 24 patients with CD30-positive lymphomas (21 with HL) who received six doses of SGN-30. Five patients with HL showed disease stabilization, and 1 patient suffering from anaplastic large-cell lymphoma (ALCL) achieved a CR.[248] It was speculated that the antibody could be used as a chemosensitizer in future trials.[249] The fully human antibody MDX-060 mediates antibody-dependent cellular cytotoxicity in vitro and xenograft models.[250] No dose-limiting toxicity was found in a phase I/II dose escalation study including patients with relapsed and refractory HL, ALCL, or other CD30-positive lymphomas. In a currently ongoing phase 2 trial, 48 patients have been treated with MDX-060 (40 patients with HL, 6 patients with ALCL, and 2 patients with other lymphomas). CR was observed in two patients (1 ALCL and 1 HL), while 3 patients showed partial response (1 ALCL and 2 HL).[251] Overall, clinical results with anti-CD30 antibodies for relapsed HL patients show some mild antitumor activity but must be considered disappointing to date.

Pfreundschuh and coworkers[252] constructed a CD16/CD30 bi-specific antibody using hybridoma technology, with one arm directed against the CD30 antigen on the HRS cells and with the other arm directed against the IgG-Fc-receptor-III on NK cells. Heavily pretreated patients with refractory HL showed some modest clinical response after intravenous infusions of the CD16/CD30 (A9/HRS-3) antibody.[217,253] Other CD30/CD64 bi-specific molecules have been developed as well.[254] Ten patients were enrolled and were evaluable for toxicity and response. Responses to the H22xKi-4 antibody included one complete remission and three partial remissions. It was concluded that the H22xKi-4 antibody could be given safely and that it showed measurable activity in heavily pretreated patients with refractory HL.

Radioimmunoconjugates

Radioimmunoconjugates are constructed by linking a monoclonal antibody to radioisotopes without significantly altering the immunologic specificity of the protein. The most important advantage of these constructs compared with all other antibody-based therapeutic strategies is that beta particles emitted by radionuclides can kill adjacent tumor cells through a crossfire effect, regardless of whether cells express the target antigen or not.

A phase I trial is investigating the safety of the ^{99}Tc-labeled anti-CD30 antibody Ber-H2 for immunoscintigraphy and possible therapy in patients with refractory HL and large-cell anaplastic lymphoma. Results obtained demonstrate the antibody conjugate is well tolerated and exhibits satisfactory efficacy for imaging purposes. One trial using an iodine-131 conjugated murine anti-CD30 antibody showed 6 responses in 22 patients.[255] Nevertheless, this treatment was associated with severe long-lasting hematotoxicity in seven patients which will make further clinical application difficult.

Vriesendorp and colleagues[256] performed a phase I/II study with ^{90}Y-labeled polyclonal anti-ferritin antibodies for refractory HL followed by autologous bone marrow transplantation. Seven of 17 patients achieved complete remissions lasting 2 to 26 months or longer, and four patients achieved partial remissions of 2 to 6 months. Twelve patients received a reduced dose (20 mCi) because of bone marrow involvement or unsuccessful marrow harvest. Complete remissions were observed in two patients, and partial remissions were achieved in five of them. Response rates were better in patients with small tumor burden. Based on these encouraging results, radioimmunotherapy appears to be a new promising option for relapsed or refractory HL patients, alone or in combination with chemotherapy or immunotherapy, or both, but toxicity is a limiting factor for an application in mostly heavily pretreated patients.

Cellular Therapy

Modulation of EBV-directed T-cell activity may be an immunotherapeutic option for the treatment of HL because approximately 40% of HL cases are positive for EBV. Heslop and colleagues[257] developed EBV-specific cytotoxic T lymphocytes (CTLs) for treatment of EBV-associated lymphoma after bone marrow transplantation. This approach was adopted for EBV-positive cases of HL where autologous EBV CTL lines containing clones reactive with LMP2 were generated in vitro and reinfused into patients.[258] Nine patients with active, relapsed HL and four patients in complete remission after first or subsequent therapy were treated with these autologous EBV-specific CTLs. A 100-fold reduction of EBV-DNA was observed in all patients; in two patients, B symptoms disappeared.[259] Five patients were in a continuous complete remission at 40 months follow-up. Of note is that this approach is limited to EBV-positive HL cases and requires establishment and preclinical testing of autologous cells for each individual to be treated. Considering immunologic approaches, it is noteworthy to mention that vaccination strategies with keyhole limpet hemocyanin (KLH) administered together with autologous anti-idiotype vaccines-similar to current phase 3 trials in follicular lymphoma-are not applicable to HL due to the lack of Ig gene expression in HRS cells.

Small Molecules

The antiapoptotic phenotype is one of the hallmarks of the malignant H-RS cells in HL.[260] It might therefore be promising to target molecules that mediate apoptosis resistance. Among those, cFLIP and XIAP were shown to inhibit the CD95-/TRAIL-mediated and mitochondria- associated apoptosis in H-RS cells, respectively. Compounds that target these molecules are available, but so far only preclinical data are available. Besides the antiapoptotic phenotype, another attractive target to attack in H-RS cells is the NF-KB signaling pathway as NFKB upregulation is one of the characteristic features of H-RS cells. Inhibition of the IKK-IKBa-NFKB cascade, using IKK inhibitors, proteasome inhibitors or direct NFKB inhibitors, might be attempted clinically. Among those, bortezomib (PS-341), a reversible inhibitor of the 26S proteasome, has been shown to be only modestly effective in about 10% of relapsed and refractory HL patients. In any instance, it will be necessary to perform prospective clinical trials with novel compounds to assess their value for the treatment of HL.

NEWER DRUGS ACTIVE IN HODGKIN LYMPHOMA

Vinorelbine is a vinca alkaloid and is a semi-synthetic analog of vinblastine. The main side effect of vinorelbine is myelosuppression. WHO grade 3 or 4 neutropenia occurs in up to 70% of patients, but it has a very short duration and low incidence of infectious complications.[261] Vinorelbine used as single-agent therapy in HL was administered in a weekly schedule at a dose of 30 mg/m^2. Devizzi and associates[262] reported 22 patients with HL refractory or resistant to at least two chemotherapy regimens; 50% (n = 11) showed an objective response (3 complete remissions, 8 partial remissions), with a median duration of 6 months, to therapy with this agent.

Gemcitabine is a derivative of deoxycytidine and thus a pyrimidine antimetabolite with unique metabolic and mechanistic properties among the nucleoside analogs. Although structurally similar to cytarabine, gemcitabine differs pharmacokinetically and pharmacologically. It acts as a competitive substrate for incorporation into the DNA, where it leads to chain termination. Based on the impressive results in solid tumors such as non–small cell lung cancer and pancreatic cancer, gemcitabine was given in a multicenter clinical phase II study to patients with multiple-relapsed or refractory HL who had received at least two prior chemotherapeutic regimens.[263] Gemcitabine was administered in a weekly schedule of 1250 mg/m^2 on days 1, 8, and 15 of a 28-day cycle. An interim analysis of this trial showed an overall response of 39%; of 23 patients, 2 had complete remissions, and 7 had partial remissions. Another 10 patients had stable disease. Myelosuppression was the main toxic side effect. In ongoing trials, classical chemotherapeutic drugs as well as novel compounds including antibodies are tested in various combinations with gemcitabine.

SELECTED READING LIST

Aleman BM, Raemaekers JM, Tirelli U, et al: Involved-field radiotherapy for advanced Hodgkin's lymphoma. N Engl J Med 348:2396, 2003.

Bhatia S, Yasui Y, Robison LL, et al: High risk of subsequent neoplasms continues with extended follow-up of childhood Hodgkin's disease: report from the Late Effects Study Group. J Clin Oncol 21:4386, 2003.

Diehl V, Franklin J, Pfreundschuh M, et al: Standard and increased-dose BEACOPP chemotherapy compared with COPP-ABVD for advanced Hodgkin's disease. N Engl J Med 348:2386, 2003.

Engert A, Schiller P, Josting A, et al: Involved-field radiotherapy is equally effective and less toxic compared with extended-field radiotherapy after four cycles of chemotherapy in patients with early-stage unfavorable Hodgkin's lymphoma: results of the HD8 trial of the German Hodgkin's Lymphoma Study Group. J Clin Oncol 21:3601, 2003.

Hasenclever D, Diehl V: A prognostic score for advanced Hodgkin's disease. International Prognostic Factors Project on Advanced Hodgkin's Disease. N Engl J Med 339:1506, 1998.

Hutchings M, Loft A, Hansen M, et al: FDG-PET after two cycles of chemotherapy predicts treatment failure and progression-free survival in Hodgkin lymphoma. Blood 107:52, 2006.

Josting A, Engert A, Diehl V, Canellos GP: Prognostic factors and treatment outcome in patients with primary progressive and relapsed Hodgkin's disease. Ann Oncol 13 Suppl 1:112, 2002.

Kuppers R, Rajewsky K: The origin of Hodgkin and Reed/Sternberg cells in Hodgkin's disease. Annu Rev Immunol 16:471, 1998

Peggs KS, Hunter A, Chopra R, et al: Clinical evidence of a graft-versus-Hodgkin's-lymphoma effect after reduced-intensity allogeneic transplantation. Lancet 365:1934, 2005.

Poppema S: Immunobiology and pathophysiology of Hodgkin lymphomas. Hematology Am Soc Hematol Educ Program 231, 2005.

Re D, Thomas RK, Behringer K, Diehl V: From Hodgkin disease to Hodgkin lymphoma: biologic insights and therapeutic potential. Blood 105:4553, 2005.

Schmitz N, Pfistner B, Sextro M, et al: Aggressive conventional chemotherapy compared with high-dose chemotherapy with autologous hemopoietic stem-cell transplantation for relapsed chemosensitive Hodgkin's disease: a randomised trial. Lancet 359:2065, 2002.

REFERENCES

For complete list of references log onto www.expertconsult.com

CHAPTER 78

THE PATHOLOGIC BASIS FOR THE CLASSIFICATION OF NON-HODGKIN LYMPHOMAS

Elaine S. Jaffe and Stefania Pittaluga

INTRODUCTION AND HISTORICAL BACKGROUND

The classification of the malignant lymphomas has undergone significant reappraisal over the past 50 years. These changes have resulted from insights gained through the application of immunologic and molecular techniques, as well a better understanding of the clinical aspects of lymphoma through advances in diagnosis, staging and treatment.

Early classifications were based on architectural and cytologic characteristics of the neoplastic elements; however, with increasing knowledge of the complexity of the immune system a more functional approach was sought.[1,2] This attempt was only partially successful, because of the limited array of tools available to the pathologist in the 1970s and 1980s. The integration of immunologic functions with morphologic descriptions of that era was best exemplified by the Kiel classification. The identification of morphologically distinct cell types within normal lymphoid tissue provided a conceptual framework into which malignant lymphomas could be placed and matched with their normal counterparts. However, the proposed differentiation scheme was not always supported by experimental evidence, and despite extensive study, the definition of lymphoid compartments in humans and movement of cells between these compartments still contain many uncertainties. Lymphomas, like most other tumors, are typically classified according to their presumed normal counterpart, to the extent possible. However, there are difficulties in defining the full extent of the neoplastic clone in individual cases of lymphoma, and some well-defined lymphoma types lack obvious normal counterparts. Consequently, although differentiation schemes provide useful conceptual frameworks for understanding lymphomas (Fig. 78–1), and suggest important new lines of research, our current understanding of both the immune system and the lymphomas appears to be inadequate to support a biologically "correct" lymphoma classification. Thus, a classification strictly based on a theoretical relationship of tumors to normal stages of differentiation is both unrealistic and unnecessary for the practical categorization of human lymphomas. Such an approach also overlooks the relationship of molecular pathogenesis to the definition of disease entities.

The International Lymphoma Study Group in 1994 concluded that the most practical approach to lymphoma categorization was to define the diseases that one can recognize with currently available morphologic, immunologic, and genetic techniques.[3] Thus, a lymphoma classification was proposed based on these principles and comprised a list of well-defined disease entities. The REAL classification departed from previous traditional schemes and represented a new paradigm for the classification of lymphomas. Each variant could be distinguished by a combination of morphologic, immunophenotypic, and genotypic analyses, and each was associated with a characteristic clinical behavior, pattern of spread, and response to therapy. In addition it stressed the distinction between histologic grade and clinical aggressiveness and emphasized that histologic grade should be applied within individual diseases and not across the entire spectrum of lymphoid neoplasms. It further noted that the site of involvement (eg, nodal vs extranodal) often was an indicator of important biological distinctions. It stressed that many disease entities are associated with distinctive clinical presentations and natural histories, even though treatment options may still be limited.

To test the validity of this approach, an International Study directed by Dr J Armitage sought to determine the applicability and reproducibility of the REAL classification among a group of independent expert pathologists.[4] Other goals included determining the role of immunophenotyping and clinical data in the diagnosis of disease entities and the usefulness of clinical groupings for clinical trials and practice. This study concluded that indeed the REAL classification enhanced diagnostic accuracy and reduced subjectivity on the part of pathologists. Immunophenotyping improved reproducibility and was essential in some specific entities such as most peripheral T cell lymphomas.[5] This study also stressed the importance of clinical factors, such as the International Prognostic Index (IPI), for predicting prognosis and providing a guide to clinical management.[6] Applying the IPI, a wide range of survival was observed across most disease entities. This observation would suggest that it can be misleading to stratify different diseases into risk groups based only on histologic criteria. Moreover, when diseases were grouped according to posttreatment survival (as previously done in the Working Formulation), it was noted that not only were the entities included in each group heterogeneous but also they required markedly different treatment modalities. It became evident that there was a need to approach each disease entity individually considering the diagnosis, the patient's risk factors, and the known idiosyncrasies of each disease with regard to treatment.

Based on these data, the World Health Organization (WHO) adopted the approach of the REAL classification for developing a classification of lymphoid malignancies (List 1)[7]; in addition a Clinical Advisory Committee (CAC) composed of expert hematologists and oncologists was formed to advise the pathologists and confirm the clinical usefulness of the new classification scheme.[8] In 2007 in preparation for a timely revision of the classification, CACs again met in Chicago, IL, and Airlie, VA, to consult on revisions and agreement regarding new entities. The WHO classification recognizes three main categories of lymphoid neoplasms: B-cell neoplasms, T- and NK-cell neoplasms, and Hodgkin lymphoma (HL).

The WHO classification represents a significant achievement in terms of cooperation, communication, and consensus among pathologists, hematologists, and oncologists. Furthermore, it recognizes, as in the REAL classification, that any classification system is an evolving process and should incorporate new data resulting from recent technologic advances in the field of hematopathology and is subjected to periodical review and revisions.

This chapter focuses on the classification of neoplasms derived from mature B cells, T cells, and NK cells with emphasis on malignant lymphomas. We provide a brief review of lymphoblastic malignancies emphasizing the solid-tissue aspects, although these diseases are discussed in greater detail in the chapters of pediatric and adult acute lymphoblastic leukemias, Chapters 62 and 65.

PRECURSOR B-CELL AND T-CELL NEOPLASMS

B-Lymphoblastic Leukemia/Lymphoma

Although most B-lymphoblastic leukemia/lymphoma (B-LBL) present as leukemia, lymphomatous presentations occur in approximately 5% to 10% of cases.[9–11] Frequent sites of involvement include

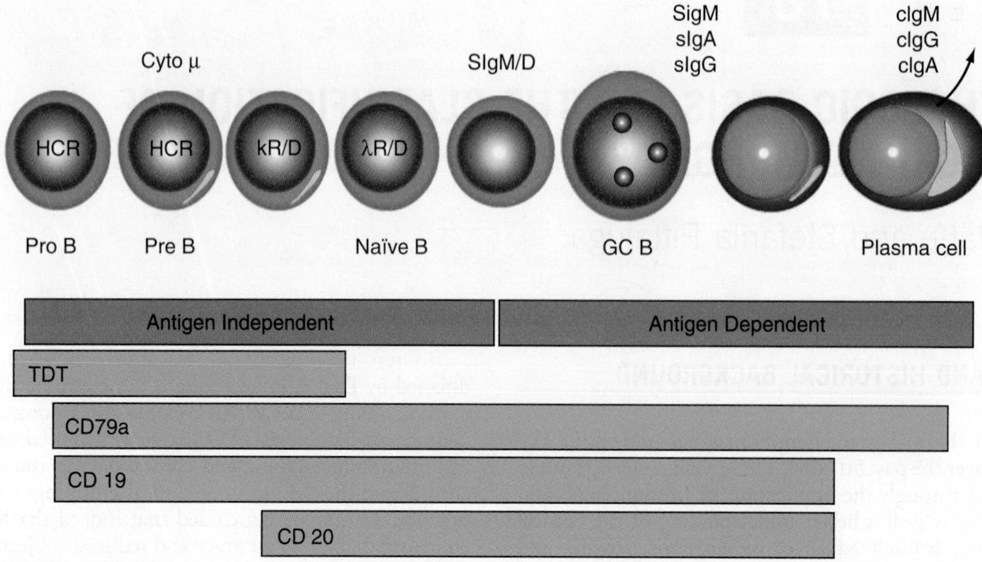

Figure 78–1 B-cell neoplasms relate to different stages of B-cell differentiation. Precursor B-cell lymphomas/leukemias are at an antigen-independent stage of differentiation. CD79a is expressed from early B cells to the plasma cell stage of differentiation. CD20 is acquired at the time of light-chain gene rearrangement. HCR, heavy-chain rearrangement; κR/D, kappa light-chain gene rearrangement/deletion; λR/D, lambda light-chain gene rearrangement/deletion; GC, germinal center; cyto μ, cytoplasmic mu heavy chain.

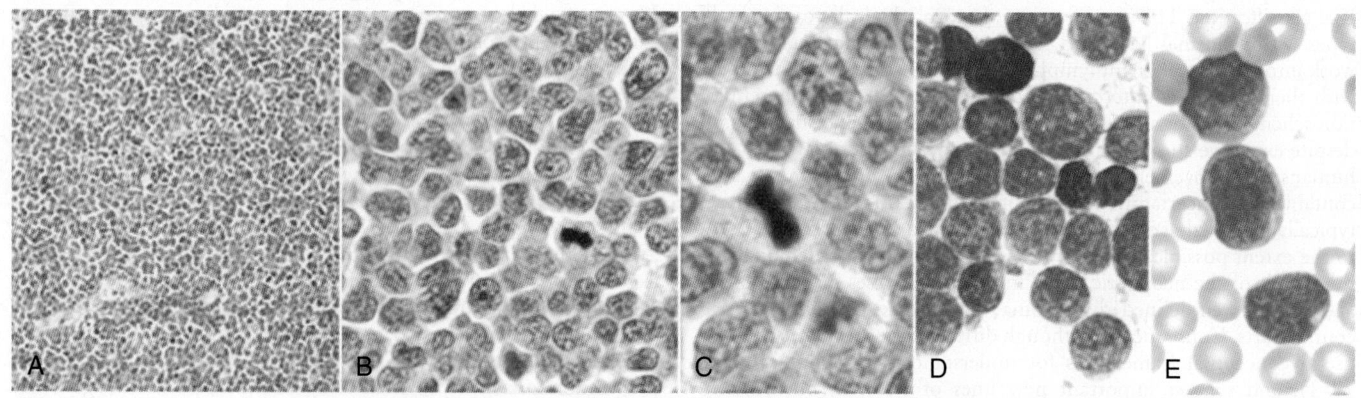

Figure 78–2 Lymphoblastic lymphoma. Low power (**A**) and higher power (**B**) showing a diffuse infiltrate of intermediate-sized cells with high mitotic rate and finely dispersed "blastic" nuclear chromatin (**C**). Touch imprints performed at the time of the biopsy (**D**) illustrate the fact that the lymphoma cells are identical to circulating lymphoblasts seen in acute lymphoblastic leukemia (**E**).

lymph nodes, skin, and bone. Skin lesions in children frequently present in the head and neck region, including the scalp.[9] Progression to leukemia will occur in the vast majority of cases if a complete remission is not obtained. The disease is most common in children and young adults.

Cytologically, it is composed of lymphoblasts that are usually somewhat larger than a small lymphocyte, but smaller than the cells of diffuse large B-cell lymphoma (Fig. 78–2). The cells have finely stippled chromatin with very sparse cytoplasm and inconspicuous nucleoli. The nuclei may be round or convoluted, and the presence or absence of nuclear convolutions is not useful in predicting immunophenotype in lymphoblastic malignancies. Mitotic figures are frequent, in keeping with the high-grade nature of this neoplasm. The differential diagnosis of B-LBL includes the blastic variant of a mantle cell lymphoma (MCL).[12] The clinical presentation is useful in that MCL is much more common in adults. In some cases immunophenotypic studies will be required for the differential diagnosis. The blastic variant of MCL is TDT$^-$ and has a mature B-cell phenotype, in contrast to B-LBL.

Although B-LBLs do not normally express immunoglobulin, other markers of B-cell lineage, such as CD19, PAX5, and CD79a will be present (Fig. 78–1).[13] These antigens are expressed at the time of heavy-chain gene rearrangement, usually indicating commitment to the B-cell lineage. The CD20 antigen is not acquired until the stage of light-chain gene rearrangement, and is expressed in approximately 50% of cases.[14] Thus, pre-B-LBL are often negative for CD20 in paraffin sections. PAX-5, a B-cell transcription factor, is a useful diagnostic marker in CD20-negative ALL[15]; however, it should be noted that PAX-5 is not restricted to B-cell lineage and it has also been described in neuroendocrine carcinomas, in particular Merkel cell carcinoma, which is often in the differential diagnosis of small blue round cell tumors involving the skin.[16]

Both T-and B-LBL may be negative for the leukocyte common antigen (CD45). In addition, they both express CD99, the *MIC2* gene product, in a high proportion of cases. This antigen is expressed in Ewing sarcoma, a nonlymphoid malignancy presenting in children and young adults, often with lytic bone lesions of the distal extremities. Because of potentially overlapping histologic and clinical features, an extensive immunohistochemical panel may be required for accurate differential diagnosis.[17]

T-Lymphoblastic Lymphoma/Leukemia

Most T-Lymphoblastic Lymphoma/Leukemias (T-LBLs) are cytologically indistinguishable from their B-cell counterparts. The cells have finely distributed chromatin, inconspicuous nucleoli, and sparse, pale cytoplasm. Nuclear irregularity is variable. This is a disease of adolescents and young adults, with an increased male-to-female ratio. Fifty to 80 percent of patients present with an anterior mediastinal mass, usually with involvement of the thymus gland. This is a high-grade lymphoma; the rapidly growing mass may be associated with airway obstruction. Bone marrow involvement is common, and progression to a leukemic picture will occur in the absence of effective therapy. This tumor also has a high frequency of involvement of the central nervous system. T-LBL is the tissue equivalent of T-cell ALL, although the lymphomatous forms usually exhibit a more mature T-cell phenotype.[18]

In lymph nodes, T-LBL has a diffuse leukemic pattern of infiltration. There is very little stromal reaction, and the cells diffusely infiltrate the lymph node parenchyma. Streaming of cells in the medullary cords may be prominent, especially around vascular structures. A starry sky pattern is seen in approximately one-third of cases. Mitotic figures are readily observed.

By immunophenotypic studies, the cells have an immature T-cell phenotype that correlates with different stages of intrathymic maturation (Fig. 78–3). The earliest T cell-associated antigen with some lineage specificity is CD7. However, it is also expressed in rare cases of acute myeloid leukemia, where it may represent evidence of lineage infidelity, often seen in primitive hematopoietic malignancies. CD3, linked to the T-cell antigen receptor, is expressed in the cytoplasm prior to its presence on the surface and thus may be negative when examined by immunofluorescence techniques on living cells.[19] In this situation, a T-cell LBL may be CD3 positive in tissue sections but negative by routine flow cytometry. However, techniques that permeabilize the cell membrane are available to detect cytoplasmic antigens by flow cytometry. It should be noted that the normal thymocytes encountered in a lymphocyte-rich thymoma are phenotypically similar to the cells of a T-cell LBL. Immunohistochemical analysis are necessary to detect the thymic epithelial cells numerous in the former condition.[20]

The classification of pre-B and pre-T LBL has attained greater precision through the application of gene expression profiling into the various cytogenetic and molecular subtypes.[21,22]

MATURE B-CELL NEOPLASMS

Chronic Lymphocytic Leukemia / Small Lymphocytic Lymphoma

Chronic lymphocytic leukemia / small lymphocytic lymphoma (CLL/SLL) usually presents in adults with generalized lymphadenopathy, frequent marrow and blood involvement, and often hepatosplenomegaly. Presentation as leukemia, that is, CLL, is more common than as lymphoma, SLL. Even in patients with a lymphomatous presentation, careful examination of the blood may disclose a circulating monoclonal B-cell component. Nevertheless, there are some patients who will present with generalized lymphadenopathy, and whereas progression to leukemia is frequent, it does not necessarily occur in all cases.[23]

Histologically, the lymph nodes involved by CLL/SLL show diffuse architectural effacement (Fig. 78–4), although occasional residual naked germinal centers may be present. In this regard, the process may simulate a mantle cell lymphoma, but usually can be readily distinguished from MCL on cytologic grounds. The predominant cell is a small lymphocyte with clumped nuclear chromatin, but a spectrum of nuclear morphology is generally seen. Pseudofollicular growth centers or proliferation centers are present in the majority of cases and contain a spectrum of cells ranging from small lymphocytes to larger prolymphocytes and paraimmunoblasts. The prolymphocytes and paraimmunoblasts have somewhat more dispersed chromatin and usually centrally placed prominent nucleoli.

In some cases, the small lymphoid cells may show nuclear irregularity. This feature has caused confusion with mantle cell lymphoma. However, the presence of pseudofollicles and paraimmunoblasts argues strongly in favor of a diagnosis of CLL/SLL over MCL. It has been shown that cases with cleaved nuclear morphology and pseudofollicles retain the indolent clinical behavior of CLL/SLL and not the more aggressive clinical course of MCL.[24,25] If needed, immunophenotypic studies can be helpful in this differential diagnosis. CLL/SLL is characterized by $CD5^+$, $CD23^+$, B cells expressing dim CD20, and usually dim surface immunoglobulin (sIg).[26] The absence of staining

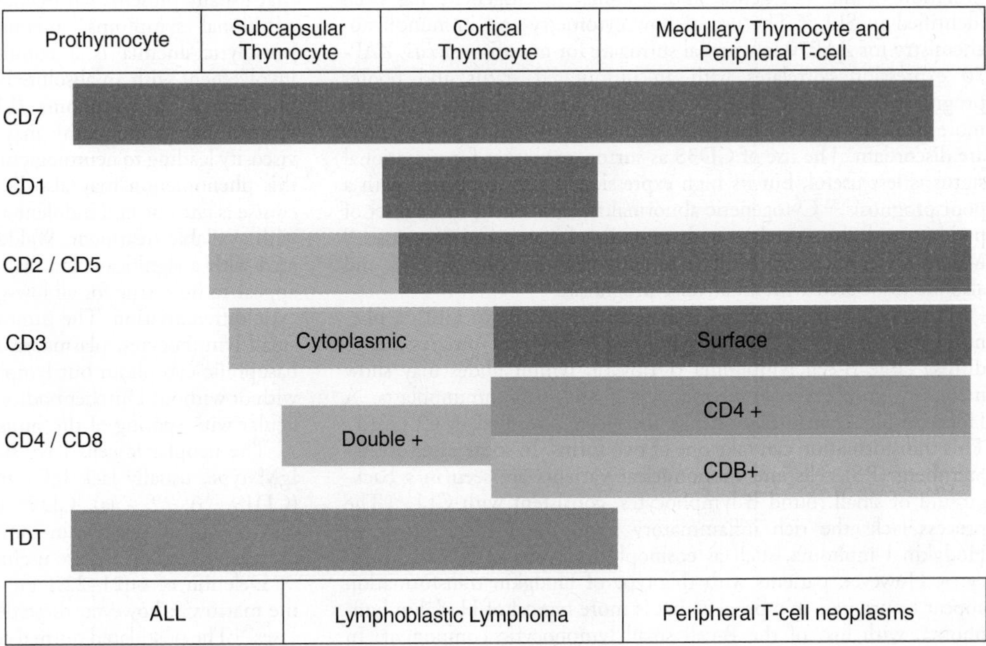

Figure 78–3 T-cell neoplasms related to stages of T-cell differentiation. ALL, acute lymphoblastic leukemia.

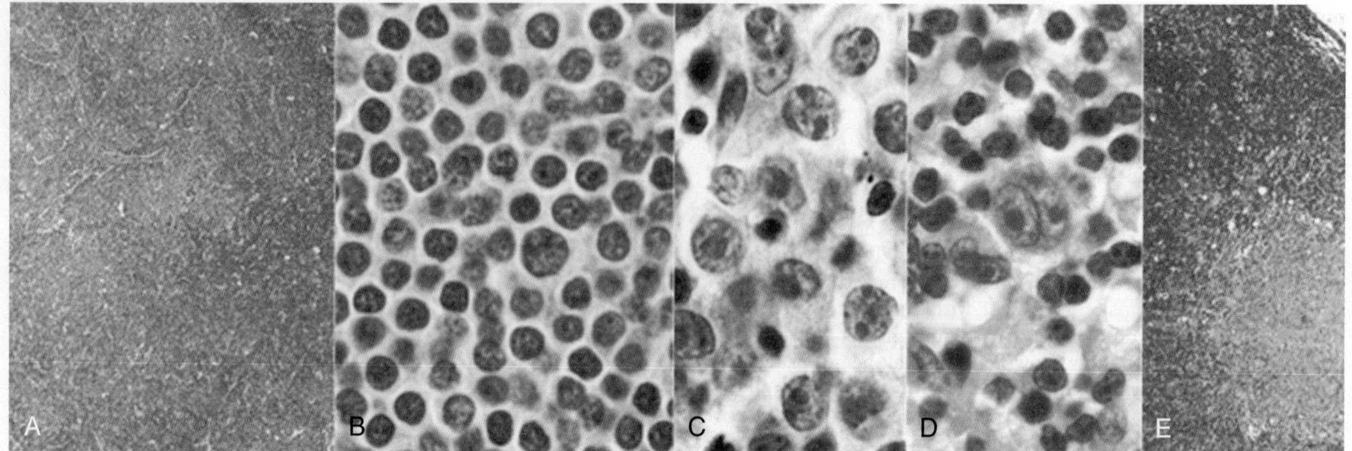

Figure 78–4 Small lymphocytic lymphoma (SLL). Low power illustrates a diffuse effacement of the lymph node. A monotonous population of small lymphocytes is seen at higher power (**B**). These have fairly round nuclear contours, condensed nuclear chromatin, and inconspicuous or absent nucleoli. Only rare larger cells are present. SLL can transform to large cell lymphoma (**C**) and occasionally to Hodgkin lymphoma (**D**). Patients can also develop worsening lymphadenopathy as a result of viral infections such as Herpes Simplex Virus, where the node typically shows focal necrosis (**E**).

Table 78–1 Differential Diagnosis of "Small" B-Cell Lymphomas

Disease	CD5	CD10	CD23	CD43	Cyclin D1	Ig Class
FL	–	+	+/–	–	–	IgM, IgG
MCL	+	–	–	+	+	IgM/IgD
CLL/SLL	+	–	+	+	–	IgM/IgD
LPL	–	–	–	+/–	–	IgM (c)
MALT	–	–	–	+/–	–	IgM (c, s)
SMZL	–	–	–	–	–	IgM/IgD
HCL	–	–	–	–	–/+	IgG

c, cytoplasmic Ig; CLL/SLL; chronic lymphocytic leukemia/ small lymphocytic lymphoma; FL, follicular lymphoma; HCL, hairy cell leukemia; Ig class, most commonly expressed heavy-chain classes; LPL, lymphoplasmacytic lymphoma; MALT; marginal-zone lymphoma of MALT type; MCL, mantle cell lymphoma; s, surface Ig; SMZL; splenic marginal zone lymphoma.

for cyclin D1 can help rule out the diagnosis of MCL (Table 78–1).[27] CLL has been shown to be heterogeneous with respect to somatic mutation of the VH genes, and a similar heterogeneity has been identified in SLL.[28] The use of flow cytometry and immunohistochemistry for ZAP70 is a partial surrogate for mutation status; ZAP-70 expression correlates with an unmutated status and poorer prognosis.[29–31] In fact, ZAP70 expression has been suggested to be more clinically relevant than mutation status, when the two markers are discordant. The use of CD38 as surrogate marker for mutational status is less useful, but its high expression is also associated with a poor prognosis.[32] Cytogenetic abnormalities also occur in a subset of patients and also correlate with mutational status and prognosis.[33] Mutations in micro-RNAS have recently been described in CLL and also are associated with an adverse prognosis.[34]

Histologic transformation over time may occur in CLL, a phenomenon known as Richter syndrome.[35] Short of progression to diffuse large B-cell lymphoma (DLBCL), lymph nodes may show increased numbers of prolymphocytes and paraimmunoblasts. A Hodgkin-like transformation has also been described in CLL/SLL. This transformation can take one of two forms. In some cases, Reed–Sternberg (RS) cells and mononuclear variants are seen in a background of small round B lymphocytes, consistent with CLL.[36] The process lacks the rich inflammatory background characteristic of Hodgkin lymphoma, such as eosinophils, plasma cells, and histiocytes. However, patients with this type of Hodgkin transformation appear to progress to a process that is more typical of Hodgkin lymphoma, with loss of the B-cell small lymphocytic component. In other instances, classical Hodgkin lymphoma of the mixed cellularity or nodular sclerosis subtype may be seen in patients with a history of CLL.[37] Studies have implicated Epstein–Barr virus (EBV) in the Hodgkin type of Richter transformation.[38] The RS cells and variants are EBV^+ and in some cases have been shown to be derived from the CLL clone.[39] In other instances, diverse clonal origins are shown.[40,40a]

In some cases of CLL/SLL, limited plasmacytoid differentiation may occur.[41] The overall cytology may resemble that of CLL/SLL, but the cells contain moderate amounts of cytoplasmic immunoglobulin. In such cases, a small monoclonal immunoglobulin spike may be detected in the serum. These cases conform to the lymphoplasmacytoid subtype of immunocytoma in the Kiel classification.[42] However, because such cases retain the immunophenotype of classical CLL, they are regarded in the WHO classification as a variant of CLL.[43]

Lymphoplasmacytic Lymphoma

This lymphoma subtype conforms in most cases to the clinical picture of Waldenstrom macroglobulinemia. This is a disease of adult life that usually presents with generalized lymphadenopathy, vague constitutional symptoms, anemia, and splenomegaly. Autoimmune hemolytic anemia is a common complication. Peripheral blood involvement with an absolute lymphocytosis is less common in lymphoplasmacytic lymphoma (LPL) than in B-cell CLL/SLL. IgM monoclonal gammopathy may be associated with increased serum viscosity leading to neurologic and vascular complications.[44] However, this phenomenon may also be observed in other lymphomas. The course is chronic and indolent and the disease is not generally curable with available treatment. Waldenstrom macroglobulinemia is associated with a significant familial disposition,[45] although this does not appear to hold true for all low-grade B-cell lymphomas with plasmacytic differentiation. The tumor consists of a diffuse proliferation of small lymphocytes, plasmacytoid lymphocytes (cells with abundant basophilic cytoplasm but lymphocyte-like nuclei), and plasma cells, with or without Dutcher bodies. The growth pattern is often interfollicular with sparing of the sinuses.[46]

The neoplastic cells have surface and cytoplasmic Ig, usually of IgM type, usually lack IgD, and express B cell-associated antigens (CD19, 20, 22, 79a), $CD5^-$, $CD10^-$, $CD43^{+/-}$; CD25 or CD11c may be faintly positive in some cases.[42,47–49] Lack of CD5 and the presence of strong cIg are useful in distinction from CLL.

Deletion of 6q21–22.1 are confirmed in most WM patients in the marrow[50]; however, these deletions were not confirmed in nodal cases.[51] The postulated normal counterpart is thought to be a memory

B cell,[49,52] based in part on the presence of somatic mutations in the Ig heavy- and light-chain variable region genes.[53] New, interesting gene expression profiling data suggest that WM has a relatively homogeneous profile and is more closely related to CLL than multiple myeloma.[54] The identification of interleukein-6 (IL-6) by this technique as a distinctive marker for WM provides additional support to the clinical observation of increased levels of serum IL-6 in these patients and its association with disease severity and tumor burden.

Mantle Cell Lymphoma

Mantle cell lymphoma (MCL) is a distinct entity that has been more precisely defined in recent years through the integration of immunophenotypic, molecular genetic, and clinicopathologic studies. Early on it was noted that this tumor tended to surround residual naked germinal centers, and a derivation from the follicular lymphoid cuff was postulated.[55,56] Tumors with a very conspicuous mantle zone pattern of growth were also termed "mantle zone lymphoma."[57]

Mantle cell lymphoma occurs in adults (median age 62), with a high male-to-female ratio. Most patients present with advanced stage at diagnosis.[58–61] Common sites of involvement include lymph nodes, spleen, bone marrow, and lymphoid tissue of Waldeyer ring. Gastrointestinal tract involvement is frequent and is associated with the picture of lymphomatous polyposis.[62] The hallmark of MCL is a very monotonous cytologic composition. In the typical case, the cells are slightly larger than a normal lymphocyte with finely clumped chromatin, scant cytoplasm, and inconspicuous nucleoli (Fig. 78–5). The nuclear contour is usually irregular or cleaved. Some cytologic variants, blastoid (blastic) and pleomorphic, tend to be associated with a more aggressive course, and adverse biological features, such as tetraploidy or p53 mutation/deletion.[12,63,64] However, because of the overall poor prognosis and the lack of statistical significance of these cytologic changes, the WHO classification considers mantle cell lymphoma and its variants as one group.[7,27] The use of morphologic variants is optional. The variant with the greatest clinical significance is the blastoid or blastic form. A high mitotic rate and high proliferative index have been found to be an adverse prognostic indicator.[65] More recently, a proliferation signature identified by gene expression profiling of MCL was shown to correlate with survival[66]; this signature has been further refined by quantitative gene expression study.[67]

Immunophenotypic and genotypic studies have been helpful in precisely defining MCL. The immunophenotype is distinctive (IgM/IgD$^+$, CD5$^+$, CD10$^-$, and CD23$^-$). The postulated normal counterpart is the CD5$^+$ "virgin" B cell, IgM$^+$, and IgD$^+$ that can be found in the blood and in the mantle of reactive germinal centers. Mutational analysis of the rearranged immunoglobulin variable region genes shows few or no somatic mutations.[68]

The chromosomal translocation t(11;14) involving *CCND1* is associated with MCL but absent in most other low-grade and high-grade B-cell malignancies.[69,70] By Northern analysis, virtually 100% of cases of MCL have shown overexpression of cyclin D1.[71,72] However, rare cyclin D1-negative cases with otherwise identical features have been identified.[73] Additional alterations involving other cell cycle regulatory molecules such as RB, p53, and CDK inhibitors (p16 and p27) have been described in the more aggressive forms of MCL.[63,74–78]

Follicular Lymphoma

Follicular lymphoma (FL) is the most common subtype of non-Hodgkin lymphoma within the United States and accounts for approximately 45% of all newly diagnosed cases. It has a peak incidence in the fifth and sixth decades, and is rare under the age of 20. Men and women are equally affected. FL is less common in black and Asian populations. Most patients have stage 3 or 4 disease at diagnosis, with generalized lymphadenopathy.[79] Staging evaluation will usually detect bone marrow involvement. Approximately 10% of patients will have circulating malignant cells.[80] However, careful immunophenotypic or molecular analyses may disclose peripheral blood involvement in a higher proportion of patients.[81] A more accurate prognostic index than the IPI, which was originally designed for aggressive B-cell lymphomas, has been recently proposed[82] and it has become widely accepted as a more accurate predictive measure for FL.

The natural history of the disease is associated with histologic progression in both pattern and cell type (Fig. 78–6). A heterogeneous cytologic composition is one of the hallmarks of FL. Usually, all of the follicle center cells are represented, but in varying proportions.[83] It should be stressed that the variation in cytologic grade is a continuum, and therefore precise morphologic criteria for subclassification are difficult to establish. Most studies have shown that sub-

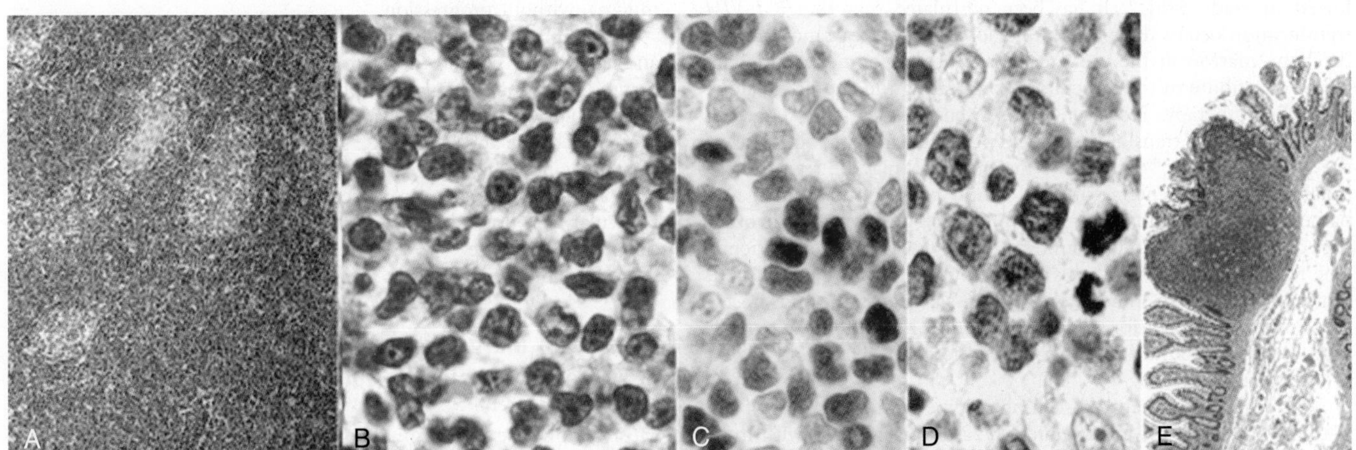

Figure 78–5 Mantle cell lymphoma (MCL). At low power mantle cell lymphoma can show a diffuse, vaguely nodular, or a mantle zone pattern. In the latter, the neoplastic mantle zones are expanded and can become confluent, leaving "naked" germinal centers (**A**). At higher power, the lymphoma cells are small or slightly enlarged. They have irregular nuclear contours, especially compared to SLL, and a dense chromatin. (**B**) Typically cases are positive for cyclin D1 expression (**C**) which is related to the t(11;14) involving IgH and *CCND1*. Some cases can develop a "blastoid" transformation (**D**), although some cases can present as a blastoid variant. Such cases are characterized by cells with an intermediate size, a high mitotic rate, and finely dispersed blastic chromatin. Sometimes when the blastoid cases develop a leukemic phase, they can be difficult to distinguish from ALL, morphologically. Flow immunophenotyping is needed to resolve the differential. Mantle cell lymphoma can also present with gastrointestinal involvement (**E**) as in lymphomatoid papulosis.

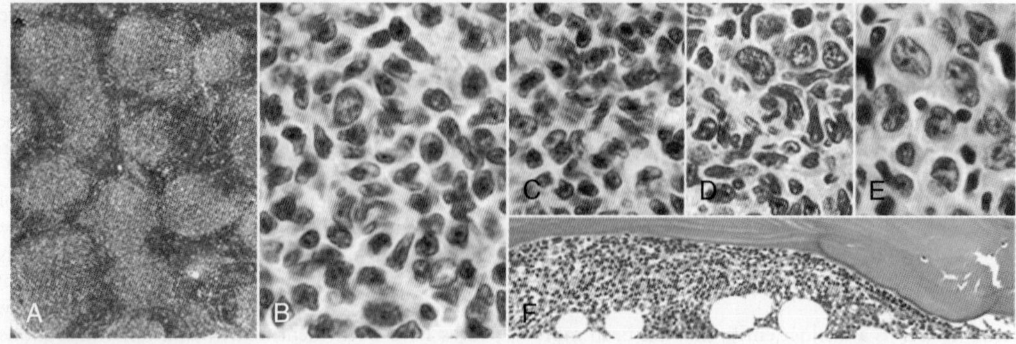

Figure 78–6 Follicular lymphoma (FL). Follicular lymphoma shows effacement of the normal lymph node architecture because of an accumulation of neoplastic lymphoid follicles that lack the features of reactive follicles (**A**). They are crowded, show back-to-back localization, lack distinct mantle zones, and show no polarity. The lymphoma cells are highly irregular (**B**) with elongated, twisted, or clefted nuclear contours and dense chromatin. Follicular lymphoma is typically graded into grade 1, 2, or 3 (**C**, **D**, and **E**) depending on the number of large cells seen at higher power (see text). Follicular lymphoma typically involves the bone marrow, with lymphoma cells spreading along the bone (**F**). This localization is termed "para-trabecular."

classification of follicular lymphoma is difficult to reproduce among groups of pathologists.

The current WHO classification (using the Mann/Berard method) maintains three major grades: grade 1 (<5 centroblasts/high power field [hpf]); grade 2 (5–15 centroblasts/hpf); grade 3 (>15 centroblasts/hpf).[84] In addition, grade 3 FL is further subdivided into grade 3a (>15 centroblasts/hpf, but centrocytes still present) and grade 3b (solid sheet of centroblasts). Recent studies indicate that FL grade 3b may be more closely related to DLBCL.[85,86] These data might provide a biological explanation for the greater curability of grade 3 FL with aggressive therapy,[87] although other studies have not found support for this hypothesis.[88] Differences in diagnostic criteria might account for this apparent discrepancy. In light of the significance of clinical and possibly genetic factors in the prognosis of FL, histologic grading is assuming less importance in clinical trials and clinical practice.[4,89,90]

The vast majority of FL (approximately 85%) are associated with a t(14;18) involving rearrangement of the *BCL2* gene.[91] This translocation appears to result in constitutive expression of Bcl-2 protein, which is capable of inhibiting apoptosis in lymphoid cells.[92] The cells of FL accumulate and are at risk to acquire secondary mutations, which may be associated with histologic progression. The proportion of FL expressing Bcl-2 protein varies with histologic grade, and is lowest in grade 3 FL.[93] It has been postulated that the *BCL2/JH* translocation occurs during immunoglobulin gene rearrangement in the bone marrow at the pre-B cell stage of development. This fact might contribute to the difficulty in eradicating the neoplastic clone with chemotherapy. However, more recent studies have suggested that the *BCL2/JH* translocation might occur in a mature B cell within the germinal center.[94,95] In some instances, FL may be restricted to isolated germinal centers within a lymph node, termed an in situ pattern of localization.[95] This pattern may be seen with FL at other sites of disease, or the only manifestation of disease in some patients. The risk for progression in this latter group is not fully established, but it appears that in some cases the *BCL2*/JH translocation is necessary but not sufficient for the development of FL. Indeed, this translocation can be found in the peripheral blood and lymphoid organs of healthy individuals.[96,97]

The cells have a mature B-cell phenotype with expression of the B-cell antigens CD19, CD20, and CD22. SIg is positive, with most commonly expression of IgM, but IgG or IgA can be seen in many cases. CD10 is positive but CD5 is negative.[98] The presence of CD10 in the interfollicular region can be a diagnostic clue, as this pattern is not seen in normal lymph nodes.[99] As evidence of the germinal center origin of FL, Bcl-6 is nearly always expressed.[100]

Follicular lymphoma was one of the first lymphomas for which an immunophenotypic derivation from a normal lymphoid equivalent was shown[98,101,102] and represent the neoplastic counterpart of the reactive germinal center cells.[103] Consistent with their normal counterpart, intraclonal heterogeneity with a high number of somatic mutations and ongoing mutations of the Ig genes was detected in these cells (Fig. 78–7).[104] In addition, the complexity of the reactive germinal center and the different components lend support to the data obtained from gene expression profiling in nodal FL on the prognostic implication of the accompanying immune cells.[105]

Most cases of FL present in lymph nodes. A subset of cases with the morphologic features of FL may present in skin.[106] Clinically, these tumors are usually localized and infrequently associated with lymph node involvement; cytologically they are predominantly composed of large centrocytes. They have an excellent prognosis, and complete remissions may be obtained with either surgical excision or local radiation therapy.[107,108] Interestingly, these cutaneous FL frequently lack the *BCL2* translocation associated with nodal FL. For these reasons both the WHO classification and the WHO-EORTC classification for cutaneous lymphoma consider this a separate variant, primary cutaneous follicle center lymphoma.[7,109]

Other unusual variants of FL have been described. There is a form of FL involving the intestinal mucosa that is often localized, with risk of local recurrence but low risk of dissemination. These cases are generally Bcl-2 protein positive and positive for the *BCL2/JHR*.[110–112] They appear to represent another form of in situ FL, because in most patients the polypoid lesions remain confined to the intestinal mucosa, without progression.

Although FL are generally rare in children, the nasopharyngeal and palatine tonsils and the gastrointestinal tract are among the most common sites of follicular lymphomas in children.[113,114] In contrast to follicular lymphomas in adults, these tumors are usually Bcl-2 protein negative and lack *BCL2* gene rearrangements. They are typically grade 3, with a predominance of centroblasts and a high mitotic rate. Pediatric FL may also present as an isolated testicular mass.[115] Follicular lymphoma in the pediatric age group is probably a biologically distinct disease.

Extranodal Marginal-Zone B-Cell Lymphoma of Mucosa-Associated Lymphoid Tissue Type

Most lymphomas of marginal-zone derivation present in extranodal sites and have the histopathologic and clinical features identified by Isaacson and Wright as part of the spectrum of mucosa-associated lymphoid tissue (MALT) lymphomas.[116,117] MALT lymphomas are characterized by a heterogeneous cellular composition that includes marginal-zone or centrocyte-like cells, monocytoid B cells, small lymphocytes, and plasma cells (Fig. 78–8A). In most cases, large transformed cells are infrequent. Reactive germinal centers are nearly always present. Therefore, it is not surprising that based on the heterogeneous cellular composition and presence of reactive follicles,

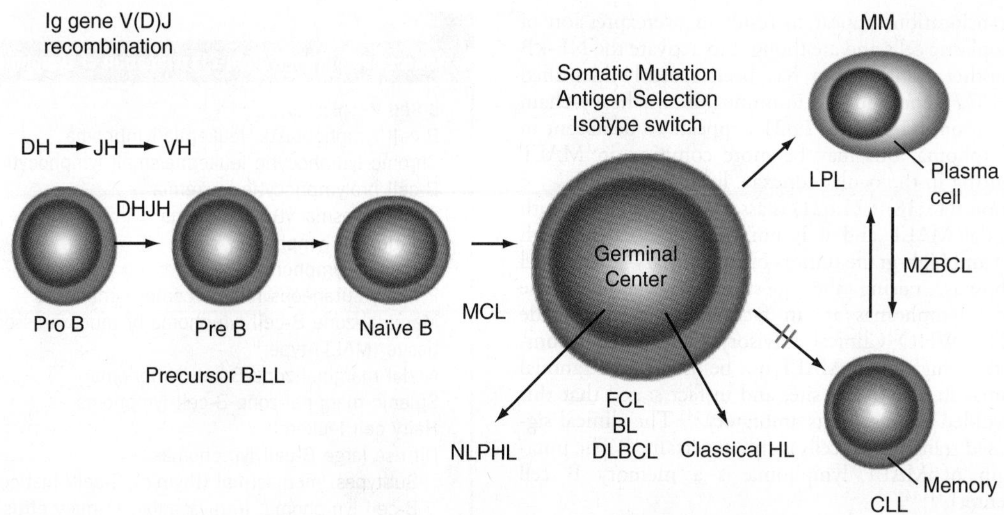

Figure 78–7 B-cell differentiation scheme and associated B-cell neoplasms. Precursor B-LL, precursor B-cell lymphoblastic lymphoma/leukemia; MCL, mantle cell lymphoma; FL, follicular lymphoma; BL, Burkitt lymphoma; DLBCL, diffuse large B-cell lymphoma; NLPHL, nodular lymphocyte-predominant Hodgkin lymphoma; MM, multiple myeloma; MZBCL, marginal-zone B-cell lymphoma; CLL, chronic lymphocytic leukemia.

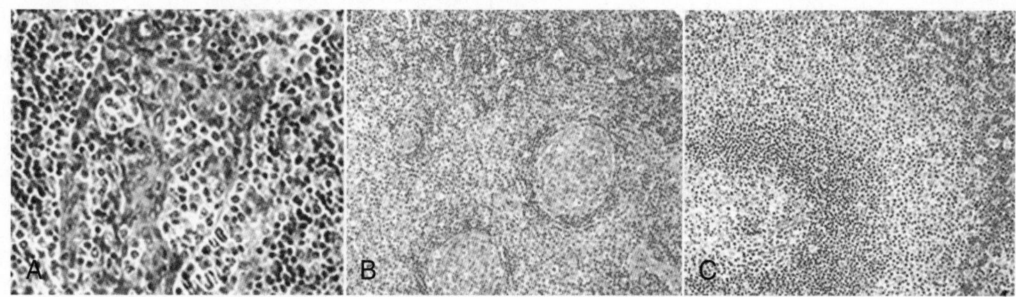

Figure 78–8 Marginal-zone lymphoma. Marginal-zone lymphomas commonly occur at extranodal sites from mucosa associated lymphoid tissue (MALT). MALT-lymphomas are composed of small- to intermediate-sized cells with abundant cytoplasm. These typically infiltrate or invade into epithelial structures resulting in lymphoepithelial lesions (**A**). Normal lymph nodes do not have a marginal zone, but primary nodal marginal-zone lymphomas (NMZL) can occur. They infiltrate the node in what would be a marginal-zone (peripheral to mantle cells) pattern (**B**). The spleen does have a normal marginal zone, and this can give rise to a splenic marginal-zone lymphoma (SMZL). Early on, these show expansion of the marginal-zone areas (**C**) but later can become more diffuse, infiltrating the red pulp. In the case illustrated, the spleen weighed 1700 g.

most MALT lymphomas were diagnosed in the past as pseudolymphomas or atypical hyperplasias. However, recent studies have shown the majority to be composed of monoclonal B cells. The follicles usually contain reactive germinal centers, but the germinal centers may become colonized by neoplastic cells. When follicular colonization occurs, the process may simulate follicular lymphoma.[118] The plasma cells are usually found in the subepithelial zones and are monoclonal in up to 50% of cases.

MALT lymphomas have been described in nearly every anatomic site but are most frequent in the stomach, lung, thyroid, salivary gland, and lacrimal gland.[52,119] Other less common sites of involvement include the orbit, breast, conjunctiva, bladder and kidney, and thymus gland.[120] Most patients present with localized disease, although regional lymph node involvement is common in gastric and salivary gland MALT lymphoma. The involved lymph nodes in those cases resemble monocytoid B-cell lymphoma, and it is thought that monocytoid B-cell lymphoma is the nodal equivalent of a MALT lymphoma.[121–124] Widespread nodal involvement is infrequent, as is marrow involvement. The clinical course is usually quite indolent, and many patients are asymptomatic. MALT lymphomas tend to relapse in other MALT-associated sites.[52]

MALT lymphomas of the salivary gland and thyroid are usually associated with a history of autoimmune diseases. Helicobacter gastritis is frequent in most patients with gastric MALT lymphomas, and it has been suggested that antigen stimulation is critical to both the development of a MALT lymphoma and the maintenance of the neoplastic state.[125] Indeed antibiotic therapy and eradication of *Helicobacter pylori* has led to the spontaneous remission of gastric MALT lymphoma in some cases.[126] Antibiotic treatment is currently advocated as first-line therapy. However, the therapy of MALT lymphomas is still controversial. Isolated lesions readily amenable to surgical excision should be removed. Systemic chemotherapy may be warranted for more widespread disease, and local radiation therapy may play a role in the control of localized tumor masses, especially for gastric and orbital MALT lymphomas.

Immunophenotype is helpful in the differential diagnosis of MALT lymphomas from cytologically similar lymphomas such as CLL/SLL and MCL. MALT lymphomas are positive for B cell-associated antigens CD19, CD20, and CD22 but are negative for CD5, in contrast to most systemic small lymphocytic malignancies. The absence of cyclin D1 is useful in ruling out MCL, especially in intestinal disease. Rare cases of MALT lymphoma have been reported to be CD5-positive, and in some but not all instances this has been associated with more aggressive disease.[127–129]

MALT lymphomas also have a commonly recurring cytogenetic abnormality the t(11;18) observed in 50% of extranodal cases.[130–133] The genes involved in the translocation have been identified as *CIAP2 (BIRC3)*, a gene encoding for an inhibitor of apoptosis, and a novel gene on 18q21 named *MALT1* (of unknown function).[134] It has been speculated that the fusion protein may lead to increased inhibition of apoptosis conferring a survival advantage to the neoplastic cells.[134] The t(1;14) involving *BCL10* is more infrequent.[135]

However, both translocations appear to result in overexpression of BCL-10 in the neoplastic cells and are thought to activate the NF-κB pathway.[136,137] Another translocation has been recently identified involving the *MALT1* gene and the immunoglobulin heavy-chain gene. This translocation, t(14;18)(q32;q21), appears to be absent in gastric MALT lymphoma, but may be more common in MALT lymphomas presenting in the ocular adnexae, liver, and skin.[138]

The translocation t(11;18)(q21;q21) is associated exclusively with low-grade extranodal MALT and it is not detected in cases with simultaneous low- and high-grade tumors or in "primary" extranodal large cell lymphomas, raising the question of whether these primary extranodal lymphomas are in fact related to low-grade MALT.[133,139–141] The WHO Clinical Advisory Committee recommended that the term high-grade MALT not be used for extranodal large cell lymphomas in a "MALT" site, and in fact stated that this term should be avoided because of its ambiguity.[142] The clinical significance of increased transformed cells is still uncertain.[143] The putative cell of origin of MALT lymphoma is a memory B cell (post–germinal center).[144,145]

Nodal Marginal-Zone B-Cell Lymphoma

The existence of primary nodal marginal-zone B-cell lymphoma (NMZL) has been controversial, with many cases representing secondary involvement by extranodal MALT lymphomas.[146–148] However, the existence of the primary extranodal disease may not be immediately apparent. Relapses in nodal sites may occur many years after primary diagnosis. However, in recent years there are several well-documented reports of primary nodal lymphomas with features of MZL.[149,150] These patients often have marrow involvement and tend to have a more aggressive clinical course than extranodal MALT.[147,149,150]

The neoplastic proliferation is polymorphous and composed of monocytoid B cells, plasmacytoid cells, with interspersed large blast-like cells. There is an expansion of the marginal-zone area, often with preservation of the nodal architecture (see Fig. 78–8B). The mantle zone may be intact, attenuated, or effaced.[146]

The immunophenotype is similar to other MZL, that is, CD20$^+$, CD5, CD10$^-$, with variable expression of IgD (weak to negative). Some nodal MZL have a morphology and immunophenotype similar to that of splenic MZL (see Splenic Marginal Zone Lymphona). These cases are IgD positive.[146] Because there are no precise immunophenotypic or genotypic markers of NMZL, the diagnosis is sometimes one of exclusion. A continuing problem is the differential diagnosis with LPL, which has overlapping morphologic and immunophenotypic features.[46] The presence of marked plasmacytic differentiation with prominent Dutcher bodies favors LPL. Clinical correlation is important in this distinction.

A morphologically similar but biologically distinct phenomenon is monocytoid B-cell differentiation in a primary nodal lymphoma. Cells resembling monocytoid B lymphocytes have been described in many low-grade lymphomas, most commonly FCL.[151] The monocytoid B-cell component appears to occupy the marginal zone. Nevertheless, the immunophenotype and genotype of the neoplastic cells is that of FCL. Monocytoid differentiation is an interesting morphologic variant, but does not yet have proven clinical or biological significance. One study suggested that cases with MZL differentiation have a more aggressive clinical course,[152] but these results have not yet been confirmed.

Splenic Marginal-Zone Lymphoma

Splenic marginal-zone lymphomas (SMZLs) present in adults and are slightly more frequent in females than males.[153] The clinical presentation is splenomegaly, usually without peripheral lymphadenopathy. The majority of patients have marrow involvement, but there is usually only a modest lymphocytosis, with elevations in the lymphocyte count usually less than that seen in CLL. Some evidence of plasmacytoid differentiation may be seen and patients may have a small M component. The abundant pale cytoplasm evident in tissue sections may also be seen in blood smears. The cytologic features may be mistaken for hairy cell leukemia. The disorder described as splenic lymphoma with villous lymphocytes (SLVL) appears closely related to SMZL.[154,155] The course is reported to be indolent, and splenectomy may be followed by a prolonged remission.[156]

Histologically, the spleen shows expansion of the white pulp, but usually some infiltration of the red pulp is present as well.[157–160] In early cases, preferential involvement of the marginal zone may be seen with residual mantle cells present (see Fig. 78–8C).[161] A characteristic

World Health Organization Classification of Lymphoid Tumors*

B-Cell Neoplasms
B-cell lymphoblastic leukemia/lymphoma
Chronic lymphocytic leukemia/small lymphocytic lymphoma
B-cell prolymphocytic leukemia
Lymphoplasmacytic lymphoma
Mantle cell lymphoma
Follicular lymphoma
Primary cutaneous follicle center lymphoma
Marginal-zone B-cell lymphoma of mucosa-associated lymphoid tissue (MALT)-type
Nodal marginal-zone B-cell lymphoma
Splenic marginal-zone B-cell lymphoma
Hairy cell leukemia
Diffuse large B-cell lymphomas
 Subtypes: mediastinal (thymic), T-cell/ histiocyte-rich large B-cell lymphoma, intravascular, primary effusion lymphoma, plasmablastic, ALK$^+$ large B-cell lymphoma, primary cutaneous diffuse large B-cell lymphoma, leg-type.
Burkitt lymphoma
Plasmacytoma
Plasma cell myeloma

T-Cell Neoplasms
T-cell lymphoblastic leukemia/lymphoma
T-cell prolymphocytic leukemia
T-cell large granular lymphocytic leukemia
Aggressive NK-cell leukemia
Hepatosplenic T-cell lymphoma
Extranodal NK- and T-cell lymphoma, nasal type
Angioimmunoblastic T-cell lymphoma
Peripheral T-cell lymphoma (unspecified)
Adult T-cell leukemia/lymphoma
Anaplastic large cell lymphoma, ALK-positive
Anaplastic large cell lymphoma, ALK-negative
Enteropathy-associated intestinal T-cell lymphoma
Subcutaneous panniculitis-like T-cell lymphoma
Primary cutaneous gamma-delta T-cell lymphoma
Primary cutaneous CD30$^+$ T-cell lymphoproliferative disorders
Lymphomatoid papulosis
Primary cutaneous anaplastic large cell lymphoma
Mycosis fungoides
Sezary syndrome

Hodgkin Lymphoma
Nodular lymphocyte-predominant Hodgkin lymphoma
Classical Hodgkin lymphoma
Hodgkin lymphoma, nodular sclerosis
Classical Hodgkin lymphoma, lymphocyte-rich
Hodgkin lymphoma, mixed cellularity
Hodgkin lymphoma, lymphocytic depletion

*Includes updates proposed in the WHO-EORTC classification of cutaneous lymphomas (2005).[109]

biphasic pattern in the neoplastic white pulp has been described,[155] in which a peripheral zone of larger cells that resembles marginal-zone cells surrounds a central zone of small lymphocytes. In this instance, the residual polytypic mantle is no longer present. Progression to diffuse large B-cell lymphoma, often involving the spleen, can be seen.[162]

In the marrow, large ill-defined non-paratrabecular aggregates are seen. A characteristic feature is the propensity of the neoplastic cells to infiltrate marrow sinusoids.[158] Splenic hilar lymph nodes usually show diffuse infiltration, often with preservation of lymph node sinuses.

Immunophenotypic studies are useful in distinguishing SMZL from CLL/SLL involving the spleen. Whereas typical CLL/SLL are $CD5^+$, SMZL are $CD5^-$.[160] Careful attention to the cytologic features in these cases indicates that the cells have somewhat more abundant cytoplasm than those of typical CLL/SLL and resemble the lymphocytes of the normal splenic marginal zone. The nuclei are usually predominantly round but may be slightly irregular. They have a moderate amount of pale cytoplasm. The phenotype of these cells resembles the other marginal-zone B-cell lymphomas; however, the IgD expression is more frequently positive.[158]

Although the molecular pathogenesis of SMZL has not been delineated, a frequent cytogenetic alteration involving deletions of the region 7q 22-32 is seen.[153,163] Studies of the Ig variable genes have also revealed the presence of mutations suggesting a postfollicular origin,[145,164] but variations in this profile have been observed.[165]

Diffuse Large B-Cell Lymphoma

Diffuse large B-cell lymphoma (DLBCL) is one of the more common subtypes of non-Hodgkin lymphoma, representing up to 40% of cases. It has an aggressive natural history but responds well to chemotherapy. The complete remission rate with modern regimens is 75% to 80%, with long-term disease-free survival approaching 50% or more in most series.[166] This lymphoma may present in lymph nodes or in extranodal sites. Frequent extranodal sites of involvement include bone, skin, thyroid, gastrointestinal tract, and lung.

Because there is variation in the responsiveness to chemotherapy, and because large B-cell lymphoma is one of the more common subtypes, there has been great interest over the years in identifying morphologic or immunophenotypic features that might be prognostically important. In most studies there is the suggestion that tumors composed predominantly of centroblasts have a better prognosis than those composed predominantly of immunoblasts.[79,167,168] However, the differences have not been consistently reproducible, possibly reflecting diverse criteria for the designation of a lymphoma as immunoblastic. At present, although morphologic features are useful in identifying the spectrum of appearances that one may encounter diagnostically, morphologic features do not appear to be important prognostically.

DLBCLs are composed of large, transformed lymphoid cells with nuclei at least twice the size of a small lymphocyte (see Fig. 78–9A,B). The nuclei generally have vesicular chromatin, prominent nucleoli, and basophilic cytoplasm, resembling the centroblasts of the normal germinal center. Marked variation in the nuclear contour may be seen, and the cells may be polylobated or cleaved.[169] The immunoblastic variant is characterized by cells with prominent central nucleoli, and abundant deeply staining cytoplasm. According to the Kiel classification, 90% of the cells must have this appearance for the tumor to be classified as immunoblastic in type.[170]

T-cell/histiocyte-rich large B-cell lymphoma is a morphologic variant of DLBCL. It has been associated with aggressive clinical behavior, and often presents with advanced stage and bone marrow involvement.[171,172–174] It may mimic classical Hodgkin lymphoma, or even peripheral T-cell lymphoma.[175] Some cases appear related to nodular lymphocyte-predominant Hodgkin lymphoma, with the neoplastic cells being epithelial membrane antigen (EMA)-positive and having a popcorn-like morphology.[176]

Cutaneous lymphomas differ in some respect from lymphomas in other sites.[109,177] Primary cutaneous follicle center lymphomas may be composed predominantly of large B cells in some cases but nevertheless have an indolent clinical course. By contrast, the entity primary cutaneous diffuse large B-cell lymphoma, leg-type, is clinically more aggressive.[178] By gene expression profiling and immunophenotype, it resembles the activated B-cell type of nodal DLBCL.[179] As with nodal DLBCL, Bcl-2 expression is an adverse prognostic factor.[180]

Acknowledging the heterogeneity of DLBCL, there is greater promise for molecular studies to dissect out biologically relevant subgroups. The use of RNA gene expression arrays has identified biologically distinct subtypes. Staudt and colleagues showed that at

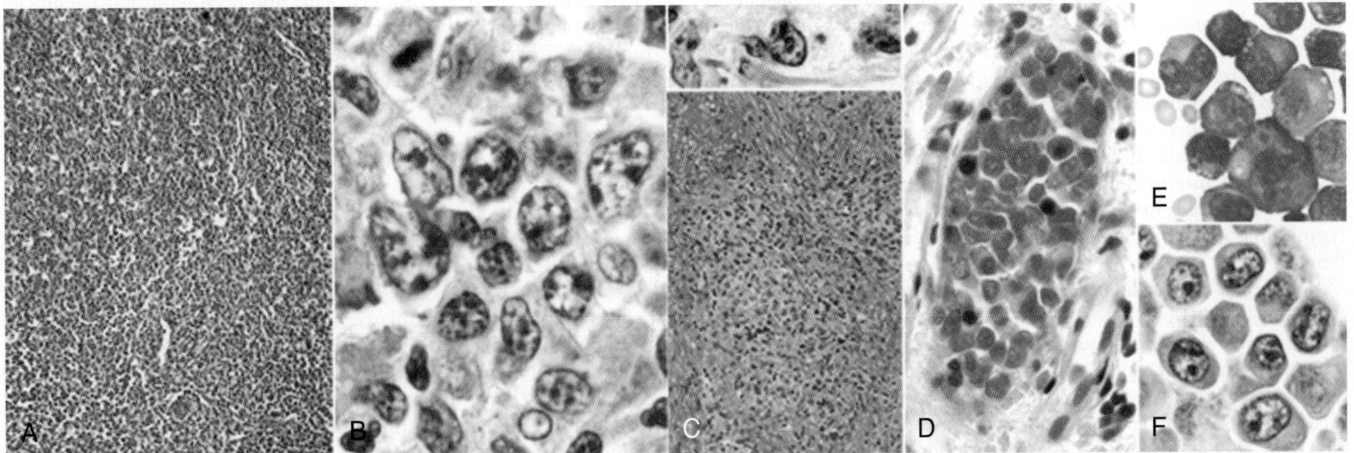

Figure 78–9 Diffuse large B-cell lymphoma (DLBCL). The low-power illustration (**A**) demonstrates the diffuse nature of the process (**A**). At high power (**B**), there are sheets of large cells with vesicular nuclear chromatin and variable numbers of nucleoli. A number of distinct types of large B-cell lymphoma have been described. These include mediastinal large B-cell lymphoma (**C**), intravascular large B-cell lymphoma (**D**), primary effusion lymphoma (**C**), and plasmablastic lymphoma (**F**). Mediastinal large B-cell lymphoma typically shows sclerosis and large B cells enmeshed in the fibrosis (**C**, top). In intravascular lymphoma, also know as angiotropic lymphoma, the large B cells are confined to the inside of vessels (**D**). Paradoxically, they do not spread to the blood. Primary effusion lymphoma must be diagnosed from cytologic preparations (**E**) and by flow cytometric and molecular techniques, as the lymphoma does not form a solid mass. Plasmablastic lymphoma cells have a distinctive appearance with large size, eccentric nuclei, and amphophilic cytoplasm (**F**), all resembling plasma cells.

least two major types of DLBCL can be identified, with expression profiles resembling either germinal center B cells (GCB) or activated B cells (ABC).[181,182] In two studies, tumors with a germinal center profile were found to have a better prognosis, irrespective of other clinical factors. Shipp et al, using a similar approach, identified a series of genes associated with treatment failure in DLBCL.[183]

The cDNA microarray-based classification of DLBCLs has been validated by an immunohistochemical approach using tissue arrays.[184] This study used immunohistochemistry to identify surrogate markers of the gene expression profile. The expression of CD10 correlated with a good prognosis, whereas the expression of MUM1/IRF4 was associated with a poor prognosis.

DISTINCT SUBTYPES OF DIFFUSE LARGE B-CELL LYMPHOMA

Mediastinal (Thymic) Large B-cell Lymphoma

Mediastinal large B-cell lymphoma (MLBCL) has emerged in recent years as a distinct clinicopathologic entity.[185–187] Cytologically, it resembles many other large B-cell lymphomas and is composed of large transformed cells that can resemble centroblasts or even immunoblasts. A constant feature is relatively abundant pale cytoplasm, often with distinct cytoplasmic membranes.[187] Many cases have fine compartmentalizing sclerosis, which may even lead to misdiagnosis as an epithelial tumor, such as thymoma (see Fig. 78–9C). The tumor appears to be derived from medullary B cells within the thymus gland.[186,188,189] These cells express CD20 and CD79a, but do not express surface Ig.[189] CD30 is often positive, and in some cases the distinction from nodular sclerosis can be difficult, so-called grey-zone lymphomas.[190] Mediastinal large B-cell lymphomas may also occur as a secondary malignancy following nodular sclerosis Hodgkin lymphoma, further supporting the potential of a biological relationship between these lymphomas.[191–193] The use of transcription factors such as Pax-5, Oct-2, BOB.1 and Pu.1 by immunohistochemistry in MLBCL may help in the differential diagnosis.[194,195]

Recently, expression of the *MAL* gene has been detected in MLBCL and not in other DLBCLs.[196] This observation further supports the distinctive nature of this lymphoma. Mediastinal large B-cell lymphoma usually lack rearrangement for *BCL2*, *BCL6*; however, *MYC* abnormalities and *REL* amplification have been described.[197,198] A common cytogenetic abnormality seen in approximately 50% of cases includes gains in 9p, which may be associated with amplification of *JAK2*. Recently, gene expression profiling studies have found that MLBCL bears a distinct molecular signature that differs from that of other DLBCLs and shares features of classical Hodgkin lymphomas.[199,200] Additionally, there are lymphomas, termed mediastinal grey-zone lymphomas, that appear to bridge the gap between MLBCL and classical Hodgkin lymphoma.[193] These cases exhibit intermediate histologic and immunophenotypic features. Interestingly, in contrast to both MLBCL and classical Hodgkin lymphoma, grey-zone lymphomas are more common in males than females.[193,201]

Clinically, mediastinal large B-cell lymphoma is much more common in females than males.[202] It is common in adolescents and young adults with a median age at presentation in the fourth decade. The clinical presentation is that of a rapidly growing anterior mediastinal mass with frequent superior vena caval syndrome and/or airway obstruction. Nodal involvement is uncommon at presentation and also at relapse. Frequent extranodal sites of involvement, particularly at relapse, include the liver, kidneys, adrenal glands, ovaries, gastrointestinal tract, and central nervous system. Earlier studies suggested that the tumor was associated with an unusually aggressive clinical course with poor responses to conventional chemotherapy. This may have been due to inadequate therapy, because the tumor usually presents with low-stage disease, Stage I or II. More recent studies have reported cure rates similar to those seen for other large B-cell lymphomas with combined chemotherapy and irradiation.[203]

Intravascular Large B-Cell Lymphoma

Intravascular large B-cell lymphoma is a rare form of DLBCL characterized by the presence of lymphoma cells only in the lumens of small vessels, particularly capillaries.[204] This lymphoma is composed of a disseminated intravascular proliferation of large lymphoid cells, nearly always of B-cell phenotype (see Fig. 78–9D). The tumor cells are large, with vesicular nuclei and prominent nucleoli, resembling centroblasts or immunoblasts. Lymph node involvement is rare, and the tumor presents in extranodal sites, most readily diagnosed in the skin.[205] Neurologic symptoms associated with plugging of small vessels in the central nervous system are common. The disease is often not diagnosed until autopsy, because of the lack of definitive radiologic or clinical evidence of disease, and diverse symptomatology.

Primary Effusion Lymphoma (HHV8/KSHV-Associated)

Primary effusion lymphoma (PEL) is a novel lymphoproliferative disorder associated with human herpesvirus 8 (HHV8) infection.[206] Most PEL develop in HIV-seropositive individuals and are usually coinfected with EBV. Most patients are young to middle-aged homosexual males.[207] The disease also occurs in areas with high seroprevalence for HHV8 infection, such as the Mediterranean, usually in elderly males.[208] Many affected patients also have a history of Kaposi sarcoma, and less commonly multicentric Castleman disease.[209] The most common sites of involvement are the pleural, pericardial, and peritoneal cavities. Some cases may present with tumor masses involving the gastrointestinal tract, soft tissue, and other extranodal sites.[210]

The cells usually have plasmablastic or immunoblastic morphology, with some cells having more anaplastic morphology (see Fig. 78–9E). The cytoplasm is very abundant and deeply basophilic. This disease should be distinguished from pyothorax-associated DLBCL, which usually presents with a pleural mass lesion, and is EBV-positive but HHV8-negative. The cells often have a "null-cell phenotype" with loss of B-cell surface markers, in keeping with a late B-cell stage of differentiation. However, sIg and cIg are often absent. Activation and plasma cell-related markers such as CD30, CD38, and CD138 are usually demonstrable.[211] Aberrant cytoplasmic CD3 expression has been reported.[212] Because of the markedly aberrant phenotype, it is often difficult to assign a lineage with immunophenotyping. Genotypic studies usually show IgH gene arrangement, but aberrant rearrangement of T-cell receptor genes has also been reported. The nuclei of the neoplastic cells are positive by immunohistochemistry for the HHV8/KSHV-associated latent protein, which is a useful diagnostic test.

Plasmablastic Lymphoma

The plasmablastic variant of DLBCL is more than a single entity.[213] The name is most commonly associated with plasmablastic lymphoma (PBL) of the oral cavity, usually diagnosed in the setting of HIV infection.[214] Most cases are EBV-positive. The tumor cells have immunoblastic or plasmablastic features but do not show evidence of ongoing plasmacytic differentiation (see Fig. 78–9F). Other rare examples of PBL may complicate multicentric Castleman disease and contain HHV8.[215] Although these lymphomas are indistinguishable from some examples of immunoblastic lymphoma on morphologic grounds, the lymphoma cells are negative for CD20 and CD45 but express plasma cell markers such as CD138.[216] Still another type of PBL is ALK-positive large B-cell lymphoma.[217] This lymphoma expressing the ALK tyrosine kinase usually expressed in T cell-derived anaplastic large cell lymphoma. The mechanism of overexpression is complex, and most cases express full-length ALK, although translocations involving the ALK gene and other partners such as clathrin and nucleophosmin have been described recently. The tumor presents in adults (M > F), with aggressive disease and frequent sinusoidal invasion in lymph nodes.

Burkitt Lymphoma

Burkitt lymphoma (BL) is most common in children and accounts for up to one-third of all pediatric lymphomas in the United States.[218] It is the most rapidly growing of all lymphomas, with 100% of the cells in cell cycle at any time. It usually presents in extranodal sites. In nonendemic regions, such as the United States, frequent sites of presentation are the ileocecal region, ovaries, kidneys, or breasts. Jaw presentations, as well as involvement of other facial bones, are common in African or endemic cases and are seen occasionally in nonendemic regions. Some cases present as acute leukemia with diffuse bone marrow infiltration and circulating Burkitt tumor cells (formerly known as L3-ALL in the FAB classification). Even in patients with typical extranodal disease, bone marrow involvement is a poor prognostic sign.

Burkitt lymphoma is one of the more common tumors associated with the human immunodeficiency virus (HIV).[219] It can present at any time during the clinical course. In some patients with HIV infection, Burkitt lymphoma may be the initial acquired immunodeficiency syndrome (AIDS)-defining illness.

The pathogenesis of Burkitt lymphoma is undoubtedly related to the translocations involving the *MYC* oncogene that are seen in virtually 100% of cases.[220,221] Most cases involve the Ig heavy-chain gene on chromosome 14. Less commonly the light-chain genes on chromosomes 2 and 22 are involved in the translocation. African Burkitt lymphoma occurs in regions endemic for malaria and it has been postulated that immunosuppression associated with malarial infection puts patients at increased risk for Burkitt lymphoma.[91] In this regard, the pathogenesis appears similar to that seen with HIV infection.

EBV is closely linked to Burkitt lymphoma in endemic regions but is less frequently seen (15%–20%) in European and North American cases.[218] In other regions, characterized by low socioeconomic status and EBV infection at an early age, Burkitt lymphoma is often EBV-positive, in the range of 50% to 70%.[222] These data support the concept that the EBV is a cofactor for the development of Burkitt lymphoma. Differences in the proportion of cases associated with the two EBV strains (types 1 and 2) have also been shown in sporadic and endemic EBV-positive Burkitt lymphomas.[223]

Cytologically, Burkitt lymphoma is monomorphic (Fig. 78–10). The cells are medium in size with round nuclei, moderately clumped chromatin, and multiple (2–5) basophilic nucleoli. The cytoplasm is deeply basophilic and moderately abundant. These cells contain cytoplasmic lipid vacuoles, which are probably a manifestation of the high rate of proliferation and high rate of spontaneous cell death. The starry sky pattern characteristic of Burkitt lymphoma is a manifestation of the numerous benign macrophages that have ingested karyorrhectic or apoptotic tumor cells.

Burkitt lymphoma has a mature B-cell phenotype. The cells express CD19, CD20, CD22, CD79a, and monoclonal surface Ig, nearly always IgM. CD10 is positive in nearly all cases, and CD5 and CD23 are consistently negative.[224]

The WHO includes three clinical variants of BL that are associated with different clinical settings: endemic BL, sporadic BL, and AIDS-associated BL. In addition, three morphologic variants are defined: classical BL, atypical BL, and BL with plasmacytoid differentiation. The last variant is most often seen in association with HIV infection, whereas the other two variants can be encountered in both endemic and sporadic clinical settings. The distinction of BL from morphologically similar aggressive B-cell lymphomas has been problematic for pathologists and clinicians. The category of small non–cleaved cell lymphoma or non-Burkitt in the working formulation was biologically and clinically heterogeneous. In addition, the *MYC* translocation as a secondary event is not associated with identical clinical consequences.[225]

The *atypical variant* of BL is composed of medium-sized Burkitt cells and shows other features of BL (high degree of apoptosis, high mitotic index). However, in contrast to classical BL, the cells show greater pleomorphism in nuclear size and shape. Nucleoli are more prominent and fewer in number. The diagnosis requires a growth fraction of 100% and the appropriate immunophenotype for BL.

Because of imprecision in the cytologic features, molecular studies to identify a *MYC* translocation are highly desirable, if not required, for diagnosis, especially in cases with atypical cytology. In the clinical setting, fluorescence in situ hybridization (FISH) is the most practical method and can be performed on routinely fixed and processed paraffin sections.[226] Recent studies have shown that BL has a characteristic gene expression profile and that infrequent cases morphologically resembling DLBCL may exhibit an identical profile.[227,228]

Although the *MYC* translocation is the hallmark of BL, it may occur as a secondary event in other lymphomas, including follicular lymphoma, mantle cell lymphoma, and DLBCL.[225,229] In follicular lymphoma, secondary *MYC* translocations have been associated with high-grade transformations showing Burkitt-like and lymphoblastic cytologies.[230–232] Mantle cell lymphomas with *MYC* deregulation are aggressive or blastic in appearance, but very rare.[233]

T- AND NK-CELL LYMPHOMAS

Overview of the Classification of T-Cell Neoplasms

Although the definition of precursor T-cell or lymphoblastic neoplasms is straightforward, the classification of peripheral T-cell lymphomas has been controversial. These are uncommon, representing less than 10% of all non-Hodgkin lymphomas. Most previously published classification schemes for the malignant lymphomas in the United States or Europe have been based on B-cell malignancies, as these are far more common than their T-cell counterparts. T- and NK-cell lymphomas show significant variation in incidence in different geographic regions and racial populations.[234]

The classification of T- and NK-cell neoplasms proposed by the WHO emphasizes a multiparameter approach, integrating morphologic, immunophenotypic, genetic, and clinical features. Clinical

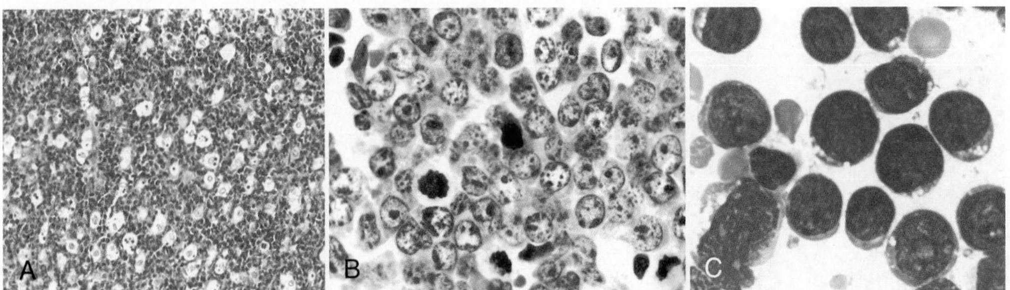

Figure 78–10 Burkitt lymphoma (BL). At low power, Burkitt lymphoma gives a classic "starry sky" appearance as a result of numerous histiocytes or tingible body macrophages with clear cytoplasm (stars), in a background of darkly stained tumor cells (sky) (**A**). At high power, the cells exhibit a very high mitotic rate, and are intermediate in size with an almost stippled nuclear chromatin (**B**). On a Wright-stained touch preparation or in the blood or bone marrow, the cells also have a characteristic appearance, with deep blue cytoplasm typically with vacuoles (**C**).

features play particular importance in the subclassification of these tumors, in part due to the lack of specificity of other parameters. T-cell lymphomas show great morphologic diversity, and a spectrum of histologic appearances can be seen within individual disease entities. The cellular composition can range from small cells with minimal atypia to large cells with anaplastic features. Such a spectrum is seen in anaplastic large cell lymphoma, adult T-cell lymphoma/leukemia, and nasal T- and NK-cell lymphoma, as selected examples. Moreover, there is morphologic overlap between disease entities. Many of the extranodal cytotoxic T- and NK-cell lymphomas share similar appearances, including prominent apoptosis, necrosis, and angioinvasion.[235]

In contrast to B-cell lymphomas, specific immunophenotypic profiles are not associated with most T-cell lymphoma subtypes. Although certain antigens are commonly associated with specific disease entities, these associations are not entirely disease-specific. For example, CD30 is a universal feature of anaplastic large cell lymphoma but can be expressed, usually to a lesser extent, in other T- and B-cell lymphomas. CD30 is of course also positive in classical Hodgkin lymphoma. Similarly, although CD56 is a characteristic feature of nasal T- and NK-cell lymphoma, it can be seen on other T-cell lymphomas, and even malignant plasma cell neoplasms.[236–238]

Presently, specific genetic features have not been identified for many of the T- and NK-cell neoplasms. One of the few exceptions is anaplastic large cell lymphoma, which is strongly associated with the t(2;5) and other variant translocations.[239,240] However, the molecular pathogenesis of most T- and NK-cell neoplasms remains to be defined. The lack of specific genetic and immunophenotypic markers increases the importance of clinical features for the mature T-cell lymphomas.

Angioimmunoblastic T-Cell Lymphoma

Angioimmunoblastic T-cell lymphoma (AILT) was initially proposed as an abnormal immune reaction or form of atypical lymphoid hyperplasia with a high risk of progression to malignant lymphoma.[241] Because the majority of cases show clonal rearrangements of T-cell receptor genes, it is now regarded as a variant of T-cell lymphoma.[242] The median survival is generally less than 5 years, so that the designation as lymphoma is warranted on clinical grounds.[243]

The nodal architecture is generally effaced, but peripheral sinuses are often open and even dilated. The abnormal infiltrate usually extends beyond the capsule into the surrounding tissue. Hyperplastic germinal centers are absent. However, there may be regressed follicles containing a proliferation of dendritic cells and blood vessels. At low power there is usually a striking proliferation of postcapillary venules with prominent arborization (see Fig. 78–11A). The cellularity of the lymph node usually appears reduced or depleted at low power. Clusters of lymphoid cells with clear cytoplasm may be seen. The neoplastic cells are admixed with a polymorphous cellular background containing small normal-appearing lymphocytes, basophilic immunoblasts, plasma cells, and histiocytes, with or without eosinophils. The abnormal cells are usually CD4-positive T cells that show expression of CD10, and sometimes BCL-6[244]—features that suggest the neoplastic cells may derive from germinal center-associated T helper cells.[245] Recently, several groups have identified increased expression of a chemokine, CXCL13, in AILT,[246,247] providing further evidence that AILT derives from follicular helper T cells. This link is also supported by recent gene expression profiling of AILT.[248]

In paraffin sections, a helpful diagnostic feature is the presence of numerous CD21^{+} dendritic reticulum cells, which are especially prominent around postcapillary venules.[249] EBV-positive large B-cell blasts are nearly always present in the background,[250,251] and progression to EBV-positive DLBCL has been reported in rare cases. The EBV-positive cells may have an RS-like appearance, simulating Hodgkin lymphoma.[252] Atypical B-cell proliferations that are negative for EBV also occur, presumably related to the function of the neoplastic cells in promoting the activation and migration of bystander B cells.[253]

Angioimmunoblastic T-cell lymphoma presents in adults. Most patients have generalized lymphadenopathy, hepatosplenomegaly, skin rash, and prominent constitutional symptoms. There are usually signs of B-cell hyperactivity, including polyclonal hypergammaglobulinemia and other hematologic abnormalities such as Coombs-positive hemolytic anemia. Rituximab has been used in some recent clinical trials, in an attempt to control some of the effects of B-cell hyperactivity in this disease.[253] Patients may also show evidence of immunodeficiency with recurrent opportunistic infections that may ultimately lead to their demise.

Adult T-Cell Leukemia/Lymphoma

Adult T-cell leukemia/lymphoma (ATLL) is a distinct clinicopathologic entity originally described in southwestern Japan that is associated with the retrovirus HTLV-1.[254,255] HTLV-1 is found clonally integrated in the T cells of this lymphoma. HTLV-1 is also endemic in the Caribbean, where clusters of ATLL have been described, predominantly among blacks.[256,257] It is seen with lesser frequency in blacks in the southeastern United States.[258] The median age of affected individuals is 45 years. Patients in the Caribbean tend to be slightly younger than those in Japan.[259] Patients may present with leukemia or with generalized lymphadenopathy. The leukemic form predominates in Japan, whereas lymphomatous presentations are more common in the western hemisphere. Other clinical findings include lymphadenopathy, hepatosplenomegaly, lytic bone lesions, and hypercalcemia.[260] The acute form of the disease is associated with a poor prognosis and a median survival of under 2 years.[258] Complete remissions may be obtained but the relapse rate is nearly 100%.

Chronic and smoldering forms of the disease are seen less commonly.[261] These are associated with a much more indolent clinical course. There is usually minimal lymphadenopathy. The predominant clinical manifestation is skin rash, with only small numbers of atypical cells in the peripheral blood. In the chronic and smoldering

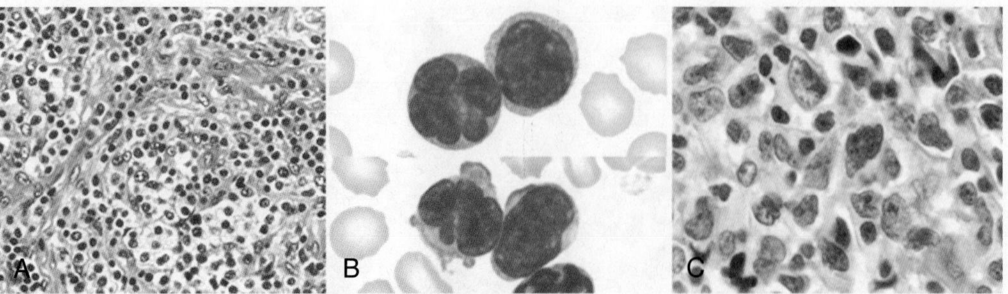

Figure 78–11 T-cell lymphoma: angioimmunoblastic T-cell lymphoma (AILT), adult T-cell leukemia/lymphoma (ATLL), and peripheral T-cell lymphoma (PTCL). In AILT the lymph node shows effacement as a result of a vascular proliferation of postcapillary venules, and clustered large cells with clear cytoplasm in the background of plasma cells, immunoblasts, and small lymphocytes (**A**). The peripheral blood in ATLL has classic "flower cells" (**B**). PTCL is heterogeneous, but typically there is a mixture of small and large neoplastic T cells (**C**).

forms, HTLV-1 virus is also found integrated within the atypical lymphoid cells.

The cytologic spectrum of ATLL is extremely diverse (see Fig. 78–11B). The cells may be small with condensed nuclear chromatin and markedly polylobated nuclear appearance.[258,262] Larger cells with dispersed chromatin and small nucleoli may be admixed and predominate in some cases. RS-like cells can be seen, simulating Hodgkin lymphoma.[263] The RS-like cells represent EBV-infected B cells, expanded secondary to underlying immunodeficiency.[264] In the smoldering form of ATLL, the cells may show minimal cytologic atypia and may even be diagnosed as small lymphocytic lymphoma. The larger cells usually show abundant cytoplasmic basophilia. Skin involvement is seen in approximately two-thirds of patients, and the cutaneous infiltrates often show prominent epidermotropism, simulating mycosis fungoides. Immunophenotypically, the neoplastic cells are positive for T cell-associated antigens, such as CD2, CD3, and CD5; they are typically $CD4^+/CD8^-$, and in almost all cases express CD25.

Peripheral T-Cell Lymphomas, Unspecified

Peripheral T-cell lymphoma (PTCL) is a diagnosis of exclusion and is admittedly a heterogeneous category. Most cases are nodal in origin. Peripheral T-cell lymphomas are characterized by a heterogeneous cellular composition. There is usually a mixture of small and large atypical lymphoid cells (see Fig. 78–11C). An inflammatory background is frequent, consisting of eosinophils, plasma cells, and histiocytes. If the epithelioid histiocytes are numerous and clustered, the neoplasm fulfills the criteria for the *lymphoepithelioid cell variant* of PTCL.[265,266] The *T-zone variant* is composed of small- to medium-sized cells that preferentially involve the paracortical regions of the lymph node.[267,268]

Clinically, PTCL most often presents in adults. Most patients exhibit generalized lymphadenopathy, hepatosplenomegaly, and frequent bone marrow involvement. Constitutional symptoms, including fever and night sweats, are common, as is pruritus. The clinical course is aggressive, although complete remissions may be obtained with combination chemotherapy.[269–271] However, the relapse rate is higher than in aggressive B-cell lymphomas, including DLBCL.[271]

Peripheral T-cell lymphoma, as defined in the WHO classification, remains heterogeneous. It is likely that individual clinicopathologic entities will be delineated in the future from this broad group of malignancies. Thus far, immunophenotypic criteria have not been helpful in delineating subtypes. Most cases have a mature T-cell phenotype, and express one of the major subset antigens: CD4 > CD8. These are not clonal markers, and antigen expression can change over time. Loss of one of the pan T-cell antigens (CD3, CD5, CD2, or CD7) is seen in 75% of cases, with CD7 most frequently being absent.[272]

Anaplastic Large Cell Lymphoma—ALK positive or ALK negative

Anaplastic large cell lymphoma (ALCL) is characterized by pleomorphic or monomorphic cells, which have a propensity to invade lymphoid sinuses (see Fig. 78–12A).[273] Because of the sinusoidal location of the tumor cells, and their lobulated nuclear appearance, this disease was previously interpreted as a variant of malignant histiocytosis. Misdiagnosis as metastatic carcinoma or melanoma was also common.

A consistent feature is the expression of the CD30 antigen, which is a hallmark of this disease.[274] The older terminology of $Ki\text{-}1^+$ lymphoma is not favored because CD30 expression is not specific for ALCL and can be seen in a variety of conditions, of course, including classical Hodgkin lymphoma (Table 78–2).[275,276] Systemic ALCL is associated with a characteristic chromosomal translocation, t(2;5)(p23;q35) involving *NPM/ALK* genes respectively.[277] A number of variant translocations have been identified that involve partners other than *NPM*. All lead to an overexpression of *ALK*, although the cellular distribution of ALK varies according to the gene partner.[278,279]

The cells of classical ALCL have large, often lobated nuclei. Nucleoli are present but tend not to be prominent and are frequently basophilic. In some cases the nuclei may be round. The cytoplasm is usually abundant, amphophilic, and there are distinct cytoplasmic borders. A prominent Golgi region is generally visible. Cells with lobulated and indented nuclei, so-called hallmark cells, are a constant feature.[240,280]

The cells exhibit an aberrant phenotype with loss of many of the T-cell associated antigens. Both CD3 and CD5 are negative in greater than 50% of cases. CD2 and CD4 are positive in the majority of cases. CD8 is usually negative. ALCL cells, despite the $CD4^+/CD8^-$ phenotype, exhibit positivity for the cytotoxic associated antigens TIA-1, granzyme B, and perforin. By molecular studies, in most of the cases a T-cell receptor rearrangement is found, confirming a T-cell origin.

Anaplastic large cell lymphoma is most common in children and young adults. A marked male predominance is noted. Although most patients present with nodal disease, a high incidence of extranodal involvement has been reported (involving skin, bone, and soft tissue). Approximately 75% of cases present with advanced-stage and systemic symptoms.[281] Although these lymphomas have an aggressive natural clinical history, they respond well to chemotherapy. Overall

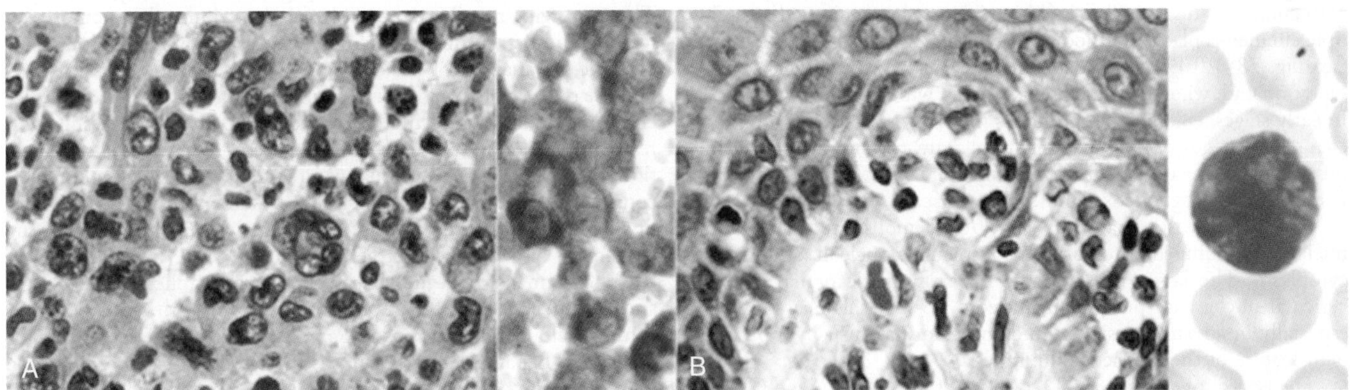

Figure 78–12 T-cell lymphoma: anaplastic large cell lymphoma (ALCL) and mycosis fungoides/Sezary syndrome (MF/SS). ATCL is characterized by a mix of pleomorphic malignant large T cells (**A**), which include "wreath cells" (*center*) and "hallmark cells" (*bottom right*). The presence of ALK staining with nuclear and cytoplasmic localization (*right*) is associated with the t(2;5). In MF there is a dermal infiltrate with some malignant T cells infiltrating into the epithelium (Pautrier microabscesses) (**B**). A Sezary cell with convoluted nuclear folding is seen to the right.

Table 78–2 Differential Diagnosis of Anaplastic Large Cell Lymphoma

Disease	CD30	CD15		LCA	CD3	TIA-1	EMA	Clu	ALK	CD20
ALCL	+	–	+	–/+	+		+		+	+
CHL	+	+	–	–	–	–	–	–		–/+
NLPHL	–	–	+	–	–	+/–	–	–	+	+
PTL	–/+	–	+	+	–/+	–	–	–	–	–
DLBCL	–/+	–	+	–	–		+/–	–	–	+

ALCL, anaplastic large cell lymphoma; cHD, classical Hodgkin lymphoma; DLBCL, diffuse large B-cell lymphoma (includes T-cell rich large B-cell lymphoma); NLPHD, nodular lymphocyte predominant HL; PTL, peripheral T-cell lymphoma, unspecified.

survival and disease-free survival are significantly better among ALK+ vs ALK− cases.[281,282,282a] Recent studies suggest that the IPI is prognostically useful, in contrast with early reports.[281,282]

Anaplastic large cell lymphoma negative for ALK represents approximately 15% to 20% of cases of ALCL, with otherwise classical morphologic and immunophenotypic criteria. Because CD30 can be expressed in a wide variety of lymphoma, stringent morphologic and immunophenotypic criteria are required for the diagnosis of ALK-negative ALCL. These include the presence of a cytotoxic T-cell immunophenotype. Although ALK-negative ALCL has a worse prognosis than ALK-positive cases, recent studies have indicated a better prognosis than PTCL-unspecified, with suggestive evidence of a plateau in the survival curve.[282a]

Primary Cutaneous Anaplastic Large Cell Lymphoma

A primary cutaneous form of ALCL is closely related to lymphomatoid papulosis, and differs clinically, immunophenotypically, and at the molecular level from the systemic form.[283–286] Lymphomatoid papulosis and cutaneous ALCL are part of the spectrum of CD30+ cutaneous T-cell lymphoproliferative diseases. Small lesions are likely to regress. Patients with large tumor masses may develop disseminated disease with lymph node involvement. However, primary cutaneous ALCL is a more indolent disease than other T-cell lymphomas of the skin. Because the skin nodules may show spontaneous regression, usually a period of observation is warranted before the institution of any chemotherapy.[287] Cutaneous ALCL is CD30+ but ALK-negative, lacking translocations involving the *ALK* gene.[285,286]

Mycosis Fungoides/Sézary Syndrome

Mycosis fungoides/Sézary syndrome (MF/SS) by definition present with cutaneous disease. Skin involvement may be manifested as multiple cutaneous plaques or nodules, or with generalized erythroderma (see Fig. 78–12B). Lymphadenopathy is usually not present at presentation and, when identified, is associated with a poor prognosis.[288] In early stages, enlarged lymph nodes may only show dermatopathic changes (Category I). If malignant cells are present in significant numbers and are associated with architectural effacement (Category II or III), the prognosis is significantly worse.[7]

Cytologically, the small cells of MF/SS demonstrate cerebriform nuclei with clumped chromatin, inconspicuous nucleoli, and sparse cytoplasm. The larger cells may be hyperchromatic or have more vesicular nuclei with prominent nucleoli. RS-like cells may be seen, especially in advanced lesions. Epidermotropism is usually a prominent feature of the cutaneous infiltrates.

The typical phenotype is CD2+, CD3+, CD5+, CD4+, and CD8−. The absence of CD7 is a constant feature but may also be seen in reactive conditions, and therefore is of limited diagnostic value.[289] Aberrant expression of other T-cell antigens may be seen but mainly occurs in the advanced (tumor) stages.

T-cell receptor genes are clonally rearranged in most cases, and the identification of clonality is clinically useful, but not entirely specific as benign cutaneous infiltrates also may be clonal by PCR.[290] Inactivation of p16 (*CDKN2A*) and *PTEN* have been identified in some cases and may be associated with disease progression.[291–293] Although Sezary syndrome is much more aggressive, the presence of common genetic pathways supports a close relationship between MF and SS.[294] Transformation to a large T-cell lymphoma may occur and is associated with an adverse prognosis. The expression of CD30 in these cases does not appear to have prognostic significance.[295] Some cases of MF may be associated with classical Hodgkin lymphoma or a T-cell lymphoma closely resembling classical Hodgkin lymphoma.[296–299]

Subcutaneous Panniculitis-Like T-Cell Lymphoma

Subcutaneous panniculitis-like T-cell lymphoma (SPTCL) usually presents with subcutaneous nodules, primarily affecting the extremities and trunk. The nodules range in size from 0.5 cm to several centimeters in diameter. Larger nodules may become necrotic. In its early stages the infiltrate may appear deceptively benign, and lesions are often misdiagnosed as panniculitis.[300,301] However, histologic progression usually occurs and subsequent biopsies show more pronounced cytologic atypia, permitting the diagnosis of malignant lymphoma.

The cytologic composition of SPTCL may vary. The lesions may contain a predominance of small- to medium-sized lymphoid cells with clear cytoplasm or larger cells with hyperchromatic nuclei. Admixed reactive histiocytes are frequently present, particularly in areas of fat infiltration and destruction. The histiocytes are frequently vacuolated, because of ingested lipid material. Vascular invasion may be seen in some cases, and necrosis and karyorrhexis are common (see Fig. 78–13A).

The neoplastic cells are CD8+ T cells, and display an activated cytotoxic immunophenotype (TIA-1+, granzyme-B+ and perforin+).[238] These proteins may be responsible for the cellular destruction seen in these tumors. In the original definition of SPTCL, cases of alpha-beta and gamma-delta T-cell derivation were included.[238,302] However, because of the worse prognosis of gamma-delta T-cell cases, and other clinical and pathologic differences, the WHO-EORTC classification restricts the definition of SPTCL to cases of alpha-beta derivation.[109,303] Primary cutaneous gamma-delta T-cell lymphoma is considered a distinct entity, which may in some cases have a panniculitis-like pattern.[304] The cells are EBV-negative but show clonal rearrangement of T-cell receptor genes.

A hemophagocytic syndrome is a frequent complication of SPTCL and is associated with an adverse prognosis in both alpha-beta and gamma-delta derived tumors.[300] Patients present with fever, pancytopenia, and hepatosplenomegaly. It is most readily diagnosed in bone marrow aspirate smears where histiocytes containing erythrocytes, platelets, and other blood elements may be observed. The cause of the hemophagocytic syndrome appears related to cytokine production by the malignant cells. Interferon gamma, tumor necrosis factor-alpha, granulocyte–monocyte colony-stimulating factor, and

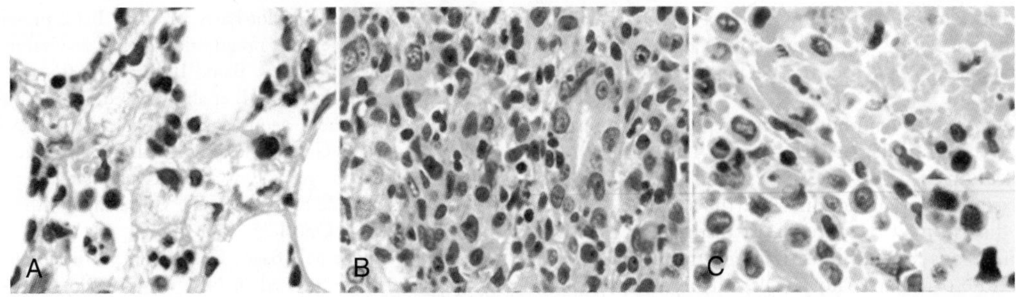

Figure 78–13 T-cell lymphoma: subcutaneous panniculitis-like T-cell lymphoma (SPTCL), enteropathy-type T-cell lymphoma (ETL), extranodal NK- and T-cell lymphoma, nasal type. A case of SPTCL is illustrated and shows an abnormal lymphoid infiltrate in the subcutaneous fat (**A**). This is associated with hemophagocytosis (*bottom left*) and necrosis. In ETL, there is an abnormal T-lymphoid proliferation with infiltration into the gastrointestinal glandular elements (*center-right*). Extranodal NK- and T-cell lymphoma typical has marked necrosis (**C**). The malignant cells are Epstein–Barr virus (EBV)-positive by in situ hybridization for EBV RNA (*insert*).

MIP-1alpha have been identified.[301,305,306] Dissemination to lymph nodes and other organs is uncommon and usually occurs late in the clinical course.

Enteropathy-Associated T-Cell Lymphoma

Enteropathy-associated T-cell lymphoma (EATL) was originally termed malignant histiocytosis of the intestine.[307] However, the demonstration of clonal T-cell gene rearrangement indicated that it was a T-cell lymphoma. The small bowel usually shows ulceration, frequently with perforation. A mass may or may not be present. Two morphologic and immunophenotypic types are recognized[308]: (a) monomorphic with small- to medium-sized cells, CD56$^+$, CD3cyto$^+$, alphabeta$^{+/-}$, CD8$^+$, CD4$^-$, CD5$^-$, CD57$^-$, TIA-1$^+$ and (b) pleomorphic with large to medium sized cells with a morphology most consistent with anaplastic large cell, CD56$^-$, CD3$^+$, CD7$^+$, CD5$^-$, CD8$^-$, CD4$^-$, TIA-1$^+$, which also express the homing receptor CD 103 (HML-1) (see Fig. 78–13B).[309] The strong association with gluten-sensitive enteropathy is seen only with the latter histologic type. Anaplastic cells strongly positive for CD30 may be present. Genetically, EATL are remarkably homogeneous and are characterized by chromosomal gain on 9q33–34, which is usually not detected in other PTCLs.[310] The cells express cytotoxic molecules, a feature shared by nearly all extranodal T-cell lymphomas and appear to be part of the innate immune system.[311] EBV is generally negative. EBV has been detected in some intestinal T- and NK-cell lymphomas in certain geographic regions, such as Mexico and Asia, but it is likely that such cases represent extranodal T- and NK-cell lymphomas involving the intestine.[312,313] The gastrointestinal tract is a common site of secondary involvement by extranodal T- and NK-cell lymphoma, nasal type.[314]

This disease occurs in adults, the majority of whom have either overt or clinically silent gluten-sensitive enteropathy. Most patients have the HLA DQA1*0501, DQB1*0201 genotype. The adjacent small bowel usually shows evidence of villous atrophy.[315] Although celiac disease is usually associated with an increase in intraepithelial gamma-delta T cells, the cells of EATL are usually of alpha-beta origin.[316] T-cell receptor beta and gamma genes are clonally rearranged. Similar clonal rearrangement may be found in adjacent intestine, suggesting that the associated increase in intraepithelial T cells constitutes a neoplastic or preneoplastic population.[317] Patients usually present with abdominal symptoms, including pain, small bowel perforation, and associated peritonitis. The clinical course is aggressive, and most patients have multifocal intestinal disease.

Hepatosplenic T-Cell Lymphoma

Hepatosplenic T-cell lymphoma presents with marked hepatosplenomegaly in the absence of lymphadenopathy.[318,319] The great majority of cases are of gamma-delta T-cell origin.[320,321] Most patients are male, with a peak incidence in young adults.[321] Although patients may respond initially to chemotherapy, relapse has been seen in the vast majority of cases, and the median survival is less than 3 years. Rare long-term survival has been seen following allogeneic hematopoietic cell transplantation.[321]

The cells of hepatosplenic T-cell lymphoma are usually moderate in size, with a rim of pale cytoplasm. The nuclear chromatin is loosely condensed, with small inconspicuous nucleoli. The liver and spleen show marked sinusoidal infiltration, with sparing of both portal triads and white pulp, respectively. Abnormal cells are usually present in the sinusoids of the bone marrow but may be difficult to identify without immunohistochemical stains. The neoplastic cells have a phenotype that resembles that of normal resting gamma-delta T cells. They are often negative for both CD4 and CD8, although CD8 may be expressed in some cases. CD56 is typically positive.[319,321] A small percentage of cases appear to be of alpha-beta origin.[322–324] The neoplastic cells express markers associated with cytotoxic T cells, such as TIA-1. However, perforin and granzyme B are usually negative, suggesting that these cells are not activated.[321,325] Isochromosome 7q is a consistent cytogenetic abnormality, and is often seen in association with trisomy 8.[326–328]

Although hepatosplenic T-cell lymphoma is a tumor of inactive or immature gamma-delta T cells, other forms of gamma-delta T-cell lymphoma exist. A gamma-delta phenotype can be seen in cases of T LBL/ALL.[329] Most tumors of activated gamma-delta T cells arise in mucocutaneous sites.[304,330] These lymphomas are positive for granzyme B, perforin, and TIA-1, and express granzyme M, characteristic of innate cytotoxic effector T cells.[311]

Extranodal NK- and T-Cell Lymphoma, Nasal-Type

Extranodal NK- and T-cell lymphoma, nasal type, is a distinct clinicopathologic entity highly associated with EBV.[331,332] It affects adults (median age 50) and the most common clinical presentation is a destructive nasal or midline facial lesion. Palatal destruction, orbital swelling, and edema may be prominent.[333] NK- and T-cell lymphomas have been reported in other extranodal sites, including skin, soft tissue, testis, upper respiratory tract, and gastrointestinal tract. Aggressive NK-cell leukemia/lymphoma is a closely related leukemic disorder.[334,335] The clinical course is usually highly aggressive, with a slightly improved median survival in patients with localized disease. However, the outcome remains poor with current chemotherapy. Radiation therapy may be effective in localized disease. A hemophagocytic syndrome is a common clinical complication and adversely affects survival in extranodal NK- and T-cell lymphoma, nasal type. It is likely that EBV plays a role in the pathogenesis of the hemophagocytic syndrome.

Extranodal NK- and T-cell lymphoma, nasal type, is much more common in Asians than in Europeans. Clusters of the disease also have been reported in Central and South America in individuals of Native American heritage, suggesting that ethnic background i.e., genetic risk factors, may play a role in the pathogenesis of these lymphomas.[336]

Extranodal NK- and T-cell lymphoma, nasal type, is characterized by a broad cytologic spectrum (see Fig. 78–13C). The atypical cells may be small or medium in size. Large atypical and hyperchromatic cells may be admixed, or may predominate. If the small cells are in the majority, the disease may be difficult to distinguish from an inflammatory or infectious process. In early stages there may also be a prominent admixture of inflammatory cells, further causing difficulty in diagnosis.[337]

Although the cells express some T cell-associated antigens, most commonly CD 2, other T-cell markers, such as surface CD3, are usually absent.[338] The cells express cytoplasmic CD3ε and are usually CD56-positive. Cytotoxic markers such as granzyme B and TIA-1 are present. Molecular studies are negative for T-cell gene rearrangement, despite clonality being shown by other methods.[338–340]

SUGGESTED READINGS

Alizadeh AA, Eisen MB, Davis RE, et al: Distinct types of diffuse large B-cell lymphoma identified by gene expression profiling. Nature 403:503, 2000.

Calin GA, Ferracin M, Cimmino A, et al: A MicroRNA signature associated with prognosis and progression in chronic lymphocytic leukemia. N Engl J Med 353:1793, 2005.

Chng WJ, Schop RF, Price-Troska T, et al: Gene-expression profiling of Waldenstrom macroglobulinemia reveals a phenotype more similar to chronic lymphocytic leukemia than multiple myeloma. Blood 108:2755, 2006.

Dave SS, Fu K, Wright GW, et al: Molecular diagnosis of Burkitt's lymphoma. N Engl J Med 354:2431, 2006.

Dave SS, Wright G, Tan B, et al: Prediction of survival in follicular lymphoma based on molecular features of tumor-infiltrating immune cells. N Engl J Med 351:2159, 2004.

Grange F, Petrella T, Beylot-Barry M, et al: Bcl-2 protein expression is the strongest independent prognostic factor of survival in primary cutaneous large B-cell lymphomas. Blood 103:3662, 2004.

Harris NL, Jaffe ES, Stein H, et al: A revised European-American classification of lymphoid neoplasms: a proposal from the International Lymphoma Study Group. Blood 84:1361–1392, 1994.

Kienle D, Katzenberger T, Ott G, et al: Quantitative gene expression deregulation in mantle-cell lymphoma: Correlation with clinical and biologic factors. J Clin Oncol 25:2770, 2007.

Krenacs L, Smyth MJ, Bagdi E, et al: The serine protease granzyme M is preferentially expressed in NK-cell, gamma delta T-cell, and intestinal T-cell lymphomas: Evidence of origin from lymphocytes involved in innate immunity. Blood 101:3590, 2003.

Nava VE, Jaffe ES: The pathology of NK-cell lymphomas and leukemias. Adv Anat Pathol 12:27, 2005.

Orchard JA, Ibbotson RE, Davis Z, et al: ZAP-70 expression and prognosis in chronic lymphocytic leukaemia. Lancet 363:105, 2004.

Savage KJ, Monti S, Kutok JL, et al: The molecular signature of mediastinal large B-cell lymphoma differs from that of other diffuse large B-cell lymphomas and shares features with classical Hodgkin lymphoma. Blood 102:3871, 2003.

Solal-Celigny P, Roy P, Colombat P, et al: Follicular lymphoma international prognostic index. Blood 104:1258, 2004.

Streubel B, Lamprecht A, Dierlamm J, et al: t(14;18)(q32;q21) involving IGH and MALT1 is a frequent chromosomal aberration in MALT lymphoma. Blood 101:2335, 2003.

Wiestner A, Rosenwald A, Barry TS, et al: ZAP-70 expression identifies a chronic lymphocytic leukemia subtype with unmutated immunoglobulin genes, inferior clinical outcome, and distinct gene expression profile. Blood 101:4944, 2003.

Willemze R, Jaffe ES, Burg G, et al: WHO-EORTC classification for cutaneous lymphomas. Blood 105:3768, 2005.

REFERENCES

For complete list of references log onto www.expertconsult.com

CHAPTER 79

CLINICAL MANIFESTATIONS, STAGING, AND TREATMENT OF INDOLENT NON-HODGKIN LYMPHOMA

John G. Gribben

Non-Hodgkin lymphoma (NHL) refers to all malignancies of the lymphoid system with the exception of Hodgkin lymphoma. Development of the lymphoid system is a highly regulated process characterized by differential expression of a number of cell-surface and intracytoplasmic proteins and antigen receptor gene rearrangements, somatic hypermutation and class switching. Dysregulation of this orderly process can result in humoral deficiency, autoimmunity, or malignancy. The indolent B cell lymphomas are mature peripheral B-cell neoplasms that exclude those diseases associated with an aggressive clinical course. Despite differences in cell of origin, molecular biology, clinical presentation, and clinical course, the indolent lymphomas share common features, including frequent localization to the principal lymphoid organs, a propensity for marrow infiltration and leukemic presentation, and generally an indolent clinical course. The classification of NHLs has been a challenge for pathologists as well as practicing physicians. A variety of classifications have been proposed over the years, leading to considerable confusion and difficulty in comparison of outcomes of clinical trials performed using different pathologic classifications. The World Health Organization (WHO) lymphoma classification[1] is based on cell of origin and pathophysiology of the lymphoma and is used throughout this chapter. The WHO classification does not include the terminology *indolent lymphoma*. This is a clinical and not pathological term and defines those lymphomas that tend to grow and spread slowly and produce few symptoms (www.nih.gov/). The frequency of the indolent lymphomas by the WHO classification is shown in Table 79–1.

The indolent lymphomas encompass the low-grade and some categories of intermediate-grade NHL in the Working Formulation. Mantle cell lymphoma was previously classified as a low-grade lymphoma and is included here although it is generally now considered a more aggressive lymphoma.

EPIDEMIOLOGY

Almost 60,000 new cases of NHL were diagnosed in the USA in 2006[2] and the incidence is similar in Europe.[3] The incidence rates increased dramatically during the second half of the twentieth century and doubled since the early 1970s to 2000. Non-Hodgkin lymphoma is extremely heterogeneous in its molecular pathophysiology, histology, and clinical course. There are major differences in the incidence of subtypes in different geographic locations and among different racial and ethnic populations. For most subtypes of NHL and particularly for the indolent lymphomas, the age-specific incidence rates are higher in men than in women, and appear higher in whites compared with blacks. Indolent lymphomas are observed much more frequently in the Western world and are rare in Asia. There are familial clusters, especially in small lymphocytic lymphoma/chronic lymphocytic leukemia, and an increased incidence in family members of affected individuals. Therefore, differentiation of complex environmental factors from true inherited factors remains difficult. The complexity of the epidemiology of NHL mirrors the complexity of the disease and the complexity of the immune system. Because lymphomas do not constitute a single disease, it should come as no surprise that there is no single etiologic factor. The influence on immune dysregulation of viruses, chemicals, radiation, diet, and aging remains unclear. Immune suppression leads to increased incidence of aggressive lymphomas, but not usually indolent lymphomas. The role of hepatitis C virus (HCV) in the pathogenesis of indolent lymphomas has been controversial. A significant association between B cell-derived NHL and HCV infection has been reported in Italian subjects[4] and subsequently confirmed by international studies.[5–7] However, discordant data appeared in northern European and North American surveys,[8–10] and it is now evident that a clear south/north gradient of prevalence exists, in part reflecting different HCV infection prevalence in the general population and suggesting the contribution of environmental and/or genetic factors.[6] A great deal of attention has been paid recently to the complex interaction between the malignant B cell, the host,[11] and the tumor microenvironment.[12–14]

CLINICAL PRESENTATION

Although specific subtypes may be associated with specific presenting features, there are many common features and the majority of patients present with lymphadenopathy. Extranodal disease is common and can affect any organ. The most common sites of extranodal disease include the marrow, skin, gastrointestinal tract, and bone. Symptoms may be nonspecific or related to the site of disease involvement. Many patients with indolent lymphomas are asymptomatic, but some, particularly those with bulky disease, may present with B symptoms defined as fever, drenching sweats, or weight loss of more than 10% of body weight. Patients may present with evidence of bowel obstruction from intraabdominal lymphadenopathy and retroperitoneal disease may manifest as obstructive uropathy. Inguinal disease may cause compression of the venous system with deep venous thrombosis. Central nervous system involvement can occur, but is uncommon in indolent lymphomas.

DIAGNOSIS OF INDOLENT LYMPHOMAS

Suggested guidelines for the diagnosis of indolent lymphomas have been outlined by the National Comprehensive Cancer Network (guidelines available at www.nccn.org/) and by the European Society for Medical Oncology.[15] In all cases diagnosis should be confirmed by excisional biopsy of an accessible lymph node with review by a hematopathologist with expertise in lymphoma diagnosis. Fine needle aspiration is not appropriate for diagnosis, and sufficient material must be obtained for immunophenotyping and genetic studies as required for diagnosis and prognostic markers. In patients without easily accessible peripheral nodes, computed tomography (CT) or ultrasound guided biopsy are typically well tolerated. Where possible, consent should be obtained for the procurement and storage of use of excess tissue from lymph node biopsies at the time of presentation and at each subsequent relapse of disease for research purposes to investigate the molecular biology of these diseases. Marrow biopsy provides essential information and should be performed routinely. The yield of bilateral marrow biopsy is moderately higher (15%) than that of unilateral biopsy.

Initial investigations are shown in Table 79–2. Physical examination should include careful examination of all peripheral lymph node

Table 79–1 Frequency of Indolent Lymphomas Among All Lymphomas in the WHO Classification

Follicular lymphoma	22.1%
Extranodal marginal zone lymphoma of mucosa-associated lymphoid tissue type	7.6%
Small lymphocytic lymphoma/chronic lymphocytic leukemia	6.7%
Mantle cell	6.0%
Splenic marginal zone lymphoma	1.8%
Lymphoplasmacytic lymphoma	1.2%
Nodal marginal zone B-cell lymphoma (±monocytoid B cells)	1.0%

groups including the cervical, supraclavicular, axillary and inguinal chains and examination of Waldeyer ring. Abdominal examination should focus on evaluation of any intraabdominal masses, with particular attention paid to detection of enlargement of the liver or spleen. The skin should be carefully examined. Patients may present with pleural or pericardial effusions, although this is less common than in the aggressive lymphomas.

Laboratory investigations should include a complete blood count to evaluate for cytopenias, which may be evidence of marrow infiltration or of autoimmunity. A white blood cell count with differential and examination of the peripheral blood smear may indicate leukemic involvement. Baseline electrolytes including calcium and phosphate, creatinine, and liver function tests are important to determine organ dysfunction that may be related to direct infiltration by lymphoma. Elevation of lactate dehydrogenase is an important prognostic factor and may be a useful indicator of transformation from indolent to aggressive lymphoma. Assessment of immunoglobulin levels and serum electrophoresis are useful, particularly in lymphoplasmacytic lymphoma, to evaluate for monoclonal protein. Cryoglobulins may also be present, particularly in marginal zone lymphoma in association with hepatitis C. A Coombs test and reticulocyte count may be indicated in patients with anemia.

Initial staging workup also includes a CT scan of the chest, abdomen, and pelvis, with particular attention to sites of bulk disease and to the number of involved sites. Gastrointestinal tract workup and biopsy are indicated in mantle cell lymphoma and in patients with mucosa-associated lymphoid tissue (MALT) lymphomas. Liver biopsy may be indicated on the basis of abnormal imaging or laboratory values.

STAGING

The Ann Arbor Classification is currently used to stage NHL (Table 79–3). CT scans have replaced lymphangiography. The impact of newer technologies such as positron emission tomography (PET), which are included in the revised guidelines for aggressive lymphomas,[16] have been much less studied in the indolent lymphomas. There is considerable heterogeneity in uptake of fluorine-18 fluorodeoxyglucose based on histology, but PET demonstrates 94% sensitivity and 100% specificity for staging in follicular lymphoma (FL).[17] Whereas there is insufficient data yet to recommend PET scans routinely in patients with indolent lymphomas, these scans can be useful to direct biopsy in cases where transformation is suspected.

Table 79–2 Initial Evaluation of Indolent Non-Hodgkin Lymphomas

Physical examination with attention to peripheral nodes, abdomen
Complete blood count, evaluation of peripheral blood
Liver function tests; lactate dehydrogenase
CT scans of chest, abdomen, pelvis
Lymph node biopsy with review by an expert lymphoma histopathologist
Bone marrow biopsy/aspirate
Other studies as indicated

Table 79–3 Ann Arbor Staging

Stage	Criteria
I	Involvement of 1 lymph node (I) or 1 extralymphatic organ or site (IE)
II	Involvement of ≥2 lymph nodes on same side of diaphragm (II) or localized extralymphatic organ or site and ≥1 involved lymph node on same side of diaphragm (IIE)
III	Involvement of lymph nodes on both sides of diaphragm (III) or same side with localized involvement of extralymphatic site (IIIE), spleen (IIIS), or both (IIIS + E)
IV	Diffuse or disseminated involvement of extralymphatic organ or tissues with or without lymph node enlargement

CLASSIFICATION OF INDOLENT LYMPHOMAS

Follicular Lymphoma

Follicular lymphoma is by far the most common of the indolent lymphomas and is the second most common subtype of lymphoma worldwide. FL accounts for approximately 20% of malignant lymphomas in adults, but 40% of all lymphomas diagnosed in the USA and in Western Europe.[18] FLs are derived from germinal center B cells and maintain the gene expression profile of this stage of differentiation.[12] Morphologically, the disease is composed of a mixture of centrocytes and centroblasts and is graded from I to III dependent on the proportion of large cells per high power field. Grades I and II are indolent disease. The rare subtype Grade IIIb is more aggressive and is managed as diffuse large B-cell lymphoma (DLBCL). FL cells express CD19, CD20, CD22, and surface immunoglobulin and 60% express CD10. A hallmark of the disease is the t(14;18) contributing to overexpression of the antiapoptotic protein BCL2. Median age at presentation is 60 years and males and females are equally affected. Patients usually present with asymptomatic lymphadenopathy, most cases are advanced stage, and 50% have marrow involvement at presentation. Lymphadenopathy may wax and wane and spontaneous remissions can occur, albeit rarely.[19] Disease transformation to a more aggressive histologic type is a common terminal event.[20] Until recently there was little evidence that the natural history of FL had changed over the last 30 years, and the median survival from diagnosis has been approximately 10 years.[21] Recent studies, however, suggest that the introduction of therapy combining monoclonal antibodies and chemotherapy has led to a longer median survival of 12 to 14 years.[22,23] The clinical course is extremely variable. Some patients have an extremely aggressive course and die within 1 year, whereas others may live for more than 20 years and never require therapy. The Follicular Lymphoma International Prognostic Index (FLIPI) is a five-factor prognostic index based on the clinical characteristics of age, stage, number of nodal sites, and hemoglobin and lactate dehydrogenase levels (Table 79–4), and defines three prognostic risk groups of almost equal numbers of patients.[24] This tool is useful in assessing the need for early treatment and potential outcome, as well as in comparing the outcomes of different clinical trials.

Marginal Zone Lymphomas

The WHO classification lists three forms of marginal zone lymphomas (MZLs) including extranodal, nodal, and splenic marginal zone

Table 79–4 Factors Having Prognostic Significance in the Follicular Lymphoma International Prognostic Index[24]

Parameter	Adverse Factor	RR	95% CI
Age	≥60 years	2.38	2.04–2.78
Ann Arbor stage	III–IV	2.00	1.56–2.58
Hemoglobin level	<120 g/L	1.55	1.30–1.88
Serum LDH level	>ULN	1.50	1.27–1.77
Number of nodal sites	>4	1.39	1.18–1.64

LDH, lactate dehydrogenase; RR, relapse rate.

Management of Follicular Lymphoma

Patients most often present with asymptomatic lymphadenopathy. The diagnosis should be made by excisional biopsy and reviewed by an expert hematopathologist. In the absence of symptoms requiring treatment, a watch and wait approach is the treatment of choice. Although in this phase of treatment, patients should be followed every 3 to 6 months, with history, physical, and laboratory examination and radiologic restaging as clinically indicated. Once a decision to treat has been made, there is no clear treatment algorithm and a number of treatment options are available. The treatment goal, whether palliative or with curative intent, is dependent on the age and performance status of patients. Enrollment in clinical trial should be a priority. For younger patients in whom high-dose therapy may be indicated later in their disease course, it is best to avoid myelotoxic regimens. The role of maintenance therapy in first remission using interferon-α remains controversial and the role of rituximab maintenance therapy in first remission remains the focus of ongoing clinical trials. The choice of therapy after first relapse is also dependent on the goal of therapy, but is also dependent on the previous therapy given and the response and duration of response. Autologous or allogeneic hematopoietic cell transplantation has a role to play in selected younger patients with this disease.

lymphomas. However, there are still uncertainties as to whether they represent a homogeneous group of tumors. These lymphomas behave differently than most indolent lymphomas and require different treatment approaches.

The marginal zone (MZ) corresponds to the outer part of secondary follicles. It is well developed and easily recognizable in the spleen, intraabdominal lymph nodes, and mucosa-associated lymphoid tissue. Most MZ cells express CD19 and CD20 and have the phenotypic profile of memory B cells and are strongly positive for IgM, IgG, or IgA, with only a small subpopulation exhibiting weak IgD staining. They also express CD21, CD27, and Bcl-2 protein, but are negative for CD5, CD10, CD23, CD43, and CD75. A subset of splenic MZ cells shares phenotypic features with mantle B elements by showing positivity for IgM, IgD, and Ki-B3 and negativity for CD21 and CD27. Most, but not all, splenic MZ B cells show somatic hypermutation of Ig genes contain point mutations of the Ig genes at frequencies found in postfollicular memory B elements. However, a small subset of the same MZ B cells displays a low load of Ig gene point mutations, as usually found in mantle B cells. Therefore, although belonging to the same anatomic compartment, splenic MZ B elements do show a certain phenotypic and molecular variability, the vast majority of them being likely part of the recirculating memory B-cell pool. Interestingly, splenic MZ B cells can bind polysaccharide antigens with one of two results, depending on the follicle microenvironment. First, they can migrate into the germinal centers (GCs) and present the antigen to GC B cells. If follicular dendritic cells have surface Ig that binds to the presented antigen, they proliferate and give rise to the GC cell reaction. Second, antigen in association with cytokines released by T cells can rapidly induce differentiation of MZ B cells into plasma cells, which in turn synthesize and release antigen-specific Ig. MALT lymphomas (extranodal marginal zone lymphomas) and monocytoid B-cell NHLs (nodal marginal cell lymphomas) are included within the WHO terminology as marginal zone lymphomas. Both types share the presence of positive surface immunoglobulin CD19, CD20, and CD22 and are negative for CD5 and CD23.[25] Monocytoid B-cell lymphoma is the nodal form of marginal zone lymphoma. These patients do well, with rates of disease-free and overall survival similar to the other low-grade lymphomas, as shown in studies conducted by the Southwest Oncology Group (SWOG).[25]

Extranodal Marginal Zone Lymphoma

In the WHO classification, the term *extranodal marginal zone lymphoma* is restricted to tumors consisting of small elements provided with centrocyte-like or monocytoid morphology and associated or not with plasmacytoid differentiation, which resemble normal MALT MZ cells and share with them phenotypic and molecular characteristics, including the IRTA-1 gene expression. In the original description, these neoplasms were called MALT lymphomas.

MALT lymphomas typically arise in the mucosal lymphoid tissue or glandular epithelium, including stomach, salivary glands, lungs, or thyroid, with gastrointestinal tract involvement being the most common presentation. There is a clear association with autoimmune diseases such as Sjogren syndrome and Hashimoto thyroiditis.[26] Molecular analysis demonstrates that extranodal MZLs are characterized by the occurrence of different chromosomal aberrations, t(11;18), t(1;14), and t(14;18), which influence invasive potential and possibly the response to therapy. t(11;18)(q21;q21) is detected in 30% to 35% of gastric extranodal MALT lymphomas producing the fusion gene *API2-MALT1*, leading to the overexpression of the *API2* gene, which inhibits apoptosis via the caspase system. Presence of the t(11;18) is associated with antibiotic resistance, a higher potential of local infiltration and metastasis and progression to a more aggressive tumor.[27] This translocation is found even more frequently in the lung than in the stomach[28] and is found also in approximately one-half of the rare examples of gastric *Helicobacter pylori* (HP)-negative MZL,[29] further supporting the concept that tumors carrying t(11;18) do not need HP stimulation for their growth and maintenance. The t(1;14)(p22;q32) is exceedingly rare and causes transfer of the *BCL10* gene close to the Ig enhancer on chromosome 14. The role of the t(14;18)(q32;q21) in MZL has been the subject of much debate in the literature, with confusion with the translocation found in FL. Although the t(14;18) of MZLs does not affect *BCL2*, it affects *MALT1* by possibly following the same pathogenetic pathway as the t(1;14). Bacterial infection with the gram-negative rod *H pylori* is associated with 92% of gastric MALT lymphomas.[30]

Large B-cell lymphoma can arise at an anatomic site containing MALT, which has been named "high-grade MZ/MALT lymphoma," a term not included in the WHO classification. There is no evidence that large B-cell lymphoma occurring de novo at a MALT site is derived from MZ cells; and the clonal relationship between an MZL and a large B-cell neoplasm simultaneously detected in the same organ should be proven molecularly, as the latter can represent the blastic phase of the former, but might also develop as a second unrelated neoplasm.

Nodal Marginal Zone Lymphoma

In the WHO classification, nodal marginal zone lymphoma (NMZL) is defined as a primary nodal B-cell neoplasm that morphologically resembles lymph nodes involved by MZ lymphoma of the extranodal or splenic type, but without evidence of extranodal or splenic disease. This suggests that the terms *extranodal, nodal,* and *splenic MZL* refer to different clinical presentations of the same disease.

Nodal marginal zone lymphoma is clinically more aggressive than the extranodal and splenic forms and has a higher incidence of advanced-stage disease and lower 5-year overall and disease-free survival.[31] In addition, 10% to 20% of cases transform into a DLBCL. Most cases display a distinct "monocytoid" appearance, and the tumor was originally termed *monocytoid B-cell lymphoma.* Molecular studies strengthen the concept of significant differences among the three types of MZL. The t(11;18) does not occur in nodal MZL. Analysis of IgV_H gene demonstrates that some nodal MZLs carry somatic mutations whereas others do not, suggesting derivation from post-GC and virgin B cells, respectively. Among mutated cases, usage of specific IgV_H gene segments seems to occur frequently and to discriminate between HCV-positive and -negative patients.[32] None of the translocations characteristically recorded in splenic MZL, including del(7q), del(13q14), and del(10)(q22,q24), has been detected in nodal MZL.

Splenic Marginal Zone Lymphoma

Splenic marginal zone lymphoma is generally characterized by splenomegaly and leukemic spread, although at times cases with disseminated disease or exclusively leukemic presentation have been reported. In approximately half of the cases, circulating neoplastic cells display cytoplasmic villous projections, which justify the term *splenic lymphoma with villous lymphocytes* used formerly. Infiltration of the marrow occurs in most if not all patients. Molecular studies have shown that splenic MZL is a heterogeneous tumor[33] with chromosomal abnormalities including del(7q), del(13q14), and del(10)(q22,q24).

Lymphoplasmacytic Lymphoma/Waldenstrom Macroglobulinemia

Lymphoplasmacytic lymphoma (LPL) is rare, accounting for less than 2% of all NHL. Lymphoplasmacytic lymphoma was defined initially as a small B-cell lymphoma with plasmacytoid or plasmacytic features. Because other types of small B-cell lymphoma, particularly marginal zone B-cell lymphoma, may exhibit plasmacytic differentiation, the WHO classification has defined LPL more narrowly to exclude other small B-cell lymphomas. Waldenstrom macroglobulinemia (WM) was combined with LPL and designated LPL/WM. The consensus group at the Second International Workshop on WM in 2002 redefined WM as a distinct clinicopathologic entity characterized by marrow infiltration with LPL and IgM monoclonal gammopathy.[34]

Variations in the immunophenotypic profile exist, but the typical immunophenotype consists of expression of CD19, CD20, CD22, cytoplasmic Igs, FMC7, BCL2, PAX5, CD38, and CD79a; CD10 and CD23 are usually absent. CD5 is variably expressed in up to 20% of cases. The immunophenotypic profile in combination with the presence of somatic mutations of IgVH genes without intraclonal diversity strongly suggests that the malignant cells originate from cells at a late stage of differentiation derived from a B cell arrested after somatic hypermutation in the germinal center and before terminal differentiation to a plasma cell. Most patients with WM have symptoms attributable to tumor infiltration or monoclonal serum protein. Lytic bone disease is rare. Extensive marrow infiltration leads to cytopenias, and progressive anemia is the most common indication for initiation of treatment. The neoplastic clone can also infiltrate other organs, including lymph nodes, liver, and spleen, presenting as organomegalies. In rare cases, diffuse lymphoplasmacytic infiltration of the lung, stomach, or bowel can occur. The Bing–Neel syndrome (long-standing hyperviscosity altering the vascular permeability and leading to perivascular malignant infiltration) consists of headache, vertigo, impaired hearing, ataxia, nystagmus, diplopia, and eventually coma. Serum hyperviscosity is the most distinguishing feature of WM, but is observed only in less than 15% of patients at diagnosis. Symptoms of hyperviscosity usually appear when the normal serum viscosity of 1.4 to 1.8 cP reaches 4 to 5 cP (corresponding to a serum IgM level of at least 30 g/L) and include constitutional symptoms, bleeding, ocular, neurologic, and cardiovascular manifestations. High-output cardiac failure may develop because of the expanded plasma volume arising from increased osmotic pressure. Abnormalities in bleeding and clotting times occur from the interaction of IgM with coagulation factors and platelets. Cryoglobulins may be detected in 20% of patients. IgM deposition can occur in the kidney, intestine, and skin, presenting as proteinuria, diarrhea, and macroglobulinemia cutis (papules and nodules). Primary amyloidosis occurs mainly in the heart, peripheral nerves, kidneys, soft tissues, liver, and lungs due to deposition of monoclonal light chains. Secondary amyloidosis is rarely seen in WM. Although most patients have detectable light chains in the urine, renal insufficiency and cast nephropathy are rare. The median survival of patients with WM ranges from 5 and 10 years. Prognostic factors include age, hemoglobin, serum albumin level, and β_2-microglobulin level. IgM levels have no prognostic value.[35]

Small Lymphocytic Lymphoma

Historically, small lymphocytic lymphoma (SLL) was considered a different disease from chronic lymphocytic leukemia (CLL). In the WHO classification, SLL and CLL are classified as different clinical manifestations of the same disease.[36] When the disease involves the blood and marrow, it is called CLL. When lymph nodes or other tissues are infiltrated by CLL cells in the absence of leukemia, it is called SLL. Only 5% of CLL/SLL patients present with clinical features of SLL without the leukemic component. The National Cancer Institute guidelines recommend that the threshold for diagnosis of CLL should require a lymphocytosis of greater than 5000/μL.[37] However, if diagnostic immunophenotypic features are clearly those of typical CLL/SLL, the diagnosis can be made in the presence of a blood lymphocyte count of less than 5000/μL. CLL/SLL is largely a disease of the elderly, with a median age at diagnosis of 70 years. It is extremely rare at less than 30 years of age, but the incidence increases with increasing age and occurs almost twice as frequently in males than females. The variation in international incidence patterns among the leukemias and lymphomas is most marked for SLL/CLL, with a 26-fold increase in incidence for men and a 38-fold increase for women in North America when compared to the incidence in Japan.[38] Genetic rather than environmental factors probably underlie these differences, because the disease is rare among Japanese Americans.[39] Among the strongest risk factors for SLL/CLL is a family history of this or other lymphoid malignancies, and a number of familial clusters of CLL/SLL have been reported.[40]

The diagnosis of SLL is made by the detection of a clonal population of small B lymphocytes in the lymph node biopsy showing cells expressing the characteristic morphology and immunophenotype. Full immunophenotype is required to make the diagnosis. Chronic lymphocytic leukemia cells express CD19, dim CD20, dim CD5, CD23, CD43, and CD79a and weakly express surface IgM and IgD. Occasional cases lack expression of CD23, and this can lead to a differential diagnosis of mantle cell lymphoma. The dim expression of CD20 and surface immunoglobulin can be useful in distinguishing SLL from mantle cell lymphoma. Expression of CD38 is variable and has prognostic significance. Detection of specific cytogenetic and molecular features can be helpful in making the definitive diagnosis.

SLL usually presents with marrow and blood involvement and typically runs an indolent course. Transformation into DLBCL (Richter syndrome) may occur. Although it is reasonable to assume that a similar profile of molecular cytogenetic lesions may characterize

SLL and CLL, no formal studies have been performed to demonstrate this conclusively. However, the molecular changes and their incidence appears identical in SLL and CLL. Fluorescence in situ hybridization studies found an approximate 50% incidence of cryptic 13q14 deletions and a 5% to 10% incidence of 17p13 deletions. Structural changes of 11q, mostly deletions involving the q22–23 segment (del(11q)), were detected in 10% to 20%. Trisomy 12 was seen in 10% to 30% of the cases and other trisomies, involving chromosomes 3 (+3) and 18 (+18) in approximately 10% of the cases. Deletions/translocations of 6q21–23 were detected in 15% to 25% of the cases and correlated with leukemic involvement by large prolymphocytoid cells. The t(14;19)(q32;q13.3) deletions/translocations 14q22 and the t(11,14)(q13;q32) were reported in several cases. Other chromosome 14q32 translocations with 1p32 and other unknown partners may be found in SLL; in general, those cases with a 14q anomaly require a precise histologic characterization because distinction from mantle cell lymphomas and marginal zone B-cell lymphomas may pose difficult diagnostic problems.

Mantle Cell Lymphoma

Mantle cell lymphoma (MCL) was recognized as a separate clinicopathologic entity in 1992. It has been previously referred to as intermediate lymphocytic lymphoma, mantle zone lymphoma, centrocytic lymphoma, and lymphocytic lymphoma of intermediate differentiation. In the Rappaport and Working Formulation classifications, the majority of cases of diffuse small cleaved cell lymphomas on re-review were found to be MCLs; however, cases were also found in the small lymphocytic and follicular categories. Histologically, MCL is composed of small cells with irregular nuclei, although the cells may be larger in the blastic variant. Immunophenotype is characterized by the coexpression of the T-cell antigen CD5, with the B-cell markers CD20, CD19, CD22, and CD79a. It is distinguished from CLL by the lack of expression of CD23, by bright CD20 and surface immunoglobulin, and by expression of cyclin D1. The t(11;14) occurs in virtually all cases of MCL. The histologic pattern of MCL may be diffuse, nodular, or mantle zone, or a combination of the three. It has been reported that there is a better prognosis for cases with a mantle zone pattern. Most cases are composed exclusively of small- to medium-sized lymphoid cells, with slightly irregular, or "cleaved," nuclei. However, the morphology can range from lymphocyte-like to large cleaved or lymphoblast-like. Despite the small size and bland appearance of these cells, there is often more mitotic activity than in other histologically low-grade lymphomas. Single epithelioid histiocytes may be present, but clusters and granulomas are not seen. Transformed cells with basophilic cytoplasm (centroblast- or immunoblast-like cells) are extremely rare or absent, aside from residual germinal centers. Mantle cell lymphoma is thought to arise from naïve cells from the follicle mantle, although a number of studies have suggested that somatic hypermutation can occur in a subset of patients.

Mantle cell lymphoma is an aggressive, generally incurable subtype of NHL that accounts for approximately 5% to 6% of all NHL cases.[18] Approximately 3000 to 4000 new MCL cases occur annually in both the USA and Europe. The median age of presentation is 65 years, with a strong male preponderance. Most cases are at an advanced stage at presentation,[41] and extranodal involvement is common, especially in the gastrointestinal tract.[42] A small number of patients who present with limited-stage disease may potentially be cured by modified extended field radiation therapy. MCL has the poorest long-term survival of all the lymphoma subtypes, and a watch and wait approach is generally not justified. Factors associated with poor prognosis include poor performance status, splenomegaly, anemia, and age.[43] The international prognostic index is of limited value in predicting outcome. Mantle cell lymphoma has one of the poorest prognoses of all NHL subtypes.[18] With standard therapies, median failure-free survival is 8 to 20 months and median survival is approximately 3 to 4 years.[25,41,44,45]

TREATMENT OF INDOLENT LYMPHOMAS

For most cases of indolent lymphoma, the goal of therapy has been to maintain the best quality of life and to treat only when patients develop symptoms. Any alteration to this approach requires demonstration of improved survival with early institution of therapy, or identification of criteria that define patients sufficiently high-risk to merit early therapy. There are many available therapies and no consensus on an optimal first-line or relapse treatment. Despite a paucity of data demonstrating any benefit for early therapy, patients are being treated earlier in their disease course. There is no clear cut treatment pathway for patients with indolent lymphomas and little or no data regarding the optimal sequencing of treatment approaches in these diseases. In the absence of such data, treatment choices remain empiric and should always involve discussion regarding patient choice and goal of therapy. Decisions concerning therapy are likely to become even more complicated because many novel agents are currently being investigated in preclinical and clinical studies, particularly, novel monoclonal antibodies and agents that alter the antiapoptotic pathways. Enrollment of patients on properly conducted clinical trials should be encouraged until we have a clear-cut established treatment approach that leads to cure for the majority of patients.

Options for treatment of low-grade lymphomas include a watch and wait approach, single-agent chemotherapy, or monoclonal antibody therapy with rituximab, combination chemoimmunotherapy, and the use of autologous or allogeneic hematopoietic cell transplantation (HCT) (Table 79–5). Patients remaining on an expectant course should be followed every 3 months with history, physical examination, and blood counts, including lactate dehydrogenase. Special attention should be paid to any change in symptoms that might be suggestive of transformation, which should be an indication for repeat biopsy to examine for histologic evidence to confirm transformation. The role of routine repeat scanning remains unclear.

Because there is no clearly defined treatment algorithm for most patients with indolent lymphomas, eligible patients should be included whenever possible in clinical trials. This ensures delivery of optimal care and helps inform design of subsequent trials, hopefully leading to cure. Information on available clinical trials can be found at www.clinicaltrials.gov.

WHEN TO INSTITUTE THERAPY

With the exception of patients enrolled in clinical trials assessing the impact of early therapy, expectant management is the treatment of

Table 79–5 Treatment Strategies for Indolent Lymphomas

Advanced Stage Disease
"Watchful waiting"
Alkylating agents
Purine analogs
Combination chemotherapy
Monoclonal antibodies
Unconjugated
Conjugated – radioimmunoconjugates and immunotoxins
Chemotherapy + monoclonal antibodies (chemoimmunotherapy)
High dose chemotherapy plus autologous/allogeneic hematopoietic cell transplantation
Reduced intensity conditioning allogeneic transplantation.
Palliative radiotherapy
Localized Disease
Radiotherapy
"Watchful waiting"

Table 79–6 Criteria for Delaying Treatment

Groupe pour l'Etude de Lymphome Folliculaire (GELF)[48]
All of the following
Maximum diameter of disease <7 cm
Fewer than three nodal sites
Absence of systemic symptoms
Spleen <16 cm on CT
No significant effusions
No risk of local compressive symptoms
No circulating lymphoma cells or marrow compromise (Hb ≤10 g/dL, WBC <1.5, or platelets <100,000/dL)
British National Lymphoma Investigation (BNLI)[49]
Absence of all of the following
B symptoms or pruritus
Rapid generalized disease progression
Marrow compromise (Hb ≤10 g/dL, WBC <3.0, or platelets <100,000/dL)
Life-threatening organ involvement
Renal infiltration
Bone lesions

Table 79–7 National LymphoCare Study Survey of Current Practice for FL in the USA[52]

"Watch and Wait"	19%
Rituximab monotherapy	13%
Chemotherapy plus rituximab	51%
R-CHOP	59%
R-CVP	19%
R-fludarabine-based	11%
R-other	11%
Chemotherapy alone	4%
Radiation alone	5%

R-CHOP, rituximab with cyclophosphamide, adriamycin, vincristine, and prednisone; R-CVP, rituximab, cyclophosphamide, vincristine, and prednisolone.

choice for asymptomatic patients with low bulk disease until clear indications for initiation of treatment are seen. This approach is based on the demonstration of no survival advantage for institution of immediate compared with deferred treatment until time of progression.[46] Three randomized trials, performed in the pre-rituximab era, confirmed no survival benefit for early therapy.[47–49] In the National Cancer Institute study in 104 newly diagnosed patients with FL, deferred treatment was compared with immediate treatment with ProMACE-MOPP followed by total nodal irradiation. An updated analysis of the data is long overdue, but there was no difference in overall survival (OS) between the two arms at the time of the last analysis.[47] The Groupe pour l'Etude de Lymphome Folliculaire (GELF) used defined criteria for patients in whom immediate therapy was not felt to be indicated (Table 79–6) and randomized 193 patients to deferred treatment or to receive prednimustine 200 mg/m²/day for 5 days per month for 18 months or interferon-alpha (IFN-α) 5 MU/day for 3 months, then 5 MU three times per week for 15 months.[48] The median OS time was not reached and was the same in all three arms of the study. The British National Lymphoma Investigation[49] compared treatment in 309 patients with asymptomatic advanced-stage, indolent lymphoma in whom 158 patients were randomized to receive immediate therapy with oral chlorambucil 10 mg per day continuously and 151 patients randomized to deferred treatment until disease progression (Table 79–6). In both arms, local radiotherapy to symptomatic nodes was allowed. There was no difference in OS or cause-specific survival between the two groups with 16 years' median follow-up. A meta-analysis of more than 2000 patients with early-stage CLL/SLL showed no difference in survival between early versus deferred therapy using alkylating agents.[50]

A major clinical trial question is whether identification of clinical or molecular risk factors can identify which patients are candidates for early therapy. A survival predictor score has also been developed from gene expression profiling studies.[12] The results from this study suggest that the molecular determinants of biological heterogeneity are already present in the diagnostic lymph node biopsies rather than by the later acquisition of secondary genetic changes. A major component of the gene expression prognostic signature is related to immune cells in the tumor microenvironment.[13,14,51] Future guidelines for treatment will likely be based on clinical staging systems, genetic profiles, and immune response signatures, but these factors do not yet help us to decide who should receive immediate therapy.

From available data, there is little to suggest that we should change our practice of "watch and wait" for asymptomatic low bulk patient, but data demonstrate that this practice is becoming much less common in the USA.[52] The National Lymphocare Study is a prospective observational study designed to assess presentation, prognosis, treatment, and clinical outcomes in newly diagnosed FL. The treating physician determines management according to clinical judgment with no prescribed treatment regimen and data regarding histology, stage, therapy, response, relapse, and death are recorded. Among 1493 patients enrolled at 237 centers, 26% of initially observed patients had switched to active therapy after a median of 2.8 months on observation since diagnosis, and by the first follow-up visit only 19% of patients continued on watch and wait at 6 months (Table 79–7). This observation is in stark contrast to the data from the British National Lymphoma Investigation (BLNI) study demonstrating that (censored for nonlymphoma death) 19% of patients and 40% for those older than 70 years who were randomized to expectant management still did not require therapy at 10 years.[49]

TREATMENT APPROACHES

Treatment is indicated in patients with symptomatic disease, bulky lymphadenopathy, and/or splenomegaly; risk of local compressive disease; marrow compromise; or rapid disease progression. Once indicated, numerous treatment approaches are available (Table 79–5). The concept that the approach can be to "do nothing" or discuss an approach with considerable morbidity and mortality such as hematopoietic cell transplantation is a confusing one for the newly diagnosed patient (as well as for the physician), and considerable consultation time is required to review available treatment approaches. Staging of response in indolent lymphomas is by the revised response criteria.[16] Depending on the treatment approach used, restaging after two to three cycles of therapy can be useful to ensure responsiveness with full restaging after completion of therapy. Whereas curative approaches are being sought in indolent lymphomas, the failure to achieve complete remission (CR) does not have the same implication in indolent lymphomas as in aggressive lymphomas, and a PR may be a sufficient response to therapy to alleviate symptoms.

Optimal first-line treatment is enrollment in randomized clinical trials. In the National Lymphocare Study,[52] academic sites are more likely than community sites to treat patients on clinical trials (12% vs 4%), but it is lamentable that such a small proportion of these patients are enrolled in clinical trials. For patients who are not eligible for or who refuse entry into clinical trials, there are data demonstrating higher response rates and longer duration of responses, and perhaps improved survival with chemoimmunotherapy. Many investigators favor alkylator- over fludarabine-based regimens for FL, based on concerns regarding the ability to obtain stem cells for later use for autologous HCT in fludarabine-treated patients.[53] It is suggested that more aggressive first-line therapy should be offered to patients who progress within 1 year of presentation, because these patients have a worse outcome.[48] Elderly patients or those with poor performance status remain candidates for single-agent chlorambucil. Single-agent monoclonal antibody therapy is appropriate for patients who chose to avoid chemotherapy and is a reasonable treatment choice based on the results of clinical trials of prolonged or maintenance therapy with rituximab. Although data suggest a survival advantage with the use of IFN-α in combination with chemotherapy, this is associated with a significant side effect profile and this agent is rarely used in the USA. Optimal results are seen when radioimmunoconjugates are used earlier in the disease course. There is no indication for the use of high-dose therapy and HCT in first remission in FL except in the context of a properly conducted clinical trial.

Data from the National Lymphocare study[52] demonstrate that chemoimmunotherapy is now the treatment of choice of physicians in the USA (Table 79–7). No randomized trials demonstrate a benefit for the addition of anthracyclines, but cyclophosphamide, adriamycin, vincristine, prednisone, and rituximab (CHOP-R) is heavily favored over cyclophosphamide, vincristine prednisone, and rituximab (CVP-R) or fludarabine-based regimens. Choice to initiate therapy was associated with FLIPI, stage, and grade but FLIPI was not associated with the decision to utilize a specific treatment approach. Significant regional and center differences were observed, strongly suggesting that physician preference is the predominant factor that drives initial therapy. For example, initial "watch and wait" was used in 31% in the Northeast, but in 13% in the Southeast, whereas fludarabine-based chemoimmunotherapy was used in 18% of patients in the Southwest and only 3% in the Northeast.

Alkylating Agents

The alkylating agents chlorambucil and cyclophosphamide with or without prednisone and CVP or CHOP, and other alkylator-based combination chemotherapy regimens, have been the standard of therapy for decades. Single-agent alkylators at different doses and schedules produce overall response (OR) rates of 50% to 75% in FL.[54,55] Comparable response rates but higher complete remission rates with longer progression-free survival (PFS) are seen with CVP compared to chlorambucil, but there is no survival advantage.[56,57] The addition of anthracyclines has not improved the response rate or duration of the response,[58,59] but its use may be associated with a lower risk of histologic transformation.[47,60] This finding has to be confirmed, particularly in the era of chemoimmunotherapy.

Purine Analogues

The purine analogues have been studied extensively in various types of indolent lymphoma. Fludarabine monotherapy produces response rates of 65% to 84%, with 37% to 47% CR in previously untreated FL patients.[61] In a randomized trial of 381 previously untreated indolent lymphoma patients, CR rates were higher with fludarabine than CVP.[62] Fludarabine combinations result in increased response rates, with 89% CR rate in an Eastern Cooperative Oncology Group trial combining fludarabine and cyclophosphamide,[63] whereas fludarabine and mitoxantrone produced a 91% overall response rate, 43% CR, and 63% 2-year disease-free survival.[64] A higher CR rate was seen with fludarabine and mitoxantrone (68%) compared to CHOP (42%) in a randomized trial.[65] The use of alkylator-based regimens or purine analog-based regimens appears to vary geographically, suggesting personal preference for the use of regimens in which the clinician has experience, rather than alterations of practice based on the results of the published studies. In CLL/SLL, fludarabine is associated with a higher response rate and longer duration of response than chlorambucil,[66] but no OS advantage. The use of fludarabine in combination with cyclophosphamide is associated with a higher response rate and longer duration of response compared with fludarabine alone in randomized trials.[67] The highest response rates have been with fludarabine, cyclophosphamide, and rituximab.[68]

Biologic Therapy

IFN-α is approved by the Food and Drug Administration (FDA) for the treatment of advanced-stage FL in combination with anthracycline-based chemotherapy, based on improved survival in a clinical trials[24,69,70] and meta-analysis of phase III trial data.[71] IFN-α has been widely used in Europe but not in the USA, where it is felt that its toxicity profile outweighs any potential benefit. In the SWOG study,[72] 571 patients with stage III and IV indolent lymphoma were treated with ProMACE-MOPP, and 279 responding patients were randomized to 24 months of observation versus treatment with IFN-α. No statistically significant difference in PFS or OS was observed between observation and IFN-α groups at 4 years.

Monoclonal Antibody Therapy

Monoclonal antibodies are the most exciting agents to emerge in the treatment of indolent lymphomas, and recent data suggest their use may finally be leading to improvement in patient survival.[22,23] The most widely used monoclonal antibody is rituximab, a chimeric unconjugated antibody against the CD20 antigen licensed by the FDA[73] and the European Agency for the Evaluation of Medicinal Products[74] for treatment of patients with relapsed or refractory, CD20-positive low-grade FL; for the first-line treatment of CD20-positive FL in combination with CVP chemotherapy; and for the treatment of CD20-positive low-grade NHL in patients with stable disease or who achieve a PR or CR following first-line treatment with CVP chemotherapy.

Following phase I studies,[75] rituximab at a dose of 375 mg/m^2 weekly for 4 weeks was selected for the pivotal phase II trial and this remains the standard dose.[76] In relapsed indolent lymphoma patients, OR was 48% and 60% in FL. Median PFS for responders was 13 months. Factors associated with lower response rates include chemoresistant disease,[76] bulky disease,[77] and treatment late in the disease course.[78] The incidence of OR was 73% in previously untreated patients with low bulk disease,[79] and some of these patients have needed no further treatment and have no evidence of polymerase chain reaction-detectable minimal residual disease after 7 years.[80] Extended use with 8 weeks instead of four is associated with improvement in OR and duration of response.[81] Comparable or even longer durations of response have been observed with retreatment.[82]

A number of trials in front-line and in relapsed/refractory patients have investigated the potential benefits of extended or maintenance rituximab treatment[83–87] and all demonstrated prolonged time to progression in patients receiving maintenance rituximab (Table 79–8). The results from the E1496 randomized trial from the Eastern Cooperative Oncology Group and the Cancer and Leukemia Group B comparing CVP alone to CVP followed by rituximab in patients with advanced-stage FL demonstrated that addition of rituximab maintenance significantly improved OS[83] and led to FDA approval for rituximab therapy in patients responding to CVP chemotherapy. A problem with interpretation of the role of maintenance therapy or in recommending a specific regimen is that there is no standard schedule and trials have been performed in rituximab-naïve patients as well as in patients treated with previous rituximab monotherapy or combination chemoimmunotherapy, as shown in Figure 79–1.

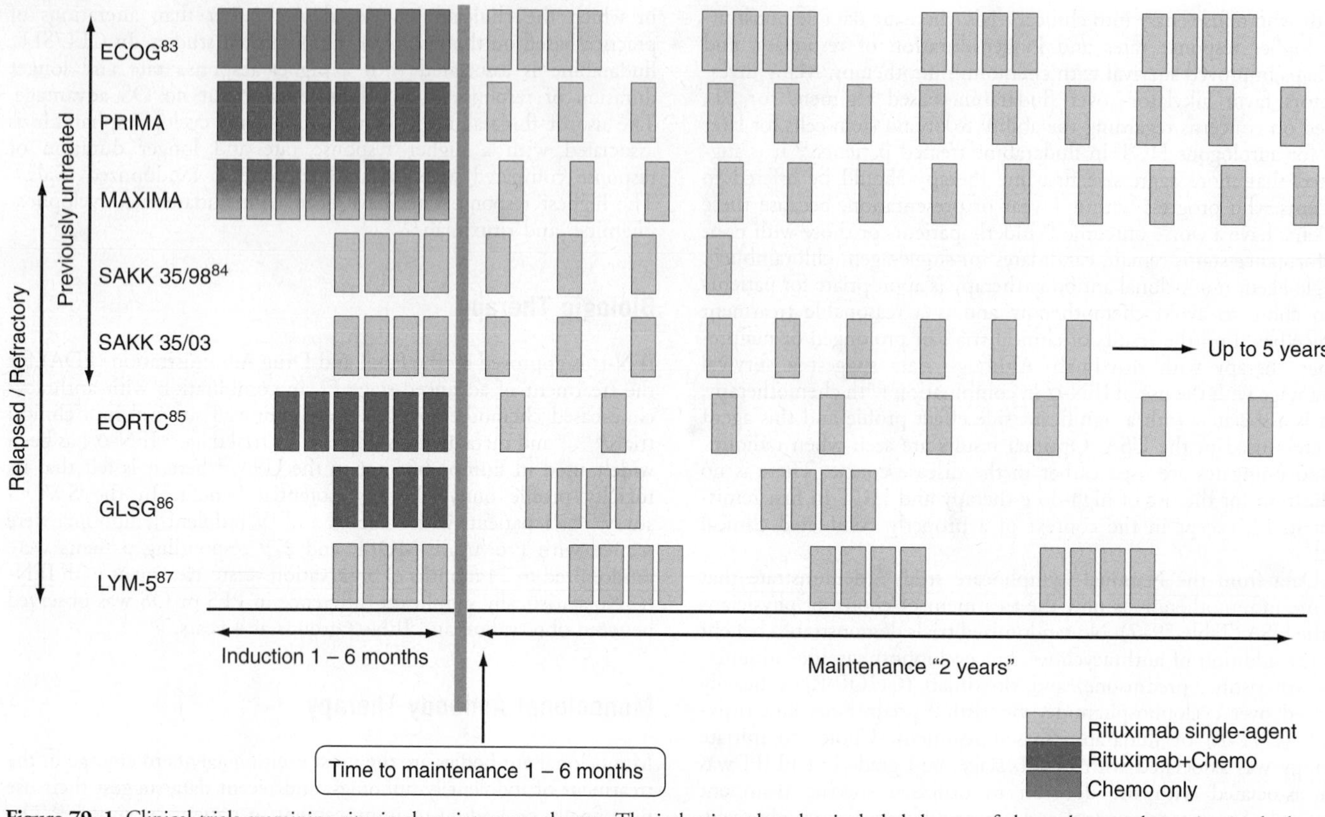

Figure 79–1 Clinical trials examining rituximab maintenance therapy. The induction phase has included the use of chemotherapy alone, rituximab alone or chemoimmunotherapy. The PRIMA and MAXIMA studies are ongoing randomized studies examining the use of chemoimmunotherapy followed by rituximab maintenance. Studies included previously untreated and treated patients.

Table 79–8 Studies of Rituximab Maintenance Therapy in Indolent Lymphomas

Trial	Disease Setting	Diseases Included	Previous Therapy
ECOG[83]	First line	Follicular Small lymphocytic	CVP
SAKK[84]	First line Relapsed/refractory	Follicular Mantle cell	Rituximab
EORTC[85]	Relapsed/refractory	Follicular	CHOP vs R-CHOP
GLSG[86]	Relapsed/refractory	Follicular Mantle cell	FCM vs R-FCM
LYM-5[87]	Relapsed/refractory	Follicular Small lymphocytic	Rituximab

CHOP, cyclophosphamide, adriamycin, vincristine, and prednisone; R-CHOP, rituximab with cyclophosphamide, adriamycin, vincristine, and prednisone; FCM, fludarabine, cyclophosphamide, mitoxantrone; R-FCM, rituximab with fludarabine, cyclophosphamide, mitoxantrone; ECOG, Eastern Co-operative Oncology Group; SAKK, Schweizerische Arbeitsgemeinschaft für klinische Krebsforschung; EORTC, European Organisation for Research and Treatment of Cancer; GLSG, German Low Grade Lymphoma Study Group; LYM-5, Lymphoma 5 trial.

Chemoimmunotherapy

In a phase II study, 40 patients with indolent lymphoma were treated with six infusions of rituximab (375 mg/m^2 per dose) in combination with six doses of CHOP chemotherapy (R-CHOP).[88] Overall response was 95%, with a CR of 55% and OR of 45% in patients with bulky disease. In a phase II study of 40 patients with indolent lymphomas, rituximab in combination with fludarabine produced OR of 90% and CR of 80%, with similar response rates in treatment-naïve and previously treated patients.[89]

A number of randomized trials show a benefit for the use of rituximab with chemotherapy compared to chemotherapy alone (Table 79–9).[85,90–93] Each study showed an improvement in time to treatment failure. More recent follow-up data suggest improved OS in patients treated with chemoimmunotherapy compared to chemotherapy alone. A meta-analysis of these trials demonstrates that OS, OR, and disease control are significantly better in those on chemoimmunotherapy compared to chemotherapy for FL and mantle cell lymphoma.[94] Data from the German Low-Grade Study Group suggest that it is the addition of rituximab that has led to the recent improvement in survival of patients with FL.[23] A recent independently assessed analysis of the clinical benefits provided by rituximab in relation to cost concluded that it is highly cost-effective.[95]

Conjugated Radiolabeled Monoclonal Antibody Therapy

Binding a radioisotope to a monoclonal antibody (radioimmunoconjugate) might be expected to improve efficacy over antibody therapy alone. Tositumomab joins ^{131}I to the anti-B1 antibody and has been studied extensively in the treatment of heavily pretreated[96] and untreated[97] lymphomas and for retreatment of indolent lymphomas.[98] Best responses are seen in previously untreated FL patients with a 95% OR and 75% CR. Eighty percent of assessable patients achieved eradication of polymerase chain reaction-detectable minimal residual disease after a single treatment course with tositumomab.[97] Median PFS was 6.1 years, with 40 patients remaining in remission for 4.3 to 7.7 years and no cases of myelodysplastic syndrome observed. A SWOG study investigated chemoimmunotherapy with six cycles of CHOP chemotherapy followed 4 to 8 weeks later by tositumomab in 90 patients with previously untreated, advanced-stage FL.[99] The OR was 91%, including 69% CR and at median

Table 79–9 Randomized Trials of Chemotherapy vs Chemoimmunotherapy

Study	Treatment, No. of Patients	Median FU, Months	OR %	CR %	Median TTF, Months	OS %
M39021[90]	CVP, 159	53	57	10	15	77
	R-CVP, 162		81	41	34	83
					$P < .0001$	$P = .0290$
GLSG[91]	CHOP, 205	18	90	17	29	90
	R-CHOP, 223		96	20	NR	95
					$P < .001$	$P = .016$
M39023[92]	MCP, 96	47	75	25	26	74
	R-MCP, 105		92	50	NR	87
					$P < .0001$	$P = .0096$
FL2000[93]	CHVP-IFN, 183	42	73	63	46%	84
	R-CHVP-IFN 175		84	79	67%	91
					$P < .0001$	$P = .029$

CR, complete remission; CHOP, cyclophosphamide, adriamycin, vincristine, and prednisone; CHVP-IFN, cyclophosphamide, doxorubicin, teniposide, prednisone, and IFN-α; CVP, cyclophosphamide, vincristine, and prednisolone; FU, follow-up; GLSG, German Low Grade Lymphoma Study Group; MCP, mitoxantrone, chlorambucil, and prednisolone; OR, overall response; OS, overall survival; R-CHOP, rituximab with cyclophosphamide, adriamycin, vincristine, and prednisone; R-CHVP-IFN, rituximab with cyclophosphamide, doxorubicin, teniposide, prednisone, and IFN-α; R-CVP, rituximab, cyclophosphamide, vincristine, and prednisolone; R-MCP, rituximab with mitoxantrone, chlorambucil, and prednisolone; TTF, time to failure.

follow-up time of 5.1 years, the estimated 5-year OS was 87% and PFS 67%. These results were significantly better than results of therapy with CHOP alone on previous SWOG protocols. Ibritumomab Tiuxetan is a ^{90}Y-labeled anti-CD20 antibody and produced an OR of 74% and CR of 15% in 57 FL patients refractory to rituximab.[100] Toxicity is primarily hematologic, with nadir counts occurring at 7 to 9 weeks and lasting approximately 1 to 4 weeks. The risk of hematologic toxicity increased with dose delivered and with degree of baseline marrow involvement.[101] An acceptable safety profile was observed in relapsed patients with less than 25% lymphoma marrow involvement, adequate marrow reserve, platelets greater than 100,000 cells/μL, and neutrophils greater than 1500 cells/μL.

High-Dose Therapy as Consolidation of First Remission

The role of high-dose therapy and autologous HCT in FL patients during first remission was explored in phase II trials,[102,103] and in three phase III randomized trials.[104–106] The German Low-Grade Study Group trial[104] recruited 307 previously untreated patients up to 60 years of age. Patients who responded after induction chemotherapy with 2 cycles of CHOP or mitoxantrone–chlorambucil–prednisone were randomized to autologous HCT or IFN-α maintenance. Among 240 evaluable patients, the 5-year PFS was 64.7% for autologous HCT and 33.3% in the IFN-α arm ($P < .0001$). Acute toxicity was higher in the autologous HCT group, but early mortality was below 2.5% in both study arms. Longer follow-up is necessary to determine the effect of autologous HCT on OS. In the Groupe Ouest Est des Leucemies Aigues et des Maladies du Sang study, 172 newly diagnosed advanced FL patients were randomized either to cyclophosphamide, doxorubicin, teniposide, prednisone (CHVP) and IFN-α or to high-dose therapy followed by purged autologous HCT.[105] Patients treated with high-dose therapy had a higher response rate than patients who received chemotherapy and IFN-α (81% vs 69%, $P = .045$) and a longer median PFS (not reached versus 45 months), but this did not translate into a better OS because of an excess of secondary malignancies after transplantation. A subgroup of patients with a significantly higher event-free survival rate could be identified using the FLIPI. The GELF-94 study enrolled 401 previously untreated advanced-stage FL patients who were randomized to receive CHVP plus IFN-α compared with four courses of CHOP followed by HDT with total body irradiation and autologous HCT. Overall response rates were similar in both groups (79% and 78%, respectively), and 87% of eligible patients underwent autologous HCT. Intent-to-treat analysis after a median follow-up of 7.5 years showed no difference between the two arms for OS ($P = .53$) or PFS ($P = .11$). Long-term follow-up demonstrated no statistically significant benefit in favor of first-line autologous HCT in patients with FL. In view of these results, autologous HCT should be used in first remission only in the setting of clinical trials.

TREATMENT OF RELAPSED INDOLENT LYMPHOMA

The treatment options after relapse remain the same as for first-line therapy (Table 79–5), and relapsed patients should ideally be treated in clinical trials. Relapsed asymptomatic disease is not necessarily an indication for treatment and patients can again be managed expectantly. A number of factors must be taken into account in planning therapy and it is not possible to define treatment at relapse without considering the goal of therapy (palliative vs potentially curative) performance status, previous therapy, response, and duration of response. Single agent rituximab is approved for relapsed lymphoma and is widely used in this setting. A multicenter randomized trial in relapsed patients has demonstrated a survival advantage for chemoimmunotherapy with CHOP-R or CHOP followed by R compared to CHOP alone, and a further benefit for rituximab maintenance therapy.[85] For younger patients who are suitable candidates for autologous HCT or reduced-intensity conditioning (RIC) allogeneic transplantation, referral to a transplant center should be considered early to discuss the potential role and timing of transplantation. Best results are seen when transplantation is considered early in the course of disease before patients become chemorefractive. Hematopoietic cell transplant approaches must be considered in the context of the improving results that are being seen with salvage therapy alone. The results of autologous HCT have been disappointing for CLL/SLL;[107] however, RIC allogeneic transplants appear promising in selected patients with this disease.[108]

The Role of Transplant in Relapsed Indolent Lymphomas

Unlike aggressive lymphomas, the use of high-dose chemotherapy with autologous HCT in the treatment of indolent lymphomas has not yet been fully established. The rationale for considering transplantation is that the disease is incurable using standard approaches, and promising results have been observed in a number of phase II studies.[109–111] Detection of minimal residual disease has been a useful surrogate marker for tracking long-term PFS in patients examining the autologous stem cells or serial samples after transplantation.[111–115] A major concern relates to the risk of secondary myelodysplasia/acute myeloid leukemia.[116] The European Bone Marrow Transplant Registry-sponsored CUP study (conventional chemotherapy, unpurged, purged autograft) is the only prospective randomized trial to assess the role of autologous HCT in patients with relapsed FL.[117] The results of the study suggest a PFS and OS advantage of autologous HCT over conventional chemotherapy, with a 4-year OS of 46% for the chemotherapy arm, versus 71% for the unpurged and 77% for the purged autologous HCT arms. The study was closed early because of slow accrual with 140 of the planned 250 patients accrued and only 89 randomized. In CLL/SLL, the use of autologous HCT was not associated with improved outcome in patients transplanted in first remission compared to those transplanted later in their disease course.[107]

Allogeneic Hematopoietic Cell Transplant

There is a trend toward increasing use of allogeneic HCT in the management of indolent lymphomas. In a report of the International Bone Marrow Transplant Registry, results after HCT are described for 904 patients with FL.[118] Among these patients, 176 patients underwent allogeneic HCT, and 131 patients underwent autologous HCT using a purged inoculum and 597 using an unpurged autologous inoculum. The treatment-related mortality (TRM) in these three groups was 30%, 14%, and 8%, respectively, disease recurrence in 21%, 43%, and 58% and 5-year OS was 51%, 62%, and 55%, respectively. The use of total body irradiation-containing regimens was associated with increased TRM but decreased risk of relapse. The use of allogeneic HCT was associated with increased TRM but significantly lower risk of disease recurrence in keeping with a graft-versus-lymphoma effect in this disease. It should be noted that the majority of allogeneic transplant recipients reported in these studies received a fully myeloablative regimen. Long-term PFS has been observed after allogeneic SCT even in patients with refractory FL.[119] In 29 FL patients, 11 of whom had refractory disease, the nonrelapse mortality was 24% and there was a 23% incidence of relapse. The 5-year OS was 58%, with 53% event-free survival. Patients who have relapsed after previous autologous HCT have a very poor prognosis. The outcome following myeloablative allogeneic HCT of 114 such patients has been reported from the International Bone Marrow Transplant Registry.[120] The TRM was 22% and the probability of disease progression was 52% at 3 years. The use of total body irradiation conditioning regimens and achievement of CR at the time of allogeneic HCT were associated with improved outcome. The use of RIC regimens appears to be associated with improved outcome. In 20 such patients, there was only one TRM from fungal infection and the 3-year progression-free survival was an excellent 95%.[121] The out-come following RIC transplant regimen incorporating alemtuzumab immunosuppressive therapy has been reported for 81 patients with lymphoma, including 41 with low grade, 37 with high/intermediate grade, and 10 patients with MCL, 31 of whom had relapsed following previous autologous HCT.[122] Patients received a conditioning regimen consisting of alemtuzumab, fludarabine, and melphalan, and received short-course cyclosporine as GVHD prophylaxis. The use of this conditioning regimen was associated with a low incidence of GVHD and TRM was decreased in patients with low-grade compared to higher-grade histology. The 3-year progression-free survival was 65% for patients with low-grade lymphoma, 50% for patients with MCL, and 34% for high-grade lymphoma ($P = .002$). Donor lymphocyte infusion was given to 36 patients, 21 for relapsed or persistent disease and 15 for persistence of mixed chimerism. Investigators hypothesize that the use of donor lymphocyte infusion to treat relapse after allogeneic HCT will stimulate an effective graft-versus-lymphoma response. In one series, seven patients with FL and SLL who had relapsed after prior allogeneic HCT received donor lymphocyte infusion. Six patients responded and four experienced CRs, which have been maintained for 43 to 89 months. The effectiveness of donor lymphocyte infusion to treat relapse after allogeneic HCT provides very strong evidence for a graft-versus-lymphoma effect that can be exploited in indolent lymphomas.[107,122]

SPECIAL CONSIDERATIONS FOR TREATMENT

Waldenstrom Macroglobulinemia

The aim of treatment in Waldenstrom macroglobulinemia is to improve the quality and duration of life with minimal adverse effects in the most cost-effective manner. Whether achievement of CR confers clinical benefit is still debatable. Treatment should be reserved for symptomatic patients and should not be initiated on the basis of serum monoclonal protein levels alone. The main choices for primary treatments are alkylating agents (chlorambucil, cyclophosphamide, melphalan), purine analogues (cladribine, fludarabine), and monoclonal antibody (rituximab). Plasma exchange is indicated for the acute management of patients with symptoms of hyperviscosity because 80% of the IgM protein is intravascular. Patients may be candidates for initial combination therapy with purine nucleoside analogues or antibody therapy.

Mucosa-Associated Lymphoid Tissue Lymphomas

Bacterial infection with the gram-negative rod *H pylori* is associated with 92% of gastric MALT lymphomas.[30] Large-scale epidemiologic studies have confirmed a statistical association between *H pylori* infection and the subsequent development of gastric MALT lymphoma,[123] suggesting that gastric MALT lymphoma is "driven" by *H pylori.* These observations have led to clinical trials of antibiotic therapy in an attempt to treat MALT lymphomas. Using a combination of antibiotics and a histamine blocker for eradication of *H pylori* produces CR rates of approximately 70% in patients with localized gastric MALT lymphomas, with some molecular CRs. Of interest, responses may occur as long as 18 months after completion of antibiotic therapy. In a series of 158 patients with gastric MALT lymphoma, 54 were found to have disseminated disease, yet antibiotic treatment resulted in equivalent CR rates (74%), independent of local or disseminated disease, with overall 5- and 10-year survival rates of 86% and 80%, respectively, and median PFS of 5.6 years.[124] The importance of this findings is the suggestion that outcome can be improved with eradication of a factor that drives proliferation of the malignant cells, although putative factors driving other indolent lymphomas have yet to be identified.

The prognosis is also good for nongastrointestinal MALT lymphomas with CRs and PRs of 79% and 21%, respectively, in patients receiving various treatment approaches, including local radiation therapy, IFN-α, and/or chemotherapy.[125]

Monitoring of these patients should be performed according to guidelines such as those shown here. Morphology represents the most effective tool to assess lymphoma regression, as polymerase chain reaction can remain positive years following therapy in the absence of any sign of disease relapse.[126]

Splenic Marginal Zone Lymphoma

No consensus has been achieved on the optimal therapeutic approach in this disease. Most studies have suggested better outcomes for those patients who underwent splenectomy, suggesting that splenectomy may be the first-line treatment choice,[127] but this can be delayed until the occurrence of symptoms or cytopenia and seems to be sufficient for correcting cytopenic manifestations, improving quality of life and increasing survival (with median values of between 9 and 13 years).[33] The utility of alternative approaches, including chemotherapy, radiotherapy, or immunotherapy, is the subject of prospective clinical trials. Adverse prognostic predictors include hemolytic anemia, immune thrombocytopenia, M-component in the serum, elevated

Management of Gastric Malt Lymphoma

For patients presenting with gastric MALT lymphoma, diagnosis is usually made by endoscopic biopsy, which should be reviewed by an expert lymphoma pathologist. The stomach specimen should be tested for *Helicobacter pylori*. The disease is staged by CT scan and marrow biopsy. Treatment with antibiotics is appropriate only if the lymphoma is confined to the stomach and infection with *H pylori* is found. If the lymphoma is more advanced and has spread to surrounding lymph nodes, radiation therapy may be added. After treatment, endoscopy with biopsy should be repeated after 3 months. For advanced-stage disease, chemotherapy may be given if there are reasons for treatment, including bleeding from stomach, vital organ damage, large tumor, steady growth of lymphoma, symptoms, or enrollment in a clinical trial. For stages III and IV, treatment is similar to that used for follicular lymphoma (FL).

Endoscopy should be repeated after 3 months. If neither lymphoma nor *H pylori* is found, no further treatment is needed. If the *H pylori* is gone but lymphoma persists, then 3 more months of observation is suggested or radiation therapy delivered to the stomach, particularly if there are symptoms. If the lymphoma is gone but *H pylori* persists, then another course of different antibiotics should be given. If both the lymphoma and *H pylori* are still present, a second course of different antibiotics can be given if the lymphoma is not growing. If it is growing, then radiation therapy to the stomach and surrounding area is suggested.

A further endoscopy and biopsy should be performed at 6 months and a similar algorithm followed. Endoscopy and biopsy should be repeated again, although the exact timing is not known. If the lymphoma has not gotten smaller and radiation therapy has not been given, then the lymphoma is treated like an FL. If antibiotics have been given, then it is treated with radiation therapy.

Summary: For localized disease with *H pylori*, treat with antibiotics. If the lymphoma is gone, no more treatment is needed. If the lymphoma returns after antibiotic therapy, radiation therapy should be given. If the lymphoma returns after radiation therapy, it should be treated with chemotherapy as for FL. If it has spread to a site away from the stomach, it should be treated with chemotherapy as for FL.

β2-microglobulin level, leukocyte count >20,000/μL, lymphocytes >9000/μL, and p53 overexpression by neoplastic cells.[33,127] Progression to DLBCL has been recorded rarely.

Mantle Cell Lymphoma

The treatment of mantle cell lymphoma merits special attention. The treatment of choice in this disease is entry into a clinical trial because there is no generally accepted therapeutic approach, treatment options are often limited, and chemoresistance is common. Therefore, novel therapies are required for relapsed and/or refractory MCL. There is widespread acceptance of the use of anthracycline-based combination chemotherapy, despite the fact that the only randomized trial examining this question showed no benefit for CHOP compared to COP.[128] Despite response rates of up to 97% with first-line standard or high-intensity chemotherapy, most patients relapse with or without autologous hematopoietic cell transplantation.[41,45,129–132] Single-agent fludarabine produces a 41% overall response rate with few CRs.[133] Single-agent rituximab has moderate activity in MCL, with response rates of 38% in both previously untreated and treated patients, with some patients achieving CR. The median duration of response was 15 months.[133] Longer survival has been reported with high-intensity

Management of Mantle Cell Lymphoma

The management of mantle cell lymphoma represents a great challenge. This disease has the worst prognosis among all of the B-cell lymphomas and carries the incurability of the indolent lymphomas with a more aggressive clinical course. Aggressive chemotherapy regimens are being explored. Rituximab with cyclophosphamide, adriamycin, vincristine, and prednisone (R-CHOP) or R-EPOCH are suitable for elderly patients, but promising results have been obtained using the R-Hyper-CVAD regimen. Once relapse has occurred, experimental treatment approaches are indicated and promising results have been obtained using bortezomib, particularly in combination with rituximab. Prolongation in progression-free survival has been observed with the use of high-dose chemoimmunotherapy and autologous hematopoietic cell transplantation. There is evidence for a graft-versus-lymphoma effect and in the setting of clinical trials, ablative and nonmyeloablative allogeneic hematopoietic cell transplantation may be indicated.

regimens such as hyper-CVAD, especially when used in combination with rituximab.[130,131] A Cochrane analysis has shown that the addition of rituximab to chemotherapy is superior to chemotherapy alone.[134] After the first relapse, prognosis is considered very poor, with median survival of less than 2 years.[41] Novel treatment approaches include the investigation of bortezomib, which shows activity in MCL,[135–138] particularly in combination with rituximab.

Several phase II studies have suggested a role for consolidation with high-dose therapy and autologous HCT.[139,140] However, on longer-term follow-up, this does not appear to be curative.[141] The European MCL Network have reported results of a randomized trial comparing consolidation with myeloablative radiochemotherapy followed by autologous HCT compared to maintenance in first remission.[142] Patients 65 years of age or younger with advanced-stage MCL were assigned to autologous HCT or IFN-α after achievement of complete or partial remission using a CHOP-like induction therapy. Among 122 patients enrolled, 62 patients proceeded to autologous HCT and 60 received IFN-α. Patients in the autologous HCT arm experienced a significantly longer PFS (median 39 months) compared with patients in the IFN-α arm (median 17 months). The 3-year OS was 83% after autologous HCT versus 77% in the IFN group ($P = .18$). The study demonstrated that consolidation by myeloablative radiochemotherapy followed by autologous HCT is feasible and results in a significant prolongation of PFS in advanced-stage MCL, but longer follow-up is needed to determine the effect on OS.

Long-lasting remissions can be achieved using allogeneic HCT, but this can be associated with high morbidity and mortality in the more elderly patients with this disease.[143] Recent results have suggested that RIC approaches prior to allogeneic transplantation may be associated with decreased mortality and good disease control.[144]

SUGGESTED READINGS

Cerhan JR, Wang S, Maurer MJ, et al: Prognostic significance of host immune gene polymorphisms in follicular lymphoma survival. Blood 109:5439, 2007.

Cheson BD, Pfistner B, Juweid ME, et al: Revised response criteria for malignant lymphoma. J Clin Oncol 25:579, 2007.

Colombat P, Brousse N, Morschhauser F, et al: Single treatment with rituximab monotherapy for low-tumor burden follicular lymphoma (FL): Survival analyses with extended follow-up of 7 years. Blood 108:147a, 2006.

Eichhorst BF, Busch R, Hopfinger G, et al: Fludarabine plus cyclophosphamide versus fludarabine alone in first-line therapy of younger patients with chronic lymphocytic leukemia. Blood 107:885, 2006.

Escalon MP, Champlin RE, Saliba RM, et al: Nonmyeloablative allogeneic hematopoietic transplantation: A promising salvage therapy for patients with non-Hodgkin's lymphoma whose disease has failed a prior autologous transplantation. J Clin Oncol 22:2419, 2004.

Fisher RI, Bernstein SH, Kahl BS, et al: Multicenter phase II study of bortezomib in patients with relapsed or refractory mantle cell lymphoma. J Clin Oncol 24:4867, 2006.

Friedberg JW, Huang J, Dillon H, et al: Initial therapeutic strategy in follicular lymphoma: An analysis from the National LymphoCare study. J Clin Oncol 24:7527a, 2006.

Ghobrial IM, Fonseca R, Gertz MA, et al: Prognostic model for disease-specific and overall mortality in newly diagnosed symptomatic patients with Waldenstrom macroglobulinaemia. Br J Haematol 133:158, 2006.

Giordano TP, Henderson L, Landgren O, et al: Risk of non-Hodgkin lymphoma and lymphoproliferative precursor diseases in US veterans with hepatitis C virus. JAMA 297:2010, 2007.

Gribben JG, Zahrieh D, Stephans K, et al: Autologous and allogeneic stem cell transplantations for poor-risk chronic lymphocytic leukemia. Blood 106:4389, 2005.

Hiddemann W, Hoster E, Buske C, et al: Rituximab is the essential treatment modality that underlies the significant improvement in short and long term outcome of patients with advanced stage follicular lymphoma: A 10 year analysis of GLSG trials. Blood 108:147a, 2006.

Kaminski MS, Tuck M, Estes J, et al: ^{131}I-tositumomab therapy as initial treatment for follicular lymphoma. N Engl J Med 352:441, 2005.

Keating MJ, O'Brien S, Albitar M, et al: Early results of a chemoimmunotherapy regimen of fludarabine, cyclophosphamide, and rituximab as initial therapy for chronic lymphocytic leukemia. J Clin Oncol 23:4079, 2005.

Parsonnet J, Hansen S, Rodriguez L, et al: *Helicobacter pylori* infection and gastric lymphoma. N Engl J Med 330:1267, 1994.

Peterson BA, Petroni GR, Frizzera G, et al: Prolonged single-agent versus combination chemotherapy in indolent follicular lymphomas: A study of the Cancer and Leukemia Group B. J Clin Oncol 21:5, 2003.

Schulz H, Bohlius J, Skoetz N, et al: Combined immunochemotherapy with rituximab improves overall survival in patients with follicular and mantle cell lymphoma: Updated meta-analysis results. Blood 108:781a, 2006.

Schulz H, Bohlius JF, Trelle S, et al: Immunochemotherapy with rituximab and overall survival in patients with indolent or mantle cell lymphoma: A systematic review and meta-analysis. J Natl Cancer Inst 99:706, 2007.

van Oers MH, Klasa R, Marcus RE, et al: Rituximab maintenance improves clinical outcome of relapsed/resistant follicular non-Hodgkin lymphoma in patients both with and without rituximab during induction: Results of a prospective randomized phase 3 intergroup trial. Blood 108:3295, 2006.

REFERENCES

For complete list of references log onto www.expertconsult.com

CHAPTER 80

DIAGNOSIS AND TREATMENT OF NON-HODGKIN LYMPHOMA (AGGRESSIVE)

Kieron Dunleavy and Wyndham H. Wilson

INTRODUCTION

The term "aggressive" non-Hodgkin lymphoma (NHL) encompasses several distinct disease entities that are defined in the World Health Organization (WHO) classification of tumors of the lymphoid system (Table 80–1). Although the approach to the diagnosis of these diseases is similar, management varies according to the lymphoma subtype, and for this reason an accurate histological diagnosis is of utmost importance.

CLINICAL FEATURES

The clinical presentation of aggressive NHL is variable and depends on a number of factors including histology, patient age and immune status. Aggressive NHL typically presents with lymphadenopathy that can range from relatively asymptomatic to causing organ compromise such as ureteral obstruction or spinal cord compression. Certain histological subtypes are associated with distinct features at diagnosis such as ileocecal involvement in Burkitt lymphoma (BL) and lymphomatoid polyposis in mantle cell lymphoma (MCL). In most aggressive NHL, bone marrow involvement is less common than with low-grade lymphomas.

Patients may have constitutional manifestations from the production of inflammatory molecules and a variety of other cytokines and chemokines produced by the lymphoma cells or host tissues. Such manifestations include weight loss, malaise, fevers, night sweats, and loss of appetite. Of these, unexplained weight loss of more than 10% of body weight and temperature higher than 38°C (100.4°F), and drenching night sweats are referred to as *B symptoms*.

INVESTIGATION

History and Physical Examination

Patients should be questioned about systemic symptoms and performance status should be assessed (Table 80–2). It is important to determine if there is a history of potential causative factors such as prior malignancy, chemotherapy or radiation treatment and/or autoimmune or immunodeficiency disease. A history of infection with, or exposure to various pathogens including HIV, hepatitis C and HTLV-1 should be excluded. A detailed physical examination should be performed with detailed attention to lymph node regions.

An accurate histological diagnosis is imperative to determine prognosis and treatment; therefore the single most important diagnostic test is a properly evaluated and technically adequate lymph node biopsy. With few exceptions, fine needle aspiration is inadequate for diagnosis. Aggressive lymphoma should be diagnosed by an experienced pathologist familiar with the nuances and pitfalls of lymphoma diagnosis.

Laboratory Investigations

Laboratory tests should include a complete blood count, serum chemistry (including lactate dehydrogenase [LDH]), human immunodeficiency virus (HIV), and hepatitis serology tests. Other viral tests such as human T-lymphocyte virus-1 (HTLV-1) should be included as indicated. Epstein Barr virus (EBV) viral loads may also be useful in specific lymphomas such as posttransplant lymphoproliferative disorders (PTLD) and nasal NK/T-cell lymphoma.[1,2] An elevated LDH has prognostic implications for certain lymphoma subtypes.

Imaging and Staging

It is important to determine sites of disease involvement (Table 80–3) Imaging studies should include chest radiography and computed tomography (CT) scanning of the chest, abdomen and pelvis. (Fig. 80–1 and 80–2) The need for additional imaging studies such as magnetic resonance imaging (MRI) and positron emission tomography (PET) scanning will depend on the clinical presentation and sites of disease. For example, if central nervous system (CNS) involvement is highly suspected, evaluation of the head by MRI may be indicated. Involvement of the bone is best evaluated by MRI and PET scans. Although PET scanning is widely used for lymphoma imaging, it does not have an established role in the initial staging of aggressive NHL.[3] However, it may be a useful adjunct to CT for staging in certain clinical situations.

While marrow involvement is highly variable in aggressive lymphomas, presence of lymphoma cells in marrow affects management and should be assessed in all patients at initial staging. Patients at increased risk of central nervous system (CNS) involvement should undergo lumbar puncture with evaluation of the cerebrospinal fluid (CSF) by cytology and flow cytometry.[4] Specifically, histological subtypes such as BL, and clinical presentations such as extranodal disease in diffuse, large B cell lymphoma (DLBCL) are associated with an increased risk of CNS disease.[5]

Aggressive NHL is staged according to the Ann Arbor staging system (Table 80–4), which was originally designed for Hodgkin lymphoma (HL). However, because of the heterogeneity and hematogenous pattern of dissemination in NHL, in contrast to contiguous lymph node spread with HL, the staging system has more limited value. At the same time, important modifications to the Ann Arbor staging system made at the Cotswold Conference have made it more applicable to NHL.[6]

Prognosis

To identify prognostic factors in NHL, an international project to correlate clinical variables and outcome in 2031 patients with untreated aggressive lymphoma was undertaken.[7] The following parameters were associated with inferior outcome: age over 60 years, Ann Arbor stage III or IV disease, serum LDH above normal range, Eastern Cooperative Oncology Group (ECOG) performance status of two or higher, and involvement of two or more extranodal sites. A clinical prognostic model, termed the International Prognostic Index (IPI) was developed using these five factors (Table 80–5). In this model, one point was allocated for each feature and nicely stratified patients into 4 groups with 5-year survivals of 73%, 51%, 43% and 26% for 0–1, 2, 3, and 4–5 risk factors, respectively, with

Table 80–1 Classification of Aggressive Lymphomas

B cell neoplasms
Precursor B-cell lymphoma
Precursor B lymphoblastic leukemia/lymphoma
Mature B-cell lymphoma
Mantle cell lymphoma
Diffuse large B-cell lymphoma
Mediastinal (thymic) large B-cell lymphoma
Intravascular large B-cell lymphoma
Primary effusion lymphoma
Burkitt lymphoma/leukemia
B-cell proliferations of uncertain malignant potential
Lymphomatoid granulomatosis
Posttransplant lymphoproliferative disorder, polymorphic
T-cell and NK-cell neoplasms
Precursor T-cell
Precursor T lymphoblastic leukemia/lymphoma
Blastic NK cell lymphoma
Mature T-cell and NK-cell lymphoma
Adult T-cell leukemia/lymphoma
Extranodal NK/T cell lymphoma, nasal type
Hepatosplenic T-cell lymphoma
Peripheral T-cell lymphoma, unspecified
Angioimmunoblastic T-cell lymphoma
Anaplastic large cell lymphoma

Table 80–2 Eastern Cooperative Group (ECOG) Performance Scale

Performance Status	Definition
0	Asymptomatic
1	Symptomatic but fully ambulatory
2	Symptomatic and in bed <50% of the day
3	Symptomatic and in bed >50% of the day
4	Bedridden

Table 80–3 Staging Evaluation

All Patients	As clinically indicated
History and physical examination	Other viral studies
CBC and chemistry (including LDH)	CT or MRI head
HIV and hepatitis B and C serology	Body PET scan
Chest radiograph	Additional imaging
CT scan of chest, abdomen, and pelvis	CSF evaluation by cytology/flow cytometry
Bone marrow aspirate and biopsy	Other tests indicated by results of staging

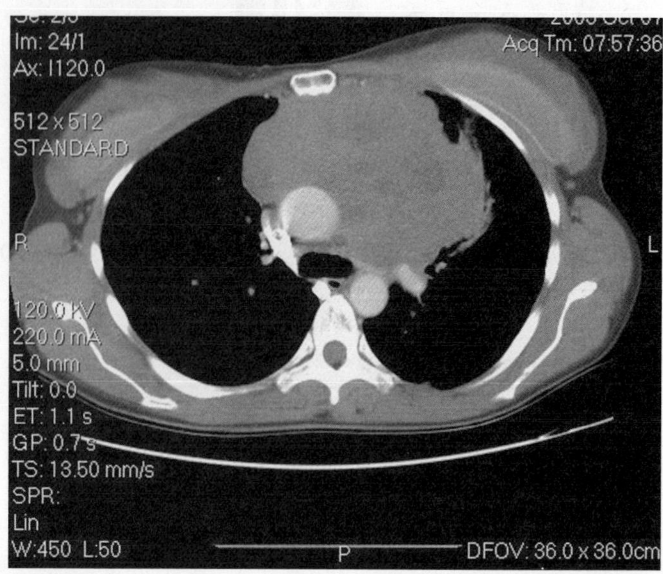

Figure 80–1 Computed tomography scan of the chest showing a large 17 cm anterior mediastinal mass. A biopsy was consistent with primary mediastinal B-cell lymphoma (PMBL).

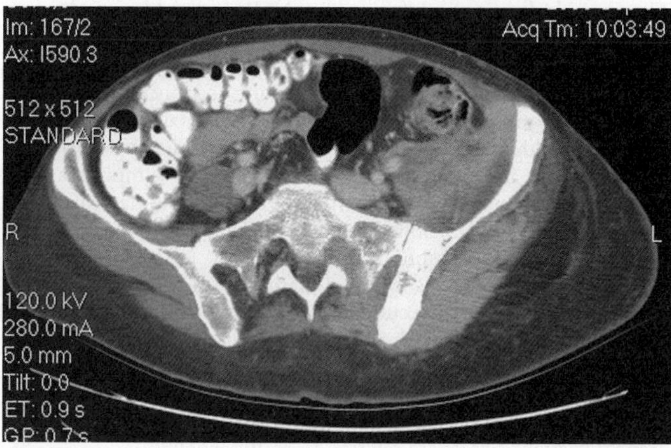

Figure 80–2 Computed tomography scan of the abdomen showing a large left-sided psoas mass. A biopsy was consistent with diffuse large B-cell lymphoma.

CHOP-based treatment.[7] Based on this model, the IPI has become the standard for assessing clinical prognosis, and treatment stratification within and comparison between clinical trials. Although it has yet to be fully revalidated in the rituximab era, a revised prognostic model for R-CHOP, termed R_{evised}-IPI, was recently published based on a limited retrospective series (Table 80–6).[8]

Although not yet routinely performed in aggressive NHL, gene expression profiling is emerging as an important prognostic tool.[9–12] In DLBCL, for example, morphologically indistinguishable tumors can show marked heterogeneity in gene expression, and these patterns of expression may be classified into signatures that correspond with the cellular origin of the lymphoma according to its stage of differentiation. On the basis of these signatures, DLBCL can be divided into at least 3 different subtypes: germinal center B-cell (GCB) like, activated B-cell (ABC) like and primary mediastinal B-cell lymphoma (PMBL). Overall survival is different in each group and superior in patients with the GCB compared to the ABC type. Using gene expression profiling, a molecular prognostic model of survival, independent of the IPI, has been also been developed for CHOP treated DLBCL.[10] This model is based on four signatures: germinal-center B cells, proliferating cells, reactive stromal and immune cells in the lymph node and major-histocompatibility-complex class II cells. This molecular prognostic model has not yet been applied to rituximab based treatment. An immunohistochemical (IHC) model has also been developed to predict GCB and non-GCB subtypes of DLBCL.[13] Although this IHC model requires further validation, its application in two recent studies suggest that the addition of rituximab to chemotherapy ameliorates the adverse outcome of non-GCB DLBCL.[14,15]

Recently, the gene expression profile of BL has been elucidated. Of note, some cases of DLBCL by histology had gene expression profiles consistent with BL.[16,17] Since BL does not respond well to CHOP based treatments, gene expression profiling may be important

Table 80–4 Ann Arbor Staging System for Lymphomas

Stage*	Cotswold Modification of Ann Arbor Classification
I	Involvement of a single lymph node region or lymphoid structure
II	Involvement of two or more lymph node regions on the same side of the diaphragm (the mediastinum is considered a single site, whereas the hilar lymph nodes are considered bilaterally); the number of anatomic sites should be indicated by a subscript (e.g., II_3)
III	Involvement of lymph node regions on both sides of the diaphragm: III_1 (with or without involvement of splenic hilar, celiac, or portal nodes) and III_2 (with involvement of para-aortic, iliac, and mesenteric nodes)
IV	Involvement of one or more extranodal sites in addition to a site for which the designation E has been used

All cases are subclassified to indicate the absence (A) or presence (B) of the systemic symptoms of significant fever (>38.0° C [100.4° F]), night sweats, and unexplained weight loss exceeding 10% of normal body weight within the previous 6 months. The clinical stage (CS) denotes the stage as determined by all diagnostic examinations and a single diagnostic biopsy only. In the Ann Arbor classification, the term pathologic stage (PS) is used if a second biopsy of any kind has been obtained, whether negative or positive. In the Cotswold modification, the PS is determined by laparotomy; X designates bulky disease (widening of the mediastinum by more than one third or the presence of a nodal mass >10 cm), and E designates involvement of a single extranodal site that is contiguous or proximal to the known nodal site.

Table 80–5 International Prognostic Index for Aggressive Lymphomas[7]

Risk Group	IPI Score	CR Rate (%)	5 year overall survival (%)
Low	0, 1	87	73
Low intermediate	2	67	51
High intermediate	3	55	43
High	4,5	44	26

*One point is given for the presence of each of the following characteristics: age >60 years, elevated serum LDH level, ECOG performance status ≥ 2, Ann Arbor stage III or IV, and more than two extranodal sites.
CR, complete response; ECOG, Eastern Cooperative Oncology Group; IPI, International Prognostic Index; LDH, lactate dehydrogenase.

Table 80–6 Revised International Prognostic Index (R-IPI)*[8]

No. of IPI Factors	IPI Score	Outcome	Overall Survival
0	0	Very Good	94%
1–2	1–2	Good	79%
3, 4, or 5	3–5	Poor	55%

*One point is given for the presence of each of the following characteristics: age >60 years, elevated serum LDH level, ECOG performance status ≥ 2, Ann Arbor stage III or IV, and more than two extranodal sites.
ECOG, Eastern Cooperative Oncology Group; IPI, International Prognostic Index; LDH, lactate dehydrogenase.

in rare cases that would otherwise be diagnosed as DLBCL. Gene expression profiling has also generated survival predictors in mantle cell lymphoma (MCL) and is being applied to T-cell lymphomas.[12,18,19] Although molecular profiling remains an experimental technique that is not widely available, it will undoubtedly help to improve pathologic diagnostic accuracy, predict outcome with greater precision and help elucidate pathways of lymphomagenesis. This should lead to the identification of novel cellular targets and subsequent personalized therapy. The integration of immunostaining and gene expression profiling into large prospective clinical trials is imperative in order to facilitate the investigation and development of new and useful prognostic models that may guide therapeutic choices.

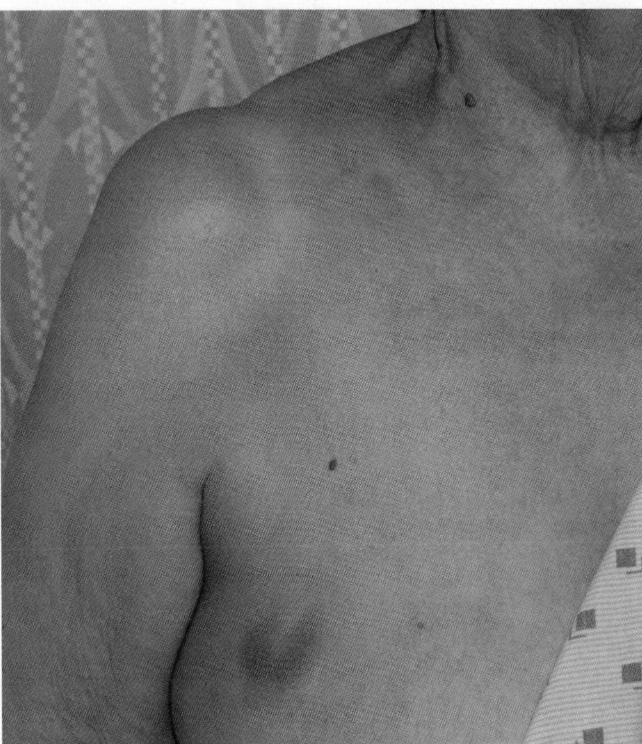

Figure 80–3 Infiltration of the right lower anterior chest wall with diffuse large B-cell lymphoma (DLBCL).

AGGRESSIVE B-CELL LYMPHOMAS

The most common aggressive B-cell lymphomas are DLBCL, BL, and MCL. They have variable natural histories and in the case of MCL, a quarter of patients have an indolent clinical course.[12] Unlike indolent B-cell lymphomas, these aggressive subtypes are more rapidly progressive and with the exception of MCL, are potentially curable. For this reason, it is imperative to promptly evaluate patients and expeditiously institute appropriate therapy.

Diffuse Large B Cell Lymphoma (DLBCL)

Diffuse large B-cell lymphoma is the most prevalent histologic subtype of NHL and compromises 30% to 40% of these diseases.[20] Though the median age at diagnosis is in the seventh decade, DLBCL affects children and adults of all ages. Patients may present with localized or disseminated disease and with nodal or extra-nodal involvement. (Fig. 80–3) Within DLBCL, there are several morphological variants that include centroblastic, immunoblastic, T-cell rich/histiocyte rich and anaplastic subtypes, and progress in molecular profiling is further advancing this taxonomy.[10,21] There are also several clinical-pathologic variants of DLBCL. Primary mediastinal B-cell lymphoma (PMBL) represents one such variant that more commonly presents in young women and usually remains localized to the mediastinum. It is important to recognize that DLBCL can also arise as a result of histologic transformation from an indolent lymphoma. Though this differentiation may not affect treatment choice initially, it will affect prognosis and natural history and therefore needs to be recognized at diagnosis.

The mainstay of treatment for DLBCL is systemic chemotherapy; radiation treatment alone is inadequate and associated with high recurrence rates.[22] For early stage disease, whether or not radiation treatment adds benefit to chemotherapy has been controversial. Based on a randomized study that showed a survival advantage of limited course CHOP plus involved field radiation compared to full course CHOP in early stage (I/II) aggressive lymphoma, combined modality therapy became the standard.[23] However, longer patient follow-up showed a convergence of the overall survival curves due to late systemic relapses in the combined modality arm—thus reopening the debate on radiation.[23,24] In this regard, a recent prospective Groupe d'Etude des Lymphomes de l'Adulte (GELA) study randomized 576 elderly patients with favorable early stage aggressive lymphoma to receive CHOP alone (4 cycles) or CHOP plus radiation and found that combined modality therapy was not superior to chemotherapy alone.[25] Given these results and the improved outcome of CHOP with rituximab (R-CHOP), it is difficult to justify the routine use of radiation in early stage disease.

A possible exception to the omission of radiation, however, is in the treatment of primary mediastinal DLBCL (PMBL), depending on the chemotherapy regimen. In a study of 50 untreated patients with PMBL who received MACOP-B followed by radiation, 66% had persistently positive gallium scans after chemotherapy, suggesting active disease. Following consolidation radiotherapy, however, only 19% of patients had a positive gallium scan and 80% were event free at 39 months median follow-up.[26] This important study suggested that radiotherapy was necessary following chemotherapy. Furthermore, there is historical evidence that dose intense regimens such as MACOP-B or VACOP-B are superior to CHOP for PMBL, raising yet another question about the optimal chemotherapy for this disease.[27–29] Recent results with the pharmacodynamically dose adjusted regimen of doxorubicin, vincristine and etoposide infused over 96 hours with bolus intravenous cyclophosphamide, rituximab and oral prednisone (DA-EPOCH-R) may be challenging the need for radiation in PMBL.[30,31] In a phase II study of DA-EPOCH-R in 26 patients with PMBL, 100% and 91% are alive and event free at a median 4.2 year follow-up, respectively, and only 2 patients required radiation treatment.[32] These results suggest that DA-EPOCH-R obviates the need for radiation in most patients with PMBL, thus eliminating the risk of long-term toxicities such as secondary malignancies and heart disease. This is particularly important given that patients afflicted with PMBL are typically young and often women, and are at increased risk of breast and other cancers as well as late term toxicities. Of course, it is possible that patients who receive R-CHOP may also not require radiation therapy, but this question needs to be carefully studied.

Systemic treatment is required for advanced DLBCL (Table 80–7). The CHOP regimen was developed some 30 years ago and established as the standard by a randomized trial which showed CHOP was equally effective to three other common albeit more

Table 80–7 Treatment Regimens for Diffuse Large B-cell Lymphoma

Study	Therapy	Patient group	Event-free Survival	Overall Survival	Reference
Phase III R-CHOP V CHOP	R-CHOP GELA	Age ≥60 y All IPI	EFS: 47% at 5 years	58% at 5 years	43, 44
Phase III R-CHOP V CHOP	R-CHOP U.S. intergroup	Age ≥60 y All IPI	FFS: 53% at 3 years	NA	45
Phase III R-CHOP-like V CHOP	R-CHOP-like* MInT	Age ≤60 y Low IPI	EFS: 79% at 3 years	93% at 3 years	47
Phase III ACVBP V CHOP	ACVBP GELA	Age ≥60 y. At least 1 IPI factor	EFS: 39% at 5 years	46% at 5 years	35
Single arm Phase II	DA-EPOCH-R NCI	Age ≥18 years All IPI	PFS: 82% at 43 months	79% at 43 months	48
Phase III: 4 arms CHOP-14, CHOP-21, CHOEP-14, CHOEP-21	CHOEP-21 DSHNHL	Age 18–60 y. Good prognosis disease	EFS: 69.2% at 5 years	NA	39
Phase III: 4 arms CHOP-14, CHOP-21, CHOEP-14, CHOEP-21	CHOP-14 DSHNHL	Age 61–75 years. All IPI	EFS: 43.8% at 5 years	53.3% at 5 years	38
Phase III: 4 arms R-CHOP-14 × 8, R-CHOP-14 × 6, R-CHOP-21 × 8, R-CHOP-21 × 6	R-CHOP-14 (X6) DSHNHL	Age ≥60 y. All IPI	EFS: 66% at 3 years	78% at 3 years	46

*CHOP like regimens included CHOP, CHOEP, MACOP-B, PmitCEBO.

ACVBP: doxorubicin, cyclophosphamide, vindesine, bleomycin, prednisone; CHOEP: cyclophosphamide, doxorubicin, vincristine, etoposide, prednisone; DA-EPOCH-R: dose-adjusted etoposide, prednisone, vincristine, cyclophosphamide, doxorubicin; DSHNHL: Deutsche Studiengruppe für Hochmaligne Non-Hodgkin' Lymphome; GELA: Groupe d'Etude Lymphomes d'Adultes; MACOP-B: methorexate, doxorubicin, cyclophosphamide, vincristine, prednisone, bleomycin; MINT: MabThera International Trial; NCI: National Cancer Institute; PmitCEBO: prednisone, mitozantrone, cyclophosphamide, etoposide, bleomycin, vincristine; R-CHOP: rituximab, cyclophosphamide, doxorubicin, vincristine, prednisone.

complex and/or toxic regimens.[33] The fact that only 44% of patients achieved complete remissions with CHOP, however, left significant room for improvement and spawned multiple studies aimed at improving treatment outcome.[33,34] Many of these studies have focused on modifications to the CHOP platform. A GELA study compared doxorubicin; cyclophosphamide, vindesine, bleomycin and prednisone (ACVBP) to CHOP in elderly patients with aggressive lymphoma and showed a superior 5 year EFS of 39% and OS of 46% compared to 29% and 38% for CHOP, respectively.[35] Much of the benefit in the ACVBP arm, however, was due to a lower incidence of central nervous system (CNS) progression, which could be attributed to the use of CNS prophylaxis with ACVB. Furthermore, a previous study of ACVBP in low IPI patients showed no benefit over m-BACOD, which was shown to be equivalent to CHOP.[36]

In aggressive lymphomas, high tumor proliferation determined by Ki-67 or MIB-1 immunohistochemistry has been shown to be an adverse prognostic finding with CHOP chemotherapy, suggesting that "kinetic" failure is a problem.[10,37] One strategy to overcome "kinetic" failure is to increase dose density through frequent chemotherapy administration. The Deutsche Studiengruppe für Hochmaligne Non-Hodgkin' Lymphome (DSHNHL) group evaluated the effect of dose density and etoposide in two four-arm studies of CHOP administered every 14 or 21 days, with or without etoposide (CHOEP), in patients older than 60 years and low-risk patients 60 years or younger.[38,39] In younger patients, CHOEP-21 showed the best overall results with a CR rate of 88% versus 79%, and EFS of 69% versus 58% at 5 years compared to standard CHOP-21, respectively.[39] In older patients, however, dose dense CHOP-14 showed the best outcome with a CR rate of 76% versus 60%, and EFS of 44% versus 33% at 5 years compared to standard CHOP-21.[38] While these studies provided the best evidence that outcome could be improved through specific changes to the CHOP chemotherapy platform, it remains unclear why optimal treatment differed in the studies given the continuum in disease biology across age.[10] The question of whether dose intensity or the addition of etoposide can improve outcome has been and continues to be addressed in various other studies.[40,41]

An alternative strategy to dose density is to increase the fractional cell kill or efficacy of chemotherapy, thereby reducing the number of tumor cells that can survive and proliferate between cycles. Longer drug exposure may take advantage of the increased sensitivity of cycling cells, and in vitro studies have shown that prolonged low concentration exposure to vincristine and doxorubicin, compared with brief higher-concentration exposure, can increase cytotoxicity by up to one log.[42] This approach was translated into the pharmacodynamically dose adjusted DA-EPOCH regimen, which showed a promising PFS and OS of 70% and 73%, respectively, at 5 years median follow-up in newly diagnosed DLBCL.[30] Interestingly, high tumor proliferation was not found to be an adverse biomarker in this study.[30]

It has been the development of rituximab that has made the single greatest impact on the treatment of DLBCL since CHOP was first introduced over 30 years ago. The first study to show the benefit of rituximab was performed by GELA where patients over 60 years were randomized to receive CHOP or CHOP with rituximab (R-CHOP).[43] In this study, the complete remission (CR) (76% versus 63%) and 5-year event free survival (EFS) (47% versus 29%) were higher with R-CHOP than CHOP, respectively, making R-CHOP the de facto standard in DLBCL.[43,44] The benefit of rituximab was later confirmed by the US intergroup study in a similar patient population.[45]

With the benefit of rituximab established, investigators have gone on to explore its use in a variety of clinical settings and treatment strategies. The DSHNHL group explored the question of whether there was a difference in outcome between six or eight cycles of treatment in a randomized study of six versus eight cycles of CHOP-14, with or without rituximab, in elderly patients with DLBCL. In that study, termed the RECOVER-60 trial, they found no difference in outcome with six versus eight cycles of treatment.[46] Although they showed an excellent 3-year EFS of 66% with R-CHOP-14 over six cycles, which is somewhat better than the GELA and US intergroup study results, one cannot conclude that R-CHOP-14 is superior to standard R-CHOP-21, given all the caveats of interstudy comparisons. The MabThera International Trial (MInT) studied the benefit of rituximab with CHOP-based treatment in younger patients (= 60 years) with favorable characteristics defined as low IPI risk; furthermore, nearly half of patients received involved field radiotherapy.[47] Similar to the other randomized rituximab studies, patients who received rituximab fared significantly better with a 3-year EFS of 79%. As an interesting aside, the MInT study also showed that rituximab obviated the benefit of CHOEP in younger patients.[47]

Rituximab has also been tested in combination with the DA-EPOCH regimen.[48] In a recent report of 72 patients, 82% and 79% of patients were progression free and alive, respectively, at the median follow-up of 43 months. Furthermore, 93% and 64% of patients in the low and high IPI risk groups, respectively, had not progressed. While one must be cautious in interpreting preliminary results, it should be noted that these findings are consistent with a recent phase II of DA-EPOCH-R in which 91% and 45% of patients with high-Intermediate and high IPI, respectively, were event free at two years.[49] Evaluation of DA-EPOCH-R versus R-CHOP in untreated DLBCL is currently ongoing in the Cancer and Leukemia Group B (CALGB) cooperative group in conjunction with microarray analysis.

While it is clear that rituximab has significantly improved the overall outcome of DLBCL, several studies suggest its benefit is limited by tumor pathobiology.[50–52] Two studies found rituximab benefit was primarily in Bcl-2 positive DLBCL, while another study showed benefit was limited to Bcl-6 negative DLBCL.[50–52] These biomarkers suggest that rituximab may primarily benefit tumors derived from a post-germinal center B cell.[10,11,53] At this point, though, it is not possible to accurately identify who will benefit from rituximab, and further progress is critical to help identify new strategies and molecular targets for patients who do not benefit from rituximab.

The role of high dose chemotherapy and autologous hematopoietic cell transplantation (HCT) in the initial treatment of DLBCL remains controversial.[54,55] Although some studies have suggested benefit, they were performed in the pre-rituximab era.[56] Autologous HCT is also associated with late toxicities, including leukemia and secondary myelodysplasia, which must be considered in the risk benefit of treatment.[57]

Primary Central Nervous System Lymphoma (PCNSL)

Primary central nervous system lymphoma (PCNSL) is a rare and highly aggressive lymphoma confined to the CNS, and is usually of diffuse large B-cell histology. (Fig. 80–4) Its unique radiographic findings presents challenges in evaluation which have been recently addressed in a report of an international workshop to standardize criteria for baseline evaluation and response.[58] The incidence of PCNSL is particularly high in the setting of HIV infection where it often presents with multifocal disease and is virtually always associated with Epstein Barr virus (EBV). In contrast, PCNSL in HIV negative patients often presents with solitary intracranial masses and is rarely associated with EBV.

Treatment of PCNSL differs from systemic DLBCL because many chemotherapy agents do not adequately penetrate the blood-brain barrier. Radiotherapy has been a mainstay of treatment because it is effective and side stepped the limitations of chemotherapy, but responses are usually short-lived and virtually all patients relapse. High-dose methotrexate (HD-MTX) on the other hand is a cytotoxic agent with good CNS penetration, but when used alone progression-free survival is a relatively short 7 months.[59] A logical step was to combine HD-MTX followed by whole brain radiotherapy and produced an impressive 82% to 88% complete remission and median progression free-survival rates of 32 to 40 months.[59–61] Unfortunately, such combined modality treatment is associated with severe long-term neurotoxicity.[59,62] For this reason, there has been much interest in developing regimens that obviate or defer the need for radiation until relapse. Most promising, in this regard are combinations of high

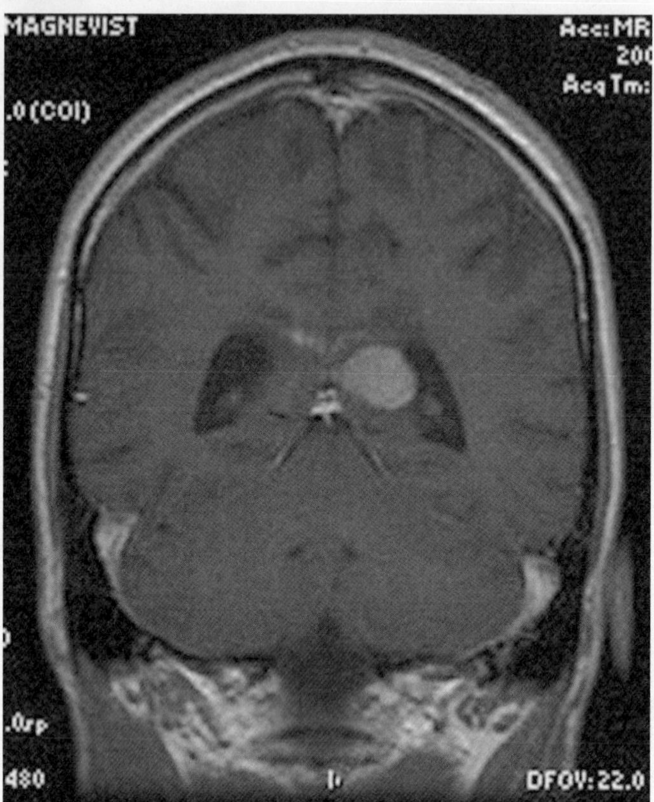

Figure 80–4 This gadolinium enhanced MRI scan of the brain shows an enhancing infiltrative mass in the major forceps of the corpus callosum. A biopsy was consistent with primary central nervous system lymphoma (PCNSL).

dose methotrexate with systemic agents that cross the blood brain barrier, such as cytarabine, vincristine and ifosfamide, particularly in patients under 60 years of age.[63] The Bonn group and others have adopted such an approach and have reported promising results with chemotherapy and deferred radiation in younger patients.[63,64] These results require further validation in trials. Studies are also addressing the role of immunochemotherapy with rituximab and other novel agents which promise to improve the outcome of PCNSL.[65]

Burkitt Lymphoma (BL)

Burkitt lymphoma (BL) most commonly occurs in the first two decades of life and accounts for some 2% of all lymphomas.[20] Burkitt lymphoma is highly aggressive as reflected by its 100% tumor proliferation by MIB-1 immunohistochemistry and high spontaneous apoptosis which accounts for its starry sky appearance. Biologically, BL is derived from a germinal center B cell as indicated by its CD20+, CD10+ and TdT negative immunohistochemical profile and gene expression profiling.[16] Three clinical variants are recognized: Endemic BL which is primarily found in equatorial Africa; Sporadic BL which presents worldwide but is the most common type in Western countries and; Immunodeficiency associated BL which is associated with HIV infection. There are important clinical differences in these variants. Endemic BL typically presents with jaw and facial bone disease and is virtually always associated with EBV. Sporadic BL usually presents with ileocecal disease and is associated with EBV in 30% to 50% of cases. Immunodeficiency associated BL usually occurs in HIV positive populations and is associated with nodal disease and is variably associated with EBV. Burkitt lymphoma may be associated with CNS involvement, particularly when there is bulky or disseminated disease. Rare cases present as acute leukemia and are included in the French-American-British (FAB) classification.[20]

Burkitt lymphoma requires chemotherapy for all disease stages. Several biological characteristics of BL have helped guide treatment strategies including its high proliferative fraction. The high tumor proliferation rate led to the use of dose intense regimens with a short cycle time to theoretically minimize tumor regrowth between cycles.[66,67] Multiple drugs, typically administered in alternating combinations, are employed and the high rate of spread to the CNS has led to the standard use of CNS prophylaxis.[68] A variety of dose-intense short duration regimens have achieved durable complete remissions in 47% to 84% of patients.[69–72] Included in these are the French LMB and German Berlin-Frankfurt-Munster (BFM) protocols and the National Cancer Institute CODOX-M/IVAC regimen. These regimens are similar in their drug composition, short cycle length and CNS prophylaxis. Although BL is most common in children, Magrath and colleagues demonstrated that adults have a similar disease outcome when treated with the same regimen.[66] Toxicity is an important clinical limitation of these regimens in adults, particularly in older patients where severe morbidity and even mortality occur. Therefore, one of the major therapeutic challenges in BL is to develop therapies that are as effective in achieving high cure rates as "standard" regimens but that improve the therapeutic index and reduce toxicity complications. This approach is being investigated in a pilot study of DA-EPOCH-R. Based on studies in DLBCL which suggested DA-EPOCH overcomes the adverse effect of high proliferation, likely due to its infusional schedule, it appeared to be a good candidate to test in adult BL.[30] Indeed, preliminary results in 17 patients with BL showed an EFS and OS of 92% and 100%, respectively, at a median follow-up of 28 months, with low toxicity compared to conventional regimens.[30,32]

Mantle Cell Lymphoma (MCL)

Mantle cell lymphoma (MCL) s a relatively rare B-cell lymphoma, which comprises some 3% of all lymphomas and has a median age of 60 years and male predominance.[21] Its pathobiology is characterized by dysregulation of the cell cycle with almost all cases showing the t(11;14) translocation and overexpression of cyclin-D1 (bcl-1). Hence, immunohistochemical detection of cyclin D1 along with CD20 and CD5 is virtually diagnostic of MCL.[20] The biological importance of cell cycle dysregulation in MCL was elegantly demonstrated by gene-expression profiling where the tumor proliferation signature was the best molecular predictor of survival.[12]

Most patients present with advanced stage disease and based on historical series have a median survival of 3 to 5 years. While overall survival appears to be improving with the development of more effective therapies, cure remains elusive for most patients.[73] Treatment approaches are constrained by the older median age of MCL with more aggressive regimens often preferred in younger patients. One of the more promising and aggressive regimens for MCL is fractionated cyclophosphamide administered with doxorubicin, vincristine, and dexamethasone (Hyper-CVAD), alternating with high-dose methotrexate and cytarabine.[74] In an initial phase II study of 45 previously treated and untreated patients, 38% achieved CR with an overall response of 94%; of these patients, 29 went on to receive autologous HCT consolidation.[74] Among the 25 previously untreated patients, EFS and OS at 3 years were 72% and 92%, respectively, which appeared significantly better than historical outcomes with CHOP based treatment.[75] Recently, a study of Hyper-CVAD with rituximab alternating with high-dose methotrexate and cytarabine was reported in untreated MCL.[76] In this study, 87% of patients achieved CR and at 3 years, 64% were failure free. Although effective, the unacceptable toxicity in older patients led the authors to recommend it only in patients younger than 66 years of age. Other studies have shown that the addition of rituximab to CHOP improves response rates and time to treatment failure, but not survival.[77,78] The DA-EPOCH-R regimen has also shown good efficacy in untreated MCL with 93% of patients achieving CR but similar to other studies, most patients ultimately relapse.[79]

There has been much interest in investigating the role of high-dose chemotherapy and autologous HCT in MCL, and several phase II studies show promising results.[80–83] While a number of these studies have shown excellent event free survival (EFS) and overall survival (OS), patient selection is by necessity biased and there is no convincing plateau on the Kaplan-Meier curves. Even in the absence of significant cures, it is possible that autologous HCT may prolong survival; however, this can only be judged in the context of a randomized study. Allogeneic HCT, frequently employing reduced intensity conditioning, has also been investigated in MCL.[84] In one study of 18 patients, 17 achieved CR, and there were only three progressions with 26 months median follow-up.[84] The 3-year EFS of 82% suggests that a graft-versus-lymphoma effect plays an important role.

Recently, the proteasome inhibitor bortezomib has shown promising activity in patients with relapsed or refractory MCL. After demonstrating activity in two small phase II studies, a large multicenter study reported a response rate of 33% with 8% CR in relapsed or refractory MCL.[85–87] The mTOR inhibitor temsirolimus has also shown interesting results with a response rate of 38%.[88] A small phase II study also reported a favorable response rate of 90% for the combination of rituximab and thalidomide.[89] Presently, combinations of bortezomib and chemotherapy are being investigated in MCL and it is likely in the near future, that other novel agents will find their way into clinical trials for untreated patients.

EBV Associated Lymphoproliferative Disorders

The loss of adequate EBV immune surveillance underlies the pathobiology of virtually all EBV associated lymphoproliferative disorders (LPD).[90] It is useful to consider the origin of the immune suppression as it affects disease biology and treatment. The most commonly recognized diseases are associated with iatrogenic immunosuppression, as exemplified by posttransplant LPD (PTLD) and MTX-associated LPD.[91,92] Diseases associated with acquired immunosuppression are heterogeneous and include senile EBV+ B-cell LPD and lymphomatoid granulomatosis.[93–95] Congenital immunodeficiencies comprise the last group and include such entities as Wiskott-Aldrich syndrome (WAS) and X-linked severe combined immunodeficiency (SCID) which are associated with EBV related LPDs.[90]

Posttransplant lymphoproliferative disorder (PTLD) encompasses a broad spectrum of diseases which occur in the setting of allogeneic hematological and solid organ transplantation; as a group, they show considerable heterogeneity.[92,94] PTLD is classically approached by withdrawal of immunosuppression, providing the possibility of organ rejection is not life threatening, and often in conjunction with rituximab. Chemotherapy, however, is frequently required, particularly in patients with monomorphic histology, where the clone is usually immune independent.[96] EBV+ LPD arising in the setting of chronic immune suppression with methotrexate can also respond to withdrawal of the offending agent, although most cases require chemotherapy.[91] Senile EBV+ B-cell LPD's are increasingly being recognized and are postulated to arise in the setting of age-related waning of EBV immune surveillance.[93] In general, they should be approached as other aggressive lymphomas while recognizing that highly localized disease with limited involvement by EBV+ large B-cells may be self-limited. Lymphomatoid granulomatosis (LYG) is a rare EBV associated LPD which primarily occurs in otherwise healthy patients who on examination have evidence of immune deficiency.[94,95] LYG virtually always involves extranodal sites and can be treated with interferon or immunochemotherapy, depending on the grade of disease.[94]

AGGRESSIVE T/NATURAL KILLER (T/NK) CELL LYMPHOMAS

Lymphomas of T/NK cells are relatively uncommon and account for approximately 15% of all NHL.[20,97] They are distributed over at least 14 different subtypes, all of which are infrequent and not well studied. Those tumor types with an identifiable clinical-pathobiology are classified by name, whereas the other cases are simply described as "peripheral T-cell lymphoma, unspecified" ($PTCL_{us}$); which by design is a heterogeneous group. Generally, T/NK cell lymphomas are clinically aggressive, though some can behave quite indolently, and unlike their aggressive B-cell cousins, most are incurable. Important exceptions to cure include anaplastic large cell lymphoma (ALCL) and early stage T/NK cell, nasal type lymphoma.

To help define the outcome of aggressive T/NK and B-cell lymphomas in the international arena, the Non-Hodgkin Lymphoma Classification Project examined all newly diagnosed cases of lymphoma over a 2-year period from multiple international centers.[98] A survival analysis predictably demonstrated a poor outcome of $PTCL_{us}$ compared with DLBCL. Similar to DLBCL, the IPI was predictive of outcome in $PTCL_{us}$. At 5 years, only one quarter of low-IPI patients were alive without disease. This is in contrast to the anaplastic large cell lymphoma (ALCL) subtype in which 80% of patients were alive at 5 years regardless of the IPI score.

Three large series of PTCL treated with CHOP-based therapy have been reported.[99–101] The overall CR varied from 49% to 65% and in all series, ALCL had a favorable outcome. Like the NHL Classification Project, IPI score predicted outcome with 5-year survivals of 60% to 80% in low (0–1), 20% in intermediate (2–3) and 0% in high (4–5) IPI patients.[102]

Anaplastic Large Cell Lymphoma (ALCL)

ALCL is a CD30 positive T-cell lymphoma with an excellent prognosis and unlike the other PTCLs, it frequently can be cured. It typically occurs in children and young adults and compromises approximately 3% of all lymphomas in adults. In some 80% of cases, ALCL is associated with the t(2;5)(p23;q35) translocation, resulting in expression of the nucleophosmin anaplastic lymphoma kinase (ALK).[103] While ALK positive ALCL has a significantly better prognosis than ALK negative cases, patients with ALK negative disease should still be approached with curative intent.[103] In adults, CHOP-based therapy is considered the standard of care and produces durable remissions in approximately 65% of ALK+ and 35% of ALK negative ALCL.[104]

Extranodal T/NK-cell Lymphoma; Nasal Type

This is a rare extranodal lymphoma characterized by a broad morphological spectrum. It is more prevalent in Asia and Central/South America and is almost always associated with EBV.[21] It has a predilection for the nasal cavity, nasopharynx, palate, skin, gastrointestinal tract, and testis. Hemophagocytic syndrome is a devastating event associated with this tumor type.[105] Disease outside the nasal cavity is usually highly aggressive and associated with a poor prognosis. Because of its rarity and lack of prospective clinical trials, optimal therapy has not been defined. However, disease localized to the nasal cavity can be cured with radiotherapy. The beneficial of chemotherapy in this setting has yet to be defined.[106]

Angioimmunoblastic T-cell Lymphoma (AILT)

Angioblastic T cell lymphoma is characterized by systemic symptoms, skin rash, organomegaly, hypergammaglobulinemia, and hemolytic anemia. It most commonly afflicts older patients and frequently presents with peripheral lymphadenopathy, hepatosplenomegaly, skin rash, and constitutional symptoms, which distinguish it from other peripheral T-cell lymphomas.[107] Patients often exhibit some degree of immunodeficiency, polyclonal hypergammaglobulinemia, and other hematological abnormalities, which are probably related to abnormal immune regulation.[108] The neoplastic T cells appear to be of germinal center origin, known as follicular B helper T (T_{FH}) cells.[109,110] A prominent histological feature of AILT is the near uni-

Table 80–8 Salvage Regimens for Aggressive Lymphoma

Therapy	Patient Group	CR Rate (%)	Overall response (%)	Survival	Reference
DHAP	Relapsed or refractory lymphoma	31%	57.5	OS: 25% at 2 years	135
ESHAP	Relapsed or refractory lymphoma	37%	70	OS: 31% at 3 years	136
EPOCH	Relapsed or refractory DLBCL	36%	70	OS: 30% at 6 years	139
R-ICE	Relapsed or refractory DLBCL	53%	88	NA	132

DHAP: dexamethasone, cytarabine, cisplatin; EPOCH: etoposide, prednisone, vincristine, cyclophosphamide, doxorubicin; ESHAP: etoposide, methylprednisone, cytarabine, cisplatin;
R-ICE: rituximab, ifosfamide, carboplatin, etoposide.

versal presence of EBV positive B cells within the lesions.[111,112] Optimal therapy has not been defined for AILT but anthracycline-based regimens and purine analogs have shown some efficacy.[107,113] Recently, novel approaches such as the use of cyclosporine and anti-angiogenesis therapies such as bevacizumab have shown activity and warrant further investigation in the future.[114,115] Unfortunately, most patients succumb from infection or disease.

Hepatosplenic T-cell Lymphoma

This extranodal T-cell lymphoma presents with marked hepato-splenomegaly and bone marrow involvement.[116] Most cases have and T-cell receptor rearrangement which if present in other PTCLs, portends a particularly poor prognosis.[20,117] The disease often afflicts younger males and occurs with increased frequency in the setting of iatrogenic immune suppression.[118] Outcome is extremely poor and is characterized by rapid progression and death, although allogeneic transplantation has been associated with prolonged remission and potential cure.[119]

Peripheral T-cell Lymphoma, Unspecified

The poor outcome of $PTCL_{us}$ has prompted the search for new strategies and targeted agents. Purine analogs are associated with good response rates but are rarely curative.[120] Alemtuzumab, a monoclonal antibody that binds CD52 is expressed on most $PTCL_{us}$ and has shown a 36% response rate in one series of heavily pretreated patients. The success of immunochemotherapy in B-cell lymphomas has led to several ongoing studies of alemtuzumab and chemotherapy.[121] Other novel agents with activity in this disorder include denileukin, diftitox, and the histone deacetylase inhibitor depsipeptide.[122,123] While autologous HCT may provide some benefit, a recent report of a graft versus lymphoma effect in PTCL suggests that allogeneic HCT may have curative potential.[124,125]

Precursor B-cell and T-cell Lymphoma

Precursor B-lymphoblastic and T-lymphoblastic lymphomas (LBL) are highly aggressive diseases with primarily nodal presentations, but are cytologically identical to acute lymphoblastic leukemia (ALL).[20] Precursor T-LBL comprises approximately 90% of lymphoblastic lymphomas and typically presents in young males with a mediastinal mass and occasional involvement of the meningeal space. A variety of chemotherapy regimens have been used including ACVBP, leukemia-based regimens and autologous HCT.[126,127] A recent study published by the British Columbia Transplant Group reported an excellent outcome with induction chemotherapy followed by stem cell transplantation; in this study, 69% of patients were event-free at four years.[127] An earlier German study evaluated an ALL-type regimen in 45 adult patients with T-LBL and reported a 62% disease-free survival at seven years.[128] These studies highlight the need for very aggressive therapies in these diseases.

PROPHYLACTIC INTRATHECAL (IT) CHEMOTHERAPY FOR AGGRESSIVE B-CELL LYMPHOMA

Although secondary involvement of the CNS (central nervous system) in aggressive B-cell lymphoma is rare, it is usually a fatal complication and strategies aimed at preventing it are important. Certain clinical risk factors are associated with an increased risk of CNS relapse and the risk benefit appears to favor prophylactic intrathecal chemotherapy in such patients.

These risk factors include a diagnosis of Burkitt lymphoma (BL) and AIDS-related lymphoma (ARL), and diffuse large B-cell lymphoma that presents with diffuse bone or bone marrow involvement, or two or more extra-nodal sites with an elevated lactate dehydrogenase (LDH). Testicular involvement is also a high-risk disease site. All patients at risk should undergo lumbar puncture with CSF evaluation and a brain MRI scan. Recent studies indicate that flow cytometry is significantly more sensitive than conventional cytology for detection of CSF involvement and should be performed. Patients with evidence of CNS disease at diagnosis receive a treatment course of IT chemotherapy.

SALVAGE THERAPY

The salvage treatment of relapsed DLBCL should be approached in an individual manner as the choice of treatment is influenced by the time to recurrence, prior therapy, medical condition and the potential for cure. While most relapsed aggressive lymphomas require combination chemotherapy for adequate disease control, it is important to recognize that patients with local disease may be salvaged with radiation therapy. Examples include primary mediastinal DLBCL, which can remain local even at relapse, and PTLDs, which may have an isolated resistant EBV clone following chemotherapy.[129]

There are a variety of active salvage chemotherapy regimens for relapsed or refractory DLBCL (Table 80–8).[130–136] Platinum containing regimens, such as ESHAP and ICE, are currently among the most widely used salvage treatment.[132,134,137] It is a commonly held notion that salvage treatment should include different agents from past treatment to avoid drug resistance. Recent evidence indicates, however, that sensitivity to apoptosis is a central cause of drug resistance and that drug-specific mechanisms are less important.[10,138] Hence, salvage regimens developed around the most active up-front agents should show high activity.[139] This concept was tested with EPOCH chemotherapy in patients who had failed after receiving similar drugs on a bolus schedule.[139] In this study of 67 patients with relapsed/refractory

HOW WE TREAT PRIMARY MEDIASTINAL B-CELL LYMPHOMA (PMBL)

PMBL predominantly affects females in the third to fourth decade. Standard treatment usually involves doxorubicin-based chemotherapy and involved field radiation. Although combined modality therapy is highly effective, the inclusion of radiation increases the late risk of secondary tumors and cardiac disease. A recent study indicates that rituximab significantly improves the survival of PMBL when combined with DA-EPOCH chemotherapy and obviates the need for radiation in 92% of patients.

Based on these results, we treat PMBL with six cycles of DA-EPOCH-R. At the completion of therapy, we perform a CT (computed tomography) and PET (positron emission tomography) scan to determine complete response. Patients with proven residual disease receive consolidation radiation treatment. It is important to note, however, that PET scan abnormalities are common on treatment completion and may not represent residual disease. Because of the low specificity of PET, we usually perform a biopsy in patients with persistent or worsening PET abnormalities before commencing radiation treatment.

de novo aggressive lymphoma, 70% responded with 36% complete remissions. The addition of rituximab appears to enhance the activity of salvage regimens as demonstrated by results with R-ICE and ICE which showed a CR of 53% and 27%, respectively.[132,137]

Patients with chemotherapy sensitive disease have the best outcome with autologous HCT and is recommended at initial relapse. Autologous HCT used as salvage therapy in chemoresponsive patients has yielded OS and EFS in the range of 40% to 50% and 30% to 40%, respectively.[132,140] Autologous HCT rarely achieves cure in BL and LBL, but it is often successful in ALK positive ALCL. Lymphomas that are rarely cured with initial treatment, such as MCL and PTCL, are less likely to benefit from autologous HCT. It is important to consider, when assessing the outcome of autologous HCT, improvements in upfront therapy from rituximab have resulted in relapse population with greater resistance. The incorporation of rituximab or radioimmunoconjugate into conditioning regimens may also enhance the benefit of autologous HCT, thus underscoring the importance of controlled autologous HCT trials in the post-rituximab era.[132,140] Patients with chemotherapy resistant disease do poorly with autologous HCT, but may still benefit from allogeneic HCT.

LATE COMPLICATIONS OF TREATMENT

It is important to recognize that successful treatment may be associated with late complications that may not appear for decades. Among the major late term complications are secondary malignancies, ischemic heart disease, anthracycline-related cardiotoxicity, and radiation or bleomycin-induced pulmonary toxicity.[141] The risk of developing myelodysplastic disorders and acute myeloid leukemia is related to alkylator and topoisomerase inhibitor use and is enhanced by radiation. Radiation therapy increases the risk of malignancy in the treatment region and in particular, breast cancer in women and lung cancer in smokers. Indeed, it is imperative to consider late-term toxicity when selecting treatment.

A general guideline for follow-up after initial therapy involves visits every three months for two years, every six months for three years, and annually thereafter. During these visits, examination of the lymph node areas, abdomen, thyroid, and skin is important. CT scans are recommended in routine follow-up. It is important to note that CT scans are associated with a relatively high radiation exposure and should not be used unnecessarily.[142] PET scans are not recommended for routine follow-up because the high rate of false positive scans is unlikely to offset the value of early detection. Indeed, the role of PET sans in the overall treatment of lymphomas requires prospective studies.[143] Routine laboratory studies with blood counts, liver function tests, and LD should be performed. Patients with disease in the chest can be followed with chest radiographs. Thyroid-stimulating hormone levels should be monitored annually in patients who received neck radiotherapy. Mammography for women should begin ten years from diagnosis of lymphoma or at age 40, whichever comes first. Patients should be immunized against influenza yearly and against pneumococcus every six years.

FUTURE DIRECTIONS

There has been marked progress in our understanding of molecular events underlying aggressive lymphomas, particularly B-cell diseases. Powerful techniques such as gene expression profiling, array-CGH, and RNAi have paved the way for the identification of new targets and the development of small molecule inhibitors. Indeed, a number of targeted agents have entered clinical trials including inhibitors of mTOR, proteasome, histone deacetylation, and bcl-2. Other approaches such as incorporation of rituximab, autologous and even allogeneic HCT into algorithms for patient treatment are likely to have an impact on prolonged remission and cure of aggressive NHL. The challenge will be to determine the priority, sequence and combination of active agents needed for initial treatment and salvage therapy through well-designed clinical trials.

SUGGESTED READING LIST

A predictive model for aggressive non-Hodgkin's lymphoma. The International Non-Hodgkin's Lymphoma Prognostic Factors Project. N Engl J Med 329:987, 1993.

Blum KA, Lozanski G, Byrd JC: Adult Burkitt leukemia and lymphoma. Blood 104:3009, 2004.

Cheson BD, Pfistner B, Juweid ME, et al: Revised response criteria for malignant lymphoma. J Clin Oncol 25:579, 2007.

Feugier P, Van Hoof A, Sebban C, et al: Long-term results of the R-CHOP study in the treatment of elderly patients with diffuse large B-cell lymphoma: a study by the Groupe d'Etude des Lymphomes de l'Adulte. J Clin Oncol 23:4117, 2005.

Fisher RI, Bernstein SH, Kahl BS, et al: Multicenter phase II study of bortezomib in patients with relapsed or refractory mantle cell lymphoma. J Clin Oncol 24:4867, 2006.

Greer JP: Therapy of peripheral T/NK neoplasms. Hematology Am Soc Hematol Educ Program. 2006:331, 2006.

Gutierrez M, Chabner BA, Pearson D, et al: Role of a doxorubicin-containing regimen in relapsed and resistant lymphomas: an 8-year follow-up study of EPOCH. J Clin Oncol 18:3633, 2000.

Habermann TM, Weller EA, Morrison VA, et al: Rituximab-CHOP versus CHOP alone or with maintenance rituximab in older patients with diffuse large B-Cell lymphoma. J Clin Oncol 24:3121, 2006.

Kewalramani T, Zelenetz AD, Nimer SD, et al: Rituximab and ICE as second-line therapy before autologous stem cell transplantation for relapsed or primary refractory diffuse large B-cell lymphoma. Blood 103:3684, 2004.

Pels H, Schmidt-Wolf IG, Glasmacher A, et al: Primary central nervous system lymphoma: results of a pilot and phase II study of systemic and intraventricular chemotherapy with deferred radiotherapy. J Clin Oncol 21:4489, 2003.

Pfreundschuh M, Trumper L, Osterborg A, et al: CHOP-like chemotherapy plus rituximab versus CHOP-like chemotherapy alone in young patients with good-prognosis diffuse large-B-cell lymphoma: a randomised controlled trial by the MabThera International Trial (MInT) Group. Lancet Oncol 7:379, 2006.

Romaguera JE, Fayad L, Rodriguez MA, et al: High rate of durable remissions after treatment of newly diagnosed aggressive mantle-cell lymphoma with rituximab plus hyper-CVAD alternating with rituximab plus high-dose methotrexate and cytarabine. J Clin Oncol 23:7013, 2005.

Rosenwald A, Wright G, Chan WC, et al: The use of molecular profiling to predict survival after chemotherapy for diffuse large-B-cell lymphoma. N Engl J Med 346:1937, 2002.

van Besien K, Ha CS, Murphy S, et al: Risk factors, treatment, and outcome of central nervous system recurrence in adults with intermediate-grade and immunoblastic lymphoma. Blood 91:1178, 1998.

Wilson WH, Grossbard ML, Pittaluga S, et al: Dose-adjusted EPOCH chemotherapy for untreated large B-cell lymphomas: a pharmacodynamic approach with high efficacy. Blood 99:2685, 2002.

Winter JN, Weller EA, Horning SJ, et al: Prognostic significance of Bcl-6 protein expression in DLBCL treated with CHOP or R-CHOP: a prospective correlative study. Blood 107:4207, 2006.nErratum in: Blood 109:2292, 2007.

CHAPTER 81

MALIGNANT LYMPHOMAS IN CHILDHOOD

John T. Sandlund, Jr. and Michael P. Link

INTRODUCTION

Malignant lymphomas are the third most common malignancy among children and adolescents.[1–4] Among children less than 15 years of age, non-Hodgkin lymphoma (NHL) is more frequent; however, in patients up to 18 years of age, Hodgkin disease is predominant.[2] NHLs in children are usually extranodal diffuse high-grade tumors, whereas low- and intermediate-grade nodal lymphomas predominate in adults.[5] These differences are speculated to reflect maturational changes in the function and composition of the immune system.[6] The different histologies explain in part the differing clinical features, disease course, and treatment strategies used in adults and children.

The differences in treatment approach and disease subtypes are less striking in adults and children with Hodgkin disease. However, there are significant challenges in the management of children with Hodgkin disease. These primarily comprise the sequelae of therapy, such as radiation-induced bone growth abnormalities, endocrine dysfunction, and chemotherapy-related sterility. Of greater concern are the radiation- and chemotherapy-related second malignancies and late cardiac deaths. Current trials are under way to examine ways to reduce the toxicity of therapy without compromising the excellent outcome generally achieved. These issues, as well as differences between children and adults in the proportion of histologic subtypes, are covered in Chapter 74, which deals with the management of Hodgkin disease in adults.

EPIDEMIOLOGY

The incidence of NHL increases steadily throughout life, in contrast to Hodgkin disease, which has a bimodal age distribution with peaks in early and late adulthood.[2] Although the NHLs may occur at any age in childhood, they occur very infrequently among children younger than 3 years of age; the median age at presentation is approximately 10 years. NHL occurs 2 to 3 times more often in boys than in girls and is almost twice as common in whites as in African Americans—the reasons for these differences have yet to be determined.[7]

Specific populations at risk for the development of NHL include those with either congenital or acquired immunodeficiency conditions.[8–12] Inherited immunodeficiency syndromes include Wiskott–Aldrich syndrome, X-linked lymphoproliferative syndrome (XLP), and ataxia-telangiectasia (AT). The recognition of these syndromes in children with newly diagnosed NHL is important for appropriate therapeutic design. For example, involved field irradiation and the use of radiomimetics should be avoided in children with AT. Additionally, children with AT are at increased risk for the development of cyclophosphamide-induced hemorrhagic cystitis; therefore, they should receive vigorous hydration and uroprotectants (eg, MESNA) when administering any dose of cyclophosphamide. XLP should be considered in any male with a high-grade B-cell lymphoma who either develops a late recurrence (second occurrence) of a high-grade B-cell lymphoma or has a brother with either a high-grade B-cell lymphoma or fatal infectious mononucleosis. Children with acquired immunodeficiency conditions that predispose to the development of NHL include those who have received posttransplant immunosuppressive therapy and those with the acquired immunodeficiency syndrome (AIDS).

There are differences in both the incidence and proportion of histologic subtypes in different parts of the world. For example, the NHLs are very rare in Japan but occur quite frequently in equatorial Africa. Burkitt lymphoma, which accounts for about one-half of all childhood cancers in equatorial Africa, is the predominant NHL histologic subtype in both equatorial Africa and northeast Brazil.[13] There are also geographic differences in both the clinical and biologic features of certain NHL subtypes.[14,15] For example, Burkitt lymphoma in equatorial Africa ("endemic" Burkitt lymphoma) is clinically characterized by frequent involvement of the abdomen, jaw, paraspinal region, orbit, and central nervous system. In contrast, Burkitt lymphoma occurring in the United States and Western Europe ("sporadic" Burkitt lymphoma) typically involves the abdomen, nasopharynx, and bone marrow. The predominant chromosome 8 breakpoints among sporadic cases occur within the MYC gene, whereas those in endemic cases usually occur upstream of the MYC gene.[16,17]

In equatorial Africa, the region of high incidence of Burkitt lymphoma overlaps with the malaria belt.[18] This observation prompted investigators to search for an infectious cause for this disease. This effort led to the discovery of the association between Epstein–Barr virus (EBV) and this tumor. Although no direct pathogenic role has been demonstrated for this virus, it has been speculated that as a B-cell mitogen, EBV increases the target pool of cells for transformation. This hypothesis is supported by the observation that Rag gene expression can be induced by EBV, an event that may theoretically increase the chance of a translocation occurring in B cells that are rearranging their immunoglobulin genes.[19] The potential role of EBV in pathogenesis is also strengthened by the observation that lymphomas develop in mice that are transgenic for EBV nuclear antigen 1 (EBNA-1).[20] Moreover, an EBNA-1 variant has been found to be associated with the majority of EBV-positive Burkitt lymphoma cases, suggesting that this mutation may provide a growth advantage to lymphoma cells by modifying EBNA-1 function in some way.[21] A more direct role for EBV in lymphomagenesis is suggested by analyses of the EBV+ Burkitt lymphoma cell line, Akata.[22] When this cell line spontaneously loses EBV episome, it loses its malignant phenotype; however, on reinfection with EBV, a malignant phenotype is again observed. EBV is associated with 90% of African (endemic) Burkitt lymphoma cases, but with only 15% of cases in the United States (sporadic).[23–28] Disrupted and aberrant expression of the EBV genome has been identified in the host genome of sporadic Burkitt lymphoma cells that appeared to be EBV-negative by conventional EBNA testing.[29] This finding, together with the 50% EBV-positive rate among Burkitt lymphoma cases in other parts of the world (eg, South America) suggests that EBV has a widespread role in the pathogenesis of this malignancy.[13,30]

CLASSIFICATION

After Thomas Hodgkin described the disease bearing his name in 1832, various schemes emerged to classify the tumors now collectively referred to as the NHLs. Several classification schemes were developed based on histopathologic features and the putative cell of origin. In an attempt to reduce the confusion of multiple classification schemes, the National Cancer Institute (NCI) sponsored a workshop to design a single classification scheme for clinical usage. This scheme published in 1982 and referred to as the NCI Working Formulation was widely accepted for almost two decades.[5] In the Working Formulation, the NHLs of childhood are predominantly diffuse high-grade tumors and can be divided among three major subgroups: lymphoblastic, small noncleaved cell, and large-cell lymphomas.

In the past decade, additional classification schemes were designed to improve on the NCI Working formulation. Because of the problems associated with attempts to classify lymphoid neoplasms into categories based on presumed normal cell counterparts, the International Lymphoma Study Group proposed a classification system for lymphoid neoplasms[31] predicated on a practical approach to categorization of these diseases using available immunologic and molecular genetic techniques in addition to the standard morphologic criteria. This Revised European-American Classification of Lymphoid Neoplasms (REAL Classification) has been endorsed by many of the world's leading lymphoma pathologists,[31,32] and it has served as the basis for the World Health Organization (WHO) classification of hematopoietic and lymphoid tumors.[33] Both the REAL and WHO classification systems include related lymphoid leukemias and recognize that NHL and acute lymphoblastic leukemia (ALL) represent different stages of evolution within specific morphologically and immunologically defined disease categories—an observation recognized by clinicians caring for children with lymphoid neoplasms and reflected in current clinical practice that prescribes similar therapies for lymphomas and leukemias of related phenotype.

In the REAL[31] and WHO[33] classification systems, the non-Hodgkin lymphomas that occur commonly in children appear in four major categories: precursor B-cell neoplasms (including precursor B-lymphoblastic leukemia/lymphoma); precursor T-cell neoplasms (including precursor T-lymphoblastic leukemia/lymphoma); mature (or peripheral) B-cell neoplasms (including Burkitt lymphoma/leukemia and the apparently related entity "high-grade B-cell lymphoma, Burkitt-like," diffuse large B-cell lymphoma and the subtype mediastinal [thymic] large B-cell lymphoma); and mature (or peripheral) T cell and NK-cell neoplasms (including anaplastic large-cell lymphoma, CD30$^+$, and T- and null-cell types).

The clinical and biologic characteristics of NHL in children are summarized in Table 81–1 and illustrated in Fig. 81–1.

Burkitt Lymphoma

The designation of "small noncleaved cell" lymphoma used in the NCI Working Formulation[5] has been replaced by the designation of "Burkitt's lymphoma" in both the REAL[31] and WHO[33] classification systems. The Burkitt lymphoma designation also includes the L3-ALL leukemia subtype (Burkitt leukemia) of the French–American–British classification system.[34] Histologically, Burkitt lymphoma is characterized by a diffuse infiltrative pattern of monomorphic small- to medium-sized cells with round nuclei, clumped chromatin, 1 to 3 nucleoli, and basophilic cytoplasm. Tingible body macrophages interspersed among lymphoma cells result in a "starry sky" appearance under low-power microscopic examination. An atypical or Burkitt-like lymphoma, which is also described in the WHO classification system, is characterized by a wider range in nuclear shape and size, and nucleoli that are larger but fewer in number.[33,35] The Burkitt-like lymphomas may be difficult to distinguish from the diffuse large B-cell lymphomas.

Burkitt lymphoma is a mature B-cell lymphoma expressing surface immunoglobulin (usually IgM, or less commonly IgA or IgG, and kappa or lambda light-chain restriction), as well as other B cell-associated antigens, including CD19, CD20, CD22, and CD79a.[33] CD10 may be detected in more than 50% of cases studied. CD21, the EBV receptor, is more frequently detected in the endemic than sporadic Burkitt subtype. There are very unusual cases of Burkitt lymphoma that express cytoplasmic mu but no surface immunoglobulin, as well as some cases that express neither.[36,37]

Cytogenetically, Burkitt lymphomas are characterized by the presence of one of three reciprocal chromosomal translocations.[38–40] The unifying feature in these translocations is the juxtaposition of the c-*myc* protooncogene on chromosome 8 with one of the three immunoglobulin genes, resulting in deregulation of the c-*myc* gene. The classical translocation t(8;14)(q24;q32), which involves the heavy-chain immunoglobulin locus, is identified in approximately 85% of cases. Each of two variant translocations, t(2;8)(p12;q24) and t(8;22)(q24;q11), involves one of the two light-chain immunoglobulin loci; these account for the remaining 15% of cases.

Expression of the c-*myc* gene is associated with cell proliferation. For example, in normal B cells, mitogenic stimulation results in increased rates of c-*myc* transcription. The c-myc protein induces cell cycle progression from G_1 to S phase through the activation of various target genes.[41] This DNA-binding protein forms heterodimers with related proteins (eg, MAX, MAD) that subsequently influence cell cycling.[42–45] In Burkitt lymphoma, it has been speculated that the deregulated expression of c-*myc* results in an increased proportion of MYC–MAX complexes, leading to tumor cell proliferation.[46]

There are various theories about the pathogenic mechanism of c-*myc* deregulation in Burkitt lymphoma.[47–50] The invariable presence of mutations (truncations or point mutations) in the translocated c-*myc* gene has led to speculation that these mutations result in deregu-

Table 81–1 Clinical and Biologic Characteristics of Non-Hodgkin Lymphoma in Children

Subtype	Proportion of Cases (%)[a]	Phenotype	Primary Site	Translocation	Affected Genes
Burkitt	39	B cell	Abdomen or head and neck	t(8;14)(q24;q32) t(2;8)(p11;q24) t(8;22)(q24;q11)	IgH-c*MYC* Igκ-c*MYC* Igλ-c*MYC*
Lymphoblastic	28	T-cell[b]	Mediastinum or head and neck	t(1;14)(p32;q11) t(11;14)(p13;q11) t(11;14)(p15;q11) t(10;14)(q24;q11) t(7;19)(q35;p13) t(8;14)(q24;q11) t(1;7)(p34;q34)	TCRαδ-*TAL1* TCRαδ-*RHOMB2* TCRαδ-*RHOMB1* TCRαδ-*HOX11* TCRβ-*LYL1* TCRαδ-*MYC* TCRβ-*LCK*
Large cell					
ALCL	10	T cell, indeterminate	Mediastinum, abdomen, head and neck, bone, soft tissue or skin	t(2;5)(p23;q35)	*NPM-ALK*
DLBCL	16	B cell	Mediastinum, abdomen, head and neck		

ALCL, anaplastic large cell lymphoma; DLBCL, diffuse large B-cell lymphoma; TCR, T-cell receptor.
[a]Proportion at St. Jude Children's Research Hospital; other histotypes account for approximately 7%.
[b]B-cell-progenitor variants have also been described.

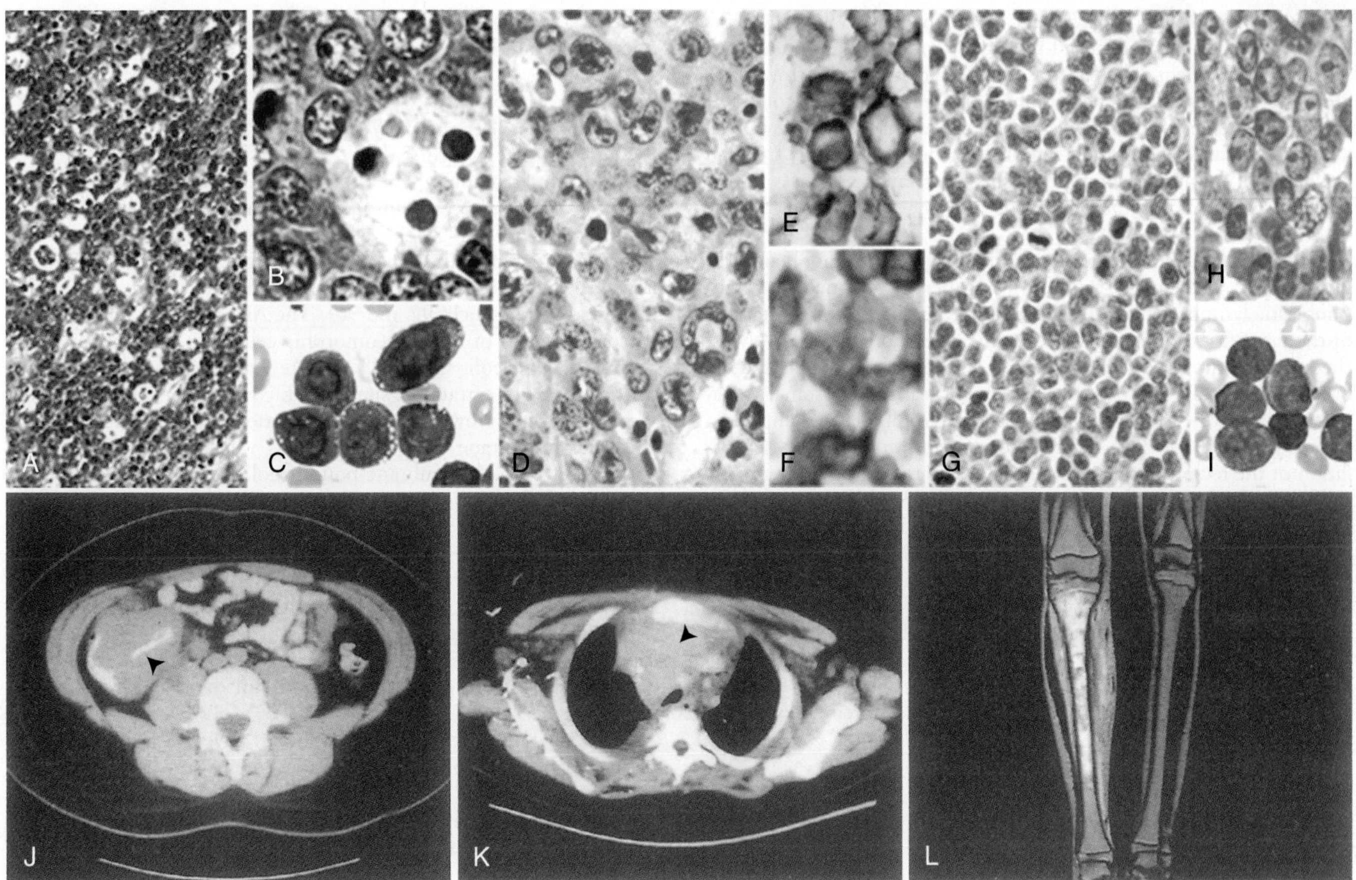

Figure 81–1 Burkitt lymphoma, anaplastic large-cell lymphoma, lymphoblastic lymphoma: **A–I**. Burkitt lymphoma (**A**) showing the classic "starry-sky" low power appearance of sheets of dark intermediate-sized lymphoma cells growing in syncytia, interspersed with scattered tingible body macrophages with abundant clear cytoplasm. At high power (**B**), the Burkitt cells have coarse chromatin, multiple nucleoli, and are adjacent to a large tingible body macrophage containing phagocytized debris. The Burkitt cells on a Wright-stained touch preparation or smear (**C**) have deep-blue cytoplasm with vacuoles. Anaplastic large-cell lymphoma (**D**) is composed of sheets of large bizarre cells including "wreath cells" (*lower right*) and "hallmark cells" (*upper middle*). These cells are CD30 (Ki-1)-positive (**E**), and ALK-positive (**F**). The ALK-positivity in the nucleus and cytoplasm corresponds to the classic t(2;5), which was present in this case. Lymphoblastic lymphoma (**G, H**) composed of sheets of small- to intermediate-sized blasts with high mitotic rate and fine chromatin. On a touch preparation (**I**), the cells are typical lymphoblasts with scant cytoplasm. The lower panels show common clinical presentations of the three histologic subtypes of lymphoma: encasement of the bowel lumen by Burkitt lymphoma on abdominal computed tomography (Panel J); airway compression by lymphoblastic lymphoma of the anterior mediastinum on computed tomography of the chest (Panel K); and bony destruction of the tibia by large-cell lymphoma on magnetic resonance imaging (Panel L). (Reproduced with permission from Sandlund JT, Downing JR, Crist WM: Non-Hodgkin's lymphoma in childhood. N Engl J Med 334:1238, 1996.)

lated expression. The mutations may occur in either the regulatory or coding regions of the gene. For example, mutations in the myc-inhibitory factor binding sites in the first intron-regulatory region negate the repressive effect of myc-inhibitory factor binding on transcription.[51] Gu et al[49] have demonstrated that in cases that contain a coding region mutation in the amino terminal transactivation domain where p107 would normally bind and block transactivation, tumor cells are no longer responsive to p107-mediated functional suppression. Other hypotheses focus on the juxtaposition of c-*myc* to the immunoglobulin loci. It has been suggested that the immunoglobulin gene usurps control over the translocated c-*myc* gene, perhaps through long-range enhancer sequences.[48,50] It is likely that multiple mechanisms deregulate c-*myc* in Burkitt lymphoma.

The apparent abrogation of the c-*myc* induction of apoptosis suggests that other factors besides deregulation of c-*myc* are involved in the pathogenesis of Burkitt lymphoma.[52] Data supporting this position have emerged from a transgenic mouse model in which insertion of a deregulated c-*myc* gene mimicking the abnormality in Burkitt lymphoma results in the development of B-cell malignancies.[53,54] The fact that these tumors are monoclonal and take 6 to 9 months to develop suggests that additional factors or molecular events are necessary for malignant transformation. The identity and potential role in pathogenesis of other oncogenes or tumor suppressor genes is currently under investigation.[52,55] In this regard, novel insights into pathogenesis have emerged from analyses of the ARF-mdm2-p53 apoptotic pathway in Eu-myc transgenic mice.[56–58] Abnormalities in this pathway, which were identified in 80% of the lymphomas that developed in these mice, included deletions of Ink34a/ARF (25%), overexpression of Mdm2 (50%), and mutations of p53 (30%). Studies of this pathway in human Burkitt lymphoma are currently under way. Abnormalities in the p53 gene have been identified in cases of human Burkitt lymphoma and B-cell acute lymphoblastic leukemia (ALL).[59,60] The mutations in these tumors differ from those seen in solid tumors such as lung, breast, and colorectal carcinomas. Beyond the mere association of p53 with these tumors, observed regulatory interactions between c-*myc* and p53 have supported the hypotheses regarding the role of p53 in pathogenesis.[60]

Lymphoblastic Lymphoma

The morphology of these tumor cells is similar to that of ALL. The distinction between lymphoblastic lymphoma and ALL is arbitrarily based on the degree of bone marrow involvement: patients with between 5% and 25% replacement of the marrow by lymphoblasts are considered to have advanced-stage lymphoblastic lymphoma with marrow involvement, whereas those with 25% or more marrow blasts are designated as ALL. The lymphoblasts are small with round or convoluted nuclei, distinct nuclear membranes, inconspicuous nuclei, and a scant rim of basophilic cytoplasm. The vast majority (>95%) are of T-cell immunophenotype. A small percentage of cases have a B-cell progenitor immunophenotype and may be associated with cutaneous involvement.[61–63]

Because of the similarities in cellular origin, immunophenotype, morphology, and clinical features, it is generally assumed that lymphoblastic lymphoma and T-cell leukemia are different presentations of the same disease process; however, this is yet to be proved.[64] Most theories regarding the pathogenesis of lymphoblastic lymphoma are based on studies of T-cell ALL. The reciprocal chromosomal translocations identified in T-cell leukemia and lymphoblastic lymphoma typically involve one of the T-cell receptor genes and result in deregulation of the reciprocal partner gene.[65–73] The reciprocal partner gene is often a transcription factor gene such as *TAL1*, which is not usually operative in T cells.[66,67,72,73] In T-cell leukemia, a submicroscopic deletion of *TAL1* can be identified in up to 25% of cases, suggesting that this deletion may also be the most common molecular abnormality in lymphoblastic lymphoma.[72] Examples of other genes involved in translocations that have been described in these T-cell malignancies include the *HOX11* transcription factor gene and the *RHOMB* genes, whose products are members of a family of proteins that contain a cysteine-rich (LIM) protein–protein interaction domain.[68,70,71]

Diffuse Large B-cell Lymphoma

Approximately one-third of the non-Hodgkin lymphomas of childhood are not classifiable as either lymphoblastic or Burkitt lymphomas and fell into the categories of large-cell lymphoma in previous classifications. Many of these are now classified as diffuse large B-cell lymphomas (DLBCL) in the REAL and WHO classifications. These tumors are composed of large cells with nuclei at least twice the size of small lymphocytes with a high proliferative fraction. The diffuse large B-cell lymphomas are thought to arise from peripheral B cells of either germinal center or post–germinal center origin, and thus express a variety of pan-B-cell antigens with or without the expression of surface immunoglobulin.[33] Recent gene expression profiling studies of DLBCL in adults[74,75] have revealed further heterogeneity among these tumors that can now be divided among germinal center B-cell-like, activated B-cell-like, and type 3 phenotypes, and this subclassification was found to be prognostically important. The validity of such a subclassification among cases of childhood DLBCL is unknown, but such studies are ongoing.

Diffuse large B-cell lymphomas occur at a variety of sites, including the gastrointestinal tract, abdomen, head and neck region,[7] as well as primary sites of involvement that are unusual in childhood non-Hodgkin lymphomas such as bone and central nervous system. Lymphomas occurring in the setting of immunodeficiency are frequently of the large B-cell type. Mediastinal presentations also occur, and primary mediastinal (thymic) large B-cell lymphoma—a presentation more common in adolescents and young adults—is included as a recognized subtype of diffuse large B-cell lymphomas in both the WHO and REAL classifications.[31,33,76,77] Dense, compartmentalizing sclerosis and Reed–Sternberg-like cells are often present, leading to possible misdiagnosis of Hodgkin disease, particularly if only a small biopsy is available for review.

There is substantial overlap in the definition of diffuse large B-cell lymphomas and the Burkitt-like lymphomas,[31] and some investigators who have advocated immunophenotype-based therapies recommend that children with DLBCL be treated on protocols designed for Burkitt lymphomas with excellent overall results. However, there are several clinical distinctions, particularly the rarity of marrow and central nervous system involvement in DLBCL as compared to Burkitt lymphoma; thus, the very intensive central nervous system-directed therapy specified in regimens designed for Burkitt lymphoma may not be necessary for children with DLBCL.

Anaplastic Large-Cell Lymphoma

Most of the remaining childhood NHLs previously classified as large-cell lymphomas fall into the category of anaplastic large-cell lymphomas (ALCLs) in the REAL and WHO classification. This entity was first described in 1986 as a clinicopathologic variant of large-cell lymphoma with a predilection for young patients[78–89] (reviewed in references 92 and 96). The ALCLs are characterized by the proliferation of large, pleomorphic cells with multiple or single prominent nucleoli. The cells preferentially involve lymph node sinuses as well as extranodal sites (notably skin, bone, and soft tissue) where the cells grow in a cohesive pattern.[31,33] The cells express epithelial membrane antigen (EMA) as well as the CD30 (Ki-1) antigen—a 120-kd membrane-bound molecule now known to be a member of the tumor necrosis factor (TNF) receptor superfamily[80,90–92]—previously found in association with Hodgkin disease. A soluble (88-kd) form of the CD30 molecule is found in high levels in the serum of virtually all patients with ALCL.[92–94] Marked elevation of the level of soluble CD30 in patients with ALCL correlates with higher risk of relapse, and levels of soluble CD30 have been found to correlate with clinical disease status, returning to normal with attainment of complete remission and increasing with disease recurrence.

The anaplastic large-cell lymphomas have been found to be associated with chromosomal rearrangements involving the long arm of chromosome 5 at position q35.[86,95] In the majority of cases, this translocation involves material from chromosome 2p23 [t(2;5)(p23;q35)] resulting in the fusion of the NPM nucleolar phosphoprotein gene on chromosome 5q35 to ALK (anaplastic lymphoma kinase), a tyrosine kinase gene on chromosome 2p23. The hybrid protein produced from the translocation links the amino terminus of nucleophosmin (NPM) with the catalytic domain of ALK.[96] Deregulated expression of the truncated ALK may contribute to malignant transformation.[97] The chimeric NPM–ALK protein is clearly oncogenic, perhaps through triggering of antiapoptotic signals via phosphatidylinositol 3-kinase/Akt,[98] although secondary molecular events may be required for lymphomagenesis.

Immunologic and molecular biologic studies reveal that the majority of cases of Ki-1$^+$ anaplastic large-cell lymphomas are derived from activated T cells, although non-T, non-B-cell (null cell) cases, and more rarely B-cell cases have been described.[84,87,99] Based on extended testing for T-cell antigens and examination of the configuration of T cell receptor genes, many of the "null" cell cases are, in fact, T lineage-derived neoplasms, although a minority may be derived from natural killer (NK) cells.[92] The diagnosis of ALCL can be difficult to establish, and many cases are initially misdiagnosed as Hodgkin disease.[84] The use of molecular techniques (RT-PCR) to detect the presence of the fusion gene produced by the t(2;5) in many cases of ALCL allows the establishment of the correct diagnosis.[96,100–102] Variant translocations where *ALK* is involved with other partner genes on other chromosomes limits the application of RT-PCR for diagnosis. However, the t(2;5) results in the expression of the NPM–ALK fusion protein, whereas the variant translocations result in upregulation of *ALK*. The expression of the normal ALK protein is restricted to rare cells in the central nervous system in normal postnatal tissues, so the expression of either ALK or the NPM–ALK fusion protein is a marker for ALCL. The ALK1 monoclonal antibody that recognizes the formalin-resistant epitope of both the NPM–ALK chimeric protein and normal ALK thus serves as a useful diagnostic reagent for identifying cases of ALCL.[92,96,103] It should be recognized that the distribution of ALK staining has been found to vary depending on the translocation.[33] Further, ALK expression is also observed in inflammatory myofibroblastic tumors (IMT) as a result of rearrangements of chromosome 2p23 that occur in this family of tumors, as well as in other mesenchymal tumors[104]; however, confusion with ALCL can be minimized by testing for other hematopoietic markers, and the distinction is usually not difficult for experienced pathologists.

ALCL is rare, accounting for approximately 8% to 12% of childhood NHLs and roughly 30% to 40% of the pediatric large-cell lymphomas.[89] Approximately one-third of the cases present with localized disease, whereas the majority have advanced-stage disease at presentation, although involvement of the bone marrow and central nervous system is uncommon.[89] A leukemic presentation of ALCL has been described but is uncommon; it may be associated with the small-cell variant of ALCL.[105] Systemic symptoms (fevers, weight loss) are frequently present in advanced-stage disease. Cutaneous lesions (which often spontaneously regress) sometimes accompany disease at other sites,[78] but skin involvement is not universal.[79] A variety of presenting sites—both nodal and extranodal—have been observed, including the mediastinum, gastrointestinal tract, and bone. The outcome of children with ALCL in most series has been good, with survivals ranging from 70% to 85%,[89,106,107] although inferior to that of children with Burkitt and diffuse large B-cell lymphomas.

Rare Subtypes

Other subtypes that are observed rarely in children deserve mention, but the rarity of these neoplasms in children makes generalizations and therapeutic recommendations difficult. Follicular lymphomas (characterized by the arrangement of malignant cells in aggregates separated by normal cells), which account for approximately 30% of NHLs seen in adults, are extremely rare in children.[108–113] Children with follicular lymphomas tend to present with cervical lymph node involvement (although primary tumors of the testis have been reported[114,115]) with early-stage disease and have an excellent prognosis.[108–113] Unlike most cases of follicular lymphoma in adults where aberrant expression of bcl-2 (usually as a result of the t(14;18) translocation) is thought to play an important role in lymphomagenesis, the majority of cases of follicular lymphomas in children demonstrate neither the t(14;18) nor bcl-2 expression. Bcl-2 expression appears to occur more frequently in older children and is associated with advanced-stage disease at presentation and a more aggressive clinical course.[113]

Marginal zone B-cell lymphomas arising in mucosa-associated lymphoid tissue (MALT) can arise in extranodal sites. They tend to present with localized disease and infrequently disseminate. Natural killer cell lymphoma and NK-like T-cell lymphomas usually involve the upper aerodigestive tract (midline lethal granuloma, angiocentric T-cell lymphoma), but can present in the skin as well.[116–118] They are rare in children, and follow a very aggressive clinical course, are often fatal, but may respond to high-dose chemotherapy with stem cell transplantation.[116] Peripheral T-cell lymphomas include a variety of neoplasms that have not yet been further specified. These lymphomas are rare in children, but advanced stage at presentation, often in association with systemic symptoms and hematophagocytic syndrome, is common, and an aggressive course is the rule.

CLINICAL FEATURES

The clinical features at presentation vary with both primary site (Table 81–2) and extent of disease spread.[7,119] There is a striking difference in primary site between the Burkitt and lymphoblastic histologic subtypes.[7] The primary site of Burkitt lymphoma may be either abdomen or head and neck, but rarely the mediastinum. In contrast, lymphoblastic lymphomas may primarily involve the mediastinum or head and neck, but rarely the abdomen. Children with large B-cell lymphoma and ALCL present with less predictable sites of involvement, although such patients may present with primary involvement of head and neck, abdomen, or mediastinum.[7] The bone marrow may be involved at diagnosis in any of the histologic subtypes.[120] The central nervous system (CNS) may be involved at diagnosis in both the Burkitt and lymphoblastic lymphomas, but rarely in large-cell lymphoma.[7,121,122]

Table 81–2 Distribution of Primary Sites of Tumor in Children and Adolescents With Non-Hodgkin Lymphoma

	St. Jude Children's Research Hospital	The Hospital for Sick Children
No. of cases	338	102
Intraabdominal	31%	40%
Mediastinal	26%	23%
Head and neck	29%[a]	11%[b]
Nodal	7%[c]	21%
Other[d]	7%	6%

[a]Includes Waldeyer ring and/or cervical lymph nodes.
[b]Includes only Waldeyer ring.
[c]Includes cases with primary nodal disease arising outside the head/neck region.
[d]Includes a variety of less common locations, including bone, skin, epidural space, thyroid.
(Modified from reference 7 with permission).

Children who have a mediastinal mass may present with a spectrum of symptoms ranging from cough to severe respiratory distress caused by direct airway compression—this condition may be worsened by an associated pleural effusion (Fig. 81–1K). Mediastinal disease may also compress the superior vena cava, resulting in swelling of the neck and shoulder (superior vena cava syndrome).

Primary involvement of the abdomen may be associated with nausea, vomiting, and abdominal pain. Abdominal lymphoma often arises from the distal ileum and may result in intestinal obstruction secondary to either intussusception or compression by an expanding mass encasing the bowel lumen (Fig. 81–1J). These tumors may invade adjacent structures and be associated with ascites and other intraabdominal sites of disease, including kidney, liver, and lymph nodes.

Involvement of the bone marrow may result in pancytopenia with associated pallor and bruising. Involvement of the CNS may be associated with cranial nerve palsies or symptoms of increased intracranial pressure such as headache and vision changes. Cutaneous involvement may also occur and is usually associated with $CD30^+$ anaplastic large-cell lymphoma[81,88]; however, lymphoblastic lymphoma (often non–T cell immunophenotype) may also involve skin.[61–63] Bone involvement may be associated with pain or limping (Fig. 81–1L).

LABORATORY EVALUATION

Initial laboratory evaluation should include a complete blood count with differential—these may identify abnormalities in children with bone marrow involvement. A chemistry profile, which should include electrolytes, blood urea nitrogen, creatinine, lactic dehydrogenase (LDH), calcium, phosphorus, and uric acid is also important, particularly for children with bulky Burkitt lymphoma, who often present with metabolic abnormalities such as hyperuricemia. A screen for human immunodeficiency virus should be performed on all patients with newly diagnosed B-cell lymphomas. These individuals may be at increased risk for therapy-related toxicity, specifically, life-threatening infections. Serologic studies for EBV infection and measurement of EBV viral load may be helpful in children in whom lymphoproliferative disease is highly suspected in the differential diagnosis.

DIAGNOSIS AND DIFFERENTIAL DIAGNOSIS

The differential diagnosis of NHL includes both benign and malignant conditions. If the blood counts are normal and there is no mediastinal mass, a single 10- to 14-day trial of antibiotics for painless enlarged peripheral adenopathy is permissible to treat presumed bacterial adenitis. Other infectious causes for adenopathy-simulating lymphoma include histoplasmosis, tuberculosis, and EBV infection, for which serologic and skin testing may be helpful. If the diagnosis of NHL is suspected, consultation with a pediatric oncologist is indicated.

The diagnosis of NHL is usually established by examination of tissue obtained by open biopsy of the involved site (see Fig. 81–1). A comprehensive characterization of the biologic features of the tissue will help to distinguish NHL from the small round blue cell tumors of childhood, including Ewing sarcoma, neuroblastoma, and rhabdomyosarcoma. Sufficient tissue should be obtained not only for histology but also for immunophenotypic, cytogenetic, and molecular studies. In some cases, a patient is too unstable to undergo anesthesia for open biopsy, as in children with large anterior mediastinal masses and associated airway compression. In such cases, the diagnosis may be established by parasternal fine-needle aspiration or biopsy with local anesthesia. If there is an associated pleural effusion, thoracentesis with cytologic examination of pleural fluid is usually diagnostic. In cases of large abdominal Burkitt tumors, direct percutaneous aspiration of the mass for cytology and cytogenetics is often diagnostic, as is cytologic examination of associated ascitic fluid obtained by paracentesis. In children with suspected NHL, a bone marrow and cerebrospinal fluid examination may be diagnostic, averting the need for more invasive procedures and possible increased morbidity.

STAGING

It is imperative that a complete staging workup be performed because therapy is determined in part by location and degree of disease spread. Additionally, because NHL in children grows very rapidly, there should be no unnecessary delay in the staging workup or in starting appropriate therapy. The staging workup should include a complete history and physical, including the documentation of the presence or absence of systemic symptoms (eg, weight loss, sweats, and fever). Diagnostic imaging studies should include computed tomography scanning of the chest, abdomen, and pelvis, and bone scanning. Gallium scanning may also be helpful in selected cases, particularly in following residual masses that were gallium positive at diagnosis. FDG positron emission tomography (PET) scanning is proving to be more sensitive and will likely supplant the Gallium scan for this purpose. The cerebrospinal fluid and bone marrow must be examined in all patients. Bilateral posterior iliac crest aspiration and biopsy increases the chance of identifying marrow involvement, thus reducing the possibility of underestimating the disease stage.[123]

On completion of the above workup, the stage of disease is usually determined according to the staging system described by Murphy (Table 81–3),[124] which was developed to accommodate the noncontiguous nature of disease spread, predominant extranodal involvement, and involvement of the bone marrow and CNS. Stages I and II are considered limited-stage disease, whereas stage III represents advanced-stage disease. Stage IV is reserved for children with the bone marrow or central nervous system involvement—presentations associated with a less favorable prognosis.

THERAPY

General Principles

The dramatic improvement in treatment outcome achieved over the past 30 years is in large part due to the refinement in multiagent chemotherapeutic strategies through sequential clinical trials.[7,89,106,107,121,125–167] A randomized trial performed by the Children's Cancer Group (CCG) that compared two of the earliest effective treatment regimens for childhood NHL (COMP [cyclophosphamide, Oncovin, methotrexate, prednisone] and LSA_2L_2) provided data supporting a stage- and histology-directed approach to treating children with NHL.[126,168] In this trial, children with limited-stage disease had an excellent outcome regardless of histology or treatment regimen used. In contrast, among children with advanced-stage disease, outcome varied with histology and therapy. Children with Burkitt lymphoma had a better outcome with the cyclophosphamide-based COMP regimen, whereas children with lymphoblastic lymphoma had a better outcome with LSA_2L_2, a regimen designed for children with ALL. Among children with large-cell lymphoma, outcome did not vary with treatment protocol. In the United States, subsequent trials built on this histology- and stage-directed approach. In Europe, and more recently in some US trials, an immunophenotype-directed approach is used. Data suggest that immunophenotype-directed therapy may be particularly important for children with advanced large-cell lymphomas.[130]

There is a minimal role for radiation therapy and surgery in the management of childhood NHL.[7] Prospective randomized trials in children with either limited- or advanced-stage disease have shown there is no improvement in treatment result when involved-field radiation is included[165,169]; in fact, this modality may only add to treatment-related morbidity. Apart from the initial diagnostic biopsy or the complete resection of an isolated peripheral node, tonsil, or ileocecal primary tumor associated with mesenteric nodes only (see discussion on staging), there is no other clear indication for the surgical management of this disease.[170,171] Of note, aggressive debulking procedures are not indicated.

To prevent the spread of disease to the CNS, prophylactic intrathecal and high-dose systemic chemotherapy are used in most children. Prophylactic intrathecal therapy may not be necessary in children with limited-stage disease outside of the head and neck region. Some groups have included cranial radiation for CNS prophylaxis in pediatric lymphoblastic lymphoma; however, this approach is controversial.[155] Among children who present with overt CNS disease, intensification of both intrathecal and systemic chemotherapy is often needed, and with the exception of Burkitt lymphoma, the addition of cranial irradiation.

Table 81–3 Stages of Non-Hodgkin Lymphoma*

Stage I
A single tumor (extranodal) or involvement of a single anatomical area (nodal), with the exclusion of the mediastinum and abdomen.
Stage II
A single tumor (extranodal) with regional node involvement. Two or more nodal areas on the same side of the diaphragm. Two single (extranodal) tumors, with or without regional node involvement on the same side of the diaphragm. A primary gastrointestinal tract tumor (usually in the ileocecal area), with or without involvement of associated mesenteric nodes, that is completely resectable.
Stage III
Two single tumors (extranodal) on opposite sides of the diaphragm. Two or more nodal areas above and below the diaphragm. Any primary intrathoracic tumor (mediastinal, pleural, or thymic). Extensive primary intraabdominal disease. Any paraspinal or epidural tumor, whether or not other sites are involved.
Stage IV
Any of the above findings with initial involvement of the central nervous system, bone marrow, or both.

*Based on the classification proposed by Murphy.[124]

Limited-Stage Disease

The excellent prognosis for children with limited stage disease has prompted investigators to develop treatment strategies that reduce treatment-related morbidity while maintaining an excellent treatment result.[125,132,133,148,151,152,169] These studies have examined various ways to reduce treatment intensity. For example, in the first of two sequential trials performed by the Pediatric Oncology Group (POG),[133,169] it was demonstrated that involved-field radiation therapy could be safely deleted from a 33-week chemotherapy regimen that comprised three courses of CHOP (cyclophosphamide, doxorubicin, vincristine, and prednisone) given over a 9-week period, followed by a 24-week maintenance phase consisting of daily oral mercaptopurine and weekly methotrexate. In the subsequent trial,[133] they demonstrated that the 24-week maintenance phase could be deleted without compromising the treatment result for those with either large cell or Burkitt lymphoma. The optimal therapeutic approach for children with limited-stage lymphoblastic lymphoma remains controversial. In the POG trial, one-third of these children treated with the 33-week regimen experienced treatment failure, but were successfully salvaged with leukemia-like therapy in most cases. French investigators have taken a different approach, treating children with limited-stage lymphoblastic lymphoma with the same regimen used for those with advanced-stage disease.[147] Although this approach may reduce the need for retreatment, it also increases the risk of treatment-related morbidity.

Table 81–4 Treatment Outcome for Advanced-Stage Burkitt Lymphoma

Protocol	Stage	No. of Patients	Event-Free Survival Rate	Reference
Total B	III	17	2-year EFS = 81%	131
	IV/B-ALL	4/8	2-year EFS = 17%	
POG 8616 (Total B)	III	64	2-year EFS = 79% (SE = 6%)	134
POG 8617	IV	34	4-year EFS = 79% ± 9%	135
	B-ALL	47	4-year EFS = 65% ± 8%	
LMB 89*	III	278	5-year EFS = 91% (95% CI, 87%–94%)	125
	IV	62	5-year EFS = 87% (95% CI, 77%–93%)	
	B-ALL	102	5-year EFS = 87% (95% CI, 79%–92%)	
BFM 90	III	169	6-year EFS = 86% ± 3%	152
	IV	24	6-year EFS = 73% ± 10%	
	B-ALL	56	6 yr EFS = 74% ± 6%	

*Includes patients with diffuse large B-cell Non-Hodgkin Lymphoma.

Advanced-Stage Disease

In the United States, efforts to improve the treatment outcome for children with advanced-stage disease have primarily examined strategies to increase treatment intensity in the framework of a histology-directed approach, whereas in Europe, an immunophenotype-directed strategy is generally used.

Burkitt Lymphoma

Advances in the treatment outcome of patients with Burkitt lymphoma represent one of the true success stories in pediatric oncology (Table 81–4). Following the CCG trial that demonstrated the efficacy of the cyclophosphamide-based COMP regimen for advanced-stage Burkitt lymphoma, improved treatment results were achieved by including high-dose methotrexate and cytarabine[129,131,134–137] even in regimens given over as short a period as 2 to 4 months.[136,140] Subsequent improvements were achieved by dose intensification of therapy and by the inclusion of additional active agents such as etoposide or ifosfamide.[125,152,154] For example, the LMB-89 regimen pioneered by the French Society of Pediatric Oncology (SFOP) has produced some of the best results to date.[125] This strategy features risk-adapted therapeutic arms of escalating intensity (groups A, B, and C). The least intensive arm (group A) is reserved for those with completely resected limited-stage disease, whereas the most intensive arm (group C) is designed for those with CNS disease or marrow involvement, with more than 70% replacement by lymphoma cells. All of the remaining patients are treated according to group B, which is of intermediate intensity. Group B features high-dose methotrexate at a dose of 3 g/m^2, whereas a dose of 8 g/m^2 is used in group C. In contrast to group C, which incorporates high-dose cytarabine and etoposide, group B features low-dose continuous-infusion cytarabine and no etoposide. The therapeutic components of Group A are restricted to vincristine, prednisone, cyclophosphamide, and doxorubicin (these agents are also included in Groups B and C). The total duration of therapy is approximately 2, 5, and 8 months for groups A, B, and C, respectively. Results from a recently completed international trial using the LMB 89 regimen confirm the excellent outcome achieved in the initial report from the SFOP and indicate that the intensity of LMB-89 therapy may be safely reduced for Group B patients,[172] whereas for Group C patients a reduction in treatment intensity was associated with a poorer outcome.[173] The German Berlin–Frankfurt–Munster (BFM) cooperative group has also achieved excellent results in the treatment of B-cell NHL and ALL with a regimen that incorporates high-dose methotrexate at a dose of 5 g/m^2, ifosfamide, etoposide, and steroids.[152] An improved outcome was also reported in an NCI trial that incorporated etoposide, high-dose cytarabine, and ifosfamide into a backbone of cyclophosphamide, doxorubicin, vincristine, and high-dose methotrexate.[154] These more aggressive therapeutic approaches, which have been effective in improving the outcome for children with Burkitt lymphoma and B-cell ALL, have also provided encouraging results when administered to adults with the same diseases.[153,157]

Lymphoblastic Lymphoma

Most of the regimens used successfully to treat lymphoblastic lymphoma are similar to or derived from those designed for children with high-risk T-cell ALL (Table 81–5).[126–128,142,143,147,150,155]

A St. Jude study demonstrated the benefit of adding teniposide and cytarabine to an otherwise conventional antimetabolite-based regimen.[142] The SFOP demonstrated that an excellent response could be achieved by incorporating courses of high-dose methotrexate into an LSA$_2$L$_2$ backbone.[147] The BFM group has incorporated a reinduction phase into their treatment strategy and, in their most recent trial, has featured high-dose methotrexate pulses (5 g/m^2) as an early consolidation with outstanding results (ie, 90% event-free survival at 3 years).[155] Although the French and German studies suggest an important role for high-dose methotrexate in the management of advanced-stage lymphoblastic lymphoma, the multiagent nature of the regimens studied to date makes the relative value of individual components uncertain. In this regard, a current Children's Oncology Group (COG) study is examining whether high-dose methotrexate can be safely eliminated from a BFM-based regimen, if replaced by extended intrathecal chemotherapy administration. L-Asparaginase is a component of most successful treatment regimens for advanced-stage lymphoblastic lymphoma. Its importance was demonstrated in a randomized trial performed by the POG that reported a survival advantage for those patients who received additional L-asparaginase.[160] Other strategies to improve outcome have included

Table 81–5 Treatment Outcome for Advanced-Stage Lymphoblastic Non-Hodgkin Lymphoma

Protocol	Stage	No. of Patients	Event-Free Survival (EFS) Rate	Reference
LSA_2L_2 (modified) CCG-551	III/IV	124	5-year EFS = 64%	126,168
BFM 90	III IV	82 19	5-year EFS = 90% ± 3% 5-year EFS = 95% ± 5%	155
X-H SJCRH	III/IV	22	4-year DFS = 73%	142
APO (Dana Farber)	III/IV	21	3-year DFS = 58% ± 23%	167
A-COP + (POG)	III	33	3-year DFS = 54% ± 9%	143
SFOP LMT81	III IV/ALL	33 43	57 mo EFS = 79% (SE, 4%) 57 mo EFS = 72% (SE, 4%)	147
CCG: LSA_2L_2 (modified) vs ADCOMP	I–IV I–IV	243 138	5-year EFS = 74% 5-year EFS = 64%	150
POG8704: no extra Asp vs extra Asp	III/IV III/IV	83 84	4-year CCR = 64% (SE, 6%) 4-year CCR = 78% (SE, 5%)	160

the incorporation of other active agents (eg, epipodophyllotoxins) and delayed intensification or reinduction phases.[142,155,160]

Large-Cell Lymphoma

The optimal approach to the treatment of advanced-stage large-cell lymphoma has been a challenge to identify, both because of the biologic heterogeneity of these tumors and the markedly varied treatment strategies reported. In the United States, children with large-cell NHL have historically been treated on histology-directed protocols (Table 81–6).[88,126,130,138,144–146]

Most of these histology-directed strategies are CHOP based, with current trials examining the benefit of adding agents such as carboplatin, high-dose cytarabine, etoposide, ifosfamide, and high-dose methotrexate. Some trials have examined the feasibility of eliminating individual agents with significant late effects, such as doxorubicin or cyclophosphamide.[138,159] In a POG trial, children with large-cell lymphomas of B-cell immunophenotype had a superior treatment result compared with those with a non-B-cell immunophenotype, suggesting that an immunophenotype-directed approach should be explored in future trials.[130] In this regard, European trials for children with large-cell NHL have generally been designed according to immunophenotype; children with B-cell tumors are treated like those with Burkitt lymphoma.[125] The SFOP reported that children with diffuse large B-cell lymphoma had an equally excellent outcome as compared to those with Burkitt lymphoma when treated with the same LMB-89 regimen.[125] However, those with mediastinal large B-cell lymphoma may have a somewhat inferior outcome compared to other diffuse large B-cell lymphomas.[77,172,174,175]

The anaplastic large-cell lymphomas account for the vast majority of large-cell lymphomas having a T-cell immunophenotype. The optimal treatment approach for patients with this type of lymphoma has yet to be elucidated, as evidenced by the wide range of treatment strategies that have been successfully implemented.[89] In the United States, children with CD30+ ALCL have generally been treated with the same regimen used for non-ALCL large-cell lymphomas, with long-term event-free survival rates ranging from 60% to 70%.[89] In a randomized trial performed by the POG, the addition of intermediate-dose methotrexate and high-dose cytarabine did not improve upon the 70% 4-year event-free survival achieved with APO alone.[176,177] The BFM have reported among the best results to date (3-year event-free survival of approximately 80%) using a Burkitt lymphoma-based strategy.[106,166] Regimens designed specifically for children with CD30+ ALCL have been developed by the French (SFOP) and German Groups.[106,107] The SFOP also reported the successful salvage of ALCL patients with the weekly administration of single-agent vinblastine.[162] The impact of incorporating vinblastine

Table 81–6 Treatment Outcome for Advanced Stage Large-Cell Non-Hodgkin Lymphoma

Protocol	Stage	No. of Patients	Event-Free Survival Rate	Reference
CHOP	III & IV	21	3-year EFS = 62% ± 11%	121
MACOP-B	III & IV	11	3-year EFS = 55% ± 16%	146
COMP vs LSA_2L_2	III & IV III & IV	42 18	5-year EFS = 52% 5-year EFS = 43%	126
APO vs ACOP+	III & IV III & IV	62 58	3-year EFS = 72% ± 6% 4-year EFS = 62% ± 7%	159

into two different front-line treatment for strategies for ALCL [the BFM B-cell approach (multinational European trial) and APO (COG trial in the United States)] is currently being studied in randomized fashion.

EMERGENCY SITUATIONS

Various emergency situations may arise in the management of the child with newly diagnosed malignant lymphoma.[178] Those with a large anterior mediastinal mass may present with severe respiratory distress secondary to direct tracheal compression, a situation that may be worsened by an associated pleural effusion. If the diagnosis has been confirmed, appropriate chemotherapy should be started as soon as possible. If the diagnosis has not been established, efforts should be made to establish it expeditiously (see section on diagnosis). If the degree of respiratory compromise requires emergency management, involved-field irradiation of the tumor mass should be considered, with sparing of peripheral portions of the tumor so that a biopsy can be obtained when the patient is stable.[179] Steroids may also be considered; however, this approach risks altering the tumor histology, making it difficult to establish the correct diagnosis.[180]

Children with a large tumor burden, particularly those with Burkitt lymphoma, are at increased risk of significant metabolic abnormalities. Specifically, they may present with hyperuricemia, hyperkalemia, hyperphosphatemia, and associated renal dysfunction. This situation may only worsen with the massive tumor cell lysis that follows administration of chemotherapy (tumor lysis syndrome).[181–183] Some of these children develop renal failure, requiring dialysis. To help prevent this complication, children at risk should be vigorously

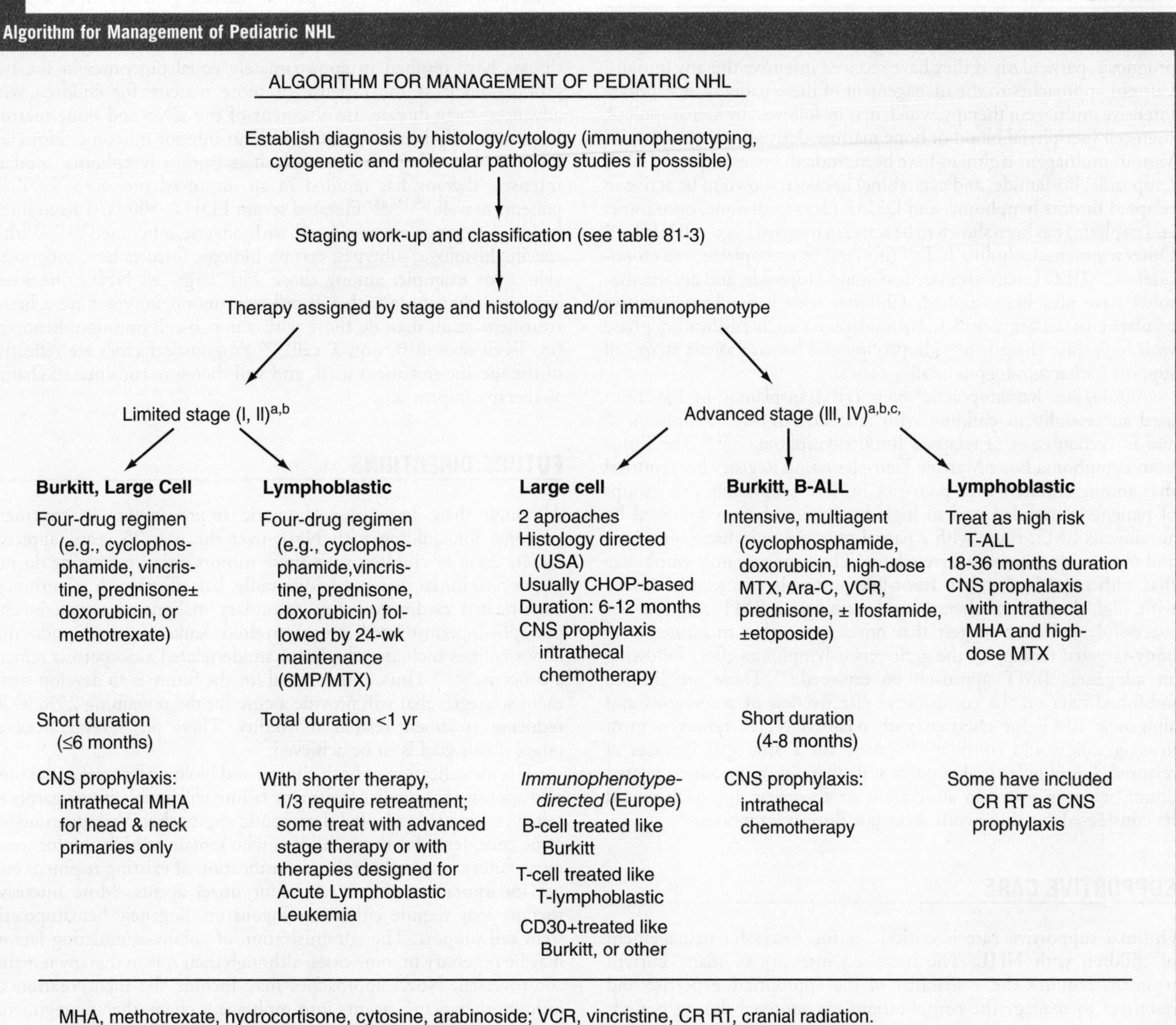

ALGORITHM FOR MANAGEMENT OF PEDIATRIC NHL
Establish diagnosis by histology/cytology (immunophenotyping, cytogenetic and molecular pathology studies if possible)
Staging work-up and classification (see table 81-3)
Therapy assigned by stage and histology and/or immunophenotype
Limited stage (I, II)a,b
Advanced stage (III, IV)a,b,c,
Burkitt, Large Cell
Four-drug regimen (e.g., cyclophosphamide, vincristine, prednisone± doxorubicin, or methotrexate)
Short duration (≤6 months)
CNS prophylaxis: intrathecal MHA for head & neck primaries only
Lymphoblastic
Four-drug regimen (e.g., cyclophosphamide,vincristine, prednisone, doxorubicin) followed by 24-wk maintenance (6MP/MTX)
Total duration <1 yr
With shorter therapy, 1/3 require retreatment; some treat with advanced stage therapy or with therapies designed for Acute Lymphoblastic Leukemia
Large cell
2 aproaches
Histology directed (USA)
Usually CHOP-based
Duration: 6-12 months
CNS prophylaxis intrathecal chemotherapy
Immunophenotype-directed (Europe)
B-cell treated like Burkitt
T-cell treated like T-lymphoblastic
CD30+treated like Burkitt, or other
Burkitt, B-ALL
Intensive, multiagent (cyclophosphamide, doxorubicin, high-dose MTX, Ara-C, VCR, prednisone, ± Ifosfamide, ±etoposide)
Short duration (4-8 months)
CNS prophylaxis: intrathecal chemotherapy
Lymphoblastic
Treat as high risk T-ALL
18-36 months duration
CNS prophalaxis with intrathecal MHA and high-dose MTX
Some have included CR RT as CNS prophylaxis
MHA, methotrexate, hydrocortisone, cytosine, arabinoside; VCR, vincristine, CR RT, cranial radiation.
aRelapses or induction failures should be treated with multiagent intensive chemotherapy; if shown to be chemosensitive, consider consolidation with haematopoietic stem cell support.
bNo involved field radiation therapy up front, but may be considered for biopsy-proven induction failure or relapse.
cBulky advanced stage Burkitt and lymphoblastic lymphoma will require prechemotherapy stabilization including vigorous hydration/alkalization/allopurinol.

Algorithm for Management of Pediatric NHL

hydrated (3–4 L/m^2/day with D5 1/4 NaCl and 40 mEq/L $NaHCO_3$; there should be no added potassium) and started on allopurinol, a xanthine oxidase inhibitor. The urine pH should be maintained at approximately 7.0; at a more alkaline pH, phosphorus is less soluble, and at a more acidic pH, uric acid is less soluble. In some cases, mannitol followed by furosemide is required to maintain urine output. Uricolytic agents (eg, uricozyme, which has been used for many years in Europe) directly cleave the uric acid molecule and result in a precipitous drop in serum uric acid levels within a few hours.[184] The use of uricolytic agents (eg, urate oxidase, uricase, rasburicase)[185–188] has proven to be superior to allopurinol to reduce rapidly the level of serum uric acid and improve renal function. This precludes the need for alkalinization, thus facilitating the excretion of phosphorus. The use of uricolytic agents and the initiation of induction therapy with a course of low-dose chemotherapy as a cytoreductive "pre-phase" have reduced the incidence of renal insufficiency from urate nephropathy in European trials.[125,151] Few children treated on recent trials for advanced-stage B-cell lymphomas conducted by the BFM Group and the SFOP have required hemodialysis during induction, and few early deaths have been encountered. A similar experience has been appreciated in recent North American trials.

Children with NHL may present with epidural masses and associated neurologic deficits caused by spinal cord compression. If the diagnosis is known, chemotherapy should be started as soon as possible. If the diagnosis is not known, or if there is a sluggish response to chemotherapy, low-dose radiation therapy may be considered in consultation with a radiation oncologist.

SALVAGE THERAPY

Children who fail initial therapy are generally considered to have a poor prognosis, particularly if they have received intensive therapy initially. Current approaches to the management of these patients incorporate intensive multiagent therapy, which may be followed by hematopoietic stem cell (peripheral blood or bone marrow-derived) transplantation. Various multiagent regimens have been studied. For example, VIPA[154] (etoposide, ifosfamide, and cytarabine) has been shown to be active in relapsed Burkitt lymphoma, and DHAP (dexamethasone, cytarabine, and cisplatin) has been shown to be active in relapsed large-cell NHL.[146] Other regimens, including ICE[189] (ifosfamide, carboplatin, and etoposide) and MIED (methotrexate, ifosfamide, etoposide, and dexamethasone) have also been studied. Children who have chemosensitive recurrent disease are considered candidates for an intensification phase with high-dose chemo- or radiotherapy and hematopoietic stem cell support (either autologous or allogeneic).

Autologous hematopoietic stem cell transplantation has been used successfully in children with relapsed large-cell lymphoma[190] and in certain cases of relapsed Burkitt lymphoma.[191,192] The European Lymphoma Bone Marrow Transplantation Registry has reported that among children with poor-risk Burkitt lymphoma, two groups of patients responded well to high-dose chemotherapy followed by autologous BMT: those with a partial response to induction therapy and those with chemosensitive relapse. These investigators emphasize that with intensive modern front-line protocols, postrelapse salvage with high-dose chemotherapy and autologous BMT may be less successful, and they suggest that novel approaches including antibody-targeted therapy or the graft-versus-lymphoma effect following an allogeneic BMT approach be explored.[193] There are limited published data on the comparative effectiveness of autologous and allogeneic BMT for children with relapsed NHL; however, most investigators would consider allogeneic BMT strategies in cases of relapsed lymphoblastic lymphoma if there is a matched related donor, whereas either an autologous or allogeneic approach would be considered for those with recurrent Burkitt lymphoma.

SUPPORTIVE CARE

Optimal supportive care is critical for the successful management of children with NHL. The increased intensity of many current regimens requires the availability of the appropriate expertise and resources to manage the complications encountered during periods of profound pancytopenia. The management of life-threatening infections requires the availability of appropriate broad-spectrum antibiotics and antifungals and an intensive care facility. The use of prophylactic trimethoprim-sulfamethoxazole is recommended in all patients to reduce the chance of *Pneumocystis carinii* pneumonitis; for patients on aggressive B-cell protocols, prophylaxis should be continued for approximately 6 months after chemotherapy is completed. Access to a blood bank that can quickly provide irradiated, leukocyte-depleted packed red blood cells and platelets is also important. The role of colony-stimulating factors such as granulocyte-CSF or granulocyte/macrophage-CSF has yet to be fully elucidated; however, the use of these cytokines provides the potential benefit of reducing the duration of neutropenia, thus reducing infectious morbidity. The placement of a permanent venous access device greatly facilitates the delivery of hydration fluids, chemotherapy, antibiotics, and blood products. Consultation with a nutritionist or nutritional support team regarding need for enteral or total parenteral nutritional support is often necessary, particularly for children on intensive advanced-stage B-cell NHL protocols, which are associated with significant gastrointestinal tract toxicity.

PROGNOSTIC FACTORS

Factors that are associated with treatment outcome include treatment era and tumor burden as reflected by both stage and serum LDH.[7] Those with limited-stage (I and II) disease generally have a better prognosis than those with advanced-stage (III and IV) disease; however, more intensive therapies for children with advanced-stage disease have resulted in approximately equal outcomes in the two groups, albeit at the expense of more toxicity for children with advanced-stage disease. Involvement of the CNS and bone marrow has historically been associated with an inferior outcome. However, for certain histologic subtypes, such as Burkitt lymphoma, modern intensive therapy has resulted in an improved prognosis for these patients as well.[125,135,152] Elevated serum LDH (>500 IU/L) and interleukin-2 receptor are associated with adverse outcome.[194,195] Within specific histologic subtypes, certain biologic features have prognostic value. For example, among those with large-cell NHL, one study suggested that those with a B-cell immunophenotype have a better treatment result than do those with a non-B-cell immunophenotype (ie, T-cell or non-B, non-T cell).[130] Prognostic factors are reflective of the specific treatment used, and will therefore continue to change as therapy improves.

FUTURE DIRECTIONS

Although there have been dramatic improvements in treatment outcome for children with NHL over the past 25 years, approximately 25% of children with these tumors either relapse or do not respond to initial therapy. Additionally, late effects such as anthracycline-related cardiomyopathy, secondary malignancies such as epipodophyllotoxin-related acute myeloid leukemia, and endocrine abnormalities such as cyclophosphamide-related azoospermia remain a concern.[196–198] Thus, a major goal for the future is to develop treatment strategies that will provide a cure for the remaining 25% while reducing treatment-related morbidity. There are several areas to target if this goal is to be achieved.

The identification of both clinical and biologic features at the time of diagnosis that predict treatment failure will enable investigators to refine existing risk-adapted therapeutic approaches. Various strategies to be considered for those children who remain at high risk for treatment failure may include the intensification of existing regimens and the incorporation of new active or novel agents. More intensive therapy may require either autologous or allogeneic hematopoietic stem cell support. The administration of colony-stimulating factors may be necessary in some cases, although their role in therapy remains controversial. Novel approaches may include the incorporation of immunotherapeutic agents into multiagent chemotherapy regimens. For example, the anti-CD20 antibody (rituximab) has been successfully used in the management of adults with B-cell lymphomas, including diffuse large B-cell lymphoma and follicular lymphomas.[199–201] A radiolabeled form of this product (Yttrium-90 Zevalin) has also yielded promising preliminary results.[202] These agents are currently under investigation in children. $CD30^+$ lymphomas such as anaplastic large cell (ALCL), mediastinal B-large cell and Hodgkin's disease are also potential candidates for antibody therapy. In this regard, a humanized anti-CD30 antibody (SGN-30) has been shown to have preclinical activity in both cell culture and xenograft mouse model systems of ALCL and Hodgkin disease.[203] Preliminary results from adult phase I and II single-agent trials of SGN-30 suggest that it is both well tolerated and active against $CD30^+$ lymphomas. Trials are currently ongoing to study this agent in children with ALCL. Novel immunotherapeutic approaches may also include the use of surface protein-specific cytotoxic T lymphocytes; this approach has been successful in both the prevention and treatment of EBV-related posttransplant lymphoproliferative disease.[204] Agents that target the specific molecular lesion are also being developed. In this regard, the use of small-molecule inhibitors for tumors such as ALCL that contain the NPM–ALK fusion gene would be very attractive; studies are currently ongoing.[205] The implementation of antiidiotype and antisense strategies are also being studied.[206]

The continued investigation of molecular abnormalities and pathogenic mechanisms of malignant transformation associated with childhood lymphomas is essential. The use of microchip gene arrays has already been shown to identify clinically relevant subtypes of large B-cell lymphomas in adults.[74,75] The results of gene array analyses of Burkitt lymphoma,[207–210] anaplastic large cell lymphoma,[211] and T-lymphoblastic disease[212] have also been reported. Similar studies are ongoing for lymphomas occurring in children, with preliminary results for those with T-lymphoblastic lymphoma recently published.[213] Comprehensive molecular characterization of childhood lymphomas may help to further refine disease classification, provide a means of detecting minimal residual disease (MRD) during clinical remission and enhance our assessment of early response. In this regard, it has been demonstrated that the level of MRD in the peripheral blood is equivalent to that in the bone marrow of children presenting with advanced-stage lymphoblastic lymphoma.[214] In a current COG study of children with this lymphoma subtype, peripheral blood samples are being analyzed at various time points during induction to measure rates of early response. Additionally, a more complete understanding of the molecular pathogenesis of pediatric NHLs will provide clues to novel and more successful treatment strategies, including those directed toward tumor-specific molecular lesions.

ACKNOWLEDGMENT

This work was supported in part by grant CA-21765 from the National Institutes of Health, and by the American Lebanese Syrian Associated Charities (ALSAC).

SUGGESTED READINGS

Cairo MS, Gerrard M, Sposto R, et al: Results of a randomized international study of high-risk central nervous system B non-Hodgkin lymphoma and B acute lymphoblastic leukemia in children and adolescents. Blood 109(7):2736, 2007.

Campana D, Coustan-Smith E, Sandlund J, Abromowitch M: A novel approach for staging and minimal residual disease detection in T-cell lymphoblastic lymphoma—A Children's Oncology Group Study. Ann Oncol 16(Suppl 5):62, 2005.

Dave SS, Fu K, Wright GW, et al: Molecular diagnosis of Burkitt's lymphoma. N Engl J Med 354(23):2431, 2006.

Goldberg JM, Silverman LB, Levy DE, et al: Childhood T-cell acute lymphoblastic leukemia: The Dana-Farber Cancer Institute acute lymphoblastic leukemia consortium experience. J Clin Oncol 21(19):3616, 2003.

Harris NL, Horning SJ: Burkitt's lymphoma—the message from microarrays. N Engl J Med 354(23):2495, 2006.

Hummel M, Bentink S, Berger H, et al: A biologic definition of Burkitt's lymphoma from transcriptional and genomic profiling. N Engl J Med 354(23):2419, 2006.

Lamant L, de Reynies A, Duplantier MM, et al: Gene-expression profiling of systemic anaplastic large-cell lymphoma reveals differences based on ALK status and two distinct morphologic ALK+ subtypes. Blood 109(5):2156, 2007.

Laver JH, Kraveka JM, Hutchison RE, et al: Advanced-stage large-cell lymphoma in children and adolescents: Results of a randomized trial incorporating intermediate-dose methotrexate and high-dose cytarabine in the maintenance phase of the APO regimen: A Pediatric Oncology Group phase III trial. J Clin Oncol 23(3):541, 2005.

Laver JH, Mahmoud H, Pick TE, et al: Results of a randomized phase III trial in children and adolescents with advanced stage diffuse large cell non-Hodgkin's lymphoma: A Pediatric Oncology Group study. Leuk Lymphoma 43(1):105, 2002.

Link MP, Shuster JJ, Donaldson SS, et al: Treatment of children and young adults with early-stage non-Hodgkin's lymphoma. N Engl J Med 337(18):1259, 1997.

Lorsbach RB, Shay-Seymore D, Moore J, et al: Clinicopathologic analysis of follicular lymphoma occurring in children. Blood 99(6):1959, 2002.

Morris SW, Xue L, et al: Alk+ CD30+ lymphomas: A distinct molecular genetic subtype of non-Hodgkin's lymphoma. Br J Haematol 113(2):275, 2001.

Patte C, Auperin A, Michon J, et al: The Societe Francaise d'Oncologie Pediatrique LMB89 protocol: Highly effective multiagent chemotherapy tailored to the tumor burden and initial response in 561 unselected children with B-cell lymphomas and L3 leukemia. Blood 97(11):3370, 2001.

Patte C, Auperin A, Gerrard M, et al: Results of the randomized international FAB/LMB96 trial for intermediate risk B-cell non-Hodgkin lymphoma in children and adolescents: It is possible to reduce treatment for the early responding patients. Blood 109(7):2773, 2007.

Quackenbush J: Microarray analysis and tumor classification. N Engl J Med 354(23):2463, 2006.

Reiter A, Schrappe M, Tiemann M, et al: Improved treatment results in childhood B-cell neoplasms with tailored intensification of therapy: A report of the Berlin-Frankfurt-Munster Group Trial NHL-BFM 90. Blood 94(10):3294, 1999.

Reiter A, Schrappe M, Ludwig WD, et al: Intensive ALL-type therapy without local radiotherapy provides a 90% event-free survival for children with T-cell lymphoblastic lymphoma: A BFM group report. Blood 95(2):416, 2000.

Sandlund JT, Downing JR, Crist WM: Non-Hodgkin's lymphoma in childhood. N Engl J Med 334(19):1238, 1996.

Stein H, Foss HD, Durkop H, et al: $CD30^+$ anaplastic large cell lymphoma: A review of its histopathologic, genetic, and clinical features. Blood 96(12):3681, 2000.

Williams DM, Hobson R, Imeson J, et al: Anaplastic large cell lymphoma in childhood: Analysis of 72 patients treated on The United Kingdom Children's Cancer Study Group chemotherapy regimens. Br J Haematol 117(4):812, 2002.

REFERENCES

For complete list of references log onto www.expertconsult.com

CHAPTER 82

RADIOIMMUNOTHERAPY FOR B-CELL NON-HODGKIN LYMPHOMA

Thomas E. Witzig

INTRODUCTION

The most significant advances in the treatment of non-Hodgkin lymphoma (NHL) in the last decade have been anti-CD20 immunotherapy and radioimmunotherapy (RIT).[1] Rituximab is an unlabeled (*cold*) monoclonal antibody that targets the CD20 antigen on benign and malignant B-cells. In 1997, rituximab became the first monoclonal antibody to be approved by the Food and Drug Administration (FDA) for the treatment of cancer. The pivotal clinical trial treated 166 patients with relapsed B-cell NHL with rituximab 375 mg/m^2 weekly for four doses and demonstrated an overall response rate (ORR) of 48% with 6% complete remission (CR) and a 13-month time to tumor progression (TTP).[2] High response rates have also been demonstrated in previously untreated patients with follicular NHL.[3,4] Randomized trials have demonstrated the superiority of rituximab chemotherapy combinations in both indolent[5,6] and aggressive NHL.[7–10] The results of rituximab chemoimmunotherapy is further discussed in Chapters 79 and 80.

Despite these impressive results with immunotherapy and chemoimmunotherapy, patients cannot be promised cure, and there is room for improvement. Unlabeled monoclonal antibodies theoretically must target each tumor cell to kill. RIT involves the linking of a radionuclide to an antibody to form a radioimmunoconjugate (RIC) (Fig. 82–1). In RIT the goal is to attach a radionuclide with high energy but short path length to the antibody to focus radiation on the target cell population while sparing the effects of radiotherapy on the nearby normal tissue. The RIC kills tumor cells by the direct effects of the antibody, such as antibody-dependent cellular cytotoxicity (ADCC), as well as the effects of ionizing radiation. The radionuclide can potentially be attached to any antibody. The choice of antibody depends on the antigenic profile of the tumor cell to be targeted. Ideal targets are those antigens that are expressed on tumor cells but not normal cells so as to avoid toxicity to normal organs. Cell surface antigens that are not internalized or shed from the cell surface are preferred. The microscopic intratumoral dosimetry of the radionuclide appears to be important.[11]

The application of RIT to treat B-cell NHL was a logical choice because it has been known for many years that NHL are sensitive to radiation delivered by conventional external sources. Indeed, radiation therapy has been a mainstay in the treatment of bulky masses that are producing normal organ compromise and is effective at relieving pain from spinal cord compression. The difficulty with applying radiation therapy to indolent NHL relates primarily to the widespread nature of these tumors even at initial diagnosis. In addition, extensive radiation damages normal marrow making it difficult to provide effective chemotherapy or to collect stem cells at a later date. For these reasons conventional external beam radiotherapy (RT) has been typically limited to involved field applications in this disease.

Initial studies of RIT in lymphoma used polyclonal antibodies;[12] however, most RIC today are murine monoclonal antibodies.[13,14] Recent studies of RIT using a variety of tumor antigen targets on NHL cells have indeed demonstrated tumor regressions with very few side effects in normal organs other than myelosuppression.[15–41] This review will focus on RIC that target CD20 that are now in clinical use for FDA-approved indications.[13,42–49] The CD20 antigen has proven to be an excellent target for RIT because CD20 expression is restricted to normal B cells, almost all B-cell NHL express CD20, the antigen is not internalized within the cell or expressed on other normal tissue (including stem cells), and depletion of normal B-cells by these antibodies has not led to significant short or long-term side effects.

RADIONUCLIDES USED IN RADIOIMMUNOTHERAPY

There are many different radionuclides that have been attached to antibodies for the treatment of cancer.[50] The most common ones in current use and that are commercially available are yttrium 90 (^{90}Y) and iodine 131 (^{131}I). Administration of a RIC is preceded by a dose of cold antibody to deplete normal blood B-cells and block nonspecific binding sites resulting in improved tumor to normal organ biodistribution. There are several differences in the two radionuclides that affect the methods of delivery of the respective RIC in the clinic (Table 82–1). To date, these differences have not translated into any apparent clinical advantages of one radionuclide over another. The ^{131}I labeled antibodies can be used for imaging and dosimetry because they are γ emitters. In contrast, as ^{90}Y is a pure β emitter, imaging is performed with γ-emitting indium 111 (^{111}In)-labeled antibodies. For ^{131}I RIC, patient-specific dosing is used because of differences in renal excretion between patients. In the case of ^{90}Y, the dose for nonmyeloablative use is determined by the weight of the patient in kilograms (with a maximum of 32 mCi) rather than from dosimetry because only 7% of ^{90}Y is excreted from the kidneys over 7 days. ^{111}In imaging is still required to ensure there is normal biodistribution. In most states in the United States, ^{131}I -labeled RIC can be administered as an outpatient; however, outside the United States patients may be required to be hospitalized briefly after administration of ^{131}I RIC. ^{90}Y RIC can be administered to patients in the outpatient setting because they do not emit γ radiation. With ^{131}I RIC oral iodine is required before and after the RIT to block the thyroid; this is not necessary with ^{90}Y.

RIT must be handled and injected by personnel certified by the Nuclear Regulatory Commission. Administration of RIT is a team effort between the hematologist/oncologist who is caring for the patient and the nuclear medicine physician or radiation oncologist who will administer the RIT.[51,52]

CHARACTERISTICS OF RADIOLABELED MONOCLONAL ANTIBODIES TO CD20

Ibritumomab Tiuxetan (Zevalin)

Ibritumomab is a murine anti-CD20 antibody from which the human chimeric antibody rituximab (Rituxan and MabThera; Biogen IDEC Cambridge, MA and Genentech, Inc, South San Francisco, CA) was engineered. Ibritumomab, a murine anti-CD20 antibody, was attached to tiuxetan, a MX-DTPA linker-chelator to form Zevalin (Biogen IDEC Cambridge, MA). Tiuxetan forms a covalent, urea-type bond with ibritumomab and chelates the radionuclide through five carboxyl groups. Zevalin is then reacted with either ^{111}In for tumor imaging and dosimetry or with ^{90}Y for therapeutic RIT.

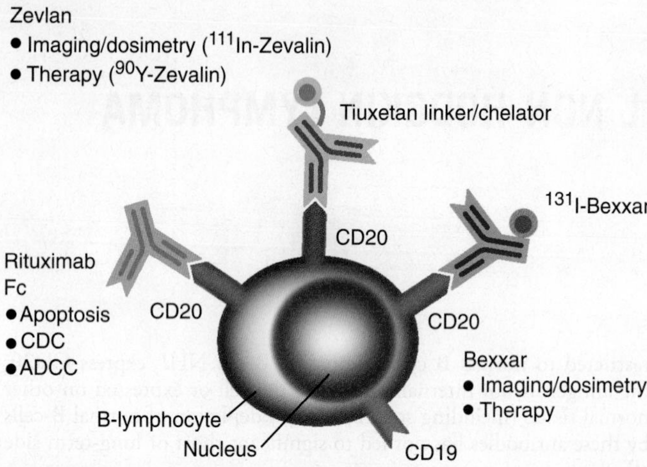

Figure 82–1. B-cell lymphoma cells express CD20, which can be targeted with unlabeled (rituximab) or labeled monoclonal antibodies. Ibritumomab tiuxetan (Zevalin) is the murine parent antibody from which the human chimeric antibody rituximab was engineered. Tiuxetan is a linker/chelator to which indium 111 (^{111}In) (for imaging and dosimetry) or yttrium 90 (^{90}Y) (for therapy) can be attached. In the case of tositumomab (Bexxar) the ^{131}I is directly attached to the murine antibody and the resulting radioimmunoconjugate used for imaging and dosimetry.

Table 82–1. Characteristics of Radionuclides Currently Used in Radioimmunotherapy

Parameter	^{131}Iodine	^{90}Yttrium
Gamma emission	Yes	No
β emission	Yes	Yes
β emission path length (mm)	0.8 mm	5 mm
Theoretical half-life	8 days	2.4 days
Free radioisotope	Thyroid/stomach	Bone
Administration	Outpatient in most states	Outpatient
Pretreatment cold antibody	Yes	Yes
Imaging	Yes	No (^{111}In required as a surrogate)

^{111}In, indium 111.

^{90}Y emits pure β radioactivity with a path length of approximately 5 mm. Because there is no γ emission, useful tumor and normal organ images cannot be obtained with ^{90}Y-Zevalin. ^{111}In emits γ rays, therefore ^{111}In-Zevalin is used to produce high-quality images of the tumor and normal organs for dosimetry and biodistribution studies.[52–56] Patients are imaged in anterior and posterior projections in a whole body area mode between day 1 (the day of ^{111}In-Zevalin injection) and day 7. In the research trials of Zevalin if the ^{111}In-Zevalin scans predicted that the delivered dose of radiation to any non-tumor organ was greater than 2000 cGy, or if the dose to the bone marrow was greater than 300 cGy, then no treatment with ^{90}Y-Zevalin was to be administered.[57,58] No patient in these trials failed dosimetry using these parameters.

The first phase I trial of Zevalin used cold ibritumomab before Zevalin and stem cells were cryopreserved in case of prolonged myelosuppression. Patients were treated with single doses of 20 to 50 mCi of Zevalin; doses equaling 40 mCi were not myeloablative.[25] The second phase I trial used rituximab 250 mg/m^2 as the unlabeled antibody before Zevalin, and patients were treated with one of three dose levels—0.2, 0.3, or 0.4 mCi/kg. If the patient weighed more than 80 kg the dose was capped at 32 mCi. Higher doses were not tested because stem cell cryopreservation was not required as part of the protocol eligibility. There was no provision for retreatment in this trial.[28] The FDA approved the Zevalin treatment program in February 2002. It delivers rituximab and ^{111}In-Zevalin on day 1 followed by one imaging session to determine biodistribution 48 to 72 hours later (images at other time points are optional). The amount of uptake of ^{111}In-Zevalin in a specific lesion is not predictive of tumor response;[59] therefore, the imaging is only performed for safety. If there is normal ^{111}In-Zevalin biodistribution, on day 8 the patient receives a second dose of rituximab followed by ^{90}Y-Zevalin over 10 minutes. The dose of Zevalin is determined by weight and baseline platelet count. If the platelet count is normal (>150,000 cells/mm^3) the recommended dose is 0.4 mCi/Kg; if the platelet count is between 100 and150,000 cells/mm^3, the dose is 0.3 mCi/Kg. The dose is capped at 32 mCi for patients weighing more than 80 kg.

Tositumomab (Bexxar)

Tositumomab is an IgG2a murine monoclonal antibody directed against CD20 (see Fig. 82–1). It was previously referred to as anti-B1[22,60] before being named tositumomab. For RIT, tositumomab has been radiolabeled with ^{131}I. Because ^{131}I emits γ as well as β radiation ^{131}I-tositumomab can be used for both dosimetry and treatment, that is, there is no need for ^{111}In.[61] The Bexxar treatment regimen consists of cold tositumomab and ^{131}I -tositumomab (GlaxoSmithKline, Research Triangle Park, NC). Tositumomab is administered intravenously on 2 treatment days with each day consisting of two separate infusions. Although both Zevalin and Bexxar require tumor imaging, for Bexxar the dosimetry is used to calculate a patient-specific therapeutic dose.[62] This is necessary because of the interpatient differences in body mass (weight), spleen size, tumor burden, and the metabolism and renal excretion of ^{131}I.[22,61–64] Because of the propensity of iodine to concentrate in the thyroid, saturated potassium iodide solution (SSKI; Lugol's) is started 1 day before the cold tositumomab and is continued for 2 weeks after the radiolabeled tositumomab. The first treatment is referred to as the *dosimetric dose.* It consists of tositumomab 450 mg over 1 hour followed by 5 mCi of ^{131}I- tositumomab. γ Scans to measure whole body counts are performed on day 1 and repeated within 2 to 4 days and 6 to 7 days after the dose. The results of the dosimetry determine the amount of radiation activity (as mCi of ^{131}I) needed for each patient to receive a specified total body absorbed radiation dose 75 cGy for patients who have platelet counts greater than 150,000 cells/mm^3 or 65 cGy for patients with platelets between 100,000 and 150,000 cells/mm^3. The therapeutic dose is given within 7 to 14 days of the dosimetric dose and consists of 450 mg of tositumomab followed by a 20-minute infusion of the patient-specific mCi amount of ^{131}I-tositumomab. The Bexxar therapeutic program can be given as an outpatient procedure for the vast majority of patients using the revised US Nuclear Regulatory Commission (NRC) regulations 10CFR 35.75, which allow outpatient release if the total effective dose equivalent to another person who is exposed to the treated patient is less than 500 mrem.[65,66]

CLINICAL RESULTS OF ANTI-CD20 RADIOIMMUNOTHERAPY FOR RELAPSED NHL

The clinical trials of the two anti-CD20 RIC that were performed to assess toxicity and efficacy have primarily been limited to patients with relapsed disease and excellent bone marrow and normal organ function. The eligibility requirements for both the Zevalin and Bexxar trials have been similar except for certain studies as mentioned below (see Phase I Bexxar Trial, Phase II Trials of Bexxar, and Pivotal Trial of Bexxar). Patients were to have measurable disease, bone marrow with less than 25% involvement with lymphoma, absolute neutrophil count ≥1500, platelet count ≥100,000 cells/mm^3, normal renal and liver function, and less than 25% of the bone marrow previously treated with external beam radiotherapy. Patients were excluded from these trials if they had CNS lymphoma, HIV infection or HIV-related NHL, chronic lymphocytic leukemia (CLL), pleural or peritoneal fluid that was positive for lymphoma, known myelodysplasia, or history of a prior allogeneic or autologous stem cell transplant. Tables 82–2 and 82–3 describe the patient population included in each of the clinical trials, Table 82–4 summarizes the efficacy results, and Table 82–5 the hematologic toxicity (Fig. 82–2). In general, both Bexxar and Zevalin as single-agents in relapsed-indolent NHL produce an ORR of 80% with 30% CR and 20% of patients achieving long-term remissions without relapse to date. These agents can produce impressive responses in both nodal and extranodal disease without damage to adjacent normal structures (Fig. 82–3). The only side effect is reversible myelosuppression; there is no solid organ toxicity.

Phase I Bexxar Trial

The phase I trial of ^{131}I-tositumomab was designed to determine a dose that could be administered without stem cell support.[22,23,67] Patients were treated with 15 to 20 mg of intravenous anti-B1 (anti-CD20) mouse monoclonal antibody trace-labeled with ^{131}I (5 mCi) over 30 minutes. The first 10 patients received ^{131}I-tositumomab without cold tositumomab pretreatment. The next eight patients were given a small dose (135 mg) of cold tositumomab pre-^{131}I-tositumomab, and another two received 685 mg pretreatment.[22]

Table 82–2. Summary of the Clinical Trials of Ibritumomab Tiuxetan (Zevalin)

Trial	N	Goal
IDEC 106-02[25]	14	• Used cold ibritumomab prior to ^{90}Y-ibritumomab • Determine MTD
IDEC 106-03[28]	51	• Determine dose of rituximab prior to ^{111}In-ibritumomab • Determine MTD
IDEC 106-04[34]	143	• Randomized trial of rituximab vs ^{90}Y-ibritumomab to determine if efficacy of ^{90}Y-ibritumomab is superior
IDEC 106-05[35]	30	• Efficacy and toxicity of 0.3 mCi/kg ^{90}Y-ibritumomab for patients with platelet count of 100K–149K × 10^6/L
IDEC 106-06[76]	54	• Efficacy and toxicity of 0.4 mCi/kg ^{90}Y-ibritumomab for patients refractory to rituximab.
Safety analysis[73]	349	• Evaluate the side effects experienced by patients treated with ^{90}Y-ibritumomab on clinical trials

IDEC, IDEC Pharmaceuticals, San Diego, CA; ^{111}In, indium 111; MTD, maximum tolerated dose; ^{90}Y, yttrium 90.

Table 82–3. Clinical Trials of ^{131}I-Tositumomab in Patients without the Use of Stem Cell Support

Trial	N	Goal
Phase I[22,23,67]	59	• Used single or multiple doses trace-labeled tositumomab prior to therapeutic ^{131}I-tositumomab • Determine MTD of ^{131}I-tositumomab
Phase II[37,68]	86	• Validate dose determined in phase I
Pivotal[32]	60	• Compared response to last qualifying chemotherapy to that obtained with ^{131}I-tositumomab
Cold versus hot[75]	48	• Establish improved efficacy of radiolabeled tositumomab compared to cold tositumomab
Rituximab-refractory[78]	38	• Evaluated response to ^{131}I-tositumomab in patients failing rituximab
Previously untreated[108]	76	• Evaluated overall and complete response rate in patients treated with ^{131}I-tositumomab as their first therapy

^{131}I, iodine 131; MTD, maximum tolerated dose.

Table 82–4. Response Rates in Trials without Stem Cell Support

Trial	Agent	N	ORR	CR	DR	DR/CR
Phase 1[22,23,67]	^{131}I-Tositumomab	59	71	34	8.9	18.3
Phase I[25]	^{90}Y-Ibritumomab	14	79	36	—	—
Phase I/II[28]	^{90}Y-Ibritumomab	51	67	26	11.7+	
Phase II[37]	^{131}I-Tositumomab	45	57	32	9.9	19.9
Phase II[68]	^{131}I-Tositumomab	41	76	49	1.3	>2.5 years
Pivotal[32]	^{131}I-Tositumomab	60	65	17	6.5	
Randomized[34]	^{90}Y-Ibritumomab	73	80	30	14.2 (0.9–28.9)	
Randomized[75]	^{131}I-Tositumomab	42	67	33	NR	
Previously untreated[108]	^{131}I-Tositumomab	76	95	74	NR	
Transformed[81]	^{131}I-Tositumomab	71	39	25	20	36.5
Rituximab refractory[76]	^{90}Y-Ibritumomab	54	74	15	6.4 (0.5–≥24.9)	
Rituximab refractory[78]	^{131}I-Tositumomab	33	58	21	17	
Expanded access[69]	^{131}I-Tositumomab	273	58	27	NR	
Phase II for patients with thrombocytopenia[35]	^{90}Y-Ibritumomab	30	83	43	11.7 (3.6–≥23.4)	

CR, complete remission; DR, duration of response; DR/CR, duration of response in the CR patients; ^{131}I, iodine 131; ORR, overall response rate; ^{90}Y, yttrium 90.

Table 82–5. Hematologic Toxicity Experienced with Anti-CD20 Radioimmunoconjugates

Study	Neutrophils		Platelets		Hemoglobin	
	Nadir × 10⁶/L	*% Grade 4 (<500 × 10⁶/L)*†	*Nadir × 10⁶/L*	*% Grade 4 (<10,000 × 10⁶/L)*††	*Nadir (g/dL)*	*% Grade 4 (<6.5 g/dL)*
Zevalin Studies						
Phase I[28]	1100	27	49,500	10	—	—
Randomized trial[34]	900	32	42,000	6	10.8	1
Phase II for patients with thrombocytopenia[35]	600	33	26,500	13	10.1	3
Rituximab-refractory[76]	700	35	33,000	9	9.9	4
Bexxar Studies						
Pivotal trial[32]	800	18	50,000	2	10.2	0
Rituximab-refractory[78]	1200	16	90,000	11	NA	
Combined analysis[71]	1060	16	70,000	2	11.1	1
Previously untreated[108]	1300	34 (grades 3/4)	83,000	0	NA	
Phase II in early relapse[68]	1200	20	78,000	5	11.3	0

†Grade 4 neutropenia is <500 × 10⁶/L.
††Grade 4 thrombocytopenia is <10,000 × 10⁶/L.

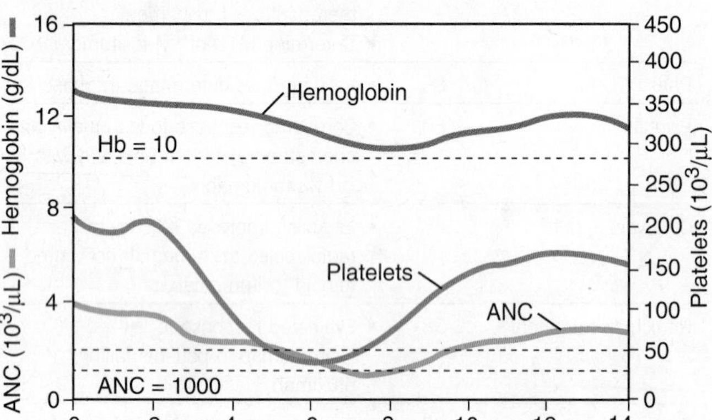

Figure 82–2. Median blood counts in 349 patients treated with ibritumomab tiuxetan (Zevalin) radioimmunotherapy.[73] ANC, absolute neutrophil count; Hb, hemoglobin.

Thirty-four patients were included in the next phase I report.[23] All patients received at least one tracer dose, and 68% (23:34) had more than one tracer dose. It was concluded that indeed the cold predose did improve tumor/normal organ biodistribution. The trial treated patients with doses calculated to deliver 25 to 85 cGy to the whole body. Of the 34 patients entering the trial, 28 (82%) received a therapeutic dose; three patients developed a human antimouse antibody (HAMA), and three had rapid progression during the tracer studies that precluded treatment.

The dose-limiting toxicity (DLT) was myelosuppression and occurred at 85 cGy when two of the three patients treated at this dose experienced grade 3 and 4 absolute neutrophil count (ANC) and platelets. The maximum tolerated dose (MTD) was therefore determined to be 75 cGy. Three patients in the trial who had been previously treated with a stem cell transplant had more severe myelosuppression. The ORR in the 28 patients receiving a therapeutic dose was 79% (22:28) with 50% CR (14:28). Six patients who had achieved a partial remission (PR) or minor response were administered a second dose, and three had a further response, but none of the three patients converted to a complete remission (CR). The disease remission (DR) for CR patients was 16.5 or more months; the DR was not reported for PR patients nor was the TTP. When patients relapsed it was in areas not previously involved by NHL in 75% (6:8) patients. Four patients were retreated at relapse, and all responded again (2 CR; 2 PR).[23]

The next report on this phase I/II trial concluded that a predose of 475 mg of cold tositumomab produced optimal tumor/normal organ biodistribution, and indeed that was the dose used in all the other trials discussed below (see Phase II Trials of Bexxar and Pivotal Trial of Bexxar).[67] The ORR was 71% (42:59) with 34% (20:59) CR. The patients with low-grade or transformed NHL had an ORR of 83% compared to 41% in those with intermediate-grade NHL. The median DR for all responders was 8.9 months (18.3 months for CR patients). Additional long-term followup of these 59 patients was described in 2000.[40]

Phase II Trials of Bexxar

Several dedicated phase II trials were conducted to validate the high ORR to Bexxar determined in the phase I/II trials.[22,23,67] Vose and colleagues[37] treated 47 patients with relapsed low-grade or transformed NHL with either 75 cGy or 65 cGy depending on baseline platelets. The calculated dose to the normal organs for patients receiving the 75 cGy total body dose was as follows: 499 cGy to the kidneys, 383 spleen, 225 liver, 214 bladder, and 183 to the lungs. The tumors were calculated to receive a mean dose of 795 cGy. The ORR was 57% (27:45) and 32% (15:45) had a CR. The median DR was 9.9 months for all responders and 19.9 months for responders that were CR. The median TTP for all patients was 5.3 months and 11.6 months for responders. There was no mention of any patient developing myelodysplastic syndrome or acute leukemia. One patient (2%) developed a HAMA.

A more recent phase II trial of single-agent Bexxar restricted the patient population to only one or two prior therapies.[68] The ORR was 76% (31:41) with 49% CR and unconfirmed/uncertain complete remission (CRu); the median DR for all responders was 1.3 years. The median DR in the CR patients has not yet been reached, but will be longer than 2.5 years. Seven of the patients had transformed histology, and the ORR was 71% (5:7) with 29% (2:7) CR/CRu. Patients with bulky disease (mass >5 cm) had a lower chance of ORR but a similar DR.

Pivotal Trial of Bexxar

The pivotal Bexxar trial enrolled 60 patients with relapsed low-grade (n = 36), transformed (n = 23), or mantle-cell (n = 1) NHL, and compared the ORR and DR to Bexxar with that achieved by the patient's last qualifying chemotherapy. The patients had received a median of four prior chemotherapies (range, 2–13 chemotherapies) and were required to have failed to respond or progressed within 6 months of the last chemotherapy regimen. The patients were a median of 54 months from initial diagnosis, 44% had an elevated

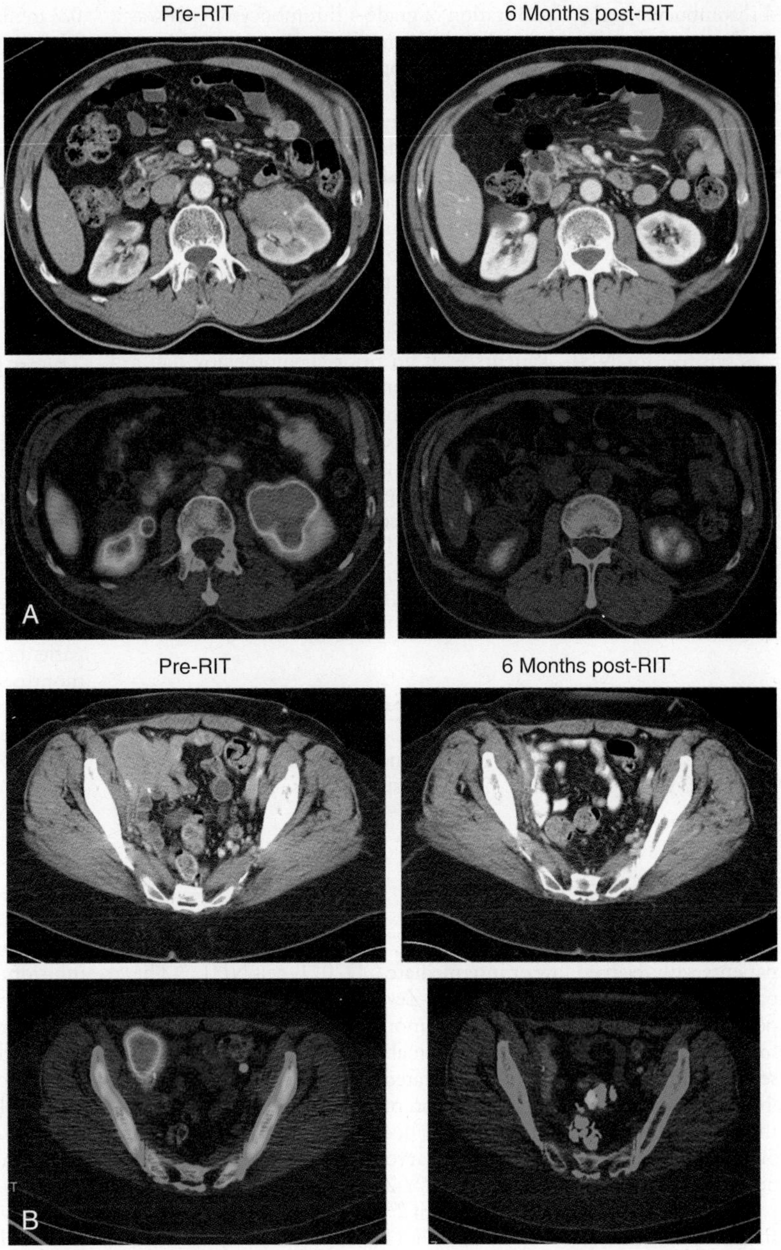

Pre-RIT 6 Months post-RIT

Pre-RIT 6 Months post-RIT

Figure 82–3. Computed tomography (CT) and positron emission tomography (PET) scans before and after ibritumomab tiuxetan (Zevalin) radioimmunotherapy in two patients with relapsed follicular lymphoma. (**A**) Extranodal disease—left renal mass that is PET-avid pretreatment is effectively treated with radioimmunotherapy. This is a good example of the clinical usefulness of RIT to treat extranodal disease with radiation with excellent preservation of underlying organ function. (**B**) Nodal disease-complete response in a bulky nodal mass in the pelvis.

lactate dehydrogenase (LDH), and 55% had bulky disease (mass = 5 cm). The primary end point was DR. Nineteen patients in the trial had responses equivalent to that of their last qualifying chemotherapy. Of the 41 cases where DR was not equivalent, 32 (78%) patients experienced a longer DR with Bexxar compared to nine (22%) patients who experienced a longer DR with chemotherapy ($P < 0.001$). The median DR from Bexxar was 6.5 months compared to 3.4 months with chemotherapy. The ORR was a secondary end point in the trial; it was 65% (39:60) with Bexxar compared to 28% (17:60) with chemotherapy ($P < 0.001$). Seventeen percent (10:60) had a CR with Bexxar compared to 3% (2:60) with chemotherapy ($P = 0.01$).[32]

After the initial trials of Bexxar demonstrated a high ORR with acceptable toxicity an expanded access study treated patients with relapsed low-grade or transformed NHL with standard doses of Bexxar (total body dose of 75 cGy for patients with platelets >150,000 cells/mm^3 and 65 cGy for platelets 100,000–150,000 cells/mm^3).[69,70] Ninety-eight percent (359:368) received Bexxar, and 273 are currently evaluable for efficacy. The ORR was 58% and 27% had a CR. The ORR in rituximab failures was 47% (55:118) with 19% CR (23:118). In patients with bulky tumors (mass >5 cm) the ORR was 47% (57:121) with 17% (20:121) CR. The TTP for all patients was 7.1 months; the median TTP and DR in responders have not yet been reached.

SAFETY OF BEXXAR RADIOIMMUNOTHERAPY

The potential adverse events with the Bexxar treatment program include a transient flu-like syndrome and bone marrow suppression. There is typically minimal infusion-related toxicity with cold tositumomab infusion, and only 7% and 2% of patients experienced an adverse event that required an adjustment to the rate of infusion during the dosimetric and therapeutic doses, respectively. The marrow toxicity has been summarized for 215 patients who received a 75 cGy total body dose.[71] The median neutrophil nadir was 1060 cells/mm^3 occurring at day 46 and recovering by day 66. Sixteen percent of patients developed grade 4 neutropenia with a median duration of 11 days. The median time to platelet nadir was 32 days, the platelet nadir was 70,000 cells/mm^3, and only 2% of patients developed grade

4 thrombocytopenia. The duration of grade 4 thrombocytopenia was 14 days, and the platelets recovered in a median time of 50 days from the day of treatment. The median hemoglobin nadir was 11.1 g/dL on day 46. Only 1% of patients developed grade 4 anemia, and the hemoglobin recovered a median of 61 days following the therapeutic dose. Seventeen percent of patients required hematologic supportive care with 8% receiving a platelet transfusion, 9% red blood cell (RBC) transfusion, and 12% growth factors (granulocyte colony-stimulating factor [GCSF], granulocyte-macrophage colony-stimulating factor [GM-CSF], or erythropoietin).

The hematologic nadirs varied by patient characteristics. For example, patients with a negative bone marrow pre-Bexxar had a 12% incidence of grade 4 neutropenia compared to 21% if the marrow was positive for NHL. Patients with no prior chemotherapy had a 5% incidence of grade 4 neutropenia compared to 21% if they had one to three prior regimens and 23% if they had four prior regimens. The need for hematologic supportive care ranged from 0% in previously untreated patients to 32% in patients with three prior therapies. There was no difference in incidence of grade 4 toxicity by age. The toxicity of Bexxar in the expanded access study showed similar results.[70] The HAMA rate was 8%. HAMA has not been reported to influence overall survival (OS) in the trials of Bexxar and Zevalin; however, in the trials of the Lym-1 RIC patients who developed HAMA actually had a superior OS.[72]

RESULTS OF CLINICAL TRIALS OF ZEVALIN

Five separate clinical trials of ^{90}Y-Zevalin have been conducted over the last 10 years (see Table 82–2). The results of these trials are briefly reviewed.

Phase I Trials of ^{90}Y-Zevalin

There were two phase I trials of Zevalin. The first study enrolled 14 patients with relapsed low or intermediate CD20$^+$ B-cell NHL.[25] The patients were imaged twice with ^{111}In-Zevalin—the first imaging was performed without unlabeled ibritumomab; the second was performed following unlabeled ibritumomab. A comparison of the two sets of ^{111}In-Zevalin images demonstrated that pre-dosing with cold ibritumomab improved biodistribution of the Zevalin. Patients were then treated with ^{90}Y-Zevalin with doses ranging from 13.5 to 50 mCi. All patients had stem cells harvested from peripheral blood or marrow prior to treatment with ^{90}Y-Zevalin; however, only two patients (both had received 50 mCi of ^{90}Y-Zevalin) required reinfusion of stem cells. The ORR was 79% (11 : 14) with 36% CR, and 43% PR.

A second phase I study of Zevalin was conducted to test the use of rituximab rather than cold ibritumomab before Zevalin. It was felt that rituximab was less likely to cause a HAMA or human antichimeric antibodies (HACA) than murine ibritumomab. An additional goal of the second phase I trial was to determine the maximum tolerated dose of ^{90}Y-Zevalin that could be given to patients without the use of stem cells or prophylactic growth factors. Fifty-one patients were enrolled, and the study demonstrated that 250 mg/m^2 was the optimal dose of rituximab to be used before ^{111}In-Zevalin imaging and ^{90}Y-Zevalin therapy.[28] Dosimetry predicted that all patients were eligible for ^{90}Y-Zevalin; that is, all normal non-tumor bearing organs were predicted to receive less than 2000 cGy and the bone marrow, less than 300 cGy.[58] The median age was 60 years, and 24% of patients were older than 70 years of age. In the low-grade group, 6% of patients had diffuse small lymphocytic, 27% follicular small cleaved, and 33% had follicular mixed lymphoma. All patients had received prior chemotherapy (median of two regimens), and 92% had received an anthracycline. Thirty-seven percent of patients had received prior external beam radiotherapy; 27% had two extranodal sites of disease; 59% had bulky disease (mass = 5 cm), and 43% had a bone marrow positive for NHL. The doses of ^{90}Y-Zevalin used in the phase I/II trial were 0.2 mCi to 0.4 mCi/kg; 5 patients received 0.2 mCi/kg, 15 received 0.3, and 30 patients received 0.4. All patients who received 0.4 mCi/kg were able to recover bone marrow function without prophylactic growth factors or stem cells. The dose was not increased to greater than 0.4 mCi/kg because substantial myelosuppression was already being obtained with 0.4 mCi/kg, and stem cells had not been collected pre-Zevalin. The efficacy portion of the phase I/II trial demonstrated a 67% ORR in all patients with 26% CR. In patients with low-grade NHL the ORR was even higher at 82% with 26% CR.[28] The median time-to-progression for responders was 15.4 months; the DR was 11.7 or more months.

Use of Zevalin in Patients with Mild Thrombocytopenia

Both of the phase I trials indicated that the DLT was reversible myelosuppression. Because of previous treatment some patients have mild thrombocytopenia and are therefore at increased risk of myelosuppression from RIT. To study this group of patients further a separate phase II trial using a reduced-dose ^{90}Y-Zevalin (0.3 mCi/kg) for patients with platelet counts between 100,000 to 149,000 × 10^6/L was designed. Thirty patients were treated in this study, and the ORR was 83% with 43% CR/CRu. The TTP was 9.4 months in all patients and 12.6 months in responders.[35] The median DR was 11.7 months (3.6–23.4 months). Hematologic toxicity was the primary toxicity with a median nadir absolute neutrophil count of 600 × 10^6/L (grade 4 in 33% of patients). The median nadir platelet count was 26,500 × 10^6/L (grade 4 in 13% of patients).

Safety of Zevalin Radioimmunotherapy

The safety of Zevalin RIT in 349 patients treated on all reported studies to date has been summarized.[73] Infusion-related toxicities were typically grade 1 or 2 and were associated with the rituximab infusion; there were no further infusion-related reactions when Zevalin was administered at the conclusion of the rituximab. No significant normal organ toxicity was noted. The main toxicity noted was myelosuppression (see Table 82–5) with the nadir hemoglobin, white blood cell (WBC), and platelet counts typically occurring at 7 to 9 weeks and lasting approximately 1 to 4 weeks depending on the method of calculation (see Fig. 82–2). Following the 0.4 mCi/kg dose, grade 4 neutropenia, thrombocytopenia, and anemia occurred in 30%, 10%, and 3% of patients, respectively, and following the 0.3 mCi/kg dose in 35%, 14%, and 8%. Bone marrow involvement with NHL at study entry was present in 146 patients (42%). Patients with any degree of bone marrow involvement had a significantly greater incidence of grade 4 neutropenia ($P = 0.001$), thrombocytopenia ($P = 0.013$), and anemia ($P = 0.040$) than patients with no bone marrow involvement. The incidence of grade 4 hematologic toxicity increased with increasing levels of bone marrow involvement at baseline.

Because in all of these trials prophylactic growth factors were not prescribed, it is not yet known whether grade 3 or 4 myelosuppression can be prevented if growth factors were integrated into the Zevalin program. Despite the substantial myelosuppression observed with RIT, only 7% of patients were hospitalized with infection (3% with neutropenia), and only 2% had grade 3 or 4 bleeding events. A recent case report documented skin necrosis after extravasation of Zevalin;[74] therefore, RIC should be considered vesicants.

RADIOLABELED RITUXIMAB

Another approach to anti-CD20 RIT is to radiolabel rituximab with ^{131}I. Leahy and colleagues[41] conducted a trial that enrolled 91 patients with relapsed CD20$^+$ B-cell NHL. The entry criteria were similar as the Bexxar and Zevalin trials except there were no restrictions on the level of marrow involvement. The ORR was 76% with 53% CR/

CRu. The median DR was 10 months (20 months for CR patients). Nine patients were enrolled with greater than 25% marrow involvement with NHL. These patients had a lower platelet nadir, but the incidence of grade 4 myelosuppression was not different than those patients with less than 25% marrow involvement.

RADIOIMMUNOTHERAPY VERSUS IMMUNOTHERAPY

At the conclusion of the initial phase I and II trials of RIT for NHL, it appeared that the ORR was higher with RIT than with the same corresponding cold monoclonal antibody. Two key trials were designed to further address the question as to whether RIT was superior to immunotherapy with the a similarly targeted antibody. The first trial, IDEC 106-04 (IDEC Pharmaceuticals, San Diego, CA), was a prospective, randomized trial of RIT verses rituximab in patients with relapsed CD20$^+$ NHL that had never received rituximab. Patients were randomized to receive either 0.4 mCi/kg (maximum of 32 mCi) ^{90}Y-Zevalin or rituximab 375 mg/kg weekly in four doses.[34] One hundred forty-three patients were randomized in this trial—73 received Zevalin and 70 rituximab. The analysis of all 143 patients found an ORR (International Workshop NHL criteria [75]) of 80% with ^{90}Y-Zevalin compared to 56% for rituximab ($P = 0.002$). The CR rate of 30% in the ^{90}Y-Zevalin arm was also higher than the 16% found with rituximab ($P = 0.04$). The median DR was 14.2 months (0.9–28.9 months). The trial was not statistically powered to detect a difference in TTP. The Kaplan-Meier estimated median TTP was 11.2 or more months (range, 0.8–31.5 or more months) for the ^{90}Y-Zevalin group compared with 10.1 or more months (range, 0.7–26.1 months) for the rituximab group ($P = 0.173$). However, the estimated time to next therapy (TTNT) for patients with nontransformed histology indicates a significantly longer TTNT for Zevalin patients (17.8+ months; range, 2.1–21.7+ months) than for rituximab patients (11.2 months; range, 1.3–19.0+ months) ($P = 0.040$).

The second key trial addressing this issue used Bexxar. Seventy-eight patients with relapsed low-grade or transformed NHL were randomized to receive Bexxar or two doses of cold tositumomab.[75] The ORR was 67% (28:42) for Bexxar compared to 28% (10:36) for those who received cold tositumomab ($P < 0.001$). The CR rate was 33% (14:42) versus 8% (3:36) ($P = 0.01$) in the Bexxar and tositumomab arms, respectively. The DR was 18 months for tositumomab and has not been reached for Bexxar. The hematologic toxicity was higher in the RIT arm—17% (7:42) had grade 4 ANC and 5% (2:42) grade 4 thrombocytopenia. The HAMA rate was 17% (7:41) in the patients treated with Bexxar and 25% (9:36) in the cold tositumomab group.

RADIOIMMUNOTHERAPY IN RITUXIMAB-REFRACTORY PATIENTS

The current treatment of new and relapsed NHL includes rituximab; therefore, the more relevant clinical question today is—will patients who are refractory to rituximab respond to an anti-CD20 RIC? Several studies have addressed this, and the answer is—yes, they respond, but the TTP is shorter than if the patient was not rituximab refractory. Rituximab-refractory is currently defined as either no response to a standard course of rituximab or a response that lasts less than 6 months. The trial of Zevalin in this patient population included 54 patients meeting this definition.[76] All were treated with a single dose of 0.4 mCi/kg of ^{90}Y-Zevalin and were followed without further therapy. The median age was 54 years (range, 34–73 years), 95% of patients had follicular NHL, 32% had bone marrow involvement, and 74% had bulky disease (mass = 5 cm). The ORR using International Workshop criteria[77] was 74% with 15% CR. The median TTP estimated by the Kaplan-Meier method is 6.8 months (range, 1.1–25.9+ months) with 30% of data censored. Median TTP in the 40 responders is 8.7 months (range, 1.7–25.9+ months), with 28% of data censored. The median DR estimated by Kaplan-Meier is 6.4 months (range, 0.5–24.9+ months).

The study by Horning and coworkers[78] administered a standard dose of Bexxar to 38 patients who had relapsed after rituximab. This trial was slightly different than the Zevalin trial discussed above (see Phase I Trials of ^{90}Y-Zevalin) in that although all patients previously had rituximab, only 24 were rituximab refractory. Thirty-eight patients were treated, and 33 were evaluable for response. Fifty-eight percent of patients responded with 21% CR. In the 24 patients who were rituximab refractory (no prior response) the ORR was 57% (21 of the 24 evaluable), and 14% obtained a CR. Twelve patients had a rituximab response but it lasted less than 6 months. In the 11 patients evaluable the ORR was 55% with 27% CR. Two patients had experienced a response to rituximab that lasted longer than 6 months and the only patient evaluable obtained a CR. The median DR was 478 days (17 months); median TTP was 182 days for the entire group and 566 days for responders. No patient developed a HAMA.

It is apparent from these two important studies that the radiation portion of the RIT is important to the efficacy of RIT. RIT can overcome resistance of rituximab-refractory tumors; however, the responses are not as durable in this more heavily treated population. It is worth noting that these studies for the most part enrolled patients who were rituximab-refractory. This patient group is not the same as patients today who are treated with rituximab-based chemotherapy upfront and then relapse several years later.

RADIOIMMUNOTHERAPY FOR PREVIOUSLY UNTREATED PATIENTS

The high ORR in relapsed patients led to the development of a phase II study of Bexxar in 76 previously untreated patients with advanced stage (stages III or IV) follicular (70% grade 1; 29% grade 2) NHL (one patient had mantle-cell NHL).[18] This is the only trial where a RIC has been used in previously untreated patients. Sixty-four percent of the patients had bone marrow involvement, 30% had an elevated LDH, and 43% had bulky disease (mass = 5 cm). The median age was 49 years (range, 23–69 years). The ORR was 95% (72:76) with 75% (57:75) CR. The 5-year progression-free survival (PFS) for all patients is 59% with a median PFS of 6.1 years. The 5-year PFS for CR patients was 77%, and 70% of the CR patients remained in CR for 4.3 to 7.7 years after treatment. Patients with only a PR had a median TTP of 7 months, and none became long-term responders. Patients with bulky disease (mass >5 cm) and marrow involvement with NHL had a lower chance of obtaining a CR. To date, no patients in this previously untreated group have developed a myelodysplastic syndrome; however, 63% developed a HAMA. Whether the HAMA will wane with time and what impact this will have on the future ability to re-treat patients is unknown. In the studies of Bexxar on previously treated patients the HAMA rate has been approximately 10%. This is likely because of the fact that when patients are previously treated with chemotherapy they are more immunosuppressed and less likely to develop a HAMA. The HAMA rate in the studies with Zevalin has been less than 1%.[73]

RADIOIMMUNOTHERAPY FOR RELAPSED LARGE-CELL LYMPHOMA

Patients with diffuse large-cell NHL that relapse after rituximab, cyclophosphamide, hydroxydaunorubicin, vincristine (Oncovin), and prednisone (RCHOP) and respond to salvage chemotherapy are typically treated with high-dose chemotherapy with stem cell support.

Therefore, the available experience of RIT in aggressive NHL is limited to relapsed refractory disease in patients relapsed after, or not eligible for stem cell transplantation. In the initial phase I/II of Zevalin the ORR was 43% for the 14 patients with intermediate-grade histology.[28] A recent update on the long-term course of patients in that study demonstrated a 58% (7 : 12) ORR for the patients with diffuse large-cell NHL with a median DR of 49.8 months (1.3–67.6+ months).[79]

A more recent study with shorter followup evaluated Zevalin in the treatment of 104 elderly patients with relapsed and primary refractory diffuse large B-cell lymphoma that were not candidates for stem cell transplantation. The ORR in the entire group was 44%.[80] Patients not treated with rituximab-based chemotherapy had a 52% ORR compared with a 19% ORR in the group that had previously been treated with rituximab. The latter group appears to have been particularly high-risk as 37% were reported to be refractory to RCHOP. Although the treatment was generally well tolerated, four patients died because of adverse events. Three of these were cerebral hemorrhages associated with grade 4 thrombocytopenia; the other case was a late hemorrhage not attributed to RIT.

RADIOIMMUNOTHERAPY FOR TRANSFORMED LYMPHOMA

Patients who transform from low-grade to large-cell NHL are a difficult group to treat. Eligible patients are typically recommended for high-dose therapy with stem cell support. However, these patients may be elderly, lack stem cell reserve, or have other comorbidities that make transplant impossible. The largest clinical experience of treating transformed NHL with RIT has been with Bexxar.[81] There were 71 patients with transformed lymphoma who had been enrolled in the five studies since 1990. In addition to the transformed histology, 28% of patients had bone marrow involvement, 70% had bulky disease (mass >5 cm), 57% had elevated LDH, and 52% had an International Prognostic Index (IPI) score of three or more. The ORR was 39% with 25% CR. The median DR was 20 months (range, 10.8 months—not reached) for all responders and was 36.5 months (range, 14.7 months—not reached) for CR patients. The median TTP for all patients was 4.3 months (3.2–10.2 months), but for those who responded to treatment the median TTP was 20.2 months (12.4 months—not reached). Five patients remain in remission beyond 40 months.

THERAPY OF CENTRAL NERVOUS SYSTEM LYMPHOMA WITH RADIOIMMUNOTHERAPY

Primary central nervous system lymphomas (PCNSLs) are difficult to treat if the patient relapses after initial therapy. Whole-brain radiation therapy is useful but can produce long-term side effects. There has been minimal use of RIT for PCNSL, but several case reports show promise. Shah and coworkers[82] reported the first successful case of PCNSL treated with single-agent Zevalin. More recently, Pitini and colleagues[83] treated two patients with relapsed PCNSL with standard Zevalin and both entered CR. After recovery from myelosuppression the patients were treated with maintenance temozolomide and remain in CR. This is clearly an area that requires further investigation.

LONG-TERM RESULTS OF RADIOIMMUNOTHERAPY

Prolonged followup of the initial studies provides useful data on the long-term prognosis of patients with relapsed indolent NHL treated with RIT.[79,84–86] Long-term responses (LTRs) have been defined as CR or PR for at least 12 months. Fisher and coworkers[84] reported results on 250 patients with relapsed or refractory low-grade or transformed NHL who had been treated with Bexxar. LTRs were achieved in 81 (32%) of 250 patients; 23% had a PFS longer than 18 months, and 21% had a PFS longer than 2 years (Fig. 82–4A and B). Patients who became long-term responders were more likely to have had a CR (77% vs. 8%, respectively) and low-bulk disease (51% vs. 31%, respectively) than those without a LTR. Other characteristics that were predictive of a LTR with Bexxar treatment were sensitivity to the last therapy, history of fewer than three previous therapies, follicular histology, normal LDH level, and modified IPI score of 2. The LTR patient population had a median DR of 45.8 months with a median followup of 61 months. Those patients who attained a CR have done especially well; the median DR has not been reached, and 47% remain in CR ranging from longer than 2.7 years to longer than 10.2 years. In the previously untreated study the only patients with extended remissions were those who had a CR.[18] A smaller series of 18 patients treated with Bexxar also demonstrated that six of the eight patients with CR/CRu remained in unmaintained remission at 46 to 70 months.[86]

Long-term responses were seen in 37% (78 : 211) of patients treated on Zevalin trials for relapsed NHL.[85] Patients with bulky disease (masses >5 cm) were less likely to become long-term responders; however, if they did respond, the DR was similar to those with low-bulk disease. The achievement of a CR/CRu was a strong positive predictor of an LTR, with an odds ratio of 7.0 (95% confidence interval, 3.4–14.5). At a median followup of 53.5 months (range, 12.7–88.9 months) the median duration of response was 28.1 months, and the median time to progression was 29.3 months. The findings in patients with follicular lymphoma (n = 59) were similar to those in the overall population of long-term responders. The estimated overall survival at 5 years was 53% for all patients treated with Zevalin and 81% for long-term responders (see Fig. 84–4C and D). It is now apparent that even in the relapsed indolent patient population that LTR can be observed with single doses of RIT. Patients who are treated early in the relapse phase of disease have a higher rate of CR and a longer TTP than those who are treated after multiple relapses.[87]

RISK OF MYELODYSPLASIA WITH RADIOIMMUNOTHERAPY

Once it was determined that myelosuppression was the primary toxicity of RIT, there has been concern that these agents might increase the risk of myelodysplastic syndrome (MDS)/acute leukemia (AL). This issue has been followed closely in all the trials of RIC. In the Bexxar database of 995 patients who received a single dose of Bexxar for relapsed NHL, MDS or AL has been documented in 35 patients (3.5%). All 35 patients had also received chemotherapy for their NHL. The annualized rate of MDS/AL was 1.6%, a rate similar to that observed in chemotherapy-alone treated patients.[88] Although followup is short, to date there have been no patients with MDS in the previously untreated group of patients treated with Bexxar.[18,88]

A recent analysis of 746 patients treated with Zevalin between 1996 to 2002 included patients in the trials discussed earlier as well as the compassionate-use trials. A total of 17 cases of MDS/AL have now been identified for an incidence of 2.3% (17 : 746). The MDS/AL occurred at a median of 5.6 years (range, 1.2–13.9 years) after the diagnosis of NHL and 1.5 years (range, 0.1–5.8 years) after RIT. The annualized rates were 0.3% (95% confidence interval [CI], 0.2%–0.4%) a year after the diagnosis of NHL and 0.7% (95% CI, 0.4%–1.0%) a year after RIT.[89]

At this juncture, now more than 10 years after the initiation of the RIT trials, there is no evidence yet that RIT increases the risk of MDS/AL over that of chemotherapy alone and no cases of MDS/AL in patients treated only with RIT. This issue will need ongoing investigation. Actually, the issue of bone marrow damage may become more relevant as RIT is used earlier in the disease course because patients will have longer OS post-RIT with more time for MDS/AL to become apparent.

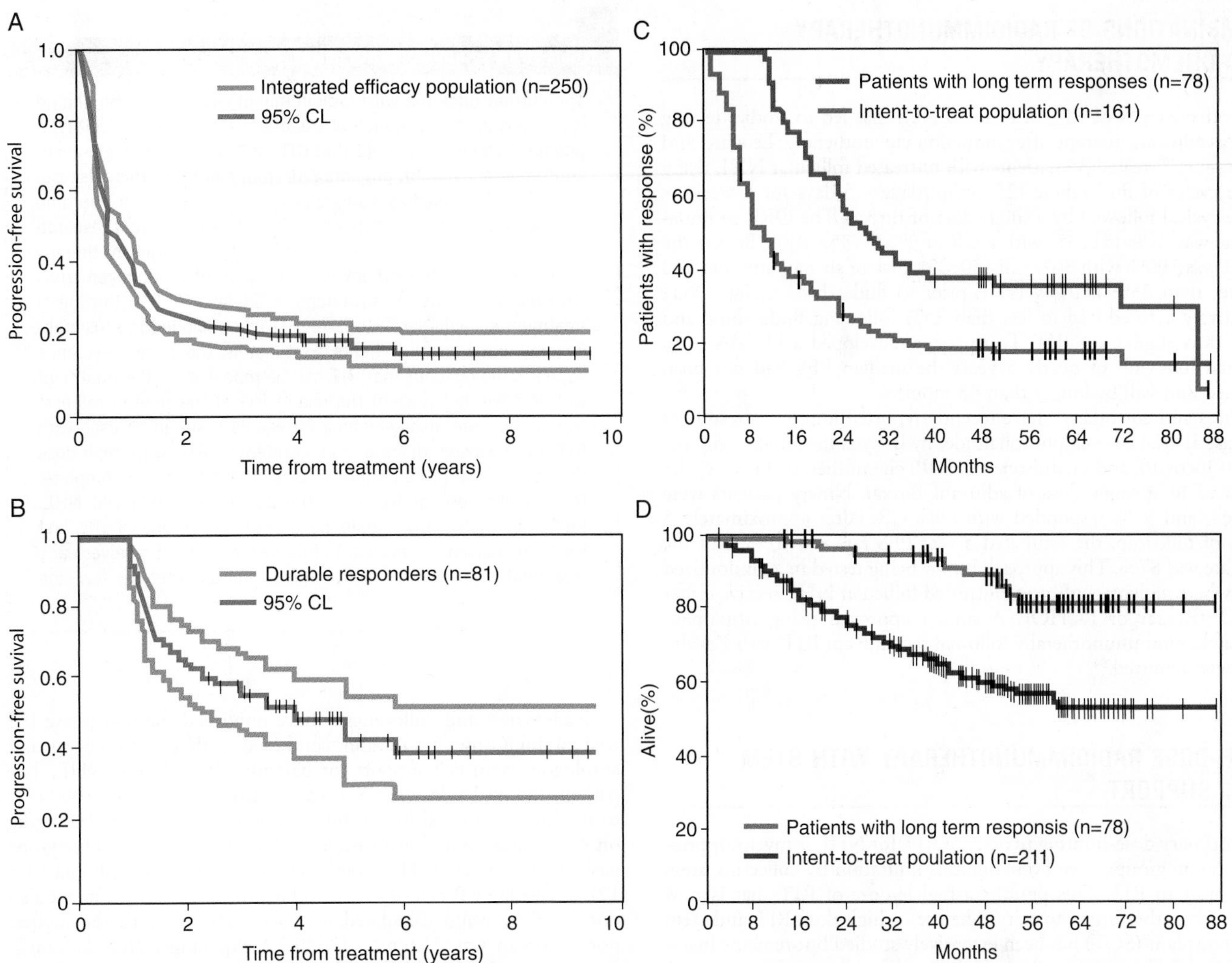

Figure 82–4. Survival results of patients with relapsed non-Hodgkin lymphoma treated with single-agent tositumomab (Bexxar) or ibritumomab tiuxetan (Zevalin) and no maintenance therapy. A long-term or durable response was defined as a response (complete or partial) that lasted longer than 1 year. **(A)** Progression-free survival of 250 patients treated on Bexxar clinical trials.[84] **(B)** Progression-free survival of the 81 patients who had a long-term response.[84] **(C)** Duration of response of all 161 responders compared to the 71 patients who achieved a long-term response after treatment on a Zevalin clinical trial. **(D)** Overall survival of the long-term response population ($n = 71$) compared to all 211 patients treated on Zevalin clinical trials. CL, confidence limits.

FEASIBILITY OF TREATMENT AFTER RADIOIMMUNOTHERAPY FAILURE

Because the CR rate with RIT when used for relapsed NHL is approximately 30%, most patients will at some point relapse and require additional therapy. The myelosuppression universally observed after RIT has raised the question of the feasibility of chemotherapy following RIT. Ansell and colleagues[90,91] examined the subsequent therapy administered to 58 patients who had relapsed after receiving 0.4 mCi/kg of ^{90}Y-Zevalin. The median number of therapies the patients had received before Zevalin was two (range, 1–7 therapies). Twenty-eight (48%) of the patients had transformed NHL—14 had the transformation before Zevalin and in 14 the transformation developed after Zevalin (8 at first relapse after Zevalin; 6 during the chemotherapy that followed Zevalin). The median WBC count at the time of the next therapy after Zevalin was 4.2×10^9/L (range, 0.9–8.7 cells), the median hemoglobin was 11.6 g/dL (range, 7.2–14.7 cells), and the median platelet count was 163,000 cells/mm^3 (range, 14,000–292,000 cells). The median number of subsequent treatments received was two (range, 1–7 treatments). Subsequent chemotherapy was feasible and tolerable. Peripheral blood stem cell collection was also feasible, with one of eight patients requiring marrow harvest after failing peripheral blood stem cell collection. All eight patients engrafted. An additional patient received an allogeneic transplant with adequate engraftment.

The issue of treatment after RIT has also recently been addressed using the Bexxar patient database. Sixty-eight patients who relapsed a median of 168 days after RIT were reviewed.[92] At the time of relapse, the median WBC was 4900 cells/mm^3 (range, 1100–24,100 cells) and the median platelet count was 130,000 cells/mm^3 (range, 9,000–440,000 cells); only the platelet count was significantly lower than the pre-RIT value. The 65% (44:68) of patients who received further chemotherapy were able to receive a median of two (range, 1–4 treatments) additional regimens using typical myelosuppressive agents. Thirteen patients went on to stem cell transplantation—3 had stem cells harvested prior to RIT; 10 after RIT.

Although these data are encouraging, it should not be interpreted that collection of stem cells will be feasible in all patients after RIT. It can be difficult to collect stem cells from patients that have received extensive chemotherapy or external beam radiation therapy even in the absence of RIT.[93] If the patient is considered to be a strong candidate for autologous transplant, stem cells should be collected before RIT.

COMBINATIONS OF RADIOIMMUNOTHERAPY AND CHEMOTHERAPY

The effectiveness of RIT in relapsed NHL has led to studies testing RIT as adjuvant therapy after induction chemotherapy. Leonard and collleagues[16] treated 35 patients with untreated follicular NHL using three cycles of fludarabine (25 mg/m^2/days × 5 days for 5 weeks × three cycles) followed by a single dose of Bexxar. The ORR to fludarabine was 89% (31:35) with a CR of 9% (3:35). After Bexxar the ORR was 100% with 86% CR (30:35). Five of six patients who had greater than 25% marrow NHL prior to fludarabine therapy were effectively cytoreduced to less than 25% following fludarabine and were thus eligible for RIT. Two patients developed a HAMA. At a median followup of nearly 5 years the median PFS had not been reached and will be longer than 48 months.

Press and coworkers[17] have recently reported long-term results of a phase II trial of cyclophosphamide, hydroxydaunorubicin, vincristine (Oncovin), and prednisone (CHOP) chemotherapy for six cycles followed by a single dose of adjuvant Bexxar. Ninety patients were treated, and 91% responded with 69% CR. After approximately 5 years of followup, the estimated 5-year PFS rate was 67%, and the OS rate was 87%. This approach is now being tested in a randomized trial where patients with new, untreated follicular NHL receive either CHOP/Bexxar or RCHOP. A similar approach using rituximab-based chemoimmunotherapy followed by adjuvant RIT with Zevalin has been reported.[94]

HIGH-DOSE RADIOIMMUNOTHERAPY WITH STEM CELL SUPPORT

The primary dose-limiting toxicity of RIT for NHL is myelosuppression. Some groups have overcome this limitation by collecting stem cells prior to RIT. This permits a higher dose of RIT that is now limited by other organ toxicity. The use of high-dose RIT and stem cell transplant (SCT) has been extensively studied but remains investigational.[95–97] In a phase I study, Press and colleagues[98] entered 43 patients, and 19 were able to receive therapeutic infusions of Bexxar. The ORR was 95% (18:19) and 84% (16:19) had a CR. An additional 25 patients were enrolled into the phase II trial,[26] and 84% (21:25) were treated. Tumor response was observed in 86% (18:21) with 76% CR. The stem cells were infused 12 to 18 days after Bexxar; the source of stem cells was bone marrow in 19 and blood stem cells in the other 2. Neutrophil recovery to greater than 500 and platelet count recovery to greater than 20,000 occurred a median of 23 days and 22 days, respectively, after stem cell infusion. HAMA was documented in 16%. Long-term followup (median 42 months) on these patients and those from the phase 1 trial demonstrated that the projected OS and PFS was 68% and 42%, respectively.[21]

These studies have been expanded to combine Bexxar with cyclophosphamide and etoposide with autologous stem cell support.[31] Fifty-two of the 55 enrolled received treatment. All patients were required to have a bone marrow that had less than 25% involvement with NHL. The study determined that a dose of Bexxar that delivered 25 Gy to critical normal organs could be safely combined with chemotherapy and stem cells. The estimated OS and PFS at 2 years was 83% and 68%, respectively. Gopal and coworkers[99] recently compared the long-term results of patients with relapsed follicular NHL treated with SCT. The 27 patients conditioned with high-dose Bexxar RIT had a superior OS and PFS compared to 98 patients treated with chemotherapy and total body irradiation or chemotherapy-alone. The estimated five-year OS and PFS were 67% and 48%, respectively, for high-dose Bexxar conditioning, and 53% and 29%, respectively, for chemotherapy alone or chemotherapy/TBI. Performing SCT with RIT-alone conditioning is well tolerated even in older adults.[100] Sixteen patients with mantle cell NHL have been treated with a similar protocol,[101] and all patients had a tumor response with 91% CR. The OS and PFS at 3 years were 93% and 61%, respectively.

WHEN TO USE RADIOIMMUNOTHERAPY?

The current dilemma with radioimmunotherapy is "when should it be used in the sequence of treatment for indolent B-cell lymphoma"? There is no doubt that RIT has the highest single-agent antitumor activity of any drug or treatment for this disease. However, when used as a single-agent for relapsed NHL the time to progression for most patients is 1 to 2 years. Current research is moving RIT to initial treatment by itself or as adjuvant therapy after debulking chemotherapy. If the current randomized trials demonstrate a survival advantage of adjuvant RIT in the initial treatment of follicular NHL, then RIT will be added to rituximab-chemotherapy for all patients. Fortunately, the current evidence supports the concept that RIT can be repeated. Initial treatment with RIT will not prevent the use of RIT at the time of relapse. Researchers are also searching for agents that can be used with RIT for relapsed disease and combining RIT with high-dose therapy with stem cell support. Until these trials are complete, the standard use of RIT is in the patient with relapsed NHL. Radioimmunotherapy should be considered as one of the first treatments given for relapse. In this way the patient receives early treatment with the most active agent, and one that has few side effects.

Nademanee and colleagues[102] have published the first phase I/II trial of high-dose ^{90}Y-Zevalin combined with chemotherapy and autologous stem cell support for patients with relapsed NHL. The patients received a dose of ^{90}Y-Zevalin calculated to deliver 1000 cGy to the highest normal organ followed by etoposide 40 to 60 mg/kg on day 4 and cyclophosphamide 100 mg/kg on day 2. Thirty-one patients were treated. Histology included follicular lymphoma (n = 12), diffuse large B-cell (n = 14), and mantle cell (n = 5). The median dose of ^{90}Y-Zevalin calculated to deliver 1000 cGy to the highest normal organ was 71.6 mCi (2649.2 MBq; range, 36.6–105 mCi; range, 1354.2–3885 MBq). Engraftment was prompt with the median times to reach an ANC greater than 500 cells/mm^3 and platelet count more than 20,000 cells/mm^3 were 10 days and 12 days, respectively. During followup there have been two deaths, and five patients have relapsed. The 2-year estimated OS is 92%, and the PFS is 78%. It is to be noted that in this trial the dose of ^{90}Y-Zevalin was not dose escalated beyond a dose calculated to deliver 1000 cGy to the liver. There is another trial combining ^{90}Y-Zevalin with BEAM conditioning chemotherapy and stem cells that is dose escalating the ^{90}Y-Zevalin in a typical phase I protocol. That trial has been published in abstract form.[103]

RETREATMENT WITH RADIOIMMUNOTHERAPY

The high ORR observed with single-agent RIT in relapsed NHL and the excellent toxicity profile has led to increased interest in retreatment. In the original phase I/II trials of Bexxar, 16 patients that responded to Bexxar and later relapsed received a second dose. The ORR with the second dose was 56% with 31% CR.[40] These encouraging results led to a multicenter, phase II trial that treated 32 patients.[19] The ORR was again 56% (18:32) with 25% of patients attaining a CR. Interestingly, 10 of the 18 responders had a DR after the second course of Bexxar that was longer than the DR with the first dose of Bexxar.

There has been limited experience with treating patients with a second dose of Zevalin.[25] Wiseman and coworkers[104] reported preliminary results on a phase I trial where all patients are treated with two sequential doses of Zevalin. The first dose was 0.4 mCi/kg, and the phase I dose levels for the second dose delivered 3 to 6 months after the first dose was 0.2 to 0.4 mCi/kg. In the report of ^{131}I-rituximab six patients with response to the first dose were re-treated at the time of relapse, and four responded with a median DR of 11 months.[41]

RADIATION THERAPY AFTER RADIOIMMUNOTHERAPY

A recent report has demonstrated that patients who relapse or progress with RIT can respond to external beam radiation. Justice and colleagues[105] reviewed 19 patients who received radiation therapy after Zevalin. They found a 90% (26:29 sites radiated) ORR with 12 (41%) CR, 7 (24%) CCR, 7 (24%) PR, and 3 (10%) stable disease. Toxicities were generally transient, reversible, and corresponded to the anatomic regions irradiated.

SUMMARY

The results of the phase I, phase II, and randomized trials demonstrate that single doses of RIT are safe and efficacious in patients with relapsed B-cell NHL. Currently, RIT is used worldwide primarily for patients with indolent NHL that has relapsed after conventional therapy.[106] RIT produces a response rate of approximately 80%, 30% of patients obtain a CR, and 20% have not yet relapsed after years of followup. The primary toxicity is myelosuppression, and this is dose-limiting if stem cell support is not used. Patient acceptance of these agents has been very high, and there is an excellent quality of life.

RIT produces a higher response rate than cold unlabeled rituximab in rituximab-naïve patients. There is also a very high (75%–80%) response rate in rituximab-refractory patients but a shorter TTP in this patient group. RIT produces a longer time to next chemotherapy than rituximab. The rate of HAMA is variable between the two agents (<2% with Zevalin and approximately 10% in Bexxar). Patients who have received RIT have developed MDS and AL following therapy. To date, all of these patients have been previously treated with chemotherapy that included alkylating agents and/or purine nucleoside analogs. Previously untreated patients who received RIT have not developed MDS/AL. At this time, calculations suggest that the rate of MDS is no different in patients who received RIT than those treated with previous chemotherapy, although the time of followup is still relatively short.

There is a lower (approximately 40%), but significance response rate in patients with relapsed large cell lymphomas. The response rate in bulky disease (mass >5 cm) is lower than those patients with nonbulky disease. Preliminary studies indicate that after patients relapse after RIT they can undergo stem cell harvest and receive additional chemotherapy once their counts have recovered from RIT. Stem cell harvest and transplants after radioimmunotherapy are feasible.

FUTURE DIRECTIONS

Current trials are focusing on moving RIT earlier in the disease course with the goal of increasing the rate of CR and prolonging OS. For example, randomized trials are testing RIT as adjuvant therapy after induction rituximab-based chemotherapy for indolent and aggressive NHL (Table 82–6). The safety and efficacy of RIT with stem cell support has led to a randomized phase III trial testing Bexxar-BEAM versus rituximab-BEAM with stem cell support. This large trial will determine if RIT adds to TTP and OS in this patient population. Trials combining agents simultaneously with RIT are somewhat more difficult because of the issue of myelosuppression. The choice of agents to combine must also be made carefully, and the results may not be predictable.[107] These combinations are now being tested in phase I trials to maximize patient safety.

Although there are many studies evaluating the role of rituximab maintenance after chemotherapy or after response to rituximab, to date, there have been no studies providing rituximab maintenance following RIT. Although this certainly is feasible, it is not known whether response can be prolonged. The results of these exciting studies will establish the role of RIT in the overall treatment plan of patients with B-cell NHL.

Table 82–6. Methods to Improve the Clinical Efficacy of Radioimmunotherapy for Non-Hodgkin Lymphoma

Initial therapy in patients with asymptomatic but advanced-stage disease
Adjuvant therapy after chemoimmunotherapy induction
Standard dose RIT with high-dose chemotherapy and stem cell transplant
High-dose RIT with high-dose chemotherapy and stem cell transplant
Addition of immunostimulatory agents to improve killing by antibodies

RIT, radioimmunotherapy.

SUGGESTED READINGS

Ansell SM, Schilder RJ, Pieslor PC, et al: Antilymphoma treatments given subsequent to Yttrium 90 ibritumomab tiuxetan are feasible in patients with progressive non-Hodgkin's lymphoma: A review of the literature. Clin Lymphoma 5:202, 2004.

Dosik AD, Coleman M, Kostakoglu L, et al: Subsequent therapy can be administered after tositumomab and iodine I-131 tositumomab for non-Hodgkin lymphoma. Cancer 106:616, 2006.

Fisher RI, Kaminski MS, Wahl RL, et al: Tositumomab and iodine-131 tositumomab produces durable complete remissions in a subset of heavily pretreated patients with low-grade and transformed non-Hodgkin's lymphomas. J Clin Oncol 23:7565, 2005.

Gopal AK, Rajendran JG, Gooley TA, et al: High-dose [131i]tositumomab (anti-CD20) radioimmunotherapy and autologous hematopoietic stem-cell transplantation for adults ≥60 years old with relapsed or refractory B-cell lymphoma. J Clin Oncol 25(11):1395, 2007.

Horning SJ, Younes A, Jain V, et al: Efficacy and safety of tositumomab and iodine-131 tositumomab (Bexxar) in B-cell lymphoma, progressive after rituximab. J Clin Oncol 23:712, 2005.

Kaminski MS, Estes J, Zasadny KR, et al: Radioimmunotherapy with iodine^{131} tositumomab for relapsed or refractory B-cell non-Hodgkin lymphoma: Updated results and long-term follow-up of the University of Michigan experience. Blood 96:1259, 2000.

Kaminski MS, Tuck M, Estes J, et al: 131I-Tositumomab therapy as initial treatment for follicular lymphoma. N Engl J Med 352:441, 2005.

Kaminski MS, Zasadny KR, Francis IR, et al: Iodine-131-anti-B1 radioimmunotherapy for B-cell lymphoma. J Clin Oncol 14:1974, 1996.

Kaminski MS, Zasadny KR, Francis IR, et al: Radioimmunotherapy of B-cell lymphoma with [131I]anti-B1 (anti-CD20) antibody. N Engl J Med 329:459, 1993.

Knox SJ, Goris ML, Trisler K, et al: Yttrium-90-labeled anti-CD20 monoclonal antibody therapy of recurrent B-cell lymphoma. Clin Cancer Res 2:457, 1996.

Nademanee A, Forman S, Molina A, et al: A phase I/II trial of high-dose yttrium-90-ibritumomab tiuxetan in combination with high-dose etoposide and cyclophosphamide followed by autologous stem cell transplantation in patients with poor-risk or relapsed non-Hodgkin lymphoma. Blood 106:2896, 2005.

Press OW, Unger JM, Braziel RM, et al: Phase II trial of CHOP chemotherapy followed by tositumomab/iodine I-131 tositumomab for previously untreated follicular non-Hodgkin's lymphoma: Five-year follow-up of Southwest Oncology Group Protocol S9911. J Clin Oncol 24:4143, 2006.

Wahl RL. Iodine-131 anti-B1 antibody therapy in non-Hodgkin's lymphoma: Dosimetry and clinical implications. J Nucl Med 39:1S, 1998.

Wiseman GA, Kornmehl E, Leigh B, et al: Radiation dosimetry results and safety correlations from 90Y-ibritumomab tiuxetan radioimmunotherapy for relapsed or refractory non-Hodgkin's lymphoma: Combined data from 4 clinical trials. J Nucl Med 44:465, 2003.

Witzig TE. Efficacy and safety of 90Y ibritumomab tiuxetan (Zevalin) radioimmunotherapy for non-Hodgkin's lymphoma. Semin Oncol 30:11, 2003.

Witzig TE, Flinn IW, Gordon LI, et al: Treatment with ibritumomab tiuxetan radioimmunotherapy in patients with rituximab-refractory follicular non-Hodgkin's lymphoma. J Clin Oncol 20:3262, 2002.

Witzig TE, White CA, Wiseman GA, et al: Phase I/II trial of IDEC-Y2B8 radioimmunotherapy for treatment of relapsed or refractory CD20+ B-cell non-Hodgkin's lymphoma. J Clin Oncol 17:3793, 1999.

Witzig T, Molina A, Gordon LI, et al: Long-term responses in patients with relapsed or refractory B-cell non-Hodgkin lymphoma treated with yttrium 90 ibritumomab tiuxetan. Cancer 109(9):1804, 2007.

REFERENCES

For complete list of references log onto www.expertconsult.com

CHAPTER 83

CHRONIC LYMPHOCYTIC LEUKEMIA

Thomas S. Lin, Farrukh T. Awan, and John C. Byrd

INCIDENCE AND EPIDEMIOLOGY OF CHRONIC LYMPHOCYTIC LEUKEMIA

Chronic lymphocytic leukemia (CLL) is one of the most common types of leukemia in the Western Hemisphere. SEER estimates for 2008 indicated that approximately 15,110 patients (8,750 men and 6,360 women) would be diagnosed in the United States and that 4,390 patients will die from CLL in 2008.[1] The median age at diagnosis for CLL was 72 years during 2000–2005 according to the SEER database. The incidence of CLL increases proportionately by decade, as shown in Fig. 83–1.[1] This figure illustrates that CLL is a very uncommon diagnosis under the age of 45 and infrequent (30% of total patients diagnosed) in patients under the age of 65. The age-adjusted incidence rate was 4 per 100,000 men and women per year; 0.46% of men and women born in 2008 are expected to be diagnosed with CLL during their lifetime.[1] The extended time of survival following diagnosis is 75.9% at 5 years, which explains the estimated prevalence of 95,123 patients living with CLL in the United States currently.[1] Similar to other types of leukemia, the risk of dying from disease-specific causes increases proportionately with increasing age. Another analysis of the SEER database comparing outcome of elderly patients with CLL to age- and sex-matched healthy controls demonstrated that CLL has the greatest impact on survival in the most elderly group of patients.[2] However, even for patients diagnosed with CLL before the age of 50, Montserrat and colleagues demonstrated that the median expected life span is only 12.3 years, compared with 31.2 years in age-matched controls.[3] Thus, CLL is a significant health problem affecting all ages of patients with this disease.

CLL is more common in men than women. Women diagnosed with CLL have 5- and 10-year overall survival (OS) rates that exceed those of men. CLL is most common in Caucasians and decreases in frequency in a descending order among blacks, Hispanics, American Indians and Native Alaskans, and Asians and Pacific Islanders. The rarity of CLL among Asians and Pacific islanders persists even in immigrants from these areas who have migrated to the Western Hemisphere. This implicates a possible genetic predisposition to the development of CLL. The relationship of environmental factors such as exposure to benzene and other chemicals to the development of CLL is not clearly defined.[4–6] However, CLL is recognized as a service-connected illness among Vietnam War veterans who were exposed to Agent Orange.[7] Occupational or environmental exposure to radiation does not appear to predispose patients to a higher risk of developing CLL.[8–11] For example, although the frequency of acute myeloid leukemia, chronic myeloid leukemia, and acute lymphoblastic leukemia were increased among survivors of the atomic bomb at Hiroshima, no increase in CLL was appreciated.[12] Recent studies of leukemia rates in inhabitants around the Chernobyl nuclear reactor accident site have supported this notion, where essentially all other types of leukemia were increased with the exception of CLL.[13,14]

FAMILIAL CLL

Up to 10% of CLL patients have a first- or second-degree relative with CLL,[15] making CLL one of the most common types of malignancy with familial predisposition. Unlike other types of familial cancer, it is very uncommon for CLL patients to have large pedigrees with many affected distant relatives throughout an extensive family tree. Rather, the more common finding is for most patients to have one or two first- or second-degree relatives with this diagnosis.[16] Large case–control studies concluded that the risk ratio (RR) for first-degree relatives of CLL probands to also have CLL was higher than that for most other cancers.[17] Although the average RR for all cancers in a US study was approximately 2.1, CLL showed an RR of 5.0, the fourth highest of all cancers.[17,18] Other studies in Swedish[19] and Icelandic populations[20] have demonstrated a similarly high RR. Relatives of patients with CLL also appear to have a higher frequency of other lymphoproliferative disorders and autoimmune diseases.[21,22] Unlike a variety of other cancers that have known predisposing genes, identification of these in CLL have been generally elusive. To date, only a single germline mutation of death-associated protein kinase (DAPK) has been convincingly linked to familial predisposition in a single CLL family.[23] Two other studies[16,24] were limited by weak evidence for linkage, and the occurrence at many loci were different between the two studies. Two loci at chromosome bands 11p11 and 13q21 were backed by statistically significant evidence, but no genes at these sites have been implicated in familial CLL. The role of anticipation in identifying other family members has been reported by several groups,[25,26] and patients with such a family history are generally diagnosed a median of 10 years earlier than other patients.[27] However, other clinical features of CLL at diagnosis do not appear to be different.[27] Thus, patients with familial CLL do not appear to be genetically or clinically different from individuals with sporadic CLL.

BIOLOGY AND GENETICS OF CLL

The complexity of the biology of CLL has become increasingly apparent as the knowledge of the basic science of this disease has expanded. Despite these advances, many questions remain unsolved, including (a) the cell of origin from which CLL is derived, (b) the existence of a CLL stem cell as occurs in other leukemias, (c) the biological etiology of the divergent natural histories of IgV_H-mutated versus unmutated CLL, and (d) the existence and identification of infectious or other naturally occurring antigens that may drive the B-cell clone in this disease. Nonetheless, significant advances in our understanding of the role of cytogenetics, immunology, and other relevant biological markers in predicting the natural history of disease progression and response to therapy in CLL make an understanding of the basic biology of CLL increasingly relevant and important to the clinician caring for CLL patients.

For many years, CLL was felt to represent a single disease that had a varied natural history. Basic research focused on understanding (a) the normal cell of origin from which CLL is derived, (b) the function of the B-cell receptor in CLL, (c) the maturational point in B-cell development at which CLL occurs, and (d) the relevance and contribution of a self- or acquired antigen to driving the disease. The normal counterpart to the cell of origin of transformed CLL remains unknown, and no stem cell for this disease has been identified. Indeed, CLL is one of the few adult leukemias that does not engraft and proliferate to recapitulate the disease when tumor cells are inoculated or transplanted into immunocompromised mice. Each of these observations are important scientific areas of active, ongoing study,

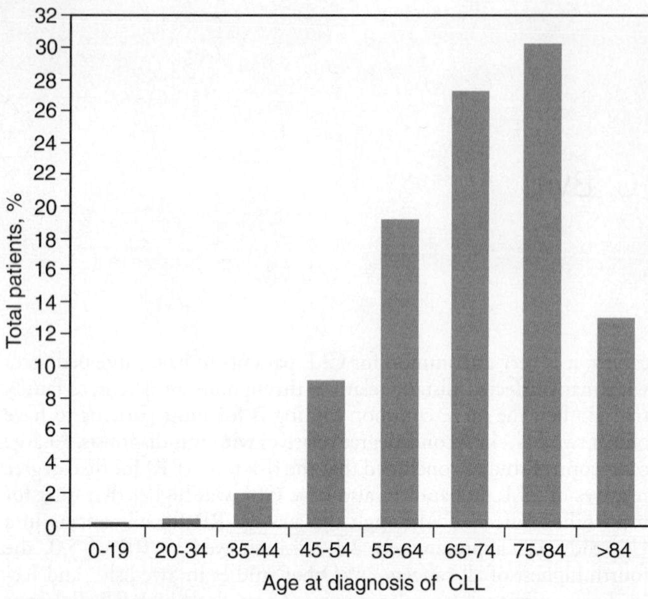

Figure 83–1 Illustration that CLL is a very uncommon diagnosis under the age of 45 and infrequent (30% of total patients diagnosed) in patients under the age of 65.

and the reader is referred to several recent definitive reviews for further information on the basic biology of CLL.[28–33] The biology and genetics covered within this chapter focuses predominately on areas relevant to the clinician who cares for patients with CLL.

IgV$_H$ Mutational Status

Two seminal manuscripts demonstrated that the IgV$_H$ gene had undergone somatic mutation, indicating that the patient's CLL arose after this point in B-cell maturation, in 60% of CLL patients at diagnosis.[34,35] The majority of IgV$_H$-unmutated CLL cells demonstrate evidence of syk activation and other essential B-cell receptor downstream activation signals following ligation of sIgM.[36] In contrast, virtually all IgV$_H$-mutated patients do not signal following ligation by sIgM but can often weakly signal through other alternative B-cell receptors, including sIgD and Ig-α. Thus, although gene expression profiling demonstrates all CLL cells to be most closely related to memory B cells,[37] IgV$_H$-unmutated and -mutated CLL cells differ significantly with respect to their ability to transduce intracellular signals following sIgM ligation.[36,38] A common repertoire of mutational changes among CLL patients has also been documented that differs significantly from that found in the normal adult B-cell repertoire.[39,40] These studies have prompted the hypothesis that CLL may represent an antigen-driven disease similar to other B-cell diseases including monocytoid B-cell lymphoma and gastric MALT lymphomas.[41]

Defective Apoptosis

Since its initial description and early characterization, CLL has been considered a disease of slow accumulation of tumor cells due to disrupted or defective apoptosis. Multiple studies have demonstrated that CLL cells overexpress several antiapoptotic proteins including bcl-2,[42,43] mcl-1,[44,45] bak,[44] and XIAP[46] and have diminished expression of compensatory proapoptotic proteins such as bax. Overexpression of bcl-2[42,43] and mcl-1[44] and an increase of the ratio of these proteins to bax[47,48] have correlated not only with disrupted apoptosis but also shortened overall survival and poor response to therapy. Why are these antiapoptotic genes overexpressed in vivo? Studies have demonstrated that CLL cells have constitutive activation of several antiapoptotic transcription factors including NF-κB,[49,50] NFAT,[51] and STAT3.[52,53] Each of these transcription factors can influence one or more of the antiapoptotic proteins that promote survival in vivo. The source of activation of these different transcription factors is not completely defined but may in part be due to autocrine and paracrine networks involving BAFF, APRIL, VEGF, IL-4, and CD40.[54–58] CLL cells are also maintained through contact with stromal cells (bone marrow and dendritic)[59–61] and nurse like cells through a complex interface of adhesion molecules and stromal survival factors such as SDF.[62–64] The importance of the in vivo environment to CLL survival is supported by the increase in apoptosis when CLL cells are cultured in vitro.

Genetic Abnormalities

Much of the advances in understanding the biology of acute leukemia has come from studying repetitively occurring cytogenetic abnormalities. Such detailed study of the genetics of CLL has been hindered by the inability to effectively induce proliferation of tumor cells for standard metaphase cytogenetic analysis and the poor response of CLL cells to B-cell mitogens. Nonetheless, several cytogenetic studies identified a variety of deletions, including del(11q22.3), del(17p13.1), del(13q14), and del(6q21-q23), as well as trisomy 12, as common abnormalities in CLL. The frequency of these abnormalities has been further refined through the use of interphase cytogenetic analysis, which does not require isolation of dividing cells. These studies have demonstrated that del(13q14) is by far the most common cytogenetic abnormality in CLL, followed by trisomy 12, del(11q22.3), del(17p13.1), and del(6q22.3). Stimulation studies with CpG oligonucleotides plus IL4 or CD40 confirmed the prevalence of these abnormalities and also identified unbalanced translocations not generally observed with traditional metaphase cytogenetics.[65] The prognostic significance of these unbalanced translocations appears to be important, yet the biological role of these translocations in the progression of CLL is not known and requires further study. Interestingly, balanced translocations, which are more frequently observed in acute lymphoblastic leukemia and acute myeloid leukemia, are generally not observed in CLL.

The presence of recurrent deletions in CLL suggests the possibility of unique tumor suppressor genes in these different regions. Extensive pursuit of such genes within the 13q14 region failed to identify a viable tumor suppressor gene candidate for many years. However, in 2002 Croce and colleagues identified miR15 and miR16, two noncoding microRNAs, in the deleted region of 13q14.[66] Noncoding RNAs range in size from 21 to 25 nucleotides and represent a newly recognized class of gene products whose function is to silence genes through binding to the 3′-untranslated region of specific genes to inhibit translation. This same group later showed that mir16 regulates expression of bcl-2, an antiapoptotic protein that is overexpressed in CLL and other B-cell lymphoproliferative disorders.[67] Other miRs have subsequently been shown to be expressed in CLL, and these miRs likely contribute to the pathogenesis of CLL.[68,69] Further study of miRs in CLL is under way to elucidate their full role in the pathogenesis and progression of CLL.

Methylation

In addition to genetic deletions and overexpression of miRs, gene expression can by modified by silencing of the promoter region through methylation. Gene silencing by methylation has been shown to regulate tumor suppressor gene expression in several types of cancer and leukemia. Recently, silencing of genes by methylation was shown to occur in CLL in a gene-specific manner that is greater than that observed in normal B cells. Select genes including ID4,[70] DERMO-1,[71] and SFRP family members[72] were found to be preferentially silenced in CLL, as compared to normal B cells. Additionally, epigenetic silencing of genes such as DAPK was recently noted to be present in 98% of CLL patients and to occur in familial CLL.[23] These

Initial Evaluation of Young Patients with Chronic Lymphocytic Leukemia

Only 10% of patients diagnosed with chronic lymphocytic leukemia (CLL) will be under the age of 50, and these patients often present a diagnostic and therapeutic dilemma to hematologists initially evaluating them. The great majority of patients diagnosed under the age of 50 will have early-stage CLL with a slightly higher predisposition to a prior first generation relative with this disease. Additionally, these patients are generally of a higher economic stature or have chronic fatigue or medical illnesses for which they have been undergoing routine blood testing, leading to diagnosis of CLL. Once the diagnosis of CLL is made, these younger patients have a more challenging time understanding how the disease will impact them. For those patients with no symptoms referable to CLL, I generally discuss complications of the disease during the first visit and have a detailed discussion regarding assessment of genetic risk factors predisposing to early disease progression, including select interphase cytogenetic abnormalities [del(17p13.1) and del(11q22.3) and IgV_H mutational status [unmutated]. During this time it is important to counsel patients that identification of high-risk genomic features can actually increase anxiety and still no treatment intervention will be considered in absence of symptoms outside of a clinical trial. In my experience, the great majority of patients desire this testing. Despite the potential benefit of allogeneic stem cell transplant in younger patients with CLL, I generally mention this as one treatment option used in this disease and do not pursue consultation or tissue typing of patient/siblings until patients are truly symptomatic from their disease. During the second visit 4 to 6 weeks later I review the results of these prognostic factors and answer additional questions that have arisen. Ultimately the majority of patients have low-risk disease, and knowing this allows patients to take partial control and move on. Serial assessment of the psychological well-being of the patient with CLL during this first year is incredibly important. At no place during the evaluation do I refer to CLL as being a good or favorable leukemia. In our experience, the most common reason for dissatisfaction toward the initial hematology evaluation is lack of explanation of the disease process or minimizing CLL as a "good leukemia to have."

For young patients presenting with other chronic medical problems and CLL who are asymptomatic, I follow the approach outlined above. More commonly these patients have fatigue, mild anemia, or other symptoms that could be referable to the CLL. Additionally, this group is more commonly overweight or obese. In either setting, it is important to first think like an internist and pursue other causes for symptoms potentially referable to CLL. In particular for fatigue, encouragement of both weight loss and a fixed exercise plan is encouraged and often improves quality of life and improvement in other medical comorbidities. It is very important to note that younger patients with CLL can often go a decade or more without therapy and early treatment of this patient group still offers no advantage. For this reason our group remains very conservative on starting therapy for the young patient with CLL.

findings provide support for the importance of epigenetic silencing of genes in CLL.

ESTABLISHING THE DIAGNOSIS OF CLL

The diagnosis of CLL, as defined by the NCI working group,[73] requires an absolute lymphocyte count of greater than 5000/μL. Morphologically, the lymphocytes must appear mature with fewer than 55% prolymphocytes (see Fig. 83–1A–E). The bone marrow aspirate smear must show greater than 30% of all nucleated cells to be lymphoid, or the bone marrow core biopsy must show lymphoid infiltrates consistent with CLL (see Fig. 83–1F, G). The overall cellularity must be normocellular or hypercellular. Immunophenotyping must reveal a predominant B-cell monoclonal population coexpressing the B-cell markers CD19, CD20, and CD23 and the T-cell antigen CD5 in the absence of other pan-T cell markers (see below section).

Table 83–1 Diseases That Can Mimic Chronic Lymphocytic Leukemia

Follicular lymphoma
Mantle cell lymphoma
Monocytoid B-cell lymphoma or splenic lymphoma with villous lymphocytes
Hairy cell leukemia
Acute lymphoblastic leukemia
T-cell prolymphocytic leukemia
Large granular natural killer or T-cell leukemia

Patients may present with tumor cells immunophenotypically consistent with CLL but have predominately lymph node disease without a peripheral B-cell lymphocyte count of 5,000/μL despite bone marrow involvement. Although these patients are considered to have small lymphocytic lymphoma (SLL) and not true CLL by the NCI criteria, the most recent World Health Organization (WHO) classification[74] considers such SLL patients to have CLL, given the similar immunophenotypic features, genetic findings, natural history, and complications of these two diseases. The clinical management of SLL patients should be similar to CLL with respect to diagnostic testing and treatment. However, SLL patients may not be eligible for some clinical studies in CLL, if those trials follow NCI criteria and mandate a peripheral B-cell lymphocyte count of 5000/μL for study entry.

The recent increase in diagnostic blood testing for other B-cell lymphoid cancers has led to recognition of a precursor to CLL called monoclonal B-cell lymphocytosis (MBL). Patients with MBL have circulating peripheral B cells immunophenotypically consistent with CLL but do not have enlarged lymph nodes, a lymphocyte count greater than 5000/μL, or bone marrow lymphoid infiltration greater than 30%.[75] The frequency of MBL increases with age; 0.3% of patients under the age of 40 years have MBL compared to 2.1% of 40- to 60-year-old patients and 5.2% of 60- to 90-year-old patients.[76] The frequency of MBL in family members of patients with a first-degree relative with CLL is significantly higher in both young and older patients alike.[76–78] Similar to the relationship of MGUS and multiple myeloma, it appears that only a small proportion of patients with MBL develop overt CLL over time.[75,79,80] Prospective studies to investigate the natural history of isolated MBL will help elucidate the relationship of this diagnosis to CLL.

IMMUNOPHENOTYPIC, CLINICAL, AND LABORATORY FEATURES OF CLL

For many years, the diagnosis of CLL was made based on morphologic examination of the peripheral blood smear, which demonstrated mature lymphocytes with an abundance of smudge cells. Despite rigorous morphology, many diseases can mimic CLL in both appearance and clinical presentation, as summarized in Table 83–1, resulting in incorrect diagnoses. With the advent of new, more effective targeted therapies in CLL and other related diseases listed in Table 83–1, determining the correct diagnosis is of great importance. Flow cytometry, or immunophenotyping, has become a widely used diagnostic test that is currently performed in most reference pathology laboratories, and the use of flow cytometry is now the standard approach to establish the diagnosis of CLL (Fig. 83–2, for example). The diagnosis of CLL relies on immunophenotypic confirmation, and flow cytometry should therefore be performed on all CLL patients at diagnosis. CLL cells have a relatively consistent immunophenotype, which differentiates CLL from mantle cell lymphoma, hairy cell leukemia, follicular center cell lymphoma, splenic lymphoma with villous lymphocytes, and other indolent B-cell malignancies. Specifically, CLL cells expresses a variety of B-cell markers, including dim sIg, CD19, dim CD20 and CD23, as well as the pan T-cell marker CD5. Kappa or lambda restriction is always present, establishing the presence of a clonal B-cell population, although sIg expression may be so dim that light chain restriction may be difficult to determine. In contrast, presence of CD10, FMC7, or CD79b (all typically absent on CLL cells) or bright expression of CD11c, CD20, or CD25 (all typically dim on CLL cells) suggests an alternative low-grade B-cell lymphoproliferative malignancy. Expression of CD5 without CD23 suggests mantle cell lymphoma, and FISH for t(11;14) should be performed to exclude mantle cell lymphoma. Some genetic subsets of CLL are predisposed to variant antigen expression, particularly patients with trisomy 12.[81,82] A scoring system based on antigen expression to definitely diagnose CLL has been proposed but is not widely used.[83] Repeating immunophenotyping after the initial diagnosis is not required unless there is a suspicion of transformation to a more aggressive histology or there is a need to assess bone marrow response, most notably the absence or presence of minimal residual disease, following treatment. Transformation of CLL (Fig. 83–3A–C) to either prolymphocytic leukemia (PLL) or large cell lymphoma (Richter transformation) is often associated with immunophenotypic drift, where CD5 is lost and FMC7 expression is acquired. Additionally, expression of CD20 and surface immunoglobulin typically becomes brighter in PLL or Richter transformation. Although the morphologic appearance of prolymphocytes or large cells in blood, bone marrow or lymph nodes is typically adequate to make the diagnosis of transformation, flow cytometry may be useful in cases where morphologic findings are less clear.

CLL patients often present with no symptoms, with the diagnosis being made as a consequence of asymptomatic enlarged lymph nodes or splenomegaly detected on physical exam or routine blood work done for another cause. Other patients present with symptoms of marrow replacement (fatigue, dyspnea or petechiae secondary to anemia and thrombocytopenia), symptomatic lymphadenopathy or hepatosplenomegaly, autoimmune complications (hemolytic anemia

When Do I Consider a Transplant Evaluation in Chronic Lymphocytic Leukemia?

With the introduction of nonmyeloablative stem cell transplant, the morbidity and mortality associated with this therapy in chronic lymphocytic leukemia (CLL) has decreased and this option thereby has been extended to young and older patients alike. Additionally, extended follow-up in several transplant series has suggested that prolonged remissions can occur with this treatment approach, potentially providing the only curative therapy option for this disease. In general, I do not consider detailed discussion of transplant or referral early in the disease. When patients become symptomatic and require therapy for their CLL, I also consider if they would qualify for transplant. Approximately 50% of patients with CLL are 75 years or younger, have acceptable end-organ function, and lack comorbidities when symptomatic disease develops. It is with this CLL patient group that a transplant consultation with HLA-tissue typing of patient and sibling is considered. For patients attaining a complete remission to initial combination chemotherapy, we would never consider a consolidative stem cell transplant. However, for those patients having only a partial response to combination therapy, remission duration is often short, and particularly in patients with high-risk genomic features such as del(17p13.1) and del(11q22.3), consolidation transplant in first partial remission might be considered. For all patients relapsing after first therapy, I strongly recommend transplant evaluation and pursuit of this option following second treatment unless a complete remission is obtained again. For patients attaining a complete remission both as initial and first relapse therapy, remission duration can be prolonged and transplant can be delayed, particularly in the absence of high-risk genomic features. Usually, patients referred for transplant beyond second-line therapy often do not eventually get to transplant treatment. Reasons for this include inability to cytoreduce for transplant, lack of time to identify unrelated donor, insurance approval delays following meeting criteria for eligibility for transplant and subsequent progression before approval can be obtained, and intervening complications of CLL or therapy that prevent moving forward with transplant. Therefore, if transplantation is to be considered for CLL patients, it should be pursued early in the course of disease.

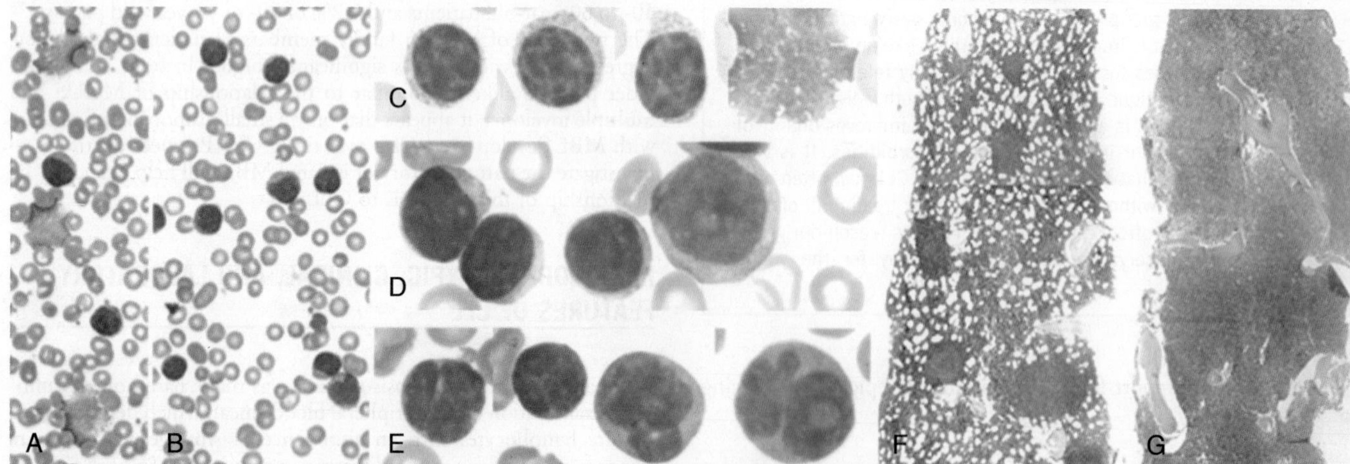

Figure 83–2 Chronic lymphocytic leukemia (**A–G**). Peripheral blood smear (**A**) typically shows lymphocytosis and increased smudge cells as a result of the fragility of the CLL cells (see also smudge cell in **C**, right side). These can be avoided by making a preparation of blood and bovine serum albumin (22%) at a ratio of 11 drops of blood and 1 drop of albumin before preparing the slide (**B**). Cytologic features of CLL cells differ. Classic cells have a small nucleus with a "soccer ball" chromatin pattern (**C**). Some cases have increased large cells, or prolymphocytes, with more open chromatin and prominent "punched-out" nucleoli (**D**; prolymphocyte, right side). Other cases, sometimes referred to as "atypical," can have clefted cells and large cells (**E**). The bone marrow can show nodular infiltrates of CLL cells (**F**), an interstitial infiltrate, or a diffuse infiltrate (**G**).

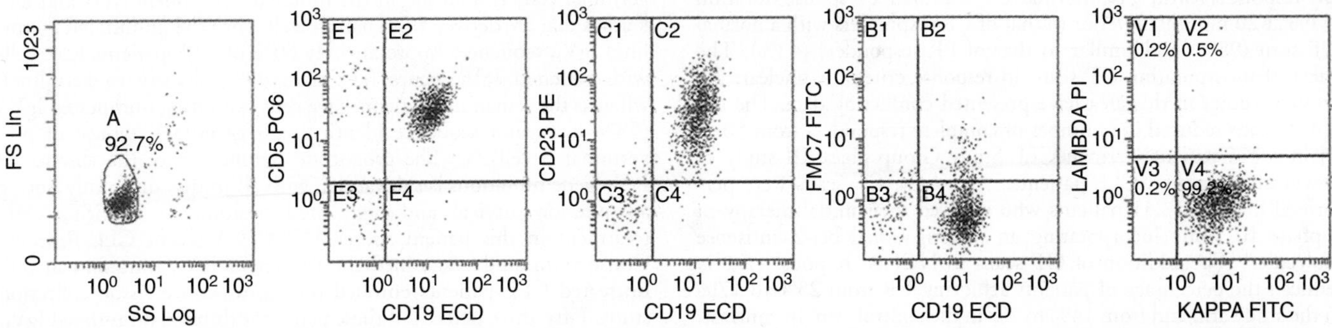

Figure 83–3 Flow immunophenotyping in chronic lymphocytic leukemia (CLL). Flow data in a typical case of CLL. The phenotype is CD19+ clonal B cells with Kappa light chain restriction (weak to moderately intense), with coexpression of CD5 and CD23, but lack of FMC-7. The cells were CD38-negative.

Table 83–2 Rai Staging System

Rai Stage at Diagnosis	Percent of Patients Never Requiring Chronic Lymphocytic Leukemia Therapy	Expected Survival in Months From Initial Diagnosis
0. Lymphocytosis >5 × 10⁹/L only	59	150
1. Lymph node (LN) enlargement	21	101
2. Spleen/liver (S/L) enlargement ± LN	23	71
3. (Anemia with hemoglobin <11 g/dL) ± LN or S/L	5	19
4. (Thrombocytopenia <100 × 10¹²/L ± LN or S/L)	0	19

Adapted from Rai KR, Sawitsky A, Cronkite EP, Chanana AD, Levy RN, Pasternack BS: Clinical staging of chronic lymphocytic leukemia. Blood 46:219, 1975.

or idiopathic thrombocytopenic purpura), or B-symptoms (fevers, night sweats, and weight loss). A small proportion of CLL patients will have pulmonary infiltrates at diagnosis that is representative of CLL involvement in some cases and active infection in others. Clearly, a wide spectrum of presentations exists for patients with CLL.

In addition to blood and bone marrow lymphocytosis, a few abnormal laboratory findings are commonly observed in CLL. Neutropenia, anemia, and thrombocytopenia can develop as a consequence of bone marrow infiltration or therapy administered to eliminate the leukemia. A positive direct antibody, or Coombs, test is observed in approximately 10% to 25% of CLL patients sometime during the course of the disease. Similarly, autoimmune thrombocytopenia or neutropenia may be present, although other causes such as marrow replacement or chemotherapy effect are much more common and should be excluded. Other nonhematologic autoimmune antibodies can rarely be present but do not appear to be more common than age-matched control patients without CLL.[84] Pure red cell aplasia can sometimes be observed with isolated anemia and absence of red cell precursor cells. Hypogammaglobulinemia is common in CLL and becomes more frequent and marked as the disease progresses. In contrast, hypercalcemia and markedly elevated LDH is not common in CLL and suggests Richter transformation.

STAGING AND PROGNOSTIC FACTORS IN CLL

Until recently patients with CLL have been staged utilizing either the Rai or Binet system.[85,86] Both of these discriminate CLL by the sites of disease and degree of cytopenias induced by leukemia marrow replacement. Patients can be categorized into three groups on the basis of these features. According to the modified Rai criteria, patients in the low-risk group (stage 0) have lymphocytosis without any other abnormality; patients in the intermediate-risk group (stages I and II) have, in addition to their lymphocytosis, enlarged lymph nodes and/or spleen or liver; and patients in the high-risk group have anemia (hemoglobin <11.0 g/dL) and/or thrombocytopenia (platelets <100 × 10^9/L). The median survival times for the Rai low-, intermediate-, and high-risk groups are similar to those of Binet stages A, B, and C: 12+, 8, and 2 years, respectively, as shown in Table 83–2.[85,86] For early-stage patients with CLL (Rai low and intermediate stage and Binet stage A and B), a significant range of time to developing symptoms of CLL exists. The lack of survival advantage with early treatment, the observation that a subset of CLL patients will never require therapy, and the varied natural history of the disease has driven research efforts in CLL to identify specific biologic or clinical prognostic factors that predict time to progression; several comprehensive reviews exist.[87–90]

Although lymphadenopathy is a common clinical feature of CLL and is incorporated into both major clinical staging systems, computed tomography (CT) scans are not standardly used to determine staging or to evaluate response to therapy according to NCI 96 criteria. However, several studies have recently examined whether the incorporation of CT scans in initial staging or response evaluation may affect the ability to predict disease progression and assessment of clinical response to therapy. A Spanish study prospectively performed abdominal CT scans on 140 consecutive patients who were diagnosed with Rai stage 0 CLL.[91] CT scans determined abnormal lymphadenopathy or splenomegaly in 27% of patients, and an abnormal CT scan correlated with 50% or more bone marrow infiltration, lymphocyte count of 30 × 10^9/L or greater, lymphocyte doubling time less than 12 months, and zeta-associated protein (ZAP)-70 expression or more. More importantly, patients with an abnormal CT scan were more likely to progress and require earlier therapy than patients with a normal CT scan (RR = 2.7; median TTP 3.5 years vs. not reached). However, no difference in 5-year OS was observed between the two groups.

The same group examined the role of CT scans in predicting response duration in 34 previously untreated CLL patients who received fludarabine, cyclophosphamide, and mitoxantrone (FCM) as initial therapy.[92] Sixty-four percent of the 69 patients treated with FCM achieved a complete response (CR), and 30% of the CR responders had residual abdominal lymphadenopathy by CT scans.

CR responders with an abnormal CT scan had a response duration (54% at 20 months) inferior to that of CR responders with a normal CT scan (95%) and similar to that of PR responders (42%). The effect of incorporating CT scans in response criteria is unclear; the limited studies in this area have presented conflicting data. The use of CT scans reduced the number of complete responders from 50 to 35 in a 375-patient German CLL Study Group phase III study of previously untreated CLL patients.[93] Similarly, CT scans were performed in 189 of 241 patients who received their initial therapy in a phase III study incorporating an investigational bcl-2 antisense molecule.[94] The addition of CT scans to NCI 96 response criteria reduced the percentage of patients achieving CR from 25% to 17% in the study arm and from 14% to 7% in the control arm. In contrast, a retrospective study of 82 patients who underwent pretherapy and posttherapy CT scans in three clinical trials at our institution concluded that CT scans did not improve the predictive power of existing NCI 96 response criteria, which do not use CT scans, in predicting progression-free survival (PFS) or overall survival (OS).[95] Thus, the use of CT scans in staging and response evaluation in CLL needs further study by well-designed, prospective clinical trials. However, CT scans should not be routinely incorporated in standard clinical use until their significance is evaluated by such trials. Although CT scans have been the focus of greatest debate, the use of positron emission tomography (PET) should also be briefly discussed. Specifically, PET scans may be useful in detecting Richter transformation (RT). In a single-institution study of 37 patients, PET scans identified 10 of 11 patients who had documented RT by tissue biopsy.[96] However, nine patients had false positive scans. Thus, PET scans appear to be sensitive for RT, with a high negative predictive value, but specificity is poor.

With recent advances in the molecular biology of CLL, some prognostic factors such as bone marrow infiltration pattern, which requires an invasive procedure at diagnosis, have not maintained their usefulness in predicting disease progression. Prognostic features outside of the traditional staging systems outlined above relative to daily practice are summarized below.

Thymidine Kinase Activity and β_2-Microglobulin

Thymidine kinase is an enzyme involved in the salvage pathway of DNA synthesis and correlates with proliferative activity. An elevated TKA has been observed to be predictive of early progression in a subgroup of untreated patients with smoldering CLL.[97] β_2-microglobulin (β_2M) is an extracellular protein component of the HLA Class I complex. β_2M has been shown to have significant prognostic relevance in lymphoma and multiple myeloma and correlates with disease burden in CLL. Hallek and colleagues examined 113 CLL and immunocytoma patients for β_2M levels and TKA and demonstrated that elevated TKA and β_2M both were independent predictors of shortened PFS.[98,99] Keating et al confirmed the prognostic value of β_2M in 622 patients, reporting that an elevated level was associated with a significantly shorter survival for both untreated and previously treated patients.[100] In this study, elevated β_2M was observed in patients with high tumor burden and extensive bone marrow infiltration. In addition to disease progression, both β_2M[101–103] and TKA[104] have been associated with short duration of remission and inferior survival following treatment.

IgV_H Mutational Status

Although the malignant cell of CLL morphologically resembles a mature lymphocyte, genetic, immunologic, and phenotypic studies suggest that this cell is better designated as either a pregerminal or postgerminal B cell. Somatic mutations in the first and second complementarity-determining regions (CDR1 and CDR2) of the IgV_H genes are thought to occur in the germinal centers. Examination of IgV_H genes in patient cells suggest that there may be two subsets of CLL: leukemias whose cell of origin has successfully traversed the germinal center, resulting in the mutated IgV_H phenotype, and leukemias that are derived from naïve B cells with the unmutated (germline) IgV_H sequence. Approximately 60% of CLL patients have cells with mutated IgV_H genes (less than 98% identity to germline), whereas the remaining patients have cells exhibiting unmutated IgV_H (98% or greater sequence identity with germline), typical of pregerminal B cells.[34,35] The prognostic significance of the absence of IgV_H gene mutations is substantial, with all studies uniformly noting an inferior survival and high predisposition to requiring early treatment in this patient subset.[34,35,105–109] A recent CLL Research Consortium study examined the impact of IgV_H mutation in 307 untreated CLL patients enrolled on a prospective tissue collection study. Fifty-three percent of these patients exhibited unmutated IgV_H genes, and this population had a significantly shorter median time to initial therapy (3.5 years) than those with mutated IgV_H (9.2 years, $P < 0.001$).[110]

Because of the difficulties in determining IgV_H gene mutational status, researchers have sought surrogate markers for this parameter. Correlation between the absence of IgV_H gene mutations and elevated expression of the cell surface molecule CD38 on CLL cells was noted in one such report.[34] In another work, ZAP-70 expression was shown to correlate with IgV_H gene mutational status.[111] ZAP-70 is a T-cell receptor associated tyrosine kinase that is aberrantly expressed in CLL cells, and ZAP-70 expression is generally found in patients with unmutated IgV_H but not in patients with mutated IgV_H.[111] These two associated biomarkers appear to tie directly to the difference in biology of CLL between these two genetic subtypes and are discussed independently. Other surrogate markers for CLL with unmutated IgV_H gene status have been reported, including methylation and subsequent silencing of *TWIST2*, a transcription factor that negatively regulates *p53*, is preferentially observed in IgV_H-mutated CLL cases.[71] Elevated levels of lipoprotein lipase and related genes[112–118] have been noted in patients with IgV_H-unmutated disease. Additionally, it has been reported that IgV_H-mutated CLL cells have long telomeres with low telomerase activity,[119–122] whereas IgV_H-unmutated patients have short telomeres with high telomerase activity. The extreme shortening of telomeres and elevated telomerase activity is associated with both genetic instability and disrupted apoptosis in other diseases.[123–125] Finally, distinct gene and miRNA expression profiles[69] have also been correlated with IgV_H gene mutational status.[111,126]

CD38 Expression

Retrospective studies have shown that CD38 is an independent prognostic marker in CLL, demonstrating that high CD38 expression is associated with both a shorter time from diagnosis to treatment and inferior survival.[34,105,127–138] CD38 functional studies using CD31 and plexin B1 transfected fibroblasts have provided a biologic explanation for this observation. CD38 interaction with its ligand CD31 in the presence of IL-2 results in upregulation of survival receptor CD100 exclusively on proliferating CLL cells. This occurs with concomitant downmodulation of CD72, a negative regulator of immune response. The interaction between CLL cells and transfected fibroblasts (CD38/CD31 and CD100/plexin B1) results in enhanced survival and growth of CLL cells. Furthermore, the presence of nurse-like cells in CLL patients expressing high levels of CD31 and plexin B1 corroborates the interplay of CD38 and CD31 and provides evidence of activation of circulating CD38-positive CLL cells.[139–141] This finding also may explain the aggressive nature of these CLL clones.

ZAP-70

ZAP-70 expression was identified as another surrogate marker for IgV_H gene mutational status by a cDNA microarray analysis of untreated CLL patients.[111] Multiple studies have subsequently confirmed this finding.[110,126,142–144] Functional studies in ZAP-70-positive cases have shown that on B-cell receptor ligation, increased phosphorylation of cytosolic proteins (Syk, BLNK, PLCγ), calcium mobilization, and degradation of IκB leads to NF-κB target gene activation.[36,110,145,146] Despite the positive data with ZAP-70 as a prognostic factor, the reproducibility of this across laboratories has been problematic.[147,148] Inconsistent measurement of ZAP-70 may be the cause, as ZAP-70 is a labile protein and laboratories have employed different methods and reagents. Given the challenges of measuring ZAP-70 protein accurately, others have attempted to identify alternative markers or more stable readouts of ZAP-70 expression. For example, Corcoran and colleagues demonstrated that methylation of a specific CpG dinucleotide of the ZAP-70 gene correlated closely with expression of ZAP-70.[149] Overall, despite the apparent usefulness of ZAP70 in research laboratories for discriminating CLL patients at high risk for progression, this test currently is not useful for clinical practice.

Chromosomal Aberrations

Conventional metaphase cytogenetics can identify chromosomal aberrations in only 20% to 50% of cases, because of the low in vitro mitotic activity of CLL cells. Abnormalities noted in descending frequency of occurrence include trisomy 12, deletions at 13q14, structural aberrations of 14q32, and deletions of 11q, 17p, and 6q.[150] In addition, a complex karyotype (three or more abnormalities) occurs in approximately 15% of patients and predicts for rapid disease progression, Richter transformation, and inferior survival.[151–153] A recent study showed that the use of CD40L or combination of IL-2 and CpG stimulation revealed translocations in 33 of 96 patients (34%). These translocations were both balanced and unbalanced, occurring in 13q14, 11(q21q25), 14q32, or in regions also seen in lymphomas such as 1(p32p36), 1(q21q25), 2(p11p13), 6(p11p12), 6(p21p25), and 18q21.[65] These data define a new prognostic subgroup of patients with significantly shorter median time from diagnosis to requiring therapy (24 vs 106 months) and OS (94 vs 346 months) compared to those without translocations.[65] The frequency of these translocations in untreated patients was less common.[65] Although of interest, these findings require prospective validation before being used as a standard prognostic tool for CLL patients and may be more relevant for studies of clonal evolution from diagnosis.

Given the limitation of standard or stimulated karyotype analysis, at the present time interphase cytogenetics of known abnormalities by fluorescence in situ hybridization (FISH) is the state-of-the-art technique for accurately distinguishing genetic subtypes of CLL. The largest study of interphase cytogenetics resulted in improved sensitivity to detect partial trisomies (12q12, 3q27, 8q24), deletions (13q14, 11q22–23, 6q21, 6q27, 17p13), and translocations (band 14q32) in more than 80% of all cases.[65] In a large study of 325 patients by Dohner and colleagues,[156] a hierarchical model consisting of five genetic subgroups was constructed on the basis of regression analysis of CLL patients with chromosomal aberrations. The patients with a 17p deletion had the median survival time of 32 months and shortest treatment-free interval (TFI) of 9 months, whereas patients with 11q deletion followed closely with 79 months and 13 months, respectively.[156] The favorable 13q14 deletion group had a long TFI of 92 months and a median survival of 133 months, whereas the group without detectable chromosomal anomalies and those with trisomy 12 fell into the intermediate group with median survival of 111 and 114 months. Their TFI was 33 and 49 months, respectively. According to this pivotal study, CLL patients are prioritized in a hierarchical order (deletion 17p13 → deletion 11q22-q23 → trisomy 12 → no aberration → deletion 13q14).[156] The hierarchical model of cytogenetic abnormalities by FISH has been further confirmed by other studies relative to predicting disease progression. Of interest, patients with high-risk interphase cytogenetic abnormalities or other complex abnormalities are almost always found to have IgV_H-unmutated CLL.[136] The impact of high-risk interphase cytogenetics relative to disease progression, outside of its association with IgV_H-unmutated CLL, is yet unknown.

p53 Inactivation in CLL

p53 gene inactivation can occur through mutation or deletion of *p53* (primary) or mutation of other p53 regulatory factors (secondary). Mutations and/or deletions of *p53* are relatively uncommon (10%–20%) in CLL, compared to other tumor types,[136] but become more frequent as the disease progresses and predict an aggressive disease course, with rapid progression to time requiring therapy and inferior survival.[107,157,158] Indirect inactivation of p53 by mutation of *ATM* can also occur.[157] Indeed, examination of both primary p53 dysfunctions (ie, *p53* mutations) in the setting of other prognostic factors has demonstrated each of these to be important in predicting outcome and this represented 15% of the patient outcome.[157] Prospective validation of primary and secondary p53 inactivation will be required before this can be routinely implemented at diagnosis for routine risk stratification.

Preliminary Prospective Validation of New Biomarkers From the German CLL Study Group

The CLL-1 Study of the German CLL Study Group (GLLSG) is a randomized phase III study of early treatment with fludarabine versus observation in newly diagnosed CLL patients.[29] Risk of progression is determined on the basis of lymphocyte-doubling time, thymidine kinase, and diffuse bone marrow pattern. Differing from other early-intervention studies, patients with disease that meet some criteria of the NCI 96 criteria (ie, lymphocyte-doubling times <1 year) may enroll. Accompanying this study is the plan to assess interphase cytogenetics, IgV_H mutations, and β_2M level to determine their independent prognostic significance compared to other variables. If shown to be of prospective importance relative to predicting early treatment progression, these laboratory tests would be incorporated into subsequent risk stratification criteria. IgV_H-unmutated disease represented 41% of patients at diagnosis. Patients with IgV_H-unmutated disease assigned to observation had a median time to symptomatic disease of only 2 years. High-risk karyotypes were present in 15% of cases, with the great majority being IgV_H unmutated. A preliminary analysis of the first 340 patients randomized to observation suggested that IgV_H-unmutated disease, high-risk interphase cytogenetics, thymidine kinase, and lymphocyte-doubling time correlated with time to first treatment. Publication of these large prospective new prognostic factors will be important to determining the risk of CLL progression.

How Should Staging and Biomarkers Be Used for CLL in Year 2008?

Our understanding of the biology of CLL has improved dramatically and many relevant biomarkers are now becoming useful for predicting when CLL will clinically progress. However, no study to date has demonstrated that earlier treatment will alter the natural history of the patient in even the higher-risk groups with high progression rates. Therefore, at the present time the use of staging and predictive biomarkers should be used only to provide patients with information relative to the expected course of their disease. Outside of a clinical trial, these results should never be used to initiate therapy in patients with asymptomatic disease and no indication for treatment. Prior to performing predictive tests, a detailed discussion of how these tests will be used with the patient should occur and the option of not performing them should be provided. In a subset of patients, significant anxiety can be produced by identifying high-risk features for which intervention remains the only observation. Table 83–3 provides an example of the initial evaluation provided by our group when seeing a newly diagnosed patient. As lymphocyte-doubling time is a prognostic feature in the progression of CLL, our approach is to follow patients every 3 months during the first year and if little

Table 83–3 Evaluation of Chronic Lymphocytic Leukemia (CLL) Patients at Diagnosis

History
B-symptom and fatigue assessment
Infectious history assessment
Occupational assessment for chemical exposure
Familial history of CLL and lymphoproliferative disorders
Preventive interventions for infections and secondary cancers
Physical Exam
Laboratory Assessment
Complete blood count with differential
Morphology assessment of lymphocytes
Chemistry, LFT enzymes, LDH
Flow cytometry assessment to confirm immunophenotype of CLL
Serum immunoglobulins
Serum β_2M levels
Interphase cytogenetics for del(17p13.1), del(11q22.3), del(13q14), del(6q21), and trisomy 12
IgV_H mutational analysis
Stimulated metaphase karyotype (if available)
Selected Tests Under Certain Circumstances
Direct antiglobulin test (DAT), haptoglobin, reticulocyte count if anemia present
CT Scan if unexplained abdominal pain or enlargement present
PET Scan and/or biopsy if large nodal mass present
Bone marrow aspirate and biopsy if cytopenias present
Familial counseling if first-degree relative with CLL
Teaching
Varicella zoster identification instruction
Skin cancer identification
Disease education (Leukemia and Lymphoma Society, CLL Topics, ACOR)

change in clinical or laboratory parameters occurs at this point, we extend this time period to every 6 months in the absence of new complaints.

INITIAL TREATMENT OF CLL

Initiation of Treatment of Newly Diagnosed or Previously Untreated Patients

Many patients are incidentally diagnosed with CLL on routine complete blood count (CBC) examination and are asymptomatic with a normal hemoglobin and platelet count at time of initial diagnosis. Expectant observation without therapy is the standard practice for such asymptomatic patients, and patients receive treatment only when their disease progresses. This practice is based on several studies that failed to show an improvement in OS when early therapeutic intervention with chlorambucil therapy was administered to asymptomatic patients.[159] A meta-analysis of 2048 patients in six trials demonstrated no difference in death rate between patients who were randomized to early therapy (42.6%) and those whose treatment was deferred (41.6%).[159] Thus, patients with asymptomatic or early-stage disease derive no therapeutic benefit from early alkylating agent therapy. However, in these studies chlorambucil was administered as initial therapy, and chlorambucil achieves CR in few patients. The past decade has seen the development of more effective treatment regimens combining monoclonal antibody therapy with purine analogs (chemoimmunotherapy), which are able to achieve a CR in a majority of previously untreated patients, and the increasing use of new molecular markers to risk-stratify newly diagnosed CLL patients. Furthermore, it is now well established that CLL undergoes genetic

Table 83–4 Modified Indications for Treatment of Chronic Lymphocytic Leukemia

Grade 2 or greater fatigue limiting life activities
B-symptoms persisting for 2 weeks or greater
Lymph nodes greater than 10 cm or progressively enlarging lymph nodes causing symptoms
Spleen or liver with progressive enlargement or causing symptoms
Anemia (Hemoglobin <11 g/dL) referable to CLL
Thrombocytopenia (Platelets <100 × 10^{12}/L) referable to CLL
Autoimmune hemolytic anemia or idiopathic thrombocytopenic purpura poorly responsive to traditional therapy
WBC > 300 × 10^9/L on two occasions two weeks apart if no alternative comorbid diseases increase morbidity of Treatment
Severe paraneoplastic (insect hypersensitivity, vasculitis, myositis, etc) process related to CLL not responsive to traditional therapies

clonal evolution with time with greater frequency in IgV_H-unmutated CLL,[160] resulting in increasing resistance to therapy. Thus, the issue of early treatment needs to be reconsidered, particularly in patients with high-risk biological or molecular markers predicting a poor long-term prognosis. Ongoing efforts within the German CLL Study Group (GCLLSG) and several US cooperative groups will hopefully determine whether early intervention with modern chemoimmunotherapy regimens will improve long-term survival in patients with high-risk CLL.

To establish uniform clinical practice standards and ensure reproducible eligibility criteria for entrance into clinical studies, an NCI-sponsored working group on CLL established guidelines for initiation of treatment in 1996.[161] Indications to begin therapy included non-autoimmune cytopenias (Rai stage III and IV), bulky or symptomatic lymphadenopathy or hepatosplenomegaly, disease-related B symptoms or fatigue, extreme lymphocytosis (greater than 300 × 10^9/L) or a rapid lymphocyte-doubling time, and autoimmune hemolytic anemia or thrombocytopenia not controlled with steroids. It is imperative to determine if a patient's symptoms are due to CLL or a comorbid medical condition, because constitutional symptoms such as fatigue are nonspecific and can be due to many etiologies in elderly patients with comorbid illnesses. In addition to the official NCI 96 criteria for therapy, increasing frequency of infections and slowly progressive anemia are other indications that can aid the practicing physician in deciding when to initiate therapy in CLL. A summary of the NCI 96 guidelines for treatment is provided in Table 83–4 with some minimal modifications used by our group, and revised guidelines are under development at this time.

A useful paradigm for clinical practice is to institute treatment in CLL only for cytopenias or directly referable symptoms. When treatment is necessary, a variety of agents have been examined in clinical trials (outlined below). In addition, several retrospective[129,162–165] and prospective trials[93,166] recently demonstrated that some of the same prognostic features that predict time to progression and therapy may also predict the outcome of treatment. The role of these biomarkers in selecting the initial treatment for CLL is currently under study by several groups. In general, patients with del(17p13.1) and del(11q22.3) generally do not respond well to traditional therapy and should be considered for more aggressive interventions as part of initial therapy. Additionally, several studies have shown that CLL patients older than 70 or who have multiple comorbid illnesses do not tolerate certain more aggressive therapies,[102,167] and this needs to be factored into treatment algorithms. Below, we summarize the findings of clinical studies of different treatments for CLL; where such data exist, we integrate genomic biomarkers as well as clinical, including age and comorbid illnesses. Different therapies are outlined below with attention to details related to their initial use in previously untreated CLL.

As many of these regimens were also developed in relapsed CLL, these data are also reviewed and later referred to in the section Treatment of Patients with Relapsed CLL.

Cytotoxic Chemotherapy

Alkylating Agents

Chlorambucil and other alkylating agents served as first-line therapy for CLL for many decades, and chlorambucil is still given as first-line therapy for some patients, particularly older patients and patients who cannot tolerate purine analog therapy.[168] Chlorambucil is generally administered as a single pulse dose 40 mg/m^2 orally (PO) every 28 days, with or without concomitant steroid therapy.[169] Chlorambucil is typically given without steroid therapy, since the addition of steroids to alkylating agent therapy has not been shown to improve survival. Although a high-dose continuous dosing schedule of 15 mg PO daily has been evaluated in several large European studies and led to results superior to those of pulse therapy, high-dose therapy is associated with greater myelosuppression and frequently requires dose reduction, particularly in older or more fragile patients in whom chlorambucil is typically considered.[170] Although high-dose therapy may be more effective if maximal cytoreduction is desired, the less intensive pulse dosing schedule should generally be used outside the setting of a clinical study. Because most studies of alkylating agent therapy predated widespread use of cytogenetic and biological risk factors, data on the effect of biomarkers on response to chlorambucil are limited. However, the existing data indicate that patients with del(11q) or del(17p13.1) have a lower response rate and a shorter remission duration to chlorambucil, as compared to patients without these abonormalities.[171] The primary advantages of chlorambucil are its well-established toxicity profile and its low cost; its primary disadvantages are its low CR rate, even in previously untreated patients, and the very low possibility of developing myelodysplasia with extended therapy. Although not typically given as a single agent, its use should be considered in older patients and other patients who may not tolerate fludarabine or monoclonal antibody therapy.

Combination Chemotherapy With Alkylating Agents

A variety of trials combining alkylating agents and other cytotoxic agents have been performed. A phase III Eastern Cooperative Oncology Group (ECOG) study of chlorambucil and prednisone (CP), with or without vincristine (CVP), demonstrated no benefit in PFS for the CVP arm.[172] The French CLL group showed that a modified CHOP regimen (cyclophosphamide, adriamycin, vincristine, prednisone) was superior to CVP and achieved similar results as fludarabine monotherapy.[173,174] A meta-analysis compared alkylating agent-based combination regimens to a single-agent regimen based on an alkylating agent and demonstrated no survival benefit.[175] Given that alkylating agent-based combination regimens are associated with more toxicity and show no benefit over fludarabine-based therapy, our approach is to use the latter for most patients. Only in rare cases of de novo CLL do we consider alkylating agent-based combination therapy (ie, a young patient without comorbid illnesses who has fludarabine toxicity that prohibits further use, or a patient with renal failure who cannot receive fludarabine). In the relapse setting, although salvage lymphoma regimens such as CHOP-R, RICE, and ESHAP-R are used to treat CLL, clinical studies of these regimens in CLL are lacking and the utility of these regimens is undefined.

Purine Analogs

The introduction of purine analogs in the 1980s revolutionized CLL therapy, and fludarabine has demonstrated significant clinical efficacy in both relapsed and previously untreated CLL.[176–183] Pentostatin was the first nucleoside analog that demonstrated clinical activity in CLL and related B-cell lymphoproliferative disorders.[184] Phase II studies of pentostatin monotherapy in heavily pretreated patients showed modest activity, limiting further trials of single-agent pentostatin.[185,186] Given its more favorable myelosuppression profile, compared to other nucleoside analogs, pentostatin has been combined with other agents and shown favorable clinical activity and toxicity in selected populations.[187–189] Two other nucleoside analogs, fludarabine and cladribine, were subsequently found to be clinically active in CLL.[190–193] Phase II–III studies of cladribine monotherapy achieved similar clinical responses as alkylating agent-based treatments (reviewed in 194, 195) but were associated with more cytopenias and immune suppression. The Food and Drug Administration (FDA) approved fludarabine for the treatment of CLL, and thus most studies of purine analog-based therapy in CLL have focused on fludarabine. The remainder of this section will focus predominately on clinical trials of fludarabine.

Fludarabine was initially approved by the FDA for alkylating agent-resistant CLL in 1991 based on two phase II studies demonstrating a high response rate to fludarabine in this patient subset.[190,196] These two studies[190,196] prompted several additional trials of fludarabine as monotherapy in relapsed and previously untreated CLL. Following the observation of high response rates and a 33% CR rate in previously untreated CLL by Keating and colleagues,[197] several large prospective randomized studies in previously untreated CLL patients compared alkylating agent-based regimens to fludarabine. These studies collectively established fludarabine as an accepted standard first-line therapy for CLL based on improved response rates and PFS.[154,198,199] These studies are summarized in Table 83–5. A multicenter European study randomized 196 evaluable patients to fludarabine or cyclophosphamide, doxorubicin, and prednisone (CAP).[154] The overall response rate (ORR) favored fludarabine (60% vs 44%), and this benefit was observed in both relapsed ($n = 96$, 48% vs 27%) and previously untreated ($n = 100$, 71% vs 60%) patients, although the difference was not statistically significant in the untreated group. Fludarabine achieved a longer median duration of response than did CAP, with a tendency toward longer OS in previously untreated patients.[154] A randomized, multicenter American study confirmed these findings in 509 previously untreated CLL patients. Patients were randomized to receive fludarabine 25 mg/m^2 IV daily for 5 days every 28 days, chlorambucil 40 mg/m^2 PO every 28 days, or fludarabine 20 mg/m^2 daily for 5 days and chlorambucil 20 mg/m^2 PO every 28 days, for up to 12 cycles.[169] Patients who failed to respond or relapse were allowed to cross over to the other arm. The combination arm was closed because of excessive toxicity. Fludarabine achieved a superior CR rate, ORR, median duration of remission, and median duration of PFS (20%, 63%, 25 months, 20 months) than did chlorambucil (4%, 37%, 14 months, 14 months). However, there was no statistically significant difference in OS (66 vs 56 months), possibly because of the crossover design. A multicenter French study randomized 938 patients with previously untreated Binet stage B and C CLL to fludarabine, CHOP, or CAP. Although fludarabine achieved better response rates than CAP, overall survival (67–70 months) was identical in all three treatment groups.[199] Thus, single-agent fludarabine achieves superior response rates and duration of PFS than alkylating agent-based regimens. The impact of prognostic factors on response rates and duration of PFS to fludarabine was recently examined; patients with high-risk cytogenetic abnormalities including del(11q22.3) and del(17p13.1) have significantly shorter remission rate abnormalities in response to fludarabine-based therapy than patients with other cytogenetic abnormalities.[166]

Combining Fludarabine With Alkylating Agent Therapy

Fludarabine was combined with cyclophosphamide (Flu/Cy) in three randomized phase III studies (summarized in Table 83–5), based on two promising pilot studies in previously untreated CLL patients, with the goal of improving response rates and hopefully long-term

Table 83–5 Selected Trials of Fludarabine-Based Regimens in Previously Untreated Chronic Lymphocytic Leukemia

Reference	Regimen	Phase	No Pts	CR	ORR	Mean PFS (Months)	Median OS (Months)
Johnson, 1996[155]	Flu	III	52	23	71	NR	NR
	CAP		48	17	60	7	54
Rai, 2000[169]	Flu	III	170	20	63	20	66
	CLB		181	4	37	14	56
	Flu + CLB		123	20	61	N/A	55
Leporrier, 2001[173]	Flu	III	341	40	71	32	69
	CHOP		357	30	72	30	67
	CAP		237	15	58	28	70
Flinn, 2000[182]	Flu + Cy	II	17	51	92	N/A	N/A
O'Brien, 2001[183]	Flu + Cy	II	34	35	88	NR	NR
Eichhorst, 2006[93]	Flu	III	182	7	83	20	NR
	Flu + Cy		180	24	95	48	NR
	Flu + Cy		136	5	59	19	NR
Catvosky, 2005[202]	CLB	III	387	7	72	N/A	N/A
	Flu		194	15	80	N/A	N/A
	Flu + Cy		196	39	94	N/A	N/A
Byrd, 2003[232]	Flu + Ritux	Ran II	51	47	90	NR	NR
	Flu then Ritux		53	28	77	NR	NR
Keating, 2005[236]	Flu + Cy + Ritux	II	300	72	94	NR	NR

CAP, cyclophosphamide, adriamycin, prednisone; CHOP, cyclophosphamide, adriamycin, vincristine, prednisone; CLB, chlorambucil; CR-complete remission; Cy, cyclophosphamide; Flu, fludarabine; N/A, not available or not reported; NR, not reached; ORR, overall response rate; OS, overall survival; PFS, progression-free survival; Ref, reference; Ritux, rituximab.

survival.[183,182] The GCLLSG randomized 375 previously untreated patients (age ≤65 years) to standard fludarabine or Flu/Cy (fludarabine 30 mg/m^2 IV and cyclophosphamide 250 mg/m^2 IV daily for 3 days) every 28 days for 6 cycles.[200] The ORR (94% vs 83%), CR rate (24% vs 7%), median PFS (48 vs 20 months), and duration of treatment-free survival (37 vs 25 months) all favored Flu/Cy, although there were more patients with cytopenias in the combination arm. Furthermore, no difference in OS was observed. EGOG randomized 278 patients to single fludarabine or fludarabine 25 mg/m^2 days 1 to 5, cyclophosphamide 600 mg/m^2 days 1, and G-CSF support every 28 days for 6 cycles.[201] Flu/Cy therapy achieved a superior ORR (74% vs 59%), rates of CR (23% vs 5%) and duration of PFS (32 vs 19 months), although no OS advantage was observed. Most recently, the United Kingdom LRF CLL4 study randomized 777 patients to oral chlorambucil, fludarabine or Flu/Cy.[202] Patients randomized to Flu/Cy enjoyed superior ORR, CR rates, and 5-year PFS rates (94%, 39%, and 33%) than did patients who received chlorambucil (72%, 7%, and 9%) or fludarabine (80%, 15%, and 14%).

Thus, three large, prospective, randomized, multicenter studies in the United States and Europe have clearly demonstrated that Flu/Cy therapy is associated with better response rates and duration of PFS than single-agent fludarabine. However, no OS advantage for upfront Flu/Cy has been observed to date. Although toxicity has generally been manageable, greater hematologic toxicity has been observed with Flu/Cy. Additionally, patients older than 65 or 70, who make up the majority of CLL patients receiving initial therapy in clinical practice, have either been excluded or minimally represented in these trials. Further studies are needed to determine if Flu/Cy is as well tolerated and active in older patients as it is in younger patients. Finally, of these patients long-term follow-up is required to determine the duration of remission, overall survival, and the incidence of potential late complications such as myelodysplasia to fully assess the utility of the Flu/Cy regimen. Examination of outcome by cytogenetic risk groups showed that patients with high-risk cytogenetic abnormalities including del(11q22.3) and del(17p13.1) had a significantly shorter remission than patients in the groups with good-risk or intermediate-risk cytogenetic findings.[166] Thus, the addition of alkylating agents to fludarabine does not appear to alter the poor prognosis associated with high-risk cytogenetic abnormalities.

Rituximab

Rituximab (Rituxan, IDEC-C2B8) is a chimeric murine monoclonal antibody that targets the CD20 antigen on the surface of normal and malignant B lymphocytes, and is the best studied and most widely used monoclonal antibody for the treatment of CLL and B-NHL. CD20, a calcium channel that interacts with the B-cell receptor complex, is an ideal target, because CD20 is expressed in 90% to 100% of CLL and B-NHL and is not internalized or shed. Rituximab induces antibody-dependent cellular cytotoxicity (ADCC) and complement-dependent cytotoxicity (CDC), activates caspase 3, and induces apoptosis in CLL and B-NHL cells.[203–206] Thus, multiple mechanisms of action likely contribute to rituximab's effectiveness in CLL.

In Phase I clinical studies in indolent B-NHL rituximab 375 mg/m^2 IV was administered weekly for 4 doses, although the dose and length of treatment were empirically determined. The pivotal phase II trial of rituximab was pursued in 166 patients with relapsed or refractory indolent B-NHL including SLL.[207] Although an ORR of 60% was achieved in indolent follicle center B-NHL, only 4 of 30 patients (13%) with SLL/CLL responded. Similarly, disappointing results were obtained in several other small studies enrolling 10 or fewer SLL/CLL patients each.[208–210] Two studies performed by the GCLLSG (n = 28 patients) and the Nordic Study Group (n = 24 patients) demonstrated an ORR of 25% and 35%, respectively, with short remission duration, as summarized in Table 83–6.[211,212]

Table 83–6 Selected Phase II Trials of Weekly Rituximab in Chronic Lymphocytic Leukemia/Small Lymphocytic Lymphoma

Reference (Authors/year)	Doses	Prior Therapy	Evaluable Patients	Response Rate (ORR)
McLaughlin et al, 1998[207]	4	Yes	30	13%
Nguyen et al, 1999[208]	4	Yes	10	10%
Winkler et al, 1999[209]	4	Yes	9	11%
Ladetto et al, 2000[210]	4	Yes	7	0%
Huhn et al, 2001[211]	4	Yes	28	25%
Hainsworth et al, 2003[217]	4	No	44	58%

Table 83–7 Summary of Alemtuzumab Studies in Chronic Lymphocytic Leukemia

Ref	No. of Patients	# Weeks of Rx	Prior Rx	% CR	% PR	% OR
Osterborg, 1996[247]	9	6–18	No	33	55	89
Osterborg, 1997[248]	29	6	Yes	4	38	43
Bowen, 1997[244]	6	6–12	Yes	0	50	50
Rai, 2003[270]	24	4–16	Yes	0	33	33
Kennedy, 2002[265]	29	NR	Yes	34	25	59
Keating, 2002[246]	92	4–12	Yes	2	31	33
Hillmen, 2006[171]	149	12	No	24	59	83

Responses in each of these studies were predominately in the blood and nodal compartment with little improvement in marrow disease. In contrast, two trials in which higher doses of rituximab weekly (up to 2250 mg/m^2 per dose) or rituximab was administered thrice weekly to relapsed CLL patients showed an improved rate of response.[213–215] Benefit in these two trials was predominately in the blood and nodal disease, although response duration approached that achieved in follicular B-NHL in prior trials. Unfortunately, no patients with del(17p13.1) responded to rituximab administered thrice weekly, indicating that single agent rituximab is ineffective in this high-risk population.[216] Nonetheless, both dose escalation and thrice-weekly dosing improved response rates and established a role for single-agent rituximab in patients with relapsed CLL and provided support for the study of rituximab in combination with other agents in relapsed CLL.

Weekly single-agent rituximab demonstrated greater clinical efficacy when given to patients with previously untreated SLL/CLL (Table 83–7). Forty-four previously untreated patients with SLL/CLL received 4-weekly doses of rituximab 375 mg/m^2; the ORR after the first course of rituximab was 51% (CR 4%). Twenty-eight patients with stable or responsive disease received additional 4-week courses of rituximab every 6 months for up to 4 cycles. However, there was only a modest increase in ORR (58%) and CR rates (9%), and the median duration of PFS of 19 months was shorter than the 36- to 40-month median duration of PFS reported by the same investigators using the same regimen in previously untreated patients with follicle center B-NHL.[217] Nonetheless, this response duration compared favorably with the response duration achieved with fludarabine in the upfront setting, suggesting that rituximab is active and may have a role in the upfront therapy of SLL/CLL.

Rituximab is selective for the B-cell antigen CD20 and therefore has a relatively favorable toxicity profile. Toxicity associated with infusion of this agent commonly occurs with the first infusion of rituximab and may be greater in patients with CLL, compared to patients with NHL. These symptoms generally include fever, rigors, transient hypoxemia, dyspnea, and hypotension, which are partly due to an inflammatory cytokine release syndrome.[218] Although initial studies suggested that patients with high lymphocyte counts may be at greater risk of this cytokine release syndrome, subsequent larger studies failed to support this finding.[218,219] Tumor necrosis factor-alpha (TNF-α) and interleukin-6 (IL-6) levels peak 90 minutes after the start of rituximab infusion and are the likely source of the cytokine release syndrome. Although poorly understood, CLL patients with platelet counts less than 50 × 10^{12}/L may experience transient, severe thrombocytopenia associated with this infusional toxicity and may require platelet transfusions with the first 1 or 2 doses of rituximab. Patients with preexisting thrombocytopenia should therefore have a posttherapy platelet count after the first 1 or 2 doses of rituximab. Another uncommon, but potentially severe, toxicity is a tumor lysis syndrome, which is generally observed in patients with a high circulating peripheral lymphocyte count.[220,221] Such patients should receive prophylactic allopurinol, hydration, and careful observation, and inpatient monitoring and administration of rituximab can be considered for the highest-risk patients. Patients who develop tumor lysis syndrome following the first dose of rituximab can safely receive subsequent doses, especially after the number of circulating CLL cells is reduced.[220] Other rare toxicities with rituximab therapy include delayed neutropenia,[222–225] hepatitis B reactivation, skin toxicity, and interstitial pneumonitis. Patients with active hepatitis should be followed closely, and prophylactic antiviral therapy should be considered. Patients who develop profound neutropenia, pulmonary, or skin toxicity with rituximab should not be challenged with repeated dosing. In general, rituximab is a very well-tolerated therapy, making it ideal for use in combination with other agents in patients with CLL.

Rituximab Chemoimmunotherapy

Given its activity and toxicity profile, rituximab has been combined with cytotoxic chemotherapy in the treatment of CLL, and clinical trials have examined several such chemoimmunotherapy regimens.[226–230] Studies of chemoimmunotherapy in CLL have focused primarily on fludarabine-based combinations, because of the established role of fludarabine therapy in this disease.[231,232]

Fludarabine and Rituximab

The CALGB 9712 study randomized 104 previously untreated CLL patients to sequential or concurrent fludarabine and rituximab (FR) therapy.[232] Patients received standard fludarabine 25 mg/m^2 days 1 to 5 every 4 weeks for six cycles, with or without concurrent rituximab 375 mg/m^2 on day 1 of each cycle, with an additional dose on day 4 of cycle 1. Patients in both arms received rituximab 375 mg/m^2 weekly for four doses beginning 2 months after completion of fludarabine; thus, patients in the concurrent arm received 11 total doses of rituximab, compared to four in the sequential arm. Patients receiving concurrent FR therapy enjoyed a superior CR rate (47% vs 28%) and ORR (90% vs 77%) than patients in the sequential arm. The median duration of response was not reached at 23 months. The 104 patients in this study experienced an improved ORR rate (84% vs 63%), CR rate (38% vs 20%), 2-year PFS rate (67% vs 45%), and 2-year OS rate (93% vs 81%), as compared to 179 previously untreated patients who received single-agent fludarabine in the prior CALGB 9011 trial.[233] Retrospective analysis of prognostic cytogenetic abnormalities demonstrated that patients with del(11q22.3) and del(17p13.1) have a shorter duration of response to this regimen. Additionally, very few patients more than the age of 75 were treated on this trial, making its relevance to elderly CLL patients uncertain.

A second multicenter European phase II study administered fludarabine 25 mg/m^2 days 1 to 5 every 4 weeks for six cycles, as well as rituximab 375 mg/m^2 on day 1 of cycles 3 to 6, to 31 evaluable CLL patients. The ORR and CR rate were 87% and 32%, respectively, with similar outcomes in previously treated (ORR 91%, CR rate 45%) and untreated patients (ORR 85%, CR rate 25%). Sixteen patients developed a total of 32 infections, and one patient died of cerebral hemorrhage resulting from prolonged thrombocytopenia.[234] The duration of PFS and the impact of age and prognostic factors were not reported with this trial.

Fludarabine, Cyclophosphamide, and Rituximab

The most active phase II results with chemoimmunotherapy have been achieved with a combination regimen of fludarabine, cyclophosphamide, and rituximab (FCR) in both previously treated and untreated CLL. One hundred seventy-seven evaluable patients with previously treated CLL received fludarabine 25 mg/m^2 and cyclophosphamide 250 mg/m^2 on days 2 to 4 of cycle 1 and on days 1 to 3 of cycles 2 to 6, in addition to rituximab 375 mg/m^2 on day 1 of cycle 1 and 500 mg/m^2 on day 1 of cycles 2 to 6.[235] An ORR of 73%, with a 25% CR rate and 16% nodular PR rate, was reported, and 12 of 37 patients (32%) in CR achieved molecular remission. The same authors administered FCR to 300 previously untreated CLL patients (Table 83–5); the ORR was 94%, with 72% of patients attaining a CR.[236] Remissions were durable, with the rates of 4-year relapse-free survival (RFS) and 4-year OS being 77% and 83%, respectively. The ability to achieve a remission with 1% or less residual CLL cells in the marrow as assessed by two-color flow cytometry significantly affected the duration of RFS and OS. Only 5 of 138 patients (4%) whose posttherapy bone marrow by immunophenotypic analysis demonstrated that 1% or less residual CLL cells relapsed, in contrast to 17 of 62 patients (27%) with more than 1% residual CLL cells by flow cytometry. Toxicity was acceptable, and infectious complications were manageable. A randomized phase III study comparing this regimen to fludarabine and cyclophosphamide in both previously treated and untreated CLL is currently ongoing. To date, data available from the phase II study outlined above suggests this regimen is not well tolerated by CLL patients older than 70 years of age. The impact of high-risk cytogenetic abnormalities on response to this regimen is also not certain.

Pentostatin, Cyclophosphamide, and Rituximab

Although the use of regimens such as FR and FCR to treat patients with have obtained excellent results, the median age of patients in these phase II studies was 63 and 58 years, respectively. In contrast, SEER data indicate that the median age of CLL patients at first treatment is 72 years. Thus, there are limited data on the toxicity profile and efficacy of chemoimmunotherapy regimens in patients more than 70 years of age. A recent phase II study of pentostatin, cyclophosphamide, and rituximab (PCR) in 64 patients with previously untreated CLL indicates that this regimen is effective and may be a particularly good choice for older patients.[237] The median age of participants in this trial was 62.5 years, and 71% of patients had unmutated IgV_H. Patients received pentostatin 2 mg/m^2 on day 1, cyclophosphamide 600 mg/m^2 on day 1, and rituximab 375 mg/m^2 on day 1 (100 mg/m^2 on day 1 and 375 mg/m^2 on days 3 and 5 of cycle 1) every 21 days for up to 6 cycles. Filgrastim was administered beginning on day 3. PCR was well tolerated and clinically active, with OR, CR, and nPR rates of 91%, 41%, and 22%, respectively, being reported. The duration of the median PFS was 33 months. The ability to achieve CR or nPR was not affected by any high-risk genetic or biological factor, with the exception that all three patients with del(17p13) failed to achieve CR or nPR. Patients aged 70 or more tolerated PCR as well as younger patients aged less than 70, with the only notable exception being that older patients required a dose delay of more than 1 week (28% vs 7%, $P = 0.03$). Grade 3 to 4 hematologic (61% vs 48%), infectious (6% vs 11%), and other nonhematologic toxicities (22% vs 28%) were similar in older and younger patients. The OR and CR rates were similar in patients aged 70 or more and those of age less than 70 (83% vs 93%, 39% vs 41%). EFS was identical for older and younger patients, with $P = 0.98$. Thus, the use of PCR should be particularly considered for previously untreated CLL patients aged 70 or more, who constitute approximately half of all patients requiring initial treatment of their CLL. Prophylactic antibiotics and G-CSF should be used as utilized in this study, in order to ensure the reproducibility of these results in CLL patients aged 70 or more.

What Is the Role of Rituximab in CLL?

Studies of rituximab to this point have demonstrated modest clinical activity in both previously untreated CLL patients using the weekly dosing schedule and in the relapsed state using more intensive dosing regimens. Rituximab does not have activity against CLL with del(17p13.1). For this reason, rituximab monotherapy is generally used in either of these settings only if more definitive therapy cannot be administered because of other comorbid conditions. Rituximab's greatest contribution is to combination therapy both in symptomatic, previously untreated CLL patients and relapsed patients receiving the FR, FCR, or PCR regimens. However, phase III studies demonstrating the clear benefit of such approach over traditional chemotherapy (FC) based treatments are required before this can be considered an established standard of care. To this point, no data exist for maintenance rituximab in CLL and this should not be considered out of the context of a clinical trial.

Alemtuzumab

Alemtuzumab (Campath-1H) is a humanized monoclonal antibody against CD52.[238–240] CD52 is a 21- to 28-kd cell-surface glycopeptide expressed on virtually all human lymphocytes, monocytes, and macrophages, a small subset of granulocytes, but not erythrocytes, platelets, or hematopoietic stem cells. CD52 is expressed on all CLL cells and indolent B-NHL cells.[241,242] Its physiological function remains unknown, but crosslinking of CD52 on B-cell and T-cell lymphoma cell lines inhibits their cell proliferation.[243] Alemtuzumab has been demonstrated to mediate apoptosis, CDC, and ADCC of CLL cells in vitro. CD52 is not shed, internalized, or modulated and is therefore an ideal antigen for targeted immunotherapy. However, the ubiquitous expression of CD52 on normal lymphocytes and monocytes is predictive of the increased neutropenia, lymphopenia, and infectious complications observed with alemtuzumab therapy.

Phase I studies of alemtuzumab has established a dose of 30 mg IV three times per week for 4 to 12 weeks. Alemtuzumab induced significantly more infusion-related toxicity than rituximab, but stepped up dosing diminished initial infusion-related toxicity and made administration of the antibody tolerable and feasible. Three milligrams is given on the first day, 10 mg on day 2, and 30 mg on day 3; after dose escalation, patients receive 30 mg thrice weekly. Several clinical studies have established a role for alemtuzumab in CLL, as summarized in Table 83–7.[244–248] In a multicenter European phase II study, alemtuzumab was administered 30 mg thrice weekly for up to 12 weeks to 29 recurrent and refractory CLL patients. The ORR was 42%, but only 1 patient (4%) achieved a CR.[248] Alemtuzumab cleared CLL cells from the peripheral blood in 97% of patients but was less effective at eliminating marrow (36%) or nodal disease (7%).

The pivotal CAM211 trial administered the same regimen of alemtuzumab therapy to 93 heavily pretreated, fludarabine-refractory CLL patients. The ORR was 33%, but only 2% of patients achieved a CR.[245] Median time to progression for responders was 9.5 months, with a median OS of 16 months for all patients and 32 months for responders. The median peripheral blood CLL count decreased by more than 99.9%, but the antibody was less effective against nodal

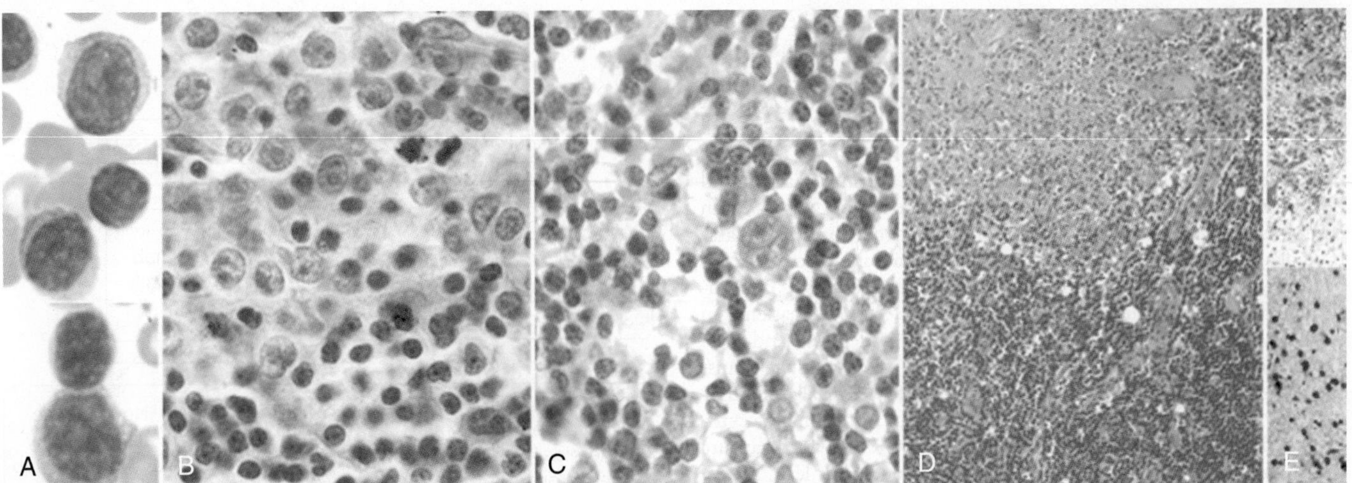

Figure 83–4 Transformation in chronic lymphocytic leukemia (CLL) (**A–E**). Some cases of CLL develop increasing numbers of prolymphocytes (**A**), and a "prolymphocytic transformation." A Richter transformation is to a large-cell lymphoma (**B**; large cells upper left, residual CLL lower right). Occasionally, cases can transform to Hodgkin lymphoma (ie, the Hodgkin variant of Richter) (**C**). With the use of fludarabine and other immunosuppressants, patient can also develop Epstein–Barr virus-related lymphadenopathies, or lymphadenopathies with large areas of necrosis due to herpes simplex virus. The case illustrated in **D** and **E** had both (**E**; upper panel shows an immunostain of HSV-1/2 and lower is EBER in situ hybridization).

disease, particularly in patients with bulky lymph nodes greater than 5 cm in diameter. Although 90% of patients with lymph nodes measuring less than or equal to 2 cm responded, with 64% achieving resolution of adenopathy, only 12% of patients with lymph nodes greater than 5 cm responded with no patients attaining resolution of their adenopathy. All patients were placed on prophylactic antibodies and antiviral agents, and treatment-related toxicity was manageable. Patients with a poor performance status did markedly worse than patients with no or minimal symptoms from their disease, likely owing to their reduced ability to tolerate the hematologic and infectious side effects of alemtuzumab, and no patients with ECOG performance status greater than 1 responded to therapy. The activity of alemtuzumab was later confirmed by a multiinstitutional, compassionate use study in 136 patients with fludarabine-refractory CLL.[249]

The German CLL Study Group has recently explored the use of subcutaneous (SC) alemtuzumab for patients with relapsed CLL in an attempt to diminish infusion-related toxicity associated with this regimen. This study administered alemtuzumab 3, 10, and 30 mg IV during week 1, followed by 30 mg SC thrice weekly for 4 to 12 weeks.[250] Forty-six heavily treated patients, with a median of 4 prior therapies, received a median of 838 mg (of the 1123 mg of the planned dose) of alemtuzumab. Despite less infusion-related toxicity, therapy was interrupted in 29 patients due to neutropenia (15), infection (8), or other cytopenias (3). Furthermore, treatment was discontinued early in 26 patients due to a lack of response (12), infection (4), or neutropenia (3). The ORR (36%), CR rate (2%), median duration of PFS (9.7 months), and median OS (13.1 months) were virtually identical to the results achieved with IV alemtuzumab in the CAM211 study. Additionally, the response rate was similar in patients with high-risk cytogenetic abnormalities with del(11q22.3) and del(17p13.1). Thus, SC administration of alemtuzumab appears to be as effective as IV dosing, with less infusion-related toxicity but significant hematologic and infectious toxicity.

Alemtuzumab's other distinguishing feature is its ability to eradicate CLL cells within the bone marrow and to achieve minimal residual disease (MRD) negativity. In a British study, alemtuzumab was administered at a dose of 30 mg IV thrice weekly for up to 16 weeks in (median 9 weeks) to 91 patients with relapsed CLL.[251] The ORR was 54% (CR 36%), and 18 patients had no evidence of disease as determined by flow-cytometric analysis. With a median follow-up of 36 months, the median treatment-free survival was significantly longer (not reached) in patients with no MRD in the bone marrow as compared to patients who achieved a CR but had MRD in the marrow (20 months) or MRD-positive PR (13 months). The 5-year OS was 84% for the 18 MRD-negative patients. However, this study also illustrated alemtuzumab's relatively poor activity as a single agent in patients with bulky nodal disease.[251] The ORR was 87% in 33 patients with no lymphadenopathy (CR 72%), compared to only 9% (CR 0%) in 11 patients with lymph nodes greater than 5 cm in size. As a result, the median OS was 30 months for patients whose largest lymph was equal to or less than 5 cm, compared to 9 months for patients with a lymph node greater than 5 cm. Thus, alemtuzumab's ability to eliminate MRD in the bone marrow translated into an improved long-term survival.

In a phase II clinical trial, alemtuzumab was administered at a dose of 30 mg SC three times per week for up to 18 weeks to 41 previously untreated patients with CLL. Except for transient grade 1–2 fever, adverse reactions after the first were minimal. The ORR was 81% on an intent-to-treat basis, and 87% of the 38 patients who received at least 2 weeks of treatment responded.[252] Alemtuzumab effectively cleared the peripheral blood (CR 95%) and bone marrow of evidence of disease (CR + nodular PR 66%) and was effective against the nodal disease (ORR 87%, CR 29%). Some patients who achieved a CR in the marrow required the full 18 weeks of therapy to do so, suggesting that prolonged administration was necessary to clear CLL cells from the marrow. The median time to treatment failure had not been reached at time of study report (18+ months). On the basis of these promising results in the upfront setting, the CAM307 study prospectively randomized 297 previously untreated CLL patients to oral chlorambucil 40 mg/m^2 every 4 weeks for 12 cycles or alemtuzumab 30 mg IV three times per week for up to 12 weeks. All patients on the alemtuzumab arm received prophylaxis for *Pneumocystis carinii* and varicella zoster. Alemtuzumab achieved a superior ORR (83% vs 55%), CR rate (22% vs 2%), and duration of PFS. Additionally, this trial prospectively demonstrated that patients with del(11q13.1) and del(17p13.1) had a superior response to alemtuzumab as compared to chlorambucil. The results of this study are still being analyzed for full publication.

Owing to the ubiquitous expression of CD52 on lymphocytes and monocytes, immunosuppression and infectious complications constitute the most concerning toxicity of alemtuzumab.[237,253,254] Although alemtuzumab also depletes B cells, CD8$^+$ T cells, natural killer (NK) cells, and monocytes, the antibody's most profound effect is its ablation of CD4$^+$ T lymphocytes.[255–257] This delayed recovery of CD4$^+$ T-lymphocytes has been observed by multiple investigators. The absolute CD4$^+$ T-cell count reached a nadir of 2/μL by week 4 and increased only to 84/μL by week 12 in the CAM211 trial.[245] Furthermore, alemtuzumab depleted CD52$^+$ myeloid peripheral blood dendritic cells, inhibiting the ability of peripheral blood mononuclear cells (PBMCs) to present antigen to purified CD4$^+$ T lymphocytes.[258] This effect may explain the ability of alemtuzumab to prevent graft-versus-host disease (GVHD) following allogeneic stem cell transplantation.[259,260]

Given this prolonged immunosuppression, alemtuzumab should be administered carefully, particularly when the antibody is given in combination with other immunosuppressive agents such as fludarabine. Patients receiving alemtuzumab are at an increased risk for bacterial, fungal, viral, and other opportunistic infections as demonstrated by multiple clinical trials. For instance, 55% of patients in the CAM211 study developed infections (27% grade 3–4), and 13% experienced septicemia.[246] Patients receiving alemtuzumab must therefore be placed on appropriate prophylaxis for *P carinii* pneumonia and varicella zoster infection/reactivation. Additionally, cytomegalovirus (CMV) infection monitoring by PCR or hybrid capture assays should be performed regularly during and for at least 2 to 3 months after therapy with alemtuzumab. Patients who reactivate CMV should be treated appropriately. With these prophylactic measures, alemtuzumab can be administered safely and with acceptable infection-related morbidity in most patients.

Infusion-related toxicity is another event that occurs predominately with IV alemtuzumab. In the CAM211 study, infusion-related events occurred in 93% of patients, although the majority of reactions were grade 1 or 2. Rigors (90% overall, 14% grade 3), fever (85% overall, 17% grade 3, 3% grade 4), and nausea (53%) were the most common infusion-related toxicities.[245] Similar rates of developing rigors (71%), fevers (65%), and nausea (45%) were reported in the multicenter, compassionate use study, and almost all infusion-related toxicities were grade 1 or 2.[249] Most toxicity was observed with the first infusion.[246] This first-dose cytokine release syndrome involves TNF-α, IFN-γ, and IL-6.[260] TNF-α is the primary cytokine in this syndrome, with an increase of greater than 1000-fold in levels after alemtuzumab infusion.[261–263] Ligation of the low-affinity Fcδ receptor for IgG, FcδRIIIa, on NK cells resulted in release of TNF-α and may play a central role in inducing this infusional toxicity.[260] Corticosteroids may be administered if the infusion-related toxicity is severe, and side effects generally abate with steroid therapy.

The ubiquitous presence of CD52 on hematopoietic cells is predictive of the significant hematologic toxicity following alemtuzumab therapy. The multicenter, compassionate use study observed that 26% of the patients developed neutropenia (22% grade 3 or 4), 35% thrombocytopenia (23% grade 3 or 4), and 21% of the patients developed anemia (11% grade 3).[249] Many patients who develop cytopenias after alemtuzumab experience grade 3 or 4 toxicity, resulting in potentially severe infectious complications. Although infusion-related toxicity can cause discomfort to patients, hematologic toxicity and infectious complications are the most serious toxicities. These toxicities are clinically manageable with proper monitoring of peripheral blood counts, appropriate antibiotic prophylaxis, and routine CMV screening. Both G-CSF and GM-CSF should be avoided, as each may increase toxicity without improving granulocyte recovery.[262,264]

Chemoimmunotherapy With Alemtuzumab

Several groups have pursued adding alemtuzumab, similar to rituximab, either concurrently or sequentially with several chemotherapeutic agents for the treatment of previously treated or symptomatic untreated CLL patients. Results of these studies have not yet translated to a standard therapy used for the treatment of patients with CLL.

Fludarabine and Alemtuzumab

A small study of six CLL patients, refractory to fludarabine alone and alemtuzumab alone, suggested that such synergy may exist clinically. Fludarabine was given at a dose of 25 mg/m^2 IV for 3 to 5 days, and alemtuzumab was administered at 30 mg IV three times weekly for 8 to 16 weeks. Five patients responded, with 1 patient achieving CR; furthermore, MRD was undetectable using flow cytometric analysis in two patients. Patients received prophylaxis for PCP and VZV, and no serious adverse events were noted.[265] A German study confirmed these findings in a phase II study of 36 relapsed CLL patients who received fludarabine 30 mg/m^2 IV and alemtuzumab 30 mg IV for 3 days every 28 days for four to six cycles based on toxicity and response. The study achieved an ORR of 83%, with 30% CR; the median time to progression (TTP) was 13 months, and the median OS was 36 months. Although one heavily pretreated patient died of a fever of unknown origin, infection-related toxicity was tolerable. Median CD4 counts did not return to near normal for 14 to 18 months, so prolonged PCP and VZV prophylaxis should be considered.

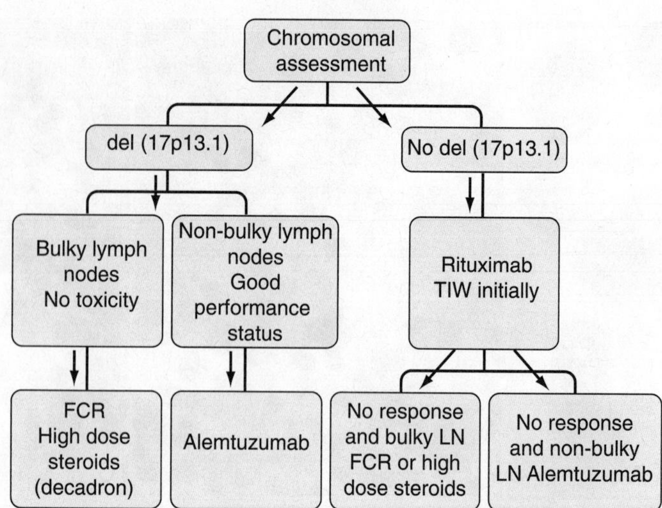

Figure 83–5 Algorithm to treatment approach to first relapsed chronic lymphocytic leukemia.

FCR + Alemtuzumab

Another phase II study added alemtuzumab to FCR, to determine if efficacy could be improved in previously treated CLL patients. Seventy-eight patients with relapsed CLL received fludarabine 25 mg/m^2 on days 2 to 4, cyclophosphamide 250 mg/m^2 on days 2 to 4, rituximab 375 mg/m^2 (cycle 1) or 500 mg/m^2 (cycles 2–6) on day 2, and alemtuzumab 30 mg IV on days 1, 3, and 5 every 28 days for up to six cycles.[266] Patients received pegfilgrastrim, as well as prophylaxis, for PCP pneumonia and CMV reactivation. Grade 3–4 neutropenia was seen in 89% of patients, and 59% developed grade 3–4 thrombocytopenia. The incidence of major infections (11%), minor infections (28%), and fever of unknown origin (36%) were similar to the same institution's historical experience with FCR in the relapsed setting. However, prophylactic valganciclovir was significantly more effective in preventing CMV reactivation (3 of 30 patients, 10%) than was prophylactic valacyclovir (25 of 48 patients, 52%). The ORR was 65%, with 24% of patients achieving CR. Median duration of PFS was 27 months for the 19 patients achieving CR, compared to only 10 months for the 32 patients attaining PR. Significantly better results were observed in patients who were sensitive to their last fludarabine regimen (ORR 74%, CR rate 36%), compared to patients refractory to fludarabine (ORR 49%, CR rate 6%). Given these promising results, a phase II study of CFAR in previously untreated patients is presently being conducted.

Alemtuzumab as Consolidation Therapy After Chemotherapy

Given the ability of alemtuzumab to clear bone marrow of CLL cells and to eliminate MRD, several investigators have examined the use of alemtuzumab as consolidation therapy after initial induction therapy with fludarabine. In one report, alemtuzumab was administered at a dose of 10 or 30 mg IV thrice weekly for 4 weeks to 58 patients who had responded to their most recent therapy but still had residual disease.[267] The ORR was 53%, and the response rate was dose dependent; 65% of patients who received 30 mg responded as compared to 39% of patients who received 10 mg. Eleven of 29 patients (38%) achieved an MRD-negative marrow, and the TTP was not reached after a median follow-up of 24 months. In addition, the TTP was significantly longer in patients who had no marrow MRD after alemtuzumab consolidation. Similar findings were reported by the GCLLSG, which randomized 21 eligible patients, who had responded to fludarabine or Flu/Cy induction therapy but still had persistent disease, to observation ($n = 10$) or alemtuzumab 30 mg IV thrice weekly for up to 12 weeks ($n = 11$). The study was discontinued early as a result of increased toxicity in the alemtuzumab arm; 6 of 11 patients experienced grade 4 hematologic toxicity, and 7 of 11 patients developed grade 3 or 4 infectious complications, including 4 patients with CMV.[268] However, five of six evaluable patients had no MRD in the marrow with alemtuzumab consolidation. After a median follow-up of 48 months, the median PFS favored the alemtuzumab arm (not reached vs 20.6 months) with only 3 of 11 patients who received alemtuzumab relapsing.[269] On the basis of these promising results, the GCLLSG FLL2i study is currently evaluating the optimal dose and schedule of alemtuzumab consolidation after initial fludarabine-based therapy.

The administration of alemtuzumab subcutaneously (SC) has also been examined in the consolidation setting. The CALGB 19901 study administered fludarabine 25 mg/m^2 IV daily for 5 days every 28 days for six cycles, followed by alemtuzumab 30 mg subcutaneously thrice weekly for 6 weeks, to 28 patients (24 evaluable) with previously untreated CLL.[270] The ORR after fludarabine induction was only 36% (CR 4%), and 18 patients with stable or responsive disease went on to receive alemtuzumab. Twelve of these 18 patients responded, and 4 of 8 patients converted from a PR to a CR, for a final intent-to-treat ORR of 50% (CR 18%). Treatment was well tolerated, with only 3 of 18 patients reactivating CMV with alemtuzumab therapy. The CALGB 10101 study is currently examining a phase II regimen of concurrent fludarabine and rituximab for six cycles, followed by SC alemtuzumab for 6 weeks as consolidation therapy.

What Is Alemtuzumab's Role in CLL?

As a result of the ubiquitous expression of CD52 on lymphocytes and monocytes, alemtuzumab causes significantly more hematologic and immune toxicity than does rituximab, and careful monitoring of and prophylaxis for potential infections is required for any administration of alemtuzumab. Nonetheless, infectious complications are manageable with adequate antibiotic prophylaxis and careful monitoring for potential CMV reactivation. Infusion-related toxicity to intravenous administration of alemtuzumab is manageable with a stepped up dosing schedule, and infusion-related toxicity usually diminishes as therapy progresses. Alemtuzumab most effectively clears CLL cells from peripheral blood and bone marrow, but has limited activity against nodal disease, particularly bulky lymph nodes. Initial studies indicate that SC administration is as effective as IV dosing; although SC dosing markedly diminishes infusion toxicity, hematologic and immune side effects remain. Despite its limitations, alemtuzumab is the only approved therapy for CLL that has clinical activity in relapsed patients with del(17p). In addition, alemtuzumab is able to eliminate MRD from the bone marrow, thereby improving long-term OS. Thus, alemtuzumab has a role in the treatment of high-risk CLL, although it should always be used carefully. Current studies are focusing on the use of alemtuzumab in combination with fludarabine, such as the CFAR protocol at the MD Anderson Cancer Center, or as consolidation therapy after fludarabine induction (CALGB 10101 study). Until the toxicity and response data from such studies are published, the use of alemtuzumab in combination regimens should be reserved for clinical trials and should not be employed in standard clinical practice.

TREATMENT OF PATIENTS WITH RELAPSED CLL

The approach to reinitiating therapy for CLL patients who have relapsed after initial therapy is similar to that applied for initial therapy assessment. Patients need not receive therapy at the first sign of relapse. Rather, patients should have an indication for treatment, as discussed above. Patients should have repeat interphase cytogenetic analysis of the peripheral blood or bone marrow aspirate, as patients may acquire additional cytogenetic abnormalities most notably del(17p13.1) as their CLL becomes more advanced. The incidence of del(17p13.1) increases from 5% of patients at initial diagnosis to nearly half of heavily treated patients with advanced CLL, and acquisition of this abnormality has profound implications on treatment, as will be discussed below. IgV_H mutational analysis does not need to be performed if such information has been obtained previously, as a patient's IgV_H mutational status does not change with time. A bone marrow should be performed if cytopenias are present, to confirm that CLL is the cause and to exclude other potential causes of cytopenias such as transformed lymphoma, prolonged marrow toxicity from prior therapy, or development of treatment-related myelodysplasia. Patients should be treated according to the indications outlined in Table 83–4. An algorithm to our treatment approach to first relapsed CLL is summarized in Fig. 83–2. In general for the patient under the age of 70 who has experienced a good remission with initial therapy (>12 months), an FCR regimen preferably in combination with an investigational agent is suggested. If a complete remission is obtained in the absence of del(17p13.1) being present, our approach at this point is to observe. If a del(17p13.1) is present or a complete response to therapy is not obtained, we generally will consider a nonmyeloablative stem cell transplant. For patients relapsing who are 70 years or older, retreatment with the same therapy or an alternative antibody or investigational agent can be considered. In general, we do not administer FCR to this patient population owing to concerns of increasing toxicity.

Stem Cell Transplantation

For many years, autologous and allogeneic stem cell transplants (SCTs) were generally used for treatment of CLL late in the course of the disease. However, trials of SCTs have indicated that patients with multiply relapsed and chemotherapy-resistant disease are at highest risk for both relapse and treatment-related morbidity and mortality (TRM). Additionally, many patients with heavily treated CLL cannot be adequately cytoreduced or disease control cannot be maintained for a sufficient period of time to obtain insurance approval, producing a selection bias that often excludes patients with the most refractory or aggressive disease from actually receiving SCT. The recognition that patients with poor prognostic features such as del(11q22.3) and del(17p13.1) and patients who fail to achieve CR after receiving regimens such as FCR have a short remission duration to initial therapy has prompted many transplant centers to consider earlier application of SCT as therapy for CLL, including as consolidation treatment after induction therapy for the highest-risk patients. Referral of high-risk CLL patients at the time of initial treatment to an experienced transplant center for evaluation, potential tissue typing of the patient and his or her siblings, and initiation of an unrelated donor search (if needed) should be considered. Although historical data on autologous SCT is reviewed in this chapter, nonmyeloablative allogeneic SCT is the preferred modality for most patients requiring a transplant unless a suitable allogeneic donor is not available.

Autologous Stem Cell Therapy

Results of studies of high-dose therapy with autologous stem cell rescue, or autologous SCT, have varied considerably as a result of patient selection and the variable use of stem cell purging. A British MRC study of autologous SCT in 65 patients attained a 5-year DFS and OS of 52% and 78%, respectively, and 16 of 20 evaluable patients achieved molecular remission.[271] In contrast, unmutated IgV_H remained an adverse prognostic factor despite autologous SCT in a retrospective German study of 58 CLL patients.[272] The median time to relapse was 37 months in the unmutated IgV_H group (n = 38), whereas only 1 of 20 mutated IgV_H patients relapsed 4 years after SCT. A retrospective case–control study matched 44 CLL patients who underwent autologous SCT with 44 similar CLL patients who did not.[272] Unmutated IgV_H was seen in 66% of patients in both cohorts. Median survival from diagnosis for unmutated IgV_H patients favored autologous SCT (139 months vs. 73 months; hazard ratio 0.31). Thus, although autologous SCT may benefit CLL patients with unmutated IgV_H, the results of autologous SCT in unmutated IgV_H patients is inferior to those achieved in mutated IgV_H patients.

The largest study of autologous SCT for CLL was performed by the Dana-Farber Cancer Institute in 137 patients, 90% of whom were IgV_H unmutated.[274] Patients received cyclophosphamide 120 mg/kg IV and 1400 cGy of total body irradiation (TBI), followed by infusion of anti-CD20-, anti-CD10-, and anti-B5-purged autologous bone marrow. The 100-day mortality was 4%, and 6-year PFS and OS were 30% and 58%, respectively. Thirteen patients (9%) developed myelodysplasia (MDS) at a median of 36 months after SCT.

Despite these promising results, autologous SCT for relapsed CLL is not routinely pursued. First, most CLL patients are poor candidates for autologous SCT because of bone marrow infiltration by CLL and contamination of the autologous stem cell product despite cytoreductive therapy.[275] Second, myelosuppression due to prior therapies such as fludarabine negatively affects autologous stem cell mobilization; in the MRC study, peripheral stem cell mobilization was unsuccessful in 33% of patients.[271] Third, secondary MDS or AML is a major concern, with 8% of patients in the MRC study and 9% in the Dana-Farber study developing MDS/AML.[271,274] Finally, no study has demonstrated a survival plateau for autologous SCT in CLL. Given these limitations, the major focus of clinical research in SCT for CLL has shifted to allogeneic SCT.

Myeloablative Allogeneic Stem Cell Therapy

Allogeneic SCT offers several theoretical advantages over autologous SCT in CLL. Contamination of the stem cell source and inadequate stem cell collection are not obstacles, and use of an allogeneic donor provides an immunologic graft-versus-leukemia (GVL) effect. Limited data suggest that TBI-containing conditioning regimens are superior to chemotherapy-only regimens in CLL transplant patients. A small study of 25 patients demonstrated a 100-day treatment-related mortality (TRM) of 57% in patients who received busulfan and cyclophosphamide (Bu/Cy; $n = 7$), compared to 17% for patients who received a TBI regimen (n = 18). Five-year actuarial survival was 56% for 14 patients transplanted with TBI regimens during 1992–1999.[276] A study of Cy/TBI in 28 CLL patients observed a 100-day TRM of 11%. Five-year PFS and OS were 78% and 78% for chemosensitive patients, compared to 26% and 31% for refractory patients.[277]

A retrospective EBMT study of 135 patients showed 54% 3-year OS and 40% 100-day TRM.[277] The IBMTR reported similar findings, with 45% 3-year OS and 30% 100-day TRM in 242 patients.[278] The high TRM may be explained in part by the late stage of the disease in many of these patients. Median time from diagnosis to SCT was 41 and 46 months in these two studies, and 37% of patients in the EBMT study were chemorefractory prior to transplant.[278,279] In a Canadian study of allogeneic SCT in 30 CLL patients, the 5-year EFS and OS were both 39%, with 48% OS for patients with sibling donors.[280] The role of unrelated donor allogeneic SCT was examined by a multicenter study in 38 patients, 92% of whom received TBI.[281] Five-year FFS and OS were 30% and 33%, and TRM was 38%. Although there are no prospective randomized studies, a retrospective comparison showed a 3-year DFS of 57% for allogeneic SCT, versus 24% for purged autologous SCT.[282] Finally, allogeneic SCT appears to overcome the adverse prognosis associated with an unmutated IgV_H; an analysis of 34 CLL patients who underwent SCT found that only 2 of 14 patients who received allogeneic SCT relapsed, compared to 13 of 20 patients who underwent autologous SCT.[283]

Thus, myeloablative allogeneic SCT may provide superior DFS to patients with CLL, as compared to autologous SCT. Although the 3-year DFS after allogeneic SCT is approximately 50%,[276–279,282] longer follow-up is needed to determine if the disease remissions are durable. However, this DFS advantage is offset by significantly higher TRM,[278,279] thus limiting the use of allogeneic SCT in CLL. Limited data indicate that Bu/Cy may be particularly toxic in this population; by contrast, TBI regimens have acceptable TRM.[276] To preserve the immunologic GVL effect while reducing TRM, the focus of clinical SCT research in CLL has turned to nonmyeloablative, or reduced-intensity, allogeneic SCT.

Nonmyeloablative Allogeneic Stem Cell Therapy

Ideally, the goal is to harness the GVL effect of allogeneic SCT for patients with CLL, while reducing TRM from acute GVHD, acute infection, and organ toxicity associated with myeloablative conditioning. Fludarabine, busulfan, and ATG were administered to 30 German CLL patients; the stem cell source was a matched related (n = 15) or unrelated (n = 15) donor.[284,285] Grade 2 to 4 acute GVHD was observed in 56% of patients, while 75% developed chronic GVHD.[285] Responses were seen in 93% of patients, with 40% achieving CR. Of note, it took up to 2 years for patients to achieve CR, suggesting a GVL effect. All patients achieved a molecular CR by PCR, but only six patients were in continued molecular CR after a median follow-up of 2 years. Two-year TRM, PFS, and OS were 15%, 67%, and 72%, respectively.[285]

The EBMT retrospectively examined 77 CLL patients who received a variety of nonmyeloablative conditioning regimens, following by allogeneic SCT.[286] The 1-year TRM was 18%, and the 2-year probability of relapse was 31%. Two-year DFS and OS were 56% and 72%, respectively. Nineteen patients received donor lymphocyte infusions (DLIs) for relapse or incomplete donor chimerism, but only seven responded to DLI (37%). Unfortunately, this study was complicated by the heterogeneity of conditioning regimens and the use of ATG or Campath-1H for T-cell depletion of the grafts in 40% of patients. A retrospective analysis of 73 CLL patients who underwent nonmyeloablative SCT and 82 patients who underwent myeloablative allogeneic SCT showed that the TRM was significantly reduced in the former group, with a hazard ratio of 0.4; however, there was no difference in EFS or OS between the two groups.[287]

Sixty-four patients received 200 cGy of TBI, with (n = 53) or without (n = 11) fludarabine, followed by an allogeneic SCT from a related (n = 44) or unrelated (n = 20) donor.[288] The 2-year DFS and OS were 52% and 60%, respectively, and the 2-year TRM was 22%. The incidence of relapse at 2 years was 26%, and the mortality due to relapse was 18%. Finally, a British study of 41 CLL patients who received fludarabine, melphalan, and alemtuzumab, followed by an allogeneic SCT from a related (n = 24) or unrelated (n = 17) donor observed a 2-year OS and TRM of 51% and 26%.[289] Eleven patients (27%) relapsed and received escalated donor lymphocyte infusions, but only three patients had a sustained response to DLI. Five patients (12%) have died of relapse.

Nonmyeloablative allogeneic SCT may be superior to autologous SCT in obtaining clinical and molecular remissions in high-risk CLL patients with unmutated IgV_H, due to a GVL effect. Seven of nine patients (78%) in a German study became negative by PCR for allele-specific IgV_H after d+100 post-SCT; attainment of molecular CR occurred after DLI or development of chronic GVHD.[290] In contrast, only 6 of 26 control CLL patients (23%) achieved a PCR-negative state after autologous SCT. Similar findings were reported by a

Spanish study of nonmyeloablative SCT in 30 CLL patients.[290] The 6-year EFS and OS were 92% and 90% patients with unmutated IgV_H or del(11q). Thus, an immunologic GVL effect appears to be important in CLL and may confer a long-term survival advantage for allogeneic over autologous SCT, given sufficient time.[291]

Investigational Agents Currently in Phase II–III Testing for Relapsed CLL

Although there are numerous therapeutic agents currently being tested in CLL, many likely will be ineffective. Attention is therefore directed toward agents that are currently in phase III registration studies based on preliminary efficacy in relapsed CLL.

HuMax CD20 (Ofatumumab)

HuMax CD20 (ofatumumab) is a fully humanized, high-affinity monoclonal antibody that targets a different epitope on CD20 molecule than rituximab. HuMax CD20 has higher affinity binding to CD20 and activates CDC more effectively than rituximab, suggesting that it may have more effective anti-tumor activity. Results of a phase I/II trial included 26 patients treated at the phase II dose and demonstrated an ORR of 46% (12 of 26 evaluable patients) with 1 nPR and 11 PR.[292] The median time to TTP was 161 days in responders, and median time to next CLL therapy was 366 days. The AUC of HuMax CD20 correlated with both TTP and time to next therapy, whereas clearance of ofatumumab (median 10 mL/h; range 3–42) correlated inversely with clinical outcome. Toxicity was predominately grade 1–2 infectious events in 48% of patients, although patient developed life-threatening interstitial pneumonitis. A phase III registration study of ofatumumab in patients with CLL resistant to alkylating agents, fludarabine, and alemtuzumab is ongoing. There are currently no data on the efficacy of HuMax CD20 in CLL patients with high-risk cytogenetic abnormalities.

Lumiliximab (IDEC-152)

CD23, a 45-kd low-affinity IgE receptor, is another potential target of monoclonal antibody therapy, as the antigen is expressed on almost all CLL cells. In vitro studies of a chimeric macaque-human anti-CD23 monoclonal antibody, Lumiliximab (IDEC-152), demonstrated that cross-linked lumiliximab was able to induce apoptosis in primary CLL cells, and that this apoptosis was enhanced by fludarabine and rituximab.[293] In an initial phase I study, 46 patients with relapsed CLL received lumiliximab 125–500 mg/m² IV weekly or thrice weekly for 4 weeks.[294] Toxicity was observed in 89% of patients, but only 15% developed grade 3 or 4 toxicity. A decrease in the degree of peripheral lymphocytosis was observed in 91% of patients, and 28% experienced more than a 50% reduction in their lymphocyte count. Reduction of nodal disease was seen in 52% of patients. A subsequent phase II study by the same investigators examined the combination of lumiliximab and FCR.[295] Thirty-one relapsed CLL patients received fludarabine 25 mg/m² and cyclophosphamide 250 mg/m² on days 2 to 4 of cycle 1 and on days 1 to 3 of cycles 2 to 6, rituximab 50 mg/m² and 325 mg/m² on days 1 and 3 of cycle 1 and 500 mg/m² on day 1 of cycles 2 to 6, and lumiliximab 50 mg/m² and 325 or 450 mg/m² on days 2 and 4 of cycle 1 and 375 or 500 mg/m² on day 1 of cycles 2 to 6, every 28 days for up to six cycles. Grade 3 or 4 toxicity, primarily hematologic, was observed in 65% of patients. The ORR was 71%, with 52% of patients attaining a CR. Patients with del(11q22.3) but not del(17p13.1) experienced high response rates and durable remissions to this therapy. On the basis of these promising results, a randomized phase III study comparing FCR alone to the combination of FCR and lumiliximab is under way.

Lenalidomide

Lenalidomide, or 3-(4-amino-1,3-dihydro-1-oxo-2*H*-isoindol-2-yl)-2,6-piperidinedione (Revlimid), is an immunomodulatory drug (IMiD) that is a more potent analog of thalidomide and targets the tumor microenvironment. At this time, the mechanism of action of this agent in CLL is uncertain. Lenalidomide 25 mg PO was given for 21 days every 28 days for up to 12 months to 45 patients with relapsed CLL.[296] A flare reaction was observed in 50% of patients (8% grade 3–4), and several patients discontinued therapy as a result of the flare reaction. The flare reaction clinically presents with sudden onset of tender enlargement of lymph nodes and/or spleen associated with fever and/or rash. Some patients can experience an increased white blood cell count. Low-dose prednisone, 20 mg daily, can alleviate the flare reaction. Hematologic toxicity associated with lenalidomide therapy was significant, with grade 3 to 4 neutropenia and thrombocytopenia occurring in 70% and 45% of patients, respectively, but only 5% of patients developed grade 3 to 4 infectious complications. The intent-to-treat ORR was 47%, with 9% patients achieving a CR. Lenalidomide was administered at a dose of 10 mg daily to 35 patients with relapsed CLL in one trial; dose escalation by 5 mg daily every 28 days was allowed, but median dose was 10 mg daily.[297] The ORR of the first 22 patients was 32%, with one patient achieving a CR. Nine additional patients had stable disease or experienced clinical benefit. In each of these two lenalidomide trials, a small number of responses were noted in CLL patients with del(11q22.3) and del(17p13.1) although data on their durability are not available. On the basis of these promising phase II clinical studies, a large, multicenter trial randomizing patients to low-dose (10 mg) or high-dose (25 mg) lenalidomide is currently under way in patients with relapsed and refractory CLL. Because of the potential for life-threatening tumor flair and other toxicity with lenalidomide, this agent should only be considered as part of a well-designed clinical trial despite its FDA approval for other indications (MDS and multiple myeloma).

Flavopiridol

Flavopiridol (alvocidib) is an *N*-methylpiperidinyl, chlorophenyl flavone that induces caspase 3-dependent apoptosis of primary CLL cells.[298] Caspase 3 acts distal to p53; thus, induction of apoptosis by flavopiridol is p53 independent.[299] Flavopiridol also induces profound reduction in Mcl-1 and XIAP expression in CLL cells in vitro.[300] Phase I clinical studies determined a safe, tolerable dose of 50 mg/m²/day given by 72-hour continuous IV infusion (CIVI).[299] Unfortunately, phase II studies administering flavopiridol by 24- to 72-hour CIVI failed to show any clinical activity. Despite plasma flavopiridol concentrations of 200 to 400 nM, apoptosis was not seen in peripheral blood mononuclear cells of patients who received this CIVI schedule.[301,302] This lack of efficacy in CIVI dosing schedules was due to increased binding of flavopiridol to human serum proteins. Free flavopiridol concentration decreased from 63%–100% to 5%–8% if human plasma was used instead of fetal calf serum when performing in vitro studies, resulting in an increase in 1-hour and 24-hour LC_{50} values from 670 and 120 nM to 3510 and 470 nM, respectively.[302,303] Thus, CIVI dosing did not achieve pharmacologically effective drug concentrations, resulting in the lack of clinical responses.[301–303] Bolus dosing achieves the necessary LC_{50}; a phase II CALGB study giving flavopiridol 50 mg/m² by 1-hour IV bolus (IVB) for 3 consecutive days to 36 relapsed patients observed 4 PR (ORR 11%), and one patient experienced a tumor lysis syndrome (TLS).

Pharmacokinetic (PK) modeling indicated that a dosing schedule of a 30-min IVB followed by 4-hour CIVI would achieve a target $C_{4.5hr}$ of 1.5 *n*/4 and induce apoptosis of CLL cells in vivo. On the basis of this PK model, investigators conducted a phase I study of flavopiridol in patients with relapsed CLL.[304] The planned dose escalation was 30 to 80 mg/m² 30-min IVB followed by 30–80 mg/m² 4-hour CIVI weekly for 4 weeks, every 6 weeks for up to six cycles. DLT was observed at dose level 2 (40 mg/m^2 30-min IVB + 40 mg/m^2 4-hour CIVI), with two of three patients developing grade 4 to 5 tumor lysis syndrome. Decreasing the dose to 30 mg/m^2 30-min IVB + 30 mg/m^2 4-hour CIVI, increased safety precautions, aggressive monitoring of serum potassium, and prompt intervention for hyperkalemia allowed safe administration of the drug. Subsequent cohorts in the phase I study demonstrated that the 4-hour CIVI could be safely escalated to 50 mg/m^2 after the initial treatment. This increase in the 4-hour CIVI dose from 30 to 50 mg/m^2 increased $C_{4.5hr}$ from 0.96 to 1.55 μM, with a concomitant increase in antitumor activity, as measured by a median rise in LDH. A tumor lysis syndrome requiring hemodialysis with first treatment dose was observed in 3% of patients with WBC less than 200 × 10^9/L, but 63% of patients with WBC counts of 200 × 10^9/L or more. Therefore, patients with extremely high peripheral lymphocyte counts should undergo cytoreduction before receiving flavopiridol. Nineteen of the first 42 patients in the phase I study responded (45%), including 5 of 12 patients (42%) with del(17p), 13 of 18 patients (72%) with del(11q), and 16 of 31 patients (51%) with bulky lymph nodes more than 5 cm in size.[305] The median duration of PFS was 12 months. Phase II studies are under way in CLL, as are clinical trials to examine flavopiridol as consolidation therapy for patients with MRD, as single-agent therapy for acute leukemias and lymphomas and as part of fludarabine-based combination regimens.

Other Agents in Clinical Trials for CLL

A variety of other therapeutic agents are currently in early phase I/II clinical trials for CLL or will be entering the clinic within the next year. Therapeutic antibodies or small modular immune pharmaceuticals (SMIP™) targeting surface antigens including CD40 (SGN40, HDC122), HLA-DR, CD19, CD20, and CD37 are under development. Additionally, therapeutic agents targeting signal transduction pathways (HSP-90 inhibitors, AKT inihibitors, PI3K-δ inhibitors, PKC-δ inhibitors, and PP2A activating agents) are in early clinical development. Finally, agents targeting epigenetic events (histone deacetylase inhibitors, hypomethylating agents, or miR-directed therapy), telomerase (GRN163), or innate immune activation (CpG oligonucleotides or IL-21) have promising preclinical data to support their ongoing early clinical investigation.

SPECIAL CONDITIONS IN CLL

Young Patients (Less Than 50 Years of Age) With CLL

As mentioned previously, CLL is a disease of the elderly, with only 10% of patients being under the age of 50 at diagnosis. Although CLL patients live for a prolonged period of time, young patients without comorbid illnesses have a great potential to have their life significantly shortened by the disease, irrespective of their cytogenetic abnormalities. Additionally, stress associated with job performance, insurance coverage maintenance, and disease-related symptoms are most significant in this age group. Special attention to psychosocial issues related to CLL should occur early in the course of the disease to allow patients to maintain or resume their normal life style as soon as possible. In the absence of impending need for therapy, our approach is generally not to empirically pursue HLA typing or examine transplant options prior to the development of symptomatic disease. Once therapy is initiated for this group of patients, consideration of aggressive intervention to promote prolonged remission duration is always a top priority. SCT is generally considered for patients in this age group with CLL with high risk cytogenetic abnormalities in first remission and for all patients who relapse after initial therapy unless high risk cytogenetic abnormalities are not present and a complete response is attained.

Patients With Fludarabine-Refractory CLL

Fludarabine-refractory CLL is generally considered to exist if a patient has not responded to a fludarabine-based therapy or relapses within 6 months of completing such a regimen. Several retrospective studies have documented a short survival (9 to 12 months) and particularly high frequency of both bacterial and opportunistic infections in this patient population.[306,307] New therapeutic agents such as alemtuzumab (currently approved for use in CLL) and new investigational agents (ofatumumab, lenalidomide, and flavopiridol) have been evaluated in this patient population. Although one group has advocated not pursuing nonmyeloablative allogeneic stem cell transplant until patients reach this state,[308] many patients have bulky lymph nodes or extensive bone marrow involvement that cannot be cleared with traditional or investigational therapies, making them a higher risk for treatment failure. Many patients also develop uncontrollable disease proliferation, Richter transformation, or infection that combined with insurance or regulatory delay prevents transition to this potentially curative intervention in a timely fashion. Therefore, although all patients under the age of 70 with fludarabine-refractory CLL should be considered for transplant, pursuit of this earlier following relapse is the approach used by our group. The complexities of complications, poor therapy options, and acute features of fludarabine-refractory CLL can put great strain on the patient, family members, and general hematologist alike. Referral of such patients to tertiary CLL centers for access to clinical trials and treatment of these specialized needs should be considered for patients with fludarabine-refractory CLL.

Richter Syndrome

Richter syndrome (RS) was described as the development of high-grade lymphoma in patients with CLL by Maurice Richter in 1928.[309] Over the years, the classification of RS has expanded to include lymphoid malignancies like Hodgkin disease, lymphoblastic lymphoma, prolymphocytic leukemia (PLL), and hairy cell leukemia (see Fig. 83–3A–C).[310] Incidence estimates range from 2.8 to 10.7%.[311,312] Recent studies have suggested that the development of RS may be related to the evolution of an abnormal clone unrelated to the underlying CLL clone.[313,314] Clearly identifiable risk factors for the development of RS are lacking, and its development has been shown to be independent of disease stage, duration of disease, type of therapy, or response to therapy.[310] However, the presence of diffuse lymphomatous involvement, advanced Rai stage, ZAP-70 expression, high LDH and β_2M levels may predict the development of RS.[315,316] The RS syndrome is characterized by sudden onset of B-symptoms (fever, night sweats, weight loss) and rapidly progressive lymphadenopathy at any anatomic site. Rarely the lymphomatous clone may arise from the bone or an extranodal site.[310] Laboratory abnormalities include anemia, neutropenia, and thrombocytopenia due to large-cell transformation in the bone marrow. A rapid increase in the serum LDH is seen in the majority of patients, with a significant proportion of patients also exhibiting paraproteinemia.[312] The diagnosis is generally made on examining the histology of a rapidly enlarging lymph node, which typically reveals large-cell lymphoma. Less commonly, the histology may be consistent with a high-grade small noncleaved cell lymphoma, lymphoblastic lymphoma, or hairy cell leukemia.[310] Even though a significant proportion of patients with advanced CLL and RS have abnormal cytogenetics, their prognostic significance has not been established.[317] Trisomy of chromosome 12 in the presence of a complex karyotype may have some correlation with aggressive disease,[318] although it is unlikely to be the only cytogenetic abnormality contributing to the lymphomatous transformation.[309] Historically, RS has been treated with regimens similar to those used for the treatment of large-cell lymphomas involving multiple agents like methotrexate, doxorubicin, cyclophosphamide, vincristine, prednisone, bleomycin, dexamethasone, cytarabine, and cisplatin (eg, MACOP-B, CHOP-B, DHAP, and VAD).[312,319] The best overall response rates of approximately 40% have been recently reported with the CFA (cyclophosphamide, fludarabine, cytarabine) and HyperCVXD-R (fractionated cyclophosphamide, vincristine, liposomal daunorubicin, dexamethasone, and rituximab) regimens.[319–322] The duration of response and the overall survival rates are dismal, with most patients likely to die within 6 months of their diagnosis despite aggressive therapy.[311] Long-term remissions and survival have been reported in a few patients following allogeneic SCT but this approach is associated with an extremely high 30-day transplant-related mortality of around 38%.[323]

Like RS, prolymphocytic transformation (PT) occurs in less than 10% of patients with CLL.[324] PT is characterized by the appearance of large, immature prolymphocytes in the peripheral blood, which make up 10% to 50% of the peripheral circulating malignant lymphoid cells.[325] These patients may be older with advanced disease and have more pronounced lymphadenopathy and splenomegaly.[326] PT is associated with a poor outcome, with limited survival beyond 1 year.[327] Therapeutic options are limited, with patients typically responding poorly to chemotherapeutic agents, including nucleoside analogs.[328] Alemtuzumab has shown promising results in patients with T-PLL, a closely related disorder.[328] Allogeneic SCT may also be utilized as a potentially curative therapeutic option.

Secondary Malignancies in CLL

CLL is associated with an increased risk of secondary malignancies. These include not only hematologic malignancies like MDS and AML associated with the use of chemotherapeutic agents[329] but also solid tumors such as Kaposi sarcoma, malignant melanoma, and laryngeal and lung cancers.[330] The increased incidence of secondary malignancies may be attributable to multiple reasons, including the immune dysfunction associated with CLL, the frequent infectious complications, the carcinogenic side effects of the various chemotherapeutic agents, and the increased and close medical surveillance that patients with CLL receive from trained oncologists.[330,331]

Hypersensitivity in CLL to Mosquitoes and Insect Bites and Treatment

CLL patients commonly exhibit an exaggerated cutaneous response to insect bites. This was first reported by Robert Weed in 1965 who documented a hypersensitivity reaction to insect bites in 8 out of 97 patients with CLL over a 13-year period.[332] The reaction is characterized histologically by the presence of a dermal infiltrate comprising a mixed population of T and B cells, eosinophils, and eosinophilic granule protein.[333] The extent of eosinophilic degranulation may also correlate with the severity of symptoms[334] Clinically, these patients present with recurrent, painful, bullous eruptions that may be traced to an insect bite in some instances.[335] Identification and avoidance of known triggers may be useful in some cases, but most patients are unable to identify the inciting exposure.[333] Treatment with a short course of steroids is usually effective, but these patients frequently relapse and may require multiple courses of therapy. Dapsone and chlorambucil may also be useful in severe, recurrent cases.[333,335]

Other cutaneous conditions are also common in CLL patients, with up to 45% reporting some form of skin involvement.[336] This includes petechial, purpural or ecchymotic lesions related to thrombocytopenia, infectious eruptions like herpes simplex and zoster, and direct leukemic involvement in less than 10% of all patients wiıh advanced disease.[336]

INFECTIONS IN PATIENTS WITH CLL

Infectious complications remain the leading cause of morbidity and mortality in patients with CLL. The incidence of infectious complications has been estimated to be as high as 80%[337,338] with a mortality of approximately 60%.[337,339] Various factors contribute to the increased incidence of infectious complications in CLL, the most important being progressive disease affecting host immunity through an impaired antibody response and hypogammaglobulinemia[340], weakened host cellular immune responses including impaired macrophage function[341], a decrease in T-regulatory cells[342], and finally the acquired defects after immunosuppressive chemotherapy.[306,343,344]

Recent studies have examined predictors of severe infections in patients with CLL. In their retrospective analysis of infection-related mortality in 280 patients, Francis and colleagues[345] identified advanced age, clinical Stage B or C disease, unmutated IgV_H, and positive CD38 status as independent predictors of both shorter time to first infection and infection-related mortality. Other risk factors that may also have an impact on development of infections include type of initial therapy and development of renal insufficiency.[345,346]

Historically, sinopulmonary infections from encapsulated bacteria like *Streptococcus pneumoniae* and *Haemophilus influenzae* have been the most common cause of infectious complications in patients with CLL.[347,348] With the recent use of more potent cytotoxic chemotherapy and the resultant profound myelosuppression, an increased frequency of severe pulmonary infections, bacteremia and gram negative infections has been reported.[337,349] Infections caused by atypical organisms like *Listeria monocytogenes*, *Nocardia* spp, *Mycobacterium* spp, and *Neisseria meningitidis* are relatively infrequent in patients who receive conventional chemotherapy.[350] Treatment for presumed infection can be initiated empirically in CLL patients who develop fever, since fever in CLL patients usually indicates an active infection.[350,351] Therapy should be tailored to the particular organ involved and the sensitivity of the organism. Prophylactic antibiotics can be initiated for debilitated patients with high-risk disease and significant immune dysfunction.

Viral infections are also commonly encountered in CLL patients (see Fig. 83–3D, E). Herpesvirus infections are especially common in patients treated with nucleoside analogs.[351,352] Chronic, indolent oropharyngeal and circumoral herpes simplex virus (HSV) outbreaks are more frequent than aggressive, disseminated visceral disease.[353] Reactivation of Epstein–Barr virus (EBV) has been implicated in some cases of Richter transformation.[354] Other viruses may cause severe systemic disease in patients with CLL. Varicella zoster virus (VZV) can cause herpes zoster, herpetic neuralgia, and rarely meningoencephalitis[306]; Parvovirus B19 can cause severe polyarthritis and pure red cell aplasia[355,356]; and JC polyoma virus has been implicated in the development of progressive multifocal leukoencephalopathy.[357,358] Management of these infections depends on early recognition of disseminated viral disease, timely initiation of antiviral therapy in cases of HSV and EBV, and a low threshold for the introduction of prophylactic acyclovir and supportive therapy. All patients should be provided instruction to identify the signs and symptoms of herpes virus infection at the time of diagnosis of CLL.

Fungal infections are not typically observed in CLL in the absence of treatment with corticosteroids or other immunosuppressive therapy for autoimmune complications arising from CLL. Cryptococcal meningitis, pneumonia, and fungemia are well recognized occurrences in patients with CLL and are associated with significant morbidity and mortality.[359] More cases of *P carinii* pneumonia, systemic candidiasis, and aspergillosis have been reported since the advent of combination nucleoside analog therapy with steroids.[337,360,361] Reactivation of parasitic infections including *Leishmania*[362] and *Strongyloides*[363] have also been reported. Treatment of the infection is dictated by the identification of the particular organism. Trimethoprim-sulfamethoxazole is routinely used as effective prophylaxis against *P carinii* infections, especially during and immediately after the use of nucleoside analogs.[346] Fungal prophylaxis with fluconazole may also be employed during protracted therapy with high dose steroids, although it should be noted that fluconazole will not cover organisms such as Aspergillus.

Prophylactic Strategies for Infections

Routine use of prophylactic antibiotics for CLL is generally not employed despite the higher frequency of infections observed in patients with this disease. Early recognition of signs and symptoms of infection and prompt initiation of empiric broad-spectrum antibiotics is probably a more feasible and cost-effective approach. When chemoimmunotherapy is used that includes a nucleoside analog or alemtuzumab therapy, prophylaxis for herpes simplex and varicella zoster should be used, particularly in older patients. Trimethoprim-sulfamethoxazole (or other alternative PCP prophylaxis) should also administered in this setting.[364,365]

Hypogammaglobulinemia is virtually always present in advanced CLL, and several studies have examined if IVIG replacement therapy can reduce the incidence and severity of infectious complications. Patients receiving IVIG in a double-blinded, placebo-controlled trial[366] experienced significantly fewer bacterial infections than the placebo group. The therapy was well tolerated with few adverse reactions, but there was no observed benefit in terms of preventing viral or fungal infections. However, other studies have shown an almost 50% reduction in the number of serious infections per year with IVIG infusions. Limited data support the use of IVIG at a higher dose of 600 mg/kg every 4 weeks to reduce the number and severity of respiratory infections.[367] However, the prohibitive cost of IVIG therapy and the fact that it has not been shown to prolong survival[368] argues against its empiric use in all patients. IVIG should be used judiciously and reserved for patients with advanced stage disease and recurrent infections. The usual dose used is 200 to 400 mg/kg every 4 to 6 weeks as needed, with the aim of keeping the trough serum IgG concentration greater than 500 mg/dL.

Among the strategies for preventing infection in this patient population is immunization. CLL patients however typically respond poorly to pneumococcal and influenza vaccines.[369,370] Advanced age, advanced disease stage, hypogammaglobulinemia, and low levels of soluble CD23 correlate with response to immunization.[371] Soluble CD23, a degradation product of membrane-bound CD23, is involved in several aspects of B-cell activation and proliferation and has a synergistic effect on histamine release. Histamine has a direct inhibitory effect on immunoglobulin production by B cells in vitro via histamine type-2 (H_2) receptors and also acts as an immune regulatory factor that can be modulated by H_2 receptor antagonists. Thus, responses to vaccines may be further enhanced by adjuvant treatment with H_2 blockers. Studies have shown that response to protein-conjugated vaccines may be enhanced by ranitidine in CLL patients to as much as 90%, compared to 43% in the control group.[372] Unfortunately, this response is not seen with polysaccharide vaccines. Recent studies have indicated that protein-conjugated vaccines may be more immunogenic, as shown by a more significant immune response to *Haemophilus influenzae* type b conjugate vaccine than to plain polysaccharide antigen.[373,374] In light of the paucity of data on an appropriate immunization schedule, we suggest a modified immunization plan based on the recommendations of the Advisory Committee on Immunization Practices.[375]

Growth factors such as granulocyte colony-stimulating factor (G-CSF) or granulocyte macrophage colony-stimulating factor (GM-CSF) can be used prophylactically in high-risk, severely neutropenic patients to shorten the duration and severity of neutropenia.[376]

AUTOIMMUNE COMPLICATIONS OF CLL

Patients with CLL have a greater predisposition to develop autoimmune hematologic complications, including autoimmune hemolytic anemia (AIHA), idiopathic thrombocytopenia purpura (ITP), and pure red cell aplasia. AIHA occurs in up to 37% of CLL patients at some time during the course of their disease. A small proportion (10%–15%) of patients may present with AIHA at diagnosis. AIHA can have a varied presentation, with patients developing signs of anemia, including weakness, lethargy, dyspnea on exertion, and dizziness over a period of months. Examination may reveal pallor, jaundice, hepatosplenomegaly and lymphadenopathy. Hemolysis can cause mild to moderate indirect hyperbilirubinemia, elevated LDH levels, and hemoglobinuria. The direct antiglobulin Coombs test is positive in up to 74% of patients with CLL,[377] but not all patients develop hemolysis. Most of the antibodies produced are warm reactive,[84] but patients can occasionally present with cold agglutination syndrome.[378] The antibodies are mostly polyclonal and usually a product of normal B cells rather than the leukemic clone.[379,380]

In contrast to the high frequency of AIHA in CLL, ITP or ITP and AIHA or Evan syndrome occurs less frequently in CLL. These events can occur throughout the entire course of CLL and is much more difficult to diagnose because of the absence of multiple implicating laboratory features as seen with autoimmune hemolytic anemia.

Given the small number of patients with AIHA, there are no data from controlled trials to guide the management of AIHA. Glucocorticoids have been used since 1940s[381] and are considered the first line of therapy. Most patients will respond to prednisone at a dose of 1 mg/kg for 10 to 14 days, followed by a slow taper over 2 to 3 months depending on the extent of hemolysis. Overall response rates of up to 90%, with 65% complete responses, have been reported with the use of steroids.[382] Unfortunately, approximately 60% of patients relapse when steroid therapy is stopped. IVIG, the next line of treatment, induces responses in 40% of patients.[382,383] Cyclosporine A (CSA) has been used for refractory AIHA at a dose of 5 to 8 mg/kg/day given in divided doses twice daily. The dose should be adjusted to maintain a serum level of around 100 to 150 μg/dL.[384–386] Rituximab has been used as treatment for AIHA with some success,[387] and studies are now examining the impact of rituximab in further reducing the incidence of AIHA when combined with conventional therapy.[388] Similarly, alemtuzumab has been used in combination with steroids or CSA or treatment of AIHA.[389–391] Alemtuzumab can also be effective as a steroid sparing agent.[390] Other treatment modalities include splenectomy[392,393] or splenic irradiation, alkylating agents, danazol, plasma exchange, immunoabsorption as an adjunct to plasma exchange,[394] and vincristine-loaded platelets.[395] Treatment of the underlying CLL is generally required for long-term control of autoimmune cytopenias. However, our practice is to first control the autoimmune process with steroids or other therapies before considering treatment of the underlying CLL. Supportive therapy with periodic red cell transfusions is also important in the management of AIHA.

There are limited data on the routine use of erythropoiesis-stimulating agents (ESA) in patients with Coombs negative anemia.[396,397] These agents are most effective in patients with low levels of endogenous erythropoietin and may improve the quality of life and reduce the frequency of transfusions in this subset of patients. However, given the recent data on the increased risk of thromboembolic events and higher sudden death rates in patients treated with these agents,[398–400] judicious use is recommended. ESAs are never recommended when rapid correction of hemoglobin is required.

Pure red cell aplasia (PRCA) is a relatively rare T-cell–dependent complication associated with CLL, but an incidence as high as 6% has been reported.[401] PRCA was first described by Dameshek and colleagues in 1967.[402] It is characterized by a hypoproliferative anemia that can be detected even in early-stage CLL and is thought to be caused by cytotoxic effects of suppressor T cells on erythroid progenitor cells.[403] Higher number of these CD3, CD8, and CD57 coexpressing cells have been shown to gradually accumulate in the bone marrow of patients with PRCA.[401] Abeloff and Waterbury described the first remission of PRCA to cyclophosphamide therapy in 1974,[404] and Chikkappa and colleagues described the first case of response to CSA.[405] Subsequent larger studies have shown a response rate as high as 63% with 300 mg daily of oral CSA.[385] Mild reversible nephrotoxicity may warrant dose adjustment in some patients. Most patients exhibit a response by having reticulocytosis within the first 10 to 14 days, but maximal response may occur an average of 10 weeks after the start of therapy. However, steroid therapy at a dose of 1 mg/kg/day of prednisone remains the first line of treatment.[382] If a response is not obtained in 4 weeks, CSA should be added to the regimen.[382,386]

Other agents that have shown promising activity in treating PRCA include rituximab,[387] IVIG,[406] alemtuzumab,[407] and antithymocyte globulin.[408] Packed red cell transfusions are usually indicated in patients who are clinically symptomatic from severe anemia.

A number of other complications, most of which are autoimmune in nature, have been reported in patients with CLL. These complications include paraneoplastic pemphigus,[409] angioedema due to acquired C1-inhibitor deficiency,[410] and nephrotic syndrome.[411] As a result of autoimmune involvement of various organs, patients with CLL may have abnormal serum chemistry profiles and liver function tests.

CONCLUSIONS

Advances in the molecular biology of CLL over the past two decades have translated into new diagnostic tests that allow better assessment of initial prognosis and also to assign treatment. Additionally, multiple new therapies have come forward and progress is being made to extend remission duration and improve quality of life of CLL patients. Additionally, medications and interventions to support complications that arise from CLL have also been introduced. Overall, the future for patients with CLL remains brighter based on these past efforts and likely will improve further with continued laboratory and clinical research ongoing in this disease.

FINANCIAL SUPPORT

This work was supported by the National Cancer Institute P01 CA95426, R01 CA095241, the American Cancer Society, the Leukemia and Lymphoma Society, and the D. Warren Brown Foundation.

SUGGESTED READINGS

Blum KA, Young D, Broering S, et al: Computed tomography scans do not improve the predictive power of 1996 National Cancer Institute sponsored working group chronic lymphocytic leukemia response criteria. J Clin Oncol 25:5624, 2007.

Borthakur G, O'Brien S, Wierda WG, et al: Immune anaemias in patients with chronic lymphocytic leukaemia treated with fludarabine, cyclophosphamide and rituximab—incidence and predictors. Br J Haematol 136:800, 2007.

Byrd JC, Lin TS, Dalton JT, et al: Flavopiridol administered using a pharmacologically derived schedule is associated with marked clinical efficacy in refractory, genetically high-risk chronic lymphocytic leukemia. Blood 109:399, 2007.

Flinn IW, Neuberg DS, Grever MR, et al: Phase III trial of fludarabine plus cyclophosphamide compared with fludarabine for patients with previously untreated chronic lymphocytic leukemia: US Intergroup Trial E2997. J Clin Oncol 25:793, 2007.

Fung SS, Hillier KL, Leger CS, et al: Clinical progression and outcome of patients with monoclonal B-cell lymphocytosis. Leuk Lymphoma 48:1087, 2007.

Gobessi S, Laurenti L, Longo PG, Sica S, Leone G, Efremov DG: ZAP-70 enhances B-cell-receptor signaling despite absent or inefficient tyrosine kinase activation in chronic lymphocytic leukemia and lymphoma B cells. Blood 109:2032, 2007.

Grever MR, Lucas DM, Dewald GW, et al: Comprehensive assessment of genetic and molecular features predicting outcome in patients with chronic lymphocytic leukemia: Results from the US Intergroup Phase III Trial E2997. J Clin Oncol 25:799, 2007.

Karlsson C, Hansson L, Celsing F, Lundin J: Treatment of severe refractory autoimmune hemolytic anemia in B-cell chronic lymphocytic leukemia with alemtuzumab (humanized CD52 monoclonal antibody). Leukemia 21:511, 2007.

Karlsson C, Hansson L, Celsing F, Lundin J: Treatment of severe refractory autoimmune hemolytic anemia in B-cell chronic lymphocytic leukemia with alemtuzumab (humanized CD52 monoclonal antibody). Leukemia 21:511, 2007.

Kay NE, O'Brien S M, Pettitt AR, Stilgenbauer S: The role of prognostic factors in assessing "high-risk" subgroups of patients with chronic lymphocytic leukemia. Leukemia 48:2412, 2007.

Kay N, Geyer SM, Call TG, et al: Combination chemoimmunotherapy with pentostatin cyclophosphamide and rituximab show significant clinical activity with low toxicity in previously untreated B chronic lymphocytic leukemia Blood 109:405, 2007.

Muntanola A, Bosch F, Arguis P, et al: Abdominal computed tomography predicts progression in patients with Rai stage 0 chronic lymphocytic leukemia. J Clin Oncol 25:1576, 2007.

Nikitin EA, Malakho SG, Biderman BV, et al: Expression level of lipoprotein lipase and dystrophin genes predict survival in B-cell chronic lymphocytic leukemia. Leuk Lymphoma 48:912, 2007.

Raval A, Tanner SM, Byrd JC, et al: Downregulation of death-associated protein kinase 1 (DAPK1) in chronic lymphocytic leukemia. Cell 129:879, 2007.

Rawstron AC: Monoclonal B-cell lymphocytosis: Good news for patients and CLL investigators. Leuk Lymphoma 48:1057, 2007.

Ries LAG MD, Krapcho M, Mariotto A, et al (eds.): SEER Cancer Statistics Review, 1975–2004, National Cancer Institute. Bethesda, MD. http://seer.cancer.gov/csr/1975_2005/ (based on November 2007 SEER data submission, posted to the SEER Web site, 2008) Accessed on April 25, 2008.

Robak T, Robak P: Current treatment options in prolymphocytic leukemia. Med Sci Monit 13:RA69, 2007.

Telle-Lamberton M, Samson E, Caer S, et al: External radiation exposure and mortality in a cohort of French nuclear workers. Occup Environ Med 64:694, 2007.

Terrier B, Ittah M, Tourneur L, et al: Late-onset neutropenia following rituximab results from a hematopoietic lineage competition due to an excessive BAFF-induced B-cell recovery. Haematologica 92:ECR10, 2007.

Van Bockstaele F, Pede V, Janssens A, et al: Lipoprotein lipase mRNA expression in whole blood is a prognostic marker in B cell chronic lymphocytic leukemia. Clin Chem 53:204, 2007.

Van der Velden AM, Van Velzen-Blad H, Claessen AM, et al: The effect of ranitidine on antibody responses to polysaccharide vaccines in patients with B-cell chronic lymphocytic leukaemia. Eur J Haematol 79:47, 2007.

Wright JR, Ung YC, Julian JA, et al: Randomized, double-blind, placebo-controlled trial of erythropoietin in non-small-cell lung cancer with disease-related anemia. J Clin Oncol 25:1027, 2007.

REFERENCES

For complete list of references log onto www.expertconsult.com

CHAPTER 84

HAIRY CELL LEUKEMIA

Anaadriana Zakarija, LoAnn C. Peterson, and Martin S. Tallman

INTRODUCTION

Hairy cell leukemia (HCL) is an uncommon chronic lymphoproliferative disorder initially described by Bouroncle and colleagues in 1958.[1] Although the cause remains unknown, the morphologic findings, clinical manifestations, and pathologic features have been well described over the past 50 years. HCL is characterized by splenomegaly, pancytopenia, and infiltration of the bone marrow with lymphocytes that have irregular cytoplasmic projections when identified in the peripheral blood (Fig. 84–1).[2,3] The disease is known to be a clonal B-cell malignancy as determined by heavy-chain immunoglobulin gene rearrangements.[4–6] Hairy cells exhibit an immunophenotype of mature B cells with expression of B-cell–associated surface antigens and monoclonal surface immunoglobulin.[7,8] Although many patients have few symptoms at diagnosis, others have life-threatening pancytopenia, symptomatic splenomegaly, or constitutional symptoms requiring treatment.[9,10]

Splenectomy, the treatment of choice for many years, leads to normalization of the peripheral blood counts in approximately one-half of all patients.[11–14] Interferon-α was first introduced for the treatment of patients with HCL in 1984,[15] and although a high overall response rate is achieved, most responses are partial.[14–21] Patients invariably relapse when the drug is discontinued. The most remarkable progress has occurred with the introduction of the two purine analogs, 2′-deoxycoformycin (2′-DCF)[22,33] and 2-chlorodeoxyadenosine (2-CdA).[24,34–44] Most patients with previously treated or untreated HCL achieve durable complete remission (CR) with either of these agents. The purine analogs appear to have changed the natural history of this disease.

EPIDEMIOLOGY

In the United States, HCL represents 2% of adult leukemias; approximately 600 to 800 new patients are diagnosed each year.[45,46] Although there have been several reports of familial HCL, there is no known genetic predisposition.[47–53] The median age of diagnosis is 52 years, and the disease occurs in men more often than in women by a ratio of approximately 4 to 1.[54] Although the incidence is similar in the United States and Great Britain,[45,46] classical HCL is rare in Japan, where a distinct variant form has been described.[55–57]

ETIOLOGY AND PATHOGENESIS

The cause of HCL is not known. Although some studies have suggested that exposure to benzene,[58,59] organophosphorus insecticides,[60] or other solvents[61] may be associated with development of the disease, this association has not been confirmed by other reports.[62] Exposure to radiation,[63] agricultural chemicals,[59] or wood dust[46] and a previous history of infectious mononucleosis[61] have also been suggested etiologies, but a causal relationship has not been firmly established.

Cyclin D1, an important cell cycle regulator, may play a role in the molecular pathogenesis of HCL. Overexpression of the cyclin D1 protein has been described in HCL patients.[64,65] Unlike mantle cell lymphoma, 11q13 rearrangements are not detected in most cases, suggesting other mechanisms of gene deregulation.[65]

CLINICAL PRESENTATION

The diagnosis is usually readily apparent in a middle-aged man who presents with splenomegaly, pancytopenia, and circulating hairy cells (Table 84–1). The initial evaluation of a patient with HCL should include a history and physical examination, a complete blood cell count with a differential cell count, review of the peripheral blood smear, routine serum electrolyte determinations, levels of blood urea nitrogen and creatinine, assays of hepatic transaminases, a bone marrow aspirate and trephine biopsy, and immunophenotyping of peripheral blood or bone marrow aspirate by flow cytometry (Table 84–2).

At the time of diagnosis, most patients present with symptoms related to anemia, neutropenia, thrombocytopenia, or splenomegaly. Approximately 25% of patients present with fatigue or weakness, 25% with infection, and 25% because of the incidental discovery of splenomegaly or an abnormal peripheral blood count.[54]

Patients usually appear well at the time of diagnosis. The most common and almost always sole physical finding is palpable splenomegaly, occurring in approximately 80% of patients.[3,54] The spleen is palpable 5 cm below the left costal margin in approximately 60% of patients. Hepatomegaly occurs in approximately 20% of patients. Unlike many other lymphoproliferative disorders, peripheral adenopathy is uncommon, with less than 10% of patients presenting with peripheral nodes larger than 2 cm in diameter. Although adenopathy is not common at diagnosis, internal adenopathy may develop after a prolonged disease course[66,67] and is present in 75% of patients at autopsy.[68] The characteristic distribution of disease in HCL probably results from the expression of the integrin receptor $\alpha_4\beta_1$ by the hairy cells and its interaction with the vascular adhesion molecule–1 (VCAM-1) found on splenic and hepatic endothelia, bone marrow, and splenic stroma.[69]

Patients with HCL are susceptible to gram-positive and gram-negative bacterial infections,[70] but they are also susceptible to atypical mycobacterial infections,[71] particularly *Mycobacterium kansasii*, and invasive fungal infections.[70] Other diseases of opportunistic infections that have been reported include Legionnaires disease,[72] toxoplasmosis,[73] and *Listeria monocytogenes* infection.[74] Infection in HCL may be attributable in part to granulocytopenia, monocytopenia, poor granulocyte reserve and abnormal mobilization,[75] T-cell dysfunction,[76] and decreased numbers of dendritic cells and antigen-presenting cells.[77]

Patients with HCL may have associated systemic immunologic disorders,[78] including scleroderma and polymyositis[79] and polyarteritis nodosa.[80] HCL has been associated with other cutaneous lesions such as erythematous maculopapules[81] and pyoderma gangrenosum.[82,83] An associated coagulopathy manifested by factor VIII antibodies has been reported.[84] Osseous involvement has also been described, primarily manifesting as lytic lesions in the axial skeleton, usually the proximal femur.[85,86] Rarely, osteolytic lesions may be associated with paraproteinemia.[87] A rare case of HCL occurring with systemic mast cell disease has been reported.[88]

LABORATORY EVALUATION

Pancytopenia is present in approximately 50% of patients with HCL at diagnosis, whereas most other patients present with suppression of

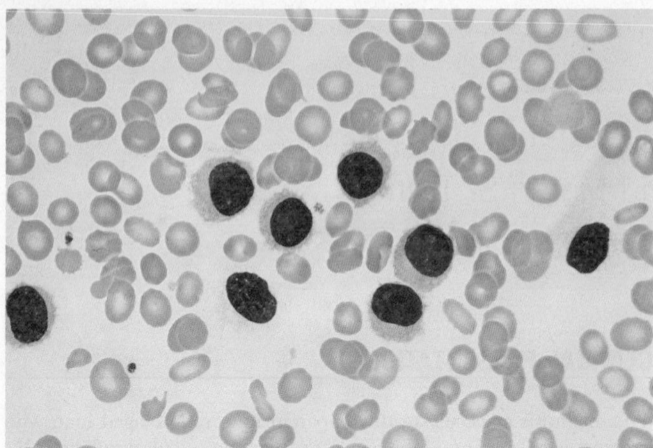

Figure 84–1 Peripheral blood smear from a patient with hairy cell leukemia. The patient was unusual in that he presented with a marked leukocytosis. The hemoglobin level and platelet count were reduced. The nuclei of the hairy cells are eccentrically located and exhibit a reticular chromatin. The cytoplasmic borders are irregular, with fine, hairlike projections (Wright-Giemsa stain, 1000×).

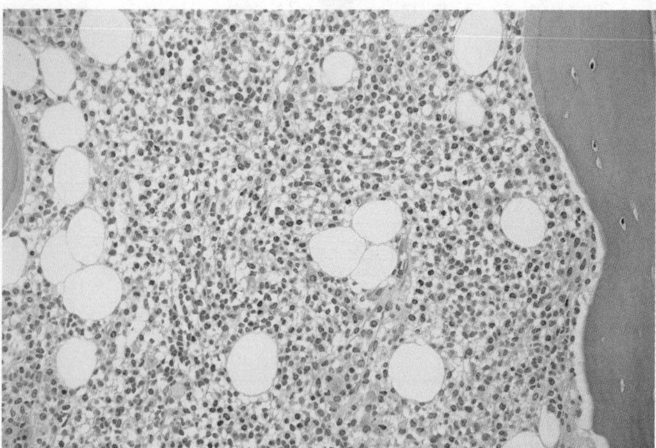

Figure 84–2 Bone marrow trephine biopsy section from a patient with hairy cell leukemia. The bone marrow is hypercellular with a diffuse infiltration by hairy cells. The hairy cell nuclei are widely spaced, separated from each other by a pale, lightly eosinophilic cytoplasm. Many extravasated red blood cells are present between the hairy cells (hematoxylin and eosin stain, 630×).

Table 84–1 Classic Presentation of a Patient with Hairy Cell Leukemia

Middle-aged man
Splenomegaly, often more than 5 cm below the left costal margin
Pancytopenia
Bone marrow usually cannot be aspirated ("dry tap")
Bone marrow trephine biopsy showing mononuclear cells separated by clear cytoplasm

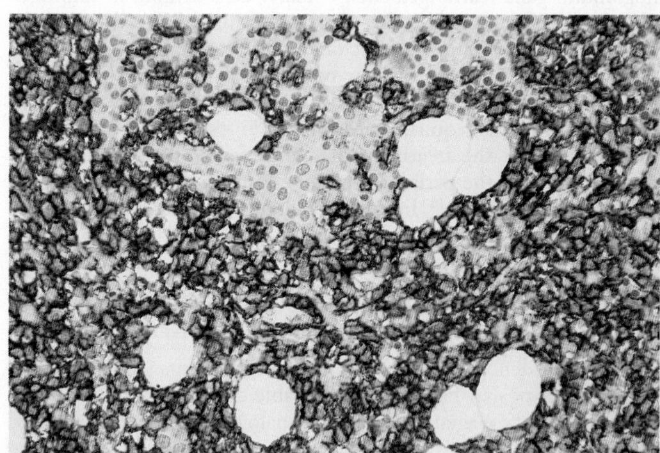

Figure 84–3 The hairy cells in the hypercellular bone marrow biopsy shown in Fig. 80–2 are accentuated by immunostaining for the B-cell antigen CD20. Residual erythroid and myeloid precursors are negative for CD20 (immunohistochemical stain for CD20, 400×).

Table 84–2 Initial Evaluation of a Patient with Hairy Cell Leukemia

History and physical examination
Complete blood cell count, differential cell count
Review of peripheral blood smear
Serum chemistries
Bone marrow aspirate and biopsy
Immunophenotyping of peripheral blood or bone marrow aspirate

only one or two cell lines.[3,54] Most patients with HCL present with leukopenia, although 10% to 20% of patients exhibit a leukemic phase with a white blood cell count higher than 10 to 20 × 10^9/L. Monocytopenia is a common, but often overlooked, finding and may be a helpful clue to the diagnosis.[1,3,54] Other laboratory findings include abnormal levels of hepatic transaminases (19%), azotemia (27%), and hypergammaglobulinemia (18%), which is rarely monoclonal.[3,87,89] Hypogammaglobulinemia is uncommon.

Hairy cells can be identified in Wright-stained peripheral blood smears from most patients with HCL. The number of circulating hairy cells varies, but is usually low. In some patients, hairy cells can be found only after a prolonged search. Bone marrow often cannot be aspirated, resulting in a so-called dry tap. However, when bone marrow aspiration is successful, hairy cells similar to those in the blood are present.

The morphologic features of hairy cells are characteristic (see Fig. 84–1). The neoplastic cells are approximately one to two times the size of a small lymphocyte. The nuclei are usually round, oval, indented, or monocytoid; rarely, they appear convoluted.[90] The nuclei are located in a central or eccentric position. The chromatin pattern is reticular or netlike in appearance; nucleoli are indistinct or absent. The amount of pale blue-gray cytoplasm varies. The cytoplasmic borders are irregular, with fine, hairlike projections or ruffled borders. Occasionally, cytoplasmic granules are present. Rarely, the cytoplasm exhibits rod-shaped inclusions that correspond to ribosomal lamellar complexes, which are observed ultrastructurally in approximately 40% of cases.[91]

Examination of the bone marrow trephine biopsy plays a critical role in the diagnosis of HCL because of its characteristic histopathologic appearance (Figs. 84–2 and 84–3).[92–95] The bone marrow is hypercellular in most patients. Hairy cell infiltration may be diffuse, patchy, or interstitial. In patients with diffuse involvement, large areas of the bone marrow are replaced by hairy cells, with complete effacement of the bone marrow in some patients. With patchy infiltration, subtle, small clusters of hairy cells are present focally or throughout the bone marrow. The hairy cells do not form well-defined, discrete aggregates; instead, they merge almost imperceptibly with the surrounding normal hematopoietic tissue. In the interstitial pattern of involvement, variable numbers of hairy cells infiltrate

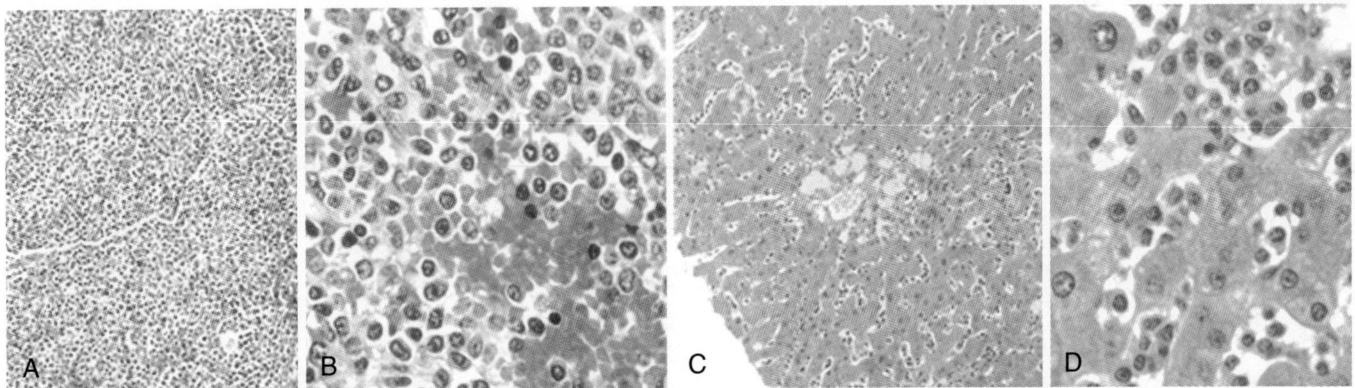

Figure 84–4 Spleen and liver in hairy cell leukemia (**A–D**). The spleen (**A, B**) shows a massive and diffuse infiltrate in the red pulp and depletion of the white pulp. The infiltrate is associated with hemorrhage, which results in red blood cell "lakes" (**B**, *lower right*). The liver (**C, D**) is frequently involved and the pattern of infiltration is predominantly sinusoidal.

between normal hematopoietic cells and fat, with preservation of the overall bone marrow architecture. The hairy cell nuclei are usually round, oval, or indented and are widely separated from each other by abundant, clear or lightly eosinophilic cytoplasm; rarely, the cells are convoluted or spindle shaped. The nuclear chromatin is lightly condensed, nucleoli are small and inconspicuous, and mitotic figures are rare. Extravasated red blood cells are frequently seen, and blood lakes, similar to those observed in the spleen, may also be present. Mast cells are often numerous. Reticulin stains of the bone marrow trephine biopsy in HCL almost always show a moderate to marked increase in reticulin fibers.

Residual hematopoietic cells are usually decreased in HCL; granulocytes are typically more severely reduced than erythroid precursors and megakaryocytes. Approximately 10% to 20% of patients exhibit a hypocellular bone marrow. The hypocellularity may be severe, with small numbers of hairy cells infiltrating around fat cells.[96] The morphology of these latter cases strongly resembles aplastic anemia.

Cytochemical or immunohistochemical demonstration of tartrate-resistant acid phosphate (TRAP) activity can aid in the diagnosis of HCL.[97] TRAP-positive cells are found in almost all cases of HCL at diagnosis, although the percentage of positive cells varies greatly among patients. TRAP positivity is not specific for HCL since a wide variety of other hematopoietic malignancies, including prolymphocytic leukemia, Sézary syndrome, and adult T-cell leukemia/lymphoma, may rarely show positive reactions. The introduction of immunophenotyping for the diagnosis of chronic lymphoproliferative disorders has made reliance on the TRAP stain much less important than it was historically.

Flow cytometric immunophenotyping is an important part of the diagnostic evaluation to identify the characteristic immunophenotypic profile of HCL and to distinguish it from other lymphoproliferative disorders. Because hairy cells exhibit distinctive light scatter pattern and a characteristic immunophenotype, they can be identified even in very low levels (<1% of lymphocytes) in the peripheral blood or bone marrow aspirate.[98] This property is useful at the time of diagnosis and after therapy to assess the blood and marrow for residual disease.[99]

Hairy cells strongly express CD45, seen as a bright signal, with increased forward and side scatter. They exhibit a mature B-cell phenotype and typically express one or more heavy chains and monotypic light chains. The heavy chain type is usually IgG, occurring alone or in combination with other types of heavy chains. The number of cases expressing κ or λ light chains is approximately equal. Surface immunoglobulin is expressed as moderate to bright intensity. Hairy cells strongly express pan-B-cell antigens, including CD19, CD20, CD22, and CD79b. They are usually negative for CD5, CD10, and CD23, but they strongly express CD11c, CD25, and FMC7. CD103, an antigen expressed on mucosal T cells and some activated T cells, is expressed in most cases of HCL.[98,100] Atypical immunophenotype with typical morphologic findings can be found in approximately 35% of patients including CD23$^+$ in 17%, and all such patients appear to respond well to purine analogs.[101]

Table 84–3 Differential Diagnosis of Hairy Cell Leukemia

Prolymphocytic leukemia
Splenic marginal zone lymphoma
Hairy cell leukemia variant
Chronic lymphocytic leukemia
Low-grade lymphoma
Agnogenic myeloid metaplasia
Systemic mastocytosis

Several B-cell–associated antibodies, including CD20, CD79a, and DBA.44, react with hairy cells in fixed, routinely processed tissue sections. None is specific for HCL, but these antibodies are useful in documenting the B-cell nature of the infiltrate and highlighting the extent of bone marrow infiltration at the time of diagnosis and after therapy.[102–105]

Splenic involvement in HCL is characterized by diffuse infiltration of the red pulp cords and sinuses, with atrophy or replacement of the white pulp (see Fig. 84–4A,B). Blood-filled sinuses lined by hairy cells are often a prominent, but not pathognomonic finding in the spleen; they have been referred to as *pseudosinuses*.[106] The liver shows sinusoidal and portal infiltration by hairy cells (see Fig. 84–4C,D). Involved lymph nodes commonly exhibit partial effacement, with hairy cells infiltrating the paracortex and medulla in a leukemic pattern. The leukemic cells often surround residual lymphoid follicles and extend through the capsule.

Clonal cytogenetic abnormalities are present in approximately two-thirds of patients with HCL. Chromosomes 1, 2, 5, 6, 11, 14, 19, and 20 are most frequently involved. Chromosome 5 is altered in 40% of patients, most commonly as trisomy 5, pericentric inversions, and interstitial deletions involving band 5q13.[107–109]

DIFFERENTIAL DIAGNOSIS

The differential diagnosis of HCL includes other small B-cell lymphoproliferative disorders associated with splenomegaly, such as prolymphocytic leukemia, splenic marginal zone lymphoma (ie, splenic lymphoma with villous lymphocytes), and HCL variant (Table 84–3 and Fig. 84–5). Patients with prolymphocytic leukemia typically present with splenomegaly, but this disorder can usually be readily

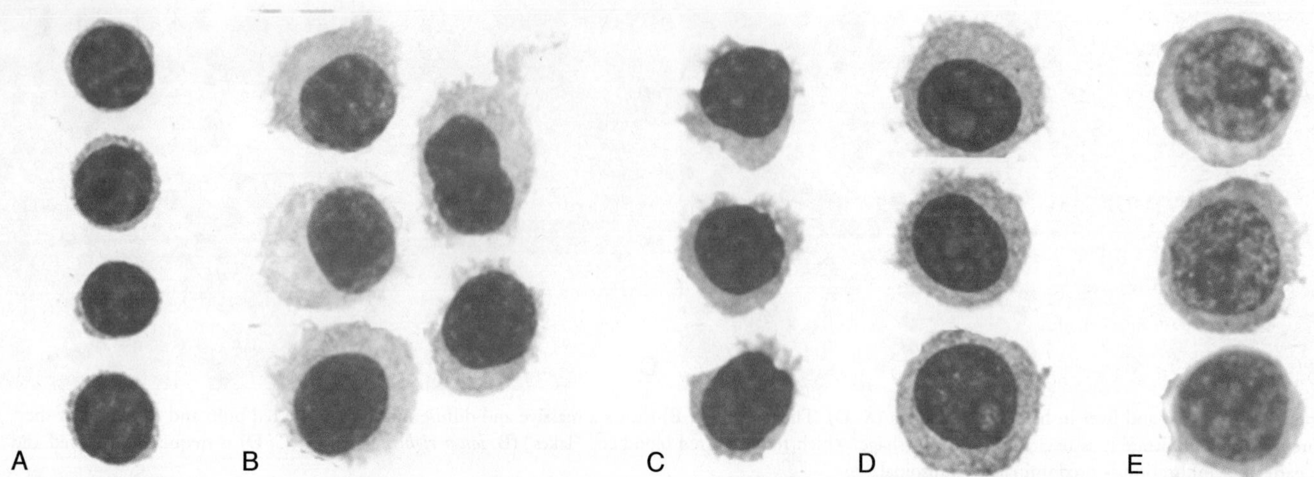

Figure 84–5 Cytologic features of hairy cells in comparison to other lymphoid leukemias to be considered in the differential diagnosis (**A–F**). Chronic lymphocytic leukemia cells (**A**), for comparison. Note small size, block-like, chromatin and scant cytoplasm. Hairy cells (**B**) have a larger nucleus, which is sometimes oval, reniform, or dumbbell-shaped, with more open chromatin and abundant pale cytoplasm with fuzzy edges. Splenic marginal zone lymphoma cells (ie, splenic lymphoma with villous lymphocytes) (**C**) are smaller and have more condensed and more blue cytoplasm with polar projections. Cell of the prolymphocytic variant of hairy cell leukemia (**D**) resemble hairy cells, although the nucleus is more condensed and nucleoli are present. Prolymphocytes (**F**) are large and have an open nuclear chromatin and prominent "punched-out" nucleoli.

distinguished from HCL by the marked elevation of the white blood cell count, the morphology of the prolymphocytes, and an immunophenotypic profile different from that of HCL.[110–113] Splenic marginal zone lymphoma exhibits some clinical and morphologic features similar to HCL, but the cells usually do not exhibit TRAP positivity, the bone marrow infiltrates are sharply demarcated, and the immunophenotypic profile differs from that of HCL, including no expression of CD103.[114–117] HCL variant exhibits morphologic features intermediate between hairy cells and prolymphocytes. HCL variant is associated with leukocytosis, lack of monocytopenia, and absence of CD25 expression.[118–122] Infiltrates of systemic mastocytosis in the bone marrow may closely resemble HCL. Immunohistochemical studies show the mast cells, unlike hairy cells, to be negative for B-cell markers and positive for tryptase.[123]

TREATMENT

Indications

HCL usually has an indolent course, with some patients surviving 10 years without requiring therapy.[124] In most patients, progressive disease eventually leads to complications resulting from anemia, bleeding, splenomegaly, or recurrent infections. Therapy is indicated when the patient has significant cytopenias, symptomatic organomegaly or adenopathy, or infections or constitutional symptoms such as fever, night sweats, or fatigue. Typical blood counts that warrant treatment include an absolute neutrophil count less than 1000/μL, a hemoglobin concentration less than 11.0 g/dL, or a platelet count less than 100,000/μL.

Role of Splenectomy

Splenectomy was the first effective therapy for HCL and remained the initial treatment of choice until the introduction of interferon and then the purine analogs.[11–14] Although splenectomy does not produce morphologic remissions in the bone marrow, all three cell lines return to normal in approximately 40% to 70% of patients.[14,125] This response is maintained for a median of 20 months in approximately two-thirds of patients, and the overall 5-year survival rate is approximately 70%.[125] There appears to be no correlation between spleen size and response to splenectomy. There may be a role for splenectomy in rare, selected patients for diagnostic reasons, in cases of splenic rupture, or when thrombocytopenia and a significant bleeding diathesis exist, because splenectomy can lead to a rapid rise in the platelet count. However, there has been little or no role for splenectomy since the introduction of the purine analogs.

Chemotherapeutic Approaches

Cytotoxic chemotherapy was used before the advent of more effective therapies in the early 1980s. A variety of agents, including anthracyclines,[126] alkylating agents (eg, chlorambucil),[127] and high-dose methotrexate,[128] demonstrated some efficacy. Combination chemotherapy, such as the CHOP regimen, was reported to produce long-lasting normalization of peripheral blood counts.[129] There is also a report in the literature of a successful syngeneic (identical twin) bone marrow transplantation in which the patient remained free of disease at least 15 years after the procedure.[124] HCL is sensitive to chemotherapy, but treatment is associated with significant myelosuppression and toxicity. Conventional chemotherapy is now only of historic interest.

Interferon

Interferon was first reported to be an effective therapy for patients with HCL in 1984.[15] Since then, numerous large studies have confirmed its activity.[15–21] The precise mechanism of action of interferon is unknown, but it may result from the reduced production of cytokines such as granulocyte colony-stimulating factor (G-CSF), granulocyte–macrophage colony-stimulating factor (GM-CSF), interleukin-3 (IL-3), and interleukin-6 (IL-6), perhaps related to the characteristic monocytopenia associated with interferon treatment.[130] Some work suggests that interferon-α results in apoptotic death of hairy cells, mediated by tumor necrosis factor-α.[131] Despite a high overall response rate of 75% to 90%, most patients achieve only partial remission (PR, defined as normalization of all peripheral blood cell counts).[18,19] Interferon is commonly administered subcutaneously at a dose of 2 million international units/m^2 three times each week for 12 to 18 months. During the first 2 months of treatment, the white blood cell count and hemoglobin level are often decreased, occasionally necessitating transfusion. The numbers of platelets normalize first in responding patients, followed by the hemoglobin concentration and the white blood cell count. An absolute neutrophil count greater than 1500/μL is achieved after a median of 5 months of therapy.

Common toxicities include flu-like symptoms, anorexia and fatigue, nausea and vomiting, diarrhea, dry skin, peripheral neuropathies, and central nervous system dysfunction. The latter usually manifests as depression or memory loss. Elevated levels of hepatic transaminases are the most common clinical abnormality other than myelosuppression. The median failure-free survival after discontinuing interferon ranges from 6 to 25 months in different series.[18–20,132] Patients with more than 30% hairy cells in the marrow or a platelet count of less than 160,000/μL at the end of treatment are at higher risk for early relapse.[18–20] Patients whose cells express the CD5 antigen appear to respond poorly to interferon.[133] One report suggests that patients can be maintained on long-term interferon at a dose of 3 million units administered subcutaneously and given three times each week with minimal toxicity. Sixty percent of patients sustain their initial response for a median of 5 years, 9% discontinue therapy early because of unexpected neurologic toxicity, and only 13% stop therapy because of progressive disease.[21] In summary, treatment of HCL with interferon is effective, resulting in normalization of the peripheral blood counts in most patients. However, CRs are uncommon, and failure-free survival is usually short after discontinuation of treatment (see box). The purine analogs have completely supplanted interferon except is very rare and unusual circumstances.

Purine Analog Therapy

Twenty-five years ago, Giblett and colleagues[137] observed that 30% of children with severe combined immunodeficiency syndrome lacked the enzyme adenosine deaminase (ADA). It appeared that the accumulation of the triphosphorylated form of deoxyadenosine was responsible for the absence of lymphocyte development.[138] The deliberate inhibition of ADA became a potentially useful antileukemic strategy. The methods to accomplish this include agents to bind irreversibly to ADA or resist the action of the enzyme. These agents affect dividing and nondividing cells.[139] After purine analog therapy, accumulation of deoxyadenosine triphosphates leads to DNA strand breaks and inhibition of DNA repair, which ultimately results in cell apoptosis.

2′-Deoxycoformycin

The first agent found to induce a significant number of CRs in patients with HCL was 2′-DCF.[22,140] This drug binds to ADA, resulting in irreversible inhibition of the enzyme,[141] which is found in all lymphoid cells and is important in purine metabolism. In most studies, CR is defined by disappearance of hairy cells in the blood and bone marrow; complete normalization of peripheral counts (hemoglobin concentration >12.0 g/L, platelets >100 × 10^9/L, and absolute neutrophil count >1.5 × 10^9/L); and resolution of splenomegaly and lymphadenopathy. A PR requires normalization of blood counts, more than 50% reduction in hairy cells in the bone marrow, and greater than 50% reduction in splenomegaly.

Several studies have demonstrated the efficacy of 2′-DCF in patients with HCL (Table 84–4).[23–33] A large, prospective, randomized study showed that the CR rate and relapse-free survival rate are significantly better with 2′-DCF than with interferon.[31] Various dosing schedules were used in early studies, but the current convention is 4 mg/m^2 given by intravenous infusion every 2 weeks until a maximum response is achieved. The median number of cycles required by patients until best response has been 6 to 12 cycles.[24,27,29,33] In one of the earlier studies conducted by the Eastern Cooperative Oncology Group, most patients achieved a maximal response within the first 6 months.[27] Therapy is relatively well tolerated; neutropenia, fever, and infections are the most common toxicities.[25,27,32] One of the largest published series with long-term follow-up was reported by the Southwest Oncology Group.[25] A total of 241 patients received 2′-DCF in a phase III trial comparing interferon with 2′-DCF; 154 were randomized to 2′-DCF initially, and 87 crossed over after failing interferon therapy. Seventy-two percent of patients achieved a CR with 2′-DCF. Long-term survival was not statistically different based on initial treatment; in both groups, the overall survival rate was 90% at 5 years and 81% at 10 years (Fig. 84–6). With longer follow-up, it has become obvious that 2′-DCF is not curative in all patients, and the relapse incidence continues to increase. Studies with follow-up longer than 5 years after treatment report relapses in 15% to 48% of patients.[23–25,30]

Management of Hairy Cell Leukemia

For patients with newly diagnosed hairy cell leukemia (HCL) who require treatment (absolute neutrophil count <1000/μL, or hemoglobin concentration <11.0 g/dL, or platelet count <100,000/μL or symptomatic organomegaly), we administer 2-chlorodeoxyadenosine (2-CdA) at a dose of 0.1 mg/kg/day by continuous intravenous infusion for 7 days as an outpatient procedure by portable pump using a midline percutaneous intravenous central catheter. Other schedules such as a 2-hour daily infusion for 5 days may be equally effective.[134] If fever of 100.5°F or higher develops while the patient is neutropenic, blood is drawn for cultures, urine culture and chest radiography are done, and oral ciprofloxacin (750 mg taken orally twice daily) or another antibiotic of similar spectrum of coverage is administered. If cultures are sterile at 24 to 48 hours, naproxen (250 mg taken orally twice daily) is added for 2 to 4 days. Treatment with 2-CdA is not discontinued. Hematopoietic growth factors are not routinely given. The platelet count is usually the first cell line to recover (within 2–4 weeks), followed by the white blood cell count and then the hemoglobin concentration. We repeat the bone marrow examination at 3 months to assess remission status. We do not administer a second cycle of 2-CdA for patients with minimal residual disease. Recent data suggest that the anti-CD20 monoclonal antibody rituximab (Rituxan) may be effective in eradicating minimal residual disease, but the benefit with respect to overall survival is not determined.[135]

Both 2′-DCF and 2-CdA are effective therapies for newly diagnosed patients with HCL. In a long-term follow-up retrospective report, CR rates (81% and 82%, respectively) and overall survival rates at 10 years (96% and 100%, respectively) were the same. With both purine analogs, relapses continue to occur.[136]

For patients with relapsed HCL who have been previously treated with splenectomy, interferon, or 2′-deoxycoformycin (2′-DCF), we administer a cycle of 2-CdA as described previously. For patients who relapse after a single cycle of 2-CdA, we administer a second cycle of 2-CdA. For patients with relapsed HCL previously treated with at least two prior cycles of 2-CdA, we consider BL22 or rituximab. 2′-DCF is considered depending on the availability or response to either BL22 or rituximab.

Food and Drug Administration–Approved Treatments for Hairy Cell Leukemia

Interferon-α: 2 × 10^6 international units/m^2 administered subcutaneously three times each week for 12 to 18 months

2′-Deoxycoformycin (2′-DCF, Pentostatin): 4 mg/m^2 given intravenously every 2 weeks until remission (usually 3 to 6 months)

2-Chlorodeoxyadenosine (2-CdA, cladribine, Leustatin): a single cycle, with 0.1 mg/kg/day given as a continuous infusion for 7 days

Table 84–4 Activity of 2′-Deoxycoformycin in Hairy Cell Leukemia

Study	No. of Patients	Previously Untreated	Median No. of Cycles	CR (%)	PR (%)	NR (%)	Median Follow-up (mo)	Relapse Rate (%)	Median Time to Relapse (mo)
Johnston et al[26]	28	18	NA	89	11	0	14	4	13.8
Ho et al[28]	33	0	NA	33.3	45.5		14.5	8	10
Rafel et al[32]	78	35	7	72	16	1	31	33	29
Cassileth et al[27]	50	19	6	64	20	16	39	14	CR: 13 PR: 31
Catovsky et al[29]	148	23	9	74.3	22.3	3.4	42	8	22
Ribeiro et al[33]	50	18	12	44	52	0	47	10	22
Grever et al[31]	154	154	NA	76	3		57	9	NA
Maloisel et al[23]	238	NA	9	79	16.6		63.5	15	NA
Dearden et al[24]	165	38	9	82	15		71	24	51.5
Kraut et al[30]	24	NA	NA	100	0	0	82	48	30
Flinn et al[25]	241	241	NA	72			112	18	NA

CR, complete response; NA, not available; NR, no response; PR, partial response.

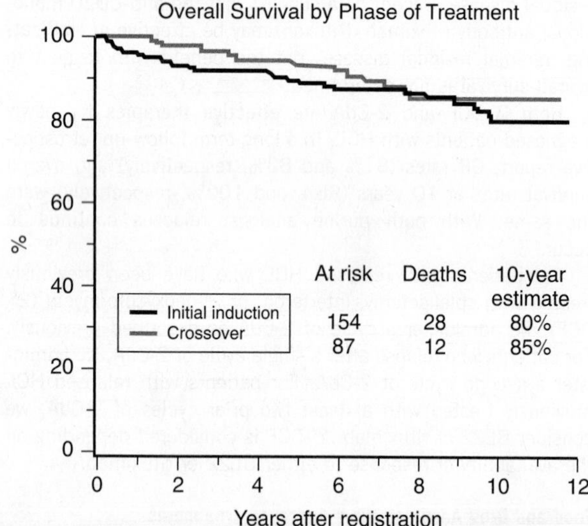

Figure 84–6 Overall survival of 241 patients with hairy cell leukemia treated with 2′-deoxycoformycin. Patients were stratified by treatment upfront or after failure on interferon. *(Data from Flinn IW, Kopecky KJ, Foucar MK, et al: Long-term follow-up of remission duration, mortality, and second malignancies in hairy cell leukemia patients treated with pentostatin. Blood 96:2981, 2000.)*

2-Chlorodeoxyadenosine

2-CdA is a purine analog that is resistant to the action of ADA. This agent accumulates in the lymphoid cells, presumably because they are rich in the enzyme deoxycytidine kinase.[141] This enzyme phosphorylates 2-CdA to the active 5′-triphosphate form, creating a deoxynucleotide that cannot readily exit the cell. This compound inhibits ribonucleotide reductase, which results in decreased synthesis of deoxynucleotides. DNA synthesis and repair are impaired.

2-CdA was first reported to be effective for HCL by Piro and colleagues in 1990.[34] Twelve patients were treated with a single cycle of 2-CdA at a dose of 0.1 mg/kg/day by continuous infusion for 7 days, and a pathologic CR was obtained in 11 of the 12 patients within 8 weeks of treatment. Subsequent studies have shown similar efficacy with the same dosing schedule (Table 84–5).[24,34–44] Clear orders for the 7-day infusion pump are critical because poor response to therapy has been attributed to underdosing of drug when 1 day's dose was administered over 7 days.[142] Alternative dosing schedules and routes have been reported with good results (Table 84–6).[143–146] In the study conducted by Von Rohr and colleagues,[146] 2-CdA was administered by subcutaneous bolus injection of 0.14 mg/kg/day for 5 days to 62 patients. The results were similar to those of previous studies, with 76% of patients achieving CRs and an overall response rate of 97%.

The most common toxicities in patients treated with 2-CdA are neutropenia and fever. Saven and colleagues[38] at the Scripps Clinic reported the largest collection of patients treated with 2-CdA. Among 349 patients who received a single cycle of 2-CdA, 87% had grade 3 or 4 neutropenia, 42% had neutropenic fever, but only 13% had documented infections, none of which was an opportunistic infection. Most of the fevers seen with administration of 2-CdA do not reflect infection but are probably caused by the release of cytokines. Because of the high incidence of neutropenic fever, Saven and colleagues[147] conducted a prospective trial on the effect of filgrastim in 35 patients treated with 2-CdA. Filgrastim was administered on days −3 through −1 and again after completion of 2-CdA until the absolute neutrophil count was more than 2×10^9/L on 2 consecutive days. When compared with historical controls, the filgrastim-treated group achieved an absolute neutrophil count greater than 1.0×10^9/L more rapidly than controls (9 vs 22 days). Despite this effect, the incidence of fever and rate of admission to the hospital were not different in the two groups, and routine use of prophylactic filgrastim therefore is not indicated for these patients.

Although responses are excellent with 2-CdA, they are not sustained in all patients. Follow-up after 2-CdA has been shorter than after 2′-DCF treatment, but the experience is similar—relapses have appeared with longer follow-up (Table 84–5). Several studies have reported quite long follow-up. After a median follow-up of 108 months, Goodman and colleagues reported that 37% of patients relapsed, with a median time to relapse of 42 months.[39] Initial PR was associated with a shorter duration of remission (Fig. 84–7). The response to retreatment remained very good; 79% of relapsed patients were retreated with 2-CdA. The overall response was 92%, including 75% with CRs.[39] Jehn and coworkers reported that among 44 consecutive patients, after a median follow-up of 8.5 years, the disease-free survival was 36% at 12 years with an overall survival or 79%.[148] At Northwestern University, among 86 consecutive patients treated with a single cycle of 2-CdA, the progression-free survival after 12 years was 54% with an overall survival after 12 years of 87%.[149] Results of one retrospective study suggested that the durability of response is greater with 2′-DCF than with 2-CdA; at 45 months of follow-up for each, the relapse rates were 9.7% and 29%, respec-

Table 84–5 Activity of 2-Chlorodeoxyadenosine in Hairy Cell Leukemia*

Study	No. of Patients	Previously Untreated	CR (%)	PR (%)	NR (%)	Median Follow-up (month)	Relapse Rate (%)	Median Time to Relapse (month)
Estey et al[40]	46	27	78	11	11	9	2	17.8
Juliusson and Liliemark[41]	16	3	75		13	12	0	
Tallman et al[42]	20	12	80	20	0	12	5	NA
Piro et al[44]	144	69	85	12	2	14	3	36
Piro et al[34]	12	3	92	8	0	15.5	0	
Seymour et al[35]	46	27	78	11	11	30	20	16
Tallman et al[36]	50	27	80	18	2	33	14	24
Jehn et al[37]	42	32	98	2	0	33	14	29
Dearden et al[24]	45	12	84	16	0	45	29	23.5
Von Rohr et al[142]	62	33	76	21	3	46	24	38
Hoffman et al[43]	49	21	76	24	0	55	24	NA
Saven et al[38]	349	179	91	7	2	58	26	CR: 30 PR: 24
Goodman et al[39]	207	119	95	5	0	108	37	42
Chadha et al[145]	85	56	79	21	0	114	36	NAH

*Dose of 2-CdA: 0.1 mg/kg/day × 7 days by continuous infusion.
CR, complete response; NA, not available; NAH, not attained; NR, no response; PR, partial response.

Table 84–6 Alternate Schedules of 2-Chlorodeoxyadenosine Therapy

Study	Dosing	Route of Administration	Responses
Juliusson et al[141]	3.4 mg/m²/day × 7 days	Subcutaneous injection	CR: 75% after 1 cycle, 85% after 2 cycles
Robak et al[142]	0.14 mg/kg/day × 5 days	2-hour IV bolus	CR: 82%, PR: 17.4%
Chacko et al[143]	0.15 mg/kg/wk × 6 weeks	3-hour infusion	CR: 100%
Von Rohr et al[144]	0.14 mg/kg/day × 5 days	Subcutaneous injection	CR: 76%, PR: 21%

CR, complete response; PR, partial response.

tively.[24] There are no randomized trials comparing the two agents that could answer this question. No plateau has been reached with either agent, and relapses continue to occur after initial treatment.

Immunosuppression with Purine Analogs

Both 2′-DCF and 2-CdA are associated with prolonged immunosuppression.[41,150–154] With 2′-DCF, a decrease in the total lymphocyte count occurs, with a greater reduction in T cells than B cells or natural killer (NK) cells.[153] The levels of CD4+ and CD8+ cells decrease to less than 200 cells/μL for at least 6 months after 2′-DCF treatment is discontinued. In a series of 15 patients treated with 2′-DCF with a long follow-up period, the median time to recovery of CD4+ lymphocyte counts to normal was 54 months.[152] Treatment with 2-CdA induces similar suppression of CD4+ lymphocyte counts.[35] The median time to recovery of CD4+ lymphocyte counts to normal levels after 2-CdA was 40 months. Treatment with 2-CdA affects two distinct subsets of CD4+ T cells. The CD4+CD45RA+ subset is significantly reduced for up to 5 years, but the CD4+CD45RO+ T cells, which secrete cytokines and enhance B-cell function, are not suppressed.[153] Recovery of CD8 and NK cells is more rapid; they normalize within 3 months of treatment with 2-CdA. This may explain why opportunistic infections, other than an occasional case of herpes zoster, are uncommon.[33,38,41,155]

Prognosis

Purine analog therapy has significantly changed the outcome of patients with HCL, who now have excellent long-term survival rates. Before the advent of interferon therapy, survival at 4 years was reported to be 68%.[156] With the use of purine analogs, durable remissions are attained, and even after relapse, retreatment produces good responses. The 5-year survival rates are more than 85%.[24,25,29,33,38,39] Flinn and coworkers[25] reported long-term results for 241 patients treated with 2′-DCF, and the overall survival rate was 90% at 5 years and 81% at 10 years (Fig. 84–7). The leading causes of death were second malignancies and infections. Only 2 of 40 deaths were attributable to HCL. Two hundred nine patients treated at the Scripps clinic with 2-CdA have been followed for at least 7 years.[39] The overall survival rate at 9 years is 97% (Fig. 84–7). Because of the indolent natural history of this disease, very long follow-up of patients treated with either purine analog will be required to determine whether one of the agents offers a substantially longer remission duration or overall survival. However, it seems unlikely that such a prospective, randomized comparison between 2-CdA and 2′-DCF

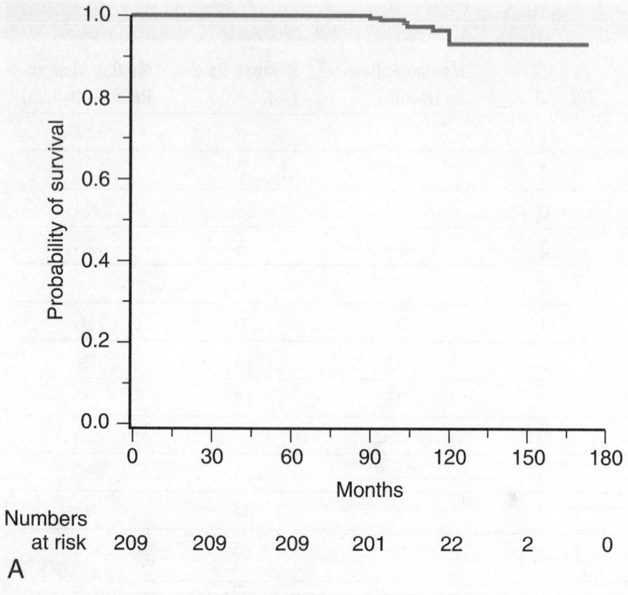

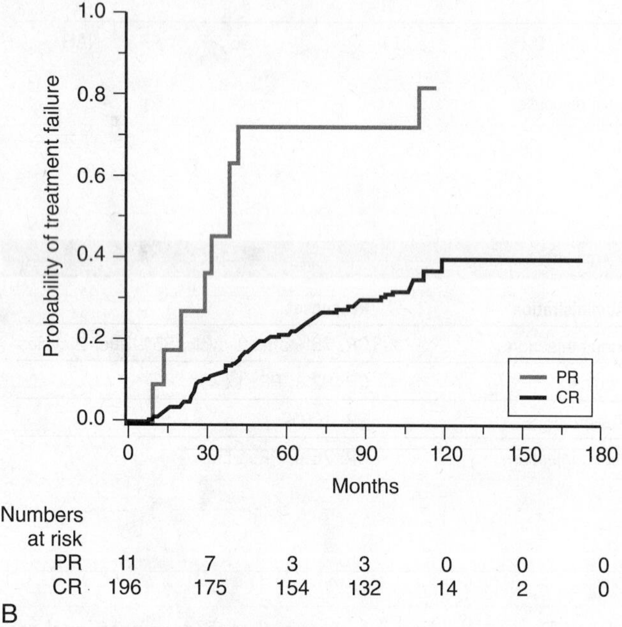

Figure 84–7 **A**, Kaplan–Meier survival curves for 209 patients with hairy cell leukemia (HCL) treated with 2-chlorodeoxyadenosine (2-CdA) and followed for at least 7 years. **B**, Time to treatment failure of 207 patients with HCL after the first course of 2-CdA, stratified by response to first course of therapy. CR, complete response; PR, partial response. *(Data from Goodman GR, Burian C, Koziol JA, Saven A: Extended follow-up of patients with hairy cell leukemia after treatment with cladribine. J Clin Oncol 21:891, 2003.)*

will ever be conducted because the CR rates with each agent are so high, and many years and resources would be required to detect even small differences.

EVALUATION OF MINIMAL RESIDUAL DISEASE

The remarkable activity of the purine analogs has led to the examination of posttreatment bone marrow biopsies to detect minimal residual disease (MRD) in patients otherwise in CR. Immunohistochemistry using anti-CD20, DBA.44, and anti-CD45RO antibodies in paraffin-embedded biopsy specimens has been used most frequently.[102–105,155–158] Techniques for MRD detection include flow cytometric immunophenotyping or consensus primer polymerase

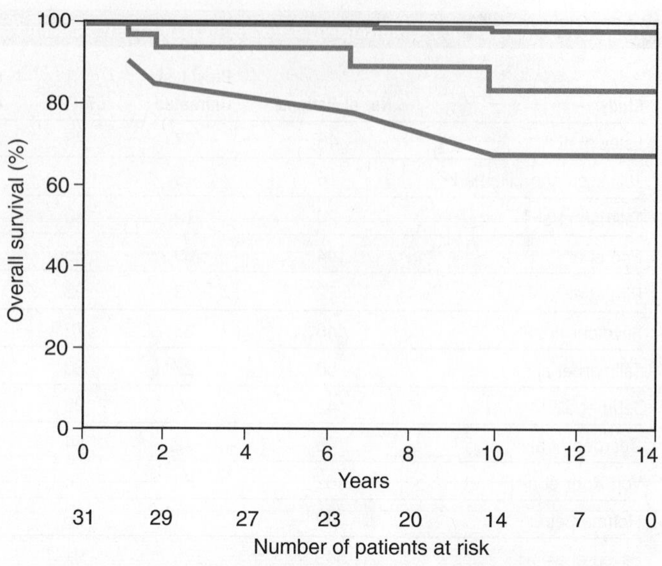

Figure 84–8 Kaplan–Meier survival curve for 31 patients with hairy cell leukemia (HCL) treated with 2-chlorodeoxyadlnosine (2-CdA) and who then sustained a relapse of their disease. Light lines represent 95% confidence limits. *(Data from Chadha P, Rademaker AW, Mendiratta P, et al: Treatment of hairy cell leukemia with 2-chlorodeoxyadenosine (2-CdA): Long-term follow-up of the Northwestern University experience. Blood 106:241, 2005.)*

chain reaction (PCR).[99] Depending on the criteria used, 13% to 51% of patients in apparent CR have evidence of MRD.[102–105,158] There has not been a statistically significant difference in the incidence of MRD between patients treated with 2′-DCF or 2-CdA.[159] The presence of MRD appears to predict relapse.[104,158] In one study evaluating MRD in 66 patients, 50% of those with MRD relapsed, whereas only 6% of patients without MRD relapsed.[158] There is no evidence to support the treatment of MRD.

TREATMENT OF RELAPSE

Relapse is often detected on bone marrow biopsy alone, and immediate retreatment is not necessary. In the study by Kraut and colleagues,[30] relapse was detected at a median of 30 months from achievement of remission with 2′-DCF, but retreatment was initiated at a median of 60 months after first remission. Five of seven patients retreated with purine analogs attained CRs. Patients with an initial response to 2-CdA also respond well to retreatment with a purine analog. In the Scripps Clinic series, 76 of 207 patients relapsed; 79% were retreated with 2-CdA. The overall response was 92%, including 75% with a CR.[39] The median duration of the second response was 35 months, which is comparable to the 42-month duration of first response. Responses continue to be seen even with a third cycle of 2-CdA in 80% of retreated patients. Patients who relapse after purine analog therapy should be retreated with 2-CdA or 2′-DCF. An alternative in relapsed or refractory cases includes enrollment in a clinical trial with newer therapies (discussed later under Monoclonal Antibody Therapies). The outcome of patients who relapsed after 2-CdA and receive other therapies or are observed is very favorable (Fig. 84–8).

RISK OF SECOND MALIGNANCIES

An association has been noticed between HCL and second malignancies, although the link is controversial. Malignancies that have been observed in HCL patients include melanoma, prostate cancer, gastrointestinal cancers, non-Hodgkin's lymphoma, and nonmelanomatous skin cancers. It is not clear whether HCL itself

Table 84–7 Antibody and Immunoconjugate Therapy

Study	Treatment	No. of Patients	Previously Treated	CR (%)	PR (%)	OR (%)
Lauria et al[163]	Rituximab	10	10	10	40	50
Hagberg and Lundholm[164]	Rituximab	11	11	55	9	64
Nieva et al[165]	Rituximab	24	24	13	13	26
Kreitman et al[167]	LMB-2	4	4	25	75	100
Kreitman et al[170]	BL22	23	23	65	18	83

CR, complete response; OR, overall response; PR, partial response.

increases risk or whether the type of therapy plays a role. Kampmeier and colleagues[160] reported a significantly increased incidence of second malignancies in HCL patients treated with interferon. The British Columbia Cancer Agency reported a 20-year follow-up of 117 patients—31% developed a second malignancy, 30% of which were diagnosed before the diagnosis of HCL.[161] The risk was elevated regardless of the type of therapy. However, this association has not been uniformly observed.[159,162] Kurzrock and colleagues[163] reported no excess of second malignancies among 350 patients treated with interferon, 2-CdA, or 2′-DCF.

Immunosuppression due to the purine analogs may play a role in the increased malignancy incidence, but the evidence is not clear. Long-term follow-up studies of patients treated with 2′-DCF have not demonstrated a statistically significant increased risk of second malignancies.[23,25] However, other studies have suggested that treatment with 2-CdA is associated with an increased cancer risk.[38,39,164] In Saven's review of the Scripps Clinic experience with 349 patients, 8% of patients had a second malignancy that developed at a median of 62 months after the diagnosis of HCL and 21 months after treatment with 2-CdA.[38] Eleven percent of the patients in this study had a diagnosis of malignancy before the diagnosis of HCL. It is still not clear whether therapy increases risk; HCL itself may have an inherent predisposition to malignancy. Continued observation will be necessary to address this question.

MONOCLONAL ANTIBODY THERAPIES

The anti-CD20 monoclonal antibody rituximab has been tested in patients with HCL refractory to other treatments.[165,166] Hagberg and associates[167] treated 11 patients with rituximab and reported an overall response rate of 64% (Table 84–7). The median duration of response in this group was 14 months. The largest published report[168] describes 24 patients treated with 4 weekly doses of rituximab. All the patients had relapsed after prior treatment with 2-CdA, and the median time since treatment was 73 months. Thirteen percent of patients had CRs, and 13% had PRs, for an overall response rate of 26%. One-third of responders relapsed after a median follow-up of 14.6 months. It appears that rituximab has activity in some patients with HCL.

CD25, also known as Tac, is the α subunit of the IL-2R and is expressed in 80% of patients with HCL.[169] LMB-2, anti-Tac(Fv)-PE38, is an immunotoxin that contains the variable heavy domain of anti-Tac fused to the amino terminus of a 38-kd truncated form of the *Pseudomonas* exotoxin.[169] It has demonstrated some efficacy in patients with CD25$^+$ hematologic malignancies. After binding to CD25, the compound is internalized and leads to apoptotic cell death. Of four patients who were refractory to standard therapies, including 2-CDA and interferon, all had a response to LMB-2, with one CR.[170] This treatment is well tolerated and appears to have no hematologic toxicity. Larger studies need to be conducted to better determine the safety and efficacy of this treatment.

Another promising immunotoxin under investigation is BL22, a recombinant immunotoxin containing anti-CD22 monoclonal antibody and PE38, the *Pseudomonas* exotoxin. CD22 is expressed by normal B cells and B-cell leukemias and lymphomas, including HCL, but it is not found on stem cells.[171] Kreitman and coworkers updated their original study[172] and presented the results of 23 HCL patients treated with BL22.[173] The overall response was 83%, with 65% of patients attaining CRs. Of the complete responders, only one had MRD determined by immunohistochemistry of the bone marrow, and none had MRD when peripheral blood was tested by PCR. The median follow-up was 12 months, and in four patients who relapsed, retreatment resulted in CRs in three. This therapy appears to be well tolerated, although two patients did have a reversible hemolytic-uremic syndrome. No other hematologic toxicity or decrease in T-cell count was observed. This is the first therapy since the purine analogs to produce a high rate of CR.

These newer therapies have efficacy in patients who are resistant or refractory to the purine analogs and therefore offer another option for therapy. The durability of effect remains to be determined in larger studies with longer follow-up.

HA22 is a second-generation recombinant immunotoxin that differs from BL22 by three animo acids, which results in increased binding of the immunotoxin to CD22.[174] Preliminary in vitro studies suggest that this agent has better cytotoxic activity in B-cell cell lines and in leukemic cells from patients with HCL.[175] Clinical studies are under way.

SUGGESTED READINGS

Arons E, Margulies I, Sorbara L, et al: Minimal residual disease in hairy cell leukemia patients assessed by clone-specific polymerase chain reaction. Clin Cancer Res 12:2804, 2006.

Cassileth PA, Cheuvart B, Spiers AS, et al: Pentostatin induces durable remissions in hairy cell leukemia. J Clin Oncol 9:243, 1991.

Catovsky D, Matutes E, Talavera JG, et al: Long term results with 2′-deoxycoformycin in hairy cell leukemia. Leuk Lymphoma 14(Suppl 1):109, 1994.

Dearden CE, Matutes E, Hilditch BL, et al: Long-term follow-up of patients with hairy cell leukaemia after treatment with pentostatin or cladribine. Br J Haematol 106:515, 1999.

Else M, Ruchlemer R, Osuji N, et al: Long remissions in hairy cell leukemia with purine analogs. A report of 219 patients with a median follow-up of 12.5 years. Cancer 104:2442, 2005.

Flandrin G, Sigaux F, Sebahoun G, Bouffette P: Hairy cell leukemia: Clinical presentation and follow-up of 211 patients. Semin Oncol 11:458, 1984.

Flinn IW, Kopecky KJ, Foucar MK, et al: Long-term follow-up of remission duration, mortality, and second malignancies in hairy cell leukemia patients treated with pentostatin. Blood 96:2981, 2000.

Golomb HM, Catovsky D, Golde DW: Hairy cell leukemia: A clinical review based on 71 cases. Ann Intern Med 89:677, 1978.

Golomb HM, Vardiman JW: Response to splenectomy in 65 patients with hairy cell leukemia: An evaluation of spleen weight and bone marrow involvement. Blood 61:349, 1983.

Goodman GR, Burian C, Koziol JA, Saven A: Extended follow-up of patients with hairy cell leukemia after treatment with cladribine. J Clin Oncol 21:891, 2003.

Kreitman RJ, Wilson W, Bergeron K, et al: Efficacy of the anti-CD22 recombinant immunotoxin BL22 in chemotherapy-resistant hairy-cell leukemia. N Engl J Med 345:241, 2001.

Quesada JR, Reuben J, Manning JT, et al: Alpha interferon for induction of remission in hairy-cell leukemia. N Engl J Med 310:15, 1984.

Saven A, Burian C, Koziol JA, Piro LD: Long-term follow-up of patients with hairy cell leukemia after cladribine treatment. Blood 92:1918, 1998.

Seymour JF, Kurzrock R, Freireich EJ, Estey EH: 2-Chlorodeoxyadenosine induces durable remissions and prolonged suppression of CD4+ lymphocyte counts in patients with hairy cell leukemia. Blood 83:2906, 1994.

Spiers A, Moore D, Cassileth P, et al: Remissions in hairy cell leukemia with pentostatin (2′-deoxycoformycin). N Engl J Med 316:825, 1987.

Tallman MS, Hakimian D, Variakojis D, et al: A single cycle of 2-chlorodeoxyadenosine results in complete remission in the majority of patients with hairy cell leukemia. Blood 80:2203, 1992.

Thomas D, O'Brien S, Bueso-Ramos C, et al: Rituximab in relapsed or refractory hairy cell leucemia. Blood 102:3906, 2003.

Wheaton S, Tallman MS, Hakimian D, Peterson L: Minimal residual disease may predict bone marrow relapse in patients with hairy cell leukemia treated with 2-chlorodeoxyadenosine. Blood 87:1556, 1996.

REFERENCES

For complete list of references log onto www.expertconsult.com

CHAPTER 85

CUTANEOUS T-CELL LYMPHOMAS

Timothy M. Kuzel, Joan Guitart, and Steven T. Rosen

The T-cell non-Hodgkin lymphomas include a wide variety of clinical disorders with different prognoses. The Revised European-American Lymphoma (REAL) classification system[1] suggests that more than 10 discrete clinicopathologic entities can be considered part of this family. This chapter focuses on the disorders that would be encompassed by the diagnosis cutaneous T-cell lymphoma (CTCL) (Table 85–1). The most common subtypes of cutaneous T-cell lymphomas are the epidermotropic variants mycosis fungoides (MF) and the related leukemic variant, Sézary syndrome (SS). Most of this chapter focuses on the approach to these more common disorders, although features that allow the clinician to exclude the distinct variants are also described.

EPIDEMIOLOGY

MF and SS are the most common primary lymphomas involving the skin.[2,3] Data collected from the Surveillance, Epidemiology, and End Results (SEER) program showed a rapidly increasing incidence from 0.2 cases per 100,000 people in 1973 to 0.4 cases per 100,000 people in 1984. This corresponds to approximately 1000 new cases each year in the United States. Whether this represented a true increase in incidence or was attributable to a better awareness and therefore more frequent recognition of this disease has not been resolved. Since that time, the incidence rate of CTCL has stabilized at 0.36 cases per 100,000 persons, and the mortality rate has declined. The incidence of MF/SS increases with advancing age, as does the incidence of non-Hodgkin lymphomas in general. The average age at presentation is approximately 50 years. Although very young patients have been reported, most patients are at least 30 years of age.[4,5] MF/SS is seen in all racial groups. There is a 1.6 : 1 ratio of black people to white people and a 2.2 : 1 ratio of men to women with this disorder. MF is less common in the Asian population. Clusters of cases of MF/SS within families have been reported.[6] An association with histocompatibility antigens AW31, AW32, B8, BW35, and DR5 has been described.[7] However, a solid genetic predisposition or inherited genetic defect has not been demonstrated.

BIOLOGY AND MOLECULAR ASPECTS

The T lymphocyte is central to the body's ability to mount an immune response and is the precursor of neoplastic cells in MF/SS. These cells spontaneously form rosettes with sheep red blood cells. Sézary cells respond to phytohemagglutinin and perform T-cell immunoregulatory functions similar to normal lymphocytes.[8,9] The clonal nature of CTCL can be demonstrated by Southern blotting or polymerase chain reaction (PCR) methods of analysis of the T-cell receptor.

The development of monoclonal antibodies directed against specific cluster of differentiation (CD) antigens has allowed for more precise identification of surface markers on the malignant cell.[10] Most cases of MF and SS are of the helper T memory or effector subset with a $CD4^{+}CD45RO^{+}$ phenotype. In most instances, the cells express the pan–T-cell antigens CD2 (the sheep erythrocyte receptor), CD3, and CD5. Early T cells may also express CD7 on their cell surface. This marker is frequently deleted in MF/SS but may also be deleted in benign dermatoses and inflammatory skin lesions. Additionally, CD26 is often deleted in cases of MF and SS. Flow cytometry provides a sensitive method for detecting early peripheral blood involvement in patients by detection of a $CD4^{+}$, $CD26^{-}$ population. Occasional cases expressing the suppressor $CD8^{+}$ phenotype have been described. Low expression of the α-chain component of the interleukin-2 receptor (CD25) is detected with heterogenous expression on the malignant cells in less than half of the patients. The implication of this finding is of uncertain significance, as both activated T cells and immunoregulatory T cells can express CD25.

Cytogenetic analyses have demonstrated numerical and structural chromosomal abnormalities in MF/SS[11] although usually in advanced-stage disease. Hyperdiploidy and complex karyotypes are common. Nonrandom deletions of chromosomes 1, 6, 8, 10, and 17 have been reported with gains in chromosome 17q and 4p occurring in more than 25% of cases. Regions of the genome that include genes encoding the T-cell receptor do not appear to be involved, suggesting that the genetic basis for malignant transformation in MF/SS appears to be different from that involved in other T-cell malignant disorders.

Modest data exist on the aberrant expression of oncogenes and suppressor genes in MF/SS. Loss of heterozygosity (LOH) is identified in 30% to 60% of patients, commonly at 9p 10q, 1p, and 17p. LOH in early stages is associated with a threefold increase in mortality.[12] Mutant forms of the P53 tumor suppressor gene are observed rarely, usually in tumor-stage and large cell transformation of MF.[13] LYT-10, a member of the NF-κB family of transcription factors associated with translocations in lymphoid malignancies, is rearranged in a small proportion of cases.[14] However, *BCL2,* a gene whose rearrangement is characteristic of follicular B-cell lymphomas and which slows programmed cell death, is overexpressed in MF. Constitutive phosphorylation of STAT3 (a member of the transcription factor family that contributes to the diversity of cytokine responses) has been reported and suggests these malignant T cells are activated.[10,15] Altered expression or release of select cytokines or their receptors including IL-1, IL-2R, IL-4, IL-5, IL-6, IL-7, IL-8, IL-12, and TGF-β receptor II has been noted.[16] IL-7 and IL-15 have been identified as growth factors for MF/SS and shown to regulate expression of the *BCL2* and *MYB* oncogenes and stimulate DNA binding of stat proteins.[17,18]

ETIOLOGY AND PATHOGENESIS

The cause of MF/SS remains unknown. It is considered to be a sporadic disease without compelling evidence of transmissibility. Several viruses have been implicated in the pathogenesis of MF/SS, including human T-cell lymphotropic virus types 1 and 2, herpes simplex virus, herpesvirus-6, and the Epstein–Barr virus. However, a viral cause of MF/SS has not been proved, and no epidemiologic evidence supports these hypotheses.

Investigators have suggested that prolonged exposure to contact allergens may lead to enhanced immune responses leading directly or indirectly to the development of MF/SS. Sézary cells respond in vitro to superantigenic exotoxins, and colonization by *Staphylococcus aureus* may influence disease activity.[19] Several reports suggested that exposure to metals or their salts, pesticides or herbicides, and organic sol-

Table 85–1 Comparison of EORTC and WHO Classifications of Primary Cutaneous Lymphoma

EORTC Classification	WHO Classification
Cutaneous T-Cell Lymphoma	
Indolent clinical behavior	Mycosis fungoides
Mycosis fungoides variants	Mycosis fungoides variants
Follicular mycosis fungoides	Follicular mycosis fungoides
Pagetoid reticulosis	Pagetoid reticulosis
CTCL, large cell, $CD30^{+}$	Primary cutaneous $CD30^{+}$ ALCA ($CD30^{+}$ lymphoproliferative disease, including lymphomatoid papulosis)
Lymphomatoid papulosis	
Aggressive clinical behavior	Sézary syndrome
Sézary syndrome	Peripheral T-cell lymphoma, unspecified (most); extranodal NK/T-cell lymphoma, nasal type
CTCL, large cell, CD-30-negative	
Provisional entities	
CTCL, pleomorphic, small/medium sized	
Subcutaneous panniculitis-like T-cell lymphoma	Subcutaneous panniculitis-like T-cell lymphoma
Cutaneous B-Cell Lymphoma	
Indolent clinical behavior	Extranodal marginal zone B-cell lymphoma
Primary cutaneous immunocytoma (marginal zone B-cell lymphoma)	
Follicle Center Cell Lymphoma (any grade)	
Intermediate clinical behavior	
Primary cutaneous large B-cell lymphoma of the leg	
Provisional Entities	
Primary cutaneous plasmacytoma	Plasmacytoma
Intravascular large B-cell lymphoma	Diffuse large B-cell lymphoma (intravascular)

ALCL, anaplastic large cell lymphoma; CTCL, cutaneous T-cell lymphoma; EORTC, European Organization for the Research and Treatment of Cancer; NK, natural killer; WHO, World Health Organization.

vents (halogenated or aromatic hydrocarbons) could be related to the development of MF/SS.[20] However, two well-designed case-control studies have failed to support these observations.[21,22]

Various theories have been advanced to explain the epidermotropism of malignant T cells in MF/SS. Organ-specific affinity to skin and other organs has been recognized in subsets of normal T cells. Homing of CTCL cells to the skin is probably mediated by more than one adhesion receptor mechanism. CTCL cells express cutaneous lymphocyte antigen (CLA), a skin homing receptor that interacts with e-selectin expressed on dermal venules.[10,23,24] Furthermore, the CLA+ T-lymphocytes also typically express the CC-chemokine receptor 4 which binds to chemokines produced in the skin, such as the CC-chemokine ligands 17 and 22. Peripheral blood mononuclear cells bind to cultured keratinocytes exposed to interferon-γ. The MHC II proteins, along with intercellular adhesion molecule 1 (ICAM-1) present on keratinocytes, attract and bind lymphocytes. Additional chemokine receptors, such as CXC-chemokine receptors 3 and 4, as well as unique integrins, have been shown to have corresponding ligands or integrin receptors on dermal Langerhans cells, suggesting a relationship between the malignant T cells and host immune cells.

An additional feature of MF/SS cells is the production of a cytokine profile consistent with T-helper-2 type cells ($T_{H}2$).[25] The $T_{H}2$ cells produce IL-4, IL-5, and IL-6 and they are inhibited by interferon-γ. The $T_{H}2$ cells are critical for stimulating antibody and eosinophil-mediated responses. Hypergammaglobulinemia and eosinophilia are often seen in advanced cases of MF/SS and are consistent with a $T_{H}2$ profile. Stimulation of $T_{H}2$ cells inhibits the $T_{H}1$ subpopulation of lymphocytes involved in cell-mediated immunity. A cause as well as a consequence of the progression of MF/SS is immune suppression as a result of depletion of this T-cell subset. The $T_{H}2$ cytokine profile may explain the decrease in tumor infiltrating lymphocytes during tumor progression. In addition to the effect of cytokines secreted by the neoplastic cells, it has been shown that the malignant $CD4^{+}$ cells express antigens (eg, FAS ligand) that may directly mediate elimination of the $CD8^{+}$ infiltrating lymphocytes by induction of apoptosis.[26]

CLINICAL PRESENTATION

Alibert reported the first case of MF in 1806.[27] His patient developed a skin eruption that progressed into mushroom-like tumors, prompting the term mycosis fungoides. Later in the nineteenth century, Bazin defined the three classic cutaneous phases (patch, plaque, and tumor stage) of the disease.[28] The recognition of the clinical triad of intensely pruritic erythroderma, lymphadenopathy, and abnormal hyperconvoluted cells in the peripheral blood led to the description of SS.[29]

More than 50% of CTCL patients have MF. The initial course of patients with MF is usually indolent. Most patients give a history of antecedent skin lesions, usually nonspecific erythematous patches that can mimic eczema or psoriasis. In many cases, there is an orderly progression from limited patches to more generalized patches, plaques, tumors, and nodal or visceral involvement. The characteristic patch lesion is typically poorly demarcated, lightly erythematous, with a predilection for sun-protected areas, such as the lower abdomen or buttocks (Fig. 85–1). Plaque lesions are more indurated, have well-demarcated margins, and some scaling (Fig. 85–2*)*. Plaques can arise from patch lesions or previously uninvolved areas of skin. Tumor lesions tend to be later lesions, frequently associated with previous patches or plaques, and often represent advanced disease, with histologic evidence and large cell transformation. They can be located on any part of the body. Ulceration of these lesions is common and secondary infection is a major cause of morbidity (Fig. 85–3). Tumors may be the initial presentation in a small percentage of patients (D'emblée presentation, Videl and Brocg, 1889).

SS patients present with generalized desquamative erythroderma, pruritus, and circulating malignant cells. Peripheral blood usually shows a significant number or percentage of hyperconvoluted atypical lymphocytes (Fig. 85–4). Approximately 5% to 10% of all newly reported cases of CTCL are SS. In its most advanced form, patients with SS suffer from alopecia, ectropion, leonine facies, hyperkeratosis, nail dystrophy, fissuring of the palms and soles, and severe pruritus and cutaneous pain. Many other entities can clinically mimic this disease including drug eruptions, atopic dermatitis, contact dermatitis, and erythrodermic psoriasis.

A number of variant presentations of CTCL have been described. The following sections discuss variants of CTCL.

CLONAL DERMATITIS

Clonal dermatitis is a term introduced by Wood and colleagues[30] that included a variety of lymphocyte-rich dermatoses, often characterized by clonal T-lymphocyte proliferations. Clinically they exhibit a myriad of cutaneous presentations from poikiloderma (atrophic patches) to hyperpigmented areas resembling pigmented purpuric dermatosis.

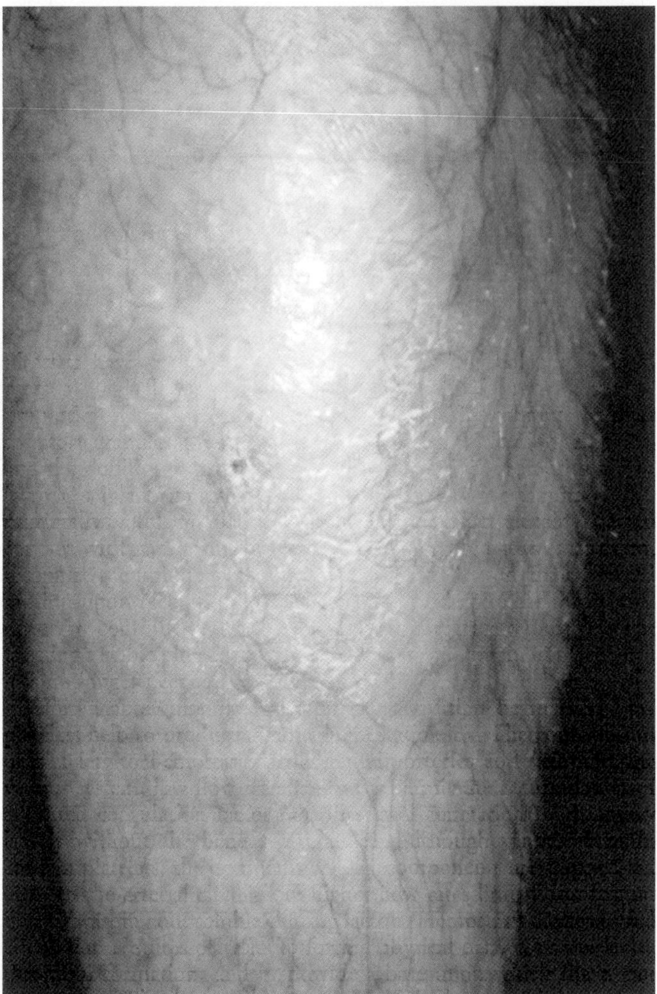

Figure 85–1 Erythematous and scaly patch lesion of mycosis fungoides.

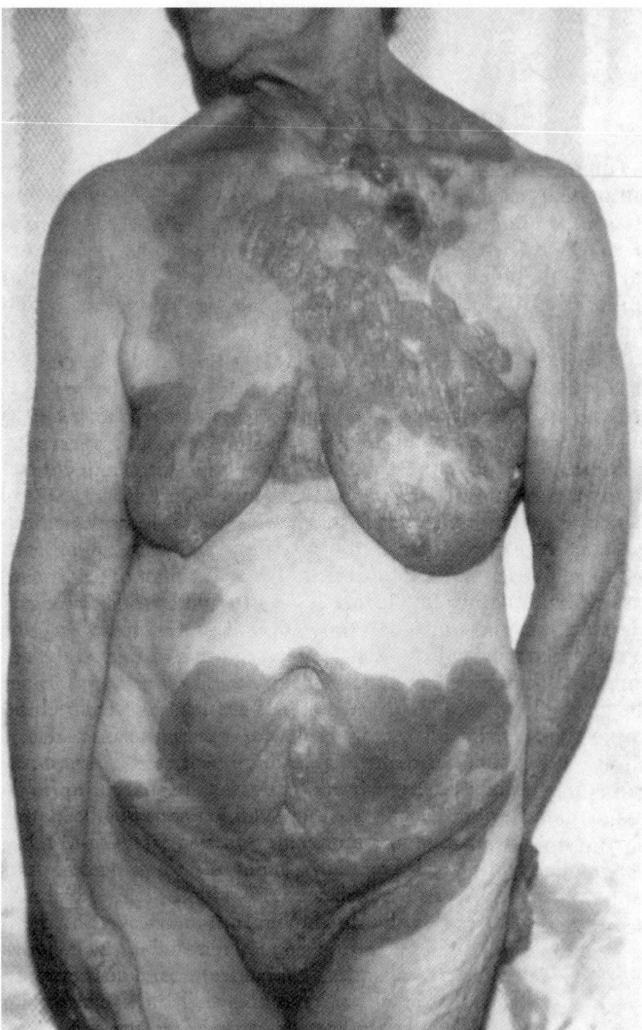

Figure 85–2 Plaque lesion of cutaneous T-cell lymphoma.

LARGE PLAQUE PARAPSORIASIS

Large plaque parapsoriasis is the classic premalignant lesion of MF. It most commonly consists of a few scattered, erythematous to brown plaques that are usually greater than 6 cm in size.[31] There is a predilection for the buttocks and intertriginous areas. Histologic examination shows a superficial lymphocytic infiltrate with minimal nuclear atypia. Epidermotropism is scant or absent and dermal fibrosis correlates with the chronicity of the process. Plaques can persist for decades before a frank evolution to MF occurs. Approximately 10% to 30% of patients ultimately develop an overt malignant transformation.

FOLLICULAR MUCINOSIS

Follicular mucinosis manifests with grouped erythematous follicular papules or boggy or indurated nodular plaques, notably devoid of hair (Fig. 85–5).[32] There is a predilection for the head and neck area, especially the forehead, which has the highest density of pilosebaceous units. Histopathologic evaluation reveals cells in sebaceous glands often associated with destruction of hair follicle structures due to infiltration by a T-lymphocytic process. This condition may be idiopathic or associated with MF. Even idiopathic cases can be associated with clonal T-lymphocytic infiltration.[33] In general, patients older than 40 with a more generalized cutaneous involvement and a chronic course are more likely to develop associated MF. No cases of MF have been reported in children with alopecia mucinosa, although few reports of Hodgkin disease have been reported in children with

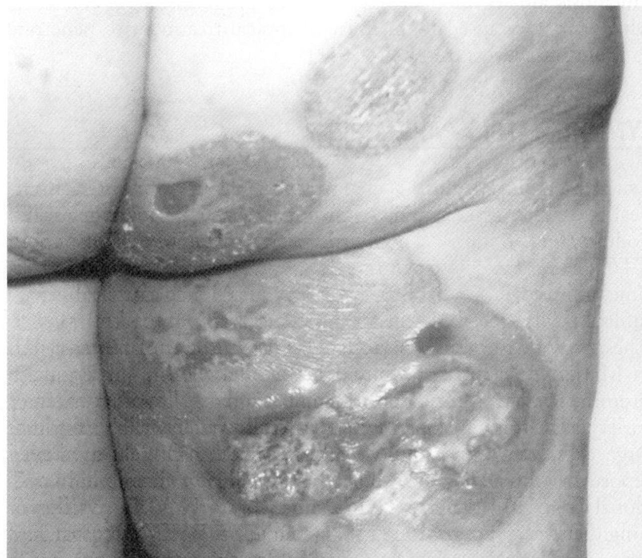

Figure 85–3 Ulcerated tumors arising from mycosis fungoides plaques.

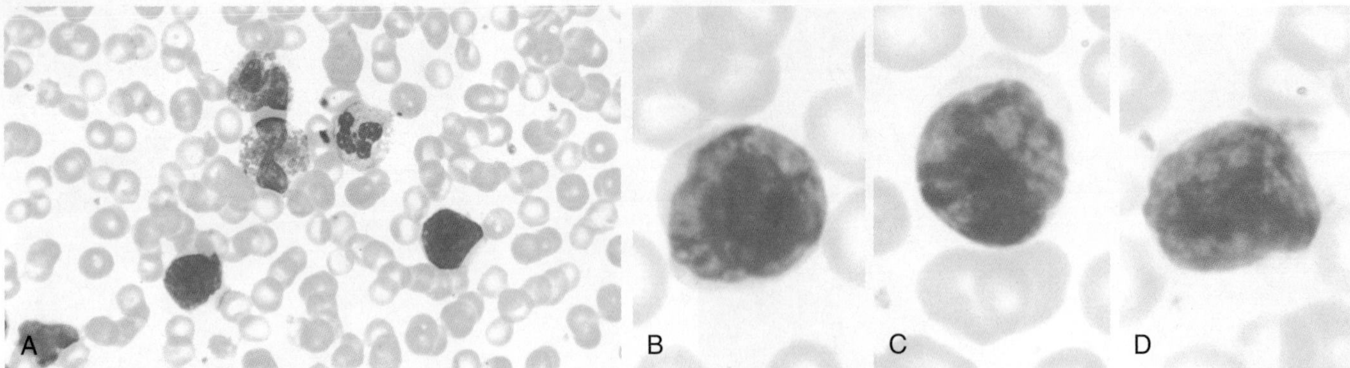

Figure 85–4 Sézary Cells **A–D**. Peripheral smear (**A**) with Sézary cells associated with eosinophilia. Note the cerebriform nuclei with fine chromatin (**B**, **C**, **D**). The hyperconvoluted nature of the nuclei is evident as complex nuclear folds seen through the chromatin.

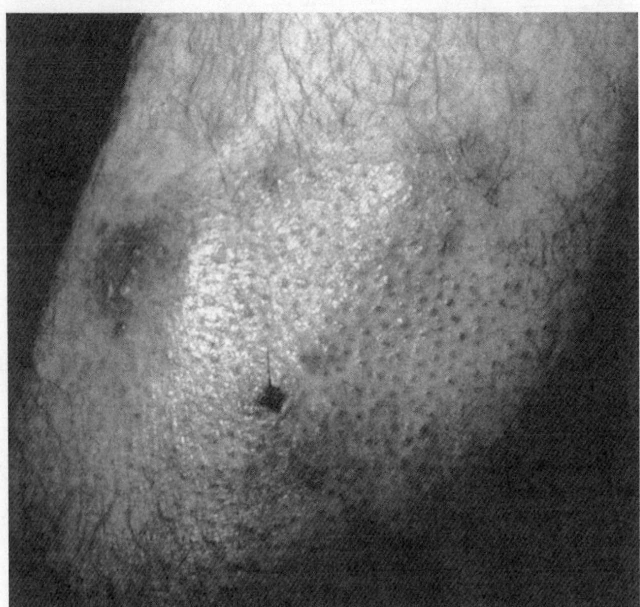

Figure 85–5 Follicular mucinosis showing a patch of alopecia with follicular prominence.

follicular mucinosis.[34] Patients with mycosis fungoides and follicular mucinosis are reported to have a worse prognosis, stage for stage, which may be caused by inability of topical treatment to penetrate to the deeper layers of the process.[35]

LYMPHOMATOID PAPULOSIS

Lymphomatoid papulosis is characterized by recurrent crops of self-healing, red-brown, centrally necrotic, asymptomatic papules and nodules (Fig. 85–6).[36] This entity represents 10% to 15% of all CTCL cases. Patients may have a few lesions or more than 100 at a time. Histologic evaluation reveals an atypical $CD4^+$ lymphocytic infiltrate with a variable mixed inflammatory infiltrate (Fig. 85–7). These may be primarily small cerebriform cells similar to those seen in MF (type B) but most often there are larger $CD30^+$ cells with prominent nucleoli resembling Reed–Sternberg cells (type A). A third variety of lymphomatoid papulosis (type C) with sheets of anaplastic large cells resembling $CD30^+$ large cell lymphoma has also been reported.[37] T-cell receptor gene rearrangement studies demonstrate a clonal origin. Although the typical course is usually indolent, spanning decades, approximately 15% of patients develop MF, Hodgkin, or non-Hodgkin lymphoma during their lifetime.[38] A direct link between lymphomatoid papulosis, CTCL, and Hodgkin disease was demonstrated in a patient with the three lymphoproliferative disorders arising from a common T-cell clone as shown by TCR gene studies.[39]

PAGETOID RETICULOSIS

Pagetoid reticulosis (ie, Woringer–Kolopp disease) is a rare condition affecting young adults. It typically manifests with a solitary, hyperkeratotic, often-verrucous plaque on the lower limb.[40] Biopsies show atypical cerebriform lymphocytes with a perinuclear halo almost exclusively localized within the intraepidermal compartment.[41] Extracutaneous dissemination is exceedingly rare. Most cases have a $CD8^+$ phenotype, although $CD4^+$ cases or double-negative ($CD4^-$/CD8) cases have been reported. Frequently the tumor cells express CD30, but T-cell receptor gene rearrangement studies are often negative. Whether pagetoid reticulosis should be considered a localized form of MF or a reactive pseudomalignant process is debatable. Although most cases have an indolent protracted course, generalized and sometimes aggressive variants have been reported.[42]

GRANULOMATOUS SLACK SKIN

In granulomatous slack-skin syndrome, an extremely rare disorder, clonal $CD4^+$ T cells elicit a reactive granulomatous response that destroys the elastic fibers, rendering skin slack, fibrotic, and inelastic (Fig. 85–8).[43] Changes characteristic of MF are often found within the epidermis and papillary dermis, and the reticular dermis contains numerous histiocytes with multinucleated giant cells and elastophagocytosis. Some patients with granulomatous MF do not have destruction of the elastic fibers with slack-skin changes. The differential diagnosis for such cases includes sarcoidosis and tuberculoid leprosy.

LABORATORY EVALUATION

The gold standard in the diagnosis of MF/SS is light microscopic examination of a skin biopsy. Characteristic findings include a band-like infiltrate involving the papillary dermis containing small, medium-sized, and occasionally large mononuclear cells with hyperchromatic, hyperconvoluted (cerebriform) nuclei and variable numbers of admixed inflammatory cells often expanding into adnexal structures (hair follicles and sweat glands).[16,44] Epidermal exocytosis of single or small clusters of neoplastic cells is a characteristic finding (Fig. 85–9 A,C,D). The presence of Pautrier's microabscesses defined as four or more atypical lymphocytes arranged in an aggregate in the epidermis is classic, but is seen only in a minority of cases. Tumor-stage lesions demonstrate a more diffuse, superficial and deep, dermal infiltrate with fewer reactive cells and an absence of epidermotropism (Fig. 85–9 B,E,F)). The malignant T-cell clone often evolves into

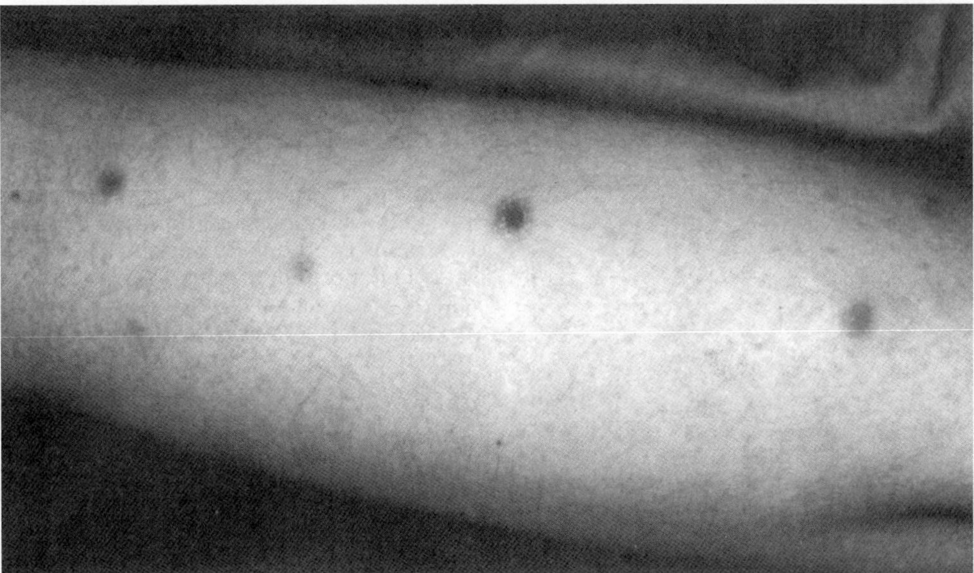

Figure 85–6 Lesions of lymphomatoid papulosis appear in crops and consist of ulcerated papules and scars.

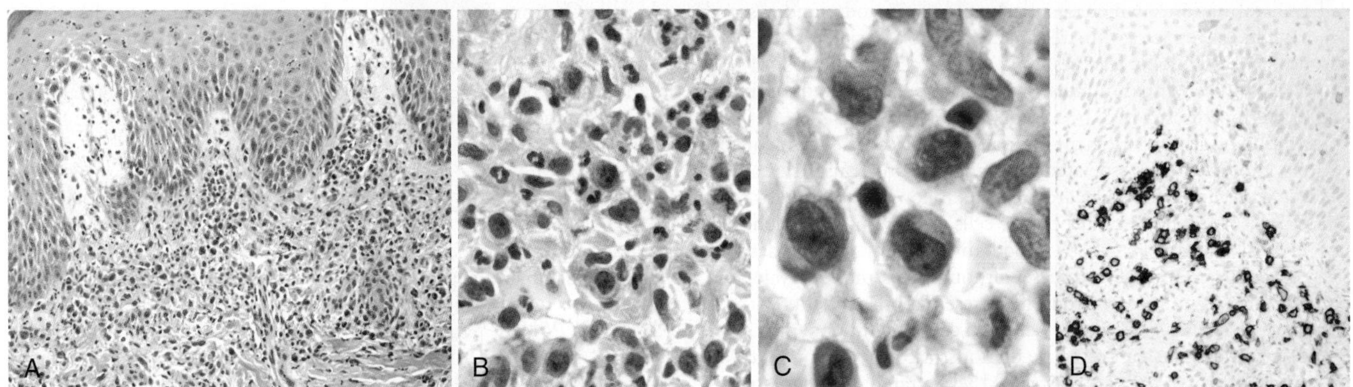

Figure 85–7 Lymphomatoid papulosis (**A–D**). Low power (**A**) shows a moderately dense dermal infiltrate of lymphoid cells admixed with inflammatory cells including neutrophils and eosinophils (**B**). The lymphoid cells are varied but include atypical large forms (**C**), which are brightly positive for CD30 (**D**). *(Case courtesy of Drs. Vesna Petrovic-Rosic and Mark Racz, University of Chicago.)*

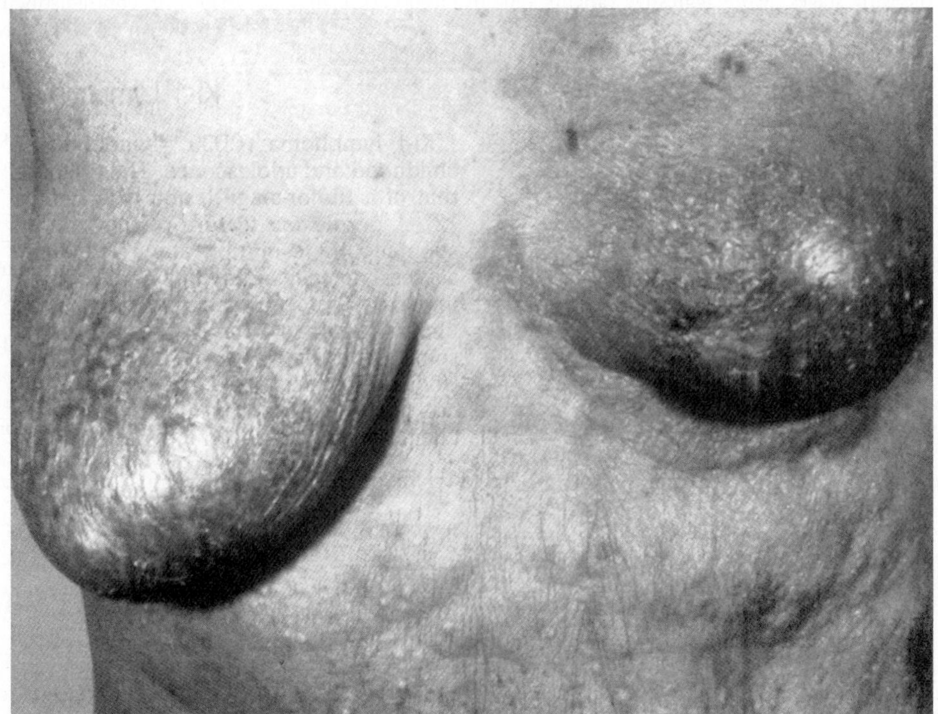

Figure 85–8 Lesions of granulomatous slack skin with destruction of the dermal elasticity.

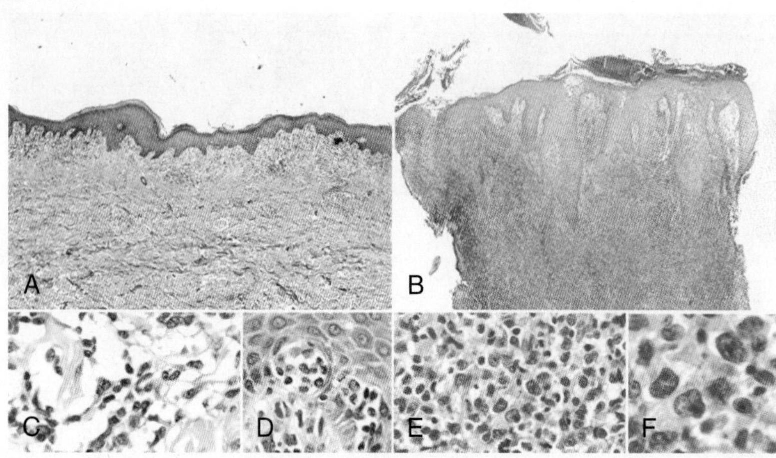

Figure 85–9 Mycosis fungoides, plaque-stage and transformed tumor-stage (**A–F**). Plaque stage (**A**, **C**, and **D**) demonstrates a band-like infiltrate (**A**, **C**) with some epidermotropism in the form of Pautrier micro-abscesses (**D**). In the tumor stage (**B**, **E**, **F**), there is a deep and dense infiltrate without significant epidermotropism. The cells are mostly large and atypical (**E**, **F**) and CD30+ (not shown). *(Case courtesy of Drs. Vesna Petrovic-Rosic and Robert Chen, University of Chicago.)*

large cell morphology during tumor progression, although rare cases show large cell morphology from the early patch lesions.[45] The presence of large cells in a skin lesion should be distinguished from "large cell transformation," which displays rapid skin, node, and visceral progression, is refractory to treatment, and is associated with poor survival. The histologic features in SS may be similar to those of MF. However, the cellular infiltrates in SS are more often monotonous, and epidermotropism may be absent.

Lymph node involvement initially involves the paracortical regions. Progression is associated with small to large clusters of atypical cells with preserved nodal architecture, followed by partial or total effacement of the node by neoplastic cells. Visceral involvement is a late clinical feature. Peripheral blood involvement can be demonstrated in all stages of skin disease, although it is most prevalent in patients with tumor or erythrodermic presentations. Patients with SS may have circulating neoplastic cells but can be lymphopenic. Bone marrow involvement can often be demonstrated in patients with SS or advanced tumor- or plaque-stage MF, but rarely influences management outside an investigational setting. We do not recommend a staging bone marrow aspirate and biopsy.

The malignant cells are typically $CD3^+$, $CD4^+$, $CD45RO^+$, $CD8^-$, and $CD30^-$ by immunohistochemistry. CD7 is often deleted from the early stages. More aggressive variants and advanced CTCL may have multiple pan–T-cell antigen deletions, especially CD2, CD5, and even CD4. T-cell receptor genes are clonally rearranged, and can be demonstrated in most cases by Southern blotting or polymerase chain reaction (PCR) assays when a sufficient malignant infiltrate exists.

Analysis of peripheral blood may reveal an elevated LDH (lactate dehydrogenase) in a small percentage of patients with bulky advanced disease. Eosinophilia and hypergammaglobulinemia are not uncommon is SS patients. A limited number of patients have an associated monoclonal gammopathy. Elevated serum β_2–microglobulin and IL-2 receptor levels have also occurred in advanced cases.

Imaging studies for classic MF/SS are generally of modest utility. CT scans of the chest, abdomen, or pelvis should be reserved for patients with SS, nodal involvement, or CTCL variants. In an investigational setting, electron microscopy, cytogenetics, and molecular analyses have shown that a higher percentage of patients have occult involvement of internal organs.

DIFFERENTIAL DIAGNOSIS

Primary CTCL represents a heterogeneous group of disorders with considerable variability in histology, phenotype, and prognosis. The Kiel Classification, Working Formulation, and the Revised European-American Lymphoma (REAL) classification system were developed for non-Hodgkin lymphomas and are not designed to provide an adequate characterization of the spectrum of CTCL. To address the deficiencies of the previously proposed systems a more clinically useful classification has been developed by the European Organization for Research and Treatment of Cancer (EORTC).[3] The World Health Organization has proposed a new classification with nearly 90% concordance with the EORTC classification (see Table 85–1). A number of other disorders in which malignant T cells infiltrate the skin should be distinguished from MF/SS. These disorders are discussed in the following sections.

CD30-POSITIVE CUTANEOUS LARGE T-CELL LYMPHOMA

Primary cutaneous $CD30^+$ large cell lymphoma ($CD30^+$LCL) typically occurs in adults presenting with solitary or localized (ulcerating) nodules or tumors (Fig. 85–10).[46] Regional lymph node involvement is seen in 25% of patients at presentation. These primary cutaneous $CD30^+$ LCLs are probably closely related to lymphomatoid papulosis, regressing atypical histiocytosis, and primary cutaneous Hodgkin disease. The tumor has a favorable prognosis and often complete or partial spontaneous regression occurs. This is in contrast to primary noncutaneous $CD30^+$ LCL, which can be seen in children or adults and which carries a poor prognosis.[47] These primary cutaneous lesions, in contradistinction from the nodal or pediatric cases, have been shown to rarely have the chromosomal translocation t(2:gene 5) associated with overexpression of the anaplastic lymphoma kinase (ALK negative). Histopathology consists of diffuse nonepidermotropic infiltrates with cohesive sheets of large $CD30^+$ tumor cells (Fig. 85–11). In most instances, the tumor cells have an anaplastic morphology, showing round, oval, or irregularly shaped nuclei; prominent (eosinophilic) nucleoli; and abundant cytoplasm. Less commonly, the neoplastic cells have a pleomorphic or immunoblastic appearance. Reactive lymphocytes are often present, but infiltrating eosinophils are often less conspicuous. The immunophenotype of this disorder is characteristically $CD4^+$, with more than 75% of neoplastic cells expressing CD30. In contrast to the poor outcome of MF that has transformed to a $CD30^+$ large cell variant, primary $CD30^+$ cutaneous large T-cell lymphomas are associated with an excellent prognosis. Radiotherapy is the preferred treatment for solitary or localized disease, with combination chemotherapy reserved for patients with generalized skin lesions or extracutaneous dissemination. Surgical excision may be adequate in many cases. In advanced cases, 5-year survival exceeds 30%.

CD30-NEGATIVE CUTANEOUS LARGE T-CELL LYMPHOMA

These lymphomas tend to have an aggressive clinical course. Patients present with localized or generalized plaques, nodules, or tumors.[48]

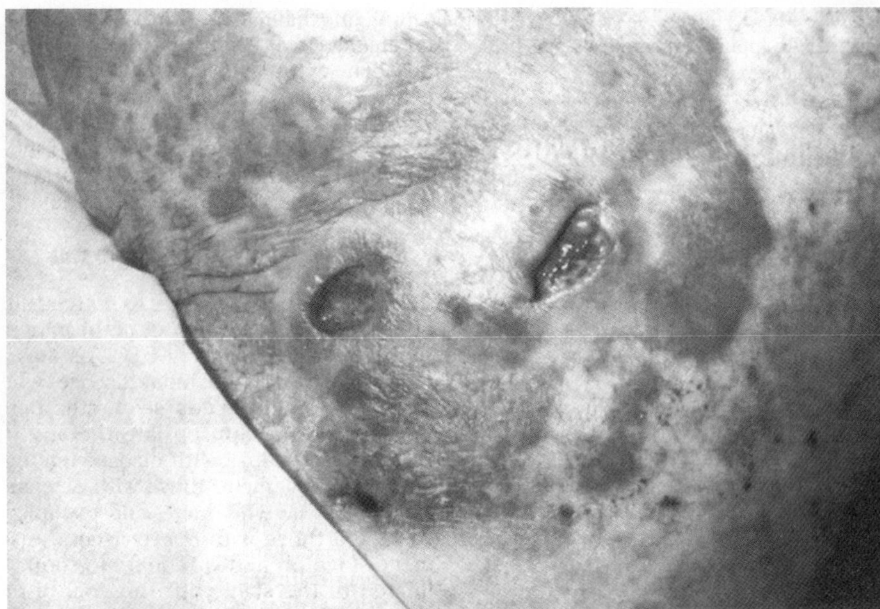

Figure 85–10 Lesions of CD30+ large cell lymphoma with ulceration.

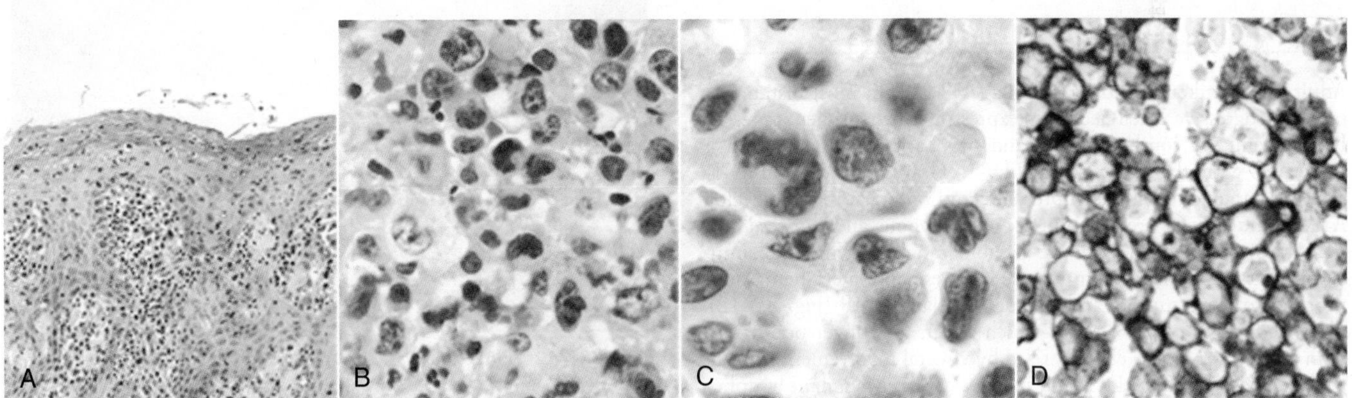

Figure 85–11 Cutaneous anaplastic large cell lymphoma (**A–D**). Sheets of tumor cells are present in the dermis (**A**) and are associated with marked pseudoepitheliomatous hyperplasia. The cells are quite varied and bizarre (**B**) and frequently show abnormal "embryoid" shapes (**C**) constituting the so-called hallmark cells. There is bright staining with CD30 (**D**). ALK-staining (not shown) is typically negative.

Histopathology demonstrates that infiltrates are nonepidermotropic with variable numbers of medium-sized to large pleomorphic T cells with or without cerebriform nuclei, and immunoblasts. The tumor cells are CD4+ with CD30 staining negative or restricted to a few scattered tumor cells. Multiagent chemotherapy is used in most instances, with radiation therapy reserved for patients with localized disease. The 5-year survival rate is less than 20%.

PLEOMORPHIC SMALL OR MEDIUM-SIZED CUTANEOUS T-CELL LYMPHOMA

This is an uncommon entity. Patients typically present with red-purplish nodules or tumors. Histopathology shows a dense, diffuse, or nodular infiltrate with small or medium-sized pleomorphic neoplastic cells within the dermis, often with extension into the subcutis.[49] The neoplastic cells are of the helper phenotype and do not express CD30. Localized disease is typically treated with radiation therapy. Prognosis for these patients is good in our experience, with rare progression to more aggressive clinical behavior. Patients with more generalized disease have been treated with regimens used for indolent non-Hodgkin lymphomas. Five-year survival rates exceed 60%.

SUBCUTANEOUS PANNICULITIS-LIKE T-CELL LYMPHOMA

Subcutaneous panniculitis-like T-cell lymphoma is a rare entity. Patients present with subcutaneous nodules and plaques.[50,51] Systemic symptoms are common, including fevers, fatigue, and anorexia. Histopathology reveals a subcutaneous infiltrate with pleomorphic T cells of variable size, mixed with benign macrophages. Tumor cell necrosis, karyorrhexis, and erythrophagocytosis are common findings. Differential diagnosis includes the frequently fatal but non-neoplastic cytophagic histiocytic panniculitis. Neoplastic infiltration of deep blood vessels can be noted in some cases.[52] Immunophenotyping reveals postthymic T-cell markers with CD4+ and CD8+ subtypes. T-cell γ/δ gene rearrangement may be present in some cases, (typically those with a cytotoxic T-cell phenotype CD8+). The prognosis is in general poor despite aggressive chemotherapy, especially when the disorder manifests concurrent with a hemophagocytic syndrome (fevers, cytopenias). Cases in which the panniculitic findings coexist with lupus erythematosus may behave in a clinically indolent fashion, however.

LYMPHOMATOID GRANULOMATOSIS

Lymphomatoid granulomatosis is a rare multiorgan disease of the lungs, nasopharynx, joints, and peripheral and central nervous systems.[53] Cutaneous involvement occurs in 25% to 50% of patients. Though nodules are most common, some patients have nonspecific macules, papules, or ulceration. Histologic evaluation reveals an angiocentric, polymorphous infiltrate of atypical lymphocytes and histiocytes surrounding and invading blood vessels within the dermis. Molecular and immunologic studies suggest a mature clonal helper T-cell process. However, reports have suggested a massive reactive T-cell infiltrate driven by a small number of clonal B cells.[54]

Epstein–Barr virus DNA sequences are frequently present, and their role in the pathogenesis of this disorder is being explored. Though the clinical course is variable, the prognosis for patients with diffuse pulmonary involvement or the appearance of high-grade lymphoma is poor, with a median survival of less than 2 years. Treatment that depends on histologic findings and extent and location of disease may include corticosteroids, radiotherapy, and chemotherapy. Interferon has shown significant activity against this disease.[55]

ADULT T-CELL LEUKEMIA AND LYMPHOMA

Adult T-cell leukemia and lymphoma (ATLL) is in most instances a rapidly progressive T-cell neoplasm expressing a helper phenotype.[56,57] It is endemic in southern Japan and the Caribbean islands and is associated with the retrovirus HTLV-1. However, most HTLV-I–infected patients remain asymptomatic and only 2% to 4% develop ATLL. The clinical presentation is polymorphous and can resemble MF or SS. Cutaneous lesions are variable, ranging from a rash simulating a viral exanthem, to annular lesions resembling erythema multiforme, to large tumors and plaques similar to MF (Fig. 85–12). Advanced stages of the disease, which affects a younger population than seen with MF, are characterized by visceral involvement, immunodeficiency, elevated LDH, and hypercalcemia. Malignant lymphocytes often have convoluted or multilobed nuclei and can be detected in the peripheral blood in 75% of patients. The neoplastic T cells express high levels of the IL-2 receptor (CD25). For purposes of treatment and prognosis, it is wise to view ATLL as a spectrum with two subgroups, acute and all others, with treatment, though inadequate, reserved for those with acute ATLL. Therapeutic options include multiagent chemotherapy and antibody or recombinant toxins directed against the IL-2 receptor. Patients with acute ATLL have poor survival rates, with a median duration of 4 to 6 months. Patients whose disease is not "acute" are considered to have "smoldering" disease and have lesions that may wax and wane in size and shape despite treatment.

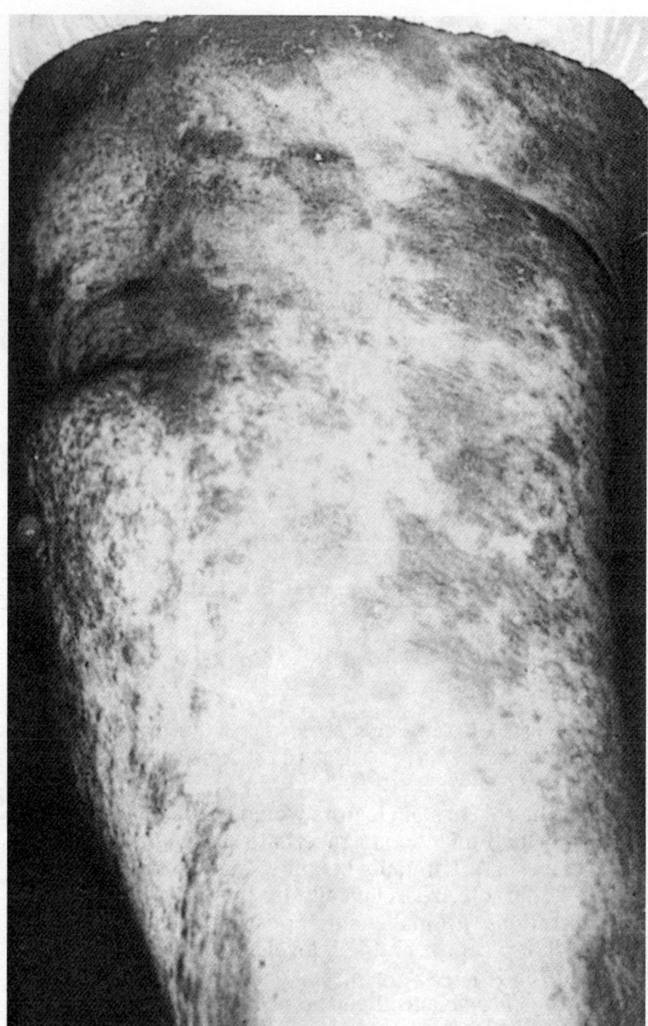

Figure 85–12 Skin lesions in adult T-cell lymphoma/leukemia syndrome.

PROGNOSIS

The goals of treatment in MF are the relief of symptoms with improved quality of life generally through prevention or delay in development of advanced skin disease, and improvement in cosmetics. Despite some uncontrolled clinical trial results that have been reported to suggest "cures" in this disease, the general perception remains that this disease is not curable with standard therapies available today. The disease behaves similarly to other low-grade lymphomas, with periods of remission gradually becoming shorter with subsequent therapeutic interventions. Unlike B-cell low-grade lymphomas, however, advanced-stage MF is associated with a relatively short median life expectancy. Patients with significant nodal involvement (LN3 or LN4) or extensive skin involvement (T4) have median life expectancies of 30 to 55 months.[58,59] A driving force in the development of treatments for this disease is the goal of altering the natural history for this group of poor prognosis patients. No clinical trial has determined that aggressive early therapy is better than sequential palliative approaches or investigational approaches,[60] and new treatments continue to be developed and tested for these patients.

Techniques such as flow cytometry, cytogenetic analysis, and determination of nuclear contour indices are specialized methods, which may also improve diagnostic and prognostic specificity. Flow cytometry and cytogenetic analysis are complementary techniques. Flow cytometry allows the detection of cell populations with the normal (diploid) number of chromosomes versus abnormal (aneuploid) numbers, and cytogenetic analysis precisely identifies the individual chromosomal structure and number. Bunn and coworkers[61] demonstrated that this can be important prognostically in MF/SS, as the presence of aneuploidy during the clinical course was associated with more aggressive behavior of the disease. Hyperdiploid cell clones were demonstrated in patients with large-cell histology, aggressive disease, and shortened survival time. Specific chromosomal deletions also have an effect on prognosis.[62]

The nuclear contour index has been used by several groups in an effort to separate "benign" cutaneous lymphocytic disorders, such as lymphomatoid papulosis and pityriasis lichenoides, from MF/SS.[63,64] Electron microscopy allows the calculation of a value based on the degree of nuclear folding; this nuclear contour index is significantly greater in patients with MF than in other benign conditions.

The density of epidermal Langerhans cells in biopsy samples, as determined by immunoperoxidase stains, has been identified as a prognostic feature.[65] Epidermal Langerhans cells are necessary for antigen recognition and processing in the normal immune response. Patients with Langerhans cell densities greater than 90 cells per square millimeter had a significantly reduced risk of death from MF/SS compared with those with lower densities. There was no prognostic significance identified for the presence or absence of CD30-positive cells. It has been noted that the presence of cytotoxic $CD8^+$ T lymphocytes in the skin infiltrate is associated with a better prognosis.[66]

Occasionally patients may develop a more clinically aggressive lymphoma concurrent with a change in the histologic appearance of the neoplastic cells and the pace of their disease. This progression from typical small, convoluted lymphocytes to larger lymphocytes, such as those associated with large-cell lymphoma, has been documented.[67,68] Whether this conversion is secondary to prior therapeutic modalities used remains uncertain.

The gold standard for the diagnosis of mycosis fungoides is still routine histopathology with adequate clinical correlation. Early lesions of MF are frequently accompanied by heavy infiltrates of benign reactive T cells, hampering the detection of abnormal T-cell clones by any laboratory method. Hence most adjuvant laboratory methods are not helpful at the precise time when they are most needed.

In 1979, the staging committee at an international workshop on MF proposed a staging system based on the international tumor-node-metastasis (TNM) system (Table 85–2).[69] This classification was based on the evaluation of 347 patients and a multivariate analysis of potential prognostic factors. This group identified several independent prognostic factors: extent of skin disease at diagnosis (T), type of lymph node (N) involvement, presence or absence of peripheral blood (PB) involvement, and presence or absence of visceral (M) involvement. The group also translated this staging into a recommended clinical staging system (see Table 85–2).

Investigators at the National Cancer Institute retrospectively analyzed 152 patients who underwent uniform pathologic staging.[70] They were able to identify three distinct prognostic groups. Good-risk patients had plaque-only skin disease without lymph node, blood, or visceral involvement, and a median survival of more than 12 years. Less than 10% of patients with stage 1A (limited patch) and less than 30% with stage 1B (extensive patch or plaque) progress to more advanced disease. Intermediate-risk patients had skin tumors, erythroderma, or plaque disease with lymph node or blood involvement (but no visceral disease) and a median survival of 5 years. Poor-risk patients had visceral disease or complete effacement of lymph nodes by lymphoma, and a median survival of 2.5 years.

Table 85–2 TNM Staging System for Cutaneous T-Cell Lymphomas

Classification	Description
T	Skin
TO	Clinically or histopathologically suspicious lesions
T1	Limited plaques, papules, or eczematous patches covering 10% of the skin surface
T2	Generalized plaques, papules, or erythematous patches covering 10% of the skin surface
T3	Tumors (one or more)
T4	Generalized erythroderma
	Pathology of T1–4 is diagnostic of a cutaneous T-cell lymphoma. When more than one T stage exists, both are recorded and highest is used for staging. Record other features if appropriate (eg, ulcers, poikiloderma, scale)
N	Lymph nodes
NO	No clinically abnormal peripheral lymph nodes
N1	Clinically abnormal peripheral lymph nodes (record number of sites)
NPO	Biopsy performed, not cutaneous T-cell lymphoma (CTCL)
NP1	Biopsy performed, CTCL
PB	Peripheral blood
PBO (≤5%)	Atypical circulating cells not present
PB1	Atypical circulating cells not present (>5%), record total white blood cell count, total lymphocyte count, and percentage of abnormal cells
M	Visceral organs
MO	No visceral organ involvement
M1	Visceral involvement (must have pathologic confirmation), record organ involved
Staging	
Stage Ia	T1, NO NPO, MO
Stage Ib	T2, NO NPO, MO
Stage IIa	T1-2, N1 NPO, MO
Stage IIb	T3, NO NPO, MO
Stage III	T4, NO NPO, MO
Stage IVa	T1-4, NO,1 NP1, MO
Stage IVb	T1-4, NO,1 NPO,1, M1

THERAPY

Therapy can be conveniently divided into two approaches: *topical* (skin directed), such as psoralens with ultraviolet light A (PUVA), topical chemotherapy application (nitrogen mustard or carmustine), and total skin electron beam radiotherapy, and *systemic* (skin and viscera directed), such as interferons, oral or parenteral chemotherapy, photopheresis, oral retinoids, and investigational new compounds (Table 85–3). No studies have demonstrated that one topical therapy is more effective than another, and patient and investigator preference remains the most important discriminating factor governing choice. However, as the biology of the neoplastic cell has become better understood,[71] it is clear that some therapies may actually have topical and systemic effects through alterations in the body's cytokine milieu and ability to mount a host response against the neoplastic cell.[72] Investigational approaches combining therapies remain active research strategies. The following sections detail the individual treatment options and discuss the mechanisms of action, rationale for use, and outcomes.

PHOTOTHERAPY

8-Methoxypsoralen (8-MOP) is a member of a family of photoactivated compounds (furocoumarin derivatives), which may inhibit DNA and RNA synthesis through formation of mono- or bifunctional thymine adducts, gene mutations, or sister chromatid exchanges.[73,74] The cross strand formed between DNA strands results in a halt in cell division as well as oxidative damage of cytoplasmic organelles and cell membranes. These drugs are only active if the tissue containing the psoralen compound is exposed to ultraviolet A rays (UVA). The mechanism of cell cytotoxicity for many cancer therapies involves the induction of apoptosis. Yoo and associates[75] demonstrated that peripheral blood mononuclear cells from Sézary syndrome patients and controls exposed in vitro to PUVA undergo apoptosis. This finding was confirmed with light microscopy, flow cytometry, and electron microscopy, and by gel electrophoresis.

Table 85–3 Therapeutic Options for Mycosis Fungoides

Topical Therapy
Ultraviolet light A with psoralen (PUVA)
Ultraviolet light B (UVB)
Total-skin electron beam radiation
Topical chemotherapy
Topical retinoids
Systemic Therapy
Photophoresis
Interferon-α
Single-agent chemotherapy
Combination chemotherapy
Oral retinoids
Investigational agents

Unfortunately, normal and neoplastic lymphocytes were equally sensitive to the apoptosis induction with PUVA (as opposed to with psoralen alone). However, macrophages appeared to be resistant to apoptosis induction and phagocytized apoptotic lymphocytes (but not nonapoptotic lymphocytes). Apoptosis induction may be the ultimate end point yielding benefit, but an immunologic effect due to monocyte phagocytosis and antigen presentation resulting from effector cells may also be present.

Photochemotherapy units with UVA lamps emit a continuous spectrum of long UVA in the range of 320 to 400 nm with peak emission between 350 and 380 nm. Initial exposure times of patients to high-output UVA are based on the degree of pigmentation before therapy, history of ability to tan, and the output of the photochemotherapy units. Exposure times are increased with each treatment depending on the patient's response, and evidence of erythema. The initial UVA dose is between 0.5 and 2.0 J/cm^2 and can be increased by approximately 0.5 J/cm^2 per treatment as tolerated. The psoralen compound is ingested 2 hours before the UVA exposure. Topical psoralen protocols are also available. UV light-blocking glasses should be worn for 24 hours after administration of 8-MOP. Therapy is typically given three times weekly until complete clearing occurs. The frequency of treatments can then be reduced, but some maintenance therapy (once every 2–4 weeks) may prolong the duration of remission. As new data emerge regarding the long-term risks of second skin malignancies after PUVA, the advisability of this maintenance therapy recommendation has been questioned.

Initial trials using PUVA noted benefit in psoriasis patients.[76] Several clinical trials with PUVA for patients with MF soon followed.[77] These studies all demonstrated high rates of remission induction in the early stage (patch or plaque stage of disease). The Scandinavian study group reported a 58% complete remission rate for these patients within 4 to 12 months of initiation of therapy.[78] Maintenance therapy allowed remission duration of up to 53 months. In these early studies, the same group also reported a surprisingly high rate of objective remission induction in tumor-stage patients of 83%.[79] In a large series, 82 patients were followed for a median of 43 months.[80] An objective response rate was observed in 95% of patients, with a 65% complete clearance rate. Ninety percent of these patients had early-stage disease (stage IA–IIA). A single patient with tumor-stage disease attained a short remission with PUVA alone. Two of six patients with generalized erythroderma cleared completely (no evidence of circulating neoplastic lymphocytes). Given the difficulty in treating advanced-stage patients with PUVA alone, we usually restrict PUVA therapy to patients with stage IA–IIA disease (see Table 85–2), monitoring patients with tumor disease closely for progression.

Side effects with PUVA are quite tolerable. Nausea or vomiting due to psoralen ingestion is observed occasionally, and erythema, pruritus, and chronic dry skin are effects of the UVA light damage to the skin. Long-term PUVA exposure has been associated with a number of late effects. These include dry skin, lichenification, keratosis, and rarely amyloid deposition in the skin.[81] Most important is the late development of iatrogenic (basal and squamous) carcinomas,[82] secondary malignant melanomas of the skin,[83] and rarely cataract formation. Because the cumulative dose of PUVA is correlated with the risks of second skin neoplasms, routine use of maintenance therapy may be less desirable, especially for patients with an excellent prognosis (stage IA). Despite these problems, the long remissions induced, the ease of administration, and the lack of interactions with other therapeutic modalities make PUVA an attractive early intervention.

Narrow-band UVB light (wavelength of 311 nm) is emerging as a valid alternative to PUVA for patients with limited patch or plaque disease. Although probably not as effective as PUVA, initial studies reported response rates near 70%.[84] The advantages of narrow-band UVB are that oral psoralen is not required and there may be less of a photocarcinogenic effect. The role for maintenance therapy has not been established.

UVA-1 is a new modality of phototherapy that uses high-energy UVA-1 (340–400 nm) output, which penetrates deep into the dermis. Resolution of tumor lesions has even been reported using this new therapeutic approach.[85] However, the reduction in circulating CD4$^+$ cells raises the possibility that chronic use of this modality could be immunosuppressive.

RADIATION THERAPY

The non-Hodgkin lymphomas in general, and the CTCL in particular, have been shown to be radiosensitive.[86] External-beam radiation has been shown to adequately control local areas of otherwise resistant MF, or provide palliation in cases of bulky tumor lesions.[87,88] Unfortunately, the cumulative dosage that can be given to patients over time is limited owing to normal organ toxicity. Side effects consisting of leukopenia, thrombocytopenia, and radiation dermatitis may prevent long-term therapy with other agents. Newer techniques involving total nodal irradiation, fractionated total-body irradiation, or hemibody irradiation may have a role to play in the development of multimodality approaches to this disease.

The limitations of external beam radiation led to increasing use of electron beam radiotherapy for cases of MF confined to the skin. Linear accelerator-generated electron beams are scattered by a penetrable plate placed at the collimator site. The energy of the electrons is reduced to 4 to 7 MeV and allows adequate field distribution. Because of this low energy level, the beam only penetrates the surface several millimeters to 1 cm into the dermis. Patients may be treated using six-field or rotational treatments.[89,90] The total skin surface can be treated without significant internal organ toxicity. Most patients are able to tolerate total doses of approximately 3000 to 3600 cGy over an 8- to 10-week period.[90]

An excellent review[91] compared results of external beam therapy at Stanford University with those achieved in Hamilton, Ontario. The results cited in this paper reflect the extensive expertise of both centers in the delivery of this therapy, and may not be applicable to centers with much less frequent use of the technique. For patients with stage IA–IIA (see Table 85–2), almost 65% to 95% of patients achieved a complete remission. Treatment delivered without adjuvant therapies is associated with a relatively high rate of relapse in patients of all stages except stage IA. Ten-year relapse-free survival rates at the two centers range from 33% to 52% for this good-prognosis group. However, for stage IB and worse disease, 10-year unmaintained remission rates are only 16% or less. Higher-risk patients may be "induced" with external beam radiation and then placed on topical chemotherapy or systemic treatments such as extracorporeal photopheresis for "maintenance." Still the benefits of therapy may extend beyond crude estimates of relapse rates or survival. Patients with tumor lesions, generalized erythroderma, peripheral blood or nodal involvement, and even visceral spread can be successfully palliated with electron beam radiation therapy, as well. Side effects, however, can be occasionally extreme, including scaling, dryness of skin, erythema, extremity edema, telangiectasia formation,

Algorithm for Care of Patients with Mycosis Fungoides or Sézary Syndrome

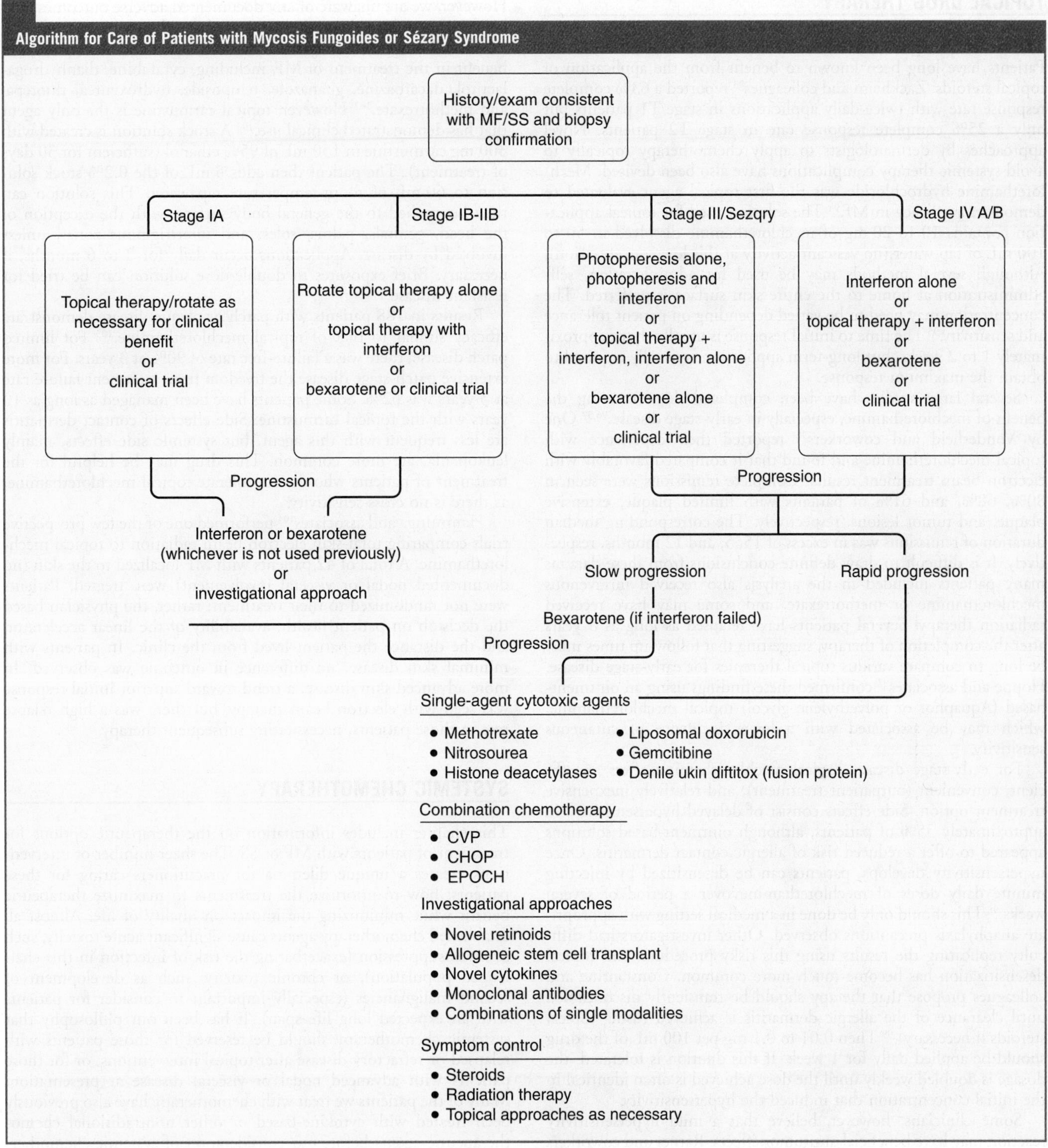

skin ulceration, and hair or sweat gland loss (usually transient but occasionally permanent). Careful radiation dosimetric techniques are required to ensure adequate skin treatment without excessive normal organ toxicity.[90] We do not use electron beam radiotherapy early in the disease because other topical therapies have been developed that yield similar response rates with less potential toxicity. The long duration of remissions observed in patients with stage IA disease does not equate with cure, as their life expectancy is essentially the same as age-matched controls, and these patients may simply have indolent biology. One group has reported their experience with multiple courses of therapy.[92] They re-treated 15 patients with relapsed MF a mean of 41 months after the initial course of electron beam therapy. All patients had received intervening therapies for disease control. Eleven of the 15 had a complete remission with their first cycle of radiation. The second course achieved six complete remissions and nine partial remissions. The median duration of initial complete remission was 11 months. The median duration of complete remission to the second course of therapy was only 3 months, suggesting radioresistance had developed between the first and second cycles in many patients. In general, toxicity was thought to be tolerable.

TOPICAL DRUG THERAPY

The earliest therapies for MF focused on treatment of the skin disease. Patients have long been known to benefit from the application of topical steroids. Zackheim and colleagues[93] reported a 63% complete response rate with twice-daily applications in stage T1 patients but only a 25% complete response rate in stage T2 patients. Novel approaches by dermatologists to apply chemotherapy topically to avoid systemic therapy complications have also been devised. Mechlorethamine hydrochloride was the first topical agent evaluated to demonstrate efficacy in MF.[94] The solution used for topical application contains 10 to 20 mg of mechlorethamine dissolved in 50 to 100 mL of tap water (no vesicant activity at this low concentration). Although several methods may be used for administration, self-administration at home to the entire skin surface is preferred. The concentration may need to be varied depending on patient tolerance and sensitivity.[95] The time to initial response is usually short, approximately 1 to 2 weeks, but long-term application is usually required to obtain the maximum response.

Several large studies have been completed demonstrating the benefit of mechlorethamine, especially in early-stage disease.[96,97] One by Vonderheid and coworkers[96] reported their experience with topical mechlorethamine and found that it compared favorably with electron beam treatment results. Complete remissions were seen in 80%, 68%, and 61% of patients with limited plaque, extensive plaque, and tumor lesions, respectively. The corresponding median duration of remissions was in excess of 15, 5, and 12 months, respectively. It is difficult to draw definite conclusions from these data, as many patients included in the analysis also received intravenous mechlorethamine or methotrexate, and some may have received radiation therapy. Several patients have relapsed as long as 8 years after the completion of therapy, suggesting that follow-up times must be long to compare various topical therapies for early-stage disease. Hoppe and associates[97] confirmed these findings using an ointment-based (Aquaphor or polyethylene glycol) topical mechlorethamine, which may be associated with a lower incidence of cutaneous sensitivity.

For early-stage disease, topical mechlorethamine offers an efficient, convenient (outpatient treatment), and relatively inexpensive treatment option. Side effects consist of delayed hypersensitivity in approximately 35% of patients, although ointment-based solutions appeared to offer a reduced risk of allergic contact dermatitis. Once hypersensitivity develops, patients can be desensitized by injecting minute daily doses of mechlorethamine over a period of several weeks.[98] This should only be done in a medical setting with appropriate anaphylaxis precautions observed. Other investigators had difficulty replicating the results using this risky procedure, and topical desensitization has become much more common. Constantine and colleagues propose that therapy should be transiently discontinued until clearance of the allergic dermatitis is achieved (using topical steroids if necessary).[99] Then 0.01 to 0.1 mg per 100 mL of the drug should be applied daily for 1 week. If this dilution is tolerated, the dosage is doubled weekly until the dose achieved is often identical to the initial concentration that induced the hypersensitivity.

Some clinicians, however, believe that a mild hypersensitivity reaction may have beneficial antitumor effects. Ratner and coworkers previously demonstrated that plaque lesions of MF cleared when exposed to topical doses of 2,4-dinitrochlorobenzene, a known universal inducer of delayed hypersensitivity responses.[100] Anergic individuals failed to improve. Other known sensitizing agents yielded similar but less dramatic responses. Some hypersensitivity may be beneficial; the generalized erythroderma and pruritus are usually poorly tolerated when severe, however, and some alteration in therapy is required.

There has been an increased risk of secondary skin cancers in patients receiving long-term mechlorethamine. Of recent concern is the safety of family members or health care workers secondarily exposed to the topical solutions. Home treatment with topical mechlorethamine has been shown to result in aerosolized drug levels, which may result in mucous membrane or ocular irritation.[101] However, we are unaware of any documented adverse outcomes, and believe this to be a theoretical concern more than a practical one.

Several other topical agents have been tested and shown to be of benefit in the treatment of MF, including, cytarabine, dianhydrogalactitol, dacarbazine, guanazole, teniposide, hydroxyurea, thiotepa, and methotrexate.[102] However, topical carmustine is the only agent that has demonstrated clinical use.[103] A stock solution is created with 300 mg carmustine in 150 mL of 95% ethanol (sufficient for 30 days of treatment). The patient then adds 5 mL of the 0.2% stock solution to 60 mL of room-temperature tap water. This solution can then be applied to the general body surface, with the exception of the head, genitals, palms, soles, and intertriginous zones, unless involved by disease. Applications occur daily for 2 to 6 months, if necessary. Brief exposures to double-dose solution can be tried for resistant disease.

Results in 188 patients with patch or plaque disease demonstrate efficacy similar to that of topical mechlorethamine.[103] For limited patch disease, there was a failure-free rate of 90% at 3 years. For more extensive patch-stage disease the freedom from treatment failure rate at 3 years was 62%. Some patients have been managed as long as 10 years with the topical carmustine. Side effects of contact dermatitis are less frequent with this agent, but systemic side effects, mainly leukopenia, are more common. This drug may be helpful for the treatment of patients who do not tolerate topical mechlorethamine, as there is no cross-sensitivity.

Hamminga and associates[104] performed one of the few prospective trials comparing total-skin electron beam radiation to topical mechlorethamine. A total of 42 patients with MF localized to the skin (no documented nodal or visceral involvement) were treated. Patients were not randomized to their treatment; rather, the physician based the decision on patient health, availability of the linear accelerator, and the distance the patient lived from the clinic. In patients with minimal skin disease, no difference in outcome was observed. In more advanced skin disease, a trend toward superior initial response was seen with electron beam therapy, but there was a high relapse rate in those patients, necessitating subsequent therapy.

SYSTEMIC CHEMOTHERAPY

This chapter includes information on the therapeutic options for treatment of patients with MF or SS. The sheer number of interventions creates a unique dilemma for practitioners caring for these patients: how to prioritize the treatments to maximize therapeutic benefit while minimizing the impact on quality of life. Almost all established chemotherapy agents cause significant acute toxicity, such as myelosuppression (exacerbating the risk of infection in this challenged population), or chronic toxicity, such as development of second malignancies (especially important to consider for patients with an expected long life span). It has been our philosophy that systemic chemotherapy should be reserved for those patients with relapsed or refractory disease after topical interventions; or for those patients with advanced nodal or visceral disease at presentation. Many of the patients we treat with chemotherapy have also previously been treated with cytokine-based or other nontraditional chemotherapeutic agents before our consideration of systemic chemotherapy. With that in mind, a number of trials have been published, reporting results using agents developed many years ago for other indications but still in use for the treatment of MF/SS today, as well as new agents being increasingly studied for specific efficacy in MF/SS based on molecular or proteonomic rationale. An example of such a family of agents is the histone deacetylase (HDAC) inhibitors. Vorinostat (aka SAHA) has recently been approved by the FDA for the treatment of the cutaneous manifestations of CTCL in patients in whom bexarotene (see Retinoids below) has failed,[105–108] and a related HDAC inhibitor depsipeptide (aka FR901228) is in late phase testing. These agents increase acetylation of histones and other nuclear factors, and alter the expression of a number of genes, including some that control growth and differentiation. Vorinostat 400 mg daily orally was tested in an open-label trial of 74 patients who had progressed on at least two prior systemic therapies. The objective response rate was 29.5%, with 1 complete and 18 partial responses. Common adverse events included diarrhea (49%) and fatigue (46%). Grade III events were less common but included fatigue (5%), deep venous thromboses/pulmonary emboli (5%), and thrombocytopenia (4%).

Reports from the National Cancer Institute with depsipeptide, another histone deacetylase inhibitor, have provided confirmatory results of the use of this class of agent for the treatment of patients with T-cell lymphomas including some with MF/SS.[109,110] In these reports of several phase I and phase II trials, 10 of 20 patients with MF/SS appeared to have had a partial response. Toxicity to depsipeptide has included alterations in the electrocardiogram that could potentially predispose to arrhythmias, and treatment of patients has required ongoing telemetry monitoring in some trials, but no evidence for acute or chronic impairment in cardiac function has been noted. Vorinostat demonstrated drug-related grade I ECG changes in five patients and grade II in one patient.

Unfortunately, depsipeptide has been shown to be a substrate for the multidrug resistance (MDR) protein (a *p*-glycoprotein) and upregulates the expression of MDR1. Preliminary molecular analysis confirmed the upregulation of MDR1. Several patients demonstrated increased surface expression of the CD-25 component of the high-affinity interleukin-2 receptor after treatment. This protein is a target for denileukin diftitox, discussed elsewhere in this chapter as a therapy for MF, suggesting strategies for combination approaches could be devised to enhance responses to both agents.

Older agents studied previously include alkylating agents like chlorambucil or cisplatin, the microtubule inhibitors etoposide, vincristine, and vinblastine, or the antitumor antibiotics, like bleomycin and doxorubicin.[111–114] In general, the response rates are modest and duration of response typically less than 6 months.

McDonald and Bertino[115] reported particularly good results with the antimetabolite methotrexate administered intravenously followed by oral citrovorum factor. Patients received 1 to 5 mg/kg of intravenous methotrexate every 5 days. If a patient tolerated the lowest dose, each subsequent dose was escalated. After 5 intravenous doses, patients were switched to oral methotrexate (25–50 mg) with oral citrovorum as weekly maintenance. All 11 patients achieved "good" or better clearing (>60%) for a median duration of 24 months. Mucositis and skin ulcerations were the most significant toxicity witnessed. Myelosuppression was mild in general. The related compound, trimetrexate, also was effective in treating CTCL.[116]

Subsequently, the benefits of adding 5-fluorouracil to the methotrexate-based regimen, exploiting the synergy between these agents, were evaluated.[117] The methotrexate was administered as a 24-hour continuous infusion at 60 mg/m^2. Immediately after this infusion, 5-flourouracil (20 mg/kg each 24 hours) was continuously infused for 36 to 48 hours. Oral citrovorum factor (10 mg/m^2) was administered intravenously 6 hours after cessation of the methotrexate infusion and then orally for five additional doses. The methotrexate dose was escalated to a maximum of 120 mg/m^2, as allowed by toxicity and response. Ten patients were treated for an average duration of 33 months (range, 3 to 78 months). The number of cycles administered ranged from 5 to 45. All patients achieved a partial remission. Initial cycles were given every 5 to 8 days. Once a good response was achieved, cycles were administered every 3 months as maintenance. Other groups anecdotally reported success with low doses of oral methotrexate. In general these regimens appear to be fairly well tolerated.

The purine antimetabolites have been shown to be active in the treatment of MF/SS. These compounds do not have a single mechanism of action, but all ultimately interfere with intracellular regulation of deoxyribonucleotide pools and this imbalance partially explains the cytotoxicity. This family of drugs includes 2-deoxycoformycin (DCF), fludarabine phosphate, and 2-chlorodeoxyadenosine (2-CdA).[118]

DCF is a transition state inhibitor of adenosine deaminase. Inhibition of this enzyme, necessary for the conversion of adenosine to inosine, results in accumulation of 2-deoxy-ATP and subsequent inhibition of the enzyme ribonucleotide diphosphate reductase necessary for DNA synthesis in dividing cells. DCF is also effective against cells in the resting state, where ribonucleotide diphosphate reductase levels are barely detectable. It has been shown that deoxy-ATP accumulation in resting lymphocytes results in increased DNA strand breaks over time; this results in the activation of Ca^{2+}/Mg^{2+}-dependent endonuclease that produces double-stranded DNA strand breaks at internucleosomal regions, and also activation of a poly-ADP-ribose polymerase that consumes NAD and adenosine triphosphate. These perturbations lead to apoptotic cell death.

Fludarabine phosphate represents the fluorinated derivative of ara-A. This compound was known to retain cytotoxic action against leukemias, and was resistant to degradation by adenosine deaminase. Solubility was poor, however, unless the 5′-monophosphate derivative was used; hence fludarabine monophosphate is the 5′-monophosphate form of F-ara-A. Similar to the mechanism of action of cytarabine or ara-A, fludarabine phosphate requires phosphorylation by deoxycytidine kinase to the active triphosphate metabolite F-ara-ATP. Again, this triphosphate derivative inhibits ribonucleotide reductase, resulting in nucleotide pool imbalances, which prevent DNA repair, and ultimately cause apoptosis.

2-CdA represents another chemical modification of deoxyadenosine, which renders the drug resistant to adenosine deaminase. After activation by deoxycytidine kinase, the triphosphate derivative similarly inhibits ribonucleotide reductase, and accumulates intracellularly perturbing the deoxyribonucleotide pool balance, resulting in DNA damage and cell death.

Enzymes such as cytoplasmic 5′-nucleotidase catalyze the degradation of the active triphosphate derivatives discussed earlier. Cells with relatively greater levels of the activation enzymes versus degradation enzymes were identified as likely clinical targets. Lymphoid disorders make good targets for these agents because they contain high levels of deoxycytidine kinase and low levels of 5′-nucleotidase and depend on polymerase-α for DNA repair. Because it was known that T-lymphoblastoid cell lines were most sensitive to these drugs, it was thought that T-lymphocyte disorders would be sensitive in vivo to these agents.

A number of studies treating patients with MF/SS have been performed with these drugs. Table 85–4 shows the results in these studies. Four studies used DCF as a single agent at doses ranging from 3.75 to 10 mg/m^2 daily for three doses every 21 to 28 days.[119–122] Twenty-five patients with MF/SS were included in the first three studies[119–121]; overall, 3 complete responses (12%) and 12 partial responses (48%) were documented. The fourth study represents the largest phase II experience reported to DCF for the treatment of MF/SS and other cutaneous T-cell lymphomas.[122] Twenty-seven eligible patients were treated for 3 consecutive days at 3.75 mg/m^2/day. Essentially, 80% of the doses in the trial were delivered at 3.75 or 5.0 mg/m^2/day. Twenty-one of 24 response-evaluable patients had

Table 85–4 Response Rates Observed in Clinical Trials with Purine Antimetabolite Agents

Drug	Overall Response Rate	Reference
DCF	66%	119
DCF	100%	120
DCF	54%	121
DCF	66%	122
Fludarabine	18%	123
2-CdA	28%	124
2-CdA	38%	125
2-CdA	18%	126
2-CdA	100%	127

DCF, deoxycoformycin; 2-CdA, 2-chlorodeoxyadenosine.

SS (14 patients), tumor-stage MF (6 patients), or large cell transformation of MF (1 patient). Patients had failed a median of three prior treatments before enrollment. The overall response rate for patients with MF/SS was 66% (five complete and nine partial responses). Most responses were short-lived as the median duration of response in patients with tumor-stage disease was 2 months (range, 1–2 months), and the median duration of response in erythrodermic disease was 3.5 months (no range given, but 2 patients had responses of at least 17 months).

The use of fludarabine for the treatment of MF/SS has also been assessed in a single, large phase II trial by von Hoff and colleagues.[123] They treated 33 patients who were good risks (ie, no prior systemic therapy) or poor risks (ie, prior systemic therapy) with fludarabine alone at doses of 25 or 18 mg/m^2 for the two groups, respectively. One complete response and five partial responses were obtained for an overall response rate of 18%.

2-CdA has been evaluated as a single agent for the treatment of MF/SS. We have treated 21 patients who had failed at least one prior therapy.[124] There were three complete and three partial responses (overall response rate of 28%). The median duration of response in this heavily pretreated group, however, was only 4 months. Three other groups have also reported results in small numbers of patients in the treatment of MF.[125–127] A total of 21 patients were reported when the studies are taken together. Seven patients achieved responses, giving an overall objective response rate of 33%, remarkably similar to results from our large, single-institution study.

The similarity in mechanism of action of these compounds would suggest that toxicity associated with the various compounds would be similar. This has definitely not been the case, however. There are distinct differences in the spectrum of acute and chronic toxicities with these agents. DCF and fludarabine are associated with higher rates of nausea or vomiting and alopecia than commonly associated with 2-CdA. The most significant toxicity with DCF and fludarabine, however, are neurotoxicity and immunosuppression. Approximately 15% of patients developed sepsis, and 10% developed an opportunistic infection, such as disseminated toxoplasmosis, cytomegaloviral infection, *Pneumocystis carinii* pneumonia, atypical mycobacterial infection, and fungemia in studies with these drugs. Another 15% developed severe neurotoxicity in the form of confusion, motor weakness, paresthesias, and central nervous system demyelination. Treatment with 2-CdA is extremely well tolerated acutely, but may result in somewhat greater myelosuppression than the other agents. This myelosuppression may even be more significant when the agent is used to treat T-lymphocyte disorders compared with B-cell diseases. In the study by Betticher and coworkers,[127] significant decrements in neutrophils and lymphocyte populations occurred in 46% and 41%, respectively. In our study of 2-CdA, we reduced the days of therapy delivered by continuous infusion to 5 days from the usual 7 because of a perception that the toxicity, primarily prolonged thrombocytopenia, was unacceptable. These results suggest that patients treated with these agents should be carefully evaluated for infectious complications, especially opportunistic infections, and that prophylactic therapy should be considered during and after therapy if significant immunosuppression is documented. Additionally, one should carefully consider the value of continuing to administer cycles of therapy if there is no evidence of further improvement in clinical response, because of the risk of suddenly developing prolonged cytopenias that may limit future therapeutic approaches. In general it is not apparent that one purine antimetabolite is dramatically better for this indication from these studies, although DCF has a slightly higher overall response rate. It has been observed repeatedly in these studies that occasional patients with SS may have striking and durable responses to treatment, but ideally other agents emerging may allow for higher response rates with less toxicity in this population.

Combination chemotherapy has often been employed for patients with advanced disease at presentation or with progression. Usually alkylator agents are used, in combination with doxorubicin, or vinca alkaloids.[128,129] Response rates of 80% to 100% have been achieved, with longer durations of remission than observed with single agent therapy. There have been no trials comparing different aggressive combination regimes. High response rates with perhaps less toxicity have been observed in treating other non-Hodgkin lymphomas using infusional combination regimens such as etoposide, vincristine, doxorubicin, cyclophosphamide, and prednisone (EPOCH regimen). A trial in CTCL suggested comparable activity to a bolus schedule, with greater risk of febrile neutropenia and bacteremia associated with indwelling catheters required for the infusion.[130]

It is our philosophy that this disease behaves similarly to other low-grade lymphomas (ie, B-cell type), with periods of remission becoming shorter with subsequent therapeutic interventions. However, as noted, advanced-stage MF is associated with a relatively short median life expectancy. Patients with significant nodal involvement or extensive skin disease (T4 in particular) have median life expectancies of 30 to 55 months.[58] A driving force in the development of treatments for this disease is the goal of altering the natural history for this group of poor prognosis patients, or for delaying the development of poor prognosis disease. There is no clinical trial of any modality that has demonstrated a survival benefit compared with a control group. Kaye and associates demonstrated more than a decade ago that combination chemotherapy (and total skin electron beam radiation therapy) did not provide better survival or even clinically significant delays in time to recurrence for patients compared with standard palliative, less aggressive therapies.[60] New drugs or approaches are still being developed with the goal of altering the disease state in poor-prognosis patients.

Because of the pressing need to identify new strategies to provide more durable remissions or even curative therapy for advanced CTCL, new drugs continue to be tested. On the basis of the clinical evidence of possible activity in early-phase testing, several drugs have been evaluated. In a phase II trial of 44 patients with relapsed MF or peripheral T-cell lymphoma (unspecified), gemcitabine was administered at 1200 mg/m^2 over 30 minutes on 3 weekly administrations every 28 days.[131] There were 5 (11.5%) complete remissions and 26 (59%) partial responses (overall response rate 70.5%). The median duration of response ranged from 15 months for complete responders to 10 months for those patients with partial response. There appeared to be no difference in response type between patients with MF or peripheral T-cell lymphomas. In a second trial at the MD Anderson Cancer Center with gemcitabine administered similarly but at a dose of 1000 mg/m^2, investigators found a 68% overall response rate (17/25), with two patients developing a complete remission.[132] Toxicity included myelosuppression in the majority of patients and development of a hemolytic-uremic syndrome in two elderly patients. Most recently gemcitabine was studied as a first-line systemic treatment in 27 patients with stage T3 or T4 MF/SS.[133] The overall response rate was 70% (19/27), with six complete remissions. The median time to progression was 10 months. Toxicity was generally mild.

The campothecins are a family of compounds that inhibit topoisomerase I, an enzyme required for unwinding strands of DNA for transcription and replication. In early phase studies it was recognized that the administration of 9-aminocampothecin (9-AC) by continuous infusion to maintain a drug concentration above a threshold level coupled with duration of exposure was important to ensure adequate inhibition of the target enzyme. In these studies at appropriate concentrations, activity was identified in non-Hodgkin lymphomas,[134] and it was therefore appropriate to study in MF/SS. We undertook a trial of infused 9-AC in patients with MF/SS.[135] The trial was prematurely closed after 12 patients received 30 cycles. There were two partial responses (17%) in a heavily pretreated population of patients; however, 6 of the 12 patients (50%) developed indwelling catheter infections, and 3 patients died 4 to 8 weeks after the last dose of 9-AC. The toxicity was deemed too excessive to justify this dose, route, and schedule of administration. This study nicely demonstrates the hazards of chemotherapy in this patient population, including the underlying risk of infection and the relative contraindication to indwelling catheters (hence a bias toward agents administered with short infusions through peripheral catheters, or oral agents, and the importance of prophylactic antibiotics if excessive invasive procedures are anticipated).

Another drug empirically tested for the treatment of MF/SS is pegylated doxorubicin based on the historic activity of doxorubicin against non-Hodgkin lymphomas. The process of encapsulating the doxorubicin in pegylated liposomes creates stable, long circulating carriers of the drug that results in greater tumor cell uptake versus normal cell uptake. This may reduce normal cardiotoxicity and myelosuppression. The drug is approved for use against Kaposi sarcoma but has been evaluated in a small group of patients with MF from Europe. Six patients in this pilot study received pegylated liposomal doxorubicin at 20 mg/m^2 every 4 weeks.[136] Four patients achieved a complete remission and one other patient achieved a partial remission. The overall response rate was 83%. The median duration of response was not reported. Grade III adverse events were few and included one patient with lymphopenia and two with anemia. No other severe adverse effects were noted. A larger retrospective multicenter report of this agent administered intravenously at 20 to 40 mg/m^2 every 2 to 3 weeks in 34 patients has also been conducted.[137] Overall, 15 patients achieved a complete remission and 15 achieved a partial remission (response rate of 88%), with event-free survival of 12 months. Toxicity was similarly manageable.

The ability to biopsy skin lesions for studies of tumor cells in MF/SS has resulted in this disease being a favored setting for the evaluation of candidate therapeutic agents and exploration of rational therapeutic development. The knowledge gained regarding the human genome and the new studies of proteonomics are increasingly allowing investigators to test new drugs at appropriate dosages, by correct schedule of administration, and to generate, prove, or refute hypotheses regarding mechanism of action or resistance. A number of studies of such agents have recently been completed and may lead to further drug testing in search of enhanced therapeutic activity in MF or perhaps achieve cure of MF.

An example of such an achievement has been the work with temozolomide for the treatment of MF/SS. This agent is an oral imidazotetrazine that has shown activity in solid tumors, such as brain tumors and melanoma. It has been determined that mechanisms of resistance to this agent include expression of high levels of the scavenger protein O^6-alkylguanine DNA alkyl transferase (AGT) in tumor cells. This protein is implicated in the recognition and repair of alkylator-induced DNA damage introduced by chloroethylnitrosourea (eg, *bis*-chloroethylnitrosourea or BCNU) or methylating agents (temozolomide).[138] The presence of the AGT protein imparts resistance by removing toxic lesions formed at the O^6 position of guanine. Chloroethylnitrosourea cross-links are prevented from forming by the removal of the chlorethyl lesion from the O^6 position before rearrangement or by the reaction with the intermediate, 1,O^6-ethanoguanine, to form a cross-link between DNA and the repair protein. The AGT protein is inactivated in the process.[139] Studies evaluating AGT levels in patients with brain tumors receiving BCNU therapy support the role of AGT in resistance to chlorethylating and methylating agents. Retrospective and prospective human studies have demonstrated a correlation between AGT concentration and clinical outcome after treatment with BCNU.[140]

Because of the unique sensitivity of MF to topical BCNU, we were interested in exploring levels of AGT in a variety of patients with various stages of MF/SS. Patients with patch or plaque lesions expressed low levels of the AGT protein compared with a number of controls with reactive dermatitis, and the level of AGT increased correlating with the stage of the patient (ie, patients with malignant lymphocytes harvested from peripheral blood or involved lymph nodes had higher levels of AGT than patch or plaque lesions).[141] Given this data, we initiated a prospective trial of temozolomide in relapsed patients with MF/SS, correlating response to levels of AGT and other known resistance proteins (such as the family DNA mismatch repair proteins).

We reported a preliminary evaluation of the trial.[142] Twenty-two patients had been treated with relapsed stage Ib–IVa disease. All patients had tumor sampled before treatment for assessment of the biologically important resistance proteins. At the time of the presentation, 5 of 19 evaluable patients had achieved a response (26% overall response rate). Preliminary analysis of the resistance proteins suggest that the optimal phenotype, which predicts for good response to therapy, would be low levels of AGT combined with normal levels of several DNA mismatch repair proteins. Interestingly, hypermethylation of these DNA repair proteins has been reported resulting in silencing of the genes, and correlating with lack of the proteins by immunohistochemical techniques in patients with MF.[143] This hypermethylation may be more prevalent in more advanced tumor lesions, and suggests that a propensity for mutations may precede clinical progression. It also suggests that patients might benefit from treatment with demethylating agent in combination with temozolomide. More patients continue to accrue to this trial, and further analysis of pretreatment tumor specimens is ongoing to provide more robust data for assessment of this agent in this disease.

STEM CELL TRANSPLANTATION

The natural evolution of the use of chemotherapy for this disease has been to use dose-intensified approaches with hematopoietic reconstruction with autologous[144] or allogeneic bone marrow.[145] There are few reports in the literature of such treatment programs. Of a total of nine patients (of whom we are aware) who received high-dose chemotherapy with or without total-body irradiation and autologous bone marrow transplants, only two had reasonable disease-free intervals (>12 months).

Given the propensity of Sézary cells to be detectable despite a lack of clinical evidence even in early-stage disease if sophisticated molecular techniques are used, it is likely that reinfusion of neoplastic cells may occur with autologous bone marrow transplantation. The lack of benefit in low-grade B-cell lymphomas for autologous bone marrow transplantation similarly suggests that this approach will not benefit patients. Allogeneic bone marrow transplantation has been presumably curative in small percentages of patients with low-grade B-cell lymphomas, and this approach should be investigated in the small subset of young patients with HLA identical siblings who have poor-prognosis disease and have demonstrated relapse or resistance to interferons and topical therapies. A single patient treated with cyclophosphamide and total-body irradiation was reported to achieve complete remission after allogeneic stem cell transplantation, but relapse occurred by day 70, necessitating additional therapy.[146] The patient remained in complete remission and alive at least 6 years after the transplantation. In light of this, we have begun to explore this approach in patients with MF/SS who are young and have matched donors available.[105] We have used marrow-derived stem cells enriched with peripheral blood-derived stem cells or peripheral blood stem cells only. In appropriate patients, this approach should continue to be explored, and older patients may benefit from strategies involving the use of so-called "mini-allogeneic" transplants that involve less myeloablative preparative regimens, and rely on the effects of the donor marrow to create a graft-versus-lymphoma effect for disease control. Recently, Molina and coworkers have reported promising data utilizing allogenic hematopoietic stem cell transplantation for patients with refractory Sézary syndrome and mycosis fungoides.[147] Each of the seven patients treated had failed a median of seven therapies. Although one patient received a myeloablative conditioning regimen, five received a reduced-intensity regimen consisting of fludarabine and melphalan. Each of the patients achieved a clinical remission and resolution of molecular and cytogenetic evidence of the disease. After a median follow-up of 56 months, six of the eight patients were alive and free of evidence of lymphoma. The two other patients died of transplant-related complications. This small study provides impetus to further development of allogeneic transplantation strategies for the treatment of advanced CTCL refractory to standard therapies. The breakthroughs in technology and basic understanding of the cell biology in patients with MF/SS suggest that chemotherapy will be a component of treatment for patients with this disease, joining the retinoids, cytokines, and targeted approaches.

PHOTOPHERESIS

An adaptation of the use of psoralen with UVA light called extracorporeal photopheresis (ECP) has been described by Edelson and associates.[148] Patients ingest 0.6 mg/kg of oral 8-methoxypsoralen before a treatment. The treatment consists of routine leukapheresis with isolation of the mononuclear cell fraction. The cells are then exposed to UVA light ex vivo within a special chamber inside the pheresis device. In the initial report, Edelson and colleagues documented an 88.5% loss of lymphocyte viability compared with control patients treated with drug alone. Overall, 64% of patients responded to therapy, with the best results in those with generalized erythroderma and, presumably, higher circulating Sézary cell levels. The mechanism is not thought to be directly cytotoxic, but rather to induce a host immune response to the reinfused altered Sézary cells possibly through activation of circulating dendritic cells.[149] This theory would explain the findings of some investigators that patients without leukemic involvement do poorly with this therapy. This treatment modality has given best results in SS patients with erythroderma of short duration and with adequate $CD8^+$ blood counts.

Several other groups have reported their experiences with photopheresis.[150,151] When the data are analyzed on an intent-to-treat basis, overall response rates of 36% to 52% are observed. Only 12% to 18% achieve complete remissions using this therapy. These investigators attempted to wean patients from therapy as clearing of lesions was documented. Ultimately, most responders developed recurrent disease. Many trials are underway combining ECP with other active modalities.

Toxicity is mild and includes occasional nausea, erythematous flares, and temperature elevations. Patients may develop hypotension during leukapheresis, which usually responds to saline infusions.

INTERFERONS

The most active agent for the treatment of MF is interferon-α.[152–156] Dosages and routes of administration have differed among studies. Initially, high-dose interferon was used, with maximum doses of 36 to 50 million IU. Bunn and colleagues[152,153] and Olsen and coworkers[153] independently demonstrated complete response rates of 10% to 27% in heavily pretreated patients. The duration of response was only 5.5 months. Later trials of untreated patients with doses of 3 to 18 million IU given subcutaneously daily have demonstrated response rates of 80% to 92%. From all these studies, it appears that a reasonable and tolerable single-agent dose is 12 million IU/m^2 administered subcutaneously daily. We recommend starting at 3 million IU and gradually increasing as treatment is tolerated by the patient.

In a single trial, the results of treatment of 16 refractory CTCL patients with interferon-γ were reported.[157] Five patients experienced partial responses (response rate 31%) with a median duration of 10 months (range, 3 to 32+ months).

Side effects of all interferons are dose-dependent. Most common adverse effects are constitutional symptoms consisting of fever, chills, myalgias, malaise, and anorexia. Rarely, cytopenias, elevations of liver function tests, renal dysfunction, cardiac dysfunction, or changes in mental status can be seen. Patients need to be monitored closely while on interferon.

RETINOIDS

Vitamin A and its natural and synthetic analogs are known as retinoids. These compounds have diverse biologic effects, influencing differentiation and proliferation of a number of structures during development.[158] Additionally, some compounds have been shown to influence immune function.[159,160] Clinically, a number of approved formulations have demonstrated efficacy in MF and SS.

Many of the trials of retinoids for MF/SS were performed decades ago with limited patient numbers. Treatment with isotretinoin (13-*cis*-retinoic acid), a nonaromatic retinoid, has been associated with clinical benefit in a number of trials. Overall objective responses have been described in 33 of 56 patients treated in three clinical trials.[161–163] A monoaromatic retinoid compound, etretinate, did not achieve similar results when tested as monotherapy for MF in several trials[164–170] but did show efficacy in a trial for the treatment of parapsoriasis en plaque.[166] A polyaromatic retinoid demonstrated efficacy in a small trial. Objective responses were observed in three of six patients (one complete and two partial responses).

There has been a resurgence of interest in retinoids for the treatment of hematologic malignancies with the approval of all-trans retinoic acid (ATRA) for acute promyelocytic leukemia. The mechanism of biologic effect for retinoids is better understood given the advances in basic sciences over the past decades. ATRA has been studied in 33 patients with relapsed MF who had not had prior exposure to oral retinoids.[167] Patients received 45 mg/m^2 daily in two divided doses for up to 2 years. In 29 evaluable patients, 5 responses were observed (1 complete, 4 partial) for an objective response rate of 17% with a median duration of response of 4.5 months. Another seven patients (24%) had stable disease. The most common toxicities included headache (37%) and mucous membrane dryness (80%). Only one patient experienced severe elevation of lipids. ATRA works through binding to specific retinoic acid receptors (RAR family α, β, and γ) that then bind to retinoic acid response elements located upstream of gene promoters, providing transcriptional control of proteins.

A second family of receptors, the retinoid X family of receptors (RXR), has been identified.[167,168] Bexarotene is a synthetic retinoid that selectively binds this family of receptors. Unfortunately, as is the case with the retinoids that bind the RAR family of receptors, it is not known ultimately which gene's expression is altered to provide the clinical benefits observed. This compound has been tested in separate trials of early- and advanced-stage patients. At the 300 mg/m^2 dosage daily (recommended dose by U.S. Food and Drug Administration), 54% of the 94 advanced-stage patients in an open-label phase II study responded to therapy (2% clinical complete response).[167] The median duration of response was 299 days. The early disease trial showed similar response rates. The toxicity spectrum is somewhat different from the RAR-specific retinoids, including more frequent severe elevations of lipids (although rarely associated with pancreatitis), hypothyroidism, and less frequent headaches and dry mucous membranes. The compound can also be used topically. A phase I/II trial of the topical bexarotene demonstrated a 63% response rate (clinical complete response 21%) in mostly early-stage patients with lesional application.[168] Toxicity was mostly local irritation with erythema.

The favorable toxicity profile has led to a number of combination modality trials using retinoids. Some of these small trials have combined retinoids with interferon-α and have reported response rates of 40% to 50%. Combinations of retinoids with PUVA have been suggested to result in clinical benefit in less time with less exposure to ultraviolet radiation. These experiences have been generally limited and often uncontrolled, making definitive conclusions impossible. Larger randomized trials would be needed to determine if routine use of such combinations should be undertaken off of an investigational trial except in rare cases.

FUSION PROTEIN-TARGETED THERAPIES

Targeted therapy has become a reality for the treatment of many types of cancer, including MF/SS. Although the most common approach has been with the use of antibodies that target antigens on the tumor cell surface (eg, rituximab), another class of compounds known as recombinant fusion proteins have been developed, the prototype being denileukin diftitox, for the treatment of CTCL.

Denileukin diftitox is a single-chain protein in which the receptor-binding domain of native diphtheria toxin is replaced by the sequences encoding the interleukin-2 (IL-2) gene.[169] Once this molecule binds to the high-affinity IL-2 receptor, the fusion toxin is internalized by receptor-mediated endocytosis and is proteolytically cleaved within endosomes to liberate the free adenosine diphosphate

(ADP)-ribosyl transferase activity of diphtheria toxin into the cytosol, where it then inhibits protein synthesis.[170,171]

In early phase I studies with denileukin diftitox, the response rate of CTCL patients who demonstrated at least 20% expression of the IL-2 receptor was 30%.[172] A phase III study comparing various dose levels of denileukin diftitox demonstrated a similar response rate, but there was significant toxicity that led to a high drop-out rate (constitutional symptoms, infusion reactions such as hypotension, chest pain or dyspnea, and a vascular leak syndrome).[173]

Because of the toxicity spectrum, we limit the use of this agent to patients who have failed several systemic agents previously, and have more threatening disease such as the presence of skin tumor lesions or nodal involvement. It is important to note that the pivotal trials did not allow concomitant use of corticosteroids to prevent nausea and infusion reactions. Subsequently, a retrospective case review of patients pretreated with corticosteroids suggested a more favorable toxicity profile, and a response rate of nearly 60%.[174] The nature of the trial limits the conclusions to be drawn, but suggests that aggressive pretreatment can make this drug a useful addition to patients with advanced relapsed mycosis fungoides.

INVESTIGATIONAL APPROACHES

Because of the chronic relapsing nature of MF, new therapies with different mechanisms of action are needed to circumvent tumor resistance. A variety of such approaches are under investigation. These include the use of existing or newly developed retinoid compounds or combinations of retinoids with other agents.[175] Other combination modalities under study include retinoids, interferons, and chemotherapy or radiation therapy[176] and total-skin electron beam radiotherapy followed by photopheresis or chemotherapy.[177] Given the lack of benefits of combination chemotherapy and radiotherapy previously, the role of such approaches should remain investigational. Another less toxic combination approach has been the simultaneous administration of interferon and phototherapy.[178] An overall response rate of 92% has been observed with this combination in all stages of patients, many of whom had been previously treated with other therapies.

Another approach to the therapy of this disease has involved new drugs to exploit the biology of these neoplastic cells. Targeted therapies against unique tumor antigens continue to be tested, such as the monoclonal antibody, Campath-1H. Knowledge of the unique cytokine milieu associated with these neoplastic T cells has led to trials testing cytokines that may inhibit the growth of these cells, such as IL-12[178] or IL-2.[179] Vaccine approaches may be practical. As molecular knowledge continues to expand regarding the biology of MF/SS, specific agents can be developed and tested. For example, data demonstrating that the activation of NF-κB in CTCL cell lines predisposes to resistance to apoptosis were cited above. Specific inhibitors of NF-κB or proteosome inhibitors that result in NF-κB inhibition may result in clinical benefits.[180]

Significant amounts of basic and practical research have been performed in an attempt to control this disease, and future treatment approaches will likely depend on further understanding of the molecular and genetic bases of these disorders. We hope that one of the strategies under development or study will lead to treatments that can control the disease and symptomatic effects or even cure this neoplasm.

SUGGESTED READINGS

Beljaards RC, Kaudewitz P, Berti E, et al: Primary cutaneous CD30-positive large cell lymphoma: Definition of a new type cutaneous lymphoma with a favorable prognosis. A European multicenter study on 47 cases. Cancer 71:2097, 1993.

Duvic M, Talpur R, Ni X, et al: Phase 2 trial of oral vorinostat (suberoylanilide hydroxamic acid, SAHA) for refractory cutaneous T-cell lymphoma (CTCL). Blood 109:31, 2007.

Duvic M, Talpur R, Wen S, Durzrock R, David CL, Apisarnthanarax N: Phase II evaluation of gemcitabine monotherapy for cutaneous T-cell lymphoma. Clin Lymphoma Myeloma 7:51, 2006.

Kuzel TM, Roenigk HH Jr, Samuelson E, et al: Effectiveness of interferon alfa-2a combined with phototherapy for mycosis fungoides and the Sézary syndrome. J Clin Oncol 13:257, 1995.

Molina A, Zain J, Arber DA, et al: Durable clinical, cytogenetic, and molecular remissions after allogeneic hematopoietic cell transplantation for refractory Sezary syndrome and mycosis fungoides. J Clin Oncol 23:6163, 2005.

Olsen E, Duvic M, Frankel A, et al: Pivotal phase III trial of two doses of DAB389IL2 (Ontak) for the treatment of cutaneous T-cell lymphoma. J Clin Oncol 19:376, 2001.

Rook AH, Gottlieb SL, Wolfe JT, et al: Pathogenesis of cutaneous T-cell lymphoma: Implications for the use of recombinant cytokines and photopheresis. Clin Exp Immunol 107(Suppl 1):16, 1997.

Siegel R, Pandolfino T, Guitart J, Rosen ST, Kuzel TM: Cutaneous T-cell lymphoma: Review and current concepts. J Clin Oncol 18:2908, 2000.

Van Doorn R, van Haselen CW, van voorst Vader PC, et al: Mycosis fungoides: Disease evolution and prognosis of 309 patients. Arch Dermatol 136:504, 2000.

Vowels BR, Cassin M, Vonderheid EC, Rook AH: Aberrant cytokine production by Sézary syndrome patients: Cytokine secretion pattern resembles murine TH2 cells. J Invest Dermatol 99:90, 1992.

Willemze R, Kerl H, Sterry W, et al: EORTC classification for primary cutaneous lymphomas: A proposal from the Cutaneous Lymphoma Study Group of the European Organization for Research and Treatment of Cancer. Blood 90:354, 1997.

Wood GS, Bahler DW, Hoppe RT, et al: Transformation of mycosis fungoides: T-cell receptor beta gene analysis demonstrates a common clonal origin for plaque-type mycosis fungoides and CD30+ large-cell lymphoma. J Invest Dermatol 101:296, 1993.

REFERENCES

For complete list of references log onto www.expertconsult.com

CHAPTER 86

AIDS-RELATED LYMPHOMAS

David T. Scadden

Non-Hodgkin lymphoma (NHL) is the most lethal complication of human immunodeficiency virus (HIV) infection. It was noted to be associated with HIV infection early in the epidemic and was added to the list of complications defining the acquired immunodeficiency syndrome (AIDS) in 1987.[1–9] The clinical landscape of HIV infection has changed since the introduction of highly active antiretroviral therapy (HAART) accompanied by modifications in both the understanding and treatment of AIDS-related lymphomas. This chapter covers current background information, evolving concepts in pathophysiology, treatment guidelines, and prospects for future development in AIDS-related lymphoma (ARL).

Lymphoid proliferation is common among many different types of immunodeficiencies. Congenital abnormalities of lymphocyte function, such as Wiskott-Aldrich syndrome, or immunosuppressive therapy employed in the setting of organ transplantation have long been known to predispose patients to developing often fatal lymphoproliferative disease. The incidence of NHL following organ transplant is related to the severity of the immunosuppressive regimen used and is more common in multiorgan transplants for that reason. Although the depth of immunosuppression enhances the likelihood of developing lymphoma, immune stimulation may also participate in the lymphomagenic process. This is supported by the association of lymphoma with autoimmune diseases considered reflective of excessive immune activation, such as sicca syndrome (Table 86–1).[10–19]

Despite a common association of immunodeficiency with lymphoma, HIV-1–induced immunosuppression and resultant lymphoma do have distinctive features. For example, the relatively high incidence of a polyclonal, prodromal phase in posttransplant patients appears to be relatively infrequent in ARL, although the issue remains controversial.[20] Epstein-Barr virus (EBV) is virtually uniformly present in the posttransplant lymphomas, whereas it is present only in approximately half of ARLs. Translocations of *c-MYC* are generally not seen in the posttransplant setting but are common in ARL. The small noncleaved cell- or Burkitt-like lymphoma seen in ARL is not an entity among the other immunodeficiency lymphomas. It is extremely rare in the posttransplant patient, strongly suggestive of unique pathophysiologic characteristics in the setting of AIDS.

The heterogeneity of lymphomas within the HIV-infected population emphasizes the complexity of tumor development. A range of different mechanisms have been evoked, including abnormal B-cell activation, excessive cytokine stimulation, altered microenvironment preferentially supporting lymphomatous cells, the predisposition to the persistence of specific chromosomal abnormalities, and perhaps most important, the inadequate immunologic control of persistent viral infections with transforming potential. Understanding how these factors can result in the manifestation of malignancy offers the potential for unraveling how immunologic function interfaces with immunologic malignancy with implications extending beyond that of the AIDS epidemic.

EPIDEMIOLOGY

An increased incidence of NHL was first noted among middle-aged unmarried men in the San Francisco area in 1984 and, with the first redefinition of the syndrome by the Centers for Disease Control and Prevention (CDC), became a criterion for defining an AIDS-related illness. This association has been reaffirmed in other epidemiologic series and includes individuals from virtually every risk group for HIV infection. Unlike the other major neoplastic complication of AIDS, Kaposi sarcoma (KS), NHL is fairly uniform across the spectrum of HIV-infected individuals.[21,22] There is a slight increase in incidence noted among hemophiliacs[21–23] that has provided an intriguing link and potential window on other contributing cofactors, but this remains simply a statistical observation at this time. Lower incidences of lymphoma among intravenous (IV) drug abusers in some series probably reflects the early death of such patients from other opportunistic diseases as well as issues related to their overall care, rather than a true biologic difference. Distinct risk appears to be biologically determined in genotypes of chemokines and their receptors. It has been noted that the presence of an inactivating mutation in the CCR5 chemokine receptor (CCR5 del32) can substantially reduce the risk of susceptibility to HIV infection and its complications. These are data indicating that heterozygosity for this gene may also affect risk for NHL in HIV disease.[24] This same study noted that polymorphisms in the noncoding region of the chemokine SDF1 (SDF103'A) was associated with an approximate increased risk for ARL of twofold for heterozygotes and fourfold for homozygotes. The variable frequency of this genotype in racial groups was thought to contribute to the higher incidence of ARL in whites in the United States.

The overall incidence of NHL in HIV-infected individuals has been variably estimated between 1.6% and 6% per year.[25–27] The discrepancy in estimates can be related to inclusion of postmortem diagnoses in the series with high estimates. The incidence of lymphoma increases with worsening immunosuppression and most often is seen in patients with long-standing HIV infection. However, lymphoma can be the presenting symptom of HIV, and consideration should be given to this possibility in patients with aggressive lymphomas. Concerns have been voiced that antiretroviral therapy can predispose to the development of lymphoma because of the potential effect of nucleoside analogs on cellular DNA synthesis. However, subsequent studies have failed to note any association and discount the notion that retroviral therapy should be withheld out of concern about induction of lymphoma.[28]

Projected increases in the incidence of NHL in AIDS as other opportunistic disease has been better controlled,[29] have not materialized. Indeed, it is now clear that the risk for lymphoma is reduced among patients treated with HAART for HIV. This effect is uneven across the types of lymphoma. For example, primary CNS lymphoma is an agonal manifestation of HIV disease and has dramatically dropped in incidence among those patients with access to antiretrovirals. A decline in incidence of systemic lymphomas is less dramatic but is estimated to be twofold to sevenfold decreased since the introduction of HAART.[30–33] In an observational cohort study of 8500 HIV-infected individuals in Europe, the reduction was apparent across all lymphoma subtypes.[34] In contrast, an international cohort study found that the decline was disproportionately great in immunoblastic and primary CNS lymphoma, the subtypes most often associated with EBV. Therefore, antiviral immunity is likely a host factor influencing the risk for ARL development, but the issue involves a more complex array of pathophysiologic processes (Fig. 86–1).

Table 86–1 Magnitude of Relative Risk of Lymphoma*

High (RR > 15)	Intermediate (RR > 2)	Low (RR ≤ 2)
Multiple transplants	Sibling transplant	Splenectomy
Cadaver transplant	Mild sicca syndrome	Sarcoidosis
Severe Sicca syndrome	Nontropical sprue	Hyperimmunization
Wiskott-Aldrich syndrome	Crohn disease	Asthma
Ataxia telangiectasia	Short-term HIV infection	Hansen disease
Long-term HIV infection	Rheumatoid arthritis	Cytotoxic drug prescription
		Systemic lupus erythematosus

HIV, human immunodeficiency virus; RR, relative risk.
*Risk of lymphoma in patients with the condition relative to a risk of 1.0 compared with individuals without the condition.
Data from Hoover RN: Lymphoma risks in populations with altered immunity: A search for mechanism. Cancer Res 52(19 Suppl):5477s, 1992.

Table 86–2 AIDS-Associated Tumors

Definite
Kaposi sarcoma
Non-Hodgkin lymphoma
Squamous cell neoplasia of uterine cervix, anus, conjunctiva
Probable
Hodgkin disease.
Leiomyosarcoma
Plasmacytoma

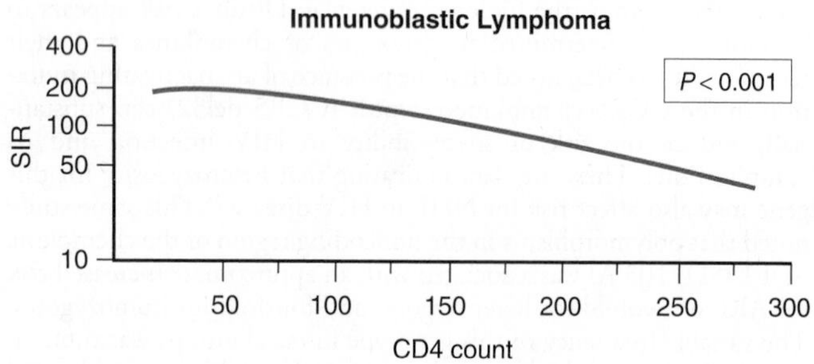

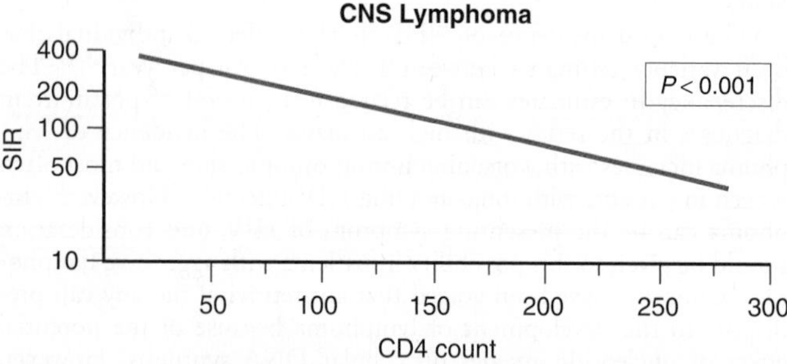

Figure 86–1 Risk of cancer in persons with acquired immunodeficiency syndrome (AIDS) by CD4 count (measured in units of cells/mm3) at AIDS onset for immunoblastic lymphoma and central nervous system lymphoma presented on a log-transformed scale as the (SIR). CNS, central nervous system. *(Data from Mbulaiteye SM, et al: Immune deficiency and risk for malignancy among persons with AIDS. J Acquir Immune Defic Syndr 32:527, 2003.)*

PATHOPHYSIOLOGY

The epidemiology of NHL is generally changing within the United States, with an increased incidence noted particularly among men. The bases for this change are poorly understood, but a contributing factor is the HIV epidemic and ARL. The epidemiology of ARL is influenced by HIV treatment and coincident associated viruses, such as EBV and the KS herpesvirus (KSHV), also known as human herpesvirus type 8 (HHV-8). There are likely other, yet undetected cofactors that account for some of the other subsets of this disease. In particular, the Burkitt or Burkitt-like lymphomas uniquely seen in AIDS and not in other immunodeficiency states represent a subset likely to yield novel insight into factors contributing to ARL.

HIV-1 itself rarely participates directly in the malignant process, but rather provides the background of immunodeficiency within which lymphomas might arise. However, rare tumors have been associated with a direct effect of HIV among the small minority of lymphomas seen in AIDS that are of T-cell origin. Molecular analysis of some of these cases has indicated that HIV was either integrated in the T cells or highly expressed in tumor-associated macrophages. The site of HIV integration into the host genome was evaluated and found to be in a common site upstream of the protooncogene, *c-fes*.[34] Aside from these relatively uncommon tumors, the transformed cells do not contain HIV-1 DNA. Rather, other mechanisms of lymphomagenesis predominate.

Potential contributing underlying abnormalities include most prominently:

1. Inadequate immunologic control of persistent viruses with transforming capability.
2. Alteration in the regulatory environment for lymphoid growth control.
3. Accumulation of genetic abnormalities in frequently activated B cells.

The issue of participating secondary infectious processes in ARL is generally supported by the spectrum of AIDS malignancies (Table 86–2). Tumors with definite or probable increased frequency in HIV disease are notable for the relatively small number of tumor types seen. Unlike tumors outside the setting of HIV disease, where a broad spectrum of epithelial neoplasms occur, the spectrum of malignancy is narrow. Unifying most of these diseases is an association with underlying infectious agents. The herpes virus KSHV is associated with both KS and a subset of NHL.[35] The squamous cell neoplasia of the uterine cervix in HIV-infected women, of the anus of homosexual men, and of the conjunctiva in individuals in Africa is associated with the human papillomavirus.[36–42] EBV is a well-known participant in a subset of lymphomas, as well as the leiomyosarcoma seen in children,[43] and in the Hodgkin lymphoma seen in the setting of HIV.[44] Therefore, viral pathogens are strongly related to the development of neoplastic complications. The specific mechanisms participating in transforming events are in the process of further evaluation. These offer the potential for novel types of therapeutic intervention, and the viral antigens associated with them offer possible immunotherapeutic targets.

The EBV genome has been reported to be present in 33% to 67% of ARLs, as opposed to 5% of high-grade lymphomas outside the setting of HIV.[45] The frequency varies depending on the cell type involved. The EBV genome is present in virtually all immunoblastic tumors of the CNS, whereas only 20% to 34% of the Burkitt-like tumors contain EBV.[46,47] Oral-cavity ARLs with T-cell markers[48] and plasmablastic lymphomas in the oral cavity[49] all appear to contain the EBV. Leiomyosarcomas occurring in children with HIV disease, but not in adults, also uniformly contain EBV within the tumor cells.[46]

EBV is thought to infect cells and induce their altered proliferation by expression of virus genes that are part of the latent (as opposed to lytic) virus phase. The pattern of EBV gene expression varies with the clinical and pathologic setting. In most patients with primary CNS lymphoma, the EBV latent gene expression pattern is identical to that of posttransplant lymphoproliferative disease, including Epstein-Barr nuclear antigen (EBNA)-2 through EBNA-5 and latent membrane protein (LMP)-1 and LMP-2.[50,51] In Burkitt lymphoma (BL), only EBNA-1 is usually detectable.[50,51–54] For some systemic ARLs, a unique combination of EBNA-1 and LMP-1 expression has been reported.[55] Molecular analysis of EBV latent genes has indicated that EBNA-1 is important for transformation because of its effects on transcription and maintenance of the EBV episome. LMP-1 is essential for primary B-cell transformation and for transforming effects on nonlymphoid cells.[56–58] LMP-1 interacts with the signaling pathway used by the tumor necrosis factor receptor family of genes through very specific molecular interactions at its carboxyl terminus.[56–59] Several mutations have been noted within the LMP-1 portion of the EBV genome, and some data have supported the possibility that these variants are associated with ARL or HIV-related Hodgkin lymphoma.[60–63] However, controversy on this continues, as some studies have indicated that LMP-1 mutations occur with similar frequency in patients with lymphoproliferative disease and in unaffected individuals.[61] The relationship of EBV to transformation is clear, but why certain individuals are more predisposed to develop lymphoma is still unknown. Molecular evolution of the virus within the host remains a tenable, but unproved, hypothesis.

An alternative possibility is that some individuals will selectively lose their immunologic reactivity to EBV or other transforming viruses. Many immunologically recognized antigens within the EBV genome have been characterized as being targets for cytotoxic T lymphocytes (CTLs).[64] These may be masked by direct effects of EBV EBNA-1 on antigen presentation through altered antigen-processing pathways[43,65,66] or through deletion of reactive CTL clones during the course of progressive immunodeficiency. Alteration of the T-cell receptor repertoire is a well-documented phenomenon in AIDS and may result in nonhomogeneous losses of reactivity to specific foreign or tumor antigens.[67] This phenomenon suggests the potential for clonal repletion as a strategy for intervention and, indeed, such an approach has been successfully demonstrated in posttransplant patients with EBV lymphoproliferation.[68–70] Adoptive transfer of T cells is complicated outside the transplant setting, however, and, therefore, reconstituting EBV immunity in HIV disease is currently left to the gradual immune regeneration following HAART. Whether this can have a therapeutic effect for EBV-related ARL is unclear, but the documentation of long-term survivors of primary CNS lymphoma in AIDS following radiation and HAART is suggestive.

The vigor of immunologic response may also be affected by oncovirus gene products. In particular, an EBV gene (BCRF-1) has homology with human interleukin 10 (IL-10) and mimics IL-10 function.[71–73] IL-10 has been noted to inhibit interferon gamma and interleukin 2 (IL-2) elaboration by T-helper cell type 1 (Th1), cells important in activating and sustaining an immunologic response.[72] Cell lines and primary tumors isolated from patients with AIDS lymphoma produce a high level of IL-10, and elevated circulating levels of IL-10 in mouse models of AIDS lymphoma have been well documented.[71,73–76] Other cytokine-related effects include the production of CD40 (a B-cell proliferation signal) by HIV-infected bone marrow endothelial cells[77] and interleukin 6 (IL-6) production by HIV-infected macrophages or by KSHV-infected cells.[78,79] Increased IL-6 levels have been noted to correlate with malignancy and increased serum CD23 (a marker of activation) to precede it.[80,81] Dysregulation of cytokines further induces alterations in B-cell biology contributing to a hyperproliferative state.

Another viral pathogen that contributes to ARL is the most recently described member of the γ-herpesvirus family, KSHV. This virus was originally identified by comparative analysis of the DNA content from KS tissue versus uninvolved tissue.[82] This genetic approach to pathogen identification revealed a virus that has now been shown convincingly to be associated with KS, but also with a subset of ARLs, Castleman disease, and perhaps plasma cell dyscrasias.[33,35,83,84] The lymphomas are generally restricted to body cavities without tumor masses and are called primary effusion lymphomas (PELs). Features of this clinicopathologic entity are discussed further in a separate section, but features of this virus are extremely interesting from the pathophysiologic perspective.

KSHV is known to be capable of infecting primary B cells[85] and is uniformly found in the transformed B cells of PELs. Mechanisms by which this virus participates in the malignant process remain speculative because in-vitro infection with KSHV does not result in B-cell transformation. However, a number of components of the KSHV genome suggest the potential for this virus to alter B-cell physiology. These include a constitutively active chemokine receptor that causes cell lines to have enhanced malignant potential when transfected, a physiologically active cyclin-D homologue, a viral IL-6 with potent biologic activity, a B cell lymphoma (BCL)-2 homologue, and CC chemokine homologues.[79,84,85–90] This constellation of different immunoregulatory proteins is highly suggestive of direct mechanisms by which the virus can perturb cell functions, but the details have not yet been clarified. Activation of STAT3 has been noted in KSHV primary effusion cells, but its relationship to KSHV is not known.[91] However, interruption of STAT3 signaling efficiently induces PEL apoptosis mediated by reduced expression of the antiapoptotic gene, survivin. Therefore, targeting this pathway may have therapeutic significance for controlling KSHV-related lymphoma. Another approach would be through immunologic response to KSHV. The nature of the response is not well understood because in-vivo reactivity appears to be at very low levels even in immunocompetent individuals. Although T-cell targets of KSHV have been defined,[92,93] the virus also encodes proteins capable of hiding infected cells from either CTL or natural killer cell attack.[93–96] The strong association of KS with immunodeficiency and the response of this tumor to immune regeneration indicates the role of immune control, but the specific details of this response, whether it can be enhanced with vaccine, and whether it participates in control of lymphoma outgrowth, remain undefined.

Many ARLs do not evidence either EBV or KSHV infection. Although it has been hypothesized that these may represent cells transformed by still-unknown infectious agents, a number of potential etiologies remain. These include the proliferative drive provided by EBV- or HIV-induced cytokine alterations as noted previously. In addition, a gross dysregulation of B-cell biology is evident early on in HIV disease, regardless of the subsequent development of lymphoma.[97] This includes the presence of hypergammaglobulinemia, which is perhaps the most common serologic abnormality among HIV-infected individuals.[98,99] As patients progress in HIV disease, lymphadenopathy with follicular hyperplasia is common and is similarly reflective of disordered regulation of the B-cell lineage.[100,101] It has been postulated that a portion of the HIV envelope may be capable of inducing T-cell–mediated B-cell activation.[102,103] This may result in particular outgrowth of HIV-specific B cells. With chronic stimulation, transformation can occur, and sporadic multiple myeloma with HIV specificity has been reported.[104–106] Characterization of the variable chain repertoire of immunoglobulins produced by B cells in patients with HIV disease has indicated that preferential use of the variable heavy chain (VH) subsets occurs early in HIV infection[107] and in ARL tumors.[108] These findings suggest that there may be an antigen-driven expansion of selected B-cell clones that can provide the mitogenetic background for mutagenesis to result in malignancy.

Many specific genetic mutations have been observed in ARL and are associated with specific tumor types.[109–111] That is, tumors of small cell, Burkitt, or Burkitt-like histology uniformly exhibit *c-MYC* gene rearrangements, have *p53* gene mutations in approximately 50% of tumors, and do not exhibit *BCL6* rearrangements.[112–116] This is in contrast with large cell lymphomas, among which approximately one-third demonstrates *BCL6* rearrangement, 40% *c-MYC,* and 25% to 40% of *p53* mutations.[116,117] The *c-MYC* rearrangement that is found most often juxtaposes *c-MYC* with the immunoglobulin heavy

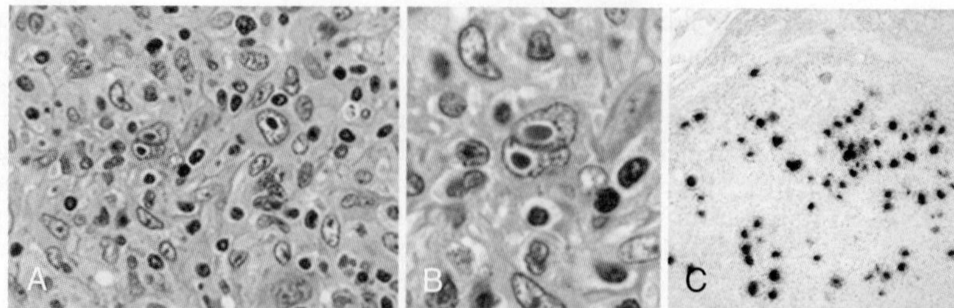

Figure 86–2 AIDS-Related Hodgkin Lymphoma. Hodgkin lymphoma (**A, B, C**): Hodgkin lymphoma of the mixed cellularity type in an HIV-positive patient (**A**) These cases commonly have some depletion of lymphocytes in the background, and increased numbers Hodgkin and Reed-Sternberg cells (**B**). Epstein Barr Virus mRNA (EBER) can usually be detected by in-situ hybridization (**C**).

chain switch region.[114,118–121] The involvement of this region suggests that the transforming event has occurred in a B cell that is undergoing transition between heavy chain isotopes: phenomena occurring at a relatively late stage in B-cell ontogeny.[22,102,103,112,113,115,122–124] The malignant cell, therefore, appears to be a relatively mature B lymphocyte. In ARL, *c-MYC* rearrangement and EBV infection are not necessarily present in association with one another.[112–115] Similarly, *BCL6* rearrangements are variably associated with the presence of EBV. It is of interest that no coincident *c-MYC* and *BCL6* rearrangements have been detected.[125] A characteristic of B cells is the ongoing mutation of the immunoglobulin locus to potentially enhance immunoglobulin affinity for antigens. This process, called *somatic hypermutation*, can target genes besides the immunoglobulin genes such as *BCL6*. Not usually seen, however, and what has now been identified in ARL is mutation in the *PIM-1* or *c-MYC* loci, genes associated with lymphoma. Somatic hypermutation may, therefore, play a role in lymphomagenesis in AIDS. Molecular abnormalities associated with low-grade lymphomas (such as the 11 : 14 rearrangement) are generally not seen in ARL.

CLINICAL MANIFESTATIONS

ARLs are generally extremely aggressive, high-grade lymphomas of B-cell origin. However, the spectrum of lymphoproliferative disease is broad and is continuing to expand. T-cell malignancies have been reported, including large granular lymphocyte disease, large-cell or anaplastic T-cell lymphoma, Sézary syndrome, and angiocentric T-cell proliferation.[106,126–133] Virus infection with human T-cell leukemia-lymphoma virus (HTLV)-1 has been noted in some cases of T-cell malignancy with coincident HIV infection.[134] In addition, HIV itself has been noted to be integrated in some of these lymphomas,[34,133] as previously discussed. Oropharyngeal T-cell lymphoma has been described in AIDS patients and is associated with the presence of EBV in the tumor cells.[48]

Castleman disease or angiofollicular lymph node hyperplasia has been reported in patients with advanced HIV disease.[35] This is typically a multicentric variant of Castleman disease that is associated with fever, peripheral adenopathy, weight loss, hepatosplenomegaly, pulmonary symptoms, and anemia or pancytopenia. Both the hyalin-vascular and plasma-cell subtypes of multicentric Castleman disease have been reported in AIDS patients. There is a very high association of this process with the presence of KSHV in the involved nodes and a high prevalence of coincident or subsequent KS.[35,84,135,136] This lymphoproliferative process is often aggressive with poor outcome, although responses to chemotherapy have been reported.[35] Anti-CD20 antibody therapy may be active in the treatment of Castleman disease, and initiation of HAART can influence the outcome.[125,137]

Plasma cell disorders appear to be increased in the setting of HIV infection. Plasmablastic lymphomas of the oral cavity have been described[138] as a relatively uncommon neoplasm, notable for the frequent absence of typical lymphoid markers such as CD45 (leukocyte common antigen) or CD20. Extramedullary plasmacytomas have been reported, as well as overt multiple myeloma.[139,140] The clinical course of these disorders is highly variable, and the clinical approach should be based on standard guidelines for these diseases outside the context of HIV infection.

Hodgkin Lymphoma

The incidence of Hodgkin lymphoma in patients with HIV infection has been variably reported, but an excess above the general age-matched population is evident and estimated to be 2.5- to 8.5-fold in magnitude.[141–143] The clinical presentation in the setting of HIV infection is often distinct in that the clinical stage is more advanced and the mixed cellularity subtype more common.[5,128,144–151] Stage III to IV disease at presentation has been noted in more than 80% of HIV-seropositive patients.[146] Extranodal disease is also more common in HIV-seropositive patients, with one series reporting a frequency of 63% compared with 29% in seronegative patients.[150] In addition, histopathologic features of Hodgkin lymphoma in AIDS are different both in the frequency of mixed cellularity and the presence of EBV (Fig. 86–2). Virtually all tumors have detectable EBV and express LMP-1.[152] A high frequency of LMP-1 molecular abnormalities has also been noted in patients with AIDS compared with patients with Hodgkin lymphoma who do not have AIDS.[152]

The clinical approach to patients with Hodgkin lymphoma in the setting of HIV infection is similar to that in other contexts with standard staging methods. Treatment strategies should be applied as appropriate for stage, similar to guidelines outside the setting of HIV infection. However, the underlying level of immunosuppression and overall performance status of the patient must be considered. A higher incidence of treatment complications can be expected if the patient has very advanced AIDS, and appropriate prophylaxis for *Pneumocystis carinii* should be undertaken. However, cure of Hodgkin lymphoma has been well demonstrated in the setting of HIV infection, and dose attenuation should be contemplated only in those patients with advanced AIDS or those who have demonstrated intolerance to the standard dose regimens.

Non-Hodgkin Lymphoma

Most lymphomas that occur in the context of HIV are of B-cell origin and are typically aggressive, high-grade malignancies (Fig. 86–3). The lymphomas can basically be broken down into two major subcategories: primary CNS lymphoma and systemic lymphoma that may or may not include CNS involvement. In the systemic disease category, a subset of patients have the primary effusion lymphoma (PEL) mentioned previously (Table 86–3) or the plasmablastic lymphoma of the oral cavity. Both these latter tumors are uncommon outside the setting of HIV disease.

These primary effusion lymphomas or body-cavity lymphomas are generally present in body fluids without associated tumor masses.[33,153] They have a common immunophenotype in that markers of B or T cells are generally absent from the cell surface, but evidence for

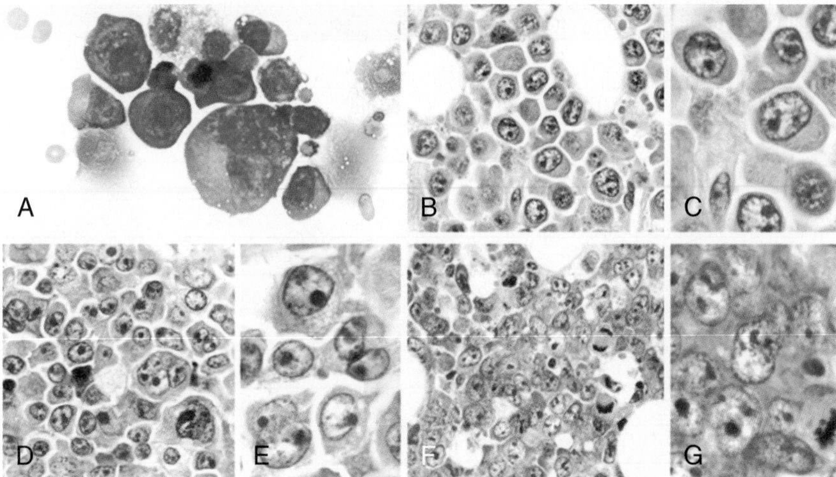

Figure 86–3 AIDS-Related Non-Hodgkin Lymphoma. Pleural effusion lymphoma (**A**), primary effusion lymphoma (PEL), or body cavity lymphomas are diagnosed by examination of the fluid on cytospin preparations and by flow cytometric and genetic studies. On the cytospin preparation the cells are large and frequently include multinucleated forms. Flow cytometric studies can be difficult to interpret as the cells lack B markers and surface immunoglobulin, but clonality can be detected by immunoglobulin gene rearrangement analysis. Plasmablastic lymphoma (**B, C**): Plasmablastic lymphomas occur in the oral cavity but can present elsewhere. They are comprised of large plasmablastic cells with eccentric nuclei and amphophilic cytoplasm. These are usually CD45- and CD20-negative but express CD138 and MUM1. Large B-cell lymphoma (**D, E**): These lymphomas resemble large B-cell lymphoma in the non-AIDS setting. Frequently they have an activated B-cell phenotype. Burkitt lymphoma (**F, G**): In AIDS patients Burkitt lymphoma sometimes has atypical morphology with plasmacytic features or more irregular nuclei than usually seen (**G**). These cases are considered variant Burkitt lymphoma. The case depicted had the typical t(8;14) associated with *c-MYC* rearrangement.

Table 86–3 Primary Effusion Lymphoma (Body-Cavity Lymphoma)
Positive fluid cytology without mass
Distinct phenotype: null cell immunophenotype with rearranged immunoglobulin genes
Human herpes virus-8–positive

immunoglobulin gene rearrangement by analysis of tumor DNA indicates that they are of B-cell origin. Gene-profile analysis has indicated that these tumors are not of germinal center or mature B-cell origin, but rather resemble immunoblasts and plasma cells and have, therefore, been considered of "plasmablast" origin.[143,154] These tumors are uniformly associated with the presence of the KSHV genome in the tumor cells. Although many also contain EBV, this finding is less uniform.[109,110] Seroepidemiologic data regarding this virus are still limited, but it is clear that the virus can be found in abundance in saliva.[154,155] Transmission is associated with sexual activity, but nonsexual transmission to young children in endemic areas is also common.[155,156]

The virus is found in subsets of the North American population with estimates ranging from 5% to 20%.[157,158] Other areas associated with the higher frequency of KS, such as the Mediterranean basin and Central Africa, have been noted to have far higher frequencies of seropositivity for KSHV.[157] Patients with PEL often have advanced immunosuppression and present with rapidly evolving pleural or pericardial effusions or ascites. The bowel can be involved,[159] and some patients will show dissemination to bone marrow and blood. This tumor generally behaves very aggressively, and the outlook with current approaches is unfavorable.

The most common histologic types of NHLs in AIDS are those also seen outside the setting of HIV disease. Among these, diffuse large B-cell lymphoma is the most common, followed by Burkitt or Burkitt-like lymphoma. Mucosa-associated lymphoid tissue lymphomas have been reported but are rare. Low-grade B-cell malignancies are a distinct minority among HIV-infected patients. Such tumors can occur but with a frequency approximately comparable with the background for the population.

Like high-grade malignancies outside the setting of HIV disease, ARL often involves sites outside the confines of the lymphatic system (Table 86–4). Extranodal disease has been estimated to occur in up to 95% of patients with ARL, with extranodal tissue frequently the source of diagnosis.[3,5,7,113,160–173] Disease that is exclusively outside the lymphatic system has been reported in up to 56% of patients.[173]

The frequency of extranodal disease emphasizes the necessity of exercising particular vigilance in evaluating these patients. Unusual symptoms must be assessed with attention to possible direct tumor involvement as the cause. ARL can also mask or be confused with other opportunistic disease. In particular, the constitutional symptoms accompanying either infection or lymphoma should be assessed for both. In addition, lymphadenopathy occurs frequently in the course of HIV infection and is often simply evidence of hyperproliferation without transformation. A high index of suspicion must be maintained, particularly for those patients who have coincident B symptoms or who have rapidly progressive asymmetric lymphadenopathy.

Sites of extratumor involvement are favored by particular histologic subtypes. For example, the small, noncleaved cell histology often favors bone marrow or meninges. In contrast, immunoblastic histology often favors the gastrointestinal (GI) tract and brain parenchyma. The most common extranodal sites of involvement are the bone marrow in approximately 25% of patients, CNS in 23%, GI tract in 15%, and liver in 13%.[4,5,7,8,113–115,160–162,164–174]

Although approximately 15% to 25% of patients will present with stage I or II disease (see Table 86–4), the sites of involvement are often extranodal. If local therapies are undertaken, it is highly likely that patients will relapse at remote sites, and, therefore, systemic therapy is generally favored, regardless of the stage at presentation.

DIAGNOSIS AND PROGNOSIS

Staging of patients with systemic ARL includes tests performed in other lymphoma populations, such as computed tomography (CT) scans of the chest, abdomen, and pelvis; bone marrow biopsy; and, if bulky mediastinal or abdominal disease is present, positron emission tomography (PET), or gallium-67 scanning. In addition, the frequency of involvement of the CNS supports the use of both

Table 86–4 Histology, Extranodal Sites, and Stage of Lymphoma in AIDS

	Histology				Extranodal Sites				Stage	
	Pts.	SNCC	IBS/ALC	LC	Gastro	Liver	CNS	Marrow	I, II	III, IV
Levine et al.[2]	27	10	13	—	6	1	8	5	7	20
Katler et al.[3]	14	7	1	5	2	2	8	4	1	13
Gill et al.[164]	22	16	6	—	5	5	3	7	1	21
Knowles et al.[165]	89	36	25	25	14	14	19	19	27	57
Ziegler et al.[7]	90	32	24	17	8	8	38	30	38	52
Bermudez et al.[166]	31	8	6	10	6	6	8	10	1	30
Lowenthal et al.[160]	43	16	8	16	11	6	11	13	9	26
Kaplan et al.[167]	84	29	36	17	7	22	10	26	14	69
Kaplan et al.[169]	30	7	16	3	?	?	?	7	12	14
Levine et al.[162]	42	17	14	4	5	11	6	6	11	24
Remick et al.[170]	18	0	7	10	5	?	?	?	5	13
Raphael et al.[173]	113	41	33	35	18	3	22	17	—	—
Kaplan et al.[176]	198	35	17	85	48	51	3	30	61	129
Sparano et al.[191]	50	22	16	12	10	20	4	16	—	—
TOTAL	851	276	222	239	145	149	140	190	187	468

AIDS, acquired immunodeficiency syndrome; ALC, anaplastic large cell; CNS, central nervous system; Gastro, gastrointestinal; IBS, immunoblastic; LC, large cell; Pts., points; SNCC, small non-cleaved cell

radiographic imaging and cerebrospinal fluid (CSF) sampling at the time of initial staging.[162]

Patients who present with constitutional or B symptoms and a low CD4 count should have a thorough microbiologic workup to address the possibility of coincident opportunistic infections. This should include isolator cultures of the blood for mycobacteria, serologic assays for cryptococcal antigen, cytomegalovirus antigen, toxoplasmosis antibody, induced sputum for *P. carinii*, and routine blood culture.

The prognostic indicator that has been most predictive in patients not on HAART with ARL is the stage of immunodeficiency as reflected by the CD4 count at the time of diagnosis. CD4 cells of less than 100 cells/cm^3 are associated with a shorter survival in several series. In addition, previous AIDS-defining diagnoses, the Karnofsky performance score, and the presence of extranodal disease have been regarded as indicators of outcome.[150,167,175–177] More recent studies evaluating patients after the introduction of HAART have indicated that the parameters of HIV infection and immunodeficiency have largely been supplanted by features common to lymphomas outside the setting of HIV disease. The International Prognostic Index (IPI) score has been shown to be highly predictive of risk in ARL, although CD4 count has not always been found to be relevant.[178,179] There are several molecular features of large cell lymphomas that have been associated with prognosis, including the overexpression of BCL2[116] and markers of a post-germinal center cell of origin; both of these are unfavorable when present. Post-germinal center markers predicting poorer outcome include MUM1/IRF4 and/or CD138/Syn-1 and the absence of CD10 or BCL-6.[180] The analysis of ARL since the advent of HAART has indicated that the molecular features of this disease are changing and that tumors in the post-HAART era bear the more favorable indications of a germinal center tumor (the expression of CD10 or *BCL6* rearrangement) and do not overexpress BCL2. Thus, the frequency of ARL is diminished with the use of HAART, and the virility of the tumor may be lessened; however, overexpression of *p53* (generally a poor prognostic indicator) is not decreased in frequency.

Other molecular features that have been associated with outcome include polyclonality, which in one study was associated with a more positive outcome.[175] This feature was particularly favorable if tumors were EBV negative and the CD4 counts more than 200 cells/cm^3. Of note, histology has generally not been predictive.[180,181] The presence of the Burkitt or Burkitt-like subtype generally thought to bode poorly outside HIV disease has generally not been a feature affecting outcome. Whether this will change in the era when patients are overall doing better with HAART is still to be determined.

The presence of PEL has generally been associated with a very poor outcome; however, the compiled number of cases with this syndrome remains relatively limited.[153]

TREATMENT

Treatment of patients with ARL should include several components that distinguish this patient population from others. These include the use of prophylaxis for *P. carinii* pneumonia at initiation of chemotherapy. This practice is generally applied because of the high potential risk during treatment-induced exacerbation of immunosuppression. The high incidence of CNS involvement in a series reported early in the epidemic[164] has led to a controversy as to whether or not CNS prophylaxis should be provided for all patients. There are no definitive data on this point, but with use of CNS prophylaxis, the previously observed frequency of CSF relapse has been diminished.[182] No clinical standard can be said to have been defined, although many centers including our own administer either cytosine arabinoside (ara-C) or methotrexate weekly for 4 weeks by intrathecal injection to at least those patients with Burkitt histology, bone marrow involvement, testis involvement, or perinasal sinus disease. In addition, EBV present in the primary tumor has been identified as a risk factor for CNS involvement and can be useful in factoring the relative risk for individual patients.[181,183]

A concern regarding myelotoxicity has led many investigators to use growth factors prophylactically. Bone marrow dysfunction is a common feature of advanced HIV disease, and those patients who present with cytopenias at diagnosis are reasonable candidates for prophylactic growth factor use. A small, randomized, prospective trial in patients receiving a cyclophosphamide, hydroxydaunomycin, vincristine (Oncovin), and prednisone (CHOP) regimen indicated that patients who received granulocyte-macrophage colony-stimulating factor (GM-CSF) had statistically significantly reduced instances of fever and neutropenia and fewer days of hospitalization than patients who received chemotherapy without growth factor support.[169]

The use of antiretroviral therapy in conjunction with chemotherapy remains controversial. Earlier in the epidemic when zidovudine (AZT) was essentially the only retroviral agent available, the myelotoxic effects of this medication generally precluded its use. Most reports of treatment in patients with ARL are patients who have not received concurrent antiretroviral therapy. A study by Levine and colleagues[177,184] assessed whether or not antiretroviral dideoxycytidine (DDC) could be given concurrently with modified methotrexate, bleomycin, doxorubicin (Adriamycin), cyclophosphamide, vincristine (Oncovin), dexamethasone (m-BACOD) chemotherapy and did not note any enhanced toxicity. In particular, neurotoxicity was not worsened, and a favorable effect on HIV p24 antigen levels was noted. Other studies have taken one of two approaches: Either dictate the antiretroviral regimen and study the pharmacokinetics, or preclude antiretrovirals and measure the immunologic and virologic consequences. Both approaches are supported by study data. A study by the AIDS Malignancy Consortium documented that CHOP could be given in conjunction with stavudine, lamivudine, and indinavir with no unexpected or unusually severe toxicities.[183,185] The pharmacokinetic data indicated an approximate doubling of the cyclophosphamide clearance time, but this was without clinical correlate and levels of doxorubicin, and indinavir metabolites were unaffected. The U.S. National Cancer Institute took the alternative approach, stopping all antiretroviral drugs or not starting them for those with newly diagnosed HIV. With the use of a continuous infusion regiment, dose-modified etoposide, prednisone, vincristine (Oncovin), cyclophosphamide, fluoxymesterone (Halotestin) (EPOCH), these authors noted reductions in CD4 not unlike what others have seen when chemotherapy was given and antivirals continued. HIV plasma levels did increase in those stopping anti-HIV medications, but both the CD4 and HIV RNA levels improved to at least baseline once the antiretrovirals were resumed after antitumor therapy was completed.[116] This approach can, therefore, be reasonable for patients willing to accept it. For many, the concept of withholding medications they view as lifesaving is simply a nonstarter. In such cases, very few drug-drug interactions have been reported. It should be noted that the P450 effects of the non-nucleoside reverse transcriptase inhibitors can be particularly potent. Drug-drug combinations must always be vigilantly assessed when combining antiretroviral and antitumor chemotherapies. Because HIV levels are generally a risk in the context of chronicity, it should also be noted that antitumor chemotherapy against these imminently life-threatening lymphomas should not be compromised to accommodate antiretroviral therapy. If antiretrovirals are to be given, they should be used at doses that maximally suppress the virus, because submaximal suppression may permit the emergence of resistant strains of the virus.

Selecting treatment for lymphoma is largely dictated by the patient's overall clinical status. Until the availability of HAART, a fair amount of skepticism existed as to whether a curative approach should be undertaken in ARL patients because they all had what was considered a uniformly fatal underlying disease-AIDS. However, with the optimism surrounding the developments in anti-HIV therapy, it is now clear that a curative approach should be undertaken except under usual circumstances. For those patients who have far-advanced AIDS, are refractory to antiretroviral therapy, and have poor performance status, a palliative approach might be appropriate. No specific guidelines in this situation can be provided except that careful consideration should be given to patients' history of antiretroviral therapy, their history of HIV-related complications, their current CD4 count, their HIV RNA levels, and, most important, their wishes regarding the level of aggressiveness of care.

Full-dose chemotherapy of regimens established in the non-HIV setting is now standard. CHOP is a mainstay and the generally standard approach. The responses to this regimen are comparable to those seen outside the context of the HIV epidemic. Efforts to improve on standard CHOP include studies of adding rituximab (a humanized anti-CD20 antibody) to CHOP similar to that found useful in the context of large-cell lymphoma outside the context of HIV. A randomized trial comparing this regimen with CHOP alone demonstrated that there was not an overall benefit of adding rituximab (Rituxan) in either complete response rate, progression-free survival or overall survival. Instead, an increased incidence of fatal infections was noted, particularly among those with fewer than 50 $CD4^+$ cells/mm^3.[186] Increased infections were seen in another report of patients receiving rituximab (Rituxan) with an infusional regimen,[187] although a phase II trial of CHOP-rituximab (Rituxan)saw no significant infections, yet strikingly good remission and overall 2-year survival outcomes (77% and 75% respectively).[188] Therefore, it remains ambiguous as to whether rituximab (Rituxan) adds benefit in this patient group. If CHOP-rituximab (Rituxan)is contemplated, additional antimicrobial prophylaxis should be considered.

An alternative to CHOP has been proposed by Little and colleagues[116] at the U.S. National Cancer Institute using a dose-modified continuous infusion regimen, dose-adjusted EPOCH. This approach has resulted in remarkably high levels of response (complete remission in 74%) and durability of response (Fig. 82–4). At 53 months, the disease-free survival was 92%, and overall survival, 60%. The activity of this regimen may in part be caused by the high proliferative nature of ARL. The tolerability of the regimen has been good, and it is now being tested in larger consortia to evaluate whether it should become the new standard of care. This regimen involves continuous infusions of etoposide (50 mg/m^2/day for 96 hours), doxorubicin

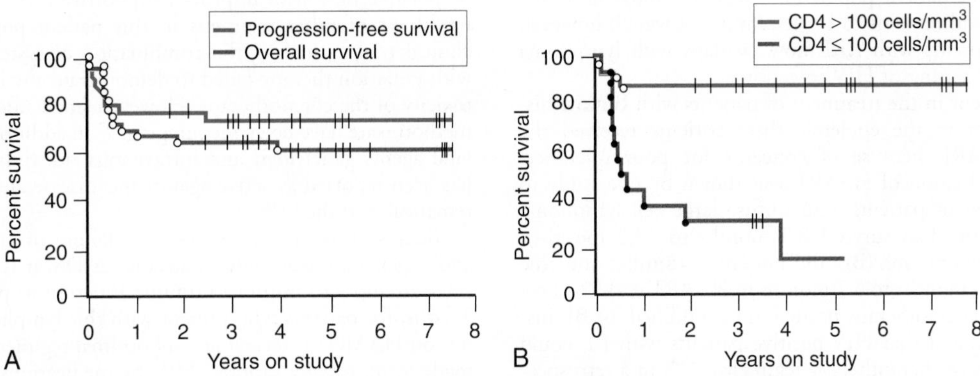

Figure 86–4 Kaplan-Meier survival curves of acquired immunodeficiency syndrome (AIDS)-related lymphoma patients treated with dose-adjusted etoposide, prednisone, vincristine (Oncovin), cyclophosphamide, fluoxymesterone (Halotestin) (EPOCH). (Data from Little RF, et al: Highly effective treatment of acquired immunodeficiency syndrome-related lymphoma with dose-adjusted EPOCH: Impact of antiretroviral therapy suspension and tumor biology. Blood 101:4653, 2003.)

(10 mg/m²/day for 96 hours) vincristine (0.4 mg/m²/day for 96 hours), bolus infusion of dose adjusted cyclophosphamide on day 5 (375 mg/m² if CD4 > 100 cells/mm³; 187 mg/m² if CD4 < 100 cells/mm³ on the first cycle; thereafter, increase by 187 mg/m² if nadir absolute neutrophil count [ANC] > 500 cells/mm³ or decrease by 187 mg/m² if ANC < 500 cells/mm³ or platelets <25,000 cells/mm³). Prednisone is given at 60 mg/m² daily days 1 through 5, and filgrastim is given at 5 μg/kg/day, beginning day 6, until the ANC exceeds 5000 cells/mm³. The cycle is repeated every 21 days or when the ANC exceeds 1000 cells/mm³ and platelets exceed 50,000 cells/mm³.

Efforts in Europe have similarly focused on alternative approaches such as cyclophosphamide, doxorubicin, vincristine and prednisone (CHOP) plus rituximab (Rituxan), and chemotherapy-intensive regimens have been assessed. In a 140-patient study conducted by a French-Italian Cooperative Group using the LNH84 regimen, 65% of patients achieved a complete remission with a relatively low relapse rate of 24%.[186] In a followup study, patients who had CD4 counts of >100 cells/mm³, no prior AIDS-defining illnesses, and good performance status were enrolled. The patients were randomized to receive either CHOP chemotherapy, or ACVB (doxorubicin [Adriamycin] 75 mg/m² day 1, cyclophosphamide 1.2 g/m² day 1, vindesine 2 mg/m² day 1, bleomycin 10 mg days 1 through 5, prednisolone 60 mg days 1 through 5) with granulocyte colony-stimulating factor (GCSF) support. More severe toxicity in the ACVB arm, but a higher response rate, has been reported.[187] Further analysis of these data is required before firm conclusions can be drawn. However, the potential for dose-intensive regimens for patients in this population with good prognostic factors is suggested and should be further explored.

Other continuous infusion regimens have been assessed for patients as first-line therapy. The CDE regimen (cyclophosphamide 800 mg/m², doxorubicin 50 mg/m², etoposide 240 mg/m², all over 4 days) to which dideoxyinosine (ddI) was added, resulted in a complete response rate of 58%, with a median response duration exceeding 18 months.[188] Although controversy remains regarding the optimal strategy for treating patients who present with AIDS-related lymphoma, each of the trials indicates the potential for durable response. These data emphasize the need to approach patients with otherwise good prognostic features in a manner focused to maximize cure. However, the fraction of patients failing to respond continues to remain high and the frequency of relapse significant. Because the use of HAART has resulted in more patients tolerating anticancer chemotherapy, autologous transplant protocols have been initiated. Several studies have indicated that this approach is tolerated, results in rapid engraftment, and can result in long-term tumor control.[189–191] Multicenter trials to test this approach also indicate favorable outcomes. The long-term results of this approach are beginning to be available and indicate that autologous stem cell transplantation may be curative. In at least one study of 20 patients the progression-free survival rate is at 85% with a median followup of 32 months.[192] Therefore, intensive chemotherapy with stem cell rescue is a reasonable approach to this patient population. Whether allogenic transplant will prove useful remains to be determined. Overall, however, the approach to patients with ARL now overlaps with lymphoma patients outside the setting of HIV infection.

This is also evident in the treatment of patients with Burkitt histology ARL. Earlier in the epidemic these patients received the therapy of other ARL because of concerns for poor tolerance. Although the introduction of HAART was shown by one study to improve the survival of patients with diffuse large cell lymphoma (DLCL) histology (median survival 8.3 months to 43.2 months), those with Burkitt lymphoma (BL) did not enjoy a similar outcome (median survival 6.4 months to 5.7 months in HAART era).[178] These data suggested that chemotherapy needed to be modified for BL histology, and it was noted that HIV-positive patients with BL could tolerate more intensive chemotherapy regimens.[193,194] In a retrospective analysis of patients with BL histology treated with either standard regimens or a more intensive regimen (similar to what this group uses for acute lymphocytic leukemia), those who received the intensive therapy had a better complete response rate and 1-year survival (65% vs. 44%).[195] Patients with HIV infection and BL should be considered for standard BL treatment approaches.

PRIMARY CENTRAL NERVOUS SYSTEM LYMPHOMA

Patients with HIV presenting with a mass lesion of the brain raise a number of diagnostic possibilities. Abscesses (toxoplasma, mycobacterial, or bacterial) or progressive multifocal leukoencephalopathy must be considered in addition to primary CNS lymphoma.[196–202] Criteria for distinguishing between these entities are not definitive without tissue sampling. However, for those patients in whom biopsy is either impossible or refused, certain parameters can raise or lower the likelihood of a lymphoma diagnosis. Perhaps the most important among these is CSF for EBV. The patient's toxoplasmosis serologic status and knowledge of whether the patient has been using trimethoprim-sulfamethoxazole as *P. carinii* pneumonia prophylaxis can also be extremely informative. The latter is highly effective for toxoplasma, and this, coupled with a negative toxoplasma titer, is strong evidence against toxoplasmosis. More commonly, patients have had previous toxoplasma exposure and have an immunoglobulin (Ig)G titer to this agent; differentiating an IgG versus IgM response can weigh the relative likelihood of an acute process. In addition, cultures for mycobacterium, fungus, and serum assay for cryptococcal antigen can be helpful in defining the nature of the CNS process. Some radiographic criteria have been described as being more suggestive of AIDS-lymphoma than toxoplasma brain abscess. These include large size (>2 cm), central location, and lack of multifocality.[174,198] Lymphoma can cross the midline, but this is extremely rare in the case of infectious causes.

Data in toxoplasma seronegative patients suggest that the presence of EBV detected by polymerase chain reaction strongly correlates with the presence of EBV-related disease (lymphoma) in the CNS.[197,199–201] In some centers, it has now become acceptable to use positive DNA polymerase chain reaction with radiographic imaging (often including thallium or PET scanning) to begin empirical therapy for lymphoma. In those patients in whom ambiguity remains, but biopsy is not possible, it is reasonable to begin an empirical trial of antibiotic therapy (sulfadiazine or clindamycin and pyrimethamine) directed against toxoplasmosis. In those patients who worsen after day 5 or fail to improve after 14 days, there is a higher likelihood that the disease not caused by toxoplasmosis.[202]

The clinical presentation of patients with primary CNS lymphoma can be extremely variable and quite subtle. This is a disease most common in late-stage AIDS, and in that patient population a high level of vigilance must be maintained for patients who present with neurologic or psychologic symptoms. Treatment of primary CNS ARL has generally been restricted to radiation therapy and steroids. The response rate to radiotherapy is high (60% to 79%), but durable remissions are relatively uncommon.[174,203–206] Patients' prognoses have often been limited by other opportunistic disease. It may be possible now with improved supportive care to better define the usefulness of other regimens in this patient population. A recent clinical trial evaluating the combination of systemic chemotherapy with radiation therapy failed to demonstrate any benefit to offset the toxicity of the chemotherapy. However, small studies with high-dose methotrexate have been encouraging.[207] In addition, combining antiviral agents ganciclovir and intravenous zidovudine with interferon has been reported as active against this disease and is now being systematically studied.[196]

Because this disease represents a failure of anti-EBV immunity and is generally seen only in advance AIDS, it is important to consider attempts to improve immune function as part of the therapy. That is, for patients who present with this lymphoma and are either not on HAART or receiving a suboptimal regimen, efforts should be made to maximally suppress HIV by medications in addition to the antitumor therapy. In such settings, there are a number of reports of patients with long-term control of the lymphoma despite having received radiation therapy alone. However, it cannot be considered sufficient to use HAART as therapy for this lymphoma.

Overall, primary CNS ARL remains a devastating and poorly treated problem. It is important that new approaches be critically evaluated, and enrollment of patients in clinical trials is strongly encouraged. If no trial is available, the approach must be clearly tailored to the overall status of the patient. Frank discussion of the generally poor prognosis (historically 2 to 5 months) in patients with end-stage AIDS should be a part of establishing a treatment plan. In patients with advanced AIDS who have failed HAART, palliative measures, such as steroids or pain medications alone, may be appropriate.

CONTROVERSY AND FUTURE DIRECTIONS

A number of areas within the context of ARL remain to be fully defined. The need for better understanding of the basis for lymphomagenesis is particularly acute in AIDS because of the potential for novel underlying infectious cofactors that can serve as therapeutic targets. Recent identification of KSHV and its clear relationship with a small subset of these tumors has provided a compelling example of this and represents considerable opportunity for new therapeutic interventions. The presence of multiple viruses now identified in ARL raises the question of what role there might be for specific antiviral medications or immunization. Why some patients develop malignancy whereas others with EBV or KSHV remain tumor-free is a puzzle rich with possibilities. Unraveling such issues will potentially point to mechanisms of screening and subsequent intervention. The molecular biologic basis of cell transformation by infectious cofactors is also a highly appealing area for investigation with potential targets for the small molecule or structurally designed pharmacologic agents currently under vigorous study by the pharmaceutical industry.

More extensive clinical investigation into the immunologic, cytokine, and viral profiles of select patient populations or in animal models with EBV-like disease[208] will likely provide significant insights into the pathology of ARL. Looking for potential interactions of virus and host by intensive laboratory study and genetic profiling may identify patients with high risk for ARL development and provide surrogate markers for early intervention.

Issues specifically related to therapy of ARL include which patients need CNS prophylaxis and what the role is for intensive retroviral therapy during ARL chemotherapy. Pursuing therapeutic trials testing agents such as additional monoclonal antibodies directed against lymphoma cells and novel infusion regimens is important. Augmentation of immunologic reactivity is compelling in a disease arising from an immunologic incompetent background; however, the specific nature of the intervention is yet to be defined. The use of specific cell-based approaches to therapy in this setting are based on the striking success of adoptively transferred lymphocytes in patients with EBV lymphoproliferative disease in the transplant setting.[69,70] Attempts employing similar approaches or efforts to immunize against tumor-related antigens in patients with ARL are planned and can offer alternative approaches to those patients refractory to standard cytotoxic agents. The potential of supplementing chemotherapy with biologically directed therapies is a focus of clinical investigation in ARL, and, if fruitful, might provide benefit not just for patients with ARL but also for non–HIV-infected lymphoma patients. The interplay between immune function and lymphomagenesis is an issue best demonstrated by ARL. Unraveling the details of this relationship will provide principles applicable well outside the scope of the AIDS epidemic.

Preferred Approach

Patients who present with NHL in the setting of AIDS should be assessed with a standard complete blood cell count and chemistry panel to which should be added a lymphocyte subset analysis and plasma HIV RNA. Patients who have "B" symptoms and a CD4 count of fewer than 200 cells/cm^3 should also have blood cultures and blood isolator tubes sent. A cytomegalovirus serum titer, toxoplasmosis titer, and cryptococcal antigen are also indicated as is sputum analysis for *P. carinii* pneumonia. Imaging studies for evaluation of the extent of lymphoma should be completed in the manner employed outside the setting of HIV disease. However, we also recommend imaging of the CNS and sampling of the CSF. Bone marrow aspiration biopsy should be obtained and special stains and cultures performed to exclude opportunistic infections.

For those patients who have a small, noncleaved, or Burkitt-like histology, paranasal involvement, bone marrow involvement, or testicular involvement, I prefer the administration of intrathecal arabinoside (ara-C) at 50 mg weekly for 4 weeks. This should be started at the initiation of chemotherapy. Chemotherapy, in patients for whom a protocol is not available or practical, is generally standard CHOP, unless patients have advanced AIDS or poor bone marrow reserve. In such cases, a modified or half-dose regimen can be justified, and is often quite effective. For patients with Burkitt histology, a Burkitt protocol should be used.

If patients have active involvement of the meninges, twice weekly ara-C is used until clearing of the CSF of lymphoma cells is achieved, and ara-C is administered monthly for 3 months. Whole-brain radiation is also added.

With relapse, there are no standard regimens available. I commonly use the EPOCH regimen, but encourage consideration of investigational protocols for such patients.

Patients who present with primary CNS lymphoma should receive dexamethasone (Decadron) 4 mg, four times daily until improvement of symptoms, and then the dose should be gradually reduced during a course of CNS radiation therapy. Steroids should be tapered as rapidly as tolerated to avoid the complications of prolonged immunosuppression. All such patients should receive antiretroviral therapy.

In general, all patients undergoing treatment for systemic NHL should have prophylaxis for *P. carinii* pneumonia. I prefer trimethoprim-sulfamethoxazole when tolerated. My policy regarding antiretroviral therapy is to use standard regimens avoiding those likely to affect myelosuppression (AZT) or drug metabolism. Alterations in drug metabolism are more likely to be encountered with the use of ritonavir or the non-nucleoside reverse transcriptase inhibitors delavirdine or nevirapine, and these should, therefore, be used with caution. Growth factor support is often required because of poor marrow reserve in patients with AIDS, but is often not needed in patients responding to HAART.

SUGGESTED READINGS

Antinori A, Ammassari A, De Luca A, Cingolani A, et al: Diagnosis of AIDS-related focal brain lesions: A decision-making analysis based on clinical and neuroradiologic characteristics combined with polymerase chain reaction assays in CSF. Neurology 48:687, 1997.

Baumgartner JE, Rachlin JR, Beckstead JH, et al: Primary central nervous system lymphomas: Natural history and response to radiation therapy in 55 patients with acquired immunodeficiency syndrome. J Neurosurg 73:206, 1990.

Boue F, Gabarre J, Gisselbrecht C, et al: Phase II trial of CHOP plus rituximab in patients with HIV-associated non-Hodgkin's lymphoma. J Clin Oncol 24(25):4123, 2006.

Bower M, Gazzard B, Mandalia S, et al: A prognostic index for systemic AIDS-related non-Hodgkin lymphoma treated in the era of highly active antiretroviral therapy [erratum in: Ann Intern Med 144(8):620, 2006; summary for patients in Ann Intern Med 16;143(4):I28, 2005]. Ann Intern Med 143(4):265, 2005.

Ciricillo SF, Rosenblum ML: Use of CT and MR imaging to distinguish intracranial lesions and to define the need for biopsy in AIDS patients. J Neurosurg 73:720, 1990.

Cortes J, Thomas D, Rios A, et al: Hyperfractionated cyclophosphamide, vincristine, doxorubicin, and dexamethasone and highly active antiretroviral therapy for patients with acquired immunodeficiency syndrome-related Burkitt lymphoma/leukemia. Cancer 94(5):1492, 2002.

Diamond C, Taylor TH, Aboumrad T, Anton-Culver H: Changes in acquired immunodeficiency syndrome-related non-Hodgkin lymphoma in the era of highly active antiretroviral therapy: incidence, presentation, treatment, and survival. Cancer 106(1):128, 2006.

Heslop HE, Ng CY, Li C, et al: Long-term restoration of immunity against Epstein-Barr virus infection by adoptive transfer of gene-modified virus-specific T lymphocytes. Nat Med 2:551, 1996.

Hoffmann C, Tiemann M, Schrader C, et al: AIDS-related B-cell lymphoma (ARL): Correlation of prognosis with differentiation profiles assessed by immunophenotyping. Blood 106(5):1762, 2005.

Kaplan LD, Lee JY, Ambinder RF, et al: Rituximab does not improve clinical outcome in a randomized phase 3 trial of CHOP with or without rituximab in patients with HIV-associated non-Hodgkin lymphoma: AIDS-Malignancies Consortium Trial 010. Blood 106(5):1538, 2005.

Lim ST, Karim R, Tulpule A, Nathwani BN, Levine AM: Prognostic factors in HIV-related diffuse large-cell lymphoma: before versus after highly active antiretroviral therapy. J Clin Oncol 23(33):8477, 2005.

Pluda JM, Yarchoan R, Jaffe ES, et al: Development of non-Hodgkin lymphoma in a cohort of patients with severe human immunodeficiency virus (HIV) infection on long-term antiretroviral therapy. Ann Intern Med 113:276, 1990.

Pluda JM, Venzon DJ, Tosato G, Lietzau J, et al: Parameters affecting the development of non-Hodgkin's lymphoma in patients with severe human immunodeficiency virus infection receiving antiretroviral therapy. J Clin Oncol 11:1099, 1993.

Spina M, Jaeger U, Sparano JA, et al: Rituximab plus infusional cyclophosphamide, doxorubicin, and etoposide in HIV-associated non-Hodgkin lymphoma: pooled results from 3 phase 2 trials. Blood 105(5):1891, 2005.

Wang ES, Straus DJ, Teruya-Feldstein J, et al: Intensive chemotherapy with cyclophosphamide, doxorubicin, high-dose methotrexate/ifosfamide, etoposide, and high-dose cytarabine (CODOX-M/IVAC) for human immunodeficiency virus-associated Burkitt lymphoma. Cancer 98(6):1196, 2003.

REFERENCES

For complete list of references log onto www.expertconsult.com

CHAPTER 87

MULTIPLE MYELOMA

Guido Tricot

Multiple myeloma (MM) is a prototype of a differentiated clonal B-cell tumor usually comprising slowly proliferating plasma cells. The disease is mainly contained within the bone marrow. The disorder is frequently accompanied by monoclonal (M) protein production and either diffuse osteoporosis or lytic bone lesions (Fig. 87–1). MM accounts for approximately 1% of all malignant diseases and 10% of hematologic malignancies. The annual incidence of myeloma is three to four per 100,000. An estimated 14,000 new cases of myeloma are diagnosed each year in the United States, and approximately 13,000 patients die of myeloma each year. A distinct feature of myeloma is the late age of onset. The median age at diagnosis for myeloma patients is approximately 69 years for men and 71 years for women; less than 5% of patients are younger than 40 years. Although myeloma can occur in people younger than 30 years, the diagnosis should be considered only after careful evaluation of all data and when other causes of monoclonal gammopathy or lytic lesions, such as a non-Hodgkin lymphoma or metastatic malignancy, have been ruled out. An excessive incidence of MM is observed among blacks and males. The incidence of myeloma in black males is approximately nine per 100,000 per year compared with six per 100,000 persons per year in black females. The incidence in white males is four per 100,000 persons per year and in white females is three per 100,000 persons per year.[1] Other ethnic groups, including Hawaiians, female Hispanics, female American Indians from New Mexico, and Alaskan Natives, also experience high myeloma rates compared with U.S. whites from the same geographic region. The Asian population has a lower incidence of myeloma compared with their white counterparts. Whereas the mortality rate for most other malignancies has slowly decreased during the past 30 years, it has increased for patients afflicted with MM and non-Hodgkin lymphoma. This finding is mainly due to the increased frequency of diagnosis in men and women aged 85 years and older. Compared with 1968 to 1990, the mortality rate due to myeloma in men and women 85 years and older has increased by approximately 45%.

ETIOLOGY

The cause of MM is largely unknown. Genetic predisposition and environmental factors likely are involved. The genetic susceptibility probably is related to the method by which individuals deal with environmental toxins and antigen exposure. A large individual variation in activity along xenobiotic metabolic pathways has been implicated in the susceptibility to childhood acute lymphoblastic leukemia.[2,3] Several of these participating enzymes metabolize environmental carcinogens. Multiple variants in genes coding for detoxification and DNA repair enzymes have been described.[4,5] Although more than 99% of human DNA sequences are the same for all individuals, variations in DNA sequence in the remaining less than 1% can have a major impact on how humans respond to environmental insults. Single nucleotide polymorphisms are the most frequent forms of DNA variation and disease-causing gene mutations.

Environmental and occupational exposures have been implicated in the etiology of myeloma. Exposure to ionizing radiation is the most convincing risk factor for MM. MM occurred after a long latent period in atomic bomb survivors exposed to high-dose radiation.[6] Studies performed on radiologists also suggest a link with long-term exposure to low-dose radiation. Several studies have indicated an increased risk of MM mortality among workers in the nuclear industry,[7–10] whereas other studies failed to show such a correlation.[11] Most excesses of MM mortality rates correlate with exposure to radiation between 10 to 15 years before diagnosis.[8,10] The role of occupational exposures to the risk of MM development remains unclear. Most occupational associations with myeloma have been related to agriculture and include dusty occupations and exposure to grain dusts, aflatoxins, and engine exhausts from farm equipment.[12–14] A 2.5-fold increased risk of development of MM has been observed with pesticide use.[15]

Exposure to various metals have been linked to myeloma. A significant risk of myeloma has been found among smelter, metallurgy,[16] and sheet metal workers.[17] An increased mortality rate due to MM was seen in workers in a Canadian nickel refinery.[18]

Benzene has been suggested as a possible etiologic agent of MM because its metabolites are known bone marrow toxins.[19,20] Epidemiologic studies correlating MM with employment as a beautician or cosmetologist have reported both positive[21,22] and negative associations.[23] Medications such as propoxyphene, phenytoin, phenobarbital, diazepam, propranolol, ibuprofen, diet drugs, stimulants, and laxatives have been implicated in an increased risk for developing MM.[24,25] MM has not been found to be strongly related to either cigarette smoking or alcohol consumption.

Familial occurrence of myeloma is well established.[26,27]

PATHOGENESIS

Normal B-Cell Development

B-cell development[28,29] occurs initially in the bone marrow and subsequently in lymphoid tissues. Terminal B-cell differentiation takes place in the bone marrow. In the bone marrow, hematopoietic progenitor cells differentiate into the earliest identifiable cell type committed to the B lineage, the *pro-B cell.* This cell undergoes rearrangement of its immunoglobulin (Ig) heavy chain genes and is called a *pre-B cell.* It is characterized by the presence of cytoplasmic μ chains. Subsequent rearrangement of the light chain enables the cell to express surface IgM and the cell becomes an *immature B lymphocyte.* These cells leave the bone marrow and, on entering the peripheral blood, start to express surface IgD and are called *virgin B cells.* They are arrested in the G_0 phase of the cell cycle. These virgin B cells enter the lymphoid tissue, where they are exposed to antigen-presenting cells, become activated, and differentiate into *short-lived low-affinity plasma* cells or *memory B cells.* These memory B cells travel from the extrafollicular area of the lymph node to the primary follicles, where they are confronted with an antigen, presented by follicular dendritic cells, resulting in the development of a secondary response. At this stage, primary follicles change into secondary follicles containing germinal centers. Through activation by an antigen, memory B cells differentiate into *centroblasts,* resulting in Ig isotype switching and somatic mutations in the variable region of the Ig with the generation of high-affinity antibodies. Centroblasts then progress to the *centrocyte* stage and reexpress surface Ig. The centrocytes with high-affinity antibodies differentiate into either memory B cells or *plasmablasts,* which subsequently move to the bone marrow and ter-

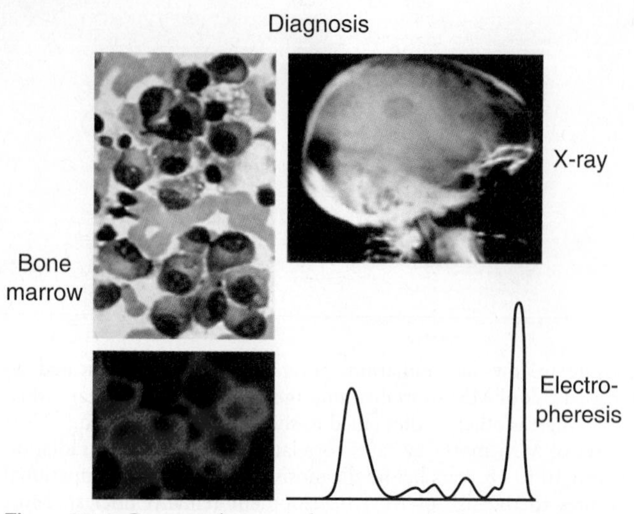

Figure 87–1 Common diagnostic features in multiple myeloma: light chain–restricted plasma cells in a bone marrow aspirate; multiple lytic lesions in a skull radiograph; large monoclonal spike in the γ-globulin area in serum electrophoresis.

minally differentiate to *plasma cells.* These bone marrow plasma cells produce most of serum Igs and have a lifespan of approximately 1 month.

Three distinct gene segments, the variable (V_H), diversity (D_H), and joining region (J_H) genes, encode the variable region of the heavy chain, whereas two segments, variable (V_κ or V_λ) and joining (J_κ or J_λ) region genes, encode the variable fraction of the light chain. The Ig heavy chain (IgH) locus on chromosome 14q32 contains an estimated 100 to 150 V_H genes, 30 D_H, and 6 J_H gene segments. Because some of the V_H genes are nearly identical, 60 to 70 V_H genes likely are available for rearrangement. These 60 to 70 genes belong to seven families (V_H1 to V_H7) whose members have more than 80% sequence homology. Of the 75 known V_κ sequences, only 36 are potentially functional, and of the 36 known V_λ sequences, only 24 are functional. Rearrangement of V gene segments is dependent on the protein products of the recombinase-activating genes RAG-1 and RAG-2. Recombination of V genes starts in lymphoid progenitors within the IgH locus of either the maternal or paternal chromosome 14. If the initial VDJ rearrangement yields a sequence that cannot be translated, then rearrangement of the IgH locus proceeds on the other allele. The presence on the B-cell surface of a fully assembled μ heavy-chain rearrangement begins when one of the V_κ genes rearranges to one of the J_κ genes. If κ light-chain rearrangement is unsuccessful on both alleles, by default λ light chains subsequently rearrange.

Ig heavy and light chains each contain three hypervariable segments (complementarity-determining regions [CDRs]), which are the areas of the Ig in direct contact with the antigen. In a process of trial and error, Igs increase their affinity for an antigen by a series of somatic mutations. CDR3 is the most variable portion of the Ig molecule because it not only contains somatic mutations, as is the case for CDR1 and CDR2, but it also encompasses the 3′ end of V_H, all of D_H, and the 5′ end of J_H. Therefore, it is an ideal marker for detecting a very small population of the malignant myeloma clone within a larger population of normal cells.

Myeloma Stem Cell

The origin of malignant plasma cell remains a mystery. Although the predominant cell in MM is the plasma cell, accumulating data show that other lymphoid cell types are involved in the malignant process. A significant number of peripheral blood lymphocytes bear the unique paraprotein idiotype found in plasma cells[30–33] and have clonal Ig gene rearrangements identical to those seen in bone marrow plasma cells.[34,35] These data strongly suggest the existence of a precursor compartment, which may contain the myeloma stem cell. Killing all myeloma stem cells will be required to completely eradicate the disease. However, in most cancers enough plasticity is present to allow more mature-appearing cells to again assume the characteristics of tumor stem cells. Little is known about the characteristics of the myeloma stem cell. It has been proposed that such a stem cell is $CD138^-$ and $CD20^+$, based on the observation that this subpopulation derived from either myeloma cell lines or primary myeloma has a greater clonogenic potential.[36] Cloning and sequencing of V_H genes in myeloma show multiple somatic mutations, characteristic of an antigen-driven process with no further intraclonal diversity with disease progression,[37,38] strongly implying that malignant clone in MM evolves from a cell in late B-cell development, which has traversed the germinal center and has been extensively exposed to an antigen.[28,38] Therefore, the cell of origin for myeloma most likely is either a memory B cell or a plasmablast. That myeloma arises in the lymph node remains somewhat counterintuitive because lymphadenopathy is not a hallmark of MM. During migration of the B cell through the germinal center, multiple DNA breaks occur at the level of the gene coding for the heavy chains of the Ig (14q32). These breaks are the consequence of VDJ rearrangements. It is also clear that somatic mutations are associated with DNA breaks. In addition, while and after the antigen-primed B cell leaves the germinal center, additional DNA breaks occur when the Ig isotype switches from IgM to either IgA or IgG. These DNA breaks lead to genetic instability and an increased chance of chromosome translocations involving 14q32.

Once malignant precursor cells leave the lymph node and enter the peripheral blood circulation, they acquire adhesion molecules and home to the bone marrow environment. Homing to the bone marrow is the consequence of the presence on the plasma cell membrane of the chemokine receptor CXCR4. The ligand for CXCR4 is CXCL12 or stroma-derived factor (SDF)-1.[39–41] Remember that hematopoietic stem cells are attracted to the bone marrow microenvironment through the same mechanism of CXCR4 expression on their cell surface. This explains why myeloma cells usually are found only in bone marrow areas, where normal hematopoiesis occurs. In addition, myeloma cells are attracted to CCL1, which is secreted by myeloma cells; this explains why myeloma cells have the tendency to form small or larger nodules.[42] The larger nodules cause the typical osteolytic lesions seen on metastatic bone survey, magnetic resonance imaging (MRI) or positron emission tomography (PET) scan. Like myeloma cells, osteoclasts are attracted to sources of CXCL12 (SDF-1). Myeloma cells are able to attract osteoclasts precursors directly via the secretion of CCL3 or macrophage inflammatory protein 1α (MIP-1α).[42]

ROLE OF THE MICROENVIRONMENT IN MULTIPLE MYELOMA

MM cells adhere to bone marrow stromal cells. The myeloma cells interact with the bone marrow stromal cells through multiple adhesion molecules. These include CD56/CD56; syndecan-1 (CD138)/collagen; intercellular adhesion molecule (ICAM)-1/leukocyte function-associated antigen (LFA)-1; CD49d/vascular cellular adhesion molecule (VCAM)-1 or fibronectin; and CD38/CD31. CD49d/VCAM-1 likely is the major pathway capable of providing effective capture of myeloma cells within the bone marrow, as has also been demonstrated for hematopoietic stem cells.[43] These adhesion molecules not only are important for binding myeloma cells to stroma, but they also cause homotypic aggregation of myeloma cells in concert with CCL1, which is secreted by myeloma cells. Interaction of myeloma cells with stromal cells leads to bone destruction as well as survival, proliferation, drug resistance, and genetic instability of myeloma cells.

Bone Destruction

Bone destruction is a prominent clinical feature of almost all patients with MM. It is responsible for many of the most debilitating clinical features of the disease, such as pain, fractures, and hypercalcemia. When myeloma cells adhere to the bone marrow stroma, stromal cells produce cytokines and inflammatory proteins such as interleukin (IL)-6,[44] IL-1,[45] tumor necrosis factor (TNF),[46] IL-11,[47] and MIP-1α.[48] In addition, myeloma cells secrete hepatocyte growth factor (HGF)[49] and parathyroid hormone-related peptide.[50] All of these factors, called osteoclast-activating factors (OAFs), cause local expression on stromal cells of receptor activator of nuclear factor (NF)-κB ligand (RANKL), also called TNF-related activation-induced cytokine (TRANCE). RANKL is a member of the TNF gene family. It activates c-Jun terminal kinase and signals through NF-κB.[51] The gene for RANKL has been mapped to chromosome 13q14. OAFs induce osteoclast formation indirectly by stimulating marrow stromal cells to express increased levels of RANKL on their surface. RANKL binds to the RANK receptor on osteoclast precursors and induces osteoclast differentiation and maturation. Osteoclasts are derived from monocytes/macrophage precursor cells. Osteoclastogenesis is induced by macrophage colony-stimulating factor 1 in combination with RANKL or TNF-α and is completely inhibited by the addition of granulocyte–macrophage colony-stimulating factor or IL-3 at the early stages of differentiation.[52] The absence of RANKL expression in mice results in severe osteopetrosis and absence of osteoclasts.[53] In contrast, overexpression of RANKL in mice induces severe osteoporosis. RANKL activity can be blocked by the naturally occurring decoy receptor osteoprotegerin (OPG), which is a member of the TNF receptor superfamily. Most cell types produce OPG. However, OPG is not a specific receptor for RANKL. It also binds TNF-related apoptosis-inducing ligand (TRAIL). Overexpression of OPG results in severe osteopetrosis, whereas absence of OPG induces osteopenia.[54] In patients with MM, OPG levels are reduced,[55,56] with an inverse correlation between OPG levels and the degree of skeletal destruction in myeloma. Myeloma cells bind, internalize, and degrade OPG.[57] The process of degradation by myeloma cells of OPG is dependent on interaction with heparan sulfates on myeloma cells. OPG has a highly basic heparan-binding domain, making interactions with heparin and heparan sulfates possible. One feature of normal and malignant plasma cells is abundant expression of syndecan-1, which is a transmembrane proteoglycan having heparan sulfate side chains.[58]

The ultimate result is a major imbalance between RANKL, the activity of which is highly increased, and OPG, the activity of which is drastically decreased. This situation switches the balance completely in the direction of bone destruction.[59] The bony matrix is a rich source of all types of cytokines, such as insulinlike growth factor (IGF), IL-6, and basic fibroblastic growth factor, which stimulate the survival and growth of myeloma cells and result in the release from the myeloma cells of OAFs such as parathyroid hormone-related peptide and MIP-1α. More myeloma cell growth will result in more release of OAFs, which will cause more production of RANKL. This becomes a vicious cycle where growth of myeloma cells leads to more bone destruction, and more bone destruction leads to more growth of myeloma cells. This cycle can be effectively blocked by administration of bisphosphonates[60] or OPG.[61] Treatment of myeloma in the SCID-hu hosts with an inhibitor of osteoclast activity (*pamidronate* or zoledronate) or with a specific inhibitor of RANKL halts myeloma-induced bone resorption but also results in inhibition of myeloma cell growth and survival.[62] Evidence has shown that MIP-1α and MIP-1β are major OAFs produced by myeloma cells.[63] Stromal cells express the receptor for MIP-1α and MIP-1β, called CCR5. Whether myeloma cells actually express RANKL is a matter of debate.[59,64] A schematic representation of bone destruction in myeloma is shown in Fig. 87–2. MIP-1α is abnormally regulated in myeloma due to imbalanced expression of acute myeloid leukemia (AML)-1A and AML-1B.[65] IL-3 also is induced by this imbalanced expression. Increased IL-3 levels in the microenvironment can increase bone destruction and myeloma cell growth.[66]

The method by which bone destruction occurs in myeloma is reasonably well known, but the reason why increased bone destruction does not result in increased bone formation as in most other malignancies involving the bone remains largely unknown. Although an increased number of osteoblasts is present in the earlier stages of myeloma, osteoblasts undergo apoptosis and ultimately almost completely disappear with progression of disease.[67] The canonical Wnt/

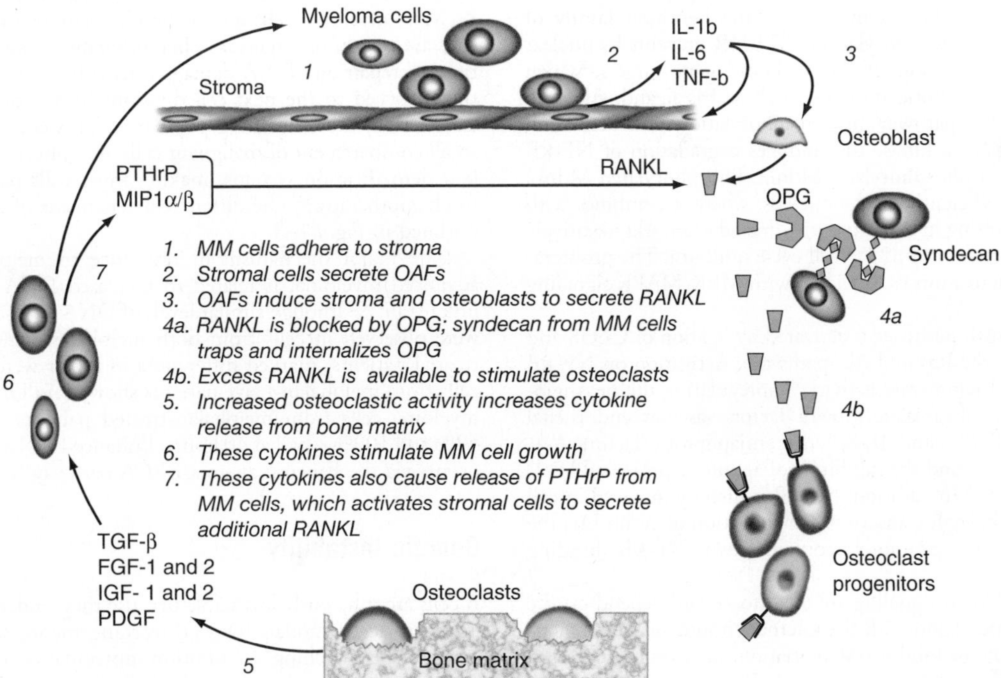
Myeloma cells
1
Stroma
2
IL-1b
IL-6
TNF-b
3
Osteoblast
PTHrP
MIP1α/β
RANKL
OPG
Syndecan
1. MM cells adhere to stroma
2. Stromal cells secrete OAFs
3. OAFs induce stroma and osteoblasts to secrete RANKL
4a. RANKL is blocked by OPG; syndecan from MM cells traps and internalizes OPG
4b. Excess RANKL is available to stimulate osteoclasts
5. Increased osteoclastic activity increases cytokine release from bone matrix
6. These cytokines stimulate MM cell growth
7. These cytokines also cause release of PTHrP from MM cells, which activates stromal cells to secrete additional RANKL
7
6
4a
4b
TGF-β
FGF-1 and 2
IGF- 1 and 2
PDGF
5
Osteoclasts
Bone matrix
Osteoclast
progenitors

Figure 87–2 Bone destruction in multiple myeloma. *(From Tricot G: New insights into the role of microenvironment in multiple myeloma. Lancet 355:248, 2000.)*

β-catenin signaling pathway plays an important role in bone formation during embryonic development by differentiation of osteoblasts from precursor cells through direct regulation of the *Runx2* gene.[68,69] Wnt signaling also negatively regulates osteoclasts formation through transcriptional repression of *RANKL*.[70] Dkk1 (Dickkopf-1) is a Wnt antagonist that negatively regulates osteoblast differentiation and bone formation.[71] Our group has shown that Dkk1 is produced by myeloma cells and is associated with the presence of myeloma bone lesions.[72] Other potential osteoblast inhibitors are secreted Frizzled-related protein 2 (sFRP-2) and IL-7.[73,74]

Growth and Survival of Myeloma Cells

Myeloma cells in the early stages of the disease are completely dependent for their survival and growth on the bone marrow microenvironment. The myeloma cell has multiple receptors on its membrane, the ligands of which are present in the microenvironment. Important receptors are the IL-6 receptor, IL-15 receptor, IGF receptor, β_1 integrins (very late antigen [VLA]-4 and VLA-5), CD38, and CD40. The ligands for β_1 integrins are fibronectin and VCAM. The ligand for C38 is CD31. Activation of these multiple receptors by their ligand results in activation of four major pathways: STAT3, Ras, Akt, and NF-κB (Fig. 87–3). STAT3 is activated by IL-6 and IL-15. It results in upregulation of the antiapoptotic factors Bcl-X_L and myeloid leukemia cell (Mcl)-1 as well as the cell cycle regulatory protein p21.[75] Activation of STAT3 is responsible for the increased level of C-reactive protein (CRP), which is frequently seen in MM and has been associated with a poor prognosis. In addition, STAT3 increases transcription of c-myc.

The Ras pathway is activated by IGF and IL-6. It results in upregulation of myc and cyclin D, and it activates the NF-κB pathway. In addition, the Ras pathway plays an important role in downregulation of the CDK inhibitor p27.[76]

The Akt pathway is activated by IL-6 and IGF and acts downstream of the phosphatidylinositol 3-kinase (PI3K). The PI3K/Akt signaling pathway is constitutively activated in MM.[77] Constitutively active Akt rescues myeloma cells from PTEN-mediated apoptosis. Akt activation results in inactivation through phosphorylation of BAD, which is a proapoptopic member of the Bcl-2 family of proteins and promotes cell death by forming a nonfunctional heterodimer with the survival factor Bcl-X_L. Phosphorylation of BAD by Akt prevents such interaction and restores Bcl-X_L antiapoptotic function. Akt phosphorylates FKHR, a member of the Forkhead family of transcription factors. Phosphorylation of FKHR prevents its nuclear translocation and activation of the Forkhead gene targets, which include several proapoptotic proteins, such as Fas ligand. Akt also activates the NF-κB pathway by phosphorylation and activation of I-κB kinase (IKK), a kinase that induces degradation of NF-κB inhibitors I-κB. Akt phosphorylates Mdm2. Phosphorylated Mdm2 translocates more efficiently to the nucleus, where it combines with wild-type p53, resulting in enhanced p53 degradation. Akt negatively influences the expression of p27, a cell cycle inhibitor. The proliferative effect of Akt activation is associated with MEK/MAPK signaling cross-talk.[78,79]

NF-κB, the fourth pathway, is activated by ligation of CD38 and CD40 but also by the Ras and Akt pathways. Activation on NF-κB results in increased telomerase activity,[80] upregulating the proangiogenic factors basic fibroblastic growth factor, vascular endothelial growth factor (VEGF), and IL-8,[81] the antiapoptotic factors A-1, Bcl-2, and Bcl-X_L,[82,83] and the inhibitors of apoptosis proteins IAP-1, IAP-2,[84] and IEX-1.[85] In addition, NF-κB is directly involved in cell cycle progression through transcriptional activation of cyclin D1; the *c-myc* protooncogene promoter contains two NF-κB binding sides.[86]

The effects of Notch signaling are pleiotropic and depend on the cell type and its interaction with the microenvironment. Notch activation may promote or inhibit differentiation, increase proliferation or trigger cell cycle arrest, induce apoptosis, or protect cells from apoptosis.[87] Jundt et al.[88] reported that Jagged1-induced Notch signaling drove proliferation of myeloma cells, whereas Nefedova et al.[89] showed that activation of Notch1 resulted in protection of myeloma cells from melphalan and mitoxantrone-induced apoptosis by upregulation of p21, resulting in cell cycle arrest. These seemingly contradictory findings can be explained by the pleiotropic activity of Notch. In the presence of stimulating signals, Notch may cause proliferation, whereas in the presence of toxic agents, Notch may cause cell cycle arrest to protect myeloma cells from apoptosis.[87] Finally, Notch promotes osteoblastic cell differentiation of multipotent mesenchymal cells.[90]

The result of activation of the different pathways is increased proliferation, increased antiapoptotic activity, and increased angiogenic activity. Figure 87–3 clearly shows the tremendous redundancy in activation of the end targets. Therefore, blocking a single pathway is unlikely to have a major lasting effect on the growth of myeloma cells. Although all of these pathways have been shown to be active either in myeloma cell lines or in fresh myeloma cells, whether all these pathways are active all the time and which of these pathways is the most important are not clear. High interpatient variability is likely.

Drug Resistance in Multiple Myeloma

In contrast to what is generally accepted, drug resistance in the early stages of the disease is mainly induced by the microenvironment and by epigenetic changes.[91] This type of resistance can be overcome by high-dose chemotherapy. However, in the end stages of disease, drug resistance is determined by major genetic alterations. The existence of cell adhesion-mediated drug resistance in myeloma has been well demonstrated.[92] The human myeloma cell line 8226, which expresses CD49d (VLA-4), is resistant to the apoptotic effect of doxorubicin and melphalan when preadhered to fibronectin but not when the same cells are grown in suspension. Adhesion of myeloma cells to the stroma induces upregulation of p27, resulting in a decrease of cells in the S phase. Evidence also indicates that Notch signaling protects myeloma cells from the apoptotic effects of chemotherapy.[89] The importance of the microenvironment in drug resistance was also shown by using a human B-cell lymphoma line.[82] After treatment with etoposide, more than 80% of the cells in culture died as a result of apoptosis. When the microenvironment was artificially recreated by ligating VLA-4 with VCAM-1, CD40 with an anti-CD40 antibody, and IL-4 receptor with IL-4, less than 25% of the cells died.

Most myeloma cells are in the G_1 phase of the cell cycle. These cells are very poor targets for chemotherapy because they have ample time to repair any DNA damage caused by alkylating agents before they proceed to the next cell division. In addition, the concept of cancer stem cells is gaining popularity. This concept assumes that a small compartment of malignant cells are noncycling and have excellent detoxification systems, making those cells particularly resistant to chemotherapy.[93] The different mechanisms of drug resistance are outlined in Fig. 87–3.

The major mechanism of resistance to melphalan, at least in advanced myeloma, is related to increased DNA interstrand cross-link repair.[94] Although similar levels of DNA interstrand cross-linking were observed in cells from both melphalan-naive and melphalan-treated patients, marked differences in repair were noted. Myeloma cells from melphalan-naive patients showed no DNA repair, whereas myeloma cells from melphalan-treated patients exhibited between 42% and 100% repair at 40 hours. Enhanced DNA repair in myeloma occurs via the Fanconi anemia/BRCA pathway (Fig. 87–4).[95]

Genetic Instability

B cells are inherently less stable because they undergo multiple DNA breaks to accommodate for VDJ rearrangements, somatic mutations, and isotype switching. In addition, upregulation of many antiapoptotic factors makes it possible for cells that have acquired a tremendous amount of genetic changes to survive, which would not be

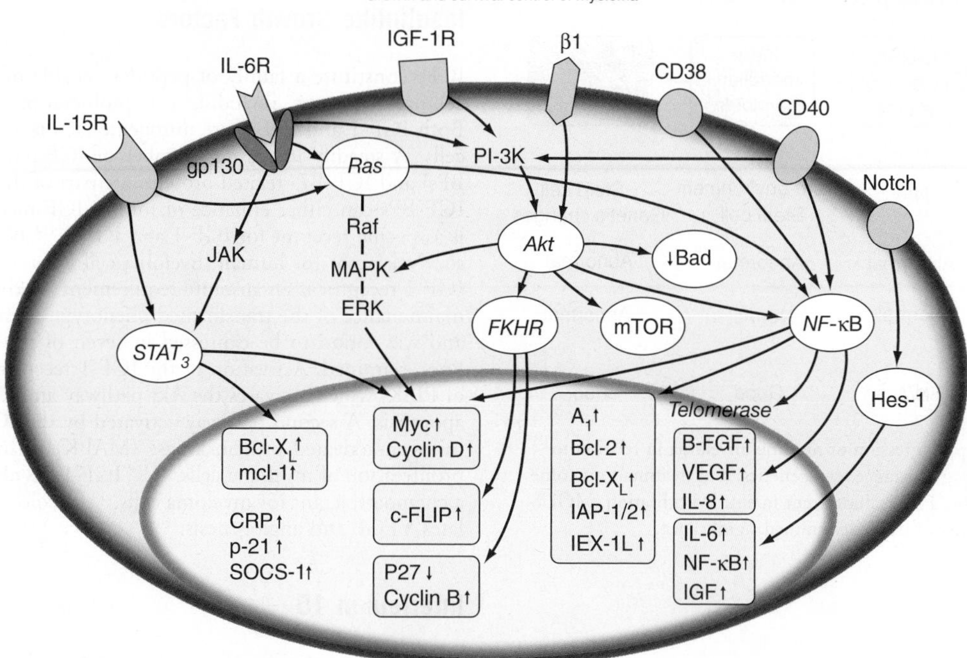

Figure 87–3 Growth and survival control of myeloma.

possible in the absence of these antiapoptotic factors. This is reflected in the complex karyotypes observed in myeloma that are reminiscent of solid tumor karyotypes rather than those seen in hematologic malignancies.

Multiple Myeloma is a Multistep Transformation Process

As is the case for chronic lymphocytic leukemia, low-grade non-Hodgkin lymphoma, chronic myeloid leukemia, and the myelodysplastic syndromes (MDS), myeloma evolves from a relatively benign process to a highly malignant transformed phase ("malignant myeloma"). The initial stage is an *indolent phase* (monoclonal gammopathy of undetermined significance [MGUS], smoldering myeloma or myeloma stage IA with stable disease, and no evidence of end-organ damage). In this phase of the disease, patients do not require any cytotoxic treatment. The growth and death rates of myeloma cells are approximately equivalent.

The second phase is the *overt phase* of myeloma, with either progressive increase in myeloma protein or the appearance of end-organ damage. In this phase, the disease is completely dependent on the bone marrow stroma for survival and growth, and it is chemosensitive. This is the optimal phase to treat patients effectively.

In the *aggressive terminal phase*, the myeloma cells become independent of the bone marrow stroma. Increased proliferation is evidenced by an increase in plasma cell labeling index (PCLI), usually to more than 1%, and in the level of lactate dehydrogenase (LDH). The bone marrow morphology is much more aggressive, having the appearance of plasmablasts. Conventional cytogenetics reveal abnormalities in most patients, who frequently also have manifestations of extramedullary disease. A PET scan probably is the best test for evaluating the presence of extramedullary disease. In this stage of the disease, the myeloma has become virtually resistant to chemotherapy due to acquisition of multiple genetic changes. Although the disease can be temporarily controlled with chemotherapy, consisting of a combination of alkylating and cell cycle-specific agents, responses are generally short lived and survival is generally poor, even with high-dose chemotherapy and autotransplants (Fig. 87–5).

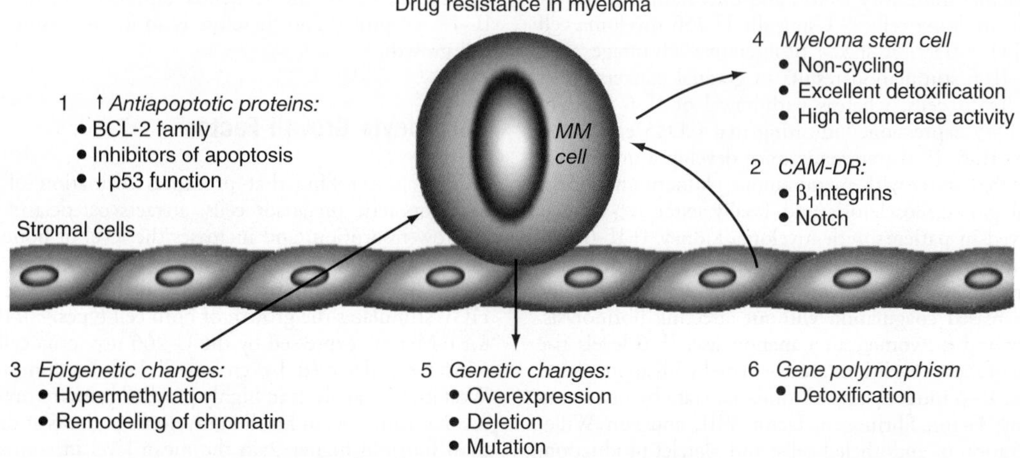

Figure 87–4 Multiple mechanisms of drug resistance in myeloma. CAM-DR, cell adhesion-mediated drug resistance; IAP, inhibitor of apoptosis; MM, multiple myeloma.

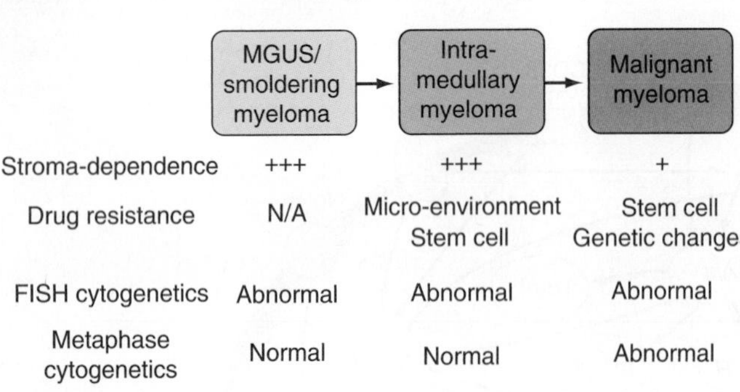

Figure 87–5 Multistep progression of multiple myeloma in relation to stroma dependence, drug resistance, cytogenetics, and treatment outcome after autotransplantation. FISH, fluorescent in situ hybridization, MGUS, monoclonal gammopathy of underdetermined significance.

ROLE OF CYTOKINES IN MYELOMA

Interleukin 6

IL-6 has always been considered the most important cytokine in myeloma. However, other cytokines are equally, if not more, important in the survival and growth of myeloma. IL-6 is essential for the proliferation of normal plasmablastic cells and for the terminal differentiation of plasmablast to nondividing plasma cells. Terminally differentiated plasma cells produce a large amount of Ig (>600 pg/cell in 24 hours).[96] In MM, IL-6 is mainly a survival factor[97] and does not induce terminal differentiation. It promotes survival through upregulation of many antiapoptotic factors (see Fig. 87–3) but also through inhibition of the JNK/SAPK pathway, resulting in inhibition of Fas-induced apoptosis.[98,99] IL-6 prevents dexamethasone-induced myeloma cell death.[100,101] IL-6 is also a growth factor for myeloma,[96] among other mechanisms through phosphorylation of the retinoblastoma (Rb) protein.[102] The major source of IL-6 production is the bone marrow stroma[103,104] although myeloma cells also produce IL-6 but to a much lesser extent.[105,106] Support for the role of IL-6 in the survival and growth of myeloma cells has been provided by the clinical application of anti–IL-6 monoclonal antibodies and IL-6 receptor antagonists.[107,108] Other cytokines using the same signal transducer (gp130) as IL-6, such as ciliary neurotropic factor, IL-11, leukemia inhibitory factor, and oncostatin M, stimulate the growth of myeloma cells.[109] Using the U-266 myeloma cell line, only the $CD45^+$ fraction shows proliferative advantage after IL-6 stimulation. IL-6 stimulation results in gradual conversion of $CD45^-$ cells to $CD45^+$ cells, whereas withdrawal of IL-6 leads to gradual loss of CD45 expression, indicating that CD45 expression can be induced by IL-6. IL-6 transgenic mice develop a progressive kidney pathology that starts with membranous glomerulonephritis, followed by focal glomerulosclerosis and finally extensive tubular damage, as observed in patients with myeloma kidney.[110] IL-6 prevents differentiation of monocytes to macrophages and dendritic cells,[111] which are functionally defective in MM.[112] Additionally, IL-6 promotes increased coagulation without affecting fibrinolysis. During pregnancy and in women after menopause, IL-6 levels rise significantly. Both of these conditions are associated with an increased risk of thrombosis. IL-6 induces a prothrombotic state by increasing expression of tissue factor, fibrinogen, factor VIII, and von Willebrand factor; activation of endothelial cells; and platelet production. It also reduces levels of inhibitors of hemostasis, such as antithrombin III and protein S.[113]

Insulinlike Growth Factors

IGFs constitute a family of peptides capable of stimulating various cellular responses, including cell proliferation and differentiation. Both IGF-1 and IGF-2 are mitogenic factors secreted by malignant cells. A steadily increasing number of IGF-binding proteins (IGF-BPs) and IGF-BP–related proteins are part of the IGF system. These IGF-BPs can either enhance or inhibit IGF-mediated effects. There is a specific receptor for IGF-1 and IGF-2.[114] IGF-1 is a growth and survival factor for human myeloma cell lines.[115] The presence of an IGF-1 receptor is an absolute requirement for the establishment and maintenance of the transformed phenotype of many malignancies[116] and was found to be expressed in seven of the eight myeloma cell lines examined. Activation of the IGF-1 receptor leads to activation of PI3K, which activates the Akt pathway and leads to inhibition of apoptosis. A second pathway activated by the IGF-1 receptor is the mitogen-activated protein kinase (MAPK) pathway, which leads to proliferation of myeloma cells.[117,118] IGF-1 has also been shown to be a chemoattractant for myeloma cells.[119] In colon cancer, IGF-1 regulates VEGF and angiogenesis.[120]

Interleukin 15

IL-15 induces proliferation and promotes cell survival of T cells, B cells, natural killer cells, and neutrophils. Constitutive expression of a functional IL-15 receptor was shown in all of the six myeloma cell lines and in the primary myeloma cells of 14 of 14 patients.[121] IL-15 transcripts were found in all six myeloma cell lines and IL-15 protein in four of the six cell lines. IL-15 transcripts were also found in eight of the 14 primary myeloma samples. This finding suggests the existence of an autocrine IL-15 loop. In addition to the autocrine loop is a paracrine loop, as IL-15 is released from the bone marrow microenvironment. Blocking IL-15 in myeloma cell lines increases the rate of spontaneous apoptosis. Furthermore, IL-15 lowers the responsiveness to Fas-induced apoptosis and to cytotoxic treatment with vincristine and doxorubicin but not with dexamethasone. In addition to preventing apoptosis of myeloma cells, IL-15 induced proliferation in four of the six primary myeloma samples.[122]

Interleukin 10

IL-10 is a potent inducer of Ig secretion by normal plasma cells. IL-10 does not induce differentiation or increased Ig synthesis in myeloma cells. However, it stimulates proliferation of primary myeloma cells and myeloma cell lines.[123] The proliferative activity of IL-10 can be abrogated by antibodies to the gp130 transducer. IL-10 induces the production of oncostatin M in myeloma cells as well as the expression of the leukemia inhibitory factor receptor and the IL-11 receptor[124] and therefore is an indirect stimulator of myeloma cell growth.

Hepatocyte Growth Factor

HGF is a cytokine that promotes formation of osteoclasts from hematopoietic precursor cells, attracts osteoclasts to sides of bone marrow resorption, and increases the level of bone resorption when in coculture with osteoblasts. The HGF receptor c-Met is expressed by the bone-forming osteoblasts and the bone-resorbing osteoclasts. HGF stimulates the growth of both cell types.[125] HGF and its receptor c-Met are expressed by the U-266 myeloma cell line. c-Met proteins were detected by enzyme-linked immunosorbent assay and Western blot analysis in highly purified primary myeloma cells.[49] The mean serum level of HGF in myeloma patients at diagnosis was more than fourfold higher than the mean level in controls. Activation of c-Met favors cell invasion, migration, and proliferation, all of which are essential in myeloma tumor progression.

Transforming Growth Factor β

Transforming growth factor (TGF)-β has pleiotropic biologic effects, including suppression of hematopoiesis by antagonizing stem cell factor as well as inhibition of wound healing and immune response. It suppresses B-cell proliferation and Ig production. In myeloma, TGF-β is produced by bone marrow stroma cells and myeloma cells. It triggers IL-6 secretion by both types of cells. It causes tumor cell proliferation indirectly, probably by upregulation of IL-6 secretion.[126] In myeloma, the Rb protein is constitutively phosphorylated. TGF-β does not alter or increase phosphorylation of Rb protein. TGF-β probably is the major factor causing suppression of normal plasma cells resulting in low levels of uninvolved Igs in patients with myeloma.

Tumor Necrosis Factor α

TNF-α is a potent mediator of inflammation and bone resorption. It induces expression of NF-κB and adhesion molecules[127] but only modestly triggers proliferation of myeloma cells. It markedly upregulates secretion of IL-6 and expression of CD11a (LFA-1), CD54 (ICAM-1), CD106, and CD49d (VLA-4).[128] The proteosome inhibitor PS-341 and thalidomide abrogate TNF-α–induced NF-κB activation as well as induction of the adhesion molecules, resulting in decreased adhesion of myeloma cells to the bone marrow stroma.

Vascular Endothelial Growth Factor

VEGF is produced by myeloma cells and bone marrow stromal cells and probably is the major factor explaining increased angiogenesis in myeloma. In human myeloma cells VEGF is upregulated by IL-6 and CD40 activation.[129,130] It promotes migration and, to a lesser extent, proliferation of myeloma cells.[131]

CYTOGENETICS IN MULTIPLE MYELOMA

Cytogenetic information obtained by conventional techniques is limited in MM because it is a malignancy composed mainly of more differentiated B cells with low proliferative activity. Abnormal karyotypes are observed in only 30% to 50% of cases.[132–134] Typically, previously treated and relapsed patients have a higher frequency of chromosome abnormalities compared with newly diagnosed patients. This finding reflects the more proliferative nature of myeloma in its advanced stages. The presence of abnormal cytogenetics by conventional karyotyping has been associated with an inferior outcome.[132,133,135] Flow cytometry-derived aneuploidy data and fluorescent in situ hybridization (FISH) analysis indicate the presence of cytogenetic abnormalities in at least 90% of myeloma patients. Therefore, most of the normal karyotypes in myeloma patients are derived from normal hematopoietic cells and not from the myeloma clone. Even at the stage of MGUS, flow cytometry and FISH analysis demonstrate aneuploidy or cytogenetic abnormalities in at least 50% of patients.[136–138] Approximately 65% of myeloma patients with abnormal cytogenetics have a hyperdiploid karyotype. Pseudodiploid and hypodiploid karyotypes are found in approximately 15% and 20% of patients, respectively. The most common abnormalities are gains of the whole chromosomes 3, 5, 7, 9, 11, 15, and 19. Every single chromosome potentially can be involved in deletions, gains, additions, or translocations in MM (Fig. 87–6).

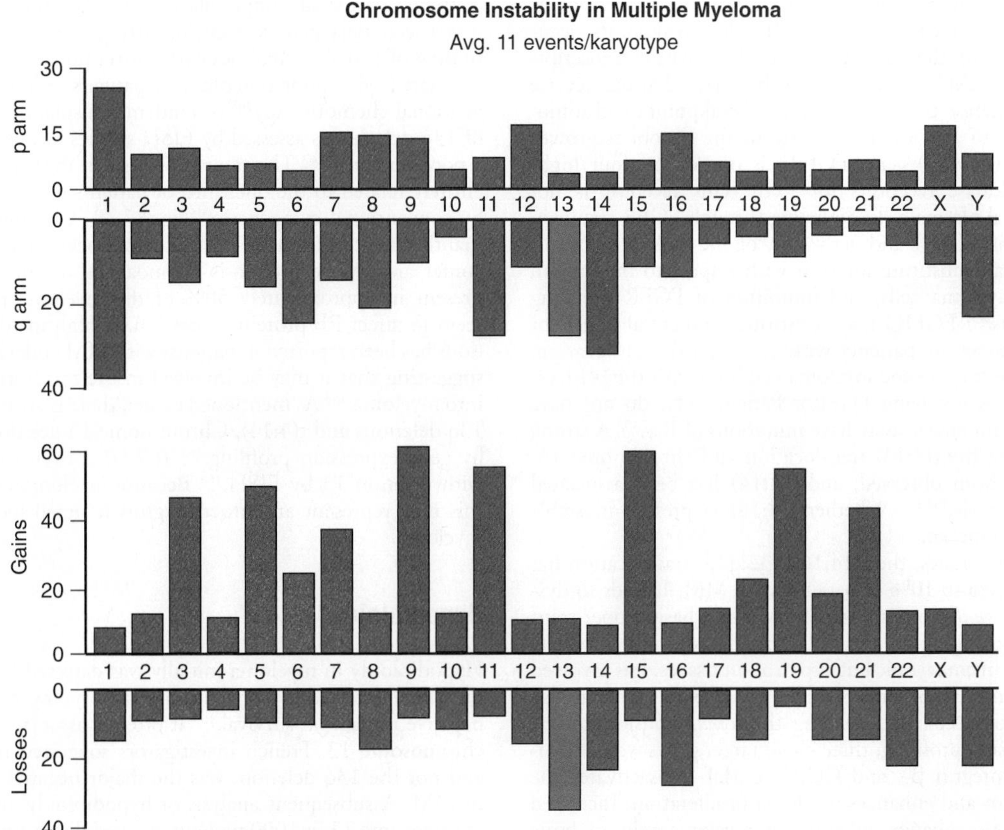

Figure 87–6 Chromosome instability in multiple myeloma.

Importance of Translocations Involving Chromosome 14q32

Chromosome 14q32 translocations involving IgH probably are an early important event in the pathogenesis of myeloma.[139] Multiple translocation partners have been identified for 14q32, several of which cannot be detected by conventional cytogenetics because they are located in telomeric positions. By interphase FISH analysis, IgH translocations are found in approximately 47% of MGUS patients, in 60% to 70% of patients with intramedullary MM, and in more than 80% of patients with primary or secondary plasma cell leukemia.[140,141] Translocations involving the λ light chain on chromosome 22 are present in approximately 17% of advanced and intramedullary myelomas. Translocations involving the κ light-chain gene on chromosome 2 are rare. The major recurrent translocation partners involving 14q32 are 4p16, 6p21, 11q13, and 16q23. Using FISH analysis, the t(11;14)(q13;32) translocation is present in approximately 15% to 20% of myeloma patients.[142,143] The breakpoint on 14q32 is located within the IgH or the switch region, compatible with the translocations caused by either somatic hypermutation or switch recombination. This is in contrast to mantle cell lymphoma, where the IgH breakpoints occur near the site targeted by VDJ recombination.[144] On 11q13, the breakpoints in myeloma are dispersed over a 330-kb region, centromeric to cyclin D1. Because of this translocation, cyclin D1 is juxtaposed to the powerful IgH 3′ enhancer on 14q32, leading to overexpression of cyclin D1. The t(11;14) translocation is also common in MGUS and primary systemic amyloidosis.[145] When detected by conventional cytogenetics, the t(11;14) translocation was associated with a poor prognosis.[146,147] However, when the t(11;14) translocation was identified by FISH, no inferior outcome was found.[148,149] Patients with the t(11:14) translocation are more likely to have lymphoplasmacytic morphology and a pseudodiploid karyotype. The labeling index usually is low.

Using FISH-based techniques, the t(4;14)(p16;q32) translocation was found in approximately 15% of MM patients.[142,150] This translocation is undetectable by conventional karyotyping because of its telomeric location. On chromosome 4p16, the breakpoints occur within the 5′ exon of the MMSET gene. The hybrid transcripts between IgH and MMSET gene are easily detected using reverse transcriptase polymerase chain reaction. The breakpoint on chromosome 4 occurs 50 to 100 kb centromeric to the fibroblast growth factor receptor 3 (*FGFR3*) gene. FGFR3 is one of the four high-affinity tyrosine kinase receptors for FGF. This receptor is not expressed in normal plasma cells. Signaling through FGFR results in phosphorylation of STAT3 and activation of the MAPK pathway. FGFR signaling can substitute for IL-6 with respect to the growth and survival of myeloma cells, and inhibition of FGFR signaling results in apoptosis.[151] FGFR3 may constitute a potential target for experimental therapies in patients with the t(4;14) translocation. Approximately one third of the myeloma cell lines with t(4:14) have activating mutations involving FGFR3. Patients who do not have activating FGFR3 mutations may have mutations of Ras.[152] A strong association between the t(4;14) translocation and chromosome 13/hypodiploidy has been observed, and t(4;14) has been associated with a poor prognosis.[153,154] Whether t(4;14) is present in stable MGUS patients is unclear.

Using FISH techniques, the t(14;16)(q32;q23) translocation has been identified in 5% to 10% of patients with MM. It leads to dysregulation of the c-*maf* protooncogene. c-Maf is a basic zipper transcription factor belonging to the AP1 superfamily and is widely expressed not only in embryonic but also in adult tissues. It is involved in the transcription of IL-6. Unexpectedly, *c-maf* expression was also observed in myeloma cell lines lacking the *c-maf* translocation.[155] Using gene expression profiling, three *c-maf* target genes were identified: cyclin D2, integrin β_7, and CCR1. c-Maf transactivates the cyclin D2 promotor and enhances myeloma proliferation. Increased levels of integrin β_7 enhance adhesion of myeloma cells to bone marrow stroma and increase production of VEGF. CCR1 is the receptor for MIP-1α and increases the chemotaxis of myeloma cells.[155] Patients with this translocation have a poor prognosis, at least with conventional chemotherapy.[156]

The t(14;20)(q32;q11) translocation results in aberrant expression of MafB, another basic transcription factor, and is present in fewer than 5% of newly diagnosed myeloma patients.[156,157] It appears to be associated with poor outcome.

The t(6;14)(p21;32) translocation results in dysregulation of cyclin D3 and has been identified in 4% of patients using metaphase chromosome analysis and in 6% of patients using gene expression profiling.[158] In approximately 20% to 25% of myeloma patients, either cyclin D1 or cyclin D3 is involved in translocations, highlighting the importance of this pathway.

The t(6;14)(p25;q32) translocation occurs downstream of the *IRF-4* gene, a member of the interferon regulatory factor family. The exact incidence of this translocation in patients with myeloma and its role in pathogenesis of myeloma are unclear. This translocation is found in approximately 18% of myeloma cell lines.[159]

The t(8;14)(q24;q32) translocation involves the protooncogene c-*myc*. This classic translocation for Burkitt lymphoma occurs very rarely in myeloma and mostly in the advanced stages of the disease.

The t(9;14)(p13;q32) translocation has been found in rare patients with myeloma. This translocation dysregulates the *PAX-5* gene at 9p13 and is seen more frequently in lymphoplasmacytoid lymphoma.[160]

Deletion 13q14 (Δ13)

By conventional cytogenetics, deletion of chromosome 13 has been detected in approximately 15% to 20% of the patients. Using interphase FISH, deletions have been detected in 50% of the patients.[161] Using 11 probes spanning the entire long arm, chromosome 13 deletions have been found in up to 86% of patients.[162] A 13q deletion by FISH is also found in 50% of patients with MGUS.[163,164] In contrast to MM, however, the 13q14 abnormality in MGUS may be restricted to a small subpopulation of cells, probably indicating that it is a secondary genetic event occurring after clonal expansion. The finding of 13q abnormalities with conventional karyotyping has been associated with poor outcomes in patients treated with either conventional chemotherapy[165] or tandem transplants.[146,166] The presence of 13q deletion as assessed by FISH studies has been associated with a poor outcome.[167] The poor prognosis in these patients probably is entirely related to the one third of patients who have a 13q deletion by conventional cytogenetics (Fig. 87–7). Chromosome 13q abnormalities are common in chronic lymphocytic leukemia but do not confer an adverse prognosis. Monoallelic deletion of the *Rb* gene, present in approximately 50% of the myeloma patients, does not seem to affect Rb protein expression. A high incidence of 13q deletions has been reported in patients with MM and a history of MGUS, suggesting that it may be involved in the transformation of MGUS into myeloma.[163] As mentioned earlier, there is an association between 13q deletions and t(4;14). Chromosome 13 deletion can be detected by gene expression profiling.[168] *IGF1R* is overexpressed in patients with deletion 13 by FISH.[168] Because myeloma cells express *IGF1*, this may represent an autocrine growth signal loop in this type of myeloma.

Hypodiploidy

Hypodiploidy in myeloma initially was detected by DNA content[138] but when detected by conventional karyotyping was found to have a negative impact on survival.[169] It often is associated with deletion of chromosome 13. French investigators suggested that hypodiploidy, and not the 13q deletion, was the major negative prognostic factor in MM. A subsequent analysis of hypodiploidy and the deletion of chromosome 13 in 1000 patients showed that both abnormalities are independently associated with poor prognoses.[170]

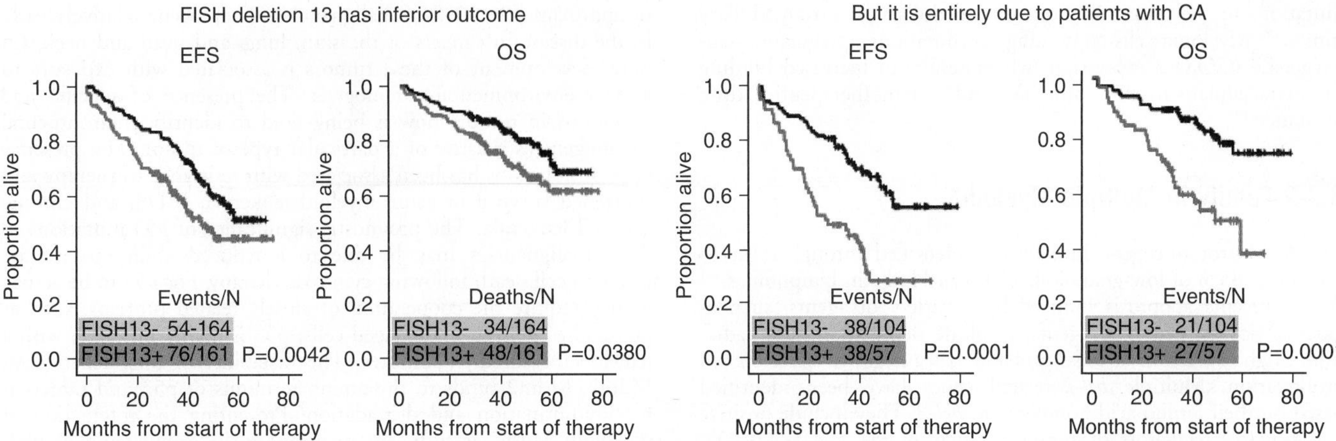

Figure 87–7 Fluorescent in situ hybridization deletion 13 (FISH 13+) occurs in approximately 50% of myeloma patients, whereas deletion of chromosome 13 by metaphase cytogenetics is seen in approximately 17% of patients. Although event-free survival (EFS) and overall survival (OS) of myeloma patients with FISH deletion, the difference in outcome is entirely due to the poor prognosis of patients who in addition to FISH deletion 13 have abnormal metaphase cytogenetics (CA). *(From Zhan F, Sawyer J, Tricot G: The role of cytogenetics in myeloma. Leukemia 20:1484, 2006.)*

Gene Expression Profiling

Metaphase and FISH chromosomal analysis are relatively crude methods for assessing DNA damage. Gene expression profiling permits quantitation of RNA expression of more than 30,000 genes, many related to important cancer features such as proliferation, apoptosis, DNA repair, and drug resistance. Based on unsupervised hierarchical clustering of highly purified plasma cells of newly diagnosed myeloma patients, seven subgroups were identified, related to either spiked gene expression as a consequence of translocations involving 14q32 or hyperdiploidy or a proliferative signature.[171] In addition to its biologic significance, the seven-group gene model had major prognostic implications, with an inferior outcome seen in patients with a proliferative signature and translocations involving *MMSET*, that is, t(4;14) or c-*maf;* t(14;16) or MafB; t(14;20). In an effort to identify gene expression patterns linked to an aggressive disease course, a model was created that included 70 genes with either very high (quartile 4) or very low expression (quartile 1) and correlating with outcome.[172] It was remarkable that 30% of these genes mapped to chromosome 1. One of these genes, *CKS1B*, maps to chromosome 1q21, which often shows gains based on comparative genomic hybridization[173] CKS1B is an essential cofactor of the SCF (Skp1-Cullin1-F-box protein) ubiquitin ligase complex that regulates p27 ubiquitination and degradation. Amplification of 1q21 (three or more signals) can be assessed by FISH. Patients with amplification of 1q21 have an inferior 5-year event-free survival (EFS) and overall survival (OS).[174] A combination of metaphase cytogenetic abnormalities and either *CKS1B* by gene array or amplification of 1q21 by FISH, after exclusion of cases with t(11;14), identifies most patients with a poor prognosis even after tandem transplants.[175] A poor prognosis was seen in all stages of the International Staging System.

Oncogenes/Suppressor Genes in Myeloma

Dysregulation of oncogenes and suppressor genes that control cellular proliferation, survival, and apoptosis contribute to the pathogenesis of most malignancies, including MM.

Loss of Function of Suppressor Genes

The *p15* and *p16* genes often are hypermethylated in MM and, therefore, deactivated,[176,177] even more frequently in advanced disease.[178,179] Whether hypermethylation of these genes is an early immortalization event in MGUS[180] or appears during progression of the myeloma is unclear.[181]

Levels of p21 and p27 protein are increased in patients with myeloma, probably as a consequence of the constitutively activated STAT3 pathway. They protect myeloma cells from apoptosis by inducing cell cycle arrest and allow subsequent DNA repair. Upregulation of expression of these gene products probably is a major factor in inducing resistance to chemotherapy and radiation therapy. Degradation of p27 occurs in the proteasome complex and is inhibited by bortezomib.

SOCS1 and *SHP1* are often hypermethylated in myeloma.[182] Suppressor of cytokine secretion (SOCS) members are induced by cytokines and are negative regulators of cytokine signaling. SHP1 is a tyrosine phosphatase. Both negatively regulate the Jak/STAT signaling pathway.

Death-associated protein (DAP) kinase promoter is hypermethylated in two thirds of primary myeloma samples.[183] DAP kinase is a cytoskeletal-associated serine/threonine kinase with death-inducing properties. Because myeloma in the early stages is a disease with very slow growth, hypermethylation of this gene may be critical in the induction and maintenance of tumor cells.

ras Oncogenes

The frequency of *ras* mutations in newly diagnosed patients with MM is approximately 40%[184] and increases significantly with disease progression. Mutations are present in most patients with terminal disease or plasma cell leukemia.[185,186] The most frequent mutation seems to be in N-*ras* at codon 61. Activating mutations of *ras* likely result in independence of myeloma cells from external cytokines such as IL-6 and IGF. It probably is one of the first mechanisms myeloma cells acquire in becoming stroma independent. Transduction of the IL-6–dependent cell line ANBL-6 with mutant *ras* makes this cell line IL 6 independent.[187]

More recently, N-*ras* mutations at codon 61 have been detected in plasma cells of all 34 myeloma patients examined, suggesting that mutational activation of N-*ras* is a mandatory event in the pathogenesis of MM.[188] *ras* Mutations are not evenly distributed among different molecular subclasses. A higher frequency of *ras* mutations is seen in patients expressing high levels of cyclin D1, whereas a low frequency of such mutations is seen in patients with t(4;14).[189] Surprisingly, in patients with paired samples of intramedullary and extramedullary myeloma, *ras* mutations were found only in the extramedullary plasmacytomas, suggesting a role of *ras* mutations in the transition from intramedullary to extramedullary tumor.[188] Myeloma cells containing *ras* mutations upregulate cyclo-oxygenase (COX)-2 expression, which results in increased binding to extracellular matrix proteins and chemotherapeutic drug resistance.[190]

Bcl-2 Family in Multiple Myeloma

The *bcl-2* protooncogene initially was identified through t(14;18) present in 85% of low-grade follicular non-Hodgkin lymphomas.[191] Bcl-2 prevents apoptosis induced by a variety of agents, such as glucocorticoids, cytotoxic agents, cytokine deprivation, and radiation. High expression of *bcl-2* probably has a negative effect on cell proliferation. Multiple *bcl-2*–related genes have been identified based on their amino acid homology to *bcl-2.* They include positive and negative regulators of apoptosis, such as Bax, Bcl-X_L, Bcl-X_s, Mcl-1, and A-1. These proteins localize to the outer membrane of the mitochondria. Bax initiates an increase in permeability of the outer mitochondrial membrane leading to cytosolic release of cytochrome C. An activation complex consisting of cytochrome C, apoptotic protease activating factor 1, and deoxyadenosine triphosphate triggers activation of caspases, which in turn effects cell demise. Antiapoptotic members of the Bcl-2 family prevent this increase in permeability of the outer mitochondrial membranes by associating with Bax. Smac/diablo is another apoptogenic protein released from the mitochondria that can induce activation of caspases and lead to cell death. Smac binds to IAPs, overcoming their inhibitory influence on various caspases.[192] Levels of Bcl-2 in myeloma usually are increased and contribute to the resistance of myeloma cells to chemotherapy. It has also been suggested that Bcl-2 expression is upregulated after exposure to chemotherapeutic agents.[193] Most myeloma cells show overexpression of Bcl-X_L and Mcl-1.[194] There seems to be a good correlation between the expression of the latter two gene products. Their expression is tightly regulated by IL-6. It appears that Mcl-1 rather than Bcl-2 or Bcl-X_L is essential to survival of myeloma cells, based on antisense strategies. Antisense oligonucleotides against Mcl-1 trigger an important decrease of viability in myeloma cell lines and in primary myeloma cells, whereas neither Bcl-2 nor Bcl-X_L antisense affected the viability of myeloma cells.[195]

Retinoblastoma Gene in Multiple Myeloma

The *Rb* tumor suppressor gene is located on chromosome 13q14 and codes for a nuclear phosphoprotein that suppresses the G_1 to S transition of the cell cycle by inhibiting E2F-mediated transactivation of a variety of genes involved in initiating DNA synthesis, such as *myc,* dihydrofolate reductase, and thymidine kinase. Hypophosphorylated or dephosphorylated Rb protein binds E2F and prevents its activity. Mutations of the *Rb* gene or protein contribute to cellular transformation in many types of malignancies. Elimination or deactivation of both *Rb* gene copies is required for manifestation of a tumorigenic phenotype. Several independent studies have concluded that *Rb* gene deletion is frequent in myeloma.[196,197] However, biallelic deletion of *Rb* is infrequent.[198] Monoallelic deletion of *Rb* does not appear to modulate expression of the Rb protein. Evidence indicates that IL-6 promotes MM cell growth through phosphorylation of the Rb protein.[102,199] Whether *Rb* deletion plays any role in myeloma transformation is unclear.

p53 Mutations

The p53 protein plays a central role in modulating cellular responses to cytotoxic agents by contributing to cell cycle arrest and programmed cell death. Loss of *p53* function usually is accomplished through mutations and leads to inappropriate cell growth, increased cell survival, and genetic instability. *p53* gene mutations are observed in approximately 50% of malignancies. They occur relatively early in the disease in cancers of the skin, lung, and head and neck. Of note, development of these tumors is associated with exposure to known environmental carcinogens. The presence of specific *p53* mutations in tumors now is being used to identify environmental carcinogens as a cause of a particular type of tumor. The presence of *p53* mutations has been associated with resistance to therapy and shortened survival in acute myeloid leukemia, MDS, and chronic myeloid leukemia. The prognostic significance of *p53* mutations in these malignancies may be due to a reduced ability to initiate program cell death following cytotoxic therapy. For *p53* to be active, it may require the cooperation of closely related proteins, such as p63 and p73.[200] In undamaged cells, p53 is highly unstable, with a half-life measured in minutes. The instability of p53 depends on Mdm2. Mdm2 binds to the amino terminus of p53 and targets it for ubiquitination and degradation. Preventing the interaction of p53 with Mdm2 is sufficient to promote the stabilization of p53. Mdm2 protein facilitates G_1 to S phase transition by activating E2F-1 and enhances cell survival by suppressing wild-type p53. Mdm2 is strongly and constitutively expressed in MM cell lines and in plasma cell leukemia cells.[201] Mdm2 enhances cell cycle progression in myeloma cells by downregulating cell cycle inhibitory proteins such as p21. p53 may be involved in transcriptional repression of the IL-6 gene during cellular differentiation and oncogenesis.[202] *p53* mutations are very uncommon in myeloma and usually are associated with the end-stages of the disease,[185,203] explaining the common occurrence of *p53* mutations in human myeloma cell lines, which are derived from end-stage patients.[204] The overall incidence of *p53* mutations probably is not more than 8% to 10%.[205] This is confirmed by the very low incidence of p53 antibodies in MM.[206] In contrast, the presence of *p53* gene deletion as measured by FISH, and which usually is monoallelic, has been detected in 10% to 33% of myeloma patients; it usually is caused by an interstitial deletion of 17p.[207] *p53* gene deletion has been associated with stage III disease and significantly shorter survival times compared with patients without the deletion.[207,208]

c-myc in Myeloma

The c-Myc protein is a nuclear phosphoprotein with DNA-binding properties. c-Myc heterodimerizes with max, a protein that cooperates with c-myc to bind specifically to core DNA sequences. c-myc participates in the regulation of gene transcription of normal and neoplastic cells. It plays a role in controlling proliferation, differentiation, and apoptosis. The classic translocations t(8;14), t(2;8), or t(8;22) juxtaposing c-myc and the IgH or Ig light-chain locus are the hallmark of Burkitt lymphoma. Although such translocations also occur in murine plasmacytomas induced by pristine, in human myeloma, the classic t(8;14) occurs in less than 5% of cases.

Transcription of c-myc in the normal plasma cells is repressed by blimp-1, an inducer of terminal B-cell differentiation. However,[209] in human MM, elevated myc expression was found in approximately 25% of myeloma patients.[210] In a subsequent study, *c-myc* gene transcripts were detected in 92% of cases (12 out of 13) with no correlation to proliferative activity, as measured by KI-67, but correlating with the extent of bone marrow plasmacytosis and percentage of plasmablasts.[211] It was shown that c-myc abrogates p53-induced G1 arrest by interfering with the inhibitory action of p21.[212] In the absence of growth factors, c-myc is an important inducer of apoptosis. Induction of apoptosis by c-myc can be counteracted by bcl-2 expression.[213] *c-myc* and cyclin D3 genes are independent targets for glucocorticoid inhibition of lymphoid cell proliferation.[214] Using FISH analysis, c-myc rearrangements have been detected in approximately 15% of myeloma patients and 55% of myeloma cell lines.[215] These translocations are often complex, frequently do not involve the IgH locus, and are typically not expressed in all the myeloma cells, suggesting that c-myc rearrangements occur late in myeloma development.

Fas Gene in Myeloma

The Fas antigen, CD95, is a transmembrane protein that induces apoptosis when engaged by Fas ligand. Point mutations of the *Fas* gene have been identified in 10% of primary myeloma samples (4/48) leading to blocking apoptosis by the Fas ligand.[216] All of the mutations identified were located in the cytoplasmic region of the Fas antigen, known to be involved in transduction of apoptotic signals. In addition, it has been shown that β_1-integrin–mediated adhesion (VLA-4) to fibronectin inhibits Fas-induced caspase 8 activation. This adhesion-dependent inhibition of Fas-mediated apoptosis correlates with enhanced c-*fas*–associated death domainlike IL-1–converting enzymelike inhibitory protein (cFLIP).[217] Expression of the Fas antigen was found in 7 of 11 primary myeloma samples. Remarkably, Fas ligand was found in all five cases with high serum LDH.[218] Myeloma cells upregulate Fas ligand,[219] leading to erythroblast apoptosis, partly explaining the anemia observed in myeloma.

TNF-Related Apoptosis-Inducing Ligand

TRAIL induces apoptosis of primary myeloma cells and of the majority of myeloma cell lines, both sensitive and resistant to dexamethasone, doxorubicin, or melphalan, and overcomes the survival effect of IL-6 on myeloma cells. It induces apoptosis of myeloma cells by interacting with a complex system of cell surface receptors, including the death signal-transducing receptors DR4 and DR5. In contrast, death receptors DR1 and DR2 lack a functional death domain and cannot transduce a proapoptotic signal and therefore are considered decoy receptors. Both NF-κB inhibitors and proteosome inhibitor PS-341 enhance the proapoptotic activity of TRAIL. TRAIL activates caspase 8 in TRAIL-sensitive myeloma cells. Sensitivity in TRAIL-resistant myeloma cells is restored by cycloheximide and the protein kinase C inhibitor bisindolylmaleimide, which lowers cFLIP and the cellular inhibitor of apoptosis protein 2.[220]

CLINICAL MANIFESTATIONS

The clinical manifestations of MM are the direct consequence of marrow infiltration by plasma cells, production of monoclonal protein in blood or urine, and immune deficiency (Fig. 87–8).

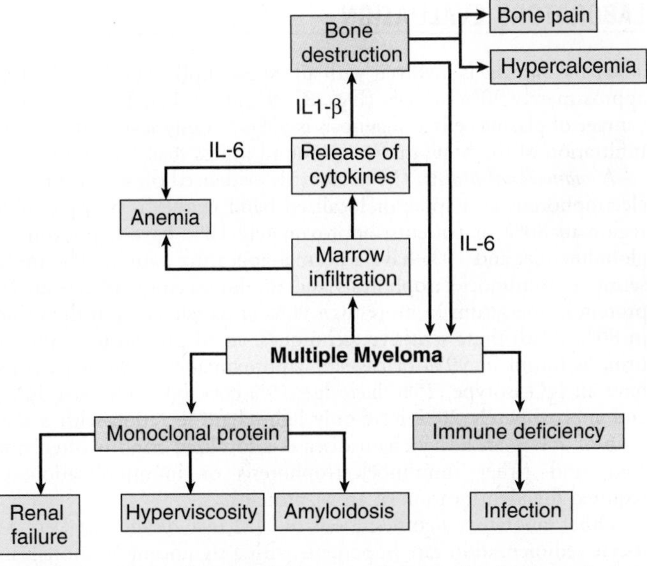

Figure 87–8 Major clinical and laboratory features of multiple myeloma.

Bone Pain

Bone pain, typically in the back (spine) or chest (ribs) and less often in the extremities, is present at diagnosis in more than two thirds of patients. The pain usually is aggravated by movement. The patient's height may be reduced by several inches because of collapse of one or more vertebral bodies.[221] Sudden onset of back pain in an individual older than 40 years, especially if the complaint is new for the patient, is sufficient to suspect the diagnosis of myeloma and should lead to a proper workup for the disease.

Renal Insufficiency

The two major causes of renal insufficiency in MM are myeloma kidney and hypercalcemia. Myeloma kidney is characterized by the presence of large, waxy, laminated casts in the distal and collecting tubules. The casts are composed mainly of precipitated monoclonal light chains and are surrounded by multinucleated syncytial epithelial cells (giant cells). The casts result in dilation and atrophy of the renal tubules. Eventually the entire nephron becomes nonfunctional, and interstitial fibrosis may occur.[222] The extent of cast formation correlates directly with the amount of free urinary light chains, but the actual mechanism of nephrotoxicity from Bence Jones proteinuria is unknown, although dehydration, associated with hypercalcemia, or radiographic contrast medium studies may precipitate myeloma kidney. Myeloma kidney is more often encountered with λ light chains.

The second most common course of renal insufficiency is hypercalcemia, resulting in hypercalciuria and osmotic diuresis, leading to volume depletion and prerenal kidney failure. Hypercalcemia also may cause calcium deposits, leading to interstitial nephritis. Hyperuricemia as well as nonsteroidal antiinflammatory drugs reduce blood flow to the glomeruli and may promote the development of renal failure. Patients with myeloma are highly sensitive to nephrotoxic medications, such as aminoglycosides, cisplatin, amphotericin B, and cyclosporine A. Plasma cell-derived (light-chain associated [AL]) amyloidosis of the kidney in myeloma patients is associated with minimal light-chain proteinuria and usually presents as nephrotic syndrome, but it can lead to renal failure with time (see Chapter 89). Probably underestimated as a cause of renal failure is Ig light-chain deposition disease, which is commonly associated with κ light-chain myeloma proteins, in which monoclonal light chains are deposited in renal glomeruli. Urinary total protein and M protein usually are minimal. The histopathologic picture resembles nodular glomerulosclerosis, but electron microscopy reveals granular, electron-dense deposits representing light chains. Myeloma involvement of the kidneys is uncommon but should be suspected in patients who have renal enlargement that is not caused by amyloidosis. IL-6 may contribute to renal failure.[110]

Bisphosphonates, especially infused over a short period, eventually may lead to renal insufficiency, usually preceded by nonspecific proteinuria in case of pamidronate but not commonly in the case of zoledronate.

Hypercalcemia

Some patients with myeloma have paraproteins that avidly bind calcium, resulting in spurious hypercalcemia. The best solution to this problem involves measuring the ionized serum calcium level. Hypercalcemia occurs in 30% to 40% of patients with MM and usually is associated with a large disease burden. Hypercalcemia is the presenting finding in 15% to 30% of patients and leads to lethargy, polyuria, polydipsia, constipation, nausea, and vomiting.[223] Levels of total serum calcium should be adjusted for serum protein concentrations, especially albumin. Pronounced hypoalbuminemia, caused by an increased level of IL-6, poor food intake, or urinary loss in the case of concomitant amyloidosis, can mask frank hypercalcemia unless an ionized serum calcium level is measured.

Neurologic Symptoms

Neurologic symptoms usually are the result of compression by a soft-tissue plasmocytoma or bone fragments of a vertebral body on the spinal cord or on a nerve. The pain usually is in the thoracic or lumbosacral area. Compression of the spinal cord must be considered an oncologic emergency requiring prompt intervention. It is best diagnosed by MRI. In addition to back pain with radicular features, weakness or paralysis of the lower extremities and bowel or bladder incontinence may occur. Peripheral neuropathy is uncommon in MM and almost always is associated with amyloidosis. It is seen in osteosclerotic myeloma and sometimes is part of the polyneuropathy, organomegaly, endocrinopathy, monoclonal protein, and skin changes (POEMS) syndrome. Intracranial plasmacytomas usually represent extensions of myelomatous lesions of the skull and may lead to cranial nerve deficits or, more infrequently, leptomeningeal infiltration (usually seen only in the terminal phases of the disease). Peripheral neuropathy, mainly sensory (numbness and paresthesias), is a common side effect of thalidomide and, to a lesser extent, bortezomib therapy.

Hyperviscosity

In contrast to Waldenström macroglobulinemia, hyperviscosity is rare in MM, occurring in less than 10% of patients. Because of a greater tendency for IgA to form polymers, patients with IgA myeloma more often have features of hyperviscosity, resulting in circulatory problems and leading to cerebral, pulmonary, and renal manifestations. Hyperviscosity often is associated with bleeding. Among patients with IgG myeloma, those with the IgG3 subclass are most likely to develop hyperviscosity. The diagnosis of hyperviscosity can be made by measuring serum viscosity or by funduscopic examination showing slow blood flow in blood vessels that often are distorted. Hyperviscosity can give the clinical and radiologic pictures of pulmonary edema and will worsen only if treated with diuretics. Plasmapheresis is the appropriate treatment of the condition.

Amyloidosis

Amyloidosis is a clinical syndrome that results from extramedullary deposition of insoluble fibrillar protein. A diagnosis of MM can be made in 20% of patients with AL amyloidosis.[221] Approximately 3% of patients with newly diagnosed MM have overt amyloidosis,[224] but the frequency of asymptomatic amyloidosis in myeloma, as diagnosed by subcutaneous fat aspiration and rectal and bone marrow biopsies, is much higher (35%).[225] The most common clinical manifestations are carpal tunnel syndrome or generalized edema due to nephrotic syndrome. Less common manifestations are cardiomyopathy, macroglossia, and extensive bruising around the eyelids. The presence of symptomatic amyloidosis in patients with MM adds to morbidity rates and has an adverse effect on survival.[224] When treated with conventional chemotherapy, the median survival duration of patients with myeloma and amyloidosis is approximately 12 months.[224] More encouraging results have been obtained with high-dose melphalan and stem cell support.[226]

Infections

Patients with MM have an increased susceptibility to develop infections because of the associated hypogammaglobulinemia. Myeloma patients are not able to mount a vigorous primary immune response and have an impaired secondary antibody response to antigens. Defects of T cells, natural killer cells, and monocytes may accelerate and contribute to humoral deficiency. The additional immunosuppressive effect of chemotherapy, especially with corticosteroids, further increases the infection risk. The average MM patient will suffer from 0.5 to 1.5 infections per year, with the highest frequency during the first 2 months of treatment. Polysaccharide-encapsulated organisms, especially *Streptococcus pneumoniae* and *Haemophilus influenzae*, initially were identified as the major causes of infection. However, now it is clear that enteric gram-negative bacilli are the most common isolates, accounting for approximately 60%; encapsulated organisms represent less than 25% of blood culture isolates. Oral thrush is the only fungal infection of significance. Other organisms, such as anaerobes, *Mycobacterium tuberculosis*, herpes simplex, cytomegalovirus, and varicella zoster, are uncommon unless patients have received transplantation. Early diagnosis and prompt initiation of broad-spectrum antibiotic therapy are critical in patients with MM. Third-generation cephalosporins or extended-spectrum penicillins are used most frequently. Infection prophylaxis with trimethoprim-sulfamethoxazole is effective in decreasing the incidence of infectious complications during the first few months of initial standard-dose chemotherapy.[227] Vaccination against influenza in patients with MM is safe and may have significant benefits.[228]

Extramedullary Disease

Extramedullary plasmacytomas have been found in the lymph nodes, skin, liver, and spleen and occasionally in the kidneys, breast, testis, and meninges. The finding usually is associated with high serum LDH levels and plasmablastic morphology (end-stage myeloma). Patients usually have poor outcomes even with more aggressive treatment approaches.

Bleeding and Anemia

Bleeding problems occur in 15% of IgG myelomas and 30% of IgA myelomas and may be due to platelet dysfunction or acquired coagulopathy. Thrombocytopenia, even with extensive bone marrow involvement, is rare in the early phases of the disease. The preserved platelet count might be related to increased IL-6 levels, which promote megakaryocyte maturation. Anemia, which is present in two thirds of myeloma patients, is the consequence of increased IL-6 production by the microenvironment, MIP-1α secretion by myeloma cells, and Fas ligand expression on their membranes, inducing apoptosis of red cell precursors. It may be spuriously aggravated by expansion of plasma volume due to large amounts of circulating Igs. Serum erythropoietin levels are low relative to the degree of anemia, a finding that probably is due to abundant production of cytokines such as IL-1β and TNF-β. Routine use of erythropoietin should be encouraged in cases of anemia.

LABORATORY EVALUATION

The *bone marrow* is involved with an excess of plasma cells (>5%) in approximately 90% of cases (Figs. 87–9 and 87–10). The mean percentage of plasma cells at diagnosis is 30%.[229] Only scattered nodular infiltration of the bone marrow is found in less than 5% of cases.

A *monoclonal protein* (M protein) is evidenced on serum protein electrophoresis as a spike or localized band in the β- or γ-globulin region in 80% of patients; approximately 10% have hypogammaglobulinemia, and 10% have a normal-appearing pattern. The more sensitive immunoelectrophoresis and immunofixation reveals an M protein in the serum in more than 90% of patients and in the urine in 80%. With these sensitive techniques, an M protein in serum or urine is found in 99% of cases.[221] Approximately 55% of patients have an IgG isotype, 25% have IgA, 1% have IgD, 1% have IgM, and approximately 20% have only light-chain secretion with a κ/λ ratio of 2:1.[230] In heavy-chain disease, a localized band is often not seen, and either immunoelectrophoresis or immunofixation is required for identification of an M protein.

Other laboratory manifestations of MM include increased erythrocyte sedimentation rate in patients with a significant M protein in the serum, elevated creatinine in approximately half of cases, and a decreased albumin level, which usually is associated with increased IL-6 activity.

A relatively new test that has rapidly gained importance measures the concentration of serum Ig free light chains. Serum concentrations of free light chains are dependent upon the balance of production by plasma cells and renal function. In cases of increased polyclonal Ig production or renal failure, both κ and λ concentrations can increase considerably, but the κ/λ ratio remains unchanged. Approximately 20% of myeloma patients have either nonsecretory or light-chain only disease. The majority of those patients have abnormal free light-chain concentrations. Among patients with a clear serum M protein, 95% have abnormal free light-chain concentrations.[231] The serum free light-chain concentration and serum M protein level do not correlate. In general, the larger the imbalance between light- and heavy-chain production, the more aggressive the myeloma, although there are exceptions. The half-life of free light chains is short (2–6 hours), compared to more than 20 days for intact IgG. Therefore, responses to therapy will be noted much more rapidly by following free light-chain concentrations than serum M protein.[232] Serum free light-chain concentrations are below the sensitivity of serum protein electrophoresis, although occasional patients have a persistent serum M protein and normal free-light concentrations and ratio. Regular followup of free light chains is a good method for detecting early myeloma relapse. Serum free light-chain concentrations are important in assessing hematologic responses in patients with AL amyloidosis and in predicting survival after therapy.[233]

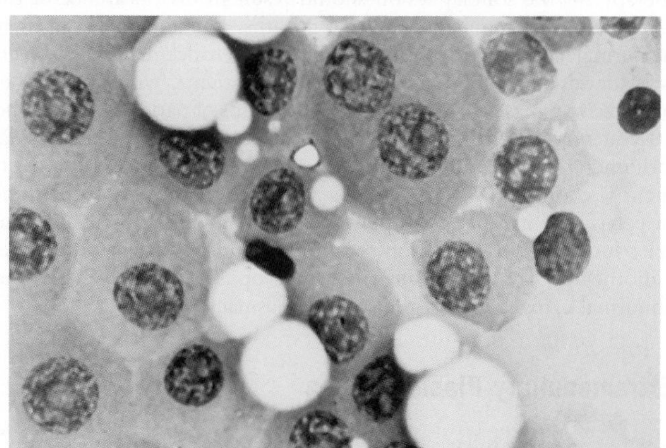

Figure 87–9 Bone marrow is invaded by plasma cells, which are more immature than normal plasma cells, as evidenced by a more delicate chromatin structure and the presence of a nucleolus in some of the cells.

DIAGNOSIS

Minimal criteria for diagnosis of overt myeloma include the presence of at least 10% abnormal plasma cells in the bone marrow or histologic proof of a plasmacytoma and at least one of the following abnormalities: serum M protein (usually >3 g/dL), M protein in the urine (usually >1 g/dL), or osteolytic lesions.[234]

If the diagnosis of MM is suspected, the physician should obtain, in addition to a complete history and physical examination, the following tests: complete blood count with differential, electrolytes, blood urea nitrogen, creatinine, calcium, phosphorus, uric acid, LDH, alkaline phosphatase, serum protein electrophoresis, quantitative Igs, serum immunoelectrophoresis, β_2 microglobulin (β_2M),

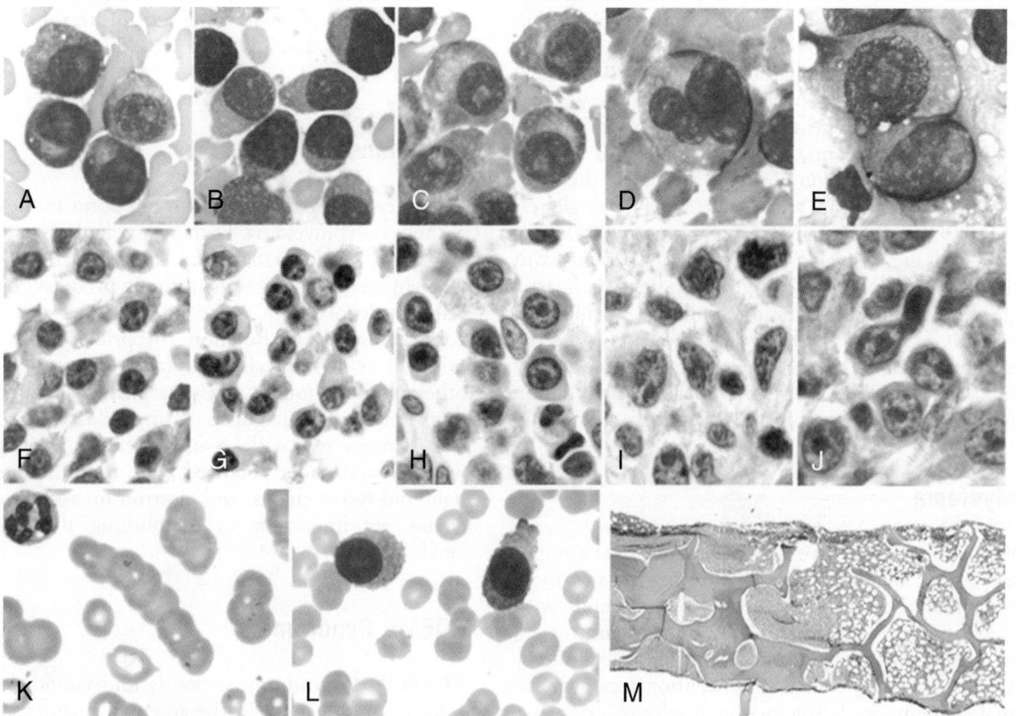

Figure 87–10 Multiple myeloma. **A–J,** Morphologic spectrum of myeloma. Multiple myeloma exhibits a wide cytologic and morphologic spectrum in the bone marrow aspirate and biopsy. **A, F,** The typical type has fairly mature appearing plasma cells with eccentric nuclei and cytoplasmic hofs. **B, G,** A lymphocytelike type has less abundant cytoplasm. **C, H,** A dyssynchronous type C, H) has mature chromatin but prominent nucleoli. **D, I,** An anaplastic type has highly irregular plasma cells that on the aspirate sometimes resembles monocytes **(D).** This type can present a diagnostic challenge if myeloma is not suspected. **E, J,** The plasmablastic type can be difficult to distinguish morphologically from immunoblastic lymphoma. **K,** Rouleau formation. The red cells resemble a stack of coins. **L,** Plasma cell leukemia. A diagnosis can be made when circulating plasma cells are greater than 2×10^9/L or when they account for greater than 20% of circulating leukocytes. **M,** Osteosclerotic myeloma. The left side of the illustration shows bone sclerosis and the marrow cavity replaced by myeloma. This patient had the polyneuropathy, organomegaly, endocrinopathy, monoclonal protein, and skin changes (POEMS) syndrome.

CRP, free light chains, radiographic survey of the bones, and bone marrow aspirate and biopsy, preferentially with PCLI and cytogenetics, and either MRI with T1 and short T1 inversion recovery images or PET/CT scan. In case of a solitary plasmacytoma, MRI of the head, spine, pelvis, shoulders, and sternum or PET/CT scan are indicated to better evaluate the extent of disease. In case of severe back pain, MRI of the spine is performed to exclude cord compression. If extramedullary disease is suspected, PET/CT scan is the preferred test.

DIFFERENTIAL DIAGNOSIS

In patients with monoclonal gammopathies associated with borderline bone marrow plasmacytosis, connective tissue diseases, chronic infections, carcinoma, and lymphoma should be excluded. In most patients, however, the diagnosis of MM is readily established. It is important to distinguish myeloma from MGUS, solitary plasmacytoma of the bone, and amyloidosis. Imaging tests such as MRI and PET/CT scan, free light chains, cytogenetics, and PCLI will help in the differential diagnosis.

Monoclonal Gammopathy of Undetermined Significance

MGUS is characterized by the presence of a serum M protein concentration usually less than 3 g/dL, less than 10% plasma cells in the bone marrow, no or only small amounts of Bence Jones protein in the urine, absence of lytic lesions or focal lesions due to myeloma cells on MRI and PET/CT scan, anemia, hypercalcemia, cytogenetic abnormalities with conventional karyotyping and renal insufficiency, and, most importantly, the presence of a stable M protein.[23] MGUS is found in approximately 3% of individuals older than 70 years. Of all patients with monoclonal gammopathies, 62% have MGUS.[235] Most patients with MGUS die of unrelated causes (52%), whereas 22% have either no substantial increase in M protein or an increase in M protein without any symptoms, and 11% progress to MM.[235] The median interval from recognition of the M protein to the diagnosis of MM is 10 years (range 2–29 years). Currently, no single test can distinguish MGUS from MM. In MGUS, PCLI is low (<0.2%), and β_2M and CRP levels are normal.[138] Fifty percent of patients with MGUS have an abnormal DNA content either by flow cytometric analysis[138] or FISH.[136] On gene expression profiling, plasma cells from patients with MGUS cluster with myeloma patients and separate from normal bone marrow cells.[236] The clinical and laboratory features of patients with MGUS with chromosomal abnormalities on FISH analysis are indistinguishable from those without.

Smoldering Myeloma

Patients with smoldering disease have a serum monoclonal component greater than 3 g/dL but usually less than 4.5 g/dL and more than 10% marrow plasmacytosis. However, they have no end-organ damage, exemplified by normal renal function and calcium levels, very mild (if any) anemia, and no lytic bone lesions on skeletal survey or CT scan. PCLI is invariably low, and conventional cytogenetic analysis is normal. Patients with smoldering myeloma may have decreased uninvolved Ig levels and a small amount of Bence Jones proteinuria.[237,238] The median time to progression to active myeloma is 26 months, with shorter times observed in patients with higher levels of monoclonal protein and Bence Jones proteinuria. Response rates and survival times after initiation of treatment are similar despite the different times to progression. Participation of patients with smoldering myeloma in clinical trials evaluating the impact of various interventions on the time to disease progression is strongly encouraged.

Solitary Plasmacytoma of the Bone

Solitary plasmacytoma of bone is uncommon; it is present in 3% to 5% of patients with plasma cell dyscrasias. The most common symptom at diagnosis is pain. The median patient age is one decade younger than that in MM.[235]

The diagnosis is based on histologic evidence of a tumor consisting of light chain–restricted plasma cells with no other lesions on skeletal survey, MRI, or PET/CT scan, a normal bone marrow without clear excess of light chain–restricted plasma cells, and absence of an M protein in blood and urine; or, if M protein is present, therapy for the solitary lesion should result in disappearance of the M protein, which may take up to 6 months. The uninvolved Igs may be normal, and no evidence of anemia or hypercalcemia is seen. Overt MM develops in approximately 50% of patients, with evidence of progressive disease within 3 years in two thirds of patients. The 5- and 10-year survival rates are 74% and 45%, respectively.[235] Tumoricidal radiotherapy with 4000 to 5000 cGy has been considered the treatment of choice. However, such doses given to a large part of the spine or pelvis may hamper attempts to collect adequate numbers of stem cells for autotransplantation. Common findings after tumoricidal radiotherapy are continuing increased uptake on PET scan and abnormal cytogenetics of the solitary plasmacytoma.

Extramedullary Plasmacytoma

Isolated extramedullary (soft-tissue) plasmacytomata occurs more frequently in the respiratory sinuses, nasopharynx, larynx, and gastrointestinal tract.[239] The diagnosis is established by detection of monoclonal plasma cells in an involved organ biopsy in the absence of other disease manifestations. The treatment of choice is local radiotherapy, which in cases of head and neck lesions should encompass the adjacent lymph nodes. Approximately 70% of patients with extramedullary plasmacytoma remain free of disease at 10 years and less than 30% develop frank myeloma or multiple extramedullary tumors.[240]

Amyloidosis

Plasma cell-derived amyloidosis can occur in the context of MM but without overt myeloma. Primary amyloidosis and amyloidosis associated with myeloma have the same underlying pathologic process whereby excessive amounts of the Ig produced by a single clone of B cells are deposited in tissues in a manner and quality sufficient to compromise organ function. In primary amyloidosis, there is a minimal or no clinically detectable increase in plasma cells and no other manifestations of myeloma, such as anemia, hypercalcemia, and bone lesions. The diagnosis of amyloidosis is made by staining tissue with Congo red with resulting classic apple-green birefringence when viewed under polarized light, immunofluorescent staining for light and heavy chains, and electron microscopy.[222] Serum free light chains are important in establishing the diagnosis of primary amyloidosis.[233]

POEMS Syndrome

The POEMS syndrome is poorly understood. Other important features not represented in the acronym include sclerotic bone lesions (see Fig. 87–10 *M*), Castleman disease, thrombocytosis, pleural effusion, edema, and ascites. The dominant clinical feature is a sensorimotor demyelinating polyneuropathy, presumably due to the toxic effects of the secreted monoclonal Ig. Endocrine abnormalities (hypogonadism, hypothyroidism, primary adrenal dysfunction, diabetes mellitus) and skin changes (hyperpigmentation, acrocyanosis, hypertrichosis, multiple hemangiomata) were reported in approximately two thirds of 99 patients included in the largest, published series from the Mayo Clinic.[241] The amount of M protein (possible subtype in all cases in this series) was relatively small (median serum M spike of 1.1 g/dL). These patients have minimal bone marrow plasmacytosis (except in areas of sclerotic bone disease) and normal renal function and calcium levels. Cytokines appear important in the disease pathogenesis. IL-1β, IL-6, and TNF-α levels are elevated; more recently, VEGF has been implicated as having a potentially pathogenetic role. Chemotherapy, not including potentially neurotoxic agents, and aggressive local measures (surgery or radiotherapy) to alleviate the bone manifestations are indicated. High-dose treatment (HDT) with stem cell support has been found effective, especially in patients with rapidly progressive polyneuropathy, but is associated with significant morbidity.[242] The overall median survival duration in the Mayo Clinic series was 165 months.[241] Survival was adversely affected by the presence of clubbing and extravascular fluid overload. Responding patients had superior survival times. Infections and cardiorespiratory failure were the most common causes of death; no patient died of progression to frank myeloma.

Plasma Cell Leukemia

Although detection of circulating plasma cells in the peripheral blood by flow cytometry is not rare, the term *plasma cell leukemia* (PCL) is used when the absolute plasma cell count is greater than 2×10^9/L or the relative number is greater than 20% of the peripheral white cells (see Fig. 87–10 *L*). PCL may be de novo, when the patient is originally diagnosed in the leukemic phase, or secondary, when a patient with previously recognized myeloma undergoes leukemic transformation. Fewer than 5% of newly diagnosed MM patients present with PCL. These patients tend to have higher tumor burdens (compared with MM patients) and higher incidences of extramedullary involvement and thrombocytopenia. Elevated LDH and β_2M levels, higher proliferative potentials (expressed by percentage of plasma cells in S phase), and hypodiploidy are observed more frequently in PCL than MM.[243,244] In one series, 11 of 13 patients with PCL analyzed by FISH had monosomy of chromosome 13,[243] OS was much worse in PCL (8 months) versus MM (36 months), but it was significantly better in PCL patients treated with more aggressive chemotherapy than in those treated with melphalan plus prednisone (MP). The higher incidence of monosomy 13 in PCL patients was confirmed in another study.[141] Timely application of HDT is indicated in de novo PCL. Patients with secondary PCL usually are refractory to chemotherapy and have a poor survival compared to patients with primary PCL (median <2 months).[245]

PROGNOSTIC FACTORS

MM is a highly heterogeneous disease, with survival ranging from a few months to several years. The median survival achieved with standard treatment is approximately 3 years; a small percentage (5%) of patients survive more than 10 years.

Attempts to better identify subgroups of patients with distinct outcomes has led to the recognition of various prognostic factors. The serum level of β_2M is one of the most important prognostic factors in myeloma. β_2M is a small protein that associates with human leukocyte antigen class I and normally is excreted by the kidneys. It reflects tumor load and renal function; however, it predicts survival irrespective of renal function and Durie-Salmon stage.[246] The exact underlying biologic significance of β_2M is unknown; possible interactions with drug resistance pathways may exist. The best cutoff level at diagnosis is 6 mg/L.[246,247] Levels of β_2M may increase during treatment with interferon-α. The significance of β_2M as prognostic factor has been confirmed in HDT trials; the best cutoff level before autologous stem cell transplant is 2.5 mg/L.[248]

Serum concentrations of CRP, as a surrogate marker of IL-6 activity, is a prognostic factor independent of β_2M. Combining the two parameters stratifies patients into three groups with distinct prognoses when treated with standard therapy: a low-risk group with CRP and β_2M less than 6 mg/L, an intermediate-risk group with either CRP or β_2M of 6 mg/L or more, and a high-risk group with CRP and β_2M of 6 mg/L or more. The median survival duration in the three groups was 54, 27, and 6 months, respectively.[249] Given that any inflammation or infection can cause significant elevations of CRP, its prognostic value is relevant only in the absence of other possible causes for elevated CRP.

The *Durie-Salmon staging* system is based on a combination of factors that correlate with myeloma burden and renal function.[250] Patients with low tumor mass and a serum creatinine concentration less than 2 mg/dL have a median survival of approximately 5 years, whereas patients with high tumor burdens and renal insufficiencies have a median survival of 15 months. This staging system has allowed more uniform subgrouping of myeloma patients and, therefore, probably a more accurate interpretation of clinical trials. However, it has significant shortcomings in categorizing lytic bone lesions and does not take into consideration important characteristics such as the proliferative rate of the disease and the patient's response to treatment.

The *International Staging System*, which was introduced in 2005, is based on clinical and laboratory data gathered on 10,750 myeloma patients.[251] Serum β_2M, albumin, platelet count, creatinine level, and age were powerful predictors of survival. A combination of β_2M and albumin provides a simple and powerful staging system. Stage 1 is defined as β_2M less than 3.5 mg/L and albumin at least 3.5 g/dL. Median survival of stage 1 patients is 62 months. Stage 3 is defined as β_2M of 5.5 mg/L or higher. Median survival of stage 3 patients is 29 months. Stage 2 is defined as neither stage 1 or 3. Median survival of stage 2 patients is 44 months. It now is widely used as a prognostic parameter. However, it does not include genetic information gained from FISH analysis, metaphase cytogenetics, or gene expression profiling.

The *PCLI* reflects the proliferative capacity of malignant cells. In the presence of PCLI, CRP level does not provide additional prognostic information.[252,253] The combination of β_2M and PCLI allows identification of distinct subgroups regarding the prognosis. Median survival time is 17 months when both markers are elevated compared with 71 months when both markers are low.[254] Although clinical and biologic parameters such as β_2M and PCLI are quantitative and reproducible and are very useful indicators of outcome in patients receiving standard treatment, they do not address the fundamental genetic abnormalities involved in myeloma.

Angiogenesis (new blood vessel formation driven by increasing growth of malignant cells) appears to be important not only in solid tumors but also in hematologic malignancies. Both angiogenesis and expression by plasma cells of various adhesion molecules such as LFA-1, VLA-4, leukocyte adhesion molecule 1, and CD44 are markedly increased in patients with active MM (vs patients with nonactive MM and MGUS).[255] A positive correlation was found between bone marrow angiogenesis (evaluated as microvessel density) and tumor proliferation (evaluated by PCLI) in patients with MGUS, and active and nonactive MM. The combination of vessel density (high, if >2% of bone marrow microvessel area) and PCLI (high, if >1%) appropriately grouped more than 85% of MM patients between rapidly and slowly progressive disease.[256] Significantly increased microvessel densities in biopsy samples from patients with deletion of chromosome 13 have been reported.[257] Myeloma patients with low microvessel densities as assessed by immunostaining of bone marrow biopsies with anti-CD34 monoclonal antibodies survived longer than did patients with higher densities (independent prognostic factor).[258]

Plasmablastic myeloma occurs in approximately 8% of newly diagnosed patients and is considered to be present when at least 2% of the bone marrow plasma cell population consists of plasmablasts.[259] A *plasma cell* is defined as a plasmablast when it has a large nuclear size (>10 μm) or large nucleolus (>2 μm), fine reticular nuclear chromatin pattern with minimal or no clumping, and cytoplasm composing less than half the nuclear area.[260] Using these morphologic criteria, plasmablastic morphology was identified as an independent adverse prognostic factor in a large study of 453 newly diagnosed patients.[259] Median OS time was 1.9 years in patients with plasmablastic morphology versus 3.7 years in patients with nonplasmablastic morphology. The significance of plasmablastic morphology was confirmed in the posttransplant setting in patients treated for relapsed or refractory myeloma.[261]

The detection of *circulating plasma cells* is associated with a poor prognosis. In a study from the Mayo Clinic, the median number of circulating monoclonal plasma cells (quantified by the presence of cytoplasmic Ig staining) was 6% of mononuclear cells.[262] Fifty-seven percent of patients had a high count (>4%). OS times were poorer among patients with high than in those with low counts (2.4 vs 4.4 years, respectively; $P < 0.001$). The presence of circulating plasma cells also predicts shorter time to progression from smoldering to active myeloma.[263]

Syndecan-1 (CD138) is a transmembrane heparan sulfate-bearing proteoglycan expressed on the surface of and actively shed by myeloma cells. Through its ability to bind to various growth factors and to mediate cell attachment to extracellular matrix, it may promote myeloma growth in vivo. It appears that the molecule in its soluble form may stimulate tumor growth and survival more effectively than in its membrane-bound form.[264] In an analysis of 138 myeloma patients, serum syndecan-1 levels emerged as an independent prognostic parameter. Patients with high soluble syndecan-1 levels had a median survival period of 20 months versus 44 months in patients with low levels.[265] Confirmatory clinical studies and further elucidation of the biologic activities of the molecule are needed.

The significance of high *serum LDH* levels (in the absence of any other cause, such as liver disease or hemolytic anemia) in predicting poor prognosis in MM has long been recognized.[266] Although rarely observed in the early phase of disease, marked elevations of LDH were detected in up to 20% of patients with disease progressing after vincristine, Adriamycin (doxorubicin), and dexamethasone (VAD) chemotherapy. High LDH levels were associated with hypercalcemia, elevated serum β_2M levels, extramedullary manifestations, plasmablastic morphology, and short OS duration, despite marked (usually very transient) antitumor responses to HDT. The same poor prognosis was noted in patients with initially normal LDH levels in whom marked LDH increments were induced by HDT, presumably resulting from tumor lysis syndrome as an indicator of rapidly proliferative myeloma.[266] This observation was confirmed in a small study of MM patients who developed tumor lysis syndrome after effective chemotherapy (usually HDT). Despite significant cytoreduction achieved immediately after treatment, the survival of this group of patients was extremely short. Close correlations with PCLI and plasmablastic morphology were confirmed in this study.[267] Elevated serum LDH levels at diagnosis also emerged as a significant prognostic factor in an analysis of 155 newly diagnosed patients who received at least one course of HDT with autologous stem cell transplantation (ASCT), irrespective of deletion of chromosome 13. The combined use of Δ13/LDH levels identified subgroups with distinct prognosis (Fig. 87–11). The median OS for patients with no Δ13/normal (<190 μ/L) LDH was 9.5 years (vs 4.7 and 4.1 years for the groups with no Δ13/high LDH and with Δ13/normal LDH, respectively).

Involvement of the central nervous system by MM, as defined by detection of malignant plasma cells in the cerebrospinal fluid in the presence of suggestive symptoms (elevated intracranial pressure, motor or sensory impairment, cranial nerve pulses), is considered extremely rare; the overall incidence is approximately 1.5% to 2%.[268] Almost all patients have cerebrospinal fluid pleocytosis and elevated protein levels. Brain MRI scans are invariably abnormal, with frequent observation of leptomeningeal enhancement. Central nervous system involvement is strongly associated with unfavorable cytogenetic abnormalities (especially translocations and deletion of the chromosome 13), high tumor mass, plasmablastic morphology, additional extramedullary myeloma manifestations, and circulating plasma cells. Despite intensive local (intrathecal chemotherapy and craniospinal irradiation) and systemic treatment, the prognosis of central nervous system myeloma is extremely poor, probably reflecting the aggressive features of the underlying systemic disease.

The role of *cytogenetics* and *gene expression profiling* as a prognostic marker has been outlined above.

THERAPY

Standard-Dose Treatment

Effective treatment of MM became available in the early 1960s when melphalan was introduced. The most commonly used standard treatment is the combination of melphalan and prednisone (MP).[269] A reasonable schedule is concomitant administration of oral melphalan 8 to 10 mg/day and prednisone 60 to 100 mg/day for 7 days, with courses repeated every 4 to 6 weeks. Unless rapid disease progression is documented, treatment should continue for at least 1 year, because responses may be delayed. Due to the erratic absorption of oral melphalan, leukocyte and platelet counts must be checked frequently after initiation of treatment, and the dose of melphalan (in the subsequent courses) should be modified, targeting nadir (days 14–21 of the cycle) absolute neutrophil count and platelet count of approximately 1 and 100 × 10^9/L, respectively.[270] Because similar hemato-

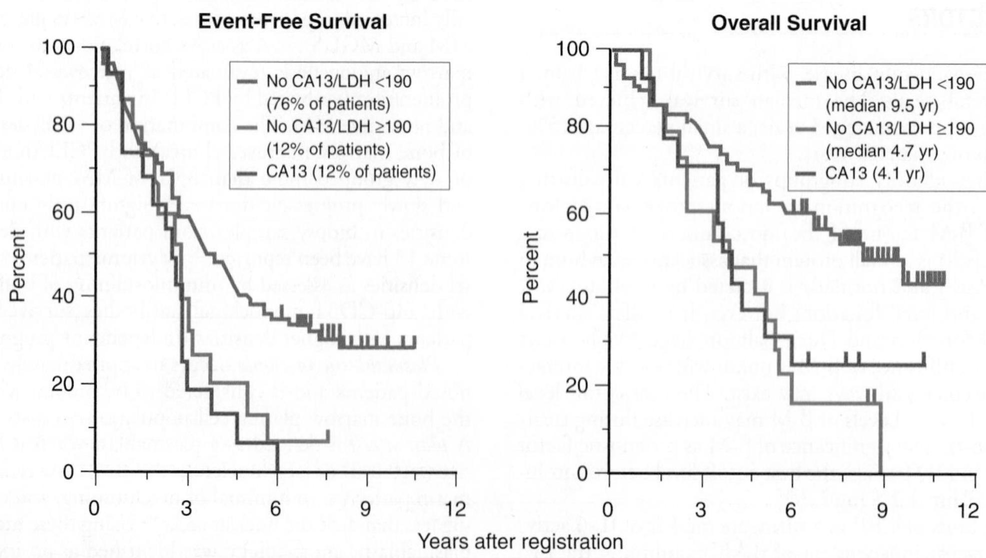

Figure 87–11 Event-free survival and overall survival based on serum lactate dehydrogenase levels at diagnosis and Δ13 in a group of 155 newly diagnosed myeloma patients treated with high-dose treatment. CA, cytogenetic abnormalities. *(From Fassas A, van Rhee F, Tricot G: Predicting long-term survival in multiple myeloma patients following autotransplants. Leuk Lymphoma 44:749, 2003.)*

logic toxicities are observed in responders and nonresponders, resistance is more likely due to inherent disease features, regardless of absorption.[271] This is further supported by the fact that response is not affected by the route of administration, that is, intravenous low-dose versus oral melphalan.[272]

The overall objective response rate (>50% reduction in paraprotein levels) to MP is approximately 50% to 60%, with a median survival of 24 to 30 months.[273] Responding patients enjoy longer survival than do nonresponders (43 vs 19 months); no survival advantage exists for complete versus partial responders.[274,275] Most responders attain a plateau phase during which the malignant clone appears to be dormant. The duration of the plateau phase is variable; the longer the plateau, the longer the median OS period.[276]

Observations that human and mouse plasmacytomata that are resistant to melphalan retained chemosensitivity to cyclophosphamide[276,277] prompted the design of various combination regimens. Vincristine, bis-chloroethyl-nitrosourea (BCNU), cyclophosphamide, and doxorubicin were used in different combinations along with melphalan and steroids. In a large meta-analysis of more than 6500 patients treated with either MP or combination regimens,[278] no survival advantage was detected for the combination chemotherapy, despite the statistically significant superior response rate (60% for the combination vs 53% for MP; $P < 0.00001$), suggesting that minor increases in dose intensity do not affect disease outcome.

In an effort to overcome the problems with the low proliferative rate of myeloma, the combination of vincristine and doxorubicin given as 96-hour continuous intravenous infusion along with three 4-day pulses of oral dexamethasone at 40 mg/day (VAD regimen) was introduced and was found to produce rapid and marked cytoreduction (>50% decrease in paraprotein levels) in at least 50% of patients who relapsed after treatment with MP.[279] Furthermore, near-maximum response occurs after two to three cycles of treatment.[279] When used up front (in previously untreated patients), it produces a response rate of approximately 50% to 60%; however, survival durations achieved with VAD last no longer when compared with MP.[280] VAD can be used safely in patients with renal insufficiency, and, in contrast to melphalan and BCNU, it is not stem cell toxic. However, it requires the insertion of a central venous catheter, potentially leading to a higher incidence of infection or thrombosis, and in rare cases leads to extravasation of the chemotherapeutic agents. Concomitant administration of prophylaxis against *Pneumocystis carinii* pneumonia as well as against viral and fungal infections is strongly recommended. Because the activity of the VAD regimen is almost entirely due to high-dose dexamethasone,[281] its failure to significantly affect survival is not surprising. Probably only mature plasma cells are killed by dexamethasone, whereas the immature, clonogenic myeloma compartment can be rescued from dexamethasone-induced apoptosis by IL-6. Actually, an increase in clonogenic myeloma cells has been observed after treatment with VAD.[282]

Newer Agents

Thalidomide

The observation that increased neovascularization occurs in bone marrow biopsies from myeloma patients and is prognostically relevant prompted the evaluation of thalidomide (at the time, the only drug available with major antiangiogenic activity) in patients with relapsed and refractory disease by the Arkansas group. In a landmark study, 90% of the 84 study patients had relapsing disease after at least one course of HDT. Thalidomide dose was escalated (from a starting dose of 200 mg/day) to a maximum of 800 mg/day. The overall response rate (>50% reduction in monoclonal component) was 32%, with a median time to response of 1 month. The median duration of response was approximately 15 months. No correlation was seen between response rate and microvessel density in the bone marrow biopsies.[283] An update of 169 myeloma patients demonstrated 2-year EFS of 20% and OS rate of 48%. Absence of cytogenetic abnormalities, low β_2M levels, and low PCLI, the same factors that predict outcome with cytotoxic therapy, were associated with superior survival as well as higher cumulative thalidomide dose.[284] Similar response rates, response durations, and survival times were reported by the Mayo Clinic group.[285] Thalidomide has also been used for treatment of indolent/smoldering myeloma.[286] Thalidomide with pulse dexamethasone yielded a 70% response rate in the remission induction phase of patients with newly diagnosed active disease.[287,288]

In a retrospective matched case-control analysis of 200 patients treated with either thalidomide/dexamethasone or VAD in preparation for autologous transplantation, thalidomide/dexamethasone resulted in a significantly higher response rate of 76% versus 52% ($P < 0.001$), with comparable numbers of patients in both groups proceeding to transplantation and no significant differences in quantity of stem cell collection.[289] Deep vein thrombosis was more frequent in the thalidomide/dexamethasone arm, whereas neutropenia was more often observed in the VAD arm. In a randomized phase III clinical trial of thalidomide plus dexamethasone compared with dexamethasone alone in newly diagnosed patients, entire study group included 207 newly diagnosed patients, the response rate to thalidomide and dexamethasone was significantly higher (63% vs 41%), but grade 3 or greater deep vein thrombosis, rash, bradycardia, neuropathy, and any grade 4 and 5 toxicity in the first 4 months were significantly higher in the thalidomide/dexamethasone arm.[290] The authors concluded that the higher response rate with this regimen must be balanced against its greater toxicity. The combination of thalidomide with dexamethasone normalizes abnormal bone remodeling through a reduction in the soluble RANKL (sRANKL)/OPG ratio.[291] Thalidomide markedly downregulates angiogenic genes in endothelial cells of active, but not of nonactive, myeloma.[292] The appropriate dose of thalidomide in myeloma is unknown. Most of its side effects (somnolence, constipation, fatigue, tremor, bradycardia, edema, neuropathy, rash) can be managed by reducing the dose. Hypothyroidism frequently complicates its use and requires thyroid hormone replacement.[293] An increased incidence of deep vein thrombosis from 5% when used as a single agent up to 25% to 30% when thalidomide is given concurrently with cytotoxic chemotherapy (especially doxorubicin-containing regimens) is observed.[294] Use of low-molecular-weight heparin can mostly prevent this risk.[295] Arterial thromboses are seen with thalidomide.[296] In one study focused on neuropathy in myeloma patients treated with thalidomide who had undergone serial nerve electrophysiologic studies, 39% already had some abnormalities at baseline on electrophysiologic studies. The study showed that the majority of patients will develop neuropathy given sufficient length of treatment with thalidomide. The actuarial incidence of neuropathy increased from 38% at 6 months to 73% at 12 months. Serial electrophysiologic studies did not reliably predict the imminent development of clinical neuropathy. To minimize the risk of neuropathy, thalidomide therapy should be limited to less than 6 months.[297] The mechanism of action of thalidomide is unclear. In addition to its antiangiogenic properties, thalidomide has potent immunomodulatory effects (induction of secretion of interferon-γ and IL-2 by cytotoxic T cells,[298] inhibition of TNF-α,[299] IL-6, and VEGF production in the bone marrow milieu, modulation of expression of several cell surface adhesion molecules,[300] inhibition of the transcription factor NF-κB[301]) and targets the cross-talk between malignant cells and stromal cells in the bone marrow microenvironment, thereby overcoming drug resistance.

Thalidomide has been combined with noncytotoxic and cytotoxic therapy. In a multicenter phase II trial, thalidomide up to 800 mg was combined with celecoxib 400 mg bid. Cyclooxygenase 2 inhibitors suppress angiogenesis and induce apoptosis and hematogenic metastases. Cyclooxygenase 2 is overexpressed in myeloma cell lines and primary myeloma cells.[302,303] Among 66 previously treated patients enrolled in the phase II study, the overall response rate was 42% and the median time to progression was 6.8 months. Because of fluid retention and decreased renal function, celecoxib was discontinued in 57% of patients.[304] More than 250 elderly patients (age 60–85 years) with newly diagnosed myeloma were randomly assigned to MP with or without thalidomide for six 4-week cycles.[305] In this study, patients in the thalidomide arm had a higher response rate than did those in the nonthalidomide arm (76% vs 48%), with complete remission (CR) and near-CR rates of 28% and 7%. The 2-year EFS was 54% vs 27% (thalidomide vs nonthalidomide; $P = 0.0006$). Grade 3 or 4 adverse events were 48% in the thalidomide arm versus 25% in the nonthalidomide arm ($P = 0.0002$). Low-dose molecular heparin reduced the risk of thromboembolic complications from 20% to 3%. In another phase II trial, thalidomide and dexamethasone were combined with pegylated liposomal doxorubicin (ThaDD) for treatment of 50 newly diagnosed patients older than 65 years.[306] CR was achieved in 34%, near-CR in 7%, and very good partial response in another 10%; 30% attained a partial remission (PR). Time to progression, EFS, and OS at 3 years were 60%, 57%, and 74%, respectively. Grade 3 to 4 infections and thromboembolic events were 22% and 14%, respectively. Thalidomide/dexamethasone has been combined with 4 days of continuous infusions of cisplatin, doxorubicin, cyclophosphamide, and etoposide in the DT-PACE regimen. Response to two cycles of this regimen was evaluated in 236 patients, of whom 63% had progressive myeloma on standard chemotherapy and 23% had chromosome 13 abnormalities by metaphase cytogenetics. Thirty-two percent achieved PR and 16% CR or near-CR. Excellent responses were also seen in patients with high LDH and chromosome 13 abnormalities. Patients who received two cycles of this regimen at 100% dose had a 49% partial response rate and a 27% CR and near-CR rate.[307]

Thalidomide has been given posttransplantation. Two months after transplantation, 597 patients younger than 65 years were randomly assigned to receive no maintenance (arm A), pamidronate (arm B), or pamidronate plus thalidomide (arm C).[308] A complete or very good partial response was achieved in 55% of patients in arm A, 57% in arm B, and 67% in arm C ($P = 0.03$). The 3-year post-randomization EFS was 36% in arm A, 37% in arm B, and 52% in arm C ($P = 0.009$). The 4-year postdiagnosis survival was 77% in arm A, 74% in arm B, and 87% in arm C ($P < 0.04$).

Lenalidomide

Lenalidomide is a thalidomide derivative. Its immunomodulatory effects include growth arrest or apoptosis of drug-resistant myeloma cell lines, abrogation of adhesion of myeloma cells to bone marrow stromal cells, and modulation of cytokines that promote growth, survival, and drug resistance of myeloma cells. It is nonteratogenic in rabbits and has a toxicity profile different from thalidomide.[309] Lenalidomide activates natural killer and natural T cells.[310,311] In a phase I dose escalation study of 27 patients, the majority of whom had received a prior transplant and thalidomide, grade 3 myelosuppression developed in all patients treated with lenalidomide 50 mg/day. Therefore, 25 mg/day was considered the maximum tolerated dose. Importantly, no significant somnolence, constipation, or neuropathy was observed.[312] In a multicenter double-blind phase III trial, 354 patients with relapsed or refractory myeloma were randomized to dexamethasone pulsing every 4 weeks with or without lenalidomide 25 mg/day on days 1 to 21. The overall response rate was greater in the lenalidomide/dexamethasone arm (59% vs 21%; $P < 0.001$). Complete responses were observe in 13% of patients in the lenalidomide/dexamethasone group versus < 1% in the dexamethasone arm. Median time to progression was 11 months in the study group versus 4.7 months in the control group. Grade 3 to 4 neutropenia (24% vs 3.5%) and thromboembolic events (15% vs 3.5%) were more frequent in the study group.[313] In a multicenter randomized phase II study of relapsed refractory myeloma, two different dose regimens of lenalidomide were evaluated. Seventy patients received either lenalidomide 30 mg once per day or lenalidomide 15 mg twice per day for 21 days of every 28-day cycle. After two cycles, dexamethasone was added for patients with progressive or stable disease. Myelosuppression was more common in the group that received 15 mg twice per day (41% vs 13%; $P = 0.03$). An additional 32 patients received 30 mg once per day. Median progression-free survival was 7.7 months in the once per day group versus 3.9 months in the twice per day group. Significant neuropathy and deep vein thrombosis each occurred in 3% of patients.[314] In 34 newly diagnosed myeloma patients, lenalidomide and dexamethasone was given as initial treatment. Lenalidomide dose was 25 mg/day on days 1 to 21 of a 28-day cycle. Thirty-one patients showed an objective response, including two who achieved CR. Another 11 patients achieved a near-CR or a very good partial response. The most common grade 3 or higher nonhematologic toxicities were fatigue (15%), muscle weakness (6%), pneumonia (6%), and rash (6%).[315] In relapsed and refractory myeloma, lenalidomide/dexamethasone is associated with an increased risk of venous thrombosis. This risk may be further increased with concomitant administration of erythropoietin.[316] The risk of thrombosis also is higher if lenalidomide is given as initial therapy, and thrombosis prophylaxis is indicated.[317]

Another thalidomide derivative CC-4047 (Actimid) has been tested in a phase I study of 24 relapsed or refractory myeloma patients. One patient developed deep vein thrombosis but was found to have a malignant melanoma; he died while the myeloma was stable. Three other patients developed thromboembolic complications after day 28. No other grade 3 or higher nonhematologic toxicities were seen. Dose-limiting neutropenia occurred in six patients a median of 3 weeks after the start of treatment. The maximum tolerated dose was considered 2 mg/day. Thirteen patients had a greater than 50% reduction in M protein, and four entered CR. All patients showed an increase in CD45RO on CD4 and CD8 cells, with a concomitant decrease in CD45RA.[318] This drug also potently blocks osteoclasts differentiation.[319] There is little doubt that lenalidomide, just like thalidomide, will be combined with conventional chemotherapy.

Bortezomib

Bortezomib is the first in a new class of pharmacologic agents that inhibit the proteasome. The proteasome is a multienzyme complex found in all eukaryotic cells that orderly degrades more than 80% of ubiquitin-tagged cellular proteins, which control cell division, survival, growth, and apoptosis. These proteins include cyclins, cyclin-dependent kinases, cyclin-dependent cyclin kinase inhibitors, oncogenes, tumor suppressor genes, and transcriptional activators or inhibitors. Bortezomib selectively and reversibly inhibits the chymotryptic but not the tryptic and post–glutamyl peptide hydrolyticlike activity of the proteasome. The major mechanism of action of bortezomib initially was thought to be related to inhibition of degradation of IκB. Its lack of degradation prevents activation and translocation of NF-κ B to the nucleus. Bortezomib was identified as an active drug in the NCI screening program. Its growth inhibitory effects correlated strongly with proteasome inhibition. Bortezomib has other activities in myeloma, such as prevention of adhesion of myeloma cells to stromal cells, induction of cytokines by the microenvironment, decrease in angiogenic activity, and direct apoptotic effect on myeloma cells.[320] In a phase II trial, 202 patients with relapsed myeloma were enrolled. As a requirement, the patients had to be refractory to their most recent chemotherapy. Patients were given bortezomib 1.3 mg/m^2 on days 1, 4, 8, and 11 every 3 weeks. In patients with suboptimal response, oral dexamethasone 20 mg was added the day of and the day after bortezomib administration. Of the evaluable patients, responses were seen in 35%, with 10% CR and near-CR. Median duration of response was 12 months. Grade 3 and 4 toxicities were thrombocytopenia (31%), neutropenia (14%), fatigue (12%), peripheral neuropathy (12%), and vomiting (8%).[321] Clinical factors predicting poor outcome with bortezomib were age 65 years and older and more than 50% plasma cell infiltration in the bone marrow for response, and thrombocytopenia, hypoalbuminemia, and more than 50% bone marrow plasma cell infiltration for time to progression. Chromosome 13 deletion and elevated β_2M levels were not predictive of poor outcome.[322] In a multicenter randomized study that included 669 relapsed myeloma patients, the efficacy of single-agent bortezomib was compared to that of dexamethasone. The response rate, including complete and partial responders, was higher in the bortezomib group (38% vs 18%;

$P < 0.001$). Complete responses were seen in 6% of the bortezomib patients versus less than 1% in the dexamethasone arm ($P < 0.001$). Median duration of response was 8 months in the bortezomib group versus 5.6 months in the dexamethasone group ($P < 0.001$).[323] Bortezomib therapy appears to be safe in patients with renal failure, although the numbers of patients studied was small.[324] Mean platelet count decreased by 60% during bortezomib treatment but recovered rapidly between treatments in a cyclical fashion. Mean percent reduction in platelets was independent of baseline platelet count. Bortezomib-induced thrombocytopenia appears to be due to a reversible effect on megakaryocytic function rather than a direct cytotoxic effect on megakaryocytes and their precursors.[325] Bortezomib was given alone or in combination with dexamethasone to 32 previously untreated myeloma patients. The response rate (CR + PR) was 88%, with CR and near-CR rate of 25%. Median time to response was 2 months. Bortezomib therapy did not influence stem cell collection. Grade 3 and 4 toxicities were sensory neuropathy in 16%, myalgia in 13%, and neutropenia in 16%.[326] In a phase I trial, bortezomib combined with pegylated liposomal doxorubicin was given to 42 patients with advanced hematologic malignancies, including 22 patients with myeloma. Eight myeloma patients achieved CR or near-CR, and another eight patients had partial responses. Maximal tolerated dose was bortezomib 1.5 mg/m^2 and pegylated doxorubicin 30 mg/m^2. Adverse events were fatigue in 88%, thrombocytopenia in 69%, peripheral neuropathy in 55%, and neutropenia in 45%.[327] Twenty-one untreated myeloma patients received a combination of bortezomib, doxorubicin, and dexamethasone (PAD) for four 21-day cycles. Patients then proceeded to autologous transplantation. The partial response rate was 95%, and the CR rate was 24%. This regimen allowed stem cell collection in 95% of patients; median number of CD34 cells per kilogram collected was 3.75 million. One patient developed grade 3 peripheral neuropathy; three patients experienced a varicella zoster infection.[328] Sixty newly diagnosed myeloma patients 65 years or older (50% older than 75 years) were treated with bortezomib plus MP. PR or better was observed in 89% of patients, and an IFE-negative complete response was seen in 32%. Results were superior to those obtained in historical controls receiving MP. Major toxicities (grade 3 and 4) were thrombocytopenia (51%), neutropenia (43%), and peripheral neuropathy (17%).[329] Response to bortezomib is associated with osteoblastic activation.[330] Bortezomib-associated neuropathy appears reversible in the large majority of patients after dose reduction or discontinuation.[331] Severe pulmonary complications after treatment with bortezomib have been reported by Japanese investigators.[332]

High-Dose Treatment and Autologous Transplantation

Application of HDT has been challenging in MM. Median patient age at diagnosis is 69 years, and almost half of patients experience some degree of renal insufficiency during their disease course. Many have inadequate hematopoietic stem cell reserve due to prolonged previous exposure to alkylating agents or radiation treatment to the spine and pelvis. Functional limitations due to skeletal pain or fractures and treatment-related immunosuppression further complicate the ability to deliver HDT to MM patients.

It has been more than 20 years since the late Tim McElwain and colleagues introduced HDT for MM. Administration of melphalan 100 to 140 mg/m^2, without stem cell support, induced biochemical and bone marrow CR in three (all previously untreated) of nine patients, which is much higher than the 3% to 5% complete response rate seen with conventional treatment.[333] Its efficacy subsequently was confirmed in larger studies.[334] However, high-dose melphalan induced prolonged aplasia and was associated with high morbidity and mortality rates.[333,335] This finding led other investigators to the concept of stem cell support and further escalation of the dose of melphalan, initially with autologous bone marrow,[336] and subsequently peripheral blood stem cells to reduce the duration of cytopenias and thereby the toxicity of the procedure. With the current use of peripheral blood stem cells, median duration of granulocytes less than 0.5×10^9/L and platelets less than 50×10^9/L is approximately 1 week (Fig. 87–12), reducing the transplant-related mortality (TRM) rate to less than 5%.[337]

In a study from the University of Arkansas group of 1000 consecutive MM patients with various lengths of preceding standard-dose treatment and intended to receive two courses of melphalan-based HDT (76% actually received two transplants), CR (defined as negative serum and urine immunofixation and <5% light chain–restricted plasma cells in the bone marrow aspirate and biopsy) rate achieved was 44%. Median duration of CR was 2.4 years. TRM was 2.7% with the first transplant and 4.8% with the second transplant.[166] Projected EFS and OS at 5 years were 25% and 40%, respectively. On multivariate analysis, CR rates were higher when standard treatment did not exceed 12 months and still was effective (chemosensitive disease), and in the absence of Δ13 abnormalities. Both EFS and OS were significantly longer in the absence of Δ13 abnormalities and with fewer than 12 months of prior standard treatment, low β_2M levels, and chemosensitive disease. Of 390 CR patients without Δ13, 35% enjoyed 5-year continuous CR compared with none of 54 patients with Δ13. The presence of Δ13 reduced the 5-year EFS from 20% to 0% and the OS from 44% to 16%. Total Therapy I was the first tandem autotransplant trial for 231 patients with newly diagnosed myeloma. With a minimum followup of 12 years, 27% of patients are still alive, and 10-year EFS and OS are 15% and 33%, respectively. OS was superior in the absence of a hypodiploid karyotype or deletion of chromosome 13, and in the presence of a low baseline CRP.[338]

The superiority of HDT over conventional treatment in terms of CR, CR duration, EFS, and OS has been shown convincingly in randomized,[339] case-control,[340] and population-based[341] studies. Attal et al.[339] compared in randomized fashion HDT followed by autologous bone marrow transplantation with standard treatment in 200 previously untreated patients younger than 65 years (IFM 90). Data were analyzed on an intention-to-treat basis. However, more than one fourth of patients randomized to HDT did not receive a transplant. Response rates (81% vs 57%), CR rates (22% vs 5%), and 5-year EFS (28% vs 10%) and OS (52% vs 12%) rates were significantly better in the transplant group. The study was criticized because of the relatively small number of patients and the poor response rate of the standard treatment arm, which compared unfavorably with other trials of standard treatment. In a multicenter UK study of 407 patients, higher CR rate (44% vs 8%), longer median progression-free survival (32 vs 20 months), and greater OS (54 vs 42 months) were found in the transplant arm compared to the standard chemotherapy arm.[342] In a nonrandomized elective single autograft study of high-dose melphalan use in 451 patients, CR and near-CR was observed in 59%. The 10-year probability of EFS and OS were 17% and 31%, respectively.[343] In a case-control study, the results of Total Therapy I were compared with the outcomes of untreated patients (matched for the major prognostic factors available) receiving standard treatment according to Southwest Oncology Group (SWOG) trials.[339] HDT induced higher response rates (85% vs 52%; $P < 0.001$) and extended EFS (49 vs 22 months; $P = 0.001$) and OS (62+ vs 48 months; $P = 0.01$). In a population-based study, the results of HDT in newly diagnosed, symptomatic patients younger than 60 years were compared with those of conventionally treated historic controls, most of whom fulfilled the criteria for HDT. Survival was prolonged in the HDT group compared with the control group (risk ratio for control group 1.62; $P = 0.001$).[341] Other studies have not confirmed the superiority of transplantation over conventional chemotherapy.[344–347] In Total Therapy II, including 668 newly diagnosed myeloma, all patients received identical intensive induction, transplantation, consolidation, and maintenance therapy but were randomized up front to either thalidomide or no thalidomide during treatment. With median followup of 42 months, the CR rate (62% vs 43%; $P < 0.001$) and 5-year EFS (56% vs 44%; $P = 0.01$) were superior in the thalidomide arm, whereas OS at 5 years was similar at approximately 65% in both arms. The shorter survival after relapse in the thalidomide arm (1.1 vs 2.7 years; $P = 0.001$) probably explains the lack of survival benefit in the thalidomide arm.[348]

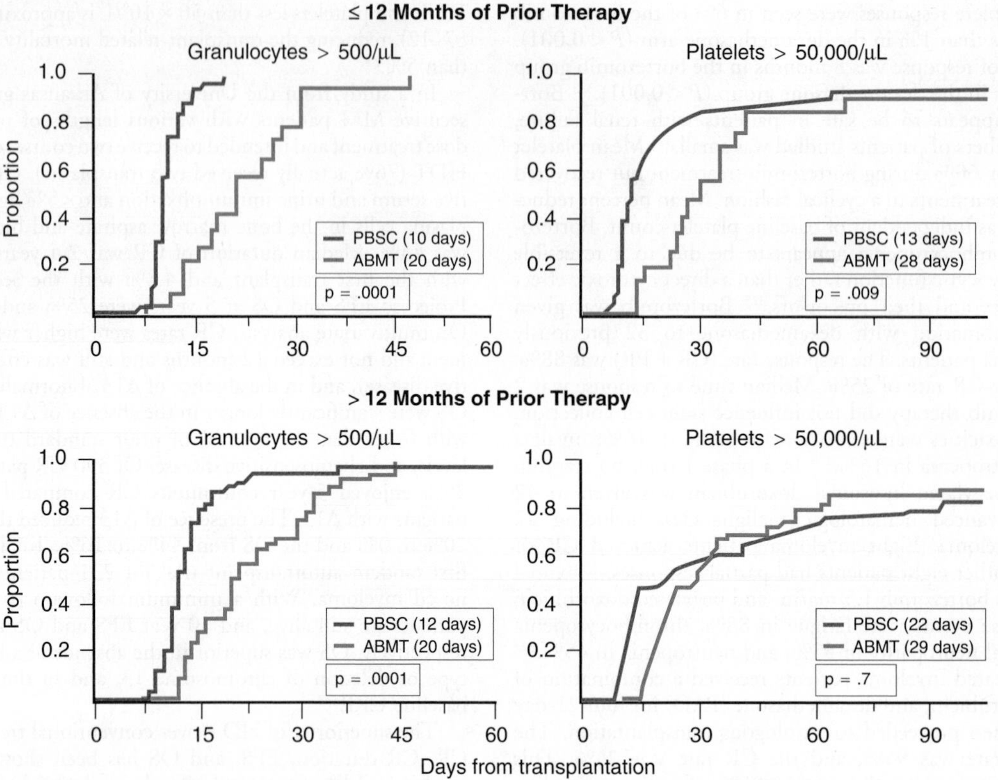

Figure 87–12 Hematologic recovery posttransplantation. ABMT, autologous bone marrow transplantation; PBSC, peripheral blood stem cell. *(From Barlogie B, Jagannath S, Tricot G, et al: Advances in the treatment of multiple myeloma. Adv Intern Med 43:279, 1998.)*

"Upfront" application of HDT has clinical benefits. More profound cytoreduction is associated with better quality of life, whereas development of drug resistance of the malignant clone is minimized. If the choice is made not to proceed with upfront standard treatment but to retain the option of HDT at relapse, hematopoietic progenitors should be collected and stored at the initiation of standard treatment, thus enabling adequate collections of stem cells and reducing damage to stem cells by long exposure to alkylating agents, thereby minimizing the risk of treatment-related MDS. The risk for treatment-related MDS is much higher when patients have received prolonged standard treatment before HDT. All seven patients with treatment-related MDS were identified from among a group of 117 transplanted patients who had received more than one cycle of conventional chemotherapy before enrollment in our transplant study. No treatment-related MDS was seen in a group of 71 patients who were transplanted after no or only one cycle of conventional chemotherapy.[349] However, since this report, some patients with minimal treatment before the first transplant subsequently developed treatment-related MDS. In the majority of cases of treatment-related MDS analyzed, the signature chromosome abnormalities of treatment-related MDS were retrospectively identified by FISH in the collected stem cell grafts, lending further support to the notion that the stem cells were already abnormal before transplantation.[350,351] A population-based survey covering two geographically distinct UK regions revealed that 57% of myeloma patients 65 years and younger do not receive transplantation for their disease.[352]

One Versus Two Courses of High-Dose Treatment

Despite the improvements achieved with application of HDT, the 7-year EFS in the IFM 90 trial was only 16% in the HDT arm, with no plateau in the survival curve.[353] Because achievement of CR or very good PR in this trial was believed to be a sine qua non for meaningful survival benefit, dose escalation subsequently was tested in a randomized fashion by the same group (IFM 94). A total of 399 untreated MM patients younger than 60 years were enrolled by 45 centers and randomized to either a single ASCT with melphalan 140 mg/m^2 and total body irradiation (TBI) or a double ASCT. The preparative regimen for the first transplant was melphalan 140 mg/m^2 and for the second was melphalan 140 mg/m^2 and TBI. A second randomization between bone marrow or peripheral blood stem cell support was performed after initial cytoreduction with VAD. Transplant-related deaths were 4% in the single ASCT arm versus 6% in the double ASCT arm; 85% of patients assigned to the single ASCT received the planned treatment versus 78% assigned to the double ASCT arm. By pooling the bone marrow and peripheral blood stem cell support data with a median followup of more than 75 months, the 7-year probabilities of EFS and OS are superior in the double transplant arm (20% and 42% vs 10% and 21%, respectively; $P < 0.03$ and $P < 0.01$, respectively). Surprisingly, no significant difference in the CR rate between the two arms was seen. Patients who had achieved at least very good PR did not benefit from a second transplant. Important prognostic factors for survival were baseline β_2M level, age, LDH, and treatment arm.[354] In the Bologna 96 trial of double versus single ASCT in previously untreated MM patients, significant prolongation of EFS was seen in the double ASCT arm (median 34 vs 25 months; $P = 0.05$). Again, no difference in the CR rate between the arms was detected. With median followup of only 3 years, no significant OS advantage has emerged yet, in keeping with the IFM 94 experience in which separation of the EFS and OS curves occurred only after 3 years.[355] In the European Group for Blood and Marrow Transplantation (EBMT) registry experience, 441 newly diagnosed, chemosensitive MM patients who received tandem autotransplants were compared with a matched group of 1380 patients who received only a single transplant. Median posttransplantation survival was 7.1 years for the tandem group and 5.6 years for the single transplant time group. Actuarial posttransplant survival rates at 7 years were 57% and 39%, respectively. Although the difference reached borderline statistical significance ($P = 0.1$) in this trial, the data taken together support the superiority of the tandem (versus single) autologous transplantation approach.[356] The optimal time to perform a second transplant is before relapse and within 6 to 12 months after the first transplant.[357] In a trial of high-risk myeloma, defined as β_2M level and FISH deletion 13, 219 patients received a first transplant with melphalan 200 mg/m^2 and a second transplant with melphalan 220 mg/m^2. Patients were randomized to either receive or not receive an anti–IL-6 monoclonal antibody (IFM 99-04). No benefit of the monoclonal antibody was seen. However, 2-year survival was superior to that in previously studied patients receiving tandem transplants but with a lower dose of melphalan. Median EFS and OS were 30 and 41 months, compared to 15 and 25 months, respectively, in a similar group of patients treated previously. The survival in this high-risk group of patients was similar to that of all patients (good and bad prognosis combined) who received tandem transplants in the IFM 94 study.[358] The same IFM group compared tandem autologous transplants (IFM 99-04) to one autologous transplant followed by a dose-reduced allotransplant in 65 high-risk patients with a human leukocyte antigen (HLA)-identical sibling donor (IFM 99-03). With a median followup of 24 months, EFS of the 166 patients receiving tandem autologous transplants was similar to that of the 46 patients who completed the entire IFM 99-03 program. with a trend for a better OS in patients receiving tandem autotransplants. No benefit from the combination of autologous transplantation followed by reduced-intensity allotransplantation in high-risk patients was seen.[359]

Primary Refractory Disease

Dose escalation has consistently increased tumor cytoreduction and extended EFS and OS even in the subset of patients with primary refractory myeloma (disease progression or <50% reduction in monoclonal protein levels with initial standard-dose regimen), as shown in single-center and Intergroup trials. In a report from Royal Marsden Hospital of 222 patients, lack of response to induction treatment did not predict poor long-term outcome because a significant proportion of primary refractory patients responded to HDT. More specifically, among 130 patients who either attained or remained in CR after one course of HDT with melphalan 200 mg/m^2, 5-year OS was independent of response to primary treatment.[360] The Mayo Clinic compared the outcome of 50 patients with primary refractory myeloma to that of 101 patients with chemosensitive myeloma. The response rate in the chemorefractory patients was 92% versus 99% in the chemosensitive patients. The CR rate was 20% in chemorefractory patients versus 35% in chemosensitive patients ($P = 0.06$). One-year progression-free survival was 70% in the chemorefractory patients and 83% in the chemosensitive patients ($P = 0.065$).[361] In another study from the MD Anderson Cancer Center, the outcome of 89 consecutive patients refractory to dexamethasone-based chemotherapy was compared to that of 45 patients who refused or were unable to receive an autotransplant for socioeconomic reasons. After autotransplantation, the response rate was 69%, including 16% CR. Survival of the CR patients was significantly better than that of PR patients (>7 years vs 4.5 years). Median survival of transplanted patients was 27 months longer than for the controls ($P < 0.01$), even though the control patients had more favorable features.[362] The feasibility and efficacy of HDT in refractory MM (relapsed and primary refractory) were also shown in an Intergroup trial.[363] In contrast to experiences in other B-cell malignancies, such as relapsed non-Hodgkin lymphoma, primary refractory patients are good candidates for HDT and ASCT.

Graft Contamination by Myeloma

Ample and convincing evidence indicates that not only bone marrow but also peripheral blood stem cell grafts are contaminated with a small amount of myeloma cells.[364,365] Using quantitative polymerase chain reaction amplification assays of patient-specific CDR III DNA sequences from bone marrow and peripheral blood mononuclear cell samples, myeloma cells have been detected in nearly all patients.[366] Reinfusion of these cells may contribute to disease relapse, as shown to be the case in other hematologic malignancies, such as acute myeloid leukemia, neuroblastoma, and chronic myeloid leukemia.[367,368] Additionally, an inverse correlation between plasma cell contamination in the peripheral blood stem cell products and disease-free survival has been demonstrated in a small prospective study of 33 patients; the presence of more than 2×10^5 tumor cells per liter predicted an early relapse[369] but probably was more a reflection of the overall higher tumor burden in these patients. Other investigators have not confirmed this observation.[370,371] Different ex vivo purging techniques, based on chemical or immunologic approaches, have been used in an attempt to obtain tumor-free products. Delayed hematologic recovery and increased infectious complications have compromised the applicability of these strategies, despite their success in substantially reducing the autograft tumor burden.[372–374]

A multicenter phase III, randomized trial compared the hematologic recovery and toxicity after autologous transplantation using either unselected or CD34$^+$-selected peripheral blood stem cells.[375] Median time to neutrophil engraftment was 12 days for patients in both arms of the study, whereas median time to platelet engraftment was slightly prolonged (by 1–2 days) for patients receiving less than 2×10^6 CD34$^+$-selected cells per kilogram. No differences in the incidence or type of infections, EFS, and OS were seen between the two arms. Given the high cost of the procedure and the potential for delayed platelet engraftment and late (>1 year posttransplant) opportunistic infections, positive selection of CD34$^+$ cells should not be routinely performed outside of the context of a clinical trial.

Indirect evidence favoring the significance of reinfusion of "clean" grafts comes from an analysis of EBMT.[376] The outcomes of 25 MM patients who received transplants from twin donors were compared in a case-matched analysis to the outcomes of 125 patients who received ASCT and of 125 patients who received allogeneic transplantation. Although the CR rate was not statistically different among the three groups, median OS tended to be better (73 vs 44 months) and EFS was significantly better (72 vs 25 months) for the twin transplants compared with ASCT, and both (twin and autologous) were significantly better than those with the allogeneic transplants. A graft-versus-myeloma effect cannot be completely excluded, as a graft-versus-hostlike disease has been reported for syngeneic transplants.[377,378]

Conditioning Regimen

Most conditioning regimens are based on melphalan either alone or in combination with TBI. However, other alkylating agents, such as busulfan, carmustine, thiotepa, and cyclophosphamide, have been used. In a report from the Spanish Registry, no statistically significant differences in OS and EFS were seen among four conditioning regimens (melphalan alone vs melphalan/TBI or busulfan vs cyclophosphamide/busulfan alone), despite a trend for better response rates and somewhat improved EFS and OS associated with use of melphalan/busulfan.[379] In a French randomized study comparing the two most commonly used regimens (melphalan 200 mg/m^2 and melphalan 140 mg/m^2 plus TBI 800 cGy), the melphalan-alone arm was shown to be less toxic and probably more effective; the investigators recommended it as the standard of care.[380] Two other nonrandomized studies have shown that use of non-TBI conditioning is associated with better survival. In the University of Arkansas experience, use of TBI combined with melphalan 140 mg/m^2 led to higher TRM and inferior EFS and OS (despite identical CR rates) rates compared to conditioning with melphalan 200 mg/m^2 alone. The investigators hypothesized that more prolonged and severe immunosuppression in the TBI-treated group may be responsible for the adverse outcome.[381] The EBMT registry analysis on prognostic factors also showed that a non-TBI preparative regimen was independently associated with superior outcome.[382] Based on the IFM 99-04 study, higher doses of melphalan result in better outcomes.[358]

High-Dose Treatment in the Elderly and in the Presence of Renal Dysfunction

Most HDT trials have included relatively young patients with normal vital organ function. However, if a major impact on the outcome in myeloma is to be achieved, the fact that more than half of MM patients are older than 65 years at diagnosis cannot be ignored. Several studies have reported contradictory findings on the influence of increasing patient age on the ability to collect adequate numbers of stem cells. In a retrospective analysis of 984 patients (106 older than 70 years), increasing age inversely correlated with $CD34^+$ cell yield. However, the overwhelming majority (85%) of elderly patients still were able to collect at least 4×10^6 $CD34^+$ cells/kg, provided the length of the previously administered standard treatment was 12 months or less and the platelet count prior to mobilization was 200,000/μL or more.[383] Encouraged by the lower toxicity seen in the recent years (due to use of peripheral blood stem cells, hematopoietic growth factors, and improved supportive care), the University of Arkansas group retrospectively examined its experience with 49 newly diagnosed and previously treated patients older than 65 years after HDT and compared their outcomes with 49 younger patients, matched for relevant prognostic features.[384] Seventy-six percent of the younger group and 65% of the older group completed a second ASCT. Hematologic recovery and TRM were comparable among younger and older patients with first and second transplants. Multivariate analysis that included both younger and older patients showed pretransplant cytogenetic abnormalities and β_2M levels as critical prognostic features for EFS and OS, whereas age was insignificant. The outcomes of 71 MM patients (median age 64 years; 53 patients >60 years) who received two or three courses of melphalan 100 mg/m^2 followed by stem cell support were compared with the outcomes of 71 pair mates, matched for age and β_2M levels, who received standard treatment with oral MP.[385] The HDT regimen was well tolerated. Median EFS was 34 months in the HDT group and 17.7 months in the standard treatment group ($P < 0.001$). Median OS was 56+ and 48 months, respectively ($P < 0.01$). Therefore, it appears that myeloma in the elderly is not biologically different from the disease in younger patients and that HDT can be safely and effectively administered to the majority of older patients. However, because of significant toxicity, lower doses of melphalan (100–140 mg/m^2) should be administered to patients older than 70 years.

The same conclusion is applicable to myeloma patients with impaired renal function (including hemodialysis-dependent patients). The pharmacokinetics of intravenous high-dose melphalan are comparable regardless of renal function.[386] The presence of renal insufficiency did not affect the quality of stem cell collections or the engraftment kinetics in a group of 81 patients treated with 140 to 200 mg/m^2 and ASCT at the University of Arkansas.[387] Probabilities of EFS and OS at 3 years were 48% and 55%, respectively. In a study of 59 patients who received autotransplants while on dialysis, 5-year EFS and OS were 24% and 36%, respectively. Dialysis duration less than 6 months prior to transplant and pretransplant creatinine clearance greater than 10 mL/min were significant predictors of renal function recovery; 33% of patients on dialysis for less than 6 months recovered renal function versus 6% of those on dialysis for more than 6 months; 38% with creatinine clearance greater than 10 mL/min recovered renal function versus 11% of the other patients.[388] One fourth of dialysis-dependent myeloma patients became dialysis independent after autotransplantation.[388] The Royal Marsden group also confirmed that the presence of renal dysfunction did not affect EFS and OS in patients treated with HDT.[389] In a Danish study of 78 patients with normal renal function at diagnosis and transplantation, 30 patients with renal failure at diagnosis but normal at transplant, and 29 patients with renal failure at diagnosis and transplant, no differences in numbers of stem cells collected, time to engraftment, or response to transplantation was observed. One third of patients with renal failure at transplantation regained normal kidney function. However, significantly longer hospitalizations, increased use of blood products, and more infections were seen in patients with renal failure at transplantation. TRM was 17% in those patients compared to 0% and 1% in the other groups. Four of the eight patients on dialysis at transplantation died.[390]

Posttransplantation Manipulations

It is appealing to consider some form of posttransplant "consolidation" or "maintenance" treatment in myeloma. The theoretical advantages are eradication of graft-contaminating malignant cells and further cytoreduction of the remaining myeloma cells by killing newly cycling cells. The available data on its efficacy are limited. The role of interferon-α as posttransplant maintenance therapy was examined in a small trial of 85 patients who were randomly assigned to treatment with interferon-α (3×10^6 U/m^2 subcutaneously three times weekly until relapse) or no further treatment.[391] Although initial analysis showed a survival benefit favoring interferon use, the difference disappeared with longer followup. Two other studies, both in abstract form, reported conflicting results. The French registry study showed no significant impact on EFS and OS, whereas the EBMT registry showed that use of interferon-α appeared to improve survival.[382,392] Applying cytotoxic chemotherapy intermittently in the post-ASCT period in myeloma patients with high-risk disease did not show a significant benefit in a pair-matched analysis, but this finding requires study in a randomized fashion.[393] In a retrospective analysis comparing outcome of patients on Total Therapy II on the no-thalidomide arm (consolidation and maintenance) to that of Total Therapy I (no consolidation, only maintenance), CR rates were similar (43% vs 41%). However, 5-year continuous CR (45% vs 32%; $P < 0.001$) and 5-year EFS (43% vs 28%; $P < 0.001$) were superior with Total Therapy II, with a trend for improved OS (62% vs 57%; $P = 0.11$). A superior OS was seen for the two thirds of patients with no cytogenetic abnormalities.[394] Thalidomide maintenance prolonged EFS and OS after transplantation.[308]

Allogeneic Stem Cell Transplantation

Allogeneic stem cell transplantation may eradicate disease and restore hematopoiesis through the use of a tumor-free graft. Furthermore, the immunologic effect of the allograft (graft-versus-myeloma effect) has been clearly demonstrated.[252,395] However (and despite the introduction of nonmyeloablative conditioning regimens), the option of allogeneic transplant is limited to a relatively small minority of patients, given the overall median age of myeloma patients, the frequent existence of comorbid conditions, and the profound immunosuppression caused by the disease and its treatment (based on corticosteroids). In several published series, the median survival time after transplant has been approximately 1.5 years, with long-term survival (7 years) less than 30%. Relapse rates are approaching 70% (not appreciably different, but somewhat delayed from the tandem autotransplant experience), with late relapses occurring up to 10 years posttransplant, contrary to the experience in acute and chronic leukemias.[396,397] The major obstacle has been the high TRM, which reaches 40% to 50% during the first year,[396,398,399] partly reflecting the fact that allogeneic transplantation was mainly used as a last resort approach to relapsing patients. The Intergroup study of newly diagnosed MM patients closed the allogeneic transplant arm after enrollment of the first 31 patients because of a 50% mortality rate in the first 3-month posttransplant period. The exception to this excessively high TRM is a trial using CD6 depletion in 61 patients, with an early TRM of only 10% due to the fact that only 17% of the patients developed grade II or greater graft-versus-host disease (GVHD).[398] The CR rate was only 22%, and median EFS and OS were 12 and 22 months, respectively. The Seattle group reported on 80 MM patients, mostly with chemoresistant disease.[398] Sixty received marrow from HLA-identical sibling donors and 20 from unrelated or mismatched donors. Conditioning was achieved with busulfan and cyclophosphamide plus TBI. Prophylaxis against GVHD was cyclosporine combined with methotrexate or prednisone. TRM was 56%; 15% of patients died of late (after day 100) complications. The CR rate achieved was 36%, and 5-year EFS and OS were 16% and 20%, respectively. In a multicenter analysis of 139 patients, a comparison was performed between TBI combined with either melphalan or cyclophosphamide. TRM at 1 year was similar with both regimens; however, the relapse/progression rate was significantly lower in the melphalan-treated patients (37% vs 81%; $P = 0.009$).[399] This study seems to indicate that the conditioning regimen is important for outcome and that the entire effect of allogeneic transplantation is not only a graft-versus-myeloma effect.

The favorable prognostic factors for long-term survival are similar to those for autologous transplant: low β_2M levels, limited previous treatment, and chemosensitive disease. Women appear to fare better, with the best combination being female donor and female recipient.[356] The EBMT Myeloma Registry performed a retrospective analysis comparing 189 allogeneic transplant patients with 189 case-matched autologous transplant controls.[396] Median survival was 18 months in the allotransplant group versus 34 months in the autotransplant group, despite the significantly higher relapse rate in the latter. The difference in relapse rate did not compensate for TRM (41% in the allogeneic transplant group vs 13% in the autologous transplant group). An update on 690 patients from EBMT reports an encouraging decrease in TRM in the period between 1994 and 1998 (approximately 25% and 30% at 6 months and 2 years, respectively) compared with the previous 10 years (1983–1993), believed to be due to decreased incidence of infections and interstitial pneumonitis and, possibly, implementation of allogeneic transplant earlier in the disease course. The improvement in TRM resulted in an actuarial survival rate of 50% at 4 years in the most recently treated group versus 30% in the previously treated group. However, no reduction in relapse rate was observed. No survival benefit was shown with use of peripheral blood stem cells compared with bone marrow.[400]

In an effort to decrease TRM, the Seattle group sought to separate the immunotherapeutic effect of the allogeneic transplant from the toxicity of the high-dose conditioning regimen. These investigators combined an autologous transplant (with low TRM) for maximal cytoreduction with a subsequent nonmyeloablative allogeneic transplant.[401] Fifty-four previously treated MM patients (median age 52 years, 52% with refractory or relapsed disease) received HDT with melphalan 200 mg/m^2 and ASCT, followed 40 to 229 days later (median 62 days) by TBI (200 cGy) and immunosuppression with mycophenolate mofetil (for 1 month) and cyclosporine (for at least 2 months) and unmanipulated peripheral blood stem cells from HLA-identical siblings. Fifty-two patients received the allografts (mostly on an outpatient basis) with minimal, if any, hematologic toxicity. All engrafted (90% and 99% of donor T-cell chimerism by postallotransplant day 28 and 84, respectively) with no late graft rejection. Eleven patients died after the allograft, three of progressive disease and eight of due to transplant-related complications. At median followup of 552 days after allograft, the OS rate is 78%. Acute GVHD (grades II–IV) developed in 38% of the patients; 46% required treatment of chronic GVHD. The overall response rate was 83%, with 57% CR. Others have reported similar results with the application of a dose-reduced conditioning regimen (melphalan, fludarabine, antithymocyte globulin) and allogeneic transplant from either a related or an unrelated donor following an autologous transplant (melphalan 200 mg/m^2).[402] Median interval between the two transplants was 4 months. Strictly defined CR rate was 73% after allografting. Thirteen of 17 patients with advanced myeloma are alive (12 progression-free) with median followup of 13 months after allogeneic transplant. The same conditioning regimen was used in 21 patients with advanced disease who received unrelated stem cell transplants. At median followup of 13 months, 2-year estimated OS and EFS are 74% and 53%, respectively.[403] In an update on 120 patients, TRM was 18%. Relapse after a preceding transplant was the most important risk factor for TRM, relapse, EFS, and OS. The risk of relapse decreased significantly in patients with chronic graft-versus-host disease. Even in the subgroup of patients with chemosensitive myeloma and no relapse prior to allotransplantation, 2-year EFS was only 60% with a related donor (n = 32) but 81% with an unrelated donor (n = 12).[404] A study from the University of Arkansas of 45 MM patients who received grafts from a sibling or an unrelated donor after dose-reduced conditioning regimens showed that chemosensitive and adequate performance status were the only significant factors for EFS and OS.[405] The EBMT reported the outcome of 229 patients who received an allograft for myeloma with reduced-intensity conditioning. Conditioning regimens were heterogeneous. TRM at 1 year was 22%. Three-year OS and progression-free survival were 41% and 21%, respectively. Inferior OS was seen in patients with chemorefractory myeloma, in those with more than one prior transplant, and in male patients with female donors. Grade II to IV acute GVHD occurred in 31%. Chronic GVHD was associated with better progression-free and OS, suggesting that a graft-versus-host effect is important. The probability of disease progression at 3 years was 50%.[406] With followup now extending to 7 years, it is clear that reduced-intensity conditioning regimens are associated with lower TRM but a higher rate of disease progression compared to myeloablative conditioning regimens. In an EBMT study, the rate of relapse after reduced-intensity conditioning was more than twice that seen with myeloablative conditioning ($P = 0.0001$).[407] KIR-ligand mismatching in the setting of reduced-intensity conditioning was found to be protective against relapse,[408] as had been shown in acute leukemia.

Is a Cure Possible with Autotransplants?

In a report from the University of Arkansas, the outcome and prognostic factors in a group of 515 consecutive newly diagnosed and previously treated MM patients intended to receive melphalan-based tandem autotransplants with followup of more than 5 years were studied. Cytogenetic abnormalities were detected in 34% of patients; 72% received two transplants less than 12 months apart. Median OS and EFS were 30 and 17 months, respectively; 121 (24%) of 515 patients had EFS for more than 5 years. On multivariate analysis, favorable factors for EFS greater than 5 years were the absence of chromosome 11 and 13 abnormalities (odds ratio 6.1), less than 12 months of preceding standard treatment (odds ratio 2.6), and pretransplant β_2M 2.5 mg/L or less (odds ratio 1.7). The EFS curve shows a rapid decline during the first 3 years, a slower decline between 3 and 7 years, and an apparently stable plateau after 7 years among 46 patients (Figs. 87–13 and 87–14). Forty patients (of the 46 on the plateau phase) had received two autotransplants, whereas two had received an allogeneic transplant as a second (consolidative) transplant. Median survivals of patients with 0, 1, 2, and 3 unfavorable factors were 37, 26, 14, and 7 months, respectively, whereas 7-year EFS was 36%, 15%, 10%, and 0%, respectively. By using a 1-year landmark analysis (and thus excluding patients who relapsed or died during the first posttransplant year), achievement of CR was not significant for EFS. Our data suggest that patients in CR more than 7 years posttransplant in all likelihood are cured, whereas non-CR patients with EFS more than 7 years may have "regressed" to an MGUS phase, with possibly very good long-term prognoses.[409]

Biologic Agents

Interferon

When used as a single agent, interferon-α has modest activity against myeloma, with an objective response rate of 10% to 20%.[410] In an attempt to improve the efficacy of first-line treatment, interferon has been combined with MP. In two randomized trials comparing MP with MP plus interferon, no survival difference was detected.[411,412] Also, no difference in survival was detected when interferon was used as maintenance after a plateau phase had been reached after standard treatment.[413] The Myeloma Trialists' Collaborative Group performed a meta-analysis of 12 induction and 12 maintenance trials, which

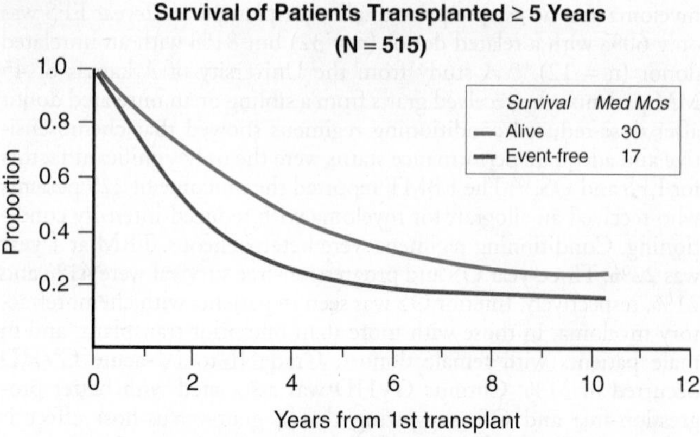

Figure 87–13 Event-free survival and overall survival of 515 patients receiving autotransplants and median followup of at least 5 years. *(From Tricot G, Spencer T, Sawyer J, et al: Predicting long-term [≥5 years] event-free survival in multiple myeloma patients following planned tandem autotransplants. Br J Haematol 116:211, 2002.)*

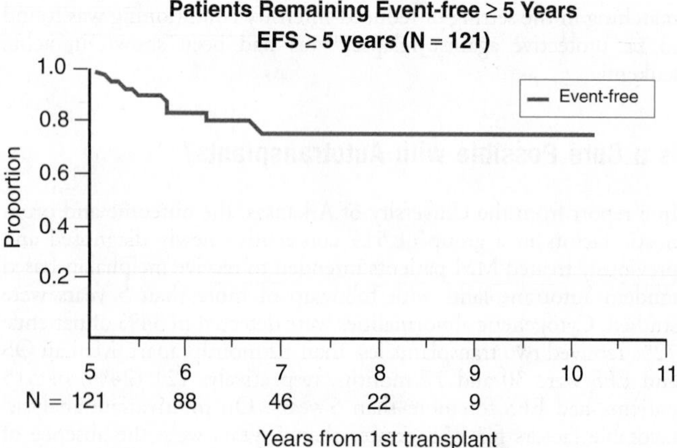

Figure 87–14 Event-free survival times of only those patients alive and without disease progression at 5 years. *(From Tricot G, Spencer T, Sawyer J, et al: Predicting long-term [≥5 years] event-free survival in multiple myeloma patients following planned tandem autotransplants. Br J Haematol 116:211, 2002.)*

included more than 4000 MM patients.[239] In induction trials, response rates were slightly better with interferon (57.5% vs 53.1%; $P = 0.01$). EFS was better with interferon (33% vs 24% at 3 years; $P < 0.00001$). Median time to progression was increased by approximately 6 months in both settings, whereas OS was slightly better with interferon (53% vs 49% at 3 years; $P = 0.01$), with median OS increased by approximately 4 months. Additionally, interferon-α did not extend survival when used as maintenance in the postautologous transplantation setting in one study,[391] but it did prolong survival in the retrospective analysis of EBMT registry, which addressed the same question.[356] Given the very modest benefit, toxicity, inconvenience, cost, and stem cell damaging potential of interferon, it should be used cautiously, if at all.

Supportive Care

Bisphosphonates

Bone involvement in MM contributes significantly to the morbidity of the disease. Bisphosphonates inhibit bone resorption in different ways: they block the development of osteoclasts from monocytes, induce osteoclast apoptosis, prevent migration of osteoclasts to the bone surface, and inhibit the production of bone-resorbing cytokines by bone marrow stromal cells.[414] In a prospective randomized trial, patients with symptomatic myeloma and at least one lytic lesion received either placebo or pamidronate 90 mg as a 4-hour intravenous infusion every 4 weeks for nine cycles in addition to antimyeloma treatment.[415] The proportion of patients who experienced any skeletal-related event (i.e., spinal cord compression, new fractures, need for radiation treatment, or surgery) was significantly lower in the pamidronate than in the placebo group (24% vs 41%; $P < 0.001$). Pain improved, and quality of life and performance status were better in patients who received pamidronate. The same results were observed after extended administration of pamidronate for 21 cycles.[416] Although OS times were not different in the two groups, pamidronate-treated patients who received salvage chemotherapy regimens lived longer than did patients on salvage treatment who did not receive the drug (21 vs 14 months; $P = 0.041$). Zoledronate (third-generation bisphosphonate) is much more potent in vitro (at least 100 times) than pamidronate and is administered as a 30-minute intravenous infusion. Zoledronate has only proved to be superior for treatment of hypercalcemia but not for prevention of skeletal-related events compared with pamidronate. Bisphosphonates are generally well-tolerated agents. Prolonged use by infusions at a more rapid rate or higher than recommended dose or frequency has caused nonspecific proteinuria and impaired renal function.[417] Focal segmental glomerulosclerosis was the underlying pathologic lesion. Even more intriguing (and perhaps more important than their bone-strengthening effects), bisphosphonates appear to have an antimyeloma effect in vivo, stimulate T-cell proliferation and function, and may modulate the adhesion molecule profile and thus overcome drug resistance by interfering with the malignant cell–extracellular matrix interactions.[418] Findings have shown that bisphosphonates inhibit production of IL-6 by marrow stromal cells and secretion of matrix metalloproteinase 1 (molecule critical for bone remodeling and tumor invasion).[419] Osteonecrosis of the jaw has been recognized as a complication of long-term bisphosphonates treatment.[420–424] Since its first description in 2003, hundreds of cases of osteonecrosis of the jaw have been reported worldwide. It is characterized by the appearance of necrotic bone in the oral cavity and affects either the mandible or the maxilla. Although it can develop spontaneously, it is more common after a surgical procedure such as dental extraction or implant.[421,424] The risk increases in patients who have been taking bisphosphonates for more than 3 years[421] and is more common in myeloma than in other cancers.[421] The risk is higher with zoledronate than with pamidronate.[421–424] The inhibitory effect of bisphosphonates on osteoclastic activity is thought to occur via suppression of bone remodeling resulting in microfractures that are not repaired, and perhaps angiogenesis. Bone histology often shows osteomyelitis, and microbiology may reveal actinomyces or mixed bacterial flora.[425] Whether a correlation exists between osteonecrosis of the jaw and avascular necrosis of the hip is unclear.

Avascular Necrosis of the Femur

Avascular necrosis of the bone is thought to be caused by a compromised blood supply. It typically occurs after trauma but may result from glucocorticoid therapy, radiation therapy, sickle cell anemia, and connective tissue diseases. The diagnosis is mainly based on MRI findings. Glucocorticoids reduce blood flow to the bone and induce apoptosis of osteoblasts and osteocytes. In a study of 553 patients with median followup of 33 months, the incidence of avascular necrosis was 9%. Median onset was 12 months. Multivariate analysis identified three major risk factors: cumulative dexamethasone dose, male gender, and younger age. It usually was asymptomatic, and only four of 49 patients with avascular necrosis required hip replacement. This complication was not more frequent in thalidomide-treated patients.[426]

Vertebroplasty and Kyphoplasty

Painful vertebral compression fractures traditionally have been managed with radiation therapy, analgesics, bed rest, and bracing.

Most patients experience limited, if any, benefits from these interventions. Cement augmentation of the vertebral body (vertebroplasty) has been used for pain relief in patients with spine involvement by various tumors, including MM.[427,428] The technique consists of percutaneous injection of low-viscosity liquid bone cement into the damaged vertebral body. Improvement in pain is reported by virtually all patients and is sustained in most patients for long periods.[429] Although significant durable pain relief is anticipated, vertebroplasty does not restore the loss of height of the vertebral body and does not correct the spinal deformity. Furthermore, a high incidence of cement leakage, especially if the bone contour is not intact, usually occurring in the paraspinal soft tissues, is seen in the majority of cases.[429] Although this leakage is of no clinical importance in the overwhelming majority of patients, it occasionally leads to nerve root compression that requires emergency decompressive surgery. Kyphoplasty is a more recently developed technique that involves the creation of a cavity in the vertebral body (through a trocar placement, drilling of a bone channel, and insertion of an inflatable balloon) and its filling with highly viscous cement. A report of 55 consecutive procedures performed in 18 MM patients (mean followup 7.4 months) showed significant pain relief, improvement in performance status, and an average 34% restoration of the vertebral body height loss. Asymptomatic cement leakage occurred in only 4% of procedures.[430] The technique is unsuitable when the posterior vertebral wall is deficient because of possible further displacement of bony fragments during the balloon inflation phase, possibly leading to spinal cord compression.

Erythropoietin

Anemia of variable severity affects more than two thirds of MM patients. Patients with MM have an inappropriate erythropoietin response for their degree of anemia. Overexpression of the Fas ligand, MIP-1α, and TRAIL by malignant cells triggers the death of immature erythroblasts.[431] In several randomized, placebo-controlled[432] and community-based studies, recombinant human erythropoietin has been shown to significantly decrease the frequency of transfusion requirements, increase the mean hemoglobin levels, and improve quality of life and performance status in anemic myeloma patients. The impact of treatment is greater in patients with limited preceding treatment. Furthermore, patients with mild anemia (Hb levels approximately 12 g/dL) should not be excluded from treatment, because the greatest incremental improvement in quality of life occurs when hemoglobin increases from 12 to 13 g/dL. Erythropoietin is well tolerated; the once-weekly epoetin alfa and darbepoetin every 2 weeks schedules are equally efficacious.[433] Administration of erythropoietin before autologous transplantation reduces transfusion requirements.[434,435] Erythropoietin may have an antimyeloma effect by decreasing hypoxemia in the tumor but also by activation of $CD8^+$ T cells.[436,437] Although it has been claimed that erythropoietin increases the risk of deep vein thrombosis when thalidomide or lenalidomide is given,[316] we did not observe such an increase in our Total Therapy II study.[438]

Approach to Therapy for Multiple Myeloma

Patients who are asymptomatic and have no end-organ damage should not be treated until clear evidence of disease progression is demonstrated by new lesions on skeletal survey, MRI, or PET scan, hypercalcemia, increase in M protein, or worsening renal failure or anemia due to myeloma. If a physician is unsure whether a patient should be treated after a complete workup has been performed, it usually is better to delay therapy and reevaluate after 6 to 8 weeks, with biweekly or weekly measurements of M protein in the blood and urine to determine the pace of myeloma progression. Remember that before any treatment is given, patients should undergo bone marrow aspirate and biopsy, skeletal survey, measurement of LDH, creatinine, complete blood count, CRP, and β_2M, serum protein electrophoresis, 24-hour urine collection to measure total Bence Jones proteinuria, serum and urine immunofixation electrophoresis, and determination of free light chains. It is important that patients undergo routine cytogenetic analyses. Cytogenetic analysis is preferable to FISH analysis. For patients who require treatment, sufficient evidence based on randomized, pair-mate historic, controlled, and population-based studies indicate that high-dose chemotherapy with stem cell support is superior to standard-dose treatment. It results in a higher CR rate and prolonged EFS and OS periods. Median OS of 10 years is realistic with optimal intensive treatment. Multiple studies have indicated that the best preparative regimen for autologous transplantation is melphalan 200 mg/m^2. Age should not be a contraindication to autologous transplantation. However, comorbid conditions, such as severely decreased cardiopulmonary function, major liver function abnormalities, and impaired mental status not due to metabolic causes, are contraindications to transplantation. Patients with renal failure also clearly benefit from autologous transplantation. In contrast with myeloma patients who are in good condition, patients with renal insufficiency and those older than 70 years do better with a reduced dose of melphalan at 140 mg/m^2. Before transplantation, patients should receive chemotherapy, including alkylating agents, but not melphalan, busulfan, or BCNU. The main goal of induction therapy is to collect a large number of stem cells that will allow up to four transplants if necessary. It probably is not appropriate to collect stem cells with growth factors in patients who have only been pretreated with VAD or dexamethasone/thalidomide. The quality of response prior to autologous transplantation is not important. The only mature study that has compared a single with tandem transplants has clearly shown a superior outcome with tandem transplants. It should be noted that the difference was evident only more than 3 years after the start of treatment. Patients without chromosome 13 deletions, without hypodiploidy, and without increased LDH levels at the time of diagnosis (75% of all patients) will do very well with tandem transplants. Median survival duration of these patients is predicted to be greater than 10 years, which is three times longer than that with conventional chemotherapy. Patients with increased LDH levels, hypodiploidy, or chromosome 13 deletion have inferior outcomes; however, among these patients, the best outcome is seen with tandem autologous transplants. In the patients who have increased LDH hypodiploidy, no benefit has been observed with allotransplantation or a combination of autologous transplantation followed by nonmyeloablative allotransplantation. Other treatment modalities for those patients must be identified and may include a combination of autotransplantation with immunotherapy such as tumor vaccination or natural killer cells. Application of the newer drugs, such as thalidomide, lenalidomide, and bortezomib, is best in the posttransplantation period after major tumor debulking, when the chances of developing resistance to these marginally active drugs is much lower. They are best used in combination with dexamethasone.

Patients who are not candidates for transplantation should be treated with combinations of cytotoxic drugs with the newer drugs, such as melphalan, thalidomide or lenalidomide or bortezomib and dexamethasone. Treatment should be continued for at least 12 months or until a clear plateau has been reached.

Supportive care in the treatment of myeloma is essential. All patients should begin receiving treatment immediately after diagnosis with monthly bisphosphonates, preferably pamidronate if renal function is preserved. Ideally, treatment should be combined with a calcium supplement and hormone replacement therapy in patients who do not have contraindications to such therapy. After 2 to 3 years of bisphosphonates therapy, the frequency should be reduced to every 3 months to decrease the risk of osteonecrosis of the jaw. Anemia should be corrected by administration of erythropoietin. Patients who do not respond to erythropoietin administration often benefit from intravenous iron administration. It is important to adequately control pain so that patients remain ambulatory and can perform their daily functions; this usually require opiates. In most cases, pain ultimately is best controlled by administration of high-dose chemotherapy and stem cell support. However, some patients will require either vertebroplasty or kyphoplasty for persistent pain. Depression is very common, especially in the early stages of the disease. Antidepressants are indicated in at least one third of myeloma patients. During the early stages of chemotherapy, it is important to provide antibiotic prophylaxis, including antiherpetic and antifungal drugs and antibiotics. After transplantation, the risk of herpes zoster remains high and will require continued administration of an antiherpetic drug. Yearly influenza vaccinations are indicated for myeloma patients. As soon as immune function has recovered adequately after transplantation, patients should be revaccinated for tetanus and pneumococcal infections.

SUGGESTED READINGS

Anderson G, Gries M, Kurihara N, et al: Thalidomide derivative CC-4047 inhibits osteoclast formation by down-regulation of PU.1. Blood 107:3098, 2006.

Attal M, Harousseau JL, Leyvraz S, et al: Maintenance therapy with thalidomide improves survival in multiple myeloma patients. Blood 108:3289, 2006.

Badros A, Weikel D, Salama A, et al: Osteonecrosis of the jaw in multiple myeloma patients: Clinical features and risk factors. J Clin Oncol 24:945, 2006.

Barlogie B, Tricot G, van Rhee F, et al: Long-term outcome results of the first tandem autotransplant trial for multiple myeloma. Br J Haematol 135:158, 2006.

Barlogie B, Kyle R, Anderson K, et al: Standard chemotherapy compared with high-dose chemoradiotherapy for multiple myeloma: Final results of phase III US Intergroup Trial S9321. J Clin Oncol 24:929, 2006.

Barlogie B, Tricot G, Anaissie E, et al: Thalidomide and hematopoietic-cell transplantation for multiple myeloma. N Engl J Med 354:1021, 2006.

Barlogie B, Tricot G, Rasmussen E, et al: Total therapy 2 without thalidomide in comparison with total therapy 1: Role of intensified induction and posttransplantation consolidation therapies. Blood 107:2633, 2006.

Bensinger WI: The current status of reduced-intensity allogeneic hematopoietic stem cell transplantation for multiple myeloma. Leukemia 20:1683, 2006.

Chang D, Liu N, Klimek V, et al: Enhancement of ligand-dependent activation of human natural killer T cells by lenalidomide: Therapeutic implications. Blood 108:618, 2006.

Dimopoulos M, Kastritis E, Anagnostopoulos A, et al: Osteonecrosis of the jaw in patients with multiple myeloma treated with bisphosphonates: Evidence of increased risk after treatment with zoledronic acid. Haematologica 91:968, 2006.

Garban F, Attal M, Michallet M, et al: Prospective comparison of autologous stem cell transplantation followed by dose-reduced allograft (IFM99-03 trial) with tandem autologous stem cell transplantation (IFM99-04 trial) in high-risk de novo multiple myeloma. Blood 107:3474, 2006.

Glaspy J, Vadhan-Raj S, Patel R, et al: Randomized comparison of every-2-week darbepoetin alfa and weekly epoetin alfa for the treatment of chemotherapy-induced anemia: The 20030125 Study Group Trial. J Clin Oncol 24:2290, 2006.

Hanamura I, Stewart JP, Huang Y, et al: Frequent gain of chromosome band 1q21 in plasma cells dyscrasias detected by fluorescence in situ hybridization: Incidence increase from MGUS to relapsed myeloma and is related to prognosis and disease progression following tandem stem cell transplantation. Blood 108:1724, 2006.

Hartmann C: A Wnt canon orchestrating osteoblastogenesis. Trends Cell Biol 16:151, 2006.

Hoang B, Zhu L, Shi Y, et al: Oncogenic RAS mutations in myeloma cells selectively induce cox-2 expression, which participates in enhanced adhesion to fibronectin and chemoresistance. Blood 107:4484, 2006.

Knight R, DeLap R, Zeldis J, et al: Lenalidomide and venous thrombosis in multiple myeloma. N Engl J Med 354:2079, 2006.

Mateos MV, Hernandez JM, Hernandez MT, et al: Bortezomib plus melphalan and prednisone in elderly untreated patients with multiple myeloma: Results of a multicenter phase I/II study. Blood 108:2165, 2006.

Migliorati C, Siegel M, Elting L: Bisphosphonate-associated osteonecrosis: A long-term complication of bisphosphonate treatment. Lancet Oncol 7:508, 2006.

Mileshkin L, Stark R, Day B, et al: Development of neuropathy in patients with myeloma treated with thalidomide: Patterns of occurrence and the role of electrophysiologic monitoring. J Clin Oncol 24:4507, 2006.

Miyakoshi S, Kami M, Yuji K, et al: Severe pulmonary complications in Japanese patients after bortezomib treatment for refractory multiple myeloma. Blood 107:3492, 2006.

Moreau P, Hullin C, Garban F, et al: Tandem autologous stem cell transplantation in high-risk de novo multiple myeloma: Final results of the prospective and randomized IFM 99-04 protocol. Blood 107:397, 2006.

Morgan G, Krishnan B, Jenner M, et al: Advances in oral therapy for multiple myeloma. Lancet Oncol 7:316, 2006.

Morvan F, Boulukos K, Clement-Lacroix P, et al: Deletion of a single allele of the Dkk1 gene leads to an increase in bone formation and bone mass. J Bone Miner Res 21:934, 2006.

Palumbo A, Bringhen S, Caravita T, et al: Oral melphalan and prednisone chemotherapy plus thalidomide compared with melphalan and prednisone alone in elderly patients with multiple myeloma: Randomized controlled trial. Lancet 367:825, 2006.

Offidani M, Corvatta L, Piersantelli MN, et al: Thalidomide, dexamethasone, and pegylated liposomal doxorubicin (ThaDD) for patients older than 65 years with newly diagnosed multiple myeloma. Blood 108:2159, 2006.

Rajkumar S, Blood E, Vesole D, et al: Phase III clinical trial of thalidomide plus dexamethasone compared with dexamethasone alone in newly diagnosed multiple myeloma: A clinical trial coordinated by the Eastern Cooperative Oncology Group. J Clin Oncol 24:431, 2006.

Ramos L, de las Heras JA, Sanchez S, et al: Medium-term results of percutaneous vertebroplasty in multiple myeloma. Eur J Haematol 77:7, 2006.

Richardson P, Blood E, Mitsiades C, et al: A randomized phase 2 study of lenalidomide therapy for patients with relapsed or relapsed and refractory multiple myeloma. Blood 108:3458, 2006.

Richardson P, Briemberg H, Jagannath S, et al: Frequency, characteristics, and reversibility of peripheral neuropathy during treatment of advanced multiple myeloma with bortezomib. J Clin Oncol 24:3113, 2006.

Tricot G, Zhan F, Huang Y, et al: Metaphase cytogenetics adds to gene expression profiling in the identification of high risk multiple myeloma. American Society of Hematology 48th Annual Meeting and Exposition, December 9–12, 2006, Orlando, Florida, Abstract 114.

Weber DM, Chen C, Niesvizky R, et al: Lenalidomide plus high-dose dexamethasone provides improved overall survival compared to high-dose dexamethasone along for relapsed or refractory multiple myeloma (MM): Results of a North American phase III study (MM-009). J Clin Oncol 24:7521, 2006.

Zangari M, Cavallo F, Prasad K, et al: Erythropoietin therapy and venous thromboembolic events in patients with multiple myeloma receiving chemotherapy with or without thalidomide. Blood [ASH poster presentation], 2006.

Zervas K, Verrou E, Teleioudis Z, et al: Incidence, risk factors and management of osteonecrosis of the jaw in patients with multiple myeloma: A single-centre experience in 303 patients. Br J Haematol 134:620, 2006.

Zhan F, Huang Y, Colla S, et al: The molecular classification of multiple myeloma. Blood 108:2020, 2006.

Zonder J, Barlogie B, Durie B, et al: Thrombotic complications in patients with newly diagnosed multiple myeloma treated with lenalidomide and dexamethasone: Benefit of aspirin prophylaxis. Blood 108, 403:2006.

REFERENCES

For complete list of references log onto www.expertconsult.com

CHAPTER 88

WALDENSTRÖM MACROGLOBULINEMIA/LYMPHOPLASMACYTIC LYMPHOMA

Steven P. Treon, Evdoxia Hatjiharissi, Xavier Leleu, Aldo Roccaro, and Giampaolo Merlini

INTRODUCTION

Waldenström macroglobulinemia (WM) is a distinct clinicopathologic entity resulting from the accumulation, predominantly in the bone marrow, of clonally related lymphocytes, lymphoplasmacytic cells (LPC) and plasma cells that secrete a monoclonal IgM protein (Fig. 88–1).[1] This condition is considered to correspond to the lymphoplasmacytic lymphoma (LPL) as defined by the Revised European American Lymphoma (REAL) and World Health Organization classification systems.[2,3] Most cases of LPL are WM, with less than 5% of cases made up of IgA, IgG, and nonsecretory LPL.

EPIDEMIOLOGY AND ETIOLOGY

WM is an uncommon disease, with a reported age-adjusted incidence rate of 3.4 per million among males and 1.7 per million among females in the United States, and a geometrical increase with age.[4,5] The incidence rate for WM is higher among Caucasians, with descendants of Africans representing only 5% of all patients. A similar incidence was reported in a European-based study: 2.0 for females and 4.2 for males per million person-years.[6] However, a recent study conducted in U.K. reported a higher rate: 5.5 (7.3 for males and 4.2 for females) per million.[7] Genetic factors appear to be an important factor in the pathogenesis of WM. Approximately 20% of WM patients have an Ashkenazi (Eastern European) Jewish ethnic background, and there have been numerous reports of familial disease, including multigenerational clustering of WM and other B-cell lymphoproliferative diseases.[8–12] In a recent study, approximately 20% of 257 serial WM patients presenting to a tertiary referral had a first-degree relative with either WM or another B-cell disorder.[9] Frequent familial associations with other immunologic disorders in healthy relatives, including hypogammaglobulinemia and hypergammaglobulinemia (particularly polyclonal IgM), autoantibody (particularly to thyroid) production, and manifestation of hyperactive B cells have also been reported.[11,12] Increased expression of the *bcl-2* gene with enhanced B-cell survival may underlie the increased immunoglobulin synthesis in familial WM.[11] The role of environmental factors in WM remains to be clarified, but chronic antigenic stimulation from infections, certain drug and Agent Orange exposures remain suspect. An etiologic role for hepatitis C virus (HCV) infection has been suggested; however, in a recent study examining 100 consecutive WM patients, no association could be established using both serologic and molecular diagnostic studies for HCV infection.[13–15]

BIOLOGY

Cytogenetic Findings

Several studies, usually performed on limited series of patients, have been published on cytogenetic findings in WM, demonstrating a great variety of numerical and structural chromosome abnormalities. Numerical losses involving chromosomes 17, 18, 19, 20, 21, 22, X, and Y have been commonly observed, although gains in chromosomes 3, 4, and 12 have also been reported.[9,16–21] Chromosome 6q deletions encompassing 6q21–22 have been observed in up to half of WM patients, and at a comparable frequency among patients with and without a familial history.[9,21] Several candidate tumor suppressor genes in this region are under study, including BLIMP-1, a master regulatory gene implicated in lymphoplasmacytic differentiation. Notable, however, is the absence of IgH switch region rearrangements in WM, a finding that may be used to discern cases of IgM myeloma where IgH switch region rearrangements are a predominant feature.[22]

Nature of the Clonal Cell

The WM bone marrow B-cell clone shows intraclonal differentiation from small lymphocytes with large focal deposits of surface immunoglobulins, to lymphoplasmacytic cells, to mature plasma cells that contain intracytoplasmic immunoglobulins.[23] Clonal B cells are detectable among blood B lymphocytes, and their number increases in patients who fail to respond to therapy or who progress.[24] These clonal blood cells possess the peculiar capacity to differentiate spontaneously, in vitro, to plasma cells. This is through an interleukin-6 (IL-6)-dependent process in cells from patients with IgM monoclonal gammopathy of undetermined significance (MGUS) and mostly an IL-6-independent process in cells from WM patients.[25] All these cells express the monoclonal IgM present in the blood and a variable percentage of them also express surface IgD. The characteristic immunophenotypic profile of the lymphoplasmacytic cells in WM includes the expression of the pan B-cell markers CD19, CD20, CD22, CD79, and FMC7.2.[26–28] Expression of CD5, CD10, and CD23 may be found in 10% to 20% of cases, and does not exclude the diagnosis of WM.[29]

The phenotype of lymphoplasmacytic cells in WM suggests that the clone is derived from a post–germinal center B cell. This conclusion is further strengthened by the results of the analysis of the nature (silent or amino acid replacing) and distribution (in framework or CDR regions) of somatic mutations in Ig heavy- and light-chain variable regions performed in patients with WM.[30,31] This analysis showed a high rate of replacement mutations, compared with the closest germline genes, clustering in the CDR regions and without intraclonal variation. Subsequent studies showed a strong preferential usage of VH3/JH4 gene families, no intraclonal variation, and no evidence for any isotype-switched transcripts.[32,33] These data indicate that WM may originate from an IgM^+ and/or IgM^+ IgD^+ memory B cell. Normal IgM^+ memory B cells are localized to the bone marrow, where they mature to IgM-secreting cells.[34]

Bone Marrow Microenvironment

Increased numbers of mast cells are found in the bone marrow of WM patients, wherein they are usually admixed with tumor aggregates.[28,35] Recent studies have helped clarify the role of mast cells in WM. Coculture of primary autologous or mast cell lines with WM LPC resulted in dose-dependent WM cell proliferation and/or tumor

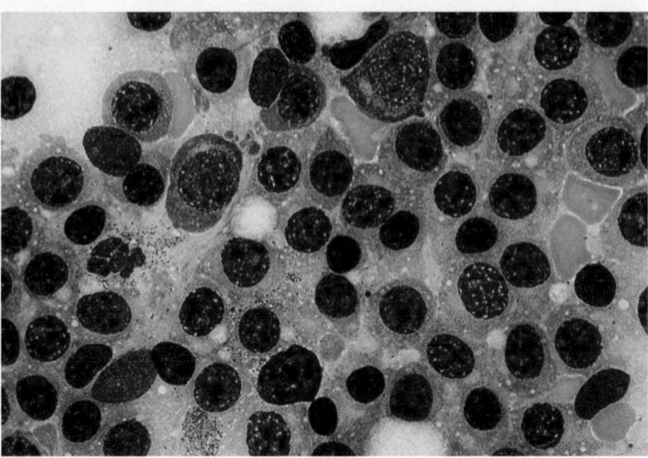

Figure 88–1 Aspirate from a patient with Waldenström macroglobulinemia demonstrating excess mature lymphocytes, lymphoplasmacytic cells and plasma cells. *(Courtesy of Marvin Stone, MD.)*

Table 88–1 Clinical and Laboratory Findings for 149 Consecutive Newly Diagnosed Patients with the Consensus Panel Diagnosis of Waldenstrom Macroglobulinemia Presenting to the Dana Farber Cancer Institute

	Median	Range	Institutional Normal Reference Range
Age (year)	59	34–84	NA
Gender (male/female)	85/64		NA
Bone marrow involvement	30%	5–95%	NA
Adenopathy	16%		NA
Splenomegaly	10%		NA
IgM (mg/dL)	2,870	267–12,400	40–230
IgG (mg/dL)	587	47–2770	700–1600
IgA (mg/dL)	47	8–509	70–400
Serum viscosity (cp)	2.0	1.4–6.6	1.4–1.9
Hct (%)	35.0%	17.2–45.4	34.8–43.6
Plt ($\times10^9$/L)	253	24–649	155–410
Wbc ($\times10^9$/L)	6.0	0.3–13	3.8–9.2
B_2M (mg/dL)	3.0	1.3–13.7	0–2.7
LDH	395	122–1131	313–618

NA, not applicable.

colony, primarily through CD40 ligand (CD40L) signaling. Furthermore, WM cells through elaboration of soluble CD27 (sCD27), induce the upregulation of CD40L on mast cells derived from WM patients and mast cell lines.[36]

CLINICAL FEATURES

The clinical and laboratory findings of patients with WM at time of diagnosis in one large institutional study[9] are presented in Table 88–1. Unlike most indolent lymphomas, splenomegaly and lymphadenopathy are prominent in only a minority of patients (≤15%). Purpura is frequently associated with cryoglobulinemia and more rarely with AL amyloidosis, whereas hemorrhagic manifestations and neuropathies are multifactorial in origin. The morbidity associated with WM is caused by the concurrence of two main components: tissue infiltration by neoplastic cells and, more importantly, the physicochemical and immunologic properties of the monoclonal IgM. As shown in Table 88–2, the monoclonal IgM can produce clinical manifestations through several different mechanisms related to its physicochemical properties, nonspecific interactions with other proteins, antibody activity, and tendency to deposit in tissues.[37–40]

MORBIDITY MEDIATED BY THE EFFECTS OF IgM

Hyperviscosity Syndrome

Blood hyperviscosity is affected by increased serum IgM levels leading to hyperviscosity-related complications.[41] The mechanisms behind the marked increase in the resistance to blood flow and the resulting impaired transit through the microcirculatory system are rather complex.[41–43] The main determinants are (1) a high concentration of monoclonal IgMs, which may form aggregates and may bind water through their carbohydrate component, and (2) their interaction with blood cells. Monoclonal IgMs increase red cell aggregation (*rouleaux* formation, see Fig. 88–2) while also reducing deformability. The possible presence of cryoglobulins can contribute to increasing blood viscosity as well as to the tendency to induce erythrocyte aggregation. Serum viscosity is proportional to IgM concentration up to 30 g/L, then increases sharply at higher levels. Increased plasma viscosity may also contribute to inappropriately low erythropoietin production, which is the major reason for anemia in these patients. Plasma viscosity may actually inhibit anemia-induced erythropoietin production.[44] Clinical manifestations are related to circulatory disturbances that can be best appreciated by ophthalmoscopy, which shows distended and tortuous retinal veins, hemorrhages, and papilledema (Fig. 88–3).[45] Symptoms usually occur when the monoclonal IgM concentration exceeds 50 g/L or when serum viscosity is >4.0 centipoises (cp), but there is a great individual variability, with some patients showing no evidence of hyperviscosity even at 10 cp.[41] The most common symptoms are oronasal bleeding, visual disturbances due to retinal bleeding, and dizziness that may rarely lead to coma. Heart failure can be aggravated, particularly in the elderly, owing to increased blood viscosity, expanded plasma volume, and anemia. Inappropriate transfusion can exacerbate hyperviscosity and may precipitate cardiac failure.

Cryoglobulinemia

In up to 20% of WM patients, the monoclonal IgM behaves as a cryoglobulin (type I), which leads to symptoms in 5% or less of the cases.[46] Cryoprecipitation is mainly dependent on the concentration of monoclonal IgM; for this reason plasmapheresis or plasma exchange are commonly effective treatment in this condition. Symptoms result from impaired blood flow in small vessels and include Raynaud phenomenon, acrocyanosis, and necrosis of the regions most exposed to cold (tip of the nose, ears, fingers, and toes), malleolar ulcers, purpura, and cold urticaria. Renal manifestations may occur but are infrequent.

Autoantibody Activity

Monoclonal IgM may exert its pathologic effects through specific recognition of autologous antigens, the most notable being nerve constituents, immunoglobulin determinants, and red blood cell antigens:

IgM-Related Neuropathy

In a series of 215 patients with WM, Merlini et al[46] reported the presence of symptomatic peripheral neuropathy in 24% of WM

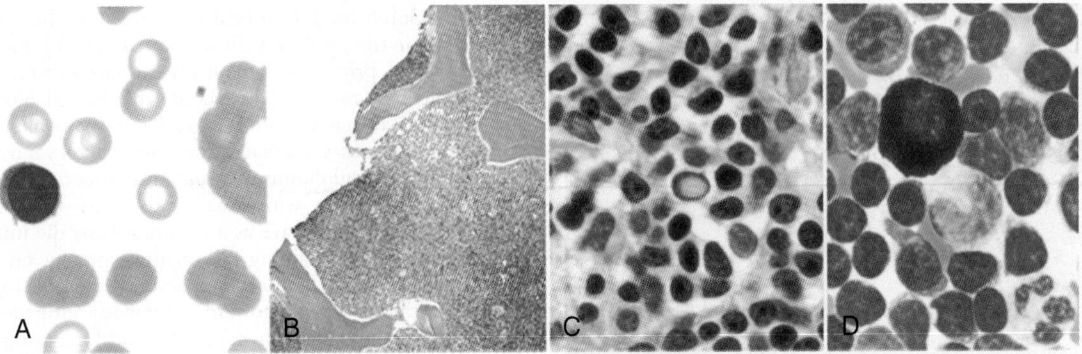

Figure 88–2 Lymphoplasmacytic lymphoma consistent with Waldenström Macroglobulinemia (**A–D**). The patient was a 78-year-old male who first presented with anemia. Serum electrophoresis demonstrated an IgM kappa monoclonal protein, and quantitative immunoglobulins showed an IgM of 5130 mg/dL. His serum viscosity was elevated at 2.9. The peripheral blood smear showed circulating lymphoma cells with slight plasmacytic appearance (**A**). There was also marked rouleaux formation of the red blood cells The bone core biopsy showed an interstitial and slightly paratrabecular infiltrate of malignant lymphoid cells (**B**), which at higher power included many with intranuclear inclusions or Dutcher bodies (**C**, *center*). The aspirate (**D**) was packed with lymphoplasmacytic cells associated with increased mast cells (*upper left*). The phenotype was CD19$^+$, CD20$^+$, IgM/kappa$^+$ with no CD5, CD10, or CD11c expression.

Table 88–2 Physicochemical and Immunological Properties of the Monoclonal IgM Protein in Waldenstrom Macroglobulinemia

Properties of IgM Monoclonal Protein	Diagnostic Condition	Clinical Manifestations
Pentameric structure	Hyperviscosity	Headaches, blurred vision, epistaxis, retinal hemorrhages, leg cramps, impaired mentation, intracranial hemorrhage
Precipitation on cooling	Cryoglobulinemia (Type I)	Raynaud phenomenon, acrocyanosis, ulcers, purpura, cold urticaria
Autoantibody activity to myelin-associated glycoprotein (MAG), ganglioside M1 (GM1), sulfatide moieties on peripheral nerve sheaths	Peripheral neuropathies	Sensorimotor neuropathies, painful neuropathies, ataxic gait, bilateral foot drop
Autoantibody activity to IgG	Cryoglobulinemia (Type II)	Purpura, arthralgias, renal failure, sensorimotor neuropathies
Autoantibody activity to red blood cell antigens	Cold agglutinins	Hemolytic anemia, Raynaud phenomenon, acrocyanosis, livedo reticularis
Tissue deposition as amorphous aggregates	Organ dysfunction	Skin: bullous skin disease, papules, Schnitzler syndrome GI: diarrhea, malabsorption, bleeding. Kidney: proteinuria, renal failure (light-chain component)
Tissue deposition as amyloid fibrils (light-chain component most commonly)	Organ dysfunction	Fatigue, weight loss, edema, periorbital purpura, hepatomegaly, macroglossia, organ dysfunction of involved organs: heart, kidney, liver, peripheral sensory and autonomic nerves.

patients, although prevalence rates ranging from 5% to 38% have been reported in other series.[47,48] An estimated 6.5% to 10% of idiopathic neuropathies are associated with a monoclonal gammopathy, with a preponderance of IgM (60%) followed by IgG (30%) and IgA (10%) (reviewed in Nemni et al[49] and Ropper and Gorson[50]). In WM patients, the nerve damage is mediated by several pathogenetic mechanisms: IgM antibody activity toward nerve constituents causing demyelinating polyneuropathies; endoneurial granulofibrillar deposits of IgM without antibody activity, associated with axonal polyneuropathy; occasionally by tubular deposits in the endoneurium associated with IgM cryoglobulin and, rarely, by amyloid deposits or by neoplastic cell infiltration of nerve structures.[51] Half of the patients with IgM neuropathy have a distinctive clinical syndrome that is associated with antibodies against a minor 100-kd glycoprotein component of nerve, myelin-associated glycoprotein (MAG). Anti-MAG antibodies are generally monoclonal IgMκ, and usually also exhibit reactivity with other glycoproteins or glycolipids that share antigenic determinants with MAG.[52–54] The anti-MAG-related neuropathy is typically distal and symmetrical, affecting both motor and sensory functions; it is slowly progressive with a long period of stability.[48,55] Most patients present with sensory complaints (paresthesias, aching discomfort, dysesthesias, or lancinating pains), ataxia and abnormal gaits, owing to lack of proprioception, and leg muscle atrophy in patients with advanced stage disease. Patients with predominantly demyelinating sensory neuropathy in association with monoclonal IgM to gangliosides with disialosyl moieties, such as GD1b, GD3, GD2, GT1b, and GQ1b, have also been reported.[56,57] Anti- GD1b and anti-GQ1b antibodies were significantly associated with predominantly sensory ataxic neuropathy.[58] These antiganglioside monoclonal IgMs present clinical features of chronic ataxic neuropathy with variably present ophthalmoplegia and/or red blood cell cold agglutinating activity. The disialosyl epitope is also present on red blood cell glycophorins, thereby accounting for the red cell cold agglutinin activity of anti-Pr2 specificity.[59,60] Monoclonal IgM proteins that bind to gangliosides with a terminal trisaccharide moiety, including GM2 and GalNac-GD1A, are associated with chronic demyelinating neuropathy and severe sensory ataxia, unresponsive to corticosteroids.[61] Antiganglioside IgM proteins may also cross-react with lipopolysaccharides of *Campylobacter jejuni*, an infection that is known to precipitate the Miller Fisher syndrome, a variant of the Guillain–Barré syndrome.[58] This finding indicates that molecular mimicry may play a role in this condition. Antisulfatide monoclonal IgM proteins, associated with sensory/sensorimotor neuropathy, have been detected in 5% of patients with IgM monoclonal gammopathy and neuropathy.[62] Motor neuron disease has been reported in patients with WM, and monoclonal IgM with anti-GM1 and sulfoglucuronyl

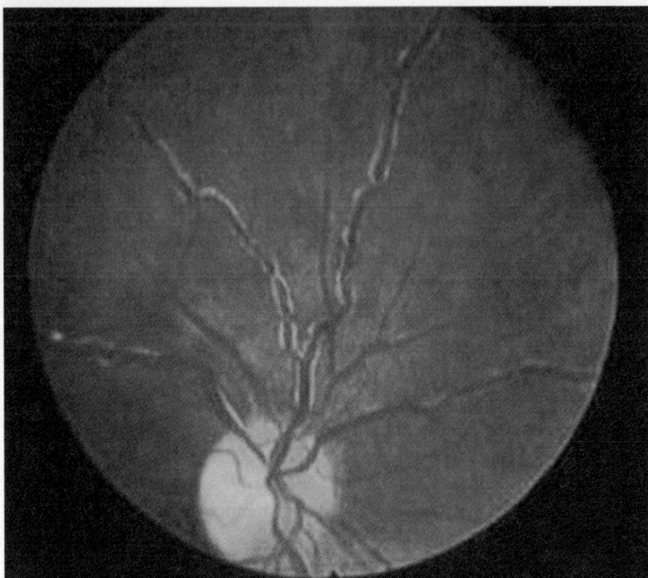

Figure 88–3 Funduscopic examination of a patient with Waldenström macroglobulinemia demonstrating hyperviscosity-related changes including dilated retinal vessels, peripheral hemorrhages, and "venous sausaging". *(Courtesy of Marvin Stone, MD.)*

paragloboside activity.[63] POEMS (polyneuropathy, organomegaly, endocrinopathy, M protein, and skin changes) syndrome is rarely associated with WM.[64]

Type II Cryoglobulinemia

The monoclonal IgM may have an autoantibody activity against the FC portion of IgG (monoclonal rheumatoid factors).[40] The cryoprecipitating property results from the size and limited solubility of the IgM–IgG immune complex. The systemic vasculitis that characterizes the disease appears to be caused by deposition of immune complexes on the walls of small vessels and subsequent activation of the complement cascade. Majority of patients with mixed cryoglobulinemias (MCs) are infected with hepatitis C virus (HCV), which is considered the triggering factor of the disease.[65] Not all patients infected with HCV have MCs, but their presence correlates with duration of the hepatitis. The cryoprecipitable immune complexes contain HCV core proteins and specific anticore IgG which are bound to IgM with rheumatoid factor activity. This large complex binds specifically to endothelial cells through the C1q receptor.[66] The monoclonal IgM rheumatoid factors are generated by an antigen-driven process. The clinical features of patients with MCs are purpura, arthralgias, weakness, liver involvement, renal involvement (cryoglobulinemic glomerulonephritis), peripheral neuropathy, and widespread vasculitis. The severity of vasculitic manifestations has little relationship with the serum level of cryoglobulins (cryocrit) or complement. Thermal amplitude, the temperature at which the immune complex precipitates, appears to be more important.

Cold Agglutinin Hemolytic Anemia

Patients with a monoclonal IgM may present with cold agglutinin activity. The IgM may recognize specific red cell antigens at low temperatures, producing a chronic hemolytic anemia. This disorder occurs in less than 10% of WM patients[67] and is associated with cold agglutinin titers greater than 1 : 1000 in most cases. The monoclonal component is usually an IgMκ and reacts most commonly with I/i antigens, with complement fixation and activation.[68,69] Mild chronic hemolytic anemia can be exacerbated by cold exposure but rarely does the hemoglobin level drop below 70 g/dL. The hemolysis is usually extravascular (removal of C3b opsonized cells by the reticuloendothelial system, primarily in the liver) and rarely intravascular because of complement mediated destruction of the red blood cell (RBC) membrane. The agglutination of RBCs in the cooler peripheral circulation also causes Raynaud syndrome, acrocyanosis, and livedo reticularis. Macroglobulins with the properties of both cryoglobulins and cold agglutinins with anti-Pr specificity have been reported. These properties may have as a common basis the immune binding of the sialic acid-containing carbohydrate present on red blood cell glycophorins and on Ig molecules. Several other macroglobulins with various antibody activity toward autologous antigens (ie, phospholipids, tissue and plasma proteins, etc) and foreign ligands have also been reported.

Tissue Deposition

The monoclonal protein can be deposited in several tissues as amorphous aggregates. Linear deposition of monoclonal IgM along the skin basement membrane is associated with bullous skin disease.[70] Amorphous IgM deposits in the dermis determine the so-called IgM storage papules on the extensor surface of the extremities—macroglobulinemia cutis.[71] Deposition of monoclonal IgM in the lamina propria and/or submucosa of the intestine may be associated with diarrhea, malabsorption, and gastrointestinal bleeding.[72,73] Kidney involvement is less common and less severe in WM than in multiple myeloma, probably because the amount of light chain excreted in the urine is generally lower in WM than in myeloma and because of the absence of contributing factors, such as hypercalcemia, although cast nephropathy has also been described in patients with WM.[74] On the other hand, the IgM macromolecule is more susceptible to being trapped in the glomerular loops where ultrafiltration presumably contributes to its precipitation, forming subendothelial deposits of aggregated IgM proteins that occlude the glomerular capillaries.[75] Mild and reversible proteinuria may result and most patients are asymptomatic. The deposition of monoclonal light chain as fibrillar amyloid deposits (AL amyloidosis) is uncommon in patients with WM.[76] Clinical findings and prognosis are similar to those of other AL patients with involvement of heart (44%), kidneys (32%), liver (14%), lungs (10%), peripheral/autonomic nerves (38%), and soft tissues (18%) occurring. However, the incidence of cardiac and pulmonary involvement is higher in patients with a monoclonal IgM than with other immunoglobulin isotypes. The association of WM with reactive amyloidosis (AA) has been documented rarely.[77,78] Simultaneous occurrence of fibrillary glomerulopathy, characterized by glomerular deposits of wide noncongophilic fibrils and amyloid deposits, has been reported in WM.[79]

Manifestations Related to Tissue Infiltration by Neoplastic Cells

Tissue infiltration by neoplastic cells is rare but can involve various organs and tissues, from the bone marrow to the liver, spleen, lymph nodes, and possibly the lungs, gastrointestinal tract, kidneys, skin, eyes, and central nervous system. Pulmonary involvement in the form of masses, nodules, diffuse infiltrate, or pleural effusions is relatively rare, since the overall incidence of pulmonary and pleural findings reported for WM is only 3% to 5%.[80–82] Cough is the most common presenting symptom in such patients, followed by dyspnea and chest pain. Chest radiographic findings include parenchymal infiltrates, confluent masses, and effusions. Malabsorption, diarrhea, bleeding, or obstruction may indicate involvement of the gastrointestinal tract at the level of the stomach, duodenum, or small intestine.[83–86] In contrast to multiple myeloma, infiltration of the kidney interstitium with lymphoplasmacytoid cell has been reported in WM,[87] whereas renal or perirenal masses are not uncommon.[88] The skin can be the site of dense lymphoplasmacytic infiltrates, similar to that seen in the liver, spleen, and lymph nodes, forming cutaneous plaques and, rarely, nodules.[89] Chronic urticaria and IgM gammopathy are the two cardinal features of the Schnitzler syndrome, which is not usually associated initially with clinical features of WM,[90,91] although evolution to WM is not uncommon. Thus, close follow-up of these patients is warranted. Invasion of articular and periarticular structures by WM malignant cells is rarely reported.[92] The neoplastic cells can infiltrate the periorbital structures, lacrimal gland, and retro-orbital lymphoid tissues, resulting in ocular nerve palsies.[93,94] Direct infiltration of the central nervous system by monoclonal lymphoplasmacytic cells as infiltrates or as tumors constitutes the rarely observed Bing–Neel syndrome, characterized clinically by confusion, memory loss, disorientation, and motor dysfunction (reviewed in Civit et al[95]).

LABORATORY INVESTIGATIONS AND FINDINGS

Hematologic Abnormalities

Anemia is the most common finding in patients with symptomatic WM and is caused by a combination of factors: mild decrease in red cell survival, impaired erythropoiesis, hemolysis, moderate plasma volume expansion, and blood loss from the gastrointestinal tract. Red cells are usually normocytic and normochromic, and rouleaux formation is often pronounced. The mean corpuscular volume as determined by an automated analyzer may be spuriously elevated owing to erythrocyte aggregation. In addition, the hemoglobin estimate can be inaccurate, that is, falsely high, because of interaction between the monoclonal protein and the diluent used in some automated analyzers.[96] Leukocyte and platelet counts are usually normal at presentation, although patients may occasionally present with severe thrombocytopenia. As reported above, monoclonal B-lymphocytes expressing surface IgM and late-differentiation B-cell markers are rarely detected in blood by flow cytometric analysis. A raised erythrocyte sedimentation rate is frequently observed in patients with WM and may be the first clue to the presence of the macroglobulin. The clotting abnormality detected most frequently is prolongation of the thrombin time. AL amyloidosis should be suspected in all patients with nephrotic syndrome, cardiomyopathy, hepatomegaly, or peripheral neuropathy. Diagnosis requires the demonstration of green birefringence under polarized light of amyloid deposits stained with Congo red.

Biochemical Investigations

High-resolution electrophoresis combined with immunofixation of serum and urine is recommended for identification and characterization of the IgM monoclonal protein. The light chain of the monoclonal IgM is κ in 75% to 80% of patients. A few WM patients have more than one M-component. The concentration of the serum monoclonal protein is very variable but in most cases lies within the range of 15 to 45 g/L. Densitometry should be utilized to serially quantitate IgM levels because nephelometry is unreliable and shows large intralaboratory as well as interlaboratory variation. The presence of cold agglutinins or cryoglobulins may affect the determination of IgM levels and, therefore, testing for cold agglutinins and cryoglobulins should be performed at diagnosis. If present, subsequent serum samples should be analyzed under warm conditions for determination of serum monoclonal IgM level. Although Bence Jones proteinuria is frequently present, it exceeds 1 g/24 hours in only 3% of cases. Although IgM levels are elevated in WM patients, IgA and IgG levels are most often depressed and do not recover even after successful treatment.[97] In recent studies by Hunter et al,[98] mutations in the receptor transmembrane activator and calcium modulator and cytophilin–ligand interactor (TACI) were demonstrated in WM patients akin to those observed in patients with common variable deficiency disorder (CVID) suggesting a possible CVID background for WM patients.

Serum Viscosity

Because of its large size (almost 1,000,000 Da), most IgM molecules are retained within the intravascular compartment and can exert an undue effect on serum viscosity. Therefore, serum viscosity should be measured if the patient has signs or symptoms of hyperviscosity syndrome. Fundoscopy remains an excellent indicator of clinically relevant hyperviscosity. Among the first clinical signs of hyperviscosity, the appearance of peripheral and midperipheral dot and blot-like hemorrhages in the retina, which are best appreciated with indirect ophthalmoscopy and scleral depression.[45] In more severe cases of hyperviscosity, dot-, blot-, and flame-shaped hemorrhages can appear in the macular area along with markedly dilated and tortuous veins with focal constrictions resulting in "venous sausaging," as well as papilledema (Fig. 88–3).

Bone Marrow Findings

The bone marrow is always involved in WM. Central to the diagnosis of WM is the demonstration, by trephine biopsy, of *bone marrow infiltration by a lymphoplasmacytic cell population* constituted by small lymphocytes with evidence of plasmacytoid/plasma cell differentiation (Figs. 88–1 88–2B–D). The pattern of bone marrow infiltration may be diffuse, interstitial, or nodular, showing usually an intertrabecular pattern of infiltration. A solely paratrabecular pattern of infiltration is unusual and should raise the possibility of the diagnosis of a follicular lymphoma.[1] The marrow lymphoid infiltration should routinely be confirmed by *immunophenotypic studies* (flow cytometry and/or immunohistochemistry) showing the following profile: sIgM $^{+}$CD19^{+}CD20^{+}CD22^{+}CD79^{+}.[26–28] Up to 20% of cases may express either CD5, CD10, or CD23.[29] In these cases, care should be taken to satisfactorily exclude chronic lymphocytic leukemia and mantle cell lymphoma.[1] Intranuclear periodic acid–Schiff (PAS)-positive inclusions (Dutcher–Fahey bodies, see Fig. 88–1C)[99] consisting of IgM deposits in the perinuclear space, and sometimes in intranuclear vacuoles, may be seen occasionally in lymphoid cells in WM. An increased number of mast cells, usually in association with the lymphoid aggregates, is commonly found in WM, and their presence may help in differentiating WM from other B-cell lymphomas (see Fig. 88–1D).[2,3]

Other Investigations

Magnetic resonance imaging (MRI) of the spine in conjunction with computed tomography (CT) of the abdomen and pelvis are useful in evaluating the disease status in patients with WM.[100] Bone marrow involvement can be documented by MRI studies of the spine in more than 90% of patients, whereas CT of the abdomen and pelvis demonstrated enlarged nodes in 43% of WM patients.[100] A Lymph node biopsy may show preserved architecture or replacement by infiltration of neoplastic cells with lymphoplasmacytoid, lymphoplasmacytic, or polymorphous cytologic patterns. The residual disease after high-dose chemotherapy with allogeneic or autologous stem-cell rescue can be monitored by polymerase chain reaction (PCR)-based methods using primers specific for the monoclonal Ig variable regions.

PROGNOSIS

Waldenström macroglobulinemia typically presents as an indolent disease though considerable variability in prognosis can be observed. The median survival reported in several large series has ranged from 5 to 10 years.[101–107] Age is consistently an important prognostic factor (>60–70 years),[101,102,104,107] but this factor is often affected by comorbidities. Anemia, which reflects both marrow involvement and the serum level of the IgM monoclonal protein (because of the impact of IgM on intravascular fluid retention), has emerged as a

Table 88–3 Prognostic Scoring Systems in Waldenstrom Macroglobulinemia

Study	Adverse Prognostic Factors	Number of Groups	Survival
Gobbi et al[101]	Hb <9 g/dL Age >70 years Weight loss Cryoglobulinemia	0–1 prognostic factors 2–4 prognostic factors	Median: 48 months Median: 80 months
Morel et al[102]	Age ≥65 years Albumin <4 g/dL Number of cytopenias: Hb <12 g/dL Platelets <150 × 10^9/L Wbc <4 × 10^9/L	0–1 prognostic factors 2 prognostic factors 3–4 prognostic factors	5 year: 87% 5 year: 62% 5 year: 25%
Dhodapkar et al[103]	β_2M ≥3 g/dL Hb <12 g/dL IgM <4 g/dL	β_2M <3 mg/dL + Hb ≥12 g/dL β_2M <3 mg/dL + Hb <12 g/dL β_2M ≥3 mg/dL + IgM ≥4 g/dL β_2M ≥3 mg/dL + IgM <4 g/dL	5 year: 87% 5 year: 63% 5 year: 53% 5 year: 21%
Application of International Staging System Criteria for Myeloma to WM Dimopoulos et al[105]	Albumin ≤3.5 g/dL β_2M ≥3.5 mg/L	Albumin ≥3.5 g/dL + β_2M <3.5 mg/dL Albumin ≤3.5 g/dL + β_2M <3.5 or β_2M 3.5–5.5 mg/dL β_2M >5.5 mg/dL	Median: NR Median: 116 months Median: 54 months
International Prognostic Scoring System for WM Morel et al[107]	Age >65 years Hb <11.5 g/dL Platelets <100 × 10^9/L β_2M >3 mg/L IgM >7 g/dL	0–1 prognostic factors* 2 prognostic factors** 3–5 prognostic factors *excluding age **or age >65	5 year: 87% 5 year: 68% 5 year: 36%

strong adverse prognostic factor with hemoglobin levels less than 9–12 g/dL being associated with decreased survival in several series.[101–104,107] The cytopenias have also been regularly identified as a significant predictor of survival.[96] However, the precise level of cytopenias that has prognostic significance remains to be determined.[104] Some series have identified a platelet count less than 100–150 × 10^9/L and a granulocyte count less than 1.5 × 10^9/L as independent prognostic factors.[101,102,104,107] The number of cytopenias in a given patient has been proposed as a strong prognostic factor.[102] Serum albumin levels have also correlated with survival in WM patients in certain but not all studies using multivariate analyses.[102,104,105] High beta-2 microglobulin levels (>3–3.5 g/dL) have been reported in several studies,[103–107] a high serum IgM M-protein (>7 g/dL)[107] as well as a low serum IgM M-protein (<4 g/dL)[105] and the presence of cryoglobulins[101] to be adverse factors. Several prognostic scoring systems have been developed based on the parameters outlined above (Table 88–3).

TREATMENT OF WALDENSTRÖM MACROGLOBULINEMIA

As part of the 2nd International Workshop on Waldenström macroglobulinemia, a consensus panel was organized to recommend criteria for the initiation of therapy in patients with WM.[104] The panel recommended that initiation of therapy should not be based on the IgM level per se, since this may not correlate with the clinical manifestations of WM. The consensus panel, however, agreed that initiation of therapy was appropriate for patients with constitutional symptoms, such as recurrent fever, night sweats, fatigue due to anemia, or weight loss. The presence of progressive symptomatic lymphadenopathy or splenomegaly provides additional reasons to begin therapy. The presence of anemia with a hemoglobin value of 10 g/dL or less or a platelet count of 100 × 10^9/L or less owing to marrow infiltration also justifies treatment. Certain complications, such as hyperviscosity syndrome, symptomatic sensorimotor peripheral neuropathy, systemic amyloidosis, renal insufficiency, or symptomatic cryoglobulinemia, may also be indications for therapy.[104]

FRONTLINE THERAPY

Although a precise therapeutic algorithm for therapy of WM remains to be defined given the paucity of randomized clinical trials, consensus panels composed of experts who treat WM were organized as part of the 2nd and 3rd International Workshop on Waldenström macroglobulinemia and have formulated recommendations for both frontline and salvage therapy of patients with WM based on the best available evidence. Among frontline options, the panels considered alkylating agents (eg, chlorambucil), nucleoside analogues (cladribine or fludarabine), the monoclonal antibody rituximab as well as combinations thereof as reasonable choices for the upfront therapy of WM.[108,109] Importantly, the panel felt that individual patient considerations, including the presence of cytopenias, need for more rapid disease control, age, and candidacy for autologous transplant therapy, should be taken into account in making the choice of a first-line agent. For patients who are candidates for autologous transplant therapy, and in whom such therapy is seriously considered, the panel recommended that exposure to alkylator or nucleoside analogue therapy should be limited.

Alkylating Agent-Based Therapy

Oral alkylating drugs, alone and in combination with steroids, have been extensively evaluated for the upfront treatment of WM. The greatest experience with oral alkylating agent therapy has been with chlorambucil, which has been administered on both a continuous (ie, daily-dose schedule) and intermittent schedule. Patients receiving chlorambucil on a continuous schedule typically receive 0.1 mg/kg per day, whereas on the intermittent schedule patients will typically receive 0.3 mg/kg for 7 days, every 6 weeks. In a prospective randomized study, Kyle et al[110] reported no significant difference in the overall response rate between these schedules, although interestingly the median response duration was greater for patients receiving intermittent versus continuously dosed chlorambucil (46 vs 26 months). Despite the favorable median response duration in this study for use of the intermittent schedule, no difference in the median overall survival was observed. Moreover, an increased incidence of developing myelodysplasia and acute myeloid leukemia was associated with the intermittent (3 of 22 patients) versus the continuous (0 of 24 patients) chlorambucil schedule, which prompted the authors to express preference for use of continuous chlorambucil dosing. The use of steroids in combination with alkylating agent therapy has also been explored. Dimopoulos and Alexanian[111] evaluated chlorambucil (8 mg/m^2) along with prednisone (40 mg/m^2) given orally for 10 days, every 6 weeks, and reported a major response (ie, reduction of IgM by greater than 50%) in 72% of patients. Non–chlorambucil-based alkylating agent regimens employing melphalan and cyclophosphamide in combination with steroids have also been examined by Petrucci et al[112] and Case et al[113] producing slightly higher overall response rates and response durations, although the benefit of these more complex regimens over chlorambucil remains to be demonstrated. Facon et al[114] have evaluated parameters predicting response to alkylating agent therapy. Their studies in patients receiving single-agent chlorambucil demonstrated that age 60, male sex, symptomatic status, and cytopenias (but, interestingly, not high tumor burden and serum IgM levels) were associated with poor response to alkylating agent therapy. Additional factors to be taken into account in considering alkylating agent therapy for patients with WM include necessity for more rapid disease control given the slow nature of response to alkylating agent therapy, as well as consideration for preserving stem cells in patients who are candidates for autologous transplant therapy.

Nucleoside Stem Cell Analogue Therapy

Both cladribine and fludarabine have been extensively evaluated in untreated as well as previously treated WM patients. Cladribine administered as a single agent by continuous intravenous infusion, by 2-hour daily infusion, or by subcutaneous bolus injections for 5 to 7 days has resulted in major responses in 40% to 90% of patients who received primary therapy, whereas in the salvage setting responses have ranged from 38% to 54%.[114–121] Median time to achievement of response in responding patients following cladribine ranged from 1.2 to 5 months. The overall response rate with daily infusional fludarabine therapy administered mainly on 5-day schedules in previously untreated and treated WM patients has ranged from 38% to 100% and 30% to 40%, respectively,[122–127] which are similar to the response data achieved with cladribine. The median time to achievement of response for patients receiving fludarabine was also similar to cladribine at 3 to 6 months. In general, response rates and the duration of response have been greater for patients receiving nucleoside analogues as first-line agents, although in several of the above studies wherein both untreated and previously treated patients were enrolled, no substantial difference in the overall response rate was reported. Myelosuppression commonly occurred following prolonged exposure to each of the nucleoside analogues, as did lymphopenia with sustained depletion of both CD4$^+$ and CD8$^+$ T lymphocytes observed in WM patients 1 year following initiation of therapy.[114,116] Treatment-related mortality due to myelosuppression and/or opportunistic infections attributable to immunosuppression occurred in up to 5% of all treated patients in some series with either nucleoside analogue. Factors predictive of response to nucleoside analogues in WM included age at start of treatment (<70 years), pretreatment hemoglobin more than 95 g/dL, platelets more than 75 × 10 g/L, disease relapsing after therapy, patients with resistant disease within the first year of diagnosis, and a long interval between first-line therapy and initiation of a nucleoside analogue in relapsing patients.[114,120,126] There are limited data on the use of an alternate nucleoside analogue to salvage patients whose disease relapsed or demonstrated resistance after cladribine or fludarabine therapy.[128,129] Three of four (75%) patients responded to cladribine therapy when used to salvage patients who progressed following an unmaintained remission to fludarabine, whereas only 1 of 10 (10%) with disease resistant to fludarabine responded to cladribine.[128] Lewandowski et al[129] reported a response in two of six patients (33%) and disease stabilization in the remaining patients to fludarabine, in spite of an inadequate response or progressive disease following cladribine therapy. The long-term safety of nucleoside analogues in WM was recently examined by Leleu et al[130] in a large series of WM patients. A sevenfold increase in transformation to an aggressive lymphoma, and a threefold increase in the development of acute myeloid leukemia/myelodysplasia was observed among patients who received a nucleoside analogue versus other therapies for their WM.

CD20-Directed Antibody Therapy

Rituximab is a chimeric monoclonal antibody that targets CD20, a widely expressed antigen on lymphoplasmacytic cells in WM.[131] Several retrospective and prospective studies have indicated that rituximab, when used at standard doses (ie, 4 weekly infusions at 375 mg/m^2), induced major responses in approximately 27% to 35% of previously treated and untreated patients.[132–138] Furthermore, it was shown in some of these studies, that patients who achieved minor responses or even stable disease benefited from rituximab as evidenced by improved hemoglobin levels and platelet counts, and reduction of lymphadenopathy and/or splenomegaly. The median time to treatment failure in these studies ranged from 8 to 27+ months. Studies evaluating an extended rituximab schedule consisting of 4 weekly courses at 375 mg/m^2/week repeated 3 months later by another 4-week course have demonstrated major response rates of 44% to 48%, with estimates of time to progression ranging from 16+ to 29+ months.[138,139]

In many WM patients, a transient increase of serum IgM may be noted immediately following initiation of treatment with rituximab. Such an increase is not indicative of treatment failure, and whereas most patients will return to their baseline serum IgM level by 12 weeks some will continue to show prolonged elevations despite demonstrating a reduction in their bone marrow tumor load.[140–142] However, patients with baseline serum IgM levels more than 50 g/dL or serum viscosity greater than 3.5 cp may be particularly at risk for developing a hyperviscosity-related event, and in such patients plasmapheresis should be considered in advance of rituximab therapy.[141] Because of the decreased likelihood of response in patients with higher IgM levels, as well as the possibility that serum IgM and viscosity levels may abruptly rise, rituximab monotherapy should not be used as sole therapy for the treatment of patients at risk for hyperviscosity symptoms.

Time to response after rituximab is slow and exceeds 3 months on the average. The time to best response in one study was 18 months.[139] Patients with baseline serum IgM levels less than 40 to 60 g/L are more likely to respond, irrespective of the underlying bone marrow involvement by tumor cells.[138,139] A recent analysis of 52 patients who were treated with single-agent rituximab has indicated that the objective response rate was significantly lower in patients who had either a low serum albumin (<35 g/L) or an elevated serum monoclonal protein (>40 g/L M-spike). Furthermore, the presence of both adverse prognostic factors was related with a short time to progression (3.6 months). Moreover patients who had normal serum albumin levels and relatively low serum monoclonal protein enjoyed a substantial benefit from rituximab, with a time to progression exceeding 40 months.[143]

The genetic background of patients may also determine the success rate with rituximab therapy. In particular, a correlation between polymorphisms at position 158 in the Fc gamma RIIIa receptor (CD16), an activating Fc receptor on important effector cells that mediate antibody-dependent cell-mediated cytotoxicity (ADCC), and rituximab response has been observed in WM patients. Individuals may encode either the amino acid valine or phenylalanine at position 158 in the FcγRIIIa receptor. WM patients who carried the valine amino acid (either in a homozygous or heterozygous pattern) had a fourfold higher major response rate (ie, 50% decline in serum IgM levels) to rituximab versus those patients who expressed phenylalanine in a homozygous pattern.[144]

Combination Therapy

Because rituximab is an active and a nonmyelosuppressive agent, its use in combination with a variety of chemotherapeutic agents has been explored in WM patients. Weber et al[145] administered rituximab along with cladribine and cyclophosphamide to 17 previously untreated patients with WM. At least a partial response was documented in 94% of WM patients, including a complete response in 18% of patients; with a median follow-up of 21 months no patient has relapsed. In a study performed by the Waldenström Macroglobulinemia Clinical Trials Group (WMCTG), the combination of rituximab and fludarabine was evaluated in 43 WM patients, 32 (75%) of whom were previously untreated.[146] Ninety-one percent of patients enjoyed at least a 25% decrease in serum IgM levels, and response rates were as follows: CR 7%; PR 74.4%, and MR 9.3%. Hematologic toxicity was common with grade III, IV; neutropenia was observed in 58% of patients. Two deaths occurred in this study, which may have been related to therapy-related immunosuppression. With a median follow-up of 17 months, 34/39 (87%) remain in remission. The addition of rituximab to fludarabine and cyclophosphamide has also been explored in the salvage setting by Tam et al, wherein four of five patients demonstrated a response.[147] In another study of a chemotherapeutic agent in combination with rituximab, Hensel et al[148] administered rituximab along with pentostatin and cyclophosphamide to 13 patients with untreated and previously treated WM or lymphoplasmacytic lymphoma. A major response was observed in 77% or patients. In a study by Dimopoulos et al,[149] the combination of rituximab, dexamethasone, and cyclophosphamide was used as primary therapy to treat 70 patients with WM. On an intent-to-treat basis, a major response was observed in 70% of patients. With a median follow-up of 24 months, 60% of patients remain progression free. Therapy was well tolerated, though one patient died of interstitial pneumonia.

In addition to nucleoside analogue-based trials with rituximab, two studies have examined CHOP (cyclophosphamide, doxorubicin, vincristine, prednisone) in combination with rituximab (CHOP-R). In a randomized frontline study by the German Low Grade Lymphoma Study Group (GLSG) involving 72 patients (71% of whom had lymphoplasmacytic lymphoma), a significantly higher response rate (94% vs 69%) was observed among patients receiving CHOP-R versus CHOP, respectively.[150] Treon et al[151] have also evaluated CHOP-R in 13 WM patients, 8 and 5 of whom had relapsed or were refractory to nucleoside analogues and single-agent rituximab, respectively. Among the 13 evaluable patients, 10 patients achieved a major response (77%), including 3 CR and 7 PR, and 2 patients achieved a minor response.

The addition of alkylating agents to nucleoside analogues has also been explored in WM. Weber et al[145] administered two cycles of oral cyclophosphamide along with subcutaneous cladribine to 37 patients with previously untreated WM. At least a partial response was observed in 84% of patients, and the median duration of response was 36 months. Dimopoulos et al[152] examined fludarabine in combination with intravenous cyclophosphamide and observed partial responses in 6 of 11 (55%) WM patients with either primary refractory disease or who had relapsed on treatment. The combination of fludarabine plus cyclophosphamide was also evaluated in a recent study by Tamburini et al[153] involving 49 patients, 35 of whom were previously treated. Seventy-eight percent of the patients in this study achieved a response, and the median time to treatment failure was 27 months. Hematologic toxicity was commonly observed and three patients died of treatment-related toxicities. Two interesting findings in this study was the development of acute leukemia in two patients, histologic transformation to diffuse large cell lymphoma in one patient, and two cases of solid tumors prostate and melanoma), as well as failure to mobilize stem cells in four of six patients.

In view of the above data, the consensus panel on therapeutics amended its original recommendations for the therapy of WM to include the use of combination therapy with either nucleoside analogues and alkylating agents, or rituximab in combination with nucleoside analogues, nucleoside analogues plus alkylating agents, or combination chemotherapy such as CHOP as reasonable therapeutics options for the treatment of WM.[109]

SALVAGE THERAPY INCLUDING NOVEL AGENTS

For relapsed patients or those who have refractory disease, the consensus panels recommended the use of an alternative first-line agent as defined above, with the caveat that for those patients for whom autologous stem cell transplantation was being seriously considered, further exposure to stem cell-damaging agents (ie, many alkylating agents and nucleoside analogue drugs) should be avoided, and a non–stem cell toxic agent such as cyclophosphamide and thalidomide should be considered if stem cell grafts had not previously been harvested.[108,109] Recent studies have also demonstrated activity of several novel agents including bortezomib, thalidomide alone or in combination, and alemtuzumab. These agents can be considered for the treatment of relapsed/refractory WM. Lastly, autologous stem cell transplant remains an option as salvage therapy of WM patients particularly younger patients who have had multiple relapses, or have primary refractory disease.

Proteosome Inhibitors

Bortezomib, a stem cell-sparing agent,[154,155] is a proteosome inhibitor that induces apoptosis of primary WM lymphoplasmacytic cells, at pharmacologically achievable levels.[156] Moreover, bortezomib may also affect the bone marrow microenvironmental support for lymphoplasmacytic cells.[157] In a multicenter study of the Waldenström Macroglobulinemia Clinical Trials Group (WMCTG),[158] 27 patients received up to eight cycles of bortezomib at 1.3 mg/m^2 on days 1, 4, 8, and 11. All but one patient had relapsed/or had refractory disease. Following therapy, median serum IgM levels declined from 4.7 g/L to 2/.1 g/L ($P < 0.0001$). The overall response rate was 85%, with 10 and 13 patients achieving a minor (<25% decrease in IgM) and major (<50% decrease in IgM) response. Responses were promptly achieved, and occurred at a median of 1.4 months. The median time to progression for all responding patients in this study was 7.9 (range 3–21.4+) months, and the most common grade III/IV toxicities occurring in 5% or more of patients were sensory neuropathies (22.2%); leukopenia (18.5%); neutropenia (14.8%); dizziness (11.1%); and thrombocytopenia (7.4%). Importantly, sensory neuropathies resolved or improved in nearly all patients following cessation of therapy. As part of an NCI-Canada study, Chen et al[159] treated 27 patients with both untreated (44%) and previously treated (56%) disease. Patients in this study received bortezomib utilizing the standard schedule until they either demonstrated progressive disease, or two cycles beyond a complete response or stable disease was documented. The overall response rate in this study was 78%, with major responses observed in 44% of patients. Sensory neuropathy occurred in 20 patients, 5 with grade III and above, and occurred following two to four cycles of therapy. Among the 20 patients developing a neuropathy, 14 patients resolved and 1 patient demonstrated a one-grade improvement at 2 to 13 months. In addition to the above experiences with bortezomib monotherapy in WM, Dimopoulos et al[160] observed major responses in 6 of 10 (60%) previously treated WM patients treated with bortezomib, whereas Goy et al[161] observed a major response in one of two WM patients included in a series of relapsed or refractory patients with non-Hodgkin lymphoma (NHL) treated with this agent.

CD52-Directed Antibody Therapy

Alemtuzumab is a humanized monoclonal antibody that targets CD52, an antigen widely expressed on WM bone marrow LPC, as well as on mast cells that are increased in the bone marrow of patients with WM. These mast cells provide growth and survival signals to WM LPC through several TNF family ligands (CD40L, APRIL,

BLYS). As part of a WMCTG effort,[162] 28 subjects with the REAL/WHO clinicopathologic diagnosis of LPL, including 27 patients with IgM (WM) and 1 with IgA monoclonal gammopathy, were enrolled in this prospective, multicenter study. Five patients were untreated and 23 were previously treated, all of whom had previously received rituximab. Patients received three daily test doses of alemtuzumab (3, 10, and 30 mg IV) followed by 30 mg alemtuzumab IV three times a week for up to 12 weeks. All patients received acyclovir and Bactrim or equivalent prophylaxis for the duration of therapy plus 8 weeks following the last infusion of alemtuzumab. Among 25 patients evaluable for response, the overall response rate was 76%, which included 8 (32%) major responders and 11 (44%) minor responders. Hematologic toxicities were common among previously treated (but not untreated) patients and included grade III/IV neutropenia 39%; thrombocytopenia 18%; anemia 7%. Grade III/IV nonhematologic toxicity for all patients included dermatitis 11%; fatigue 7%; and infection 7%. CMV reactivation and infection was commonly seen among previously treated patients and may have been responsible for one death. With a median follow-up of 8.5+ months, 11/19 responding patients remain free of progression. High rates of response with the use of alemtuzumab as salvage therapy have also been reported by Owen et al[163] in a small series of heavily pretreated WM patients (with a median of four prior therapies who received up to 12 weeks of therapy (at 30 mg IV TIW) following initial dose escalation. Among the seven patients receiving alemtuzumab, five patients achieved a partial response and one patient a complete response. Infectious complications were common, with CMV reactivation occurring in three patients requiring ganciclovir therapy, and hospitalization for three patients for bacterial infections. Opportunistic infections occurred in two patients and were responsible for their deaths. An upfront study by the WMCTG examining the role of alemtuzumab in combination with rituximab is anticipated given the efficacy results reported in the above studies.

Thalidomide and Lenalidomide

Treatment with thalidomide as a single agent, and in combination with dexamethasone and clarithromycin, has also been examined in patients with WM, in view of the success of these regimens in patients with advanced multiple myeloma. Dimopoulos et al[164] reported a major response in 5 of 20 (25%) previously untreated and treated patients who received single-agent thalidomide. Dose escalation from the starting dose of 200 mg daily was hindered by development of side effects, including the development of peripheral neuropathy in five patients, requiring discontinuation of therapy or dose reduction. Low doses of thalidomide (50 mg orally daily) in combination with dexamethasone (40 mg orally once a week) and clarithromycin (250 mg orally twice a day) have also been examined, with 10 of 12 (83%) previously treated patients experiencing at least a major response.[165] However, in a follow-up study by Dimopoulos et al[166] using a higher thalidomide dose (200 mg orally daily) along with dexamethasone (40 g orally once a week) and clarithromycin (500 mg orally twice a day), only 2 of 10 (20%) previously treated patients responded. In a previous study, thalidomide and its analogue lenalidomide significantly augmented rituximab-mediated antibody-dependent cell-mediated cytotoxicity (ADCC) against lymphoplasmacytic cells.[167] Moreover, an expansion of natural killer cells has been observed with thalidomide, which in previous studies have been shown to be associated with a response from rituximab.[168,169] In view of these data, the WMCTG has conducted two phase II clinical trials in symptomatic patients with WM combining thalidomide or lenalidomide with rituximab.[170] Therapy consisted of thalidomide administered at 200 mg daily for 2 weeks, followed by 400 mg daily thereafter for 1 year. Patients received four weekly infusions of rituximab at 375 mg/m^2 beginning 1 week after initiation of thalidomide, followed by four additional weekly infusions of rituximab at 375 mg/m^2 beginning at week 13. Twenty-three of 25 patients were evaluable in this study and responses included: CR (n = 1); PR (n = 15); MR (n = 2); SD (n = 1) for an overall (ORR) and a major response rate of 78% and 70%, respectively. Median serum IgM levels decreased from 3. 7 (0.91–8.1 g/L) to 1.6 (.36–5.2 g/L) ($P < 0.001$), whereas the median hematocrit level rose from 33.0 (23.6%–42.6%) to 37.6% (29.3%–44.3%) ($P = 0.004$). With a median follow-up of 42+ months, the median TTP for evaluable patients on this study was 35 months, and 38+ months for responders. Responses were associated with a median cumulative thalidomide dose: CR/PR/MR (29,275 mg) vs SD/NR (7400 mg); $P = 0.004$. Responses were unaffected by FcγRIIIA-158 polymorphism status (81% vs 71% for VV/FV vs FF); IgM (78% vs 80% for <6000 mg/dL vs ≥6000 mg/dL); and B_2M (71% vs 89% for <3 g/dL vs ≥3 g/dL). Reduction of thalidomide dose occurred in all patients and led to discontinuation in 11 patients. Among 11 patients experiencing grade II or more neuroparesthesias, 10 demonstrated resolution to grade I (n = 3) or complete resolution (n = 7) after a median of 6.7 months (range 0.4–22.5).

In a phase II study of lenalidomide and rituximab in WM,[171] patients were treated with lenalidomide at a dose of 25 mg daily wherein therapy was administered for 3 weeks, followed by a 1 week pause for 48 weeks. Patients received 1 week of therapy with lenalidomide, after which rituximab (375 mg/m^2) was administered weekly on weeks 2 to 5, then 13 to 16. Twelve of 16 patients were evaluable and responses included: PR (n = 4); MR (n = 4); SD (n = 3); NR (n = 1) for an overall and a major response rate of 67% and 33%, respectively, and a median TTP of 15.6 months. In two patients with bulky disease, a significant reduction in node/spleen size was observed. An acute reduction in hematocrit was observed during the first 2 weeks of lenalidomide therapy in 13/16 (81%) patients, with a median hematocrit reduction of 4.4% (1.7%–7.2%), resulting in hospitalization in four patients. Despite reduction in starting doses to 5 mg daily, anemia continued to be problematic without evidence of hemolysis or more general myelosuppression. Therefore, the mechanism for pronounced anemia in WM patients receiving lenalidomide remains to be determined and the use of this agent among WM patients remains investigational.

HIGH-DOSE THERAPY AND STEM CELL TRANSPLANTATION

The use of transplant therapy has also been explored in patients with WM. Desikan et al[172] reported their initial experience of high-dose chemotherapy and autologous stem cell transplant, which has more recently been updated by Munshi et al.[173] Their studies involved eight previously treated WM patients between the ages of 45 and 69 years, who received either conditioning prior to transplant with melphalan at 200 mg/m^2 (n = 7) or melphalan at 140 mg/m^2 along with total body irradiation. Stem cell grafts were successfully collected in all eight patients, although a second collection procedure was required for two patients who had extensive prior nucleoside analogue exposure. There were no transplant-related mortalities and toxicities were manageable. All eight patients responded, with seven of eight patients achieving a major response, and one patient achieving a complete response, with duration of response ranging from 5+ to 77+ months. Dreger et al[174] investigated the use of the DEXA-BEAM (dexamethasone, BCNU, etoposide, cytarabine, melphalan) regimen followed by myeloablative therapy with cyclophosphamide, and total body irradiation and autologous stem cell transplantation in seven WM patients, which included four untreated patients. Serum IgM levels declined by more than 50% following DEXA-BEAM and myeloablative therapy for six of seven patients, with progression-free survival ranging from 4+ to 30+ months. All three evaluable patients, who were previously treated, also attained a major response in a study by Anagnostopoulos et al[175] in which WM patients received various preparative regimens and showed event-free survivals of 26+, 31, and 108+ months. Tournilhac et al[176] recently reported the outcome of 18 WM patients in France who received high-dose chemotherapy followed by autologous stem cell transplantation. All patients were previously treated with a median of three (range 1–5) prior regimens.

Table 88–4 Summary of Updated Response Criteria from the 3rd International Workshop on Waldenström Macroglobulinemia[174]

Complete response (CR)	Disappearance of monoclonal protein by immunofixation; no histological evidence of bone marrow involvement, and resolution of any adenopathy/organomegaly (confirmed by CT scan), along with no signs or symptoms attributable to WM. Reconfirmation of the CR status is required at least 6 weeks apart with a second immunofixation.
Partial response (PR)	A ≥50% reduction of serum monoclonal IgM concentration on protein electrophoresis and ≥50% decrease in adenopathy/organomegaly on physical examination or on CT scan. No new symptoms or signs of active disease.
Minor response (MR)	A ≥25% but <50% reduction of serum monoclonal IgM by protein electrophoresis. No new symptoms or signs of active disease.
Stable disease	A <25% reduction and <25% increase of serum monoclonal IgM by electrophoresis without progression of adenopathy/organomegaly, cytopenias or clinically significant symptoms due to disease and/or signs of WM.
Progressive disease (PD)	A ≥25% increase in serum monoclonal IgM by protein electrophoresis confirmed by a second measurement or progression of clinically significant findings due to disease (ie, anemia, thrombocytopenia, leukopenia, bulky adenopathy/organomegaly) or symptoms (unexplained recurrent fever ≥38.4°C, drenching night sweats, ≥10% body weight loss, or hyperviscosity, neuropathy, symptomatic cryoglobulinemia, or amyloidosis) attributable to WM.

Therapy was well tolerated with an improvement in response status was observed for seven patients (six PR to CR; one SD to PR), whereas only one patient demonstrated progressive disease. The median event-free survival for all patients without progressive disease was 12 months. Tournilhac et al[176] have also reported the outcome of allogeneic stem cell transplantation in 10 previously treated WM patients (ages 35–46) who received a median of three prior therapies, including three patients with progressive disease despite therapy. Two of three patients with progressive disease responded, and an improvement in response status was observed in five patients. The median event-free survival for nonprogressing, evaluable patients was 31 months. Concerning in this series was the death of three patients owing to transplantation-related toxicity. Anagnostopoulos et al[177] have also reported a retrospective review of WM patients who underwent either autologous or allogeneic transplantation. Seventy-eight percent of patients in this cohort had two or more previous therapies, and 58% of them were resistant to their previous therapy. The relapse rate at 3 years was 29% in the group receiving autografts and 24% in the group receiving allografts. Nonrelapse mortality however was 40% in the allogeneic group, and 11% in the autologous group in this series. In view of the high rate of nonrelapse mortality associated with high-dose chemotherapy and allogeneic stem cell transplantation, Maloney et al[178] have evaluated the use of nonmyeloablative allogeneic stem cell transplantation in five patients with refractory WM. In this series, three of three evaluable patients (all of whom had matched sibling donors) responded with two CR and one in PR at 1 to 3 years posttransplant. In view of the above data, the consensus panel on therapeutics for WM has recommended that autologous stem cell transplantation in WM be considered in the relapsed setting, particularly among younger patients who have had multiple relapses or primary refractory disease, whereas allogeneic and reduced intensity conditioning followed by allogeneic stem cell transplantation should be undertaken ideally in the context of a clinical trial.[108,109]

RESPONSE CRITERIA IN WALDENSTRÖM MACROGLOBULINEMIA

Assessment of response to a treatment option by WM patients has not always been judged using uniform criteria. As a consequence studies using the same regimen have reported significantly different response rates. As part of the second and third International Workshops on WM, consensus panels developed guidelines for uniform response criteria in WM.[179,180] The category of minor response was adopted at the Third International Workshop of WM, given that clinically meaningful responses were observed with newer biological agents and is based on a ≥25 to <50% decrease in serum IgM level, which is used as a surrogate marker of disease in WM. In distinction, the term *major response* is used to denote a response of ≥50% in serum IgM levels, and includes partial and complete responses.[180] Response categories and criteria for progressive disease in WM based on consensus recommendations are summarized in Table 88–4. An important concern with the use of IgM as a surrogate marker of disease is that it can fluctuate, independent of tumor cell killing, particularly with newer biologically targeted agents such as rituximab and bortezomib.[140–142,158,181] Rituximab induces a spike or flare in serum IgM levels that can last for months, whereas bortezomib can suppress IgM levels apparently independent of tumor cell killing in certain patients. In circumstances where the serum IgM levels appear out of context with the clinical progress of the patient, a bone marrow biopsy should be considered in order to clarify the patient's underlying disease burden. Soluble CD27 is currently being investigated by Ho et al[36] as an alternative surrogate marker in WM.

SUGGESTED READINGS

Anagnostopoulos A, Zervas K, Kyrtsonis M, et al: Prognostic value of serum beta 2-microglobulin in patients with Waldenstrom's macroglobulinemia requiring therapy. Clin Lymph Myeloma 7:205, 2006.

Anagnostopoulos A, Hari PN, Perez WS, et al: Autologous or allogeneic stem cell transplantation in patients with Waldenstrom's macroglobulinemia. Biol Blood Marrow Transplant 12:845, 2006.

Chen CI, Kouroukis CT, White D, et al: Bortezomib is active in patients with untreated or relapsed Waldenstrom's macroglobulinemia: A phase II study of the National Cancer Institute of Canada Clinical Trials Group. J Clin Oncol 25:1570, 2007.

Dimopoulos MA, Anagnostopoulos A, Kyrtsonis MC, et al: Primary treatment of Waldenstrom's macroglobulinemia with dexamethasone, rituximab and cyclophosphamide. J Clin Oncol 25:3344, 2007.

Hunter ZR, Boxer M, Kahl B, et al: Phase II study of alemtuzumab in lymphoplasmacytic lymphoma: Results of WMCTG trial 02-079. Proc Am Soc Clin Oncol 24:427s, 2006.

Hunter Z, Leleu X, Hatjiharissi E, et al: IgA and IgG hypogammaglobulinemia are associated with mutations in the APRIL/BLYS receptor TACI in Waldenstrom's macroglobulinemia (WM). Blood 108:228, 2006.

Kimby E, Treon SP, Anagnostopoulos A, et al: Update on recommendations for assessing response from the Third International Workshop on Waldenstrom's Macroglobulinemia. Clin Lymphoma Myeloma 6:380, 2006.

Leleu X, O'Connor K, Ho A, et al: Hepatitis C viral infection is not associated with Waldenstrom's macroglobulinemia. Am J Hematol 82:83, 2007.

Leleu XP, Manning R, Soumerai JD, et al: Increased incidence of disease transformation and development of MDS/AML in Waldenstrom's

Macroglobulinemia patients treated with nucleoside analogues. Proc Am Soc Clin Oncol 25:445s, 2007.

Menke MN, Feke GT, McMeel JW, Branagan A, Hunter Z, Treon SP: Hyperviscosity-related retinopathy in Waldenstrom's macroglobulinemia. Arch Opthalmol 124:1601, 2006.

Morel P, Duhamel A, Gobbi P, et al: International prognostic scoring system (IPSS) for Waldenstrom's macroglobulinemia. Blood 108:42a, 2006.

Soumerai JD, Branagan AR, Patterson CJ, et al: Long term responses to thalidomide and rituximab in Waldenstrom's macroglobulinemia. Proc Am Soc Clin Oncol 25:445s, 2007.

Strauss SJ, Maharaj L, Hoare S, et al: Bortezomib therapy in patients with relapsed or refractory lymphoma: Potential correlation of in vitro sensitivity and tumor necrosis factor alpha response with clinical activity. J Clin Oncol 24:2105, 2006.

Tournilhac O, Santos DD, Xu L, et al: Mast cells in Waldenstrom's macroglobulinemia support lymphoplasmacytic cell growth through CD154/CD40 signaling. Ann Oncol 17:1275, 2006.

Treon SP, Hunter ZR, Matous J, et al: Multicenter clinical trial of bortezomib in relapsed/refractory Waldenstrom's macroglobulinemia: Results of WMCTG Trial 03-248. Clin Cancer Res 13:3320, 2007.

Treon SP, Hunter ZR, Aggarwal A, et al: Characterization of familial Waldenstrom's macroglobulinemia. Ann Oncol 17:488, 2006.

Treon SP, Gertz MA, Dimopoulos M, et al: Update on treatment recommendations from the Third International Workshop on Waldenstrom's Macroglobulinemia. Blood 107:3442, 2006.

REFERENCES

For complete list of references log onto www.expertconsult.com

CHAPTER 89

IMMUNOGLOBULIN LIGHT-CHAIN AMYLOIDOSIS (PRIMARY AMYLOIDOSIS)*

Morie A. Gertz, Martha Q. Lacy, Angela Dispenzieri, and Suzanne R. Hayman

BACKGROUND

In 1858, Rudolf Virchow described the reaction of amyloid deposits with iodine and sulfuric acid.[1] This reaction was considered a marker for starch; hence Virchow used the term *amyloid*, meaning "starch-like," to describe the deposits. At approximately the same time, Professor Carl Rokitansky in Vienna had recognized lardaceous deposits in the viscera of patients with tuberculosis or syphilis.[2] The white shiny appearance of these deposits led him to conclude that they were of fat origin. Later, Carl Friedreich recognized that the waxy spleen described by Virchow contained no material structurally similar to cellulose and determined that the deposits were probably albuminoid.[3] Sir Samuel Wilks, the first physician to use bromide in the treatment of epilepsy, reported on a patient who had lardaceous changes of the liver with no obvious cause.[4] This may have been the first reported patient with primary amyloidosis (AL).

Congo red staining of amyloid was introduced by Bennhold in 1922,[5] and in 1927 Divry and Florkin described the green birefringence of amyloid under polarized light.[6] In 1959, Cohen and Calkins[7] recognized that all forms of amyloid had a fibrillar structure when viewed with the electron microscope. In 1968, Eanes and Glenner[8] reported that unlike normal proteins, which have an α-helical configuration, amyloid deposits form a β-pleated sheet, rendering them resistant to the action of solvents. The first purification of amyloid was described by Pras et al[9] in 1968. The first amyloid protein was sequenced in 1970 by Glenner et al,[10] who recognized it as the N-terminus of an immunoglobulin light chain. In 1974, Isobe and Osserman[11] first recognized that the Bence Jones proteins had a role in the pathogenesis of AL.

CLASSIFICATION

All forms of amyloid stain positively with Congo red, and this is the sine qua non for the diagnosis of this disorder. Amyloid deposits appear amorphous and extracellular when stained with hematoxylin and eosin. False-positive results have been reported with Congo red staining, however, and some experience with the technique is desirable.[12] All forms of amyloid are fibrillar in nature; the fibrils are rigid and nonbranching. In the early and mid-20th century, amyloidosis was classified by the anatomic distribution of the amyloid deposits and was assigned to one of three categories.

Familial amyloidosis was recognized by its presentation, which was usually a painful peripheral neuropathy with an autosomal-dominant inheritance pattern.[13,14] Mutations in a number of plasma proteins including transthyretin (TTR), apolipoprotein AI and AII, fibrinogen A α-chain, and lysozyme are associated with hereditary systemic amyloidosis. TTR amyloidosis is the most common and is usually associated with peripheral neuropathy. Mutations in the other proteins usually have no neuropathic consequences and instead principally cause renal and cardiac amyloidosis.

The secondary form of amyloidosis was characterized by the associated long-standing inflammatory disorder. One hundred years ago, this usually represented tuberculosis, leprosy, syphilis, and chronic infection such as bronchiectasis and osteomyelitis. Today, in Western countries, amyloidosis is commonly associated with chronic inflammatory polyarthritis syndromes such as ankylosing spondylitis and juvenile rheumatoid arthritis. It is also associated with Castleman disease and Crohn disease.

Fifty years ago, all forms of amyloidosis that were not secondary or familial were considered "primary." In the original terminology, "primary" meant "idiopathic" and most likely contained a heterogeneous combination of multiple forms of amyloidosis. Today, the term *primary amyloidosis*, or AL, refers to a systemic disorder with amyloid deposits consisting of immunoglobulin light chains or their fragments or heavy chains.

All forms of AL are associated with a clonal disorder of plasma cells, which may range from a small clonal population of 5% plasma cells or less in the bone marrow to overt multiple myeloma. Table 89–1 contains a modified classification of the more frequently described forms of amyloidosis.

PATHOPHYSIOLOGY

Amyloid fibrils can be produced in vitro by peptic digestion of purified monoclonal human immunoglobulin light chains. The light chains of patients with AL have an abnormal sequence and an abnormal tertiary structure that favors the β-pleated sheet configuration. Investigation of the thermodynamic properties of light chains that form fibrils and those that remain stable have shown an inverse relationship between thermodynamic stability and fibrillogenic potential. Structural parameters and overall thermodynamic stability contribute to the fibril-forming propensity of immunoglobulin light chains.[15] When injected into mice, immunoglobulin light chains purified from the urine of patients with AL produce human AL deposits,[16] whereas light chains from patients with multiple myeloma (and not AL) do not.

Two-thirds of patients with monoclonal gammopathy of undetermined significance or multiple myeloma have κ immunoglobulin light chains. Three-fourths of patients with amyloidosis who have a light chain have λ, which reflects the intrinsic "amyloidogenicity" of λ immunoglobulin light chains. The λ_{VI} is always associated with amyloid, suggesting that unique amino acid structures render these proteins amyloidogenic.[17]

A comparison of monoclonal proteins in AL and multiple myeloma is shown in Fig. 89–1. Amyloid-associated germline gene segments have been identified[18]; the λ_{III} family is found most frequently in amyloidosis. Two germline genes, 3r and 6a, belonging to the λ_{III} and λ_{VI} families contributed equally to encode 42% of amyloid variable λ regions. These same two gene segments have a strong association with amyloidosis and are most likely responsible for the λ light-chain overrepresentation typical of amyloidosis.[18]

The reason that patients with AL present with amyloid disease displaying organ tropism is unknown. The renal tropism of some chains was investigated.[19] Patients with clones derived from the 6a

*Portions of this manuscript were originally included in Gertz MA, Lacy MQ, Dispenzieri A, Hayman SR, Kumar S. Transplantation for amyloidosis. Curr Opin Oncol 2007;19:136–41. Used with permission.

Table 89–1 Nomenclature of Amyloidosis

Protein	Precursor	Clinical characteristics
AL or AH	Immunoglobulin light or heavy chain	Primary or localized; myeloma- or macroglobulinemia-associated
AA	SAA	Secondary or familial Mediterranean fever, familial periodic fever syndromes
ATTR	Transthyretin	Familial and senile
A Fibrinogen	Fibrinogen	Familial renal amyloidosis (Ostertag)
Aβ_2M	β_2-Microglobulin	Dialysis-associated; carpal tunnel syndrome
Aβ	ABPP	Alzheimer disease
A Apo A-I/A-II	Apolipoprotein A-I Apolipoprotein A-II	Proteinuria Cardiac Neuropathy
A Lysozyme	Lysozyme	Gastrointestinal tract Liver Renal

ABPP, amyloid β protein precursor; SAA, serum amyloid A.
From Gertz MA, Lacy MQ, Dispenzieri A: Immunoglobulin light chain amyloidosis (primary amyloidosis, AL). In Gertz MA, Greipp PR (eds.): Hematologic Malignancies: Multiple Myeloma and Related Plasma Cell Disorders. New York, Springer-Verlag, 2004, p 157–195. Used with permission of Mayo Foundation for Medical Education and Research.

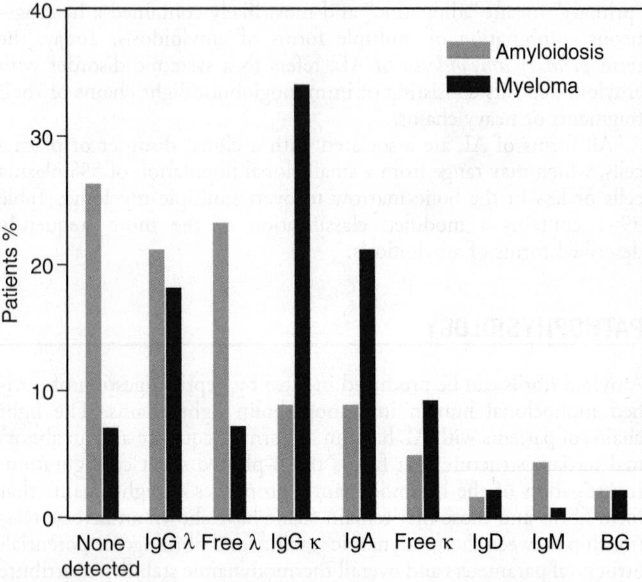

Figure 89–1 Distribution of serum monoclonal protein in patients with amyloidosis ($N = 270$) or multiple myeloma ($N = 1000$). The κ:λ ratio in amyloidosis is 1:3.6. BG, biclonal gammopathy; Ig, immunoglobulin. *(From Gertz MA, Lacy MQ, Dispenzieri A, et al: Transplantation for amyloidosis. Curr Opin Oncol 2007; 19:136–41.)*

variable λ_{VI} germline gene were more likely to present with renal involvement. Those with clones derived from the 1c, 2a2, and 3r variable λ genes were more likely to present with dominant cardiac and multisystem disease. Patients with variable κ clones were more likely to have dominant liver involvement.[19]

The classification of AL among patients with and without myeloma is usually made on the basis of clinical criteria, but considerable clinical overlap exists. The presence of multiple myeloma bone disease, such as lytic lesions, multiple compression fractures, or pathologic fractures of long bones, is rare in AL. Patients with AL and renal insufficiency rarely have myeloma cast nephropathy. Renal failure in these patients is usually tubular atrophy from glomerular amyloid and long-standing albuminuria. The percentage of bone marrow plasma cells is useful in making the distinction between AL and myeloma. We have arbitrarily defined patients as having multiple myeloma-associated amyloidosis if the bone marrow plasma cells exceed 30%.[20] Amyloidosis rarely evolves into overt multiple myeloma; it occurs in less than 0.5% of patients.[20]

The incidence of amyloidosis is 8 per million persons per year and is not increasing with time.[21] Amyloidosis is one-fourth as common as multiple myeloma but has an incidence similar to those of nodular sclerosing Hodgkin disease, Philadelphia chromosome-positive chronic myeloid leukemia, and polycythemia vera.

Chromosomal anomalies are seen often in the bone marrow plasma cells of patients with AL.[22] Studies of bone marrow samples found trisomies of chromosomes 7, 9, 11, 15, and 18 in 42%, 52%, 47%, 39%, and 33% of patients, respectively. Trisomy X was seen in 13% of women and 54% of men. Monosomy of chromosome 18 was seen in 72%. This aneuploidy supports the neoplastic nature of the disorder even though it is not proliferative over time. Fluorescence in situ hybridization analysis of the plasma cells of AL patients showed that 16 of 29 (55%) had a definite immunoglobulin heavy-chain translocation, and 5 additional patients (17%) had a pattern compatible with heavy-chain translocation.[23] Sixteen of 21 patients were confirmed to have t(11;14)(q13;q32), accounting for 76% of all immunoglobulin heavy-chain translocations.[24] Fifteen of 16 patients with an 11;14 translocation had cyclin D1 overexpression.

CLINICAL FEATURES

The most common presenting symptoms of amyloidosis are fatigue, dyspnea, edema, paresthesias, and weight loss.[25] The symptoms are generally not specific and not particularly helpful in formulating the differential diagnosis. Weight loss usually results in an investigation for occult malignancy. The fatigue can be misdiagnosed as functional or stress related. Patients with dyspnea on exertion regularly undergo coronary angiography; in most, no coronary artery disease is seen and the evaluation is halted. Lightheadedness is common but nonspecific. Hypotension is seen in patients with nephrotic syndrome because the hypoalbuminemia results in reduced oncotic pressure and contraction of the plasma volume. In cardiac AL, the stiffened heart has poor diastolic filling.[26] The stroke volume decreases, resulting in a decrease in systolic blood pressure. Amyloid autonomic neuropathy also produces orthostatic lightheadedness and occasionally syncope.[27]

The physical findings of amyloidosis can be highly specific but are only present in a minority of patients. Amyloid purpura is typical but is seen in only one-sixth of patients. The purpura occurs above the nipple line and is seen in the webbing of the neck, the face, and the eyelids (Fig. 89–2). The purpura may be subtle and limited to eyelid

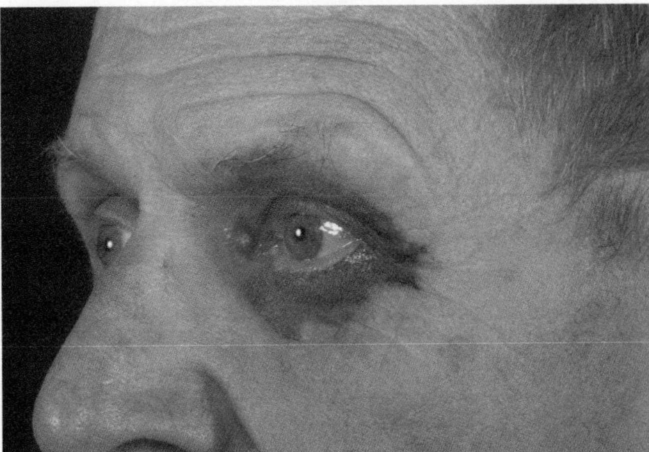

Figure 89–2 Classic periorbital purpura associated with amyloidosis.

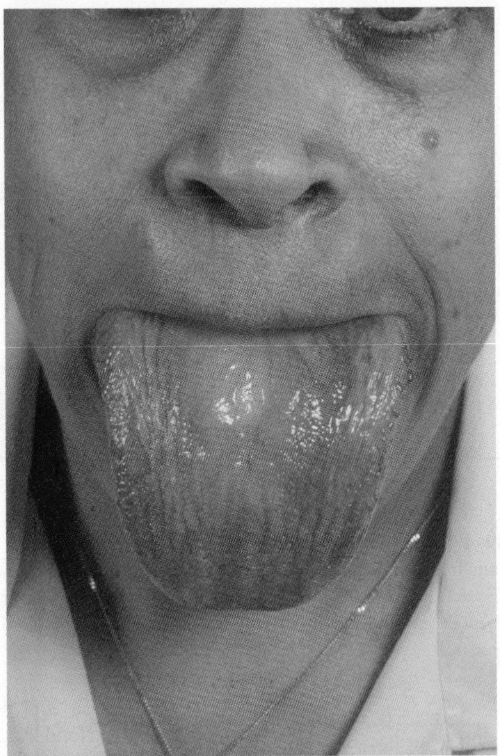

Figure 89–3 Massive enlargement of the tongue due to amyloid infiltration. This patient had severe obstructive sleep apnea, was unable to swallow solid food, and had obstructed eustachian tubes leading to bilateral serous otitis media.

petechial lesions. Hepatosplenomegaly is seen in one-fourth of patients but is located more than 5 cm below the right costal margin in one-tenth of patients.[28] The presence of macroglossia is highly specific for AL[29]; it is not seen in familial, secondary, or senile systemic amyloidosis. Only 1 patient in 11 has an enlarged tongue; it can be overlooked because the most common finding is dental indentations on the underside of the tongue, which may not be inspected during a routine physical examination. If the tongue is enlarged, the submandibular salivary glands are also palpable (Fig. 89–3), which can be misinterpreted as submandibular lymph nodes. Salivary gland infiltration with amyloid can produce a sicca syndrome, and patients can be misdiagnosed as having Sjögren syndrome.[30]

Patients can be seen with diffuse vascular involvement without obvious visceral disease. Involvement of the small vessels supplying blood to major muscle groups can produce vascular occlusion and ischemic symptoms that include jaw,[31] calf, and limb claudication. Involvement of the coronary arteriolar system can produce true exertional angina without evidence of large vessel coronary disease. In one study, obstructive intramural coronary amyloidosis was found in 63 of 96 patients.[31] Myocardial ischemia was more common in patients with obstructive intramural coronary amyloidosis than those without (86% vs 52%). Syndromes of myocardial ischemia affected 25% of patients with obstructive intramural coronary amyloidosis.[32] For 11% of these patients, a syndrome of ischemia consisting of acute myocardial infarction or angina was the first manifestation of AL.

Most patients with AL and cardiac involvement have obstructive intramural coronary amyloidosis and associated changes of myocardial ischemia.[31] The presence of jaw claudication has led to an incorrect diagnosis of polymyalgia rheumatica.[33] Other manifestations of nonvisceral soft tissue infiltration include skeletal muscle pseudohypertrophy, which can produce the shoulder-pad sign.[34] Despite the enlargement of the muscles, patients frequently have diffuse muscular weakness and atrophy.[35] The creatine kinase concentration may be increased, which results in a polymyositis or inflammatory myopathy syndrome.

ESTABLISHING THE DIAGNOSIS OF AMYLOIDOSIS

The subjective symptoms associated with amyloidosis are vague.[36] The physical findings with AL may be highly specific but are present in only 15% of patients. Given that AL is rare, when should a clinician suspect this diagnosis and begin a diagnostic evaluation to confirm the diagnosis? The eight most common clinical syndromes associated with amyloidosis are (a) infiltrative cardiomyopathy manifesting as a spectrum from fatigue to overt congestive heart failure; (b) albuminuria with or without renal insufficiency; (c) peripheral neuropathy with demyelinating or axonal features; (d) unexplained hepatomegaly; (e) carpal tunnel syndrome; (f) enlargement of the tongue; (g) weight loss associated with intestinal symptoms of pseudo-obstruction or malabsorption; and (h) "atypical myeloma" (Table 89–2). If any of these syndromes are seen in an adult, AL enters the differential diagnosis.

Table 89–2 Syndromes in Primary Amyloidosis

Syndrome	Patients, %
Nephrotic or nephrotic and renal failure	30
Hepatomegaly	24
Congestive heart failure	22
Carpal tunnel	21
Neuropathy	17
Orthostatic hypotension	12

From Gertz MA, Lacy MQ, Dispenzieri A: Amyloidosis. In: Mehta J, Singhal S (eds.): Myeloma. London, Martin Dunitz Ltd., 2002, p 445–463. Used with permission.

Because of the presence of a monoclonal protein, patients are often extensively evaluated for multiple myeloma but are found to have less than 10% plasma cells and no lytic bone lesions, and a diagnosis of AL frequently is not considered by the clinician. By definition, patients with AL have a clonal population of plasma cells that produces the immunoglobulin light chain comprising the amyloid deposits. The finding of a monoclonal protein in a patient with a compatible syndrome would be compelling evidence for pursuing a diagnosis of AL (Fig. 89–4).

If a patient has one of the clinical syndromes outlined above, a sensitive and noninvasive screening test for AL should be used. Simple serum protein electrophoresis is not an adequate screen. The monoclonal proteins in patients with AL are frequently either small or limited to free light chains that do not produce a peak in the

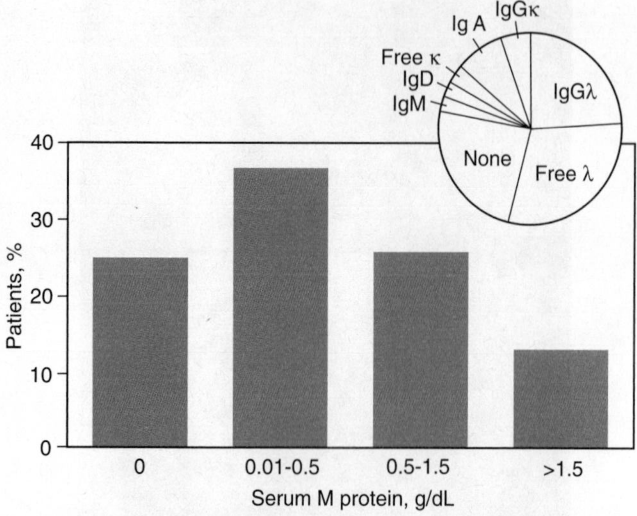

Figure 89–4 Serum monoclonal protein concentration in patients with primary amyloidosis. Pie chart shows distribution of serum immunofixation results. *(From Gertz MA, Lacy MQ, Dispenzieri A: Amyloidosis. In Mehta J, Singhal S [eds.]: Myeloma, London, Martin Dunitz Ltd, 2002, p 445–463. Used with permission.)*

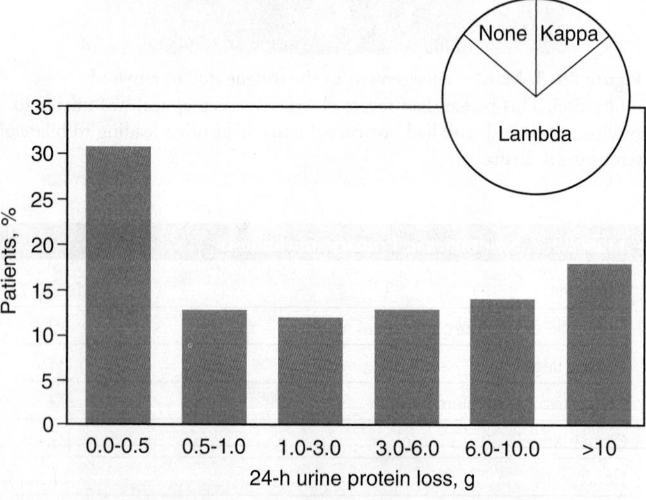

Figure 89–5 Distribution of urinary protein excretion in patients with primary amyloidosis. Pie chart shows results of urine immunofixation. *(From Gertz MA, Lacy MQ, Dispenzieri A: Amyloidosis. In Mehta J, Singhal S [eds.]: Myeloma, London, Martin Dunitz Ltd, 2002, p 445–463. Used with permission.)*

electrophoretic pattern. In addition, a high proportion of patients has significant albuminuria, which can obscure the presence of small monoclonal proteins in the urine (Fig. 89–5).

A serious consideration of AL requires immunofixation of serum and urine; urine immunofixation is mandatory because a fourth of patients do not have detectable light chains in the serum by immunofixation. By this method, a monoclonal light chain will be detected in 90% of patients with AL. Adding the free light-chain nephelometric assay increases the detection rate to 99%. An automated immunoassay for free light chains is more sensitive than immunofixation by at least a factor of 10. Quantification of monoclonal free light chains by nephelometry is more sensitive than immunofixation in serum samples from patients with AL and light-chain deposition disease. This method allows quantification of free light chains in patients who have no detectable serum or urine monoclonal protein concentration.[37]

Immunofixation of serum and urine combined with a free light-chain assay is the single best noninvasive screening panel when a patient is seen with a suggestive clinical syndrome. In patients who do not have a detectable light chain in the serum or urine, a bone marrow specimen will almost always demonstrate a clonal population of plasma cells by immunohistochemistry or immunofluorescence.

Because the production of immunoglobulin light chains by the plasma cells in AL is at a low level, a monoclonal protein occasionally may not be found. Presumably, the light chains are present, but the amounts are below the level of detection by conventional techniques. This may be a result of low-level production or rapid migration from the plasma compartment into the amyloid deposits. Occasionally, the light-chain fragments do not express epitopes recognizable by commercial light-chain antisera, which are directed against the entire immunoglobulin light-chain protein.

Virtually all patients with AL have a monoclonal protein in the serum or urine or clonal bone marrow plasma cells. If no immunoglobulin light chain is found in a patient with proven amyloidosis, other types of amyloidosis should be suspected, including familial, secondary, and localized. The presence of a monoclonal protein does not unequivocally prove that the amyloidosis type is AL. Three percent of patients older than 60 years have an incidental monoclonal gammopathy of undetermined significance.[38] It is therefore reasonable to believe that 3% of patients older than 60 years with localized, secondary, and familial amyloidosis have an incidental monoclonal protein in the serum. Case reports exist of patients with low-level monoclonal gammopathies associated with a nonimmunoglobulin form of amyloidosis. The possibility, albeit uncommon, of an incidental monoclonal gammopathy unrelated to the patient's amyloidosis must be kept in mind.

A nephelometric technique for analyzing circulating immunoglobulin light chains in the serum recognizes only free immunoglobulin light chains and not those that are part of the intact immunoglobulin molecule.[39,40] A study of approximately 100 patients, using antibodies specific for free immunoglobulin light chains, showed a sensitivity of nearly 90% for the nephelometric technique.[41] The sensitivity was the same for patients with κ and λ amyloid. In patients who had a known monoclonal light chain in the urine but negative serum immunofixation results, free light chains were detected in 85% of patients with κ and 80% of patients with λ. In a carefully evaluated group of patients with definite AL who had no detectable monoclonal protein in the serum or urine by immunofixation, a free light chain was found in 86% and a free λ light chain in 30%.[41]

The nephelometric method is a convenient assay for free light chain detection and allows classification of patients with amyloidosis as having AL.[42] Patients with familial, secondary, or localized amyloidosis are not expected to have an abnormal ratio of free light chains in the serum. If the serum free light-chain assay and serum and urine immunofixation results are all negative or normal, the likelihood of a diagnosis of AL is small.

The free light-chain assay also is useful in assessing the outcome of treatment of amyloidosis. Eighty-six patients whose abnormal free light-chain concentration decreased by more than 50% after chemotherapy had a 5-year survival of 88% compared with only 39% among patients for whom the free light-chain concentration did not decrease similarly.[43] The conclusion was that decrease in the free light chain by more than 50% after chemotherapy is associated with a substantial survival benefit.

The amyloid P component is a glycoprotein that comprises as much as 10% of the amyloid fibril by weight.[44] All forms of amyloid contain the P component. The amyloid P component is related structurally to C-reactive protein, an acute-phase reactant used in the screening of patients at risk for coronary artery disease. The amyloid P component is not irreversibly bound to the amyloid fibril but is in dynamic equilibrium with the normal plasma amyloid P component compartment.[45] It is found in all humans and maintains a stable plasma level throughout life.

Radiolabeled amyloid P component—with iodine 123[46] or iodine 131[47]—is a useful imaging agent for indicating amyloid deposits. Serialized serum amyloid P scintigraphic scans have been used to assess the response to therapy and have shown regression of established amyloid deposits after successful interruption of immunoglobulin light-chain production.[48] This scan does not distinguish AL from the other forms of amyloidosis. Imaging indicates deposits in the spleen, liver, and kidneys in 87%, 60%, and 25% of patients, respectively.[49] Because of the cardiac blood pool, this technique is not useful in detecting myocardial amyloid deposits and is usually used in conjunction with echocardiography. The diagnostic sensitivity of serum amyloid P scintigraphy for AL is 90%, and specificity is 93%.[50] Myocardial uptake is not visualized in any patient. Splenic amyloid is present in 80% of patients, even though it is rarely detected clinically (14%). Tracer uptake in the liver and kidneys correlates with abnormal liver function and proteinuria. Bone marrow uptake is specific for AL but is only seen in 21%.[50]

Plasma clearance of the amyloid P component has been shown to correlate with survival. Rapid plasma clearance is associated with high body burdens of amyloid and shortened survival. Scintigraphic scans have shown that the distribution of amyloid within organs is nonhomogeneous, and imaging studies do not correlate well with the clinical degree of organ dysfunction.[51] Most patients have hepatic involvement by serum amyloid P scan, but palpable hepatomegaly with increased concentration of alkaline phosphatase is seen in no more than 15% of patients. Therapeutic clinical trials of agents that prevent the binding of amyloid P component to the amyloid fibril have been started.[52] The rationale is that inhibition of P component binding may destabilize the fibrillar structure of amyloid and result in more rapid catabolism by the body.

Although the presence of immunoglobulin free light chains, positive immunofixation results, or positive amyloid P component scans is highly suggestive of the diagnosis of AL, these findings are not substitutes for histologic confirmation of the disease. Amyloidosis is a serious life-threatening disorder, and some of the currently available therapies carry a considerable morbidity and mortality risk. Given the serious prognosis and potential for administering toxic therapies, a biopsy-proven diagnosis is vital. Although the presence of renal, cardiac, hepatic, or peripheral nerve amyloid is easily established by direct biopsy of these tissues, invasive diagnostic biopsies of these tissues are generally not required. Amyloidosis is a widespread disorder at diagnosis, with involvement of blood vessels even in the absence of clinical symptoms. Any biopsy that samples blood vessels can less invasively establish the diagnosis effectively and at a lower risk to the patient.

At Mayo Clinic, if a patient has a compatible clinical syndrome and screening suggests the presence of a free or monoclonal immunoglobulin light chain, the first diagnostic technique is generally subcutaneous fat aspiration[53] combined with bone marrow biopsy. The fat aspiration procedure performed by our nursing staff is risk free, and no infection at the site of puncture has occurred. Results are generally available in 24 to 48 hours, and the technique has a sensitivity of nearly 80% (Table 89–3). Thorough examination of three fat smears showed a sensitivity of 93% and a specificity of 100% for the test. The clinical utility of fat tissue aspiration was greater than that of rectal biopsy.[54] Fat aspiration is the preferred method for detecting amyloidosis, with a sensitivity of 80% using a routine approach and 90% with a thorough assessment by experienced interpreters.[54] Bone marrow biopsy shows amyloid deposits in half of patients if the biopsy specimen contains blood vessels.[55] A bone marrow biopsy is generally required because once a monoclonal protein has been found, determining the percentage of bone marrow plasma cells is vital to exclude the diagnosis of multiple myeloma (Fig. 89–6). In our experience, 90% of patients with AL have positive results of the subcutaneous fat aspiration and bone marrow biopsy.

Others have reported success using rectal biopsies[56] (Fig. 89–7), gingival biopsies, and minor salivary gland biopsies.[57] If noninvasive biopsies do not establish the diagnosis, biopsy of the affected organ can generally be performed quite safely. Endomyocardial biopsy is an outpatient procedure and can be done with low risk in experienced centers. Despite reports to the contrary, liver biopsy is exceedingly safe, with no reported fatalities in our experience with more than 100 liver biopsies and a bleeding risk of 4%, which required transfusion in 2%. Biopsy of uninvolved skin has been shown to be positive in 70% of patients with AL.[58]

The most common clinical presentation at Mayo Clinic is that of a patient referred to a nephrologist for nephrotic syndrome. Immunofixation of the serum and urine and free light-chain assay indicate presence of a light chain; fat aspiration is performed and is positive. Positive fat aspiration results eliminate the need for a renal biopsy in nearly 90% of patients, which results in reduced cost, eliminates the need for hospitalization, and decreases the risk to the patient.

The diagnosis of amyloidosis requires positive Congo red staining of tissues, but use of the Congo red stain is not simple.[59] False-positive results have been reported[60] because of overstaining of tissue or misinterpreting Congo red–positive fibrils of collagen and elastin as being amyloid. Conversely, we have seen patients whose rectal biopsy specimens were interpreted as collagenous colitis,[61] only later to be identified as AL. By routine hematoxylin and eosin staining, amyloid deposits in the glomerulus can be misinterpreted as hyalin. In our routine clinical practice, our cardiac pathologists prefer the sulfated alcian blue stain[62] for recognition of amyloid deposits in the myocardium. In our peripheral nerve laboratories, pathologists screen biopsy specimens with crystal violet and, if positive, subsequently confirm the diagnosis by using Congo red.

Table 89–3 Noninvasive Biopsy Results in 233 Patients with Primary Amyloidosis

Finding	No. of Patients (%)
Fat + Marrow +	138 (59)
Fat + Marrow –	30 (13)
Fat – Marrow +	38 (16)
Fat – Marrow –	27 (12)

Modified from Gertz et al.[292] Used with permission.

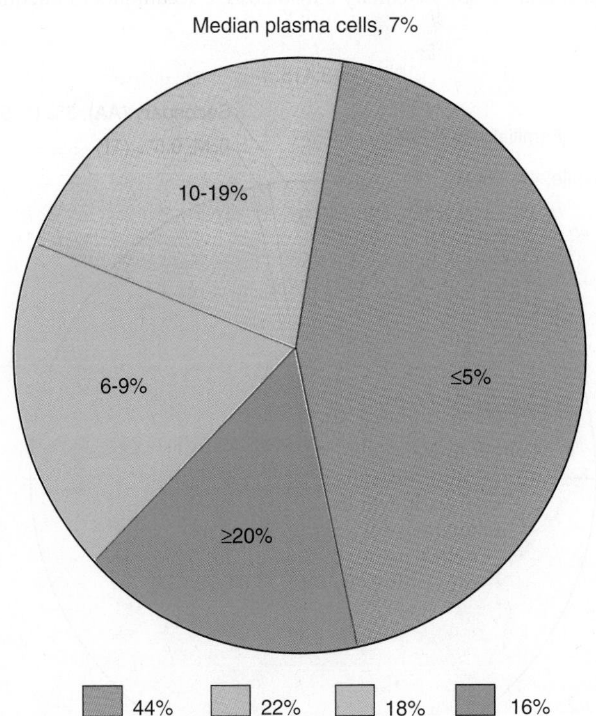

Figure 89–6 Distribution of bone marrow plasma cells in patients presenting with primary amyloidosis. *(From Gertz MA, Lacy MQ, Dispenzieri A: Amyloidosis. Hematol Oncol Clin North Am 13:1211–1233, 1999. Used with permission.)*

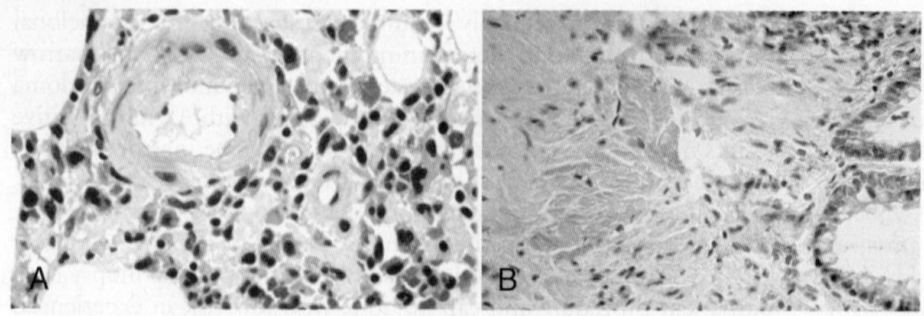

Figure 89–7 **A,** Bone marrow biopsy specimen showing thickened large and small vessels due to amyloid deposition. **B,** Rectal biopsy specimen demonstrates amyloid deposits (left) with Brunner glands (right). (Congo red; original magnification, ×100)

DISTINGUISHING PRIMARY AMYLOIDOSIS FROM OTHER FORMS OF AMYLOIDOSIS

After a diagnosis of amyloidosis has been established, it is imperative to be certain that the amyloidosis is of the immunoglobulin light-chain type. Localized, familial, secondary, and senile systemic forms of amyloid are structurally dissimilar to that in AL, and the therapeutic approach is substantially different for each (Fig. 89–8). Only systemic AL has an underlying bone marrow plasma cell dyscrasia responsible for fibril deposition.

It is possible to misdiagnose hereditary amyloidosis as AL. Among 350 patients with amyloidosis in whom AL was suspected, 34 (9.7%) were found to have mutations consistent with familial amyloidosis, most often fibrinogen-A α-chain mutations and TTR mutations.[63] A low-grade monoclonal gammopathy was detected in 8 of the 34 (24%), which easily could have led to a misdiagnosis of AL. A genetic cause should be sought in all patients with amyloidosis in whom AL cannot be unequivocally confirmed by immunohistochemistry of the amyloid deposits.

The possibility of familial amyloidosis with an incidental monoclonal gammopathy must be kept in mind.[63] In 178 consecutive patients referred for amyloidosis, 54 were screened with primers to detect TTR, apolipoprotein, fibrinogen, and lysozyme variants.[64] Three patients had both a monoclonal gammopathy and an amyloid-associated mutation, were thought to have apparent AL, and were later found to have hereditary amyloidosis.[64] Techniques to unequivocally identify TTR amyloidosis include immunoaffinity chromatography and immunoprecipitation combined with mass spectrometry.[65] Matrix-assisted laser desorption ionization/time-of-flight mass spectrometry can also quickly detect TTR variants with small changes in molecular weight.[66]

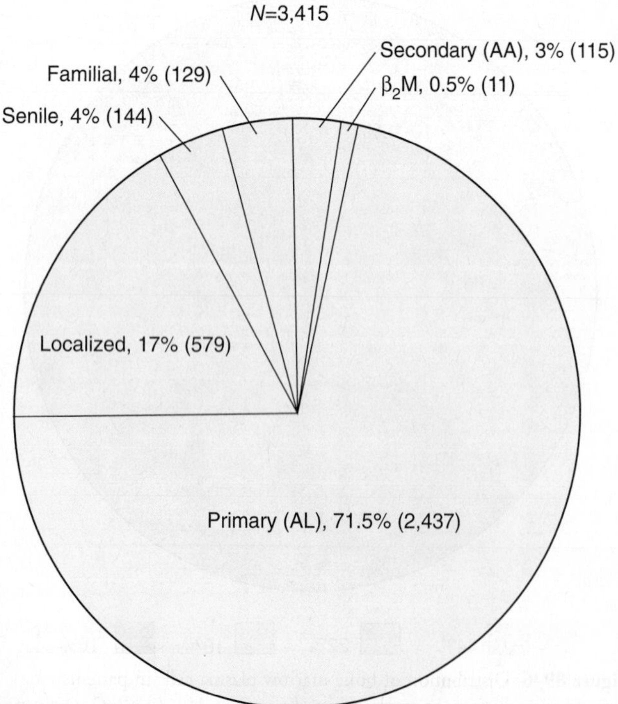

Figure 89–8 Distribution of the various forms of amyloidosis seen in patients at Mayo Clinic. β_2M, β_2-microglobulin.

Patients with localized amyloidosis can often have serious clinical problems such as hematuria, respiratory compromise, and visual disturbances. Patients with localized amyloidosis do not have development of widespread systemic vascular amyloid deposition. Localized forms of amyloidosis most commonly are derived from immunoglobulin light chains, but a bone marrow plasma cell dyscrasia is not present, and it is presumed that there was a localized synthesis of fibrillar material. Most patients with localized amyloidosis have involvement of the respiratory tract, genitourinary tract, or skin.

Amyloidosis involving the respiratory tract can be divided into tracheobronchial, pulmonary nodular, and pulmonary diffuse interstitial. The first two of these are forms of localized amyloidosis, and the third is a manifestation of systemic AL disease. In tracheobronchial amyloidosis, submucosal deposits (composed of immunoglobulin light chains) can produce obstruction, cough, dyspnea, wheezing, and hemoptysis. The most common site of involvement is the larynx and false vocal cords. The diagnosis is usually established bronchoscopically in a patient who presents with hoarseness. The treatment entails surgical excision[67] or the use of yttrium–aluminum–garnet laser resection of the tissue.[68] If extensive airway obstruction prevents passage of a bronchoscope, external beam radiotherapy (2000 cGy) can lead to dramatic improvement in symptoms, effort tolerance, bronchoscopic appearance, and forced expiratory volume in 1 second. If amyloidosis involves the pulmonary tissues, it can manifest as solitary nodules.[69] The diagnosis is usually made at thoracotomy or transthoracic needle biopsy, because these nodules are noncalcified and pulmonary malignancy must be excluded.[70]

Amyloid in the urinary bladder, urethra, or ureter is usually localized. Clinically, patients present with hematuria, and the cystoscopic findings of these bladder deposits are usually suspicious for transitional cell cancer.[71] Treatment consists of transurethral resection, fulguration, or partial cystectomy. We have experience with the use of intravesicular dimethylsulfoxide (DMSO) and have seen substantial regression of deposits in patients who were not candidates for surgical resection because of extent of disease. Amyloid in the ureter,[72] renal pelvis,[73] and urethra[74] usually presents with obstruction and colicky pain or hematuria; the preoperative diagnosis is usually malignancy. Recognition of ureteral amyloidosis is important because it prevents an unnecessary nephrectomy.

Amyloidosis of the skin can be classified into lichen, macular, or nodular.[75] The first two of these are localized forms of amyloid that never become systemic. Nodular amyloidosis may be a cutaneous manifestation of systemic AL. The deposits in macular and papular amyloidosis appear to be degenerated keratin protein.[76] Local therapy, including dermabrasion, is beneficial. An underlying inflammatory skin condition is usually present. Macular and lichen amyloidosis are benign conditions. Nodular amyloidosis is often an important clinical clue to a more serious life-threatening AL.

Amyloid found in the carpal tunnel may represent either a localized form or be part of AL.[77] Of 124 patients who had carpal tunnel syndrome as an isolated syndrome, the median survival was 12 years, and systemic AL developed in only two. Localized carpal tunnel amyloid is composed of TTR.

Diagnostic Pathway for Primary Amyloidosis

Consider primary amyloidosis in patients with
- Nephrotic-range proteinuria (nondiabetic)
- Cardiomyopathy (no ischemic history)
- Hepatomegaly (no filling defects on imaging)
- Peripheral neuropathy (nondiabetic)
- Atypical myeloma

Heighten suspicion
- Immunofixation of serum and urine, free light-chain assay

Confirm diagnosis histologically
- Fat aspirate and marrow biopsy stain with Congo red (90% sensitive)

Assess prognosis
- Echocardiography required (Doppler important)
- Brain natriuretic peptide and troponin

Treat
- Melphalan and prednisone
- High-dose corticosteroids
- Stem cell transplantation
- Organ transplantation

From Gertz MA, Lacy MQ, Dispenzieri A: Amyloidosis. In Mehta J, Singhal S (eds.): Myeloma, London, Martin Dunitz Ltd, 2002, p 445–463. Used with permission.

Amyloid may also be localized to the conjunctiva, orbits, or extraocular muscles. Conjunctival amyloid is best treated with surgical excision.[78] Localized amyloid has also been described in the breast, mesenteric lymph nodes, colon polyps, thyroid, ovary, and retroperitoneum. We have seen 4 patients with colon deposits of amyloid that resulted in bleeding, all of whom were followed up for more than 5 years without other manifestations developing. These patients had no evidence of a plasma cell dyscrasia. Finding traces of amyloid in surgical specimens from total hip arthroplasty is common.[79] Similar deposits can be seen at the time of knee arthroplasty[80] and are never associated with systemic disease.

Secondary amyloidosis (AA) also must be distinguished from AL.[81] AA can involve organs in a manner indistinguishable from AL but is not associated with an immunoglobulin light-chain disorder or clonal plasma cell disorder. AA is a consequence of long-standing uncontrolled systemic inflammation. Typically, elevation of the acute-phase proteins in the serum, serum amyloid A protein, or C-reactive protein parallel the activity of the underlying inflammatory process. In the Third World, AA is common because it can follow long-standing tuberculosis, lepromatous leprosy, malaria, and untreated syphilis. The most common clinical manifestation of AA is nephrotic-range proteinuria. Therefore, it is not easily distinguished clinically from AL.

In the West, AA is rare and found in only 2% of patients with amyloidosis at Mayo Clinic.[82] The most common causes are poorly controlled inflammatory polyarthropathies including ankylosing spondylitis,[83] juvenile rheumatoid arthritis,[84] psoriatic arthritis,[85] and rheumatoid arthritis.[86] The median duration of the arthritis is 15 years before the diagnosis of amyloidosis, and the underlying cause is usually obvious.[87]

In a 10-year study of 1000 patients with rheumatoid arthritis, 3.1% died of AA.[88] Amyloidosis can be seen in Crohn disease,[89] long-standing bronchiectasis,[90] cystic fibrosis, or chronic osteomyelitis.[91] The most common clinical manifestation is proteinuria followed by diarrhea and amyloid goiter. In these patients, the chronic, inflammatory, or infectious condition is usually present for many years and is easily recognized. These patients do not have a detectable immunoglobulin light chain or clonal plasma cell disorder. AA has been described in drug users who inject illegal substances subcutaneously.[92] The result is multiple skin abscesses that can produce the inflammation characteristic of AA.[93] Instances of AA have been described in Hodgkin disease[94] and in association with renal cell cancer.

Castleman disease (especially the plasma cell variant) complicated by AA has been reported. These patients typically present with a mesenteric mass; with successful abdominal surgery, proteinuria decreases and disappears.[95–97] Resection of the Castleman tumor has been documented to produce regression of the amyloid syndrome, even in advanced cases. AA has been seen in patients with paraparesis as a consequence of chronically infected decubitus ulcers[98] or chronic infection of the urinary tract, a consequence of urinary retention or a long-standing indwelling urinary catheter.[99] At autopsy, AA has been found in more than half of those with sustained spinal cord injuries in excess of 10 years. The presence of an amyloid goiter is characteristic of AA and is rarely seen in the other forms of amyloidosis.

AA amyloidosis can also be a consequence of hereditary periodic fevers characterized by recurrence of fever and inflammation separated by symptom-free intervals. Familial Mediterranean fever is the most frequent entity in this group, but hyperimmunoglobulinemia-D with periodic fever, tumor necrosis factor receptor-associated periodic syndrome, and cryopyrin-associated periodic syndrome are also seen.[100–102]

Familial amyloidosis is more common than AA in the United States. A clinical distinction for this variant can be difficult. These patients can present with cardiomyopathy,[103] peripheral or autonomic neuropathy,[104] and nephrotic syndrome.[105] The patients do not have a monoclonal gammopathy or plasma cell dyscrasia unless they have an incidental monoclonal gammopathy of undetermined significance. It is important to use immunostains on amyloid-containing tissues in an attempt to determine the protein subunit within the fibril. Typical immunostains include κ and λ immunoglobulin light chain, amyloid A antisera, TTR, fibrinogen, lysozyme, and apolipoprotein.

The most commonly reported forms of familial amyloidosis are a result of mutations of the TTR gene. More than 80 mutations in the TTR gene have been described and are associated with the development of either amyloid peripheral neuropathy or amyloid cardiomyopathy.[106] Half of the patients identified at Mayo Clinic with familial amyloid polyneuropathy do not have a positive family history, and lack of a family history is not useful in making the distinction.[107] Frequently, the history includes a family member dying of an obscure illness that is suspicious but has not been verified to be amyloidosis. Any patient with amyloidosis who does not have a detectable monoclonal protein or plasma cell dyscrasia should be carefully evaluated for the presence of familial amyloidosis.

Cardiac amyloidosis can be caused by mutations in the TTR gene and can also be seen with deposition of wild-type TTR in the heart.[108] So-called senile systemic amyloidosis usually manifests as amyloid cardiomyopathy in the elderly. Analysis of the cardiac deposits shows normal TTR that can be found in 8% to 25% of persons older than 80 years.[109] Familial amyloid cardiomyopathy was first recognized 45 years ago in a Danish kindred but has since been detected in pedigrees throughout the world. Onset of symptoms typically begins after age 60 years, which decreases the suspicion of a familial disorder. The clinical manifestations of both senile systemic amyloidosis and familial amyloid cardiomyopathy are quite similar: congestive heart failure or intractable rhythm disturbances. In one autopsy series, 21% of those older than 90 years had amyloid deposits.[109] Patients with senile systemic amyloidosis are older than those with AL. Proteinuria is generally not present in senile systemic amyloidosis, and the left ventricular wall thickness is substantially greater in senile systemic amyloidosis despite these patients' having less severe heart failure. The median survival has been reported to be 75 months.[110]

An important mutation of the TTR protein at position 122 was described in a 68-year-old African American man.[111] The allele responsible for this mutation is carried by 3.9% of African Americans—1.3 million people in the United States. This mutation is a major cause of cardiac amyloidosis among black Americans.[112] The finding of cardiac amyloidosis in an older adult in the absence of a monoclonal gammopathy should raise the possibility of familial amyloid cardiomyopathy or senile systemic amyloidosis.

Other mutant proteins have been shown to produce amyloidosis. Familial renal amyloidosis has been reported with deposition of a mutant fibrinogen α chain[113] or due to mutant lysozyme.[114] The clinical course in these patients is more indolent than in patients with nephrotic syndrome due to AL. We have seen such patients with slowly progressive proteinuria for more than a decade without development of extrarenal manifestations of amyloidosis and renal failure. There are no other clinical distinguishing features. Renal amyloidosis has been described in patients with mutations of apolipoprotein A-I[115] and A-II.[116] The clinical presentation is indistinguishable from that of AL; the main difference is the lack of a monoclonal immunoglobulin disorder.

Distinguishing familial amyloidosis from AL is critical because liver transplantation has been used successfully in more than 500 patients with familial amyloidosis.[117,118] In the forms of familial amyloidosis due to mutations of the TTR gene, TTR is produced in only the liver and choroid plexus, and subsequent liver transplantation induced regression of amyloid deposits.[119] The outcome of transplantation appears to be best for patients with a TTR Val30Met mutation. Liver transplantation is not curative in all. Morbidity is high in patients with significant nutritional disability before transplantation or neuronal dropout on a pretransplantation peripheral nerve biopsy. Progressive cardiac amyloidosis after liver transplantation has been reported.[120] The theory is that preexistent amyloid deposits in the myocardium, even when asymptomatic, can serve as the nidus for further deposition of wild-type TTR and progressive cardiac dysfunction and failure.[121]

Early liver transplantation can improve survival in familial amyloid polyneuropathy. For transplant recipients with a modified body mass index (which is multiplied by serum albumin level) greater than 600 kg · g · m^{-2} · L^{-1}, improved survival has been noted compared with historical controls without transplantation. It is important for these patients to undergo transplantation when their nutritional status is good.[122] Domino liver transplantation, in which the recipient's liver is in turn given to another recipient, has been used for patients with familial amyloidosis, in one reported case resulting in the transmission of amyloidosis.[123]

In summary, any patient with amyloidosis who lacks a monoclonal protein in the serum and urine and does not have a plasma cell dyscrasia should be evaluated for the presence of localized, secondary, senile, or familial amyloidosis. Rarely, a patient with amyloidosis and a monoclonal gammopathy can also have a nonimmunoglobulin form of amyloidosis, and immunohistochemical staining of the amyloid deposits is warranted to exclude this possibility.

CLINICAL PRESENTATION OF PRIMARY AMYLOIDOSIS

A distinct male predominance in amyloidosis has been noted for more than 30 consecutive years. In Mayo Clinic patients with AL, 67% are male, whereas males comprise 52% of all multiple myeloma patients. The median age of patients with amyloidosis seen at Mayo Clinic is 67 years. The median age of patients with AL from Olmsted County, however, is 73 years, which may reflect referral bias of younger patients to an institution that has expertise in the disorder.

When patients are classified by a dominant organ manifestation, cardiac amyloidosis is the most common and is seen in 37.4% of patients (Fig. 89–9). Overt congestive heart failure is found in only half of patients with demonstrable cardiac amyloidosis. The others have manifestations that include fatigue, arrhythmia, or syncope. The widespread use of echocardiography has increased the recognition of cardiac amyloidosis.[124] Dominant renal amyloidosis is seen in 27.8% of patients. The most common manifestation is nephrotic-range proteinuria (albuminuria). Amyloid peripheral neuropathy is seen in 15.3%. Hepatomegaly is found in 17.7% of amyloidosis patients, but liver amyloidosis presenting as the dominant manifestation is seen in only 4.6%. Gastrointestinal tract amyloidosis manifested by intestinal bleeding, pseudo-obstruction, or diarrhea is seen in 7.1% of patients, and the other patients (7.8%) have a heterogeneous mix of soft tissue, vascular, tongue, periarticular, and interstitial amyloidosis.

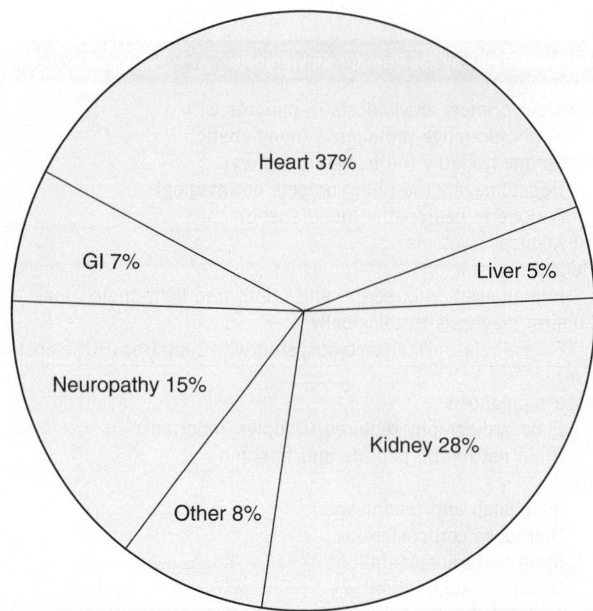

Figure 89–9 Distribution of dominant syndromes in patients with amyloidosis. GI, gastrointestinal.

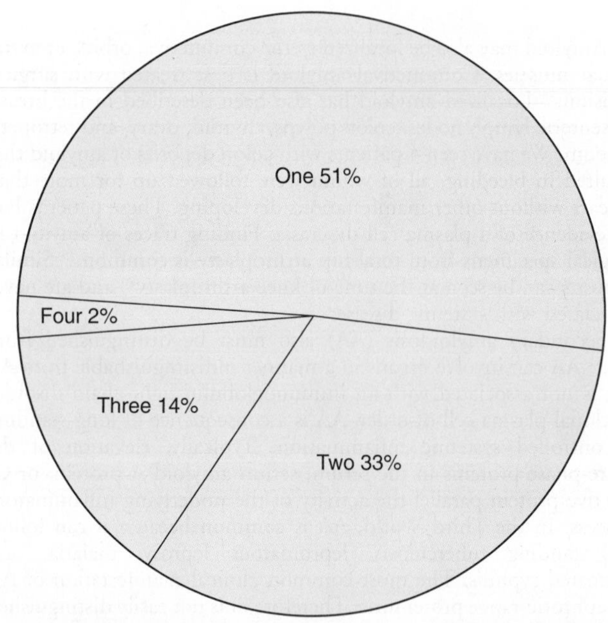

Figure 89–10 Number of organs involved at presentation in Mayo Clinic patients with amyloidosis.

In our patient population,[125] 49% presented with two or more organs involved (Fig. 89–10). In assigning a dominant organ of involvement, the designation is occasionally arbitrary because it is often difficult to distinguish which of the organs is responsible for the presenting symptoms. The organ most likely to be associated with additional visceral involvement was the liver.

If presentation with purpura alone is excluded, only 2.3% of patients presented with significant bleeding, 16.4% had carpal tunnel syndrome, and 19.6% had clinically overt congestive heart failure.[126] Symptoms included edema in 44.8% and fatigue in 46.4%. Nephrotic-range proteinuria was seen in 21%, orthostatic hypotension in 12%, lower extremity paresthesias in 34.9%, and weight loss in 51.7%. Anemia is uncommon in AL; 90% of patients have a hemoglobin value greater than 10 g/dL.[126] Only 1.5% of patients had

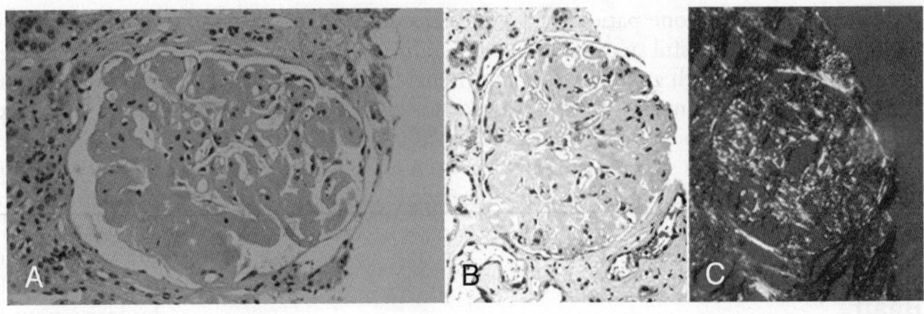

Figure 89–11 **A,** Amyloid deposits in the glomerulus. Note the amorphous nature that could easily be confused with hyalin degeneration (Hematoxylin and eosin; original magnification, ×100). **B,** A second case showing amyloid deposits (×100); **C,** Congo red stain with "apple-green" birefringence (×100).

a hemoglobin value less than 8 g/dL, and this was usually a sign of active intestinal tract hemorrhage or the anemia of renal failure. The median platelet count was 257 × 10^9/L; only 5.5% had a platelet count greater than 500 × 10^9/L. Thrombocytosis usually is seen with hepatic amyloidosis and hyposplenism.

A serum creatinine concentration greater than 2 mg/dL is present in 13.6% of patients at presentation.[126] An alkaline phosphatase concentration of 2 times the institutional normal value, which reflects hepatic involvement, is present in 6.7%. The median number of bone marrow plasma cells is 7% (range, 1%–30%) (Fig. 89–6); 11.3% of patients with AL have more than 20% plasma cells in the bone marrow without any other signs of multiple myeloma. The median 24-hour urine protein loss for all patients was 790 mg/24 h (Fig. 89–5). The monoclonal light chain is λ in 70%, κ in 19%, and no monoclonal protein is found in 11%. When an immunoglobulin (Ig) heavy chain was detectable in the serum, it was IgG in 58%, IgA in 10%, and IgM in 8% (Fig. 89–4). It is important to remember that amyloidosis is associated with IgM monoclonal gammopathies.[127] Waldenström macroglobulinemia has also been reported to be associated with amyloid arthropathy presenting as bilateral symmetric polyarthritis.[128]

Echocardiographic findings in the entire patient population demonstrate a median septal thickness of 14 mm.[126] The septal thickness is less than 15 mm in 53% and 15 mm or greater in 47%, reflecting a high proportion of patients with cardiac amyloidosis at diagnosis. The median survival of all patients is approximately 12 months. The 2- and 5-year survival rates are 33.6% and 15%, respectively. Variables important in survival prediction include the patient's performance status on the Eastern Cooperative Oncology Group scale, the presence of heart involvement as the dominant syndrome, and the involvement of two or more organs at presentation.

Kidney

When free monoclonal light chains are found in the urine, the differential diagnosis of the proteinuria is cryoglobulinemia,[129] amyloidosis, light-chain deposition disease,[130,131] and myeloma cast nephropathy. Immunofixation of the urine is important in the diagnostic evaluation whenever protein is present. Renal involvement is seen in 28% of patients,[126] but in the Italian Intergroup the frequency of renal involvement was nearly 50%.[132] In nondiabetic adults with nephrotic syndrome, amyloid is seen in 12% of biopsies. Survival is associated with the serum creatinine value at diagnosis.[133] The median survival of patients with a creatinine value less than and greater than 1.3 mg/dL was 25.6 and 15 months, respectively. Patients with increased protein excretion do not have shorter survival but do have a shorter time to the development of end-stage renal disease.[134] Fewer than 5% of patients with AL have urinary protein loss less than 150 mg/day. Two-thirds of patients have a light chain detectable in the urine and two-thirds a detectable light chain in the serum. In AL patients with greater than 1 g of proteinuria, a light chain can be found in as many as 86%. The ratio of κ to λ light chains in patients with nephrotic syndrome is 1 : 5. The median urinary protein loss in κ light-chain amyloidosis is 1.1 g/day; in λ light-chain amyloidosis, it is 4.6 g/day. There is no difference in the frequency of renal insufficiency in κ and λ light-chain amyloidosis.

Long-standing proteinuria results in hypoalbuminemia, which leads to decreased intravascular oncotic pressure. The clinical end result is transudation of fluid into the extracellular space with refractory edema. The use of diuretics can aggravate intravascular volume contraction and hypotension and reduces renal blood flow. In patients with advanced anasarca, bilateral catheter embolization of the renal arteries has been used.[135] The continuous loss of protein into the urine produces tubular atrophy and damage. Median time from the diagnosis of AL nephrotic syndrome to dialysis is 14 months; median survival from the start of dialysis in AL patients is 8 months. The cause of death in most is the development of cardiac amyloidosis. We have not recognized a difference in outcome between patients undergoing hemodialysis and peritoneal dialysis; 1-year survival is 68% after initiation of dialysis. The most important extrarenal complications of AL are heart failure, heart arrhythmias, and hypotension. Dialysis is regularly complicated by hypotension.

The amount of proteinuria is poorly correlated with the extent of amyloid deposits on biopsy (Fig. 89–11). Most patients with AL have normal-sized kidneys by ultrasonography. The urinary sediment shows fat but no casts or red blood cells. In a study of 118 patients with monoclonal gammopathies, 30% of those having a renal biopsy had AL.[136] Median survival in the group was 24 months, with death largely due to cardiac amyloidosis. Predictors of survival included age less than 70 years and high serum calcium and creatinine concentrations at presentation. It is rare for renal amyloidosis to develop if it is not present at diagnosis. We have seen four patients in whom nephrotic-range proteinuria developed after cardiac transplantation for amyloidosis. Presumably, in the past, these patients would not have survived long enough for renal amyloidosis to develop.

The cause of the proteinuria in AL is amyloid deposits disrupting the glomerular basement membrane. Immunotactoid (fibrillary) glomerulopathy is a fibrillar deposition in the kidney that can be confused with AL.[137] On electron microscopy, the fibrils of fibrillary glomerulopathy are twice the width of amyloid fibrils, and the deposits do not stain with Congo red. Light-chain deposition disease (Randall-type) represents the deposition of nonamyloid immunoglobulin light chains in a granular fashion on the tubular or glomerular basement membrane.[138] It can produce nephrotic syndrome and renal failure. Amyloidosis and light-chain deposition disease have been reported in the same patient.

Few reports exist of renal transplantation for AL. In a report on 12 patients, 2 of whom had AL, 4 were alive at 2 years, and in 2 of these 4, the renal biopsy showed recurrent amyloid.[139] In another report, 11 patients received transplants, and 3 showed recurrent amyloid deposits in the allograft at 11, 28, and 37 months.[140] In 45 patients with amyloidosis who received a renal transplant, the 3-year survival was 51%, which is inferior to the outcome of renal transplantation for primary renal disease.[141] The estimate for recurrent amyloidosis in a recipient of a renal transplant is approximately 20% at 1 year. On scintigraphy, uptake of radiolabeled serum amyloid was seen in 4 of 10 renal transplant recipients. Of 22 patients with renal amyloidosis, 7 had adrenal insufficiency and 4 died of hypoadrenalism.

We performed living donor kidney transplantation followed by autologous stem cell transplantation for AL patients with end-stage renal disease.[142] Two patients had complications and died 3 and 10 months later. Two patients had development of subclinical acute cellular rejection, and one patient had acute rejection, all reversible. Six patients had successful stem cell harvest, and five underwent stem cell transplantation with good engraftment. Renal function stabilized after stem cell transplant in four and was decreased in one. The feasibility of donor kidney transplant with an autologous stem cell transplant for carefully selected patients has been established.[142] It is unclear whether stem cell transplant should precede or follow kidney transplantation.[143]

Heart

The heart is prognostically the most important determinant of outcome in AL. Patients present with infiltrative cardiomyopathy that leads to restricted ventricular filling and may present with disabling fatigue and unexplained weight loss. These patients have early diastolic dysfunction and no systolic dysfunction.[144] Chest radiography does not show cardiomegaly or pulmonary vascular redistribution. The ejection fraction is preserved on echocardiography. As a result of poor diastolic filling and normal contractility, the ejection fraction is normal, but end-diastolic volume is decreased as a result of poor filling, and this results in low cardiac output.[145] Electrocardiography typically shows low voltage, which is frequently overlooked.[146] Patients can be misdiagnosed as having ischemic heart disease because of the pseudoinfarction pattern seen in amyloidosis, with loss of the R wave in leads V1 through V3. Coronary arteriography is commonly performed during evaluation and is invariably normal.[147] Echocardiography shows thickening as a result of infiltration, but this can easily be misinterpreted as concentric left ventricular hypertrophy[148] or asymmetric septal hypertrophy (Fig. 89–12).

A patient with diastolic heart failure or restrictive hemodynamics should be evaluated for the presence of a monoclonal protein in the serum or urine.[149] The noncompliant left ventricle due to infiltration is referred to as the "stiff heart."[150] There is minimal effect on systolic function, and the ejection fraction is preserved until late in the course

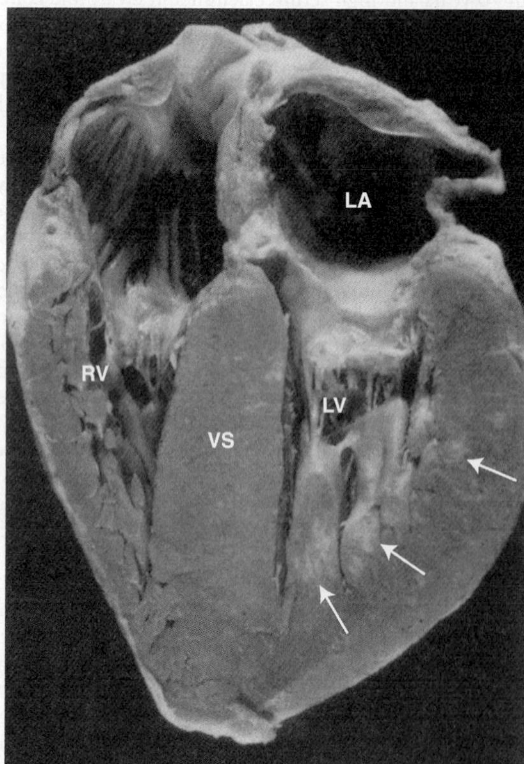

Figure 89–12 Autopsy specimen of cardiac amyloidosis. Arrows indicate the white deposits of amyloid that Rokitansky thought were "lardaceous." LA, left atrium; LV, left ventricle; RV, right ventricle; VS, ventricular septum.

of the disease. Echocardiography can be frankly misleading owing to the normal ejection fraction and a lack of focal or segmental wall motion abnormalities.[151] The infiltration of the myocardial wall does result in thickening, but electrocardiography does not show the voltage changes of ventricular hypertrophy. Instead it shows low voltage or the pseudoinfarction pattern.

Doppler studies are required to assess myocardial function in AL because Doppler echocardiography best demonstrates restriction to inflow during diastole.[152] The Doppler filling patterns closely relate to the extent of amyloid infiltration. Patients with early cardiac amyloidosis show abnormal relaxation. Patients with advanced cardiac AL show a short deceleration time consistent with restrictive physiology. The combination of decreased fractional shortening of less than 20% and a mean left ventricular wall thickness of 15 mm is associated with a median survival of only 4 months. A short deceleration time on Doppler echocardiography indicates restrictive physiology, and these patients have shortened survival compared with patients whose deceleration time exceeds 150 milliseconds.

The recent introduction of echocardiographic strain imaging demonstrated its ability to show functional abnormalities before any morphologic echocardiographic abnormalities were present.[153] When combined with tissue Doppler imaging, cardiac involvement can be detected in early stages.[153] Magnetic resonance imaging has also been applied to early detection of cardiac amyloidosis. The combination of widespread myocardial enhancement on delayed postcontrast inversion recovery T1-weighted images with features of restrictive cardiac disease is highly suggestive.[154]

Sudden death is a well-recognized complication of cardiac amyloidosis[155] whether or not the patient receives digoxin. Digoxin has never been demonstrated conclusively to increase the risk of sudden death in AL. Digoxin provides rate control in the presence of atrial fibrillation and is unlikely to improve myocardial performance because systolic function is so well preserved in AL.[156] The mainstay of supportive care in cardiac AL is the use of diuretics.[157,158] The presence of orthostatic hypotension and intravascular volume contraction can make diuretic therapy difficult and may cause syncope or an increase in the creatinine value. Pacemaker implantation is commonly required in patients with cardiac amyloidosis and syncope. The use of angiotensin-converting enzyme inhibitors, a standard for the management of heart failure, has an uncertain role in AL. The high frequency of hypotension associated with angiotensin-converting enzyme inhibitors limits their value in AL. The use of implantable cardioverter-defibrillator therapy has been reported. A defibrillator cannot consistently prevent cardiac death from amyloidosis.[159,160]

Of 204 patients with AL seen at Mayo Clinic, the median septal thickness was 14 mm.[161] The most common echocardiographic features are thickened right ventricular wall, interventricular septum, and left ventricular free wall. Typically, the left ventricular cavity size is decreased. Cardiac involvement is present on echocardiography in 41% of patients at presentation; overt congestive heart failure is present in 20%. If the interventricular septal thickness is 15 mm or greater, median survival is less than 1 year. If the septal thickness is less than 15 mm, the median survival can approach 4 years. Exercise-induced syncope has been associated with a median survival of 2 months and is presumed due to complex ventricular arrhythmias.[162] Any patient presenting with symptoms of a cardiomyopathy that does not have a clear-cut ischemic basis should have immunofixation of the serum and urine.

The pseudoinfarction pattern seen on electrocardiography may misdirect the evaluation toward coronary disease. Low voltage is seen on electrocardiography in nearly two-thirds of patients with cardiac AL.[163] Cardiac amyloidosis is characterized by atrial systolic failure and dilatation of the right ventricle. Thickening of the mitral and tricuspid valves is common and is an important clue to the diagnosis. Doppler examination regularly demonstrates clinically insignificant valvular regurgitation.[164] Atrioventricular pacing does not improve cardiac hemodynamics.

Restrictive cardiomyopathy can be confused with pericardial disease causing restriction.[165] Little clinical benefit has been reported from pericardiectomy in patients with AL. An endomyocardial biopsy establishes the diagnosis of AL 100% of the time if at least three biopsy specimens are obtained.[166] Owing to poor contractility, the development of thrombi in the ventricular chambers is common. These can be sources of cardiac embolism resulting in stroke or arterial insufficiency of a lower extremity.[167] Atrial standstill is recognized in amyloidosis and is an indication for long-standing anticoagulation therapy. Rarely, patients can have occlusive deposition of amyloid in small-caliber coronary arterioles. These patients can have ischemic symptoms including exertional angina and true myocardial infarction.[32] Large-caliber coronary arteries show no abnormalities on angiography. Exercise testing regularly confirms ischemia, but the diagnosis is difficult to establish premortem.

We have seen 11 patients who presented with angina or unstable coronary syndromes.[31] Low voltage on electrocardiography was seen in only 2, and the median time from symptomatic angina to death was 18 months. Most diagnoses of cardiac AL with coronary artery occlusion were made at autopsy. Obstructive coronary amyloidosis is present in 66% of patients with cardiac involvement. None of these patients have obstruction of epicardial coronary arteries. Myocardial ischemia affects 25% of patients with obstructive intramural coronary amyloidosis. These patients present with ischemia and have normal angiographic studies but have small arteriolar amyloid disease.[31]

All patients with cardiac amyloidosis do not have AL. Familial forms of amyloid cardiomyopathy due to mutations at position 122 of TTR are commonly seen in older African American men. These patients do not have a monoclonal protein in serum or urine. Senile cardiac amyloidosis is associated with cardiac deposition of wild-type TTR.[168] The echocardiographic features of these forms of cardiac amyloidosis are indistinguishable, and all three show Congo red–positive deposits. One-fourth of patients older than 90 years have amyloid deposits in the heart. Failure to find an immunoglobulin light chain in the serum or urine should redirect the evaluation toward non–light chain forms of amyloid. Clues to senile systemic amyloidosis include male sex, advanced age, pronounced thickening of the interventricular septum (frequently greater than 20 mm), and TTR immunostaining of the endomyocardial biopsy.

Liver

Hepatomegaly is found by physical examination in one-fourth of patients and may be due to cardiac failure and hepatic congestion. Symptomatic hepatic involvement is present in 16% of patients. The most common clinical presentations are unexplained hepatomegaly and unexplained increase in the serum alkaline phosphatase value. There is high concordance between hepatic and renal involvement, and if the liver is involved, the kidney is the next most commonly involved organ. Half of patients with hepatic amyloidosis have greater than 1 g of protein in the urine in 24 hours. Proteinuria in a patient with hepatomegaly and an increased alkaline phosphatase value is an important clinical clue to the diagnosis of AL.[169]

Four clinical clues permit the prebiopsy recognition of hepatic amyloidosis: (a) presence of proteinuria; (b) monoclonal protein in the serum or urine; (c) Howell-Jolly bodies in the peripheral blood, which reflect splenic replacement with amyloid; and (d) hepatomegaly out of proportion to the degree of abnormality on liver function tests. Most patients have only an increased alkaline phosphatase value. The concentrations of aspartate aminotransferase and alanine aminotransferase are typically less than twice normal at diagnosis. The bilirubin value is normal. The finding of an increased bilirubin value in a patient with hepatic amyloidosis is usually a preterminal finding.[170] Rarely, hepatic amyloidosis occurs from splenic rupture with intraabdominal hemorrhage and, rarely, hepatic rupture.[171] Hepatic rupture has been diagnosed in AL, with computed tomography of the abdomen demonstrating subcapsular hematoma.[172] At the time of diagnosis of hepatic amyloidosis, the median liver span is 7 cm below the right costal margin; 50% of patients have a span between 5 and 9 cm.[173]

Ten percent of patients with hepatic amyloidosis on liver biopsy do not have palpable hepatomegaly and are diagnosed because of an unexplained increase in alkaline phosphatase concentration.[173] Splenomegaly is seen in 11% of these patients and nephrotic-range proteinuria in 36%. At diagnosis, the median elevation of the alkaline phosphatase value is 2.3 times the upper limit of normal. Patients with hepatic amyloidosis have a significantly higher level of C-reactive protein than do patients without hepatic amyloidosis. There is no difference in the ratio of κ to λ light chains in hepatic amyloidosis compared with other forms of amyloidosis.

Liver biopsy is not a high-risk procedure in these patients, and although reports of hepatic rupture have appeared in the literature, the bleeding incidence is 4%, with a transfusion need of 2%. We recently reported our updated experience with hepatic amyloidosis.[174] Seventy-two percent of patients had involuntary weight loss leading to an evaluation for occult malignancy. Clinicians considered amyloidosis in the differential diagnosis in only 26% before liver biopsy. Predictors of a poor prognosis included heart failure, an elevated bilirubin level, and thrombocythemia.[174]

Cholestatic jaundice is a preterminal finding.[175] Portal hypertension with varices and gastrointestinal tract bleeding is rarely seen.[176] Presumably, patients succumb to the effects of extrahepatic amyloid deposits before portal hypertension can develop. Ascites is commonly seen but is usually a consequence of concomitant nephrotic syndrome with hypoalbuminemia or of severe congestive heart failure rather than portal hypertension.[177] Liver biopsy shows perisinusoidal and portal deposition in most patients. Vascular involvement of the portal triads is common but not clinically important. The median survival after diagnosis was 8.5 months.

Radionuclide scintigraphy in amyloidosis is nonspecific, showing irregular distribution of the radionuclide[178] and absence of splenic uptake.[179] This form of imaging is not clinically useful. Angiography is also nonspecific, demonstrating luminal irregularity and abrupt changes in the caliber of the branches of the hepatic artery.[180] The hepatic artery is presumed to be compressed by sinusoidal amyloid deposition. Although hepatic biopsy is a safe technique, biopsy of the subcutaneous fat or the bone marrow yields a correct diagnosis in 90% of patients, so only a few patients should be subjected to transcutaneous liver biopsy.

Patients with hepatic AL have been treated with transjugular intrahepatic portal systemic shunting.[181] This can decrease portal pressures, ascites, and hydrothorax. In one patient, bilateral nephrectomy for uncontrolled nephrotic syndrome resulted in an improvement in liver function and normalization of hyperbilirubinemia.[182] The presence of hepatic involvement in amyloidosis does not adversely affect survival on multivariate statistical analysis. As noted, hepatomegaly may be from causes other than direct infiltration of the organ. In one report, hepatomegaly was due to passive congestion of the liver without hepatic amyloid deposits in three of nine patients.[183] A second study found that 20% of patients with amyloidosis and palpable hepatomegaly did not have parenchymal amyloid deposits at autopsy.[184]

The presence of hyposplenism on the peripheral blood film is highly specific for a diagnosis of amyloidosis. Conversely, hyposplenism is not a sensitive indicator of splenic involvement.[185] In one report, 12 patients with diffuse splenic involvement at autopsy did not have peripheral blood film evidence of hyposplenism.[185] Technetium scanning can indicate a decrease in splenic blood flow, but this correlates poorly with the findings on the peripheral blood film.

In summary, the cardinal features of hepatic AL are (a) hepatomegaly with increased concentration of alkaline phosphatase and minimal change in aspartate and alanine aminotransferases, (b) proteinuria, (c) a monoclonal light chain in the serum or urine, and (d) hyposplenism on peripheral blood film or technetium scanning.

Gastrointestinal Tract

Anatomic deposits of amyloid are seen in the gastrointestinal tract of most patients by screening rectal biopsy or upper endoscopy. These deposits tend to be vascular, are in the submucosa, and are not associated with symptoms or clinical signs. Less than 5% of patients with AL present with symptoms referable to the gastrointestinal tract. The presence of anorexia and weight loss generally is not associated with substantial gastrointestinal tract deposits, and the cause of the weight loss is unrelated. Malabsorption defined by steatorrhea or a low serum carotene value is seen in less than 5% of amyloidosis patients. The symptoms of advanced intestinal amyloidosis include intestinal pseudo-obstruction,[186] and patients have been reported for whom exploratory laparotomy resulted in unnecessary morbidity. Some patients have severe intestinal dysmotility with vomiting and alternating diarrhea and constipation that can be managed only with long-term parenteral nutrition.[187] Abdominal distension and pain are common. Nausea is seen even with fasting. Cisapride has been reported to be effective for treating chronic intestinal pseudo-obstruction, but we have found it to be of limited value. The mechanism underlying gastrointestinal tract dysmotility can be a consequence of either direct mucosal infiltration or autonomic nerve damage.

We reviewed the cases of 19 patients seen at Mayo Clinic with small-bowel biopsy proof of AL; these patients represented only 1% of our total patient population with AL.[188] The most common presenting symptoms were diarrhea, anorexia, dizziness, and abdominal pain. The median weight loss was 30 lb. Half had orthostatic hypotension. A prolonged prothrombin time due to vitamin K malabsorption was seen in one-fourth. Depressed levels of factor X were also seen in a fourth of patients, but only one patient had less than 30% activity. Less than a third of the patients had an increased serum alkaline phosphatase value. Only 15% had hepatomegaly.

Barium studies of the upper gastrointestinal tract showed esophageal dysmotility or gastroesophageal reflux.[189] Dilatation of the small bowel has been seen only rarely. Small bowel barium studies show thickening or nodularity, dilatation with delayed transit, and fluid accumulation. Computed tomography is not helpful, showing mild splenomegaly or lymphadenopathy. Endoscopy demonstrates esophagitis, duodenitis, and gastritis but is frequently normal.[190] The median time from the onset of intestinal symptoms to a histologic diagnosis of AL is 7 months, but in one instance the diagnosis was delayed by 4 years. Laparotomy was performed in 4 of 19 patients, and even when the surgical tissue was obtained in 3 of the 4, Congo red stains were not performed initially. The most important features predicting survival were the hemoglobin level at diagnosis and the extent of weight loss. Patients who had weight loss greater than 20 lb had a median survival of 10 months, and the most common cause of death was nutritional failure (55%). A fourth died of cardiac amyloidosis.

The diarrhea of amyloidosis can be managed with loperamide and diphenoxylate; injections of long-acting octreotide also have been used. Ingested polyethylene glycol appears in the stool of amyloidosis patients 10 times faster than in normal subjects. These patients typically have autonomic neuropathy, which is most likely the cause of rapid transit. The severe chronic diarrhea is mediated by extremely rapid transit of chyme and digestive secretions.[191] The nausea is difficult to manage, even with phenothiazines or ondansetron. The most common preintestinal biopsy diagnosis is inflammatory bowel disease.

AL can present as ischemic colitis.[192] In this circumstance, deposits obstruct the vessels of the lamina propria and muscularis mucosa, and this leads to mucosal ischemia with sloughing of the lining and bleeding[193] (Fig. 89–13). Radiographic studies demonstrate luminal narrowing, thickening of mucosal folds, and ulcerations. The most common site of ischemia is the descending and rectosigmoid colon. Duodenal perforation due to vascular obstruction has been reported. After intestinal pseudo-obstruction develops, therapy for the underlying amyloidosis does not result in recovery of intestinal motility. Extensive replacement of the muscularis propria by amyloid deposits is particularly prominent in the small intestine.

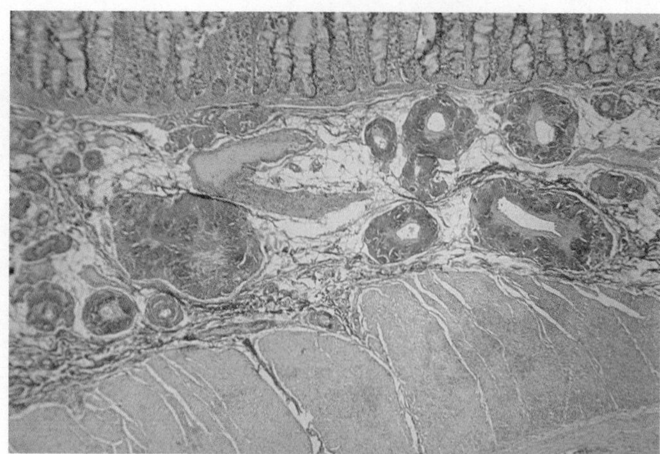

Figure 89–13 Rectal mucosal biopsy specimen demonstrates marked thickening of submucosal vessels with amyloid deposits. (Congo red; original magnification, ×100)

Nervous System

Amyloid involvement of the peripheral nervous system was first described in 1938.[194] The frequency of neuropathy in AL is 15% to 20%. Most patients are minimally symptomatic, and the clinical picture is dominated by cardiac or renal involvement. If patients present with a predominant neuropathic syndrome, the possibility of a familial amyloidosis syndrome must be kept in the differential diagnosis.[195] A monoclonal protein in the serum or urine would not be expected in patients with nonimmunoglobulin forms of amyloidosis. A diagnosis of amyloid neuropathy can be confirmed by sural nerve biopsy, but most patients with clinical and electromyographic evidence of neuropathy can be diagnosed by a fat aspirate, rectal biopsy, or bone marrow specimen.

The most common symptoms of amyloid neuropathy are paresthesias, muscle weakness, numbness, pain, orthostatic hypotension, urinary retention, and impotence. Syncope is seen in 12% of patients. The peripheral neuropathy has a characteristic dysesthetic feature with distal burning. The lower extremities are involved before the upper extremities in 90% of patients, and symptoms of autonomic failure are seen in two-thirds. Cranial nerve involvement is rare but has been reported.[196] Carpal tunnel syndrome is present in half of patients with neuropathy. One-third have significant weight loss. Atypical presentations of amyloid neuropathy can include mononeuropathy multiplex, painful sensory neuropathy, and primary demyelinating polyneuropathy.[197]

Echocardiography is abnormal in 44% of patients with neuropathy. Renal involvement is uncommon, occurring in only 5%. The neuropathy of AL may be demyelinating and results in an increased concentration of cerebrospinal fluid protein in one-third. Electromyography shows decreased amplitude of muscle action potentials, decreased or absent sensory responses, slowing of nerve conduction velocity, and fibrillation potentials on needle examination.[198] Axonal degeneration is detected by electromyography in 96% of patients.

On sural nerve biopsy, deposits of amyloid surround endoneurial capillaries or are found in the epineurium. Examination of teased fibers shows a decrease in myelin fiber density and axonal degeneration.[199] The median survival of patients presenting with AL neuropathy is 25 months.[200] Standard-dose chemotherapy rarely results in clinical improvement in the neuropathic symptoms. The neuropathy is progressive over time, and three-fourths of patients ultimately have restricted mobility, with one-third becoming bedridden. Survival is predicted by the serum albumin value of these patients at presentation. Patients whose serum albumin concentration is less than 3 g/dL have a median survival of 18 months, compared with 31 months if the albumin value is greater than 3 g/dL.

Associated autonomic neuropathy is an important diagnostic clue to AL as the cause of peripheral neuropathy.[201] Urinary dysfunction is a common manifestation of autonomic failure. Voiding difficulties are due to detrusor weakness and impaired bladder sensation. There is also evidence of detrusor denervation supersensitivity. This urinary dysfunction implicates postganglionic cholinergic and afferent somatic nerves.[202] Only diabetes mellitus generally produces a substantial autonomic component in patients with peripheral neuropathy.

The diagnosis of AL neuropathy is commonly delayed. The median duration of symptoms before diagnosis is 29 months. It is important that all patients with a peripheral neuropathy of unknown cause have immunofixation of serum and urine and an immunoglobulin free light-chain assay to search for a light chain.

The differential diagnosis of neuropathy associated with a monoclonal protein includes monoclonal gammopathy of undetermined significance–associated neuropathy, POEMS syndrome (osteosclerotic myeloma), and cryoglobulinemia. Amyloidosis preferentially causes the loss of small myelinated fibers and unmyelinated fibers. Electromyography detects changes in large myelinated fibers. Therefore, patients can have symptoms with paresthesias and normal electromyography results. The sural nerve biopsy is not 100% sensitive for the diagnosis. Of nine patients who had a sural nerve biopsy, the specimen did not show amyloid in six.[203] Amyloid can deposit proximally in the nerve root and lead to distal demyelination, and amyloid deposits will not be seen in a sural nerve biopsy specimen.

Respiratory Tract

Most patients with histologic deposits of amyloid in the respiratory tract are asymptomatic.[204] Most patients with pulmonary involvement also have cardiac involvement that dominates the clinical picture. If alveolar or interstitial amyloid is present, gas exchange is usually preserved until quite late in the disease.[205] Of 55 patients seen at Mayo Clinic with lung biopsy proof of amyloidosis, 20 had localized forms of pulmonary amyloidosis, predominantly nodular pulmonary amyloidosis.[206] These patients had a benign prognosis. Patients with tracheobronchial amyloidosis have been treated with neodymium : yttrium–aluminum–garnet laser therapy and external beam radiotherapy. Thirty-five of the 55 patients had pulmonary AL. These patients presented with radiographic findings of an interstitial or reticulonodular pattern with or without effusion. The median survival after diagnosis was 16 months. Bronchoscopic lung biopsy was safe and effective and was not associated with bleeding.

Chest radiography in pulmonary AL is nonspecific, showing an interstitial process that can be interpreted as lower lobe fibrosis.[207] Involvement of minor salivary glands is common and results in xerostomia.[208] These patients can be misdiagnosed as having Sjögren syndrome. Patients with amyloidosis associated with an IgM monoclonal protein have a higher prevalence of pulmonary involvement than patients with non-IgM amyloidosis. A monoclonal gammopathy is not associated with tracheal, bronchial, or nodular pulmonary amyloidosis and is seen exclusively in diffuse interstitial amyloidosis. Long-term observation for nodular pulmonary amyloidosis is justifiable. These patients can remain stable for long periods of time without requiring resection of the lung.[209] Patients with dyspnea from interstitial amyloidosis benefit from low doses of prednisone, even though this does not produce radiographic change.[210]

At autopsy, pulmonary involvement was reported in 11 of 12 deceased patients.[211] Amyloid deposition was in blood vessel walls and alveolar septum. Of the 12, dyspnea was present in 4, and pulmonary amyloidosis was directly responsible for death in only 1. Hemoptysis has been reported.[211] Ventilatory failure has been reported due to muscular infiltration of the diaphragm.[212]

Amyloid infiltration of skeletal muscles and the diaphragm has been reported.[213] Pleural infiltration can produce effusions.[214] Pulmonary hypertension with right-sided cardiac failure can be seen as a rare complication.[215] These patients have occlusive amyloid deposits in the pulmonary arteriolar circulation. None of these patients had echocardiographic evidence of amyloid deposition. In the presence of pulmonary hypertension, the median survival was 2.8 years. Treatment included calcium-channel blockers; however, patients tolerated these medicines poorly owing to concomitant orthostatic hypotension.

Coagulation System

Bleeding is a serious complication of amyloidosis. Factors contributing to the abnormal bleeding include coagulation factor deficiencies, hyperfibrinolysis, platelet dysfunction, and increased fragility of blood vessels.[216] Deficiency of factor X is well recognized.[217] The most common manifestation of bleeding is purpura due to fragile blood vessels infiltrated with amyloid.[218] Factor X deficiency is seen in less than 5% of patients. In a recent review, 8.7% of patients had factor X levels less than 50% of normal; serious bleeding is seen only in those with factor X levels less than 25% of normal.[219] Factor X deficiency is associated with extensive hepatic and splenic amyloidosis. Improvement in factor X levels has been reported with splenectomy,[220] use of oral melphalan and prednisone, and stem cell transplantation.[221] The use of recombinant human factor VIIa in the management of amyloid-associated factor X deficiency was reported in a 63-year-old woman with levels from 4% to 10% of normal.[222] Recombinant human factor VIIa was administered preoperatively and every 3 hours postoperatively for 48 hours to permit safe splenectomy. This was an effective means of controlling bleeding to allow for definitive surgical intervention.[222] Recombinant factor VIIa has now been widely used to treat intractable life-threatening hematuria, severe bleeding, and to support a hemicolectomy.[222–224]

The most common hemostatic abnormality in vitro is prolongation of the thrombin time.[225] This may be related to the low serum albumin values seen in patients with amyloidosis. Others have suggested the presence of an inhibitor to fibrin polymerization. Abnormal platelet aggregation has been reported, as have decreased levels of α_2-plasmin inhibitor and increased levels of plasminogen. Life-threatening bleeding is rare in AL, except for those few patients with severe factor X deficiency or ischemic colitis due to vascular obstruction. Bleeding in amyloidosis has also been reported as a result of a deficiency of factor V.[226] This deficiency was not due to acquisition of a factor V inhibitor. The bleeding in this case was fatal and unresponsive to fresh frozen plasma. At autopsy, massive hepatic deposits of amyloid were seen.[226]

Thirty-six patients underwent extensive coagulation profiling[225]; hemorrhagic manifestations were mild to moderate in nine and severe in only one. The most frequent in vitro abnormalities were prolongation of the thrombin time and reptilase time. Severe depression of factor X was seen in only one. The prothrombin times were prolonged in 8, and the activated partial thromboplastin time was prolonged in 25. None had a lupus anticoagulant.

We reviewed the medical records of 2132 patients with AL to identify patients with thromboembolism.[227] We identified 21 men and 19 women with a median age of 65 years. In 11 of 40, thromboembolism preceded the diagnosis of AL. In 9 of the 11, the event occurred 1 month or more before the diagnosis of AL. In 20 of 40 patients, thromboembolism occurred 1 month or more after diagnosis. Twenty-nine had a venous thrombosis and 11 had arterial clots. Thirty-seven of the 40 patients had an additional risk factor for thrombosis: nephrotic syndrome in 20, immobilization in 13, tobacco in 6, heart failure in 8, estrogens in 1, obesity in 4, aortic aneurysm in 1, and prosthetic material in 4. Two of the patients had an associated disseminated intravascular coagulation, and 5 had detectable activated protein C resistance. Eight of the 40 patients died within a month after the thrombotic event. Eighteen of the 40 died within 1 year. There were no associations with the type of heavy or light chain.[227]

PROGNOSIS

When a patient has a syndrome compatible with amyloidosis and is found subsequently to have a monoclonal protein or clonal plasma cell population, and the diagnosis is confirmed histologically, the next step is to assess prognosis. In a group of 153 patients with AL, the median survival was 20 months, with a 5-year survival of 20%.[228] Patients with congestive heart failure had a median survival of 8 months and a 5-year survival of 2.4%.[228] The best outcome occurred in patients with amyloid neuropathy as the sole manifestation of the disease: a median survival of 40 months and a 5-year survival of 32%. Patients may be classified clinically into five groups: heart failure or cardiomyopathy, nephrotic syndrome, peripheral neuropathy, liver, and other. Women have slightly better survival than men.

In a review of 229 patients with AL, heart failure and orthostatic hypotension were associated consistently with a median survival of less than 1 year.[25] With heart failure and nephrotic syndrome patients excluded, patients with peripheral neuropathy had a median survival of 56 months. Jaw claudication can be seen in as many as 9%. These patients have a survival of 42 months.[229] Patients with jaw claudication have predominantly vascular deposits and sparing of the viscera. They frequently have associated amyloid arthropathy and tongue enlargement.

The presence of hyposplenism on peripheral blood film was associated with a median survival of 4.4 months, reflecting advanced splenic and hepatic involvement.[230] The median survival of 80 patients diagnosed by a liver biopsy was 9 months, and 5-year survival was 13%.[169] The cause of death in most patients with amyloidosis was cardiac related—either heart failure or fatal arrhythmia. Echocardiography is important in the assessment of the patient's prognosis.[231] Although only 17% to 20% of patients have heart failure at presentation, nearly 40% have evidence of cardiomyopathy on echocardiography.[232] Early cardiac amyloidosis is characterized by abnormalities of relaxation. Advanced cardiac amyloidosis shows restrictive filling and a shortened deceleration time.[233] With Doppler echocardiography, patients can be divided into two groups on the basis of deceleration time greater or less than 150 milliseconds. The 1-year survival of patients with a deceleration time of 150 milliseconds or less was 49% compared with 92% for a deceleration time greater than 150 milliseconds. Doppler studies of right ventricular function correlate well with the degree of amyloid infiltration.[234]

Findings on renal biopsy have been reported to have prognostic value.[235] A lower percentage of glomerular capillary wall thickening, a higher incidence of amyloid deposits in vessels but not glomerular capillaries, and deposits of IgG and C3 in mesangial and glomerular capillary walls are all associated with a better prognosis. Urinary light-chain excretion and serum creatinine values are also important prognostic indicators. Increased serum creatinine values are associated with a median survival of 15 months.

Exertional syncope is an ominous finding and is associated with a high incidence of sudden death. This is usually an indication for consideration of an implantable defibrillator. Most patients with exertional syncope die within 3 months.[236]

The plasma cell labeling index measures the proliferative potential of the bone marrow plasma cells in AL. More than 95% of patients with AL have a demonstrable clonal excess of plasma cells in the bone marrow. The median survival of patients whose plasma cell labeling index was 0 (no proliferative plasma cells) was 30 months. Patients with a plasma cell labeling index greater than 0 had a median survival of 15 months.[237] Analysis of peripheral blood mononuclear cells in 147 patients with AL showed 16% of the patients to have detectable circulating plasma cells.[238] The median survival of patients with circulating plasma cells was 10 months compared with 29 months for patients without circulating plasma cells. In a multivariate analysis, the presence of circulating plasma cells and the serum β_2-microglobulin level were independent prognostic indicators of survival.[239]

The median survival of patients with an increased serum β_2-microglobulin value at presentation was 11 months, compared with 33 months in patients with a normal β_2-microglobulin value.[240] β_2-Microglobulin value is an independent predictor of survival, even in the presence of heart failure and renal failure. When the serum β_2-microglobulin value is combined with the presence or absence of circulating plasma cells, patients can be classified into three separate groups with median survivals of 4 months (circulating cells and increased β_2-microglobulin), 42 months (no circulating cells and normal β_2-microglobulin), and 21 months (one of the two variables abnormal).[239]

The time between diagnosis and referral for evaluation remains an important prognostic variable. When all patients seen at Mayo Clinic are assessed, the median survival is 2 years. However, when only patients seen within 1 month of diagnosis are considered, the median survival decreases to 13 months. This suggests significant referral bias, favoring patients physically able to come to a large amyloidosis treatment center. This information is important when interpreting the results of clinical trials from single centers.[126]

In a multivariate analysis of prognostic factors, the median survival of the entire group was 12 months, ranging from 4 months for those with overt heart failure to 15 months for those with peripheral neuropathy.[241] Heart failure, urinary monoclonal light chain, hepatomegaly, and multiple myeloma were all adverse factors influencing survival within 1 year after diagnosis. After the first year, increased serum creatinine concentration, multiple myeloma, orthostatic hypotension, and a monoclonal serum protein predicted poor survival.[241] Stratification for the impact of variables with an adverse effect on survival is important when comparing studies of therapy among various centers.

Recently, measurement of cardiac biomarkers has been shown to be critically important in assessing the prognosis of patients with amyloidosis. Brain natriuretic peptide (BNP) is a marker of ventricular dysfunction and has been used to assess prognosis in heart failure. When N-terminal pro-BNP (NT-pro-BNP) was quantified at diagnosis in 152 patients with AL and compared with echocardiography, two groups were distinguished on the basis of NT-pro-BNP levels.[242] Survival was vastly different in patients with elevated and normal NT-pro-BNP levels. This model for assessing prognosis was superior to echocardiography. Serum cardiac troponin value measurements combined with the NT-pro-BNP values were used in the development of a staging system for patients with amyloidosis.[243] Patients who had abnormal values for both parameters (stage III) had a median survival of 3.5 months, those with normal values for both parameters (stage I) had a survival of 26.4 months, and those with 1 of 2 abnormal values (stage II), 10.5 months.[243,244] The staging system using troponins and NT-pro-BNP was subsequently verified in a cohort of patients undergoing stem cell transplantation.[244] The three stages had median survivals of 66.1, 66.1, and 26.1 months, respectively.[245] Forty-nine percent of transplant patients were in stage I, 38% in stage II, and 13% in stage III. Levels of circulating cardiac biomarkers are the most powerful tool for staging patients with AL undergoing stem cell transplantation.[245]

Not only has the immunoglobulin free light chain been found to be important in classifying the type of amyloidosis and providing a method for assessing response, it has also been found to be of prognostic value.[244] Patients with higher baseline free light-chain levels had a significantly higher risk of death. Baseline free light chain correlated with serum cardiac troponin levels, and higher free light chain levels were associated with more organs with amyloid involvement. The absolute level of free light chain achieved after therapy predicted survival. Normalization of free light-chain level after transplantation predicted both organ response and complete hematologic response. Free light-chain measurements before and after treatment are important predictors of patient outcome.[244]

In summary, all patients being assessed for amyloidosis require echocardiography, including measures of diastolic performance, ejection fraction, and mitral deceleration time. The serum β_2-microglobulin concentration, the presence of overt congestive heart failure, and circulating plasma cells remain important measures affecting outcome. BNP and troponin levels are an essential part of the diagnostic evaluation of patients with AL.

THERAPY

Supportive Therapy for Primary Amyloidosis

Cardiac Amyloidosis

The primary modality of therapy for cardiac AL remains diuretic agents.[246] Diuretics decrease extravascular volume, which reduces the peripheral edema that limits these patients. Diuretic therapy helps decrease preload; filling pressures tend to be extremely high in patients with amyloidosis because of the restriction to cardiac inflow. Diuretic therapy is limited by hypotension, which, if associated with hypoalbuminemia from renal amyloidosis, can be difficult to manage.[247] Furosemide doses of 120 mg three times per day may be necessary for edema control. Metolazone can be beneficial in mobilizing fluid. Spironolactone has been shown to decrease mortality in patients with chronic heart failure, although it has not been specifically tested in amyloid cardiomyopathy. Digoxin has little beneficial effect on the diastolic heart failure seen in amyloidosis[248] but can be useful in controlling heart rate in patients with atrial fibrillation, which is generally difficult to convert to sinus rhythm. Nifedipine and diltiazem can precipitate congestive heart failure in patients with AL.[249,250] The use of angiotensin-converting enzyme inhibitors can reduce the afterload in patients with cardiac amyloidosis and has been shown to decrease mortality in patients with ischemic cardiomyopathy. In addition, lisinopril has been reported to reduce proteinuria in renal amyloidosis.[251]

Orthostatic hypotension in amyloidosis can be a major problem.[252] The use of a fitted thigh-high elastic leotard can actually decrease dependence on medications. If medications are necessary, fludrocortisone acetate 0.1 mg two to three times daily can be effective, but it produces some fluid retention and can aggravate supine hypertension.[253] Midodrine can be used in doses ranging from 2.5 to 10 mg two times daily.[254] Dosing should take place during the day to avoid nocturnal supine hypertension. This agent is rapidly absorbed from the intestinal tract, and peak serum values occur in 30 minutes. The maximum recommended dose is 30 mg per day, and the medication comes in 2.5- and 5-mg tablets. If renal insufficiency is present, the dose should be decreased because active metabolites are excreted renally. Adverse effects of midodrine include tachycardia, hypertension, and restlessness. In a patient who did not respond to midodrine and fludrocortisone, subcutaneous erythropoietin resulted in resolution of symptoms related to orthostatic hypotension unassociated with improvement of anemia.[255]

Cardiac transplantation has been used for patients with advanced cardiac AL. A survey of seven patients with a mean age of 46 years reported recurrent amyloidosis in two patients at 3½ and 4 months, one of whom died 13 months after transplantation.[256] Five patients were alive at 32 months. A follow-up study of 10 patients showed recurrent amyloidosis in the graft in four of nine survivors.[257] One patient with AL survived 9 years after cardiac transplantation.[258] Ten patients (mean age, 54 years) received heart transplants; two died postoperatively, and the mean follow-up in the remaining eight patients was 50 months. Recurrent amyloid deposits in the cardiac allografts were demonstrable in 5 patients at 5 to 30 months (median, 12 months) after transplantation. Seven patients died at a median of 32 months; four of the seven died of extracardiac amyloidosis. The 1-year actuarial survival was 60%, and 5-year actuarial survival was 30%.[258]

A 47-year-old woman with AL cardiac amyloidosis received a heart transplant, followed 6 months later by a stem cell transplant in an attempt to prevent recurrent disease.[259] The patient died 2 years after stem cell transplantation, and the myocardium showed mild deposits of amyloid.[259] In 13 cardiac transplant patients with AL at Mayo Clinic, the actuarial 5-year survival was 50%.[260] We have performed stem cell transplantation in 11 patients who were recipients of cardiac transplants; 5 died and 6 were alive at 18, 19, 22, 23, 59, and 82 months after stem cell transplantation.

One study queried the United Network for Organ Sharing database and found 69 patients with amyloidosis who had cardiac transplants.[261] Five operative deaths occurred, and 29 late deaths occurred at a mean follow-up of 40 months. Nine patients died of amyloid-related complications, and graft vasculopathy developed in 1. The 1-year survival was 84% for men and 64% for women.[261] In a report from the United Kingdom, 24 patients had amyloid heart disease, 17 of whom had AL.[262] Survival of 10 patients was 50% at 1 year and 20% at 5 years after heart transplant. Amyloid recurrence in the grafts occurred at a median of 11 months. Extracardiac amyloid contributed to mortality in 70%. Seven patients with AL who also had chemotherapy had 1- and 5-year survival rates of 86% and 64%. The survival was less than after transplant for other indications. Progression of the AL contributed to the increased mortality.[262]

In a single-center report of five patients with cardiac AL, three were dead and two were alive at 60 and 41 months after transplant.[263] Two patients died of sudden death after 23 months and one of multiorgan failure because of progression of AL.[263] Because recurrent amyloidosis is such a common cause of morbidity, the use of stem cell transplantation to prevent disease recurrence after heart transplantation has been reported. Five patients had stem cell transplants after heart transplant, and three of the five were well without evidence of recurrent amyloid.[264] Two patients died at 33 and 90 months after heart transplant after relapse of the amyloidosis.[264]

Renal Amyloidosis

Diuretics can manage the edema of nephrotic syndrome. For patients in whom renal failure eventually develops, hemodialysis support is required. The results of dialysis in AL patients are inferior to those in patients with primary kidney disease.[265] In 61 patients with amyloidosis who had dialysis, 18 died within a month after starting therapy and 43 underwent dialysis for more than 1 month. Younger patients had better 5-year survival. The most important complications after initiation of dialysis were the subsequent development of cardiac and intestinal amyloidosis. Survival was not different between amyloidosis patients who received hemodialysis and those who received peritoneal dialysis.[265] Two-thirds of the deaths in our patient population were due to extrarenal amyloidosis progression, primarily cardiac.[133]

The use of lisinopril has been reported to decrease proteinuria in patients with nephrotic syndrome and can result in significant hyperkalemia. Enalapril has been reported to be effective in reducing proteinuria in steroid-resistant nephrotic syndrome.[266] The mechanism of action is thought to be hemodynamic and is potentially effective in amyloidosis as well.

Renal transplantation has been used in AL. Recurrent amyloidosis in the graft remains a major problem, however. We have performed renal transplantation in eight patients, six of whom had stem cell harvest; five of these underwent stem cell transplant.[142] Stable renal function was present in four. Sequential kidney and stem cell transplantation is feasible.[142] Others have argued that stem cell transplantation should precede kidney transplantation in an effort to produce a complete response before placement of the new organ.[143]

Survival is linked to the development of amyloidosis in the graft; it has been estimated that 1-year survivors have a 20% chance of amyloidosis developing in the transplanted kidney. Fifteen patients with renal amyloidosis underwent transplantation and had 42 to 216 months of follow-up (median, 73 months).[267] The grafts remained normal in all patients whose underlying amyloidogenic disorder had remitted. If the underlying precursor protein production had not remitted, abnormal uptake of radiolabeled serum amyloid P was found, reflecting the development of amyloid in the transplanted kidney. Patients with evidence of renal amyloid by serum amyloid P scan also had evidence of graft dysfunction.[267]

Three patients were reported who received kidney transplants after monoclonal light chain synthesis was suppressed by chemotherapy.[267] The response to chemotherapy was documented by eradication or reduction of immunoglobulin light-chain production. Three patients were alive at 4, 11, and 16 years after transplantation. Renal function in the AL patients remained normal. Renal transplantation is therefore appropriate for patients whose light-chain production can be suppressed.[266]

Hepatic Amyloidosis

As is the case for all other types of AL, the mainstay of therapy for hepatic amyloidosis is suppression of the underlying plasma cell clone with chemotherapy. However, liver transplantation has been reported for the management of AL. A 61-year-old man was hospitalized for spontaneous splenic rupture.[268] Shortly after splenectomy, liver failure with jaundice, ascites, and hyponatremia developed. A subsequent hepatorenal syndrome with hepatic encephalopathy developed over 3 weeks. Hepatic transplantation was performed, and the patient was dismissed from the hospital with normal hepatic and kidney function. At 1-year postoperative follow-up, liver function was normal, although a liver biopsy showed amyloid deposits in the hepatic allograft.[268] Another patient with progressive hepatic failure from AL received a liver allograft.[269] The patient had development of recurrent amyloidosis that led to stem cell transplantation in an effort to suppress amyloid precursor protein production. After a second (tandem) transplantation procedure, the patient had no clinical evidence of recurrent amyloidosis at 28 months. Liver transplantation can be considered for patients with amyloidosis, but suppression of light-chain production is essential to prevent recurrent disease.[269]

Gastrointestinal Tract Amyloidosis

The most frequent symptoms related to amyloidosis of the gastrointestinal tract are diarrhea and constipation. In most patients, this is due to autonomic failure, but in some patients massive deposits develop in the mucosa and submucosa and result in a malabsorption syndrome. Loperamide, diphenoxylate, tincture of opium, and paregoric are used regularly and produce variable results. Octreotide in a long-acting formulation can decrease diarrhea when given in doses ranging from 10 to 30 mg every 4 weeks for 2 months, and then every 4 weeks, according to the response of the diarrhea. Rarely, ostomies are required for diarrhea control. Occasionally, widespread vascular obstruction of blood supply to the bowel develops, leading to massive bleeding and infarction for which surgical intervention is the only option. For nausea, abdominal distension, and pain, cisapride has been reported to provide symptomatic relief.[270]

Noncytotoxic Chemotherapy for Primary Amyloidosis

The primary approach to therapy has been to decrease production of the amyloidogenic light chain with therapy directed against the plasma cell population. DMSO has been used because of in vitro data suggesting an ability to solubilize amyloid deposits.[271] The benefit of DMSO is unproven, and it is infrequently used today to treat amyloidosis.[272] Colchicine has been shown to be effective in the treatment of AA associated with familial Mediterranean fever, a disorder characterized by recurrent peritonitis, pleuritis, synovitis, and rash. Before the introduction of colchicine, the 5-year survival of patients with familial Mediterranean fever was 20%. Nephrotic-range proteinuria and dialysis-dependent renal failure developed in these patients. Two double-blind, placebo-controlled trials showed that colchicine was effective in preventing attacks of serositis and reduced the frequency of amyloidosis.[273]

Given the success of colchicine for familial Mediterranean fever amyloidosis,[274] it was used in patients with AL. Fifty-three patients with AL received colchicine and were compared with retrospective controls.[275] The median survival of colchicine-treated patients was 7 months, compared with 1 year in melphalan-treated patients.[275] Today, colchicine is rarely used for AL. Colchicine is not effective for any of the hereditary periodic fever syndromes including hyperimmunoglobulinemia-D with periodic fever, tumor necrosis factor receptor–associated periodic syndrome, and cryopyrin-associated periodic syndrome.[102]

Cytotoxic Chemotherapy for Primary Amyloidosis

The same chemotherapy drugs used to treat amyloidosis have been used for the management of multiple myeloma. These include oral melphalan and prednisone; oral dexamethasone; combination chemotherapy, including vincristine, carmustine, melphalan, cyclophosphamide, and prednisone; and infusional vincristine, doxorubicin, and dexamethasone, thalidomide, and lenalidomide. These low-toxicity therapies can decrease the plasma cell burden to some degree. Many patients die of the disease before adequate time has elapsed to determine if they will achieve a response. Two prospective randomized studies have demonstrated a survival benefit for oral melphalan and prednisone compared with colchicine.[276,277] Unfortunately, the median survival is prolonged to only 17 or 18 months.

Responders to melphalan and prednisone have significantly prolonged survival compared with nonresponders.[228] Patients who have nephrotic syndrome have a better outcome in terms of response rate than those who have peripheral neuropathy or cardiac involvement. It is unclear whether clinical regression is associated with histologic regression because follow-up biopsies are done infrequently. However, the use of serum amyloid P component scanning has definitely indicated decreased uptake of the isotope at sites of previously known disease, which suggests resolution of the amyloid deposits. Melphalan is leukemogenic, and the risk of myelodysplasia developing is substantial.[278]

We have reported that even in the presence of significant cardiac amyloidosis, survival of more than 5 years was seen in 8 of 153 patients.[279] All long-term survivors received chemotherapy. All but 1 had a demonstrable response to chemotherapy. Continuous oral melphalan has been administered as a single agent for patients with cardiac amyloidosis who could not tolerate prednisone or stem cell transplantation. Seven of 13 evaluable patients achieved a partial hematologic response, 3 achieved a complete hematologic response, and 6 survived for longer than 1 year. Continuous low-dose oral melphalan can induce hematologic responses.[280]

Responses to melphalan and prednisone are uncommon if the serum creatinine value exceeds 3 mg/dL, if hyperbilirubinemia is present, or if the alkaline phosphatase value increases to more than 4 times the institutional normal.[228] In patients who have isolated nephrotic syndrome, a normal serum creatinine value, and a normal echocardiogram, the response rate to melphalan can exceed one-third of patients. It is rare to see symptomatic improvement in peripheral neuropathy after melphalan and prednisone therapy. The median time to response with melphalan is 1 year.[228]

In a 21-year period at Mayo Clinic, 841 patients with AL were evaluated.[281] The actuarial survival for the 810 patients diagnosed premortem was 51% at 1 year, 16% at 5 years, and 4.7% at 10 years (Fig. 89–14). We reported on 30 patients with survival for 10 years after diagnosis, all of whom received melphalan-based therapy.[281] Fourteen had complete eradication of the light chain from serum and urine. Of 10 patients with nephrotic syndrome, 4 had a greater than 50% reduction in proteinuria. Heart failure, older age, a creatinine value greater than 2 mg/dL, and bone marrow plasma cells greater than 20% were poor prognostic factors for long-term survival.[279,280]

Four patients in whom alkylating agents had failed were treated subsequently with vincristine, doxorubicin (Adriamycin), and dexamethasone (VAD) as a 96-hour infusion.[282] Two of the patients had a 50% decrease in the serum monoclonal protein. The VAD regimen could be considered for patients with AL and has been reported as an induction treatment to decrease the plasma cell burden before stem cell transplantation.[282] The use of VAD resulted in improvement in patients' conditions, allowing them to receive high-dose chemotherapy and stem cell transplantation with reduced risk.[282] A series of patients from a single institution had successful use of VAD induction followed by melphalan-based stem cell transplantation.[283,284]

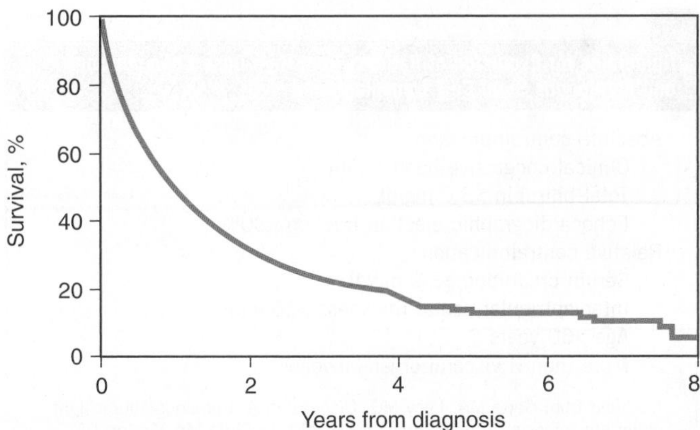

Figure 89–14 Overall survival of patients seen at Mayo Clinic with amyloidosis.

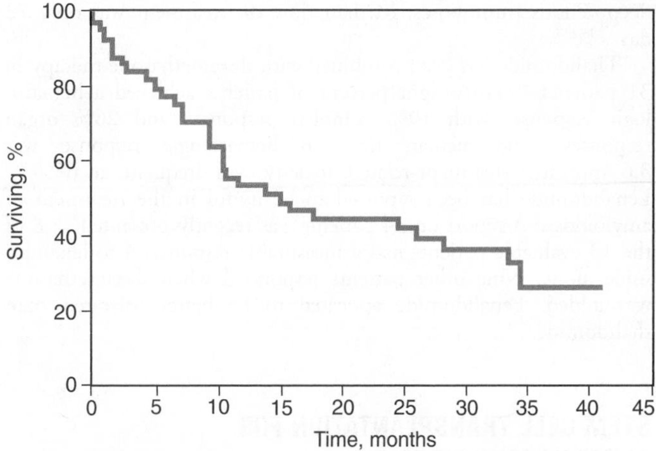

Figure 89–15 Survival of 55 patients with amyloidosis treated with high-dose dexamethasone.

In a three-arm study that accrued 219 patients over 10 years, patients were randomly assigned to receive colchicine, or melphalan and prednisone, or melphalan, prednisone, and colchicine.[276] Patients were stratified by age, sex, and major clinical manifestation of amyloidosis. Half had nephrotic-range proteinuria, and 20% had heart failure. The colchicine group survived a median of 8½ months, and the melphalan-containing regimens resulted in survivals of 17 months. Similar results were reported in patients treated with melphalan at Boston University.[277] We reported on the development of myelodysplasia in 10 of 153 patients who were treated with melphalan for AL.[278] Eight of the 10 died as a result of the myelodysplasia, including acute leukemia and progressive pancytopenia due to myelodysplasia. This group represents 7% of all patients treated with melphalan; the actuarial risk for survivors at 3½ years was 21%. The median survival after the diagnosis of myelodysplasia or acute leukemia was 8 months.

In one patient, the diagnosis of amyloidosis was established, and the patient received 28 months of oral melphalan, prednisone, and colchicine.[285] Five years later, he had dialysis-dependent renal failure with no other evidence of amyloidosis and received a renal transplant. He survived for 7 years; pancytopenia developed with bone marrow that showed dysplastic red blood cells but no acute leukemia. Cytogenetics were complex but included a 5q abnormality. Myelodysplasia developed 12 years after his diagnosis of amyloidosis.

High-dose dexamethasone as a single agent given at 40 mg on days 1 to 4, 9 to 12, and 17 to 20 every 5 weeks has been reported.[286] Responding patients received maintenance dexamethasone at 40 mg per day, 4 days per month for 1 year. Improvement in amyloid organ involvement was seen in eight of nine patients, and six of seven had a greater than 50% decrease in urinary protein loss with a median time to response of 4 months. Patients with heart failure did not benefit. Median survival of the cohort was 31 months. In a report on 93 patients treated with this regimen, 2-year overall survival was 60% and event-free survival was 52%.[287] Heart failure and β_2-microglobulin levels were the predictors of adverse outcome.[287] We treated 19 patients with high-dose dexamethasone therapy,[288] and 3 showed objective organ response. The median survival of the entire group was 11.2 months, but 3 were alive at 110, 116, and 119 months. Dexamethasone should be considered as an option for patients who are not suitable candidates for transplantation. Dexamethasone has also been used for patients in whom melphalan therapy had previously failed.[289] The objective response rate was 12% (Fig. 89–15). One patient was alive at 104 months.

Because high-dose dexamethasone therapy can be toxic in patients with AL, a lower-dose schedule has been reported: 40 mg on days 1 through 4 every 21 days for up to eight cycles.[290] Overall, 8 of 23 patients had a median time to response of 4 months (range, 2–6 months). This regimen has been used as a first-line therapy. This same group reported on the combination of low-dose melphalan and modified high-dose dexamethasone therapy.[290]

Melphalan has been combined with high-dose dexamethasone in patients with AL who were ineligible for stem cell transplantation, primarily because of cardiomyopathy.[291] Of 46 patients, a complete response was seen in 15 (33%) and a hematologic response in 31 (67%). Twenty-two patients (48%) showed an improvement in organ dysfunction. There was a strong correlation between hematologic and organ response. If the hematologic response was complete, the organ response rate was 87%. If the hematologic response was greater than 50%, organ function improved in 56%; patients with no hematologic response had no organ functional improvement. The 100-day mortality with this regimen was 4%. Cardiac failure resolved in 6 of 32 patients. The median time to response was 4.5 months, and only 11% had adverse effects.[291]

We studied 101 patients with AL; half received melphalan and prednisone and half received vincristine, carmustine, melphalan, cyclophosphamide, and prednisone.[292] Seventy-six of the 101 patients died, and the median overall survival for the entire group was 26.4 months, with no difference between the two arms. In this group of 101, 18 ultimately required dialysis therapy; 15 of the 18 have since died. The most common cause of death was intractable hypotension related to cardiac involvement while on dialysis. The three surviving dialysis patients have been alive for 87, 94, and 103 months. A myelodysplastic syndrome was documented in eight patients, all of whom have died, including one who received an allogeneic bone marrow transplant. The overall survival of these eight patients ranged from 18 to 90 months, with a median of 43 months. We also studied 45 patients who received the agent iodo-deoxydoxorubicin and found a response rate of 15%.[293]

Thalidomide has been shown to be active in the treatment of AL. In the initial report, six patients with AL were treated with thalidomide.[294] All patients had renal amyloidosis and were treated previously. The duration of thalidomide therapy was 3 to 9 months (median, 5 months). Four also received oral corticosteroids. An improvement was reported in five patients. Proteinuria decreased by more than 50% in two, and the serum albumin concentration improved in three. Two patients died, and four were alive and remained on therapy.[294]

In another report of 12 patients receiving thalidomide, 8 patients had renal, 4 had cardiac, 3 had liver, and 2 had soft-tissue amyloidosis.[295] Ten had received a prior stem cell transplant. The median maximum tolerated thalidomide dose was 500 mg. No patient had a 50% decrease in serum or urine monoclonal proteins. Five of 11 patients had a 25% to 50% improvement. Three patients had stable disease and three had progressive disease.[295] We have found thalidomide difficult to administer, and initial doses should not exceed 50 mg. It is unusual for patients with amyloidosis to tolerate more than 200 mg per day long term, and the toxicity is substantially greater in this population. We encountered edema and cognitive difficulties in 75%; dyspnea, dizziness, and rash in 50%; and two deep venous thromboses. Median time on treatment was only 72 days.[296,297]

Thalidomide has been combined with dexamethasone therapy in 31 patients.[298] Forty-eight percent of patients achieved a hematologic response, with 19% complete responses and 26% organ responses. The median time to hematologic response was 3.6 months. Treatment-related toxicity was frequent at 65%.[298] Lenalidomide has been reported to be useful in the treatment of amyloidosis. A report on 34 patients was recently presented[299]; 8 of the 13 evaluable patients had a measurable response, 4 to lenalidomide alone. Nine other patients responded when dexamethasone was added. Lenalidomide appeared to be better tolerated than thalidomide.[299]

STEM CELL TRANSPLANTATION FOR PRIMARY AMYLOIDOSIS

The use of high-dose chemotherapy and stem cell transplantation for patients with amyloidosis remains controversial because this modality of therapy is associated with a high treatment-related mortality (Table 89–4).[300–313] Transplant-related mortality can range from 11% to 43%. Moreover, mortality has even been reported during stem cell mobilization using granulocyte colony-stimulating factor (G-CSF); these deaths were attributed to noncardiogenic pulmonary edema,[314] cardiac ischemia, or sudden rhythm disturbances with ventricular fibrillation. The significant visceral organ dysfunction that accompanies amyloidosis places patients at a high risk for complications developing. The number of organs involved at the time of transplantation is predictive of outcome. Patients who have one organ involved fare better than those who have two, and those who have more than two organs involved have an even poorer outcome.[315] Causes of treatment-related mortality in AL include gastrointestinal tract bleeding,[316] cardiac rhythm disturbances, and multiorgan failure.

At Mayo Clinic, high-dose chemotherapy and autologous stem cell transplantation has been performed in 270 patients with AL. The median age was 57 years. The median serum albumin level was 2.8 g/dL, which reflects a high prevalence of nephrotic-range proteinuria. Ten percent of patients had serum creatinine levels greater than 1.8 mg/dL. Alkaline phosphatase levels greater than twice normal, a marker for liver amyloidosis, were observed in 19% of patients. The median serum monoclonal protein concentration was 0.3 g/dL. A serum monoclonal protein component was found in 196 of the 270 patients. The median 24-hour urine protein excretion was 3.4 g/day (interquartile range, 0.24–7.1 g/day). Fifty-four percent had urinary protein loss greater than 3 g/day. Only 6% had monoclonal light-chain excretion of greater than 1 g in 24 hours. One-, two-, and three-organ amyloid involvement was seen in 48%, 38%, and 14% of patients, respectively.

Stem cell mobilization in patients with amyloidosis was achieved with G-CSF alone without prior cytotoxic chemotherapy. The median number of apheresis collections required to collect an adequate stem cell product was 3 (interquartile range, 2–4 aphereses). The median number of $CD34^+$ cells collected was 6.5×10^6/kg (range, 2.0–50.9 $\times$ 10^6 cells/kg). Hematopoietic growth factors were not administered after transplantation because of their ability to produce fluid retention in patients with cardiac and renal amyloidosis.

The 100-day mortality rate of these 270 patients was 11%, which compares favorably with reports from other institutions where morality rates as high as 40% have been reported.[307] Mortality (before day 100) at Mayo Clinic has progressively decreased over the years: from 12.1% of stem cell transplant recipients before 2004, to 10 of 107 consecutive transplant recipients (9.3%) since January 1, 2004.

Sixty-two percent of patients received conditioning therapy with melphalan at a dose of 200 mg/m^2, 26% received melphalan at 140 mg/m^2, and the rest received lower doses because of advanced cardiac amyloidosis. The intensity of chemotherapy delivered appears to be predictive of outcome.[317] Patients receiving full-dose melphalan fare better, although patients selected for full-intensity therapy tend to have less advanced disease and are somewhat younger.[317]

Bias is inherent in selecting patients for transplantation and the intensity of their conditioning. At Mayo Clinic, only one-fourth of patients encountered with amyloidosis ultimately go on to receive a stem cell transplant. Transplant recipients survive longer than patients not selected for transplant. In a case-matched control study, 63 transplant patients were compared with 63 conventionally treated patients matched for age, sex, cardiac function, creatinine, urinary protein loss, and liver involvement. An overall survival advantage for the patients undergoing transplant was observed.[318] In a report from the American Bone Marrow Transplant Registry of 107 patients treated with high-dose chemotherapy and autologous stem cell transplant at 48 centers,[319] the 30-day treatment mortality was 18%, and the response rate was 34%, with 33% having stable disease.[319] Only 11% of patients had posttransplant disease progression. The projected median survival was 47 months. Experienced transplant groups

Guidelines for Exclusion of Patients from High-Dose Chemotherapy and Autologous Stem Cell Transplantation

Absolute contraindication
- Clinical congestive heart failure
- Total bilirubin >3.0 mg/dL
- Echocardiographic ejection fraction <30%

Relative contraindication
- Serum creatinine >2.0 mg/dL
- Interventricular septal thickness >15 mm
- Age >60 years
- More than 2 visceral organs involved

Modified from Gertz MA, Lacy MQ, Dispenzieri A: Immunoglobulin light chain amyloidosis (primary amyloidosis, AL). In Gertz MA, Greipp PR (eds.): Hematologic Malignancies: Multiple Myeloma and Related Plasma Cell Disorders. New York, Springer-Verlag, 2004, p 157–195. Used with permission of Mayo Foundation for Medical Education and Research.

Risk-Adapted Approach to Primary Amyloidosis Therapy

Good risk
- One or two organs involved
- No cardiac involvement
- Creatinine clearance ≥51 mL/min
- Any age

Intermediate risk
- Younger than 61 years
- One or two organs involved
- Asymptomatic or compensated cardiomyopathy
- Creatinine clearance <51 mL/min

Poor risk
- Three organs involved
- Advanced cardiac involvement

Melphalan dosing as a function of risk group and age

Good risk	*Intermediate risk*	*Poor risk*
200 mg/m^2 if ≤60 years	140 mg/m^2 if ≤50 years	Standard therapy
140 mg/m^2 if 61–70 years	100 mg/m^2 if 51–60 years	Clinical trials
100 mg/m^2 if ≥71 years		

From Gertz MA, Lacy MQ, Dispenzieri A: Immunoglobulin light chain amyloidosis (primary amyloidosis, AL). In Gertz MA, Greipp PR (eds.): Hematologic Malignancies: Multiple Myeloma and Related Plasma Cell Disorders. New York, Springer-Verlag, 2004, p 157. Used with permission of Mayo Foundation for Medical Education and Research.

Table 89–4 Results of High-Dose Chemotherapy and Autologous Stem Cell Transplantation for Amyloidosis

Reference	Patients, no.	100-Day Treatment-Related Mortality	Overall Survival (Intention-to-Treat)	Evaluable, no.	Follow-up	Hematologic Response	Amyloid Organ Disease Involvement
Majolino et al[300]	1	1/1 (100%) CMV pneumonitis	0 at 74 days	1	74 days	PR at 2 weeks	Not reported
van Buren et al[301]	3 (1 syngeneic)	0/3 (0%)	2/2 (100%) at 24 months	2	12 months	2/2 (100%) CR	2/2 (100%) PR
Gillmore et al[302]	16 (too early to analyze)	1/16 (6%) GI bleeding	Not reported	0	NA	NA	NA
Amoura et al[303]	9	3/9 (33%) ARF, sepsis, arrhythmia	5/9 (55%); median, 12.6 months	5	Mean, 8.9 months	Not reported	4/5 (80%), 1/5 CR, 3/5 PR
Moreau et al[304]	21 (June 1993, March 1997)	9/21 (43%) multiorgan failure, bleeding, arrhythmia	12/21 (57%) at median of 14 months	12	Median, 14 months	3/12 (25%) CR	10/12 (83%) PR + CR
Schulenburg et al[305]	1	1/1 (100%) GI perforation	0 at 4 days	0	NA	NA	NA
Patriarca et al[306]	1	0	1/1 (100%) at 22 months	1	22 months	1/1 (100%) CR	1/1 (100%) PR
Saba et al[307]	9	7/9 (78%) (3 during mobilization) arrhythmia, CHF, hypotension	2/9 (22%) at >6 months after referral	2	Not reported	Not reported	2/2 (100%) PR
Sezer et al[308]	1	0	1/1 (100%) at 3 months	1	3 months	1/1 (100%) CR	1/1 (100%) renal and cardiac PR
Gertz et al[309]	23 (3 never had transplant)	4/20 (20%) pneumonia, multiorgan system failure, sudden death	13/23 (57%) at median of 16 months	20	Median, >13 months	8/20 (40%) CR	12/20 (60%) PR
Reich et al[310]	4	2/4 (50%) acute MI, diffuse alveolar hemorrhage	2/4 (50%) at 7 and 19 months	2	7 and 19 months	1/2 (50%) PR	2/2 (100%) PR
Sanchorawala et al[311]	205 (20 never had transplant)	22/185 (12%)	115/152 (76%) at >12 months	115 at >12 months	>12 months	54/115 (47%) CR	18/50 (36%) renal CR at 12 months
Perz et al[312]	13	2/13 (15%)	10/13		10.5 months	3/7	
Blum et al[313]	10	0	18.5 months			6/7	

ARF, acute renal failure; CHF, congestive heart failure; CMV, cytomegalovirus; CR, complete response; GI, gastrointestinal; MI, myocardial infarction; NA, not available; PR, partial response.

Modified from Gertz MA, Lacy MQ, Dispenzieri A: Immunoglobulin light chain amyloidosis (primary amyloidosis, AL). In Gertz MA, Greipp PR (eds.): Hematologic Malignancies: Multiple Myeloma and Related Plasma Cell Disorders. New York, Springer-Verlag, 2004, p 157–195. Used with permission of Mayo Foundation for Medical Education and Research.

appear to be able to achieve similar results as those of centers with a special interest in amyloidosis and transplantation.[320]

The 270 Mayo Clinic patients with amyloidosis received their transplants a median of 4.2 months after histologic diagnosis: one-fourth within 3 months and three-fourths within 7.2 months. The median actuarial survival for the entire group was 75 months. Predictors of survival included weight gain of greater than 2% during stem cell mobilization and an absolute lymphocyte count at day 15 of greater than 500/μL.[321] The number of organs involved appeared to be relevant to successfully predicting outcome (Fig. 89–16). Patients with two-organ involvement have a survival of 55 months; those with three-organ involvement, 25.5 months. The serum creatinine, troponin-T, and BNP levels (Fig. 89–17) and septal thickness were all significant predictors of outcome.

Stem cell transplantation has not yet been established as the therapy of choice for patients with amyloidosis. In a French multicenter randomized trial (MAG and IFM Intergroup), patients with amyloidosis received either high-dose chemotherapy and autologous stem cell transplantation or melphalan/dexamethasone therapy.[322] The median survival was 57 months in the melphalan/dexametha-

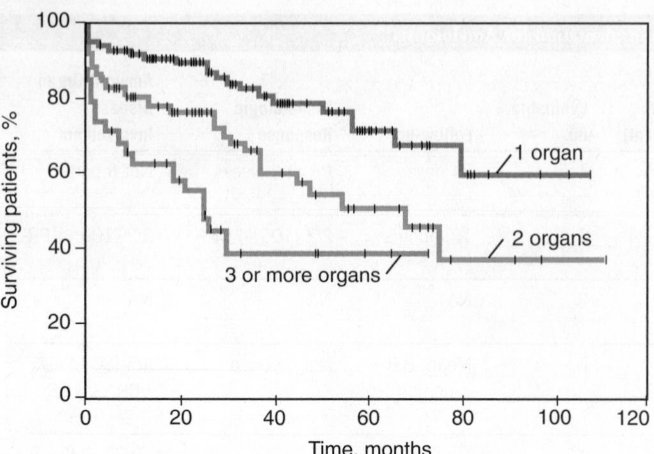

Figure 89–16 Kaplan–Meier curves estimating survival in 270 Mayo Clinic patients with amyloidosis on the basis of number of organs involved at presentation. Tick marks indicate censored patients (alive). *(From Gertz MA, Lacy MQ, Dispenzieri A, et al: Transplantation for amyloidosis. Curr Opin Oncol 2007;19:136–41. Use with permission.)*

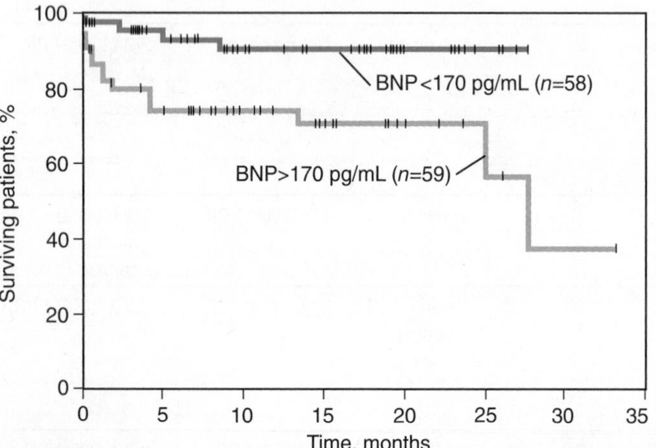

Figure 89–17 Kaplan–Meier curves estimating survival in 117 Mayo Clinic patients with amyloidosis on the basis of brain natriuretic peptide (BNP) concentration greater or less than 170 pg/mL ($P = 0.008$). *(From Gertz MA, Lacy MQ, Dispenzieri A, et al: Transplantation for amyloidosis. Curr Opin Oncol 2007;19:136–41. Used with permission.)*

sone group and 49 months in the transplant group. Transplant patients received conditioning chemotherapy with either 140 or 200 mg/m^2 melphalan. The hematologic response rates were similar for both groups (65% vs 64%). These results suggest that overall survival may not be superior following stem cell transplantation as compared with melphalan/dexamethasone therapy.[322] The results of this study must be interpreted with caution because of the short median follow-up (29 months) and high transplant-related mortality (24%).

After transplant, responders to autologous stem cell transplantation have a superior survival as compared with nonresponders. Overall survival is linked to pretransplant free light-chain levels and the number of organs involved.[244,317] In centers performing stem cell transplantation, treatment-related mortality has ranged from 6% to 18%, hematologic complete responses from 16% to 50%, and organ responses from 34% to 64%.[323] Organ responses are time-dependent and may be delayed for up to 36 months after transplantation. The use of induction therapy with two cycles of melphalan and prednisone before stem cell transplant did not improve the rate of hematologic or organ response.[324]

Table 89–5 Selected Treatment-Related Toxicities (SWOG Grade >2) in Patients with Primary Amyloidosis Who Received Stem Cell Transplant

	No. of patients (%)	
Toxicity	**Melphalan, 200 mg/m^2 (n = 23)**	**Melphalan, 100 mg/m^2 (n = 27)**
Nausea/vomiting	19 (83)	14 (52)
Diarrhea	15 (65)	13 (48)
Mucositis	21 (91)	10 (37)
Non-GI bleeding	4 (17)	0 (0)
GI bleeding	5 (22)	2 (7)

GI, gastrointestinal tract; SWOG, Southwest Oncology Group.

Data from Gertz MA, Lacy MQ, Dispenzieri A: Immunoglobulin light chain amyloidosis (primary amyloidosis, AL). In Gertz MA, Greipp PR (eds.): Hematologic Malignancies: Multiple Myeloma and Related Plasma Cell Disorders. New York, Springer-Verlag, 2004, p 157–195. Used with permission of Mayo Foundation for Education and Research.

Deaths have been reported during stem cell mobilization with cyclophosphamide plus G-CSF or G-CSF alone.[325] Hypoxia and hypotension may develop even in patients without cardiac involvement and may reflect a variant of pulmonary leukostasis syndrome. Excessive fluid accumulation during stem cell mobilization is an important predictor of 1-year survival.[326]

Toxic megacolon is a complication of high-dose chemotherapy.[327] Others have also reported fatal cardiac arrhythmias after infusion of DMSO-cryopreserved stem cell grafts.[328,329] The absolute numbers of $CD4^+$ T cells is significantly reduced after stem cell transplantation, raising the theoretical risk of serious opportunistic infections developing after transplantation. In a series of six patients, four had acute renal failure, one had splenic rupture, and one had severe gastrointestinal bleeding.[330,331] In a multicenter study of 15 transplant patients, there was no treatment-related mortality and 67% of patients experienced complete hematologic responses, which suggests the feasibility of performing stem cell transplantation at experienced transplant centers not associated with major amyloidosis referral centers.[332]

Amyloid-related cardiomyopathy is associated with a high rate of early mortality post transplant.[333] The median survival of patients with cardiac amyloidosis was 2 years. The overall median survival was 5.5 years, and the relapse rate of complete responders was only 5%.[333]

Most conditioning regimens used to treat patients with AL undergoing transplant include melphalan; currently, melphalan alone is preferred to melphalan plus total body irradiation. Complete hematologic response rates appear to be related to the dose of melphalan: 55% at 200 mg/m^2 and 35% at 100 or 140 mg/m^2.[317] Gastrointestinal tract bleeding is a frequent complication.[316] It is assumed that amyloid infiltration of the submucosa of the gastrointestinal tract followed by chemotherapy-induced mucosal erosion leads to exposure of amyloid-laden blood vessels, with resultant bleeding.

Despite the high mortality and morbidity associated with transplantation (Table 89–5), the hematologic and organ response rates far exceed the prior experience with conventional-dose melphalan. Improvement in quality of life has also been reported in melphalan-treated patients undergoing stem cell transplantation.[334] The best responses to transplant are seen in patients who have renal amyloidosis and nephrotic syndrome. We believe that the dose of melphalan used for conditioning must be modified according to patient risk factors. Clearly, patients with more than two major organs involved or severe cardiomyopathy are at a high risk when receiving melphalan doses of 200 mg/m^2 (Fig. 89–18). Patients with one or two organs involved, younger patients, and those without advanced cardiac disease are favorable candidates for stem cell transplants. A risk-

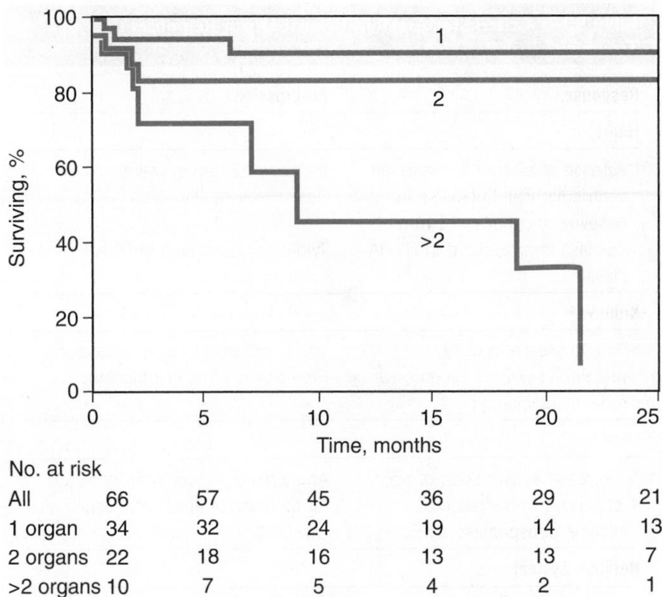

No. at risk						
All	66	57	45	36	29	21
1 organ	34	32	24	19	14	13
2 organs	22	18	16	13	13	7
>2 organs	10	7	5	4	2	1

Figure 89–18 Survival of patients with amyloidosis receiving stem cell transplantation according to the number of organs involved. *(From Gertz et al.[315] Used with permission.)*

adapted stratification has been useful in selecting patients for therapy and assigning melphalan dose.[317]

The use of both conventional and high-dose chemotherapy has been shown to normalize factor X deficiency associated with amyloidosis.[335] Dose-intensive melphalan therapy improves nephrotic syndrome in patients with AL, but the benefit is limited to patients achieving eradication of the plasma cell dyscrasia.[336] A randomized study was performed comparing autologous stem cell transplantation with therapy with two cycles of oral melphalan and prednisone followed by stem cell transplantation.[337] The overall survival of patients 1 year after randomization was higher for those who went directly to transplantation.

The role of tandem transplants and nonmyeloablative conditioning regimens has yet to be defined in this setting. Tandem transplantation has been reported in four patients, all with nephrotic syndrome.[338,339] Two died, one of sudden death and one, who had sepsis with gastrointestinal tract bleeding, of complications of renal failure. Two of the patients are alive and in good health.

Patients who receive transplants for AL are highly selected on the basis of age, performance status, number of organs involved, absence of severe cardiomyopathy, and preserved renal function. The superiority of high-dose chemotherapy and autologous stem cells has never been demonstrated in a prospective study. Dispenzieri et al[340] reviewed an amyloidosis patient database to identify patients who might have been eligible for stem cell transplantation. The inclusion criteria of biopsy-proven amyloidosis, symptoms of amyloidosis, absence of multiple myeloma, restrictions on age, and adequate cardiac function led to the selection of 229 of 1,288 patients. The median survival of this group was 45 months, with 5- and 10-year survival rates of 36% and 15%, respectively (Fig. 89–19). Predictors of survival were size of the monoclonal protein component in the urine, number of organs involved (Fig. 89–20), serum alkaline phosphatase value, performance status, and weight loss. Being eligible for stem cell transplantation but not actually receiving the transplant was associated with a better outcome than not being eligible for transplantation.

In summary, with appropriate patient selection, stem cell transplantation is feasible but is associated with risks of higher morbidity and mortality than stem cell transplantation for other disorders.

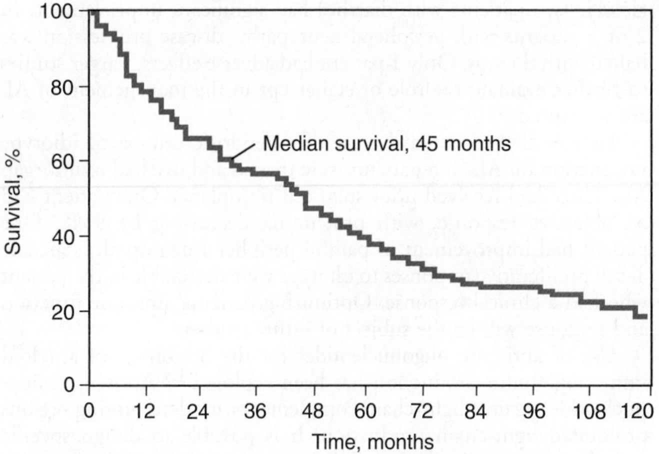

Figure 89–19 Kaplan–Meier curve estimating survival of patients with amyloidosis who would have been eligible for stem cell transplantation by Mayo Clinic criteria but were treated conventionally. *(Modified from Dispenzieri et al.[340] Used with permission.)*

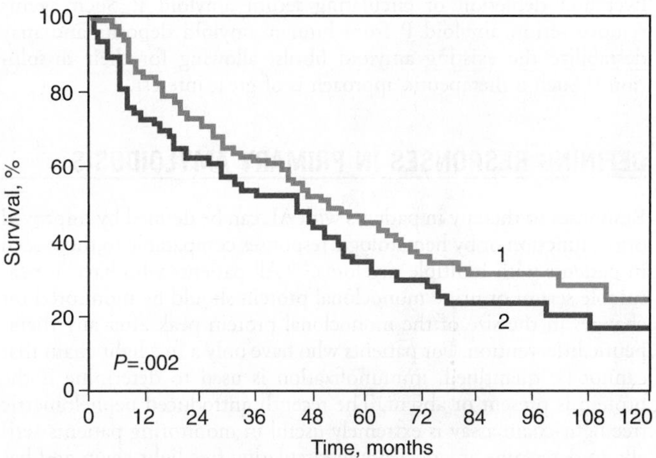

Figure 89–20 Kaplan–Meier curve estimating survival of stem cell transplant–eligible patients with amyloidosis who were treated conventionally, according to the number of organs involved at the time of diagnosis. *(Modified from Gertz MA, Lacy MQ, Dispenzieri A: Immunoglobulin light chain amyloidosis [primary amyloidosis, AL]. In Gertz MA, Greipp PR [eds.]: Hematologic Malignancies: Multiple Myeloma and Related Plasma Cell Disorders. New York, Springer-Verlag, 2004, p 157–194. Used with permission of Mayo Foundation for Medical Education and Research.)*

INVESTIGATIONAL THERAPIES

In an experimental model in which mice are injected with human AL proteins, amyloidomas result.[341] When these animals receive injections of an anti–light chain monoclonal antibody having specificity for an amyloid-related epitope, the amyloidomas rapidly resolve. This monoclonal antibody is directed toward a β-pleated sheet conformational epitope expressed by AL proteins. The amyloidolytic response appears to be associated with the release of proteolytic factors. AL resolution can be induced by passive administration of amyloid reactive antibodies.[341] This approach is currently under evaluation.

Fourteen patients with AL received etanercept, an anti-TNF receptor monoclonal antibody, at 25 mg subcutaneously twice weekly.[342,343] Of 10 patients with adequate follow-up, 2 died and 8 are stable. One patient had an improved septal wall thickness. Three patients experienced a 25% to 50% decrease in the degree of macroglossia. Two patients with diarrhea had significant improvement. In 2 of 5 patients with peripheral neuropathy, disease progression was halted with therapy. Only 1 patient had adverse effects. Larger studies to further evaluate the role of etanercept in the management of AL are warranted.[342]

Lacy et al[344] reported the use of a dendritic cell–based idiotype vaccination for AL. Ten patients were treated and five had multiorgan AL. Three had received prior stem cell transplants. One patient had an objective response, with proteinuria decreasing by 95%. One patient had improvement of painful peripheral neuropathy. Specific T-cell proliferative responses to idiotype were detectable in the patient who had a clinical response. Optimizing patients' immune function and response will be the subject of future studies.

Use of antisense oligonucleotides for the inhibition of amyloid immunoglobulin production has been explored.[345] Antisense oligonucleotides against light-chain complementarity-determining regions prohibited light-chain production. It is possible to design specific complementary oligonucleotides, suggesting that treatment with antisense oligonucleotides could represent a rational approach to improve treatment outcomes in AL.[345]

Serum amyloid P binds to all forms of amyloid deposits. Drugs have been developed that act as competitive inhibitors of serum amyloid P binding to amyloid fibrils.[52] Such compounds dimerize serum amyloid P molecules, leading to their rapid clearance by the liver and depletion of circulating serum amyloid P. Such agents remove serum amyloid P from human amyloid deposits and may destabilize the existing amyloid fibrils, allowing for their dissolution.[52] Such a therapeutic approach is of great interest.

DEFINING RESPONSES IN PRIMARY AMYLOIDOSIS

Responses to therapy in patients with AL can be defined by improved organ function or by hematologic responses comparable to those seen in patients with multiple myeloma.[346] All patients who have a measurable serum or urine monoclonal protein should be monitored for changes in the size of the monoclonal protein peak after any therapeutic intervention. For patients who have only a free light chain that cannot be quantified, immunofixation is used to determine if the protein is present or absent. The recently introduced nephelometric free light-chain assay is extremely useful in monitoring patients serially to determine any decrease in circulating free light chain and has made the evaluation of response much easier.[41]

The utility of the free light-chain assay in predicting outcome has been validated as noted earlier in this chapter, with 5-year survival rates of 88% for responders and 39% for nonresponders.[43] In our experience, normalization of the free light-chain level was a better predictor of survival than was achievement of a complete hematologic response or normalization of the free light-chain ratio.[244] These results have been verified in a series of 25 patients with sequential free light-chain analyses.[347] All patients with a normalized κ to λ free light-chain ratio had a good prognosis.[347] The fraction of patients with serum free light-chain responses has been suggested to be higher in patients receiving high-dose melphalan than in those who receive conventional therapy.[348]

Free light-chain responses also seem to parallel decreases in NT-pro-BNP levels in cardiac responders to therapy. For patients in whom free light chain decreased by more than 50%, the NT-pro-BNP concentration decreased by a median of 48%, whereas in patients without such a free light-chain decrease, the NT-pro-BNP concentration increased by 47%.[349] The NT-pro-BNP decrease was greater in complete responders than in other responders. The decrease of free light chains translates to a simultaneous decrease of NT-pro-BNP and improved survival. Cardiac function in AL can improve due to a decrease in circulating amyloidogenic precursor, despite the amount of cardiac amyloid deposits remaining unaltered as measured by echocardiography.[349]

Organ-based response criteria have been defined for patients with amyloid nephrotic syndrome (Table 89–6).[350] Requirements for definition as an "organ response" include a 50% decrease in the 24-hour albumin excretion without an increase in serum creatinine value. For hepatic involvement, a 50% decrease in an increased serum alkaline phosphatase concentration with no increase in liver size is required. Echocardiographic regression of amyloidosis is difficult to assess because of variability in estimates of the interventricular septal wall thickness. Typically, a decrease in septal thickness of at least 2 mm is required. Neurologic responses can be documented by electromyography demonstrating improved nerve conduction velocities. A consensus panel has defined what constitutes organ involvement and treatment response in patients with AL.[350]

Table 89–6 Criteria for Amyloid-Related Organ Responses to Treatment*

Response	Progression
Heart	
Decrease of ≥2 mm in mean left ventricular wall thickness from baseline thickness >11 mm	Increase ≥2 mm in wall thickness
Two-class improvement in NYHA class	Two-class worsening in NYHA class
Kidneys	
>50% decrease in daily proteinuria without progressive renal insufficiency	>50% increase in daily proteinuria Progressive renal insufficiency
Liver	
A decrease in liver span of >50% A concomitant decrease of alkaline phosphatase by 50%	An increase in liver span of >25% An increase of alkaline phosphatase by 50%
Nervous System	
Autonomic: normalization of orthostatic vital signs and symptoms, resolution of gastric atony	Autonomic: progression of orthostatic vital signs and symptoms, increasing gastric atony
Peripheral neuropathy: resolution of symptoms	Peripheral neuropathy: progression of symptoms

NYHA, New York Heart Association.
*If organ function neither improves nor worsens, it is graded as stable.

CONCLUSION

AL is a disease for which therapy remains inadequate. The diagnosis should be suspected whenever a patient is seen with unexplained nephrotic syndrome, heart failure, neuropathy, or hepatomegaly. The first screening test should be immunofixation of serum or urine and the free light-chain assay. If a monoclonal protein is found, bone marrow biopsy and fat aspiration should be performed to obtain tissues for Congo red staining. Prognosis should be assessed by two-dimensional echocardiography and BNP and troponin level measurements. Monitoring therapy includes the use of immunoglobulin free light-chain assays by nephelometry. Systemic chemotherapy is appropriate for most patients. The response rates observed with stem cell transplantation are higher than those seen with standard therapy, and transplantation should be strongly considered if patients fulfill eligibility criteria. The use of solid organ transplantation remains investigational. The ideal treatment of AL remains unknown, but early diagnosis is essential to ensure superior outcome.

SUGGESTED READINGS

Benson MD: Ostertag revisited: The inherited systemic amyloidoses without neuropathy. Amyloid 12:75, 2005.

Dispenzieri A, Gertz MA, Kyle RA, et al: Serum cardiac troponins and N-terminal pro-brain natriuretic peptide: A staging system for primary systemic amyloidosis. J Clin Oncol 22:3751, 2004.

Dispenzieri A, Kyle RA, Lacy MQ, et al: Superior survival in primary systemic amyloidosis patients undergoing peripheral blood stem cell transplantation: A case-control study. Blood 103:3960, 2004. Epub 2004 Jan 22.

Dispenzieri A, Lacy MQ, Katzmann JA, et al: Absolute values of immunoglobulin free light chains are prognostic in patients with primary systemic amyloidosis undergoing peripheral blood stem cell transplantation. Blood 107:3378, 2006. Epub 2006 Jan 5.

Falk RH: Diagnosis and management of the cardiac amyloidoses. Circulation 112:2047, 2005.

Gertz MA, Lacy MQ, Dispenzieri A, et al: Transplantation for amyloidosis. Curr Opin Oncol 19:136, 2007.

Gillmore JD, Goodman HJ, Lachmann HJ, et al: Sequential heart and autologous stem cell transplantation for systemic AL amyloidosis. Blood 107:1227, 2006. Epub 2005 Oct 6.

Greipp PR, Kyle RA, Bowie EJ: Factor-X deficiency in amyloidosis: A critical review. Am J Hematol 11:443, 1981.

Hazenberg BP, van Rijswijk MH, Piers DA, et al: Diagnostic performance of ^{123}I-labeled serum amyloid P component scintigraphy in patients with amyloidosis. Am J Med 119:355.e15, 2006.

Jaccard A, Moreau P, Lebond V, et al: Autologous stem cell transplantation (ASCT) versus oral melphalan and high-dose dexamethasone in patients with AL (primary) amyloidosis: Results of the French Multicentric Randomized Trial (MAG and IFM Intergroup). Blood 106:142, 2005.

Lachmann HJ, Booth DR, Booth SE, et al: Misdiagnosis of hereditary amyloidosis as AL (primary) amyloidosis. N Engl J Med 346:1786, 2002.

Leung N, Griffin MD, Dispenzieri A, et al: Living donor kidney and autologous stem cell transplantation for primary systemic amyloidosis (AL) with predominant renal involvement. Am J Transplant5:1660, 2005.

Palladini G, Anesi E, Perfetti V, et al: A modified high-dose dexamethasone regimen for primary systemic (AL) amyloidosis. Br J Haematol 113:1044, 2001.

Palladini G, Lavatelli F, Russo P, et al: Circulating amyloidogenic free light chains and serum N-terminal natriuretic peptide type B decrease simultaneously in association with improvement of survival in AL. Blood 107:3854, 2006. Epub 2006 Jan 24.

Palladini G, Perfetti V, Obici L, et al: Association of melphalan and high-dose dexamethasone is effective and well tolerated in patients with AL (primary) amyloidosis who are ineligible for stem cell transplantation. Blood 103:2936, 2004. Epub 2003 Dec 18.

Rajkumar SV, Gertz MA, Kyle RA: Prognosis of patients with primary systemic amyloidosis who present with dominant neuropathy. Am J Med 104:232, 1998.

Sanchorawala V, Wright DG, Seldin DC, et al: An overview of the use of high-dose melphalan with autologous stem cell transplantation for the treatment of AL amyloidosis. Bone Marrow Transplant 28:637, 2001.

REFERENCES

For complete list of references log onto www.expertconsult.com

CHAPTER 90

ATYPICAL IMMUNE LYMPHOPROLIFERATIONS

Timothy C. Greiner and Thomas G. Gross

The development of modern classification systems for hematologic malignancies resulted from the recognition that specific histologic and cytologic patterns correlated with prognosis.[1] The Working Formulation for Clinical Usage predicted prognoses in many of the subtypes of lymphoma but was limited by the lack of immunophenotype and molecular data that the Revised European and American classification system proposed and the WHO classification system now provides.[1–3] These lymphoma classification systems can be reliably applied to most clinically relevant neoplastic lesions, but some lymphoproliferations are not addressed because they do not meet the pathologic definition of malignancy. No unifying system exists for classifying atypical or preneoplastic lymphoproliferations that provides prognostic information to predict whether a patient will have a self-limited illness or progress to lymphoma or death.

WHAT CONSTLTUTES AN ATYPLCAL LYMPHOPROLIFERATION?

The tremendous complexity of the immune system and its various responses to challenges has led to recognition of certain hyperplastic responses that are clearly benign and manifest specific histologic patterns when biopsied.[4] Examples of benign hyperplastic immune responses include follicular hyperplasia, in which B-cell areas of the lymph node increase in size and number. As a nonspecific diagnosis, follicular hyperplasia may be seen in a wide range of clinical presentations, from bacterial infections to generalized lymphadenopathy of acquired immunodeficiency syndrome (AIDS).[4] Sinus histiocytosis, in which benign histiocytes distend lymph node sinuses,[4] is seen in reaction to particulates and organisms in the hilar lymph nodes and in lymphoid drainage sites of carcinomas. Clearly benign or malignant lesions can be easily diagnosed by biopsy, clinicopathologic correlation, and the exclusion or establishment of clonal rearrangements.

A significant group of patients present with unusual clinical features, and their biopsies result in pathologic diagnoses that prompt the use of terms such as *atypical* or *suspicious for malignant lymphoma*, leaving the physician with incomplete information on how to treat the condition. Some disorders manifest with clinical features that suggest a malignant process but show characteristic histologic features that correlate with a benign outcome. Most of these processes are related to an abnormal immune response to some inciting stimulus. Others may sometimes result in the death of the patient, by progression to malignancy or by damage to or by the immune system. Accurate diagnosis requires careful correlation of immunohistologic, karyotypic, virologic, and genotypic analyses with the clinical findings. The more commonly encountered "atypical lymphoproliferations" related to viruses, drugs, genetic abnormalities, and unknown causes will be discussed (Table 90–1).

VIRUS-ASSOCIATED ATYPLCAL LYMPHOPROLIFERATIONS

Epstein–Barr Virus: Fatal Infectious Mononucleosis

Biologic Aspects

The prototypical cause of atypical lymphoproliferations is the ubiquitous Epstein–Barr virus (EBV).[5] EBV causes the well-characterized clinical syndrome of infectious mononucleosis (IM) (Chapter 54).[6] This discussion will not specifically address IM but will cover those lesions that fall outside the usual clinical spectrum of self-limited IM.

EBV, a large herpesvirus (172,000 base pairs), preferentially infects B cells in humans and causes lifelong infection.[6,7] The key to understanding atypical responses to EBV involves the relationship that is established between the virus and the immune system after primary infection.[8] Primary infection by EBV results in two main responses, depending on the age of the individual or the maturity of the immune system.[8] If the primary infection occurs in early childhood, the immune response and clinical symptoms are almost always silent, but about two-thirds of infected older children and adults will develop IM.[6] Once infected by EBV, an individual maintains a lifelong relationship with the virus in which a virus-driven B-cell proliferation is kept in check by the host immune surveillance. A low level of virus production occurs in the oropharyngeal region by unknown mechanisms; approximately 1 in 10^6 B cells in peripheral blood carries EBV.[9,10] The intimate association of oropharyngeal epithelium with oropharyngeal lymphoid tissue results in a constant cycle of circulating infected B cells. Disease results when the immune system is depressed, by iatrogenic means or by concurrent infections with other agents (Fig. 90–1).[8] The resulting immune suppression allows escape of EBV-infected B cells and resultant lymphoproliferation.[5,7,8,11] The self-limited course of IM contrasts with the atypical responses that can occur, such as fulminant infectious mononucleosis (FIM).[8,11] In FIM, the EBV nonspecific response, primarily the cellular response, is uncontrolled. FIM is characterized by extensive infiltration of parenchymal organs by polymorphous lymphoid cells (Fig. 90–2), primarily $CD8^+$ cells in various degrees of transformation and histiocytes with surprisingly few B cells.[8,11] The cells infected by EBV in FIM are usually T cells and may become clonal.[12,13] The extent of T-cell and histiocytic reactions in FIM is often dramatic and hemophagocytosis is common.[8,11–14]

Epidemiology

FIM occurs in approximately 1 in 3000 IM cases, or approximately 40 cases annually in the United States.[5,8] The explosive lymphoproliferation that occurs in FIM mimics that in certain hematologic neoplasms, such as lymphoid leukemia, and can obscure recognition

Table 90–1 Infectious and Immunodeficiency Causes of Atypical Lymphoid Hyperplasia

Infectious
Cat-scratch fever
Epstein–Barr virus
Human herpes virus-8
Human immunodeficiency virus
Human T-cell leukemia/lymphoma virus
Postvaccination
Toxoplasmosis
Primary Immunodeficiency
Ataxia telangiectasia
Autoimmune lymphoproliferative syndrome
Bruton agammaglobulinemia
Common variable immunodeficiency
Severe combined immunodeficiency
Wiskott–Aldrich syndrome
X-linked lymphoproliferative disease
Autoimmune
Rheumatoid arthritis
Sjögren syndrome
Systemic lupus erythematosus
Unknown
Angioimmunoblastic lymphadenopathy
Castleman disease
Kikuchi disease
Rosai–Dorfman disease

of FIM as a cause of death.[5,8,11–14] The median age at presentation is 13 years, with a 1 : 1 male/female ratio.[14]

Clinical Manifestations

Patients who progress to FIM initially present with the usual signs and symptoms of IM, including fever, sore throat, malaise, anorexia, nausea, vomiting, and a maculopapular rash, but these symptoms are usually more extensive than those of IM.[8,14] Patients initially present with an atypical lymphocytosis but subsequently develop severe, persistent pancytopenia, hepatic dysfunction resulting in fulminant hepatitis, meningoencephalitis, and various degrees of myocarditis.[5,8,11–15] The development of hepatic dysfunction, often with coagulation abnormalities secondary to liver failure or disseminated intravascular coagulation, and pancytopenia is an ominous sign, as are other signs of hemophagocytic syndromes, such as hypofibrinogenemia and elevated triglycerides.[8,11,15,16] The course and progression of the disease are variable, ranging from presentation in multiorgan failure developing over hours to persistent or recurring symptoms of IM for months.

Laboratory Diagnosis

The diagnoses of EBV-associated atypical lymphoproliferations and of FIM can be difficult, because the usual EBV antibody responses may be lacking or unusually high, and the clinical picture may resemble an acute leukemia, another malignancy, or overwhelming sepsis.[5,8,11–14] Reactive lymphocytes may be seen in the peripheral blood. An accurate diagnosis may require performing serologic studies

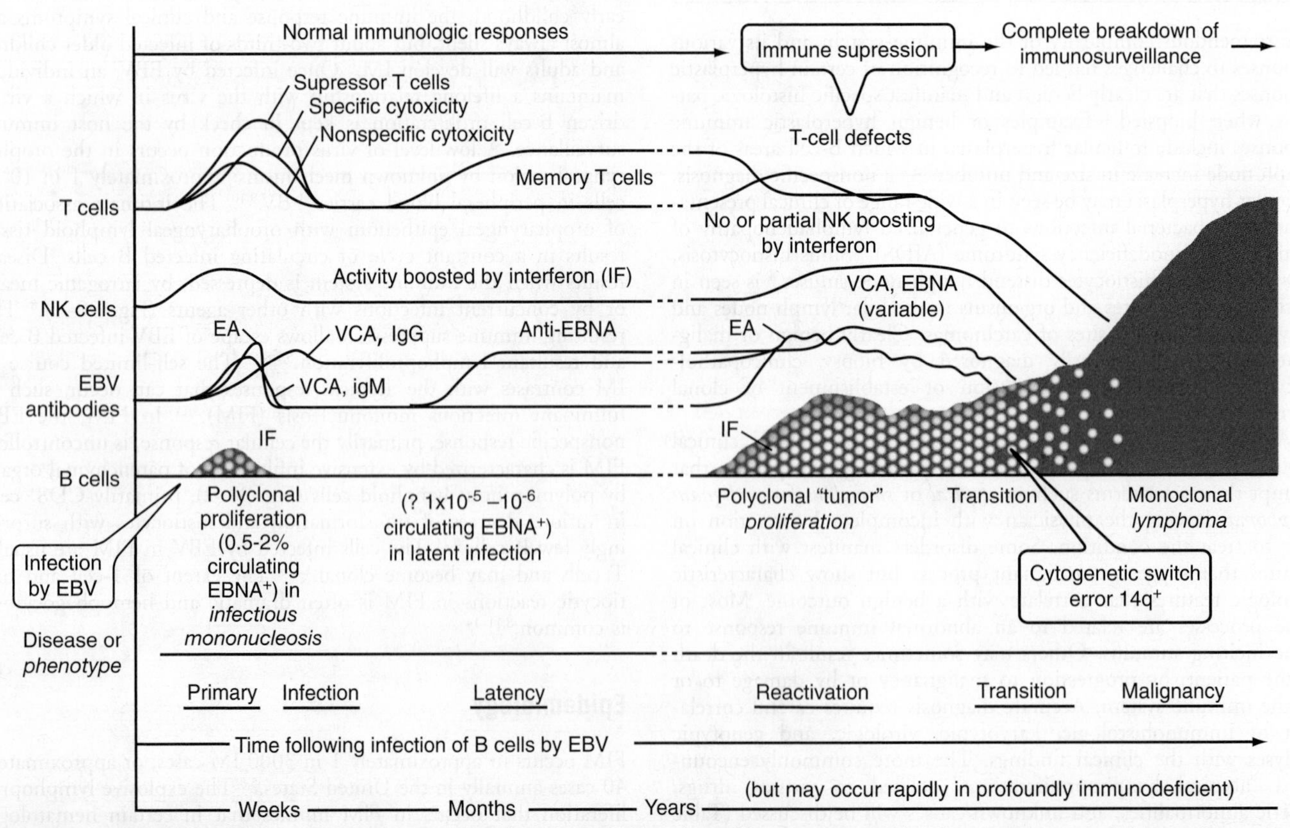

Figure 90–1 The EBV-immune system relationship and the development of lymphoproliferations associated with various immune deficits or diseases.

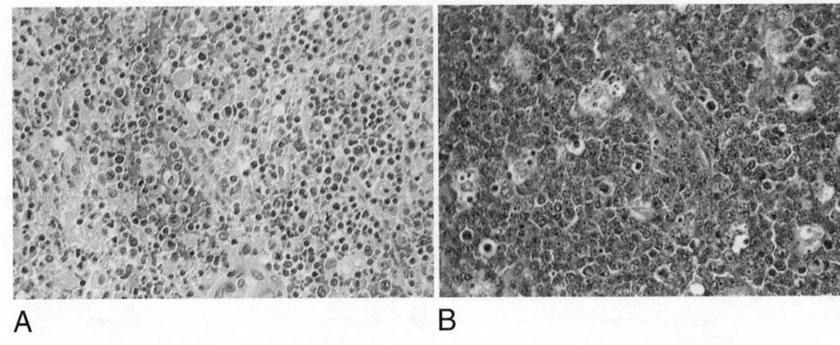

Figure 90–2 A, Florid fatal infectious mononucleosis involving a lymph node shows a polymorphous, immunoblastic infiltrate (H & E × 400). **B,** Burkitt type non-Hodgkin lymphoma, in contrast, shows a monomorphous infiltrate (H & E × 400).

of the EBV-specific antibodies to the viral capsid antigen (VCA), early antigen (EA), and EBV nuclear-associated antigen (EBNA). In situ hybridization is more sensitive than immunohistochemical staining of lymphoid tissue for latent membrane protein (LMP)-1.[17] Molecular analyses, such as Southern blot hybridization can be used to determine clonal integration, and quantitative viral load can be performed by polymerase chain reaction (PCR) studies.[18–20] Because FIM is rare, a search for a heritable immune deficiency in family members is mandatory.[8,11,15,16] Although FIM is the most common manifestation of males affected with X-linked lymphoproliferative disease (XLP), FIM can occur outside the context of XLP.[5,8,14–16] Clinically, FIM is indistinguishable from other viral-associated hemophagocytic syndromes (VAHS), familial hemophagocytic lymphohistiocytosis, and the accelerated phase of Chédiak–Higashi syndrome.[8,11,16]

Therapy

Treating FIM is difficult and often unsuccessful, with a median survival time of approximately 4 weeks.[15,21] Antiviral drugs, immunoglobulins, IL-2, IFNα, IFNγ, plasmapheresis, corticosteroids, and most cytotoxic drugs have been ineffective.[8,11] There is one report of 20 patients with IM and hemophagocytosis, without severe symptoms of FIM, successfully treated with chloroquine.[22] The most consistent success in the treatment of FIM is with the early use of etoposide, which reduces the activity of stimulated macrophages in vitro, in combinations with intravenous immunoglobulins or immunosuppression with corticosteroids and cyclosporin A or tacrolimus (FK506).[11,21,23–25] Therapy may be required for 6 to 12 months. These patients are profoundly immunocompromised from their disease and the therapy. Therefore, a successful outcome is dependent on the control of FIM symptoms, while preventing and treating life-threatening infectious complications. Even with remission of symptoms, recurrences are common and for those cases, the prognosis is poor. Allogeneic blood/marrow transplantation (BMT) is recommended for patients where the disease can be controlled and results in cures in up to half of the patients.[25–27]

Prognosis

Patients who develop FIM succumb to severe and progressive multiorgan failure, apparently brought on by anomalous cytotoxic T-cell and natural killer cell activities, which nonselectively destroy uninfected hepatocytes, bone marrow elements, skin, and other organs during the unrestricted polyclonal immune response initiated by the EBV infection.[5,8,11,13–15] Until recently, the median survival was 4 weeks.[15,21] However, with immunochemotherapy with etopside and allogeneic BMT as many as half of patients can survive.[25–27]

OTHER PRESENTATIONS OF EPSTEIN–BARR VIRUS LYMPHOPROLIFERATIONS

Rarely, elderly patients, malnourished patients, and those with cancer also develop EBV-associated atypical lymphoproliferations.[28] These patients usually have a secondary immunodeficiency. Most of them will have had a prior infection with EBV and will have achieved a virus-immune system balance before acquiring the immune deficiency, which then allows the virus to escape the defective immune surveillance mechanisms. Lymphoproliferations ranging from IM to FIM to overt lymphoma (see Fig. 90–2B) can then occur.[5,14] Patients with the acquired immunodeficiency syndrome also experience virus reactivation because the T-cell arm of the immune system is selectively attacked by the AIDS virus, resulting in loss of control over the persistent EBV infection.[5] Various lesions, including polyclonal immunoblastic proliferations, hairy leukoplakia of the tongue, leiomyosarcoma and lymphoma have all been associated with EBV.[29–31] Children with AIDS often develop lymphoid interstitial pneumonitis resulting from EBV-induced polyclonal B-cell proliferation.[32] Highly active antiretroviral therapy (HAART) has reduced the incidence and improved the outcome for HIV patients with lymphoma.[33–35]

CYTOMEGALOVIRUS

Cytomegalovirus (CMV), also a herpesvirus, can cause the mononucleosis syndrome but is usually latent until unmasked by immune deficiency, pregnancy, multiple drug exposures, or immune suppression. CMV causes less of a lymphoproliferative response than EBV, and activation often results in more extensive inflammation and tissue necrosis.[36] Diagnosis is made by appropriate serologic studies, by identification of characteristic nuclear inclusions in cytologic or tissue biopsy specimens (Fig. 90–3A) immunoperoxidase studies (see Fig. 90–3B), or by molecular techniques, including in situ hybridization and PCR.[36,37] Therapy includes the use of current antiviral agents, such as ganciclovir, foscarnet, or cidofovir.

VIRUS-ASSOCIATED HEMOPHAGOCYTIC SYNDROME

Introduction and Epidemiology

Virus-associated hemophagocytic syndrome (VAHS) is also included in the spectrum of atypical lymphoproliferations and usually occurs in the setting of immunodeficiency.[15,25,38] The syndrome was originally described in patients with viral infections but has subsequently been encountered in patients with fungal, bacterial, and parasitic infections; in immunodeficient patients; and in patients with T-cell lymphomas.[38] VAHS has now been classified as a secondary form of type-II histiocytic disease, termed histiocytic lymphohistiocytosis

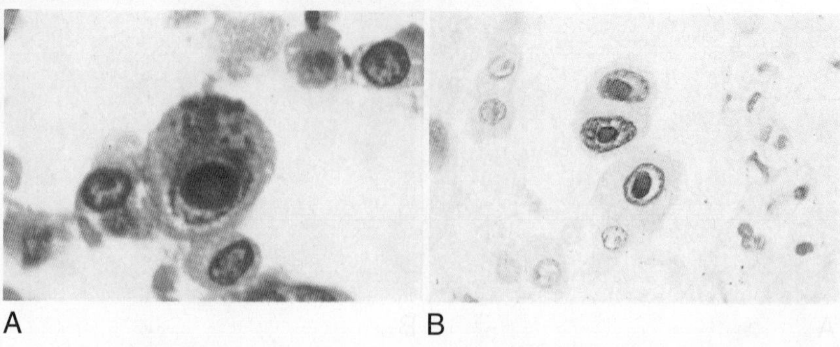

Figure 90–3 Cytomegalic inclusion disease. **A,** Characteristic cytomegalovirus (CMV) nuclear inclusion and cytoplasmic inclusions are evident (H & E × 1000). **B,** Immunoperoxidase with anti-CMV confirms the presence of cytomegalovirus (dilute hematoxylin counterstain × 400).

(HLH).[25] A familial form of HLH also occurs, called familial erythrophagocytic lymphohistiocytosis (FEL), which is an autosomal recessive condition, and has been associated with mutations in the genes encoding perforin, Munc 13–4, and syntaxin.[16] Evidence of viral infection does not rule out a genetic etiology of HLH.

Clinical Manifestations

Approximately 80% of patients with FIM exhibit clinicopathologic findings consistent with VAHS.[11,15,39] Patients with VAHS present with hepatosplenomegaly, abnormal liver function tests, fever, rashes, lymphadenopathy, coagulopathy, and pancytopenia, but may also present with central nervous system and pulmonary abnormalities.[11,16,39]

Laboratory Diagnosis

Early in the course of VAHS, the bone marrow appears normal, but myeloid hyperplasia, lymphocytic infiltration, cellular necrosis, and increased macrophages subsequently appear.[39] Marked sinus histiocytosis with prominent erythrophagocytosis[39] (Fig. 90–4) is evident throughout the reticuloendothelial system of affected patients, and hyperplasia of the spleen can result in splenic weights in excess of 1 kg.[39] Histologic examination of lymph nodes, especially in HLH, shows lymphoid proliferation early in the disease, which is followed by lymphoid depletion at later stages. At necropsy, activated macrophages exhibiting phagocytosis, can be seen infiltrating areas of hemorrhagic necrosis.[15,16,39] The disease often terminates in a hemophagocytic syndrome with pancytopenia, jaundice, and marked erythrophagocytosis.

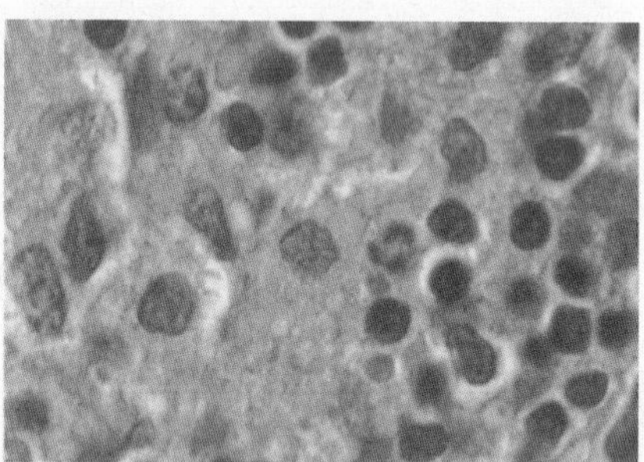

Figure 90–4 Virus-associated hemophagocytic syndrome. Extensive histiocytic erythrophagocytosis is evident in sinusoids of the lymph node. Histiocyte cytoplasm is distended by numerous red blood cell "ghosts" (H & E × 400).

RETROVIRUSES AND LYMPHOPROLIFERATIONS

Human Immunodeficiency Virus

During the past decade, the RNA retroviruses have been implicated in a spectrum of lymphoproliferations. The AIDS retrovirus, human immunodeficiency virus (HIV), does not transform lymphocytes but selectively destroys helper T cells.[40] During acute HIV infection, a mononucleosis-like syndrome often occurs, and the virus can cause chronic, persistent lymphadenopathy characterized by florid follicular hyperplasia, follicular lysis, or follicular involution.[40] In situ hybridization of lymph nodes will demonstrate HIV sequences. Often EBV-positive cells will be increased 5- to 10-fold in lymphoid tissues of HIV-infected patients compared with those of non-HIV-infected patients. The T-cell immunodeficiency caused by HIV permits opportunistic viral, bacterial, protozoal, and fungal infections.

HUMAN T-CELL LEUKEMIA/LYMPHOMA VIRUS TYPE I

The most extensively studied transforming retrovirus is the human T-cell leukemia/lymphoma virus type I (HTLV-I), which is implicated in the endemic form of adult acute T-cell leukemia/lymphoma (ATL) in Japan and the Caribbean basin.[41] This virus has the capacity to selectively immortalize T cells in vitro, but HTLV-I infection alone is insufficient to cause malignancy, because only 1 in 2500 chronic viral carriers develop the T-cell malignancies after a long latent period.[41] HTLV-I infection is transmitted during sexual intercourse or by blood transfusion. The viral infection probably increases the likelihood of further cytogenetic events by stimulating T-cell lymphoproliferation. Seropositive asymptomatic carriers of the virus exhibit subtle signs of immunodeficiency.[41] Those who progress to ATL have HTLV-l-positive serology, generalized lymphadenopathy, hepatosplenomegaly, skin lesions, and distinct involvement of peripheral blood by a spectrum of malignant T cells ranging from small lymphocytes to bizarre hyperlobated forms.[41] Not all patients present with a leukemic phase. The prognosis for ATL patients is poor. If untreated, the median survival is weeks and even with chemotherapy expected survival is only months to a couple of years.[42] Of the many HTLV-infected patients who do not develop ATL, most are asymptomatic, but a small group may develop an early benign transient lymphocytosis; if subacute or chronic lymphocytosis persists, the risk of progression to ATL increases.

DRUG-ASSOCIATED LYMPHOPROLIFERATIONS

Although some drugs permit activation of latent viral infections such as EBV by causing immunosuppression, other drugs cause atypical lymphoid responses by a hypersensitivity reaction or by unknown mechanisms (Table 90–2). This results in lymphadenopathy mimicking lymphoma or skin lesions mimicking mycosis fungoides. Diphenylhydantoin (Dilantin) is a rare but well-documented cause of such responses.[43,44] The clinical presentation is similar to that of a viral infection and includes fever, rash, lymphadenopathy, and eosinophilia. Acquired immunoglobulin A deficiency may develop. The symptoms usually abate when the drug is stopped. The lymph node pathology may contain florid follicular hyperplasia, or it may be similar to that in infectious mononucleosis or paracortical expansion by a polymorphous immunoblastic infiltrate, which is sometimes mistaken for lymphoma.[43,44] Focal necrosis and Reed–Sternberg-like

Table 90–2 Drug-Associated Lymphadenopathy and Lymphoid Proliferations in the Skin

	Lymphadenopathy	Skin Lesion
EBV Proliferation Associated		
Corticosteroids	X	
Cyclosporine	X	
FK506	X	
Methotrexate	X	
Antithymocyte globulin	X	
Azathioprine	X	
Hypersensitivity or Unknown Mechanism		
Dilantin	X	X
Carbamazepine	X	X
Cyclosporine		X
Gleevec		X

cells may be evident. Hodgkin disease and non-Hodgkin lymphoma have been reported in association with diphenylhydantoin therapy.[44] Other hyperplastic lymphoid responses to drugs have been reported, including a hypersensitivity response to carbamazepine[45] that produces immunoblasts, which may be mistaken for peripheral T-cell lymphoma.[46–48] The immunosuppressive drugs, including cyclosporine, steroids, antilymphocyte globulin, tacrolimus, and cytotoxic agents usually unmask latent viral infections. Drug-induced atypical lymphoid infiltrates in the skin mimicking mycosis fungoides have been described with diphenylhydantoin, cyclosporine, and, most recently, imatimib.[49–51]

POSTTRANSPLANT LYMPHOPROLIFERATIVE DISORDERS

Blood/marrow (BMT) and solid organ transplant (SOT) recipients are exposed to a variety of immunosuppressive agents, including prednisone, antimetabolites (azathioprine, methotrexate, and or mycophenolate mofetil) polyclonal antilymphocyte globulin, monoclonal antibodies (including anti-CD3, anti-CD25, etc), calcineurin inhibitors (cyclosporine, tacrolimus, etc), and/or mTOR inhibitors, such as rapamycin. These patients are at increased risk for malignancy, lymphoproliferative disease being most common following BMT and second only to nonmelanomatous skin cancer following SOT. Posttransplant lymphoproliferative disease (PTLD) includes predominantly atypical B-cell lymphoproliferations and, rarely, Hodgkin disease and T-cell lymphomas.[52–55] This discussion will be largely confined to the EBV-positive B-cell PTLDs.

Epidemiology

Over 90% of early (<1-year posttransplant) PTLDs are EBV-positive, whereas EBV is less frequently associated in late (>2 years) PTLDs.[56–58] The incidence of PTLD correlates with low T-cell immunity against EBV post-BMT[59] and in young children following SOT, which likely reflects EBV-naïve patients acquiring EBV infection.[60] Among bone marrow transplant recipients, those receiving T cell-depleted bone marrow allografts or anti-T cell therapy appear to be at particularly high risk for EBV-associated lymphoproliferation.[56] The prevalence and the posttransplantation interval that precedes development of PTLD vary with the type of organ transplanted and the immunosuppressive agents administered, though EBV naivety pretransplant and therefore young age appear to be the strongest risk factors for PTLD development.[57]

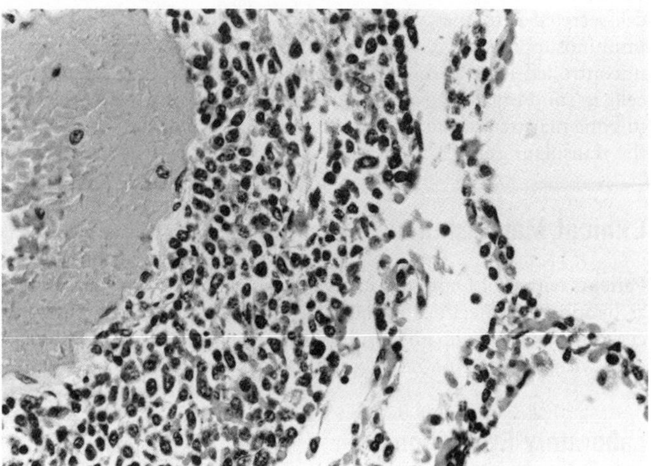

Figure 90–5 Posttransplant lymphoproliferative disorder, polymorphous, expanding the perivascular space (H & E × 200).

Table 90–3 Categories of Posttransplant Lymphoproliferative Disease*

Early
Plasmacytic hyperplasia Infectious mononucleosis-like disease
Polymorphic Monomorphic
B cell
Diffuse large B-cell lymphoma Burkitt and Burkitt-like lymphomas Plasma cell myeloma Plasmacytoma-like lesions
T cell
Peripheral T-cell lymphoma, not otherwise specified Hodgkin lymphoma and Hodgkin lymphoma-like lesions

HL, Hodgkin lymphoma; PTLD, posttransplant lymphoproliferative disease.
*Adapted from Jaffe ES, Harris NL, Stein H, et al: Pathology and Genetics of Tumours of Haematopoietic and Lymphoid Tissues. Lyon, IARC Press, 2001, p 264.

Biology and Molecular Aspects

These atypical lymphoproliferations can be aggressive with continued immunosuppression, even when polyclonal or oligoclonal, as defined by immunoperoxidase in situ hybridization or gene rearrangement studies. The clonal ambiguity has led to difficulties in diagnosis, nomenclature, and therapy.[61,62] A classification of PTLD, by Knowles, describes three main subgroups: plasmacytic hyperplasias, polymorphous PTLDs (Fig. 90–5), and monomorphous PTLDs, which include lymphoma and multiple myeloma.[63] This classification system is reflected in the recent WHO classification of hematologic malignancies, which includes PTLD (Table 90–3).[3] The monomorphous PTLDs have a higher incidence of clonal heavy-chain or light-chain immunoglobulin gene rearrangements. However, this subgroup also has a low incidence of chromosomal translocations and mutations in p53, compared with non-transplant-related lymphomas.[63] Deletions in LMP-1 do not predict for an aggressive tumor.[64] It has been proposed that bcl-6 mutations predict for poor survival; however, this finding has yet to be confirmed.[65]

The pathogenesis of PTLD is related to a disruption of the host's EBV immune surveillance by immunosuppression (see Fig. 90–1). During the first 6 months after transplant, the cytotoxic T-lymphocyte response to EBV is often absent.[59,66] In addition, patients on immunosuppression, such as cyclosporine, have an imbalance of T cell-secreted cytokines, favoring B-cell proliferation.[67] Therefore, if immunosuppression is continued, EBV-infected B cells proliferate uncontrolled. The B-cell origin appears to be predominantly host cells in solid organ transplant patients[68] but are usually donor origin in bone marrow transplant patients.[68] The source of the virus is often the transplant graft.[69,70]

Clinical Manifestations

Patients with PTLD present in several ways: single mass lesions, such as lymphoma, infectious mononucleosis with tonsillar enlargement, cervical lymphadenopathy or hepatitis, or both, or a septic appearance with fever but no radiologically detectable mass.[52,61,62,71]

Laboratory Evaluation

Radiology studies may reveal a mass, a miliary pattern of PTLD may be seen in the lungs, or there may be no lesion at all. Peripheral blood will sometimes reveal circulating plasmacytoid lymphocytes or plasma cells. Quantitative measurements of EBV load in the peripheral blood often rise before the rapid development of PTLD lesions.[72,73] However, caution is advised as some patients do not develop increased levels of EBV and the diagnosis of PTLD, therefore, cannot always be predicted.[74] Tissue biopsy should be performed for immunophenotyping and in situ hybridization for EBV sequences, because LMP-1 protein will be negative in 25% of cases.[17] Typically, the lymphoid tissue is composed of plasmacytoid B cells, with few T cells and often regional areas of necrosis. Distinguishing between a polyclonal and a monoclonal PTLD often requires lymphoid receptor gene analysis, because up to 50% of PTLDs do not express surface immunoglobulin.[61]

Therapy and Prognosis

Mortality rates among patients with PTLD are as high as 50% to 90%, with about half of patients succumbing to tumor and 30% to 50% dying from treatment-related complications, including allograft rejection, infections, and end organ toxicity from cytotoxic therapies.[56–58,75–77] Successful treatment of PTLD is a therapeutic challenge, in part because of the patients' increased toxicity from chemotherapy, increased susceptibility to life-threatening infections, and the necessity to maintain the allograft, especially with vital organs (heart, lung, or liver). Reduction of immunosuppression is the most widely used approach.[57,78,79] Many times this is sufficient in controlling the disease, especially in localized, polyclonal cases or cases that manifest as infectious mononucleosis. Patients who do not tolerate reduction of immunosuppression (ie, graft rejection), or do not respond to immunosuppression reduction, require more aggressive therapy and have a much poorer prognosis. Antiviral agents (acyclovir or ganciclovir), and intravenous immunoglobulin (IVIG) have been used extensively for the prophylaxis and treatment of PTLD.[57,79] The efficacy of antivirals and IVIG is difficult to assess because reduction of immune suppression is almost always initiated simultaneously.

Surgery or radiotherapy are very effective in curing localized disease, but this represents only a small percentage of patients.[57,79] Monoclonal antibodies are attractive because of the favorable toxicity profile. In the past, anti-CD21 and anti-CD23 and more recently anti-CD20 (rituximab) have been successful in curing PTLD in both the BMT and SOT setting. Response rates with anti-B cell monoclonal antibodies results are variable, with complete response rates ranging from 25% to 75% and overall survival usually approximately 50%.[80–84]

Because virus-specific cytotoxic T cells (CTL) are critical in the control of EBV-driven B-cell proliferations, adoptive T-cell therapy is a logical approach.[85] To overcome potential risks of graft-versus-host disease or rejection, ex vivo generated EBV-specific CTLs have been used. This approach has been very successful at preventing and treating PTLD after BMT without significant GVHD.[86] However, the issue of using adoptive cellular therapy (DLI) in solid organ transplant (SOT) patients with PTLD is complex. First, cadaveric organs are most widely used; therefore, donor leukocytes are often not available and the use of closely matched relatives' leukocytes runs the risk of rejection and GVHD. Recent studies have demonstrated that recipient EBV-specific CTLs can be generated ex vivo and administered safely. As opposed to BMT, following SOT patients receiving EBV-specific CTLs have a less pronounced effect on reduction of viral load in peripheral blood and do not persist, which may necessitate multiple infusions to obtain a remission.[87,88]

The use of chemotherapy for a PTLD does not require waiting for the progression to the standard pathologic criteria for diagnosis of lymphoma because the polymorphous hyperplasia subgroup of PTLD can be equally lethal. Chemotherapy has been efficacious in treating PTLD in some patients. The intensive, multidrug regimens (ie, anthracycline-based) traditionally used to treat high-grade lymphomas are usually immunosuppressive enough to maintain the organ graft, but treatment-related death resulting from toxicity and infection has been in the 30% to 50% range in most series and the 1-year survival rate is only 40% to 45%.[75,76,89,90] A low-dose chemotherapy approach has demonstrated little toxicity and approximately 67% disease-free survival in children with PTLD following SOT.[91]

ATYPICAL LYMPHOPROLIFERATIVE DISEASE IN PATIENTS WITH AUTOIMMUNE DISORDERS

Other disorders of immune regulation have an increased prevalence of lymphoid neoplasia. Patients with autoimmune collagen-vascular disease (ie, rheumatoid arthritis) can develop non-Hodgkin lymphomas, which often arise in the setting of reactive lymphadenopathy.[92,93] These patients develop atypical lymphoid hyperplasia and non-Hodgkin lymphoma during methotrexate or azathioprine therapy.[94–96] Case reports describe spontaneous resolution on discontinuance of methotrexate.[95,96] Individuals with Sjögren syndrome also show a progression of lymphoid hyperplasia to frank neoplasia, with a risk 44 times that observed in the general population.[97]

GENETICALLY LINKED IMMUNODEFICIENCY AND LYMPHOPROLIFERATIONS

Subsequently, the triad of autoimmunity, immunodeficiency, and lymphoproliferation has been defined in an increasingly large group of patients with inherited and acquired immunodeficiency disorders. Below are described some of the more well characterized.

THE X-LINKED LYMPHOPROLIFERATIVE DISEASE

XLP disease illustrates the spectrum of lymphoproliferations that can occur in hereditary immune deficiencies—ranging from benign or fatal IM to non-Hodgkin lymphoma.[5,8,12–15] After EBV infection, chronic or fatal IM, acquired hypogammaglobulinemia, or agammaglobulinemia, pure red cell aplasia, necrotizing lymphoid vasculitis, or non-Hodgkin lymphoma ensues.[15,21]

Biologic and Molecular Aspects

The gene responsible for XLP, SH2D1A, was discovered in 1998.[98–100] The SH2D1A gene codes for a protein of 128 amino acid residues that consists of an SH2 domain and a 25-amino acid C-terminal tail.[98,99] SH2D1A is expressed throughout thymocyte development, as well as in $CD4^+$ and $CD8^+$ peripheral T cells.[100] The function of the SH2D1A protein appears to be in the regulation of immune responses. The SH2D1A protein interacts with several proteins, including SLAM (CD150, signaling lymphocyte activating protein), and has also been called SLAM-associated protein (SAP).[99] Other proteins SH2D1A/SAP has been demonstrated to interact with are members of the CD2 superfamily of molecules, including CD2, CD4, CD583, CD84, Ly-9, 2B4, and with a new family of RasGAP adapter proteins such as p62Dok (Dok-1, downstream of kinases-1), p56Dok (Dok-2), and Dok-3.[101–105] The immunologic effects of SH2D1A interactions with these proteins is under investigation. Recent studies from sh12da-deficient mice demonstrate a phenotype that recapitulates that observed in affected males, that is, an exuberant and lethal CD8 T-cell response following lymphocytic choriomeningitis virus (LCMV).[106] In vitro studies have demonstrated that CD8 cytotoxic T cells from XLP males are deficient in killing autologous EBV B-cell lines.[107] As well, recent studies with sh2d1a-deficient mice over time develop problems with immunoglobulin class switching and defective memory humoral immune responses and ultimately hypogammaglobulinemia even without LCMV infection, again analogous to what is observed in affected males.[108] To date, however, it has not been demonstrated that sh2d1a-deficient mice have a high incidence of lymphoma or cytopenias.

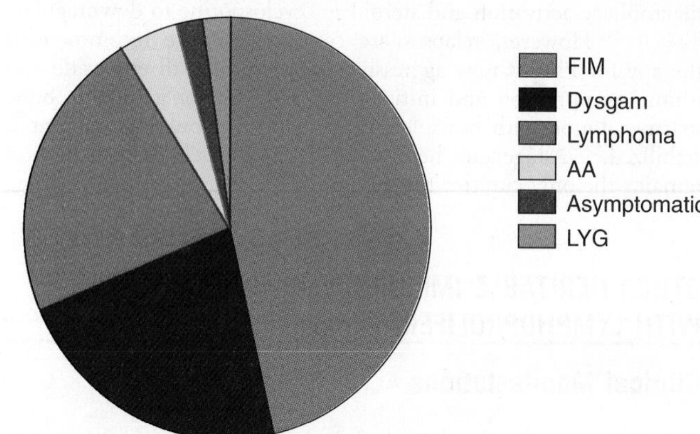

Figure 90–6 Frequency of phenotypes in X-linked lymphoproliferative disease. AA, Aplastic anemia; Dysgam, dysgammaglobulinemia; FIM, fulminant infectious mononucleosis; LYG, lymphoid granulomatosis/vasculitis.

CLINICAL MANIFESTATIONS

Initially, three phenotypes were described in XLP patients and these continue to characterize most patients: fulminant infectious mononucleosis (FIM or EBV-HLH), malignant lymphoma (LPD), and dysgammaglobulinemia.[15] Less commonly reported manifestations include disorders such as vasculitis, pulmonary lymphomatoid granulomatosis, and hematologic cytopenias, including aplastic anemia and pure red cell aplasia.[15,21] The "disease state" is capricious because it may feature a single phenotype, or two or more phenotypes, which may develop sequentially in susceptible individuals.[21] Reflecting the ubiquitous nature of EBV infection, FIM is the most common XLP phenotype affecting approximately 50% of patients. FIM or EBV-HLH observed in XLP is indistinguishable clinically from disease observed in patients without XLP and treatment and prognosis is identical.[8,11–16,27] Other than FIM, a lymphoproliferative disorder (LPD) develops in approximately 25% of XLP patients. Most lymphomas are of B-cell phenotype and are characterized by a small noncleaved (Burkitt) or diffuse large-cell histology.[109] Karyotypic analysis has not been extensively performed; however, the t(8;14) associated with Burkitt lymphoma is rare.[110,111] Approximately 10% of LPDs are not of B-cell phenotype.[21] There have been a small number of patients with Hodgkin disease or T-cell lymphoproliferative disorders, including lymphoblastic lymphoma, lymphomatoid granulomatosis, or angiocentric immunoproliferative lesions.[112] As in other immunodeficiencies, the role of EBV in the LPD of XLP is unclear, because about one half of the boys with LPD have no evidence of prior EBV infection, and EBV is detectable in only 25% of tumor specimens.[21]

Initially, it was believed that males affected with XLP only present with symptoms after primary EBV infection. Although IM is by definition caused by EBV, other XLP phenotypes can developed in EBV-seronegative patients.[21,113] Data from the XLP Registry demonstrated that at least 12.5% of affected boys will present with symptoms of XLP before exposure to EBV.[21] There is no difference of age at onset of clinical symptoms between males that have or have not been previously exposed to EBV.[21] Therefore, prevention of EBV infection in boys with XLP will not avert clinical manifestations. It is also curious that approximately 40% of the boys develop FIM after primary infection with EBV, but 60% never develop FIM but instead dysgammaglobulinemia, hematologic cytopenias, and a few have no symptoms at all.[21] These data suggest that other genetic or environmental factors, or both, influence host susceptibility to EBV and are important in the determination of the clinical phenotype of XLP. The disease should be suspected in families in which maternally related boys develop FIM, acquired hypogammaglobulinemia, agammaglobulinemia, or malignant lymphoma (Fig. 90–6).

The main differential diagnosis in these patients involves lymphoma versus florid IM. Patients who develop malignant lymphoma usually present with discrete mass(es), often extranodal, with or without dissemination at the time of diagnosis.[112] In contrast, patients with severe or fatal IM have a disseminated lymphoproliferation that may or may not present with generalized lymphadenopathy but does involve lymphocytic infiltration of multiple organ sites, including the skin, liver, spleen, lung, bone marrow, and brain.[11,15] Although most boys will not have a detectable immune defect prior to EBV infection, it has been shown that the cytotoxic T cells from affected males have a defect in killing autologous EBV-transformed cell lines,[108] and all boys over time will evidentially develop dysgammaglobulinemia even if not infected with EBV.[15,21]

LABORATORY EVALUATION

Before the isolation of SH2D1A, the gene known to be absent or mutated in XLP, it was often difficult to make a diagnosis of XLP based solely on clinical or laboratory features.[15] Now the diagnosis can more easily be made on the basis of the identification of an abnormal SH2D1A gene sequence or protein expression.[21,114] One might predict that mutations that delete the XLP gene or truncate the protein would be more likely to be associated with a severe phenotype, whereas missense mutations would occur preferentially in mildly affected patients. However, it is not uncommon to observe different phenotypes with identical mutations, even within the same family. No significant differences have been observed in the phenotypes or severity of disease based on the type (missense, nonsense, truncating) or localization of SH2D1A mutations. The age of onset of clinical manifestations of XLP varied considerably, from younger than 1 to 40 years, and there was no correlation with the type of mutation. Therefore, genetic analysis does not predict the phenotype or severity of disease.[21]

Therapy and Prognosis

Complete remissions (CR) at rates as high as 80% can be achieved in XLP boys presenting with lymphoma using standard lymphoma protocols; however, relapses or other manifestations (ie, hypogammaglobulinemia) are very common.[21] Boys with dysgammaglobulinemia receive monthly IgG infusions, but this does not prevent EBV infection and its sequelae. Several boys have developed FIM and died while receiving IgG supplementation.[15] Because FIM is essentially indistinguishable from other hemophagocytic syndromes (ie, HLH) it is now recommended that boys receive aggressive chemotherapy, to quell the immunologic anarchy of uncontrolled T-lymphocytes and macrophages, with etoposide (VP-16) to quench macrophage activation and steroids or cyclosporine to downregulate T cells.[25] However, relapses are common, so the recommended therapy for FIM is now aggressive intervention with etoposide and immunosuppression and initiation of a search for a suitable bone marrow donor, with transplantation performed once the patient is stabilized.[27] Allogeneic hematopoietic stem cell transplantation remains the only curative therapy for XLP.[24]

OTHER HERITABLE IMMUNODEFICIENCY DISEASES WITH LYMPHOPROLIFERATIONS

Clinical Manifestations

A complete review of genetically linked diseases manifesting lymphoproliferation is beyond the scope of this discussion, but certain conditions have been sufficiently characterized to allow recognition (see Table 90–1). Both reactive lymphoproliferations and malignant transformation can be observed in these patients and more extensive evaluations, such as clonality and molecular genetics for oncogene activation may be required. As mentioned previously, there are genetic immunodeficiencies that primarily present as HLH, that is, perforin, munc13–4, and syntaxin 11.[16] One recent report suggests that perforin deficiency also increases the risk of lymphoma.[115] Chediak–Higashi syndrome also can manifest as an "accelerated phase" following EBV infection, which is indistinguishable from other EBV–HLH and patients are at increased risk for lymphoma.[16,116] Autoimmune lymphoproliferative syndrome (ALPS) is a recently described entity in which patients present as early as infancy with generalized lymphadenopathy, hepatosplenomegaly, hypergammaglobulinemia, and usually B-cell lymphocytosis. The autoimmune characteristics include hemolytic anemia, Guillain–Barrè syndrome, urticarial rash, glomerulonephritis, and idiopathic thrombocytopenia.[117] Recently, it has been demonstrated that a significant number of patients diagnosed with Evan syndrome have fas mutations or ALPS.[118] The risk of developing lymphoma, both Hodgkin and non-Hodgkin, is significantly increased for the life of patients with ALPS.[119] As in XLP, many of the lymphomas in patients with inherited immunodeficiencies are B-cell phenotype and associated with EBV, but this is not universal, suggesting the defect lies in more than an inability to control a viral infection, but in immunosurveillance against aberrant lymphoproliferation in general.[116]

Epidemiology

The incidence of cancer is greatly increased in patients with genetic immunodeficiencies, and lymphoproliferations are common.[116] Patients with primarily antibody deficiencies, such as X-linked agammaglobulinemia (XLA) and combined variable immune deficiency (CVID), also have an increased risk of epithelial cancers and adenocarcinomas.[116] Lymphomas predominate in diseases with a significant T-cell defect, such as XLP, severe combined immunodeficiency (SCID), Wiskott–Aldrich syndrome, ataxia-telangiectasia, X-linked hyper-IgM (CD40 ligand deficiency), Chediak–Higashi syndrome, perforin deficiencies, and autoimmune lymphoproliferative syndrome (fas deficiency).[116,118]

In autoimmune lymphoproliferative syndrome (ALPS), the pathology is characterized by an expansion of double-negative T cells ($CD3^+$, $CD4^-$, $CD8^-$) in lymph nodes, accompanied by a polymorphous infiltrate composed of plasma cells, small lymphocytes, and immunoblasts. Florid follicular hyperplasia is frequently present. Reduced apoptosis and an increased percentage of proliferative cells are seen.[119] The etiology of most patients with ALPS is impairment of apoptosis due to inherited heterozygous (Type O) or heterozygous mutations (Type 1) in the fas gene (CD95), or fas ligand.[116,120,121] Rare cases have been described of ALPS type II with mutations in caspase 10 or capase 8. In Type III, wherein no germline mutation of buccal mucosa has been identified,[121,122] heterozygous fas mutations have been observed in double-negative ($CD4^-$, $CD8^-$) T cells.[123]

Laboratory Evaluation

The diagnosis of lymphoma can be difficult in these patients, who frequently have reactive lymphoid hyperplasia or chronic granulomatous inflammation. Demonstration of EBV in lesions is helpful in evaluating a lymphoid lesion, but is not synonymous with lymphoma. EBV-positive cells can be found in greater than normal numbers in benign nodes, and EBV is not found in all the lymphomas.[124,125]

Therapy and Prognosis

Although complete remissions can be achieved in these patients, the outcomes for patients with primary immunodeficiencies and lymphoma compared with immunocompetent patients with lymphoma have been poor.[116,126] One reason is death due to chemotherapy toxicities, especially in conditions with DNA repair defects as well, that is, ataxia telangectesia or Bloom syndrome. Deaths due to infections and sepsis are also frequent, and relapses are also common.[116,124,126] Therefore, induction of remission with reduced-intensity or standard-dose chemotherapy followed by correction of the underlying immune defect (ie, allogeneic stem cell transplantation, if a suitable donor can be identified) offers the greatest chance of long-term survival.

ATYPLCAL LYMPHOPROLIFERATIONS OF UNKNOWN CAUSE ANGIOFOLLICULAR LYMPH NODE HYPERPLASIA

Epidemiology

Angiofollicular lymph node hyperplasia (AFH), or Castleman disease, has many other names, including giant lymph node hyperplasia, angiomatous lymphoid hamartoma, lymph node hamartoma, and lymph node hyperplasia of Castleman.[127] There is no gender or age preference, and most patients present with asymptomatic mediastinal masses, which are discovered on routine chest radiographic examinations. There are two types of localized AFH, the more common hyaline vascular (90%) and the plasma cell type (10%).[127]

Multicentric lesions have been identified in a subgroup of patients and may herald a higher risk of subsequent development of overt lymphoma.[127,128] Most reports in the literature favor the concept that the hyaline vascular type of AFH is a reactive chronic lymphoid hyperplasia.[129,130] The plasma cell type is considered to have an inflammatory pathogenesis, through chronic antigenic stimulation (ie, infection) or by an autoimmune mechanism. The plasma cell group tends to affect younger persons and has higher rates of mesenteric and retroperitoneal tumors.[127]

Clinical Manifestations

When symptomatic, the hyaline vascular subgroup of patients present with mass-related symptoms, such as pain, chronic cough, and obstruction. Clinical symptoms associated with the plasma cell type include fever, sweats, weight loss, and fatigue. Patients with multicentric disease can be extremely ill with malaise and cytopenias.[127,128]

Laboratory Evaluation

Associated laboratory abnormalities include anemia, an elevated erythrocyte sedimentation rate, hypergammaglobulinemia, hypoalbuminemia, hyperferritinemia, and hypertransferrinemia.[127] The hyaline-vascular type has a histologic pattern characterized by follicular hyperplasia distributed evenly throughout the lymph node.[127] The follicles are unusually small, and their germinal centers are often penetrated by radial capillaries, which are surrounded by collagen or hyaline material, hence the name (Fig. 90–7).[127,128] The germinal centers are surrounded by multiple concentric layers of lymphocytes (see Fig. 90–7A).[127,129] In the plasma cell type, which is less common (10%) and may represent an earlier stage of the lesion,[127] the germinal centers are larger, the peripheral cuffs of mature lymphocytes are not as prominent, and their interfollicular areas are occupied by extensive sheets of plasma cells, occasionally including some atypical forms (see Fig. 90–7B). Immunohistochemical and gene rearrangement studies have identified clonal cell populations in some cases of multicentric AFH.[131,132]

BIOLOGY

Hypotheses for the causes of Castleman disease have included autoimmunity, disorder of cytokine production, and infection with the human herpes virus-8 (HHV-8). HHV-8, also called Kaposi sarcoma herpes virus (KSHV), has been associated with the multicentric form of Castleman disease in 25% of cases but not in pediatric patients or patients with the more common subtypes.[133,134] Because HHV-8 produces a viral form of the cytokine IL-6, it is relevant to Castleman disease. Experimental and clinical data indicate that IL-6 plays a pivotal role in the biogenesis of multicentric Castleman disease.[135] The hyperplastic germinal centers of these patients have been shown to produce excessive quantities of IL-6.[136]

Therapy

Localized Castleman disease is usually a self-limited process, curable with local surgical resection.[127,135,137,138] After local excision, there is frequently total disappearance of systemic symptoms with only rare local recurrences. Multicentric Castleman disease is a systemic disease associated with an aggressive, often fatal course associated with infectious complications, and a risk of developing malignancies, such as lymphoma or Kaposi sarcoma.[137] The median survival of patients with multicentric Castleman disease has been reported to be 29 months.[135] Twenty-six percent of patients in one series died within the first year of diagnosis.[135] A limited body of information is available regarding the treatment of multicentric Castleman disease.[133,135,139] A reduction in the quantity of involved tissue surgically or by radiation therapy may be an effective strategy to control the systemic signs and symptoms.[135] High doses of corticosteroids have been reported to result in sustained remissions, although continuous high-dose prednisone therapy is frequently required.[135] Chemotherapy with single agents or combination therapy used to treat non-Hodgkin lymphoma has resulted in partial responses, although occasionally patients may enjoy durable complete remissions.[135,140] Alleviation of the systemic manifestations of this disorder has been achieved with an anti-IL-6 monoclonal antibody and a humanized form of an anti-IL-6 receptor antibody.[139,141] Other therapies have included retinoic acid administration and bone marrow transplantation.[142–144] The use of rituximab has also been used with success.[145]

ANGIOIMMUNOBLASTIC LYMPHADENOPATHY WITH DYSPROTEINEMIA IS OFTEN A PERIPHERAL T-CELL LYMPHOMA

Clinical Manifestations

Angioimmunoblastic lymphadenopathy with dysproteinemia (AILD) is the preferred term for a condition that occurs more often in elderly patients and is characterized by generalized lymphadenopathy, hepatosplenomegaly, fever, night sweats, weight loss, anemia (frequently caused by antibody-mediated hemolysis), and hypergammaglobulinemia and pruritic skin rashes.[146,147] Other terms for AILD include immunologic aberrations in idiopathic reticuloses, atypical lymph node hyperplasia with fatal outcome (immunodysplastic disease), diffuse plasmacytic sarcomatosis, chronic pluripotential immunoproliferative syndrome, immunoblastic lymphadenopathy, and lymphogranulomatosis X.[146,147] Most cases are now regarded as peripheral T-cell lymphoma-angioimmunoblastic type, in the WHO classification.[3]

Laboratory Evaluation

Biopsies of lymph nodes affected by AILD show complete effacement of the architecture, a prominent vascular proliferation, a florid immunoblastic proliferation, abundant plasma cells in clusters or sheets, burned-out germinal centers, focal necrosis, eosinophilic material, a background of mature lymphocytes, and, occasionally, eosinophils and neutrophils (Fig. 90–8).[146,147] Although AILD is considered a T-cell malignancy in most cases, the main differential diagnosis is lymphadenopathy secondary to a drug side effect of a hypersensitivity response. Serum protein electrophoresis reveals a polyclonal hypergammaglobulinemia, and a CBC shows mild to moderate anemia. The Coombs test is frequently positive. Clonal T-cell gene rearrangements are present in many cases supporting a diagnosis of peripheral T-cell lymphoma. Trisomy 3, trisomy 5, and an additional X chromosome are the most frequent chromosome aberrations in peripheral T-cell lymphoma-AILD. The unrelated clones have been hypothesized to be the consequence of increased genetic instability and an immune defect resulting in impaired clearing of damaged cells.[148,149]

Therapy

The median survival time of patients with AILD is 30 months.[146] Most patients are treated with prednisone or combination chemotherapy. The most important prognostic factor in AILD is achievement of complete remission. Randomized prospective treatment trials

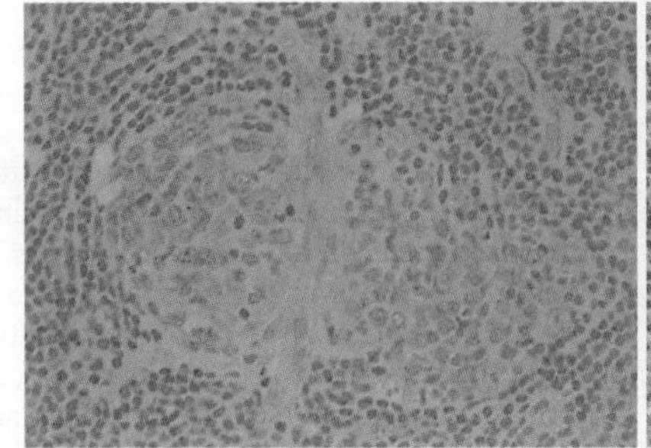

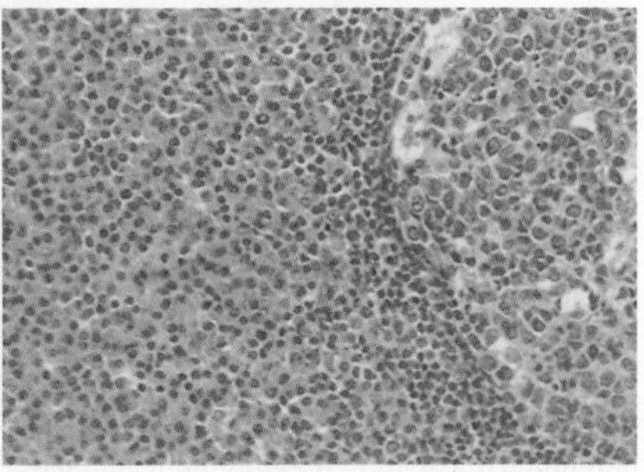

Figure 90–7 Castleman disease. **A**, The hyaline vascular subtype is characterized by small, sclerotic germinal centers, penetrated by a radial artery and surrounded by a cuff of lymphoid cells with onion skinning (H & E × 400). **B**, The plasma cell subtype shows larger germinal centers, with sheets of plasma cells in the interfollicular areas (H & E × 400).

are needed to determine optimal treatment. Although aggressive courses are observed in most patients, some patients experience a more indolent course or even spontaneous remissions. A prospective evaluation of standardized treatment in patients with AILD has been reported.[150] In this study, patients initially received prednisone therapy followed by five cycles of COPBLAM (cyclophosphamide, vincristine, prednisone, bleomycin, doxorubicin, and procarbazine) followed by two cycles of ifosfamide, methotrexate (IM) and VP-16. The combination chemotherapy was administered to patients who did not achieve a complete remission with prednisone or relapsed after prednisone therapy. Prednisone therapy was skipped in patients who presented with rapidly progressive life-threatening disease. Initial prednisone therapy led to resolution of B symptoms and reduction in tumor load in most patients.[150] The complete remission rate with prednisone only was 29%, and more than 60% of these patients eventually relapsed. In contrast, the complete remission rates after primary and secondary chemotherapies were 56% and 64%, respectively. Siegert and colleagues have concluded that primary chemotherapy is superior to sequential therapy with prednisone with or without chemotherapy. In their series, the projected event-free survival rate was 32% at 36 months, and no relapses occurred after 12 months.[150] Because of the high death rate resulting from *Pneumocystis carinii* and aspergillosis during treatment with prednisone or combination chemotherapy, strong consideration should be given to prophylactic therapy with trimethoprim-sulfamethoxazole and oral antifungal agents.[150]

Prognosis

Many apparent cases of AILD actually represent early T-cell lymphomas as clonal populations of T cells have been identified by Southern blot analysis and PCR.[151] Cytogenetic analysis and fluorescent hybridization demonstrate the clonal nature in many instances.[148,151] The overt malignant T-cell lymphoma is defined by the presence of clusters, islands, or diffuse infiltrates of monomorphic immunoblasts and has a much graver prognosis than AILD without evidence of clonality.[4,146,150]

HISTIOCYTIC NECROTIZING LYMPHADENOPATHY

Histiocytic necrotizing lymphadenitis (Kikuchi disease) is a pseudolymphomatous lesion that manifests as cervical lymphadenopathy and occurs predominantly in young women, often of Asian descent. Patients usually present with a cervical mass, but are otherwise asymptomatic and do not show evidence of IM.[151–153] The process usually resolves spontaneously in 1 to 4 months without further therapy.[153–155] These patients do not have an increased risk of lymphoma, and surgical excision is curative. Although the cause of histiocytic necrotizing lymphadenitis is unknown, its histologic and clinical features are similar to those of systemic lupus erythematosus,[156] and the disease may, in fact, reflect a self-limited autoimmune condition resembling systemic lupus erythematosus. Therefore, an autoimmune disorder, such as lupus, must be ruled out clonality when a pathologic diagnosis of Kikuchi disease is made.

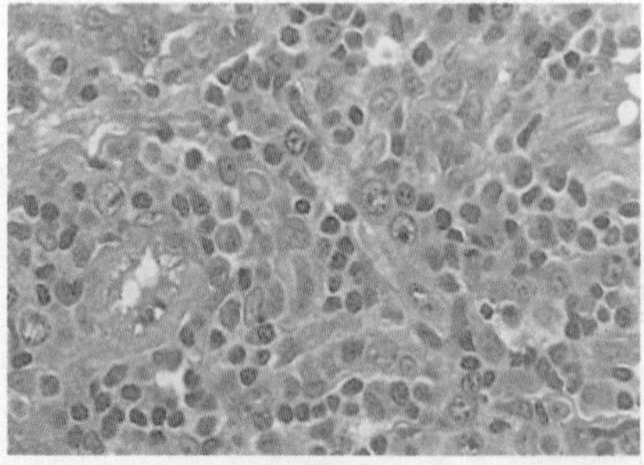

Figure 90–8 Angioimmunoblastic lymphadenopathy. A marked vascular proliferation with endothelial hyperplasia, small- and intermediate-sized immunoblasts, mature background lymphocytes, and reactive-appearing plasma cells are evident (H & E × 400).

SINUS HISTIOCYTOSIS WITH MASSIVE LYMPHADENOPATHY

Clinical Manifestations

Patients with sinus histiocytosis with massive lymphadenopathy (Rosai–Dorfman disease) usually present with bilateral lymphadenopathy predominantly affecting the cervical region, and they usually exhibit some systemic symptoms, including fever, polyclonal hypergammaglobulinemia, and an increased erythrocyte sedimentation rate.[155,156] The disease occurs more frequently in black children.[157,158] The cause of the disease remains obscure. A relationship to an underlying immunodeficiency has been postulated.[159]

An Approach to the Diagnosis of Atypical Lymphoid Hyperplasias

Clinical

Accurate diagnosis of atypical lymphoproliferations requires a systematic approach. The patient's history and physical examination often suggest a malignant process, which requires a biopsy for confirmation. If the clinical features and biopsy findings are suggestive of a viral process, serology and virologic assays may be confirmatory, and the patient can be observed without further workup. If the family history and clinical features suggest a heritable immune defect, then pedigree and immunologic analyses of the patient and family members are mandatory. Conditions that have a characteristic histologic appearance (eg, Castleman disease) can be accurately diagnosed with histologic examination alone, but most patients will require application of more sophisticated diagnostic procedures on appropriately prepared specimens.

Laboratory

To obtain optimal results from a lymph node biopsy in the settings described in this chapter, close cooperation between the referring physician, surgeon, and pathologist is required. In our practice in the Nebraska Lymphoma Study Group, we sometimes see patients who have had one or more biopsies that have had improper handling of the tissue, negating the opportunity to perform adjunctive studies. These procedures require fresh tissue. The practice of placing the entire lymph node biopsy specimen in formalin is to be condemned for it is a frequent cause of a second biopsy. Therefore, a protocol to handle lymphoid tissue is mandatory to evaluate these difficult lesions. It is imperative for the referring physician to communicate the differential diagnosis of lymphoma, atypical immune response, transplant status, and recent drug history to the surgeon and pathologist so that fresh tissue is appropriately partitioned. At the Nebraska Lymphoma Study Group, fresh lymph node tissue is routinely frozen for possible molecular gene rearrangement analyses after routine histology. Other laboratories choose to form cell suspensions for flow cytometry. In addition, cytogenetic analysis is performed on a portion of the fresh tissue. Case records are maintained for each patient in our lymphoma registries. In situ hybridization for Epstein–Barr virus is performed in all cases of suspected immune deficiency. After a diagnosis of Epstein–Barr virus-positive lymphoproliferation, new masses are biopsied to rule out transformation to non-Hodgkin lymphoma.

Laboratory Evaluation

Biopsies reveal pericapsular fibrosis, dilatation of sinuses, numerous intrasinusoidal histiocytes, and abundant plasma cells. The most striking histiologic feature is the presence of lymphocytes and other hematopoietic cells within the cytoplasm of the sinus histiocytes called emperipoiesis.

Therapy and Prognosis

Clinically, in most of the patients the concern is to rule out non-Hodgkin lymphoma. However, the disease has a protracted but benign course; spontaneous regression of the lymphadenopathy and total recovery will occur in most cases.[157,158] Surgery or the administration of antibiotics, radiation, antituberculin therapy, or steroids have little impact on the course of the disease.[157,158]

CONCLUSION

Atypical lymphoproliferations occur in a variety of clinical settings in response to a variety of stimuli. Accurate diagnosis of these processes is made by careful clinicopathologic correlation and in some cases by genetic, immunologic, virologic, and molecular techniques. In many of these conditions, emphasis should not be placed on whether this is a malignant lymphoma but, rather, whether this is a lethal clinical condition requiring optional staged therapy.

SUGGESTED READINGS

Choquet S, Leblon V, Herbrecht R, et al: Efficacy and safety of rituximab in B-cell post-transplantation lymphoproliferative disorders: Results of a prospective multicenter phase 2 study. Blood 107:3053, 2006.

Clementi R, Locatelli F, Dupre L, et al: A proportion of patients with lymphoma may harbor mutations of the perforin gene. Blood 105:4424, 2005.

Gross TG, Bucuvalas J, Park J, et al: Low dose chemotherapy for the treatment of refractory post-transplant lymphoproliferative disease in children. J Clin Oncol 23:6481, 2005.

Henter JI, Horne A, Arico M, et al: HLH-2004: Diagnostic and therapeutic guidelines for hemophagocytic lymphohistiocytosis. Pediatr Blood Cancer 48:124, 2007.

Henter JI, Samuelsson-Horne A, Arico M, et al: Treatment of hemophagocytic lymphohistiocytosis with HLH-94 immunochemotherapy and bone marrow transplantation. Blood 100:2367, 2002.

Holzelova E, Vonarbourg C, Stolzenberg MC, et al: Autoimmune lymphoproliferative syndrome with somatic Fas mutations. N Engl J Med 351(14):1409, 2004.

Okano M, Gross TG: Epstein-Barr virus-associated hemophagocytic syndrome and fatal infectious mononucleosis. Am J Hematol 53:111, 1996.

Papadopoulos EB, Ladanyi M, Emanuel D, et al: Infusions of donor leukocytes to treat Epstein-Barr virus-associated lymphoproliferative disorders after allogeneic bone marrow transplantation. N Engl J Med 330:1185, 1994.

Paya CV, Fung JJ, Nalesnik MA, et al: Epstein-Barr virus-induced posttransplant lymphoproliferative disorders. Transplantation 68:1517, 1999.

Poppema S, Maggio E, van den Berg A: Development of lymphoma in Autoimmune Lymphoproliferative Syndrome (ALPS) and its relationship to Fas gene mutations. Leuk Lymphoma 45:423, 2004.

Quintanilla-Martinez L, Kumar S, Fend F, et al: Fulminant EBV$^+$ T-cell lymphoproliferative disorder following acute/chronic EBV infection: A distinct clinicopathologic syndrome. Blood 96:443, 2000.

Rooney CM, Smith CA, Ng CC, et al: Infusion of cytotoxic T cells for prevention and treatment of Epstein-Barr virus-induced lymphoma in allogeneic transplant recipients. Blood 92:1549, 1998.

Sayos J, Wu C, Morra M, et al: The X-linked lymphoproliferative-disease gene product SAP regulates signals induced through the co-receptor SLAM. Nature 395:462, 1998.

Teachey DT, Manno CS, Axsom KM, et al: Unmasking Evans syndrome: T-cell phenotype and apoptotic response reveal autoimmune lymphoproliferative syndrome (ALPS). Blood 105:2443, 2005.

REFERENCES

For complete list of references log onto www.expertconsult.com

CHAPTER 91

CLINICAL APPROACH TO INFECTIONS IN THE COMPROMISED HOST

Jo-Anne H. Young and Daniel J. Weisdorf

The clinical approach to infections occurring among hematology patients involves understanding host immune system defects and anatomic barrier disruption that predispose patients to infection. This chapter reviews specific hematologic conditions for their unique host defense defects and associated infections (Table 91–1), the host defense defects, and the differential diagnoses of common infectious pathogens (Table 91–2). To demonstrate how periods of predictable anatomic defects combine with severe immune compromise, the prevention, diagnosis, and management strategies for infections occurring in the hematopoietic stem cell transplantation (HCT) recipient are presented as models.

HEMATOLOGIC CONDITIONS PREDISPOSING TO INFECTION

Malignant Hematologic Disorders

Antineoplastic Therapy

During antineoplastic treatment, cytotoxic agents frequently are administered in combination with other immunosuppressive therapies, such as corticosteroids or radiation therapy. Several cytotoxic agents, notably methotrexate, cyclophosphamide, 6-mercaptopurine, and azathioprine, impair cell-mediated immunity.[1–3] Many of the drugs themselves (e.g., cyclophosphamide) can impair other immune parameters, including humoral responses, and can produce quantitative phagocyte defects.

Exogenous administration of glucocorticoids leads to increased susceptibility to infection. The degree of immunosuppression and the relative risk of infection depend on the dose and duration of use.[4] The major effect of steroids on granulocyte function is a decrease in chemotactic activity.[5,6] This accounts, in part, for the clinical observation that the signs and symptoms of severe infections may be masked or greatly reduced in patients receiving steroids. Steroids may enhance susceptibility to infection by means of negative effects on wound healing, skin fragility, monocyte and lymphocyte function, production of cytokines, and humoral immune responses.

Radiation therapy has been associated with granulocyte dysfunction and delayed wound healing.[7] Defects in cell-mediated immunity may persist for more than 1 year after intensive radiation therapy or after hematopoietic cell transplant.[8,9]

Interleukin (IL)-2 administration depresses host defense. Granulocyte function studies in patients receiving IL-2 demonstrate decreased production of superoxide, decreased chemotaxis, and decreased Fc γ receptor III (FcγRIII) expression.[10] Patients receiving high-dose IL-2 therapy have a predictable increased incidence of significant gram-positive infections, particularly those due to *Staphylococcus aureus*, so antibacterial prophylaxis is routinely added during IL-2 administration.[11,12]

Acute Leukemias

In patients with acute leukemias, infection is a major cause of morbidity due to drug-associated mucositis and therapy-induced neutropenia. Substantial improvements in supportive care management over the past 2 decades have allowed patients to complete adequate courses of antineoplastic treatment without succumbing to major infectious complications.[13] Most infections occurring during neutropenia are bacterial,[14,15] but patients with prolonged neutropenia are at additional risk for development of yeast and mold infections. The broad-spectrum antibacterial agents that are used empirically during neutropenia should achieve serum bactericidal levels against *Pseudomonas aeruginosa* in particular.[15,16] Patients with acute leukemia who progress to advanced therapies, such as hematopoietic cell transplant, have added risk for infections associated with acquired deficiencies in cell-mediated and humoral immunity, such as *Pneumocystis jiroveci* and cytomegalovirus (CMV) infections.

Chronic Leukemias

Patients with chronic myeloid leukemia do not have prominent host defense impairments, so infections are limited unless patients proceed to aggressive chemotherapy or HCT.[17] Host defense defects with tyrosine kinase inhibitors, such as imatinib or dasatinib, have not been described. Chemotherapy for blast crisis resembles therapy for acute leukemia.

Patients with chronic lymphocytic leukemia (CLL) are predisposed to infection due to immunodeficiency related to the leukemia itself (humoral and cellular immune dysfunction) and to therapy-related immunosuppression. In early B-cell CLL, the infectious risk is mainly related to unbalanced immunoglobulin chain synthesis and resultant hypogammaglobulinemia. In patients with advanced CLL, particularly after the introduction of therapy with purine analogues and monoclonal agents (e.g., rituximab, alemtuzumab[18–20]), neutropenia and defects in cell-mediated immunity are other factors predisposing to infection.[18–24] Fludarabine, the major first line therapy, results in prolonged and profound defects in cell-mediated immunity, thereby increasing susceptibility to *Pneumocystis*, yeast, and herpes group viruses (herpes simplex virus [HSV], varicella-zoster virus [VZV], and CMV). The risk of infectious complications increases with the duration of CLL, reflecting the cumulative immunosuppression related to its treatment.[25] The incidence of infection correlates with the serum levels of immunoglobulins (particularly IgG), which may be further impaired by use of rituximab. Patients with CLL should receive pneumococcal vaccination. Prophylaxis with pooled intravenous immunoglobulin (IVIg) decreases the incidence of minor or moderately severe bacterial infections,[26] but this benefit is challenged by the very high cost and the effect of such therapy.[27] Routine prophylaxis with IVIg is not recommended.

Lymphomas

Hodgkin and non-Hodgkin lymphoma are commonly associated with impaired cell-mediated immunity.[28–30] Although the degree of immune impairment may correlate with the extent of disease and often is compounded by administration of immunosuppressive therapy, the intrinsic impairment of cell-mediated immunity in Hodgkin lymphoma can persist even after apparent cure. Splenectomy-related infections occur with sepsis due to encapsulated bacte-

Table 91–1 Malignant and Select Nonmalignant Hematologic Diseases and Their Associated Infection-Predisposing Host Defects

Hematologic Condition	Infection-Predisposing Host Defects
Acute myeloid leukemia	Neutropenia; therapies such as dose-intensive chemotherapy and hematopoietic cell transplant may result in additional anatomic disruptions, cell-mediated defects, and humoral defects
Acute lymphocytic leukemia	Neutropenia; therapy effects similar to acute myeloid leukemia
Hairy cell leukemia	Neutropenia (also monocytopenia); abnormal humoral immunity; T-cell suppressing therapy
Chronic lymphocytic leukemia	Hypogammaglobulinemia; abnormal cell-mediated immunity
Chronic myeloid leukemia	No prominent host defects unless aggressive therapy, advanced stage, or postsplenectomy
Multiple myeloma	Hypogammaglobulinemia; other host defects may occur with aggressive therapy or advanced stage
Hodgkin/non-Hodgkin lymphomas	Abnormal cell-mediated immunity, therapy-related neutropenia, splenic dysfunction (if splenectomy or radiation)
Myelodysplastic syndromes	Functional or absolute neutropenia
Aplastic anemia	Neutropenia; abnormal cell-mediated immunity from immunosuppressive therapies (e.g., steroids, antithymocyte globulin, cyclosporine, hematopoietic cell transplantation)
Paroxysmal nocturnal hemoglobinuria	Deficient Fc receptor may contribute to abnormal cell-mediated immunity
Hemolytic states (thalassemia)	Gallstones may serve as a nidus for infection; splenic dysfunction or splenectomy
Sickle cell disease	Can be neutropenic with aplastic crisis; bone infarcts may serve as a nidus for infection; splenic dysfunction with poor complement activation and opsonization from autosplenectomy

rial organisms at a median of 22 months but sometimes many years after surgery.[31] Patients who progress to HCT are at additional risk for infections associated with peritransplant neutropenia and delayed immune reconstitution.[32,33]

Myelodysplastic Syndrome

Neutrophils and band forms from patients with myelodysplastic syndrome are functionally defective and probably are derived from a malignant clone of myeloid precursor cells.[34] Neutrophils from patients with myelodysplastic syndrome have deficiencies in myeloperoxidase,[35] elastase,[36] and integrins.[37] Lowered expression of granulocyte colony-stimulating factor receptor may be a partial explanation for neutropenia, although impaired maturation and accelerated apoptosis impair neutrophil production.[38] More than half of patients with myelodysplastic syndrome die within 3 years of diagnosis from infections, bleeding complications, or progression to acute leukemia.

Multiple Myeloma

Malignant plasma cells induce production of a macrophage protein that selectively suppresses B-cell function, so multiple myeloma is frequently associated with a variety of defects in humoral immunity.[39] Patients having myeloma with IgG paraprotein have an increased rate of catabolism of normal and clonal IgG. They also may have defects in complement and granulocyte function. Cell-mediated immunity is not impaired by the disease but is compromised by corticosteroids or cytotoxic therapy.[40]

Patients with multiple myeloma should receive pneumococcal vaccination. Antibody titers may rise after administration of the vaccine, but postimmunization titers may not reach a protective level.[39] In addition, postimmunization antibody levels fall rapidly in this population, in part because of the increased catabolism of immunoglobulins.[8] Revaccination should be considered but not sooner than 6 years after administration of the initial vaccine because revaccination may be associated with Arthus reactions or systemic reactions.[8] Prophylaxis with passive administration of immunoglobulin is not recommended.

Uncommon Malignancies

Patients with hairy cell leukemia develop mycobacterial disease relatively often, especially infection with atypical mycobacteria.[41] Reversal of host cellular immune defects with effective therapy can lead to rapid clinical response with eradication of mycobacterial infection.[42]

Defects in cell-mediated immunity have been postulated to explain the incidence of infection caused by intracellular pathogens in patients with the relatively rare T-cell malignancies mycosis fungoides[43] and T-cell CLL.

Nonmalignant Hematologic Disorders

Aplastic Anemia

This blood dyscrasia is associated with decreased peripheral blood cell counts due to marrow failure. The severity of pancytopenia is variable. Chronic neutropenia is the main cause of recurrent bacterial and fungal infections among patients. Periodontal infections are particularly common.[44] Treatment of the underlying hematologic disease is required to stop recurrent infections and cure some chronic infections. Therapy with immunosuppression or HCT is associated with the attendant risks of acquired defects in cell-mediated and humoral immunity, requiring careful attention to supportive measures that reduce infection risk.[45,46]

Paroxysmal Nocturnal Hemoglobinuria

Paroxysmal nocturnal hemoglobinuria is an acquired clonal expansion of marrow stem cells that are deficient in the phosphatidylinositol-linked complement regulatory protein decay-accelerating factor. Patients with paroxysmal nocturnal hemoglobinuria are at some increased risk for bacterial infection due to a deficiency of this glycoprotein on the membrane of neutrophils.[47] In addition, neutrophils from some patients with paroxysmal nocturnal hemoglobinuria show a deficiency for FcγRIIIb,[48] but this receptor can be functionally replaced by FcγRII.[49] Modest and progressive granulocytopenia

Table 91–2 Host Defense Impairments and Their Associated Infectious Pathogens

Host Defense Defect	Pathogen Categories
Neutropenia	Enteric gram-negative organisms Gram-positive staphylococci and streptococci Anaerobes Yeast, particularly *Candida* species Molds, particularly *Aspergillus* species
Abnormal cell-mediated immunity	Atypical bacteria: *Legionella, Nocardia* *Salmonella* species *Mycobacteria* (*M. tuberculosis* and atypical mycobacteria) Disseminated infection from live bacilli Calmette-Guérin (BCG) vaccine Environmental fungi, including *Cryptococcus neoformans, Histoplasma capsulatum, Coccidioides immitis* Endogenous yeast, particularly *Candida* species Herpesviruses Infections from live-virus vaccines *Pneumocystis (carinii) jiroveci* *Toxoplasma gondii* *Cryptosporidium* *Strongyloides stercoralis*
Immunoglobulin abnormalities	Gram-positive *Streptococcus pneumoniae, Staphylococcus aureus* Gram-negative *Haemophilus influenzae, Neisseria* species, enteric organisms Enteroviruses Disseminated infections from live-virus vaccines *Giardia lamblia*
Complement abnormalities C3, C5	Gram-positive *S. pneumoniae*, staphylococci Gram-negative *H. influenzae, Neisseria* species, enteric organisms
Complement abnormalities C5–C9	*Neisseria* species
Anatomic Disruption	**Pathogen Categories**
Oral cavity	α-Hemolytic streptococci, oral anaerobes *Candida* species Herpes simplex virus
Esophagus	*Candida* species Herpes simplex virus, cytomegalovirus
Lower gastrointestinal tract	Enterococcus, gram-negative enteric organisms Anaerobes (*Bacteroides fragilis, Clostridium perfringens*) *Candida* species *Strongyloides stercoralis*
Skin (IV catheter)	Gram-positive staphylococci and streptococci, *Corynebacteria, Bacillus* Atypical mycobacteria
Urinary tract	Enterococcus Gram-negative enteric organisms *Candida* species
Splenectomy	Encapsulated organisms: *S. pneumoniae, H. influenzae, Neisseria* *Capnocytophaga canimorsus* *Salmonella* (especially sickle cell disease) *Babesia*

progression to aplasia or leukemia may compound these risks. Vaccination against meningococcus is required prior to treatment with the complement inhibitor eculizumab.

Granulocytic Phagocyte Disorders

Defects in phagocyte numbers, structure, and function predispose patients to infection. Infections resulting from qualitative or quantitative defects in neutrophil production tend to be prolonged, recurrent, and respond slowly to antimicrobial therapy.

The clinical approach to infections is specific to each of these disorders and is beyond the scope of this chapter. However, chronic granulomatous disease is discussed because patients with this congenital immunodeficiency who survive into adulthood are at risk for severe infections. Chronic granulomatous disease results from defective or malfunctioning oxidative metabolism capacity of neutrophils. Recurrent infections with bacteria and fungi are common and occasionally life threatening despite optimal antimicrobial therapy. Infections with *Staphylococcus* species and *Aspergillus* species can be particularly aggressive. Granulomata may form in response to infection, especially in the gastrointestinal and genitourinary tracts. Antibiotic prophylaxis has decreased the rate of bacterial infections. Important adjuncts to antimicrobial therapy may include interferon γ, colony-stimulating factors, granulocyte transfusions, and possibly gene therapy.[50,51]

Erythrocyte Disorders

Glucose-6-phosphate dehydrogenase deficiency is a sex-linked disorder. Both heterozygous females and homozygous males are protected against malaria. In contrast to this protective function, the enzyme deficiency is associated with excessively severe rickettsial infections.[52,53] Deficiency of this enzyme limits glucose metabolism through the hexose monophosphate shunt, resulting in an abnormal respiratory burst in neutrophils. Bacterial infections can occur if the deficiency is severe.

Hemoglobin Gene Variants

Patients with chronic hemolytic states may develop bilirubin gallstones, which can serve as a nidus for infection.[54,55] Defects in cell-mediated immunity have been described in patients with thalassemia.[56–58] Patients with sickle cell disease have an increased susceptibility to bacterial infections.[59] Defective alternative pathway function, especially in conjunction with asplenia, contributes to the propensity to bacterial infection.[60] Splenic involution results in depressed synthesis of alternate pathway factor(s) of complement and decreased phagocytic clearance of bacteria.[61] Phagocytosis of *Streptococcus pneumoniae* is abnormal, in part because of an inability to use the alternate pathway for C3 fixation as a means of opsonization. An increased risk for *Salmonella* infection appears to be unique to the sickle cell population. Patients with sickle cell anemia have been found to have anergy in association with zinc deficiency and decreased nucleoside phosphorylase activity.[62] Suppurative arthritis can occur after repeated episodes of hemarthrosis among patients with sickle cell disease. Patients with sickle cell disease die more frequently from infection than from any other cause.[63] Early pneumococcal vaccination and aggressive therapy, particularly of respiratory infections, are essential.

Coagulation Disorders

Hemophilias are sex-linked deficiencies of clotting factor VIII or IX. Septic arthritis should be considered in the differential diagnosis of any hemophiliac with repeated episodes of hemarthrosis whose articular signs and symptoms fail to improve quickly after administration of appropriate coagulation factor replacement.[64] Hemophiliacs who have acquired infection with human immunodeficiency virus (HIV)-1 from plasma-derived factor replacement therapy may develop severe impairment of cell-mediated immunity after this retroviral infection progresses to acquired immunodeficiency syndrome (AIDS). Abnormalities in cell-mediated immunity have been described in HIV-1–seronegative patients with hemophilia who have received factor VIII concentrates.[65,66]

Blood Groups

The Duffy blood group antigen serves as a receptor for *Plasmodium vivax* to invade erythrocytes.[67] Blood group O is associated with *Helicobacter pylori* infection and an associated increase in peptic ulceration because the Lewis(b) blood group antigen mediates *H. pylori* attachment to human gastric mucosa.[68]

Host Defense Impairment and Associated Infection Issues

Granulocytopenia

Profound or absolute granulocytopenia can occur in patients with aplastic anemia or leukemia or from chemotherapy used for treatment of various malignant diseases. Infection rates increase when granulocyte counts fall below 1000/mm^3, but the patient is most at risk for spontaneous infection when the count is below 100/mm^3.[69] The patient who is granulocytopenic from cytotoxic therapy can serve as a basic model for predicting infections that could occur in other patients with qualitative or quantitative granulocyte defects.

Granulocytopenia is defined as a cell count less than 500 neutrophils plus band forms per cubic millimeter. Profound granulocytopenia (<100/mm^3) often requires prophylactic broad-spectrum antibiotic therapy. Granulocytopenia predisposes to the development of bacterial and fungal infections but does not appear to increase the incidence or severity of viral and parasitic infections. Patients with moderate granulocytopenia (i.e., absolute granulocyte counts in the range from 500–2000/mm^3 that are not falling precipitously) should not receive prophylactic antimicrobial agents. These patients include those with myelodysplastic syndromes, newly diagnosed leukemias, early engraftment after hematopoietic cell transplant, and marrow suppression from various drugs, such as ganciclovir.

Colony-stimulating factors (granulocyte colony-stimulating factor [G-CSF; filgrastim pegylated filgrastim], granulocyte-macrophage colony-stimulating factor [GM-CSF, sargramostim]) are routinely used in the management of hematologic disorders. A number of functional granulocyte parameters may be enhanced by G-CSF or GM-CSF, including enhanced per cell phagocytosis, oxidative metabolism, microbicidal activity, and antibody-dependent cytotoxicity. However, G-CSF or GM-CSF administration may decrease the motility of granulocytes, impair in vivo migration, and decrease bacteria-induced chemotaxis. The clinical significance of any of these effects remains to be established but is generally believed to be insignificant in light of the potency of these agents in shortening the depth and duration of therapy-induced neutropenia.

Defects in Cell-Mediated Immunity

Cellular immune dysfunction occurs in patients with lymphomas, in those with hematologic malignancies undergoing hematopoietic cell transplant, and patients with AIDS. T-cell function may be required for macrophage activation and subsequent microbicidal activity. The most frequently encountered pathogens are intracellular organisms because they can survive and even replicate inside macrophages in a nonimmune individual or in the absence of T-cell immunity. Other pathogens associated with infection in patients with cell-mediated immunity include bacteria (including *Mycobacterium tuberculosis*, atypical mycobacteria, *Salmonella, Legionella, Nocardia*, and *Listeria*); fungi (including the yeasts *Candida* and *Cryptococcus*; molds such as *Aspergillus*; endemic dimorphic fungi such as *Histoplasma* and *Coccidioides*; and *Pneumocystis*); viruses (including herpes group viruses [HSV, VZV, CMV] and respiratory viruses); and protozoa (*Toxoplasma gondii*, *Cryptosporidium*, and *Strongyloides stercoralis*).

Patients with defects in cell-mediated immunity or who are about to receive hematopoietic cell transplant should undergo risk factor assessment for reactivation of tuberculosis. Patients with a known history of an untreated but positive Mantoux test should receive prophylactic isoniazid to prevent reactivation and potential dissemination of tuberculosis. Patients without a prior Mantoux test but with risk factors for tuberculosis should undergo the Mantoux test before starting the conditioning regimen for HCT.[70–72]

Patients with defects in cell-mediated immunity are at risk for the development of disseminated infection due to live vaccines, even when the vaccine contains attenuated organisms. Accordingly, these patients should not receive vaccines containing bacillus Calmette-

Guérin (BCG), vaccinia/smallpox, measles, mumps, rubella, yellow fever, or oral polio. Hematopoietic cell transplantation recipients are eligible for revaccination with some of the live virus vaccines at the 2-year anniversary visit, provided the patient does not have graft-versus-host disease (GVHD) or is not receiving ongoing pharmacologic immunosuppression.

Defects in the Humoral Immune System

Immunoglobulin and complement are components of the humoral immune system. Immunoglobulin and complement both have associated phonic, lytic, and neutralizing activities, predominantly against bacterial infection. Patients with primary or secondary defects or deficiencies in humoral immunity are susceptible to recurrent pyogenic infections from polysaccharide-encapsulated bacteria, such as *Streptococcus pneumoniae, Haemophilus influenzae*, and *Neisseria* species. Hematopoietic cell transplant recipients who continue to receive immunosuppressants more than 100 days after transplantation should be given antimicrobial prophylaxis with coverage for encapsulated bacteria until immunosuppression is discontinued. Patients are also at risk for infections from enteroviruses and *Giardia lamblia*. Patients with low levels of circulating IgG may benefit from IVIg infusions, although use of IVIg infusions for routine prophylaxis must be weighed against the expense of this approach.

Abnormalities in Splenic Function

A number of hematologic disorders are complicated by either intrinsic splenic impairment or splenectomy. The spleen removes organisms from the blood that have been ineffectively opsonized by complement, serving an adjunctive role in fighting infection. It is involved in the regulation of the alternate complement pathway, and low levels of immunoglobulin and properdin have been reported in patients after splenectomy.[73,74] A decrease in the opsonic peptide tuftsin has been reported after splenectomy.[75] Alternate pathway defects may be particularly important in patients with splenic dysfunction associated with sickle cell disease.[76]

Asplenic or splenectomized patients are at increased risk for serious bacterial infections, primarily for infections caused by *S. pneumoniae, H. influenzae, Neisseria, Babesia*, and *Capnocytophaga canimorsus*. The initial presentation of even overwhelming infection can be subtle, with fever often the only sign. Accordingly, all asplenic patients with underlying hematologic disease who present with fever should be managed initially as potentially septic. Overwhelming infection after splenectomy occurs in approximately 7% of postsplenectomy patients, with 50% of infection-related deaths occurring in the first 3 months.[77] Prophylaxis against pneumococcal infection is used for asplenic patients who are small children or for those with increased immune impairment from malignant disease.

Pneumococcal, *H. influenzae* type b, and meningococcal vaccines should be administered to asplenic patients.[78] Patients with an intact spleen may respond better to pneumococcal polysaccharide vaccine than do splenectomized patients, so immunization is recommended as early as possible before elective surgery.[79] Additionally, immunization before splenectomy can result in protective pneumococcal antibody titers immediately after the operation. For patients with Hodgkin lymphoma, the antibody response to pneumococcal vaccine may not be affected by the timing of immunization relative to splenectomy.[80] Immunizations do not eliminate the risk of serious infection with encapsulated bacteria.

Anatomic Alterations in Host Defense

Immunocompromised patients frequently have disruptions in the skin and mucosa, which are important primary physical barriers against endogenous and exogenous sources of infections. Disruption of skin and mucosa may result from invasion by malignant cells, from the effects of chemotherapy or radiation therapy, from use of invasive diagnostic or therapeutic procedures (e.g., intravenous catheters), and from the effects of local infections, such as oral HSV. Such alterations may provide a nidus for microbial colonization, a focus for localized infection, and a portal of entry for systemic invasion. Organisms associated with defects in skin or mucosal surfaces depend on the site of breakdown, local colonizing flora, and other factors. Gram-positive organisms are associated with isolated disruption of the skin from an indwelling intravenous catheter, usually with coagulase-negative staphylococci, but also with *Corynebacterium jeikeium, Bacillus* species, and occasionally atypical mycobacteria.

Gastrointestinal mucosal integrity is frequently disrupted by chemotherapeutic agents. Because the gastrointestinal tract normally is colonized by a multitude of organisms, this state can lead to infection by aerobic gram-negative enteric and anaerobic bacteria, viruses, and yeast. Mucosal damage can allow normal flora to invade and become pathogens. Lower gastrointestinal ulcerations permit infections with *Bacteroides fragilis* or *Streptococcus bovis*.

Oral lesions are associated with HSV reactivation, ulceration, and possible bloodstream infection with other common oral flora such as α-hemolytic streptococci. Individuals with intact oral mucosa can experience periodic episodes of transient α-hemolytic or viridans streptococcal bacteremia secondary to toothbrushing.

The genitourinary tract mucosa may be disrupted by tumors, invasive procedures, or cytotoxic therapy, with subsequent colonization and the potential for local or invasive infection. The most common urinary tract pathogens are enteric gram-negative bacilli, enterococci, and *Candida albicans*. Viral reactivation is common, predominantly from adenovirus and polyomavirus (BK virus) but also from the herpesviruses (HSV and CMV).

The lung, genitourinary tract, biliary tract, and auditory canal are potential sites of mechanical obstruction, increasing the risk of localized infection. Obstruction may lead to stasis of local body fluids, with resultant overgrowth of potentially pathogenic colonizing organisms. Patients with chronic hemolytic states are prone to gallstones that can become a nidus for infection.

Anatomic alteration can predispose to infection simply by providing a nidus for growth of organisms. Many patients with sickle cell anemia and hemophilia have underlying anatomic abnormalities of the bones and joints as a result of vasoocclusive crises causing infarction of marrow, bony cortex, or synovium. In turn, these changes may predispose to infection such as osteomyelitis or arthritis.[81,82] Decreased local blood flow and increased bacterial adherence may be other contributing factors. Foreign bodies, such as prosthetic devices, can lead to persistent infection after even transient bacteremia.

Infection in Chemotherapy or Transplantation Patients with Acute Profound Neutropenia and Lymphopenia

This section outlines predictable infections that can present during acute profound neutropenia/lymphopenia.

Pulmonary Infiltrates

Pulmonary infections are common in the immunocompromised host (see box on Approach to Pulmonary Infiltrates). Chest radiography is a good initial screen, and it may provide useful information in terms of characterizing the nature of an infiltrate and assist the pulmonologist in determining where to direct the bronchoscope for highest yield. A specific infectious and noninfectious differential diagnosis exists for certain radiologic signs (Table 91–3).[83,84] For example, consolidative focal airspace disease most typically is associated with a bacterial pneumonia. A halo of interstitial changes around a pulmonary nodule or an air crescent above a pulmonary nodule most likely is due to aspergillosis. Although 90% of pulmonary nodules are due to fungal pneumonia (mainly aspergillosis), 10% have various etiologies, including septic bacterial emboli, *Nocardia*,[85] *Legionella*,[86] myco-

Approach to Pulmonary Infiltrates

Pulmonary infiltrates can be divided into three general categories: consolidative, interstitial, and nodular. A consolidative infiltrate may be bacterial, even polymicrobic, so sampling of the infiltrate through sputum or endotracheal tube suctioning for bacterial and fungal cultures is required. If either of these methods does not provide an adequate sample from a consolidative infiltrate or if these methods do not lead to a diagnosis, immediate bronchoscopy is indicated. If interstitial or nodular infiltrates are not peripheral (i.e., within the range of the bronchoscope), they should also be evaluated with timely bronchoscopy. An advantage of bronchoscopy, in addition to the ability to obtain a deep specimen, is that the samples usually are sent for a broad range of diagnostic tests. These tests usually are ordered from preprinted order sheets, which reduces errors. Most preprinted order sheets for bronchoalveolar lavage fluid will test for the following:

- Cytology, with the attendant Fite and Gomori methenamine silver stains
- Bacterial (gram) stain and aerobic culture
- Mycobacterial (acid fast bacillus) stain and culture
- Fungal (potassium hydroxide or calcofluor) stain and culture
- *Nocardia* culture
- *Legionella* culture
- Viral cultures for herpes viruses and respiratory viruses
- Rapid test for cytomegalovirus (shell vial or polymerase chain reaction [PCR])
- Rapid test for respiratory viruses during respiratory virus season (pooled respiratory virus shell vial, respiratory syncytial virus antigen, influenza A/B antigen)

Optional tests that can be requested from bronchoalveolar lavage fluid, some at significant extra expense, include the following:

- Stat mycobacterial stain (requires separate 5-mL volume that cannot be used later for culture)
- *Mycoplasma* pneumoniae PCR
- *Chlamydia* pneumoniae PCR
- Human herpes virus type 6 PCR
- Human metapneumovirus PCR
- *Aspergillus* galactomannan antigen
- Any of the above first-tier tests that your institution does not send on a routine basis (e.g., *Nocardia* or *Legionella*)

Invasive sampling may be the only definitive means for making a diagnosis of peripheral nodules. The two main options are percutaneous fine-needle aspiration or open lung biopsy (usually obtained through video-assisted thoracoscopic surgical procedure). In toto sampling of a lung nodule permits enough material for the whole range of the above diagnostic tests as well as histopathology. Of note, fewer lobectomies of unilateral pulmonary nodular infiltrates have been reported in recent years, probably a result of the frequent use of a broad range of less toxic antifungal medications.

bacterial infection (with cavitation),[70] Epstein-Barr virus (EBV)-related lymphoproliferative disease, relapsed malignancy, and pulmonary embolism (pleural based). Interstitial infiltrates can be caused by either respiratory viruses during the winter season (except for parainfluenza virus, which is nonseasonal), herpes viruses, *Pneumocystis*, edema, or idiopathic. A complete differential of causes of interstitial pneumonitis, a pulmonary syndrome often associated with HCT, is given in Chapter 113.

Pulmonary and sinus infections from inhaled molds are more likely occurrences as the duration of neutropenia lengthens, particularly beyond an initial 21-day window. For that reason, among hematopoietic cell transplant recipients without graft failure, invasive tissue mold infections occur at a low rate less than 3% before engraftment due to the environmental measures taken for air filtration.[87,88]

Table 91–3 Pulmonary Infiltrates and Their Association with Specific Infectious and Noninfectious Etiologies

Radiologic Sign	Differential Diagnosis
Interstitial infiltrates	Pulmonary edema Diffuse alveolar damage Idiopathic pneumonia syndrome Respiratory viruses: Respiratory syncytial virus, parainfluenza, influenza, adenovirus, enterovirus Herpes viruses: Cytomegalovirus, herpes simplex virus, varicella zoster virus, human herpes virus type 6 *Pneumocystis* pneumonia
Focal airspace disease	Bacterial pneumonia Fungal pneumonia
Nodules	Fungal pneumonia (aspergillosis) *Nocardia* *Legionella* Septic bacterial emboli Mycobacterial infection (with cavitation) Epstein-Barr virus lymphoproliferative disorder Relapsed malignancy Pulmonary embolism (pleural based)
Halo sign or air crescent sign	Aspergillosis

However, if endogenous aspergillosis infections are present on a subclinical level before hematopoietic cell transplant, the infection can rapidly escalate when the immune system is profoundly suppressed by the preparative regimen. This phenomenon manifests as early invasive aspergillosis (before day 40).[89] Therefore, patients at risk for occult mold infections in the lungs, sinuses, and, at times, the oral cavity (aplastic anemia, Fanconi anemia, myelodysplastic syndrome, heavily pretreated pneumonia) should have computed tomography (CT) scans of the lungs and sinuses before the onset of any profoundly immunosuppressive regimens, such as hematopoietic cell transplant and select nontransplantation regimens. High-risk patients may be given antimicrobial agents with activity against molds to either prevent or suppress invasive mold infections.

Fever

Despite the specific prophylactic measures directed against common pathogens, many fevers occur in neutropenic patients after transplantation or chemotherapy. Fever can be divided into three categories: infectious fever with an obvious source, infectious fever without an obvious source, and noninfectious fever. Risk factor assessment should include knowledge of the temporal relationship to blood product infusions; recent exposure to contagious infection; degree of fever and whether the fever is accompanied by chills, rigors, or diaphoresis; and response to antipyretics. Symptom assessment should include evaluation to assess sinus drainage, sore throat, ear pain, cough, sputum production, shortness of breath, diarrhea, and dysuria.

Daily examination of any severely immunocompromised patient should include vital signs, mental status, oral cavity, indwelling catheter exit site, skin, lungs, heart, and abdomen. The physical examination is helpful in determining the cause of fever among hematologic malignancy patients because particular infections, such as mucositis, line infections, sinusitis, and pneumonia, occur predictably among severely immunocompromised patients. When fever is present, the examination should be expanded to include the sinuses (especially if the patient recently underwent any nasal manipulations), neurologic system, genitourinary system, and possibly the perineal area, looking for tenderness (neutropenic patient) or abscess (patient with neutrophils).[90]

The initial workup of fever, regardless of whether an infectious or noninfectious source is suspected, is identical and includes blood culture, culture of symptom-related sites even if there is no obvious source (e.g., sputum, urine, with/without stool, with/without cerebrospinal fluid), review of medication list for potential contributors to drug fever, review of recent transfusions, chest radiograph, and CT scan of any symptom-related body systems. Many times blood cultures are drawn through an existing indwelling line without being drawn from a peripheral site concurrently. Indications for drawing a peripheral culture include new heart murmur and recent access of an older IV access site.

Two common anaerobic infections occur during neutropenia at sites where biopsy is difficult or contraindicated. Typhlitis is preceded by fever, abdominal pain, and tenderness. CT scan of the abdomen shows signs of right-sided colonic inflammation.[91–95] Excessive soft-tissue swelling of the neck during mucositis can present as a Ludwig angina variant. Broadly active antianaerobic, aerobic, and possibly antifungal antimicrobial agents should be added for either of these clinical findings.

Bacteria

Because many fevers are caused by bacterial infections, broad-spectrum antibacterial prophylaxis is used during absolute neutropenia.[96,97] The exact agents used vary. Institutional protocols and resistance patterns drive selection of specific prophylactic agents. Implementation of prophylaxis with first fever or commencement of neutropenia and substitution of oral agents for intravenous agents among low-risk, febrile individuals has been suggested.[98]

Mucositis, with breakdown of oral and gastrointestinal mucosal barriers, is common during this period.[99,100] This condition can predispose to sepsis from colonizing mouth/gut, bacterial/fungal, and normal flora organisms. Bacteremia from *Streptococcus viridans* is common during the first several weeks of HCT, so prophylaxis with penicillin or cefazolin is routinely continued until approximately 21 days after transplantation.[101–105] Acute, fatal sepsis from gram-negative organisms is common if not prevented, so the minimum acceptable broad-spectrum prophylaxis standard involves monotherapy with an agent active against gram-negative bacilli.[106] Quinolone-resistant viridans group streptococci and gram-negative bacteria can be found in the oropharynx of neutropenic patients after brief exposures to quinolones.[107]

Central venous catheter placement through the skin can lead to blood infection from colonizing gram-positive skin organisms, despite sterile, operative placement of these catheters and antisepsis cleansing procedures.[108] Because the gram-positive bacteremias, including those caused by coagulase-negative *Staphylococcus* species, usually are not immediately life threatening, direct prophylactic coverage often is not immediately provided.[105,109,110] During workup of a new fever, some centers recommend administration of vancomycin for several days until blood cultures demonstrate no gram-positive bacteremia.

Once a gram-positive bacterial infection is identified, vancomycin therapy is used empirically until the susceptibility profile is available. At this point the regimen is tailored to a single agent. If the patient is known to be colonized with vancomycin-resistant enterococcus and the Gram stain indicates gram-positive organisms in chains, therapy for empiric vancomycin-resistant enterococcus is appropriate until the bacterial identification and susceptibility profile is available.

Once a gram-negative infection is identified, empiric therapy that includes *Pseudomonas* coverage is continued until the susceptibility profile is available. For many infections, the regimen then can be tailored to a single agent and continued for 2 weeks after the last positive culture in clinically responding patients. If the organism is known to have an inducible β-lactamase enzyme (e.g., *Enterobacter*), therapy is tailored to two agents with two different mechanisms of action.

For bloodstream infections, blood cultures should be followed daily for several days to determine the date of last positive culture. Removal of central venous catheters may be required for most, but not all, infections.[111] At the end of a 14-day treatment course beyond the last positive culture, the patient should continue a gram-negative prophylaxis regimen if still neutropenic.

Antimicrobial agents with anaerobic activity should be added for typhlitis, enlargement of neck soft tissues during mucositis (Ludwig angina variant), or culture-documented anaerobic infection. Antifungal agents should be part of the treatment regimen for typhlitis.[93–95]

Infrequently, tuberculous and nontuberculous mycobacteria are responsible for infections in the bloodstream, catheters, and pulmonary tree.[70,112,113] Nontuberculous (i.e., atypical) mycobacterial infections of central catheters or catheter tunnels require a high index of suspicion as well as specific culture media.[114] Organism identification and drug sensitivities may take several weeks. Tuberculous disease can be empirically treated based on risk factors. For patients without risk factors for tuberculosis, recovery of acid-fast bacilli will prompt therapy for suspected nontuberculous mycobacteria, usually with clarithromycin and either a quinolone or ethambutol until specific susceptibility information is available. Tailored therapy often continues for 3 to 6 months.

Viruses

Only one viral infection, herpes simplex, is common during the preengraftment phase of HCT or intensive, nontransplant therapy. Herpes simplex reactivation infections are treated with low doses of acyclovir adjusted for renal function (e.g., 5 mg/kg IV every 8 hours) or similar drugs, whereas VZV infections are treated with higher doses (e.g., 10 mg/kg IV every 8 hours or oral valacyclovir). Use of acyclovir to prevent reactivation of HSV will also prevent VZV reactivation.[115] Because many patients have not been exposed to acyclovir chronically (except for patients previously treated with recurrent courses of acyclovir for frequent outbreaks of genital herpes), there is little reason to expect resistance to acyclovir. However, HSV infections that appear or persist through acyclovir prophylaxis should be considered acyclovir resistant until viral sensitivity testing can be performed, and consideration should be given to initiating treatment with foscarnet or cidofovir. Reports of acyclovir-resistant varicella are extremely rare.[116] Foscarnet infusions affect calcium homeostasis, so monitoring of ionized calcium and phosphorus levels is required during clinical use of the drug. Cidofovir is well tolerated with probenecid and hydration, although renal toxicity has been recognized. Cidofovir, when combined with aggressive supportive measures, is considered an adjunct in treatment of several of the viruses associated with hemorrhagic cystitis[117,118] and disseminated adenovirus infections.[119] When clinically significant CMV infection occurs during neutropenia the antigenemia test cannot be used for diagnosis or monitoring of response to therapy. and DNA polymerase chain reaction (PCR) methods are preferred.[120,121]

Human herpesvirus type 6 (HHV-6) infection can manifest most commonly as fever or pancytopenia. Other recognized clinical syndromes include pneumonitis and encephalitis. Infection is diagnosed by quantitative PCR. Patients who undergo cord blood transplantation have a higher incidence of infection than do those who undergo unrelated bone marrow transplantation (87% vs 19%, $P < 0.0001$), although this analysis requires confirmation.[122] Virus detection at week 3 following transplant may be associated with early skin rash and acute GVHD but also may be asymptomatic. Prospective large-scale studies are needed to determine the role of HHV-6 infection. HHV-6 has 60% DNA homology with CMV, and treatment of documented infection usually is initiated with induction doses of foscarnet or ganciclovir. Responses to antiviral therapy are not universal, and benefits of foscarnet versus ganciclovir have not been determined.[123]

Respiratory virus infections are seasonal, except for parainfluenza.[83,84] A frequent pathogen with clinical significance is respiratory syncytial virus, although influenza, parainfluenza, adenovirus, enteroviruses, the herpesviruses (including HHV-6), human metapneumovirus, and rhinovirus also produce diffuse interstitial infiltrates and pneumonitis. HHV-6 and human metapneumovirus are not recovered with the usual tests ordered at the time of bronchoscopy, so a high suspicion for infection is required to order specific PCR testing.[124,125] Documented infection prompts contact and droplet isolation precautions. Treatment components may include aerosolized ribavirin, IVIg, and, in some cases, monoclonal antibody therapy. However, proof of efficacy of these treatments remains elusive. With respiratory syncytial virus infections, aerosolized ribavirin treatment appears safe, and trends of decreasing viral loads have been reported.[126] Secondary graft failure associated with parainfluenza virus infection has been reported following transplantation.[127]

Fungi

Most yeast infections are caused by *Candida*.[128] Candidal organisms that colonize the mouth and gut proliferate when antibacterial agents suppress the coexisting bacterial flora population. The current standard in the United States for more than a decade has been use of fluconazole to prevent *C. albicans* bloodstream and hepatosplenic infection among allogeneic hematopoietic cell transplant recipients.[87,88,129] However, fluconazole does not have activity against nonalbicans yeasts (e.g., *Candida glabrata, Candida krusei*) and all molds (e.g., *Aspergillus, Fusarium*, the Zygomycetes). Among patients colonized with yeast species other than *C. albicans* and among heavily pretreated patients who may have incubating mold infection, prophylaxis using an advanced-generation azole or an echinocandin is preferred.[130,131] Empirical treatment of yeast recovered from a sterile site should include coverage for a nonalbicans *Candida* species until the species is identified.

Use of twice weekly serum *Aspergillus* galactomannan enzyme-linked immunosorbent assay (ELISA) for the detection of invasive aspergillosis is a highly specific diagnostic tool. When used regularly, the galactomannan ELISA may allow for earlier diagnosis of invasive aspergillosis in some patients. The test is troubled by a low sensitivity and high frequency of false negative tests.[132–135] Several reports have described a high rate of false-positive galactomannan ELISA results for patients treated with piperacillin-tazobactam.[136] Administration of β lactams containing galactomannan is responsible for false-positive diagnostic results, even up to 5 days after cessation of treatment.

For bloodstream and other invasive tissue fungal isolates, the susceptibility profile should be reported with the following drug options: amphotericin, fluconazole, itraconazole, voriconazole, posaconazole, and caspofungin. After the susceptibility profile is available, the regimen can be tailored to a single agent. Long-term treatment with newer azoles may be valuable in responding patients. Echinocandins cannot be used to treat *Cryptococcus* or Zygomycetes. The Zygomycetes are susceptible to amphotericin and posaconazole. Echinocandin agents may be fungistatic, rather than fungicidal, in the case of mold infections because interruption of fungal cell wall synthesis is limited to areas of hyphal branch points and growing hyphal tips. Because susceptibility testing for the echinocandin agents is of uncertain reliability, use of an echinocandin after the susceptibility profile has returned should be limited to nonneutropenic patients with uncomplicated candidemia[137] or salvage therapy for aspergillosis. At present, the efficacy of combination drug therapy is unproven, but such therapy is often used in situations associated with high mortality. Clinical experience, but little clearly documented evidence, supports the value of extended combination antifungal therapy. Molds that often are resistant to amphotericin but may be susceptible to voriconazole or posaconazole include *Fusarium, Scedosporium* or *Pseudallescheria*, and *Trichosporon* (see box on Use of Antifungal Agents in Combination).

Use of Antifungal Agents in Combination

The development of new antifungal drugs gives the clinician more options for prophylaxis and therapy than in previous years. There is an overall level of simplicity to the drug choices once their mechanisms of action are understood. The polyenes, including amphotericin products and nystatin, attach onto ergosterol in the fungal cell membrane and are considered fungicidal, because cytoplasm leaks out and individual cells die. The azoles, including fluconazole, itraconazole, voriconazole, and posaconazole, prevent the formation of new ergosterol. Azoles are considered fungistatic, because removal of the drug permits cell regrowth. Theoretically, use of an azole together with a polyene may have an overall static effect for an established infection as the ergosterol target for the fungicidal polyene is depleted. The echinocandins, including caspofungin, micafungin, and anidulafungin, prevent interaction of the catalytic and regulatory subunits of the β glucan synthesis enzyme, so less β glucan is formed for the cell wall. The scaffolding for the fungal cell wall is not maintained, and a dividing cell may burst open when trying to extend the new cell wall over daughter cells. The echinocandins are considered fungicidal for yeasts but fungistatic for molds, as not every mold cell in a large tangle of fungal hyphae is actively dividing. Combination therapy may have the most effect when a cell wall agent (an echinocandin) is used together with a cell membrane agent (a polyene or an azole). There is no role for three-drug therapy (an echinocandin, a polyene, and an azole). The clinical response to combination therapy has been variable; however, the mortality rate appears to be lower with combination therapy than with monotherapy. Controlled trials are needed to determine the role of combination therapy.

Fever Without an Obvious Infectious Source

If there is no obvious source of infection in a hematopoietic cell transplant patient receiving standard antimicrobial prophylaxis before engraftment, then further systematic review of the patient is required. Figure 91–1 presents an 11-step guide to reviewing the HCT recipient for other infectious sources to ensure an appropriate evaluation. The basic differential diagnosis of noninfectious fever includes secondary malignancy (including posttransplantation lymphoproliferative disorders), transfusion of blood products, drug fever (including febrile response to growth factor), autoimmune phenomena, and endocrine disorders (e.g., as malignant hyperthermia). Transfusion-related fever and drug fever probably are the most commonly encountered causes of noninfectious fever in hematologic practice. Transfusion-related fever typically is self-limited.

Pulmonary infections are common in the immunocompromised patient (see Table 91–3).[83,84] Chest radiography is a good initial screen, but it may be more useful for characterizing the nature of an infiltrate and assisting the pulmonologist in determining where to direct the bronchoscope for the highest diagnostic yield of bronchoalveolar lavage. Although 90% of pulmonary nodules among transplantation recipients are due to fungal pneumonia (mainly aspergillosis), 10% have various etiologies, including *Nocardia*,[85] *Legionella*,[86] septic bacterial emboli, mycobacterial infection (with cavitation),[70] EBV-related lymphoproliferative disease, relapsed malignancy, and pulmonary embolism (pleural based).

A drug may cause fever by increasing metabolism, mimicking endogenous pyrogens, evoking a cellular or humoral immune response, interfering with heat dissipation peripherally, or damaging tissue. Drug-induced fevers typically begin 7 to 10 days after drug administration is initiated, are low grade, persist for as long as the drug is continued, cause eosinophilia in up to 20% of cases, and may be associated with a rash. Fever disappears soon after stopping an offending drug, usually over the course of 2 to 3 days. Certain drugs

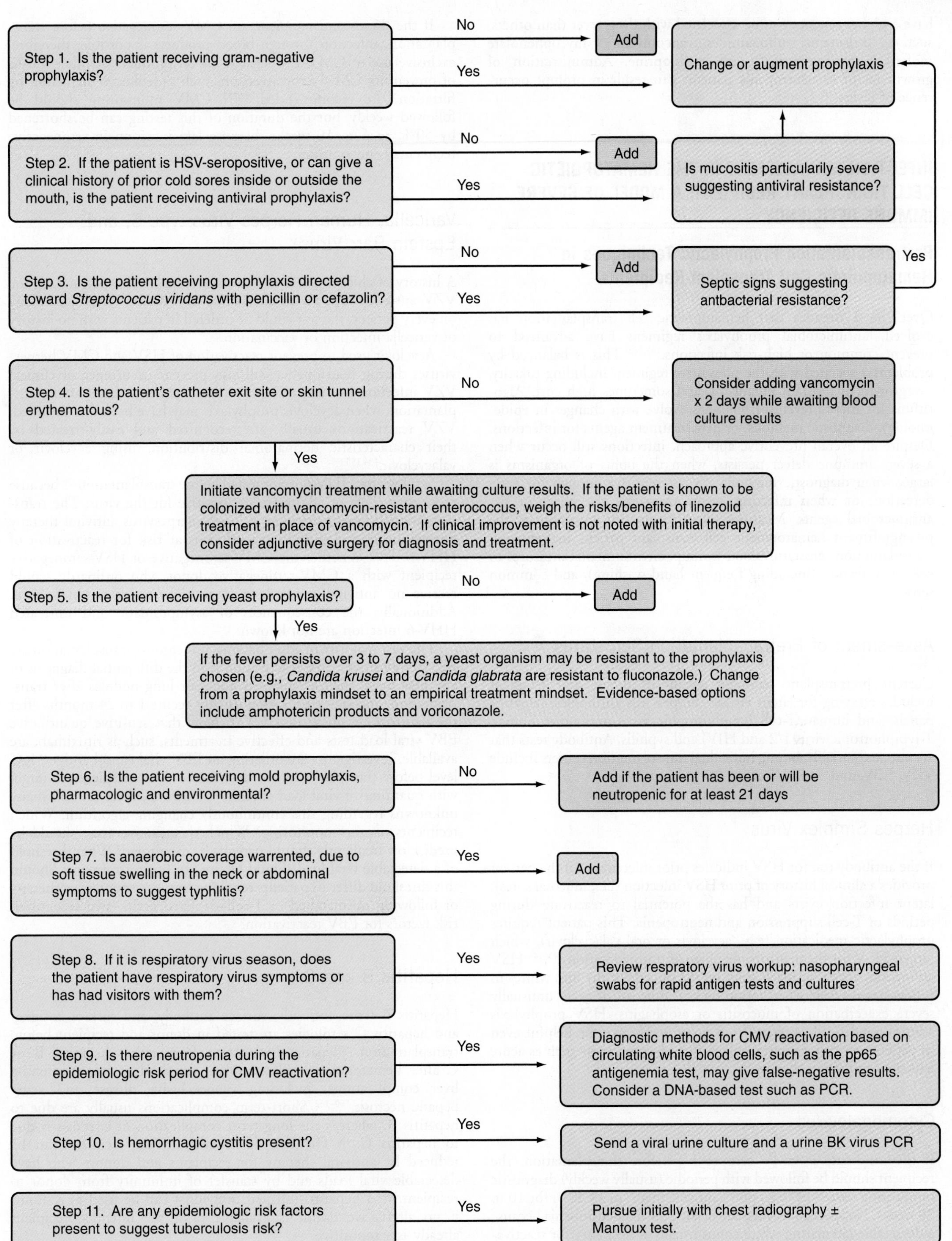

Figure 91–1 Systematic approach to causes of fever and infection in the high-risk hematology patient without an obvious source. This algorithm can be used for hematopoietic cell transplantation patients before engraftment or for patients who are receiving conventional, high-dose therapy for hematologic malignancies and are profoundly neutropenic. BK virus BK polyomavirus; CMV, cytomegalovirus; HSV, herpes simplex virus; PCR, polymerase chain reaction.

have a higher tendency to be associated with drug fever than others, such as β lactams, sulfonamides, vancomycin,[138] mycophenolate mofetil,[139] hydroxyurea,[140] and azathioprine. Administration of growth factor to neutropenic patients can result in prompt occurrence of fevers.

INFECTION MANAGEMENT IN THE HEMATOPOIETIC CELL TRANSPLANT RECIPIENT: A MODEL OF SEVERE IMMUNE DEFICIENCY

Pretransplantation Prophylactic Techniques in Hematopoietic Cell Transplant Recipients

Over the 4 decades that hematopoietic cell transplantation has evolved, antimicrobial prophylaxis regimens have advanced to prevent common or high-risk infections.[141,142] This is balanced by problems associated with the preventive regimen, including toxicity, overgrowth of resistant organisms, and sometimes high cost. Algorithms for these preventive regimens evolve with changes in epidemiology, diagnostic methods, or new treatment agents for infections. Despite an overall preventive approach, infections still occur when a severe immune defect persists, when the bolus of organisms is large, when diagnostic methods are not sensitive enough for early detection, or when infecting agents overcome the effect of the antimicrobial agents. Measures taken to prevent infection in the preengraftment hematopoietic cell transplant patient include pretransplantation serostatus blood workup, environmental measures to prevent infection (including frequent hand washing), and common sense.

Assessment of Pretransplantation Serostatus

Current pretransplant serologic testing of donor and recipient includes assaying for latent viruses (herpesvirus antibodies, hepatitis panels, and human T-cell lymphotrophic virus antibodies human T-lymphotropic virus 1/2 and HIV) and syphilis. Antibody tests that are checked variably among individual transplantation centers include VZV, EBV, and *Toxoplasma.*

Herpes Simplex Virus

If the antibody test for HSV indicates prior infection or if the patient provides a clinical history of prior HSV infection (i.e., mucosal sores), latent infection exists and has the potential to reactivate during periods of T-cell suppression and neutropenia. This patient requires prophylactic medication (e.g., acyclovir or oral valacyclovir), which targets HSV for the neutropenic phase of transplantation.[143–146] HSV lesions can appear as black scabs on the outside of the lips, white- to yellow-based ulcers when found on oral mucosa, or as an unusually severe exacerbation of mucositis or esophagitis. HSV prophylaxis administered until recovery from neutropenia may be helpful even in patients receiving nontransplantation chemotherapy such as acute leukemia induction therapy.[147]

Cytomegalovirus

If the candidate is CMV seropositive before transplantation, the recipient should be followed with periodic (usually weekly) diagnostic monitoring tests[148,149] (e.g., pp65 antigenemia[150] or PCR[151]) for 10 to 20 weeks. No special measures are needed during neutropenia because a detectable circulating white count usually is necessary for reactivation of CMV. If the patient is CMV seronegative before transplantation but the donor is seropositive, the same monitoring algorithm used for the CMV-seropositive patient is needed.

If the donor and recipient are CMV seronegative before transplantation, infection through blood products is possible; therefore, exclusive use of CMV-seronegative blood products or other means of preventing CMV seroconversion, such as leukocyte depletion by filtration, are recommended.[152,153] CMV monitoring should be followed weekly, but the duration of this testing can be shortened by 50%, to 6 to 10 weeks, because late infection in seronegative recipients is uncommon.

Varicella, Human Herpes Virus type 6, and Epstein-Barr Virus

A history of chickenpox is an adequate surrogate for performing the VZV antibody test. As an alternative to ordering varicella serology on every patient, the test could be ordered in patients with no history of varicella infection or vaccination.

Acyclovir used to prevent reactivation of HSV and CMV herpesviruses during neutropenia will also prevent occurrence of clinical VZV infection in most transplantation recipients. Later after transplantation, when acyclovir prophylaxis may have been discontinued, VZV reactivations usually are recognized and easily treated by their characteristic dermatomal distribution, using acyclovir or valacyclovir.[154,155]

Serology for HHV-6 is not tested before transplantation[156] because more than 95% of adults are seropositive for the virus. The transplantation recipient receiving minimal herpesvirus antiviral therapy during the transplantation procedure is at risk for reactivation of HHV-6.[123,157] Whether the CMV-seronegative or HSV-seronegative recipient with a CMV-seronegative donor who ordinarily would receive no antiviral prophylaxis is at highest risk is not known. Additionally, the consequences of asymptomatic and untreated HHV-6 infection are not known.

The vast majority of adult patients undergoing transplantation are EBV seropositive. EBV reactivation is in the differential diagnosis of any new mass, such as enlarged nodes or lung nodules after transplantation, and this reactivation usually occurs 1 to 24 months after the neutropenic phase of HCT.[158] Now that sensitive quantitative EBV viral load tests and effective treatments, such as rituximab, are available, investigators are ordering an EBV viral capsid antigen IgG level before transplantation to determine which recipients to target with quantitative viral load studies.[159] However, there are still many unknowns regarding this continuously changing algorithm. Which recipients require monitoring? Which quantitative assay should be used? How frequently should patients be monitored? What threshold of a detectable viral load should be used to begin treatment? Should this threshold differ in patients receiving immunosuppressive therapy or following mismatched or T-cell–depleted grafts, two recognized risk factors for EBV reactivation?

Hepatitis B and C

Hepatitis B (core antibody, surface antibody, and surface antigen) and hepatitis C serologies are tested in donor and recipient before transplantation. Hepatic dysfunction from either hepatitis B or C after hematopoietic cell transplant can lead to life-threatening liver complications, including venoocclusive disease and acute hepatic necrosis.[160–162] Short-term complications usually are due to hepatitis B, whereas the long-term complication of cirrhosis is due to hepatitis C.[163] The risk of hepatitis in the recipient can be reduced by antiviral therapy for recipients and donors who have detectable viral loads and by transfer of immunity from donor to recipient.[160] A hepatitis-infected individual can be used as a donor if no alternative donor is available or if the intended recipient already is seropositive.

The risk of transmission is small when the hepatitis B-seropositive donor has an undetectable viral load; however, careful followup of recipients is recommended.[164] A surface antigen-positive hepatitis B donor with a high viral load should be treated with lamivudine or another agent to reduce the circulating viral load before transplantation.[165] High circulating hepatitis C viral load in the seropositive donor for a seronegative recipient is an indication for interferon or other antiviral therapy of the donor before HCT.[166]

If the potential recipient has serologic evidence of infection with hepatitis B or C before transplantation, viral load levels should be checked before and monitored after HCT. High hepatitis B viral load (>10^5 copies/mL) is the most important risk factor for reactivation in patients positive for surface antigen undergoing HCT.[164] High circulating hepatitis B viral load in the intended recipient is an indication for lamivudine.[164,165] There is no evident correlation between hepatitis C genotype and type or severity of liver disease after transplantation.[167] There is no effective therapy for hepatitis C in the HCT recipient.

Human Immunodeficiency Virus

A positive donor HIV test for a recipient candidate not known to be seropositive is a contraindication for donation. If the screening test for HIV is positive, a Western blot study should be completed to confirm the result because of the potential for false-positive testing. Appropriate counseling should be provided when a positive HIV test result is conveyed to a patient.[168]

Syphilis

Some screening tests indicate a need for therapy.[169] If the indirect screening test for syphilis returns positive and is confirmed by a direct test, high-dose penicillin treatment should be given for 10 days after transplantation, then *Streptococcus viridans* prophylaxis agent resumed until 21 days after transplantation.[170,171]

Toxoplasma

Historically, 15% of patients who undergo transplantation in the United States are seropositive for *Toxoplasma*, but this percentage may be higher for European centers.[172] The risk of reactivation among seropositive patients is 2%, for an overall incidence of less than 1% of HCT recipients.[172,173] It is suspected that sulfa-based regimens in low dose, such as those used to prevent *Pneumocystis* pneumonia, may be effective in preventing *Toxoplasma*.[173,174]

Review of Commonsense Measures to Prevent Infection

Commonsense measures that should be discussed before transplantation or aggressive nontransplantation chemotherapy include attention to diet, travel, crowds, and pets.[175] Additionally, a history of family or social exposure to tuberculosis should be used to guide whether or not a Mantoux test is applied before therapy.

Diet should be reviewed for herbal supplements or restricted foods.[175] Patients may not recognize that most supplements will have to be discontinued after HCT.[176] Ground meat products need to be thoroughly cooked so that bacteria, distributed onto meat in the grinding process, are killed. Any fruits or vegetables that cannot be peeled should be washed. Salad bars are associated with occasional transmission of infections. Food products that inherently contain infectious organisms should be avoided, including undercooked eggs. For example, Beano, pepper, and miso paste for soup[177] are known to have recovery of *Aspergillus* organisms when cultured. Blue cheeses have molds spiked into the cheese wheel as they are curing and should be avoided. Soft cheeses carry the potential risk of *Listeria* infection. Yogurt contains *Lactobacillus* that, rather than causing gut problems, has been found to cause infection in other sites,[178] including the lungs after aspiration events.

There are no particular travel restrictions, but strategies to minimize transmission of infectious diseases have been summarized.[175] Some social situations, such as sitting in a crowded movie theater or classroom, increase the risk of acquiring a viral illness. Turning away from individuals who are coughing or sneezing may be helpful in preventing the transmission of infections in this situation. Patients need instruction to remember to complete the cycle of infection prevention by washing their hands as soon as possible after being close to such an individual. Given outbreaks of Noroviruses (Norwalk-like viruses) on cruise ships and other types of outbreaks (e.g., *Staphylococcus*) commonly associated with the close living quarters during this type of vacation, cruise ships should be avoided.[179,180]

Healthy dogs and cats are considered acceptable pets. However, the immunosuppressed patient should not be responsible for scooping cat litter because of potential *Toxoplasma* cyst exposure. Similarly, the patient should not play in sandboxes because these areas are concentrated sites that feral outdoor cats may use as litter boxes. Because reptiles of many sorts have been reported to be infected with *Salmonella*, patients should not touch these animals or the insides or outsides of their cages or tanks. The heated water of tropical fish tanks carry *Mycobacterium marinum*. *Cryptococcus* and *Chlamydophila* (formerly *Chlamydia*) *psittaci* can be transmitted from large pet birds.

Environmental Measures to Prevent Infection

Persons entering the patient's room to perform an examination or touch the patient (including visitors as well as health care workers) should wash their hands outside the room.[181] Ideally, the institution will have handwashing sinks in the hallways outside patient rooms for this purpose. During respiratory virus season, the infection control department often adds extra signs to doorways and other places in the wards to remind visitors of the importance of hand washing. Staff and visitors without control of body secretions should not be permitted to have direct patient contact.

Some infectious situations require special isolation procedures.[181] Contact isolation (gloves and gowns) is used for patients with adenovirus, methicillin-resistant *S. aureus*, or *Clostridium difficile* infection. Droplet precautions are added to contact precautions for respiratory virus or varicella infection. Carriers of vancomycin-resistant enterococcus are placed in contact isolation until they meet defined criteria for discontinuation of isolation.

Laminar airflow is a cumbersome and expensive isolation technique that has been largely outmoded with advances in airflow and isolation technology as well as current antimicrobial therapy. Historically, it has been most commonly used for patients with aplastic anemia[46] or those receiving T-cell–depleted transplants.

High-efficiency particulate air (HEPA) filtration has replaced laminar airflow as the means for preventing infection through ventilation.[181] With at least 12 air exchanges per hour, HEPA filters are capable of removing particles greater than 0.2 μm in diameter, such as mold spores. Patients often ask if they should purchase portable HEPA filters for the home or apartment they will occupy after hospitalization. In the broadest sense, this is an extra measure that can be used on an individual basis. If portable HEPA filters are used, they should be obtained for each of the rooms that the patient will occupy during the day and night, and each unit should be sized for the individual room. A beneficial effect of HEPA filtration in the outpatient setting has not been demonstrated.

Hemorrhagic Cystitis

Hemorrhagic cystitis is hematuria that results from diffuse bladder inflammation and is not confined to the preengraftment period. If blood clots form, bladder irrigation may be required to break up an obstructive uropathy. Massive bladder hemorrhage can be a serious clinical problem with a high mortality rate. Common causes include chemotherapeutic agents (cyclophosphamide or ifosphamide), radiation, viral infection, and rarely GVHD. Although CMV can be associated with hemorrhagic cystitis after hematopoietic cell transplant, adenovirus and polyomavirus infection (specifically BK viruria) often are responsible, especially when hemorrhagic cystitis lasts longer than 7 days.[182,183] Diagnosis is made by urine viral culture to rule out adenovirus and quantitative urine BK virus PCR.[184] Intravesical instillation of cidofovir has resulted in clinical improvement of both adenovirus- and BK virus-associated intractable hemorrhagic cystitis and is an attractive alternative to intravenous administration of cidofovir.[185,186]

Infection in the Hematopoietic Cell Transplant Recipient After Engraftment

Viral infections that reactivate after engraftment often are related to defective T-cell–mediated immunity.[187] Outpatient HCT recipients inhale mold spores and *Pneumocystis* cysts from the environment, so common exogenously acquired infections include aspergillosis and *P. jiroveci* (previously *carinii*).[187–189]

Cytomegalovirus

Use of prophylactic ganciclovir at engraftment usually is avoided because it leads to myelosuppression and possibly a higher incidence of late CMV disease.[150] Instead, the patient is treated with ganciclovir when weekly PCR or pp65 antigenemia monitoring test meets a positive threshold. Initial viral load levels do not predict disease.[190] CMV infections are treated with an induction ganciclovir regimen followed by approximately 6 weeks of a maintenance regimen (half the induction dose). The duration of induction (1–3 weeks) varies by institution, but in general 1 week is used for low-grade infection, 2 weeks for high-grade infection, and 3 weeks for end-organ disease. A rising viral load when checked weekly during the first month of preemptive therapy signals the need for continued induction dosing or repeat induction dosing.[191]

When the end-organ manifestation of CMV is pneumonitis (recovery of CMV from a deep lung specimen along with an infiltrate on chest radiograph), IVIg is added on an every-other-day basis for the duration of induction.[192,193] When CMV manifests in an end organ other than the lungs, use of IVIg is not as clearly useful. Some centers add IVIg when the patient's total IgG level falls below 400 mg/dL. Dosing schedules vary from IVIg given once weekly for 3 weeks to every other day for the duration of induction, similar to therapy for pneumonitis.[194] Ganciclovir resistance is uncommon.[195]

Varicella-Zoster Virus

Varicella-zoster virus reactivations from latency (zoster) usually are recognized by their characteristic dermatomal distribution. No temporal pattern is seen, viremia can occur concurrently, and multiple episodes are possible but uncommon. For patients who have been treated for a zoster episode after HCT, some centers provide acyclovir prophylaxis until 1 year after HCT. Less common VZV clinical manifestations that can result in severe infection and may require molecular testing[196] or viral culture for diagnosis include hemorrhagic pneumonia, hepatitis,[197] central nervous system disease,[198] thrombocytopenia, and retinal necrosis.[199]

Hematopoietic cell transplant recipients with a negative or unknown VZV disease history and a significant exposure to active varicella are susceptible to primary VZV infection. For these patients, varicella-zoster immune globulin should be provided within 96 hours of exposure. Patients with positive serology can become clinically reinfected after exposure and should be provided with acyclovir prophylaxis; however, such patients do not require varicella-zoster immune globulin.[200]

Epstein-Barr Virus

EBV causes asymptomatic but detectable viremia, hemophagocytic syndrome, or posttransplant lymphoproliferative disorder. Quantitative EBV viral load diagnostic testing is relatively new and not standardized, so the algorithms for monitoring and initiation of treatment vary. Recognition of greater than 1000 viral copies/mL of blood requires investigation, repeated testing, and possibly treatment, especially in high-risk patients. Some EBV reactivations are subclinical and require no therapy. Direct antiviral agents have limited impact on reducing detectable EBV viral loads. Posttransplant lymphoproliferative disorder after allogeneic transplantation most often is of donor origin. General treatment approaches involve reduction of immunosuppression plus rituximab. Both monomorphic and polymorphic histology (and immunophenotyping) may be seen. Monoclonal histology predicts an unfavorable prognosis.[201] The incidence of EBV-related complications is higher in mismatched donors, T-cell–depleted transplants, and patients receiving intensive immunosuppression (e.g., antithymocyte globulin).[202]

Invasive Mold Infections

Among HCT recipients studied at autopsy, yeast and mold infections were common, seen in more than 25% of deaths.[203] The probability of survival is higher in recent years, likely due to newer and safer treatment agents as well as nonmyeloablative conditioning.[189] Posaconazole is effective in preventing invasive fungal infections during GVHD.[204] Mold spores may initiate a localized infection in the lungs or sinuses that, after intensive immunosuppression for GVHD, may disseminate to the skin, abdominal organs, or central nervous system.[89,205] Treatment of central nervous system infections should include voriconazole, which attains cerebrospinal fluid levels approximately 50% those of plasma or central nervous system tissue levels approximately 200% those of plasma. Infection with Zygomycetes organisms has a later onset than infection with *Aspergillus* (after day 90) and possibly lower mortality.

Pneumocystis

The most common presenting symptoms of *Pneumocystis* infection are dyspnea, cough, and fever.[206] Diagnosis requires demonstration of the organism in silver-stained specimens (bronchoalveolar lavage or lung biopsy). Disease occurs by both new infection and activation of latent infection. Most patients present between day 40 and day 80 after HCT,[207] but cases as early as day 12[208] and as late as 42 months after HCT have been reported.[209] Once lymphocyte function is more fully reconstituted, *Pneumocystis* infections are rare. Prophylaxis options include trimethoprim-sulfamethoxazole, aerosol pentamidine, dapsone,[210,211] and atovaquone.[212] Among patients treated with dapsone after transplantation, increased red blood cell and platelet transfusion requirements are noted.[210] Prophylaxis is generally discontinued 1 to 2 years after HCT, or longer if immunosuppression is ongoing.

Parasitic Infections

Toxoplasma gondii is a ubiquitous pathogen that causes significant morbidity and mortality. Although relatively uncommon, toxoplasmosis is recognized as a cause of cerebral, ocular, and lung disease in immunocompromised patients.[173] Disseminated toxoplasmosis has resulted in graft failure in a cord blood transplant recipient.[213]

Accurate diagnosis of this treatable infection is critical. PCR-based testing has become an adjunct method for diagnosis, occasionally replacing tissue biopsy.

Infection Issues in the Late Posttransplantation Period

Encapsulated Organism Prophylaxis

Penicillin prophylaxis has decreased the incidence of infection-related morbidity and mortality from polysaccharide-encapsulated bacteria (*S. pneumoniae, H. influenzae* type b, *Neisseria meningitidis*). Penicillin-resistant pneumococcal infection has been reported, prompting consideration of alternate prophylaxis, such as a change from penicillins to quinolones.[214,215] Prophylaxis is generally discontinued 2 years after HCT, or later if GVHD and immunosuppression are ongoing at the 2-year time point. Once the patient is ready for vaccinations, conjugate pneumococcal, meningococcal, and *H. influenzae* type b vaccines are given.

Vaccination

Recipients of HCT frequently lose antibody responses to viral and bacterial pathogens previously targeted by childhood vaccination. Although practice varies among transplantation centers, killed-virus vaccines are often given at 1 year after HCT and live-virus vaccines approximately 2 years after HCT for patients without GVHD. For adults, Tdap (formulation of reduced-antigen, combined diphtheria-tetanus-acellular pertussis vaccine) has replaced Td (diphtheria-tetanus booster vaccine) as a means for decreasing the adult reservoir of pertussis.[216] For protection against hepatitis, the combined vaccine providing protection against both hepatitis A and B can be used.[217] The efficacy of vaccination is influenced by the time elapsed since transplantation, the nature of the hematopoietic graft, the presence of GVHD, and the use of serial immunization.[218,219] Despite this evidence, a national survey of HCT immunization practices revealed that vaccines are underused, and schedules for revaccination vary.[220,221]

SUGGESTED READINGS

Boeckh M, Englund J, Li Y, et al: Randomized controlled multicenter trial of aerosolized ribavirin for respiratory syncytial virus upper respiratory tract infection in hematopoietic cell transplant recipients. Clin Infect Dis 44:245, 2007.

Boeckh M, Gooley TA, Myerson D, et al: Cytomegalovirus pp65 antigenemia-guided early treatment with ganciclovir versus ganciclovir at engraftment after allogeneic marrow transplantation: A randomized double-blind study. Blood 88:4063, 1996.

Bowden RA, Slichter SJ, Sayers M, et al: A comparison of filtered leukocyte-reduced and cytomegalovirus seronegative blood products for the prevention of transfusion-associated CMV infection after marrow transplant. Blood 86:3598, 1995.

Brunstein CG, Weisdorf DJ, DeFor T, et al: Marked increased risk of Epstein-Barr virus-related complications with the addition of antithymocyte globulin to a nonmyeloablative conditioning prior to unrelated umbilical cord blood transplantation. Blood 108:2874, 2006.

Cornely OA, Maertens J, Winston DJ, et al: Posaconazole vs. fluconazole or itraconazole prophylaxis in patients with neutropenia. N Engl J Med 356:348, 2007.

Cullen M, Steven N, Billingham L, et al: Antibacterial prophylaxis after chemotherapy for solid tumors and lymphomas. N Engl J Med 353:988, 2005.

Freifeld AG, Sepkowitz KA, Martino P, et al: Antibacterial prophylaxis in patients with cancer and neutropenia. N Engl J Med 354:90, 2006.

Dykewicz CA: Summary of the guidelines for preventing opportunistic infections among hematopoietic stem cell transplant recipients. Clin Infect Dis 33:139, 2001.

Goodman JL, Winston DJ, Greenfield RA, et al: A controlled trial of fluconazole to prevent fungal infections in patients undergoing bone marrow transplantation. N Engl J Med 326:845, 1992.

Henning KJ, White MH, Sepkowitz KA, Armstrong D: A national survey of immunization practices following allogeneic bone marrow transplantation. JAMA 277:1148, 1997.

Limaye AP, Huang ML, Leisenring W, et al: Cytomegalovirus (CMV) DNA load in plasma for the diagnosis of CMV disease before engraftment in hematopoietic stem-cell transplant recipients. J Infect Dis 183:377, 2001.

MacMillan ML, Goodman JL, DeFor TE, Weisdorf DJ: Fluconazole to prevent yeast infections in bone marrow transplantation patients: A randomized trial of high versus reduced dose, and determination of the value of maintenance therapy. Am J Med 112:369, 2002.

Martin SI, Marty FM, Fiumara K, et al: Infectious complications associated with alemtuzumab use for lymphoproliferative disorders. Clin Infect Dis 43:16, 2006.

Patel SR, Ortin M, Cohen BJ, et al: Revaccination with measles, tetanus, poliovirus, Haemophilus influenzae type B, meningococcus C, and pneumococcus vaccines in children after hematopoietic stem cell transplantation. Clin Infect Dis 44:625, 2007.

Reed EC, Bowden RA, Dandliker PS, et al: Treatment of cytomegalovirus pneumonia with ganciclovir and intravenous cytomegalovirus immunoglobulin in patients with bone marrow transplants. Ann Intern Med 109:783, 1988.

Sullivan KM, Dykewicz CA, Longworth DL, et al: Preventing opportunistic infections after hematopoietic stem cell transplantation: The Centers for Disease Control and Prevention, Infectious Diseases Society of America, and American Society for Blood and Marrow Transplantation Practice Guidelines and beyond. Hematology Am Soc Hematol Educ Program 1:392, 2001.

Ullmann AJ, Lipton JH, Vesole DH, et al: Posaconazole or fluconazole for prophylaxis in severe graft-versus-host disease. N Engl J Med 356:335, 2007.

Upton A, Kirby KA, Carpenter P, et al: Invasive aspergillosis following hematopoietic cell transplantation: Outcomes and prognostic factors associated with mortality. Clin Infect Dis 44:531, 2007.

van Burik J-A, Leisenring W, Myerson D, et al: The effect of prophylactic fluconazole on the clinical spectrum of fungal diseases in bone marrow transplant recipients with special attention to hepatic candidiasis: An autopsy study of 355 patients. Medicine (Baltimore) 77:246, 1998.

van Burik JA, Ratanatharathorn V, Stepan DE, et al: Micafungin versus fluconazole for prophylaxis against invasive fungal infections during neutropenia in patients undergoing hematopoietic stem cell transplantation. Clin Infect Dis 39:1407, 2004.

Wald A, Leisenring W, van Burik JA, Bowden RA: Epidemiology of *Aspergillus* infections in a large cohort of patients undergoing bone marrow transplantation. J Infect Dis 175:1459, 1997.

Weinstock DM, Boeckh M, Sepkowitz KA: Postexposure prophylaxis against varicella zoster virus infection among hematopoietic stem cell transplant recipients. Biol Blood Marrow Transplant 12:1096, 2006.

Zerr DM, Corey L, Kim HW, et al: Clinical outcomes of human herpesvirus 6 reactivation after hematopoietic stem cell transplantation. Clin Infect Dis 40:932, 2005.

REFERENCES

For complete list of references log onto www.expertconsult.com

CHAPTER 92

NUTRITIONAL SUPPORT OF PATIENTS WITH HEMATOLOGIC MALIGNANCIES

Polly Lenssen and Paula M. Charuhas

Patients with hematologic malignancies are highly heterogeneous in terms of their nutritional needs and requirement for nutritional intervention. Patients with aggressive leukemias and lymphomas receive the most intensive of oncologic therapies and frequently experience significant oral and gastrointestinal toxicities, decreased dietary intake, and weight loss. Patients with good-risk acute lymphocytic and chronic leukemias less commonly encounter significant nutritional problems, although the problem of overnutrition has been increasingly recognized in survivors of childhood acute lymphocytic leukemia (ALL).

Use of total parenteral nutrition (TPN) to prevent or treat malnutrition in cancer patients carries significant risks, and in the last decade more attention has focused on feeding patients by the enteral route. This chapter addresses the appropriate use of TPN, tube feeding, and other dietary intervention strategies, such as low microbial diets and high-dose vitamin supplementation, in patients with hematologic malignancies, with special focus on patients undergoing hematopoietic stem cell transplantation (HSCT).

NUTRITIONAL PROBLEMS

Protein-Calorie Malnutrition

Significant weight loss is not common in most patients with hematologic malignancies. In a classic study, DeWys et al.[1] reported that only 4% of patients with acute myeloid leukemia (AML), 10% with favorable-prognosis non-Hodgkin lymphoma, and 15% with unfavorable-prognosis non-Hodgkin lymphoma presented with more than 10% weight loss during the 6 months before initiation of chemotherapy. In children with newly diagnosed acute leukemia, primarily ALL, several large cohort studies found approximately 7% had malnutrition, defined as body mass index (BMI) ≤2 standard deviations compared with reference data or less than 90% weight for height.[2,3]

The risk for development of malnutrition subsequent to diagnosis depends on the toxicity of the therapy administered and the progression of the disease. For patients with hematologic malignancies who go on to HSCT, malnutrition is more prevalent. Deeg et al.[4] categorized a large cohort of adult and pediatric marrow graft recipients by weight status and found that except for chronic myelogenous leukemia in chronic phase and low-risk pediatric ALL, 8% to 28% of patients had mild to moderate malnutrition before transplantation (Table 92–1).

Limited data about the effect of protein-calorie malnutrition on outcome in hematologic malignancies are available. DeWys et al.[1] found that weight loss before diagnosis had no influence on survival in patients with AML but was associated with a significant decrease in survival in patients with favorable-prognosis and unfavorable-prognosis non-Hodgkin lymphoma. Sala et al.[5] reviewed the effect of malnutrition on outcome in pediatric cancer and found mixed results, with the largest cohort (1025 children with ALL) having no relation between nutritional status based on BMI and prognosis (P = 0.72). Likewise, BMI was not associated with prognosis in 621 consecutive patients treated for ALL at St. Jude's, nor did it affect the intracellular levels of thioguanine nucleotides and methotrexate polyglutamates or the systemic clearance of methotrexate, teniposide, etoposide, and cytarabine.[6] On the other hand, in an analysis of 768 children with AML, of whom 10.9% were lower than 10th percentile BMI and 14.8% greater than 90th percentile BMI, the underweight patients were less likely to survive than were patients with BMI in the more normal range (hazard ratio 1.85; P = 0.006) and more likely to experience treatment-related mortality (hazard ratio 2.66; P = 0.003). Similarly, overweight children with AML were less likely to survive (hazard ratio 1.88; P = 0.002) and more likely to have treatment-related mortality (hazard ratio 3.49; P < 0.001).[7] During HSCT, underweight patients are at increased risk for early death. Among adults, survival to day 150 after transplantation is significantly worse for patients at 85% to 95% ideal body weight (IBW; P = 0.004) or less than 85% IBW (P = 0.0001) than for patients at 95% to 140% IBW status. Underweight children had a less marked but similar decrease in survival compared with well-nourished children (P = 0.22 for < 85% IBW vs 95%–140% IBW, and P = 0.01 for 85%–95% IBW vs 95%–140% IBW).[4]

Weight loss of 10% to 15% correlates with a 20% loss of protein mass and clinically significant impairment of physiologic function.[8] Morbidity associated with malnutrition has included increased length of hospital stay and infectious complications. Horsley et al.[9] reported that malnourished HSCT patients, as defined by the patient-generated subjective global assessment tool, experienced an increased length of hospital stay (P = 0.002) compared to well-nourished patients in a prospective study of 66 patients. The adverse consequences of malnutrition on immunity, especially T-cell function, phagocytosis, and complement-mediated defenses, are well described.[10] The effects of malnutrition on gastrointestinal function and immunity may be particularly relevant during the intense treatment of hematologic malignancies, in which the breaching of the gastrointestinal barrier has been implicated as a source of bacteremias and sepsis.[11,12] Although the role of dietary variables in actual bacterial translocation and clinical infections has not been established in humans,[13,14] data in children with cancer support the adverse consequences of malnutrition on infection rates and anergy.[5,7]

Obesity

The concern about excess mortality as a result of inappropriate doses of cytotoxic therapy in obese patients has gained more interest as the prevalence of obesity has increased worldwide in adults and children. Adjusting doses down may result in insufficient tumor kill, whereas dosing on actual weight may result in too much organ toxicity. In a retrospective study of 4356 patients with ALL enrolled in Children's Cancer Group studies, Butturini et al.[15] reported that in patients aged 10 years or older, obesity was associated with an increased risk of leukemia relapse, whereas in patients younger than 10 years, no effect of obesity on disease outcome was observed. In a smaller cohort of Hispanic children with ALL (n = 322), obesity at diagnosis was not associated with decreased overall survival (hazard ratio 1.40) or event-free survival (hazard ratio 1.08).[16] Several studies have implicated obesity as contributing to mortality in pediatric AML[7] as well as in HSCT, including autografting[17–19] and allografting.[20,21] Deeg et al.[4] failed to find any association of obesity and mortality in the largest

Table 92–1 Patients with Malnutrition Before Marrow Grafting

	Adults		Children	
Diagnosis	**Total N**	**N < 95% IBW (%)**	**Total N**	**N < 95% IBW (%)**
AML, low risk	114	15 (13.2)	43	7 (16.2)
AML, high risk	307	40 (13.0)	105	24 (22.8)
ALL, low risk	35	4 (11.4)	21	0
ALL, high risk	158	28 (25.9)	217	25 (11.5)
CML, chronic phase	372	16 (4.3)	23	3 (13.0)
CML, other	206	32 (15.5)	33	8 (24.2)
Lymphoma, remission	92	7 (7.6)	18	4 (22.2)
Lymphoma, relapse	159	23 (14.5)	25	7 (28.0)

ALL, acute lymphocytic leukemia; AML, acute myelogenous leukemia; CML, chronic myelogenous leukemia; IBW, ideal body weight.

Data from Deeg HJ, Seidel K, Bruemmer B, et al: Impact of patient weight on nonrelapse mortality after marrow transplantation. Bone Marrow Transplant 15:461, 1995.

cohort (n = 2238) of adult and pediatric patients undergoing allogeneic or autologous HSCT. These data provide little firm ground on which to inform patients about risks associated with obesity or to make recommendations about healthy weight loss options in anticipation of HSCT.

Obesity as a consequence of therapy has been intensively investigated in childhood ALL Prevalence rates exceed 50% in children treated for ALL. A variety of contributing factors have been identified, including cranial radiation, treatment with prednisone and dexamethasone, decreased physical activity levels, younger age, female gender, and lower than expected total daily energy expenditures.[22–24] In young children aged 30 months or younger at the time of diagnosis, adiposity rebound occurs prematurely, possibly contributing to the high prevalence of obesity in long-term survivors.[25] Adiposity rebound, when BMI increases after its nadir in childhood, is a critical period for regulation of energy balance and adult obesity risk. The metabolic syndrome has been well described in obese survivors of ALL.[22,26–28] Effective interventions to reduce the risk of premature cardiovascular disease have not been defined; however, a rational approach focuses on minimizing excess weight gain by counseling patients on the benefits of proper diet and exercise during and after therapy.

Altered Metabolism

The metabolism of malignant bone marrow is markedly accelerated. Energy expenditure averages 35% to 50% higher than predicted in pediatric and adult patients with leukemia.[29–32] Rates of whole-body protein synthesis and breakdown are almost twice normal.[30,32] Similar derangements in energy and protein metabolism have not been found in patients with lymphoma.[32] Energy expenditure decreases in patients with acute leukemia within days of starting chemotherapy[31,33] providing further evidence that the leukemia itself induces the high metabolic rate. Analogously, maintenance chemotherapy in children with ALL in remission appears to exert no significant adverse effects on energy metabolism.[34,35]

During induction chemotherapy[31] or HSCT,[36] energy expenditure and protein losses appear to increase, although this finding is not consistent.[37] It is likely that the variability of diseases, treatments, and complications after transplantation make it impossible to generalize about the impact of HSCT on energy needs.

Several investigators have reported lower than expected resting metabolic rate in long-term obese survivors of ALL.[38–40]

Toxicities of Oncologic Treatment

The nutritionally relevant toxicities of oncologic treatment are summarized in Table 92–2. Aggressive multimodal treatment often produces multiple toxicities; when prolonged, it can lead to significant nutritional deficits, particularly in children. The nutritional consequences of biologic response modifiers are associated with anorexia and mild to moderate gastrointestinal disturbances.

ASSESSMENT OF ALTERED NUTRITION STATUS

Basic Evaluation

Initial and serial nutritional evaluation and screening are indicated in all patients with hematologic malignancies (see Algorithm for Nutrition Assessment and Intervention below). Early identification of poor dietary intake or depleted weight status (rapid weight loss or inadequate reserves compared with an IBW estimate or reference BMI for age and gender) may avert the morbidity associated with moderate to severe malnutrition. In a survey of 173 pediatric oncology patients of whom 45% had leukemia or lymphoma, Tyc et al.[41] found that poor oral intake, even as a subjective report, was the single best predictor of need for intervention with TPN or enteral tube feeding. In this cohort the mean length of time after diagnosis for nutrition support intervention was 33 weeks, suggesting that earlier identification of poor oral intake often may allow sufficient time to implement earlier intervention programs to increase caloric intake, including nutritional counseling and behavioral therapies. Earlier intervention potentially may circumvent the need for more invasive and costly nutrition therapies.

Weight assessment as an index of body composition is of less value in states of fluid imbalance (edema, dehydration, iatrogenic fluid overload). Weight must be interpreted with caution in metabolically stressed patients, such as those experiencing infectious complications or organ dysfunction with induction therapy or stem cell grafting.[42] Actual nutrient intake as documented by the dietitian often provides the best guide for judging nutritional adequacy during periods of stress. In many institutions, bedside metabolic monitors that measure energy expenditure and help establish the energy goals of nutrition therapy are available.

Measurements of serum albumin, prealbumin, and transferrin seem to reflect metabolic stress, not the adequacy of recent nutrient intake, in patients with leukemia undergoing induction chemotherapy[31,43] or HSCT.[36,44] Serum creatinine may be a surrogate for nutritional status in children. In 37 children with ALL, serum creatinine strongly correlated with serum creatinine and lean body mass (r = 0.83 at diagnosis, r = 0.77 on therapy, r = 0.56 off therapy).[45]

Pediatric Assessment

Accurate serial weight and height measurements are required for assessment of growth and development in children and adolescents. Weight for length in infants and children up to age 3 years and BMI for age in children older than 3 years are the appropriate tools for assessing adequacy of body reserves, using standardized charts.[46] Children less than the fifth percentile for length/height, weight, weight for length, or BMI for age require in-depth assessment and development of a nutrition care plan to improve nutritional status. Likewise, children who are not gaining and growing or who are experiencing weight loss require immediate dietary evaluation and intervention.

Serial heights should also be plotted on velocity charts.[47] Decreased height velocity has been observed in children with hematologic malignancies treated at all ages before puberty and with radiation, chemotherapy alone, and a variety of conditioning regimens with HSCT. The greatest risk factors are younger age, cranial irradiation, single-dose total body irradiation, and male gender.[48–51] The role of chronic nutrient deficiencies has not been investigated, although poor

Table 92–2 Nutritional Problems Associated with Treatment of Hematologic Malignancies

Treatment	Complications
Chemotherapy	
Alkylating agents[a]	Anorexia, nausea, vomiting Diarrhea: Carboplatin, carmustine, cisplatin, dacarbazine, lomustine, mechlorethamine, melphalan, streptozocin Hepatotoxic: Busulfan, carboplatin, carmustine, dacarbazine, lomustine, mechlorethamine, melphalan, streptozocin, thiotepa Hypoglycemia: Streptozocin Nephrotoxic: Carboplatin, carmustine, cisplatin, ifosfamide, lomustine, streptozocin Metallic taste: Cisplatin, melphalan Stomatitis: Carmustine, chlorambucil, ifosfamide, lomustine, mechlorethamine, thiotepa Taste disturbances: Carboplatin, cisplatin
Antitumor antibiotics[b]	Anorexia, nausea, vomiting, stomatitis, diarrhea Gastrointestinal ulceration: Dactinomycin, doxorubicin Hepatotoxic: Idarubicin, mitomycin C, mitoxantrone, plicamycin Nephrotoxic: Mitomycin C, plicamycin Taste disturbances: Bleomycin, dactinomycin, daunorubicin
Antimetabolites[c]	Anorexia, nausea, vomiting, mucositis, diarrhea Constipation: Cladribine, fludarabine, gemcitabine, hydroxyurea, pentostatin Hepatotoxic: Capecitabine, cytarabine, fluorouracil, mercaptopurine, methotrexate, thioguanine Malabsorption: Mercaptopurine, methotrexate Nephrotoxic: Cytarabine, pentostatin, mercaptopurine, methotrexate, thioguanine Taste disturbances: Methotrexate
Plant alkaloids[d]	Stomatitis, nausea, vomiting, diarrhea Anorexia: Etoposide, topotecan, vincristine Constipation, ileus: Vinblastine, vincristine Hepatotoxic: Etoposide, paclitaxel, vinblastine, vincristine, vinorelbine Nephrotoxic: Irinotecan, paclitaxel
Other[e]	Anorexia, diarrhea, fluid and electrolyte disturbances Diarrhea: L-Asparaginase, imatinib mesylate, pegaspargase, procarbazine Hyperglycemia: L-Asparaginase, pegaspargase Nausea, vomiting: Procarbazine Nephrotoxic and/or hepatotoxic: L-Asparaginase, pegaspargase, procarbazine Pancreatitis: L-Asparaginase Stomatitis: Procarbazine
Hormones[f]	Muscle and bone loss, hypokalemia, fat deposition and weight gain, sodium and fluid retention, glucose intolerance, hyperphagia, increased thirst, hypercalcemia, hyperlipidemia, osteoporosis, gastrointestinal upset, negative nitrogen balance Anorexia: Diethylstilbestrol, letrozole, tamoxifen Diarrhea: Letrozole Hepatotoxic: Tamoxifen Increased growth velocity: Fluoxymesterone
Irradiation	
Head and neck	Stomatitis, xerostomia, odynophagia and dysphagia, anorexia, taste alterations, dysosmia, osteonecrosis
Esophageal	Esophagitis, esophageal stricture
Stomach	Anorexia, gastritis, nausea, vomiting
Abdominal	Enteritis, diarrhea, steatorrhea, malabsorption, stenosis, obstruction, fistula formation, protein-losing enteropathy, fluid and electrolyte imbalances
Total body	Stomatitis, nausea, vomiting, diarrhea, taste alterations, xerostomia, growth failure
Biologic Agents[g]	
	Anorexia, nausea, vomiting, diarrhea Angioedema: Rituximab Hepatotoxic: Aldesleukin, interferon, interleukin Nephrotoxic: Aldesleukin Stomatitis: Aldesleukin
Hematopoietic Stem Cell Transplantation	
	Stomatitis, esophagitis, gastrointestinal ulceration, diarrhea, taste alterations, xerostomia Venoocclusive disease; Hepatic, renal, pulmonary dysfunction; multiple organ failure Acute and chronic graft-versus-host disease Infectious enteritis

[a]Busulfan, carboplatin, carmustine, chlorambucil, cisplatin, cyclophosphamide, dacarbazine, ifosfamide, lomustine, mechlorethamine, melphalan, streptozocin, thiotepa.
[b]Bleomycin, dactinomycin, daunorubicin, doxorubicin, epirubicin, idarubicin, mitomycin C, mitoxantrone, plicamycin.
[c]Azacytidine, capecitabine, cladribine, cytarabine, fludarabine, fluorouracil, gemcitabine, hydroxyurea, mercaptopurine, methotrexate, pentostatin, thioguanine.
[d]Docetaxel, etoposide, irinotecan, paclitaxel, teniposide, topotecan, vinblastine, vincristine, vinorelbine.
[e]L-Asparaginase, imatinib mesylate, mitoxantrone, pamidronate, pegaspargase, procarbazine, zoledronic acid.
[f]Glucocorticoids.
[g]Aldesleukin, alemtuzumab, gemtuzumab ozogamicin, interferons, interleukins, rituximab, trastuzumab, tretinoin.

nutritional status before HSCT was associated with decreased height velocity at 1 year after transplantation.[52] Optimizing nutritional intake is essential for children with hematologic malignancies to maximize their growth potential along the entire continuum of care for their disease (see Algorithm for Nutrition Assessment and Intervention below).

NUTRITIONAL INTERVENTION

Dietary Recommendations and Modifications

Dietary recommendations during periods of treatment toxicities and prolonged anorexia are accessible elsewhere,[53] including recommendations specific for pediatric[54] and adult[55] patients undergoing HSCT.

Appetite and taste perception can be influenced by central nervous system changes as well as by peripheral mechanisms associated with insults to chemosensory structures resulting from chemotherapy, radiation, poor oral health, altered salivary flow, and oral mucositis.[56] Up to 70% of patients receiving chemotherapy report changes in taste and smell. Cisplatin, cyclophosphamide, doxorubicin, carboplatin, 5-fluorouracil, levamisole, and methotrexate are associated with taste changes (see Table 92–2). In 284 adults surveyed by questionnaire after chemotherapy, taste changes were most often associated with xerostomia, nausea, and decreased appetite.[57] Taste changes may influence interest in eating and diet quality from several days to several weeks after HSCT. Mattsson et al.[58] reported significant hypogeusia immediately after HSCT in 10 patients compared with 10 control subjects, which can adversely impact oral intake at a time when nutritional requirements are elevated. Epstein et al.[59] surveyed 50 patients 90 to 100 days after HSCT and reported that 65% of patients still complained of changes in taste, ranked as mild, moderate or severe, at the time of the survey; smell changes and xerostomia were significantly correlated with changes in taste. However, these taste changes were reported to have a limited impact on perceived quality of life. Proper assessment and considerations of taste and smell alterations are essential to provide individualized diet recommendations.

Diet modifications may include changes in consistency, texture, temperature, taste, and smell of food, especially when patients experience mucositis, esophagitis, xerostomia, or dysgeusia. Reduction of fat and lactose content may decrease nausea or diarrhea. A dietetics professional can recommend appropriate nutritional supplements for patients who exhibit malabsorption or show an inability to gain weight. During hospitalization, a food service that is individualized and that includes frequent followup by trained nutrition staff best meets the needs of patients undergoing intense oncologic therapy.

Diet Guidelines for Immunosuppressed Patients

Historically, HSCT patients were treated with gastrointestinal decontamination in ultraisolation or high-efficiency particulate air (HEPA)-filtered environments and were served diets of varying microbial restrictions, ranging from "sterile" to "cooked food only."[60,61] Sterile diets are rarely served by institutions today because of high production costs[61] and the shift to ambulatory clinic treatment and care. Most hospitals acknowledge the need to impose dietary restrictions to limit pathogen exposure in patients with compromised immune function and routinely provide some form of low microbial food service to patients with neutropenia or who are undergoing HSCT.[62–64]

The protective benefit of low microbial diets against infection has not been established because of a lack of randomized controlled trials.[62,65] Nonetheless, the possibility that food may serve as a source of infection is evidenced by reports implicating food as sources of pathogenic organisms in immunosuppressed patient populations, including HSCT recipients.[66–74] Safdar et al.[75] suggested an association between reactivation of acute human cytomegalovirus infection in HSCT recipients and subsequent *Listeria monocytogenes* infection due to human cytomegalovirus–associated dysfunction in host cellular immune response. Other immunosuppressive conditions that diminish cellular immunity may increase the risk of listeriosis.[69,71–73] During a 15-year period that included 20,612 hospital admissions, Mora et al.[76] reported listeriosis infections in five children (three with leukemia, one with lymphoma, and one with a brain tumor), all of whom recovered after antibiotic treatment. Case reports of *L. monocytogenes* and *Clostridium botulinum* infections in HSCT recipients have proved difficult to attribute to contaminated foodstuffs.[70,71,74,75] The incubation period for *L. monocytogenes* (onset up to 30 days) as well as other foodborne illness organisms may be such that suspect foodstuffs have been discarded, and an accurate food intake history to identify the potential contaminated food is difficult. Furthermore, most *L. monocytogenes* infections in HSCT patients have been detected in the ambulatory care setting, making it more difficult to trace to specific food intake.[71,74,75] Fungal infections are common in the immunosuppressed host but difficult to link with food-originated infection. Numerous foods, such as aged cheeses, fermented products (e.g., miso, tempeh), and naturopathic substances,[77] may serve as sources of fungal infections. Bouakline et al.[78] examined the prevalence of fungal organisms in nonheat-sterilized foods. *Aspergillus* species were detected in 100% of black pepper and regular tea samples (unbrewed sample), 12% to 66% of fruits, 27% of herbal teas (unbrewed sample), and 20% of freeze-dried soup samples (not reconstituted). All soft cheese samples were contaminated by *Geotrichum* and yeast (*Candida norvegensis*), but processed cheeses were free of fungal organisms. The raw produce in this study was not washed before culturing, nor were the food cultures taken after brewing or cooking.

Low microbial or cooked food diets vary widely in terms of food choices (e.g., exclusion or inclusion of raw produce) and bacterial content and are generally empirically formulated, although some institutions culture foods and assess food acceptability when developing such diets.[61] Moe[79] cultured 198 foods prepared by conventional methods. Although 80% of beverages, starches, cooked meats and entrees, and frozen vegetables were acceptable, only 36% of pasteurized dairy products and 42% of dessert and snack items met minimal microbiologic criteria. Up to 17 different species of gram-negative rods in concentrations as high as 10^6 colony-forming units (CFU)/mL in milk, pudding, and ice cream were identified. Ayers et al.[66] found that serving foods containing only *Bacillus* resulted in transient colonization with *Bacillus* species in 41% of patients studied, but no infections occurred.

Fresh fruits and vegetables historically have been excluded from low microbial diets, placing patients at risk for micronutrient deficiencies.[65] Organisms routinely found on washed raw fruits and vegetables do not appear to be common sources of infection in immunosuppressed patients. At the Fred Hutchinson Cancer Research Center, 29 cultures of assorted raw, washed fruits showed gram-positive cocci and gram-negative rods (<4000 CFU/mL) that are commonly found in food (SN Aker, Unpublished Data, 2003). One of three strawberry cultures and two of three apricot cultures showed a range from 200 to 2000 CFU/mL of five mold types. Thirty-six samples of raw, washed vegetables resulted in a broader variety of gram-positive and gram-negative organisms at levels ranging from less than 200 to too numerous to count per milliliter, with few yeasts or molds. The organisms cultured from these fruits and vegetables are not representative of common infections routinely seen in immunosuppressed cancer and HSCT patient populations. Except for infrequent reports such as cyclosporiasis associated with imported fresh raspberries[80] and *Escherichia coli* 0157:H7 contamination of unpasteurized fruit juices[81] and raw vegetable sprouts, food outbreaks associated with raw, washed domestic fruits and vegetables are rare.

Use of strict isolation laminar airflow environments has been largely replaced with single and occasionally HEPA-filtered hospital rooms that use strict hand washing only for the neutropenic oncology

Algorithm for Nutrition Assessment and Intervention

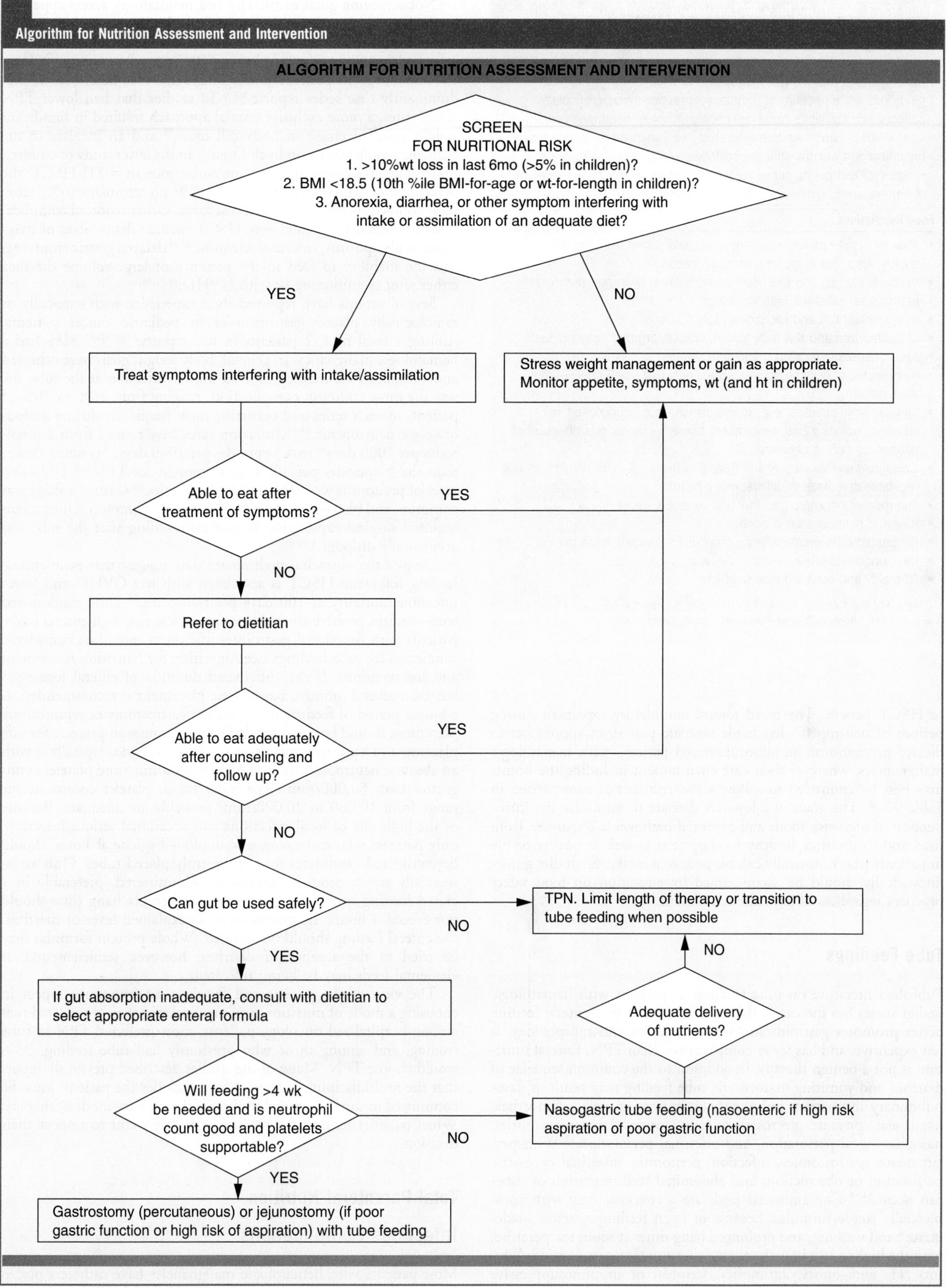
ALGORITHM FOR NUTRITION ASSESSMENT AND INTERVENTION
SCREEN
FOR NUTRITIONAL RISK
1. >10%wt loss in last 6mo (>5% in children)?
2. BMI <18.5 (10th %ile BMI-for-age or wt-for-length in children)?
3. Anorexia, diarrhea, or other symptom interfering with
intake or assimilation of an adequate diet?
YES
NO
Treat symptoms interfering with intake/assimilation
Stress weight management or gain as appropriate.
Monitor appetite, symptoms, wt (and ht in children)
Able to eat after
treatment of symptoms?
YES
NO
Refer to dietitian
Able to eat adequately
after counseling and
follow up?
YES
NO
Can gut be used safely?
TPN. Limit length of therapy or transition to
tube feeding when possible
NO
YES
NO
If gut absorption inadequate, consult with dietitian to
select appropriate enteral formula
Adequate delivery
of nutrients?
Will feeding >4 wk
be needed and is neutrophil
count good and platelets
supportable?
Nasogastric tube feeding (nasoenteric if high risk
aspiration of poor gastric function
NO
YES
Gastrostomy (percutaneous) or jejunostomy (if poor
gastric function or high risk of aspiration) with tube feeding

Table 92–3 Diet Guidelines for Immunosuppressed Patients

These diet guidelines restrict high-risk foods as *potential* sources of organisms known to cause infection in immunosuppressed persons. It is recommended that the following groups of patients use these diet guidelines while undergoing immunosuppressive therapy: oncology patients with low white blood cell counts (absolute neutrophil count <1.0 × 10^3 μL) and hematopoietic stem cell transplant recipients for a minimum of 4 months after transplantation (autologous, allogeneic, syngeneic) and during subsequent immunosuppressive drug treatment of chronic complications (all transplant types).

Food Restrictions

- *Raw and undercooked* meat (including wild game), fish, shellfish, poultry, eggs, hot dogs, tofu, sausage, bacon
- Ready-to-eat deli and luncheon meats, salami, sausages, precooked ham (unless reheated until steaming)
- Cold smoked fish and lox, pickled fish
- *Unpasteurized* and raw milk, yogurt, cheese, or other dairy products
- Aged cheeses (e.g., bleu, Roquefort, Stilton)
- Refrigerated cheese-based salad dressings, (e.g., bleu cheese), not shelf stable
- Mexican-style cheeses (e.g., queso blanco fresco); uncooked soft cheeses, including brie, camembert, farmer's cheese, feta cheese; hot pepper–containing cheeses
- *Unwashed* raw vegetables and fruits and those with visible mold; all raw vegetable sprouts (e.g., alfalfa, mung bean)
- Commercial *unpasteurized* fruit and vegetable juices
- Raw and nonheat-treated honey
- Fermented miso products (e.g., miso soup), tempeh, maté tea
- Raw, uncooked brewer's yeast
- All moldy and outdated food products

Courtesy of the Nutrition Services Department, Seattle Cancer Care Alliance, and Fred Hutchinson Cancer Research Center, Seattle, WA.

or HSCT patient. The trend toward ambulatory treatment during periods of neutropenia has made obsolete past strict approaches to dietary precautions. Immunosuppressed patients with hematologic malignancies, wherever their care environment including the home, may best be counseled to follow a low-risk diet as summarized in Table 92–3. The goals of a low-risk diet are to minimize the introduction of high-risk foods and potential pathogenic organisms from food and to promote healthy food options as well as quality of life in patients who historically exhibit poor oral intake. Such diet guidelines ideally should be accompanied by education on food safety practices regardless of patient environment.

Tube Feedings

Published literature on tube feedings in patients with hematologic malignancies has increased, driven by the belief that enteral feeding better promotes gastrointestinal tract function and morphology, is less expensive, and has fewer complications than TPN. Enteral nutrition is not a benign therapy. In addition to the common sequelae of diarrhea and vomiting, nasoenteric tube feeding may result in nasopulmonary intubation, pulmonary aspiration, epistaxis, rhinorrhea, nasal alar pressure necrosis, sinusitis, otitis, laryngeal injuries, nasopharyngeal perforation, and intestinal perforation.[82] With percutaneous gastrostomies, infection, peritonitis, intestinal or gastric perforation or obstruction, and abdominal wall migration of tubes can occur.[83,84] Contaminated feeds are a concern, even with commercially sterile formulas, because of open feeding systems, inadequate hand washing, and prolonged hang times at room temperature, with the highest risk in patients receiving antacids, gastric acid inhibitors, H_2 antagonists, antibiotics, steroids, or immunosuppressive therapy.[85]

Not achieving goals of therapy and maintaining access appear to be the biggest obstacles with enteral feeds, leading to undernutrition or the need for supplementation with partial TPN. The inability to infuse adequate nutrition has led to TPN "rescue" rates ranging from 14% to 100% in patients undergoing HSCT as described in predominantly case series reports.[86–96] In studies that had lower TPN rescue rates, a more exclusive enteral approach resulted in significant weight loss,[92] decrease in body cell mass,[86] and an increase in the frequency of malnutrition in children.[93] In the latter study of children undergoing allogeneic (n = 42) or autologous (n = 11) HSCT, the percentage of patients less than 85% IBW pretransplant (6%) more than doubled to 14% at hospital discharge. Other reported complications of enteral feeds following HSCT include deficiencies of magnesium, phosphorus, zinc, and selenium,[87,93] delayed gastric emptying, and the inability to feed in the presence of large-volume diarrhea either after conditioning or with GVHD.[88,91,93]

Several groups have reported their experience with surgically or radiologically placed gastrostomies in pediatric cancer patients. Among a total of 152 patients in five reports,[89,90,97–99] 31% had a hematologic malignancy. In general, body weight goals were achieved and complications were considered minor. Infection at the tube site was the most common complication, ranging from 40% to 70% of patients in each series and occurring most frequently during periods of severe neutropenia.[88,91] Infection rates have ranged from 1.6 episodes per 1000 days[88] to 4.5 episodes per 1000 days,[92] generally lower than the 5 episodes per 1000 days reported for TPN.[100] Only two cases of peritonitis were reported in these series.[90] Gastric leakage was common, and bleeding at the tube site was less common. One patient required surgical exploration to control bleeding after the tube was accidentally dislodged.[98]

Despite the obstacles, preliminary data suggest that early enteral feeding following HSCT is associated with less GVHD and lower infection mortality at 100 days posttransplant.[96] Until randomized trials confirm positive clinical benefit and less risk with enteral feeds, patients with functional gastrointestinal tracts should be considered candidates for tube feedings (see Algorithm for Nutrition Assessment and Intervention). If the anticipated duration of enteral feeding is less than several months, nasoenteric placement is recommended. If a longer period of feeding is expected, a gastrostomy or jejunostomy placement should be considered. The most common practice for safe placement of a gastrostomy either surgically or endoscopically is with an absolute neutrophil count of 500 to 1000/mm^3 and platelet count greater than 50,000/mm^3. For nasal tubes, platelet counts in the range from 10,000 to 20,000/mm^3 probably are adequate. Because of the high rate of local infections and occasional serious infection, only patients who can manage scrupulous hygiene at home should be considered candidates for permanently placed tubes. Only commercially sterile products should be administered, preferably in a closed feeding system. In open systems, formula hang time should not exceed 4 hours. In patients with unexplained fever or diarrhea, the enteral feeding should be cultured. Whole-protein formulas may be tried in the absence of diarrhea; however, semielemental or elemental feeds may be better tolerated.

The view of the patient and family is an important aspect in choosing a mode of nutrition support. Scolapio et al.[101] reported that among hospitalized oncology patients, most preferred TPN to tube feeding, and among those who previously had tube feeding, 93% would choose TPN. Many of the studies described previously report that the multidisciplinary team, which includes the patient, must be committed to support enteral feeding as the primary mode of therapy. When patients refuse tube feeding, it is important to respect their decision.

Total Parenteral Nutrition

Infectious Complications

Most patients with hematologic malignancies have catheters placed for central venous access. In patients provided with TPN, an increase in infection rates has been observed compared with patients with central catheters not on TPN.[44,100,102] In 310 children with cancer and central venous lines (including 244 patients with acute leukemia), administration of TPN was associated with a 2.4-fold increase in the risk of infection ($P < 0.001$), defined as documented catheter-related septicemia, catheter exit site, port or tunnel infection, or sepsis of unknown origin.[100] Among 104 adult and pediatric recipients of allogeneic marrow grafts, Weisdorf et al.[44] documented bacteremias in 72% of patients randomized to TPN versus 48% randomized to hydration therapy during the first posttransplantation month ($P < 0.001$). Lough et al.[102] demonstrated similar findings in a smaller study of 29 allogeneic and autologous transplant patients in which 57% of the patients randomized to TPN developed positive blood culture compared with less than 7% randomized to maintenance hydration for 14 days ($P < 0.05$). No deaths were attributed to the infectious complications described in these reports.

The association between TPN and infectious complications has been linked to a variety of etiologic factors, including excessive dextrose and total calorie infusion, inadequate glycemic control, lipids, insufficient glutamine, and lack of enteral stimulation of gut immunity. Elevated serum glucose levels impair neutrophil and complement function and predispose patients to *Candida* infections.[103,104] Interest in controlling blood sugar levels has grown since the publication of findings that intensive insulin therapy that maintained blood glucose level at or below 110 mg/dL reduced bloodstream infections by 46% and mortality by 34% in critically ill surgical patients.[105] In patients in a medical intensive care unit, however, insulin therapy was associated with greater mortality.[106] In the absence of data specific to patients with hematologic malignancies, strategies to control blood sugar in addition to insulin therapy involve matching the TPN prescription to metabolic needs (determined by indirect calorimetry or estimated by experienced clinician) and substitution of a greater proportion of dextrose energy with lipid.

Lipids have long been a concern in terms of infection risk. It appears that only large doses (up to 4 g/kg) or very fast infusion rates (100–200 mL/hour of 20% emulsions) cause any adverse effect on neutrophil, phagocyte, and reticuloendothelial system function.[107] No evidence indicates that lipids affect humoral immunity or the complement system, although their impact on T-cell lymphocyte activities is not clearly established.[108] In general, infusion of moderate amounts of lipids (25%–30% of total calories) over a minimum of 12 hours is considered prudent and safe practice. A large randomized trial failed to show an association between a moderate dose of lipid (25%–30% of total energy) versus a low dose (6%–8% of total energy to prevent essential fatty acid deficiency) and bacterial and fungal infections during the first hospitalization in patients undergoing HSCT.[109] Lipids containing medium-chain triglycerides are popular in Europe because they have improved bloodstream clearance and are purported to have immunologic benefits, but they are not approved for use in the United States. No clinical benefit was observed with use of a 50% medium-chain triglycerides/50% long-chain triglyceride mixture versus a 100% long-chain triglyceride–based lipid emulsion when provided as 30% of nonprotein calories in 36 patients undergoing HSCT, and fewer days of febrile neutropenia and antibiotic use were observed with the long-chain triglyceride group.[110]

The addition to TPN of pharmacologic doses of intravenous glutamine, a nonessential amino acid oxidized by stimulated lymphocytes and macrophages and intestinal mucosal cells, has been postulated to maintain the gut mucosal barrier during periods of gut rest and prevent infection associated with bacterial translocation, as has been described in animal models of methotrexate or radiation-induced intestinal injury.[111–113] In a Cochrane review of available trials in humans, TPN with glutamine was associated with a decrease in positive blood infections.[114] However, careful analysis of the data reveals that the Cochrane review counted colonization cultures from stool and other sites as blood infections. These studies are perhaps not as strong as suggested,[115,116] and other reviews caution against routine use until more studies demonstrate efficacy (Table 92–4).[91,117] In patients with AML undergoing chemotherapy, neutrophil recov-

Table 92–4 Summary of Randomized Trials of Glutamine in Patients Undergoing Hematopoietic Stem Cell Transplantation with Myeloablative Regimens

Study	No. of Autograft Patients	No. of Allograft Patients	Mucositis	TPN	Days of Infection	GVHD	Relapse	Long-term Survival
Intravenous Glutamine								
Zeigler et al.[115] 1992		45	ND	ND	+	ND	?	?
Schloerb and Amare[116] 1993	14	15	ND	ND	ND	?	?	?
Pytlik et al.[119] 2002	40		–	ND	ND	Not applicable	-	-
Piccirillo et al.[157] 2003	27		ND	+	?	?	?	
Sykorova et al.[120] 2005	54		?	?	?			–
Oral Glutamine								
Jebb et al.[152] 1995	24		ND	ND	?	Not applicable	ND at 6 months	?
Anderson et al.[153] 1998	87	55 sibling 51 URD	+ Auto – Sibling ND URD	ND	ND	ND	?	ND[a]
Schloerb and Skikne[154] 1999	48	18	ND	ND	ND	ND	?	ND
Coughlin Dickson et al.[155] 2000	34	24	ND	ND	?	?	ND	ND
Acquino et al.[156] 2005	54	66	ND	+	ND	?	?	

[a]Day 28 survival was significantly better for the glutamine group, but no difference was seen by day 100.

GVHD, graft-versus-host disease; ND, no difference between glutamine and placebo; TPN, total parenteral nutrition; URD, unrelated donor; +, benefit of glutamine over placebo; –, benefit of placebo control over glutamine; ?, not reported.

Adapted from the American Society for Parenteral and Enteral Nutrition (ASPEN): Nutrient support in hematopoietic cell transplantation. JPEN J Parent Enteral Nutr 25:223, 2001.

ery was more rapid ($P = 0.052$) in patients receiving TPN supplemented with glycyl-glutamine dipeptide than in patients receiving nonsupplemented TPN; however, no difference in the occurrence of neutropenic fever, the recovery of $CD4^+$ or $CD8^+$ lymphocytes, or monocyte activation was observed.[118] Two clinical trials using alanyl-glutamine dipeptide described significantly more relapses in patients undergoing autologous HSCT randomized to glutamine supplementation.[119,120] Although infection data were not specifically reported, these data generate concern for the effect of glutamine supplementation on long-term survival in patients with hematologic malignancies. Glutamine enhances the synthesis of the intracellular antioxidant glutathione, such that pharmacologic doses given in the peritransplantation period could protect the tumor. To examine the key endpoints of relapse and survival, Powell-Tuck et al.[121] suggested that a glutamine study would require in excess of 160 patients, far more than any study published to date.

Efficacy

Do the benefits of weight maintenance and provision of macronutrient and micronutrient substrates outweigh the infectious risks of TPN? Expert reviews have generally concluded that TPN should not be a routine part of care for patients undergoing chemotherapy or radiation because of the complications associated with TPN. It is recommended only in patients with malnutrition and in children unable to grow and develop normally or with weight loss greater than 5% when oral or enteral feedings fail.[117,122–124] Many of the studies forming the basis of these reviews were performed several decades ago, when energy prescriptions were excessive. The efficacy of adjunctive TPN during therapy has not been adequately investigated in the current era, and the clinician must exercise judgment based on expected toxicities, ongoing surveillance of nutritional status, and ability of the family and team to overcome any barriers to alternatives, adequate volitional oral intake, or tube feeding.

Weisdorf et al.[44] reported TPN increased survival after HSCT. When data from other studies were combined in a meta-analysis, a nonsignificant trend for TPN to decrease mortality compared with intravenous hydration was noted.[114] The overall interpretation of the collective data is equivocal with a variety of published recommendations, including the routine use of TPN when prolonged gastrointestinal failure is expected,[114] more specifically in myeloablative conditioning regimens or refractory GVHD,[117] and finally leaving its use to the judgment of the responsible clinician.[123] As other supportive measures have altered the toxicity profile of HSCT and as reduced-intensity and nonmyeloablative conditioning regimens have been established as viable treatment options, the role of TPN and its substitution with enteral feedings requires reexamination.

Implementation and Formulations

Safe and appropriate TPN may be initiated and monitored in consultation with a hospital nutrition support service or with a nutrition support-certified or oncology dietitian. Table 92–5 outlines an approach to implementation of TPN.

Research on the pharmacologic applications of nutritional support has intensified with accumulating evidence on the modulation of physiologic, immune, and endocrine functions by nutrients. TPN solutions enriched with branched-chain amino acids have been investigated as a fuel source designed to blunt the muscle catabolism and obligatory nitrogen losses associated with HSCT, with mixed success.[36,125] Taurine, another nonessential amino acid not contained in adult TPN solutions, also may be deficient after HSCT.[126] Taurine conjugates hepatotoxic bile acids and improves bile acid secretory rates.[127] Glutamine-supplemented TPN was discussed earlier (see Infectious Complications above).

NUTRITION SUPPORT IN HEMATOPOIETIC STEM CELL TRANSPLANTATION

Standard supportive care during the first month after transplantation with myeloablative regimens has included TPN, and many patients with slow gastrointestinal healing or GVHD have relied on TPN to some degree for extended periods in the ambulatory setting. Among patients who are at increased risk for GVHD, early TPN intervention helps prevent significant weight loss before the onset of acute or chronic GVHD when metabolic needs appear higher and may be more difficult to achieve.[128] Less need for TPN has been described in patients whose source of stem cells was peripheral blood compared with bone marrow,[129] treatment occurred at home compared with the hospital setting,[130] or conditioning regimen was of reduced intensity.[131]

The decision to terminate TPN may depend on a constellation of clinical factors, including nutritional status, severity of gastrointestinal toxicities, ability to sustain or progress with oral intake, and the physiologic and psychological impact of TPN. In a large, double-blind trial that included adult and pediatric allogeneic and autologous transplant patients, Charuhas et al.[132] compared the effect of continuing TPN or changing to hydration fluids on the time to resumption of adequate oral intake in patients who were not able to eat 70% of estimated maintenance energy needs at the time of hospital discharge. Patients randomized to hydration fluids met oral calorie goals a median of 6 days sooner than did patients on TPN ($P = 0.049$) without evidence of adverse consequences, such as increased hospital readmissions or clinically significant weight loss, when TPN was withheld for up to 1 month. Discontinuation of TPN appears safe when patients are eating 30% of estimated energy needs at hospital discharge unless a clinical condition, such as malnutrition, malabsorption, or significant gastrointestinal toxicities, warrants otherwise.

Total energy and protein (oral plus TPN) support is recommended at stress levels (see Table 92–5) after myeloablative conditioning and during the neutropenic period based on the well-described losses of nitrogen and body cell mass.[36,44,133] Patients who still require TPN after engraftment and are otherwise without infectious problems or GVHD may be supported at maintenance needs. Use of specialty formulations was discussed earlier (see Implementation and Formulations above).

Few studies characterize micronutrient status after HSCT. Serum levels of the antioxidants vitamin E and β carotene in patients on TPN are markedly depressed, but the clinical significance is unknown.[134] Depleted antioxidant status is associated with increased free radical activity after transplantation[135,136]; however, no correlations have been established between these findings and the degree of toxicities observed with cytoreductive therapy nor the effect on tumor cell killing. In experimental models, vitamin C at therapeutic doses protects bone marrow cells.[137] In a prospective study, Bruemmer et al.[138] observed that pretransplantation intakes of more than 500 mg vitamin C and more than 400 mg vitamin E were associated with increased mortality or relapse in HSCT patients treated for acute leukemia. These studies suggest cautious use of antioxidants in the peritransplantation period (see box on Complementary and Alternative Nutritional Therapies).

Manganese toxicity that manifested as a Parkinson-like syndrome with brain magnetic resonance imaging suggestive of manganese accumulation has been described in a patient with cholestatic liver disease who received supplementation with manganese 0.3 mg/day during 2 months of TPN.[139] These investigators found elevated serum manganese levels in eight other transplant patients with liver disease, suggesting the need for manganese restriction in the presence of cholestasis.[139]

Oral and Gastrointestinal Complications

The degree of mucosal toxicity is regimen specific and has been characterized in four phases: an inflammatory phase caused by the

Table 92–5 Approach to TPN Management

1. Determine Macronutrient Requirements (Protein, Dextrose, Lipid, and Fluid)

Nutrient	Adult	Adolescent	Children
Protein (g/kg)			
Available as crystalline amino acids 4 kcal/g protein			
Maintenance	1.0	1.0	1.2 (7–10 years) 1.5 (4–6 years) 1.8 (1–3 years)
Stress	1.5–2.0	2.0	2.4 (7–10 years) 3.0 (1–6 years)
Energy (kcal/kg)			
Maintenance 1.2–1.3 × basal needs	25–30	40–50	50–60 (7–10 years) 60–70 (4–6 years) 70–85 (1–3 years)
Rehabilitation/stress 1.5 × basal needs	40–45	45–65	65–75 (7–10 years) 75–90 (4–6 years) 90–100 (1–3 years)
Carbohydrate (mg/kg/min)[a]	<5	<7–10	<10–15
Available as dextrose monohydrate 3.4 kcal/g			
Lipid	% of total kcal:	1–4 g/kg	
Available as long-chain triglycerides (soybean or safflower oil, egg yolk phospholipid) in 10% (1.1 kcal/mL) and 20% (2 kcal/mL) solutions; 30% (3 kcal/mL) solutions available for 3:1 compounding only; 20% and 30% lipids preferred because of lower phospholipid content	Minimum 6%–8% Maximum 60%		
Maintenance fluid	1500 mL/m^2	1500 mL/m^2	100 mL/kg up to 10 kg +50 mL/kg for each kg 11–20 kg +20 mL/kg for each kg 21–40 kg

2. Provide Electrolytes, Vitamins, and Trace Elements Daily, Altering Requirements Based on Organ Function

Electrolyte or Micronutrient	Adult	Adolescent	Children
Potassium[b]		1–2 mEq/kg	2–4 mEq/kg
Available as phosphate, chloride, acetate salts. Increased needs with amphotericin, thiazide diuretics, foscarnet, steroids, anabolism, GI losses. Decreased needs with spironolactone, renal dysfunction, tumor lysis syndrome.			
Sodium[b]		1–2 mEq/kg	2–4 mEq/kg
Available as chloride, acetate, or phosphate salts. Increased needs with GI losses, syndrome of inappropriate antidiuretic hormone secretion. Decreased needs with pulmonary edema, congestive heart failure, venoocclusive disease.			
Calcium	10–15 mEq	10–30 mEq	1–2.5 mEq/kg
Available as gluconate salt. Increased needs with foscarnet. Decreased need with renal dysfunction, tumor lysis syndrome, multiple myeloma, metastatic breast cancer.			
Phosphorus		10–40 mM	0.5–2 mM/kg
Available as potassium or sodium salts. Increased needs with diuretics, cyclophosphamide, cisplatinum, foscarnet, anabolism.			
Decreased needs with renal dysfunction.			
Magnesium		16–32 mEq	0.25–0.5 mEq/kg
Available as sulfate salt. Increased needs with amphotericin, cyclosporine, tacrolimus, cisplatinum, foscarnet, GI losses, anabolism.			
Decreased needs with renal dysfunction, tumor lysis syndrome.			
Zinc		2.5–5 mg	100 μg/kg[c]
Available as chloride or sulfate salt in both single-entity and combination preparation. Increased needs with GI losses (5–10 mg/L of stool) wound healing.			

Table 92–5 Approach to TPN Management—cont'd

Electrolyte or Micronutrient	Adult	Adolescent	Children
Copper Available as sulfate salt in both single-entity and combination preparation. Increased needs with GI losses. Decreased needs with cholestasis.		300–500 mg	20 μg/kg[c]
Manganese Available as chloride salt in both single-entity and combination preparation. Decreased needs with cholestasis.		60–150 μg	40–100 mcg
Chromium Available as chloride salt in both single-entity and combination preparation.	10–15 μg		5–15 mcg
Selenium Available as selenious acid in both single-entity and combination preparation.		30–60 μg	3 μg/kg (maximum 30 mcg)
Molybdenum Available as ammonium molybdate as single entity.	20–120 μg	5-10 mcg	0.25 μg/kg (maximum 5 mcg)
Vitamins Available as adult and pediatric multivitamin combinations of water- and fat-soluble vitamins or single infusions of cobalamin, folate, thiamine, pantothenic acid, pyridoxine, ascorbic acid, vitamin K. A D E B_1 (thiamine) B_2 (riboflavin) Niacin Folic acid B_5 (pyridoxine) Pantothenic acid Biotin[d] B_{12} (cobalamin) C K	3300 IU (990 RE) 200 IU (5 RE) 10 IU (6.7 RE) 6 mg 3.6 mg 40 mg 600 μg 4 mg 15 mg 60 μg 5 μg 200 mg 150 mg		2300 IU (690 RE) 400 IU (10 RE) 10.4 IU (7 RE) 1.2 mg 1.4 mg 17 mg 140 μg 1 mg 5 mg 20 μg 1 μg 80 mg 200 μg
Iron Available as iron dextran.	Contraindicated in patients with hematologic malignancies		
3. Monitor for Special Managements Issues			
Hyperglycemia	If preexisting diabetes or refractory to insulin, limit dextrose to <3 mg/kg/min in adults, <7–10 mg/kg/min in children; increase lipids to 50% total energy		
Hypertriglyceridemia	>500 mg/dL: Limit lipids to 4%–8% total energy to provide essential fatty acids >1000 mg/dL: discontinue lipids to decrease risk of pancreatitis		
Fluid overload	Provide concentrated dextrose, lipid, amino acid solutions to maximize nutrient support		
Altered liver function	Avoid overfeeding, provide balance of lipids and dextrose, provide some enteral feeds		
4. Monitor Ability to Eat, Transition to Tube Feeding, or Both, As Soon As Feasible			

[a]To calculate carbohydrate dose, divide total mg dextrose per day by 1440 min/day/kg weight. For example, 1700 mL 25% dextrose in a 70-kg patient = 425 g dextrose × 1000 mg/g ± 1440 min/day/70 kg = 4.2 mg/kg/min dextrose.

[b]After determining phosphate needs, remainder provided primarily as chloride salt (except in presence of metabolic acidosis) to meet chloride needs.

[c]Up to 5 years; older than 5 years, use lower limit of guidelines for adolescent and adult.

[d]Currently available multivitamin combinations do not contain biotin.

GI, gastrointestinal; IU, international unit; RE, retinol equivalent; TPN, total parenteral nutrition.

Mirtullo J, Canada T, Johnson D, et al: Safe practices for practical nutrition. JPEW J Parent Enteral Nutr 28:539, 2004.

Complementary and Alternative Nutritional Therapies

Many patients elect to use complementary and alternative therapies, the most common of which include supplementation with vitamins and minerals. When cancer is diagnosed, significant lifestyle alterations often occur, and "wellness" recommendations are embraced. Diets and supplements may be used as an adjunct to primary treatment, to mitigate the side effects of the therapy, or to reduce the risk for disease recurrence. Above all else, complementary therapies appear to give patients hope.

It is a challenge for the oncologist to determine the safety and efficacy of "pharmacologic" doses of supplements when combined with conventional therapies. Antioxidants present a special conundrum because competing hypotheses rage. Experimental models support the idea that antioxidants may improve the efficacy of cancer treatment by increasing tumor response and decreasing toxic effects on normal cells and that antioxidants may decrease the efficacy of treatment by protecting cancer cells. A member of the oncology team must stay abreast of the results of ongoing clinical trials integrating alternative with conventional treatments. By providing patients with the latest evidence-based information and showing respect for their beliefs and choices, the clinician can help guide the level of alternative therapy that is reasonable. When a patient elects to use an alternative therapy, adverse effects or interactions with conventional treatments must be monitored.

We advise our patients to avoid the use of antioxidants in excess of or, for some nutrients, below the tolerable upper limits of the dietary reference intakes during treatment with irradiation or chemotherapy that relies on free radicals and reactive oxygen species as mediators of cytotoxicity: anthracyclines, bleomycin, dactinomycin, epipodophyllotoxins (i.e., topoisomerase II inhibitors such as etoposide or teniposide), platinum compounds, alkylating agents, and agents without established molecular pharmacology (e.g., plicamycin, tamoxifen, aromatase). These agents, as do isoflavonoids and many herbs (e.g., garlic, ginger, *gingko biloba*, ginseng), may further diminish platelet function and aggregation and must be used cautiously by patients with thrombocytopenia. To avoid excess intake, patients should not take an oral multivitamin or mineral supplement while receiving intravenous vitamins and minerals in parenteral nutrition.

Our Practice During High-Dose Chemotherapy or Irradiation.

Antioxidant	*Age*	*Dietary Intake (RDA or AI)*	*Reference Intake (RDA or AI)*	*Tolerable Upper Limit*
Vitamin A	Birth–6 months	400 µg[a]	600 µg	Limit intake to tolerable upper limits
	7–12 months	500 µg		
	1–3 years	300 µg		
	4–8 years	400 µg	900 µg	
	9–13 years	600 µg	1700 µg	
	14–18 years, male	900 µg	2800 µg	
	14–18 years, female	700 µg		
	19+ years, male	900 µg	3000 µg	
	19+ years, female	700 µg		
Vitamin C (L-ascorbic acid)	Birth–6 months	40 mg	ND	40 mg
	7–12 months	50 mg		50 mg
	1–3 years	15 mg	400 mg	250 mg
	4–8 years	25 mg	650 mg	
	9–13 years	45 mg	1200 mg	
	14–18 years, male	75 mg[b]	1800 mg	500 mg
	14–18 years, female	65 mg[b]		
	19+ years, male	90 mg[b]	2000 mg	
	19+ years, female	75 mg[b]		
Vitamin E[c] (as α tocopherol)	Birth–6 months	4 mg	ND	4 mg
	7–12 months	5 mg	5 mg	
	1–3 years	6 mg	200 mg	50 mg
	4–8 years	7 mg	300 mg	
	9–13 years	11 mg	600 mg	
	14–18 years	15 mg	800 mg	
	19+ years	15 mg	1000 mg	60 mg
Selenium	Birth–6 months	15 mg	45 µg	
	7–12 months	20 µg	60 µg	Limit intake to dietary reference intake
	1–3 years	20 µg	90 µg	
	4–8 years	30 µg	150 µg	
	9–13 years	40 µg	280 µg	
	14+ years	55 µg	400 µg	

[a]1 µg = retinol activity equivalent; convert to international units (IU) by multiplying by 3.33.

[b]Add 35 mg if the patient is a smoker.

[c]If the patient is receiving anticoagulant therapy, measure the prothrombin time 1–2 weeks after starting vitamin E therapy.

AI, adequate intake; ND = not determined; RDA = recommended dietary allowance.

Data from references 138, 204, 205, 206. Web sites (www.nccam.nih.gov/, www3.cancer.gov/occam) can provide updated information on research in alternative therapies for cancer.

release of cytokines during conditioning therapy; an epithelial phase, when cells cease dividing and die; an ulcerative phase when microbes and endotoxins translocate into the bloodstream; and a healing phase, which can be prolonged with deep lesions and is more complex in the gut than in the mouth.[140] The severity of oral mucositis is increased in patients treated with total body irradiation[141] or who receive methotrexate as prophylaxis against GVHD.[142] Patients have identified the associated mouth pain as the single most debilitating side effect of HSCT.[143]

Characterizing the severity of lower gut toxicity is more difficult. Permeability studies and absorption studies are more objective approaches than are clinical symptoms. Increased gut permeability appears to precede clinical symptoms[144]; likewise, normal digestion and absorption appear impaired for prolonged periods, even in the absence of GVHD, as evidenced by abnormal d-xylose and Schilling test results at 4 months after transplantation,[145–147] suggesting a risk for subclinical nutrient deficiencies. However, with reduced-intensity regimens that included chemotherapy with fludarabine and antithymocyte globulin with busulfan or cyclophosphamide, intestinal permeability remained intact.[148]

The symptoms associated with mucosal injury (nausea, vomiting, diarrhea, oropharyngeal mucositis) inhibit oral intake for 1 month or longer (Fig. 92–1). Nutrition interventions have included ice chips or ice pops[149–151] and oral glutamine (see Table 92–4).[151–157] Six randomized studies of glutamine supplementation included patient groups heterogeneous for transplant type, diagnosis, and conditioning therapy, making interpretation of endpoints problematic. One study demonstrated oral glutamine supplementation reduced mucositis in a subset of patients receiving allografts, whereas patients receiving autografts who were provided glutamine in the same study experienced worse mucositis.[153]

In patients who received glutamine-enriched TPN solutions, only one study showed a decrease in the daily mucositis score. Thornley et al.[158] demonstrated reduced prevalence and severity of mucositis ($P = 0.008$ and $P = 0.004$, respectively) using a multiagent strategy consisting of ursodeoxycholic acid, folinic acid, and vitamin E in a pilot study of 37 pediatric transplant recipients.

Organ Complications

Sinusoidal Obstructive Syndrome (Venoocclusive Disease)

Insidious weight gain typically is the first sign of sinusoidal obstructive syndrome or hepatic venoocclusive disease (VOD). If it progresses, more severe symptoms of liver failure occur, including encephalopathy, coagulopathy, and renal failure,[159] all of which complicate nutrition management. Because fluids are limited to minimize edema and ascites, intravascular volume depletion and deterioration of renal function may occur. Conversely, repletion of the intravascular space often results in pulmonary edema and massive ascites. Use of continuous renal replacement therapy is helpful for removing fluid while providing nutrition support.

Determination of daily weights and frequent serum bilirubin levels in the immediate posttransplantation period facilitates early detection of disease in patients at increased risk. Nomograms for six time intervals between 1 day before transplantation and 16 days after transplantation that estimate the probability of developing severe VOD using total serum bilirubin and percent weight gain above baseline have been reported.[160] In patients with weight gain and decreased urinary sodium excretion, restriction of total fluid and sodium may decelerate fluid accumulation. Concentrated TPN solutions are indicated if renal perfusion is adequate. The capacity to eliminate intravenous lipids from the bloodstream should be monitored in patients with severe VOD. If encephalopathy develops, the benefits of HepatAmine (an amino acid solution with lower aromatic amino acids, tryptophan, and methionine content) have not been established.[161] If hyperbilirubinemia persists for more than 1 week, the biliary-excreted trace elements copper and manganese should be removed from TPN. Measurement of energy needs with indirect calorimetry, if available, may avert additive hepatotoxicity associated with overfeeding as well as the risks of debilitation with prolonged underfeeding.

Contraindicated Herbals During Therapy

- Alfalfa
- Borage
- Chaparral
- Chinese herbs
- Coltsfoot
- Comfrey
- DHEA
- Dieter's tea (including senna, aloa, rhubarb root, buckthorn, cascara, castor oil)
- Ephedra or ma huang
- Groundsel or life root
- Heliotrope or valerian
- Kava kava
- Laetrile (apricot pits)
- Licorice root
- Lobelia
- L-Tryptophan
- Maté tea
- Pau d' arco
- Pennyroyal
- Sassafras
- St. John's wort
- Yohimbe and yohimbine

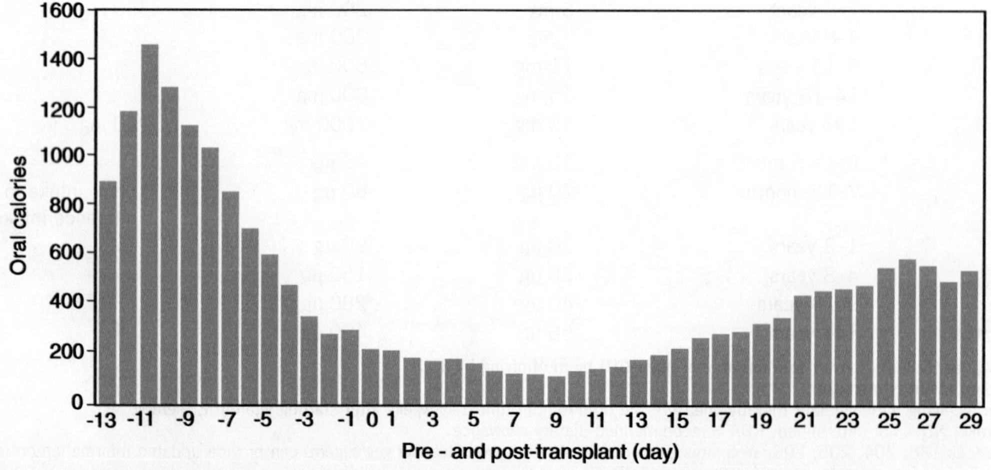

Figure 92–1 Average daily oral calorie intake of adult marrow transplant recipients undergoing myeloablative conditioning (n = 295).

Several case studies have described therapeutic responses to glutamine and vitamin E for VOD.[158,162,163] One prospective study described improvement in markers of hepatic function, protein C, and albumin when patients were provided glutamine compared with an isonitrogenous mixture of amino acids in TPN, although no cases of VOD occurred in either group.[164] Whether nutritional therapies play an adjunctive role in VOD management is not firmly established.

Renal Disease

Renal insufficiency typically is multifactorial and associated with total body irradiation, chemotherapy, drug toxicities, sepsis, and especially liver toxicity.[165] Renal damage manifested as doubling of the baseline creatinine level occurs in up to 75% of allograft patients.[166] An elevated blood urea nitrogen level, however, may be partially caused by nonrenal factors, including increased protein intake, gastrointestinal bleeding, or hypercatabolism. Prolonged protein restriction to minimize a rise of blood urea nitrogen should be avoided to ensure that adequate calorie and protein support are provided.

Maintaining intravascular volume and correcting electrolyte imbalances are essential in the management of renal complications. The large fluid load necessitated by TPN is problematic in the oliguric patient and if continuous renal replacement therapy is contraindicated requires daily manipulation, depending on urine output and clinical signs of fluid overload. Hypervolemic hyponatremia is treated with water restriction to prevent congestive heart failure. General indications for hemodialysis or continuous renal replacement therapy after HSCT are extracellular fluid volume expansion, acidemia, hyperkalemia, and azotemia. The primary goal of nutritional therapy for acute renal failure is to minimize uremia toxicity and other metabolic derangements and yet prevent malnutrition. Protein levels typically are restricted before dialysis by the TPN volume tolerated. During dialysis, protein intake should meet stress needs as defined in Table 92–5. Serum triglyceride levels must be monitored weekly because clearance of intravenous lipids may be reduced.[167] Water-soluble vitamins that are lost in the dialysate and the continuous renal replacement therapy circuit should be provided while standard intravenous multivitamins are decreased in an effort to prevent excessive serum vitamin A levels.[168]

Pulmonary Disease

Pulmonary edema due to increased capillary permeability after cytoreduction therapy may be compounded by iatrogenic fluid overload. Management includes reducing total sodium from oral intake, TPN, and medications, and using concentrated TPN solutions. During ventilator dependency, adequate TPN or tube feeding should be provided to preserve muscle reserves.

Graft-Versus-Host Disease

Acute Graft-Versus-Host Disease

Whether lipids favorably modulate GVHD by suppressing production of inflammatory cytokines through prostaglandin E_2-mediated pathways has interested several investigators. In a study of lipids and infection outcome, the secondary outcome of grade II to IV GVHD incidence was not different in patients receiving 25% to 30% or 6% to 8% of total calories as lipids, occurring in 77% and 75% of patients, respectively.[109] Time to acute GVHD (before 80 days posttransplantation), censored for death, relapse, and treatment failure, also did not differ. Other investigators compared very high doses of lipid (80% of total energy) to lipid-free TPN in 66 allograft recipients. Although incidence and median day of onset were similar between the groups, lethality of GVHD was decreased in the lipid group.[169] In a small study of oral eicosapentaenoic acid supplemented at 1.8 g/day from day 21 to day 180 posttransplantation, three patients who received eicosapentaenoic acid (n = 7) experienced grade II to III GVHD and all survived, whereas in the control group (n = 9), six experienced grade II to IV GVHD, and five died.[170]

In the most severe form of acute intestinal GVHD, voluminous diarrhea is a prominent manifestation, with the volume corresponding to the extent of mucosal damage. The diarrheal fluid is green and watery, with ropy strands of mucus, protein, and cellular debris, and often contains occult blood. Protein content is high, as evidenced by falling plasma protein levels or by measurements of fecal α_1 antitrypsin in fecal water.[171] Associated symptoms include anorexia, nausea, vomiting, and crampy abdominal pain, which may be related to food ingestion or may occur spontaneously because of the secretory nature of the diarrhea. Other causes of diarrhea should always be ruled out because enteric pathogens and late-onset toxicities due to the conditioning regimen may occur with signs and symptoms similar to acute intestinal GVHD.[172] Biopsy findings range from necrosis of individual intestinal crypt cells to total mucosal denudation.[173,174] Fluid and electrolyte management may be problematic in patients with large-volume diarrhea (>2.5–3.0 L/day). In severe disease, the patient initially is dependent on TPN because complete bowel rest helps decrease diarrhea. Additional daily zinc is recommended at 10 mg/L of stool volume in excess of 1 L. When diarrheal volumes diminish and abdominal pain subsides, isotonic oral liquid supplements are introduced to stimulate intestinal regeneration and assess absorption. Guidelines for the introduction of oral intake have been empirically derived using a five-phase regimen that emphasizes foods low in lactose, fat, fiber, and total acidity.[175] Antidiarrheal agents are generally contraindicated because of the risk for ileus and abdominal distension. Use of octreotide acetate has been reported to control diarrhea but may lower serum cyclosporine levels.[176–178] Ippoliti et al.[179] advocate administration of octreotide early in the course of GVHD as soon as onset of diarrhea is noted and discontinuation as soon as diarrhea resolves to prevent constipation and development of an ileus. If no benefit is seen in 4 to 7 days, then octreotide probably will not help.

Weisdorf et al.[180] described a syndrome of upper intestinal GVHD presenting clinically as anorexia, dyspepsia, food intolerance, nausea, and vomiting. Prolonged nausea and vomiting beyond day 20 posttransplantation and failure to progress with oral dietary intake constitute indications for endoscopic evaluation to establish a diagnosis of stomach or upper intestinal GVHD.[181] Upper gut GVHD is very responsive to steroids, and hyperphagia supplants anorexia.

The oral mucosa may be involved in acute GVHD. Oral examination reveals erythema and lichenoid changes that cannot be differentiated from conditioning-induced mucositis until approximately 3 weeks posttransplantation.[182,183] It may evolve into a chronic form, and patients may develop taste fatigue with prolonged use of oral supplements and bland foods, experiencing significant weight loss unless supported with TPN or tube feeding.

Acute liver GVHD is characterized by abnormal liver function tests, jaundice, and mild hepatomegaly. Hepatic synthesis and enterohepatic circulation of bile salts may be diminished or inhibited, resulting in steatorrhea and the need for fat restriction. In severe disease, encephalopathy and ascites ensue, with nutritional management similar to VOD.

Adequate nutrition is a vital adjunct to immunosuppressive drugs for treatment of acute GVHD. Energy needs during acute GVHD have been predicted at 45 to 50 kcal/kg in adults and 65 kcal/kg in children.[129] Drug therapy for GVHD often has a profound effect on nutritional status and may require nutritional intervention as summarized in Table 92–6.

Chronic Graft-Versus-Host-Disease

Clinical manifestations of chronic GVHD that may adversely affect nutritional status include anorexia, mucositis, xerostomia, dysphagia, esophageal stricture, cholestatic liver disease, diarrhea or steatorrhea,

Table 92–6 Nutritional Consequences of Graft-Versus-Host Disease Immunosuppression

Immunosuppressive Agent	Nutritional Effects	Recommended Interventions
Corticosteroids	Muscle wasting	Early intervention with physical therapy if exercise level low; high protein intake (twice normal requirements)
	Sodium and fluid retention	Low-sodium diet if edema limits mobility
	Hyperphagia and weight gain	Regular exercise, dietary counseling
	Hyperglycemia	Insulin therapy, blood glucose monitoring, dietary counseling to limit overfeeding and excessive total carbohydrate intake; oral agents have not been shown to be safe or efficacious
	Hyperlipidemia	Lipid-lowering agent if patient with history of pancreatitis or very high levels, reassess plasma lipids several months after discontinuation of drug to assure return to baseline level
	Bone loss, fracture risk	Vitamin D: 400–800 IU/day
Cyclosporine, tacrolimus	Renal insufficiency	Maintenance fluid or more via oral ± intravenous; routine monitoring serum creatinine
	Magnesium wasting	Magnesium replacement via oral ± intravenous route; oral dosing often limited by diarrhea (protein complex forms may be better tolerated); routine monitoring serum magnesium level
	Hyperglycemia	May exacerbate hyperglycemia observed with corticosteroids (see corticosteroids)
	Hyperlipidemia	Usually not to same degree as with corticosteroids (see corticosteroids)
	Hyponatremia	Limit free water, encourage fluid with solute
Mycophenolate mofetil	Diarrhea, vomiting	Rule out other causes of diarrhea; otherwise antiemetic therapy and adequate hydration status
Sirolimus	Hyperlipidemia	Monitor serum lipids frequently; if on total parenteral nutrition, provide lipid only for essential fatty acids; lipid-lowering agent if very high levels

Table 92–7 Nutrition-Related Problems 1 Year After Bone Marrow Grafting

	Chronic GVHD Status[a]		
Sign or Symptom	None (%)	Limited (%)	Extensive (%)
Weight loss	27	19	33
Weight gain	14	28	34
Oral sensitivity	7	14	41
Xerostomia	10	11	27
Stomatitis	3	3	14
Anorexia	3	6	13
Reflux symptoms	1	6	12
Diarrhea	3	3	12
Steatorrhea	1	0	9
Dysgeusia	0	0	6
Esophageal stricture	0	0	2
Dyspnea	0	0	7
Contractures	0	0	2

GVHD, graft-versus-host disease.

[a]Among 192 allogeneic transplant recipients, the percentage of total number of patients is shown.

Adapted from Lenssen P, Sherry ME, Cheney CL, et al: Prevalence of nutrition-related problems among long-term survivors of allogeneic marrow transplantation. J Am Diet Assoc 90:835, 1990.

dyspnea and limited exercise tolerance, restricted joint mobility, and generalized wasting (Table 92–7).[184] Weight loss can be profound, in one review as high as 34% of the pretransplantation weight. Among 93 patients evaluated a median of 2.4 years posttransplantation, 29% had moderate malnutrition (BMI 18.5–21.9 kg/m^2) and 14% had severe malnutrition (BMI < 18.5 kg/m^2), with patients with active chronic GVHD having significantly lower BMI than patients with inactive disease.[185] Only dysphagia and abdominal pain resulted in an increased likelihood of weight loss, whereas oral sensitivity, nausea, and anorexia did not, leading the authors to hypothesize a cachexia-like syndrome in chronic GVHD. The resting energy expenditure was measured in 13 patients with stable chronic GVHD who had suffered a maximum weight loss of 22% after transplantation and regained 15% of body weight at the time of measurement at day 518 ± 261 posttransplantation. All patients had chronic skin disease and sicca syndrome involving the eyes and salivary glands, and half also had involvement of the liver (n = 4) or lung (n = 3). Energy expenditure and fat oxidation were found to be significantly higher and carbohydrate oxidation significantly lower than in controls matched for sex, age, weight, and height.[186] Studies of weight loss are complicated by the finding of weight gain in many patients because of steroids and concomitant fluid and fat gain, which may explain why weight loss has not been a prognostic indicator.[187]

Oral disease is common, with frank stomatitis occurring in a significant portion of patients. Pain, burning, and loss of taste have been described as prodromes of chronic GVHD.[188] In severe cases, only bland liquids and soft foods may be tolerated. Complete nutritional supplements and nutrient-dense carbohydrate polymers are important dietary adjuncts in patients experiencing weight loss. If significant weight loss occurs, gastrostomy feeding may be indicated.

Esophageal webbing or stricture can result in severe swallowing difficulties.[189] Typical symptoms include pain and difficulty in swallowing food and pills as well as retrosternal pain caused by esophageal thinning. Webs and strictures are managed with periodic dilation. Diet tolerance varies widely and may be limited to liquids in patients with extensive webbing. Gastrostomy tubes may be indicated when the passage of food is obstructed.

Intestinal involvement presents with diarrhea, nausea and vomiting, and often complete dependence on enteral nutrition or TPN. In one series the incidence was 7.3% of all patients transplanted.[190] Bacterial overgrowth, medications, chronic liver GVHD, and pancreatic insufficiency may contribute to diarrhea or steatorrhea. When weight loss occurs in chronic liver GVHD, the relative contributions of deficient energy intake and malabsorption must be determined. Patients often are anorectic, yet others have good dietary intake but significant stool nutrient losses. A malabsorption workup may include quantitative stool fat collection, Sudan black stain for stool fat, stool for fecal elastase, serum carotene, serum xylose or Schilling test, or serum 25-hydroxyvitamin D. Vitamin D status is of special concern because inadequate hepatic and renal hydroxylation to the active metabolite may occur. In patients with malabsorption, moderate fat restriction, calorie supplementation with medium-chain triglycerides, and mineral and water miscible fat-soluble vitamin supplementation may be necessary interim measures. Some patients respond to pancreatic enzymes. In patients who fail to gain weight, a gastrostomy feeding should be considered given the known slow resolution of the disease.

Vitamin D and calcium status are jeopardized by use of sun-blocking agents to diminish photoactivation of skin GVHD and the almost universal use of steroids for treatment. Loss of vertebral bone mass at 1 year posttransplantation was described by Stern et al.[191] in a small series of patients treated with cyclosporine and corticosteroids. In another series of 39 patients followed for a median of 30 months (range 5–64 months), the allograft patients (n = 29) lost 11.7% of femoral neck and 3.9% of spinal bone mineral density compared with a nonsignificant decrease of 1.1% and an increase of 1.5% in the autograft patients (n = 10). Bone loss correlated best with the cumulative steroid dose, with spinal bone loss of 4% per 10 g of prednisolone and femoral neck bone at 9% per 10 g of prednisolone.[192] Several studies have described the prevalence of bone loss in children with chronic GVHD exceeding 50%.[193,194] The rate of bone loss appears to be highest in the first 6 months after HSCT,[195,196] and early intervention with calcium and vitamin D and aggressive ambulation is encouraged.

With the multiple problems that can interfere with a balanced nutrient intake, the need to avoid sun exposure, and drug-nutrient deficiencies (e.g., folic acid, trimethoprim-sulfasoxazole), a multivitamin and mineral supplement is recommended for all patients. In most cases, iron-free formulas are recommended, unless the patient has documented iron-deficiency anemia, because iron overload is a frequent finding in long-term survivors.[197,198] Iron-free or low-iron infant formulas are also recommend for young children. When skin disease is treated with psoralen plus ultraviolet A radiation, supplemental β carotene, which protects against ultraviolet radiation,[199] should be discouraged.

Children with extensive chronic GVHD represent a special risk group. Growth failure and studies of growth hormone efficacy have been reviewed by Brennan and Shalet,[200] who concluded that the data on catchup growth after steroid therapy were inconsistent and that other factors such as GVHD itself might play a role. The role of growth hormone is not fully delineated because of the lack of randomized controlled studies with documentation of final height for predicting the gain in stature. Although the contribution of poor nutrient intake as a factor in growth failure after HSCT has not been adequately investigated, children displaying weight loss, inappropriate weight gain, or growth failure deserve thorough nutritional evaluation to rule out treatable dietary deficiencies. Height should be monitored every 3 months posttransplantation for the purpose of early detection of growth failure.

Children may experience long-term metabolic alterations following HSCT that may adversely affect nutritional status.[201,202] Taskinen et al.[201] reported a 39% incidence of combined hyperinsulinemia and hypertriglyceridemia in pediatric transplant patients compared to 8% in leukemia patients and none in healthy controls ($P = 0.0015$) as a late effect following HSCT. An increased incidence of diabetes mellitus has been reported in long-term survivors of pediatric HSCT.[201,203] In a retrospective review of more than 700 transplant survivors, the prevalence of diabetes mellitus type 1 was 0.52%, or three times higher than the prevalence in the general U.S. population, whereas the prevalence of diabetes mellitus type 2 was 9% among leukemia survivors and 2% among aplastic anemia survivors, both higher than expected.[203] Patients should be educated and monitored for the development of diabetes, with appropriate therapy instituted.

SUGGESTED READINGS

ASPEN Guidelines for the Use of Parenteral and Enteral Nutrition in Adult and Pediatric Patients. JPEN J Parenter Enteral Nutr 26(1s):82SA, 2002.

Charuhas PM: Pediatric hematopoietic stem cell transplantation. In Hasse JM, Blue LS (eds.): Comprehensive Guide to Transplant Nutrition. Chicago, American Dietetic Association, 2002, p 226.

Jacobson DA, Margolis J, Doherty J, et al: Weight loss and malnutrition in patients with chronic graft-versus-host disease. Bone Marrow Transplant 29:231, 2002.

Lenssen P, Aker SN: Adult hematopoietic stem cell transplantation. In Hasse JM, Blue LS (eds.): Comprehensive Guide to Transplant Nutrition. Chicago, American Dietetic Association, 2002, p 123.

Lenssen P, Bruemmer B, McDonald GB, Aker S: Nutrient support in hematopoietic cell transplantation. JPEN J Parent Enteral Nutr 25:219, 2001.

Oeffinger KC, Mertens AC, Sklar CA, et al: Obesity in adult survivors of childhood acute lymphoblastic leukemia: A report from the Childhood Cancer Survivor Study. J Clin Oncol 21:1359, 2003.

Sefcick A, Anderton D, Byrne JL, et al: Naso-jejunal feeding in allogeneic bone marrow transplant recipients: Results of a pilot study. Bone Marrow Transplant 28:1135, 2001.

Tyc VL, Vallelunga L, Mahoney S, et al: Nutritional and treatment-related characteristics of pediatric oncology patients referred or not referred for nutritional support. Med Pediatr Oncol 25:379, 1995.

Weiger WA, Smith R, Boon H, et al: Advising patients who seek complementary and alternative medical therapies for cancer. Ann Intern Med 137:889, 2002.

Weisdorf SA, Lysne J, Wind D, et al: Positive effect of prophylactic total parenteral nutrition on long-term outcome of bone marrow transplantation. Transplantation 43:833, 1987.

REFERENCES

For complete list of references log onto www.expertconsult.com

CHAPTER 93

PSYCHOSOCIAL ASPECTS OF HEMATOLOGIC DISORDERS

Ruth McCorkle and Elizabeth Cooke

Major changes in the understanding and treatment of cancer have led to a wider range of treatment options and increasing length of survival for people diagnosed with hematologic cancers. Regardless of the advances and concomitant survival increase, a diagnosis of a hematologic malignancy can have great impact on the psychosocial aspects of the lives of cancer survivors and their families because diseases of the blood are widely perceived as serious and often fatal. Psychological, social, economic, cognitive, and existential stressors are common experiences for cancer survivors. Despite the increasing focus of long-term survivorship issues within the past 20 years by providers, policymakers, and the general public, ongoing progress must continue to provide interventions and services to meet the psychosocial aspects of quality cancer care for patients and their families.[1,2] Psychosocial interventions and services are those that enable patients, their families, and health care providers to optimize health care and health care outcomes by managing the psychological, social, and behavioral aspects of cancer and its consequences.

Psychosocial aspects associated with cancer may be intensified in patients with hematologic malignancies because of their association with an uncertain prognosis, a prolonged treatment course often involving numerous hospitalizations, and the systemic nature of the diseases.[3] Discomfort from painful medical procedures, body image disturbances because of hair loss, central line catheters, sexual dysfunction related to fatigue and fertility, and role and relationship disruptions resulting from lengthy hospitalizations and fear of premature death are just a sampling of the issues that confront patients with hematologic malignancies, highlighting the necessity for monitoring of and attention to the psychosocial needs that accompany all aspects of these diseases. Involvement with a complicated and fragmented health care delivery system, the need for episodic and aggressive treatment, remissions and exacerbation of acute and uncomfortable symptoms, family separation, financial burden, functional limitations, and role disruptions are a few of the issues that characterize the life of patients with hematologic malignancies, not to mention the threat to life imposed by these diagnoses. Many nonmalignant hematologic conditions are associated with chronic morbidity, shortened survival, and many of the issues just listed.

This chapter provides information on factors that affect psychosocial adjustment among patients with hematologic malignancies, the wide range of psychological responses that are possible throughout the illness trajectory, and the efficacy of various modes of psychosocial interventions and services to minimize distress and promote adaptation. Some practical guidelines regarding patient management and identification of patients who may require formal psychiatric consultation are offered.

ACCOMPANYING TRENDS IN PSYCHOSOCIAL ISSUES

Within the last 20 years has been a shift to include quality-of-life components in the care of cancer survivors. This shift is due, in part, to the birth of the survivorship moment. Since the inception of the National Coalition for Cancer Survivorship in 1985, there has been increasing growth in legislation, education, and advocacy of cancer survivors. This movement has continued with new definitions of the word "survivor" by the Center for Disease Control, Lance Armstrong Foundation, National Cancer Institute, and the Institute of Medicine report released in 2006.[4] Patients with a hematologic cancer experience a wide range of psychosocial issues as cancer survivors. For example, one study with more than 600 hematopoietic stem cell transplantation (HSCT) survivors found that, relative to healthy controls, survivors reported poorer physical, psychological, and social functioning with changes that were long-lasting and had a profound impact over several years.[5]

CLINICAL COURSE OF HEMATOLOGIC MALIGNANCIES

In contrast to many solid tumor cancers, treatment of hematologic malignancies often involves numerous and lengthy hospitalizations and ongoing outpatient monitoring of the patient's condition. The clinical course of cancer typically follows one of several possible trajectories (Fig. 93–1).[6] A number of patients respond to the curative attempt with long-term remission, remain well, and, after a period, are considered cured. Some patients have a positive response to a curative attempt but then relapse. Other patients begin treatment with a hope for cure but do not respond and progressively decline. In some patients, the disease is too far advanced when diagnosed, and they experience a rapid progression of their disease.[6]

This model is useful in understanding the medical consequences of the cancer and its treatment, but a number of other models have been developed to classify the cancer course from a patient management perspective. One model is the cancer control continuum, which describes the stages of prevention, early detection, diagnosis, treatment, survivorship, and end-of-life care.[7] Another model from the patient's perspective is Mullan's three seasons of survival: acute, extended, and permanent.[8] Mullan's conceptualization was expanded by Dow[9] to include the following: surviving the diagnosis and treatment, extended survival, surviving with uncertainty, and permanent survival. Dow's model[9] combined with the cancer control continuum provides a template for this chapter and the cancer experience for patients diagnosed with hematologic cancers.

Acute Season: Time of Diagnosis

Being diagnosed with a hematologic malignancy can be devastating. The time of diagnosis has been described by a cancer survivor as a lightening bolt through a stop sign.[10] It is a time of intense stress and likened to a personal disaster in the patient's and family's life.[9] Often these patients describe vague symptoms such as fatigue for weeks, even months, or they are treated in urgent care centers for bronchitis or other infections only to be diagnosed with an unexpected catastrophic illness such as leukemia. The period from time of diagnosis through initiation of treatment is characterized by sometimes fast-paced medical evaluation and treatment, the development of new relationships with unfamiliar medical personnel, and the need to integrate a barrage of information that is at best frightening and confusing. Within the context of this anxiety-provoking situation, a decision must be made regarding treatment. As one man aptly stated, "a decision upon which my very life or death might be based." This statement illustrates the tremendous responsibility, concern, and isolation that many people experience during this period.[11]

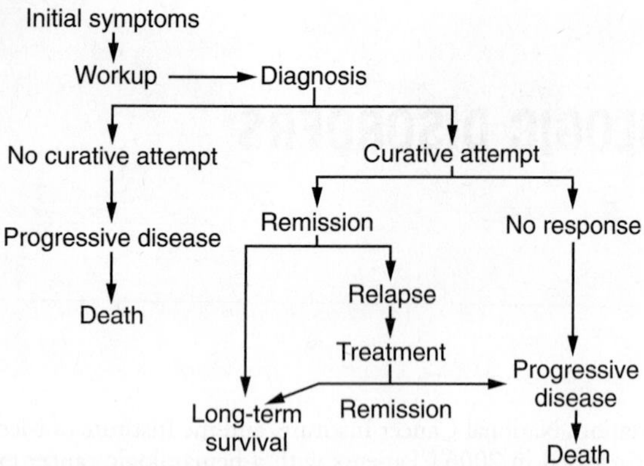

Figure 93–1 Clinical course of a patient with a hematologic malignancy. (Adapted from Lesko LM: Hematopoietic dyscrasias. In Holland JC [ed.]: Psychooncology. New York, Oxford University Press, 1998, p 408.)

Initial response to a diagnosis may be profoundly influenced by a person's prior association with cancer.[6] Those with memories of close relatives with cancer often demonstrate heightened distress, particularly if the relative died or had negative treatment experiences. During the diagnostic and early treatment periods, patients may search for explanations or causes for their cancer and may struggle to give personal meaning to their experience.[12] Because many clinicians are guarded about disclosing information until a firm diagnosis is established, patients may develop highly personal explanations that can be inaccurate and provoke intensely negative emotions. Ongoing involvement and accurate and repeated information from key health care providers help to minimize patients' uncertainty and the development of maladaptive coping strategies based on erroneous beliefs.

Because the time of diagnosis usually is a time of crisis, care must be given to assess multiple areas of the patient's psychosocial status. Weissman and Worden[13] described the first 100 days after diagnosis as the period of an "existential plight." They documented that patient concerns initially focused on existential issues of life and death more than on concerns related to health, work, finances, religion, self, or relationships with family and friends. Although extreme and sustained psychological reactions as the first response to a cancer diagnosis are unusual, careful assessment of the nature of the patient's reaction remains important. Initial reactions often are predictive of later adaptation.[14,15] Early assessment by clinicians can help to identify people who are at risk for later adjustment problems and in greatest need of ongoing psychosocial support.[16–20] (see box on Factors That May Predict Poor Coping in Patients with Cancer). Major depression and depressive symptoms occur frequently in patients with cancer, with a prevalence rate of 10% to 25%.[21,22] Both anxiety and depression are easy to assess in the patient and family, and timely referral for assistance during this period may lay a foundation of adequate coping throughout the cancer trajectory. During this time, many providers are conveying large amounts of information to patients and family members. It is not always easy for patients to differentiate the importance of each communication and prioritize their problem-solving behaviors. Consequently, providers must repeat information at several contacts and inquire about the patient's and families' understanding of facts and treatment options. Often patients and families describe that they are in a state of numbness and that information is not really understood, comprehended, or processed.

Although the literature substantiates the devastating psychological impact of a cancer diagnosis, it is also well documented that many patients cope effectively. Positive coping strategies, such as taking action and finding favorable characteristics in the situation, have been reported as effective. Maintaining optimism[23] and having an active determination to recover have been associated with positive adjustment. Contrary to the beliefs of many clinicians, denial has also been found to assist patients in coping effectively with a diagnosis of cancer, unless used to an excessive degree. With the firm establishment of the cancer diagnosis, planning for treatment begins. If patients have been given a clear explanation of their condition while encouraged to maintain hope, the initial reaction of shock, fear, and desperation can give way to a sense of optimism. Health care providers have an important role in monitoring and possibly mediating psychosocial adjustment. Keeping patients informed and actively involved in their care and being aware of the unique meaning that people may associate with a diagnosis of cancer are vital. Patients who have a pervasive and unyielding negative affect that persists long after the crisis of diagnosis may require ongoing psychosocial monitoring and referral for services and supportive interventions throughout their treatment and disease course.[24]

Factors that May Predict Poor Coping in Patients with Cancer

- Past psychiatric history
- Limited social support
- Alcohol or drug abuse
- Recent losses
- Advanced disease
- Uncontrolled symptoms
- Pessimistic outlook on life
- Multiple obligations
- Avoidance coping
- Lower functional status
- Smoking cessation
- Higher regimen-related toxicity

Acute Phase: The Treatment Decision

Psychosocial factors are critical parameters in considering which treatment is best for a particular patient.[25] The development of a treatment plan should include information about all aspects of medical/surgical treatments as well as what is known about the psychosocial sequelae. Often, patients react to a diagnosis of cancer with feelings of fear and helplessness. Patients look to the primary oncologist for a curative treatment that also can preserve their quality of life. Patients may feel vulnerable and believe that complete reliance on the oncologist is essential. Combating feelings of helplessness during this period can help patients alleviate painful anxiety. This is best done by a member of the health care team who has established a treatment alliance with the patient. The health care provider must make the patient feel like a partner in everything that takes place. This is especially true regarding decisions about treatment options. Giving information to patients and families often alleviates anxiety and uncertainty because patients feel more in control.

Active treatment of cancer usually initiates another acute phase of the cancer experience. It can occur while a patient is receiving treatment or as a complication of treatment. An important standard of clinical practice, based on extensive research, is to provide patients with information that will prepare them on what to expect during their treatment. Research by Johnson provides convincing evidence that patients who receive specific information about the nature, pattern, and timing of treatment side effects report less disruption in activity than those who are not given this detailed information.[26,27] Some providers wait until patients complain about potentially expected side effects. When this happens, patients may become skeptical about the completeness or accuracy of any future information given by the person. This potential distrust has important implications for decision making, patient choice of care setting in the future, and recommendations made by patients to others who are seeking a source of cancer care.

Often during the treatment phase increasing burdens are placed on the immediate caregiver and family to support the patient's schedule for treatment, multiple admissions, and increasing dependency.[28]

Often the patient is unable to work, and financial stressors accumulate. Sensitivity and awareness by providers to social, economic, and relationship stresses are needed to assist with referral for social services or psychological assistance. Support groups with other patients can be helpful during this time. Evidence clearly indicates that sharing a common experience in a support group can have psychological benefit.[29]

Decision for Hematopoietic Stem Cell Transplantation

HSCT is becoming a standard treatment of many hematologic malignancies and nonmalignant diseases. Both autologous and allogeneic transplant numbers are increasing worldwide.[30] Although mortality has improved over the years since transplants began in the 1970s, treatment-related mortality continues to cause significant anxiety in patients and families. The procedure for transplantation is complex, can cause intense psychological distress, and extreme social strain on the patient's caregiver, friends and family members. Often the psychological and social issues can be more challenging for the health care team than the medical issues. Because HSCT is an intense and distinctive experience for patients and families and has the potential to cause prolonged psychological distress unlike other experiences with oncology patients, the issues unique to this population warrant a separate discussion.[31]

HSCT patients face physical and psychological stresses of hospitalization and social isolation for weeks to months during their initial recovery; therefore, a thorough pretransplant psychosocial evaluation to identify those patients at risk for development of psychosocial morbidity and to initiate timely interventions to optimize adaptation is recommended. The time of transplantation when the infusion of cells occurs can be a special moment for patients, with patients often referring to the date of transplant as a "birthday" or special anniversary date. Often family members are gathered at the bedside to celebrate the long awaited event of the transplant. However, the weeks following transplant can be difficult psychologically. The threat of death continues to be real, and patients experience social isolation, bodily discomfort, major body image changes, and a sense of loss of control. These issues lead to a myriad of emotions; including hope, anger, depression, anxiety, anticipation, guilt, and joy.[31] Prieto et al.[19] assessed 220 inpatients after transplantation and found that the psychiatric disorder incidence after admission followup was approximately 22%. They identified the following variables as risks factors for psychiatric morbidity: younger age, women, past psychiatric history, lower functional status, pain, smoking cessation, and higher regimen-related toxicity. They reported that although the isolation period has decreased substantially over the last decades, patients still experience anxiety from isolation. They also reported high anxiety when the isolation is lifted and patients are "exposed" to a "germ-filled" environment with all its implications.[19]

Often patients are not prepared for the slow gradual speed of recovery after transplantation. Patients are more familiar with recovery after surgery that takes days to weeks, and they are unprepared and overwhelmed with the long recovery that can take weeks to months or even months to years. Heinonen et al.[32] studied allogeneic patients during the first 3 years after transplantation and found that patients perceived their quality of life worst after the first year than prior to transplant. During this time, patients continue to feel functional limitations, and both autologous and allogeneic patients report usual somatic symptoms, such as fatigue, as the most common distressing occurrences after transplantation.[33–35] Periods when patients are particularly psychologically vulnerable during the first year include admission workup, directly before transplant, discharge from the inpatient setting, between 3 and 5 months, and between 6 and 9 months.[15,36–38] Other factors that have been identified as related to psychological distress and poor health after transplantation are the following: pre-HSCT psychological and psychological status, anxiety, depression, poorer quality of life, disease recurrence, negative mood, type of transplant, locus of control, low social support, presence of graft-versus-host disease (GVHD), and caregiver/family distress.[31,34,39]

The financial burden for patients who undergo bone marrow transplantation (BMT) can be overwhelming, including medical expenses for the patient and marrow donor in the case of an allogeneic BMT, potential travel expenses, and loss of income for other family members.[40] Patients and their immediate families often are far from their usual support systems because of the distance to the BMT center. In some cases, family members who have not been close in the past may be forced by the situation to interact with each other, leading to additional stress.

The first few years after transplantation, patients and family members may continue to experience physical and psychological sequelae from the transplant, although the literature is clear that most patients return to a productive life with high quality of life. Heinonen et al.[32] identified the following factors that predicted a poorer quality of life in patients 1 to 5 years after transplant: age, long-term sequelae, chronic GVHD, and short followup by the treatment center.[32] Patient and families are ready to put the experience behind them, only to discover that the experience of transplant has forever changed the patient's outlook, priorities, and family network. Fear of recurrence and feelings of uncertainty related to future relationships, work, and financial strain continue.[29] There is discordance between the patients' pre-HSCT expectations and the everyday symptoms that limit their physical abilities. Besides fatigue, which continues to be the dominant symptom, another distressing issue is cognitive dysfunction as patients return to the workplace and reenter school.[29] Educating patients about some expected common short-term side effects can reduce anxiety. Neurocognitive side effects of treatment can be long term in high-risk patients but are mostly temporary, including diminished concentration, short-term memory loss, decreased speed of information, and loss of effective problem-solving abilities. Sexuality issues are another area of great concern for patients in the posttransplant period. Barriers for discussion and lack of referrals for supportive services in this area may be related to the patient's embarrassment, the clinician's lack of knowledge, or the focus on other issues that may be interpreted as more critical. Common sexual issues after transplant include vaginal dryness and distressing menopausal symptoms in women and erectile dysfunction in men.[41]

Patients who experience long-term physical symptoms after transplantation may be at risk for long-term psychological distress.[28] Despite the fact that patients are followed by transplant physicians longer than are patients with nonhematologic malignancies; this population often is referred back to primary care physicians 1 to 2 years after transplant. Primary care clinicians do not have the knowledge or experience to tie physical complications to the effects of chemotherapy, radiation, and GVHD, so ongoing communication between the providers and the transplant team and center is imperative. Long-term effects may include persistent viral, bacterial, and fungal susceptibility, GVHD, oral dental caries, muscle atrophy, pneumonitis, gonadal dysfunction, sexual dysfunction, endocrine abnormalities, cataracts, ocular sicca syndrome, reduced bone mass, secondary malignancies, and cognitive dysfunction.[42] In addition to monitoring physical complications, the American Society for Blood and Marrow Transplantation consensus statement recommends annual evaluation of patients' psychological status. Health care providers must have a high level of vigilance to assess depression in both the family caregiver and the patient years after transplant, with clinical assessments recommended annually after transplant. Gruber et al.[43] assessed 163 patients for long-term psychosocial effects as far as 16 years posttransplant and found that the majority of patients had serious problems with "physical fitness," followed by pain and fear/psychological stress. Thirty percent of these patients did not return to work, and the subgroup of unemployed patients had higher scores for pain, depression, sleep disorders, depression, impairment in social functioning partnership, and family life. In spite of the range of problems, only 9.8% of these patients reported accessing psychological support.

The concept of posttraumatic growth (PTG) after transplantation has been evolving. By definition, the potential for PTG requires that patients experience a stressful event and subsequently experience positive psychological outcomes or benefits. As early as 1996, Fromm identified positive sequelae possible after transplantation, including the development of a new philosophy of life, greater appreciation of life, making changes in personal characteristics, and improving relationships with family and friends. Potential predictors of PTG among posttransplant patients include good social support, little avoidance coping, younger age, less education, greater use of positive reinterpretation, problem solving, seeking alternative rewards, more stressful appraisal of the experience, and more negatively biased recall of pretransplant levels of psychological distress.[18,44] Discussing the PTG potential with patients and making referrals for counseling to experienced clinicians who are aware of the potential for PTG are essential. Although patients report long-term psychosocial effects after transplantation, they may be reluctant to accept help and fail to access psychological resources and social support.[43] These patients must be encouraged to use resources and seek psychological support, because this experience may impair the patient's and families' ability to cope with life after transplant. In an article about HSCT patients' experiences with a support group, Sherman et al.[29] identified the themes of meaning and changing of perspectives as patients expressed their struggles with redefining themselves, their priorities, and their values.[29] Some patients wanted to change their former values and behaviors. The support group experience may be therapeutic for patients who often do not have physical signs of transplant to the untrained eye but continue to experience increasing or unresolved psychological and physical issues.[28] Sharing a common experience may encourage patients to believe that their symptoms and feelings are not unique and may decrease their feelings of isolation.

Extended Phase: Surviving Diagnosis and Treatment

As the treatment and acute side effects improve and subside, patients often feel that the whirlwind has passed, only to be confronted with uneasy silence. Weeks and months of clinic and physician appointments, infusions, and admissions stop or trickle to a small steam of appointments. Families that have been functioning on a grinding schedule of crisis mode find the change almost paralyzing. Adding to this halt of activity, health care providers have a tendency to limit their contacts when patients' physical statuses have stabilized. This is a critical time when psychosocial interventions and supportive services from other members of the health care team must be instituted for patients and family members to deal with the uncertainty and anxiety of waiting. Fears and anxieties change from fighting the disease to returning to life.[9] Because of less contact with the primary treatment oncologists, patients and families perceive a withdrawal of support from the medical team. Therefore, there is a need to establish mechanisms to monitor these patients and family members for ongoing and increasing psychological distress, including anxiety and depression.

Extended Phase: Relapse of the Disease

The time of recurrence of cancer has been reported to be more distressing for patients and family members than the initial diagnosis. The recurrence of the disease can plunge the patient and family into despair and crisis as the realization that death may occur despite the ongoing fight to live. The psychosocial issues experienced by the person with cancer depend in part on the clinical course of the disease process. As the disease progresses, the person often reports an upsetting scenario that includes uncertainty, frequent pain, disability, increased dependence, and diminished functional ability.[6]

The development of a relapse after a disease-free interval can be especially devastating for patients and those close to them. The medical workup often is difficult and anxiety provoking, and psychosocial problems experienced at the time of diagnosis frequently resurface, often with greater intensity.[6] Shock and depression often accompany relapse and require patients and family members to reevaluate the future. In spite of the overwhelming nature of the psychosocial responses, however, most patients do cope effectively with progressive disease, and it is important to recognize that intense emotions do not necessarily equate with maladaptive coping. Investigators studying quality of life in patients with cancer have demonstrated a clear relationship between a person's perception of their quality of life and the presence of discomfort.[45,46] As uncomfortable symptoms increase, perceived quality of life diminishes. An important goal in the psychosocial treatment of patients with advanced cancer centers on optimal symptom control.

An issue that repeatedly surfaces among patients, family members, and professional care providers is the use of aggressive treatment protocols[47] in the presence of relapse and progressive disease. Patients and families often request participation in experimental protocols, even when there is little likelihood of extending survival. Controversy continues about the efficacy of such therapies and the role health care providers can play in facilitating patients' choices about participating.

The need for health care providers to establish structured dialogue among patients, family members, and other providers regarding treatment goals and expectations is essential. That certain patients respond to investigational treatment with increased hope, despite progressive disease, should be a consideration in treatment planning. The need to separate and clarify the values, thoughts, and psychological reactions of care providers, patients, and families to these delicate issues is important if individualized care with attention to the particular patient's psychosocial needs is to be provided.

Permanent Phase: Survivorship

The definition of a long-term survivor has changed radically. Initially, individuals who had survived cancer-free for longer than 5 years were considered "survivors and cured." More recently the term has been used to define individuals who have completed the acute phase of illness. Others use the term for all patients diagnosed with cancer. Some people would prefer changing the term to "thrivers," champions, or fighters.[4] In this chapter, the term *survivor* is used to define a person who is diagnosed with cancer and the *permanent phase* as the phase when therapy has been completed permanently.

Successful treatment of hematologic malignancies has resulted in cure for many patients and progressively longer lives for others. However, longer survival is not without significant psychological sequelae.[48–53] Innovative and new treatments may produce long-term physiologic consequences, such as infertility, treatment-related toxicity, persistent side effects, and organ system failure that can magnify and exacerbate the psychological issues initially associated with diagnosis and treatment.[45,54] The overwhelming evidence from the literature involving survivors with hematologic malignancies is that, on the average, most do very well after the initial adjustment in the first 1 to 3 years after treatment.[50,55,56] Most long-term BMT survivors express satisfaction with their quality of life and describe themselves as productive, stable, and well adjusted without significant physical, functional, psychological, and social problems related to their disease or BMT treatment. However, there is a group of patients with a high rate of psychosocial morbidity who are vulnerable to ongoing and intermittent psychosocial distress. Empirical evidence showed that as many as 9% to 30% of long-term survivors with hematologic malignancies experience significant psychological distress, including anxiety, depression, and posttraumatic distress symptoms.[48,52,57]

Psychological aspects of survivorship may include concern over termination of treatment, fear of relapse, preoccupation with somatic symptoms, reentry into previous roles, lingering affinity with death, and financial, job, and insurance difficulties. These issues may manifest in a variety of ways, including denial of past illness, leading to medical compliance issues; ongoing problems with anxiety, panic, and depression; and inability to reenter or modify previous roles. Fear of recurrence by both patients and family members can severely impact quality of life.[8] In her classic article "The enduring seasons in survival," Dow[9] stated that the season of extended survival is dominated by fear of recurrence. In fact, Baker et al.[58] showed in a group of cancer survivors that "being fearful my illness will return," "concern

Table 93–1 Long-term Consequences of Therapies for Hematologic Cancers

Anxiety
Depression
Fear of recurrence
Disfigurement
Conditioned nausea and vomiting
Unemployment
Denial of life insurance
Denial of health benefits
Increase in life insurance rates
Difficulty changing health care coverage
Breakdown of marriage or relationship
Decline in participation in leisure activities
Diminution of support from others
Disruption in sexual functioning
Fertility

about relapsing," "fears about the future," and "difficulty making long-term plans" were a problem 68%, 60%, 58% and 41% of the time.

There is increasing interest in patients' experiences with posttraumatic stress disorder (PTSD). Studies have consistently described a higher incidence of PTSD in patients with hematologic malignancies than in the average population.[59–62] Predictors of PTSD severity among patients with hematologic diagnosis include higher levels of distress and high avoidance coping coupled with low social support.[18] These researchers describe how providers can assess coping and presence of family support and potentially mitigate the effects of a distressing experience with the cancer diagnosis. Considerable evidence indicates that the wide range of surgical, chemotherapeutic, and radiation therapies leaves permanent damage to organs and physiologic functioning and disfigurement across the different hematologic diagnoses (Table 93–1). Health care providers should be mindful of psychological sequelae among patients, even within the context of remission and a hopeful prognosis, and refer patients and family members to a mental health specialist for further evaluation, as needed.

Permanent Phase: Terminal Stage and End-of-Life Care

Technologic advances in health care have improved the potential for cure of many previously fatal hematologic malignancies. However, many patients still have disease that is unresponsive to treatment, continues to progress, and is considered incurable. When cure is acknowledged to be impossible and alternative efforts to combat the progress of disease are exhausted, patients are recognized as terminally ill or dying. In this situation, some authors advocate a palliative care approach with no active treatment and a shift in the emphasis of medical care from the pursuit of cure to supportive and hospice care, including the provision of care and comfort, control of distressing symptoms, and maintenance of quality of life at an optimal level.[63–65] However, this paradigm currently is shifting in the field of palliative care to initiate palliative care alongside curative treatment with the philosophy that it should be implemented across the illness trajectory, with the promotion of quality of life through the relief of suffering.[66] The new World Health Organization definition states "Palliative care is an approach to care which improves quality of life of patients and their families facing life-threatening illness, through prevention, assessment and treatment of pain and other physical, psychological, and spiritual problems."[67]

The root of palliative care began with the hospice movement. Since the concept of hospice was first introduced in England in the 1960s, hospice care has been recognized as the state-of-the-science end-of-life care, and hospice services now are available around the world. However, hospice care has not been integrated into the care of patients dying with hematologic malignancies.[68,69] Despite the strong emphasis of providing end-of-life care in accordance with patients' wishes[70] and empirical studies[70,71] showing that most terminal patients prefer spending their final days of life and dying at home, hematologic malignancy is the only diagnosis that has been repeatedly and consistently shown to predict hospital death.

The reasons for such insufficiency have been attributed to patient and family difficulties in acknowledging and accepting the poor prognosis and imminent death, health care providers' attitudes toward aggressive treatment for hematologic malignancies and reluctance to shift to end-of-life care, and profound symptom distress and dramatic changes in physical conditions experienced by patients at the end of life.[72] Health care providers, first and foremost, must examine their own attitudes toward death and dying and avoid imposing their own values on patients and their families. Respecting patient and family wishes, appropriately managing and alleviating distressing symptoms, and providing care tailored at meeting patients' needs can help patients dying of hematologic malignancies reach the end of life with peace and dignity.

FACTORS THAT INFLUENCE PSYCHOSOCIAL ADJUSTMENT

Psychosocial responses to cancer vary widely and are influenced by several factors that clinicians should bear in mind when considering the responses of individual patients. A review of the literature points to key factors that may have an impact on psychosocial adjustment. They include demographic and disease factors, previous coping strategies and psychological stability, and the existence of social support.

Demographic and Disease Factors

Gender, age, type of treatment, and time interval after treatment have been consistently documented as important predictors for psychosocial adjustment and quality of life for patients with hematologic malignancies. A significantly higher anxiety score,[73] constant fatigue,[74] sleep problems,[75] no return to work,[76] and more impaired quality of life[74] were observed more in women than in men. The presence of current sleep problems[75] and fatigue[74,77] were associated with older age at BMT. Poor quality of life after treatment[78,79] was associated with higher age of the recipient at the time of the transplant, poorer self-image and overall cognitive functioning,[51] and inability to return to work.[73]

Different treatment modalities introduce different degrees of side effects, symptoms, and impact on quality of life. Significant differences were found between transplant groups with regard to loss of appetite, physical and role functioning, symptom distress, sexual impairment, infertility, mood, and overall quality of life.[15,54,55,79–82] Without exception, the greatest difficulties in psychosocial adjustment were observed among patients who underwent allogeneic BMT, followed by autologous BMT recipients and patients who received conventional or maintenance chemotherapy. The latter groups experienced the least impairment in quality of life and psychological distress. Patients who underwent transplant also had more psychiatric morbidity if they experienced lower functional status and higher regimen-related toxicity[19]

Time since BMT or completion of treatment was an important factor for facilitating psychosocial adjustment and improving quality of life. In general, during the first year after BMT, patients perceived their physical and overall well-being as being worst, experienced more anxiety and total mood disturbance, and reported the highest degree of illness intrusiveness in every aspect of life.[15,54,55,79–82] Improvement in functional status and quality of life, significant decrease of anxiety and depression, and levels of satisfaction with life were frequently observed with the passage of time after BMT.

Previous Coping Strategies and Psychological Stability

One of the key predictors of psychosocial adjustment to cancer is the psychological stability of the person before diagnosis. People with a history of poor psychosocial adjustment before development of cancer are at highest risk of psychological decompensation and should be monitored closely throughout all phases of treatment.[83] This is particularly true of people with a history of a major psychiatric syndrome, psychiatric hospitalization, or both.[19]

Because a person's coping style is determined relatively early in life and remains stable over time and across situations, it serves as a useful predictor of adjustment to cancer. Several investigators have identified specific personality characteristics, coping strategies, and life experiences that enhance or inhibit positive adjustment to cancer.[84,85] Empirical evidence also demonstrated the beneficial impact of positive coping strategies and personality attributes on long-term survival.[86–88] Coping strategies found to be most effective include a "fighting spirit," hopefulness and acceptance of the situation, a belief that life has purpose and coherence, and having a feeling of control over events, resulting in active participation in treatment and engagement in daily life. By contrast, poor adjustment and even PTSD have been associated with avoidant coping strategies, anxious preoccupation and high distraction, prior negative sexual experiences, body image problems, and inhibition in discussing personal and sexual problems.[18] One study showed that patients who smoke are at higher risk for psychiatric morbidity, perhaps due to the potential development of depression and or anxiety with withdrawal symptoms.[19] It is important to include smoking history in the patient's assessment of substance control use when preparing patients for treatment.

Existence of Social Support

Social support, network size, satisfaction with social support, and reliance on formal and informal social ties have consistently been found to influence a person's psychosocial adjustment to cancer.[89,90] The ability and availability of significant others in dealing with a diagnosis and discussion of treatment options can significantly affect the patient's view of himself or herself. Patients diagnosed with all types of life-threatening chronic disorders experience a heightened need for interpersonal support. Those who are able to maintain close connections with family and friends during the course of illness are more likely to cope effectively with the disease than are those who are not able to maintain such relationships.[56,87,89]

Living with a chronic illness often requires continuing care and management by a team of specialists. Use of supportive care services has been tied to improved quality of life; therefore, it is in the patient's best interest to access services needed for psychological distress.[89] Care usually is provided through followup visits to ambulatory or outpatient clinics and consulting rooms, rather than through hospitalization. However, several barriers that may impair the outpatient cancer survivor from accessing health care services include economic and financial constraints.[91]

Traditionally, patients are not referred to home nursing care routinely once they are discharged from the hospital. An initial home nursing visit can be invaluable in assisting patients and families with the transition, in addition to identifying areas in which ongoing assistance is needed. Home care referral can assist families that are increasingly relied on within the current health care system to be the major providers of care outside the hospital (see box on Caregiver Burden).[92]

Caregiver Burden

The phenomenon of caregiver burden acknowledges that cancer affects not only the patient but also members of the family.[92] The burden that caregiving places on the family highlights the family's needs and the importance of targeting education and support information that can help reduce caregiver burden. Helping to arrange respite care for family members primarily responsible for the care of patients also aids in relieving caregiver burden.

DIFFERENTIATING PSYCHIATRIC COMPLICATION FROM EXPECTED PSYCHOLOGICAL RESPONSES

Most patients do not react to a diagnosis and treatment for cancer by developing a clinically diagnosable psychiatric condition. However, in some cases a psychiatric syndrome does occur. If the patient's problems become severe, that is, if the provider believes that supportive measures are insufficient and ineffective in controlling psychological distress, referral to a psychiatric clinician is indicated. Factors that can prevent adjustment to cancer and its treatment include a history of significant depression, manic-depressive illness, schizophrenia, neuroses, organic mental conditions, personality disorders, lack of social support, and inadequate control of physical discomfort.

Because transient symptoms of anxiety and depression are common in patients with cancer, the ability of health care providers to distinguish expected reactions from more severe psychiatric complications is crucial. Anxiety and depression are common symptoms that are particularly evident at transition points during the clinical course of cancer. These symptoms usually subside within 2 to 4 weeks and are responsive to supportive reassurance and information regarding what to expect during the course of treatment. For a proportion of patients, psychological distress does not subside with usual interventions. Unfortunately, nonpsychiatric care providers often miss clinically relevant and severe psychiatric syndromes. Detecting serious psychiatric problems in patients can be difficult because several of the diagnostic criteria used to evaluate the presence of severe depression (e.g., lack of appetite, insomnia, decreased sexual interest, diminished energy) may overlap with usual disease and treatment effects. It is not unusual for health care providers to confuse their own fears about cancer with the psychological reactions of their patients (i.e., "I too would be extremely depressed if I were in a similar situation"; see box on Screening for Psychological Distress).

Most patients manifest transient psychological symptoms that are responsive to support, reassurance, and information about what to expect regarding the cancer course and its treatment. Some require more aggressive psychotherapeutic interventions, such as pharmacotherapy and ongoing psychotherapy. The following guidelines can assist the clinician in identifying those patients who exhibit behavior suggesting the presence of a psychiatric syndrome.

General guidelines designed to assist in distinguishing patients who should be referred for evaluation by a trained psychiatric clinician include the following:

1. History of psychiatric hospitalization or significant psychiatric/personality disorder
2. Persistent refusal, indecisiveness, or noncompliance with regard to needed treatment
3. Persistent symptoms of anxiety and depression that are unresponsive to usual support from health care providers or family members;

Screening for Psychological Distress

A number of tools have been developed to screen for psychological distress, but they have not been consistently incorporated into clinical care.[93,94] One tool that is easy to administer and that patients report as capturing their problems is the *distress thermometer*.[95] The tool is similar to pain measurement scales that ask patients to rate their pain on a scale from 0 to 10 and consists of two parts. The first part is a picture of a thermometer, and patients are asked to mark their level of distress. A rating of 4 or above indicates that a patient has symptoms indicating a need for evaluation by a mental health professional and potentially has a need for referral for services. The patient then is handed a second part of the tool and is asked to identify which items from a six-item problem list (illness-related, family, psychological, practical, financial, or spiritual effects) relate to the patient's distress (Fig. 93–2).[95,96] Lee et al. [97] found that the distress thermometer was a useful tool for screening transplant patients before admission. Pretransplant distress appeared to be highly predictive of distress posttransplant and was a feasible marker to target screening and intervention programs.

symptoms may present in the form of constant fear associated with treatment and procedures or excessive crying and hopelessness that worsen rather than improve with time
4. Abrupt, unexplained change in mood or behavior
5. Insomnia, anorexia, diminished energy out of proportion to expected treatment effects
6. Persistent suicidal ideation
7. Unusual or eccentric behavior or confusion (may be indicative of an organic mental disorder)
8. Excessive guilt and self-blame for illness
9. Evidence of dysfunctional family coping or complex family issues

After referral to a psychiatric specialist, one or a combination of several therapeutic modalities may be used. Cancer and its treatment may precipitate an exacerbation of an underlying mental illness to which a patient was predisposed and that may require extensive treatment (e.g., hospitalization for a psychosis, ongoing pharmacotherapy or psychotherapy). A discussion of these specialized forms of treatment is not given here, but the interested reader can consult appropriate standard texts.[20]

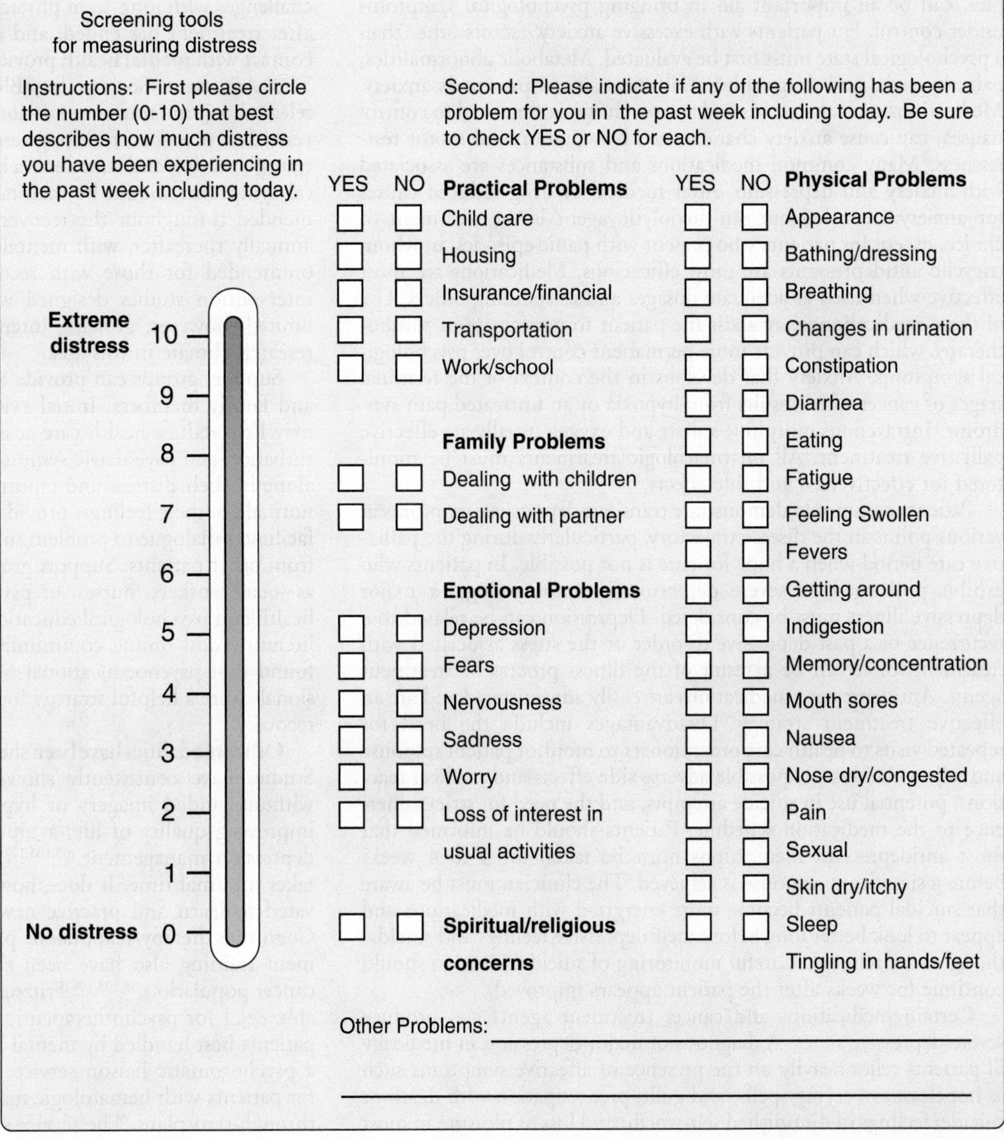
Screening tools for measuring distress

Instructions: First please circle the number (0-10) that best describes how much distress you have been experiencing in the past week including today.

Extreme distress 10 — 9 — 8 — 7 — 6 — 5 — 4 — 3 — 2 — 1 — No distress 0

Second: Please indicate if any of the following has been a problem for you in the past week including today. Be sure to check YES or NO for each.

YES	NO	Practical Problems	YES	NO	Physical Problems
☐	☐	Child care	☐	☐	Appearance
☐	☐	Housing	☐	☐	Bathing/dressing
☐	☐	Insurance/financial	☐	☐	Breathing
☐	☐	Transportation	☐	☐	Changes in urination
☐	☐	Work/school	☐	☐	Constipation
			☐	☐	Diarrhea
		Family Problems	☐	☐	Eating
☐	☐	Dealing with children	☐	☐	Fatigue
☐	☐	Dealing with partner	☐	☐	Feeling Swollen
			☐	☐	Fevers
		Emotional Problems	☐	☐	Getting around
☐	☐	Depression	☐	☐	Indigestion
☐	☐	Fears	☐	☐	Memory/concentration
☐	☐	Nervousness	☐	☐	Mouth sores
☐	☐	Sadness	☐	☐	Nausea
☐	☐	Worry	☐	☐	Nose dry/congested
☐	☐	Loss of interest in usual activities	☐	☐	Pain
			☐	☐	Sexual
			☐	☐	Skin dry/itchy
☐	☐	**Spiritual/religious concerns**	☐	☐	Sleep
			☐	☐	Tingling in hands/feet

Other Problems: ______________________

Figure 93–2 National Comprehensive Cancer Network (NCCN) Distress Management Guideline DIS-A-Distress Thermometer. (From the National Comprehensive Cancer Network 1.2005 Distress Management, The Complete Library of NCCN Clinical Practice Guidelines in Oncology [CD-ROM]. Jenkintown, PA, National Comprehensive Network, 2005.)

MANAGEMENT OF PSYCHOSOCIAL PROBLEMS

Interventions for these patients center on the uniqueness of the experience. In the initial phase of the experience, 50% of patients have psychological distress, including both anxiety and depression.[96] A growing body of literature provides evidence that patients may experience PTSD.[98] Increased length of survival from time of diagnosis has highlighted the need for psychopharmacologic, psychotherapeutic, and behaviorally oriented interventions to reduce distress, promote adjustment, and improve quality of life for patients with hematologic malignancies. Because of the increasing complexity of patient care, a multidisciplinary approach that includes regular avenues and options for communication about patient management and status updates is imperative. Numerous studies have documented the efficacy of a variety of modalities in managing psychosocial problems for such patients. Problems that can be managed effectively include psychological distress such as anxiety and depression; sexual dysfunction; body image disturbances; marital and family difficulties; noncompliance, pain, and neurologic complications such as delirium and dementia induced by brain metastasis or treatment; anticipatory and posttreatment nausea and vomiting; and anorexia and feeding problems.

Pharmacologic Interventions

Pharmacotherapy, as an adjunct to one or more of the psychotherapies, can be an important aid in bringing psychological symptoms under control. For patients with excessive anxiety, factors other than a psychological state must first be evaluated. Metabolic abnormalities, pain, hypoxia, and drug withdrawal states all can present as anxiety. Medications such as steroids and antipsychotics, often used to control nausea, can cause anxiety characterized by agitation and motor restlessness. Many common medications and substances are associated with anxiety and depression. After medical or drug-induced causes for anxiety are ruled out, an anxiolytic agent is the treatment of choice, except for patients who present with panic episodes, in whom tricyclic antidepressants are most efficacious. Medications are most effective when used at adequate dosages and as standing orders. Use of these medications may assist the patient to participate in psychotherapy, which can provide more permanent control over psychological symptoms. Anxiety that develops in the context of the terminal stages of cancer often results from hypoxia or an untreated pain syndrome. Intravenous morphine sulfate and oxygen usually are effective palliative treatment. All pharmacologic treatments must be monitored for effectiveness and side effects.

Patients commonly demonstrate transient depressive symptoms at various points in the disease trajectory, particularly during the palliative care period when a hope for cure is not possible. In patients who exhibit prolonged or severe depressive symptomatology, a major depressive illness must be considered. Depression can be related to a recurrence of a past depressive disorder or the stress associated with treatment, or it can be a result of the illness process or treatment agents. Antidepressant medications are easily administered and are an effective treatment strategy. Disadvantages include the need for repeated visits to health care practitioners to monitor patient response and adjust the dosage, possible adverse side effects and medical reactions, potential use in suicide attempts, and the need for strict adherence to the medication schedule. Patients should be informed that most antidepressant medications must be taken for 3 to 4 weeks before a significant response is achieved. The clinician must be aware that suicidal patients become more energized with medications and appear to look better long before their depressive feelings and suicidal thoughts are relieved. Careful monitoring of suicidal ideation should continue for weeks after the patient appears improved.

Certain medications and cancer treatment agents can produce severe depressive states. A diagnosis of major depression in medically ill patients relies heavily on the presence of affective symptoms such as hopelessness, crying spells, and guilt; preoccupation with death or suicide; feelings of diminished self-worth; and loss of pleasure in most activities such as being with friends and loved ones. The neurovegetative symptoms that usually characterize depression in physically healthy individuals are not good predictors of depression in the medically ill because disease and treatment can also produce these symptoms. A combination of psychotherapy and antidepressant medication often proves useful in treating major depression in medically ill patients.[99] Antidepressant medications may take 2 to 6 weeks to produce their desired effects. Patients may need ongoing support, reassurance, and monitoring in the period before the antidepressant effects of medication are achieved. Patients must be monitored closely by a consistent provider during the initiation and modification of psychopharmacologic regimens.

Psychotropic drugs are highly effective for treatment of anxiety, depression, agitation, and confusion in patients with hematologic malignancies.[100] It is beyond the scope of this chapter to include the current medications recommended for common psychiatric disorders. A comprehensive discussion of psychotropic drugs by classification is summarized in the quick pocketbook reference for oncology clinicians.[100] Medications specific for the management of anxiety, depression, and delirium also are presented.[101]

Psychotherapeutic Modalities

"Returning to normal" is a prominent theme in the clinical management of patients but is not always possible for patients with hematologic malignancies.[102,103] Survivors of cancer continue to face challenges with long-term physical and psychological symptoms long after treatment has ended, and data indicate that they report more contact with mental health providers than do people without cancer.[91] The American Society for Blood and Marrow Transplantation released a joint recommendations statement on screening and preventative practices for long-term survivors of hematopoietic cell transplantation and state that "a high level of vigilance for psychological symptoms should be maintained. Clinical assessment is recommended throughout the recovery period, at 6 months, 1 year and annually thereafter, with mental health professional counseling recommended for those with recognized deficits."[42] The number of intervention studies designed with the hematologic population is limited; however, growing interest in survivorship is changing the research climate in this area.

Support groups can provide a therapeutic experience for patients and family members. Initial evidence suggests that support groups may help reduce health care costs along with depression, mood disturbance, and psychiatric symptoms in patients.[104] Patients often feel alone in their distress and report that sharing a common experience normalizes their feelings, provides an avenue for emotional support, facilitates dialogue to problem solve, and offers opportunities to learn from other patients. Support groups facilitated by professionals such as social workers, nurses, or psychologists can provide a forum for health and psychological education and provide patients with printed literature and online community-based resources. Sherman et al.[29] found that psychoeducational support groups facilitated by professionals were a helpful strategy for patients' post-HSCT psychological recovery.

Other modalities have been shown to be effective with patients.[103,104] Studies have consistently shown that relaxation training with or without guided imagery or hypnosis may have some benefit with improving quality of life, symptom management, and anxiety and depression management.[103,105,107] It is a skill taught to patients that takes minimal time. It does, however, require that patients be motivated to learn and practice new techniques and a way of coping. Cognitive therapy/reappraisal, problem solving, and stress management training also have been shown to be helpful in the general cancer population.[98,103,106] Fritzsche et al.[107] identified that a considerable need for psychotherapeutic treatment of inpatient hematology patients best handled by mental health professionals. They described a psychosomatic liaison service that provided psychosocial support for patients with hematologic malignancies, including patients going through transplant. The service screened patients for anxiety, depres-

Table 93–2 Therapeutic Modalities Useful for Patients and Family Members

Modality	Selected Indications	Goals and Advantages	Comments
Individual psychotherapy	Prolonged adverse reactions to diagnosis, treatment, and other aspects of chronic illness (e.g., anxiety, depression)	Supports patient and enhances ability to cope with distressing feelings Short-term therapy; focused and goal directed	Pharmacotherapy and family involvement are useful adjuncts in some cases
Support groups	Patients desire contact with others who are experiencing chronic illness	Supports patient and enhances coping ability Usually does not involve a fee Patients benefit by observing coping strategies of others	Expands social network of patients with limited support systems
Family and marital therapy	Relationship problems secondary to illness (e.g., family tension, role changes, conflict, sexual problems)	Assists couples to clarify problems and facilitates solving them together Addresses role changes in the family system	Problems, issues, and concerns about relationships including children can be addressed
Mind–body therapies, including progressive muscle relaxation, yoga, guided imagery, Reiki, meditation, hypnosis, biofeedback	Patients desire assistance with control of pain, anxiety, anticipatory and posttreatment nausea and vomiting, fears associated with medical procedures	Increases sense of control and participation in treatment Individualized to meet patient's preferences and circumstances Time limited and goal directed Evaluated in terms of observable changes in symptoms	Realistic goals should be stated explicitly (some patients may view these therapies as a cancer cure)

sion, poor coping, quality of life, and psychosocial openness for support and provided psychotherapy, relaxation training, or group therapy as interventions. Although all transplant patients received support from the team, 23% on the hematology patients on the general ward received additional psychosocial interventions.

Other evidence-based interventions that have been found to be helpful in the general oncology population include individual and group counseling, family therapy, music, and art therapy. In comparison to patients with solid cancers, there should be a low threshold for referral for psychosocial support for patient and families faced with a hematologic malignancy because the primary treatment is intense and long and associated with sensitivity to potential barriers such as economic constraints, including lost of insurance. It has been estimated that one of six cancer survivors with mental health problems who need services are unable to access those services due to cost.[91] If cost is prohibitive and referral to a psychologist is not feasible, both patients and providers must investigate other potential providers, such as chaplains, art therapists, music therapists, social workers, and psychiatric advanced-practice nurses who might be able to see patients as part of their work responsibilities. Other possibilities include online support groups and advocacy organizations, including local wellness communities.

Depending on the nature of the problem, the treatment modality may take the form of individual psychotherapy, group therapy, family therapy, marital therapy, behaviorally oriented therapy, or some combination.[108] Increasing evidence supports use of an aerobic exercise program for patients with hematologic malignancies.[109–111] Researchers have concluded that fatigue and loss of physical performance in patients undergoing BMT may improve with exercise.[110] Others have found increased muscle strength after allogeneic BMT.[111] Table 93–2 outlines the major psychotherapeutic modalities and their advantages, goals, and indications.

CONCLUSION

The psychosocial issues faced by people diagnosed and treated for hematologic malignancies are influenced by sociocultural, medical, family, and individual factors. Although involvement in decision making clearly is a positive aspect of current cancer therapies, great care should be taken to ensure the communication of timely, repeated, and relevant information consistent with the patient's needs, tolerance, and comprehension. A multidisciplinary approach is essential to guarantee the communication of timely and essential information to all patients. Patients should be given the opportunity to speak with multiple members of the interdisciplinary treatment team and other patients who have experienced similar management and treatment protocols. Care should be taken to provide needed information from a variety of expert perspectives while respecting the unique characteristics, psychosocial profiles, needs, and desires of each individual. In treatment settings with limited resources, every effort should be made to enlist the help and support of providers and services that can assist patients with their complex treatment decisions. Referral to community resources and support services after discharge from the hospital often is helpful, even for patients who cope well with initial treatment.[20]

Most patients undergoing cancer treatment, as well as their families, experience expected periods of psychological turmoil that occur at transition points along the clinical course of cancer. In a small proportion of patients more severe psychiatric complications may occur, warranting referral to a psychiatric specialist, including psychiatrists, social workers, psychologists, and psychiatric nurses. Screening for ongoing psychiatric problems must become standard care. A variety of psychotherapeutic modalities are useful for helping patients work through the expected psychological responses to cancer as well as more severe responses.[24] Supportive psychotherapeutic measures should be used routinely because they minimize distress and enhance feelings of control and mastery over self and environment. For these reasons alone, their value in the care of patients with cancer is paramount. For patients who are not responsive to routine support and information, referral to a psychiatric specialist may be indicated.

Throughout the clinical course of cancer, the patient's relationship with health care providers and the presence of a supportive social network are important factors that can ensure successful negotiation of the many physical and psychosocial demands imposed by a cancer diagnosis and treatment. As scientific inquiry continues to produce vast but sometimes conflicting information regarding etiology and treatment of cancers, concurrent research regarding the psychosocial aspects of hematologic malignancies is crucial. This line of inquiry will, at the very least, assist in promoting psychosocial well-being in patients and family members faced with an extreme and unexpected life crisis. At best, expanding the knowledge base relative to the psychosocial aspects of cancer may provide some "missing links" regarding psychosocial adaptation and quality of life and their impact on survival. Their results underscore the recommendations of the recent Institute of Medicine report that all cancer care should ensure the provision of appropriate psychosocial health sevices.[108] Minimally, patients must be screened for emotional distress and evaluated for additional services.

SUGGESTED READINGS

Claessens JJM, Beerendonkk CCM, Schattenberg AVMB: Quality of life, reproduction and sexuality after stem cell transplantation with partially T-cell-depleted grafts and after conditioning with a regimen including total body irradiation. Bone Marrow Transplant 37:831–836, 2006.

Cooke L, Grant M, Eldredge D: Hematopoietic cell transplantation: The trajectory of quality of life. In Ezzone S, Schmit-Pokorny K (eds.): Blood and Marrow Stem Cell Transplantation, 3rd ed. Sudbury, MA, Jones and Bartlett Publishers, 2007, p 391.

Coyle N: Introduction to palliative nursing care. In Ferrell BR, Coyle N (eds.): Textbook of Palliative Nursing, 2nd ed. New York, Oxford University Press, 2006, p 1.

Fleishman SB, Greenberg DB: Pharmacological interventions. In Holland JC, Greenberg DB, Hughes MK (eds.): Quick Reference for Oncology Clinicians: The Psychiatric and Psychological Dimensions of Cancer Symptom Management. Charlottesville, VA, IPOS Press, pp. 26–32, 2006.

Frick E, Ramm G, Bumeder I, et al: Social support and quality of life of patients prior to stem cell or bone marrow transplantation. B J Health Psychol 11(Pt 3):451, 2006.

Haylock PJ: The shifting paradigm of cancer care. Am J Nurs 106:16, 2006.

Hewitt M, Sheldon G, Stovall E (eds.): From Cancer Patient to Cancer Survivor: Lost in Transition. Washington, DC, National Academy Press, 2006.

Institute of Medicine (IOM): Cancer Care for the Whole Patient: Meeting Psychosocial Health Needs, Nancy Adler & Ann Page, eds. Washington, DC, Natural Academy Press, 2008.

Jacobsen P: State of the Science: Psychological Well-Being and Survivorship. Survivorship Education for Quality Cancer Care Conference, City of Hope, Duarte, CA, July 2006.

Lim J, Zebrack B: Social networks and quality of life for long-term survivors of leukemia and lymphoma. Support Care Cancer 14:185, 2006.

McQuellan RP, Danhauer SC: Psychosocial rehabilitation in cancer care. In Chang AE, Ganz PA, Hayes DF, et al. (eds.): Oncology: An Evidence-Based Approach. New York, Springer Verlag, 2006, p 1942.

NCI: Cancer Control Continuum. http://www.cancercontrol.cancer.gov/od/continuum.html. Accessed November 16, 2006.

Paice JA, Fine PG: Pain at the end of life. In Ferrell BR, Coyle N (eds.): Textbook of Palliative Nursing, 2nd ed. New York, Oxford University Press, 2006, p 131.

Pirl WF: Screening instruments. In Holland JC, Greenberg DB, Hughes MK (eds.): Quick Reference for Oncology Clinicians: The Psychiatric and Psychological Dimensions of Cancer Symptom Management. Charlottesville, VA, IPOS Press, pp. 6–18, 2006.

Prieto JM, Blanch J, Atala J, et al: Stem cell transplantation: Risk factors for psychiatric morbidity. Eur J Cancer 72:514, 2006.

Rizzo JD, Wingard JR, Tichelli A, et al: Recommended screening and preventive practices for long-term survivors after hematopoietic cell transplantation: Joint recommendations of the European group for blood and marrow transplantation, the Center for International Blood and arrow Transplant Research, and the American Society of Blood and Marrow Transplantation. Biol Blood Marrow Transplant 12:138, 2006.

Valentine AD: Common psychiatric disorders. In Holland JC, Greenberg DB, Hughes MK (eds.): Quick Reference for Oncology Clinicians: The Psychiatric and Psychological Dimensions of Cancer Symptom Management. Charlottesville, VA, IPOS Press, pp. 39–71, 2006.

REFERENCES

For complete list of references log onto www.expertconsult.com

CHAPTER 94

PAIN MANAGEMENT AND ANTIEMETIC THERAPY IN HEMATOLOGIC DISORDERS

Craig D. Blinderman, Bridget Fowler, and Janet L. Abrahm

Relieving the pain of patients who have hematologic disorders requires a multifaceted approach.[1,2] An understanding of the taxonomy of pain, basic pain pathophysiology, and a systematic evaluation of the pain complaint will provide a rational basis for treatment decisions. After the source of the pain has been identified, appropriate nonpharmacologic and pharmacologic therapies can be initiated. The neurosurgical and anesthetic procedures for the management of cancer pain are not discussed in this chapter; those interested in these techniques are referred to several excellent reviews.[1–6]

TAXONOMY OF PAIN

Although there is no one standardized classification system for cancer pain, several systems have been proposed.[7–14] Cancer pain syndromes, and thus by analogy pain syndromes in hematologic disorders, may be classified temporally, pathophysiologically, etiologically, or according to distinct clinical-anatomical entities, or any combination thereof. Clinically, it is useful to determine both the etiology and inferred pathophysiology in the assessment of the pain complaint, as this may suggest the use of specific therapies. A conceptually useful taxonomy therefore categorizes pain as *nociceptive* (somatic or visceral), *neuropathic*, or *idiopathic*. Nociceptive pain refers to pain that is sustained predominantly by tissue injury or inflammation. Nociceptive somatic pain is described as sharp, aching, stabbing, throbbing, or pressure-like. Nociceptive visceral pain is poorly localized and is usually described as crampy pain (eg, obstruction of hollow viscus), or as aching and stabbing (eg, pain secondary to splenomegaly). Neuropathic pain is sustained by abnormal somatosensory processing in the peripheral or central nervous system. Sensations described as "burning," "shock-like," and "electrical" typically suggest neuropathic pain. On physical examination, patients may have allodynia (pain induced by nonpainful stimuli) and hyperalgesia (increased perception of painful stimuli). In the absence of evidence sufficient to label pain as either nociceptive or neuropathic, we may use the term *idiopathic*. However, in patients with hematologic disorders, this term should lead to additional workup and a search for an underlying etiology and pathophysiology.

BASIC PAIN PATHOPHYSIOLOGY

Pain is defined as an unpleasant sensory and emotional experience associated with actual or potential tissue damage, or described in terms of such damage.[15] For a patient to feel pain,[1] a signal arising from a noxious stimulus in the periphery must be transmitted to the centers in the brain that create the experience of pain. After activation of peripheral receptors by chemical, thermal, or mechanical stimuli, the signal passes along unmyelinated A-delta or C fibers and enters the spinal cord via the dorsal root ganglion. Chemicals released at the site of tissue injury mediate or modulate the transmission of the pain signal. Arachidonic acid metabolites, bradykinin, adenosine, serotonin, nitric oxide, prostaglandins, and lipoxygenase products have all been identified as playing a role in initiating or increasing the transmission of the pain signal in peripheral nociceptors.[16]

The dorsal horn of the spinal cord is where the peripheral signals are received and modulated. The excitatory amino acids (eg, glutamate and aspartate) and neuropeptides (eg, substance P and calcitonin gene-related peptide) enhance transmission of the peripheral signal.[1,17] But a complex interaction of other neurotransmitters (ie, γ-aminobutyric acid [GABA], glycine, adenosine, bombesin, cholecystokinin, dynorphin, enkephalin, neuropeptide-Y, neurotensin, substance P, somatostatin, and vasoactive intestinal peptide) determines whether the signal will proceed up the spinothalamic tract.[1] The signals that are transmitted ascend in one of the two contralateral spinothalamic tracts: the paleospinothalamic tract, which mediates the "suffering" and autonomic reactions to pain, or the neospinothalamic tract, which localizes the pain and records its intensity.[1]

Descending pathways originating in the central nervous system can inhibit transmission of the pain signal. A modulatory network with major relays in the midbrain periaqueductal gray and rostral ventromedial medulla exerts control over dorsal horn nociceptive transmission and is the central substrate of opioids-both endogenous and exogenous.[18] This major pain-modulating pathway involves regions of the frontal lobe, amygdala and hypothalamus, all of which have projections to the periaqueductal gray. The periaqueductal gray inhibits spinal nociceptive neurons via connections in the rostral ventromedial medulla and the dorsolateral pontine tegmentum. The neurotransmitters involved in this and other central inhibitory pathways include serotonin, norepinephrine, cholecystokinin, neurotensin, acetylcholine, cannabinoids, and the endogenous opiates β-endorphin, enkephalin, and dynorphin.[18]

Opiate receptors for endogenous and exogenous opioids are present in the dorsal horn of the spinal cord, in those ventromedial thalamic nuclei that transmit signals from the paleospinothalamic tract, in the periaqueductal gray, the periventricular diencephalon, and the amygdala.[18] The analgesic affects of opioids is thought to be due to the reduction of neurotransmitter release (eg, glutamate, substance P, and others) from presynaptic nociceptive fibers as well as postsynaptic inhibition of neurons transmitting the painful signal to the brain.[17]

The *N*-methyl-D-aspartate (NMDA) receptor at the level of the spinal cord plays an important role in chronic painful states. Chronic pain or long-term opioid therapy may result in activation of the NMDA receptors. Activation of the NMDA receptor initiates intracellular processes that lead to several neuronal plastic changes that in turn result in enduring increases in neuronal excitability.[19] Antagonists of these receptors, for example, ketamine[20] and dextromethorphan,[21] may enhance analgesia and reduce the amount of opioid analgesics required. Further studies are necessary to determine the clinical role of NMDA antagonists.

Several reviews have described the diverse pathophysiologic processes involved in neuropathic pain.[22,23] Most neuropathic pain syndromes are the result of peripheral nerve injury. Following injury, changes occur at the molecular level, within the nerve itself, and within the spinal cord and brain. At the molecular level, there is upregulation in the expression of both tetrodotoxin-sensitive (TTX-S) and tetrodotoxin-resistant (TTX-R) Na channels. These Na channels are the targets for many of the adjuvant medications used to treat neuropathic pain, for example, local anesthetics, antiarrhythmics, anticonvulsants, and tricyclic antidepressants.[24] Other cellular components that are thought to play a role in neuropathic pain include TRPV-1 channels, N and P/Q type voltage-gated calcium channels, purine receptors (P2X), TrkA, proton receptors, and cannabinoid receptors (CB1, CB2).[22] Additional changes take place within the nerve itself. Following injury to peripheral nerves, there is a subsequent change in the phenotype of the nerves by de novo gene expression.[25] Both injured and unaffected nerves develop a sensitivity to a number of factors to which they were previously insensitive, and also respond to subthreshold stimuli. Such sensitization may lead to ectopic and spontaneous activity in tissue nociceptors, perhaps explaining paroxysmal episodes of pain. A host of chemical and inflammatory mediators further alter the gene expression of nerves, leading to increased sensitivity. At the level of the spinal cord, several processes occur that alter the way sensory nerves function, thus maintaining a pathologic pain state. These processes can be described as reorganization, sensitization, and disinhibition.[24] Reorganization refers to the phenomenon of new connections being established in the laminae of the spinal cord, for example, A-beta fibers (which normally transmit light touch) sprout into lamina II of the dorsal horn, replacing C-fibers that transmit nociceptive information to second-order neurons. Dorsal horn neurons also become sensitized as a result of repeated firing from peripheral nerve fibers. The release of substance P, CGRP, and other neuropeptides lead to the activation of the NMDA receptor, release of nitric oxide postsynaptically, with subsequent excitation of pain transmission neurons. Microglia activation also plays a role in sensitizing and maintaining pathologic pain states.[26] Finally, disinhibition at the level of the spinal cord is thought to be a result of interneuron death in lamina II, downregulation of GABA and opioid receptors, and increased production of cholecystokinin.[24]

Table 94–1 Common Pain Syndromes in Hematologic Malignancies

Procedure-related Pain	
Bone marrow biopsy	
Central catheter placement	
Lumbar puncture headache	
Therapy-related Pain	
Myalgias (eg, from corticosteroid withdrawal)	
Myopathy	
Oropharyngeal mucositis	
Postherpetic neuralgia	
Osteoporosis	
Peripheral Neuropathies (eg, secondary to chemotherapy agents)	
Visceral pain syndromes (eg, typhlitis, hemorrhagic cystitis, enteritis)	
Pain from Hematologic Malignancy	
Pain Syndrome	**Cause(s)**
Bone Pain	Bone marrow expansion/infiltration Bone infarct/necrosis Osteomyelitis Compression fracture Hemarthrosis
Visceral Pain	Tumor involvement Splenomegaly Lymphadenopathy/lymphadenitis
Headache	Meningeal infiltration, infection Brain metastasis or primary tumor
Neuropathic Pain	Paraproteins with antimyelin properties Amyloid infiltration Peripheral nerve compression Spinal cord compression

EVALUATION OF THE PAIN COMPLAINT

Initial Evaluation

Effective pain management requires a comprehensive assessment of the patient's pain. Pain reports by patients should be believed. The clinician may not be aware that the clinical presentation of a patient suffering from chronic pain is very different from that of a patient in acute pain. If a patient does not manifest the common autonomic manifestations of acute pain (eg, tachycardia, sweating, elevated blood pressure) or facial grimacing, the clinician might doubt that the patient is suffering from severe pain. A patient with severe but chronic pain does not manifest these autonomic findings, but often is withdrawn, quiet, depressed, or irritable and can move very little spontaneously but complains of discomfort when moved. When the pain is relieved, these patients often exhibit completely different behaviors, becoming mobile, engaged, and involved with other people. The first component in the assessment is to believe the patient's complaint.

Patient reports of pain are valid, reliable, and reproducible.[1] A variety of assessment tools that can be completed within 5 to 10 minutes are available.[1,27,28] The pain complaint should be characterized by a number of descriptors: pain location, intensity, quality, onset, and duration; location and patterns of radiation; and what relieves or exacerbates the pain and its functional consequences, including how the pain affects the patient's ability to sleep or eat and how it affects physical activity, relationships with others, emotions, and concentration. Most patients with chronic cancer pain also experience periodic flares of pain, or "breakthrough pain."[29] An important subtype of breakthrough pain is "incident pain," which is caused by voluntary activity. The initial evaluation should determine the extent to which the patient suffers from breakthrough pain and if it is provoked by movement (nociceptive) or tends to be paroxysmal in nature (neuropathic). This subjective information, combined with the physical examination and diagnostic studies, may identify a specific pain syndrome and its implied pathophysiology.

In the patient with a hematologic disorder, the cause of pain may be: the disease itself, the specific therapy for the disease, diagnostic procedures related to the disease, or unrelated disorders (Table 94–1). Splenomegaly, bone injury (eg, infarction, infection, hemarthroses, infiltration), leptomeningeal infiltration, and spinal cord compression frequently accompany hematologic diseases. Chemotherapy and radiation therapy can cause mucositis, typhlitis, hemorrhagic cystitis, and peripheral neuropathy; corticosteroid withdrawal may cause myalgias.[30] Immunosuppression, caused by the diseases themselves or by the therapies used to treat them, may lead to painful infections such as perirectal abscesses, herpetic or candidal esophagitis, and herpes zoster. Patients with sickle cell disease have a number of causes for both acute and chronic pain (Table 94–2).

Distress, however, may arise from nonanatomic sources. The pain complaint may represent the patient's only means of expressing nonspecific feelings of distress to the physician. Chapman[31] recognized three categories of this distress: anxiety, arising from fear of disfigurement or of uncontrollable pain, fear of loss of social position or of self-control, or fear of death; anger at the failure of the physicians to provide a cure; and depression from the loss of physical ability, a sense of helplessness, and the impact of financial problems. In addition to these psychological, social, and financial contributions, spiritual concerns may exacerbate any concomitant painful sensations.[32] Alleviating them may significantly reduce distress and decrease the need for pain medications or other interventions.[33]

For the patient whose complaint of pain does not seem to have a straightforward explanation or who has not responded well to the therapeutic maneuvers outlined subsequently, additional questions must be asked to uncover the source of the distress. Patients may deny their disease and use the complaint of pain to justify their incapacity. Their denial is demonstrated by answers to the following types of questions. *How would life be different without the pain?* Such patients give unrealistic assessments of the extent of their abilities "if only the pain were gone." Answering another question may reveal hidden fears, resentments, and distrust of the physician: *What do you think is causing the pain?* Unrealistic expectations of pain treatment

Table 94–2 Classification of Pain Syndromes in Sickle Cell Disease

Pain Secondary to the Disease Itself
Acute pain syndromes
Acute chest syndrome
Calculus cholecystitis (pigment stones)
Hand–foot syndrome (in children)
Hepatic crisis
Priapism
Pulmonary infarction
Recurrent acute painful episode
Splenic sequestration (in children)
Chronic pain syndromes
Arthropathies/arthritis
Avascular necrosis
Chronic osteomyelitis
Intractable chronic pain
Pain secondary to therapy
Loose prosthesis (in patients post arthroplasty for avascular necrosis)
Opioid withdrawal
Postoperative pain
Pain due to Comorbid Conditions
Leg ulcers
Neuropathic pain

Adapted from Ballas SK: Pain management of sickle cell disease. Hematol Oncol Clin N Am 19:785, 2005.

may be revealed by answers to the following question: *To what extent do you expect your pain to be relieved?* The patient may expect that taking one pill each day will provide total relief, whereas the physician expects that even a multimodality regimen will relieve only 75% of the pain. A "contract" detailing the expectations of the patient and physician may be formulated once these unspoken assumptions are understood. Other sources of confusion in the way the patient communicates the type of pain experienced can be clarified by the answer to the following question: *Do you seem to show your feelings about the pain to the same extent that your family and friends do?* Patients may come from cultural backgrounds different from the person reporting the pain, and people with cultural differences often report pain very differently.[34–36] For example, patients from a "stoic" cultural upbringing may not communicate their distress to their spouse, who may then question the patient's need for opioid pain medication (ie, if they themselves were in that much pain, they would be sure to tell their spouse). Unless the cultural differences are explored, adequate pain control may not be achieved.

Continued Assessment

A standardized measurement tool, for example, verbal rating scale or a visual analog scale, should be consistently used during follow-up visits. These measurements are thought to be more accurate than mere qualitative descriptors, such as "the pain is better." Using, for example, a scale of 0 (*no pain*) to 10 (*the worst pain one can imagine*), a decrease in pain intensity from 10 to 8 indicates that the patient needs a stronger pain medication, whereas a decrease from 10 to 3 suggests that the current medication regimen is effective. This inference can be confirmed by asking the patient, "Is this level of pain relief acceptable to you?"[1] The ongoing assessment should also pay attention to changes in the phenomenology of the pain, new occurrences of pain, or a change in the location of pain—all of which may suggest progression of disease in the patient with a hematologic disorder.

The successful outcome of pain therapy should be more than simply the lowering of pain intensity scores. Passik and Weinreb developed a useful mnemonic device for the assessment of pain therapy in chronic nonmalignant pain known as the "4 A's": analgesia, activities of daily living, adverse events, and aberrant drug-taking behaviors (eg, repeated dose escalation or noncompliance, hoarding drugs, acquiring drugs from other medical sources).[37] By focusing on these relevant domains in the continued assessment of the pain therapy, the clinician is able to determine if the therapy makes a true difference in the patient's life, stabilizes or improves psychosocial functioning, manages side effects, and provides a means of assessing for aberrant drug behaviors. Ultimately, the goal should be to lower the pain *to a level acceptable to the patient* and to improve the patient's level of functioning.

THERAPY

A major component of pain therapy is an attempt to ameliorate the underlying cause of the pain. Surgery, chemotherapy, radiation therapy, and antibiotics may all be employed. However, the pain can still be treated effectively during diagnostic testing to define the cause, during specific therapy, or after all disease-related therapies are exhausted.

The goal of pain management is to relieve pain while preserving the patient's ability to perform normal activities. This requires expertise on the part of health care personnel, who seek to maximize the relief obtained while minimizing side effects and alterations in daily routines. A multifaceted approach is required that includes nonpharmacologic approaches, correct use of a variety of medications and anesthetic techniques so that pain will be relieved with a minimum of side effects, and patient and family education at each step to foster communication and cooperation with the therapeutic plan.

NONPHARMACOLOGIC METHODS OF PAIN MANAGEMENT

Cognitive–Behavioral Interventions

Education and Reassurance

Patients with serious hematologic disorders are often required to undergo extensive diagnostic testing, which can include painful procedures. A rehearsal of the planned test or procedure, including a discussion (or view) of the appearance of the room and the length of time to be spent in the test apparatus, can minimize the patient's anxiety. Such explanations, offered preoperatively, lessen the need for postoperative medication and shorten the patient's hospital stay.[38] If conscious sedation is not planned, a pleasant distraction may be helpful to divert attention from certain procedures (eg, bone marrow aspiration or biopsy) that take place in the physician's office or in the patient's room.[39] For example, the physician might encourage the patient to bring in a CD or MP-3 player with earphones so that the patient can listen to a favorite piece of music or a book on tape while the procedure is taking place. Alternatively, the physician might turn on the television or radio in the patient's room and encourage the patient to pay attention to that, rather than to the procedure. Patients with a good imagination can pretend to be in a place they have previously enjoyed (eg, at the beach or in the mountains). They can dissociate themselves[40] from the procedure by concentrating on those pleasant memories and thereby diminishing the painfulness of the procedure.

Hypnosis

Practitioners with formal training in hypnosis can use more elaborate hypnotic techniques to help their patients deal with painful procedures or conditions.[39,40] Hypnosis takes advantage of the natural ability to enter a trance-like state. An athlete "playing through the pain" is an example of the spontaneous induction of such a state. Patients who are trained to enter a trance can modify their perception of pain and diminish sleeplessness, anxiety, and the anticipation of discomfort.[41] Hypnotic training of patients with sickle cell anemia or hemophilia decreases the frequency and pain intensity of painful crises[42] or bleeding episodes,[43,44] respectively.

Even in the absence of a formal hypnotic induction, the words used by the practitioner to describe procedures are very important. For example, the suggestion that skin coolness and numbness will persist after application of an alcohol swab may markedly diminish the discomfort of starting an intravenous line. Using the phrase "You will feel something; I'm not sure what you will feel, because everyone feels this a little differently" in place of "This is going to hurt a lot!" gives the patient permission to alter the sensation and may also diminish the experience of pain.

Cognitive–Behavioral Techniques and Counseling

The cognitive–behavioral approach addresses a number of psychosocial and behavioral factors that contribute to the patient's experience of pain.[45] These techniques have demonstrated clinical utility for patients with a wide range of chronic pain syndromes.[45] Psychological counseling, as part of a multidisciplinary approach to pain treatment, provides education, support, and skill development for patients with pain. It can improve patients' abilities to communicate their pain to health care personnel and may be effective in overcoming anxiety and depression. Spiritual counseling may help patients who have lost hope, can find no meaning in their lives, or feel they are being punished or have been forsaken by God.[46] They may interpret their pain in light of these feelings. Through counseling, they can regain a sense of worth and belonging. As they recast the pain in its true light, its intensity is often diminished.

Cutaneous Techniques

Acupuncture, massage, vibration, and applying cold or heat to the skin over injured areas are often very effective. Cold wraps, ice packs, or cold massage using a cup filled with water that has frozen into a solid piece of ice relieve the pain of muscles that are in spasm from nerve injury. Heat from heating pads, hot wraps, or paraffin treatments can soothe injured joints but should not be used over areas of vascular insufficiency.[47] Transcutaneous electrical nerve stimulation devices are indicated for patients with dermatomal pain, such as postherpetic neuralgia or radiculopathy from spinal cord compression.[48] For optimal effect, a physiatrist or physical therapist familiar with the device should train the patient in its use.

EMLA, a cream containing two topical anesthetics (2.5% lidocaine and 2.5% prilocaine) is used, especially in children, to decrease the pain of superficial cutaneous procedures (eg, venous cannulation or skin anesthesia before lumbar puncture, bone marrow aspiration, or biopsy).[49–51] In adults, it is used before access of implanted vascular access devices or central nervous system ports. To achieve anesthesia, the EMLA cream must be applied 1 to 1.5 hours before the planned procedure in a mound under a semipermeable dressing such as Opsite or Tegaderm.[52,53] When EMLA is used as directed, methemoglobinemia has not been a problem even in infants as young as 3 months old.[54,55] Skin blanching occurs, sometimes exceeding or equaling the frequency of that found with placebo moisturizing cream placed under the occlusive dressing.[53,56] ELA-Max, a cream containing 4% lidocaine, is available over the counter and is an alternative to EMLA cream. Because it does not contain prilocaine, there is no risk of methemoglobinemia.

Lidocaine patches can be used over areas of hyperesthesia, as can occur in patients with postherpetic neuralgia or nerve entrapment by vertebral body collapse.[57] The patch is applied to the affected area for no more than 12 consecutive hours a day and can be cut to size. Use should be avoided over areas of broken skin and in patients undergoing radiation therapy. Extended application of lidocaine patches has been safely applied for up to 24 hours/day for up to 4 days with minimal systemic absorption in healthy volunteers and in postherpetic neuralgia patients.[58]

Radiation Therapy

Radiation therapy is commonly used in the management of painful bone lesions, spinal cord compression, bulky lymphadenopathy, and symptomatic splenomegaly in patients with hematologic malignancies.[59] Radiotherapy is the treatment of choice for local metastatic bone pain in most situations; however, patients with underlying pathologic fractures may require surgical fixation prior to radiotherapy. Randomized trials have shown that single-fraction radiotherapy is as effective as multifraction radiotherapy in relieving pain due to metastases. However, there are higher rates of retreatment, and single-fraction radiotherapy may not prevent pathologic fractures or spinal cord compression.[60] In patients with poor performance status or a short life expectancy, a single dose (8 Gy) of radiation or a hypofractionated course (20 Gy/5 fractions) may be preferable and less burdensome.

Surgery

Surgical intervention is often required in patients with impending or actual pathologic fractures or an unstable spine.[61,62] The patient's functional status and quality of life are important considerations regarding the appropriateness and timeliness of surgical intervention.

Vertebroplasty and Kyphoplasty

Vertebroplasty and kyphoplasty are relatively new surgical techniques used to stabilize vertebral compression fractures and reduce pain. Vertebroplasty is a procedure where bone cement, usually polymethylmethacrylate, is injected into the vertebral body. With kyphoplasty, a balloon is first inserted into the vertebral body, followed by inflation then deflation, before cement is added. Balloon kyphoplasty has been shown to stabilize pathologic vertebral fractures caused by multiple myeloma and to significantly reduce pain.[63,64]

Anesthetic Techniques

Trigger-point injections, nerve blocks, and neurolytic procedures are useful for acute and chronic localized pain. After excisional biopsy of an axillary lymph node, for example, a burning, constricting pain in the posterior arm and chest wall may develop; this pain is often promptly relieved by trigger-point injection.[65,66]

Lymphoma or myeloma may involve the spine and lead to vertebral collapse or pain from progressive disease that is refractory to antineoplastic therapy. Such pain is often particularly difficult to manage. Insertion of temporary or permanent indwelling epidural or intrathecal catheters to deliver opioids, local anesthetic agents, clonidine, or combinations of these and other agents can be very effective, especially in relieving lower thoracic or lumbar spine pain, as well as pelvic and lower extremity pain.[67–69] Those interested in the indications for and techniques of the anesthetic and neurolytic procedures are referred to several reviews.[5,6,70]

PHARMACOTHERAPY

Drugs useful for pain relief include nonopioid analgesics, opioids, and adjuvant analgesics. Most patients require a combination of medications for optimal pain relief (Fig. 94–1).

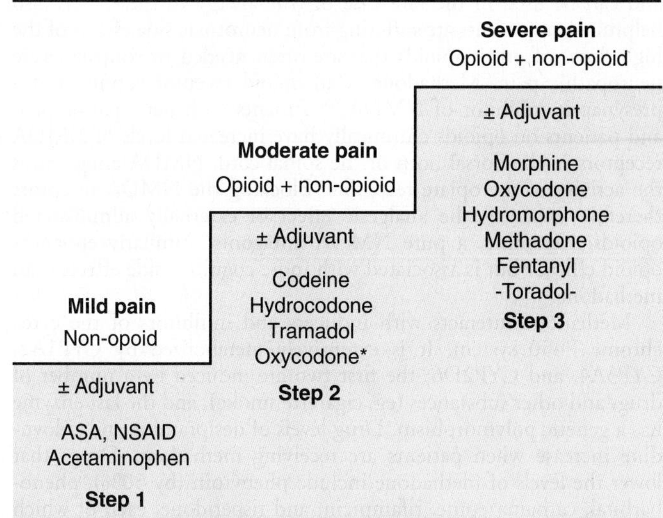

Figure 94–1 Strategy for pharmacologic management of pain using the WHO analgesic ladder. Multiagent therapy is usually required for optimal pain management. Patients with mild pain should be started on a nonopioid analgesic, and those with moderate pain on a step 2 opioid. Many patients can benefit from the addition of a nonopioid to the opioid (eg, for bone pain) or an adjuvant agent to the opioid (eg, for neuropathic pain). If this combination does not produce adequate relief or the patient presents with severe pain, step 3 opioids should be begun initially. Toradol (Ketorolac) is an NSAID with the pain-relieving potency of a step 3 opioid. Many patients can benefit from the addition of nonopioid analgesics or adjuvants, if indicated. ASA, aspirin; NSAID; nonsteroidal antiinflammatory drug.

Nonopioid Analgesics

Nonopioid analgesics should be given to patients with mild to moderate pain. Tramadol, which both weakly inhibits norepinephrine and serotonin reuptake and weakly binds to mu-opioid receptors and has opioid-induced side effects, but is not an opioid, also relieves mild to moderate pain. A dose of 100 mg is more effective than 60 mg of codeine.[71] Aspirin and nonsteroidal antiinflammatory drugs (NSAIDs) including COX-2 inhibitors are especially useful as antiinflammatory agents as they decrease local prostaglandin release through the inhibition of cyclooxygenase (though the mechanisms for their analgesic properties are not as clear).[72,73] Acetaminophen is an effective analgesic but only a weak antiinflammatory agent. Higher doses than that used for analgesia may be needed for its antiinflammatory effect. Acetaminophen's weak inhibition of cyclooxygenase may be due to the presence of high concentrations of peroxides found in inflammatory lesions.[74,75] It is important to prescribe an adequate dose of each drug at regular intervals, switching to another nonopioid analgesic only when maximal doses of the first have become ineffective.

Ketorolac tromethamine (Toradol) is an NSAID of particular value in relieving moderate to severe acute bone pain.[76] A dose of 30 mg of ketorolac given intramuscularly equals the pain-relieving potency of 15 mg of morphine intramuscularly, and acute toxicity is minimal if the total daily dose is under 100 mg.[77] Intravenous administration is less painful and equally effective as an intramuscular injection. Ketorolac may also be given orally, although it has a delayed peak response and is considered less potent. However, ketorolac has all the side effects of the NSAIDs and is not recommended for use beyond 5 days.[78] If that degree of pain relief is needed chronically, an opioid agent should be substituted.

Because the NSAIDs can cause renal insufficiency in a significant number of patients, renal function should be assessed 1 or 2 weeks after initiation of any of these agents. NSAIDs should be used with caution in patients with a history of aspirin allergy or asthma because they can precipitate bronchospasm in as many as 20%.[79] Significant edema can occur in patients with cirrhosis or congestive heart failure.[79,80] The relatively selective COX-2 inhibitors, such as etodolac, meloxicam, celecoxib, and nabumetone, should not, and apparently do not, cause gastrointestinal side effects with the same frequency as nonselective NSAIDs.[80] If NSAIDs are required in patients with a history of significant gastritis or ulcer disease or who are older than 70 years, COX-2 inhibitors or concomitant proton-pump inhibitors should be considered.[81,82]

The nonopioid analgesics should be continued in appropriate cases when opioid analgesics are added, because they can potentiate the pain-relieving effect of the opioid (see Fig. 94–1).[83] However, when aspirin or acetaminophen is included in a fixed drug combination (eg, Percodan, Percocet), toxicities may develop if the patient takes the pills more often than the prescription indicates. The metabolism of salicylates is limited by the capacity of the hepatic microsomal system. Once that is saturated, salicylate levels are dependent on renal clearance. Small increases in maintenance doses can lead to serious salicylism.[84] Patients with low albumin levels or acid urine are particularly susceptible to the development of salicylate toxicity.[85] Daily intake of acetaminophen should not exceed 4 g because of the potential hepatic toxicity.

Opioid Analgesics

Patient Education

Opioid analgesics are the mainstay of therapy for moderate to severe pain of malignant or nonmalignant origin. To ensure patient compliance with an opioid prescription, however, education of other members of the health care team, the patient, and the family is often required to dispel the many misconceptions associated with opioid therapy. Even physicians who are cancer specialists may hesitate to prescribe opioids as needed for patients with severe pain.[86]

Fear of addiction is a common cause of inadequate dispensing of opioids[87] and a barrier to their acceptance by patients.[86] The physician can increase compliance by providing a full explanation of the differences between addiction and physical dependence, along with reassurance that research has repeatedly indicated that patients with malignancies who take opioids do not become addicts.[88,89] Patients may also fear that if they take opioid medications for moderate pain, the medications will no longer be effective if more severe pain occurs. Because this fear, if unexpressed, can lead to undertreatment, the topic should be addressed even if the patient does not raise the question. A functional goal of therapy, such as returning to a favorite hobby or reinstituting normal activities of everyday life, may enable the patient and the family to accept the opioid. Misconceptions about religious teachings may prevent health care personnel, patients, and their families from giving or accepting adequate pain medication. Catholics, for example, may not be aware of the Church's position, as stated in the current catechism, that opioids may be used at the approach of death, even if their use ultimately shortens the patient's life.[90,91] The Church does not consider this use of pain medication to be a means of suicide or euthanasia.[92]

Choice of Medication

Because a wide variety of medications is available, pharmacokinetic considerations and side-effect profiles should be considered when choosing opioid agents. Intermittent moderate to severe pain lasting hours to several days is amenable to oral analgesics with short half-lives (3–4 hours) with appropriate potency (eg, immediate-release oxycodone, morphine, hydromorphone [Dilaudid], or oxymorphone (when available)). Severe pain of relatively constant intensity should be treated with oral sustained-release morphine or oxycodone (taken every 8 or 12 hours[93,94]), methadone (taken every 8 hours), or transdermal fentanyl (renewed every 48 to 72 hours). Twelve- to 24-hour

Management of Severe Pain

Opioid therapy is the cornerstone of management of the patient presenting with severe pain. Our practice is to begin with reassurance of patients and their families. We tell them that to relieve the pain as quickly as possible, we will initiate the use of intravenous opioid medications immediately, but that we will begin oral pain medication as soon as the pain is well controlled. Without this explanation, patients have misinterpreted a "morphine drip" as an indication that they were considered terminal. The starting dose is calculated from the patient's baseline opioid requirement (10% of their 24-hour opioid dose) or weight (eg, 0.05 mg/kg/hour of morphine). The patient is monitored continuously and given an opioid bolus dose. If the patient was on standing opioid medication, the medication is continued, when possible, or converted to an intravenous drip, if necessary. Pain is reassessed every 20 minutes after the patient receives a bolus dose. If the pain remains severe (7, 8, or 9/10), the bolus dose is doubled. If the pain has decreased to moderate (4, 5 or 6), another bolus at the same dose as the immediately previous dose is used. If the pain is less than 4, the patient is carefully monitored. At 4 to 8 hours, either a continuous infusion is begun or the ongoing infusion rate is adjusted upward according to the amount of opioid taken as boluses during that period. There is no maximal opioid dose; we give whatever is required to relieve the pain. If the patient falls asleep, this is usually an indication that pain relief has been achieved, not that the dose should be lowered. We lower the dose if the respiratory rate falls to below 10 to 12 breaths per minute.

Agents to prevent side effects are begun along with the opioid. All patients are given a stool softener and an irritant agent such as senna one or two tablets orally daily, up to a maximum of eight pills per day. If a more laxative effect is needed, lactulose (15–30 mL) or polyethylene glycol (17 g) is added. In opioid-naive patients, prochlorperazine [Compazine] (10 mg, taken orally two or three times daily) is ordered as needed to treat the common development of nausea. In patients with bone or nerve pain, appropriate adjuvants are added.

When pain relief is adequate, the patient is converted to an equivalent dose of oral or transdermal opioid. If morphine is used, for example, the patient will need three times the parenteral dose that was effective (see the box on Relative Potencies of Commonly Used Opioids). For example, a patient who requires 10 mg of morphine per hour (ie, 240 mg/24 hours, given intravenously) will need 720 mg/day of the oral sustained-release agent (240 mg × 3). This can be given orally as 360 mg every 12 hours. Two hours after the oral opioid is begun, the drip is discontinued. Short-acting immediate-release morphine should be available for rescue dosing at 10% of the total daily dose. For this patient, 60 to 90 mg is recommended. If the amount of opioid taken as a rescue dose is significant (>25% of the daily dose) for 1 or 2 days, the total dose of long-acting agent is adjusted upward accordingly.

formulations of oral morphine (eg, Kadian, Avinza) are available; for patients unable to take pills, the capsule can be opened and the pellets sprinkled on food or suspended in water and given through a feeding tube[95] (see the boxes on Relative Potencies of Commonly Used Opioids and Choice of Medication).

Practical Considerations When Using Opioids

Although methadone is not a new drug, it is increasingly used for patients with moderate to severe pain. It is by far the least expensive of the opioids[98]; can be given by oral, rectal, intravenous, or epidural routes; and has particular usefulness in patients with neuropathic pain.[99] Methadone is structurally unrelated to morphine and fentanyl and can be used in the rare case of true allergy to these. It is also helpful when patients are suffering from neurotoxic side effects of the high doses of other opioids that are often needed to control severe neuropathic pain. Methadone is an opioid receptor agonist and a presynaptic inhibitor of NMDA.[100] Patients with neuropathic pain and patients on opioids chronically have increased levels of NMDA receptors in the dorsal horn of the spinal cord. NMDA antagonizes the activity of the opiate receptors. Blocking the NMDA receptors therefore enhances the analgesic effect of externally administered opioids. Ketamine, a pure NMDA antagonist, similarly enhances opioid efficacy but is associated with more cognitive side effects than methadone.[9]

Methadone interacts with inducers and inhibitors of the cytochrome P450 system. It is extensively metabolized by CYP1A2, CYP3A4, and CYP2D6; the first two are induced by a number of drugs and other substances (eg, cigarette smoke), and the last enzyme has a genetic polymorphism. Drug levels of desipramine and zidovudine increase when patients are receiving methadone. Drugs that lower the levels of methadone include phenytoin (by 50%), phenobarbital, carbamazepine, rifampicin, and risperidone, each of which has precipitated withdrawal symptoms.[100] Drugs that raise the serum methadone levels include ketoconazole, fluconazole, and the selective serotonin reuptake inhibitors (SSRIs) (except venlafaxine), which raise methadone levels in CYP2D6-positive patients (rapid metabolizers).[99]

Methadone can cause prolongation of the QT interval. A mean methadone dose of 400 mg/day (SD = 283 mg) was found in 17 patients with torsades de pointes.[101] In an evaluation of reports of methadone-related adverse events to the FDA, approximately 1% of the greater than 5000 reports were of QT prolongation or torsades de pointes. The median dose was 345 mg, with a range of 29 to 1680 mg.[102] Drugs that also prolong the QT interval, such as metoclopramide and olanzapine, should be used with caution in patients receiving significant doses of methadone. Gabapentin, the drug used most often as a neuropathic pain adjuvant, does not interact with methadone metabolism.

Other difficulties with using methadone lie in its variable and long biologic half-life and the controversy about its equianalgesic dosing range. Some studies have reported that the equianalgesic dose of morphine to methadone varies as the dose of morphine increases.[103] Dose ratios vary from 4 : 1 at morphine doses of 30 to 90 mg, to 6 : 1 at 90 to 300, and to 8 : 1 at doses of more than 300 mg of morphine. Other studies report a ratio of 20 : 1 for doses of oral morphine equivalents greater than 1000 mg.[104] Some physicians advise a 3-day conversion to methadone. The first day, the dose of the old opioid is reduced by one-third, and one-third of the calculated dose of methadone is given; the second day, the dose of the remaining opioid is reduced by one-half, and only rescue doses of methadone are given every 4 hours; the third day the old opioid is discontinued, and the standing dose of methadone is adjusted to reflect the rescue doses.[99] When converting patients directly from intravenous fentanyl to intravenous methadone, a conversion ratio of 25 μg/hour of fentanyl to 0.1 mg/hour of methadone has been found in a pilot study to be a safe and effective initial infusion rate.[105]

A new opioid to the US market that is now available in both extended release and immediate release is oxymorphone. Oxymorphone extended release has been found to provide safe and effective pain relief for cancer pain.[106,107] Oxymorphone extended release is dosed twice daily and is approximately twice as potent as oxycodone.[108]

Levorphanol, which is chemically similar to dextromethorphan (an NMDA antagonist and cough suppressant), is a potent opioid that may be considered for patients with severe cancer pain. It was originally synthesized as an alternative to morphine more than 40 years ago. It has a greater potency than morphine, approximately 5 times as potent in its oral formulation. Analgesia is achieved through its agonistic activity at mu, delta, and kappa opioid receptors, as well as by its antagonism of NMDA receptors. Levorphanol can be given orally, intravenously, and subcutaneously.[109]

Buprenorphine has long been used to treat patients with addiction as an alternative to methadone. The new buprenophine patch has been found to be effective in patients with cancer and noncancer pain.[110,111] Postmarketing surveillance has indicated that 81% of patients achieve good or very good pain relief and approximately 50% of patients did not require additional medications for breakthrough pain.

Meperedine is 8 to 10 times less potent than morphine and has a short duration of action, approximately 2 to 3 hours. Normeperidine, an active metabolite that induces dysphoria, is excitatory to the central nervous system and can cause agitation, tremors, myoclonus and seizures, especially in high doses, with prolonged use, or in renal failure.[112] Normeperidine has a half-life of 13 to 24 hours, which can lengthen with renal failure.[113] The seizure incidence is further increased if the opioid antagonist naloxone (Narcan) must be given.[114] Therefore, meperidine is not recommended for chronic use in patients with long-lasting moderate to severe pain.[1]

Routes of Delivery

Opioids can be delivered noninvasively (orally, rectally, transmucosally, or transdermally) or invasively (subcutaneously, intravenously, or by spinal infusion). For patients switched from oral or rectal to parenteral or spinal medication, or vice versa, the dose must be altered accordingly to avoid overdose or undertreatment (see the box on Relative Potencies of Commonly Used Opioids). No matter which route is chosen, patients experiencing continuous pain should receive the analgesics regularly and be awakened, if necessary, to administer medications that will prevent recurrence of the pain.[1]

Oral Route

Most patients can achieve excellent pain relief with short-acting or sustained-release oral opioid preparations. The typical onset of short-acting opioids via the oral route is 45 minutes to an hour, with a typical duration of action of around 3 to 4 hours. When tablets and capsules are not feasible, many liquid forms are available in various concentrations. Some solutions do contain alcohol, which can be irritating to patients with oral lesions.

Rectal Route

Rectal opioids (eg, morphine and hydromorphone) replace subcutaneous or intramuscular injections in patients who are suddenly unable to take oral medications. They have about the same potency and half-life as orally administered agents[115–118] and must therefore be administered frequently. Although not approved by the US Food and Drug Administration (FDA), in single-dose bioavailability studies of sustained-release morphine preparations, despite delayed absorption from the rectal route, total morphine absorption over 24 hours was equivalent, whether the drug was given orally or rectally.[115–118]

Transdermal Route

The transdermal fentanyl patch delivers the lipophilic fentanyl into the fat-containing areas of the skin. The drug diffuses continuously from the patch's reservoir through a rate-controlling membrane and is absorbed from the skin depot into the bloodstream, where it is rapidly metabolized.[119] The onset of pain relief is delayed approximately 12 hours and a relatively constant plasma concentration of fentanyl is not reached until approximately 14 to 20 hours after the initial patch is placed.[119] Liberal rescue medication must therefore be provided during the first 24 hours of use of the patch.[120] Similarly, if a patient develops signs of fentanyl overdose, naloxone (Narcan) must be given until the skin reservoir has become depleted.[121] Approximately 50% of the drug is still present 24 hours after patch removal.[122] Converting patients from oral or parenteral medication to the patch is easily accomplished[123] (see the box on Relative Potencies of Commonly Used Opioids). A new patch is applied every 72 hours, although up to 25% of patients require a new patch every 48 hours.

The transdermal system is an effective method of delivering pain relief for patients with a stable level of chronic moderate to severe pain, no oral route available, or no desire to take pills. Side effects include those due to the contact adhesive, along with those commonly associated with other opioids, but may be better tolerated than those caused by morphine.[122–124]

The transdermal system should not be used in septic patients, those experiencing acute pain, those with markedly fluctuating opioid requirements, cachectic patients, or individuals with significant dermatologic insults (ie, skin grafts-versus-host disease or diffuse varicella). When the patient's temperature rises to 40°C, drug absorption from the skin can increase by as much as 35%.[119] If hepatic function is impaired or sepsis or shock develops and blood flow to the liver decreases, plasma concentrations may rise sharply.[122] Patients with cachexia lack the subcutaneous tissue necessary for formation of a drug reservoir. Lower doses may also be required in elderly patients[125] or in those with respiratory insufficiency.

Transmucosal Route

Oral transmucosal fentanyl citrate (Actiq) induces rapid analgesia with a short duration of affect, and is an effective treatment in the management of breakthrough pain.[126,127] A new commercially available fentanyl buccal tablet (Fentora) employs an effervescent delivery technology to enhance the rate and extent of absorption through the buccal mucosa. It was found to be both efficacious and safe in the treatment of cancer-related breakthrough pain.[128]

Subcutaneous and Intravenous Routes

Continuous subcutaneous or intravenous administration of opioids can provide pain relief in the shortest amount of time, with a minimum of oversedation. The drugs can be delivered by portable infusion pump and initiated or continued in the home.[129–131] Guidelines for their use are available.[132,133] Patient-controlled analgesia (PCA) systems for subcutaneous or intravenous drug delivery have the advantage of responding to the individual patient's threshold for pain while eliminating delays when nurses must administer supplemental medication.[134] The pumps administer a continuous fixed infusion of the opioid chosen and allow the patient to self-administer boluses of additional medication at frequencies chosen by the physician. By recording the additional amounts of self-administered medication, the devices also facilitate the adjustment of the continuous dose required for pain relief.

Spinal Route

Epidural or intrathecal opioid infusions, which include the option of patient-controlled epidural analgesia, can be helpful for select patients.[135] The infused opioids block pain transmission by binding to receptors in the dorsal horn of the spinal cord.[17] Because the drug is being infused in close proximity to the receptors, only a small amount of opioid is needed and the systemic side effects are reduced. Problems with this delivery system in patients who are not opioid naive[136] are listed in Table 94–3. If tolerance to the opioid develops and higher doses are required for relief, the incidence of side effects will approach that of systemically administered opioids. Addition of local anesthetic or alpha-adrenergic agent (eg, clonidine)[137] or other agents[67–69] to the epidural opioid infusion allows for fairly rapid lowering of the opioid concentration and reestablishment of opioid sensitivity.[136,138]

Adjuvant Analgesics

Adjuvant analgesics are a diverse class of medications, which typically have indications for conditions other than pain. They have analgesic properties and are often used when an opioid regimen is unable to provide sufficient analgesia or is associated with dose-limiting side effects.

Neuropathic Pain

Adjuvant agents are often needed for patients with neuropathic pain. Several classes of medications may be considered for the treatment of neuropathic pain. Anticonvulsants, antidepressants, alpha-2-adrenergic agonists, corticosteroids, topical agents, GABA agonists, and NMDA receptor antagonists have some evidence for the pharmacologic management of neuropathic pain.[139–142] However, the analgesic antidepressants and anticonvulsants are typically preferred for treating neuropathic pain secondary to cancer.[144]

The anticonvulsant gabapentin (Neurontin) has the fewest side effects and is very effective for patients with neuropathic pain from tumor, peripheral neuropathy from tumor or treatment, and postherpetic neuralgia.[139–142] In spite of its name, it has no effect on GABA, but rather binds to the alpha-2-delta subunit of the N-type calcium channels in neurons within the dorsal horn, thus inhibiting calcium influx and diminishing neuronal hyperactivity.[143] To minimize sedation, doses should be low at first (eg, 100 mg three times daily or 300 mg at bedtime) and should be increased as tolerated every 3 to 5 days until analgesia is achieved. The effective dose varies between 900 and 3600 mg daily in divided doses. The pharmacokinetics of gabapentin are unique in that it has a ceiling effect related to a saturable transport mechanism in the gut, such that the effects of this drug may plateau during dose escalation.[144] The most common dose-limiting side effect is sedation. Gabapentin needs to be renally dosed in patients with decreased creatinine clearance. Peripheral edema related to gabapentin may require diuretics. Pregabalin (Lyrica) has the same mechanism of action as gabapentin and has been found to be effective in patients with neuropathic pain.[145,146] Pregabalin can be started at 50 mg BID or TID, with the usual effective dose between 150 and 300 mg BID. Pregabalin is more efficiently absorbed through the gastrointestinal tract and the absorption is proportional to the dose throughout the effective dose range[146] making titration simpler. In addition to the gabapentinoids (gabapentin and pregabalin), there is some evidence for the use of other anticonvulsants (eg, phenytoin, carbamazepine, lamotrigine, topiramate, tiagabine) for neuropathic pain syndromes.[142,144]

Tricyclic antidepressants (eg, amitriptyline, nortriptyline) are effective agents for neuropathic pain.[147] The tricyclics, when used as adjuvant analgesics, are effective faster and at lower doses than when they are used as antidepressants (eg, amitriptyline is effective within 2–3 days at 50–100 mg/day).[147] However, because of their anticholinergic side effects, they should be used with caution in the elderly or in patients who have cardiac conduction abnormalities or bladder outlet obstruction. Selective serotonin and norepinephrine reuptake inhibitors (SSNRIs), for example, venlafaxine and duloxetine, have been shown to be analgesic for a number of neuropathic pain syndromes.[148–152] There is less evidence supporting the use of selective serotonin reuptake inhibitors (SSRIs) for neuropathic pain.

Table 94–3 Adverse Effects from Spinal Infusions: Catheter-Related Effects

Opioid	Anesthetic	Epidural	Subarachnoid
Respiratory depression	Hypotension	Insertion related (eg, hematoma)	Insertion related (eg, hematoma)
Sedation		Fibrosis Skin abscess	Cerebrospinal fluid leak Meningitis

Data from Paice JA, Williams AR: Intraspinal drugs for pain. In McGuire DB, Yarbro CH, Ferrell BR (eds.): Cancer Pain Management, 2nd ed. Boston, Jones & Bartlett, 1995, p 131.

Corticosteroids given epidurally, intravenously, or orally are useful as antineoplastics (eg, in leukemia, lymphoma, and myeloma) and can also provide nonspecific relief for patients with spinal cord compression and plexus infiltrations. Doses of 16 to 100 mg of dexamethasone are needed to reduce vasogenic edema in spinal cord compression,[153] but lesser doses (6–20 mg/day) can be helpful in patients with plexus injuries.[30] Patients must be monitored for the development of oral or esophageal candidiasis and steroid-induced delirium.

Bone Pain

Adjuvants for bone pain include NSAIDs, corticosteroids, bisphosphonates[154,155] and the radiopharmaceuticals, strontium chloride (^{89}Sr)[156] and samarium153-lexidronan.[157] Multiple studies have demonstrated the efficacy of bisphosphonates in reducing skeletal complications and pain from bone metastases.[158–161] Pamidronate and zolendronate are recommended for patients with multiple myeloma and other hematologic malignancies with painful bone lesions.[162,163] However, the long-term use of bisphosphonates is associated with a small but meaningful risk of osteonecrosis of the jaw.[164] The limitations of radiopharmaceuticals include cost and cytopenias.[80] Given the limited evidence available, a recent Cochrane review did not support the use of calcitonin for control of pain from bone metastases.[165]

Management of Opioid-Related Side Effects

Sedation

The addition of 2.5 to 7.5 mg of dextroamphetamine or methylphenidate[166–168] (taken orally twice daily) has been shown to reduce opioid-induced sedation and at times allow for escalation of opioid doses without sedation. These medications also improve cognitive function and symptoms of depression. Methylphenidate may also enhance the analgesic effects of opioids.[168] They should be avoided in patients with anxiety, moderate to severe hypertension, agitation, thyrotoxicosis, tachyarrhythmias, severe angina pectoris, and closed-angle glaucoma. Modafinil (Provigil), a novel psychostimulant with a mechanism of action different than the amphetamine derivatives (approved for narcolepsy and fatigue related to multiple sclerosis), has also been found to be effective for opioid-related sedation.[169]

Constipation

Constipation is the most common opioid-induced side effect.[170] Laxatives should therefore be given routinely, not on an as-needed (PRN) basis,[1,170,171] to patients treated with any of the drugs listed in the box on Relative Potencies of Commonly Used Opioids. Detailed bowel preparation recommendations can be found,[171,172] but no regimen has been studied in a controlled fashion. Commonly used stool softeners and stimulants include docusate sodium, senna, lactulose, and polyethylene glycol. A combination of a stool softener and laxative seems to be a rational choice for patients on chronic opioids, for example, docusate sodium with senna. Promotility agents most directly counter the mechanism of opioid-induced constipation. Continuous subcutaneous or intravenous infusion of metoclopramide (to 60 mg/day)[173] reverses the "opioid bowel syndrome,"[174] enabling patients to continue with oral opioids. Bulk-forming laxatives such as psyllium and methylcellulose should be avoided as they increase stool volume without promoting peristaltic action. For refractory opioid-induced constipation, a trial of oral naloxone, methylnaltrexone, or alvimopan may be initiated.[175,176] These mu-opioid receptor antagonists act locally to reverse the effects of opioids on the gut. There is minimal systemic absorption and subsequently a low risk for precipitating opioid withdrawal or worsening pain with use of these medications.

Nausea

Prochlorperazine (10 mg taken two to three times daily) or metoclopramide (10 mg taken three to four times daily) can prevent the nausea that occurs in most patients during the first days of opioid therapy. Relieving constipation or changing the opioid (eg, from morphine to oxycodone) often eliminates the later development of nausea. Rarely, patients need oral or intravenous ondansetron (8 mg taken two or three times daily).[177]

Insomnia

Antidepressants such as nortriptyline, mirtazapine, and trazodone are preferred sleep medications for patients on opioids. Benzodiazepines (eg, temazepam, 15–30 mg before sleeping) may also be used effectively. These patients should be monitored for daytime somnolence and mental status changes. Barbiturates and chloral hydrate are not good first-line choices, as these drugs can produce excessive daytime sedation.

Respiratory Depression

Naloxone (Narcan), given intravenously, reverses opioid-induced respiratory depression, although repeated doses are often required.[30] Respiratory depression can occur in patients with mild to moderate pain during the initial use of opioids, although it is rare in patients with severe pain or in those chronically receiving opioids. Caution should be exercised before administering naloxone to the patient who is chronically receiving opioids to avoid precipitation of severe pain and withdrawal. In such cases, it is inadvisable to administer the usual 0.4 mg/mL dose; rather, 0.4 mg of naloxone should be diluted with 9 mL of saline and 1 to 2 mL of this dilute mixture given every 2 to 3 minutes until the patient is rousable and breathing at least 10 times/minute. Do not give enough to fully waken the patient or withdrawal is likely to ensue.[1] In a comatose patient, endotracheal tube placement is recommended to prevent aspiration from the salivation and bronchial spasm that will be induced.[1] Naloxone should not be administered to an alert patient.

SPECIFIC CLINICAL PROBLEMS

Oral Complications

Oral complications of chemotherapeutic and marrow transplant regimens can be frequent causes of pain. A thorough dental evaluation and prompt treatment of infections can minimize the discomfort arising from underlying periodontal disease and caries; secondary bacterial, viral, and fungal infections; and mucositis.[178] Preventive regimens include saline, sodium bicarbonate, or chlorhexidine gluconate rinses, acyclovir, antifungals, and ice.[179] Sucralfate,[180] capsaicin,[181] and granulocyte colony-stimulating factor[182] diminish the incidence, duration, and intensity of chemotherapy-induced mucositis. Viscous lidocaine (Xylocaine) or a slurry of sucralfate, dyclonine, or Kaopectate in diphenhydramine provides symptomatic treatment of mucositis pain.[179] For individual lesions, benzocaine in Orabase can be helpful. Milk of magnesia, which dries out the mucosa, is not recommended.[178] The more severe cases, occurring in marrow transplant recipients, usually require infusional opioid therapy, delivered by standard drip or PCA.[183] Pilocarpine (5–7.5 mg three or four times daily 1 hour before meals) reverses xerostomia from neck irradiation[184] and opioids. Sugar-free hard candy is also useful for opioid-induced xerostomia and dysgeusia.

Coagulation Disorders

Patients with inherited or acquired disorders of coagulation may have excessive risks of bleeding if aspirin-containing pain relievers are used.[185,186] If acetaminophen is not effective, these patients may obtain significant relief from the nonacetylated salicylates, such as salsalate (Disalcid) or choline magnesium trisalicylate (Trilisate), which do not prolong the bleeding time.[186–188] Because these agents share aspirin's ability to compete with warfarin for albumin binding,[85] the careful monitoring of patients' coagulation parameters is recommended when these drugs are started or stopped.

Celecoxib, in phase II[189] and two phase III placebo-controlled trials enrolling patients with arthritis,[190] showed no "meaningful" effect on platelet aggregation or thromboxane B_2 levels.

Postherpetic Neuralgia

Postherpetic neuralgia can be a difficult problem for patients with hematologic disorders and has been the subject of several reviews.[139,141,191] Most patients with symptoms for less than 6 months experience spontaneous resolution of pain.[101] For those with long-term symptoms, gabapentin is the agent of choice.[139,140] If the patient cannot tolerate gabapentin or pregabalin, amitriptyline is effective in 60% to 70% of patients.[192,193] Elderly patients, however, often do not tolerate the anticholinergic side effects well. Nortriptyline (Pamelor), a less anticholinergic tricyclic antidepressant, may be useful in these patients. Sustained-release oxycodone or morphine, topical lidocaine gel, or ointment (5% to 10%)[194] and EMLA[195] may also be effective. Topical capsaicin (0.075%), which depletes substance P, has shown efficacy in a multicenter, double-blinded, randomized, placebo-controlled trial.[196] Capsaicin (0.075%) is also used for musculoskeletal discomfort. Transcutaneous electrical nerve stimulation devices provided relief for 1 year in 50% of postherpetic neuralgia patients, and 30% were pain free at 2 years.[48] Patients with severe pain refractory to these therapies may benefit from a combination of intrathecal methylprednisolone and lidocaine. Acute herpes zoster pain may be diminished by a combination of acyclovir and prednisone.[197]

Sickle Cell Anemia

Patients with sickle cell anemia suffer from chronic and episodic pain despite optimal medical therapy.[198] Chronic arthritic pain can be treated with physical therapy and full doses of antiarthritic medication, but some patients require low doses of chronic opioid therapy to maintain independent functioning. Several studies have confirmed the safety and efficacy of long-term opioids in the treatment of pain of nonmalignant origin.[199–202] In some cases, joint replacement may be required.

Sixty percent of sickle cell patients will have an episode of severe pain each year.[198] When a patient with sickle cell anemia experiences a severe episode of pain, it is always important to attempt to define the precise cause of the pain before attributing it to a vasoocclusive crisis. To manage crisis pain, except in patients with renal failure, nonopioid analgesics are used to treat bone pain (see Fig. 94–1). Preliminary studies have shown inhaled nitric oxide to be a potentially effective treatment for acute pain crises.[203]

Treating patients with sickle cell pain is complex and requires understanding that much of the pain in adults with this illness is chronic, with intermittent, recurring painful episodes. In fact, the frequency of painful crises may increase as the patient ages and is subject to progressive damage of bones, joints, and tissues. Uncontrolled pain accounts for more than 90% of hospital admissions in adults with sickle cell disease.[204] Using short-acting analgesics on an as-needed basis exposes the patient to periods of insufficient analgesia, anticipation and anxiety, and may lead to drug-seeking behavior.[199] Thus, intravenous analgesics should be started as a continuous infusion or with patient-controlled pumps.[199,205] Once adequate analgesia is obtained, a long-acting opioid, or a sustained-release opioid, may be initiated with intermittent use of rescue medication. In adult patients with frequent episodes of painful crisis, the use of long-acting opioid medications reduces visits to the emergency department and hospitalizations and shortens the lengths of stay in hospital.[199,206]

Relative Potencies of Commonly Used Opioids

Drug	Epidural	SC/IV (mg)	PO (mg)
Morphine	1	10	30
Codeine		130	200
Oxycodone		N/A	20
Hydromorphone	0.15	1.5	7.5
Methadone*		*	
Oxymorphone		1	10
Levorphanol		2	4
Fentanyl		0.1	N/A
Meperidine (Demerol)**	75		300

*Methadone is approximately half as potent orally as it is intravenously. It is usually not given subcutaneously because of local irritation

**Not recommended for patients with chronic pain

Conversions Between the Transdermal Fentanyl Patch and Morphine

	Morphine (mg/24 hour)	
Fentanyl (µg/hour)	Oral	IM/IV
25	50	17
50	100	33
75	150	50
100	200	67
125	250	83
150	300	100

Data from: Miaskowski C, Cleary J, Burney R, et al. Guideline for the Management of Cancer Pain in Adults and Children, APS Clinical Practice Guidelines Series, No. 3. Glenview, IL, American Pain Society, 2005.

Using Opioids With Short or Long Half-Lives[96]

Short

"Rescue Doses"

Incident pain, eg, with movement

Breakthrough pain: Pain that recurs between regularly scheduled doses

Dosing: 10% of the total 24-hour opioid dose

For example, rescue dose for patient on 300-mg sustained-release morphine twice a day

300 mg + 300 mg = 600 mg; 10% of 600 mg = 60 mg

Elderly patients

Impaired renal function

Impaired hepatic function

Long (eg, Methadone)

Patients with a history of drug abuse

For basal opioid therapy if not using sustained-release or transdermal opioids

Management of Opioid Side Effects

Adverse Effect	Management Considerations
Allergic reaction	True allergic reactions are rare (ie, IgE involvement). Symptoms are usually secondary to mast cell activation and subsequent histamine release. Selection of another opioid class is usually necessary only if the patient has had a true allergic reaction (eg, rash, hives, difficulty breathing) and not simply a sensitivity to histamine release. Opioid Structural Classification: *Phenanthrenes*—codeine, hydrocodone, hydromorphone, levorphanol, morphine, oxycodone, oxymorphone *Phenylpiperidines*—fentanyl, meperidine, sufentanil *Diphenylheptanes*—methadone, propoxyphene
Delirium, confusion, hallucinations	Dose reduction Use different opioid Neuroleptic therapy: Haloperidol 0.5 to 1 mg PO/IV BID-TID *or* Olanzapine 2.5 to 5 mg QD-BID
Constipation	Begin bowel regimen when opioid therapy is initiated. Include a mild stimulant laxative ± stool softener as routine prophylaxis. eg, Senokot 1 to 4 tabs PO QHS-BID ± Colace 100 mg PO BID-TID Consider adding Lactulose or Miralax when necessary. In patients who are NPO, consider metoclopramide 10 mg IV q 6 hours.
Myoclonis	Dose reduction Use different opioid Pharmacologic therapy: Clonazepam 0.25 to 0.5 mg PO TID *or* Baclofen 5 to 10 mg PO TID
Nausea/vomiting	Tolerance may develop Antiemetic therapy: fixed schedule for a few days, then PRN dosing Prochlorperazine 10 mg PO q 6 to 8 hours or 25 mg PR q 12 hours *or* Metoclopramide 10 to 40 mg PO/IV q 6 hours *or* Haloperidol 0.5 to 2 mg q 6 to 12 hours *or* Phenergan 6.25 to 12.5 mg PO/IV q 6 hours *or* Scopolamine patch change every 3 days
Pruritus	Pruritus in the absence of evidence of rash/allergic reaction is a central mu-related phenomenon (not histamine) Pharmacologic Treatment: Nubain 5 mg IV q 6 hours prn Consider switching opioids for refractory pruritus.
Respiratory depression	Hold opioid Supportive measures Consider dilute naloxone: Dilute 0.4 mg (1 mL) of naloxone in 9 mL of saline to yield 0.04 mg per mL. Administer to patient in 1- to 2-mL increments (0.04–0.08 mg) at 2- to 3-minute intervals until response. If no change in respiratory depression after 0.4 mg naloxone has been titrated, consider etiologies other than opioid-induced
Sedation	Tolerance typically develops Hold sedatives/anxiolytics Hold opioid Dose reduction; if persistent Consider CNS stimulants (eg, increase caffeine intake, methylphenidate, or dextroamphetamine 2.5 to 5 mg daily, or QAM and at noon).

Meperidine should be avoided in this population and has been associated with seizures in 1% to 12% of these patients.[207]

Patients With Opioid Addiction

A team approach, including the patient's family and drug counselor, maximizes the coordination of care for these patients. Opioid requirements may be significantly higher, and dosing intervals are shorter in the addict.[208,209] In patients on methadone maintenance, therapeutic dosing must be provided over and above their baseline dose.[208] In all cases, the goal should be to deliver adequate medication to relieve the patient's pain. It has been recommended that the physician always work from a written treatment plan, that one physician prescribe all psychotropic medication, that information about the patient's drug use be obtained from additional sources, and that when the question of addiction first arises, consultation be obtained from an addiction medicine specialist.[209] If opioids are needed, patients should be given limited quantities of long-acting or sustained-release medications on a scheduled basis.

Former opioid abusers themselves and the physicians caring for them hesitate to use opioids for pain relief, as they fear inducing a relapse of the addiction.[210] This concern is based on the observation that once a receptor has been habituated to the opioid, it retains its avidity for opioids, even after a long period of abstinence.[208] In addition to those previously described, suggested techniques to minimize these risks include discussion of the individual's concerns and increased involvement by the patients in their recovery programs.[208]

Graft-Versus-Host Disease

For patients who have undergone bone marrow transplantation, graft-versus-host disease (GVHD) can be a significant problem.[211] Of the usual triad of hepatitis, dermatitis, and gastroenteritis, it is the intestinal involvement that usually causes the greatest physical pain. Abdominal cramping and voluminous diarrhea are the hallmarks of bowel GVHD. Treatment often begins with intravenous opioids given through a patient-controlled analgesia pump. Addition of octreotide continuous infusion at 50 to 100 µg/hour or intermittent dosing at 500 µg every 8 hours may be effective in decreasing the volume of diarrhea and level of abdominal pain.[212]

Peripheral Neuropathy Due To Chemotherapy Agents

Several chemotherapy agents used in the treatment of hematologic malignancies can cause painful peripheral neuropathy. The vinca alkaloids, most notably vincristine, are neurotoxic, but they are not always associated with painful neuropathy. Thalidomide, lenalidomide, bortezomib, cisplatinum, oxaliplatin, and paclitaxel are all commonly used agents that carry a significant risk of causing painful peripheral neuropathy. The most common mechanism of neuropathy is damage to the axons starting with the most distal branches. This is the result of chemotherapy's ability to damage DNA replication, leading to apoptosis.[213]

Studies have evaluated numerous agents for prevention of painful peripheral neuropathy, although there have not been any magic bullets. Most of the research has focused on taxane and platinum-based chemotherapy agents. Amifostine and leukemia-inhibitory factor do not prevent neurotoxicity induced by these agents.[213] Magnesium and calcium infusions have been shown to prevent neurotoxic symptoms associated with oxaliplatin without affecting its antitumor activity.[214] Glutathione at doses of 1500 mg/m^2 administered prior to each dose of oxaliplatin for 12 cycles prevented grade 2 to 4 toxicities compared to placebo with no effect on response rate.[215] Vitamin E has been shown to prevent neurotoxicity associated with cisplatin in small open-label evaluations.[216,217] Glutamine 10 g three times daily for 4 days has had positive results as a neuroprotective agent in paclitaxel-treated patients.[218] Acetyl-l-carnitine 1 g three times daily has been reviewed in the treatment of cisplatin- and paclitaxel-induced peripheral neuropathy, although there have been no randomized studies.[219,220]

Treatment of chemotherapy-induced painful peripheral neuropathy includes the usual agents used for patients with neuropathic pain from any etiology (ie, anticonvulsants, tricyclic antidepressants, and occasionally tramadol or opioids). In addition to treating these painful symptoms of neuropathy, the doses of the chemotherapy often require reduction or even discontinuation of therapy.[221]

Problems of the Elderly

Pain management in the elderly is complicated by difficulties in pain assessment and by the altered pharmacokinetics of opioids and of psychotropic adjuvant medications.[222] Elderly patients may underreport pain.[223] Physicians may ascribe observed limitations in social contacts and physical activities to age-related changes when they are pain-induced limitations.[224] Family members can be crucial to the success in managing an elderly patient's pain.

Elderly patients are particularly susceptible to the side effects of NSAIDs and opioids, and patients taking them should be monitored closely.[224] In elderly patients (70 to 89 years old), the volume of distribution for opioids is generally smaller, the drugs have longer plasma half-lives, and renal and hepatic clearances are decreased, all of which can prolong the duration of effect.[224] The effective doses for these patients are one-half to one-fourth of those needed in younger patients.[222,224] Drugs with short half-lives (eg, morphine, oxycodone, hydromorphone) should be used, and initial doses should be low.[224] Patients should be monitored carefully for the development of sedation or confusion, especially if they are receiving antihistaminic agents (eg, famotidine, diphenhydramine), drugs with anticholinergic activity, or hypnotics.

The acute urinary retention due to opioids (especially in patients with prostatic hypertrophy) and the hypotension and tachycardia caused by tricyclic compounds can occur more frequently and be more clinically severe in this population. The starting dose of nortriptyline should be low (usually 10 mg at bedtime), and the dose should be slowly increased as tolerated. Treatment of opioid-related urinary retention may include generic (Proscar) (5 mg daily) in patients with benign prostatic hypertrophy and bethanechol (10–50 mg three times daily) to help increase bladder smooth-muscle tone.

ANTIEMETIC THERAPY

A number of effective antiemetic therapies are used to prevent the nausea and vomiting induced in patients by treatment of their hematologic disorders with chemotherapy or radiation therapy. These antiemetic therapies markedly improve patients' quality of life. The vast majority of patients can expect complete control of vomiting,[225] and most patients also are free of nausea.

PATHOPHYSIOLOGY OF NAUSEA AND VOMITING

Nausea is the subjective sensation that precedes vomiting. It is caused by stimulation of one or more of four sites—the gastrointestinal tract, the vestibular system, the chemoreceptor trigger zone in the area postrema of the floor of the fourth ventricle, or higher centers in the central nervous system (Fig. 94–2). The gastrointestinal tract can activate the vomiting center by stimulation of mechanoreceptors or chemoreceptors on glossopharyngeal or vagal afferents (cranial nerves IX and X) or by release of serotonin from gut enterochromaffin cells, which in turn stimulates serotonin (5HT3) receptors on vagal afferents. The vestibular system activates the vomiting center when stimulated by motion or disease (eg, labyrinthitis) or when sensitized by medication (eg, opioids). Histamine (H1) and acetylcholine M1 receptors are present on vestibular afferents. Endogenous or exoge-

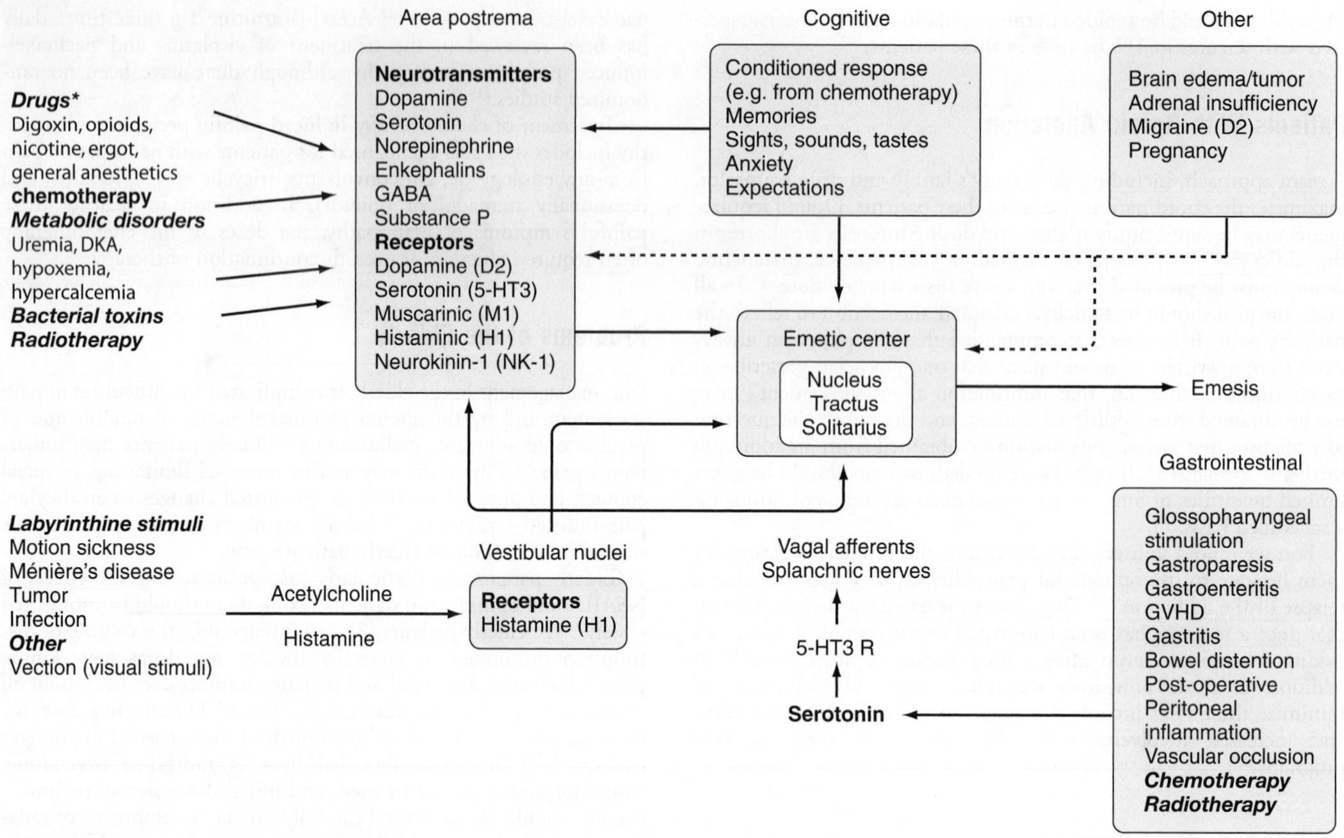

Figure 94–2 Pathophysiology of nausea and vomiting.

nous blood-borne toxins may activate chemoreceptors in the area postrema of the floor of the fourth ventricle via dopamine type 2 receptors. Finally, higher central nervous system centers may activate or inhibit the vomiting center. In addition, there may be direct activation of H1 receptors in the meninges, secondary to increased intracranial pressure.[226]

The means by which chemotherapy agents induce vomiting are still incompletely understood but the most likely mechanism is believed to include stimulation of the chemoreceptor trigger zone. Other causes of nausea and vomiting in the hematologic patient include stimulation of the cerebral cortex, gastritis and GERD, delayed gastric emptying, radiation enteritis, constipation, esophageal candidiasis, inner ear processes, hypoadrenalism, hypercalcemia, changes in taste and smell, and anticipatory nausea.[226,227]

Although the sites of emetic action of the chemotherapeutic agents have not been identified, blocking agents directed against type 3 serotonin receptors (5-HT$_3$ receptors), dopamine (D$_2$) receptors, and neurokinin (NK$_1$) receptors have been effective in inhibiting chemotherapy-induced nausea and vomiting (CINV).[227] Higher centers in the brain, such as the cortex, are also believed to be involved in producing anticipatory nausea and vomiting. Cognitive therapy, as well as antianxiety and amnesic agents, may provide effective antiemesis.

EVALUATION

Risk factors for developing CINV include age less than 60 years, female gender, history of motion sickness, and hyperemesis gravidarum.[228] Patients who have a history of alcohol intake of more than five alcoholic drinks per day (>100 g of alcohol) tend to have less nausea and vomiting. This has been studied carefully in patients receiving high-dose cisplatin therapy[227,229] but has been anecdotally observed in patients receiving other agents.

Anticipatory

Anticipatory nausea and vomiting (ANV) is believed to be a classic conditioned response.[230] Chemotherapy administration (the unconditioned stimulus) results in nausea and vomiting (the unconditioned response). Clinic sights, smells, and sounds are the conditioned stimuli. After frequent pairings of chemotherapy administration and the clinic sights, smells, and sounds, the responses (nausea and vomiting) can be triggered in the absence of any chemotherapy by the clinic sights, smells, or sounds or simply by seeing clinic personnel, even at a location distant from the site of treatment.

Patients who are at risk for developing ANV are those who have already experienced posttreatment nausea and vomiting. The risk of developing ANV increases with the increasing frequency, severity, and duration of the symptoms.[230] Other possible predisposing factors include susceptibility to motion sickness,[231,232] awareness of tastes or odors during infusions, younger age, lengthier infusions, greater autonomic sensitivity, and general anxiety or emotional distress.[230]

Acute and Delayed Chemotherapy-Induced Nausea and Vomiting

Acute CINV is defined as nausea or vomiting, or both, occurring within 24 hours of administration of the agent. The emetogenic potential of the drugs[233,234] is shown in the box on the Emetic Risks of Chemotherapy. Although most drugs produce emesis 1 to 2 hours after they are given (in patients who have never before received chemotherapy), the onset of emesis from high-dose intravenous cyclophosphamide is delayed until 9 to 18 hours after treatment,[235] and nausea and vomiting from high total doses of cisplatin can occur 24 to 72 hours later.[236]

Combination Antiemetic Regimens

Highly Emetogenic
Prophylactic

5HT3 RA PO/IV 30 minutes before chemotherapy each day for the duration of chemotherapy +
Dexamethasone, 12 to 20 mg PO/IV 30 minutes before chemotherapy each day for the duration of chemotherapy +
Aprepitant, 125 mg PO 1 hour before chemotherapy (use 12-mg dose of dexamethasone)

To prevent or manage delayed nausea and vomiting after chemotherapy

For 2 to 5 days after chemotherapy:
Dexamethasone, 8 mg PO each day
Aprepitant, 80 mg PO each morning on days 2 and 3 (see above)

Moderately Emetogenic
Prophylactic

5HT3 RA PO/IV 30 minutes before chemotherapy ±
Dexamethasone 8 to 12 mg PO/IV 30 minutes before chemotherapy

To prevent or manage delayed nausea and vomiting

Dexamethasone 8 mg PO once daily for days 2 and 3

Low Emetogenic Potential
Dexamethasone 8 mg PO/IV 30 minutes before chemotherapy as needed *or*
Metoclopramide 10 to 20 mg PO/IV 30 minutes before chemotherapy as needed *or*
Compazine10 mg PO/IV 30 minutes before chemotherapy as needed

(From: Kris MG, Hesketh PJ, Sommerfield MR, et al: American Society of Clinical Oncology guideline for antiemetics in oncology: Update 2006. J Clin Oncol 24:2932, 2006.)

Emetic Risks of Chemotherapy

High (>90%)
Carmustine (>250 mg/m²)
Cisplatin
Cyclophosphamide (>1500 mg/m²)
Dacarbazine (>500 mg/m²)
Dactinomycin
Mechlorethamine
Streptozocin
Moderate (30%–90%)
Carboplatin
Cyclophosphamide (<1500 mg/m²)
Cytarabine (>1 g/m²)
Doxorubicin
Epirubicin
Idarubicin
Irinotecan
Ifosfamide
Oxaliplatin

Low (10%–30%)
Aldesleukin (IL-2)
Asparaginase
Bortezomib
Cetuximab
Cytarabine (<1 g/m²)
Docetaxel
Etoposide
Fluorouracil
Gemcitabine
Methotrexate
Mitomycin
Mitoxantrone
Paclitaxel
Pemetrexed
Temozolomide
Topotecan
Thiotepa
Trastuzumab

Minimal (<10%)
Bleomycin
Bevacizumab busulfan
Capecitabine
Fludarabine
Rituximab
Vincristine
Vinblastine
Vinorelbine

THERAPY

Anticipatory Nausea and Vomiting

The best way to prevent ANV is to give aggressive antiemetic therapy and to treat anxiety with the appropriate agents. However, in patients for whom this approach has not been successful and in whom ANV develops, a variety of behavioral techniques have been helpful. These include hypnosis,[237] progressive muscle relaxation with guided imagery,[238] systemic desensitization,[239] and distraction.[240] Results may be optimized if a therapist trained in these techniques works with the patient, but patients can use progressive muscle relaxation with guided imagery on their own.[238]

Acute and Delayed Chemotherapy-Induced Nausea and Vomiting

Most studies of the potent antiemetic agents have been conducted in patients receiving therapy with cisplatin, a drug of high emetic potential. Although cisplatin is not generally used to treat patients with hematologic malignancies, the data are included in the following discussion, as the findings can probably be extrapolated to other drugs of equivalent or less emetogenic potential. When available, data regarding efficacy in patients receiving radiation therapy or emetogenic drugs commonly used to treat hematologic disorders are reviewed. The choice of antiemetic agents depends on the emetogenic potential of the chemotherapy or radiation therapy regimen, the side-effect profiles of the antiemetic agents, and patient preferences and characteristics.

The emetogenic potentials of commonly used chemotherapeutic agents are outlined in the box on the Emetic Risks of Chemotherapy. Risks of specific side effects help to guide antiemetic choice. Younger patients have a higher incidence of CINV and of metoclopramide-related acute dystonic reactions; trismus or torticollis was seen in only 2% of patients older than 30 years of age but in 27% of younger patients.[241] Even if they are receiving only moderately emetogenic therapy, they should be given an antiemetic regimen; for high-emetogenic drugs.[242] Younger patients find cannabinoids (such as Marinol) more effective than do older patients because they can better tolerate the side effects associated with the therapeutic doses of these agents.[243] Elderly patients also have high risks of extrapyramidal side effects and are more susceptible to anticholinergic and sedating side effects.[242] 5-HT_3 receptor antagonists are therefore preferred to regimens containing metoclopramide and diphenhydramine.

5-HT_3-Receptor Antagonists: Ondansetron, Granisetron, and Palonosetron

Ondansetron, granisetron, and palonosetron are the best studied of the 5-HT_3-receptor antagonists (5HT RA). This class also includes the drugs dolasetron and tropisetron. Several studies of patients receiving regimens that included cyclophosphamide, methotrexate, or doxorubicin showed significant efficacy and the superiority of ondansetron over placebo.[244–246] Ondansetron also demonstrates efficacy in patients with emesis (induced by non–cisplatin-containing chemotherapy) that has been refractory to standard antiemetics, with complete control achieved in 50% of these patients.[247,248] When dexamethasone is added, the rate of control is as high as 91%.[249]

Ondansetron effectively prevents nausea and vomiting in patients treated with highly emetogenic agents for acute leukemia,[250,251] for multiple myeloma (ie, high-dose melphalan),[252] or who are being prepared for bone marrow transplantation with cyclophosphamide and total-body irradiation.[253,254] In the transplantation recipients, 83% of patient-days were without any vomiting or retching, and in another 10%, there were no more than two emetic episodes. Ondansetron is also effective in preventing emesis induced by single- or multiple-fraction radiation therapy.[255,256] Ondansetron is as effective as metoclopramide in preventing nausea induced by cisplatin[257–259] or by cyclophosphamide alone or with doxorubicin chemotherapy.[260–262]

Oral granisetron has shown equivalence to ondansetron in studies of patients receiving cisplatin- or carboplatin-based regimens.[225,263,264] In patients receiving moderately emetogenic therapy, oral granisetron with dexamethasone was as effective as intravenous ondansetron and dexamethasone.[265,266] Oral or intravenous granisetron and dexamethasone were effective in a bone marrow transplantation program in which patients were treated with Cytoxan and total body irradiation,[267] and these agents, along with oral prochlorperazine, were also effective in patients undergoing peripheral blood stem cell transplantation for which patients received Cytoxan, VP-16 or thiotepa, and cisplatin.[268]

Palonosetron is a second-generation 5-HT_3 receptor antagonist with higher potency, stronger receptor-binding activity, and longer half-life than the other drugs in this class. Palonosetron 0.25 mg intravenous has been studied in moderately and highly emetogenic chemotherapy. Current guidelines do not designate palonosetron as superior although several subgroup analyses of the registrational noninferiority trials have been reported in which palonosetron was superior. Current studies seek to find palonosetron's place in therapy. Ondansetron and the other 5-HT_3 receptor antagonists have far fewer side effects than high-dose metoclopramide. Reports of extrapyramidal reactions are rare,[269] and sedation, dystonic reactions, akathisia (eg, severe restlessness, "ants in pants" feeling), and tardive dyskinesias do not occur. Patients can develop constipation, mild headache, and elevated levels of transaminases.[225]

The therapy of choice for moderately or highly emetogenic chemotherapy is therefore a 5-HT_3 receptor antagonist plus a corticosteroid (usually dexamethasone).[225]

Corticosteroids

The mechanism of the antiemetic action of corticosteroids remains undefined. Corticosteroids are effective when used alone to prevent emesis induced by agents of moderate or low emetogenic potential.[270–272] They are also a useful component of antiemetic therapy regimens that include ondansetron, granisetron, or metoclopramide and add efficacy in randomized controlled trials.* Dexamethasone and methylprednisolone are the best-studied agents, but no trials have demonstrated the superiority of one corticosteroid over another.

Metoclopramide

Metoclopramide is a substituted benzamide that promotes gastric motility and reduces the emetic activity of chemotherapy agents by blocking dopamine receptors (at low to moderate doses) and 5-HT_3 receptors (at high doses) in the chemoreceptor trigger zone. Owing to a more favorable side-effect profile, 5HT_3 antagonists have replaced high-dose metoclopramide. At lower doses, metoclopramide is useful in treating mild to moderate and delayed nausea and vomiting. Delivery of the drug on a schedule that maintains adequate levels during expected emesis appears to be important.[225]

The side effects, which may be caused by the interaction of metoclopramide with dopamine receptors, can be quite troublesome. They include akathisia, dystonic reactions (age related), sedation, and diarrhea. Benzodiazepines such as lorazepam can prevent or reverse the akathisia, and diphenhydramine or benztropine can prevent or reverse the dystonias.[274] However, these agents induce additional side effects, including dry mouth and sedation. Short-term, high-dose metoclopramide or the long-term use of the drug has been associated with persistent and disabling movement disorders, especially tardive dyskinesias.[275,276] Metoclopramide finds its role in low-dose (10–20 mg taken two to four times daily) prevention and management of mild to moderate nausea and vomiting.

NK-1 Inhibitors

Substance P can cause emesis,[277] and it appears to play a role in chemotherapy-related nausea and vomiting. Its effects are mediated through NK-1 receptors.[278] Agents that cross the blood–brain barrier and inhibit NK-1 activity (eg, aprepitant) are more effective than granisetron and dexamethasone alone in moderating acute chemotherapy-related nausea and vomiting, and they are particularly effective in decreasing delayed nausea and vomiting occurring after cisplatin chemotherapy.[279] The need for continued dexamethasone with the NK-1 inhibitor has not yet been determined, and comparisons with the metoclopramide and dexamethasone regimen for delayed nausea and vomiting have not yet been performed. Aprepitant is an inhibitor of CYP3A4, and therefore may cause elevation of chemotherapy agents primarily metabolized by this route; however these elevations are not considered clinically significant and there are no recommend dose adjustments. Aprepitant can cause significant decreases in the prolongation of the international normalized ratio induced by warfarin.

*References 225, 263, 264, 266, 268, and 273.

Combination Antiemetic Therapy

For drugs with low or moderately low emetogenic potential, no antiemetic drug, or dexamethasone alone may be sufficient. For drugs with higher emetogenic potential, standard antiemetic treatment usually includes combinations of several antiemetic agents along with agents designed to treat anxiety, cause amnesia, or prevent known side effects. These combinations frequently include a 5-HT_3 receptor antagonist such as ondansetron, a corticosteroid such as dexamethasone, and optional lorazepam for anxiety-related symptoms. For drugs with high emetogenic potential, it is important to give antiemetic therapy for an adequate period before administering chemotherapy agents and to continue to prevent emesis for approximately 24 to 72 hours after the drugs have been given. For highly emetogenic combination chemotherapy with significant incidences of delayed nausea and vomiting, such as cisplatin-containing regimens, aprepitant (NK-1 inhibitor) should be added to the antiemetic combination.[280] Transdermal scopolamine adds efficacy when added to a standard regimen of metoclopramide and dexamethasone.[281]

Benzodiazepines

The benzodiazepine lorazepam has only mild antiemetic activity, when used as a single agent.[274] It is used frequently in the treatment and prevention of nausea and vomiting, in particular when there is anxiety associated with the nausea and vomiting. It markedly decreases the akathisia and anxiety associated with metoclopramide therapy and induces a dose-related memory loss and marked sedation.[274,282,283]

Other Drugs

Other agents that are more active than placebo include the butyrophenones haloperidol and droperidol,[284] the phenothiazine prochlorperazine,[285] and the cannabinoids dronabinol (THC) and nabilone.[225,286,287] These agents are less effective drugs than the agents previously mentioned, and all cause sedation. The butyrophenones produce dystonic reactions, akathisia, and occasionally hypotension. The cannabinoids cause ataxia, dry mouth, orthostatic hypotension and dizziness, euphoria or dysphoria, and a feeling of being "high."[288] Scopolamine, a centrally acting anticholinergic, can be effective for patients with a vertiginous component to their nausea. (see box on Combination Antiemetic Regimens).

Patient preferences regarding degree of alertness can help the health care provider choose an antiemetic regimen, as can the level of anxiety the provider observes in the patient. Some patients do very well with regimens that include no antianxiety agents; others may benefit from the inclusion of those agents, despite the somnolence that accompanies their use.

SUGGESTED READINGS

Bajwa ZH, Warfield CA: Nonpharmacologic therapy of cancer pain. UpToDate online 15.1, 2006.

Bajwa ZH, Warfield CA: Interventional approaches to the management of cancer pain. UpToDate online 15.1, 2006.

Breivik H: Local anaesthetic blocks and epidurals. In McMahon SB, Koltzenberg M (eds.): Wall and Melzack's Textbook of Pain, 5th ed. Philadelphia, Elsevier/Churchill Livingstone, 2006, p 507.

Campbell JN, Meyer RA: Mechanisms of neuropathic pain. Neuron 52:77, 2006.

Chang VT, Janjan N, Jain S: Update in cancer pain syndromes. J Palliat Med 9:1414, 2006.

Cherny NI: The assessment of cancer pain. In McMahon SB, Koltzenberg M (eds.): Wall and Melzack's Textbook of Pain, 5th ed. Philadelphia, Elsevier/Churchill Livingstone, 2006, p 1099.

Fields HL, Basbaum AI, Heinricher MM: Central nervous system mechanisms of pain modulation. In McMahon SB, Koltzenberg M (eds.): Wall and Melzack's Textbook of Pain, 5th ed. Philadelphia, Elsevier/Churchill Livingstone, 2006, p 125.

Flatters SJ, Xiao WH, Bennett GJ: Acetyl-L-carnitine prevents and reduces paclitaxel-induced painful peripheral neuropathy. Neurosci 397:219, 2006.

Kris MG, Hesketh PJ, Sommerfield MR, et al: American Society of Clinical Oncology guideline for antiemetics in oncology: Update 2006. J Clin Oncol 24:2932, 2006.

Martinez-Zapata MJ, Roque M, Alonso-Coello P, Catala E: Calcitonin for metastatic bone pain. Cochrane Database Syst Rev 1, 2007.

McDonald A, Portenoy RK: How to use antidepressants and anticonvulsants as adjuvant analgesics in the treatment of neuropathic cancer pain. J Support Oncol 4:43, 2006.

McMahon SB, Koltzenberg M (eds.): Wall and Melzack's Textbook of Pain, 5th ed. Philadelphia, Elsevier/Churchill Livingstone, 2006.

McMahon SB, Bennett DLH, Bevan S: Inflammatory mediators and modulators of pain. In McMahon SB, Koltzenberg M (eds.): Wall and Melzack's Textbook of Pain, 5th ed. Philadelphia, Elsevier/Churchill Livingstone, 2006, p. 49.

Mystakidou K, Katsouda E, Parpa E, Vlahos L, Tsiatas ML. Oral transmucosal Fentanyl citrate: Overview of pharmacological and clinical characteristics. Drug Deliv 13:269, 2006.

Pappagallo M et al: Difficult pain syndromes. In Berger A, Portenoy RK, Weissman DE. (eds.): Principles and Practice of Palliative Care, 3rd ed. 2006.

Pfugmacher R, Kandziora F, Schroeder RJ, Melcher I, Haas NP, Klostermann CK: Percutaneous balloon kyphoplasty in the treatment of pathological vertebral body fracture and deformity in multiple myeloma: A one-year follow-up. Acta Radiol 47:369, 2006.

Portenoy RK, Taylor D, Messina J, Tremmel L: A randomized, placebo-controlled study of fentanyl buccal tablet for breakthrough pain in opioid-treated patients with cancer. Clin J Pain 22:805, 2006.

Prommer E: Oxymorphone: A review. Support Care Cancer 14:109, 2006.

Prommer E: Levorphanol: The forgotten opioid. Support Care Cancer 15:259, 2006.

Rodriguez P: Comparison of gene expression profiles in neuropathic and inflammatory pain. J Physiol Pharmacol 57:401, 2006.

Stillman M, Cata JP: Management of chemotherapy-induced peripheral neuropathy. Curr Pain Headache Rep 10:279, 2006.

Turk DC, Flor H: The cognitive-behavioural approach to pain management. In McMahon SB, Koltzenberg M (eds.): Wall and Melzack's Textbook of Pain, 5th ed. Philadelphia, Elsevier/Churchill Livingstone, 2006, p 339.

Yeh HS, Berenson JR: Myeloma bone disease and treatment options. Eur J Cancer 42:1554, 2006.

Zeppetella G, Ribeiro MD: Opioids for the management of breakthrough pain in cancer patients. Cochrane Database Syst Rev 25(1):CD004311, 2006.

REFERENCES

For complete list of references log onto www.expertconsult.com

CHAPTER 95

PALLIATIVE CARE

Janet L. Abrahm and Joanne Wolfe

Palliative care in children and adults is centered on the wishes and goals of patients and their families. Palliative care practitioners require expertise in communication, in treatment of physical symptoms, and in relieving sources of social, psychological, and spiritual distress. Each section of this chapter will first review core elements of palliative care for children and then for adults.

PEDIATRIC PALLIATIVE CARE

> *I just wish that I had armfuls of time.*
>
> —*(4-year-old child)*[1]

Pediatric palliative care is an emerging frontier in the comprehensive care of children. The recent Institute of Medicine Report *When Children Die: Improving Palliative and End-of-Life Care for Children and Their Families*[2] (Table 95–1) highlights its critical importance. In the last few years, a powerful statement by the American Academy of Pediatrics,[3] the findings of a comprehensive British report on children with life-threatening and terminal conditions,[4] and two earlier Institute of Medicine studies[5,6]—as well as other documentation[7–10]—set the stage for this seminal report. A comprehensive definition is:

> *Palliative care for children and young people with life-limiting conditions is an active and total approach to care, embracing physical, emotional, social, and spiritual elements. It focuses on enhancement of quality of life for the child and support for the family and includes the management of distressing symptoms, provision for respite, and care through death and bereavement.*[4]

As this field develops, there is much debate about the terms *life-limiting* and *life-threatening*. Life-threatening is a broader concept, in that it includes illnesses for which cure is possible, although the threat of a fatal outcome exists (eg, childhood malignancies). Of course, an illness may begin as life-threatening and convert into a life-limiting condition, as when a child relapses and curative options no longer exist. Life-limiting conditions are those for which there is no reasonable chance of cure from the outset; even if children survive for years and decades, they will not live out a normal life expectancy.

In addition to end-of-life care for the child (and bereavement follow-up for the family), pediatric palliative care includes care throughout the trajectory of the child's illness, including respite as an important component. This is one major difference from traditional adult cancer-based end-of-life care. Other differences from adult palliative care include:[4,11]

Smaller numbers of dying children than adults mean that there is less professional expertise and underrepresentation of children in palliative care protocols.

The heterogeneity of illnesses, many rare, requires the involvement of many disciplines and specialists.

Many children have genetic diseases so there may be more than one affected child in a family.

The time course of some illnesses is extremely variable. Pediatric palliative care may extend over years, even decades.

A broad developmental spectrum is represented, including changes in the individual child through time.

The underlying principles and ethics of palliative care are universal across the life span. However, as in all specialties, children bring with them unique issues and dilemmas.

A child or adolescent diagnosed with a life-threatening or life-limiting illness throws an assumed sequence out of order. A time of role reversal is expected, when children will care for dying parents. When parents instead find themselves watching their child face death, a sense of tragic absurdity prevails. Not only is time shortened, but its order is shattered. A child or adolescent with a life-threatening illness represents a premature separation to the family. Even before the child has become a differentiated individual through a natural developmental sequence, that child is wrenched away. There is little preparation for separation by death when a psychological separation has not yet been effected. The adolescent who is beginning to negotiate an independent existence is often the hardest to face when that "moving forward" is irreversibly halted, or at least disrupted. A child has not even had the time to begin to form life goals.[12]

The necessity for palliative care—the concept and the clinical approach—may emerge at different points in the illness trajectory, depending on the prognosis for the child, the decisions that must be made in choosing treatment options, and always, the management of pain and suffering in the provision of optimal quality of life. One of the foremost goals is to initiate palliative care for children earlier in the illness trajectory—in a proactive manner—so that effective care planning can be implemented. Care of the family, with a particular focus on the young siblings, is a priority.

COMMUNICATION

Good communication can dispel fears of abandonment. Breaking bad news and discussing prognosis with patients with advanced disease are occasions when physicians can demonstrate their commitment to an ongoing partnership with patients and families. Conversations must demonstrate respect for cultural differences[13–15] and the conviction that growth can occur even at the end of life.[16] If done well, the groundwork will be laid for further discussions of patient hopes and fears, goals, values, and spiritual concerns that form the basis of decisions about resuscitation and artificial life support.[17]

Communication with a child . . .

> *When I first heard my diagnosis, one question kept going around and around in my head: "How long do I have, Doc?"*
>
> —*(12-year-old child)*[1]

Children with serious hematologic disorders have usually lived with the illness over a prolonged period of months or years. Their knowledge, understanding, and awareness of their precarious life situation are often profound, at physical, cognitive, and emotional levels.

Table 95–1 Summary of the Institute of Medicine Report: When Children Die: Improving Palliative and End-of-Life Care for Children and Their Families

Improve Organization and Delivery of Care
Emphasis is placed on the development of care guidelines and protocols in all pediatric settings, the development of regional information programs and resources in rural areas, and policies and procedures for involving children in decision making.
Reform Financing of Palliative Services and Hospice Care
Vast changes in public and private health coverage: add hospice, change eligibility rules, provide outlier payments, extend coverage for counseling family members and for bereavement follow-up.
Better Prepare Health Professionals
Create educational experiences and curricula that will provide basic and advanced competence in palliative, end-of-life, and bereavement care.
Strengthen Research Base for Effective Care
Emphases include appropriate quality-of-life measures, effective symptom management, impact of perinatal death on parents and siblings, impact of sudden death on family and professional caregivers, efficacy of bereavement interventions, models for provision of care, financing alternatives, effective strategies for educating professionals.

From Institute of Medicine: When Children Die: Improving Palliative and End-of-Life Care for Children and their Families. Washington, DC, National Academy Press, 2003.

Table 95–2 Breaking Bad News

1. Make yourself, the patient, and the family comfortable.
2. Find out what they know.
3. Indicate that you are planning to tell them something that is unpleasant and may be disturbing.
4. Find out whether they want to be told, or whether they want someone else to be told.
5. Find out how much they want to know (ie, the big picture versus all the details).
6. Tell them in words they can understand, allowing time for questions along the way.
7. Respond to their feelings.
8. Let them know that this is only the first of many discussions with you.
9. Ask them to summarize what they heard you say; ask if they have further questions.
10. Arrange your next meeting with them.

Data from Abrahm JL: Update in palliative medicine and end-of-life care. Annu Rev Med 54:53, 2003.

The doctors think my bone marrow is fine for now—and for now is for now.

—(8-year-old child)[12]

The protective stance of the past stated that disclosure to the child of his or her prognosis (and even, in some instances, the diagnosis) would cause increased anxiety and fear. Since the 1980s, however, a shift toward open communication has been evident.[18] To shield the child from the truth may only heighten anxiety and cause the child to feel isolated, lonely, and unsure of whom to trust.

In communication with the life-threatened child at any juncture in the illness, "The truth is not a principle nor a duty nor a rule. The truth is an atmosphere of exchange, of listening, and of respect for the child and his needs. The truth is a state."[19] The precedent for a climate that enables such honest interchange is created from the time of diagnosis. The individual child's competence and vulnerability serve as the context for decisions regarding disclosure at any point in the illness trajectory. Considerations about what, or how much to tell, include the child's age, cognitive and emotional maturity, family structure and functioning, cultural background, and history of loss.[1] These same factors determine at the end-of-life, with extreme sensitivity to how the parents have chosen to inform the child throughout the illness experience, how the child has understood and processed information up to this time, and what the child is now asking—implicitly and explicitly—about his or her situation.

BREAKING BAD NEWS

Table 95–2 contains an outline of the suggested steps to take when breaking bad news.[20–22] For adult patients with advanced disease, the goal is to establish or strengthen trust and reassure them that the physician is committed to caring for them. To do this well, physicians need to believe that they have not failed the dying patient, medicine has.

PROGNOSIS AND DECISION MAKING

Surveys of bereaved parents indicate that physician communication about prognosis is not optimal.[23] At the same time, emerging data suggest that bereaved parents consider high-quality communication as the top value when reflecting on physician quality of care.[24] Parents value clear information that is communicated sensitively, and inclusive of the child, when developmentally appropriate. When it comes to discussing prognosis, a majority of parents want as much information as possible.[25] Furthermore, although many parents find prognostic information about their child upsetting, they still want prognosis to be discussed. The data suggest, however, that parents are overly optimistic about the child's chances of cure in comparison to physicians, and this is especially true when the prognosis is uncertain.[26] Being aware of these trends may help physicians to discuss prognosis with greater clarity.

One side of my head says: "Think optimistic." The other side says: "What if this treatment doesn't work?"

—(11-year-old-child)[1]

The child is often aware of the diminishing curative or life-prolonging options that he or she faces. It is at this time that the child may ask anxiously: "What if this medicine doesn't work? What will you give me next?" The child experiences a profound sense of loss of control. It is at this time that families are confronted by a series of decisions regarding the nature and intensity of medical interventions they wish to pursue. This process can be excruciating: they do not want their child to suffer more, yet they often cannot tolerate the thought of "leaving any stone unturned" in the quest for a cure or prolonged time, however minuscule the chance. The physician and team's role shifts from leadership in recommending a curative treatment plan to the clarification of experimental and palliative options and consequences. In most instances, the parents make the decision; however, to varying degrees, the child may be involved in such discussions.[1,12,27] Hinds and colleagues have demonstrated that when asked in a sensitive manner, children as young as 10 years of age are able and willing to talk about their experiences and end-of-life decisions.[27]

During the last decade, there has been increased recognition of the child's participation in making treatment decisions. Crucial to this process is an assessment of the child or adolescent's ability to appreciate the nature and consequences of a specific medical decision. This becomes particularly complex when the wishes of the child differ from those of the parents. Because actual assessment tools are only in the early stages of development[28,29] professionals must rely exclusively on their clinical judgment to assess children's understanding of the contingencies they are facing. This is often a juncture when input from members of the interdisciplinary team can be crucial: children often express their understanding, awareness, and thoughts about treatment options and living or dying to individuals other than their parents or primary physician.

The following example illustrates the remarkable capacity of a young child to address the transition to palliative care.

A 7-year-old girl told her parents that she was too tired to fight anymore, and that she wanted to give up. She added: "If I have to continue suffering, I would rather be in heaven." These statements were major determinants in the parents' choosing a palliative care plan without any further attempts at life-prolonging treatment. She went home on hospice care and died peacefully several weeks later.[1]

ADULT PATIENTS

Adult patients and families want to be prepared. The vast majority (80%–98%) want to be able to name someone to make decisions, know what to expect about their physical condition, have financial affairs in order, know that the doctor is comfortable talking about death and dying, feel that the family are prepared for their death, have funeral arrangements in place, and have treatment preferences in writing.[30] For this to happen, physicians must tell patients how long they are likely to have left to live. Because prognoses are shrouded in uncertainty, however, the natural tendency is to avoid the discussion altogether.[31]

Physicians may assume that patients who want to know their prognosis (or their caregivers) will raise the subject with them. There are no data, however, on how often patients with advanced refractory disease ask about their prognosis. Sometimes patients fail to report unrelieved pain[32] or their preferences about resuscitation.[33]

There are significant benefits from having a discussion of prognosis with a relatively asymptomatic patient with a limited time left to live and his or her caregivers. Patient preferences for resuscitation are affected by the likely outcome of treatment, especially bad functional or cognitive outcomes,[34] and by his or her understanding of their prognosis. Caregivers, similarly, are usually unaware that the patient is incurable or that he or she would benefit from hospice care until they hear it directly from their physician.[35] For them to choose, therefore, physicians must provide the most accurate data they can. It is equally important that patients with very poor prognoses understand how limited they really are. Patients who thought they had a greater than 10% chance of surviving 6 months, for example, usually wanted to be resuscitated. Patients who thought they had a less than 10% chance of surviving 6 months overwhelmingly chose comfort care and did not want to be resuscitated.[36]

What should be the approach, however, for patients too sedated to participate in the discussion? When decisions need to be made about continued support or allowing natural death, should their sedation be lessened in hopes they could take part in the conversation? Several authors have suggested that if a patient has a terminal, irreversible illness, waking would likely involve physical, psychological, and spiritual suffering, and the patient or surrogate has clearly stated the wish to allow natural death in these circumstances, the patient need not be awakened before life-sustaining treatment is withdrawn.[37,38] All agree that the decision should be reached through a joint decision-making process with the family, surrogate decision maker, and medical team and relevant others (social workers, chaplains who knew the patient). The focus then changes to intensive comfort care for the patient and the family with special attention to spiritual needs, cultural values, privacy, and physical comfort.[39]

Cultural Considerations

Consensus evidence and case series suggest that communication difficulties may be avoided if physicians and nurses explore with patients and families both the context and the structure of discussions about end-of-life care.[40] African Americans and non-Hispanic whites differ in who they want present (extended family, friends, and pastor versus immediate family only), focus and tempo of the discussion (spiritual concerns, lack of trust, concerns about DNR orders and hospice, allowing adequate time for decisions and not feeling pressure to make them vs concerns about prognosis, irreversibility of the illness, quality of life, financial concerns, and medical choices),[41,42] and having durable power of attorney or living will in place (more common in non-Hispanic whites),[40,42,43] or knowing about hospice programs.[43] More patients not of non-Hispanic white or African American descent prefer to have surrogates informed of their prognosis and make treatment decisions for them. Some patients from Asian, Bosnian, or Italian American cultures may perceive the frank communication of a serious illness or prognosis as "at a minimum, disrespectful, and more significantly, inhumane."[40] In addition to culture, "Patients' functional and cognitive abilities, age, racial and ethnic backgrounds, and desire to avoid burdening loved ones may influence attitudes and definitions of autonomy."[44] To respond to the vast cultural and spiritual variation in disclosure, decision making, and "quality living," clinicians should query into the *preferences* of patients and families before confronting them with bad news and critical decisions regarding end-of-life care, and remain sensitive to their changing needs and preferences by adopting a case-by-case approach. It is important to determine from the patient whether he or his designees, therefore, are to be involved in these discussions, and to respect that choice as the exercise of that patient's autonomy. To ensure such clear communication, therefore, every effort should be made to provide a qualified translator in conversations about prognosis and goals of care where the clinician is not a fluent speaker of the patient's language.[40]

Impact on Hope

The rigors of treatment regimens and the physical and emotional demands of the complex care required for advanced disease tend to isolate patients and their families and focus all their hopes on disease remission. They may have forgotten how to hope for anything else. Physicians and the teams they work with can help patients with advanced hematologic diseases develop new kinds of hope by encouraging them to reintegrate into activities that were meaningful before their disease began and they rearranged their lives around treatment schedules. Most patients hope for time to say their good-byes, to bring closure to their lives, and to leave their legacies: videotapes, scrapbooks, letters, DVDs, and presents for children or grandchildren for events far into the future.

As disease progresses, despite ongoing treatment, patients who have begun to reengage in nontreatment-related activities and who have developed a broader relationship with their physicians are more likely to understand that the physician is not abandoning them when he or she says that the goals of treatment should be comfort. Such patients do not complain that stopping treatment is "waiting around to die" because they have other activities to fill their days.

CAREGIVERS

Families and other nonprofessional caregivers provide the vast majority of care for patients with advanced cancer, which is thought to be worth the equivalent of more than $250 billion a year.[45] Caregivers of patients with advanced illness are stressed by the patient's disability and degree of suffering, the lack of coordination of care, and underlying family, work, or financial pressures.[46] Increased stress occurs at transition points, such as placing patients in a nursing home or deciding to change the focus of care to intensive comfort or, when necessary, to withdraw life-sustaining technology.[46] Caregiving can take a physical and psychological toll on the caregivers, with increased prevalence of depression, decrease in self-care and preventive care, and perhaps increased mortality. For caregivers of cancer patients,

Caregiver Support

Sources of caregiver stress
- Patient disability
- Degree of patient suffering
- Lack of coordination of care
- Underlying family, work, or financial pressures
- Periods of increased stress
- Symptom exacerbation

Transitions
- Moving patient to a nursing home
- Changing the focus of care to intensive comfort

Consequences of caregiver stress
- Depression
- Decrease in self- and preventive care
- Fatigue
- Increased mortality (data equivocal)

Supportive measures
- Decreasing patient suffering
- Management of symptoms and other sources of distress

Decrease/share care burden
- Hospice home health aides
- Hospice volunteers
- Friends and family members
- Availability for questions

Education
- Safety and use of medications (especially opioids)
- Anticipated potential emergencies
- Dying process

Skill building
- Physical care
- Transfers

Counseling
- Mental health providers
- Chaplains

fears of addiction and side effects of pain medications and the presence of unrelieved pain are associated with increased rates of depression. Caregiver satisfaction and quality of life are improved when caregivers are able to have questions answered. Providing information and increasing coping skills can improve caregiver knowledge and skill but even providing respite care has not lessened the sense of burden or depression.[46] As many as 32% of caregivers either have a major psychiatric condition (panic disorder, major depression, posttraumatic stress disorder, or generalized anxiety disorder) or access mental health services after the patients' diagnosis.[45] Caregivers are likely to need the support of many members of the team, therefore, to continue in their difficult role.

RELIEF OF SUFFERING

Suffering includes physical, psychological, social, and spiritual dimensions.

Symptom Management in Children

Therapist: If you could choose one word to describe the time since your diagnosis, what would it be?

Child: PAIN.[1]

Maintaining patient comfort is a critical issue throughout treatment, as well as during the end stages of life. Although effective pain control is a hallmark of palliative care, pain is only one of many distressing symptoms.[8,10,11] The spectrum of physical symptoms includes (although it is not limited to) dyspnea, fatigue, seizures, loss of appetite, nausea and vomiting, constipation, and diarrhea. Several comprehensive studies,[47–49] in which bereaved parents were interviewed regarding their children's end-of-life care, indicated that optimal symptom management is still far from being achieved, even in major pediatric teaching centers. Liben[11] presents a succinct overview of symptom management in pediatric palliative care. Relief of a child's end-of-life distress may have long-lasting implications for bereaved parents, who are negatively affected by the child's experience of pain years beyond their child's death.[49]

Psychological symptoms such as depression and anxiety are also prevalent in children at the end of life.[47] Hinds and colleagues have shown that children also experience existential concerns.[50] Creating opportunity for communication around these sources of distress involves using creative strategies that incorporate the developmental stage of the child. Strategies may involve verbal communication using open-ended questions, such as "What are you hoping for?" and "What are you worried about?"[51] However, many children communicate best through nonverbal means such as through artwork and music. Children may be more willing to "talk things over" with puppets or stuffed animals rather than real people. Importantly, euphemistic expressions about death can be confusing or even frightening (for instance, equating death with sleep may result in the child's being afraid of going to bed) and should be avoided.

Needless to say, parents of children with life-limiting conditions also experience distressing symptoms such as anxiety, depression, and spiritual concerns.[52,53] Recognition by the pediatric clinician may serve families well while the child is alive and during bereavement.

Symptom Management in Adults

Pain and antiemetic therapy for adults is reviewed elsewhere in this volume. Anxiety, depression, delirium, and control of symptoms occurring in the last days of life are reviewed subsequently. Interested readers are referred to other references for reviews of assessment and management of other common troubling symptoms and syndromes in adults (eg, PTSD, substance abuse, major psychiatric illnesses, personality disorders, or demoralization).[54–59]

Among social sources of distress are financial concerns and, with increasing debility, the loss of roles in the community, the workplace, and even in the family.[60] Worries about burdening the family or that the family will fail them when they really need them may lead patients to request physician-assisted suicide.[61,62] Social workers are the key team members who can help alleviate or at least ameliorate these sources of distress and can help the caregivers cope.

Physicians should also explore religious and spiritual concerns and understand what rituals will be important at the end of life. For these patients "spiritual distress and spiritual crisis occur when individuals are unable to find sources of meaning, hope, love, peace, comfort, strength and connection in life or when conflict occurs between their beliefs and what is happening in their life".[63] Patients who use "positive" religious coping (eg, prayer, feeling a sense of connectedness to a religious community, having a positive relationship with God) have been found to have better mental health status, growth with stress and in the spiritual dimension, as well as a better overall quality of life.[64] Patients who use "negative" religious coping (eg, ascribe their illness to a punishing God or one who has abandoned them) have a poorer quality of life. Clinicians should therefore include either a formal or informal[63] spiritual assessment for all patients diagnosed with life-limiting diseases.[63–67] Psychological, spiritual, or religious counseling may be needed to help these patients reconnect and find what they have lost.

PSYCHOLOGICAL CONCERNS

As Dr Susan Block states in her 2006 review of psychological issues in end-of-life care, "Grief, sadness, despair, fear, anxiety, loss and loneliness are present, at times, for nearly all patients facing the end of their lives."[58] For patients to cope with the diagnosis and its implications, they need "good communication and trust among patient, family, and clinical team, the ability to share fears and concerns, as well as meticulous attention to physical comfort and psychological and spiritual concerns."[58] For a thorough discussion of the patient assessment, which includes "developmental issues; meaning and impact of illness; coping style; impact on sense of self; relationships; stressors; spiritual resources; economic circumstances; physician-patient relationship,"[58] please refer to Dr Block's review.[58]

Anxiety and Depression

It is noteworthy that the psychological states of depression and anxiety are often not recognized as symptoms in children and, in many instances, are inadequately addressed. Significant anxiety is found in approximately 25% of adult patients with cancer.[58] Patients with panic disorders, agitated depression, phobias, obsessive–compulsive disorder, delirium, posttraumatic stress disorder, or with adjustment disorders can all present with anxiety.[58] Anxiety in dying patients may arise from worries about the future (uncontrolled symptoms, family concerns or concerns about death); isolation from loved ones; sepsis; hypoxia; metabolic abnormalities; withdrawal from alcohol,[68] opioids, or benzodiazepines; drug reactions (eg, akathisia from metoclopramide, phenothiazines, and butyrophenones); paradoxical agitation from benzodiazepines and olanzapine;[69,70] and uncontrolled pain). Nonpharmacologic treatments, such as relaxation training, hypnosis, supportive psychotherapy, and counseling, are very effective.[54] Pharmacologic treatments usually include benzodiazepines (eg, the short-acting lorazepam 0.5–2 mg every 2 hours as needed or long-acting clonazepam 0.5 mg PO three times daily), selective serotonin reuptake inhibitors (see later in this section), and, when there is evidence of delirium, neuroleptics (see in Delirium). A Cochrane review, however, did not feel there was adequate systematic evidence for the effectiveness of pharmacologic therapy of anxiety in patients at the end of life.[71]

At least 7% of patients with advanced cancer meet criteria for a major depressive disorder, 41% of whom had a previous history of major depressive disorder.[72] It can be difficult to discern which patients with advanced disease are depressed or grieving. The usual somatic signs of depression or grief (eg, anorexia, sleep disturbances, fatigue, or weight loss) are common in this population. Depressed patients, however, will be anhedonic, and feel worthless, guilty, hopeless, or helpless.[73] Grieving patients, in contrast, are very sad, but they are able to find happiness in some circumstances and can plan for the future.[58] Pain, a past or family history of substance abuse, depression, or bipolar illness are major risk factors for depression.[58] Terminally ill patients responding "Yes" to the screening question "Are you depressed?" are very likely to be confirmed as depressed in a more comprehensive evaluation.[58,74] Useful follow-up questions include "How do you see your future?" "What do you imagine is ahead for yourself with this illness?" "What aspects of your life do you feel most proud of, most troubled by?"[73]

As part of the treatment of depression, pain must be brought under control.[73] Counseling can explore patient fears, provide emotional support, help patients review their lives, and find the meaning and areas of accomplishment in them. A variety of models of therapy are used and none has been shown to be superior over the others.[58] The psychostimulants dextroamphetamine and methylphenidate (2.5–5 mg, 8 AM and noon; maximum dose 60–90 mg daily) often act within a few days.[75] The selective serotonin uptake inhibitors (SSRIs) are the first choice when immediate onset is not needed because they usually take several weeks to show effect. Useful agents include citalopram (Celexa) and paroxetine (Paxil) (10 mg PO daily initially; maximum 60 mg PO daily); escitalopram (Lexapro) (10 mg PO daily initially, maximum 20 mg PO daily); sertraline (Zoloft) (50 mg PO daily initially, maximum 200 mg PO daily); fluoxetine (5 to 10 mg PO daily initially, maximum 60 mg PO daily); venlafaxine (Effexor) (37.5 mg PO twice daily initially, maximum 225 mg PO daily) inhibits norepinephrine, serotonin, and dopamine reuptake. Major side effects of the SSRIs include hyponatremia, sexual dysfunction or loss of libido, and gastrointestinal complaints (eg, nausea, diarrhea, and foul-smelling flatus). Modafinil may also be an effective adjuvant agent to reduce SSRI-related sedation.[76] The exact mechanism of action of mirtazapine (Remeron) (15 mg PO at bedtime initially; maximum 45 mg PO at bedtime) is unknown.

If the patient is expected to live longer than weeks to a few months, a stimulant and an SSRI should be started simultaneously, and the stimulant can be titrated off several weeks later. Tricyclic antidepressants are less useful in these patients because of their side-effect profile.

If the patient does not respond to first-line agents, a psychiatrist should be consulted. Referral to a psychiatrist is also necessary when the physician is unsure of the diagnosis; the patient is psychotic, confused or delirious; the patient previously had a major psychiatric disorder; the patient is suicidal or requesting assisted suicide; or there are dysfunctional family dynamics.[73]

Delirium

Delirium occurs in up to 80% of dying patients.[77] Delirious patients can be agitated or hypoactive or vacillate between the two.[78] Symptoms of delirium include insomnia and daytime somnolence, nightmares, restlessness or agitation, irritability, distractibility, hypersensitivity to light and sound, anxiety, difficulty in concentrating or marshaling thoughts, fleeting illusions, hallucinations and delusions, emotional lability, attention deficits, and memory disturbances.[79]

Validated delirium screening and severity tools are available,[80] but a comprehensive psychiatric evaluation is recommended to exclude other disorders, such as anxiety, minor depression, anger, dementia, or psychosis.[78] The cause of delirium is determined in approximately 43% of cases,[81] and it is often multifactorial.[81,82] Medications, especially opioids, NSAIDs, and high-dose corticosteroids, often contribute.[81,82] Opioid-induced CNS toxicities are more common in patients with renal dysfunction, on high doses of opioids for long periods of time, with impaired cognition before starting the opioids, with dehydration, or taking other psychoactive drugs.[83] Other causes include metabolic abnormalities (hypercalcemia, hyperglycemia, or uremia), malnutrition, dehydration, hypoxia, fever, infection, uncontrolled pain, hepatic failure, primary brain tumor, and brain metastases.[79,81]

Treatment for delirium should begin while the underlying cause(s) are being treated. In addition to the medications listed in Table 95–3, it is helpful to make the patient's surroundings as familiar as possible, restore aids to hearing and sight if they are needed, reorient the patient frequently, and have family members, friends, or well-known caregivers present.

MANAGEMENT CONCERNS DURING THE LAST DAYS OF LIFE

For some families, there is the possibility of planning ahead and choosing a setting for their child's death-home, hospice, or hospital. The child may express a preference about where he or she feels safe, or prefers to be. Clear information about how the child is likely to die and professional support to validate the family's choice are crucial. Even more important is the explicitly stated "permission" from all members of the professional team that the family may change their choice freely at any time—that all options remain open and that no decision is irrevocable. Although in the current zeitgeist, there is

Table 95–3 Delirium

Drug	Dose	Comment
Antipsychotics		
Haloperidol	0.5–5 mg PO, IM, SC, IV*	Do not exceed 20 mg in 24 hours
	Repeat q 2–12 hours as needed	Maintain the patient on the effective dose (divided into a bid dose) then taper over 2 weeks, as tolerated
Quetiapine	25–250 mg PO tid	Particularly useful in elderly patients with evening delirium
		Start 25 mg h.s. for 3–4 days
Olanzapine	2.5–15 mg PO qd	Start 2.5–5 mg PO bid (2.5 mg for elderly); also antiemetic
Risperidone	0.5–3 mg PO bid	Start 1 mg PO bid (0.5 mg in elderly)
Chlorpromazine	25–50 mg PO/IV/PR q 6–8 hours	Sedating; in very agitated patients, may give q 1 hour until sedated
Sedatives		
Lorazepam	0.5–2 mg PO, SL, IV q 1–4 hours	Add to haloperidol for patients with an agitated delirium
		Tablets can be used PR for terminal delirium.
Diazepam	10–30 mg PO, PR qd	Useful PR for patients unable to take oral medication
Clonazepam	0.5–2 mg PO bid–tid	Tablets have been used PR for terminal delirium; do not exceed 20 mg/24 hours
Midazolam	30–100 mg IV, SC over 24 hours	IV drip or SC infusion for terminal delirium

*Oral doses are half as potent as parenteral doses.

Data from Massie MJ, Holland J, Glass E: Delirium in terminally ill cancer patients. Am J Psychiatry 140:1048, 1983; Breitbart W, Bruera E, Chochinov H, et al: Neuropsychiatric syndromes and psychological symptoms in patients with advanced cancer. J Pain Symptom Manage 10:131, 1995; and Ingham JM, Caraceni A: Delirium. In Berger AM, Portenoy RK, Weissman DE [eds.]: Principles and Practice of Palliative Care and Supportive Oncology, 2nd ed. Philadelphia, Lippincott Williams & Wilkins, 2002, p 555.

strong advocacy for children to die at home, professionals must bear in mind that for some children and families, the hospital is a better option, and that choice must be respected. In the past, siblings were rarely included in these discussions, and were often inadequately prepared for the eventuality of a child dying at home. It is only recently that their voices are beginning to be heard.

The Dying Child

Therapist: Are you in any pain? Does anything hurt?
Child: My heart.
Therapist: Your heart?
Child: My heart is broken. . . . I miss everybody.[84]

The distillation of anticipatory grief to its essence marks the imminence of death. At times imperceptibly, at other times dramatically, the child who has been living with the illness is transformed into a dying child.

The end point of the terminal phase is often marked by a turning inward on the part of the child, a pulling back from the external world. Cognitive and emotional horizons narrow, as all energy is needed simply for physical survival. A generalized irritability is not uncommon. The child may talk very little, and may even retreat from physical contact. Although such withdrawal is not universal, a certain degree of quietness is almost always evident. The child is pulling into himself or herself, not away from others. This behavior is a normal and expectable precursor to death—a form of preparation for the ultimate separation that lies ahead.[1]

Adults

Physical symptoms that occur in the last week to days before an adult's death include the following: pain, 70%; noisy or moist breathing, restlessness/agitation/delirium, 60%; urinary incontinence or retention, 50%; dyspnea, 20%; and nausea and vomiting, 10%.[54] Patients may also experience fatigue. Hunger and thirst are unusual.[85] Treatments for problems at the end of life are reviewed in Table 95–4.

HOSPICE PROGRAMS

In the United States, most hospice care takes place in the home, although patients can be admitted to nursing homes for brief periods (usually 5 days) to provide a respite for the family caregivers, or to the hospital (usually for up to 14 days) if symptoms cannot be controlled at home. The Medicare Hospice Benefit does not require a do not resuscitate (DNR) status, but does requires that the attending physician and the hospice medical director certify that the patient has a prognosis of 6 months or less to live, if the disease follows its usual course.[86] Medicare reimburses hospice programs approximately $130 per day per patient to provide the routine care described in Table 95–5. Therefore, the cost of transfusions typically required for many patients with hematologic malignancies, even at the end of life, may make it difficult for hospice programs to enroll patients insured by Medicare alone. Other insurance programs, thankfully, often will allow their patients to receive transfusions and hospice care. Early referral to hospice can decrease the risk of major depressive disorder and better quality of survival.[87] Notably, many children are not referred to hospice because their illness experience is inconsistent with hospice specifications—prognosis is uncertain; there is a blending of goals, which can result in more costly health care; and providers' lack of pediatric expertise. In a survey of 632 pediatric oncologists, Fowler and colleagues demonstrated that continued disease-directed therapy was cited as the most common reason for not making a referral, especially when the hospice did not admit children receiving chemotherapy.[88] Thus, despite the availability of this medical benefit adults and children are often left without the intensive support needed to receive end-of-life care in the home.

BEREAVEMENT

Bereavement follow-up by the professional team is an intrinsic component of comprehensive pediatric palliative care. Bereaved families often express the sentiment of a double loss: loss of their child and loss of their professional "family"—the treatment team whom they have known and trusted, often over months and years.[2,89] Parental grief has been recognized as more intense and longer-lasting than other types of grief.[90] Contact from a team member after the child's death not only assuages the family's sense of abandonment; it can

Table 95–4 Treatment of Problems at the End of Life

Problem	Agent(s)	Routes, Doses	Comment
Baseline pain	Morphine, hydromorphone, oxycodone SL oral concentrates, SQ infusions	Scheduled Individualized	
	Fentanyl	Transdermal, individualized	
Breakthrough pain	Concentrated oxycodone or morphine solutions	Individualized	Intermittent
"Death rattle"	Scopolamine	Gel; Transderm Scop patch 1–3 q 3 days	
	Hyoscyamine	0.125–0.25 SL tid to qid	
	Glycopyrrolate	0.1–0.2 mg IV tid to qid	
Delirium	Haloperidol	2–4 mg PO, PR or 1–2 mg SQ, IV q 1–2 hours	
	Olanzapine	2.5–10 mg PO bid, Start 2.5 mg for elderly	
	Chlorpromazine	25–50 mg PO, IV, PR q 4–8 hours	
	Midazolam	2–3 mg IV load; 0.5–1 mg/hour initial	Palliative sedation
	Pentobarbital	3 mg/kg IV load; 1–3 mg/kg/hour IV drip	Palliative sedation
		120–200 mg PR q 4 hours	
Dyspnea (anxiety)	Lorazepam	1 mg PO, SL, IV q 2 hours	
Dyspnea (other)	Morphine/oxycodone	5–10 mg SL oral concentrate q 2 hours	
	Morphine	2–3 mg IV q 2 hours	
	Chlorpromazine	25–50 mg PO, IV, PR q 4–12 hours	
Nausea	Combinations of lorazepam, metoclopramide, dexamethasone, and/or haloperidol as indicated	Compounded suppositories with desired agents (depending on presumed cause of nausea) PR q 6 hours	
Anxiety	Lorazepam	1 mg PO, SL, IV q 2 hours	

Adapted from Abrahm JL: A Physician's Guide to Pain and Symptom Management in Cancer Patients, 2nd ed. Baltimore, Johns Hopkins University Press, 2005, p 408.

Table 95–5 Hospice Services

Personnel
Medical director, nurses, social workers, home health aides, chaplains, volunteers, administrative personnel, medical consultants, occupational therapists, physical therapists, speech therapists, and bereavement counselors
Items Needed for Palliation of Terminal Illness
Prescription medications
Durable medical equipment and supplies
Oxygen
Laboratory and diagnostic procedures
Radiation and chemotherapy
Transportation when medically necessary for changes in level of care (ie, inpatient or "respite" in nursing home)

serve a crucial preventive role by identifying families at particular risk and identifying resources for them.[91]

Each bereaved person's loss is unique, but many people manifest similar symptoms of grief, some of which become less persistent as they rebuild their lives.[92,93] Recurrent intense symptoms typically occur at the anniversary of the death of the patient, but can occur at unpredictable times, induced by reminders of the deceased. Just as in the patients described above, survivors' grief must be differentiated from depression. Survivors appreciate calls or letters from the patient's physician and nurses.[94] For patients enrolled in hospice, a formal bereavement program is offered for the family throughout the first year after the patient's death. After the formal program ends, the bereaved are welcome to continue to participate in any bereavement activities that have been meaningful to them.

At the time of death, survivors may seem numb, confused, or dazed, and experience disbelief.[94,95] By the second month after the death, yearning has replaced disbelief.[87] During the next months, disbelief, depressed mood, and yearning decline gradually, and by 6 months after the death, most people will have accepted the reality of the death and begin to think about reengaging in relationships and work, and discover new meaning and purpose.[87] By a year or two, most survivors have accommodated to their loss.[87,92] They become aware of the changes that must be made if they are to resume old relationships and responsibilities or to establish new ones and risk recurrent loss.[92]

Approximately 10% to 20% of survivors, however, suffer either from depression or from a symptom complex called "complicated grief." Patients with depression manifest "symptoms of sadness, impassivity, and psychomotor retardation"[87] but they are not yearning for the deceased or unable to accept the death. Depressed survivors benefit from counseling and consideration of pharmacologic treatment.[87,96] Patients with Prolonged Grief Disorder, in contrast, have grief that causes serious functional impairments, with profound yearning for the deceased as well as feelings of "numbness, feeling that part of oneself has died, assuming symptoms of the deceased, disbelief, or bitterness."[87,97] Such patients are at increased risk of medical and psychiatric illness[98] and should be referred for psychiatric or spiritual counseling. Persons at higher risk for this disorder include those with a history of attachment disorders (childhood abuse, childhood separation anxiety), aversion to lifestyle changes, being unprepared for the death and unsupported after it. Additional risks include a "dependent, close, confiding" relationship with the deceased.[87] Unfortunately, although there is no randomized controlled trial of a pharmacotherapy that is effective for the extreme grief symptoms,[87,97] there is a novel effective psychotherapy developed specifically for this disorder that is superior to standard interpersonal psychotherapy.[99]

INTERDISCIPLINARY TREATMENT TEAM

Thank you for giving me aliveness.

—(6-year-old child)[1]

Palliative care demands the combined expertise of an interdisciplinary treatment team to address medical, psychological, social, and spiritual concerns of the child, siblings, parents, and close family. This knowledge-based expertise must be provided within a context of ongoing accessibility and availability to the family, granting them a sense of the team's abiding presence.

Yet, even while providing this steady care for the patient and family, professional caregivers are often experiencing their own distress in a sort of parallel process.[1,2,12,89,100] The professional often feels anguish and helplessness in witnessing a child endure pain and suffering—physical or psychic. He or she often identifies with the parents of the child. This reaction intensifies when the caregiver is also a parent, especially if his or her healthy child is of the same age as the patient. For the caregiver who does not yet have children, the specter of a fatally ill child may loom threateningly. In a survey,[89] staff cited the personal pain of losing a child as the most difficult experience in their work with dying children.

For all these reasons, the professionals who engage in this extraordinarily rich and demanding work articulate significant needs for support themselves.[2,89] Otherwise, the toll of cumulative unresolved grief exacts a heavy toll in their personal and professional lives. A cohesive team and/or the opportunity for individual and group consultation are crucial for those who are intimately engaged in repeated cycles of attachment and loss with dying children and their families.

SUGGESTED READINGS

Ballon JS, Feifel D: A systematic review of modafinil: Potential clinical uses and mechanisms of action. J Clin Psychiatry 67:554, 2006.

Berger AM, Schuster K, Von Roenn JH, (eds.): Principles and Practice of Palliative Care and Supportive Oncology, 3rd ed. Philadelphia, Lippincott Williams & Wilkins, 2007.

Block SD: Psychological Issues in End-of-Life care. J Palliat Med 9:751, 2006.

Fowler K, Poehling K, Billheimer D, et al: Hospice referral practices for children with cancer: A survey of pediatric oncologists. J Clin Oncol 24(7):1099, 2006.

Hebert R, Schulz R: Caregiving at the end of life. J Palliat Med 9:1174, 2006.

Jalmsell L, Kreicbergs U, Onelov E, Steineck G, Henter JI: Symptoms affecting children with malignancies during the last month of life: A nationwide follow-up. Pediatrics 117(4):1314, 2006.

Mack JW, Cook EF, Wolfe J, Grier HE, Cleary PD, Weeks JC: Understanding of prognosis among parents of children with cancer: Parental optimism and the parent-physician interaction. J Clin Oncol 25(11):1357, 2007.

Mack JW, Wolfe J, Grier HE, Cleary PD, Weeks JC: Communication about prognosis between parents and physicians of children with cancer: Parent preferences and the impact of prognostic information. J Clin Oncol 24(33):5265, 2006.

Ogawa M, Shinjo T, Tei Y, Morita T: Uncommon underlying etiologies of reversible delirium in terminally ill cancer patients. J Pain Symptom Manage 32:205, 2006.

Robinson MR, Thiel MM, Backus MM, Meyer EC: Matters of spirituality at the end of life in the pediatric intensive care unit. Pediatrics 118(3): e719, 2006.

Tarakeshwar N, Vanderwerker LC, Paulk E, Pearce MJ, Kasl SV, Prigerson HG: Religious coping is associated with the quality of life of patients with advanced cancer. J Palliat Med 9:646, 2006.

Zhang B, El-Jawahri A, Prigerson HG: Update on bereavement research: Evidence-based guidelines for the diagnosis and treatment of complicated bereavement. J Palliat Med 9:1188, 2006.

REFERENCES

For complete list of references log onto www.expertconsult.com

CHAPTER 96

INDWELLING ACCESS DEVICES

Douglas E. Brandoff and Janet L. Abrahm

Indwelling devices that permit chronic access to the venous and central nervous systems have permitted novel and more comfortable forms of treatment for children and adults. Indwelling central venous access devices are useful for patients who require frequent withdrawal of blood specimens or administration of blood or blood products, peripheral stem cell apheresis, parenteral nutrition, or infusional therapy with medications such as chemotherapeutic agents, deferoxamine, amphotericin, or pain medications. These devices also facilitate therapies in the outpatient and home settings. Similarly, through the use of indwelling epidural or intrathecal catheters and Ommaya reservoirs, prolonged access to the cerebrospinal fluid (CSF) may be obtained for the delivery of chemotherapy, antibiotics, antifungal agents, or pain medications. The choice of the appropriate device and application of careful maintenance procedures can minimize the associated complications and maximize the patient's quality of life. As therapies continue to become more intensive, maintenance of adequate, reliable venous access is a critical issue for the management of many patients with hematologic diseases. Since 1973, when the Broviac catheter was first introduced, the sizes and uses of indwelling central venous access devices (CVADs) have expanded dramatically. It is estimated that more than 5 million CVADs are placed in patients in the United States every year.[1]

INDWELLING CENTRAL VENOUS ACCESS DEVICES

Chronic venous access devices can minimize the physical and psychological discomforts of repeated venipuncture; prevent venous thrombosis, phlebitis, and vesicant infiltration; maintain patient mobility; and minimize hospital stays. Certain patients with hematologic diseases are at increased risk for the development of thrombophlebitis from standard (peripheral) intravenous lines and may therefore be best served by an indwelling access device. Factors associated with this increased risk include age of the patient (>60 years); certain characteristics of the solutions being infused (eg, hypertonicity of the solution, irritating diluents such as alcohol, highly acidic or alkaline pH, particulate matter in the solution); type of drugs infused (vesicant chemotherapy, certain antibiotics, dexamethasone, furosemide, phenytoin); factors associated with the catheter itself and its insertion (size and composition, traumatic insertion, microbial contamination); and duration of infusion (85% of cases of phlebitis occur 24 to 48 hours after placement of the intravenous line).[2–6] Because patients with these risk factors or with visibly poor peripheral venous access can usually be identified before therapy begins, early placement of an indwelling device is reasonable. To minimize the occurrence of septic episodes, the devices should be placed before the administration of agents that induce neutropenia.[7–9] With platelet transfusions, catheters and ports can be safely placed surgically or radiologically in patients whose thrombocytopenia (platelet count <50,000/mm^3) is caused by conditions other than disseminated intravascular coagulation.[9,10]

DEVICE TYPES

Catheters

In all indwelling catheters used for prolonged central venous access, the proximal capped portion of the catheter exits from a subcutaneous tunnel on the chest or abdominal wall while the distal tip is indwelling in a central vein (Fig. 96–1).[11] All catheters are composed of radiopaque elastomeric hydrogel, polyurethane, or silicone elastomer but differ in types of opening and internal diameter.[12] Catheter design varies among manufacturers with some catheters having end openings at the distal tip, others having side openings, and some having end and side openings.[13]

Catheters with a simple opening at the distal tip include those placed at the bedside (ie, midline catheters and peripherally inserted central catheters [PICCs]) and the tunneled Hickman, Broviac, and apheresis catheters, which are surgically inserted. Hickman catheters can have single, double, or triple lumens and have an anchoring cuff in subcutaneous tissue. Broviac catheters have a smaller internal lumen diameter than Hickman catheters. Midline catheters, which do not extend into the veins beyond the arm itself, come in 28 to 16 gauges and are 3 to 8 inches long with single or double lumens. Their use is restricted to nonirritating and nearly isoosmotic therapies, and has fallen increasingly out of favor.[6,12,14,15] The PICCs, which terminate in the superior vena cava, vary in size from 1.9 French (Fr) to 6 Fr for the single-lumen catheters and 3 Fr to 7 Fr for double-lumen catheters, and they are 15 to 27 inches long.[12,14,16,17] The tunneled catheters range from 2.7 Fr to 12.5 Fr and are 29.5 to 42.7 inches long.[12] For apheresis (eg, for peripheral stem cell harvest, for preoperative exchange transfusions or vasoocclusive crisis in patients with sickle cell disease[18]), 8.4 Fr to 13.5 Fr catheters are available and are 5.4 to 18 inches long.[12,19]

Valved catheters (eg, Groshong, PASV) are available in a variety of internal diameters and are designed to prevent the reflux of blood into the catheter tip. The valve allows the catheter to be flushed with saline solution rather than heparin. The PASV has a pressure-sensitive valve at the proximal end, and the Groshong three-position slit valve is adjacent to a closed distal tip. The valve remains closed at rest but opens outward for infusion when positive pressure is applied and opens inward for aspiration when negative pressure is applied.[20] Valved catheters are also available as peripherally inserted devices.

For patients requiring multiple simultaneous therapies, nutritional support or infusional therapy along with blood sampling and blood product administration, all the previously mentioned catheters are available with double lumens, and there is a triple-lumen tunneled catheter available.[12,21] Double-lumen devices have 1.3-mm internal diameters or 1.0-mm and 1.6-mm internal diameters; those with triple lumens have 1.0-mm, 1.0-mm, and 1.25-mm internal diameters.

Implantable Central Venous Devices (Ports)

In the United States, more than 200,000 ports are implanted annually and their use is increasing.[22] Totally implantable central venous access devices consist of single- or dual-lumen ports that may be round, square, oval, or hexagonal[12] and are connected to a radiopaque silicone elastomer or polyurethane catheter (Fig. 96–2).[11,12] Ports are also available in low profile (less depth) designs. The port includes a self-sealing silicone septum with a body of plastic or metal, both of which can cause an artifact on magnetic resonance imaging (MRI).[12] The artifact effect is greater with stainless steel than with plastic. Many ports now available are marketed as being MRI compatible.

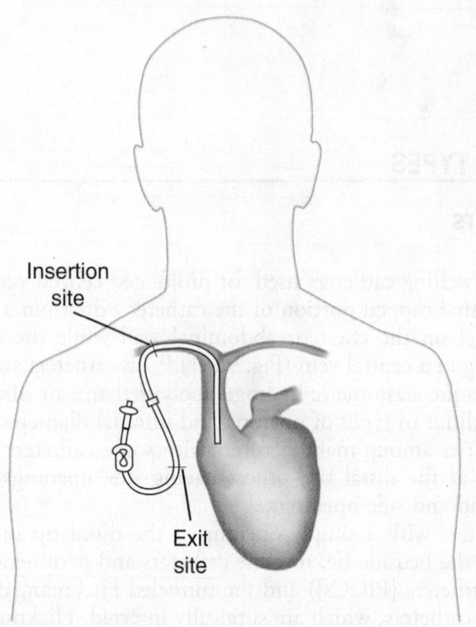

Figure 96–1 Schematic diagram of an indwelling central venous catheter in place. *Insertion site* refers to the insertion of the proximal end of the catheter into the chest wall. Clamp attached to the catheter is shown next to the Luer-Lok cap at the distal end. *(Adapted from Hickman Subcutaneous Port, Use and Maintenance, and How to Care for Your Hickman or Broviac Catheter. Cranston, RI, Davol Inc.)*

No portion exits onto the chest wall. This port is surgically placed in a subcutaneous pocket, and the catheter is inserted into a central vein. The single or double port is connected to a standard or valved catheter. Attached catheters range from 4 Fr to 12 Fr and from 19.7 to 34.5 inches long.[12] Ports are available as one- or two-piece systems. The position of the distal tip of the two-piece system is more easily adjusted during insertion as it can be shortened at the port pocket before connection to the reservoir. However, with the two-piece system there is the potential for disconnection of the port from the catheter with resultant infiltration into the port pocket.

The Vortex port is designed with a tangential rather than perpendicular outlet tube to promote more efficient and thorough flushing of the port chamber. This design appears to inhibit buildup of thrombus or drug residuals in the port chamber, resulting in fewer complications than those associated with traditional ports.[22] The OmegaPort allows access from multiple angles rather than at 90 degrees only.[23] The CathLink port is designed with a series of panels with centrally located openings replacing its silicone septum and without a reservoir. The CathLink is accessed by standard 20-gauge over-the-needle peripheral intravenous catheters.[9]

Ports that can be placed in the antecubital fossa are also available (eg, the PAS).[8,12,24–26] The peripherally implanted ports are smaller and flatter than the standard port and have 3 Fr to 7 Fr catheters.

Other implantable devices have self-contained pumps. These devices and guidelines for their use are discussed elsewhere.[27–30]

DEVICE CHOICE

Patient characteristics and preference, as well as the duration of use, purposes for which the device is required, and relative complication rates all aid in deciding among the types of catheters and in choosing between catheters and ports (Table 96–1).[6,8,11,21,31–37]

Patient Characteristics and Preference

The peripheral devices are helpful in patients with chest wall abnormalities that preclude the use of centrally placed catheters or ports (eg, subcutaneous carcinoma of the chest wall, open wounds, tracheostomies, or fibrosis induced by radiation therapy).[9,21]

Valved catheters that do not require heparin for maintenance are particularly appropriate for patients with known heparin allergy, for

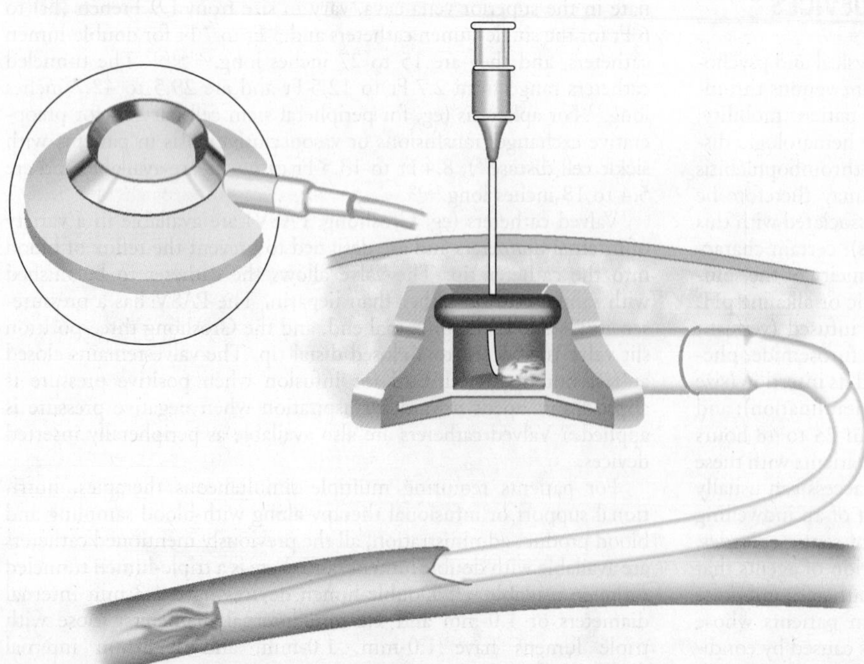

Figure 96–2 Totally implanted Hickman subcutaneous (central venous access) port with a noncoring needle in place. *(Adapted from Hickman Subcutaneous Port, Use and Maintenance, and How to Care for Your Hickman or Broviac Catheter. Cranston, RI, Davol Inc.)*

Table 96–1 Choices of Indwelling Venous Access Devices

	Peripheral		Tunneled	
Patient Characteristics	*PICC*	*Port*	*Catheter*	*Port*
Chest wall problem	X	X		
Outpatient	X	X		X
Age: child or adolescent				X
Thrombocytopenia	X		X	
Duration of use				
<3 months	X			
<6 months		X	X	
>6 months				X
Purpose				
Frequent access			X	
Rapid infusion			X	X
Vesicant infusion	X		X	X

PICC, peripherally inserted central catheter.

those who develop heparin-induced thrombocytopenia (HIT) from heparin flushes, and in whom continuation of a CVAD is desirable. Although rare, HIT from catheter flushes alone has been documented with heparin flush doses as low as 60 units per day.[38] Valved catheters require somewhat less care than standard catheters and may be preferred for patients unable to care for a Hickman or Broviac catheter at home.[20,39,40]

Children and adolescents have lower risks of complications with ports than with catheters.[33] Four prospective, nonrandomized studies indicated a significantly lower complication rate for the ports than for the catheters, especially in the youngest children.[31,33,41] Implantable devices have several advantages for children in particular: they are cosmetically acceptable, cause less limitation of activities, are at less risk of accidental dislodgment or damage, and require less care when not in active use.[42] Ports also have a lower rate of infectious complications in adult patients.[1,43–45] Ports are also useful for adult patients who are unable to care for a catheter or who do not wish to do so, and for those who prefer a less visible access device.

Port systems are less successful in patients with hematologic malignancies as there is an increased risk for developing any type of complication (eg, infection, thrombosis). Ports are also less successful when placed outside the cervical or infraclavicular areas; this may be caused by factors such as tendencies for groin infections or catheter thrombosis in low-flow vessels.[46]

In obese patients and in patients with thrombocytopenia, the subcutaneous location of the ports poses a problem. In the obese patient, it may be difficult to access a port placed deep in the antecubital fossa or chest wall. Needle stability may also be an issue for obese patients. If the needle length is not sufficient, it may be displaced or lifted out of the port by shifting flesh (ie, if the patient lies on the affected side). For the patient with chronic thrombocytopenia (platelet count <20,000/mm^3), neither type of port may be satisfactory because of the risk of hematoma associated with the recurrent needle punctures required for access.

For hemophiliac patients, consensus recommendations for central venous access devices (CVAD) have been published to help guide clinicians in patient selection. Ports are recommended both for patients with and without inhibitors, in part to minimize infectious risks. CVADs can be advantageous for small children requiring frequent factor infusions; to facilitate home-based treatment and/or prophylaxis; rapid and reliable response to a spontaneous bleeds or for administration of immune tolerance therapy.[47]

For sickle cell patients requiring chronic apheresis red cell exchange, reported experiences have been limited but poor with permanent access devices such as Vortex ports and double/dual ports. They have proven unable to accommodate the flow rates required by apheresis machines.[48]

Duration of Use

Because a surgical procedure is not needed, midline catheters and PICCs are useful for patients needing only short-term access, usually several weeks to months. The average PICC is in place for 2 to 10 weeks, but they have functioned for more than 300 days.[6,16,49,50] In patients needing a longer duration of infusion and more extensive supportive care, surgically placed catheters and ports are generally preferred. Catheters and ports have remained in place safely for months to years.[51,52] Most ports remain in place until the patient dies. Of 707 ports studied in an oncology population, 72.4% were still in place at the patient death (2 to 1960 days), and only 13.5% were removed at the end of therapy.[46]

There are significant differences in costs among the different types and methods of insertion (ie, peripherally inserted versus radiologically placed versus surgical placement).[15] Although the initial installation cost is greater for the ports than for the tunneled or nontunneled catheters, the replacement and maintenance costs of the catheter make it more expensive after 6 months of use.[33–35] The peripherally placed port is even more cost-effective than a standard port because it does not require fluoroscopy, an operating room, or a physician for placement; physician assistants can place them safely.[12,53–55]

Purpose for which the Device is Required

PICCs are used for antifungal therapy, hyperalimentation, or infusion of chemotherapy regimens that may include vesicant agents.[14,40,56,57] Their smaller bore makes them less useful for blood drawing or transfusion. Contraindications to PICCs include ipsilateral local cellulitis, thrombophlebitis, conditions that affect venous return (eg, lymphedema, previous axillary node dissection, hypercoagulopathy).[15,58] Peripheral ports are not recommended when fluids or blood products must be given rapidly, because the flow rate may be significantly less than that of standard central lines or ports placed in the chest.[55] They have only a single lumen and therefore have limited usefulness for complex multidrug therapies or simultaneous infusions. The smaller septum also tolerates fewer punctures (100 to 500 versus up to 4000), depending on the needle size.[14,59]

In general, surgically implanted catheters are more useful than ports or PICCs in patients in whom frequent access to the device or frequent blood drawing or blood product administration is needed.[8] The larger-bore catheters are more useful for blood drawing and blood product administration, because the incidence of clotting after such use is lower with them than with smaller-bore devices.[51] If a port or a PICC is chosen, the catheter with the largest bore is recommended. In the larger-gauge PICCs, which collapse easily, blood drawing is usually more successful if a syringe is used instead of a vacuum tube collection system.[56]

Continuous vesicant infusion may be more safely accomplished with catheters, as they avoid the danger of needle dislodgment and disconnection of the catheter from the septum associated with the implanted ports.

For support during autologous or allogeneic bone marrow transplantation, double- or triple-lumen catheters are used.[60,61] In transplantation patients undergoing peripheral stem cell apheresis, silicone apheresis or the largest-bore standard catheters is preferred, because the internal diameter of the smaller catheters may not support the apheresis procedure.[62] The complication rates for the large-bore catheters in transplantation recipients are similar to those of other central venous catheters used for pheresis or transplantation, or both.[63]

RELATIVE COMPLICATION RATES

Midline catheters are associated with lower rates of phlebitis than short peripheral catheters and with lower infection rates and lower costs than PICCs or tunneled catheters.[6] PICCs cause more phlebitis than tunneled catheters, and earlier reports indicated that the infection rates associated with their use were also higher than those for tunneled catheters. Some studies, however, suggest that the infection rates may be the same for PICCs and tunneled catheters.[6,9] One prospective study of 351 oncology patients found a relatively high complication rate with PICCs; 33% of catheters were removed because of complications, including infection, thrombus, phlebitis, occlusion, leakage or broken catheter, and accidental removal.[64]

Conflicting data have been reported regarding the relative complication rates seen with tunneled catheters and ports, although the overall complication rate is probably less for the ports than for the catheters. Five of six prospective, randomized trials and all retrospective studies, including one cohort study and one matched study, found significantly higher rates of complications with tunneled catheters than with ports.[6,8,65,66] Only catheter occlusion is no more likely with catheters than with ports.[8] Patients with ports also reported fewer restrictions in activity and hygiene.[65] In one study, PASV ports had fewer instances of poor blood return and less nursing access time compared to nonvalved devices.[67]

In HIV-infected patients, retrospective studies demonstrate that catheters[68–70] appear to cause more infectious complications than ports (0.47 to 0.97 cases per 100 days versus 0.17 to 0.39 cases per 100 days).[70,71] Patients receiving infusional ganciclovir through catheters for cytomegalovirus retinitis who had neutrophil counts of less than 1000/mm^3 were at particular risk for early septicemia.[70]

Hemophiliacs have higher infection rates than the oncology population for external and implanted venous access devices (71% versus 41%). Hemophilia patients with fully implanted CVADs were 31% as likely to develop an infection as those with external devices.[47] The presence of inhibitors seems to increase the infection rate, though the incidence of infection in inhibitor patients with ports was only 33% of that with external catheters.[47,72–74] There has been debate over potential bleeding risks into a port pocket, with associated infectious risk, versus ample risk reduction with newer recombinant hemostatic regimens such as activated prothrombin complex concentrate or rFVIIa. Given these considerations, this meta-analysis supported the use of fully implantable ports for hemophiliacs with inhibitors.[47]

Sickle cell patients may also have higher complication rates of sepsis and thrombosis than the oncology patient. This may be due to the hypercoagulable state and frequent admissions with resultant antibiotic resistant colonization.[75] Because of a high rate of complications (0.4 cases per 100 patient-days in this small study), one institution has discontinued the use of implanted ports in its sickle cell population.[76]

In children with cancer, one observational study showed risk factors for central venous catheter (CVC)-related complications included having a hematologic malignancy Risk Ratio (RR 3.0) and being younger than 6 years of age at time of insertion (RR 2.5). Single-lumen Hickman/Broviac catheters had fewer complications and greatest catheter survival, compared to double-lumen catheters or PASV.[77]

Choice of Device

We recommend indwelling venous access devices based on patient characteristics and preference, anticipated duration of use, purpose(s) for which the device is required, and relative complication rates among catheters and ports.

PICCs are an appropriate choice when patients have chest wall problems, have outpatient-based treatments, and/or have thrombocytopenia. PICCs can be selected when duration of use will be 3 months or less. They allow for vesicant infusions, antifungal therapies, and hyperalimentation.

Peripheral ports are appropriate for patients with chest wall problems receiving outpatient-based treatments. They may be used longer than PICCs, but not longer than 6 months.

Tunneled catheters may be chosen for patients with thrombocytopenia who require frequent access, rapid infusion, or administration of vesicants. Valved catheters that do not require heparin are useful for patients who should not receive it. Like peripheral ports, they may be used for up to 6 months.

Ports are appropriate for outpatients, particularly children or adolescents, but they may be problematic in patients who are obese, especially if they are thrombocytopenic. They are used for rapid infusions and administration of vesicants, and, if they have more than one lumen, hyperalimentation. They allow for the longest duration of use of the various devices (>6 months).

DEVICE INSERTION

Catheters

Catheters can be inserted nonsurgically or surgically. Midline catheters and PICCs are placed nonsurgically in the hospital or in the home by appropriately trained physicians, nurses, or physician assistants.[12,40,56] Insertion failure can occur in 8% to 22% of attempts, although the failure rate decreases with experience.[16] After careful skin preparation using a sterile technique (and for large-gauge introducers, local anesthesia), the catheter is inserted 1 to 2 inches above or below the antecubital fossa into the basilic, cephalic, or median cubital vein. PICC catheters are advanced into the superior vena cava (or, less frequently, the axillary, innominate, or subclavian vein) and secured by sutures or sterile tape. Placement above the antecubital fossa is more acceptable to patients and interferes less with patients' activities of daily living.[78] Radiologic confirmation of tip placement should be obtained before initiating therapy.[79]

Tunneled Hickman, Broviac, and valved catheters (and ports) are inserted surgically in an operating suite or minor procedure room, physician's office, radiology suite,[80] or at the bedside.[9] All catheter insertion techniques include creating a subcutaneous tunnel on the anterior chest wall, pulling the catheter up through the tunnel, and positioning the catheter cuff in it, leaving its remaining proximal portion with the Luer-Lok tip exiting from the tunnel on the chest wall (see Fig. 96–1).[8,20,31,81] The distal catheter tip is then usually placed percutaneously or by a cutdown technique into the central circulation through the axillary, subclavian, internal jugular, or cephalic vein[29,82] and threaded into the superior vena cava under fluoroscopic guidance.[12] Cutdown technique greatly diminishes the possibility of pneumothorax or hemothorax as the vessel is cannulated under direct visualization.[45] Literature from the dialysis population and a retrospective study of oncology patients suggest that there is a lower incidence of symptomatic venous thrombosis when the catheter is inserted through the internal jugular vein.[83,84]

The catheter position in the superior vena cava at the right atrial junction[9] should be confirmed by chest radiography. In patients expected to need crutches for a prolonged period, catheters should be inserted through the internal or external jugular vein or in the subclavian vein lateral to the midclavicular line to prevent pinching the catheter in the costoclavicular space, which leads to catheter pinch-off and fracture.[37]

No significant differences have been found in time to failure or in infection or obstruction rate of catheters inserted percutaneously ("blind" or landmark technique) rather than under direct visualization.[29,85,86] Real-time ultrasound-guided insertion techniques are associated with fewer placement failures and complications compared with landmark techniques.[87] One study of 589 blind placements had a 92% success rate, with 2.9% of catheters requiring repositioning.[88] Especially thin or obese patients are identified as higher risks for insertion failure and complications when the landmark technique is used. Other patients at higher risk are those who have had previous major surgery or previous central venous access devices.[89]

Catheters should be inserted by experienced personnel, however, as complication rates fall with increasing experience in catheter insertion.[51,90,91] Long-term central venous access devices are increasingly placed with interventional radiology techniques. These image-guided techniques have a 99% success rate at a lower cost than surgical placement and with a comparably low infection rate.[92,93] Placement using interventional radiology is often obtainable in a more timely manner than surgical placement.[94] If the chest wall or the vessels of the upper body are not usable, an alternative site is the inferior vena cava, which is accessed through the femoral or saphenous vein or by a translumbar approach directly into the inferior vena cava.[29,45,62,95–98]

Ports

Ports are surgically inserted into the antecubital fossa or chest or abdominal wall with the patient under local anesthesia.[99] If possible, they should be placed in the nondominant arm or in the side of the chest near it to minimize the probability of needle dislodgment or coring of the port septum during continuous access.[28]

The peripheral port can be inserted at the bedside by physicians or physician assistants.[9,53–55] It consists of an implantable port with an attached polyurethane radiopaque catheter, the distal tip of which contains an electromagnet. The port is placed percutaneously in a pocket in the antecubital fossa. The venous catheter is introduced using the same techniques as described earlier for PICCs without attached ports.[53–56] Fluoroscopy is unnecessary, as the progress of the catheter toward the right atrium can be externally tracked with a hand-held sensor wand (Cath-Finder) that detects the electromagnet in the distal tip.[12] A chest radiograph to verify catheter position is still recommended before infusion.[79]

The chest wall ports are placed into a subcutaneous pocket in the infraclavicular space, and the attached catheter is placed under fluoroscopic guidance into the subclavian, jugular, or cephalic vein and threaded through the superior vena cava to the junction with the right atrium (see Fig. 96–2). No portion of the device remains visible.

DEVICE MANAGEMENT

Catheters

Care of nontunneled and tunneled catheters is begun by the nurses and later taught to patients and their families. To minimize infectious complications, it is preferable to assign this responsibility (as well as infusions and blood sampling through the catheter) to nurses expert in catheter care and use.[6,31,100,101] Standard procedures are available and should be adopted by each institution, to be followed by all who care for the patient.[14,21,40,56]

Patient and family education in catheter care is required to maintain patency, to prevent damage to the external portion of the catheter, to prevent air embolization, and to reduce the risk of infection.[20,32,40,56,102] Instructions should cover permissible activities, techniques of dressing changes, heparin instillation, and changing the Luer-Lok plug, as well as emergency care in the event of damage to the external portion of the catheter. This educational program should be started well in advance of patient discharge to ensure patient and family competence; it may be reinforced by an educational booklet,[103] by attendance at a "hands-on" class, or by nurses sent into the home, at least initially, to verify compliance with procedures. Patients with catheters or ports in place should be given written information about the device[28] as well as a medical alert card, necklace, or bracelet indicating its location and type of access and a person to be contacted if problems arise.[40]

Dressing changes for surgically inserted catheters require a sterile technique for 2 weeks after insertion, until fibrous growth into the cuff is complete.[11,32] The catheter exit site is cleaned with an antiseptic solution. Povidone iodine has been commonly used in the United States, but chlorhexidine-based solutions may be preferable because they have been shown to reduce the risk of catheter colonization and catheter-related bloodstream infection (CRBSI).[104,105]

A formulation of chlorhexidine with isopropyl alcohol has been approved by the US Food and Drug Administration (FDA) for catheter site use and has been available for over-the-counter purchase since 2005.[106,107] Sterile dressing changes are done every 3 to 7 days for 2 to 3 weeks after insertion, depending on the dressing materials used (more frequently for povidone iodine and less frequently for chlorhexidine).[11,21,32,105]

The type of dressing, if any, needed to cover the site once the incision is healed is controversial.[14,21,32,40,108] One prospective, randomized study indicated that when a rigorous cleaning protocol was followed, the incidence of site infection was not different whether standard gauze and povidone iodine, a transparent polyurethane dressing (eg, OpSite, Tegaderm) permeable to water vapor, or no dressing was applied.[109] Another study, however, found an increased risk of infection when transparent dressings were used.[110] A chlorhexidine-impregnated sponge dressing decreased the risk of catheter colonization and catheter-related infection in a prospective, randomized study.[111] The advantages and disadvantages of transparent dressings, gauze, or no dressing have been reviewed.[40]

Dressings should be replaced whenever damp, loosened, or soiled.[43] Moisture vapor-occlusive dressings are strongly recommended for patients with tracheostomies or open wounds near the catheter site. After 2 to 3 weeks, a clean technique is used in some institutions for nonneutropenic patients, and a Band-Aid or small gauze dressing may be used to cover the exit site.[11,112] More complete guidelines for access and maintenance of surgically inserted catheters are available.[6,14,21]

The effectiveness of antibiotic or iodine ointment used at the exit site in the prevention of infection has not been conclusively proved. Any ointment used should be checked for compatibility with the catheter material. Some ointments may allow fungal growth. For these reasons, their routine use is not recommended.[43,108]

The catheter is not usually considered to be securely anchored in place until 10 to 21 days after catheter placement, although insertion site stitches are usually removed after 10 days. Even then, catheters should not be allowed to hang freely; instead, they should be taped to the chest wall or inserted into a brassiere cup.[40] A clamp should be immediately available in the event of any breaks in the line. Some manufacturers include a clamp placed on the catheter. Patients should be advised to keep the catheter out of the reach of pets or small children who could inadvertently dislodge the catheter by pulling on it.

Because a thrombus on the catheter tip can be the nidus for a bacterial or fungal infection,[113,114] every effort should be made to prevent one from forming. Heparin should be instilled in nonvalved catheters after each episode of blood drawing or blood product administration and when the catheters are not being used for intravenous therapy. A wide variety of flushing regimens are reported in the literature with various concentrations and volumes of heparin and frequencies although few regimens are based on research. Based on a review of the available research-based practice, a flushing regimen of 5 mL of 10 units/mL heparin one or two times per week is recommended.[115] In one study, twice-weekly flushing, rather than daily, resulted in a 33% decrease in catheter-related bacteremia without an increase in thrombus or intraluminal clots.[116] A further decrease in intraluminal infection rate in immunocompromised, nonneutropenic patients with tunneled catheters may be provided by adding vancomycin to the heparin flush.[117,118] However, the antibiotic flush has been associated with increased antibiotic resistance and allergic reactions.[108] Recommendations for PICC flushes range from 3 mL of heparin (100 units/mL daily) to 3 mL of 10 units/mL three times per week.[14] The dose of heparin used to flush the catheter should not alter the patient's clotting factors. At a minimum, the flush should be twice the volume of the catheter plus any add-on devices.[119]

The use of the heparin flush alters coagulation tests if blood is drawn through the catheter.[120] The first 10-mL sample shows spurious elevations in levels of fibrin degradation products, prothrombin times, partial thromboplastin times, and spuriously low fibrinogen levels. Elevations in the prothrombin time and partial thromboplastin time will persist in the second 10-mL sample.

Valved catheters require a 5-mL to 10-mL normal saline flush weekly or after use.[11,20,21,39] The Groshong-type valve can be kept in the open position by small clots or solid residues from medications, allowing blood to flow back into the catheter, forming a clot.

Investigators have examined the potential role for using thrombophylaxis for cancer patients with central venous access devices. The most recent data show no proven role for using mini-dose warfarin or low molecular weight heparin. Their use has been shown to be safe and well-tolerated in such patients with hematologic malignancies and pronounced thrombocytopenia.[121] Some experts still advocate thrombophylaxis for patients at high risk for developing catheter-related complications. One study suggested fewer clinical and asymptomatic thrombotic events in patients treated with continuous infusion of unfractionated heparin (UFH) 100 international units/kg/day versus placebo (1.5% vs 12.6%)[122] Dalteparin prophylaxis using 5000 international units once daily did not reduce frequency of central venous catheter-related thrombosis in cancer patients.[123]

For apheresis catheters used for peripheral stem cell harvest, a regimen of aspirin (325 mg/day) begun the day after catheter placement led to a greater number of thrombosis-free apheresis procedures than were observed with historic control subjects.[124] More detailed guidelines for nursing education and practice regarding maintenance of catheters are available.[14,119]

Ports

Ports can be used immediately after insertion. However, because postoperative edema and discomfort often delay any attempts at access for several days, patients should be sent from the operating room with the Huber needle in place and ready for use.[14,28,40] Incisions should have a dressing until the sutures are removed. If skin closure is accomplished with surgical adhesive, a dressing is not required after the operative day and the site may get wet after the first day although it may be preferable to delay this longer.[108]

To access a port that has no needle in place, the skin is prepared with antiseptic; povidone-iodine or chlorhexidine are recommended.[14,43] Anesthetic agents that may be applied include ice or a cold pack for a few minutes, a freezing agent (ethylene dichloride), or topical anesthetic cream (EMLA), which must be applied one hour before needle insertion.[125] A 19- to 22-gauge Huber needle (depending on the product to be infused) is inserted (see Fig. 96–2).[28] This steel needle has a deflected point and side opening, designed to prevent coring of the septum.[27] The needle is primed with saline, attached to a saline-containing syringe and then inserted perpendicular to the septum.[126] Correct placement in the port can be confirmed by aspiration for blood return. However, aspiration for blood may be unsuccessful, usually because the needle is misaligned or a fibrin sheath has formed, creating a ball-valve effect. If there is no swelling, the port flows well to gravity and there is no other symptom to suggest a potential problem, the needle can be assumed to be correctly placed and the port safely used for nonvesicant infusions.[11] If access is difficult, it may be helpful to palpate the site while comparing it with a recent radiograph. Access may also be accomplished under fluoroscopy if standard technique by palpation is unsuccessful. Detailed accessing procedures for drawing blood and for administering drugs and blood products are available.[14,28,119,126]

During use, the port is covered with a sterile dressing. A transparent, occlusive dressing may be preferable to help stabilize the needle and prevent inadvertent dislodgment. Dressing guidelines for external catheters can be followed for ports. The needle is changed weekly. After each use or every 4 weeks, implanted access devices also require heparin instillation or a 20-mL saline flush for valved ports.[11,27,40] A variety of heparin concentrations and volumes have been reported. Use and maintenance of the peripheral port are essentially the same as for ports implanted in the chest wall.[24] More detailed guidelines for nursing education and practice regarding the maintenance of implanted ports and reservoirs are available.[14,119,127] Ongoing discussion continues regarding optimal maintenance procedures. One author suggested that assessments may be possible at a lesser frequency than every month, with greater cost-effectiveness, equal patient safety, and greater convenience.[128]

DEVICE REMOVAL

Device removal should be considered when it is no longer needed, in part to minimize risks of thrombosis and infection. Nontunneled catheters are removed nonsurgically by applying steady tension. If the catheter appears to be stuck, measures should be taken to reverse vasospasm (eg, application of warm compresses, flushing with normal saline).[12] If the catheter remains fixed, a cutdown on the venous insertion site to remove thrombotic material is usually effective.[9] Tunneled catheters should be removed by surgical cutdown around the cuff, which should be entirely removed.[9] For cases in which bacterial studies of the internal catheter tip are desired, blunt dissection of the cuff, with transection of the catheter above it and sterile removal of its inner portion, can be performed under local anesthesia.[129,130] Ports, including the reservoir, catheter, and all suture materials, are removed surgically with the patient under local anesthesia.[9]

COMPLICATIONS

Complications of indwelling vascular access devices include those occurring during the initial placement, cutaneous reactions to standard care materials, mechanical problems, phlebitis and infiltration, infection, hemorrhage, catheter occlusion of nonthrombotic or thrombotic origin, and vesicant drug extravasation.

Children

Pediatric-specific studies have cited age (younger than 5 years in one, younger than 2 years in another), use of multilumen catheters, absence of skin exit site suture, and platelet transfusion at time of insertion as the most common reasons for premature catheter removal.[131,132] Pediatric cancer patients with external catheters had more complications requiring device removal compared with port devices (23% vs 9%; infection occurred in 6% ports and 16% external catheters); occlusive events requiring removal occurred in 1.5% ports and 4.5% external catheters; fewer occlusive events in patients receiving urokinase vs heparin (23% vs 31%).[133]

Initial Placement

Rarely, patients who have had a midline catheter composed of a hydrogel elastomer inserted and flushed experience an anaphylactoid reaction (5% of which are complicated by cardiac arrest).[6,134] This reaction was not seen when silicone midline catheters were used.[135] Approximately 1% to 4% of patients in whom a central catheter is inserted percutaneously develop a pneumothorax.[9] Other surgical complications include hemothorax, arterial venous or cardiac perforation, brachial plexus injury, air embolism, and pericardial tamponade.[9,87]

Cutaneous Reactions

Approximately 5% of patients develop skin reactions to the products used in caring for the devices.[136] These reactions include erythema, urticaria, exanthematous or purpuric eruptions, and skin peeling or abrasion. These skin abnormalities must be distinguished from exit-site infections by appropriate culturing of the site for bacteria. In uninfected patients, changes in the dressing material, tape, and local skin care regimen are effective in reversing the skin abnormalities.[136] Skin reactions may be compounded when the patient has received radiation therapy to the area covered by the dressing.

Skin erosion over the implanted ports, caused by malnutrition, separated wound edges, local infection, or carcinoma metastatic to the skin, occurs in 3% to 10% of patients, and removal of the port is always required.[40,137] Peripheral ports may cause this complication more frequently than ports placed on the chest or abdominal wall.[9]

In very thin patients, the risk of erosion may be lower when a low profile rather than standard depth port is used.[59]

MECHANICAL PROBLEMS

Catheters

Damage to the external segment of the tunneled catheter includes separation between the Luer-Lok connection and the tubing; cracks caused by repeated cross-clamping, if rubber-tipped forceps are not used; and cuts made by scissors mistaken for clamps.[11] Catheter repair kits should therefore be available. Patients should also be instructed to contact their physicians or the oncology nursing staff immediately if the catheter is damaged at home.

Catheter fractures and emboli occur in about 0.2% of subclavian catheter insertions.[9] The internal portion of the catheter usually fractures at the junction of the clavicle and first rib,[138] and angiographic studies reveal the pathognomonic catheter pinch-off sign.[139] Catheter pinch-off occurs when catheters inserted medially to the midclavicular line become compressed by shoulder movements.[139] The resulting fragments migrate to the right heart or pulmonary artery and cause thromboses, cardiac arrhythmias, and fatal emboli; extravasation of fluids, lymph, or vesicant agents may also ensue at the site of breakage.[9,138] Patients complain of pain or swelling at the port or vein insertion site, chest pain, cough, or palpitations.[138] Catheter fragments are usually retrievable with interventional radiology techniques.[138,140,141]

PICC lines can also embolize if they are sheared by needles, sutures, or surgical instruments while they are being inserted. If the fragment cannot be prevented from migrating more proximally by applying local pressure at the break site or by placing a tourniquet proximal to the site, it can be removed by venous cutdown.[138,142] If it has migrated, percutaneous techniques or a thoracotomy will be required,[138,142] but some fragments are never retrieved. Apheresis catheters placed in the inferior vena cava can also develop fractures of the external segment, with visible leakage,[62] and they can be repaired using the kits mentioned earlier. Fractures of the internal portion of the catheter, however, require catheter removal. Most of these fractures can be detected by injecting radiologic contrast material through them and observing the flow of the dye fluoroscopically.[62]

Ports

The port may migrate or flip within its pocket because of defective suturing or excessive arm movement, or because of manipulation by the patient.[40,143] This malposition can be surgically corrected.

PHLEBITIS AND INFILTRATION

Phlebitis and infiltration are uncommon complications associated with properly positioned centrally placed access devices but are noted with the peripheral port[9] and in 2.2% to 23% of patients with PICCs.[6,25,56,144,145] Two studies of cancer patients with PICCs had comparable rates of phlebitis at 6.6% and 7%, respectively.[36,64] A randomized, controlled trial compared the complications associated with steel needles; small-bore, short Teflon catheters; and PICCs.[146] PICCs were associated with the highest incidence of phlebitis (27%) and the lowest incidence of infiltration (8.1%), steel needles were associated with the lowest incidence of phlebitis (8%) and the highest incidence of infiltration (45%), and Teflon catheters fell in between, with 19% to 20% incidences of phlebitis and infiltration. An aseptic phlebitis may occur within the first week after PICC insertion. It can be prevented by administration of nonsteroidal antiinflammatory agents[53] or treated with warm compresses applied for 48 to 72 hours.[15,56] Catheter removal is usually not required.

Infection

Definitions

The Centers for Disease Control and Prevention have established the following definitions for catheter- and port-associated infections.[43]

Localized catheter colonization: Significant growth of a microorganism (>15 CFU) from the catheter tip, subcutaneous segment of the catheter, or catheter hub.

Exit-site infection: Erythema, or induration within 2 cm of the catheter exit site, in the absence of concomitant bloodstream infection (BSI) and without concomitant purulence.

Clinical exit-site infection (or tunnel infection): Tenderness, erythema, or site induration of more than 2 cm from the catheter exit site along the subcutaneous tract of a tunneled catheter (ie, Hickman or Broviac) in the absence of concomitant BSI.

Pocket infection: Purulent fluid in the pocket of a totally implanted intravascular catheter that may or may not be associated with spontaneous rupture and drainage or necrosis of the overlaying skin in the absence of concomitant BSI.

Infusate-related bloodstream infection: Concordant growth of the same organism from the infusate and blood cultures (preferably percutaneously drawn) with no other identifiable source of infection.

Catheter-related bloodstream infection: Bacteremia or fungemia in a patient with an intravascular catheter with at least one positive blood culture obtained from a peripheral vein, clinical manifestations of infections (eg, fever, chills, or hypotension), and no apparent source for the BSI except the catheter. One of the following should be present: a positive semiquantitative (>15 CFU/catheter segment) or quantitative (>10^3 CFU/catheter segment) culture whereby the same organism (species and antibiogram) is isolated from the catheter segment and peripheral blood; simultaneous quantitative blood cultures with a 5:1 ratio for central venous catheter (CVC) versus peripheral; or differential period of CVC culture versus peripheral blood culture positivity of more than 2 hours.

INFECTION

Incidence

When expressed as infection rate per 1000 patient days, the highest risk exists with peripheral catheters placed by surgical cutdown; the next highest risk is with peripheral steel needles. Cuffed catheters and cuffed implantable devices have lower risks of infection than uncuffed ones. Cuffed devices share the lower rates of infection with outpatient, PICC and peripheral IV catheters, as well as ports.[147] Increasingly, standardized infection control procedures are utilized to help reduce CRBSI, as published by the CDC in 2005.[148]

Between 1% and 9% of patients experience infection at the exit site, tunnel, or pocket. Retrospective and prospective studies showed exit-site infections to be responsible for 39% to 45.5% and tunnel infections for 20.3% to 22% of all catheter-related infections.[51,149] Most catheter-related bloodstream infections for catheters in place for less than 10 days are of cutaneous origin from the insertion site, and gain access extraluminally, whereas for long-term devices in place for more than 10 days, luminal colonization is the major mechanism of CRBSI.[150] Prophylactic antibiotics have not consistently proven beneficial in preventing these infections, and their use is not recommended.[6,32,51] Catheters and cuffs coated or impregnated with antimicrobial or antiseptic show some promise in decreasing CRBSI. The compounds used are chlorhexidine/silver sulfadiazine, minocycline/rifampin, and platinum/silver, but there are concerns about the emergence of resistant organisms with these catheters.[43] The evidence supporting use of these compounds to reduce risk for CRBSI is equivocal for short-term CVCs and inconclusive for long-term CVCs in place longer than 10 days.[151] One randomized controlled study found low-dose unfractionated heparin via continuous infusion (100 units/kg/day) helped decrease fibrin deposition and decreased rates of CRBSI to 6.8% from 16.6%.[152] However, use of heparin remains controversial with questions of physical compatibility, chemical stability, and condition-limiting factors such as HIT.[153]

Infections are generally prevented by meticulous insertion and maintenance techniques.[100,154] PICCs inserted at the bedside versus those inserted by interventional radiologists show a higher rate of infection, probably because of insertion conditions (aseptic technique at the bedside versus sterile technique in the interventional radiology suite).[64,155] With maximal barrier precautions, however, catheter insertion at the bedside is associated with no higher infection incidence than placement in the operating room.[6]

The incidence of device-associated infection varies depending on the type of device inserted and the medical disorder of the patient. Conditions associated with CVC infections are more anecdotal and based on weaker evidence.[154] Overall, the incidence of midline catheter-associated infections is 0.8 per 1000 days of patient use[134] and that of tunneled catheters is approximately 1 to 3 per 1000 days of patient use.[32] Cumulative incidence of PICC-related BSI is 2.1 per 1000 PICC-days (range 0–6.5). The risk of PICC-related BSI per 100 PICCs is 3.2 overall; 2.5 in adults and children, and 3.8 in neonates.[156] The use of multiple-lumen catheters probably increases the infection rate significantly.[6] In one study, the sepsis rate for double- and triple-lumen catheters was comparable at 13% and 16%, respectively, but infections occurred significantly earlier with the triple-lumen catheters (a mean of 54 days vs 141).[45] There are fewer catheter-related bacteremias in TIVADs (totally implantable venous access devices) than tunneled catheters. Valved catheters have not altered the rate of infectious complications. Several social conditions contribute to greater risk of indwelling venous access device infections, including poor hygiene, and low socioeconomic status. For pediatric cancer patients, increased risk of infection is associated with language barriers limiting parental understanding of how to care for CVC.[154] The infection rate with implanted ports is lower, 0.2 to 0.3 per 1000 patient-days for ports inserted on the chest wall and 0.8 per 1000 patient-days for PAS Ports.[32,44,157,158] A prospective study of chest implanted ports revealed infection rates of 2.1% for local infections (ie, with cellulitis around the insertion site or reservoir), 2.2% for port pocket infections, and 4.4% sepsis.[46]

Neutropenic patients, particularly with a hematologic malignancy, have a near 14% greater risk of developing CRBSI.[159] Patients with HIV infection[68–71] and those receiving a bone marrow transplant,[60,61,160] have significantly higher rates of catheter- and port-related infections. Patients with hemophilia had a pooled incidence of 0.66 infections per 1000 CVAD days; age greater than 6 years and the use of fully implanted CVADs significantly reduced the risk of infection, while the presence of inhibitors significantly increased the risk.[47] For adult patients with sickle cell disease, bacterial infections are a leading cause of mortality, and one study cited a greater incidence of bloodstream infections (BSI) in younger patients with HbS disease, on transfusion and/or desferrioxamine programs, and in patients with a central venous catheter. Of all BSI episodes in these sickle cell patients, 41% were attributed to a venous catheter, and device infection occurred in 77% of patients with tunneled implantable ports.[161]

Patients with acute leukemia have a higher rate of infection than other patients with a cancer diagnosis, in part due to greater numbers of manipulations of the catheters, and possibly also due to longer periods of neutropenia.[35,154,162] They are also at higher risk for developing septicemia as a consequence of prolonged neutropenia.[163] The presence of a CVC increases the risk of infection in the early phases of low-intensity ALL treatment in pediatric patients.[164] Some tunneled catheters have a silver-impregnated collagen cuff in addition to the Dacron cuff to decrease infection rates but its usefulness is not definitive.[165] One prospective study cited a difference between CVAD-related infections in outpatients versus inpatients (25-fold higher incidence rate during hospital stay) for pediatric oncology patients. The cumulative incidence of CVAD-related BSI for these pediatric oncology inpatients was 2.21/1000 utilization days (UD) for Broviacs and 3.73/1000 UD for ports.[166]

Organisms

The most common organisms associated with hospital-acquired CRBSI are coagulase-negative staphylococci (37%), *Staphylococcus aureus* (13%), enterococci (13%), and *Candida* (8%).[43] Staphylococcal and candidal organisms adhere to the fibrin or fibronectin sheaths surrounding indwelling catheters, and some staphylococci produce a "slime" that further promotes bacterial proliferation on the catheter surface as the slime protects the organisms from phagocytes, antibodies and antibiotics.[106,114,167] Catheters with siliconized latex and polyvinyl chloride catheters have been shown to have more bacterial adherence than catheters made from other materials.[154] Coagulase-negative staphylococci also adhere to polymer surfaces more readily than other organisms. Other gram-negative organisms, including *Pseudomonas*, also cause infection.[9,168] *Pseudomonas* is particularly problematic when showering or swimming has been allowed. *Xanthomonas* (*Stenotrophomonas maltophilia*) infections can be particularly troublesome because of increasing multidrug resistance, formation of biofilm, and their prevalence in immediate post-CVC insertion setting and longer term indwelling setting. They are more prevalent in cancer patients with three independent risk factors: pneumonia, neutropenia at onset of bacteremia, and admission to ICU within one month of onset of bacteremia.[169,170]

A reported 5.4% to 9.9% of infecting organisms are fungal, three-fourths of which are *Candida* species,[5,32,51,171,172] although nosocomially acquired cutaneous infections with *Aspergillus flavus* have been noted at the sites of insertion and along the subcutaneous tract of Hickman catheters.[173–175] *Candida* infections in the oncology or bone marrow transplantation population are associated with a high mortality rate.[106] Infection with drug-resistant non-*C. albicans* is increasing in frequency in patients with CVCs.[176,177] In HIV-positive patients, staphylococci are the most common infecting organisms,[68–70] but *Pseudomonas* species causing fatal septicemia,[68,70,178–181] other gram-negative organisms,[182] and lactobacilli[183] are increasingly reported. Liposomal amphotericin B was successful in eradicating a port-associated fungemia from *Fusarium oxysporum* in an HIV-infected patient.[184] Septicemia due to catheter infection by typical or atypical *Mycobacterium* species has also been noted.[31,185–188]

S. aureus is the most common organism infecting ports of patients with hemophilia, especially those with inhibitors.[72,189] Other implicated organisms in hemophilia patients include *Pseudomonas* species, *Enterobacter cloacae*, *Escherichia coli*, *Klebsiella* species, *Serratia liquefaciens*, and *Acinetobacter* species.[47]

In adult sickle cell patients with CVADs, infections were seen with *Staphylococcus aureus*, *Escherichia coli*, *Acinetobacter* species, and *Pseudomonas*.[161]

INDICATIONS FOR REMOVAL

Debate continues over cost-effectiveness and salvage rates for catheters once CRBSI is documented.[190]

Exit-Site and Tunnel Infections

Exit-site infections caused by bacteria rarely require catheter removal for resolution, because most (69% to 100%) respond to antibiotics alone.[51,90,91,149,191] These infections are most often caused by *Staphylococcus epidermidis*.[29,32] Similarly, with implanted ports, infections of the skin pocket have been found to resolve in about 70% of cases without removal of the device.[31,32,52,99,191]

Tunnel infections or port pocket abscess, by contrast, usually do not respond to antibiotics; they have been reported to resolve without catheter removal in only 25% to 50% of cases.[1,51,90,91,149] Catheters were removed from all patients with cutaneous *Aspergillus* infection,

INFECTIOUS INDICATIONS FOR DEVICE REMOVAL[1,166]

Venous Access Devices

Tunnel infection or port pocket abscess

Catheter-related bacteremia caused by *Staphylococcus aureus, Xanthomonas, Pseudomonas* spp, mycobacteria, *Bacillus and Corynebacterium* species

Catheter-related fungemia

Septic thrombosis

Endocarditis

Osteomyelitis

Sepsis with signs of shock/persistent end-organ dysfunction

Central venous thrombosis

Central Nervous System Access Devices

Deep catheter track or epidural space infection

Mermel LA, Farr BM, Sheretz R, et al: Guidelines for the management of intravascular catheter-related infections. J Intraven Nurs 24:180, 2001.

Simon A, Bode U, Beutel K. Diagnosis and treatment of catheter-related infections in paediatric oncology: an update. Clin Microbiol Infect 12:606, 2006.

six of whom recovered after antifungal therapy and local wound care[172] (see box on Infectious Indications for Device Removal). Resolution of leukopenia was required for infection resolution. Similarly, *Mycobacterium*[31] and atypical mycobacterial infection of the tunnel or exit site requires catheter removal as well as excision of infected tissue.[188]

Septicemia

In a patient with septicemia and a catheter or port in place, it is often difficult to determine whether the catheter itself is truly infected or whether the bacteremia is from another source. Quantitative culture is the most sensitive technique,[6] but the semiquantitative roll-plate method is most often used to diagnose catheter-related infections.[192,193] Both, however, require that the catheter be removed. Quantitative blood culture techniques can be used with a catheter in place. If the colony count in cultures of blood drawn from the catheter is 5 to 10 times greater than the count in cultures of peripherally drawn blood, the infection is very likely to be catheter related.[6] For presumed *Candida* infection, it has been suggested that molecular analyses of material from various anatomic sites may help determine the true source of the infection (eg, sputum versus blood) and prevent needless device removal.[194]

In assessing the cause of infection in a patient with a port, care must be taken not to draw blood for culture through a possibly infected port pocket unless the Huber needle is already in place. Accessing a port through an infected port pocket could introduce organisms into the reservoir and from there into the systemic circulation.[40,191,195] To determine whether a port is truly infected, material within the port should also be cultured after it is removed.[196]

When another source is definitely identified, however, the catheters can usually be left in place, because the incidence of hematogenous colonization is low (1%).[51,81] When there is no thrombophlebitis, even when the catheter is believed to be the source of the infection, or when no source is clearly identified, resolution of bacterial septicemia occurs in 75% of episodes without removal of the catheter.[32,197]

The possibility of clearing the infection without catheter removal, however, is much lower in patients with septic thrombophlebitis, occluded catheters, exit-site infections, or bacteremia due to *S. aureus*, *Xanthomonas*, or *Pseudomonas* or fungal septicemia.[9,32,70,198,199] In one retrospective review, adult cancer patients with candidemia did just as well with catheters left in place as those whose catheters were removed;[200] and in one pediatric study, *Candida* fungemia was treated successfully with the line left in place.[7] In other studies, children and adults with catheter-related candidemia had higher rates of treatment failure, secondary complications, and mortality if the catheters were left in place during antifungal treatment.[201–203] Line removal is recommended when the fungemia is line related.[204] Successful surgical removal of right atrial thrombi superinfected with *Candida tropicalis* or *S. epidermidis* has been reported in several patients, including those with sickle cell anemia.[205,206] Replacement of catheters on the contralateral side within 1 to 3 days after removal is usually not associated with recurrent catheter infection.[81,99]

Antibiotic lock therapy (ALT), with and without concomitant parenteral therapy, has shown success in the prevention and treatment of catheter-related bacteremia when intraluminal infection is likely. Several trials have reported catheter salvage without relapse.[1,106] It involves instillation of an antibiotic solution, at a concentration of 1 to 5 mg/mL, into the catheter hub. The solution remains in place for a predetermined amount of time and is withdrawn before the next dose of intravenous antibiotic or medication. ALT itself allows much higher concentration and longer duration of activity of antibiotics at the colonized intraluminal/infected catheter surface without the potential side effects of systemic exposure. It also helps eradicate biofilm-forming bacteria. The goals include prolonging catheter life and reducing patient morbidity and costs associated with catheter-related infections. ALT can also be an option for salvaging venous access when venous access is otherwise limited, and patients have a CRBSI that has not progressed to septicemia and does not involve tissue infection at insertion or tunnel site.[153] ALT has been less effective for treating infections of implantable ports than infections from other types of CVCs.[153]

The most efficacious concentration and duration of ALT remains unclear, though the Infectious Disease Society of America recommends catheter locking for 14 days, with daily changing, in addition to 7-day systemic administration of antibacterial treatment for uncomplicated catheter-related bacteremias. It should be combined with systemic treatment for at least the first 72 hours.[166] At this time, no evidence-based recommendations are available regarding optimal concentration or intraluminal dwell time.[166] Combination ALT including minocycline/vancomycin, minocycline/rifampin, vancomycin/rifampin, is more effective in vitro against biofilm-forming coagulase negative staphylococci.[153,166] M-EDTA (minocycline plus EDTA) has demonstrated activity against gram-positive and gram-negative bacteria, as well as *Candida* species. A randomized control trial is needed to judge its efficacy for long-term CVC infections.[151] In general, ALT has not been as successful for fungal infections.[1,106]

In existing studies, several factors limit how best to use ALT. These include a lack of data from large, randomized control trials, comparing the efficacy of ALT to systemic antibiotics for treatment of line infections. Additionally, differences in antibiotics used for ALT, heterogeneity in study populations tested, presence or absence of heparin, and inconsistent definitions of catheter-related sepsis further complicate the generalizability of existing data. Overall, it appears ALT alone shortens the length of hospital stay, compared with systemic antibiotic therapy for treatment of line infections.

Taurolidine has been found to have broad bactericidal and fungicidal efficacy in vitro. It is active against methicillin-resistant *Staphylococcus aureus* (MRSA) and vancomycin-resistant enterococcus (VRE) and is felt not to select antibiotic-resistant microorganisms. It also might inhibit biofilm formation. Experiences are limited and require more study.[166]

Hemorrhage

Despite the frequent occurrence of thrombocytopenia in patients with indwelling access devices, few bleeding complications are associated with their placement or with the placement of the larger apheresis catheters.[81,90] Capillary fragility from prolonged steroid therapy, however, may contribute to perioperative hemorrhage.[90] Pressure dressings and platelet transfusions given pre- and postoperatively usually control local oozing.[81] However, in patients with uncontrolled disseminated intravascular coagulation, excessive bleeding has occurred with catheter insertion; many groups consider disseminated intravascular coagulation an absolute contraindication to catheter placement.[32,81,90] In contrast, catheters and ports have been placed without excessive bleeding in patients with hemophilia when factor levels were maintained at 100% preoperatively and for 5 days postoperatively.[189,207]

CATHETER OCCLUSION

Nonthrombotic Causes

Although a clot is the most common cause of occlusion,[167] inability to aspirate blood from the port or catheter does not necessarily mean that it has clotted. Other causes include a malpositioned Huber needle, catheter abutment against the wall of the vein, catheter kinking, catheter pinch-off, precipitation of drug solutions in the catheter lumen, development of fibrin sheaths, and catheter migration with resultant malposition of the tip.[40,167,208] Tip migration secondary to growth, especially during periods of growth spurts, is a problem specific to the pediatric population. Tip placement should be evaluated regularly as the child grows in height.[209] Algorithms for the evaluation and treatment of catheter occlusion are available.[167]

Catheter abutment may resolve by changing the patient's position or by performing a Valsalva maneuver.[21,28,40] Pinch-off occurs when the catheter is placed too medially and is compressed between the clavicle and first rib. Repositioning patients with catheter pinch-off often relieves the compression and reestablishes catheter function; but this is impractical for long-term catheter use, and the catheter usually needs to be repositioned.[138]

Precipitation of incompatible solutions occurs with etoposide, calcium, diazepam, phenytoin, heparin, and total parenteral nutrition (TPN) infusions.[167] Catheter blockage due to precipitation of calcium carbonate was reported at from 8 to 24 weeks in 50% of patients with metastatic colon carcinoma receiving once weekly 24-hour infusions of high-dose 5-fluorouracil (2600 mg/m^2) and leucovorin (500 mg/m^2).[210] Although precipitates may occasionally resolve with warm soaks over the tunnel site, dilute solutions of hydrochloric acid have successfully cleared precipitates from TPN solutions alone or with lipids, etoposide, calcium salts plus sodium bicarbonate, and heparin with incompatible antibiotics.[9,167] A solution of 0.1 normal HCl to equal the volume of the catheter is instilled and allowed to stand for 20 to 60 minutes.[141,167] Febrile reactions may occur. Sodium bicarbonate has resolved phenytoin, ticarcillin clavulanate, and oxacillin precipitates.[211,212] Lipid buildup or occlusions may respond to 70% ethanol instilled for 1 to 2 hours or sodium hydroxide (0.1N).[14,141]

Fibrin may start depositing on a catheter within 24 hours of insertion and may be present in as many as 67% of catheters.[213,214] Withdrawal occlusion secondary to the ball-valve effect of a fibrin sheath accounts for 10% to 57% of catheter occlusions.[11,29,208,215] The fibrin sleeve itself may embolize.[216,217] Presence of a fibrin sheath increases the risk of infection.[108] Techniques using nonlytic and lytic agents to remove the sheaths have been described.[28,40] Lytic therapy is discussed later.

Maintaining correct position of the catheter tip can help prevent numerous complications. Catheter migration occurs in 5.5% to 29% of insertions when the subclavian approach is used.[218] Review of the patient's chest radiograph most commonly shows the malpositioned catheter tip to be in the ipsilateral jugular vein, axillary vein, or in the contralateral brachiocephalic vein. When the catheter is in the jugular vein, patients often complain of a whooshing or gurgling sound when the line is flushed.[14] Venous thrombosis can occur as a result of damage to the endothelium, turbulence created by the tip at venous branching points, or insufficient dilution of infusate that causes thrombophlebitis. Catheter erosion through the vessel or cardiac wall can produce extravasation, fistula formation, and pericardial tamponade.[138] Catheters inserted into the left internal jugular or subclavian veins have also eroded into the bronchi; the ensuing venobronchial fistulas were associated with cough, pneumonia, and respiratory failure.[219] Repositioning the catheter can usually be done by interventional radiologists without catheter removal.[208,218]

PICC malposition ranges from 21% to 55%.[138] PICCs should be well secured at the insertion site to prevent "pistoning" in the vein, which increases the possibility of phlebitis or infection.[141] The catheters can usually be repositioned by trained nurses employing simple bedside techniques.[134] Migration of the apheresis catheter in the subcutaneous space also manifests as access failure, because the catheter tip is pulled back to the wall of the inferior vena cava or out of the intravascular space.[62] Intravascular malposition can be corrected by tip deflectors or J-wires.[220]

Thrombosis

Thrombosis can occur in the catheter itself or in the superior vena cava or veins of the upper extremity. While asymptomatic thromboses have been reported in rates up to 60%, most recent studies show an incidence of symptomatic catheter-related DVT to be lower than 6%, with similar rates of catheter-related DVT for access achieved through the subclavian and jugular veins.[221] Almost all central indwelling venous access devices become coated with a fibrin sheath within days of insertion, and accordingly, the majority of CVC-related thrombi arise within 30 days of initial placement.[222]

Several potential risk factors for indwelling access catheters and cancer patients have been studied. Catheter tip placement has been implicated in the formation of extraluminal thrombosis, with location high in the SVC accounting for a greater incidence of thrombosis than placement in the distal SVC or right atrium (62%–78% vs 16%).[45,46] Thrombogenicity was shown to be lesser in silicone and polyurethane CVC compared to polyvinylchloride and polyethylene CVC. Studies have yielded contrasting and inconclusive results regarding the impact of underlying thrombophilic states. In one study, factor V Leiden (FVL) and the prothrombin G20210A mutation (PGM) increased risk of CVC-related thrombosis threefold and led to a disproportionately high percentage of CVC thrombotic episodes.[223] In another study, neither PGM nor FVL were associated with thrombosis in cancer patients with ports, although a positive association was noted with elevated homocysteine levels.[224] Additional risk factors include greater than one attempt at insertion, a previous catheter (with vessel wall trauma and endothelial damage), ovarian cancer, and left-sided insertion site. There were no clear differences in the rate of CVC-related thrombosis with regard to chemotherapy administration methods (push/bolus vs infusion).[221,225] A threefold increased rate of catheter failure from thrombosis was noted for triple-lumen compared to double-lumen Hickman catheters.[222]

More clearly, a bidirectional impact of infection and thrombosis has been well-documented. One study reported a RR of 17 for developing clinical thrombosis manifestations after an episode of CVC-related infection, with 57% risk after an episode of CVC-associated septicemia versus 27% risk in patients with local CVC-infection only. Even in those patients with subclinical thrombosis, CVC-related infection occurred in 92%, compared with 7% without thrombosis.[226]

For pediatric patients, those with ALL receiving L-asparaginase and external catheters had 3.9 fold higher risk of CVC-thrombosis compared to children with implanted ports. Children with leukemia, neuroblastoma, and Hodgkin lymphoma with FVL, protein C deficiency, and high lipoprotein (a) levels had a significant association with symptomatic CVC-related thrombosis.[122]

For hemophilia patients, thrombosis has been a relatively rare event. A pooled incidence thrombosis of 0.056 per 1000 CVAD days has been cited, with no cases documented of superior vena cava syndrome or catheter-associated pulmonary embolism. Furthermore, neither age nor the presence of inhibitors significantly altered the thrombotic incidence. However, because thrombotic complications have been documented less extensively for hemophiliac patients (especially compared with infectious complications), the true extent of subclinical and clinical complications is unknown.[47]

For sickle cell patients, although the condition itself is considered hypercoagulable, it remains unclear how this, coupled with the presence of indwelling access devices, affects the incidence of clinically significant and symptomatic thrombosis.

A particularly vexing problem has been with frank development of upper extremity DVT (UEDVT). Spontaneous UEDVT has been reported to be 2.6-fold to 2.8-fold more likely in patients with active cancer, with the additional presence of an indwelling venous access device increasing the risk further. Clinical UEDVT has been reported to occur in 0% to 9% of patients with chest ports and 2% to 30% with arm ports. All told, central venous access devices account for 75% of all cases of UEDVT.[227] Another consideration is the postphlebitic and postthrombotic syndrome following UEDVT. Reported rates among cancer patients range from 4% to 30%.[121,122,222]

Noninvasive methods used for diagnosis of catheter-related thrombosis and/or UEDVT, including duplex ultrasound,[228–230] Doppler imaging,[228,231] and plethysmography,[228] have low sensitivity or have not been reliable. Color Doppler duplex sonography has been shown to have sensitivity 78% to 100% and specificity 82% to 100% for diagnosis of UEDVT. The primary difficulty remains the presence of overlying bones which may make difficult the visualization and direct assessment via compression techniques.[232] Nuclear scans can confirm patency of the line and vein, rule out superior vena cava syndrome, confirm catheter tip placement, demonstrate collateral circulation, and assess the presence of a fibrin sheath at the tip of the central line.[233] Spiral computed tomography (CT) can be helpful for suspected catheter-related thrombosis involving the brachiocephalic vein or superior vena cava (SVC), and for those with suspected pulmonary embolus.[122] Magnetic Resonancy Venography (MRV) has been studied but not proven to be a reliable alternative. Flow scintigraphy can be done faster than conventional venography, at lower cost, with lower radiation exposure, and with lower procedural risk (eg, reaction to iodinated contrast).[233] If venous obstruction is demonstrated, intraluminal versus extraluminal obstruction may be further defined by venography if clinically warranted.[52,62,228,233] In patients with prior central venous catheterization associated with deep venous thrombosis, preprocedural duplex ultrasound may be useful to predict the success of repeat catheter placement.[234]

THERAPY

The course of action is unclear in patients undergoing high-intensity antineoplastic therapy who develop asymptomatic subclavian, or innominate vein thromboses. Patients with symptomatic upper extremity deep venous thrombosis (DVT) require therapy. They may develop septic thrombophlebitis,[32,51] superior vena cava syndrome, major long-term upper extremity disability, venous gangrene, and pulmonary emboli. In one retrospective study and review, 12% of patients with catheter-induced upper extremity DVT developed pulmonary emboli, 40% of which occurred in patients receiving anticoagulant therapy.[228] A 16% incidence of pulmonary emboli was found in a prospective study of patients with upper extremity DVT in whom lung scans were performed within 24 hours of venographic diagnosis of the thrombosis.[235] Patients with polyurethane and siliconized catheters had a significantly lower incidence of emboli than those with polyvinyl chloride or polyethylene catheters (7% vs 26%).[235]

The National Comprehensive Cancer Networld (NCCN) published guidelines in late 2006 for catheter-related UEDVT to help guide clinicians in evaluation and treatment.[236] They suggest anticoagulation be used if DVT is present, the catheter is required, and there are no relative contraindications to anticoagulation. Suggested duration of therapy includes all time with the catheter in place, and for 1 to 3 months following its removal. If DVT symptoms or presence of clot persist despite this therapy, the catheter should be removed. If anticoagulation is contraindicated, then the catheter should be removed, the patient followed for any changes in relative contraindications, and anticoagulation initiated if otherwise permissible. A minimum of 3 to 6 months for DVT, 6 to 12 months for PE, and indefinite anticoagulation if active cancer or persistent risk factors, was recommended.

Management of Catheter Occlusion

Catheter occlusion, whether partial (sluggish flow), complete (inability to infuse or withdraw), or withdrawal type, have all been successfully treated with thrombolytic agents. Streptokinase, urokinase, and recombinant alteplase (t-PA) have all been used. Bolus thrombolytic therapy has reopened occluded catheters in 85% to 90% of episodes, and removal of the catheter is not usually required.[237–241] No excessive bleeding has been noted, even in patients with hemophilia.[189] Streptokinase is not commonly used because of its antigenic properties and associated allergic and anaphylactic reactions.[242] Urokinase was commonly used at a dose of 5000 units/2 mL until 1999, when the FDA reported the potential for viral contamination and it was removed from distribution.[243] No fevers, coagulation abnormalities, or other adverse reactions have been noted with urokinase. It is available again in recombinant form and has demonstrated efficacy for lysis of intraluminal thrombosis. Alteplase (t-PA) has demonstrated superiority and has become the preferred therapeutic option. A randomized trial comparing bolus urokinase (10,000 units) with t-PA (2 mg) suggested marked superiority for t-PA. Twenty-five of 28 t-PA–treated versus 13 of 22 urokinase-treated catheters returned to normal function; 17 versus 7 were normal radiographically; and 13 versus 4 needed only one drug instillation.[241] Alteplase is available for catheter clearance in a 2 mg/2 mL vial, a volume sufficient to fill most catheter lumens. The technique is to fill the catheter lumen plus 0.2 mL to ensure that the t-PA has close contact with any fibrin/clot at the distal tip of the catheter. It should dwell for 30 minutes to 2 hours and then be withdrawn. The dose may be repeated if withdrawal is unsuccessful.[212,242,244,245] If this is unsuccessful, an infusion of TPA 2 mg/50 mL infused over 4 hours may be used.[165] One Phase II trial examined Alfimeprase (recombinant fibrolase) because of its ability to cleave fibrin independently of plasminogen activation, as is necessary for t-PA, urokinase, and streptokinase.[246] Further study is planned.

For extraluminal thrombi refractory to the bolus administration of thrombolytics, options to dissolve the thrombus include infusions of t-PA, urokinase, or streptokinase through a catheter placed at or within the clot.[141,237,247] High-dose streptokinase therapy is effective[247] but expensive and is associated with a high incidence of bleeding. It is not recommended for patients with such bleeding risks as thrombocytopenia or mucositis. Infusion of urokinase for 24 to 72 hours restored catheter patency in 74% of patients (81% of those with clots present less than 7 days and 56% of those with clots present more than 7 days).[237] Infusion into the superficial venous circulation of the involved extremity was not effective. Even though a low infusion concentration was used (5000 international units/hour of streptokinase or 500 to 2000 international units/kg/hour of urokinase), a systemic lytic state was documented. Urokinase infusion should not be undertaken in patients with contraindications to systemic fibrinolytic therapy.[248] Another regimen for refractory clots involves an infusion of urokinase (40,000 units/hour) for 6 hours. This regimen led to dissolution of thrombi in 90% of patients; a repeat 6-hour infusion raised the dissolution rate to 95%.[249,250] Infusions as short as 1 to 3 hours were successful in one half the cases studied.[251] Addition of heparin to the 1- to 12-hour infusion did not improve the results.[251] No bleeding complications were seen. In patients with catheter tips placed below the carina and not adherent to the venous wall, there is a low risk of reocclusion; these catheters need not be removed.[251] Successful clot resolution with urokinase was reported for 50% to 87% of patients.[31,99]

Once patency is restored, heparin is usually given for 5 to 7 days. Studies have shown an increased risk of recurrent DVT/PE in cancer patients. Currently there is no sound evidence to guide duration of anticoagulant therapy in these patients. The recommended practice is to continue treatment while there is evidence of active cancer and while the patient is receiving antineoplastics.[252]

Vesicant Drug Extravasation

It is very unusual for a spontaneous leak to form in a large-bore catheter, but an attempt to irrigate an occluded catheter with a small syringe can cause a rupture through which the drug can extravasate.[11,81] Occlusion of the catheter tip by a fibrin sheath may force drugs back up the sheath and through the exit site of the catheter.[52,140,253] This so-called back-tracking appears to be more common with percutaneously placed access devices.[138]

Leaks may develop if the catheter is disconnected from the reservoir or if the catheter is punctured by mistake by the Huber needle.[40] Outpatients using a port for continuous infusion of chemotherapy can experience drug extravasation if the Huber needle is dislodged from the septum.[129,254–256] Even usually nonvesicant drugs can produce skin necrosis severe enough to warrant removal of the port.[129] Use of the Port-A-Cath port, which has a thicker septum than the Mediport and Infus-A-Port devices, has been associated with only a 3% to 4% incidence of extravasation.[99,254–256] The thickness of the septum has been postulated to be responsible for the low incidence of needle displacement noted with the Port-A-Cath,[256] but no randomized trials have compared complications associated with the three devices. Selection of an appropriate length Huber needle and securing the needle to the chest wall with tape or a transparent occlusive dressing can provide some protection against dislodgment. If infusion pumps are used, attention must be paid to minimizing tension between the needle and the infusion tubing.

CENTRAL NERVOUS SYSTEM ACCESS DEVICES

In patients with hematologic disorders, devices that permit chronic access to the CNS are useful for a variety of purposes. The available devices include temporary or permanent epidural catheters, ports with attached silicone elastomer catheters, implanted pumps with attached silicone elastomer catheters, and Ommaya reservoirs. The choice of device is determined by a number of factors, including available routes, duration of therapy, cost, efficacy for the therapy planned (eg, antineoplastics vs pain medications), and the ability of the patient and family to care for the device.[265]

Treatment of Vesicant Drug Extravasation

Treatment protocols for vesicant drug extravasation, including those recommended by the Oncology Nursing Society,[257] are outlined in Table 96–2.[258–263] When these protocols were used, 89% of vesicant extravasations were reported to resolve without additional therapy.[258] However, 30% of anthracycline extravasations progressed to ulceration. A prospective uncontrolled study of anthracycline extravasation showed that the application of DMSO four times each day for 4 days prevented progression to ulceration in all patients.[264]

At many centers, it is recommended that an extravasation kit be kept in units in which vesicant drugs are given. The kit includes the appropriate medications, as well as order sheets preprinted for immediate use. For most vesicant drugs there is no proved antidote or local care measures. The antidote for vinca extravasation, hyaluronidase, is no longer commercially available. In general, whether an antidote is to be administered through the device or not, as much of the residual drug as possible should be aspirated from the needle, tubing, and tissues. Any antidote may then be administered. If swelling or pain persists for 72 to 96 hours after drug administration, a plastic surgeon should be consulted.

Catheters

Local anesthetics alone or combined with fentanyl, other opioids, and medications given through temporary epidural catheters (in place for less than 5 days), have successfully managed the pain and have improved oxygenation in children with sickle cell crisis.[266] Chronic epidural access has become widely available since the development of a permanent epidural catheter that can be placed percutaneously.[267] The catheters are most commonly used for pain control. Some catheters are one piece, and others consist of three pieces: two radiopaque silicone rubber catheters, an epidural segment (1.3-mm outer diameter), and an exteriorized line (3.1-mm outer diameter, 0.68-mm inner diameter) with an external Luer connector and a subcutaneous Dacron cuff and a splice segment that joins the two catheter segments.[267]

Insertion

Catheter insertion is done under local anesthesia or conscious sedation.[267] A paravertebral incision is made at the level of the L2 dorsal spine, and the epidural portion of the catheter is inserted through a 14-gauge Hustead or Tuohy needle to the desired spinal cord level. Epidural placement is verified by fluoroscopy and sensory blockade. The exteriorized line is then tunneled from a subcostal location on the mid-nipple line around to the lower end of the paravertebral incision, and the splice segment is secured to the two catheters and then to the supraspinous tissue to avoid kinking. A Millex-OR 0.22-μm filter is attached to the Luer connector, and a locking Luer injection cap is connected to the filter.

Access and Management

The catheter can be used immediately. Bolus doses can be given from a syringe, or the catheter can be connected to external pumps that deliver continuous infusion opioid with bolus rescue doses or combinations of opioids and local anesthetics. Only preservative-free solutions should be used. Wound and catheter exit-site cleaning and dressing changes are recommended until the last sutures are removed, usually after 3 weeks. After that, the exit site is cleaned every other day with povidone iodine, and the filter and injection port are changed weekly using sterile technique.[14,267] More detailed nursing protocols for accessing and managing these catheters and for monitoring patients receiving epidural opioids are available.[14] Patient and family education in catheter care can be effectively supplemented by referral to a home health care or hospice agency.[265]

Complications

The catheters can remain safely in place for months,[268] but even temporary catheters can rarely cause serious infections if left in place for days to weeks.[269] Complications include those attributable to the opioids being infused, pain during injection,[270] myoclonus,[271] epidural fibrosis,[272] obstruction and dislocation,[270,273] and infection.[268,270,274,275] Patients whose catheters take longer to insert have higher infection rates.[275] Exit-site and superficial catheter track infections occur infrequently (in approximately 10% of patients).[268,274] The epidural space infection rate has been reported as 1 in 1702 days of catheter use, similar to the infection rate of 1 in 1045 per days of use associated with the Hickman catheter.[269] *S. aureus* and *S. epidermidis* account for two-thirds of all infections.[268,269] Exit-site and superficial catheter track infections may be cleared without catheter removal,[268,274] but catheter removal is required for patients with deep catheter track or epidural infections (see Table 96–3 and the box on Infectious Indications for Device Removal).[268]

Table 96–2 Management of Vesicant Drug Extravasation

Drug Therapy	Local Care	Antidote Administration
Antibiotics		
Doxorubicin	Cold/ice pack for 15–20 min qid for 24–48 hours	Apply 1–2 mL of 99% DMSO to site every 6 hours.
Mitomycin-C		Apply 1–2 mL of 99% DMSO to site every 6 hours.
Vinca alkaloids		
Vincristine	For all vincas, elevate and apply warm pack for 15–20 min at least qid for 24–48 hours.	
Vinblastine		
Vindesine		
Vinorelbine		
Taxane		
Paclitaxel	Cold/ice pack 15–20 minutes qid for 24–48 hours.	
Alkylating agents		
Mechlorethamine		Mix 1.2 mL of 25% sodium thiosulfate with 8.4 mL of sterile water for injection. Through existing IV line, inject 2 mL of antidote for each 1 mg of drug extravasated. Remove needle and inject subcutaneously around site.
Cisplatin (only if >20 mL of 0.5 mg/mL concentration infiltrates)		Use sodium thiosulfate as above, 2 mL for each 100 mg of cisplatin infiltrated.

From: Scheiner JD, Van den Abbeele AD: Flow scintigraphy: Surgical lines and their associated veins. Clinical Nuclear Medicine Workshop, Harvard Medical School Department of Continuing Education, Boston, MA, 1996.

Povoski SP, Zaman SA. Selective use of preoperative venous duplex ultrasound and intraoperative venography for central venous access device placement in cancer patients. Ann Surg Oncol 9:493, 2002.

Monreal M, Raventos A, Lerma R, et al: Pulmonary embolism in patients with upper extremity DVT associated to venous central lines: A prospective study. Thromb Haemost 72:548, 1994.

Wagman LD, Baird MF, Bennett CL, et al. Venous thromboembolic disease clinical practice guidelines in oncology. J Natl Compr Canc Netw 4:838, 2006.

Fraschini G, Jadeja J, Lawson M, et al: Local infusion of urokinase for the lysis of thrombosis associated with permanent central venous catheters in cancer patients. J Clin Oncol 5:672, 1987.

Hurtubise MR, Bottino JC, Lawson M, McCredie KB: Restoring patency of occluded central venous catheters. Arch Surg 115:212, 1980; Glynn MFX, Langer B, Jeejeebhoy KN: Therapy for thrombotic occlusion of long term intravenous alimentation catheters. JPEN J Parenter Enteral Nutr 4:387, 1980.

Lawson M: Partial occlusion of indwelling central venous devices. J Intraven Nurs 14:157, 1991.

Table 96–3 Important Pathogens in Central Venous Access Device-related Infections.

Pathogen	Source	Notable Complications
Gram-positive bacteria	Hub; skin at exit site of device	
Coagulase-negative staphylococci		
Methicillin-resistant *S. aureus*		Local/systemic suppurative complications
Staphylococcus epidermidis		
Enterococci, including vancomycin-resistant *Enterococcus*	Intestines	
α-hemolytic streptococci	Oropharynx	
Gram-negative bacteria		
Pseudomonas aeruginosa		
Klebsiella spp.		

Epidural Ports and Implanted Pumps

Epidural ports (eg, Port-A-Cath) and implanted pumps (eg, Infusaid, Medtronic) have also been used to deliver bolus or continuous infusions of opioids into the epidural or intrathecal space to relieve pain of malignant or nonmalignant origin.[271,274] Subarachnoid infusions using the implanted pumps are recommended as efficacious and cost-effective for patients with a relativel long life expectancy (>3 months).[271] The use of implanted pumps has been reviewed elsewhere.[276]

Complications include those previously described for implanted ports and pain on injection of morphine, pump pocket seromas, CSF leaks, CSF hygromas, and postspinal headache.[271,277] But the use of injection ports appears to reduce the rate of complications associated with percutaneously inserted epidural catheters. A retrospective comparison of catheters with or without associated injection ports indicated that those attached to ports became dislodged much less frequently and were associated with one-half the infection rate per 1000 patient-days.[278] Port removal rates for infection were similar to removal rates of ports used for vascular access (10%).[277] Because the seromas act as growth media for bacterial contamination, they should be monitored carefully. The management of hygromas and postspinal headache is reviewed elsewhere.[271] Ports and pumps can also erode through the skin.[14] Detailed access and management procedures for epidural ports and implanted pumps and for monitoring patients receiving opioids through them are available.[14,30]

Ommaya Reservoir

The Ommaya reservoir device was first described in 1963 by Ommaya,[279] and with minimal changes, it is still used for access to the spinal fluid within the cerebral ventricle. The reservoir is used to remove CSF for culture, cytology, or measurement of drug levels; to drain cysts in craniopharyngiomas and astrocytomas; to administer antibiotics or antifungal agents; to administer intraventricular chemotherapy to treat leukemic or carcinomatous meningitis; to administer interferon or lymphokine-activated killer cells directly into a tumor; and to administer opioid pain medications.[265,280]

The device consists of a dome- or mushroom-shaped capsule with a top made of a self-sealing silicone elastomer that can be punctured numerous times without leaking. The flat base of the capsule, by contrast, is composed of firm polypropylene and is not easily punctured. An outlet arm connected to a ventricular catheter is attached at the base, laterally or in the center, extending downward. Capsules range from 12 mm in diameter (for babies) to 30 mm. Those commonly used for adults have an internal volume capacity of 1.45 to 2.4 mL.

Insertion

The Ommaya reservoir is placed subcutaneously by a neurosurgeon.[281] Before insertion, CT is generally required to evaluate ventricular size and placement. Presoaking the device in bacitracin to prevent subsequent infection has been advocated.[282] For placement, the ventricular catheter is passed through a burr hole into the frontal horn of the right lateral ventricle or, if necessary, into that of the left lateral ventricle or the ventricle body. The catheter end is connected to the base or side arm of the capsule, which then is fitted into the burr hole or a subgaleal pocket. The Silastic skirt of the reservoir may be sutured to the periosteum. A postoperative CT scan is suggested to verify the catheter tip position. Stereotactic techniques are used when the ventricle is small or misplaced.[283]

Accessing the Device

The Ommaya reservoir can be used immediately postoperatively for sampling CSF or for injection of drugs. Usually, however, it is not accessed until the third postoperative day.[280] The thoroughly cleaned, gently shaved scalp is prepared with three iodine scrubs, and with the use of a sterile technique, the reservoir is accessed obliquely with a 23- or 25-gauge butterfly needle inserted with the bevel downward.[280] The CSF can be directly aspirated, or antibiotics or chemotherapeutic agents can be administered through a second syringe attached to the butterfly needle. After removal of the needle, the injected medication can be gently pumped into the spinal fluid by emptying the capsule using repeated pressure, but to allow CSF to refill the reservoir, the clinician should avoid steadily compressing the device.[284] After the incision has healed and the stitches have been removed, no special local care or flushing is required. The device can remain in place for months or years. More detailed accessing and management guidelines are available.[14]

Complications

Infection

In general, the Ommaya reservoir has proved very safe, with a complication rate of 9% to 20%,[281,282,285–287] although higher rates were reported in the past.[288] The most common complication is infection, which occurs in about 1% to 15% of patients,[286,287] especially those who have undergone radiation therapy or who required a second surgical procedure for revision of the catheter.[281] Most infections have been caused by *S. epidermidis*, but infections from numerous other gram-positive and gram-negative bacteria and fungal organisms have been documented.[286,289] In general, the device is not removed, and patients are treated as though they had meningitis. For infections with *S. epidermidis*, vancomycin is given intravenously[290] or, in refractory cases, instilled into the reservoir.[291] Removal of the reservoir is sometimes required.

Miscellaneous Complications

Neurologic complications are rare when the catheter is placed into the nondominant ventricle, but a variety of other complications, which occur infrequently, have been reported. These include intraventricular hemorrhage or subdural hematoma shortly after catheter placement; leakage of CSF around the catheter, primarily in patients with increased intracranial pressure, which caused backflow of fluid along the catheter and produced a subgaleal collection[288,292]; reservoir leaks after repeated use[285]; occlusion by cellular debris or, when a catheter is placed directly into a tumor, by very proteinaceous tumor fluid[285]; obstruction by lodging of the catheter in brain tissue or abutment against a ventricle wall[285]; seizures immediately after injection of medications[285]; white matter disease (leukoencephalopathy or brain necrosis), most often due to methotrexate injection through the Ommaya device, although found with systemic administration of methotrexate as well[285,293]; and tumor growth around the cannula. In one case, the catheter may have permitted the spread of Burkitt lymphoma cells from the meninges into the cerebral tissue, where the tumor was found.[294]

SUGGESTED READING LIST

Agnelli G, Verso M: Therapy insight: venous-catheter-related thrombosis in cancer patients. Nat Clin Pract Oncol 3:214, 2006.

Boktour M, Hanna H, Ansari S, et al: Central venous catheter and *Stenotrophomonas maltophilia* bacteremia in cancer patients. Cancer 106:1967, 2006.

Cunningham MS, White B, Hollywood D, O'Donnell J: Primary thromboprophylaxis for cancer patients with central venous catheters: a reappraisal of the evidence. Br J Cancer 94:189, 2006.

Gaitini D, Beck-Razi N, Haim N, Brenner B: Prevalence of upper extremity deep venous thrombosis diagnosed by color Doppler duplex sonography in cancer patients with central venous catheters. J Ultrasound Med 25:1297, 2006.

Ho KM, Litton E: Use of chlorhexidine-impregnated dressing to prevent vascular and epidural catheter colonization and infection: a meta-analysis. J Antimicrob Chemother58:281, 2006.

Karthaus M, Kretzschmar A, Kroning H, Biakhov M, et al: Dalteparin for prevention of catheter-related complications in cancer patients with central venous catheters: final results of a double-blind, placebo-controlled phase III trial. Ann Oncol 17:289, 2006.

Lai CH, Wong WW, Chin C, et al: Central venous catheter-related *Stenotrophomonas maltophilia* bacteraemia and associated relapsing bacteraemia in haematology and oncology patients. Clin Microbiol Infect 12:986, 2006.

Lee, AY, Levine MN, Butler G, et al: Incidence, risk factors, and outcomes of catheter-related thrombosis in adult patients with cancer. J Clin Oncol 24:1404, 2006.

Linenberger ML: Catheter-related thrombosis: risks, diagnosis, and management. J Natl Compr Canc Netw 4:889, 2006.

Moll S, Kenyon P, Bertoli L, et al: Phase II trial of alfimeprase, a novel-acting fibrin degradation agent, for occluded central venous access devices. J Clin Oncol 24:3056, 2006.

Simon A, Bode U, Beutel K: Diagnosis and treatment of catheter-related infections in paediatric oncology: an update. Clin Microbiol Infect 12:606, 2006.

Snydman DR: Prevention of catheter and intravascular device-related infections: a quality-of-care mandate for institutions and physicians. Mayo Clin Proc 81:1151, 2006.

Swerdlow PS: Red Cell Exchange in Sickle Cell Disease. Hematology Am Soc Hematol Educ Program. 2006;48–53.

Wagman LD, Baird MF, Bennett CL, et al: Venous thromboembolic disease clinical practice guidelines in oncology. J Natl Compr Canc Netw 4:838, 2006.

Zarrouk V, Habibi A, Zahar J-R, et al: Bloodstream infection in adults with sickle cell disease: association with venous catheters, staphylococcus aureus, and bone-joint infections. Medicine 85:43, 2006.

REFERENCES

For complete list of references log onto www.expertconsult.com

CHAPTER 97

LATE COMPLICATIONS OF HEMATOLOGIC DISEASES AND THEIR THERAPIES

Wendy Landier and Smita Bhatia

Survival of patients with hematologic malignancies has improved markedly over the past 3 decades. The population of long-term cancer survivors continues to grow. Sixty-six percent of adults and 79% of children with malignancies survive 5 years after diagnosis.[1] It is estimated that there are more 10 million 5-year cancer survivors in the United States, and approximately 15% of these survivors have been alive for 20 years.[2]

With this success comes the need to consider the long-term morbidity and mortality associated with the treatments responsible for increased survival. Late effects among individuals treated for cancer have been the topic of numerous reviews.[3–8] Disease- or treatment-specific subgroups of long-term survivors have been shown to be at risk for developing adverse outcomes, including premature death, second neoplasms, organ dysfunction (e.g., cardiac, pulmonary, gonadal), reduced growth and development, decreased fertility, impaired intellectual function, difficulties obtaining employment and insurance, and overall reduced quality of life.

Hematopoietic cell transplantation (HCT) is the treatment of choice for patients with hematologic malignancies experiencing recurrent disease after therapy with conventional regimens and for those with disease characteristics associated with a very poor prognosis when treated with conventional chemotherapy and radiation regimens. Complications observed after HCT often have a multifactorial origin encompassing issues related to prior cancer therapy, intensity of the preparative regimen, graft-versus-host disease (GVHD), and other posttransplantation complications.[9–16]

This chapter summarizes select long-term adverse outcomes in individuals treated with conventional therapy and HCT for hematologic malignancies. Recommendations for providing ongoing followup care to this population of survivors are reviewed.

CARDIAC EFFECTS

Chronic cardiotoxicity after therapy for hematopoietic malignancies usually manifests as cardiomyopathy, congestive heart failure, or pericarditis. The anthracyclines, notably doxorubicin and daunorubicin, are well-known causes of late-onset cardiomyopathy, characterized by increased afterload followed by development of a dilated, thin-walled left ventricle that eventually becomes poorly compliant. A review of 30 published studies determined that the frequency of clinically detected anthracycline-related congestive heart failure among survivors treated for cancer during childhood ranged from 0% to 16%.[17] In an analysis across reported studies, the type of anthracycline (e.g., doxorubicin) and the maximum dose given in a 1-week period (i.e., >45 mg/m^2) was found to explain a large portion of the variation in the reported frequency of anthracycline-induced congestive heart failure. The incidence of anthracycline-induced cardiomyopathy, which is dose dependent, may exceed 30% among survivors who received cumulative doses in excess of 600 mg/m^2.[18] Moreover, a cumulative anthracycline dose greater than 300 mg/m^2 administered during childhood has been associated with an 11-fold increased risk for clinical heart failure, compared with a cumulative dose of less than 300 mg/m^2, with the estimated risk of clinical heart failure increasing with time from exposure and approaching 5% after 15 years.[18]

The incidence of subclinical anthracycline-related myocardial damage has been the subject of considerable interest. A review of the literature on subclinical cardiotoxicity among children treated with an anthracycline found that the reported frequency of subclinical cardiotoxicity varied considerably across the 25 studies reviewed (frequency range 0%–57%).[17] Steinherz et al.[19] found that 23% of 201 patients who had received a median doxorubicin cumulative dose of 450 mg/m^2 had echocardiographic abnormalities a median of 7 years after therapy. In a group of childhood leukemia survivors who received a median doxorubicin cumulative dose of 334 mg/m^2, progressive elevation of afterload or depression of left ventricular contractility was present in approximately 57% of patients.[20] Because of marked differences in the definition of outcomes for subclinical cardiotoxicity and because of the heterogeneity of the patient populations investigated, accurate evaluation of the potential long-term outcomes within anthracycline-exposed patient populations or the potential impact of the subclinical findings is difficult.

Among anthracycline-exposed patients, the risk for cardiotoxicity can be increased by mediastinal irradiation,[21] uncontrolled hypertension,[22,23] underlying cardiac abnormalities,[24] exposure to chemotherapeutic agents other than anthracyclines (e.g., cyclophosphamide, dactinomycin, mitomycin C, dacarbazine, vincristine, bleomycin, and methotrexate),[23,25,26] and electrolyte imbalances such as hypokalemia and hypomagnesemia.[27] Risk also is increased for survivors who are female,[28] who are African American,[29] and who were very young (age <5 years) at the time of therapy.[30]

Chronic cardiac toxicity associated with radiation alone most often manifests as pericardial effusions or constrictive pericarditis, sometimes in association with pancarditis. This risk is associated with radiation dose and volume and is lifelong; absolute risk increases with length of time since exposure.[31] Although a 40-Gy dose of total heart irradiation appears to be the usual threshold, pericarditis has been reported after doses as low as 15 Gy, even in the absence of radiomimetic chemotherapy.[32] Symptomatic pericarditis, which usually develops 10 to 30 years after irradiation, is found in 2% to 10% of patients.[33] Subclinical pericardial and myocardial damage as well as valvular thickening may be common in this population.[34] Coronary artery disease has been reported after radiation to the mediastinum, although mortality rates have not been significantly higher in patients who receive mediastinal irradiation than in persons in the general population.[35]

Data regarding late cardiotoxicity after HCT are scarce, with studies limited because of small sample size and short followup.[9,36] Late cardiac dysfunction after HCT is multifactorial in origin. Factors that may increase the risk for its development include prior therapy with anthracyclines, total body irradiation (TBI), cyclophosphamide, and other cardiotoxic drugs. Damage often is subclinical and may not be detected by routine methods of investigation. More invasive methods, such as radionuclide angiography, may be required.

Comorbidities resulting from cancer treatment may increase the risk for cardiovascular disease in survivors. Oeffinger et al.[37] found that 62% (16/26) of young adult survivors of childhood acute lymphoblastic leukemia (ALL) had at least one cardiovascular risk factor (obesity, dyslipidemia, increased blood pressure, insulin resistance) potentially related to their cancer treatment. Patients treated with cranial radiation therapy had an increased incidence of obesity and dyslipidemia compared with those who received chemotherapy alone.

Given the known acute and long-term cardiac complications of cancer therapy, prevention of cardiotoxicity is a focus of active investigation. Previous reports have suggested that doxorubicin-induced cardiotoxicity can be prevented by continuous infusion of the drug.[38–40] Lipshultz et al.[41] compared cardiac outcomes in children with leukemia who received bolus or continuous infusion doxorubicin and reported that continuous doxorubicin infusion over 48 hours did not offer a cardioprotective advantage over bolus infusion. Both regimens were associated with progressive subclinical cardiotoxicity.

Agents such as dexrazoxane, which remove iron from anthracyclines, have been investigated as cardioprotectants. Clinical trials of dexrazoxane have been conducted, with encouraging evidence of short-term cardioprotection among children.[42] In a study of 206 children with ALL who were randomly assigned to receive doxorubicin with or without dexrazoxane, Lipshultz et al.[43] demonstrated that patients treated with doxorubicin alone were significantly more likely to have elevated troponin T levels, indicative of myocardial injury, than those who received doxorubicin with dexrazoxane, with no difference in event-free survival at 2.5 years. However, comprehensive long-term followup is required to document that dexrazoxane does have a cardioprotective effect while maintaining comparable event-free survival.[44,45] No peer-reviewed, published, randomized controlled trials have addressed the efficacy of dexrazoxane for preventing cardiac toxicity in adult patients receiving doxorubicin-based therapy for malignancies other than breast cancer. The long-term avoidance of cardiotoxicity with use of dexrazoxane has yet to be sufficiently determined.

PULMONARY EFFECTS

Compromise of pulmonary function among survivors of hematologic malignancies has been reported after conventional therapy for Hodgkin lymphoma[46–48] and leukemia[49,50] and after HCT.[10,11,51] Impairments evident by pulmonary function testing include reductions in total lung capacity, forced vital capacity, forced expiratory volume, and gas transfer, suggesting obstructive and restrictive defects. Risk factors include exposure to certain chemotherapeutic agents (particularly bleomycin), radiation to the chest, underlying lung disease, and younger age at exposure to the pulmonary-toxic therapeutic agents.

Significant late toxicities involving the airway and lung parenchyma, including restrictive and chronic obstructive lung disease and bronchiolitis obliterans, are observed in 15% to 40% of patients after HCT. Restrictive lung disease is related to pretransplant chemotherapy as well as therapeutic exposures used during conditioning.[52] Bronchiolitis obliterans has a strong correlation with chronic GVHD, has been reported in up to 14% of allogeneic transplantation recipients, and carries a mortality rate of 50%.[53]

ENDOCRINOLOGIC EFFECTS

Thyroid

Patients with hematologic malignancies who are treated with cranial, craniospinal, or mantle irradiation are at increased risk for thyroid complications. Among survivors of Hodgkin lymphoma (and, to a lesser extent, leukemia), abnormalities of the thyroid gland, including hypothyroidism, hyperthyroidism, and thyroid neoplasms, have been reported to occur at rates significantly higher than those found in the general population.[54–56] Hypothyroidism is the most common nonmalignant late effect involving the thyroid gland. After exposure to radiation at doses greater than 15 Gy, laboratory evidence of primary hypothyroidism is evident in 40% to 90% of patients with Hodgkin lymphoma and non-Hodgkin lymphoma.[55,57,58]

In an analysis of 1791 5-year survivors of pediatric Hodgkin lymphoma (median age at followup 30 years), Sklar et al.[54] reported the occurrence of at least one thyroid abnormality in 34% of subjects. The risk of hypothyroidism was increased 17-fold compared with sibling controls. Increasing dose of radiation, older age at diagnosis of Hodgkin lymphoma, and female gender were identified as significant independent predictors of increased risk. The actuarial risk of hypothyroidism for subjects treated with 45 Gy or more was 50% at 20 years after diagnosis of Hodgkin lymphoma. Hyperthyroidism was reported to occur in only 5%.

In another large cohort of 1677 patients with Hodgkin lymphoma treated with irradiation involving the thyroid at Stanford University Hospital between 1961 and 1989 (mean age at diagnosis 28 years, mean duration of followup 9.9 years), the actuarial risk of developing thyroid disease was 52% at 20 years and 67% at 26 years after treatment. In this population, the actuarial risk of developing overt or subclinical hypothyroidism was 44% by 25 years after therapy; the risk of developing thyroid cancer was 1.7% (15.6 times the expected risk).[55]

Most cases of overt hypothyroidism after HCT result from primary hypothyroidism caused by radiation injury. The incidence of hypothyroidism after HCT depends on the type of myeloablative conditioning regimen, ranging from as high as 90% after exposure to single-dose TBI to 10% to 15% after fractionated TBI.[13,14]

Thyroid nodules are common in patients treated with neck radiation for Hodgkin lymphoma, but the majority of these nodules do not undergo malignant transformation.[59,60] In a study of 647 children treated for Hodgkin lymphoma, 67 developed thyroid nodules during or after therapy (median time between diagnosis of Hodgkin lymphoma and thyroid nodule 10.5 years, range 0.2–24.8 years). All but one of these patients had received neck radiation as part of their therapy, with a median dose to the thyroid of 35 Gy. Seven (10%) of the 67 nodules were malignant.[59]

Growth

Poor linear growth and short adult stature are common complications after successful treatment of hematologic malignancies in childhood. The adverse impact of central nervous system (CNS) irradiation on adult final height among childhood leukemia patients has been well documented, with final heights below the fifth percentile in 10% to 15% of survivors.[61–64] The effects of cranial irradiation appear to be related to age and gender, with females and children younger than 5 years at the time of therapy being more susceptible. The precise mechanisms by which cranial irradiation induces short stature are not clear. Disturbances in growth hormone production have not been found to correlate well with observed growth patterns in these patients.[65,66] The phenomenon of early onset of puberty in girls receiving cranial irradiation may play some role in the reduction of final height.[67,68] Results regarding the impact of chemotherapy on final height in childhood leukemia survivors not treated with cranial irradiation are conflicting.[62,69]

Impaired linear growth after HCT likely is due to an interaction of multiple factors, including host characteristics (young age), treatment exposures (prior cranial irradiation, TBI), and post-HCT complications, such as chronic GVHD.[14] Findings suggest that final height is unaffected in children who receive busulfan or cyclophosphamide as pretransplant conditioning.[70]

Obesity

An increased prevalence of obesity has been reported among survivors of childhood ALL.[71] In an analysis from the Childhood Cancer Survivor Study, Oeffinger et al.[72] compared the distribution of body mass index of 1765 adult survivors of childhood ALL with that of 2565 adult siblings of childhood cancer survivors. Survivors were significantly more likely to be overweight (body mass index 25–30) or obese (body mass index ≥30). Risk factors for obesity were cranial irradiation, female gender, and age 0 to 4 at diagnosis of leukemia. Females diagnosed before age 4 years who received a cranial radiation dose more than 20 Gy were found to have a 3.8-fold increased risk for obesity. Obesity has the potential to adversely impact the overall health status of survivors and is associated with insulin resistance, diabetes mellitus, hypertension, and dyslipidemia. Growth hormone deficiency related to cranial radiation may predispose adult survivors of childhood ALL, particularly females, to metabolic syndrome.[73]

Gonadal Dysfunction

Treatment-related gonadal dysfunction has been well documented in male and female patients after therapy for hematologic malignancies. A reasonable body of research provides a basis for counseling patients regarding the long-term gonadal effects of radiation and chemotherapy.

Radiation effects on the ovary are age and dose dependent. It has been estimated that 50% depletion in oocytes occurs after the ovaries are exposed to 2 Gy.[74] Amenorrhea develops in approximately 68% of prepubescent females treated with ovarian doses of 12 to 15 Gy for Hodgkin lymphoma, whereas 100% of adult females older than 40 years sustain irreversible ovarian failure after doses of 4 to 7 Gy.[75] Spinal irradiation for treatment of childhood leukemia appears to result in clinically significant ovarian damage in some survivors.[76] Cranial irradiation in young girls is associated with an increased risk for premature puberty.[77]

The effects of radiation on testicular function, including germ cell number and Leydig cell function, have been investigated. Reduced sperm production has been observed after testicular doses of 1 to 6 Gy and follows a dose-dependent pattern.[78] Azoospermia has been reported among patients with Hodgkin lymphoma with calculated testicular irradiation exposures ranging from 1 to 3 Gy.[79] Testicular doses between 4 and 6 Gy have been associated with prolonged azoospermia and decreased testicular volume.[80] The limited data on the long-term outcomes of very young males treated for Hodgkin lymphoma suggest germ cell effects similar to those seen in older patients with Hodgkin lymphoma.[81] Leydig cells, although also impacted by radiation in a dose-dependent fashion, require higher exposure levels to sustain damage than those seen for the germ cells.[82] Testicular dose of 24 Gy among prepubertal males have been reported to be associated with delayed pubertal development and abnormal testosterone and gonadotropin levels.[83–85]

Ovarian and testicular damage can result from chemotherapeutic agents, with alkylating agents showing the strongest association. Effects of chemotherapy on gonadal function typically are gender, age, and dose dependent. The ovaries tend to be less sensitive to the effects of alkylating agent exposure than are the testes. Ovarian dysfunction has been well documented in patients with Hodgkin lymphoma treated with alkylating agents, singly or in combination (e.g., MOPP regimen consisting of mechlorethamine, Oncovin [vincristine], procarbazine, and prednisone or a COPP regimen consisting of cyclophosphamide, Oncovin [vincristine], procarbazine, and prednisone).[86,87] MOPP and COPP regimens have been reported to result in azoospermia in more than 90% of exposed males.[88] Even with a reduction in the dose of cyclophosphamide in the hybrid COPP/ABV regimen for treatment of Hodgkin lymphoma, the majority of young males are infertile, likely due to the procarbazine component of this regimen.[89]

Young boys and adolescent males with aplastic anemia who receive standard-dose cyclophosphamide alone (200 mg/kg) as the pretransplant conditioning regimen appear to retain normal Leydig cell function, as do males who receive busulfan and cyclophosphamide, with normal plasma concentrations of luteinizing hormone (LH) and testosterone and normal progression through puberty.[14] Germ cell damage can occur and is more likely among patients treated after puberty.[90] Semen analyses have been normal in approximately two thirds of men after high-dose cyclophosphamide, and several men have fathered normal children. Men treated with TBI-based regimens who have not received prior testicular irradiation generally retain normal Leydig cell function, regardless of their age at treatment.[90] Germ cell dysfunction occurs in all men treated with TBI-based regimens, and azoospermia is the rule.

Female patients treated with high-dose cyclophosphamide alone retain normal ovarian function, regardless of age at exposure, although these subjects may be at increased risk for early menopause as they reach the third decade of life.[91] These individuals can sustain a normal pregnancy resulting in normal offspring. Females treated with busulfan and cyclophosphamide are at very high risk for ovarian failure and premature menopause.[92] The outcome of ovarian function after TBI appears to be determined by the age at exposure. Approximately 50% of prepubertal girls receiving fractionated TBI enter puberty spontaneously, and premature ovarian failure is seen in all patients older than 10 years of age when treated with TBI.[14] Pregnancies among survivors of TBI are at increased risk for spontaneous abortion.[93]

Pregnancy Outcomes

Offspring of survivors of childhood hematologic malignancies do not appear to be at increased risks for cancer or congenital malformations.[94] In a study of 593 adult survivors of childhood ALL, 15.7% (93/593) of survivors (mean age 22.6 years) had given birth to or fathered a total of 140 liveborn offspring, compared with 29.8% (122/409) of sibling controls (mean age 25.2 years). There was no significant difference in the rate of birth defects between offspring of survivors (3.6% [5/140]) versus sibling controls (3.5% [8/228]; relative risk 1.02; 95% confidence interval 0.34–3.05).[95]

MUSCULOSKELETAL EFFECTS

Avascular necrosis (osteonecrosis) is seen in pediatric and adult survivors of hematologic malignancies. Most often it is a consequence of therapy with corticosteroids, particularly dexamethasone, and occurs in up to 10% of patients.[96–98] This complication usually develops during or shortly after completion of therapy but may progress over time. Avascular necrosis of bone after allogeneic marrow transplantation is a frequent complication, with the reported incidence as high as 8% to 10% in long-term survivors.[99] Identified risk factors include prolonged steroid therapy for GVHD, male gender, and TBI. The mean latency period is 18 months. The hip is the most commonly involved joint (80%); however, the knee, wrist, and ankle joints also are affected in some patients. The probability of a patient requiring total hip replacement after diagnosis of AVN of the femoral head is 80% at 5 years.[100]

Osteopenia is commonly seen in survivors of hematologic malignancies.[101–103] Risk factors include therapy with corticosteroids, methotrexate (given at higher doses), and cranial irradiation with resultant pituitary insufficiency or gonadal dysfunction. Survivors of HCT are at increased risk for reduced bone mineral density. Identified risk factors in these patients include treatment with corticosteroids for chronic GVHD, prior cranial irradiation (resulting in growth hormone deficiency), and gonadal failure.[14] Lifestyle factors that increase the risk for osteopenia include lack of regular weight-bearing exercise, inadequate calcium and vitamin D intake, smoking, and excessive alcohol consumption.[104,105]

Radiation to the trunk (e.g., thoracic, abdominal, spinal) or TBI administered before skeletal maturity is achieved are risk factors for development of scoliosis and kyphosis.[106] Patients at highest risk are those who were very young at the time of radiation and those with a coexisting history of abdominal or thoracic surgery.

NEUROCOGNITIVE EFFECTS

Among survivors of childhood leukemia, neurocognitive late effects represent one of the more intensively studied topics.[107–110] Early curative regimens for childhood ALL relied heavily on cranial irradiation, usually in doses of 24 Gy.[107] Results from studies of neurocognitive outcomes in early populations of ALL survivors (particularly younger children) are directly responsible for the marked reduction in the use of cranial irradiation, which currently is reserved for treatment of very-high-risk subgroups or patients with CNS involvement. As a general rule, neurocognitive deficits usually become evident within several years after CNS-directed therapy and tend to be progressive in nature. Leukemia survivors treated at a younger age (i.e., <6 years) may experience significant declines in intelligence quotient (IQ) scores.[111] However, reductions in IQ scores typically are not global but reflect specific areas of impairment, such as attention and other nonverbal cognitive processing skills.[112,113] Affected patients may experience information processing deficits resulting in academic difficulties. These patients are particularly prone to problems with receptive and expressive language, attention, and visual and perceptual motor skills, most often manifested as academic difficulties in the areas of reading, language and mathematics. Assessment of educational needs and subsequent educational attainment have demonstrated that survivors of childhood leukemia are significantly more likely to require special educational assistance but have a high likelihood of successfully completing high school if they receive appropriate educational services.[114,115] Chemotherapy- or radiation-induced destruction of normal white matter partially explains intellectual and academic achievement deficits.[116] The pathogenesis of CNS damage is only partially understood. Evidence suggests that therapy-related direct effects on intracranial endothelial cells and brain white matter, as well as immunologic mechanisms, play roles.

A spectrum of neuropathologic syndromes related to leukoencephalopathy[117] may occur in survivors of childhood hematologic malignancies, including radionecrosis, necrotizing leukoencephalopathy, mineralizing microangiopathy and dystrophic calcification, cerebellar sclerosis, and spinal cord dysfunction, manifesting clinically as ataxia, spasticity, dysarthria, hemiparesis, or seizures. Imaging abnormalities are not always evident in these patients. Leukoencephalopathy has been primarily associated with methotrexate-induced injury of white matter. However, cranial irradiation may play an additive role through disruption of the blood–brain barrier, allowing greater exposure of the brain to systemic therapy. Although some abnormalities have been detected by diagnostic imaging studies, the abnormalities observed have not been well demonstrated to correlate with clinical findings and neurocognitive status.

Many survivors of adult-onset hematologic malignancies experience impairments of neurocognitive function, including memory loss, distractibility, and difficulty performing multiple tasks. These patients may concurrently suffer from mood disturbances and symptoms that compromise their ability to function adequately, including fatigue and pain.[118]

Survivors of hematopoietic stem cell transplantations are at risk for neurocognitive late effects. Prospective, longitudinal evaluations of intellectual and adaptive functioning of children receiving a transplant have revealed declines in intellectual function, particularly among those younger than 6 years of age at the time of transplantation.[119] Among the adult populations, studies in general have reported good levels of function and well-being in long-term survivors of transplantation, although there are increasing reports of fatigue, lack of energy, sleep problems, sexual dysfunction,[120] and cognitive dysfunction[121–124] (see box on Neuropsychological Sequelae after Hematopoietic Cell Transplantation in Adults).

Neuropsychological Sequelae after Hematopoietic Cell Transplantation in Adults

The few studies describing neurocognitive sequelae in adults undergoing hematopoietic cell transplant (HCT) suggest that these patients are at risk for developing adverse sequelae related to neuropsychological functioning, such as slowed reaction time, reduced attention and concentration, and difficulties in reasoning and problem solving[121]; memory impairment[122–124,194]; problems with executive functioning and processing speed[123]; and cognitive impairment.[121–123] Reduced memory function is associated with older age, longer interval since HCT, chronic graft-versus-host disease, and long-term cyclosporine use.[195] Other predictors include fatigue and poor physical functioning. Lower education level and poorer social functioning appear to impact cognitive performance.[123] Therefore, it is prudent to query post-HCT patients regarding perceived deficits in neuropsychological functioning and to refer patients with these problems to a neuropsychologist who is experienced in the followup care of HCT patients.

OTHER TOXICITIES

Ocular Effects

Survivors of hematologic malignancies are at risk for development of cataracts as a consequence of therapy with corticosteroids, cranial irradiation,[125,126] TBI,[127] or busulfan.[128] Hoover et al.[126] evaluated 82 ALL survivors, all of whom received treatment with prednisone (3.4–10.2 g/m^2/year) and cranial irradiation (1800–2800 cGy). At a mean of 32 months after completion of therapy, 52% of patients had evidence of posterior subcapsular cataracts; however, the cohort had minimal ocular morbidity, with median visual acuity of 20/20 in the affected eyes (range 20/15 to 20/50). Holmstrom et al.[128] studied a cohort of 45 children who were followed for 2 to 10 years after HCT; 95% (20/21) of children conditioned with TBI and 21% (5/24) of children conditioned with busulfan developed cataracts. Belkacemi et al.[129] studied 1063 patients who underwent HCT for acute leukemia; the overall 10-year incidence of cataracts in this group of patients was 50%. Single-dose TBI was associated with a 60% incidence of cataracts. Fractionated TBI was associated with a 43% incidence in those receiving six or fewer fractions and a 7% incidence for those receiving more than six fractions. Factors independently associated with increased risk for cataract formation in this cohort were older age (>23 years), allogeneic blood marrow transportation, higher dose rate (>0.04 Gy/min), and steroid administration for more than 100 days. Xerophthalmia may occur as a late complication due to decreased lacrimation resulting from damage to the lacrimal gland during radiation or, in HCT patients, from chronic GVHD.[130]

Audiologic Effects

Survivors of hematologic malignancies who received platinum chemotherapy, those who underwent cranial irradiation at a young age (especially during infancy),[131] and those who required supportive therapy with aminoglycoside antibiotics[132] are at risk for therapy-related hearing loss. Hearing loss associated with ototoxic agents generally is sensorineural in origin and usually is irreversible. Although a low incidence of hearing loss has been reported in survivors of hematopoietic cell transplant performed in childhood, the risk is elevated threefold to fourfold over that in the general population.[127]

Dental Effects

Children whose teeth have not completely developed at the time of cancer treatment are most vulnerable to dental complications, and treatment with chemotherapy during early childhood may result in qualitative problems with enamel and root development.[133] However, patients of all ages who received radiation therapy involving the head or neck (including cranial irradiation and TBI) are susceptible to dental complications, most often manifesting as increased susceptibility to dental caries and gingivitis as a result of diminished salivary gland function. Patients who have undergone HCT are at increased risks for dental caries and gum disease; abnormalities of tooth development are seen in survivors who underwent HCT during childhood.[134] Younger age at transplantation (especially <6 years) and TBI doses greater than 10 Gy are associated with the greatest risk.[135]

Hepatic Effects

Although acute hepatic dysfunction may be seen with certain chemotherapeutic agents, including antimetabolites and anthracyclines, late hepatic toxicity has not generally been seen. However, reports of chronic hepatotoxicity and portal hypertension have emerged in survivors of childhood ALL who received 6-thioguanine–based maintenance therapy,[136–138] and these survivors require long-term surveillance for this complication.[139] Chronic viral hepatitis, resulting from transfusion of contaminated blood or serum products, should be considered in the differential diagnosis of all survivors with persistently elevated alanine aminotransferase levels. Hepatitis C is the most prevalent type of hepatitis seen in survivors transfused before universal screening of the blood supply for this infection (implemented in the United States in July 1992). Cirrhosis and hepatocellular carcinoma are potential sequelae of untreated chronic viral hepatitis and potential causes of morbidity and mortality in this population. In a cohort of 431 pediatric patients in Italy who were diagnosed with leukemia or lymphoma before 1990 and completed treatment before August 1994, 17.2% (74/431) were anti–hepatitis C virus positive.[140] Hepatocellular carcinoma or progression to liver failure was not seen in this group of patients after a 14-year median followup; however, due to the natural history of this disease, a longer followup is required to clearly define the risk of chronic hepatitis C virus infection in this population. In a study of 3721 survivors of HCT,[141] the cumulative incidence of cirrhosis was estimated at 0.6% after 10 years and 3.8% after 20 years. The major risk factor for development of cirrhosis in this cohort was chronic hepatitis C infection, evident in 81% (25/31) of patients with cirrhosis. These Seattle investigators estimate that approximately 30% to 35% of their patients transplanted before 1991 were infected with hepatitis C and are at risk for development of cirrhosis and related complications.

Second and Subsequent Malignancies

A *second cancer* is defined as a histologically distinct cancer that develops after the first cancer. In total, 95,000 of the approximately 1.2 million new cancers diagnosed every year in the United States are second cancers. Second cancers account for approximately 6% to 10% of all cancer diagnoses and are the fourth or fifth most common cancer in the United States.[142,143]

Several large epidemiologic studies have attempted to determine the magnitude of the burden of second cancers after primary cancers in adulthood. For example, 470,000 cancer patients registered between 1953 and 1991 in Finland were followed for the development of a second cancer.[144] Overall, the cohort was not at increased risk for developing a second cancer compared with the risk of cancer in an age- and gender-matched healthy population. However, patients younger than 50 years at the time of diagnosis of their primary cancer had a 1.7-fold increased risk for developing a second cancer. Another cohort of 633,964 cancer patients diagnosed between 1958 and 1996 in Sweden and followed for the development of subsequent cancers revealed a modestly increased risk (less than twofold) compared with the general population.[145] A third cohort of 250,000 patients followed for the development of a second cancer in the United States revealed that cancer patients had a 1.3-fold increased risk for developing a second cancer compared with the general population.[146] However, when determining second cancers after cancers occurring in childhood or adolescence, a clearer and somewhat different picture emerges.

Several studies following large cohorts of childhood cancer survivors have reported a threefold to sixfold increased risk for a second cancer compared with the background incidence of cancer in the general population, and this risk continues to increase as the cohort ages. Followup of a Nordic cohort of 30,880 patients diagnosed with their first cancer at 21 years of age or younger between 1943 and 1987 resulted in the identification of 247 second cancers.[147] The estimated cumulative incidence of second cancers in this cohort was 3.5% at 25 years, and the cohort was at a 3.6-fold increased risk for developing a second cancer compared with an age- and gender-matched healthy population. In a report, a retrospective cohort of 13,581 children diagnosed with common cancers in the United States before age 21 years between 1970 and 1986 and who survived at least 5 years was followed for the development of second cancers. The estimated cumulative incidence of second cancers was 3.2% at 20 years. Overall, the cohort was at a 6.4-fold increased risk for developing a second cancer. The relative risk of developing a second malignancy was significantly increased for survivors of non-Hodgkin lymphoma (relative risk 3.2), leukemia (relative risk 5.7), and Hodgkin lymphoma (relative risk 9.7). However, only 1.9 excess malignancies occurred per 1000 years of patient followup; therefore, even though the incidence of a second cancer is greater in those whose first cancer occurred in early life, the annual excess risk of second cancers in this group still is very small.[148]

Second cancers are conventionally categorized into two major types: acute leukemia and myelodysplastic syndromes or solid tumors. The latency between diagnosis and treatment of the primary cancer and the development of a secondary leukemia is generally short, whereas nonhematopoietic malignancies or solid tumors seem to have a longer latency, and the risk continues to rise for 2 or more decades.[149]

Evaluations of large cohorts of patients diagnosed with childhood ALL and entered into therapeutic trials of the Children's Cancer Group have shown that the cumulative incidence of second and subsequent malignancies is only approximately 2% at 15 years from diagnosis and treatment of ALL.[150,151] CNS tumors, the most common second malignancy observed among survivors of childhood ALL, are predominantly associated with exposure to cranial irradiation.[148] Histologically, radiation-related late-occurring neoplasms include high-grade gliomas, (glioblastomas and malignant astrocytomas), peripheral neuroectodermal tumors, ependymomas, meningiomas, and basal cell carcinomas.[150–153] Potential risk factors for secondary CNS tumors include younger age at radiation, inherited genetic predisposition to cancer, and genetic profile with regard to genetic polymorphisms involved in metabolizing enzymes. An example of a polymorphism that has been found to be predictive of the risk of secondary CNS tumors in childhood ALL is thiopurine *S*-methyl-transferase.[154] Other commonly reported second cancers within the population of ALL survivors include thyroid cancer, lymphoma, and acute myeloid leukemia (AML). Secondary thyroid malignancies, typically papillary carcinoma, are generally associated with radiation exposure to the thyroid gland as part of CNS irradiation, either prophylactic or for treatment of CNS leukemia. Thyroid malignancy has been reported to represent between 6% and 17% of secondary cancers among large cohorts of ALL survivors[148,150,151] and typically develops 10 or more years from treatment. As is true of *de novo* thyroid malignancy, the long-term outcome of survivors diagnosed with a secondary thyroid malignancy is excellent. The risk of secondary AML after therapy for ALL is generally low, except among patients treated with epipodophyllotoxin therapy in whom a cumulative risk of 3.8% at 6 years has been reported.[155] Secondary AML associated with topoisomerase II inhibitors is characterized typically by a shorter latency period (3–5 years from therapeutic exposure) than that seen for secondary AML after alkylating agents, lack of a myelodysplastic phase, and the presence of 11q23 rearrangements with mutations in the *MLL* gene. Epipodophyllotoxin-associated secondary AML depends more on the schedule of drug administration than on total cumulative dose.[156]

Because the survival rate for pediatric patients with Hodgkin lymphoma has been high for more than 3 decades, a considerable amount of outcomes-based research is focused on the occurrence of second malignancies in this population. Survivors of pediatric and adolescent Hodgkin lymphoma clearly represent one of the subgroups of cancer survivors who are at very high risk for secondary cancer. This is particularly true for patients who received earlier regimens with predominantly radiation-based therapies in whom an approximate 10-fold increased risk has been reported.[148] A number of studies, including cohorts ranging from 499 to 5925 patients with Hodgkin lymphoma, have reported cumulative risks of second malignancies ranging from 7.6% at 20 years to 18.0% at 30 years.[148,149,157–159] Early studies of survivors of Hodgkin lymphoma identified the increased risk of secondary leukemias among patients treated with MOPP-based therapy, which included mechlorethamine and cyclophosphamide.[160,161] These alkylating agent-associated secondary leukemias are characterized as having a relatively short latency period (mean approximately 7 years), presence of monosomy 5 or monosomy 7, and often preceded by a phase of myelodysplasia.[162] The risk of therapy-related leukemia usually does not extend beyond the first 10 to 15 years after therapeutic exposure.

There is increasing interest in the investigation of the associations between therapy-related myelodysplasia or acute leukemia and polymorphisms in specific drug-metabolizing enzymes capable of metabolic activation or detoxification of anticancer drugs, such as NAD(P)H:quinone oxidoreductase (NQO1), glutathione *S*-transferase (GST)-M1 and -T1, and CYP3A4.[163–165] Evidence indicates that the NQO1 polymorphism is significantly associated with the genetic risks of therapy-related acute leukemia and myelodysplasia. Individuals with the CYP3A4-W genotype may be at increased risk for treatment-related leukemia by increasing the production of reactive intermediates that might damage DNA.

Breast cancer is the most commonly reported second malignancy among female survivors of childhood Hodgkin lymphoma treated with mantle field irradiation, and the risk remains markedly elevated for many decades after exposure.[148,149,157–159] An update of the Late Effects Study Group cohort found female survivors had a 55-fold increased risk for breast cancer compared with the general population, and the cumulative incidence of developing a secondary breast cancer approached 20% at age 45 years.[166] Moreover, 40% of identified cases were found to have developed contralateral disease. Secondary thyroid cancer, the second most common solid tumor reported among survivors of childhood Hodgkin lymphoma, is strongly associated with radiation therapy, occurs more frequently in females, and is associated with an approximately 36-fold increased risk over the general population. As the cohort of pediatric survivors of Hodgkin lymphoma continues to age, an increasing number of other forms of malignancy associated with an excess risk likely will emerge. Extended followup of early cohorts have already reported excess risks for lung and gastrointestinal cancers.[166–170]

HCT recipients have a fourfold to sevenfold increased risk for developing a second cancer, particularly Epstein-Barr virus-related posttransplantation lymphoproliferative disease, myelodysplastic syndromes, and a variety of solid nonhematopoietic tumors.[171–173] Research indicates that the determinants of risk of second cancers are multifactorial. Second cancers are more likely to develop in survivors who were diagnosed with cancer at a younger age, after exposure to high-dose radiation therapy and certain chemotherapeutic agents, and in those with a known genetic predisposition to cancer.[148–150,174,175] Although we have begun to understand some of the causes of second cancers, we still have much to learn about the nature of the interactions among the treatments given for the initial cancer, genetic susceptibility to cancer, medical complications, and an individual's lifestyle choices in the genesis of subsequent new cancers.

Late Mortality

Late recurring disease as well as sequelae of treatment of hematologic malignancies can have a direct or indirect impact on overall mortality. Several large studies of late mortality among 5-year survivors of childhood cancer have been conducted.[176,177] In a study of 5-year survivors in the United States,[176] the probability of survival 25 years after diagnoses of leukemia, Hodgkin lymphoma, and non-Hodgkin lymphoma was 87%, 81%, and 90%, respectively. The standardized mortality ratio (SMR; i.e., observed deaths to expected deaths) for death due to subsequent cancer, cardiac complications, or pulmonary conditions was statistically significantly elevated among leukemia patients (SMR from 3.8 for cardiac complication to 17.4 for second cancer), Hodgkin lymphoma patients (SMR from 12.0 for pulmonary condition to 24.0 for second cancer), and non-Hodgkin lymphoma patients (SMR from 6.5 for cardiac complication to 15.6 for second cancer).

Late mortality due to recurrent disease and complications of therapy has been described among patients who underwent HCT for hematologic malignancies.[178,179] Socie et al.[178] reported that among 6691 individuals who underwent allogeneic transplant for hematologic malignancies and were free of disease 2 years after transplantation, the probability of living for 5 more years was 89%. The authors concluded that the disease probably is cured in patients who receive an allogeneic stem cell transplantation as treatment for AML, ALL, chronic myeloid leukemia (CML), or aplastic anemia and who remain free of their original disease 2 years later. However, for many years after transplantation, the mortality rate among these patients is higher than that in a normal population. Bhatia et al.[179] assessed late mortality in 854 survivors who underwent autologous HCT for hematologic malignancies and survived 2 or more years after transplant. At a median followup of 7.6 years. overall survival was 68.8% ± 1.8% at 10 years, and the cohort was found to be at a 13-fold increased risk for late death compared with the general population. Relapse of primary disease (56%) and subsequent malignancies (25%) were leading causes of late death.

Psychosocial Effects

Survivors of hematopoietic malignancies are at risk for adverse psychosocial outcomes that may impact the overall quality of life, including anxiety, depression, posttraumatic stress disorder, and barriers to accessing the health care system due to problems obtaining health insurance coverage. The impact of cancer therapy on psychosocial functioning is dependent on many variables, including intensity and duration of therapy, treatment-related complications, family functioning, developmental processes, and treatment-specific sequelae such as altered cognitive and physical functioning.[180]

Results from an analysis of 5736 long-term survivors of childhood leukemia and lymphoma demonstrated that although a relatively low proportion reported symptoms indicative of depression (4.6%) and somatic distress (10.8%), they were significantly more likely to report these symptoms compared with sibling controls.[181] Long-term survivors of adult-onset Hodgkin lymphoma report poorer health-related quality of life, primarily in physical health, compared with a healthy general population.[182] Survivors of Hodgkin lymphoma also appear to be at increased risk for psychosocial distress compared with acute leukemia survivors; areas of greatest impact for these patients include impaired family and sexual functioning.[183] There is growing interest in the reported occurrences of fatigue and sleep disturbances among cancer survivors, particularly those with Hodgkin lymphoma,[6,184,185] which may contribute to depression.

Fatigue, psychological distress, psychiatric symptoms, mood disturbances, and sexual difficulties are commonly reported by HCT survivors.[186] Risk factors for impaired health-related quality of life include older age, advanced disease at transplantation, presence of chronic GVHD, and lower level of education. Fatigue and sleep disturbances have been reported in up to 65% of patient cohorts studied,[187] and sexual disturbances are prevalent in 25% of HCT survivors[188] (see Evaluating Survivors for Potential Late Effects below).

POTENTIAL LATE EFFECTS BY DIAGNOSIS

Therapeutic approaches to hematologic malignancies vary widely depending on the patient's age at diagnosis, biologic subtype and staging of disease, year (era) of diagnosis, and physician/institutional preference. Even though two patients may share an identical diagnosis, their risks for late effects may differ significantly due to differences in therapy, age at exposure to therapy, or individual variations in the ability to handle the therapy (polymorphisms in drug-metabolizing enzymes). General associations of late effects with conventional treatment of common hematologic malignancies are reviewed in Tables 97–1 to 97–3. The risk for specific late effects in survivors who have undergone HCT depends on the conditioning regimen, donor source, complications experienced during the transplantation

Table 97–1 Late Effects Associated with Conventional Therapy for Acute Lymphoblastic Leukemia and Non-Hodgkin Lymphoma

Common Therapeutic Exposures	Potential Late Effects
Vincristine	Peripheral neuropathy, Raynaud phenomenon
Corticosteroids	Cataracts, osteopenia, osteoporosis, avascular necrosis
Asparaginase	No known late effects
Mercaptopurine	Hepatic dysfunction (rare)
Thioguanine	Portal hypertension, hepatotoxicity (when used continuously in maintenance therapy)
Methotrexate (systemic)	Osteopenia, osteonecrosis, renal dysfunction (rare), hepatic dysfunction (rare)
Methotrexate (intrathecal) Cytarabine (high-dose)	Neurocognitive deficits, clinical leukoencephalopathy
Cranial or craniospinal irradiation	Neurocognitive deficits, clinical leukoencephalopathy, cataracts, hypothyroidism, second malignant neoplasm in radiation field (e.g., skin, thyroid, brain), short stature, scoliosis or kyphosis, obesity
Anthracyclines	Cardiomyopathy, arrhythmias, subclinical left ventricular dysfunction, secondary AML
Cyclophosphamide	Hypogonadism, hemorrhagic cystitis, dysfunctional voiding, bladder malignancy, secondary AML or myelodysplastic syndrome
Blood products	Chronic viral hepatitis, human immunodeficiency virus

AML, acute myeloid leukemia.

Table 97–2 Late Effects Associated with Conventional Therapy for Acute Myeloid Leukemia

Common Therapeutic Exposures	Potential Late Effects
Anthracyclines	Cardiomyopathy, arrhythmias, subclinical left ventricular dysfunction, secondary acute myeloid leukemia
Corticosteroids	Cataracts, osteopenia, osteoporosis, avascular necrosis
Asparaginase	No known late effects
Cytarabine (high dose)	Neurocognitive deficits, clinical leukoencephalopathy
Blood products	Chronic viral hepatitis, human immunodeficiency virus infection

process, presence or absence of GVHD, and prior cancer therapy. Transplantation-related sequelae have been reviewed throughout the text of this chapter.

Acute Lymphoblastic Leukemia

ALL, like most hematologic malignancies, is a heterogeneous disease. Therapy for ALL ranges from a relatively innocuous, antimetabolite-based approach for low-risk childhood ALL[189] to marrow-ablative therapy followed by HCT for very-high-risk disease in all age groups.[190,191] The risk of long-term complications in individual survivors varies widely and is dependent on the specific therapy received as well as the patient's age at the time of treatment. Potential late effects that may occur as a consequence of conventional therapy for ALL are listed in Table 97–1.

Acute Myeloid Leukemia

Therapy for AML is generally more intense and of shorter duration that that used for treatment of ALL. Higher doses of anthracycline

Evaluating Survivors for Potential Late Effects

To diminish the incidence and severity of untoward late effects and to improve the quality of survival for patients with hematopoietic malignancies, systematic evaluation of outcomes with subsequent modification of current and future therapies is required. To decrease late morbidity and mortality rates and to meet the specialized health care needs of this group of patients, ongoing comprehensive followup care with attention to early detection and intervention for late effects are essential.

Patients are generally eligible to enter formal long-term followup care when the risk of relapse of their primary disease is minimal. For most hematologic malignancies, this occurs when a patient is free of disease for 5 or more years and is at least 2 years off therapy. When a patient enters long-term followup, the focus of care shifts from management of the acute toxicities of therapy and vigilant surveillance for disease recurrence to a survivorship model of health maintenance or promotion and management of treatment-related late effects. Effective management of these late effects requires ongoing surveillance, early intervention, and, when possible, prevention.

The long-term complications of treatment for which an individual survivor is at risk are determined by several factors, including the patient's diagnosis, age at treatment, specific chemotherapeutic agents received (including cumulative doses), specific radiation fields and doses, therapy-related complications, degree of psychosocial support received, genetic predisposition, and current health-related behaviors (e.g., diet, physical activity, tobacco and alcohol use). Because of the impact of cytotoxic agents on growing tissues and organs, survivors treated during childhood or adolescence appear to be at higher risk for late complications than are those who received treatment after achieving physical maturity.

Table 97–3 Late Effects Associated with Conventional Therapy for Hodgkin Lymphoma

Common Therapeutic Exposures	Potential Late Effects
Anthracyclines	Cardiomyopathy, arrhythmias, subclinical left ventricular dysfunction, secondary AML
Corticosteroids	Cataracts, osteopenia, osteoporosis, avascular necrosis
Bleomycin	Pulmonary dysfunction
Vincristine, vinblastine	Peripheral neuropathy, Raynaud phenomenon
Procarbazine, mechlorethamine, dacarbazine	Hypogonadism, infertility, secondary AML or MDS
Cyclophosphamide	Hypogonadism, infertility, hemorrhagic cystitis, dysfunctional voiding, bladder malignancy, secondary AML or MDS
Mantle irradiation	Hypothyroidism, premature cardiovascular disease, cardiovalvular disease, cardiomyopathy, arrhythmias, carotid artery disease, scoliosis or kyphosis, second malignant neoplasm in radiation field (e.g., thyroid, breast), pulmonary dysfunction
Inverted Y irradiation	Hypogonadism, infertility, adverse pregnancy outcome, second malignant neoplasm in radiation field (e.g., gastrointestinal)
Splenectomy	Acute life-threatening infections
Blood products	Chronic viral hepatitis, human immunodeficiency virus

AML, acute myeloid leukemia; MDS, myelodysplastic syndrome.

chemotherapy are often used, as is consolidation therapy with HCT. Typically, patients with AML receive less CNS-directed therapy than do those with ALL. Examples of potential late effects associated with conventional therapy for AML are listed in Table 97–2.

Hodgkin Lymphoma

Therapy for Hodgkin lymphoma relies heavily on the use of alkylating agents, antitumor antibiotics (including anthracyclines and bleomycin), corticosteroids, and radiation therapy. Many survivors are asplenic as a consequence of surgical staging. Examples of potential late effects associated with conventional therapy for Hodgkin lymphoma are listed in Table 97–3.

Non-Hodgkin Lymphoma

The potential late effects after therapy for non-Hodgkin lymphoma are therapy specific and similar to those experienced by survivors of ALL (see Table 97–1). Patients whose treatment included HCT are also at risk for transplantation-related sequelae.

Chronic Myeloid Leukemia

Long-term survivors of CML usually either have undergone HCT or are receiving imatinib mesylate (Gleevec) long term. Although therapy for CML differs from therapy for AML in that it generally does not require intensive pretransplantation chemotherapy; nevertheless, there is a significant risk for late effects as a result of the transplantation conditioning regimen as well as the treatment for and sequelae of GVHD.[15] As new therapies (e.g., imatinib mesylate [Gleevec]) for CML continue to emerge, potential late effects of these therapies in survivors will require study (see box on Late Effects Research: What Is Needed and Providing Clinical Care to Survivors above).

Late Effects Research: What is Needed

Medical Issues Faced by This Population

Cancer survivors are at increased risk for adverse outcomes, including the following:

- Premature death
- Second neoplasms
- Organ dysfunction (e.g., cardiac, pulmonary, gonadal)
- Impaired growth and development
- Decreased fertility
- Neurocognitive impairment
- Difficulties obtaining employment and insurance
- Overall reduced quality of life

Options for Physicians Providing Care to This Population

- Models of care delivery:
  - Pediatric oncology-based
  - Adult oncology-based
  - Community medicine-based
- Guidelines for ongoing screening and management:
  - Screening for potential complications
  - Health protective counseling or interventions
  - Management of identified complications

Major Clinical and Research Challenges

Cancer survivorship research continually changing because of new:

- Therapeutic agents and combinations of agents
- Radiation oncology techniques
- Surgical procedures
- Supportive care techniques

Future Directions

Much of the available information relates to outcomes within the first decade after treatment, and only minimal data address the longer-term outcomes that may occur later.

Research is needed to more clearly define the survivors at greatest risks for specific outcomes.

Research is needed to identify genetic predispositions to certain key outcomes and the roles of gene–environment interactions.

Research is needed to identify the role of lifestyle choices (e.g., alcohol, tobacco, diet, exercise) in terms of modification of the risks for these late outcomes.

Research is needed to understand the potential long-term impact of cancer therapy to effectively counsel survivors and offer effective intervention strategies to prevent or minimize the impact of adverse late effects.

Interventions are needed to include scientifically valid, evidence-based recommendations for clinical followup of survivors, which should include screening for potential late effects and application of proven approaches for health promotion.

PROVIDING CLINICAL CARE TO SURVIVORS

A comprehensive treatment summary should be prepared for each patient entering long-term followup (Table 97–4) and a copy given to each survivor with instructions to share this information with all

Table 97–4 Comprehensive Treatment Summary

Topic	Specific Information To Include
Demographics	Name Record number or patient identification number Date of birth Gender Race or ethnicity
Diagnosis	Date or age at diagnosis Referring physician or institution Treating physician or institution Presenting symptoms Past medical history Family history (including cancer in first- or second-degree relatives) Physical examination findings at presentation Initial diagnostics (complete blood cell count, chemistry panel, radiographic studies) Diagnostic procedures (biopsies, cytologic studies) Pathology (morphology, histology, cytochemistry, flow cytometry) Cytogenetics Central nervous system status (if applicable) Stage (if applicable) Metastatic sites (if applicable) Initial response to therapy (e.g., rapid early response [RER], slow early response [SER], date first complete remission achieved) Relapse(s) dates, age at relapse(s), relapse site(s)
Treatment	Date of initial treatment (initiated and completed) Date(s) for treatment of relapse (initiated and completed) Final off-therapy date Chemotherapy agents received, including route of administration (list all) Cumulative doses (in mg/m^2) and age at treatment for all alkylators, anthracyclines, and heavy metals Dose ranges for cytarabine and methotrexate (e.g., standard dose vs high dose ≥1000 mg/m^2) Radiation fields, doses, shielding, age at treatment Surgical procedure(s) Transfusion(s), including all blood or serum products Stem cell transplantation(s), including donor source, preparative regimen, GVHD prophylaxis or treatment
Acute complications	Significant therapy-related complications (e.g., tumor lysis, septic shock, typhlitis, acute GVHD) Significant treatment required for complications (e.g., hemodialysis, amphotericin, aminoglycosides)
Complications after therapy	Significant complications after completion of therapy (e.g., herpes zoster, acute life-threatening infection after splenectomy)

GVHD, graft-versus-host disease.
Adapted from Children's Oncology Group Summary of Cancer Treatment, 2006 (www.survivorshipguideline.org).

health care providers. Survivors should undergo annual comprehensive, multidisciplinary health evaluations (Fig. 97–1) with special attention to the detection of potential late effects specific to the patient's diagnosis and treatment history (Table 97–5). Guidelines for long-term followup of survivors of hematologic malignancies and those who underwent hematopoietic cell transplant in childhood, adolescent, or young adulthood have been developed by the Children's Oncology Group[192] (available at www.survivorshipguidelines.org). Because certain late effects have prolonged asymptomatic intervals before becoming clinically evident (e.g., late-onset congestive heart failure as a result of anthracycline-induced cardiomyopathy), ongoing evaluation is important for identifying and providing early intervention for these potential complications. Health education regarding potential health risks and risk reduction measures should be provided to each survivor. Targeted health education materials related to potential late complications of therapy during childhood, adolescence, or young adulthood have been developed by the Children's Oncology Group[193] (available at www.survivorshipguidelines.org). After completion of each annual evaluation, identified late effects should be systematically recorded, and recommendations for any additional testing and for health maintenance and promotion should be shared with the patient and his or her primary health care provider. To optimize future followup care for all survivors, patients should be invited to participate in any relevant research studies for which they are eligible (see box on Late Effects Research: What Is Needed).

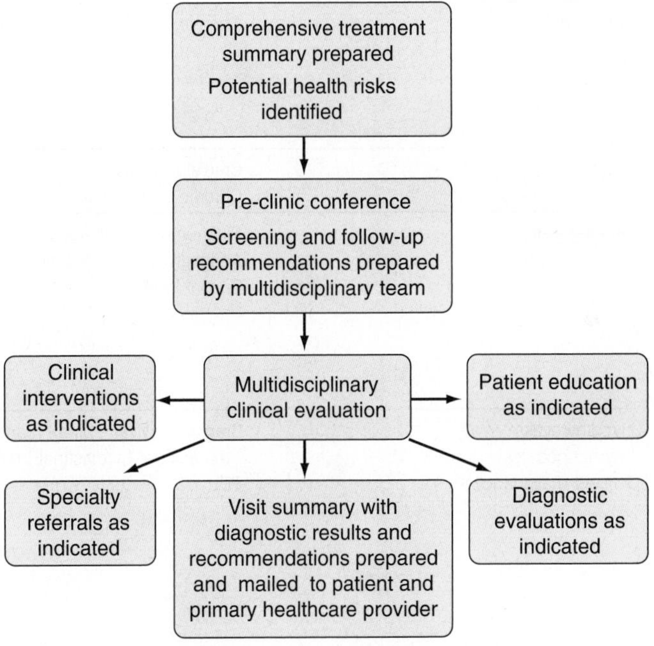

Figure 97–1 Annual comprehensive multidisciplinary health evaluation for the cancer survivor.

Table 97–5 Monitoring for Potential Late Effects

Potential Late Effects	Therapeutic Exposure	Recommended Monitoring	Suggested Interventions
Adverse psychosocial effects (e.g., depression, anxiety, posttraumatic stress disorder, limitations in health care access)	Diagnosis and treatment of hematologic malignancy	Clinical evaluation: yearly	Psychological or social work consultation if indicated
Dental abnormalities (abnormal tooth development; increased susceptibility to caries and gum disease)	Chemotherapy Cranial irradiation TBI	Dental examination: every 6 months	Professional dental cleaning every 6 months; use of fluoridated toothpaste; topical fluoride applications as indicated; Panorex radiograph before orthodontic or dental procedures for patients treated before completion of tooth development
Peripheral neuropathy Raynaud phenomenon	Vincristine Vinblastine	Neurologic examination if symptomatic	Physical therapy if indicated; advise patient to protect against precipitating factors (e.g., cold environment)
Neurocognitive deficits	Methotrexate (intrathecal, high-dose systemic) Cytarabine (high-dose systemic) Cranial irradiation TBI	Formal neuropsychological testing: baseline on entry to long-term followup; repeat as clinically indicated if evidence of impaired performance Clinical evaluation: yearly, including assessment of educational and vocational progress	Referral for specialized educational services, curricular modifications, or vocational training programs if indicated
Clinical leukoencephalopathy	Methotrexate (intrathecal, high-dose systemic) Cytarabine (high-dose systemic) Cranial irradiation	Clinical evaluation: yearly Brain MRI or CT if clinically indicated	Neurology consultation if clinically indicated
Cataracts	Corticosteroids Busulfan Cranial irradiation TBI	Funduscopic examination and visual acuity evaluation: yearly Ophthalmologic examination: yearly for patients who received TBI or cranial radiation ≥30 Gy; every 3 years for cranial radiation <30 Gy	Ophthalmology consultation if abnormalities detected
Xerophthalmia	Chronic GVHD related to HCT	History and eye examination: yearly	Artificial tears, ophthalmology Consultation if indicated
Xerostomia	Cranial irradiation Chronic GVHD related to HCT	Dental evaluation: every 6 months	Meticulous oral hygiene Artificial saliva products if indicated
Hearing loss	Platinum chemotherapy Aminoglycoside antibiotics Cranial irradiation	History and physical examination: yearly Audiogram: baseline at entry into long-term followup, then as clinically indicated; every 5 years for cranial radiation dose ≥30 Gy	Audiology consultation if indicated
Hypothyroidism Thyroid nodules Thyroid malignancy	Cranial, cervical, spinal, mantle, thoracic, or mediastinal irradiation TBI	Free T_4, TSH, thyroid examination: yearly	Endocrine or surgical referral as indicated

Table 97–5 Monitoring for Potential Late Effects—cont'd

Potential Late Effects	Therapeutic Exposure	Recommended Monitoring	Suggested Interventions
Cardiomyopathy Arrhythmias Subclinical left ventricular dysfunction	Anthracyclines Chest or thoracic irradiation (e.g., mantle, mediastinal)	Detailed history of exertional tolerance (e.g., dyspnea on exertion, chest pain): yearly ECG (for evaluation of QT interval): baseline on entry into long-term followup; echocardiogram: baseline on entry to long-term followup, then every 1 to 5 years as indicated based on age at therapy and total anthracycline or radiation dose	Cardiology consultation if indicated; additional cardiology evaluation of patients who are pregnant or planning to become pregnant if patient received ≥300 mg/m^2 of an anthracycline, radiation dose ≥30 Gy, or any dose of anthracycline combined with irradiation
Pericarditis Pericardial fibrosis Valvular disease Premature atherosclerotic heart disease	Chest or thoracic irradiation (e.g., mantle, mediastinal)	Consider cardiology consultation 5–10 years after irradiation to evaluate risk for coronary artery disease in patients who received doses ≥40 Gy Fasting glucose and lipid profiles: every 3–5 years	Cardiology consultation if indicated; additional cardiology evaluation in patients who are pregnant or planning to become pregnant if patient received anthracycline combined with radiation, ≥300 mg/m^2 anthracycline, or radiation dose ≥30 Gy
Pulmonary dysfunction (fibrosis, interstitial pneumonitis)	Bleomycin Busulfan Chest/thoracic irradiation TBI Chronic GVHD related to HCT	Pulmonary function testing and chest radiograph: baseline at entry into long-term followup and as clinically indicated for patients with progressive dysfunction	Pulmonary consultation for symptomatic patients; influenza and pneumococcal vaccine; counsel patients to avoid smoking and avoid scuba diving
Thrombosis Vascular insufficiency Infection of retained cuff or line tract	Central venous catheter	History and physical examination: yearly as clinically indicated	Surgical referral as indicated
Hepatic dysfunction	Mercaptopurine, thioguanine, methotrexate (systemic) HCT	ALT, AST, bilirubin: baseline on entry into long-term followup; repeat if clinically indicated	If abnormal results on baseline studies, obtain prothrombin time (to assess hepatic synthetic function) and viral hepatitis screening
Chronic viral hepatitis	Blood products	Hepatitis C antibody and HCV-RNA by PCR: once if transfused before universal screening of blood supply (1992 in the United States) Hepatitis B surface antigen and core antibody: once if transfused before universal screening of blood supply (1972 in the United States)	Gastroenterology or hepatology consultation and annual AFP for patients with chronic hepatitis; hepatitis A and B immunizations in patients lacking immunity
HIV infection	Blood products	HIV-1 and HIV-2 antibodies: once if transfused before universal screening of blood supply (1985 in the United States)	Infectious disease consultation for patients with confirmed infection
Life-threatening infection	Splenectomy Splenic radiation ≥40 Gy Chronic active GVHD	Physical examination at time of febrile illness to evaluate degree of illness and for potential source of infection	Administer parenteral antibiotics and continue close medical observation in patients with temperature ≥38°C (101°F) or other signs of serious infection; immunize with pneumococcal, meningococcal, and HIB vaccines

Continued

Table 97–5 Monitoring for Potential Late Effects—cont'd

Potential Late Effects	Therapeutic Exposure	Recommended Monitoring	Suggested Interventions
Iron overload	HCT (and patients requiring multiple red blood cell transfusions)	Serum ferritin: at entry into long-term followup	If abnormal, consider chelation, or repeat as clinically indicated until within normal limits
Bowel obstruction Chronic enterocolitis Fistulas and strictures	Abdominal surgery Abdominal or pelvic irradiation Chronic GVHD related to HCT (esophageal strictures, vaginal stenosis)	History and physical examination: yearly and as clinically indicated Serum protein and albumin levels: yearly in patients with chronic diarrhea or fistula	Surgical and gastroenterology consultations as clinically indicated
Renal insufficiency	TBI Abdominal or splenic irradiation Ifosfamide Platinum chemotherapy Methotrexate	Blood pressure: yearly Urinalysis: yearly BUN, creatinine, electrolytes, calcium, magnesium, phosphorus baseline and repeat as clinically indicated	Nephrology consultation for proteinuria, hypertension, progressive renal insufficiency
Hemorrhagic cystitis Bladder fibrosis Dysfunctional voiding Bladder malignancy	Cyclophosphamide Ifosfamide Irradiation of abdomen, pelvis, iliac, inguinal sites	Urinalysis: yearly Voiding history: yearly	Urology consultation for incontinence, dysfunctional voiding, macroscopic hematuria (culture negative)
Growth hormone deficiency	Cranial irradiation TBI	Height, weight: every 6 months during puberty until growth is complete Obtain bone age in poorly growing children	Endocrine referral for patients failing to follow normal growth curve
Overweight/obesity	Cranial irradiation	BP, growth percentile, BMI: yearly	Endocrine referral as indicated
Metabolic syndrome	TBI	Fasting glucose, lipid profile, and insulin levels every 2–5 years	
Hypogonadism Infertility	Alkylating agents Cranial irradiation Abdominal or pelvic irradiation Testicular irradiation Spinal irradiation >25 Gy TBI	Menstrual history, sexual function, height, weight: yearly Pubertal history, Tanner stage: yearly until maturity FSH, LH, estradiol or testosterone: baseline at age 13 years (females) or 14 years (males) or at entry into long-term followup and for clinical symptoms of estrogen or testosterone deficiency Semen analysis: as indicated or requested by patient	Endocrine referral for hypogonadal patients (for hormone replacement therapy); reproductive endocrinology referral for patients desiring evaluation of fertility options
Precocious puberty	Cranial irradiation	Physical examination, height, weight, Tanner stage: yearly until maturity LH, FSH, estradiol or testosterone: as clinically indicated in patients with accelerated pubertal progression Obtain bone age in rapidly growing prepubertal children	Endocrine referral as indicated
Adverse pregnancy outcomes (e.g., spontaneous abortion, premature delivery, low birth weight infant)	Irradiation of abdomen, pelvis, iliac, inguinal, paraaortic sites TBI	History: yearly and as clinically indicated	High-risk obstetric care

Table 97–5 Monitoring for Potential Late Effects—cont'd

Potential Late Effects	Therapeutic Exposure	Recommended Monitoring	Suggested Interventions
Osteopenia, osteoporosis	Corticosteroids Methotrexate (high-dose systemic) HCT	Bone density study (DEXA scan or quantitative CT scan): baseline at entry into long-term followup, repeat as clinically indicated	Calcium and vitamin D supplementation; weight-bearing exercise; treatment of exacerbating conditions (e.g., hypogonadism); consider pharmacologic intervention (e.g., bisphosphonates)
Avascular necrosis	Corticosteroids HCT	History: yearly; MRI if clinically indicated	Orthopedic consultation if indicated
Scoliosis/kyphosis	Irradiation of trunk (e.g., mantle, spine, abdomen, pelvis)	Physical examination of spine: yearly (every 6 months during pubertal growth spurt) Radiologic imaging of the spine if clinical evidence of scoliosis or kyphosis	Orthopedic referral
Joint contractures	Chronic GVHD related to HCT	Physical examination: yearly	Orthopedic referral if indicated
Chronic infection	Chronic GVHD related to HCT	History: yearly	Prophylactic antiinfective agents; infectious disease consultation if indicated
Vitiligo Scleroderma Joint contractures Nail dysplasia Dysplastic nevi Skin cancer Secondary benign or malignant neoplasms in radiation field	Chronic GVHD related to HCT Irradiation (any field)	Physical examination: yearly Careful physical examination, inspection and palpation of irradiated skin and soft tissues: yearly	Dermatology or rehabilitation consultation if clinically indicated Dermatology or surgical referral and radiographs if indicated for any suspicious lesions
Bone malignancies Brain tumor	Cranial irradiation	History and physical examination: yearly Brain MRI: baseline at maturity for all patients and as clinically indicated	Neurosurgical consultation as indicated
Breast cancer	Chest or thorax irradiation ≥20 Gy (mantle radiation field)	Clinical breast examination: yearly until age 25 years, then every 6 months Mammogram: yearly beginning at age 25 or 8 years after irradiation (whichever comes last)	Teach breast self-examination; instruct patient to perform monthly self-examination and report changes immediately; surgical consultation if clinically indicated
Gastrointestinal malignancy	Abdominal, pelvic, spinal irradiation ≥30 Gy	Colonoscopy every 5 years beginning 10 years after radiation or at age 35 years, whichever comes last; or more frequently as clinically indicated	Surgical consultation if indicated
AML (preceding myelodysplastic phase associated with alkylating agents)	Anthracyclines Epipodophyllotoxins Alkylating agents Stem cell priming with etoposide Autologous transplantation for NHL or Hodgkin lymphoma	Physical examination, CBC and differential: yearly for 10 years after therapy Bone marrow evaluation if clinically indicated	Counsel patient to report fatigue, bruising, bleeding, bone pain

AFP, α-fetoprotein; ALT, alanine aminotransferase; AML, acute myeloid leukemia; AST, aspartate aminotransferase; BMI, body mass index; BP, blood pressure; BUN, blood urea nitrogen; CBC, complete blood cell count; CT, computed tomography; DEXA, dual-energy x-ray absorptiometry; ECG, electrocardiogram; FSH, follicle-stimulating hormone; GVHD, graft-versus-host-disease; HCT, hematopoietic cell transplantation; HCV, hepatitis C virus; HIB, *Haemophilus influenzae* type B; HIV, human immunodeficiency virus; LH, luteinizing hormone; MRI, magnetic resonance imaging; NHL, non-Hodgkin lymphoma; PCR, polymerase chain reaction; T_4, thyroxine; TBI, total body irradiation; TSH, thyroid-stimulating protein.

Adapted from Children's Oncology Group Long-Term Follow-Up Guidelines for Survivors of Childhood, Adolescent, and Young Adult Cancers, Children's Oncology Group, 2006 (www.survivorshipguideline.org).

CONCLUSION

As therapies for hematopoietic malignancies continue to improve, followup care for survivors of these diseases must be provided in a comprehensive manner. To minimize treatment-related sequelae and provide early intervention for identified late effects, the risks of long-term complications for each individual survivor must be evaluated; however, it is important to keep these risks in perspective. In reality, most survivors of hematologic malignancies have the potential to lead full lives with excellent performance status and minimal to no physical limitations. The overall goal of followup care is to assist each patient to maximize his or her full potential for a healthy life while balancing the small, but real, risk of potential complications that may arise. Providing this type of ongoing comprehensive followup care to survivors of hematologic malignancies is an essential service.

SUGGESTED READINGS

Baker KS, Gurney JG, Ness KK, et al: Late effects in survivors of chronic myeloid leukemia treated with hematopoietic cell transplantation: Results from the Bone Marrow Transplant Survivor Study. Blood 104:1898, 2004.

Bhatia S, Blatt J, Meadows AT: Late effects of childhood cancer and its treatment. In Pizzo PA, Poplack DG (eds.): Principles and Practice of Pediatric Oncology, 5th ed. Philadelphia, Lippincott Williams & Wilkins, 2006, p 1490.

Bhatia S, Sather HN, Pabustan OB, et al: Low incidence of second neoplasms among children diagnosed with acute lymphoblastic leukemia after 1983. Blood 99:4257, 2002.

Bhatia S, Robison LL, Francisco L, et al: Late mortality in survivors of autologous hematopoietic-cell transplantation: Report from the Bone Marrow Transplant Survivor Study. Blood 105:4215, 2005.

Bhatia S, Yasui Y, Robison LL, et al: High risk of subsequent neoplasms continues with extended follow-up of childhood Hodgkin's disease: Report from the Late Effects Study Group. J Clin Oncol 21:4386, 2003.

Fraser CJ, Bhatia S, Ness K, et al: Impact of chronic graft-versus-host disease on the health status of hematopoietic cell transplantation survivors: A report from the Bone Marrow Transplant Survivor Study. Blood 108:2867, 2006.

Hewitt ME, Greenfield S, Stovall E (eds.): From Cancer Patient to Cancer Survivor: Lost in Transition. Washington, DC, The National Academies Press, 2006.

Hewitt ME, Weiner SL, Simone JV (eds.): Childhood Cancer Survivorship: Improving Care and Quality of Life. Washington, DC, The National Academies Press, 2003.

Hancock SL, Cox RS, McDougall IR: Thyroid diseases after treatment of Hodgkin's disease. N Engl J Med 325:599, 1991.

Hudson MM: Late complications after leukemia therapy. In Pui CH (ed.): Childhood Leukemias, 2nd ed. Cambridge, Cambridge University Press, 2006, p 750.

Kremer LCM, van Dalen EC, Offringa M, et al: Frequency and risk factors of anthracycline-induced clinical heart failure in children: A systematic review. Ann Oncol 13:503, 2002.

Landier W, Bhatia S, Eshelman DA, et al: Development of risk-based guidelines for pediatric cancer survivors: The Children's Oncology Group Long-Term Follow-Up Guidelines from the Children's Oncology Group Late Effects Committee and Nursing Discipline. J Clin Oncol 22:4979, 2004.

Loge JH, Kaasa S: Medical and psychosocial issues in Hodgkin's disease survivors. In Chang AE, Ganz PA, Hayes DF, et al. (eds.): Oncology: An Evidence-Based Approach. New York, Springer-Verlag, 2006, p 1804.

Oeffinger KC, Mertens AC, Sklar CA, et al: Obesity in adult survivors of childhood acute lymphoblastic leukemia: A report from the Childhood Cancer Survivor Study. J Clin Oncol 21:1359, 2003.

Pui C-H, Cheng C, Leung W, et al: Extended follow-up of long-term survivors of childhood acute lymphoblastic leukemia. N Engl J Med 349:640, 2003.

Sklar C, Boulad F, Small T, et al: Endocrine complications of pediatric stem cell transplantation. Front Biosci 6:G17, 2001.

Socie G, Salooja N, Cohen A, et al: Non-malignant late effects after allogeneic stem cell transplantation. Blood 101:3373, 2003.

Socie G, Stone JV, Wingard JR, et al: Long-term survival and late deaths after allogeneic bone marrow transplantation. N Engl J Med 341:14, 1999.

Syrjala KL, Martin P, Deeg HJ, et al. Medical and psychosocial issues in transplant survivors. In Chang AE, Ganz PA, Hayes DF, et al. (eds.): Oncology: An Evidence-Based Approach. New York, Springer-Verlag, 2006, p 1902.

Zebrack BJ, Zeltzer LK, Whitton J, et al: Psychological outcomes in long-term survivors of childhood leukemia, Hodgkin's disease and non-Hodgkin's lymphoma: a report from the Childhood Cancer Survivor Study. Pediatrics 110:42, 2002.

REFERENCES

For complete list of references log onto www.expertconsult.com

PART VII

TRANSPLANTATION

CHAPTER 98

OVERVIEW OF CELL- AND IMMUNE-BASED THERAPIES

Philip McGlave

INTRODUCTION

The use of cell- and immune-based therapies to treat hematologic disorders has come of age. Over the last 50 years hematopoietic cell transplantation has evolved into curative therapy for a variety of marrow failure states, hematologic malignancies, immune deficiencies, and inborn errors of metabolism. Appreciation of the graft versus tumor effect has provided a foundation for the treatment of hematologic malignancies with donor leukocyte infusions that exploit the allogeneic response of donor T lymphocytes, and experimentation with infusion of other allogeneic effector cell populations such as natural killer cells (see Fig. 98–1). During this era, investigators have made remarkable progress in the use of reduced-intensity conditioning, alternative donors for transplantation and measures to prevent and treat graft-versus-host disease (GVHD) and infections. Parallel studies have demonstrated the efficacy of humanized monoclonal antibodies used alone or conjugated to radioactive isotopes to treat hematologic malignancies. Collectively, these advances have expanded the population eligible for cell- and immune-based therapies to include nearly all children and adults. This chapter provides a brief overview of principles underlying the treatment of hematologic disorders with cell and immune-based therapies. These topics are discussed in depth in Chapters 98 to 113.

ALLOGENEIC HEMATOPOIETIC CELL TRANSPLANTATION

Transplant Terminology

The first successful hematopoietic cell transplants in humans were performed by infusion of hematopoietic progenitor and stem cells derived from the marrow of identical twins (syngeneic transplant). Application of transplant therapy broadened with the use of hematopoietic cells obtained from either related or unrelated donors (allogeneic transplant) suitably matched at the human leukocyte antigens (HLA), or even with a patient's own hematopoietic cells (autologous transplant). Although the term *bone marrow transplantation* (BMT) is historically applied to the field, *hematopoietic cell transplantation* (HCT) may be more appropriate because stem and progenitor cells are needed for prompt and complete engraftment in the clinical arena, and their source may be not only marrow but peripheral blood (PB), umbilical cord blood (UCB), or even fetal liver.[1,2]

Allogeneic Transplant Principles

Successful allogeneic HCT depends on principles demonstrated first in animals and then in the human clinical setting. Hematopoietic stem and progenitor cells obtained from donor marrow or other sources are infused intravenously, home to the recipient's hematopoietic microenvironment, and engraft.[3,4] Under optimal circumstances the recipient's immune system will tolerate engraftment of donor cells so that neither nonengraftment nor late graft failure occurs. Immune effector cells from the donor will interact with recipient cells and tissue in a fashion that ensures sustained engraftment and does not provoke fatal GVHD. Eventually, reconstitution of B lymphocyte, T lymphocyte, and natural killer (NK) cell function occurs, a stable chimeric state predominates, and a long-lasting graft-versus-tumor (GVT) effect is sustained.[5–7]

Donor–Recipient Histocompatibility

Transplantation of allogeneic cells requires careful matching of donor and recipient. Failure to do so is associated with delayed or incomplete engraftment and with GVHD. Graft failure and GVHD can occur when immunocompetent cells of host or donor origin respectively respond to alloantigens encoded on the major histocompatibility complex (MHC) and peptides presented in association with these antigens.[8,9] The MHC is located on chromosome 6 in humans and contains two distinct human HLA families implicated in alloreactivity. HLA class I antigens are encoded by three dominant loci termed HLA-A, HLA-B, and HLA-C. HLA class II antigens are encoded by three loci termed HLA-DR, HLA-DP, and HLA-DQ. Historically, HLA antigens were defined by serologic testing. More recently, families of alleles corresponding to the HLA antigens have been identified by molecular methods, and donor–recipient HLA characterization now depends heavily on these molecular methods.[10]

In both the related and unrelated donor transplant setting, optimal clinical results are achieved when donor and recipient are matched at HLA class I and HLA class II. Successful allogeneic transplantation can occur, however, even with some degree of HLA mismatch.[11] For example, successful transplant of HLA haploidentical related donor hematopoietic cells after T lymphocyte depletion has been reported,[12,13] and some degree of donor–recipient HLA mismatch is common in adult, volunteer unrelated donor transplant and unrelated umbilical cord blood transplant.[14] Both graft failure and GVHD can occur even in cases where apparent MHC matching is achieved, and in some cases mismatch of antigens not recognizable with current testing methods may have clinically relevant consequences.[15]

Graft-Versus-Host Disease

GVHD is the most important cause of mortality, morbidity, and diminished quality of life after allogeneic HCT. Early observations suggested that GVHD occurred when immune effector T lymphocytes engrafted and subsequently attacked host tissue. Recent observations have characterized a more complex process underpinned by host tissue damage and release of inflammatory factors, involvement of host as well as donor cells implicated in inflammation, antigen presentation, and immune effector function and modulation by regulatory T (Treg) cells and other cell populations.[16–19] Acute GVHD occurs in the first few months after engraftment, whereas a somewhat different clinical syndrome termed chronic GVHD typically evolves later in the transplant course. Chronic GVHD often appears as a sequela of acute GVHD and can be a chronic illness resulting in physical stigmata as well as malabsorption, chronic infection, failure to thrive, and generalized debility. GVHD can be exacerbated by HLA mismatch, infection, prior host tissue damage associated with the underlying disease, previous therapy, or tissue damage associated with the preparative regimen.[20–24]

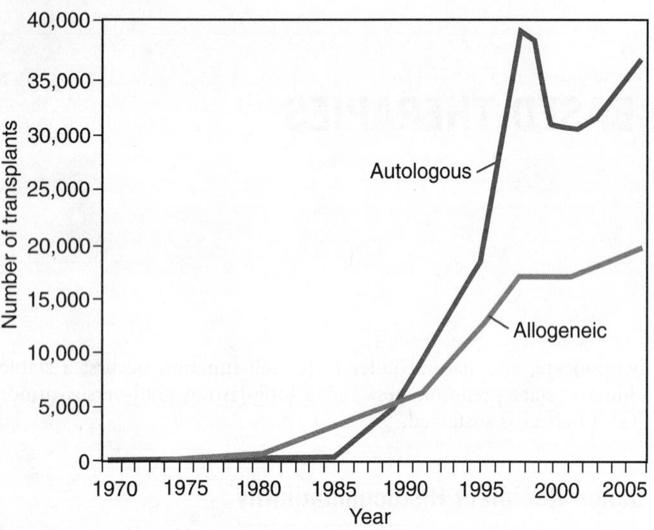

Figure 98–1 Annual numbers of hematopoietic cell transplants worldwide. There are now an estimated 50,000 to 60,000 autologous and allogeneic hematopoietic cell transplants performed each year. (Adapted from CIBMTR Summary Slides, 2007.)

Cyclosporine has become the backbone of in vivo GVHD prophylaxis and treatment. This compound inhibits calcineurin cell membrane flux and has a specific suppressive effect on T lymphocyte function. Cyclosporine, tacrolimus, or related calcineurin inhibitors may be used alone or in combination with other agents that have specific effects on lymphocytes such as sirolimus, agents with general immunosuppressive functions such as steroids, methotrexate or antithymocyte globulin, or with promising agents such as rituximab, whose mechanism of action in GVHD is not entirely understood.[25]

Acute GVHD can also be prevented or ameliorated by ex vivo depletion of T lymphocytes (T-cell depletion) from the hematopoietic stem and progenitor cell inoculum. Ex vivo T-cell depletion can be accomplished by negative selection of T cells with monoclonal antibodies used alone, conjugated to toxins (immunotoxins) or by physical methods such as elutriation.[26] Alternatively, positive selection of hematopoietic cells based on physical properties such as CD34 expression (CD34 selection) can provide an inoculum enriched for hematopoietic progenitors and depleted of T lymphocytes. Antibodies specifically targeting T cells can also be used for in vivo T-cell depletion.[27]

Graft-Versus-Tumor Effect

Early investigators postulated that effective antitumor therapy with hematopoietic cell transplantation might require not only an ablative effect of the preparatory conditioning regimen but also an ongoing allogeneic graft versus tumor (GVT) or graft versus leukemia (GVL) effect.[28] Subsequent reports of a high incidence of relapse after T cell-depleted related donor transplant therapy for chronic myelogenous leukemia (CML), and of the reinduction of cytogenetic and molecular remissions after donor leukocyte infusion (DLI) supported the importance of the GVT effect.[29,30] Recent studies implicate an interplay of donor and recipient T lymphocytes and, possibly, a role for NK cells in the GVT effect.[31–34] In any case, the GVT effect plays an important role in the long-term suppression of malignant clones of host origin, which sometimes survive even the most rigorous preparative regimens.

Conditioning Regimens for Allogeneic Transplantation

Historically, recipients were treated with an immunosuppressive conditioning regimen to ensure engraftment of donor hematopoietic stem cells. A regimen of high-dose cyclophosphamide (CY) used alone was immunosuppressive and could be used successfully to condition patients with nonmalignant conditions such as severe aplastic anemia, immunodeficiencies, or inborn errors of metabolism for HCT.[35] Regimens containing high-dose cyclophosphamide used first in combination with total body irradiation (CY/TBI) or subsequently with busulfan (BU/CY) were considered "ablative" and were used to provide immunosuppression and tumor suppression in patients receiving HCT therapy for a variety of malignancies.[36–39] Acceptance of the GVT effect led to speculation that "reduced-intensity conditioning" (RIC) regimens could be employed to treat hematologic malignancies with HCT. Such regimens provided adequate immunosuppression for engraftment, relied on the GVT effect for ongoing tumor suppression, and spared patients the toxicity associated with ablative conditioning.[40,41] Reduced-intensity conditioning regimens may use cyclophosphamide or TBI, but at markedly reduced doses. Other immunosuppressive agents such as antithymocyte globulin or fludarabine may also be effective.[42,43] Reduced-intensity conditioning is often used in older, debilitated, or heavily pretreated patients in whom the toxicity associated with ablative conditioning would be unacceptable.

Alternative Donors

Application of allogeneic HCT has broadened as investigators demonstrate that donors other than HLA-identical or 1 antigen mismatched siblings can be used successfully. Recently, there has been resurgent interest in the use of HLA haploidentical related donors for HCT. HLA haploidentical transplant is appealing because a suitable related donor is usually available. However, such transplants require aggressive immunosuppression, and effects on engraftment, GVHD, and immune reconstitution are not yet fully understood.[12,13] Adult volunteer unrelated donors (URD) have been used successfully as a source of hematopoietic cells for transplantation for more than 30 years.[44–47] Results with an HLA-matched URD transplant performed in younger patients are comparable to HLA-matched sibling transplant.[48] The process of donor identification and hematopoietic cell procurement has been vastly aided by the development of international registries such as the National Marrow Donor Program (NMDP), with more than 30,000 transplants facilitated from 1987 to 2007.[49,50]

Perhaps the most exciting recent development in the field of HCT has been the successful use of umbilical cord blood (UCB) derived from related or (more commonly) unrelated donors as a source of donor stem and progenitor cells.[51,52] The establishment of a worldwide network for UCB cell procurement, typing, and storage has resulted in the collection and cryopreservation of more than one-quarter million cords and has facilitated more than 7000 unrelated donor UCB transplants. Recent clinical studies suggest that the use of pooled cells from two cords (double cord blood transplant), each partially or completely HLA-matched with the recipient, can provide timely engraftment even in larger, unrelated recipients.[53] Most recently, UCB transplant after RIC has been tested successfully.[54] Collectively, these advances in the use of alternative donors combined with standard ablative or RIC regimens suggests that transplants will be available for the majority of children and adults who are otherwise suitable candidates for such therapy.

Clinical Application

The first successful use of human hematopoietic cell transplantation was reported in the late 1950s by E. Donnall Thomas and colleagues, who demonstrated that marrow cells from identical twin donors could reconstitute hematopoiesis after supralethal irradiation therapy for acute lymphocytic leukemia.[55] Subsequently, other groups used HCT to restore immune function in children with immune deficiencies and to attempt correction of inborn errors of metabolism.[56,57]

By the late 1970s, Thomas and his group had ushered in the era of successful antitumor therapy with hematopoietic cell transplantation when they reported that HLA-matched sibling transplantation could be used to correct refractory cases of acute leukemia.[58] A similar story unfolded in the treatment of CML and other hematologic malignancies, as well as severe aplastic anemia and other marrow failure states.[59–63] Dramatic improvement in transplant outcome occurred when investigators realized that transplant therapy was most effective when used early in the disease course, rather than as a "last resort."[64]

Broad acceptance of alternative donors by the transplant community has greatly broadened the pool of eligible transplant recipients.[65,66] Successful use of RIC approaches has also opened transplant to older and more debilitated patients and seems to be particularly useful in CML and some low-grade lymphoid malignancies. Collectively, these advances now permit allogeneic transplant therapy for the majority of suitable candidates in ages ranging from infancy to the eighth decades.

AUTOLOGOUS HEMATOPOIETIC CELL TRANSPLANTATION

Autologous Transplant Principles

Autologous hematopoietic cell transplantation is most commonly used to reestablish hematopoiesis after high-dose cancer chemotherapy or radiation therapy. This approach permits the use of antitumor agents in doses much higher than can be provided in a conventional therapy setting. Autologous HCT is most useful in circumstances where a correlation exists between increased therapy dose and tumor response, and where the dose-limiting feature of therapy is hematopoietic suppression.

In selected cases, autologous HCT may have advantages over allogeneic transplant. There is no need to identify an HLA-compatible related or unrelated donor. Immunologic complications of allogeneic transplantation such as graft failure and GVHD are avoided. The use of immunosuppressive agents for transplant preparation, GVHD prophylaxis, and GVHD treatment is unnecessary. Not surprisingly, transplant mortality is low. Older patients tolerate the autologous transplant procedure relatively well. Hospital stay and convalescence periods are shorter. With the judicious use of prophylactic and empiric antimicrobial therapy, nutritional support, a state-of-the-art clinic facility and dedicated caregivers, many autologous transplants may even be performed in the outpatient setting.[67]

Unfortunately, autologous transplant has important drawbacks. The benign hematopoietic stem and progenitor populations may be reduced or damaged by previous therapy, resulting in delayed or partial engraftment.[68] The inoculum, whether derived from marrow or blood, may be contaminated with clonogenic malignant cells capable of re-establishing primary tumor growth in the transplanted patient.[69] The risk of relapse is compounded because autologous HCT does not produce an ongoing GVT effect analogous to that observed after allogeneic transplant. Finally, autologous transplant may increase the risk of secondary, therapy-related myeloid leukemias or myelodysplastic syndromes.[70]

Priming and Mobilization

The priming process facilitates collection by apheresis of a mobilized peripheral blood mononuclear cell population enriched for hematopoietic progenitors. In some cases, priming is performed with growth factor alone or, in some cases, with a combination of chemotherapy and growth factors.[71,72] The use of chemokines in the CXCR family during the mobilization process may further enhance the yield of hematopoietic progenitors. These agents interfere with adhesion of hematopoietic progenitors in the microenvironment and promote their circulation in the peripheral blood.[73] The use of these various mobilization approaches can result in WBC and platelet engraftment within 2 weeks. The shortened time to engraftment associated with peritransplant use of hematopoietic growth factors, antimicrobial agents, and transfusions have resulted in a shift to outpatient-based autologous HCT.[67]

> **A Primer On Terminology**
>
> The field of blood and bone marrow transplantation is changing rapidly, and so is the terminology. In fact, we now use the term *hematopoietic cell transplant* (HCT) instead of *bone marrow transplant* because we often obtain hematopoietic stem and progenitor cells from the peripheral blood after mobilization, or even from *umbilical cord blood* rather than from the marrow. Some terms have not changed, however. *Syngeneic transplants* require an identical twin donor whereas *allogeneic transplants* draw on other related or unrelated human donor sources. Of course, we can also use the recipient as a source of his or her own cells in the *autologous transplant* process. We can prepare recipients for HCT with an *ablative* conditioning regimen. However, *reduced-intensity conditioning* or even *nonmyeloablative conditioning* regimens may have advantages in some settings and can be effective because we now realize that donor cells exert a *graft-versus-leukemia* or *graft-versus-tumor* effect. This beneficial immune-mediated effect of allogeneic HCT must be distinguished from acute or chronic *graft-versus-host disease* resulting from an interaction of donor immune or effector cells with host cells and tissue, and leading to a variety of often serious clinical problems.

Clinical Application

Autologous HCT therapy for selected subsets of patients with acute myelogenous leukemia (AML) in first remission as well as some cases of Hodgkin and non-Hodgkin lymphoma can result in long-term disease-free survival.[74–76] Autologous transplant therapy can also prolong survival when used as therapy for myeloma.[77] Innovative trials with tandem autologous transplants or autologous followed by RIC allogeneic HCT (auto/allo transplant) in the treatment of myeloma have been undertaken; however the roles of single auto, tandem auto, or "auto/allo" tandem HCT in the treatment of myeloma have not yet been determined definitively.[78–81] As noted above, there is an unexpectedly high incidence of myelodysplastic syndrome and other hematologic malignancies after autologous HCT. It is not known if this is a result of an underlying predisposition for hematologic malignancies in these patients, damage to hematopoietic progenitors during the conventional and autologous transplant therapy, or a combination of these factors.[82–84]

NEWER APPROACHES TO CELL- AND IMMUNE-BASED THERAPIES

Effector Cells

Although there has been a long-standing acceptance of the GVT effect, clinical application was first demonstrated in 1990 when Kolb infused donor leukocytes into relapsing allogeneic transplant recipients.[29] In these cases, and in scores of cases reported subsequently, DLI produced a rapid reversal of the relapsing hematologic malignancy.[85–87] Optimal timing, number, and cell dose of the DLI is not known. GVHD and graft failure can complicate DLI therapy, especially if there is limited donor chimerism at the time of DLI.[88,89] Donor leukocyte infusion may be more effective in the treatment of some relapsing diseases such as CML and low-grade lymphoid malignancies and less effective in the treatment of other hematologic malignancies.

Investigators have speculated that natural killer (NK) cells may have an antitumor effect.[90,91] Recent reports suggest that "killer immunoglobulin receptors" (KIRs) found on NK cells are implicated in killing of host leukemia cells after HCT, although the importance of KIR is not fully understood.[33,92] Clinical trials of allogeneic NK infusion without allogeneic HCT have also demonstrated unexpected remissions in refractory AML patients.[93] Collectively, these observations suggest that allogeneic NK cells may be useful in the treatment of select hematopoietic malignancies, even in the nontransplant setting.

Antibody and Radioimmunotherapy

The development of rituximab, a humanized monoclonal antibody that recognizes the CD20 receptor on benign and malignant B-cells, has had a profound effect on the therapy of B-cell lymphoma. This antibody has efficacy in both low-grade and aggressive lymphomas and can be used successfully alone and in combination with conventional chemotherapy, even in the elderly.[94,95] Recently, anti-CD20 antibody has been conjugated to either ^{90}Yttrium or ^{131}Iodine. Both radioimmunoconjugates have activity against a spectrum of B-cell lymphomas.[96,97] Efforts are now focused on determining the optimal treatment strategies for the use of rituximab and of anti-CD20 radioimmunoconjugates alone or in conjunction with conventional chemotherapy.[98] It seems likely that the development of these and other antibodies and immunoconjugates recognizing specific cell surface receptors on malignant cells will change our approach to the treatment of hematologic malignancies including choice of initial therapies, approach to refractory or recurrent disease, and timing of HCT.[99,100]

Long-Term Effects and Quality of Life

As the field evolves, investigators have begun a systematic attempt to understand the impact of cell- and immune-based therapies not only on the disease process but on the quality of life and on well-being in long-term survivors (see Fig. 98–2). Such studies have demonstrated significant problems with growth and retardation in children, the development of second tumors, long-lasting adverse effects on physical and mental health, sexual function, capacity to return to work, and even overall economic status.[101–103] These important observations are being incorporated into the informed consent process and should lead to judicious choices of initial therapy and increased efforts to provide ongoing medical, counseling, and financial help for patients receiving cell- and immune-based therapies.[104,105]

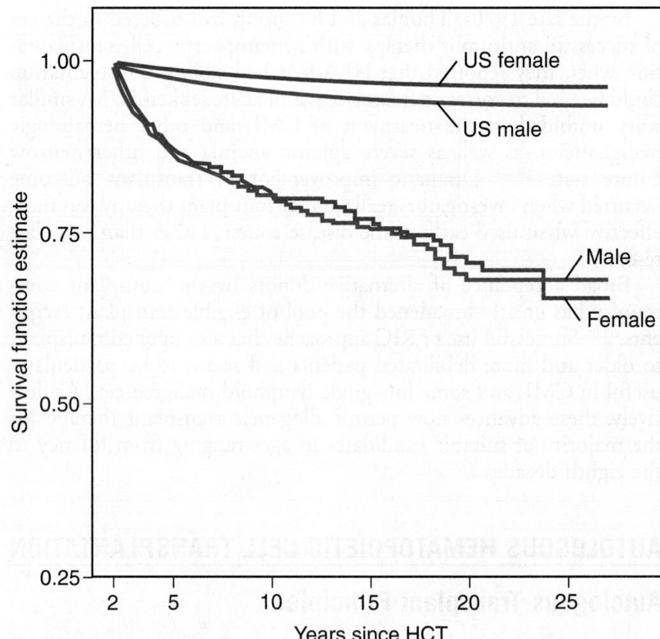

Figure 98–2 Assessment of late mortality in 1479 allogeneic HCT recipients surviving more than 2 years from transplant. Transplant survivors have a significantly higher mortality rate than that of the general population, even after 15 years. Leading causes of death are relapse and complications of chronic GVHD. (Data from Bhatia S, Francisco L, Carter A, et al: Late mortality after allogeneic hematopoietic cell transplantation and functional status of long-term survivors: Report from the BMT survivor study. Blood 110:3784, 2007.)

SUGGESTED READINGS

Barker JN, Weisdorf DJ, DeFor TE, et al: Transplantation of two partially HLA-matched umbilical cord blood units to enhance engraftment in adults with hematologic malignancy. Blood 105:1343, 2005.

Bhatia S, Francisco L, Carter A, et al: Late mortality after allogeneic hematopoietic cell transplantation and functional status of long-term survivors: Report from the BMT survivor study. Blood 110:3784, 2007.

Bruno B, Rotta M, Patriarca F, et al: A comparison of allografting with autografting for newly diagnosed myeloma. N Engl J Med 356:1110, 2007.

Brunstein CG, Barker JN, Weisdorf DJ, et al: Umbilical cord blood transplantation after nonmyeloablative conditioning: Impact on transplant outcomes in 110 adults with hematological disease. Blood 110:3064, 2007.

Dreyling M, Trumper L, von Schilling C, et al: Results of a national consensus workshop: Therapeutic algorithm in patients with follicular lymphoma-role of radioimmunotherapy. Ann Hematol 86:81, 2007.

Fernandez-Aviles F, Carreras E, Urbano-Ispizua A, et al: Case-control comparison of at-home to total hospital care for autologous stem-cell transplantation for hematologic malignancies. J Clin Oncol 24:4855, 2006.

Ferrara JL, Reddy P: Pathophysiology of graft-versus-host disease. Semin Hematol 43:3, 2006.

Gluckman E, Broxmeyer HA, Auerbach AD, et al: Hematopoietic reconstitution in a patient with Fanconi's anemia by means of umbilical-cord blood from an HLA-identical sibling. N Engl J Med 321:1174, 1989.

Hansen JA, Petersdorf EW, Lin MT, et al: Genetics of allogeneic hematopoietic cell transplantation. Role of HLA matching, functional variation in immune response genes. Immunol Res 41:56, 2008.

Khouri I, Keating M, Korbling M, et al: Transplant lite: Induction of graft-versus-leukemia using fludarabine-based nonablative chemotherapy and allogeneic blood progenitor cell transplantation as treatment for lymphoid malignancies. J Clin Oncol 16:2817, 1998.

Kolb HJ, Mittermuller J, Clemm C, et al: Donor leukocyte transfusions for treatment of recurrent chronic myelogenous leukemia in marrow transplant patients. Blood 76:2462, 1990.

Quesenberry PJ, Colvin G, Abedi M: Perspective: Fundamental and clinical concepts on stem cell homing and engraftment: A journey to niches and beyond. Exp Hematol 33:9, 2005.

Reddy P: Pathophysiology of acute graft-versus-host disease. Hematol Oncol 21:149, 2003.

Ruggeri L, Mancusi A, Capanni M, et al: Donor natural killer cell allorecognition of missing self in haploidentical hematopoietic transplantation for acute myeloid leukemia: Challenging its predictive value. Blood 110:433, 2007.

Shankar SM, Carter A, Sun CL, et al: Health care utilization by adult long-term survivors of hemopoietic cell transplant: Report from the Bone Marrow Transplant Survivor Study. Cancer Epidemiol Biomarkers Prev 16:834, 2007.

Shlomchik WD: Graft-versus-host disease. Nat Rev Immunol 7:340, 2007.

Speck B, Zwaan FE, van Rood JJ, et al: Allogeneic bone marrow transplantation in a patient with aplastic anemia using a phenotypically HLA-A identical unrelated donor. Transplantation 16:24, 1973.

Thomas ED, Lochte HL Jr, Cannon JH, et al: Supralethal whole body lethal irradiation and isologous marrow transplantation in man. J Clin Invest 38:1709, 1959.

Yakoub-Agha I, Mesnil F, Kuentz M, et al: Allogeneic marrow stem-cell transplantation from human leukocyte antigen-identical siblings versus human leukocyte antigen-allelic-matched unrelated donors (10/10) in patients with standard-risk hematologic malignancy: A prospective study from the French Society of Bone Marrow Transplantation and Cell Therapy. J Clin Oncol 24:5695, 2006.

REFERENCES

For complete list of references log onto www.expertconsult.com

CHAPTER 99

HEMATOPOIETIC STEM CELL TRANSPLANTATION FOR ACQUIRED NONMALIGNANT DISEASES AND MYELODYSPLASTIC SYNDROME

Bart L. Scott and H. Joachim Deeg

BACKGROUND

Systematic research into the possibility of marrow (hematopoietic cell) transplantation (HCT) began after the observations of the medical effects of radiation exposure at Hiroshima and Nagasaki.[1] Studies on total body irradiation (TBI) in animal models showed that shielding of the spleen during TBI, implantation of autologous or syngeneic spleen or infusion of syngeneic marrow following TBI rescued animals from the radiation induced marrow syndrome.[2,3] The most effective way of hematopoietic reconstitution was by intravenous (IV) injection of hematopoietic cells. By a mechanism now termed "homing" and mediated by a series of receptors and counter-receptors on cells and vascular endothelium, injected cells reached the marrow cavity and other hematopoietic organs and settled in supportive niches. Studies in several animal models then showed that hematopoiesis in lethally irradiated animals was restored by parabiosis with a normal animal, proving in principle the presence of circulating stem cells in peripheral blood.

While the infusion of autologous or syngeneic hematopoietic cells rescued marrow-ablated animals without complications, animals given cells from histoincompatible (allogeneic) donors developed "secondary disease," now known as graft-versus-host disease (GVHD).[3] These observations showed convincingly that transplantation of spleen or marrow cells not only resulted in hematopoietic reconstitution, but also conveyed immune effects.[4] The development of moderate GVHD was associated with improved survival in mice with leukemia, due to what has been termed a graft-versus-leukemia (GVL) effect.[5] However, no such benefit could be expected in recipients transplanted for nonmalignant disorders.

The first modern transplant attempts, beginning in 1957, were in patients with end-stage leukemia, and results were discouraging: Patients transplanted from syngeneic (monozygotic twin) donors did well immediately posttransplant but died from progressive leukemia; patients transplanted from allogeneic donors died with severe GVHD.[2,6] Beginning in the late 1950s, Dausset and others, showed that, similar to observations in mice, differences in major histocompatibility complex (MHC) antigens triggered immune reactions of the donor cells against the patient.[7] These insights, considerable work in animal models, and pioneering work by Thomas, Good, Santos and others, ushered in the modern era of hematopoietic cell transplantation (HCT).[2]

Table 99–1 lists acquired nonmalignant disorders that have been treated by HCT. The indications for HCT are continuously under revision as new treatment strategies evolve. While the number of separate disease entities amenable to transplantation is considerable, the large majority of transplants are currently performed to cure malignancies, and a smaller proportion for nonmalignant disorders.

RATIONALE FOR HEMATOPOIETC CELL TRANSPLANTATION FOR NONMALIGNANT DISEASES

HCT may serve as a rescue procedure generally in patients with malignant disorders treated with high-dose cytotoxic regimens or as replacement therapy in patients with missing, aberrant, or defective lymphohematopoietic cells, including marrow failure and autoimmune disorders.[8,9] In both situations, however, HCT also has immunotherapeutic effects, which may provide important signals to eradicate the patient's disease. In addition, HCT serves as a vehicle for gene therapy (Chapter 101)[10] and possibly as a strategy to establish tolerance for solid organ transplantation.

DONOR SELECTION

Potential donor categories are listed in Table 99–2. The preferred donor is a genotypically HLA-identical sibling, available in approximately 25% to 30% of patients who have living siblings. In addition, about 1% of patients have phenotypically HLA-matched donors within the family, and a few patients will have identical twin donors. A haploidentical donor (such as a parent or child) would be available for most patients, but HLA and non-HLA differences may result in major morbidity and mortality due to GVHD and rejection, although recent work shows that it is possible to overcome those hurdles.[11]

Approximately 70% to 75% of patients, who could benefit from HCT, lack a suitably matched related donor. This need has driven (a) efforts at improving the techniques of autologous transplantation, and (b) the development of unrelated donor registries. Thanks to the efforts of the National Marrow Donor Program (NMDP; www.marrow.org) and registries in Great Britain, France, Germany, Japan, Taiwan and other countries, there are now about ten million volunteer donors who have been typed for HLA-A and -B antigens, and many also for HLA-C, DRB1, and DQB1 antigens, a rapidly growing proportion of them by "high resolution" typing, ie, by DNA sequencing. Computer inquiries based on the patient's HLA typing quickly generate an idea as to the probability of identifying unrelated donors. In North America, the probability of finding a suitably matched unrelated donor is about 75% for whites; the probability is lower for patients of different ethnicity.[12]

An autologous stem cell approach may be possible with acquired disorders. Granulocyte colony-stimulating factor (G-CSF) mobilized peripheral blood progenitor cells (PBPCs) have been harvested and transplanted even in patients with severe acquired aplastic anemia. In patients with paroxysmal nocturnal hemoglobinuria (PNH) normal ($CD34^+$, $CD50^+$, $CD59^+$) hematopoietic precursors are present, and the possibility of using those for transplantation has been suggested.[13] Results in animals, eg, with experimental allergic encephalomyelitis, suggest that transplantation of autologous stem cells depleted of T lymphocytes can even restore neurologic function by eliminating Vβ-8positive autoreactive T cells.[14] Transplantation for various autoimmune disorders is a rapidly developing area of research, and new insights are likely to advance this field in the near future.[15,16]

Regardless of the stem cell source, problems with hematopoietic reconstitution may be encountered in patients whose disease is associated with defects in the marrow microenvironment.

Table 99–1 Acquired Disorders Treated by HCT

Aplastic anemia
Pure red cell aplasia
Paroxysmal nocturnal hemoglobinuria
Myelodysplastic syndrome
Autoimmune disorders
Acquired immunodeficiency syndrome
Langerhans cell histiocytosis

HCT, hematopoietic cell transfusion.

Table 99–2 Potential Marrow or Stem Cell Donors

		Histocompatibility Barrier	
		Minor	**Major**
Autologous	Patients are their own donors	–	–
Syngeneic	Monozygotic (identical) twin	–	–
Allogeneic	HLA genotypically identical donor	+	–
	HLA phenotypically identical donor		
	—Related	+	–/+
	—Unrelated	+++	–/+
	HLA-nonidentical donor		
	—Related	+	++
	—Unrelated	+++	++
Xenogeneic	Different species donor	+++	+++

HLA, human leukocyte antigen

PREPARATION FOR HEMATOPOIETIC CELL TRANSPLANTATION

Rationale for Conditioning

In preparation for HCT, patients generally receive cytotoxic or immunosuppressive treatment "conditioning" with the following objectives:

1. To eradicate or at least reduce the number of abnormal or defective cells below detectable levels; this applies to allogeneic, syngeneic, and autologous transplantation.
2. To suppress the patient's immunity, natural or acquired through allosensitization, to prevent rejection of donor cells; this applies to allogeneic but not to autologous cells (which constitute an "autoplantation" rather than a transplantation) or to syngeneic cells, which should not encounter a histocompatibility barrier. However, immunosuppression is needed in preparation for some syngeneic transplants in many patients with aplastic anemia, apparently to eliminate autoimmune reactivity, which may interfere with sustained hematopoietic reconstitution.
3. The concept that conditioning is required to create space for donor cells is no longer tenable, as there is good evidence that donor cells create the space required for their engraftment and expansion.[17] However, observations in patients who are prepared for HCT with reduced-intensity conditioning (RIC) or nonmyeloablative regimens have shown that a certain degree of "debulking" of patient cells is required to provide an advantage to donor cells so that they can progressively replace patient cells.[18]

Exceptions to the requirement of conditioning exist in patients with severe immunodeficiency disorders in whom even HLA-haploidentical stem cells may engraft without conditioning.[19]

Modalities of Conditioning

Various therapeutic modalities are being used to prepare patients for transplantation. In principle, they comprise:

1. **Irradiation**: Irradiation is given in several forms: external beam total body irradiation (TBI), total lymphoid irradiation (TLI) or modifications thereof delivered at various exposure rates, fractionation schedules and total doses have been used extensively. There is a strong trend to avoid or reduce the radiation dose in patients who are transplanted for nonmalignant disorders. With transplants from HLA-nonidentical or unrelated donors, TBI is often used at higher total doses, eg, 11 × 120 or 6 × 200 cGy given over 3 to 4 days. TBI doses as low as 200 cGy, often combined with chemotherapy, have been used in reduced intensity conditioning (RIC) or nonmyeloablative regimens. For some malignant disorders, bone seeking isotopes (eg, holmium) have proven useful. Yet another strategy has employed radioisotopes such as^{131} I or^{90} Y, conjugated to monoclonal antibodies directed to lymphoid or myeloid antigens (eg, CD20, CD45).[20]
2. **Chemotherapy**: Chemotherapy, particularly cyclophosphamide ([CY] 120–200 mg/kg over 2–4 days), is included in many regimens. In patients with aplastic anemia and Fanconi anemia, CY has been used successfully as single agent for transplant conditioning. Others have combined CY with busulfan ([BU] ± antithymocyte globulin [ATG]). Busulfan, when given orally, may show considerable variations in plasma levels, which may result in significant differences in toxicities and clinical responses.[21] These variations can be minimized by monitoring of steady state plasma levels of BU (BUss), and dose adjustments to target BUss to predetermined plasma levels.[22] Recent trials using once-a-day rather than every 6 hours dosing with the IV preparation suggest that this is a well-tolerated and practical approach.[23] Another increasingly used agent is fludarabine, given either in combination with BU[24] or treosulfan[25]or in RIC as part of nonmyeloablative approaches in combination with low-dose TBI or with melphalan.[18,26,27]
3. **Biologics**: Biological reagents, such as ATG, a polyclonal heterologous antibody preparation generated in horses or rabbits, or monoclonal antibodies directed at T-cell antigens or adhesion molecules are employed primarily to suppress recipient immunity. Specific monoclonal antibodies targeted at cancer cells, such as radiolabeled anti-CD45[28] are also under active investigation for conditioning. Similarly, monoclonal antibodies (eg, anti-CD33) conjugated to chemotherapeutic agents have been tested in transplant conditioning regimens.[29]
4. **Cellular Therapy**: Viable donor buffy coat in addition to marrow cells has been used to facilitate engraftment in patients with aplastic anemia but has been abandoned because of a high incidence of GVHD.[30] The observation that broad T-lymphocyte depletion of donor marrow increased the probability of graft failure has led to protocols of partial T-cell-depletion, selective T-cell add back or, more recently, the infusion of NK cells[31] or regulatory T cells, to assure engraftment, prevent disease recurrence, or modulate GVHD.

Other procedures include plasmapheresis of the patient to remove isoagglutinins directed at the donor's ABO blood group or, conversely, removal of plasma from the donor marrow to remove isoagglutinins directed at recipient cells. Alternatively, the donor red blood cells with which recipient antibodies may react are removed, thus minimizing the risk of hemolysis and possibly accelerating the tempo of erythroid reconstitution. With the use of PBPCs, such procedures are usually not required since these preparations are largely red blood

Table 99–3 Sources of Stem Cells[a]

Bone marrow
Peripheral blood
Cord blood
Fetal liver[b]

[a]Preclinical studies on the use of embryonic stem cells as a source for transplantation are ongoing.
[b]Very infrequently used.

cell depleted and of small volume, so that isoagglutinin amounts may be negligible.

TRANSPLANT PROCEDURE

Sources of Hematopoietic Stem Cells

Hematopoiesis during embryogenesis evolves from a mesodermal (yolk sac), a hepatosplenic, and a medullary stage. At the time of birth, the bone marrow has generally become the only site of hematopoiesis. In adult humans extramedullary hematopoiesis occurs only under pathologic conditions (eg, chronic myelogenous leukemia, myelofibrosis). Accordingly, hematopoietic stem cells can be obtained from fetal (but not adult) livers, whereas an adult donor usually can donate stem cells only in the form of bone marrow or from peripheral blood where some stem cells circulate (Table 99–3).

a. Bone Marrow
In the adult human, bone marrow is the major reservoir of hematopoietic stem cells, which might also have potential as adult organ-specific stem cells (stem cell plasticity).[32,33] Marrow is harvested with the donor under anesthesia, and under sterile conditions. Generally multiple small-volume aspirates of marrow are obtained from both posterior iliac crests.[34]

b. Peripheral Blood Progenitor Cells (PBPC)
Under steady state conditions, only low numbers of hematopoietic stem cells circulate in peripheral blood.[35] However, peripheral blood contains dramatically increased numbers of early hematopoietic precursors during the recovery phase following cytotoxic therapy.[36] A single leukapheresis on a normal donor may suffice to harvest the numbers of cells required for a transplant, generally at least 5×10^6 $CD34^+$ cells/kg of recipient weight. The use of G-CSF mobilized PBPCs rather than marrow is associated with more rapid hematopoietic recovery. However, there is convincing evidence that the incidence of chronic GVHD is higher than with marrow cells, and PBPC should not be used indiscriminately as a source of hematopoietic stem cells in patients with nonmalignant diseases.

c. Umbilical Cord Blood
Umbilical cord blood is another source of hematopoietic stem cells.[37] Cord blood cells maybe less immunocompetent than adult cells and might carry a lower risk of inducing GVHD than adult marrow cells, although this notion has recently been challenged. While the concentration of stem cells in cord blood is high (frequency of long-term culture-initiating cells approximately 1:100 as compared to 1:500 in peripheral blood), the small volume usually available (50–150 mL) may limit the use of these cells for transplantation, particularly to adult patients. Recent trials suggest that the transplantation of two cord blood units may overcome this problem.[38] Additional studies will determine whether expansion of available cells in vitro will be feasible and useful.

d. Fetal Liver
For several months during fetal development, the liver is physiologically part of the hematopoietic system, and fetal liver cells, a mixture of hepatocytes and hematopoietic stem cells can be used for transplantation. Fetal liver cells have been studied extensively in experimental models and have been shown clinically to reconstitute successfully both hematopoietic and immunologic systems in children with congenital immunodeficiencies.[39] Because of ethical concerns and the development of alternative approaches, fetal liver cells are currently used only by a few investigators and for selected indications.

PERI- AND POSTTRANSPLANT CARE

Complications of HCT are related to the underlying disease, therapy given before transplantation, the preparative regimen (regimen-related toxicity [RRT]), the interactions of donor cells with recipient tissues (GVHD), and prophylactic and therapeutic measures administered after HCT.

Many transplant recipients have received therapy for extended periods of time before HCT. Patients with aplastic anemia who have HLA-identical related donors and are no more than 45 years of age generally receive a transplant as first-line therapy; all others are initially treated with immunosuppressive therapy, transfusions and hematopoietic growth factors. Only when these attempts fail and an alternative, usually unrelated, donor is identified, will HCT be considered. As a result, patients become allosensitized and frequently are platelet transfusion refractory. Over prolonged periods of neutropenia and immunosuppression, many patients become colonized by fungal organisms. While only hematopoietic reconstitution can eradicate these organisms, aggressive antibacterial and antifungal therapy must be given in the peritransplant period. In heavily transfused patients iron overload is the rule, and chelation therapy should be instituted (for ferritin >1000 ng/mL). Recent reports indicate that transplant outcome is inferior in patients with iron overload.[40,41]

Except for patients who are prepared with nonmyeloablative regimens, all patients experience pancytopenia before hematopoietic reconstitution from the transplanted (donor-derived) stem cells occurs. Pancytopenia may last 3 weeks with marrow cells, but possibly only 10 to 12 days with PBPCs. With single-unit cord blood transplants, recovery may take 5 to 6 weeks. The administration of growth factors such as G-CSF or granulocyte/macrophage colony-stimulating factor (GM-CSF) early after marrow transplantation has been shown to accelerate granulocyte recovery, although treatment with growth factor is not considered standard.[42] After transplantation of mobilized PBPCs, growth factors may show little or no acceleration of hematopoietic recovery as the transplanted cells were already "activated" by G-CSF mobilization. Whether a different effect will be seen with cells mobilized by the CXCR4 antagonist AMD3100 remains to be determined.[43] Virtually all marrow recipients conditioned with conventional regimens will need transfusion support with platelets and red blood cells. Erythropoietin administration may slightly speed reticulocyte recovery and moderately reduce red blood cell transfusion requirements.[44] Thrombopoietin (megakaryocyte growth and differentiation factor) and interleukin-11 can enhance platelet production; however, side effects are considerable and both have had only a limited impact on HCT.

Infection prophylaxis consists primarily of systemic broad spectrum antimicrobials. The indications for granulocyte transfusions, eg, in granulocytopenic patients in whom bacterial or fungal infections are not controlled by antimicrobials, have remained controversial. Treatment of patients in laminar air flow rooms and with gastrointestinal decontamination may reduce the frequency of infections and the duration of febrile episodes.[45] Because of an 80% to 90% risk of reactivation of herpes simplex virus (HSV), prophylaxis with acyclovir is given for at least 2 to 3 months after HCT. Some protocols also include the infusion of IV immunoglobulins on a weekly basis, although available data indicate that this strategy will benefit only patients with IgG levels <400 mg/L. Trimethoprim/sulfamethoxazole is administered primarily for *Pneumocystis jiroveci* prophylaxis but also reduces the incidence of other infections, in particular in patients with chronic GVHD. Fluconazole is administered as antifungal prophylaxis for 2 to 3 months (or longer), and has a long-term protective effect against *Candida* related morbidity and mortality.[46] Ongoing trials are aimed at determining the place for newer agents, such as caspofungin and posaconazole.[47] Ganciclovir and valacyclovir provide good prophylaxis and are effective as preemptive therapy in patients with evidence of cytomegalovirus (CMV) reactivation. Epstein-Barr virus (EBV) reactivation is more frequently seen in patients who receive T cell depleted, HLA-nonidentical transplants, and in vivo anti–T cell reagents. Anti-CD20 antibodies, eg, rituximab, at doses of 375 mg/m^2, have been effective in controlling the rise of EBV DNA titers in blood.

Because of mucositis and gastroenteritis, many patients are unable to eat early posttransplant and require parenteral nutrition and hydration. Oral intake is less of a problem in patients prepared with RIC regimens.

All allogeneic transplant recipients receive some form of GVHD prophylaxis.[48] Modalities involve administration of immunosuppressive agents such as methotrexate (MTX), cyclosporine (CSP), FK506 (tacrolimus), mycophenolate mofetil (MMF), rapamycin (sirolimus), and others, either alone or in combination. Currently, the two most widely used regimens are combinations of MTX, 10 mg/m^2 IV on day 1, 3, 6, and 11 (or 15 mg/m^2 on day 1, and 10 mg/m^2 on days 3, 6, and 11), and CSP or tacrolimus, given daily starting on day −1 (or −3), and continued at gradually tapering doses for 6 to 12 months.[49,50] It is recommended that plasma levels for both CSP and tacrolimus be monitored as frequently as twice a week during the early course after HCT, to maintain therapeutic but nontoxic levels. As an alternative or adjunct to immunosuppressive therapy, T lymphocytes, responsible for triggering GVHD, are depleted from the donor marrow in vitro before infusion.

CLINICAL RESULTS

Aplastic Anemia

The term "aplastic anemia," is actually a misnomer since, as originally described by Ehrlich, not only erythropoiesis but all cell lineages are defective, and the marrow appears empty.[51] T-cell–mediated destruction or suppression of bone marrow hematopoietic cells plays a central role in most cases. The differential diagnosis may be difficult, and the distinction from a hypoplastic myelodysplastic syndrome (MDS; refractory anemia [RA]) may be impossible. However, patients with clonal cytogenetic abnormalities (approximately 50% of patients with MDS) should be treated as MDS because transplant regimens as used for aplastic anemia have been unsuccessful.[52]

Historically, the course of aplastic anemia, was considered as progressively, inexorably, and more or less rapidly fatal. In the past 30 years, morbidity and mortality from aplastic anemia have been reduced significantly as a better understanding of the disease pathophysiology has led to effective therapies, ie, immunosuppressive treatment[53,54] and allogeneic HCT.

Hematopoietic recovery is often incomplete after immunosuppressive treatment, but tends to be complete and stable after HCT (with the exception of an occasional patient who rejects the donor cells). Nevertheless, ex-vivo studies suggest that at the level of hematopoietic precursor cells recovery may not be complete with either approach.[55] However, although the development of clonal hematopoietic disorders, such as PNH or MDS, is extremely rare after HCT, it has been observed in 15% to 30% of patients given immunosuppressive therapy.[56] For this reason, HCT from HLA-identical siblings is the treatment of choice for patients younger than 45 or 50 years of age, despite treatment-related morbidity and mortality. Older patients and patients without HLA-identical related donors generally receive first-line therapy with immunosuppressive drugs.

Syngeneic Transplants

Infusion of genetically identical hematopoietic stem cells without pretransplant conditioning should correct marrow function if marrow failure simply resulted from a lack of or a defect in stem cells. Conversely, if marrow failure was due to an active immune process, that process may also affect the transplanted genotypically identical donor cells. In this case, effective therapy would require conditioning of the patient even in the absence of histocompatibility barriers. If marrow failure was secondary to defects in the marrow microenvironment, it is unlikely that HCT would correct the defect unless donor-derived cells contribute to the microenvironment. In about half of the 100 identical twin transplants for aplastic anemia, transplantation was successful without conditioning. The remaining patients achieved long-term hematopoiesis only when given high-dose immunosuppression with cyclophosphamide or other agents.[57]

Allogeneic Transplants

Progress in the prevention and treatment of graft rejection, and acute and chronic GVHD has resulted in significant improvements in long-term outcome. In young patients with aplastic anemia who have HLA-identical sibling donors, HCT is the treatment of choice. Opinions in regard to the upper age limit of patients differ, although 45 to 50 years is accepted by many transplant centers.

In early trials, 30% to 60% of previously transfused and, thereby, allosensitized patients who were conditioned with cyclophosphamide failed to achieve sustained donor cell engraftment, and only about 40% survived long-term. In contrast, among untransfused patients, only 5% failed to engraft, and 81% survived with sustained donor-derived hematopoiesis.[58] The infusion of viable donor leukocytes in addition to the marrow or the use of TBI (eg, 300 cGy) or TLI (400–750 cGy) given in combination with cyclophosphamide, reduced the incidence of graft failure to 5% or less even in transfused patients, and 70% to 80% of patients survived with sustained engraftment.[59,60] However, one disadvantage of the addition of donor leukocytes, which contain immunocompetent peripheral blood T lymphocytes, was an increased incidence of chronic GVHD (as high as 50% even in children), and the enthusiasm for this approach has decreased.[59] The use of irradiation, in particular limited field irradiation, has been associated with an increased risk of posttransplant malignancies.[61] Furthermore, radiation exposure is associated with impaired growth and development in children and infertility in adults.[62,63]

Studies in patients who rejected a first marrow graft after conditioning with cyclophosphamide showed that a combination of equine ATG and cyclophosphamide was effective in the majority of patients in securing sustained engraftment of a second marrow infusion.[64] Based on these results, this regimen (cyclophosphamide 4 × 50 mg/kg plus ATG 3 × 30 mg/kg, both given IV) was, therefore, introduced as conditioning for first transplants. With this strategy, 95% of patients engrafted and approximately 88% survived long term (Fig. 99–1). The incidence of chronic GVHD, still a major problem after transplantation, was also reduced.[65]

Progressively improving survival figures (Fig. 99–2) have also been reported in retrospective studies by the IBMTR and EBMT groups.[60,66] While changes in conditioning regimens have contributed to these improvements, the use of leukocyte-depleted transfusion products, thereby reducing the frequency of allosensitization, advances in antibiotic therapy, and improved methods for the prevention and treatment of GVHD were equally important.[65–67] Results of representative trials are summarized in Table 99–4.

Unfortunately, only 25% to 30% of patients have HLA-matched related donors. The remaining patients first receive immunosuppressive therapy and are transplanted only if this approach fails.[68–70]

Representative trials are summarized in Table 99–5. A report from the Fred Hutchinson Cancer Research Center showed that 30% to 45% of patients who were transplanted from HLA-nonidentical

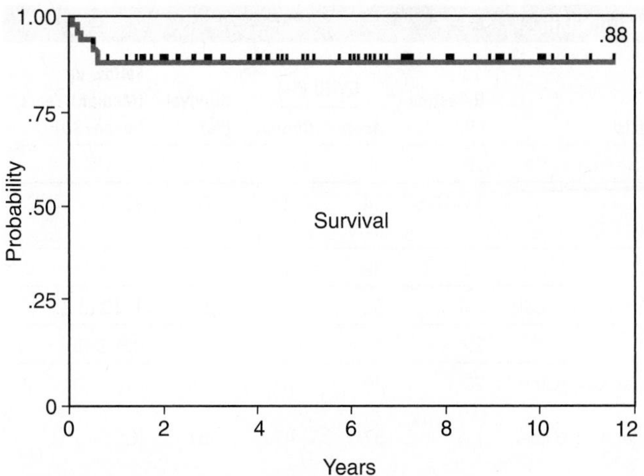

Figure 99–1 Kaplan-Meier probability of survival among 94 patients with aplastic anemia transplanted from HLA-identical related donors. *(From: Storb R, Blume KG, O'Donnell MR, et al: Cyclophosphamide and antithymocyte globulin to condition patients with aplastic anemia for allogeneic marrow transplantations: the experience in four centers. Biol Blood Marrow Transplant 7:39, 2001, used with permission.)*

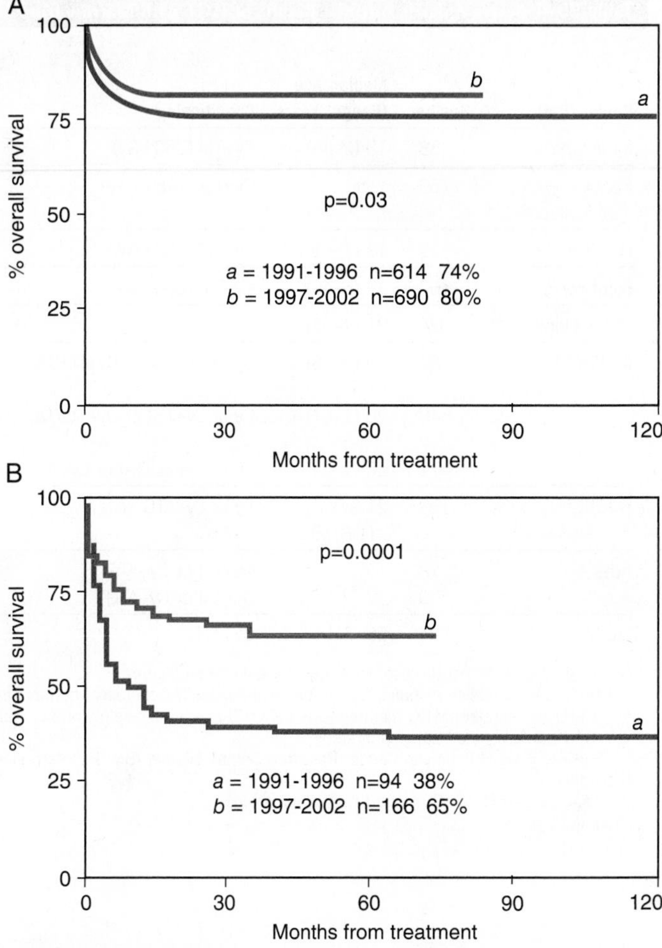

Figure 99–2 Actuarial survival of patients undergoing HCT from HLA-identical siblings (**A**) or from alternative donors (**B**) by time period (1991–1996 and 1997–2002). Results have improved significantly over time for patients transplanted both from HLA-identical siblings (74% versus 80%, $P = 0.03$) and from alternative donors (38% versus 65%, $P = 0.0001$). *(From: Locasciulli A, Oneto R, Bacigalupo A, et al; on the Behalf of the Severe Aplastic Anemia Working Party of the European Blood and Marrow Transplant Group: Outcome of patients with acquired aplastic anemia given first line bone marrow transplantation or immunosuppressive treatment in the last decade: a report from the European Group for Blood and Marrow Transplantation. Haematologica 92:11, 2007.)*

related donors after conditioning without the use of TBI failed to achieve engraftment, and only 15% to 35% survived. With the use of TBI (eg, 6 × 200 cGy) in addition to cyclophosphamide, engraftment was generally achieved, and 50% of patients survived long term, albeit with considerable morbidity.[68]

The establishment of registries of HLA typed unrelated donors has provided the option of HCT for patients without related donors, and the use of high resolution HLA typing has allowed for the search and selection of unrelated donors who are matched with a given patient at the molecular level. The outcomes with unrelated donor HCT has remained somewhat inferior to that obtained with HLA genotypically identical sibling donors. Among 298 patients, reported to the IBMTR, who received matched unrelated donor transplants between 1991 and 1997, the 5-year probability of survival was 44% for those 20 years of age or younger, and 35% for those 21 to 40 years of age.[71] A retrospective analysis of 141 patients transplanted under the auspices of the NMDP yielded similar results and showed that patients transplanted within a year of diagnosis had a much higher probability of long-term survival than patients transplanted later in their disease course. The most important factor, however, was HLA matching by high resolution typing.[72] A more recent prospective NMDP-sponsored trial involving 87 patients was aimed at optimizing the transplant conditioning regimen (Fig. 99–3A and B).[69] Patients were conditioned with cyclophosphamide and ATG as used for HLA-identical sibling transplants[65] and, in addition, received TBI in deescalating doses (from 3 × 200 to 1 × 200 cGy). All patients had failed to respond (or lost their response) to nontransplant immunosuppressive therapy. Graft failure occurred in less than 5% of patients. With donors who were identical for HLA-A, -B, -C, -DRB1, and -DQB1 by high-resolution typing, best results were obtained with a TBI dose of 200 cGy, which resulted in long-term survival of 66%. Among patients less than 20 years old at HCT who received 200 cGy of TBI (in addition to ATG and cyclophosphamide), 5-year survival was 78%. Among 23 patients transplanted from less than completely HLA-matched donors, 45% and 50% are surviving after TBI doses of 200 and 400 cGy, respectively. The TBI dose-limiting toxicities were pulmonary complications.

An alternative source of stem cells may be cord blood. Laughlin et al reported results in 562 cord blood recipients including 21 patients with aplastic anemia. Among 19 patients able to be evaluated patients, eight patients had sustained engraftment.[73] However, more recent data from Europe and the US in larger numbers of patients indicate a higher success rate.[38]

Autologous HCT

If aplastic anemia was a stem cell disorder, autologous HCT would not be an option. However, if the disease is immune mediated and residual normal stem cells are present, it is possible that treatment with G-CSF to mobilize stem cells, and "conditioning" treatment given before reinfusion of those stem cells, so that autoreactive (and marrow-suppressive) lymphocytes are eliminated, the reinfused cells meet growth conditions that allow hematopoietic repopulation. Some data to that effect have been reported.[74] Similarly, there are data to show that patients can recover hematopoiesis following the infusion of high doses of cyclophosphamide, without stem cell administration,[54] although this approach has remained controversial.[75]

Pure Red Cell Aplasia

As discussed in Chapter 31, pure red cell aplasia is associated with various disorders, eg, with parvovirus B19 infection, chronic lympho-

Table 99–4 Severe Aplastic Anemia: Results of HCT with Marrow from HLA-Identical Siblings

Center (Ref)	Number	Median Age (Range) Years	Conditioning[a]	GVHD Prophylaxis[b]	Rejection (%)	GVHD (%) Acute	GVHD (%) Chronic	Survival (%)	Follow-up (Median) Years [mean±SD]
Minneapolis[156]	58	18 (2–45)	Cy+TLI (750 cGy)	MTX+ATG+Pred	5	38	12–54	70	<0.5–8
EBMT Bacigalupo[66]	1759	1–50	Cy±TLI, TAI, or TBI	MTX or CSP	11–18%	24 II–IV	23	65	<1–6
UCLA[157]	29	19 (1–41)	Cy+TLI (300 cGy)	MTX/CSP	23	22	NA	78	0.5–5 (2)
Saint Louis[158]	107	19 (5–46)	Cy+TAI (600 cGy)	MTX, CSP or MTX+CSP	3	32	55	62	1–10 (3.7)
Johns Hopkins[159]	24	21 (4–53)	Cy	CSP	29	4.5	0	79	0.8–8 (5)
IBMTR[60]	186	19 (2–56)	Cy or Cy+TBI or Cy+TLI/TAI	MTX±Other, CSP±Other, etc.	20	39	37	48	(6)
	648	20 (1–57)	Cy or Cy+TBI or Cy+TLI/TAI	MTX±Other, CSP±Other, MTX+CSP	11	37	47	61	(6)
	471	20 (1–51)	Cy or Cy+TLI/TAI or Cy+ATG	CSP±Other, MTX+CSP	16	19	32	66	(5)
FHCRC[58]	168	21.9 (1.8–53.5)	Cy or Cy+ATG or buffy-coat +ATG	MTX, or CSP or MTX+CSP	11	31	40	69	1–15 (5.2)
Ades[160]	78 30	*	Cy+TAI or Cy+ATG Cy+TAI or Cy+ATG	MTX; CSP; or MTX+CSP MTX+CSP	NA	NA	58	59[1]	[13.6±7]
Storb[65]	94	26 (2–59)	CY+ATG	MTX+CSP	4	29	32	88	1–6.5

GVHD, graft-versus-host disease; HLA, human leukocyte antigen.
[a]ATG, antithymocyte globulin; Cy, cyclophosphamide; TAI, thoracoabdominal irradiation; TBI, total body irradiation; TLI, total lymphoid irradiation.
[b]CSP, cyclosporine; MTX, methotrexate; MTX±Other, methotrexate alone or with a second agent (not CSP); Pred, prednisone.
[c]Only nontransfused patients in study.
FHCRC, Fred Hutchinson Cancer Research Center, Seattle; IBMTR, International Bone Marrow Transplant Registry; NA, Not available; UCLA, University of California, Los Angeles.
*Age range <15 to >30 years (median not given).
1At 10 years.

cytic leukemia, and immune diseases. It usually responds to steroids and immunosuppressive therapy. Some patients who present with red cell aplasia of undetermined etiology and who do not respond to treatment with glucocorticoids or other nontransplant regimens aimed at the underlying disorder have undergone HCT. These patients are transplanted with conditioning regimens as used for aplastic anemia. No large series has been reported. Registry data suggest that problems with sustained engraftment may be more common than with other marrow failure states.[76]

Paroxysmal Nocturnal Hemoglobinuria (PNH)

PNH is an acquired clonal disorder of hematopoiesis resulting from the expansion of a clone that arises by somatic mutations in the X-linked PIG-A gene in pluripotent hematopoietic stem cells. This gene encodes a protein that affects the synthesis of glycosylphosphatidylinositol (GPI), an anchor for numerous cell surface antigens, eg, CD59. Recent data indicate that various genes that are involved in the expression of the anchor protein can be mutated and lead to similar phenotypes. These mutations are necessary but may not be sufficient to cause the PNH disorder. Autoreactive cytotoxic T cells target GPI in normal hematopoietic stem cells, while PNH cells "escape" damage and tend to expand.[77] Patients with PNH classically present with hemolytic anemia, venous thrombosis, and deficient hematopoiesis associated either with marrow aplasia or with a cellular marrow. Some patients show evolution into MDS or acute leukemia. PNH clones may also be present in patients who present with the classic features of aplastic anemia or MDS.[78]

Allogeneic HCT is effective therapy for PNH patients with either aplastic or cellular marrows. Transplantation corrects hematopoiesis and resolves thrombotic complications.[79,80] HCT from syngeneic donors without preceding conditioning failed to correct the underlying disease. This observation confirms the assumption that the PNH clone has a survival and proliferative advantage, and requires cytotoxic therapy for elimination.[81] In at least one syngeneic transplant recipient with PNH "recurrence" molecular analysis revealed that a new PNH clone had arisen.[82]

Investigators of the IBMTR presented information on 57 patients with PNH transplanted between 1978 and 1995.[83] Two patients were transplanted from monozygotic twin donors and were alive 8 and 12 years after HCT, respectively. The 2-year survival among 48 patients transplanted from HLA-identical siblings was 56%. Among 7 patients transplanted from alternative donors, there was one survivor at 5 years. Major complications were graft failure and infections. Nonmyeloablative HCT may further improve results in patients with PNH.[80,84]

It has been suggested that normal $CD34^+CD38^-$ hematopoietic precursors can be collected from the blood of patients with PNH and used as a source for autologous transplantation after separation of $CD34^+/CD38^-/CD59^-$ cells.[13] This strategy would offer the possibility of HCT with normal autologous cells in patients with PNH, although it might be difficult to collect sufficient numbers of normal precursors because of the majority of precursors in circulation after G-CSF mobilization are clonal.[85]

Myelodysplastic Syndrome (MDS)

MDS is one of the most common hematopoietic disorders in older adults. There are an estimated 15,000 to 20,000 new cases annually in the US. Among 70-year-old individuals (average age at diagnosis), the incidence is estimated at 20 to 40 per 100,000 per year.[86] The number of new cases will likely increase because of the increasing proportion of older adults (primary MDS), and because of increasing numbers of patients who survive after treatment for cancer or other diseases (secondary MDS). Clinically, MDS comprises a group of disorders in which the clonal proliferation of pluripotent

Table 99–5 Transplants for Severe Aplastic Anemia Using HLA-Nonidentical Related or Unrelated (Alternative) Donors

Center (Ref)	Number of Patients	Median Age (Range) Years	Donor (Rel/URD)	Conditioning[a]	GVHD Prophylaxis[b]	Rejection (%)	GVHD (%) Acute	GVHD (%) Chronic	Survival (%)	Follow-up (Median) Years
EBMT[66]	46[c]	35	REL (26≠)	Cy (±Pro)[d]	CSP	30	35	NA	45 (=)	1.3–7
		11	URD	Cy+TBI/TLI	MTX		(III/IV)		25 (1 Ag≠)	
				Other	TCD				11 (>1 Ag≠)	
5 Centers[161]	40[e]	19 (1–41)	URD	Cy±TBI/TLI	MTX; CSP,	18	86	NA	28 (=)	0.7–13 (4.5)
IMUST	15[f]	13 (5–38)	URD		MTX+CSP	28	50	NA	50 (=)	
					TCD					
Milwaukee[162]	13	9	URD	Cy	MTX	23	10	15	53	0.7–8
		4	URD	Cy+TBI	CSP					
				Cy+AraC+	CSP+TCD					
				TBI+MP						
FHCRC[68]	40	15 (2–44)	9=	CY	MTX	0	33	67	89	3–18
			15≠	CY	MTX+CSP	71	100	100	0	1.5–11.3
			16≠	CY+TBI	Pred+MTX	14	79	75	50	
					(±CSP)TTX+CSP					
Deeg et al[69]	87	19 (1–53)	URD 55=	CY+ATG+TBI[1]	MTX+CSP	4	69	52	55[g]	1.2–10.2 (7)
			23≠						40	
Kojima et al[163]	154	17 (1–46)	URD 79=	TBI+Cy+ATG	MTX+CSP	11	10	22	75	0.25–6.8 (2.5)
			74≠	LFI+Cy+ATG	MTX+TAC		15	23	61	
				TBI+Cy	Other		29	34	53	
				LFI+Cy			18	35	24	
NMDP[72]	141	18 (0.9–47)	URD (91=)	Cy±Chemo	MTX+CSP±Other	18	53	31	42 (=)	1–8 (3)
			(50≠)	TBI±Chemo	CSP±Other				20 (≠)	
				Cy±LFI	TCD					
					Other					
NMDP[72]	34	18 (3–46)	URD (27=)	Cy+ATG+	MTX+CSP	0	55	41	55	0.3–3.5 (2)
			(7≠)	FTBI						

GVHD, graft-versus-host disease; HLA, human leukocyte antigen.

[a]ATG, antithymocyte globulin; Cy, cyclophosphamide; FTBI, fractionated TBI; REL, related donor; TAI, thoracoabdominal irradiation; TBI, total body irradiation; TLI, total lymphoid irradiation; URD, unrelated donor; "=" indicates HLA match, "≠" HLA-nonidentical

[b]CSP, cyclosporine; LFI, limited field irradiation; MTX, methotrexate; MTX±Other, methotrexate alone or with a second agent (not CSP); Pred. prednisone; TAC, tacrolimus; TCD, T-cell depletion.

[c]Includes 14 patients with Fanconi anemia.

[d]Pro, procarbazine.

[e]Retrospective.

[f]Prospective.

[g]66% for patients who received 1×200 cGy of TBI (78% for patients <20 years old).

[1]Nine patients who did not tolerate ATG received Cy, 2 × 60 mg/kg, and TBI, 6 × 200 cGy over 3 days.

hematopoietic cells results in a very heterogeneous clinical syndrome characterized by ineffective hematopoiesis and a propensity to progress to marrow failure with severe pancytopenia or to transform into acute myeloid leukemia (tAML). Clinical and possible pathophysiologic overlap with aplastic anemia, myeloproliferative disorders, and acute leukemia can make the differential diagnosis challenging.

While several therapeutic strategies are being pursued, the only current therapy with proven curative potential for patients with MDS is HCT. However, MDS often has a protracted course, and many patients are in their 60s, 70s, or older, and the morbidity and mortality associated with HCT may be prohibitive. A decision-making analysis by Cutler et al suggested that patients with advanced/high-risk MDS (IPSS intermediate-2 or high-risk groups) had the best life expectancy if HCT was carried out without delay (assuming the patient was a candidate for HCT and a donor could be identified); patients in the low risk group did benefit from initial conservative management followed by HCT if and when the disease showed signs of progression.[87] For patients in the intermediate-1 risk group, there was little difference between early and late HCT, and decisions should probably be made on a case-by-case basis, dependent on disease manifestations. For example, patients with isolated severe neutropenia or thrombocytopenia may have a poor prognosis (without HCT) even though they may fall into IPSS categories low or intermediate-1. In addition, recent data show that red blood cell transfusion dependence is an important negative risk factor for survival.[88] Whether transfusion dependence also adversely affects transplant outcome remains to be determined.

Transplant outcome in patients with MDS is related to disease stage (marrow myeloblast count), prognostic score (IPSS), cytogenetic findings,[89] possibly remission status before transplantation, iron overload, source of stem cells, comorbid conditions, and preparative regimen.[40,90–93] In early clinical trials, transplant success showed a strong inverse correlation with patient age. Age continues to be a relevant factor for transplant success, but less so than in the past, and the development of reduced intensity nonmyeloablative conditioning strategies has further attenuated the impact of age.[94,95]

Less Advanced/Low-risk MDS

The best results with HCT are achieved in patients with low myeloblast counts in the marrow (less <5%) and in patients who lack high-risk cytogenetic markers; these are generally patients with low IPSS scores. The European Group for Blood and Marrow Transplantation (EBMT) reported results on 131 patients with MDS transplanted from HLA-identical sibling donors. The 5-year relapse-free

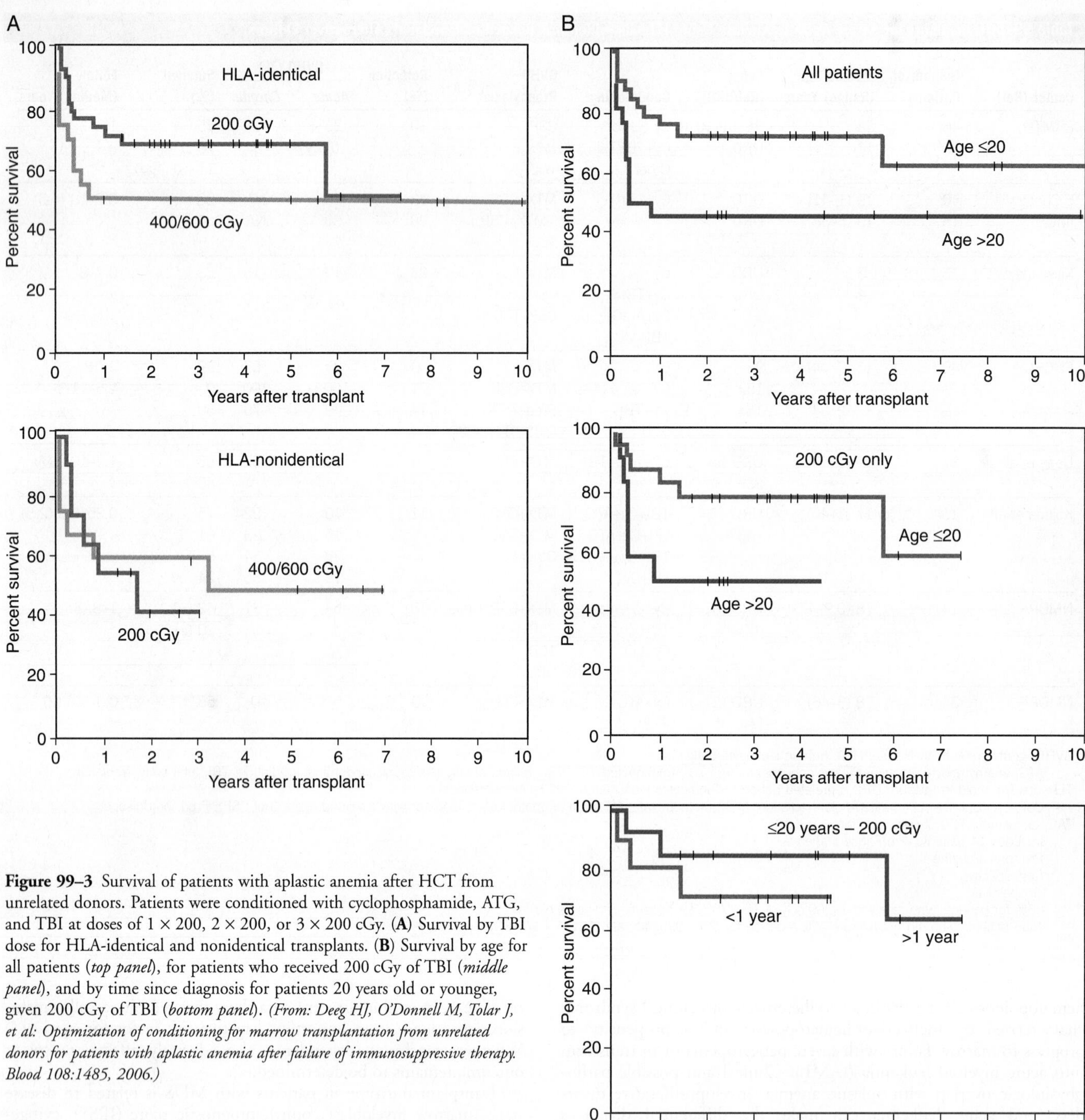

Figure 99–3 Survival of patients with aplastic anemia after HCT from unrelated donors. Patients were conditioned with cyclophosphamide, ATG, and TBI at doses of 1 × 200, 2 × 200, or 3 × 200 cGy. (**A**) Survival by TBI dose for HLA-identical and nonidentical transplants. (**B**) Survival by age for all patients (*top panel*), for patients who received 200 cGy of TBI (*middle panel*), and by time since diagnosis for patients 20 years old or younger, given 200 cGy of TBI (*bottom panel*). *(From: Deeg HJ, O'Donnell M, Tolar J, et al: Optimization of conditioning for marrow transplantation from unrelated donors for patients with aplastic anemia after failure of immunosuppressive therapy. Blood 108:1485, 2006.)*

survival (RFS) was 52%, and the relapse rate was 13%.[96] The same group reported a RFS of 24% at 2 years with a relapse rate of 13% for patients transplanted from unrelated HLA-matched donors.[97] The International Bone Marrow Transplant Registry (IBMTR) reported results in 452 patients with MDS transplanted from HLA-matched siblings, showing a 3-year RFS of 40%, although only 140 patients (31%) had less than 5% blasts at HCT. Treatment-related mortality (TRM) was 37%, and the relapse rate was 23%. High marrow blast count and high IPSS score were significantly correlated with relapse. Relapse-free survival was 72% for patients younger than 18 years.[98] In a cohort of 510 patients with MDS transplanted from unrelated donors, those conditioned with busulfan and cyclophosphamide (BUCY) fared better than patients conditioned with other regimens, in particular regimens containing high-dose TBI.[90] A study at the FHCRC in patients conditioned with a targeted BUCY regimen showed a 3-year RFS of 68% with related donors and 70% with unrelated donors. Among 69 patients with RA/RARS, the non-relapse mortality rate (NRM) was 31%, and relapse occurred in 5% of patients.[99] Survival in patients 55 to 66 years of age was comparable to that in younger patients.

In several studies, improved survival was independently associated with higher donor cell dose, recipient CMV seronegativity, shorter interval from diagnosis to HCT, and transplantation in more recent years.

Advanced/High-risk MDS

The success rates of HCT decline as the nontransplant prognosis of MDS worsens, particularly with an increase in the marrow myeloblast count above 5%. Intensification of conditioning regimens aimed at reducing the relapse risk has been associated with higher rates of NRM, and no improvement in survival.[93] The IBMTR reported results in 352 patients with high-risk MDS transplanted from HLA-matched sibling donors; most were conditioned with TBI-based regimens. The 3-year RFS was 63% for patients younger than 18 years and 33% for older patients.[98] The EBMT reported a 5-year RFS for patients transplanted from related donors of 34%, 19%, and 26% for RAEB, RAEB-T, and tAML, respectively; the relapse rate was approximately 50% for the entire cohort. The 2-year RFS for patients transplanted from HLA-matched unrelated donors was 27%, 8%, and 27% for RAEB, RAEB-T, and tAML, respectively.[96,97] A study from the FHCRC center in patients with RAEB transplanted after conditioning with targeted BUCY showed 3-year RFS of 45% with related donors and 40% with unrelated donors. The corresponding figures for RAEB-T/tAML were 33% and 17%, respectively. The data also indicate that the IPSS correlates strongly with outcome; patients with low IPSS scores had the highest probability of RFS and the lowest rates of relapse (Fig. 99–4A and B).[92]

Another trial examined a combination of BU and TBI without high-dose CY. Sixty patients with advanced MDS, tAML or CMML were transplanted from related (n = 20) or unrelated (n = 40) donors with a 3-year Kaplan-Meier estimate of survival of 26% and a relapse rate of 25%.[99] This was comparable to an earlier trial examining the combination of BUCY and TBI.[100] However, NRM was 38% at 100 days.[99] This observation suggested that further increases in the conditioning intensity (with the aim of reducing relapse frequency) were unlikely to improve overall survival.

In an effort to reduce toxicity, the tolerability and efficacy of fludarabine in combination with BU has been tested.[23,101] Bornhauser et al prepared 42 patients with high-risk hematologic neoplasms (38 with MDS) with a fludarabine plus oral BU combination for HCT from related (n = 16) or unrelated (n = 26) donors. The probabilities of overall survival and RFS at a median follow up of 18 months were 42% and 35%, respectively. All patients achieved engraftment, and the day 100 mortality was 7%.[101] Similarly, the M.D. Anderson group used a regimen of IV BU and fludarabine given consecutively for 4 days to treat patients with advanced myeloid malignancies (22 patients had MDS). The 1-year RFS and TRM were 52% and 3%, respectively.[23] Encouraging studies such has these have stimulated interest in further modifications of conventional conditioning regimens to reduce toxicity while maintaining efficacy.

Generally, patients who received G-CSF mobilized PBPC had superior outcome compared to patients who received marrow stem cells in all subgroups of MDS, although differences were often not significant.[92,102] Thus, there has been progress with related and unrelated transplants for advanced and less advanced MDS. However, while early nonrelapse mortality has been reduced to 10% or less, 3-year mortality has remained in the range of 25% to 35%.

Reducing Transplant-related Toxicity

Major efforts have been directed at preventing or attenuating transplant-related complications. This is particularly important in patients with MDS who tend to be older and often have significant comorbidities. Nonmyeloablative/reduced intensity conditioning regimens in preparation for allogeneic HCT (also referred to as "mini-transplants") have been developed by several groups.[103] The basic principle behind these regimens is to provide sufficient immunosuppression to secure donor cell engraftment and then rely on the graft-vs-tumor effect mediated by donor-derived cells to eradicate the underlying disease. Initial regimens consisted of low dose busulfan ± other agents or low dose (200 cGy) TBI ± fludarabine.[104,105] Subsequently, many groups have adopted similar regimens but have increased the intensity. Conventional conditioning regimens have been attenuated, leading to a broad spectrum of regimens aimed at eradicating the patient's disease while minimizing NRM.[106]

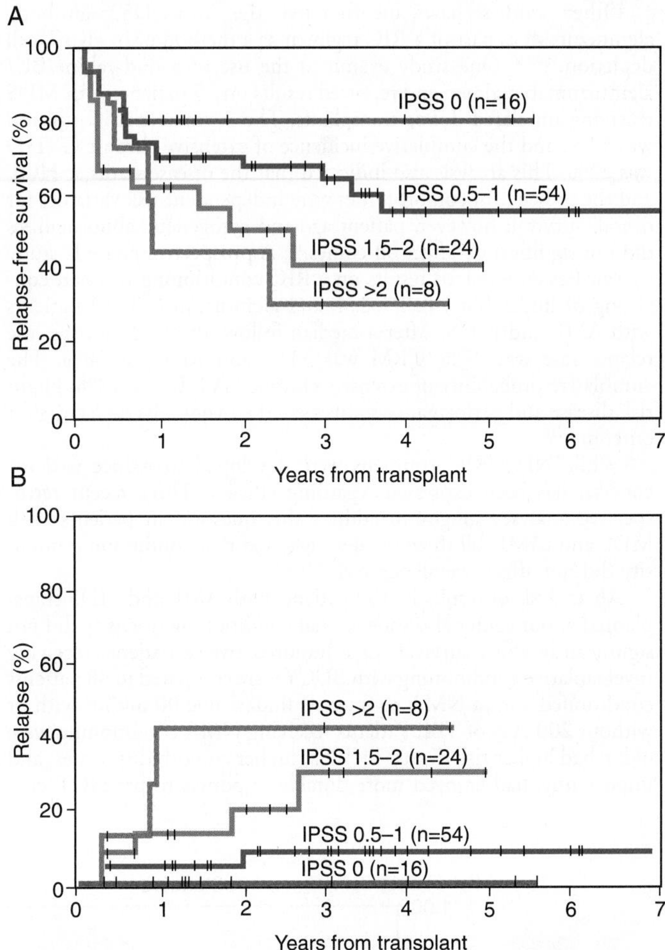

Figure 99–4 Impact of IPSS score on transplant outcome in patients with MDS. The + indicates censored patients; in 7 patients, an IPSS score could not be assigned. (**A**) relapse-free survival. (**B**) Cumulative incidence of relapse. *(From: Deeg HJ, Storer B, Slattery JT, et al. Conditioning with targeted busulfan and cyclophosphamide for hemopoietic stem cell transplantation from related and unrelated donors in patients with myelodysplastic syndrome. Blood 100:1201, 2002.)*

A multicenter study examined the use of NMA conditioning to transplant patients with MDS (n = 77) or MPD (n = 14) from related (n = 49) or unrelated donors (n = 42). The median patient age was 59 (range 6–72) years, and conditioning consisted of fludarabine and 200 cGy of TBI. With a median follow-up of 2 years, the estimated overall survival for the entire cohort was 37%, with a relapse rate of 43%. Patients with advanced MDS had a higher relapse rate than those with low-risk disease.[105]

Several groups have tested combinations of fludarabine and BU as part of RIC regimens.[107,108] Kroger et al reported on 37 patients with MDS or tAML conditioned with such a regimen from related (n = 19) or unrelated donors (n = 18). TRM was 27%, and with a median follow-up of 20 months, the 3-year estimated disease-free survival was 38%, with a relapse rate of 32%.[107] Spanish investigators reported results on 37 patients with MDS or AML transplanted from HLA-identical siblings following a fludarabine/BU conditioning regimen. The 1-year TRM and RFS were 5% and 66%, respectively.[108]

Other studies have incorporated the anti-CD52 antibody alemtuzumab as part of a RIC regimen as a method of in vivo T-cell depletion.[109,110] One study examined the use of a fludarabine/BU/alemtuzumab regimen and reported results on 75 patients with MDS receiving unrelated donor transplants. The 3-year actuarial survival was 43%, and the cumulative incidence of extensive chronic GVHD was 22%. This analysis also indicated that the disease status at HCT and the presence of comorbidities were independent risk variables for overall survival; however, patient age and cytogenetic abnormalities did not significantly affect outcomes.[109] A prospective phase II study by van Besien reported results on a RIC conditioning regimen consisting of fludarabine, melphalan, and alemtuzumab in 52 patients with AML and MDS. After a median follow-up of 18 months, the relapse rate was 27%, TRM was 33%, and RFS was 38%. The cumulative probability of extensive chronic GVHD was 18%. High-risk disease and performance status were the major adverse factors for outcome.[110]

While NMA/RIC regimens were developed to reduce toxicity, concern has been expressed regarding efficacy. Three recent retrospective analyses sought to address this question in patients with MDS and tAML; all three studies suggested that conditioning intensity did not affect overall survival.[93,111,112]

An analysis of results in 150 patients with AML and MDS transplanted at our center also showed that conditioning intensity did not significantly affect survival. One hundred twelve patients receiving myeloablative conditioning with BUCY were compared to 38 patients conditioned with a NMA regimen of fludarabine 90 mg/m^2 with or without 200 cGy of TBI. Patients receiving NMA conditioning were older, had higher risk disease by IPSS, higher comorbidity scores, and importantly, had enjoyed more durable responses to pre-HCT chemotherapy. The 3-year RFS and overall survival did not differ significantly between the two groups.[111]

Alyea et al carried out a retrospective analysis of 136 patients transplanted for MDS and tAML. Outcomes among 97 patients receiving myeloablative conditioning with CY combined with either BU or 1400 cGy TBI were compared to those among 39 patients receiving NMA conditioning with fludarabine and low-dose BU. This study also showed no statistically significant difference in overall survival and RFS between the two groups. Of note was that patients receiving NMA conditioning had higher rates of relapse, but the impact on survival was counterbalanced by a higher rate of TRM in patients receiving myeloablative conditioning.[112] Martino et al recently reported the results of an analysis in 836 patients with MDS, comparing high-dose (n = 621) with reduced-intensity (n = 215) regimens (Fig. 99–5A and B).[93] For all age and MDS categories, treatment-related mortality was lower but relapse rates were higher with RIC, and relapse-free survivals were comparable for the two cohorts, 35% and 39%, respectively.

Since patients selected for RIC as compared to more conventional myeloablative regimens were not comparable in regards to risk factors in these retrospective studies, conclusions must be drawn cautiously. Only prospective randomized trials will provide definitive answers. Furthermore, it would be wrong to simply contrast myeloablative to NMA/RIC regimens. As emphasized in several recent reviews,[106,113] a broad spectrum of conditioning regimens using various modalities has been developed. It is quite likely that what is "optimal" for one disease category may be "suboptimal" (either too intense or insufficient) for another, and what may yield superior results in patients whose disease is in remission at the time of HCT, may lead to disappointing outcomes in patients with disease burden at HCT.

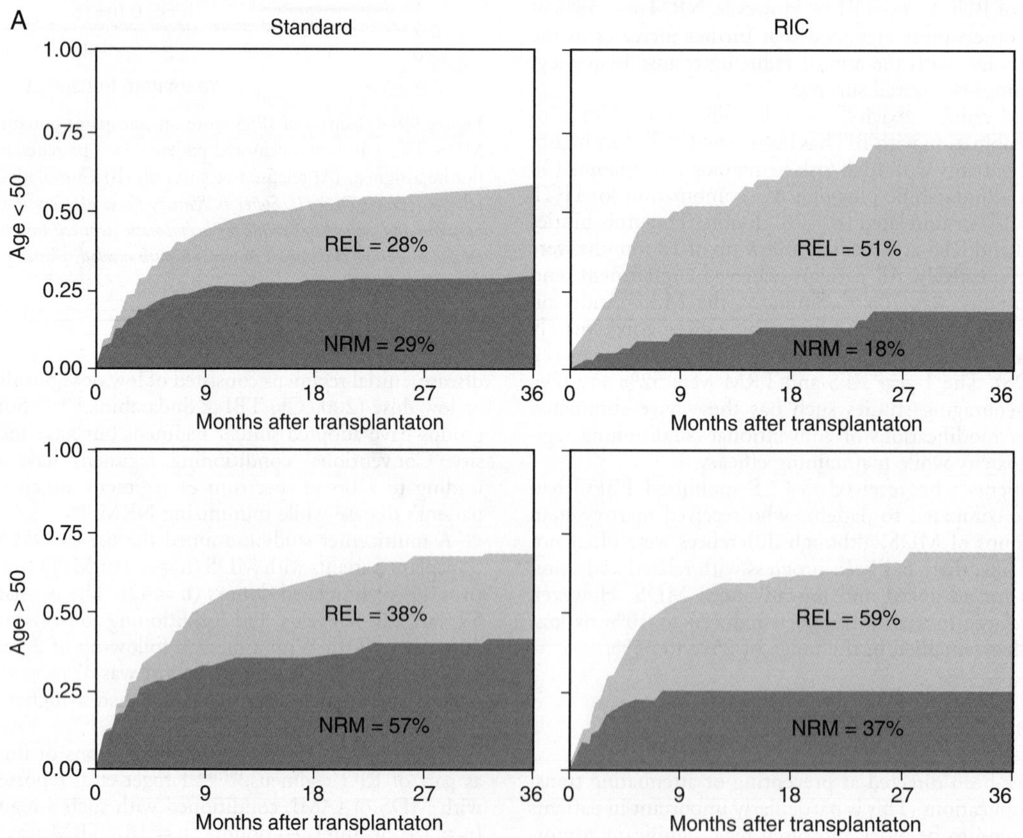

Figure 99–5 Incidence of relapse (REL) and non–relapse mortality (NRM) in patients with MDS conditioned with conventional regimens (standard) or reduced intensity regimens (RIC) and transplanted from HLA-identical sibling donors. **A**) Outcome by age (years). **B**) Outcome by pretransplant chemotherapy: no therapy (*top panel*), therapy but not achieving complete remission (*middle panel*), and achieving complete remission (*bottom panel*). *(From: Martino R, Iacobelli S, Brand R, et al; for the Myelodysplastic Syndrome subcommittee of the Chronic Leukemia Working Party of the European Blood and Marrow Transplantation Group: Retrospective comparison of reduced-intensity conditioning and conventional high-dose conditioning for allogeneic hematopoietic stem cell transplantation using HLA-identical sibling donors in myelodysplastic syndromes. Blood 108:836, 2006).*

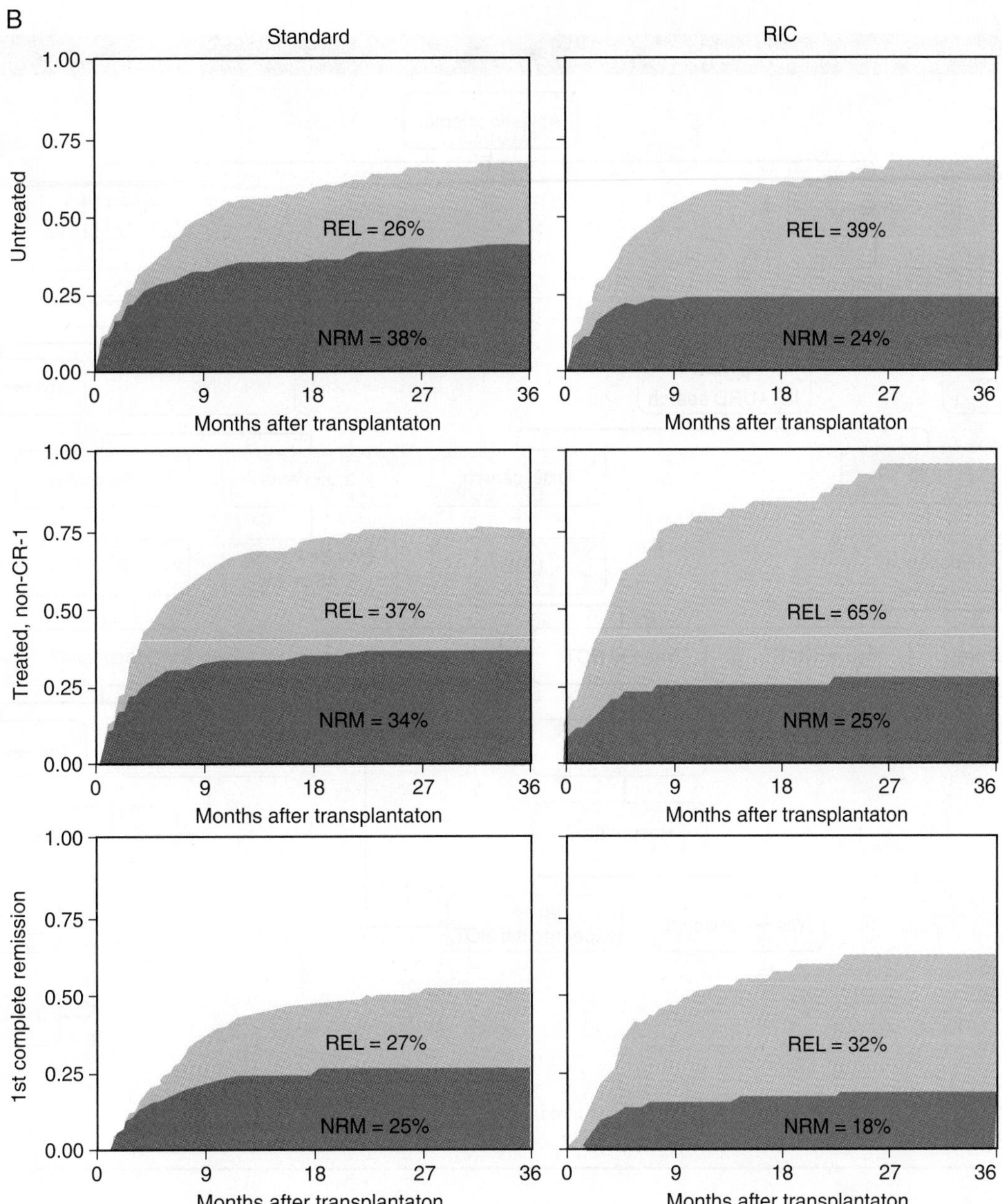

Figure 99–5, cont'd

Autologous HCT

In MDS marrow, normal and clonal hematopoietic precursors coexist. If sufficient normal precursors could be harvested without contamination by clonogenic MDS cells, autologous HCT should be feasible. The EBMT group reported autologous transplant results in 79 patients with MDS or tAML who achieved complete remissions after induction chemotherapy, and showed a 2-year relapse-free survival, relapse rate, and treatment-related mortality of 34%, 64%, and 5%, respectively.[114] Among 19 patients with MDS, the 2-year disease-free survival, relapse rate, and treatment-related mortality were 40%, 58%, and 5%, respectively. De Witte and colleagues also presented a comparison in 184 patients with MDS or tAML who received either allogeneic or autologous HCT after induction chemotherapy, dependent on sibling donor availability. The overall survival and relapse-free survival rates in the autologous group were 33% and 27%, compared with 36% and 31% in the allogeneic group, respectively. In a prospective study assessing feasibility of autologous HCT after conditioning with BU/CY, Wattel et al showed that among 24 patients who were in complete remission after induction chemotherapy, 50% were alive at 8 to 55 months; median disease-free survival was 33 months.[115] These data suggest that autologous HCT can result in long-term remission in some patients and can be considered as an option for transplant candidates without HLA-matched allogeneic donors.

Autoimmune Disorders

Proof that HCT may offer effective treatment for severe autoimmune disorders came from observations in patients who received HCT for other indications, and were also cured of concurrent autoimmune disorders, eg, rheumatoid arthritis.[116] Subsequently, Yasumizu et al showed that diabetes in NOD mice was curable by allogeneic HCT from an autoimmune resistant donor strain, but not by syngeneic HCT.[117] Other groups presented similar results in mice with autoimmune encephalomyelitis and renal disorders.[118,119] However, HCT

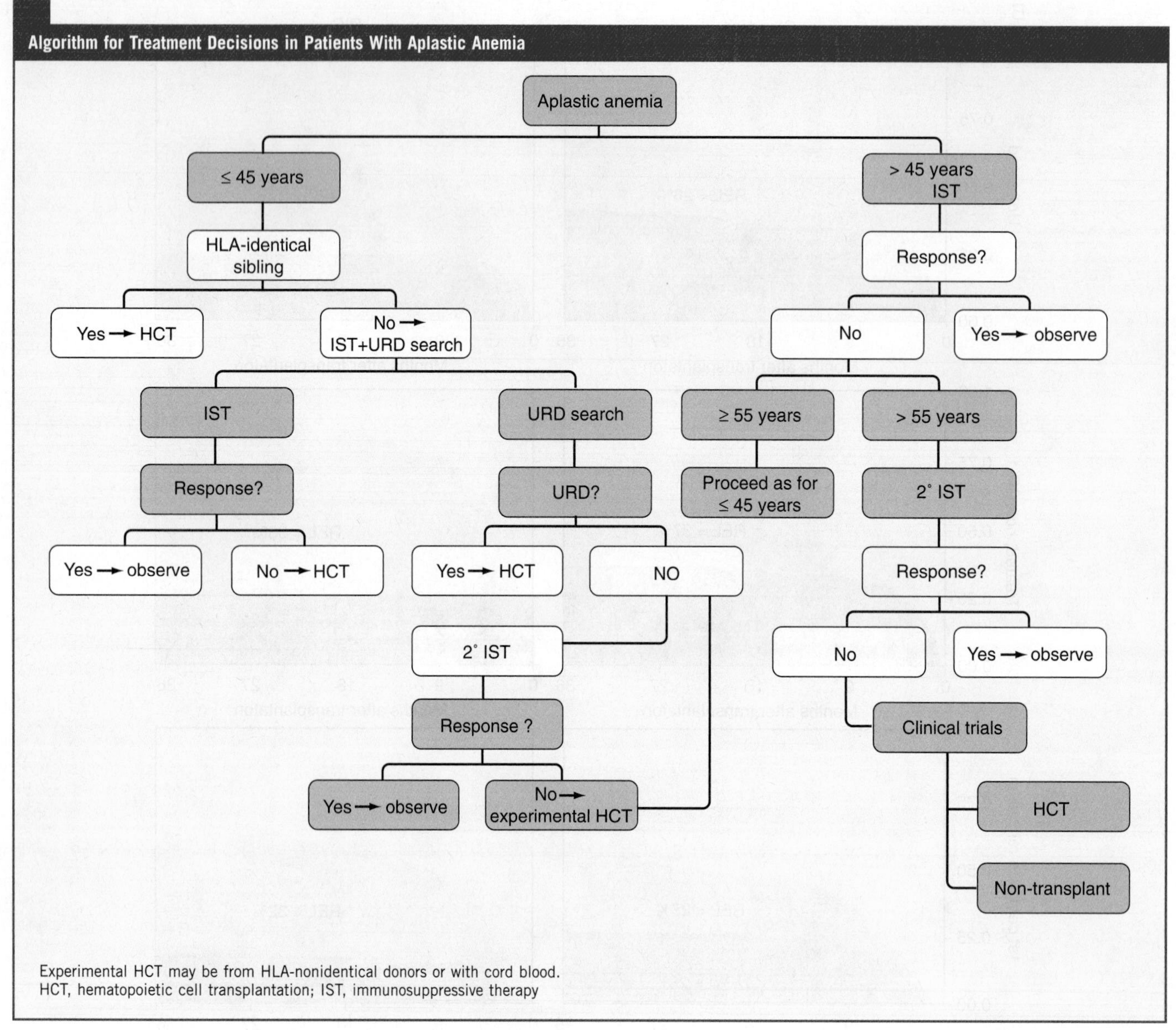

was effective only if given at an early stage of the disease, when there was no significant end-organ damage.[120]

Autologous HCT

Systemic sclerosis (SSc): The European cooperative (EBMT) group reported results of a multicenter phase I/II trial of autologous HCT in 41 patients with SSc.[121] Patients had predominantly diffuse skin disease, and various transplant regimens (mainly CY/ATG/TBI based) were used. Twenty of 29 evaluable patients (69%) had improvements in skin scores of more than 25%. Disease progression occurred in seven patients (19%) at a median followup of 67 (range 49–255) days. Eleven patients (27%) died, seven apparently from treatment-related toxicity. The probability of survival at one year was 73%. Lung function and pulmonary hypertension did not improve significantly, but stabilized. Nash et al recently reported results of a phase II, single arm North American study of high-dose immunosuppressive conditioning therapy and autologous CD34-selected HCT in 34 patients with diffuse cutaneous SSc.[122] Conditioning included TBI (800 cGy) with lung shielding, cyclophosphamide (120 mg/kg) and equine ATG (90 mg/kg). Neutrophil and platelet counts recovered by 9 (7–13) and 11 (7–25) days after HCT, respectively. Seventeen of 27 (63%) evaluable patients who survived at least 1 year after HCT had sustained responses at a median follow-up of 4 (range 1–8) years. Major improvement was noted in skin (modified Rodnan skin score −22.08; $P < 0.0001$) and overall function ($P < 0.0001$). Importantly, skin biopsies showed a statistically significant decrease in dermal fibrosis compared to baseline ($P < 0.0001$). Lung, heart, and kidney function remained clinically stable. There were 12 deaths during the study (8 transplant-related and 4 related to SSc). The estimated progression-free survival at 5 years was 64%. Thus, sustained responses, including decrease in dermal fibrosis, were observed exceeding those reported with other therapies. Prospective randomized trials are planned.

Multiple sclerosis (MS): MS may have a relative benign course or may progress rapidly with devastating clinical effects. Earlier data suggested that these patients may benefit from high-dose immunosuppressive therapy and autologous HCT.[123,124] Several updates have been published recently. A retrospective analysis of results in 183 patients by the EBMT group showed stabilization or improvement in 63% of patients at a median follow-up of 42 months.[124] Treatment-related mortality was 5% among patients transplanted before 2000. Subsequently, no toxic deaths were observed in patients conditioned with a BEAM (carmustine, etoposide, cytosine-arabinoside, melphalan)/ATG regimen. Progression-free survival rates of 60% to 65% at 4 to 5 years have also been reported by others.[125] T-cell depletion did not offer an advantage.[126] One among 26 patients who were treated at other major centers died with a post-transplant lymphoproliferative disorder.[127] All reports indicate some EDSS improvement. Because of concern about neurological flare-up during G-CSF stem cell mobilization, administration of either cyclophosphamide or prednisone has been added to G-CSF. Overall, these results suggest that autologous HCT has some efficacy in stabilizing progressive MS. Results may be comparable or superior to currently available alternative treatment options. Randomized studies are underway.

Systemic lupus erythematosus (SLE): SLE in many patients is a crippling disease and great hopes have been placed on HCT.[128] A recent report summarizes results in 50 patients.[129] All patients were refractory to "standard" therapy and had life-threatening organ involvement. Patients were conditioned with cyclophosphamide, 200 mg/kg, and equine ATG, 90 mg/kg, and given $CD34^+$ selected autologous cells that had been harvested after mobilization with cyclophosphamide and G-CSF. Among 48 evaluable patients, one died from treatment-related toxicity, and with a median follow-up of 29 months, the projected 5-year survival was 84%, "disease-free" survival 50%. Renal function stabilized and various parameters, including carbon monoxide diffusion improved. These data suggest that controlled prospective trials should be conducted.

Rheumatoid arthritis: Rheumatoid arthritis was one of the first autoimmune disorders shown to improve with HCT albeit with allogeneic cells.[116] Subsequent studies showed that autologous HCT were also beneficial. Compared to other autoimmune diseases, the mortality of autologous HCT for rheumatoid arthritis has been as low as 1%. The EBMT registry reported the largest cohort of 70 patients with rheumatoid arthritis who received autologous HCT. This study showed that while most patients responded initially, relapses occurred in at least 50% of patients.[130] Generally, the conditioning regimens involved CY only, or BU/CY.

Autologous HCT has been carried out for additional autoimmune/inflammatory disorders, such as Crohn disease, resulting in remissions and prolonged disease quiescence.[131]

Allogeneic HCT

Allogeneic HCT for the treatment of autoimmune diseases was mainly a by-product of treatment for other hematological disorders. Many of these cases involved patients with rheumatoid arthritis who developed gold therapy-related aplastic anemia, and subsequently were cured by allogeneic HCT.[116] However, many patients with severe autoimmune diseases, such as SLE, SSc, already have extensive vital organ damage, and are not good candidates for such treatment. Nevertheless, Nash et al recently reported on two patients with SSc who were conditioned with busulfan, cyclophosphamide, and equine ATG and transplanted with marrow cells from HLA-identical siblings.[132] Although one patient died at 17 months with GVHD and infections, one is alive and well at 5 years with nearly complete resolution of dermal fibrosis and marked improvement in physical function.

AIDS

The initial experience with allogeneic HCT in patients with AIDS was with AIDS related lymphoma.[133,134] While short term eradication of HIV was observed, there were no long-term survivors. Vilmer and colleagues reported on three patients who had developed AIDS at 8 to 56 months after marrow transplantation for aplastic anemia or leukemia,[135] who were given six sequential lymphocyte infusions from the original marrow donor combined with interferon IFN-α and later IFN-γ. All three patients showed hematologic and immunologic improvement. Numerous additional attempts were reported,[136] but overall HCT has not been successful.

The introduction of highly active antiretroviral therapy (HAART) has improved the prognosis of patients with AIDS, including those who have developed lymphoproliferative disorders.[137] A report summarizing results in 62 patients with AIDS-related lymphoma indicates that 38 achieved complete remissions with autologous HCT, and overall survival ranged from 50% to 85% at 9 to 32 months.[137]

Ho et al proposed to use stem cells transfected with retroviral vectors containing the gene for a hairpin ribozyme capable of cleaving HIV-1 RNA. In vitro studies showed, indeed, that transfected cells were resistant to infection by HIV.[138] Ongoing studies are exploring the possibility of combining a hematopoietic stem cell transplant with cytotoxic T cells specific for HIV-1.[139]

Langerhans Cell Histiocytosis (LCH)

LCH, formerly called histiocytosis X, is an uncommon disorder of childhood. Children whose disease progresses to the disseminated form have a poor prognosis. Since the originator cell of the disease is thought to be marrow-derived, marrow-ablative therapy and transplantation should provide effective therapy. Both autologous and allogeneic HCTs have been carried out.[140,141] After conditioning with chemotherapy (eg, etoposide and cyclophosphamide) and TBI engraftment is achieved, with about half of the patients surviving free of disease.[142]

POSTTRANSPLANT COMPLICATIONS AND THERAPEUTIC INTERVENTIONS

Graft-Versus-Host Disease (GVHD)

GVHD is the most frequent complication of allogeneic HCT.[48] Methods of GVHD prevention are listed in Table 99–6. With a combination of CSP (given daily) and MTX (given on days 1, 3, 6, and 11) as prophylaxis, acute GVHD occurs in 10% to 50% of patients after HLA-identical transplants and in 50% to 90% of patients transplanted from alternative donors. The corresponding figures for chronic GVHD are 20% to 50% and 30% to 60%, respectively. Acute GVHD is the single most important risk factor for the development of chronic GVHD.[143] In patients prepared with conventional conditioning regimens, acute GVHD usually presents within a month of transplantation. With HLA-nonidentical transplants, the presentation may be "hyperacute" within days of HCT. In patients prepared with nonmyeloablative regimens, clinical manifestations of typical acute GVHD may develop 4 to 5 months (or even later) after transplantation. Conversely, clinical and histologic features of chronic GVHD may be present as early as 50 to 60 days after HCT. A new classification of GVHD has recently been presented.[144]

The main target organs of GVHD are the immune system, skin, liver and intestinal tract, although other organs can be involved. The result of interactions between donor and host cells is an activation and clonal expansion of donor T cells (afferent phase of the graft-versus-host reaction/GVHD), leading to a complex pattern of cytokine release, recruitment of secondary effector cells, and destruction of recipient target cells and tissues (efferent phase). These interactions occur not only in recipients who differ from the donor for MHC class I or class II antigens, but even between HLA-matched individuals, because of differences for non-HLA or "minor" antigens encoded for by genes outside of but presented by the MHC. The chronic GVHD syndrome has prominent features of autoreactivity, and T

HCT for Patients with MDS Is an Evolving Field.

The algorithm provides some guidance regarding consideration of patient age, comorbid conditions, disease stage (and the possible advisability of induction therapy) when deciding upon a conditioning regimen. For patients with high-risk disease and with reduced-intensity/nonmyeloablative transplant regimens, G-CSF mobilized peripheral blood progenitor cells (G-PBMC) are currently the preferred source of stem cells. Posttransplant manipulations depend on the type of transplant, the degree of donor cell chimerism that is achieved, and the remission status.

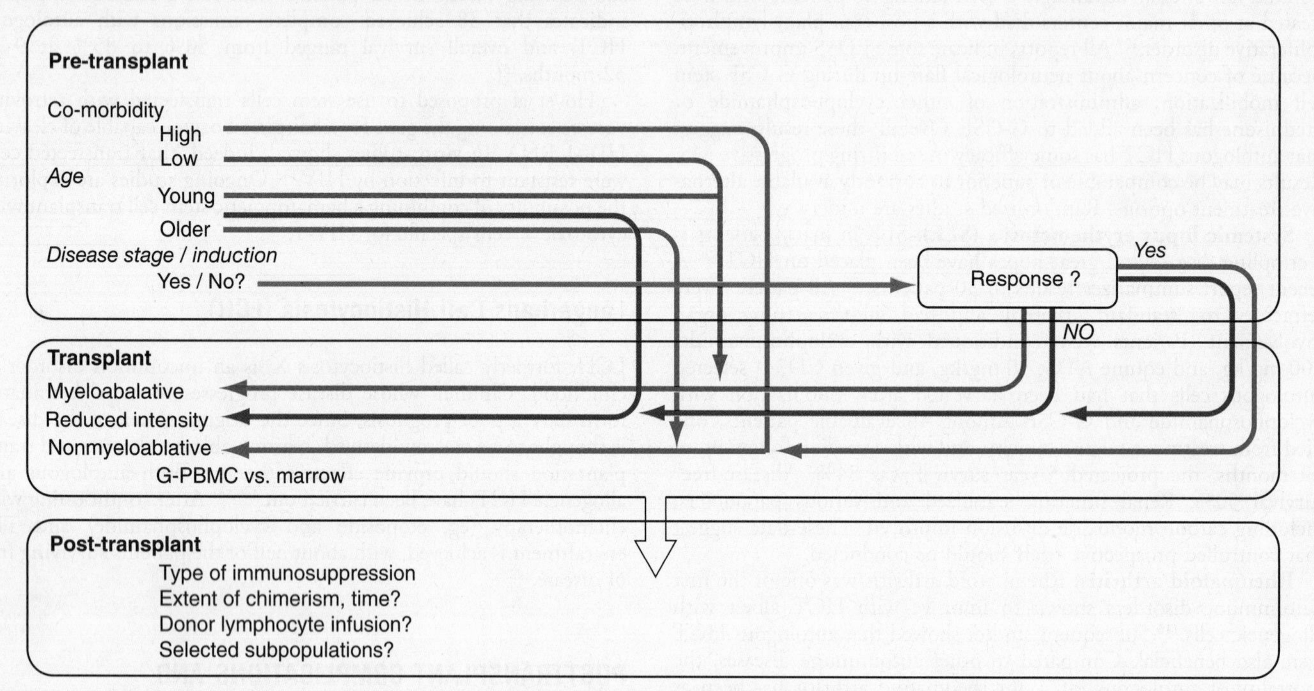

Table 99–6 Modalities of GVHD Prevention

Selection of histocompatible donors
T lymphocyte elimination or inactivation —in the donor cell inoculum —in the patient posttransplant
Cytokine blockade
Gnotobiosis
Establishment of mixed chimerism (?)

GVHD, graft-versus-host disease.

lymphocytes with abnormal cytokine profiles (secreting, eg, IL-4 and IFN-γ) may be present.[48]

In patients with malignant disorders, graft-versus-host reactivity may be beneficial in the form of a GVL effect. In nonmalignant disorders, however, GVHD is undesirable. Methods of GVHD prophylaxis are summarized in Table 99–6. Combination regimens of MTX and CSP or MTX and tacrolimus offer the most effective currently available prophylaxis.[49,145] Other promising agents, such as mycophenolate mofetil (MMF) and rapamycin (sirolimus), are under active investigation. In vivo administration of monoclonal antibodies (murine, humanized or human) against the interleukin-2 (IL-2) receptor or antibodies neutralizing TNF-α have only been of transient benefit.[146] Gnotobiosis (treatment in a sterile environment) has been effective in some trials.

T-cell depletion of donor marrow by 2–4 log, clearly effective in reducing the incidence of GVHD, is complicated by an increased incidence of graft failure.[147,148] Since failure of sustained engraftment is a potential problem in patients with aplastic anemia even with unmanipulated marrow, T-cell depletion has generally not been applied to this patient group. Of note is the observation in several studies that the incidence of GVHD was lowest in patients who showed "mixed chimerism," ie, the coexistence, at least transiently, of donor and host lymphohematopoietic cells postgrafting.[149] The mechanism is not clear. Recent studies aimed at inducing mixed chimerism by design, in particular in the setting of nonmyeloablative transplants, have shown a reduction of GVHD incidence in some, but not in other studies, although GVHD manifestation may be less severe.[150]

GVHD is the most important risk factor for long-term morbidity and mortality after HCT. Therefore, if GVHD develops, it requires aggressive therapy for both the acute and chronic form. Current therapy for acute GVHD includes glucocorticoids, CSP, monoclonal antibodies, immunotoxins, and cytokine blockade.[146]

Graft Failure

Graft failure and rejection may be due to allosensitization of the recipient, HLA disparities between patient and donor,[151] or defects in the recipient microenvironment. This may be the case in about 5% of patients with aplastic anemia; it also occurs in MDS. Certain anti–human monoclonal antibodies (eg, Campath IG), or immuneglobulin conjugates, thymoglobulin (rabbit ATG) administered during the peritransplant period may reduce the graft failure rate without increasing toxicity.[148,152]

Table 99–7 Delayed Complications

Chronic GVHD
Immunodeficiency and infections
Airway and pulmonary disease
Autoimmune dysfunction
Impaired growth and development
Neuroendocrine dysfunction
Sterility
Cardiac disease
Ocular problems
Musculoskeletal disease
Dental problems
Gastrointestinal and hepatic complications
Posttransplant malignancies
Central and peripheral nervous system impairment
Psychosocial dysfunction

GVHD, graft-versus-host disease.

Infections

Infections in recipients of HCT are a major cause of transplant-related morbidity and mortality. In the peritransplant phase, neutropenia is the most important risk factor, particularly for bacterial infections. All patients receive broad-spectrum antibiotics (eg, ceftazidime or quinolone) when the neutrophil count declines to <500/μL. In addition, acyclovir and fluconazole are given as prophylaxis. As hematopoiesis recovers, GVHD may develop and viral, eg, CMV, respiratory virus, and invasive fungal infections (*Candida, Aspergillus*) may occur. Iron overload of the patient may increase the risk of invasive fungal infections.[41] Close monitoring for reactivation of organisms or new infections is important to allow prompt institution of (preemptive) therapy, especially in patients with GVHD. All patients should receive trimethoprim/sulfamethoxazole for *P. jiroveci* prophylaxis.

Delayed Complications

The longest surviving HCT recipients have now been followed for almost four decades, and many are leading normal lives; some, however, have developed late complications (Table 99–7). Complications are related either to pretransplant events, the conditioning regimen (irradiation) or transplant-associated events (chronic GVHD, immunodeficiency).[153] Potentially life-threatening problems include infections and pulmonary dysfunction, particularly bronchiolitis obliterans which is usually associated with chronic GVHD.[154] Autoimmune disorders may develop due to adoptive transfer (from a donor who is affected), may be related to GVHD, or may be idiopathic.[155]

The omission of high-dose TBI as part of the conditioning regimen has reduced the frequency and severity of transplant-related complications such as interstitial pneumonitis, cataracts, impairment of growth and development.[63] It is desirable to avoid irradiation completely, at least in very young children, in whom growth and development of the skeleton and the central nervous system occur at an exponential rate.

Systematic psychosocial studies investigating the effects of HCT on personal development, family dynamics and partner-relationships are only now being pursued. Active rehabilitation is necessary in many instances.

SUMMARY

HCT has been developed into curative therapy for many nonmalignant disorders. Best results are achieved with HLA-identical sibling transplants. However, there has been considerable progress with molecular HLA typing, also allowing for close matching of patients and unrelated donors. Selection of donors on that basis has significantly improved transplantation outcome for these patients. For example, outcome in patients with aplastic anemia and MDS who received transplants from molecularly matched unrelated donors is comparable to that in patients who were transplanted from HLA-identical sibling donors. A major problem in all patients is GVHD, especially with its chronic manifestations, which are also responsible for systemic or organ-specific late complications. Because with nonmalignant diseases, there is no potential benefit of GVHD in the form of a GVL effect, every effort must be directed at preventing GVHD. There is limited data on a graft-vs-tumor effect in patients with MDS. To what extent the application of nonmyeloablative conditioning to patients with nonmalignant disorders and MDS will improve outcome, remains to be determined.

SELECTED REFERENCES

Ades L, Mary JY, Robin M, et al: Long-term outcome after bone marrow transplantation for severe aplastic anemia. Blood 103:2490, 2004.

Burt RK, Traynor A, Statkute L, et al: Nonmyeloablative hematopoietic stem cell transplantation for systemic lupus erythematosus. JAMA 295:527, 2006.

Cornetta K, Laughlin M, Carter S, et al: Umbilical cord blood transplantation in adults: results of the prospective Cord Blood Transplantation (COBLT). Biol Blood Marrow Transplant 11:149, 2005.

Cutler CS, Lee SJ, Greenberg P, et al: A decision analysis of allogeneic bone marrow transplantation for the myelodysplastic syndromes: delayed transplantation for low-risk myelodysplasia is associated with improved outcome. Blood 104:579, 2004.

de Lima M, Couriel D, Thall PF, et al: Once-daily intravenous buslfan and fludarabine: clinical and pharmacokinetic results of a myeloabltive, reduced-toxicity conditioning regimen for allogeneic stem cell transplantation in AML and MDS. Blood 104:857, 2004.

Deeg HJ, Maris MB, Scott BL, Warren EH: Optimization of allogeneic transplant conditioning: not the time for dogma. Leukemia 20:1701, 2006.

Deeg HJ, O'Donnell M, Tolar J, et al: Optimization of conditioning for marrow transplantation from unrelated donors for patients with aplastic anemia after failure of immunosuppressive therapy. Blood 108:1485, 2006.

Deeg HJ, Storer BE, Boeckh M, et al: Reduced incidence of acute and chronic graft-versus-host disease with the addition of thymoglobulin to a targeted busulfan/cyclophosphamide regimen. Biol Blood Marrow Transplant 12:573, 2006.

Doney K, Leisenring W, Storb R, Appelbaum FR, for the Seattle Bone Marrow Transplant Team: Primary treatment of acquired aplastic anemia: outcomes with bone marrow transplantation and immunosuppressive therapy. Ann Intern Med 126:107, 1997.

Flowers MED, Deeg HJ: Delayed complications after hematopoietic cell transplantation. In Blume KG, Forman SJ, Appelbaum FR, (eds.): Thomas' Hematopoietic Cell Transplantation. 3rd ed. Oxford, UK, Blackwell Publishing Ltd, 2004, p 944.

Hegenbart U, Niederwieser D, Forman S, et al: Hematopoietic cell transplantation from related and unrelated donors after minimal conditioning as a curative treatment modality for severe paroxysmal nocturnal hemoglobinuria. Biol Blood Marrow Transplant 9:689, 2003.

Ishiyama K, Chuhjo T, Wang H, Yachie A, Omine M, Nakao S: Polyclonal hematopoiesis maintained in patients with bone marrow failure harboring a minor population of paroxysmal nocturnal hemoglobinuria-type cells. Blood 102:1211, 2003.

Jang YY, Collector MI, Baylin SB, Diehl AM, Sharkis SJ: Hematopoietic stem cells convert into liver cells within days without fusion. Nat Cell Biol 6:532, 2004.

Malcovati L, Porta MG, Pascutto C, et al: Prognostic factors and life expectancy in myelodysplastic syndromes classified according to WHO criteria: a basis for clinical decision making. J Clin Oncol 23:7594, 2005.

Martino R, Iacobelli S, Brand R, et al: Retrospective comparison of reduced-intensity conditioning and conventional high-dose conditioning for allogeneic hematopoietic stem cell transplantation using HLA-identical sibling donors in myelodysplastic syndromes. Blood 108:836, 2006.

Musto P, D'Arena G, Cascavilla N, Carotenuto M: Normal G-CSF-mobilized CD34+ peripheral blood stem cells in paroxysmal nocturnal hemoglobinuria: a perspective for autologous transplantation. Leukemia 11:890, 1997.

Nash RA, McSweeney PA, Nelson JL, et al: Allogeneic marrow transplantation in patients with severe systemic sclerosis: resolution of dermal fibrosis. Arthritis Rheum 54:1982, 2006.

Saccardi R, Kozak T, Bocelli-Tyndall C, et al: Autologous stem cell transplantation for progressive multiple sclerosis: update of the European Group for Blood and Marrow Transplantation autoimmune diseases working party database. Mult Scler 12:814, 2006.

Slavin S, Nagler A, Naparstek E, et al: Nonmyeloablative stem cell transplantation and cell therapy as an alternative to conventional bone marrow transplantation with lethal cytoreduction for the treatment of malignant and nonmalignant hematologic diseases. Blood 91:756, 1998.

Storb R, Blume KG, O'Donnell MR, et al: Cyclophosphamide and antithymocyte globulin to condition patients with aplastic anemia for allogeneic marrow transplantations: the experience in four centers. Biol Blood Marrow Transplant 7:39, 2001.

REFERENCES

For complete list of references log onto www.expertconsult.com

CHAPTER 100

HEMATOPOIETIC STEM CELL TRANSPLANTATION FOR IMMUNE DEFICIENCIES AND GENETIC DISORDERS

Sarita A. Joshi and Stella M. Davies

The first successful studies of hematopoietic cell transplantation for treatment of any disease were performed for treatment of the genetic disorder severe combined immunodeficiency (SCID).[1] This transplantation established proof of principle that engraftment of hematopoietic stem cells was possible and could correct a genetic disorder. Children with immunodeficiencies were obvious subjects for these investigations because they have a limited capacity to reject a graft, and the early successes were a result of an emerging understanding of human leukocyte antigen (HLA) typing.

Use of hematopoietic cell transplantation therapy for indications other than immunodeficiencies has required the development of immunosuppressive and myeloablative therapies. These strategies have extended the applicability of hematopoietic cell transplantation to individuals with intact immune systems. It has been shown that achievement of engraftment from related and unrelated HLA-matched donors is possible in that setting. Currently, most hematopoietic cell transplantations are performed for treatment of hematologic malignancies. Over the last 20 years, however, a growing body of literature has described the application of allogeneic transplantation for correction of inborn errors of metabolism. In these disorders, a single gene defect leads to the absence of a key protein, which causes the clinical phenotype of disease. Allogeneic hematopoietic cell transplantation provides a means for replacing the missing protein, potentially improving the clinical phenotype. The most significant experience has been with treatment of mucopolysaccharidoses (MPS) and leukodystrophies, although case reports have described transplantation therapy for many other genetic disorders.

This chapter reviews the development and current status of hematopoietic cell transplantation for genetic immunodeficiencies, MPS, and leukodystrophies, discusses use of hematopoietic cell transplantation for less frequent disorders, and describes future directions for the field.

IMMUNE DEFICIENCIES

Severe Combined Immunodeficiency

SCID is a rare syndrome of profoundly impaired cellular and humoral immune system function (see Chapter 51).[2] Although both X-linked recessive and autosomal recessive forms of SCID are recognized, the X-linked form is the most frequent. Patients with X-linked SCID typically have very low numbers of T cells and natural killer (NK) cells, whereas B cells are often found in relatively high numbers even though specific antibody responses are deficient (B^+ SCID). A less common variant of SCID in which the numbers of T and B cells are low (B^- SCID) has an autosomal recessive inheritance. The true incidence of SCIDs is not known; however, they are estimated to occur in approximately one of every 10,000 live births. Infants with SCID have lymphopenia, and recognition of this abnormality can lead to early diagnosis. The lymphocytes of these babies are functionally abnormal and fail to proliferate in vitro or on challenge with mitogens, antigens, or allogeneic cells. Typically, levels of immunoglobulin are low or undetectable, thymus-dependent areas of the spleen are devoid of lymphocytes, and lymph nodes and tonsils usually are absent. SCID requires immediate treatment. Unless hematopoietic cell transplantation or, in a small number of cases, gene therapy succeeds, death occurs during infancy. Early reports of transplantation for treatment of SCID involved the use of HLA-matched family member donor cells, and current data indicate excellent outcomes with this therapy. A review of hematopoietic cell transplantation therapy for immunodeficiencies at Duke University covering a period of more than 16.5 years demonstrated that all 12 recipients of HLA-identical donor grafts were surviving.[3]

Use of Alternative Donors

The majority of patients with SCID do not have an HLA-matched related donor available. Alternative approaches (e.g., T-cell–depleted HLA-haploidentical parental hematopoietic cell transplantation and identification of unrelated donors from registries) have been used aggressively. Use of haploidentical grafts has the advantage of almost immediate availability and availability for essentially all infants because the mother or father of the child can be a donor. This strategy has the disadvantage of delayed, sometimes incomplete, immune system recovery as a consequence of the aggressive T-cell depletion that is needed to reduce the risk of graft-versus-host disease (GVHD). Buckley et al.[3] reported outcomes in 77 infants with SCID receiving T-cell–depleted HLA-haploidentical parental grafts at Duke University. Sixty of the 77 patients (78%) were surviving 3 months to 16.5 years after transplantation. T-cell function became normal approximately 3 to 4 months after transplantation, and the majority of long-term survivors had normal T-cell function, with all T cells in the blood being of donor origin. B-cell function remained abnormal in many of the recipients of haploidentical marrow, and most of these patients continue to receive intravenous immunoglobulin as support.

A large multicenter series of hematopoietic cell transplantation therapy for immunodeficiencies has been reported from Europe.[4] This study included data from 37 centers in 18 countries that participated in a European registry for stem cell transplantation for SCID and other immunodeficiency disorders. The registry includes 1082 transplantations performed in 919 patients; 566 transplantations were performed in 475 SCID patients. One hundred four SCID patients receiving an HLA-identical related donor transplantation were included in this series, and the survival rate was 77%. Of note, the analysis showed that similarly positive outcomes could be achieved with unrelated donor cells, with a survival rate of 81% in recipients of genotypically identical related donor cells, 72% in phenotypically matched related donors, and 63% in phenotypically matched unrelated donors. Significant improvements in survival after HLA-identical and HLA-nonidentical hematopoietic cell transplantations have occurred over time (Fig. 100–1). Cox regression multivariate analysis of risk factors for mortality showed only the age at the time of transplantation and use of trimethoprim-sulfamethoxazole prophylaxis had a significant effect on survival after transplantation from a related HLA-identical donor. Younger age was associated with an improved prognosis, with survival of 85% at 3 years in patients who underwent transplantation at an age less than 6 months. Survival of patients receiving an HLA-mismatched graft was 54%. SCID phenotype had an effect on survival after HLA-nonidentical stem cell transplantation. SCID patients without B cells had a poorer prognosis than did SCID patients with B cells, in accordance with a previous report.[5] In

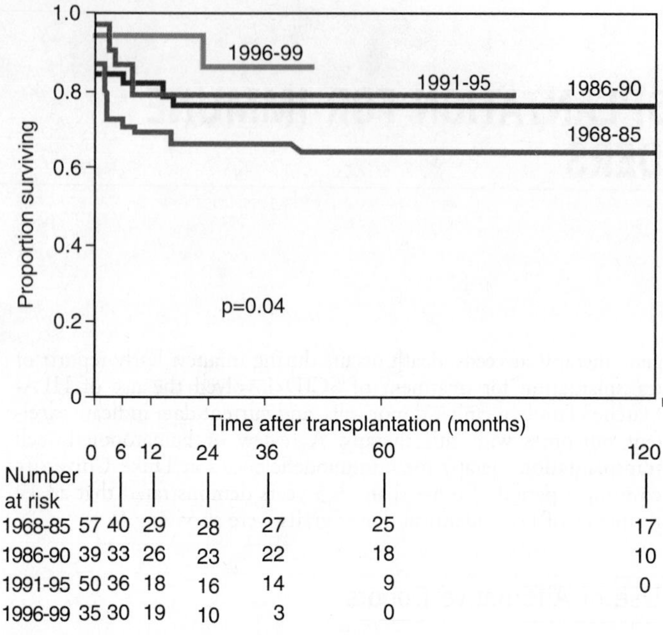

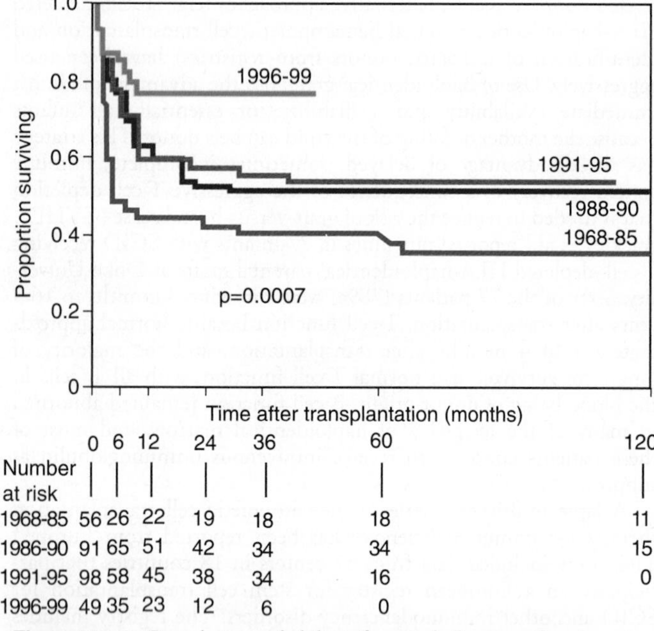

Figure 100–1 Cumulative probability of survival after transplant in patients with severe combined immunodeficiency disease, according to donor source (related or unrelated) and human leukocyte antigen matching and year of transplantation. (From Antoine C, Muller S, Cant A, et al: Long-term survival and transplant of haemopoietic stem cells for immunodeficiencies: Report of the European experience, 1968–99. Lancet 361:553, 2003.)

the HLA-nonidentical setting, use of a myeloablative conditioning regimen had a positive effect on survival in SCID patients without B cells but did not reach significance in other SCID groups. Independent predictors of increased mortality in SCID patients given a graft from a related HLA-mismatched donor included the SCID without B-cell phenotype, absence of a protected environment, and presence of pulmonary infection before transplantation.

The study of Antoine et al.[4] explored a center-size effect, segregating data from experienced centers (at least 50 procedures). In the more experienced centers, the survival rate after HLA-nonidentical transplantation was significantly better (57% vs 43%; $P = 0.009$). Moreover, the frequency of acute GVHD decreased over time after haploidentical transplantation, from 35% to 40% before 1996 to 22% thereafter ($P < 0.009$), perhaps because more effective methods of T-cell depletion are now used. This might contribute to the observed improvements in survival over time.

Debate continues regarding the relative merits of transplantation using haploidentical stem cells, commonly immediately available from the child's parents, or conducting an unrelated donor search to find perhaps more closely HLA-matched stem cells from an unrelated donor. Data from two transplant centers (Hospital for Sick Children, Toronto, Canada, and University of Brescia Spedali Civili, Brescia, Italy) were combined in a study designed to address this question.[6] This study showed improved survival with matched unrelated donor stem cells compared with mismatched family member stem cells (80.5% vs 52.5%; $P = 0.03$). In addition, long-term reconstitution of a full T-cell repertoire was achieved more frequently after unrelated donor transplant compared with mismatched family member donor transplantation (94% vs 61.1%; $P = 0.02$).

Use of Cord Blood

Umbilical cord blood, from either siblings or unrelated donors, stored in cord blood banks is being used increasingly for hematopoietic cell transplantation therapy for immunodeficiencies. Cord blood is an attractive stem cell source because recipients with immunodeficiencies typically are small; therefore, cell doses likely will be adequate. In addition, search commonly can be completed and a suitable unit identified in a period of a couple of weeks.[7]

Knutsen and Wall[8] reported the outcomes of umbilical cord blood transplantation in eight children with severe primary T-cell immunodeficiency disorders. Three patients had SCID, one had reticular dysgenesis, one had Nezelof syndrome, two had combined immunodeficiency, and one had Wiskott-Aldrich syndrome (WAS). In this series, all patients received a preparative regimen of busulfan and cyclophosphamide, and all achieved complete donor chimerism, although one child required a second transplantation after rejecting the initial graft. In this study, the early appearance of T-cell immunocompetence was observed, likely due to engraftment of memory T cells. In addition, proliferative responses to mitogens and alloantigens were normal. Similarly, Bhattacharya et al.[9] reported results of umbilical cord transplants in 14 children ((two from siblings, 12 from unrelated donors) with immune deficiency, including eight children with SCID. Outcomes were excellent; all children achieved donor cell engraftment, and 12 of 14 children were surviving at the time of the report. Although these results are encouraging, continuing followup of these patients is necessary to evaluate long-term outcomes and determine the optimal stem cell source for treatment of patients with SCID. It remains possible that umbilical cord blood stem cells, typically not exposed to prior viral infections, may be inferior in achieving rapid control of viral pathogens in children with infection acquired before or during transplantation.

Timing of Transplant

A number of studies have shown that the best outcomes in children with SCID are achieved with transplantation performed as early as possible. Kane et al.[10] performed a retrospective review of patients with SCID who underwent transplantation in the neonatal period between 1987 and 1999 at a center in the United Kingdom and described excellent outcomes. Thirteen patients received 18 hematopoietic cell transplantations. Stem cell sources included marrow (n = 4), umbilical cord blood (n = 1), parental T-cell–depleted haploidentical marrow (n = 10), and T-cell–depleted unrelated donor marrow (n = 3). Patients were conditioned with busulfan and cyclophosphamide. All patients were surviving 6 months to 11.5 years after transplantation. Of note, five patients required additional hematopoietic cell infusions to achieve adequate and stable immune system recovery. Multiple hematopoietic cell infusions are not infrequent in transplantation therapy for SCID, particularly if grafts are given without a preparative regimen. Myers et al.[11] also addressed the value of early transplantation in a report describing a subset of the Duke University experience reported by Buckley. This study compared immune system function in 21 SCID infants receiving transplantations in the neonatal period with function in 70 SCID infants undergoing transplantations at an older age. Lymphocyte phenotypes, response to mitogens, immunoglobulin levels, and T-cell receptor circles were evaluated before transplantation and sequentially thereafter. Of the 21 SCID patients who underwent transplantation in the neonatal period, 95% were surviving. The infants who underwent transplantation in the neonatal period developed higher lymphocyte responses to phytohemagglutinin and higher numbers of $CD3^+$ and $CD45RA^+$ T cells in the first 3 years of life than those who received transplantations later. T-cell receptor circles peaked earlier and with higher values in the neonatal transplants than in the later transplants. These authors proposed that improved outcomes for SCID could be achieved with universal newborn screening for lymphopenia so that children with SCID would be diagnosed early and transplantation performed under the most favorable circumstances.

In Utero Transplant

A logical extension of the reports describing improved outcome with younger age at the time of transplantation has been the investigation of in utero transplantation for treatment of SCID. Flake et al.[12] reported successful treatment of a fetus with X-linked SCID by in utero transplantation of paternal marrow cells enriched with hematopoietic cell progenitors by $CD34^+$ cell selection. Three transabdominal injections of hematopoietic stem cells were given to the fetus in utero. At birth, the patient had no evidence of GVHD, and hematologic and immune system function appeared normal. Notwithstanding the success of this case, the clinical experience with in utero hematopoietic stem cell transplantation has been otherwise disappointing, and in most cases engraftment was not achieved. Touraine et al.[13,14] reported the treatment of one patient with bare lymphocyte syndrome and another patient with SCID by in utero transplantation of hematopoietic cells from fetal liver. Multiple prenatal and postnatal fetal liver transplantations were performed, and the evidence of engraftment in these two patients was limited. Whether benefit was gained from the in utero component of the therapy was unclear. Additional work in this field is needed before in utero transplantation becomes an accepted therapy.

Reduced-Intensity Regimens

The need for a preparative regimen prior to transplantation therapy for SCID is variable. Many patients with little residual NK cell or lymphocyte function will achieve engraftment without a preparative regimen. Avoiding use of a preparative regimen significantly reduces the late effects of transplantation. No clinical test can categorically predict graft rejection. A common approach is to attempt engraftment in the absence of a preparative regimen but to resort to hematopoietic cell infusion with a preparative regimen if engraftment fails. The greater the degree of HLA mismatch between donor and recipient, the more difficult will be achieving engraftment and the greater the likelihood of needing a preparative regimen. An alternative to a full preparative regimen, particularly suitable for children with significant organ dysfunction, is use of a nonmyeloablative regimen. Rao et al.[15] reported 33 consecutive unrelated donor transplants in children with primary immune deficiencies, including six children with SCID, using a reduced-intensity preparative regimen that included fludarabine, melphalan, and antilymphocyte globulin or alemtuzumab (Campath). All patients had successful initial engraftment with predominantly donor chimerism, and early toxicity was low. Thirty-one of 33 children were surviving 1 year after transplantation. Mixed chimerism occurred at later time points, with 55% of children full donor chimeras at 1 year, and 39% with likely adequate levels of donor chimerism. Two of the 33 children had low-level chimerism requiring prophylactic medication and likely retransplantation. The authors of this study compared these results with those of ablative transplants performed for a similar patient population at the same institution. Incidences of engraftment and GVHD were similar between the two groups. Overall survival was notably superior in the reduced-intensity preparative regimen group (94% vs 53%; $P = 0.014$) compared with the myeloablative group, although it should be noted that the majority of the myeloablative transplants were performed in earlier years. Viral reactivation was common after reduced-intensity conditioning but was controllable with careful monitoring and preemptive treatment.

Reduced-intensity preparative regimens likely will provide an attractive option for transplantation for SCID in the future. Transplantation with no conditioning regimen has been used widely because late adverse effects are reduced in children who can achieve adequate immune reconstitution. However, this approach may result in graft failure, and the time course of T-cell reconstitution may be prolonged or recovery limited in some patients.[16,17] Use of a conditioning regimen appears to improve cell recovery in particular SCID phenotypes, and it is anticipated that better tolerated reduced-intensity regimens may increase enthusiasm for use of preparative therapy.[18]

Wiskott-Aldrich Syndrome

WAS is a lethal hematologic disease characterized by platelet and lymphocyte dysfunction, microthrombocytopenia, and a tendency to autoimmunity and lymphoreticular malignancies (see Chapter 51). WAS has a worldwide distribution, with an estimated incidence between one and 10 per million live male births. In the past it was diagnosed based on the triad of microthrombocytopenia, eczema, and recurrent infections. WAS is a consequence of mutation in the WAS (also called WASP) gene at Xp11.22–11.23.[19] *WASP* encodes a 502-amino-acid protein that is selectively expressed in hematopoietic stem cell-derived lineages and is a key regulator of cell signaling and cytoskeletal reorganization. Mutations in the WASP gene can result in classical WAS or in a less severe form of X linked thrombocytopenia that may present at birth or during the first few months of life with petechiae, bruising, and bloody diarrhea. Excessive hemorrhage after circumcision is an early diagnostic sign, particularly when associated with eczema during infancy and childhood. Correlation of genotype with phenotype has shown that complete absence of expression of WASP protein is associated with greater susceptibility to infection, severe eczema, tendency to hemorrhage, and malignancy.[20] Children who expressed some WASP protein have a less severe phenotype, and commonly these children have missense mutations.[21] Boys with deletions or insertions commonly have the more severe WASP-negative phenotype.

The current mainstays of supportive care for WAS are splenectomy and intravenous immunoglobulin infusion.[22,23] With these treatments, patients with WAS remain at high risk for overwhelming sepsis due to an inherent deficiency of antibody production to polysaccharide antigens in combination with splenectomy. In addition, boys who do not achieve safe platelet counts are restricted in their activities. Immune system complications of WAS are commonly managed by long-term corticosteroid therapy or, in extreme cases, by palliative organ transplantation for end-stage renal failure or liver disease.[24,25] Development of lymphoma, which occurs frequently in the second decade of life in untransplanted boys, is associated with poor outcomes.

Transplant Outcome

Two large registry series have described the outcome of hematopoietic cell transplantation for patients with WAS. Filipovich et al.[26] analyzed outcomes reported to the International Bone Marrow Transplant Registry (IBMTR) and the National Marrow Donor Program (NMDP). This study included 170 hematopoietic cell

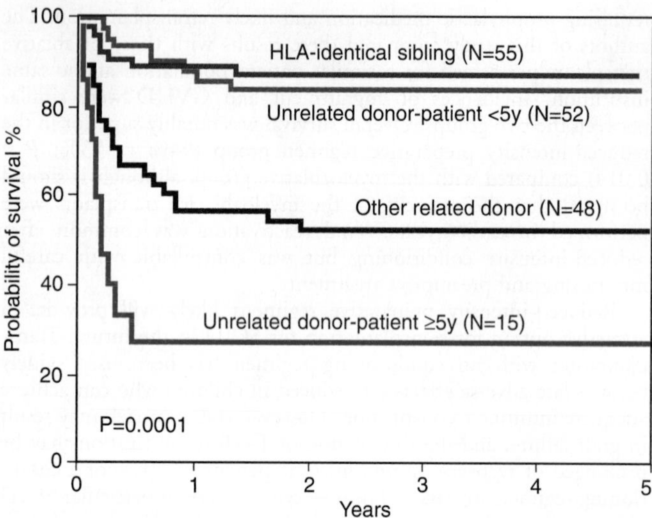

Figure 100–2 Probabilities of survival by donor type and recipient age for 170 patients receiving hematopoietic cell transplantations for treatment of Wiskott-Aldrich syndrome. There was no significant difference in the risk of mortality after human leukocyte antigen (HLA)-matched sibling–donor transplantations and after unrelated-donor transplantations in children younger than 5 years. A significantly worse rate of survival was associated with use of related donors other than HLA-identical siblings, regardless of recipient age, and with use of unrelated donors in patients older than 5 years. (From Filipovich AH, Stone JV, Tomany SC, et al: Impact of donor type on outcome of bone marrow transplant for Wiskott-Aldrich syndrome: Collaborative study of the International Bone Marrow Transplant Registry and the National Marrow Donor Program. Blood 97:1598, 2001.)

transplantations for patients with WAS performed between 1968 and 1996. Fifty-five were from HLA-identical sibling donors, 48 from other relatives, and 67 from unrelated donors. The 5-year probability of survival for all subjects was 70%. Probabilities differed by donor type: 87% of recipients of HLA-identical sibling donor grafts survived compared with 52% of recipients of other related donor grafts. Seventy-one percent of patients who received unrelated donor transplantations survived. Multivariate analysis indicated that boys older than 5 years had significantly lower survival rates when receiving transplants from related donors other than HLA-identical donors or from unrelated donors compared with transplantations from HLA-identical sibling donors. Boys receiving unrelated-donor transplantation before age 5 years had survival rates similar to boys receiving HLA-identical transplantation (Fig. 100–2). Detailed data regarding chimerism and immune system reconstitution were not available in this multicenter registry series. Other studies have indicated that early mixed chimerism in patients with WAS often is stable because of a survival advantage for stem cells and hematopoietic precursors bearing the normal WAS gene.[27]

European registry data indicate similarly good results with genotypically identical transplantations.[4] This study included 32 patients with WAS who received a genotypically identical graft, and 81% were surviving. Survival was inferior for recipients of HLA-mismatched related grafts, with 45% surviving (n = 43). Although data for WAS cases were not shown separately for non-SCID immunodeficiency patients, there was no difference in survival between recipients of genotypically HLA-identical and HLA-matched unrelated-donor transplantations. In this study, 75% of patients with unrelated donors were considered "HLA-identical" to their donors. The level of resolution of HLA typing and the loci included to define "identical" were not stated in the report. A case series of 57 boys with WAS transplanted in a number of centers in Japan also describes excellent outcomes for young patient transplanted with related or matched unrelated donor stem cells.[28] This study includes transplants performed between 1985 and 2004 and included 11 boys transplanted from HLA-matched related donors, 10 from mismatched related donors, 21 from unrelated bone marrow donors, and 15 from unrelated cord blood units. The overall 5-year survival rate for patients receiving bone marrow from unrelated donors and those receiving cord blood from unrelated donors was 80% in both groups. Univariate factors associated with poorer survival included age over 5 years, transplantation from an HLA-mismatched donors, and use of a preparative regimen other than busulfan, and cyclophosphamide, with or without antithymocyte globulin. Only the preparative regimen remained significant in a multivariate analysis. Similar observations have been reported by investigators from the University of Brescia, Italy, who described their single-center experience of 23 transplants for WAS, spanning the years 1990 to 2005.[29] This report described similar excellent outcomes in recipients of unrelated donor marrow stem cells, with 81.2% (13/16) surviving; deaths occurred only in recipients of mismatched related stem cells or in children with severe symptomatology at the time of transplantation.

Taken together, these data show that early hematopoietic cell transplantation using genotypically or phenotypically matched donor–recipient pairs is excellent therapy for boys with WAS. Transplantation before age 5 years is associated with the best outcome. These data should encourage earlier referral of suitable candidates for transplantation.

Table 100–1 Classification and Underlying Conditions of Hemophagocytic Lymphohistiocytosis

Genetic HLH
Familial HLH (Farquhar disease[a])
Known gene defects (perforin, Munc13-4, syntaxin 11)
Unknown gene defects
Immune deficiency syndromes
Chédiak-Higashi syndrome
Griscelli syndrome
X-linked lymphoproliferative syndrome
Acquired HLH
Exogenous agents (infectious organisms, toxins)
Infection-associated hemophagocytic syndrome
Endogenous products (tissue damage, metabolic products)
Rheumatic diseases
Macrophage activation syndrome
Malignant diseases

[a]Familial hemophagocytic lymphohistiocytosis (HLH) was first described by Farquhar and Claireaux in 1952.

Adapted from Janka G, zur Stadt U: Familial and acquired hemophagocytic lymphohistiocytosis. Hematology 2005 American Society of Hematology Education Book, 82, 2005.

Hemophagocytic Lymphohistiocytosis

Hemophagocytic lymphohistiocytosis (HLH) is a life-threatening immune system disorder characterized by fever, massive hepatosplenomegaly, pancytopenia, hypertriglyceridemia, hypofibrinogenemia, and central nervous system disease, commonly manifested as seizures and encephalopathy (see Chapter 52).[30] Historically, HLH has been categorized as primary or secondary. The primary form, also known as *familial erythrophagocytic lymphohistiocytosis*, typically has a symptomatic presentation at infancy. Inheritance usually is autosomal recessive. Secondary HLH often is associated with Epstein-Barr virus infections and typically manifests at an older age. Clinical findings similar to those seen in HLH also occur in children with Chédiak-Higashi syndrome, Griscelli syndrome, and X-linked lymphoproliferative disorder (Table 100–1). Children with these genetic disorders who manifest HLH will generally require prompt transplant for disease control.

Table 100–2. Gene Mutations Identified in Hemophagocytic Lymphohistiocytosis.

Disease	Chromosome Location	Associated Gene	Gene Function
FHLH1	9q21.3–22	Unknown	Not known
FHLH2	10q21–22	PRF1	Induction of apoptosis
FHLH3	17q25	UNC13D (Munc)	Vesicle priming
FHLH4	6q24	STX11	Vesicle transport; t-SNARE
GS-2	15q21	RAB27A	Vesicle transport; small GTPase
CHS-1	1q42.1–q42.2	LYST	Vesicle transport, not further defined
XLP	Xq25	SH2D1A	Signal transduction and activation of lymphocytes

CHS, Chédiak-Higashi syndrome; FHLH, familial hemophagocytic lymphohistiocytosis; GS, Griscelli syndrome; XLP, X-linked lymphoproliferative syndrome.

Adapted from Janka G, zur Stadt U: Familial and acquired hemophagocytic lymphohistiocytosis. Hematology 2005 American Society of Hematology Education Book, 82, 2005.

Most patients with familial HLH have complete lacking of or impaired NK cell function. The specific underlying genetic cause can now be discerned in approximately 50% to 60% of cases. The most common genetic defects in patients with FHL involve the perforin gene (*PRF1*) on chromosome 10q21 and the *Munc13-4* gene on chromosome 17q25 (Table 100–2).[31,32] Mutations of *PRF1* account for approximately 30% to 40% of patients, defined as the FHL2 subtype, and *MUNC13-4* mutations are identified in an additional 25% to 30% of cases (FHL3). The proteins encoded by both genes are implicated in the killing machinery of cytotoxic lymphocytes.[32,33] Perforin is a protein expressed in the cytoplasmic granules of cytotoxic T lymphocytes and NK cells. Perforin may be principally responsible for translocation of granzyme B from cytotoxic cells into target cells. Granzyme B then can migrate to the target cell nucleus and participate in triggering of apoptosis.[34]

Munc13-4, a protein essential for cytolytic granule fusion to the cell surface membrane, is a direct partner of rab27a.[32,33] The two proteins are highly expressed in cytotoxic T lymphocytes and mast cells, where they colocalize on secretory lysosomes. This complex is an essential regulator of secretory granule fusion with the plasma membrane in hematopoietic cells.

More recently, mutations in the syntaxin11 gene (6q24) have been reported in a small group of patients (FHL4) of common Kurdish origin.[35] This defect is thought to alter intracellular vesicle trafficking of the phagocytic system, but the exact functions are unknown. In addition, a small number of male patients with the clinical syndrome of HLH have germline mutations in SH2D1A/SAP, the gene associated with X-linked lymphoproliferative disorder.[36]

The clinical features of HLH are due to widespread infiltration of the liver, spleen, marrow, and central nervous system with activated lymphocytes and macrophages. Expansion of these cells represents a failure of regulation of the immune system response, particularly by NK cells. NK cells primarily use the perforin/granzyme pathway to eliminate virus-infected or transformed cells and achieve cytotoxicity. Flow cytometric analyses of intracytoplasmic perforin expression and surface CD107a, a marker of granule exocytosis (expressed at the surface of NK cells after their interaction with suitable target cells), as a surrogate for Munc13-4 defects have been used to identify cases with these mutations.[37] Therapeutic options have evolved along t he principles of control of exaggerated clinical manifestations of inflammation, eradication of pathogen-infected antigen-presenting cells, and stem cell transplantation to replace the defective immune system.

Transplant Outcomes

An analysis of 122 HLH patients treated with chemotherapy alone revealed a very poor 5-year survival rate of 10.1%.[38] In contrast, the 5-year survival rate for allogeneic hematopoietic cell transplantation recipients was 66%. The majority of patients in this report received transplants from HLA-matched sibling donors. As with any genetic disease, use of matched sibling donor marrow cells for transplantation raises the concern that the sibling donor also might have HLH. Differences in age at onset of at least 3 years between siblings have been described. Potential donors from affected families should be studied carefully for evidence of latent HLH. In light of the emerging genes being associated with HLH, every effort must be made to identify these mutations in probands so that similar mutations can be sought in sibling donors prior to transplantation. If similar outcomes can be achieved with unrelated donor hematopoietic cell transplantation, this might be a more attractive option that avoids this uncertainty in families without a defined gene mutation. A survival rate of 44% was reported in HLH patients receiving unrelated-donor hematopoietic cell transplantation (n = 16) treated at two institutions.[39] This report also noted that survival was poor in patients not in clinical remission at the time of transplantation, with only one of six patients surviving. These data emphasize the need to make the best possible attempt to achieve a remission prior to transplantation.

An international study of the treatment of HLH with a uniform chemotherapy and transplantation protocol (HLH 94) supports the value of hematopoietic cell transplantation for patients with HLH.[40] In 1994, the Histiocyte Society initiated a prospective international collaborative therapeutic study aimed at improving survival. One hundred thirteen patients younger than 15 years with persistent, recurring, or familial disease received a chemotherapy regimen of etoposide, corticosteroids, cyclosporine, and, in selected patients, intrathecal methotrexate, followed by hematopoietic cell transplantation. All patients either had an affected sibling or fulfilled the Histiocyte Society diagnostic criteria for HLH. At a median followup of 3.1 years, the estimated overall 3-year probability of survival was 55%, and in familial cases the probability of survival was 51%. The 3-year probability of survival in patients who underwent transplantation was 62%.

A separate report dissected in detail the transplant outcomes of children receiving transplantation according to the HLH 94 study.[41] Eighty-six children, 29 with familial HLH, were included in the report. Overall 3-year survival post transplant was 64%, with similar outcomes in recipients of matched related or matched unrelated donor stem cells (71% and 70%, respectively) and inferior survival in recipients of family haploidentical donors or mismatched unrelated donors (50% and 54%, respectively). Outcomes were improved in children with inactive disease at the time of transplant, although some children with persistent active disease were survivors post-transplant.

Reduced-Intensity Regimens

The majority of deaths posttransplant in HLH 94 were due to regimen-related toxicity, raising interest in less toxic preparative regimens. The Great Ormond Street Hospital team reported outcomes of reduced-intensity conditioning transplants in 12 children with HLH, using a variety of fludarabine-based regimens and stem cell sources.[42] Nine of 12 children were surviving, three of whom had mixed chimerism ranging from 2% to 84% donor cells. The patient with 2% donor cell engraftment remains in clinical complete remission 73 months from transplantation; however, the adequacy of such low-level chimerism for long-term disease control remains uncertain. A proportion of children transplanted for HLH will have graft failure (i.e., completely absent donor chimerism), particularly when mismatched or haploidentical stem cells are used, raising the question of whether a second attempt at transplant is indicated in children with quiescent disease. Ardeshna et al.[43] reported three children with HLH and graft rejection. After a period of disease quiescence lasting 4 months to 8 years, disease recurrence and subsequent death occurred in each case, suggesting that further transplantation should be offered in such cases. Further long-term followup is needed to define the level of mixed chimerism that is acceptable in HLH, and this number may vary in different children with different genetic and infectious etiologies of disease.

Control of CNS Disease

An important challenge in the management of HLH is the control of CNS disease. Thirty-two percent of children enrolled in HLH 94 had neurologic alterations at onset, secondary to an inflammatory meningoencephalopathy. CNS involvement with HLH can lead to severe and perhaps permanent CNS dysfunction. As survival improves, CNS impairment is being increasingly identified as a long-term sequela of HLH. In the HLH 94 protocol, early intensification with systemic chemotherapy as well as intrathecal methotrexate was recommended for children with CNS involvement. Sixty-seven percent of children receiving intrathecal methotrexate achieved resolution of CNS symptoms, but a similar proportion of children with CNS disease who did not receive IT therapy had resolution of symptoms, leaving uncertainty regarding the importance of IT therapy.[40] Of note, patients with HLH-related CNS insults who underwent stem cell transplantation did not generally have radiologic resolution of CNS lesions; however, there was a suggestion of disease stabilization by magnetic resonance imaging with functional and cognitive correlates. Other reports cite stabilization of neurologic function and frequent reversal of neurologic deficits within 1 to 3 years after a successful graft.[44] Ouachee-Chardin et al.[45] reported 48 patients with HLH treated between 1982 and 2004. The report highlights a 28% incidence of veno-occlusive disease (VOD) among younger recipients of haploidentical grafts and antithymocyte globulin during conditioning. The overall survival of patients followed for a median of 5.8 years was 58.5 %. A sustained remission was noted in all patients, and donor chimerism greater than 20% was seen in these patients. In contrast to the development of myglodysplastic syndrome and acute myelogenous leukemia (MDS/AML) in three patients with HLH treated with the HLH 94 protocol, none of the patients treated with combination immunotherapy and hematopoietic stem cell transplantation in the French study developed this phenomenon.[45] Patients studied here also demonstrated stabilization of neurologic disease without development of new lesions or CNS reactivation.

MUCOPOLYSACCHARIDOSES

MPS I (Hurler Syndrome)

MPS comprises a group of recessively inherited lysosomal storage diseases characterized by specific enzyme deficiencies, tissue accumulation of glycosaminoglycans leading to musculoskeletal deformities, organ involvement, and mental retardation of varying severity (see Chapter 53).[46] Experience with hematopoietic cell transplantation therapy is greatest in cases of Hurler syndrome (MPS I), the prototypical MPS disease. MPS I is caused by deficiency of lysosomal α-L-iduronidase. Affected children appear normal at birth but subsequently develop coarse facial features, hepatosplenomegaly, short stature, persistent rhinitis, corneal clouding, claw hands, coronary artery stenosis, hydrocephalus, progressive mental retardation, and a variety of well-defined musculoskeletal abnormalities known as *dysostosis multiplex*. Untreated patients will have progressive mental retardation with development of severe kyphosis. Such patients typically die of cardiopulmonary insufficiency and/or complications of progressive mental retardation.

Transplant Outcomes

A 9-month-old boy was the first child treated with hematopoietic cell transplantation for MPS I in 1980.[47] This patients is surviving 20 years later, fully engrafted with cells from his mother's marrow; he has stable intelligence in the low-to-normal range.[48] This initial favorable experience has encouraged further investigation of transplantation therapy for MPS I. In the largest series to date, Peters et al.[49] reported outcomes of hematopoietic cell transplantation for MPS I in 54 children using data collected by the Storage Disease Collaborative Study Group. The patients in this study had a median age of 1.8 years at the time of transplantation (range 0.4–7.9 years). Transplantations were performed between 1983 and 1995. Thirty-nine of the 54 patients (72%) had engraftment after the first hematopoietic cell transplantation. This is a much lower frequency of engraftment than would be expected in other disorders and indicates that patients with MPS I have particular difficulty perhaps with stem cell homing or adhesion. The actuarial probability of 5-year survival was 75% for recipients of genoidentical grafts and 53% for recipients of related HLA-mismatched donor grafts. Survival for all patients who achieved engraftment was 53%.

This large study provided the opportunity for the authors to examine cognitive outcomes. Baseline and posthematopoietic cell transplantation neuropsychological data were available for 26 of 30 engrafted survivors. Of 14 patients who underwent transplantation before age 24 months, nine demonstrated developmental trajectories that were normal or somewhat slower than normal. In contrast, only three of 12 patients who underwent transplantation after age 24 months showed developmental trajectories that were normal or somewhat slower than normal ($P = 0.01$). For children with a baseline Mental Developmental Index (MDI) greater than 70, there was a significant correlation between the MDI at followup study and leukocyte α-L-iduronidase enzyme activity ($P = 0.02$). Children were more likely to maintain normal cognitive development if they received transplants from a donor with homozygous normal leukocyte α-L-iduronidase enzyme activity compared with a heterozygous carrier of MPS I. These data indicate the importance of early transplantation in children with MPS I (typically before age 2 years) to optimize cognitive outcome.

A companion paper described the outcome of 40 children with MPS I who received unrelated-donor hematopoietic cell transplantations.[50] The children in this report had a median age of 1.7 years (range 0.9–3.2 years) and underwent transplantation between 1989 and 1994. Only 25 of the 40 patients achieved donor cell engraftment, again emphasizing the difficulty in engraftment in this patient population. An estimated 49% percent of patients were alive at 2 years. Sixty-three percent had evidence of allogeneic donor engraftment, and 37% had recovery of autologous hematopoiesis. When graft failure occurs in this population, recovery of autologous hematopoiesis is usual, rather than aplasia. Higher hematopoietic cell dose correlated with both improved donor cell engraftment and superior survival. Neither T-cell depletion of the marrow nor inclusion of irradiation as part of the conditioning regimen influenced the incidence of engraftment, although the power of the study to identify an effect was modest. Similar results were reported in a large single-center study from France describing transplantation in 27 children with MPS I, using mostly unrelated donors, 23 of whom were surviving, 21 with functional grafts.[51] Similar to other reports, the incidence of primary graft failure was high (16%).

Use of Cord Blood

The rapid availability of umbilical cord blood units for transplantation makes cord blood an attractive therapeutic option. Staba et al.[52] reported outcomes of 20 consecutive children with MPS I who received unrelated cord blood transplants after a chemotherapy-based preparative regimen. They described survival rates similar to those reported with bone marrow as a stem cell source (17/20 alive) and amelioration of the disease phenotype. Umbilical cord blood transplantation allows rapid transplantation to halt substrate deposition in MPS I. An alternative approach is active substrate depletion with enzyme replacement therapy prior to transplantation. Commercial availability of enzyme (Aldurazyme; Genzyme) is allowing many transplant centers to explore this approach. Early reports indicate that this strategy is well tolerated, although the optimal duration of replacement prior to transplantation and the value of posttransplant therapy remain unclear.[53,54] Children with MPS I have a high incidence of pulmonary hemorrhage after transplantation, and use of enzyme for substrate depletion from the lungs might reduce this clinically very significant toxicity, although data are still early.[55,56] Use of reduced-intensity conditioning therapy is also being explored and might similarly reduce pulmonary toxicity.[57]

Assessment of Transplant Outcomes

Assessment of cognitive outcomes is a vital component of evaluating the success of transplantation for genetic disorders. Peters et al.[49,50] assessed the MDI before and after transplantation in 11 engrafted survivors. Eight children had a baseline MDI of greater than 70 at the time of transplantation. Of these cases, six patients showed stability in the age equivalence scores; two patients were too early to evaluate. Four of the children were acquiring skills at a pace equal to or slightly below age peers, and two children had shown either a plateau in their learning or extreme slowing in their learning process. Posttransplantation evaluation of engrafted children with baseline MDI less than 70 (typically older children) indicated that two children had shown deterioration in their developmental skills, whereas the remaining three children maintained their skills and were adding to them at a variable rate. The authors concluded from this study that MPS I patients with baseline MDI greater than 70 who achieve engraftment will have favorable long-term outcomes, with cognitive function close to or within the normal range. A further report of adaptive functions in a cohort of 41 posttransplant children with MPS I examined communication, daily living skills socialization, and motor skills and described long-term slow improvement in functional outcomes, with best outcomes in children with good cognitive function before transplant.[58] Again, these data emphasize the need for early transplantation in MPS I patients before the occurrence of significant loss of cognitive function.

Biochemical studies have shown a close correlation between mean posttransplant enzyme level and residual substrate, indicating that higher levels are likely to yield better functional outcomes.[59] This observation is of particular importance in families with an HLA-matched sibling donor who is a heterozygote and has reduced levels of α-L-iduronidase. Results of well-matched unrelated donor transplants have improved due to better HLA typing, larger registries, and better supportive care, making this a potentially better donor source than a heterozygous sibling donor.

The low frequencies of engraftment described in these studies are a common feature of transplantation for MPS I cases. A proportion of children who fail to engraft can be rescued with a second allogeneic transplantation. Grewal et al.[60] described outcomes in 11 MPS I patients who received a second transplantation after initial graft failure. The median age at second transplantation was 25 months (range 16–45 months), and the median time from the first transplantation was 8 months (range 4–18.5 months). The conditioning regimen consisted of cyclophosphamide and total body irradiation, with or without antithymocyte globulin. The source of hematopoietic cells was an unrelated donor in six cases, an HLA-matched sibling in four cases, and an HLA-mismatched related donor in one case. Five of the 11 grafts were T-cell–depleted prior to infusion. Actuarial survival was 50% over 4 years. All surviving patients show sustained donor engraftment with normalization of α-L-iduronidase levels. Neuropsychological function stabilized after the second transplantation in three of five evaluable patients.

Long-term followup after transplantation for MPS I has shown that although donor cell engraftment can stabilize neurocognitive decline, continuing complications secondary to accumulation of glycosaminoglycans occur as the children mature. In particular, orthopedic abnormalities, including acetabular dysplasia, kyphoscoliosis, carpal tunnel syndrome, trigger finger, and genu valgum, tend to progress. Typically, multiple surgeries are required in the first decade after transplantation.[61,62]

The management of children with MPS during transplantation can be complex. Cardiac involvement due to deposition of glycosaminoglycan in coronary arteries causing stenosis can lead to sudden death during anesthesia or cardiac failure secondary to cardiomyopathy.[63–65] These manifestations improve significantly after engraftment is achieved. However, as the children grow, deposition of glycosaminoglycan in the poorly vascularized cardiac valves continues despite the presence of donor enzyme. Some long-term transplantation survivors have required cardiac valve replacement. Patients with MPS commonly have deposition of glycosaminoglycan in the upper airway and can be particularly difficult to intubate.[64,66] Belani et al.[64] described 141 episodes of anesthesia in children with MPS. In children with MPS I, the incidence of odontoid dysplasia was 94%, and 38% demonstrated anterior C1–2 subluxation, illustrating the need for great care during anesthesia. Intubation was noted to be more difficult, with the vocal cords frequently not visible, and there was a high frequency of airway obstruction after extubation. Two children required reintubation to support their airway. In this series, two deaths occurred secondary to severe and extensive coronary obstruction, and the study noted that cardiac catheterization could underestimate the degree of coronary stenosis. Ocular abnormalities associated with MPS may progress after successful transplantation, and careful efforts to optimize vision with surgery or refraction are important to optimizing developmental progress.[67,68] Lifelong observation of all aspects of the child's growth and development is essential to achieve the highest possible level of function. Significant improvements can be achieved with frequent and aggressive speech, physical, and occupational therapy.

MPS VI (Maroteaux-Lamy Syndrome)

MPS VI (Maroteaux-Lamy syndrome) is characterized by defective degradation of dermatan sulfate due to deficiency of *N*-acetylgalactosamine IV sulfatase.[69] The clinical severity of MPS VI is highly variable, with a continuum from mildly affected to severely affected patients.[70] Affected individuals typically have bony dysplasia hepatosplenomegaly, airway narrowing, deposition of dermatan sulfate on cardiac valves, and deposition in subcutaneous tissues leading to restriction in movement. MPS VI patients typically have a normal intellect, although cognitive deterioration, perhaps in association with hydrocephalus, can occur later in life. Patients usually die in their teens or early adult life, often of cardiopulmonary failure. Experience with transplantation in MPS VI is limited because of the rarity of this disease and the variable phenotype. The first human hematopoietic cell transplantation for MPS VI was reported in 1984, when Krivit et al.[71] described the outcome of sibling donor transplantation in a 13-year old girl with a severe form of MPS VI. This patient had severe life-threatening upper airway obstruction leading to obstructive sleep apnea. A subsequent report of her clinical status 40 months later described resolution of the sleep apnea, improvement in hepatosplenomegaly, and improvement in range of motion due to resolution of soft-tissue changes.[72] Of note, no radiographic improvement in bone pathology and no increase in height were observed. The patient had severe corneal clouding that did not resolve and required corneal transplantation.

Subsequent case reports have observed that some aspects of the MPS VI phenotype will be improved by transplantation.[73,74] Herskhovitz et al.[74] described four patients who underwent transplantation for MPS VI, with followup periods ranging between 1 and 9 years. The indications for transplantation were cardiomyopathy in three patients and severe obstructive sleep apnea in one. In all engrafted patients, facial features have become less coarse. Cardiac manifestations improved or remained stable, and three of the four patients were being educated in mainstream schools. However, skeletal changes persisted or even progressed, although posture and joint stability improved, and all patients remained ambulatory and active. These data support the role of transplantation therapy in prolonging survival and improving quality of life in MPS VI patients. However, careful selection of patients whose condition is most likely to improve with transplantation is necessary.

MPS II (Hunter Syndrome)

MPS II (Hunter syndrome) is an X-linked disorder caused by deficiency of iduronate sulfatase enzyme activity.[70] MPS II has a wide range of clinical severity, from the early-onset severe form (MPS IIA) to the milder later onset form (MPS IIB). Boys with MPS IIA exhibit significant somatic features, such as coarse facial features, progressive hearing loss, hepatosplenomegaly, cardiomyopathy, dysostosis multiplex, macrocephaly, central nervous system deterioration, and neuropsychological impairments. As in cases of MPS I, clinical features of the disease are due to deposition of storage material. Neuropsychological consequences of MPS IIA are similar to those of MPS I, except that behavioral abnormalities may be more marked. In general, male subjects with MPS IIB experience milder signs and symptoms with great variability in age of onset and severity, with survival as long as 40 years reported. The variable phenotype and life expectancy of patients with MPS II make the decision to submit a patient to the risks of transplantation very difficult. In addition, some cases of children who underwent transplantation for MPS II and who suffered continuing neurologic deterioration despite achievement of adequate engraftment have been reported.[75,76] Vellodi et al.[76] described a series of 10 patients who underwent transplantation as treatment for Hunter syndrome. The donor was an HLA-identical sibling in two cases, an HLA-nonidentical relative in six cases, a volunteer unrelated donor in one case, and unknown in one case. Only three of the 10 patients survived more than 7 years posttransplantation. In two of these cases, patients experienced steady progression of physical disability and mental handicap, although one patient maintained normal intellectual development with only mild physical disability. These authors and others have suggested a role for transplantation in carefully selected boys with Hunter syndrome.[77–80] This issue is controversial. If such transplantations are undertaken, careful attention should be given to the process of informed consent and to long-term followup to document the benefits achieved.[81–83]

MPS VII (Sly Syndrome)

MPS VII (Sly syndrome) is an autosomal recessive disorder caused by an inherited defect in the lysosomal hydrolase β-glucuronidase. The enzyme defect causes accumulation of undegraded glycosaminoglycans. Approximately 40 cases of MPS VII have been reported worldwide, and there is considerable experience in transplantation of mouse models in this disease.[84–86] Animal models have also been used in an investigation of brain-directed gene therapy, with encouraging preliminary results.[87] One detailed case report of transplantation in a 12-year-old girl with Sly syndrome has been reported.[88] This child had significant improvement in mobility and in apnea associated with upper airway obstruction after engraftment. Of note, the patient's mental retardation was not reversed by transplantation, which is in agreement with the findings in animal models.[89]

LEUKODYSTROPHIES

Adrenoleukodystrophy

X-linked adrenoleukodystrophy (ALD) is a demyelinating disorder of the central nervous system with highly variable clinical presentation.[90–93] The gene responsible for ALD encodes for the peroxisomal membrane protein adrenoleukodystrophy protein (ALDP), which is a member of the ABC (ATP-binding cassette) transporter superfamily.[94] Individuals with ALD are deficient in lignoceroyl-CoA ligase, an enzyme needed for degradation of very-long-chain fatty acids. Elevated levels of very-long-chain fatty acids in blood, particularly C24 and C26, are useful for diagnosing ALD. Approximately half of individuals with a mutation in this gene have the rapidly progressive childhood cerebral form of the disease, which is associated with an inflammatory response in the brain. Boys with childhood-onset cerebral adrenoleukodystrophy (COCALD) commonly experience rapid neurologic deterioration progressing to death 2 to 3 years after diagnosis, although a minority survive for a prolonged period in a semivegetative state. Within the same kindreds, however, 25% or more of individuals have a milder form of the disease called adrenomyeloneuropathy. Adrenomyeloneuropathy progresses slowly, involves the spinal cord, and shows little or no inflammatory response. Adrenomyeloneuropathy is compatible with a near-normal lifespan. In addition, within the same kindred, individuals can be carriers of a gene mutation but be asymptomatic or they can have Addison disease in isolation.[90] The phenotypic variability of ALD and the discordance in severity even within families make the decision to offer a therapy that is associated with significant morbidity and mortality, such as hematopoietic cell transplantation, a difficult one.[91] In addition, in symptomatic boys with COCALD, the rapid, often stepwise progression of the disease and the deterioration that can occur after transplantation may lead to severe disability, even in children who are successfully engrafted. Identifying the benefits that can be achieved with hematopoietic cell transplantation for COCALD and identifying the optimal patients for with transplantation remain a challenge. It is desirable to identify boys destined to manifest COCALD at the earliest stage of their disease and offer transplantation. It is not desirable to offer transplantation to those destined to have adrenomyeloneuropathy or isolated Addison disease. Data suggest that neuropsychological testing may predict early progression of a symptomatic case of COCALD.[95] In addition, monitoring progression of lesions detected by magnetic resonance imaging, with scoring according to the Loes scale, may assist in patient selection.[96]

The largest experience with transplantation for COCALD reported pooled data from 43 transplant centers worldwide, including transplants performed between 1982 and 1999.[97] One hundred twenty-six boys were included in the report, and complete data were available for 94 transplants. Overall survival was 56%, and the leading cause of death was disease progression. Neurologic function prior to transplantation was a key predictor of outcome, with 92% survival in boys with no or one neurologic deficit and a low magnetic resonance imaging severity score prior to transplant. Similar findings were reported in a single-center study of 12 transplants for COCALD, with poor outcomes in boys with poor or rapidly progressing neurologic function prior to transplantation.[98]

A single-center study described late neurologic outcomes in 12 patients with COCALD who were followed for 5 to 10 years after transplantation.[99] The findings indicated variable levels of improvement. Magnetic resonance imaging showed complete reversal of abnormalities in two patients and improvements in one. All patients who showed continued radiologic demyelination early after transplantation were stabilized and remained unchanged thereafter. Motor function remained normal or was improved after transplantation in 10 patients, verbal intelligence remained within the normal range for 11 patients, and performance abilities were improved or were stable in seven patients. The authors concluded that hematopoietic cell transplantation had long-term beneficial effects when the procedure was performed at an early stage of the disease. Identifying boys with known ALD based on elevated levels of very-long-chain fatty acids at the start of the decline that will lead to symptomatic COCALD is an important goal in the continuing investigation of transplantation for ALD.

Early diagnosis of ALD is commonly not possible for the first affected child in a family. Boys commonly present with behavioral difficulties and a decline in school performance that is mistaken for attention deficit disorder, and diagnosis is commonly delayed until gait abnormalities appear. Immunosuppressive approaches are currently being explored in boys with neurologic disease too far advanced to allow successful transplantation. Future transplantation series should continue careful monitoring of short- and long-term complications to ensure that the therapy gives maximum benefit and least harm.

Metachromatic Leukodystrophy

Metachromatic leukodystrophy (MLD) is an autosomal recessive inherited disorder caused by a deficiency of arylsulfatase A activity, which leads to accumulation of galactosyl sulfatide. Clinical symptoms vary depending on the patient's age at onset of the disease.[100] MLD can be classified clinically as infantile (onset at 6 months to 2 years), early juvenile (onset at 4–6 years), late juvenile (onset at 6–16 years), and adult (onset after 16 years of age). The juvenile- and early-onset presentations are characterized by progressive mental regression, loss of speech, quadriplegias, peripheral neuropathy, and death within a few years of onset. The adult-onset forms are more typically associated with psychiatric symptoms, particularly in the early stages of the disease.[101] Presentation commonly includes a change in personality, poor school or job performance, emotional instability, disorganized thinking, and impairment of memory. Diagnoses of hypomania, depression, or psychosis are common until additional clinical signs prompt magnetic resonance imaging examination, which will show diagnostic white matter changes.[102] Late-onset MLD can manifest as polyneuropathy because a progressive peripheral neuropathy is an important cause of morbidity in this disorder.

In 1985, Bayever et al.[103] reported transplantation for late infantile MLD using an HLA-identical sibling donor. In the 33 months after the procedure, progression of the patient's neurologic deterioration appeared to be halted. In 1990, Krivit et al.[104] reported a second case of late infantile MLD with transplantation from a matched sibling donor. In this case, progression of neurologic deterioration appeared to be delayed. Subsequent case reports support the belief that transplantation can retard the progression of disease in early cases.[105–115] However, the peripheral neuropathy associated with MLD appears likely to progress even in the presence of full donor engraftment. Experience with transplantation in cases of adult-onset MLD remains limited. Case reports of this disorder also suggest a halting of neurologic deterioration, although there is no evidence of any gain in function after successful engraftment.

Investigators are studying the role of umbilical cord blood transplantation for treatment of early-onset rapidly progressive infantile MLD. Identification and procurement of suitable donor cells can proceed more quickly with an umbilical cord blood source than with an adult volunteer unrelated donor. Determination of the degree of specific and measurable benefit of the umbilical cord blood transplantation approach and appropriate patient selection will require long-term followup.

Globoid Cell Leukodystrophy (Krabbe Disease)

Globoid cell leukodystrophy (Krabbe disease) is an autosomal recessive disease caused by diminished or absent activity of the lysosomal enzyme glucocerebrosidase.[100,116] Globoid cell leukodystrophy is characterized by progressive loss of central and peripheral myelin and by spasticity, dementia, and peripheral neuropathy.[117] Globoid cell leukodystrophy typically progresses to a chronic vegetative state and premature death. The most frequent form of globoid cell leukodystrophy has onset in early infancy and is rapidly progressive, typically leading to death within 2 years. The late-onset form, which begins in later childhood, has a more insidious onset and progresses over several years to death. Data describing the outcome of transplantation therapy for patients with globoid cell leukodystrophy are sparse. Krivit et al.[118] described five children with globoid cell leukodystrophy treated with allogeneic hematopoietic cell transplantation. Four of the patients received marrow from an HLA-identical sibling, and one was treated with unrelated umbilical cord blood with one HLA DR mismatch. Engraftment of donor-derived hematopoietic cells occurred in all patients and was followed by a return to normal glucocerebrosidase levels. In the four patients with later-onset disease, central nervous system deterioration was halted. In the patient with the infantile form of the disease, which was diagnosed biochemically prior to development of symptoms, signs and symptoms of neurologic deterioration had not appeared by the time of reporting. Of note, some of the patients in this series achieved significant reversal of symptoms of globoid cell leukodystrophy. This observation contrasts with the findings of most transplantation studies of metabolic disease in which halting of deterioration is achieved but few, if any, patients show gain in function.

Transplantation in children with the rapidly progressive infantile form of globoid cell leukodystrophy is controversial.[119,120] Early transplantation reports described difficulty in achieving engraftment and early death from GVHD without reversal of symptomatic disease. Prompt transplantation in the immediate postnatal period or even in utero offers the possibility of reversal or control of disease. Umbilical cord blood allows rapid transplantation once the diagnosis has been made. An initial report of cord blood transplantation in 11 asymptomatic newborns and 14 symptomatic infants with infantile globoid cell leukodystrophy showed that although engraftment could be achieved, no substantial improvement was seen in children treated after onset of symptoms.[121] In contrast, some benefit was seen in asymptomatic children, some of whom retained normal cognitive and motor skills while others had mild-to-moderate delays in expressive language and mild-to-severe delays in gross motor function. The long-term results of this therapy remain to be determined, and such investigations should be performed within the context of a carefully monitored clinical investigation because the long-term benefits and risks currently are unknown.

OTHER RARE DISEASES

Case reports have described the role of hematopoietic cell transplantation in the treatment of patients with a range metabolic disorders. Successful outcomes of transplantation have been reported for patients with diseases such as α-mannosidosis, Wolman disease, and Niemann-Pick type 1A disease.[122–126] In light of the small number of cases reported for these diseases, it is difficult to make firm recommendations about therapy. In addition, positive outcomes are more likely to be reported than are negative outcomes. There is a continuing role for registries such as the IBMTR and disease-specific registries for reporting the outcomes of consecutive series of cases.

FUTURE DIRECTIONS

Partial correction of a clinical phenotype (e.g., patients with MPS I) is a significant limitation to the success of hematopoietic cell transplantation as therapy for metabolic diseases. Transplantation fails to deliver adequate levels of enzyme to areas of the body that are poorly vascularized, such as cardiac valves, bone, and cartilage. A potential strategy to address this problem is use of mesenchymal as well as hematopoietic stem cells. Mesenchymal stem cells are cells with the potential to differentiate into mesodermal cells, such as cartilage and bone. Data have shown that after a hematopoietic cell transplantation, the stromal cells of the marrow remain of host origin.[127] The addition of mesenchymal stem cells cultivated ex vivo might achieve donor cell engraftment, improve delivery of enzyme to bone and cartilage, and improve disease course. Additionally, animal models suggest that coinfusion of mesenchymal stem cells can facilitate engraftment of allogeneic cells and reduce GVHD.[128,129] Although these studies are in their early stages, they have shown that it is possible to grow mesenchymal stem cells ex vivo and infuse them without toxicity. Krivit et al.[130] infused mesenchymal stem cells into children with MLD who had previously successfully undergone transplantation. In these children, peripheral neuropathy had progressed despite successful halting of central nervous system disease by hematopoietic cell transplantation. Preliminary data indicate improvement in nerve conduction times after infusion of mesenchymal stem cells grown from the original hematopoietic cell donor. There likely will be significant continuing efforts in this area, using genetically modified and unmodified mesenchymal stem cells to an attempt to optimize correction of the phenotype.

An additional limitation of transplantation as therapy for metabolic disorders is, in general, the inability to reverse central nervous system damage that occurred before transplantation. A potential and likely feasible approach to solving this problem is newborn screening for storage disorders to enable transplantation at the earliest possible time. Newborn screening programs performed using heel-stick cards currently used to screen for other disorders have been proposed.[131–134] Such programs would identify affected patients in the first month of life and allow early transplantation before severe central nervous system damage has occurred.

Significant morbidity is associated with the intensive myeloablative conditioning regimens used for bone marrow transplantation. Reduced-intensity preparative therapies that combine powerful immunosuppression with fludarabine with moderate myeloablation with alkylating agents have been explored. Preliminary results suggest that the approach may achieve adequate engraftment with reduced regimen-related toxicity and may improve long-term outcomes.[135,136]

An exciting alternative approach to hematopoietic cell transplantation for treatment of genetic disorders is use of gene therapy, in which autologous cells are transduced with a normal copy of the defective gene. This approach is attractive because the issues of donor identification and GVHD are removed. A large amount of preclinical work has been performed addressing the use of this strategy. Significant issues and technical questions remain to be addressed, however, before gene therapy is a viable option in humans. Chief among these are the relative inefficiency of gene transduction and the challenges related to regulation and durability of gene expression using these strategies. An additional challenge has arisen recently because one of the examples of successful use of human gene therapy, treatment of children with γ-chain SCID, has been associated with insertional leukemogenesis in a significant number of patients.[137,138] However, analysis of the insertion sites and better understanding of the biology of this event may show that the phenomenon is specific to this particular transgene or therapeutic approach.[139–142] Similar studies using vectors and transduction strategies with relatively minor differences have not shown the same tendency for leukemogenesis.[143] Further understanding of the mechanism by which this occurred is essential for the development of future gene therapy studies (see Chapter 110).

SUGGESTED READINGS

Antoine C, Muller S, Cant A, et al: Long-term survival and transplant of haemopoietic stem cells for immunodeficiencies: Report of the European experience, 1968–99. Lancet 361:553, 2003.

Buckley RH: Primary immunodeficiency diseases: Dissectors of the immune system. Immunol Rev 185:206, 2002.

Buckley RH, Schiff SE, Schiff RI, et al: Hematopoietic stem-cell transplant for the treatment of severe combined immunodeficiency. N Engl J Med 340:508, 1999.

Cooper, N, Rao K, et al: Stem cell transplantation with reduced-intensity conditioning for hemophagocytic lymphohistiocytosis. Blood 107:1233, 2006.

Cox-Brinkman J, Boelens JJ, et al: Haematopoietic cell transplantation (HCT) in combination with enzyme replacement therapy (ERT) in patients with Hurler syndrome. Bone Marrow Transplant 38:17, 2006.

Escolar ML, Poe MD, et al: Transplantation of Umbilical-cord blood in babies with infantile Krabbe's disease. N Engl J Med 352:2069, 2005.

Filipovich AH, Stone JV, Tomany SC, et al: Impact of donor type on outcome of bone marrow transplant for Wiskott-Aldrich syndrome: Collaborative study of the International Bone Marrow Transplant Registry and the National Marrow Donor Program. Blood 97:1598, 2001.

Filipovich AH: Life-threatening hemophagocytic syndromes: Current outcomes with hematopoietic stem cell transplantation. Pediatr Transplantation 9:87, 2005.

Grunebaum E, Mazzolari E, et al: Bone marrow transplantation for severe combined immune deficiency. JAMA 295:508–518, 2006.

Henter JI, Samuelsson-Horne A, Arico M, et al: Treatment of hemophagocytic lymphohistiocytosis with HLH-94 immunochemotherapy and bone marrow transplant. Blood 100:2367, 2002.

Horne A, Janka G, Egeler RM, et al: Haematopoietic stem cell transplantation in haemophagocytic lymphohistiocytosis. Br J Haematol 129:622, 2005.

Jacobsohn DA, Duerst R, Tse W, Kletzel M: Reduced intensity haemopoietic stem-cell transplantation for treatment of non-malignant diseases in children. Lancet 364:156, 2004.

Koc ON, Day J, Nieder M, et al: Allogeneic mesenchymal stem cell infusion for treatment of metachromatic leukodystrophy (MLD) and Hurler syndrome (MPS-IH). Bone Marrow Transplant 30:215, 2002.

Krivit W, Shapiro EG, Peters C, et al: Hematopoietic stem-cell transplant in globoid-cell leukodystrophy. N Engl J Med 338:1119, 1998.

Mullen CA, Chan KW: Ethical considerations in allogeneic hematopoietic cell transplant for children with slowly fatal conditions. Bone Marrow Transplant 26:1030, 2000.

Peters C, Charnas LR, Tan Y, et al: Cerebral X-linked adrenoleukodystrophy: the international hematopoietic cell transplantation experience from 1982 to 1999. Blood 104:881, 2004.

Peters C, Shapiro EG, Anderson J, et al: Hurler syndrome: II. Outcome of HLA-genotypically identical sibling and HLA-haploidentical related donor bone marrow transplant in fifty-four children. The Storage Disease Collaborative Study Group. Blood 91:2601, 1998.

Rao, K, Amrolia PJ, Jones A, et al: Improved survival after unrelated donor bone marrow transplantation in children with primary immunodeficiency using a reduced-intensity conditioning regimen. Blood 105:879, 2005.

Shapiro E, Krivit W, Lockman L, et al: Long-term effect of bone-marrow transplant for childhood-onset cerebral X-linked adrenoleukodystrophy. Lancet 356:713, 2000.

Staba SL, Escolar ML, Poe M, et al: Cord-blood transplants from unrelated donors in patients with Hurler's syndrome. N Engl J Med 350:1960, 2004.

REFERENCES

For complete list of references log onto www.expertconsult.com

CHAPTER 101

OUTCOMES OF ALLOGENEIC HEMATOPOIETIC CELL TRANSPLANTATION FOR HEMATOLOGIC MALIGNANCIES IN ADULTS

Parameswaran Hari and Mary Horowitz

BACKGROUND

Allogeneic hematopoietic cell transplantation (HCT) offers the potential for cure in many hematologic malignancies. Thomas et al.[1,2] were the first to report long-term leukemia-free survival (LFS) after HLA (human leukocyte antigen)-identical sibling transplantation in patients with refractory acute leukemia. Better outcomes subsequently were demonstrated in patients transplanted in first complete remission (CR1) or second complete remission (CR2).[3–6] Durable cytogenetic remissions and long-term LFS after identical twin and allogeneic bone marrow transplantation for chronic myelogenous leukemia (CML) were reported in the late 1970s and early 1980s.[7–9] Use of allogeneic HCT for treatment of leukemia increased dramatically in the 1980s. By 1985, approximately 75% of allogeneic transplantations were performed for leukemia, with approximately equal numbers for CML, acute myelogenous leukemia (AML), and acute lymphoblastic leukemia (ALL). In the 1990s, allogeneic HCT was increasingly considered an effective salvage treatment strategy for patients with lymphoma or myeloma that failed to respond to conventional chemotherapy and/or autologous HCT.

Allogeneic transplantation involves administration of a preparative regimen of chemotherapy, immunosuppressive drugs, and/or radiation followed by infusion of donor hematopoietic cells. Most patients receive prolonged (≥3 months) therapy with immunosuppressive drugs posttransplant to prevent or treat graft-versus-host disease (GVHD). The purpose of the preparative or conditioning regimen is twofold: to eradicate malignant cells and to eliminate host immune cells capable of rejecting donor cells. The ability to restore hematopoiesis with donor hematopoietic stem cells permits administration of substantially higher (myeloablative) doses of cytotoxic therapy than is otherwise possible. Although originally regarded primarily as a way of rescuing patients from therapy-induced marrow aplasia, it now is accepted that graft-versus-tumor effects conferred by alloreactive donor cells contribute substantially to cancer eradication.

PATIENT POPULATION

Accompanying the growth of HCT has been a coordinated international effort to collect and analyze data on transplant outcomes through the International Bone Marrow Transplant Registry (IBMTR), which was established in 1972. The IBMTR affiliated with the United States (U.S.) National Marrow Donor Program (NMDP) in 2004 to become the Center for International Blood and Marrow Transplant Research (CIBMTR). CIBMTR currently collects data on HCT outcomes from more than 400 transplant centers worldwide and received information on more than 7000 allogeneic HCTs in 2006. These data show that hematologic malignancies (and premalignant conditions) are the most common indications for allogeneic HCTs (Fig. 101–1). In 2006, AML accounted for 33% of allogeneic HCTs, ALL 16%, CML 6%, other leukemias and preleukemias 18%, Hodgkin lymphoma and non-Hodgkin lymphoma (NHL) 12%, and multiple myeloma 3%. Use of allogeneic HCT for hematologic malignancies in the 1980s and early 1990s was largely restricted to young patients ≤45 years with an HLA-identical sibling donor. Less intensive conditioning regimens and improved GVHD prophylaxis and supportive care have increased use of allogeneic HCT in older patients. Only 4% of allogeneic HCT recipients in 1987 to 1992 were older than 50 years. In 2006, 33% were older than 50 years and 11% were older than 60 years. Application of HCT in patients without HLA-identical siblings was facilitated by establishment of large unrelated donor registries. In 1987 to 1992, less than 10% of HCTs for hematologic malignancies used unrelated donors; in 2006, this figure was greater than 40%.

CONDITIONING REGIMENS

The purpose of the preparative or conditioning regimen is to eradicate malignant cells and to suppress host immune competent cells. Historically, these regimens included myeloablative doses of cytotoxic drugs with or without radiation. Myeloablative regimens used for hematologic malignancies often involve a combination of cyclophosphamide (commonly 60 mg/kg/day for 2 days) and total body irradiation (TBI; 8–15 Gy, single or fractionated doses).[3] Many regimens use busulfan (typically 4 mg/kg/day for 4 days if given orally or 3.2 mg/kg/day if given intravenously) in place of TBI in combination with cyclophosphamide (most commonly 60 mg/kg/day for 2 days). Reported posttransplant survival rates with cyclophosphamide and TBI and with cyclophosphamide and busulfan are similar, although some data suggest advantages for TBI-containing regimens in ALL.[10–12] Other drugs have been added to or substituted for cyclophosphamide and/or busulfan, including etoposide, melphalan, and cytarabine, in a variety of regimens to provide better, generally disease-specific, antineoplastic activity.[13–23] Large trials comparing efficacy of these regimens are lacking. A CIBMTR study suggested better outcomes for patients with ALL in CR2 with either higher doses of TBI or substitution of cyclophosphamide by etoposide in a standard-dose TBI regimen.[24] Table 101–1 lists the most commonly used myeloablative conditioning strategies by disease. Table 101–2 lists doses and schedules for the most frequently used myeloablative conditioning regimens.

High-dose conditioning regimens are associated with significant risks of regimen-related toxicity. An important strategy for decreasing early regimen-related morbidity and mortality is reduced-intensity conditioning. This approach uses immunosuppressive but submyeloablative doses of drugs and radiation to allow donor cell engraftment. It relies primarily upon immune-mediated effects of donor cells to eradicate malignancy (see Chapter 106). Reduced-intensity regimens are designed to cause less host tissue damage and less inflammatory cytokine secretion, with the intent of lowering the risk of transplant-related mortality (TRM) and, possibly, severe GVHD.[25,26] The intensity of these regimens varies considerably, ranging from low (200 cGy) doses of TBI that do not induce cytopenia to combinations of fludarabine, busulfan, and/or melphalan that induce significant (although reversible) cytopenia.[27–33] A list of common reduced-intensity regimens, grouped in general order of intensity, is given in Table 101–3.

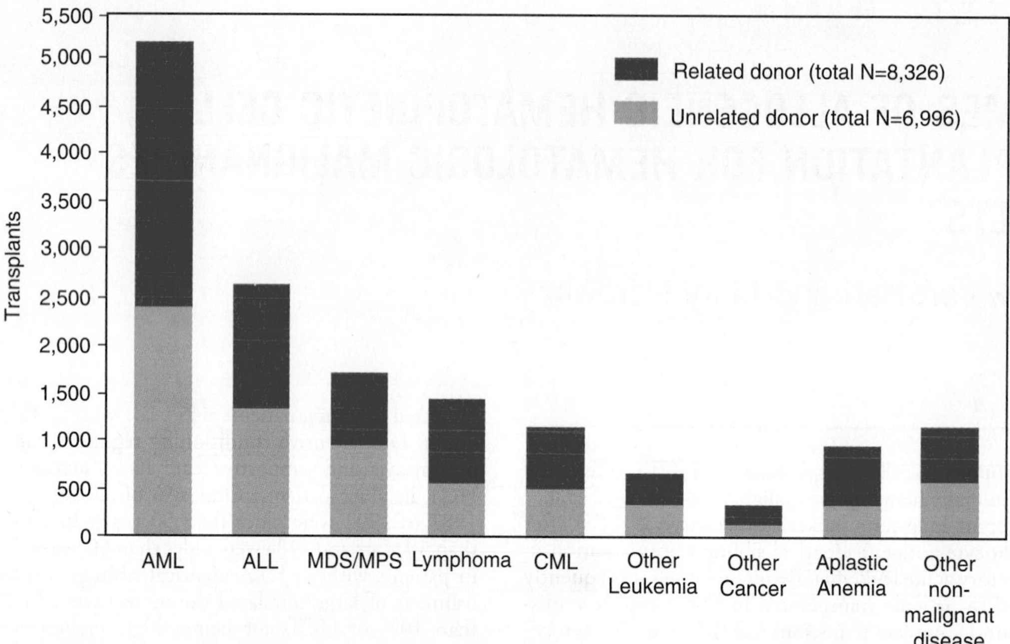

Figure 101–1 Indications for allogeneic hematopoietic cell transplants by donor type and disease status from 2005–2006.

Table 101–1 Common Myeloablative Conditioning Regimens by Disease

Disease	Regimens Used in Order of Frequency Reported to Center for International Blood and Marrow Transplant Research
Acute myelogenous leukemia	Busulfan + cyclophosphamide TBI + cyclophosphamide Other TBI combinations Other busulfan combinations
Acute lymphoblastic leukemia	TBI + cyclophosphamide Busulfan + cyclophosphamide TBI + other agents (not cyclophosphamide) TBI + cyclophosphamide + other agents
Chronic myelogenous leukemia	TBI + cyclophosphamide Busulfan + cyclophosphamide TBI + other agents
Non-Hodgkin lymphoma	TBI + cyclophosphamide Busulfan + cyclophosphamide

For chronic lymphocytic leukemia and multiple myeloma, the majority of allogeneic transplants currently are performed after reduced-intensity conditioning protocols.
See Table 101–2 for details of the regimens used.
TBI, total body irradiation.

Reduced-intensity regimens have less antitumor activity than conventional myeloablative regimens. However, they also induce less immune compromise as the duration and depth of neutropenia are reduced and host-derived immunocompetent cells are not immediately eliminated. They also may facilitate faster recovery of a T-cell repertoire that is more complex and robust than the early T-cell repertoire of patients receiving myeloablative regimens.

Less peritransplant immune compromise, neutropenia, and organ toxicity make reduced-intensity regimens attractive for use in patients not eligible for conventional high-dose regimens because of advanced age or comorbidities.[31,34,35] Whether these benefits outweigh the risks of reduced antitumor effects in patients eligible for traditional conditioning regimens remains an important research question. However, reduced-intensity regimens are increasingly used in patients of all ages receiving both related and unrelated donor transplants, as is shown in Fig. 101–2 depicting data from the CIBMTR.[36–38]

GRAFT SOURCES

Historically, hematopoietic cells for transplantation were collected directly from the marrow, and marrow is still the graft source used for many allotransplants. Collection of hematopoietic cells from peripheral blood by leukapheresis after administration of hematopoietic growth factors was introduced in 1981.[39] Use of umbilical cord blood as a source of hematopoietic stem cells was introduced in 1988.[40] Grafts from marrow, peripheral blood, and cord blood differ in the total numbers of cells available, the proportion of pluripotent stem cells to lineage-committed late progenitor cells, and the characteristics of immune reactive cells.[41] Marrow is the primary source (approximately 55% of transplants) of allogeneic donor cells for transplantation in children; peripheral blood is the main source (80% of transplants) in adults. Among patients receiving grafts from unrelated donors, umbilical cord blood is used for 40% of transplants in children (younger than 20 years) and 5% of transplants in adults.

The CIBMTR, in collaboration with the European Group for Blood and Marrow Transplantation (EBMT), examined long-term outcomes after peripheral blood and marrow transplantation in adults with acute and chronic leukemia. The first report,[42] with a median followup of 1 year, showed higher chronic GVHD rates in patients receiving peripheral blood grafts. Among patients transplanted for advanced leukemia, those receiving peripheral blood grafts had lower TRM and higher LFS rates. Long-term followup data (median followup >6 years) were obtained for the patients who were alive at the time of the initial report.[43] Consistent with the initial report, chronic GVHD was more frequent after peripheral blood transplantation than after bone marrow transplantation; relapse rates were similar in the two groups. An LFS advantage for peripheral blood was seen in patients receiving HCT for advanced CML (33% vs 25%) but a disadvantage in those with CML in first chronic phase (41% vs 61%). Long-term LFS was similar with peripheral blood and bone marrow transplants in patients with acute leukemia. The Stem Cell Trialists collaborative group conducted a meta-analysis using data from nine randomized trials of related donor peripheral blood versus bone marrow transplants enrolling 1111 adult patients.[44] Patients receiving

Table 101–2 Commonly Used Myeloablative Conditioning Regimens for Hematologic Malignancies

Drugs and Total Doses	Schedule (days)	Comments and References
Classic Regimens		
"Cy/TBI"		Used in myeloid and lymphoid malignancies
Cyclophosphamide 120 mg/kg	-6, -5	Extensive experience over 30 years[309,310]
TBI 12–14.4 Gy	-3, -2, -1	
"BU/Cy"		Developed as an alternative nonradiation regimen
Busulfan 16 mg/kg PO	-9, -8, -7, -6 q6h	Used primarily for myeloid malignancies[10]
Cyclophosphamide 200 mg/kg	-5, -4, -3, -2	
"BU/Cy-2"		Derived from Bu/Cy above
Busulfan 16 mg/kg PO	-7, -6, -5, -4 q6h	Most common current nonradiation regimen used for wide variety of myeloid and lymphoid malignancies[11]
Cyclophosphamide 120 mg/kg	-3, -2	
Other Standard Regimens		
"TBI/VP"		Alternative to Cy/TBI
Etoposide 60 mg/kg	-3	Randomized study showed no differences in advanced leukemia outcomes[311,312]
TBI 12–13.2 Gy	-7, -6, -5, -4	
"Ara-C/TBI"		Used for myeloid and lymphoid leukemias[18]
Ara-C 36 g/m^2	-9, -8, -7, -6, -5, -4	
TBI 12 Gy	-3, -2, -1	
"Bu/MEL"		Active in a wide variety of myeloid and lymphoid malignancies as well as myeloma[17,21]
Busulfan 16 mg/kg PO	-5, -4, -3, -2	
Melphalan 140 mg/m^2	-1	
"Thiotepa/Cy"		Active against advanced leukemia and hematologic malignancies[14]
Thiotepa 15 mg/kg	-7, -6	Thiotepa has also been combined with busulfan
Cyclophosphamide 120–150 mg/kg	-4, -3, -2	
Intensified Regimens With Additional Agents Added to the Standard		
"Cy/TBI/VP"		Primarily used in acute leukemia to improve therapeutic efficacy of Cy/TBI but no randomized comparisons[15]
Cyclophosphamide 120 mg/kg	-6, -5	
Etoposide 30–60 mg/kg	-4	
TBI 12–13.75 Gy	-3, -2, -1	
"TBI/Thiotepa/Cy/ATG"		Used in acute leukemias in an attempt to increase conditioning intensity
TBI 13.75 Gy	-9, -8, -7, -6	Current multicenter acute myelogenous leukemia trial explores this regimen with T-cell–depleted grafts[23]
Thiotepa 10 mg/kg	-5, -4	
Cyclophosphamide 120 mg/kg	-3, -2	
± ATG (dose depends on type used)	-5, -4, -3, -2	
"BU/Cy/VP"		Used in advanced hematologic malignancy[22]
Busulfan 16 mg/kg PO	-7, -6, -5, -4 q6h	
Cyclophosphamide 120 mg/kg	-3, -2	
Etoposide 60 mg/kg	-3	
"Cy/TBI/Ara-C"		Intensified combination used in advanced leukemia and with T-cell–depleted grafts[16,19]
Ara-C 18–36 g/m^2	-14, -13, -12, -11, -10, -9	
TBI 12–14 Gy	-7, -6, -5, -4, -3	
Cyclophosphamide 60–90 mg/kg	-2	
"Bu/Cy/Ara-C" (BAC)		Primarily used in high-risk myeloid malignancies for dose intensity[13]
Busulfan 16 mg/kg PO	-7, -6, -5, -4 q6h	
Cyclophosphamide 120 mg/kg	-3, -2	
Ara-C 8 g/m^2	-5, -4	
"CBV"		Used in non-Hodgkin lymphoma, chronic lymphocytic leukemia[20]
Cyclophosphamide 6 g/m^2	-6, -5, -4, -3	
BCNU 450 mg/m^2	-6, -5, -4, -3	
Etoposide 1600 mg/m^2	-6, -5, -4, -3	

Ara-C, cytosine arabinoside; ATG, antithymocyte globulin; BCNU, carmustine; BU, busulfan; Cy, cyclophosphamide; Gy, Gray; MEL, melphalan; TBI, total body irradiation; VP, etoposide.

peripheral blood grafts had faster neutrophil and platelet engraftment, a lower relapse rate if transplanted for hematologic malignancy, and higher overall and disease-free survival if transplanted for late-stage disease. However, peripheral blood was associated with a significantly increased risk of extensive chronic GVHD and conferred no survival advantage for patients with early-stage disease. In the unrelated donor setting, a CIBMTR analysis of 917 transplants facilitated by the NMDP suggests that survival is similar with bone marrow and peripheral blood grafts but that chronic GVHD is more frequent with peripheral blood.[45] A large randomized trial of unrelated bone marrow versus peripheral blood HCT for hematologic malignancies is being conducted by the United States Blood and Marrow Transplant Clinical Trials Network (BMT CTN).

One important obstacle to allografting is identifying a donor for the 70% of patients without an HLA-identical sibling (see Chapter 103). Despite increasing numbers of volunteer HLA typed donors available through national and international donor registries, many patients, especially non-Caucasian patients, do not find suitable donors.[46,47] Also, the unrelated donor search process can be time consuming, raising the risk of disease progression before transplanta-

Table 101–3 Commonly Used Reduced-Intensity Conditioning Regimens

Regimen	Disease(s)	Donor	Graft-versus-Host Disease Prophylaxis	Comments	References
Low-Dose TBI Based					
TBI 2 Gy	Hematologic malignancies	MRD	CsA/FK + MMF	Widely used in HLA-identical sibling transplants More immunosuppressive than myeloablative	90, 228
TBI 2 Gy ± Flu 90 mg/m²	Hematologic malignancies	MUD, MRD	CsA/FK + MMF	Widely used More immunosuppressive than myeloablative	30, 32
TBI 4–5.5 Gy ± Cy 80–120 mg/kg	Hematologic malignancies	MUD	CsA ± MMF ± MTX ± steroid	Used in advanced malignancies with unrelated donor HCT TRM 19% in good-risk patients and 42% in poor-risk patients at 2 years	313
TBI 8 Gy + Flu 120 mg/m² ± ATG	AML	MUD, MRD	CsA ± MTX	Increasing myeloablation and immunosuppression Used in AML with TRM 8% in good-risk patients	314
TBI 8 Gy + Cy 80–120 mg/kg + Flu 120 mg/m² ± ATG	CML	MUD, MRD	CsA + MTX	Reported in early-phase CML in elderly patients, with TRM 29% at 1 year	315
Thymic radiation + Cy 150–200 mg/kg + ATG	Hematologic malignancies	MRD	CsA	33% disease-free survival at 1 year in refractory hematologic malignancies	316
Fludarabine and Cyclophosphamide Based					
Flu 90–125 mg/m² + Cy 2–3.6 g/m²	NHL, HL, AML, CML	MUD, MRD	FK/CsA ± MMF/ rapamycin ± MTX	Reduced-intensity regimen with more chemotherapy-related toxicity TRM 0%–30% at 1 year	317–319
Flu 90–125 mg/m² + Cy 2–2.5 g/m² + rituximab ± ATG	NHL, indolent lymphoma	MUD, MRD	FK + MTX	Popular reduced-intensity regimen for NHL CD20-expressing NHL	28, 268
Busulfan (IV or PO) Based					
Flu 120–150 mg/kg + BU 3.2–10 mg/kg	AML, MDS, hematologic malignancies	MUD, MRD	CsA/FK + MTX	Increasingly used combination for myeloid malignancies Busulfan IV equivalent used commonly	320
Flu 120–180 mg/kg + BU 8 (PO) or 6.4 (IV) mg/kg ± ATG	AML, MDS	MUD, MRD	CsA ± MMF + MTX	TRM 3%–8% at 2 years Busulfan IV also dosed at 130 mg/m²/day × 4 Primarily used in AML and MDS	27, 33, 321
Flu 150–180 mg/kg + BU 8 mg/kg + Campath	AML, MDS, hematologic malignancies	MUD, MRD	CsA ± MTX	TRM 12.5%–33% at 1 year	322, 323
Flu 200 mg/kg + BU 8 (PO) mg/kg + TBI	AML, MDS	MUD, MRD	CsA + MMF	Increasing myeloablation TRM 25% at 1 year	324
Flu 125–240 mg/kg + BU 6.6–12 mg/kg ± Ara-C	CML including advanced phase	MUD, MRD	CsA ± MMF ± MTX	Least immunosuppressive and most ablative 41% disease-free at 562 days	325
Melphalan Based					
Flu 90–180 mg/m² + MEL 70–180 mg/m² ± ATG	Hematologic malignancies	MRD, MUD	CsA/FK + MTX	TRM 18%–26% at 1 year Significant myeloablation from MEL	29, 282, 326
Flu 150 mg/m² + MEL 140 mg/m² ± Campath	Hematologic malignancies	MUD, MRD	CsA/FK + MTX	TRM 11%–38% at 1 year Used in lymphoid and myeloid malignancies	327, 328
Cladribine 60 mg/m² + MEL 140–180 mg/m²	Hematologic malignancies	MUD, MRD	FK + MTX	Excessive toxicity reported and used only in clinical trials	329

AML, acute myelogenous leukemia; Ara-C, cytosine arabinoside; ATG, antithymocyte globulin; BU, busulfan; CML, chronic myelogenous leukemia; CsA, cyclosporine; Cy, cyclophosphamide; FK, tacrolimus; Flu, fludarabine; Gy, Gray; HCT, hematopoietic cell transplantation; HLA, human leukocyte antigen; MEL, melphalan; MMF, mycophenolate; MRD, matched related donor; MTX, methotrexate; MUD, matched unrelated donor; NHL, non-Hodgkin lymphoma; TBI, total body irradiation; TRM, transplant-related mortality. HL, Hodgkin lymphoma; MDS, myelodysplastic syndrome.

tion can be performed.[48] Umbilical cord blood offers several advantages as a source of hematopoietic stem cells for unrelated donor transplantation (see Chapter 105). It is readily available and entails little or no risk to the donor. Current data also indicate that HLA-matching criteria for cord blood transplantation need not be as stringent as for adult donor transplantation, greatly increasing the likelihood of finding a suitably matched graft for most patients.[49,50] The major drawback of cord blood transplants is the limited number of cells in each cord blood unit leading to slow rates of hematopoietic recovery relative to bone marrow or peripheral blood transplants. Numbers of cord blood transplants have increased steadily over the past decade (Fig. 101–3). Few controlled comparisons of cord blood and marrow grafts in hematologic malignancies and no randomized trials are available. A CIBMTR analysis compared HLA-matched (at the allele level for A, B, C, and DR) marrow transplants with matched and mismatched (intermediate resolution for A and B, allele level for DR) cord blood transplants in children with leukemia.[51] The highest survival was seen in children receiving HLA-matched cord blood, although this group was small. No difference in outcome between HLA-matched marrow and 5/6 HLA-locus matched cord blood

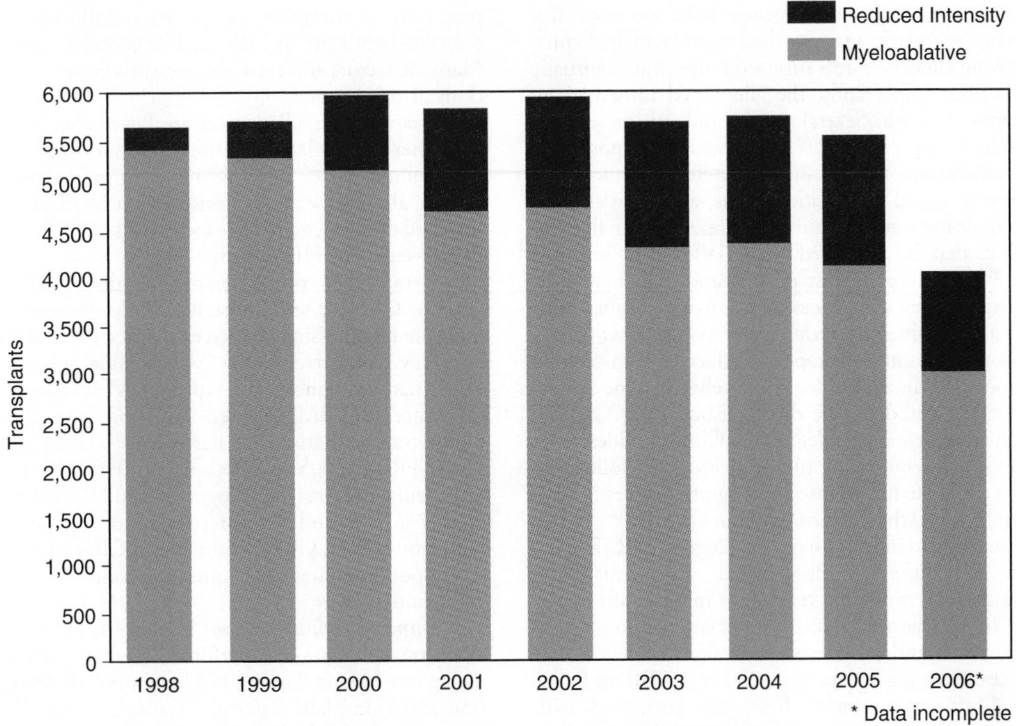

Figure 101–2 Proportion of myeloablative and reduce-intensity constitioning regimens a year.

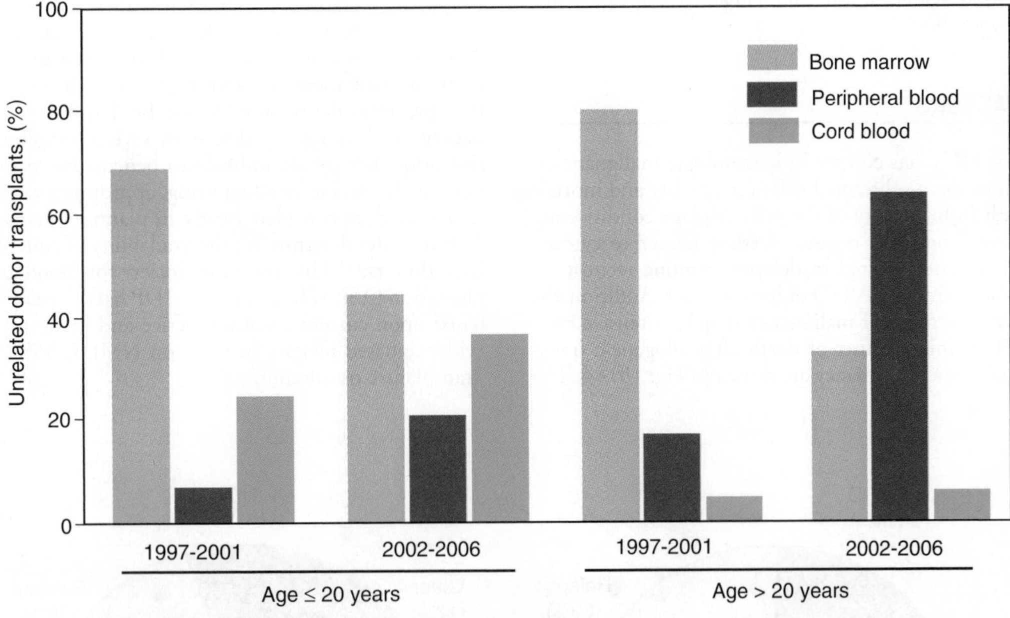

Figure 101–3 Allogeneic stem cell sources by donor type versus recipient age from 1997–2006.

transplants was observed, provided the cord blood cell dose was greater than 3×10^7 kg. Several studies have compared bone marrow transplants and cord blood transplants in adults.[52–56] Results are mixed; some show similar survival between HLA-mismatched cord blood units and HLA-matched bone marrow and some show an advantage for HLA-matched marrow. The data consistently show slower hematopoietic recovery but less GVHD with cord blood grafts. Results from all studies indicate that a one or two HLA-antigen mismatched cord blood transplant may be an acceptable alternative for patients with hematologic malignancies who need HCT but do not have an HLA-identical adult donor, assuming a unit of adequate cell dose can be identified. Studies developing approaches to facilitate engraftment with limited cord blood cell doses, including use of multiple units and cell expansion techniques, are in progress.

GRAFT-VERSUS-MALIGNANCY EFFECTS

Substantial laboratory and clinical evidence indicate that alloreactive cells exhibit potent anticancer activity (see Chapter 107). Barnes et al.[57] studied leukemic mice treated with high-dose TBI and compared those receiving syngeneic and allogeneic bone marrow infusions. Mice receiving syngeneic marrow died quickly of leukemia, whereas those receiving allogeneic cells survived longer but eventually developed fatal GVHD. Importantly, the allografted mice had no evidence of leukemia at death. Several canine and murine experiments have reproduced these results.[58–60] Mathé et al.[61] proposed the term *adoptive immunotherapy* for the antitumor effect of allogeneic cells. Antitumor effects could be specific, that is, after sensitization of the donor or the donor's cells to antigens present on malignant cells, or nonspecific, that is, associated with GVHD, an immune reaction of donor lymphocytes against normal and malignant host cells presumably triggered by differences in histocompatibility antigens.[62–65] Bortin et al.[58,66] coined the term *graft versus leukemia* (GVL) to indicate the adoptive immunotherapeutic effect of transplanted allogeneic hematopoietic cells against leukemia cells. In some animal models, the GVL effect could not be distinguished from GVHD, whereas in others the two were separable.[58,59,67–70] Clinical evidence for the importance of GVL in eradicating tumor includes the following: (a) lower incidence of leukemia relapse in allograft recipients with acute and/or chronic GVHD than in those without GVHD[60,63–65,71–75]; (b) higher relapse rates after identical twin versus allogeneic HCT[65,76,77]; (c) high relapse rates after T-cell–depleted transplants[65,78–82]; (d) durable cytogenetic and molecular remissions induced after posttransplant relapse by infusion of donor leukocytes without other antileukemia therapy[83–89]; and (e) durable remissions achieved after very low doses of conditioning agents (e.g., 200-cGy TBI) and allogeneic HCT.[90,91] Graft–versus-tumor effects are associated with GVHD, and measures that prevent or suppress GVHD may allow more relapse, but significant anticancer effects are demonstrable even in the absence of clinically significant GVHD, especially in AML and CML.[92,93] The efficacy of immune-mediated antitumor effects vary by disease but are most evident in myeloid leukemias and some subtypes of lymphoma.[87,89,94–102]

PROGNOSTIC FACTORS

Although allogeneic HCT has efficacy in hematologic malignancies, the procedure itself carries a substantial risk of morbidity and mortality. TRM may result from toxicity of the pretransplant conditioning regimen to lung, liver, and other organs, bleeding related to cytopenias, GVHD, and infection related to delayed immune reconstitution, especially in the setting of GVHD or its treatment. Additionally, many patients have recurrence of malignancy despite intensive conditioning and GVL. Primary causes of death after allogeneic transplantation for hematologic malignancy are shown in Fig. 101–4. The prognosis of transplant recipients is influenced by several factors associated with risk of TRM and/or cancer recurrence or progression. Many of factors these are disease specific and discussed in later sections of this chapter.

Donor Factors: TRM rates are lower after HLA-identical sibling than after other related or unrelated donor transplants because of less graft failure, faster immune reconstitution, and less GVHD.[103–111] Among alternative donor transplants, those from more closely HLA-matched donors tend to have lower risks of GVHD and TRM.[105,108–111] Donor-recipient HLA mismatching is associated with increased risk of posttransplant complications, including graft rejection, acute and chronic GVHD, and mortality. Risks increase progressively with multiple HLA mismatches (see Chapter 103). With modern molecular HLA typing techniques (which allow selection of more closely HLA-matched donors) and current GVHD prevention strategies, the difference in TRM between HLA-matched sibling and unrelated donor transplantation has narrowed.[112] Using data reported to the CIBMTR for 2005 to 2006, day 100 TRM rates for patients with acute leukemia receiving allografts from HLA-identical sibling donors were 5%, 7%, and 9% for patients transplanted in first complete remission (CR1), CR2 or subsequent CR, or not in CR, respectively. Corresponding rates after unrelated donor transplantation were 8%, 10%, and 12%.

Timing of Transplantation: In general, HCT outcomes are better when transplantation is performed earlier in the course of a malignancy (see box on Timing of Hematopoietic Stem Cell Transplantation and Transplant Referral). Transplantation for advanced disease is associated with higher risks of both relapse and TRM. High TRM in the setting of advanced disease likely reflects the poorer clinical status and more extensive prior treatment of these patients. Because some hematologic malignancies have excellent prognosis with nontransplant therapy (e.g., children with standard-risk ALL or adults with acute promyelocytic leukemia), appropriate timing of transplantation requires consideration of likely outcomes with transplant and nontransplant therapies. However, even when not used as first-line therapy, transplants should not be inordinately delayed because patients with refractory disease or severe complications from extensive prior therapy are unlikely to benefit. For patients with diseases potentially curable by allografting, appropriate timing of transplantation should be considered early in planning management strategies. This includes determining the availability of suitable related or unrelated donors.[113] The American Society for Blood and Marrow Transplantation (ASBMT) and the NMDP have developed joint guidelines based upon current clinical practice and literature review, including evidence-based reviews (see box on NMDP-ASBMT Guidelines for Transplant Consultation).[114]

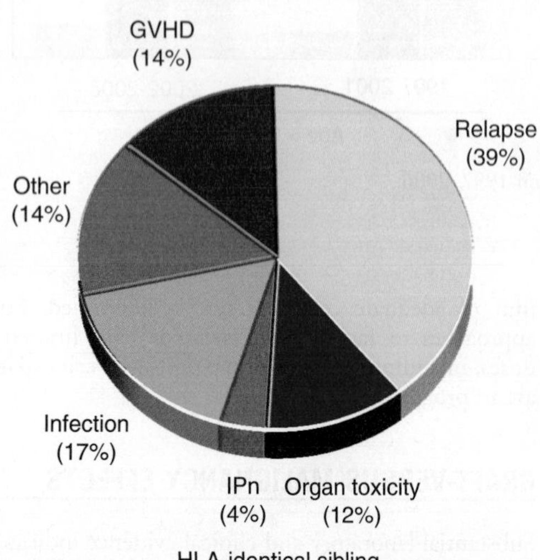

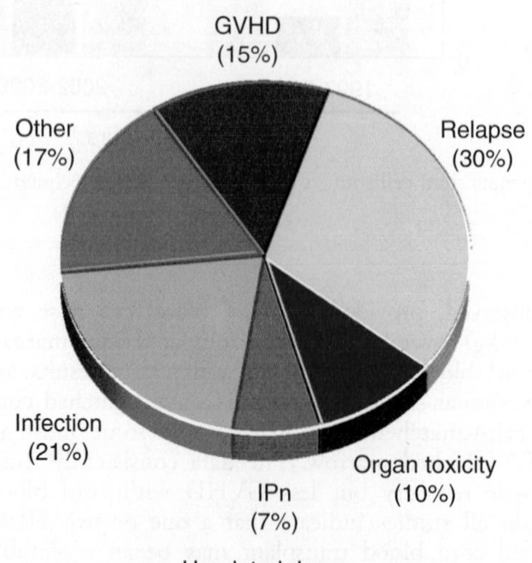

Figure 101–4 Causes of death after transplants performed in 1998–2004.

Timing of Hematopoietic Cell Transplantation and Transplant Referral

General Principles

- HCT outcomes are better when performed earlier in the course of hematologic malignancies.
- HCT for advanced disease is associated with higher TRM and relapse.
- Appropriate timing of HCT requires consideration of likely outcomes with nontransplant and transplant therapies.
- Even when not considered as front-line therapy, inordinate delay in HCT is to be avoided.
- For patients who are potentially curable by allogeneic HCT, consideration of HCT should be addressed early in the treatment plan. This includes HLA typing and identification of suitable donors.

Patient- and Disease-Related Factors: TRM is lower and, consequently, survival is higher in patients who are young, are cytomegalovirus negative, and have good performance scores and no active infection.[115–117] Age poses a significant barrier to application of allogeneic HCT, as older patients are at significantly higher risk for regimen-related toxicity and GVHD. Consequently, the median age of transplant recipients is substantially lower than the median age at diagnosis of the diseases for which transplantation is performed (Table 101–4). In most settings, factors associated with increased likelihood of relapse or progression after conventional therapy also predict increased risk of posttransplant relapse or progression. Importantly, patients whose disease does not respond to conventional therapy are significantly less likely to have durable remissions after transplantation than those with responsive disease. However, HCT may cure a significant proportion of patients with diseases considered incurable with nontransplant therapy.

ACUTE MYELOID LEUKEMIA

The incidence of AML increases with age, varying from 12 per million in persons 20 to 44 years old to 150 per million in persons older than 65 years.[118] Median age at diagnosis is 67 years, with only approximately 33% of patients younger than 55 years at diagnosis and 15% between the ages of 55 and 65 years.[119] Although 50% to 75% of adults with AML achieve CR, only 20% to 30% achieve long-term LFS with conventional chemotherapy approaches.[120,121] The curative potential of allogeneic HCT in AML is well established, and AML currently is the most common indication for allogeneic HCT, accounting for approximately one third of allografts in 2006. However, variation is considerable among countries and physicians with regard to the timing of and the strategy for applying HCT, that is, consolidation versus salvage therapy.[122–125] In the United States, approximately 25% of AML patients younger than 70 years undergo an allogeneic HCT. Median age at transplantation is 45 years; 75% of HCT recipients are younger than 55 years.

Approximately 2400 allogeneic transplantations for AML were registered with the CIBMTR in 2006; approximately 40% were from unrelated donors.[126] Sixty percent of HLA-identical sibling transplants were performed as consolidation therapy in patients in CR1, 15% in CR2 or subsequent CR, and 25% in patients with active disease (induction failure or relapse). Thirty percent of unrelated donor transplants were done in CR1, 30% in CR2 or subsequent CR, and 37% in patients with active disease. Myeloablative conditioning regimens were used for 75% of transplants in patients younger than 55 years and in 60% of transplants in patients older than 55 years; the remainder received a variety of reduced-intensity regimens.

Major predictors of HCT outcome in AML are remission state at the time of transplantation, donor type, and age. The CIBMTR has data on approximately 10,000 recipients of allogeneic HCT for AML performed between 1998 and 2004. Among 6092 patients receiving transplants from HLA-identical siblings, 5-year probabilities of relapse, LFS, and overall survival were 34%, 44%, and 47%, respectively. Patients in CR1 have the best posttransplant outcomes; those with more advanced disease have higher risks of both relapse and TRM. Among adults who received HLA-identical sibling transplants following myeloablative conditioning between 1998 and 2004, 5-year probabilities of survival were 55% for 2369 patients transplanted in CR1, 42% for 611 patients transplanted in CR2 or subsequent CR, and 21% for 1,113 patients transplanted with active disease (Fig. 101–5A). Among children (younger than 20 years), 5-year probabilities of survival were 59% for 804 children transplanted in CR1, 56% for 174 transplanted in CR2 or subsequent CR, and 25% for 165 transplanted with active disease (Fig. 101–5B). Nine hundred sixteen

NMDP-ASBMT Guidelines for Transplant Consultation

Adult Acute Myelogenous Leukemia

High-risk acute myelogenous leukemia, including

- Antecedent hematologic disease (e.g., myelodysplasia)
- Treatment-related leukemia
- Induction failure

CR1 with poor-risk cytogenetics (see text for details)

CR2 and beyond

Adult Acute Lymphoblastic Leukemia

High-risk acute lymphoblastic leukemia, including

- Poor-risk cytogenetics (see text for details)
- High white blood cell count (>30,000–50,000) at diagnosis
- Central nervous system or testicular leukemia
- No CR within 4 weeks of initial treatment
- Induction failure

Second complete remission or beyond

Non-Hodgkin Lymphoma

Follicular lymphoma

- Poor response to initial therapy
- Initial remission duration <12 months
- Second relapse
- Transformation to diffuse large B-cell lymphoma

Diffuse large B-cell lymphoma

- First or subsequent relapse
- CR1 for patients with high or high–intermediate IPI
- No CR with initial treatment

Mantle cell lymphoma

- Following initial therapy

Hodgkin Lymphoma

No initial CR

First or subsequent relapse

Multiple Myeloma

After initiation of therapy

At first progression

Chronic Myeloid Leukemia (European LeukemiaNet Guidelines)[211]

Imatinib as first-line therapy in all cases

Allogeneic HCT to be considered in the following scenarios:

For patients in early chronic phase

Intolerance/excess toxicity from imatinib

Failure on imatinib *or* "warning features" at presentation (defined in Baccarani et al.[211])

Accelerated phase or early blast crisis

Initial imatinib therapy followed by HCT

Available online at http://www.asbmt.org/policystat/policy.htm.

Table 101–4 Impact of Age at Diagnosis on Allogeneic Hematopoietic Stem Cell Transplantation

Disease	Proportion of Patients Aged >65 Years at Diagnosis	Matched Sibling HCT Recipients Aged >65 Years	Unrelated Donor HCT Recipients Aged >65 Years
Acute myelogenous leukemia	23%	2%	1%
Acute lymphoblastic leukemia	2%	<1%	<1%
Chronic myeloid leukemia	35%	<1%	<1%
Chronic lymphocytic leukemia	71%	3%	0%
Non-Hodgkin lymphoma	50%	1%	1%
Hodgkin lymphoma	10%	0%	2%
Multiple myeloma	60%	1%	0%

HCT, hematopoietic cell transplantation.

Data from SEER database: Ries L, Harkins D, Krapcho M, Miller B, Mariotto A, Feuer E: SEER Cancer Statistics Review, 1975–2003 National Cancer Institute. Bethesda, MD. http://seer.cancer.gov/csr/1975_2003/, based on November 2005 SEER data submission, posted to the SEER web site, 2006. Accessed August 1, 2007; and CIBMTR database.

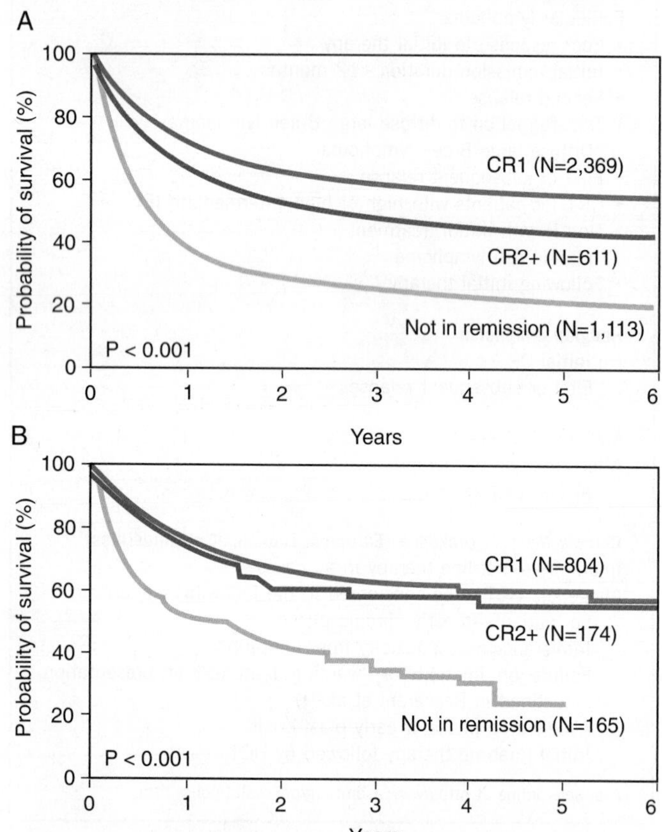

Figure 101–5 Probability of survival after human leukocyte antigen (HLA)-identical sibling transplants with myeloablative conditioning for acute myelogenous leukemia (AML), age ≥ 20 years, 1998–2004, by disease status. **B**, Probability of survival after HLA-identical sibling transplants with myeloablative conditioning for AML, age <20 years, 1998–2004, by disease status.

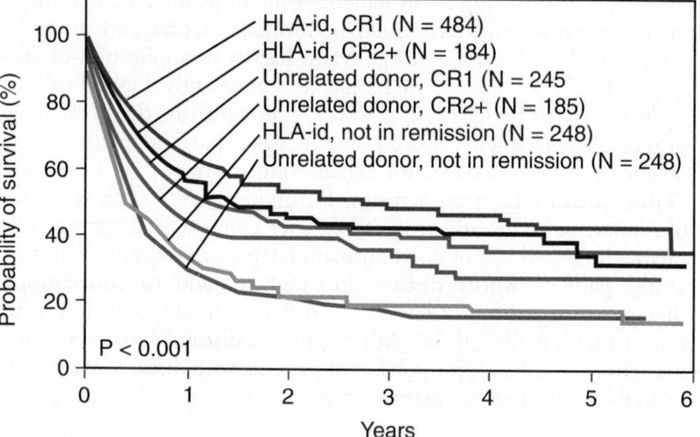

Figure 101–6 Probability of survival after allogeneic transplants with reduced-intensity conditioning for acute myelogenous leukemia, age ≥ 20 years, 1998–2004, by donor type and disease status.

transplants for AML reported to the CIBMTR in 1998 to 2004 used reduced-intensity conditioning. These patients were older and more likely to have significant comorbidities than patients receiving myeloablative regimens. Among adults receiving HLA-identical sibling transplants with reduced-intensity conditioning, 5-year probabilities of survival were 42% for 484 patients transplanted in CR1, 35% for 184 patients transplanted in CR2 or subsequent CR, and 17% for 248 patients transplanted in relapse (Fig. 101–6).

Unrelated donor transplantation is associated with higher TRM but somewhat lower relapse rates than HLA-identical sibling transplantation. Among 4097 recipients of unrelated donor transplants reported to the CIBMTR between 1998 and 2004, 5-year probabilities of relapse, LFS, and overall survival were 34%, 29%, and 30%, respectively. Among adults receiving unrelated donor transplants following myeloablative conditioning, 5-year probabilities of survival were 41% for 833 patients transplanted in CR1, 36% for 733 transplanted in CR2 or subsequent CR, and 16% for 1015 transplanted with active disease (Fig. 101–7A). Among children (younger than 20 years), 5-year probabilities of survival were 38% for 345 children transplanted in CR1, 47% for 427 transplanted in CR2 or subsequent CR, and 21% for 293 transplanted with active disease (Fig. 101–7B). Reduced-intensity conditioning is also used for unrelated donor HCT for AML, again more commonly in older patients with significant comorbidities. Among adults receiving unrelated donor HCT following reduced-intensity conditioning in 1998 to 2004, 5-year probabilities of survival were 35% in 245 patients transplanted in CR1, 27% in 185 transplanted in CR2 or subsequent CR, and 15% in 248 transplanted with active disease (see Fig. 101–6).

One of the most powerful prognostic indicators in conventional therapy of AML is the cytogenetic profile.[127–129] The commonly used Southwest Oncology Group (SWOG)/Eastern Cooperative Oncology Group (ECOG) classification[130] identifies three risk groups for cytogenetic abnormalities:

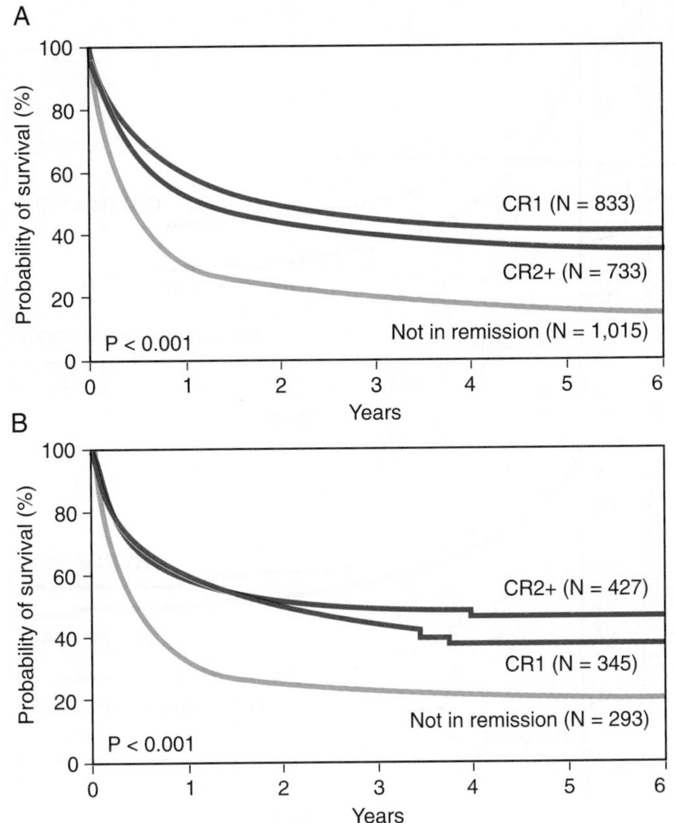

Figure 101–7 **A**, Probability of survival after unrelated donor transplants with myeloablative conditioning for acute myelogenous leukemia (AML), age ≥ 20 years, 1998–2004, by disease status. **B**, Probability of survival after unrelated donor transplants with myeloablative conditioning for AML, age <20 years, 1998–2004, by disease status.

- Favorable: inv[16]t(16;16)/del(16q) with or without other chromosome anomalies and t(8;21) without either del(9q) or as part of a complex karyotype
- Intermediate: +8, −Y, +6, del(12p) and normal karyotype
- Unfavorable: −5/del(5q), −7/del(7q), inv(3q)/t(3;3), abnormal 11q, 20q, or 21q, del(9q), t(6;9), t(9;22), abnormal 17p, and complex karyotype (>3anomalies)

Several new cytogenetic and molecular characteristics (FLT-3 mutations, NPM mutations, and c-kit mutations) are also associated with prognosis of AML treated with chemotherapy.[131]

Disease factors, such as cytogenetics, that predict prognosis with conventional chemotherapy may or may not affect HCT outcomes. Cytogenetics appears to be important in the HLA-matched related donor HCT setting.[127,132,133] An EBMT analysis of 500 recipients of sibling allografts for AML in CR1 showed that adverse cytogenetics had a strong impact on the risk of relapse and survival in multivariate analysis.[133] An earlier IBMTR study of 708 patients transplanted in CR1 from sibling donors also demonstrated similar increased risks of relapse and treatment failure for patients with poor prognosis cytogenetic abnormalities.[127] However, given the possibility of varying susceptibility of different cytogenetic risk groups to the immune effects of HCT, the current cytogenetic risk grouping schemes may not be ideal for patients undergoing HCT. A large single-center study suggested the utility of a novel transplant-specific risk classification scheme based on cytogenetics over other disease- or transplant-related factors.[134]

In contrast to these studies, among 560 patients receiving unrelated donor transplants for AML in CR1 or CR2 between 1988 and 2002, LFS rates were not significantly associated with cytogenetic profile.[135] Among 261 patients transplanted in CR1, 5-year LFS rates were 29%, 30%, and 27% for patients with favorable, intermediate, and unfavorable cytogenetics, respectively. Among 266 patients transplanted in CR2, corresponding 5-year LFS rates were 42%, 38%, and 37%. The outcome for patients with unfavorable cytogenetics is superior to that reported with conventional consolidation chemotherapy; these patients should be considered for allogeneic transplantation early in their treatment course.

Posttransplant Relapse

The optimal therapy for patients whose AML recurs after allogeneic HCT is not defined, and most therapies have limited utility. Although combination chemotherapy can induce remission in 30% to 40% of patients, the remissions usually are of short duration.[136,137] Some patients may be successfully treated with donor lymphocyte infusions (DLI), with or without prior chemotherapy, to induce a GVL effect, although DLI alone rarely results in long remissions.[87,88,99] Second allogeneic transplantation with myeloablative conditioning is associated with very high TRM, ranging from 40% to 50%.[138,139] Relapse rates are high, and the procedure is generally not considered useful unless the initial posttransplant remission is longer than 1 year. The role of second HCT with reduced-intensity conditioning is uncertain.

Timing of HCT for AML

Despite numerous studies, the question of whether allogeneic HCT is superior to consolidation chemotherapy or autologous transplantation for AML in CR1 is controversial. Five cooperative group trials have compared allogeneic BMT to other postremission therapies for AML in CR1.[140–144] Despite large numbers of enrolled patients, interpretation of results is difficult for several reasons: biologic rather than random assignment to the allogeneic transplant arm (based on availability of an HLA-matched donor), poor compliance with transplant assignment, absence of studies specifically designed to address the question in high-risk patients, ongoing redefinition of high-risk subgroups as new markers are discovered, and variation in analytical approaches.[145–148] There is general agreement that most patients younger than 55 years who do not respond to conventional therapy and who have good performance status are best treated with allogeneic transplantation if an appropriate related or unrelated donor is available.[149–152]

The National Comprehensive Cancer Network (NCCN) guidelines, widely used to guide cancer therapy in the United States, endorse allogeneic HCT with HLA-identical sibling or unrelated donors as consolidation therapy for patients with poor-risk cytogenetics, therapy-related AML, or AML with antecedent myelodysplasia.[149] However, the NCCN AML panel did not reach consensus on a single preferred postremission strategy for patients without poor-risk cytogenetics. A risk-based approach was recommended using factors such as patient age, comorbid conditions, features of the disease at diagnosis, and number of cycles of induction therapy needed to achieve remission to guide selection of chemotherapy versus transplant approaches. The long-term toxicities of allogeneic HCT were considered prohibitive for patients with good-risk cytogenetics; the panel recommended reserving this option for patients who relapsed after initial nontransplant treatment. Transplant-based options using either sibling or autologous stem cell sources were recommended for patients with intermediate-risk cytogenetics. The joint NMDP and ASBMT guidelines recommend a transplant evaluation for all patients with high-risk AML (defined as AML preceded by another hematologic disorder, treatment-related leukemia, and primary induction failure) and for patients in CR2 or beyond.[114]

ACUTE LYMPHOBLASTIC LEUKEMIA

The incidence of ALL is 1.5 per 100,000 persons. Median age at diagnosis is 13 years. Approximately 60% of patients are younger than 20 years and 15% are older than 55 years at diagnosis.[119] More than 70% of children with ALL are cured with chemotherapy regimens. The outcome of adults with ALL has improved in recent years, with more than 75% achieving initial CR,[153–155] but long-term survival of adults is less than 40%.[156–163] Prognosis is influenced by patient and disease characteristics such as age, performance status, phenotype, and genotype. Allogeneic HCT for ALL is generally reserved for patients who do not respond to conventional therapy, that is, they relapse or are in CR2 or subsequent CR. It also is an option for patients in CR1 with factors predicting a high risk of failure.[155,164] In the United States, approximately 15% of ALL patients younger than 70 years receive an allogeneic HCT (CIBMTR, unpublished data).

In 2006, approximately 1300 allogeneic HCTs for ALL were registered with the CIBMTR; about half were from unrelated donors. Median age at transplantation was 22 years; only 15% were performed in patients older than 55 years. Among patients younger than 20 years receiving HLA-identical sibling transplants, 40% were performed in CR1, 50% in CR2 or subsequent CR, and 10% in children with active disease. Corresponding probabilities for children receiving unrelated donor transplants were 30%, 60%, and 10%. Among adults 20 years or older receiving HLA-identical sibling transplants, 60% were performed in CR1, 20% in CR2 or subsequent CR, and 20% in patients with active disease. Corresponding probabilities for adults receiving unrelated donor transplants were 40%, 30%, and 30%. Most (90%) transplantations were done using myeloablative conditioning.

Major predictors of HCT outcome in ALL are remission state at time of transplantation, donor type, and age. The CIBMTR has data on approximately 6000 recipients of allogeneic HCT for ALL between 1998 and 2004. Among patients receiving transplants from HLA-identical siblings, 5-year probabilities of relapse, LFS, and overall survival were 39%, 37%, and 42%, respectively. Among adults receiving HLA-identical sibling transplants, 5-year probabilities of survival were 42% for 879 patients in CR1, 29% for 323 in CR2 or subsequent CR, and 16% for 360 with active leukemia (Fig. 101–8A). Among children receiving HLA-identical sibling HCT, 5-year probabilities of survival were 56% for 589 children transplanted in CR1, 48% for 880 children transplanted in CR2 or subsequent CR, and 27% for 185 with active leukemia (Fig. 101–8B).

Among 3212 patients receiving unrelated donor transplants between 1998 and 2004, 5-year probabilities of relapse, LFS, and overall survival were 31%, 29%, and 31%, respectively. Among adults receiving unrelated donor transplants, 5-year probabilities of survival were 36% for 519 patients transplanted in CR1, 24% for 380 in CR2 or subsequent CR, and 8% for 392 transplanted with active disease (Fig. 101–9A). Five-year probabilities for children receiving unrelated donor transplants were 45% for 466 children transplanted in CR1, 36% for 1221 children in CR2 or subsequent CR, and 17% for 244 transplanted with active disease (Fig. 101–9A).

The major cause of mortality after allogeneic transplantation for ALL is TRM, which is higher with unrelated donor transplants. The reported TRM in prospective trials ranges from 15% to 26% after HLA-identical sibling transplants and from 30% to 37% after unrelated donor transplants.[165–167] The ECOG/Medical Research Council (MRC) study reported 5-year overall survival of 55% for HLA-identical sibling and 46% for unrelated donor HCT (restricted to patients with bcr-abl–positive ALL).[166] In the German Multicentre ALL study 6/99, survival at 2 years was 53% with HLA-identical sibling donor and 44% with unrelated donor HCT.[167] CIBMTR data also indicate higher TRM with unrelated versus HLA-identical sibling transplants (approximately 40% vs approximately 25%.) Although some of this difference derives from a tendency for delayed transplantation in the unrelated donor setting, TRM rates differ even after stratification by disease state. Among patients transplanted in CR1, 5-year TRM rates are 19% with HLA-identical sibling and 34% with unrelated donor transplants. Corresponding rates for patients transplanted with advanced disease are 30% and 47%.

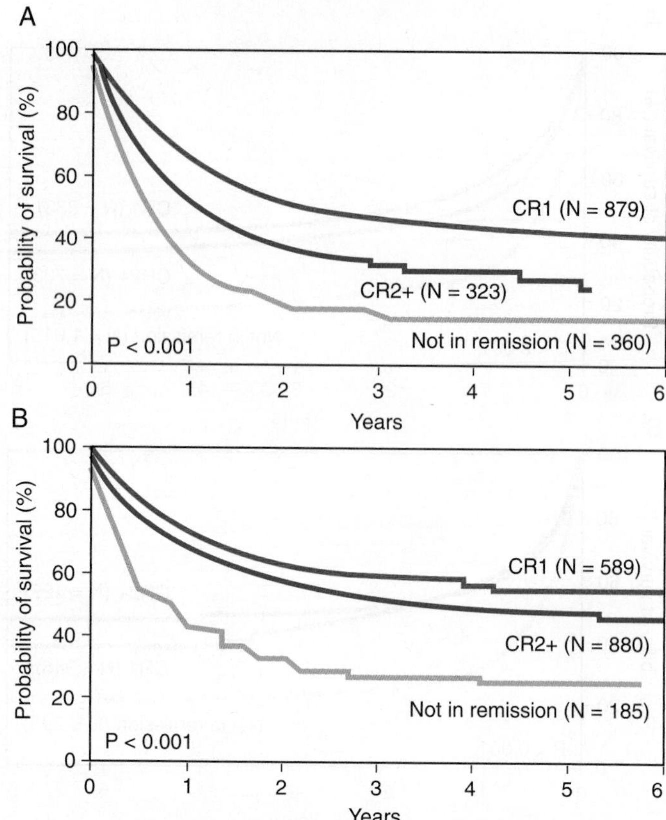

Figure 101–8 **A**, Probability of survival after human leukocyte antigen (HLA)-identical sibling transplants for acute lymphoblastic leukemia (ALL), age ≥ 20 years, 1998–2004, by disease status. **B**, Probability of survival after HLA-identical sibling transplants for ALL, age <20 years, 1998–2004, by disease status.

As in AML, prognosis in ALL is influenced by cytogenetic profile. In the most definitive study of cytogenetic risk in adult ALL, the outcomes of 1522 patients enrolled in the UKALLXII/ECOG 2993 study were analyzed.[168] The Philadelphia chromosome [t(9;22)(q34;q11.2)]/*BCR-ABL* fusion [Ph$^+$, t(4;11)(q21;q23), t(8;14)(q24.1;q32)], complex karyotype (five or more chromosomal abnormalities), or high hypodiploidy/near triploidy were associated with inferior rates of event-free and overall survival. In contrast, patients with high hyperdiploidy or a del(9p) had significantly better outcome. Multivariate analysis demonstrated that the prognostic relevance of t(8;14), complex karyotype, and low hypodiploidy/near triploidy was independent of sex, age, white blood cell count, and T-cell status among Philadelphia chromosome–negative (Ph$^-$) patients. Too few patients in the prognostically relevant cytogenetic subgroups underwent allogeneic HCT in the study to assess the impact of cytogenetics on transplantation. In Philadelphia chromosome–positive (Ph$^+$) ALL, long-term remissions are rare with chemotherapy despite CR rates of up to 90%. Related or unrelated HCT in CR1 is recommended. Although adverse cytogenetics are also associated with increased risk of relapse after HCT, allogeneic transplantation cures 20% to 40% of patients with Ph$^+$ and other high-risk cytogenetic abnormalities.[169–172]

Posttransplant Relapse

Overall, few patients who relapse after allogeneic HCT are long-term survivors.[136,137] In a series of 130 patients who relapsed after HCT for treatment of ALL, 94 patients underwent salvage therapy.[136] Relapse more than 1 year after HCT and isolated extramedullary relapses were associated with a higher probability of subsequent

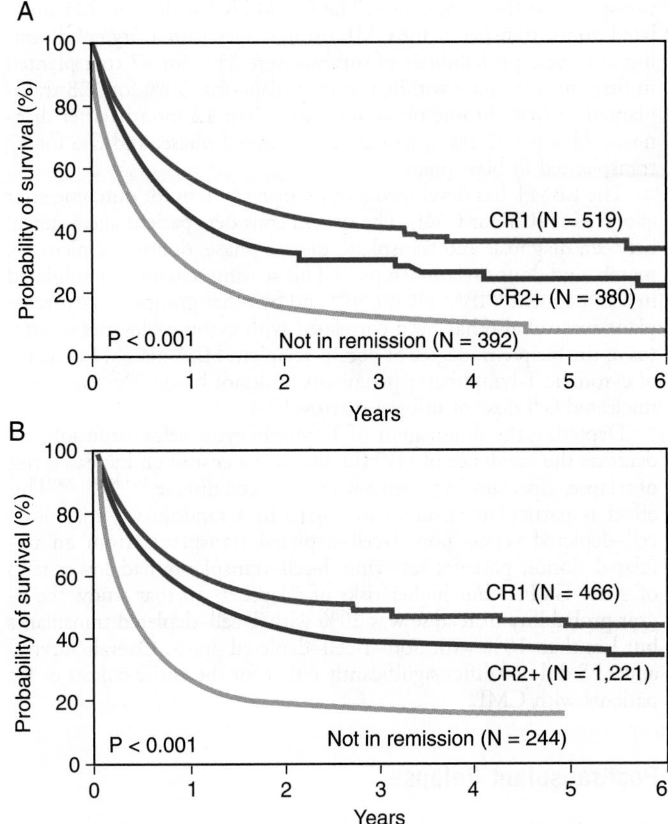

Figure 101–9 **A**, Probability of survival after unrelated donor transplants for acute lymphoblastic leukemia (ALL), age ≥ 20 years, 1998–2004, by disease status. **B**, Probability of survival after unrelated donor transplants for ALL, age <20 years, 1998–2004, by disease status.

remission. However, of the 52 patients who achieved a remission, only three became long-term leukemia-free survivors. DLIs and second HCT also are considerations in patients who relapse late after HCT. In a series of 15 patients who relapsed after HCT, a second allogeneic HCT was associated with TRM of 36% at day 100, and only 8% had long-term disease-free survival.[173] DLIs rarely produce long-term disease-free survival in ALL.[87]

Timing of Allogeneic HCT in ALL

Allogeneic HCT in CR1 from related or unrelated donors is generally accepted as the most effective available therapy for patients with Ph^+ ALL.[169–172] In children with standard-risk ALL, HCT is an accepted therapy for those in CR2.[174] For adults with Ph^- ALL, the appropriate timing of HCT is more controversial. Some prospective and retrospective comparative studies fail to show a significant advantage for allogeneic HCT in adults, with lower relapse rates offset by high TRM.[175,176] Two studies showed an advantage for allogeneic HCT in specific subsets of patients: one in patients with high-risk features [t(9;22), null or undifferentiated phenotype, high leukocyte count, age >30 years at onset, and >4 weeks to achieve first remission] and the other in adults younger than 50 years at the time of treatment.[163,177] The combined ECOG/MRC International ALL study compared postremission strategies in adult ALL.[178] Patients with HLA-matched sibling donors had higher overall and event-free survival and lower relapse rates than did patients assigned to other therapies. However, this advantage was confined to standard-risk patients (defined as bcr-abl negative, age <35 years, and without high leukocyte counts at presentation). In high-risk patients, high TRM abrogated the reduction in relapse risk. Two-year probability of TRM was 39% in high-risk patients and 20% in standard-risk patients. Despite these findings, allogeneic transplantation currently is considered by expert consensus[164] as the best curative therapy for adult patients with high-risk features such bcr-abl–positive ALL or those with a poor response to initial induction therapy[177,179] and among adults with t(4;11) ALL.[180]

No published comparisons of unrelated donor HCT with conventional therapy for ALL are available. In an analysis performed by the German Multicentre ALL Study group, patients with ALL in CR1 receiving HLA-identical sibling and unrelated donor transplants had similar LFS.[181] Other studies have shown superior LFS with unrelated donor transplants compared to autotransplants in high-risk subgroups of patients, particularly those beyond first remission.[182,183] A CIBMTR comparison of unrelated donor and autologous transplantation in ALL showed similar survival rates (40% and 32%, respectively), although the unrelated donor recipients included more patients with high-risk features such as unfavorable karyotype and high white blood cell count at diagnosis.[183] High TRM (>40%) offset the benefit of lower leukemia relapse in the unrelated donor cohort. In practice, most unrelated donor transplants are reserved for patients who do not respond to conventional therapy or with poor prognosis cytogenetic abnormalities such as bcr-abl–positive ALL.

The NMDP and ASBMT joint committee recommends transplant evaluation in patients with ALL in CR2 and at diagnosis in patients with high-risk ALL, such as patients with poor-risk cytogenetics (Ph chromosome or 11q23 abnormalities), high leukocyte count (>30,000–50,000), CNS or testicular leukemia, or patients who do not achieve CR within 4 weeks of initial induction treatment.[164]

CHRONIC MYELOID LEUKEMIA

The incidence of CML is 1.5 per 100,000 persons per year. Median age at diagnosis is 67 years; approximately 33% of patients are younger than 55 years at diagnosis and 14% are between 55 and 64 years old.[119] Allogeneic HCT is an established curative therapy for CML. Thousands of patients have been followed for more than 10 years (many for more than 15 and 20 years) after allogeneic HCT, with sustained hematologic and molecular remissions noted.[184–186] However, dramatic changes in practice occurred after targeted tyrosine kinase inhibitors were introduced for CML treatment. From 1999 to 2003, the numbers of allogeneic HCTs for CML decreased by approximately 40% in Europe[186] and by approximately two thirds in the United States.[187] CML accounted for more than 25% of allogeneic HCTs performed in the United States in 1998 to 1999 but fewer than 10% in 2006. Despite these changes, there is consensus that HCT is a valuable treatment for some patients with CML, affording the possibility of cure in patients with high-risk disease or those not responding to imatinib or other tyrosine kinase inhibitor therapy.[149]

Approximately 500 allogeneic transplantations for CML were registered with the CIBMTR in 2006; approximately 40% were from unrelated donors. Median age at HCT was 35 years; approximately 10% were older than 55 years and 10% younger than 20 years. Fifty-five percent were performed in patients in first chronic phase, 35% in patients in a subsequent chronic phase or in accelerated phase, and 10% in patients in blast phase. More than 80% had received imatinib prior to HCT. Myeloablative conditioning regimens were used for 85% of transplants in patients younger than 55 years and in 60% of transplants in patients older than 55 years; the remainder received a variety of reduced-intensity conditioning regimens. As in acute leukemia, major predictors of HCT outcome in CML are disease status, donor type, and age. Additionally, among patients transplanted in chronic phase, disease duration is important. The CIBMTR has data on 5229 patients receiving HLA-identical sibling transplants for CML performed from 1998 to 2004. Five-year probabilities of relapse, LFS, and overall survival were 24%, 52%, and 63%, respectively. Among patients receiving HLA-identical sibling transplants after myeloablative conditioning, 5-year probabilities of survival were

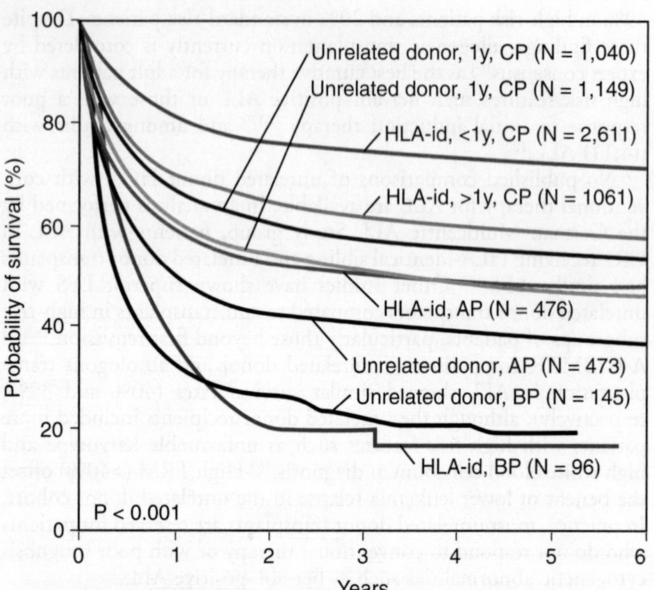

Figure 101–10 Probability of survival after allogeneic transplants with myeloablative conditioning for chronic myelogenous leukemia, 1998–2004, by disease status and donor type.

72% for 2611 patients transplanted in first chronic phase within 1 year of diagnosis, 58% for 1061 transplanted in first chronic phase but more than 12 months after diagnosis, 47% for 476 transplanted in accelerated phase, and 19% for 476 transplanted in blast phase (Fig. 101–10). Seven hundred one transplants for CML reported to the CIBMTR from 1998 to 2004 used reduced-intensity conditioning regimens. Among those receiving HLA-identical sibling transplants with reduced-intensity conditioning, 5-year probabilities of survival were 73% for 183 transplanted in first chronic phase within 1 year of diagnosis, 48% for 147 transplanted in first chronic phase but more than 12 months after diagnosis, and 46% for 63 transplanted in accelerated phase. The EBMT has reported outcomes in 187 patients who received reduced-intensity conditioning followed by allogeneic HCT for CML between 1994 and 2002.[188] Median age was 50 years; 61% received a transplant from an HLA-identical sibling, 25% from an unrelated donor, and the remainder from HLA-mismatched related donors. TRM was only 6% at 100 days but rose to 23% by 2 years posttransplant. Grade II to IV acute GVHD occurred in 32% of patients and chronic GVHD in 43%. Among patients transplanted in first or second chronic phase, overall survival rate and LFS rate at 3 years were 69% and 57%, respectively. Two-year probabilities of survival for patients transplanted in accelerated or blast phase were only 24% and 8%, respectively. Progressive CML was the major cause of death.

Overall survival rates of 35% to 45% 3 years after unrelated donor HCT for CML are reported.[16,105,106,108,189–193] In a series of 1423 transplants for CML facilitated by the NMDP, 3-year LFS was 43% in 914 patients transplanted in first chronic phase.[193] Although severe acute GVHD rates were high (43% grade II–IV, 33% grade III–IV), relapse rates were low at 6%, indicating a strong GVL effect. Among patients receiving unrelated donor HCT for CML after myeloablative conditioning from 1998 to 2004 and reported to the CIBMTR, 5-year probabilities of survival were 54% for 1040 transplanted in first chronic phase within 1 year of diagnosis, 48% for 1149 transplanted in first chronic phase but more than 12 months after diagnosis, 37% for 473 transplanted in accelerated phase, and 19% for 145 transplanted in blast phase (see Fig. 101–10). The largest single-center series of HCT for CML, including 196 patients transplanted at the Fred Hutchinson Cancer Center in Seattle, Washington, reported 5-year survival rates of 57%.[108] In that study, among patients 50 years or younger who received HCT within 1 year of diagnosis from an HLA-A, HLA-B, and HLA-DRB1 matched unrelated donor, 5-year survival was 74%, similar to that observed after HLA-matched sibling transplants at the same center. The CIBMTR has data on 231 unrelated donor transplants for CML using reduced-intensity conditioning. Five-year probabilities of survival were 55% for 47 transplanted in first chronic phase within 1 year of diagnosis, 50% for 128 transplanted in first chronic phase but more than 12 months after diagnosis, 43% for 39 transplanted in accelerated phase, and 6% for 17 transplanted in blast phase.

The EBMT has developed a risk scoring system for outcome after allogeneic HCT for CML. The system considers patient age, interval between diagnosis and transplant, disease phase, donor–recipient sex match, and donor relationships.[115] This scoring scheme was validated in a subsequent CIBMTR study[194] and by other groups.[195] Posttransplant survival also has been correlated with cytomegalovirus serostatus of the recipient, degree of donor–recipient HLA match, frequency of cytotoxic T-lymphocyte precursors in donor blood,[105,196] and total nucleated cell dose of infused marrow.[193]

Depleting the donor graft of T lymphocytes before infusion can decrease the incidence of GVHD, but at the cost of an increased risk of relapse, especially in patients with advanced disease.[16,189,197–200] This effect is particularly evident in CML. In a randomized trial of T-cell–depleted versus non–T-cell–depleted transplants from an unrelated donor, patients receiving T-cell–transplants had lower risks of acute GVHD but higher risks of relapse.[189] In that study, the 3-year probability of relapse was 20% with T-cell–depleted transplants but less than 10% with non–T-cell–depleted grafts. Overall survival and LFS did not differ significantly either for the entire cohort or for patients with CML.

Posttransplant Relapse

The probability of relapse at 5 years is approximately 20% for patients receiving HLA-identical sibling transplants for CML in first chronic phase.[65,74,77,82,201,202] The risk is higher for patients transplanted in accelerated or blast phase. Therapeutic options for patients who relapse following allogeneic HCT include DLI, second transplants with reduced-intensity or myeloablative conditioning, and imatinib or other tyrosine kinase inhibitor or interferon-α. Numerous studies support use of DLI to exploit GVL effects for inducing complete molecular remissions.[84,86–88,97,98,203,204] Durable complete remission can be established in up to 75% of patients, especially when DLI is performed in early cytogenetic relapse. In an analysis reported by Collins et al.,[87] complete responses were seen in 76% of patients receiving DLI for molecular or chronic phase hematologic relapse compared to 33% in patients with accelerated phase relapse and 17% in patients with blast phase relapse. Although response rates are higher in patients with GVHD, durable molecular responses occur in many patients without clinically evident GVHD. Second HCT with full or reduced-intensity conditioning is sometimes used for posttransplant relapse but is associated with high rates of TRM, especially if the interval between the first and second transplant is less than 1 year. This approach is generally reserved for young patients who have accelerated or blast phase relapse more than 1 year after a first transplant.

Imatinib is reported to be effective for treatment of posttransplant CML relapse in small case series.[205–209] Olavarria et al.[208] reported outcomes in 128 patients receiving imatinib after relapsing after allogeneic HCT. Fifty-one patients were in chronic phase, 31 in accelerated phase, and 46 in blast crisis. Fifty patients had not responded to treatment with DLI prior to imatinib. The overall hematologic response rate was 84%. The complete cytogenetic response rate was 58% for patients in chronic phase, 48% for those in accelerated phase, and 22% for those in blast crisis. Twenty-five (26%) patients had complete molecular responses. With median followup of 9 months, the estimated probabilities of 2-year survival were 100%, 86%, and 12% for patients treated in chronic phase, accelerated phase, and blast crisis, respectively. These results are encouraging, but longer followup is necessary. It is likely that the newer tyrosine kinase inhibitors will also be used in the posttransplant relapse setting, although efficacy data are not available.

Timing of Transplantation

As recently as 1999, CML treatment guidelines recommended early HCT within 1 to 2 years of diagnosis in young patients with an HLA-identical donor.[210] Imatinib is now the initial therapy of choice for CML, although national[149] and international guidelines[211] recommend consideration of allogeneic transplantation in some newly diagnosed patients. An early consultation with a transplant physician is important to evaluate the potential role of HCT (including performing a preliminary related and unrelated donor search), to formulate a strategy for HCT in the event of imatinib failure or discovery of resistant bcr-abl mutations, and to agree upon a strategy for monitoring the patient's progress. Early HCT is indicated for patients whose initial presentation is in blast phase and should be considered for those with a suboptimal response to imatinib. HCT is also a consideration for patients whose CML progresses after an initial response or have bcr-abl mutations that predict for nonresponse to tyrosine kinase inhibitors. A monitoring plan for early signs of progression is indicated because outcomes are significantly better if HCT is performed prior to transformation to accelerated or blast phase. Definitions of suboptimal response and failure with imatinib, guidelines for monitoring patients receiving imatinib, and indications for initiating alternative therapy, including HCT, have been developed and published by a consensus panel sponsored by the European LeukemiaNet[211] and the United States NCCN consensus panel.[149]

CHRONIC LYMPHOCYTIC LEUKEMIA

Chronic lymphocytic leukemia (CLL) is the most common leukemia in the Western world, affecting 3.8 per 100,000 population in the United States.[119] It is primarily a disease of older adults. Median age at onset is 72 years; only approximately 10% of patients are younger than 55 years at diagnosis and 20% between 55 and 65 years. Many patients have prolonged survival with observation alone or conservative therapy. The role and timing of allogeneic transplantation are controversial. Patients requiring therapy can achieve good responses and prolonged survival with a variety of modalities, such as chemotherapy, monoclonal antibodies, or autologous transplantation.[212–216] However, these approaches are not curative.[216] Allogeneic transplantation is a consideration for younger patients with high-risk features predicting short survival, such as patients with Rai stage II to IV disease or those not responding to or relapsing after fludarabine-based therapy.[217] Currently CLL accounts for approximately 4% of allogeneic HCTs.

Biologic predictors of high-risk disease in CLL include specific cytogenetic abnormalities (e.g., 17p13 abnormalities), ZAP-70 expression, high CD38 expression, and unmutated immunoglobulin heavy chain variable (Ig V_H) gene status of the tumor clone (see Chapter 83).[218–222] Poor-risk CLL is characterized by resistance to conventional chemotherapy, including fludarabine-based regimens and, typically, short duration of responses.[223–226] Allogeneic HCT can induce long-term clinical remissions in patients with CLL even in the presence of fludarabine resistance and some biologic risk factors and in these patients may offer the best option for long-term disease control.[227–229] In contrast to other CLL therapies, late relapses are uncommon after allografting.[217,230] T-cell depletion of the donor graft is associated with increased risk of relapse, whereas development of chronic GVHD is associated with reduced relapse risk.[214,231] The latter data as well as the efficacy of DLI[229,232] in inducing durable molecular responses after allotransplant relapse suggest that GVL plays a role in the efficacy of allogeneic HCT in CLL.

Approximately 260 allogeneic transplantations for CLL were registered with the CIBMTR in 2006; approximately 40% were from unrelated donors. Median age at transplantation was 55 years. Approximately 70% were in patients older than 50 years; only 30% were in patients older than 60 years. Median interval between diagnosis and transplantation was 5.5 years. Ten percent of patients had their disease for more than 10 years before transplantation. Most transplants for CLL used reduced-intensity conditioning regimens; only 45% of patients younger than 55 years and 25% of patients older than 55 years received myeloablative conditioning in 2006.

A review of 54 myeloablative HLA-identical sibling transplants for CLL performed in 1984 to 1992 reported to the IBMTR or the EBMT showed 46% survival at 3 years.[233] TRM was high at 46%. Most of these patients had long-standing or advanced disease with multiple courses of chemotherapy. The authors concluded that transplantation should be considered for young patients with poor prognosis with chemotherapy. The Fred Hutchinson Cancer Center reported their early experience in 25 patients with CLL transplanted in 1980 to 1999.[234] TRM at day 100 was unacceptably high at 57% for patients receiving busulfan and cyclophosphamide conditioning but only 17% for those receiving TBI regimens. Five-year survival was 32%. Results of HCT with myeloablative conditioning in 38 patients receiving unrelated donor transplants in 1993 to 1999 were reported by the NMDP/CIBMTR.[235] Twenty-one of the patients were chemotherapy refractory, and 89% had received fludarabine. Conditioning included TBI in 92% of patients. Five-year survival, TRM, and relapse rates were 33%, 32%, and 38%, respectively.

Data suggest that reduced-intensity conditioning regimens are effective and less toxic than myeloablative regimens in allogeneic HCT for CLL. A report describing heavily pretreated patients with advanced CLL receiving reduced-intensity conditioning demonstrated 2-year overall and disease-free survival rates of 60% and 52%, respectively.[228] In another study of 30 patients with advanced CLL who received allogeneic HCT after reduced-intensity regimens, 4-year survival, TRM, and relapse rates were 69%, 15%, and 30%, respectively.[229] The EBMT compared the outcomes of 73 patients with CLL transplanted with reduced-intensity regimens with 82 similar patients transplanted after standard myeloablative conditioning during the same time period.[231] The patients who received reduced-intensity conditioning had 2-year survival, TRM, and relapse rates of 70%, 19%, and 28%, respectively. Corresponding rates for patients who received myeloablative conditioning were 70%, 26%, and 11%. Although reduced-intensity regimens were associated with significantly less TRM, no difference in event-free or overall survival between the two groups was observed given the higher incidence of relapse in the reduced-intensity group.

Among 684 patients receiving HLA-identical sibling transplants for CLL in 1998 to 2004, 5-year probabilities of survival were 46% for 318 patients receiving myeloablative conditioning and 45% for 366 receiving reduced-intensity regimens. Corresponding LFS rates were 29% and 8%. Among 317 patients receiving unrelated donor transplants during this period, 5-year probabilities of survival were 26% for 138 patients receiving myeloablative conditioning and 29% for 179 receiving reduced-intensity regimens (Fig. 101–11). Corresponding LFS rates were 19% and 19%. For older patients or those

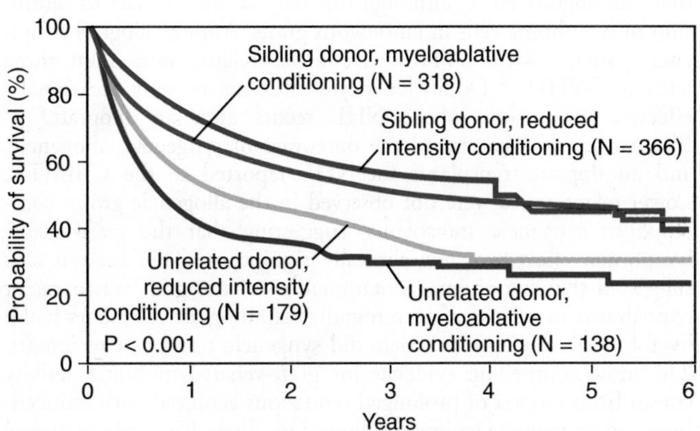

Figure 101–11 Probability of survival after allogeneic transplants for chronic lymphocytic leukemia, 1998–2004, by donor type and regimen intensity.

with significant comorbidities that increase the risk of TRM, reduced-intensity regimens appear to be an appropriate choice, especially if the CLL is chemosensitive. Whether myeloablative regimens is preferable in younger patients with poorly controlled disease is not clear.[236]

Current NCCN or ASBMT guidelines do not address the role of HCT in CLL. However the EBMT consensus group has recommended allogeneic HCT as a reasonable treatment option for younger patients with nonresponse or early relapse (within 12 months) after purine analogue therapy.[237] Patients who relapse within 24 months after having responded to purine analogue-based combination therapy or autologous transplantation and patients with p53 abnormalities requiring treatment are also considered candidates for transplant evaluation.

NON-HODGKIN LYMPHOMA

The NHLs are a heterogeneous group of malignancies with an incidence of 19.1 per 100,000 persons (see Chapter 80). Median age of onset is 67 years, with only 30% younger than 55 years at diagnosis.[119] Treatment choices, prognosis, and the role of allogeneic HCT in NHL depend on histologic subtype as well as patient characteristics such as age and comorbidities. Although nontransplant therapies are the mainstay of treatment for follicular NHL, these treatments rarely cure the disease. Autologous HCT cures a substantial proportion of patients with relapsed or high-risk diffuse large cell lymphoma but is less effective for follicular, mantle cell, and lymphoblastic lymphomas.[238] A tumor-free graft and the potential for immune-mediated graft-versus-lymphoma effects are the major advantages of allogeneic over autologous HCT in NHL. Disadvantages are the risks of TRM, GVHD, and donor restrictions.[239] Fewer than 700 allogeneic HCTs were performed for NHL in the United States in 2006, much fewer than the 3000 autologous HCTs performed for NHL and considerably less than the more than 50,000 cases of NHL diagnosed each year. Autologous HCT is an accepted therapy for patients who do not respond to nontransplant treatment or as initial consolidation therapy in patients with a high risk of failure. Allogeneic HCT is generally reserved for patients with a high likelihood of relapse after autografting or from whom an adequate autologous graft cannot be obtained.[238,240,241] This includes patients with follicular or lymphoblastic NHL, patients with lymphoma refractory to conventional chemotherapy, and patients with extensive marrow involvement, coexisting myelodysplasia, poor marrow reserve, or prior pelvic irradiation. Some patients relapsing after an autograft for NHL can achieve long-term disease-free survival with allogeneic transplantation.[242]

Graft-versus-lymphoma effects are less well defined in lymphoma than in leukemia but may play a role in preventing relapse after transplants for NHL.[243–246] Relapse rates are lower after allogeneic than autologous HCT, although this may be due in part to reinfusion of lymphoma cells in autologous grafts. Among allograft recipients, patients with GVHD have lower relapse rates than those without GVHD.[244] Donor leukocyte infusions are only occasionally effective in persons whose NHL recurs after an allograft.[87,247] Bierman et al.[248] compared the outcomes of syngeneic, allogeneic, and autologous transplants for NHL reported to the CIBMTR. Lower relapse rates were not observed in the allogeneic group compared to syngeneic transplants, suggesting that the graft-versus-lymphoma effect was not clinically significant. This analysis also suggested that lymphoma contamination of the graft was a major contributor to relapse after autografts, as autograft recipients had a fivefold higher relapse risk than did syngeneic transplant recipients. The most compelling evidence for graft-versus-lymphoma activity comes from reports of prolonged remissions achieved with reduced-intensity preparative regimens followed by allografting, where disease control would not be expected from the conditioning regimen alone. The effect appears to be strongest in follicular and mantle cell lymphoma.[30,249,250]

Diffuse Large Cell Lymphoma

The most common lymphoma subtype is diffuse large B-cell (non-Hodgkin) lymphoma (DLBCL). Population-based studies indicate that DLBCL is curable in approximately 50% of cases in the current era.[251] Among patients who relapse, those with chemosensitive lymphoma have a 40% to 50% chance of long-term disease-free survival with autologous HCT.[252,253] No randomized studies have compared allogeneic with autologous transplants in relapsed DLBCL. An EBMT study comparing allogeneic and autologous transplants in NHL failed to show a difference in progression-free survival or relapse in the intermediate-grade NHL subset.[244] A CIBMTR study comparing patients receiving HLA-identical sibling allografts for DLBCL with patients matched on disease- and patient-related risk factors who received autotransplants showed higher TRM and no beneficial effect on risk of progression with allografting.[254] Allografts are often recommended for patients who relapse after an autograft.[242] Several single-center studies with small numbers of patients give conflicting results for allogeneic HCT in this setting.[25,255,256] A CIBMTR analysis of 114 patients who received a myeloablative allograft for treatment of relapse following autologous transplantation between 1990 and 1999 showed 5-year survival of 24% and disease-free survival of 5%.[257] TRM was high in all of these studies, and current approaches increasingly use reduced-intensity conditioning to ameliorate this problem.[258–260] Long-term data on outcome are lacking.

Forty-five percent of the 250 allografts for DLBCL registered with the CIBMTR in 2006 were in patients who never achieved first remission; only half of these patients had chemotherapy-sensitive disease. Fifteen percent of transplants were performed as consolidation therapy for DLBCL in first or subsequent remission, 20% in resistant or untreated relapse, and 20% in chemosensitive relapse. Thirty percent of patients had a prior autograft. Median age at HCT was 50 years. Reduced-intensity conditioning was used in 40% of transplants. Among 440 recipients of HLA-identical sibling transplants for DLBCL performed in 1998 to 2004, 3-year probabilities of actuarial survival were 39% for 323 patients with chemotherapy-sensitive disease and 21% for 117 with resistant disease. Corresponding progression-free survival rates were 33% and 15%. Among 129 recipients of unrelated donor transplants for DLBCL performed in this period, the 3-year probabilities of actuarial survival were 28% for 86 patients with chemotherapy-sensitive disease and 14% for 43 with resistant disease. Corresponding progression-free survival rates were 25% and 6%.

Follicular Lymphoma

Follicular lymphoma is the second most common lymphoma in the United States (see Chapter 79).[261] The natural history of this disease is marked by repeated chemosensitive relapses of progressively shorter duration and ultimately death from progressive disease.[262] Currently no nontransplant options are considered curative, but prolonged survival with good quality of life is possible for most patients. Autologous and allogeneic HCT are alternative approaches aimed at long-term survival and potential cure in patients for whom nontransplant therapy fails.[263] Although none of the trials were randomized, multiple studies show substantially lower risks of relapse with allogeneic compared to autologous HCT.[246,264,265] A CIBMTR analysis compared the outcomes of 131 patients with follicular NHL who underwent myeloablative allogeneic HCT with 597 who received autologous HCT (n = 597).[265] The risk of relapse was significantly lower in the allogeneic HCT group ($P < 0.001$): 19% at 1 year with very few relapses thereafter versus 36% at 1 year and 58% at 5 years after autografting. However, the benefit of lower relapse rates was offset by higher TRM; 5-year probabilities of overall survival were similar after allogeneic and autologous transplantation (52% and 55%, respectively). These results are very similar to a large single-center report from the University of Nebraska.[266]

The low recurrence rate with allogeneic HCT shows the potential for cure of follicular lymphoma. However, the toxicity of allogeneic

HCT is a major barrier to the general applicability of this approach to most patients with follicular lymphoma. Current clinical practice recommends allogeneic HCT for younger patients with recurrent follicular lymphoma who have suitable sibling donors because they may tolerate treatment-related toxicity better.[267] There is also considerable interest in using reduced-intensity regimens for follicular lymphoma because of an apparent greater graft-versus-lymphoma effect for this histology.[240] The best reported outcomes with reduced-intensity regimens have been demonstrated in single-center studies in patients with chemotherapy-sensitive relapses.[268] An EBMT study of 52 patients with low-grade NHL receiving allografts reported 2-year progression free and overall survival rates of 54% and 65%, respectively, with a 2-year TRM rate of 31%.[250]

Of the approximately 250 allogeneic transplants for follicular lymphoma registered with the CIBMTR in 2006, 81% were performed in patients with chemotherapy-sensitive disease. Sixty-percent were performed using a reduced-intensity conditioning regimen. Among 747 HLA-identical sibling transplants for follicular lymphoma performed in 1998 to 2004, 5-year probabilities of survival were 58% in 426 patients receiving standard myeloablative conditioning and 66% in 321 receiving reduced-intensity conditioning. Corresponding probabilities of progression-free survival were 42% and 44%. Among 209 recipients of unrelated donor transplants for follicular lymphoma performed during this period, 5-year probabilities of actuarial survival was 39% for 99 patients receiving myeloablative conditioning and 47% for 110 receiving reduced-intensity conditioning. Corresponding progression-free survival rates were identical at 34%.

Mantle Cell Lymphoma

Mantle cell lymphoma accounts for 6% of cases of adult NHL and is primarily a disease of older men (median age at onset 65 years).[269,270] The natural history of the disease is characterized by response to initial chemotherapy followed by refractory relapse and median survival of approximately 3 years. The role of autologous and allogeneic HCT is poorly established, although common clinical options include combination chemotherapy followed by autologous HCT in first remission and autologous or allogeneic HCT in relapse.[149] Among 175 allogeneic HCTs registered with the CIBMTR in 2006, 20% were performed in first remission; 20% of patients had a prior autograft. Seventy percent were performed using a reduced-intensity conditioning regimen. Reduced-intensity conditioning regimens are increasingly used in mantle cell NHL. Because autologous transplants are not curative, most patients are of advanced age at diagnosis, and a graft-versus-tumor effect appears to exist.[271] Two-year overall survival of 64% and disease-free survival of 60% were demonstrated using reduced-intensity conditioning allogeneic HCT in a single-center study.[30] Relapse and TRM rates were 9% and 24%, respectively. Among 488 patients receiving allogeneic HCT for mantle cell NHL in 1998 to 2004 reported to the CIBMTR, 3-year probabilities of survival were 50% and 34% after 375 HLA-identical sibling transplants and 113 unrelated donor transplants, respectively. Reduced-intensity conditioning was used in 40% of cases and yielded similar survival outcomes to myeloablative conditioning.

Current U.S. NCCN guidelines recommend consideration of allogeneic HCT as an adjunct to initial therapy, preferably on a clinical trial.[149]

Rare Subtypes of NHL

The lymphoblastic lymphomas account for only approximately 2% of NHLs.[269] They usually are of precursor T-cell origin and occur most commonly in children and young adults. Both autologous and allogeneic HCTs have been used in patients with lymphoblastic lymphoma; reported overall survival rates are 56% to 80% for patients who received transplants in CR1.[157,244,272,273] In a CIBMTR analysis, HLA-identical sibling allogeneic HCT for lymphoblastic lymphoma was associated with fewer relapses than autologous HCT, but higher TRM of allogeneic HCT abrogated any survival benefit.[274]

The role of allogeneic HCT in relapsed or chemotherapy-refractory anaplastic large cell lymphoma is not defined. In case reports, allogeneic HCT has been shown to be effective in patients with multiple relapses of ALK-positive anaplastic large cell lymphoma or even with chemotherapy-refractory disease.[275] The existence of a graft-versus-anaplastic large cell lymphoma effect also has been postulated. Fewer than 150 allogeneic HCTs for anaplastic large cell lymphoma were reported to the CIBMTR between 1989 and 2006.

HODGKIN LYMPHOMA

The incidence of Hodgkin lymphoma is 2.7 per 100,000 persons in the United States. Median age at onset is 37 years, and 75% of patients are younger than 55 years at diagnosis.[119] There is a bimodal peak in the incidence of HD, with most patients between the ages of 15 and 30 years, followed by another peak in adults older than 55 years. Most patients with Hodgkin lymphoma are cured with conventional chemotherapy (with or without radiation).[276,277] Autologous HCT is an accepted and effective salvage therapy for the 20% to 30% patients who do not respond to conventional chemotherapy. Two randomized studies and several retrospective studies support the use of autologous HCT in relapsed and refractory Hodgkin lymphoma, especially in chemotherapy-sensitive patients.[278,279] In 2006, 928 autologous transplants for Hodgkin lymphoma were registered with CIBMTR but only 240 allogeneic HCTs. About half of the allogeneic transplants were in patients who had relapsed after a prior autotransplant. Median age was 33 years; 70% used reduced-intensity conditioning regimens. Potential advantages of allogeneic transplants in advanced Hodgkin lymphoma are that donor hematopoietic cells have not been exposed to chemotherapy, there is no risk of lymphoma cells contaminating the graft, and there may be a graft-versus-lymphoma effect. However, relatively few allogeneic transplants for Hodgkin lymphoma are performed; 80% are from related donors. As in NHL, most are performed in heavily pretreated and often chemotherapy-refractory patients.[280]

An IBMTR analysis of 100 HLA-identical sibling transplants for Hodgkin lymphoma performed between 1982 and 1992 showed high TRM (61%) and 3-year disease-free survival of 15%.[280] A matched pair analysis of autologous and allogeneic transplants for Hodgkin lymphoma showed fewer relapses but more transplant-related deaths with allografts; survival was similar.[281] Reduced-intensity conditioning regimens for reducing TRM have been explored. An early single-center study reported TRM of 22% at 18 months in 40 heavily pretreated patients.[282] Overall survival at 18 months was 61%, with progression-free survival of 32%.

Three hundred eighty allogeneic HCTs for Hodgkin lymphoma were reported to the CIBMTR between 1998 and 2004. Among patients receiving HLA-identical sibling transplants, 3-year probability of survival was identical (38%) in 141 patients receiving myeloablative conditioning and 93 patients receiving reduced-intensity conditioning. The outcomes of 146 unrelated donor transplant recipients for Hodgkin lymphoma using reduced-intensity conditioning and reported to the CIBMTR between 1999 and 2004 have been evaluated.[283] Overall survival, progression-free survival, and TRM rates were 38%, 20%, and 33% at 2 years. Most (90%) of these patients had relapsed after a prior autograft, and 50% had chemotherapy-resistant disease at transplantation. A comparison with 38 unrelated donor transplants using myeloablative conditioning did not show statistically significant differences in TRM, survival, or relapse risk.

National consensus guidelines do not currently recommend allogeneic HCT in relapsed or refractory Hodgkin lymphoma; therefore, this treatment should ideally be performed as part of a clinical trial.[149]

MULTIPLE MYELOMA

Multiple myeloma is a disease of older adults. Median age at onset is approximately 70 years.[119] Two thirds of patients are 65 years or older; only 15% are younger than 55 years. The most common treatment strategy for multiple myeloma involves initial therapy with corticosteroid-based combination regimens followed by single or planned tandem autologous peripheral blood stem cell transplantation in transplant-eligible patients. Currently, myeloma is the most common indication for HCT in the United States, although most HCTs use autologous cells. Approximately 4000 autologous and 350 allogeneic HCTs for myeloma were performed in the United States in 2006. Approximately 20% of allogeneic HCTs were from unrelated donors. Median ages of autologous and allogeneic HCT recipients were 58 and 54 years, respectively; fewer than 10% of allograft recipients were older than 60 years. Eighty percent of the allogeneic HCTs were in patients who had a prior autotransplant.

Two prospective randomized clinical trials have shown that high-dose therapy with autologous HCT is superior to conventional chemotherapy in prolonging survival.[284,285] Unfortunately, the vast majority of patients eventually relapse after autologous HCT, including after planned sequential autotransplant.[286] Several studies show that allogeneic HCT produces durable molecular remissions in myeloma, with a significantly lower risk of relapse than autologous HCT.[274,287–289] Other evidence for a graft-versus-myeloma effect of allogeneic HCT include reports of lower relapse rates in patients developing GVHD and the success of DLI in reinducing remission in some patients who relapse after allogeneic transplantation.[102,290–292] Unfortunately, TRM rates after allogeneic HCT done with conventional myeloablative conditioning have been high, leading to significantly inferior overall survival rates compared to autotransplants.[293,294] Nevertheless, some allotransplant recipients have prolonged disease-free survival and may be cured of their myeloma.[295] The allotransplant arm of the U.S. Intergroup S9321 study demonstrated a long-term (7-year) plateau in the survival curve at 39%, although the very high initial TRM (40%) led to premature termination of this arm.[295] Data from the EBMT indicate that TRM after myeloablative HCT decreased significantly to approximately 20% over the past 10 years; the change was attributed to improved supportive care and better patient selection.[296]

In practice, most allogeneic HCTs for myeloma now use reduced-intensity conditioning. An analysis by the EBMT of 320 patients is the largest reported experience with reduced-intensity conditioning in multiple myeloma.[297] Most of the patients had undergone a prior autograft (23% as a planned tandem procedure), were in a complete or partial response (72%) prior to transplant, had HLA-matched sibling donors (82%), and had received fludarabine-based conditioning (86%) with the addition of melphalan, busulfan, or TBI. Compared to 196 patients who received myeloablative conditioning for myeloma, patients who received reduced-intensity conditioning were older and more likely to have progressive disease. TRM rates at 2 years in the reduced intensity and myeloablative groups were 24% and 37%, respectively. Three-year probabilities of survival were similar at 38% and 50%, whereas progression-free survival was lower in the reduced-intensity group (19% vs 34% in the myeloablative group). In multivariate analysis, progressive disease at transplantation and use of alemtuzumab were associated with worse outcomes. Current studies do not indicate that lower early TRM with reduced-intensity conditioning translates into a survival plateau, with relapse risks as high as 60% in the first 3 years, especially in patients with high-risk disease (e.g., adverse cytogenetics).[298–300] The best results with reduced-intensity conditioning seem to occur in patients with chemosensitive disease[301] without adverse markers such as chromosome 13 abnormalities[302] or high β_2-microglobulin levels[300] or in patients who had an autotransplant in the preceding year.[303]

Allogeneic HCT with reduced-intensity conditioning can be performed may as an initial transplant approach, for relapse after autologous transplantation, or after autologous transplantation in a planned sequential approach. The Seattle group who pioneered the latter approach reported initial results in three groups of patients[304,305]: relapsed patients who had not responded to prior autologous HCT (n = 14), relapsed patients who had not received prior autotransplant (n = 19), and patients who had received planned sequential autologous allogeneic transplants (n = 84). Four-year overall survival probabilities were 40%, 35%, and 70%, respectively. TRM was 2% at day 100 and 17% overall. The strategy of initial autologous transplantation for tumor reduction followed by allogeneic HCT from related and unrelated donors after reduced-intensity conditioning to provide a graft-versus-myeloma effect is increasingly used. A study from Italy indicates significantly higher progression-free and overall survival rates with sequential auto-allotransplants (using HLA-identical sibling donors) versus tandem autologous transplants.[306] A large trial testing this strategy is underway in the United States.

Among 1152 HLA-identical sibling HCTs for multiple myeloma performed in 1998 to 2004 and reported to CIBMTR, 5-year probabilities of survival were 38% for 532 patients receiving myeloablative conditioning and 39% for 620 receiving reduced-intensity conditioning. Among 340 unrelated donor HCTs performed during the same time period, 5-year probabilities of survival were 16% for 130 patients receiving myeloablative conditioning and 21% for 210 patients receiving reduced-intensity conditioning. Twenty-five percent of those receiving myeloablative conditioning and 64% of those receiving reduced-intensity conditioning had undergone a prior autotransplant (Fig. 101–12).

The NCCN guidelines do not distinguish between myeloablative and nonmyeloablative allogeneic HCT in myeloma. All indications are considered a category 2A recommendation (reflecting uniform NCCN consensus, based on lower-level evidence including clinical experience, that the recommendation is appropriate).

LATE EFFECTS IN SURVIVORS OF ALLOGENEIC TRANSPLANTS

Patients who survive the first 5 years after HCT are likely to survive long term, with mortality rates eventually approaching that of the general population.[184,307] However, some survivors experience late complications of HCT. Baker et al.[307] studied the long-term risks and benefits of HCT for CML. Two hundred forty-eight recipients of HCT for CML who had survived at least 2 years post-HCT were compared to 317 normal siblings. Subjects completed a 238-item survey on medical late effects. Compared with sibling controls, survivors had higher risks of ocular, oral health, endocrine, gastrointestinal, musculoskeletal, neurosensory, and neuromotor impairments. Chronic GVHD is a major risk factor for hypothyroidism, osteoporosis, cardiopulmonary, neurosensory, and neuromotor impairments and late deaths.[184,307] These data show the need for continued monitoring and medical intervention in these patients.

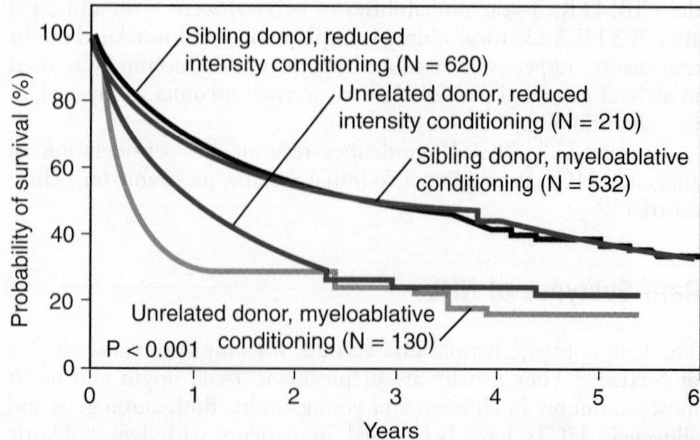

Figure 101–12 Probability of survival after allogeneic transplants for multiple myeloma, 1998–2004, by donor type and regimen intensity.

Disappointingly, HCT survivors do not seem more likely than the general population to seek regular medical care or follow routine personal health guidelines. Education on the importance of such followup should be an integral part of posttransplant care. The CIBMTR and EBMT have published guidelines for long-term followup of transplant recipients.[308]

SUGGESTED READINGS

Baccarani M, Saglio G, Goldman J, et al: Evolving concepts in the management of chronic myeloid leukemia: Recommendations from an expert panel on behalf of the European LeukemiaNet. Blood 108:1809, 2006.

Beatty PG, Boucher KM, Mori M, Milford EL: Probability of finding HLA-mismatched related or unrelated marrow or cord blood donors. Hum Immunol 61:834, 2000.

Blume KG, Forman SJ, Appelbaum F (eds.): Thomas' Hematopoietic Cell Transplantation, 3rd ed. Oxford, Blackwell Publishing, 2003.

Bortin MM, Truitt RL, Rimm AA, Bach FH: Graft-versus-leukaemia reactivity induced by alloimmunisation without augmentation of graft-versus-host reactivity. Nature 281:490, 1979.

Bruno B, Rotta M, Patriarca F, et al: A comparison of allografting with autografting for newly diagnosed myeloma. N Engl J Med 356:1110, 2007.

Burnett AK: Current controversies: Which patients with acute myeloid leukaemia should receive a bone marrow transplantation?—An adult treater's view. Br J Haematol 118:357, 2002.

Cassileth PA, Harrington DP, Appelbaum FR, et al: Chemotherapy compared with autologous or allogeneic bone marrow transplantation in the management of acute myeloid leukemia in first remission. N Engl J Med 339:1649, 1998.

Collins R Jr, Shpilberg O, Drobyski W, et al: Donor leukocyte infusions in 140 patients with relapsed malignancy after allogeneic bone marrow transplantation. J Clin Oncol 15:433, 1997.

Diaconescu R, Flowers CR, Storer B, et al: Morbidity and mortality with nonmyeloablative compared with myeloablative conditioning before hematopoietic cell transplantation from HLA-matched related donors. Blood 104:1550, 2004.

Eapen M, Rubinstein P, Zhang MJ, et al: Outcomes of transplantation of unrelated donor umbilical cord blood and bone marrow in children with acute leukaemia: A comparison study. Lancet 369:1947, 2007.

Gribben JG, Zahrieh D, Stephans K, et al: Autologous and allogeneic stem cell transplantations for poor-risk chronic lymphocytic leukemia. Blood 106:4389, 2005.

Hahn T, Wall D, Camitta B, et al: The role of cytotoxic therapy with hematopoietic stem cell transplantation in the therapy of acute lymphoblastic leukemia in adults: An evidence-based review. Biol Blood Marrow Transplant 12:1, 2006.

Horowitz MM, Gale RP, Sondel PM, et al: Graft-versus-leukemia reactions after bone marrow transplantation. Blood 75:555, 1990.

Hunault M, Harousseau JL, Delain M, et al: Better outcome of adult acute lymphoblastic leukemia after early genoidentical allogeneic bone marrow transplantation (BMT) than after late high-dose therapy and autologous BMT. A GOELAMS trial. Blood 104:3028, 2004.

Kantarjian HM, O'Brien S, Cortes JE, et al: Imatinib mesylate therapy for relapse after allogeneic stem cell transplantation for chronic myelogenous leukemia. Blood 100:1590, 2002.

Kolb HJ, Mittermuller J, Clemm C, et al: Donor leukocyte transfusions for treatment of recurrent chronic myelogenous leukemia in marrow transplant patients. Blood 76:2462, 1990.

Laughlin MJ, Eapen M, Rubinstein P, et al: Outcomes after transplantation of cord blood or bone marrow from unrelated donors in adults with leukemia. N Engl J Med 351:2265, 2004.

Rizzo JD, Wingard JR, Tichelli A, et al: Recommended screening and preventive practices for long-term survivors after hematopoietic cell transplantation: Joint recommendations of the European Group for Blood and Marrow Transplantation, the Center for International Blood and Marrow Transplant Research, and the American Society of Blood and Marrow Transplantation. Biol Blood Marrow Transplant 12:138, 2006.

Slavin S, Nagler A, Naparstek E, et al: Nonmyeloablative stem cell transplantation and cell therapy as an alternative to conventional bone marrow transplantation with lethal cytoreduction for the treatment of malignant and nonmalignant hematologic diseases. Blood 91:756, 1998.

Socie G, Stone JV, Wingard JR, et al: Long-term survival and late deaths after allogeneic bone marrow transplantation. Late Effects Working Committee of the International Bone Marrow Transplant Registry. N Engl J Med 341:14, 1999.

Sorror ML, Maris MB, Storer B, et al: Comparing morbidity and mortality of HLA-matched unrelated donor hematopoietic cell transplantation after nonmyeloablative and myeloablative conditioning: Influence of pretransplantation comorbidities. Blood 104:961, 2004.

Stem Cell Trialists' Collaborative Group: Allogeneic peripheral blood stem-cell compared with bone marrow transplantation in the management of hematologic malignancies: An individual patient data meta-analysis of nine randomized trials. J Clin Oncol 3:5074, 2005.

Thomas ED, Buckner CD, Banaji M, et al: One hundred patients with acute leukemia treated by chemotherapy, total body irradiation, and allogeneic marrow transplantation. Blood 49:511, 1977.

Wagner JE, Thompson JS, Carter SL, Kernan NA: Effect of graft-versus-host disease prophylaxis on 3-year disease-free survival in recipients of unrelated donor bone marrow (T-cell Depletion Trial): A multi-centre, randomised phase II-III trial. Lancet 366:733, 2005.

Yakoub-Agha I, Mesnil F, Kuentz M, et al: Allogeneic marrow stem-cell transplantation from human leukocyte antigen-identical siblings versus human leukocyte antigen-allelic-matched unrelated donors (10/10) in patients with standard-risk hematologic malignancy: A prospective study from the French Society of Bone Marrow Transplantation and Cell Therapy. J Clin Oncol 24:5695, 2006.

REFERENCES

For complete list of references log onto www.expertconsult.com

CHAPTER 102

AUTOLOGOUS TRANSPLANTATION FOR HEMATOLOGIC MALIGNANCIES

Jeffrey R. Schriber, Amrita Krishnan, and Stephen J. Forman

In the last 30 years, combination chemotherapy regimens have been developed for treatment of the majority of hematologic malignancies and solid tumors. These regimens typically utilize agents with relatively nonoverlapping toxicities and different mechanisms of action to decrease the potential for drug resistance.[1] Such regimens are designed to maximize objective clinical responses while minimizing toxicity.

Although most malignancies demonstrate significant disease responsiveness to conventional dose chemotherapy, many such responses are incomplete or not durable. One strategy to overcome the lack of response is dose intensification. In laboratory models, delivery of the highest possible doses of chemotherapy is a frequent requirement for achieving long-term disease control.[2] These studies also indicate that disease resistance to a variety of cytotoxic agents can, in some tumor systems, be overcome with a 5- to 10-fold escalation in drug dose. The ability to overcome drug resistance by dose intensification is one of the fundamental requirements for autologous transplantation to be successful.

The second fundamental requirement is the ability to overcome the toxicity of dose-intensive therapy. By choosing agents where the primary dose limiting toxicity is hematologic, it is possible to harvest either marrow or peripheral blood stem cells to shorten or eliminate the duration of hematologic toxicity. Table 102–1 shows the list of commonly used chemotherapy drugs used in autologous transplant regimens with the organ-limiting toxicity when autologous stem cell support is provided.

RATIONALE FOR HIGH-DOSE THERAPY

Hyriniack and Bush introduced the concept of dose intensity (drug dose administered in mg/m²/week) for the purposes of being able to quantify the dose–response effect.[3] The dose–response effect is defined as the correlation of the effect of a drug with increasing doses. It was their hypothesis that dose intensity correlated with response, which in turn correlated with survival. Several assumptions are inherent in this hypothesis and include the following:

1. All drugs in a given regimen are therapeutically equivalent.
2. Synergy and cross-resistance between drugs do not play an active role.
3. The area under the curve is more important than peak drug concentrations.
4. Scheduling has no importance other than what is reflected in total dose intensity.

This suggests that chemotherapy regimens should be designed to maximize dose intensity and focus on the overall dose administered over time rather than achieving the highest peak dose. Laboratory models and clinical observations have demonstrated a dose–response relationship against a variety of tumors, leading to the concept that the highest possible doses should be incorporated into the design of the regimen.[4,5] Where possible, combinations of active, non-cross-resistant agents should be used to decrease the emergence of drug resistance. This latter consideration is based on studies by Skipper that estimate a spontaneous rate of mutation conferring resistance to a single drug to be in the order of 1 in 10^6 or 1 in 10^7 cancer cell.[2] The implication of this is that spontaneous mutations are highest in patients at diagnosis or at relapse (high tumor burden). The agents used in the regimen need to have different dose-limiting toxicities to avoid dose reduction and prevent additive toxicity. This would facilitate the delivery of full single-dose therapies of the drug. To minimize the rapid emergence of resistance, combinations of drugs in high-dose regimens with different mechanisms of action would limit the emergence of cross resistance.

Table 102–2 lists the malignant hematologic diseases for which utilizing high-dose chemotherapy or chemoradiotherapy and autologous transplant have been studied and showed improved outcome for patients. Unlike allogeneic transplant, where the high-dose preparatory regimen provides both cytoreduction to reduce or eliminate the tumor burden and immunosuppression to facilitate engraftment and a graft-versus-tumor effect, the regimen used for autologous transplant is designed to provide maximal antitumor activity limited only by the nonhematologic toxicity of the regimen.

CONTRIBUTION OF THE GRAFT TO RELAPSE

Despite the success of transplantation, the major cause for failure following autologous transplantation continues to be disease relapse. Relapsed disease can theoretically be due to the inability of the chemotherapy to eliminate the tumor burden that had remained in the body or due to tumor cells that may reside in the reinfused stem cell product. Even when there is no potential for the graft to be responsible for relapse, that is, a syngeneic (identical twin) graft, the cure rate is far from 100% and emphasizes that it is the tumor burden and its sensitivity to treatment that is responsible for the majority of relapses.[6]

In diseases where the bulk of the disease resides in the marrow, such as acute myelogenous leukemia (AML) and myeloma, the high likelihood of reinfusing tumor cells has led to the development of methods designed to eradicate tumor cells with the goal of achieving results comparable to syngeneic transplantation. Intuitively it would seem that all sources of autologous stem cells from patients with hematologic malignancies might contain cells that contribute to relapse, and studies of stem cell products have documented the presence of tumor cells in the grafts, including leukemia, myeloma, lymphoma, and breast cancer.[7–10]

Although tumor cells can be found in the stem cell product, what is critical is whether these cells are in fact clonogenic. Brenner et al have provided direct evidence that infusion of autologous tumor cells contributes to relapse following autologous transplantation. They incubated a third of harvested marrow from two children undergoing hematopoietic cell transplantation (HCT) for AML with the L and L-6 retroviral vector.[11] This vector contained the selectable neomycin resistance gene, which marked approximately 5% of cultured progenitor cells. Patients underwent transplantation with infusion of both marked and unmarked marrow cells. At the time of the relapse, some of the leukemia cells contained the neomycin resistance gene, demonstrating that these leukemia cells were present in the reinfused graft and could be detected at relapse.

Most of the phase II trials that have purged the graft use either chemotherapeutic agents (AML), monoclonal antibodies against differentiation antigens on B cell hematopoietic tumor cells (B-cell lymphoma), or enrichment devices that enrich stem cells and reduce tumor cell contamination of the graft. These studies suggest that

Table 102–1 Agents Used in Autologous Transplant Regimens and Their Dose-Limiting Toxicity

Agent	Dose-Limiting Toxicity
Etoposide	Mucositis, dermatitis
Cyclophosphamide	Cardiac failure, pulmonary failure, hemorrhagic cystitis
Cisplatinum	Renal failure, hearing loss
Carmustine (BCNU)	Interstitial pneumonitis, seizures
Total body irradiation	Interstitial pneumonitis, enteritis, mucositis
Melphalan	Mucositis
Busulfan	Venoocclusive disease of the liver Interstitial pneumonitis Seizures
Thiotepa	Mucositis
Mitoxantrone	Cardiac failure
Taxol	Neuropathy
Carboplatin	Neuropathy

Table 102–2 Autologous Transplantation for Hematologic Malignancy

1.	Acute myelogenous leukemia: First and second remission
2.	Hodgkin lymphoma: Induction failure, second remission and relapse
3.	Non-Hodgkin lymphoma: Intermediate with high-risk features in first remission, chemoresponsive relapse
4.	Low grade B-cell lymphoma: Second remission or chemosensitive relapse
5.	Mantle cell lymphoma: First remission, mantle cell in second, complete remission
6.	Peripheral T-cell lymphoma: First or second remission
7.	Multiple myeloma: Chemosensitive, responsive disease
8.	Chronic lymphocytic leukemia: In remission

purging reduces the number of clonogenic cells but often delays engraftment.[12–14]

Studies in lymphoma patients have correlated the ability to deplete contaminating malignant lymphoma cells from the graft with overall disease-free survival following transplant.[15] What is not clear is whether purging itself in this instance reduces the relapse rate or if the ability to purge the tumor is simply an indication of lower tumor burden, which may correlate with improved disease survival. In addition, strategies such as treatment of the patient with monoclonal antibody prior to peripheral blood stem cell collection reduce tumor cell contamination and in some circumstances such as B-cell lymphoma obviate the need for in vitro purging.[17,18]

Laboratory studies have shown purging to reduce tumor cell contamination in vitro. The benefit of purging of tumor cells in human transplant studies however has remained controversial and unproven. Retrospective analyses give some indication as to the potential value of purging; however, no prospective randomized trials addressing the efficacy of ex vivo purging have been reported.[12,14] Although tumor contamination clearly can play a role in relapse, the relative contribution compared to the total body burden of tumor cells appears to be low and definitive randomized trials would require huge numbers of patients and are impractical to consider at this time.

AUTOLOGOUS TRANSPLANTATION FOR HEMATOLOGIC MALIGNANCY

The first successful case of autologous HCT was reported in 1959. The case described a 2-year-old girl with recurrent acute lymphoblastic leukemia (ALL) who received total body irradiation (TBI) and followed by reinfusion of marrow, which had been obtained while she was in a remission. At the time of her therapy she was bedridden and a marrow showed 98% lymphoblasts.[18] Despite her advanced stage, she eventually recovered and 3 months later remained in remission. Since this case, tens of thousands of patients have undergone this therapy for a variety of diseases. This chapter summarizes the currently understood benefits and limitations of autologous transplant for hematopoietic malignancy.

ACUTE MYELOGENOUS LEUKEMIA

Initially, autologous transplant applied the same clinical approach previously utilized for patients undergoing allogeneic transplant. Patients with advanced disease were treated with high-dose chemotherapy and then received infusion of their own marrow, typically collected during remission rather than marrow from a human leukocyte antigen (HLA)-identical sibling. Although this approach produced a high remission rate, there were few, if any, cures. Similar to the strategy that evolved with allogeneic transplant, autologous HCT was subsequently used earlier in the clinical course of the disease (first complete remission), for those who lacked a histocompatible sibling donor or who were ineligible for allogeneic transplantation. The high-dose chemoradiotherapy regimens used for autologous HCT in AML are generally derived from those utilized for allogeneic transplant, the most common of which include TBI and cyclophosphamide, TBI, etoposide and cyclophosphamide, busulfan and etoposide, or busulfan and cyclophosphamide.[19–23]

Studies utilizing unpurged marrow, purged marrow, and peripheral blood stem cells have reported disease-free survivals for patients with AML transplanted in first remission ranging between 34%–70%, 41%–76%, and 35%–80% respectively.[24] Although these trials demonstrate the efficacy of autologous transplant, they have been criticized for including patients with a mixture of disease subtypes, cytogenetic risk factors, and pretransplant therapy. In addition, differences in the stem cell product source, manipulation, and in preparative regimens make comparisons between trials and conventional therapy difficult.

Despite the differences, numerous phase II and phase III trials have shown that autologous HCT is a useful alternative for patients who are not allogeneic HCT candidates, especially those with normal cytogenetics. Currently patients with AML with good-risk cytogenetics (8:21; inversion 16) do relatively well with repeated doses of high-dose ARA-C, whereas patients with poor-risk cytogenetics are best treated with an allogeneic approach. Many trials show a similar outcome for autologous HCT compared with allogeneic HCT and a higher cure rate compared with chemotherapy.[25] In one such trial, the European Organization for Research and Treatment of Cancer (EORTC) conducted a prospective randomized trial comparing three postremission treatment strategies in patients who were in a complete remission (CR) after induction therapy.[26] After receiving intensive consolidation therapy, patients with HLA-identical siblings were assigned to the allogeneic transplant arm. The remainder were randomized to receive high-dose treatment followed by autologous BMT or a second course of intensive chemotherapy. Two hundred fifty-four patients were randomized to autologous BMT using cyclophosphamide and either TBI or busulfan or to intensive therapy with high dose ARA-C and daunorubicin. Figure 102–1 shows the Kaplan–Meier estimates of disease-free survival by group. Patients who received intensive therapy had a predicted 4-year disease-free survival of 30% versus 48 and 55% for the autologous and allogeneic bone marrow transplantation (BMT) groups.

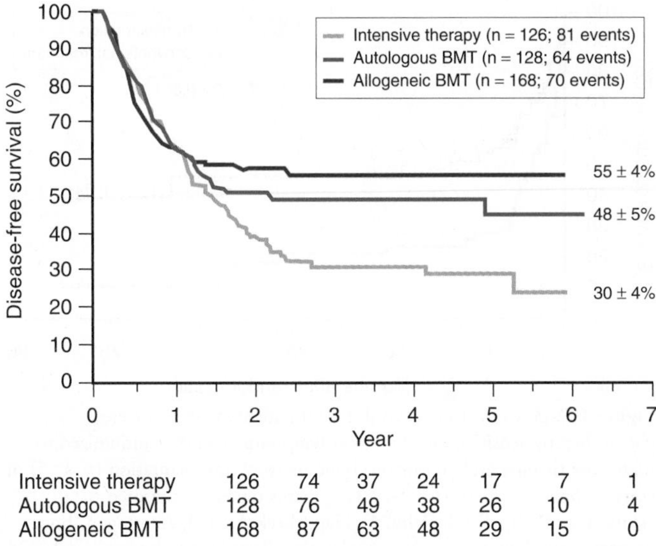

Figure 102–1 Kaplan–Meier estimates of disease-free survival for patients assigned to allogeneic bone marrow transplantation (BMT) (dotted line, n = 168), autologous BMT (dashed line, n = 128), or intensive consolidation chemotherapy (solid line, n = 126). Percentages represent estimated disease-free survival rates ± standard error. (Data from Zittoun RA, Mandelli F, Willemze R, et al: Autologous or allogeneic bone marrow transplantation compared with intensive chemotherapy in acute myelogenous leukemia. European Organization for Research and Treatment of Cancer (EORTC) and the Gruppo Italiano Malattie Ematologiche Maligne dell'Adulto (GIMEMA) Leukemia Cooperative Groups. N Engl J Med 332:217, 1995.)

Despite the apparent improvement over conventional therapy with autologous HCT, the most common cause for failure is relapse. Better definition of the risk factors that predict patients who will relapse and studies that examine patients prospectively based on these factors will further define the role of autologous HCT in patients who are in first remission. The detection of quantifiable minimal residual disease after achieving a remission is one approach being studied to determine the need and timing of transplant.[27]

The role of autologous HCT in second remission is better defined than in first remission as the cure rate with conventional therapy—regardless of the initial leukemic cell characteristics—for such patients is extremely low.[28] Patients have undergone transplant utilizing either chemically or immunologically purged marrow, or utilizing stem cells collected in first remission after achieving second remission. One study comparing autologous transplantation to unrelated donor transplant for advanced leukemia showed that although relapse rates were lower with unrelated donor transplantation, disease-free survival was not significantly different between the two types of transplant.[29]

For patients with acute promyelocytic leukemia in second remission, an analysis of the quantity of leukemic cells in the stem cell product can predict the outcome following autologous transplant. Those patients whose stem cells remain positive for the 15;17 translocation by polymerase chain reaction (PCR) have a high likelihood of relapse, whereas those patients whose reinduction therapy allowed the collection of a PCR-negative stem cell product are often cured by the autologous transplant. These studies indicate that autologous transplant with a PCR-negative stem cell product is a reasonable alternative for patients who do not have a suitable donor and for older patients who achieve a second remission and may not be candidates for allogeneic transplantation.[30]

Patients with newly diagnosed AML have significantly higher chances of long-term disease-free survival presently than two decades ago, largely as a result of better induction and consolidation chemotherapy regimens, supportive care, and the selective use of allogeneic and autologous transplantation. Importantly, knowledge of the cytogenetic and molecular biological characteristics of the patient's leukemia can be used to determine the appropriate therapy and whether the transplant should be performed during first or subsequent remission.

ACUTE LYMPHOBLASTIC LEUKEMIA

Improvements in induction and consolidation therapy for both adults and children with ALL have resulted in improved disease-free survival, particularly those with certain subgroups of disease.[31–33] For those patients with high-risk features, including the Philadelphia chromosome, high white count at diagnosis, and longer time to achieve remission, allogeneic transplantation has also been successfully utilized to prevent disease recurrence.[34] However, many patients with high-risk ALL or those with second CR do not have a readily available histocompatible related or unrelated donor and are candidates for autologous transplant. Despite this, the experience of autologous transplant, both in single institutional studies and larger randomized trials, has been disappointing.[35] At present, there is no clear role for autologous HCT for patients with ALL outside of a clinical trial designed to reduce relapse.

CHRONIC LYMPHOCYTIC LEUKEMIA

Although a large number of patients have undergone autologous transplant for acute leukemia, myeloma, lymphoma, and Hodgkin lymphoma, there have been relatively few studies addressing the issue of autologous transplant in CLL.[36–38] The role of transplant has been limited by the older age of the patient population, and difficulty collecting sufficient stem cells that are not contaminated with leukemic cells. Therefore, patients undergoing transplant represent a highly selected group who have had a very good response to therapy. Although the complete response rate after transplant is high, the overall impact on disease-free survival is difficult to ascertain, with no studies showing a disease-free survival plateau.[39] Nevertheless, studies suggest that it is feasible to perform in selected patients and may extend the duration of remission.[40,41] Recent progress in the initial treatment of CLL, particularly with the addition of anti-CD20 monoclonal antibodies, has increased the number of patients who achieve a complete morphologic remission and may expand the possibility of successful autologous transplant in patients with CLL.

HODGKIN LYMPHOMA

Hodgkin lymphoma, even when advanced, can often be cured with standard doses of combination chemotherapy. However, patients who relapse can achieve further remissions with chemotherapy or radiation treatment but rarely are cured with standard therapy alone. The use of high-dose therapy followed by autologous transplant can produce long-term disease-free survival in selected patients with advanced Hodgkin lymphoma.[42] Reports from single institutions and cooperative group trials indicate that between 30% and 65% of selected Hodgkin lymphoma patients can become long-term disease-free survivors after autologous transplant,[43–49] including some patients with primary refractory disease.[50,51]

A large randomized phase III trial comparing high-dose chemotherapy and stem cell rescue versus standard salvage chemotherapy in patients with relapsed Hodgkin lymphoma was conducted to determine the role of dose intensity on disease response and survival.[52] In this trial, 161 patients with relapsed Hodgkin lymphoma were randomized to receive two cycles of Dexa-BEAM followed by either two subsequent courses of Dexa-BEAM or high dose BEAM and stem cell rescue for all patients with evidence for chemosensitive disease. One hundred seventeen patients were deemed chemosensitive and 56

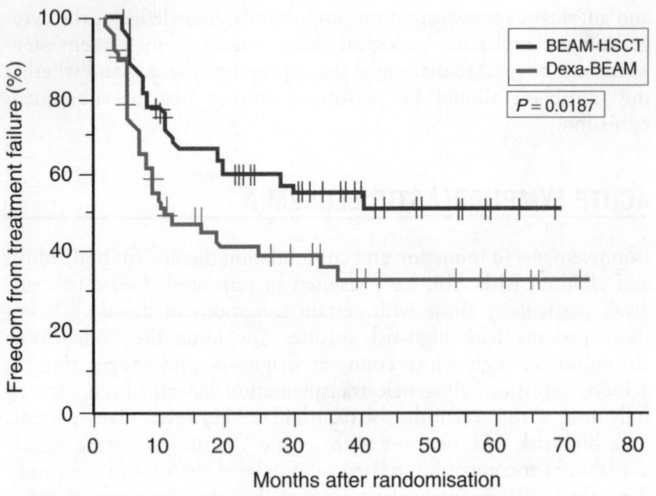

Number of patients							
BEAM-HSCT	61	43	34	25	13	8	7	0
Dexa-BEAM	56	27	20	15	10	8	5	1

Figure 102–2 Freedom from progression for patients with relapsed chemosensitive Hodgkin lymphoma randomized to conventional therapy (Dexa BEAM) or high dose therapy and autologous stem cell rescue (BEAM HSCT). (Data from Schmitz N, Pfistner B, Sextro M, et al: Aggressive conventional chemotherapy compared with high-dose chemotherapy with autologous haematopoietic stem-cell transplantation for relapsed chemosensitive Hodgkin's disease: A randomised trial. Lancet 359:2065, 2002.)

underwent standard therapy, with 61 randomized to the high-dose chemotherapy arm. Freedom from treatment failure as shown in Fig. 102–2 was significantly better (55 vs 34%) for patients who underwent autologous transplantation ($P < 0.019$). This treatment advantage was maintained for patients who had early or late relapses. The median time to treatment failure for those patients who received standard chemotherapy was 12 months and has not been reached for the high-dose arm (median follow-up 39 months). There were however no differences as yet in overall survival between the two groups. Of note, 8 of the 17 relapses that occurred following standard chemotherapy had since proceeded to autologous transplantation. This report confirmed the results of a smaller randomized trial performed by the British National Lymphoma group.[53]

An international effort analyzing a large number of patients with Hodgkin lymphoma suggested that there are disease characteristics that predict a high likelihood of relapse after conventional therapy. Several factors were identified, each of which reduced tumor control by 7% to 8%.[54] Among these poor prognostic factors at diagnosis are anemia (Hb < 10.5 g/dL), stage IV disease, male sex, age over 45, albumin less than 4 mg/dL, WBC greater than 15,000/μL, lymphocyte count less than 600/μL (or <8%). Patients with four or more of these features have a poor prognosis and could potentially benefit from early autologous transplantation. Pilot trials for the use of high-dose chemotherapy and transplantation as part of the initial management of Hodgkin lymphoma have been conducted with very optimistic results.[55] To date, no randomized trials comparing early versus late transplant have been performed to answer this question in this group of patients at high risk for relapse.

The preparative regimens used in autologous transplantation for Hodgkin lymphoma have depended on combination chemotherapy, most commonly combinations of Carmustine (BCNU), VP-16 with either cyclophosphamide (CBV) or cytarabine and melphalan (BEAM).[44–52] Augmented CBV regimens have been shown to improve long-term disease control in phase II trials. Given its known effectiveness in the treatment of Hodgkin lymphoma, some programs have also used TBI or total lymphoid irradiation.[48] However, many patients who require transplant have had prior mediastinal mantle radiation, thus precluding the use of TBI as a component of the

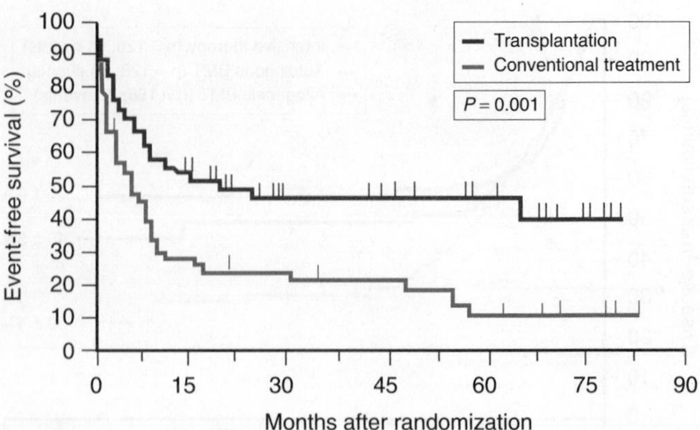

Figure 102–3 Event-free survival in 109 patients with recurrent, chemotherapy-sensitive non-Hodgkin lymphoma (NHL) randomized to high-dose therapy and autologous bone marrow transplantation ($n = 55$) or conventional treatment ($n = 54$). Tick marks represent censored data. (Data from Philip T, Guglielmi C, Hagenbeek A, et al: Autologous bone marrow transplantation as compared with salvage chemotherapy in relapses of chemotherapy-sensitive non-Hodgkin's lymphoma. N Engl J Med 333:1540, 1995.)

treatment regimen. The combination of TBI and prior mantle radiation increases prohibitively the risk of cardiac and pulmonary toxicity and likely increases the risk for subsequent development of myelodysplastic syndrome (MDS) or AML. In some cases, irradiation directed to site of bulky or refractory disease can be used following transplantation, to help reduce the chance of relapse in those areas.

NON-HODGKIN LYMPHOMA

Like other tumors, the basis for high-dose chemotherapy and autologous stem cell transplant in non-Hodgkin lymphoma (NHL) is that resistance to standard therapy can be overcome by escalation of doses of drugs or radiation beyond limiting marrow toxicity. The initial reports of successfully incorporating high-dose therapy with autologous transplant were from the National Cancer Institute, where BACT (carmustine, cytarabine, cyclophosphamide and thioguanine) chemotherapy followed by autologous bone marrow transplantation eradicated lymphoma in some patients with "high grade" lymphoma previously considered incurable.[56] These observations led to the development of several trials, including a randomized trial documenting the efficacy of autologous transplant in patients with lymphoma.

INTERMEDIATE GRADE B CELL LYMPHOMA

Several investigations have reported a cure rate of 35% to 40% of patients with chemotherapy-sensitive diffuse aggressive non-Hodgkin lymphoma with high-dose therapy and autologous transplant.[57] These studies were received with great enthusiasm because under ordinary circumstances, less than 10% of patients with relapsed lymphoma can be cured with conventional salvage therapy. Eventually an international randomized trial demonstrated that second-line chemotherapy with cisplatin, cytarabine, and decadron (DHAP) followed by consolidation with high-dose chemotherapy with carmustine, etoposide, cytarabine, and cyclophosphamide (BEAC) and autologous transplant was more effective than continued conventional chemotherapy alone.[58] Patients randomized to the transplant arm had significantly higher CR rates (84% vs 44%). At 5 years, event-free survival (46% vs 12%; $P = .001$) and OS (53% vs 32%; $P = .038$) were significantly superior in transplanted patients (Fig. 102–3). This study was limited to patients under the age of 60 who had achieved a CR after primary therapy and who had no known

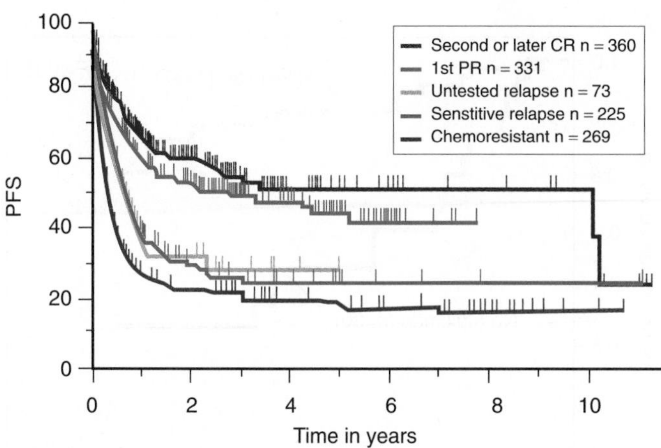

Figure 102–4 Progression-free survival of all adult non-Hodgkin lymphoma (NHL) patients after HDC by status at time of HDC. (Data from Armitage JO: Bone marrow transplantation. N Engl J Med 330:827, 1994.)

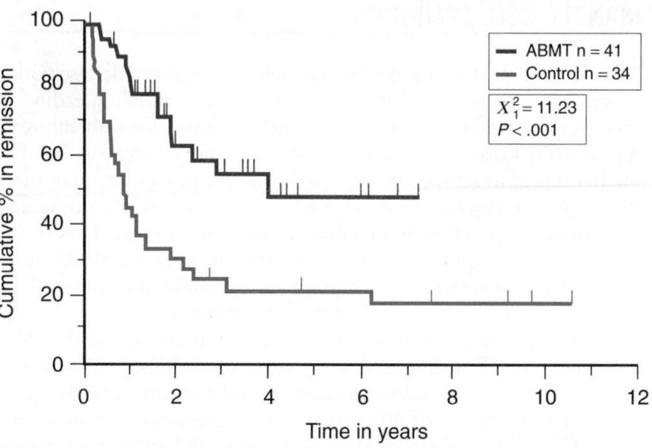

Figure 102–5 Freedom from progression curve in 41 patients with follicular lymphoma in second remission treated with CY/TBI plus autologous bone marrow transplantation compared with 34 historical control patients treated with chemotherapy at St. Bartholomew's Hospital. (Data from Rohatiner AZ, Johnson PW, Price CG, et al: Myeloablative therapy with autologous bone marrow transplantation as consolidation therapy for recurrent follicular lymphoma. J Clin Oncol 12:1177, 1994.)

marrow or CNS involvement and had responded to second-line therapy.

The issue of chemosensitivity appears to play an important part in the overall long-term disease-free survival of patients with lymphoma who undergo autologous transplant. Patients refractory to initial therapy often responded to transplant but suffered a relapse relatively quickly.[59] In addition, those patients with lymphoma who had responded to primary treatment but proved resistant to second-line treatment also had a relatively low response rate. In contrast, patients responding to conventional therapy did well after subsequent autologous transplant. Figure 102–4 shows the long-term disease-free survival for patients with advanced lymphoma depending upon the remission status and sensitivity to chemotherapy.

Some investigators have attempted to identify patients who had poor prognostic features at diagnosis and who were at high risk for relapse even with achievement of a complete remission. These phase II studies showed that early transplant while in first remission resulted in high disease-free survival in patients who would be expected to have had a greater chance of relapse with standard therapy.[60] A large phase III trial comparing chemotherapy alone to chemotherapy followed by transplant in patients with intermediate high-grade lymphoma who had one or more unfavorable prognostic features did not show a significant difference in event-free overall survival in the study arms.[61] However, an analysis limited to poor risk subsets demonstrated significant benefit in disease-free survival for patients with high-dose therapy and autologous transplant.[62] The transplant arm had significantly higher disease-free (55% vs 39%; $P < .02$) and overall survival rates (64% vs 49%; $P < .04$) compared to the sequential chemotherapy arm. Another smaller study randomized high-risk patients to MACOP B for 12 weeks versus high-dose sequential (HDS) therapy and autologous transplantation.[63] At a median 55-month follow-up, the CR rate was 96% in the HDS group, compared with 70% in the MACOP-B group ($P = .001$). Rates of freedom from disease progression (84% vs 49%; $P < .001$), freedom from relapse (88% vs 70%; $P = .055$), and event-free survival (76% vs 49%; $P = .004$) were all significantly superior in the HDS group. Overall survival at 7 years favored the HDS group (81% vs 55%; $P = 0.09$). Currently a large national trial is being conducted to determine if patients with high-risk lymphoma undergoing treatment in the era of rituxan treatment have improved survival if transplanted early or at the time of relapse.[64]

Patients with primary refractory NHL represent a very difficult subset to treat. Fortunately, true refractoriness is relatively rare. Kewalramani et al[65] examined the outcomes of 85 patients who underwent second-line chemotherapy with ICE following failure with first-line induction therapy. Patients were classified as induction partial responders (IPR) or induction failures (IF) according to their response to initial therapy. Forty-three (51%) had chemosensitive disease with no difference in response seen between those who were IPR or IF. Of 42 patients who ultimately underwent ABMT, the 3-year OS and EFS rates were 53% and 44%, respectively, suggesting that even patients with induction failure, as long as they remain chemosensitive, can be cured with transplantation. An analysis of the Autologous Blood and Marrow Transplant Registry study led to similar conclusions.[66]

LOW GRADE B-CELL LYMPHOMA

A number of phase II trials have been conducted to determine the curative potential of high-dose therapy and autologous transplant in patients with "low grade" lymphomas.[67–70] Even if the approach was noncurative, the prolongation of remission itself would be a worthwhile goal for this group of patients. Similar to diffuse aggressive high-grade lymphoma, selection of appropriate patients is key for the success of high-dose therapy and autologous transplant in low-grade lymphoma. The long natural history of patients with low-grade lymphoma makes it difficult to determine if a proportion of patients are cured or had their survival prolonged by high-dose therapy and autologous transplant. Figure 102–5 illustrates what is considered to be the best available historical comparison for patients with recurrent low-grade lymphoma. This analysis from St. Bartholomew's Hospital in London showed that freedom from recurrence and survival for patients treated with CY and FTBI plus purged autologous marrow were improved compared with chemotherapy controls matched for remission status. Although there was a statistically significant advantage in disease control with a high-dose approach, this did not translate into a survival benefit.[67]

Similar to large-cell lymphoma, several groups have attempted to identify patients with low-grade lymphoma with poor-risk features who should undergo transplant during first remission. Disease-free survival in these studies was extended compared to remission durations expected with chemotherapy, and overall survivals to date have been excellent.[71,72] However, based on available data, patients with low-grade lymphoma who have brief initial remission (less than 1 year) and who are responsive to chemotherapy with standard treatment represent a group of patients with very short survivals after relapse and are the most appropriate candidates for high-dose therapy and autologous transplant.

MANTLE CELL LYMPHOMA

Mantle cell lymphoma is a relatively newly recognized disease with a unique phenotype and characteristic genetic abnormality leading to increased expression of cyclin D_1, which accounts for only approximately 6% of cases of adult NHL (see Chapters 79 and 80).[73,74] The median age of onset is 65 years, and the disease predominates in men. Although the disease often responds well to initial chemotherapy, remissions are short, with a median survival of 3 to 4 years. No chemotherapeutic regimen has been shown to be curative, which leads to further investigations of high-dose chemotherapy followed by autologous HCT in first or subsequent remission.[73,74]

There have been a number of single-center trials that have studied autologous HCT in first and subsequent remissions.[75–77] Studies at the University of Nebraska evaluated clinical outcomes and prognostic factors in a group of 40 patients who underwent high-dose chemotherapy and autologous HCT for mantle cell lymphoma between 1991 and 1998.[76] In this report with a median follow-up of 24 months, the 2-year EFS was 36% and the OS was 65%. The only factor that was associated with the poor EFS rate was the number of prior chemotherapy regimens, similar to the prognostic features observed in transplantation for low-grade lymphoma. Those patients who had received 3 or more prior therapies had a 2-year EFS of 0% as compared to 45% for those who had received fewer than 3 therapies ($P = .004$).[76]

A larger, retrospective analysis was performed using data from the EBMT and ABMTR registries on the outcome of 195 mantle cell lymphoma patients who had received an autologous HCT.[78] After a median follow-up of 3.9 years, the 2-year and 5-year PFS rates were 55% and 33%, and OS rates were 76% and 50%, respectively. Patients with chemosensitive disease who were not in a first CR were 2.99 times more likely to succumb to their disease over time than patients transplanted in first CR ($P < .001$), confirming the results observed by many institutions. These reports suggest that patients treated with autologous HCT in first CR have better outcome than patients receiving autologous HCT in subsequent relapses, because of better disease control and decreased disease relapse.

On the basis of these observations, the European Mantle Cell Lymphoma Network performed a prospective randomized trial comparing myeloablative radiochemotherapy followed by autologous HCT to an interferon-α maintenance program in patients in first CR. In their study, 122 patients were assessable; 62 proceeded to autologous HCT and 60 received interferon-α. The patients who underwent the transplantation had a significantly longer PFS, with a median of 39 months compared with 17 months in the interferon arm ($P = .01$). In a subset analysis, patients undergoing transplantation in CR had the greatest benefit. Although longer follow-up is required to determine the difference in OS, collectively, the data suggest that autologous HCT may improve prognosis when performed as part of a first-line treatment strategy in patients with mantle cell lymphoma. However, many patients continue to relapse and as a result autologous HCT does not appear to be curative in the majority of patients. The apparently strong GVL affect seen in mantle cell lymphoma has led to the consideration of reduced-intensity allogeneic transplant in patients in relapse or who fail to achieve a CR with initial therapy.[79,80]

RITUXIMAB AND AUTOLOGOUS STEM CELL TRANSPLANT

Rituximab, a chimeric IgG1 monoclonal antibody that targets CD20, has revolutionized the treatment of B-cell NHL. Two randomized trials have shown that rituximab improves the response rate and survival in patients with advanced-stage DLCL-B when administered in combination with standard chemotherapy (see Chapters 89 and 90). Given its efficacy in depleting B cells with limited toxicity, rituximab has been incorporated into HDT and autologous HCT for DLCL-B as in vivo purging, as part of a high-dose regimen or as maintenance therapy posttransplant to prevent relapse.[82–84]

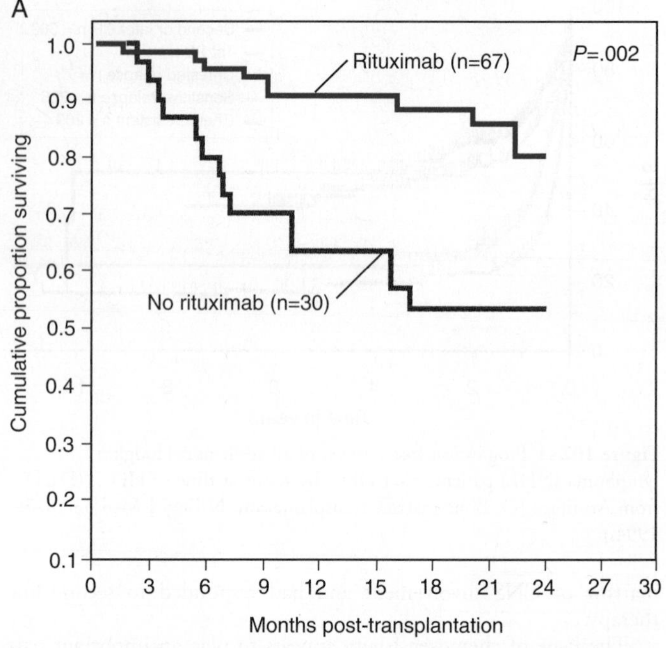

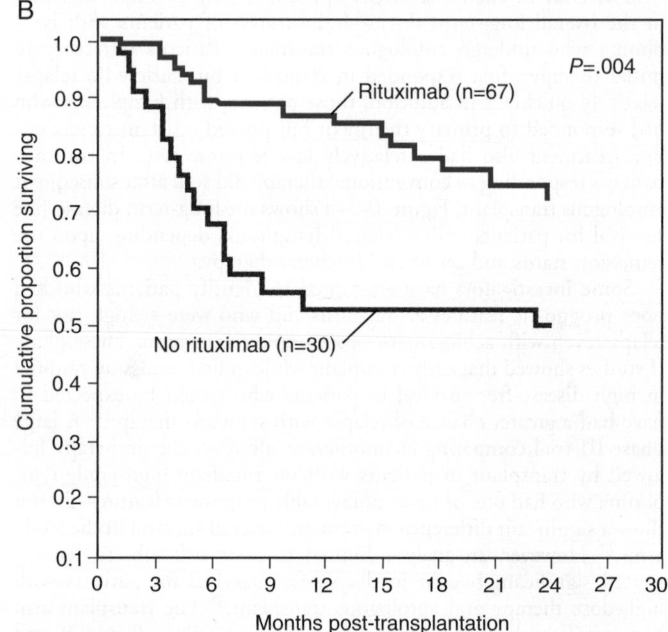

Figure 102–6 Kaplan–Meier estimates of survival (A) and disease free suivival (B) for patients with non-Hodgkin lymphoma by treatment group. (Data from Khouri IF, Saliba RM, Hosing C, et al: Concurrent administration of high-dose rituximab before and after autologous stem cell transplantation for relapsed aggressive B cell non-Hodgkin's lymphomas. J Clin Oncol 23:2240, 2005.)

Khouri et al evaluated the efficacy and safety of administering high-dose rituximab in combination with high-dose BEAM and autologous HCT in 67 patients with recurrent aggressive B-cell NHL.[84] Rituximab was administered during stem cell mobilization at 375 mg/m^2 1 day before chemotherapy and 1000 mg/m^2 7 days after chemotherapy and on days 1 and 8 after transplant. The results of this treatment were retrospectively compared with a historical control group receiving the same preparative regimen without rituximab. With the median follow-up time for the study group of 20 months, the 2-year OS was 80% for the study group compared with 53% for the control group ($P = .002$). The 2-year disease-free survival rates were 67% and 43%, respectively, for the study group and the control group ($P = .004$) (Fig. 102–6). The median time to neutrophil recovery of more than 500 cells/μL was 11 days in the rituximab group and 10 days for the matched control group ($P = .001$).

Horwitz et al evaluated the feasibility and toxicity of rituximab post autologous HCT in 35 patients with B-cell NHL (25 DLCL-B) who underwent HDT followed by refulling a purged autologous graft.[85] Rituximab schedule was 4 weekly infusions (375 mg/m^2) starting on day 42 and repeated for a second course at 6 months after transplant. With a median follow-up of 30 months, the 2-year EFS rate was 83% and the OS rate was 88%. For 21 patients with relapsed or refractory DLCL-B, the EFS and OS rates were 81% and 85%, respectively. Grade 3 to 4 neutropenia occurred in 54% of patients; however, the incidence of infection was not increased. Delayed B-cell recovery was observed in all patients and suppressed immunoglobulin G level and low pneumococcal titer were observed in a subset of patients. These results are promising and further studies are required to establish whether posttransplant rituximab can improve cure rates in patients with relapsed or refractory DLCL-B.

RADIOIMMUNOTHERAPY-BASED TRANSPLANT FOR B-CELL LYMPHOMA

Recently, radioimmunotherapy (RIT) has been utilized to improve disease control in patients with B-cell lymphoma. Radioisotope-labeled monoclonal antibodies provide a mechanism by which radioactivity can be directly targeted to tumor sites while sparing normal tissues (see Chapter 82). B-cell lymphomas are attractive targets for RIT because of their radiosensitivity, their well-defined surface antigens, and the availability of multiple monoclonal antibodies to those antigens. There are two US Food and Drug Administration-approved radioisotope-labeled monoclonal antibodies for treatment of relapsed or refractory B-cell NHL: the yttrium 90-labeled ibritumomab tiuxetan (^{90}Y-Zevalin, Biogen Idec, San Diego, CA) and the iodine 131-labeled tositumomab (Bexxar, Corixa, Seattle, WA). In an attempt to deliver target radiation to tumor sites, RIT has been evaluated in myeloablative trials with and without high-dose chemotherapy. Press et al pioneered the use of high-dose RIT in conjunction with autologous HCT in two different trials.[86,87] The first trial used high-dose ^{131}I-tositumomab with autologous bone marrow rescue in 43 patients with B-cell lymphoma in relapse.[86]

Nineteen patients received therapeutic infusions of 234 to 777 mCi of ^{131}I-labeled antibodies followed by autologous marrow infusion. Sixteen patients achieved a CR, two a partial response, and one a minor response. Nine of 16 complete responders have remained in CR for 3 to 53 months. Toxicities included myelosuppression, nausea, infection, and two episodes of cardiopulmonary toxicity. The second study was a phase I/II trial of high-dose ^{131}I-tositumomab, etoposide, and cyclophosphamide and autologous HCT in 52 (38 indolent, 14 aggressive) NHL patients.[87] The maximum tolerated dose of ^{131}I-tositumomab that could be safely combined with high-dose etoposide and cyclophosphamide delivered 25 Gy to critical normal organs. The regimen was well tolerated, with a 15% incidence of grades III and IV toxicity. The estimated OS and PFS at 2 years were 83% and 68%, respectively. The results compared favorably with those in a nonrandomized control group of patients who underwent autologous HCT using TBI, etoposide, and cyclophosphamide during the same period (53% OS and 36% PFS at 2 years) (Fig. 102–7).

Nademanee et al[88] evaluated high-dose ^{90}Y-ibritumomab tiuxetan in combination with high-dose etoposide 40 to 60 mg/kg and cyclophosphamide 100 mg/kg in 31 patients with poor-risk or relapsed B-cell NHL, including 14 patients with DLCL-B.[88] The median number of prior chemotherapy regimens was two (range, 1–6). All but two had received rituximab either alone ($n = 8$) or in combination with chemotherapy ($n = 21$). The median ^{90}Y-ibritumomab tiuxetan dose delivered was 72 mCi (range, 37–105) to deliver a target dose of 1000 cGy to the highest normal organ. The treatment was well tolerated, with mucositis and neutropenic fever being the most

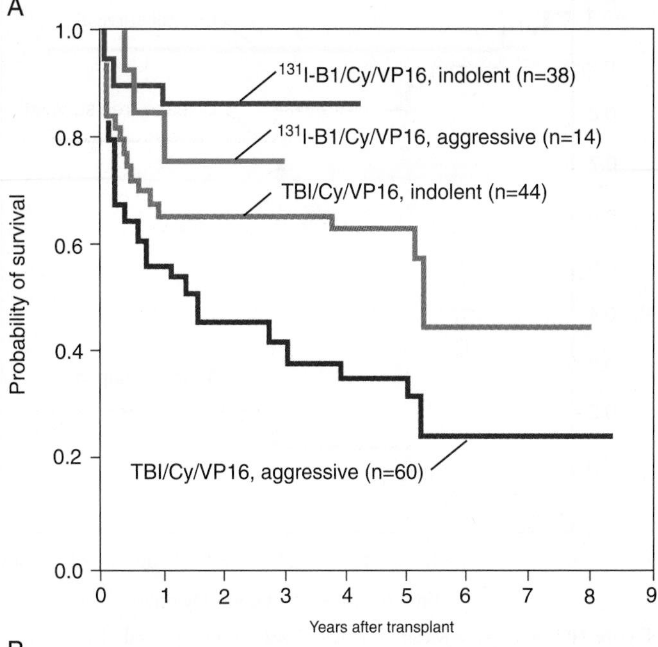

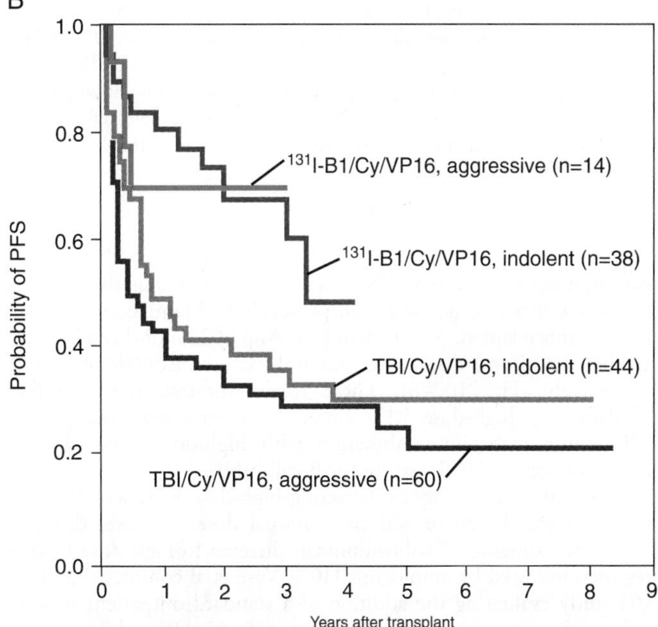

Figure 102–7 Survival analyses according to type of lymphoma. **A**, Overall survival in 38 patients with relapsed indolent lymphomas and 14 patients with relapsed aggressive lymphomas treated with ^{131}I-tositumomab, etoposide, cyclophosphamide, and ASCT and in 44 patients with relapsed indolent lymphomas and 60 patients with relapsed aggressive lymphomas treated with external-beam TBI (1.5 Gy twice a day for 4 days), etoposide (60 mg/kg), cyclophosphamide (100 mg/kg), and ASCT. **B**, Progression-free survival in 38 patients with relapsed indolent lymphomas and 14 patients with relapsed aggressive lymphomas treated with ^{131}I-tositumomab, etoposide, cyclophosphamide, and ASCT and in 44 patients with relapsed indolent lymphomas and 60 patients with relapsed aggressive lymphomas treated with external-beam TBI (1.5 Gy twice a day for 4 days), etoposide (60 mg/kg), cyclophosphamide (100 mg/kg), and ASCT. (Data from Press OW, Eary JF, Gooley T, et al: A phase I/II trial of iodine-131-tositumomab (anti-CD20), etoposide, cyclophosphamide, and autologous stem cell transplantation for relapsed B-cell lymphomas. Blood 96:2934, 2000.)

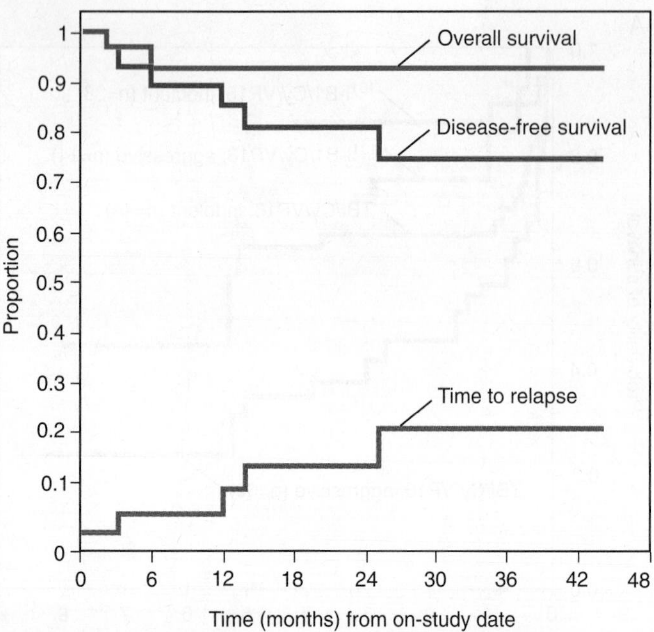

Figure 102–8 Kaplan–Meier estimated 2-year overall survival, disease-free survival, and relapse for 31 patients who received high-dose ^{90}Y-ibritumomab tixetan etoposide and cyclophosphamide plus ASCT in NHL. (Data from Nademanee A, Forman S, Molina A, et al: A phase 1/2 trial of high-dose yttrium-90-ibritumomab tiuxetan in combination with high-dose etoposide and cyclophosphamide followed by autologous stem cell transplantation in patients with poor-risk or relapsed non-Hodgkin's lymphoma. Blood 106:2896, 2005.)

common acute toxicities. There was no delay in engraftment. All patients with active disease at transplant achieved remission, although five patients relapsed. At a median follow-up of 22 months, the 2-year estimated OS and disease-free survival rates were 92% and 78%, respectively (Fig. 102–8). These results indicate the feasibility of delivering high-dose RIT, either ^{90}Y-ibritumomab tiuxetan or ^{131}I-tositumomab, in combination with high-dose chemotherapy in an autologous HCT setting for B-cell NHL.

Given the complexity of delivering high-dose RIT, several investigators have chosen to add conventional doses or lower doses of ^{131}I-tositumomab or ^{90}Y-ibritumomab tiuxetan to high-dose BEAM regimen followed by autologous HCT. Vose et al conducted a phase I/II study evaluating the addition of a standard outpatient dose of ^{131}I-tositumomab in four doses cohorts (30, 45, 60, and 75 cGy) to the BEAM regimen in 23 patients with chemotherapy-refractory or multiply relapsed aggressive B-cell NHL.[89] The treatment was well tolerated without additional toxicity. The CR rate after transplantation was 57% and the overall response rate was 65%. At a median follow-up of 38 months, the 3-year EFS was 39% and OS was 55%. Winter et al evaluated escalating doses of ^{90}Y-ibritumomab tiuxetan to deliver 100, 300, and up to 1300 cGy to normal organs followed by high-dose BEAM and autologous HCT.[90] Thirty-five patients with B-cell NHL were treated, including 16 with DLCL-B and 7 with transformed NHL. The median number of chemotherapy regimens was three. All patients received individualized RIT doses, which ranged from 100 to 1300 cGy. Thirteen patients received ^{90}Y-ibritumomab tiuxetan doses of 0.5 mCi/kg or higher. There was no delay in hematopoietic recovery. One patient experienced asymptomatic decreases in diffusion capacity less than 50% and one had grade IV hepatotoxicity. At a median follow-up of 14 months, the median survival had not been reached. Three-year OS and PFS were 65% and 42%, respectively. Krishnan et al evaluated the combination of standard-dose ^{90}Y-ibritumomab tiuxetan 0.4 mCi/kg and high-dose BEAM followed by autologous HCT in 24 older patients (median age 60 years) with relapsed aggressive B-cell NHL (10 DLCL, three transformed).[91] Median granulocytes and platelet engraftment occurred at days 11 and 13, respectively. At a median follow-up of 13 months, OS and PFS were 98% and 74%, with a relapse rate of 21%. The regimen was well tolerated even in these older patients and toxicity was similar to high-dose BEAM. These studies suggest that a standard dose of RIT can be added to high-dose chemotherapy in the autologous HCT setting without additional toxicity. Additional studies with RIT and autologous HCT are ongoing and preliminary results suggest that these approaches may be superior to conventional high-dose regimens.

PERIPHERAL T-CELL LYMPHOMA

Mature T- and natural killer cell lymphomas constitute a rare and heterogeneous group of neoplasms. Their incidences vary according to the geographic region and ethnic origin of the population. In general, peripheral T-cell lymphomas are defined by their postthymic origin, in comparison to precursor T-cell lymphomas, which includes lymphoblastic lymphoma. The importance of the T-cell phenotype as well as the other subtypes of the disease is being increasingly recognized as separate clinical-pathologic entities, with the primary chemotherapy and transplant approaches being evaluated in light of this new knowledge. The revised European/American Lymphoma Classification utilizes information regarding morphology, phenotype, and molecular and clinical information to provide a more unified scheme for all lymphoid malignancies, and included peripheral T-cell lymphoma. This provided the basis for the recently published WHO classification with the important separation of cutaneous, systemic, and anaplastic types of T lymphomas. Reports based on earlier classifications did not distinguish prognosis among B- and T-cell lymphomas. However comprehensive studies in recent years demonstrated that the T-cell phenotype has a negative impact in overall survival. (See Chapters 78–80 for details of treatment and classification of peripheral T-cell lymphoma).

Similar to research work in distinguishing the various histologies and molecular characteristics of B-cell lymphomas and their impact on treatment, the same approach has now been conducted in the analysis of peripheral T-cell lymphomas. For example, anaplastic large-cell lymphoma, identified by its very pleomorphic appearance and expression of CD30 on tumor cells, can be separated into those that demonstrate overexpression of the anaplastic lymphoma kinase (ALK) and those that do not. The abnormal expression is due to a characteristic acquired genetic abnormality that leads to overexpression of the ALK gene on chromosome 2. This results in a different clinical outcome with a 5-year overall survival for patients with ALK-positive, systemic anaplastic T-cell lymphoma, between 65% and 90% compared with 30% to 40% for a group of patients whose tumor was ALK-negative. In addition, the International Prognostic Index (IPI) utilized to define prognosis among patients with B-cell lymphoma is also applicable to patients with T-cell lymphoma. Given the varying prognosis among patients with these diseases, transplantation has also been utilized in patients who present with poor prognosis disease and with patients with relapsed disease.

With the poor outcome in most patients with peripheral T-cell lymphomas utilizing CHOP-type treatment, several studies have been conducted to study autologous HCT as consolidation therapy with patients with peripheral T-cell lymphoma, including anaplastic large-cell lymphoma.[92–94] In one study made up of predominantly young patients, an encouraging 5-year overall survival of 80% was reported after initial chemotherapy followed by autologous transplant.[93] A recent study of patients with advanced disease and a high IPI showed the 2-year overall survival and disease-free survival at 83% for patients transplanted after achievement of remission, compared with 45% for those patients transplanted beyond first remission, with little differences between the various types of T-cell lymphoma, including anaplastic large-cell lymphoma, peripheral T-cell lymphoma, and angioimmunoblastic lymphadenopathy.[95] Patients with relapsed peripheral T-cell lymphoma who demonstrate chemosensitivity appear to have approximately a 35% disease-free survival rate.

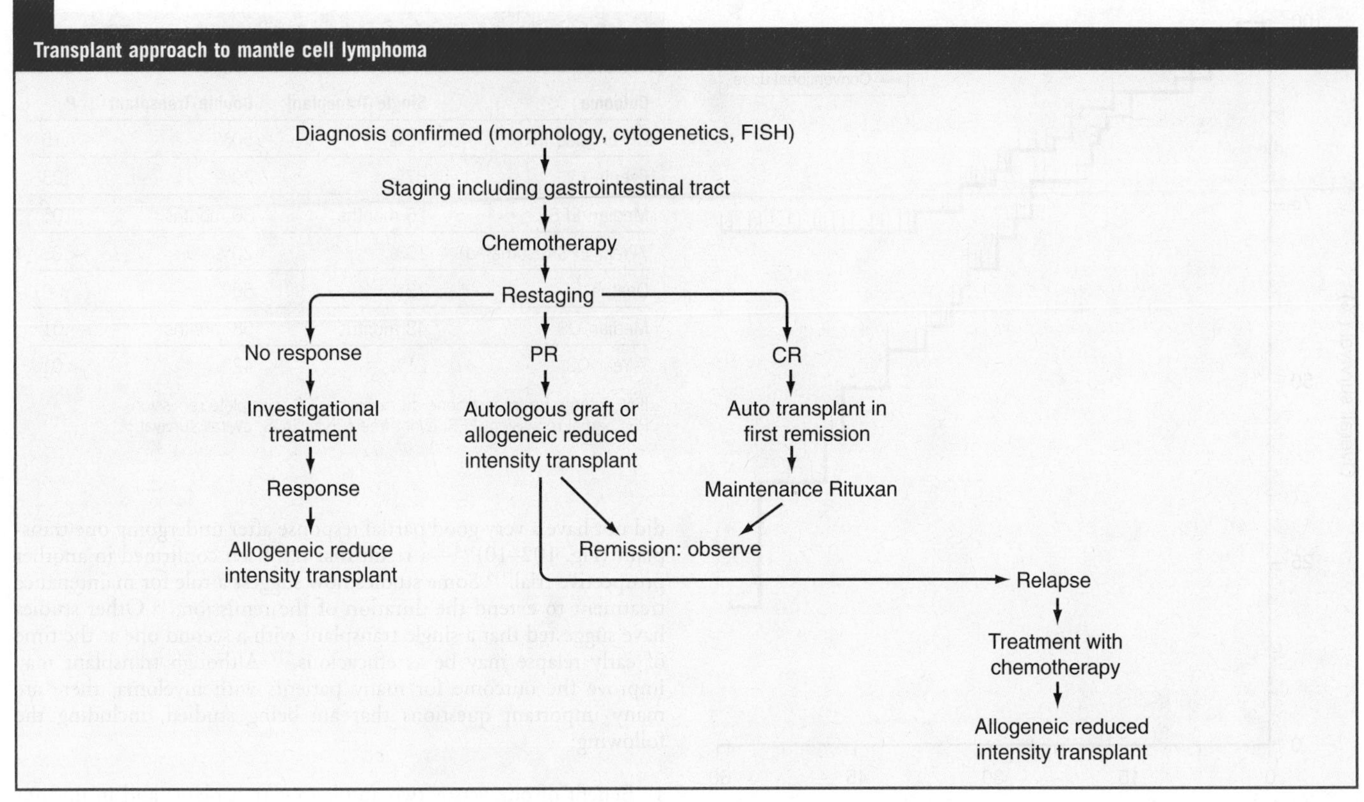

Patients with refractory disease have much less favorable outcome, very similar to what is seen in relapsed B-cell lymphoma. Although the studies are smaller than have been conducted with B-cell lymphoma and randomized trials are limited, the data suggest that those patients with peripheral T-cell lymphoma with a high IPI or ALK-negative disease are reasonable candidates for treatment with autologous HCT early in the course of disease. For patients with relapsed disease, a transplant may be the only curative option.

MULTIPLE MYELOMA

Multiple myeloma is part of a spectrum of disorders referred to as plasma cell dyscrasias that includes benign conditions such as monoclonal gammopathy (see Chapter 87) and accounts for approximately 10% of hematologic tumors with a median presentation age of approximately 65 years. Symptomatic multiple myeloma (MM) requires initiation of systemic therapy utilizing combination chemotherapy, most commonly with thalidomide and dexamethasone, with new combination therapy showing improved response and depth of remission using agents such as thalidomide, lenalidomide and bortezomib.[96] Very few patients achieve a true complete remission and the median survival is approximately 36 months.

High-dose cytotoxic therapy combined with autologous transplant was first considered for MM in 1986, resulting in some patients' having prolonged survival with minimal disease activity.[97] In 1983, investigators from the Royal Marsden Hospital explored high-dose melphalan alone at a dose of 140 mg/m².[98] The observation of true complete remissions following this procedure performed without hematopoietic growth factor and stem cell support led to the introduction of autologous transplant in the mid-1980s initially in support of higher-dose melphalan or melphalan combined with TBI.[99,100] An underlying hypothesis in these trials was that the reinfusion of typically hypoproliferative tumor cells with low in vitro clonogenic potential would not contribute significantly to disease recurrence despite their presence in the marrow graft. This led to studies focused on high-dose therapy given during the early phase of disease as well as the exploration of multiple cycles of high-dose therapy, each supported by stem cells.

A number of phase II studies indicated a high response rate as well as apparent improved disease-free survival in patients undergoing high-dose therapy for MM.[101–103] These studies have achieved a 40% to 50% complete remission rate with a median duration of progression-free survival of 24 to 36 months.[104] Patients with chemosensitive tumor cells or who are less heavily pretreated have the most favorable outcome. The major favorable prognostic features associated with EFS and OS after autologous HCT include low levels of β2M and CR prior to transplantation; the absence of "unfavorable cytogenetics" (ie, abnormalities of chromosomes 11 and 13); less than 12 months of standard therapy preceding transplantation; and non-IgA myeloma. Combinations of these important prognostic variables allow a risk-based therapeutic approach of MM patients.[105]

In 1995 Attal et al published a French trial of 200 patients with MM, demonstrating the efficacy of high-dose therapy in improving the outcome of patients with myeloma.[106] In this trial, patients received two courses of vincristine, melphalan, cyclophosphamide, and prednisone (VMCP) alternating with vincristine, carmustine, doxorubicin, and prednisone (VBAP) and were then randomized to receive either conventional chemotherapy (eight additional courses of VMCP/VBAP) or high-dose therapy (melphalan and TBI) followed by autologous transplant. The transplant patient demonstrated significantly higher response rates, event-free survival (EFS), and overall survival (OS) compared with conventional therapy. Response rates in the high-dose and conventional arms were 81% and 57%, respectively. The 5-year probability of EFS and OS was 28% and 52% in recipients of high-dose therapy, and only 10% and 12% in patients treated with conventional therapy: the treatment-related mortality was comparable between the two groups (Fig. 102–9). Attempts to improve on this outcome including the use of autologous either depleted of tumor cells or processed to select normal hematopoietic progenitor cells have not improved outcomes although several log tumor depletion is obtained. This and other similar trials make

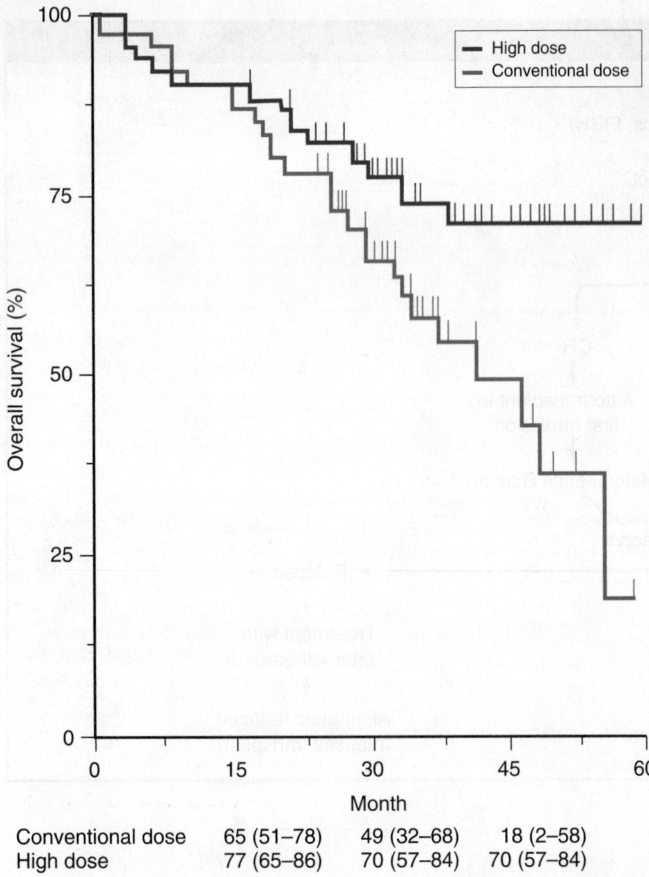

Figure 102–9 Overall survival according to treatment group in patients with multiple myeloma 60 years old or less who were treated with either conventional dose or high dose chemotherapy. (Data from Attal M, Harousseau JL, Stoppa AM, et al: Autologous bone marrow transplantation versus conventional chemotherapy in multiple myeloma: A prospective, randomized trial. N Engl J Med 335:91, 1996.)

autologous transplantation part of the standard of care for most patients with symptomatic myeloma, even with high-risk features.[107] At many centers it is now the most common indication for autologous transplantation.

There are still a number of issues that remain regarding transplant for MM. One key issue is the timing of transplantation. One study collected stem cells upfront on patients and then randomized them to early versus late (at time of disease progression) transplantation.[108] The patients in the late-transplant arm received chemotherapy with VMCP and were transplanted if they had disease progression or relapse following a plateau phase. One important characteristic is that patients did not have further therapy to ensure disease sensitivity but rather went directly to transplantation. In this trial, there was no difference in the median survival rates between the two groups.

Myeloma, like many malignancies, tends to be more common in older patients. Importantly, several studies have now demonstrated that patients over the age of 60 have comparable outcomes to younger patients.[109–111] In addition, it appears that patients with renal failure on the basis of myeloma also show similar benefits from high-dose therapy.[112]

Several centers have been utilizing a tandem autologous transplant approach in attempts to improve the overall disease-free survival in patients with myeloma. An update of one trial suggested that patients who undergo a second transplant have increased the 7-year event-free survival to 20% and the overall survival to 42%, representing a doubling of the results obtained with a single transplant (Table 102–3).[113] A recent update of a study of single versus double transplant suggested that the double cycle was most effective in those patients who

Table 102–3 Final Results of IFM Trial of Single vs Double Transplant in Multiple Myeloma Patients Under 60 Years of Age

Outcome	Single Transplant	Double Transplant	*P*
CR or good PR	42%	50%	.15
Events	87%	79%	.03
Median EFS	25 months	30 months	.05
7-Year EFS (estimated)	10%	20%	<.03
Deaths	72%	56%	.001
Median OS	48 months	58 months	.01
7-Year OS	21%	42%	<.01

IFM, intergroup francophone du myélome; CR, complete remission; PR, partial remission; EFS, event-free survival; OS, overall survival.

did not have a very good partial response after undergoing one transplant (Fig. 102–10)[114]—a result that has been confirmed in another prospective trial.[115] Some studies now suggest a role for maintenance treatment to extend the duration of the remission.[116] Other studies have suggested that a single transplant with a second one at the time of early relapse may be as efficacious.[117] Although transplant may improve the outcome for many patients with myeloma, there are many important questions that are being studied, including the following:

1. Benefit of one versus two autologous transplants and in upfront treatment
2. Timing of autologous transplant (early vs late)
3. Impact of remission prior to or after first transplant on the need for a second autologous transplant
4. Role of maintenance therapy after autologous transplant—which regimens, and for how long?
5. Does maintenance therapy obviate the need for a second autologous transplant?
6. Impact of gene array and cytogenetic analysis on the benefits of transplant or maintenance therapy.
7. Optimal transplant regimen
8. Potential for immunotherapy after transplant.

AMYLOIDOSIS

Primary amyloidosis is a clonal plasma-cell dyscrasia in which systemic disease results from extracellular deposits of proteinaceous material in end organs such as the heart, kidneys, and the peripheral nervous system (see Chapter 89). In contrast to myeloma, the percentage of plasma cells in the bone marrow tends to be low. Owing to its pattern of end-organ damage, autologous HCT for amyloid has been associated with a 4 to 8 times higher mortality than for myeloma. The presence of cardiac amyloid contributes most significantly to the mortality. The amyloid protein can diffusely infiltrate the GI tract and, therefore, GI bleeding is also a significant cause of transplant-related mortality. Attempts to reduce mortality have included a risk-adapted approach, with stratification based on the extent of end-organ involvement, although this may be at the cost of lower response rates.[118–120]

LONG-TERM COMPLICATIONS OF AUTOLOGOUS TRANSPLANTATION

Most patients will recover from the acute effects of the high-dose regimens used in the treatment of the disease. This has been facilitated by the use of mobilized stem cells, growth factors and optional use of antibiotics, antifungal agents and transfusion support. However,

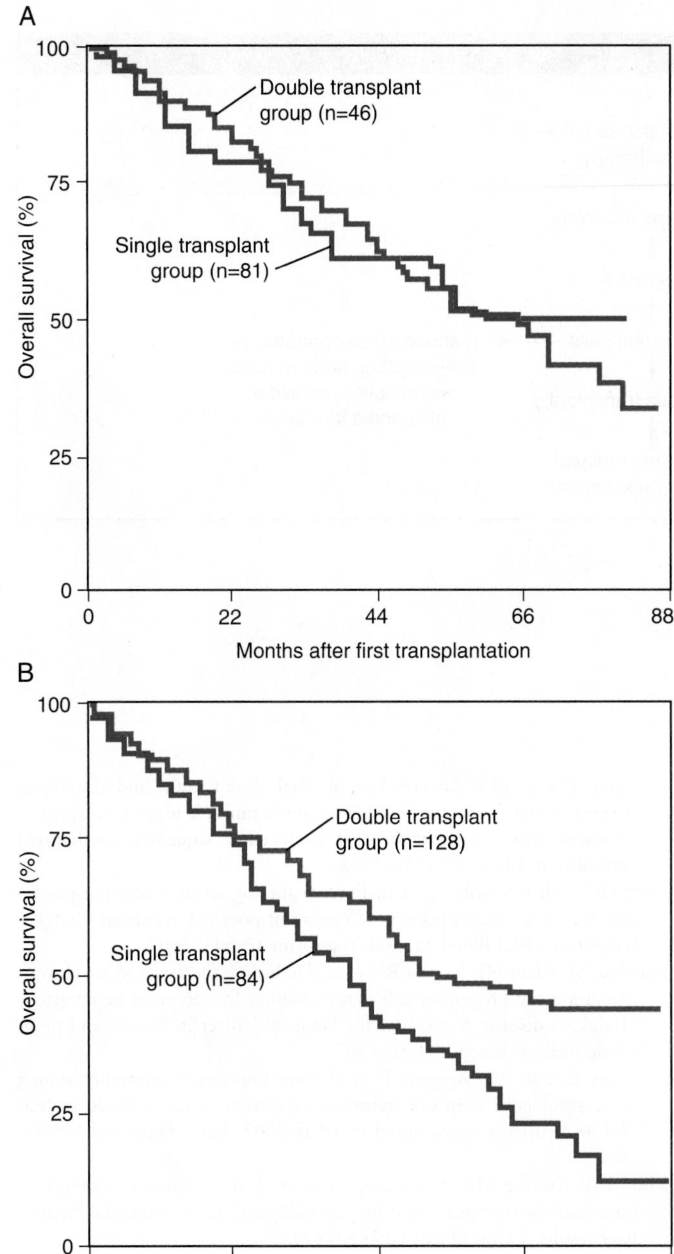

Figure 102–10 Single vs double HCT for multiple myeloma. (Data from Attal M, Harousseau JL, Facon T, et al: Single versus double autologous stem-cell transplantation for multiple myeloma. N Engl J Med 349:2495, 2003.)

all patients are at risk for long-term problems that require follow-up and care.[121]

Cataracts

Cataracts are usually a complication that results from the use of TBI in the preparatory regimen. An analysis from the European Bone Marrow Transplant Registry indicated that cataracts developed only in those patients who received TBI.[122,123] Depending on the degree of impairment of visual acuity, lens replacement can be performed with excellent results.

Secondary Malignancies

The most important long-term complication of autologous HCT is the development of MDS or secondary leukemia.[124–126] The incidence of secondary acute leukemia and MDS, although difficult to assess, appears to be substantially lower in patients undergoing transplant for AML than those receiving similar preparative regimens for lymphoma and Hodgkin lymphoma. This finding has been attributed to the type of prior therapy that is utilized in patients with Hodgkin lymphoma, lymphoma, and myeloma (alkylating agents, topoisomerase I and II inhibitors) as opposed to patients with acute leukemia whose therapy is built around the use of anthracycline and cytosine arabinoside. MDS is reported to occur in 6% to 15% of patients undergoing autologous HCT for lymphoma or Hodgkin lymphoma.[127,128] A second factor that has been implicated has been the type of stem cells (marrow versus peripheral blood) that are reinfused. Some studies have suggested that patients who receive peripheral blood cells rather than marrow grafts have higher incidences of MDS, as well as patients who had their stem cells mobilized using VP16 and have the 11q23 abnormality that is seen following topoisomerase exposure. The third factor that has been implicated as a potential risk factor for the development of MDS in many studies is the use of a TBI-based transplant regimen.[128]

Further investigation is still necessary and it is clear that patients who have had high previous alkylator exposure should be carefully evaluated for the presence of MDS prior to proceeding with autologous transplantation. For patients who are noted to have abnormalities prior to transplant or those who develop this complication secondary to transplant, allogeneic HCT is the best option for treatment.

Infertility

One of the major complications of high-dose chemoradiotherapy for the treatment of hematologic malignancy is infertility, a frequent concern expressed by young patients who are being evaluated for transplant.[129] With current methods, men are sometimes able to collect viable sperm for future use and women are able, under some circumstances, to cryopreserve fertilized ova for implantation following transplantation. New techniques involving the harvesting of and storage of ova prior to fertilization will further expand the possibilities for female patients. Despite these technical advances, the expense is often limiting and there is not always sufficient time to collect sperm or fertilized eggs prior to proceeding to urgently needed antitumor therapy. For patients who wish to consider a family, it is imperative that this is addressed early in the course of their disease well before transplant is anticipated because often the therapy prior to transplantation can reduce the quality and quantity of viable sperm necessary for storage.

Impairment of ovarian function after radiation depends on the radiation dose and the patient's age.[130] Patients who are young and receive TBI can, on rare occasions, recover ovarian function and fertility. Nevertheless, for the vast majority of patients receiving high-dose radiotherapy-containing regimens, infertility is a long-term problem.

For men given TBI, more than 90% of patients are azoospermic and have elevated follicle-stimulating hormone levels. There is less effect on testosterone levels, with some patients having normal luteinizing hormone levels and normal levels of testosterone. However, some patients demonstrate hypogonadism requiring replacement therapy (transdermal testosterone patches or intramuscular injections). Women who develop an early menopause can usually be treated with hormone replacement therapy to avoid secondary problems of osteoporosis and sexual dysfunction. The effect of these therapies on sexual satisfaction is also an important one. As the number of long-term survivors undergoing autologous transplant increases, the issues of fertility and normal sexual function are becoming increasingly important problems that require sensitive attention.[129,131]

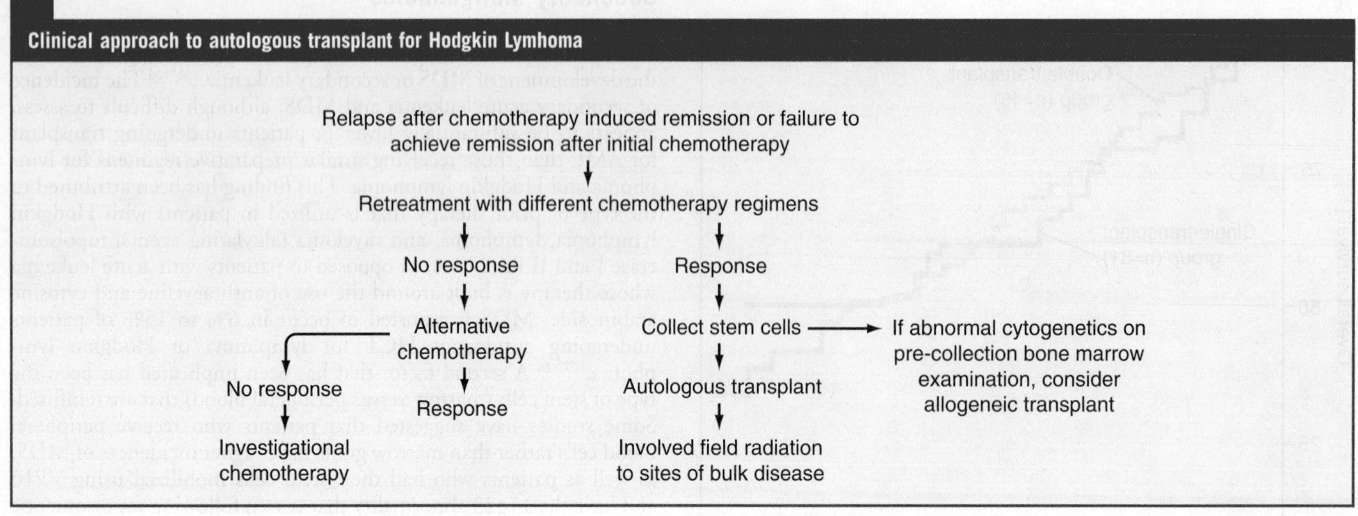

FUTURE DIRECTIONS

Although autologous HCT represents an important component of cancer care, relapse continues to be the major cause for failure regardless of the underlying disease. It is likely that in the future, rather than being seen as a treatment that stands alone autologous HCT be seen as part of an overall treatment plan for individual malignancies, with both pretransplant and posttransplant strategies affecting the outcome. Because its main efficacy is derived by tumor debulking, it may be possible to activate the immune system using combinations of growth factors (IL 2, GM CSF), tumor-based vaccines, and dendritic cells or other immune-based or -targeted therapy that may be most effective when there is a low tumor burden, such as monoclonal antibodies, antiangiogenic factors, and genetically modified T cells. Another possibility that is being actively explored is combining the relative safety of autologous transplant to largely debulk tumors and then utilizing nonmyeloablative allogeneic transplants with less toxicity to derive the benefit of a graft-versus-tumor effect, as has been reported in MM.[132] Some combination of these or similar approaches will enable continued improvement in survival to these devastating illnesses.

SUGGESTED READINGS

Attal M, Harousseau J, Facon T, et al: Double autologous transplantation improves survival of multiple myeloma patients: Final analysis of a prospective randomized study of the "Intergroupe Francophone du Myelome." Blood 100:6a, 2002.

Attal M, Harousseau JL, Facon T, et al: Single versus double autologous stem-cell transplantation for multiple myeloma. N Engl J Med 349:2495, 2003.

Attal M, Harousseau JL, Stoppa AM, et al: Autologous bone marrow transplantation versus conventional chemotherapy in multiple myeloma: A prospective, randomized trial. N Engl J Med 335:91, 1996.

Bruno B, Rotta M, Patriarca F, et al: A comparison of allografting with autografting for newly diagnosed myeloma. N Engl J Med 356:1110, 2007.

Doroshow J: Pharmacological basis for high-dose chemotherapy. In Blume KG, Forman SJ, Appelbaum FR (eds.): Thomas' Hematopoietic Cell Transplantation, 3rd ed. Boston, Blackwell Science, Inc., 2004, p 130.

Fermand JP, Ravaud P, Chevret S, et al: High-dose therapy and autologous peripheral blood stem cell transplantation in multiple myeloma: Up-front or rescue treatment? Results of a multicenter sequential randomized clinical trial. Blood 92:3131, 1998.

Fung HC, Stiff P, Schriber J, et al: Tandem autologous stem cell transplantation for patients with primary refractory or poor risk recurrent Hodgkin lymphoma. Biol Blood Marrow Transplant 13:594, 2007.

Horning SJ, Chao NJ, Negrin RS, et al: High-dose therapy and autologous hematopoietic progenitor cell transplantation for recurrent or refractory Hodgkin's disease: Analysis of the Stanford University results and prognostic indices. Blood 89:801, 1997.

Jantunen E, Itala M, Siitonen T, et al: Late non-relapse mortality among adult autologous stem cell transplant recipients: A nation-wide analysis of 1,482 patients transplanted in 1990–2003. Eur J Haematol 77:114, 2006.

Khouri IF, Keating MJ, Vriesendorp HM, et al: Autologous and allogeneic bone marrow transplantation for chronic lymphocytic leukemia: Preliminary results. J Clin Oncol 12:748, 1994.

Khouri IF, Lee MS, Saliba RM, et al: Nonablative allogeneic stem-cell transplantation for advanced/recurrent mantle cell lymphoma. J Clin Oncol 21:4407, 2003.

Nademanee A, Forman S, Molina A, et al: A phase 1/2 trial of high-dose yttrium-90-ibritumomab tiuxetan in combination with high-dose etoposide and cyclophosphamide followed by autologous stem cell transplantation in patients with poor-risk or relapsed non-Hodgkin lymphoma. Blood 106:2896, 2005.

Press OW, Eary JF, Gooley T, et al: A phase I/II trial of iodine-131-tositumomab (anti-CD20), etoposide, cyclophosphamide, and autologous stem cell transplantation for relapsed B-cell lymphomas. Blood 96:2934, 2000.

Rodriguez J, Conde E, Gutierrez A, et al: The results of consolidation with autologous stem-cell transplantation in patients with peripheral T cell lymphoma (PTCL) in first complete remission: The Spanish Lymphoma and Autologous Transplantation Group experience. Ann Oncol 18:652, 2007.

Stein AS, O'Donnell MR, Slovak M, et al: Interleukin-2 after autologous stem-cell transplantation for adult patients with acute myeloid leukemia in first complete remission. J Clin Oncol 21:615, 2003.

Stone RM, Neuberg D, Soiffer R, et al: Myelodysplastic syndrome as a late complication following autologous bone marrow transplantation for non-Hodgkin's lymphoma. J Clin Oncol 12:2535, 1994.

Tierney DK: Sexuality after hematopoietic cell transplantation. In Blume KG, Forman SJ, Appelbaum FR (eds.): Thomas' Hematopoietic Cell Transplantation, 3rd ed. Boston, Blackwell Science, Inc., 2004, p 519.

Vandenberghe E, Ruiz de Elvira C, Loberiza FR, et al: Outcome of autologous transplantation for mantle cell lymphoma: A study by the European Blood and Bone Marrow Transplant and Autologous Blood and Marrow Transplant Registries. Br J Haematol 15:283, 2004.

Vose JM, Bierman PJ, Enke C, et al: Phase I trial of iodine-131 tositumomab with high-dose chemotherapy and autologous stem-cell transplantation for relapsed non-Hodgkin's lymphoma. J Clin Oncol 23:461, 2005.

Yuen AR, Rosenberg SA, Hoppe RT, et al: Comparison between conventional salvage therapy and high-dose therapy with autografting for recurrent or refractory Hodgkin's disease. Blood 89:814, 1997.

REFERENCES

For complete list of references log onto www.expertconsult.com

CHAPTER 103

UNRELATED DONOR HEMATOPOIETIC CELL TRANSPLANTATION

Effie W. Petersdorf and Claudio Anasetti

The outcomes of unrelated donor hematopoietic cell transplantation (HCT) have greatly improved as a result of better understanding of the diversity of genes that give rise to host-versus-graft (HVG) and graft-versus-host (GVH) allorecognition. Development of robust typing methods that define functional variation of human leukocyte antigen (HLA) and killer immunoglobulin-like receptor (KIR) genes have greatly accelerated understanding of gene–gene interactions that lead to graft failure, graft-versus-host disease (GVHD), and graft-versus-leukemia (GVL). Elucidation of which HLA molecules are the ligands for KIR receptors of natural killer (NK) cells and discovery of the pivotal role played by NK alloreactivity are opening up new avenues for potential antitumor therapy. Continued growth of registries of volunteer donors worldwide now provides the potential for identifying suitable donors for up to 80% of Caucasian patients in need of a transplant. The major challenges are to increase the safety and efficacy of unrelated donor HCT therapy through improved prevention and treatment of GVHD, while leveraging control of leukemia through GVL effects. For unrelated HCT to be more widely applied to patients of diverse ethnic and racial background, more information on permissible HLA mismatches is needed so that mismatched donors can be safely used when matched donors are not available. This chapter chronicles genotyping methods used for donor selection and the clinical results of unrelated donor HCT in the era of DNA typing for HLA and KIR genes.

VOLUNTEER REGISTRIES

The field of allogeneic transplantation has witnessed a rapid growth in the use of unrelated donors over the last 15 years. In an European Group for Bone Marrow Transplantation (EBMT) survey, unrelated donor transplants accounted for the largest increase among allogeneic transplants in Europe.[1] A total of 24,168 first transplants were performed yearly, of which 37% were allogeneic and 14% from unrelated donors. The primary indications for unrelated donor HCT were leukemia (acute myeloid leukemia [AML], acute lymphoblastic leukemia [ALL], chronic myeloid leukemia [CML], chronic lymphocytic leukemia) 63%, myelodysplastic syndrome (MDS) 10%, lymphoma 9%, and nonmalignant disorders 8%. In the United States, unrelated donor transplants are performed for treatment of leukemia (65%), MDS (8%), lymphoma (10%), and nonmalignant disorders (9%) (http://www.marrow.org). In 2006 alone, more than 1000 transplants were performed in patients 50 years and older.

Unrelated HCT has been made feasible by the establishment of registries of volunteer donors worldwide. The Anthony Nolan Appeal was the first effort to demonstrate the feasibility of donor recruitment.[2] Now known as the Anthony Nolan Research Institute, this registry was the first to promote access to HLA-matched marrow donors for patients around the world. In the United States, early efforts for donor recruitment were spearheaded by individual centers.[3] Growing interest in unrelated donor HCT led the U.S. Congress to authorize the creation of a national registry comprising a network of donor centers, transplant centers, and a national coordinating center through the Transplant Act of 1984. Two years later, a federal contract to establish a national registry was awarded to the National Marrow Donor Program (NMDP) (http://www.nmdp.org).[4] In the Netherlands, Professor Jon J. van Rood led the Europdonor Foundation in the collection of HLA data from donor registries around the world and in the formation of a database of HLA phenotypes known as Bone Marrow Donors Worldwide (BMDW) (http://www.bmdw.org).[5] Continued growth in registry size worldwide has increased the chances that well-matched donors can be identified. The NMDP registers 25,500 new donors each month and more than 300,000 each year (www.marrow.org). Today, more than six million donors are available through the NMDP, and more than five million donors are available through international cooperative agreements with registries around the world. With this database of 11 million donors, the average likelihood of identifying a potential donor for bone marrow (BM) or peripheral blood stem cells (PBSC) is 84%.

The median time from initiation of a formal unrelated donor search to a request for a donation is 51 days (http://www.marrow.org). Although more than half of all U.S. patients who initiate a search will have 10 or more suitably matched NMDP donors, efficiency of the search process is highly dependent on the racial and ethnic background of the recipient and the composition of the registry.[6] A Dutch study of 549 unrelated donor searches conducted between 1987 and 2000 showcased the differences between median search times for patients of Northwestern and non-Northwestern European descent.[7] Whereas almost 60% of Northwestern European patients received a transplant within a median time of 4.4 months from the start of the search, only 32% of non-Northwestern European patients were able to identify suitable donors, and half did not have a compatible donor. For all patients, the efficiency with which the unrelated donor search is conducted is critical, and guidelines for planning transplantation as well as approaches for surmounting the unique challenges of finding donors are available (http://www.asbmt.org/policystat/policy.html).[7,8]

DONOR EVALUATION AND SELECTION

Selection of unrelated donors includes consideration for the level of the HLA tissue type match with the recipient and the presence of recipient antidonor antibodies, which place the patient at high risk for nonengraftment.[9,10] Criteria other than HLA are considered for donor selection when more than one HLA-identical match is available for a given patient. An NMDP analysis designed to study donor variables associated with transplant outcome examined 6978 transplants performed between 1987 and 1999.[11] Improved recipient survival and disease-free survival (DFS) were observed with use of young BM donors; these transplant recipients experienced lower risks of both acute and chronic GVHD. With each increasing decade of donor age, the risk of acute and chronic GVHD increased by 10%. This study did not find any effects of donor gender on engraftment, acute GVHD, or survival. However, transplantation from parous female BM donors was associated with increased risk of chronic GVHD. Among female parous donors, the relative risk was 1.19 with a history of a single pregnancy and increased to 1.40 with two or more pregnancies. In general, larger (male) donors provide larger BM and PBSC cell doses compared to smaller (female) donors.[6,12] Donor ABO blood type does not affect the risk of GVHD or mortality. In an updated NMDP analysis of 7043 transplants performed between 2000 and 2004, the donor–recipient HLA match status and younger

Table 103–1 Common Definitions in HLA Genetics

Term	Definition	Example
Allele	Unique sequence of an HLA gene defined by molecular methods	DRB1*0401 allele is a unique sequence defined as DR4 by serologic methods
Antigen	Antibody-defined protein	DR4 antigen is a serologically defined protein product of an HLA gene
Haplotype	HLA genes inherited as a chromosomal unit	HLA-A1, HLA-B8, HLA-DR3 is a common haplotype among white populations
Genotype	Molecularly defined HLA allele or sequence	Genotypically matched donor and recipient are identical for the HLA alleles at a given HLA gene (e.g., HLA-DRB1*0401)
Phenotype	Serologically defined HLA protein or antigen	Phenotypically matched donor and recipient share the same HLA antigen (e.g., HLA-DR4)

HLA, human leukocyte antigen.

donor age were the two variables significantly associated with clinical outcome.[6]

Evaluation of unrelated donors includes a screening medical history, physical examination, and laboratory testing for risks associated with transmissible elements akin to blood transfusion donors. Special focus is placed on risks of transmission of hepatitis, human immunodeficiency virus (HIV), malaria, West Nile virus, transmissible spongiform encephalitis (Creutzfeldt-Jacob disease), and Chagas disease. Donor screening includes blood tests for human immunodeficiency virus 1 and 2, hepatitis B virus, hepatitis C virus, *Treponema pallidum*, human T-cell lymphotrophic virus I and II, and cytomegalovirus.

The importance of a "backup" donor has been increasingly recognized.[8] In a Dutch study of 502 unrelated donor evaluations, 46 were canceled, 78% were deferred due to medical reasons, and 22% were deferred due to nonmedical reasons. In half of the cases for which a backup donor was already identified, the delay in scheduling the transplant was less than 2 weeks. However, when no backup donor was available, the median delay to transplant was 18 weeks. Identification of backup donors is particularly important for patients with high-risk hematologic malignancies, whose disease tempo does not afford delays in transplantation.

PROCESS OF IDENTIFYING A SUITABLE UNRELATED DONOR

HLA Typing and Donor Matching in the DNA Era: Genetics of the HLA Complex

The advent of molecular techniques has made possible the definition of unique sequence variants (alleles) that encode each HLA molecule that is recognized by an antibody (antigen; Table 103–1). Polymorphism ensures that a large array of foreign peptides can be presented to the immune system by HLA molecules.[13] As of April 2007, more than 469 HLA-A, 794 HLA-B, 244 HLA-C, 525 HLA-DRB1, 71 HLA-DQB1, and 124 HLA-DPB1 alleles have been defined in diverse human populations (http://www.ebi.ac.uk/imgt/hla; Table 103–2).[14] DNA genotyping was adopted as standard technique for selection of HLA-matched unrelated donors because unrelated individuals who are matched for HLA antigens may not necessarily share the same HLA sequences. If HLA alleles can be expressed in any combination and if inheritance of alleles were random, then the total estimated number of possible five-locus HLA-A, HLA-B, HLA-C, HLA-DRB1, and HLA-DQB1 genotypes would be more than 1×10^{23}. Clinical experience demonstrates that some patients have been able to find a matched donor even in a relatively small file of unrelated donors. Donor identification is successful because HLA alleles are found in association with each other at an observed frequency that exceeds their expected frequency, a phenomenon known as *linkage disequilibrium* (LD).[15,16] The probability of identifying a matched donor for a given patient is higher when the patient and donor share a similar ethnic background.[5,17–27] Linked HLA genes are inherited from each parent as a haplotype in classical Mendelian fashion (see Assessment of HLA Haplotypes below). HLA gene and haplotype frequencies provide important data for estimating optimal registry size and composition (www.allelefrequencies.net).[18,19,24]

Table 103–2 Polymorphism of HLA Genes

	Antigens	Alleles
HLA-A	24	469
HLA-B	50	794
HLA-C	9	244
HLA-DRB1	15	525
HLA-DQB1	9	71
HLA-DPB1	6	124

HLA, human leukocyte antigen.
Available at http://www.ebi.ac.uk/imgt/hla/.

Table 103–3 Definition of Matching for Alleles and Antigens

Designation	Match Status	Examples[a]	
		Donor	*Recipient*
Matched	Antigen matched	HLA-B44	HLA-B44
	Allele matched	HLA-B*4402	HLA-B*4402
Allele[b] mismatched	Antigen matched	HLA-B44	HLA-B44
	Allele mismatched	HLA-B*4402	HLA-B*4403
Antigen[c] mismatched	Antigen mismatched	HLA-B44	HLA-B27
	Allele mismatched	HLA-B*4402	HLA-B*2705

[a]Human leukocyte antigen (HLA) alleles and antigens are designated according to the World Health Organization Nomenclature for Factors of the HLA System.
[b]Defined by DNA sequencing.
[c]Defined by serology.

Given the polymorphism of allele sequences that encompass variants of a single serologically defined antigen, it is not surprising that antigen-matched donor and patient pairs may differ for their alleles (Table 103–3).[28–32] A study by the NMDP defined the extent of allele mismatching among serologically typed recipients and their transplant donors.[33] Among HLA-A, HLA-B, HLA-DRB1 serologically matched pairs, as many as 29% encoded allele mismatches at HLA-A, HLA-B, or HLA-DRB1; 89% of HLA-A, HLA-B, HLA-DRB1

Table 103–4 International Histocompatibility Workshops and Conferences

Workshop	Year	Chairman	Venue	Advances	Reference
First	1964	D.B. Amos	Durham, North Carolina	Definition of "Hu-L," "LA," and "Four" antigen specificities	40
Second	1965	J.J. Van Rood	Leiden, The Netherlands	Mixed lymphocyte culture testing	41
Third	1967	R. Ceppellini	Turin, Italy	Family studies HLA in renal transplantation	42
Fourth	1970	P. Terasaki	Los Angeles, California	Definition of 27 HLA-A, HLA-B, and HLA-C specificities	43
Fifth	1972	J. Dausset	Evian, France	Worldwide typing of 49 populations	44
Sixth	1975	F. Kissmeyer Nielsen	Aarhus, Denmark	Description of Dw specificities	45
Seventh	1977	W. Bodmer	Oxford, England	Definition of DR1-7 specificities HTC testing	46
Eighth	1980	P. Terasaki	Los Angeles, California	Definition of HLA-MB (DQ) MT (DR52/53) HLA in renal transplantation and disease association	39
Ninth	1984	E. Albert/ W. Mayr	Munich, Germany Vienna, Austria	New class I and II specificities HLA class II in renal transplantation	48
Tenth	1987	B. Dupont	Scanticon, New Jersey New York, New York	Establishment of RFLP/T cell clones and HTC methods Creation of panel of homozygous cell lines	49
Eleventh	1991	T. Sasazuki K. Tsuji	Yokohama, Japan	HLA class I PCR typing anthropology	50
Twelfth	1996	D. Charron	Saint-Malo, France Paris, France	Sequencing Class I DNA typing/HLA in medicine	51
Thirteenth	2002	J. Hansen	Victoria, British Columbia, Canada Seattle, Washington	Virtual DNA analysis Identification of SNP markers HLA in anthropology, disease association, HCT	http://www.ihwg.org
Fourteenth	2005	J. McCluskey	Melbourne, Australia	MHC and anthropology, disease, infection, HCT, cancer Nonclassical genes, NK-KIR, cytokine genes	http://www.ihwg.org

HCT, hematopoietic cell transplantation; HLA, human leukocyte antigen; HTC, homozygous typing cells; KIR, killer immunoglobulin-like receptor; MHC, major histocompatibility complex; NK, natural killer; PCR, polymerase chain reaction; RFLP, restriction fragment length polymorphism; SNP, single nucleotide polymorphism.

allele-identical pairs encoded additional mismatches at HLA-C and HLA-DP. Early donor selection criteria did not include consideration for HLA-C, so many donors who were serologically or even sequence matched for HLA-A and HLA-B antigens were later found to be mismatched at the HLA-C locus.[30] The overall frequency of allele mismatching is lower if the recipient has a common haplotype.[31] Because the frequencies of HLA alleles and haplotypes reflect the ethnicity and race of the patient and donor population, donor–recipient HLA mismatches can be ethnogeographically distinct (www.allelefrequencies.net).[29,34–36] In Caucasian transplant populations, for example, donor–recipient allele disparity is frequent for the A2, B27, B35, B39, and DR4 antigens.[29,31]

HLA TYPING METHODS

Serology and Cellular Assays

Serologic reagents have served as the gold standard for HLA antigen typing since the early 1960s.[37–39] Development of standardized tissue typing reagents and methods of nomenclature for HLA genes have been facilitated by a series of 14 international histocompatibility workshops (Table 103–4).[40–51] Serologic typing methods use a complement-dependent microcytotoxicity assay with alloantisera containing antibodies against polymorphic HLA specificities.[37] A public specificity is shared by distinct HLA molecules, whereas a private specificity is unique to a single HLA molecule. HLA molecules can share one or more public epitopes and differ for private epitopes. The combination of HLA antigens of an individual defines their phenotype, and the alleles define their genotype. All serologically defined alloantigens have been characterized at the allele level; however, not all sequenced-defined alleles have an equivalent phenotype studied by serology. Hence, a nomenclature has been developed to translate serologically defined antigens and DNA-defined alleles.[52]

The most commonly used cellular assay for the class II region is the mixed lymphocyte culture (MLC), in which disparity between the donor and the recipient for the antigens encoded by HLA class II region genes (also known as the HLA-D region) leads to lymphocyte activation and proliferation.[53,54] Although the strength of the proliferation measured in an MLC correlates roughly with the degree of HLA-D region incompatibility,[55] MLC is poorly predictive of GVHD and therefore has limited clinical utility for donor selection.[56–58]

The limiting dilution assay is a technique for determining the frequency of donor antihost cytotoxic T-lymphocyte precursors and helper T-lymphocyte precursors. These assays have proved useful in predicting the risk of GVHD and mortality prior to transplantation in some reports and may provide a means for selecting a suitable unrelated donor when more than one equally matched donor is available.[21,59–67] High frequencies of cytotoxic T-lymphocyte precursors have been observed with class I donor–recipient mismatching; helper T-lymphocyte precursor has been shown to detect class II disparity.[21,60,61,65] The frequency of donor cytotoxic T-lymphocyte precursor reactivity against recipient targets is correlated with the risk of acute GVHD after unrelated donor HCT when ex vivo or in vivo T-cell depletion is used for GVHD prophylaxis.[59,62,64,66,67] In T-cell–replete transplantation, significant associations between frequency of cytotoxic T-lymphocyte precursors and acute GVHD have not been identified.[68–70]

DNA Methods

The advent of polymerase chain reaction (PCR) in the 1980s revolutionized donor typing and matching and has greatly accelerated understanding of the HLA barrier in transplantation. Guidelines for typing volunteer donors using DNA-based methods are available.[71–73] To transition from serologic to DNA-based methods, development of dictionaries of HLA alleles and antigen equivalents has become a necessity because many donors in the registries have been typed only by serologic assays.[74] Interpretation and use of molecular typing data for donor search and selection has required the development of informatics programs.[75,76]

Low-resolution DNA-based typing methods can define groups of alleles that are serologic equivalent (e.g., HLA-A*02 is DNA defined and is equivalent to HLA-A2 that is serologically defined). Intermediate-resolution DNA typing methods provide additional information, but not to the level of the complete DNA sequence that distinguishes one allele from another (e.g., the information is sufficient to delineate one group of alleles that include HLA-A*0201 and another that include HLA*0205, but cannot definitely assign the allele). High-resolution typing defines the unique DNA sequence of an allele (e.g., HLA-A*0201). The term "6/6" matched refers to recipients and donors who share the same low-resolution-defined HLA-A, HLA-B, and HLA-DR genes. The term "8/8" refers to high-resolution matching at the four loci HLA-A, HLA-B, HLA-C, and HLA-DRB1. When HLA-DQB1 is added, "10/10" refers to high-resolution matching at the five loci. When HLA-DPB1 is added, "12/12" refers to donor–recipient pairs that are allele matched at all six genetic loci.

Several PCR-based HLA typing approaches are widely used by clinical tissue typing laboratories in support of unrelated HCT programs. The sequence-specific primer method uses a panel of primers to amplify the HLA locus or alleles.[77–82] The PCR products are electrophoresed on a gel, and assignment of an HLA type is made by examining the composite pattern of positive and negative PCR reaction methods.

The sequence-specific oligonucleotide probe hybridization (SSOPH) method uses a solid phase support[83–95] to immobilize PCR-amplified products. Nonradioactive-labeled oligonucleotide probes are allowed to hybridize to the support. Probes with sequences complementary to the target DNA will hybridize, whereas probes with as few as one nucleotide difference will fail to hybridize. Alternatively, SSOPH methods can use probes that are immobilized to the solid phase support and allow PCR-amplified target DNA to hybridize to the support.

A variation of the SSOPH method is oligonucleotide array technology.[96] Arrays can simultaneously query multiple regions of polymorphisms in many HLA genes. Oligonucleotide probes can be designed to all four potential nucleotides, thereby enabling detection of new sequence polymorphisms with the same sensitivity and specificity as sequencing-based typing. Redundancy of probe sequences allows combinations of alleles to be distinguished in heterozygous individuals. Finally, sequencing methods provide high resolution of HLA alleles and are the definitive method for characterizing novel HLA sequences.[97–102]

ASSESSMENT OF THE VECTOR OF MISMATCHING

The "vector" or "direction" of HLA compatibility between a donor and a recipient has biologic relevance in defining the risks of graft failure and GVHD. The concept of the vector was first demonstrated in cases of haploidentical related mismatched transplantation and defines HVG and GVH alloreactivity.[103] The presence of donor alleles not shared by the recipient determines HVG allorecognition, whereas the presence of recipient alleles not shared by the donor provides the immunologic basis for GVH allorecognition (Table 103–5). "Bidirectional" mismatching refers to the situation in which both HVG and GVH vectors are present at a given HLA locus. "Unidirectional" mismatching describes the situation in which either the donor or the recipient is homozygous for the same allele at the mismatched locus. A unidirectional GVH vector mismatch occurs when the donor is homozygous and the recipient is heterozygous and shares one allele with the donor (e.g., patient DRB1*0101, *0410 vs donor DRB1*0101, *0101). A unidirectional HVG vector mismatch occurs when the patient is homozygous and the donor is heterozygous and shares one allele with the patient (e.g., patient DRB1*0101, *0101 vs donor DRB1*0101, *0401). Clinical outcomes analyses that evaluate the association between HLA disparity and risk of graft failure or GVHD should specify the vector of incompatibility that is used to define the comparison groups.

Table 103–5 Vector of Mismatch

Vector	Definition	Examples	
		Donor	*Recipient*
HVG	Presence of donor alleles not present in the recipient	DRB1*0101,0401[a]	DRB1*0101,0410
		DRB1*0101,0401[b]	DRB1*0101,0101
GVH	Presence of recipient alleles not present in the donor	DRB1*0101,0401[a]	DRB1*0101,0410
		DRB1*0101,0101[b]	DRB1*0101,0410

[a]These combinations contain bidirectional (both HVG and GVHD) mismatch vectors.
[b]Unidirectional mismatches.
GVH, graft versus host; HVG, host versus graft.

ASSESSMENT OF HLA HAPLOTYPES

Patients who are candidates for allogeneic transplantation undergo a pedigree analysis to determine the availability of potential HLA genotypically identical siblings who could serve as a donor. The family study, which includes typing of the propositus' mother, father, and all full siblings, provides an internal verification of the patient's HLA haplotypes. Because HLA genes segregate in classical Mendelian fashion, the probability that a sibling inherits the same parental haplotypes is 25% (genotypically identical). The probability that a sibling inherits one identical paternal or maternal haplotype plus one nonshared haplotype is 50% (haploidentical). The probability of inheriting neither of the same haplotypes is 25% (complete mismatch).

When no related donor is available or suitable, a search for an unrelated donor is initiated. A search of all available international registries today includes consideration of more than 11 million donors worldwide (www.nmdp.org; www.worldmarrow.org). In the assessment of every unrelated donor, matching for each HLA genetic locus allele is considered. However, gene-by-gene identity for HLA-A, HLA-B, HLA-C, HLA-DR, and HLA-DQ between two unrelated individuals does not necessarily signify that the HLA alleles are linked on the same chromosomal haplotype.[104] Hence, it is possible for two unrelated individuals who share the same HLA genotype to have different HLA haplotypes. The clinical significance of haplotype matching is described next.

CLINICAL IMPORTANCE OF DONOR HLA MATCHING IN CASES OF UNRELATED DONOR HCT

The first successful human allogeneic marrow transplantations were performed in 1968.[105,106] Early clinical experience in allogeneic transplantation identified both HLA and non-HLA factors as important in defining posttransplantation complications. Donor HLA mismatching was identified as a risk factor for graft failure after HCT from relatives.[9] Non-HLA factors associated with an increased risk of graft failure included transplantation of a lower marrow cell dose,[107] use of T-cell–depleted marrow,[108] and transplantation of marrow from a cross-match–positive donor (presence of antidonor lymphocyte antibodies in the patient's serum pretransplant).[103] HLA mismatching was also shown to increase the incidence and severity of acute GVHD.[109]

Use of HLA-matched unrelated donors as the source of marrow was first applied in the case of a patient with severe aplastic anemia.[110] Durable engraftment and immunologic reconstitution were early barriers to successful unrelated donor HCT.[111–115] As clinical experience matured and tissue typing methods became more robust, unrelated donor HCT was established as a therapeutic approach for treatment of hematologic disorders when an HLA-identical sibling is not available. DNA-based methods have become established as the gold standard for HLA testing, as serologically identical recipients and potential unrelated donors can be mismatched for one or more alleles that are identified by DNA testing methods.[30,32,116]

Retrospective analysis of transplant donors and recipients that test the hypothesis that allele disparity confers biologic significance on transplant outcome should include examination of pairs that are fully typed for HLA-A, HLA-B, HLA-C, HLA-DRB, HLA-DQB1, and HLA-DPB1 at the sequence level. Many non-HLA variables have an impact on the same clinical endpoints that are also affected by HLA disparity. Hence, multivariable models should adjust for all clinical variables that are known to affect outcome. Finally, the study should have sufficient statistical power to detect a significant difference in outcome when one truly exists. Very large numbers of transplants are required to adjust for HLA and non-HLA variables (see box on Criteria for an Interpretable Study on the Role of HLA Matching in Cases of Unrelated Donor Transplantation). Studies meeting these criteria have demonstrated that patients had superior DFS after HLA-matched unrelated HCT.[117–123] When allele-matched donors are not available, the criteria for prioritization of mismatched donors come into focus. The current criteria for donor selection are as follows. (i) When feasible, "8/8" HLA-A, HLA-B, HLA-C, and HLA-DRB1 matching predicts for best patient survival. (ii) When a matched donor cannot be identified, use of a donor mismatched for a single allele can be considered. Under these circumstances, matching for HLA-DQB1 should also be considered, as mismatch for DQB1 alone seems forgiving, but mismatch for DQB1 plus another locus appears to increase mortality.[124,125] (iii) Multiple mismatches are less well tolerated and should be limited, (iv) Permissible HLA mismatches have been proposed as defined by polymorphism for selected HLA class I residues that participate in peptide repertoire or direct contact with the T-cell receptor. (v) HLA haplotype matching between donors and recipients may lower the risk of severe acute GVHD. (vi) Polymorphisms outside of the classical HLA loci may be clinically significant (Table 103–6).

Criteria for an Interpretable Study on the Role of HLA Matching in Cases of Unrelated Donor Transplantation

DNA-based methods have become established as the gold standard for HLA testing. It now is evident that serologically identical recipients and potential unrelated donors can be mismatched for one or more alleles that are identified by DNA testing methods. Therefore, retrospective analysis of transplant donors and recipients that test the hypothesis that allele disparity confers biologic significance on transplant outcome should include examination of pairs that are fully typed for HLA-A HLA-B, HLA-C, HLA-DRB1, HLA-DQB1, and HLA-DPB1 at the sequence level. In this way, the relative risks of HLA disparity on a given clinical endpoint can be more accurately measured. Many non-HLA variables have an impact on the same clinical endpoints that are also affected by HLA disparity; hence, multivariable models should adjust for all clinical variables that are known to affect outcome. Finally, the study should have sufficient statistical power to detect a significant difference in outcome when one truly exists. Very large numbers of transplants are required to adjust for HLA and non-HLA variables.

HLA-MATCHED UNRELATED DONOR HCT

The impact of more complete and precise donor HLA matching is dramatic. Overall survival after transplantation for treatment of AML, MDS, ALL, and CML from an 8/8 matched unrelated donor can approach the results observed after HLA-identical sibling transplantation (http://www.marrow.org).[117–119,123,126–130] For all modalities, the underlying disease diagnosis, and stage of disease at transplantation remain the most important prognostic features that affect DFS. The impact of HLA mismatching with respect to these clinical variables is coming into better focus.[125] The development of reduced-intensity conditioning regimens has expanded the clinical indications of HCT to patients of older age or patients who have underlying medical conditions that preclude the use of myeloablative regimens.[131,132]

In an analysis of patients transplanted for treatment of acute or chronic leukemia or NHL from HLA-identical siblings, patients positive for HLA-DR15 had lower recurrence of disease posttransplant and improved survival compared to patients who were DR15 negative.[133] Additional reports of HLA-A3 and HLA-DR1 and GVHD risk after sibling transplantation suggest that the immunogenicity of the specific alleles may directly influence GVHD risk.[134–136] Because the siblings were HLA identical, these observations cannot be explained by HLA disparity. These data have significance not only in the setting of HLA-identical related HCT but also for unrelated and mismatched related donor HCT. In addition to HLA allele mismatch-specific risk after unrelated HCT, new evidence suggests that risk can arise from mismatching for HLA haplotypes (see Importance of MHC Haplotypes later). The risk associated with haplotype mismatching after unrelated donor HCT can be assessed with haplotyping tools.

Table 103–6 Principles of Donor HLA Matching Using High-Resolution DNA Typing Methods

1. When feasible, four-locus HLA-A, HLA-B, HLA-C, and HLA-DRB1 matching is optimal.
2. When a matched donor cannot be identified, use of a single allele or single antigen mismatched donor can be considered. Avoid double mismatches including HLA-DQB1.
3. Multiple mismatches are less well tolerated and should be limited.
4. Permissible HLA mismatches can be defined by specific class I and class II residues that participate in peptide repertoire or direct contact with the T-cell receptor.
5. Haplotype matching of HLA-A, HLA-B, HLA-C, HLA-DRB1 allele-identical donors and recipients may lower posttransplant risks of clinically severe acute graft-versus-host disease.

HLA, human leukocyte antigen.

SINGLE-LOCUS MISMATCHED UNRELATED HCT

Early studies of patients receiving HLA antigen-matched, MLC-compatible unrelated donor HCT uniformly reported a relatively high incidence of acute GVHD and transplant-related mortality (TRM) compared with transplantations from HLA-identical siblings.[137–140] The possibility that undetected donor–recipient mismatching for HLA allele variants could be responsible for increased complications in cases of unrelated donor HCT suggested that the safety and success of unrelated donor transplantations could be improved by further advances in HLA typing and donor matching and prompted close examination of serologically identical unrelated transplant pairs using DNA typing methods. The HLA variation that is identifiable using DNA methods is functional.[29,36,131,141,142] DNA-based methods can detect differences in allele sequences among serologically identical unrelated donor–recipient pairs, and the risk of mortality is increased with mismatching for a single HLA allele. Most posttransplant complications associated with donor HLA mismatching occur within the first 6 months after transplantation,[29,36,141,143,144] but some occur quite late.[145]

The risks of graft failure, GVHD, and mortality associated with mismatching were not contributed equivalently by all HLA loci. Because DNA-based laboratory methods were first developed for class II genes, clinical information on donor mismatching for HLA-DRB1, HLA-DQB1, and HLA-DPB1 preceded that for HLA-A, HLA-B, and HLA-C. As a result, donor selection criteria included consideration for donor class II matching in the early 1990s, followed by refined criteria inclusive of class I (see box on HLA Selection Criteria for Unrelated Donors). Early studies of class II allele matching were performed in study populations typed by serology for class I antigens. As a result, the risks attributed to DRB1 or DQB1 mismatching may have included the risk related to additional undetected class I disparities. In one of the earliest studies of patients with hematologic malignancy transplanted from HLA-A, HLA-B, HLA-DR serologically matched unrelated donors, DRB1 and DQB1 allele mismatching was associated with increased risk of severe acute GVHD.[146] Several large studies extended the findings of class II disparity and risk of clinically significant acute GVHD.[141,147–150] An NMDP analysis of 831 CML transplants found that the HLA-DRB1 effects were significant when class II allele matching was evaluated in a good-risk subset of patients transplanted during the first chronic phase from class I serologically matched unrelated donors.[150]

HLA Selection Criteria for Unrelated Donors

DNA typing can uncover additional allele disparity between HLA-A, HLA-B, HLA-DR phenotypically matched unrelated donors and recipients. Both GVHD and mortality are increased with use of phenotypically matched unrelated donors compared with related donor–recipient pairs. The difference in outcome can be attributed in part to the effects of mismatching for HLA-A, HLA-B, HLA-C, and HLA-DRB1 alleles and to the degree of HLA-A, HLA-B, HLA-DRB1 haplotype identity between the donor and recipient. Routine testing of potential donors should include DNA typing for HLA-A, HLA-B, HLA-C, and HLA-DRB1 at the intermediate resolution (antigen-equivalent) level. After the best-matched unrelated donors are identified, routine testing should include allele (sequence)-level typing for these genes. When a matched donor is not available, then the number of mismatches should be limited to one or two, with a single HLA-DQB1 mismatch being the best tolerated.

HLA-C: Discovery of a Classical Transplantation Antigen

Among the earliest clinical observations implicating class I was the demonstration that HLA-C is capable of eliciting an alloantibody immune response.[151] HLA-C antigens could be recognized by cytotoxic T lymphocytes and present peptides to T cells.[152–154] Demonstration of HLA-C as a classical transplantation antigen did not occur until the 1990s.[155,156] HLA-C mismatching was identified as an independent risk factor for graft failure, particularly in patients receiving myeloablative conditioning regimens followed by T-cell–replete transplantations for treatment of CML.[156] Increased risk of graft failure was also associated with HLA-A and/or HLA-B mismatching and low marrow cell dose.

The importance of unrelated donor matching for HLA-C was confirmed by two large analyses from the Japan Marrow Donor Program (JMDP)[36] and the NMDP (Table 103–7).[141] In the JMDP study, both HLA-C and HLA-A allele disparities were independent risk factors for severe acute GVHD, and HLA incompatibility for HLA-C was associated with reduction of leukemia relapse after HCT, a so-called GVL effect. Mismatching at the HLA-C locus in combination with mismatching at HLA-A/B and/or HLA-DR/DQ was associated with a lower 3-year relapse rate compared with mismatching at HLA-A/B or HLA-DR/DQ alone. In an expanded dataset, the JMDP demonstrated that HLA-A, HLA-B, HLA-C, and HLA-DRB1 are each independent risk factors for grade III and IV acute GVHD.[143] In the NMDP study, DNA from donors and recipients were typed for HLA-A, HLA-B, HLA-C, HLA-DRB, HLA-DQA1, HLA-DQB1, HLA-DPA1, and HLA-DPB1 alleles using high-resolution methods.[141] After accounting for clinical variables and mismatching at HLA-A, HLA-B, and HLA-DR, multivariate analysis revealed that HLA-C allele disparity conferred a statistically significantly increased relative risk on mortality (see Table 103–7). These data demonstrate that prospective evaluation of unrelated donors should include consideration for compatibility at HLA-C.

Models for Understanding Alloreactivity

HLA-B and HLA-DP have served as models for understanding the structural basis for allorecognition, where specific amino acids residues of class I and II molecules contribute to eliciting the immune response.[157–159] Donor-derived cytotoxic T lymphocytes isolated from a patient with graft rejection selectively recognized the patient-mismatched HLA-B44 allele (B*4402 vs B*4403),[160] indicating that class I allele differences may evoke donor–antihost responses and

Table 103–7 Mortality by HLA Mismatch

Locus	Relative Risk	95% Confidence Interval	*P* Value
A[a]	1.3	1.2–1.6	0.0002
B[a]	1.2	1.1–1.4	0.007
C[b]	1.2	1.1–1.4	0.005
DR[a]	1.2	1.0–1.5	0.01
DQ[b]	1.0	0.8–1.1	0.80
DP[b]	1.1	0.9–1.3	0.50

[a]Antigen or low-resolution mismatch.

[b]Mismatch detectable by any DNA method (high, intermediate, or low resolution).

HLA, human leukocyte antigen.

From Flomenberg N, Baxter-Lowe LA, Confer D, et al: Impact of HLA class I and class II high resolution matching on outcomes of unrelated donor bone marrow transplantation: HLA-C mismatching is associated with a strong adverse effect on transplant outcome. Blood 104:1923, 2004.

supporting the hypothesis that allelic variants of the same HLA antigen can be functionally relevant. A parallel story emerged for HLA-DP.[36,141,161–167] Population studies have shown that HLA-DP is unique among other HLA genes because of very weak LD between HLA-DP and HLA-A, HLA-B, HLA-C, HLA-DR, and HLA-DQ. As a result, less than 20% of HLA-A, HLA-B, HLA-C, HLA-DRB1, and HLA-DQB1–matched unrelated donor pairs are also matched for HLA-DP. Retrospective examination of HLA-DP has required very large transplant populations so that sufficient numbers of HLA-DP matched pairs could be compared with mismatched pairs. Furthermore, the measured effects attributed to single loci in early studies likely measured additive effects of HLA-DP with HLA-A, HLA-B, and HLA-DR. HLA-DP does function as a classical transplantation antigen with respect to GVHD.[161,166–168] Mismatching for two DPB1 allele increases the risk of acute GVHD compared to one or no HLA-DP mismatch.[161] Analysis of the structural basis of HLA alloreactivity shed light on specific epitopes encoded by HLA-DP exon 2 that are responsible for increased GVHD risk.[158] This study showcases the importance of functional studies side-by-side genetic analysis to better understand the residues that define alloreactivity.

The hypothesis that donor-recipient mismatching at certain amino acid substitutions in the class I HLA molecule may be associated with higher post-transplant risks compared to mismatching at other residues was first tested by Ferrara et al.[157] Amino acid mismatching at residue 116 was found to be associated with significantly increased risks of acute GVHD and transplant-related mortality compared to matching at this residue. Recently, the JMDP has evaluated 5210 Japanese recipients of unrelated donor transplants to identify mismatched residues of HLA-A, -B, -C, -DRB1, -DQB1 or -DPB1 molecules that correlate with clinical outcome.[149] Analysis of each allele-defined mismatch yielded 4 HLA-A, 1 HLA-B, 7 HLA-C, 2 HLA-DR/DQ, and 2 HLA-DP mismatch combinations to be significantly associated with increased post-transplant complications. Each allele was subsequently defined by its putative amino acid sequence, and all polymorphic donor-recipient mismatched positions at each locus were individually analyzed for associations. Donor-recipient mismatching for Tyr9–Phe9 of HLA-A and for Tyr9–Ser9, Asn77–Ser77, Lys80–Asn80, Tyr99–Phe99, Leu116–Ser116, and Arg156–Leu156 of HLA-C were identified to be clinically significant. When the study group was restricted to pairs matched at HLA-C for positions 77 and 80 that define KIR ligands, donor-recipient mismatching at positions 9, 99, 156, and 163 were found to correlate strongly with GVHD risk. This study demonstrates that mismatching for positions of HLA-A or C that participate in peptide binding is functional and provides a basis for defining non-permissive HLA allele mismatches. Statistical models have been developed to predict peptide binding of HLA molecules as an approach to predict those HLA alleles that lead to diverse binding of peptide and which may consequently affect T cell recognition of HLA and its minors.[170]

DOES MISMATCH FOR ALLELES OR ANTIGENS POSE THE SAME RISKS?

With the availability of molecular methods for defining the HLA alleles of transplant recipients and donors, it now is possible to evaluate the impact of the location and number of mismatched amino acid residues as potential factors defining the permissibility of a mismatch. In a single-center study of graft failure after myeloablative unrelated HCT, donor–recipient mismatching for HLA-A, HLA-B, or HLA-C antigens conferred greater risk for graft failure than did single allele mismatches at these loci.[142] Recipient homozygosity for alleles or antigens was also significantly associated with graft failure among patients with a single class I antigen mismatch. Graft failure occurred in one of two homozygous recipients and in none of 47 heterozygous recipients mismatched for a single allele ($P = 0.04$), whereas graft failure occurred in four of five homozygous recipients and in seven of 51 heterozygous recipients mismatched for a single antigen ($P = 0.004$). The allele and antigen mismatches represented in this study population differed in the number of nonsynonymous substitutions and in the location of the mismatch in the α_1 and α_2 domains of the molecule. Single class I allele disparity encoded from 0 to 14 (median 2) substitutions in the α_1 and α_2 domains. In contrast, single antigen mismatched pairs had involvement of 1 to 27 (median 13) substitutions. These data series, highly enriched for mismatches at HLA-C, suggest that multiple mismatches for residues that affect peptide binding and T-cell receptor contact might have been instrumental in evoking T-cell responses that led to graft failure in these patients.

Table 103–8 Impact of HLA-A, B, C, DR Matching on Mortality: 8/8 Model

	N	RR	95% CI	P Value
Matched	1840	1.00	—	—
HLA-A, Mismatch	274	1.36	1.17–1.59	<0.0001
HLA-B, Mismatch	116	1.16	0.92–1.47	0.20
HLA-C, Mismatch	478	1.19	1.05–1.35	0.006
HLA-DR, Mismatch	117	1.48	1.19–1.85	0.0005

HLA, human leukocyte antigen; N, number; RR, relative risk; CI, confidence interval. (From Lee SJ, Klein J, Haagenson M, et al: High-resolution donor-recipient HLA matching contributes to the success of unrelated donor marrow transplantation. Blood 110:4576, 2007.)

Two studies have examined allele and antigen mismatches in large populations and the risks conferred by each kind of mismatch on TRM and survival. A single-center analysis from Seattle indicated that an isolated allele or antigen mismatch was similarly detrimental to survival.[125] Among low-risk patients, no single-locus mismatch with the exception of HLA-DQ appeared tolerable. HLA-C mismatches were particularly detrimental, whether patients had low- or high-risk malignancy. An analysis by the NMDP measured risks associated with single-locus mismatches in a large population of HLA allele-typed pairs (Table 103–8).[124] Each HLA-A, HLA-B, HLA-C, or HLA-DRB1 mismatch was found to confer a 9% to 10% lower overall survival compared to a baseline of 8/8 allele matches. Among all single-locus mismatches, disparity for HLA-A or HLA-DRB1 was associated with higher mortality than disparity at HLA-B or HLA-C. Mismatching at HLA-A, HLA-B, and HLA-C each was associated with increased risk of GVHD. As in the previous NMDP analysis,[141] allele and antigen mismatches were similarly detrimental except for the case of HLA-C, where allele disparities did not contribute to the risk. These data are consistent with the graft failure study discussed earlier,[142] in which a predominance of HLA-C mismatches and allele disparities did not contribute to increased risk. These studies demonstrate that when measuring the effects of HLA mismatching, large well-characterized populations are needed, and variables known to affect clinical outcome should be accounted for. Avoidance of HLA-A, HLA-B, HLA-C, and HLA-DRB1 allele mismatches may lower risks of posttransplant complications.

MULTILOCUS MISMATCHED UNRELATED DONOR HCT

The effects of HLA disparity on risk of graft failure, GVHD, and mortality can be measured by the total number of detectable mismatches. As the number of HLA disparities increases, so does risk for these complications. In the JMDP study of 1298 patients,[143] the overall incidence of graft failure increased with increasing numbers of mismatched HLA loci: 1.7% matched; 4.8%, 4.1%, and 4.8% of single HLA-A/B, HLA-C, and HLA-DR/DQ, respectively; 10.4%, 8.9%, and 6% in two-locus HLA-A/B plus HLA-C, HLA-A/B plus HLA-DR/DQ, and HLA-C plus HLA-DR/DQ, respectively; and 10.6% in three-locus incompatible transplants. In patients who received unrelated donor HCT for treatment of CML,[29] single allele mismatch at HLA-A, HLA-B, or HLA-C did not increase the risk of

Table 103–9 Three-Year Survival after Unrelated Donor Hematopoietic Cell Transplantation for Standard Risk Diseases: The Japan Marrow Donor Program Experience

Match Status	Survival (%)	*P* value
Matched	65.4	—
A/B	39.9	<0.001
C Mismatch	68.9	NS
DR/DQ	70.9	NS
A/B + C	51.5	0.10
A/B + DR/DQ	50.0	0.09
C + DR/DQ	50.6	0.06
A/B + C + DR/DQ	39.1	<0.001

From Morishima Y, Sasazuki T, Inoko H, et al: The clinical significance of human leukocyte antigen (HLA) allele compatibility in patients receiving a marrow transplant from serologically HLA-A, HLA-B, and HLA-DR matched unrelated donors. Blood 99:4200, 2002.

graft failure compared to matched recipients (2%); however, multiple HLA-A, HLA-B, and/or HLA-C allele mismatches were associated with a 29% incidence of graft failure.

Quantitative effects of multiple class I, multiple class II, or simultaneous class I and II mismatching can be associated with acute GVHD risk.[36,141,143,146–148,171] Pronounced effects of two-locus HLA-DRB1, HLA-DQB1 mismatching on risk of grade III and IV acute GVHD can be discerned (22% matched; 43% single-locus mismatches; 64% two-locus mismatches).[148] In HLA-A, HLA-B, HLA-DR serologically matched unrelated pairs who received unmodified grafts,[147] matching for both HLA-DRB1 and HLA-DQB1 reduced the rate of GVHD from 73% (any mismatch) to 38% (matched for both genes; $P = 0.02$).

JMDP data provide information on the quantitative effects of HLA mismatching on GVHD risk.[143] Not only were multiple class I disparities a risk factor for GVHD, but HLA-C disparity in the presence of mismatching at any other HLA locus (class I and/or class II) was associated with significantly increased incidence of grades II through IV GVHD: 60.9%, 55.7%, and 64.3% for HLA-C plus HLA-A/B, HLA-C plus HLA-DR/DQ, and HLA-C plus HLA-A/B and HLA-DR/DQ, respectively, compared with 34.5%, 54.9%, 42.7%, and 34.4% for matched, HLA-A/B mismatched, HLA-C mismatched, and HLA-DR/DQ mismatched, respectively. The JMDP experience demonstrates that multilocus mismatching is associated with a decreased rate of survival (Table 103–9). In some pediatric series, children tolerate higher degrees of disparity with use of certain immunosuppressive regimens.[172]

IMPORTANCE OF MHC HAPLOTYPES

The MHC is the most diverse region in the human genome known to date.[173] The MHC is residence of the classical HLA and nonclassical genes, including HLA-E, HLA-F, HLA-G, MICA, and MICB. Of the known genes, data suggest a role for HLA-E in transplant outcome.[174,175] Increased risk for bacterial infections and corresponding TRM at day 180 posttransplant were found in recipients transplanted from HLA-E*0101,0101 homozygous unrelated donors.[174] HLA-E*0103,0103 homozygosity among HLA-identical siblings conferred protection against acute GVHD and TRM, leading to increased overall survival. These data point to the potential involvement of the innate immune system in GVHD.

In addition to the nonclassical HLA genes, more than 100 loci within the extended 7.6 megabase (Mb) MHC region have immune function.[173] One approach that has been taken to discover putative novel transplantation determinants is LD mapping. The MHC is characterized by LD of discrete segments or blocks of sequences that reside between HLA genes.[176–179] Although the specific content of these blocks is under investigation, donor–recipient matching for these regions is associated with superior clinical outcome.[179,180] If these data point to the importance of non-HLA MHC variation in transplantation, then new approaches for querying the MHC that take advantage of the strong LD would be immensely helpful in localizing functional variation. Currently, gene-by-gene matching between recipients and unrelated donors is performed to approximate the haplotype matching that is feasible between genotypically identical sibling pairs. However, HLA-matched unrelated donors and recipients are not related to one another, and given the extreme diversity of the MHC, haplotype-associated variation among HLA-matched transplant pairs may exist. To test the hypothesis that the HLA haplotype serves as a tool for querying such areas outside of classical loci, a novel long-range phasing technique has been developed.[104] By physically linking HLA-A with HLA-B with HLA-DR on the same strand of DNA, this technique has been applied to test the hypothesis that HLA-identical unrelated donors and recipients encode different HLA haplotypes, and, furthermore, haplotype mismatching is associated with increased posttransplant risks conferred by variation that is linked to the different haplotypes.[181] In this study, a homogeneous population of HLA-A, HLA-B, HLA-C, HLA-DRB1, HLA-DQB1 allele-matched unrelated transplants were characterized using the phasing method. Of these pairs, 20% were found to have different physical linkage of HLA-A, HLA-B, and HLA-DR. Haplotype mismatching was associated with significantly increased risk of grade III to IV acute GVHD. The increased risk of GVHD was offset by lower relapse, leading to similar overall survival. This study demonstrates that variation linked to the haplotype is functional and that the HLA haplotype can be used as a surrogate marker for GVHD risk. Prospective donor matching for HLA haplotypes in addition to HLA genes may lower risks of acute GVHD.

In the future, haplotypes can be used to map putative transplantation determinants, as the map of the MHC continues to be refined for single nucleotide polymorphisms, the most common kind of variation in the human genome (http://www.sanger.ac.uk/HGP/Chr6?MHC). If such variation is functional, it may explain the increased risks of GVHD observed after HLA-matched unrelated donor HCT compared to sibling transplantation. Laboratory approaches for capturing MHC diversity include direct sequencing and high-throughput platforms for single nucleotide polymorphism genotyping. Traditionally, microsatellite (Msat) markers have been a robust tool for mapping disease-causing variation in many model systems, including autoimmunity and cancer.[182–184] Msats provide indirect information because Msats themselves are not functional. Their LD with putative functional genes, however, provides the basis for its application in estimating optimal donor registry size and composition[185,186] and for donor selection.[187] Two studies have used Msats to query the MHC region for novel determinants.[184,185] Tumor necrosis factor (TNF) variation within the class III region of the HLA complex was associated with lower survival among patients who developed GVHD.[185] These studies provide the impetus for further exploration of the MHC.

KIR RECEPTORS

Elucidation of the genetic diversity of the *KIR* family of genes and their functional role as receptors for HLA class I offers a novel approach for use of HLA class I mismatched donors to decrease risks of GVHD and relapse.[188–193] KIRs are inhibitory or activating. Both types are expressed on NK cells and other cell types, including T cells; however, inhibitory KIRs are dominant. HLA and KIR genes are encoded on chromosomes 6 and 19, respectively, and segregate independently. However, HLA serves a dominant role in selection of the peripheral repertoire of NK cell inhibitory KIRs. Thus, HLA-mismatched siblings, haploidentical relatives, and mismatched unrelated donors have different repertoires of NK cell inhibitory KIRs. In some HLA-mismatched pairs, the recipient is missing the appropriate ligands for donor NK cell inhibitory KIR. A recipient who lacks the appropriate HLA ligand for the donor KIR will trigger NK-mediated killing of host target cells.[194] In HCT for malignancy, such a combination is desirable, as killing of target host leukemia cells would lead to lower risk of relapse after transplantation. Some pairs of HLA-identical individuals encode distinct KIR sequences and can express distinct KIR on their peripheral NK cells. Recipients lacking the specific HLA ligand for donor KIR could enjoy enhanced antitumor activity after HCT.

The specificity of the dominant inhibitory KIR receptors for its ligand is governed by residues 77 and 80 of HLA-C and by the HLA-Bw4 epitope present on some HLA-B and HLA-A molecules.[195] For HLA-C, ligands are classified into two groups, named C1 and C2. Inhibitory KIR2DL2 and 2DL3 receptors recognize Ser77 and Asn80 present in the following C1 ligands: HLA-Cw1; Cw3 (except Cw*0307, 0310, 0315); Cw7 (except Cw*0707, 0709); Cw8; Cw12 (except Cw*1205,12041/2); Cw13; Cw14 (except Cw*1404); Cw*1507; and Cw16 (except Cw*1602). The KIR2DL1 receptor recognizes Asn at position 77 and Lys at position 80 of the following C2 ligands: HLA-Cw2; Cw*0307; Cw*0315; Cw4; Cw5; Cw6; Cw*0707, Cw*0709; Cw*1205 Cw*12041/2; Cw15 (except Cw*1507); Cw*1602; Cw17; and Cw18. The HLA-Bw4 epitope serves as a ligand for the inhibitory KIR3DL1 receptor. The following HLA-B antigens and alleles are Bw4 positive: B5, B13, B17, B27, B37, B38, B44, B47, B49, B51, B52, B53, B58, B59, B63, B77, B*1513, B*1516, B*1517, B*1523, and B*1524. Based on high-resolution typing of HLA class I alleles of the recipient, the presence or absence of ligands and whether the recipient is C1/C2 heterozygous, C1/C1 homozygous, or C2/C2 homozygous is determined.

The concept of donor NK-mediated killing of recipient antigen-presenting cells was demonstrated in mice and suggested by a study in patients who underwent HLA haplotype-incompatible T-cell–depleted mismatched transplantation for high-risk AML or ALL.[188] These patients received a high CD34+ cell dose and no postgrafting immunosuppression, a regimen that promotes rapid NK recovery.[193] AML patients who received transplants from KIR ligand–mismatched donors had significantly improved 5-year survival rates compared with patients who received KIR ligand–matched transplants (60% vs 5%; $P = 0.0005$). Donor KIR ligand mismatching was associated with no graft failure, no acute GVHD, and a 0% 5-year probability of relapse in cases of transplantation for AML. Relapse of ALL was not associated with KIR mismatching, presumably because NK cells do not express adhesion receptors to LFA-1–deficient ALL cells. In contrast, KIR ligand mismatching was an independent risk factor for poor transplantation outcome (15.5% incidence of graft failure, 13.7% incidence of acute GVHD, and 75% 5-year probability of relapse). Patients carrying the diagnosis of ALL were not protected against relapse with use of KIR ligand–mismatched donors (90% in KIR ligand matched vs 85% in KIR ligand mismatched at 5 years).

These original observations have been reproduced in some but not all studies.[188,196,197] Extension of the original concepts of KIR ligand mismatch in the haploidentical transplant model to HLA-matched sibling donor and unrelated donor populations has yielded heterogeneous results and may reflect the vastly different conditioning and immunosuppressive regimens that promote T-cell and NK-cell reconstitution early after transplantation.[194,196,198–204] In one study, HLA genotypes were analyzed in a large population of T-replete unrelated donor transplants.[202] Lower posttransplant relapse was observed among HLA-mismatched recipients who were homozygous for HLA-Bw6 and HLA-C KIR ligand groups. This association was not observed among HLA-matched recipients. A population of T-replete allografts for ALL, AML, MDS, and CML was examined, and three groups were established based on HLA genotypes ligand and 14 KIR genes: HLA class I antigen matched (KIR ligand matched), class I antigen mismatched but KIR ligand matched, mismatch at both HLA class I and inhibitory KIR-ligand mismatched.[205] The overall survival at 1 year posttransplant for these three groups differed significantly (59%, 49%, and 30%, respectively). The mismatched groups had lower overall survival and event-free survival compared to the matched group. Furthermore, the group with both HLA and KIR mismatching had higher relapse and TRM than the other groups. A detrimental effect was observed for patients who lacked inhibitory KIR receptors. Among HLA-matched cases, those who lacked C1 or C2 HLA ligand had lower overall survival compared to patients with either present. Patients who lacked C1 or C2 had higher TRM compared to patients who had all ligands present. Therefore, for T-replete unrelated donor HCT, inhibitory KIR ligand mismatching and missing inhibitory KIR ligands confer higher risk to patients.

A large analysis by the JMDP sheds further light on the importance of KIR ligand matching.[206] This study included 1790 T-replete unrelated donor transplants. Donor–recipient HLA-C disparity was associated with reduced relapse among patients with ALL. HLA-DPB1 mismatches were associated with lower relapse among CML transplants. Mismatching for the KIR2DL ligand in the GVH vector was associated with an increased risk of relapse for ALL. An increased risk of rejection was observed for KIR2DL ligand mismatches in the HVG vector. The risk of acute GVHD was increased with disparity for HLA-A, HLA-B, HLA-C, HLA-DPB1, and KIR ligand mismatching in the GVHD vector. Mismatching for HLA-A, HLA-B, HLA-DQB1, and KIR ligand in the GVH vector increased mortality. In summary, this analysis demonstrated an important role for HLA-C, HLA-DPB1, and KIR ligand mismatching in GVHD vector on posttransplant relapse. As a whole, KIR ligand mismatching had adverse effects on acute GVHD and rejection and had no survival benefit for patients undergoing T-replete unrelated HCT.

The KIR family of genes displays allelic and haplotypic polymorphism. KIR genes are organized into two broad groups of haplotypes known as "group A" and "group B" haplotypes.[195,207–213] Group A haplotypes encode primarily inhibitory receptors and the activating KIR2DS4 gene. Group B haplotypes tend to exhibit more diversity, encoding more activating genes including KIR2DS1, KIR2DS2, KIR2DS3, KIR2DS5, and KIR3DS1. The clinical relevance of KIR haplotypes has been explored and reveals that the number of activating KIR genes is a determinant of relapse and DFS.[214] In this analysis, patients received myeloablative in vivo antithymocyte globulin T-cell–depleted unrelated transplants. The study population was evaluated according to the presence of donor Group A haplotypes (inhibitory receptors with one activating KIR2DS4) and donor Group B haplotypes (more activating KIRD KIR2DS1, KIR2DS2, KIR2DS3, KIR2DS5, and KIR3DS1). KIR ligand mismatching was associated with significantly higher TRM, lower overall survival, and lower DFS compared to ligand matching. Transplantation from donors with group A KIR haplotypes or donors with lower numbers of activating KIR genes was associated with reduced relapse and improved DFS among AML/MDS recipients and to lesser extent among CML patients. No haplotype effects were observed in patients with ALL. This study indicates not only that the HLA ligand is an important factor but that the composition of donor KIR haplotypes (i.e., group A KIR haplotypes) influences risk of relapse and improved DFS. These observations point to the potential usefulness of prospective integration of recipient and donor KIR genotype information into donor selection to fully maximize NK-driven antileukemic effects.

UNRELATED DONOR TRANSPLANTATION FOR SELECTED HEMATOLOGIC MALIGNANCIES

Acute Leukemia

Historical clinical experience with use of unrelated donor HCT for treatment of acute leukemia demonstrated superior DFS when HCT was performed for patients in remission or early first relapse.[140,215–220] In early studies of patients receiving transplants for AML or ALL in relapse, the presence of circulating blasts in the peripheral blood and the presence of more than 30% blasts in the marrow both were associated with poor outcome.[216] For patients carrying the diagnosis of AML, a higher marrow cell dose was associated with improved DFS of 54% at 5 years.[221] An analysis from Japan illustrated the importance of disease stage at transplantation as a important variable influencing DFS. Patients with ALL in first complete remission (CR1), second complete remission (CR2), third complete remission (CR3), and no complete remission (CR) had DFS of 56%, 33%, 22%, and 12%, respectively. Rates for patients with AML were 71%, 55%, 43%, and 12%, respectively.[222] Similar results demonstrating lower relapse and higher DFS with transplantation for early disease provided the basis for recommendations for initiation of an unrelated donor search as soon as possible after the diagnosis of high-risk leukemia is made if a suitable family donor is not identified.[223–225] Furthermore, these data demonstrated that if an HLA-matched unrelated donor is found, transplantation should be carried out during remission or early after relapse. A much larger worldwide experience has provided the opportunity to refine indications for allogeneic transplantation for acute leukemia and specific approaches to optimize transplant results for patients with AML and ALL. For patients with active leukemia, the availability of high-throughput HLA typing laboratory support has decreased the time required to identify well-matched donors. Depending on the recipient's genotype, it currently is feasible to offer transplantation for high-risk patients within 3 months.

Acute Myeloid Leukemia

Allogeneic transplantation for patients with high-risk AML might improve survival compared to chemotherapy alone or autologous transplantation, but prospective trials of unrelated donor HCT are lacking.[226] When an HLA-identical sibling is available to serve as donor, high-risk patients with unfavorable cytogenetics have improved survival after HCT compared to chemotherapy alone.[227] If a matched related donor is not available, CIBMTR data demonstrate that transplantation for high-risk CR1 disease yields survival rates at least as good as those observed after related donor HCT (http://www.cimbtr.org). Cytogenetics are predictive of remission rates, remission duration, and long-term DFS,[228–230] but heterogeneity of data merits further longitudinal analysis.[231] After transplantation in CR1 from matched or mismatched unrelated donors, patients with unfavorable cytogenetics had a 28% 5-year survival rate, 26% DFS, and 25% relapse rate.[229] These outcomes compare favorably with the 5% to 15% survival observed for high-risk CR1 patients who receive chemotherapy only and with outcome after sibling transplantation. This clinical experience indicates that transplantation in CR1 for patients with unfavorable cytogenetics should be considered if possible. Delay of transplantation for patients with "good-risk" cytogenetics may be reasonable until there is evidence of disease recurrence with careful molecular monitoring of marrow function. In these patients, initiation of an unrelated donor search in CR1 would prevent delay in scheduling transplantation when disease recurs. Patients with intermediate-risk cytogenetics remain the most challenging and require both careful assessment of comorbidities and close monitoring of disease for planning the appropriate time for transplantation.

Three-year DFS greater than 40% can be achieved when unrelated HCT for high-risk patients can be performed in remission.[232] The combination of busulfan and melphalan for conditioning has yielded 3-year DFS of 61% for advanced leukemia.[233] For patients with chromosome 5 or 7 abnormalities, relapse remains the primary reason for transplant failure, with higher rates of relapse observed after related donor compared to unrelated donor HCT; however, 3-year survival rates of 25% are observed.[234] Higher nonrelapse mortality has been observed after related donor transplantation for pediatric AML/ALL compared to unrelated donor HCT.[235] Strategies for lowering regimen-related toxicity have included the development of safer myeloablative conditioning regimens using pharmacokinetics-targeted busulfan[236] and intravenous busulfan.[237–239] For older patients and patients with coexisting medical issues that preclude the use of myeloablative conditioning, the availability of reduced-intensity and nonmyeloablative regimens for AML patients has provided high-risk AML patients the option for cure.[132,240–259] For patients transplanted in CR1, overall survival at 2 years may exceed 60%.[132] Primary causes of failure after transplant are relapse and infectious complications.[260] For patients at high risk for disease recurrence, prophylactic donor lymphocyte infusions after transplantation has yielded superior outcomes: 87% overall survival with a cumulative incidence of leukemic death of 8% and nonrelapse mortality of 17% at 1 year.[259]

Acute Lymphoblastic Leukemia

The most common stage of ALL patients referred for unrelated donor HCT is CR2, but mounting evidence indicates that high-risk patients should be considered early for transplantation in CR1. Factors associated with poorer outcome after chemotherapy include high-risk cytogenetic abnormalities including t(9;22) and t(4;11) translocation and hypodiploid DNA. For patients in CR1 with such high-risk features and no HLA-identical sibling donor, striking a balance between the increased TRM associated with unrelated HCT and the probability of survival with conventional chemotherapy alone is required for each patient.[260–265] For Philadelphia chromosome–positive (Ph$^+$) ALL, use of donors with limited HLA mismatches has been shown to be acceptable and is associated with decreased leukemic relapse post-transplant, indicating the presence of GVL effects, albeit with higher rates of acute GVHD, which obviates any advantages for survival.[215] More recently, a survival advantage favoring related HCT has been shown for Ph$^+$ recipients in either CR1 or CR2 and a potential benefit of unrelated HCT with a 37% to 49% DFS at 2 years.[266,267] For Ph chromosome–negative (Ph$^-$) ALL, the probability of cure is 30% with chemotherapy alone. Transplantation in CR1 for high-risk patients may afford DFS of 56%.[261]

When an HLA genotypically identical sibling is not available, transplantation from unrelated donors has been associated with a 44% to 46% overall survival compared to 53% to 55% after sibling transplantation.[268–270] The overall outcomes between these two populations in some series are becoming more similar to one another.[271,272] In an evidence-based review, transplantation for high-risk ALL in CR1 was recommended, but not for standard-risk ALL.[273] Striking a balance between the toxicities associated with unrelated donor transplantation and the beneficial GVL feasible with alternative donors remains a major clinical challenge.[274,275] For high-risk T-cell ALL in one series, overall survival was comparable after sibling, unrelated donor, or mismatched related donor transplantation.[276] DFS was 67% for CR1 compared to 42% for patients receiving chemotherapy alone. Overall survival 5 years after HCT was 67% compared to 47% for patients receiving chemotherapy only. Relapse remained the major cause of failure after sibling HCT; TRM was the major cause of failure after unrelated donor/mismatched related donor transplantation. In a study of high-risk patients with t(1;19)- and t(4;11)-positive ALL, allogeneic transplantation in CR1 provided opportunity for DFS.[277]

Compared to autologous transplantation, unrelated donor HCT provides a greater antileukemic effect (40% 3-year overall survival for unrelated donor vs 32% for autologous transplantation) and is the treatment of choice in patients with CR2 at high risk for relapse.[275] In an analysis of a large Medical Research Council/Eastern Cooperative Oncology Group trial, autologous transplantation was no better than standard chemotherapy for ALL.[278] In a series of Ph$^+$ ALL adults, a 34% overall survival rate for CR1 and 21% rate for CR2 or beyond was achieved. Improved survival was associated with younger age, CR at HCT, use of total body irradiation, and a sibling donor.[279] Severe acute GVHD increased TRM but did not lower the relapse rate. Chronic GVHD was associated with lowered relapse and did not increase TRM. New approaches to optimizing transplant and immunosuppressive regimens through lower regimen-related toxicity and increased GVL are promising. The addition of rituximab to a cyclophosphamide–total body irradiation regimen in adults with ALL was well tolerated and resulted in 30% DFS, 24% TRM, and 47% overall survival at 2 years.[280] Full donor chimerism and GVL can be achieved with use of reduced-intensity conditioning, and this modality has provided a transplant option to patients who otherwise are not candidates for standard regimens.[281]

Transplantation for pediatric ALL suggests greater tolerability of HLA mismatching in this population.[282,283] Overall outcome for patients transplanted in CR3 showed 3-year event-free survival of 35%, 42% relapse, and 23% TRM.[283] No significance differences in outcomes between mismatched unrelated and matched unrelated donors were observed. Both short CR1 and extramedullary relapse at first relapse were identified as poor risk factors. In an analysis by the CIBMTR that included transplants for AML or ALL from sibling and unrelated donors, TRM was 6% for siblings and 15% for unrelated donors.[284] DFS at 3 years for these two groups was 49% and 54% for patients in CR1, respectively, and 20% and 30% for patients with advanced disease. The risks of relapse, mortality, and DFS were associated with disease stage at the time of transplant. Relapse was lowest after unrelated donor HCT for CR1, but overall survival and DFS were similar after sibling and unrelated HCT.

Myelodysplastic and Myeloproliferative Syndromes

There has been an increased appreciation of the considerable heterogeneity of disorders formally classified as MDS and their multifactorial etiologies.[285–287] New information on the significance of the Jak2 mutation provides the basis for considering myeloproliferative syndromes including polycythemia vera, essential thrombocythemia, and chronic idiopathic myelofibrosis as clinical diseases distinct from refractory anemia (RA) and RA with excess blasts in transformation (RAEB-t).[288,289] Criteria used in the evaluation of MDS include extent and nature of peripheral blood cytopenia, evidence for dysplasia on marrow morphology, and presence and kind of cytogenetic abnormalities.[290,291]

Allogeneic transplantation is the only known cure for MDS and myeloproliferative disorders, including chronic myelomonocytic leukemia.[140,292–294] Transplantation outcome is related to disease morphology, blast count, neutrophil count, disease duration, patient age, and cytomegalovirus serostatus.[294] The International Prognostic Scoring System (IPSS) stage at transplantation, which includes cytogenetics, and therapy-related MDS strongly correlate with risk of posttransplant disease recurrence and is useful for determining patients who might benefit from HCT early after diagnosis.[295] Given the average unrelated donor search time, consideration of HCT should be made for patients with RAEB or RAEB-t at the time of diagnosis because of the short median survival and high incidence of transformation to AML among patients with blasts. Decision analysis algorithms suggest that transplantation is indicated for patients with MDS diagnoses carrying higher risk according to IPSS definitions.[296] In general, patients with MDS are older and often have accompanying medical issues that potentially can increase morbidity. These factors frequently require additional medical evaluation and treatment and must be taken into account when planning transplantation.

In general, improved DFS is associated with good-risk cytogenetic markers and shorter disease duration,[297] whereas longer disease duration and lower neutrophil count at the time of HCT are associated with increased risk of nonrelapse mortality. Unrelated donor HCT for higher-risk MDS or secondary AML is an option, particularly for younger patients.[298] In a single-center study of patient transplanted for RAEB using targeted busulfan-cyclophosphamide conditioning, 40% DFS was achieved; DFS for more advance diseases was 33% for RAEB-t and 17% for transformed AML; and lower IPSS scores were associated with the highest DFS and lowest relapse rates.[299] Overall transplant outcome may be optimized with use of pretransplant chemotherapy for secondary MDS.[300,301]

Use of busulfan-cyclophosphamide is associated with higher survival than with other myeloablative regimens.[302] Compared to regimens containing total body irradiation, transplant outcome after busulfan-cyclophosphamide conditioning is effective,[303] with DFS at 3 years approaching 70% for unrelated transplants with early-stage (or low-risk) MDS.[297] Fludarabine in combination with targeted oral busulfan has yielded an overall survival rate of 42% and DFS of 35% at 18 months in advanced MDS, and a modified fludarabine-busulfan regimen up to 74% DFS for AML in remission.[236] Intravenous busulfan-fludarabine has been shown to be an effective regimen with low toxicity for conditioning patients with AML or MDS.[304] Transplantation for chronic myelomonocytic leukemia (CMML) after myeloablative conditioning has achieved 41% 4-year DFS and 23% incidence of relapse.[305] Little difference in overall survival was observed between unrelated and related recipients after treosulfan-fludarabine conditioning for secondary AML/MDS.[257]

Attempts to increase the intensity of the conditioning regimen in order to lower the relapse rate have led to increased regimen-related toxicity and nonrelapse mortality. Because TRM remains a major cause of failure for low-risk MDS,[299,306] new approaches to reduce toxicity from the transplant procedure have been explored.[297,299,307] Reduced-intensity regimens lower regimen-related toxicity while providing beneficial GVL effects.[308–314] The combination of the anti-CD52 antibody alemtuzumab with reduced-intensity conditioning has demonstrated a 43% 3-year overall survival rate, with a 22% incidence of chronic extensive GVHD.[315] In an analysis of patients with AML in remission, RA, RAEB, RAEB-t or refractory/untreated AML, DFS of 75%, 46%, 33%, and 11%, respectively, were observed after conditioning with 550-cGy total body irradiation with cyclophosphamide. The overall incidence of relapse was 7%, and TRM was 37%.[251] An optimal conditioning regimen has not been determined.[309,316,317]

Chronic Myeloid Leukemia

With the availability of specific bcr-abl targeting agents capable of producing clinical and cytogenetic remissions for CML, HCT has moved to second-line therapy. The efficacy of tyrosine kinase inhibitors (imatinib) to induce CR and, in some patients, durable remission has been shown in phase I, II, and III clinical trials.[318–322] This has led to a decline in the number of allogeneic transplants performed for good-risk early CML.[323] Although imatinib as front-line therapy for CML in chronic phase appears to be more efficacious than transplantation within the first 2 years of disease diagnosis,[324] some patients who develop resistance to imatinib may be salvaged with allogeneic transplantation.[325] Given that allogeneic transplantation remains a proven curative modality for CML,[326] the availability of imatinib and other targeting agents opens the question about optimal timing of HCT. An expert panel convened by the European LeukemiaNet put forward recommendations for the preferred upfront treatment of newly diagnosed CML, developed criteria for monitoring hematologic, cytogenetic, and PCR-defined responses, and provided considerations for optimal timing of allogeneic transplantation.[327] When an HLA genotypically matched sibling is not available, balancing the risks and benefits of unrelated donor HCT is required, with careful attention to the time required for the donor search. With increasingly more patients deferring allogeneic transplantation in favor of upfront bcr-abl tyrosine kinase targeted therapy, an area of active investigation is the impact of the time from diagnosis to HCT on overall transplant outcome. Several studies provide evidence that pretransplant imatinib therapy does not adversely affect the outcome of subsequent allogeneic transplantation.[328–331] Comparison of transplant results between patients receiving imatinib for at least 3 months before HCT and patients who did not receive imatinib demonstrated no increase in early hepatotoxicity, delay in engraftment, or differences in overall survival, DFS, relapse, or nonrelapse mortality. However, patients who had a suboptimal response or loss of response to imatinib had a higher hazard of mortality compared to patients who achieved a complete cytogenetic remission or a major cytogeneic response.[331]

The historic transplant experience in the era before imatinib demonstrated a 45% 2-year DFS rate for patients with chronic phase disease who underwent transplantation within 1 year of diagnosis, 36% for patients who underwent transplantation more than 1 year from diagnosis, 27% for patients who underwent transplantation in the accelerated phase of disease, and 0% for patients who underwent transplantation in the blast phase of disease.[332] An expanded analysis of 1423 unrelated donor HCT showed that graft failure occurred in 9.9% of patients and grade III to IV acute GVHD occurred in 33%.[333] For patients receiving HCT in chronic phase, 5.7% developed hematologic relapse 3 years posttransplantation. Factors identified as associated with improved DFS included disease phase (chronic phase) at transplantation within 1 year of diagnosis, recipient age younger than 35 years, cytomegalovirus seronegative recipient, and development of no or mild acute GVHD. Such patients had a 63% DFS rate at 3 years. Single-institution results of unrelated donor transplantation for CML patients receiving T-cell–depleted BM with anti-CD52 monoclonal antibody (alemtuzumab [Campath])[334] showed that the probability of graft failure was 16%, probability of grade III and IV acute GVHD was 24%, and probability of clinically extensive chronic GVHD at 1 year was 38%. Clinical relapse occurred in 20% of patients who underwent transplantation in the first chronic phase. Survival and DFS rates were 52% and 41%, respectively, at 3 years for patients who underwent transplantation in chronic phase, and 28% and 26% for patients who underwent transplantation in accelerated phase. Patients with chronic phase disease who were younger than 40 years who underwent transplantation from HLA-matched donors had survival and DFS rates of 73% and 49%, respectively. Two-year survival rates of 77% have been achieved for patients 35 years and younger in early chronic phase.[335] Similar results were reported by the NMDP in a matched-cohort comparison of unrelated donor and HLA-identical sibling donor transplantations.[336] When unrelated donor HCT was performed in chronic phase (within 1 year from diagnosis), the 5-year DFS rates of unrelated versus matched sibling donors were 61% and 68% for patients younger than 30 years, 57% and 67% for patients 30 to 40 years, and 46% and 57% for patient older than 40 years. Compared to patients receiving a transplant for CML prior to 1997, current patients have a 10% to 15% overall better outcome.[120,336–344] Good-risk patients have achieved the greatest improvement in transplant outcome, with an overall survival rate of 80% and TRM of 17%. Updated outcomes confirm that disease phase at the time of transplantation remains the single most important predictor of relapse and DFS,[336,345] and transplantation in cytogeneic remission remains highly favorable for long-term survival.[346]

The extent of donor–recipient matching for HLA has historically correlated with transplant outcome. Comprehensive donor matching for class I and II HLA alleles is associated with increased survival after unrelated donor HCT for CML. In an NMDP study of 831 donor–recipient pairs, survival rates for HLA-A, HLA-B serologically matched transplantations were significantly better with HLA-DRB1 allele matching of the donor than with HLA-DRB1 mismatching.[150] Other transplantation centers have reported similar results, with an estimated cumulative incidence of clinical or cytogenetic relapse at 5 years of 10% for patients transplanted in chronic phase.[344] Overall 3-year survival rates for chronic phase, accelerated phase, blast phase, and blast phase/second chronic phase patients who underwent transplantation from an HLA-A, HLA-B, HLA-DRB1–matched donor were 62%, 34%, 9%, and 27%, respectively. Among patients younger than 50 years old who underwent transplantation from an HLA-A, HLA-B, HLA-DRB1–matched donor less than 1 year or more than 3 years from diagnosis, the probability of surviving 5 years was 74% and 50%, respectively. Among patients who underwent transplantation in chronic phase, the risk of acute GVHD was significantly higher across an HLA-DR serologic mismatch, with a trend for a higher incidence of grade II to IV acute GVHD with use of an HLA-A or HLA-B cross-reactive group (CREG) antigen-mismatched donor. The cumulative incidence of clinically extensive chronic GVHD was 67% among patients surviving disease free for more than 100 days. No significant difference in the risk of clinically extensive chronic GVHD between HLA-matched and HLA-mismatched cases was noted.

Reduced-intensity and nonmyeloablative conditioning for patients with CML is better tolerated, sustained engraftment is feasible, and overall survival statistics are approaching 65% for good-risk patients.[1,347–353] An EBMT review of clinical outcome following allogeneic transplantation has shown that the results of reduced-intensity conditioning (fludarabine, busulfan, antithymocyte globulin) approach those of conventional transplants.[351]

With the lowered up-front toxicity of reduced-intensity and nonmyeloablative conditioning, the risk of posttransplant disease recurrence and the role of donor lymphocyte infusion and posttransplant imatinib remain important questions.[354,355] Furthermore, potential differences in outcome between BM and PBSC sources demonstrate the need to balance potential up-front benefits with long-term morbidities.[341,356–359] PBSC has been associated with faster engraftment; however, its use increased the risks of grade III to IV acute GVHD, chronic and chronic extensive GVHD, which led to lower relapse, higher DFS, and higher overall survival.[358] In a CIBMTR analysis,[357] a higher incidence of acute and chronic GVHD with PBSC compared to BM did not lead to different relapse risks. TRM in the first 9 months was similar among PBSC and BM recipients. However, among patients who survived 9 months, TRM was higher with PBSC than with BM, which led to poorer overall survival with PBSC, especially in good-risk patients. This CIBMTR analysis suggests that the early advantages of PBSC should be put into the context of potential late risks stemming from chronic GVHD.

Strategies for monitoring disease recurrence after transplantation for CML remain important for identifying patients at high risk for relapse who would benefit from ancillary antileukemic therapy.[360–363] Posttransplant monitoring of bcr-abl transcripts using quantitative reverse transcriptase PCR (RT-PCR) after transplantation has been used to measure risk of relapse.[363] Ongoing research into the mechanisms leading to new mutations[364] and development of new laboratory tools[365] remain important questions.

CONCLUSION

The HLA and KIR genetic systems regulate the transplantation barrier. Clinical outcome after unrelated donor transplantation can be achieved with donor matching for the highly polymorphic HLA loci. When HLA disparity cannot be avoided, judicious selection of a donor with the fewest HLA mismatches and avoidance of certain loci may provide patients with the opportunity for lifesaving transplantation. Disease stage remains a strong predictor of overall transplant outcome, and expediency in timing of transplantation for patients with high-risk disease is paramount. New research avenues include identification of novel MHC resident genetic variation that may contribute to risks of GVHD and TRM and the precise role of the KIR systems in preventing transplant complications and disease relapse.

SUGGESTED READINGS

Anasetti C, Amos D, Beatty PG, Appelbaum FR, et al: Effect of HLA compatibility on engraftment of bone marrow transplants in patients with leukemia or lymphoma. N Engl J Med 320:197, 1989.

Beatty PG, Clift RA, Mickelson EM, et al: Marrow transplantation from related donors other than HLA-identical siblings. N Engl J Med 313:765, 1985.

Farag SS, Bacigalupo A, Eapen M, et al: The effect of KIR ligand incompatibility on the outcome of unrelated donor transplantation: A report from the Center for International Blood and Marrow Transplant Research, the European Blood and Marrow Transplant Registry, and the Dutch Registry. Biol Blood Marrow Transplant 12:876, 2006.

Flomenberg N, Baxter-Lowe LA, Confer D, et al: Impact of HLA class I and class II high resolution matching on outcomes of unrelated donor bone marrow transplantation: HLA-C mismatching is associated with a strong adverse effect on transplant outcome. Blood 104:1923, 2004.

Hansen JA, Gooley TA, Martin PJ, et al: Bone marrow transplants from unrelated donors for patients with chronic myeloid leukemia. N Engl J Med 338:962, 1998.

Hows JM, Passweg JR, Tichelli A, et al: Comparison of long-term outcomes after allogeneic hematopoietic stem cell transplantation from matched sibling and unrelated donors. Bone Marrow Transplant 38:799, 2006.

Hsu KC, Gooley T, Malkki M, et al: KIR-ligands and prediction of relapse after unrelated donor hematopoietic cell transplantation for hematologic malignancy. Biol Blood Marrow Transplant 12:828, 2006.

Hurley CK, Fernandez-Vina M, Hildebrand WH, et al: A high degree of HLA disparity arises from limited allelic diversity: Analysis of 1775 unrelated bone marrow transplant donor-recipient pairs. Hum Immunol 68:30, 2007.

Kernan NA, Bartsch G, Ash RC, et al: Analysis of 462 transplantations from unrelated donors facilitated by The National Marrow Donor Program. N Engl J Med 328:593, 1993.

Kollman C, Howe CWS, Anasetti C, et al: Donor characteristics as risk factors in recipients after transplantation of bone marrow from unrelated donors: The effect of donor age. Blood 98:2043, 2001.

Kroger N, Binder T, Zabelina T, et al: Low number of donor activating killer immunoglobulin-like receptors (KIR) genes but not KIR-ligand mismatch prevents relapse and improves disease-free survival in leukemia patients after in vivo T-cell depleted unrelated stem cell transplantation. Transplantation 82:1024, 2006.

Morishima Y, Yabe T, Matsuo K, et al: Effects of HLA allele and killer immunoglobulin-like receptor ligand matching on clinical outcome in leukemia patients undergoing transplantation with T-cell-replete marrow from an unrelated donor. Biol Blood Marrow Transplant 13:315, 2007.

Parham P: MHC class I molecules and KIRs in human history, health and survival. Nat Rev Immunol 5:201, 2005.

Petersdorf EW, Gooley TA, Anasetti C, et al: Optimizing outcome after unrelated marrow transplantation by comprehensive matching of HLA class I and II alleles in the donor and recipient. Blood 92:3515, 1998.

Kawase T, Morishima Y, Matsuo K, et al: High-risk HLA allele mismatch combinations responsible for severe acute graft versus host disease and implication for its molecular mechanism. Blood 110:2235, 2007.

Petersdorf EW, Hansen JA, Martin PJ, et al: Major-histocompatibility-complex class I alleles and antigens in hematopoietic-cell transplantation. N Engl J Med 345:1794, 2001.

Petersdorf EW, Malkki M, Gooley TA, Martin PJ, Guo Z: MHC haplotype matching for unrelated hematopoietic cell transplantation. PLoS Med 4: e8, 2007.

Ruggeri L, Capanni M, Urbani E, et al: Effectiveness of donor natural killer cell alloreactivity in mismatched hematopoietic transplants. Science 295:2097, 2002.

Sasazuki T, Juji T, Morishima Y, et al: Effect of matching of class I HLA alleles on clinical outcome after transplantation of hematopoietic stem cells from an unrelated donor. N Engl J Med 339:1177, 1998.

Lee SJ, Klein J, Haagenson M, et al: High resolution donor—recipient HLA matching contributors to the success of unrelated donor marrow transplantation, Blood 110:4576, 2007.

REFERENCES

For complete list of references log onto www.expertconsult.com

CHAPTER 104

HAPLOIDENTICAL HEMATOPOIETIC CELL TRANSPLANTATION

Bimalangshu R. Dey and Thomas R. Spitzer

PRINCIPLES AND RATIONALE

The complex innate and adaptive human immune systems are well equipped to withstand major antigenic challenges. Transgressing major histocompatibility barriers has been a particularly severe challenge, and the experience of haploidentical hematopoietic cell transplant (HCT) has underscored the problems of this approach. Our understanding of the basic immunobiology of HCT across major histocompatibility complex (MHC) barriers has increased dramatically over the past 2 to 3 decades; however, the translation of those discoveries into clinical practice has evolved more slowly. The most formidable complications of HCT across human leukocyte antigen (HLA) barriers, namely, graft rejection and graft-versus-host disease (GVHD), have been more effectively prevented and treated with modern pharmacologic interventions and manipulations of the hematopoietic graft.

Restoration of competent immunity remains a major obstacle to the long-term success of haploidentical HCT. With vigorous ex vivo depletion of a graft containing a high number of $CD34^+$ progenitor cells (the "megadose" approach) and sufficiently immunosuppressive conditioning, high rates of sustained engraftment with minimal GVHD have been achieved.[1] However, severe, potentially fatal opportunistic infections and recurrent malignancy are impediments to the successful application of this approach to many patients.

Realization of the potential of allogeneic HCT has one major limitation: the lack of an HLA-matched related donor in the majority of families. The HLA genes are tightly linked and inherited in a genetic unit called a *haplotype*. Haplotypes can be determined by testing for alleles at three loci: HLA-A, HLA-B, and HLA-DR. Every child inherits one haplotype from each parent. Two siblings have a 25% chance of inheriting the same two parental haplotypes and thus of becoming HLA-*genotypically* identical. There is always an excellent chance of finding a family member who shares with the patient at least one HLA haplotype but differs in the second haplotype. If the donor's different haplotype is by chance *phenotypically* identical for HLA-A, HLA-B, and HLA-DR to the recipient's, the results of transplantation following HLA-phenotypically matched related donors are comparable to that after HLA-genotypically identical related donors. However, only approximately 30% of patients have an HLA-genotypically or phenotypically matched related donor. In approximately 60% of cases without a family donor, an HLA-matched unrelated donor can be identified. In reality, in a substantial proportion of situations an unrelated, HLA-compatible adult donor cannot be identified in the needed time frame. Related donors matched for one haplotype but mismatched for the alleles of the other haplotype (haploidentical donors) are virtually always readily available.

The successful performance of haploidentical HCT would mean that most patients will have an immediately available donor both for the transplant and potentially for future modulation of the cellular environment by administration of selected donor cell populations. At least in preclinical animal models, a stronger graft-versus-tumor (GVT) effect has been demonstrated when MHC barriers are crossed.[2] A primary reason for treatment failure after HCT for advanced hematologic malignancies, particularly with use of reduced-intensity conditioning, is recurrent malignancy.[3–5] One way to address the risk of relapse would be to capture the potentially more potent GVT effect of a haploidentical transplant. Finally, the lessons of haploidentical HCT will be important for strategies to induce donor specific tolerance through mixed lymphohemapoietic chimerism.[6,7]

COMPLICATIONS OF HAPLOIDENTICAL HCT

Although the theoretical rationale for haploidentical HCT is clear, the application of this strategy has been limited by three major complications: GVHD, graft rejection, and prolonged immunodeficiency. These problems are discussed as a prelude to the historical clinical experience of haploidentical HCT and the attempts that have been made to overcome these complications.

Graft-Versus-Host Disease

Not surprisingly, the risk of acute (and perhaps chronic) GVHD is substantially higher after T-cell–replete haploidentical HCT than HLA-matched related donor transplantation.[8–10] The frequency and severity of a "hyperacute GVHD" syndrome with pharmacologic prophylaxis was well demonstrated by Powles et al. [8] in an early experience with T-cell replete haploidentical bone marrow transplantation (BMT) for advanced acute leukemia. Powles et al. reported 35 patients with advanced acute myeloid leukemia (AML) or acute lymphoblastic leukemia (ALL) who received 1–3 HLA antigen-mismatched related BMT following cyclophosphamide/total body irradiation (TBI) or cyclophosphamide/melphalan conditioning and cyclosporine with or without methotrexate GVHD prophylaxis. Twelve of these patients died of a syndrome consisting of pulmonary edema, seizures, intravascular hemolysis, and/or acute renal failure. Ten patients had primary graft failure requiring a second transplant from the same donor. This life-threatening syndrome probably reflects an inflammatory cytokine cascade associated with a potent graft-versus-host alloresponse (or, in some cases, possibly graft rejection) and illustrates the potentially catastrophic consequences of crossing HLA barriers with pharmacologic GVHD prophylaxis alone.

Beatty et al.[9] at the Fred Hutchinson Cancer Research Center also showed in an early retrospective analysis of transplant outcomes that the incidence of acute GVHD was significantly higher after 1–3 HLA antigen-mismatched BMT compared to HLA-genotypically identical sibling donor transplants. Despite a higher incidence of GVHD, however, overall survival was not significantly different following HLA-matched and single antigen-mismatched donor BMT, likely due to a stronger GVT effect of single antigen-mismatched BMT balancing the harmful effects of acute GVHD. Although the number of patients who received a 2 or 3 HLA antigen-mismatched transplant was too small to reach meaningful conclusions, the survival of those patients was poor and indicated that the mortality risk of transplants was unacceptably high in donor–recipient pairs with more than a single antigen mismatch.

Use of ex vivo T-cell depletion of the haploidentical hematopoietic graft can result in a substantially lower incidence of GVHD, albeit in some experiences with a greater risk of engraftment failure.[11] With "megadose" peripheral blood stem cells (PBSCs) obtained by stimulation of the donor with high-dose granulocyte colony-stimulating factor (G-CSF) and vigorous ex vivo T-cell depletion, the probability of sustained engraftment after haploidentical transplant was high (100/101 patients in one series),[1] and the probability of acute GVHD was very low (8 %) in that same series. However, the complications of severe opportunistic infection and disease relapse, reflecting inadequate immune reconstitution, persist with this approach.[12,13]

Graft Rejection

A strong association between the degree of HLA incompatibility and graft failure was well demonstrated by Anasetti et al[14] in an analysis of 269 myeloablative BMTs for leukemia or lymphoma. The overall rate of graft failure for transplants from haploidentical donors was 12.3% compared to 2.0% for transplants from genotypically identical sibling donors. The graft failure rate also correlated with the degree of histocompatibility with 9% and 21% graft failure rates for transplants from single locus mismatched and two loci mismatched donors, respectively. Incompatibility at both the B and D loci and a positive cross-match for antidonor lymphocytotoxic antibody independently predicted graft failure.

With T-cell depletion of bone marrow grafts, graft failure rates after haploidentical HCT have been very high.[15] The problem of graft failure has been overcome in large part by the use of very-high-dose G-CSF–mobilized PBSC, as discussed in the Principles and Rationale section.[1] A "veto" function of CD34$^+$ cells and selected CD8$^+$ cells likely has contributed to the high rate of sustained engraftment with this strategy.[16,17]

Nonmyeloablative haploidentical HCT approaches have been explored more recently. Higher rates of graft failure have been observed with T-cell–replete bone marrow versus T-cell–depleted G-CSF–mobilized PBSC.[18,19] Posttransplant high-dose cyclophosphamide also has been used to deplete alloreactive (in both the GVH and host-versus-graft directions) T cells with a high rate of sustained engraftment following nonmyeloablative haploidentical BMT.[20]

Prolonged Immunodeficiency

The well-known serious consequences of haploidentical HCT, including relapse and delayed immune recovery with resultant risk of fatal infectious complications, are complicated by the rigorous T-cell depletion that is necessary to prevent fatal GVHD. Delayed immune recovery after T-cell–depleted haploidentical HCT has been associated with a very high risk for bacterial, fungal, viral, and other opportunistic infections.[21,22] With refinements in transplant strategy, including the use of "megadose" CD34$^+$ cells, the rate of donor engraftment has improved with a very low incidence of GVHD, but infectious complications have remained a substantial problem.[23] In this important study, the mortality from causes other than leukemic relapse was 40%. The high incidence of infectious complications, which occurred despite the use of antibacterial, antifungal, and antiviral prophylaxis, resulted in 59% of all nonleukemic deaths. Of note, CD4$^+$ T-cell counts were below 200/μL for as long as 16 months. Immune recovery was faster in patients who received 10 times as many T cells, but that resulted in an increased incidence of GVHD.[24]

Delayed immune recovery results from the degree of HLA disparity, the low numbers of T cells infused, the use of T-cell–depleting serotherapy (e.g., antithymocyte globulin [ATG]), the intensity of the conditioning regimen, and impaired thymic function.[25,26] Development of a fully functional immune system requires recovery of both innate and adaptive immune responses. Whereas the innate system, represented by natural killer (NK) cells, neutrophils, dendritic cells, monocytes, and macrophages, is restored relatively rapidly, the recovery of the adaptive system, represented by a broad functional T- and B-cell repertoire, is markedly delayed following T-cell–depleted haploidentical-HCT. T-cell reconstitution occurs through two main pathways: *early reconstitution* via a thymic-independent pathway known as *homeostatic peripheral expansion*, which involves expansion of mature T cells that survive the conditioning and/or are retained within the allograft, and *late reconstitution* via a thymic-dependent pathway. Although a broad T-cell repertoire presumably resulting from donor precursor cells emigrating from the thymus (i.e., via thymopoiesis) provides optimal T-cell reconstitution, effective immune reconstitution can occur relatively early through homeostatic peripheral expansion alone conferring protection against disease progression and infectious pathogens. However, this recovery is effectively eliminated by T-cell depletion in the haploidentical HCT setting. Impaired thymic function as a result of toxicity of the conditioning regimen or GVHD further contributes to delayed immune recovery.[26–28] Lamb et al.[22] demonstrated NK cell recovery as early as 1 month posttransplant, with B- and T-cell recovery at 6 months and more than 2 years, respectively, in patients who received T-cell–depleted haploidentical HCT.

HISTORICAL CLINICAL EXPERIENCE OF HAPLOIDENTICAL HCT

The first reported successful allogeneic transplants were performed in children with primary immunodeficiency syndromes who received HLA-matched sibling donor bone marrow.[29,30] Based on this initial encouraging experience, T-cell–depleted parental donor haploidentical BMT was attempted. This strategy subsequently was shown to be successful in a number of primary immunodeficiency disorders, including severe combined immunodeficiency disease and Wiskott-Aldrich syndrome.[31,32] Despite the early successes of HLA-matched BMT and the realization that only sustained lymphoid chimerism was necessary for functional cure of these diseases, it was quickly learned that more aggressive conditioning was required to overcome HLA barriers in the haploidentical BMT setting.[33,34]

The early clinical experience with myeloablative T-cell–replete BMT with pharmacologic GVHD prophylaxis for treatment of hematologic malignancies was remarkable for a significantly higher incidence of GVHD compared to HLA-matched related donor transplants[9] and a high incidence of early and severe ("hyperacute") GVHD.[8] The comparable survival of patients in the Beatty report who received an HLA-matched versus a single antigen–mismatched donor BMT despite a higher incidence of acute GVHD in the latter patient population was believed to result from a stronger GVT effect of HLA single antigen–mismatched BMT balancing the harmful effects of acute GVHD. Too few patients received a 2 or 3 HLA antigen-mismatched transplant to reach meaningful conclusions, but the poor outcomes of those patients suggested that the mortality risk of transplants involving donors who were more than a single antigen mismatch with their recipient was unacceptably high.

An International Bone Marrow Transplant Registry (IBMTR) analysis of transplant outcomes following HLA-matched and HLA-mismatched related and unrelated donor BMT for AML, ALL, and chronic myeloid leukemia (CML) added to our understanding of transplant outcomes according to degree of histocompatibility. In this analysis, transplant-related mortality was significantly higher after a 1 or 2 HLA antigen-mismatched related or matched or single antigen-mismatched unrelated donor BMT than after HLA-matched sibling BMT.[10] The large number of patients also permitted an analysis of outcomes according to leukemia status at the time of transplant. Among patients with early leukemia (AML or ALL in first complete remission or CML in chronic phase), transplants from non–HLA-matched related donors were associated with a higher risk for transplant-related mortality than were matched donor transplants. The risk of treatment failure also was higher following alternative donor BMT. For patients with more advanced leukemia, treatment failure risk was similar for HLA-matched donor transplants and single antigen-mismatched related donor transplants and lower than the treatment failure risk following matched unrelated donor and 2 HLA antigen-mismatched related donor BMT. Although this study demonstrated the importance of leukemia status and the impact of HLA matching on treatment failure risk and survival outcomes, the analysis was limited by the heterogeneous groups of patients (including, for example, both T-cell–depleted and T-cell–replete transplants) and the exclusive use of serologic methods of HLA typing (thus underestimating the HLA disparity that now can be identified by molecular methods).

Drobyski et al.[35] compared the transplant outcomes of 139 patients with hematologic malignancies who underwent T-cell–depleted BMT from HLA-matched unrelated, single antigen-mismatched unrelated and related haploidentical donors. No significant differences in rates of engraftment or cumulative incidences of acute or chronic GVHD were observed among the three groups. Surprisingly, a higher 2-year cumulative relapse probability was observed after haploidentical BMT, and transplant-related mortality risk was higher in both the haploidentical and single antigen-mismatched unrelated donor groups. Overall survival was significantly higher in the HLA-matched unrelated donor group.[35]

RECENT HAPLOIDENTICAL HCT APPROACHES

In an effort to overcome the complications of haploidentical HCT and to improve disease-free and overall survival, a number of strategies have been developed (Table 104–1). Both myeloablative and nonmyeloablative (reduced-intensity) conditioning regimens have been evaluated. The most successful approaches have been those that address and modulate the T-cell content (or function) of the graft and provide sufficient immunosuppression to allow for sustained engraftment.

Table 104–1 Relent Haploidentical HCT Stratreles

Center	Disease	Conditioning *GVHD Prophylaxis*	GVHD (%) *Acute*	 *Chronic*	NRM	EFS or DFS/OS
Non-Ex Vivo T-cell–Depleted Haploidentical Hematopoietic Cell Transplantation						
Royal Marsden[8] (N = 35)	AML/ALL	TBI/CY or TBI/MEL CYA ± MTX	80%	18%	34%	NS/31% at 6 months to3 years
Boston Children's[44] (N = 12)	Leukemia, NHL, NMD	TBI/CY Ex vivo T-cell anergization	27%	20%	50%	42%/42% at 4.5–29 months
Multicenter (China)[45] (N = 135)	Leukemia, MDS	BU/CY/ARA-C/MECCNU/ATG CYA/MTX/MMF	55%	74%	22%	64%/71% at 2 years
University of Tokyo[171] (N = 12)	Leukemia, MDS, NHL	TBI/CY/VP-16 or BU/FLU + alemtuzumab CYA/MTX	18%	25%	17%	42%/58%
Multicenter (Japan)[103] (N = 35)	Leukemia, NHL	Myeloablative (n = 24) Nonmyeloablative (n = 11) Microchimeric NIMA-mismatched donor SCT/tacrolimus ± other drugs	56%	57%	31%	40%/43% at 20 months
Osaka/Hyogo[46] (N = 12)	Leukemia, MDS, NHL	BU/FLU/ATG Tacrolimus/methylprednisolone	19%	25%	15%	55%/55% at 1.8 years
Johns Hopkins[20] (N = 13)	Leukemia, MDS	TBI/CY/FLU post-BMT CY CYA, MMF	54%	50%	8%	38%/46% at >6 months
Ex Vivo T-cell–Depleted Haploidentical Hematopoietic Cell Transplantation						
University of South Carolina[38] (N = 201)	AML, ALL	TBI/VP-16/CY/ARA-C, ATG, CYA Partial TCD, steroids, ATG/MP	13%	15%	51%	18%/19% at 5 years
Basel University Hospital[11] (N = 10)	AML, CMLm, MDS	TBI/VP-16/CY or BU/CY ± ATG CYA ± OKT3	30%	NS	40%	30%/30% at 3– 24 months
University of Perugia[1] (N = 104)	AML, ALL	TBI/TT/FLU/ATG TCD PBSC	8%	7%	40%	48% (AML)[a] 46% (ALL)[a]
Multicenter (Canada)[12] (N = 11)	AML[a]	MEL/TT/FLU/ATG TCD PBSC	0%	0%	55%	9%/9% at 9+ months
Emory University[13] (N = 28)	HM	ATG based TCD PBSC	NS	NS	64%	NS/7%
Children's University Hospital, Teubingen[40] (N = 63)	HM, NMD	TBI or BU + CY/TT ± FLU TCD PBSC	8%	13%	29%	48% at 3 years (ALL, NHL in CR)/NS
Catholic University of Korea (Seoul)[170] (N = 11)	AML	TBI or MEL + BU/ATG/FLU TCD PBSC	0%	0%	36%	36%/36% at 6 months
Bristol Children's Hospital[43] (N = 34)	AML, ALL, CML, MDS	TBI/CY ± ATG TCD PBSC ± CYA ± alemtuzumab	13%	12%	35%	36%/36% at 6 months
Duke University Medical Center[56] (N = 49)	HM, solid	MEL/TT/FLU/ATG MMF ± CYA	16%	14%	31%	43%/31% at 1 year
Massachusetts General Hospital Medical Center[18] (N = 12)	AML, lymphoma	CY, anti-CD2 Mab, thymic XRT CYA (≥35 days) ± ex vivo TCD PBSC	25%	NS	25%	17%/25% at 15– 34 months

[a]AML/ALL in remission, EFS only.

ALL, acute lymphoblastic leukemia; AML, acute myeloid leukemia; ARA-C, cytarabine; ATG, antithymocyte globulin; BMT, bone marrow transplantation; BU, busulfan; CML, chronic myeloid leukemia; CR, complete remission; CY, cyclophosphamide; CYA, cyclosporine; DFS, disease-free survival; EFS, event-free survival; FLU, fludarabine; GVHD, graft-versus-host disease; HM, hematologic malignancy; Mab, monoclonal antibody; MDS, myelodysplastic syndrome; MECCNU, methyl-CCNU; MEL, melphalan; MMF, mycophenolate mofetil; MP, methylprednisone; MTX, methotrexate; NHL, non-Hodgkin lymphoma; NIMA, noninherited maternal antigen; NMD, nonmalignant disease; NRM, nonrelapse mortality; NS, not stated; OS, overall survival; PBSC, peripheral blood stem cell; SCT, stem cell transplantation; TBI, total body irradiation; TCD, T-cell depletion; TT, thiotepa; VP-16, etoposide; XRT, irradiation.

Myeloablative Haploidentical HCT: Ex Vivo T-cell Depletion

An abundant preclinical experience[36] and an early randomized clinical trial in patients undergoing HLA-matched BMT[37] showed that GVHD could be effectively prevented following ex vivo T-cell depletion of the graft. However, increased rates of graft failure and disease recurrence showed important limitations of this strategy.

Henslee-Downey et al.[38] in a series of haploidentical BMT clinical trials evaluated TBI-based myeloablative conditioning with partial (1–1.5 log reduction) T-cell depletion of the allograft and posttransplant cyclosporine-based pharmacoprophylaxis. Ex vivo T-cell depletion was accomplished with either a T10B9 (anti-αβ T-cell receptor) monoclonal antibody or OKT3 (anti-CD3) monoclonal antibody. Sustained engraftment occurred in more than 90% of their transplants, which was attributable to an intensified conditioning regimen and the incomplete T-cell depletion. The incidence of acute GVHD was low in one report (13% grade > I GVHD), and an encouraging long-term survival probability of 20% in patients with advanced hematologic malignancy was observed.

Using high numbers of PBSC to address the problem of graft loss and more vigorous T-cell depletion to prevent GVHD, Aversa et al.[23] demonstrated a very low incidence of GVHD and impressive event-free and overall survival probabilities following myeloablative haploidentical HCT in patients with acute leukemia. Conditioning therapy consisted of TBI, thiotepa, fludarabine, and ATG. Ex vivo T-cell depletion was performed using $CD34^+$ cell selection (most recently with a Miltenyi CD34 cell selection device). With "megadose" PBSC containing a median of 13.6×10^6 (range $5.1–29.7 \times 10^6$) $CD34^+$ cells/kg, sustained engraftment was reliably achieved with minimal acute or chronic GVHD. In a published experience, 104 patients with AML (n = 67) or ALL (n = 37) received a haploidentical T-cell–depleted HCT using this regimen. Engraftment ultimately was achieved in 100 of 101 evaluable patients. Eight patients had grade II or higher acute GVHD, whereas five of 70 patients developed chronic GVHD. A 38% nonrelapse mortality risk, predominantly due to opportunistic infection, occurred. Killer cell immunoglobulin-like receptor (KIR) ligand mismatching in the GVH direction was shown to be associated with strikingly less relapse following transplantation for AML.[39] No difference in relapse probability was observed for ALL, according to KIR ligand compatibility.

Several pediatric experiences have demonstrated high rates of sustained engraftment and a low incidence of GVHD following vigorously T-cell–depleted HCT for nonmalignant hematologic disorders and hematologic malignancy.[40–42] Using positive selection of stem cells with $CD34^+$- or $CD133^-$-coated magnetic microbeads or, more recently, depletion of T and B cells using $CD3^-$- and $CD19^-$-coated microbeads, Lang et al. reported primary engraftment in greater than 70% of their patients. 41 of 63 patients transplanted with $CD34^+$- or $CD133^+$-selected cells, 83% achieved stable primary engraftment (which increased to 98% after retransplant). Grade II to IV acute GVHD occurred in less than 10% of patients. Disease-free and overall survival probabilities for patients with nonmalignant disease and hematologic malignancy (non-Hodgkin lymphoma or ALL in complete remission) were 60% and 48%, respectively. A less than 10% incidence of fatal viral infections in recently transplanted patients was observed, suggesting favorable immune reconstitution in this population of pediatric patients.

Marks et al. [43] treated 34 children having acute leukemia and other hematologic malignancies with TBI/cyclophosphamide and alemtuzumab or ATG followed by T-cell–depleted (either by $CD34^+$ cell selection or ex vivo treatment with alemtuzumab) megadose PBSC transplantation. Cyclosporine as sole GVHD prophylaxis was used only for children who did not receive $CD34^+$ cell-selected grafts. Twenty-four patients (71%) died of relapse or infection. Actuarial overall survival at 2 years was 26%. Of the nine patients with refractory AML, there were no long-term survivors.

The experience with myeloablative ex vivo T-cell–depleted (by $CD34^+$ cell selection) "megadose" PBSC transplantation for hematologic malignancy has not been universally favorable. High early nonrelapse mortality rates due to impaired immune reconstitution (resulting in a high incidence of opportunistic infections or recurrent malignancy) have been reported with this approach. Waller et al.[13] reported a mortality rate of 93% (26/28 patients), mostly due to infection or relapse, following ATG-based myeloablative conditioning and high dose $CD34^+$ cell-selected PBSC. In a Canadian multicenter trial using myeloablative conditioning and $CD34^+$ cell-selected PBSC grafts, 10 (91%) of 11 patients died of infection or recurrent leukemia.[12] The reasons for the inferior survival outcomes in these trials are unclear but may reflect patient selection (i.e., transplantation of patients with more advanced disease) or modifications of the treatment regimen.

Ex Vivo T-cell Anergization

Given the impaired reconstitution following nonselective T-cell–depleted HCT and based on experiments showing ex vivo induction of alloantigen-specific anergy by coculturing of host and donor bone marrow mononuclear cells in the presence of cytotoxic T lymphocyte antigen 4 immunoglobulin (CTLA4Ig), Guinan et al.[44] conducted a trial of ex vivo anergized haploidentical BMT in an attempt to induce alloantigen specific tolerance. Anergy was demonstrated by measuring precursor T-cell frequencies before and after ex vivo treatment of the marrow graft. A multiple log decrease in antirecipient precursor helper T-cell frequency was demonstrated after ex vivo anergization. Anti–third party precursor helper T-cell frequency was not significantly changed by ex vivo treatment of the graft. Twelve patients with advanced hematologic malignancy received TBI-based myeloablative conditioning and ex vivo anergized BMT. Three patients developed acute gastrointestinal GVHD. Five of 12 patients were alive and disease free from 4.5 to 29 months following transplant.

Myeloablative Haploidentical HCT with In Vivo T-cell Depletion

Because of the very high incidence of GVHD and transplant-related mortality following non–T-cell–depleted haploidentical HCT, most of the recent efforts in this field have focused on ex vivo T-cell or T-cell subset depletion. Recently, however, several groups have reported impressive, acceptably low transplant-related mortality and favorable survival probabilities following non–T-cell–depleted PBSC transplantation. Common to these strategies, however, has been the use of polyclonal ATG for in vivo T-cell depletion.

Lu et al.[45] treated 135 patients having a variety of hematologic malignancies with busulfan, cytarabine, cyclophosphamide, rabbit ATG (on days −5 through −2), and non ex vivo T-cell–depleted bone marrow and/or PBSC transplantation. GVHD prophylaxis consisted of mycophenolate mofetil, cyclosporine, and methotrexate. All patients had full donor chimerism at day 30 posttransplant. The cumulative incidence of grades II to IV acute GVHD was 40%, and the 2-year incidence of transplant-related mortality was 22%. The probability of relapse at 2 years was 18%. Infectious complications included cytomegalovirus virus (CMV) interstitial pneumonitis and hemorrhagic cystitis in 17% and 35% of patients, respectively. Two-year leukemia-free and overall survival probabilities were 64% and 71%, respectively.

Ogawa et al.[46] used reduced-intensity conditioning (busulfan, fludarabine, and rabbit ATG) as preparation for 2–3 HLA antigen-mismatched non–ex vivo T-cell–depleted PBSC transplantation in 26 patients with high-risk hematologic malignancies. GVHD prophylaxis consisted of tacrolimus and corticosteroids. Serum soluble interleukin-2 receptor (sIL-2R) levels were followed, and tapering of corticosteroids was based partly on the results of these assays. Twenty-five of the 26 patients achieved full donor chimerism. Five patients developed grade II acute GVHD, and five of 20 evaluable patients developed chronic GVHD. Transplant-related mortality was 15%

(4/26 patients). CD4+ cell recovery was slow, with a median count greater than 100/μL at 9 months. Fifteen (58%) of the 26 patients were alive and in complete remission at a median of 664 days posttransplant.

The surprisingly low incidence of GVHD in these series compared to historical experiences of non–ex vivo T-cell–depleted HCT likely reflects the use of ATG for in vivo T-cell depletion, improved GVHD prophylaxis strategies, and better prevention and treatment of opportunistic infections. The importance of genetic factors (i.e., heterogeneity of the population) and other factors, such as use of donors mismatched for noninherited maternal antigens, remains to be determined in future clinical trials of non–ex vivo T-cell–depleted haploidentical transplant.

Nonmyeloablative Conditioning for Haploidentical HCT

Nonmyeloablative (reduced-intensity) conditioning for HCT is associated with significantly less transplant-related morbidity and mortality than is myeloablative conditioning, thus permitting the transplantation of older patients and patients with significant pretransplant comorbidity.[3–5,47] A variety of postulated mechanisms, including less proinflammatory cytokine production and preservation of host "regulatory" cellular elements observed after nonmyeloablative transplants, may account for less clinical evidence of GVHD.[48] A potent GVT effect may be achieved, following either spontaneous or donor lymphocyte infusion (DLI)-induced conversion of mixed to full donor lymphohematopoietic chimerism.[4,49]

Nonmyeloablative Haploidentical HCT Strategies Using In Vivo T-cell Depletion

Pelot et al.[49] showed in murine MHC-mismatched transplant models that mixed lymphohematopoietic chimerism can be reliably induced following nonmyeloablative conditioning, in vivo T-cell depletion with anti-CD4 and anti-CD8 monoclonal antibodies, and thymic irradiation. Remarkably, these mixed chimeric mice are resistant to in-duction of GVHD following delayed DLI, despite a potent lymphohematopoietic graft-versus-host response, which converts their mixed chimerism to full donor hematopoiesis. A more potent GVT effect has been demonstrated in mixed chimeric mice that convert to full donor chimerism after DLI, compared to full donor chimeras given DLI (with the enhanced antitumor effect shown to result from the preservation of host professional antigen-presenting cells).[50,51]

Based on these murine models, a series of haploidentical nonmyeloablative HCT clinical trials have been conducted at the Massachusetts General Hospital. The initial trials involved cyclophosphamide, equine ATG for in vivo T-cell depletion, and pretransplant thymic irradiation.[52] Cyclosporine was given as GVHD prophylaxis and was tapered and discontinued by 5 weeks posttransplant in the absence of GVHD. DLIs were given to patients with mixed chimerism and without GVHD in an attempt to maximize the GVT effect. Because of a high incidence of severe acute GVHD in the initial group of patients, the monoclonal anti-CD2 antibody MEDI-507 was substituted for ATG in an effort to effect a more complete T-cell depletion.[18] A series of protocol changes have since been made, including the use of ex vivo T-cell depleted G-CSF–mobilized PBSC (rather than bone marrow), changes in the dose and schedule of MEDI-507, and the addition of fludarabine to address the problems of GVHD and graft failure. Mixed "split lineage" lymphohematopoietic chimerism has been achieved in all of the patients treated with ex vivo T-cell–depleted PBSC, with an early predominance of donor granulocyte chimerism and a much lower percentage of donor T-cell chimerism. In the majority of these patients, mixed chimerism in all lineages has converted to full or nearly full donor chimerism, either with tapering of immunosuppression or following DLI. Although GVHD has occurred in the majority of patients following conversion to full donor chimerism, it has been manageable in most cases. Striking antitumor responses in selected patients with chemorefractory aggressive lymphomas also have been achieved.

An unexpected observation in these clinical trials as well as HLA-matched nonmyeloablative HCT trials at the Massachusetts General Hospital was that durable antitumor responses in some patients with chemorefractory hematologic malignancies occurred despite loss of the hematopoietic graft.[53] Nine (41%) of 22 patients who received an HLA-matched or haploidentical nonmyeloablative HCT achieved a response after loss of their graft. Six patients were alive from 2.5 to 5.5 years posttransplant; four of these patients were in a sustained complete remission. The observation of ongoing tumor regression following serial DLI in a patient who lost his graft, accompanied by "spikes" in circulating host CD8+ T cells, raised the intriguing possibility that a host specific antitumor response was induced. In an effort to elucidate the mechanism of these antitumor responses, Rubio et al.[54,55] established a murine nonmyeloablative transplant model in which recipient lymphocyte infusions were administered in order to cause rejection of the graft, followed by tumor challenge with host strain-specific malignant cells. A survival benefit was observed in the mice that developed mixed chimerism followed by recipient lymphocyte infusion–induced graft rejection compared to mice that received conditioning only, conditioning and transplant, or conditioning and recipient lymphocyte infusions alone. The antitumor response has been shown to be mediated by recipient lymphocyte infusion–derived interferon-γ–producing CD8+ cells and recipient CD4+ cells.

Rizzieri et al.[56] at Duke University Medical Center have used anti-CD52 monoclonal antibody therapy (alemtuzumab) for both ex vivo and in vivo T-cell depletion in a clinical trial of haploidentical nonmyeloablative HCT for hematologic malignancies and selected solid tumors. Conditioning consisted of fludarabine, cyclophosphamide, and alemtuzumab, followed by infusion of alemtuzumab-treated PBSC. GVHD prophylaxis consisted of mycophenolate mofetil with or without cyclosporine. DLI were given to patients with persistent disease. Of 49 patients, 8 (16%) developed grade II to IV acute GVHD, and 7 (8%) developed chronic GVHD. Three patients (6%) experienced primary graft failure, and 4(8%) had secondary graft failure. The complete remission rate was 75%; relapse-free and overall survival probabilities at 1 year were 43% and 31%, respectively.

Nonmyeloablative Haploidentical HCT with Posttransplant High-Dose Cyclophosphamide

Based on canine experiments in which high-dose posttransplant cyclophosphamide was effective in depleting alloreactive T cells in both the GVH and host-versus-graft directions, O'Donnell et al.[20] performed a phase I trial to determine the minimal conditioning needed to achieve stable engraftment after 1–3 HLA antigen-mismatched BMT. Thirteen patients with hematologic malignancy received low-dose TBI, fludarabine with or without cyclophosphamide conditioning, and high-dose cyclophosphamide on day +3 posttransplant. Nine of 13 patients achieved sustained engraftment. Six of 13 patients developed acute GVHD. Six of 13 patients were alive, five in complete remission, at a median of 191 days posttransplant.

In an updated report of their experience of 84 patients treated with this protocol, 16 (19%) patients experienced graft rejection; 14 of those patients recovered autologous hematopoiesis. Seven of the 16 patients who had graft loss achieved an antitumor response, including three of 6 patients with myelodysplastic syndrome, two of three patients with CML, and both patients with chronic myelomonocytic leukemia.[57]

Selective Allodepletion

Nonselective depletion of T cells from the allograft prior to transplantation effectively prevents severe acute GVHD but invariably predisposes the recipient to loss of the graft, disease relapse, and an increased incidence of infectious complications. Unmanipulated T-cell add-backs likely will not be effective in preventing these problems without causing GVHD because the frequency of alloreactive T cells in the peripheral blood is far greater than that of either specific antiviral or antileukemic T cells. One approach to overcoming these adverse outcomes is to selectively deplete the graft of the GVHD-causing alloreactive T cells identified by upregulation of activation markers while conserving cells mediating GVT and antimicrobial immune responses. Several methods of selective removal of alloreactive T-cells have been reported that rely on ex vivo stimulation of donor T cells by recipient peripheral blood mononuclear cells in a unidirectional mixed lymphocyte reaction culture. Host-reactive donor T cells can be identified by their expression of activation markers (CD25, CD69, CD71), proliferative potential, or preferential retention of photoactive dyes. They subsequently can be targeted for depletion using a variety of methods, including an immunotoxin,[58,59] immunomagnetic bead separation,[60–63] fluorescence-activated cell sorting,[64,65] photodynamic purging,[66,67] or Fas–Fas ligand-mediated apoptosis.[68] These selective allodepletion methods have yielded 70% to 95% reductions in alloreactivity in vitro, with retention of immune responses against third-party and infectious organisms. Several methods even allow retained alloreactivity against leukemia cells.[66,69–71] Although this promising approach has been shown to be feasible in clinical trials,[72,73] several concerns have been raised, including contamination of recipient peripheral blood mononuclear cells by leukemic cells, loss of antileukemic activity, and induction of clinically significant GVHD. In a clinical trial, Amrolia et al.[74] used different cell doses for allodepleted (via immunotoxin) T-cell add-back. At a dose level of 10^5 $CD3^+$ cells/kg, patients exhibited significantly more rapid recovery of T cells at 3 to 5 months after haploidentical HCT than did patients who received 10^4 $CD3^+$ cells/kg. The incidence of GVHD was very low, and the median time to reach a $CD4^+$ cell count greater than 300/μL was 4 months in patients at dose of 10^5 $CD3^+$ cells/kg compared with more than 6 months in patients at a dose of 10^4 $CD3^+$ cells/kg and 8 months in the series by Eyrick et al.[75] without allodepleted T-cell add-back. A similar improvement in immune reconstitution without GVHD has been demonstrated by another group that used photodynamic therapy for selective depletion of alloreactive T cells.[76] Bear in mind that however small the alloreactive T-cell subset of the total T-cell population (<0.1% in the HLA-matched sibling setting; 1%–5% in the HLA-mismatched setting), their complete elimination may be difficult, and doses of unmanipulated T cells as low as 3×10^4 kg can be associated with severe GVHD following haploidentical HCT. Mielke et al.[77] at the National Institutes of Health demonstrated that selective depletion of alloreactive T cells preserves a $CD25^-CD4^+Foxp3^+$ fraction of T cells that is capable of undergoing marked expansion posttransplant to T regulatory cells (Tregs), which can provide protection against GVHD.

CHOICE OF DONORS FOR HAPLOIDENTICAL HCT: SPECIAL CONSIDERATIONS

Exploiting KIR Ligand Mismatching in the GVH Direction

NK-cell alloreactivity in the GVH or host-versus-graft direction can be a powerful means of optimizing the efficacy and safety of haploidentical HCT. NK cells are a unique $CD56^+CD3^-$ cell population composing approximately 10% of peripheral blood lymphocytes[78,79] and are involved in innate antiviral and antitumor immune responses.[80–83] They compose a heterogeneous population of different cell subsets with distinct phenotypic and functional characteristics. The majority (90%) are highly cytotoxic $CD56^{dim}$ cells likely functioning as efficient effector cells, whereas a minority (10%) are immunoregulatory $CD56^{bright}$ cells producing cytokines.[84,85] Following HCT, including haploidentical transplant with selected $CD34^+$ cells, NK cells recover as early as 2 to 3 weeks posttransplant by rapid differentiation from engrafted $CD34^+$ cells.[14,22,86]

The "missing self" recognition concept was hypothesized 2 decades ago by Klas Karre. He suggested that, unlike T and B cells, NK cells are activated by the absence of self MHC class I molecules on the surface of target cells.[87–90] Expression of self MHC molecules on target cells delivers an inhibitory signal to NK cells via inhibitory KIRs. In the absence of this inhibitory signal, NK cell alloreactivity, manifested by NK cell-mediated target cell lysis, proceeds by default. When NK-cell inhibitory receptors are engaged by KIR-specific epitopes, killing is inhibited, whereas killing of target cells occurs when NK-cell inhibitory receptors are not engaged, due to either absence of MHC class I or MHC mismatch. Because virally infected cells and tumor cells downregulate MHC expression to escape adaptive immune surveillance, the ability of NK cells to identify "missing self" is critical in (innate) immune response against viruses and tumor cells.[91,92] Essentially all NK cells express at least one inhibitory receptor that is specific for a self MHC class I epitope, thereby preventing autoreactivity.[93] NK cells also have activating receptors, most notably NKG2D and NKp46, which can trigger NK-cell alloreactivity when they are engaged by appropriate antigens on virally infected cells and tumor cells.[94–97] Although inhibitory signals are believed to dominate over activating signals, NK cell activity is regulated by quantitative differences in cumulative inhibitory and activating signals transmitted via KIRs. Therefore, the presence or absence of the respective ligands on recipient cells determines if NK cells will be primed to be alloreactive and kill the targets.[79,98]

By selecting haploidentical stem cell donors whose NK cells are not fully inhibited by recipient MHC class I ligands, that is, there is a KIR ligand mismatch in the GVH direction, the graft NK-cell alloreactivity may be used to optimize a GVT effect. As discussed in the Myeloablative Haploidentical HCT: Ex Vivo T-cell Depletion section, Ruggeri et al.[39,99] found that HLA (KIR ligand) mismatching in the GVH direction following T-cell–depleted haploidentical HCT is associated with strong NK-cell alloreactivity leading to (a) a dramatically reduced relapse in patients with AML, (b) a lower rate of graft rejection, and (c) a reduction in GVHD. As supported by their animal studies, the reduction in GVHD is due to donor NK-mediated depletion of host antigen-presenting cells that are crucial in priming alloreactive donor T cells and hence in the pathogenesis of GVHD, and donor NK cells that attack host hematopoietic cells and spare epithelial GVHD target tissues.[39,99,100] The lower rates of graft rejection were shown to be due to donor NK-mediated lysis of host residual T cells, thereby preventing them from rejecting the graft. Furthermore, in their murine transplant model they showed that pretransplant transfer of NK cells into mice improved engraftment after transplantation, allowing durable full donor chimerism following reduced-intensity conditioning. This NK-cell conditioning prevented GVHD well enough to allow for safe infusion of otherwise lethal doses of allogeneic T cells, which were given to facilitate immune reconstitution.

Fetomaternal Microchimerism

Several transplant centers have developed haploidentical HCT strategies based on the principle of tolerance induction as a result of in utero exposure to maternal antigens and the development of long-lasting fetomaternal microchimerism.[101] A large IBMTR analysis by van Rood et al.[102] showed that the incidence of grade II or higher acute GVHD following non–T-cell–depleted haploidentical HCT was related to haplotype inheritance. Transplants from a noninherited maternal antigen-mismatched sibling were associated with significantly less acute GVHD. Moreover, transplant-related mortality was significantly higher in transplants from a maternal or a paternal donor. Several Japanese transplant centers have performed non–T-cell–depleted transplants following either myeloablative or nonmyeloablative conditioning from microchimeric noninherited maternal antigen-mismatched donors.[103–106] Although the overall incidence of grade II or higher acute GVHD incidence was high (56% of 34 evaluable patients) in one series, a significantly lower risk of acute GVHD was observed in patients who received a transplant from a donor who was noninherited maternal antigen mismatched in the GVH direction.

IMMUNE RECONSTITUTION FOLLOWING HAPLOIDENTICAL HCT

Transfer of a functional lymphohematopoietic system from donor to recipient in a timely fashion determines in large part the eventual success of HCT. Given the problem of delayed immune reconstitution with resultant risk of infectious complications and disease relapse following haploidentical transplantation, particularly after ex vivo T-cell–depleted HCT, new strategies are required to limit the severity and duration of this immunodeficiency. Both adoptive cellular therapy approaches and strategies using soluble factors are being investigated.

Immunotherapy involving both cellular and soluble factors can be guided by two distinct concepts: (a) enhancement of general immune reconstitution relative to enhancement of antigen specific responses, and (b) expansion of beneficial cell subsets and depletion of harmful effectors cells. New approaches aimed at facilitating engraftment and reducing GVHD while preserving GVT effects have been developed using regulatory T cells and mesenchymal stem cells (MSCs). In mice, two types of regulatory T cells, $CD4^+CD25^+$ T cells (Tregs) and NK T cells (NK/Tregs), have been shown to prevent acute GVHD.[107–111]

Tregs represent approximately 5% to 10% of peripheral $CD4^+$ T-cells in mice and humans and are identified by their capacity to suppress both $CD4^+$ and $CD8^+$ T-cell activation. Tregs have been shown to promote engraftment and reduce acute GVHD without loss of GVT effects.[107,108,112] In murine models, Tregs can be successfully expanded ex vivo by in vitro stimulation with allogeneic splenocytes plus IL-2. When added to the donor inoculum containing alloreactive T cells, the Treg population can prevent GVHD, enhance immune reconstitution, and reduce the risk of infection while the GVT effect is well preserved.[113] Preliminary experience with expanded Tregs in humans is promising,[114] although clinically meaningful expansion of this small effector cell population and its beneficial use outside of acute GVHD[115] are not defined. Composing only 1% to 3% of all T cells in the spleen in normal mice, NK/Tregs of either donor or host type have the unique capacity to prevent acute GVHD in mice by secreting IL-4, which prompts donor T cells to acquire an antiinflammatory, IL-4–secreting helper T cell 2 (T_H2) phenotype.[110,111,116] NK/Tregs-mediated GVHD prevention strategy was evaluated clinically by Lowsky et al.,[117]who showed an apparent reduction in the rate of acute GVHD in patients with lymphohematopoietic malignancies while permitting GVT effects after HLA-matched HCT. Preliminary evidence also suggests that this strategy may be effective in the haploidentical HCT setting.[118] MSCs, which are multipotential nonhematopoietic progenitors and constitute only 0.001% of nucleated cells in human bone marrow,[119] have been extensively evaluated for their regenerative and immunomodulatory properties. Human MSC have a high in vitro proliferative potential and have the capacity to differentiate into a number of mesenchymal tissues, such as bone, cartilage, and fat. MSCs have been demonstrated to inhibit T-cell alloreactivity[120–124] and prolong skin allograft survival.[121] In addition, ex vivo expanded MSCs have the potential to prevent and treat acute GVHD when used after HLA-matched or HLA-mismatched HCT.[125,126] Although the exact mechanism of immune modulation by MSC is not clearly defined, they appear to mediate their immunomodulatory effects by inhibiting interferon-γ secretion from T_H1 and NK cells, increasing IL-10 secretion from Tregs and increasing IL-4 secretion from T_H2 cells, thereby promoting a $T_H1 \rightarrow T_H2$ shift.[123]

Cytokines and Chemokines

A number of cytokines and chemokines and their associated monoclonal antibodies can be applied to influence effector cell development, activation, trafficking, and thereby transplant outcomes, including engraftment, GVHD, immune reconstitution, and antitumor effects.[127–129] Use of G-CSF posttransplant accelerates neutrophil recovery, but studies have shown deleterious effects on immune restoration, namely, by inhibition of NK-cell and T-cell function.[130–132] Given their excellent capacity to enhance in vivo expansion of NK and T cells after T-cell–depleted HCT, IL-2[133–136] and IL-18[137] potentially could improve immune reconstitution after haploidentical transplant. However, caution must be taken because, depending on the timing of administration of these cytokines, unfavorable outcomes such as exacerbation of GVHD may occur.[138,139] In one murine model, IL-7 improved immune reconstitution by enhancing thymopoiesis in addition to expanding peripheral T cells, NK cells, NK/Tregs, B cells, monocytes, and macrophages.[140] However, in another model this cytokine enhanced the development of acute GVHD.[141] Keratinocyte growth factor has been shown in a murine model to improve thymic and peripheral T-cell recovery after transplant.[142] Monoclonal antibodies specific for selective cytokines and chemokines to prevent GVHD[44,143,144] and optimize GVT effects are being evaluated.[128]

Enhancement of Antigen-Specific Immune Responses

Prevention and treatment of opportunistic viral, fungal, bacterial, and parasitic infections remain formidable challenges after haploidentical HCT. For example, the failure to successfully treat viral infections, which is partly due to the limited number of nontoxic antiviral drugs, constitutes a major cause of treatment failure following haploidentical transplant. Both $CD4^+$ and $CD8^+$ cells are critical in maintaining CMV, Epstein-Barr virus, adenovirus, polyomavirus, and herpes virus in their latent phase. Therefore, adoptive immunotherapy with ex vivo expanded virus-specific cytotoxic T lymphocytes (CTLs) is being explored. Infusion of donor-derived allogeneic CMV-specific T-cell clones into recipients for prevention or treatment of CMV-related disease, without causing GVHD, has shown promising potential.[145–148] These studies also demonstrated that CMV-specific $CD4^+$ cells are important for reconstitution and maintenance of $CD8^+$ CTL responses. Encouraging early results have been achieved when ex vivo expanded allogeneic CTL clones specific for Epstein-Barr virus were used for prophylaxis and management of Epstein-Barr virus–associated diseases, including posttransplant lymphoproliferative disorder.[149–152] The identification of antigens that are specifically expressed by leukemia cells, such as PR1 by CML and AML cells, and can be recognized by T cells has led to successful ex vivo generation of leukemia-specific donor T cells (PR1-CTL) that may promote a GVT effect.[153–155] Notwithstanding the promise of these novel approaches, the large-scale therapeutic potential of adoptive transfer of ex vivo expanded antigen-specific effector cells has not yet been fully realized for a number of reasons. One reason is the short survival of the effector cells, which likely is due to factors intrinsic to the cells themselves or to the host environment into which the cells are infused.

OPTIMIZATION OF GVT EFFECT: ADOPTIVE CELLULAR THERAPY VIA DLI

Adoptive cellular immunotherapy using DLI has been shown experimentally and clinically to be a potent means of inducing a GVT effect by converting mixed to full donor chimerism after allogeneic transplant.[156–158] In patients with recurrent CML after HLA-matched HCT, complete clinical and molecular remissions are achieved in the majority of patients following unmodified DLI.[159,160] A high incidence of GVHD (and marrow aplasia) has tempered the use of this approach and has led to a revision of DLI strategies, such as lowering the dose of infused T cells or giving T-cell subsets such as $CD8^+$–

depleted DLI.[161] The GVHD risk likely is higher after alternative donor transplantation, and considerably smaller doses of T-cells have been used in the haploidentical HCT setting.[162,163] Lewalle et al.[162] reported the outcomes of escalating DLI doses after haploidentical transplantation. $CD3^+$ T-cell doses greater than 1×10^4 kg every 3 months (given to convert mixed to full chimerism) caused significant GVHD in recipients of T-cell– and B-cell–depleted myeloablative haploidentical HCT. Or et al.[163] treated 28 patients (six prophylactic and 22 therapeutic) with HLA-mismatched DLI. The dose range of T cells in the DLI was 1×10^2 to 1.5×10^9 kg. GVHD (median peak grade 2) occurred in 13 of the 28 patients. A higher incidence of GVHD unexpectedly occurred in recipients of 5/6 HLA-matched DLI compared to recipients of a 3/6 HLA-matched DLI. In our nonmyeloablative HCT trial, in which vigorous ex vivo and in vivo T-cell depletion are used, $CD3^+$ T-cell doses greater than 1.0×10^6 kg were given in some circumstances. Because GVHD occurred in the majority of cases (most often skin-limited GVHD), future strategies will use a smaller initial DLI dose.[18] Additional dose finding studies are required to establish the safest and most effective DLI T-cell dose and schedule following haploidentical HCT. Critical to the success of HCT will be the identification of specific cellular populations that can be administered as adoptive cellular immunotherapy (e.g., pathogen- or tumor-specific CTL) and that are capable of optimizing the separation of GVHD and GVT.

HAPLOIDENTICAL HCT: NEW APPLICATIONS

Combining Haploidentical PBSCs with Umbilical Cord Blood for Facilitation of Engraftment

Umbilical cord blood transplantation has been complicated by slow hematologic recovery and delayed immune reconstitution due in part to the relatively low number of hematopoietic progenitor cells collected and transplanted. In an attempt to facilitate hematologic recovery and reduce the complications associated with impaired immune recovery, Fernandez et al. cotransplanted 11 patients with umbilical cord blood cells and $CD34^+$ cell-selected haploidentical PBSC.[164] Rapid neutrophil recovery occurred at a median of 10 days (range 9–17 days) days. Chimerism studies showed a predominance of the haploidentical genotype in the granulocyte and mononuclear lineages early posttransplant, followed by progressive replacement by cells of umbilical cord donor origin. Grade II or higher GVHD occurred in 4 (36%) of the 11patients. Five of the 11 patients were alive and in complete remission 6 to 43 months posttransplant. Evaluation of immune reconstitution in this patient population demonstrated early recovery of NK cells and B cells and delayed but eventually complete recovery of $CD4^+$ and $CD8^+$ cells.[165]

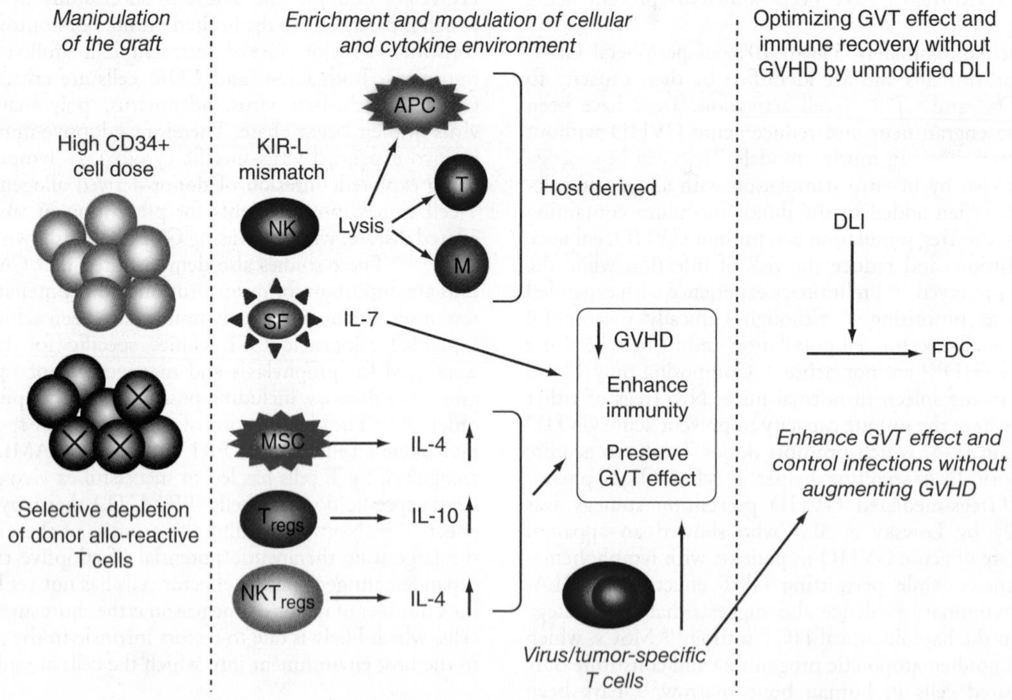

Figure 104–1 Schema of a strategy for optimizing outcomes of haploidentical HCT. Graft Manipulation: High $CD34^+$ cell dose likely will improve donor engraftment by overcoming host-mediated resistance. Selective ex vivo depletion of donor alloreactive T cells may reduce the incidence of severe acute graft-versus-host disease (GVHD) while preserving graft-versus-tumor (GVT) effect and improving immune recovery. Enrichment and Modulation of Cellular and Cytokine Environment: KIR ligand mismatching in the graft-versus-host (GVH) direction will prompt donor natural killer (NK) cells to promote engraftment by attacking host T cells (T), diminish acute GVHD by depleting host antigen-presenting cells (APC) while eliminating host-derived malignant cells (M). Ex vivo expanded NK cells, mesenchymal stem cells (MSCs), T regulatory cells (Tregs), NK Tregs, and soluble factor (interleukin-7) will further augment donor engraftment, innate and adaptive immune responses, and reduce GVHD while not impairing GVT effects. MSC and NK Tregs, via IL-4 production, will skew donor T cells toward an antiinflammatory T_H2 phenotype that is associated with reduced GVHD. Optimizing GVT Effect and Immune Recovery Without GVHD by unmodified Donor Leukocyte Infusion (DLI): Ex vivo engineered tumor antigen- and pathogen (virus)-specific donor-derived T cells (both cytotoxic T lymphocytes [CTLs] and CD4 cells) can be used to prevent and/or treat relapse of an underlying malignancy and opportunistic infections, respectively. In some circumstances, unmodified DLI may be used to convert mixed chimerism to full donor chimerism (FDC), probably enhancing a GVT effect without augmenting GVHD.

Specific Tolerance Induction

Induction of donor-specific tolerance has important implications for the field of organ transplantation, which currently is limited by the complications of lifelong immunosuppressive therapy. Multiple preclinical small and large animal models have shown that sustained specific tolerance can be induced after induction of even transient mixed lymphohematopoietic chimerism.[166,167] Based on these preclinical discoveries, we have conducted clinical trials of combined related donor bone marrow and kidney transplantation for patients with end-stage renal disease. In the first of these trials, combined HLA-matched bone marrow and kidney transplantation was performed in patients with multiple myeloma and end-stage renal disease. This experience was notable for the achievement of complete remissions in four of six patients and the occurrence of renal graft rejection (transient and reversible) in only one patient. All six patients were alive from approximately 3 to 8 years posttransplant.[7,168]

In order to broaden the application of this strategy, we initiated a trial of combined haploidentical bone marrow and kidney transplantation for patients with end-stage renal disease but no associated malignancy. The preparative therapy is one that we used in earlier trials of haploidentical HCT for hematologic malignancies and was notable for the uniform development of transient mixed chimerism followed by graft rejection.[18] Of the first five patients who received a combined haploidentical bone marrow and kidney transplant, four are no longer receiving immunosuppressive therapy. In vitro evidence of specific tolerance also has been demonstrated.[169]

The proof of principle of sustained donor-specific tolerance induction through mixed lymphohematopoietic chimerism has been demonstrated clinically. Future trials will include the transplantation of other organs, including cadaveric organs, and the inclusion of fully HLA-mismatched related donors.

FUTURE DIRECTIONS

The promise of haploidentical HCT, specifically the opportunity to offer allogeneic transplantation to virtually everyone who requires it and to take advantage of the powerful GVT effect that it affords, has yet to be fully realized. Although the complications of severe GVHD and graft rejection have been overcome in large part by the use of "megadose" T-cell–depleted hematopoietic progenitor cells, prolonged immunodeficiency remains a formidable problem. Reduced-intensity conditioning has ameliorated early transplant-related morbidity and perhaps mortality but has been associated with a higher relapse probability and no clear advantage in terms of restoration of effective immunity. Vigorous pan–T-cell depletion of the graft dramatically reduces the incidence of acute GVHD but delays immune reconstitution, resulting in a high incidence of opportunistic infections and disease relapse.

The future of haploidentical HCT relies on the ability to modulate the cellular content of the graft and the posttransplant cellular environment, to separate GVHD and GVT, and to rapidly restore effective immunity (shown schematically in Fig. 104–1). Strategies such as selective allodepletion of the graft or enrichment for (or addition of) cell populations such as Tregs or MSC to the graft may achieve effective protection from GVHD while imparting effective antitumor and antiinfective immunity.

Following the transplant, administration of specific cellular populations or soluble factors may affect the separation of GVHD and graft-versus-malignancy effect. Unmanipulated DLI may still be considered at certain time points to convert the mixed chimerism to full donor hematopoiesis in an effort to achieve an early GVT effect and facilitate early reconstitution. The adoptive transfer of allogeneic cytotoxic T cells that are specific for viral or tumor antigens may be other strategies for addressing the problems of infection and disease relapse. Other cellular populations, such as NK or NK T cells or MSC, may favorably influence the balance of GVHD and immune reconstitution. The future of haploidentical transplant depends on our expanding knowledge of the cellular populations and soluble factors that determine the separation of GVHD and GVT effect and our ability to modulate the cellular content of the graft and the posttransplant environment to improve disease-free and overall survival probabilities.

SUGGESTED READINGS

Aggarwal S, Pittenger MF: Human mesenchymal stem cells modulate allogeneic immune cell responses. Blood 105:1815, 2005.

Alpdogan O, Schmaltz C, Muriglan SJ, et al: Administration of interleukin-7 after allogeneic bone marrow transplantation improves immune reconstitution without aggravating graft-versus-host disease. Blood 98:2256, 2001.

Amrolia PJ, Muccioli-Casadei G, Huls H, et al: Adoptive immunotherapy with allodepleted donor T-cells improves immune reconstitution after haploidentical stem cell transplantation. Blood 108:1797, 2006.

Aversa F, Terenzi A, Tabilio A, et al: Full haplotype-mismatched hematopoietic stem-cell transplantation: a phase II study in patients with acute leukemia at high risk of relapse. J Clin Oncol 23:3447, 2005.

Beatty PG, Clift RA, Mickelson EM, et al: Marrow transplantation from related donors other than HLA-identical siblings. N Engl J Med 313:765, 1985.

Chen BJ, Cui X, Liu C, Chao NJ: Prevention of graft-versus-host disease while preserving graft-versus-leukemia effect after selective depletion of host-reactive T cells by photodynamic cell purging process. Blood 99:3083, 2002.

Edinger M, Hoffmann P, Ermann J, et al: $CD4^+CD25^+$ regulatory T cells preserve graft-versus-tumor activity while inhibiting graft-versus-host disease after bone marrow transplantation. Nat Med 9:1144, 2003.

Fehse B, Frerk O, Goldmann M, Bulduk M, Zander AR: Efficient depletion of alloreactive donor T lymphocytes based on expression of two activation-induced antigens (CD25 and CD69). Br J Haematol 109:644, 2000.

Guinan EC, Boussiotis VA, Neuberg D, et al: Transplantation of anergic histoincompatible bone marrow allografts. N Engl J Med 340:1704, 1999.

Ichinohe T, Uchiyama T, Shimazaki C, et al: Feasibility of HLA-haploidentical hematopoietic stem cell transplantation between noninherited maternal antigen (NIMA)-mismatched family members linked with long-term fetomaternal microchimerism. Blood 104:3821, 2004.

Karre K, Ljunggren HG, Piontek G, Kiessling R: Selective rejection of H-2-deficient lymphoma variants suggests alternative immune defence strategy. Nature 319:675, 1986.

Le Blanc K, Rasmusson I, Sundberg B, et al: Treatment of severe acute graft-versus-host disease with third party haploidentical mesenchymal stem cells. Lancet 363:1439, 2004.

Mapara MY, Kim YM, Wang SP, Bronson R, Sachs DH, Sykes M: Donor lymphocyte infusions mediate superior graft-versus-leukemia effects in mixed compared to fully allogeneic chimeras: a critical role for host antigen-presenting cells. Blood 100:1903, 2002.

O'Donnell PV, Luznik L, Jones RJ, et al: Nonmyeloablative bone marrow transplantation from partially HLA-mismatched related donors using posttransplantation cyclophosphamide. Biol Blood Marrow Transplant 8:377, 2002.

Peggs KS, Verfuerth S, Pizzey A, et al: Adoptive cellular therapy for early cytomegalovirus infection after allogeneic stem-cell transplantation with virus-specific T-cell lines. Lancet 362:1375, 2003.

Powles RL, Morgenstern GR, Kay HE, et al: Mismatched family donors for bone-marrow transplantation as treatment for acute leukaemia. Lancet 1:612, 1983.

Ruggeri L, Capanni M, Urbani E, et al: Effectiveness of donor natural killer cell alloreactivity in mismatched hematopoietic transplants. Science 295:2097, 2002.

Shlomchik WD, Couzens MS, Tang CB, et al: Prevention of graft versus host disease by inactivation of host antigen-presenting cells. Science 285:412, 1999.

Spitzer TR, McAfee S, Sackstein R, et al: Intentional induction of mixed chimerism and achievement of antitumor responses after nonmyeloablative conditioning therapy and HLA-matched donor bone marrow transplantation for refractory hematologic malignancies. Biol Blood Marrow Transplant 6:309, 2000.

Sykes M, Preffer F, McAfee S, et al: Mixed lymphohaemopoietic chimerism and graft-versus-lymphoma effects after non-myeloablative therapy and HLA-mismatched bone-marrow transplantation. Lancet 353:1755, 1999.

REFERENCES

For complete list of references log onto www.expertconsult.com

CHAPTER 105

UMBILICAL CORD BLOOD TRANSPLANTATION

Claudio G. Brunstein and John E. Wagner, Jr.

Transplantation of allogeneic hematopoietic stem cells (HSC) derived from bone marrow (BM) or peripheral blood has been used successfully to treat high-risk or relapsed hematologic malignancies, marrow failure syndromes, selected hereditary immunodeficiency states, and metabolic disorders. However, the availability of suitable donors remains a major limitation, often preventing the application of hematopoietic cell transplantation (HCT). Because only 30% of patients have an HLA-matched sibling donor, adult volunteer unrelated donor (URD) registries have been created.[1] Currently more than 11 million donors are registered worldwide, with more than eight million donors typed at the HLA-A, B, and DR loci and approximately 870,000 typed by high-resolution molecular techniques *(www.bmdw.org)*. The National Marrow Donor Program (NMDP) has more than six million registered donors, with approximately 410,000 having undergone high-resolution HLA-A, B, and DR typing (S. Spellman and D. Weisdorf, Personal Communication, May 2007). However, only 40% of caucasians and a far greater proportion of those of racial and ethnic minority descent are able to find a suitable HLA-matched donor.[1,2] Furthermore, data from marrow donor registries have consistently reported a 3- to 4-month median interval from initiation of the search to transplantation. During the search process, transplant candidates may die of disease progression or related complications (i.e., infections, treatment toxicities) or become ineligible for HCT. Although great efforts have been made to improve donor availability,[3,4] there remains a need to investigate alternative sources of HSCs to alleviate the shortage of suitable URDs and reduce the length of the donor search process. New strategies are needed to reduce the high risk of mortality that currently limits the successful application of adult volunteer URD HCT therapy intended to replace a diseased or damaged hematopoietic compartment and immune system.

The concept of using umbilical cord blood (UCB) as a clinical source of HSC was first considered in the late 1960s. Recognizing the potential value of UCB, Ende and Ende[5] were among the first to apply UCB to the treatment of a child with leukemia. In the first published report, freshly procured UCB samples from eight donors were infused over a 17-day period in a 16-year-old boy with acute lymphocytic leukemia who previously had been treated with 6-mercaptopurine and prednisone. Although long-term reconstitution was not demonstrated, Ende and Ende documented a transient alteration in red cell antigens in the peripheral blood, suggesting a transient mixed chimerism from at least one if not several of the units. Additional studies performed by Koike[6] and Vidal[7] in the late 1970s and early 1980s suggested that UCB may contain sufficient numbers of hematopoietic progenitor cells for transplantation. Preclinical studies compared numbers of hematopoietic progenitors in UCB and marrow. The authors concluded that if a sufficient volume of cord blood could be collected, the number of BM progenitors would be adequate to reconstitute hematopoiesis in transplant recipients.[6,7] In anticipation of possible clinical application, Koike[6] subsequently showed that UCB progenitors could be cryopreserved without significant loss of viability and proliferative capacity. The conclusion was that "(cryopreserved) cord blood cells . . . may be useful as a source of hemopoietic progenitor cells for marrow transplantation."

Hal Broxmeyer, Ted Boyse, Gordon Douglas, and Lewis Thomas in collaboration with Pablo Rubinstein were instrumental in further development of the concept that UCB could be a clinically applicable source for HSCs and progenitors useful for transplantation. The Broxmeyer laboratory systematically evaluated the hematopoietic potential of human UCB in vitro and developed practical and efficient methods for large-volume collections and storing UCB in anticipation of its clinical use.[8–11] This work ultimately led to a collaboration between Henry Friedman, Joanne Kurtzberg, and Arleen Auerbach, who cared for a child with Fanconi anemia, Hal Broxmeyer and Gordon Douglas who collected and stored the cord blood unit from the patient's sibling, and Eliane Gluckman, Agnes Devergie, Hélène Esperou, Gérard Socie, and Pierre Lehn, the transplant team. The first human UCB transplant took place on October 6, 1988 in Paris.[12] Complete chimerism was sustained long term after transplantation in both myeloid and lymphoid lineages. Thus, these investigators were the first to demonstrate that pluripotent HSC existed in human UCB. The recipient of this first UCB HCT remains alive and well with complete chimerism 19 years later (J. Kurtzberg, Personal Communication, June 2007).

After this initial report, several investigators started to explore the potential of UCB as a source of HSC for transplantation. At first many questions were raised: Would this HSC source engraft larger recipients or patients with diseases other than Fanconi anemia? Would lethal graft-versus-host disease (GVHD) occur because of maternal lymphocyte contamination, previously shown to occur in some neonates with congenital immunodeficiency? Would naive lymphocytes in the UCB unit really be less likely to cause GVHD? Would these naive UCB lymphocytes mount an effective graft-versus-leukemia (GVL) response? Could UCB be used as a source of HSC in the URD setting, rather than in the relatively rare situation of sibling HCT? Some of these questions would not be resolved for another decade.

Based on the early successes with sibling donor UCB transplantation,[12–15] public cord blood banks (CBBs) were created. The first was founded in 1992 by Pablo Rubinstein at the New York Blood Center. Today, at least 38 CBBs collecting UCB units for public use worldwide. As of May 2007, more than 260,000 HLA-A, B, and DRB1 typed UCB units were registered with Bone Marrow Donors Worldwide (www.bmdw.org). However, a significant proportion of the UCB units, particularly those collected in the early years, have limited usefulness based on the number of cells stored and the quality controls (i.e., infectious disease screen) applied at the time. Despite these limitations, UCB from siblings and URDs has been used to reconstitute hematopoiesis in at least 7000 patients with malignant and nonmalignant disorders, including more than 2500 adult recipients. This chapter reviews the current state of knowledge regarding UCB biology as well as clinical results with UCB transplantation and current research initiatives with this unique source of HSC.

ATTRIBUTES OF UMBILICAL CORD BLOOD HEMATOPOIETIC PROGENITOR CELLS

Recognition of the potential clinical utility of UCB prompted numerous laboratory studies to reassess the biologic characteristics of the primitive hematopoietic progenitors found in UCB. Ontologically, hematopoiesis begins in the ventral aspect of the fetal aorta and primitive yolk sac early after conception. Following a brief hepatic phase, at the end of the second trimester it enters the marrow space, where it remains throughout adulthood. It has long been recognized that human UCB contains a high frequency of hematopoietic progenitor cells, at least equal to that of colony-forming unit granulocyte-macrophage (CFU-GM) progenitor cells in adult BM.[8–10,16] The reason for the presence of these cells in the circulation is not known but may relate to growth factors released by the placenta. Within hours of birth, however, the progenitors leave the neonatal circulation and subsequently are present only at very low frequency in unmobilized peripheral blood.

Primitive hematopoietic progenitor cells in UCB express both CD34 and HLA-DR, suggesting that they are phenotypically distinct from those of adult BM.[17] In contrast to HLA-DR, Hao et al.[18] and Cardoso et al.[19] found that CD38 distinguishes subpopulations of hematopoietic progenitor cells in UCB. The $CD34^+CD38^-$ immunophenotype defines a rare, quiescent $CD34^+$ subpopulation in both UCB and adult BM that can be distinguished functionally from the $CD34^+CD38^+$ population by sustained clonogenicity in extended long-term culture assay (>8 weeks). However, in comparison to $CD34^+CD38^-$ cells in adult marrow, Hao et al.[18] showed that UCB $CD34^+CD38^-$ cells continue to proliferate well beyond 8 weeks. In addition, UCB $CD34^+CD38^-$ cells proliferate more rapidly in response to cytokine stimulation in vitro, and each $CD34^+$ cell generates a significantly greater number of progeny compared to adult marrow counterparts.

Lansdorp et al.[20] compared the proliferative responses of purified candidate stem cell populations in adult marrow, fetal liver, and UCB. When cells with the $CD34^+CD45RA^{lo}CD71^{lo}$ phenotype were cultured in serum-free media supplemented with a mixture of cytokines including interleukin (IL)-3, IL-6, stem cell factor, and erythropoietin, striking differences were observed. Throughout the culture period, the number of $CD34^+$ BM cells remained relatively constant, whereas $CD34^+$ UCB cells increased several hundred-fold, and $CD34^+$ fetal liver cells increased several thousand-fold. Additionally, Carow et al.[21] demonstrated that UCB CFU-granulocyte, erythrocyte, megakaryocte, macrophage (GEMM) progenitors had extensive replating capacity, which contrasts with that of adult marrow. Addition of UCB plasma to the culture medium resulted in extensive secondary replating potential, suggesting that other factors were present in UCB plasma not found in adult plasma or in artificial media supplemented with recombinant growth factors. These properties suggest that UCB may be more amenable than BM to in vitro manipulation for the purposes of genetic manipulation or ex vivo expansion.

Broxmeyer et al.[10] assessed the potential suitability of UCB as a graft for adult recipients. Although the numbers of nucleated cells (NC) and progenitors in UCB specimens were substantially lower than that of allogeneic marrow grafts, they postulated that the progenitors in UCB had a greater capacity for expansion than did BM. Work performed in this laboratory and others supported this claim. Cardoso et al.[19] showed that the total CFU-GM production of UCB $CD34^+CD38^-$ cells was 7.6-fold greater than that in a corresponding population in adult marrow. Similarly, Lewis and Verfaillie[22] demonstrated a higher frequency of both myeloid and lymphoid progenitors at day 0 and enhanced proliferative capacity at 5 weeks in both contact and noncontact culture conditions with UCB compared to mobilized adult peripheral blood.

Consistent with these in vitro findings, UCB was also found to have a higher engrafting capability in vivo using a murine model than did cells derived from adult marrow.[23] Although no validated in vitro or animal model in vivo assay for true pluripotential HSC exists, it is clear that UCB $CD34^+$ cells contain a higher frequency of mouse severe combined immunodeficient (SCID) repopulating cells (SRC). Through limiting dilution analysis, the frequency of SRC in UCB is 1 in 9.3×10^5 cells, in marked contrast to 1 in 3×10^6 found in adult BM and 1 in 6×10^6 found in mobilized adult peripheral blood. Although there is one SRC per 660 $CD34^+CD38^-$ UCB cells, Yahata et al.[24] demonstrated an SRC frequency of 1 in 44 $CD34^+CD38^-$ cells using the technique of intrabone marrow injection rather than conventional tail vein injection. Using the same technique, Wang et al.[25] also demonstrated that UCB contains $CD34^-$ cells that have SCID-repopulating activity.

In summary, UCB appears to contain an increased concentration of primitive hematopoietic progenitors with greater proliferative capacity compared to adult marrow. These unique biologic features may explain in part the higher than expected rate of engraftment observed in UCB transplant recipients despite the low absolute numbers of $CD34^+$ cells and CFU-GM infused. Interestingly, other studies suggest that UCB progenitors may also be "less mature" by virtue of telomere length.[26] How these attributes affect engraftment or the capacity of UCB stem and progenitor cells to be expanded or genetically modified in ex vivo culture remains to be determined.

ATTRIBUTES OF THE NEONATAL IMMUNE SYSTEM

Adult URD marrow transplantation is limited by the lack of suitable donors, particularly in certain ethnic and racial minorities, and by the risk of life-threatening complications such as GVHD and opportunistic infection, particularly when donor and recipient are not HLA matched. To address this problem, efforts over the last 3 decades have focused on enlarging the URD pool and developing new immunosuppressive drugs. However, although a reduction in T-cell number can reduce the incidence of severe acute GVHD, T-cell depletion (TCD) increases the risks of graft failure, viral infection, and relapse.[27,28] These complications offset the advantage of reduced GVHD. Other strategies are required to improve survival in the setting of URD HCT.

In this context, the unique neonatal immune system associated with UCB may be advantageous. Clinical results with UCB transplantation show a less than expected incidence of GVHD given the use of HLA-disparate grafts. The precise explanation for the reduced alloreactive response is unclear. The median $CD3^+$ cell dose of approximately 8×10^6/kg in UCB grafts[29,30] compares to 30 to 40×10^6 $CD3^+$ cells/kg recipient body[28] weight in a typical marrow allograft and can be equated with a BM graft after modest TCD. Because a $CD3^+$ cell dose less than 0.1×10^6 $CD3^+$ cells/kg is required to eliminate the risk of severe acute GVHD, the T-cell dose delivered in UCB should be capable of inducing significant GVHD, particularly in the setting of HLA mismatch. Therefore, the more likely explanation for the reduced incidence of GVHD with UCB transplant is qualitative and functional differences found with UCB lymphoid cells.

Rainaut et al.[31] reported that, compared to adult peripheral blood, UCB has (a) a significantly greater absolute number of lymphocytes per milliliter (two to threefold greater), (b) a significantly lower percentage of $CD8^+$ T cells, and (c) a significantly greater CD4/CD8 ratio.[31] Hannet et al.[32] further characterized UCB lymphocytes, reporting phenotypic characteristics suggestive of T-cell "immaturity". These authors found that the majority of $CD4^+$ UCB lymphocytes coexpressed CD45RA (91% vs 40% of adult $CD4^+$ lymphocytes), fewer $CD3^+$ T cells expressed IL-2 receptors (8% vs 18%), and fewer $CD3^+$ T cells expressed the activation marker HLA-DR (2% vs 10%). Clement et al.[33] found that virtually all UCB $CD4^+$ T cells coexpress CD38 (95%) and CD45RA (>90%).[33] They also demonstrated that $CD4^+CD45RA^+$ UCB T cells have no detectable helper function and that their dominant immunoregulatory activity is suppression.

Roncarolo et al.[34] reported investigations of the functional immunologic properties of UCB lymphocytes. Purified UCB T cells were found to proliferate vigorously when activated by allogeneic antigens in primary mixed lymphocyte reactions, indicating that UCB cells respond normally to activation by alloantigens. In addition, strong proliferative responses were observed when UCB T cells were activated by cross-linked anti-CD3 monoclonal antibodies. However, UCB cells had a reduced capacity to stimulate allogeneic cells in primary mixed lymphocyte reactions, suggesting reduced antigen-presenting capacity. UCB cells are impaired in their capacity to generate allogeneic cytotoxic activity in primary mixed lymphocyte reactions. Whether this defect is intrinsic to cytotoxic T cells or due to other factors preventing the generation of alloantigen-specific cytotoxic T cells is not known.

The alloreactive T-cell repertoire present in UCB is composed of unprimed cells, compared to the repertoire of T cells in adult BM or peripheral blood in which more than 50% of alloreactive T cells are of the primed memory phenotype. Studies by Roncarolo et al.[34] indicate that repeated activation of unprimed UCB T cells with alloantigens in vitro results in the inability of these cells to proliferate or produce cytokines following restimulation with the same antigens. Furthermore, although these authors showed that the natural killer (NK) activity of purified CD56$^+$ UCB NK cells against NK-sensitive targets is comparable to that observed with adult NK cells, El Marsafy et al.[35] showed that UCB NK cells can exhibit suppressor activity inhibiting autologous UCB T-cell responders in mixed lymphocyte cultures.

Roncarolo et al.[34] demonstrated that IL-2, IL-6, and tumor necrosis factor-α production by UCB mononuclear cells following activation was comparable to that observed with adult peripheral blood mononuclear cells. However, in contrast, interferon-γ and IL-10 production was significantly decreased, and IL-4 and IL-5 were absent. Granulocyte-macrophage colony-stimulating factor levels were generally higher in the supernatants of UCB cells.

In addition, Godfrey et al.[36] demonstrated a high frequency of regulatory T cells in UCB. These cells, characterized by coexpression of CD4, CD25, and FOXP3, have already been shown to be critically important in self-tolerance and prevention of autoimmunity.[37–42] Numerous investigators have shown that regulatory T cells markedly impair the activation and expansion of alloreactive CD4$^+$ and CD8$^+$ T cells and GVHD lethality.[37–41] Whether these cells are responsible for the reduced risk of severe GVHD typically observed in recipients of UCB, even when highly HLA mismatched, is not known. This T-cell subpopulation is under active investigation.

Of interest is the finding that fetal immune cells are tolerant to noninherited maternal HLA antigens and that this tolerance is reduced over the first year of life.[43] At birth, UCB cells were observed to be immunologically nonreactive with cells from mother and minimally reactive with cells from father. Although the neonatal blood was capable of mediating NK lysis, the infant did not develop the ability to generate an alloantigen-specific cytotoxic response until sometime between birth and 6 months of age. The concept of partial fetal tolerance to the noninherited maternal allele (NIMA) was first proposed on the basis of outcomes observed in recipients of parental renal allografts.[44,45] How such "tolerance" develops is unknown, but this phenomenon is particularly intriguing in view of the clinical results observed in haploidentical sibling donor–recipient pairs. If the immune cells in the UCB graft are partially tolerant to HLA antigens on NIMA, this finding could have significant implications in defining what is an "acceptable" donor in both the related and URD setting, which heretofore has not been explored.

Today, the unique attributes of the neonatal immune system permit the clinical application of HLA-mismatched UCB without increased risk of GVHD. Although the mechanisms remain to be discovered, work is ongoing to isolate and expand unique lymphocyte populations to enhance engraftment, reduce GVHD, or augment the GVL response.

SIBLING DONOR UMBILICAL CORD BLOOD TRANSPLANTATION

The first multiinstitutional registry report detailing the transplant outcomes after UCB transplantation from HLA-matched and HLA-mismatched sibling donors was published in 1995[13] and updated in 1998.[15] For the 74 patients transplanted with sibling donor UCB, the median recipient age was 4.9 years (range 0.5–16.3 years). Of these patients, 56 received a 0–1 HLA antigen-mismatched graft and 18 a 2–3 HLA antigen-mismatched graft. Prophylaxis for acute GVHD most often consisted of cyclosporine alone or in combination with methylprednisolone or an anti–T-cell antibody. The median cell dose infused was 4.7 (range 1.0–33.0), with half of patients receiving prophylactic granulocyte colony-stimulating factor or granulocyte-macrophage colony-stimulating factor. For recipients of 0–1 HLA antigen-mismatched sibling donor UCB grafts, the probability of neutrophil recovery (defined as absolute neutrophil count $>5 \times 10^8$/L) was 91% (±2%) at 60 days posttransplantation at a median of 22 days (range 9–46 days). Platelet recovery after transplantation (defined as platelet count $>5 \times 10^{10}$/L untransfused for 7 days) was achieved at a median of 51 days (range 15–117 days). Although the engraftment rate was high for the group as a whole, there was a trend toward a greater risk of graft failure in recipients with a history of a marrow failure syndrome, hemoglobinopathy, or storage disease. All patients receiving transplant as therapy for a malignancy engrafted. Of note, use of hematopoietic growth factor was not associated with more rapid myeloid recovery or better engraftment. This first analysis led to several critical conclusions in terms of engraftment: (a) UCB appears to be a reliable source of HSC at least for children, (b) hematopoietic growth factor has no clear effect upon rate or durability of engraftment, and (c) no clear cell dose effect suggested that the number of hematopoietic cells infused was still above the threshold number of cells needed for consistent engraftment.

Gluckman et al.[46] on behalf of the Eurocord Transplant Registry subsequently reported transplant outcomes in 74 recipients of related donor UCB. The median age of the population was 5 years (range 0.2–20 years); 46 patients had malignancy, 17 BM failure syndromes, eight hemoglobinopathy, and seven inborn errors of metabolism. Sixty of the 74 patients received HLA-identical grafts. In contrast to the report by Wagner et al,[15] the probability of neutrophil engraftment was 79%, and platelet engraftment was 62% by day 60. Myeloid recovery and engraftment were favorably influenced by younger recipient age ($P = 0.02$), lower recipient body weight ($P = 0.02$), and HLA identity ($P = 0.04$), with a trend toward better outcome in those with a higher NC dose ($P = 0.06$). Furthermore, in univariate analysis platelet recovery was favorably influenced by lower recipient body weight ($P = 0.04$) and HLA identity ($P < 0.001$). In the setting of related donor UCB transplantation, this was the first report suggesting a possible relationship between NC dose of the UCB graft and speed and likelihood of myeloid engraftment. This finding for the first time suggested that a lower threshold might be identifiable for which the risk of graft failure or markedly delayed myeloid recovery might be considered excessive.

In terms of acute GVHD, the incidence has been consistently low in recipients of 0–1HLA antigen-mismatched sibling donor UCB transplants. In the first report by Wagner et al,[13,15] the probability of grade II to IV and grade III to IV GVHD was only 3% (±2%) and 2% (±2%), respectively, by day 100 after UCB transplantation. Of the cohort of patients with a 0–1 HLA antigen-disparate sibling donor, chronic GVHD was reported in only three patients; no patient had extensive disease. Interestingly, severe GVHD was observed infrequently in the 15 evaluable patients with haploidentical sibling donors.[15] Of the 15 evaluable patients, two were mismatched at two HLA antigens and 13 were mismatched at three HLA antigens. Although patient numbers were small, donor–recipient pairs mismatched at the NIMA appeared to be less likely to develop grade II to IV acute GVHD than donor–recipient pairs mismatched at the paternal allele. This observation supported the hypothesis that partial tolerance to the NIMA might develop during gestation, as suggested by van Rood et al.[47] and subsequently supported by other reports in recipients of haploidentical BM. Gluckman et al.[46] also observed a low incidence of acute GVHD, with 18% of the entire cohort having grade II to IV disease. In this study, the probability of acute GVHD was 9% in recipients of HLA-matched UCB and 50% in recipients of HLA-mismatched units ($P < 0.001$). Chronic GVHD was observed in eight of 56 patients surviving beyond day 100 after transplantation.

Wagner and Kurtzberg[15] reported a survival rate of 61% (±12%) in recipients of 0–1HLA antigen-mismatched UCB grafts at median followup of 2 years. Causes of death were multifactorial, including graft failure, relapse, organ failure, infection, and bleeding. For the entire cohort, GVHD was listed as a cause of death in only one patient with an HLA 3 antigen-mismatched donor graft. The probability of disease-free survival (DFS) in those treated for malignancy was 41% (±11%). Similarly, Gluckman et al.[46] reported a survival of 63% at 1 year. Factors that favorably influenced survival were younger age ($P < 0.001$), lower recipient body weight ($P < 0.001$), HLA identity ($P < 0.006$), and negativity of recipient cytomegalovirus (CMV) serology ($P = 0.002$). Lower body weight was associated with improved outcome, but cell dose had yet to be identified as a key factor in terms of survival.

These observations led to a comparison of sibling UCB transplants and marrow transplants using BM from HLA-matched sibling donors. Therefore, in a joint study of the International Bone Marrow Transplant Registry and Eurocord, Rocha et al.[48] reported the results of an analysis comparing outcomes in 2052 recipients of HLA-matched marrow and 113 recipients of HLA-matched UCB from sibling donors. UCB recipients were transplanted between 1990 and 1997 and received grafts containing a median cell dose of 4.7×10^7 NC/kg. Myeloid recovery after UCB transplantation (median 26 days, 89% by day 60) was inferior to that observed after BM (median 18 days, 98% by day 60; $P < 0.001$). However, UCB transplantation was associated with a significantly lower incidence of grade II to IV acute GVHD (14% vs 24%, $P = 0.02$), with less frequent grade III to IV acute GVHD and less chronic GVHD. Importantly, survival rates after UCB and BM transplantation were similar at 3 years (64% vs 66%, $P = 0.93$). Causes of death between the two cohorts were similar, with no significant differences in the number of deaths from relapse, suggesting that risk of relapse may be similar. Although only suggestive, these data indicated that the GVL effect of the allograft still might be intact despite the apparent reduction in risk of acute and chronic GVHD.

In summary, these data suggested that survival after sibling UCB transplantation was comparable to that observed with sibling donor BM. Although the rate of hematopoietic recovery and probability of engraftment were inferior to those of marrow, risks of acute and chronic GVHD were superior. The data supported the routine use of sibling donor UCB when available. More importantly, these data supported the development of both private and public CBBs, as it was becoming increasingly clear that directed UCB collections (i.e., for a sibling with a disease amenable to hematopoietic cell transplantation) would obviate the need for harvesting marrow from an appropriately HLA-matched sibling. Investigators speculated that UCB might offer significant advantages over marrow or peripheral blood as a source of HSCs and progenitor cells for both children and adults in need of URD HCT. The stage was set for large-scale banking of UCB and UCB transplantation using partially HLA-matched URDs.

UNRELATED DONOR UMBILICAL CORD BLOOD TRANSPLANTATION: OUTCOMES IN CHILDREN

As a result of the early successes with sibling donor UCB transplantation, programs for the banking of URD UCB were initiated in many countries around the world. Currently CBBs are located throughout North America, South America, Europe, Asia, and Australia. Known benefits of banked UCB include (a) rapid availability, (b) absence of donor risk, (c) absence of donor attrition, and (d) very low risk of transmissible infectious diseases, such as CMV and Epstein-Barr virus (EBV). The attributes of UCB compared with BM are summarized in Table 105–1.

The literature on the use of URD UCB transplantation in children is summarized in Table 105–2. The first two reports of URD UCB transplantation in children were published simultaneously in 1996.[49,50] These two studies demonstrated that hematopoietic recovery and sustained engraftment could be expected in the majority of patients. Furthermore, risk of acute GVHD was low, a particularly striking finding given the use of HLA 1 and 2 antigen-mismatched units in the majority of patients. Gluckman et al.[46] subsequently reported the outcomes of 65 patients (median age 9 years; 49 with hematologic malignancy) transplanted with URD UCB. The probability of myeloid recovery was 87%. Notably, recipients of an UCB unit containing greater than 3.7×10^7 NC/kg were more likely to have faster myeloid recovery (25 days vs 35 days) and higher probability of myeloid recovery (94% vs 76%), more clearly demonstrating the importance of NC dose compared to prior reports with sibling donors. More recent analyses of the Eurocord dataset, including more than 500 patients, reported a 74% incidence of myeloid recovery by day 60 after UCB transplantation.[51] In multivariate analysis, neutrophil engraftment was positively influenced by HLA-matched, cryo-

Table 105–1 Comparison of Umbilical Cord Blood and Bone Marrow as Hematopoietic Stem Cell Sources for Unrelated Donor Transplantations

Factor	Bone Marrow Graft	Umbilical Cord Blood Graft
Available pool	Adult volunteer donors Estimated 11 million	Cryopreserved Estimated 260,000
Typing in database	68% HLA A, B, DRB1	100% HLA A, B, DRB1
Current standard for HLA match	8/8 A, B, C, DRB1 (allele level)	4–6/6 A, B, DRB1 (A and B antigen level, DRB1 allele level)
Median search time	4 months	1 month
Major factors limiting availability	HLA match Donor attrition	Cell dose
Minimum total nucleated cell needed for transplantation	~2.0×10^8/kg	~2.5×10^7/kg
Ease of changing transplantation date	Difficult	Flexible
Access to additional stem cells or lymphocytes	Yes	No
Potential disease transmission CMV or EBV Congenital disease	 Yes No	 No Yes
Risk to donor	Uncommon (potential complications related to anesthesia, surgery, growth factor, or needed for central access) Median time to return to normal activity: 7 days	None

Table 105–2 Unrelated Umbilical Cord Blood Transplantation for Children

	N	Median Age in Years (Range)	Cell Dose $\times 10^7$/kg (Range)	Median Time to Neutrophil Recovery in Days	Neutrophil Engraftment (%)	Platelet Engraftment (%)	Acute GVHD II–IV (%)	Acute GVHD III–IV (%)	GVHD Chronic (%)	TRM (%)	Survival (%)
Wagner et al.[50] 1996 (Minnesota and Orange County)	18	2.6 (0.1–21.3)	4.1 (1.4–40.0)	24	100	77	50	11	NA	39	65% at 6 months
Kurtzberg et al.[49] 1996 (Duke)	25	7 (0.8–24)	3.0 (0.7–11)	22	92	NA	43	10	10	44 at 6 months	64% at 100 days
Gluckman et al.[46] 1997 (Registry)	65	9 (0.3–45)	3.7 (0.7–30)	30	87	39 at 60 days	40	NA	0	NA	29% at 1 year
Rubinstein et al.[238] 2000 (Registry)	864	NA (79% < 18)	NA	NA	93	NA	48	24	31	NA	27% at 3 years (leukemia), 48% at 3 year (genetic disease), 29% at 3 year (BM failure)
Wagner et al.[30] 2002 (Minnesota)	102	7 (0.2–57)	3.1 (0.7–58)	23	88	65 at 180 days	39	11	10	30 at 1 year	58% at 1 year, 70% at 1 year if dose >1.7 × 10^5 CD34+/kg, 60% at 2 years (nonmalignant disease), 38% at 2 years (malignant disease)
Gluckman et al.[51] 2004 (Registry)	550	9.4 (4.5–21.1)	3.11 (1.9–5.2)	NA	76	43 at 60 days	36	20	26	34	34% at 3 years
Kurtzberg et al.[29] 2007 (COBLT)	193	7.7 (0.9–17.9)	5.1 (1.5–23.7)	27	80	50 at 180 days	42	20	20	17 at 100 days	57% at 1 year, influenced by CMV serostatus, ABO match, gender, HLA match, TNC

BM, bone marrow; CMV, cytomegalovirus; GVHD, graft-versus-host disease; NA, not available; TNC, total nucleated cell dose; TRM, treatment-related mortality.

preserved NC dose 4 × 10^7/kg or greater and administration of hematopoietic growth factors.[51]

Rubinstein et al.[52,53] subsequently summarized the results using UCB facilitated by the CBB at the New York Blood Center. In this study, patients had a hematologic malignancy (n = 581 [67%]), genetic disease (n = 209 [24%]), or acquired BM failure (n = 79 [9%]); the majority of patients (79%) were children. In contrast to the report by Gluckman et al., engraftment was 93% overall. One of the most important aspects of this report was identification of the cell dose threshold. Although a stepwise increase in graft NC dose was associated with a progressively shortened time to myeloid recovery, the incidence of myeloid recovery did not significantly change once the NC dose exceeded 2.5 × 10^7/kg. For the first time, the clinical data clearly established a cell dose threshold of 2.5 × 10^7/kg recipient body weight (based on the number of cells cryopreserved). In addition, HLA match (HLA 0 vs >1 mismatch) was associated with improved engraftment. The median time to myeloid recovery in recipients of 6/6 HLA-matched UCB unit was 23 days compared to 28 days in those transplanted with HLA-mismatched units ($P = 0.0027$).

Several studies failed to detect any association between HLA match and risk of acute GVHD,[51,54] but Rubinstein et al.[53] discerned a relationship. In the latter analysis, 3 (8%) of 36 recipients of 6/6 HLA-matched UCB, 42 (19%) of 227 recipients of 5/6 HLA-matched UCB, and 92 (28%) of 323 recipients of less than 4/6 HLA-matched UCB transplants developed severe acute GVHD ($P = 0.006$). Gluckman et al.[51] reported survival in 34% of patients at 1 year, with older recipient age, female gender of recipient, and advanced disease stage being adverse risk factors for survival. Notably, neither degree of HLA mismatching nor cell dose was shown to influence survival in this study. Rubinstein and Stevens[53] reported 3-year survival for each disease category, with 48% (95% confidence interval [CI] 40–55) of patients with genetic disease alive and 27% (95% CI 40–55) of patients with hematologic malignancy alive. Risk factors for adverse transplant-related events (defined as autologous reconstitution, requirement for a second graft, and death) were low cell dose and HLA mismatch.[53] Risk factors for relapse were advanced stage of disease at time of transplant and absence of acute GVHD after UCB transplantation.

In addition to registry analyses, several single-institution series have been reported. Between 1994 and 2001, outcomes in the first 102 consecutive patients (median age 7.4 years) transplanted at the University of Minnesota have been reported.[55] All patients received a myeloablative preparative regimen for treatment of malignant (n = 65) or nonmalignant (n = 37) disease. UCB grafts contained a median infused NC dose of 3.1 × 10^7/kg, CD34 cell dose 2.8 × 10^5/kg, and CD3 cell dose of 8.0 × 10^6/kg. Eighty-six percent of the UCB units were 1–3 HLA antigen-mismatched with the recipient. Median time to myeloid recovery (absolute neutrophil count >5 × 10^8/L) was 23 days (range 9–54 days), with 88% of patients recovering by day 42. Of note, CD34+ cell dose less than 1.7 × 10^5 cells/kg was associated with markedly inferior engraftment, higher treatment-related mortality (TRM), and lower probability of survival compared to higher cell doses. In Cox regression, HLA match, higher CD34+ cell dose, and absence of grade III-IV acute GVHD after transplantation were associated with improved survival.

Results of the Cord Blood Transplantation (COBLT) study, a national trial in the United States sponsored by the National Heart, Lung, and Blood Institute, have been reported.[29] This prospective, multiinstitutional study benefited by the use of standardized eligibility criteria, treatment plan, and evaluation criteria. Similar to prior reports, this cohort was primarily pediatric, and most patients had a malignancy. Of the 191 patients with malignancy in the pediatric age range (<18 years), the median age was 7.7 years (range 0.9–17 years), the median weight 25.9 kg (range 7.5–118.4 kg); 40% were Caucasian. The UCB units contained a median NC, CD34, and CD3 cell dose of 5.1 × 10^7/kg, 1.9 × 10^5/kg, and 7.9 × 10^6/kg, respectively. Although 9% of donor–recipient pairs were 6/6 HLA-matched (at antigen level HLA-A and B, and allele level HLA-DRB1), 30% and 58% were matched at 5/6 and 4/6 loci, respectively. In this report, engraftment was observed in 79.9% (75–85) at a median of 27 days (range 11–90 days). In Cox regression, HLA match and higher NC dose were favorable risk factors. In terms of acute and chronic GVHD, grade II to IV disease was observed in 41.9% (95% CI 34%–49%) and grade III to IV disease in 19.5% (95% CI 14%–26%) by day 100, and chronic GVHD was observed in 20% at 1 year. Of note, more closely matched pairs (6/6 and 5/6) were less likely to have acute GVHD. Of the 191 patients with malignancy, overall survival was 57.3% (50–64) at 1 year. In Cox regression, negative recipient CMV, male gender, ABO match, and higher NC dose were favorable risk factors.

As the experience with URD UCB transplantation widened, analyses of outcomes within specific disease categories became possible. Acute leukemia represents the single largest group for which children require allogeneic HSC transplantation. DFS rates range from 35% to 60% after UCB transplantation (Table 105–3).[56–62] Locatelli et al.[63] analyzed risk factors potentially influencing outcomes in children with acute leukemia who received UCB from either related (n = 42) or unrelated BM (n = 60) donors. In this study, 66 patients were defined as good risk (transplant in first or second complete remission), whereas 36 were transplanted in more advanced stages and were considered poor risk. Overall, the probability of event-free survival (EFS) at 2 years was 30%, with 49% survival for good-risk patients and 8% in those with more advanced disease. As expected for recipients of BM, multivariate analysis demonstrated that disease status at the time of transplant was the most significant risk factor. Similarly, Michel et al.[59] reported 2-year leukemia-free survival (LFS) of 42% and overall survival of 49% in children with acute myeloid leukemia undergoing UCB transplantation. Again, multivariate analysis only found disease status as a risk factor for both outcomes. Wagner et al.[30] observed a probability of survival of 50% at 2 years specifically for patients with acute leukemia in remission. In contrast, survival was 30% at 2 years for those with more advanced disease. Regardless of risk group, outcomes were similar for patients with acute lymphoblastic leukemia and acute myeloid leukemia.

Several reports have focused on acute lymphocytic leukemia. A report from the Eurocord Registry revealed a 36% DFS rate at 2 years for children in complete remission and 15% for those in relapse.[64] More recently, Sawczyn et al.[61] reported results in 26 children with acute lymphocytic leukemia undergoing myeloablative UCB trans-

Table 105–3 Umbilical Cord Blood Transplantation for Children with Acute Leukemiaa

Reference	No./Source of HSC	Median Age (years)	Disease/No.	TRM	EFS/LFS/RFS Relapse	OS
Pediatric Umbilical Cord Blood Transplantation						
Locatelli et al.[58] 1999	42/REL UCB 60/URD UCB	5	ALL: 70 AML: 32	50% at 1 year 30% at 1 year	2-year relapse: 28% 2-year relapse: 46%	42% at 1 year
Arcesse et al.[57] 1999[a]	14/URD UCB	11	ALL: 11 AML: 2	3/6	3-year LFS: 53%	64% at 3 years
Ohnuma et al.[56] 2001[a]	39/URD UCB	3.1	ALL: 21 AML: 15	26 %	3-year EFS 49%	50% at 3 years
Wagner et al.[30] 2002[a]	102/URD UCB	7.4	ALL: 28 AML: 26	35% at 2 years	2-year relapse: 37%[e]	47% at 2 years[e]
Michel et al.[59] 2003[c]	95/URD UCB	4.8	AML: 95	20% at 100 days	2-year LFS: 42%	49% at 2 years
Jacobsohn et al.[60] 2004[d]	26/URD UCB 23/REL HSC	6 4	ALL: 26 ALL: 23	19% at 100 days 13% at 100 days	3-year EFS: 61% 3 year EFS: 60%	65% at 3 years 64% at 3 years
Gluckman and Rocha[64] 2004[c]	195/URD UCB	7	ALL: 195	39% CR 58% relapsed	LFS 36% CR 15% relapsed	NA
Wall et al.[62] 2005*	32/URD UCB	1.6	ALL: 14 AML: 13	NA	2-year RFS: 31%[b]	47% at 1 year
Sawczyn et al.[61] 2005	25/URD UCB 1/REL UCB	8.5	ALL: 26	6/10 patients	2-year EFS: 62% at 548 days CR1: 78% CR2: 56% CR3: 38%	NA

The column labeled "No./Source of HSC" reflects all patients reported in the study regardless of diagnosis. The column labeled "Disease/No." reflects only patients with different forms of acute leukemia and its respective number in that cohort.

[a]Some reports included in this table reported on cohorts of patients, which included diseases other than acute leukemias.

[b]Outcome for all patients.

[c]The 95 patients with acute myelogenous leukemia are reported in both references.

[d]Study compared outcomes of UCB with other hematopoietic stem cell sources.

[e]For patients with ALL, relapse at 2 years was 10% for patients with standard-risk disease (n = 14) and 43% for high-risk disease (n = 14).

For patients with high-risk AML (n = 22), the incidence of relapse was 47%, and one of four patients with standard-risk disease relapsed. In patients with ALL, the survival rate was 55% for standard-risk patients and 32% for high-risk patients. For patients with AML, the survival rate was 33% for high-risk patients, and two of four with standard-risk disease survived.

ALL, acute lymphoblastic leukemia; AML, acute myeloid leukemia; CR, complete remission; EFS, event-free survival; HSC, hematopoietic stem cell; LFS, leukemia-free survival; NA, not available; OS, overall survival; REL, related; RFS, relapse-free survival; TRM, transplant-related mortality; UCB, umbilical cord blood; URD, unrelated donor.

Table 105–4 Umbilical Cord Blood Transplantation for Children with Nonmalignant Diseases

Study	Diagnosis	No./Source	Median Age	Conditioning Regimen	Immunosuppression	Neutrophil Engraftment	Survival/Comment
Knutsen et al.[72] 2000	T-cell ID	8/URD	2 weeks to 8 years	NA	NA	6/8 patients	6/8 patients
Knutsen et al.[71] 2003	WAS	3/URD	1.9–7.9 years	BU/CY/ATG	CsA/Steroid	100%	100%
Locatelli et al.[76] 2003	β-thal SCD	44/REL	5 years	NA	NA	NA	100%
Fang et al.[69] 2004	β-thal	9/REL	5.5 years	BU/CY/ATG ± MEL	CsA/Steroid CsA/MTX	7/9 patients	8/9 patients at 49 months
Walters et al.[79] 2005[b]	β-thal SCD	22/REL	NA	NA	NA	NA	80% EFS with median followup of 12 months
Bhattacharya et al.[66] 2005	8: SCID 6: other ID	12/URD 2/REL	3.5 months	BU/CY: 7 patients ALEN/FLU/MEL: 2 patients No chemo: 5 patients	CsA ± Steroid	100%	86% achieved immune reconstitution
Staba et al.[70] 2004[a]	Hurler's syndrome	20/URD	16 months	BU/CY/ATG	CsA/Steroid	18/20 patients	85% at 905 days
Adamkiewicz et al.[75] 2005	SCD	7/URD	NA	MA: 4 patients NMA: 3 patients	CsA/Steroid FK506/Steroid FK506/MMF	4/7 patients	NA
Vibhakar et al.[65] 2005	S-D syndrome	3/URD	1.5 years 8 years 11 months	MEL/VP-6/ATG/TLI	CsA/Steroid	3/3 patients	3/3 patients (309–2029 days)
Jaing et al.[67] 2005	β-thal	5/URD	2.3–11.4 years	BU/CY/ATG	CsA/Steroid.	100%	100% at 303 days
Escolar et al [68] 2005[a]	Krabbe's disease	11/newborns 14/infants All URD	12–352 days	BU/CY ± ATG	CsA/Steroid	100%	Newborns: 100% Infants: 43% at 3 years $P = 0.01$
Martin et al[81] 2006[a]	Lysosomal/ peroxisomal storage diseases	69/URD	1.8 years	BU/CY/ATG	CsA/Steroid	84%	72% at 1 year
Kobayashi et al.[77] 2006	WAS	15/URD	1.1 years	BU/CY ± ATG: 8 patients Other: 7 patients	CsA ± Steroid	13/15 patients	80% at 5 years

[a]Of the patients reported in Martin et al.81 2006, 14 with Hurler's syndrome and 4 with Krabbe's disease previously had been reported in Staba et al. 2004 and Escolar et al. 2005, respectively.

[b]Study describes experience of the Sibling Donor Cord Blood Program, which includes hematologic malignancies that are not included in this table.

ALEN, Alemtuzumab; ATG, antithymocyte globulin; β-thal, β-thalassemia; BU, busulfan; chemo, chemotherapy; CsA, cyclosporine; CY, cyclophosphamide; FLU, fludarabine; ID, immunodeficiency disease; MA, myeloablative; MEL, melphalan; MMF, mycophenolate mofetil; MTX, methotrexate; NMA, nonmyeloablative; REL, related; SCD, sickle cell disease; SCID, severe combined immunodeficiency disease; S-D, Shwachman-Diamond; TLI, total lymphoid irradiation; URD, unrelated donor; VP-16, VePesid (etoposide); WAS, Wiskott-Aldrich syndrome.

plantation. Survival was 62% with a median follow-up of 36 months for the surviving patients. In multivariate analysis NC dose was the only independent predictor of EFS. In this analysis, disease stage and HLA match were not significant variables bearing on outcome. EFS in recipients of a UCB unit containing greater than 3×10^7 NC/kg was 90% compared to 15% for recipients of $\leq 3 \times 10^7$/kg.[61]

More recently are reports on the use of UCB for treatment of nonmalignant diseases such as metabolic diseases, hemoglobinopathies, and immune deficiencies. Most of these transplants were performed in children. Outcomes are summarized in Table 105–4.[65–78] Reports of UCB transplantation for treatment of children with sickle cell disease and β-thalassemia have shown high rates of engraftment and encouraging survival.[67,69,74–76] Walters et al.[79] reported that engraftment and survival rates are similar in patients transplanted with UCB and BM from HLA-matched donors. This work has supported the further development of directed donor UCB banking efforts, particularly for ethnic and racial minorities at higher risk for hemoglobinopathies.[79]

Allogeneic HCT has been successfully applied to treatment of selected metabolic diseases.[80] In contrast to other transplant indications, the goal in this setting is adoptive transfer of missing or defective enzymes. As hematopoietic elements circulate throughout the body, including the central nervous system, partial or complete chimerism often is associated with stabilization (and in some cases improvement) in the central and peripheral manifestations of these disorders. In the COBLT study, which included a patient population with lysosomal and peroxisomal storage diseases, 1-year survival was 72%.[81] However, results vary with stage of disease and age of the recipient.[68,70] Escolar et al.[68] reported outcomes of UCB transplantation in infants with Krabbe disease diagnosed in utero or during the early neonatal period and transplanted shortly after birth. Early results suggest very high survival rates. Similarly, Staba et al.[70] reported high survival rates in children with Hurler syndrome if UCB transplant occurred early in the course of the disease.

Experience with UCB HCT for treatment of relatively rare immune deficiency states is growing. Early reports are promising, with high rates of engraftment and survival in excess of 80%.[66,71,72,77] Importantly immunologic recovery was observed in the majority of patients.[66,72]

Larger numbers of patients and longer followup are needed to determine the true benefit of UCB in the setting of nonmalignant disease. Comparative studies are required to determine how outcomes after UCB transplant compare to those after BM transplant. Whether UCB offers advantages remains to be proven. However, it is unequivocally clear that UCB is (a) associated with less GVHD, which has no beneficial effect in this setting (in contrast to the setting of malignant disease), and (b) more rapidly available, which is particularly critical for rapidly progressive neurologic diseases. However, bear in mind that graft rejection does occur after UCB transplantation, and the donor is not available for reharvesting or donor lymphocyte collection.[69] However, data increasingly demonstrate the impact of HLA match and cell dose on engraftment,[82] such that better selection of units may reduce the risk of graft failure in the future (see Umbilical Cord Blood Graft selection below). Overall, the available clinical data support use of UCB as a source of HSC for transplantation in children with nonmalignant diseases.

In summary, increasing body of evidence supports front-line use of URD UCB in children. In a report by the Institute of Medicine of the U.S. National Academy of Sciences, UCB use now matches that of BM as a source of HSCs for URD transplantation in children.[83]

UNRELATED DONOR UMBILICAL CORD BLOOD TRANSPLANTATION: OUTCOMES IN ADULTS

After the initial success in children, URD UCB transplant was explored in adults. The literature on use of URD UCB transplantation in adults is summarized in Table 105–5. The first reports of URD UCB transplantation in adults were published in 1996.[49,50,84] Laporte et al.[84] reported on a case of a 26-year-old patient with chronic myelogenous leukemia who had not responded to interferon and was in second chronic phase after myeloid blast crisis. The patient received cyclophosphamide, antithymocyte globulin (ATG), and total body irradiation (TBI) conditioning followed by infusion of a 5/6 HLA-matched unrelated UCB unit with NC dose of 1×10^7/kg. The patient had myeloid recovery by day 23 and platelet recovery by day 48. At the time of the report, the patient was 8 months from transplantation with donor-derived hematopoiesis, with no cytogenetic evidence of the Philadelphia chromosome. Wagner et al.[50] reported on two 21-year-old patients, one with Fanconi anemia and refractory anemia and another with adrenoleukodystrophy. The patient with Fanconi anemia received a 3/6 HLA-matched UCB graft with NC dose of 2×10^7/kg. The conditioning regimen consisted of cyclophosphamide and TBI as well as GVHD immunoprophylaxis with cyclosporine and prednisone. The patient died shortly after transplant. The other patient with adrenoleukodystrophy received a 5/6 HLA-matched graft with a cell dose of 1.7×10^7/kg. The conditioning regimen consisted of busulfan, cyclophosphamide, and TBI. GVHD immunoprophylaxis included cyclosporine and prednisone. The patient had myeloid recovery at day 24 with full chimerism but remained platelet transfusion dependent and had developed grade II acute GVHD at the time of the report. Kurtzberg et al.[49] described a 23-year-old patient with Fanconi anemia and untreated acute myeloid leukemia. The patient received a 5/6 HLA-matched UCB unit with NC dose of 3.7×10^7/kg. The conditioning regimen consisted of cyclophosphamide, TBI, and ATG with cyclosporine immunoprophylaxis. The patient engrafted, developed grade III acute GVHD, and was alive for more than 1 year at the time of the report. These studies were the first to demonstrate the potential of hematopoietic recovery and sustained engraftment in adults after URD UCB transplant.

In 2001, the first series on the use of URD UCB for treatment of adults was reported.[85,86] Laughlin et al.[85] described 68 adult patients (median age 31 years, range 17–58 years) with hematologic diseases who received 3/6 to 6/6 HLA-matched UCB grafts. The median NC dose was 1.6×10^7/kg. The probability of myeloid recovery was 90%, at a median time to neutrophil and platelet recovery of 27 and 99 days, respectively. The incidence of grade II to IV acute GVHD was 60% and grade III to IV was of 16%. There was no association between the development of acute GVHD and HLA match, CMV seropositivity, or conditioning regimen. Thirty-three percent of evaluable patients developed chronic GVHD. The 100-day TRM was 50%, and EFS was 26%. Patients who received CD34$^+$ cell dose ≥ 1.2×10^5/kg had better EFS. Neither age nor HLA match was a predictor of EFS. Rocha et al.[86] reported on 108 adult patients (median age 26 years, range 15–53 years) with hematologic malignancies who underwent URD UCB transplantation. Median NC dose infused was 1.7×10^7/kg. Median time to neutrophil and platelet recovery were 32 and 129 days, respectively. Grade II to IV acute GVHD was observed in 41% of patients and chronic GVHD in 26%. TRM was 54%, and the 1-year survival rate was 27%.

These and other early reports on the efficacy of UCB transplant in adults generally demonstrated poor engraftment and high TRM. Reasons for poor outcomes included patient selection and low UCB graft cell dose. During the early period of UCB transplantation in adults, 1×10^7 NC/kg was frequently cited as the lower acceptable dose limit.[85–88] However, markedly delayed time to myeloid recovery was consistently noted with median durations of neutropenia up to 32 days.[85–88] In addition, graft failure was a common event, with rates as high as 40%.[86,87,89] Acute GVHD also tended to be higher than typically reported in pediatric populations (30%–70% grade II–IV acute GVHD).[85–88] The reasons for higher GVHD in adult UCB recipients included older recipient age, greater use of HLA-mismatched UCB units, and higher proportion of patients with CMV-positive serostatus.[90] Delayed hematopoietic recovery, higher incidence of graft failure, and GVHD contributed to TRM incidences reported to be as high as 50%.[85–88] However, patient selection may have played an important role, as UCB transplant candidates had experienced delay in transplantation (failed a prior marrow donor search), had extensive prior therapy, and had advanced disease. In the COBLT study[89] performed between 1999 and 2000, 15% of patients were in relapse at the time of UCB transplant, and 12% died during the preparative therapy prior to UCB infusion. Survival rates ranged from 20% to 30%.[85–88]

Since the first successful URD UCB transplant in an adult with chronic myelogenous leukemia in 1996,[84] an estimated 2500 UCB transplants have been performed in adults older than 18 years. Most adult recipients of UCB have had acute leukemia.[85,87–89,91–97] For patients with acute leukemia, EFS is between 15% and 50%[85,87–89,91,92,94,95,97]; some small series report EFS up to 70%[93,96] and overall survival between 17% and 45%.[85,88,89,91,92] Better outcomes are associated with younger age,[87,88] higher CFU-GM, CMV-negative serostatus,[92] and leukemia in complete remission.[91,98]

Results of URD UCB transplant used as therapy for other hematologic diseases in adults are starting to emerge. Overall survival for UCB transplant therapy of chronic myeloid leukemia ranges from 20% to 50%.[91,99,100] For lymphoma, 1-year progression-free survival (PFS) ranges from 50% to 63%. Of note, most patients with lymphoma typically received a nonmyeloablative conditioning regimen in contrast to patients with leukemia. Reasons for use of a nonmyeloablative regimen include extensive prior therapy, failed prior autologous HCT, and older age.[101–103] One study in patients with Hodgkin lymphoma reported PFS of 25%.[103]

In summary, interest in use of UCB as a source of HSC for URD transplantation in adults has been growing. Limited availability of units with adequate cell doses has been the principal obstacle. New strategies for addressing the cell dose limitation are detailed in Strategies for Augmenting Cell Dose section.

UMBILICAL CORD BLOOD VERSUS OTHER HEMATOPOIETIC STEM CELL SOURCES

Hematopoietic cell transplant using BM or peripheral blood from HLA-matched related and URDs as a source of stem cells has

Table 105–5 Studies of Adults Undergoing Myeloablative Umbilical Cord Blood Transplantation

Reference	N	Median Age (Years)	Infused Nucleated Cell Dose (×10⁷/kg)	Median Time to ANC ≤ 500/µL (Days)	Median Time to Platelet Recovery (20 or 50 × 10⁹/L)	Grade II–IV Acute GVHD (%)	Extensive Chronic GVHD (%)	DFS/LFS/ Relapse	TRM (%)	EFS/OS	Comment
Rocha et al.[86] 2000	108	26	1.7 (0.2–6.0)	32	129 (20)	41	26	NA	24	1-year OS: 27%	• None
Sanz et al.[87] 2001	22	29	1.7 (1.0–5.0)	22	69 (20)	73	45	1 year DFS: 53%	43 at 100 days	NA	• Patients <30 years have better DFS • Alive at 1 year without disease: AML 3/3, MDS 1/1, CML 5/12
Laughlin et al.[85] 2001	68	31	1.6 (0.6–4.0)	27	99 (50)	60	33	22-month DFS: 26%	50 at 100 days	OS: 28% at22 months[a]	• Higher CD34+ cell dose improves EFS
Ooi et al.[94] 2001	7	38	2.2 (2.1–4.0)	24	49(50)	2/7	1/6	Relapse 2/7	NA	OS: 5/7 at 12 months[a]	• None
Long et al.[88] 2003	57	31	1.5 (0.5–2.8)	28	84 (20)	30	32	3-year EFS: 15%	50 at 100 days	3-year OS: 19%	• Patients <31 years have better EFS
Ooi et al.[96] 2004	18	43	2.5[c] (1.2–5.5)	23	49 (50)	65	NA	2-year LFS: 77%	NA	14/18 pts	• De novo AML
Iori et al.[92] 2004	42	12	3.2 (1.3–10.9)	29	63 (20)	21	20	4-year LFS: 47% 4-year relapse: 28%	28 at 4 years	4-year EFS: 46% 4-year OS: 45%	• Relapse for AML:1/13 • Higher CFU-GM and negative CMV serology associated with improved OS
Kai et al.[120] 2004[b]	11	33	3.9[c] (2.8–4.8)	21	53 (50)	44	Zero	NA	NA	NA	• Abstract
Barker et al.[98] 2005[b]	23	24	3.5 (1.1–6.3)	23	71% (50) at 6 months	65	23	1-year DFS: 57%	22	NA	• 1-year DFS for patients in remission 72%; in relapse" 25%
Cornetta et al.[89] 2005	34	34	2.3[c] (1.4–5.5)	31	117 (20)	34	21	1-year relapse: 46%	NA	1-year OS: 17%	• COBLT
Ooi et al.[239] 2006	22	40	2.4[c] (1.8–4.1)	21	49 (50)	33	42	4-year DFS: 76% Relapse: 4/22	NA	NA	• Myelodysplastic syndrome
Konuma et al.[93] 2006	11	51	2.5[c] (2.1–3.5)	19.5	42 (50)	4/10	2/8	2-year DFS: 73% Relapse: 3/11	0	OS: 8/11 at 24 months[a]	• Patients 50–55 years undergoing myeloablative conditioning
Arcese et al.[91] 2006	171	29	2.1 (0.8–7.3)	28	84 (20)	25	36	2-year DFS: 27% 2-year relapse: 22%	51% at 2 years	2-year OS: 33%	• 2-year DFS for AML" 34%; MDS: 25%, CML: 19%; sAML: 22% • 2-year relapse for CML: 5.5%; MDS: 31% • Advanced disease and non-CML have higher relapse risk • Advanced disease, patient female gender, and major ABO incompatibility have poorer DFS

[a]Median followup.
[b]Double umbilical cord blood unit graft.
[c]Cryopreserved cell dose.
AML, acute myeloid leukemia; ANC, absolute neutrophil count; CFU-GM, colony-forming unit granulocyte-macrophage; CML, chronic myelogenous leukemia; COBLT, Cord Blood Transplantation study; DFS, disease-free survival; EFS, event-free survival; GVHD, graft-versus-host disease; LFS, leukemia-free survival; MDS, myelodysplastic syndrome; NA, not available; OS, overall survival; sAML, secondary acute myeloid leukemia; TRM, treatment-related mortality.

represented the standard of care for patients with various hematologic diseases, cancers, BM failure syndromes, and metabolic disorders. UCB has gradually emerged over the past decade as an alternative source for hematopoietic cells for use in transplant of patients unable to identify a suitably matched marrow or peripheral blood donor. Increasing use of UCB is principally due to the favorable results in children, increased availability of units with larger cell doses, rapid donor identification and cell acquisition, and less restriction of donor/recipient HLA matching. Because use of UCB as a source of stem cells for transplant may have certain advantages, comparison of UCB transplant outcome with that of more conventional marrow or peripheral blood HCT is of interest.

Umbilical Cord Blood Versus Related Donor Hematopoietic Cell Transplantation

Analyses comparing outcomes after unrelated UCB transplant and HLA-matched and HLA-mismatched related donor HCT have been reported (Table 105–6).[60,103–106] Comparing results of recipients of UCB (n = 26) and related donor grafts (n = 23) after myeloablative conditioning, Jacobsohn et al.[60] reported prolonged time to myeloid recovery in recipients of UCB (median 29 vs 16 days, $P < 0.001$), similar incidences of acute and chronic GVHD, and similar TRM, EFS, and overall survival rates. In multivariate analysis the authors were unable to find any independent predictors of short- and long-term outcomes, suggesting that UCB transplant had outcomes comparable to related donor HCT.

In another single-institution study, Takahashi et al.[106] compared outcomes in recipients of unrelated UCB transplant (n = 100) and HLA-matched (n = 54) or HLA-mismatched (one locus: n = 11; two loci: n = 6) related donor HCT after a myeloablative preparative regimen. All UCB grafts were HLA mismatched (one locus: n = 16; two loci: n = 54; three loci: n = 28; four loci: n = 2). Recipients of related donor grafts received either BM (n = 55) and/or peripheral blood stem cells (n = 21). Except for the degree of HLA matching, pretransplant characteristics between the two groups were similar. Despite longer time to neutrophil and platelet recovery after UCB transplantation, engraftment was comparable (UCB 94% vs 98% related donor). As reported by Jacobsohn et al.,[60] incidences of acute and chronic GVHD, TRM, and relapse and probability of survival were similar between cohorts.

In a registry-based retrospective study,[105,107] Rocha et al. compared outcomes in patients with advanced acute myeloid and lymphocytic leukemia who received unrelated UCB or haploidentical, related donor T cell depleted (TCD) marrow grafts. Again, time to myeloid recovery was longer (23 vs 13 days, $P < 0.001$) and incidence of grade II to IV acute GVHD was higher (23% vs 5%, $P < 0.001$) in recipients of UCB. TRM was similar between groups regardless of diagnosis. Interestingly, LFS in patients with acute myeloid leukemia was similar (UCB 30% vs haploidentical TCD marrow 24%, $P = 0.39$). However, in patients with acute lymphoblastic leukemia, LFS was statistically higher in those transplanted with UCB (36% vs 13%, $P = 0.01$).

Investigators at the University of Minnesota have studied the use of reduced-intensity conditioning (RIC) regimens in UCB transplant. They compared outcomes in recipients of unrelated UCB and HLA-matched sibling donors for adult patients with (a) advanced Hodgkin lymphoma[103] and (b) acute myeloid leukemia.[104] In both studies, no significant differences could be discerned between the UCB and the sibling donor groups with regard to incidence of myeloid recovery, acute GVHD, or TRM. In the series of heavily pretreated patients with Hodgkin lymphoma, neither PFS (UCB 25% vs sibling 20%, $P = 0.67$) nor survival (UCB 51% vs sibling 48%, $P = 0.93$) was significantly different.[103] Among patients with de novo or secondary acute myeloid leukemia, only disease status at the time of transplantation and preexisting comorbidities affected outcome, with no significant difference between the two HSC sources. Relapse rates (UCB 35% vs sibling 35%, $P = 0.72$) and survival (UCB 31% vs sibling 32%, $P = 0.62$) were similar for the two cohorts.

Umbilical Cord Blood Versus Unrelated Donor Hematopoietic Stem Cells: Children

Several studies have compared outcomes of UCB and unrelated marrow transplants in pediatric recipients (Table 105–7). One of the first reports was a matched-pair analysis (matching age, diagnosis, and disease stage) at the University of Minnesota that compared the outcomes in pediatric patients transplanted with either 0–3 HLA-A, B, DRB1-mismatched UCB or HLA-A, B, DRB1-matched BM.[108] Recipients of UCB received cyclosporine and methylprednisolone as GVHD prophylaxis. BM recipients received either cyclosporine and methotrexate (BM-MTX) or T-cell depletion (BM-TCD). Although myeloid recovery was significantly slower after UCB transplantation, incidence of recovery by day 45 was similar (UCB 88% vs BM-MTX 96%, $P = 0.41$; UCB 85% vs BM-TCD 90%, $P = 0.32$). Likewise, incidences of platelet recovery and acute and chronic GVHD were similar. Overall, the probability of survival after UCB transplantation was 53% versus 41% in BM-MTX recipients ($P = 0.40$) and 52% after UCB transplantation versus 56% in BM-TCD recipients at 2 years ($P = 0.80$). This study suggested that despite increased HLA disparity in recipients of UCB, survival rates were similar to rates of recipients of HLA-matched URD BM.

Rocha et al.[109] similarly performed a comparative study in pediatric patients with acute leukemia transplanted with UCB (n = 99), unmanipulated BM (n = 262), or TCD BM (n = 180). In their study, UCB recipients were more likely to have high-risk features (e.g., history of early relapse, short interval from diagnosis to transplant, and prior transplantation). Compared to outcomes in recipients of unmanipulated BM, UCB recipients had delayed neutrophil and platelet recovery ($P < 0.01$) and increased TRM prior to day +100 ($P < 0.01$). UCB and TCD BM recipients both had decreased incidences of acute GVHD. Recipients of TCD BM (but not recipients of UCB) had an increased incidence of relapse. After day 100, compared to recipients of unmanipulated BM, both UCB ($P = 0.002$) and TCD recipients ($P = 0.0001$) had a decreased incidence of chronic GVHD, with risk of relapse and mortality higher only in TCD BM recipients. Differences in patient characteristics (not accounted for in adjusted analysis) as well as differences in supportive care and transplant center effect could have contributed to the findings of this study.

A collaboration of the New York Blood Center and the Center for International Blood and Marrow Transplant Research (CIBMTR) compared the outcomes of children receiving HLA-matched and HLA-mismatched UCB (n = 503) or allele-matched URD BM (n = 116), which is the current standard of care worldwide.[110] All patients had acute leukemia, were younger than 16 years, and were undergoing myeloablative transplantation. In this study, the UCB recipient pairs were HLA matched at A and B loci at the antigen level and DRB1 at the allele level, whereas URD BM recipient pairs were HLA matched at A, B, C, and DRB1 loci at the allele level (n = 116). For the purpose of analysis, UCB patients were segregated into those that had HLA-matched units (n = 35), one-locus HLA-mismatched units (n = 201), or two-locus HLA-mismatched units (n = 267). TRM was lowest (6%) and LFS highest (60%) in recipients of HLA-matched UCB. Relapse rates were statistically lower in recipients of HLA-mismatched UCB (20%), with lowest rates in UCB recipients mismatched at two loci. Five-year LFS was similar in recipients of UCB mismatched at one or two loci to that of allele-matched BM transplants. Outcome was superior in recipients of HLA-matched UCB. For recipients of 8/8 allele HLA-matched marrow, 6/6 antigen HLA-matched UCB, 5/6 antigen HLA-matched UCB (cell dose $>3.0 \times 10^7$ NC/kg), and 4/6 antigen HLA-matched UCB (any cell dose), adjusted LFS rates were 38%, 60%, 45%, and 33%, respectively (Fig. 105–1).

Table 105–6 Umbilical Cord Blood Versus Related Donor Hematopoietic Cell Transplantation

Reference	HSC Source	No.	Median Age (Range)	Infused NCD × 10^7/kg (Range)	Median Time to ANC > 500/μL (Days)	Median Time to Platelet Count >20 × 10^9/L (Days)	Graft Failure (%)	Acute GVHD II–IV (%)	Chronic GVHD (%)	Relapse Rate (%)	TRM (%)	Outcome (%)
Myeloablative Conditioning												
UCB Versus Related Donor Transplant												
Jacobsohn et al.[60] 2004	UCB	26	6.0	5.8	29	NA	NA	19	33	15	19	EFS 61
	REL	23	4.4	25	16	NA	NA	22	40	25	13	EFS 60
			0.90*	<0.001*	<0.001*			0.71*	0.66*	0.72*	0.71*	NA
Rocha et al.[105,107] 2005	AML											
	UCB	66						23		24	46	DFS 30
	Haplo	154						5		18	58	DFS 24
			31	NA	23	NA	NA	<0.001*	NA	0.44*	0.23*	0.39*
	ALL		38	NA	13	NA	NA		NA			
	UCB	73						26		23	41	DFS 36
	Haplo	75						8		38	49	DFS 13
								0.004*		0.07*	0.55*	0.01*
Takahashi et al.[106] 2007	UCB	92	38	2.4[a]	22	39	NA	52	23	18 at 3 years	9	DFS 71
	REL	55 marrow 16 PBSC	40	33	17	22	NA	52	30	23 at 3 years	13	DFS 60
Hazard ratio (95% CI)/*P* value			NA/0.83*	NA/ < 0.01*	0.14 (0.10–0.22)/ < 0.01*	0.19 (0.13–0.28)/ < 0.01*		1.09 (0.71–1.68)/ 0.69*	0.49 (0.29–0.85)/ 0.09*	0.72 (0.37–1.41)/ 0.34[b]*	0.49 (0.19–1.24)/ 0.13[b]*	0.74 (0.44–1.25)/ 0.26[b]*
Reduced-Intensity Conditioning												
Brunstein et al.[104] 2006	UCB	43	53	3.6	19	NA	19	51	19	35	23	PFS 31
	REL PBSC	21	54	93.4	10	NA	Zero	62	19	35	38	PFS 27
			0.77*	< 0.01*	< 0.01*		0.01*	0.85*	0.73*	0.72*	0.60*	0.50*
Majhail et al.[103] 2006	UCB	9	28	3.8	10	NA	NA	67	11	NA	22	PFS 25
	REL PBSC	12	42	10.0	7	NA	NA	58	33	NA	25	PFS 20
			0.02*	< 0.01*	0.02*			0.70*	0.24*		0.88*	0.67*

**P* value

[a]Cryopreserved nucleated cell dose.

[b]Multivariate HR (95% CI). Related donor was reference value (1.0). Relapse was adjusted for disease status (high-risk disease HR 5.0, 95% CI 2.07–12.1, P < 0.01) and diagnosis of primary disease (ALL HR 2.37, 95% CI 1.20–4.70, P = 0.03). TRM was adjusted for age (≥45 years HR 2.66, 95% CI 1.12–6.30, P = 0.03) and disease status (high-risk disease HR 4.91, 95% CI 1.43–16.8, P = 0.01). DFS was adjusted for disease status (high-risk disease HR 5.37, 95% CI 2.54–11.4, P < 0.01).

ALL, acute lymphoblastic leukemia; AML, acute myelogenous leukemia; ANC, absolute neutrophil count; CI, confidence interval; DFS, disease-free survival; EFS, event-free survival; GVHD, graft-versus-host disease; Haplo, haploidentical donor; HR, hazard ratio; HSC, hematopoietic stem cell; NA, not available or not applicable; NCD, nucleated cell dose; NS, not significant; PBSC, peripheral blood stem cell; PFS, progression-free survival; REL, related donor; TRM, treatment-related mortality; UCB, umbilical cord blood.

Table 105–7 Umbilical Cord Blood Versus Unrelated Hematopoietic Cell Transplantation in Children

Reference	HSC Source	No.	Median Age Years (Range)	Infused NCD × 10⁷/kg (range)	Median Time to ANC > 500/μL(Days)	Median Time to Platelet count >20 × 10⁹/L (Days)	Graft Failure (%)	Acute GVHD II–IV (%)	Extensive Chronic GVHD (%)	Relapse Rate (%)	TRM (%)	Survival or DFS (%)
Rocha et al.[240] 2001	UCB	99	6 (2.5–12)	3.8 (2.4–36)	32	81	NA	33	25	38 at 2 years	39 at 100 days	35 at 2 yeas
	URD marrow	262	8.0 (5–12)	42 (30–60)	18	29	NA	56	46	39 at 2 years	19 at 100 days	49 at 2 years
	URD TCD marrow	180	8.0 (6–12)	38 (14–56)	16	29	NA	34	12	47 at 2 years	14 at 100 days	41 at 2 years
P value			0.0004	0.0001	<0.001	<0.001	NA	<0.001[b]	<0.001[b]	UCB 0.47[b] TCD 0.18[b]	UCB < 0.01[b] TCD 0.19[b]	UCB 0.55[b] TCD 0.07[b]
Barker et al.[241] 2001	UCB	26	4.5 (0.2–18)	3[a] (1.0 to 28)	29	66	8	42	5		27 at 100 days	53 at 2 years
	URD marrow	26	4.7 (0.2–18)	20 (19 to 40)	22	30	4	35	20		15 at 100 days	41 at 2 years
P value			NS	<0.05	0.03	0.12	NS	0.80	0.12		0.35	0.40
	URD	31	5.8 (0.2–18)	3[a] (1 to 28)	27	61	16	36	7		23 at 100 days	52 at 2 years
	URD TCD marrow	31	6.8 (0.5–17)	5 (2 to 20)	14	59	10	35	13		16 at 100 days	56 at 2 years
P value			NS	NS	<0.01	0.74	NS	>0.80	0.32		0.60	>0.80
Eapen et al.[110] 2006	UCB 6/6[c]	35	<16	4.5 (1–20)	25	59	NA	24	30	34	6	60
	UCB 5/6[high]	157		2.2 (1–30)				42	18	31	29	45
	UCB 5/6[low]	44		6.9 (3–35)				36	18	21	43	36
	UCB 4/6	267		4.8 (0.1–32)				41	15	20	49	33
	URD marrow Matched	116	<16	42 (<10–80)	19	27	NA	46	32	40	21	38
	URD marrow Mismatched	166		38 (<10–90)				60	40	31	31	37
P value			NA	NA	NA	NA	NA	*d*	*d*	*d*	*d*	NA

[a]Cryopreserved nucleated cell dose.

[b]Adjusted P values where unrelated donor marrow is the reference group.

[c]6/6, HLA-matched UCB; 5/6[high], one-locus HLA-mismatched UCB with high cell dose; 5/6[low], one-locus HLA-mismatched UCB with low cell dose; 4/6, two-locus HLA-mismatched UCB.

[d]Multivariate analysis with matched marrow as reference group. *Acute GVHD grades II–IV*: Matched marrow vs mismatched marrow RR 1.51 (1.08–2.13), P = 0.01; matched marrow vs matched UCB RR 0.45 (0.22–.96), P = 0.04. No other significant differences. *Chronic GVHD*: Matched marrow vs mismatched marrow RR 1.90 (1.14–3.17), P = 0.01. No other significant differences. TRM: 5/6[low] UCB vs matched marrow RR 1.88 (1.01–3.47), P = 0.05; 4/6 UCB vs matched marrow RR 2.31 (1.47–3.62), P = 0.0003. No other significant differences. *Relapse*: 4/6 UCB vs matched marrow RR 0.54 (0.36–0.83), P = 0.0045. No other significant differences.

ANC, absolute neutrophil count; DFS, disease-free survival; GVHD, graft-versus-host disease; HSC, hematopoietic stem cell; NA, not available; NCD, nucleated cell dose; NS, not significant; RR, relative risk; TCD, T-cell depleted; TRM, treatment-related mortality; UCB, umbilical cord blood; URD, unrelated donor.

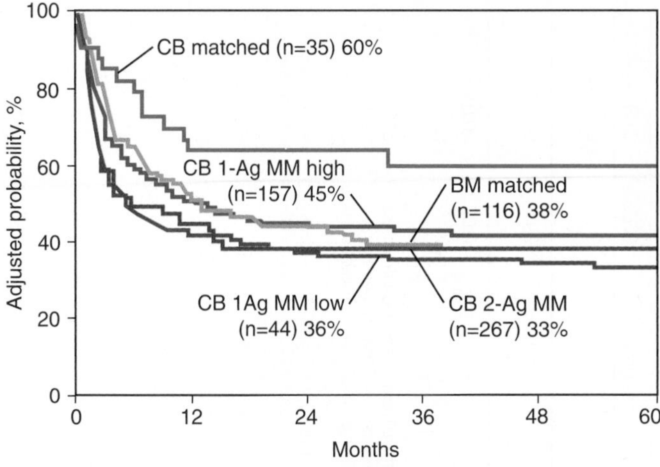

Figure 105–1 Leukemia-free survival (LFS) rates were highest after transplantation of matched cord blood (CB): 60% at 5 years. LFS rates were similar after transplantation of 1- and 2-antigen mismatched (Ag MM) CB and allele-matched bone marrow (BM). Five-year probabilities of LFS rates were 38% after matched BM; 45% after 1-AG MM CB, high cell dose; 36% after 1-AG MM CB, low cell dose; and 33% after 2-AG MM CB.

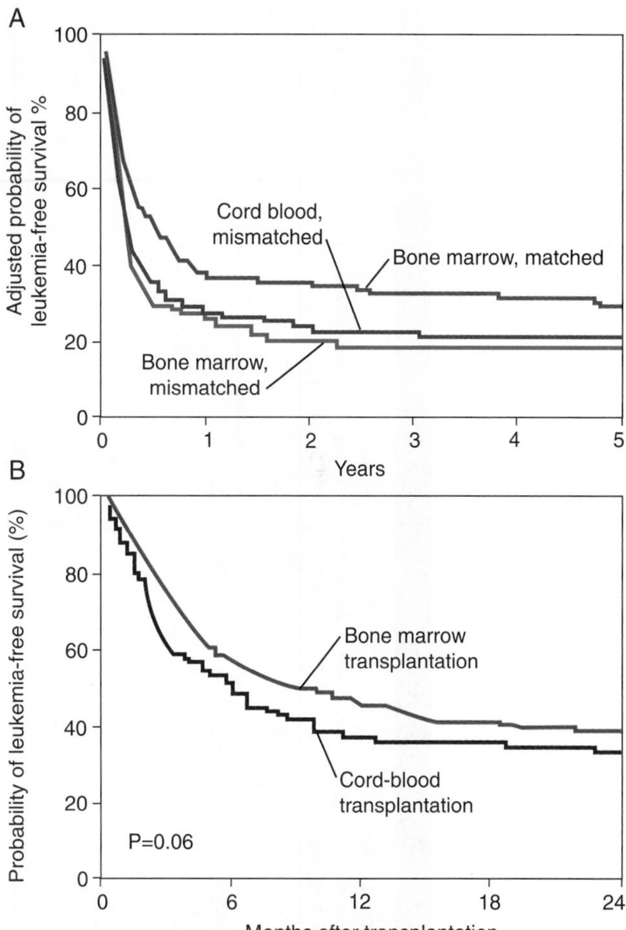

Figure 105–2 Registry-based analysis probability of leukemia-free survival for adult patients after myeloablative conditioning with unrelated umbilical cord blood versus matched or mismatched unrelated donor transplantation. (*From Laughlin MJ, et al: Outcomes after transplantation of cord blood or bone marrow from unrelated donors in adults with leukemia. N Engl J Med 351:2265, 2004, and Rocha V, et al: Transplants of umbilical-cord blood or bone marrow from unrelated donors in adults with acute leukemia. N Engl J Med 351:2276, 2004.*)

Umbilical Cord Blood Versus Unrelated Donor Hematopoietic Cell Transplantation: Adults

More recently, registry and single-institution studies have compared outcomes after UCB and unrelated marrow or peripheral blood transplantation in adult recipients (Table 105–8). Rocha et al.[111] reported a matched-pair analysis comparing outcomes in adult acute leukemia patients receiving UCB (n = 81) or BM (n = 162) transplants. In their study, patients were matched for variables including age, diagnosis, status of disease at transplant, and use of TBI. All BM grafts were matched at HLA-A, B (antigen level), and DRB1 (allele level), whereas 90% of UCB grafts were mismatched at one to three HLA antigens. As previously observed in children, myeloid recovery was significantly delayed after UCB transplantation (median 28 days vs 19 days), and duration of neutropenia after UCB transplantation could be correlated with the cryopreserved cell dose. UCB transplantation was associated with less acute GVHD (31% vs 41%, $P = 0.05$). Incidences of chronic GVHD, TRM, and relapse were comparable between groups. DFS was 26% in recipients of UCB and 33% in recipients of BM ($P = 0.28$). The authors concluded that UCB units matched at 4/6 to 6/6 HLA antigens and with a cell dose at least 1.0×10^7 NC/kg should be considered an acceptable alternative to HLA-matched URD BM for transplant of adults with acute leukemia.

Two seminal registry reports[112,113] and one single-center study[114] comparing outcomes in adult recipients of URD UCB and unrelated marrow transplant were published in 2004 (Table 105–9). All three studies demonstrated delayed neutrophil and platelet recovery after UCB transplantation.[112–114] Despite a higher degree of HLA mismatch for recipients of UCB grafts, all three studies demonstrated lower or similar incidences of grade II to IV acute GVHD after UCB transplantation.[112–114] However, survival rates differed among the three studies. Whereas survival and LFS after UCB transplantation was inferior to HLA-matched marrow in the report by Laughlin et al.[112] (Fig. 105–2A), survival and LFS were similar or superior for recipients of UCB in the reports by Rocha et al.[113] (Fig. 105–2B) and Takahashi et al.,[114] respectively. Hwang et al.[115] performed a meta-analysis and suggested that the differences in survival could not be entirely explained by HLA match, as most of the subjects in the report by Takahashi et al.[114] were 4/6 matched. Of note, Rocha et al.[113] included only patients transplanted after 1998 because they wished to avoid the "learning curve" with lower survival rates prior to 1998. Whether this influenced the outcomes reported by Laughlin et al.[112] is unknown.

In summary, these three reports support the general use of URD UCB transplant in adults. UCB transplant is particularly suited to patients for whom a suitably HLA-matched unrelated volunteer donor cannot be identified in the time interval mandated by the individual patient's disease status.

STRATEGIES FOR AUGMENTING CELL DOSE

Achievement of an adequate cell dose is one of the limiting factors that prevents increased use of UCB for transplantation. Furthermore, data from many clinical studies suggest that low cell dose compounds the deleterious effect of HLA mismatch and contributes to delayed hematopoietic recovery, poor engraftment, high TRM, and poor survival. Therefore, novel strategies are needed to augment the cell dose of the UCB graft. Several possible approaches can be considered, the most obvious being ex vivo expansion culture. Clinical trials with expanded UCB products have not yet demonstrated any obvious impact on time to neutrophil or platelet recovery. Alternative strategies being explored to enhance rate of hematopoietic recovery include (a) use of two partially HLA-matched UCB units, (b) ex vivo expansion of UCB progenitors, (c) coinfusion of mesenchymal stem cells

Table 105–8 Umbilical Cord Blood Versus Unrelated Hematopoietic Cell Transplantation in Adults

Reference	HSC Source	No.	Median Age Years (Range)	Infused NCD × 10^7/kg (Range)	Median Time to ANC > 500/μL (Days)	Median Time to Platelet Count >20 × 10^9/L (Days)	Graft Failure (%)	Acute GVHD II–IV (%)	Extensive Chronic GVHD (%)	Relapse Rate (%)	TRM (%)	Survival or DFS (%)
Laughlin et al.[112] 2004	UCB	150	(16–60)[a]	2.2 (1.0–6.5)	27	60(20)	NS	41	33	17	63	26
	URD marrow	367	(16–60)[a]	24 (0.2–170)	20	29(20)	NS	48	52	23	46	35
	URD MM marrow	83	(16–60)[a]	22 (0.1–58)	18	29(20)		51	71	14	65	20
P value					<0.001	<0.001	0.29	[c]	0.03	[c]	[c]	[c]
Rocha et al.[113] 2004	UCB	98	25 (15–55)	2.3 (0.9–6.0)	26		20	26	30	23	44	36
	URD marrow	584	32 (15–59)	29 (<10–90)	19		7	39	46	23	38	42
P value					0.001		NA	0.008	0.07	0.71	0.13	0.08
Takahashi et al.[114] 2004	UCB	68	36 (16–53)	2.5[b] (1.1–5.3)	22	40 (20)	8	30	13	16	9	DFS 74
	URD marrow	45	26 (16–50)	33 (6.6–50)	18	25(20)	Zero	30	14	25	29	DFS 44
P value					0.01	0.01	NA	[d]	[d]	[d]	0.02	<0.01

[a]Age reported in intervals of 16–20,21–30,31–40,41–50,51–60. No median available.

[b]Cryopreserved nucleated cell dose.

[c]Multivariate analysis for acute GVHD showed HR = 0.81 ($P = 0.17$) for UCB vs matched unrelated marrow, and 0.66 ($P < 0.04$) for UCB vs mismatched unrelated marrow. Relapse showed HR = 0.85 ($P < 0.61$) for mismatched unrelated marrow vs matched unrelated marrow, 0.73 ($P < 0.16$) for UCB vs matched unrelated marrow, and 0.85 ($P = 0.65$) for UCB vs mismatched unrelated marrow. TRM showed HR = 1.91 ($P < 0.001$) for mismatched unrelated marrow and 1.89 ($P < 0.001$) for UCB vs matched unrelated marrow, and 0.99 ($P = 0.96$) for mismatched unrelated marrow vs UCB. Adjusted probability of 3-year survival showed no difference between mismatched unrelated marrow and UCB ($P = 0.62$), but superior 3-year survival for recipient matched unrelated marrow ($P < 0.001$).

[d]Multivariate analysis of UCB vs unrelated marrow for acute GVHD grades II–IV showed HR = 0.61 ($P = 0.05$), for extensive chronic GVHD HR = 0.60 ($P = 0.18$), and for relapse HR = 0.76 ($P = 0.73$).

ANC, absolute neutrophil count; DFS, disease-free survival; GVHD, graft-versus-host disease; HR, hazard ratio; HSC, hematopoietic stem cell; MM, mismatched; NA, not available; NCD, nucleated cell dose; TRM, treatment-related mortality; UCB, umbilical cord blood; URD, unrelated donor.

Table 105–9 Umbilical Cord Blood Transplantation After Reduced Intensity Conditioning

Reference	No.	Preparative Regimen	Median Age (Range)	Infused NCD × 10^7/kg (Range)	Infused CD34 Cell Dose ×10^5/kg (Range)	Median Time to ANC > 500/μL (Days)	Graft Failure (%)	Median Time to Platelet Count Recovery(Days) (>20 × 10^9)	Acute GVHD II–IV (%)	Chronic GVHD (%)	Relapse Rate (%)	TRM (%)	Survival (%)
Barker et al.[170] 2003[a,b]	21	BU/FLU/TBI	49 (22–65)	2.6 (1.6–3.8)	3.7 (1.1–8.1)	26	24	24% (20) at 6 months	44	21	NR	48 at 100 days	39 at 1 year
	22	Cy/FLU/TBI	49 (24–58)	3.2 (1.1–5.1)	4.3 (1.1–10)	9.5	6	80% (20) at 6 months			NR	28 at 100 days	
Miyakoshi et al.[173] 2004	30	FLU/MEL/TBI	59 (20–70)	3.1 (2.0–4.3)	0.7 (0.2–2.5)	17.5	7	39	27	23	11	27	33 at 1 year
Morii et al.[174] 2005	14	Cy/FLU/TBI BU/FLU/TBI	57 (31–72)	2.6 (2.1–3.8)	NR	21	14	43	21	50	NR	19	37% at 1 year
Missawa et al.[176] 2006	12	Cy/FLU/TBI	49 (19–63)	2.55 (2.26–3.33)	0.91 (0.6–2.0)	17	16	32	62.5	33	NR	41.7	NR
Rocha et al.[177] 2006	65	Multiple[d]	47 (16–76)	2.4	NR	20	12[d]	35	27	NR	NR	46	NR
Ballen et al.[178] 2007[b]	21	FLU/MEL/rATG	49 (24–63)	4.0 (2.9–5.1)	1.9 (0.6–9.7)	20	14	41	40[c]	12	5	19 at 180 days	71
Brunstein et al.[171] 2007[a]	110	Cy/FLU/TBI	51 (17–69)	3.7 (1.1–5.3)	4.7 (0.7–18.8)	12	15	49	59	23	31	26 at 3 years	45 at 3 years

[a]The 22 patients who receive Cy/FLU/TBI in the series by Barker et al. are included in the series by Brunstein et al.

[b]Study included patients receiving multiple-unit UCB grafts.

[c]The incidence of grade II–IV acute GVHD for patient who received tacrolimus/sirolimus posttransplantation immunosuppression was 29%.

[d]Cy/FLU/TBI 2 Gy (TBI) was given to 33 patients, FLU/Cy or MEL in 11, FLU + busulfan (<8 mg/kg) associated or not to other drugs in 13, FLU/TBI (2 Gy) in 3, and other regimens in 5.

Antithymocyte globulin/antilymphocyte globulin was added in 26% of cases. The probability of neutrophil recovery was 88% of the 33 patients who received the Cy/FLU/TBI conditioning regimen and 65% for patients receiving other regimens ($P < 0.01$).

ANC, absolute neutrophil count, BU/FLU/TBI, busulfan, fludarabine, and total body irradiation; Cy/FLU/TBI, cyclophosphamide, fludarabine, and total body irradiation; FLU/MEL/TBI, fludarabine, melphalan, and total body irradiation; GVHD, graft-versus-host disease; NCD, nucleated cell dose; TRM, treatment-related mortality. NR, not reported; ATG, rabbit anti-thymocyte globulin.

or regulatory T cells to suppress graft resistance, and (d) strategies to reduce nonspecific losses of UCB HSC and enhance homing to the marrow microenvironment (e.g., intrabone marrow injection, treatment with parathyroid hormone [PTH]).

Multiple Unit Umbilical Cord Blood Transplantation

Among the many strategies currently being explored to enhance engraftment is the use of two partially HLA-matched UCB units as the graft source (Tables 105–5, 105–6, and 105–9).[98,116–118] Despite initial concerns regarding the possibility of bidirectional immunologic rejection between the two UCB units from two immunologically functional, HLA-mismatched donors, engraftment was consistently observed in practice. This strategy, initially pioneered at the University of Minnesota, has been studied in both the myeloablative and reduced-intensity settings.

In the myeloablative setting, a pilot study of 23 patients demonstrated the safety and feasibility of "double UCB transplantation."[98] In the first report, the conditioning regimen consisted of cyclophosphamide 120 mg/kg, fludarabine 75 mg/m^2, and fractionated TBI 1320 cGy. The median recipient age was 24 years (range 13–53 years), median weight was 73 kg (range 48–120 kg), and median infused NC dose of the two units was 3.5×10^7 (range 1.1–6.3 NC/kg). Median time to myeloid recovery was 23 days, and all patients who survived more than 21 days achieved sustained engraftment (Fig. 105–3). Interestingly, nearly one third of patients demonstrated "double chimerism" at day 21 (i.e., evidence of engraftment from each donor), with one donor predominating over time. Cell dose, HLA match, ABO match, and order of infusion does not predict which unit will predominate. Analysis clearly indicates that adult recipients of double UCB transplantation have engraftment rates similar to or better than the rates observed in children despite significantly higher median weight and greater use of HLA-mismatched units.[119] An update of 58 patients treated with this strategy reveals a median time to engraftment of 22 days and an overall incidence of myeloid recovery of 91% at 42 days. Although engraftment using double UCB transplant appears to have improved engraftment, risk of grade II to IV acute GVHD may be higher (57% at 100 days). The incidence of grade III to IV acute GVHD is 16% and TRM at 6 months is low at 18%. At 2 years, overall survival is 57% and DFS is 55%. Other investigators also considered the use of double UCB transplantation, with similar results.[120] Pilot studies using more than two UCB units have been reported.[121,122]

In addition to evaluating the impact on engraftment and GVHD, Verneris et al.[123] evaluated the impact of double UCB transplantation on the risk of relapse in patients with acute leukemia. As the use of two units was restricted to patients with an inadequate single UCB unit, recipients of a double UCB graft were significantly older (median age 24 years vs 8 years) and heavier (median weight 70 kg vs 32 kg). In 80% of double UCB transplants, at least one unit was mismatched at two HLA antigens with the recipient. Compared to recipients of a single UCB unit, double UCB recipients with acute leukemia transplanted in first or second complete remission experienced a 10-fold lower incidence of relapse. Although risk of grade II to IV acute GVHD was higher in recipients of two units, no other factor could be associated with relapse risk other than the use of two units.

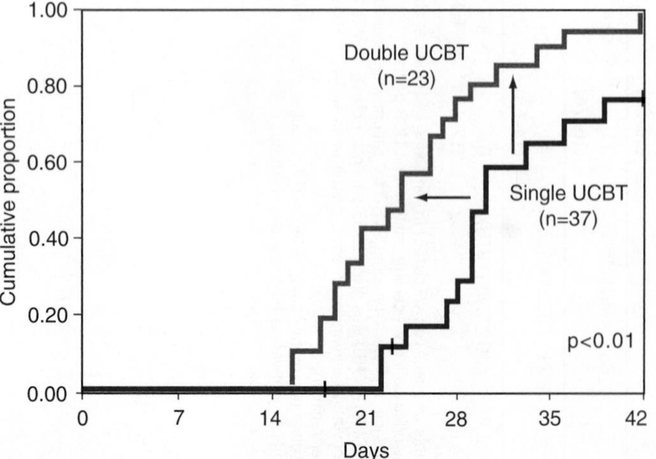

Figure 105–3 Time to neutrophil engraftment after myeloablative transplantation for adult patients with hematologic malignancy who received one (historical controls) or two umbilical cord blood units at the University of Minnesota.

Based on these results, the BMT Clinical Trials Network (CTN) initiated two phase II trials of double UCB transplantation in adults and one prospective phase III clinical trial in children comparing single versus double UCB transplantation. Although the primary endpoint of the phase II trials in adults is hematopoietic recovery, the primary endpoint of the phase III trial in children is 1-year LFS. In each of these trials, incidences of GVHD, TRM, and leukemia relapse as well as pace of immune recovery are among the secondary endpoints that will be assessed.

In summary, the data suggest that use of two partially HLA-matched UCB units in the myeloablative setting is safe as measured by the high incidence of donor engraftment, timely myeloid recovery, and low incidences of severe acute GVHD and TRM.

Ex Vivo Expansion of Umbilical Cord Blood Stem and Progenitor Cells

Because the cell dose contained in a single unit has been the single most important limitation of UCB, particularly for adult patients,[116] various ex vivo expansion culture strategies have been the evaluated over the past 10 years.[124–129] Although these studies have not shown any significant toxicity related to infusion of ex vivo expanded cells, they also have not yet shown clear evidence of clinical benefit. This may be due in part to treatment design. In most studies, a single UCB unit was used both as a graft and as a source of HSC for ex vivo expansion. After thawing, a portion of the UCB was sent for ex vivo expansion for periods of up to 2 weeks, whereas the remaining proportion of the unit was administered unmodified on day 0. This study design led to two major problems in interpretation of the results: (a) because the ex vivo expanded units were infused at a later time, there was reduced chance of observing an impact on myeloid recovery, and (b) it was not possible to determine if the engrafted cells were derived from the unmodified or the ex vivo expanded portion of the graft (because there was no genetic marker to distinguish unexpanded from expanded cells).

In an attempt to identify potentially efficacious ex vivo expansion culture strategies, new trial designs are being considered, including (a) use of UCB units that have been divided prior to cryopreservation so that one portion of the of the unit can be expanded and infused together with the unexpanded portion, (b) use of the double UCB model with coinfusion of expanded product from one UCB and unexpanded product from the other UCB, and (c) infusion of an expanded product alone, with one or two UCB units as a backup to be infused at a preestablished time in the event of graft failure.

In summary, trials with ex vivo expanded UCB cells have failed to demonstrate clear impact upon engraftment. New expansion strategies are promising and are under development and testing.[130–132] Combined with newer trial designs, identification of promising strategies for expanding the number of UCB stem and progenitor cells will be forthcoming.

Intrabone Marrow Injection

Considering that cell dose is the most significant limitation for UCB transplantation, injection of the graft directly into the BM space theoretically could lead to improved homing and avoid trapping of hematopoietic progenitors in tissues that do not support hematopoiesis.[24,25,133–135] Murine models have shown that less than 20% of HSC infused intravenously ultimately reach the BM space; most are trapped in organs with extensive capillary beds such as the lungs.[136] In addition, when hematopoietic progenitors are injected directly into the BM space, better donor engraftment at the site of injection and improved colonization of other bones occur.[25,135] Clinical data on this approach are limited.[137,138] However, one small clinical trial randomized patients undergoing related donor allogeneic transplants to receive the grafts either intravenously or through intrabone marrow injection.[137] Although well tolerated, no demonstrable impact on clinical outcome was observed. Raiola et al.[139] reported on 12 adult patients who received a single UCB transplantation through direct intrabone marrow injection after myeloablative conditioning. The median NC dose infused was 2.7×10^7/kg (range 1.6–3.5/kg). All patients engrafted at a median of 20 days for neutrophils and 30 days for platelets. Only two patients developed grade II acute GVHD. The finding of rapid repopulation and differentiation at the site of injection is intriguing.

At the University of Minnesota, a phase I to II clinical trial evaluating the safety and potential efficacy of intrabone marrow injection is underway. In this study, two partially HLA-matched UCB units are transplanted with one randomly assigned to intrabone marrow injection and the other administered intravenously. Because of genetic differences between units, it will be possible to discern a competitive advantage to cells administered by intrabone marrow injection. To date, nine patients have been enrolled. Although all patients have engrafted, median time to myeloid recovery is 22 days. In contrast to the report by Raiola et al., GVHD has been observed in five of five patients who are at least 100 days after transplantation. The study remains open.

Coinfusion of Mesenchymal Stem Cells

An alternative approach to enhancing engraftment is coinfusion of mesenchymal stem cells that actively participate in normal hematopoiesis through production of growth factors and cytokines and provision of direct cell–cell interactions.[140,141] In NOD/SCID mouse transplant models, mesenchymal stem cells have been shown to facilitate engraftment of human UCB hematopoietic cells.[142,143] Early clinical reports suggest that mesenchymal stem cells may suppress immune reactions and indirectly enhance engraftment (inhibition of host resistance) in addition to preventing GVHD.[144–146] A report suggests that the immune modulation of MSC is mediated at least partly through regulatory T cells.[147]

One clinical study at the University of Minnesota has explored coinfusion of parental haploidentical ex vivo expanded MSC with unrelated UCB.[148] No serious adverse events were observed. Although neutrophil and platelet recoveries appeared to be more rapid, a randomized trial with a larger numbers of patients would be required to provide definitive proof that use of MSC is beneficial in this unrelated UCB transplant setting.

Coinfusion of Purified Partially Hematopoietic Progenitors

A novel approach for shortening the period of neutropenia after UCB transplantation is coinfusion of partially HLA-matched, T-cell–depleted peripheral blood stem cells from related donors.[149,150] The goal is to promote a transient myeloid recovery derived from these partially HLA-matched cells as a bridge before permanent recovery and engraftment from the UCB unit. This approach has markedly shortened the time to an absolute neutrophil count greater than 0.5 × 10(9)/L to 10 days, with no obvious deleterious effect on UCB engraftment.[149] Chimerism studies reveal an initial predominance of cells derived from the haploidentical cells in both the granulocyte and mononuclear cell fractions but progressive replacement by cells derived from the UCB graft.

Parathyroid Hormone Treatment

Osteoblastic cells are a regulatory component of the hematopoietic stem niche.[151] Coinfusion of osteoblasts purified from murine long bones promoted engraftment and provided long-term survival in fully ablated mice.[152] Osteoblast function and proliferation may be regulated by many different pathways, including Notch1 and BMP.[151,153–155] Calvi et al.[153] showed that stimulation with PTH increased the number of osteoblasts, with high expression of the Notch ligand jagged1. The authors showed both in vitro and in vivo that PTH stimulation led to expansion of the number of HSC. In an allogeneic transplant murine model, PTH treatment led to an increased number of primitive hematopoietic cells and markedly improved survival.[153] The same group showed that administration of PTH to mice increased the number of circulating HSC and protected HSC from repeated exposure to cyclophosphamide.[156] A phase II clinical trial studying administration of PTH to enhance engraftment after UCB transplantation is being initiated (K. Ballen, Personal Communication, December 2007).

UMBILICAL CORD BLOOD TRANSPLANTATION AND REDUCED-INTENSITY CONDITIONING

Because the median age of diagnosis in patients with hematologic malignancies is the fifth and sixth decades of life,[157] regimen-related toxicities and, consequently, TRM are high.[158,159] In addition, older age is associated with increased incidence of comorbidities at the time of transplant, further increasing the risk of morbidity and mortality.[160] Together with a history of extensive therapy and use of autologous or allogeneic transplant comes a need to develop less toxic therapies for patients not able to tolerate a conventional myeloablative conditioning regimen.[161–163] Therefore, experience with using RIC regimens prior to related and unrelated blood and BM transplantation is rapidly growing, and results have been encouraging.[164169]

UCB is an adequate source of cells with sufficient numbers of HSC and alloreactive T cells to mediate sustained donor engraftment after an RIC regimen.[170–177] Results with UCB transplantation after RIC are summarized in Table 105–9. Although original series used single UCB units in the context of RIC,[173,174,176,177] experience with double UCB transplantation after RIC is growing.[171,178] In these series, the median age at transplantation typically is older (range 47–59 years) than in reports of myeloablative UCB transplantation. The median infused NC dose is 2.4 to 4.0×10^7/kg, with higher cell doses reflecting increased availability of larger UCB units and use of the double UCB platform. Notably, the median time to myeloid recovery has ranged from 9.5 to 26 days and platelet recovery (>20 × 109/L) from 32 to 43 days. The time to myeloid recovery is affected by the intensity of the conditioning regimen used, with shorter periods of neutropenia observed in recipients undergoing less intense regimens. Graft failure overall has been observed in 10% to 20% of patients.

Reported rates of acute and chronic GVHD after RIC and UCB transplantation vary widely (Table 105–9). The incidence of grade II to IV acute GVHD has been reported between 20% and 60% and chronic GVHD between 20% and 50%.[171,173–177] Grade II (and not grade III–IV) acute GVHD may be higher among recipients of double UCB grafts, although this remains to be proven.[179] In terms of TRM, the risk in the setting of UCB transplant and RIC relates primarily to the intensity of conditioning and presence of o-morbidities and not the age of recipients. Overall, TRM in available reports has ranged from 14% to 46%.[171,173–177] Reported rates of relapse have ranged from 5% to 30%.[171,173,175] In one study of recipients of RIC and single UCB transplantation, favorable risk factors for DFS were greater HLA match, higher NC dose (>2.4 × 10^7/kg), use of cyclophosphamide/fludarabine/TBI 200 cGy conditioning, and diagnosis of lymphoma.[177] Overall, survival rates after RIC and single UCB transplant have ranged from 33% to 37%.[173,174] Studies that included patients receiving double UCB unit grafts have reported overall survival rates ranging from 44% to 74%.[171,178]

At the University of Minnesota, more than 170 UCB transplants after RIC have been performed, primarily in older adults. The first 110 patients received a single conditioning regimen that consists of fludarabine 40 mg/m^2/day for 5 days, cyclophosphamide 50 mg/kg/day for 1 day, and low-dose TBI (200 cGy) in a single fraction without shielding.[171] For this cohort, the median patient age was 51 years. Patients were eligible for a single UCB unit graft if the cell dose exceeded 3.0 × 10^7/kg; otherwise, they were eligible for two partially HLA-matched UCB units. Ninety-three (84%) patients received double UCB graft in order to achieve the minimum target cell dose. The median total infused NC dose was 3.7 × 10^7/kg and CD34 cell dose was 4.7 × 10^5/kg, with no significant differences between recipients of single and double UCB grafts. Sixty-five percent of patients transplanted with one UCB received a two-locus HLA-mismatched unit compared to 78% of patients transplanted with two UCB units in which one or both units were mismatched at two loci. For this cohort, the incidence of primary myeloid recovery was 92% at a median of 12 days (range 0–32 days). The incidence of platelet recovery (>50 × 10^9/L) was 65% (95% CI 54%–76%) by day 180 and occurred at a median of 49 days (range 0–134 days). Sustained donor engraftment was achieved in 85% (95% CI 77%–92%). Logistic regression analysis showed a significantly higher risk of graft failures among patients who received at least one unit with a two-locus HLA-mismatched. Notably, no influence of total NC dose or number of units used on neutrophil engraftment was observed. Similar to observations in the myeloablative setting,[98] only one unit contributed to long-term hematopoiesis in all patients. However, early recovery was most often host in origin, with gradual switch to donor-derived hematopoiesis over 100 days. Incidences at day 100 of grade II to IV acute GVHD was 59% (95% CI 49%–69%) and grade III to IV acute GVHD 22% (95% CI 14%–30%). In Cox regression analysis, patients who received double-unit UCB grafts and those who did not receive ATG treatment experienced a higher relative risk of grade II to IV acute GVHD, consistent with reported findings in a larger cohort.[179] Overall cumulative incidence of TRM was 19% (95% CI 12%–26%) at day 180. The only risk factor for TRM in Cox regression analysis was the presence of comorbidities. For this heterogeneous group of older adults or patients with comorbidities or extensive prior therapy, the probability of survival was 45% and PFS was 38% (95% CI 28%–248%). In multivariate analysis, presence of comorbidities adversely influenced PFS, and use of two UCB units was associated with a trend toward improved PFS (P = 0.06; Fig. 105–4).

Since the introduction of nonmyeloablative UCB transplantation is recent, a few series on disease-specific outcomes are available.[102–104] One study included 20 patients with advanced Hodgkin lymphoma and non-Hodgkin lymphoma.[102] In this study, the median age was 47 years, and six of 20 patients had previously undergone autologous transplant. The incidence of TRM was 40%; 1-year PFS was 50%. In another analysis of 16 patients with chronic lymphocytic leukemic (CLL), mantle cell lymphoma, or follicular lymphoma, 1-year PFS was 60%.[101] As noted elsewhere in Umbilical Cord Blood versus Related Donor Hematopoietic Cell Transplantation section, two reports of UCB transplantation after RIC in patients with Hodgkin lymphoma and acute myeloid leukemia demonstrated 2-year survival of 25% and 31%, respectively.

In summary, UCB appears to be an effective HSC source in the setting of RIC. Fludarabine is a typical part of the conditioning regimen.[170,171,173,174,177,180] Based on the report by Rocha et al.[177] to date the combination of cyclophosphamide/fludarabine/TBI 200 appears to be the most effective in terms of engraftment and survival. Additional treatment strategies need to be explored, but combined use of UCB and RIC markedly extends the availability of transplant therapy.

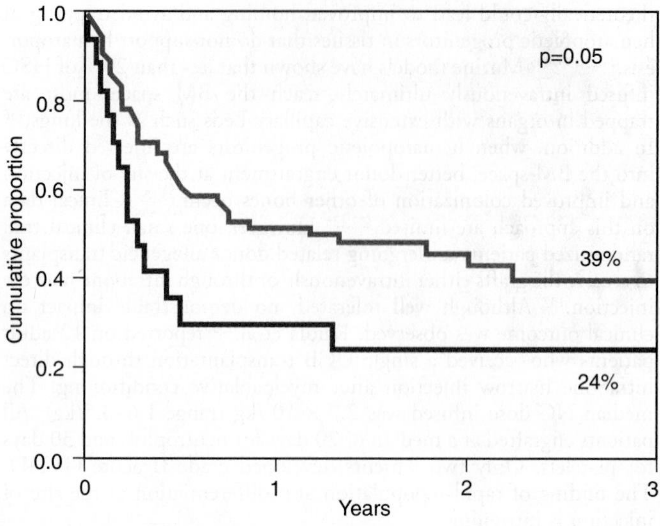

Figure 105–4 Progression-free survival after nonmyeloablative transplantation with one (n = 17) or two (n = 93) umbilical cord blood unit grafts at the University of Minnesota.

IMMUNE RECONSTITUTION AFTER UMBILICAL CORD BLOOD TRANSPLANTATION

Thomson et al.[181] reported on the immune reconstitution of 27 children receiving URD UCB transplantation. Lymphocyte recovery occurred at 2 months for NK cells, 6 months for B cells, 9 months for CD8$^+$ T cells, and 12 months for CD4$^+$ T cells. Similar findings were reported by Niehues et al.[182] in 63 pediatric UCB transplantation recipients (14 related, 49 unrelated; median age 4 years; median cell dose 6.1 × 10^7 NC/kg). Recovery occurred at 3 months for NK cells, 6 months for B cells, 8 months for CD8$^+$ T cells, and 12 months for CD3$^+$ and CD4$^+$ T cells. Factors favoring T-cell recovery were related donor, higher NC dose, and positive recipient CMV serology, whereas recovery was delayed by acute GVHD. As a further measure of T-cell recovery, new thymic emigrants, as measured by T-cell receptor excision circles (TREC), were detected at normal levels starting at 12 months after UCB transplantation.[183] In contrast, TRECs were not detected in adults until 18 months after UCB transplantation and then only at a threefold lower level than expected for age.

Moretta et al.[184] compared immune reconstitution after UCB transplant with 23 matched BM transplant recipient controls. Donors were either sibling (n = 11) or unrelated (n = 12). UCB transplant recipients showed a marked increase in the number of B lymphocytes than did BM transplant recipients. The absolute number of CD3$^+$, CD8$^+$ T cells, and NK cells as well as T-cell proliferative response to mitogens recovered similarly in UCB transplant and BM transplant recipients, with URD UCB transplant showing superior recovery of CD4$^+$ T cells. Similarly, Talvensaari et al.[185] reported on T-cell recovery in related donor transplantation by comparing 10 UCB transplant recipients to 19 age- and GVHD-matched BM transplant controls. During the first year after transplant, both TREC values and T-cell repertoire were low in both groups. However, at 2 years TREC values and T-cell repertoire were higher in UCB transplant recipients than in BM transplant recipients. In contrast, Hamza et al.[186] reported that, compared to matched URD BM transplant, lymphocyte counts recovered slower in the first 2 months after UCB transplantation. However, by 1 year after UCB transplantation lymphocyte counts were in the normal range, whereas for matched URD BM transplant lymphocyte counts still were below normal. They reported a significantly higher risk of bacterial infection during the first 50 days after UCB transplant than in matched URD BM transplant, but without significant difference between the two groups beyond 50 days. No difference was observed between the two groups with regard to the incidence of fungal or viral infections at any time after transplantation.

Weinberg et al.[187] reported that the greatest determinant of thymic function after HCT is the occurrence of GVHD. In their study, serial CD4+ and CD8+ TREC levels were measured in 12 UCB transplant recipients. In the 12 to 24 months after transplant, TREC levels rose to normal or above normal levels for age in many of the recipients and were similar to the values seen with BM. As with BM the presence of GVHD suppressed thymic output in UCB transplant recipients. However, TREC levels rose in three patients even though immunosuppression was continued for at least 6 months after transplant in the absence of GVHD. This finding suggested that active GVHD is a more potent suppressor of thymic output than is immunosuppressive therapy.

Giraud et al.[188] studied the lymphocyte subset recovery and immunoglobulin levels of eight children after unrelated UCB transplantation. They reported recovery of absolute B-cell numbers at 9 months. T cells were delayed until 12 months, particularly the subset of CD3+CD8+ compared to CD3+CD4+. The relative number of NK cells was elevated in the first 6 months, but the absolute number remained in the normal range. IgA and IgM levels returned to normal by 6 months, whereas IgG levels required 9 months. Finocchi et al.[189] reported on six children after unrelated UCB transplantation and showed recovery of T-cell, B-cell, and NK-cell absolute number by 12 months. Remarkably, three fourths of patients had a diversified polyclonal T-cell population. However, CD4+ T-cell receptor diversity recovered faster than that of CD8+ T cells.

Cohen et al.[190] studied the development of antigen-specific lymphocytes in 153 children who participated in the COBLT study. They found that antigen-specific T cells against herpesviruses (CMV, varicella zoster virus, and herpes simplex virus) could be detected as early as 1 to 2 months after UCB transplantation. Overall, 66 children were able to develop responses to one or more herpesvirus during the evaluation period. The probability of developing an antigen-specific response was not different for patients who were serologically positive or negative for the three viruses studied. No association was found between the development of antigen-specific T-cell and immunophenotypic reconstitution, NC dose, primary disease, or development of acute and chronic GVHD. In a smaller study that included 16 children who received either a related or unrelated UCB graft, Montagna et al.[191] found that despite a low absolute number of CD3+ cells T cells, this population recovered proliferative capacity in response to an anti-CD3+ monoclonal antibody, CMV, and *Candida albicans* antigens as early as 3 to 5 months after transplantation. In addition, T-cell polyclonal responses were documented. Interestingly, recipient-derived T cells were found to contribute to the observed response.[191] However, the limited number of patients does not allow firm conclusions regarding differences between recipients of sibling or unrelated UCB donor grafts.

Additional studies are needed to determine quantitative and qualitative differences in immune recovery between UCB and other sources HSCs for transplantation. In addition, correlation between immune reconstitution and susceptibility to infections would be instructive. Life-threatening infection is a significant risk after allogeneic transplantation, and approaches to augment immune reconstitution without increasing the incidence of GVHD are of great interest.

INFECTIOUS COMPLICATIONS AFTER UMBILICAL CORD BLOOD TRANSPLANTATION

Immune recovery after UCB transplant has been postulated to be delayed or incomplete, and such inadequate immune reconstitution might predispose recipients to inordinate risk of infection.[192] Reports regarding the incidence of infections after UCB transplantation can be largely grouped into case reports, reports of infections present at the time of death, retrospective small series focusing on a specific type of infection, and retrospective reports comparing prevalence of infections in UCB and in other stem cell sources.[193]

Bacterial infections are the most frequent source of serious infections after UCB transplantation, and the risk is higher for patients with graft failure.[27,186,194] However, serious and life-threatening infections were not clearly higher in patients with delayed myeloid recovery. Before 100 days, bacterial infections were more frequent after UCB transplantation compared to URD BM transplant, primarily caused by coagulase-negative staphylococci and gram-negative bacilli.[194] Among gram-negative bacteria, the most frequent were Pseudomonas, Acinetobacter, and *Escherichia coli*. Among gram-positive bacteria, the most frequent were coagulase-negative Staphylococci, Enterococcus, and *Staphylococcus aureus*.[27,194,195] Mycobacterial infections were rare events, and UCB graft recipients do not appear to be at particularly high risk.[27,194,196,197] Other case reports of rare bacterial infections after UCB transplantation are reported in the literature.[198–201]

Fungal infections have been reported to occur in 30% to 40% of patients transplanted with UCB. Aspergillus species were responsible for approximately 50% to 70% of fungal infections; Candida species represent most of the remaining fungal infections.[27,194] Development of severe acute GVHD, delayed myeloid recovery, and use of ATG for treatment of GVHD have been reported to be risk factors for fungal infections.[194]

Herpesvirus infections have been frequently observed after UCB transplantation. Among patients who are seropositive for herpes viruses prior to UCB transplantation, the incidence of reactivation rate is approximately 25% for herpes simplex,[202] 63% for varicella,[203] 80% for human herpesvirus type 6 (HHV-6),[204–206] and 30% to 100% for CMV.[194,207,208]

Whereas most of these infections tend to occur after engraftment and are associated with development of GVHD, HHV-6 reactivations occur early after UCB transplantation.[204–206] Guidelines for HHV-6 monitoring and treatment are not yet established.

The importance of CMV lies in its reported adverse effect on TRM and survival after UCB transplantation.[30,46,58] One comparative study reported earlier onset of CMV viremia after UCB transplantation compared to URD grafts, although no significant difference in the incidence of CMV reactivation or disease between HSC sources was observed.[194] Others report that CMV reactivation may be more frequent among recipients of UCB compared to other adult HSC sources,[207,208] suggesting CMV-specific immunity may be delayed after UCB transplantation.[207] CMV disease, although infrequent, is associated with pretransplantation positive serostatus and prior viremia.[194]

Review of the literature indicates the incidence of EBV viremia is between 29% and 65% in the standard (non-UCB) allogeneic HCT setting.[209–214] The incidence of EBV-associated posttransplant lymphoproliferative disease is 2% to 4% after UCB transplantation.[215,216] However, a significantly higher risk of EBV-associated posttransplant lymphoproliferative disease has been reported after UCB when a nonmyeloablative regimen including ATG was used. At the University of Minnesota, the incidence of EBV reactivation or posttransplant lymphoproliferative disease in recipients of RIC with and without ATG and with myeloablative conditioning with and without ATG has been reported as 21%, 2%, 3.3%, and 0%, respectively.[216] Others have also observed a higher risk of EBV complications after administration of ATG.[210,217] In the subset of patients who undergo UCB transplantation after a nonmyeloablative conditioning and ATG, EBV viremia monitoring should be considered with plans for therapy should EBV reactivate.[216]

UMBILICAL CORD BLOOD AS A SOURCE OF EFFECTOR CELLS

Umbilical Cord Blood–Derived Regulatory T Cells

Regulatory T cells are a subset of CD4+ T cells that coexpress CD25 (IL-2Rα chain) and high levels of FOXP3.[36] Regulatory T cells are dependent on IL-2 despite the fact that they do not produce it like other T cells.[218] Regulatory T cells have been shown to be involved with self-tolerance and prevention of autoimmunity.[37–42] Infusion of ex vivo expanded regulatory T cells prevents development of GVHD and suppresses established GVHD.[37,38,40,42,219,220] In addition, $CD4^+CD25^+$ T cells promote hematopoietic engraftment after allogeneic transplantation.[41,221] In murine models, a graft-versus-tumor effect against most acute myeloid leukemia and leukemia/lymphoma cell lines persists after infusion of regulatory T cells.[42,219,220]

The frequency of $CD25^+$ cells appears to be lower in adult human blood (2%–5% of $CD4^+$ T cells) compared to mouse lymph node T cells (5%–10% of CD4's).[222,223] Moreover, delineation of a clear population of $CD4^+CD25^+$ cells is more difficult in humans. FOXP3 transcriptional activation and expression appears to be crucial to human regulatory T-cell function.[36,224,225] The isolation and functional properties of UCB regulatory T cells have been reported.[36,224,226–228] UCB provides a highly reproducible source of potently suppressive regulatory T cells.[36] UCB-derived regulatory T cells appear to be functionally mature despite a naive phenotype.[226] Compared with thymic regulatory T cells, UCB-derived regulatory T cells have broader suppressive activity, perhaps due to further maturation in the circulation.[224]

Ex vivo expanded and activated UCB-derived regulatory T cells are being tested in humans undergoing UCB transplant in order to determine the safety and efficacy of these cells in promoting engraftment and reducing the risk and/or severity of GVHD. If results of these early clinical trials suggest that infusion of UCB regulatory T cells is safe, it is possible that UCB-derived regulatory T cells will be used for treatment of autoimmune diseases or in the setting of solid organ transplantation as a means to ameliorate immune response.

UCB-Derived Natural Killer Cells

Treatment options for advanced and particularly refractory acute myeloid leukemia are limited. NK cells have been shown to contribute to the antitumor effect after allogeneic transplantation.[229] Miller et al.[230,231] studied the administration of ex vivo expanded and activated NK cells for treatment of advanced leukemia. They observed a 25% complete remission for patients with chemotherapy-refractory acute myeloid leukemia who received haploidentical NK cells after immunosuppressive chemotherapy.[230] Compared to peripheral blood, UCB is rich in NK precursors. This led to the development of a new strategy involving ex vivo expansion and activation of UCB-derived NK cells for treatment of chemotherapy-refractory acute myeloid leukemia in the context of a myeloablative double UCB transplant.[232] After a myeloablative conditioning regimen containing cyclophosphamide 120 mg/kg, fludarabine 125 mg/m², and TBI 1320 cGy starting at day −19, patients subsequently receive a CD3-depleted UCB-derived NK cell product from one UCB unit, followed by six doses of IL-2. The UCB-derived NK cells are KIR ligand mismatched whenever possible. On day 0, patients receive a double UCB unit transplant followed by cyclosporine and mycophenolate mofetil immunosuppression for GVHD prophylaxis. Early results suggest that patients will tolerate NK infusion without major toxicity. The effect of UCB-derived NK infusion on short- or long-term suppression of leukemia is not known.

Umbilical Cord Blood–Derived Pluripotent Stem Cell Populations

Reports suggest that progenitors with pluripotent capacity are present in UCB.[233–236] A population of $CD45^-$ UCB-derived cells has been shown to differentiate into osteoblast, chondroblasts, adipocytes, hematopoietic cells, and neural cells, with tissue reconstitution and long-term engraftment in murine models.[234,236] These pluripotent unrestricted somatic cells have been shown not only to be a potential source of cellular therapy for tissue repair[233] but also to support expansion of hematopoietic progenitors.[235]

UMBILICAL CORD BLOOD GRAFT SELECTION

Insufficient information is available to make definitive recommendations guiding the choice of BM versus UCB as a source of hematopoietic stem and progenitor cells for URD transplantation. However, observations on the feasibility and efficacy of UCB transplantation suggest that a simultaneous search for unrelated BM and UCB donors should be performed for transplant candidates who do not have an HLA-matched sibling donor. Donor selection should be based on the underlying diagnosis, urgency of transplant, availability of an HLA A, B, C, and DRB1-matched BM donor(s), NC dose of UCB unit(s), and degree of HLA-disparity between UCB unit(s) and recipient HLA type (Fig. 105-5). Data still support the first use of an HLA-matched BM donor for specific diseases, such as Fanconi anemia and severe aplastic anemia, based on (a) track record and experience with BM and (b) ability to wait out the donor search in most cases. Use of an unrelated adult BM or peripheral blood donor also may be favored in nonurgent chronic myelogenous leukemia cases because of the potential availability of donor lymphocyte infusions following transplantation. However, the majority of URD HCT candidates do not have a suitably matched adult volunteer URD, and many patients

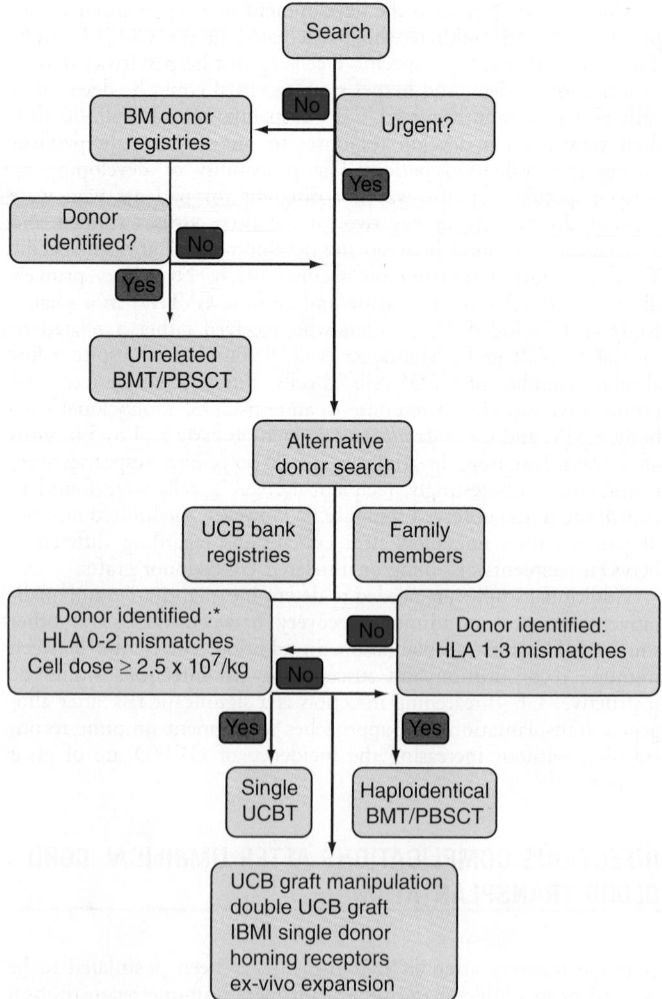

Figure 105–5 Search strategy for unrelated donor grafts: unrelated volunteer donor versus umbilical cord blood.

cannot wait 3 to 4 months for completion of a donor search. For these patients, UCB transplant often is a reasonable option. At the University of Minnesota, we have been able to identify suitable UCB donors in 93% of cases; however, this reflects the institutional practice of using two partially HLA-matched UCB units for patients who do not have a single unit with an adequate cell dose.

Currently, there is no uniform approach for selecting the "optimal" UCB graft. HLA match and cell dose are the most important factors. Disease type also may play a role in UCB donor selection. The analysis by Eapen et al.[110] demonstrates a higher TRM with every increment in HLA mismatch; however, it also demonstrates greater GVL in pediatric patients with malignancy, resulting in comparable LFS rates in patients with one-locus and two-locus mismatches. Although a two-locus mismatch may be perfectly acceptable for a child with leukemia in whom a GVL effect may be important, these data suggest that a two-locus HLA mismatch should be avoided if possible in a child with nonmalignant disease.

Historically, HLA A and B mismatches have been preferentially selected over mismatches at HLA DRB1, and two mismatches at the same antigen have been avoided. (Rocha et al. personal Communication, March 2008) have shown that mismatches at both DR antigens result in poorer results. Conversely, improved engraftment and survival have been observed in cases where the mismatches have occurred only in the rejection vector.[237]

Despite differences in unit selection preferences, most experienced UCB transplant teams would agree that the minimum graft cell dose

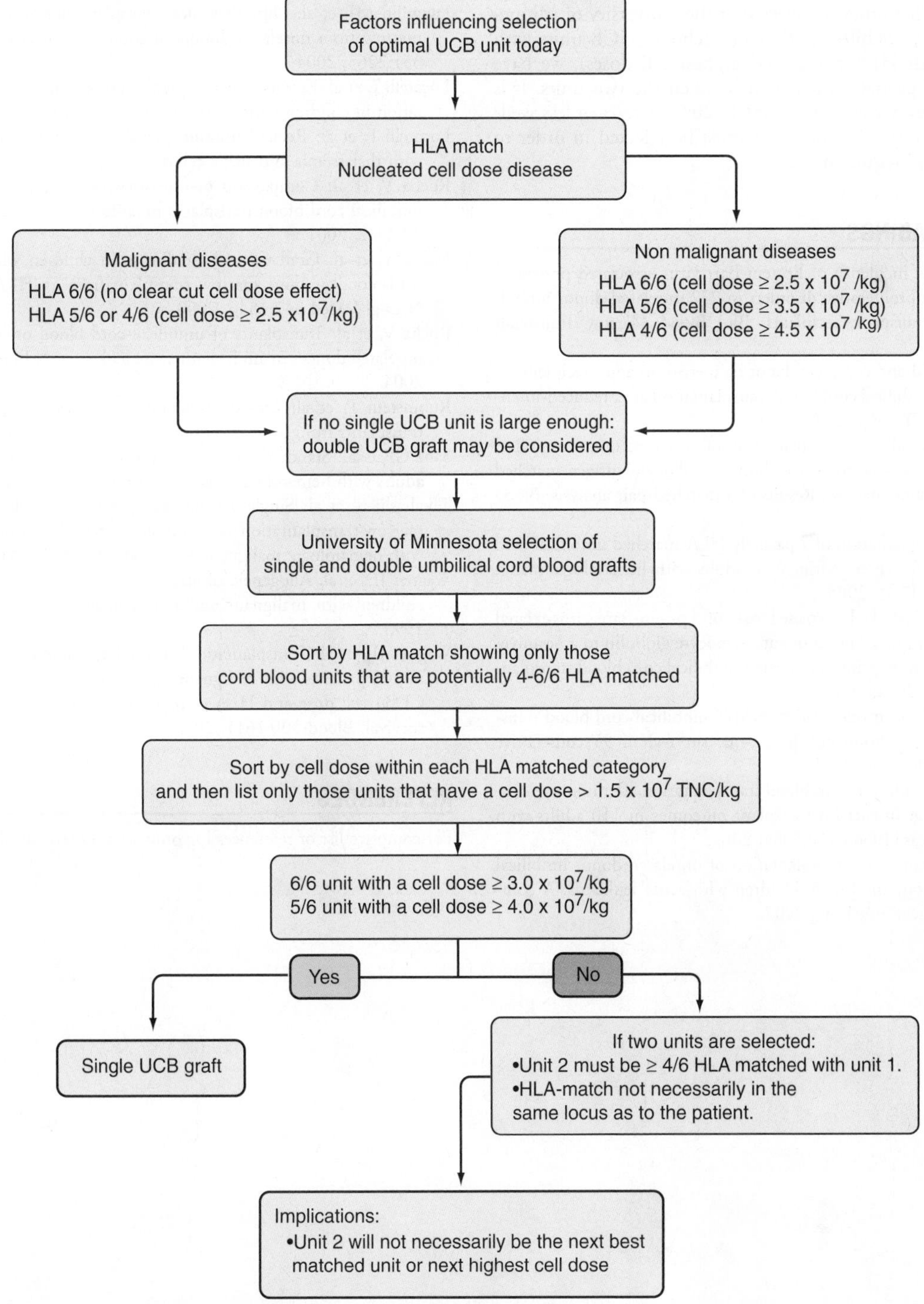

Figure 105–6 Factors influencing selection of optimal umbilical cord blood units today.

is 2.5×10^7 NC/kg actual recipient body weight, and the minimum HLA match is four of six antigens for "routine" transplant (HLA "match" is based on antigen level A and B typing and allele level DRB1 and no matching requirement for C, DP, or DQ). However, the question still remains how to balance cell dose and HLA match. Higher cell doses can ameliorate the negative effect of HLA mismatch, but the doses have to be substantially higher. In a study by Rubinstein et al,[238] an increase of 30×10^6/kg NC/kg would be needed to make a 4/6 matched graft comparable to a 5/6 matched graft. Numerous factors that play a role in UCB graft selection, and the authors have proposed a selection algorithm (Fig. 105–6). Points to consider are also shown because they may alter the general recommendations

Unit selection is even more complicated for programs considering double UCB transplantation. Although even less data on how to choose the two best units are available, the algorithm shown in Fig. 105–6 details how the units are selected at the University of Minnesota. Although the principles are the same (choose UCB units with best donor–recipient HLA match and highest cell doses), we have arbitrarily required partial HLA match between the two units. It is important to realize that in approximately 20% of cases, a less well-matched unit or lower cell dosed unit must be selected in order to fulfill this "arbitrary" requirement.

SUGGESTED READINGS

Barker JN, et al: Low incidence of Epstein-Barr virus-associated posttransplantation lymphoproliferative disorders in 272 unrelated-donor umbilical cord blood transplant recipients. Biol Blood Marrow Transplant 7:395, 2001.

Barker JN, et al: Rapid and complete donor chimerism in adult recipients of unrelated donor umbilical cord blood transplantation after reduced-intensity conditioning. Blood 102:1915, 2003.

Barker JN, et al: Survival after transplantation of unrelated donor umbilical cord blood is comparable to that of human leukocyte antigen-matched unrelated donor bone marrow: Results of a matched-pair analysis. Blood 97:2957, 2001.

Barker JN, et al: Transplantation of 2 partially HLA-matched umbilical cord blood units to enhance engraftment in adults with hematologic malignancy. Blood 105:1343, 2005.

Brunstein CG, et al: Marked increased risk of Epstein-Barr virus-related complications with the addition of antithymocyte globulin to a nonmyeloablative conditioning prior to unrelated umbilical cord blood transplantation. Blood 108:2874, 2006.

Brunstein CG, et al: Non-myeloablative (NMA) umbilical cord blood transplantation (UCBT): Promising disease-free survival in 95 consecutive patients. Blood 106:166a, 2005.

Brunstein CG, et al: Umbilical cord blood transplantation after nonmyeloablative conditioning: Impact on transplant outcomes in 110 adults with hematological disease Blood 110:3064, 2007.

Eapen M, et al: Outcomes of transplantation of unrelated donor umbilical cord blood and bone marrow in children with acute leukemia: A comparison study. Lancet 369:1947, 2007.

Fernandez MN, et al: Unrelated umbilical cord blood transplants in adults: Early recovery of neutrophils by supportive co-transplantation of a low number of highly purified peripheral blood $CD34^+$ cells from an HLA-haploidentical donor. Exp Hematol 31:535, 2003.

Gluckman E, et al: Hematopoietic reconstitution in a patient with Fanconi's anemia by means of umbilical-cord blood from an HLA-identical sibling. N Engl J Med 321:1174, 1989.

Gluckman E, et al: Outcome of cord-blood transplantation from related and unrelated donors. Eurocord Transplant Group and the European Blood and Marrow Transplantation Group. N Engl J Med 337:373, 1997.

Kurtzberg J, et al: Results of the Cord Blood Transplantation Study (COBLT): Clinical outcomes of unrelated donor umbilical cord blood transplantation in pediatric patients with leukemia. J Clin Oncol In press, 2008.

Laughlin MJ, et al: Hematopoietic engraftment and survival in adult recipients of umbilical-cord blood from unrelated donors. N Engl J Med 344:1815, 2001.

Laughlin MJ, et al: Outcomes after transplantation of cord blood or bone marrow from unrelated donors in adults with leukemia. N Engl J Med 351:2265, 2004.

Locatelli F, et al: Factors associated with outcome after cord blood transplantation in children with acute leukemia. Blood 93:3662, 1999.

Locatelli F, et al: Related umbilical cord blood transplantation in patients with thalassemia and sickle cell disease. Blood 101:2137, 2003.

Rocha V, et al: Comparison of outcomes of unrelated bone marrow and umbilical cord blood transplants in children with acute leukemia. Blood 97:2962, 2001.

Rocha V, et al: Graft-versus-host disease in children who have received a cord-blood or bone marrow transplant from an HLA-identical sibling. N Engl J Med 342:1846, 2000.

Rocha V, et al: Transplants of umbilical-cord blood or bone marrow from unrelated donors in adults with acute leukemia. N Engl J Med 351:2276, 2004.

Rubinstein P, et al: Outcomes among 562 recipients of placental-blood transplants from unrelated donors. N Engl J Med 339:1565, 1998.

Sanz GF, et al: Standardized, unrelated donor cord blood transplantation in adults with hematologic malignancies. Blood 98:2332, 2001.

Takahashi S, et al: Single-institute comparative analysis of unrelated bone marrow transplantation and cord blood transplantation for adult patients with hematologic malignancies. Blood 104:3813, 2004.

Wagner JE, et al: Allogeneic sibling umbilical-cord-blood transplantation in children with malignant and non-malignant disease. Lancet 346:214, 1995.

Wagner JE, et al: Transplantation of unrelated donor umbilical cord blood in 102 patients with malignant and nonmalignant diseases: Influence of CD34 cell dose and HLA disparity on treatment-related mortality and survival. Blood 100:1611, 2002.

REFERENCES

For complete list of references log onto www.expertconsult.com

CHAPTER 106

PREPARATIVE REGIMENS FOR HEMATOPOIETIC CELL TRANSPLANTATION

Marcos de Lima, Amin Alousi, and Sergio Giralt

The combination of chemical and physical agents used as antineoplastic or as immunosuppressive agents prior to autologous or allogeneic hematopoietic cell transplant (HCT) is known as the preparative or conditioning regimen. The preparative regimen is the sole provider of antineoplastic activity in the autologous transplant setting and, in addition, provides most of the immunosuppressive activity in allogeneic transplants. Preparative regimens vary among institutions, and comparison of safety and efficacy is difficult (Table 106–1). Furthermore, differences in supportive care, graft-versus-host disease (GVHD) prophylaxis, donor–recipient human leukocyte antigen (HLA) compatibility, and source of hematopoietic cells also should be considered when analyzing outcomes achieved after transplant with different preparative regimens. The lack of standardization makes comparisons of published results difficult. Frequently the choice of a preparative regimen is made on the basis of institutional and personal experience. Here we review the development of commonly used preparative regimens for hematopoietic cell transplant.

CLASSIFICATION OF PREPARATIVE REGIMENS

In the allogeneic transplant setting, the preparative regimen provides treatment for the underlying disease and provides the immunosuppression needed to prevent graft rejection. The intensity of immunosuppression required depends on the immunocompetence of the recipient, donor–recipient histocompatibility, and the composition of the transplanted hematopoietic cell product. Delivery of high-dose therapy is the major purpose of the preparative regimen in autologous transplant. Rescue from marrow suppression induced by the high-dose preparative regimen is provided by previously procured and stored autologous hematopoietic cells.

Preparative regimens may be classified by the use of total body irradiation (TBI), as chemotherapy-only, or as TBI-based (either TBI alone or combined with chemotherapy). If the preparative regimen is "myeloablative," patients generally do not resume normal marrow function unless rescued by autologous or allogeneic hematopoietic cell transplant. Alternatively, the preparative regimen may be "nonmyeloablative." Nonmyeloablative regimens allow for autologous recovery of hematopoiesis in most patients even if autologous or allogeneic hematopoietic cells are not administered. As proposed by Champlin and colleagues, a nonmyeloablative regimen should not eradicate host hematopoiesis and should allow hematopoietic recovery in less than 28 days without hematopoietic cell transplant.[1] On engraftment, mixed chimerism should be present. If there is graft rejection, autologous hematopoiesis should occur. The nonmyeloablative preparative regimen does not completely eliminate host malignant cells, and will rely on an allogeneic graft-versus-tumor effect to eradicate the disease. A myeloablative regimen requires hematopoietic cell transplant, and donor cells should persist after engraftment. Finally, a "reduced intensity ablative" regimen requires a transplant for hematologic reconstitution, and if rejection occurs, prolonged aplasia will be observed, particularly in heavily pretreated patients or those with marrow involvement.

Outcomes after transplant are influenced by a variety of factors other than the preparative regimen. Recipient's age, extent of prior treatments, and disease stage, for example, may affect regimen-related mortality after transplant (Table 106–2).

LANDMARKS IN THE DEVELOPMENT OF HEMATOPOIETIC CELL TRANSPLANTATION

Evidence that animals could be protected from otherwise lethal doses of radiation by shielding hematopoietic tissues emerged in the 1920s. In most cases, marrow was used as a hematopoietic cell source. Interestingly, the first (unsuccessful) attempt to perform hematopoietic cell transplant in a human was in 1939, to treat gold-induced marrow aplasia.[2] In the 1940s and early 1950s, a rapid evolution in the knowledge of radiation effects occurred, and the development of hematopoietic cell transplant concepts paralleled the investigations on radiation. Jacobson and colleagues demonstrated that shielding the spleen protected mice against radiation-induced aplasia. In 1952, it was observed that marrow aplasia could be prevented by injection of spleen cells from syngeneic mice.[3,4] In 1955, Barnes and Loutit reported that leukemia-bearing mice exposed to lethal doses of radiation and treated with isologous myeloid tissue died after 1 month with overt leukemia. Animals treated with homologous marrow cells, however, survived for longer periods without leukemia but died of a wasting syndrome with diarrhea. The wasting syndrome was more intense and occurred earlier among recipients of marrow and spleen cells, as opposed to recipients of marrow cells alone. They proposed that an immune antitumor effect could be present (graft-versus-leukemia), associated with the wasting syndrome (later defined as GVHD).[5] The secondary disease or runting syndrome (as opposed to primary disease, caused by radiation, which induced effects such as skin and gastrointestinal damage) was further characterized in the late 1950s, including the documentation that T lymphocyte-mediated GVHD targeted lymphoid organs, skin, gut, and liver.[6–8] Mixed chimerism (the coexistence of hematopoietic cells from the donor and recipient) was also characterized using erythrocyte antigens, mononuclear cell sex chromatin and sex chromosomes, and specific tolerance to donor skin grafts.

Thomas and coworkers took these concepts to the clinic and used allogeneic hematopoietic cell transplant after preparation with radiation and chemotherapy to treat end-stage patients with malignancies.[9] In 1958, five Yugoslav victims of an atomic reactor accident were treated with marrow transplant by Mathe and colleagues. Four survivors had evidence of transitory chimerism without GVHD. Mathe and colleagues also documented complete engraftment, development of acute and chronic GVHD, and survival of more than 1 year in a patient after allogeneic bone marrow transplant from six different donors in the early 1960s.[10]

The possibility of rescuing dogs exposed to lethal doses of TBI with previously collected and cryopreserved autologous stem cells was elegantly demonstrated in the early 1960s.[11] Studies in dogs also showed that progressively higher TBI doses are needed in order to engraft related, unrelated, or mismatched donors.[12] Furthermore, canine investigations provided insights into histocompatibility issues and on the use of immunosuppressants for GVHD prophylaxis.[13–16]

The description of the HLA system and the realization of the importance of immunologic matching provided another cornerstone for the development of hematopoietic transplant.[17] Children with severe combined immunodeficiency and a patient with Wiskott–Aldrich syndrome were successfully transplanted in 1968. The patient with Wiskott–Aldrich syndrome received immunosuppressive therapy

Table 106–1 Preparative Regimens for Hematopoietic Cell Transplantation

Regimen	Indications	Autologous Transplants	Allogeneic Transplants	Regimen Intensity	References
Cyclophosphamide and TBI (CyTBI)	Acute leukemias, lymphoid malignancies, CML, myelodysplastic syndromes	Yes	Yes	Ablative	40, 50, 87
Melphalan and TBI	Multiple myeloma	Yes	Less often used	Ablative	62
Etoposide and TBI	Acute (mostly ALL) and chronic leukemias	Yes	Yes	Ablative	88
Cyclophosphamide, etoposide, and TBI (CyVPTBI)	Leukemias, lymphomas	yes	Yes	Ablative	89
Busulfan (PO 16 mg/kg) and cyclophosphamide (BuCy2)	Myeloid leukemias, myelodysplastic syndromes	Yes	Yes	Ablative	29
Busulfan (IV, 3.2 mg/kg daily × 4 days) and cyclophosphamide (IV BuCy)	Myeloid leukemias and myelodysplastic syndromes; less often used for lymphoid malignancies	Yes	Yes	Ablative	33
Cyclophosphamide ± ATG	Aplastic anemia (HLA-identical sibling donors; ideal regimen for engraftment of unrelated donor stem cells is unclear). Recent results of randomized trial investigating role of ATG did not indicate benefit.	No	Yes	Ablative	90, 91
Carmustine, etoposide, cytarabine, melphalan (BEAM) ± rituximab	Non-Hodgkin lymphoma and Hodgkin lymphoma (autologous transplants)	Yes	Yes, but less often used	Ablative	92
High-dose melphalan	Multiple myeloma (autologous transplants)	Yes	No	Ablative	93
Cyclophosphamide, carmustine, etoposide (CBV)	Non-Hodgkin lymphoma and Hodgkin lymphoma (autologous transplants)	Yes	No	Ablative	94,95
Fludarabine and IV busulfan 130 mg/m² (4 doses)	Myeloid malignancies, other malignancies	No	Yes	Ablative	38, 34, 38
Thiotepa, fludarabine and melphalan ± ATG	Myeloid and lymphoid malignancies	Less often used	Yes. Donors: related matched and haploidentical, unrelated (including UCB)	Ablative	96
Fludarabine and cyclophosphamide (FC) ± rituximab or campath	Lymphoid malignancies	No	Yes	Nonmyeloablative	85, 97
Low-dose TBI ± fludarabine	Myeloid and lymphoid malignancies	No	Yes	Nonmyeloablative	84
Total-lymphoid irradiation (TLI)	Myeloid and lymphoid malignancies	No	Yes	Reduced intensity	86
Fludarabine and melphalan (FM) ± ATG or campath	Myeloid malignancies, multiple myeloma	No	Yes	Reduced intensity	98, 99, 100
Fludarabine, busulfan (8 mg/kg total dose) and ATG	Myeloid malignancies	No	Yes	Reduced intensity	101
Low-dose TBI, fludarabine, cyclophosphamide or oral busulfan and ATG	Myeloid and lymphoid malignancies	No	Yes; highly immunosuppressive; UCB transplants	Reduced intensity	102

ALL, acute lymphocytic leukemia; ATG, anti-thymocyte globulin; UCB, umbilical cord blood; CML, chronic myelogenous leukemia; HLA, human leukocyte antigen; TBI, total body irradiation. Adapted from Mangan KF: Choice of conditioning regimens. In Ball ED, Lister J, Ping L (eds.): Hematopoietic Stem Cell Therapy, 1st ed. New York, Churchill Livingstone, 2000, p 403, ch 35.[103]

before marrow infusion.[18,19] Incorporation of methotrexate, and subsequently the combination of cyclosporine and methotrexate as standard GVHD prophylaxis, allowed patients with malignant and nonmalignant diseases to be considered for allogeneic transplant. In 1977, the Seattle group reported a series of cases of refractory acute leukemia treated successfully with allogeneic hematopoietic cell transplant.[20–22]

CYCLOPHOSPHAMIDE AND THE COMBINATION OF BUSULFAN AND CYCLOPHOSPHAMIDE

Animal models were used extensively in the development of chemotherapy regimens for hematopoietic cell transplant. Cyclophosphamide emerged as an effective preparative agent that allowed successful

Table 106–2 Factors Other Than the Preparative Regimen That May Influence Outcomes Post–Hematopoietic Cell Transplants

Factors
Patient-related factors
Age (increased treatment-related mortality with older age), comorbid conditions, performance status
Disease-related factors
Diagnosis (malignant versus nonmalignant disease, for example), susceptibility to the graft-versus-tumor effect, stage of disease (increased treatment-related mortality with advanced stage), responsiveness to salvage treatment, duration of first remission (AML, non-Hodgkin lymphomas), time from diagnosis to transplant
Donor–recipient factors
Donor-recipient HLA compatibility (also, sibling versus nonsibling), number of pregnancies
Peritransplant period
GVHD prophylaxis regimen, other prophylactic drugs
Graft
Source of stem cells, graft engineering (T-cell depletion increases the relapse and rejection rates), cell dose
Posttransplant
Duration of follow-up, median follow-up, further immune manipulations (donor lymphocyte infusion, for example)
Study design
Degree of censoring in the data analysis, type of study (randomized or nonrandomized, etc)

engraftment of transplanted allogeneic hematopoietic cells. Furthermore, incorporation of antilymphocyte globulin to chemotherapy regimens decreased the engraftment failure rate. The addition of busulfan to cyclophosphamide resulted in better engraftment in the rat with lower doses of cyclophosphamide.[23–26]

Santos and coworkers investigated the optimal dose of cyclophosphamide and busulfan as a non-TBI-containing preparative regimen for allogeneic hematopoietic cell transplants. The combination of busulfan (16 mg/kg) and cyclophosphamide (200 mg/kg) (BuCy) was effective but carried a high treatment-related mortality. The combination of busulfan (16 mg/kg) and cyclophosphamide (120 mg/kg) (BuCy2) was developed to minimize toxicity and quickly became a popular preparative regimen for allogeneic hematopoietic cell transplant and an alternative to cyclophosphamide and TBI-containing regimens (Cy-TBI).[27–29]

Oral administration of busulfan, however, is limited by the erratic absorption of the drug. High plasma levels are associated with increased incidence of hepatic venoocclusive disease (VOD) and other toxicities, whereas low levels are associated with loss of therapeutic efficacy. The use of careful and frequent monitoring of drug levels after oral administration minimizes this problem.[30] Deeg and collaborators reported on 109 patients with myelodysplastic syndrome prepared with oral busulfan targeted to plasma concentrations of 800 to 900 ng/mL and cyclophosphamide 120 mg/kg followed by related (n = 45) or unrelated (n = 64) donor hematopoietic cell transplants. Three-year relapse-free survival was 56% for related and 59% for unrelated recipients, and nonrelapse mortality at 100 days was 12% for related and 13% for unrelated recipients.[31] Improved results of allogeneic transplant therapy for patients with chronic myelogenous leukemia (CML) receiving a preparative regimen consisting of oral busulfan at doses targeted to achieve effective plasma levels and intravenous cyclophosphamide were also reported by the Seattle group.[32]

Recently, the development of an intravenous busulfan formulation has circumvented most of the problems generated by unpredictable plasma drug levels associated with oral administration. An equivalence rate of 0.8 mg of intravenous busulfan to 1 mg given orally has been proposed and is widely used. Preliminary results suggest a decreased rate of hepatic VOD, possibly by elimination of the "first pass" effect in hepatic sinusoids.[33–35] Busulfan and one of the final metabolites of cyclophosphamide, acrolein, are metabolized by glutathione-S-transferase conjugation. Exchanging cyclophosphamide for fludarabine may improve the safety margin of the combination.[36] Furthermore, there is evidence that the nucleoside analog, fludarabine, potentiates alkylator-induced cell killing through inhibition of DNA-damage repair. A preparative regimen using fludarabine and single daily dosing of intravenous busulfan (130 mg/m^2) appears to be effective and safe. There is no interdose accumulation and the single daily dosing schedule delivers a higher systemic peak concentration of busulfan without additional toxicity (median daily AUC of 4871 µmol/min). Patients with acute myeloid leukemia (AML) and myelodysplastic syndrome (MDS) (n = 96) treated with this regimen had a low regimen-related mortality rate of 3% at 1 year, with only two cases of moderate, reversible hepatic VOD. The MD Anderson Cancer Center experience also suggests that there is a reduction in acute GVHD rates with this combination, which has improved survival for patients with AML and MDS transplanted in complete remission, when compared to historic controls that received IV BuCy2.[37,38]

TOTAL BODY IRRADIATION-BASED REGIMENS

In 1977, Thomas and coworkers reported results of allogeneic transplant therapy in 54 patients with acute myelogenous leukemia (AML) and 46 with acute lymphoblastic leukemia (ALL). Patients received hematopoietic cells obtained from the marrow of an HLA-identical sibling. A combination of cyclophosphamide (120 mg/kg) and TBI (10 Gy) was used as a preparative regimen in these heavily pretreated patients. Of the 94 patients engrafted, only 1 patient rejected the graft. Thirteen patients became long-term leukemia-free survivors. Survival was superior among patients with a better performance status at the time of transplant. This study demonstrated that hematopoietic cell transplant could be considered earlier in the management of patients with acute leukemia who have an HLA-matched sibling donor.[39] Thomas and colleagues also investigated preparative regimens containing TBI given in fractions (fractionated TBI) to minimize extramedullary toxicity, especially interstitial pneumonia. Patients who received 2 Gy/day for 6 days had a better outcome than subjects who were treated with 10 Gy in a single dose (Fig. 106–1).[40]

Studies of allogeneic hematopoietic cell transplant therapy for AML in first complete remission and CML in chronic phase demonstrated that increasing the dose of TBI decreased the leukemia relapse rate; higher transplant-related mortality and toxicity were observed.[41,42] When compared to patients receiving 12-Gy TBI in their preparative regimen, patients treated with 15.75 Gy had a higher incidence of hepatic VOD, interstitial pneumonia, renal failure, mucositis, and death. The incidence of grade II or greater acute GVHD was also higher after 15.75 Gy of TBI (Figs. 106–2 and 106–3). The complex interaction between preparative regimen, patient age, disease stage, and donor–recipient compatibility is also illustrated in a report by Cornelissen and associates.[43] They analyzed 127 adult patients with high-risk ALL receiving matched unrelated donor hematopoietic cell transplants reported to the National Marrow Donor Program. Sixty-four patients were transplanted in first remission, 16 in second or third remissions, and 47 patients had relapsed ALL or primary induction failure. All but 12 patients received cyclophosphamide and TBI-based preparative regimens. One-year treatment-related mortality was 50% for patients in first remission, and more than 60% for the others. Survival of patients in first remission was 40% at 2 years, and results were better for donor–recipient pairs matched at *HLA-DRB1* loci using high-resolution typing. Accordingly, better HLA typing is affecting treatment-related mortality, and incorporation of high-resolution molecular typing for class I alleles is expected to improve results further in the unrelated donor transplant setting.

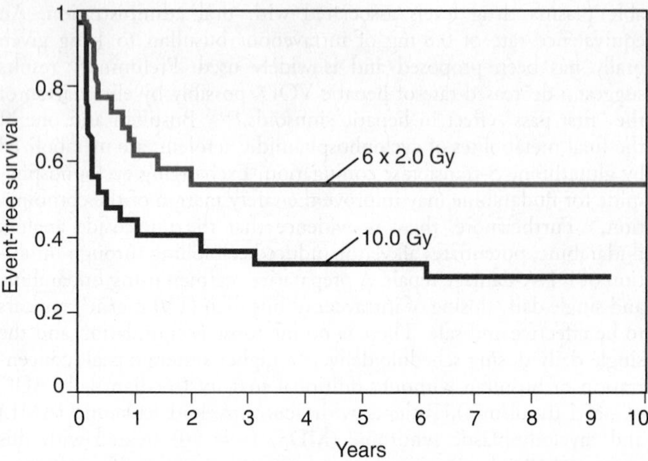

Figure 106–1 Kaplan–Meier product limit estimates for event-free survival of patients with acute myelogenous leukemia in first remission, given 60 mg/kg cyclophosphamide on each of 2 days, randomized to receive 2 Gy total body irradiation (TBI) on each of 6 days ($n = 26$) or 10 Gy TBI ($n = 27$) in one exposure followed by an infusion of hematopoietic stem cells from an HLA-identical sibling. Fractionated TBI elicited improved event-free survival. (Data from Thomas ED: Total body irradiation regimens for marrow grafting. Part 1. J Radiat Oncol Biol Phys 19:1286, 1990.)

The reader is urged to keep in mind that there is significant heterogeneity in the delivery of TBI. These include different energy sources, dissimilar shielding practices, schedules and concomitant chemotherapy. However, some form of fractionation is used at most US centers.

A preparative regimen containing cyclophosphamide (120 mg/kg) and TBI (920–1575 cGy) provides enough immunosuppression for engraftment of hematopoietic cells obtained from HLA-identical siblings, HLA-matched unrelated donors, and unrelated donor umbilical cord blood.[44] Addition of antithymocyte globulin to the preparative regimen may improve engraftment and contribute to the prevention of GVHD after transplant of hematopoietic cells from donors other than HLA-identical siblings.[45] The combination of TBI and cyclophosphamide is the most frequently used regimen for the treatment of ALL. There is little evidence, however, for or against the use of busulfan and cyclophosphamide for this disease.

RANDOMIZED COMPARISONS OF PREPARATIVE REGIMENS CONTAINING BUSULFAN AND CYCLOPHOSPHAMIDE (BuCy) VERSUS TOTAL BODY IRRADIATION AND CYCLOPHOSPHAMIDE (Cy-TBI) FOR THE TREATMENT OF LEUKEMIAS WITH ALLOGENEIC HEMATOPOIETIC CELL TRANSPLANTATION

The choice of the ideal preparative regimen for hematopoietic cell transplant therapy of myeloid leukemias has been an ongoing issue since busulfan and cyclophosphamide (BuCy) was developed as an alternative to TBI-containing regimens. Several randomized studies have been published, comparing outcomes after TBI and cyclophosphamide (Cy-TBI) and BuCy preparation for HLA-identical sibling hematopoietic cell transplants. The Nordic group enrolled patients receiving allogeneic hematopoietic cell transplant therapy for AML, lymphoid malignancies, and CML, and found improved disease-free survival with less toxicity among patients with advanced-stage disease receiving a Cy-TBI-containing preparative regimen. A long-term analysis of the Nordic study showed an increased risk of chronic GVHD, obstructive bronchiolitis, hemorrhagic cystitis, and hepatic VOD after transplant with the BuCy preparative regimen.[46] Blaise

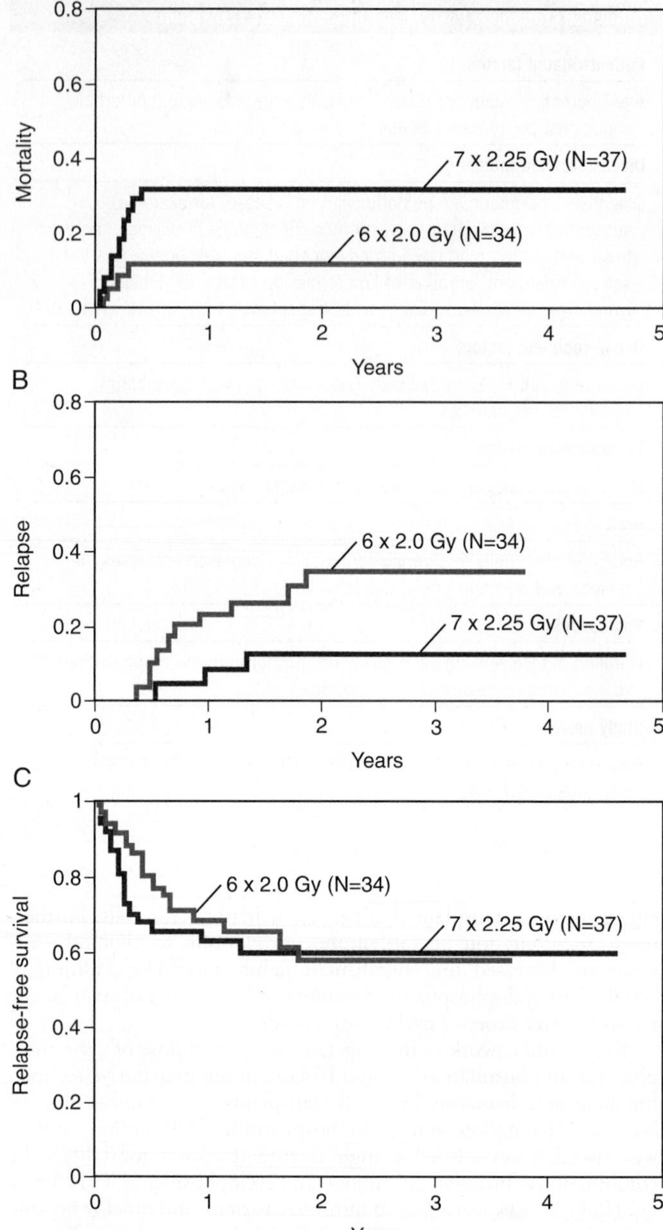

Figure 106–2 The preparative regimen with higher doses of total body irradiation (TBI) reduced probability of relapse at the expense of increased mortality. **A**, Mortality in patients not relapsing after stem cell transplantation ($P = .04$). Patients who relapsed were censored at the time of relapse. **B**, Probability of relapse ($P = .06$). **(C)** Probability of surviving relapse-free after transplantation. (Data from Clift R, Buckner C, Appelbaum F, et al: Allogeneic marrow transplantation in patients with acute myeloid leukemia in first remission: A randomized trial of two irradiation regimens. Blood 76:1869, 1990.)

and colleagues reported a study with AML patients in first remission. They found better disease-free and overall survival and decreased treatment-related mortality and relapse rate in hematopoietic cell transplant recipients prepared with Cy-TBI rather than with BuCy. In 2001, Blaise published extended follow-up data from the 1992 study of AML patients in first remission. The BuCy preparative regimen was associated with poorer outcome than the Cy-TBI regimen. Failure in the early post-transplant period, including more transplant-related deaths and relapses, occurred in the BuCy group. Late events, such as secondary cancers, had a similar incidence in

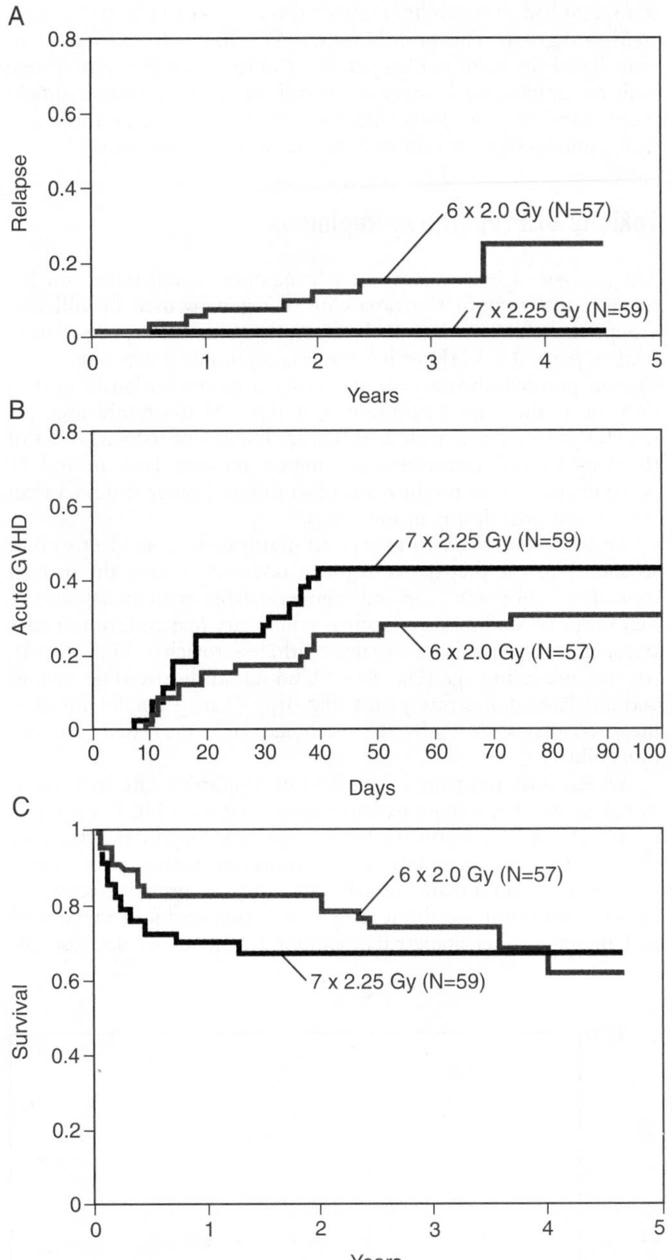

Figure 106–3 Increasing the dose of total body irradiation (TBI) reduced the relapse rate, but was associated with higher acute graft-versus-host disease (GVHD) and toxicity rates. **A**, Probability of relapse after transplantation during the chronic phase of chronic myelogenous leukemia (CML) for patients receiving 12 Gy or 15.75 Gy TBI ($P = .08$). **B**, Probability of developing grade II or worse acute GVHD after transplantation in the chronic phase of CML for patients receiving 12 Gy or 15.75 Gy TBI ($P = .15$). **C**, Probability of survival after transplantation during chronic phase of CML for patients receiving 12 Gy or 15.75 Gy TBI. (Data from Clift R, Buckner C, Appelbaum F, et al: Allogeneic marrow transplantation in patients with acute myeloid leukemia in the chronic phase: A randomized trial of two irradiation regimens. Blood 77:1663, 1991.)

both groups of patients. Interestingly, a French multicenter study showed that these preparative regimens were equivalent for the treatment of patients with CML in chronic phase.[47–50] A major weakness of these reports is that the researchers did not monitor busulfan blood levels. It is possible that at least some of the differences in toxicity and diminished efficacy of the busulfan-containing regimen could be related to undetected high or low blood levels, respectively. Clift and colleagues reported a long-term analysis of outcomes that confirmed that the two regimens had similar efficacy and nonrelapse mortality. BuCy, however, was better tolerated than Cy-TBI.[48] A Southwest Oncology Group study compared VP-16 (etoposide) and TBI with BuCy for the treatment of patients with AML not in first remission.[51] No difference in disease-free survival was documented.

Socie and associates reported consolidated long-term follow-up results of the studies described above for patients with AML (n = 172) and CML (n = 316).[52] Among patients with CML, no statistically significant difference in overall and disease-free survival was detected. Ten-year survival estimates were 65% and 63% with BuCy and Cy-TBI, respectively. In patients with AML, a 10% lower survival rate was observed after BuCy (10-year actuarial survival of 51% and 63% with BuCy and Cy-TBI, respectively); however, this difference was not statistically significant. Long-term complications, such as avascular necrosis of the femur, were associated with chronic GVHD and steroid use, and to a lesser extent with the preparative regimens.

These studies illustrate the inherent differences in response of various leukemias to the preparative regimens, as well as the need for pharmacokinetic studies and long-term follow-up when comparing preparative regimens.

AUTOLOGOUS TRANSPLANTS

Choice of Agents for Autologous Hematopoietic Cell Transplantation

The alkylating agents are the most commonly used class of antineoplastic agents in the preparative regimen for hematopoietic cell transplant. Other agents are not considered for dose escalation due to extramedullary toxicity occurring at lower doses or at the same dose levels where myelosuppression occurs. The maximum tolerated dose with autologous hematopoietic cell transplant support may be as high as 30 times the standard dose for the alkylating agent thiotepa.[53]

Tumors are heterogeneous in terms of chemotherapy or radiation sensitivity, and preparative regimens containing chemotherapy combinations may provide a way to act at different sites within cancer cells. Choice of chemotherapeutic agents is generally based on relative lack of overlapping toxicity or cross-resistance, effectiveness, and achievable fold dose escalation. Most of the preparative regimens used in autologous transplant employ combination chemotherapy or chemotherapy and radiation. More recently, the explosion of new biologic knowledge has led to the development of new classes of agents with anticancer properties. Monoclonal antibodies are becoming part of preparative regimens designed to target diseases expressing a wide range of epitopes, such as CD20 (non-Hodgkin lymphomas), as discussed below. It is to be expected that the regimens will progressively change in order to incorporate these novel agents.

Mobilization Regimens

Collection of peripheral blood stem cells for hematopoietic cell transplant in the steady state is ineffective because of the small number of hematopoietic progenitors in the peripheral blood. Several regimens for mobilization of autologous hematopoietic cells have been proposed, based on the observation that the number of these cells increase in the circulation during hematologic recovery after chemotherapy and that hematopoietic growth factors increase the numbers of circulating stem cells. Combinations of chemotherapy and growth factors are used successfully in a variety of regimens and doses.[54,55–57] Allogeneic donors are mobilized with growth factors alone whereas autologous donors may receive chemotherapy followed by growth factors.[59] AMD3100, a CXCR4 antagonist may become part of future mobilization strategies.[58] There are few formal comparisons of mobilization regimens, and various regimens have been used.

Preparative Regimens for Autologous Transplant in Multiple Myeloma

Multiple myeloma is one of the few hematologic malignancies for which there is a series of randomized studies comparing different preparative regimens for autologous transplant. It is instructive to review the results of some of these comparisons.

Response rate after conventional therapy such as oral melphalan and prednisone is 50% to 60%, with a 5% complete remission rate. Responders have a median survival of 3 years, and prognosis is based on a variety of features identified at diagnosis. Evidence has accumulated showing a dose–response relationship in the treatment of this disease. High-dose TBI-based preparative regimens coupled with autologous hematopoietic cell transplant were shown to be superior to standard dose chemotherapy in randomized trials. A French study reported complete remission and 5-year survival rates of 22% and 52% in the autologous transplant arm versus 5% and 12% in the standard therapy arm.[59] Increasing the dose of melphalan from 100 mg/m^2 to 400 mg/m^2 (200 mg/m^2 for each transplant procedure), which is delivered in some tandem transplant programs, increases the complete remission rate from 6% to 15%–25% in refractory patients, and to 20%–45% in recently diagnosed individuals. Early harvesting of mobilized peripheral blood progenitor cells (preferably during the first year of chemotherapy) allows for the collection and storage of more cells that can be used to support tandem transplants.

Moreau and colleagues reported a randomized comparison of melphalan (200 mg/m^2) versus melphalan (140 mg/m^2) plus TBI (8 Gy) as the preparative regimen for autologous transplant in patients with newly diagnosed disease.[61] All patients received four cycles of vincristine, doxorubicin (Adriamycin), and dexamethasone (VAD) prior to the high-dose preparative regimen and autologous hematopoietic cell transplant.[60] Patients treated without TBI had less toxicity, shorter hospitalization, and faster recovery than those receiving melphalan and TBI. Whereas event-free survival was similar, 45-month survival was 46% in the TBI arm and 66% in the non-TBI arm. Moreau and colleagues pointed out that although better salvage regimens were probably responsible for the difference in survival, toxicity was significantly reduced in the non-TBI arm. Barlogie and colleagues employed tandem transplants preceded by three cycles of VAD chemotherapy, cyclophosphamide (6 gm/m^2) with GM–CSF for peripheral blood stem cell harvesting, and EDAP (etoposide, dexamethasone, cytosine arabinoside, cisplatin) for one cycle.[61] The high-dose preparative regimen consisted of melphalan (200 mg/m^2) in the first transplant. Patients achieving at least a partial remission received a second transplant with the same preparative regimen, whereas nonresponders were prepared with melphalan (140 mg/m^2) and TBI. All patients received interferon maintenance until relapse. Among the 231 patients treated (median age 51 years), more than half had Durie–Salmon stage III disease and 30% had β2 microglobulin levels greater than 3 mg/L, strong predictors of poor prognosis. Seventy-one percent of the patients received the second transplant as intended. The complete remission rate increased from 5% after VAD, to 30% after the first transplant and to 41% after completion of two autologous transplants. Treatment-related mortality was 1% after the first and 4% after the second transplant, respectively. Median actuarial 5-year survival was 58 months. The role of double autologous transplants was investigated in a protocol of the Intergroupe Francophone du Myelome. Attal and coworkers randomized 399 untreated patients younger than 60 years to receive a single transplant after a preparative regimen consisting of melphalan (140 mg/m^2) and TBI (8 Gy) or tandem transplant after preparation with melphalan (140 mg/m^2) followed by the TBI–melphalan regimen, respectively.[62] Response rate was similar, but overall and event-free survival were significantly improved in the tandem transplant arm. Seven-year postdiagnosis probability of overall and event-free survival was 42% and 20% in the tandem transplant group and 21% and 10% in the single transplant group. Patients that did not achieve a very good partial remission within 3 months after the first transplant had a probability of survival at 7 years of 11% in the single transplant group. This probability was 43% in the double transplant arm. Based on these results, patients younger than 60 years treated with the autologous hematopoietic cell transplant approach should receive tandem transplants, and every effort should be performed to store autologous stem cells early in the course of the disease.

Toxicity of Preparative Regimens

The analysis of toxicity data after hematopoietic cell transplant has to take into account the variability of regimens used by different groups and the scoring system used to describe the results. Drugs used to prevent GVHD or infectious complications may alter toxicity, and prophylaxis practices may differ from institution to institution, or at the same institution over time. Methotrexate used for GVHD prevention is such an example. The use of reduced doses of the drug ("mini" methotrexate, 5 mg/m^2 on days 1, 3, 6, and 11 posttransplant) may produce less mucositis and other toxicities than more traditional dosing of this agent.[63]

Regimen-related toxicity may be arbitrarily defined as adverse event secondary to the preparative regimen occurring during the first 30 days after transplant.[64] Several regimen-related toxicities, however, may occur beyond 30 days (such as pulmonary toxicity). Autologous transplants are usually associated with less toxicity (Fig. 106–4), whereas increasing age (Fig. 106–5), advanced disease (Fig. 106–6) and unrelated donor transplants (Fig. 106–7) are generally linked to increased rates of adverse reactions and decreased survival probability.

Several improvements in the field of supportive care have minimized many of the acute toxicities associated with HCT. Examples include the incorporation of selective type three 5-hydroxytryptamine (5-HT3) receptor antagonists for prevention and treatment of nausea, palifermin (recombinant human keratinocyte growth factor) to prevent and minimize the severity of radiation-induced mucositis[65] and mesna (2-mercaptoethane sodium sulfonate) to decrease the

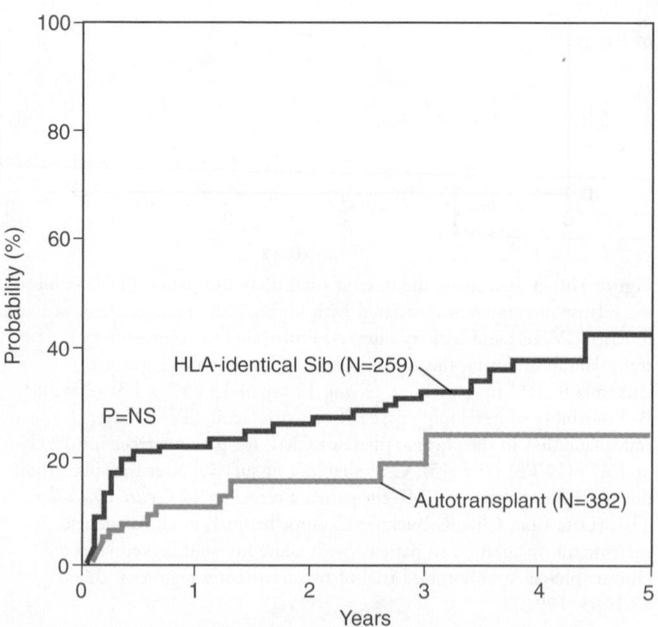

Figure 106–4 Probability of transplant-related mortality after allogeneic hematopoietic stem cell transplantation for acute myelogenous leukemia (AML) patients in second complete remission. Patients receiving autologous transplantations tend to have lower rates of treatment-related mortality than recipients of allogeneic transplants, as exemplified here by patients with AML treated with busulfan and cyclophosphamide. (Cases reported to the International Bone Marrow Transplant Registry (IBMTR), unpublished data, courtesy of the IBMTR.)

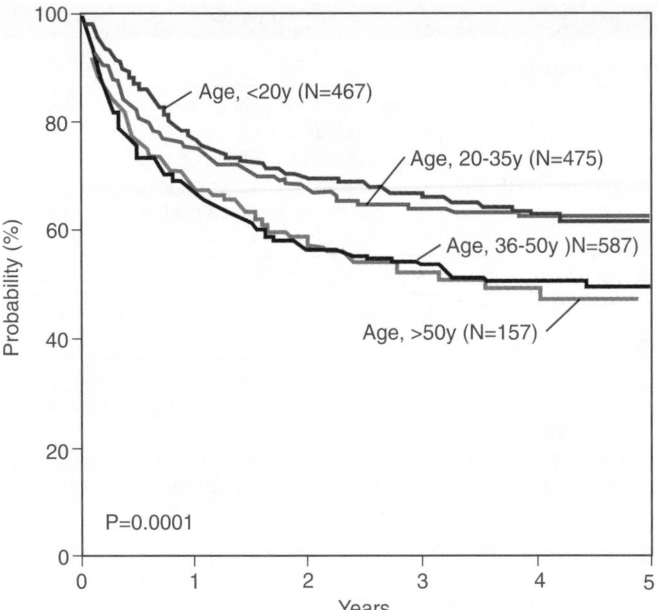

Figure 106–5 Probability of survival after human leukocyte antigen (HLA)-identical sibling transplants for patients with acute myelogenous leukemia (AML) in remission is affected by recipient's age. Kaplan–Meier survival curves of patients that received busulfan and cyclophosphamide as conditioning regimen show decreased survival probability for older patients. (Data from the International Bone Marrow Transplant Registry (IBMTR), on cases reported from years 1996–2000, unpublished data, courtesy of the IBMTR.)

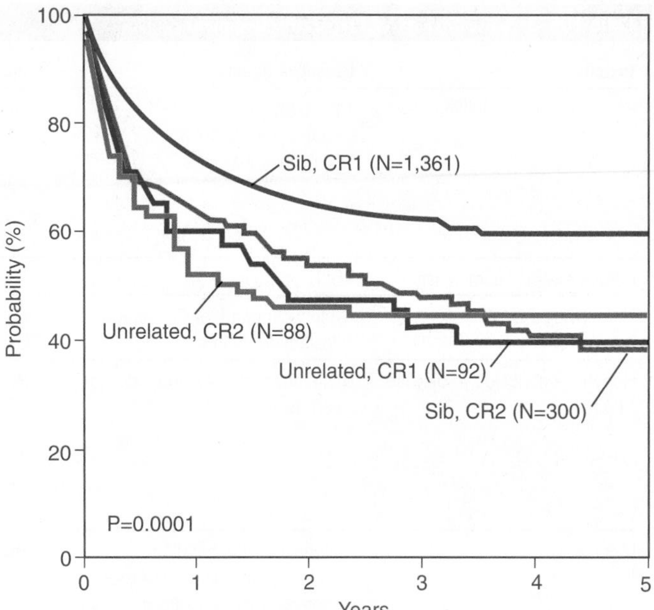

Figure 106–7 Donor type influences survival after allogeneic hematopoietic transplantations: probability of survival after matched unrelated donor and human leukocyte antigen (HLA)-identical sibling bone marrow transplant for acute myelogenous leukemia (AML). All patients received busulfan and cyclophosphamide and were treated from 1996 to the year 2000. Sib = sibling. (Cases reported to the International Bone Marrow Transplant Registry, unpublished data, courtesy of the IBMTR.)

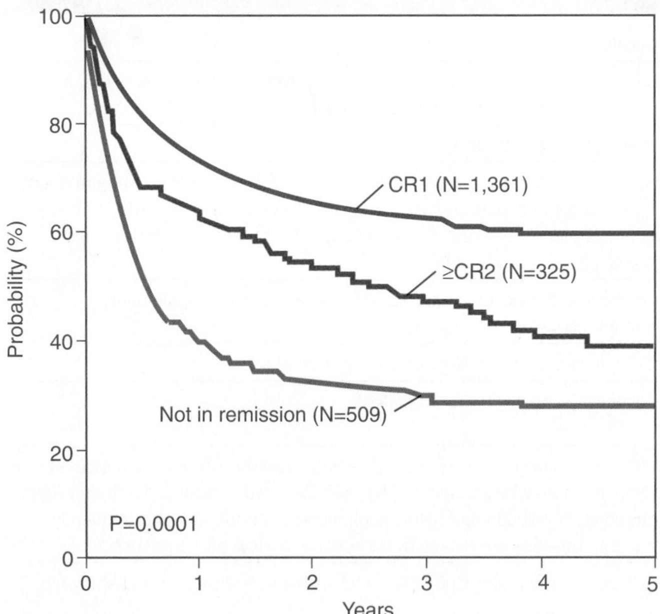

Figure 106–6 Probability of survival after allogeneic human leukocyte antigen (HLA)-identical sibling transplants for acute myelogenous leukemia (AML) is affected by the disease status at transplant. Probability of survival for patients treated with busulfan and cyclophosphamide is shown as a function of remission status. CR1 = first complete remission; CR2 = second complete remission. (Cases reported to the International Bone Marrow Transplant Registry (IBMTR) from years 1996–2000, unpublished data, courtesy of the IBMTR.)

occurrence of regimen-related hemorrhagic cystitis. Long-term toxicities are generally more difficult to prevent, and increased awareness and surveillance are highly recommended (such as for hypothyroidism after TBI). An intervention that is likely to be of benefit for selected individuals is the use of biphosphonates to prevent bone loss after transplant, although long-term benefits are largely assumed but not proven, and some serious side effects have been reported.

Second malignancies may occur following hematopoietic cell transplants, and are more common in patients conditioned with TBI-based regimens.[66] The risk of secondary cancers was 6.7% at 15 years posttransplant among 3,200 patients who survived for at least 5 years after HCT.[67] Incidence of cancers of the brain, thyroid, liver, bone, oral cavity and connective tissue were significantly increased. Incidence increased with the dose of radiation and decreased with non-TBI-containing regimens.

Posttransplant lymphoproliferative disorder represents a group of Epstein–Barr virus-related clinical syndromes that may include very aggressive non-Hodgkin lymphoma. HLA-mismatching, T-cell depletion of the graft, use of antilymphocyte antibodies in the conditioning regimen, and use of potent or multiple immunosuppressive treatments for GVHD are well-recognized risk factors. Tables 106–3 and 106–4 describe commonly reported regimen-related toxicities.

MONOCLONAL ANTIBODIES

The feasibility and efficacy of supplementing high-dose chemotherapy protocols with rituximab, an anti-CD20 mouse/human chimeric monoclonal antibody (MAb) active against various lymphoid malignancies has been documented by several groups. The goal is to achieve in vivo purging during mobilization and to eliminate minimal residual disease after transplant.[68,69] The MD Anderson Cancer Center experience using high-dose rituximab (1000 mg/m^2) after mobilization chemotherapy and on days 1 and 8 post–autologous transplant was reported by Khouri and colleagues.[70] Forty-two patients with CD20 expressing non-Hodgkin lymphoma were

Table 106–3 Acute Toxicity of Preparative Regimens

Toxicity	Causative Agents	Incidence and Comments
Interstitial pneumonitis	Total body irradiation (TBI), carmustine, busulfan, cyclophosphamide	Higher in patients who received radiation to the chest prior to bone marrow transplantation. Allogeneic transplants > autologous transplants. Fractionated doses of TBI minimize extramedullary toxicity. Busulfan (IV, 3.2 mg/kg) and cyclophosphamide (IV) (BuCy) < TBI. Acute and chronic forms. Idiopathic pneumonia syndrome classically described as occurring at a median of 50 days posttransplant.
Diffuse alveolar hemorrhage	TBI	May occur with different regimens. Allogeneic transplants > autologous transplants.
Hemorrhagic cystitis	Cyclophosphamide, TBI, etoposide, ifosfamide, holmium	Higher in cyclophosphamide-containing regimens. May lead to chronic urinary tract strictures and severe bladder dysfunction.
Hepatic venoocclusive disease (VOD)	Busulfan, cyclophosphamide, tbi, carmustine	Possibly higher incidence among patients with active viral hepatitis and iron overload. High mortality with severe forms (ascites, severe weight gain, jaundice, painful hepatomegaly) Fractionated doses of TBI minimize extramedullary toxicity. Use of IV formulation of busulfan appears to reduce the risk (better control of area under the concentration curve versus time).
Mucositis	Melphalan, TBI, busulfan, cyclophosphamide, etoposide, thiotepa, methotrexate	Higher among heavily pretreated patients, and patients who received prior radiation to the cervical and mediastinal areas. Methotrexate used for graft-versus-host disease (GVHD) prophylaxis may worsen mucositis.
Diarrhea	Melphalan, TBI, cyclophosphamide	
Seizures	Busulfan	Prophylactic use of anticonvulsants minimizes the risk. Incidence higher in children than in adults
Renal failure	TBI, carmustine, ATG, ifosfamide	Often multifactorial
Encephalopathy	Carmustine, ifosfamide	Often multifactorial

Acute GVHD and its treatment may worsen regimen-related toxicities.

Table 106–4 Delayed Toxicity of Preparative Regimens

Side effect	Regimen	Incidence / Comments
Hypothyroidism	TBI	Single fraction TBI, up to 73% incidence of thyroid dysfunction; fractionated TBI, 15%–25% (mean time to development of hypothyroidism, 49 months)[104,105]
Growth/development delay	TBI	Steroid use may worsen growth delay.
Sterility	TBI, chemotherapy-containing regimens	Women receiving TBI in doses greater than 10 cGy have higher incidence of permanent ovarian damage. Older age increases the likelihood of menopause post-BMT.[106] Sperm production is usually severely decreased post-TBI, but less so after busulfan-based regimens.
Chronic pulmonary damage	TBI, carmustine-containing regimens	Bronchiolitis obliterans caused by chronic GVHD may cause severe pulmonary dysfunction in the allogeneic setting.
Cataracts	TBI, Busulfan	Fractionated TBI, incidence of >30%. Steroid use also a factor
Osteoporosis	TBI, chemotherapy-containing regimens	Prevalence unknown (probably underestimated)
Myelodysplasia	Cyclophosphamide/TBI, etoposide containing regimens, other chemotherapy-ontaining regimens	Rare occurrence after allogeneic BMT (eg, represents disease relapse). Incidence after autologous transplant may be as high as 18% ± 9% at 6 years post-BMT. Contribution of hematopoietic stem cell damage by previous therapy is important and frequently chromosomal abnormalities are detected in the bone marrow prior to transplant.[107–109]
Alopecia	BuCy, cyclophosphamide/TBI and other regimens	Alopecia was more common after BuCy than after CyTBI in one randomized study.[110]

Development of chronic GVHD and its treatment may overlap with, precipitate, or worsen regimen-related toxicities. For explanation of abbreviations, see Table 106–1.

treated, using high-dose chemotherapy with the BEAM regimen. Two-year survival was 80% (there were no treatment-related deaths) versus 53% for a historical control group. The use of high-dose rituximab, however, remains controversial, and most groups use lower doses.

Similarly, MAb may contribute to the treatment of myeloid leukemias. A phase I/II study was conducted at the MD Anderson Cancer Center adding gemtuzumab ozogamicin (Mylotarg) 2 or 4 mg/m^2 to the reduced-intensity preparative regimen of fludarabine and melphalan 140 mg/m^2. Gemtuzumab ozogamicin is a monoclonal antibody that targets the CD33 antigen commonly present in myeloid cells. A group of 52 patients received allogeneic transplantation with this regimen (49 with refractory and/or refractory CD33-positive myeloid leukemias). The lower dose was safely added to the regimen, and a comparison with historic controls indicated a prolongation of survival.[71]

The CD52 MAb alemtuzumab (Campath) targets a glycoprotein that is highly expressed on normal T- and B-lymphocytes and on a significant proportion of malignant lymphoid cells. Graft T cell depletion using this MAb prevents acute and chronic GVHD, but it is unclear if this benefit is offset by increased relapse rates. Alemtuzumab is under intense investigation as part of the preparative regimen in several centers worldwide, especially in the context of mismatched-related, haploidentical, or unrelated donor transplants.[72]

RADIOIMMUNOTHERAPY

The principle of attaching radioactive particles to MAb is referred to as radioimmunotherapeutics (RIT). It is expected to increase both efficacy and safety by delivering irradiation directly to the target on the tumor cell with relative sparing of normal tissue. In addition, high-energy particles can kill surrounding tumor cells that do not directly bind the antibody through a bystander effect. Currently two radioimmunoconjugates (RICs) are approved by the U.S. Food and Drug Administration for the treatment of CD20+ expressing lymphoma: iodine-131 (I-131) tositumomab and yttrium-90 (Y-90) ibritumomab tiuxetan. Ibritumomab tiuxetan (Zevalin) is a murine anti-CD20 IgG1 kappa monoclonal antibody linked to tiuxetan and to the beta-emitting radioisotope Ytrium-90 (therapeutic) or to Indium-111 (for imaging). A phase I/II trial using etoposide (40–60 mg/kg on day −4), cyclophosphamide (100 mg/kg on day −2), and Zevalin has been reported.[73] Dosimetry was performed on day −21 with 5 mCi ^{111}In-ibritumomab tiuxetan, followed by Zevalin (40–100 mCi) with ytrium ibritumomab tiuxetan. Eighteen patients received hematopoietic cells when the radiation dose was estimated to be less than 5 cGy. There were no treatment-related deaths and median time to engraftment of neutrophils was 10 days, illustrating the safety of this approach.

The first phase 1 RIT study with stem cell support was conducted by Press and coworkers in 1993 with I-131-labled anti-CD20 (B1, 1F5) and anti-CD37 (MB-1) to treat relapsed lymphoma.[74] The anti-CD20 antibody was found to be superior to the anti-CD37 antibody in terms of dosing, distribution, and toxicity. Patients treated with 23.75 Gy or less to normal organs experienced minimal nonhematologic toxicity. Two patients experienced grade 3 cardiopulmonary complications after receiving doses that resulted in 27.25 and 30.75 Gy to the lung. A subsequent phase 2 study by the same investigators and trials performed by other groups confirmed the activity of regimens combining chemotherapy and RIT. A relatively common long-term toxicity has been a rise in thyroid-stimulating hormone, although acute toxicities have been similar to those observed without the RIC. I-131-tositumomab has been administered in a standard total body dose (rather than dosimetry determined) combined with the BEAM regimen, again without excessive side effects.[75] Clinical trials are underway investigating RIT as part of preparative regimens for allogeneic transplants to treat lymphoma.

Targeting radiation to the marrow is an attractive approach to minimize the toxic effects of γ radiation. Radionuclides that emit β radiation have a particle emission range that is much greater than the size of the cells, with the potential for more side effects and the need for higher doses of radioactivity. The α-emitting radionuclides may be a suitable alternative to target the hematopoietic system because of the high-energy particles that distribute the irradiation over smaller distances. In a canine model of nonmyeloablative allogeneic transplantation, a preparative regimen consisting of bismuth 213, an α-emitting radionuclide, combined to an anti-CD45 monoclonal antibody (CD45 is a broadly expressed hematopoietic surface antigen) was well tolerated and produced stable mixed chimerism.[76]

Three different antibodies have been tested—anti-CD33, -CD45, and -CD66—attached to one of four radionuclides (^{131}I, ^{90}Y, ^{188}Re, or ^{213}Bi). Various phase 1 and 2 trials have investigated the addition of one of these RIC either to fully ablative (Cy-TBI or BuCy2) or reduced-intensity conditioning regimens and are reviewed elsewhere by Kotzerke and collaborators.[77]

Matthews and coworkers reported the use of an anti-CD45 antibody incorporated into a conditioning regimen for patients with advanced acute leukemia and MDS. A total of 34 patients received the ^{131}I- anti-CD45 antibody administered in a dose estimated to deliver an absorbed dose of radiation to the liver (the highest uptaking normal organ in all but one patient) ranging from 3.5 Gy (dose level 1) to 12.25 Gy (level 6). The RIC was combined with Cy (120 mg/kg) and TBI (12 Gy divided into six fractions) followed by autologous or allogeneic transplant. The MTD (mucositis) was determined to be 10.5 Gy. This strategy resulted in supplemental doses of radiation of 24 and 50 Gy to the marrow and spleen. DFS was 29% with nonrelapse mortality and relapse rate of 18% and 50%, respectively. A phase 1/2 trial was then conducted in 46 patients with intermediate or poor risk cytogenetics AML in first remission using the ^{131}I- anti-CD45 antibody combined with targeted oral Bu (AUC of 600–900 ng/mL) and Cy 120 mg/kg, followed by matched related donor transplant.[78,79] Four patients safely received a dose at level 1 that targeted 3.5 Gy to normal organs, with all subsequent patients receiving dose level 2 of 5.25 Gy. This resulted in mean doses of 11.3 and 29.7 Gy to the bone marrow and spleen, respectively. Grade II mucositis occurred in all patients and 71% of evaluable patients developed hypothyroidism. The estimated 3-year DFS and nonrelapse mortality was 61% and 21%, respectively. These results reported by the Seattle group indicate the potential of RIC to increase the intensity of the conditioning regimen without added toxicity.

The use of skeletal targeted therapy with ^{166}HoDOTMP (Holmium), a tetraphosphonate radiotherapeutic agent that emits beta particles, was investigated by Giralt and colleagues in a group of 83 patients with multiple myeloma. Holmium was used in combination with melphalan 140 mg/m^2, 200 mg/m^2, or melphalan 140 mg/m^2 with TBI (800 cGy). Nominal doses of radiation delivered to the bone marrow ranged from 20 to 40 Gy. Autologous transplant was performed 7 to 10 days after the radioisotope was given. There were two early deaths and 23 patients developed hemorrhagic cystitis, and thrombotic microangiopathy occurred in 7 patients who were treated at 40 Gy. The kidney is the excretion organ of ^{166}HoDOTMP. Complete responses occurred in 38% of the patients, whereas 31% achieved a partial remission. The authors recommended a dose of 30 Gy or less with bladder irrigation to prevent hemorrhagic cystitis. The response rate compared favorably with that observed after other preparative regimens for autologous transplants in multiple myeloma.[80] Logistics and costs of RICs however are potential obstacles for the widespread use of these promising agents in HSCT.

NONMYELOABLATIVE HEMATOPOIETIC CELL TRANSPLANTATION

Many of the treatment failures after allogeneic hematopoietic cell transplant are due to the intensive preparative regimens traditionally used for myeloablation and immunosuppression. Furthermore, the

RATIONALE APPROACH TO CHOOSING A CONDITIONING REGIMEN

Case	Questions to ask
Case 1: 66-year-old woman with 2ry acute myeloid leukemia (AML) in first complete remission (CR1) has a human leukocyte antigen (HLA)-compatible unrelated donor. History of prior autologous transplant for lymphoma, compensated diabetes, and hypertension. Performance status is 1 and she is independent in activities of daily living	Is she a transplant candidate? Yes, phase 2 data suggests benefits for these patients. No phase 3 data available. Should she receive a reduced intensity regimen? Yes, high comorbidity score would suggest lower nonrelapse mortality (NRM) and improved survival with a reduced intensity conditioning (RIC) regimen. Is a specific regimen recommended? No, no randomized trials have been performed comparing different RIC regimens. Registry analysis has not shown a benefit of one regimen over another in the unrelated donor setting (Giralt et al).
Case 2: 55-year-old man with myelodysplastic syndrome (MDS) and an HLA-compatible sibling donor. No comorbidities.	Is he a transplant candidate? Yes, phase 2 data suggests benefits for these patients. No phase 3 data available Should he receive a reduced-intensity regimen? No, comorbidity score would suggest similar NRM for RIC and ablative regimens in this setting. Standard of care would be full-dose busulfan-based regimen with pharmacologic monitoring.

incidence of GVHD is, to some extent, related to the intensity of the regimen. Thus allogeneic hematopoietic cell transplant has been restricted to younger patients with good performance status. Many candidates are excluded because of advanced age or comorbid conditions. The peak incidence of most hematologic malignancies for which allogeneic transplant is used is in patients in their 60s and 70s; therefore, most of the patients who might benefit from hematopoietic cell transplant are ineligible.

The existence of a graft-versus-tumor (GVT) effect in humans is supported by indirect evidence, such as the lower rate of relapse in patients who develop GVHD or the higher relapse rates after syngeneic transplants or among recipients of T cell-depleted allografts. Direct evidence comes from the observation that donor lymphocytes can induce remission in patients relapsing after allogeneic transplant.[81] A less intensive preparative regimen that is sufficiently immunosuppressive to prevent graft rejection may be used to explore the graft-versus-tumor effect. In addition, achievement of stable mixed or complete hematopoietic donor chimerism may be curative for several nonmalignant genetic diseases without resorting to complete marrow ablation.[82]

Diseases that can be classified as highly sensitive to the graft-versus-tumor effect include CML, low-grade lymphoma, mantle cell lymphoma, and chronic lymphocytic leukemia. AML, intermediate-grade lymphoma, multiple myeloma, and Hodgkin lymphoma can be classified as of intermediate sensitivity, whereas ALL and the high-grade lymphomas are relatively insensitive.[1] Accordingly, the likelihood of success after nonmyeloablative transplants is highly influenced by the diagnosis and disease stage. The low intensity of the preparative regimen and the relatively delayed time for the graft-immune effect to be effective render rapidly progressing malignancies less likely to benefit from nonmyeloablative hematopoietic cell transplant.

Truly nonmyeloablative preparative regimens include fludarabine–cyclophosphamide, fludarabine–idarubicin–cytarabine, and 2-Gy TBI-based regimens, whereas reduced-intensity ablative regimens include combinations of fludarabine with intermediate doses of melphalan or busulfan (see Table 106–1 and Fig. 106–8).[83–85]

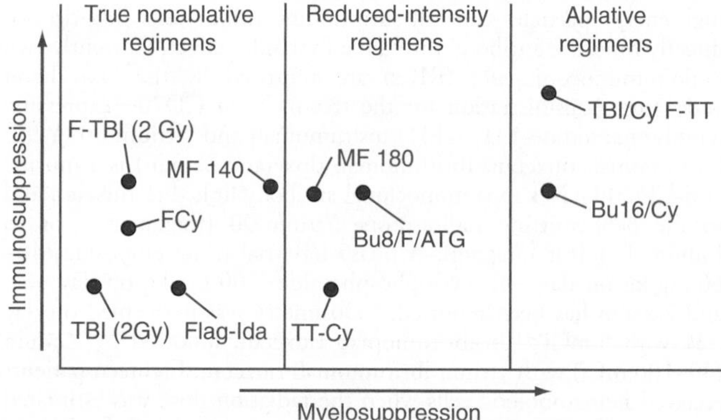

Figure 106–8 Commonly used nonablative or reduced-intensity regimens. Nonablative regimens do not completely eradicate host hematopoiesis; autologous recovery occurs if the graft is rejected. Many reduced-intensity regimens are ablative, as only donor-derived cells are generally detected posttransplant, and graft rejection results in prolonged pancytopenia. Progenitor cells from donors other than HLA-identical siblings will require greater immunosuppression to prevent rejection. Rapidly progressing malignancies generally require increased degree of myelosuppression. Bu16/Cy, busulfan (16 mg/kg)/cyclophosphamide; FCy, fludarabine/cyclophosphamide; Flag-Ida, fludarabine, cytarabine–idarubicin; F-TBI, fludarabine–total body irradiation; Bu8/F/ATG, busulfan (8 mg/kg)/fludarabine/antithymocyte globulin; MF, melphalan–fludarabine (with melphalan 140 or 180 mg/m^2); TBI/Cy F-TT, fludarabine/thiotepa; TT-Cy, thiotepa/cyclophosphamide. (Data from Champlin R, Khouri I, Anderlini P, et al: Nonmyeloablative preparative regimens for allogeneic hematopoietic transplant. Biology and current indications. Oncology [Huntingt] 17[1]:94, 2003.)

Furthermore, the intensity of the preparative regimen may be reduced if enough cytoreduction and some degree of immunosuppression is achieved by a preceding autologous transplant. This strategy of "auto-allo" transplant is under investigation in the therapy of multiple myeloma, non-Hodgkin lymphoma, and Hodgkin lymphoma.

Another less myelotoxic approach was reported by Lowsky and colleagues, using a conditioning regimen with 10 doses of total lymphoid irradiation (80 cGy each) plus antithymocyte globulin. Thirty-seven patients with lymphoid malignancies or acute leukemia were treated, and only two had acute GVHD. Antitumor effects were documented in patients with lymphoid malignant diseases.[86]

CONCLUSION

Incorporation of new drugs, antibodies, and radioimmunoconjugates in the preparative regimen, as well as graft engineering, is likely to modify the way we perform hematopoietic cell transplant. Further improvements in supportive care and the prophylaxis of GVHD will most certainly contribute to the evolution of the knowledge and practice of hematopoietic cell transplant. Pharmacogenetics data will allow individualization of doses and guide the choice of less toxic agents. The foundations of autologous and allogeneic transplant have been established over the last 50 years. The role of this form of treatment will most certainly change in the next decade to incorporate the advances in the field of immunology, cellular biology, pharmacology, and genetics.

SUGGESTED READINGS

Anagnastopoulos A, Giralt S: Critical review on non-myeloablative stem cell transplantation. Crit Rev Oncol Hematol 44:175, 2002.

Andersson B, Couriel D, Madden T, et al: Busulfan systemic exposure relative to regimen-related toxicity and acute graft vs. host disease; defining a therapeutic window for IV BuCy2 in chronic myelogenous leukemia. Biol Blood Marrow Transplant 8:477, 2002.

Bearman SI, Appelbaum FR, Back A, et al: Regimen-related toxicity and early posttransplant survival in patients undergoing marrow transplantation for lymphoma. J Clin Oncol 7:1288, 1989.

Clift R, Buckner C, Appelbaum F, et al: Allogeneic marrow transplantation in patients with acute myeloid leukemia in first remission: A randomized trial of two irradiation regimens. Blood 76:1867, 1990.

de Lima M, Couriel D, Thall PF, et al: Once-daily intravenous busulfan and fludarabine: Clinical and pharmacokinetic results of a myeloablative, reduced-toxicity conditioning regimen for allogeneic stem cell transplantation in AML and MDS. Blood 104:857, 2004.

Lowsky R, Takahashi T, Liu YP, et al: Protective conditioning for acute graft-versus-host disease. N Engl J Med 353:1321, 2005.

Moreau P, Facon T, Attal M, et al: Comparison of 200 mg/m^2 of melphalan and 8 Gy total body irradiation plus 140 mg/m^2 melphalan as conditioning regimen for peripheral blood stem cell transplant in patients with newly diagnosed multiple myeloma: Final analysis of the Intergroupe Francophone du Myelome 9502 randomized trial. Blood 99:731, 2002.

Press OW, Eary JF, Appelbaum FR, et al: Phase II trial of 131I-B1 (anti-CD20) antibody therapy with autologous stem cell transplantation for relapsed B cell lymphomas. Lancet 346:336, 1995.

Ringden O, Remberger M, Ruutu T, et al for the Nordic Bone Marrow Transplantation Group: Increased risk of chronic graft-versus-host disease, obstructive bronchiolitis, and alopecia with busulfan versus total body irradiation: long-term results of a randomized trial in allogeneic marrow recipients with leukemia. Blood 93:2196, 1999.

Thomas ED, Storb R, Clift RA, et al: Bone-marrow transplantation (first and second parts). N Engl J Med 292:832, 1975.

REFERENCES

For complete list of references log onto www.expertconsult.com

CHAPTER 107

GRAFT-VERSUS-HOST DISEASE AND GRAFT-VERSUS-LEUKEMIA RESPONSES

Pavan Reddy and James L. M. Ferrara

INTRODUCTION

The ability of allogeneic hematopoietic cell transplantation (HCT) to cure certain hematologic malignancies is widely recognized. An important therapeutic aspect of HCT in eradicating malignant cells is the graft-versus-leukemia (GVL) effect. The importance of the GVL effect in allogeneic HCT has been recognized since the earliest experiments in stem cell transplantation. Forty years ago, Barnes and colleagues noted that leukemic mice treated with a subtherapeutic dose of radiation and a syngeneic (identical twin) graft transplant were more likely to relapse than mice given an allogeneic hematopoietic cell transplant.[1,2] They hypothesized that the allogeneic graft contained cells with immune reactivity necessary for eradicating residual leukemia cells. They also noted that recipients of allogeneic grafts, though less likely to relapse, died of a "wasting syndrome" now recognized as graft-versus-host disease (GVHD). Thus, in addition to describing GVL, these experiments highlighted for the first time the intricate relationship between GVL and GVHD. Since these early experiments, both GVHD and the GVL effect have been studied extensively.[3] This chapter reviews the pathophysiology, clinical features, and treatment of GVHD and summarizes current understanding of the relationships between GVHD and the GVL effect.

GRAFT-VERSUS-HOST DISEASE: CLINICAL AND PATHOLOGIC ASPECTS

Ten years after the work of Barnes and Loutit, Billingham formulated the requirements for the development of GVHD: the graft must contain immunologically competent cells, the recipient must express tissue antigens that are not present in the transplant donor, and the recipient must be incapable of mounting an effective response to destroy the transplanted cells.[4] According to these criteria, GVHD can develop in various clinical settings when tissues containing immunocompetent cells (blood products, bone marrow, and some solid organs) are transferred between persons. The most common setting for the development of GVHD is following allogeneic HCT; without prophylactic immunosuppression, most allogeneic HCTs will be complicated by GVHD. GVHD occurs secondary to mismatches in histocompatibility antigens between the donor and recipient. Matching of the major histocompatibility complex (MHC) antigens speeds engraftment and reduces the severity of GVHD.[5] The MHC contains the genes that encode tissue antigens and were first identified functionally in murine models as transplantation antigens responsible for rejection of tissue grafts. In humans, the MHC region lies on the short arm of chromosome 6 and is called the human leukocyte antigen (HLA) region.[6] The HLA region includes many genes, not all of which are involved in immune activation. It is divided into two classes, Class I and Class II, each containing numerous gene loci that encode a large number of polymorphic alleles. MHC class I molecules are involved in the presentation of peptides to $CD8^+$ T cells, and class II molecules present peptides to $CD4^+$ T cells.[6]

Each MHC antigen is composed of two polypeptide chains. Class I antigens are made up of a heavy chain that contains the polymorphic regions and the nonpolymorphic light chain, beta-2 microglobulin. The class I HLA antigens include HLA A, B, and C antigens. These are expressed on almost all cells of the body at varying densities,[6] Both chains of class II antigens contain polymorphic regions and are encoded in the MHC. The class II antigens are further divided into DR, DQ, and DP antigens. Class II antigens are expressed on B cells, dendritic cells and monocytes and their expression can be induced on many other cell types following inflammation or injury.[6,7] The determination of HLA types has become much more accurate with molecular techniques that replace earlier serologic or cellular methods. In patients whose ancestry involves extensive interracial mixing, the chances of identifying an HLA-identical unrelated donor are diminished.[8]

Despite HLA identity between a patient and donor, substantial numbers of patients still develop GVHD as a result of differences in minor histocompatibility antigens that lie outside the HLA loci. Most minor antigens are expressed on the cell surface as degraded peptides bound to specific HLA molecules, but the precise characterization of many human minor antigens is yet to be accomplished.[9] In the United States, the average patient has a 25% chance of having an HLA match among his biological full siblings.[8] Patients who lack a suitably HLA-matched related donor may seek unrelated adult unrelated or umbilical cord blood (UCB) donors.

ACUTE GRAFT-VERSUS-HOST DISEASE

Acute GVHD can occur within days (in recipients who are not HLA-matched with the donor or in patients not given any GVHB prophylaxis) or as late as 2 months after transplantation. The incidence ranges from less than 10% to more than 80%, depending on the degree of histoincompatibility between donor and recipient, the number of T cells in the graft, the patient's age, and the GVHD prophylactic regimen.[10] The principal target organs include the immune system, skin, liver, and intestine. GVHD occurs first and most commonly in the skin as a pruritic maculopapular rash, often involving the palms, soles, and ears; it can progresses to total-body erythroderma, with bullae formation, rupture along the epidermal–dermal border, and desquamation in severe cases.[10] Gastrointestinal (GI) and liver manifestations often appear later and rarely represent the first and only findings. Intestinal symptoms include anorexia, nausea, diarrhea (sometimes bloody), abdominal pain, and paralytic ileus.[10] Liver dysfunction includes hyperbilirubinemia and increased serum alkaline phosphatase and aminotransferase values. Coagulation studies may become abnormal, and hepatic failure with ascites and encephalopathy may develop in severe cases.[10–12] Hepatic GVHD can be distinguished from hepatic venoocclusive disease (VOD) by weight gain or pain in the right upper quadrant in the latter.[12] Acute GVHD also results in the delayed recovery of immunocompetence.[10] The clinical result is profound immunodeficiency, and susceptibility to infections, often further accentuated by the immunosuppressive agents used to treat GVHD.[10]

Pathologically, the sine qua non of acute GVHD is selective epithelial damage of target organs.[13,14] The epidermis and hair follicles are damaged and sometimes destroyed. Small bile ducts are profoundly affected, with segmental disruption. The destruction of intestinal crypts results in mucosal ulcerations that may be either patchy or diffuse. Other epithelial surfaces, such as the conjunctivae, vagina, and esophagus, are less commonly involved. A peculiarity of GVHD histology is the frequent paucity of mononuclear cell infiltrates; however, as the disease progresses the inflammatory component may be substantial. Recent studies have identified inflammatory cytokines as soluble mediators of GVHD and have suggested that direct contact between target cells and lymphocytes may not be required for target cell destruction (see following sections). GVHD lesions are not evenly distributed in the target tissues. In the skin, damage is prominent at the tip of rete ridges; in the intestine, at the base of the crypts; and in the liver, in the periductular epithelium. These areas contain a high proportion of stem cells, giving rise to the idea that GVHD targets may be undifferentiated epithelial cells with primitive surface antigens.[15]

The histologic severity of a given lesion is at best semiquantitative, and consequently the severity of pathologic findings is not used in the grading of GVHD. As it is often difficult to obtain an adequate tissue biopsy, the physician is left to use clinical judgment. It can be very difficult to distinguish GVHD from other post-BMT complications such as drug eruptions and infectious complication by histologic criteria.

A recent multicenter phase 3 trial used an independent committee to assess the presence and severity of GVHD. The incidence of GVHD as determined by investigators was substantially higher than the review committee could confirm.[16] Nevertheless, for an experienced clinician a combination of physical and laboratory findings in the appropriate context provides a working diagnosis of GVHD that is satisfactory to produce a meaningful prognostic scale based on the clinical grading system. [12,17] Standard grading systems generally include clinical changes in the skin, GI tract, liver, and performance status (Table 107–1).[18] Although the severity of GVHD is sometimes difficult to quantify, the overall grade correlates with disease outcome. Whereas mild GVHD (grade I or II) is associated with little morbidity and almost no mortality, higher grades are associated with significantly decreased survival.[18,19] With grade IV GVHD, the mortality is almost 100%.[19]

Table 107–1 Glucksberg Criteria for Staging of Acute Graft-Versus-Host Disease[a]

Overall grade	Skin	Liver		Gut
I	1–2	0		0
II	1–3	1	and/or	1
III	2–3	2–4	and/or	2–3
IV	2–4	2–4	and/or	2–4

[a]See this table for individual organ staging. Traditionally, individual organs are staged without regard to attribution. The overall grade of graft-versus-host disease (GVHD), however, reflects the actual extent of GVHD.

Clinical Features of Acute Graft-Versus-Host Disease

The clinical features and staging and grading of acute GVHD are summarized in Tables 107–1 and 107–2.

In a comprehensive review of patients receiving therapy for acute GVHD, Martin et al[20] found that 81% had skin involvement, 54% had GI involvement, and 50% had liver involvement at the initiation of GVHD therapy. After high-intensity (conventional) conditioning, acute GVHD generally occurs within 14 to 35 days of stem cell infusion. The time of onset may depend upon the degree of histocompatibility, the number of donor T cells infused, and the prophylactic regimen for GVHD. A "hyperacute" form of GVHD may occur in patients with severe HLA mismatches and in patients who receive T-cell replete transplants without or with inadequate in vivo GVHD prophylaxis.[21] It is, however, important to note that this hyperacute form is pathophysiologically distinct from the hyperacute rejection after solid organ allografting. This form of GVHD is manifested by fever, generalized erythroderma and desquamation, and often edema. It typically occurs about one week after stem cell infusion and may be rapidly fatal. In patients receiving more conventional (in vivo) GVHD prophylaxis, such as a combination of cyclosporine (CSP) and methotrexate, the median onset of GVHD is typically 21 to 25 days after transplantation; however, after in vitro T cell depletion of the graft the onset may be much later.[21] Thus, the findings of rash and diarrhea by one week after transplantation would very likely be hyperacute manifestations of GVHD if minimal or ineffective prophylaxis were administered; the same kinetics would be very unlikely with the use of calcineurin inhibitors or in vitro T cell depletion of the stem cell inoculum. A less ominous syndrome of fever, rash, and fluid retention occurring in the first 1 to 2 weeks after stem cell infusion is the "engraftment syndrome." These manifestations may be seen with either allogeneic or autologous transplantation. Although the pathophysiology is poorly understood, it is thought to be due to a wave of cytokine production as the graft starts to recover. This is related to, but distinct from, the "cytokine storm"[21,22] that is thought to contribute to acute GVHD in that there is no concomitant T cell-mediated attack. This syndrome responds immediately to steroids in most patients and it typically presents earlier than acute GVHD.[16] In autologous transplantation the differential diagnosis is of little relevance, but in allogeneic transplant recipients it must be distinguished from the hyperacute manifestations of GVHD. A prompt response to steroids would argue in favor of an engraftment syndrome, although some patients with GVHD will also respond.

Table 107–2 Clinical Manifestations and Staging of Acute GVHD

Organ	Clinical Manifestations	Staging
Skin	Erythematous, maculopapular rash involving palms and soles. May become confluent. Severe disease: bullae	Stage 1: <25% rash Stage 2: 25%–50% rash Stage 3: generalized erythroderma Stage 4: bullae
Liver	Painless jaundice with conjugated hyperbilirubinemia and increased alkaline phosphatase	Stage 1: bili 2–3 mg/dL Stage 2: bili 3.1–6 mg/dL Stage 3: bili 6.1–15 mg/dL Stage 4: bili > 15 mg/dL
Gastrointestinal (GI) tract	Upper: nausea, vomiting, anorexia Lower: diarrhea, abdominal cramps, distention, ileus and bleeding	Stage 1: diarrhea > 500 mL/day Stage 2: diarrhea > 1000 mL/day Stage 3: diarrhea > 1500 mL/day Stage 4: ileus, bleeding

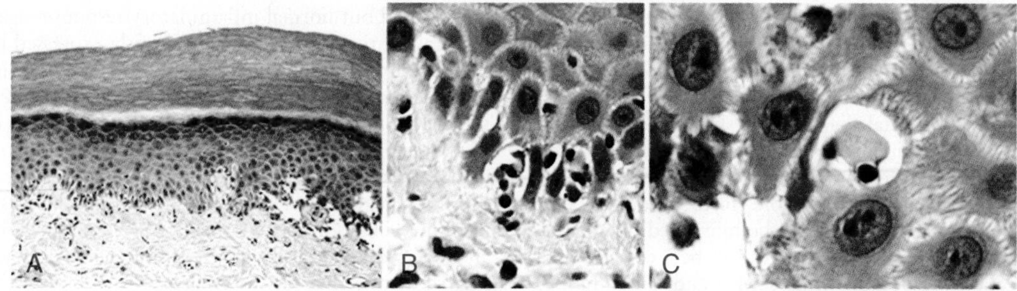

Figure 107–1 Graft-versus-host disease, skin biopsy (**A–C**). This 40-year-old man with a history of relapsed Hodgkin lymphoma was status-post allogeneic stem cell transplant with donor lymphocyte infusion. He developed painful oral ulcers, and a macular-papular rash on the arms, hand, and chest. The skin biopsy is from the palmar surface of the hand (**A**). It shows a scant lymphoid infiltrate in the dermis with a developing subepithelial blister (*right*). There is basal vacuolar change (**B**) with single lymphocytes in the epithelium, and apoptotic keratinocyte accompanied by lymphocytes (**B**, and detail, **C**). (*Case courtesy of Drs. Vesna Petronic-Rosic and Mark Racz, University of Chicago.*)

Skin

Skin is the most commonly affected organ (Fig. 107–1). In patients receiving transplants after myeloablative conditioning, the skin is usually the first organ involved, and GVHD often coincides with engraftment. However, the presentation of GVHD is more varied following nonmyeloablative transplants or donor lymphocyte infusions.[23] The characteristic maculopapular rash can spread throughout the rest of the body but usually spares the scalp, and is often described as feeling like a sunburn, with tight or pruritic skin. In severe cases the skin may blister and ulcerate.[24] Histologic confirmation is critical to rule out drug reactions or viral infections. Apoptosis at the base of dermal crypts is a characteristic histologic finding. Other features include dyskeratosis, exocytosis of lymphocytes, satellite lymphocytes adjacent to dyskeratotic epidermal keratinocytes, and dermal perivascular lymphocytic infiltration.[23,25]

Gastrointestinal Tract

Gastrointestinal (GI) tract involvement of GVHD may present as nausea, vomiting, anorexia, diarrhea, and/or abdominal pain.[25] It is a panintestinal process, often with differences in severity between the upper and lower GI tracts. Gastric involvement gives rise to postprandial vomiting that is not always preceded by nausea. Although gastroparesis is seen after hematopoietic cell transplant, it is usually not associated with GVHD. The diarrhea of GVHD is secretory. Significant GI blood loss may occur as a result of mucosal ulceration and is associated with a poor prognosis.[26] In advanced disease, diffuse, severe abdominal pain and distention is accompanied by voluminous diarrhea (>2 L/day).[19,27]

Radiologic findings of the GI tract include lumenal dilatation with thickening of the wall of the small bowel and air/fluid levels suggestive of an ileus on abdominal flat plates or small bowel series. Abdominal computed tomography may show the "ribbon" sign, of diffuse thickening of the small bowel wall.[24] Little correlation exists between the extent of disease and the appearance of mucosa on endoscopy, but mucosal sloughing is pathognomonic for severe disease.[28] Nevertheless, some studies have shown that antral biopsies correlate well with the severity of GVHD in the duodenum and in the colon even when the presenting symptom is diarrhea.[28] Histologic analysis of tissue is imperative to establish the diagnosis. The histologic features of GI GVHD are the presence of apoptotic bodies in the base of crypts, crypt abscesses, crypt loss, and flattening of the surface epithelium.[27,29]

Liver

Liver function test abnormalities are common after hematopoietic cell transplant and occur secondary to venoocclusive disease, drug toxicity, viral infection, sepsis, iron overload, and other causes of extrahepatic biliary obstruction.[12] The exact incidence of hepatic GVHD is probably underreported because many patients do not undergo liver biopsies. The development of jaundice or an increase in the alkaline phosphatase and bilirubin are the initial features of acute GVHD of the liver. The histologic features of hepatic GVHD are endothelialitis, lymphocytic infiltration of the portal areas, pericholangitis and bile duct destruction and loss.[19,30]

Other Organs

Whether GVHD affects organs other than the classic triad of skin, liver, and gut has remained a matter of debate. However, numerous reports suggest additional organ manifestations. The most likely candidate is the lung. Lung toxicity, including interstitial pneumonitis and diffuse alveolar hemorrhage, may occur in 20% to 60% of allogeneic transplant recipients but in fewer autologous transplant recipients. Causes of pulmonary damage other than GVHD include engraftment syndrome, infection, radiation pneumonitis, and chemotherapy-related toxicity (eg, methotrexate, busulfan).[21,31] At least one retrospective analysis failed to link severe pulmonary complications to clinical acute GVHD.[32] The mortality due to pneumonia increases with the severity of GVHD, but this association does not necessarily imply that GVHD, as opposed to immunosuppression given for therapy, is causative.[21] A particular histopathologic syndrome of lymphocytic bronchitis has been attributed directly to GVHD,[31] although this association has not been confirmed by others.

Despite the fact that kidneys and heart can be targets for allogeneic damage, as evidenced by their rejection after renal and cardiac transplants, respectively, there is no convincing evidence for direct renal or cardiac damage from acute GVHD that is not secondary to drugs or infection. Similarly, neurologic complications are also common after transplantation but most can be attributed to drug toxicity, infection, or vascular insults.

Differential Diagnosis

Acute GVHD must be distinguished from any process that causes a constellation of fever, erythematous skin rash, and pulmonary edema that may occur during neutrophil recovery. This picture may reflect the dysregulated production of inflammatory cytokines and cellular responses to these molecules, and has been termed *engraftment* or *capillary leak syndrome*.[33,34] The picture is most clearly recognized after autologous transplantation where, theoretically, GVHD should not occur. In allogeneic transplant recipients, distinction from acute GVHD is difficult. This engraftment syndrome is thought to reflect cellular and cytokine activities during early recovery of (donor-derived) blood cell counts and/or homeostatic proliferation of lymphocytes, but a precise delineation of the offending cells and mechanisms has not been accomplished. Engraftment syndromes may be associated with increased mortality, primarily from pulmonary failure but also (other) multiorgan dysfunction. Corticosteroid therapy may be effective particularly for the treatment of pulmonary manifestations.[35] The differential diagnosis of skin rashes, diarrhea and liver function abnormalities can be difficult to resolve. Skin rashes may reflect delayed reactions to the conditioning regimen, antibiotics, or infections and furthermore histopathologic skin changes consistent with acute GVHD can be mimicked by chemoradiotherapy and drug reactions.[21,36] Diarrhea can be a consequence of TBI, viral infections, especially with CMV and other herpes viruses, parasites, *Clostridium difficile*, nonspecific gastritis, narcotic withdrawal, and drug reactions: all of which mimic GVHD of the gut. Liver dysfunction can be due to parenteral nutrition, venoocclusive disease, viral or drug-induced hepatitis, or mechanical obstruction of the biliary tract.

PATHOPHYSIOLOGY OF ACUTE GRAFT-VERSUS-HOST DISEASE

It is helpful to remember two important principles when considering the pathophysiology of acute GVHD. First, acute GVHD represents exaggerated but normal inflammatory responses against foreign antigens (alloantigens) that are ubiquitously expressed in a setting where they are undesirable. The donor lymphocytes that have been infused into the recipient function appropriately, given the foreign environment they encounter. Second, donor lymphocytes encounter tissues in the recipient that have been often profoundly damaged. The effects of the underlying disease, prior infections, and the intensity of conditioning regimen all result in substantial changes not only in the immune cells but also in the endothelial and epithelial cells. The allogeneic donor cells rapidly encounter not only a foreign environment but one that has been altered to promote the activation and proliferation of inflammatory cells. Thus, the pathophysiology of acute GVHD may be considered a distortion of the normal inflammatory cellular responses that, in addition to the absolute requirement of donor T cells, involves multiple other innate and adaptive cells and mediators.[37] The development and evolution of acute GVHD can be conceptualized in three sequential phases (Fig. 107–2) to provide a unified perspective on the complex cellular interactions and inflammatory cascades that lead to acute GVHD: (a) activation of the antigen-presenting cells (APCs), (b) donor T cell activation, differentiation and migration and (c) effector phase.[37] It is important to note that the three-phase description as discussed below allows for a unified perspective in understanding the biology. It is, however, not meant to suggest that all three phases are of equal importance or that

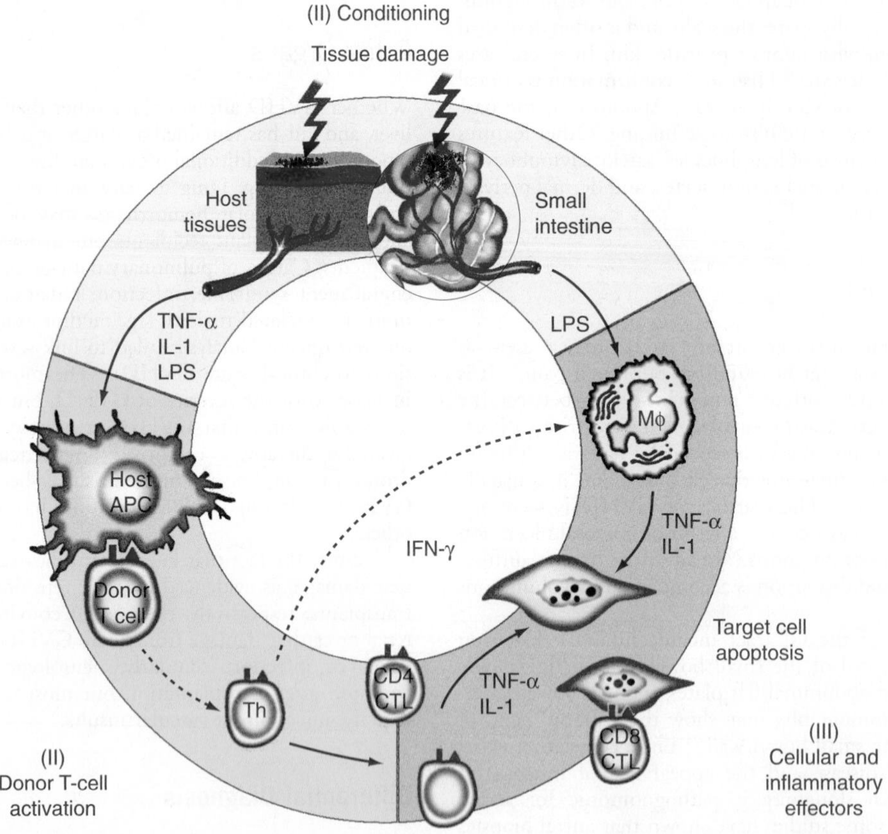

Figure 107–2 Pathophysiology of graft-versus-host disease (GVHD). During step 1, irradiation and chemotherapy both damage and activate host tissues, including intestinal mucosa, liver, and the skin. Activated cell hosts then secrete inflammatory cytokines (eg, TNF-α and IL-1), which can be measured in the systemic circulation. The cytokine release has important effects on antigen-presenting cells (APCs) of the host, including increased expression of adhesion molecules (eg, ICAM-1, VCAM-1) and of MHC class II antigens. These changes in the APCs enhance the recognition of host MHC and/or minor antigens by mature donor T cells. During step 2, donor T-cell activation is characterized by proliferation of GVHD T cells and secretion of the Th1 cytokines IL-2 and IFN-γ. Both of these cytokines play central roles in clonal T-cell expansion, induction of CTL and NK cell responses, and the priming of mononuclear phagocytes. In step 3, mononuclear phagocytes primed by IFN-γ are triggered by a second signal such as endotoxin (LPS) to secrete cytopathic amounts of IL-I and TNF-α. LPS can leak through the intestinal mucosa damaged by the conditioning regimen to stimulate gut-associated lymphoid tissue or Kupffer cells in the liver; LPS that penetrate the epidermis may stimulate keratinocytes, dermal fibroblasts, and macrophages to produce similar cytokines in the skin. This mechanism results in the amplification of local tissue injury and further production of inflammatory effectors such as nitric oxide, which, together with CTL and NK effectors, leads to the observed target tissue destruction in the transplant host. CTL effectors use Fas/FasL, perforin/granzyme B, and membrane-bound cytokines to lyse target cells.

GVHD occurs in a stepwise and sequential manner. The spatiotemporal relationships between the biological processes described below, depending on the context, are more likely to be chaotic and of varying intensity and relevance in the induction, severity and maintenance of GVHD.

Phase 1: Activation of Antigen-Presenting Cells

The earliest phase of acute GVHD is initiated by the profound damage caused by the underlying disease and infections and further exacerbated by the BMT conditioning regimens (which include total body irradiation [TBI] and/or chemotherapy) that are administered even before the infusion of donor cells.[38–42] This first step results in activation of the APCs.[7] Specifically, damaged host tissues respond with multiple changes, including the secretion of proinflammatory cytokines, such as TNF-α and IL-1, described as the cytokine storm.[40,41,43] Such changes increase expression of adhesion molecules, costimulatory molecules, MHC antigens and chemokines gradients that alert the residual host and the infused donor immune cells.[41] These danger signals activate host APCs.[44,45] Damage to the GI tract from the conditioning is particularly important in this process. Such damage results in systemic translocation of immunostimulatory microbial products such as lipopolysaccharide that further enhance the activation of host APCs. The secondary lymphoid tissue in the GI tract is probably the initial site of interaction between activated APCs and donor T cells.[41,46,47] Of interest, an increased risk of GVHD is associated with intensive conditioning regimens that cause extensive injury to epithelial and endothelial surfaces with a subsequent release of inflammatory cytokines and increases in expression of cell surface adhesion molecules.[41,42] The relationship among conditioning intensity, inflammatory cytokine, and GVHD severity has been supported by elegant murine studies.[43] Furthermore, the observations from these experimental studies have led to two recent clinical innovations to reduce acute GVHD: (a) reduced intensity conditioning (RIC) to decrease the damage to host tissues and thus limit activation of host APC and (b) natural killer (NK) cell killer immunoglobulin receptor (KIR) mismatches between donor and recipients to eliminate host APCs by the alloreactive NK cells.[48,49]

Host type APCs that are present and have been primed by conditioning, are critical for the induction of this phase; recent evidence suggests that donor type APCs exacerbate GVHD, but, in certain experimental models, donor type APC chimeras also induce GVHD.[45,50–52] In clinical situations, if donor-type APCs are present in sufficient quantity and have been appropriately primed, they too might play a role in the initiation and exacerbation of GVHD.[53–55] Among the cells with antigen-presenting capability, dendritic cells (DCs) are the most potent and play an important role in the induction of GVHD.[56] Experimental data suggest that GVHD can be regulated by qualitatively or quantitatively modulating distinct DC subsets.[57–62] Langerhans cells were also shown to be sufficient for the induction of GVHD when all other APCs were unable to prime donor T cells, although the role for Langerhans cells when all APCs are intact is unknown.[63] Studies have yet to define roles for other DC subsets. In one clinical study persistence of host DC after day 100 correlated with the severity of acute GVHD, whereas elimination of host DCs was associated with reduced severity of acute GVHD.[54] The allostimulatory capacity of mature monocyte-derived DCs (mDCs) after reduced-intensity transplants was lower for up to 6 months compared to the mDCs from myeloablative transplant recipients, thus suggesting a role for host DCs and the reduction in danger signals secondary to less intense conditioning in acute GVHD.[64] Nonetheless, this concept of enhanced host APC activation explains a number of clinical observations such as increased risks of acute GVHD associated with advanced-stage malignancy, conditioning intensity, and histories of viral infections.

Other professional APCs such as monocytes/macrophages or semiprofessional APCs might also play a role in this phase.[7] For example, recent data suggest that host-type B cells might play a regulatory role under certain conditions.[65] Also host- or donor-type nonhematopoietic cells, such as mesenchymal stem cells or stromal cells, when acting as APCs have been shown to reduce T cell allogeneic responses, although the mechanism for such inhibition remains unclear. The relative contributions of various APCs, professional or otherwise, remain to be elucidated.

Phase 2: Donor T-Cell Activation, Differentiation and Migration

The infused donor T cells interact with the primed APCs, leading to the initiation of the second phase of acute GVHD. This phase includes antigen presentation by primed APCs, and the subsequent activation, proliferation, differentiation, and migration of alloreactive donor T cells. After allogeneic HCT, both host- and donor-derived APCs are present in secondary lymphoid organs.[66,67] The T-cell receptor (TCR) of the donor T cells can recognize alloantigens either on host APCs (direct presentation) or donor APCs (indirect presentation).[68,69] In direct presentation, donor T cells recognize either the peptide bound to allogeneic MHC molecules or allogeneic MHC molecules without peptide.[69,70] During indirect presentation, T cells respond to the peptide generated by degradation of the allogeneic MHC molecules presented on self-MHC.[70] Experimental studies demonstrated that APCs derived from the host, rather than from the donor, are critical in inducing GVHD across MiHA mismatch.[7,68] Recent data suggest that presentation of distinct target antigens by the host- and donor-type APCs might play a differential role in mediating target organ damage.[7,71,72] In humans, most cases of acute GVHD developed when both host DCs and donor DCs are present in peripheral blood after HCT.[54]

Costimulation

The interaction of donor lymphocyte TCR with the host allopeptide presented on the MHC of APCs alone is insufficient to induce T-cell activation.[7,73] Both TCR ligation and costimulation via a second signal through interaction between the T-cell costimulatory molecules and their ligands on APCs are required to achieve T-cell proliferation, differentiation, and survival.[74] The danger signals generated in phase 1 augment these interactions and significant progress has been made on the nature and impact of these second signals.[75,76] Costimulatory pathways are now known to deliver both positive and negative signals, and molecules from two major families, the B7 family and the TNF receptor (TNFR) family, play pivotal roles in GVHD.[77] Interruption of the second signal by blockade of various positive costimulatory molecules (CD28, ICOS, CD40, CD30, 4–1BB, and OX40) reduces acute GVHD in several murine models, whereas antagonism of the inhibitory signals (PD-1 and CTLA-4) exacerbates the severity of acute GVHD.[78–84] The various T cell and APC costimulatory molecules and the impact on acute GVHD are summarized in Table 107–3. The specific context and the hierarchy in which each of these signals play a dominant role in the modulation of GVHD remain to be determined.

T-Cell Subsets

T cells consist of several subsets whose responses differ according to antigenic stimuli, activation thresholds, and effector functions. The alloantigen composition of the host determines which donor T-cell subsets proliferate and differentiate.

CD4$^+$ and CD8$^+$ Cells

CD4 and CD8 proteins are coreceptors for constant portions of MHC class II and class I molecules, respectively.[85] Therefore MHC class I (HLA-A, HLA-B, HLA-C) differences stimulate CD8$^+$ T cells and MHC class II (HLA-DR, HLA-DP, HLA-DQ) differences

Table 107–3 T Cell–APC Interactions

T cell	APC
Adhesion	
ICAMs	LFA-1
LFA-1	ICAMs
CD2 (LFA-2)	LFA-3
Recognition	
TCR/CD4	MHC II
TCR/CD8	MHC I
Costimulation	
CD28	CD80/86
CD152 (CTLA-4)	CD80/86
ICOS	B7H/B7RP-1
PD-1	PD-L1, PD-L2
Unknown	B7-H3
CD154 (CD40L)	CD40
CD134 (OX 40)	CD134L (OX40L)
CD137 (4–1BB)	CD137L (4–1BBL)
HVEM	LIGHT

HVEM, HSV glycoprotein D for herpesvirus entry mediator; LIGHT, homologous to lymphotoxins, shows inducible expression, and competes with herpes simplex virus glycoprotein D for herpes virus entry mediator (HVEM), a receptor expressed by T lymphocytes.

stimulate CD4+ T cells.[85–88] But clinical trials of CD4+ or CD8+ depletion have been inconclusive.[89] This perhaps is not surprising, because GVHD is induced by MiHAs in the majority of HLA-identical HCT, which are peptides derived from polymorphic cellular proteins that are presented by MHC molecules.[90] Because the manner of protein processing depends on genes of the MHC, two siblings will have many different peptides in the MHC groove.[90] Thus in the majority of HLA-identical transplants, acute GVHD may be induced by either or both CD4+ and CD8+ subsets in response to minor histocompatibility antigens.[89] The peptide repertoire for class I or class II MHC remains unknown and might even be different in different individuals.[91] But it is plausible that only a few of these peptides might behave as immunodominant "major minor" antigens that can potentially induce GVHD. In any event, such antigens remain to be identified and validated in a large patient population.

Naïve and Memory Subsets

Several independent groups have found that the naïve (CD62L(+)) T cells were alloreactive and caused acute GVHD but not the memory (CD62L(−)) T cells across different donor/recipient strain combinations.[92–95] Furthermore, expression of naïve T cell marker CD62L was also found to be critical for regulation of GVHD by donor natural regulatory T cells.[96] By contrast, another recent study demonstrated that alloreactive memory T cells and their precursor cells (memory stem cells) caused robust GVHD.[97,98] It remains as yet unknown whether the reduced GVHD potential of memory type T cells from a naïve murine donor, in contrast to their ability to cause greater solid organ allorejection,[99] is due to a consequence of the intense conditioning regimen and/or altered trafficking or from a restricted repertoire and/or from T-cell intrinsic defect.

Regulatory T Cells

Recent advances indicate that distinct subsets of regulatory CD4+D25,+ CD4+D25−L10+ Tr cells, DN− T cells, NK, T cells and regulatory DCs control immune responses by induction of anergy or active suppression of alloreactive T cells.[58,59,100–108] Several studies have demonstrated a critical role for the natural donor CD4+D25+ Foxp3+ regulatory T (Treg) cells, obtained from naïve animals or generated ex vivo, in the outcome of acute GVHD. Donor CD4+D25+ T cells suppressed the early expansion of alloreactive donor T cells and their capacity to induce acute GVHD without abrogating GVL effector function against these tumors.[109,110] CD4+D25+ T cells induced or generated by immature or regulatory host-type DCs and by regulatory donor-type myeloid APCs were also able to suppress acute GVHD.[58] One of the clinical studies that evaluated the relationship between donor CD4+D25+ cells and acute GVHD in humans after matched sibling donor grafts found that in contrast to the murine studies, donor grafts containing larger numbers of CD4+CD25+ cells developed more severe acute GVHD.[111] These data suggest that coexpression of CD4+ and CD25+ is insufficient because an increase in CD25+ T cells in donor grafts is associated with greater risks of acute GVHD after clinical HCT. Another recent study found that Foxp3 mRNA expression (considered a specific marker for naturally occurring CD4(+)CD25+regs) was significantly decreased in peripheral blood mononuclear cells from patients with acute GVHD.[112,113] But Foxp3 expression in humans, unlike mice, may not be specific for T cells with a regulatory phenotype.[114] It is likely that the precise role of regulatory T cells in clinical acute GVHD will therefore not only depend upon identification of specific molecular markers in addition to Foxp3 but also on the ability for ex vivo expansion of these cells in sufficient numbers. Several clinical trials are under way in the United States and Europe with attempts to substantially expand these cells ex vivo and use for prevention of GVHD.

Host NK1.1+ T cells are another T-cell subset with suppressive function that has been shown to suppress acute GVHD in an IL-4-dependent manner.[107,108,115] By contrast, donor NKT cells were found to reduce GVHD and enhance perforin mediated GVL in an IFN-γ dependent manner.[116,117] Recent clinical data suggest that enhancing recipient NKT cells by repeated TLI conditioning promoted Th2 polarization and dramatically reduced GVHD.[108] Experimental data also show that activated donor NK cells can reduce GVHD through the elimination of host APCs or by secretion of transforming growth factor-β (TGF-β) secretion.[117] A murine HCT study using mice lacking SH2-containing inositol phosphatase (SHIP), in which the NK compartment is dominated by cells that express two inhibitory receptors capable of binding either self or allogeneic MHC ligands, suggests that host NK cells may play a role in the initiation of GVHD.[118]

T-Cell Apoptosis

Deletional mechanisms of tolerance fall into two categories: (a) central (thymic) deletion and (b) peripheral deletion.[119] Central deletion is an effective way to eliminate continued thymic production of alloreactive T cells. To this end, lymphoablative treatments have been used as a condition to create a mixed hematopoietic chimeric state in murine transplant models.[120] In this strategy, donor cells seed the thymus and maturing donor-reactive T-cell clones are deleted through intrathymic apoptosis.[121,122] The proportion of the peripheral T-cell repertoire that can respond to allogeneic MHC antigens can play a critical role in the development of tolerance.[123] In the case of MHC-mismatched transplantation, the frequency of alloreactive T cells is at least five orders of magnitude greater than the frequency of peptide-specific T cells responding to a nominal antigen.[123,124] The pathways of T cell apoptosis by which peripheral deletion occurs can be broadly categorized into activation-induced cell death (AICD) and passive cell death (PCD).[123] An important mediator of AICD in T cells is the Fas receptor.[125] Activated T cells expressing the Fas molecule undergo apoptotic cell death when brought into contact with cells expressing Fas ligand. A critical role for Fas mediated AICD has been clearly demonstrated in attenuation of acute GVHD by several Th1 cytokines.[126–130]

PCD or "death by neglect" illustrates the exquisite dependence of activated T cells upon growth factors (eg, IL-2, IL-4, IL-7, and/or IL-15) for survival; apoptotic cell death in this instance is largely due to rapid downregulation of Bcl-2.[131–133] Transplantation of Bcl-xL T cells into nonirradiated recipients significantly exacerbates GVHD; however, no difference in GVHD mortality is observed in animals that have been lethally irradiated.[134] Selective elimination of donor T cells in vivo after HCT using transgenic T cells in which a thymidine kinase (TK) suicide gene is targeted to T cells has also been shown to attenuate the severity of acute GVHD.[134–137] Another recent approach to prevent GVHD is the selective depletion of alloantigen-specific donor T cells by a photodynamic cell-purging process wherein donor T cells are treated with photoactive 4,5-dibromorhodamine[123] and subsequently exposed to visible light.[138] Thus several deletional mechanisms have been shown to reduce acute GVHD but the conditions under which one or another of these deletional mechanisms plays a predominate role remain to be determined.

Cytokines and T-Cell differentiation

APC and T cell activation result in rapid intracellular biochemical cascades that induce transcription of many genes including cytokines and their receptors. The Th1 cytokines (IFN-γ, IL-2 and TNF-α) have been implicated in the pathophysiology of acute GVHD.[139–141] IL-2 production by donor T cells remains the main target of many current clinical therapeutic and prophylactic approaches. Such approaches include administration of cyclosporine, tacrolimus, and monoclonal antibodies (mAbs) against IL-2 and its receptor.[142,143] Of note, emerging data indicate an important role for IL-2 in the generation and maintenance of $CD4^+D25^+$ Foxp3+ Tregs, suggesting that prolonged interference with IL-2 may inadvertently hinder the development of long-term tolerance after allogeneic HCT.[144–147] Similarly the role of other Th1 cytokines as regulators or inducers of GVHD severity depends on the degree of allomismatch, the intensity of conditioning, and the T-cell subsets that are involved after HCT.[148–150] Thus, although the cytokine storm initiated in phase 1 and amplified by the Th1 cytokines correlates with the development of acute GVHD, early Th1 polarization of donor T cells to HCT recipients can attenuate acute GVHD, suggesting that physiological amounts of Th1 cytokines are critical for GVHD induction whereas inadequate production (extremely low or high) could modulate acute GVHD through a breakdown of negative feedback mechanisms for activated donor T cells.[130,141,150–152] Th2 polarization by cytokines as well as by rapamycin and the secretion of IL-4 by $NK1.1^+$ T cells can reduce acute GVHD.[153–160] But Th1 and Th2 subsets cause injury to distinct acute GVHD target tissues and some studies failed to show a beneficial effect of Th2 polarization on acute GVHD.[161] Thus the Th1/Th2 paradigm of donor T cells in the immunopathogenesis of acute GVHD has evolved over the last few years and its causal role in acute GVHD is complex and incompletely understood. IL-10 plays a key role in suppression of immune responses, and its role in regulating experimental acute GVHD is unclear.[162] Recent clinical data demonstrate an unequivocal association of IL-10 polymorphisms with the severity of acute GVHD.[163] TGF-β, another suppressive cytokine, was shown to suppress acute GVHD but to exacerbate chronic GVHD.[164] The roles of some other cytokines, such as IL-7 (that promotes immune reconstitution) and IL-13, remain unclear.[165–168] The role for Th17 cells, a recently described novel T-cell differentiation in many immunologic processes, is not yet known.[169] In any case, experimental data collectively suggest that the timing of administration, the production of any given cytokine, the intensity of the conditioning regimen, and the donor–recipient combination may all be critical to the eventual outcome of acute GVHD.

Leukocyte Migration

Donor T cells migrate to lymphoid tissues, recognize alloantigens on either host or donor APCs, and become activated. They then exit the lymphoid tissues and traffic to the target organs and cause tissue damage.[170] The molecular interactions necessary for T-cell migration and the role of lymphoid organs during acute GVHD have recently become the focus of a growing body of research. Chemokines play a critical role in the migration of immune cells to secondary lymphoid organs and target tissues.[171] T-lymphocyte production of macrophage inflammatory protein-1 alpha is critical to the recruitment of $CD8^+$ but not $CD4^+$ T cells to the liver, lung, and spleen during acute GVHD.[172] Several chemokines such as CCL2–5, CXCL2, CXCL9–11, CCL17, and CCL27 are overexpressed and might play a critical role in the migration of leukocyte subsets to the target organs liver, spleen, skin, and lungs during acute GVHD.[170,173] $CXCR3^+$ T and $CCR5^+$ T cells cause acute GVHD in the liver and intestine.[170,174–176] CCR5 expression has also been found to be critical for Treg migration in GVHD.[177] In addition to chemokines and their receptors, expression of selectins and integrins and their ligands also regulates the migration of inflammatory cells to target organs.[171] For example, interaction between α4β7 integrin and its ligand MadCAM-1 are important for homing of donor T cells to Peyer patches and in the initiation of intestinal GVHD.[46,178] αLβ2/ICAM-1, -2, -3 and α4β1/VCAM-2 interactions are important for homing to the lung and liver after experimental HCT.[170] The expression of CD62L on donor Tregs is critical for their regulation of acute GVHD, suggesting that their migration in secondary tissues is critical for their regulatory effects.[67] The migratory requirement of donor T cells to specific lymph nodes (eg, Peyer patches) for the induction of GVHD might depend on other factors such as the conditioning regimen and the inflammatory milieu.[46,179] Furthermore, FTY720, a pharmacologic sphingosine-1-phosphate receptor agonist, inhibited GVHD in murine but not in canine models of HCT.[180,181] Thus, there might also be significant species differences in the ability of these molecules to regulate GVHD.

Phase 3: Effector Phase

The effector phase that leads to GVHD target organ damage consists of a complex cascade of multiple cellular and inflammatory effectors that simultaneously or sequentially modulate each other's responses. Effector mechanisms of acute GVHD can be grouped into cellular effectors (eg, cytotoxic T lymphocytes or CTLs) and inflammatory effectors such as cytokines. Inflammatory chemokines expressed in inflamed tissues upon stimulation by proinflammatory effectors such as cytokines are specialized for the recruitment of effector cells, such as CTLs.[182] Furthermore, the spatiotemporal expression of the cytochemokine gradients might determine not only the severity but also the unusual cluster of GVHD target organs (skin, gut, and liver).[170,183]

Cellular Effectors

Cytotoxic T cells are the major cellular effectors of GVHD.[184,185] The Fas–Fas ligand (FasL), the perforin–granzyme (or granule exocytosis) and TNFR-like death receptors (DR), such as TNF-related apoptosis-inducing ligand (TRAIL: DR4, 5 ligand) and TNF-like weak inducers of apoptosis (TWEAK: DR3 ligand) are the principal CTL effector pathways that have been evaluated after allogeneic BMT.[185–190] The involvement of each of these molecules in GVHD has been tested by using donor cells that are unable to mediate each pathway. Perforin is stored in cytotoxic granules of CTLs and NK cells, together with granzymes and other proteins. Although the exact mechanisms remain unclear, following the recognition of a target cell through the TCR–MHC interaction, perforin is secreted and inserted into the cell membrane, forming "perforin pores" that allow granzymes to enter the target cells and induce apoptosis through various downstream effector pathways such as caspases.[191] Ligation of Fas results in the formation of the death-inducing signaling complex and also activation of caspases.[192,193]

Transplantation of perforin deficient T cells results in a marked delay in the onset of GVHD in transplants across MiHA disparities only, both MHC and MiHA disparities,[126] and across isolated MHC I or II disparities.[185,194–198] However, mortality and clinical and histologic signs of GVHD were still induced even in the absence of perforin-dependent killing in these studies, demonstrating that the perforin–granzyme pathway plays a minor role in target organ damage. A role for the perforin–granzyme pathway for GVHD induction is also evident in studies employing donor-T cell subsets. Perforin- or granzyme B-deficient CD8+ T cells caused less mortality than wild-type T cells in experimental transplants across a single MHC class I mismatch. This pathway, however, seems to be less important compared to the Fas–FasL pathway in CD4-mediated GVHD.[197–199] Thus, it seems that CD4+ CTLs preferentially use the Fas–FasL pathway, whereas CD8+ CTLs primarily use the perforin–granzyme pathway.

Fas, a TNF-receptor family member, is expressed by many tissues, including GVHD target organs.[200] Its expression can be upregulated by inflammatory cytokines such as IFN-γ and TNF-α during GVHD, and the expression of FasL is also increased on donor T cells, indicating that FasL-mediated cytotoxicity may be a particularly important effector pathway in GVHD.[185,201] FasL-defective T cells cause less GVHD in the liver, skin and lymphoid organs.[196,199,201] The Fas–FasL pathway is particularly important in hepatic GVHD, consistent with the keen sensitivity of hepatocytes to Fas-mediated cytotoxicity in experimental models of murine hepatitis.[185] Fas-deficient recipients are protected from hepatic GVHD but not from other organ GVHD, and administration of anti-FasL (but not anti-TNF) MAbs significantly blocks hepatic GVHD damage occurring in murine models.[185,202,203] Although the use of FasL-deficient donor T cells or the administration of neutralizing FasL MAbs had no effect on the development of intestinal GVHD in several studies, the Fas–FasL pathway may play a role in this target organ, because intestinal epithelial lymphocytes exhibit increased FasL-mediated killing potential.[204] Elevated serum levels of soluble FasL and Fas have also been observed in at least some patients with acute GVHD.[205,206]

The utilization of a perforin–granzyme and FasL cytotoxic double-deficient (*cdd*) mouse provides an opportunity to address whether other effector pathways are capable of inducing GVHD target organ pathology. An initial study demonstrated that *cdd* T cells were unable to induce lethal GVHD across MHC class I and class II disparities after sublethal irradiation.[195] However, subsequent studies demonstrated that cytotoxic effector mechanisms of donor T cells are critical in preventing host resistance to GVHD.[189,207] Thus when recipients were conditioned with a lethal dose of irradiation, *cdd* CD4+ T cells produced similar mortality to wild-type CD4+ T cells.[189] These results were confirmed by a recent study demonstrating that GVHD target damage can occur in mice that lack alloantigen expression on the epithelium, preventing direct interaction between CTLs and target cells.[190]

The participation of another death ligand receptor signaling pathway, TNF/TNFRs, has also been evaluated. Experimental data suggest that this pathway is crucial for GI GVHD (discussed more below). Recently, several additional TNF family apoptosis-inducing receptors/ligands have been identified, including TWEAK, TRAIL, and LTβ/LIGHT, that have been proposed to play a role in GVHD and GVL responses.[78,208–214] However whether these distinct pathways play a more specific role for GVHD mediated by distinct T-cell subsets in certain situations remains unknown. Intriguingly, recent data suggest that none of these pathways might be critical for mediating the rejection of donor grafts.[208,215] Thus it is likely that their role in GVHD might be modulated by the intensity of conditioning and by the recipient T-cell subsets. Existing experimental data suggest that perforin and TRAIL cytotoxic pathways are associated with CD8+ T cell-mediated GVL.[185] The available experimental data are strongly skewed toward CD8+ T cell-mediated GVL based on the dominant role of this effector population in most murine GVT models; however, CD4+ T cells can mediate GVL and might be crucial in clinical BMT depending on the type of malignancy and the expression of immunodominant antigens.

Taken together, experimental data suggest that different lytic pathways may be implicated in the development of GVHD in specific target organs and for the generation of a GVL effect. However, the clinical importance of these observations is not known.

Inflammatory Effectors

Inflammatory cytokines synergize with CTLs, resulting in the amplification of local tissue injury and further promotion of inflammation, which ultimately leads to the observed target tissue destruction in the transplant recipient.[22] Macrophages, which had been primed with IFN-γ during step 2, produce inflammatory cytokines TNF-α and IL-1 when stimulated by a secondary triggering signal.[216] This stimulus may be provided through Toll-like receptors (TLRs) by microbial products such as lipopolysaccharide and other microbial particles, which can leak through the intestinal mucosa damaged by the conditioning regimen and gut GVHD.[217,218] It is now apparent that immune recognition through both TLR and non-TLRs (such as NOD) by the innate immune system also controls activation of adaptive immune responses.[217,219] Recent clinical studies of GVHD suggested the possible association with TLR/NOD polymorphisms and severity of GVHD.[220–222] Lipopolysaccharide and other innate stimuli may stimulate gut-associated lymphocytes, keratinocytes, dermal fibroblasts, and macrophages to produce proinflammatory effectors that play a direct role in causing target organ damage. Indeed experimental data with MHC mismatched HCT suggest that under certain circumstances these inflammatory mediators are sufficient in causing GVHD damage even in the absence of direct CTL induced damage.[50] The severity of GVHD appears to be directly related to the level of innate and adaptive immune cell priming and release of proinflammatory cytokines such as TNF-α, IL-1, and nitric oxide (NO).[50,218,223–225]

The cytokines TNF-α and IL-1 are produced by an abundance of cell types during processes of both innate and adaptive immunity; they often have synergistic, pleiotrophic, and redundant effects on both activation and effector phases of GVHD.[141] A critical role for TNF-α in the pathophysiology of acute GVHD was first suggested over 20 years ago when mice transplanted with mixtures of allogeneic BM and T cells developed severe skin, gut, and lung lesions that were associated with high levels of TNF-α mRNA in these tissues.[226] Target organ damage could be inhibited by infusion of anti-TNF-α MAbs, and mortality could be reduced from 100% to 50% by the administration of the soluble form of the TNF-α receptor (sTNFR), an antagonist of TNF-α.[40,43,224] Accumulating experimental data further suggest that TNF -a is involved in a multistep process of GVHD pathophysiology. TNF-α can (a) cause cachexia, a characteristic feature of GVHD; (b) induce maturation of DCs, thus enhancing alloantigen presentation; (c) recruit effector T cells, neutrophils, and monocytes into target organs through the induction of inflammatory chemokines; and (d) cause direct tissue damage by inducing apoptosis and necrosis. TNF-α is also involved in donor T-cell activation directly through its signaling via TNFR1 and TNFR2 on T cells. TNF–TNF1 interactions on donor T cells promote alloreactive T-cell responses and TNF–TNFR2 interactions are critical for intestinal GVHD.[211,227] TNF-α also seems to be an important effector molecule in GVHD involving skin and lymphoid tissue.[226,228] Additionally, TNF-α might also be involved in hepatic GVHD, probably by enhancing effector cell migration to the liver via the induction of inflammatory chemokines.[229] An important role for TNF-α in clinical acute GVHD has been suggested by studies demonstrating elevated serum levels of TNF-α or elevated TNF-α mRNA expression in peripheral blood mononuclear cells in patients with acute GVHD and other endothelial complications, such as hepatic venoocclusive disease (VOD).[229–232] Phase 1–2 trials using TNF-α antagonists reduced the severity of GVHD, suggesting that it is a relevant effector in causing target organ damage.[233,234]

The second major pro-inflammatory cytokine that appears to play an important role in the effector phase of acute GVHD is IL-1.[235] Secretion of IL-1 appears to occur predominantly during the effector phase of GVHD of the spleen and skin, two major GVHD target organs.[236] A similar increase in mononuclear cell IL-1 mRNA has been shown during clinical acute GVHD. Indirect evidence of a role for IL-1 in GVHD was obtained with administration of this cytokine to recipients in an allogeneic murine HCT model. Mice receiving IL-1 displayed a wasting syndrome and increased mortality that appeared to be an accelerated form of disease. By contrast, intraperitoneal administration of IL-1ra starting on d 10 posttransplant was able to reverse the development of GVHD in the majority of animals, providing a significant survival advantage to treated animals.[237] However, the attempt to use IL-1ra to prevent acute GVHD in a randomized trial was not successful.[238]

As a result of activation during GVHD, macrophages also produce NO, which contributes to the deleterious effects on GVHD target tissues, particularly immunosuppression.[225,239] NO also inhibits the repair mechanisms of target tissue destruction by inhibiting proliferation of epithelial stem cells in the gut and skin.[240] In humans and rats, the development of GVHD is preceded by an increase in serum levels of NO oxidation products.[241–244]

Existing data demonstrate important role for various inflammatory effectors in GVHD. The relevance of currently studied or as yet unknown specific effectors might however be determined by other factors, including the intensity of preparatory regimens, the type of allograft, the T cell subsets and the duration of HCT. In any event, both experimental and clinical data suggest an important role for both the cellular and inflammatory mediators in GVHD induced target organ damage.

Prevention of Acute Graft-Versus-Host Disease

Elimination of T cells with monoclonal antibodies, immunotoxins, lectins, CD34 columns, or physical techniques are effective at reducing GVHD. A typical unmanipulated marrow transplant entails the infusion of $\sim 10^7$ T cells per kg of recipient weight. A reduced T cell dose of $<10^5$ per kg has been associated with complete control of GVHD.[245] More recently the combination of very high stem cell numbers and $<3 \times 10^4$ CD3 cells/kg allowed haploidentical transplantation without GVHD.[246] Presumably host immune cells that survive the initial conditioning are responsible for graft rejection. When the stem cell source contains a large numbers of T cells, the GVH reaction further reduces the residual population capable of alloreactivity, thus decreasing graft rejection. To some degree the higher graft failure rates may be controlled by increasing the intensity of the immunosuppression of the conditioning regimen,[247,248] or adding back T cells.[249] Overall there been no improvement in survival that can be definitively attributed to T cell depletion.

Treatment of established GVHD with specific T cell antibodies has produced mixed results. Although antithymocyte globulin has definite activity in established GVHD, the nonspecific clearance of T cells may result in increased opportunistic infections and no improvement in survival.[20,250,251] More specific therapy with humanized anti-IL-2 receptor antibody, daclizumab[252,253] or the humanized anti-CD3 antibody, visilizumab[254,255] are promising, because they offer selective removal of T cell subsets. However, an increased risk of infection may still be observed.[256]

The first generally prescribed GVHD preventive regimen was the administration of intermittent low dose methotrexate as developed in a dog model by Thomas and Storb.[257] The principle of this approach was to administer a cell-cycle specific chemotherapeutic agent immediately after the transplant, when the T cells have started to divide in response to allogeneic antigens. Subsequently, the addition of antithymocyte globulin, prednisone or both resulted in incremental improvement in the GVHD rate but no improvement in survival.[258,259] Ultimately the course of methotrexate was abbreviated and combined with a T cell activation inhibitor, such as cyclosporine or tacrolimus. The introduction of cyclosporine in the late 1970's was a significant advance in GVHD prevention. A similar agent, tacrolimus, has been shown to control GVHD.[260] As a single agent cyclosporine was about as effective as methotrexate.[261] However, in combination with methotrexate, there was a significant reduction in the incidence of GVHD and an improvement in survival.[262] Subsequent trials of tacrolimus and methotrexate compared with cyclosporine and methotrexate showed no advantage for either combination.[260] The addition of prednisone to the conventional two-drug regimen resulted in similar rates of GVHD and no improvement in survival.[263]

Sirolimus (rapamycin) is a macrocyclic lactone immunosuppressant that is similar in structure to tacrolimus and cyclosporine. All three drugs bind to immunophilins; however, sirolimus complexed with FKBP12 inhibits T cell proliferation by interfering with signal transduction and cell cycle progression and can prevent GVHD.[264] Because Sirolimus acts through a separate mechanism from the tacrolimus-FKBP complex (and cyclosporine-cyclophilin complex), it is synergistic with both tacrolimus and cyclosporine. More recently, mycophenolate mofetil (MMF) has been studied. It is the prodrug of mycophenolic acid (MPA) a selective inhibitor of inosine monophosphate dehydrogenase, an enzyme critical to the de novo synthesis of guanosine nucleotide. Because T lymphocytes are more dependent on such synthesis than myeloid or mucosal cells, MPA preferentially inhibits proliferative responses of T cells.[265]

One hypothesis that flows from the three step model of GVHD is that reduction of intestinal colonization with bacteria could prevent GVHD. Animal studies in germ free environments support this notion, where GVHD was not observed until mice were colonized with gram negative organisms.[266] Later, gut decontamination and use of a laminar air flow environment was associated with less GVHD and better survival in patients with severe aplastic anemia.[267] Similarly, studies of intestinal decontamination in patients with malignancies have shown less GVHD in some[268,269] but not all studies.[270] Finally, another recent approach to GVHD prevention has been the use of nonmyeloablative conditioning transplants. A less intensive preparative regimen decreases the tissue toxicity and subsequent release of cytokines in animal models.[43,271] Patients generally experience mild toxicity in the initial peritransplant period and develop little or no GVHD, although many develop GVHD later, especially after donor lymphocyte infusions. In fact, the rates of GVHD are often higher than with conventional transplants, and GVHD is associated with a significant portion of the GVL effect.[272,273]

An important role for TNFα in clinical acute GVHD has been suggested by studies demonstrating elevated levels of TNFα in the serum of patients with acute GVHD and other endothelial complications such as venoocclusive disease.[274–277] Therapy of GVHD with humanized anti-TNFα (infliximab)[278,279] or a dimeric fusion protein consisting of the extracellular ligand-binding portion of the human TNFα receptor (TNFR) linked to the Fc portion of human IgG1 (etanercept)[280] have shown some promise. The second major proinflammatory cytokine that appears to play an important role in the effector phase of acute GVHD is IL-1. Secretion of IL-1 appears to occur predominantly during the effector phase of GVHD in the spleen and skin, two major GVHD target organs.[281] IL-1 receptor antagonist (IL-1RA) is a naturally occurring pure competitive inhibitor of IL-1 that is produced by monocytes/ macrophages and keratinocytes. Interestingly, the IL-1RA gene is polymorphic and the presence in the donor of the allele that is linked to higher secretion of IL-1RA was associated with less acute GVHD.[282] Two phase 1–2 trials showed promising data that specific inhibition of IL-1 with either the soluble receptor or IL-1RA could result in remissions in 50% to 60% of patients with steroid-resistant GVHD.[283,284] But a subsequent randomized trial of the addition of IL-1RA or placebo to cyclosporine and methotrexate beginning at the time of conditioning and continuing through day 14 after stem cell infusion did not show any protective effect of the drug, despite the attainment of very high plasma levels.[238,285] Thus, at least as administered in this study, IL-1 inhibition was insufficient to prevent GVHD in humans. IL-11 was also able to protect the GI tract in animal models and prevent GVHD, but it did not prevent clinical GVHD.[285] Thus, not all preclinical strategies successfully translate to new therapies.

Therapy for Acute GVHD

Glucocorticoid steroids are the initial therapy for acute GVHD. The mechanisms by which steroids work are multifactorial; they act as lympholytic agents and inhibit the release of inflammatory cytokines such as IL-1, IL-2, IL-6, gamma interferon, and TNF-α. Because of its intravenous availability, methylprednisolone is the steroid most commonly given for acute GVHD. Various dosing regimens have been used, none of which is clearly superior. High-bolus doses (10–20 mg/kg or 500 mg/m^2) have higher initial response rates, but flares on tapering and opportunistic infections are common. Both the Seattle and Minnesota transplant groups have found that treatment with steroids was as effective as, or more effective than, other therapies or combination of therapies, with 20% to 40% of patients having durable long-term responses.[286,287] Long-term salvage rates for patients who did not respond to steroids were 20% or less; most patients eventually died from infection, acute GVHD, and/or chronic GVHD. More recently, a randomized trial demonstrated that topical therapy with oral budosenide can have prednisone sparing effects and is efficacious in treatment of GI GVHD.[288] Clinically, two types of failure of corticosteroid treatment of acute GVHD can be distinguished: true steroid resistance, that is, progression of GVHD symptoms and manifestations while patients are receiving full-dose corticosteroid treatment, and steroid dependence, that is, reoccurrence (or flare) of GVHD during or after tapering of steroid treatment.[289] In general, the prognosis with true steroid-resistant GVHD is worse than the prognosis of steroid-dependent patients.[289] A comparison of trials dealing with steroid-resistant GVHD is hampered by variable inclusion of both patient groups in many of these trials. A variety of agents has been tested, including chemical immunosuppressants such as MMF, ATG, anti-CD3 anti-T cell antibodies as well as more specific agents directed against activation or adhesion molecules anti-CD25, anti-CD147, cytokines or extracorporeal photopheresis.[289,290] To date, there are no randomized trails testing one versus the other in this clinical situation.

Other Supportive Approaches

Infections are the main cause of death in patients with steroid-refractory acute GVHD, and careful surveillance and control of infections is mandatory in patients with acute GVHD. Fungal infections, especially aspergillosis, are the leading complication. Prophylaxis and early aggressive treatment should be facilitated by the introduction of new azoles (voriconazole and posaconazole) or echinocandins (caspofungin, micafungin), which broaden therapeutic efficacy with acceptable toxicity. A variety of further supplementary approaches have been suggested; for example, large volumes of diarrhea might be controlled by the use of octreotide[291] and oral beclomethasone (or budesonide).[288]

CHRONIC GRAFT-VERSUS-HOST DISEASE

Chronic GVHD was initially defined as a GVHD syndrome presenting more than 100 days after transplant; its onset occurred either as an extension of acute GVHD (progressive), after a disease-free interval (quiescent), or with no precedent (de novo).[292,293] Chronic GVHD may be limited or extensive (Table 107–3). Any grade of acute GVHD increases the probability of chronic GVHD, although no singular pathologic feature of the former predicts the development of the latter. Its incidence ranges from 30% to 60% after transplantation with the bone marrow, although it may be higher after peripheral blood progenitor transplants.[294]

As with acute GVHD, the immune system appears to be affected in all patients, who are highly susceptible to bacterial, viral, fungal, and opportunistic infections. Specific abnormalities of cellular immunity include decreases in the production of antibodies against specific antigens, defects in the number and function of CD4$^+$ T cells, and increases in the number of nonspecific suppressor cells, which further diminish lymphocyte responses. Eighty percent of patients have skin changes resembling widespread lichen planus with papulosquamous dermatitis, plaques, desquamation, dyspigmentation, and vitiligo.[273,295] Destruction of dermal appendages leads to alopecia and onychodysplasia. Severe chronic GVHD of the skin can resemble scleroderma, with induration, joint contractures, atrophy, and chronic skin ulcers. Chronic cholestatic liver disease occurs in 80% of patients and often resembles acute GVHD; it rarely progresses to cirrhosis. Severe mucositis of the mouth and esophagus can result in weight loss and malnutrition. Intestinal involvement, however, is infrequent.[273,295] Chronic GVHD also produces a sicca syndrome, with atrophy and dryness of mucosal surfaces caused by lymphocytic destruction of exocrine glands, usually affecting the eyes, mouth, airways, skin, and esophagus.[24,295,296] The hematopoietic system may also be affected, and thrombocytopenia is an unfavorable prognostic factor in patients with chronic GVHD.[273] Important predictors of unfavorable outcome are progressive onset, lichenoid skin changes, elevated serum bilirubin level, continued thrombocytopenia, and failure to respond to 9 months of therapy.[273,297–299] Among patients with none of these risk factors, 70% are expected to survive, compared with less than 20% with two or more of these risk factors.[299]

Histologic examination of the immune system reveals involution of thymic epithelium, disappearance of Hassall corpuscles, depletion of lymphocytes, and absence of secondary germinal centers in lymph nodes.[300] Pathologic skin findings include epidermal atrophy with changes characteristic of lichen planus and striking inflammation around eccrine units. Sclerosis of the dermis and fibrosis of the hypodermis subsequently develop. GI lesions include localized inflammation of the mucosa and stricture formation in the esophagus and small intestine.[295] Histologic findings in the liver are often similar to those that occur in acute GVHD but are more intense, with chronic changes such as fibrosis with hyalinization of portal triads, obliteration of bile ducts, and hepatocellular cholestasis.[273] The endocrine glands of the eyes, mouth, esophagus, and bronchi show destruction focused on centrally draining ducts, with secondary involvement of alveolar components.[300] Findings of bronchiolitis obliterans, similar to those that occur in rejection of lung transplants, are now generally considered a pulmonary manifestation of chronic GVHD, although the pathogenesis of this process remains unclear.[300]

Clinical Manifestations of Chronic GVHD

Chronic GVHD can present with a plethora of clinical manifestations. Because of its unpredictable pattern and the late onset when patients are no longer receiving care at their transplant center, the diagnosis is often delayed or not recognized. The staging of chronic GVHD is summarized in Table 107–4. However, the recently developed NIH Consensus Criteria, upon validation, might soon become the standard for diagnosing and evaluating responses for chronic GVHD.[301,302]

Dermatologic

Skin involvement in chronic GVHD presents with varied features. Lichenoid chronic GVHD presents as an erythematous, papular rash that resembles lichen planus with no typical distribution pattern.[24] Sclerodermatous GVHD may involve the dermis and/or the muscular fascia and clinically resembles systemic sclerosis. The skin is thickened, tight, and fragile, with very poor wound healing. Either hypopigmentation or hyperpigmentation may occur. In severe cases, the skin may become blistered and ulcerate. Hair changes can include increased brittleness, premature graying, and alopecia. Fingernails and toenails may also be affected by chronic GVHD. Destruction of sweat glands can cause hyperthermia.[303]

Table 107–4 Commonly Administered Drugs for GVHD Prophylaxis and Treatment

Drug	Mechanism	Adverse Effects
Corticosteroids	Direct lymphocyte toxicity, suppress pro-inflammatory cytokines such as TNF-α	Hyperglycemia, acute psychosis, severe myopathy, neuropathy, osteoporosis, cataract development
Methotrexate (MTX)	Antimetabolite, inhibits T cell proliferation	Significant renal, hepatic, and gastrointestinal toxicities
Cyclosporine (CSP)	IL-2 suppressor, blocks Ca^{2+}-dependent signal transduction distal to TCR engagement	Renal and hepatic insufficiency, hypertension, hyperglycemia, headache, nausea and vomiting, hirsutism, gum hypertrophy, seizure with severe toxicity
Tacrolimus (FK506)	IL-2 receptor, blocks Ca^{2+}-dependent signal transduction distal to TCR engagement	Similar to CSA
Mycophenolate mofetil (MMF)	Inhibits de novo purine synthesis	Body aches, abdominal pain, nausea and vomiting, diarrhea, neutropenia
Sirolimus	mTOR inhibitor	Thrombocytopenia, hyperlipidemia, TTP
Antithymocyte globulin (ATG)	Polyclonal immunoglobulin	Anaphylaxis, serum sickness

Ocular

Ocular GVHD usually presents with xerophthalmia or dry eyes. Irreversible destruction of the lacrimal glands results in dryness, photophobia, and burning. Local therapy with preservative-free tears and ointment or the placement of punctal plugs by an ophthalmologist might be required. Conjunctival GVHD, a rare manifestation of severe chronic GVHD, has a poor prognosis.[24,303]

Oral

Oral GVHD causes xerostomia and/or food sensitivity.[303] More advanced disease may cause odynophagia as a result of esophageal damage and strictures, although esophageal involvement occurs rarely without oral disease. Physical examination may reveal only erythema with a few white plaques, prompting a misdiagnosis of thrush or herpetic infections. Lichenoid changes in advanced disease can cause extensive plaque formation.[24]

Gastrointestinal

Patients with chronic GVHD have GI complaints that mimic other disease states, including acute GVHD, infection, dysmotility, lactose intolerance, pancreatic insufficiency, and drug-related side effects. In one retrospective review of the intestinal biopsies of patients with chronic GVHD and persistent GI symptoms, a majority of patients had evidence of both acute and chronic GVHD, and only 7% of the patients had isolated chronic GVHD.[24,295] Thus although chronic GVHD may involve the GI tract alone, it may be difficult to diagnose in those circumstances without concurrent acute GVHD.

Hepatic

Hepatic disease typically presents as cholestasis with elevated serum levels of alkaline phosphatase and bilirubin. Isolated hepatic chronic GVHD has become more common with the increasing use of donor lymphocyte infusions.[11] Liver biopsy is required to confirm the diagnosis of chronic hepatic GVHD in patients with no other target organ involvement.

Pulmonary

Bronchiolitis obliterans is a late and serious manifestation of chronic GVHD. Patients typically present with a cough or dyspnea.[303] Severe sclerotic disease of the chest wall may also give rise to similar symptoms, with no intrinsic pulmonary disease. Pulmonary function tests demonstrate obstructive physiology and a reduction in DLCO. Chest computed tomography results may be normal or may show hyperinflation with a ground glass appearance. Overall, patients with bronchiolitis obliterans have minimal response to therapy and a very poor prognosis. Patients with chronic GVHD are also at risk for chronic sinopulmonary infections but symptoms may be minimal.[24]

Hematopoietic

Cytopenias in chronic GVHD are common. This may be a result of stromal damage, but autoimmune neutropenia, anemia, and/or thrombocytopenia are also seen. Thrombocytopenia at the time of chronic GVHD diagnosis is associated with poor prognosis. However, thrombocytopenia posttransplant is a poor prognostic factor regardless of GVHD and eosinophilia is occasionally seen with chronic GVHD.[303]

Immunologic

Chronic GVHD is inherently immunosuppressive. Functional asplenia with an increased susceptibility to encapsulated bacteria is common, and circulating Howell–Jolly bodies can be seen on peripheral blood smear. Patients are also at risk for invasive fungal infections and *Pneumocystis carinii* pneumonia.[303] Hypoglobulinemia is common and patients with levels below 500 mg/dL should be supplemented with intravenous immunoglobulin.[303]

Musculoskeletal

Fascial involvement in sclerodermatous GVHD is usually associated with skin changes. Fasciitis in joint areas can cause severe restriction of range of motion. Muscle cramps are a common complaint in patients with chronic GVHD, but myositis with elevated muscle enzymes is rare. Many patients with chronic GVHD are on steroid therapy and have low levels of sex hormone posttransplant. Avascular necrosis, osteopenia, and osteoporosis are also frequent complications.[303]

Whether kidneys, which are primary targets in some animal models of chronic GVHD, are also involved in the human syndrome is yet to be determined in large studies.[304] Among the myriad clinical features of chronic GVHD, three definitive signs appear to be risk factors for increased mortality: (a) extensive skin GVHD involving more than 50% of the body surface area; (b) platelet count of more than 100,000/μL; and (c) progressive onset and acute GVHD that continues uninterrupted beyond day 100.[305] Historically, it has been difficult to make a definitive diagnosis of chronic GVHD. Recent criteria established by NIH consensus conference might prove to be beneficial in establishing uniform criteria for diagnosis, treatment, and response.[302] The NIH consensus criteria are currently in the process of being evaluated.

Differential Diagnosis

The distinction between chronic and acute GVHD has been traditionally based on the time of onset. The NIH Working Group has added two subcategories to the two main categories of GVHD. The broad category of acute GVHD includes (a) classic acute GVHD (maculopapular rash, nausea, vomiting, anorexia, profuse diarrhea, ileus, or cholestatic hepatitis) occurring within 100 days after transplantation or DLI (without diagnostic or distinctive signs of chronic GVHD) and (b) persistent, recurrent, or late acute GVHD: features of classic acute GVHD without diagnostic or distinctive manifestations of chronic GVHD occurring beyond 100 days of transplantation or DLI (often seen after withdrawal of immune suppression). The broad category of chronic GVHD includes (a) classic chronic GVHD without features characteristic of acute GVHD and (b) an overlap syndrome in which features of chronic and acute GVHD appear together. In the absence of histologic or clinical signs or symptoms of chronic GVHD, the persistence, recurrence, or new onset of characteristic skin, GI tract, or liver abnormalities should be classified as acute GVHD regardless of the time after transplantation. With appropriate stratification, patients with persistent, recurrent, or late acute GVHD or overlap syndrome can be included in clinical trials with patients who have chronic GVHD.

CHRONIC GRAFT-VERSUS-HOST DISEASE: PATHOPHYSIOLOGY

The pathophysiology of chronic GVHD is less well understood than that of acute GVHD and has undergone less intensive experimental modeling.[24] It is important to recognize that chronic GVHD was originally defined as a temporal rather than a clinical or pathophysiological entity. The initial clinical reports of chronic GVHD described abnormalities that occurred at least 150 days after stem cell infusion.[306,307] By convention, day 100 after stem cell infusion is used as an arbitrary divider between acute and chronic GVHD. But some manifestations of acute GVHD occur after day 100 and some manifestations of chronic GVHD may occur before day 100.[24,303] Thus it is preferable to consider the clinical symptoms and signs per se rather than their timing of the onset.

Relatively little is known about the pathophysiology of chronic GVHD. This is due in part to the absence of appropriate animal models that can capture the kinetics and the protean manifestation of chronic GVHD.[308] On the basis of certain clinical features, chronic GVHD has been considered to be an autoimmune disease. Some experimental data suggest that chronic GVHD results from defective central negative selection, leading to the generation of autoreactive clones that escape tolerogenic mechanisms operating in the periphery.[309,310] This would suggest that the nonpolymorphic antigens expressed in both the donor and recipient rather than MiHA antigens are the likely targets. In contrast to T cells from animals with acute GVHD that are specific for host alloantigens, T cells from animals with chronic GVHD are specific for a public (common) determinant of MHC class II molecules.[311,312] These T cells are considered autoreactive because they recognize public MHC class II determinants that are common to both donor and recipient rather than polymorphic histocompatibility antigens that are specific for the host. The autoreactive cells of chronic GVHD are associated with a damaged thymus, which can be injured by several mechanisms including acute GVHD, the conditioning regimen, or age-related involution and atrophy. In chronic GVHD, the ability of the thymus to delete autoreactive T cells (negative selection) and to induce tolerance is impaired.[24,313,314] However, no clear data exist on the isolation of autoreactive donor-derived T-cell clones that equally recognize nonpolymorphic antigens from the donor and recipient cells. This, however, does not directly preclude the existence or a causative role for autoreactive T cells. Chronic GVHD could also be a product of T cells that have undergone relatively chronic antigen stimulation owing to the presence of inexhaustible and ubiquitous MiHA antigens. Allo-T cells under circumstances of chronic MiHA antigen stimulation can induce syndromes resembling those induced by the chronic antigen stimulation in autoimmune diseases. This concept is also consistent with the proposal of acute GVHD as a risk factor for chronic GVHD. The antigens targeted in chronic GVHD could be the same dominant ones targeted in acute GVHD, but the reactive T cells could be different; for example, they may secrete transforming growth factor-β. But antigens other than those that were initially immunodominant, even those not initially targeted but introduced through epitope spread could be important. It is also conceivable that regulatory mechanisms may frequently fail in allo-HCT, resulting in activation and expansion of T cells that recognize both nonpolymorphic and MiHA epitopes. One recent murine study suggested that development of a chronic GVHD-like syndrome is target antigen-dependent.[71] Furthermore, chronic GVHD pathogenesis could, in part, be a consequence of T cell priming by donor-derived APCs.[72] In some patient subsets, responses to rituximab, presence of MiHA-specific antibodies, and the presence of chronic GVHD after T-cell depletion allo-BMT would indicate that in addition to donor T cells, donor B cells might either have a direct effector role or prime T cells as APCs.[315,316] It is important to understand that given the many clinical presentations of chronic GVHD that tend to occur at variable time after HCT, it is possible that separate pathogenic mechanisms might be involved in causing distinct manifestations and that no single mechanism is sufficient to cause chronic GVHD.

THERAPY FOR CHRONIC GRAFT-VERSUS-HOST DISEASE

Chronic GVHD has a major impact on both quality of life (QOL) and survival, frequently involves multiple organs, and necessitates prolonged immunosuppressive therapy.[317] One report noted that 15% of cancer-free transplant recipients were still receiving immunosuppressive therapy after 7 years.[318] The more severe forms of chronic GVHD are clearly associated with a lower disease-free survival. Thus, the potential benefit of a graft-versus-leukemia effect is shadowed by significant treatment-related mortality.[318]

Current therapies for chronic GVHD are of limited efficacy, and there is no long-term satisfactory regimen for patients who fail front-line steroid-based therapy. Indeed, there is no Food and Drug Administration (FDA)-approved medication for use in chronic GVHD. The lack of standardized response criteria to measure therapeutic efficacy poses a major obstacle to pursuing therapeutic trials in chronic GVHD. Overall survival and / or discontinuation of systemic immunosuppression are accepted long-term endpoints in chronic GVHD trials. The recent National Institutes of Health (NIH)-sponsored consensus project provided for the first time a set of standardized measures and definitions to use as response criteria in chronic GVHD.[301,302] Nonetheless, these recommendations are yet be tested and validated in prospective studies. The NIH Consensus Conference has defined response measures classified in 2 main groups: clinician-assessed and patient-reported (see next page).[308]

The prevention of acute GVHD has not consistently resulted in a lower incidence of chronic GVHD. A clear example is the use of reduced-intensity transplants, consistently associated with a lower incidence of acute GVHD but with no a major impact on chronic GVHD.[319,320] The extended use of GVHD prophylaxis with cyclosporine, or variations in the cyclosporine dosage used, showed no beneficial effects on the incidence of chronic GVHD.[317,321] The addition of thalidomide to cyclosporine and methotrexate prophylaxis, the administration of IV Ig, or early treatment based on biopsy findings of subclinical GVHD in an attempt to treat chronic GVHD preemptively were unsuccessful.[317] The most commonly used thera-

Measure	Clinician-Assessed	Patient-Reported
I. Chronic GVHD-specific core measures		
Signs	Organ-specific measures	Not applicable
Symptoms	Clinician-assessed symptoms	Patient-reported symptoms
Global rating	Mild, moderate, or severe 0 to 10 severity scale 7-point change scale	Mild, moderate, or severe 0 to 10 severity scale 7-point change scale
II. Chronic GVHD nonspecific ancillary measures		
Function	Grip strength 2-minute walk time	Patient-reported function
Quality of life	—	Patient-reported health-related quality of life

From the NIH consensus Conference.[308]

pies to treat chronic GVHD are cyclosporine and prednisone. Sullivan et al[322] reported that prednisone alone is superior to prednisone plus azathioprine for primary treatment of patients with chronic GVHD. However, in patients classified as high-risk on the basis of platelet counts below 100,000/μL, treatment with prednisone alone resulted in only 26% 5-year survival. When a similar group of patients was treated with alternating-day cyclosporine and prednisone, 5-year survival exceeded 50%.[323] A recent randomized study of 287 patients with extensive GVHD found no statistically significant difference in nonrelapse death at 5 years or in cumulative incidence of secondary therapy at 5 years when prednisone alone was compared to prednisone plus cyclosporine.[24] For chronic GVHD that recurs or fails to respond to initial therapy, there is no standard treatment. Experimental therapies currently under evaluation include psoralen plus ultraviolet light, MMF, thalidomide, total lymphoid irradiation, plaquenil, extracorporeal photopheresis, pentostatin, and acetretin.[297] Table 107–4 lists the commonly used GVHD drugs and their common side effects.[324]

SYNGENEIC GRAFT-VERSUS-HOST DISEASE

A GVHD-like syndrome that is usually self-limited and predominantly affects the skin can occur in recipients of syngeneic or autologous transplants.[325] It is also possible that some of the cases of syngeneic GVHD reflected a mistaken assumption that the donor was syngeneic without extensive molecular confirmation. It is primarily manifest as a rash that usually responds promptly to corticosteroid therapy. Although the level of severity may be grade II or III, the disease generally resolves promptly with the administration of glucocorticoids and is not life-threatening. Virtually all patients in whom a GVHD-like syndrome develops after syngeneic transplantation have been prepared with intensive conditioning regimens, usually involving irradiation. Experimental studies suggest that such conditioning is essential for the induction of thymic dysfunction, which is necessary for the development of the disease. Generation of autoreactive cells (a defect in thymic negative selection) as well as elimination of regulatory cells appear to be the requirements for the development of this disease.[314] An additional hypothesis is that in some individuals, maternal cells transmitted to them during their fetal development remain present throughout adult life.[326] These observations suggest the possibility that in some instances small numbers of HLA incompatible cells (derived from the donor's mother) may be transmitted with HLA-identical transplants. Transplacentally transferred maternal cells may also play a role in the development of neonatal GVHD.[326]

Transfusion-Associated Graft-Versus-Host Disease

Most blood products administered to immunocompromised patients are now irradiated or at least leukocyte depleted to avoid the transfusion of viable alloreactive T cells. With most homologous blood products, the MHC incompatibility between donor and recipient results in rapid clearance of transfused T cells by the recipient's immune system. However, occasionally transfusions from donors who are homozygous for one of the recipient's MHC haplotypes are not recognized as foreign by the recipient.[327–329] These cells can survive, "engraft," and may mount an immunologic attack against the unshared haplotype in the patient, resulting in transfusion-induced GVHD.[329] This syndrome of transfusion-associated GVHD differs from GVHD occurring after transplantation in regard to its kinetics but also in regard to its manifestations insofar as the recipient marrow is a major target.[328] Because the number of stem cells in the offending blood product is inadequate, there is no hematopoietic recovery from donor cells. This syndrome is generally fatal owing to refractory pancytopenia in addition to other organ involvement.

GRAFT-VERSUS-LEUKEMIA RESPONSES

The GVL response after allogeneic HCT comes from the immunologic attack of the host tissue and, by extension, the leukemia/tumor. This response represents a potent form of immunotherapy that circumvents some of the immunoediting mechanisms used by tumor cells to develop in the hosts. The power of the alloimmune response to eliminate malignancy was first reported more than 50 years ago in experimental models by Barnes and Loutit.[1] However, the entity GVL and its close association with GVHD was not established another 15 years.[330]

CLINICAL FEATURES

Clinical evidence that the donor graft mediates important antileukemic effect comes from higher relapse rates for recipients of syngeneic stem cells than recipients of HLA-matched sibling grafts.[331] These findings have also been confirmed in a multicenter analysis of HCT recipients with acute myelogenous leukemia (AML) in first remission and subsequent retrospective analyses by the International Bone Marrow Transplant Registry (IBMTR).[332–334] The second IBMTR analysis also showed that the magnitude of this GVL effect is greater for patients with CML and AML and not statistically significant for patients with ALL in first remission.[335,336]

Several case reports of patients with relapse of leukemia after allogeneic HCT noted remissions of the malignancy either after abrupt withdrawal of immunosuppression or during a flare of acute GVHD.[337–340] Patients who develop GVHD after allogeneic HCT experience relapse less frequently than similar patients who do not develop clinical disease. GVHD is protective against relapse both for HCT recipients with advanced leukemia[341–343] and for patients who receive transplants in earlier stages of malignancy.[344] Additional analyses also suggest that the magnitude of the GVL effect appears to be disease and stage specific.[344–346] Initial reports suggested that chronic GVHD was most protective against relapse,[343] but other analyses demonstrate that acute GVHD is also protective.[344] On the basis of these reports, newer trials of immunotherapy are designed to include cessation of immunosuppressive therapy (without taper) to induce a GVL reaction for patients whose malignancy has relapsed after HCT. Furthermore, Childs et al demonstrated that the graft-versus-tumor effect also plays an important role in inducing remissions from a nonhematologic malignancy, renal cell carcinoma.[347]

Another line of clinical evidence regarding the GVL effect of allogeneic HCT and its tight linkage to GVHD comes from the studies employing T-cell depletion of the donor graft. Donor T cells included in the stem cell graft are critical for acute GVHD, and T-cell depletion by various strategies is one of the most successful means of reducing the incidence and severity of GVHD after allogeneic HCT.[348–354] Unfortunately, although T-cell depletion results in less treatment-related morbidity and mortality, improved overall survival rates have not been reliably demonstrated. This failure is due in large part to a reciprocal increase in the subsequent relapse rate after T-cell depletion, as well as to graft failure and other complications.[346,355,356]

T-cell depletion increases relapse rates particularly in CML.[344,346,357] This observation provides further strong, albeit indirect, evidence that allogeneic donor T cells are important mediators not only of GVHD but also of the GVL properties of the allogeneic stem cell graft. Finally the most compelling evidence of donor T cells in mediating GVL comes from the observations made from donor lymphocyte infusions.

Genetic Basis

The immunotherapeutic effect that occurs in an allo-BMT setting is primarily mediated by allogeneic donor T or NK cells directed against the alloantigens shared by the recipient tumor and target tissues and/or tumor-specific antigens that have the advantage of not being subjected to tolerance mechanisms by the host tumor.[358–360] Understanding of the exquisite specificity of T-cell responses led to attempts to identify specific antigens that are responsible for the GVL effect. Much of the focus has been on the identification of (a) certain oncogenic viral proteins because these are absent in normal cells but expressed by transformed tumor cells (certain EBV peptides such as EBNA-1, LMP-1, LMP, and LCL), (b) antigens that are expressed in a tissue-specific fashion (melanoma-specific proteins), and (c) proteins that are overexpressed in tumors (*WT1*, *proteinase 3*, survivin, telomerase reverse transcriptase, CYPB1 and Her-2/neu).[90,359] Although these antigens are specific, most T-cell responses to these antigens are limited because of the poor immunogenicity of these proteins, expression on normal cells, defects in the processing or presentation of tumor antigens or by production of factors that disable T-cell responses. Thus, clinical attempts to obtain high specificity of T-cell responses have been offset with difficulties in obtaining enough sensitivity and vice versa. Furthermore, given the current concepts of stem cell origins of leukemia and cancers, identification of the immunogenic proteins that are specifically expressed in the malignant stem cells and harnessing T-cell responses to those antigens will be needed for the optimal GVL effect to cure malignancy.[361,362]

In contrast to the tumor-specific or associated antigens discussed above, alloantigens are not subjected to tolerance mechanisms. Vaccination strategies with autologous T cells utilizing tumor-associated or -specific antigens have yielded disappointing clinical antitumor responses.[363] By contrast, allogeneic HCT has met with remarkable GVL responses, perhaps because of recognition of minor alloantigens in addition to the tumor-associated antigens.[364] This concept has been demonstrated by recent murine studies, which showed that alloantigen on the tumor cells is required for GVL responses and that the principal targets of GVL are the immunodominant allogeneic MiHAs rather than the tumor-associated antigens.[52,365] Thus T cells specific for MiHA antigens could provide a potent GVL effect. Significant progress has been made in the identification of MiHAs that are specifically expressed in the host hematopoietic tissues and therefore might allow for a GVL response without causing GVHD.[90] Together, these results suggest that, in addition to tumor-specific proteins, expression of alloantigens and cognate interactions between donor T cells and the tumor tissues are required for the effective induction of the majority of GVL responses. However, T cells specific for some MiHAs are also responsible for GVHD, and a means of consistently separating the beneficial GVL effect from GVHD has not yet been clinically achieved.

KIR Polymorphisms

Two competing models—mismatched and missing ligand models—for HLA-KIR allorecognition have been supported by clinical observations of GVL responses in different patient and transplant populations.[49,366] The former model has been shown to separate GVL and GVHD responses in the context of T-cell depleted (TCD) haploidentical HCT for AML.[367,368] Even though this model is supported by elegant laboratory studies, it was found to be invalid for ALL and also for AML after unrelated donor HCT with immunosuppression.[367] Recent retrospective clinical data suggest that GVHD and GVL can be separated by the "missing ligand" model in CML/AML and MDS patients after TCD HLA-identical sibling HCT.[366,368,369] Further validation of either models by clinical prospective studies and the a better understanding of the balance between the inhibitory and activating receptor - ligand interaction of the NK cells are needed to adequately exploit the interface between HLA - KIR genetics to separate GVHD from GVL.[370,371]

IMMUNOBIOLOGY OF GRAFT-VERSUS-LEUKEMIA RESPONSES

Given the tight association of clinical GVHD and GVL and the common biological principles governing these responses after allogeneic HCT, we will discuss below the similarities and distinctions between them in the context of the three cellular phases of GVHD.[372]

Phase 1: Activation of Antigen-Presenting Cells

The concept that tumor eradication after allogeneic HCT might not require toxic chemoradiotherapy and could be achieved primarily by the immunotherapeutic effect from the GVL responses has led to the clinical development of non-myeloablative HCT for hematologic and nonhematologic malignancies.[373] Phase 1 is characterized by the development of 'cytokine storm' generated 'danger signals' from the conditioning regimen and the subsequent activation of APCs.[372] Experimental data suggested that the reduction in conditioning would attenuate the 'cytokine storm', lead to the development of mixed donor-host chimerism and confine the GVH response primarily to secondary lymphoid organs, thus cause less severe GVHD without impairing GVL responses.[374–376] However, non-myeloablative HCT has delayed the kinetics but did not reduce the overall incidence of GVHD and a significant numbers of patients either failed to respond or relapsed.[21] Furthermore, recent murine and human studies have suggested that homeostatic expansion of T cells in a lymphopenic environment induced by conditioning (as opposed to mere immunosuppression) improves the antitumor efficacy of adoptively transferred syngeneic or autologous T cells by increasing the availability of space, enhancing the memory responses and reducing the competition for homeostatic cytokines (such as IL-7 and IL-15) for transferred T cells while eliminating regulatory T cells.[377–379] Thus low intensity HCT clearly demonstrate the principle of GVL effect, but the role of 'cytokine storm', and homeostatic expansion of allogeneic T cells in shaping the intensity of GVL responses is not known.

Host and donor APCs are critical for the induction and severity of GVHD.[7] Activation of APCs is the key step in Phase 1 of GVHD.[372] Significant progress has been made in understanding the role of APCs in GVL. Recent experimental evidence demonstrate a crucial role for professional host APCs in the induction of GVL responses mediated by donor T cells even when the tumor cells showed some features of APCs.[52,380] Tumors that merely express costimulatory molecules may still be unable to stimulate an effective immune response because of their various 'immunoediting' processes that cause ineffective antigen presentation.[381] However, when the tumor cell itself functions as a professional APC, as with CML, it can generate an effective GVL response.[382,383] By contrast, cancers such as acute leukemias that seldom differentiate into APCs generate poor GVL responses. Data also demonstrated that given sufficient time and a low tumor burden, cross-presentation of tumor-associated antigens and/or alloantigens by professional donor APCs can occur, and may promote or sustain GVL responses by maintaining or expanding alloreactive T cells after initial priming on host APCs.[52,383] This concept is consistent with clinical GVL responses in CML in which the final stage of a GVL response to CML may be the result of donor T cells responding not directly to the small number of CML stem cells or progenitors (which would be undifferentiated and therefore poor APCs) but to tumor antigens cross-presented on professional donor APCs. But it is unclear if such cross-presentation is sufficient to elicit effective GVL responses against acute or advanced leukemia. These data, however, suggest that GVL responses generated after low intensity conditioning may not be as robust as those after full intensity HCT and highlight the need for a clearer understanding of the effects of 'cytokine storm' and lymphopenia generated danger signals on the activation of APCs in mediating GVL.

Phase 2: Donor T-Cell Activation

The core of GVL responses, as with GVHD, is also dependent on the activation of appropriate numbers of T cells. The 'second signals' from professional APCs (or certain tumor cells that function as effective APCs) are critical for generating an effective GVL response.[78] Several of the costimulatory pathways that modulate GVHD have also been evaluated in mediating GVL responses.[78] Blockade of CD28 costimulation preserved GVL responses but reduced GVHD in murine studies.[384] However, when the tumor cells also expressed B7 molecules, such blockade reduced the GVL responses.[382] Ex vivo blockade of CD40-CD40L interaction has been shown to reduce GVHD by generating Tregs but preserve GVL.[78,100,385] By contrast blockade of the 4–1BB pathway reduced both GVHD and GVL.[82] The other costimulatory molecules (OX40 and ICOS) and the inhibitory molecules (CTLA-4 and PD-1) also modulate antitumor responses.[83,84] A better understanding of the context (ie, low intensity or DLI) and of the hierarchy of timing, duration and extent of costimulatory requirements of donor T cell subsets might result in approaches which balance the intensity of GVL and GVHD responses. Clinical and experimental evidence suggest that donor T cells numbers correlate with the severity of GVHD and GVL responses. TCD grafts have reduced GVHD but increased disease relapse suggesting a role for T cell numbers in GVL responses as well.[386] Clinical attempts to separate GVHD and GVL by regulating allogeneic T cell dose have met with limited success. For example, administration of 1×10^5 T cells/kg after HLA-matched sibling transplantation did not mediate GVL effects and yet was associated with a measurable incidence of GVHD. Thus infusion of adequate numbers of donor T cell effectors is crucial for GVL responses.[386] This has been demonstrated by durable responses that are observed in CML and other malignancies after donor leukocyte infusion (DLI, see later) despite the experimental evidence that host APCs stimulate a stronger GVL response than donor APCs.[52,383] The lack of immunosuppression after DLI increases the likelihood of a GVH response, and DLI are almost always associated with clinical GVHD. The delivery of additional allogeneic effector cells in DLI also increases the effector: target ratio compared to the time of initial HCT. This is underscored by a more effective GVL response to DLI against minimal residual disease (bcr-abl positivity by PCR) compared to the response against high leukemic burden (e.g., blast crisis) in CML patients.[383] Thus DLI provides the proof in principle for the concepts that sufficient T cell numbers and appropriate antigen presentation are required for both GVHD and an effective GVL response.

T-Cell Subsets

Most experimental studies have implicated donor CD8⁺ T cells as the primary mediators of GVL, but there are no clinical data for CD8⁺ mediated GVL responses in the absence of CD4 T cells.[185,359,383] Moreover, some clinical data suggest a role for greater CD4 mediated GVL responses without an increase in GVHD after allogeneic HCT and DLI.[380,387–390] But it is unclear whether CD4⁺ T-cell–initiated GVL responses occur in the absence of generation of MiHA specific CD8⁺ T cells. Given the critical requirement of alloantigens for most GVL responses, the specific requirement of either CD4 and/or CD8 T cells for GVL and GVHD is likely to be determined by the expression of the relevant immunodominant MiHAs and/or tumor associated proteins. Therefore it is unlikely that GVHD and GVL responses can be separated under all circumstances merely by depletion of either subset of alloreactive T cells. However, experimental data suggest it might be possible to separate GVHD and GVL when certain donor T cell subsets are either depleted or infused (DLI) at the appropriate interval after transplant.[380] But the optimal interval for such infusions has not been identified.

Because of recent identification and understanding of the role of various T cell subsets in mediating immune responses, depletion of specific T cell subsets to separate GVHD and GVL remains an area of active investigation. For example, recent experimental data suggest that CD62L expressing naïve T cells home to secondary lymph nodes and are critical for initiating GVHD.[93] By contrast, CD62L negative effector memory T cells with enhanced reactivity to recall antigens mediated GVL responses with minimal GVHD.[93] An important caveat to these data is that the lack of *a priori* knowledge of the repertoire of human memory T cells would make it difficult to predict if these cells might cross-react only with tumor associated antigens and/or with recipient's alloantigens. Using CD62L status alone as determinant of GVHD potential can also have other unintended consequences as recent studies have demonstrated that its expression is critical for the regulation of GVHD by Tregs (see later). Moreover it is not known whether the behavior of human memory T cells parallels that of murine memory T cells in their migratory, functional and cytolytic capabilities. Although Tregs reduce antitumor immunity in murine models and in human subjects experimental data suggest that administration of donor type Tregs either at the time of HCT or when delayed reduced GVHD but preserved CD8⁺ mediated perforin dependent GVL responses.[109,391] Similar preservation of experimental GVL was also observed by harnessing donor NKT function with GCSF analogues.[116,117] However, whether these observations are valid after clinical HCT when the GVL responses might not be entirely dependent on CD8 T cells remains unclear.

T-Cell Migration

It is conceivable that manipulation of these interactions to focus the alloimmune response to lymphohematopoietic tissues would enhance GVL responses but not GVHD. For example, blockade of CCR9 ligand TECK or CCR5, and CCL17 may prevent the migration of donor T cells to GI tract and skin respectively, but preserve GVL.[170] Pharmacologic manipulation with the immunosuppressive agent FTY720 has recently provided the proof in principle for this approach.[180] Given the redundancy, strategies to modulate the chemokine biology for separation of GVHD and GVL will require greater understanding of these networks in modulating the migration of not only specific T cell subsets but also of the other immune cells in the context of different conditioning regimens.

Phase 3: Effector Phase of Graft Versus Leukemia

The effector arm of GVL is also characterized primarily by the antigen specific cellular and less by the inflammatory components of alloresponse. Experimental data demonstrate that neutralization of IL-1-a reduced GVHD preserved GVL.[281] By contrast donor TNF-α secretion contributes to both GVHD and GVL effects and in some cases, antagonism of TNF-α, reduced GVHD and GVL responses.[224,392,393] Nonetheless antagonism of non-specific inflammatory effectors such as either IL-1 or TNF-α appears to regulate GVHD to a greater extent than GVL responses after experimental allogeneic HCT.[393]

Several lines of experimental and clinical data demonstrate that antigen specific donor T cell subsets and NK cells are the key effectors of GVL.[359] The cytotoxic pathways that are operative in the NK and T cell mediated antitumor responses have been well characterized.[359] Fas ligand mediated CTL of tumor targets is utilized by both NK and T (mostly Th1) cells. But most murine experiments with FasL deficient donor T cells suggested that FasL is a key effector molecule for causing GVHD but not for GVL.[185] However one study found that FasL is required for CD4+ mediated GVL against myeloid leukemia.[394,395] By contrast, even though perforin mediated CTL pathways are also utilized by T (mostly Th2) and NK cells, experimental data with perforin deficient donor T cells demonstrated a loss of GVL with a diminution in the severity of GVHD.[185] In some other experimental models, perforin was required only for GVL but not GVHD.[185] Recent data showed that TRAIL mediated CTL had no effect on GVHD severity but was required for optimal GVL.[209] Therefore strategies that increase donor T cell TRAIL expression or enhance the susceptibility of tumors to TRAIL mediated CTL (such as HDAC inhibitors) may promote a robust GVL effect without exacerbating GVHD.[396–398] Thus significant progress has been made in recent understanding of the CTL pathways employed by donor T cells for GVL responses, but, the role and context of utilization of these pathways by donor NK and NKT cells after allogeneic HCT are not known.

DONOR LEUKOCYTE INFUSIONS

Until recently the evidence for an important GVL effect in clinical transplantation was strong but largely circumstantial. The use of donor leukocyte infusion (DLI) to treat relapses after allogeneic HCT has now provided direct evidence of the GVL effect.[399–401] Kolb et al. first reported three patients with relapsed CML who achieved complete cytogenetic remission after treatment with IFN-α and DLI from the original donors.[402] Subsequently these findings have been confirmed in several reports.[403–405] Two large retrospective studies of DLI have been reported from Europe and North America.[401,406] Although the treatment protocols varied slightly among institutions, the results have been remarkably consistent. When results from these trials are combined, the complete remission rate for patients treated for relapsed CML is consistently 60–80%.[399] In many patients with CML the response to DLI is not immediate. The average time to obtain a molecular remission is between 4 to 6 months but disease free survival after DLI depends on the stage of CML.[407,408] Complete cytogenetic and molecular responses are achieved in almost 80% of patients treated with either early relapse (cytogenetic or molecular) or hematologic relapse of chronic phase.[336] Patients with more advanced CML (accelerated phase or blast crisis) are less likely to respond. Two recent analyses suggest that the outcome after unrelated DLI is similar to matched sibling DLI in CML patients.[401,406]

DLI has also produced remissions in acute leukemias. Several retrospective studies have reported response rates in AML ranging from 20–65%.[336,406,409–411] A prospective study of 65 patients with advanced myeloid leukemia who received cytarabine and GCSF primed DLI showed that 47% of the patients achieved complete remission with an overall survival of 19% at two years.[412] A recent EBMT analysis of DLI in patients with relapsed AML showed a response rate of 41% that did not change if chemotherapy was used prior to DLI.[413] Generally, DLI produces lower response rates and higher relapse rates in patients with AML than with CML.[336,383,406,409–411] Extramedullary relapses at multiple regions that are usually not considered sanctuary sites for leukemia have been observed after DLI.[411]

Although GVL responses to ALL after allogeneic HCT have been noted, DLI for ALL has generally been ineffective.[414] Reports both from Europe and from America found little benefit for DLI in ALL patients.[383,406,409,410] Furthermore Ruggeri et al found that following TCD haploidentical HCT where the donors had antirecipient NK cells, the probability of relapse was 85% for ALL in contrast to 0% for AML.[367,415]

The experience with DLI for other hematologic malignancies such as NHL and multiple myeloma is much more limited. Case reports and small series demonstrate responses to DLI in patients with posttransplant relapses of low-grade lymphoma and CLL and also after low-intensity HCT.[416,417] In multiple myeloma, complete responses to DLI were observed in 25% of the patients in two small series.[383,418,419] DLI has also been shown to induce complete remission in a majority of patients with posttransplant lymphoproliferative disorders (PTLD) after allogeneic HCT.[403,420] Viral infections may be treatable with DLI, and adoptive immune therapy with T cells specific for EBV and CMV have been shown to both treat and prevent these complications.[421–425]

Complications of Donor Leukocyte Infusion

Adoptive immunotherapy with DLI causes significant morbidity. The major complications are myelosuppression and GVHD. Myelosuppression with anemia/ thrombocytopenia/leukopenia or pancytopenia occurs in 34% of the patients.[408] Marrow aplasia presumably results from the destruction of host leukemia cells before recovery of normal donor hematopoiesis. This idea is supported by the observation that patients treated with donor mononuclear cell infusions for cytogenetic or molecular relapse rarely experience pancytopenia.[401] Occasionally, marrow aplasia has been persistent,[403,404,426] although this toxicity has been successfully reversed with the infusion of additional donor stem cells in some patients.[403,404] If pancytopenia is associated with chronic GVHD then immunosuppression might be the most appropriate therapy.[427] Acute and chronic GVHD have been the major direct complications from DLI. In retrospective and prospective studies, acute or chronic GVHD has been reported in 40% to 60% of patients (see Fig. 107–1). In most studies, GVHD correlates with GVL activity and response.[401,406] In the North American analysis, over 90% of complete responders developed acute GVHD and 88% of responders developed chronic GVHD. Of 23 patients who did not experience GVHD, only 3 achieved a complete remission. In 92 patients who had no response, only 35% had acute GHVD and only 13% had chronic GVHD. In the EBMT analysis, 41% of DLI recipients developed grade II–IV acute GVHD.[401] It should be noted, however, that many patients who fail to respond to GVL induction will die shortly of progressive disease and may not survive long enough for GVHD to develop. This is particularly important for patients with acute leukemia. It is also important to emphasize that a number of complete responses were seen in patients without any sign of GVHD. The GVL effect in the absence of clinical GVHD provides important evidence for GVL activity separate from GVHD.

In general, GVHD that occurs after DLI has been mild to moderate and has been responsive to immunosuppressive therapy. This observation is important because the dose of T cells often administered with DLI may be 10- to 100-fold higher than the T-cell dose administered at the time of transplant, and DLI is given without additional immunosuppression. At the time of transplant, if immunosuppression is withheld or a similar dose of donor T cells are given as are used for DLI (to augment GVL), toxicity is unacceptable.[428,429] This may be because the effects of GVHD are more tolerable when separated from the acute transplant toxicity. GVHD can be stimulated and exacerbated by the "cytokine storm" that can accompany transplantation. Tissue damage from the intensive conditioning regimen, infections, and other physiological insults result in a cascade of events that ultimately augment the GVHD reaction.[235] When GVHD is induced independent of other transplant-related toxicity, it may be more manageable with appropriate immunosuppression. Nevertheless, in some cases DLI-induced GVHD may be quite severe; as shown in Table 107–1, 20% to 35% of DLI recipients can be anticipated to develop grade III–IV acute GVHD. Furthermore, acute GVHD has contributed to death in almost 10% of patients.[430] Chronic GVHD occurs in 30% to 60% of recipients of unmanipulated DLI.

It is notable that the clinical presentation of GVHD after DLI is somewhat different than after myeloablative allogeneic HCT. For instance, the onset of GVHD may be later after DLI. The median time to onset of acute GVHD is approximately 32 to 42 days[406,431] compared to a median time to onset of 16 to 20 days following myeloablative T-replete transplantation.[260,432] Therefore, not only can the severity of GVHD be influenced by the use of intensive conditioning, the tissue damage and inflammatory cytokine release may influence the pace of GVHD development as well. This possibility is supported by the finding that time to onset of acute GVHD is also delayed following reduced-intensity transplantation.[433] The target organs of acute GVHD following DLI are the same as those seen following HCT, but the clinical manifestations may differ. A hepatitic variant of liver GVHD characterized by marked elevations of serum aminotransferase levels more than 10 times the upper limit of normal was observed in 11/73 (15%) patients who received DLI at Johns Hopkins University.[273] Characteristic skin, liver, and intestinal acute GVHD manifestations can be seen following DLI, but their frequency and severity has not been well described. In a study of 81 patients who received DLI for relapse, mixed chimerism, or prophylaxis following reduced-intensity HCT, skin, liver, and intestinal GVHD developed in 26%, 8%, and 14%, respectively.[434] Likewise, characteristic findings of chronic GVHD can be seen following DLI,[434] and on occasion both acute and chronic GVHD can develop simultaneously following DLI.[435]

In recent years, DLI has been utilized in the context of reduced-intensity allogeneic HCT. When conditioning is minimal and GVHD has not already occurred, DLI is often required to either reverse mixed chimerism or treat persistent disease.[434,436,437] GVHD after DLI following nonmyeloablative setting develops 19% to 45% of the time, whereas chronic GVHD develops 28% to 34% of the time. In two studies of a combined 134 subjects who received DLI after reduced-intensity transplantation, 37 (28%) patients developed acute GVHD, 15 (11%) developed grade 3–4 GVHD, and 8 (6%) died from GVHD.[434,436] There was no statistically significant relationship between DLI dose and GVHD in either study. The clinical features of GVHD after DLI following reduced-intensity HCT are similar to the GVHD that occurs after DLI is used to treat relapse following myeloablative HCT. The similarity between GVHD after DLI in either setting suggests that the reduction of tissue damage associated with either no chemotherapy (as in DLI for relapse following prior myeloablative HCT) or reduced-dose chemotherapy (as in DLI after reduced-intensity HCT) may be an important common theme.

It is likely that effector cells responsible for the GVL and GVHD effects of HCT will similarly be responsible for the GVL effect associated with DLI, although this assumption has not been formally proven. The administration of select subsets of donor mononuclear cell fractions is the ideal setting in which to dissect the cellular mechanisms responsible for GVL induction, and strategies that delay the infusion of these various cellular subsets will help define the mechanisms and enhance the efficacy of DLI.

SUMMARY

Complications of HCT, particularly GVHD, remain major barriers to the wider application of allogeneic HCT for a variety of diseases. Recent advances in the understanding of genetic polymorphisms, the chemocytokine networks, several novel cellular subsets including regulatory T cells and of the direct mediators of cellular cytotoxicity have led to improved understanding of this complex disease process. Animal studies show that modulation of several mediators of the complex GVHD cascade may reduce the undesirable inflammatory aspects of GVHD while preserving the benefits of GVL. However, most of the laboratory observations remain to be studied in well-controlled clinical trials. Multiple cellular effectors may be involved in GVL, although donor T-cell recognition of host antigens is an important element of this process. Cellular immunotherapy such as DLI offers a strategy for separating GVHD and the GVL effect. Both experimental and clinical data suggest that posttransplantation cellular immunotherapy can be performed relatively safely and effectively, and optimization of patient selection, cell dose, and timing of administration may all serve to limit toxicity and enhance the potential GVL effects.

SUGGESTED READINGS

Bleakley M, Riddell SR. Molecules and mechanisms of the graft-versus-leukaemia effect. Nat Rev Cancer 4:371, 2004.

Filipovich AH, Weisdorf D, Pavletic S, et al: National Institutes of Health consensus development project on criteria for clinical trials in chronic graft-versus-host disease: I. Diagnosis and staging working group report. Biol Blood Marrow Transplant 11:945, 2005.

Holler E, Rogler G, Brenmoehl J, et al: Prognostic significance of NOD2/CARD15 variants in HLA-identical sibling hematopoietic stem cell transplantation: effect on long-term outcome is confirmed in 2 independent cohorts and may be modulated by the type of gastrointestinal decontamination. Blood 107:4189, 2006.

Kaplan DH, Anderson BE, McNiff JM, Jain D, Shlomchik MJ, Shlomchik WD. Target antigens determine graft-versus-host disease phenotype. J Immunol 173:5467, 2004.

Martin PJ, Weisdorf D, Przepiorka D, et al: National Institutes of Health Consensus Development Project on Criteria for Clinical Trials in Chronic Graft-versus-Host Disease: VI. Design of Clinical Trials Working Group report. Biol Blood Marrow Transplant 12:491, 2006.

Merad M, Hoffmann P, Ranheim E, et al: Depletion of host Langerhans cells before transplantation of donor alloreactive T cells prevents skin graft-versus-host disease. Nat Med 10:510, 2004.

Miller JS, Cooley S, Parham P, et al: Missing KIR-ligands are associated with less relapse and increased graft versus host disease (GVHD) following unrelated donor allogeneic HCT. Blood 109:2058, 2007.

Petersdorf EW. Immunogenomics of unrelated hematopoietic cell transplantation. Curr Opin Immunol 18:559, 2006.

Reddy P, Maeda Y, Liu C, Krijanovski OI, Korngold R, Ferrara JL. A crucial role for antigen-presenting cells and alloantigen expression in graft-versus-leukemia responses. Nat Med 11:1244, 2005.

Welniak LA, Blazar BR, Murphy WJ. Immunobiology of Allogeneic Hematopoietic Stem Cell Transplantation. Annu Rev Immunol 25:139, 2006.

Yilmaz OH, Valdez R, Theisen BK, et al: Pten dependence distinguishes haematopoietic stem cells from leukaemia-initiating cells. Nature 441:475, 2006.

Zhang Y, Joe G, Hexner E, Zhu J, Emerson SG. Host-reactive CD8+ memory stem cells in graft-versus-host disease. Nat Med 11:1299, 2005.

REFERENCES

For complete list of references log onto www.expertconsult.com

CHAPTER 108

PRACTICAL ASPECTS OF STEM CELL COLLECTION

Scott D. Rowley and Michele L. Donato

Hematopoietic stem cell (HSC) products for autologous or allogeneic transplantation are available from bone marrow, peripheral blood, or umbilical cord blood (UCB) sources. Bone marrow was the original source of cells for transplantation because of the ease and reliability of collecting adequate numbers of cells for transplantation, and it remains the standard to which other sources of HSC are compared. Because of the relative immunologic naivete of the donor with the feasibility of multiple-antigen mismatched transplantation, UCB has found an important niche in the treatment of patients undergoing unrelated donor transplantation who lack an appropriate related or unrelated volunteer donor.[1] The primary limitations of UCB transplantation derive from the small cell dose collected, which can result in a longer time to hematologic recovery and a higher risk of primary engraftment failure. This same relative immunologic incompetence of the donor results in a greater risk of posttransplant opportunistic infections. Peripheral blood stem cells (PBSC) have virtually replaced bone marrow as the HSC component for autologous transplantation and are widely used for allogeneic transplantation. The rapid engraftment kinetics of PBSC compared to bone marrow are widely recognized. Median times to achieve an absolute neutrophil count greater than 500/μL and platelet transfusion independence after PBSC transplantation typically are approximately 11 to 14 days.[2–7] The improvement in engraftment kinetics reduces the cost of autologous transplantation (Table 108–1).[8–11] Although graft-versus-host disease (GVHD) prophylaxis with methotrexate will slow engraftment, the kinetics of engraftment for the allogeneic PBSC recipient is similar to that experienced by the autologous PBSC recipient.[12–18] A number of phase III studies involving either autologous or allogeneic HSC transplantation have confirmed the more rapid engraftment kinetics for recipients of PBSC (Table 108–2).[19–25] This effect is not limited to HSC collected from the peripheral blood because cytokine administration to the patient or donor before marrow harvesting will also increase the number of HSC collected and result in quicker hematologic recovery (Table 108–2).[26–30] The disadvantages to use of PBSC components compared to bone marrow or UCB for autologous or allogeneic transplantation include the usual need for multiple days of collection (especially for autologous transplantation), the inability to collect adequate components from all patients and donors, and a possibly higher risk for GVHD or the occurrence of GVHD that is more difficult to control.[31–33]

COLLECTION OF BONE MARROW FOR TRANSPLANTATION

Background

Most bone marrow products are collected from the posterior iliac crests using virtually the same techniques used to obtain diagnostic samples in the clinic as originally described by Thomas and Storb.[34] The primary differences between obtaining diagnostic specimens and cell quantities adequate for transplantation are the volume of blood and marrow removed, which requires attention to fluid replacement during the procedure and the need for appropriate anesthesia. Bone marrow harvesting from healthy donors presents little risk of serious morbidity, permitting the ethical recruitment of allogeneic donors including unrelated and pediatric bone marrow donors.[35,36]

Bone Marrow Collection Techniques

Bone marrow typically is harvested from the posterior iliac crests. Multiple aspirations are performed with collection of approximately 5 mL of marrow from each puncture site. If properly spaced, no more than two to three skin puncture sites per side usually are required. Other harvest sites, such as the anterior iliac crests or sternum, can be used, but at increased risk of complications from accidental laceration or perforation of contiguous anatomic structures. Extending the harvest to the anterior crests or sternum is unusual, used for less than 10% of patients undergoing autologous collections[37] and much less commonly for volunteer donors. For patients with a history of radiation or tumor involvement of one pelvic crest, adequate cells can be harvested from the anterior and posterior crests of the other side.

Marrow is collected in the day surgery suite using either general or regional anesthesia.[37] With proper fluid and blood replacement, overnight hospitalization should not be required. For the healthy donor, the risks of serious complications from either general or regional anesthesia are about the same. Spinal or epidural anesthesia avoid the nausea that may occur with general anesthesia, especially for young women, but hypotension from loss of vascular tone in the lower extremities often occurs as the volume of marrow is collected. General anesthesia is preferable for the donor with comorbid disorders such as cardiovascular or cerebral vascular disease because of the better control of donor airway and lower risk of hypotension during the harvest procedures. Local anesthesia is acceptable only if a very limited harvest is being performed, as large quantities of lidocaine are cardiotoxic and local anesthesia does not achieve anesthesia of the marrow space. The operating room is an intensive care unit, which is preferable to blood stem cell harvesting in an outpatient apheresis unit for the patient with serious comorbid illnesses.

Evaluation of Bone Marrow Donors

Anesthesia and blood loss present the greatest risks of serious complications, and patients and donors must undergo a thorough medical examination. Most marrow harvesting is performed under general anesthesia, which requires intubation for control of the airway for a surgical procedure performed on a prone patient. Regional (spinal or epidural) anesthesia may not be effectively established, so patients and donors who express a preference for this anesthesia must be counseled about the potential need for general anesthesia. The health assessment must include questioning about a history of joint disease of the cervical spine and mandible and examination of the mouth if general anesthesia requiring intubation is chosen. Patients and donors with comorbid conditions, such as aortic stenosis sensitive to changes in blood volume and blood pressure, may require anesthesia consultation and plans for invasive monitoring during the surgical procedure. A history of marrow fibrosis, pelvic irradiation, or pelvic tumor involvement may exclude a patient from marrow harvesting.

Table 108–1 Costs of Autologous Transplantation by Source of Hematopoietic Stem Cell

Study	No. of Patients		Days to Engraftment: *ANC >500/uL*	Days to Engraftment: *Platelet >20,000/uL*	Hospital Stay (Days)	Costs
Hartmann et al.[8]	BM	65	12	36.5[a]	31	$28,429
	PBSC	64	8	17.5	24	$23,591
Smith et al.[9]	BM	31	14	23	23	$59,314
	PBSC	27	11	16	17	$45,792
Vellenga et al.[10]	BM	42	26	18	34	$17,668
	PBSC	76	15	13	27	$13,954
van Agthoven et al.[11]	BM	29	15	18	34	€19000
	PBSC	62	10	13	27	€15008

[a]Days to platelet count > 50,000.
ANC, absolute neutrophil count; BM, bone marrow; PBSC, peripheral blood stem cell.

Table 108–2 Randomized Studies Comparing Marrow and PBSC as HSC sources[a]

	No. of Patients		CD34+ Cell Dose		ANC >500/μL			Platelet >20,000/μL			Acute Graft-Versus-Host Disease		
	BM	*PBSC*	*BM*	*PBSC*	*BM*	*PBSC*	*P Value*	*BM*	*PBSC*	*P Value*	*BM*	*PBSC*	*P Value*
Allogeneic BM vs PBSC													
Blaise et al.[19]	52	48	2.4	6.6	21	15	<0.001	21[a]	13[a]	<0.001	42%	44%	NS
Bensinger et al.[20]	91	81	2.4	7.3	21	16	<0.001	19	13	<0.001	57%	64%	0.35
Couban et al.[21]	118	109	2.4	6.7	23	19	<0.001	22	16	<0.001	44%	44%	>0.9
Schmitz et al.[22]	116	163	2.7	5.8	15	12	<0.001	20	15	<0.001	39%	52%	0.013
G-BM vs PBSC													
Morton et al.[27]	28	29	2.6	7.2	16	14	<0.1	14	12	<0.1	52%	54%	<0.6
Autologous BM vs PBSC													
Beyer et al.[23]	23	24	2.5[a]	13.1[a]	11	10	<0.01	17	10	<0.01			
Schmitz et al.[24]	31	27	Not stated	2.8	14	11	0.005	23	16	0.02			
Hartmann et al.[25]	65	64	Not stated	92.7[a]	12	8	<0.001	27[a]	12[a]	<0.001			
G-BM vs PBSC													
Damiani et al.[29]	36	19	0.6	3.3	12	11	0.22	13	11	0.24			

[a]Shown are number of patients enrolled in each arm of the study, quantity of CD34+ cells × 10^6/kg (CFU-GM × 10^4/kg for reports by Beyer and Hartman), days after transplantation to achieve a peripheral blood absolute neutrophil count >500/μL and platelet count >20,000/μL (25,000/μL for report by Blaise and 30,000/μL for report by Hartmann), and percentage of patients developing acute graft-versus-host disease.
ANC, absolute neutrophil count; BM, bone marrow, G-BM, granulocyte colony-stimulating factor–stimulated bone marrow, PBSC, peripheral blood stem cell.

Patients undergoing autologous bone marrow collection and transplantation are not at risk for transmitting disease to themselves, but the laboratory must be notified of the infectious disease status of the patient because some viruses can cross-contaminate other products stored in the liquid phase of nitrogen. All allogeneic bone marrow (and PBSC) donors must be evaluated using the criteria currently applied to blood donors, including a targeted history regarding behaviors exposing the donor to virus infection, recent and concurrent illnesses, and medication use.[38,39] Some groups advocate age-specific screening for all donors because of the higher risk of malignant diseases in older donors.[40,41] Numerous infectious diseases that would not exclude the donor from blood donation, such as cytomegalovirus, may be transmitted with the allograft.[42] However, donors who otherwise would be excluded for health reasons from donating blood for transfusion (e.g., individuals with a history of hepatitis) still may be selected to donate bone marrow if the needs of the recipient outweigh the risks and consequences of disease transmission. Guidelines regarding the management of patients and donors with hepatitis virus infection have been published.[43] Procedures involving donors with acute infectious illnesses should be delayed, if at all possible, because of the risk of disease transmission.[44] Hematopoietic disorders, such as hemoglobinopathies, will be transmitted to the recipient as a direct consequence of stem cell engraftment. Cancer can be transmitted, as illustrated by the transmission of donor leukemia not detected during initial evaluation of the donor.[45] The United States Food and Drug administration has not established donor health criteria for bone marrow donors, but criteria for PBSC donors can be applied to the marrow donor. Criteria for donor selection are established by the National Marrow Donor Program for evaluation and selection of unrelated donors and by volunteer accreditation programs such as the Foundation for Accreditation of Cellular Therapies and the American Association of Blood Banks. Use of a donor who does not meet eligibility criteria and poses a risk for transmission of disease requires appropriate informed consent both from the donor (to allow disclosure of this confidential health information and counseling of the recipient) and from the recipient (for use of the stem cell product).

Toxicity of Bone Marrow Collection

Anesthesia complications present the major health risk to the donor; marrow aspiration is generally well tolerated. Major complications occur in approximately 0.27% of healthy allogeneic donors[46] and up to 0.97% of autologous transplant patients.[47] Complications include hemorrhage and infections at skin puncture sites. Severe hematomas and neuralgias rarely occur, but attention to pelvic anatomy is required to decrease the risk of damage to vessels and nerves lying under or adjacent to the iliac crest harvest sites. Irritation of the sacral nerves may result from needle penetration through the pelvic bone or from blood tracking into the nerve roots and requires several months of convalescence. Localized pain is common, may last for several days, and may require a brief period of medication with opioid/acetaminophen combinations.[48] In a survey of almost 500 donors for unrelated marrow transplantation, the average time for recovery was 15.8 days, although 10% of donors required more than 30 days for self-reported complete recovery.[35] Most donors are able to return to routine activities 1 to 2 days after harvesting. In a study of related donors, an equivalent level of pain was reported by donors undergoing bone marrow harvesting and those receiving filgrastim for mobilization of PBSC.[49]

The usual volume harvested from healthy donors is approximately 10 to 15 mL of marrow per kilogram of recipient body weight to achieve the desired nucleated cell and CD34$^+$ cell doses. This results in an average blood loss of 800 to 1000 mL for donors providing for an adult recipient. The quantity of marrow harvested from autologous patients may be greater, reflecting previous chemotherapy given to these patients. Donors for pediatric recipients will lose proportionately less blood. Most patients and donors receive blood transfusions to alleviate symptoms of volume depletion. With proper preharvest autologous blood storage, use of homologous blood for healthy allogeneic donors should be extremely rare. For a blood loss of less than 10 mL/kg of donor weight, salt solutions are acceptable replacement. Colloid solutions, such as hydroxyethyl starch, also can be used to avoid homologous blood transfusion. Homologous blood transfusions must be irradiated to prevent transfusion-associated GVHD in the recipient. Donors undergoing second harvest shortly after the first harvest are more likely to require homologous blood.[50] Oral iron supplements should be considered for healthy donors.

Quantity of Bone Marrow Cells for Transplantation

Cell dose normally is used as a surrogate for the stem cell content of the marrow product because the definition of adequate HSC products predated the availability of flow cytometric analysis of HSC content, and nucleated cell counting is the only quality control measure easily performed during the collection procedure. For autologous transplantation, cell doses of 1×10^8 nucleated cells per kilogram are adequate. Based on early reports that smaller quantities increased the risk of engraftment failure, most centers target 3×10^8 nucleated cells per kilogram of recipient weight for allogeneic transplantation.[51] However, those early reports were of patients being treated for aplastic anemia, in which engraftment failure is a more common event. A study of 100 patients who received allogeneic transplantation for treatment of acute leukemia found that cell dose per kilogram of recipient body weight (range $0.5–13.0 \times 10^8$) did not predict the likelihood of successful engraftment.[52] A review of unrelated donor transplantation found that recipients of higher cell doses experienced faster neutrophil and platelet engraftment as well as better leukemia-free survival.[53] Pretreatment of the marrow donor with either sargramostim (granulocyte-macrophage colony-stimulating factor [GM-CSF]) or filgrastim (granulocyte-macrophage colony-stimulating factor [G-CSF]) may increase the number of myeloid progenitor cells harvested and decrease the period of post-transplant aplasia to that achievable by PBSC transplantation (see Table 108–2).[54] CD34$^+$ cell dose now is being correlated with transplant outcomes, with more rapid engraftment kinetics, possibly lower transplant-related mortality, and better overall survival, for example, in recipients of allogeneic products containing higher quantities of CD34$^+$ cells. This assay should be a routine component of bone marrow product quality control.[55–57]

COLLECTION OF UMBILICAL CORD BLOOD STEM CELLS FOR TRANSPLANTATION

Cord Blood Collection Techniques

UCB is collected from the placental vein after delivery of the infant and transection of the cord. UCB can be collected before delivery of the placenta by the obstetrician or by laboratory personnel after delivery of the placenta. Published reports conflict regarding the volume of UCB collected and the likelihood of obtaining a product inadequate for storage with either in utero or ex utero collection.[58–60] The timing of cord clamping after delivery of the infant is associated with the volume of cord blood collected. Greater volumes are collected with earlier clamping. UCB usually is collected by cannulation of the umbilical cord veins. Collection of cord blood into open containers has an unacceptable 12.5% rate of bacterial contamination,[61] and the collection techniques should be viewed as the first step in a manufacturing process with adequate quality control and improvement. However, successful "remote site" collection is feasible for parents intending to collect cells for family use.[62]

Many cord blood units are discarded because of small cell doses.[63] Investigators from the Madrid UCB Bank found that perfusion of the placenta with 50 mL of saline increased the numbers of nucleated cells collected from approximately 1×10^9 to 1.26×10^9, an increase of 15%.[64] A 36% increase was achieved by limiting the processing to UCB units of at least 0.8×10^9 nucleated cells, resulting in an average cell content of $1.46 \pm 0.52 \times 10^9$ nucleated cells. A pressure device applied to the placenta increased the yield of blood by an additional 14.3 ± 7.8 ml ($26.5\% \pm 15.1\%$).[65] Although an increase in nucleated cells was not observed, the later fractions contained increased proportions of CD34$^+$ cells, including CD34$^+$CD38$^-$ cells, which is considered a more immature phenotype. Whether perfusion of the placenta with cytokines or chemokines will affect the numbers or types of cells that can be collected for transplantation has not been reported.

Quantity of Cord Blood Cells for Transplantation

Cell dose is an important predictor of outcome after UCB transplantation. The importance of cell dose to transplant outcome is discussed in Chapter 106. Two studies of cell quantities in approximately 8000 and 1000 UCB units, respectively, found strong correlations between nucleated blood cells, colony-forming unit granulocyte-macrophage (CFU-GM), and CD34$^+$ cells contents.[66,67] Greater cell quantities were found for infants with greater birth weight, but no difference was found based on gender or gestational age. Ethnic background is important, with smaller quantities of cells collected from ethnic minorities compared to Caucasian ethnicity.[68] Many cord blood banks volume reduce the product by red cell and plasma depletion to minimize storage space for the many units to be stored and reduce possible infusion-related toxicities from mature blood cells contained in unfractioned cord blood units.[69] UCB will maintain viability for periods of at least 15 years if appropriately cryopreserved.[70]

COLLECTION OF PERIPHERAL BLOOD STEM CELLS FOR TRANSPLANTATION

Background

The presence of HSC in the peripheral circulation was suggested by animal studies as early as 1951.[71] Although the nature of the survival agent was not recognized at that time, parabiosis experiments dem-

Table 108–3 Relationship Among Mobilization Therapy, Dose of Progenitor Cells, and Engraftment Kinetics for Autologous Peripheral Blood Stem Cell Transplantation

			Progenitor Cell Dose		Engraftment Kinetics	
Author	**No. of Patients**	**Mobilization Therapy**	***CFU-GM (×10⁴/kg)***	***CD34⁺ (×10⁶/kg)***	***ANC >500/μL***	***Platelet >20,000/μL***
To et al.[6]	43	Chemotherapy	86.6	ND	11 (9–17)	13.5[a] (9–NR)
Fermand et al.[76]	8	Chemotherapy	5.5	ND	16 (10–25)	34 (10–90)
Juttner et al.[75]	8	Chemotherapy	127.2	ND	11 (9–14)	12[a] (10–28)
Kessinger et al.[78]	10	Steady-state	8.0[b]	ND	22 (11–58)	23 (14–36)
Nademanee et al.[84]	30	Steady-state	ND	1.2	20 (9–458)	31 (8–441)
Nademanee et al.[84]	39	G-CSF	ND	6.2	10 (7–40)	15.5 (7–63)
Sheridan et al.[5]	29	G-CSF	21.0	ND	6 (4–10)	11 (9–136)
Weaver et al.[90]	692	Chemotherapy + G-CSF	30.8[c]	9.9[c]	9 (5–38)	9 (4–53)[a]
Bensinger et al.[89]	124	Chemotherapy + G-CSF	ND	9.4	11 (4–20)	10 (6–65)

Shown are mean values for progenitor cell quantities infused and median times to achieve the particular endpoint of engraftment.
[a]Time to achieve >50,000 platelets/μL.
[b]Colony-forming unit granulocyte-macrophage (CFU-GM) cultures performed on thawed cells.
[c]Median value.
ANC, absolute neutrophil count; G-CSF, granulocyte colony-stimulating factor; ND, not measured; NR, not reached.

onstrated that some factor in the blood of a healthy animal was able to rescue another animal from the effects of lethal irradiation. Subsequently, a number of animal models demonstrated the presence of HSC in the peripheral blood and the use of these cells to rescue animals from the marrow-lethal effects of radiation.[72,73] Experience in human PBSC transplantation began for patients with chronic myelogenous leukemia because of the high number of clonogenic cells circulating in the peripheral blood of those patients.[74] The concentration of HSC in the peripheral blood normally is very low. Thus, very large quantities of blood must be processed to collect a quantity of HSC equivalent to what could be collected in a bone marrow harvest. For this reason, PBSC transplantation initially was limited to a few centers that explored this source of HSC for patients who otherwise were ineligible for marrow harvesting. Some transplant centers used the transient increase in circulating HSC during recovery from marrow hypoplasia-producing chemotherapy.[75–77] Other centers collected cells from the patient or donor without any preceding perturbation of the host.[78–80] These early reports noted that engraftment could be faster after infusion of PBSC components compared to marrow cell transplantation. However, because of the occasionally limited quantity of HSC that was collected from the peripheral blood, the kinetics of engraftment for some patients was considerably slower (Table 108–3). Moreover, the desired quantity of cells could not be collected from a significant proportion of patients. The effective mobilization of HSC into the peripheral blood and the reliability of flow cytometric technique in assessing within hours the quality of the collection are the direct bases for the rapid and widespread adoption of PBSC as a source of HSC for transplantation.

Mobilization of Hematopoietic Stem Cells into Peripheral Blood

The discovery that administration of hematopoietic cytokines caused a transient increase (mobilization) of HSC in the peripheral blood enabled the collection of much greater numbers of PBSC for transplantation or to ensure quick recovery after repetitive cycles of nonmarrow-ablative chemotherapy.[2,81–83] No randomized studies comparing the engraftment of cytokine-mobilized HSC to those collected during steady state or after chemotherapy mobilization have been reported, although retrospective studies demonstrated much quicker engraftment of cytokine-mobilized HSC (see Table 108–3).[84] Cytokine-mobilized PBSC components contain much greater numbers of cells expressing the CD34 antigen ($CD34^+$ cells) that, along with myeloid progenitor cells grown in culture (CFU-GM), serve as surrogate markers for the engraftment capacity of the stem cell component. Whether it is merely the quantity of cells or some other characteristic imparted by chemotherapy or cytokine mobilization that accounts for the rapid engraftment cannot be stated with certainty. $CD34^+$ cells isolated from the peripheral blood have many characteristics different from those isolated from marrow,[85] and effective mobilization requires both an expansion in the number of cells as well as release of these cells from the marrow compartment. The mechanisms involved in mobilization of HSC into the peripheral blood with cytokine or chemokine administration are only now being elucidated.[86,87] Multiple adhesion molecules appear involved in the homing and tethering of HSC in the bone marrow. Disruption of stromal cell-derived factor-1 (SDF-1) and CXCR4 interaction appears to be a critical step in HSC mobilization by G-CSF (and new chemokine agents currently in development); proteinases released by neutrophils are one possible cause. The diversity of mobilizing agents, including chemotherapy, cytokines, and some chemokines, suggests a common mechanism of action despite the distinct targets of these agents.[88] However, the dose of $CD34^+$ cells infused predicts the kinetics of engraftment. Patient groups that receive higher quantities show a higher probability of quicker recovery of neutrophil and platelet counts.[89,90] Although most transplant centers probably will accept components containing at least 1×10^6 to 2×10^6 $CD34^+$ cells per kilogram of recipient weight, cell doses of 2.5×10^6 to 5×10^6 $CD34^+$ cells per kilogram are desirable, and quicker engraftment will be observed with even higher doses.[89,90] Administration of G-CSF after transplantation will further speed the recovery of granulocytes[91–93] but may have a detrimental affect on platelet engraftment in patients receiving components containing low numbers of $CD34^+$ cells.[89]

A variety of mobilization schemes have been developed for both patients and donors. Before the availability of hematopoietic cytokines, marrow hypoplasia-producing chemotherapy, such as that used as induction therapy for acute leukemia, was noted to result in a transient increase in the number of HSC circulating in the peripheral blood. A variety of transplant programs used this approach to obtain PBSC for patients with leukemia or other diagnoses. Juttner et al.[75] demonstrated rapid engraftment in patients receiving chemotherapy-mobilized PBSC (median 11 and 12 days to achieve an absolute neutrophil count ANC >500/μL and platelet count >50,000/μL) as long as the dose of CFU-GM exceeded 63.0×10^4/kg. The finding that the quantity of CFU-GM infused roughly correlated with the speed or success of engraftment was also found by Fermand et al.[76] for chemotherapy-mobilized patients with multiple myeloma and by Brice et al.[77] for patients with non-Hodgkin lymphoma and Hodgkin lymphoma. However, Juttner et al.[75] also described a proportion of patients who received low doses of CFU-GM and experienced prolonged posttransplant aplasias or a secondary drop in blood counts 3 to 4 weeks after infusion. Moreover, some patients, mostly those with progressive disease, marrow infiltration, or extensive prior exposure to alkylating agents or radiation therapy, failed to exhibit this response to chemotherapy and had inadequate collections for transplantation.[77,94] The timing of apheresis was considered crucial, with maximal numbers of CFU-GM in the peripheral blood when leukocyte and platelet counts rose simultaneously during early recovery from chemotherapy.[95,96]

Administration of GM-CSF or G-CSF during recovery from chemotherapy subsequently was discovered to increase the numbers of circulating progenitor cells as much as 1000-fold higher than the level in the blood before treatment.[2,81–83] This finding started the exploration of efficacious mobilization regimens using hematopoietic cytokines, cytokine combinations, chemotherapy plus cytokines, or chemokines alone or in combination with cytokines.

Cytokine Mobilization

The ability of recombinant hematopoietic cytokines to increase the level of myeloid progenitor cells in the blood as well as mature blood cells was reported in 1988 by different groups for both G-CSF and GM-CSF.[82,83] Subsequently, a number of different investigators reported the collection of PBSC from patients after chemotherapy and GM-CSF or G-CSF mobilization.[4,81,97,98] Chemotherapy is not required to increase the numbers of HSC in the peripheral blood, and many patients and all donors are treated with hematopoietic cytokines alone. Various recombinant human hematopoietic cytokines, including fusion molecules, increase the quantity of CD34+ cells in the peripheral blood (see Other Hematopoietic Cytokines below). few studies have directly compared cytokines with regard to their ability to mobilize CD34+ cells. Furthermore, many of the single-arm cytokine studies were conducted in patient groups, and the effects of prior therapy on HSC mobilization is a confounding variable that hinders the comparison of these phase II studies.

Granulocyte Colony-Stimulating Factor

G-CSF is the cytokine most commonly used because of its efficacy compared to other cytokines and its relatively benign toxicity profile. Recombinant methionyl human G-CSF (filgrastim) and recombinant human G-CSF (lenograstim) are the two forms of this cytokine available for clinical use.[99] There is slight, if any, difference between these two cytokines in their ability to mobilize PBSC. Watts et al.[100] studied 20 healthy volunteers and found that peak levels of CFU-GM in the peripheral blood were 28% higher after treatment with the glycosylated molecule (lenograstim). Hogland et al.[101] found a similar comparative effect in 32 healthy male donors, with an average of 104 versus 82 CD34+ cells per microliter of blood ($P < 0.0010$) on the fifth day of administration of either drug at a dose of 10 μg/kg/day. The glycosylated molecule has a higher specific activity that may account for this difference. De Arriba et al.[102] treated 30 women with breast cancer in a randomized study of these two drugs using dosages containing bioequivalent units of activity and found no difference in mobilization of CD34+ cells. The two forms have otherwise similar biologic activity and are not further distinguished in this discussion.

Mobilization of Hematopoietic Stem Cells Using Granulocyte Colony-Stimulating Factor

G-CSF is the most potent cytokine currently available for mobilization of HSC. In a randomized study of healthy volunteers comparing G-CSF, GM-CSF, and the combination of both, Lane et al.[103] reported an average 0.99% CD34+ cells in the peripheral blood of healthy donors treated with 10 μg/kg/day of G-CSF compared to 0.25% for donors treated with the same dose of GM-CSF. The quantity of CD34+ cells in the peripheral blood before treatment averaged 1.6/μL. After GM-CSF treatment, the level increased to 3/μL, but with G-CSF, the level increased to 61/μL. Each group underwent one leukapheresis on the fifth day of treatment, and the collections from donors treated with G-CSF averaged 119 × 10^6 CD34+ cells compared to 12.6 × 10^6 for the donors treated with GM-CSF.

The appearance of CD34+ cells during administration of G-CSF follows a distinct time course, with the maximal level of CD34+ cells occurring on day 5 after daily G-CSF administration.[104,105] Smaller numbers of CD34+ are present on days 4 and 6, and the level falls rapidly on subsequent days despite a continual rise in white blood cell (WBC) count.

The number of CD34+ cells collected after G-CSF treatment is proportional to the number of these cells in the peripheral blood before initiation of the cytokine.[17] Although doses as low as 5 μg/kg/day have been used for allogeneic PBSC transplantation,[106] there is a dose response to G-CSF, with higher average levels of CD34+ cells achieved with 10 μg/kg/day compared to 5 μg/kg/day.[107] The average collection from one group of healthy donors treated with 10 μg/kg/day averaged 4 × 10^8 CD34+ cells.[107] With this dose of G-CSF and appropriate apheresis technique, adequate numbers of CD34+ cells can be collected in one procedure for transplantation of most patients. A similar dose response is observed in autologous patients and may extend to doses as high as 40 μg/kg/day.[108] Waller et al.[109] studied twice-daily administration of G-CSF to healthy donors and found greater yields of CD34+ cells in the apheresis component. However, the total amount of G-CSF administered also was doubled, so whether the twice-daily administration or the higher dose is responsible for this finding is not clear. Anderlini et al.[110] compared administration of 6 μg/kg given twice daily to 12 μg/kg given once daily and found no differences in CD34+ cells per liter of blood processed or the yield of CD34+ cells per kilogram collected. In contrast, a second trial enrolling primarily pediatric subjects noted better results with the twice-daily schedule.[111] Patients, especially those previously treated with chemotherapy or radiotherapy, will generally have lower quantities of CD34+ cells mobilized. However, previous treatment with chemotherapy does not preclude the use of G-CSF. De Luca et al.[112] noted a median 76-fold increase in CFU-GM in a population of 30 patients who previously had received extensive treatment for B-cell malignancies. Older donors have lower levels of CD34+ cells mobilized into the peripheral blood after G-CSF administration.[113]

Lymphocytes are also increased in the peripheral blood.[114] Murine studies suggest that G-CSF priming changes the cytokine response of these cells,[115] may decrease the risk of acute GVHD,[116] and may increase the graft-versus-leukemia effect.[117] The potential influence of these changes in outcome of allogeneic (or autologous) transplantation is not clear.

Toxicity and Complications of Granulocyte Colony-Stimulating Factor

The toxicity of G-CSF has been most clearly defined in studies of allogeneic donors.[106,107,118,119] The autologous patient will experience a similar toxicity profile, but with the added complications of the underlying malignancy and its treatment.

Almost all recipients of G-CSF will develop somatic complaints, of which skeletal pain is most prominent (Table 108–4). The somatic complaints are generally tolerable, and few donors will require reduction in dose or discontinuation of the medicine. At present, there appear to be minimal, if any, long-term health risks for the donor. Few serious complications of the mobilization regimen and donation process have been reported.[120,121] Splenic rupture that occurred in a healthy donor appeared to be temporally related to the donation

Table 108–4 Incidence of Somatic Complaints for Normal Donors Treated with Granulocyte Colony-Stimulating Factor

	Anderlini et al.[118]	Stroncek et al.[107]	Bishop et al.[106]
No. of donors	43	85	41
G-CSF dose (μg/kg/day)	6	2–10	5
Symptom (%)			
Malaise	82	86	83
Headache	70	28	44
Fatigue	20	14	NR
Fever	0	NR	27
Chills	NR	NR	22
Nausea	10	11	22

Shown are reported proportions of donors experiencing the somatic complaint.
G-CSF, granulocyte colony-stimulating factor; NR, particular complaint not reported in the series.

process, and a small study of normal donors showed an average increase in spleen size of 1.1 cm.[122] Another donor with known coronary artery disease experienced a myocardial infarction after the first of two intended donations. A third donor died of a cerebrovascular accident several days after donation and discontinuation of the cytokine. Although filgrastim induces a hypercoagulable state, any relationship of these events to the donation process in these last two donors remains unclear because similar events have not been reported for autologous donors or others receiving these cytokines.[123,124] Patients with autoimmune disorders may experience a flare of their disease during administration of filgrastim.[125] A variety of case reports of ophthalmologic and other adverse events have been reported for healthy donors or patients treated with filgrastim.[126–129] Also of concern is the possibility that cytokine administration will increase the risk of marrow dysplasia or malignancy. Although this is a theoretical concern in that the cytokines used are known to stimulate growth of leukemia cells, no clinical evidence indicates that these agents will induce abnormalities in the hematopoietic cell. An increased risk of myelodysplasia or hematologic malignancies in either healthy donors or patients who have been treated with short courses of G-CSF has not been reported.

G-CSF administration results in a number of changes in blood counts and chemistries in addition to the coagulation factor changes.[107,118] Alanine aminotransferase, lactate dehydrogenase, and alkaline phosphatase levels increase, and the levels of blood urea nitrogen and bilirubin may decrease. The elevation in alkaline phosphatase level is primarily of bone origin; γ-glutamyl transferase levels remain normal. These abnormalities of serum chemistries resolve within 2 weeks after discontinuation of the medication. G-CSF administration also will result in a decrease in platelet count, especially if the cytokine is administered over 5–10 days.[107,119] WBC counts fall rapidly after discontinuation of G-CSF. In approximately 10% of donors, the WBC count may fall to abnormal levels (but generally will remain above 1000/μL), reaching a nadir 10 to 14 days after discontinuation of the cytokine before stabilizing at normal levels.

Granulocyte-Macrophage Colony-Stimulating Factor

Much of the early experience with the use of hematopoietic cytokines for mobilization of HSC involved GM-CSF and chemotherapy.[2,81,83] The increase in CFU-GM in the peripheral blood can increase by as much as 1000-fold in this setting.[2] For some patients, the combination of cyclophosphamide (CY) and GM-CSF is more effective than is mobilization with G-CSF alone.[130] GM-CSF is not as potent as G-CSF (see Granulocyte Colony-Stimulating Factor above). Haas et al.[131] treated 12 patients with 250 μg/m²/day of GM-CSF and observed only an 8.5-fold increase in the number of CFU-GM in the peripheral blood (to median of 1347 CFU-GM/mL). As with G-CSF, there is a dose response in mobilization of PBSC with GM-CSF over a range from 0.3 to 20 μg/kg/day, without a plateau.[132] In this latter study, however, the average increase in CFU-GM in the blood at this highest dose level again was only 8.4-fold. In a randomized study comparing GM-CSF to G-CSF or both drugs used in sequence after chemotherapy administration, patients had faster recovery of counts, required less supportive care including transfusions, and achieved greater collections of CD34⁺ cells if given one of the G-CSF–containing regimens.[133]

Administration of GM-CSF results in similar somatic complaints and hepatic function abnormalities reported after G-CSF administration.[134] In addition, 44% to 80% of patients experience fever, sometimes after each dose, and generalized or local skin reactions. Lieschke and Burgess[135] noted that doses greater than 20 μg/kg/day are poorly tolerated because of fluid retention, pleural and pericardial inflammation, and venous thrombosis. A "first-dose reaction" characterized by hypoxia and hypotension occurring within 3 hours of administration has been described for some recipients, especially after IV administration.[136]

Other Hematopoietic Cytokines

Recognition of the mobilization potential of G-CSF led many investigators to study other hematopoietic cytokines for their capacity to mobilize HSC into the peripheral blood. Used as single agents, these cytokines resulted in only an approximately 5- to 10-fold increase in circulating CFU-GM or CD34⁺ cells. These cytokines are not currently used for HSC mobilization, and the mechanism(s) of HSC mobilization with these other cytokines is less well elucidated.

M-CSF: Few studies have investigated the efficacy of M-CSF in the mobilization of PBSC. In one study involving six patients with acute myelogenous leukemia (AML) treated with two cycles of consolidation therapy, no significant difference in the number of CFU-GM in the peripheral blood was observed after either cycle despite the addition of M-CSF at a dose of 8×10^6 U/day during the second.[137] Based on this experience, M-CSF likely does not have a major effect on the mobilization of HSC, but interpretation of this study is hindered by the facts that the study was not randomized, all patients received the cytokine only during the second consolidation cycle, and the chemotherapy regimens differed for the two consolidation cycles.

Erythropoietin: Recombinant human erythropoietin (Epo) has a mild mobilization effect. Pettengell et al.[138] treated 11 patients with malignant lymphoma with either 300 or 450 IU/kg thrice weekly for 2 weeks and found a 4.6-fold increase in CD34⁺ cells. The peak level of these cells was found on days 5 to 8 of administration of this cytokine.

Interleukin-3: Interleukin (IL)-3 has been studied primarily as a component of sequential cytokine mobilization with either GM-CSF or G-CSF.[139–141] In the nonhuman primate treated with 33 μg/kg/day, IL-3 administration results in an approximately 12-fold increase in the number of circulating CFU-GM.[142] In contrast, Ganser et al.[139] treated patients who had advanced malignancies with 60 to 250 μg/m²/day of IL-3 for 15 days and found minimal increase in circulating CFU-GM on day 8 and a decrease in some patients on day 15. Geissler et al.[141] reported similar findings.

PIXY 321: This fusion molecule of GM-CSF and IL-3 was studied by Bishop et al.[143] in 13 patients with malignant lymphoma in a phase I study involving doses ranging from 250 to 750 μg/m²/day by continuous infusion. Peak levels of CFU-GM in the blood were found on days 4 to 6 of treatment. A mild increase in CFU-GM in the blood was observed, but no consistent increase in CD34⁺ cells.

Stem Cell Factor: Most clinical studies of stem cell factor (SCF) report the use of this agent in combination with other cytokines (see Combinations of Cytokines below). Limited reports of use of SCF by itself are available. This cytokine appears to result in a dose-dependent 6- to 10-fold mobilization of CFU-GM.[144,145]

MOBILIZATION AND COLLECTION OF PBSC FOR AUTOLOGOUS TRANSPLANTATION

Four important considerations when prescribing a mobilization regimen for collection of PBSC for autologous transplantation are as follows. (a) A regimen of chemotherapy followed by G-CSF results in higher numbers of circulating CD34+ cells than will be found with G-CSF alone. (b) The choice of chemotherapy (or cytokine alone mobilization) should be appropriate to the disease and stage of disease for the patient. (c) Each cycle of prior chemotherapy or previous treatment with radiotherapy will decrease the response to mobilization therapy. (d) Tumor infiltration of the marrow will increase the probability of circulating tumor cells and will decrease the response to mobilization therapy. With these considerations in mind, elective collection of PBSC either before extensive treatment or after a limited number of cycles of debulking chemotherapy should be considered. If tumor contamination is found, additional components can be collected after additional rounds of chemotherapy. The timing of apheresis after chemotherapy and G-CSF mobilization is best guided by measurement of the level of peripheral blood CD34+ cells. Daily or every other day quantification of these cells can be initiated after the WBC count reaches 1000/μL. Patients with poor mobilization of CD34+ cells should be considered for large-volume apheresis to reduce the costs associated with daily doses of G-CSF, laboratory testing, apheresis procedures, and cryopreservation. Patients who fail to mobilize often will have successful collections if given a 2-week drug holiday and then undergo mobilization with high-dose G-CSF without chemotherapy.

Considerable dose-dependent toxicity, including angioedema, urticaria, pruritus, and laryngospasm, presumably from degranulation of mast cells, has been observed.[146,147]

Combinations of Cytokines

The mechanisms by which any of these cytokines causes mobilization of PBSC is not known. Multiple mechanisms probably are involved, including both an effect on proliferation of HSC as well as release of these cells from the marrow. Therefore, it is conceivable that combining different cytokines could result in an additive or synergistic effect. Limited studies have been conducted to date, with considerable potential to explore different cytokines with variations in both dose and schedule.

G-CSF + GM-CSF: Addition of G-CSF to GM-CSF greatly increases the number of HSC mobilized. The converse is not true. Winters et al.[148] treated patients who had a variety of malignancies with regimens of GM-CSF or G-CSF (both at 5 μg/kg/day) to which the other cytokine was added at day 7 of treatment and both continued through day 12. A third group of patients received both cytokines (at 5 μg/kg/day) simultaneously throughout the treatment. Apheresis was conducted on days 5, 7, 11, and 13. Simultaneous use of both cytokines achieved much greater mobilization of CFU-GM on day 5 than either of cytokine used singly to that point. Addition of GM-CSF on day 7 resulted in greater numbers of CFU-GM collected in subsequent apheresis procedures than were collected on day 5, although the effect was not very great. In contrast, addition of G-CSF on day 7 to patients treated with GM-CSF resulted in a strong release of CFU-GM 4 days later. Ho et al similarly studied the administration of GM-CSF or G-CSF at doses of 10 μg/kg/day or of the two cytokines together at doses of 5 μg/kg/day each and found that G-CSF alone achieved greater mobilization than GM-CSF or both drugs given in combination at a lower dose.[149] Among healthy allogeneic donors, sequential combination of GM-CSF 10 μg/kg/day for 3 days followed by G-CSF 10 μg/kg/day for 2 to 3 days yielded superior CD34+ cell collections compared to GM-CSF at the same dose or concurrent G-CSF and GM-CSF (both at 5 μg/kg/day).[150]

SCF + G-CSF: SCF by itself is a relatively weak mobilizing agent. Studies in dogs and baboons found that animals administered the combination of SCF and G-CSF had a 3.5- to 21.6-fold increase in progenitor cells in the blood.[151,152] The clinical effect has been much more modest. Moskowitz et al.[153] reported 38 patients with NHL randomized to SCF at 5 to 20 μg/kg/day plus G-CSF 10 μg/kg/day or to G-CSF alone. They found no difference between the cohorts with regard to mononuclear cells, CD34+ cells, or CFU-GM contents of the components collected by apheresis. However, patients with extensive prior therapy had increased numbers of CD34+ cells if given combination therapy, although the difference was not significant for this small number of patients. Begley et al.[154] conducted a similar phase I study of concurrent SCF and G-CSF in 62 women with early-stage breast cancer. In contrast, they found a significantly higher level of CD34+ cells in the blood of recipients treated with G-CSF plus SCF at 10 or 15 μg/kg/day compared to G-CSF alone or in combination with SCF at 5 μg/kg dose. The duration of mobilization for patients given the combination therapy was much broader, with high levels of CFU-GM still released into the blood several days after discontinuation of the cytokines. Sequential therapy with SCF given 3 days before initiation of G-CSF was even more efficacious, but even for this cohort of patients the increase in CD34+ cell levels averaged only twofold greater than for recipients of G-CSF alone. The combination of SCF and G-CSF also is effective after CY mobilization chemotherapy.[155] SCF plus G-CSF resulted in higher circulating CD34 counts on days 6 to 9 and a higher probability of collecting more than 2.5×10^6 CD34 per kilogram than G-CSF alone.[156] Side effects were mild flulike symptoms.

IL-3 + G-CSF: Geissler et al.[139] treated six patients with G-CSF at 5 μg/kg/day for 5 days, then a second course of IL-3 at a dose of 5 μg/kg/day for 7 days, followed by G-CSF again at a dose of 5 μg/kg/day for 5 days. They reported a 21-fold increase in CFU-GM in the peripheral blood after G-CSF alone, no increase after the course of IL-3, but a 56-fold increase after the combination. Peak levels of the progenitors in the blood were found on day 5 of G-CSF administration when given alone but on day 3 if the patient was first treated with IL-3.

IL-3 + GM-CSF: Brugger et al.[139] treated 32 patients with etoposide, ifosfamide or CY, and cisplatin. The chemotherapy was followed by GM-CSF for 15 days in one group, by IL-3 for 5 days and then GM-CSF for an additional 10 days in a second group, or with no cytokines for a third group. The dosages of the cytokines were not noted. The median peak numbers of CD34+ cells per microliter in the blood were 46 for the patients who did not receive either cytokine. The median for patients treated with GM-CSF alone was 426 CD34+ cells per microliter and for the group treated with both IL-3 and GM-CSF was 418 CD34+ cells per microliter. The peak numbers of CFU-GM in the blood of the group receiving both cytokines was almost twofold greater than for the group treated with GM-CSF alone.

Epo + G-CSF: In a retrospective comparison, Olivieri et al.[157] studied the addition of Epo 50 U/kg/day to G-CSF 5 μg/kg/day after mobilization chemotherapy with CY, etoposide, or epirubicin. The experimental group consisted of 18 patients with a variety of malignancies. The control group included 16 patients who received G-CSF alone. The groups were matched for diagnosis, previous chemotherapy, disease status, and mobilization chemotherapy agent. Olivieri et al. found a 2.8-fold increase in the peak number of CD34+ cells for the group that received both cytokines and a 1.7-fold increase in the number of CD34+ cells collected during apheresis. A randomized study of 50 women with ovarian cancer treated with epirubicin, paclitaxel, and cisplatin with either G-CSF or G-CSF and Epo showed a reduced number of apheresis procedures and increased PBSC collection for patients treated with the combination.[158] In contrast, the combination of Epo plus G-CSF was not found to enhance CD34+ cells in normal sibling donors and even may have been deleterious, with fewer total nucleated cells and CFU-GM collected compared to donors receiving G-CSF alone.[159]

Other Combinations: Compared to G-CSF alone, the combination of thrombopoietin and G-CSF yielded higher CD34+ cell doses (4.1 vs 0.8 × 10^6/kg) and thus fewer collections to meet the apheresis cell collection targets.[160] A limited pilot study of eight patients treated with chemotherapy followed by G-CSF with IL-11 demonstrated successful collection of CD34+ cells with a median of one apheresis procedure to collect the target dose of 5 × 10^6 CD34+ cells per kilogram.[161] The potential for chemokines in conjunction with cytokines is discussed below.

Chemotherapy Plus Cytokine Mobilization

The number of CFU-GM in the peripheral blood is greatly increased during the early hematologic recovery phase after marrow hypoplasia-producing chemotherapy.[6,75–77,94–96] A variety of chemotherapeutic regimens have been used for mobilization of PBSC, including DAT (daunorubicin, cytosine arabinoside, thioguanine),[6,75,96] high-dose CY,[94] low-dose CY,[162] (mitoguazone, ifosfamide, methotrexate, etoposide) MIME,[77] CAV (cyclophosphamide, adriamycin, vincristine),[76] DCEP (dexamethasone cyclophosphamide, etoposide, platinum),[163] and CY and etoposide.[164,165] To et al.[94] demonstrated a 14-fold increase of CFU-GM (compared to levels in healthy donors) in patients with non-Hodgkin lymphoma treated with a single dose of CY at 4 gm/m². However, only 69% of treatment courses achieve the desired mobilization of CFU-GM. As with any mobilization regimen, considerable variation between patients in their response to this treatment was observed.

Chemotherapy plus cytokine generally mobilizes greater numbers of PBSC than either agent alone.[166] Alegre et al.[130] compared the treatment of patients who had multiple myeloma with CY 4 g/m² followed by GM-CSF at 8 μg/k/day to a second group of patients treated with G-CSF alone at a dose of 10 μg/kg/day. Although G-CSF is the more potent mobilizing cytokine, the patients treated with chemotherapy plus GM-CSF achieved greater numbers of CD34+ cells per apheresis procedure, demonstrating the additive potential of chemotherapy mobilization. This finding was confirmed in a randomized study comparing CY followed by G-CSF versus G-CSF alone in which higher numbers of CD34 cells were found for the patients treated with the chemotherapy-based regimen.[167] However, no differences in the degree of tumor cell contamination of PBSC components, engraftment kinetics, or survival were found. In a randomized crossover design trial, Koc et al.[168] demonstrated that high-dose CY plus G-CSF resulted in mobilization of more progenitors than did GM-CSF plus G-CSF when tested in the same patient, regardless of sequence of administration. This trial suggests that patients who fail to mobilize with cytokine alone might be salvaged with chemotherapy-based mobilization but that the reverse might not be effective.

A wide variety of different chemotherapy regimens have been used successfully for mobilization of HSC into the blood. The primary consideration is that the choice of chemotherapy used must meet the treatment needs of the patient. However, evidence also indicates that the choice of chemotherapy regimens will affect the mobilization of HSC. Schwartzberg et al.[164] reported an average daily apheresis yield of 4.0 × 10^7 CD34+ cells in 395 apheresis components collected from 61 patients treated with CY and average yields of 8.3 × 10^7 CD34+ cells in 218 collections from 33 patients treated with both CY and etoposide. (Another group of 24 patients was treated with this latter chemotherapy regimen but also received 6 μg/kg/day of G-CSF. The average CD34+ cell contents for 122 collections from these patients were significantly higher at 38.8 × 10^7.) The average quantities of CFU-GM paralleled the numbers of CD34+ cells collected. Similarly, Demirer et al.[169] studied the effect of different chemotherapy regimens for mobilization of HSC for patients with breast cancer. Four regimens were used, all involving CY, but including etoposide with or without cisplatin, or paclitaxel. All patients also received G-CSF. The median quantity of CD34+ cells collected on the first day of apheresis after CY mobilization was 0.9 × 10^6 per kilogram of patient weight. The addition of etoposide and then of etoposide and cisplatin increased the yield to 8.1 × 10^6 and 3.5 × 10^6 CD34+ cells per kilogram, respectively. The median number of CD34+ cells harvested on the first day of apheresis after CY plus paclitaxel was 11.1 × 10^6/kg. More than 50% of the women mobilized with this last regimen achieved the target dose of CD34+ cells in one apheresis procedure. Of the 100 women studied, 94 achieved the target dose of greater than 5 × 10^6 CD34+ cells per kilogram. Only four patients failed to reach a lower but acceptable dose of 2.5 × 10^6 CD34+ cells per kilogram.

Chemokines

Chemokines (chemoattractant cytokines) are a family of approximately 40 related small proteins that influence leukocyte (and malignant cell) migration and function.[170,171] Chemokines with varying effects on different WBC populations have been identified, as have a number of chemokine receptors. The roles of chemokines and chemokine receptors in the trafficking of HSC into and from the bone marrow compartment are under active investigation.[172–178]

In a preclinical study, administration to both mice and rhesus monkeys of a modified CXC chemokine GRO-β after 4 days of G-CSF resulted in a fivefold increase in the number of circulating stem and progenitor cells compared to G-CSF alone, with a much shorter time course measured in hours.[179] Furthermore, more rapid recovery of hematopoietic function was observed for animals given similar quantities of cells collected after administration of the chemokine and cytokine combination.[179,180] IL-8, a related ligand for the CXCR2 receptor, mobilizes stem cells within 15 to 30 minutes of injection into mice,[181] which appears to involve increased matrix metalloproteinase-9 activity detectable immediately before the appearance of HSC in the peripheral circulation. Murine studies demonstrate a mobilizing effect of the chemokine SDF-1 and its receptor CXCR4 that can be blocked by neutralizing antibodies to either.[176] The bicyclam molecule AMD3100 disrupts SDF-1/CXCR4 binding and has been shown to result in mobilization of HSC in murine, canine, and nonhuman transplant models.[182–184]

Similar signaling pathways are used for mobilization and homing of normal and malignant hematopoietic cells. Although PBSC products collected after G-CSF mobilization generally contain fewer detectable tumor cells than does bone marrow harvested from the same patient, the effects of chemokine treatment on the degree of PBSC contamination and on disease relapse after autologous transplantation remain to be elucidated. Tavor et al.[185] demonstrated that acute myelogenous leukemia cells express CXCR4 in varying levels and that homing of primary human AML cells into NOD/SCID mice is CXCR4 dependent, similar to normal human stem cells. Similar studies of chemokine control on tumor cell growth, migration, and metastasis are being reported from a number of laboratories.

AMD3100

Clinical studies of HSC mobilization using AMD3100 with or without G-CSF priming are being reported in both healthy donors and patients undergoing autologous HSC transplantation. In a study involving normal volunteers, a single dose of AMD3100 was equal in mobilization to administration of a standard 5-day course of G-CSF.[186] However, a single dose of AMD3100 on day 5 of G-CSF administration resulted in a further 3.8-fold increase in circulating CD34+ cells (as well as B and T cells, which may be important in allogeneic transplantation). A nontransplant study of patients with either myeloma or non-Hodgkin lymphoma demonstrated a rapid increase in circulating WBC and CD34+ cells 4 and 6 hours after AMD3100 given at a dose of either 160 or 240 μg/kg.[187] CD34+ cells increased from a mean of 2.6 ± 0.7/μL to a mean of 16.2 ± 4.3/μL at 6 hours after injection. A subsequent crossover study compared collection from patients given a daily dose of G-CSF 10 μg/kg/day, with up to four apheresis procedures starting on day 4 of G-CSF

PHYSICIAN PRESCRIPTION FOR APHERESIS AND PBSC PROCESSING

The attending physician should be aware of apheresis and laboratory procedures in order to maximize the value of PBSC components. The choices of venous access, anticoagulant(s), blood volume processed, target dose of CD34+ cells, and cryopreservation volumes can be individualized. Apheresis unit staff may ask for guidance regarding pain medications, concurrent medications, and blood transfusions (although it is advisable to avoid transfusion during the apheresis procedure because of citrate or other reactions and because changes in the hematocrit may affect the efficiency of the collection). Adequate numbers of CD34+ cells can be collected for more than one cycle of chemotherapy. It is important to communicate with the cryopreservation facility if PBSC components will be used to support more than one cycle of chemotherapy or if DMSO toxicity is of concern. Current cytometric techniques for quantification of CD34+ cells require at least 1 hour of processing, so it is generally not practical to prescribe the number of CD34+ cells to be frozen in each bag. However, it is possible to divide the component into the number of bags equaling the number of anticipated infusions so that equal numbers of CD34+ cells will be available for each.

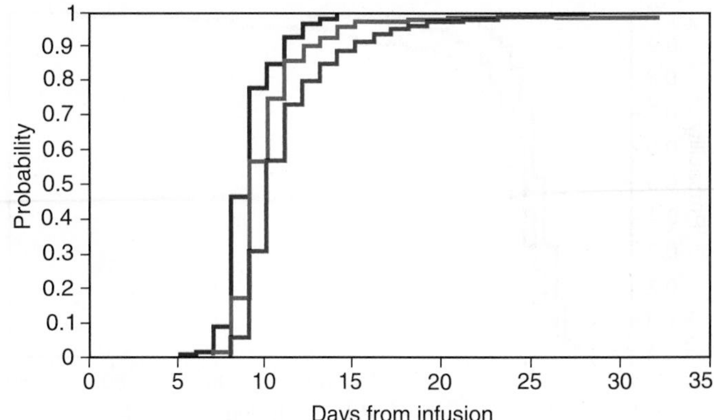

Figure 108–1 Kaplan-Meier probability of achieving ≥0.5 × 10^9 neutrophils/L for < 5.0 × 10^6 (–), > 5.0 to 10.0 × 10^6 (..), and > 10 × 10^6 (—) CD34+ cells per kilogram (P = 0.0001). (From Weaver CH, Hazelton B, Birch R, et al: An analysis of engraftment kinetics as a function of the CD34 content of peripheral blood progenitor cell collections in 692 patients after the administration of myeloablative chemotherapy. Blood 86:3961, 1995.)

administration, followed, after a 2-week washout period, with a second attempt at PBSC collection after the same schedule and dose of G-CSF with AMD3100 160 to 240 µg/kg/day given on day 4 of cytokine administration and continuing daily until the target quantity of CD34+ cells was met.[188] Of the 25 patients enrolled in the study, two with the highest quantities of CD34+ cells mobilized by G-CSF showed nonsignificant (1.1-fold) increases in CD34+ cells after treatment with the combination. Overall, however, the number of CD34+ cells circulating in the blood increased a median of 2.9-fold. Fourteen of the 25 patients collected greater than 2.0 × 10^6 CD34+ cells per kilogram on the first collection after the combination drug treatment compared to only five patients treated with the G-CSF mobilization cycle. A provocative finding of this study was the observation that nine patients who failed to reach the target goal of 2 × 10^6 CD34+ cells per kilogram after four apheresis procedures using priming with G-CSF alone each met or exceeded this target after treatment with G-CSF in combination with AMD3100. This finding suggests that the combination decreases the interpatient variability seen with cytokine mobilization and may be a treatment option for patients treated with cytokines who fail to collect adequate quantities of PBSC for transplantation.

STRATEGIES FOR THE DIFFICULT TO MOBILIZE PATIENT

Most patients achieve the targeted dose of CD34+ cells after processing of 20 to 30 L of blood in one to three apheresis procedures. However, approximately 5% to as many as 30% of patients in various series have inadequate collections because only small numbers of HSC are present in the peripheral blood despite the administration of hematopoietic cytokines. Different chemotherapy and cytokine regimens affect the mobilization of HSC (see Cytokine Mobilization). Patient-specific factors predictive of poor mobilization include older age, marrow disease, prior radiotherapy, and prior chemotherapy.[29,189–192] Specifically, previous administration of marrow-toxic drugs suppresses subsequent mobilization of HSC.[193–196] Approximately 50% of patients who fail to achieve the targeted dose of CD34+ cells will achieve this goal on a second attempt.[197] High-dose (15 mg/kg bid) G-CSF after a 2- to 4-week drug holiday to allow marrow recovery is one strategy. Combination cytokine therapy is also of potential value in this situation, and the combination of SCF with G-CSF may be effective for patients who reside in countries where the former drug is available.[198,199] Initial experience with AMD3100 suggests that the agent may be effective when used in combination with G-CSF for collection of PBSC from patients who failed a prior mobilization attempt. Repetition of a chemotherapy plus cytokine regimen also will be effective but may be associated with increased toxicity.[192] Bone marrow can be harvested, but the poor mobilization of PBSC predicts for a poor marrow harvest,[200] although G-CSF administration before marrow harvesting may be effective in increasing the number of CD34+ cells collected.[201,202] Consideration should be given to infusing a lower dose of CD34+ cells (as low as 1 × 10^6 CD34+ cells per kilogram) because, although the risk of delayed engraftment is incurred,[89,90] failure of engraftment has not been reported.[192,203]

Consideration should be given to collection of PBSC early in the course of treatment for patients who later may be candidates for autologous HSC transplantation but who are advised to receive multiple courses of therapy or therapy involving alkylating agents or radiation therapy. HSC can be collected and cryopreserved before extensive therapy while the patient has good marrow function and stored for years without obvious progressive loss of engraftment potential.[204]

DEFINITION OF ADEQUATE COMPONENT(S)

The quantity of CD34+ cells in a PBSC component varies greatly and is dependent upon the number in the peripheral blood at the time of apheresis, the volume of blood processed, and the efficiency of the apheresis device. Therefore, any definition of an adequate component cannot include a set number of CD34+ cells to be contained in any single apheresis component. Instead, one or more components will be collected to meet the appropriate dose of these cells for transplantation. The dose of CD34+ cells required for infusion depends upon the intended treatment regimen. For marrow-ablative regimens, increasingly higher CD34+ doses results in greater likelihood of rapid engraftment (Figs. 108–1 and 108–2).[89,90] Lower doses of CD34+ cells appear satisfactory for nonablative regimens.[205–208] For example, Bokemeyer et al.[207] infused 1 × 10^6 CD34+ cells per cycle for patients treated with high-dose ifosfamide and doxorubicin. Despite an overall doubling of the ifosfamide dose in this phase I study, the median times between cycles did not differ.

Many transplant programs have used quantification of hematopoietic progenitors by cell culture in an attempt to determine the adequacy of the bone marrow or PBSC collections for transplantation.[78,94,209] Based on delayed engraftment failure in some patients, Juttner et al [75] recommended a minimum CFU-GM dose of 6.3 × 10^5 per kilogram of recipient weight. Others have suggested lower doses of 2 to 5 × 10^5 CFU-GM per kilogram.[210] Patients who receive

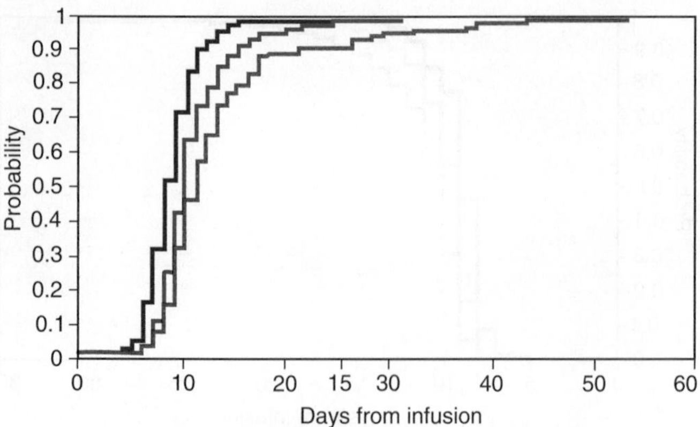

Figure 108–2 Kaplan-Meier probability of achieving ≥20.0 × 10^9 platelets/L for < 5.0 × 10^6 (–), > 5.0 to 10.0 × 10^6 (..), and > 10 × 10^6 (—) CD34⁺ cells per kilogram ($P = 0.0001$). (From Weaver CH, Hazelton B, Birch R, et al: An analysis of engraftment kinetics as a function of the CD34 content of peripheral blood progenitor cell collections in 692 patients after the administration of myeloablative chemotherapy. Blood 86:3961, 1995.)

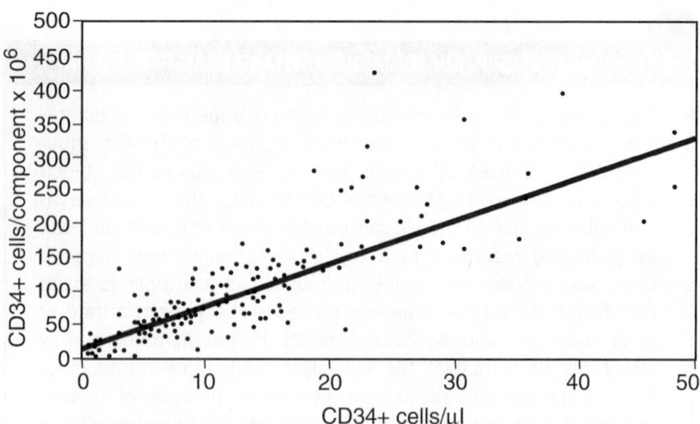

Figure 108–3 Relationship between quantity of $CD34^+$ cells in the peripheral blood and number collected by apheresis using apheresis and flow cytometric techniques.[3,89,334] Data shown are limited to peripheral blood $CD34^+$ cell numbers <50.0/µL (n = 157, r = 0.82, $P < 0.001$).

a dose of $CD34^+$ cells (or CFU-GM) above a certain threshold will engraft. At lower doses of $CD34^+$ cells there is considerable heterogeneity in engraftment speed, especially for platelet engraftment. Why this heterogeneity exists is not known, but it may reflect a weakness in the correlation between $CD34^+$ cells and the cells responsible for engraftment or, more simply, a greater degree of error in the measurement of $CD34^+$ cells at the lower cell concentrations. As the dose of $CD34^+$ cells increases, the engraftment speed becomes more consistent for the population studied.[89,90] Several investigators showed more rapid granulocyte and platelet engraftment for recipients of products containing a quantity of $CD34^+$ cells above a dose of approximately 2 to 3 × 10^6 per kilogram of recipient weight.[190,191,211] Investigators at the Fred Hutchinson Cancer Research Center found a threshold of 5 × 10^6 $CD34^+$ cells per kilogram achieved reliably prompt platelet engraftment,[212] and studies that included large patient populations found that higher doses of $CD34^+$ cells resulted in even higher proportions of patients achieving quick engraftment.[90] Investigators at the Hutchinson Center noted that the dose of $CD34^+$ cells infused was more important than the type of mobilization therapy. In a study of allogeneic transplant recipients, Singhal et al.[213] reported higher transplant-related mortality for patients who received a $CD34^+$ cell dose less than 2 × 10^6/kg, regardless of the source of HSC.

The incidence of acute GVHD does not appear to be proportionately greater after PBSC compared to bone marrow transplantation. However, one group reported, in retrospective analysis, greater risk of acute GVHD in recipients of cells from donors, with a greater response to PBSC mobilization.[214] Allogeneic transplant recipients may have a higher risk of chronic GVHD with higher $CD34^+$ cell doses independent of the dose of T lymphocytes infused.[215]

TIMING OF APHERESIS

A major problem with chemotherapy-based mobilization regimens is the difficulty in determining the optimal time to commence HSC collection. Apheresis devices can collect only those $CD34^+$ cells actually circulating in the peripheral blood. It is possible to estimate the quantity of $CD34^+$ cells that will be collected during apheresis by multiplying the quantity of $CD34^+$ cells in the blood by the total volume of blood processed during the apheresis procedure and by the efficiency of the apheresis device in collecting these cells. If the device has an efficiency of 50% and the patient undergoes a 10-L exchange, approximately 5 × 10^7 $CD34^+$ cells will be collected for a peripheral blood level of 10 $CD34^+$ cells per microliter and 5 × 10^8 $CD34^+$ cells for a blood level of $CD34^+$ cells that is 10-fold higher. Although many protocols call for initiation of apheresis after chemotherapy mobilization when the WBC count has recovered to greater than 1000/µL, there is a poor, if any, correlation between the peripheral blood white cell or mononuclear cell counts and the $CD34^+$ cells in the peripheral blood. Characteristics that suggest a higher $CD34^+$ cell level are rapidly rising WBC count, shift in differential to immature myeloid cells, circulating nucleated red cells, and platelet transfusion independence. These features may be more valuable in a homogeneous patient population receiving a uniform mobilization regimen.[216] However, it is much more cost effective to obtain an actual measurement of $CD34^+$ cells in the blood and to time the apheresis collection when these cells are present in adequate numbers. The published experience from many transplant centers describes a correlation between $CD34^+$ cells in the peripheral blood and in the harvested component.[190,211,217,218] Figure 108–3 shows such a relationship for patients with lower concentrations of $CD34^+$ cells in the peripheral blood and illustrates the very poor collections obtained when the peripheral blood $CD34^+$ count is less than 10/µL. Although there is considerable error in the enumeration of $CD34^+$ cells at levels less than 5/µL, these finding is not clinically relevant because even doubling the $CD34^+$ cells in this low range still results in a very poor apheresis yield.

The level of $CD34^+$ cells in the peripheral blood at which to start apheresis is a clinical decision. Although levels in the range from 50–100/µL or greater will reduce the number of apheresis procedures necessary to achieve a target goal of $CD34^+$ cells, each day's delay in initiating apheresis incurs the costs of additional cytokine administration and blood testing. In some patients who previously had undergone extensive treatment and who may show a slowly rising WBC count, multiple apheresis procedures may be necessary to achieve the target goal. No patient should undergo apheresis if the peripheral blood count is less than 5/µL (see Fig. 108–3). For patients with $CD34^+$ cell counts in the range from 10/µL to 20/µL, it is possible to process more blood per day using large-volume leukapheresis (LVL) techniques and thereby reduce the numbers of days the patients is required to return to the apheresis unit. Most patients have a rising $CD34^+$ cell count in the peripheral blood, so starting apheresis the day after the patient has achieved a desirable $CD34^+$ level generally is feasible.[218]

The timing of apheresis after G-CSF mobilization differs from the timing after chemotherapy and cytokine mobilization. For both patients and healthy donors, the peak concentration of $CD34^+$ cells occurs on day 5 of G-CSF administration (after four daily doses).[104,105] Lower levels are present on day 4, and the concentration continues to fall after day 6 even if cytokine administration is continued and despite a continued rise in WBC count. Thus, PBSC collection should be initiated on day 4 or 5 of G-CSF administration. The kinetics of $CD34^+$ cells in the peripheral blood for patients and donors mobilized with G-CSF alone are so reliable that monitoring of peripheral blood levels is not necessary unless there is concern that

MANAGEMENT OF PATIENTS WHO FAIL INITIAL HSC COLLECTION

Patients donating cells for autologous use are much more likely than are healthy donors to fail collection because of marrow infiltration by tumor and the HSC-toxic effects of previous chemotherapy and radiotherapy. Patients who fail initial collection attempts frequently will fail subsequent attempts, and transplantation of these patients may require use of below optimal quantities of cells with resulting delayed or incomplete hematologic recovery. A healthy donor who does not meet the target goal of PBSC can undergo bone marrow harvesting. Patients who fail an initial attempt of PBSC collection using filgrastim can undergo another attempt, preferably after a brief 1- to 2-week holiday and, possibly, with use of cyclophosphamide- or ifosfamide-based mobilizing chemotherapy. Higher doses of filgrastim (>20 μg/kg/day) given in a twice-daily schedule may be more effective. If clinically available, combinations of filgrastim and SCF may be effective. Other cytokine combinations such as filgrastim and sargramostim do not appear more effective than filgrastim alone. The combination of filgrastim with a chemokine agent is promising in early trials, and these agents are expected to be clinically available in the near future. Bone marrow collection can be attempted for patients who fail PBSC collection, and treatment of patients with filgrastim may result in a higher $CD34^+$ cell content. Bone marrow collection of patients should be delayed until the platelet count has increased to greater 100,000/μL after prior chemotherapy.

the patient has failed to mobilize cells and it is practical to obtain the cell count rapidly enough to initiate apheresis on the same day.

Apheresis Technology

Apheresis technology is widely used for collection of platelets from healthy donors and is considered to be without major risk to the donor. The important safety considerations for PBSC collection are the same as for platelet collection and include the venous access to be used for the procedure, the extracorporeal volume of blood during the procedure, and the solutions administered to the donor. Of note, however, PBSC collection for autologous transplantation involves patients with underlying medical conditions who may require considerable nursing care during the procedure. In a retrospective review of more than 5000 plasmapheresis procedures in 627 patients for treatment of a variety of diseases, complications of apheresis were observed in 12% of procedures, and 40% of patients experienced at least patients one complication during a course of therapy.[219] Most of the complications were mild and transient, such as fever, chills, urticaria, hypotension, and reactions to citrate anticoagulants. In contrast, patients and donors undergoing PBSC collection do not require the replacement fluids used during plasmapheresis and will not experience the toxicities associated with plasma protein infusions. However, rare anaphylactic reactions may occur in pediatric patients who require blood priming of the extracorporeal circuit, in patients treated with angiotensin-converting enzyme inhibitors with use of albumin priming solutions,[220] or those allergic to ethylene oxide used to sterilize the apheresis disposable set.[221] Goldberg et al.[222] studied the complications occurring during 554 PBSC collections from 75 consecutive patients. Patient diagnoses and the mobilization treatment regimens were varied. All but one patient had subclavian or jugular venous system catheters placed for apheresis. A median of nine collections per patient was performed using a discontinuous flow apheresis device. The most common problems were related to the venous catheters; 50% of patients developed at least one occlusion. Hypocalcemia occurred in 14.6% of patients and hypotension in 13.3%. Sixteen percent of patients experienced infectious complications during the PBSC collection period.

Staffing of the apheresis unit should be appropriate for the medical condition of the patients undergoing apheresis. Staffing must include nurses familiar with the care of the oncologic patient who may be recovering from marrow hypoplasia complicated by neutropenic fever requiring multiple medications and with the care of a central line. Collection of PBSC by apheresis performed in the outpatient setting should never be assumed to be a safer alternative for the healthy donor or patient with a comorbid illness than marrow harvesting conducted in the intensive care setting of the operating room without careful review of the medical support requirements for the individual patient or donor.

Venous Access

Adequate venous access is required for optimal apheresis technique. Continuous-flow apheresis devices require two-lumen access with a stable blood flow capacity generally greater than 20 mL/min. Single-lumen access may be used with discontinuous-flow apheresis devices, although at a much slower rate of blood processing. The great majority (≈90%) of adult allogeneic PBSC donors have adequate arm veins for the procedure to be conducted "vein to vein." Some allogeneic donors, especially those with small veins and undergoing several daily procedures, may require placement of a temporary venous catheter. Venous access for the patient undergoing collection for autologous PBSC transplantation is much more heterogeneous. Vein-to-vein procedures can be performed, even on several consecutive days, with proper phlebotomy technique and postcollection care of the phlebotomy site. Most patients received previous chemotherapy or are proceeding directly to transplantation, conditions for which tunneled access is commonly placed. Ideally, this venous access should be appropriate both for the apheresis procedures and the subsequent transplant. Length, lumen size, and wall stiffness all affect the blood flow that can be achieved through a catheter. For this reason, the commonly used dual-lumen Hickman or Broviac catheters usually are unsuitable for apheresis as are all subcutaneously placed ports.[223] Most triple-lumen catheters are inadequate because of the small lumen size. If such access is already in place, consideration can be given to replacement with a shorter, stiffer tunneled catheter or to placement of a temporary percutaneous dialysis/apheresis catheter.[224,225] The catheters designed for dialysis and apheresis have adequate wall thickness to prevent collapse during aspiration of blood as well as a tip design that decreases local recirculation of blood and the resulting decrease in apheresis efficiency. Catheters of 10 F or larger size are appropriate for adult patients. Pediatric patients whose blood flow rates are considerably slower may use catheter sizes of 5 to 7 F.[226]

Problems directly related to venous access account for a considerable amount of the toxicity associated with PBSC collection. Mobilization with GM-CSF has been suggested to increase the incidence of catheter occlusion.[227] Haird et al.[228] suggested that catheters placed in the subclavian vein in particular were associated with a high incidence of thrombosis, a complication seen less frequently with translumbar inferior vena cava placement. Goldman et al.[222] reported this complication in 50% of patients. In contrast, Alegre et al. reported an only 1.8% incidence of thrombosis or clotting of catheters,[224] possibly because of differences in cytokine or catheter type and care. Catheter thromboses are easily managed with streptokinase, urokinase, or recombinant tissue plasminogen activator instillation by the apheresis unit staff. One randomized study reported that low doses of warfarin decreased the incidence of venous thrombosis associated with indwelling catheters, but this study did not address catheter patency, nor were the patients enrolled in this study treated with hematopoietic cytokines.[229] Consultation with apheresis unit staff about venous access for an individual patient is appropriate. For example, for patients with adequate peripheral veins, a needle can be placed in one arm of the patient for blood draw with simultaneous use of both lumens of a tunneled catheter for return of the blood, thereby avoiding the need for placement of another venous access device.

Apheresis Devices

A number of apheresis devices are available for separating HSC from the peripheral blood. The devices may be classified as continuous flow (e.g., Fenwal CS3000, COBE Spectra, Fresenius AS104) or discontinuous flow (e.g., Haemonetics family of equipment). Discontinuous-flow devices have the advantage of requiring only a single venous access. Continuous-flow devices require two access lines for aspiration and return of blood, but they process much larger volumes of blood in a shorter period of time. Devices now available enrich the HSC-containing mononuclear cell fraction, reducing the quantities of granulocytes and platelets collected that may interfere with cryopreservation or other laboratory processing.

All apheresis devices collect HSC. The choice of apheresis device used by the collection center depends primarily on the needs and experience of the center. The CS3000 achieves a greater enrichment of mononuclear cells than does the COBE Spectra,[230] reducing the number of granulocytes in the component, but without a difference in the collection efficiency for $CD34^+$ cells. In contrast, the Spectra allows a much higher blood-to-anticoagulant ratio because additional anticoagulant solution can be added to the collect bag at the initiation of the procedure, thereby avoiding much of the citrate toxicity that may occur with processing large volumes of blood during PBSC collection.[231] Continuous-flow devices are more efficient in the collection of PBSC and are preferred over discontinuous-flow devices. In a randomized study comparing the Haemonetics MCS-3P with the COBE Spectra, Morton et al.[232] found that the latter device processed significantly more blood in a shorter period of time and collected over twice as many $CD34^+$ cells and CFU-GM.

Anticoagulation

Anticoagulants are added to the blood during apheresis to prevent clotting of the extracorporeal circuit and clumping of cells in the component. Citrate anticoagulants have a proven record of safety in the apheresis of healthy platelet donors and are used extensively for collection of PBSC. The major drawback is the risk of a symptomatic decrease in the level of ionized calcium ("citrate toxicity"), especially during processing of large volumes of blood.[233,234] Citrate ions chelate calcium ions (and other divalent cations such as magnesium), making them unavailable for Ca^{2+}-dependent metabolic reactions. ACD-A contains 10.67 g of citrate per 500-mL volume in the form of trisodium citrate and citric acid. Citrate is diffused throughout the extravascular space, and this diffusion probably is the first defense against citrate toxicity. Metabolism by liver, kidney, and muscle also reduces the concentration of citrate. Metabolism of citrate becomes more important during prolonged apheresis procedures such as LVL. The initial signs of citrate toxicity include circumoral or acral paresthesias and may progress to nausea, vomiting, loss of consciousness, tetany, and seizures. Fatal cardiac dysrhythmias have been reported (rarely) for patients undergoing plasmapheresis.[235] Citrate infusions may depress myocardial function, and it has been suggested that this effect may be worsened by the use of calcium channel-blocking medications, although reports of such complications in patients or donors undergoing apheresis have not been published.[233] Because pediatric patients may not be able to relate the initial symptoms of the condition, citrate toxicity should be considered as the cause of any change of behavior, such as crying, during the apheresis procedure. Citrate toxicity is prevented by limiting the quantity of citrate infused either by decreasing the blood flow rate through the apheresis device or changing the blood to citrate ratio. For example, the COBE Spectra limits the blood flow rate so that the amount of citrate infused is a maximum of 1.1 ml/min/L of patient blood volume as calculated from the patient's gender and size. However, these machine parameters do not account for alterations in electrolytes, plasma protein levels, muscle mass, or renal or hepatic function that may occur in patients receiving chemotherapy. The processing of blood of patients experiencing the initial symptoms of citrate toxicity should be temporarily halted until the symptoms abate and then resumed at a slower rate. The benefit of oral calcium supplements for these patients is not certain. Heparin can be used as a replacement for some or all of the citrate, although additional citrate is added to the component bag to prevent clumping of platelets.[3,236] Some centers that use citrate anticoagulants also administer intermittent or continuous infusions of calcium gluconate during the procedure, especially if large volumes of blood are being processed.[237,208] However, excessive calcium replacement can induce cardiac dysfunction.[233] "Point of care" devices that measure the ionized calcium within minutes are available and greatly simplify obtaining this test.[238,239]

Large-Volume Leukapheresis

The apheresis device has a uniform and fairly reproducible efficiency of collection. Thus, for a consistent quantity of blood processed through the machine, the quantity of $CD34^+$ cells collected is directly related to the number present in the peripheral blood. Greater quantities of $CD34^+$ cells can be collected by increasing the number of these cells in the peripheral circulation or by increasing the volume of blood processed by the device. For patients with lower $CD34^+$ cell levels, multiple apheresis procedures will be required to achieve the target dose of $CD34^+$ cells needed for transplantation. An alternate approach is to process the same total quantity of blood but in fewer, longer procedures. LVL is not standardly defined but in general usage refers to processing of more than two or three times the patient's blood volume.[239–248] Typically, the quantity of blood processed is six or more times the patient's blood volume, often 25 to 36 L of blood. The advantage of LVL is that it reduces the number of days of cytokine administration and apheresis, with associated reduced costs of laboratory processing and testing. The apheresis techniques are the same as those used for processing of smaller volumes of blood, although blood flow rates may be increased to reduce the time required. The risks of LVL are the increased time required and the higher risk of citrate (or other anticoagulant) toxicity. Patients will also incur a proportional drop in platelet counts and may become profoundly thrombocytopenic.

Most reports of LVL describe the collection of more $CD34^+$ cells than are calculated to be present in the peripheral blood at the initiation of the apheresis procedure. Release of cells from the marrow replaces those cells removed by apheresis. Apheresis of $CD34^+$ cells is a three-compartment system consisting of the extracorporeal circuit of the apheresis device (including the collection bag), the peripheral blood, and the marrow. However, it is not obvious that the apheresis technique itself consistently "mobilizes" $CD34^+$ cells, as suggested by some reports. Initial investigation of LVL in dog and rhesus monkey models and in human patients and healthy donors not receiving cytokine mobilization demonstrated an increased number of CFU-GM collected such that a doubling of these cells in the circulation must have occurred during the apheresis procedure.[242,245,249,250] The experience with patients and donors treated with cytokines or chemotherapy plus cytokine is much more variable, with reports describing an increase,[241,242,244,245] no change,[239,247,248] or even an exhaustion of $CD34^+$ cells from the peripheral blood.[247,251] Animals receiving hematopoietic cytokine stimulation have a diminished apheresis-associated increase in circulating CFU-GM compared to animals collected without any mobilization treatment.[250] This increase also may not be evident in patients with subsequent poor marrow function because they previously had received extensive treatment with chemotherapy.[246]

Clinically most important is the possibility of exhaustion of HSC such that the processing of large blood volumes exposes the patient to the risks of anticoagulant toxicity and thrombocytopenia without achieving an increased collection of HSC. However, studies at the Fred Hutchinson Cancer Research Center demonstrated continuous release of $CD34^+$ cells from the marrow (and, presumably, return to the marrow space).[231] Patients having higher levels of $CD34^+$ cells in the peripheral blood appeared to have a greater number of these cells circulating between the marrow and peripheral blood compartments (Table 108–5). In this model the apheresis device merely serves as a

Table 108–5 Replenishment of CD34+ Cells During Large-Volume Leukapheresis

	CD34+ Cells				
UPN	*Blood (per μL)*	*Blood Total*	*Harvest Total*	*Released Total*	*Released (per min)*
10605	6.8	34.9	123.5	88.6	0.3
10698	15.6	603.3	1438.1	540.8	2.1
10849	30.7	109.7	211.1	62.6	0.3
10920	37.9	214.2	952.8	57.0	1.6
11128	66.1	280.6	1010.8	532.7	1.9

Shown are numbers of CD34+ cells in the peripheral blood or apheresis component for five patients with acute myelogenous leukemia or multiple myeloma undergoing large-volume leukapheresis after granulocyte colony-stimulating factor (G-CSF) or chemotherapy plus G-CSF mobilization treatment. Blood volumes processed were six times the calculated blood volume of the patient. Peripheral blood stem cell collection was performed on the COBE Spectra as previously described.[3] The total number of CD34+ cells in the blood (third column) was calculated from the level of CD34+ cells in the blood and the estimated blood volume of the patient. The total number of CD34+ cells released (fifth column) was calculated from the total number in the apheresis component and the number in the peripheral blood after collection minus the total number in the peripheral blood at the start of the collection procedure. All CD34+ cells quantities (except blood levels reported per μL) are $\times 10^6$.

Full data are given in Rowley et al.[231]

siphon, removing these cells from the blood as they are released from the marrow. If this description of CD34+ cell kinetics is accurate, it may be possible to deplete these cells from the blood and marrow by prolonged processing, but probably only if limited numbers of these cells are present in the marrow compartment. Also, the model suggests that higher blood flow rates used to shorten the apheresis procedure may be counterproductive for patients with low CD34+ cell levels in the blood because of the slower rate of release of CD34+ cells in these patients.

The explanation for the increase in CFU-GM circulating in the peripheral blood during the procedure reported by some investigators is obscure. Murea et al.[244] suggested that this phenomenon may be related to a decrease in divalent cations resulting from the citrate anticoagulant. Divalent cations are necessary for the function of some but not all cell adhesion molecules.[252] A progressive decrease in ionized calcium levels in some patients during the prolonged LVL procedure could result in an increase in circulating HSC. This may explain why some investigators using heparin-containing anticoagulation solutions or concomitant infusion of calcium solutions have not observed this phenonmenon.[247,248,251]

LVL is appropriate management for the patient or donor who needs to complete apheresis in a limited number of procedures. The quality of the component collected by LVL does not differ from that collected by the processing of smaller volumes of blood, and patients experience the same rapid kinetics of engraftment after infusion of these components.[244]

PEDIATRIC DONORS AND PATIENTS

PBSC can be collected from pediatric patients, including infants. The special challenges of the pediatric patient arise from the fixed extracorporeal blood volume of the apheresis device, the need for venous catheters for blood access, and the management of a patient who may be unwilling or unable to rest quietly for the period of apheresis. It is especially important in management of the pediatric patient that timing of apheresis be optimal to minimize the number of procedures required to achieve the desired quantity of PBSC. Given these considerations, a number of centers have reported successful collection of PBSC from pediatric patients and donors.[208,236,251,253–260]

Almost all pediatric patients undergo insertion of a venous catheter adequate for the flow rates expected, although older patients(>12 years) may tolerate vein-to-vein procedures. The whole blood flow rate for the pediatric patient is much reduced compared to adult patients, and catheters as small as 5 F may be adequate.[226] Some centers have used arterial catheters for blood access.[256]

Appropriate management of fluid balance during the apheresis procedure is critical for the smaller patient. The volume of red blood cells contained in the extracorporeal circuit of continuous flow apheresis device could represent 30% to 50% of the red cell mass of a pediatric donor. Although discontinuous-flow devices are appealing because of the feasibility of performing apheresis with a single-lumen venous access, they may result in even higher extracorporeal volumes and should be avoided in the smallest patients. The obvious solution to this problem is to prime the apheresis device with ABO-compatible, irradiated, red blood cells (leukocyte-depleted and cytomegalovirus-negative blood may also be desirable) when the blood in the extracorporeal circuit is expected to exceed 15% of the patient's blood volume. Packed red blood cell units can be diluted with saline or albumin to reduce the loss of this plasma protein that may occur. The red cells remaining in the extracorporeal circuit at the completion of the run need not be returned ("rinse-back"),[261–263] although if performed slowly with monitoring of vital signs, rinse-back may actually increase the hematocrit after the procedure and otherwise reduce the need for red cell transfusions for these patients. Körbling et al.[258] collected and stored the red cells remaining in the machine after the first day's apheresis for use in priming for the second day's procedure for allogeneic donors requiring 2 days of apheresis, thereby avoiding the use of homologous blood transfusion. For the intermediate-size pediatric patient (weight 25–50 kg), the apheresis device can be primed with a 5% albumin solution. This steep will reduce the albumin loss that otherwise would occur. However, clotting proteins and other proteins not contained in this solution may decrease with repetitive apheresis.

The pediatric patient may not exhibit or relate the prodromal symptoms associated with citrate toxicity. Continuous calcium gluconate infusion can be incorporated into the procedure, or heparin can be added to the citrate anticoagulant solution or used as the sole anticoagulant.[3,243,244,251] Some centers report the use of sedating medications, such as chloral hydrate, during the procedure.[254,208,258] Sedation of the pediatric patient is not necessary, however,[253,257,260] and hinders the ability to recognize the symptoms of citrate toxicity. (Some patients may require antihistamine premedication if the apheresis device is primed with red blood cells.) Centers routinely performing pediatric PBSC collection should design an environment conducive to the management of pediatric patients and develop support procedures that recognize the unique physical and cognitive features of pediatric patients.[264]

The range in blood volumes for pediatric donors of differing ages is greater than for adult donors. Therefore, most centers set a goal for volume processed based on the individual's blood volume instead of a set volume (e.g., two blood volumes vs 6 L of blood) for all patients. The pediatric patient may undergo LVL to achieve the target goal of HSC with fewer procedures.[251,259] Blood flow rates for pediatric patients are slower than for adults to minimize the risk of citrate reaction. As with adults, the timing of apheresis can be optimized by monitoring the quantity of CD34+ cells in the peripheral blood.[265]

ALLOGENEIC DONORS

Multiple centers have reported their experience with the use of PBSC for syngeneic or allogeneic HSC transplantation.[12–22,266] These reports consistently describe more rapid engraftment kinetics than observed with marrow transplantation (see Table 108–2). The incidence of acute GVHD appears to be equivalent to that after marrow transplantation despite the 10-fold higher number of T lymphocytes infused.[12,13] However, chronic GVHD may be more common after PBSC transplantation, or it may be more difficult to control.[31–33] The differing reports about acute and chronic GVHD may reflect the GVHD prophylactic regimens used in these clinical trials. The reports of improved survival of patients who undergo PBSC transplantation similarly may be particular to transplant regimens or patient selection.[20] Peripheral blood mononuclear cell components collected from donors either with or without treatment with G-CSF also are effective in the immunotherapy of patients with progressive disease after allogeneic transplantation.[267–269]

The apheresis procedure is well tolerated by the allogeneic PBSC donor. In contrast to the collection of PBSC intended for autologous transplantation, the collection for allogeneic transplantation usually is performed on a healthy donor. Almost all allogeneic donors are treated with G-CSF for mobilization of PBSC, and the toxicities incurred with the use of this cytokine are discussed in the section above (cytokine mobilization). Adverse events associated, at least temporally, with the collection procedure include myocardial infarction, cerebral vascular accident, and rupture of the spleen.[121–129] Anderlini et al.[120] suggested that G-CSF specifically not be administered to patients with a history of inflammatory ocular disorders, venous thrombosis, autoimmune disorders, or malignancy treated with chemoradiotherapy. In an interim analysis of an ongoing study of healthy donors receiving one of two different doses of G-CSF, Beelen et al.[270] reported 478 acute adverse events for the first 150 donors enrolled. Most (80%) of these adverse events were transient bone pain or headache, and no persistent hematologic or nonhematologic events were recorded. The discomfort of PBSC donation measured using open-ended pain scales is rated as equivalent to that experienced by marrow donors enrolled in a randomized trial comparing marrow to PBSC transplantation, although the PBSC donor reports more rapid resolution of symptoms.[49] Similar findings regarding pain and comparable high levels of anxiety were reported for a subset of donors enrolled in a separate trial comparing marrow to PBSC donation.[271] However, Switzer et al.[272] conducted for the National Marrow Donor Program a retrospective analysis of donor experiences for donors who underwent PBSC donation after a prior bone marrow donation. They reported that donors found the marrow harvest procedure physically more difficult, time consuming, and inconvenient. The risks to the allogeneic PBSC donor conferred by apheresis should not differ greatly from the risks to the platelet donor if the apheresis techniques are similar, although the PBSC donor may undergo larger volume and repetitive exchanges with different anticoagulants compared to the platelet donor. The risk of larger-volume exchange is citrate toxicity if the donor is small or if the blood flow rate is increased to achieve this volume in a shorter period of time. Also, larger-volume and repetitive exchanges will result in platelet depletion, although the platelets can be separated from the component for infusion back to the donor.[107,118] The platelet count may reach its nadir several days after completion of the apheresis collections and discontinuation of G-CSF, and donors should be counseled in this regard.[107,119]

Most donations can be obtained using a vein-to-vein procedure. Some donors, especially pediatric donors, may require placement of a temporary central venous catheter. The risks of catheter placement are well known and are not discussed here.

Older donors will have more underlying medical conditions,[273] and the risks to the donor with underlying health problems must be fully considered before subjecting the donor to mobilization and apheresis. Published standards describe evaluation of the donor for the risk of the donation process as well as the risk of transmission of disease to the recipient.[274,275] Collection of PBSC is generally an outpatient procedure conducted in the clinic setting. In contrast, marrow harvesting has the luxury of the intensive support capability of the operating room. PBSC collection should never be viewed as a safer alternative to marrow harvesting for the donor with underlying health problems.

Management of Red Blood Cell Incompatibility

Management of red blood cell incompatibility between the PBSC donor and recipient is the same as for bone marrow transplantation.[276] Marrow processing to reduce the quantity of red cells and careful transfusion practices are used to prevent acute or delayed hemolytic transfusion reactions from infusion of incompatible red blood cells or immunocompetent B lymphocytes. Eventually, recipient red cells and isoagglutinins are replaced by donor type. Red cell incompatibility is classified into two categories: one in which the recipient has antibodies directed against donor red cells with the potential for acute hemolysis upon infusion of the component (major incompatibility), and one in which the donor has antibodies against the recipient. Although the latter rarely causes difficulty during infusion of incompatible plasma, B lymphocytes carried in the component can form isoagglutinins, resulting in a delayed transfusion reaction 7 to 12 days after transplantation. Apheresis devices are commonly used to remove red cells from marrow component for major red cell incompatibility.[277] Red blood cell quantities no more than 10 mL appear to be tolerable. Therefore, secondary processing of a PBSC component collected by the same technology used for depletion of red cells from marrow grafts and already containing low quantities of red cells is not required. Minor ABO incompatibility can result in delayed transfusion reactions that may be fatal if appropriate blood transfusion support (avoiding the infusion of donor-type red cells) is not initiated before transplant. Two case reports of severe red cell hemolysis after allogeneic PBSC transplantation have been reported. In the first, transfusion support before the event was not described.[278] The second patient received recipient-type red cells on day 7 after transplantation,[279] which is the point at which donor-derived isoagglutinins will be increasing in the recipient. Although both author groups discussed the much greater numbers of B cells in PBSC components as a possible factor in these events, it is not clear from these reports that delayed-type transfusion reactions will be more likely or of greater severity in PBSC recipients. The risk of delayed-type reaction may be reduced by the use of multi-agent posttransplant immunosuppressive medications. The Seattle transplant program found no delayed transfusion reactions in a large retrospective review of patients undergoing PBSC transplantation and who received cyclosporine and methotrexate.[280]

CELL COUNTING, PROCESSING, AND CRYOPRESERVATION

Tumor Cell Contamination

The probability that tumor cell contamination of the component could contribute to relapse was demonstrated by Brenner et al. and others in studies involving the transplantation of genetically marked marrow cells.[281–283] Sensitive immunocytostaining techniques, clonal assays, flow cytometric analysis, and polymerase chain reaction amplification of malignant genetic material detect tumor cells in the PBSC components of many patients with a variety of malignancies.[284–287] In general, the incidence of contamination (number of patients with positive components) and the level of contamination (number of tumor cells per number of normal cells) is much less for PBSC than for marrow components,[284] although this has not been a consistent finding in all studies.[285] Whether patients transplanted with PBSC have a lower relapse rate compared to patients receiving bone marrow is not well defined, and appropriate phase III studies of this question will be difficult to design and enroll with patients. In a retrospective study, Sharp et al.[288] demonstrated similar probabilities of relapse-free survival in recipients of PBSC or marrow components if the components were free of lymphoma cells. In that study, patients with marrow involvement by lymphoma were assigned to transplantation with PBSC. The authors concluded that PBSC transplantation is a sensible approach to the patient with overt marrow involvement. However, Brugger et al.[289] demonstrated that patients with breast cancer involvement of the marrow at the time of chemotherapy mobilization were likely to mobilize tumor cells into the blood. The most disturbing finding of this study is that the tumor cells were detected in the peripheral blood at the same time as $CD34^+$ cells. Similarly, Pecora et al.[290] found a relationship between the ability to detect tumor in PBSC components and in bone marrow samples, but they also found a higher incidence of positive PBSC components for patients who required greater numbers of apheresis procedures to achieve the target dose of CD34$^+$ cells. Investigators at The Johns Hopkins Oncology Center found no difference in the incidence of tumor contamination of PBSC components between patients treated with chemotherapy and cytokines or cytokines alone.[291] The probability of tumor contamination of PBSC components decreases after induction chemotherapy.[292] Patients with marrow involvement may benefit from several cycles of debulking (in vivo purging) chemotherapy before collection of PBSC, with the caveat that extensive chemotherapy will decrease the subsequent yield of PBSC. Tumor cells in the HSC inoculum likely will not benefit the patient, but until further data are available, it is advisable that reports of tumor contamination in the collections for individual patients be interpreted with caution.

Purging of Hematopoietic Stem Cell Components for Autologous or Allogeneic Transplantation

PBSC components can be purged of tumor cells or T lymphocytes using the same techniques developed for marrow, although the larger cell quantities collected and the multiple days of collection will increase the cost of processing. Because of the commercial availability of devices that enrich CD34$^+$ cells, most purging studies involving PBSC components have focused on this technology. The CD34 glycoprotein is an approximately 115-kd molecule found on lymphohematopoietic stem and progenitor cells, including malignant cells derived from these, vascular endothelium, and possibly other tissues.[293] The presence of this marker on hematopoietic stem and progenitor cells enables the enrichment of these cells from peripheral blood, cord blood, or marrow. Enriched populations of CD34$^+$ cells then can be used for transplantation or further component manufacturing, such as gene therapy or cell expansion. Numerically, simple enrichment of CD34$^+$ cells from levels less than 1% to levels from 70% to 95% results in greater than 90% to 99% depletion of CD34$^-$ cells, leading many investigators to explore CD34$^+$ cell enrichment as a technique of T-cell depletion to prevent GVHD in allogeneic cell recipients[294–297] or tumor depletion to decrease the risk of relapse for autologous component recipients.[298–301] Engraftment does not appear to be affected by CD34$^+$ cell enrichment unless low quantities of CD34$^+$ cells are infused.[298]

Positive enrichment of HSC achieves nonspecific tumor-cell depletion as CD34$^+$ cells are separated from antigen-negative cells. Because this depletion is nonspecific, the degree of purging achieved will equal the depletion of other CD34$^-$ cells such as lymphocytes. Typically, depletion ranges from 99% to 99.99%. By itself, CD34$^+$ cell enrichment will reduce the number of tumor cells below the level of detection of some assay systems. For example, Shiller et al.[298] reported that five of eight components were negative for myeloma cells after processing, but Lemoli et al.[301] found the persistence of detectable disease in five of six patients tested. The median purity of CD34$^+$ cells actually was greater in the latter study (77% vs 89.5%). Phase III studies of CD34 enrichment for patients undergoing treatment of myeloma show the feasibility of CD34$^+$ cell enrichment of PBSC components, although these studies were not powered to demonstrate efficacy in control of disease.[302] CD34$^+$ cells can be successfully enriched after thawing using the same techniques used for prefreeze separations.[303–305] Cell recovery is lower compared to prefreeze processing, but the postthaw processed samples do not undergo the potentially damaging osmotic shock that occurs with the infusion of cells cryopreserved in dimethylsulfoxide (DMSO). Greater depletion of tumor cells can be achieved with combinations of CD34$^+$ cell enrichment followed by depletion of tumor cells. Few clinical trials of combination purging techniques currently were conducted, so the usefulness of this purging cannot be assessed at this time.

Microbial Contamination of Hematopoietic Stem Cell Components

The incidence of culture-positive PBSC components is considerably less than that for marrow.[306–308] In a prospective study conducted by Attarian et al.[306] of 1263 PBSC components from 376 sequential patients, bacteria were detected in only three. Most of these patients were treated with chemotherapy mobilization, and approximately 50% were still receiving antibiotics for treatment of neutropenic fevers at the time of apheresis. None of the components collected from the patients receiving antibiotics were culture positive. The collection of cells from febrile patients appears acceptable if they are clinically stable for apheresis, the timing of apheresis is appropriate as determined by enumeration of CD34$^+$ cells in the blood, and the patients are receiving appropriate anti-microbial therapy. The collecting facility should arrange for microbial culture of the component. Skin flora are the bacteria usually isolated, and contaminated components need not be destroyed. Infusion of these components is generally without clinical sequelae, although serious infections have occurred after infusion of components contaminated during processing.[306–311] Any decision regarding the disposition of culture-positive HSC must be made by the patient's transplant physician after considering the type of contamination, the anticipated risks from use of the component, and the ability to replace the culture-positive component(s) in a timely manner.

Quantitation of CD34$^+$ Cells

Quantification of CD34 antigen-positive cells by flow cytometry has become the standard of care for management of the PBSC donor because it provides a rapid and clinically relevant assessment of HSC content in the peripheral blood or the PBSC component. This antigen is found on HSCs and limited populations of other blood cells[293] and can be identified using a variety of commercially available antibodies. If antibodies directly conjugated with dyes are used, the technique requires only about 1 hour of preparation time. Cell viability using propidium iodide (PI) or 7-aminoactinomycin D (7-AAD) exclusion can simultaneously be determined if the cells are analyzed while still fresh,[312] or the cells can be fixed after staining for analysis at a later date. Other antibodies can be added for analysis of CD34 subsets if desired (and if the flow cytometer has proper detectors to detect the different emission wavelengths of the fluorochromes used).[81] Many centers are finding strong correlations between the numbers of CD34$^+$ cells and CFU-GM in the sample, but with ratios of 5 : 1 to 20 : 1.[217,313] Thus, CD34 analysis will provide data similar to that obtainable with cell cultures, except that the latter demonstrates the viability of the progenitor cells.

The major difficulty with analysis of CD34$^+$ cells is the low frequency of these cells. Clinical decisions to initiate apheresis are being made for CD34$^+$ cell levels as low as 10/μL. This may represent a cell frequency that is 0.01% or less of the nucleated cells in the specimen. This enumeration is possible because of multidimensional measurements obtained by flow cytometry. Most cytometers can measure at least five characteristics of each cell, including size, granularity, and the presence of up to three different fluorochromes. Thus, the cells of interest can be separated in five-dimensional space, achieving discrimination of cells as rare as 1 : 10,000. The difficulties arise from developing an adequate technique that makes optimal use of the cytometer to measure these rare cells. Sources of errors include (a) sampling of the component, (b) cell counting, (c) cytometer calibration and operation, (d) choice of antibody and fluorochrome, (e) lysis technique, and (f) gating strategy. Skilled operators will avoid many of these errors by selecting appropriate antibodies and properly operating the cytometer. However, cytometry provides a proportion of cells, which must be multiplied by the cell count to obtain an absolute number. The steps involved in preparing a specimen for cytometry may alter the proportion of cells in the sample, and this error will be translated into an error in the absolute number.[314] The direct relationship between the number of events (CD34$^+$ cells counted) and the precision of this count dictates that large cell numbers be analyzed.[315] Serke et al.[315] found a coefficient of variation of 30% in counting of CFU-GM colonies and 10% in flow cytometric counting of CD34$^+$ cells. The coefficient of variation in CD34$^+$ cell enumeration could be as high as 65% for specimens containing few cells. This variation was decreased by analysis of larger cell samples. Clinically, this imprecision may explain some of the range in engraftment kinetics observed for patients receiving low doses of CD34$^+$ cells.

A variety of different cytometric techniques are used for measuring CD34$^+$ cells. They may involve only one antibody, although other techniques use two antibodies for better discrimination between CD34$^+$ and CD34$^-$ cells.[316–318] Gating on cells that are CD45$^+$ helps separate nucleated cells from red blood cells, platelets, and debris, a step that is otherwise performed using the light scatter characteristics of the cells.[318] Alternately, gating on CD14$^-$ cells allows the separation of CD34$^+$ cells from monocytes that nonspecifically bind the CD34 antibody. However, there is considerable variation in results even between laboratories using the same cytometric technique, and no cytometer-based technique has proven to have a lower interlaboratory variability.[317]

Subset analysis will provide additional information but does not appear to be clinically useful at this time. Pecora et al.[319] reported that the quantity of CD34$^+$CD33$^-$ cells infused was identified as an independent factor predictive of engraftment kinetics. Dercksen et al.[320] reported better correlation between the number of CD34$^+$CD33$^-$ cells and time to granulocyte engraftment and between the number of CD34$^+$CD41$^+$ cells and time to platelet engraftment than found with the overall number of CD34$^+$ cells. This group reported a similar finding for the number of CD34$^+$L-selectin$^+$ cells infused and platelet engraftment.[321] Given the limited range in recovery times when adequate numbers of CD34$^+$ cells are collected and infused, however, this additional information is of limited clinical value.

There is considerable disagreement about which flow cytometry technique is best for the measurement of CD34$^+$ cells. Any particular technique may have advantages over the others in specific settings, but no technique will be adequate if the cytometer is not calibrated and is not clean, if adequate events are not obtained for "rare event" analysis, and if a uniform gating strategy is not followed. These issues will become moot with the development of automated devices that provide quick and reproducible enumeration of CD34$^+$ cells, leaving the flow cytometer for research use. The ideal technique will provide an actual count of CD34$^+$ cells (instead of a percentage) and be sensitive to CD34$^+$ cell levels at least as low as 10/μL (levels below this are generally not clinically relevant). Single platform devices that provide an actual count of CD34$^+$ cells have been evaluated.[322,323] It may be possible to adopt some hematology analyzers to this purpose.[324]

Progenitor Cell Cultures

Hematopoietic progenitor cells committed to granulocytic (CFU-GM), erythroid (burst-forming unit-erythroid), or mixed granulocytic and erythroid (CFU-granulocyte, erythrocyte, megakaryocyte, macrophage; CFU-Mix) lineages can be identified using a variety of culture techniques. These techniques require expertise and equipment not available in many clinical laboratories, and they have other drawbacks that may limit their utility as routine quality control. Other than availability of equipment and expertise, the major limitation is that progenitor cell assays require 10 to 14 days of culture before the results are available. Thus, progenitor cell cultures cannot be used in the day-to-day management of the PBSC donor or the immediate quality control of bone marrow products. As with quantitation of CD34$^+$ cells, the lack of standard culture technique adopted by all laboratories complicates comparisons between laboratories of progenitor cell quantities harvested and infused. The clinical relevance of the culture technique to the transplant population must be determined if the data obtained are to be used in the management of individual patients.

Unlike other measures of component quality, progenitor cell cultures demonstrate the functional capacity of the cells. Progenitor cell cultures are the only currently available relevant assay of HSC viability other than actual engraftment of the recipient and should be available at the HSC processing facility for use in quality control or if questions about the viability of a particular component are raised.

Cryopreservation

HSC harvested from the peripheral blood, bone marrow, or UCB are frozen and stored using the same techniques. The general parameters include cryopreservation in DMSO and a source of plasma protein with or without hydroxyethyl starch, cooling at 1 to 3°C/min, and storage at −80°C or colder.[325] Variations on this technique include the concentration at which the cells are frozen, the amount and source of the plasma protein, and the cooling techniques used.[326,327] Most of these variations probably have little effect on the survival of HSC, as shown by the consistent engraftment of cryopreserved components. However, cryopreservation results in loss of an undefined but potentially substantial proportion of HSC, and delay in engraftment can occur if the component being frozen has borderline quantities of HSC.[328,329] A considerable incidence of generally minor toxicity associated with infusion of cryopreserved cells must be considered when developing cryopreservation techniques.[330]

PBSC differ from marrow components in their much larger cell quantity, frequently exceeding 4 × 10^{10} cells. Cryopreservation of these cells at a set cell concentration, especially if multiple days of collection are performed, may result in large volumes of cryopreserved material to be infused. DMSO itself has a variety of pharmacologic effects,[331] which may be compounded by the presence of lysed blood cells, foreign proteins from tumor-cell purging procedures, or contaminants from nonpharmaceutical grades of reagents used in the processing. The LD_{50} values (amount of DMSO required to kill 50% of test animals) reported for intravenous infusion of DMSO are 3.1 to 9.2 g/kg for mice and 2.5 g/kg for dogs.[332] The acute toxic dose of DMSO for humans has not been determined. A report cited two instances of encephalopathy after infusion of cryopreserved PBSC components.[333] The components for both patients were cryopreserved with a final DMSO concentration of 10%. The volumes infused were 2254 and 1198 mL, containing 249.7 and 132.7 g of DMSO, respectively. Patient weights were not provided in this report, but the dosage of DMSO probably neared or exceeded 2 g/kg of patient weight, at least for the first patient. For this reason, the volume of DMSO infused should be limited to 1 g/kg/day. Patients with larger volumes can receive the cells over more than 1 day.

Cryopreservation of these cells at the concentrations frequently used for bone marrow (5–10 × 10^7 nucleated cells per milliliter) could result in component volumes greater than 400 mL for each collection. To minimize the volume infused, PBSC can be concentrated before cryopreservation. In one series, the average cell concentration of cryopreserved PBSC was 5.59 × 10^8 nucleated cells per milliliter.[334] High concentrations of red cells and platelets also were frozen. No detrimental effect of cryopreservation at these high cell concentrations on the recovery of nucleated cells, mononuclear cells, or CD34$^+$ cells was found. No clinical studies have addressed the effect of cell concentration on engraftment speed or toxicity of infusion. Of concern, however, is that several patients infused at that center developed alterations in mental status, including seizures, after infusion of PBSC concentrated before cryopreservation.[335] These events very likely were not related to the small volumes of DMSO infused but may be related to the concentration of cells frozen.

PBSC can be frozen in solutions using reduced concentrations of DMSO. A large (294 patients) randomized phase III study comparing engraftment after autologous transplantation of PBSC frozen using either 10% DMSO or 5% DMSO with 6% hydroxyethyl starch showed faster granulocyte recovery in patients receiving cells frozen using the combination cryoprotectant solution.[336] No difference in platelet recovery speeds was found, suggesting a lineage-specific benefit. These investigators did not report on infusion-related toxicity, although others have suggested that infusion-related toxicities are proportional to the quantity of DMSO infused.[337]

Alternately, the cells can be washed after thawing, with removal of most of the DMSO.[338] The risk is that of cell loss, so a strategy ensuring that not all cells are at risk during a single processing should be adopted. An effect of postthaw washing on the speed or success of engraftment after infusion of marrow or PBSC components has not been published.

Nonfrozen Storage

Cryopreservation is not required for short-term storage of HSC. Nonfrozen storage is a less costly alternative, especially for immediate transportation of products and for transplantation of patients conditioned with brief courses of chemotherapeutic agents with short in vivo half-lives. Although most products are infused or processed within a few hours of collection, products collected for unrelated donor hematopoietic cell transplant may be shipped over long distances, sometimes requiring more than 24 hours of transit time. Similarly, products intended for autologous hematopoietic cell transplant may be transported to regional processing centers, requiring 24 to 48 hours of transit time before processing.[339,340] The major advantages of cryopreservation are the lack of progressive loss of HC over time and the greater flexibility in timing of hematopoietic cell transplant relative to collection of HSC, including the ability to modify or postpone a transplant conditioning regimen already started.

Progressive loss of HSC occurs during nonfrozen storage. One author reported a 61% loss of myeloid colony-forming progenitor cells (CFU-GM) from marrow after 72 hours of storage at 4°C.[341] However, another found only a 3% loss of CFU-GM from marrow stored for 96 hours, but a 95% loss if the source of the cells was peripheral blood.[342] Preti et al.[343] compared the survival of mature hematopoietic progenitor cells isolated from marrow during frozen or nonfrozen storage and reported an immediate loss of myeloid (CFU-GM) progenitors of 33% during cryopreservation and thawing. In contrast, cells stored at 4°C showed progressive, linear loss of total nucleated cells, cell viability, and HSC cloned in vitro. The quantity of erythroid colony-forming progenitor cells (burst-forming unit-erythroid BFU-E) in these nonfrozen samples became significantly less than cryopreserved samples after only 5 days of storage. The difference for myeloid progenitor cells (CFU-GM) was not yet significant even after 9 days of storage. These differing reports demonstrate that storage conditions such as concentration of cells, chemicals added, product volume, storage bag, and temperature of storage affect the survival of cells kept in nonfrozen storage.[344]

Most published reports of noncryopreserved storage describe storage at 4°C. This condition provides a stable temperature compared to storage at ambient temperatures, which can be quite variable (and which must be considered during the shipping of products). The optimal temperature is not known and probably depends on factors such as prestorage processing, quantity and concentration of mature blood cells, buffering capacity of the solution, and gas diffusion capacity of the storage container. Beaujean et al.[340] reported a much lower pH for PBSC products stored overnight at room temperature compared to storage at 4°C. Although they did not find a difference in recovery of progenitor cells in their experiments, this effect may be damaging to HSC under other circumstances. None of these studies entailed marrow reconstitution as the experimental endpoint. The conflicting reports about optimal storage temperatures are difficult to interpret. Storage conditions for nonfrozen storage have not been tested in an engraftment model, so proper storage conditions are not adequately defined. For laboratories intending to store stem cell products, particularly PBSC components, for prolonged periods without freezing, rigorous validation of the storage conditions must be pursued.

Regulatory Aspects of Stem Cell Collection and Processing

The United States Food and Drug Administration (FDA) developed a regulatory strategy that encompasses the wide range of cellular- and tissue-based products being developed without requiring an extensive number of focused regulations specific for each possible cell source or derived product. In 1997 the FDA proposed an approach for regulation of cellular- and tissue-based products using a continuum of regulation that is intended to enable the FDA to meet its task of protecting public health without being unfair to specific practitioners of this field of medicine or stifling the development of novel uses of these products.[345] The proposed rigor of control is proportional to the extent of risk involved, with the level of regulation dictated by five considerations: prevention of disease transmission, processing controls to prevent contamination and maintain product integrity and function, clinical safety and efficacy, labeling and promotion, and communication with and monitoring of the tissue industry. The regulatory approach taken by the FDA addresses facility registration, selection and evaluation of the tissue donor, and manufacturing of the product. The FDA views cell processing as a manufacturing activity. Therefore, the FDA expects that donor evaluation and the collection, processing, and distribution of HSC-derived components will comply, at least, to Current Good Tissue Practices (CGTP), with the much more detailed Current Good Manufacturing Practices (CGMP) required for extensively manipulated products. CGMP and CGTP differ in the level of control over the manufacturing pathway required to prevent contamination or loss of potency of the final product The FDA developed Part 1271 of Chapter 21 of the Code of Federal Regulations (CFR) for these regulations. Part 1271 does not replace CGMP regulations for drugs and medical devices found elsewhere in Chapter 21 of the CFR. Cell therapy products that combine cell products with devices or drugs must comply with Part 1271 *and* with the applicable CGMP regulations.

The CGTP regulations are designed to prevent the introduction, transmission, and spread of communicable diseases. For example, compliance with CGTP requires precautions such as cleaning facilities and equipment, storage procedures designed to prevent product mix-ups, and controls over processing to prevent product contamination and impairment to function or integrity. CGTP includes, at a minimum, requirements for the appropriate collection, processing, labeling, storage, and distribution of cellular products to ensure maintenance of the product's function and integrity but does not require the rigorous environmental and manufacturing controls inherent in CGMP.

In the final rule enacting establishment registration, the FDA defined products regulated solely under this section (lowest level of regulation) if they are (a) minimally manipulated, (b) intended for homologous use only (i.e., serves same basic function as cells being replaced), (c) not combined with a drug or a device, except for a sterilizing, preserving, or storage agent, and (d) either without a systemic effect[1] and not dependent upon the metabolic activity of living cells or has a systemic effect or is dependent upon the metabolic activity of living cells for its primary function but is for autologous use or for allogeneic use in a first-degree or second-degree blood relative.[346] This includes most HSC transplantation excluding transplantation of HSC from unrelated PBSC or cord blood donors (the FDA does not regulate bone marrow products). Products not meeting this description still are subject to the core requirements found in Part 1271 but also are subject to more stringent requirements, including the requirement for premarketing approval (gained through submission of data from preclinical and clinical studies demonstrating safety and efficacy for the use being requested) and CGMP manufacturing requirements, as described in the regulatory approach for somatic cell therapy products.[347]

---

[1]Systemic effect is not defined in the proposed regulations but is clearly distinct from tissues such as bone grafts used for local effect.

SUGGESTED READINGS

Ballen KK: New trends in umbilical cord blood transplantation. Blood 105:3786, 2005.

Confer DL, Miller JP: Optimal donor selection: Beyond HLA. Biol Blood Marrow Transplant 13(Suppl 1):83, 2007.

Cottler-Fox MH, Lapidot T, Petit I, et al: Stem cell mobilization. Hematology Am Soc Hematol Educ Program 419, 2003.

Laurence AD: Location, movement and survival: The role of chemokines in haematopoiesis and malignancy. Br J Haematol 132:255, 2006.

Papayannopoulou T: Current mechanistic scenarios in hematopoietic stem/progenitor cell mobilization. Blood 103:1580, 2004.

Stroncek DF, Holland PV, Bartch G, et al: Experiences of the first 493 unrelated marrow donors in the National Marrow Donor Program. Blood 81:1940, 1993.

Thomas ED, Storb R: Technique for human marrow grafting. Blood 36:507, 1970.

REFERENCES

For complete list of references log onto www.expertconsult.com

CHAPTER 109

GRAFT ENGINEERING AND CELL PROCESSING

Adrian P. Gee

The last decade has seen growth in the use of hematopoietic cell transplant, with or without high-dose chemotherapy or radiotherapy, for treatment of marrow failure syndromes, certain genetic disorders, and cancers that are refractory to conventional dose therapy. The collection and characterization of marrow or peripheral blood stem cell products used for such transplants is described in Chapter 108. In the majority of cases the marrow or peripheral blood stem cell graft is infused after characterization (see Chapter 108) with minimal manipulation. However, in some cases the product undergoes more extensive manipulation to deplete or positively select certain cell types. In addition the cell processing facility often supports more novel cell therapies used either in the adjuvant setting posttransplant or as investigational therapy in clinical trials. These products are subject to different regulations that influence the facility, processing methodology, and release testing.[1,2]

REGULATORY ISSUES WITH CELL PROCESSING

Over the past 15 years the United States Food and Drug Administration (FDA) has been developing a regulatory approach that could be applied to cellular therapy products and would include some products traditionally used in hematopoietic progenitor cell (HPC) transplantation. The evolution of these regulations provides insight into how the FDA formulates laws and develops its regulatory position; however, an extensive discussion is outside the scope of this chapter. In brief, manufacturers of cellular therapy products need to determine whether they fall under Investigational New Drug (IND) regulations, which require manufacturing of the product under Good Manufacturing Practices (GMP); whether they fall under Part 1271 of Title 21 of the Code of Federal Regulations (21CFR) "Human Cells, Tissues, and Cellular and Tissue-based Products (HCT/Ps)," which require manufacturing of the product under Good Tissue Practices (GTP); or whether the product is exempt from these regulations.[3]

Stratification of regulations is based upon the relative degree of risk that is posed to the donor, the recipient, and the product during ex vivo processing.[2] The newer GTP regulations, which came into effect in May 2005, were established nominally to prevent the introduction, transmission, and spread of communicable diseases by HCT/Ps. This was based on the presumption that the majority of posttransplant infections and admissions to the intensive care unit were attributable to the receipt of contaminated products. The basis of this statement is open to question, but the regulations provide a framework for screening, performing ex vivo processing, storing and distributing HCT/Ps, and providing the FDA with an overview of current activities by an annual registration of collection and processing facilities. The Part 1271 regulations effectively filled a gap in the law where few regulations could be applied to HCT/Ps that were minimally manipulated (e.g., were not cultured ex vivo, genetically modified, activated ex vivo), that were intended for homologous use, and/or were not combined with another article (e.g., a matrix or gel) for administration. In addition, the HCT/Ps should not exert a systemic effect and should not be dependent upon the metabolic activity of living cells for its function; or for autologous use, or for use in a first or second-degree blood relative, or for reproductive use. Cellular products that fall into this classification are referred to as Type 361 products. These regulations do not apply to vascularized organs for transplantation, whole blood or blood components, and, importantly for this discussion, minimally manipulated bone marrow for homologous use and not combined with another article.

With the exceptions noted, most other cellular therapy and HPC transplant products fall under IND regulations and are referred to as Type 351 products. These products have been cultured, ex vivo, transduced or transfected, or activated ex vivo and, therefore, are more than minimally manipulated. The facility processing these cells is required to operate under GMP,[4] which is a set of regulations originally developed for the pharmaceutical industry to ensure that drugs are manufactured under a controlled and auditable process that ensures their safety, purity, and potency. The FDA has indicated that the application of GMP follows a continuum, such that products that are prepared for a phase I/II clinical trial under IND are not expected to be prepared under full GMP. As the trial proceeds the expectation is that the application of GMP will become more rigorous, such that a phase III product would be well characterized and would be manufactured using a fully validated process.

Implementation of Part 1271 regulations has had an impact on the "routine" laboratory that prepares cells primarily for hematopoietic transplantation.[5] Laboratories that use cells other than bone marrow now must register annually with the FDA, ensure that donors meet eligibility requirements (or document why noneligible donors are used), and manufacture, store, and distribute the cells under GTP. If the laboratory has previous experience manufacturing products for IND studies under GMP conditions, it already will be familiar with most of the features of GTP. In general, these cover personnel, procedures, facilities, environmental control and monitoring, equipment, supplies and reagents, recovery, processing and process controls, process changes, process validation, labeling controls, storage receipt, predistribution shipment and distribution, records, tracking, and complaints. Implementation of the components of either GMP or GTP operations is a time-consuming process that requires the development, implementation, and maintenance of numerous components and generates a considerable volume of paperwork. Professional societies, such as the Foundation for the Accreditation of Cellular Therapy (FACT)[6] and the AABB (formerly the American Association of Blood Banks),[7] have developed an accreditation process that takes into account GTP regulations and provides a framework around which compliance can be built.

One of the most important components of both GMP and GTP regulations is the establishment and maintenance of a quality program. This should ensure that the appropriate regulations are being followed on an ongoing basis, that mechanisms are in place for monitoring, reviewing, and remediating errors and deviations from regulations, policies, and procedures, and that an audit program will be developed and implemented. Evidence of the work of the quality program should be documented, and the program should be staffed by individuals who are not involved in hands-on manufacturing of the products.

Each year facilities are required to register their establishment with the FDA and provide a listing of the types of products they prepare. Holders of INDs should provide the agency with an annual report on the protocol and include a listing of the products administered and those that have been prepared but not used. In addition, cell processing facilities should be prepared to assist in reporting to the

FDA information on products that have been associated with severe adverse reactions in the recipients. For Type 361 products, the facility is also required to report as Biological Product Deviations any contaminated products that have been administered to a patient.

PROFESSIONAL STANDARDS

Regulations issued by the FDA have the power of law. Standards are voluntary recommendations that are published by professional societies. They can be enforced through a voluntary inspection and accreditation process that usually involves an on-site inspection. The two major accrediting organizations for cellular therapies are FACT[6] and the AABB.[7] FACT offers accreditation of collection, processing, and clinical use of cellular therapy products, whereas the AABB focuses on collection and laboratory processing. Both organizations inspect based on standards that are published every 18 months to 3 years. In the case of FACT, the standards are published in collaboration with the Joint Committee on Accreditation in Europe (JACIE). FACT also publishes separate standards in collaboration with NetCord that cover cord blood banking.[8] Both organizations have worked to harmonize their standards with American, Canadian, and European regulatory agencies; therefore, accreditation by either organization is of great assistance on the pathway to regulatory compliance. A number of other professional organizations accredit particular aspects of operations within the cell processing facility. They include the College of American Pathologists (CAP), which inspects general laboratories, hematology, and flow cytometry; the American Society for Histocompatibility and Immunogenetics (ASHI); and the European Federation for Immunogenetics (EFI), which accredits histocompatibility testing laboratories. Some organizations, such as CAP, also provide proficiency testing services for laboratory staff.

MANIPULATION OF HEMATOPOIETIC STEM CELL TRANSPLANTATION PRODUCTS

Manipulation of a product intended for hematopoietic stem cell rescue is intended to remove a component that is unwanted or may cause adverse effects, or to positively select a desired population such as CD34 cells (Fig. 109–1).

Routine Minimal Manipulation for Volume Reduction or ABO incompatibility

The most widely form of manipulation in the HPC processing facility probably is removal of erythrocytes or plasma to overcome ABO incompatibility between donor and recipient. This process is performed using techniques that were developed by the blood banking industry. Plasma depletion to remove donor antibodies that may react with recipient cells is achieved by centrifugation of the graft, usually in a transfer pack. The pack then is placed in a plasma expresser, which compresses the product so that plasma can be forced out and into a separate collection bag. Plasma depletion is also used to reduce the volume of ABO-compatible grafts when the donor is large and the recipient small.

Red cell depletion removes incompatible donor erythrocytes to prevent the donor from mounting a reaction to them upon administration. Most facilities establish a maximum volume of incompatible red cells that can be infused with HPC; exceeding this limit can result in hemolysis and a transfusion reaction. Depletion of erythrocytes can achieved most simply by centrifugation in which the product is centrifuged and the leukocyte-rich buffy coat is collected at the interface between the plasma layer and the red cells. Similar results can be achieved by sedimenting erythrocytes using hetastarch, which promotes rouleaux formation by red cells, resulting in more rapid sedimentation without centrifugation. The most rigorous erythrocyte

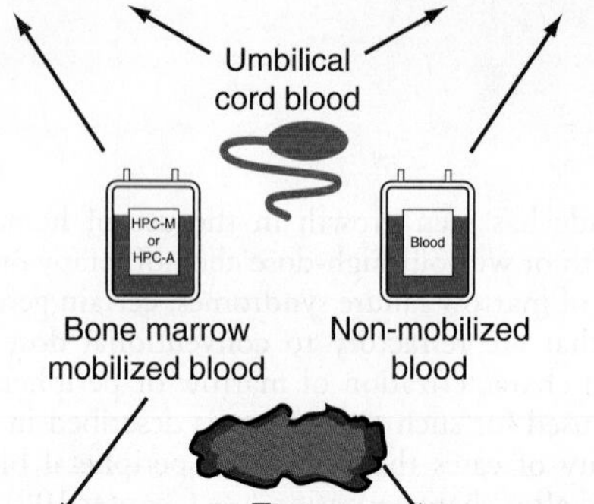

Figure 109–1 Processing methods for hematopoietic cell transplantation and immunotherapy products.

depletion is achieved by centrifugation of the collection on a Ficoll-Hypaque density gradient. This process enriches mononuclear cells at the interface between the gradient and the layered collection following centrifugation. As a result of enrichment for mononuclear cells, the overall nucleated cell recovery is lower than with other techniques.

Purging of Autologous Grafts

Autologous HPC can be used for recipients lacking a human leukocyte antigen (HLA)-matched related or unrelated donor. Debate is ongoing as to whether occult tumor cells collected with the graft and returned to the patient is in a viable state, acting as the source for disease relapse.[9] Gene marking studies have suggested this possibility.[10–12] As a result, much effort has been exerted to develop methods for the detection and removal of tumors from autologous grafts. Methods have ranged from use of chemotherapeutic drugs such as 4-hydroperoxycyclophoshamide, photosensitizing agents, and antisense oligonucleotides to methods that use tumor-directed monoclonal antibodies to identify the cells and effect their removal.[13–15] Antibody-coated tumor cells can be eliminated by adding serum complement or by linking them to a solid phase, such as a column matrix, plastic sheet, or magnetic particles. These particles may be large (5-μm diameter) so that they can be collected, with the attached tumor cells, in a standard magnetic field, or they may be much smaller, such as nanoparticles or ferrofluids, which coat the cells that are collected on a metal matrix placed in a field generated by permanent magnets. Such systems are capable of depleting 4 to 6 logs of tumor cells from a graft. However, even at such high efficiencies and given the limits of our ability to detect residual tumor cells, the clinical value of purging autologous grafts is debated. Concomitant with the potential benefits of the graft-versus-tumor (GVT) effect detected in recipients of allogeneic grafts has been a declining interest in tumor techniques.

T-Cell Depletion of Allogeneic Products

T cells in HPC grafts have the potential to cause severe or lethal graft-versus-host disease (GVHD) or to exert a potentially beneficial GVT effect (discussed in Chapters 107 and 111).[16] Considerable work has been done to determine whether these opposing effects are produced by distinct subpopulations of T lymphocytes.[17] This would allow ex vivo manipulation of allogeneic grafts to remove GVHD-producing T cells while sparing those that produce GVT responses. Various subpopulations of T cells have been identified as candidate effector subpopulations; however, there is no widespread consensus as to which populations should be targeted.[18,19]

Methods are available for eliminating T cells from grafts using approached similar to those used for purging tumor cells.[20] Early approaches included use of soybean agglutinin to aggregate the majority of nonprogenitor cells and resetting of sheep erythrocytes with T cells to increase their density and facilitate their removal.[21] Although successful, these techniques are not "FDA friendly" and do not offer the specificity that likely is required to engineer T-cell subpopulations in allogeneic grafts. This is possible by use of monoclonal antibodies directed toward the antigens that currently are used to identify T-lymphocyte subpopulations. The target population then can be removed with high efficiency using immunomagnetic separation, as described previously for purging autologous graft of tumor cells. The challenge remains to identify the target population and to source clinical grade monoclonal antibodies for these procedures. A number of potential target antigens have been identified and separation techniques implemented. They range from pan–T-cell depletions using antibodies to CD3 and CD2, to depletions of helper and suppressor T cells using monoclonals against CD4 and CD8, to stimulation and removal of alloreactive populations by targeting activation antigens.[19,22–27]

Methods that eliminate or physically remove either T cells or tumor cells from grafts are referred to as *negative selection techniques*. They are affected by variables such as target antigen expression, detection technologies, and other technical hurdles. They may be difficult to manipulate to achieve the ideal composition of the graft. For many years the goal was to replace these techniques with one in which HPC populations could be specifically enriched by positive selection. This would effectively deplete T cells and tumor cells from allogeneic and autologous graft respectively. The problem was the lack of a method for identifying the target HPC until the CD34 antigen was identified on a small population of progenitor cells, including the pluripotent cells required for transplantation.[28,29] The subsequent availability of monoclonal antibodies directed against this antigen made possible the development of techniques for enrichment of cells. Immobilization of the antibodies on a matrix (e.g., plastic sheets) and cellulose and magnetic particles was used as the primary approach, and a number of devices were commercially developed. The two most widely used are marketed by Miltenyi: the Baxter Isolex 300i, which uses Dynal 5-μm magnetic beads as the separation modality and releases CD34+ cells from the beads using a competitive binding peptide, and the CliniMACS system, which uses anti-CD34 nanoparticles to effect separation, with these biocompatible particles remaining on the HPC (Fig. 109–2). The Isolex is approved for use in the United States and Europe. The CliniMACS currently has only European regulatory approval.

One concern expressed about positive selection techniques is that they remove from the graft certain cells that are of potential benefit to the recipient. They include some stromal elements, GVT-mediating T cells, and other subpopulations that may facilitate engraftment. As our understanding of the identity of these populations improves, it may be possible to recover them from the nonpositively selected fraction and add them back to the CD34+ cells.

Table 109–1 lists various methods of direct T-lymphocyte depletion and indirect depletion by hematopoietic cell enrichment.

EVALUATION OF MANIPULATED GRAFTS

Most allograft engineering has focused on T0lymphocyte depletion and has emphasized quantitative versus qualitative removal. The

Table 109–1 Methods for T-Cell Depletion

Destruction In Situ	Physical Separation
Monoclonal antibody-based	Monoclonal antibody-based
Antibody + complement	Immunomagnetic separation
Immunotoxins	Negative selection
Panning and immunoaffinity columns	Enrichment of CD34+ cells
Cytotoxic drugs (4-hydroperoxycyclophosphamide [4HC])	Isolex 300i and CliniMACS systems
Photopheresis	Rosetting with sheep erythrocytes
	Soybean agglutinin
	Centrifugal elutriation

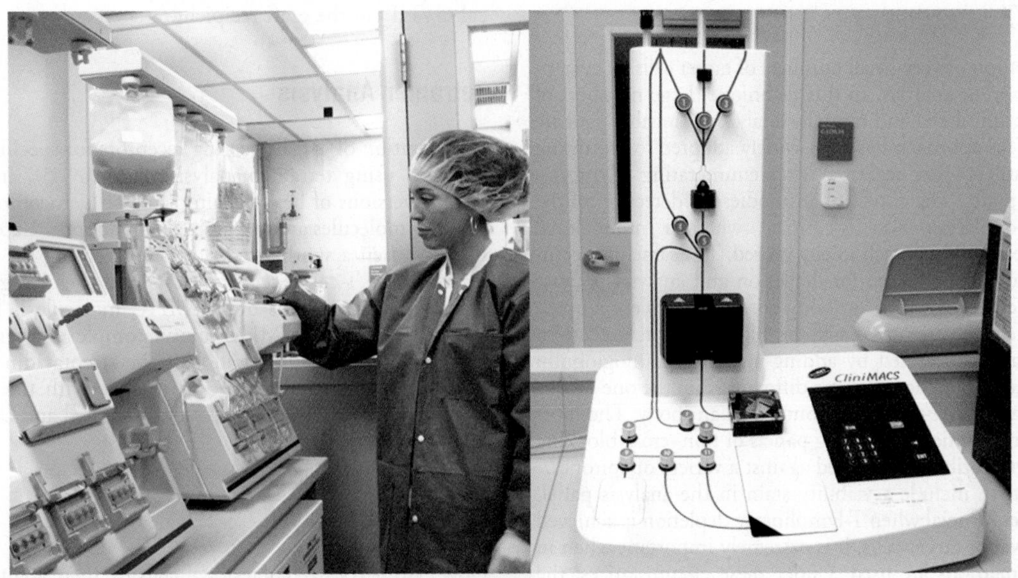

Figure 109–2 Immunomagnetic separators for enrichment of CD34+ cells. **Left**, Baxter Isolex 300i separator. **Right**, Miltenyi CliniMACS separator.

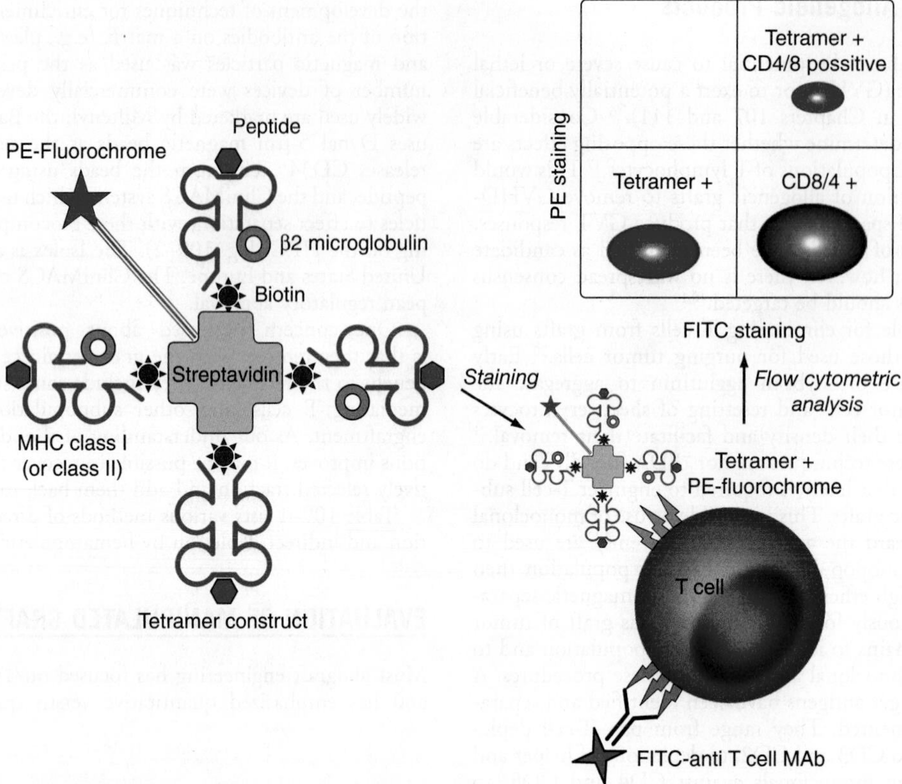

Figure 109–3 Tetramer staining to detect antigen-specific T cells (see text for details).

majority of allografts are infused immediately on preparation rather than after cryopreservation and storage, and the implications of infusing large numbers of T lymphocytes can be severe or lethal. Therefore, it is important to have available methods that can rapidly enumerate the numbers of T lymphocytes within the graft. Although early methods used detection of E-rosette–forming cells or manual immunofluorescence following staining with pan–T-lymphocyte–directed monoclonal antibody, most laboratories currently rely on flow cytometry. This technology is widely used in routine clinical laboratories; however, some precautions must be taken when it is used for T-depleted allografts.

Flow Cytometry

Accurate enumeration of very small numbers of target cells by cytometry requires rare event analysis. In this technique, large numbers of events must be accumulated and carefully analyzed if reliable data are to be obtained. This approach has been widely adopted for counting $CD34^+$ cells but still is often neglected when enumerating T lymphocytes in depleted grafts. The choice of antibodies for detection of the T-lymphocyte population also is critical when a monoclonal antibody-mediated depletion technology is used. The same monoclonal antibody should not be used for depletion and analysis because cells that became coated with the antibody during the depletion phase but were not effectively removed will be blocked from detection. However, they can be detected by adding an antiimmunoglobulin antibody conjugated to a fluorochrome different from the one conjugated to the T-lymphocyte–directed monoclonal antibody. The most sensitive detection is achieved by using panels of non–cross-blocking anti–T-lymphocyte antibodies directed against a variety of epitopes.

It is important to include a viability stain in the analysis panel. Although this is less crucial when T-lymphocyte depletion is achieved by physical removal of target cells, it is extremely important when in situ elimination methods are used. Under these circumstances, the depleted allograft may contain dead or dying T lymphocytes that will be detected by flow but may not contribute to postinfusion events. Suitable viability stains include propidium iodide and 7-aminoactinomycin. Analysis of cell viability after ex vivo depletion is not straightforward. Cell death may not be expressed immediately but may develop in the hours or days after processing and infusion. It may be possible to obtain a more accurate estimate by incubating the cells for a period before analysis. This has been particularly true in the case of depletion by immunotoxins that require the cells to divide in order to exert their toxic effects.[30] Stimulation of cells with interleukin (IL)-2 and ex vivo culture also has been used to facilitate detection of the residual T lymphocytes by flow cytometry. In some cases, this process has provided a correlation between the numbers of T lymphocytes in the cultured sample and the development of clinical GVHD in the graft recipient.

Tetramer Analysis

Enumeration of T cells bearing receptors for specific antigens can be achieved using tetramer analysis (Fig. 109–3). In this procedure, soluble versions of heavy chain of major histocompatibility complex (MHC) molecules are synthesized and adopt the appropriate conformation when a synthetic peptide representing the epitope is recognized by the T-cell receptor (TCR) and β_2-microglobulin is added. The carboxyl-terminus of the MHC molecule is biotinylated, and four of these peptide/MHC–biotin complexes assemble into a tetramer when streptavidin is added. The streptavidin is tagged with a fluorochrome; therefore, T cells reactive with the chosen peptide–MHC complex become fluorescently stained and can be detected by flow cytometry,

Functional Assays

Flow cytometry detects residual cells by their ability to bind monoclonal antibodies. Routine flow does not provide information on the functional capacity of these cells, which may be important when assessing the graft for it potential to mediate GVHD or GVT. For this purpose a number of assays have been developed. They include limiting dilution analysis, in which a range of dilutions of the graft are plated out and assessed for the ability of T cells to form colonies in response to the addition of stimulants, such as phytohemagglutinin and IL-2. Based on the proportion of colony-forming wells at the various dilutions, it is possible to determine by the Poisson distribution the number of T cells present in the original graft.

Another approach is use of an enzyme-linked immunosorbent spot (ELISpot) assay, in which cells are stimulated to produce an analyte that is characteristic of their normal function.[31] The cells are plated onto a surface that has been coated with an antibody directed against that analyte and incubated for a fixed period. The secreted analyte binds to this antibody, and the cells and any other unbound material are washed away. The surface is incubated with a biotinylated antibody directed against the analyte, and washed and incubated with alkaline phosphatase linked to streptavidin. After washing the plate is incubated with a substrate solution. A blue-black precipitate will appear at sites were the analyte was produced, with each spot representing an analyte-secreting cell. The spots can be enumerated manually or using an ELISpot reader.

CELLULAR THERAPY PRODUCTS

A number of cellular therapy products, including some that have been genetically modified, are being evaluated in the clinic. To date, clinical trials have examined the safety and efficacy of different cell populations, including, but not limited to, unmanipulated leukocyte infusions from bone marrow donors, cytokine-induced T cells, lymphokine activated killer cells, tumor-infiltrating lymphocytes (TILs), mesenchymal cells, natural killer (NK) cells, and antigen-specific T cells. Detailed accounts of the scientific basis for such studies as well as results of clinical trials are given in Chapters 110 and 111. This section focuses on processing and product evaluation issues.

Cells that have been more than minimally manipulated must be prepared under GMP conditions.[3] This requires that manufacturing be performed by trained staff following formal standard operating procedures. These procedures will have been submitted to the FDA as part of the IND application and will specify how the product is prepared, the reagents and materials that will be used, and the criteria for the release of the product for clinical use. Release criteria are test specifications that are designed to ensure that the product is sterile and pure, and they may include assays for functionality. The specific tests for sterility and purity that have been approved by the FDA are described in 21CFR and a number of guidances issued by the FDA. Some of these assays are dated, but it is important to obtain clearance from the FDA before substituting alternative tests. In the normal release mechanism for a cellular therapy product, the quality unit reviews the production records and issues a certificate of analysis. This document details the testing that was performed, who performed the tests, the specification required by the FDA, and the actual results obtained. Routine testing required for most cellular therapy products consists of aerobic, anaerobic, and fungal sterility, endotoxin levels, mycoplasma, identity/purity by flow cytometry (and in some cases HLA typing), and, for products in later stages of evaluation, functionality (e.g., cytotoxic activity toward target cells or secretion of specific bioactive products). In most cases, regulatory agencies also like to see some form of stability testing program that evaluates the stability of the cellular product over time in storage in the frozen state and when thawed for administration.

Phase I studies are designed to assess the safety of the product and should include assessment of reactions to infusion, risks for contamination during preparation, and delayed effects following administration. Clinical efficacy is evaluated during phase II/III. At this time, progress should be made toward the development of some in vitro assay for functionality that correlates with clinical efficacy. This can be problematic because most in vitro assays currently used are unreliable as predictors of the clinical value of the product, and some form of surrogate marker has been substituted.

Donor Leukocyte Infusions

The ability of donor leukocyte infusion (DLI) to effect antitumor responses initially was described in patients with chronic myeloid leukemia in hematologic relapse after allogeneic SCT,[16] but lymphomas and Hodgkin lymphoma also are sensitive to the effects of DLI.[32,33] DLI has been most successful in patients with chronic myeloid leukemia who relapse after transplant (70%–80% cytogenetic remission rate) or with Epstein-Barr virus (EBV)–associated lymphoproliferative disease (up to 90%).[16,34,35] In general response rates are higher in patients with Hodgkin lymphoma or low-grade lymphoma than in those with high-grade lymphoma.[36,37] Moderate success has been achieved with use of DLI after relapse in other malignancies such as acute myeloid leukemia (15%–40%), low-grade lymphomas (≈60%), and metastatic multiple myeloma (40%–60%). Less than 5% of patients with relapsed acute lymphoblastic leukemia respond to DLI alone. Although the etiology is unclear, the reason could be lack of antigenic expression, downregulation of T-cell recognition molecules, and/or overall tumor burden at the time of treatment.

The regulatory situation for DLI is complicated and probably is in transition. At present, they are classified as Type 361 products and fall under Part 1271 of 21CFR. It is possible that they will be reclassified as Type 351 products requiring an IND application. This is currently the case for DLI that have been manipulated ex vivo in any way (e.g., by targeting them to specific antigens). Donors of minimally manipulated DLI must be screened for eligibility, and the required infectious disease test sample must be obtained at the time of collection of the cells or up to 7 days before or after collection. Release criteria normally consists of evaluating the sterility of the final product. This provides results after the product has been infused. Formal procedures should be in place to inform the recipient's physician if a positive result is subsequently received. The contaminant should be speciated and antibiotic sensitivities obtained and communicated to the physician. Gram staining of the product prior to administration can be used, but this assay is notoriously insensitive, except in cases of gross contamination.

Natural Killer Cells

NK cells are effectors from the innate immune system that also mediate antiviral and antitumor immunity. Studies have shown that haploidentical NK cells infused after lymphodepleting chemotherapy can have antitumor effects.[38] Most facilities use a simple positive selection with clinical-scale immunomagnetic methods involving CD56 selection and/or CD3 depletion for such products.[39,40] These procedures should be done under an IND because of lack of commercially available devices or reagents for this indication. Although clinical-grade anti-CD3 is commercially available, magnetic beads and the Isolex device currently are not approved for this application. The Miltenyi device must be used under IND in the United States because it does not have regulatory approval for any indication at the present time.

When preparing an IND application for NK cell enrichment, care should be taken to ensure that the monoclonal reagents are of the highest quality available. Certificates of analysis for these reagents should be submitted with the IND application, and the agency probably will require detailed information on their manufacturing (i.e., to ensure that the process includes procedures for virus inactivation/removal). The same type of information may be required for any ancillary reagents (e.g., materials that are used to release NK cells from magnetic beads). Preclinical data demonstrating that the enrichment technique is effective should be provided and accompanied by data from clinical scale validation enrichments providing evidence that the NK cells can be enriched with an acceptable viability, purity, and yield for the proposed study. The Chemistry Manufacturing and Controls (CMC) section of the IND application should include information on the methods used to store, label, and administer the cells.

Ex Vivo Expanded Cell Therapy Products

Autologous T-Cells Nonspecifically Activated Ex Vivo

T cells can be expanded ex vivo through polyclonal activation using phytohemagglutinin, OKT3 (anti-CD3 antibody), or a combination of OKT3 and anti-CD28 antibody. Several groups have evaluated whether such expanded T cells have antitumor activity. Over the past few years several studies have correlated faster recovery of lymphocyte counts with improved outcome after autologous transplant for both non-Hodgkin lymphoma and Hodgkin lymphoma.[41,42] This led to a phase I study evaluating infusion of autologous CD3/CD28 activated cells after a CD34-selected stem cell graft.[43] Preliminary results suggested that this approach is associated with rapid recovery of lymphocyte counts.[43] The investigators subsequently combined this approach with a seven-valent pneumococcal conjugate vaccine in a phase I/II study of patients undergoing autologous stem cell transplantation for myeloma.[44] Patients who received vaccine-primed T cells early after transplant had better antipneumococcal humoral response and better $CD4^+$ proliferative response to the vaccine carrier protein than did other treatment groups. Another strategy uses interferon-μ, IL-2, and OKT3 to generate large numbers of $CD3^+CD56^+$ cytokine-induced killer T cells, which are a unique population of cytotoxic T lymphocytes (CTLs) with a characteristic $CD3^+CD56^+$ phenotype. These cells can mediate non–MHC-restricted cytotoxicity thorough NKG2D. In a phase I trial of patients with relapsed lymphoma, no toxicity or transient response was observed in a minority of patients.[45]

Cells prepared for these types of studies generally are Type 351 products because they are cultured ex vivo and they may have undergone some form of activation. Manufacturing must be carried out under GMP, and the clinical studies must be performed under an IND. The IND application must describe the procedure for manufacturing the cells and the criteria that will be used to determine whether they can be released for clinical use. Many manufacturing procedures use reagents and materials that are not approved for human use, and the application should include information about these materials and what testing will be performed before they can used in manufacturing the clinical product.

The release criteria for autologous T-cell products are similar to those described for generic Type 351 products. They include tests for sterility, endotoxin, mycoplasma, and identity and purity (i.e., by flow cytometry); some test of functionality is recommended but not usually required for phase I studies. A draft certificate of analysis, which will be used for release, should be included in the IND submission

Tumor-Infiltrating Lymphocytes

TILs are cells harvested from tumor sites and are expanded ex vivo with IL-2.[46] As the cells are being expanded, increased tumor specificity is achieved by pulsing the cells with tumor-specific peptides or exposing the lymphocytes to a retrovirus encoding a tumor-specific TCR. Although a major limitation is that patients must have preexisting lymphocytes that can both respond to tumor and be expanded ex vivo, in one study transfer of these cells led to tumor regression in 50% of lymphodepleted patients with metastatic melanoma.

A number of methods have been developed for isolation of TIL from tumors. They include mechanical, enzymatic, and differential centrifugation approaches and positive immunomagnetic selection. The method of choice depends on the type of tissue from which the cells are to be extracted and the availability of reagents, such as monoclonal antibodies, targeting the T-cell population of interest. As with T-cell depletion of allogeneic grafts, the predominant effector TIL cell population is not fully characterized, and the availability of this information should facilitate the design of more effective separation techniques. A number of approved enzymes and centrifugation media can be used, and several companies have monoclonal antibodies that have been prepared under GMP conditions but have not been submitted for FDA approval.

The extracted cells are expanded ex vivo, usually starting in semiopen systems such as cluster plates. The initial populations may be tested in a cytotoxicity assay in an attempt to identify the effector population, which then is selected for expansion. The expansion phase usually progresses through a number of types of cultures as cell numbers increase. They may progress from plates to T flasks and gas-permeable bags to hollow fiber and culture bag bioreactors. The culture medium contains IL-2 as the primary cytokine, although other agents alone and in combination may be used to promote outgrowth of specific cell subpopulations. Some investigators have used irradiated tumor cells to restimulate TILs during culture; others have performed selective separations to enrich the effector cells during expansion. Highly characterized tissue culture media, such as the serum-free lymphocyte medium AIM V, have been used for expansion. The goal is to use the simplest medium with the fewest additives that will support cell growth. Where possible the media should be free of animal serum and proteins in order to simplify the regulatory issues. However, the FDA is aware that complex media and serum combinations may be required to support growth of some cell types and is willing to consider them, particularly if the cells can be washed into an approved carrier for administration.

Initiation of a phase I study using TIL or TIL subpopulations will not require complete characterization of the effector cell population, but some preliminary information should be available that allows quantification of the putative effectors for dosing. In most cases flow cytometric analysis will be used, and the target antigens may be pan–T-cell markers or specific combinations of T subset markers. In the case where other constituents of the product may adversely affect the activity of effector cells, it may be necessary set an upper limit for contamination by these cells in the clinical product. Most facilities perform some type of functional assay as a part of the release process, which in the case of TIL may be cytokine release or cytotoxic activity toward tumor cells of the appropriate histologic type.

Allodepleted Cells

The major drawback of DLI is the significant risk of GVHD, which is the most important source of treatment-related mortality. Given that the frequency of tumor or viral antigen-specific T cells in most cases is considerably lower than that of alloreactive T cells,[47] it is necessary to expand antigen-specific T cells ex vivo not only to enhance antitumor activity but also to separate GVHD from GVT effect. An alternative method for separating GVHD from GVT effect is to selectively deplete alloreactive donor T cells ex vivo. Selective allodepletion is performed by removing donor T cells that express activation markers following coculture with nonleukemic recipient cells. Activation markers investigated include CD25[48,49] and CD69,[50] and the increased sensitivity of activated T cells to photosensitizing dyes.[51] A number of phase I/II studies using immunotoxin directed against CD25 have demonstrated the feasibility of this approach, with accelerated reconstitution of virus-specific and total T-cell numbers and low rates of severe GVHD.[48,49,52] Relapse rates remained high in these studies, which likely reflects the high-risk nature of the patient population.

Potential recipients of allodepleted cells often receive a CD34-selected HPC graft. As a part of the CD34 selection process a negatively selected population of cells that includes T cells becomes available. However, this fraction usually is not used as the source of cells for allodepletion. These cells usually have been obtained from donors who received granulocyte-macrophage colony-stimulating factor for mobilization of peripheral blood progenitor cells, and during processing for CD34 selection they were exposed to anti-CD34 monoclonal antibody. Therefore, it is preferable to obtain cells for allodepletion from a peripheral blood draw of the donor prior to administration of growth factor for mobilization. The T-cell fraction usually is obtained by centrifugation on a Ficoll-Hypaque density cushion. The cells are washed and coincubated with irradiated recipient mononuclear cells, which act as stimulators. A convenient source for stimulator cells is obtained by generation of a cell line from the donor by infection of his or her peripheral blood mononuclear cells with a laboratory strain of EBV. The coincubation step produces stimulation of alloreactive donor T cells with resulting expression of activation markers, which then can be targeted to remove the alloreactive population. Methods for elimination include cytotoxic drugs (such as methotrexate), anti-CD25 monoclonal antibody conjugated to the toxin ricin, and immunomagnetic selection. Allodepleted cells can be cryopreserved for storage until required for administration.

All of the regulatory issues associated with the manufacturing and release of Type 351 products apply to allodepleted T cell products. Release criteria include routine assays for sterility and purity. HLA typing may be included as a confirmation that the cells in the product are of donor origin. Functional assays may include demonstration that the allodepleted cells fail to proliferate when cultured in a primary mixed lymphocyte reaction (MLR).

Antigen-Specific Cytotoxic T Lymphocytes

Two major prerequisites for generating antigen-specific CTL are the identification of appropriate viral or tumor target antigens and the availability of suitable antigen-presenting cells (APCs).[53] Once identified, CTL lines can be generated by coculturing T cells with APC that express the target antigen. These lines are expanded by restimulation with the antigen of choice and the addition of cytokines such as IL-2 (Fig. 109–4).

Use of ex vivo expanded antigen-specific T cells was first reported in 1992 by Riddell et al., who showed that $CD8^+$ T-cell clones specific for cytomegalovirus administered prophylactically after allogeneic transplantation could reconstitute cytomegalovirus-specific CTLs in vivo.[54,55] Subsequent studies using EBV-specific CTLs confirmed that donor-derived CTLs could provide effective prophylaxis and therapy against posttransplant lymphoproliferative disease.[56,57] Since then many other groups have confirmed the activity of CTLs specific for these two viruses.[58–61] An approach has been developed in which multivirus-specific CTLs generated ex vivo provide protective immunity against adenovirus, cytomegalovirus, and EBV in recipients.[62]

To generate antigen-specific CTLs, it is necessary to have a good source of APCs and a source of antigen to present to T cells. A variety of APCs have been evaluated, including fibroblasts,[55] monocytes,[60] and dendritic cells (DCs),[63–65] with different types using different sources of antigen, including virus lysate[63] or lysate of antigen-positive cells, peptides,[64] or transduction of the APC with an immunodominant antigen.[65] Use of lysates as the antigen source can be problematic because they are likely to be variable and difficult to standardize, and many processing laboratories may not be experienced in handling virus and virus-infected cells.

Lymphoblastoid cell lines (LCL) prepared using laboratory strains of EBV (as described above) make excellent APCs for use in manufacturing EBV-specific T cells. They present EBV antigens efficiently, and they express high levels of costimulatory molecules. The normal procedure for generating the LCL is coincubation with EBV derived from the tamarin B95-8 cell line. This line has undergone extensive testing and is allowed for use as a source of "clinical" EBV. The resulting LCLs are cultured in media containing acyclovir to eliminate any residual EBV. The LCLs are used to repeatedly stimulate T cells (a mononuclear cell fraction of peripheral blood leukocytes), resulting in a population that is directed toward the immunodominant EBV antigens (see Fig. 109–2). These CTLs can be frozen while release testing is performed. They are delivered frozen to the bedside, where they are thawed and administered intravenously. Release testing consists of the routine tests described earlier. For allogeneic CTL, functionality usually is assessed by cytotoxicity assays, which must demonstrate less than 10% killing of autologous phytohemagglutinin (PHA) blasts.

One limitation of this approach is that expansion of virus-specific T cells to achieve adequate dose levels is extremely time consuming. All of these procedures requires several weeks to generate APCs. One means of overcoming this problem is to manufacture banked allogeneic EBV-specific CTLs so that an "off the shelf" product is available. Clinical responses have been described for some patients who received partially matched allogeneic CTL. However, immunosuppressive drug dosage was reduced and some patients also received other therapies, so how much the allogeneic CTLs contributed to the observed

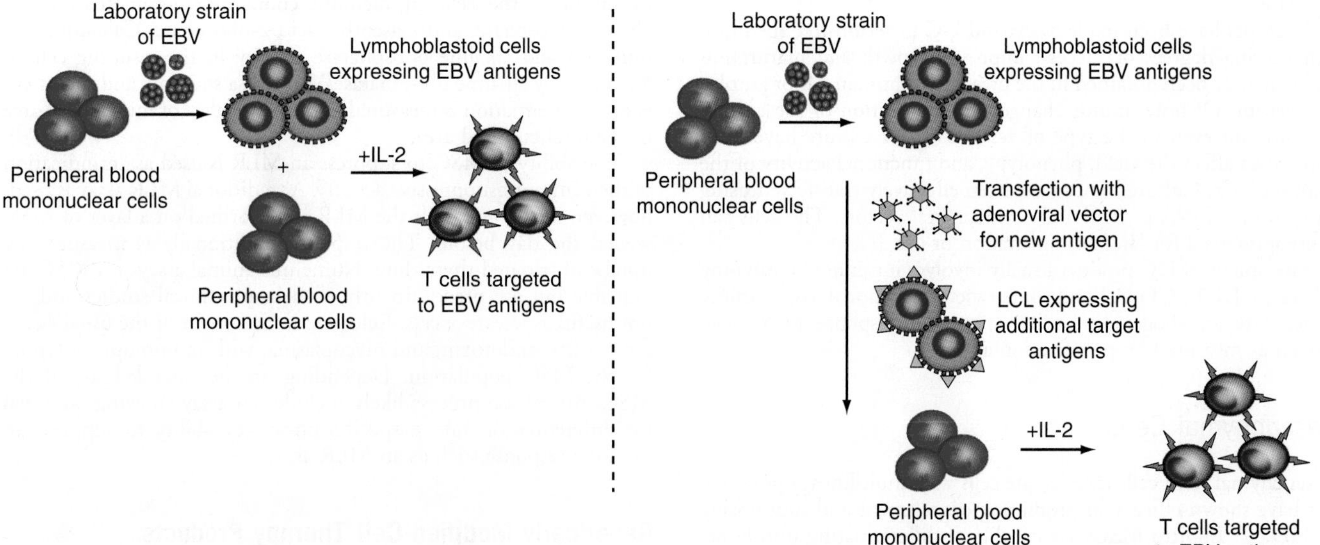

Figure 109–4 Generation of virus-specific T cells. **Left**, Use of lymphoblastoid cell line (LCL) to present Epstein-Barr virus antigens. **Right**, Use of transfected LCL to present additional antigens to T cells.

responses is unclear.[66–68] The generation of banks of CTL will require careful donor screening and HLA typing and generation of products from a sufficiently wide range of donors to allow at least partial matching with the intended recipient.

Another method for overcoming this limitation is use of rapid selection techniques such as tetramer selection and γ-interferon capture. A potential problem is the more restricted specificity of the product.

Processing and Testing Issues

Dendritic Cell Immunotherapy

DCs are powerful APCs that can be used in vitro or in vivo to elicit immune response to the antigen they are presenting.[69] A number of studies have evaluated tumor antigen-primed DCs for treatment of hematologic malignancies and solid tumors. Antigen-primed DCs are used to target T cells in vitro toward specific antigens. These cells then can be used therapeutically to eliminate viruses or tumor cells bearing that antigen. DC can be derived from bone marrow, cord blood, and mobilized and resting peripheral blood obtained from normal donors and patients.[70] The normal procedure consists of enriching monocytes from the source material, which has been accomplished by plastic adherence or CD14-based immunomagnetic selection (or by depletion of $CD19^+$ B cells and $CD2^+$ T cells). An alternative approach is use of elutriation to collect an enriched monocyte fraction from the donor. A purpose-built elutriation system for collection of monocytes is available. This method also has been used successfully to enrich monocytes from cryopreserved mobilized apheresis collections.[71]

The monocyte fraction can be cultured in polystyrene tissue culture flasks or gas-permeable bags in culture medium containing IL-4 and granulocyte-macrophage colony-stimulating factor to induce DC differentiation. This is followed by culture in medium containing proinflammatory mediators to accelerate maturation. A number of supplements have been used during this phase, including CD40 ligand or poly(I:C), interferon-γ, tumor necrosis factor-α, IL-6, IL-1β, and prostaglandin E_2. Some protocols add proinflammatory mediators at the initiation of the cultures rather than after induction of differentiation. One issue for facilities is finding clinical or GMP cytokines and growth factors. Some sources now are available, and many manufacturers will assist centers by providing information on test procedures and stability information. This information is submitted as part of the IND application, and the FDA will determine whether non-GMP reagents can be used for the specific application.

Attempts have been made to expand DC in serum-free medium, with varying degrees of success; improved growth and maturation have generally been obtained in the presence of human AB or autologous serum. Of note, minor changes in composition of the culture medium and even in the type of vessel used for culture have been reported to affect the yield, phenotype, and functional activity of the resulting DCs. Cultured DCs have been effectively transfected using native tumor DNA or lentiviral or adenoviral vectors. The cells can be cryopreserved for later administration or use.

Assessment of DC product usually involves immunophenotyping ($CD1a^+$, $CD80^+$, $CD83^-$) and some type of functional assay (ability to generate an allogeneic T-cell response or response to a recall antigen as measured by proliferation assay).

Mesenchymal Cells

Mesenchymal stem cells (MSCs) are cells with multilineage potential that have shown efficacy in promoting engraftment and suppressing GVHD.[72,73] In vitro MSCs are capable of differentiating into bone, cartilage, cardiac and skeletal muscle, neuronal cells, adipose and connective tissue, and tendons. The cells are not inherently immunogenic and do not appear to be recognized by allogeneic T cells or NK cells. They express very low levels of MHC class II and intermediate levels of class I antigens. They appear to be able to suppress in vitro T-cell proliferation and function of both memory T and naive T cells and to inhibit the development of monocyte-derived DCs in vitro.

A number of technical variables affect MSC culture and expansion ex vivo.[74] They include culture medium, passaging density, serum type and concentration, population selection, culture vessel, and use of growth factors. The following is a basic procedure. MSCs usually are isolated from bone marrow collected from the iliac crest. The cells are diluted, and the mononuclear fraction is isolated using a Ficoll-Hypaque density cushion. This fraction is plated into culture flasks to enrich for adherent cells. The nonadherent population is removed after approximately 7 days of incubation. The adherent cells are washed and detached by incubation with trypsin/ethylenediaminetetraacetic acid (EDTA) and then cultured and passaged at weekly intervals. In a study designed to optimize culture conditions, the best results were obtained when cells were cultured in low-glucose Dulbecco modified Eagle medium (DMEM)-based media containing 10% fetal bovine serum and GlutaMAX instead of L-glutamine. The cells also proliferated better when plated at low cell densities (5000–10,000 cells/cm^2) and grown in Falcon flasks. Use of basic fibroblast growth factor as a growth supplement was found to be effective; however, it caused HLA-DR induction and upregulated HLA class I expression. This did not affect the immunosuppressive capabilities of the cells. An increase in osteogenic and adipogenic potential was noted, whereas neurogenesis and CD34 engraft support were slightly suppressed. A number of media specifically designed for culture of MSC are commercially available. Various investigators have reported success growing MSCs in serum-free media, using platelet lysate, autologous serum, or human AB serum as alternatives to fetal bovine serum.

MSC can be characterized by their expression of CD105, CD73 and CD90 and their lack of expression of CD45, CD34, CD14 or CD11b, CD79a or CD19, and HLA-DR. They must be plastic adherent under standard culture conditions and must be capable of differentiating into osteoblasts, adipocytes, and chondroblasts in vitro. Differentiation assays involve growing MSCs under specific conditions that promote differentiation along the specific pathway. For neurogenic differentiation the medium contains linoleic acid, platelet-derived growth factor, and epidermal growth factor. Neural cells are identified by immunostaining with antibodies against tubulin BIII, synaptophysin, galactocerebroside, neurofilament M, and neuronal nuclei (NeuN). To assess adipogenic potential the medium contains dexamethasone, isobutylmethylxanthine, and indomethacin. The lipid droplets in the generated adipocytes are visualized by staining with Sudan Black IV. Osteogenic differentiation is measured by culturing the cells in medium containing dexamethasone, b-glycerol phosphate, and L-ascorbic acid 2-phosphate. Calcium accumulation and alkaline phosphatase activity in the resulting cells is visualized by alkaline phosphatase/Von Kossa staining, and the osteogenic differentiation is measured as the percentage of mineralized area in the total cultured area.

The ability of MSC to suppress an MLR is used as an indication of their immunosuppressive activity. A traditional MLR assay is used, however, in the test wells the MLR is performed on a layer of MSC seeded the day before. The response traditionally is measured by uptake of tritiated thymidine. Numerous animal assays for MSC are available but are predominantly used in preclinical studies and are not useful as release assays. Release criteria consist of the usual assays for sterility, endotoxin, and mycoplasma, with immunophenotyping for the MSC population. Depending on the intended use of the MSC, the release process likely includes an assay showing potential for differentiation into a specific lineage or ability to suppress an immune response such as an MLR assay.

Genetically Modified Cell Therapy Products

Many cell therapy approaches involve genetic modification of either APCs or effector cells. This therapy requires a source of vector that has been manufactured to meet regulatory requirements. Vector specifications changed markedly after the death of a gene therapy patient in Philadelphia, and they continue to evolve. Manufacturers must maintain close contact with the FDA to ensure that their products meet current specifications. Manufacturing and testing of viral vectors are extremely expensive, and use of genetically modified products requires additional monitoring of recipients. Use of vectors to transduce or transfect cellular therapy products ex vivo usually requires additional testing of the product, which may include detection of replication competent virus and checking the functionality of the introduced vector (by detecting expression of the gene product).

Suicide Gene Transduced Lymphocytes

Although treatment with DLI has led to remission in patients with disease after hematopoietic stem cell transplantation, unmanipulated cells also contain alloreactive T cells and can induce GVHD. The incidence of GVHD ranges from 55% to 90% and is associated with a treatment-related mortality rate of 20%. Approaches that maintain the GVT effect while decreasing the incidence of GVHD have been evaluated and include transduction of donor T cells with a "suicide gene." Genes can be introduced into DLI to express the herpes simplex virus-1 thymidine kinase (HSV-tk). This can be activated, with resulting suicide of the donor leukocytes, by administration of ganciclovir to the recipient if GVHD develops.[75–77]

The drawbacks of this system include the reduced immune function of transduced cells,[78] the immunogenicity of HSV-tk,[79] and the occurrence of truncated HSV-tk due to cryptic splice donor and acceptor sites that render the cells resistant to ganciclovir.[80] Addition of CD28 costimulation to CD3 activation helps to preserve the immune competence of T cells.[81,82] Alternative suicide genes based on the dimerization of Fas[83] or caspase-9[84] in the apoptotic pathway have been developed to circumvent the problem of immunogenicity of HSV-tk.

T Cells Transduced with Antigen Receptors

T cells can be transduced with genes encoding a different antigen receptor: either physiologic αβ TCR heterodimers or artificial chimeric TCRs.[85,86] Several αβ TCR heterodimers specific for tumor antigens have been evaluated in the clinic, and responses have been seen in some cases.[87] Although some inefficiency from heterologous pairing between endogenous and transduced TCR chains is expected, primary T cells transduced with cloned α and β TCR chains do mediate antitumor activity in vitro.[88–90] The main drawback of cloned TCR is HLA restriction, which limits its use to a subset of patients with a particular HLA type. Chimeric TCRs recognize target antigens on tumor cell surface through an extracellular domain, which most commonly is derived from the variable domains of an immunoglobulin. The extracellular domain is linked via a spacer to the intracellular signaling domain, which triggers T-cell activation. The latter consists of either the ζ-chain of the TCR complex or the γ-chain from FcεRI.

These studies require considerable upfront work to develop the TCR construct and to evaluate the construct for satisfactory expression. The producer cell line then must be prepared using a Master Cell Bank (e.g., of PG13 cells) and the vector generated as a supernatant from the line, purified, and tested extensively prior to use for transduction. This is a labor-intensive and expensive process that usually is beyond the expertise of cell processing facilities. Preparation of the cell product can be complex, depending on the specific protocol. Some form of stimulation may be necessary to expand the T cells and achieve the doses required. This may involve addition of immobilized or fluid phase antibody or third party cells.

Tumor Vaccines

Tumor vaccines as an approach to inducing immunity have been evaluated. Various techniques have been evaluated, including use of DCs pulsed with a tumor-associated antigen preparation and use of the entire tumor cell as an immunogen, either unmodified and/or transduced with immunostimulatory genes, aimed at eliciting a broad-based, robust immune response. This method has been used in two patient populations. In the first study, the patient's autologous Chronic Lymphocyric Leukemia or acute leukemia cells were used as the immunogen after transduction with CD40 ligand and IL-2. The results demonstrated induction of immunity and some clinical responses.[91–93] In the second study, a transduced allogeneic tumor cell line was used as the immunogen.[94]

From the manufacturing perspective, the autologous product is much more of a challenge because a stable tumor cell line must be isolated from each patient. This can be extremely difficult process. Many isolated lines do not expand well in culture, or they change phenotype over time. In some patients the line cannot be generated; other patients progress clinically before the vaccine is available and are excluded from the study. As a result, the autologous approach has a relatively high "failure rate," making it difficult to accrue a sufficient number patients into study and adding to the cost of manufacturing. The allogeneic cell line approach is technically easier because a line is selected prior to the study and can be used as the generic immunogen. This line must be tested extensively for infectious agents and should pass the FDA testing criteria for Master and Working Cell Banks. Currently testing of this type costs $100,000–$200,000 for each line. Scientifically, the drawback is that the selected line may not adequately express the antigen or range of antigens located on each patient's tumor. In addition, the choice of immunostimulatory molecules that are expressed or enhanced by transduction of the cell line may not be those that would most effectively evoke an immune response. These products are relative expensive to produce, involving not only the costs of testing the tumor cell line but also the expense of manufacturing and testing the vectors used for transduction. However, these are one-time costs because the same vaccine is used for all patients in the study.

Release testing involves testing for sterility, endotoxin, and mycoplasma, with immunophenotyping of the cells and some form of test demonstrating that the line has been effectively transduced (e.g., flow cytometry for CD40 ligand and IL-2 production in the examples described earlier). Because the product will be stored cryopreserved over the course of the study and thawed for administration to each patient, the requirement for an ongoing stability study should be anticipated.

FUTURE DIRECTIONS

Immunotherapy is undergoing a resurgence in interest. Improvements in our understanding of immune responses, targeting, immunomodulation, T-lymphocyte biology, and antigen presentation all have contributed to the revival, as has the new area of regenerative medicine using pluripotent progenitors capable of differentiation along multiple pathways. These two fields will ensure the future of cell-based therapies. The development of a new regulatory framework that applies to both areas has added to the complexity of manufacturing cell therapy products for clinical trials. This emphasizes the need for close collaboration among basic scientists, manufacturing staff, clinical researchers, and regulatory agencies. These rapidly moving areas of medicine require a flexible approach that facilitates the generation of fundamental data while allowing prompt incorporation of new findings as they emerge. This is a challenge to all involved, and the only way to meet that challenge is to open and maintain lines of communication. From the manufacturing perspective we must ensure patient and donor safety and the highest quality of the products. We face the scientific hurdles of preparing cell products that frequently are poorly characterized with regard to effector cell content and for which almost no in vitro functional assays reflecting clinical efficacy are available. Methods for separating, expanding, manipulating, and storing these products are at a relatively early stage of development, and the market opportunities for many products presently do not warrant interest from commercial entities. In spite of these hurdles, much remains to be learned from this field, and these lessons should benefit basic science, manufacturing technologists and clinicians, and hopefully many patients.

SUGGESTED READINGS

Banchereau J, Palucka AK: Dendritic cells as therapeutic vaccines against cancer. Nat Rev Immunol 5:296, 2005.

Dotti G, Heslop HE: Current status of genetic modification of T cells for cancer treatment. Cytotherapy 7:262, 2005.

Dudley ME, Rosenberg SA: Adoptive-cell-transfer therapy for the treatment of patients with cancer. Nat Rev Cancer 3:666, 2003.

FACT-JACIE International Standards for Cellular Therapy Product Collection. Processing and Administration, 3rd ed. Omaha, NE, FACT, 2007.

Gee AP: Regulatory issues in cellular therapies. Expert Opin Biol Ther 3:537, 2003.

Hernandez-Fuentes MP, Warrens AN, Lechler RI: Immunologic monitoring. Immunol Rev 196:247, 2003.

Heslop HE, Stevenson FK, Molldrem JJ: Immunotherapy of hematologic malignancy. Hematology Am Soc Hematol Educ Program 331, 2003.

Horwitz EM, Andreef M, Frassoni F: Mesenchymal stromal cells. Biol Blood Marrow Transplant 13S1:53, 2007.

Jacobsen E, Freedman A: B-cell purging in autologous stem-cell transplantation for non-Hodgkin lymphoma. Lancet Oncol 5:711, 2004.

McKenna DH Jr, Sumstad D, Bostrom N, et al: Good manufacturing practices production of natural killer cells for immunotherapy: A six-year single-institution experience. Transfusion 47:520, 2007.

NETCORD-FACT International Standards for Cord Blood Collection, Processing, Testing, Banking, Selection and Release, 3rd ed. Omaha, NE, FACT, 2007.

Standards for Cellular Therapy Product Services, 2nd ed. Bethesda, MD, AABB, 2007.

Tey SK, Brenner MK: The continuing contribution of gene marking to cell and gene therapy. Mol Ther 15:666, 2007.

Wagner JE, Thompson JS, Carter SL, Kernan NA: Effect of graft-versus-host disease prophylaxis on 3-year disease-free survival in recipients of unrelated donor bone marrow (T-cell Depletion Trial): a multi-centre, randomised phase II-III trial. Lancet 366:733, 2005.

REFERENCES

For complete list of references log onto www.expertconsult.com

CHAPTER 110

GENE TRANSFER FOR HEMATOLOGIC DISORDERS

Katherine A. High and Malcolm K. Brenner

Gene transfer is a novel area of therapeutics in which the active agent is a nucleic acid sequence, rather than a protein or small molecule. Originally conceived as a method for treating genetic disease by supplying a normal copy of a missing or defective gene, the therapeutic possibilities have been extended to include enhancement of natural protective mechanisms (eg, tumor vaccines) and augmentation of response to conventional therapies (eg, gene transfer of thymidine kinase to render tumor tissue sensitive to ganciclovir). Clinical experience with gene transfer began in 1990 when two children with severe combined immunodeficiency disease due to adenosine deaminase (ADA) deficiency underwent gene modification of lymphocytes that were then reinfused into the peripheral circulation. Since that time, over 4000 patients have been enrolled in gene transfer studies,[1] with many clear successes and two fatalities directly attributable to the gene transfer event.[2–4] There are at this time, however, no licensed gene transfer products in the United States and the field remains a developmental one, with most ongoing studies in early phase testing.

All gene transfer strategies consist of three basic elements—a therapeutic gene to be transferred in, commonly referred to as the transgene; a method of delivering the gene, termed a vector; and a physiologically relevant target cell or tissue. The disease entity itself and its pathophysiology generally determine the target cell: for sickle cell disease, hematopoietic cells; for cystic fibrosis, respiratory epithelium, etc. In hematology, the detailed elucidation of the pathophysiology of disease at the molecular level has made it fertile ground for the pursuit of gene transfer approaches to disease, because in many cases the defective gene has been identified and the cloned cDNA is available. The major limitation to progress in gene transfer at this point lies with the vectors, which have a series of shortcomings that have limited successful application. A comprehensive discussion of vector technology is beyond the scope of this chapter, but the subject has been recently reviewed,[5,6] and some of the more troublesome limitations are listed in Tables 110–1 and 110–2.

Vectors are often divided into viral and nonviral classes. Nonviral vectors, although theoretically quite attractive, have generally been characterized by low efficiency, which has limited their application in clinical settings. The viral life cycle is well suited for gene transfer, and viruses have been extensively adapted for use as vectors. This generally involves removing some or all of the viral genome and replacing it with genes of therapeutic interest. Viral genes required for replication are then supplied in *trans* during vector manufacture, with only the therapeutic gene cassette being packaged into the viral capsid. Such vectors are capable of a single round of infection but not of additional rounds of replication in the host.

Most of the clinical experience with gene transfer has been with viral vectors. Both viral and nonviral vectors can be delivered either ex vivo, where the target cells are removed from the host, transduced in the laboratory, and then reinfused, or in vivo, where the vector is injected directly into the recipient. Ex vivo transduction has been extensively explored using hematopoietic cells, either $CD34^+$ cells or their later progeny, as target cells, and much of the progress in gene transfer over the last decade has involved methods for achieving more efficient transduction of hematopoietic cells.

In an ideal setting, the donated gene persists for the duration needed (which may range from days to a lifetime), whereas the gene delivery vehicle is present only transiently. Toxicities associated with gene transfer can arise from the vector itself or from the transgene product; the distinction is worth making, because it informs future work with both components. Clinical studies in the last decade have been key to defining the safety and toxicity profiles of the available classes of vectors. Toxicities arising from the transgene product are gene-specific and defy generalizations except that there is a growing recognition that certain classes of genes, including those encoding growth factors, their receptors, signal transduction molecules, and transcription factors, may represent a higher level of risk than those encoding proteins with more narrowly circumscribed functions, such as globins or coagulation factors. The field has been more successful at identifying toxicities arising from vectors; these include problems related to the immune response, to complications arising from integration of the donated gene sequence into the target cell DNA, and to the risk of germline transmission of the donated gene sequences, if the vector transduces unintended target cells (oocytes or spermatocytes). Toxicity arising from an immune response to a viral vector is illustrated by the response to systemic infusion of adenoviral vectors, which routinely leads to fevers, myalgias, nausea, and occasional vomiting.[7] Evidence suggests that this is primarily an innate immune response to the viral capsid, because a similar toxicity profile is seen in animals even with infusion of UV-irradiated adenoviral vector.[8,9] The potential consequences of a vector-directed immune response include immune-mediated destruction of transduced cells, promotion of an adaptive immune response to the transgene product, and systemic inflammatory response syndrome, which can be fatal. Viral vectors differ widely in their propensity for triggering harmful immune responses; this is an area of ongoing investigation. The risks arising from integration of the vector into the target cell DNA are clearly illustrated by the development of an acute lymphoblastic leukemia (ALL)-like complication in five children who had been treated for X-linked severe combined immunodeficiency (SCID) by retroviral transduction of $CD34^+$ cells.[10] In these cases, the proliferative clone of cells was characterized by a proviral integration event occurring near a gene encoding a component of a hematopoietic transcription factor complex (vide infra). Vectors differ widely in terms of integrating capacity; however, even in the case of those that are classified as nonintegrating, it should be noted that foreign DNA that enters a cell always carries the potential to integrate. Investigation of integration sites, mechanisms, and consequences is also an area of active research in the field.[11–13] The inclusion of flanking insulator elements that can block promoter activity from an integrated vector sequence may reduce the risk associated with this feature of integrating vectors.[14]

The risk of germline transmission from systemic infusion of a vector at this point remains theoretical, although there have been cases where DNA extracted from semen of recipients has been transiently positive by polymerase chain reaction (PCR) for vector sequences.[15–17] Expression of the donated gene in a fetus, or altered expression of an endogenous gene at a site of integration, could theoretically disrupt the normal program of development and lead to fetal malformation or death and also raises ethical concerns arising from lack of consent. The risk of germline transmission depends on the route of administration of the vector and whether the vector efficiently transduces germ cells. Obviously, ex vivo transduction of target cells reduces this risk considerably.

Table 110–1 Limitations of Current Vector Technology
Low transduction efficiencies
Limiting tissue tropisms
Size of insert that can be accommodated
Difficulty in achieving regulated expression
Risk of insertional mutagenesis
Toxicity related to the vector capsid or viral proteins

Other limitations of current vector technology need to be addressed. These include vector-specific tissue tropisms that limit the cell types that can be transduced, and limitations on the size of the insert that can be accommodated (Tables 110–1 and 110–2). The development of promoters that can be precisely regulated by orally administered small molecules is underway, and will be an important prerequisite for safe delivery of some transgenes.

To those outside the field, the pace of development of clinical gene transfer has appeared slow. For novel classes of therapeutics, however, early clinical studies are perforce time-consuming, as key safety issues are uncovered and addressed. The fruit of the first decade of clinical studies in gene transfer was the identification of most of the critical safety issues. None of these are yet judged to be insuperable obstacles, and the potential benefits of gene transfer, which are considerable, still appear to outweigh the problems. Strides in vector manufacturing and standardization have resolved the issue of whether a biologic product as complex as a multicomponent viral vector can be reliably and reproducibly produced. What remains an issue is whether the human immune response, particularly to viral vectors, can be managed so as to achieve optimal responses in human subjects. Work over the next decade is likely to provide the answer.

GENE TRANSFER FOR GENETIC DISEASE

Hematologists have played a leading role in the field of gene transfer. In principle, any inherited genetic disorder that can benefit from transplantation of normal hemopoietic stem cells (see Chapter 100) could benefit from genetic correction of autologous stem cells as well. When Moloney-derived vectors were all that were available for clinical protocols, concerns about inefficient gene transfer and poor expression, the lack of selective advantage for transduced cells, and risks of oncogenesis all served to limit clinical investigation even of promising preclinical studies. With the successful development of lentiviral derived vectors (see also gene transfer for hemoglobinopathies and thalassemia) and the realization that submyeloablative treatment of patients can permit engraftment of gene-modified cells, there are now several efforts underway to treat a broader range of inherited metabolic disorders using gene-modified hematologic progenitor cells. Other hematologic disorders, such as hemophilia or porphyrias, will likely require the use of different target cells, eg, liver. This section will review the progress and problems over the last several years in three classes of genetic disease, hereditary immunodeficiency states, hemoglobinopathies and thalassemias, and hemophilia. These have been chosen because there is a considerable body of data available and because they illustrate well the problems presented by gene transfer and the strategies that have been used to overcome them. It should be noted that other disorders, such as Fanconi anemia, have been approached by gene transfer techniques; for overviews of these, the reader is referred to the literature.[18]

Gene Transfer Using Hematopoietic Cells as Targets—Immunodeficiency Diseases

X-Linked Severe Combined Immunodeficiency

The first example of therapeutic gene transfer in a clinical setting was reported in 2000, when Alain Fischer and colleagues reported reconstitution of T, NK, and B cell function in children with X-linked severe combined immunodeficiency disease following retroviral transduction of CD34$^+$ cells from affected infants.[19] X-linked SCID is a rare disorder affecting less than 1 in 100,000 births and is due to a mutation in the gene encoding the γc subunit of the cytokine receptor for IL-2, -4, -7, -9, -15, and -21. In the absence of the receptor, differentiation of hematopoietic stem cells to mature T and NK cells does not occur; B-cell immunity is thus also affected. The disease is lethal without treatment but is cured by bone marrow transplant from an HLA-identical donor. For those who lack an HLA-matched donor, a haploidentical transplant (eg, from a parent) results in a 78% survival rate (at the most experienced centers[20]), but survival is generally complicated by poor B-cell function, requiring monthly infusions of intravenous immunoglobulin (IVIg). In the study by Fischer and colleagues, marrow CD34$^+$ cells from infants and young children without an HLA-identical donor were transduced daily for 3 days with a retroviral vector expressing the γc subunit. T-lymphocyte counts began to rise approximately 30 days after infusion of the transduced cells and had reached normal levels within a few months. Detailed studies of T-cell function and response to primary vaccination documented reconstitution of immune function.[19,21] In all, the group treated 11 boys with X-linked SCID, and in follow-up in early 2002, 9 of 11 had had an excellent response,[22] and were well on no treatment. One teenager and one infant who had disseminated bacilli Calmette–Guerin infection at the time of gene transfer failed to reconstitute T-cell function and, in the case of the infant, went to bone marrow transplant. Failure of the procedure in the 16-year-old patient likely reflected poor thymic function, because efficient transduction of his CD34$^+$ T cells was documented.[23] Similar success was attained in a gene transfer trial in London, with 10 of 10 treated subjects well up to 59 months after initial treatment.[13] The key features contributing to the success of this work included the disease itself, where there is a strong in vivo proliferative advantage for transduced cells compared with nontransduced cells,[24] and the series of incremental advances in retroviral transduction of human hematopoietic stem cells (HSCs) that occurred in the 1990s, including improved techniques for isolating CD34$^+$ cells, identification of combinations of early-acting cytokines that could induce cell proliferation without loss of repopulating capacity and recognition of the utility of colocalizing vector particles and HSCs using fibronectin fragments.[25]

Compared with a haploidentical bone marrow transplant, gene transfer appeared to provide a better outcome, because there were no fatalities and those with a positive response had complete reconstitution of immune function (vs continued requirement for IVIg infusions in bone marrow transplantation [BMT]). In addition, reconstitution appeared to occur more quickly with gene transfer, sometimes a critical issue in children gravely ill with infections. However, the analysis of risk–benefit changed approximately 3 years after the first subjects were treated, when one of these developed a T cell-proliferative syndrome characterized by lymphocytosis (WBC 300,000) and splenomegaly. Molecular analysis of these cells revealed a monoclonal population of αβ T cells characterized by a single integration event on chromosome 11, in which the retroviral-encoded sequence was positioned in reverse orientation within the first intron of the *LMO-2* gene, which encodes a protein involved in transcription factor complex assembly.[3,26] This integration event was associated with increased expression of LMO-2 in the circulating T-cell population (LMO-2 is normally expressed only in earlier progenitors), a finding that has been reported previously in acute lymphoblastic leukemia, usually in association with a t(11:14) translocation.[27] Within months a second patient presented with similar findings,

Table 110–2 Characteristics of Gene Delivery Vehicles

	Viral Vectors								Non-Viral Vectors			
Features	***Retroviral***	***Lentiviral***	***Adenoviral***	***AAV***	***Human Foamy Virus***	***HSV-1***	***SV-40***	***Alphaviruses***	***Transposon/ Transposase System***	***Liposomes***	***Naked DNA***	***Site Specific Integrase***
Viral Genome	RNA	RNA	DNA	DNA	RNA	DNA	DNA	RNA	N/A	N/A	N/A	N/A
Tissue Tropism	Various	Various	Various	Muscle, liver, brain	Various	Neurons	Various	Various (CNS)	Various	Various	Various	Various
Cell Division Requirement	Yes	G1phase	No	No	No	No	No	No	No	No	No	No
Packaging Limitation	8 Kb	8 Kb	8–30 Kb	5 Kb	8.5 Kb	40–150 Kb	5 Kb	5 Kb	Undetermined probably large	Undetermined probably large	Undetermined probably large	Undetermined probably large
Pre-existing Immunity	No	Yes if HIV+	Yes	Yes	No	Yes	No	No	No	No	No	No
Immune Responses	Few	Few	Extensive	Few	Few	Few in recombinant virus	Few	Few	No	No	No	No
Genome Integration	Yes	Yes	Poor	Poor	Yes	No	Poor	No	Yes	No	No	Yes
Long-term Expression	No	Yes	No	Yes	Yes	No	No	No	Yes	No	No	Undetermined
Numbers of Clinical Trials Worldwide	293	8	322	46	0	43	1	0	0	99	230	0
Main Advantages	Persistent gene transfer in dividing cells	Persistent gene transfer in transduced tissues	Highly effective in transducing various tissues	Elicits few inflammatory responses, non-pathogenic	Persistent gene expression in both dividing and non-dividing cells	Large packaging capacity with persistent gene transfer	Wide host cell range; lack of immunogencity	Limited immune responses against the vector	Transfects many cell types with long term gene expression	Transfects many cell types. Large holding capacity to enable a high number of base pairs	Efficient in gene transfer, limited immunogenecity	Specific integration site
Main Disadvantages	Theoretical risk of insertional mutagenesis (occurred in 2 cases)	Might induce oncogenesis in some cases	Viral capsid elicits strong immune responses	Limited packaging capacity	In need of a stable packaging system	Residual cytotoxicity with neuron specificity	Limited packaging capacity	Transduced gene expression is transient	Early Stage in development	Expensive to produce	Transient and low level expression	Early stage in development

including a clonal population of cells showing proviral integration adjacent to the *LMO-2* locus, and since that time an additional three subjects have also developed a leukemia-like syndrome.[3,10] A puzzling aspect of this serious complication of therapy is that a similar X-linked SCID trial carried out in London had initially reported no instances of leukemia or lymphoproliferative disorders in any of their 10 successfully treated subjects; recently, however, one of these subjects also developed a leukemia-like syndrome. A comprehensive study of retroviral integration sites in these subjects[12,13] has demonstrated that the retroviral insertion sites in the transduced CD34+ progenitor cells differ from those detected in engrafted CD3+ cells. This suggests that vector integration sites may influence cell survival, engraftment, or proliferation.

Clinical gene transfer experiments started in 1990, and hundreds of patients have received cells transduced with retroviral vectors. The question thus arises as to why the subjects in the X-linked SCID trial developed this complication whereas so many others did not. Several factors may have contributed. The cytokine receptor is required for T and NK cell maturation; there is thus a powerful and stringent in vivo selection for and expansion of the transduced cells, a situation that does not occur in most other hematologic diseases for which hematopoietic stem cell gene transfer has been attempted. Second, in this case, the transgene product is essentially a growth factor receptor; genes encoding growth factors, their receptors, signal transduction molecules, and transcription factors, may represent a higher level of risk (in terms of altering cell growth) than genes with more narrowly defined functions.[28] Finally, two of the patients who developed this complication were among the youngest treated, and received a higher dose of cells per kg body weight than other subjects, reflecting the fact that their CD34+ cells expanded rapidly in culture. Whether cells from young infants are in some way different from those of older children (eg, related to differences in cord blood CD34+ vs adult CD34+ cells) in terms of abundance and identity of open chromatin remains to be explored. At the time of writing, the federal regulatory agencies in the United States have advised against the use of retroviral transduction of CD34+ cells in the setting of X-linked SCID, although exceptions may be made for those without other treatment options. Continued follow-up of children who have already received gene-modified cells for this disease will define the frequency of deleterious consequences of retroviral integration in this setting.

Adenosine Deaminase–Severe Combined Immunodeficiency

Severe combined immunodeficiency due to ADA deficiency is of special interest, since the first clinical gene transfer trials were conducted in children with this disorder. The absence of functioning ADA results in accumulation of large amounts of deoxyadenosine, an ADA substrate, which is converted to a toxic metabolite in T cells, with resulting loss of function. The disease is cured by HLA-matched bone marrow transplantation. Those who lack an HLA-matched donor can be treated, generally less successfully, with a haploidentical transplant and/or with polyethylene glycol-conjugated bovine ADA. It had been postulated that gene-corrected cells have a survival advantage, and a report of reconstitution of the immune system in a patient with ADA deficiency after a spontaneous gene reversion event[29] supports this hypothesis. Moreover, the observation that immunologic reconstitution occurred in patients who achieved only donor T-cell engraftment after BMT suggested that transduction of T cells alone would be adequate for clinical improvement. Finally, because most patients experience some increase in circulating numbers of T cells after PEG-ADA therapy, it is possible to test the efficacy of T-cell transduction by harvesting and transducing these cells.

The first clinical gene transfer trial took place in 1990 in two children with ADA-SCID; both children lacked an HLA-matched donor and failed to achieve full immune reconstitution on PEG-ADA administered for at least 9 months. T cells were harvested from peripheral blood and transduced with a retroviral vector encoding ADA. Cells were expanded in culture and infused after 9 to 12 days, with no selection to enrich for transduced cells and no myeloablation prior to cell infusion. Each patient received a total of approximately 10^{11} cells, although the number of *transduced* cells was approximately 10-fold higher in the first patient compared to the second. Both patients were continued on PEG-ADA therapy at doses in the range of 10–14 U/kg/week. The first full-length report of results[30] documented increased T-cell count and ADA enzyme activity in the first patient; the second patient showed an improvement in T-cell count but no measurable ADA activity above baseline. A follow-up report[31] documented that 10 years after gene transfer, 20% of the circulating T cells in the first patient were still positive for the donated gene by real-time PCR, with multiple integration sites documented on Southern, whereas only 0.1% were positive in the second patient. This report is important in that it provides evidence supporting the long-term safety of retroviral transduction of T cells. It also documents their long lifespan in the periphery, and the fact that the Moloney retroviral promoter is resistant to silencing in vivo. However, interpretation of efficacy in this setting has been complicated by the continuation of PEG-ADA infusion therapy, so that it is not clear what contribution gene transfer made to the patients' clinical courses.

Kohn and colleagues[32] assessed this issue in a trial in which PEG-ADA therapy was reduced and then stopped in one patient. In their study, cord blood CD34+ cells from three infants with ADA-SCID were transduced with a retroviral vector expressing ADA and reinfused. Children were also treated with PEG-ADA at doses ranging from 30 to 60 U/kg/week. In subject 1, who had the highest levels of gene marking (1%–3% PBMCs, 10%–30% of T cells) and of T-lymphocyte numbers, PEG-ADA was gradually reduced starting at 30 months post gene transfer, and stopped altogether at 48 months. Over the ensuing 2 months, there was a more than 100-fold decline in plasma ADA level, a 100-fold increase in levels of erythrocyte deoxyadenosine nucleotides, and large decreases in numbers of B and NK cells. The proliferative response to tetanus toxoid, previously demonstrated to be present, was lost entirely, although absolute numbers of CD4+ and CD8+ T cells remained constant. Two months after stopping PEG-ADA, the child presented with an upper respiratory tract infection, sinusitis documented on X-ray, and oral monilia. PEG-ADA was restarted, with resolution of infection and return of immunologic parameters to baseline. Although these data are from a single patient, they strongly suggest that the levels of gene transfer and expression achieved in this instance were not adequate to support immune function.

More recently, Alessandro Aiuti, Maria Grazia Roncarolo, and colleagues have reported clinical success in the setting of ADA-SCID after two key changes to the protocol.[33] First, the five subjects received nonmyeloablative conditioning with busulfan 2 mg/kg/day × 2 days prior to infusion of the gene-modified cells, to facilitate engraftment of the gene-modified cells. Second, the subjects were not treated with PEG-ADA at any point after gene transfer, conferring a survival advantage on the transduced cells. With these modifications, all subjects showed marked improvement in levels of circulating peripheral blood lymphocytes, with 70% to 100% of circulating T cells shown to contain vector.[11] All subjects have shown reconstitution of immune function, and were able to return home on no treatment, with documented gains in growth. Either or both of the modifications to the protocol may have been critical to success; studies in which one but not both of these maneuvers (myelosuppression, withdrawal of PEG-ADA) are carried out may help to answer this question.

In terms of safety, at a median follow-up of 3.1 years, there have been no adverse events related to gene transfer in the ADA-SCID trial.[11–13] In a recent study of retroviral integration sites in these patients, the investigators confirmed a bias toward gene-dense regions, with a preference for the region around transcriptional start sites and highly expressed genes, in both preinfusion transduced CD34+ cells and in lymphoid and myeloid progeny from blood and bone marrow at a series of time points after transduction. The investigators identified insertion sites proximal to protooncogenes and genes controlling cell growth, including *LMO-2*, but there was no associated clonal selection or expansion noted.[11] One can speculate that the difference in outcome for ADA-SCID versus X-linked SCID reflects some contribution from the transgene itself in the case of X-linked SCID, but definitive proof is lacking. Clearly, the results in the ADA-SCID trial are at this writing the best example of safe and effective gene transfer for genetic disease. It will be important to confirm that these findings can be safely extended to larger numbers of patients.

OTHER IMMUNODEFICIENCIES

Inherited disorders in which there is no selective advantage to cells expressing the corrective gene represent more of a challenge to gene therapy, given the inefficiency of most gene transfer vectors. Nonetheless, recent data from patients treated for chronic granulomatous disease (CGD) have shown success even in the absence of selection.[34] CGD is a disorder of the innate immune system, in which there is a deficiency of the oxidative microbial activity due to mutations in the X-linked gene encoding gp91^{phox}, a component of the oxidase complex. Affected individuals suffer persistent infection with organisms such as staphylococci that are normally killed after phagocytic ingestion. In an initial report on 2 patients (a third was treated subsequently), Ott et al[34] showed that administration of myeloreductive chemotherapy provided sufficient "space" for engraftment of gene-modified stem cells. Newly emergent gene-modified neutrophils were able to substantially improve the patients' infections, even to the extent of healing a persisting lung abscess. Though extremely encouraging for efforts to broaden the application of stem cell gene therapy, two subsequent observations have led to caution. First, analysis of the proviral integration site showed that there was progressive selection of clones with integrants close to a restricted number of genes (MDSI-EVI1, PRDM16 and SETBPI), which became activated. Given the experience in X-SCID, this is clearly concerning. It implied that a selective growth advantage had developed because of disruption of normal growth-regulating mechanisms and raised the specter of progression to monoclonality and then malignancy. Indeed, 3 years after treatment 2 patients developed myelodysplasia, one of whom has received a stem all transplant (Grez, personal communication). Another concern is that one of the treated patients subsequently died of infection, implying that correction may have been incomplete. Clearly, cautious treatment of additional patients will be needed to obtain a true risk–benefit assessment.

Gene Transfer for Hemoglobinopathies and Thalassemias

Sickle cell disease and thalassemia have attracted considerable interest as disease targets for gene transfer approaches: current treatment for both entities is unsatisfactory, the globin genes are available, the diseases are well-characterized at the molecular level, and the target levels of expression required for improvement of disease phenotype are relatively modest—around 20% of normal levels of expression of the β-globin genes. Despite these advantages as a model, gene transfer for these diseases has proven to be a complex undertaking, with progress stalled until more efficient (lentiviral) vectors were developed. The current state of the field is cautious optimism, the optimism based on long-term improvement in mouse models of the diseases,[35,36] the caution based on the results in the X-linked SCID trial (vide supra). Clinical trials of gene transfer for these diseases have been initiated, but results have not yet been reported.

Early studies documented that murine retroviral vectors expressing the β-globin genes could transduce murine and human hematopoietic stem cells, but levels of expression were low.[37–39] Concurrent studies revealed that the regulation of the β-globin locus depended on a 25-kb sequence located approximately 60 kb upstream of the adult β-globin gene; this locus control region (LCR) was required for high-level expression in transgenic mice.[40] Molecular analysis of the LCR identified smaller regions that were sufficient for high-level expression, but retroviral vectors composed of these LCR fragments and globin gene sequences failed to achieved integration of unrearranged copies of the transgene in target cells at high frequency.[41] A decade of research uncovered factors responsible for this, including cryptic splice sites that resulted in internal deletions in the LCR/globin minigene[42,43]; the quiescence of hematopoietic stem cells, an obstacle given the requirement of retroviruses for nuclear mitosis to gain access to nuclear chromatin; in *human* HSCs, the low level of receptor protein needed for retroviral entry into the cell,[44–46] position-dependent levels of expression following integration[43,47,48]; and silencing of gene expression over time. Solutions to several of these problems have been demonstrated (Table 110–3), but a substantial breakthrough awaited the development of a vector with improved transduction characteristics. In 2000, Michel Sadelain and colleagues designed and produced a lentiviral vector that achieved long-term "cure" in a mouse model of thalassemia.[36] Success in this case depended on several unique features of their vector. Lentiviral vectors have a higher packaging capacity than retroviral vectors, and Sadelain et al used this to incorporate larger fragments of the LCR, which helped to overcome position effects. The HIV rev protein acts to suppress splicing of the viral RNA genome; its inclusion prevented LCR/globin splicing. The lentiviral vector was pseudotyped with an alternative envelope protein (vesicular stomatitis virus-G, VSV-G), allowing higher transduction rates into murine HSCs. For reasons that are not entirely clear, silencing of expression occurs less frequently with lentiviral vectors than with retroviral vectors. In Sadelain's experiment, lethally irradiated recipient mice were transplanted with lentiviral-transduced cells from syngeneic mice.[36] Expression of human β-globin was high-level and persistent, so that at 24 weeks, tetramers composed of mouse α-globin and human β-globin constituted 13% of total hemoglobin. The same experiment in β^0-thalassemic heterozygote mice resulted in long-term clinical improvement, including increased hemoglobin and hematocrit and

Table 110–3 HIV Gene Therapy

Cells Given	Proposed Benefit	Type of Study	Outcome
Autologous T cells expressing nonfunctional Rev M10 or wild-type M10[97]	Cells should resist HIV infection if nonfunctional Rev M10 present	Phase I	Safe. Improved short-term survival of cells with nonfunctional M10
Autologous T cells expressing Rev M10 or nonfunctional M10[98]	As above	Phase I	Safe. Cells combining mutant Rev M10 survived up to 140 days. No change in viral load
HIV-specific CD4 and CD8$^+$ T cells transduce to express chimeric CD4-zeta T-cell receptors[99]	Modified T cells inhibit viral replication and kill virus-infected cells in vitro	Phase II	Gene-modified cells persistent and produced reduction in two of four viral reservoirs and tend toward fewer recurrent viremias
T cells from identical twin discordant for HIV infection expressing chimeric CD4/CD3-zeta chimeric receptor[100]	Cells have lytic activity against virus-infected cells	Phase I	Safe. Prolonged persistence when CD4 and CD8$^+$ cells infused together

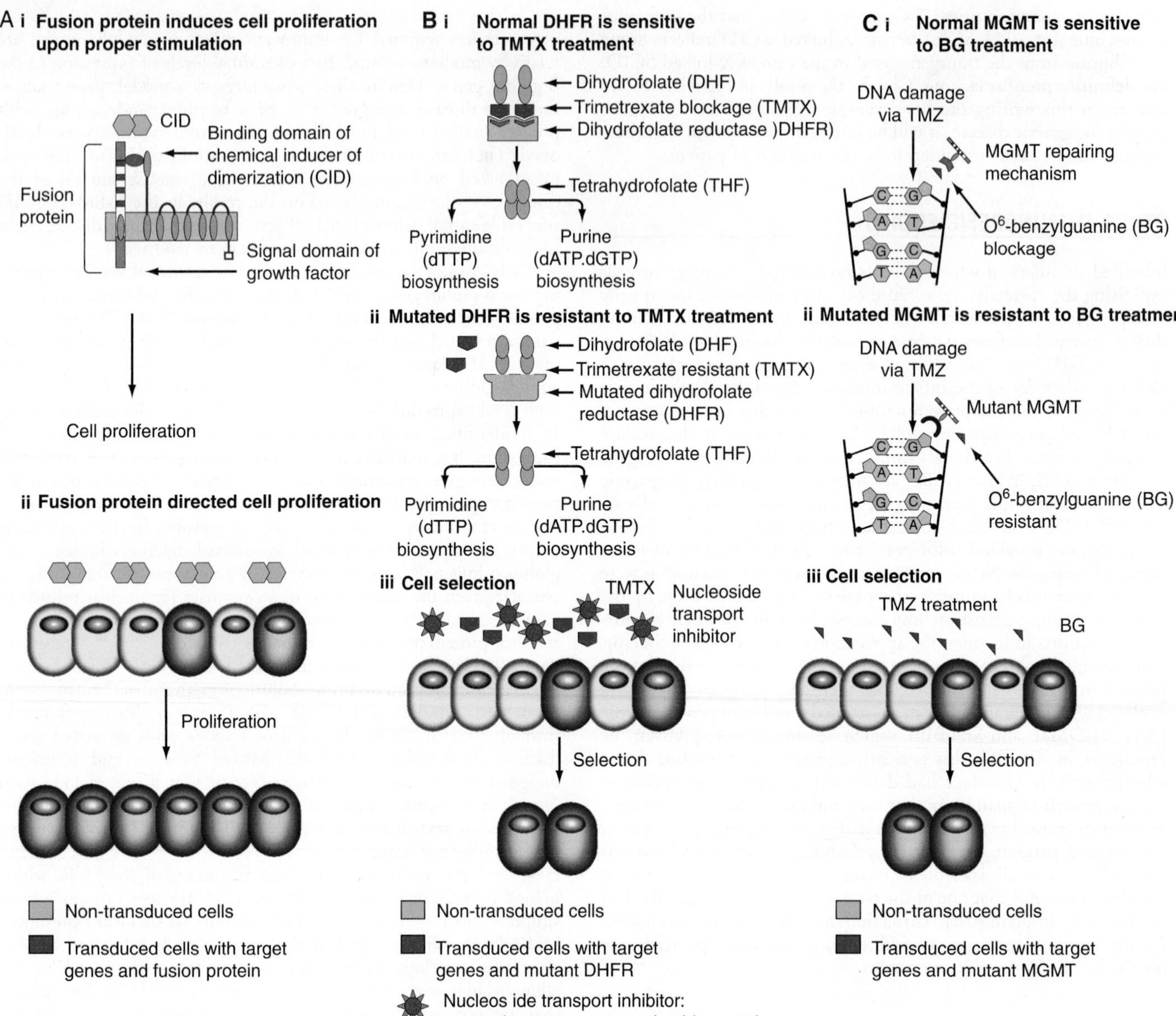

Figure 110–1 Experimental strategies for providing survival or proliferative advantages to transduced cells. **A,** Cells are transduced with sequences encoding a transmembrane fusion protein with an intracellular domain that signals cell growth, and extracellular domains that, when induced to dimerize by a small molecule (orally delivered) drug, result in growth of the transduced cell. **B,** Cells are transduced with a vector expressing a mutant dihydrofolate reductase, which is resistant to methotrexate, an inhibitor that blocks the endogenous nucleotide synthesis pathway. When cells are treated with TMTX along with a nucleoside transport inhibitor, the transduced cells enjoy a survival advantage over nontransduced cells. **C,** Cells are transduced with a vector expressing a mutant MGMT, which is resistant to BG, an inhibitor that blocks the DNA-repairing ability of MGMT. When cells are treated with TMZ, which induces DNA damage, in the presence of BG, the transduced cells enjoy a survival advantage over nontransduced cells.

a drop in the reticulocyte count. This group has now extended their findings to a novel mouse model of β^0-thalassemia major, with similar impressive results.[49] The robustness of the findings is attested to by the fact that success using a similar vector was achieved by another group in a different disease model. Leboulch and colleagues transplanted lethally irradiated mice with murine HSCs transduced with a lentiviral vector expressing an antisickling β-globin variant. Transduction and transplantation of cells from normal mice resulted in 16% of circulating hemoglobin comprised of tetramers containing the variant β chain, whereas in two different murine models of sickle cell disease they constituted 10% or 48% of total hemoglobin, with accompanying improvement in all hematologic parameters.[35]

These recent results are encouraging in a field where progress had seemed slow over the last decade. Translation of these findings to the clinic will require a few additional components that are not yet in hand. For example, complete myeloablation, as occurs when mice are lethally irradiated, is not an acceptable risk in most patients with sickle cell disease or thalassemia. Several strategies that confer a survival advantage (such as occurs naturally in immunodeficiency diseases) on transduced cells are under development (Fig. 110–1[50–52]); one that shows safety and efficacy in large animal models and humans would facilitate gene transfer for hemoglobinopathies and thalassemias. Lentiviral vectors have been extensively engineered to reduce the risk of recombination events that can lead to replication-competent virus, and transcriptional regulatory sequences have been deleted from the 3' LTR, so that the integrated proviral genome lacks viral regulatory sequences that can interfere with transgene expression or promote expression of adjacent genes. The question has been raised about whether the adverse events in the X-linked SCID trial should halt development of gene transfer into hematopoietic cells; it seems likely in that case that a number of disease- or protocol-specific factors (vide supra) may have contributed to the outcome. Whether or not additional adverse events are observed in those who have undergone retroviral transduction of HSCs, it may be prudent to incorporate insulator elements,[14] which can block effects of distal enhancers, into new vectors. Clinical studies addressing the safety of lentiviral vectors in humans are now underway in patients with HIV (see below) or with adrenoleukodystrophy.

Gene Transfer for Hereditary Disease Using Nonhematologic Target Cells—Hemophilia as a Model

Hemophilia differs from the other hematologic disorders discussed here in that the target cell is generally not one of hematopoietic origin; rather, target cells have included liver, skeletal muscle, and fibroblasts (in the clinic), and the GI tract, endothelial cells, and other cell types (in preclinical studies). Hemophilia has been an attractive model for studying gene transfer for several reasons; there is latitude in the choice of target tissue, because biologically active clotting factors can be made in many different cell types, and improvement of circulating levels of F.VIII or F.IX by even a modest amount is likely to improve the phenotype of the disease. Moreover, the existence of genetically engineered mice and of naturally occurring dog models of the disease, coupled with the availability of the murine and canine F.VIII and F.IX genes, offers the possibility of evaluating gene transfer strategies for safety and efficacy before moving to the clinic. Finally, the biologically relevant endpoint for most hemophilia gene transfer strategies is the circulating plasma level of Factor VIII or Factor IX; this endpoint is easily measured in most hospital coagulation laboratories and is known to correlate well with disease symptoms. Patients with levels lower than 1% normal have severe disease with frequent spontaneous hemorrhage; those with levels of 1% to 5% are more moderately affected; and those with levels 5% or higher are only mildly affected.

The attractiveness of hemophilia as a model and the relatively large numbers of affected patients initially resulted in active interest and the initiation in the United States of five clinical studies using five different gene transfer strategies. In the first of these, a plasmid carrying a selectable marker and a truncated form of the *F8* gene, with a deletion of the B domain, was introduced by ex vivo electroporation into autologous fibroblasts cultured from skin biopsies of affected patients. Clones expressing high levels of F.VIII were selected and expanded, then reimplanted onto the omentum of patients in a laparoscopic procedure. Results in the first six subjects showed evidence for a clinical response in terms of reduced frequency of spontaneous bleeds, reduced number of factor infusions, and levels of F. VIII activity above baseline (but not >2% in most cases) in 3 of 6 subjects.[53] These markers of gene expression were detected for a period of months but eventually returned to baseline in all subjects. Possible explanations for the decline in circulating levels include fibrosis surrounding the site of cell implantation, senescence or immune-mediated destruction of the genetically modified cells, or loss of promoter activity. A preliminary report detailed results from six additional subjects with severe hemophilia A who underwent this procedure; these did not differ substantially from those reported in full-length form. This is a potentially useful approach, particularly if the F.VIII levels could be increased, either through implantation of more cells or higher F.VIII expression per transfected cell, but it is also labor-intensive and will likely require repeat administration. This approach is not currently being actively pursued.

Retroviral vectors have also been evaluated as an approach to gene transfer for hemophilia. A major obstacle for in vivo gene transfer with retroviral vectors in the setting of hemophilia is the requirement for a dividing target cell. Kay and coworkers initially explored this approach for Factor IX deficiency in the hemophilia B dog model.[54] To induce replication in the target cells (hepatocytes), they first carried out a two-thirds partial hepatectomy in recipient animals, followed by portal vein infusion of vector. This resulted in long-term expression of canine F.IX in these animals, but at levels too low to improve disease phenotype (<1%). Vanden Driessche et al subsequently showed that one could achieve therapeutic levels of Factor VIII in mice by injecting a retroviral vector (4×10^9 cfu/kg) during the neonatal period when the rate of hepatocyte replication is still high,[55] and Ponder and colleagues have recently extended these findings to the large animal model of hemophilia B, showing that intravenous infusion of retroviral vector doses of approximately 1×10^{10} transducing units (TU)/kg into newborn hemophilic puppies results in long-term expression of Factor IX at levels higher than 10% normal.[56] Several groups have shown that pretreatment of adult mice with hepatocyte growth factor results in increased transduction of hepatocytes,[56–59] but this finding has not yet been extended to large animals. A clinical study of intravenous infusion of a retroviral vector expressing B-domain deleted F.VIII in 13 adults with severe hemophilia A documented safety of the infusion at doses up to 8×10^8 TU/kg,[60] but there was no evidence of long-term expression at levels greater than 1%; the animal studies suggest that higher doses combined with some method to induce hepatocyte replication would be required for efficacy in adults. On the basis of animal studies one would predict that infusion of vector into newborns would be more likely to demonstrate efficacy, but such an approach would require much more extensive safety studies, in animals and in adult humans, before it is undertaken.

The use of adeno-associated viral vectors has also been explored in gene transfer for hemophilia, using both skeletal muscle and liver as target tissues. AAV vectors can accommodate only a relatively small insert, so clinical studies for hemophilia have thus far been confined to hemophilia B. However, multiple preclinical studies have demonstrated that the F8 gene can be delivered by an AAV vector, either by using two distinct vectors that subsequently concatemerize as DNA in the nucleus[61] or that encode separate protein subunits that assemble in the cell,[62] or by using a very short promoter in a single vector.[63] The first AAV-mediated clinical gene transfer study for hemophilia B used skeletal muscle as the target.[64,65] As shown in Table 110–2, AAV has tropism for liver, muscle and brain, and preclinical studies in mice and hemophilic dogs had demonstrated efficacy when an AAV-Factor IX vector was administered either to skeletal muscle by IM injection[66,67] or to liver via portal vein injection.[68–70] However, at the time that the first study was undertaken, there was no previous experience with parenteral administration of AAV in humans, and it was thus decided to begin with peripheral (intramuscular) rather than systemic (intravascular) administration. Also in favor of a muscle-directed approach is the high prevalence of hepatitis C infection in the adult hemophilia population, making the liver a less attractive target organ for initial studies. Preclinical studies in mice[67] and hemophilic dogs[66] showed that doses in the range of approximately 1×10^{13} vg/kg were required to achieve therapeutic levels in animals when vector was delivered to muscle. In the clinical study, AAV-F.IX was administered at intramuscular sites in the legs and arms in a dose escalation design, but the highest doses administered (2×10^{12} vg/kg) fell short of those required for efficacy in animal studies. The practical obstacle to dose escalation was the number of injections required; the low efficiency of the required posttranslational modifications in skeletal muscle,[71] and the propensity for inhibitory antibody formation as the dose/site was raised[72] meant that dose escalation required injection of progressively larger numbers of intramuscular sites, rather than higher doses/site. An advantage of muscle as a target tissue is that it is easily sampled, and muscle biopsy at sites of injection showed gene transfer (on Southern blot) and expression of Factor IX (on immunofluorescent staining) in all eight subjects injected with AAV-F.IX, at time points as late as 3.5 years after vector injection.[73] Circulating levels were generally not higher than 1%, however. Improved delivery techniques that allow transduction of more extensive areas of skeletal muscle by introducing vector into muscle by a vascular route have been developed and tested in large animals, and will be required for further development of a muscle-based approach for hemophilia.

Infusion of AAV into the portal vein results in high-level expression of F.IX in mice and in hemophilic dogs.[68–70,72] Using a liver-specific promoter, circulating F.IX levels in the range of 5% to 10% are observed after a vector dose of approximately 1×10^{12} vg/kg.[72] Thus, compared to muscle, there is a decided dose advantage (>10-fold) in favor of liver, probably because of the hepatocyte's efficient secretion of F.IX into the circulation. In addition, more recent data in mice[74] and data in hemophilia B dog models suggest that AAV-mediated expression of F.IX in hepatocytes can promote tolerance to F.IX by inducing regulatory $CD4^+$ T cells that can suppress anti-F.IX antibody formation after adoptive T-cell transfer. These considerations and the safety data from the original muscle trial supported the safety of a proposed AAV-mediated, liver-directed gene transfer trial for hemophilia B. An early problem encountered in the clinical study was the observation of vector sequences (detected by a sensitive PCR assay) in semen samples of all treated subjects.[16,75] Additional animal studies suggested that AAV does not readily transduce spermatocytes, and that vector sequences are cleared from the semen over time, suggesting that this is a phenomenon of vector shedding rather than transduction of precursor cells,[76] with the attendant risk of germline transmission. In fact, all seven human subjects who underwent vector infusion have shown complete clearing of the semen over time. Results from this study[75] showed that the third dose cohort tested (2×10^{12} vg/kg) resulted in circulating levels of F.IX in the range of 10% for 4 to 5 weeks after infusion, but this was followed by a gradual reduction in levels to the pretreatment baseline (<1%). Accompanying the fall in F.IX levels was a transient asymptomatic transaminitis that resolved fully several weeks after it began. Subsequent study of another subject revealed that vector infusion triggered expansion of a pool of circulating capsid-specific $CD8^+$ T cells,[77] followed by contraction of these as the transaminitis resolved. The fact that such cells are not detected in the circulation of experimental animals after infusion of the same dose of vector suggests that humans, the only natural hosts for AAV infection, may harbor a population of memory $CD8^+$ T cells to AAV capsid. Because memory T cells are more readily activated than naïve T cells, this may account for the difference in observed outcomes (short-term vs long-term expression) in humans versus other species. Upcoming trials will test the hypotheses that this $CD8^+$ T-cell response to capsid can be managed by a short course of immunosuppression or avoided by use of an AAV vector engineered from a serotype that does not normally infect humans.[78]

Adenoviral Vectors

Certain features of adenoviral vectors make them attractive as potential gene delivery vehicles, for hemophilia A in particular. The vector is relatively straightforward to manufacture in high titer, and it can accommodate large inserts. Kay et al[54] and Connelly et al[79–81] exploited these characteristics early on to demonstrate high-level expression of canine clotting factors in the hemophilia dog models. However, expression was short-lived, and work by a number of other groups established that the immune response to the vector, characterized by a cytotoxic T-lymphocyte response against cells harboring the vector, prevents long-term expression from early-generation adenoviral vectors.[82,83] Moreover, systemic administration of early-generation adenoviral vectors in dogs and humans has been associated with substantial toxicity, including an early thrombocytopenia, a biphasic hepatotoxicity, and an acute systemic inflammatory response syndrome as noted above.[2] The subsequent development of fully deleted adenoviral vectors[84] raised the possibility of using these later-generation vectors as an approach for hemophilia A, since Morral et al[85] demonstrated that fully deleted adenoviral vectors could direct expression of α_1-antitrypsin for as long as 1 year in baboons (compared to only weeks for earlier-generation adenoviral vector) and that the hepatotoxicity (although not the thrombocytopenia) was greatly reduced by the use of these fully deleted vectors.[86,87] Their work also demonstrated though that over the course of 12 months there was an inexorable decline in circulating levels of α_1-antitrypsin in the baboons[86]; this highlights what may be a limiting feature of this vector, even under optimal circumstances, for genetic diseases where long-term expression is required.

The use of helper-dependent or "gutted" adenoviral vectors to treat hemophilia A was explored by Zhang and colleagues.[88] They first demonstrated that a fully deleted adenoviral vector expressing the full-length human FVIII cDNA under the control of a 12.5-kb albumin promoter could correct the phenotype of mice with hemophilia A. Injection of a dose of 8×10^{12} vp/kg resulted in circulating levels of 100 to 800 ng/mL FVIII (normal levels are 100–200 ng/mL) in 3 of 8 mice; the other mice rapidly developed antibodies to the human transgene product, and FVIII levels could no longer be measured. Vector administration in mice was not associated with any hepatotoxicity. Subsequent experiments in nonhuman primates yielded circulating levels of 3% to 8% with doses of 4.2×10^{12} vp/kg (although it should be noted that interpretation of these experiments was complicated by the use of the human transgene in the nonhuman primates, with subsequent development of antibodies to the foreign protein making it difficult to reliably measure factor levels). This dose also resulted in transient transaminitis and thrombocytopenia in nonhuman primates, although a dose of 1.4×10^{12} vp/kg did not. A phase I dose escalation study of a fully deleted adenoviral vector for hemophilia A enrolled a single subject at a dose of 4.3×10^{10} vp/kg in 2001; but in contrast to the cynomolgus primates, the subject experienced transient thrombocytopenia and transaminitis even at this low dose. A critical issue in analysis of results with fully deleted adenoviral vectors is the presence of contaminating helper adenovirus, which supplies gene products required for assembly of the fully deleted adenoviral vector. Contamination of vector preparations with helper virus can alter the toxicity profile of the vector. Differences in duration of expression and in toxicity have been observed using different preparations of fully deleted adenoviral vector. Additional studies will be required to analyze whether fully deleted adenoviral vectors will be of use for treatment of genetic disease.

GENE THERAPY FOR MALIGNANT DISEASES

To date, the widest use of gene transfer has been in patients with cancer, including those with hematologic malignancies. More than a thousand cancer gene therapy protocols exist, and most fit into one of three major approaches:

1. Modifying the tumor cell itself either by "repairing" one or more of the genetic defects associated with the malignant process or by delivering a prodrug-metabolizing enzyme that will render the tumor sensitive to the corresponding cytotoxic agent. This approach has an attractive elegance but is handicapped by the inefficiency of current vectors and their lack of targeting.
2. Modifying normal host tissues, delivering cytotoxic drug-resistance genes, thereby increasing the therapeutic index of chemotherapy. This approach also is hampered by the inefficiency of the gene transfer technology, which makes it difficult to protect sufficient cells in all organ systems that are damaged by conventional cytotoxic drugs.
3. Modifying the immune response to the tumor, by altering the specificity or effector function of immune system cells, or by transducing a small proportion of the tumor cells with immunostimulatory genes, thereby generating an immune response to tumor-associated or tumor-specific antigens. This last approach makes use of the efficiency of the immune system and its capacity to target specific cell types to compensate for the limitations of current vectors.

In addition, gene-marking studies have been used to track normal or malignant cells in vivo to monitor the effects of treatment, and conditionally replication-competent viruses that have been genetically modified to be able to replicate in and destroy malignant but not normal cells have been used for tumor oncolysis. Neither approach is described here, but both are reviewed elsewhere.[89,90]

TUMOR MODIFICATION

Tumor Correction

There is an attractive elegance to the strategy of introducing genetic material into a malignancy to correct the specific genetic defects contributing to the neoplastic phenotype. Multiple mutant oncogenes and fusion transcripts have been identified that are certainly specific to the malignant clone and frequently form a critical component of the malignant process. Unfortunately, this approach is technologically demanding, because all malignancies result from a multiplicity of genetic abnormalities. Unless correction of a single defect is subsequently lethal to the malignant cell, transfer of an individual corrective gene to a patient with 10^{11} to 10^{12} tumor blasts will leave a multiplicity of premalignant cells, with a high risk of later transformation. Present methods of gene transfer also are inefficient. Even if it were possible to transfer genes to 90% or more of malignant cells in vivo—a feat currently beyond the capability of any available vector—it would be insufficient to produce more than transient clinical benefit. Moreover, many relevant gene defects result in molecules with transdominant effects that will continue to produce a malignant phenotype, even if a wild-type gene is introduced. Under these circumstances, it would be necessary to neutralize the genes by destroying their function using ribozymes, antisense RNA, or with use of RNA interference.[91–93]

These limitations notwithstanding, several tumor correction protocols have been proposed. For example, efforts are being made to neutralize fusion transcripts such as *BCR-ABL* in patients with chronic myeloid leukemia *or* activated oncogenes such as *MYB*, using ribozymes, antisense RNA, or wild-type genes.[94] More extensive experience has been obtained with efforts to replace nonfunctioning tumor suppressors such as p53 in patients with localized solid tumors. In patients with head and neck cancers and those with bronchial carcinoma, striking tumor responses have been obtained using adenoviral vector-mediated wild-type p53 gene transfer. These benefits have been seen with even low levels of gene transfer, and there is increasing evidence for "bystander" activities that may include effects on tumor vasculature, the immune system, and intercellular signaling. A p53 adenoviral vector has received a product license in China[95] and it is estimated that well over 10,000 patients have been treated. The outcomes analyses are eagerly awaited. Meanwhile, in the United States, a long-delayed Biologics License Application is still awaited in 2008 for Ad-p53 treatment of recurrent/resistant squamous cell carcinoma of the head and neck. Approvability will be based in large part on the agent's ability to prolong survival.[96]

Interest also is increasing in targeting the gene pathways involved in regulating apoptosis, because even minor perturbations in these pathways can greatly modify the sensitivity of cancer cells to chemotherapy.[97] Because of problems with targeting, these approaches that directly correct the tumor cell itself will likely continue to be used primarily for treating localized solid tumors, rather than for hematologic malignancies, which are almost invariably widely distributed.

Increasing Tumor Sensitivity to Cytotoxic Drugs

Prodrug-metabolizing enzyme (PDME) genes encode enzymes able to convert harmless prodrugs into lethal cytotoxins.[98] More than a dozen have been described, of which the thymidine kinase (TK) gene has been the most widely used. TK itself phosphorylates the prodrugs acyclovir, valacyclovir, and ganciclovir to toxic nucleoside, and as for other PDME approaches, tumor selectivity requires either the vector or the prodrug product to be targeted to the malignant cell. Initial therapeutic study of *TK* gene transfer was made in patients with primary or secondary brain tumors; in this context, there is a particularly clear distinction between tumor cells (which divide and are destined to be killed following DNA incorporation of the phosphorylated nucleoside) and normal neurons (which do not divide and should escape unharmed). Retroviral vectors offer additional tumor specificity in this system because they function only in dividing cells and therefore do not transduce normal neurons. Later studies have used less selective vectors, such as adenoviruses, and have relied on preferential transduction of malignant targets and increased proliferation of malignant versus normal tissues to provide the desired therapeutic index.

Even when only a small percentage of tumor cells are transduced, administration of ganciclovir can produce large-scale destruction of the tumor cell population. This bystander effect is most evident in tumor cells that have gap junctions, so it probably represents the transfer of a toxic metabolite or an apoptotic signal. An immunologic bystander effect might also occur in vivo: once the tumor cell is killed by the toxic metabolite and is processed and presented by antigen-presenting cells, the host may be immunized against tumor development.

A significant added attraction of the Tk system is that the enzyme allows transduced cells to sequester radiolabeled nucleoside analogues (such as ^{131}I-labeled 2'-fluoro-2'-deoxy-1-β-D-arabinofuranosyl-5-iodouracil [FIAU]), which can then be detected by PET imaging.[99,100] The ability to assess gene transfer and expression noninvasively and in real time (rather than by analysis of biopsies) provides a much more convenient way of assessing the effectiveness of different gene transfer approaches. Insertion of the TK gene is conditionally replication competent. PDME gene transfer with the *TK* gene is now being used for the treatment of localized or recurrent prostate, bladder, breast, and colon cancer and for retinoblastoma. Although hematologic applications are more limited because of the problems of targeting widely distributed tumor cells in vivo, successful ex vivo retroviral transduction of Tk into donor T lymphocytes has provided a contingent "suicide" gene to increase the safety of these cells following adoptive immunotherapy after allogeneic hemopoietic stem cell transplantation.[101–103] The potential benefits of these T cells (reduced infection and relapse after stem cell transplant) can be preserved, with the option of destroying them should they produce unwanted graft-versus-host disease. Following promising single center data, this approach has extended to a large Phase III multicenter trial.[102]

INCREASING HOST RESISTANCE TO CYTOTOXIC DRUGS

Instead of attempting to modify the malignant cells by gene transfer, it is possible to target normal tissues by transferring genes that protect normal host tissues from the toxicity of chemotherapy. Although many different systems have been developed and studied preclinically, it is the multidrug resistance gene mutidrug resistance 1 (*MDR1*) that has been the most widely studied in humans. Its product, P-glycoprotein, functions as a drug efflux pump and confers resistance to many chemotherapeutic agents. The feasibility of using *MDR1* to protect hematopoietic cells has been demonstrated by in vitro and in vivo murine experiments, and it is likely that other drug resistance genes could function analogously.[104]

The clinical application of drug resistance gene transfer has several potential pitfalls. The low efficiency of stem cell transduction and poor gene expression observed in the earliest clinical protocols resulted in no selection of gene-modified cells and hence no in vivo protection. Although improved transduction technology is beginning to result in measurable in vivo protection in humans (albeit not yet to clinically useful levels), many problems remain.[105] There is a risk of transferring the genes to neoplastic cells to produce drug-resistant relapse, and toxicity to unprotected organs, including gut, heart, and lungs, may rapidly supervene when marrow resistance allows intensification of cytotoxic drug dosages. Moreover, expression of drug resistance genes such as *MDR1* or dihydrofolate reductase in primitive normal cells has proved leukemogenic in mice and primates, an effect of particular concern.[106,107] Hence, the approach will come to full fruition only when it becomes possible to target all sensitive normal tissues in vivo, to transduce them with high efficiency, and to prove after extensive animal testing that the approach is safe. Because of these concerns, more recent attention has shifted to alternative drug resistance genes such as O^6-methylguanine-DNA-methyltransferase (*MGMT*). This enzyme protects against toxicity to nitrosourea compounds, (such as temozolomide) that may be used for treatment of brain tumors, and occasionally for hematologic malignancies such as Hodgkin disease. Clinical trials using this approach have begun.

MODIFYING THE IMMUNE RESPONSE TO THE TUMOR

Most human cancers kill because of metastatic disease, not because of uncontrolled growth of the primary tumor. The lack of targeting of current vectors and their inefficiency mean that gene therapy aimed directly at modifying the tumor will work best on local, not systemic, disease, with limited value for hematologic malignancy. Accordingly, there has been great interest in combining gene transfer techniques with the inherent efficiency and targeting capacity of the immune system. Human tumors express tumor-associated or tumor-specific antigens that even if originally intracellular, may be processed and presented in association with major histocompatibility complex (MHC) antigens on the cell surface, where they can be targets for immune attack. There also is ample evidence, albeit primarily in studies of hematologic malignancy and melanoma, that immune intervention can eradicate even extensive malignant disease.[108–111]

Gene transfer may be used in several ways to augment the antitumor activity of the immune system.

Tumor Vaccines

To enhance immune recognition of poorly immunogenic tumors, investigators have evaluated the effect of genetically modifying tumor cells directly, or antigen-presenting cells modified to express tumor-derived antigens. Genetic modifications are aimed at enhancing recruitment of an effective (usually cellular) immune response, and include expression of cytokines such as GM-CSF and IL2, lymphotactic chemokines, allogeneic MHC molecules, or costimulatory molecules such as B7.1 or CD40 ligand. More recent efforts have focused on modifying the functionality of antigen-presenting cells by incorporating genes that counteract the normal inhibitory processes that limit the duration and degree of stimulation the cells produce. In murine model systems, the transfection of tumor cell lines with these molecules has shown that injection of neoplastic cells in doses that would normally establish a tumor instead recruits immune system effector cells, which eradicate the injected tumor cells. Often, the animal is then resistant to challenges by further local injections of nontransduced parental tumor. The transduced tumor has therefore acted like a vaccine. In some models, established, nontransduced, parental malignant cells also are eradicated.

Tumor vaccines are being evaluated in more than 300 different clinical trials. Despite gloomy prognostications,[112] positive results are being obtained in lymphoma and chronic lymphocytic leukemia as well as in solid tumors such as prostate cancer, melanoma, renal cell carcinoma, and neuroblastoma. Immunized patients may develop peripheral blood eosinophilia, a rise in natural killer (NK) and activated killer (AK) cell number and activity, and an increase in tumor-specific cytotoxic T-lymphocyte precursor frequency.[113–116] Substantial and sustained clinical responses in tumor sites/circulating malignant cells have been reported, sometimes in association with autoimmune phenomenon, which have so far been mild. Of note, an antigen-presenting cell vaccine expressing transgenic GM-CSF for the treatment of locally recurrent prostate cancer was recommended for approval by an FDA Advisory Committee, on the bass of benefits to overall survival in a phase II randomized trial. The FDA, however, has required additional clinical data. If finally successful, this application will be the first approved cell/gene therapeutic. Ultimately vaccines may have their greatest value as adjuvants to prevent relapse in patients with presumed minimal residual disease, although studies to validate this approach will need to be both large and lengthy.

Bypassing Immune Evasion Strategies

Tumor cells may fail to generate a specific immune response because they lack expression of HLA molecules, or express tumor-associated antigens that are only weakly stimulatory to the immune system and/or because they possess active defenses that thwart the immune system. Gene transfer may be used to combat both obstacles. For example, the malignant cells of Epstein–Barr virus (EBV)-associated Hodgkin disease expresses EBV-associated antigens that either are poorly processed (eg, Epstein-Barr virus nuclear antigen-1 [EBNA-1]) for presentation to CD8+ cytotoxic effector cells or are only weakly stimulatory to the immune system (such as latent membrane proteins LMP-1 and LMP-2). These malignant cells also have several active immune evasion strategies directed toward inhibition of antigen presentation, induction of an inhibitory T-cell response, and inhibition of any cytotoxic response that arises. As a consequence, adoptively transferred EBV-specific cytotoxic T cells that are highly effective against EBV-infected B lymphocytes of immunoblastic lymphoma are much less active against EBV-associated Hodgkin disease.[117] Similar active and passive immune evasion strategies are used by other hematologic and solid organ malignancies, probably contributing to the frequent failure of immunotherapy.

One way in which gene transfer can enhance the response to a weak tumor-associated antigen is exemplified by the tumor vaccine studies described in the preceding section. An alternative is to transduce professional antigen-presenting cells, such as dendritic cells or their precursors, with a vector encoding the weak tumor antigen.[118] This approach ensures that a high level of a weak antigen is expressed in an environment that favors an immune response. Alternatively, inhibitory signals for DC activation such as SOCSI may be knocked down.[118a] Gene transfer can also overcome active immune evasion strategies. For example, many tumor cells (including those of Hodgkin disease) secrete TGF-β, which inhibits cytotoxic T-cell proliferation and function. Cytotoxic T cells specific for tumor-associated antigens can be transduced with a dominant negative mutant of the TGF-receptor that renders them entirely resistant to inhibition mediated by the cytokine.[119,120]

As we learn more about the molecular basis of tumor immune evasion, it should prove possible to design effective countermeasures, and ultimately to generate immune T lymphocytes specific to even weak tumor antigens that are resistant to active tumor evasion.

Chimeric T Cells

Tumor-specific T lymphocytes can also be produced by genetically modifying human T cells to express tumor antigen-specific chimeric immune receptors that are based on antibody molecules (T-bodies) or on transgenic alpha and beta chains of the T-cell receptor.[121–123] Chimeric antibody receptors can be generated by joining the heavy- and light-chain variable regions of a monoclonal antibody, expressed as a single-chain Fv (scFv) molecule, to the T-cell receptor-ζ (TCR-ζ) (see Fig. 110–1), or Fc immune receptor domain. Antigen stimulation of the extracellular component of the chimeric receptor results in tyrosine phosphorylation of immune-receptor activation motifs present in the cytoplasmic domain, initiating T-cell signaling to the nucleus. Human T lymphocytes genetically engineered to express the recombinant receptor genes lyse tumor cells expressing the relevant target antigens, and adoptively transferred chimeric receptor-transduced cells are protective in murine tumor models.

T cells transduced to express chimeric antibody receptors have numerous potential advantages over immunotherapies based on monoclonal antibodies or T lymphocytes alone. They can be directed toward any native tumor- or virus-associated antigen for which a monoclonal antibody exists, making this strategy applicable to a wide variety of malignancies and viral diseases. Because chimeric T-cell receptors provide T-cell activation in an MHC-unrestricted manner, they permit the immune system to recognize tumors that have downregulated HLA class I molecules or that have defects in antigen processing. Chimeric receptors have been developed for a variety of antigens associated with solid tumors of breast, colon, and kidney, including Neu/HER2, folate-binding protein (FBP), carcinoembryonic antigen (CEA), TAG-72, and renal tumor-associated antigen, as well as for antigens associated with hematologic malignancy (CD30 and CD33), and the pediatric tumors neuroblastoma and Ewing sarcoma. Unfortunately, these cells have proved clinically disappointing, because they are short-lived or are rapidly inactivated in the circulation.[124–126] Clearance of modified T effector cells by immune effector mechanisms may be delayed by humanization of currently available hybridoma antibodies, or by the generation of fully human single-chain antibodies by phage display technology. Enhanced and sustained function may require chimeric receptor molecules that are coupled to the intracellular signaling mechanisms of costimulator molecules such as CD28, and clinical trials adopting this approach have begun in B-CLL.[123]

Artificial receptors based on the αβ chains of the T-cell receptor have also been exploited. Until recently, technical limitations associated with cross-pairing of transgenic and endogenous TCR, as well as competition for the limiting numbers of "chaperone" molecules that enable TCR transport and expression, has limited the functionality of this approach. Recent advances that have served to increase receptor affinity and favor appropriate rather than cross αβ-chain linkage have enabled a clinical trial in patients with melanoma using receptors specific for the melanoma-associated antigen MART-1. Four of 33 patients had tumor responses, including two complete remissions.[109]

ULTIMATE VALUE OF GENE THERAPY FOR CANCER

With recent results from the study of dendritic cell vaccines in prostate cancer, gene therapy for cancer has finally been able to show prolonged patient survival in a randomized phase III clinical trials. All the approaches we have described are now clearly feasible and are producing numbers of responses that are clearly greater than anecdotal, albeit still below the consistency and robustness desired. One of the most important characteristics of gene therapy for cancer is that it represents a series of treatment approaches that are generally not cross-resistant with other treatment modalities. Hence, the real value of the approach will become evident when it is combined with preexisting treatments. Clinical data already suggest that radiation and gene therapy approaches for recurrent prostate cancer may be superior to either alone, and combinations of low-dose chemotherapy agents and tumor vaccines may increase the response rate in patients with otherwise resistant disease. If these results are confirmed, the challenge over the next few years will be to design—and fund—studies to optimize these combination approaches.

HUMAN IMMUNODEFICIENCY VIRUS INFECTION AND ACQUIRED IMMUNODEFICIENCY SYNDROME

The treatment of HIV infection in the developed world changed dramatically with the advent of highly active antiretroviral therapy (HAART), with monitoring of viral load. Successful treatment means undetectable viral loads, increased CD4$^+$ counts, and few opportunistic infections or other complications of AIDS. The increasing effectiveness and simplicity of HAART has substantially reduced the impetus to develop gene therapies for the disease, because the quality and duration of life are now so much better for patients in whom treatment has been successful. Nonetheless HAART remains expensive and induces many adverse effects. It is not curative, and resistant strains of HIV may emerge. These and other reasons have ensured continuation of efforts to develop and clinically test gene therapy for the disease.[127]

Cellular Targets

For successful gene therapy of HIV infection, both T cells and macrophages should be permanently protected against infection, which currently requires an integrating murine retroviral or lentiviral vector. Peripheral mature T cells can be transduced, expanded ex vivo to large numbers (10^{10} to 10^{11}), and then reinfused into patients, as in reported clinical trials.[128] This strategy has several limitations:

- It is technically challenging.
- Less than 1% of the circulating T cells are typically transduced.
- Transgene expression can be lost.
- The average half-life of the T cells is unknown.

An alternative target is the HSC, which would serve as a T-cell, monocyte/dendritic cell, and microglial progenitor. Submyeloablative therapy will likely be sufficient for adequate repopulation. Because thymic architecture is progressively destroyed during HIV infection, however, it is unknown whether T-cell functionality will be completely restored.

Most clinical protocols to date have used modified lentiviral vectors based on HIV itself as the means of gene transfer, and these clinical safety and efficacy data are helping to broaden the applications in which such lentiviral vectors can be used.

POTENTIAL TARGETS FOR GENE THERAPY

Viral Receptors

HIV requires both CD4 and a coreceptor on the cell surface for productive infection. More than a dozen chemokine receptors function as HIV coreceptors in vitro, but the two most critical for the replication of T-cell-tropic and macrophage-tropic isolates in vivo are CXCR4 and CCR5, respectively. The latter is an attractive target because persons who are homozygous null (the so-called D32 mutation) are phenotypically normal but relatively resistant to HIV infection.[129] Downregulation of the CCR-5 coreceptor on the cell surface of CD4$^+$ cells was accomplished by transgenic expression of intrakines. These are modified chemokines (including MIP-1a and RANTES) that bind the endoplasmic reticulum (known as intrakines) and sequester intracellularly the newly synthesized CCR-5, preventing its transport to the cell surface. Alternatively, CCR5 knockdown can be obtained by stably expressing transgenic ribozymes or small interfering RNAs that act on CCR5 mRNA. Such genetically modified T lymphocytes are resistant to HIV-1 infection.[130]

Viral Transcription

HIV encodes a transcriptional transactivator (Tat) that acts at the level of RNA elongation in conjunction with cellular factors. A stem-loop RNA element, TAR, is recognized by Tat as well as by cyclin T1. This complex recruits the cyclin-dependent kinase CDK9 to hyperphosphorylate the carboxyl-terminal (C-terminal) domain of RNA polymerase II and increase enzyme activity. Anti-Tat single-chain variable-fragment antibodies (intrabodies) interfere with Tat function intracellularly; anti-TAR ribozymes cleave TAR, and polymeric TAR decoys compete with TAR for Tat binding.[131] Transdominant mutants of Tat also have been developed[132] that sequester cellular cofactors, including cyclin T1 and CDK9, but in general these mutants produce only limited inhibition of HIV replication and remain to be evaluated in clinical trials.

Viral RNA Transport

The HIV gene *rev* directs the export of intron-containing viral messenger RNAs from the nucleus to the cytoplasm and interacts with the Rev response element (RRE), an RNA stem-loop structure found within the *tat-rev* intron. In the presence of both Rev and the RRE, competition between the host's splicing apparatus and Rev allows export of intron-containing viral mRNAs. Anti-Rev intrabodies, similar to those against Tat, have been tested, as have RRE decoys.[133] Dominant negative Rev mutants such as Rev M10 bind to the RRE, thereby interfering with wild-type Rev RNA export. Escape mutants have rarely, if ever, been observed. Although rev M10 has now been introduced into clinical trials, effects to date have been limited.

Combination Therapy

Single gene transfer approaches to treat HIV, like single antiviral small molecules, rapidly select for resistant strains of the virus. Newer gene transfer strategies therefore target two or more anti-HIV genes at once, choosing those that are implicated at different phases of viral replication. For example, multimeric TAR decoys bearing a trans-dominant or antisense GAG sequence synergistically inhibited HIV replication, although combination of an anti-Rev intrabody with an RRE ribozyme blocked HIV replication in established T cells for prolonged periods of time. With improved technology, a single lentiviral vector can now transfer an anti-CCR5 ribozyme, an siRNA for Tat/Rev, and a TAR RNA decoy.[134] Although untested in vivo, these types of strategy are among the most promising.

Clinical Trials of Human Immunodeficiency Virus Gene Therapy and Their Ultimate Value

It is uncertain whether gene therapy will ever be used successfully against HIV infection. A multiplicity of small-molecule antiretroviral agents are currently approved by the Food and Drug Administration (FDA), and many more probably will be approved in the coming years. Many technologic barriers remain before gene therapy can contribute. These include the identification of genes that will protect against HIV at high levels of virus and the development of integrating vectors able to safely and efficiently transduce potential target cells. Ultimately, as with cancer, gene therapy may supplement rather than supplant vaccines and conventional small molecule therapeutics.

SUGGESTED READINGS

1. Cavazzana-Calvo M, Fischer A: Gene therapy for severe combined immunodeficiency: Are we there yet? J Clin Invest 117:1456, 2007.
2. Cavazzana-Calvo M, Lagresle C, Hacein-Bey-Abina S, Fischer A: Gene therapy for severe combined immunodeficiency. Annu Rev Med 56:585, 2005.
3. Verma IM, Weitzman MD: Gene therapy: Twenty-first century medicine. Annu Rev Biochem 74:711, 2005.
4. Sorrentino BP: Gene therapy to protect haematopoietic cells from cytotoxic cancer drugs. Nat Rev Cancer 2:431, 2002.
5. Manno CS, Pierce GF, Arruda VR, et al: Successful transduction of liver in hemophilia by AAV-Factor IX and limitations imposed by the host immune response. Nat Med 12:342, 2006.
6. Sadelain M, Riviere I, Brentjens R: Targeting tumours with genetically enhanced T lymphocytes. Nat Rev Cancer 3:35, 2003.
7. Tey SK, Brenner MK: The continuing contribution of gene marking to cell and gene therapy. Mol Ther 15:666, 2007.
8. Dropulic B, June CH: Gene-based immunotherapy for human immunodeficiency virus infection and acquired immunodeficiency syndrome. Hum Gene Ther 17:577, 2006.
9. Ott MG, Schmidt M, Schwarzwaelder K, et al: Correction of X-linked chronic granulomatous disease by gene therapy, augmented by insertional activation of MDS1-EVI1, PRDM16 or SETBP1. Nat Med 12:401, 2006.
10. McCormick F: Future prospects for oncolytic therapy. Oncogene 24:7817, 2005.

REFERENCES

For complete list of references log onto www.expertconsult.com

CHAPTER 111

EXPERIMENTAL CELL THERAPY

Jeffrey S. Miller and Robert S. Negrin

INTRODUCTION

Cell-based therapies are attractive alternatives to conventional treatment modalities. The exquisite functional specificity of cellular populations, identification of precursor and stem cell populations as well as advances in our basic understanding of cell and molecular biology have generated enthusiasm for future treatment concepts. Technical progress in cytokine biology, cellular manipulation, cell separation, expansion, and purification have made the idea of isolating a specific cell type, expanding relatively pure populations of cells that are active and functional, a reality. Several such concepts have been extended to the clinic and are in routine clinical use whereas others are under active exploration, with encouraging results. This chapter focuses on the cellular populations and immunological mechanisms underlying successful transfer of immune functions for the treatment of infectious diseases and malignancies focused on patients with hematologic diseases. The clinical settings in which cell therapy has been applied in hematologic practice are outlined in Table 111–1. The general concepts discussed here have broad clinical implications, with the potential to treat a wide variety of other clinical disorders such as autoimmune diseases, degenerative disorders, neurologic diseases, vascular diseases, and possibly traumatic injuries.

HISTORICAL CONSIDERATIONS

Hematopoietic Cell Transplantation

The concept of cellular therapy in hematologic practice is not new. The best example in clinical medicine is the field of hematopoietic cell transplantation (HCT). HCT developed from seminal studies in murine and canine models, which established the role of the bone marrow in protecting animals from the lethal effects of radiation.[1] These early studies also demonstrated the unexpected potential adverse effects of donor-derived cells, namely that of graft-versus-host disease (GVHD). Further investigation demonstrated that long-term surviving animals not only had a fully intact hematopoietic system but were also tolerant to tissue grafts from the donor animals.[2] These studies, and many others, ushered in the modern era of HCT. Initially, the beneficial effects of allogeneic HCT were thought to result from the high-dose chemotherapy and radiation therapy used prior to the transplant. Subsequent studies have demonstrated that HCT is more complex, with much of the benefit being derived from the transfer of immunoreactive cells capable of exerting a graft-versus-tumor (GVT) effect. The existence of a GVT phenomenon was initially based on the observation that relapse rates were lower in those patients who developed some degree of GVHD, especially chronic GVHD.[3,4] Further documentation of the GVT effect came from clinical situations where it is absent, such as following an identical twin or syngeneic transplantation[5,6] or following rigorous T-cell depletion.[7,8] Direct demonstration of the GVT effect following the transfer of donor-derived lymphocytes has been an important advance in HCT and further demonstration of the powerful therapeutic benefits of cellular therapy.[9] These studies have led to the development of nonmyeloablative allogeneic transplantation, which has allowed for the treatment of older or medically infirm patients with diseases who would otherwise benefit from this form of therapy.[10,11] Coincident with these developments has been the exploration of a number of different cellular populations with different therapeutic potential.

Donor Leukocyte Infusions for Treatment and Prevention of Disease Relapse

A clear example of the potential effectiveness of cellular therapy is in the application of donor leukocyte infusions (DLIs). The use of DLI to treat patients who have suffered a relapse following allogeneic HCT has been a well-established use of cellular therapy, which further documents the importance of GVT reactions. Two large retrospective analyses of DLI for post-HCT relapse have been reported from Europe and North America. The results of the European Group for Blood and Marrow Transplantation have further documented the beneficial effects of DLI.[12] In a series involving 27 transplant centers, 84 relapsed HCT patients had CML and of these 54 (73%) were induced into complete remission (CR) with DLI. Many of these patients who entered a hematologic CR also achieved molecular remissions assessed by polymerase chain reaction analysis of *bcr/abl* transcripts. However, DLI has been much less effective for patients with other diseases, where only five (29%) of the AML patients developed a CR, and none of the 22 patients with ALL had a CR. A major limitation with the use of DLI is the risk of GVHD, and 52 patients (41%) developed clinically significant GVHD following DLI. Seventeen patients (12.6%) died of causes other than their underlying leukemic disorder.

A similar review of 25 North American bone marrow transplant programs evaluated 140 HCT recipients with relapsed disease who underwent DLI.[13] Again CML patients responded most favorably, with a CR rate of 60% following DLI. Responses were better for those patients with cytogenetic and chronic-phase relapses only as compared to those patients with accelerated or blastic disease. Responses were durable as actuarial probability of remaining in CR at 2 years was 89.6% for those patients who achieved a CR. Longer-term results have confirmed that patients who achieve a molecular remission following the administration of DLI have remarkably durable responses, with the majority of patients continuing to have molecular remissions with long-term follow-up.[14] Results were not as favorable for HCT patients with relapsed AML (15.4% CR) or ALL (18.2% CR). Complications included GVHD (60%) and pancytopenia (18.6%).

Overall, these results indicate that DLI has substantial efficacy in the control of relapse following allogeneic HCT. This is especially true in patients with CML detected while in either cytogenetic or early hematologic relapse.[15] Upon progression to accelerated or blastic phase of the disease, DLI has clearly much less efficacy. With the resurgence of allogeneic transplantation for patients with multiple myeloma, DLI has also been used successfully for patients with progressive disease following allogeneic HCT for this disease.[16] DLI has been less effective for the treatment of patients with leukemia and lymphoid malignancies who suffer a relapse although responses have been noted.[17,18] In patients with acute leukemia the poorer results may be due to the more rapid proliferative capacity of the leukemic cells. Chemotherapy is often used to gain control of the disease before

Table 111–1 Clinical Applications of Cell Therapy in Hematology

Donor leukocyte infusions for treatment of relapse following allogeneic transplantation
Ex vivo activated cellular therapy for treatment of malignancies Natural killer and lymphokine activated killer cells Cytokine induced killer cells and activated T cells Cytotoxic T lymphocytes Gene-modified T cells Cytotoxic cell lines Antigen-pulsed dendritic cells
Cellular therapy of viral infections
Immunoregulatory Cells Regulatory T cells Mesenchymal stromal cells
Gene Delivery

administering DLI. The mechanism(s) through which DLI controls malignancies is not clear. Cytotoxic T lymphocytes (CTL) directed against minor histocompatibility antigens have been found in some patients, and their presence can be correlated with disease response.[19] B-cell maturation antigen has been identified as a potential target antigen in some of the responses in myeloma patients.[20] DLI has also been utilized to treat patients who develop Epstein–Barr virus-induced lymphoproliferative disease (EBV-LPD) which occurs in a minority of patients following allogeneic HCT, especially in those patients who have undergone T-cell depletion.[21]

Despite the durable clinical responses noted in many patients, the use of DLI has been limited by the risk of GVHD following infusion. One strategy has been to utilize dose escalation of T cells for infusion. In one study, a dose of 1×10^7 T cells/kg resulted in a low incidence of GVHD despite an obvious antitumor cell response. Using escalating numbers of T cells for those patients who do not have a complete antitumor response may decrease the risk of GVHD assuming the disease is sufficiently indolent.[22] However, the concept of T cell dose-limited GVHD risk has been challenged.[23] Other groups have attempted to deplete $CD8^+$ cells in an effort to reduce the incidence of GVHD while retaining GVL activity.[24,25] These studies are difficult to interpret because of patient and disease heterogeneity.

The "suicide gene strategy" is an elegant approach to reduce the risk of clinically significant GVHD, which involves genetically modifying the donor lymphocytes so that they can be eradicated with otherwise well-tolerated drugs in the event that the patient develops GVHD. For example, donor lymphocytes have been transfected with the herpes simplex virus tyrosine kinase (HSV-TK) gene by retroviral-mediated gene transfer, and those transfected donor lymphocytes have been infused into patients who have relapsed or developed an EBV-induced lymphoma. In one study of eight patients, the transferred lymphocytes survived for up to 12 months and resulted in antitumor activity in five of the patients. Three patients developed GVHD, which could be controlled by treating the patients with gancyclovir.[26] These exciting data pave the way for engineering cell types with specific functions whose activities can be controlled with certain drug treatments. A limitation of this approach has been the immunogenicity of HSV-TK, and other suicide gene strategies are under active investigation.

The other major complication associated with DLI has been myelosuppression and in some instances severe pancytopenia, requiring retransplantation. The more severe cases have been observed in patients who have no evidence of donor-derived hematopoiesis at the time of DLI.[27] Because of these limitations, improvements in DLI are needed. Because DLI contain dendritic cells, T and natural killer (NK) cells, one possibility is to gain a better understanding of the individual components comprising the DLI product, as discussed below.

IMMUNOLOGIC EFFECTOR CELLS

The evaluation of immune-reactive cells capable of recognizing and lysing virally infected cells and tumor cell targets has been the subject of intense investigation. Effective cellular populations can be mechanistically divided into two broad categories termed innate (NK cells and antigen-presenting cells) and adaptive (T-cell and B-cell) immunity. Cell populations capable of innate immunity are genetically poised to perform their biological functions, whereas cells of the adaptive immune response generally require activation, expansion, and education. These two general categories of immune-reactive cells interact, however, to expand and enhance an antigen-specific immune response.

THE ROLE OF NATURAL KILLER CELLS IN INNATE IMMUNITY

Basic Biology

Unlike T cells, NK cells are innate immune effectors capable of direct lysis of targets and cytokine production. NK-cell functions are regulated by a complex balance of activating and inhibitory signals transferred via several classes of receptors, including killer immunoglobulin-like receptors (KIRs).[28] Several inhibitory KIRs recognize ligands that are MHC class I molecules, where ligation protects a target from being killed. This may explain why NK cells with established lytic function do not damage normal tissues recognized as "self." The loss of KIR-ligand expression by an infected or malignant target renders it susceptible to NK-cell lysis. NK cells can kill tumors without requiring prior sensitization, can be easily isolated from donor lymphapheresis products, and do not cause GVHD when infused. These characteristics make NK cells an attractive cell population to exploit for antitumor immunotherapy. Several clinical strategies have been developed using alloreactive NK cells for therapeutic benefit.

NK cells are large granular lymphocytes that were first described in 1975 by their ability to lyse virally infected and tumor targets without MHC restriction or prior sensitization.[29,30] They were further characterized for their ability to mediate the rejection of allogeneic or parental-strain hematopoietic grafts in lethally irradiated mice,[31] a function that was first noted in 1971 when the phenomenon of "hybrid resistance" was defined.[32,33] Although they have no known capacity for sensitization or memory, NK cells express a diverse array of inhibitory and activating receptors that mediate recognition and lysis of a variety of infected and transformed cells. Human NK cells are found in the marrow, spleen, lymph nodes, and peripheral blood, where they comprise approximately 10% to 15% of the lymphocyte pool. NK cells are defined phenotypically by their expression of CD56 and by their lack of T-cell markers (CD3, CD4, and T-cell receptors) and are distinct from $CD3^+CD56^+$ lymphocytes. Peripheral blood NK cells are further categorized by their level of CD56 expression, which correlates with their effector functions. Approximately 10% of NK cells are CD56(bright), a subset that is more proliferative and produces more cytokines (especially interferon gamma [IFN-γ]), whereas the CD56(dim) subset is more cytotoxic and bears Fc receptors to mediate antibody-dependent cellular cytotoxicity.[34] Cytokine-activated cells, sometimes referred to as lymphokine-activated killer cells, show more proliferation, increased cytokine production, and higher cytotoxicity to kill targets than do resting NK cells.[35] NK cells respond to IL-2, IL-15, and IL-21, all of which signal via the IL-2 receptor γ chain,[36–38] as well as the combination of IL-12 and IL-18, which is an especially strong stimulant to increase IFN-γ production.[39]

NK cells are major producers of several cytokines such as granulocyte colony stimulatory factor, granulocyte–monocyte colony stimulatory factor, IL-5, TNF, IFN-γ, and transforming growth factor-beta. These, in turn, can stimulate or inhibit hematopoiesis and the effects of other immune cells. These cytokines and cell–cell interactions may stimulate dendritic cells (DC) to activate both NK cells and T cells, providing a link between the innate and adaptive immune system.[40,41] The interaction between DC and NK cells leads to mutual coactivation of each cell type.

NK cells have demonstrated in vivo antitumor cytotoxicity against both hematologic malignancies and a wide variety of solid tumors, including breast, ovarian, hepatocellular, and colon cancer,[42–45] as well as against virally infected cells. Most NK cells kill directly using perforin and granzyme, but they can also use Fas ligand (FasL) and tumor necrosis factor-related apoptosis-inducing ligand pathways.[46] In addition, NK cells mediate antibody-dependent cellular cytotoxicity via CD16 (FcRγIII), the Fc receptor that recognizes Ig-coated targets.[47] The recognition and response to a wide array of foreign damaged, malignant, and virally infected cells are regulated through a complex network of cell–cell interactions. NK cells express $\beta 2$ integrins and CD2, which bind to target adhesion molecules such as ICAM-1 and LFA-3. In addition, NK cells express several classes of activating and inhibitory receptors that are both MHC class I-specific and nonspecific. The net balance of signals, dependent on both the target phenotype and the NK cell receptor repertoire, determines whether or not a target is lysed.

Natural Killer Cell Receptors

Human NK cells express KIRs, type I transmembrane molecules belonging to the Ig superfamily that are all are encoded on chromosome 19. KIRs are named by the number of extracellular immunoglobulin domains (2D or 3D) and the length of the intracellular tail, which determines whether they are stimulatory (Short) or inhibitory (Long). A nomenclature committee has assigned a cluster of designation (CD) number of CD158 for the KIR genes with individual loci designated by a small letter ± a number (eg, KIR3DL1 = CD158e1).[48] All individuals contain the framework genes KIR3DL3, KIR2DL4, and KIR3DL2. In addition, a variable number of activating and inhibitory genes are inherited and population studies show diverse evolutionary patterns.[49] Individuals with only one activating receptor are referred to as having an A KIR haplotype. Individuals with more than one activating receptor are referred to as having a B KIR haplotype. These genes are highly polymorphic and new alleles continue to be reported. Some of these polymorphisms are functionally important. For example, KIR3DL1*004 is not expressed on the surface, so it cannot function to recognize its respective Bw4 ligand.[50] Murine NK cells do not express KIR, but do express Ly49 receptors of the same class.[51] Although the ligands for many KIRs are unknown, the inhibitory receptors KIR2DL1, KIR2DL2/KIR2DL3, and KIR3DL1 bind HLA class I C2, C1, and Bw4 alleles, respectively. The KIR repertoire is determined primarily by KIR genotype and at steady state is only minimally affected by class I HLA (KIR-ligand) genes, which segregate independently (chromosome 6). The recognition of self-class I HLA by the higher-affinity inhibitory receptors suppresses NK-cell effector responses, including cell-mediated lysis and cytokine release.[52] Both human and murine NK cells express CD94, which heterodimerizes with the NKG2 family of C-type lectin receptors. They are either inhibitory (NKG2A) or activating (NKG2C/E) receptors that recognize nonclassical HLA-E.[53] NKG2D is unique in that it does not heterodimerize with CD94 and it recognizes stress-induced molecules such as MHC class I polypeptide-related sequence A/B (MICA and MICB) and the class I-like CMV-homologous ULBP proteins that are often upregulated on tumor or virally infected cells.[54–56] NK cells also express Ig-like transcript (ILT) receptors, some of which bind HLA-G expressed in the placenta and on fetal tissue. Several other receptors have been identified that regulate killing of MHC class I-negative targets, including but not limited to the natural cytotoxicity receptors NKp30, NKp46, and NKp44, 2B4 (which binds CD48), and DNAM-1 (CD226) (which recognizes PVR [CD155] and Nectin-2 [CD112] as their ligands).[57]

In 1985 Ljunggren and Karre described the phenomenon of "missing self," by which the loss of MHC class I expression renders

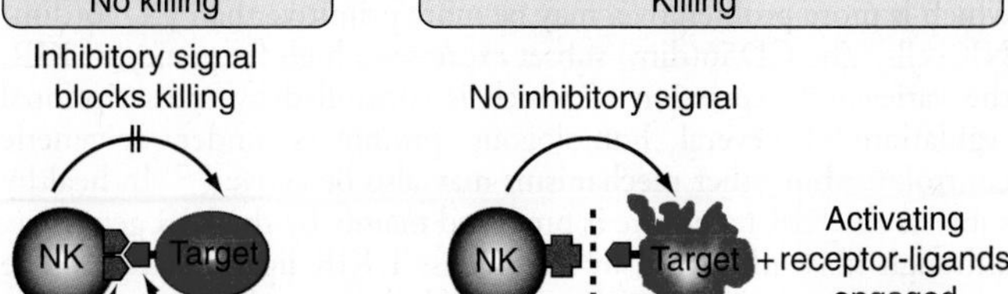

Figure 111–1 Natural killer (NK) cell alloreactivity is determined by a balance between activating and inhibitory signals. NK cells recognize targets when appropriate activating receptors are engaged by their corresponding ligands. For killing to occur (right side of figure), the activating signals must not be inhibited by recognition of "self" which can occur when MHC is downregulated by viral infection or malignant transformation or when KIR are mismatched with their respective cognate ligands. Normal tissues are protected from lysis by the lack of activating ligands or the recognition of "self" inhibitory ligands (left side of figure).

autologous targets more sensitive to NK-mediated killing, providing a mechanism by which these innate killer cells can recognize tumor or virally infected cells.[58] The discovery of class I-specific inhibitory KIR and the observation that cloned NK cells all express self-inhibitory receptors[59] led to the belief that mature peripheral blood NK cells must express "at least one" inhibitory NK receptor for self-MHC class I to prevent autoreactivity.[60] Although recent reports of murine[61] and human[62,63] NK cells lacking self-inhibitory receptors challenge this model of autoreactivity, the concept remains important for clinical applications involving alloreactive NK cell clones that may be generated by using donor NK cells expressing inhibitory KIR for which the recipient lacks the appropriate ligand (Fig. 111–1).

The stepwise evolution of the innate and adaptive immune systems in response to viral pathogens is illustrated by the example of murine cytomegalovirus (MCMV). Although the downregulation of MHC class I expression in infected cells allows them to evade recognition by T cells, it makes them good NK-cell targets. MCMV also upregulates the expression of the m144 gene, a mimic of MHC class I, which is recognized by NK cell inhibitory receptors, protecting the cell. In response, murine NK cells express Ly49H, an activating receptor that recognizes the MCMV glycoprotein m157.[64,65] This case in point provides proof of principle that activating receptors may recognize viral proteins. A similar role for human activating receptors is supported by studies of patients with HIV showing an association between AIDS progression and the activating receptor KIR3DS1.[66] However, precise mechanisms for this association remain complex because KIR3DS1 does not directly recognize Bw4 as its cognate ligand. Although antigen peptide bound to MHC is not required for recognition by KIR, it remains possible that some peptides modulate KIR interactions. Infectious natural ligands for activating KIR will likely be discovered, and it may be that activating KIR are analogous to the role of conserved pathogen-associated microbial proteins (PAMPs) and Toll-like receptors[67] expressed on other cells of the innate immune system.

Human NK cells are derived from CD34$^+$ hematopoietic progenitors found in many tissues, including bone marrow, thymus, and umbilical cord blood, and can be derived from human embryonic stem cells.[68–70] Their maturation is induced by IL-15, fms-like tyrosine kinase 3 (flt3) ligand, c-kit ligand or stem cell factor (SCF), IL-7, and IL-3.[71–73] Discrete stages of NK-cell development in lymphoid tissues are defined by the acquisition of IL-15-responsiveness[74] and a number of developmental intermediates.[75] The CD56(bright) subset, which is more proliferative, may be more primitive than CD56(dim) NK cells. The CD56(dim) subset expresses a high frequency of KIR, the variegated expression of which is controlled by transcriptional regulation of several homologous promoters under epigenetic control,[76,77] but other mechanisms may also be active.[78,79] In healthy subjects the KIR repertoire is predicted mainly by the KIR genotype, although it is influenced by HLA class I KIR ligand status.[80] The wide allelic variation in KIR genes includes several common alleles exhibiting poor or no surface expression.[50,81–83] Interestingly, KIR expression is decreased on NK cells reconstituting in patients after allogeneic HCT in whom dysregulated KIR expression correlates with clinical outcomes.[84,85]

Development of Natural Killer Cell Self-Tolerance

The developmental mechanism by which NK cells acquire self-tolerance has been referred to as NK-cell education. This has been one of the most widely debated topics in NK-cell biology over the past several years. Several models have been proposed to explain the integration of inhibitory receptor expression with the acquisition of effector functions. These concepts differ in their implied mechanisms and whether the process is one of activation or loss of function. *Disarming* refers to the suppression of effector function in maturing NK cells that receive stimulatory signals unopposed by inhibitory signals via self-MHC receptors, analogous to the development of T-cell anergy.[86,87] Licensing describes a terminal differentiation step by which NK cells acquire mature function only when they receive an appropriate signal via an inhibitory receptor ligating with self-MHC.[88,89] What is agreed on between these and other models is that human NK cells lacking inhibitory receptors are hyporesponsive.[62,63] Therefore, rather than being autoreactive, they are self-tolerant. Although the exact mechanism remains unknown, self-tolerance may be the result of a coordinated genetic developmental sequence during which mature NK function is synchronized with the acquisition of adequate expression of self-inhibitory molecules.

Autologous Natural Killer Cell Strategies

The first therapeutic trials using adoptive immunotherapy were performed in the 1980s when several groups tested autologous lymphokine-activated killer cells to treat a variety of malignancies. Peripheral blood mononuclear cells were stimulated ex vivo with IL-2 and then reinfused with high-dose IL-2 to treat immune-sensitive malignancies, including melanoma, lymphoma, and renal cell cancer. Although it was shown that the cytotoxicity was mainly mediated by NK cells, limited clinical benefit was seen.[90] The significant toxicity of the capillary leak syndrome induced by high-dose IL-2 led to trials using low-dose subcutaneous IL-2, either alone or in combination with activated NK cells. These strategies failed to show efficacy in patients with lymphoma and breast cancer.[91]

Subsequent discoveries may explain the failure of autologous lymphokine-activated killer- and NK-cell-based therapies. Such failures may occur because host lymphocytes compete with infused cells for access to cytokines[92] or possibly because infused autologous NK cells are suppressed by regulatory T cells.[93] A favorable milieu for adoptive transfer may optimally require adequate lymphodepletion or "clearing of space."[94] Rosenberg's group at the NIH developed a successful therapy for melanoma using cyclophosphamide (60 mg/kg/day × 2) followed by fludarabine (25 mg/m^2/day × 5 days) to induce T-cell lymphopenia prior to the infusion of cytotoxic T cells.[95] Although the induction of lymphopenia prior to the adoptive transfer of NK cells may enhance their expansion, autologous NK-cell strategies were abandoned after the discovery of inhibitory KIRs and their role in preventing NK-cell killing of "self" MHC-expressing tumor cells. The inherent self-tolerance of autologous NK cells was a good explanation to previous failures, leading to studies exploring the use of allogeneic donor sources. The hypothesis is that allogeneic donors will have a high frequency of alloreactive cells capable of killing tumors.

Allogeneic Natural Killer Cell Strategies

The current generation of therapeutic trials is based on a better understanding of the biologic concepts that regulate the antitumor activity of NK cells. Tumors that express ligands for activating NK receptors are more responsive to NK-cell killing, and although an attractive strategy, it is difficult to alter tumor phenotype in vivo. Therefore, more interest has been focused on ways to manipulate the interactions between inhibitory KIR and their ligands. The selection of NK-cell or stem-cell donors on the basis of their KIR ligand (HLA) status in relation to the patient has led to finding higher numbers of alloreactive NK cells in donors who express a KIR ligand lacking in the recipient.[96]

The two main strategies to harness the therapeutic power of alloreactive NK cells are (a) stem cell transplantation and (b) adoptive transfer of NK cells. Each approach has its own advantages and disadvantages. Advantages to adoptive transfer include minimal toxicity because NK cells are not believed to induce GVHD. However, the efficacy of adoptive transfer protocols is limited by the transient nature of the NK antitumor effect. Alternatively, the beneficial effects of alloreactive NK cells can be incorporated into HCT protocols by selecting donors based on one of several KIR mismatch algorithms. Although these strategies assume the risks of HCT (higher treatment-related mortality, GVHD, etc) they provide a permanently engrafted potentially alloreactive NK-cell pool that can provide ongoing antitumor activity, presuming the alloreactive cells do not become tolerant after infusion. Although NK cells are the first lymphocyte population to reconstitute after HCT, the use of exogenous IL-2 to boost their activity posttransplant is potentially dangerous as it may exacerbate GVHD. A third option may be to incorporate advantages of both strategies while lessening the cumulative toxicity associated with two separate procedures.

Regardless of the treatment strategy, the first step is to select a suitable allogeneic donor. The subtleties among the various methods by which KIR alloreactivity between donor and recipient has been defined have caused confusion (Table 111–2). The Perugia group used the KIR-ligand mismatch or KIR-ligand incompatibility model, which predicts that donor-derived NK cells will be alloreactive in the GvH direction when recipients lack C2, C1 or Bw4 alleles that are present in the donor. In this model, no alloreactivity is predicted for the approximately one-third of recipients who express all three KIR ligands. A KIR ligand match calculator based on this model, which requires knowledge of both the donor and recipient HLA types, is available on the Immuno Polymorphism Database (IPD) www.ebi.ac.uk/ipd/kir/ligand.html.[97] Alternatively, the KIR-ligand absence model categorizes recipients based on their C2, C1, and Bw4 allele status with no regard to the donor status. As most human populations have high frequencies of inhibitory KIR specific for C2, C1 and Bw4 alleles, it is assumed that most donor-derived NK cells will express inhibitory KIR and that alloreactive potential is based on the number of KIR ligands a recipient lacks. The receptor-ligand model accounts for inhibitory KIR and recipient KIR ligand status. As KIR genes have multiple alleles with variable function and expression levels, this model may be more precise if based not just on donor KIR genotype but on functional measures of KIR phenotype. This model allows for NK alloreactivity in HLA-identical transplants where recipients lack KIR ligands for inhibitory KIR expressed on self-tolerant clones in donors who may be alloreactive in the posttransplant setting.

Many groups are testing the clinical efficacy of selecting donors for HCT on the basis of their predicted alloreactivity against the host using one of the models discussed above. Potential benefits include (a) decreased rates of GVHD as host dendritic cells are killed by donor NK cells,[98,99] (b) decreased rates of graft rejection mediated by NK-cell lysis of host T cells, (c) decreased relapse via direct cytotoxcity,[46] (d) improved engraftment mediated by NK-cell release of hema-

Table 111–2 Models to Predict KIR Alloreactivity

Name	Information Needed	Model	Assumptions and Implications
KIR Ligand Mismatch *or* KIR ligand incompatibility	Donor class I HLA typing Recipient class I HLA typing (recipient KIR ligand status)	NK cells derived from donors who possess KIR ligands that are absent in the recipient (C2, C1 or Bw4) will be alloreactive in the GvH direction	Assume that NK cells will express inhibitory KIRs for all of their class I KIR ligands (C2, C1, and Bw4) Assume that donor class I HLA type predicts donor KIR expression No potential for NK alloreactivity for recipients who express C2, C1, and Bw4 (approximately one-third of patients)
KIR ligand absence	Recipient class I HLA typing (recipient KIR ligand status)	As the gene frequency for inhibitory KIRs that recognize C2, C1, and Bw4 is high in most populations, most donors will express those KIRs and alloreactivity can be estimated by recipient ligand status alone	Assume the respective inhibitory KIR genes are present in the donor Assume the donor KIR allele is expressed and functional
Receptor ligand	Donor KIR genotype (for inhibitory KIR) Recipient class I HLA typing (recipient KIR ligand status)	Both the donor KIR profile and recipient KIR ligand status are needed to accurately predict alloreactivity	Allows for NK alloreactivity in HLA-identical transplants if self-tolerant donor clones expressing KIR for which they lack the ligand become alloreactive in the posttransplant setting

KIR, killer immunoglobulin-like receptor; NK, natural killer.

topoietic cytokines,[100,101] and (e) enhanced immune reconstitution and decreased infectious complications mediated by NK-cell antiviral activity. The Perugia group demonstrated that alloreactive NK-cell clones were detected in patients after stem cell engraftment in KIR-mismatched patients and correlated KIR mismatch with improved engraftment, less relapse, and less GVHD.[96] In a recently published update, however, the only significant effect of KIR mismatch was a reduction in the relapse rates and prolonged survival in patients transplanted while in CR.[102] Results were not as good in patients who were transplanted in relapse. Additional clinical trials have supported the finding that KIR ligand mismatch is associated with these favorable clinical outcomes in myeloid malignancies, especially when T cells are depleted in vivo with antithymocyte globulin.[103] However, other studies looking at outcomes after KIR ligand-mismatched T cell-replete transplants did not achieve the same effect,[104,105] perhaps because T cells in the graft interfere with NK-cell development and KIR reconstitution after unrelated donor transplant.[85] Even in the T cell-depleted setting, some investigators have found worse outcomes in the KIR-mismatched transplants.[106] Analyses based on KIR ligand absence have also shown conflicting results. Improved survival has been reported for patients with myeloid malignancies undergoing HLA-matched sibling HCT[107] and for patients with myeloid and lymphoid malignancies after HLA-mismatched unrelated HCT.[108] Another study of unrelated HCT found that KIR ligand absence was associated with decreased relapse in early myeloid leukemias, but that patients with early CML had more GVHD.[109] Taken together, these results suggest that NK cells play a role in allogeneic transplant but the complexities of the KIR system and the heterogeneity of AML and other transplanted diseases result in some confusion. Clinical trials incorporating extensive KIR genetic analysis of donor–recipient pairs may result in better donor selection to improve transplant outcome.

Another way to promote antitumor activity with alloreactive NK cells is through adoptive transfer. This can be achieved using several strategies. One approach is based on ex vivo NK cell expansion but there are several potential limitations. Most importantly, NK cells stimulated by supraphysiologic concentrations of cytokines may undergo apoptosis when removed from ongoing stimulation and may not persist or expand in vivo. In addition, marked size changes occur with activation, which may alter homing characteristics in vivo. Consequently, developing strategies for in vivo NK-cell expansion may be optimal. The safety and success of this approach was established in a trial using in vivo expanded haploidentical, related-donor NK-cell infusions to treat 43 patients with metastasic melanoma, renal cell carcinoma, refractory Hodgkin disease, and refractory AML.[110] The trial, which tested three preparative chemotherapy regimens of differing intensity confirmed that successful NK cell expansion was only seen in the AML cohort who received the fully lymphodepleting cyclophosphamide and fludarabine regimen used by Rosenberg. Patients received NK cell infusions on day 0 following 1 or 2 doses of intravenous cyclophosphamide (60 mg/kg) days −4 and −5 and daily intravenous fludarabine (25 mg/m^2) days −5 to −1, followed by 10 million units of subcutaneous IL-2 administered over 2 weeks. Successful expansion was only seen after the high-dose cyclophosphamide-containing regimen (Hi-Cy/Flu), which was the only regimen to induce pancytopenia. In addition, it was the only one to induce a surge of endogenous IL-15 after chemotherapy. A significant inverse correlation was seen between the IL-15 levels and the absolute lymphocyte count, and high levels correlated with successful NK-cell expansion, supporting the importance of IL-15 for NK-cell homeostasis.[111]

In vivo expansion of NK cells was assessed using a PCR-based chimerism assay, with successful expansion defined by the presence of measurable donor NK cells at 2 weeks, following the IL-2 therapy. Eight of 15 evaluable patients had successful in vivo NK-cell expansion, and the circulating donor-derived NK cells were functional in standard cytotoxicity assays. Clinical efficacy correlated with in vivo NK expansion and KIR ligand mismatch. Of the 19 patients with poor prognosis AML, five achieved CRs. The remission patients had significantly higher proportions of circulating NK cells that were significantly more cytotoxic against K562 targets, suggesting that the observed clinical efficacy was mediated in part by the in vivo-expanded allogeneic donor NK cells. In this small cohort, 4 of the 19 NK donors were predicted to exhibit alloreactivity on the basis of KIR ligand mismatch in the GvH direction. CR was achieved in three of the four (75%) KIR ligand mismatch and only 2 of 15 (13%) KIR ligand match recipients, supporting a role for KIR ligand mismatching in the treatment of AML.

Adoptive transfer of allogeneic NK cells is being studied in several other disease settings on the basis of their ability to lyse targets in vitro including breast cancer,[112] non-Hodgkin lymphoma (NHL), multiple myeloma, hepatocellular carcinoma, melanoma, and renal cell carcinoma.[113–115] Another approach to achieve the benefits of NK alloreactivity has been to incorporate adoptive transfer of allogeneic NK cells into standard HCT protocols. NK-cell products are infused either prior to or during the early recovery phase. Other variables include cell source, and studies are in progress using haploidentical umbilical cord blood based on the high frequency of lymphoid precursors found in umbilical cord blood. Other groups are using NK-cell DLIs after haploidentical HCT to consolidate engraftment in adults with AML[116] or children with leukemia and solid tumors.[117] Conclusions from these studies await well-designed clinical trials with definitive clinical and biologic endpoints to understand the role of NK cells in this process.

Natural Killer Cell Therapeutic Limitations and Future Directions

There are several limitations to the therapeutic potential of adoptively transferred allogeneic NK cells. The NK-cell yield from lymphapheresis collections is limited. Although NK cells can be successfully expanded in vivo, the success is unpredictable and the expanded cell population is transient. In addition, the homing signals needed to direct NK cells to tumor sites are not fully understood. Furthermore, the alloreactivity of in vivo expanded NK-cell populations may be heterogeneous because of variable KIR repertoire expression or to differences in NK cell or accessory cell subsets. The use of monoclonal antibodies that block NK-cell inhibitory receptors may increase antitumor killing,[118] and more sophisticated techniques for subset selection of NK-cell products may affect the interaction between the innate and adaptive immune responses. For example, removing regulatory T cells that can suppress NK-cell proliferation and killing may improve the immune effector functions of the expanding NK cells.[93] NK-cell expansion may be improved by refining the use of lymphodepleting chemotherapy or the use of concurrent exogenous cytokine therapy. Irradiated cell lines such as NK92 and KHYG-1 may provide an inexhaustible supply of highly cytotoxic NK cells, but their in vivo survival is not well known.[119,120] Ex vivo expanded cells from any source can be genetically modified to express tumor-specific receptors. For example the NK92 cell line has been transfected with a chimeric antigen receptor for HER2/neu, which conferred superior cytotoxicity against HER2/neu positive targets.[120] Lastly, the antitumor activity of NK cells depends not only on the KIR ligand mismatch status, but also on tumor expression of appropriate activating ligands. For example, the lack of efficacy of KIR-mismatched transplants in lymphoid leukemias may be due to their low expression of LFA-1 or NKG2D-ligands. Additional strategies to enhance activating ligand expression on tumor cells are needed to increase tumor susceptibility to NK cell-mediated lysis. Other avenues of research for NK-cell immunotherapy include engineering NK cells with transferred genes, incorporating NK cells into dendritic cell vaccine therapies, and combination therapy with immunomodulatory drugs such as thalidomide, Toll-like receptor agonists, and monoclonal antibodies to target antibody-dependent cellular cytotoxicity.

DENDRITIC CELLS

The dendritic cell (DC) population initiates immune responses through the presentation of appropriate peptides in the context of major histocompatibility complexes (MHC) along with the expression of costimulatory molecules. There has been much interest in the adoptive transfer of DC populations that are primed with specific antigens in vitro. A number of different strategies have been explored for the isolation, expansion, activation, and priming of DC populations. To date there is no unanimity on what is the best population for clinical application, nor on the optimal priming approach. Some strategies include the use of tumor antigens, peptides, whole tumor lysates, or RNA for DC priming.

Dendritic cells are capable of presenting endogenous peptides on HLA class I proteins, or peptides derived from extracellular material or pathogens on HLA class II proteins. These peptides, typically 8 to 11 amino acids long, must have the appropriate structure to fit precisely into the peptide binding groove on HLA class I and II molecules. Using known peptide binding rules, it is possible to deduce possible peptides that might bind to an appropriate HLA molecule by defined algorithms and then search for possible responses in the blood or tissues of patients.

Dendritic cells have been isolated directly from peripheral blood or lymphoid organs or expanded in culture. Dendritic cells can be mobilized into the peripheral blood following cytokine treatment.[121] Clinical grade products have been prepared using centrifugation techniques.[122] Alternatively, DCs can be expanded from monocyte and hematopoietic progenitor precursors by the timed addition of different cytokines such as IL-4, granulocyte–monocyte colony stimulatory factor, TNF-α, and others.[123,124] Dendritic cells can be pulsed with peptides, protein, tumor lysates, RNA, or DNA in an effort to introduce and present peptide antigens of interest. Determining the optimal methodology for DC preparation, expansion and presentation of peptide antigens continues to be an area of much research activity, and no definitive approach has been developed. Alternatively, tumor cells themselves of hematopoietic origin can be activated and expanded from precursor populations, which in turn may present specific tumor-associated peptides.[125]

Dendritic cell-based treatment strategies have been extended to the clinic. One approach has been to utilize idiotype proteins in an effort to generate an immune response directed at B-cell malignancies such as NHL or multiple myeloma. Id-pulsed DCs were first used to treat patients with follicular lymphoma. In these initial studies, human DCs were harvested from peripheral blood by differential centrifugation and pulsed with patient-specific idiotype antigen.[126] The Id-pulsed DCs were then infused into patients with low-grade NHL. Impressive responses have been observed, with improvement in outcome for those patients who appeared to respond.[127] A randomized trial of newly diagnosed patients with low-grade NHL comparing chemotherapy plus idiotype vaccination to chemotherapy alone has completed accrual. A limitation of this approach has been the need to isolate patient-specific idiotype, which can be challenging and labor intensive although the fact that it could be developed for a randomized clinical trial is encouraging. Secreted idiotype can also be utilized, for example, in patients with multiple myeloma (MM). In this disease, secreted paraprotein can be readily isolated and used for DC pulsing. Initial clinical trials using this approach, for example, following autologous HCT have been performed, demonstrating feasibility and safety.[128] Unfortunately, tumor-specific responses have only been noted in a minority of patients and it is yet unclear what clinical impact these immunological responses may have.[128,129] This may be due to the often relatively large amounts of paraprotein that persist in these patients even after treatment. Alternatively, patients may be tolerant of their idiotype protein. An alternative approach is to perform idiotype-based DC vaccinations utilizing DCs isolated from the healthy HLA-matched donors or vaccinate donors with idiotype proteins followed by allogeneic HCT. Such approaches are currently being tested in early-phase clinical trials.[130,131] DC-pulsed vaccination approaches have also been applied in a number of other clinical settings of solid tumors; these are not reviewed here.

Once DCs are generated and loaded with antigen, the route of administration may be an important variable. Traditional routes of administration have included intravenous and subcutaneous injections. Relatively little is known about the trafficking of injected DCs to nodal sites or about their survival in vivo. Intradermal administration of DCs has also been explored in a dose-escalation format using between 10^6 and 10^9 tumor lysate pulsed DCs. No grade III or IV toxicities or autoimmune reactions were observed.[132] Other studies have demonstrated links between innate and adaptive immunity. The lysis of tumor cell targets by NK cells may enhance presentation of tumor-specific antigens by DCs.[133,134] Therefore, an alternative strategy may be to use a combined cellular approach of both NK cells

Use of Donor Leukocyte Infusions

Donor leukocyte infusion (DLI) is an effective treatment for patients who suffer a relapse following allogeneic HCT, yet is associated with GVHD and graft failure. Chimerism should first be checked to ensure that adequate donor hematopoiesis persists, because the presence of donor cells decreases the risk of graft failure following DLI. Lower doses of DLI can be effective for relapse of indolent diseases and avoid the risk of GVHD. Higher DLI doses may be required for effective treatment of more aggressive disease. Therefore, patients with CML, CLL, low-grade NHL and MM who relapse following allogeneic HCT can be treated initially with DLI containing a calculated T-cell dose of 1×10^7 $CD3^+$ T cells/kg. If no response is noted within 4 to 6 weeks, a second infusion of 5×10^7 $CD3^+$ T cells/kg followed by a third dose of 1×10^8 $CD3^+$ T cells/kg may be indicated. Patients with more aggressive diseases such as acute leukemias should be treated with higher-dose DLI (1×10^8 $CD3^+$ T cells/kg or higher). Induction chemotherapy should also be considered for patients with more aggressive leukemias because DLI alone is rarely effective.

and DCs. This combined approach is in the early phases of investigation. As with all of the approaches discussed, technical feasibility and practical and regulatory issues can be daunting.

ADAPTIVE IMMUNITY

Basic Biology

The adaptive immune response is characterized by selection of specific populations of B and T cells with appropriate activity, priming of clonal populations of cells, expansion and stimulation of effector function through the production of antibodies, or direct cytotoxic attack through DC populations, which initiate an adaptive immune response.[135]

Cytotoxic T cells are particularly attractive for clinical use owing to their exquisite specificity and direct lytic capabilities. The mechanistic aspects of CTLs have been characterized in great detail. CTLs recognize their targets through engagement of the T-cell receptor (TCR), which specifically binds to HLA class I (CD8 T cells) and II (CD4 T cells) molecules expressing an appropriate peptide.[136] In order for a productive interaction to occur, accessory and costimulatory molecules are also necessary.[137] In the absence of costimulatory molecules, anergy results, however, if the TCR is engaged along with costimulatory molecules, a productive interaction results in the synthesis of cytokines such as IL-2 and clonal expansion.[138] The best characterized system of costimulatory molecules are the CD28-B7 system, of which at least two members, B7.1 and B7.2, have been cloned and extensively studied.[137] Other costimulatory molecules, including CD2/LFA-3, are also important.

In addition to these protein molecules, adhesion molecules such as LFA-1 and its counterreceptor ICAM-1 play important roles in CTL function.[139] Binding of the TCR results in an increased affinity of LFA-1 toward ICAM-1 for a finite period of time, which allows for a stable interaction with the target cell.[140] Cytotoxic granule contents are then recruited along the cytoskeleton and released into the space between the two cells, resulting in pore formation by perforin and induction of apoptosis by granzymes.[141,142] For perforin to function properly, Ca^{2+} is required. In addition to granzyme/perforin-mediated lysis, a Ca^{2+}-independent pathway mediated through fasL–fas interactions also play important roles in CTL-mediated cytotoxicity.[143,144] Many tumor cell targets express fas, and fasL has been found to be upregulated on activated NK cells and T cells, which may be an important mechanism of tumor evasion (see Mechanisms of Tumor Cell Escape). CTL-based immunotherapy has been applied in a number of clinical settings for the treatment of hematologic malignancies and infectious complications that develop following allogeneic transplantation. These studies vary from the use of relatively diverse cellular populations to highly purified clonal populations of cells, which will be discussed below.

Activated T Cells

T cells can be activated and expanded in the laboratory prior to infusion. The use of anti-CD3 plus IL-2 activated lymphocytes has been extended to clinical trials. Limited toxicity has been observed following infusion.[145,146] A randomized clinical trial has been performed in the setting of patients with hepatoma following surgical resection where patients were randomized to receive several courses of activated lymphocytes or no further therapy. Those patients who received the T-cell immunotherapy had a reduced risk of disease relapse and improved progression-free survival.[147]

Another protocol utilizes interferon pretreatment followed by anti-CD3 and IL-2 exposure in extended culture for 14 to 21 days. The expanded cells have been termed cytokine-induced killer (CIK) cells. In these cultures, the cells with the greatest cytolytic activity have the phenotype $CD3^+D16^-D56^+$.[148] CIK cells are lytic to a broad range of tumor cells, including autologous tumors, and recognize target cells through an NKG2D-mediated mechanism.[149,150] The effector cells contain granzymes and perforin, which are released in the presence of tumor cell targets or by crosslinking of CD3.[151] The in vivo activity of CIK cells has been tested in a variety of animal models of human disease in mice with severe combined immunodeficiency, as well as syngeneic and allogeneic murine models.[148,152–155] Interestingly, allogeneic CIK cells have a markedly reduced capacity for GVHD induction, at least in part due to the production of high levels of interferon-γ.[154] Using a bioluminescent imaging system, luciferase-labeled CIK cells could be visualized tracking to the tumor within 3 days of injection and persisting at the site for at least 8 to 10 days.[156] An attractive approach has been to infect the CIK cells with oncolytic viruses, which are then delivered to the tumor site and released, triggering lysis and upregulation of NKG2D ligands.[157] CIK cells have been shown to be expandable from patients with a variety of hematologic malignancies and to lyse autologous and allogeneic acute myeloid leukemia cells.[158,159] Preliminary clinical trials have been performed with CIK cells, demonstrating the feasibility and tolerability of this approach.[145,146] The potential advantages of this form of immunotherapy are that the cells are readily expandable, have rapid in vivo activity without the requirement for exogenous IL-2 administration, and appear to have a reduced propensity for GVHD induction. Clinical trials in both the autologous and allogeneic transplant settings are underway in an effort to reduce the risk of tumor relapse.

Another approach of T-cell activation includes the use of anti-CD3 and anti-CD28 costimulation. The induction of CD4 T cells with capacity for T-cell help as well as the production of cytokines that may enhance the generation and survival of tumor or viral-reactive CTLs underlies the principles of potential therapy. The simultaneous activation of CD3 and costimulation through CD28 has been achieved with beads displaying these two MAbs.[160] Clinical trials using this novel strategy are currently ongoing in a number of clinical settings.[161] A particularly promising approach has been to utilize the adoptive transfer of costimulated T cells early after transplantation in a setting of lymphodepletion (Fig. 111–2). Vaccination demonstrated that earlier time points were optimal to generating an effective immune response, which could be applied to tumor-based vaccinations in the future.[162]

Cytotoxic T Lymphocytes

The specificity of CTLs has made their clinical application an attractive goal. A number of groups have attempted to identify and expand

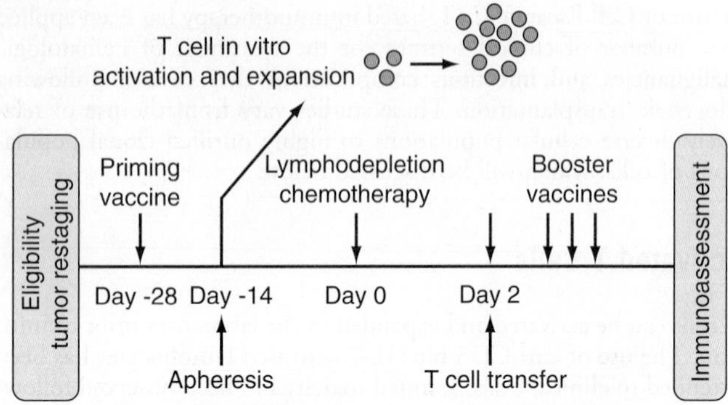

Figure 111–2 Schema for adoptive transfer of autologous, vaccine-primed, in vitro expanded T cells. As shown here, eligible patients are primed with vaccine on day −28, followed by lymphocyte harvest on day −14. The autologous T cells undergo polyclonal in vitro activation and expansion, and are reinfused on day 2 after lymphodepleting chemotherapy. Antigen-specific immune function is measured after the administration of booster vaccines. (Adapted from Cooley S, June CH, Schoenberger SP, *Miller JS*: Adaptive Therapy with T Cells/NK Cells. Biol. Blood and Marrow Transpl. 13:33–42, 2007.)

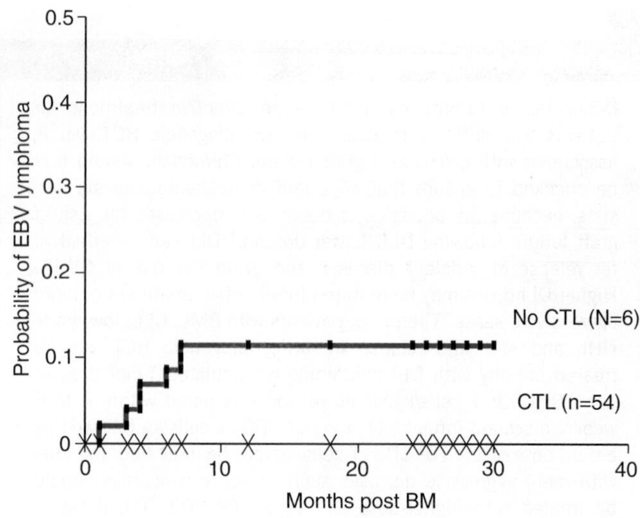

Figure 111–3 Reduced risk of Epstein–Barr virus-associated lymphoproliferative disorders in patients receiving cytotoxic T lymphocytes as compared to historical experience (H. Heslop, unpublished observations).

CTL populations capable of lysing target cells. CTL-based immunotherapy has been applied clinically for the recognition of virally infected cells and tumor cell targets. Developing viral-specific CTLs is theoretically a simpler proposition owing to the exogenous nature of the viral infection and the ability to replicate such interactions in vitro. The clinical settings that have been explored for CTL therapy most extensively are EBV and CMV infection.

Human EBV-specific CTLs have been selected from PBL isolated from seropositive donors and expanded ex vivo. These CTLs exhibit strong EBV-specific and HLA-restricted activity in vitro and in animal models. Clinical application has been explored both in the setting of treatment of patients with EBV-associated lymphoproliferative disorders or in the prophylaxis of high-risk patient populations. Clinical responses have been noted in the former setting with trafficking of marked CTLs to the tumor sites.[163,164] Prophylaxis has been very effective in reducing the risk of EBV-associated LPD (Fig. 111–3).[165] Because a significant percentage of patients with Hodgkin disease harbor latent EBV viral sequences and often express viral gene products, this strategy has been extended to the treatment of relapsed HD or for the prevention of relapse following autologous transplantation.[166] In this initial report, 14 patients with recurrent EBV$^+$ HD were treated with EBV CTL lines. Using gene marking studies, it was determined that these CTLs were well tolerated, expand in vivo, and functioned. An extension of this work has been to introduce the CD30 chimeric antigen receptor (CAR) into the CTLs because most malignant Reed–Sternberg cells express CD30. In a murine xenograft model, the CD30 CAR$^+$ CTLs induced antitumor effects against EBV$^-$CD30$^+$ tumors.[167] These elegant studies clearly demonstrate the potential of specific CTLs in the clinic.

Cytotoxic T-cell clones have also been generated against CMV-infected cells. These CD8$^+$ CTLs were isolated from the blood of the patient's donor. In the first study using this concept, CTLs were infused into recipients beginning at 30 to 40 days after allogeneic bone marrow transplantation. In these patients, cellular immunity against CMV was monitored before, during, and after the infusions of the CTLs.[168] The infusion of the CTLs did not result in significant toxicity and the transferred cells persisted for up to 12 weeks. None of these patients developed clinical CMV disease.[168] A similar study of eight patients refractory to antivirals showed clinical responses in seven patients with a reduction in CMV viremia.[169] A problem with the use of CD8$^+$ CTL clones has been the relatively short persistence of these cells following injection. Different strategies such as infusion of IL-2 or coinfusing CD4$^+$ helper T cells have been considered. In addition, this approach is technically challenging for routine use. More rapid expansion techniques are under development.[170] Other potential targets for T cell-based therapies such as aspergillosis,[171,172] papilloma viruses, adenovirus,[173] and HIV, to name a few, are actively being pursued. A clever approach has been to generate genetic modification of antigen-presenting cells to generate CTLs against multiple pathogens simultaneously.[174] More rapid selection techniques have made these approaches more feasible and clinically applicable.

The positive results of CTL-mediated immunotherapy demonstrate not only feasibility but also that these effects can be persistent and have clear biological activity. Despite these successes, there are considerable obstacles that need to be overcome to make CTL-based therapies feasible options for the routine treatment of patients. The isolation and expansion of CTLs is laborious and costly. Another major drawback in the application of CTL-based immunotherapy of cancer has been the lack of tumor-specific antigens that can be recognized by T cells. Significant advances have been made in this field, and there are a number of putative human tumor antigens expressed on solid tumors and hematologic malignancies that are recognized by T cells.[175–177] A variety of novel techniques to identify new tumor antigens are being actively pursued.[178]

A number of groups have attempted to generate CTLs against leukemic cells. In one study, two such CTL lines were cloned by limiting dilution and were found to be HLA class I and II restricted.[179] These studies demonstrate the feasibility of generating CTLs against these types of malignancies, but underscore the general difficulty in obtaining such clones and expanding them to a sufficient number of cells for clinical use. An alternative approach has been to use CTLs that are reactive against minor histocompatibility antigens and determine whether these cells will also recognize clonogenic leukemic cells. Faber and colleagues have performed such studies and demonstrated that the CD8$^+$ CTL clones were able to recognize minor histocompatibility antigen HA-1 and HA-2.[180] However, these minor histocompatibility antigens are also expressed on immature hematopoietic progenitor cells.

Another approach has been to extract tumor tissue from the patient and culture infiltrating lymphocytes (TIL cells). The cells with the majority of activity in these cultures are typical CTLs with the phenotype of CD3$^+$D8$^+$D56$^-$ and are MHC restricted.[181,182] TILs have been reported to be more potent than lymphokine-activated killer cells; however, the generation of sufficient numbers of TIL cells with significant antitumor activity is difficult. Nonetheless, this approach was used to treat a series of patients with metastatic melanoma following treatment with chemotherapy similar to that used in the nonmyeloablative transplant setting. Significant proliferation of the TILs was associated with clinical responses and in some instances the development of vitiligo.[183] This study underscored the concept of using cytoreductive chemotherapy to induce lymphopenia in an effort to stimulate in vivo expansion of the infused lymphocytes through homeostatic mechanisms.

A number of reports have suggested that tumor cells may lack the appropriate costimulatory molecules necessary for a productive interaction between the tumor cell and the CTLs. In an attempt to overcome this, follicular lymphoma cells were preactivated with CD40, which is known to upregulate expression of costimulatory molecules including the B7 proteins. Using this approach, autologous TILs could be generated by the addition of IL-2 and further expanded in the presence of IL-4, IL-7, and interferon.[184] These activated T cells showed cytotoxicity against follicular lymphomas in four of five patients tested. These studies suggest that CTLs may be present but are not stimulated owing to the lack of expression of the appropriate costimulatory molecules that may be upregulated ex vivo to enhance the generation of CTLs. In fact, many tumor cells do not express the costimulatory molecules B7–1 and B7–2.[185,186] To overcome this, several groups have attempted to introduce these costimulatory molecules into the tumor cells by transfection. This has been performed successfully and results in enhanced recognition or rejection of transfected tumor cells using in vivo model systems.[187] These observations have been extended to hematopoietic tumors such as murine AML cells that have been found not to express B7–1. When B7–1 was transfected into the tumor cells with a B7–1-containing retrovirus, the resulting transduced AML cells were used in murine models that induced immunity against the wild-type AML cells.[188] It should be pointed out, however, that these studies were performed in animals that had not previously been exposed to the leukemic cells. It remains to be seen whether the injection of B7-expressing tumor cells into diseased hosts or patients will be able to overcome the potential of T-cell anergy.

An alternative strategy has been to introduce receptors into T cells in an effort to redirect cytolytic responses to shared antigens expressed by tumor cells.[189] For example, T cells capable of recognizing and lysing CD19-expressing acute lymphocytic leukemia cells or CD20-expressing lymphoma cells could be used to treat patients with these disorders.[190] A variety of other potential receptors could be introduced in this fashion.[191] A potential problem may be the long lifespan of the T cells reactive toward normal cells also expressing these antigens. Nonetheless, these approaches are being explored in the clinic for the treatment of a variety of malignancies.

Immunoregulatory T Cells

Control of immune reactions has been an area of intense investigation. The best-characterized population of T cells capable of immune regulation are CD4$^+$ T cells that coexpress the IL2R (CD25). These CD4$^+$D25$^+$ regulatory T cells (T_{reg}) express a specific transcription factor FoxP3 and are capable of suppressing the mixed lymphocyte reaction in vitro and a variety of immune reactions in vivo. Most relevant to this discussion is the ability of T_{reg} to suppress GVHD in animal models from a number of different laboratories.[192–194] Coadministration of T_{reg} and defined numbers of conventional CD4$^+$ and CD8$^+$ T cells has resulted in the control of GVHD with maintenance of GVT responses.[195] The ability of T_{reg} to separate GVHD from GVT appears to be due at least in part to the ability of T_{reg} to suppress the proliferation of alloreactive T cells required for GVHD. T_{reg} are rare populations of cells, typically approximately 10% of CD4$^+$ T cells or 1% of peripheral blood lymphocytes; therefore, the isolation of sufficient numbers of cells for clinical application is difficult.[196] T_{reg} can be expanded using similar techniques to those described for the expansion of T cells, such as CD3 plus CD28 and IL-2.[197] The addition of rapamycin may help reduce the expansion of conventional T cells that also expand under these culture conditions.[198] The adoptive transfer of T_{reg} is an exciting area of clinical research that several groups are pursuing.

Another population of immunoregulatory lymphocytes that share phenotypic expansion and functional attributes of both of NK and T cells has been described. These cells, termed NK-T cells, have demonstrated immunoregulatory and cytotoxic capabilities.[199,200] NK-T cells have been separated into two broad categories based on the TCR expression profile. Some NK-T cells express an invariant TCR (Vα14Jα281 in murine systems and Vα24Vβ11 in humans). These cells express CD3 and the NK markers NK1.1 in murine cells and CD154 in humans.[200–202] The population of NK-T cells expressing the invariant TCRs interacts with the nonpolymorphic HLA molecule CD1. CD1-expressing cells in turn present nonprotein lipopolysaccharides. On activation, this population of NK-T cells play important immunoregulatory functions in large part related to cytokine production, in particular, IL-4. These NK-T cells typically either express CD4 or are CD4$^-$CD8$^-$.[203] Although the adoptive transfer of NK-T cells has not been pursued as aggressively as with T_{reg}, certain preparatory regimens, for example using total lymphoid irradiation and antithymocyte globulin, may alter the ratio of conventional to NK-T cells, with an apparent reduction in acute GVHD risk.[204]

A second population of NK-T cells that express a broad array of TCRs has also been described.[205] These NK-T cells are not regulated by CD-1 and do not produce IL-4 on activation. Instead, these cells appear to have primarily cytolytic functions. This population of cells is readily expandable unlike NK cells.

Mechanisms of Tumor Cell Escape

These more basic biological and mechanistic studies not only suggest strategies for therapeutic intervention but also demonstrate the complexity of the cells and cellular interactions. They also highlight mechanisms by which tumor cells may escape immune recognition (Table 111–3). With respect to NK cell-mediated killing, tumor cells may merely inactivate the effector cells through the appropriate expression of MHC molecules. The fact that many investigators have demonstrated autologous cytolysis of tumor cell targets suggests that this inhibition can be overcome. Other mechanisms of escape include the production of inactivating cytokines such as TGF-β[206] and others, as well as molecules that may inactivate perforin and granzymes. More recently, some tumor types have been found to produce and secrete ligands for NKG2D that may inactivate and help evade recognition and lysis by NK cells.[207] In regard to CTL recognition of tumor cell targets, there are a number of possible mechanisms of escape. First, there may be a lack of tumor-specific antigens expressed by a particular tumor cell that can be recognized by CTLs. There has been an intensive search for tumor-specific Ags that have been identified for a minority of malignant cells.[176] Second, if tumor cells do not express costimulatory molecules, anergy results. In fact, this mechanism has been shown to be operative in a number of tumor cell types, suggesting that the tumor itself can downregulate response directed toward it.[186] Third, tumor cells may be relatively resistant to apoptotic signals. Finally, evidence has indicated that certain tumor cell types express fasL. FasL expression that was initially demonstrated on melanoma cells, however, has subsequently been found on a variety of other tumor cell types, including those of hematopoietic malignan-

Table 111–3 Possible Mechanisms of Tumor Cell Evasion of the Immune System

Inhibition of NK cell function through the appropriate expression of HLA molecules
Lack of expression of tumor-specific antigen or peptide
Lack of costimulatory and/or adhesion molecule expression by the malignant cells
Resistance to apoptosis
Expression of fas-ligand on the tumor cell, thereby inactivating fas-expressing effector cells
Release of inhibiting cytokines or receptor ligands

Use of Allogeneic Natural Killer Cells in Patients With Advanced Myeloid Malignancies

Chemotherapy refractory leukemia remains a clinical challenge. Hematopoietic cell transplantation (HCT) studies suggest a role for the endogenous antileukemia activity of alloreactive natural killer (NK) cells. This activity is predicted by donor–recipient killer immunoglobulin-like receptor (KIR)–ligand mismatch or incompatibility. In this setting, donor NK cells expressing inhibitory KIR will result in better tumor kill if they are not inhibited by MHC class I ligands on residual recipient tumor cells. Progress has been made in adoptive transfer of allogeneic NK followed by in vivo expansion and activation as an alternative to HCT. This strategy is dependent on a high-dose chemotherapy regimen consisting of cyclophosphamide and fludarabine chemotherapy along with IL-2 administration. This lymphodepleting chemotherapy alters the milieu in vivo resulting in a surge of endogenous IL-15 and IL-7, which probably contributes to in vivo expansion of donor NK. Although promising, treatment of patients with advanced malignancy using allogeneic NK cells and IL-2 is still experimental and should be performed only in a clinical trial setting. Exploiting NK cell therapy alone or in combination with HCT is being actively pursued. Other strategies to maximize this effect, such as KIR genotyping for better donor selection, are also being explored.

cies.[208,209] Therefore, tumor cells expressing fasL could inactivate CTLs or NK cells by inducing apoptosis of the effector cell through engagement of fas. The significance of these various mechanisms of tumor cell escape and the development of strategies designed to overcome them is an area of intense basic and clinical investigation.[177]

NONHEMATOPOIETIC IMMUNOREGULATORY CELLS

Mesenchymal Stromal Cells

Nonhematopoietic stem cells (embryonic and adult tissue derived), capable of giving rise to a variety of somatic tissues, have been of great interest in regenerative medicine. Among the first adult derived cells described from bone marrow and other tissues are mesenchymal stromal cells (MSCs), which are fibroblast-like plastic adherent cells of nonhematopoietic cell origin.[210] Although they are termed mesenchymal stem cells by several investigators, the International Society for Cellular Therapy position paper encouraged a name change to mesenchymal stromal cells to accurately reflect the fact that many reports do not qualify these cells as stem cells and because not all MSCs are alike.[211] Comparing MSC populations characterized in different laboratories is difficult because of differences in culture techniques and the lack of distinct surface antigens that accurately distinguish developmental maturity or differentiating capacity. The major interest in MSCs in HCT is their potential immunomodulatory effects.

Mesenchymal stromal cells produce a number of cytokines[212] that suppress allogeneic T-cell stimuli in mixed lymphocyte reaction assays or by other nonspecific stimuli.[213] More detailed in vitro studies show that MSCs can alter the cytokine secretion profile of DCs, T cells, and NK cells to induce a tolerant phenotype.[214] Specifically, MSC can mature type 1 DC to decrease TNF-α secretion, mature type 2 DC to increase the suppressive factor IL-10, and can cause an increase in regulatory T cells. These changes lead to a shift from TH1 to TH2 responses in T cells and a decrease in interferon-γ production by NK cells. Taken together, these reports as well as studies transplanting human cells into immunodeficient mice[215,216] suggest that MSCs may play a role in facilitating engraftment and modulating GVHD much like the Treg discussed above. One concern about these reports is whether all the in vitro findings will be important in vivo. This concern is highlighted by a study evaluating the effects of mouse MSC. Although these mouse MSCs have potent suppressive effects on T cells in vitro, they had no clinical benefit on the incidence or severity in a bone marrow transplant model. Clinical trials using human MSC are under study in several centers.

The first report of clinical use of human MSC was by Koc et al, in which autologous MSCs were infused in women with breast cancer.[217] Conclusions from this study were MSC infusions were safe and hematopoietic recovery was rapid but this phase I–II study could not definitively compare effects on engraftment. In 2004, LeBlanc and colleagues first reported clinical benefit in treating grade IV GVHD of the gut and liver after 2 infusions of 1 to 2 × 10^6 haploidentical MSCs.[218] A follow-up study by this group in eight patients showed six responses demonstrating the potential promise of this therapy.[219] MSCs have been safely coinfused with HCT after sibling transplant[220] and other trials are in progress. In summary, MSCs remain a promising cellular therapy to enhance the safety of or to treat complications of HCT.

CONCLUSIONS

The use of cellular therapy for the treatment of a variety of conditions is an area of intense laboratory and clinical investigation. Some forms of cellular therapy are part of routine clinical care whereas others are just being developed. The rapid expansion in basic biological understanding of the types of effector cells, role of accessory cells and molecules, as well as the cytokines that expand and activate these cells has resulted in renewed optimism. Clinical successes have been evident in controlling infectious and malignant disease using adoptive therapy approaches. Ongoing and future clinical studies will determine where and how this novel therapeutic approach will be best applied in clinical medicine.

SUGGESTED READINGS

Anfossi N, Andre P, Guia S, et al: Human NK cell education by inhibitory receptors for MHC class I. Immunity 25:331, 2006.

Choudhury A, Gajewski JL, Liang JC, et al: Use of leukemic dendritic cells for the generation of antileukemic cellular cytotoxicity against Philadelphia chromosome-positive chronic myelogenous leukemia. Blood 89:1133, 1997.

Cooley S, Burns LJ, Repka T, Miller JS: Natural killer cell cytotoxicity of breast cancer targets is enhanced by two distinct mechanisms of antibody-dependent cellular cytotoxicity against LFA-3 and HER2/neu. Exp Hematol 27:1533, 1999.

Cooley S, McCullar V, Wangen R, et al: KIR reconstitution is altered by T cells in the graft and correlates with clinical outcomes after unrelated donor transplantation. Blood 106:4370, 2005.

Dazzi F, Szydlo RM, Cross NC, et al: Durability of responses following donor lymphocyte infusions for patients who relapse after allogeneic stem cell transplantation for chronic myeloid leukemia. Blood 96:2712, 2000.

Edinger M, Hoffmann P, Ermann J, et al: CD4(+)CD25(+) regulatory T cells preserve graft-versus-tumor activity while inhibiting graft-versus-host disease after bone marrow transplantation. Nat Med 9:1144, 2003.

Freud AG, Yokohama A, Becknell B, et al: Evidence for discrete stages of human natural killer cell differentiation in vivo. J Exp Med 203:1033, 2006.

Heslop HE, Ng CY, Li C, et al: Long-term restoration of immunity against Epstein-Barr virus infection by adoptive transfer of gene-modified virus-specific T lymphocytes. Nat Med 2:551, 1996.

Igarashi T, Wynberg J, Srinivasan R, et al: Enhanced cytotoxicity of allogeneic NK cells with killer immunoglobulin-like receptor ligand incompatibility against melanoma and renal cell carcinoma cells. Blood 104:170, 2004.

Kiessling R, Petranyi G, Klein G, Wigzel H: Genetic variation of in vitro cytolytic activity and in vivo rejection potential of non-immunized semi-syngeneic mice against a mouse lymphoma line. Int J Cancer 15:933, 1975.

Leung W, Iyengar R, Triplett B, et al: Comparison of killer Ig-like receptor genotyping and phenotyping for selection of allogeneic blood stem cell donors. J Immunol 174:6540, 2005.

Martin MP, Qi Y, Gao X, et al: Innate partnership of HLA-B and KIR3DL1 subtypes against HIV-1. Nat Genet 39:733, 2007.

Miller JS, Soignier Y, Panoskaltsis-Mortari A, et al: Successful adoptive transfer and in vivo expansion of human haploidentical NK cells in patients with cancer. Blood 105:3051, 2005.

Rapoport AP, Stadtmauer EA, Aqui N, et al: Restoration of immunity in lymphopenic individuals with cancer by vaccination and adoptive T-cell transfer. Nat Med 11:1230, 2005.

Raulet DH: Missing self recognition and self tolerance of natural killer (NK) cells. Semin Immunol 18:145, 2006.

Ruggeri L, Capanni M, Urbani E, et al: Effectiveness of donor natural killer cell alloreactivity in mismatched hematopoietic transplants. Science 295:2097, 2002.

Ruggeri L, Mancusi A, Capanni M, et al: Donor natural killer cell allorecognition of missing self in haploidentical hematopoietic transplantation for acute myeloid leukemia: Challenging its predictive value. Blood 110:433, 2007.

Shlomchik WD, Couzens MS, Tang CB, et al: Prevention of graft versus host disease by inactivation of host antigen-presenting cells. Science 285:412, 1999.

Takayama T, Sekine T, Makuuchi M, et al: Adoptive immunotherapy to lower postsurgical recurrence rates of hepatocellular carcinoma: A randomised trial. Lancet 356:802, 2000.

Walter EA, Greenberg PD, Gilbert MJ, et al: Reconstitution of cellular immunity against cytomegalovirus in recipients of allogeneic bone marrow by transfer of T-cell clones from the donor. N Engl J Med 333:1038, 1995.

REFERENCES

For complete list of references log onto www.expertconsult.com

CHAPTER 112

STEM CELLS FOR TISSUE REPAIR

Felipe Prosper and Catherine M. Verfaillie

BACKGROUND

Stem cells have become a major area of discussion in the scientific, public, and clinical arena.[1] The characterization of human embryonic stem cells[2] and the demonstration of their pluripotentiality as well as the isolation of stem cells derived from adult somatic and germinal tissues have expanded our perspective of how cell therapy may be useful for patients with a variety of diseases. The past decade has seen enormous progress in our understanding of the specific requirements of stem cells and of their potential plasticity in the context of multiple tissues including the bone marrow, the central nervous system, the cardiovascular system, and almost any other tissue. Mechanisms regulating self-renewal and differentiation of stem cells have been described. Growth factors and substrates have been discovered that guide differentiation and proliferation of stem cells into specified lineages in vitro. However, the behavior of stem cells in tissue culture does not reflect fully how these cells will act when grafted into the living host, where multiple factors both intrinsic (intracellular) and extrinsic (environmental) govern the interaction of cells and the extracellular matrix, instructing them to adopt specific cellular fates. In this chapter we focus on defining the characteristics that define a cell as stem cell, the different types of stem cells and their potential. We also discuss the current applications of stem cells for tissue repair and finally address the concept of stem cell plasticity and transdifferentiation.

CHARACTERISTICS AND DEFINITION OF STEM CELLS

Stem cells are defined functionally as clonogenic cells that can undergo self-renewal as well as differentiation to committed progenitors and eventually to differentiated, functional tissues. We will explore three aspects of the stem cell: (a) self-renewal capacity: stem cells can proliferate and give rise to cells identical to each other. Although most somatic cells can be cultured in vitro for a limited number of duplications (60 duplications) it is reasonable to say that a cell that can undergo over 100 duplications without oncogenic transformation or senescence has an extensive proliferative capacity. This proliferative potential does not mean that a cell is "immortal." (b) A second parameter to define stem cells refers to the concept of clonality, which means that a single stem cell has the potential to create new stem cells. We also refer to clonality when a population of cells with different or even the same characteristics are all derived from a single unique cell (stem cell in this case). (c) Stem cells have the potential to provide a variety of differentiated cell types. According to their potential, stem cells have been clarified as totipotent (capable of giving rise to both embryonic and extraembryonic tissues), pluripotent (may differentiate into tissues derived from any of the three germ layers) or multipotent (limited differentiating capacity to cells of a given tissue only). Finally, stem cells should differentiate not only in vitro but also in vivo, contributing robustly to the reconstitution of a given tissue after transplantation.

ORIGIN OF STEM CELLS

Stem cells can be subdivided according to their tissue of origin. Embryonic stem cells are derived from the embryo, germ stem cells from germinal tissue, and tissue-specific stem cells from differentiated tissue such as cardiac, neural, or hematopoietic sites.

Embryonic Stem Cells

Embryonic stem cells (ESCs) are derived directly from the inner cell mass of preimplantation embryos at the blastocyst stage and were first isolated from mice in 1981.[3,4] Embryonic stem cells are pluripotent; they have the capacity to contribute to all somatic lineages and to produce germ line chimeras in mice. The extensive proliferative capacity as well as the pluripotentiality of ESCs have made them particularly attractive as a source of cells for tissue repair. The derivation of the first human ESC lines in 1998 and the new cell lines derived more recently[5] has raised the possibility that ESCs will provide the basis for new cell therapies useful in the treatment of many diseases.[6]

Embryonic stem cells have been extensively tested in vitro and in different animal models with very promising results; however, a number of obstacles currently prevent the widespread application of ESC therapy. It is not yet known whether it will be possible to obtain efficient differentiation of ESCs to yield pure cultures of the desired type of cells and not a mixed population. The presence of undifferentiated cells in the graft has been invariably associated with the development of teratomas,[7] as would be expected from a pluripotent stem cell. The use of promoters for specific genes expressed in the differentiated tissues of interest with a selectable cassette (fluorochrome, cell surface antigen, or antibiotic resistance gene) has allowed the effective selection of the desired cells.[8] However, it remains to be seen whether this system will be readily applicable to the clinic. The other major limitation for clinical application of ESCs is the problem of immune rejection due to donor-recipient HLA differences. Although there are some suggestions that ESCs are immune-privileged, once ESCs differentiate to mature tissues they are subjected to the same process of immune rejection.[9] Establishing ESC lines from blastocysts derived by nuclear transfer has been advocated as a way of tailoring grafts to individual patients, thus eliminating the problem of graft rejection. While nuclear transfer is a reality in several small mammals, it is not yet known whether nuclear transfer can be applied efficiently and safely to human cells. The development of enough cell lines covering the majority of the human HLA repertoire has also been advocated as a means to prevent graft rejection.

At the blastocyst stage of early embryonic development, a population of primordial germ cells (PGCs) can be identified near the epiblast. Primordial germ cells migrate to the genital ridges where they produce mature germ cells. Pluripotent stem cells have also been isolated from the genital ridges giving rise to embryonic germ cells that share many of the characteristics of ESCs with respect to their differentiation capacity and their contribution to the germ line of chimeric animals.[10,11] Although embryonic germ cells are pluripotent, recent studies indicate that primordial germ cells have already initiated epigenetic reprogramming so that erasure of imprinting starts at the early stage after conception (before 10.5 dpc in mice).[12,13] Embryonic germ cells can be obtained from PGC before extensive epigenetic reprogramming of the genome occurs and that is followed by progressive downregulation of some pluripotency-specific genes.[14] Embryonic germ cells have the same limitations of ESCs with regard to teratoma formation and immune rejection, as embryonic germ cells are derived from PGC that have already repressed part of the somatic differentiation program. This may have an impact on their differentiation potential despite expression of the right pluripotent genes Nanog, Sox2, or Oct-4.[14]

Adult Somatic Stem Cells

The existence of stem cells in adult tissues has been recognized for more than 50 years with the first proof of concept that bone marrow contains cells that can rescue animals or humans from marrow failure.[15,16] However, complete identification and characterization of hematopoietic stem cells (HSCs) is yet to be achieved in humans despite the significant advances in the isolation of HSCs in mice.[17] Current evidence demonstrates that a single murine HSC can reconstitute all blood cell types following transplantation into a lethally irradiated animal and that the progeny of such cells can reconstitute secondary recipients, thus fulfilling all the characteristics of a stem cell derived from an adult tissue.[18]

More recently, several other tissue-specific cells have been identified, including neural,[19] epidermal,[20] gastrointestinal,[21] skeletal muscle,[22] cardiac,[23] liver,[24] pancreas,[25] or lung stem cells[26] among others. In some cases, such as neural stem cells, prospective isolation has been possible; however, this has not yet been achieved for all stem cells. Tissue-specific stem cells are multipotent, that is, they have the potential to differentiate into cells present in the tissue of origin but not other cells types. However, this concept has been challenged by a large number of studies suggesting that cells originating from one germ layer (eg, mesoderm) can generate cell types derived from a second germ layer (eg, ectoderm or endoderm).[27,28] Moreover, different studies have suggested that some adult tissues may harbor pluripotent stem cells capable of giving rise to tissues derived from all three germ layers.[29–34] The great enthusiasm generated from these studies has been paralleled by a healthy skepticism surrounding the concept of adult stem cell plasticity and pluripotency.[35–37] It is not our goal to discuss all studies and the different arguments against or in favor of stem cell plasticity but rather to provide a general view of the possible explanations of these observations.

Mesenchymal Stem Cells

Beside HSCs, BM also contains stem cells that have been termed mesenchymal stem cells (MSC or marrow stromal cells).[38] In 1976, Friedenstein et al described that fibroblastic colonies could be obtained from BM cells selected by their adherence to plastic in the presence of fetal calf serum.[39,40] Further work indicated that these cells could differentiate into bone, cartilage, and adipocytes in vitro and were transplantable.[41–43] Plastic adherent cells are a very heterogeneous population, and about 30% of these cells can be considered MSCs.[38] More recent studies by Caplan and colleagues have identified a set of surface markers that are expressed by MSCs, including SH2, SH3, CD29, CD44, CD71, CD90, and CD106. A number of hematopoietic markers are not present on MSC (CD34, CD45 or CD14).[44,45] In vitro, human, and mouse MSCs can differentiate into functional mesodermal-derived tissues. MSCs differentiate into osteoblasts, chondroblasts, adipocytes, and skeletal myoblasts.[44,46] Ring cloning[44] as well as single cell sorting strategies[47] have been used to demonstrate that single MSCs give rise to all these different lineages. A recent study also suggested that MSCs differentiate in cardiac myoblasts: injection of MSCs into an infarcted pig heart resulted in differentiation to cells staining positive for certain cardiac muscle markers and improvement of cardiac function.[48,49]

When human MSCs were transplanted by intraperitoneal injection into preimmune and immune fetal sheep, contribution to different tissues was detected by PCR for human-specific β2 microglobulin[50] and by immunohistochemical staining for chondrocytes, adipocytes, myocytes, cardiomyocytes, stromal marrow cells, and thymic stroma combined with in situ hybridization for human-specific DNA. The potential of MSCs to differentiate into mesenchymal lineages has been exploited clinically in patients with osteogenesis imperfecta undergoing allogeneic hematopoietic cell transplant. Similar to what was shown for murine BM cells[51] transplantation of whole BM was associated with osteoblast engraftment between 1% and 2% and improvement in symptoms associated with the underlying disease.[52]

Several studies have suggested that MSCs may also differentiate into neuroectoderm-derived tissues.[53–55] In vitro, both rat and human MSCs can be induced to express neuronal markers such as enolase, NeuN, neurofilament, and tau.[54] However, these studies did not demonstrate that cells with neuroectodermal staining profile also acquired functional characteristics of neurons or glial cells. When MSCs were injected into the ventricle of neonatal mice, cells migrate throughout the forebrain and cerebellum without disrupting the brain architecture, and may acquire markers of astrocytes and possibly neurons,[53,54] although again no functional data are available. In one study, MSCs were transplanted in a mouse model of Parkinson's disease. Survival of cells and acquisition of tyrosine hydroxylase expression were demonstrated. Furthermore, animals transplanted with MSCs intrastriatally had improved functional recovery compared with saline-injected animals.[55] Despite their mesodermal multipotentiality and possible neuroectodermal differentiation ability, MSCs do not differentiate into endoderm-derived tissues and thus cannot be consider pluripotent. MSCs may be a useful resource for clinical application in a number of diseases, both for regenerative therapy as well as a gene therapy vehicle.[45]

Adipose-Derived Stem Cells

Adipose tissue is a mesoderm-derived organ that has demonstrated an unexpected plasticity and potential for tissue regeneration based on the existence of a remarkable population of adipose-derived stem cells (ADSCs). Like marrow-derived mesenchymal stem cells (also frequently referred to as marrow stromal cells), adipose tissue contains a stromal population comprised of microvascular endothelial cells, smooth muscle cells, and stem cells. These cells have many properties that suggest considerable potential utility in cellular therapy for a variety of disorders. These cells can be enzymatically digested out of adipose tissue (commonly from lipoaspirate) and separated from the abundant adipocytes by centrifugation given a more homogeneous population termed ADSC. Adipose tissue-derived stem cells share many of the characteristics of their counterpart in marrow, including extensive proliferative potential and the ability to undergo multilineage differentiation.[56]

Adipose tissue-derived stem cells have been characterized by their phenotype and their potential to differentiate into mesoderm-derived tissues. The cell surface phenotype of human ADSCs is quite similar to bone marrow-derived MSCs.[45,57] It is worth noting some of the key similarities and differences between these cells. For instance, CD105, STRO-1, and CD166 (ALCAM) are three common markers used to identify cells with multilineage differentiation potential and are consistently expressed on ADSCs and MSCs. Adipose tissue-derived stem cells and MSC express adhesion molecules such as CD29 (β1 integrin), CD44 (hyaluronate receptor, which is crucial in the development of neo-extracellular matrix and plays a role in numerous pathologic and physiologic events) and CD49e (alpha-5 integrin, important for cell adhesion to fibronectin). Adipose tissue-derived stem cells also express high levels of CD54 (ICAM-1), a member of the immunoglobulin supergene family that can be upregulated in response to numerous inflammatory mediators and cytokines. Adipose tissue-derived stem cells lack the expression of known hematopoietic and endothelial markers such as CD3, CD4, CD11c, CD14, CD15, CD16, CD19, CD31, CD33, CD38, CD56, CD62p, CD104, and CD144. Less than 1% of ADSCs express the HLA-DR protein, and the majority express MHC Class I molecules.[58] The differentiation potential of ADSCs is remarkable. Besides differentiation along classical mesenchymal lineages, adipogenesis, chondrogenesis, osteogenesis, and myogenesis,[57,59] differentiation into other mesoderm-derived tissues like endothelial and cardiac cells and non-mesenchymal stem cells such as neural progenitors has been described.[60–62] These attributes make ADSCs a very promising population of stem cells for tissue repair.

PLASTICITY, CELL FUSION, AND ADULT STEM CELLS

Although there is yet no "official" definition of stem cell plasticity, it could be defined as the capacity of a given cell to acquire phenotypic and functional characteristics of cells in a tissue different from the one from which the cell is originally derived. True stem cell plasticity should include the following criteria: a single tissue-specific adult stem cell, for instance an HSC, thought to be committed to a given cell lineage can under certain microenvironmental conditions acquire the ability to differentiate to cells of a different tissue. The differentiated cell types should be functional in vitro and in vivo. Engraftment should be robust and persistent in the presence (and absence) of tissue damage. Most reports of adult stem cell plasticity have not fulfilled all of these criteria.

The idea of "stem cell plasticity" originated over 100 years ago when it was recognized that epithelial changes, for instance from squamous to columnar epithelium, occur in response to different stresses. Such changes occur in the esophagus in response to gastric reflux. Furthermore numerous examples of lineage switch exist in lower species like Drosophila in which the imaginal discs can give rise to different organs depending on the position where the discs are placed.[63] What are then the mechanisms that may explain the capacity of stem cells to transdifferentiate (stem cell plasticity)?

One possibility is that pluripotent stem cells persist after birth in the BM or even in multiple organs. These embryonic remnants may under certain in vitro culture conditions acquire proliferative potential and when stimulated either in vitro or in response to local cues in vivo, differentiate into the tissues in which they engraft. It is not unreasonable to think that only under very special circumstances in vivo they would undergo proliferation-differentiation. This would not really be transdifferentiation but rather true pluripotency. However, there is currently very little evidence that such stem cells remain in adult tissues either in animals or humans. Two recent studies have described the isolation of a population of stem cells with such pluripotent characteristics.[29,64] Very small embryonic-like cells (VSELs) have been defined as a population of $CXCR4^{+}C133^{+}D34^{+}$ in $D45^{-}$ mononuclear cells derived from umbilical cord blood and are a counterpart of a similar pluripotent stem cell population found in mice. VSEL cells express embryonic transcription factors such as Oct-4 and Nanog and differentiate into tissues derived from all germ layers. A similar population named pre-MSC has been isolated from mice BM based on the expression of SSEA-1 that also express markers and behaves as pluripotent stem cells.[29] Although other cells with phenotypic and functional characteristics of pluripotent stem cells have been isolated from cord blood (USSC),[65] bone marrow,[31,33] mouse testis,[34] or amniotic fluid,[66] all these cell populations are obtained after in vitro culture. Whether they represent a true stem cell population existing in the adult tissues or are induced after culture remains to be demonstrated.

A second possibility is that a tissue-specific stem cell may undergo genetic reprogramming in culture. This is similar to what occurs in the cloning process induced by specific culture conditions. In other words, organ-specific stem cells overcome their intrinsic restrictions when exposed to a novel microenvironment.[67,68]

It has been demonstrated that apparent plasticity can be the result of cell fusion.[69–71] Some of the original descriptions of stem cell plasticity[72] are the result of cell fusion between stem/progenitor cells and local resident differentiated cells. Fusion has been demonstrated in vitro and in vivo, particularly in studies of liver regeneration but also in other organs such as the heart and the brain (Purkinje cell).[70,73] Although the phenomenon of cell fusion has long been known and exploited (formation of hybridomas for antibody production), the extent of cell fusion's role in plasticity and the potential to use cell fusion therapeutically are not known.

Finally, it is possible that some examples of plasticity can be attributed to presence of multiple stem cells in BM, or other organs. The cell population responsible for giving rise to different tissues may, in fact, be composed of multiple stem cells with different potential (muscle stem cells, neural stem cells, liver stem cells).[74,75] Strictly speaking, this phenomenon cannot be considered "stem cell plasticity"; however, such cell populations might still have therapeutic potential.

We do not yet understand which of these mechanisms (probably several of them) underlie the phenomena of stem cell plasticity. However, stem and progenitor cell populations other than HSCs have already been used to treat a variety of diseases and comprise a very active area of research for tissue repair and cell therapy. Embryonic stem cells eventually may be used therapeutically; however, only adult stem cells have been used for tissue repair or as vehicles for gene therapy to date. We will limit our discussion to therapy with stem and progenitor cell progenitors derived from adult humans.

THERAPY WITH STEM CELLS

Multipotent adult stem cells obtained from human BM have been used therapeutically for at least 50 years, and analyses of allogeneic BM, peripheral blood, and umbilical cord blood transplants have definitively demonstrated that HSCs contribute to long-term and complete hematopoiesis after myeloablation.[76,77] The use of stem and progenitor cell populations other than HSCs to repair their tissue of origin as well as other tissues is now entering an intense phase of investigation.

Stem Cells for Cardiac Repair

The idea of repairing the diseased heart using different types of stem cells has gained widespread attention recently, leading not only to a number of preclinical studies but also to early phase I–II and even randomized clinical trials.[78,79] Efforts have been made to restore function of the damaged heart by transplanting nonresident stem cells like fetal cardiomyocytes,[80] ESCs,[8] skeletal muscle cells,[81] bone marrow-derived MSCs,[82] or ADSCs.[83] These efforts have met with variable success.

Initial studies demonstrated that fetal cardiomyocytes grafted in noninfarcted hearts can integrate into the cardiac muscle and establish gap junctions, which allows electrical conductance between the host cells and the donor cells. Both murine and human ESCs can differentiate into functional cardiomyocytes,[84] and a number of studies have shown that like fetal cardiomyocytes, ESC-derived cells can integrate into the heart muscle of both normal hearts and infarcted areas.[8,85] However, grafting of ESC-derived cardiomyocytes in ischemic areas of the heart leads to very poor survival of cells.

Other cells used to treat heart disease in preclinical models include skeletal muscle cells, a number of BM-derived or adipose-derived cells as well as putative cardiac stem cells.[78] In contrast to ESCs, there is no convincing evidence that cells from postnatal tissues other than the heart can generate functional cardiomyocytes in vivo. Nevertheless, a number of cell populations, including BM mononuclear cells, enriched hematopoietic stem and progenitor cells,[86] EPCs,[87] BM MSC[88] and adipose MSC,[83] and skeletal myoblasts have been grafted in models of chronic as well as acute myocardial infarction.[79] Improved function has been seen in a number of studies without evidence that the cells contributed to a large degree to cardiac muscle itself. As a consequence of these preclinical studies, a large number of clinical trials in patients with chronic as well as acute MI using mostly bone marrow cells[89] (freshly isolated total BM, mononuclear cells, cultured cells to increase putative endothelial progenitor cells, CD34, or AC133 selected cells) but also skeletal myoblasts[90] have been developed. These clinical trials are predominantly phase I/II.[91,92] More recently, a phase III randomized trial has been initiated.[93] The largest experience has been gained in patients with acute MI using BM-derived cells. Although some trials suggest a benefit from cell transplant in patients with acute MI, other studies do not find any effect due to cell therapy.[93–96] The differences have been attributed to the heterogeneity of the type of cells used in each trial, the type of patients, or even the endpoints.

Most clinical investigators have postulated that delivery of the appropriate cells would repair a damaged heart via active myocardial regeneration resulting from transdifferentiation of the administered cells; however, alternative mechanisms may be at play: (a) exogenous cells may stimulate proliferation of endogenous cardiac precursors or stem cells through neovascularization or paracrine signaling actions facilitating the ability of the heart to heal itself[97]; (b) exogenous cells may lead to cardiac repair via fusion of donor cells with host cardiomyocytes as has been demonstrated in animal models[98]; and (c) the effect of therapeutic cells could also be mediated by altering the mechanical properties of the scar, thereby preventing deterioration in cardiac function.[99]

Recent work from several laboratories indicates that the adult heart contains a resident population of progenitor cells with cardiomyogenic potential.[100–102] Beltrami et al isolated clusters of multipotent cardiac stem cells (CSCs) expressing the cell surface antigen Sca-1, KIT, and/or multidrug resistance transporter gene 1 (MDR1) localized throughout the myocardium and, more particularly, at the atria and lower region of the left ventricle of the heart, termed apex.[100] Cardiac stem cells possess the ability to self-renew and differentiate into myocytes, smooth muscle cells, and endothelial cells. These are the main cell components of the myocardium contributing to the maintenance of heart homeostasis, and repair of myocardial tissue after injury in animal models of infarction.[100,103] A second population of cardiac progenitor cells was isolated on the basis of the expression of Sca-1 antigen.[104] When these cells were injected into mouse 6 hours after infarction, they engrafted and differentiated into cells expressing the cardiac markers sarcomeric actin and troponin I. Using a Cre-Lox model, it could be demonstrated that half of the donor-derived cells had fused with the host cardiomyocytes while the other half had differentiated directly without fusion. A third population of cardiac stem cells was described on the basis of the isolation and differentiation potential of side population (SP) cells expressing the stem cell marker ABCG2.[105] Less information is available in terms of functional cardiac potential of this population of cardiac progenitor cells. Recently, a candidate progenitor population has been described both from human and mouse heart as cells expressing the transcription factor islet-1.[102,106,107] During development, Isl1$^+$ cells contribute to a second wave of cardiomyocyte formation. These cells are also present at birth and, to a lesser extent, during adulthood. Isl1$^+$ cells can be isolated and expanded in vitro and differentiated into all three lineages—cardiomyocytes, endothelial cells, and smooth muscle cells—required for the development of the heart.[106] There is currently little evidence, however, that these cardiac progenitor populations have a major in vivo role as robust progenitors capable of regenerating the damaged heart.

Stem Cells for Muscle Repair

Skeletal muscle has the capacity for complete regeneration and restoration of the cellular architecture in response to repeated injuries. This regenerative capacity is attributed to muscle stem cells, also known as satellite cells.[108] This ability to withstand multiple injuries implies that the satellite cell pool is replenished during the regenerative process and suggests the presence of a cycling pool of satellite cells. This pool may be analagous to the transit amplifying cell (TAC) population described in other lineages (ie, skin and gut)[109,110] and maintained by a residual pool with self-renewal capacity.[111,112]

Although recent studies establish that the majority of the satellite cells are derived from the somite (Pax3$^+$/Pax7$^+$ cells located in the central region of the myotome),[113,114] other stem cell/progenitor cell populations that contribute to the satellite cell pool and muscle regeneration have been described. These stem cell populations either reside in skeletal muscle or may be recruited from nonmuscle pools in response to signals or cues associated with injury and regeneration and include muscle-derived stem cells (MDSCs),[32] side population cells,[115] bone marrow cells (hematopoietic stem cells),[116] mesenchymal stem cells,[117] multipotent adult progenitors cells,[118] or mesangioblasts.[119]

The satellite cells have a specialized niche in adult skeletal muscle between the basal lamina and the sarcolemma and are characterized by size (ie, small), high nuclear-to-cytoplasm ratio, relative absence of cytoplasmic organelles, and increased nuclear heterochromatin representing a quiescent state of the cell. At the molecular level, satellite cells lack expression of the myogenic regulatory factors, including members of the MyoD family.[120] Recently, investigators have utilized an array of transgenic and gene disruption strategies to identify and further characterize the satellite cell population. Factors that have a restricted expression pattern and serve as markers for the satellite cells in adult skeletal muscle include cell surface receptors (c-met),[121] adhesion proteins (M-cadherin and NCAM),[122] and transcription factors such as Pax3 and Pax7.[123] These cells are usually in a quiescent state, and when muscle regeneration is required they enter an active state of proliferation in which muscle-specific transcription factors are upregulated in an orchestrated fashion, eventually leading to the formation of myofibers and restoration of the normal architecture of the muscle. It is likely that a stem cell/progenitor cell hierarchy comparable to the hematopoietic system exists for the satellite cell pool (ie, stem cells vs transit amplifying progenitors vs progenitors).[124] The definition of this satellite cell hierarchy will serve as a platform for cell-based therapies.

The myogenic potential of other cell populations has recently been established. Investigators have demonstrated the presence of a population of stem cells with myogenic potential in the skeletal muscle characterized by the expression of the CD45$^+$ Sca-1$^+$ that rapidly expands following injury to the muscle. The myogenic potential of this population is dependent on the activation of the Wnt signaling.[125]

In an interesting report, Qu-Petersen et al. isolated different populations of muscle-derived stem cells from mice based on the adhesion and proliferation characteristics of the cells.[32] One of these populations named muscle-derived stem cell (MDSC) was characterized by expression of muscle markers (MyoD) and hematopoietic markers (Sca-1 and CD34) as well as lack of expression of MHC class I. MDSCs could be maintained for more 60 population doublings without evidence of genomic abnormalities and when transfected with LacZ and transplanted into the muscle of mdx mice, contributed to generation of muscle progenitors from MDSC, indicating their self-renewal capacity. MDSCs could differentiate in vitro but also in vivo to endothelium, muscle, and neural lineages.[32]

Side population (SP) cells constitute a stem cell/progenitor cell population that resides in adult tissues including bone marrow[126] and skeletal muscle[127] and that can be identified based on their ability to efflux the Hoechst 33342 dye because of the presence of the multidrug resistance protein ABCG2.[105] Recent studies performed in chick and mouse reveal that the majority of limb muscle satellite cells arise from cells expressing Pax3. At least a subpopulation of skeletal muscle SP cells is derived from Pax3$^+$ hypaxial somitic cells,[128] establishing a relation between muscle SP cells and satellite cells. Although cultures of purified muscle SP cells fail to differentiate into muscle cells,[115] transplantation studies have demonstrated that the muscle SP population contains cells that are capable of differentiating into regenerated fibers.[129] This cell population can give rise to satellite cells in regenerating muscle following transplantation, suggesting that myogenic differentiation only develops in response to the muscle environment. Interestingly, myogenic specification of muscle SP cells was observed in vitro following coculture with primary myoblasts, indicating the inability of muscle SP cells to undergo myogenic specification unless induced by myogenic specific signals.[115]

The bone marrow is a source of stem cell populations that have myogenic potential. Genetically labeled marrow-derived mouse cells have been recruited to injured muscle and generate fully differentiated myofibers.[130] Bone marrow-derived multipotent adult progenitors cells (MAPCs) are capable of forming differentiated myotubes in vitro and in vivo following delivery into murine muscle[33,118] while studies published recently have demonstrated that GFP-labeled bone marrow-derived cells become satellite cells that are capable of myogenesis and formation of labeled myofibers.[116]

Mesoangioblasts comprise another population of multipotent progenitors of mesodermal tissue with myogenic potential.[131,132] Mesoangioblasts are vessel-associated progenitors isolated from the embryonic dorsal aorta and defined by the expression of the key marker VEGFR-2 (Flk-1). Recent evidence suggests that this type of progenitor cell can also be isolated from the bone marrow.[119] Using a dog model of Duchenne muscular dystrophy, it has been reported that intraarterial delivery of wild-type canine mesoangioblasts (vessel-associated stem cells) results in an extensive recovery of dystrophin expression, normal muscle morphology, and function (confirmed by measurement of contraction force on single fibers) with a remarkable amelioration of clinical abnormalities and preservation of active motility. These data indicate that mesoangioblasts are future candidates for stem cell therapy of patients with Duchenne's muscular dystrophy.[133]

Stem Cells for Skin Diseases

The skin epidermis is composed of pilo-sebaceous units containing a hair follicle, sebaceous gland, and interfollicular epidermis.[109] The interfollicular epidermis is a stratified squamous epithelium with a basement membrane that contains resident basal stem cells responsible for maintaining homeostasis of the interfollicular epidermis by continually replenishing the suprabasal terminally differentiating cells. The hair follicle is formed during embryogenesis as an appendage of the epidermis. Postnatally, the base of the follicle forms the hair bulge that contains multipotent stem cells responsible for differentiation into all epithelial cell lineages residing in the tissue.[134] In skin, they not only serve as a reservoir of cells for regeneration during the normal cyclic periods of hair growth but also in conditions of hyperproliferation of sebaceous glands[135] and in the repair of the interfollicular epidermis following wounding.[136]

Cell-based therapy with keratinocytes has been practiced successfully for many years. Reconstitution of a functional epidermal barrier with regeneration of the papillary dermis has been accomplished with autologous epidermal layers in patients with skin burns as well as other skin diseases. Since the first description of cultivation of human keratinocytes in 1975,[137] it took Green and his coworkers over 8 years before the first transplant of cultured autologous keratinocytes was performed.[138] The technology has been successfully used to treat hundreds of patients with extensive burns.

A combination of cell therapy using keratinocyte stem cells (known as holoclones) with gene therapy has recently been used to treat a patient with a mutation in the gene encoding the basement membrane component laminin 5 that causes junctional epidermolysis bullosa.[139] Epidermal stem cells from this patient were transduced with a retroviral vector expressing LAMB3 cDNA (encoding LAM5-b3) and used to prepare genetically corrected cultured epidermal grafts. Transplantation of epidermal grafts induced the formation of normal epidermis for up to a year after treatment as well as the synthesis of normal levels of functional LAM5. This may provide a new therapeutic approach for patients with epidermolysis bullosa.

Orthopedic Applications of Stem Cells

The initial description of the existence of a population of stem cells in the bone marrow termed mesenchymal stem cells (MSCs) (also marrow stromal cells)[38] was made by Friedenstein et al. in 1976.[39,40] Subsequently, a large body of evidence has demonstrated that these cells can differentiate into bone, cartilage, and adipocytes in vitro and are transplantable.[44] These findings constitute the bases for the application of MSC therapy in orthopedic diseases.[140] In the case of orthopedic applications of stem cells for regenerative therapy, it has been clearer that the reconstruction of any tissue requires not only a population of repair cells (ie, MSCs) but also adequate scaffolds where the implanted MSCs can proliferate and interact with specific growth factors and cytokines.

On the basis of in vitro observations, it has become apparent that MSCs can differentiate into osteocytes and chondrocytes. Marrow-derived MSCs have been seeded on extracellular matrices such as hydroxyapatite and then implanted in vivo into NOD/SCID mice or in animals with segmental bone defects, demonstrating the formation of new bone.[141] Marrow-derived MSCs have been transplanted into mice with osteogenesis imperfecta, a genetic disorder of mesenchymal tissues and also in children with osteogenesis imperfecta undergoing bone marrow transplant, demonstrating not only engraftment without side effect but also an increase in the number of osteoblasts and the formation of new lamellar bone and the total body mineral content, reducing the frequency of fractures and contributing to enhanced body growth rate.[52]

Particularly promising for orthopedic applications, especially for bone formation, is the use of natural or synthetic biomaterials as carriers for MSC delivery.[142] Newer materials such as biodegradable polymers poly-L-lactide (PLA) and poly-L-lactide-*co*-glycolide (PLGA) facilitate adhesion, proliferation, and differentiation of cells.[143] These observations have resulted in the development of clinical studies in which scaffolds loaded with in vitro expanded autologous bone marrow-derived MSCs were successfully implanted in patients with large bone defects.[144] More recently, an extended mandible discontinuity was successfully repaired through a heterotopic bone induction with biomaterials and patient's marrow cells and growth factors.[145]

The use of chondrocytes to treat cartilage lesions was reported for the first time in 1994.[146] The potential of MSCs to differentiate into chondrocytes and the possibility of obtaining large numbers of cells has led to the use of MSCs to repair joint cartilage defects in animal models using various carrier matrices.[147] Injection of mesenchymal stem cells in combination with hyaluronic acid in goats after meniscectomy has resulted in regeneration of the meniscus, a decrease in bone resorption, subchondral bone remodelling, osteophyte formation and cartilage destruction, as well as a better preservation of the joint. In other cases, repair of full-thickness defects of joint cartilage was observed after transplantation of autologous MSCs using a gel of type I collagen as carrier[148] or sponges of calcium phosphate and hyaluronic acid loaded with autologous marrow-derived MSCs.[149]

Synthetic polymers, particularly PLA and PLGA, have been developed that offer the possibility of using tridimensional scaffolds in combination with MSCs and growth factors to reconstruct joint cartilage defects.[150] Recently, autologous marrow-derived MSCs have been applied in patients with cartilage lesions.[151] Mesenchymal stem cells were injected on the medial femoral condyle and covered with autologous periosteum. The results in 12 cases were compared to control patients treated with the same procedure but without receiving MSCs. Patients treated with MSCs had better arthroscopic and histological grading scores, although the clinical improvement was not significantly different between the two groups.[151] However, this study shows the feasibility, safety, and potential efficacy of MSC therapy for cartilage repair.

Vision Restoration with Stem Cells

Stem cell transplantation has gained significant support across the medical and scientific communities as a new therapy to restore visual function. The eye is derived from three types of embryonic tissue: the neural tube (neuroectoderm), from which arise the neurosensory retina and the retinal pigment epithelium; the mesoderm, from which the corneoscleral and uveal tunics develop; and the surface ectoderm, which gives rise to the lens. Understanding cellular and molecular mechanisms that drive differentiation of early progenitors into adult competent cells in this complex environment is essential to develop approaches for stem cell therapies to treat ocular diseases. There is now well-documented evidence that the adult human eye harbors various sources of stem cells, although characteristic markers to identify individual cell types have not been clearly established. Adult stem cells that contribute to major structural ocular tissue have so far been identified in the limbal region,[152] the pars plana and pars plicata of the retinal ciliary margin,[152] and the neural retina.[153] The potential for stem cell-based therapies to treat a variety of ocular diseases is well acknowledged, particularly the successful use of limbal stem cells to treat corneal diseases. Limbocorneal epithelial stem cells (LSCs) are located in the basal layer of the limbus between the cornea and the conjunctiva and have a high capacity for self-renewal. However, no specific markers for LSCs have been clearly identified and although the expression of p63 and the transporter ABCG2 has been associated with stem cells, these markers can also be expressed by committed cells.

Transplantation of LSCs has been recognized as a therapeutic option for patients with diseases characterized by limbal stem cell insufficiency such as Stevens–Johnson syndrome, chemical or thermal injury, chronic limbitis, limbal surgery, and contact lens keratopathy.[154,155] Pioneering studies from the group of Tseng demonstrated that transplants of cultured autologous limbal epithelium in patients with unilateral limbal stem cell deficiency can restore normal corneal function.[156] Given our understanding that the stem cell niche environment is important for LSC survival and function, the amniotic membrane has been used as a "surrogate" niche for the ex vivo expansion of LSCs.[157] Transplantation of LSCs to restore visual function caused by corneal defects is at present the only recognized stem cell-based therapy in the ophthalmic field that has been clinically validated and the only one with immediate prospects for widespread use.

Fish and amphibians can regenerate the neural retina throughout life, and the existence of neural retinal stem cells in humans during fetal development and in the adult eye in both the ciliary body and the neural retina has recently been demonstrated.[158] Retinal stem cell lineage analysis studies in small vertebrates indicate that retinal neurons share a common progenitor that is multipotent and present during all stages of retinal histogenesis. This suggests that there is not a restricted lineage giving rise to specific retinal cells and that if neural retinal progenitors could be isolated and expanded from adult human tissue, they might be used for cell replacement therapy to regenerate all types of retinal neurons as has been indicated by recent studies.[159] In that sense, stem cell-based therapies offer for the restoration of sight in individuals whose visual function has been irreversibly damaged in diseases that are associated with the loss of retinal neurons, such as macular degeneration. One recent study indicates that transplantation of committed photoreceptor progenitors may be useful for retina repair, at least in a mouse model.[159] Although isolation and cultivation of adult retinal stem cells may prove feasible, at present lack of knowledge on the conditions that promote their survival and axonal integration within the neural circuit remain obstacles to grafting and constitute a major subject of intensive research.

Stem Cells for Diabetes

Replacement of insulin-producing cells in patients with diabetes has become a major goal in regenerative therapy. Promising strategies have included therapy with cells that have the potential to generate insulin-producing β cells by expansion of existing β cells, differentiation of embryonic stem (ES) cells to β cells, and conversion of either pancreatic or nonpancreatic adult stem/progenitor cells to β cells. Alternatively, investigators have tested pharmacological agents that regenerate β cells in the pancreas, either by replication of existing β cells or by the generation of β cells from other cell types.

In vitro, β-cells with the capacity to secrete insulin have been successfully derived using different types of cells, including pluripotent stem cells (ESCs), pancreatic-derived progenitors, or nonpancreatic progenitor cells such as bone marrow or peripheral blood-derived cells.[160,161] Recent studies have demonstrated that insulin-producing β cells capable of sensing glucose levels can be derived from human ESCs.[162] However, it is yet to be established whether these cells could restore normal pancreatic function in vivo.

Other studies have focused on the potential of pancreatic progenitors to proliferate and regenerate islets and insulin-producing cells. Although some authors have favored the concept that pancreatic ductal epithelial cells have the potential to regress to a less differentiated progenitor cell capable of producing new islets and acini,[163] others have supported the potential of acinar cells to transdifferentiate to islets.[164] Alternatively, beta cells may dedifferentiate to a mesenchymal-like cell type that can be extensively expanded and then redifferentiated.[165] However, lineage-tracing studies in mouse have shown that mesenchymal cells growing in such cultures are not of endodermal origin.[166] Yet others have suggested that like in the liver, beta cells can undergo cell divisions and may be responsible for regeneration.[167] Additional studies will be needed to identify which stem and progenitor cell populations may exist in the pancreas and will be available to repair endocrine pancreatic tissue.

The possibility that adult stem cells from sources other than the pancreas may be used to treat diabetes has also been studied. Some studies have suggested that marrow cells can become glucose-responsive, insulin-secreting cells in islets in vivo.[168] Others have not been able to replicate these results. Alternatively, marrow cells may contribute to the endothelium of damaged pancreas, leading to the production of cytokines and growth factors that stimulate β-cell neogenesis, β-cell proliferation, or increased survival of the residual β cells.[169,170] Another approach to the generation of β cells is transdifferentiation of differentiated cells of endodermal origin, such as liver or intestinal cells,[171,172] as those cells are derived from the same germ layer as pancreatic cells. This may be accomplished by introducing one or more transcription factors implicated in pancreatic and endocrine pancreatic commitment such as Pdx1 and/or Ngn3.[173]

The in vitro evidence for stem–progenitor cell differentiation into insulin-producing cells is clear. However, it is not yet clear that these cells closely resemble normal β cells, which are very well characterized with regard to their gene expression, metabolism, growth potential, and secretory function. Furthermore, insulin-producing cells destined for therapeutic replacement must match the extraordinary performance of normal β cells, with their ability to store large quantities of insulin and secrete it precisely to meet the complex demands of meals, exercise, and fasting.

CNS Disorders

Diseases of the CNS, although a very attractive target for cell therapy, represent a significant challenge for cell-based strategies of repair owing to the complexity of the interactions between different types of cells and the required need for integration in the different CNS structures. During prenatal development in the mammalian CNS, the neural stem cells (NSCs) and their progenitors expand and produce functional neurons and glial cells that constitute the growing brain.[174] Unlike the more classical view sustaining the lack of regenerative capacity of the CNS, a number of studies during the last 15 years have clearly demonstrated that in the adult CNS of mammals, a small number of NSCs are also able to self-renew and generate different neural cell lineages including neurons, astrocytes, and oligodendrocytes under specific microenvironmental stimuli.[175] The subventricular zone of the lateral ventricles and the subgranular zone of the hippocampal dentate gyrus in the adult contain stem cell-like precursors capable of driving neurogenesis and gliogenesis.[176] These regions have been defined as highly specialized CNS germinal niches which contain slowly-proliferating putative CNS stem cells immunoreactive for glial fibrillary acidic protein (GFAP).[176]

The regulation of proliferation, maturation, and/or migration of adult NSCs is mediated by a large array of growth factors that include EGF, bFGF, SHH, Wnt/b-catenin, Notch 1 ligand jagged 1, platelet-derived growth factors (PDGFs), ciliary neutrophic factor, NGF, neuregulins, and BMPs, among others.[176–178] This knowledge has been used to develop several novel methods for in vitro expansion and differentiation of embryonic and adult NSCs. This information also constitutes the basis for new therapeutic strategies aimed to stimulate adult neurogenesis in vivo by supplying growth factors involved in neural development or in cell proliferation such as EGF, bFGF, or BDNF. This strategy may be used to restore the impaired functions in numerous damaged brain areas after ischemia, seizures, and traumas or in degenerative disorders.[179,180] For instance, it has been recently reported in a rat model of ischemic brain injury that the intraventricular infusion of recombinant bFGF and EGF recruited novel endogenous neuronal progenitors that contributed to a massive regeneration of hippocampal pyramidal neurons.[181] Observations such as these have led to speculation that delivery of NSCs or their progenitors in brain regions could represent an effective strategy for the treatment of neurologic diseases such as stroke and spinal cord injuries as well as neurodegenerative disorders, including Huntington disease, Parkinson disease, and Alzheimer disease.

Besides NSCs, other types of stem cells are endowed with the potential to differentiate into neurons and glia. One example is ESCs.[182–185] Transplantation of both ESCs and ESC-derived neural (neuronal or glial) progenitors[186] promotes CNS regeneration in preclinical models of stroke,[187] myelin deficiency,[188] acute spinal cord injury,[189] and Parkinson disease.[190] Terminal neural differentiation can also be seen with non-CNS-derived multipotent somatic stem cells, such as marrow stem cells,[191] mesenchymal stem cells,[192] placental cord blood stem cells,[65] skin stem cells,[193] and adipose tissue stem cells.[194] Most of these studies are based on the potential of nonneural stem cells to acquire certain "neural" markers in vitro after treatment with certain cytokines or factors that induced neural differentiation.[54] However, recent studies have started to address whether putative neural progeny from MSCs or other stem cells have functional characteristics consistent with neurons.[195] The evidence for in vivo differentiation and functional integration is even less conclusive as none of the published studies have demonstrated beyond reasonable doubt that nonneural cells contribute to neural regeneration.[196] For instance, MSCs themselves, and even more so when engineered to express neurotrophic factors, promote functional recovery and decrease the infarct size following middle artery occlusion.[197] Potential mechanisms responsible for the functional benefit have been described such as induced angiogenesis in models of stroke,[198,199] paracrine production of cytokines, or recruitment of endogenous stem cells.[200,201]

Parkinson Disease

The motor dysfunction that is associated with Parkinson disease results from the progressive loss of dopaminergic neurons in the substantia nigra pars compacta, a region of brain that controls muscle movement. Cell replacement therapy that delivers new dopaminergic neurons represents a promising strategy for the treatment of this neurodegenerative disease.[202] Clinical studies have focused on implanting fetal midbrain cells, which include those destined to become dopaminergic neurons, into the neostriatum. Yet despite promising studies in experimental models, such fetal cell grafts into adult patients with Parkinson disease have yielded poor results characterized by limited clinical efficacy and significant morbidity, the latter manifested as refractory, medication-independent dyskinesias.[203] Despite the lack of success with this approach, other sources of stem cells have been used at least in preclinical models of Parkinson disease. Mouse and human ESCs can be differentiated into functional midbrain dopaminergic neurons in vitro,[204] and when implanted in animal models of Parkinson disease (mice and primates) there is a functional and histological recovery of the nigrostriatal pathway.[185,205] However, the development of tumors as well as the immune suppression required in these transplants remains significant hurdles for clinical application in humans.

Spinal Cord Injuries

Spinal cord injuries have also been an attractive target for cell-based therapies. Because the major cause of neurologic disability in spinal cord injuries is oligodendrocyte death, leading to demyelization and axonal degeneration, rescuing the oligodendrocytes and preserving myelin should result in a significant improvement in the functional outcome after such injuries. Again the use of growth factors involved in proliferation and differentiation of oligodendrocytes, such as sonic hedgehog (Shh), bFGF, and PDGF, might result in the differentiation of endogenous NSCs into oligodendrocyte progenitor cells (OPCs) in vitro and/or in vivo. However, because spinal cord injury is associated with the loss of both neurons and glia, cell-based strategies for reconstituting the injured spinal cord must accommodate the need to replace multiple cell types.

The use of neural stem cell implants into the injured spinal cord is based on the possibility that regionally appropriate phenotypes can be generated in response to local cues. Unfortunately, this approach has provided limited success.[206] Recently, investigators have demonstrated some functional benefit from NSC transplant in animal models of spinal cord injury, likely associated with local neurogenesis and suggesting a trophic effect more than true regeneration.[207] Because the sensory tracts of the posterior columns are frequently affected in spinal cord injuries, transplantation of glial progenitors has been an especially appealing strategy for treating spinal cord injury.[208] Other sources of adult stem cells have been used in preclinical models, namely mesenchymal stem cells from the marrow[209,210] and glial cells from the olfactory bulb,[211] with promising results.

There is evidence that NSC can survive after transplantation, migrate, and maintain their multipotency; however, there are very limited data to support the concept that these cells give rise to terminally differentiated neural cells able to sustain a program of CNS repair through significant cell replacement and tissue integration.[212] Furthermore, recovery obtained by stem cell transplant does not correlate with absolute numbers of transplant-derived, newly generated, terminally differentiated neuronal cells. Several mechanisms other than classical engraftment and differentiation of the stem cell may contribute to whatever efficacy has been observed. These include the release of growth factors and neurotrophins that can stimulate endogenous stem cells or prevent further loss of neurons and glia by releasing survival factors, increasing angiogenesis, or reducing the inflammation that ensues after the acute insult.[213]

CONCLUSIONS

Intrinsic mitogenic signaling cascades that are activated in mammalian embryonic, fetal, and adult stem cells during the normal process of self-renewal and differentiation have been identified. These cellular events may also be implicated in the regenerating process after tissue injuries. These observations hold great promise that stem and progenitor cells will be feasible and useful for the therapy of diverse degenerative disorders. Further in vitro and in vivo investigations with embryonic, fetal, umbilical cord blood, and adult stem cells and their more differentiated progenitors are required to determine their physical characteristics, interactions with the microenvironment, and respective therapeutic roles in the repair and restoration of tissue and organ function.

SUGGESTED READINGS

Bonner-Weir S, Weir GC: New sources of pancreatic beta-cells. Nat Biotechnol 23:857, 2005.

Goldman S. Stem and progenitor cell-based therapy of the human central nervous system. Nat Biotechnol 23:862, 2005.

Ito M, Liu Y, Yang Z, et al: Stem cells in the hair follicle bulge contribute to wound repair but not to homeostasis of the epidermis. Nat Med 11:1351, 2005.

Keirstead HS, Nistor G, Bernal G, et al: Human embryonic stem cell-derived oligodendrocyte progenitor cell transplants remyelinate and restore locomotion after spinal cord injury. J Neurosci 25:4694, 2005.

Laflamme MA, Murry CE: Regenerating the heart. Nat Biotechnol 23:845, 2005.

Langston JW: The promise of stem cells in Parkinson disease. J Clin Invest 115:23, 2005.

Lerou PH, Daley GQ: Therapeutic potential of embryonic stem cells. Blood Rev 19:321, 2005.

MacLaren RE, Pearson RA, MacNeil A, et al: Retinal repair by transplantation of photoreceptor precursors. Nature 444:203, 2006.

Martin GR: Isolation of a pluripotent cell line from early mouse embryos cultured in medium conditioned by teratocarcinoma stem cells. Proc Natl Acad Sci U S A 78:7634, 1981.

Martino G, Pluchino S: The therapeutic potential of neural stem cells. Nat Rev Neurosci 7:395, 2006.

Nussbaum J, Minami E, Laflamme MA, et al: Transplantation of undifferentiated murine embryonic stem cells in the heart: teratoma formation and immune response. FASEB J 21: 1345, 2007.

Sampaolesi M, Blot S, D'Antona G, et al: Mesoangioblast stem cells ameliorate muscle function in dystrophic dogs. Nature 444:574, 2006.

Shi X, Garry DJ: Muscle stem cells in development, regeneration, and disease. Genes Dev 20:1692, 2006.

Thomson JA, Itskovitz-Eldor J, Shapiro SS, et al: Embryonic stem cell lines derived from human blastocysts. Science 282:1145, 1998.

Vassilopoulos G, Wang PR, Russell DW: Transplanted bone marrow regenerates liver by cell fusion. Nature 422:901, 2003.

Wagers AJ, Weissman IL: Plasticity of adult stem cells. Cell 116:639, 2004.

Weissman IL: Stem cells—scientific, medical, and political issues. N Engl J Med 346:1576, 2002.

REFERENCES

For complete list of references log onto www.expertconsult.com

CHAPTER 113

COMPLICATIONS AFTER HEMATOPOIETIC CELL TRANSPLANTATION

Navneet Majhail and Daniel Weisdorf

The high-dose therapy used in hematopoietic cell transplantation (HCT) results in toxicities induced directly by the treatment and secondarily by the prolonged immunodeficiency and extended recovery process. Recognition of risk factors for particular complications allows the design of risk-specific supportive care regimens that reduce the rates of morbidity and mortality accompanying transplantation. HCT-related complications can be broadly classified into infections, early noninfectious complications (within 3 months of HCT), late noninfectious complications (after 3 months of HCT), and graft-versus-host disease (GVHD) (Table 113–1).

INFECTIONS

Infections are among the foremost causes of nonrelapse mortality in HCT recipients and can cause significant morbidity, both in the early and late transplant periods (Table 113–2). Immune defects occurring in the posttransplant period can be divided into predictable phases based on time from engraftment (sustained absolute neutrophil count >500/μL), with characteristic infections in each phase (Fig. 113–1). Antimicrobial prophylaxis regimens tailored to address the risk of specific infections during these time periods are effective in decreasing the incidence of posttransplant opportunistic infections (Table 113–3).

Engraftment generally occurs within 7 to 14 days in autologous HCT recipients and 14 to 28 days in allogeneic HCT recipients. Unrelated donor transplant recipients tend to engraft later compared to sibling donors, and 5% to 10% of unrelated donor transplant recipients may fail to engraft, leading to prolonged neutropenia. The main risk factors for infection during the preengraftment phase are disruption of mucocutaneous barriers and indwelling venous catheters. Bacterial infections can occur in up to 30% of transplant recipients during the initial period and usually arise from normal flora of the skin (coagulase-negative *Staphylococcus*), oropharynx and gastrointestinal tract (*Streptococcus viridans*, *Enterococcus* spp. and enteric gram-negative bacilli).[1] Colonizing yeasts invade because of neutropenia and disruption of normal host flora and can lead to systemic mycotic infections in 10% to 15% of patients.[2] Reactivation of herpes viruses can occur in the absence of prophylaxis. Patients with prolonged neutropenia are at risk for developing infections due to *Aspergillus* spp. The Centers for Disease Control, the Infectious Disease Society of, America and the American Society of Blood and Marrow Transplantation have published a joint guideline for preventing infections in HCT recipients.[3]

The predominant defects seen in the early to late postengraftment period are impairments of cellular and humoral immune systems.[4] This state of underlying severe immune dysfunction is enhanced and prolonged by acute and chronic GVHD and by corticosteroids and immunosuppressants used for GVHD treatment.[5,6] The incidence of late opportunistic infections is much lower in autologous HCT recipients because of quicker immune reconstitution. Immune reconstitution can take up to 2 years to recover in allogeneic HCT recipients. Patients needing long-term immunosuppression for ongoing chronic GVHD are particularly at risk and are susceptible to infections by encapsulated bacteria (*Streptococcus pneumoniae*, *Neisseria meningitides*, and *Haemophilus influenzae*), fungi (*Aspergillus* spp., *Candida* spp., and *Pneumocystis jiroveci*), and viruses (cytomegalovirus [CMV] and varicella-zoster virus).[7] Additional factors that can prolong these immune deficiencies include donor–recipient human leukocyte antigen (HLA) disparity, graft manipulation with depletion of T cells, and use of unrelated donors and possibly umbilical cord blood as a graft source.[5,8,9] Antimicrobial prophylaxis should continue beyond the initial posttransplant period, typically at least 3 to 6 months after cessation of all immunosuppression, especially in patients being treated for chronic GVHD. Some centers use total T-cell ($CD3^+$) or CD4 cell levels as surrogate markers of T-cell immunity and to guide decisions regarding antimicrobial prophylaxis. Supplemental immunoglobulin administered intravenously has been considered for patients with persistent hypogammaglobulinemia (immunoglobulin [Ig]G levels <400 mg/dL), but its prophylactic use is costly, does not prevent late infections, and may impair humoral immune reconstitution.[10] Patients with GVHD and those with indwelling venous access undergoing dental procedures should receive antibiotics for endocarditis prophylaxis.[11] Published guidelines are available for immunization of HCT survivors.[3] Vaccinations should begin 12 months posttransplant, or later if the patient is receiving chronic immunosuppression (Table 113–4).

Following HCT using nonmyeloablative or reduced-intensity preparative regimens, early experience suggests a decreased incidence of bacterial infections, most likely due to shorter duration of posttransplant neutropenia.[12] However, risks of invasive aspergillosis[13,14] and CMV reactivation remain unchanged.[15] The incidence and pattern of infections seen after unrelated umbilical cord blood transplantation are similar to those seen with adult unrelated marrow or blood graft sources.[16,17]

The approach to managing posttransplant infections is generally similar to that for infections in patients with cancer, especially leukemia (see Chapter 91). However, certain infections, particularly those due to viruses and fungi, are unique to the HCT population and are discussed in further detail here.

Febrile Neutropenia

A large proportion of patients develop fever in the early posttransplantation period, although an infectious pathogen is identified in only 50% of patients. Fever also may be due to tissue inflammation (oropharyngeal or enteric mucositis), transfusions, amphotericin, or other drug fever. Bacterial infections due to aerobic bacteria, such as coagulase-negative staphylococci, *Viridans* streptococci, and enteric gram-negative bacilli, are the primary concern during this neutropenic phase, although risk of infections with yeasts is ongoing. Prophylactic strategies can include suppressive antimicrobials against both bacteria and yeasts. Although antibiotics for bacterial prophylaxis reduce rates of bacteremia, they have not reduced infection-related mortality.[18–20] Antifungal agents, including fluconazole, have been very effective in preventing systemic candidiasis, although resistant species (*Candida krusei* or *Candida tropicalis*) have emerged as secondary pathogens.[21,22] Newer antifungal agents with activity against molds (mold-specific azoles [voriconazole, posaconazole] and echinocandins [caspofungin, micafungin, anidulafungin]) are being investigated for antifungal prophylaxis. In addition to antimicrobial prophylaxis, a few centers keep patients in a pathogen-free environment using laminar flow isolation, gut sterilization, and special diets

Table 113–1 Major Complications of Hematopoietic Cell Transplantation

	Complication	Incidence
Infections	Bacterial infections	
	Gram-positive bacteremia	20%–30%
	Gram-negative bacteremia	5%–10%
	Viral infections	
	Cytomegalovirus	5%–40% in high risk patients[a]
	Herpes simplex virus	5%–10% in seropositive patients
	Varicella-zoster virus	10%–50% in seropositive patients
	Respiratory viruses	10%–20%
	Fungal infections	
	Candida	5%–10%
	Aspergillus and other molds	5%–15%
	Pneumocystis jiroveci	<1%
	Other infections	
	Toxoplasma gondii	2%–7% in seropositive patients
Early noninfectious complications (0–3 months)	Regimen-related toxicity	
	Mucositis	60%–75%
	Hemorrhagic cystitis	5%–10%
	Venoocclusive disease	5%–40%
	Pneumonitis	10%–20%
	Alveolar hemorrhage	5%–10%
	Graft failure	2%–10%
	Adverse drug reactions	Common
Late noninfectious complications (>3 months)	Organ-specific late effects	
	Cataracts	25%–40%
	Hypothyroidism	30%–50%
	Sterility/hypogonadism	50%–90%
	Growth disturbances	30%–50% in prepubertal children
	Osteoporosis/avascular necrosis	5%–20%
	Malignant relapse	Variable
	Second cancers	2%–12%
Graft-versus-host disease	Acute	20%–50% with related, 40%–90% with unrelated donors
	Chronic	20%–40% with related, 40%–70% with unrelated donors

[a]Cytomegalovirus (CMV)-seropositive hematopoietic cell transplantation recipients or CMV-seronegative recipients with a CMV-seropositive donor.

to reduce the risk of infections. These intensive isolation measures are both cumbersome and expensive and have not proven to be helpful in preventing early posttransplant mortality.

Empiric therapy with broad-spectrum antibiotics usually is started at fever onset along with appropriate clinical and microbiologic evaluation. Choice of antibiotics depends on prior and current antibiotic usage modified by local resistance patterns and can be based on recommendations available for treatment of febrile neutropenia in general cancer patients.[23] Invasive fungal infections are a common cause of persistent febrile neutropenia, that is, fever without an identified focus that continues despite 3 to 5 days of therapy with appropriate broad-spectrum antibiotics.[24] Initiating empiric antifungal therapy with amphotericin or more commonly a mold active agent such as voriconazole or caspofungin is generally recommended at this stage.[23] Repeated vigorous investigation to identify sources of infection, even for fever recurring after initial defervescence, is essential. Although administration of myeloid growth factors (granulocyte colony-stimulating factor [G-CSF] or granulocyte-macrophage colony-stimulating factor [GM-CSF]) reduces the duration of neutropenia and accelerates engraftment, they have not been demonstrated to reduce mortality from early posttransplant infections.[25]

Cytomegalovirus Infection

Epidemiology and Risk Factors

Despite the introduction of effective antiviral therapies, CMV infection continues to be a major cause of infection-related morbidity and mortality in HCT recipients. The risk of CMV reactivation spans both the early and late transplant periods, especially in patients with GVHD on prolonged immunosuppression. Although the incidence of early CMV disease has declined to 3% to 6% with use of antiviral drug therapy, late-onset CMV infection still is seen in up to 20% to 40% of patients.[26–29]

Seropositivity of the recipient is the most important risk factor for CMV infection in HCT recipients, and reactivation of latent virus is the most important mechanism resulting in CMV disease.[29–31] Nearly all CMV infections (<5%) in seronegative recipients are the result of exogenous exposure (primary CMV infection), either from a seropositive stem cell donor or from cellular blood products from CMV seropositive donors. Early CMV reactivation also may be observed in recipients with false-negative serology. CMV infection and especially end-organ disease are more frequent following allogeneic HCT, with CMV infections occurring in less than 5% of autograft recipients.[32,33] Among patients undergoing allogeneic transplantation, the risk may be greater with unrelated donors compared to related donors.[34] Although the prevalence of donor seropositivity is nearly zero in umbilical cord blood grafts, the risk of posttransplant CMV infection may be similar because recipient CMV status still is the predominant risk factor for infection[35] and CMV-naive umbilical cord blood graft confers no latent protective immunity against CMV. Other factors that delay immune reconstitution may increase the risk for CMV infection, including older recipient age, increasing donor–recipient HLA mismatch, acute or chronic GVHD, and need for prolonged immunosuppression, especially with high-dose corticosteroids.[26,32,36–38]

Table 113–2 Common Infections in Hematopoietic Cell Transplantation Recipients

Pathogen	Risk Period After HCT	Risk Factors	Common Clinical Syndromes	Treatment
Gram-positive cocci	1–4 weeks	Neutropenia Mucositis Central venous catheters Skin breakdown	Bacteremia	Antibiotics based on susceptibility testing
Enterobacteriaceae spp.	1–4 weeks	Neutropenia Skin breakdown GI mucosal breakdown	Bacteremia	Antibiotics based on susceptibility testing
Clostridium difficile	1–8 weeks	Antibiotics	Colitis	Metronidazole Oral vancomycin
Encapsulated bacteria[a]	>12 weeks	Chronic GVHD Chronic immunosuppression	Sinusitis Pneumonia	Antibiotics based on susceptibility testing
Candida spp.	1–4 weeks	Neutropenia Skin breakdown GI mucosal breakdown	Candidemia Mucocutaneous Hepatosplenic	Azoles Echinocandins Amphotericin
Aspergillus spp.	1–4 weeks >8 weeks	HLA disparity CMV infection Acute or chronic GVHD Chronic immunosuppression High-dose corticosteroids	Sinusitis Pulmonary nodules or infiltrates	Mold-specific azoles Echinocandins Amphotericin
Pneumocystis jiroveci	>4 weeks	Chronic GVHD Chronic immunosuppression	Pneumonia	Trimethoprim-sulfamethoxazole Dapsone Pentamidine
CMV	>4 weeks	Recipient or donor seropositivity HLA disparity Acute or chronic GVHD Chronic immunosuppression	Viremia Enteritis Interstitial pneumonitis	Ganciclovir Foscarnet Valganciclovir
Herpes simplex virus	1–4 weeks	Recipient seropositivity	Oropharyngeal Esophagitis	Acyclovir Valacyclovir Foscarnet
Varicella-zoster virus	>4 weeks	Recipient seropositivity History of chicken pox HLA disparity Acute or chronic GVHD Chronic immunosuppression	Cutaneous Interstitial pneumonitis Hepatitis	Acyclovir Valacyclovir Foscarnet
Epstein-Barr virus	>4 weeks	HLA disparity T-cell depletion	Viremia Posttransplant lymphoproliferative disorder	Rituximab Reduce immunosuppression Cytotoxic chemotherapy

[a]Includes *Streptococcus pneumoniae, Haemophilus influenzae, and Neisseria meningitides.*

CMV, cytomegalovirus; GI, gastrointestinal tract; GVHD, graft-versus-host disease; HCT, hematopoietic cell transplantation; HLA, human leukocyte antigen.

Clinical Presentation and Diagnosis

The most common manifestation of CMV infection is asymptomatic reactivation noted by screening antigenemia or DNA polymerase chain reaction (PCR) testing. CMV organ infection and disease are most often pneumonia and enteritis. CMV is the most common cause of interstitial pneumonitis and is responsible for up to 50% of cases.[39] Infection at other sites, such as retinitis, hepatitis, and central nervous system disease, are less common and usually are seen in late-onset CMV infection.[26] Indirect effects of CMV infection include increased risks of graft rejection and bacterial and fungal superinfection.[26,29] The presence of posttransplant CMV viremia is a strong predictor of subsequent clinical disease.[38,40,41] CMV pneumonia develops in 60% of patients with untreated asymptomatic viremia, and treatment of viremia can reduce the incidence of CMV pneumonia to less than 5%.[40,42–44] Although autologous HCT recipients have a lower risk of developing CMV infection, the severity of infection (e.g., pneumonia), if it develops, is similar to that observed in recipients of allogeneic transplantation.

The diagnosis of CMV can be made either by demonstration of characteristic cytopathic effects in tissue culture or by use of more sensitive molecular methods that detect viral protein or DNA. Commonly used molecular assays include CMV DNA detection methods and the pp65 antigenemia assay. Detection of the CMV pp65 antigen in leukocytes has been a commonly used method for CMV surveillance after HCT but is ineffective during early post-HCT leukopenia. However, direct detection of CMV DNA by either PCR or DNA hybrid capture assay is the most sensitive method for detecting CMV.[45–48] Plasma CMV DNA PCR, although not as sensitive as whole-blood PCR, can be a valuable tool for monitoring CMV during periods of neutropenia when CMV antigenemia testing is unreliable. Viral cultures of urine, saliva, blood, or bronchoalveolar lavage (BAL), using either rapid shell-vial or routine culture techniques, have limited clinical utility because they are less sensitive than antigen or DNA detection techniques and take much longer to report. Shell-vial cultures of CMV from BAL fluid are less specific for CMV pneumonia and can be positive in asymptomatic seropositive patients without pneumonia who are shedding CMV in oral or

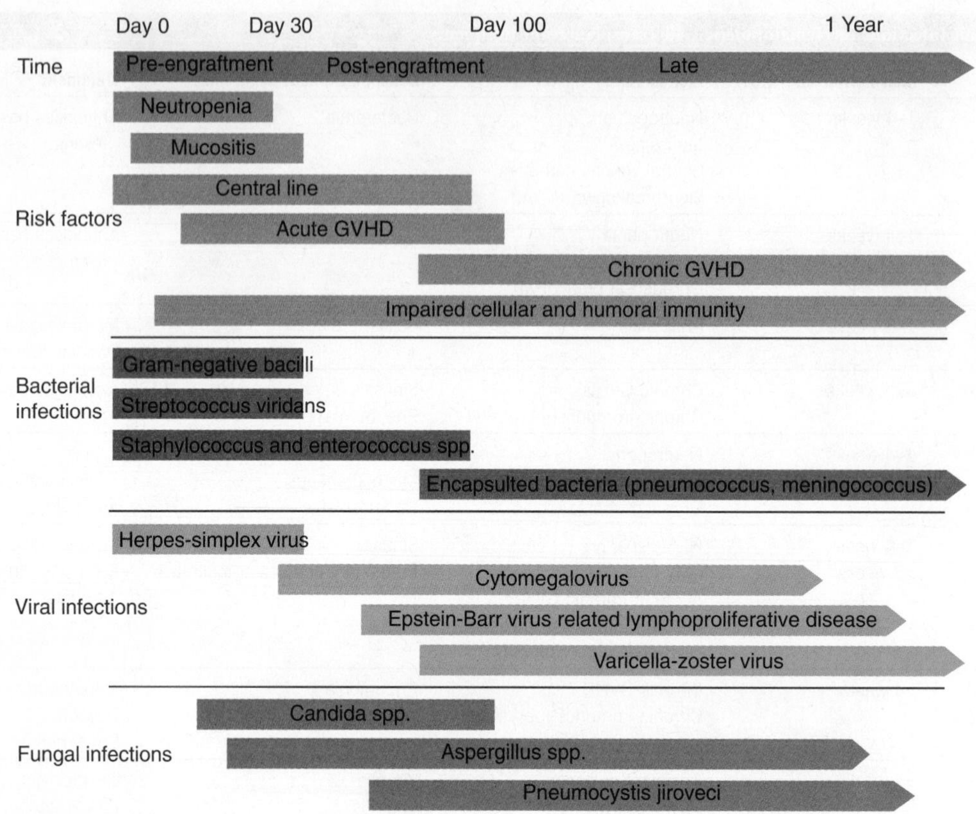

Figure 113–1 Common infections in hematopoietic cell transplantation recipients. GVHD, graft-versus-host disease.

Table 113–3 Recommended Antimicrobial Prophylaxis Against Common Infections

Pathogen	Preventing Early Disease (0–100 Days After HCT)	Preventing Late Disease (>100 Days After HCT)
Bacterial infections	No specific recommendations[a]	Antibiotics (based on local resistance patterns) to prevent infectious due to encapsulated bacteria (*Streptococcus pneumoniae, Haemophilus influenzae, N. meningitidis*) in patients on chronic immunosuppression
CMV	Prophylaxis or preemptive treatment with ganciclovir in high-risk patients[b]	Preemptive treatment with ganciclovir in high-risk patients[b]
HSV	Acyclovir in seropositive patients	Acyclovir in patients with recurrent HSV infections
Yeast infections	Fluconazole	Fluconazole in patients on chronic immunosuppression
Mold infections	No specific recommendations[c]	No specific recommendations[a]
Pneumocystis jiroveci	Trimethoprim-sulfamethoxazole (preferred) or dapsone or pentamidine	Trimethoprim-sulfamethoxazole (preferred) or dapsone or pentamidine in patients on chronic immunosuppression

[a]Limited data favor fluoroquinolones such as levofloxacin. No impact on infection-related mortality.
[b]CMV-seropositive HCT recipients or CMV-seronegative recipients with a CMV-seropositive donor.
[c]Limited data available. Prospective testing of voriconazole and posaconazole suggests possible benefit as prophylaxis. No impact on mold-related mortality.
CMV, cytomegalovirus; HCT, hematopoietic cell transplantation; HSV, herpes simplex virus.

respiratory secretions.[49] Despite this lack of specificity, even in asymptomatic people, finding CMV in BAL fluid is a strong predictor for the development of subsequent CMV pneumonia, and such patients should be treated.

Prevention and Treatment

For seronegative recipients, use of seronegative donors and blood products is the mainstay of prevention of CMV disease (see box on Approach to Prevention and Treatment of Cytomegalovirus Infection). Probably as effective as use of seronegative products, removal of white blood cells from transfused unscreened blood products by filtration is an alternative in the prevention of primary CMV infections.[50–52] For high-risk patients (seropositive recipients or seropositive donors of seronegative recipients), two general strategies can be used, both of which have been effective in reducing early CMV infection rates to less than 10%.[26,43,44,53–55] The first is the "preemptive" approach, which involves prompt treatment of early CMV viremia with ganciclovir or foscarnet before the infection leads to clinical

Table 113–4 Recommended Vaccinations for Hematopoietic Cell Transplantation Recipients

Vaccine or Toxoid	Time After Transplant[a]
Tetanus diphtheria acellular pertussis	12, 14, and 24 months
Haemophilus influenzae type b conjugate	12, 14, and 24 months
23-valent pneumococcal polysaccharide	12 and 24 months
Inactivated polio	12, 14, and 24 months
Hepatitis B[b]	12, 14, and 24 months
Influenza[c]	Lifelong, seasonal administration
Measles, mumps, and rubella[d]	24 months

[a]Vaccinations are deferred in patients with chronic graft-versus-host disease until discontinuation of immunosuppression.
[b]Recommended for all susceptible persons aged ≤18 years and for adults at high-risk for hepatitis B infection.
[c]Vaccination of household contacts may be valuable.
[d]Live attenuated vaccine not to be administered to patients with graft-versus-host disease or patients taking pharmacologic immune suppression.

disease. The second is the "general prophylaxis" approach, in which all at-risk patients are treated with ganciclovir irrespective of CMV viremia status. The former approach requires availability of reliable and rapid early diagnostic tests. The latter approach can reduce the rate of early CMV infection but does not reduce the incidence of mortality or the risk for late CMV infection and is associated with a higher incidence of ganciclovir-induced myelosuppression and secondary infections.[44,53,56] Both approaches require aggressive surveillance to allow prompt detection of infection. High-dose acyclovir or valacyclovir, although not as effective as ganciclovir, also reduces the incidence of CMV viremia, but continued surveillance for CMV still is required, with prompt initiation of preemptive therapy with ganciclovir or foscarnet in case viremia develops.[57–59] Unlike ganciclovir, which must be administered intravenously, its prodrug valganciclovir has excellent oral bioavailability and is being investigated for prophylaxis and preemptive therapy of CMV infection.[60–63] An additional role for preventing exogenous exposure in high-risk CMV seropositive patients through choosing seronegative donors or blood products is not proven. Because autologous HCT recipients have a lower risk of CMV disease, the preemptive approach to preventing CMV infection usually is sufficient. Surveillance for CMV is continued weekly until at least day 100 posttransplant for high-risk patients and longer for patients with chronic GVHD on high-dose immunosuppression.

CMV disease, especially pneumonia, must be diagnosed and treated promptly. If patients already are ventilator dependent when therapy for CMV pneumonia is instituted, the therapy almost always is ineffective, and mortality rate is nearly 100%.[32] The combined use of ganciclovir and immunoglobulin has been the most successful treatment of CMV pneumonia, with resolution in 50% to 75% of nonventilator-dependent patients.[32,64,65] Prolonged therapy (>2 months) with the combination of ganciclovir and immunoglobulin is indicated because shorter treatment regimens have been associated with recurrence of CMV pneumonia. Foscarnet can be effective in clinical settings where ganciclovir fails or is associated with excess toxicity, usually myelosuppression.[66] Although treatment is generally similar, with ganciclovir or foscarnet plus immunoglobulin, CMV enteritis, hepatitis, and retinitis are variably responsive.[26,67] The efficacy of valganciclovir for treatment of CMV organ disease is being investigated. Adoptive cellular therapy also is being explored as a treatment strategy.[68–70]

Approach to Prevention and Treatment of Cytomegalovirus Infection

Prevention

1. Seronegative Recipient with Seronegative Donor (Allogeneic and Autologous): Transfuse only cytomegalovirus (CMV)-safe blood products. Leukocyte depletion by filtration and blood from CMV-seronegative donors are clinically equivalent alternatives.
2. Seronegative Recipient with Seropositive Donor (Allogeneic): Deliver only CMV-safe blood products (seronegative or leukocyte depleted), but administer chemoprophylaxis as well to prevent reactivation of donor-derived endogenous virus.
3. Seropositive Recipient: Prophylaxis with acyclovir appears to be somewhat useful. Use of immunoglobulin may be beneficial. No proven role for seronegative blood products. Ganciclovir is highly effective when given prophylactically but is myelosuppressive. Patients who must interrupt the course of ganciclovir because of leukopenia are at risk for development of CMV pneumonia. Ganciclovir is the current best prophylaxis in high-risk patients but is not indicated for autologous recipients.
4. All patients require periodic (weekly) monitoring for CMV antigenemia or CMV DNA for 8 to 12 weeks posttransplantation. Longer-duration (beyond 12 weeks) surveillance is appropriate for allograft recipients, especially those with graft-versus-host disease.

Treatment

1. Asymptomatic Infections (Allogeneic and Autologous): Ganciclovir treatment of asymptomatic infection detected in blood or bronchioalveolar lavage (BAL), by either molecular detection or antigenic methods, is recommended to prevent development of CMV pneumonia. Intensive induction treatment (2 weeks) followed by a maintenance phase of 5–7 days/week therapy for an additional 4 to 8 weeks is necessary.
2. CMV Pneumonia: Ganciclovir in combination with immunoglobulin is recommended and should be instituted promptly. Once the disease has progressed to cause respiratory failure and ventilator dependence, survival is limited.

No Treatment

1. Empiric CMV therapy for interstitial pneumonitis is not indicated in seronegative recipients with seronegative graft and blood donors. Diagnostic evidence of CMV infection should be obtained.
2. Empiric CMV therapy for interstitial pneumonitis also is not indicated in patients whose BAL is negative for CMV by direct staining and molecular testing. However, BAL CMV studies have a small (<5%) false-negative rate, and close followup and monitoring are required.
3. Asymptomatic CMV viruria does not require therapy but does need close followup and serial blood viral testing for surveillance of systemic disease.

Fungal Infections

Invasive fungal infections are among the leading causes of mortality in HCT recipients. The vast majority of fungal infections in this setting are caused by yeasts (*Candida* spp.) or molds (*Aspergillus* spp.).

Candida infections

Candida albicans has been the leading cause of yeast infections in HCT recipients, but the current widespread use of azole prophylaxis in the early transplant period has led to the emergence of a variety of non-*albicans* species, such as *Candida tropicalis*, *Candida krusei*, and *Candida glabrata*, as important pathogens.[71] These yeasts are normal inhabitants of the skin and the oral and gastrointestinal mucosa. Breakdown of these mucosal surfaces due to radiation and chemotherapy, compounded by neutropenia in the preengraftment period, can greatly increase the risk of invasion and systemic infections. Presence of indwelling central venous catheters and alteration of normal surface flora due to antibiotics are additional risk factors for *Candida* infections.[2,72]

Clinical manifestations can range from localized mucocutaneous to disseminated deep-tissue infection. A high index of suspicion is needed for the diagnosis of *Candida* infections, especially in patients with persistent febrile neutropenia, because blood cultures usually are not very sensitive for isolation and identification of *Candida* spp. Oral and esophageal candidiasis frequently occur in the early posttransplant period and should be treated aggressively because they can serve as portals for subsequent systemic infection. Venous catheter infections can be difficult to eradicate with antifungal agents alone and require removal of the central line. Patients with candidemia are at risk for endovascular infections such as endocarditis and thrombophlebitis. Hepatosplenic candidiasis is the most common manifestation of disseminated candidiasis but is increasingly rare with widespread use of effective anticandida azoles and echinocandins. Specific signs or symptoms related to organ involvement may be absent, and the diagnosis frequently must be made by abdominal imaging using computed tomographic scan.

Prophylaxis with an azole, particularly fluconazole, is recommended in the preengraftment and early postengraftment periods and has been shown to be effective in reducing the incidence of invasive infections due to sensitive *Candida* spp from 30% to less than 10%.[21,22,73] Micafungin, itraconazole, voriconazole and posaconazole are other agents that have been shown to be effective for yeast prophylaxis in HCT recipients; they also have antimold activity.[74–77] Mucocutaneous infection can be treated with fluconazole. *Candida krusei* and *C. glabrata* are intrinsically resistant to fluconazole, and nonazole agents should be considered for their management. Patients with invasive disease should be treated with an echinocandin such as caspofungin or an amphotericin formulation, especially when infection occurs in the setting of ongoing fluconazole prophylaxis. The preferential hierarchy of the newer azoles and echinocandins for prophylaxis and therapy for yeast infections is not known and is under study.

Aspergillus Infections

Most mold infections in HCT recipients are due to *Aspergillus fumigatus*, *Aspergillus flavus*, and *Aspergillus niger*, which gain entry through breakdown of skin or mucosal surfaces or through the nasal passages and respiratory tract. *Aspergillus* infections can occur early after HCT (during the neutropenic phase) or later, especially complicating the immunosuppression associated with acute or chronic GVHD.[78,79] Risk factors for *Aspergillus* infections include allogeneic (more than autologous) HCT, prolonged neutropenia, and GVHD.[13,78–80] Transplantation for certain diseases, such as chronic granulomatous disease, aplastic anemia, and myelodysplastic syndrome, is associated with a higher than usual risk of aspergillosis. History of *Aspergillus* infection has been observed to be a risk factor for reactivation after HCT.[81]

Aspergillus occurring in the posttransplant setting can be difficult to diagnose premortem. Hence, a high index of suspicion and an aggressive approach are required to establish its diagnosis and initiate therapy. Because nasal passages and the tracheobronchial tree are the most common portals of entry for *Aspergillus* spp., these two sites are also the most common sites of infection. Sinusitis frequently is symptomatic, and more advanced disease can be associated with erosion and necrosis of surrounding structures. Pulmonary manifestations typically include nodular infiltrates, usually distributed along the lung periphery, with pleuritic pain or cough as an initial symptom. Frank consolidation or cavitary lesions can be seen in more advanced stages of pulmonary involvement. *Aspergillus* has angioinvasive properties and can present with hemoptysis or with intravascular dissemination of the skin or brain.

Blood cultures have very low sensitivity in detecting *Aspergillus*. Diagnosis must rely on demonstration of typical fungal morphology on culture or histopathology or on tests to detect fungal components or nucleic acids. Nasal and bronchial washings for *Aspergillus* may not be sensitive, and lung biopsy may be required to obtain a definitive diagnosis.[82] The galactomannan assay is an enzyme-linked immunosorbent assay that detects the *Aspergillus* cell wall glycoprotein. It has a high specificity but low sensitivity for diagnosing invasive aspergillosis and has not been validated in well-designed trials.[83–85] Molecular methods for diagnosis, including PCR for *Aspergillus* DNA, are undergoing development.[86]

Use of high-efficiency air filters has reduced the nosocomial acquisition of *Aspergillus*.[71] Pharmacologic measures for preventing aspergillosis include prophylactic low-dose amphotericin, inhaled amphotericin, and early empiric use of amphotericin, itraconazole, or voriconazole; however, the relative effectiveness of these approaches is not yet defined.[87–89] Newer antifungal agents, including micafungin and posaconazole, have demonstrated activity as mold prophylaxis, but this role requires confirmation in more clinical trials.[74,77] Agents with significant mold activity, including voriconazole and caspofungin, are available. These drugs have a more favorable side-effect profile compared to amphotericin formulations, and many experts consider voriconazole to be the drug of choice for treatment of *Aspergillus* infection in HCT recipients. Patients with disease that progresses with a single antimold drug might require combination therapy with two antimold agents. The role of adjunctive measures such as cytokine growth factors, immunoglobulin infusion, or granulocyte transfusion remains undefined.

EARLY NONINFECTIOUS COMPLICATIONS

High-dose chemotherapy and radiation regimens are used before transplantation for their antineoplastic and immunosuppressive effects. However, these treatments can damage host tissue, resulting in significant morbidity.[90] Early HCT-associated complications frequently can simulate infections or be compounded by concurrent infections. In addition, because epithelial tissue repair may be delayed by ongoing neutropenia and local microinvasive infection, delay in hematopoietic engraftment can exaggerate and prolong these toxicities.

Graft Failure

Failure to establish hematologic engraftment (primary graft failure) and loss of an established graft (late graft failure) are serious complications of both autologous and allogeneic HCT. Delayed or poor graft function can exaggerate and prolong the risks of infection and increase the risk of peritransplant mortality. Failure to engraft can occur if an insufficient number of hematopoietic progenitors is infused. Approximately 2×10^4 colony-forming cells from marrow per kilogram recipient weight are needed to establish autologous engraftment. This is accomplished by infusing approximately 1×10^8 autologous marrow mononuclear cells/kg. Most investigators recommend infusion of a minimum of at least 2×10^8 mononuclear cells/kg to ensure establishment of an allogeneic graft. Umbilical cord blood-derived hematopoietic grafts can engraft with a lower number of cells.[91] Stem cells and progenitors can be damaged by cryopreservation or by ex vivo purging, and additional cells are required if intensive purging, especially with alkylators, is performed.

Use of hematopoietic stem cells and progenitors harvested from the blood by apheresis rather than from the bone marrow has become widely prevalent for both autologous and allogeneic HCT. Autologous blood hematopoietic cell grafts are collected after mobilization of marrow-derived progenitors into the blood by cytokine (G-CSF or GM-CSF) therapy or during recovery from myelosuppressive chemotherapy, often in combination with growth factors.[92–95] Allogeneic grafts are mobilized from healthy donors using growth factors alone, nearly exclusively G-CSF. Progenitor content of blood or marrow grafts is assayed by quantitation of mononuclear cells expressing the hematopoietic progenitor-associated surface marker CD34.

Graft failure is uncommon if 2×10^6 $CD34^+$ cells/kg or more are collected, cryopreserved, and later infused as an autologous graft.[93,94] The minimum CD34 content for an allogeneic graft is less well defined, but more than 5×10^6 $CD34^+$ cells/kg is frequently cited as a target collection for a sibling donor allograft.[96–98] Mobilized peripheral blood-derived stem cells yield satisfactory and more rapid trilineage hematopoietic recovery than do grafts from marrow-derived cells.[98–101] Similar to marrow grafting, late graft failure is possible but unlikely (<5%) after transplantation using peripheral blood derived stem cells. Infusion of a sufficient graft cell dose (nucleated or $CD34^+$ cells) may be the most important controllable factor limiting the risk of graft failure.

Recipient myelofibrosis or splenomegaly can interfere with engraftment. Splenomegaly can delay hematologic recovery, presumably because both progenitors and mature blood cells are sequestered in the spleen.[102] The presence of moderate or severe myelofibrosis also delays engraftment, perhaps because of faulty homing of stem cells in the marrow microenvironment.[103,104]

Posttransplantation therapy can jeopardize engraftment. Graft failure or poor graft function with continuing pancytopenia has been associated with use of methotrexate, antithymocyte globulin (ATG), acyclovir, ganciclovir, trimethoprim-sulfamethoxazole (TMP-SMX), and mycophenolate mofetil (MMF). Posttransplant complications, such as CMV, human herpes virus-6 or fungal infections, acute and chronic GVHD, and, rarely, Epstein-Barr virus-associated posttransplant lymphoproliferative disorder, can compromise successful engraftment.

Allogeneic HCT, especially using unrelated or mismatched donors, poses unique engraftment problems. Transplants between siblings completely matched at HLA-A, HLA-B, and HLA-DR loci are rarely (1%–3%) associated with graft failure. However, the probability of graft failure in the related donor transplantation setting increases to almost 10% with greater degrees of donor-recipient HLA incompatibility.[105–108] The problem is frequent (5%–15%) in the unrelated donor setting, where primary or secondary graft failure may occur even after transplantation from donors well matched at the HLA-A, HLA-B, and HLA-DR loci.[107–110] In some cases, failure of unrelated donor stem cells to engraft may result from reactivity against other important histocompatibility determinants, including HLA-C.[111] Early failure of an allogeneic graft can be accompanied by emergence of cytotoxic T lymphocytes of host origin, presumably representing immune-mediated graft rejection.[112,113] T-lymphocyte depletion of donor marrow performed as GVHD prophylaxis can adversely affect engraftment, even from matched sibling donors.[106,114] Ex vivo marrow manipulation can deplete stem cells. T-cell depletion can render the graft immunoincompetent and functionally less capable of preventing graft rejection.

Compared to related or unrelated allografts, time to neutrophil recovery is significantly delayed in patients receiving umbilical cord blood grafts. Additionally, the overall incidence of graft failure is somewhat greater.[115–118] The most critical determinant of engraftment following umbilical cord blood transplantation is cell dose, and units with a total nucleated cell dose of at least 2×10^7 cells/kg have a greater probability of successful engraftment.[117–119] Because each umbilical cord blood unit has a limited number of hematopoietic progenitor cells, methods for overcoming this limitation of cell dose are being investigated. They include transplantation using multiple umbilical cord blood units, ex vivo expansion to increase the number of progenitor cells, and intra-bone marrow injection of the graft. Increasing overall cell dose with transplantation of two umbilical cord blood units has been shown to be feasible and lead to successful engraftment.[120,121]

Use of recombinant G-CSF or GM-CSF, which stimulate myelopoiesis, has improved the treatment of graft failure.[122] Improvement in myelopoiesis can be seen in 50% to 60% patients with poor graft function within 14 to 21 days after initiation of growth factor therapy. Myeloid growth factor therapy can increase peripheral blood leukocyte recovery but has no effect on platelet reconstitution. Recombinant human thrombopoietin has been tested in conjunction with myelosuppressive nontransplant chemotherapy and for stimulation of platelet recovery after HCT, but it is not available for clinical trials to confirm its efficacy.[123–125] Limited experience suggests the value of recombinant erythropoietin in reducing red blood cell transfusion needs.[126]

A second stem cell infusion can be useful if graft failure occurs. In the case of a failed autograft, infusion of previously harvested and frozen marrow or blood cells frequently reestablishes a graft. Procurement and storage of "backup" stem cells should be considered for autograft protocols in which a high rate of graft failure is anticipated. In the case of graft failure after related-donor transplantation, a second infusion of donor marrow or cytokine-stimulated peripheral blood stem cells may allow successful engraftment.[127] In some cases, reconditioning with reduced doses of cytotoxic agents or further immunosuppression with ATG, corticosteroids or cyclosporine is used to prepare the recipient for a second infusion.

Treatment of graft failure after unrelated donor transplantation poses special problems. Unrelated donors may not be available for a second marrow harvest or blood stem cell apheresis. In experimental settings where graft failure risks are high, storing autologous stem cells from patients undergoing unrelated donor transplantation is a prudent practice but is rarely done. The original donor is unavailable in recipients of unrelated umbilical cord blood grafts, and the only treatment option for graft failure in this setting is a second transplant using umbilical cord blood cells from a different donor or other unrelated donor allograft, or reinfusion of autologous backup cells.

Hepatic Venoocclusive Disease

Hepatic venoocclusive disease (VOD), also known as *sinusoidal obstruction syndrome*, is a serious liver disorder characterized by jaundice, ascites, fluid retention, and hepatomegaly. It complicates up to 5% to 50% of HCTs, with different incidences based on the stringency of definition of the clinical diagnosis.[128–131] The primary initiating event is thought to be portal hypertension due to obstruction of hepatic sinusoids and venules, which secondarily leads to damage to surrounding centrilobular hepatocytes.[132–134] Chemotherapy and total body irradiation (TBI) used in pretransplant conditioning regimens lead to sinusoidal endothelial injury, and subsequent deposition of fibronectin and factor VIII/von Willebrand factor at the site of damaged endothelium can lead to activation of the coagulation system and subsequent sinusoidal obstruction.[135] Such changes are often associated with depressed plasma protein C levels and other signs of procoagulant activity, including lower antithrombin III levels and elevated factor VIII and fibrinogen levels.[136–140] Cytokines such as tumor necrosis factor (TNF)-α and alterations in the levels of nitric oxide and matrix metalloproteinases may also have a role in its pathogenesis.[141–144]

Risk factors associated with the development of VOD include history of pretransplant hepatitis or liver injury, intensive preparative regimens, increased TBI dose and dose rate, and increased busulfan dose.[128–131,134,145–148] VOD may be more frequent after mismatched related or unrelated donor transplantation.[129–131] Prior therapy with gemtuzumab ozogamicin increases the risk of posttransplant VOD.[149]

Signs of VOD usually occur within 1 month after hematopoietic graft infusion but may be recognized much sooner, even during administration of the preparative regimen. Clinical evidence of VOD includes hyperbilirubinemia, hepatomegaly, ascites, and weight gain.[128,130,134] More advanced stages can be associated with encephalopathy and renal, pulmonary, and multiorgan failure. Establishing a definite diagnosis of VOD is difficult because the diagnosis is primarily based on clinical criteria. Most investigators require the presence of jaundice, with either hepatomegaly, weight gain, and/or ascites within 2 to 3 weeks of stem cell infusion.[128,150] However, other causes of hyperbilirubinemia and weight gain early after transplantation (e.g., drugs, hepatitis, capillary leak, cardiac failure, and salt and colloid overloading) can complicate the differential diagnosis. Percutaneous or transabdominal needle biopsy of the liver is hazardous in severely thrombocytopenic transplant recipients and should be avoided. Transvenous biopsies may provide sufficient histologic material for diagnosis and may allow determination of hepatic wedge pressure product (>10 mm is associated with VOD) but may be associated with hemorrhagic complications.[151] Ultrasonographic Doppler flow studies demonstrating reversal of portal flow or a higher portal vein resistive index have been suggested as a noninvasive means of confirming the diagnosis, but their validity has been questioned.[152–154] VOD can be graded from mild to severe depending on the degree of hyperbilirubinemia and weight gain. Severe VOD is almost universally fatal within several weeks of onset.[130,155]

Effective methods for prevention and treatment of VOD have not been defined. Limited understanding of the cellular and microvascular pathophysiology of VOD has confounded development of more rational approaches to its prevention and treatment. Possible approaches include preventive therapy with low-dose heparin,[156–158] prostaglandin E,[159] pentoxifylline (a TNF-α blocking agent),[160,161] or ursodiol,[162,163] although none has proved effective in carefully performed prospective trials. Recombinant tissue plasminogen factor has been used successfully to treat established VOD; however, thrombolytics are associated with substantially increased risk of hemorrhage.[164–167] Transjugular portosystemic shunts have been used with some success.[168,169] Early experience with defibrotide, a single-stranded polyribonucleotide with fibrinolytic, antithrombotic, and antiischemic properties, has been favorable; 30% to 40% of patients with severe VOD have achieved complete resolution and improvement in survival.[170–173] Its efficacy in the prophylaxis and management of severe VOD is being investigated in larger clinical trials.

Interstitial Pneumonitis

Interstitial pneumonitis is a common and frequently fatal complication, affecting up to 35% of allogeneic transplant recipients, although advances in supportive care have led to substantial reductions in this risk.[174,175] Interstitial pneumonitis is notably less common after autografting.[176] It is characterized by diffuse, nonbacterial interstitial inflammation accompanied by hypoxemia, dyspnea, and nonproductive cough, sometimes with fever. Risk factors associated with development of interstitial pneumonitis include use of methotrexate for GVHD prophylaxis, older age at transplant, severe GVHD, interval from diagnosis of hematologic disease to HCT of 6 months or greater, poor pretransplant performance status, and use of higher TBI dose rate (>4 cGy/min).[174,175] Remarkably, one study reported the risk of interstitial pneumonitis was 8% when none of these risk factors was present, compared to 94% when all six factors were present.[174] It has been hypothesized that unrelated donor transplantation is more immunosuppressive and thus associated with more severe opportunistic infections and greater risk of interstitial pneumonitis, but this has not been rigorously investigated.

The course of interstitial pneumonitis often is catastrophic, manifesting as rapidly progressive tachypnea, hypoxemia, and hemodynamic compromise. Therefore, therapeutic intervention most frequently occurs before the return of definitive results of diagnostic tests and must be initiated based on the assessment of clinical risk factors and the underlying clinical setting (see box on Approach to Interstitial Pneumonitis).

Infectious Causes of Interstitial Pneumonitis

Infections are the most common cause of interstitial pneumonitis in HCT recipients. CMV and *Aspergillus* are the most common infections associated with interstitial pneumonitis (see CMV Infections, Fungal Infections). Other important but relatively uncommon infections to consider are *Pneumocystis jiroveci*, respiratory syncytial virus (RSV), and similar respiratory viruses.

Pneumonitis caused by *Pneumocystis* has a typical bilateral distribution, with a "butterfly" pattern on chest radiograph and prominent hypoxemia.[177] The previously reported 5% to 15% risk of *Pneumocystis* pneumonia has been largely eliminated by routine use of prophylaxis with TMP-SMX (first choice), dapsone, or inhaled pentamidine.[178,179] Prophylaxis with TMP-SMX virtually eliminates *Pneumocystis* pneumonia from the differential diagnosis, but only if patient compliance with therapy is certain. Diagnosis requires cytologic evaluation of silver-stained preparations of BAL cells or sputum, although transbronchial lung biopsy may slightly increase the diagnostic yield of a bronchoscopic examination. *Pneumocystis* pneumonia is effectively treated with TMP-SMX or parenteral pentamidine. Prophylaxis against *Pneumocystis* pneumonia should be continued through the period of immunosuppression (6 months to 1 year post-transplantation) and for the duration of any therapy for chronic GVHD.

RSV is a potentially fatal cause of interstitial pneumonitis and typically occurs in the fall and winter months.[180] RSV should be suspected if the patient presents a history of rhinorrhea and if RSV has been frequently recognized in the community or in the hospital. Diagnosis can be made by rapid antigen testing on nasal washings or BAL specimens. Because of the possibility of horizontal transmission, patients with RSV should be isolated. Inhaled ribavirin is used for treatment of RSV-associated pneumonia.[181] Other community-acquired viruses, such as parainfluenza or influenza, also can cause interstitial pneumonitis in the transplant recipient. Their presentation is clinically indistinguishable from RSV, although parainfluenza pneumonitis is not seasonal and is seen year round. Yearly influenza vaccination for HCT recipients and especially their household contacts may be effective in reducing risks of this infection.

Noninfectious Causes of Interstitial Pneumonitis

Idiopathic Interstitial Pneumonitis

Idiopathic interstitial pneumonitis is a diagnosis of exclusion based on typical findings and by ruling out infectious causes. Its timing is somewhat earlier than other causes of interstitial pneumonitis, typically occurring within the first 2 to 7 weeks after HCT.[39,182] Recognized risk factors for idiopathic interstitial pneumonitis include older age at transplant, extensive pretransplant chemotherapy, high-dose cyclophosphamide, TBI (higher total dose and dose rate), blood transfusions, administration of methotrexate, and GVHD.[183–186]

The observation that idiopathic interstitial pneumonitis is as frequent among syngeneic as among allogeneic recipients and has an equally high incidence in T-cell–depleted grafts suggests that immunosuppression is less of a risk factor for idiopathic interstitial pneumonitis than it is for infectious interstitial pneumonitis.[187,188] Clinical observations support a toxic cause for idiopathic interstitial pneumonitis. Radiation-induced lung damage appears to be the major contributor, especially use of high-dose TBI.[189,190] Effective therapy has not been established, although high-dose corticosteroids are often administered. Inflammatory cytokines, including interleukin (IL)-1 and TNF-α, have been implicated in lung injury.[191,192] The TNF-α binding protein etanercept has been reported to improve lung function in patients with idiopathic interstitial pneumonitis and is undergoing evaluation in clinical trials.[193]

Approach to Interstitial Pneumonitis

The presentation of interstitial pneumonitis after hematopoietic cell transplantation (HCT) should be considered an urgent medical situation. Empiric broad-spectrum therapy must be initiated early. The choice of therapy is influenced by the following factors:

1. Timing: Within the first 3 weeks after HCT, interstitial pneumonitis is more likely to be idiopathic (including diffuse alveolar hemorrhage) or fungal than due to cytomegalovirus (CMV) infection. Beyond 6 weeks, idiopathic pneumonitis is unusual, and the cause more likely is infectious. *Pneumocystis jiroveci* pneumonia is rare beyond 1 year after transplantation, except in patients with ongoing chronic graft-versus-host disease. Respiratory syncytial virus (RSV) infections are seasonal (fall and winter), and community outbreaks can be prevalent. Influenza also is seasonal, whereas parainfluenza can occur year round.
2. CMV Serology and Prophylaxis: If a seronegative recipient has received a seronegative graft and noninfective (seronegative or leukocyte-depleted) blood, CMV pneumonia is unusual. Seropositive recipients are at higher risk, although the risk is markedly reduced with ganciclovir prophylaxis. Other prophylactic regimens for CMV, such as acyclovir or intravenous immunoglobulin, still are associated with significant risk for serious CMV infection in the seropositive recipient. Serial negative testing for CMV antigenemia or DNA polymerase chain reaction (PCR) makes CMV pneumonitis less likely.
3. Prolonged Neutropenia: This factor is associated with infectious causes, particularly with fungal pneumonias.
4. Type of Transplant: Diffuse alveolar hemorrhage is seen less frequently in patients undergoing autologous HCT. CMV pneumonia is unusual (2%–3%) in autologous recipients but has a high case fatality rate. All infectious causes are more common after allogeneic hematopoietic cell transplantation. More intensive conditioning regimens (e.g., higher total body irradiation, carmustine) are associated with more frequent pneumonitis.
5. Compliance and Prophylaxis: A thorough assessment of what prophylaxis the patient has actually been receiving (e.g., trimethoprim-sulfamethoxazole, penicillin, CMV prophylaxis, transfusions outside the transplant center) is critical for risk assessment.
6. Chest Radiograph: The pattern and distribution of the infiltrate may narrow the differential diagnosis. Cardiac enlargement or pleural effusions may suggest pulmonary edema. A chest computed tomographic scan is useful, especially if nodularity, pleural involvement, or cavitary lesions (possibly fungal) are suspected.
7. Epidemiology: Identification of the causes of other recent cases can be most helpful with infections that are horizontally transmitted (e.g., RSV) or have common environmental risk factors (e.g., *Aspergillus* infection associated with construction).
8. Bronchoalveolar Lavage: This can be extremely useful to establish a specific diagnosis or to exclude others. CMV rarely causes pneumonia without positive bronchoalveolar lavage (BAL) findings (either direct staining of CMV-associated antigens in BAL cells or DNA PCR). BAL also usually detects RSV, *Pneumocystis jiroveci*, and other respiratory viruses, although not as rapidly, but is required to identify alveolar bleeding. It is less sensitive for diagnosis of fungal pneumonias.
9. Lung Biopsy: This is the gold standard for definitive diagnosis of most possible causes of interstitial pneumonitis, but it often can be avoided by use of the clinical diagnostic measures listed. It may be necessary for definitive diagnosis of fungal pneumonias, pulmonary changes associated with chronic graft-versus-host disease (bronchiolitis obliterans), or idiopathic interstitial pneumonitis.
10. Ventilator Therapy: Progressive respiratory failure after HCT rarely is reversible, especially in adults. Although aggressive diagnostic and therapeutic measures are essential, some centers offer patients and their families the option of foregoing mechanical ventilatory support, if survival is not expected. Preliminary discussion of this possible complication in pretransplant patient counseling can facilitate decision making if respiratory failure does occur.

Diffuse Alveolar Hemorrhage

Alveolar hemorrhage is a clinical syndrome of acute onset of pulmonary infiltrates and hypoxemia with a progressively bloodier BAL on bronchoscopy.[194] Alveolar hemorrhage due to noninfectious causes has been called *diffuse alveolar hemorrhage* but often is difficult to distinguish from infection-associated pulmonary hemorrhage, especially in the early posttransplant period.[195] The reported incidence of diffuse alveolar hemorrhage ranges from 2% to 5% in autologous and 5% to 10% in allogeneic HCT recipients.[194–198] Its pathogenesis is not known but it most likely develops as result of a complex interaction of a variety of factors, including alveolar injury from radiation and chemotherapy, inflammatory damage due to neutrophils and cytokines, and underlying infections. Older age at transplant, use of allogeneic donor source, and GVHD are risk factors for the syndrome.[195,197] The risk is similar with nonmyeloablative and myeloablative conditioning regimens.[196] Onset typically occurs within the first 3 months of transplantation with dyspnea, hypoxia and cough, although late-onset alveolar hemorrhage is not uncommon. Hemoptysis usually is absent, and bronchoscopy with BAL is required to confirm the diagnosis and to exclude infectious etiologies. The syndrome is very serious, and the majority of patients develop severe respiratory failure with mortality rates of more than 70%.[195,198] Hemorrhage occurring in the periengraftment period is associated with a better outcome compared to later-onset hemorrhage. Treatment includes correction of any coagulopathy and aggressive ventilatory support. High-dose corticosteroids have been used for its management, but their efficacy has not been clearly proven.[194,195,198] Small case series have reported successful use of recombinant factor VIIa and aminocaproic acid, but their efficacy requires confirmation in clinical trials.[199–201] Cytokine antagonists (e.g., anti–TNF-α) might have a therapeutic role, but this has not yet been investigated.

LATE NONINFECTIOUS COMPLICATIONS

Improvements in transplantation techniques and supportive care have led to an increasing number of long-term HCT survivors. These survivors remain at risk for late transplant-associated complications, which include organ specific dysfunction, second cancers, infections due to ongoing immunodeficiency, and functional impairments and changes in quality of life (Table 113–5).[202–207] Guidelines for screening and prevention of late effects in HCT survivors have been published.[11] In addition, following general population guidelines for screening and prevention of cancers and chronic diseases and promoting a generally healthy lifestyle are recommended for all HCT survivors.

Organ-Specific Late Effects

A variety of exposures, both before and during transplantation, can lead to organ-specific late toxicity. In general, transplant-related risk

Table 113–5. Selected Late Complications of Hematopoietic Cell Transplantation

Complication	Risk Factors	Monitoring and Prevention
Endocrine		
Hypothyroidism	TBI/radiation	Periodic assessment of
Hypogonadism	Chronic GVHD	thyroid and gonadal
Growth retardation	Chemotherapy	function
Ocular		
Cataracts	TBI/radiation	Periodic ophthalmic
Keratoconjunctivitis sicca	Corticosteroids	examination
	Chronic GVHD	
Oral		
Dental caries	TBI/radiation	Periodic dental
Dry mouth	Chronic GVHD	assessment
Cardiovascular		
Coronary artery disease	TBI/radiation	Periodic clinical
Cerebrovascular disease	Chemotherapy	evaluation
		Modification of risk factors
Respiratory		
Bronchiolitis obliterans	TBI/radiation	Periodic clinical
Interstitial pneumonitis	Chronic GVHD	evaluation
	Infections	Smoking cessation
Hepatic		
Cirrhosis	Hepatitis B or C	Periodic hepatic
Iron overload	Transfusions	function tests
		Serum ferritin level
Renal		
Nephropathy	TBI/radiation	Periodic serum creatinine and
	Chemotherapy	urinalysis
	Cyclosporine	Control hypertension
Skeletal		
Osteoporosis	TBI/radiation	Periodic bone
Avascular necrosis	Corticosteroids	densitometry
Second cancers	TBI/radiation	Periodic cancer
	Chemotherapy	screening
	Chronic GVHD	

GVHD, graft-versus-host disease; TBI, total body irradiation.

factors for delayed complications include use of TBI in conditioning, GVHD, and protracted use of corticosteroids or calcineurin inhibitors.[205,208] Although any organ system can be involved, certain organs have a greater predilection for late-onset problems post-HCT. Cataracts develop in more than one third of patients by 5 years posttransplantation and often require surgical therapy.[209] Hypothyroidism can be seen in up to 50% and hypogonadism in up to 90% of HCT survivors.[210–212] The majority of HCT survivors become permanently sterile, although HCT without TBI can spare fertility in nearly one third of men and women.[211,213] Prepubertal children may retain fertility, although secondary sexual development may be delayed. Up to 50% of children undergoing HCT develop growth retardation.[214] Musculoskeletal complications including osteoporosis and avascular necrosis can be particularly debilitating. An increased incidence of cardiovascular events and diabetes has been reported.[206,215] The risk for most organ-specific late complications continues to increase with time, and continued surveillance for these problems is indicated in all HCT survivors. Education of both patients and their primary care providers may be most effective in establishing this surveillance.

Second Cancers

Compared to the general population, HCT survivors have a fourfold to 13-fold higher risk for developing secondary leukemias, lymphoproliferative disorders, and solid tumors.[207,216–229] Secondary leukemias and myelodysplastic syndrome are limited to recipients of autologous HCT, typically have a short latent period, and occur relatively early, with a peak incidence between 2 to 5 years posttransplant. Older age at HCT, exposure to alkylating agents or topoisomerase II inhibitors pretransplant, and use of TBI in conditioning have been associated with increased risk for this complication.[216,228,230–235] Posttransplant lymphoproliferative disorder and secondary lymphomas tend to develop in the early posttransplant period, with a peak incidence in the first 1 to 2 years. Specific risk factors for posttransplant lymphoproliferative disorder include use of HLA-mismatched donor, chronic GVHD, and T-cell depletion, either in vitro or in vivo with ATG.[218,222,236] In contrast to secondary leukemias and posttransplant lymphoproliferative disorder, solid cancers have a longer latency period, and their incidence continues to increase over time post-HCT. Factors that increase the risk for secondary solid tumors are young age at HCT, use of TBI in conditioning, and chronic GVHD.[217,222,223,225,229]

Quality of Life After Transplantation

Despite the early morbidity associated with HCT, the majority of transplant survivors attain high levels of physical and psychological quality of life and return to full-time employment by 3 to 5 years posttransplant.[205,237–244] However, up to 20% of long-term survivors continue to have functional impairments years after HCT. The major risk factors for poor quality of life are older age and advanced disease at transplantation, chronic GVHD, and presence of medical late effects.[238,239,241,245] Although chronic GVHD is a strong predictor of poor quality of life, the patient's overall health and functional status improves with resolution of GVHD and eventually reaches a level comparable to that seen in patients with no history of chronic GVHD.[245,246] Gender-specific differences in quality of life have been observed, with females more likely to report impairments in psychological and sexual domains.[238,247] Cognitive deficits, particularly involving executive function, memory, and motor skills, have been reported in 30% to 60% of HCT survivors.[248–252] The risk of developing these neuropsychological sequelae is increased in patients receiving transplantation at an older age, use of TBI-based conditioning regimens, and cyclosporine.

GRAFT-VERSUS-HOST DISEASE

GVHD is a clinicopathologic syndrome of T-cell–mediated alloreactivity that commonly occurs as a complication of allogeneic HCT and leads to significant morbidity and mortality. It usually is classified as *acute* GVHD (within 3 months of HCT) or *chronic* GVHD (after 3 months of HCT), but considerable overlap can exist between acute and chronic GVHD. There has been increasing emphasis on use of clinical manifestations to distinguish acute and chronic GVHD.[253]

Current understanding of the pathogenesis of GVHD suggests that alloreactive donor T lymphocytes recognize histocompatibility antigens on host cells and initiate secondary inflammatory injury, leading to the clinical symptoms of GVHD.[254,255] The alloreactive response can be initiated or accelerated by conditioning regimen-induced tissue injury with release of proinflammatory cytokines, primarily IL-1 and TNF-α.[256–259] GVHD is more frequent and more severe in recipients of partially matched or histoincompatible transplants, suggesting that major histocompatibility complex encoded molecules are the prime antigenic targets initiating the alloreactive T-cell response.[108,110,260] Minor histocompatibility antigens also play an important role in its pathogenesis, especially in HLA-identical sibling donor grafts.[261] Activated donor-derived T cells produce IL-2 and interferon-γ, expand and differentiate into effector cells, and recruit mononuclear phagocytes and neutrophils, ultimately leading to host tissue destruction.[254,255,258,262–264] T-cell depletion of the graft reduces the risk of acute and chronic GVHD, albeit at the cost of increasing risks of disease relapse due to blunting of the graft-versus-tumor response.[265,266] Alternative mechanisms possibly involved in the pathogenesis of chronic GVHD include autoreactivity, loss of self-tolerance, and B-cell dysregulation.[254,267,268]

Acute Graft-Versus-Host Disease

Risk Factors and Clinical Features

Up to 50% of patients receiving HLA-identical sibling donor HCT and up to 90% of patients receiving unrelated donor HCT develop acute GVHD.[108,110,260,269] Donor–recipient HLA disparity is the most important risk factor for acute GVHD.[108,270] Additional risk factors include increasing recipient and donor age,[260,269,271,272] use of alloimmunized donors such as parous women,[271,272] and HCT from unrelated instead of sibling donors.[108,271] Use of peripheral blood stem cells instead of bone marrow as the graft source may be a particular risk for chronic GHVD.[273,274] Skin, liver, and gastrointestinal tract are the most common sites of GVHD. Acute GVHD of the skin is characterized by a maculopapular rash that, when severe, can lead to bullae or even resemble toxic epidermal necrolysis. Hepatic involvement manifests as cholestatic hepatitis with marked elevation of serum bilirubin and alkaline phosphatase but usually only mild transaminase alterations. Hepatocellular function (e.g., protein synthesis and coagulation factor production) is not impaired. In the intestine, upper gastrointestinal tract GVHD can produce nausea, vomiting, and anorexia, whereas small bowel and colon GVHD produces large-volume secretory diarrhea. The diagnosis is established by the clinical symptomatology but frequently requires histologic confirmation to distinguish it from other frequent toxicities in the early posttransplantation period (e.g., hypersensitivity drug rash, drug-induced cholestasis, infectious enteritis). The histologic hallmark of acute GVHD is apoptosis of the proliferative and regenerative cell layer of the epidermis or intestinal or biliary epithelium. This manifests as basal epidermal cell vacuolization with dyskeratosis, exocytosis, and, when more advanced, dermal–epidermal clefting with bullae formation. Similarly, the basal cells of the intestinal glands or the colonic crypts show single epithelial cell degeneration, satellite cell necrosis, and sometime crypt abscesses progressing to mucosal sloughing. In hepatic portal tracts, single cells of the bile ducts are affected first, with eventual disruption or disappearance of the bile ducts.

Acute GVHD is graded according to organs involved (skin, liver, gastrointestinal tract) and the extent of each organ involvement.[275,276] Mild to moderate (grade I or II) GVHD is characterized by limited organ involvement and carries an excellent prognosis. Severe (grade III or IV) GVHD has extensive multiorgan involvement with significant morbidity and poor survival, commonly progresses to chronic GVHD, and is associated with an increased risk of secondary opportunistic infections.[277,278]

Prophylaxis of Graft-Versus-Host Disease

The most effective techniques for GVHD prevention have involved ex vivo depletion of donor T lymphocytes, most often coupling immunologic recognition (monoclonal anti–T-cell antibodies) with depletion techniques (immunomagnetic beads, complement cytotoxicity, or toxin immunoconjugates). Although vigorous T-cell depletion prevents acute GVHD, it also increases the risk of graft failure and neoplastic relapse after transplantation.[265]

Pharmacologic immunosuppression administered in the first several months after transplantation can prevent or blunt the initiating T-cell recognition and proliferative response that triggers GVHD and can allow development of immune system tolerance and complete lymphohematopoietic chimerism. Methotrexate, corticosteroids, ATG, cyclosporine, tacrolimus, MMF, and sirolimus have been used for prophylaxis of GVHD and have successfully reduced both the frequency and severity of clinical GVHD.[269,277,279–286] Despite the potential role of inflammatory cytokines in the initiation and amplification of GVHD, clinical blockade of IL-1, IL-2, or TNF-α has not been effective in GVHD prophylaxis.[287–289]

Treatment of Acute Graft-Versus-Host Disease

Therapy for acute GVHD requires immunosuppression to blunt T-cell–induced tissue injury and appropriate supportive care. Therapy should be intensified to achieve a complete response to GVHD therapy because effective treatment of acute GVHD can both protect against chronic GVHD and improve survival. Corticosteroids are the mainstay of initial therapy for acute GVHD.[277,290,291] GVHD involving limited areas of the skin can be treated with topical corticosteroids alone. Oral beclomethasone can be used to treat early-stage GVHD of the gastrointestinal tract.[292] Regimens using a tapering schedule of corticosteroids starting with methylprednisolone 1 to 2 mg/kg/day are used for more advanced GVHD with systemic or multiorgan involvement. Approximately 30% to 50% of patients will achieve a response to therapy with corticosteroids.[293–295] Patients with lesser severity and single-organ involvement tend to be more responsive to therapy, although some reports suggest that GVHD following unrelated donor HCT is more resistant to therapy.[277,290,296] Alternative treatment regimens include cyclosporine or ATG alone or in combination with corticosteroids; however, no regimens have shown a consistent increase in response rates or improvement in survival compared to corticosteroids alone.[293,297,298] Newer immunosuppressive agents under clinical investigation as initial therapy in addition to corticosteroids include MMF, pentostatin, the TNF-α receptor blocker etanercept, and the IL-2 receptor inhibitor denileukin diftitox.[280,299]

Prognosis is serious for patients with steroid-resistant disease, which is GVHD that does not respond to initial therapy with corticosteroids. From 10% to 40% of patients will respond to salvage therapy with ATG or other drugs such as sirolimus, tacrolimus, MMF, pentostatin, or cyclosporine, either as a single agent or in combination.[300–303] Monoclonal antibodies and immunotoxins directed against T cells or inflammatory cytokines have been investigated, although their effectiveness has not been demonstrated outside of small case series. Specific agents with reported activity in steroid-refractory acute GVHD include pentostatin,[304] etanercept and infliximab (TNF-α receptor blockers),[305–307] daclizumab and denileukin diftitox (IL-2 receptor inhibitors),[308–310] and visilizumab (anti-CD3 antibody).[311] Extracorporeal photochemotherapy has been reported to have some efficacy in cutaneous and hepatic steroid-refractory acute GVHD.[312]

In addition to effective immunosuppression, successful management of acute GVHD involves attention to supportive care. Infections are a leading cause of death in patients with GVHD. Infection surveillance and prophylaxis directed against fungi, encapsulated bacteria, CMV, and PCP are essential components of GVHD therapy. Hyperalimentation is frequently needed for patients with advanced GVHD, especially in those with involvement of the gastrointestinal tract.

Chronic Graft-Versus-Host Disease

Risk Factors and Clinical Features

Chronic GVHD is a complex syndrome in recipients of allogeneic HCT. It typically occurs between 3 to 7 months posttransplant, but it can begin after 2 years. Its incidence ranges from 30% to 50% in HLA-matched sibling donor transplants to 50% to 70% in HLA-matched unrelated donor transplants. It is the leading cause of non-relapse late mortality in allogeneic HCT survivors.[204,313–317] Chronic GVHD occurs most frequently in patients with preceding acute GVHD, but it can manifest de novo without any preceding acute

Table 113–6. Clinical Manifestations of Chronic Graft-Versus-Host Disease

Organ System	Clinical Manifestations
Cutaneous	Poikiloderma, lichen planus, dermal sclerosis, morphea-like features, hypopigmentation or hyperpigmentation, ichthyosis, nail dystrophy, onycholysis
Ocular	Keratoconjunctivitis sicca, conjunctivitis, corneal ulcerations
Oral	Lichen planus, hyperkeratotic plaques, xerostomia, mucosal atrophy, ulcers, restriction of mouth opening from sclerosis
Pulmonary	Bronchiolitis obliterans, bronchiolitis obliterans-organizing pneumonia
Gastrointestinal	Esophageal web and strictures, malabsorption syndrome, exocrine pancreatic insufficiency
Hepatic	Cholestasis
Genitourinary	Vaginal stenosis or scarring, lichen planus
Musculoskeletal	Fasciitis, joint contractures from sclerosis, myositis or polymyositis, arthritis
Hematopoietic	Thrombocytopenia, eosinophilia, lymphopenia, hemolytic anemia, hypogammaglobulinemia

GVHD. The distinction between acute and chronic GVHD has been based on the time of onset of GVHD (within or after 100 days of transplantation). More recent guidelines for the diagnosis of chronic GVHD emphasize the presence of typical clinical signs and symptoms instead of time of onset. Acute GVHD can occur later in patients receiving reduced-intensity preparative regimens or after donor lymphocyte infusions).[253] Acute and chronic GVHD can coexist simultaneously.

Acute GVHD is the most important risk factor for development of subsequent chronic GVHD.[316,318] Use of mismatched or unrelated donors and transplantation using peripheral blood derived hematopoietic stem cells instead of bone marrow increases risk.[273,317,319,320] Other reported risk factors for chronic GVHD include older recipient age, use of female donor, CMV seropositivity, high graft $CD34^+$ cell count, treatment with donor lymphocyte infusions, and underlying diagnosis of chronic myeloid leukemia or aplastic anemia.[314–318] Similar to acute GVHD, in vitro or in vivo T-cell depletion of the graft can reduce the incidence of chronic GVHD.[281,321–323] Lower rates of chronic GVHD have been observed following umbilical cord blood grafts.[91,118]

Chronic GVHD can affect any organ system; however, certain pathognomonic clinical signs and symptoms must be present to establish its diagnosis (Table 113–6).[253] Other clinical manifestations, although not diagnostic of chronic GVHD, can be characteristic, but they may resemble acute GVHD as well. Additional investigations, including biopsies, might be needed to verify the diagnosis and to rule out other etiologies, such as infections, drug effects, and malignancies.[324] The skin, mouth, eyes, and liver are the most commonly involved sites of chronic GHVD. Cutaneous manifestations resemble autoimmune disease and can include poikiloderma, lichen planus-like eruptions, or scleroderma (sclerosis). Inflammatory dermatitis can progress to severe dermal and periarticular fibrosis with loss of skin appendages (hair and sweat glands) as well as significant skin tightness, fasciitis, and loss of joint flexibility. Additional manifestations include dry eyes and dry mouth, which can resemble Sjögren syndrome clinically and histologically; enteritis with anorexia, early satiety, malabsorption, weight loss, and failure to thrive; and cholestatic jaundice. Pulmonary involvement in the form of bronchiolitis obliterans is an uncommon manifestation but can be particularly debilitating. The profound immune dysfunction associated with chronic GVHD due to hypogammaglobulinemia, impaired cellular immunity, and functional asplenia, greatly increases the risk of secondary infections from bacteria, viruses, and fungi. After onset of chronic GVHD, 25% to 40% of patients die within 2 years, often of secondary infections.[313,314,316]

Chronic GVHD can be classified as mild, moderate, or severe, depending on the number of organs involved and the degree of individual organ involvement.[253] In general, factors associated with an adverse prognosis include thrombocytopenia, progressive onset from acute GVHD, poor performance status, lack of response to initial therapy, and extensive skin or lung involvement.[313,314,325]

Treatment of Chronic Graft-Versus-Host Disease

Although acute GVHD is one of the strongest predictors for chronic GVHD, strategies to limit acute GVHD, such as prolonging or intensifying initial immunosuppression, have not been consistently effective in preventing subsequent chronic GVHD.[326,327] Experience with T-cell depletion, both mechanical and pharmacologic, shows decreased rates of both acute and chronic GVHD but increased risks of relapse due to blunting of the graft-versus-tumor effect; thus, T-cell depletion has not improved survival.[265]

As with acute GVHD, the specific immunosuppressive therapy for chronic GVHD most often is corticosteroids, usually in combination with cyclosporine.[328,329] The ongoing and long-lasting nature of the syndrome demands use of reduced doses and, if possible, alternate-day steroid therapy to minimize chronic complications of prolonged corticosteroid therapy. Typical corticosteroid regimens start with daily prednisone 1 mg/kg/day. In patients who respond, the dosage is tapered down to 0.5 to 1 mg/kg every other day and this dosage continued for 6 to 9 months beyond any active GVHD symptoms, followed by a slow withdrawal of immunosuppression. Longer therapy may be required for some patients, and early withdrawal of therapy frequently has been accompanied by flares of chronic GVHD. Salvage therapies, including high-dose corticosteroids, sirolimus, tacrolimus, MMF, rapamycin, thalidomide, azathioprine, and hydroxychloroquine, have been attempted, with limited response rates.[315]

Newer approaches being investigated as potential therapies for chronic GVHD include modulation of T-cell function, B-cell depletion, induction of immune tolerance, and cytokine blockade.[326] Small uncontrolled studies have reported the use of pentostatin, alemtuzumab, and ATG to inhibit T-cell function and rituximab to eliminate B cells, with response rates of 30% to 50%.[321,323,330,331] T-cell immunomodulation using extracorporeal photopheresis has been shown to have some activity, especially in sclerotic cutaneous chronic GVHD.[332,333] Preliminary studies using daclizumab, etanercept, and infliximab for blockade of the cytokine-mediated inflammatory response have shown short-term responses.[305,334]

Treatment of chronic GVHD, even more than acute GVHD, demands particular attention to prophylaxis and aggressive therapy for secondary opportunistic infections. Consequently, ongoing antibacterial, antifungal, and antiviral prophylaxis should be continued. Intravenous immunoglobulin support should be considered, but only for patients with recurring infections and persistent hypogammaglobulinemia. Most successful strategies for treating chronic GVHD incorporate long-term reduced-dose immunosuppressive therapy, aggressive antimicrobial prophylaxis, and nutritional support.

FUTURE DIRECTIONS

Complications of HCT are one of the major barriers to the wider application of transplantation for a variety of diseases. The impact of newer transplantation modalities, including the use of nonmyeloablative or reduced-intensity conditioning regimens, alternative donor transplantation with umbilical cord blood, and incorporation of immune-based therapies within transplantation regimens, on early and late complications are areas of vigorous current investigation.

Better tools for predicting the risk of post-HCT complications and nonrelapse mortality are needed.[335,336] Genomic and proteomic approaches for monitoring and predicting HCT complications are being investigated.[337,338] Although they are some years from use in clinical practice, these approaches potentially could have many applications in transplantation, including prediction of risk for complications and GVHD, refining donor selection, and utilization of pharmacogenomic data to individualize conditioning regimens and immunosuppression, all to improve the safety and effectiveness of HCT.

SUGGESTED READINGS

Antin JH: Clinical practice. Long-term care after hematopoietic-cell transplantation in adults. N Engl J Med 347:36, 2002.

Baker KS, Gurney JG, Ness KK, et al: Late effects in survivors of chronic myeloid leukemia treated with hematopoietic cell transplantation: Results from the Bone Marrow Transplant Survivor Study. Blood 104:1898, 2004.

Barker JN, Hough RE, van Burik JA, et al: Serious infections after unrelated donor transplantation in 136 children: Impact of stem cell source. Biol Blood Marrow Transplant 11:362, 2005.

Boeckh M, Leisenring W, Riddell SR, et al: Late cytomegalovirus disease and mortality in recipients of allogeneic hematopoietic stem cell transplants: Importance of viral load and T-cell immunity. Blood 101:407, 2003.

Champlin RE, Schmitz N, Horowitz MM, et al: Blood stem cells compared with bone marrow as a source of hematopoietic cells for allogeneic transplantation. IBMTR Histocompatibility and Stem Cell Sources Working Committee and the European Group for Blood and Marrow Transplantation (EBMT). Blood 95:3702, 2000.

Cornely OA, Maertens J, Winston DJ, et al: Posaconazole vs. fluconazole or itraconazole prophylaxis in patients with neutropenia. N Engl J Med 356:348, 2007.

Curtis RE. Rowlings PA, Deeg HJ, et al: Solid cancers after bone marrow transplantation. N Engl J Med 336:897, 1977.

Filipovich AH, Weisdorf D, Pavletic S, et al: National Institutes of Health consensus development project on criteria for clinical trials in chronic graft-versus-host disease: I. Diagnosis and staging working group report. Biol Blood Marrow Transplant 11:945, 2005.

Guidelines for preventing opportunistic infections among hematopoietic stem cell transplant recipients. Biol Blood Marrow Transplant 6:659, 2000.

Lee SJ, Vogelsang G, Flowers ME: Chronic graft-versus-host disease. Biol Blood Marrow Transplant 9:215, 2003.

Majhail NS, Parks K, Defor TE, Weisdorf DJ: Diffuse alveolar hemorrhage and infection-associated alveolar hemorrhage following hematopoietic stem cell transplantation: Related and high-risk clinical syndromes. Biol Blood Marrow Transplant 12:1038, 2006.

Marr KA, Seidel K, Slavin MA, et al: Prolonged fluconazole prophylaxis is associated with persistent protection against candidiasis-related death in allogeneic marrow transplant recipients: Long-term follow-up of a randomized, placebo-controlled trial. Blood 96:2055, 2000.

Metayer C, Curtis RE, Vose J, et al: Myelodysplastic syndrome and acute myeloid leukemia after autotransplantation for lymphoma: A multicenter case-control study. Blood 101:2015, 2003.

Parody R, Martino R, Rovira M, et al: Severe infections after unrelated donor allogeneic hematopoietic stem cell transplantation in adults: Comparison of cord blood transplantation with peripheral blood and bone marrow transplantation. Biol Blood Marrow Transplant 12:734, 2006.

Richardson PG, Murakami C, Jin Z, et al: Multi-institutional use of defibrotide in 88 patients after stem cell transplantation with severe veno-occlusive disease and multisystem organ failure: Response without significant toxicity in a high-risk population and factors predictive of outcome. Blood 100:4337, 2002.

Rizzo JD, Wingard JR, Tichelli A, et al: Recommended screening and preventive practices for long-term survivors after hematopoietic cell transplantation: Joint recommendations of the European Group for Blood and Marrow Transplantation, the Center for International Blood and Marrow Transplant Research, and the American Society of Blood and Marrow Transplantation. Biol Blood Marrow Transplant 12:138, 2006.

Rocha V, Labopin M, Sanz G, et al: Transplants of umbilical-cord blood or bone marrow from unrelated donors in adults with acute leukemia. N Engl J Med 351:2276, 2004.

Sorror ML, Maris MB, Storer B, et al: Comparing morbidity and mortality of HLA-matched unrelated donor hematopoietic cell transplantation after nonmyeloablative and myeloablative conditioning: Influence of pretransplantation comorbidities. Blood 104:961, 2004.

Upton A, Kirby KA, Carpenter P, Boeckh M, Marr KA: Invasive aspergillosis following hematopoietic cell transplantation: Outcomes and prognostic factors associated with mortality. Clin Infect Dis 44:531, 2007.

van Burik JA, Weisdorf DJ: Infections in recipients of blood and marrow transplantation. Hematol Oncol Clin North Am 13:1065, 1999.

Wagner JE, Barker JN, DeFor TE, et al: Transplantation of unrelated donor umbilical cord blood in 102 patients with malignant and nonmalignant diseases: Influence of CD34 cell dose and HLA disparity on treatment-related mortality and survival. Blood 100:1611, 2002.

Wagner JE, Thompson JS, Carter SL, Kernan NA: Effect of graft-versus-host disease prophylaxis on 3-year disease-free survival in recipients of unrelated donor bone marrow (T-cell Depletion Trial): A multi-centre, randomised phase II-III trial. Lancet 366:733, 2005.

REFERENCES

For complete list of references log onto www.expertconsult.com

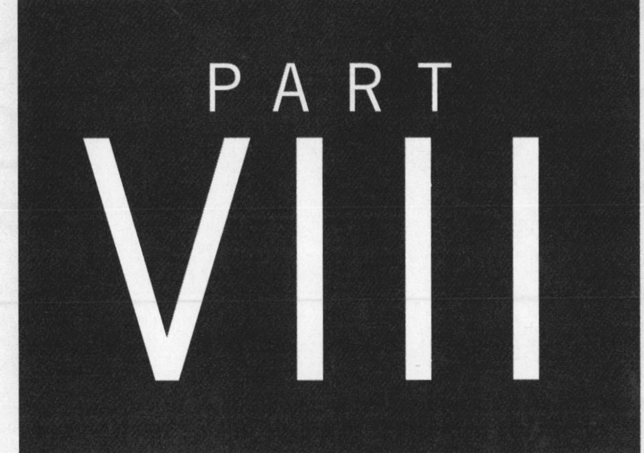

Hemostasis and Thrombosis

CHAPTER 114

MEGAKARYOCYTE AND PLATELET STRUCTURE

Joseph E. Italiano, Jr. and John H. Hartwig

Platelets are small anucleate fragments that are formed from the cytoplasm of megakaryocytes and have a characteristic discoid shape. To assemble and release platelets, megakaryocytes become polyploid by endomitosis and follow a maturation program that results in the conversion of the bulk of their cytoplasm into multiple long processes called *proplatelets*. To produce its quota of 1000 to 2000 platelets, a megakaryocyte may protrude as many as 10 to 20 proplatelets, each of which begins as a blunt protrusion that over time thins and branches repeatedly. Platelets form selectively at the ends of proplatelets. As platelets develop, their content of granules and organelles is delivered to them in a stream of individual particles moving from the megakaryocyte cell body to the nascent platelet buds at the proplatelet tips. Once the nascent platelet is filled with its components and a single microtubule (≈100 μm in length) is rolled into a peripheral coil, it releases into the circulation. Platelet formation can be arbitrarily divided into two phases. The first phase takes days to complete and requires megakaryocyte-specific growth factors. Massive nuclear proliferation to 16 to 32 × N and enlargement of the megakaryocyte cytoplasm occur as the platelet is filled with cytoskeletal proteins, platelet-specific granules, and sufficient membrane to complete the platelet assembly process. The second phase is relatively rapid and can be completed in hours. During this phase, proplatelets are extended and mature discoid platelets are released.

MEGAKARYOCYTE DEVELOPMENT

Endomitosis

Hematopoietic stem cells, which are endowed with the genetic capacity to differentiate into multiple lineages, are induced down the pathway to become megakaryocytes by their exposure to certain growth factors.[1] Megakaryocytes become polyploid (i.e., 4N, 16N, 32N, 64N) through repeated cycles of DNA replication without cell division.[2–5] Normally ploidy ranges from four to 64 times the haploid DNA complement, but the majority of cells fall within three ploidy classes (8N, 16N, and 32N), with 16N being dominant.[6,7] Ploidy number appears to be a predetermined event, possibly signifying genetic diversity among megakaryocyte populations. Megakaryocyte polyploidization results in a functional gene amplification whose likely function is an increase in protein synthesis.[8] This process, called *endomitosis*, is a shortened mitosis caused by a block in anaphase.[9,10] Megakaryocytes proceed from prophase to anaphase A, but they do not enter anaphase B or telophase or undergo cytokinesis. During polyploidization of megakaryocytes, the nuclear envelope breaks down, and an abnormal spherical mitotic spindle forms. The spindle has attached chromosomes that align from a position equidistant from the spindle poles. Sister chromatids segregate and move toward their respective poles (anaphase A). However, the spindle poles fail to move apart and do not undergo the microtubule-driven separation typically observed during anaphase B. Individual chromatids are not moved to the poles, and subsequently a single nuclear envelope encapsulates the entire set of sister chromatids.[9,10] In most cell types, checkpoints and feedback controls ensure that DNA replication and cell division are tightly coupled. Megakaryocytes appear to be an exception to this rule, indicating they have managed to deregulate this process. Proposed mechanisms for regulating endomitosis include a reduction in mitosis-promoting factor[11,12] or decreased expression of cyclin B.[12–15] Cyclins appear to play a critical role in directing endomitosis. Cyclin D3 is overexpressed in the G_1 phase of maturing megakaryocytes,[16] but a triple knockout of cyclins D1, D2, and D3 in mice does not appear to affect megakaryocyte development.[17] Cyclin E-deficient mice exhibit a profound defect in megakaryocyte development.[18] The molecular programming involved in endomitosis is characterized by the mislocalization or absence of at least two critical regulators of mitosis: the chromosomal passenger proteins Aurora-B/AIM-1 and survivin. AIM-1, a serine/threonine kinase in the Aurora family that is implicated in mitosis, is downregulated as megakaryocyte polyploidization occurs, suggesting its loss may lead to the abortive mitosis and polyploidization.[19,20] One explanation for endomitosis could be inhibition of microtubule-based forces in anaphase B. Spindle pole separation during anaphase B is believed to be powered by the sliding of antiparallel interdigitating microtubules past each other[21] by the mitotic kinesin-like protein 1 that localizes at regions of overlapping microtubules during anaphase B and has been shown to slide microtubules past one another in vitro.[22] Therefore, lack of spindle pole separation during endomitosis may result from failure of megakaryocytes to undergo normal spindle orientation and/or the absence of signals that localize or activate a kinesin motor molecule that provides force for sliding.

Cytoplasmic Maturation

Megakaryocytes, the largest of the hematopoietic cells, undergo a pronounced cytoplasmic maturation to attain their large volumes (15,000 fL). Cytoplasmic maturation begins during endomitosis and increases considerably after all DNA amplification has ended (Fig. 114–1). Megakaryocytes enlarge dramatically as they mature, reaching sizes of 100 to 150 μm in diameter in culture and in bone marrow. During this process, the megakaryocytic cytoplasm rapidly fills with platelet-specific proteins, organelles, and membrane systems that ultimately are subdivided and packaged into platelets (Fig. 114–2). Their cytoplasmic space expands and, except for the most cortical regions, becomes densely filled with internal membranes that subsequently serve as the repository for the plasma membrane to be regurgitated for coating proplatelets as they extend.[23] This internal membrane system is one of the most striking features of a mature megakaryocyte and has been referred to as the demarcation membrane system (DMS). The DMS, first described by Yamada[24] in 1957, consists of an extensive, tortuous, branching network of membrane channels composed of flattened cisternae and tubules. Initially, the DMS was proposed to play an essential role in platelet formation by defining preformed "platelet territories" or "platelet fields" within the megakaryocyte cytoplasm.[25,26] Release of individual platelets was postulated to occur by massive fragmentation of the megakaryocyte cytoplasm along DMS fracture lines between these fields. However, studies demonstrating that platelets are primarily assembled and released from proplatelet ends (see Platelet formation section) are inconsistent with this notion and indicate instead that the DMS functions predominantly as a membrane reserve for proplatelet formation.[23,27] Direct visualization of mature DMS containing phosphatidylinositol 4,5-bisphosphate suggests that it is the source of proplatelet membranes.[28] Maturing megakaryocytes, like other gran-

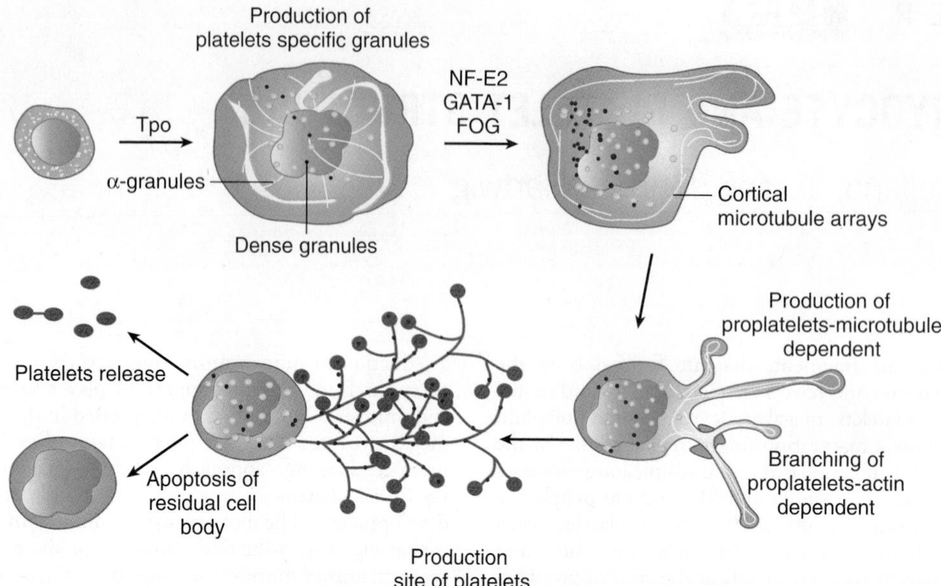

Figure 114–1 Summary of the major events that lead to platelet formation and release from megakaryocytes. Hematopoietic stem cells are converted into megakaryocytes by exposure to the specific growth factor thrombopoietin (TPO). TPO initiates a maturation program that amplifies the megakaryocyte DNA and leads to synthesis of platelet-specific proteins. In particular, cytoskeletal elements, membrane systems, and receptor proteins are made in bulk, and the megakaryocyte becomes filled with platelet-specific granules. Platelet production begins when microtubules aggregate in the cell cortex, and one pole of the megakaryocyte spontaneously elaborates pseudopodia. These begin as large blunt pseudopodia, which subsequently thin and branch into proplatelets. The branching reaction is dependent on a localized assembly of actin and is inhibited by drugs that disrupt actin filaments. Platelets are assembled primarily at the ends of the proplatelets. Intracellular organelles are delivered to the platelet buds along microtubule tracks in the shafts. Platelets are released from the ends of proplatelets.

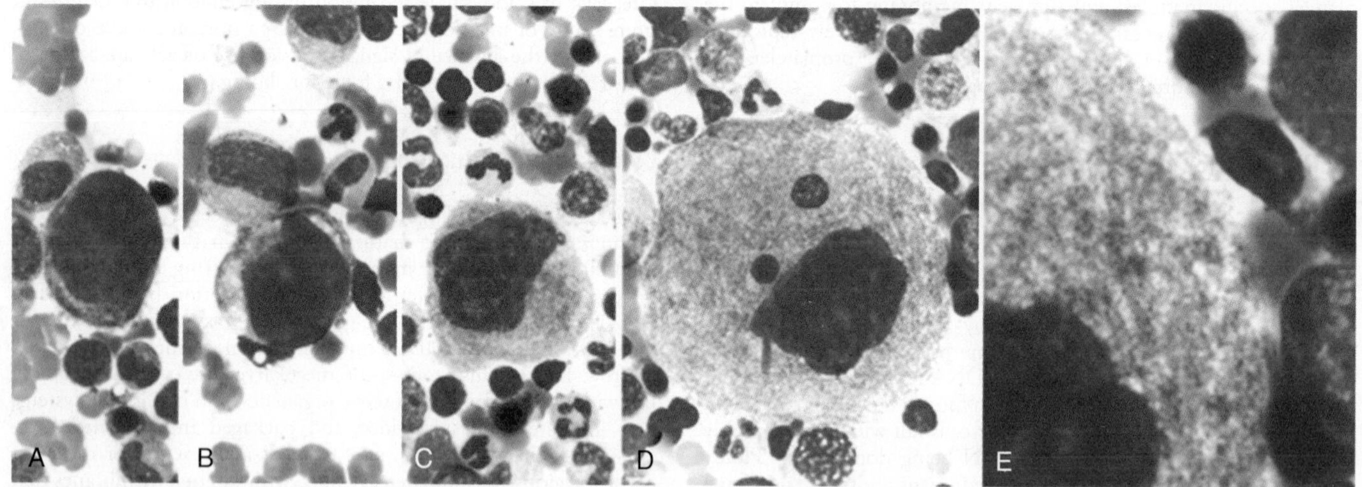

Figure 114–2 Platelet production in the megakaryocyte: **A**, Immature polyploid megakaryoblast with little differentiation. **B**, Megakaryocyte with early Golgi zone. **C**, Early platelet production in cytoplasm. **D**, Late-stage megakaryocyte with abundant internal membranes, organelles, and platelet-specific proteins. **E**, Early formation of demarcation membranes.

ulated cells, contain an abundance of ribosomes and rough endoplasmic reticulum, where protein synthesis occurs. During this phase of megakaryocyte development, the cytoplasm fills with cytoskeletal proteins, platelet-specific receptors and secretory granules, and normal cellular organelles such as mitochondria and lysosomes.

One of the hallmark features of the mature megakaryocyte is its abundance of platelet-specific secretory granules. The two specific granules destined for platelets are α granules and dense granules. α-Granules are the more abundant and larger of the two (200–500 nm in diameter). They contain proteins that enhance the adhesion of platelets, promote cell–cell interactions, regulate angiogenesis, and stimulate vascular repair. α Granules store matrix proteins and contain glycoprotein receptors in their membranes (see Fig. 114–5, *A*). The bulk of cellular P-selectin and a portion of $\alpha_{IIb}\beta_3$ and the glycoprotein Ib/IX/V complex (GPIb-IX-V; a receptor for von Willebrand factor [vWF]) are expressed in the membranes of α granules. Adhesion molecules within the granules include vWF, fibrinogen, fibronectin, vitronectin, and thrombospondin. α-Granule proteins can derive from different origins. Some proteins, such as β-thromboglobulin and vWF, are synthesized by megakaryocytes.[29] However, fibrinogen, also a major component of α granules, is not synthesized by megakaryocytes and is taken up from plasma by an endocytic mechanism requiring fibrinogen binding by $\alpha_{IIb}\beta_3$.[30–32] Although little is known about the intracellular trafficking of proteins in megakaryocytes, experiments using cryosectioning and immunoelectron microscopy suggest that multivesicular bodies are an essential intermediate stage in the formation of platelet α granules.[33] During megakaryocyte development, large (≈0.5 μm) multivesicular bodies

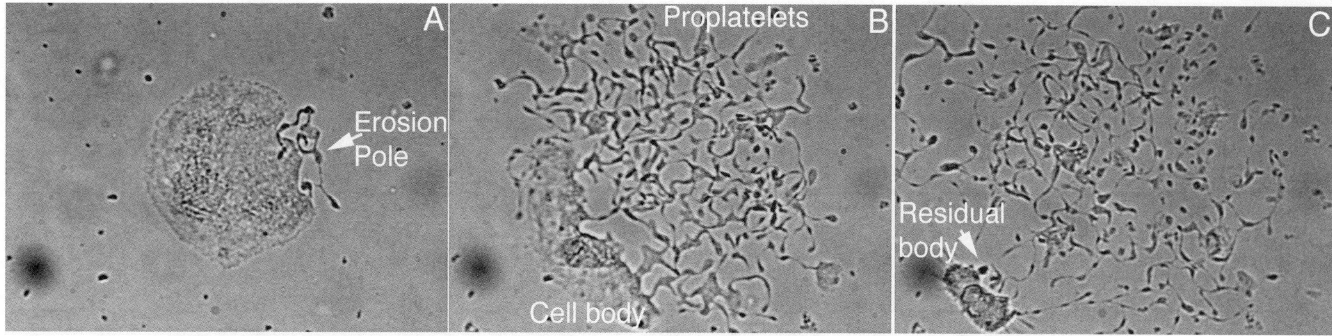

Figure 114–3 Formation of proplatelets by a mouse megakaryocyte. Time-lapse sequence of a maturing megakaryocyte showing the events that lead to elaboration of proplatelets in vitro. **A**, Platelet production begins when the megakaryocyte cytoplasm starts to erode at one pole (arrow). **B**, The bulk of the megakaryocyte cytoplasm has been converted into multiple proplatelet processes that continue to lengthen and form swellings along their length. These processes are highly dynamic and undergo bending and branching. **C**, Once the bulk of the megakaryocyte cytoplasm has been converted into proplatelets, the entire process ends in a rapid retraction that separates the released proplatelets from the residual cell body.

undergo a gradual transition from granules containing 30- to 70-nm internal vesicles to granules containing secretion concentrates. The second and smaller type of platelet granule is the dense granule. Platelets contain a small number of dense granules, which are approximately 150 nm in diameter. Dense granules have electron opaque cores and function primarily to recruit additional platelets to sites of vascular injury. Dense granules contain the soluble activating agents serotonin and ADP as well as divalent cations. When the megakaryocyte reaches a certain point of maturation, proplatelet production begins, and dense granules are sent into the proplatelets destined for platelets.

REGULATION OF MEGAKARYOCYTE DEVELOPMENT

The development of megakaryocytes and the process of platelet biogenesis occur within a complex bone marrow environment where both cytokines and adhesive interactions play an essential role. Megakaryocytes are imprisoned within the subendothelial layer of the bone marrow sinuses where development and platelet biogenesis are regulated at multiple levels by several cytokines. Thrombopoietin (Tpo), which is synthesized in bone marrow and liver, is the principal regulator of thrombopoiesis.[34] Tpo also plays a central role in hematopoietic stem cell survival and proliferation. Circulating levels of Tpo induce proliferation and maturation of megakaryocyte progenitors by binding to the c-Mpl receptor and signaling induction. Tpo regulates all stages of megakaryocyte development, from the hematopoietic stem cell stage through cytoplasmic maturation.[35] Tpo increases platelet production by increasing both the number and size of individual megakaryocytes. c-Mpl activation is regulated by a complex array of signaling molecules that turn on specific transcription factors (see Transcriptional Regulation of Platelet Formation section) to drive megakaryocyte proliferation and maturation. Although Tpo appears to function as the main regulator of megakaryocyte development, it is not exclusive in this action. The cytokine stem cell factor, granulocyte-macrophage colony-stimulating factor, FLT ligand, interleukin (IL)-3, IL-6, IL-11, and erythropoietin also can regulate megakaryocyte development but appear to function mainly in concert with Tpo.[36–40] Mice that lack Tpo or its receptor c-Mpl have approximately 15% of the normal platelet count.[41,42] The discovery of Tpo in 1994 and the development of primary megakaryocyte or mouse embryonic stem cell cultures that can be induced to faithfully reconstitute platelet formation have provided systems for studying megakaryocytes in the act of making platelets in vitro.[43–45] Megakaryocytes isolated from mouse fetal liver and incubated with Tpo for 4 to 5 days mature into huge polyploid cells that are capable of generating and releasing large numbers of platelets.[46] In similar fashion, mouse embryonic stem cells can be induced to mature into large polyploid megakaryocytes in the presence of stromal cells and Tpo, IL-6, and IL-11.[44] This process requires 10 to 12 days, during which the conversion of embryonic stem cells into hematopoietic stem cells very likely occurs in the first half of the period and the maturation of hematopoietic stem cells into proplatelet-producing megakaryocytes in the second half. Human embryonic stem cells can be coaxed to differentiate into mature megakaryocytes, although the process takes several more days in culture.[47]

PLATELET FORMATION

Proplatelets and the Cytoskeletal Mechanics of Platelet Formation

The discovery of Tpo and the development of megakaryocyte cultures that reconstitute platelet formation in vitro have allowed visualization of megakaryocytes in the act of forming platelets. The actual mechanical process of platelet production begins when mature megakaryocytes begin to elaborate proplatelets (Figs. 114–1 and 114–3).[48–52] This process is distinguished by the erosion of one pole of the megakaryocyte cytoplasm (Fig. 114–3).[27] Multiple thick pseudopodia are extended and subsequently elongate to yield thin tubules. As these slender tubules grow, they branch repeatedly and develop periodic densities along their length that impart a beaded appearance. The first insight into the cytoskeletal mechanics of platelet formation dates from the work of Tablin et al.,[53] who showed that proplatelet formation is dependent on microtubules, that is, proplatelet elaboration is inhibited by microtubule poisons. Microtubule poisons are effective because the extension of proplatelets from the megakaryocyte is mediated by the assembly of microtubules and their reorganization into cortical bundles. Cortical bundles align in the shafts of proplatelets, and proplatelet elongation is driven by sliding movements between microtubules composing these bundles. The microtubule bundles form loops at the end of each proplatelet, and ultimately a single microtubule is rolled into a coil at the proplatelet end to define the platelet territory. Cytoplasmic tubulin in solution is an $\alpha\beta$ dimer that reversibly polymerizes into microtubules, which are long hollow cylinders with an outer diameter of 25 nm. Several studies reveal an essential role in platelet biogenesis for β_1 tubulin, a divergent and lineage-specific β tubulin, which is a major component of the megakaryocyte proplatelet cytoskeleton and marginal microtubule coil of the platelet.[54] β_1 Tubulin is expressed exclusively in platelets and megakaryocytes during late stages of megakaryocyte development and is essential for the production of normal platelet numbers as well as the discoid shape of the platelet as judged by a number of criteria. First, mRNA subtraction between wild type and NF-E2-deficient megakaryocytes demonstrates that β_1 tubulin is a downstream effector of the megakaryocyte transcription factor NF-E2 and is absent from NF-E2-deficient megakaryocytes.[46] Second, genetic elimination of the β_1-tubulin gene in mice results in

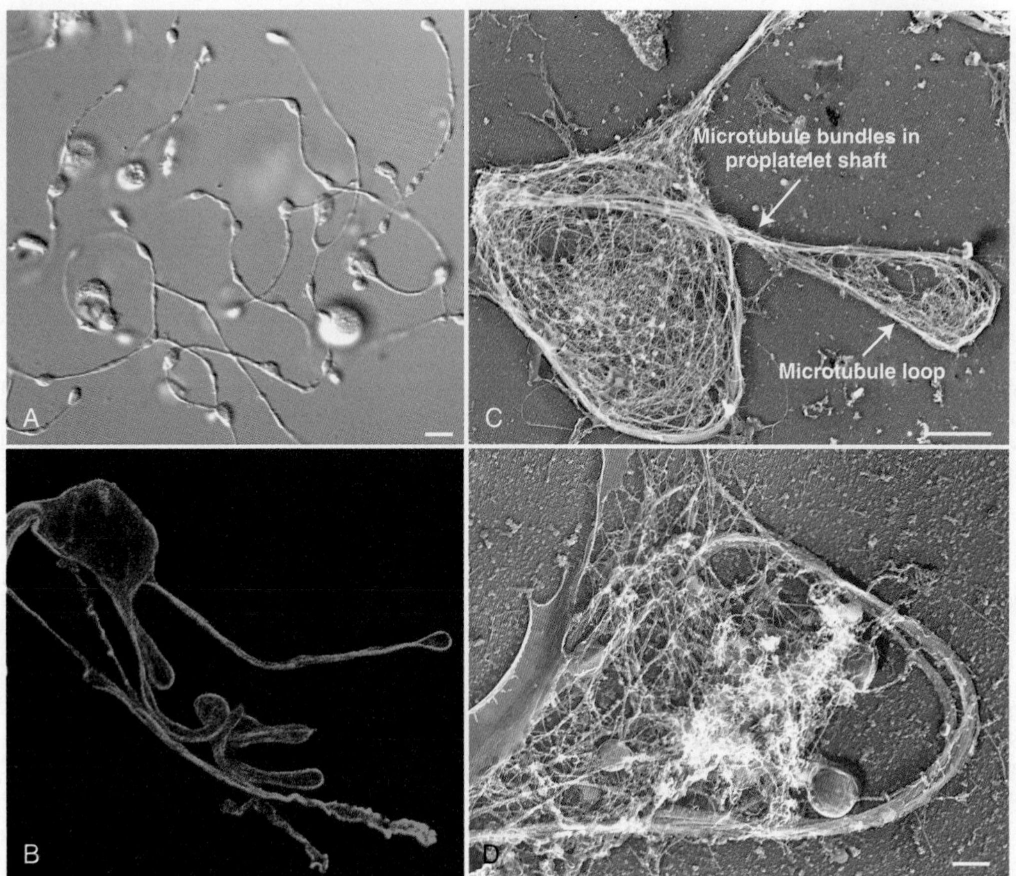

Figure 114–4 Structure of proplatelets. **A**, Differential interference contrast image of proplatelets elaborated by mouse megakaryocytes in culture. (Bar = 5 μm.) **B**, Staining of proplatelets with Alexa 488 antitubulin IgG reveals that the microtubules line the shaft of the proplatelet and form loops at the proplatelet tips. (Bar = 5 μm.) **C**, **D**, Organization of microtubules in the tips of proplatelets. **C**, Microtubules form bundles in the proplatelet shafts. (Bar = 2 μm.) **D**, Microtubules loop in the proplatelet ends and reenter the proplatelet shafts. (Bar = 0.2 μm.)

thrombocytopenia.[55] Third, megakaryocytes isolated from β_1-tubulin knockout mice fail to form proplatelets *in vitro* and instead extend only a small number of blunt protrusions.

The first event that signals proplatelet production is the consolidation of microtubules into large bundles at the megakaryocyte cortex that subsequently are reorganized into parallel bundles in the shafts of the proplatelets (Fig. 114–4). Microtubule bundles are thick near the body of the megakaryocyte as they enter the proplatelet shaft but thin progressively throughout the shaft, such that only five to 10 microtubules remain at the end of the proplatelet. Importantly, the microtubule bundles that run down the proplatelet shaft make characteristic U turns in the tips and reenter the shaft, forming teardrop-shaped structures (Fig. 114–4). This observation demonstrates a bipolar orientation of bundles in the vicinity of the proplatelet tip, a geometry required to explain the observation of bidirectional granule and organelle traffic in proplatelets.[56] The looped arrangement of microtubules in proplatelet tips also places constraints on the elongation mechanism used to grow proplatelets and indicates that assembly of microtubules at the end of the process does not elongate proplatelets because of an insufficient number of free microtubule ends to nucleate this reaction.

Direct visualization of microtubule dynamics in living megakaryocytes using green fluorescent protein (GFP) technology has provided insights into how microtubules orient to power proplatelet elongation (Fig. 114–5, *A* and *B*).[57] End-binding protein 3 (EB3), a microtubule plus end-binding protein associated only with growing microtubules, fused to GFP was retrovirally expressed in murine megakaryocytes and used as a marker to locate microtubule plus ends and follow plus end dynamics. Immature megakaryocytes without proplatelets use a centrosomal-coupled microtubule nucleation/assembly reaction, which appears as a prominent starburst pattern when visualized with EB3-GFP. Microtubules assemble only from the centrosome and grow outward into the cell cortex, where they turn and run in parallel with the cell edges. However, just before proplatelet production begins, centrosomal assembly ends and microtubules release and consolidate into the cortex as bundles. Fluorescence time-lapse microscopy of living, proplatelet-producing megakaryocytes expressing EB3-GFP reveals that as proplatelets elongate, microtubules assemble continuously throughout the entire proplatelet. EB3-GFP studies also reveal that microtubules polymerize in both directions in proplatelets, that is, toward both the tips and cell body, demonstrating that microtubules composing the bundles have a mixed polarity.

Even though microtubules are continuously assembling at their plus ends in proplatelets, polymerization per se does not provide the force for proplatelet elongation. First, the rates of microtubule polymerization (average 10.2 μm/min) are approximately 10-fold faster than the proplatelet elongation rate. Second, proplatelets continue to elongate even when microtubule polymerization is blocked by drugs that inhibit net assembly, suggesting an alternative mechanism for proplatelet elongation. Third, proplatelets possess an inherent microtubule sliding mechanism. Dynein, a minus end microtubule molecular motor protein, localizes along the microtubules of the proplatelet and appears to directly contribute to microtubule sliding, as inhibition of dynein through disassembly of the dynactin complex prevents proplatelet formation. Microtubule sliding can be reactivated in detergent-permeabilized proplatelets. Adenosine triphosphate, known to support the enzymatic activity of microtubule-based molecular motors, activates elongation in permeabilized proplatelets that contain dynein and its regulatory complex dynactin. Thus, dynein-facilitated

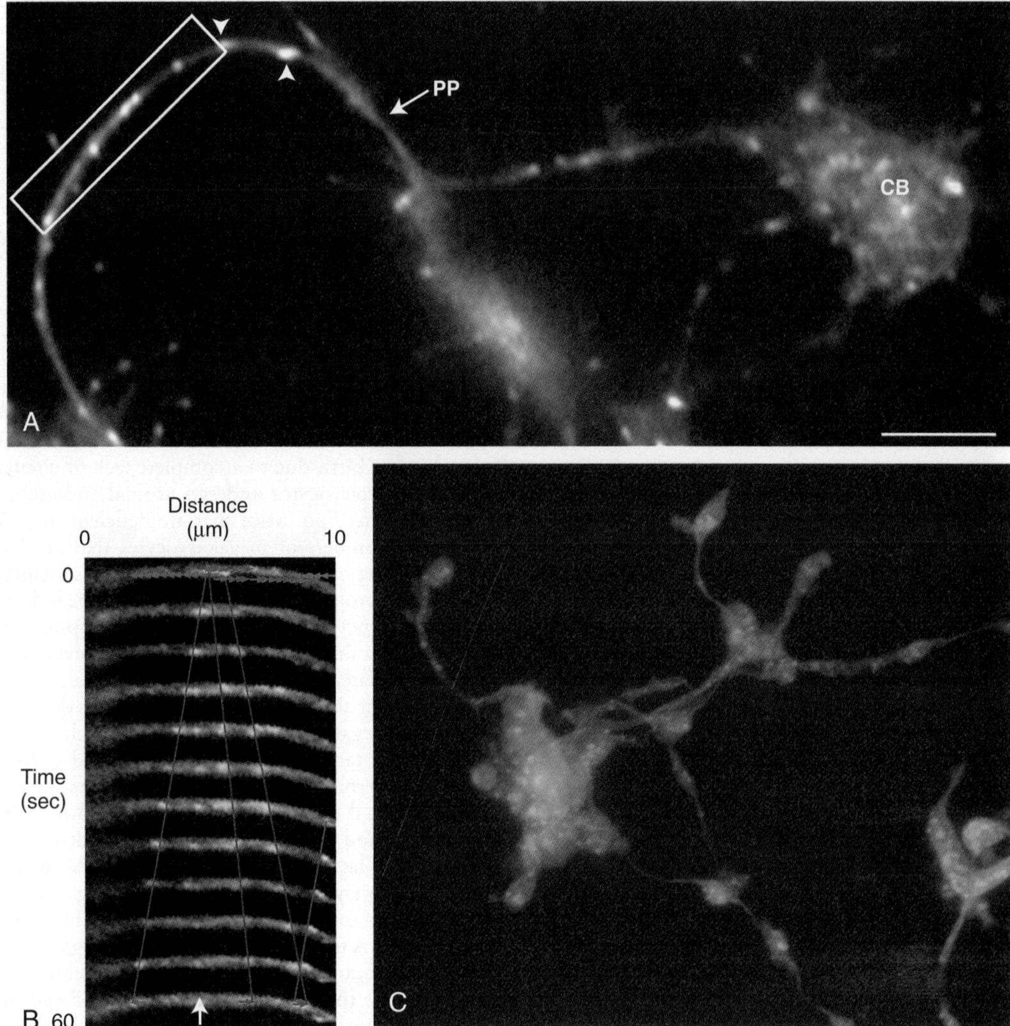

Figure 114–5 Microtubule dynamics during proplatelet formation. **A**, Visualization of plus end microtubule assembly in living megakaryocytes expressing end-binding protein 3 (EB3)-green fluorescent protein (GFP). First frame from the time-lapse sequence (shown in B) of a living megakaryocyte that was retrovirally directed to express EB3-GFP. The cell body (CB) is at the right of the micrograph and proplatelets (PP) extend to the left. EB3-GFP labels growing microtubule plus ends in a characteristic "comet" staining pattern that has a bright front and a dim tail. **B**, The kymograph shows movement over time. Images are every 5 seconds. EB3-GFP comets undergo bidirectional movements in proplatelets, demonstrating that microtubules are organized as bipolar arrays. Some EB3-GFP comets move toward the tip and are highlighted in green; others that move toward the cell body are highlighted in red. **C**, Distribution of α granules in megakaryocytes and proplatelet projections visualized by fluorescence microscopy. α Granules are stained with Alexa 568 (red)-labeled anti–von Willebrand factor antibodies. The proplatelets have been costained with Alexa 488 (green) antitubulin antibodies to highlight the microtubules.

microtubule sliding appears to be the key event in driving proplatelet elongation.

Nascent platelets form only at the bulbous ends of proplatelets as defined by the rolling of a single microtubule into a coil having the same diameter as the coil found in the mature platelet.[27] Given that maturation of the platelet is limited to these sites, efficient platelet production requires a large number of proplatelet ends. Megakaryocytes use a unique mechanical process to repeatedly bifurcate the shafts of the proplatelet and hence amplify the number of ends. To accomplish this task, the shaft of elongating proplatelets is bent upon itself and a new proplatelet grows out of the bend, a process that results in bifurcation of the shaft. Whereas proplatelet elongation is mediated by microtubules, the bending and branching of proplatelet shafts are mediated by actin. Actin filament assemblies decorate branch points, and agents that disrupt actin assembly, such as the cytochalasins, abolish proplatelet branching.[27] One possibility is that proplatelet bending and branching are powered by the actin-based molecular motor myosin. Myosin II is an ATPase motor that makes up 2% to 5% of the total platelet protein.[58,59] Myosin II binds to actin filaments and generates force for contraction. Each myosin has two heads and a long, rod-like tail whose function is to permit the molecules to assemble into bipolar filaments. Interestingly, a mutation in the tail domain of the nonmuscle myosin heavy chain A gene in humans results in several diseases, including May-Hegglin anomaly, Sebastian syndrome, and Fechtner syndrome. These rare autosomal platelet disorders are characterized by thrombocytopenia with giant platelets.[60–62] Because bipolar filament assembly is crucial for the function of myosin II, the hematologic phenotype of May-Hegglin may be due to a block in the polymerization of myosin II into filaments during megakaryocyte development and platelet formation.

In addition to playing an essential role in proplatelet elongation, the microtubules lining the shafts of proplatelets serve a secondary function: transport of membrane, organelles, and granules into proplatelets and assembling platelets at proplatelet ends (see Fig. 114–5, *C*).[56] Individual organelles are sent individually from the cell body into the proplatelets, where they move bidirectionally until they are captured at proplatelet tips. Immunofluorescence and electron microscopic studies indicate that organelles are intimately associated with microtubules, and actin poisons do not diminish organelle motion. Thus, movement appears to involve microtubule-based forces. Bidirectional organelle movement is conveyed in part by the bipolar arrangement of microtubules within the proplatelet, as kinesin-coated latex beads move in both directions over the microtubule arrays of permeabilized proplatelets. Of the two major microtubule motors, kinesin and dynein, only the plus end-directed kinesin is localized in a pattern similar to organelles and granules and likely is responsible for transporting these elements along microtubules. It appears that a twofold mechanism of organelle and granule movement occurs in platelet assembly: first, organelles and granules travel along microtubules; and second, the microtubules themselves slide bidirectionally in relation to other motile filaments, indirectly moving organelles along proplatelets in a piggyback manner.

Platelet Maturation at the Proplatelet Tip

Platelet maturation at proplatelet tips finalizes when a single microtubule detaches from the microtubule bundle and is rolled into a coil.[27] To complete its construction of mature platelets, once the fundamental cytoskeletal components have been delivered to and assembled in the platelet buds, the buds must fill with their organelle and granule content.

Granules are sent to nascent platelets on the microtubule tracks of the proplatelets. The concentration of this cargo in the platelet occurs by an end-trapping mechanism as granules and organelles, which enter the nascent platelet, continue to move in the tip but do not return to the proplatelet shaft.

Release of Mature Platelets

Details of how mature platelets release from the proplatelet tips are lacking. In vitro, maturation of proplatelets ends in a rapid retraction that separates a variable portion of the proplatelets from the residual cell body, leaving behind a naked, denuded nucleus (see Fig. 114–3, *C*). [27] Activation of apoptotic pathways in the cell body has been shown to be coincident with this event.[63–69] In vivo, the finished platelet may be shed into blood as a mature disc or released in a "preplatelet form," perhaps having a long cytoplasmic projection directly related to its previous attachment to the proplatelet process. This cytoplasmic bridge would either be subsequently shed or be absorbed into the platelet body. Because platelet buds appear discoid and contain microtubule coils, it is likely that discoid shape is established prior to shedding, and unlikely that elongated shapes are generated that have an uncoiled microtubule, although it is possible that platelets release with a portion of their microtubule uncoiled.[45] It also is likely that the microtubule motors that drive proplatelet extension are involved in aspects of platelet release as well as in the process of microtubule coiling. Sliding of an uncoiled portion of the microtubule relative to the rigid microtubule bundle in the proplatelet tip would provide a simple mechanism to effect platelet release and would explain the variable morphology of a small but reproducible percentage (<5%) of dumbbell-shaped platelets that are present in blood.

Location of Platelet Release

Although studies on megakaryocytes in culture have provided insight into the mechanics of platelet production, whether proplatelet elaboration follows the same rules in situ remains unclear. Megakaryocytes are produced in the bone marrow and certainly some undergo fragmentation into platelets at this location. The function of proplatelets has been suggested to provide a mechanism for extension into the bone marrow sinusoids, allowing release of platelets directly into circulation. Megakaryocytes have been identified in intravascular sites within the lung, leading to a theory that some platelets are formed from their parent cell in the pulmonary circulation.

Transcriptional Regulation of Platelet Formation

Megakaryocyte development and platelet formation are controlled by the coordinated action of transcription factors that specifically turn on the genes of megakaryocyte precursors or suppress gene expression that supports other cell types. Genetic approaches involving gene targeting in mice have revealed several genes that are crucial for megakaryocyte development and platelet formation. Leading the list of transcription factors that play an essential role in megakaryocyte maturation and platelet biogenesis is the basic leucine zipper heterodimer NF-E2.[70] NF-E2 is a protein composed of a ubiquitously expressed 18- to 20-kd small-Maf subunit and a p45 subunit restricted to the erythroid and megakaryocytic lineages. NF-E2 originally was thought to be a transcription factor that specifically drove the expression of genes essential for erythropoiesis, but mice lacking p45 NF-E2 do not exhibit defects in erythropoiesis. Instead, mice deficient in the p45 subunit or two of the small-Maf subunits die of hemorrhage shortly after birth due to a complete lack of circulating platelets.[71,72] These megakaryocytes undergo normal endomitosis and proliferate in response to Tpo. Mice that are deficient in p45 NF-E2 produce increased numbers of megakaryocytes that are larger than normal, contain fewer granules, exhibit a highly disorganized DMS, and fail to generate proplatelets in vitro, a phenotype indicative of a late block in megakaryocyte maturation.[46] NF-E2 appears to control the transcription of a limited number of genes involved in cytoplasmic maturation and platelet formation. Shivdasani et al.[55] generated a subtracted cDNA library that is enriched in transcripts downregulated in NF-E2 knockout megakaryocytes, and this approach has started to define the downstream targets of NF-E2 and allowed analysis of their precise role in the terminal stages of megakaryocyte differentiation. Putative transcriptional targets of NF-E2 include β_1 tubulin,[55] thromboxane synthase,[73] and proteins that regulate inside-out signaling via $\alpha_{IIb}\beta_3$ integrin.[74] The zinc finger protein GATA1 is also a transcription factor that plays a critical role in driving the expression of genes essential for megakaryocyte maturation. However, unlike NF-E2, which appears to drive the later stage of megakaryocyte development, GATA1 functions at multiple stages of development. GATA proteins initially were thought to regulate red blood cell maturation because genetic disruption of the GATA1 gene in mice results in embryonic lethality due to a block in erythropoiesis.[75] However, several observations also implicate GATA1 as an important regulator of megakaryocyte differentiation. First, forced expression of GATA1 in the early myeloid cell line 416b induced megakaryocyte differentiation of these cells.[76] Second, Shivdasani et al.[77] used targeted mutagenesis of regulatory elements within the GATA1 locus to generate mice with a selective loss of GATA1 in the megakaryocyte lineage. These knockdown mice expressed sufficient levels of GATA1 in erythroid cells to circumvent the embryonic lethality caused by anemia. GATA1 deficiency in megakaryocytes leads to severe thrombocytopenia. Platelet counts are reduced to approximately 15% of normal, and the small number of circulating platelets typically are round and significantly larger than usual. These mice have an increased number of small megakaryocytes that exhibit an increased rate of proliferation. The small cytoplasmic volume of GATA1-deficient megakaryocytes typically contains an excess of rough endoplasmic reticulum, very few platelet-specific granules, and an underdeveloped or disorganized DMS, suggesting that maturation of megakaryocytes is arrested in GATA1-deficient megakaryocytes.[78]

A family with X-linked dyserythropoietic anemia and thrombocytopenia due to a mutation in GATA1 has been described.[79] A single nucleotide substitution in the amino-terminal zinc finger of GATA1 inhibits the interaction of GATA1 with its essential cofactor, friend of GATA1 (FOG). Although the megakaryocytes in affected family members are abundant, they are unusually small and exhibit several abnormal features, including an abundance of smooth endoplasmic reticulum, an underdeveloped DMS, and a lack of granules. These observations suggest an essential role for FOG1–GATA1 interaction in thrombopoiesis. Genetic elimination of FOG in mice unexpectedly resulted in specific ablation of the megakaryocyte lineage, suggesting a GATA1-independent role for FOG in the early stages of

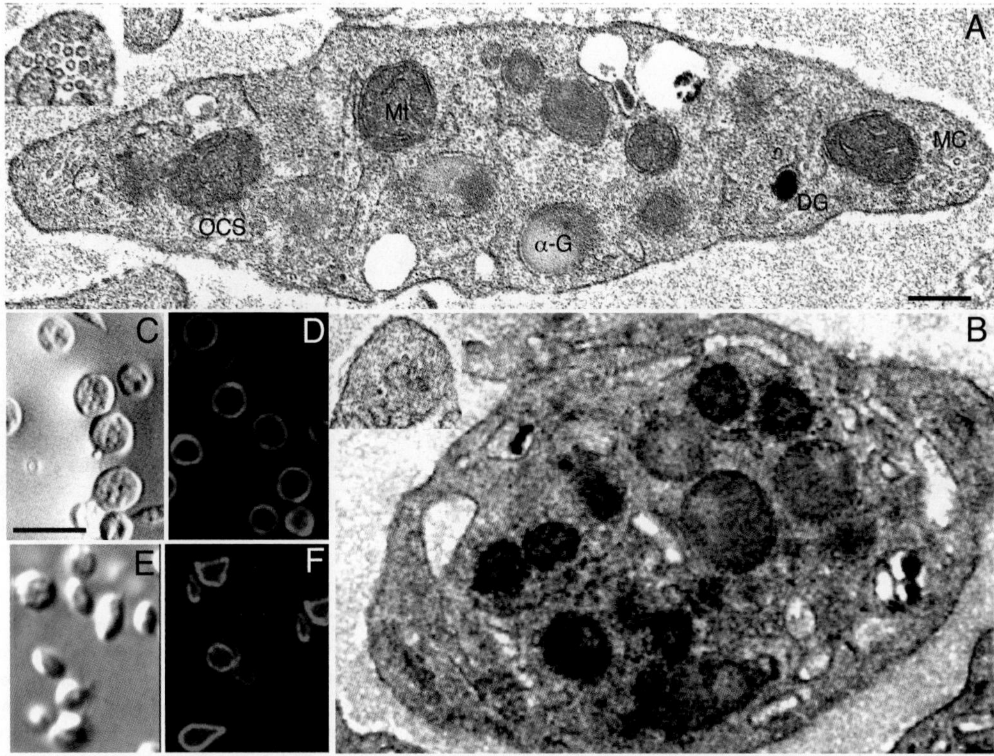

Figure 114–6 Structure of normal mouse platelets (**A**, **C**, **D**) compared to platelets lacking β_1 tubulin (**B**, **E**, **F**). **A**, Electron micrograph of a resting mouse platelet. This platelet was sectioned through its thin axis. The cut plane reveals the microtubule coil (MC) at the cell periphery. The inset shows a high-magnification cross-section through the microtubule coil of the resting platelet. The microtubule is wound 11 times in this platelet, forming the coil. The cytoplasmic space embeds mitochondria (MT), α granules (α-G), and dense granules (DG). The spaces created by the open canalicular system (OCS) are apparent. **B**, Electron micrograph of a thin section through a platelet isolated from a mouse lacking β_1 tubulin.[55] (Bar = 0.2 μm.) Platelets from these animals are spherical (E) and have only a rudimentary microtubule coil (inset). In this platelet the microtubule is twisted twice. **C**, Differential interference contrast image of resting platelets shows them to be flat discs. **D**, Microtubule coil of the resting mouse platelet. Staining of fixed mouse platelets with Alexa 488 antitubulin IgG reveals the microtubule coil. This coil resides at the periphery of the platelet. **E**, Differential interference contrast image of platelets lacking β_1 tubulin. **F**, Staining of fixed mouse β_1-tubulin–deficient platelets with Alexa 488 antitubulin IgG reveals the coil is defective and bent in a number of places throughout the platelets. (C–F are the same magnification; bar = 5 μm.)

megakaryocyte development.[80] GATA1 and FOG are required to generate megakaryocytes from a common bipotential progenitor.[80,81]

Several knockout mice also indicate a role for additional transcription factors in megakaryocyte development. Mice carrying a null mutation in Fli-1, a member of the ETS family of winged helix-turn-helix transcription factors that bind purine-rich sequences in gene promotors, exhibit defects in megakaryocyte development. Megakaryocytes cultured from mice lacking Fli-1 contain reduced numbers of α granules, disorganization of the demarcation membranes, and a reduction in size.[82,83] Mice lacking the hematopoietic zinc finger (Hzf) protein, a transcription factor that is predominantly expressed in megakaryocytes, have reduced numbers of α granules in megakaryocytes and platelets.[84] Therefore, Hzf may regulate the transcription of genes involved in the synthesis of α-granule components and/or their packaging into α granules. SCL, a basic helix-loop-helix transcription factor initially identified in a subset of human T-cell leukemia with multilineage characteristics, also appears to be critical for megakaryopoiesis. Deletion of SCL in mice indicates this transcription factor is required for proper erythroid and megakaryocyte development.[85,86]

PLATELETS

Structure of the Resting Platelet

Megakaryocyte development culminates with the release of mature discoid platelets having dimensions of approximately 3.0 × 0.5 μm and a cytoplasmic volume of 7 fL. The evolutionary explanation for the discoid shape of the platelet is unknown. Discoid shape may permit more efficient flow or dispersion of clot-promoting elements or may simply reflect the microtubule-based mechanism by which platelets are produced. In humans, platelets, once released from the ends of proplatelets, normally circulate for 7 to 10 days. Given that nearly one trillion platelets circulate in an adult human, each day an adult produces approximately 100 billion platelets.

The precise morphology of newly released platelets is unknown. However, once released into the circulation or maintained in culture, platelets have a very reproducible structure, although they are heterogeneous in size as a population in blood presumably due to changes in size as they age. Platelets have discoid shapes with flat, featureless surfaces (Figs. 114–6, *A* and 114–7, *A*) that are interrupted only by pit-like openings into the open canalicular system (OCS). The OCS is an extensive system of internal membrane conduits that serves as a passageway to the outside world into which granular contents release. It also is a reservoir of plasma membrane, membrane receptors, and proteins. For example, approximately 30% of the thrombin receptors are localized in the OCS of the resting cell, awaiting movement to the surface of the activated cells. Although contiguous with the plasma membrane, not all proteins on the cell surface can enter the OCS. Factors controlling movement into the OCS remain to be defined but likely depend on the actin cytoskeleton. Entry restriction, however, occurs at the necks of OCS infoldings. The third function of the OCS is to serve as a source of redundant plasma membrane for cell spreading. OCS membrane initially is disgorged to the surface following cell activation. When cells are activated in solution, much of this membrane subsequently is reabsorbed into the remnants of the OCS.

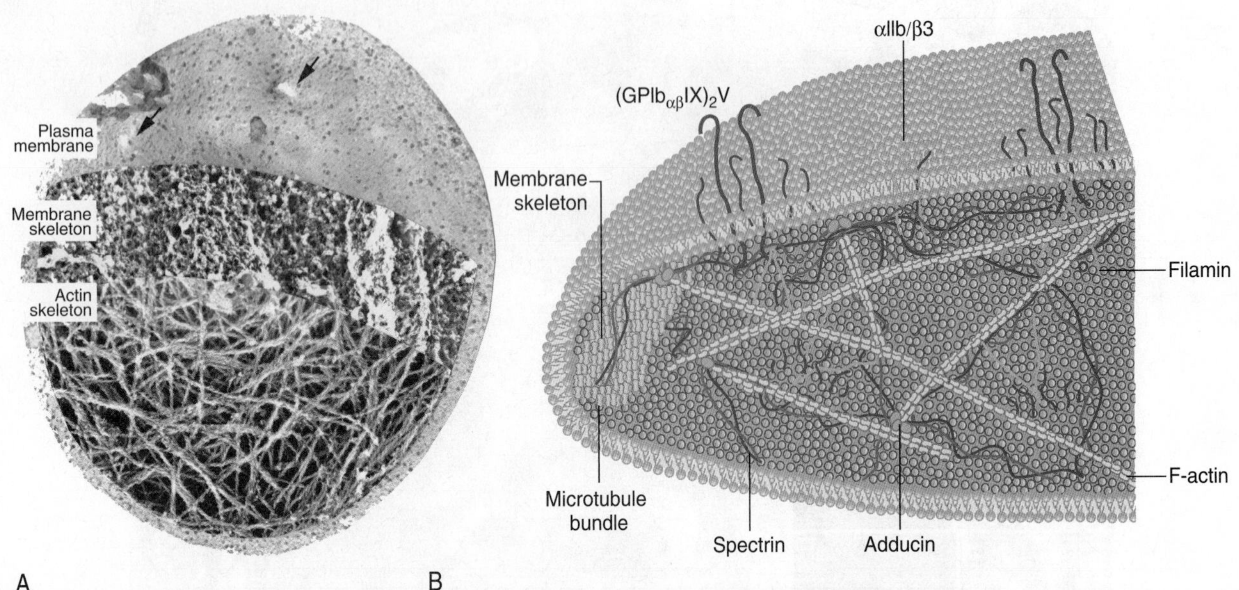

Figure 114–7 Structure of the resting human blood platelet and its actin-based cytoskeleton. **A**, Composite illustrating the major actin cytoskeletal layers of the resting platelet. Plasma Membrane: The plasma membrane of the resting cell is flat and featureless, except for periodic invaginations that lead into the open canalicular system (OCS) (arrows). Membrane Skeleton: The plasma membrane of the platelet is supported by a submembranous spectrin-based skeleton. This network is composed primarily of spectrin molecules, which are tetramers with actin binding sites at the ends. Actin filament ends dock on spectrin to complete the network. The association between spectrin and F actin is promoted by adducin. Actin Cytoskeleton: As discussed above, the spectrin network is both directly and indirectly attached to the underlying actin filaments. Filament ends interconnect spectrin molecules, while the filamin links run from the filament sides to the plasma membrane receptor $(GPIb_{\alpha\beta}IX)_2V$. The cytoplasmic space has a dense filling of actin filaments. Actin filaments from the cell center radiate outward. As the filaments approach the plasma membrane, they turn and run in parallel with it. The actin filaments have been decorated using myosin subfragment 1 (S1), which gives them a twisted cable-like appearance in frozen samples. Myosin S1 labeling reveals the polarity of the actin filament. "Pointed" and "barbed " ends are definable. The ends of actin filaments are bound by the ends of spectrin molecules on the edges of the membrane network (arrowhead). A microtubule coil composed of a single long microtubule resides just beneath the plasma membrane at the periphery of the thin axis of the platelet (not shown). (Bar = 0.5 μm.) **B**, Schematic showing the structural features of the resting blood platelet cytoskeleton. Resting cells have discoid shapes. Structural elements that support this shape are (1) a marginal microtubule coil, (2) a spectrin-based membrane skeleton, and (3) a rigid network of cross-linked cytoplasmic actin filaments (only a small number of the actin filaments have been added to this illustration so that they will not obscure the rest of the structures in the cell). Platelets have a specialized membrane skeleton composed of spectrin, actin, and many associated proteins. Spectrin tetramers (200 nm long and 5 nm wide) have actin filament binding sites at each molecular end. The membrane skeleton is held in compression between the plasma membrane and the cytoplasmic actin by filamin connections from the sides of actin filaments to the cytoplasmic tails of $GPIb_\alpha$ subunit of the membrane glycoprotein complex that binds to von Willebrand factor $(GPIb_{\alpha\beta}IX)_2V$ complex. Greater than 98% of the barbed ends of actin filaments are capped by adducin and capZ in the resting platelet.

A small thin zone of cytoplasm separates the plasma membrane of the resting platelet from a marginal microtubule coil and the general intracellular space, which contains all inclusion bodies and the internal cytoskeleton of the cell. This zone is filled with the spectrin-based membrane skeleton (see Fig. 114–7, *A*). Beneath this zone sits a microtubule coil. Then follows the cytoplasmic space, which is filled with filaments of actin that embed granules, organelles, the OCS, and other specialized membrane systems such as smooth endoplasmic reticulum.

Platelets actively recruit other bloodborne cells to areas of vascular damage by releasing mediators packaged in intracellular granules (described earlier in Cytoplasmic Maturation) that initiate secondary homeostatic interactions and that express a "sticky" apical surface after the platelets adhere. In the resting platelet, granules are juxtaposed together and are in intimate association with the membranes of the OCS. The release reaction of platelet granules differs from that of other cells. Granules rarely fuse with the plasma membrane; instead they exocytose into the OCS. Platelets also contain lysosomes and a few mitochondria, which are easily identified under the electron microscope by their internal system of membrane cristae.

Cytoskeleton of the Resting Platelet

Although both microtubule- and actin-based forces have been considered in the elaboration and branching of proplatelets, respectively, it is the integration of the microtubule and actin cytoskeletal elements that uniquely defines the shape of the mature platelet.

One of the most distinguishing features of the resting platelet is its marginal microtubule coil (see Fig. 114–6).[87] αβ–Tubulin dimers assemble into microtubule polymers under physiologic conditions. In resting platelets, tubulin is equally divided between dimer and polymer fractions. In many cell types, αβ-tubulin subunits are in a dynamic equilibrium with microtubules such that reversible cycles of assembly–disassembly of microtubules are observed. Microtubules are long hollow polymers (24 nm in diameter) that are responsible for many types of cellular movements, such as segregation of chromosomes during mitosis and transport of organelles across the cell. The microtubule ring of the resting platelet, initially characterized in the late 1960s by White and Krivit,[88] has been described as a single microtubule approximately 100 μm long and is coiled eight to 12 times inside the periphery of the platelet.[89] The primary function of the microtubule coil is to maintain the discoid shape of the resting platelet. Disassembly of platelet microtubules with drugs such as vincristine, colchicine, or nocodazole causes platelets to round and lose their discoid shape.[88] Cooling the platelets also causes disassembly of the microtubule coil and loss of the discoid shape.[87] Mice lacking the major hematopoietic β-tubulin isoform (β_1 tubulin) produce platelets that lack their characteristic discoid shapes and have defective marginal bands.[90] Genetic elimination of β_1 tubulin in mice results in thrombocytopenia with circulating platelet counts below 50% of normal. β_1-Tubulin–deficient platelets are spherical in shape,

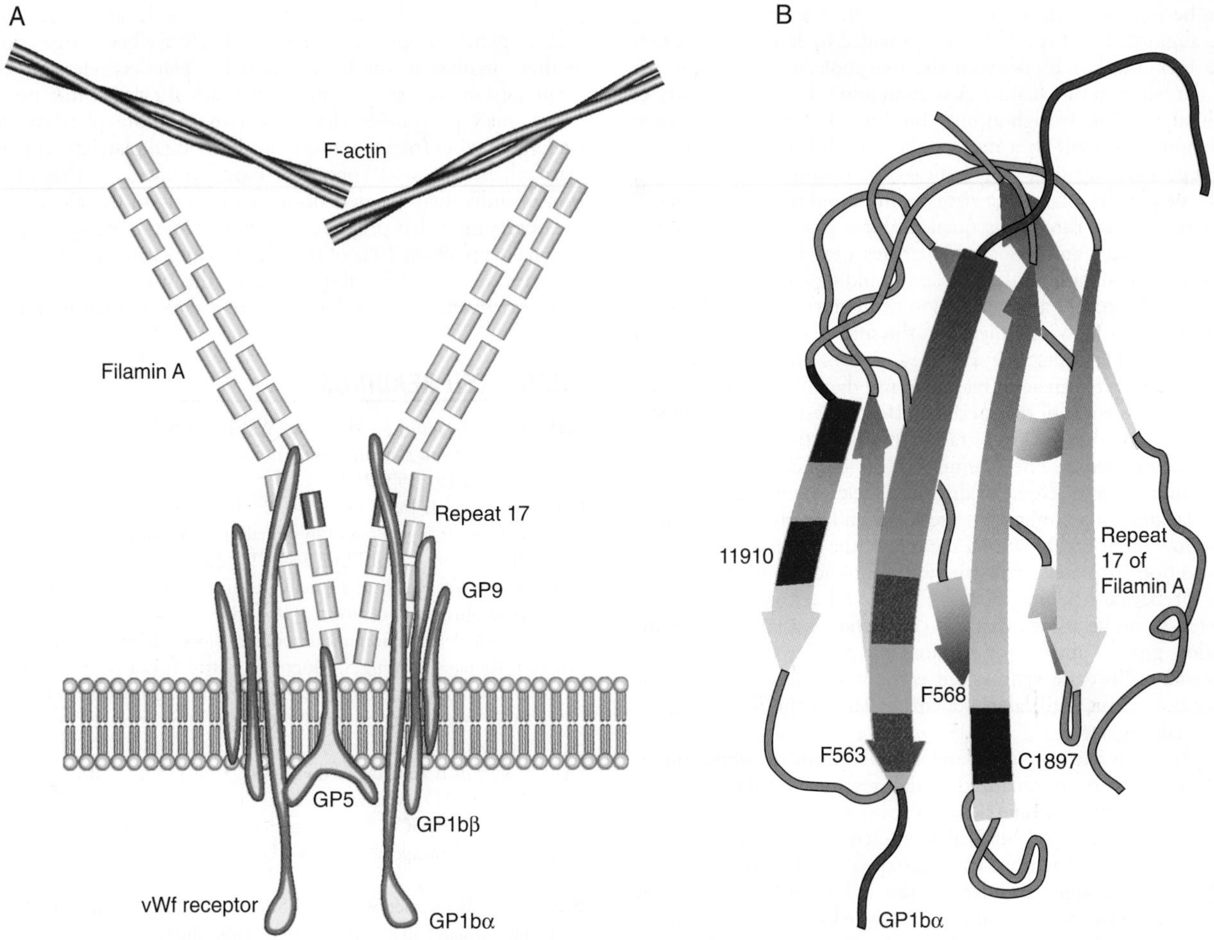

Figure 114–8 Interaction of filamin A with the von Willebrand factor receptor (vWFR). **A**, Model showing the orientation of filamin A when interacting with the GPIbα chain of the vWFR and cytoplasmic actin filaments. For tight binding of filamin A to vWFR, both GPIbα chains of the receptor must be engaged by a single filamin A molecule. **B**, Ribbon diagram showing the interface between filamin A repeat 17 and the filamin A binding region of the GPIbα tail (residues 556–577). Critical residues that provide the lock-and-key interaction between the two domains are indicated.

apparently due to shortened marginal bands with fewer coilings. Whereas normal platelets possess a marginal band that consists of eight to 12 coils, β_1-tubulin knockout platelets contain only two to three coils.[91] A human β_1-tubulin functional substitution (AG→CC) inducing both structural and functional platelet alterations has been described.[92] Interestingly, the Q43P β_1-tubulin variant was found in 10.6% of the general population and in 24.2% of 33 unrelated patients with undefined congenital macrothrombocytopenia. Electron microscopy revealed enlarged spherocytic platelets with a disrupted marginal band and structural alterations. Interestingly, platelets with the Q43P β_1-tubulin variant showed mild platelet dysfunction, with reduced ATP secretion, thrombin receptor-activating peptide (TRAP)-induced aggregation, and impaired adhesion to collagen under flow conditions. A more than doubled prevalence of the β_1-tubulin variant was observed in healthy subjects not undergoing ischemic events, suggesting it could confer an evolutionary advantage and a protective cardiovascular role.

Actin is the most abundant of all the platelet proteins, with two million molecules expressed per platelet.[59] Of these molecules, 800,000 assemble to form the 2000 to 5000 linear actin polymers that exist in the resting cell (see Fig. 114–7, *A*).[93] The rest of the actin is maintained in storage as a 1:1 complex with β_4 thymosin,[94] which can be converted to filaments during platelet activation to drive cell spreading. All evidence indicates that the filaments of the resting platelet are interconnected at various points into a rigid cytoplasmic network, as platelets express high concentrations of actin cross-linking proteins, including filamin[95,96] and α actinin.[97] Both filamin and α actinin are homodimers in solution. Three filamin genes are located on chromosomes 3, 7, and X. Filamin A (X)[98] and filamin B (3)[99] are expressed in platelets. Filamin A is expressed greater than 10-fold more than filamin B. Filamin subunits are elongated strands composed primarily of 24 repeats, each approximately 100 amino acids in length that are folded into IgG-like β barrels.[100,101] Each strand has an amino-terminus actin binding site that shares homology with other actin-binding proteins, two rod domains that are end-to-end assemblies of the repeat units, interrupted by two hinge domains between repeats 15 and 16, and 23 and 24, and a C-terminal self-association site (Fig. 114–8, *B*). Subunits assemble to form V-shaped bipolar molecules, that is, the self-association site is the vertex of the V, and the actin binding sites are on the free ends. Inclusion of the first hinge in filamin depends on alternative RNA splicing. Filamin now is recognized to be a prototype "scaffolding molecule" that collects binding partners and localizes them adjacent to the plasma membrane.[102] Partners bound by filamin members include the small GTPases RalA, Rac, Rho, and Cdc42, with RalA binding in a GTP-dependent manner[103]; the exchange factors Trio and Toll; kinases such as PAK1; phosphatases; and transmembrane proteins. Most partner proteins are bound within the carboxyl-terminal portion of filamin.[102]

Central to the structural organization of the resting platelet is an interaction between filamin and the cytoplasmic tail of the GPIbα subunit of the GPIb-IX-V complex. The second rod domain (repeat 17) of filamin has a binding site for the cytoplasmic tail of GPIbα.[104] The interaction between filamin A and GPIbα occurs at the atomic level.[105] Repeat 17 of filamin A has a groove between certain β-sheet strands that forms a pocket for the GPIbα tail (see Fig. 114–8).

Binding between filamin A and GPIbα is driven by entropic forces, and the alignment and specificity are provided by large residues that create a lock-and-key fit between the two molecules. Whereas the interaction between one filamin A subunit and GPIbα has affinity of approximately 10 μM, high-affinity binding (10 nM) results when each filamin A subunit in a molecule and both GPIbα chains in a vWF receptor are engaged. Biochemical experiments have shown that the bulk of platelet filamin (>90%) is in complex with GPIbα.[106] This interaction has three consequences. First, it posits filamin's self-association domain and associated partner proteins at the plasma membrane while dangling filamin's actin binding sites into the cytoplasm. Second, because a large fraction of filamin is bound to actin, it aligns the GPIb-IX-V complexes on the surface of the platelet over the underlying filaments (see Fig. 114–7, *B*). Third, because the filamin linkages between actin filaments and the GPIb-IX-V complex pass through the pores of the spectrin lattice, it restrains the molecular movement of the spectrin strands in this lattice and holds the lattice in compression. The filamin–GPIbα connection is essential for the formation and release of discoid platelets by megakaryocytes; platelets lacking this connection are large and fragile and are produced in low numbers. However, the role of the filamin–vWF receptor connection in platelet construction is unknown. Because a low number of Bernard-Soulier platelets form and release from megakaryocytes, it can be argued that this connection is a late event in the maturation process and is not required for platelet shedding. Both filamin and GPIbα are synthesized early, but linkage between the two may not occur until later, perhaps as late as the final stages of platelet shedding.

The platelet is the only cell besides the erythrocyte whose membrane skeleton has been visualized at high resolution. Like the erythrocyte, the platelet membrane skeleton is a self-assembly of elongated spectrin strands (see Fig. 114–7) that interconnect through binding to actin filaments. Platelets express approximately 2000 spectrin molecules.[93,107,108] Although considerably less is known about how the spectrin–actin network forms and is connected to the plasma membrane in the platelet relative to the erythrocyte, certain differences between the two membrane skeletons have been defined. First, the spectrin strands composing the platelet membrane skeleton interconnect using the ends of long actin filaments instead of short actin oligomers.[93] These ends arrive at the plasma membrane originating from filaments in the cytoplasm. Hence, the spectrin lattice is assembled into a continuous network by its association with actin filaments. Second, tropomodulins are not expressed at sufficiently high levels, if at all, to have a major role in capping the pointed ends of the platelet actin filaments. Instead, biochemical experiments have revealed that a substantial number (≈2000) of these ends are free in the resting platelet. Third, although little tropomodulin protein is expressed, α and γ adducin are abundantly expressed and appear to cap many of the barbed ends of the filaments composing the resting actin cytoskeleton.[109] Adducin is a key component of the membrane skeleton, forming a triad complex with spectrin and actin. Capping of barbed filament ends by adducin also serves the function of targeting them to the spectrin-based membrane skeleton, as the affinity of spectrin for adducin–actin complexes is greater than for either actin or adducin alone.[110–112] Platelet glycoproteins involved in attaching spectrin to the membrane remain to be defined.

Relationship Between Structure of the Circulating Platelet and That of Nascent Platelets Released by Megakaryocytes

Because the final phase of platelet birth has not been visualized, the size and shape of platelets released are unknown. Given that young platelets in animals made thrombocytopenic are larger than the normal platelet population, platelets likely are born large and shrink as they circulate in the blood. Whether platelets release as discs, as essentially discoid shapes but with residual cytoplasmic protrusion, or as small proplatelet chains of two or more platelets that can undergo further fragmentation into individual platelets remains to be clarified. Behnke and Forer[113,114] have hypothesized that the formation of individual platelets occurs exclusively in the blood, based on the observation that proplatelet-like structures circulate in blood and can make up 5% to 20% of the platelets in plasma. Dumbbell-shaped particles are found in abundance in the media of megakaryocyte cultures, which suggests that they are a preferred release form.

SUGGESTED READINGS

Barkalow K, Italiano J Jr, Matsuoka Y, Bennett V, Hartwig J: Alpha-Adducin dissociates from F-actin filaments and spectrin during platelet activation. J Cell Biol 161:557, 2003.

Clarke M, Savill J, Jones D, Noble B, Brown S: Compartmentalized megakaryocyte death generates functional platelets committed to caspase-independent death. J Cell Bbiol 160:577, 2003.

Freson K, De Vos R, Wittevrognel C, et al: The β1-tubulin Q43P functional polymorphism reduces the risk of cardiovascular disease in men by modulating platelet function and structure. Blood 106:2356, 2005.

Gaur M, Kamata T, Wang S, Moran B, Shattil S, Leavitt A: Megakaryocytes derived from human embryonic stem cells: A genetically tractable system to study megakaryocytopoiesis and integrin function. J Thromb Haemost 4:436, 2006.

Geng Y: Cyclin E ablation in the mouse. Cell 114:431, 2003.

Hall M, Curtis D, Metcalf D, et al: The critical regulator of embryonic hematopoiesis, SCL, is vital in the adult for megakaryopoiesis, erythropoiesis, and lineage choice in CFU-S. Proc Natl Acad Sci U S A 100:992, 2003.

Italiano J Jr, Bergmeier W, Tiwari S, et al: Mechanisms and implications of platelet discoid shape. Blood 101:4789, 2003.

Kozar K: Mouse development and cell proliferation in the absence of D-cyclins. Cell 118:477, 2004.

Mikkola H, Klintman J, Yang H, et al: Hematopoietic stem cells retain long-term repopulating activity and multipotency in the absence of stem cell leukemia SCL/tal-1 gene. Nature 421:547, 2003.

Nakamura F, Pudas R, Heikkinen O, et al: The structure of the GP1b-filamin A complex. Blood 107:1925, 2005.

Pang L, Weiss M, Poncz M: Megakaryocyte biology and related disorders. J Clin Invest 115:3332, 2005.

Patel S, Hartwig J, Italiano J Jr: The biogenesis of platelets from megakaryocyte proplatelets. J Clin Invest 115:3348, 2006.

Raslova H, Roy L, Vourc'h C, et al: Megakaryocyte polyploidization is associated with a functional gene amplification. Blood 101:541, 2003.

Richardson J, Shivdasani R, Boers C, Hartwig J, Italiano J Jr: Mechanisms of organelle transport and capture along proplatelets during platelet production. Blood 106:4066, 2005.

Schulze H, Korpal M, Hurov J, et al: Characterization of the megakaryocyte demarcation membrane system and its role in thrombopoiesis. Blood 107:3868, 2006.

REFERENCES

For complete list of references log onto www.expertconsult.com

CHAPTER 115

THE MOLECULAR BASIS OF PLATELET FUNCTION

Charles S. Abrams and Edward F. Plow

Platelets ordinarily circulate in blood vessels as individual cells that do not interact with other platelets or other cell types. A transition from this nonadhesive to an adhesive state can be rapidly initiated if platelets are exposed to a stimulatory agonist. Platelet adhesive reactions that may be initiated in response to an injury to a blood vessel wall, as exemplified by rupture of an atherosclerotic plaque, are shown in Fig. 115–1. Disruption of the endothelial cell lining of the vessel exposes constituents within the subendothelial matrix, including a variety of adhesive proteins that can support initial platelet attachment. After attachment, platelets may undergo a spreading reaction that permits formation of multiple and tight contacts between the cell surface and the matrix. These additional contacts may be critical in stabilizing the association of the platelets with the matrix in flowing blood. In conjunction with these adhesive reactions, the cells encounter agonists in the microenvironment that can trigger platelet secretion. The platelet secretory response results in the release of contents of intracellular storage granules. Granule constituents include substances, such as adenosine diphosphate (ADP), which can stimulate circulating platelets and cause them to acquire new adhesive properties. These stimulated platelets interact with one another, during platelet aggregation, to form an effective plug that seals the injured vessel wall and prevents excessive blood loss. This series of platelet responses (attachment, spreading, secretion, and aggregation) is essential for the hemostatic function of platelets. Nevertheless, these same events, occurring on an injured endothelial cell or on an atherosclerotic plaque, may result in the formation of a platelet-rich thrombus, which can compromise the patency of the blood vessel and lead to thrombosis. At the other extreme, abnormalities in platelet adhesive reactions of either a genetic (e.g., Glanzmann thrombasthenia or Bernard-Soulier syndrome; see Chapter 141) or an acquired origin (e.g., drug-induced thrombocytopenia; see Chapter 140) can result in bleeding. Thus, platelet adhesive reactions and secretion are central events in health and disease processes. Bleeding, hemostasis, and thrombosis are in delicate balance and are regulated by these platelet functions.

This chapter addresses the molecular basis of platelet adhesive reactions and secretory responses. Great strides have been made in defining the mechanisms that govern these functional responses. At the heart of these platelet responses are ligand–receptor interactions. The platelet has often served as a model cell type for studying ligand–receptor interactions and establishing basic mechanisms of cell adhesion and secretion.

MOLECULAR BASIS OF PLATELET ADHESION

Studies in vitro, particularly under flow conditions (i.e., in closed chambers permitting whole blood or isolated components to flow across a selected matrix at selected shears), and in vivo experiments using transgenic mouse models in which specific molecules have been deleted, mutated, or overexpressed have demonstrated the complexity of the reactions leading to thrombus formation, growth, and stability. For simplicity, we dissect these events; however, in reality these events occur very rapidly and often in overlapping fashion.

Substrates for Platelet Attachment and Spreading

Some of the major subendothelial matrix proteins that support platelet attachment or spreading reactions are listed in Table 115–1. From the extent of this list, it is clear that the platelet can adhere to a variety of substrates once the endothelium has been disrupted. The endothelium must also create an effective barrier to prevent circulating platelets from reaching the matrix and initiating thrombus formation. In addition to serving as a physical barrier, endothelial cells synthesize and elaborate components, notably prostaglandin I_2, nitric oxide, and an enzyme termed CD39 that degrades ADP, which prevent platelet activation and impart a nonthrombogenic character to the normal endothelium (see Chapters 116 and 117).

Studies of mice deficient in individual matrix proteins have documented the involvement of multiple adhesive proteins in the formation, growth, and stability of platelet-rich thrombi.[1–4] Several considerations affect the role of individual matrix constituents in mediating platelet adhesion:

1. Not all of the adhesive proteins listed in Table 115–1 support the same spectrum of platelet adhesive responses. For example, under some conditions, platelets attach to, but do not spread on, laminin,[1] whereas von Willebrand factor (vWF) and fibronectin support cell attachment and spreading.[5–7] Collagen not only supports the attachment and spreading of platelets but can provoke a secretory response.[8] Of the multiple forms of collagen, types I, III, and VI are regarded as particularly important in supporting platelet adhesion.
2. A wealth of evidence indicates that the phenotypic properties of endothelial cells from different blood vessels vary, as does the composition of the subendothelial matrix. The characteristics of the endothelial cells may differ even within the same vessel. Areas of turbulent flow, which occur at bifurcations of vessels, are prone to development of atherosclerotic lesions, and shear-responsive elements in the promoters of certain genes can lead to changes in the expression of endothelial proteins[9,10] and alterations in their adhesive properties.[11,12] Thus, certain proteins may play a dominant role in supporting platelet adhesion in certain blood vessels.
3. Shear rate developed by flowing blood varies with vessel caliber and greatly influences platelet adhesion. Shear is particularly important in defining the contribution of vWF to platelet adhesion. Patients with von Willebrand disease (see Chapter 129) have a major bleeding diathesis, attesting to the importance of vWF in supporting platelet function. However, in vitro experiments show a role for vWF in platelet adhesion at high but not at low shear rates.[6,13] In contrast, a role for fibronectin in supporting platelet adhesion can be demonstrated at both high and low shear.[14,15] Both proteins have been implicated in thrombus formation.[2,4]
4. A variety of adhesive proteins interact with one another. For example, vWF, fibronectin, and thrombospondin all bind to collagen[16–18] (although they exhibit differential reactivity with different collagen types). These interactions may bridge the platelet to a matrix protein or may modulate the adhesive properties of a matrix protein.
5. Several adhesive proteins are present in platelet secretory granules, plasma, or both, as well as being matrix constituents. vWF and

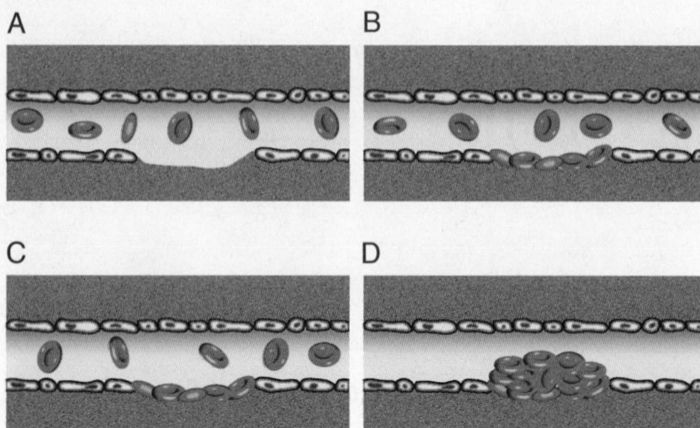

Figure 115–1 Hemostatic response of platelets to injury. **A**, Disruption of the endothelial cell lining of the blood vessel exposes constituents of the subendothelial matrix. **B**, Platelets attach to, and spread on, the matrix constituents. **C**, Platelet secretion may be initiated. **D**, Released platelet constituents can activate additional platelets, which aggregate and form a thrombus.

Table 115–1 Some Major Subendothelial Matrix Constituents That Support Platelet Adhesion

Matrix Constituent	Comment
Collagens	Large family of proteins with certain members supporting platelet adhesion, aggregation, and secretion
von Willebrand factor	Large multimeric protein critical for hemostatic function of platelets
Fibronectin	Dimeric or multimeric protein that supports attachment and spreading of platelets
Thrombospondin-1	Trimeric protein exhibiting both adhesive and antiadhesive properties
Laminins	Proteins supporting platelet attachment
Microfibrils	Fibular bundle of protein constituents found in certain matrices

Table 115–2 Platelet Receptors for Adhesive Proteins

Ligand	Receptor(s)	Other Common Designations
Collagen	GPIa-IIa, $\alpha_2\beta_1$	VLA-2
	GPIIb-IIIa, $\alpha_{IIb}\beta_3$	GPIIIb
	GPIV	CD36
	GPVI	
Fibrinogen	GPIIb-IIIa, $\alpha_{IIb}\beta_3$	
	Vitronectin receptor, $\alpha_v\beta_3$	
Fibronectin	GPIc-IIa, $\alpha_5\beta_1$	VLA-5
	GPIIb-IIIa, $\alpha_{IIb}\beta_3$	
Thrombospondin	Vitronectin receptor, $\alpha_v\beta_3$	GPIIIb
	GPIV	CD36
	Integrin-associated protein	IAP
Vitronectin	Vitronectin receptor, $\alpha_v\beta_3$	
	GPIIb-IIIa, $\alpha_{IIb}\beta_3$	
von Willebrand factor	GPIb-V-IX	
	GPIIb-IIIa, $\alpha_{IIb}\beta_3$	
Laminin	GPIc-IIa region, $\alpha_6\beta_1$	VLA-6

GP, glycoprotein; VLA, very late antigen.

fibronectin are present in all three locations, and thrombospondin is a major platelet granule constituent.[19,20] Proteins from all three sources (matrix, platelet, and plasma) contribute to platelet adhesion. The adhesive proteins derived from these different sources may be functionally distinct because they are not structurally identical. For example, the degree of vWF and fibronectin multimerization differs for molecules derived from plasma and the matrix. With fibronectin, the splice forms of the molecules derived from plasma and platelets differ.[21]

6. Matrix proteins are subject to degradation by a variety of proteolytic enzymes. Such proteolysis can modulate the adhesive properties of the matrix proteins. In some cases, cryptic adhesive sequences can be exposed that interact with additional sets of platelet adhesion receptors.[22,23]

Overall, the subendothelial matrix should be viewed as a dynamic and mutable interface that provides multiple substrates that support platelet adhesion.

Platelet Adhesion Receptors

The individual adhesive proteins come in contact with the platelet by serving as ligands for specific cell surface receptors (Table 115–2). Because several nomenclature systems have been used to identify the membrane proteins of the platelet, the same receptor may have multiple designations. One of the most widely used nomenclatures is based on electrophoretic mobility of the membrane proteins on polyacrylamide gel systems, in which the higher-molecular-weight proteins move more slowly. This separation gave rise to glycoprotein (GP) I, II, III, and so on, with GPI having the highest molecular weight. As the gel systems used became more discriminating, several proteins were discerned in the GPI position, hence GPIa, GPIb, and GPIc, and so forth.[24] Further refinement still is required; for example, there are at least three distinct polypeptides in the GPIc position. Several of the membrane proteins exist on the platelet surface as noncovalent complexes; thus, GPIb-V-IX-V, GPIc-IIa, and GPIIb-IIIa can be regarded as single-membrane proteins. Several of these membrane proteins are members of the integrin family of adhesion receptors (see Integrin Family of Adhesion Receptors), and the integrin nomenclature now tends to prevail in designating these particular membrane proteins (e.g., GPIc-IIa now is most commonly referred to as $\alpha_5\beta_1$ and GPIIb-IIIa as $\alpha_{IIb}\beta_3$). Other nomenclature systems have arisen from the fact that several platelet membrane proteins are present and have been assigned different names on other cell types. This is the basis for the VLA (very late antigen) designations for some of the platelet membrane proteins. Similarly, certain proteins also have extracellular matrix (ECM) and leukocyte differentiation antigens (CD) designations. Some receptors have been named based on their function (e.g., vitronectin, fibrinogen, and fibronectin receptors). Although functional designations seem highly appropriate from a descriptive standpoint, at least two membrane proteins on platelets can serve as receptors for vitronectin, fibrinogen, and fibronectin (see Table 115–2), and several platelet constituents have been referred to as collagen receptors (see Collagen Receptors). With the exception of the CD identifications, the latter nomenclature systems now are rarely used compared to the GP and integrin nomenclature but still may be encountered in reference to particular membrane proteins in the older platelet literature. Beyond creating a nomenclature complexity, the redundancy of the platelet receptors enables the cell to establish multiple contacts with a single matrix constituent; thus, a single ligand may initiate several distinct functional responses by engaging different receptors.

Integrin Family of Adhesion Receptors

Many of the adhesive protein receptors on platelets are members of the integrin family. The integrins are a broadly distributed family of

Table 115–3 Platelet integrins

Integrin	Major Ligands
$\alpha_2\beta_1$ (GPIa-IIa, VLA-2)	Collagen
$\alpha_5\beta_1$ (GPIc-IIa, VLA-5)	Fibronectin
$\alpha_{IIb}\beta_3$ (GPIIb-IIIa)	Fibrinogen, fibronectin, vitronectin, von Willebrand factor, CD40L
$\alpha_V\beta_3$ (Vitronectin receptor)	Fibrinogen, fibronectin, vitronectin, von Willebrand factor, thrombospondin, osteopontin
$\alpha_6\beta1$ (GPIc-IIa region)	Laminin

GP, glycoprotein; VLA, very late antigen.

heterodimeric (two subunits) cell surface molecules that share certain structural, immunochemical, and functional properties.[25–33] The β subunits, of which eight are known, are highly homologous to one another, exhibiting at least 35% to 45% identity at the primary amino acid sequence level and a common structural organization. The α subunits, of which 14 are known, also are similar to one another but exhibit less extensive sequence identity.[34,35]

The α subunits fall into two categories: those with and those without I (also called A) domains. Integrin I domains are inserted domains of approximately 200 amino acids that frequently are involved in ligand binding of the integrins containing them.[36] Only one of the major integrins on platelets, $\alpha_2\beta_1$, a collagen receptor, contains an I domain in its α subunit. The α subunits are synthesized as single-chain polypeptides; some, such as α_{IIb}, are proteolytically processed to a two-chain form.[37–40] Each β subunit combines in a noncovalent complex with an α subunit to form a functional adhesive protein receptor. A single β subunit can combine with several α subunits.

Platelets express two major β subunits, β_1 and β_3 (β_2 has been reported to be present at low levels but this requires confirmation),[41] and five α subunits (Table 115–3). Of the integrins expressed on blood cells, $\alpha_{IIb}\beta_3$ is the most narrowly distributed and is restricted predominantly to platelets/megakaryocytes. $\alpha_{IIb}\beta_3$ plays a prominent role in platelet aggregation and many other platelet responses, including the association of platelets with tumor cells, an interaction important to the metastatic dissemination of neoplastic cells.[42–44]

Role of GPIb-V-IX in Platelet Adhesion

GPIb-V-IX is a notable example of a cell surface molecule involved in platelet adhesion that is not a member of the integrin family.[45] Platelets from patients with Bernard-Soulier syndrome lack GPIb-V-IX, and patients with this syndrome have a marked bleeding diathesis (see Chapter 141).[46–48] A major role of GPIb-V-IX in hemostasis can be traced directly to its function as a receptor for vWF. vWF is composed of multiple functional domains, including the 24-kd A1 domain that binds to the amino-terminus of GPIbα and interacts, along with the A3 domain, with matrix constituents such as collagen and microfibrils (see Chapter 128).[16,49–55] Thus, by associating with matrix proteins, vWF directly mediates rapid and reversible platelet adhesion that promotes the rolling of these cells along the surface of vascular injury.[56] This rolling may transiently bridge the cells to subendothelial matrix components until a more stable adhesive bond forms. Integrins are the most likely receptors responsible for the stable platelet-adhesive bond that permanently halts the rolling of the platelet. In vitro, vWF does not interact directly with GPIb on platelets. An interaction can be measured in the presence of ristocetin, an antibiotic, or botrocetin, a snake venom peptide. Altered forms of vWF, such as asialo-vWF (protein treated to remove sialic acid residues from its carbohydrate moieties) and bovine vWF, can interact directly with platelets.[57–59] High shear appears to serve as the physiologic counterpart of ristocetin or botrocetin in humans. High shear alters the conformation of vWF, permitting their high-affinity interaction.[60,61] Such high shear stress can be attained in the microcirculation or in narrowed arteries.

Several laboratories have reported the structures of the vWF A1 domain as well as A1 domain mutants interacting with the GPIbα complex.[62–64] The globular vWF A1 domain interacts with the amino-terminus of GPIbα. This vWF-binding region of GPIβα is composed of two β loops flanking a backbone composed of eight leucine-rich repeats. This entire interaction depends on the displacement of the termini of the vWF A1 domains, an event that likely occurs under shear conditions present at the sites of vascular injury.

The role of GPIb in hemostasis is not restricted to its vWF binding function. GPIb also can serve as a binding site for thrombin,[65,66] and this activity plays an important role in the generation of platelet microparticles and procoagulant activity.[67–70] GPIb also is a target for certain drug-induced platelet antibodies[71] and is a counter-receptor for $\alpha_M\beta_2$ (CD11b/CD18 [Mac-1]) leukocyte integrin, an interaction that helps to mediate platelet-leukocyte conjugates.[72] The full primary structures of GPIb,[73,74] GPIX,[75] and GPV[76] were determined from cDNA cloning approaches in the 1980s. GPIb is composed of a heavy chain (α) and a light chain (β), both of which span the platelet membrane. GPIbα associates with the cytoskeleton within the platelet.[46,77–79] This chain is highly susceptible to proteolysis, and a large proteolytic fragment, glycocalicin, can be detected in the plasma of some patients with thrombocytopenic disorders.[80] GPIX is a small, single-chain polypeptide with a molecular weight of 20,000 Da. The contribution of GPIX to the function of GPIb-V-IX is uncertain. GPV also is deficient in Bernard-Soulier platelets and forms a loose association with GPIb-V-IX.[48,67,68] Platelets from mice deficient in GPV show enhanced sensitivity to thrombin, which may reflect a role of GPV in controlling the thrombin-binding function of GPIb.[81] An important consequence of occupancy of GPIb-V-IX by vWF is the induction of intracellular signaling events that ultimately lead to activation of $\alpha_{IIb}\beta_3$ and then platelet aggregation (see Aggregation response of platelets).[46,82] Such communication between adhesion receptors is a repeating theme for platelets as well as other cells. Key events in this communication between platelet receptors may include changes in the phosphorylation of the cytoplasmic tails of GPIb-V-IX and their association with the signaling molecule 14.3.3.[83,84]

Collagen Receptors

Subendothelial collagen has been long recognized as an important initiator of platelet responses, serving both as a substrate for platelet adhesion and as a potent platelet agonist. Three different receptors have been implicated in platelet responses to collagen.[85] The first receptor is the GPIb-V-IX complex. The second receptor, $\alpha_2\beta_1$ (also known as VLA-2, platelet GPIa-IIa), is a member of the integrin family of adhesion receptors and primarily serves as an anchor for platelets to attach to collagen exposed after disruptions in the vascular endothelial layer.[86] A patient with an acquired deficiency of this integrin exhibited a mild bleeding diathesis.[87,88] In addition to binding collagen with high affinity, $\alpha_2\beta_1$ binds laminins, E-cadherins, matrix metalloproteins, C1q, echovirus, and rotavirus. The identification of a patient with a mild bleeding diathesis who had normal amounts of $\alpha_2\beta_1$ but marked reduced amounts of platelet GPVI suggested that GPVI also served as an important collagen receptor.[89] It also can serve as a collagen adhesion receptor (at least under low shear conditions). Mice that lack GPVI on the surface of their platelets have a complete loss of collagen-induced platelet activation and a profound defect in collagen adhesion.[90] The deficiency of GPVI on platelets can be generated by inactivating either GPVI or Fc receptor γ-chain (FcRγ) genes. The latter forms a complex with GPVI and is required for surface expression of GPVI.[88] In contrast, $\alpha_2\beta_1$ serves primarily as an auxiliary receptor for platelet adhesion to collagen and functions as an agonist receptor only under unusual circumstances.[86]

Experiments using receptor-blocking antibodies, heterologously expressed receptors, and genetically altered mice have elucidated the

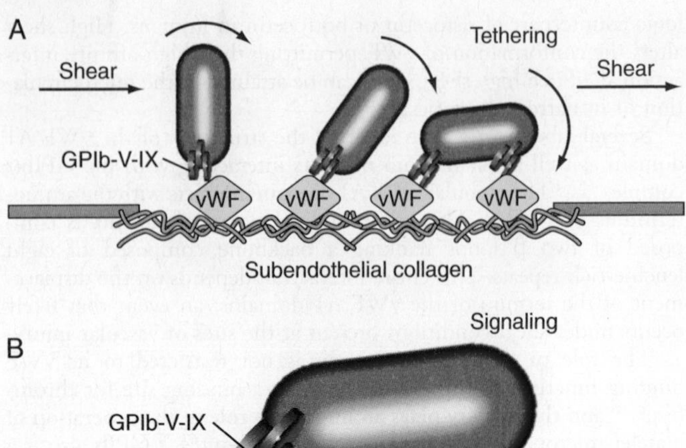

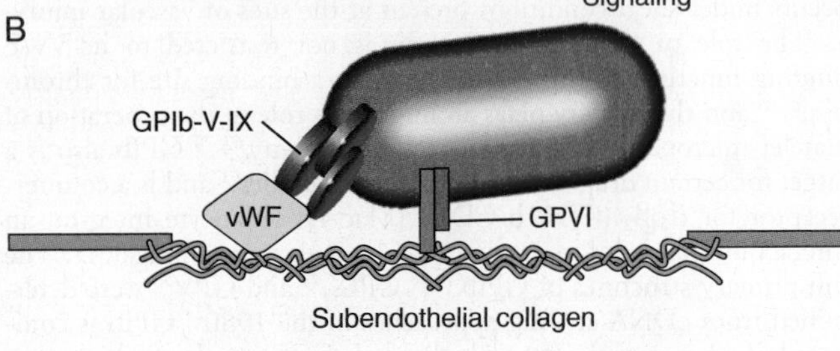

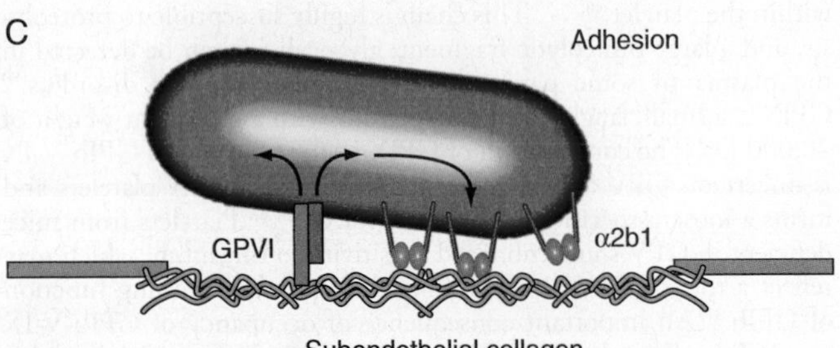

Figure 115–2 Adhesion to collagen is a multistep process. **A**, Once exposed to an injured vascular wall, von Willebrand factor adheres to subendothelial collagen and undergoes a conformational change that allows it to bind to the platelet receptor glycoprotein Ib/V/IX (GPIb-V-IX). This rapidly formed bond is quickly broken and reestablished, causing the platelet to roll along the injured vascular wall. **B**, The rolling process slows down the platelet and allows the platelet signaling receptor GPVI to bind collagen. **C**, This process induces a cascade of signaling events that ultimately activate the integrin $\alpha_2\beta_1$. This final association between the platelet and collagen is stable and allows the platelet to firmly adhere to the vessel wall.

relative roles of each of these proteins.[86,90–93] Platelet adhesion to collagen is a multistep process (Fig. 115–2). Initially platelets adhere to collagen-immobilized vWF via platelet GPIb-V-IX. This is a rapidly formed but short-lived interaction that only transiently tethers the platelet. The interaction repeatedly forms and breaks, thereby causing the platelet to slowly roll along the surface of vWF immobilized upon exposed collagen. Ultimately, GPVI directly interacts with collagen. GPVI is a low affinity receptor, but is capable of stimulatory intracellular signaling pathways. As a result of this signaling cascade, $\alpha_2\beta_1$ is induced to bind collagen with high affinity. This latter interaction promotes the stable association of platelets with collagen. The interaction between platelets and collagen is complex, and whether pharmacologic inhibition of either platelet collagen receptor has a therapeutic benefit is not known.

Reorganization of the Actin Cytoskeleton

One of the more dramatic events during platelet activation is the metamorphosis that occurs when platelets adhere and spread on exposed collagen fibrils or become activated in the circulation by soluble factors such as thrombin or ADP. In either case, platelets lose their distinct discoid shape and acquire an irregular morphology with multiple filopodial projections.[94] This transformation is associated with, and largely due to, cytoskeletal rearrangements within the platelet.[95] The proteins are arranged in three major structures: a cytoplasmic actin network, a rim of membrane-associated cytoskeleton, and a marginal band consisting of a microtubule coil.[96] Together, these structures lend support to the platelet plasma membrane and give shape to both resting and activated platelets.

The cytoplasmic actin network is composed of actin filaments and associated proteins. Actin is a 42-kd protein that accounts for as much as 20% of total platelet protein.[96] In resting platelets, 40% to 50% of the actin is present as filamentous F-actin; the remainder is present as globular monomeric G-actin.[97,98] The shift to increase the proportion of F-actin to 70% to 80% during platelet activation involves a coordinated sequence of events in which the actin filaments present in resting platelets are severed and the resultant smaller fragments are used as the nidus for new, longer actin filaments. This process is thought to be regulated in part by the increase in levels of a phosphatidylinositol-4,5-bisphosphate (PIP_2) that accompanies platelet activation.[99,100] At the same time, myosin is phosphorylated by myosin light chain kinase and becomes associated with F-actin, forming filaments that are anchored to the platelet plasma membrane by attachment (via actin-binding protein) to the glycoprotein Ib/V/IX complex.[101,102]

The cytoskeletal rim is composed of actin, filamin, P235 (talin), vinculin, spectrin, α actinin, and several membrane glycoproteins. Filamin is an elongated 280-kd protein that is present in platelets and functions as an actin-binding protein.[103] In resting platelets, filamin is part of a semirigid array that helps maintain the platelet's discoid shape and limits the lateral movement of GPIb.[77,104,105] This role is analogous to that performed by spectrin in erythrocytes.[78] When platelets are activated, actin filaments form and attach to actin-binding protein. Later the rising cytosolic Ca^{2+} concentration activates calpain, which cleaves actin-binding protein, severing the link to GPIb.[104,106,107]

The third major structural element in platelets is the marginal microtubule band.[96] This microtubule coil is a tightly wound polymer of tubulin that encircles the platelet perimeter and helps maintain its discoid shape.[108] During platelet activation, the microtubule coil contracts. That contraction of the marginal band is required for stable adhesion of platelets under arterial shear pressures has been proposed; however, this theory remains controversial.[109,110]

PLATELET SECRETION

The foregoing discussion has emphasized the adhesive functions of platelets in mediating the physical closure of breaks in blood vessels. Another important function of platelets is the release of a variety of substances that stimulate or inhibit platelets or other blood and vascular cells, which can covalently modify the thrombus and affect its mechanical properties, as well as regulate coagulation, contribute to cell adhesive events, and modulate the growth of cells of the vessel wall. Thus, the platelet is not simply the stop plug of the vasculature; it also has the capacity to signal its presence in a thrombus and modify the hemostatic response in a variety of ways. In addition, although platelets do not contain a nucleus, they do contain mRNA and may synthesize some proteins.[111,112] Although such synthesis had long been regarded as a vestigial activity of megakaryocytes, data indicate that a restricted repertoire of proteins, which are related to apoptosis and inflammation, are produced,[113] and a functional importance to the platelet "transcriptome" has been suggested.[112] Most of these substances that are actively and selectively secreted from platelets are packaged in preformed storage granules, or are synthesized de novo from membrane phospholipids. Platelets contain three types of granules: (a) dense granules containing platelet agonists that serve to amplify platelet activation, (b) α granules containing proteins that enhance the adhesive process, and (c) lysosomal granules containing glycosidases and proteases that have an unclear function in platelet biology.[114] In addition, factors in the platelet cytoplasm released as a

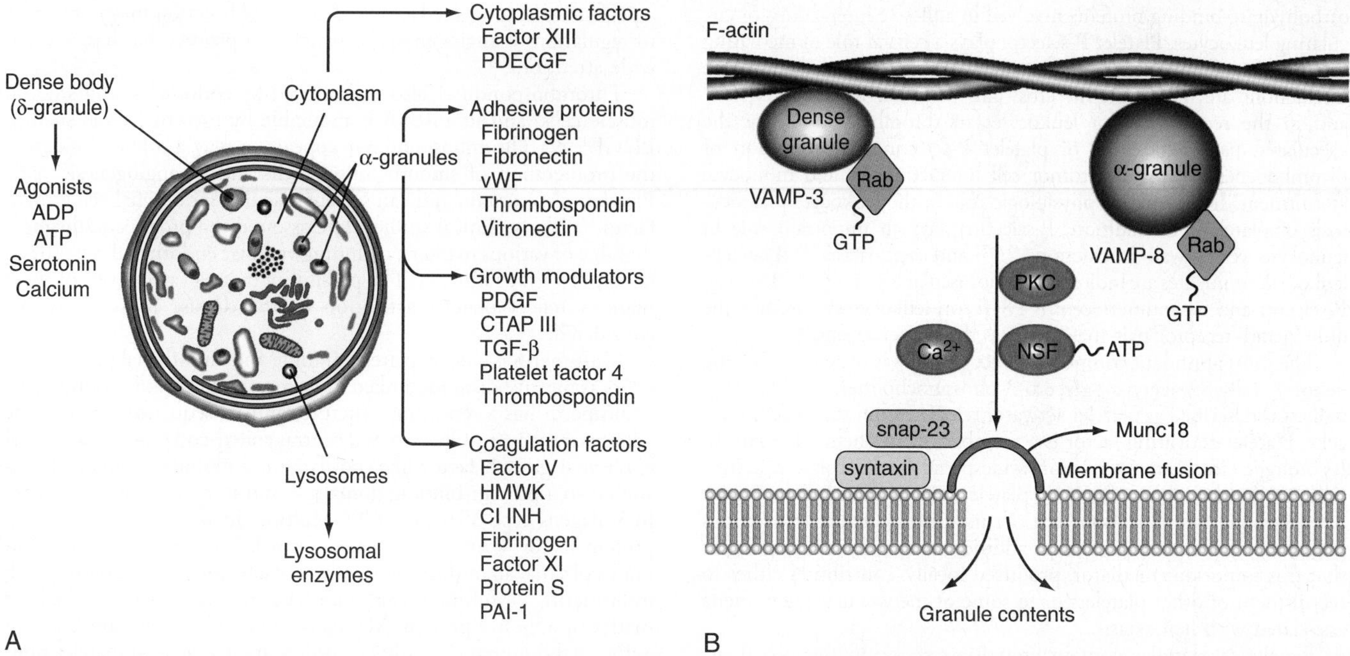

Figure 115–3 **A**, Substances released by platelets and their intraplatelet sources. Illustrated are some of the bioactive substances released from dense bodies, α granules, lysosomes, cytoplasm, and platelet membrane. **B**, In resting platelets, the actin cytoskeleton must be disassembled prior to platelet secretion. Secretion of α and dense granules occurs through a complex signaling pathway dependent on small GTPases, protein kinases, and members of the SNARE/SNAP family. These signaling pathways are highly homologous to those used during neuronal cell exocytosis. C1 INH, C1 inhibitor; CTAP, connective tissue-activating peptide; HETEs, hydroxyeicosatetraenoic acids; HMWK, high-molecular-weight kininogen; PAF, platelet-activating factor; PAI-1, plasminogen activator inhibitor 1; PDECGF, platelet-derived endothelial cell growth factor; PDGF, platelet-derived growth factor; TGF-β, transforming growth factor-β; vWF, von Willebrand factor.

result of minor degrees of platelet lysis during hemostasis can have effects on thrombus structure or vascular cell growth. Some of these factors and their intraplatelet sources are shown in Fig. 115–3, *A*.

Dense Granules

The dense bodies and platelet membranes are a source of rapidly secreted mediators. These mediators either are quickly inactivated or are promptly diffused away from the site of the thrombus; thus, they function for only a brief period of time. Their rapid effects on surrounding cells serve to modulate the behavior of platelets as well as the behavior of vessel wall cells (particularly with regard to vascular tone.)

Platelets contain approximately three to eight dense granules that are the most rapidly secreted of platelet organelles.[115] The granules contain ADP (which is a potent agonist to recruit other platelets); upon activation the granules release ADP as well as adenosine triphosphate (which is an agonist for other cells of the blood).[116,117] In addition, they release biogenic amines such as serotonin, which can influence vascular tone, and divalent cations. The physiologic role of released dense body calcium is not clear; however, one could speculate it serves to ensure adequate calcium for some of the calcium-dependent enzymes involved in coagulation or cross-linking of the thrombus.

α Granules

A large number of plasma proteins involved in cell adhesion and coagulation are present in platelet α granules. Some of the proteins found within α granules are synthesized only in megakaryocytes (e.g., β thromboglobulin and platelet factor 4); other molecules are less specific for platelets and megakaryocytes. Platelets contain approximately 80 α granules that contain adhesive plasma proteins including vWF, fibrinogen, fibronectin, and vitronectin as well as the platelet and cellular adhesive protein thrombospondin-1.[20,118] Platelet vWF is concentrated in the platelets, megakaryocytes synthesize it,[119] and the platelet form is enriched in the larger, presumably more hemostatically effective multimers.[120] Megakaryocytes clearly take up fibrinogen, but its biosynthesis by megakaryocytes remains controversial.[121] Platelet fibronectin appears to be enriched in alternatively spliced forms that are relatively lacking in plasma,[21] suggesting a possible role for platelet fibronectin in events such as matrix assembly. Vitronectin is present in platelets[122]; however, its concentration suggests that it probably is passively taken up from the plasma. Nevertheless, studies have suggested a role for platelet and plasma vitronectin in thrombus formation.[123,124] Plasminogen activator inhibitor type 1 (PAI-1) binds vitronectin,[125] and these two proteins are released as a complex.[126] Consistent with this observation, mice lacking vitronectin, PAI-1, or both have a similar deficiency in thrombosis formation.[127] A wide variety of procoagulant and anticoagulant enzymes and cofactors have been reported in platelet granules. Although controversial,[128] it appears that megakaryocytes can synthesize at least some factor V,[129–131] and more factor V is present in platelet α granules[132] than can be accounted for by nonspecific uptake from plasma. Moreover, platelet factor V appears to be distinct from plasma factor V[133] and plays a clear role in assembling the platelet prothrombinase,[134] which is involved in the final step of blood coagulation (i.e., generation of thrombin). Platelets also contain the cofactors protein S[135] and PAI-1.[136] Protein S is a cofactor for action of activated protein C (see Chapter 120), and PAI-1 is an inhibitor of urokinase and tissue plasminogen activators (see Chapter 119). Thus, the concentrations of these proteins in platelets suggest that platelets may be a favored site for the anticoagulant action of protein C, a tempting idea considering the local concentration of factor V, a protein C substrate, on the platelet surface. Similarly, local release of PAI-1 from platelets may play a role in modulating fibrinolytic events in the vicinity of thrombi.[137,138]

P-selectin[139–142] (GMP-140, GPIIa, PADGEM, CD62) is an α-granule membrane protein that is absent from the surface of resting platelets. It is structurally similar to E- and L-selectins,[143] a family of carbohydrate-binding proteins involved in adhesive interactions of circulating leukocytes. Platelet P-selectin plays a central role in mediating interactions of monocytes and neutrophils with platelets.[143] These interactions are important in "cross-talk" between these cell types[144] and in the recruitment of leukocytes to thrombi.[145] Some of the speculated pathologic roles of platelet P-selectin are promotion of thrombogenesis,[145] platelet–tumor cell interactions,[146] and monocyte recruitment. It may play a physiologic role in the leukocyte phagocytosis of platelets. In addition, P-selectin plays an important role in leukocyte–vessel wall interactions[142,147] and hemostasis.[148] Platelet–leukocyte conjugates are indicative cardiovascular events.[149,150] However, P-selectin and its counterreceptor PSGL on leukocytes[151] are not the only ligand–receptor pair that mediates these interactions.[152]

The most abundant component of α granules is platelet-activating factor[153] (alkyl-2-acetyl-*sn*-glycero-3-phosphocholine), which originally was described as platelet activator released from stimulated mast cells. Platelet-activating factor is a member of the chemokine family. Its biologic effects are much more widespread than on platelet activation,[154–156] although its effects on platelets clearly play a role in some of the platelet sequestration that occurs during allergic injury. It is produced by a variety of cells in addition to platelets. It is possible that this important mediator, produced locally, contributes either to recruitment of other platelets or to some of the vascular phenomena associated with hemostasis.

Platelet α granules contain growth-arrest specific gene 6 (Gas-6).[157,158] Gas-6 is similar to protein S, but it is a ligand for certain growth factor receptors, such as Axl.[159] Because platelets express the Axl receptor, it is speculated that secreted Gas6 functions to accelerate platelet recruitment and activation. Consistent with this hypothesis, mice lacking Gas6 have a platelet defect.[133,157]

Platelets are the major peripheral blood source of β-amyloid precursor protein (APP).[160] APP is a membrane protein, thought to be localized to α granules,[161] that serves as the precursor of the approximately 40 residue peptides found in amyloid deposits in the brains of patients with Alzheimer disease. APP is a protease inhibitor and is processed by proteolytic cleavage. Its inhibition of factors Xa, XIa, and IXa[162,163] suggests a possible role as a natural anticoagulant. The effects of platelet APP on the spectrum of coagulation and fibrinolytic proteases are of interest, as is its potential role in deposits of amyloid in the brain.

Platelets contain a wide variety of peptides and proteins, primarily in α granules, that can modulate the growth and patterns of gene expression of cells of the vessel wall. The first of these to be described was platelet-derived growth factor[164] (PDGF), which has three isoforms and two distinct receptors on smooth muscle cells and fibroblasts.[165] PDGF probably plays an important role in the smooth muscle cell proliferation that may occur consequent to platelet interaction with the vessel wall. Platelet-secreted PDGF may play a critical role in angiogenesis.[166] PDGF receptors are transmembrane tyrosine kinase-type receptors, and signal transduction from this receptor[167] is similar to that from other tyrosine kinase receptors such as insulin and epidermal growth factor receptors. Another α-granule growth factor is connective tissue-activating peptide (CTAP) III, which stimulates fibroblast proliferation. CTAP III is a probable precursor of β thromboglobulin,[168] and its structure is related to another α-granule protein, platelet factor 4. Both platelet factor 4 and CTAP III are members of a large protein family involved in growth control and inflammation.[169] Interleukin-1 is expressed on the surface of activated platelets,[170] but the mechanism explaining its presence there is unclear.

Transforming growth factor (TGF)-β was first isolated from platelets.[171] Platelets are a rich source of this peptide mediator, which is a potent stimulus for the biosynthesis of matrix molecules and their receptors. TGF-β has complex effects on cell proliferation, stimulating cellular proliferation in some cell systems but inhibiting cellular proliferation in other systems. In addition, thrombospondin-1 is present in and secreted from platelet α granules. Released thrombospondin-1 is believed to play a role in stabilizing platelet aggregates via its interaction with platelet cell surface receptors and fibrinogen bound to integrin $\alpha_{IIb}\beta_3$.[172] Another additional important role of thrombospondin-1 is its function as an activator of TGF-β[173] and as a potent antiangiogenic factor.[174] This latter function may contribute to regulation of angiogenesis by platelets, a process that has received wide attention.[175]

Thrombospondin-1 also is produced by endothelial and smooth muscle cells, and its mRNA is inducible by growth factors such as PDGF.[176,177] Thrombospondin-1 appears to play a role in regulating the proliferation of smooth muscle cells and in angiogenesis.[178–180] Platelets also contain and can secrete vascular endothelial cell growth factor.[181] Many clinical studies have assessed the prognostic/diagnostic value of various markers, including vascular endothelial cell growth factor, in various diseases. The possibility that elevated levels of these markers reflect platelet activation in the disease must always be considered.

Multimerin is a novel platelet granule and endothelial protein that exists as massive disulfide-linked multimers of a 155-kd subunit.[182,183] Multimerin has a repeating structure, and its sequence contains the adhesive motif Arg-Gly-Asp-Ser, central coiled-coil sequences, several epidermal growth factor-like motifs, and a globular domain that is similar to a protein-binding domain found in complement C1q and in collagens type VIII and X.[184] Multimerin binds the coagulation protein factor V and its activated form factor Va. In platelets, but not in plasma, all of the biologically active factor V is complexed with multimerin.[185] Multimerin also may have functions as an extracellular matrix or adhesive protein. Members of two Canadian families with autosomal dominant bleeding disorders are deficient in platelet multimerin.[185] This large granule protein may have important roles in platelet procoagulant activity and platelet adhesion.

Lysosomal Granules and Platelet Cytosol

Platelets contain a few primary and secondary lysosomes[31,114] whose enzymes are released. However, compared with neutrophils, platelets probably are a minor source of lysosomal hydrolases in the blood. Platelet-associated heparatinase,[186] which probably is a lysosomal enzyme, can cleave vascular endothelial cell surface glycosaminoglycans, producing an antiproliferative fragment.

Factor XIII is a major transglutaminase contained in the platelet cytosol.[187] It catalyzes the formation of isopeptide bonds between the γ-glutaminyl residues and the E amino groups of lysines, forming stable covalent cross-links between proteins. Factor XIII functions in the cross-linking of fibrin as well as the cross-linking of other components of a thrombus, such as fibronectin[188] and α_2 antiplasmin,[189] to fibrin (see Chapter 118). Moreover, platelet factor XIII has been suggested to play a role in cross-linking and stabilizing cytoskeletal elements.[190,191] It is likely that small quantities of platelet factor XIIIα are released into thrombi, where it may affect their stability. Transglutaminases also have been implicated in the signaling events associated with occupancy of G protein-coupled receptors,[192,193] and many of the agonist receptors, which activate platelets, are members of this family of receptors.

Secretion

Secretion of platelet granules occurs through mechanisms analogous to those required for exocytosis of granules from neurons and mast cells. Platelet secretion is triggered by a variety of strong agonists, such as thrombin. Induction of secretion by weak agonists (e.g., ADP) occurs when the cells are brought into close contact, as occurs during aggregation.[114,194,195] The latter secretory mechanism is clearly dependent on thromboxane A_2 (TXA_2) generated as a consequence of arachidonic acid release.

Granule Exocytosis

α Granules and dense bodies, the two morphologically prominent platelet storage granules, contain a variety of substances important in platelet function. Because these granules have a limiting membrane, the final secretory event likely involves exocytosis[196] (i.e., fusion of the secretory granule membrane with the plasma membrane). This process has been observed in dense body secretion.[197,198]

Building upon lessons learned about the role of the soluble *N*-ethylmaleimide soluble factor attachment receptor (SNARE) complex in neuronal cell exocytosis, there has been a substantial increase in our understanding of platelet secretion. Platelets have the three basic components of the SNARE machinery: t-SNAREs (target receptors), v-SNAREs (vesicle-associated membrane receptors), and soluble components (including NSF and NSF-attachment proteins).[114,195] Through a pathway involving Rab-GTPase, protein kinase C, and intracellular calcium, the SNARE machinery regulates the association and subsequent fusion of vesicles with membranes (see Fig. 115–3, *B*). Mice deficient in one of these SNAREs, VAMP-8, show defects in platelet secretion,[199,200] and certain single nucleotide polymorphisms in VAMP-8 are associated with increased susceptibility to acute myocardial infection.[201]

Platelet microparticles are vesicles that are shed from the membrane of stimulated platelets. In addition to membrane lipids, they are enriched in certain platelet membrane proteins.[202] This property allows their detection by flow cytometry.[203] They are highly procoagulant and may contribute to clinical thrombosis in diseases such as heparin-induced thrombocytopenia (see Chapter 140),[204] and their presence in blood has been correlated with coronary artery disease.[205–207]

In addition to the outward movement of granules toward the cell surface is substantial inward membrane traffic in platelets.[208–211] This inward traffic can serve to clear adhesive and procoagulant proteins from the cell surface and hence limit prothrombotic events.[212]

Eicosanoids and Arachidonate

In addition to exocytosis of platelet granules, passive release of TXA_2 from platelets is another mechanism for amplifying platelet activation. Eicosanoids are formed from the arachidonate released from membrane phospholipids by phospholipase A_2 during platelet activation.[213–215] Because the availability of arachidonate is the rate-limiting step in this process, phospholipase A_2 is tightly controlled. Platelet phospholipase A_2 is stimulated by the rise in cytosolic Ca^{2+} that accompanies platelet activation.

Once released from membrane phospholipids, arachidonate can be metabolized to TXA_2 by cyclooxygenase 1 (COX-1).[216] Aspirin acetylates COX-1, causing it to be irreversibly inactivated.[217] Because platelets lack the ability to synthesize significant amounts of protein, inactivation of COX-1 by aspirin blocks TXA_2 synthesis until new platelets are formed. Hence, aspirin is the drug most commonly used for antithrombotic therapy. A subset of patients may be "aspirin resistant," but the molecular basis of this disorder, and a universally accepted definition for this term, is uncertain.[218,219] Aspirin resistance can lead to undermedication of patients and, therefore, an increased risk for recurrent thrombotic events. Nonsteroidal antiinflammatory drugs also inactivate COX-1 but without covalently modifying the enzyme.[220]

Once formed, TXA_2 can diffuse across the plasma membrane and activate other platelets through signaling pathways. This process leads to platelet shape change, aggregation, secretion, phosphoinositide hydrolysis, protein phosphorylation, and an increase in cytosolic Ca^{2+}, with little effect on cyclic AMP formation (see Chapter 116).[221] Like ADP, TXA_2 amplifies the initial stimulus for platelet activation and helps recruit additional platelets. This process is effective locally but is limited by the short half-life of TXA_2 in solution, which helps confine the spread of platelet activation to the original area of injury.

MOLECULAR BASIS OF PLATELET AGGREGATION

Aggregation Response of Platelets

Platelets in blood, in plasma, or as an isolated cell population do not interact with one another. If an appropriate agonist is added, rapid

Table 115–4 Common Platelet Aggregating Agonists

Agonist	Comment
Adenosine diphosphate (ADP)	Released from platelet α-granule; acts synergistically with many other agonists
Thrombin	Formed by activation of the coagulation system
Collagen	In subendothelial matrix
Epinephrine	May allow for hormonal regulation of hemostasis
Calcium ionophore	Not naturally occurring; mobilizes calcium in platelets
Arachidonate + metabolites	Active metabolites are formed and released from stimulated platelets
Serotonin	Released from platelets, may primarily sensitize platelets to other agonists
Platelet-activating factor	Lipid mediator produced by other cells that can activate a variety of cells, including platelets

aggregation of the platelets can ensue. Some agonists that can initiate this response are listed in Table 115–4. Of particular physiologic relevance are the platelet-derived agonists ADP, serotonin, platelet-activating factor, and arachidonate metabolites, which provide a means for stimulated platelets to recruit additional cells; collagen, which supports platelet adhesion and secretion as well as aggregation; thrombin, which links platelets and the blood coagulation system in thrombus formation; epinephrine, which permits hormonal regulation of platelet function; and vWF upon its binding to GPIb-V-IX. These agonists activate platelets by interacting with specific receptors, many of which are members of the G protein-coupled receptor class. Receptor occupancy triggers a complex series of intracellular reactions (see Chapter 116) that ultimately converge to a set of common steps that permit the cells to aggregate. Platelet aggregation is energy dependent and can be distinguished on this basis from platelet agglutination induced by ristocetin or certain platelet antibodies.

At normal blood concentrations of 1 to 3×10^8/mL, platelet suspensions are opalescent. Upon addition of an agonist, a stirred suspension of normal platelets aggregates, and a visible decrease in turbidity can be observed. Platelet aggregometers are dedicated instruments that measure the changes in light transmission through platelet suspensions and are used extensively in clinical laboratories to evaluate platelet function (see Chapter 122). Certain instruments also provide simultaneous measurements of other platelet functions, such as secretion.[194] Although the information gained from aggregometry can be extremely useful, aggregation in vitro does not necessarily reflect platelet function in vivo. In particular, clinical bleeding and the aggregation response of platelets do not necessarily coincide. This disparity reflects the importance of platelet adhesion in thrombus formation, a reaction that is not detected by aggregometry. For this reason, several instruments, which consider platelet adhesion under shear or are more quantitative for more efficient monitoring of antiplatelet therapy,[222–224] are used, but aggregometry remains a mainstay of the clinical coagulation laboratory.

A typical aggregometer tracing obtained with a suspension of isolated human platelets is shown in Fig. 115–4, *A*. From this pattern, the three essential components required for this functional response can be identified. The first component is the *platelet agonist*. The agonist used in the setup shown in Fig. 115–4 is ADP. This agonist induces platelet shape change, from a discoid to a more spherical form, a transition that can be detected in the aggregometer as a decrease in light transmission. This transformation is not a prerequisite for platelet aggregation. Epinephrine aggregates platelets but does not induce a shape change that is recordable in most conventional

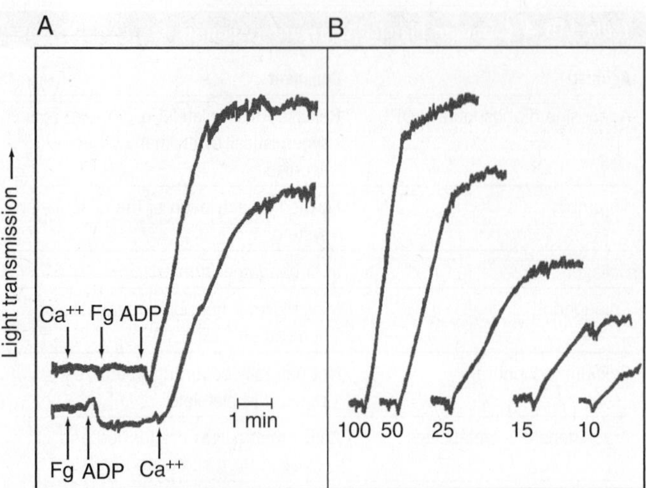

Figure 115–4 Aggregation response of human platelets. **A**, To aggregate, isolated human platelets require divalent ions (Ca^{2+}), an agonist (adenosine diphosphate [ADP], and an adhesive protein (fibrinogen [Fg]). Shape change is observed as a slight decrease in light transmission induced by ADP and is followed by an increase in transmission as the platelets aggregate. **B**, Both the rate and extent of platelet aggregation depend on the concentration of fibrinogen. The concentration of fibrinogen (in μg/mL) is indicated below each tracing.

aggregometers. At the molecular level, shape change reflects a reorganization of the platelet's actin cytoskeleton. The second component is *divalent cations*. Calcium and magnesium, as well as some other but not all divalent cations, support platelet aggregation.[225–227] The third component is *fibrinogen*. Fibrinogen not only is a major plasma protein; it also is present in and secreted from platelets (see Chapter 118).[228,229] By virtue of its capacity to form fibrin and support platelet aggregation, fibrinogen plays a dual role in thrombus formation. These activities, as well as the contribution of fibrinogen to blood viscosity, are believed to account for the increased risk of cardiovascular disease associated with elevated levels of fibrinogen.[230–232] Certain single nucleotide polymorphisms in fibrinogen have been associated with enhanced risk of myocardial infarction in some, but not all, studies.[233–235] The dependence of platelet aggregation on fibrinogen concentration is evident from the tracings shown in Fig. 115–4, *B*.

Although not evident in conventional aggregometers, vWF plays a central role in platelet aggregation and in the more complex process of thrombus formation, which entails platelet adhesion as well as aggregation. The role of vWF in platelet aggregation becomes apparent in certain pathologic circumstances such as platelet-type von Willebrand disease and type IIB von Willebrand disease (see Chapters 128 and 129).[236–240] In the setting of vascular injury in vivo, it is clear that both fibrinogen and vWF,[1–3] as well as other identified and as yet unidentified plasma and platelet molecules,[4,241] contribute to thrombus formation and stability.

Molecular Mechanisms Involved in Platelet Aggregation

The basis for the requisite roles of the agonist, calcium, and fibrinogen/vWF in platelet aggregation is well understood at the molecular level. Fibrinogen and vWF are ligands for integrin $\alpha_{IIb}\beta_3$. The absence of this integrin or its ligand binding function from the surface of platelets leads to the bleeding syndrome Glanzmann thrombasthenia, and platelet aggregation cannot be demonstrated. Further evidence for the critical role of $\alpha_{IIb}\beta_3$ in platelet aggregation and thrombus formation comes from genetically modified mice that are unable to express this receptor. These mice are unable to form a thrombus,[242] whereas mice that lack ligands for this receptor still can form a thrombus[1,2,3,4] (although excessive bleeding still occurs in these mice). Agonist is necessary to convert $\alpha_{IIb}\beta_3$ from the resting state on circulating platelets in which the integrin is unable to bind its plasma protein ligands to an activated state in which the ligands bind rapidly. All the platelet agonists listed in Table 115–4 can initiate platelet aggregation through this pathway. Calcium is needed for fibrinogen and vWF to bind to activated$\alpha_{IIb}\beta_3$. Activation of $\alpha_{IIb}\beta_3$ by agonists is very rapid. The platelet can become fully competent to bind fibrinogen/vWF via the receptor within seconds after its initial encounter with an appropriate agonist. More than 40,000 fibrinogen molecules can be bound to the platelet surface via engagement of $\alpha_{IIb}\beta_3$.[225,243–245] Fibrinogen is a dimer and vWF is a multimer. By virtue of their repeating and large structures, these ligands can bind to $\alpha_{IIb}\beta_3$ on adjacent platelets and bridge the cells together, leading to the formation of a platelet aggregate.[227,246–249]

$\alpha_{IIb}\beta_3$: Structure–Function Relationships

The resting platelet has 40,000 to 80,000 copies of $\alpha_{IIb}\beta_3$ on its surface.[250] Platelet activation can increase this number by up to 100% as a result of expression of internal pools of the receptor.[251] Each $\alpha_{IIb}\beta_3$ is capable of binding one fibrinogen molecule. $\alpha_{IIb}\beta_3$ is a typical integrin, composed of an α subunit and a β subunit, which combine to form a heterodimer.[32,34] The α subunit, α_{IIb} (GPIIb), is expressed primarily by cells of the platelet/megakaryocyte lineage, although its expression by various solid tumors and mast cells has been reported.[252–254] The β_3 subunit, GPIIIa, forms a complex not only with α_{IIb} but also with the α_V subunit to form $\alpha_v\beta_3$.[255] $\alpha_v\beta_3$ is expressed by a variety of cell types, including platelets, megakaryocytes, and endothelial cells.[256–258] These two sister receptors bind many of the same ligands and antagonists, but their specificities are not identical.[259] Complete amino acid sequences of both α_{IIb} and β_3 subunits were deduced from their cDNAs sequences.[35,38] The carbohydrate side chains and disulfide linkages also were located.[260–263] α_{IIb} is synthesized as a single chain in megakaryocytes, but it becomes proteolytically processed to the two-chain form during its transit to the cell surface.[264]

Structural biologic studies have provided significant insights into the molecular basis of the functions of $\alpha_{IIb}\beta_3$ and $a_V\beta_3$. The crystal structure of the extracellular domain of $\alpha_V\beta_3$ was solved with and without a bound peptide ligand.[265,266] A schematic model illustrating the domain organization of derived from these crystal structures is shown in Fig. 115–5. The extracellular domain of each subunit is composed of several domains, and at least one domain from each subunit directly contacts bound ligand. The primary ligand contact domain in the α subunit is the *β-propeller domain*, which is composed of seven "blades." Homologous structures are found in G proteins. In the β subunit, an A domain, also called an I domain, contacts ligand. When the β-propeller domain and the A domain come into close proximity, they form a globular head that is apparent on electron micrographs of isolated $\alpha_{IIb}\beta_3$.[267] Within the A domain of the β_3 subunit are three divalent cation-binding sites. One of these sites, termed the MIDAS, is intimately involved in ligand binding. One of the coordination sites for the cation bound within the MIDAS can be provided by an aspartic acid within the ligand. Thus, occupancy of the MIDAS cation establishes the role of divalent ions in ligand binding and platelet aggregation (Fig. 115–5). Located within the α_{IIb} and β_3 stalks, which extend out from the globular head, is a "genu," which allows bending such that the head domain can approach the cell membrane. It was this bent structure that was observed in the $\alpha_V\beta_3$ crystal structures. Subsequently, several crystal structures of portions of the extracellular domain of $\alpha_{IIb}\beta_3$ were solved.[268] They included several crystals with antagonists bound to the receptor, thus providing a clear picture as to how low-molecular-weight ligands can bind to $\alpha_{IIb}\beta_3$.

Structures for the transmembrane domains and the cytoplasmic tails have been observed or modeled.[269–273] The transmembrane segment of each subunit is composed of an α helix,[273] and evidence is clear that these transmembrane helices can interact with one

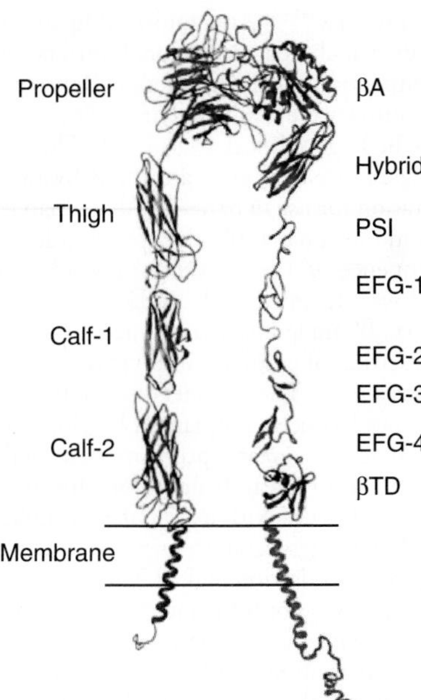

Figure 115–5 Model showing the structural organization of a β_3 integrin. The model is based on the crystal structure of the extracellular domain of $\alpha_V\beta_3$ and the cytoplasmic tails on the nuclear magnetic resonance structure of $\alpha_{IIb}\beta_3$. (Adapted from Xiong JP, Stehle T, Goodman SL, Arnaout MA: Integrins, cations and ligands: Making the connection. J Thromb Haemost 1:1642, 2003,[361] and Qin J, Vinogradova O, Plow EF: Integrin bidirectional signaling: A molecular view. PLoS Biol 2:e169, 2004.[362])

another.[274] The helices extend beyond the membrane boundary into the cytoplasm, and they also interact with one another through multiple hydrophobic and electrostatic contacts.[270]

Activation of $\alpha_{IIb}\beta_3$

$\alpha_{IIb}\beta_3$ activation is initiated by a platelet agonist and involves transmission of a signal induced by engagement of the agonist receptor to the cytoplasmic tail of the integrins. The signal is transmitted from the cytoplasmic tails through the transmembrane helices and ultimately induces a change in the extracellular domain, rendering the integrin functional. The signaling process responsible for this transformation is referred to as "inside-out" signaling.[275–277] A model for the structural basis of inside-out signaling is emerging. An integrin activator binds to the cytoplasmic tail of $\alpha_{IIb}\beta_3$ and disrupts the complex between the subunits.[270,278,279] The dissociation triggers a conformational change that is transmitted into or across the transmembrane segments and disturbs their interaction.[274] These events are transmitted to the extracellular region, allowing for acquisition of ligand competence. Within the transmembrane region, disassembly of the intramolecular interactions between helices can initiate homo-oligomerization between like subunits.[273,274,280] Consequently, the integrin heterodimers become clustered. Such clustering in itself can lead to and/or enhance activation by enhancing the avidity of the clustered extracellular domains for ligand and/or by altering the conformation of the extracellular domain.[281–283]

The crystal structures of the extracellular domain of $\alpha_V\beta_3$ are bent, with the head domain in proximity to the cell membrane.[265] This configuration was unanticipated because most electron micrographs suggested that the head domain resided at the end of long straight stalks.[267] These seemingly disparate results were reconciled in a "switchblade hypothesis," which suggested flexibility such that the integrin could exist between a bent and an extended conformation. Detailed micrographic studies supported the notion that the integrin could transit from these extreme states and could also exist in intermediate states between the fully bent and the fully extended conformation. It was further suggested that the extended conformation coincided with the activated integrin and that, in the bent state, the integrin was resting. This model provided an attractive mechanism accounting for activation of $\alpha_{IIb}\beta_3$ and integrins in general.[283] However, in a subsequent crystal structure, a macromolecular ligand, a fragment of fibronectin, was observed bound to the $\alpha_V\beta_3$ in a bent conformation.[284,285] Thus, the transition of $\alpha_{IIb}\beta_3$ from a bent to an extended conformation may occur and contribute to, but may not essential for, activation. From crystal structures of $\alpha_{IIb}\beta_3$, with or without bound ligands, differences are noted in the positioning of helices, in divalent ions in the β_3 A domain, and in movements of domains adjacent to the β_3 A domain. Such movements of structural elements relative to one another may provide local regulation of ligand binding.

Talin, a large protein intracellular protein, has been strongly implicated as a trigger of integrin activation.[286,287] Talin binds to two sites in the cytoplasmic tail of the β_3 subunit: the NPLY sequence in the midsegment of the cytoplasmic tail and a sequence in the membrane proximal region.[288–290] Its interaction with the two sites may be sequential. Its binding to the membrane proximal segment may be "unclasping," triggering separation of β_3 from the α_{IIb} cytoplasmic tail and resulting in activation.[289,290] Mice containing point mutations in the talin-binding regions of β_3 exhibit a bleeding phenotype.[291] Several other proteins bind to the NPLY sequence, and whether these function as coactivators or suppressors remains to be resolved.[292–294] Molecules that bind to the C-terminal region of β_3 or to the α_{IIb} cytoplasmic tail may regulate activation.[292] Talin itself must undergo activation in order for $\alpha_{IIb}\beta_3$ activation to be regulated, and multiple pathways involving talin activation have been identified. Thus, at this juncture, the mechanism by which inside-out signaling triggers activation of $\alpha_{IIb}\beta_3$ appears to be complex.[104,287,295–297]

Several mechanisms can be envisioned to explain how fibrinogen binding to $\alpha_{IIb}\beta_3$ results in platelet aggregation. The simplest possibility is that a single fibrinogen molecule, by virtue of its dimeric structure, bridges two $\alpha_{IIb}\beta_3$ molecules symmetrically on adjacent platelets. Evidence supporting this possibility is available.[298–300] Because multiple sites within each fibrinogen molecule can be recognized by $\alpha_{IIb}\beta_3$ (see Recognition Specificity and Antagonism of $\alpha_{IIb}\beta_3$), asymmetric variations of direct bridging can be envisioned. Still another possibility is that changes subsequent to fibrinogen binding are required for platelet aggregation. Irreversible fibrinogen binding,[227] conformational changes in bound fibrinogen[203,301] and in occupied $\alpha_{IIb}\beta_3$,[302] clustering of fibrinogen/$\alpha_{IIb}\beta_3$,[303] and additional interactions of the receptor with the cytoskeleton of the cells[304–306] occur after initial binding of fibrinogen to the cells. Moreover, a series of intracellular signaling events, including tyrosine and serine/threonine kinase and phosphatase activation, are initiated and propagated as a consequence of receptor occupancy and platelet aggregation.[275,276] These events are referred to as "outside-in" signaling. Whether such postreceptor occupancy events play a direct role in platelet aggregation is unknown, However, circumstances in which fibrinogen is bound to $\alpha_{IIb}\beta_3$ without induction of platelet aggregation have been described,[275] and mice in which the tyrosine phosphorylation sites in the β_3 subunit have been mutated showed decreased thrombus stability,[307] which implies a role for outside-in signals in platelet aggregation.

Recognition Specificity and Antagonism of $\alpha_{IIb}\beta_3$

Linear amino acid sequences define the recognition specificity of $\alpha_{IIb}\beta_3$ (Table 115–5). One peptide corresponds to the extreme COOH-terminus of the γ chain,[298,308] one of the three constituent chains of fibrinogen. The recognized amino acid sequence may be as small as the extreme six amino acid residues.[309] The second peptide is as small as four amino acids and contains the following three amino acids in sequence: arginyl-glycyl-aspartic acid (RGD).[310–313] RGD sequences occur in two sites within the Aα chain of fibrinogen.[314] RGD sequences are also found in a variety of other proteins, including several that bind to $\alpha_{IIb}\beta_3$. In addition, several other integrin receptors recognize RGD sequences within their ligands.[32,315–319]

Table 115–5 Recognition Peptides of $\alpha_{IIb}\beta_3$[a]

Peptide Designation	Structure[b]
Fibrinogen γ-chain	-XXKQAGDV
RGD	RGDX

[a]The naturally occurring sequences in human fibrinogen; S (serine) or F (phenylalanine) at the COOH-terminus of the two RGD sequences within the α chain; and H (histidine)—H-L (leucine)—G-G-A at the NH_2-terminus of the γ-chain peptide.

[b]Amino acids: K, lysine; Q, glutamine; A, alanine; G, glycine; D, aspartic acid; V, valine; X, one of several amino acids.

Thus, the RGD amino acid sequence is a broadly used recognition code in cellular adhesive reactions. RGD with specific flanking residues can react selectively with individual integrins, and it was one such peptide that was crystallized in complex with $\alpha_V\beta_3$.[266] In contrast, the γ-chain sequence appears to be unique to fibrinogen. Synthetic peptides containing either the γ-chain peptide sequence or the RGD sequence interact directly with $\alpha_{IIb}\beta_3$ and bind to the same or mutually exclusive sites within the receptor.[320,321] Crystal structures of $\alpha_{IIb}\beta_3$ with mimetics of these two peptide sequences suggest a similar binding mechanism,[268] but allosteric effects for additional binding sites for each cannot be excluded,[322] and allosteric inhibitors of ligand binding to integrins have been identified.[323] The preponderance of evidence indicates that the COOH-terminus of the γ chain is critical for fibrinogen binding to $\alpha_{IIb}\beta_3$.[324–326] Nevertheless, in the design of $\alpha_{IIb}\beta_3$ antagonists, the RGD sequence has often served as the starting compound because of its smaller size.[327] The characterization of these two sequences does not exclude that other sequences are involved in fibrinogen binding to $\alpha_{IIb}\beta_3$. Evidence indicates that additional sequences are involved in the recognition of fibrinogen by $\alpha_{IIb}\beta_3$.[328]

Fibrinogen is not the only ligand that binds to $\alpha_{IIb}\beta_3$. Several other adhesive proteins that can serve as ligands are listed in Table 115–2. All of these adhesive proteins contain at least one RGD sequence. RGD peptides interfere with binding of fibronectin[310,313] and bind of vitronectin[329] to platelets. Because plasma fibrinogen concentrations are 10-fold higher than its dissociation constant for $\alpha_{IIb}\beta_3$, under physiologic conditions, the receptor is nearly saturated with fibrinogen. Thus, fibrinogen is the dominant ligand for $\alpha_{IIb}\beta_3$ in this environment. However, all of these ligands, except fibrinogen, are present in subendothelial cell matrices, and these other interactions may dominate in this microenvironment. Because vWF is bound to platelets via GPIb-V-IX, it resides in close proximity to $\alpha_{IIb}\beta_3$ on the platelet surface, and this proximity may favor its engagement by $\alpha_{IIb}\beta_3$. In addition to its role in platelet aggregation, $\alpha_{IIb}\beta_3$ may be involved in platelet adhesion, particularly in stabilizing cell–matrix interactions.[330] It may be in this latter function that these other $\alpha_{IIb}\beta_3$ ligands play a key role. Thrombospondin-1 associates with the surface of resting and stimulated platelets.[331–333] On the surface, it plays an auxiliary role in platelet aggregation by stabilizing platelet aggregates.[334] This activity may arise from its capacity to bind to fibrinogen.[172,335] Several candidate receptors for thrombospondin have been proposed,[305,336–339] and the interaction may be mediated by a complex of several of these candidate receptors, including CD36, integrin-associated protein, and $\alpha_{IIb}\beta_3$.[340] Complexation of $\alpha_{IIb}\beta_3$ with other platelet membrane proteins (e.g., CD9,[341–343] CD40L,[241] Gas6[157]) also may play a role in controlling its activation, ligand-binding functions, and platelet responses in general. Increasing evidence indicates that a number of these and other membrane proteins in platelets can influence the adhesive responses of platelets in vitro and in vivo.[344]

Throughout the 1980s, a number of compounds that bound to $\alpha_{IIb}\beta_3$ and inhibited platelet aggregation were described. Furthermore, bleeding in patients with Glanzmann thrombasthenia was noted to be relatively mild. These observations led to the notion that blockade of $\alpha_{IIb}\beta_3$ might represent a new antithrombotic strategy. This realization spawned development programs throughout the pharmaceutical industry.[345,346] Antagonists of ligand binding to $\alpha_{IIb}\beta_3$ that were identified included monoclonal antibodies, small peptide ligands, and nonpeptidic ligand mimetics. Representatives of these classes of antagonists were evaluated in various animal models of thrombosis and in large clinical trials.[347–354] Three such agents, all intravenous drugs, ultimately were approved by the U.S. Food and Drug Administration for use in patients. Abciximab is a Fab fragment of a humanized monoclonal antibody; eptifibatide is a cyclic peptide based on the sequence of a snake venom peptide; and tirofiban is a nonpeptide that was designed with RGD as a starting structure. In 2007, all three $\alpha_{IIb}\beta_3$ antagonists continued to be used in patients, primarily in the setting of coronary interventions to prevent periprocedural thrombosis.[355,356] The broader use of these agents in acute coronary syndromes has been supplanted by clopidogrel and anticoagulants.[357,358] There was great optimism that orally active $\alpha_{IIb}\beta_3$ antagonists would be of great benefit for chronic antithrombotic therapy. A number of drugs with excellent pharmokinetic properties were developed. However, several drugs tested in clinical trials proved to be ineffective or even detrimental.[359] The reason for the failure of these oral antagonists was not fully understood. One explanation that received broad acceptance is that patients were underdosed to avoid safety issues, but this in itself would not explain detrimental effects. Another suggestion was that these drugs leave $\alpha_{IIb}\beta_3$ in an activated state as they dissociate from the receptor.[360] Regardless of the explanation, the initial clinical trials dampened the entire effort throughout the pharmaceutical industry to develop orally active $\alpha_{IIb}\beta_3$ antagonists, and all such programs were abandoned. It does appear that the intravenous $\alpha_{IIb}\beta_3$ antagonists are effective in preventing acute thrombosis in the context of coronary interventions. With approximately 800,000 such procedures performed annually, use of the approved $\alpha_{IIb}\beta_3$ antagonists remains significant.

SUGGESTED READINGS

Agah R, Plow E, Topol E: AlphaIIb beta3 (GPIIb-IIIa) antagonists. In Michaelson AD (ed.): Platelets, 2nd ed, Elsevier/Academic Press, San Diego, CA, 2006.

Brass LF, Jiang H, Wu J, Stalker TJ, Zhu L: Contact-dependent signaling events that promote thrombus formation. Blood Cells Mol Dis 36:157, 2006.

Francis J: The platelet function analyzer (PFA)-100. In Michelson AD (ed.): Platelets, 2nd ed. Elsevier/Academic Press, San Diego, CA, 2006.

Han J, Lim CJ, Watanabe N, et al: Reconstructing and deconstructing agonist-induced activation of integrin alphaIIbbeta3. Curr Biol 16:1796, 2006.

Hartwig JH: The platelet: Form and function. Semin Hematol 43:S94, 2006.

Iismaa SE, Begg GE, Graham RM: Cross-linking transglutaminases with G protein-coupled receptor signaling. Sci STKE 2006:pe34, 2006.

Ma YQ, Qin J, Plow EF: Platelet integrin alpha(IIb)beta(3): Activation mechanisms. J Thromb Haemost 5:1345, 2007.

Kiema T, Lad Y, Jiang P, et al: The molecular basis of filamin binding to integrins and competition with talin. Mol Cell 21:337, 2006.

Mackman N, Tilley RE, Key NS: Role of the extrinsic pathway of blood coagulation in hemostasis and thrombosis. Arterioscler Thromb Vasc Biol 27:1687, 2007.

Oki T, Kitaura J, Eto K, et al: Integrin alphaIIbbeta3 induces the adhesion and activation of mast cells through interaction with fibrinogen. J Immunol 176:52, 2006.

Petrich BG, Fogelstrand P, Partridge AW, et al: The antithrombotic potential of selective blockade of talin-dependent integrin alpha(IIb)beta(3) (platelet GPIIb-IIIa) activation. J Clin Invest 117:2250, 2007.

Plosker GL, Lyseng-Williamson KA: Clopidogrel: A review of its use in the prevention of thrombosis. Drugs 67:613, 2007.

Ren Q, Barber HK, Crawford GL, et al: Endobrevin/VAMP-8 is the primary v-SNARE for the platelet release reaction. Mol Biol Cell 18:24, 2007.

Shah PK: Thrombogenic risk factors for atherothrombosis. Rev Cardiovasc Med 7:10, 2006.

Shiffman D, Rowland CM, Louie JZ, et al: Gene variants of VAMP8 and HNRPUL1 are associated with early-onset myocardial infarction. Arterioscler Thromb Vasc Biol 26:1613, 2006.

Steinhubl S: The VerifyNow System. In Michelson AD (ed.): Platelets, 2nd ed. Elsevier/Academic Press, San Diego, CA, 2006.

Stone GW, McLaurin BT, Cox DA, et al: Bivalirudin for patients with acute coronary syndromes. N Engl J Med 355:2203, 2006.

Uitte DEWS, Doggen CJ, MC DEV, Bertina RM, Rosendaal FR: Haplotypes of the fibrinogen gamma gene do not affect the risk of myocardial infarction. J Thromb Haemost 4:474, 2006.

van der Zee PM, Biro E, Ko Y, et al: P-selectin- and CD63-exposing platelet microparticles reflect platelet activation in peripheral arterial disease and myocardial infarction. Clin Chem 52:657, 2006.

von Hundelshausen P, Petersen F, Brandt E: Platelet-derived chemokines in vascular biology. Thromb Haemost 97:704, 2007.

Wegener KL, Partridge AW, Han J, et al: Structural basis of integrin activation by talin. Cell 128:171, 2007.

REFERENCES

For complete list of references log onto www.expertconsult.com

CHAPTER 116

THE MOLECULAR BASIS OF PLATELET ACTIVATION

Lawrence F. Brass

Platelets have evolved as a means to respond to holes in a high-pressure, high-flow circulatory system. Many of the most pertinent properties of platelets, including their shape, the contents of their secretory granules, their high density of regulated adhesion receptors, and their ability to promote thrombin generation, are optimized to form a stable hemostatic plug under high-flow conditions. To be maximally useful, circulating platelets must be able to sustain repeated contact with the normal vessel wall without premature activation, recognize the unique features of a damaged wall, cease their forward motion upon recognition of damage, adhere despite the forces produced by continued arterial blood flow, and aggregate to each other, forming a stable plug of the correct size that can remain in place until it is no longer needed.

This chapter discusses how platelet activation begins and how platelets help to produce a stable hemostatic plug. The contribution of platelets to hemostasis is different in arteries and veins. In the venous system, low flow rates and stasis permit the accumulation of activated coagulation factors and the local generation of thrombin largely without the benefit of platelets. Although venous thrombi contain platelets, the dominant cellular components are trapped red cells. In the arterial circulation, higher flow rates limit fibrin formation by washing out soluble clotting factors. Hemostasis in the arterial circulation requires platelets to form a physical barrier, to accelerate thrombin formation, and to provide a base upon which fibrin can accumulate. Platelets work best under high shear conditions. As a result, thrombi formed in the arterial circulation are enriched in platelets as well as fibrin.

THREE STAGES IN PLATELET PLUG FORMATION

Platelet activation can be divided into three overlapping stages: initiation, extension, and perpetuation (Fig. 116–1). *Initiation* can occur in more than one way. In the setting of trauma to the vessel wall, it may occur because circulating platelets are captured and then activated by exposed collagen decorated with von Willebrand factor (VWF) multimers, thereby forming a monolayer that supports thrombin generation and the subsequent piling on of additional platelets. A key to these events is the presence of receptors on the platelet surface that can support the VWF-dependent capture of tumbling platelets (glycoprotein Ib/IX/V [GPIb-IX-V] and, to a lesser extent, $\alpha_{IIb}\beta_3$) and the subsequent intracellular signaling (via GPVI and $\alpha_2\beta_1$) that causes captured platelets to spread on the vessel wall and provide a nidus for subsequent platelet–platelet interactions. Imagine a flexible patch in which the surface in contact with the vessel wall optimizes its ability to stick to collagen, while the luminal surface acquires the ability to stick to other platelets, forming a plug. Platelet activation, particularly in thrombotic or inflammatory disorders, can also be initiated by thrombin, which activates platelets via G protein-coupled receptors (GPCRs) in the protease-activated receptor (PAR) family. *Extension* occurs when additional platelets are recruited and activated, sticking to each other and accumulating on top of the initial monolayer. Thrombin can play an important role at this point, as can secreted adenosine diphosphate (ADP) and released thromboxane A_2 (TxA_2). Each of these agonists is able to activate phospholipase C (PLC), causing an increase in the cytosolic Ca^{2+} concentration within platelets. The receptors that mediate this response are also members of the GPCR superfamily. The signals that they engender support the activation of integrin $\alpha_{IIb}\beta_3$, making possible the cohesive interactions between platelets that are critical to the formation of the hemostatic plug. ADP receptors have proved a fruitful target for antiplatelet agents, just as inhibition of TxA_2 generation has been a clinically useful target for aspirin. *Perpetuation* refers to the late events of platelet plug formation, when the intense, but often time-limited, signals arising from GPCRs may have faded. These late events help to stabilize the platelet plug and prevent premature disaggregation. Such events typically occur after aggregation has begun and are facilitated by close contacts between platelets. Examples include outside-in signaling through integrins and other cell adhesion molecules, and signaling through receptors whose ligands are located on the surface of adjacent platelets.

The platelet surface is crowded with receptors that are critical for hemostasis. Those that are directly involved in binding to collagen, VWF, or fibrinogen are expressed in the greatest numbers. Approximately 80,000 copies of integrin $\alpha_{IIb}\beta_3$ and 15,000 to 25,000 copies of GPIb-IX-V are present on the surface of human platelets. In contrast, receptors for thrombin, ADP, and TxA_2 range from a few hundred to a few thousand per platelet (Table 116–1). Many of these receptors float within the lipid bilayer; others are anchored via interactions with the membrane skeleton. Receptor distribution rarely is uniform. Some receptors tend to accumulate in cholesterol-enriched microdomains.[1–5] This position may increase the efficiency with which platelets are activated. Lateral mobility also may allow adhesion and cohesion receptors to accumulate at sites of contact.

Stage I: Initiation Platelet Activation

Although many molecules have been shown to cause platelet activation in vitro, platelet activation in vivo typically is initiated by collagen and thrombin. This may take place at a site of acute vascular injury where platelet plug formation serves to stop bleeding, but the same platelet responses can be invoked in pathologic states in which thrombin or other platelet-activating molecules are formed or exposed. Thrombin is generated at sites of vascular injury after exposure of tissue factor that is sequestered within the vessel wall, upregulated on the surface of activated monocytes and endothelial cells, or carried in the circulation on microvesicles. In pathologic states, tissue factor expression can be upregulated on the surface of endothelial cells or monocytes. Tissue factor may also be present on circulating, monocyte-derived microvesicles that bind to activated platelets at sites of injury.[6–8]

Under static conditions, collagen is able to capture and activate platelets without the assistance of cofactors, but under the flow conditions that exist in the arterial circulation VWF plays an essential role in supporting platelet adhesion and activation. Platelets can adhere to monomeric collagen but require the more complex structure found in fibrillar collagen for optimal activation. Four receptors for collagen have been identified on the surface of human and mouse platelets. Two bind directly to collagen ($\alpha_2\beta_1$ and GPVI). The other two bind to collagen via VWF ($\alpha_{IIb}\beta_3$ and GPIb-IX-V; Fig. 116–2). Of these four receptors, GPVI is the most potent in terms of initiating signal generation. The structure of GPVI places it in the immunoglobulin domain superfamily.[9] The ability of GPVI to generate signals rests

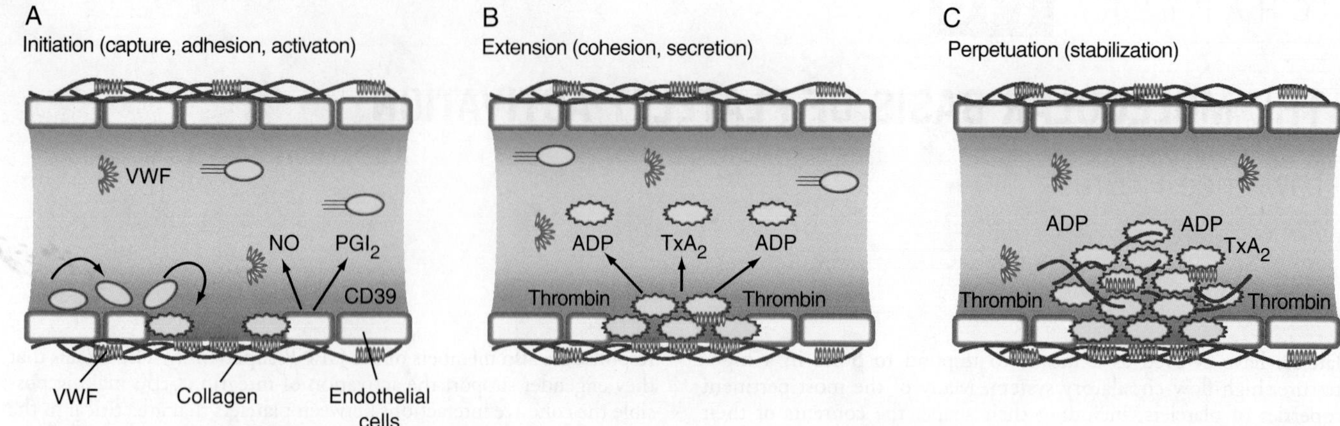

Figure 116–1 Stages in platelet plug formation. Prior to vascular injury, platelet activation is suppressed by endothelial cell-derived inhibitory factors. They include prostaglandin I_2 (PGI_2 [prostacyclin]), nitric oxide (NO), and CD39, an ADPase on the surface of endothelial cells that can hydrolyze trace amounts of ADP that otherwise might cause inappropriate platelet activation. **A,** Initiation. Development of the platelet plug is initiated by thrombin and by the collagen–von Willebrand factor (VWF) complex, which captures and activates moving platelets. Platelets adhere and spread, forming a monolayer. **B,** Extension. The platelet plug is extended as additional platelets are activated via the release or secretion of thromboxane A_2 (TxA_2), ADP, and other platelet agonists, most of which are ligands for G protein-coupled receptors on the platelet surface. Activated platelets stick to each other via bridges formed by the binding of fibrinogen, fibrin, or VWF to activated $\alpha_{IIb}\beta_3$. **C,** Perpetuation. Close contacts between platelets in the growing hemostatic plug, along with a fibrin meshwork (shown in red), help to perpetuate and stabilize the platelet plug.

Table 116–1 G Protein-Coupled Receptors Expressed on Human Platelets

Agonist	Receptor	G protein Families	Approximate Number of Copies Per Platelet
Thrombin	PAR1	G_q, G_i, G_{12}[a]	2000
	PAR4	G_q, G_{12}[a]	?
ADP	$P2Y_1$	G_q, G_{12}	150
	$P2Y_{12}$	G_i (particularly G_{i2})	600
TxA_2	$TP\alpha/\beta$	G_q, G_{12}	1000
Epinephrine	α_{2A}-adrenergic	G_i (particularly G_z)	300
PGI_2	IP	G_s	?

[a]The assignment of G_q and G_{12} but not G_i family members to PAR4 is by inference. Selective PAR4 agonists cause platelet aggregation and shape change but do not appear to inhibit adenylyl cyclase. In contrast, PAR1 has been shown to couple to G_i in platelet membrane preparation but appears to do so less well in intact platelets.

ADP, adenosine diphosphate; PAR, protease-activated receptor; PGI_2, prostaglandin I_2; TxA_2, thromboxane A_2.

on its constitutive association with the Fc receptor γ chain. Platelets that lack either GPVI or the γ chain have impaired responses to collagen, as do platelets in which GPVI has been depleted or blocked.[10–13] The $\alpha_2\beta_1$ integrin also appears to be necessary for optimal interaction with collagen. Human platelets with reduced expression of $\alpha_2\beta_1$ have impaired collagen responses,[14,15] as do mouse platelets that lack β_1 integrins when the ability of these platelets to bind to collagen is tested at high shear.[13,16]

According to current models, collagen causes clustering of GPVI. This leads to phosphorylation of FcRγ by tyrosine kinases in the Src family, creating a tandem phosphotyrosine motif recognized by the Src homology 2 (SH2) domains of Syk. Association of Syk with the GPVI/γ-chain complex activates Syk and leads to phosphorylation and activation of PLCγ2. Much of the initial response of platelets to agonists consists of activating PLC. PLCγ2, like other PLC isoforms, hydrolyzes phosphatidylinositol-4,5-bisphonate (PIP_2) to form 1,4,5-inositol triphosphate (IP_3) and diacylglycerol. IP_3 opens Ca^{2+} channels in the platelet-dense tubular system, raising the cytosolic Ca^{2+} concentration and triggering Ca^{2+} influx across the platelet plasma membrane. The changes in cytosolic Ca^{2+} concentration that occur when platelets adhere to collagen under flow can be visualized in real time.[17,18] Diacylglycerol activates the conventional and novel protein kinase C (PKC) isoforms that are expressed in platelets, allowing regulatory serine/threonine phosphorylation events.

Collectively, collagen receptors support the capture of fast-moving platelets at sites of injury, cause activation of captured platelets, and stimulate cytoskeletal reorganization that allows the previously discoid platelets to flatten out and adhere more closely to the exposed vessel wall. VWF supports this process by increasing the density of potential binding sites for collagen per platelet, especially under the conditions of flow, which stretches out VWF multimers and exposes the platelet binding sites on each monomer. This increases the likelihood that platelets will encounter an available binding site and, once bound, will be able to increase the number of contacts with collagen by bringing additional receptors into play. It appears likely that only GPVI and GPIb-IX-V are able to bind collagen and VWF, respectively, without prior platelet activation, However, once activation begins, $\alpha_2\beta_1$and $\alpha_{IIb}\beta_3$ are able to bind their respective ligands as well. Some integrin-activating signaling occurs downstream of GPVI, but growing evidence indicates that the GPIb-IX-V complex also can signal, as can $\alpha_2\beta_1$ and $\alpha_{IIb}\beta_3$ once they are engaged. Given these findings, it is perhaps not surprising that impairment of platelet receptors for collagen or loss of functional VWF produces defects in hemostasis that range from modest to profound, depending on the degree of impairment or the extent of VWF deficiency.

Stage II: Extension of the Platelet Plug

The formation of a platelet monolayer following exposure of collagen and VWF is sufficient to initiate platelet plug formation but is not sufficient to prevent bleeding. The next step is extension of the platelet plug by having one platelet stick to another, a process that technically is termed *cohesion* but commonly is referred to as *platelet aggregation* when it is studied ex vivo with the platelets in suspension. Recruitment of additional platelets beyond those in the collagen-bound monolayer is made possible by local accumulation of agonists that are secreted or released from platelets, such as ADP and TxA_2, and by local generation of thrombin (Fig. 116–1, *B)*. Contacts between platelets are maintained by a variety of cohesive interactions, of which the most essential is the binding of fibrinogen or VWF to activated $\alpha_{IIb}\beta_3$. Circulating or locally secreted catecholamines can

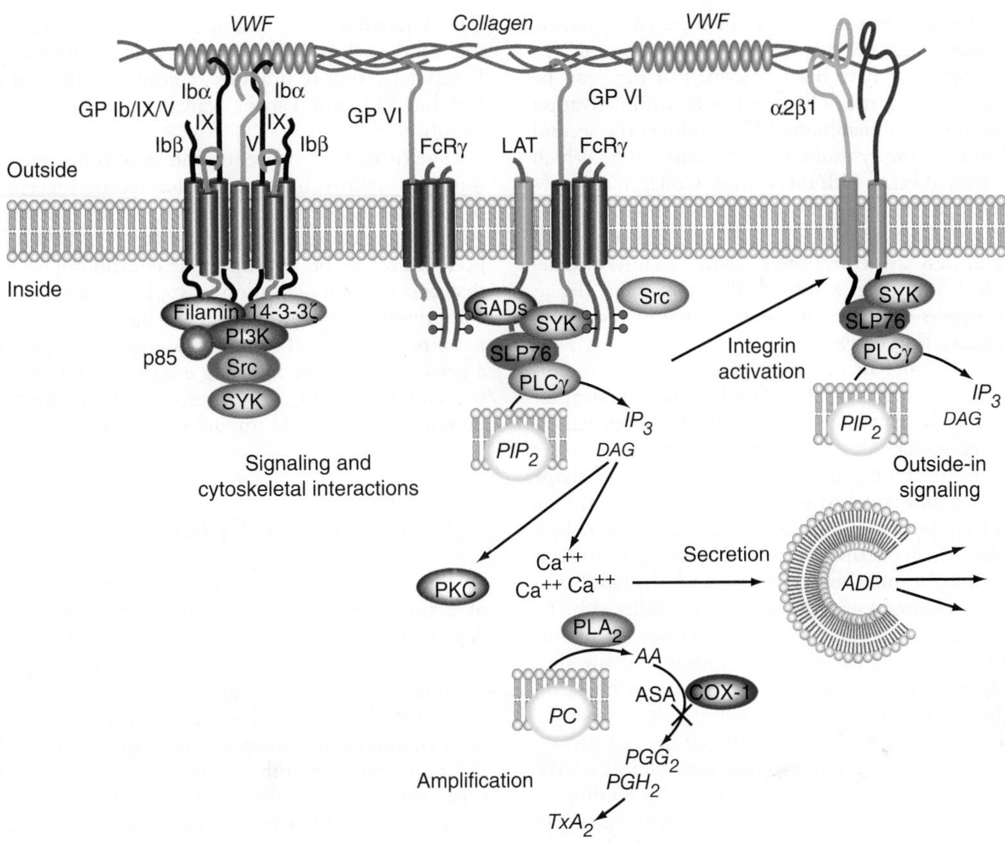

Figure 116–2 Platelet activation by collagen. Platelets use several different molecular complexes to support platelet activation by collagen. They include von Willebrand factor (VWF)-mediated binding of collagen to the glycoprotein Ib/IX/V (GPIb-IX-V) complex and integrin $\alpha_{IIb}\beta_3$, a direct interaction between collagen and both the integrin $\alpha_2\beta_1$, and the GPVI/γ-chain complex. Clustering of GPVI results in phosphorylation of tyrosine residues in the γ chain, followed by binding and activation of the tyrosine kinase Syk. One consequence of Syk activation is phosphorylation and activation of phospholipase Cγ, leading to phosphoinositide hydrolysis, secretion of ADP, and production and release of thromboxane A_2 (TxA_2). AA, arachidonic acid; ADP, adenosine diphosphate; ASA, aspirin; COX-1, cyclooxygenase 1; DAG, diacylglycerol; GP, glycoprotein; IP_3, inositol triphosphate; PC, phosphatidylcholine; PG, prostaglandin; PI3K, phosphatidylinositol 3-kinase; PIP_2, phosphatidylinositol-4,5-bisphosphate; PKC, protein kinase C; PLA_2, phospholipase A_2; PLCγ, phospholipase Cγ; VWF, von Willebrand factor.

cause vasoconstriction but also can promote platelet activation by potentiating the effects of other platelet agonists. Inherited or acquired defects in cohesion can produce significant risk of bleeding. Two examples are Glanzmann thrombasthenia, in which affected patients lack functional $\alpha_{IIb}\beta_3$ and therefore cannot bind fibrinogen or other cognate ligands, and administration of $\alpha_{IIb}\beta_3$ antagonists, which work as antiplatelet agents by blocking ligand binding.

Most of the agonists that extend the platelet plug do so via GPCRs. The properties of these receptors make them particularly well suited for this task. First, most GPCRs bind their ligands with high affinity. Second, they typically are composed of a single subunit, although receptor dimerization can affect the ligand preferences of the receptor. Third, they are constitutively associated with G proteins, reducing the time that otherwise would be required to recruit them into signaling complexes.[19] Fourth, because they act as guanine nucleotide exchange factors, each occupied receptor theoretically can activate multiple G proteins and, in some cases, more than one class of G proteins. This allows amplification of a signal that might begin with a relatively small number of receptors. It also potentially allows each receptor to signal via more than one effector pathway. Finally, because several mechanisms exist that can limit the activation of GPCRs, platelet activation can be regulated, a property that may be useful when platelet activation is inappropriate and must be controlled.

GPCRs are composed of a single polypeptide chain with seven transmembrane domains, an extracellular N-terminus, and an intracellular C-terminus.[20] Binding sites for agonists may involve the N-terminus, the extracellular loops, or a pocket formed by the transmembrane domains. The G proteins that act as mediators for these receptors are αβγ heterotrimers. The β subunit forms a propeller-like structure that is tightly associated with the smaller γ subunit. The α subunit contains a guanine nucleotide binding site that normally is occupied by guanosine 5′-diphosphate (GDP). Receptor activation causes the replacement (exchange) of the GDP by guanosine 5′-triphosphate (GTP), altering the conformation of the α subunit and exposing sites on both G_α and $G_{\beta\gamma}$ for interactions with downstream effectors. Hydrolysis of GTP by the intrinsic GTPase activity of the α subunit restores the resting conformation of the heterotrimer, preparing it to undergo another round of activation and signaling. Regulator of G-protein signaling (RGS) proteins accelerate the hydrolysis of GTP by α subunits, shortening signaling duration.[21]

Human platelets express at least 10 forms of G_α that fall into the $G_{s\alpha}$, $G_{i\alpha}$, $G_{q\alpha}$, and $G_{12\alpha}$ families. This includes at least one $G_{s\alpha}$ family member, four $G_{i\alpha}$ family members ($G_{i1\alpha}$, $G_{i2\alpha}$, $G_{i3\alpha}$, and $G_{z\alpha}$), three $G_{q\alpha}$ family members ($G_{q\alpha}$, $G_{11\alpha}$, and $G_{16\alpha}$), and two $G_{12\alpha}$ family members ($G_{12\alpha}$ and $G_{13\alpha}$). Much has been learned about the critical role of G protein α subunits in platelets. Much less is known about the $G_{\beta\gamma}$ isoforms that are expressed in platelets and the selectivity of their contributions to platelet activation.[22]

G Protein-Mediated Signaling In Platelets

The signaling events that underlie platelet activation have not been fully identified. Large gaps remain in signaling maps that attempt to connect receptors on the platelet surface with the most characteristic platelet responses: shape change, aggregation, and secretion. In general terms, the events that have been described to date can be divided into three broad categories. The first begins with activation of PLC, which by hydrolyzing membrane PIP_2 produces the second messengers needed to raise the cytosolic Ca^{2+} concentration. Which isoform of PLC is activated varies with the agonist. Collagen activates PLCγ2 using a mechanism that depends on adaptor molecules and protein tyrosine kinases. Thrombin, ADP, and TxA_2 activate PLCβ isoforms using G_q and (less efficiently) the G_i family as intermediaries. Regardless of which isoform is activated, the subsequent rise in Ca^{2+} concentration triggers downstream events, which include integrin activation and generation of TxA_2.

The second broad category of necessary events involves monomeric G proteins in the cdc42/Rac/Rho family, whose activation triggers reorganization of actin cytoskeleton and allows the formation of filopodia and lamellipodia. Along with changes in the platelet's circumferential microtubular ring, this step is the essence of shape change. Most platelet agonists can trigger shape change, with the notable exception of epinephrine. The soluble agonists (thrombin, ADP, and TxA_2) that trigger shape change typically act through receptors that are coupled to members of the G_q and G_{12} families.

A third category of required events for platelet is mediated by G_i family members and includes suppression of cyclic adenosine monophosphate (cAMP) formation and activation of phosphatidylinositol 3-kinase (PI3K). Suppression of cAMP synthesis relieves a block on platelet signaling that otherwise limits inopportune platelet activation, particularly in the presence of endothelial cell-derived prostaglandin (PG) I_2 and nitric oxide. The agonists that inhibit cAMP formation in platelets (ADP and epinephrine) do so by binding to receptors coupled to the G_i family members. Suppression of adenylyl cyclase is critical when cAMP levels are elevated, but whether it is necessary under basal cAMP conditions is less clear.

Platelet Activation In vivo

Slicing the events of platelet activation into individual pathways that are activated or suppressed by individual agonists is a didactic convenience. In vivo, however, platelet activation typically results from contact with more than one agonist. The initial injury may expose collagen, but it also will produce thrombin. Similarly, tissue and red cell damage will release ADP, as will activated platelets, which will also synthesize and release TxA_2. Remember that different agonists couple to different pathways with differing efficiencies, and it is the combined effect of multiple agonists that produces the most robust platelet activation. Even thrombin, one of the most potent platelet agonists, relies on its ability to induce ADP and TxA_2 release to yield maximal platelet activation when used at lower concentrations in vitro. This is particularly important because endogenous antagonists of platelet activation, including PGI_2, antithrombin III, the *ecto*-ADPase CD39, and the diluting effects of continued blood flow, work against the accumulation of platelet agonists and limit the ability of platelets to respond.

G_q and Activation of Phospholipase Cβ

Agonists whose receptors are coupled to G_q can provide a strong stimulus for platelet activation by activating PLCβ. PLCβ hydrolyzes membrane PI-4,5-P_2 to produce 1,4,5-IP_3 and diacylglycerol (Fig. 116–3). IP_3 formation triggers an increase in cytosolic Ca^{2+}. Diacylglycerol activates PKC. In resting platelets, the cytosolic Ca^{2+} concentration is maintained at approximately 100 nM by limiting Ca^{2+} influx and by pumping Ca^{2+} out of the cytosol across the plasma membrane or into the dense tubular system. The latter is a closed membrane compartment within platelets thought to be derived from megakaryocyte smooth endoplasmic reticulum. In activated platelets, the cytosolic free concentration can exceed 1 μM (a 10-fold increase over baseline) with potent agonists such as thrombin. Activation of PLC also releases membrane-associated proteins that bind to PI-4,5-P_2 via their pleckstrin homology (PH) domains. PLCβ-activating α subunits typically are derived from G_q in platelets, but PLC also can be activated by $G_{\beta\gamma}$ derived from G_i family members.

The rising Ca^{2+} concentration in activated platelets is a trigger for numerous events, but one that has received recent attention is Ca^{2+}-dependent activation of the Ras family member Rap1B via the guanine nucleotide exchange protein Cal-DAG GEF.[23] Rap1B has been shown to be an important contributor to signaling pathways that converge on activation of $\alpha_{IIb}\beta_3$ in platelets.[24–26] PKC isoforms are serine/threonine kinases. PKC has been identified as the cellular receptor for the lipid second messenger diacylglycerol; therefore, it is a key enzyme in the signaling events that follow activation of receptors coupled to PLC. PKC isoforms phosphorylate multiple cellular proteins on serine and threonine residues.

G_q, G_{13}, and Actin Cytoskeleton

At least two effector pathways are involved in the reorganization of actin cytoskeleton that accompanies platelet activation: Ca^{2+}-dependent activation of myosin light chain kinase downstream of G_q family members and activation of low-molecular-weight GTP-binding proteins in the Rho family, which occurs downstream of G_{12} family members (Figs. 116–3 and 116–4).[27,28] Several proteins having both G_α-interacting domains and guanine nucleotide exchange factor (GEF) domains can link G_{12} family members to Rho family members. One example is p115RhoGEF, but others exist as well.[29] With the exception of ADP, shape change persists in platelets from mice that lack $G_{q\alpha}$[30] but is lost when $G_{13\alpha}$ expression is suppressed, alone or in combination with $G_{12\alpha}$.[31,32] Put somewhat differently, loss of $G_{q\alpha}$ expression prevents shape change when mouse platelets are activated by ADP. Loss of $G_{13\alpha}$ expression (but not loss of $G_{12\alpha}$ expression alone) suppresses shape change in response to thrombin and TxA_2.

These results indicate that for most platelet agonists, G_{13} signaling is essential for shape change and that the events underlying shape change are invoked by a combination of G_{13}- and G_q-dependent signals. A combination of inhibitor and genetic approaches suggests that G_{13}-dependent Rho activation leads to shape change via pathways that include the Rho-activated kinase p160ROCK and LIM kinase.[27,33,34] These kinases phosphorylate myosin light chain kinase and cofilin, helping to regulate both actin filament formation and myosin (see Fig. 16–4). ADP, on the other hand, depends more heavily on G_q-dependent activation of PLC to produce shape change and is able to activate G_{13} only as a consequence of TxA_2 generation, hence the loss of ADP-induced shape change when G_q signaling is suppressed.

G_i Family Members and Their Effectors

Rising cAMP levels turn off signaling in platelets, and an increase in cAMP synthesis is one of the mechanisms by which endothelial cells prevent inappropriate platelet activation. Regulatory molecules released from endothelial cells cause $G_{s\alpha}$-mediated increases in adenylyl cyclase activity (PGI_2) and inhibit hydrolysis of cAMP by phosphodiesterases (nitric oxide). When added to platelets in vitro, PGI_2 can cause a 10-fold or greater increase in the platelet cAMP concentration, but even relatively small increases in cAMP levels (twofold or less) can impair thrombin responses.[35] Many platelet agonists inhibit PGI_2-stimulated cAMP synthesis by binding to receptors that are coupled to one or more G_i family members (Fig. 116–5). Human platelets express four members of the G_i family: G_{i1}, G_{i2}, G_{i3}, and G_z. Deletion of the genes encoding $G_{i2\alpha}$ or $G_{z\alpha}$ increases the basal cAMP concentration in mouse platelets. Conversely, loss of PGI_2 receptor (IP) expression causes a decrease in basal cAMP levels, enhances responses to agonists, and predisposes mice to thrombosis in arterial injury models.[36,37]

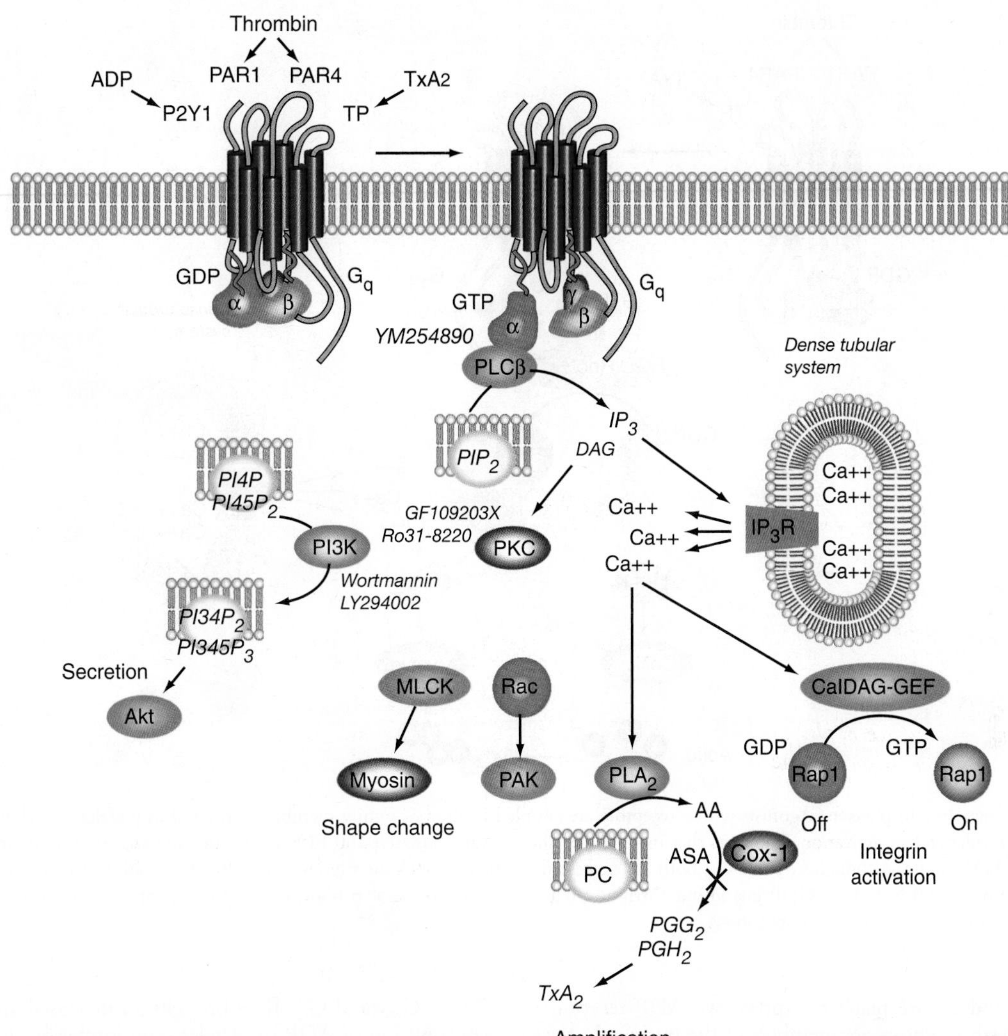

Figure 116–3 G_q signaling in platelets. Agonists whose receptors are coupled to G_q are able to activate phospholipase Cβ (PLCβ) via $G_{q\alpha}$. The potency with which activation occurs varies depending on the agonist, with thrombin and thromboxane A_2 (TxA_2) providing a stronger stimulus for PLCβ-mediated phosphoinositide hydrolysis than adenosine diphosphate (ADP). Thrombin activates two G_q-coupled receptors on human platelets, protease-activated receptor 1 (PAR1) and protease-activated receptor 4 (PAR4), which differ somewhat in the kinetics of PLC activation. YM254890 inhibits PLC activation by G_q.[140,141] GF109203X and Ro31–8220 are protein kinase C (PKC) inhibitors.[142] Wortmannin and LY294002 are phosphatidylinositol 3-kinase (PI3K) inhibitors. AA, arachidonic acid; ASA, aspirin; COX-1, cyclooxygenase 1; DAG, diacylglycerol; GDP, guanosine 5′-triphosphate; GTP, guanosine 5′-triphosphate; IP_3R, receptor for 1,4,5-inositol triphosphate; MLCK, myosin light chain kinase; PAK, p21-activated kinase; PG, prostaglandin; PI3K, phosphatidylinositol 3-kinase; PIP_2, phosphatidylinositol-4,5-bisphosphate; PLA_2, phospholipase A_2; PLCβ, phospholipase Cβ.

Although the G_i family members in platelets are most commonly associated with suppression of cAMP formation, this is not their only role. The defect of platelet function seen in mice that are missing $G_{i\alpha}$ family members cannot be reversed by adenylyl cyclase inhibitors.[36] In addition to providing $G_{\beta\gamma}$ heterodimers that can activate PLCβ, the downstream effectors for G_i family members in platelets include PI3K, Src family members, and Rap1B (see Fig. 116–5).[26,38–40] PI3Ks phosphorylate PI-4-P and PI-4,5-P_2 to produce PI-3,4-P_2 and PI-3,4,5-P_3. Human platelets express the α, β, γ, and δ isoforms of PI3K. PI3Kγ is activated by $G_{\beta\gamma}$.

Much of what is known about the role of PI3K in platelets comes from studies with inhibitors such as wortmannin and LY294002 or from studies of gene-deleted mouse platelets.[41] Those studies established that PI3K activation can occur downstream of both G_q and G_i family members and that effectors for PI3K in platelets include the serine/threonine kinase Akt[38] and Rap1B.[42] Loss of the PI3Kγ isoform causes impaired platelet aggregation.[43] Loss of PI3Kβ impairs Rap1B activation and thrombus formation in vivo, as do PI3Kβ-selective inhibitors.[42] Deletion of the gene encoding Akt2 results in impaired thrombus formation and stability and inhibits secretion.[38] Loss of Akt1 has been reported to inhibit platelet aggregation, suggesting that these are not redundant molecules.[44] Although it seems clear that PI3K activation leads to activation of Akt in platelets, what happens next is less clear. There are many established and predicted substrates for Akt, but, with the exception of GSK3β, the Akt substrates in platelets have not been identified, and much remains to be learned.

ADP: Two Receptors with Distinguishable Functions

ADP is stored in platelet dense granules and released upon platelet activation. ADP also is released by erythrocytes and damaged tissues at sites of vascular injury. When added to platelets in vitro, ADP causes TxA_2 formation, protein phosphorylation, increased cytosolic Ca^{2+} concentration, shape change, aggregation, and secretion. It also inhibits cAMP formation. These responses are half-maximal at approximately 1 μM ADP. However, even at high concentrations, ADP is a comparatively weak activator of PLC. Instead, its usefulness as a platelet agonist rests more upon its ability to activate other path-

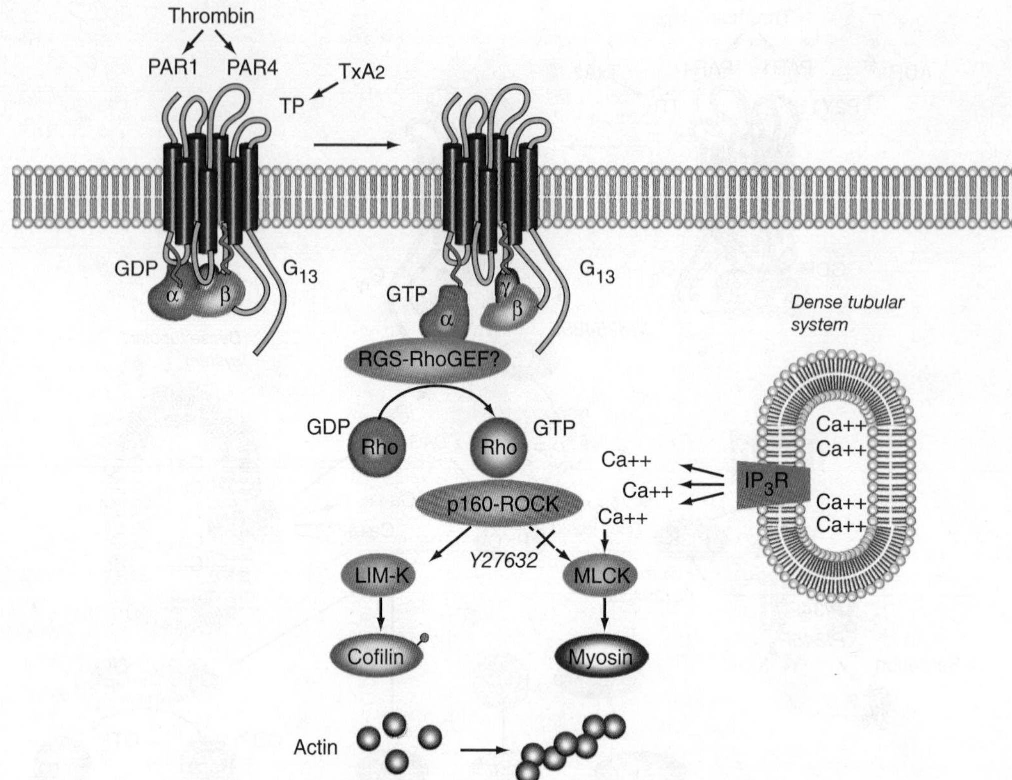

Figure 116–4 $G_{12/13}$ signaling in platelets. Agonists whose receptors are coupled to the G_{12} family members expressed in platelets are able to trigger shape change, in part by Rho-dependent activation of kinases that include the Rho-activated kinase p160 ROCK and the downstream kinases myosin light chain kinase (MLCK) and LIM kinase. Although G_{12} and G_{13} both are expressed, based on knockout studies, G_{13} is the dominant G_{12} family member in mouse platelets. Y27632 inhibits p160 ROCK.[143] GDP, guanosine 5′-triphosphate; GTP, guanosine 5′-triphosphate; IP_3R, receptor for 1,4,5-inositol triphosphate; PAR, protease-activated receptor; TxA_2, thromboxane A_2.

ways.[45,46] Human and mouse platelets express two ADP receptors: $P2Y_1$ and $P2Y_{12}$. Both receptors are members of the purinergic class of GPCRs (Table 116–1 and Fig. 116–6).[47–51] $P2Y_1$ receptors couple to G_q. $P2Y_{12}$ receptors couple to G_{i2} (see Figs. 116–3 and 116–5). Optimal responses to ADP require both. The third purinergic receptor on platelets, $P2X_1$, is an ATP-gated Ca^{2+} channel.[52–55] Platelet dense granules contain ATP as well as ADP, and studies suggest that $P2X_1$ activity is essential for platelet activation under certain conditions.[56–58]

When $P2Y_1$ is blocked or deleted, ADP still can inhibit cAMP formation, but its ability to cause an increase in cytosolic Ca^{2+} concentration, shape change, and aggregation is greatly impaired. $P2Y_1^{-/-}$ mice have a minimal increase in bleeding time and show some resistance to thromboembolic mortality after injection of ADP. Primary responses to platelet agonists other than ADP are unaffected. ADP, when combined with serotonin, which is a weak stimulus for PLC in platelets, still can cause aggregation of $P2Y_1^{-/-}$ platelets. Taken together, these results show that platelet $P2Y_1$ receptors are coupled to $G_{q\alpha}$ and are responsible for activation of PLC. $P2Y_1$ receptors also can activate Rac and the Rac effector p21-activated kinase (PAK),[59] but they do not appear to be coupled to G_i family members.

$P2Y_{12}$ receptors were characterized functionally before they actually were identified.[50,51] As predicted by the phenotype of a patient lacking functional $P2Y_{12}$,[60] platelets from $P2Y_{12}^{-/-}$ mice do not aggregate normally in response to ADP.[61] $P2Y_{12}^{-/-}$ platelets retain $P2Y_1$-associated responses, including shape change and PLC activation, but they lack the ability to inhibit cAMP formation in response to ADP. The G_i family member associated with $P2Y_{12}$ appears to be primarily G_{i2}, as platelets from $G_{i2\alpha}^{-/-}$ mice have an impaired response to ADP, whereas those lacking $G_{i3\alpha}$ or $G_{z\alpha}$ do not (Table 116–2).[36,62,63]

Identification of the receptors that mediate platelet responses to ADP, the development of antagonists that target each of the known receptors, and the successful knockouts of the genes encoding $P2Y_1$, $P2Y_{12}$, $G_{q\alpha}$, and $G_{i2\alpha}$ have brought an increased appreciation of the contribution of ADP to platelet plug formation in vivo. Absence of $P2Y_{12}$ produces a hemorrhagic phenotype in humans, albeit a relatively mild one.[50,60,64] Because the receptors for thrombin and TxA_2 can cause robust activation of PLC, the contribution of ADP when thrombin or TxA_2 is present appears to be largely due to the its ability to activate G_{i2}. Two antiplatelet agents, ticlopidine and clopidogrel, are irreversible antagonists of $P2Y_{12}$.

Thrombin: Two Receptors with Overlapping Functions

Thrombin is able to activate platelets at concentrations as low as 0.1 nM. Although other platelet agonists also can cause phosphoinositide hydrolysis, none appears to do so as efficiently as thrombin. Within seconds of the addition of thrombin, the cytosolic Ca^{2+} concentration increases 10-fold, triggering downstream Ca^{2+}-dependent events, including activation of phospholipase A_2. All of these responses, but not shape change, are abolished in platelets from mice lacking $G_{q\alpha}$.[65] Thrombin also activates Rho in platelets, leading to rearrangement of the actin cytoskeleton and shape change, responses that are greatly reduced or absent in mouse platelets that lack $G_{13\alpha}$.[31] Finally, thrombin is able to inhibit adenylyl cyclase activity in human platelets, either directly (via a G_i family member) or indirectly (via released ADP).[66–68]

Platelet responses to thrombin are mediated by members of the PAR family of GPCRs. The PAR family consists of four members. Three (PAR1, PAR3, and PAR4) can be activated by thrombin. PAR1 and PAR4 are expressed on human platelets; mouse platelets express PAR3 and PAR4 (see Table 116–1). Receptor activation occurs when thrombin cleaves the extended N-terminus of each of

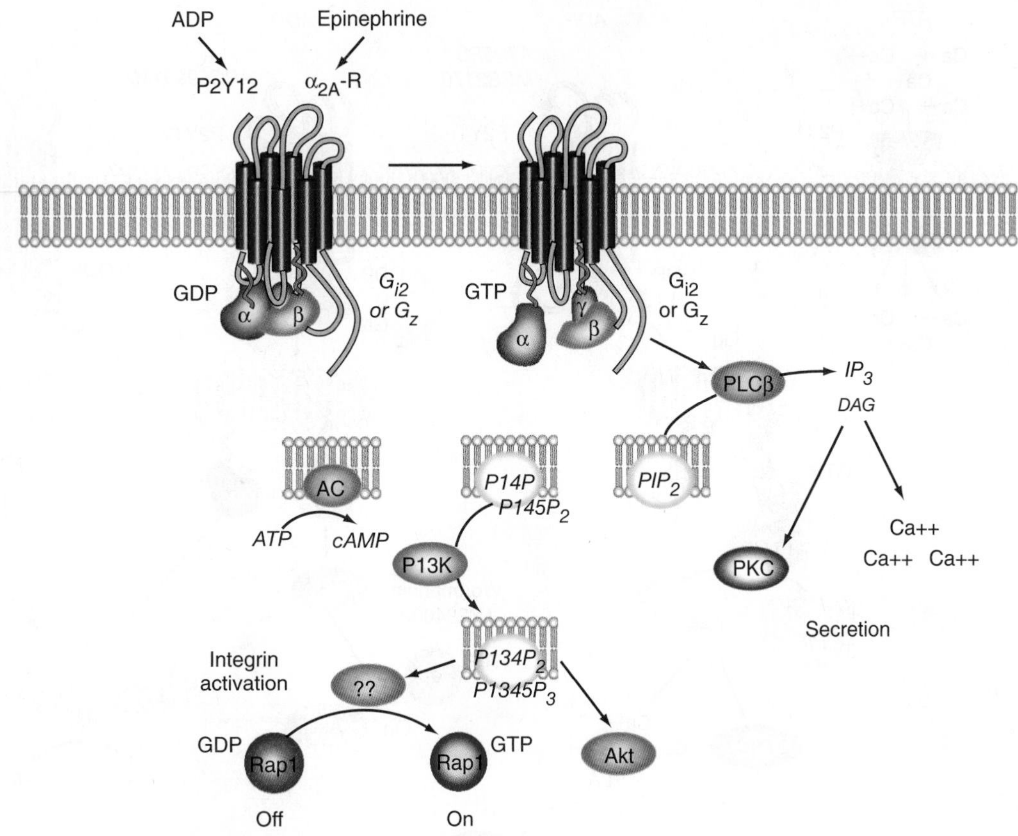

Figure 116–5 G_i signaling in platelets. G_{i2} is the predominant G_i family member expressed in human platelets. In addition to inhibiting adenylyl cyclase (alleviating the repressive effects of cyclic adenosine monophosphate [cAMP]), G_{i2} couples $P2Y_{12}$ ADP receptors to phosphatidylinositol 3-kinase (PI3K), Akt phosphorylation, and Rap1B activation. Other effectors may exist as well. The role of G_z in platelets appears to be limited to interactions with α_{2A}-adrenergic receptors and responses to epinephrine. Epinephrine appears to be primarily a potentiator of the effects of other platelet agonists, inhibiting cAMP formation and promoting activation of Rap1B and PI3K. AC, adenylyl cyclase; ADP, adenosine diphosphate; ATP, adenosine triphosphate; cAMP, cyclic adenosine monophosphate; DAG, diacylglycerol; GDP, guanosine 5′-triphosphate; GTP, guanosine 5′-triphosphate; IP_3, inositol triphosphate; PIP_2, phosphatidylinositol-4,5-bisphosphate; PKC, protein kinase C; PLCβ, phospholipase Cβ.

Table 116–2 Platelet Phenotypes of G_α Knockout Mice

Family	G_α	Platelet Phenotype
$G_{i\alpha}$	$G_{i2\alpha}$	Reduced aggregation and inhibition of cAMP formation with ADP. Normal shape change.
	$G_{i3\alpha}$	No apparent effect.
	$G_{z\alpha}$	Impaired aggregation and suppression of cAMP formation by epinephrine. Resistance to disseminated thrombosis initiated with collagen plus epinephrine but not with collagen plus ADP. Normal shape change. Increased bleeding time in one of two studies.
$G_{q\alpha}$	$G_{q\alpha}$	Predisposed to bleed. Absent aggregation with all agonists tested but normal shape change. Resistance to disseminated thrombosis initiated with collagen plus epinephrine.
	$G_{11\alpha}$	No apparent effect on platelet function.[a]
	$G_{15\alpha}$	No apparent effect on platelet function.[a]
$G_{12\alpha}$	$G_{12\alpha}$	No apparent effect on platelet function.[a]
	$G_{13\alpha}$	Embryonic lethal due to vascular defects but decreased platelet shape change and aggregation when limited to hematopoietic cells.

[a]Our unpublished observations.
ADP, adenosine diphosphate; cAMP, cyclic adenosine monophosphate.

these receptors, exposing a new N-terminus that serves as a tethered ligand.[69] Synthetic peptides based on the sequence of the tethered ligand domain of PAR1 and PAR4 are able to activate the receptors, mimicking at least some of the actions of thrombin. Approximately half of $PAR1^{-/-}$ mice die in utero, but this appears to be due to loss of receptor expression in the vasculature rather than in platelets.[70] Human PAR3 can signal in response to thrombin, whereas mouse PAR3 appears to primarily serve to facilitate cleavage of PAR4.[71] Activation of PAR4 requires higher concentrations of thrombin than PAR1, apparently because it lacks the hirudin-like sequences that can interact with thrombin's anion-binding exosite and facilitate receptor cleavage.[71–74] Kinetic studies in human platelets suggest that thrombin signals first through PAR1 and subsequently through PAR4.[75,76]

Peptide agonists for either PAR1 or PAR4 cause platelet aggregation and secretion. Conversely, simultaneous inhibition of human PAR1 and PAR4 abolishes responses to thrombin,[77] as does deletion of the gene encoding PAR4 in mice.[78] Thus, PAR family members are necessary. The picture has emerged that thrombin responses in human platelets require PAR1 and PAR4 (Fig. 116–7), whereas those in mice are mediated by PAR3-facilitated cleavage of PAR4. Abundant evidence, including studies in knockout mice, shows that PAR1 and PAR4 are coupled to G_q and G_{13}. However, a requirement for PAR family members does not preclude the involvement of other participants. One long-standing candidate is GPIb. GPIb is a heterodimer composed of disulfide-linked α and β subunits that exist in a complex with GPIX and GPV. Together they provide a binding site for VWF and an anchor for the platelet cytoskeleton. GPIbα has a high-affinity thrombin binding site located within residues 268–

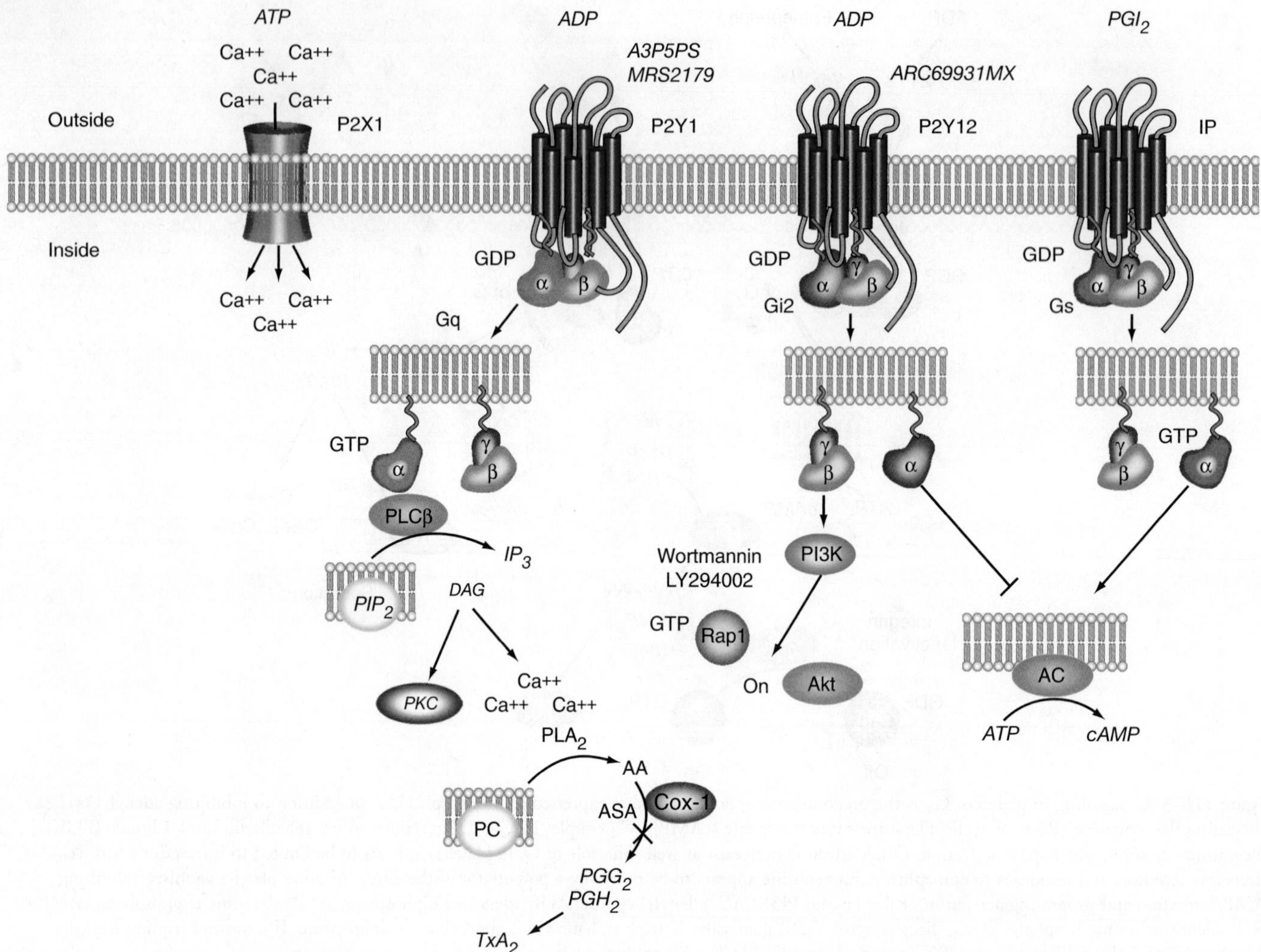

Figure 116–6 Adenosine diphosphate (ADP) receptors. Three receptors that can be activated by adenine nucleotides have been identified in platelets: $P2Y_1$ and $P2Y_{12}$ are ADP-activated, G protein-coupled receptors coupled to G_q and G_{i2}. $P2X_1$ is an adenosine triphosphate (ATP)-gated cation channel that can allow Ca^{2+} influx. A3P5PS and MRS2179 are $P2Y_1$-selective antagonists. ARC69931MX is a $P2Y_{12}$-selective antagonist. AA, arachidonic acid; AC, adenylyl cyclase; ASA, aspirin; cAMP, cyclic adenosine monophosphate; COX-1, cyclooxygenase 1; DAG, diacylglycerol; GDP, guanosine 5′-triphosphate; GTP, guanosine 5′-triphosphate; IP_3, inositol triphosphate; PG, prostaglandin; PI3K, phosphatidylinositol 3-kinase; PIP_2, phosphatidylinositol-4,5-bisphosphate; PKC, protein kinase C; PLCβ, phospholipase Cβ; TxA_2, thromboxane A_2.

287.[79] Deletion or blockade of this site reduces platelet responses to thrombin, particularly at low thrombin concentrations, and has been shown to impair PAR1 cleavage on human platelets.[80–84] VWF binding to GPIb leads to intracellular signaling that supports platelet activation. This also may occur when thrombin binds.

Epinephrine: Potentiator of Other Agonists

Compared to thrombin, epinephrine is a weak activator of human platelets when added on its own. Nonetheless, human families in which members have a mild bleeding disorder associated with impaired epinephrine-induced aggregation and reduced numbers of catecholamine receptors have been reported.[85,86] Platelet responses to epinephrine are mediated by α_{2A}-adrenergic receptors (see Table 116–1). In both mice and humans, epinephrine is able to potentiate the effects of other agonists so that the combination is a stronger stimulus for platelet activation than either agonist alone. Potentiation usually is attributed to the ability of epinephrine to inhibit cAMP formation; however, as discussed previously, other effects clearly are mediated by G_i family members as well. In contrast to other platelet agonists, epinephrine has no detectable direct effect on PLC and does not cause shape change, although it can trigger phosphoinositide hydrolysis indirectly by stimulating TxA_2 formation.[87]

The inability to stimulate phosphoinositide hydrolysis and shape change suggests that platelet α_{2A}-adrenergic receptors are coupled to G_i but not to G_q or G_{12} family members (see Fig. 116–5). Gene deletion studies have confirmed and extended this conclusion. Human and mouse platelets express four members of the G_i family. Of the four, the sequence of $G_{z\alpha}$ is the most distinct. $G_{z\alpha}$ also has the slowest rate of intrinsic GTP hydrolysis and is the only $G_{i\alpha}$ family member that is not a pertussis toxin substrate. Platelet responses to epinephrine were abolished when the gene encoding $G_{z\alpha}$ was removed. Loss of $G_{i2\alpha}$ or $G_{i3\alpha}$ had no effect.[36,62] Therefore, it appears that, in mouse platelets, α_{2A}-adrenergic receptors couple to G_z but not to G_{i2} or G_{i3}. G_z also appears to be responsible for the ability of epinephrine to activate Rap1B.[26,36]

Thromboxane A_2: Twin Receptors Coupled to G_q and $G_{12/13}$

TxA_2 is produced from arachidonate in platelets by the aspirin-sensitive cyclooxygenase 1 pathway. When added to platelets in vitro, thromboxane analogues such as U46619 cause shape change, aggregation, secretion, phosphoinositide hydrolysis, protein phosphorylation, and an increased cytosolic Ca^{2+} concentration while having

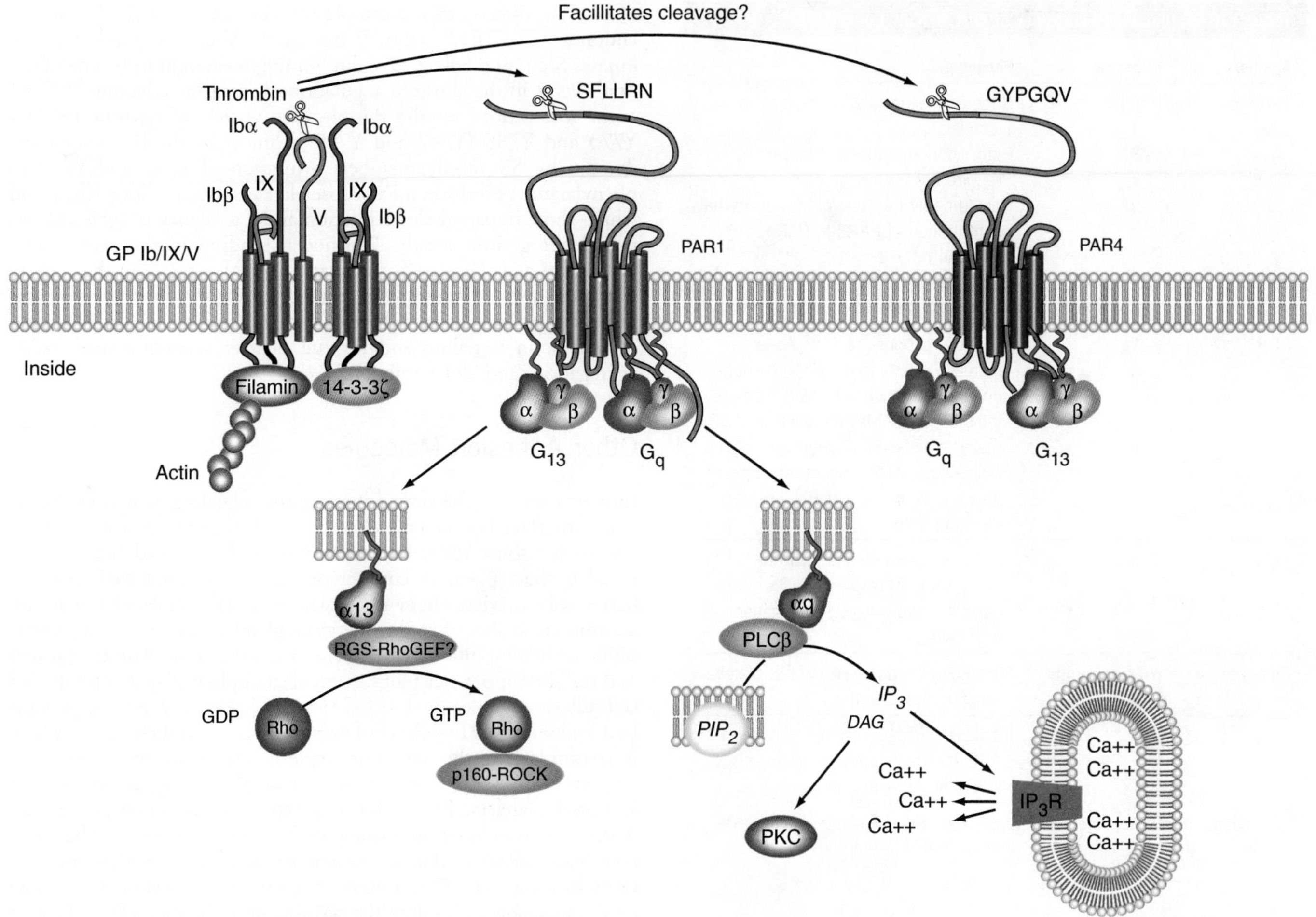

Figure 116–7 Thrombin receptors. Platelet responses to thrombin are mediated largely by members of the protease-activated receptor (PAR) family. Human platelets express PAR1 and PAR4, which collectively are coupled to G_q- and G_{13}-mediated effector pathways. Secretion of adenosine diphosphate (ADP) acts as a further activator of G_i-mediated pathways via the receptor $P2Y_{12}$. Cleavage of PAR1 by thrombin appears to be facilitated by binding of thrombin to glycoprotein Ibα (GPIbα) in the GPIb-IX-V complex. DAG, diacylglycerol; GDP, guanosine 5′-triphosphate; GTP, guanosine 5′-triphosphate; IP_3, inositol triphosphate; IP_3R, inositol triphosphate receptor; PIP_2, phosphatidylinositol-4,5-bisphosphate; PKC, protein kinase C; PLCβ, phospholipase Cβ.

little, if any direct, effect on cAMP formation. Once formed, TxA_2 can diffuse outward and activate other platelets, amplifying the initial stimulus for platelet activation (see Fig. 116–1, *B*). This process is effective locally but is limited by the short half-life of TxA_2, which helps confine the spread of platelet activation to the original area of injury.

Only one gene encodes TxA_2 receptors, but two splice variants (TPα and TPβ) that differ in their cytoplasmic tails are produced (see Table 116–1). Human platelets express both.[88] TxA_2 receptors appear to be mapped to G_q and G_{13} but not to G_i (see Table 116–2). Biochemical studies have shown that platelet TxA_2 receptors are physically associated with $G_{q\alpha}$ and $G_{13\alpha}$ and are able to activate G_{12} family members.[89–91] Loss of $G_{q\alpha}$ abolishes U46619-induced IP_3 formation but not shape change.[65] Loss of $G_{13\alpha}$ abolishes TxA_2-induced shape change.[31] Although thromboxane receptors in cells other than platelets have been shown to couple to pertussis toxin-sensitive G_i family members,[92] in platelets the inhibitory effects of U46619 on cAMP formation appear to be mediated by secreted ADP.

Loss of TxA_2 signaling impairs platelet function. $TP^{-/-}$ mice have a prolonged bleeding time. Their platelets are unable to aggregate in response to TxA_2 agonists (Table 116–3) and show delayed aggregation with collagen, presumably reflecting the role of TxA_2 in platelet responses to collagen.[93] A group of Japanese patients with impaired platelet responses to TxA_2 analogues have proved to be either homozygous or heterozygous for an R60L mutation in the first cytoplasmic loop of TP.[94] However, the most compelling case for the contribution of TxA_2 signaling in human platelets comes from the successful use of aspirin as an antiplatelet agent. When added to platelets in vitro, aspirin abolishes TxA_2 generation and impairs, but does not abolish, responses to thrombin and ADP.

Stage III: Perpetuation (Stabilization) of the Platelet Plug

Signaling from collagen receptors and GPCRs is responsible for initiation and extension of the platelet plug, but additional signaling and adhesive events affect the continued growth and stability of the platelet mass once it begins to form (see Fig. 116–1, *C*). These events are facilitated and, in some cases, made possible by the close contacts between platelets that can occur only once platelet aggregation begins. Electron micrographs show the close proximity of the plasma membranes of adjacent platelets within an aggregate but do not show the adherens and tight junctions that are typical of contacts between endothelial cells. Estimates of the gap between adjacent platelets range from as little as zero to as much as 50 nm, making it possible for molecules on the surface of one platelet to bind to those on an adjacent platelet. This interaction can be direct, as when one cell adhesion molecule binds to another in *trans*. The interaction also can

Table 116–3 Platelet Phenotypes of GPCR Knockout Mice

Agonist	Receptor	Phenotype
Thrombin	PAR1	None (not expressed on mouse platelets).
	PAR3	Higher concentrations of thrombin required to elicit responses, presumably because of loss of normal contribution of PAR3 to PAR4 activation.
	PAR4	Complete loss of thrombin responsiveness.
ADP	$P2Y_1$	Impaired response to ADP. Absent increase in cytosolic Ca^{2+} and shape change in response to ADP. Normal inhibition of cAMP formation by ADP.
	$P2Y_{12}$	Greatly diminished aggregation in response to ADP. Absent inhibition of adenylyl cyclase by ADP. Increased bleeding time.
TxA_2	$TP\alpha/\beta$	Prolonged bleeding time, absent aggregation in response to TxA_2 agonists, and delayed aggregation with collagen.
Epinephrine	α_{2A}-adrenergic	Mice have been developed but platelet function not reported.
PGI_2	IP	Increased aggregation in response to ADP. Increased rate of thrombosis following vascular injury.

ADP, adenosine diphosphate; cAMP, cyclic adenosine monophosphate; GPCR, G protein-coupled receptor; PAR, protease-activated receptor; PGI_2, prostaglandin I_2; TxA_2, thromboxane A_2.

be indirect, as occurs when multivalent adhesive proteins link activated $\alpha_{IIb}\beta_3$ on adjacent platelets. In either case, these interactions theoretically can provide both an additional adhesive force and a secondary source of intracellular signaling. The narrowness of the gap between platelets can restrict the inward diffusion of molecules such as plasmin and the outward diffusion of platelet activators, allowing higher local concentrations to be reached and maintained.[95]

Clot retraction is a platelet-dependent event in which a fibrin clot gradually pulls in upon itself, shrinking to a smaller volume after platelet activation and fibrin deposition are well underway. Clot retraction depends on the interaction between actin–myosin complexes and the cytoplasmic domain of $\alpha_{IIb}\beta_3$, as well as the binding of fibrinogen or VWF to the extracellular domain of the integrin. The absence of clot retraction is one of the hallmarks of platelets from patients with Glanzmann thrombasthenia, a condition in which platelets lack $\alpha_{IIb}\beta_3$. In the context of platelet–platelet interactions, clot retraction can be viewed as a mechanism for narrowing the gaps between platelets and increasing the local concentration of soluble ligands for platelet receptors.[96]

Integrins, Adhesion, and Outside-In Signaling

Activated $\alpha_{IIb}\beta_3$ bound to fibrinogen, fibrin, or VWF provides the dominant cohesive strength that holds platelet aggregates together. Outside-in signaling refers to the intracellular signaling events that occur downstream of activated integrins once ligand binding has occurred.[97] Integrin signaling depends in large part on the formation of protein complexes that link to the integrin cytoplasmic domain. Some of the protein–protein interactions that involve the cytoplasmic domains of $\alpha_{IIb}\beta_3$ help regulate integrin activation; others participate in outside-in signaling and clot retraction. Proteins that are capable of binding directly to the cytoplasmic domains of $\alpha_{IIb}\beta_3$ include β_3 endonexin,[98] CIB1,[99] talin,[100] myosin,[101] Shc,[102] and the tyrosine kinases Src[103] and Syk.[104,105] Talin binding is thought to be one of the final events in the allosteric regulation of integrin activation.[100,106–108] Some interactions require the phosphorylation of tyrosine residues Y773 and Y785 (Y747 and Y759 in mice) in the β_3 cytoplasmic domain by Src family members. Mutation of Y747 and Y759 to phenylalanine produces mice whose platelets tend to disaggregate and which show impaired clot retraction and a tendency to rebleed from tail bleeding time sites.[109] Fibrinogen binding to the extracellular domain of activated $\alpha_{IIb}\beta_3$ stimulates a rapid increase in the activity of Src family members and Syk. Studies of platelets from mice lacking these kinases suggest that these events are required for the initiation of outside-in signaling and for full platelet spreading, irreversible aggregation, and clot retraction.[110–113]

Other Adhesion Molecules

Integrins are not the only adhesion and signaling molecules found at the interface between platelets. Some of these molecules have been known for some time, but they have newly assigned functions in platelets that appear to counter original ideas about their roles. A better way to view them is as platelet surface molecules that can accumulate at sites of contact between platelets and enter into homophilic or heterophilic interactions in *trans* that modulate the growth and stability of platelet plugs. A good example is platelet endothelial cell adhesion molecule 1 (PECAM-1; CD31). PECAM is perhaps best known for its high level of expression on endothelial cells, where it accumulates at the junctions between cells. However, as its name suggests, PECAM-1 is also expressed on the surface of resting and activated platelets. PECAM-1 is a type 1 transmembrane protein with six extracellular immunoglobulin (Ig) domains.[114] The most membrane-distal Ig domain is able to support homotypic interactions in *trans*. The C-terminus contains phosphorylatable tyrosine residues capable of binding the tyrosine phosphatase SHP-2. Loss of PECAM-1 expression causes increased responsiveness to collagen in vitro and increased thrombus formation in vivo. The data are consistent with a model in which tyrosine phosphorylation of PECAM-1 brings the phosphatase near its substrates, including the GPVI signaling complex.[115–117] This finding suggests that, despite being named as an adhesion molecule, PECAM-1 can provide a braking effect on collagen-induced signaling and thereby help prevent either unwarranted platelet activation or the overly exuberant growth of platelet thrombi that otherwise might occlude the vessel lumen and cause ischemia.

Junctional adhesion molecules (JAMs) are members of the CTX family of Ig domain-containing cell adhesion molecules. Three have been identified: JAM-A (JAM-1; F11R), JAM-B (JAM-2; VE-JAM), and JAM-C (JAM-3).[118,119] Platelets express JAM-A and JAM-C. JAMs have an extracellular domain with two Ig domains, a single transmembrane region, and a short cytoplasmic tail that terminates in a PDZ domain binding site. JAM-A localizes to tight junctions of endothelial and epithelial cells. It also is found on monocytes, neutrophils, and lymphocytes. JAM-C has been found on endothelial cells, lymphatic vessels, dendritic cells, and natural killer cells. JAM-A contributes to cell–cell adhesion by forming *trans* interactions involving the N-terminal Ig domain. However, JAMs also support heterotypic interactions, including binding to integrins via their membrane proximal Ig domain.[120,121] Other CTX family members that have been identified on platelets include ESAM and CD226.[122–124] Their functional significance has yet to be determined.

Signaling lymphocytic activation molecule (SLAM; CD150) and CD84 are members of the CD2 family of homophilic adhesion molecules that have been studied extensively in lymphocytes; however, now they have been shown to be expressed in platelets as well.[125–127] The members of the family are type 1 membrane glycoproteins in the Ig superfamily. Among them are notable differences in the cytoplasmic domain, which supports binding interactions with a variety of adaptor/partner proteins. SLAM and CD84 become tyrosine phosphorylated during platelet activation, but only if aggregation is allowed to occur.[125] Mice that lack SLAM have a defect in platelet aggregation in response to collagen or a PAR4-activating peptide but have a normal response to ADP and a normal bleeding time. In a mesenteric vascular injury model, female (but not male) SLAM$^{-/-}$ mice showed a marked decrease in platelet accumulation.

Receptor–Ligand Interactions at the Platelet–Platelet Interface

Direct contacts between platelets can promote signaling by more than one mechanism. In addition to signaling events that occur downstream from cell adhesion molecules, there are receptors that interact in *trans* with cell surface ligands. One example is the family of Eph receptor tyrosine kinases and their ligands, known as *ephrins*. Ephrins are cell surface proteins with either a glycophosphatidylinositol anchor (the ephrin A family) or a transmembrane domain (the ephrin B family). The cytoplasmic domains of the ephrin B family members include phosphorylatable tyrosine residues and a PDZ target domain. Contact between an ephrin-expressing cell and an Eph-expressing cell causes bidirectional signaling. Human platelets express EphA4, EphB1, and ephrinB1. Clustering of ephrinB1 promotes platelet aggregation. Blockade of Eph–ephrin interactions leads to reversible platelet aggregation at low agonist concentrations and limits the growth of platelet thrombi on collagen-coated surfaces under arterial flow conditions. It also impairs β_3 phosphorylation, which inhibits clot retraction.[128] EphA4 colocalizes with $\alpha_{IIb}\beta_3$ at sites of contact between aggregated platelets. Collectively, these observations suggest a model in which the onset of aggregation brings platelets into close proximity and allows ephrinB1 to bind to EphA4 and EphB1. Signaling downstream of both the receptors and the kinases then promotes further integrin activation and integrin signaling.[128–130] A second example of ligand–receptor interactions made possible by close contacts between platelets is the binding of the ligand semaphorin 4D (sema4D) to its receptors CD72 and plexin B1. sema4D is an integral membrane protein in the semaphorin family. Signaling downstream of CD72 and plexin B1 promotes platelet activation by collagen. Loss of sema4D expression in mice inhibits platelet function in vitro and thrombus formation in vivo.[131]

A somewhat different paradigm of a ligand–receptor interaction that is facilitated by platelet–platelet contacts is binding of growth arrest-specific gene 6 (Gas-6) to its receptors. Gas-6 is a vitamin K-dependent protein related to protein S. In rodent platelets, Gas-6 is found in α granules.[132–134] Secreted Gas-6 is a ligand for the receptor tyrosine kinases Tyro3, Axl, and Mer,[135,136] all of which are expressed on platelets.[133] Because Tyro3 family members have been shown to stimulate PI3K and PLCγ, a reasonable hypothesis is that secreted Gas-6 can bind to its receptors on the platelet surface and cause signaling that promotes platelet plug formation and stability. Consistent with this hypothesis, platelets from Gas-6$^{-/-}$ mice were found to have an aberrant response to agonists in which aggregation terminates prematurely.[133] Platelets from receptor-deleted mice also failed to aggregate normally in response to agonists.[137–139] Secretion of Gas-6 into the spaces between platelets in a growing thrombus would be expected to allow it to achieve higher local concentrations and provide protection from being washed away.

CONCLUSION

The intracellular signaling that underlies platelet activation is a dynamic process in which different receptor and effector pathways are dominant at different phases in the initiation, extension, and perpetuation of platelet plugs. The main objective throughout normal hemostasis is to activate integrin $\alpha_{IIb}\beta_3$ so that it can bind adhesive proteins and then maintain it in an active (bound) state so that a platelet plug of the appropriate size will remain in place long enough for healing to occur. In general, this requires the activation of PLC- and PI3K-dependent pathways. It also involves the suppression of inhibitory mechanisms that normally are designed to prevent platelet activation, including the formation of cAMP by adenylyl cyclase. If the initial stimulus for platelet activation is the exposure of collagen, then $\alpha_{IIb}\beta_3$ activation is accomplished by a process that involves activation of PLCγ. If the initial stimulus is the generation of thrombin, then a G protein-dependent mechanism results in a more rapid and robust activation of PLCβ. Once $\alpha_{IIb}\beta_3$ has been activated and platelet aggregation has occurred, then a third wave of signaling is facilitated by the close contacts that form between platelets within a hemostatic plug or thrombus.

SUGGESTED READINGS

Brass LF, Zhu L, Stalker TJ: Minding the gaps to promote thrombus growth and stability. J Clin Invest 115:3385, 2005.

Chrzanowska-Wodnicka M, Smyth SS, Schoenwaelder SM, Fischer TH, White GC 2nd: Rap1b is required for normal platelet function and hemostasis in mice. J Clin Invest 115:680, 2005.

Del Conde I, Shrimpton CN, Thiagarajan P, Lopez JA: Tissue-factor-bearing microvesicles arise from lipid rafts and fuse with activated platelets to initiate coagulation. Blood 106:1604, 2005.

Falati S, Patil S, Gross PL, et al: Platelet PECAM-1 inhibits thrombus formation in vivo. Blood 107:535, 2006.

Fung CY, Brearley CA, Farndale RW, Mahaut-Smith MP: A major role for P2X1 receptors in the early collagen-evoked intracellular Ca2+ responses of human platelets. Thromb Haemost 94:37, 2005.

Gross PL, Furie BC, Merrill-Skoloff G, Chou J, Furie B: Leukocyte versus microparticle-mediated tissue factor transfer during arteriolar thrombus development. J Leukoc Biol 78:1318, 2005.

Jackson SP, Schoenwaelder SM, Goncalves I, et al: PI 3-kinase p110beta: A new target for antithrombotic therapy. Nat Med 11:507, 2005.

Lopez JA, del Conde I, Shrimpton CN: Receptors, rafts, and microvesicles in thrombosis and inflammation. J Thromb Haemost 3:1737, 2005.

Maguire PB, Foy M, Fitzgerald DJ: Using proteomics to identify potential therapeutic targets in platelets. Biochem Soc Trans 33:409, 2005.

Nanda N, Andre P, Bao M, et al: Platelet aggregation induces platelet aggregate stability via SLAM family receptor signaling. Blood 106:3028, 2005.

Offermanns S: Activation of platelet function through G protein-coupled receptors. Circ Res 99:1293, 2006.

Pandey D, Goyal P, Bamburg JR, Siess W: Regulation of LIM-kinase 1 and cofilin in thrombin-stimulated platelets. Blood 107:575, 2005.

Prevost N, Woulfe DS, Jiang H, et al: Eph kinases and ephrins support thrombus growth and stability by regulating integrin outside-in signaling in platelets. Proc Natl Acad Sci U S A 102:9820, 2005.

Quinton TM, Kim S, Jin J, Kunapuli SP: Lipid rafts are required in Galpha(i) signaling downstream of the P2Y12 receptor during ADP-mediated platelet activation. J Thromb Haemost 3:1036, 2005.

Ratnikov BI, Partridge AW, Ginsberg MH: Integrin activation by talin. J Thromb Haemost 3:1783, 2005.

Soulet C, Hechler B, Gratacap MP, et al: A differential role of the platelet ADP receptors P2Y and P2Y in Rac activation. J Thromb Haemost 3:2296, 2005.

Zhu L, Bergmeier W, Wu J, et al: Regulated surface expression and shedding support a dual role for semaphorin 4D in platelet responses to vascular injury. Proc Natl Acad Sci U S A 104:1621, 2007.

REFERENCES

For complete list of references log onto www.expertconsult.com

CHAPTER 117

THE BLOOD VESSEL WALL

Aly Karsan and John M. Harlan

The vasculature plays a major role in conveying and distributing hematopoietic cells, nutrients, gases, metabolites, and various chemical mediators.[1] The interior of the vessel wall is lined by the endothelium, comprising more than 10^{12} endothelial cells, covering a surface of approximately 500 m^2 and weighing approximately 1 kg in total.[2,3] The endothelium forms a continuous monolayer at the interface between blood and tissue. Thus it contributes significantly to sensing and transducing of signals between blood and tissue, trafficking of hematopoietic cells, and maintenance of a nonthrombogenic surface permitting flow of blood. Normally quiescent, with cell turnover measured on the order of years, endothelial cells have a remarkable capacity to proliferate and vascularize tissues in physiologic (menstrual cycle) and pathologic (tumorigenesis, diabetic retinopathy) situations.[4] The endothelium is critical for initiating and potentiating the inflammatory response. The pathogenesis of several disorders, such as atherosclerosis, hypertension, diabetic angiopathy, and microangiopathic hemolytic anemias, involves dysfunction of the endothelial lining. The complexity and the vast array of its functional responses have led to the description of the endothelium as a distributed organ.[5] This chapter provides a conceptual framework of the structure and development of the vessel wall and the physiologic functions of the endothelium as it relates to the hematopoietic system.

STRUCTURE OF THE VESSEL WALL

The circulatory system has traditionally been divided into the macrovasculature (vessels >100 μm in diameter) and the microvasculature.[6] The arterial system transports blood to tissues, resists changes in blood pressure proximally, and regulates blood flow distally. Veins return blood to the heart and act as capacitance vessels, as they contain approximately 70% of the total blood volume. Venules with luminal diameters less than 50 μm are structurally similar to capillaries.[6] Capillaries, and microvessels in general, are particularly important in the exchange of gases, macromolecules, and cells between blood and tissue. Although large vessels play an important role in maintaining vascular tone, a significant proportion of peripheral resistance arises from the capillaries.[7] Capillary endothelial cells also have a metabolic role, as in the conversion of angiotensin and hydrolysis of lipoproteins. Finally, sprouting of new vessels is initiated in the microvasculature.

Macrovasculature

Large vessels are composed of three layers: intima, media, and adventitia.[6,8] The intima comprises the endothelium and the subendothelium. The endothelial cells of large vessels contain a distinct rod-shaped organelle, measuring approximately 3 μm × 0.1 μm, called the *Weibel-Palade body.*[9] Ultrastructural studies indicate the presence of a single membrane around the Weibel-Palade body with tubular structures within. This organelle contains von Willebrand factor (vWF), and P-selectin has been reported to be present on the surrounding membrane.[10–12] The abluminal face of the endothelium rests on a basement membrane, which supports the endothelial cell and can act as a secondary barrier against the extravasation of blood.[2] The subendothelial matrix contains occasional smooth muscle cells and scattered macrophages. Both smooth muscle cells and endothelial cells contribute to the extracellular matrix (ECM) of the intima.[13,14] In large vessels the media is separated from the intima by a layer of elastin, the internal elastic lamina. The medial layer is composed primarily of concentric layers of smooth muscle cells and their secreted matrix, which is a complex mix of glycoproteins and proteoglycans. This layer is responsible for the structural integrity of the wall and for maintaining vascular tone. Mutations of the fibrillin-1 gene, a microfilament protein in elastic fibers, result in disruption of the media in Marfan syndrome.[12] Defects of type III collagen can cause aortic rupture in patients with Ehlers-Danlos syndrome type IV.[14] An attenuated band of elastic fibers, the external elastic lamina, separates the adventitia from the media. The adventitia is composed of loose connective tissue, and the outer portion of the media contains small nerves and nutritive blood vessels, the vasa vasorum. The external limit of the adventitial layer is loosely defined and becomes continuous with the surrounding connective tissue of the organ.[6,8]

Microvasculature

Capillaries and postcapillary venules are composed of two cell types: endothelial cells and pericytes.[15] Pericytes and endothelial cells are invested with a basement membrane and, depending upon the vascular bed, variable amounts of matrix separate the two cell types. Both cell types contribute to secretion of basement membrane proteins. Long pericyte processes extend over the abluminal surface of the endothelial cell, and reciprocal extensions of the endothelial cell make contact with the pericyte. Pericytes and endothelial cells communicate via gap junctions.[16] A variety of functions has been ascribed to the pericyte, including[15,17,18] (a) a contractile function, which regulates blood flow; (b) multipotential capabilities resulting in differentiation to adipocytes, osteoblasts, phagocytes, and smooth muscle cells; and (c) regulation of capillary growth. The best evidence probably exists for the last function. In animal models[19,20] and human disease (diabetic microangiopathy, hemangiomata),[21] a lack of pericytes is associated with microaneurysms and disordered microvasculature. In addition, there is a temporal correlation between pericyte contact and cessation of vessel growth in wound healing,[22] and pericyte contact suppresses endothelial cell migration and proliferation in vitro.[15]

Endothelial Structure and Function

In contrast to circulating blood cells and vascular smooth muscle cells but similar to epithelial cells, the endothelium exhibits polarity manifested by the asymmetric distribution of cell surface glycoproteins and by the unidirectional secretion of some ECM proteins and chemical mediators.[23,24] Although in cultured endothelial cells, an apical–basal polarity is established prior to confluence, intercellular junctions may have a role in maintaining the asymmetry in vivo.[23,25]

Four types of intercellular junctions between adjacent endothelial cells have been described[25,26]: tight junctions, gap junctions, adherens junctions, and syndesmos. Their distribution varies along the vascular tree, with tight junctions occurring more frequently in the larger arteries and brain vasculature, correlating with a more stringent requirement for permeability control. The molecular structure of endothelial *tight junctions* is similar to that of epithelial cells, consisting of a network of fibrils, with the integral membrane components composed of occludin, claudin-5, and junctional adhesion molecules (JAMs), which associate with various structural and signaling proteins on the cytoplasmic face.[27] The distribution of *gap junctions* tends to follow that of tight junctions. Connexin37, connexin40, and connexin43 are gap junction proteins that have been detected in endothelial cells. Gap junctions mediate communication between adjacent endothelial cells and between endothelial cells and pericytes or smooth muscle cells; they also may contribute to the endothelial barrier. *Adherens junctions* are formed by transmembrane glycoproteins called *cadherins,* which make the link between cell-to-cell contacts and the cytoskeleton. Several different types of cadherins are expressed in endothelial cells. The endothelial-specific cadherin *vascular endothelial cadherin* (VE-cadherin [cadherin-5]) is expressed on virtually all types of endothelium.[26] Similar to other cadherins, VE-cadherin forms homotypic contacts with VE-cadherin on adjacent cells. Within the cell VE-cadherin complexes with catenins, which, through other proteins, contact the actin cytoskeleton. Homotypic engagement of VE-cadherin results in density-dependent inhibition of endothelial proliferation, which appears to be mediated by association of vascular endothelial growth factor receptor 2 (VEGFR-2) with VE-cadherin, thereby sequestering VEGFR-2 at the membrane and preventing its internalization into signaling compartments.[28] The structure of the fourth type of junction, the *syndesmos,* is not well elucidated.

Other membrane proteins that are located at interendothelial junctions include platelet endothelial cell adhesion molecule 1 (PECAM-1), which may be important in directing the formation of junctions, and the integrins (particularly $\alpha_2\beta_1$ and $\alpha_5\beta_1$).[29] In addition to the functions listed previously, intercellular contacts are important in maintaining cell survival.[30]

On the luminal side, endothelium is exposed to blood elements and, under pathologic conditions, to circulating molecules such as cytokines and bacterial products. Engagement of endothelial receptors by these humoral factors activates a well-described series of responses. including the recruitment and transmigration of leukocytes and changes in endothelial cell coagulant activity (see The Endothelium as a Nonthrombogenic Surface). Biomechanical forces resulting from pulsatile blood flow have been shown to mediate striking changes in endothelial morphology and metabolism. Vessels must withstand three types of physical forces: radial distension (tension), longitudinal stretch, and tangential shear stress. In response to flow (shear stress), endothelial cells reorganize their cytoskeletal architecture, rearrange focal contacts at the *basal* surface, and align in the direction of flow.[31–33] Some endothelial cell responses following exposure to physical forces occur within seconds, such as activation of potassium channels and increased release of nitric oxide (NO), resulting in vasodilation. Other endothelial cell responses to flow are related to changes in gene expression and occur after a delay of a few hours. Elements in the promoters of various adhesion molecule and growth factor genes have been shown to contain sequences that respond to shear stress (in a positive or negative fashion) and have been referred to as the *shear stress response element.*[31–33]

Endothelial cells vectorially secrete certain ECM proteins to the abluminal face. The matrix molecules that are secreted by endothelium include several types of collagen, elastin, fibronectin, laminins, and proteoglycans (e.g., heparan sulfate, dermatan sulfate). The exact composition of the subendothelium varies with location in the vascular tree, age, and disease states.[2,14,34] Endothelial cells bind to the ECM via heterodimeric cell surface glycoproteins—the integrins—which link and integrate matrix proteins to the cytoskeleton, at sites referred to as focal contacts.[35] The integrins detected in resting endothelium include $\alpha_6\beta_1$, $\alpha_5\beta_1$, $\alpha_2\beta_1$, and $\alpha_v\beta_3$.[36] Interestingly, endothelial cells express integrins on luminal as well as abluminal surfaces.[36] The ECM serves several important functions: (a) it serves as a barrier to macromolecules in the event of disruption of the endothelium; (b) it sequesters growth factors and mediates their high-affinity binding to endothelial cells (e.g., heparan sulfate binds to fibroblast growth factor [FGF]); (c) it acts as a counterstructure for the binding of endothelial cell integrins.[14,34,37] This binding of endothelial cells to the ECM serves at least four purposes: (i) Certain matrix molecules provide a physical scaffold, whereas others act as haptotactic agents, inducing endothelial cells to migrate.[14] (ii) Clustering of integrins at focal adhesion contacts by certain matrix molecules can transduce survival or differentiation signals by causing phosphorylation of various proteins and lipids.[37] Fibronectin and vitronectin provide survival signals, whereas laminins appear to signal differentiation.[38–40] (iii) By maintaining cell shape, integrin-mediated cell spreading provides an antiapoptotic signal independent of direct integrin-initiated signal transduction.[41] (iv) By anchoring the cell, the matrix provides a mechanism whereby blood flow at the luminal surface of the endothelium creates shear stress, which also transmits signals to cells.[31]

Endothelial Heterogeneity

Despite their common features, quiescent endothelial cells in vivo represent a widely heterogeneous population, with their phenotype depending on vessel caliber and location. Exposure to different physical forces (e.g., arteries vs veins) and the different functions served by vessels of different caliber are reflected in different endothelial phenotypes.[42] However, study of the molecular basis of the heterogeneity of these different populations is just beginning. Experiments using serial analysis of gene expression and in vivo delivery of phage display peptide libraries have revealed organ- and tumor vasculature-specific molecules that will help to elucidate the molecular basis of endothelial heterogeneity.[43–45] Within the microvasculature is a structural heterogeneity of capillaries, depending on the organ supplied. Even within a single organ endothelial cells exhibit different phenotypes, depending on their functional role. When microvessels from different organs are harvested and cultured in vitro, they lose some of their distinctive characteristics with progressive passaging. Some specialization of the different endothelial cells can be retained if they are cocultured with cells or matrix from the organ from which they are derived. Thus, matrix proteins, soluble factors from the organ, or heterotypic contacts with parenchymal cells or pericyte/smooth muscle cells are believed to be important factors in specifying endothelial cell phenotype.[46] Conversely, emerging evidence indicates that endothelial cells in turn provide instructive morphogenic cues during organogenesis and in the adult.[47] Specific examples of microvessels found in hematopoietic tissues are discussed in the following sections.

High Endothelial Venules

Lymphocyte migration into secondary lymphoid sites, such as lymph nodes, Peyer patches, and chronically inflamed nonlymphoid tissues, occurs at specialized postcapillary venules.[48] The endothelial cells of these venules exhibit a plump/cuboidal morphology (hence the name *high endothelial venule*), display intense biosynthetic activity, and are encircled by a continuous basal lamina. They secrete a thick glycocalyx of which a proportion is glycosylation-dependent cell adhesion molecule 1, a ligand for L-selectin.[49] CD34 is another high endothelial venule "addressin" on peripheral lymph node endothelial cells. Endothelium of mesenteric lymph nodes and Peyer patches express mucosal addressin cellular adhesion molecule 1 (MAdCAM-1) as a ligand for L-selectin and $\alpha_4\beta_7$ integrin. Expression of these different addressins may recruit specific subpopulations of lymphocytes to different lymphoid tissues (i.e., they facilitate the "homing" of lymphocytes). Several other proteins, including the chemokine receptor DARC (Duffy antigen receptor for chemokines) and the antiadhesive matrix protein Hevin, have been identified as being preferentially expressed by the high endothelial venule.[50] Tight junctions are present at intermittent spots, and extensive overlap between the membranes of adjacent cells prevents macromolecules from interendothelial transit. However, when lymphoid cells transit to the high endothelial venule, there is a temporary breach in the barrier.[49] Evidence suggests that the high endothelial venule not only plays a critical role in homing and recruitment of immune cells but also can influence the outcome of the immune response.[51]

Bone Marrow Sinuses

Much less is known about the marrow sinuses than about the high endothelial venule. The marrow sinus endothelial cell is flat, in contrast to that of the high endothelial venule, and the basal lamina is discontinuous. It has been suggested that hematopoietic cells traverse pores present at attenuated areas of the endothelium rather than moving by an interendothelial route.[52] Clearly, the marrow sinus endothelial cell is specialized given the regulated egress of cells from the marrow. For example, if a red cell that still is nucleated begins to enter the circulation, the body of the cell is allowed to cross and is released as a reticulocyte, while the nucleus is retained extravascularly. The adventitial reticular cell (similar to a pericyte) is also thought to play an important role in controlling hematopoietic cell egress.[53] Stromal cell-derived factor 1 (SDF-1, also called CXCL12) and chemokine receptor CXCR4 interactions are essential for stem cell homing, mobilization, and transendothelial migration into the bone marrow.[54,55] SDF-1 activates the integrins lymphocyte function-associated antigen 1 (LFA-1 [$\alpha_L\beta_2$]), very late antigen 4 (VLA-4 [$\alpha_4\beta_1$], and very late antigen 5 (VLA-5 [$\alpha_5\beta_1$]). Vascular cell adhesion molecule 1 (VCAM-1), which is expressed on marrow endothelial cells (and spleen endothelial cells in the mouse), appears to be the major bone marrow addressin for hematopoietic progenitor cells expressing VLA-4, whereas intercellular adhesion molecule 1 (ICAM-1) binds LFA-1.[55,56] Endothelial selectins also have been implicated in promoting hematopoietic progenitor homing to the bone marrow.[57] Factors such as CD44, cytoskeletal rearrangement, and matrix metalloproteases are other key players in the homing process related to the endothelium.[55] The marrow endothelium also is involved in regulating hematopoiesis (see Relationship between Vascular Development and Hematopoiese).

VASCULAR DEVELOPMENT AND DIFFERENTIATION

The human embryo develops a vascular system by the third week, when its nutritional needs are no longer met by diffusion.[58] Vascular development proceeds in several ways. *Vasculogenesis* is the process whereby blood vessels form de novo from the differentiation of mesodermal precursors. *Angiogenesis* is the outgrowth of new capillaries from preexisting vessels and is thought to be the major mode of new vessel development in the adult. *Arteriogenesis*, or collateral development, is the rapid enlargement of preexisting collateral arterioles after occlusion of a supply artery. *Lymphangiogenesis* is the development of lymphatic vessels, which are required for transportation of extravasated lymph and lymphoid cells. Finally, in some neoplasms, tumor cells rather than endothelial cells form vascular channels or a portion of some vessels, a process termed *vasculogenic mimicry*.[59] A similar nonendothelial cell lining of vascular channels can be created by placental cytotrophoblasts forming hybrid fetal–maternal vessels in the endometrium.[59]

Vasculogenesis

Vasculogenesis in the yolk sac proceeds initially by the differentiation of mesodermal cells into angioblasts.[60] Angioblasts are vascular cells that express some, but not all, endothelial markers. These cells arise from mesodermal cells resting on the endoderm (splanchnopleuric mesoderm) but not from the mesoderm adjacent to the ectoderm (somatopleuric mesoderm). Thus, it is believed that the endoderm positively regulates vascular development, whereas the ectoderm negatively regulates vasculogenesis. Organs that are primarily of ectodermal origin (e.g., brain and kidney) are vascularized by angiogenesis and not by vasculogenesis. The mesodermal cells migrating outward from the endoderm form primitive structures termed *blood islands*. The cells at the center of the blood island are hematopoietic precursors, whereas those arranged peripherally are angioblastic precursors. Vasculogenesis within the embryo begins shortly after that in the yolk sac, again in close association with endoderm.[61] However, except for a region on the ventral aspect of the embryonic aorta, intraembryonic vascular development occurs in solitary angioblasts rather than blood islands. Angioblasts differentiate in situ and form primary capillary plexuses with lumens, or they migrate and fuse with other angioblasts or capillaries. Fusion of angioblasts or blood islands results in the formation of a capillary plexus that undergoes extensive remodeling over the developmental period.[60]

Vasculogenesis in the Adult

Although initially said to occur primarily in the embryo, vasculogenesis may also play a role in promoting vascular development in the adult. The identification of circulating bone marrow-derived vascular precursors and the demonstration that these precursors can integrate into the vasculature at sites of angiogenesis describe an adult form of de novo vessel development.[62] Two distinct marrow-derived precursors with the ability to differentiate into vascular cells have been identified: (a) accumulating evidence points to a single precursor, the hemangioblast, which can differentiate into either hematopoietic or endothelial cells[63]; and (b) a multipotent nonhematopoietic adult progenitor cell, which is thought to represent a bone marrow mesenchymal stem cell. When injected intravenously into adult mice, these mesenchymal stem cells differentiated into vascular cells, hematopoietic cells, as well as several epithelial cell types.[64,65] Both types of multipotential precursor populations express CD133, a cell surface marker that is lost upon further maturation.[66] However, only the hemangioblast expresses CD34. Whether mesenchymal stem cells are able to circulate and thus contribute to neovascularization outside the marrow remains to be shown. Various stresses, including neoplasia, sepsis, burns, and trauma, have been suggested to induce mobilization of marrow-derived endothelial precursors, which express CD133, CD34, and VEGFR-2.[66] Cytokines that reportedly induce mobilization of marrow-derived endothelial precursors include VEGF-A and granulocyte-macrophage colony-stimulating factor.[66] The contribution of bone marrow-derived vascular precursors to angiogenic vessels in tumors is highly variable, depending on the study, the model used, and the tumor cell type used.[67] The degree of endothelial precursor incorporation into the angiogenic vasculature is highly controversial; several groups suggest negligible if any involvement by distant precursors.[67] The problem arises in part from the poor definition of a circulating endothelial precursor cell. Many, if not all, of the markers used to define this rare cell population are shared with hematopoietic stem or progenitor cells, and the distinction between the endothelial and hematopoietic precursor has not been rigorously addressed in the majority of studies. More recent work has suggested that marrow-derived, perivascular CD11b$^+$ hematopoietic cells secreting angiogenic cytokines have been misidentified as endothelial precursor cells.[68,69]

Angiogenesis

In the normal adult, angiogenesis occurs primarily in the female reproductive system. However, angiogenesis is a process that has a major impact in several pathologic situations. Probably the best-known and studied example of pathologic neovascularization occurs during tumor progression. Angiogenesis also is important in chronic inflammation, ischemia, and wound healing.

Capillary sprouts from the existing microvasculature form secondary to an inciting stimulus that results in increased vascular permeability, accumulation of extravascular fibrin, and local proteolytic degradation of the basement membrane.[70–72] Endothelial cells overlying the disrupted region become "activated," change shape, and extend elongated processes into the surrounding tissue. Filopodia extending from the specialized endothelial cells at the tip of the vascular sprout guide the migration of the nascent vessel.[73] Directed migration toward the angiogenic stimulation results in the formation of a column of endothelial cells. Just proximal to the migrating tip of the column is a region of proliferating endothelial cells. These proliferating cells cause an increase in the length of the sprout. In the region of proliferation, up to 20% of endothelial cells may enter the cell cycle. This is in marked contrast to quiescent endothelium, of which less than 0.01% of cells are cycling. Proximal to the proliferative zone, the endothelial cells undergo another shape change, adhere tightly to each other, and begin to form a lumen. Evidence suggests that endothelial lumina arise through the formation and fusion of intracellular vacuoles.[74] Secondary sprouting from the migrating tip results in a capillary plexus, and fusion of individual sprouts at their tips closes the loop and circulates blood into the vascularized area. Activated macrophages and platelets, by secreting growth factors, cytokines, proteases, and protease inhibitors, can influence all phases of the angiogenic process.[75]

The morphologic features described are characteristic of sprouting angiogenesis. *Intussusceptive microvascular growth* refers to vascular network formation by insertion of interstitial tissue columns, called *tissue pillars* or *posts,* into the vascular lumen and subsequent growth of these columns, resulting in partitioning of the vessel lumen. The mechanisms of intussusceptive angiogenesis are less well described, but hemodynamic factors appear to be involved.[76]

Recruitment of Periendothelial Cells

Whether formed by vasculogenesis or angiogenesis, maturation of new vessels requires recruitment of smooth muscle cells or pericytes to reestablish vessel integrity. Periendothelial cells provide structural support, assist in production of the ECM, provide contractile function so as to modulate vessel caliber, and maintain the cells in a quiescent state. Genetically altered mice that fail to invest their vessels with pericytes develop microaneurysms.[19] In the embryo, periendothelial cells are thought to be derived from locally available mesenchymal cells as endothelial cells invade organ rudiments. Local derivation of periendothelial cells may be one mechanism that allows for tissue-specific phenotype of the vasculature.[15] Evidence suggests that embryonic endothelial cells may transdifferentiate into vascular smooth muscle cells.[77] Evidence also indicates that some periendothelial cells are derived from the neural crest during embryogenesis and from marrow-derived precursors in the adult.[78–81] Although some studies have shown pericytes to be potential antivascular targets for tumor therapy,[80,82] other work has suggested that pericytes act to limit tumor metastasis.[83]

Extracellular Matrix

It is thought that interstitial collagens (e.g., collagen I) and provisional plasma-derived fibronectin/fibrin matrices stimulate endothelial tubular morphogenic events, whereas laminin-rich matrices lead to endothelial differentiation and stabilization events.[75] Mice deficient in fibronectin die during embryogenesis and show vascular defects. Type I collagen-deficient mice die of circulatory failure just before birth. Although most tumor vessels are covered by basement membrane, this layer has multiple structural abnormalities consistent with ongoing vascular activation in tumors.[84] ECM proteins and/or their proteolytic fragments have been shown to inhibit angiogenesis.

Dissolution of the underlying matrix by matrix metalloproteases and heparanases allows endothelial cells to migrate at the initiation of angiogenesis.[85,86] Matrix-bound growth factors are also released as a consequence of ECM degradation. The balance between positive and negative regulators is the basis of tight control in this process. Tissue plasminogen activator (tPA) and urokinase plasminogen activator, by generating plasmin, can activate collagenases and other matrix metalloproteinases. Plasminogen activator inhibitors may block angiogenesis at this step. Action of the matrix metalloproteinases is required for angiogenesis, and the tissue inhibitors of metalloproteinases regulate their function.[87]

Cell Adhesion Molecules

Of the various classes of cell adhesion molecules involved in angiogenesis, the integrins have been the most studied.[14,88,89] Although it is universally accepted that integrins and integrin ligands function in angiogenesis, their exact actions remain unclear. In particular, substantial controversy surrounds the role of $\alpha_v\beta_3$ integrin.[14,88,90] Immunohistochemical studies localize this integrin to the tips of sprouting vessels. Neutralizing antibodies abrogate angiogenesis and induce vascular cell apoptosis in vivo. However, mice lacking α_v show extensive angiogenesis, and mice and humans (Glanzmann thrombasthenia) lacking β_3 integrin also show normal angiogenesis. Notwithstanding the discrepancies outlined, preclinical studies have validated $\alpha_v\beta_3$ and potentially other integrins ($\alpha_v\beta_5$, $\alpha_1\beta_1$, $\alpha_2\beta_1$, $\alpha_5\beta_1$, $\alpha_6\beta_4$) as therapeutic antiangiogenic targets, and clinical trials with combination therapy are currently in progress.[91] One of the integrin receptors for fibronectin, $\alpha_5\beta_1$, has been shown to be necessary for vascular development, whereas $\alpha_2\beta_1$ seems important for the formation of tubes by endothelial cells in vitro. However, there likely is a dynamic regulation of β_1 integrins during angiogenesis because constitutive activation of this integrin inhibits endothelial sprouting in vitro and angiogenesis in vivo.[92] The junctional proteins VE-cadherin and PECAM-1, and possibly JAM-1, are expressed early in development and have a role in assembling the vasculature.[28,93,94]

Guidance Molecules

Similar to the nervous system, the vascular system forms a highly ordered, branching network. The ordering of this patterned network is dependent on multiple attractive and repulsive cues, many of which are common to both the nervous and vascular systems.[95,96] $VEGF_{165}$ acts as an attractive cue to the tip cell of the endothelial sprout, whereas Netrin1 signals to UNC5b on the vasculature act as a repulsive cue. Other guidance pathways implicated in vascular patterning and angiogenesis are ephrinB2-EphB4, plexinD1-semaphorin, and Slit-Robo interactions, as well as the neuropilins. Patterning and specification of small arteries along peripheral nerves in the skin of the embryonic limb involves nerve-derived VEGF; in other situations, neuronal patterning is dependent on the vasculature.[97,98] Thus, the congruent patterning of the neural and vascular systems likely is due to use of common signals and may require cross-talk between the two systems.

Remodeling, Regression, and Apoptosis

Even though the vasculature is laid down before circulation begins, hemodynamic forces are important for maintenance and remodeling. Most of the vessels laid down during vasculogenesis regress or are remodeled. Following neovascularization (e.g., during wound healing), the vessels regress when no longer needed. A chronic decrease in blood flow results in narrowing of the vessel lumen. This change in vessel caliber is dependent on an intact and functional endothelium.[99] Remodeling, which involves loss of some vessels as well as changes in lumen diameter and wall thickness, requires both cell death and proliferation (as well as remodeling of the ECM). In addition to survival signals transmitted by integrins, shear stress is important for endothelial survival and vessel healing following injury.[100–102] Oxygen tension is important in vascular maintenance. Hypoxia increases levels of VEGF, which provides signals for vessel maintenance and neovascularization.[103] Hyperoxia, on the other hand, inhibits VEGF expression, which leads to regression and death of retinal vessels.[104] In some models, regression of vessels occurs by

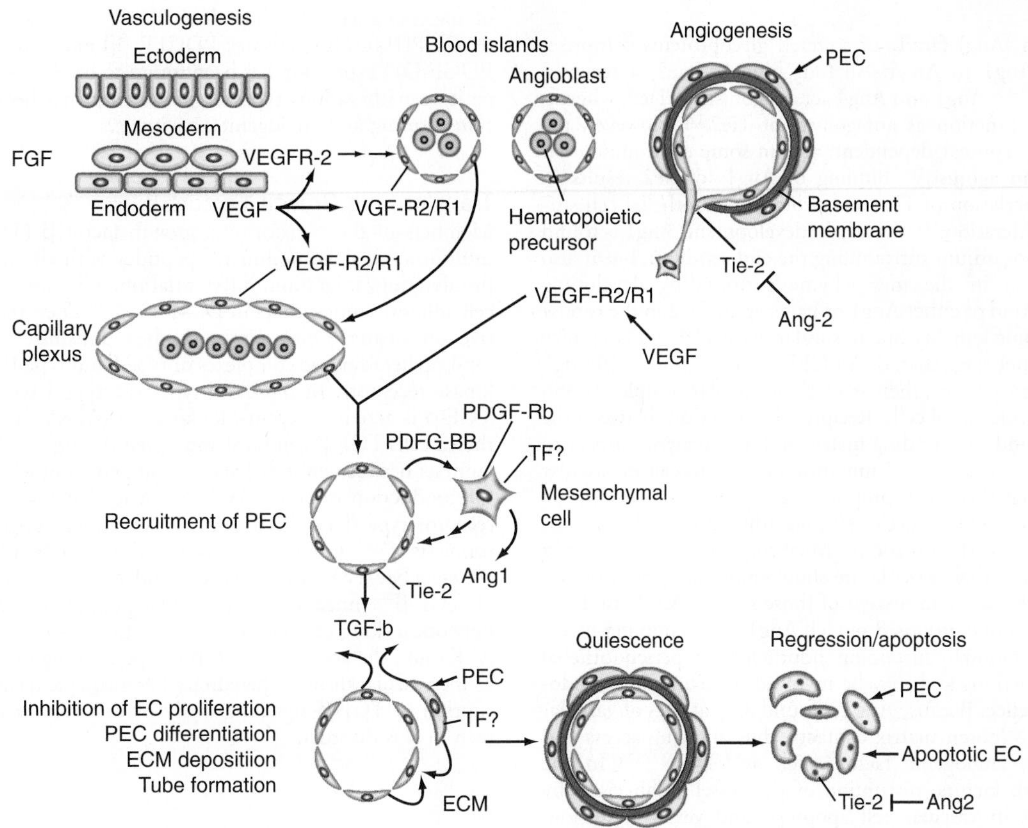

Figure 117–1 Model for vascular development. The role of secreted proteins and membrane receptors in vascular development is highlighted, but other factors such as cell adhesion molecules and extracellular matrix components also contribute significantly. Ang, angiopoietin; ECM, extracellular matrix; FGF, fibroblast growth factor; PDGF, platelet-derived growth factor; PEC, periendothelial cell (smooth muscle cell, pericyte); TF, tissue factor; TGF-β, transforming growth factor β, VEGF, vascular endothelial cell growth factor; VEGF-R, vascular endothelial cell growth factor receptor.

apoptosis of vascular cells.[105,106] Endothelial cells express several anti-apoptotic molecules in order to maintain viability when quiescent and when stressed.[107,108] Most likely, an intricate balance between cell death and proliferation is maintained by activators and inhibitors of both processes.

Role of Ligand–Receptor Interactions

Numerous factors regulate vascular development and differentiation in a positive or negative fashion. Some of the key molecules and their receptors are discussed here. A model for vascular development is shown in Fig. 117–1.

Inducers of Angiogenesis

Fibroblast Growth Factors

The role of FGFs in vascular development remains murky.[109–111] Because of possible functional redundancy in the numerous family members, assigning specific roles to the various members of the FGF family has been difficult. Evidence suggests that FGF receptors signal an inductive pathway by upregulating VEGFR-2 in differentiating mesoderm prior to vascular morphogenesis.[111–113] FGF2 may induce neovascularization in adults indirectly through activation of the VEGF–VEGFR pathway.[114]

Vascular Endothelial Growth Factors

Six members of the VEGF family have been identified[70,109,111,115–119]: VEGF-A (also called vascular permeability factor), VEGF-B, VEGF-C, VEGF-D, VEGF-E (a viral ortholog), and placental growth factor. Three members of the receptor tyrosine kinase family[109,118,119]—VEGFR-1 (flt-1), VEGFR-2 (flk-1/KDR), and VEGFR-3 (flt-4)—respond differentially to individual members of the VEGF family. In addition, the coreceptors for VEGF, neuropilin 1 and neuropilin 2, have been identified on arterial and venous endothelial cells, respectively. Neuropilin 1 is a coreceptor for VEGFR-2 that enhances binding of the VEGF-A isoform $VEGF_{165}$ to VEGFR-2.[118] VEGF-A functions as a homodimer. However, it also heterodimerizes with VEGF-B and placental growth factor, and it has a crucial dose-dependent effect on vasculogenesis[70,109,111,118,119] VEGF-A binds VEGFR-1 and VEGFR-2, whereas VEGF-C binds VEGFR-2 and VEGFR-3. Placental growth factor specifically activates VEGFR-1, whereas VEGF-E binds only VEGFR-2.[111,118,119] Lack of VEGFR-2 prevents the development of endothelial cells and a hematopoietic system because cells lacking VEGFR-2 do not reach the correct location to form blood islands.[120] Mice that have been rendered deficient for VEGFR-1 have normal hematopoietic progenitors and abundant endothelial cells, but they do not form capillary tubes or functional vessels.[121] Both VEGFR-2– and VEGFR-1–deficient mice die at an early embryonic stage, as do neuropilin 1– and neuropilin 2–deficient mice. In von Hippel Lindau disease, development of hemangioblastomas may be due to stabilization of VEGF mRNA.[122] VEGF is also believed to play a key role in propagating tumor angiogenesis. Tip cell migration has been shown to be dependent on a gradient of VEGF-A, whereas endothelial proliferation in the lengthening vascular stalk is dependent on the absolute concentration of VEGF-A, although both processes require VEGFR-2[73] Finally, injection of VEGF is capable of relieving limb ischemia by the generation of collateral vessels.[72] VEGF appears to collaborate with the angiopoietins to stimulate vascular development, whereas VE-cadherin acts to temper the VEGF response.[28]

Angiopoietins

The angiopoietin (Ang) family of secreted glycoproteins comprises four members: Ang1 to Ang4. All four bind to Tie2, a receptor tyrosine kinase.[123–126] Ang1 and Ang4 act as agonists of Tie2, whereas Ang2 and Ang3 function as antagonists of Tie2.[126] However, the action of Ang2 is context dependent, and in some environments it may behave as an agonist.[126] Binding of Ang1 to Tie2 results in tyrosine phosphorylation of Tie2 and promotes endothelial cell survival but not proliferation.[123,126] Early in development, Ang1 is found mainly in the myocardium surrounding the endocardium, but it also becomes expressed in the mesenchyme surrounding developing vessels.[123] Disruption of either Ang1 or its receptor Tie2 in the mouse results in embryonic lethality due to similar defects.[124,127] These mice die at a slightly later stage than do VEGFR-deficient mice. Although endothelial cells are present, there is a lack of vascular complexity and a scarcity of periendothelial cells. Reciprocal interactions between the endothelial cells and surrounding matrix and mesenchyme appear to be disrupted. An activating Tie2 mutation in humans causes vascular malformations that show a disproportionate number of endothelial cells compared to smooth muscle cells, resulting in dilated, tortuous vascular channels in certain tissues.[128] Mice engineered to overexpress Ang2 specifically in their vasculature show embryonic lethality and vascular defects that are reminiscent of those seen in Ang1- or Tie2-null embryos.[125] In one proposed model, Ang1–Tie2 coupling mediates vascular maturation by sustaining endothelial cell–periendothelial cell–matrix interactions and may be involved in maintaining endothelial cell quiescence. Because Ang2 is found only at sites of vascular remodeling, Ang2 loosen matrix contacts, thus allowing access and responsiveness to angiogenic factors such as VEGF.[125,126] In the absence of growth factors, disruption of the vessel architecture by Ang2 may result in vascular cell apoptosis and vessel regression. However, Ang2-deficient mice are born alive, and the major defect appears to be lymphatic development.[126] Thus, despite major advances the data are conflicting. The response of endothelial cells to angiopoietins likely is context dependent and endothelial cell type specific.[126]

Tie1 is a receptor tyrosine kinase that exhibits structural similarities to Tie2. A ligand for Tie1 has not yet been identified.[109,129] Disruption of the Tie1 gene in mice results in lethality at a much later point in development; Tie1-null mice may survive up to birth.[127,130] Tie1$^{-/-}$ mice die of hemorrhage and edema, implicating Tie1 in signaling the control of fluid exchange across capillaries and in maintenance of vessel integrity under hemodynamic stress. Chimeric mice that express Tie1$^{-/-}$ and Tie1$^{+/-}$ endothelial cells show underrepresentation of Tie1$^{-/-}$ cells in vessels primarily derived by angiogenesis but not in embryonic vessels derived by vasculogenesis, suggesting a differential function for Tie1 in angiogenesis.[131] Evidence also implicates a role for Tie1 in combination with Ang1 in establishing vascular polarity.[132]

Platelet-Derived Growth Factors

The platelet-derived growth factor (PDGF) family is composed of four chains. PDGF-A and PDGF-B can associate in a homodimeric or heterodimeric fashion.[133] Similarly, the receptors α and β are receptor tyrosine kinases that can form homodimers or heterodimers. PDGF-BB can bind the receptors PDGFR-ββ or PDGFR-αβ, but PDGFR-ββ binds only PDGF-BB and not PDGF-AA or PDGF-AB.[109] Mice null for PDGF-B die perinatally of renal, hematologic, and cardiovascular abnormalities.[134] The large vessels and heart of these mice are dilated, and microvessels exhibit microaneurysms due to lack of pericytes.[19,134] PDGFR-β knockout mice do not show an overtly abnormal cardiovascular phenotype, but generation of chimeric mice demonstrates that PDGFR-β$^{-/-}$ cells are underrepresented in all muscle lineages (smooth, cardiac, and skeletal).[135,136] Thus, it appears that PDGF-BB elaborated by the endothelial cell provides a signal to recruit mesenchymal periendothelial cells as part of the maturation process of vascular morphogenesis. Two novel PDGF chains, PDGF-C and PDGF-D, have been identified.[137] PDGF-CC can bind PDGFR-ββ or PDGFR-αβ, exhibits greater mitogenicity of mesenchymal cells than does PDGF-AA, and promotes wound repair. PDGF-DD activates PDGFR-ββ and possibly PDGFR-αβ. PDGF-DD expression has been found to be elevated in the serum of patients with various types of tumors and has been shown to have transforming and angiogenic activity.[137]

Transforming Growth Factors β

Members of the transforming growth factor β (TGF-β) family are multifunctional homodimeric peptides with diverse effects on cell proliferation, migration, differentiation, adhesion, and expression of cell adhesion molecules and ECM.[109,138,139] They are secreted as inactive precursors. Once activated, they transmit signals to cells by binding heteromeric complexes of type I and type II serine/threonine kinase receptors. In most cell types the type I receptor engaged by TGF-β is activin receptor-like kinase 5 (ALK5). However, in endothelial cells TGF-β can bind and signal through ALK5 and ALK1.[140] Contact between endothelial cells and periendothelial cells is required for production of active TGF-β.[15] Mice lacking TGF-β or TGF-β receptor type II exhibit similar defects in vasculogenesis and hematopoiesis.[138,139] Endothelial proliferation is not affected, but poor contacts between endothelial cell and mesothelial layers in embryos of TGF-β$^{-/-}$ mice result in a disorganized and reduced vascular network lacking capillary tubes. Mutations in two TGF-β receptors, ALK1 and the accessory TGF-β receptor endoglin, have been linked to the vascular disorder hereditary hemorrhagic telangiectasia.[140] Disruption of TGF-β signaling likely plays a role in the telangiectasia seen in this disorder.

Notch

The Notch family comprises four receptors (Notch1 through Notch4) and five ligands (Jagged1 and Jagged2, and Delta-like 1 [Dll1], Dll3, and Dll4). Ligand engagement results in a series of proteolytic clips that release the Notch intracellular domain, which then translocates to the nucleus where it effects transcriptional activation via the DNA-binding protein CSL (also called RBP-Jκ or CBF1).[141] Gene targeting studies have revealed a critical role for Notch1, Dll1, Dll4, and Jagged1 in vascular development and remodeling.[141] Dll4–Notch1 signaling between endothelial cells within the angiogenic sprout serves to restrict tip cell formation in response to VEGF.[142–144] Consequently, inhibition of Dll4 in adult mice results in increased endothelial proliferation, sprouting, and branching and increased tumor vascularity.[145,146] However, the vasculature is disorganized and poorly perfused; thus Dll4 blockade inhibits tumor growth in several models.[145,146]

Coagulation Factors

Tissue factor (TF) is a member of the cytokine receptor superfamily. In addition to its role in initiating coagulation as a cofactor for factor VII, TF may be involved in intracellular signaling. TF knockout mice have abnormalities of their large vessels and microvasculature secondary to defects in mesenchymal cell/periendothelial cell accumulation and function.[20] Elevated TF expression in various tumors and the associated angiogenic endothelium has been reported.[147] Expression of mutant oncogenes (K-*ras,* EGFR) or tumor suppressor genes (PTEN, p53) leads to increased TF expression and activity, and this may link tumor angiogenesis and the hypercoagulable states manifested in cancer.[147] Abnormal development of the vasculature also affects 50% of mice that are deficient in factor V. The affected mice die in utero, and the 50% embryonic lethality is similar to that observed in thrombin receptor-deficient mice that die without obvious coagulation defects.[148] Factor V-dependent generation of thrombin may be important for early vascular development by signaling through the thrombin receptor.[149] Thrombin can promote angiogenesis through a mechanism that is independent of fibrin formation.[149,150] Studies have suggested that thrombin can stimulate release of angiogenic factors (e.g., VEGF-A) from tumor cells and platelets as well induce VEGFR-2 on endothelial cells.[150]

Clinical trials have revealed that treatment with low-molecular-weight heparins improves the survival time of cancer patients receiving chemotherapy, an effect that appears to be independent of the anticoagulant properties of the low-molecular-weight heparins.[151,152] Although antiangiogenic effects of specific heparinase-generated fragments of unfractionated heparins have been demonstrated in vitro, the mechanism of the antitumor effect remains to be defined.

The potential involvement of fibrinolytic factors in angiogenesis has been mentioned. Interestingly, fragments 1 and 2 of prothrombin have been reported to inhibit angiogenesis, and various other fragments of coagulation and fibrinolytic proteins also may inhibit angiogenesis.[153]

Other Factors

Various other families of ligand–receptor pairs play a role in angiogenesis. They include Ephrin-Eph, Wnt-Frizzled, and Sonic Hedgehog-Smoothened. Various chemokines have been shown to modulate angiogenesis in either a positive or negative fashion.

Inhibitors of Angiogenesis

As with the angiogenesis inducers, multiple factors have been reported to negatively regulate vascular morphogenesis.[72,153] Of interest is a class of endogenous angiogenesis inhibitors that are fragments of larger proteins that have little or no angiogenesis-related activity in their intact form. They include fragments of ECM proteins such as fibronectin, collagen type IV α_3 chain (tumstatin), and collagen type XIII (endostatin), as well as coagulation protein fragments such as plasminogen (angiostatin) and antithrombin.[153] The mechanism of action of these protein fragments depends on the particular polypeptide, but the functional effect usually is inhibition of endothelial proliferation and/or induction of apoptosis.[153–155] Other endogenous inhibitors include interferons, chemokines, and interleukin-12 (IL-12).

More than 100 compounds are in clinical trials attempting to cause regression of tumors by inhibiting angiogenesis.[156] These compounds can be broadly divided into those that act directly by targeting the angiogenic endothelial cell and those that act indirectly by targeting activators of angiogenesis. The latter category includes targeting of oncogenes (e.g., mutant EGFR or Her2), as many aberrantly activated oncogenes have been shown to induce expression of angiogenic factors. The first clear-cut evidence of efficacy in clinical trials of an angiogenic inhibitor for tumor therapy came from regimens directed against the VEGF pathway (e.g., bevacizumab).[157,158] Because of the short improvement in overall and progression-free survival with the addition of VEGF inhibitors over standard chemotherapy, it is likely that heterogeneity and inherent instability of tumor cell populations result in the selection of malignant cells that feed their vasculature through factors other than VEGF. In this regard, use of indirect angiogenic inhibitors still suffers from the likelihood of tumors becoming resistant to the therapy.

Whether the mechanism of action of these inhibitors is truly due to the abrogation of a functional vascular supply is an open question. VEGF inhibitors "normalize" the aberrant, leaky tumor vasculature. Other than in renal cancer, VEGF inhibitors have shown effect only when used in combination chemotherapy regimens, which has led to the proposal that VEGF pathway inhibition improves vessel functionality and perfusion, thus facilitating delivery of chemotherapeutic agents.[157,158] VEGF–VEGFR signaling also acts in autocrine fashion within some tumor cell populations, raising the possibility that positive outcomes may have as much to do with direct tumor kill as with an antiangiogenic effect. Finally, as with organogenesis, the vasculature may provide a juxtacrine or paracrine role in supporting tumor viability and proliferation, independent of the provision of a circulatory system for delivery of nutrients and oxygen.[47]

Some of the more common side effects observed with use of VEGF-A inhibitors were not predicted a priori but may be understandable in retrospect. For instance, hypertension and arterial thrombosis are common side effects. Two possible reasons may explain the hypertensive side effect. One is that VEGF directly activates endothelial nitric oxide synthase (eNOS) and thus may be responsible in part for basal production of NO.[159] Another potential explanation is that podocyte-derived VEGF is required for proper glomerular function throughout life.[47] Heterozygous loss of podocyte VEGF results in hypertension and proteinuria in adult mice.[47] Given that proteinuria is also commonly seen in patients treated with VEGF inhibitors, the latter explanation would tie two of the side effects seen. The reasons for arterial thrombosis are less obvious. Because arterial circulation is more dependent on VEGF, it is possible that arterial endothelial apoptosis serves as a nidus for localized activation of coagulation and platelet aggregation. Apoptotic endothelial cells have been shown to increase thrombin-generating capacity and bind to unactivated platelets and leukocytes.[160–162]

More recently the use of PDGF inhibitors to target pericytes has been shown to be a potentially effective antiangiogenic strategy, particularly in combination with antiendothelial (anti-VEGF) molecules.[80,82] "Metronomic" or low-dose, frequent scheduling of traditional cytotoxic agents also is reported to have an antiangiogenic effect and has proven efficacious in animal studies.[163] Antivasculogenic therapy directed against recruitment of bone marrow-derived vascular precursors may have a role in future cancer therapeutic regimens, but thus far the evidence is weak at best.[66]

Arteriogenesis

Arteriogenesis is a term coined to distinguish the development of collateral vessels in the adult from the process of angiogenesis.[164,165] Remodeling of a preexisting collateral arteriole is thought to be due to flow-induced changes secondary to occlusion of a supply artery. The consequent increase in shear stress through the collateral arteriole activates endothelial cells, resulting in monocyte recruitment and infiltration into the media. Elaboration of various cytokines, growth factors, and proteases from monocytes and endothelial cells causes matrix degradation, smooth muscle cell proliferation, and rapid enlargement of the preexisting arteriole. Factors thought to promote arteriogenesis include FGF-2, placental growth factor, PDGF-BB, TGF-β1, monocyte chemoattractant protein 1, and granulocyte-macrophage colony-stimulating factor.[165,166]

Lymphangiogenesis

The lymphatics comprise a low-flow, low-pressure system that collects extravasated fluid from the tissues and transfer it back to the venous system via the thoracic duct. Lymphatic vessels also serve an immune function by transporting lymphoid and antigen-presenting cells to lymphoid organs.[167] Lymphatic vessels share features with blood vessels, but they also exhibit differences. Lymphatic vessels develop shortly after blood vessels and may arise de novo from precursor mesenchymal cells (lymphangioblasts) in a process akin to vasculogenesis.[168] Alternatively, other studies suggest that specific venous endothelial cells differentiate to lymphatic endothelium in response to signals that have yet to be determined.[169] VEGF-C and VEGF-D, by activating VEGFR-3 and Ang2 potentially through Tie2 activation, are growth factors necessary for lymphatic vessels.[170] The $\alpha_9\beta_1$ integrin also is necessary for proper lymphatic development, and the homeobox transcription factor Prox1 appears to induce transdifferentiation of venous to lymphatic endothelial cells.[169–171] Lymphedema can be caused by congenital defects, parasitic (filariasis) or neoplastic obstruction, or surgical resection. Congenital lymphedema (Milroy disease) is linked to inactivating mutations of VEGFR-3.[167] Whether lymphatic vessel density in human tumors correlates with disease progression is not clear, but in animal models induction of lymphangiogenesis by VEGF-C or VEGF-D promotes lymph node metastasis.[167]

Relationship Between Vascular Development and Hematopoiesis

Hematopoietic cells and endothelial cells are intertwined in several ways. First, there is the likely existence of a common precursor (see Vasculogenesis above). Second, the endothelium is intimately involved in hematopoiesis, having a supportive role structurally and nutritionally. Finally, the endothelium organizes the controlled egress and ingress of hematopoietic cells in hematopoietic and other tissues. The last issue is covered in Interaction of Blood Cells with the Vessel Wall section.

Bone marrow stromal cells secrete cytokines, produce ECM, and are in direct cellular contact with hematopoietic cells, thereby providing a microenvironment suitable for hematopoietic proliferation, differentiation, and self-renewal.[172] Many studies demonstrate the supportive role of endothelium in hematopoiesis.[173–175] The physical proximity of endothelium and hematopoietic precursors within the marrow and the requirement of blood cells to transit marrow endothelium to reach the circulation is presumptive evidence of an important role for endothelium. Marrow endothelial cells constitutively express high levels of IL-6, stem cell factor, granulocyte colony-stimulating factor, and granulocyte-macrophage colony-stimulating factor.[173] Both yolk sac and marrow endothelial cells support long-term proliferation and differentiation of hematopoietic cells in vitro.[173] However, endothelial cells also have been reported to inhibit hematopoiesis.[176]

Significant evidence now indicates that hematopoietic stem and progenitor cells are not randomly distributed in the marrow but rather are spatially and possibly physically associated with the endosteum and the blood vessels.[175] Functional differences between the osteoblastic and vascular niches have been described. It has been suggested that the osteoblastic niche maintains quiescence of hematopoietic stem cells, whereas stem/progenitor cells that are activated for differentiation and mobilization reside at the vascular niche.[174] Translocation of megakaryocyte progenitors to the vicinity of the marrow sinuses is sufficient to induce megakaryocyte maturation and platelet production.[175] However, a study has identified CXCL12 (SDF-1)-abundant reticular cells that are located in close proximity to the sinusoidal endothelium as well as the endosteum.[177] The authors confirmed that the CXCL12–CXCR4 signaling axis is required for maintenance of hematopoietic stem cells in the marrow, and these findings raise the possibility that the vascular and osteoblastic niches may not be that different.[177] In all likelihood, endothelial cells and osteoblasts, in concert with other stromal cells, provide a finely tuned system to modulate hematopoiesis in the marrow such that differentiation, proliferation, and self-renewal occur in a regulated fashion.

Human endothelial cells have been reported to express receptors for IL-3, stem cell factor, erythropoietin, and thrombopoietin and show functional responses to IL-3 and erythropoietin.[178–180] The shared responses to growth factors, combined with the importance of macrophages in angiogenesis and the production of cytokines by monocytes/macrophages, suggest that hematopoietic cells play a reciprocal role in maintaining the endothelium.

PHYSIOLOGIC FUNCTIONS OF THE ENDOTHELIUM

The Endothelium as a Barrier

The microvessels (capillaries and postcapillary venules) act as the exchange vessels of the circulation. However, as with other endothelial functions, vessel permeability is dependent on the type of vessel and its location. Movement of lipophilic and low-molecular-weight hydrophilic substances between blood and tissue is virtually unimpeded, but the vessels are selectively permeable to macromolecules. This semiselective barrier is necessary to maintain the fluid balance between intravascular and extravascular compartments, yet antibodies, hormones, cytokines, and other molecules must have access to the interstitial space for the initiation and potentiation of various processes, including inflammation, immune response, and wound repair.

Movement of macromolecules across the vessel wall is governed by (a) hydrostatic and oncotic pressure gradients; (b) physicochemical properties of the molecule, such as size, shape, and charge; and (c) properties of the barrier. The barrier of the vessel wall is formed by the cellular components, endothelial cells, and pericytes, as well as by the charge and compactness of the matrix components, glycocalyx, and basement membrane. Macromolecules can pass either directly through the endothelial cell (transcellular path) or between adjacent endothelial cells (paracellular path). Surprisingly, the mechanisms of macromolecular movement remain controversial, and data generated by physiologists, morphologists, and cell biologists have not been consolidated in a model that satisfies the findings of the different groups.[181]

To explain cellular transport in endothelium, physiologists have proposed the existence of two sets of "pores" based on experiments measuring the movement of dextran and other macromolecules: a small pore of radius 3 to 5 nm for transport of water and small hydrophilic molecules, and a large pore of radius 25 to 60 nm for macromolecular transport.[181–183] Although water mainly moves across the continuous endothelium via the paracellular route, a significant proportion (up to 40%) can traverse the endothelium via the transcellular route by water-transporting membrane channels, the aquaporins.[184] Macromolecular transport into cells can proceed by receptor-mediated systems, such as clathrin-coated pits, in which the molecules usually are targeted to the lysosome, but may be transported through the cell. Alternatively, molecules can be moved across the cell by plasmalemmal vesicles or caveolae, which are abundant in capillary endothelial cells. Caveolae are 50- to 100-nm membrane invaginations that can participate in transcytosis as well as in the translocation of glycosylphosphatidylinositol-linked proteins into the cytoplasm and in transmembrane signaling.[185] Because of the known leakiness of tumor microvasculature, investigators have studied these microvessels and identified a structure designated the vesiculovacuolar organelle.[186] These organelles are grape-like clusters of interconnecting uncoated vesicles and vacuoles that span the entire thickness of vascular endothelium, thereby providing a potential transendothelial connection between the vascular lumen and the extravascular space.[186] Interestingly, their function is enhanced by injection into normal skin of VEGF, which is known to increase the permeability of vessels.[186] Localization of caveolin to vesiculovacuolar organelles suggests that this structure is a fusion of caveolae.[186]

During inflammation, binding of neutrophils to the endothelium results in the generation of oxidants that can mediate endothelial cell injury and increase permeability.[187] Upon adhesion of neutrophils to the endothelium, leukocyte CD18 (β_2 integrin)-mediated signals trigger the release of the neutrophil cationic protein called heparin-binding protein/CAP37/azurocidin, which in turn induces formation of gaps between endothelial cells and macromolecular efflux.[188] Thrombin, an inflammatory mediator, can increase endothelial permeability by several mechanisms resulting from activation of its receptor on endothelial cells.[189–191] First is an increase in transcellular vesicular permeability. Second is increased paracellular permeability that results from phosphorylation of endothelial cell nonmyosin light chains and contractile activity generated by movement of actin and myosin filaments past each other. The contraction and retraction of endothelial cells are accompanied by "loosening" of intercellular junctions and focal integrin contacts with the ECM. Finally, thrombin may alter the repulsive effect of the negatively charged glycocalyx. An increase in paracellular permeability may result from alteration of cell–cell contacts present at tight junctions and adherens junctions, secondary to posttranslational modification of components of these junctions such as claudins and VE-cadherin.[181] Pericyte contractility also has been hypothesized as a mechanism for increasing permeability in inflammatory states.[191]

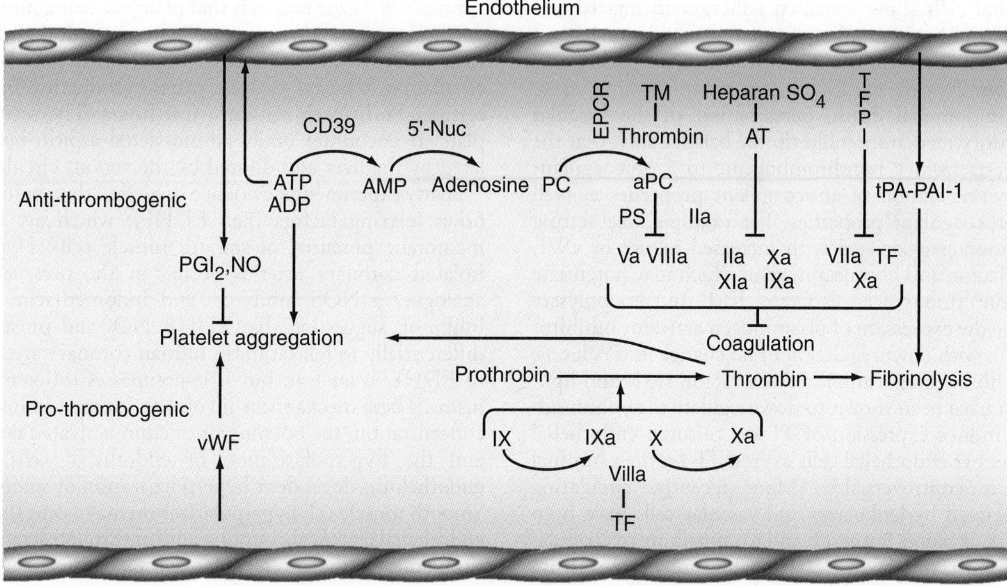

Figure 117–2 Overview of endothelial function in coagulation. ADP, adenosine diphosphate; AMP, adenosine monophosphate; AT, antithrmbin; ATP, adenosine triphosphate; EPCR, endothelial protein C receptor; NO, nitric oxide; 5′-Nuc, ecto-5′-nucleotidase; PAI-1, plasminogen activator inhibitor 1; PC, protein C; PGI_2, prostaglandin I_2 (prostacyclin); PS, protein S; TF, tissue factor; TFPI, tissue factor pathway inhibitor; TM, thrombomodulin; tPA, tissue plasminogen activator; vWF, von Willebrand factor.

The Endothelium as a Nonthrombogenic Surface

The molecular mechanisms of hemostasis and thrombosis are addressed in Chapters 115 and 116 and 118 through 120. This section places the endothelium in the appropriate context in these processes. An overview of endothelial cell contributions to the anticoagulant and procoagulant states is shown in Fig. 117–2. Normal unperturbed endothelium presents a nonthrombogenic surface to the circulation by inhibiting platelet aggregation, preventing the activation and propagation of coagulation and enhancing fibrinolysis.[192–196] These activities are accomplished by both passive and active processes. Conversely, when injured or under inflammatory conditions, the endothelium may become procoagulant.

When in close proximity to endothelial cells, platelets become unresponsive to agonists. This inhibition of platelet aggregation is accomplished by secretion of prostacyclin (prostaglandin I_2 [PGI_2]) and NO and by surface expression of an ecto-adenosine phosphatase (ADPase)/CD39/nucleoside triphosphate diphosphohydrolase (NTPDase-1).[195,197] Prostacyclin is synthesized mainly by vascular endothelial and smooth muscle cells as a product of arachidonic acid metabolism. It inhibits platelet activation, secretion, and aggregation, and monocyte interactions with endothelial cells. It also causes vascular smooth muscle cell relaxation. NO similarly has a wide range of functions, including inhibition of platelet adhesion, activation, and aggregation. Most of the NO released from endothelial cells is elaborated abluminally, where it acts on the smooth muscle cell to cause vasodilation. However, some NO may enter the lumen and thereby diffuse into platelets. Prostacyclin and NO can act synergistically to reverse platelet aggregation.[195] The released platelet agonist, ADP, can be inactivated by endothelial membrane-associated CD39.[197] Metabolism of ATP and ADP to AMP by CD39 eliminates platelet recruitment and returns platelets to their resting state. Adenosine, which is generated by hydrolysis of AMP by ecto-5′-nucleotidase, acts to inhibit platelet aggregation and cause vasodilation. ATP/ADP can stimulate purinoreceptors on endothelial cells, resulting in synthesis and release of PGI_2 and NO.[198]

Endothelial cells use three main pathways to inhibit thrombin generation and limit coagulation: the antithrombin system, the protein C system, and tissue factor pathway inhibitor (TFPI).[192,194,199,200] (a) *Antithrombin system.* Heparan sulfate proteoglycans are secreted onto the luminal surface of endothelial cells and into the subendothelium. Heparan sulfates are capable of binding and activating antithrombin III, thereby accelerating inactivation of several procoagulant serine proteases, including thrombin, factor Xa, and factor IXa. (b) *Protein C.*[201] Thrombomodulin on the surface of endothelial cells binds thrombin. This coupling inhibits the coagulant properties of thrombin and increases its affinity for protein C, which it cleaves and activates. Activation of protein C by the thrombin–thrombomodulin complex is augmented by its binding to the endothelial cell protein C receptor. Protein S, which is thought to be synthesized primarily by the endothelial cell, acts as a cofactor for protein C but itself also has anticoagulant properties. Independent of the presence of activated protein C, free protein S is able to inhibit the prothrombinase and intrinsic tenase complexes and interact directly with factors Va and VIIIa. (c) *TFPI.*[202] TFPI is a Kunitz-type serine protease inhibitor that modulates TF-initiated coagulation. TFPI binds to and directly inhibits the tissue factor/factor VIIa/factor Xa complex. It is mainly produced by and bound to endothelial cells, likely to surface glycosaminoglycans. There is also a plasma pool bound to low-density lipoprotein.

If coagulation occurs despite the many anticoagulant mechanisms, endothelial cells also provide proteins to promote fibrinolysis.[194] Endothelium is a major source of tPA.[203,204] Approximately 40% of tPA is bound to its inhibitor, plasminogen activator inhibitor 1, which is also secreted by endothelial cells. Stresses such as exercise, acidosis, hypoxia, shear forces, increased venous pressure, and thrombin will cause release of tPA[203,204] and presumably activate plasminogen. Receptors for plasminogen and tPA are present on the endothelial cell surface, allowing for effective localized production of fibrinolytic activity.

Although intact endothelium is necessary to maintain blood in a fluid state and inhibit coagulation under normal conditions, injured endothelium can rapidly downregulate its anticoagulant functions and become procoagulant, even without overt vascular damage as occurs with trauma or surgery. Further tissue injury or vascular pathology also leads to exposure of the underlying matrix, which is procoagulant by virtue of its binding to and activation of platelets. Endothelial cells that have been induced to undergo apoptosis in vitro become procoagulant. Apoptotic endothelial cells expose phosphatidylserine on their surface and downregulate their anticoagulant properties. Apoptotic endothelial cells and vascular smooth muscle cells also increase thrombin formation in recalcified citrated plasma, and apoptotic endothelial cells show increased adhesion to unactivated platelets.[160,161,205] Thrombosis resulting from procoagulant changes induced by endothelial apoptosis could contribute to the pathogenesis of diverse diseases.[206]

Even without endothelial death, perturbation of the vascular lining by inflammatory mediators could tip the balance such that the endothelium converts from a nonthrombogenic to a procoagulant surface due to downregulation of anticoagulant properties as well as induction of procoagulant properties. For example, the setting of acute inflammation is associated with increased release of vWF, platelet-activating factor, and fibronectin, all of which may potentiate thrombus formation. Tumor necrosis factor, IL-1, and lipopolysaccharide can increase the expression of plasminogen activator inhibitor 1 in endothelial cells with downregulation or no change in tPA levels, thereby impairing fibrinolysis. Tumor necrosis factor, IL-1, and lipopolysaccharide also have been shown to downregulate thrombomodulin as well as to induce expression of TF on cultured endothelial cells. However, whether endothelial cells express TF on their luminal surface in vivo is controversial.[207] More recently, circulating microparticles generated by leukocytes and vascular cells have been shown to be a source of blood-borne TF and to contribute to coagulation.[208] Although most microparticles probably are derived from platelets and monocytes, endothelial-derived microparticles may be an important source of circulating TF under conditions of drastic activation.[208,209]

Control of Vascular Tone

Control of vascular tone is orchestrated primarily by a balance between endothelium-derived vasodilators [NO, PGI_2, and endothelium-derived hyperpolarizing factor [EDHF]) and vasoconstrictors (endothelin 1 [ET-1] and superoxide). In addition to inhibiting platelet aggregation, NO and PGI_2 act as vasodilators.[210,211] NO is produced by conversion of l-arginine to l-citrulline by NO synthase (NOS). Three forms of NOS exist: a constitutive NOS in neuronal tissue; an inducible enzyme found in macrophages and other cells that plays a role in NO-induced cytotoxicity; and a constitutively active endothelial form, NOSIII (eNOS).[212] The inducible form of NOS also is present in endothelial cells and may be responsible for the uncontrolled vasodilation seen in septic shock.[212] Injection into the forearm of L-arginine analogues that inhibit NOS causes substantial vasoconstriction. Conversely, eNOS-deficient mice are hypertensive, suggesting that NO release is crucial for maintaining basal vasodilation.[210,211] The major physiologic stimulus for continuous production of NO in vivo is shear stress. The action of NO on platelets (antiaggregatory), endothelial cells, and smooth muscle cells (relaxation) is due to activation of guanyl cyclase and formation of cyclic guanosine 3′,5′-cyclic monophosphate. Whereas NO is quite unstable, the formation of *S*-nitrosothiols in the presence of oxygen and thiols provides a stable reservoir of NO.[213] Hemoglobin is an avid scavenger of NO, which may account for the vasoconstriction observed with administration of cell-free, hemoglobin-based red cell substitute.[214] Physiologically, however, *S*-nitrosohemoglobin acts as a regulator of blood flow. Deoxygenation is accompanied by an allosteric change in *S*-nitrosohemoglobin that releases the NO group, relaxing blood vessels to bring blood flow in line with local oxygen requirements.[215]

Prostacyclin (PGI_2), on the other hand, does not appear to have as global a role in vasodilation as does NO. PGI_2 is synthesized mainly by endothelial cells and acts locally at sites of injury. It may counterbalance the vasoconstriction induced by the platelet-produced arachidonic acid metabolite thromboxane A_2 (TXA_2). Most PGI_2 is released luminally, where it has an antiplatelet effect. Prostacyclin transduces a cellular signal by increasing the levels of cyclic AMP, whereas TXA_2 signals via the phosphoinositol pathway and lowering of cyclic AMP levels. Synthesis of prostaglandins begins by the action of cyclooxygenases (COX-1 and COX-2) on arachidonic acid. Aspirin inhibits cyclooxygenase irreversibly in both platelets and endothelial cells. However, the clinical effect is seen primarily in platelets for two reasons.[211,212] One reason is that platelets, being nonnucleated, cannot synthesize new cyclooxygenase, whereas endothelial cells can. Therefore, TXA_2 synthesis recovers only when new platelets enter the circulation, whereas cyclooxygenase production by endothelial cells restores PGI_2 levels within a few hours. The second reason is that platelets encounter orally administered aspirin before it is deacetylated by the liver and diluted by the venous circulation.

Early experimental evidence suggested that endothelial cells release other relaxing factors (i.e., EDHF), which act by increasing the membrane potential of smooth muscle cells. Hyperpolarization of isolated coronary arteries occurs in the presence of an arginine analogue, a NOS inhibitor, and indomethacin, a cyclooxygenase inhibitor, suggesting that EDHF, NO, and prostanoids contribute differentially to relaxation in human coronary arteries.[216] The nature of EDHF is unclear, but it encompasses different biologic mechanisms. These mechanisms involve an increase in intracellular calcium concentration, the opening of calcium-activated potassium channels, and the hyperpolarization of endothelial cells, resulting in an endothelium-dependent hyperpolarization of smooth muscle cells.[217] Smooth muscle cell hyperpolarization may occur through direct myoendothelial electrical coupling and/or through accumulation of potassium ions in the intercellular space. Findings suggest that EDHF represents cytochrome P450-linked arachidonate metabolites in some blood vessels, but also lipoxygenase derivatives and hydrogen peroxide.[217]

ET-1 is a 21-amino-acid peptide, released preferentially at the abluminal surface of endothelial cells, that exhibits potent vasoconstrictor activity.[218,219] Of the three known endothelins, only ET-1 is produced by endothelial cells. At least two receptors (ET-A and ET-B) bind to all three endothelins. ET-A is abundantly expressed on smooth muscle cells, whereas ET-B is predominantly expressed on endothelial cells. The vasoconstrictor activity of ET-1 is preferentially mediated by ET-A receptors on smooth muscle cells. Engagement of ET-B on endothelial cells by ET-3 may paradoxically cause a transient vasodilation. Little evidence indicates that ET-1 plays a role in essential hypertension, but it might contribute to pregnancy-induced hypertension and may play a role in reperfusion injury following ischemia.[219] ET-1 does appear to play a role in pulmonary arterial hypertension, and the dual endothelin receptor antagonist bosentan has been approved for treatment of this disease.[220]

Another seemingly important regulator of vascular tone is the superoxide anion.[210,221] The source of this free radical may be the endothelium itself or inflammatory cells that have been recruited to sites of injury or inflammation. Interaction of superoxide radicals and NO produces peroxynitrite and reduces the concentration of NO. Peroxynitrite can oxidize low-density lipoprotein and deleteriously modify other proteins, thereby causing endothelial dysfunction. Increased production of superoxide inhibits synthesis of PGI_2 but not that of TXA_2.[221]

The endothelium expresses angiotensin-converting enzyme at its surface; this enzyme converts angiotensin I to angiotensin II, a potent vasoconstrictor. The interaction among endothelin, angiotensin II, and α-adrenergic agonists in the pathogenesis of hypertension is complex.[222] An altered balance of the vasoactive substances described in this section has been proposed to cause endothelial dysfunction and the attendant vascular pathology observed in atherosclerosis, hypertension, and diabetes mellitus. Alteration of vascular function in these diseases then may perpetuate endothelial dysfunction and, consequently, worsen disease.

Interaction of Blood Cells with the Vessel Wall

Leukocytes

In the absence of any inflammatory stimulus, neutrophils circulate freely and do not interact significantly with the endothelium. This contrasts with continuous, low-level physiologic traffic of monocytes and lymphocytes across the vessel wall. Monocytes emigrate from the bloodstream to develop into tissue macrophages that may exhibit

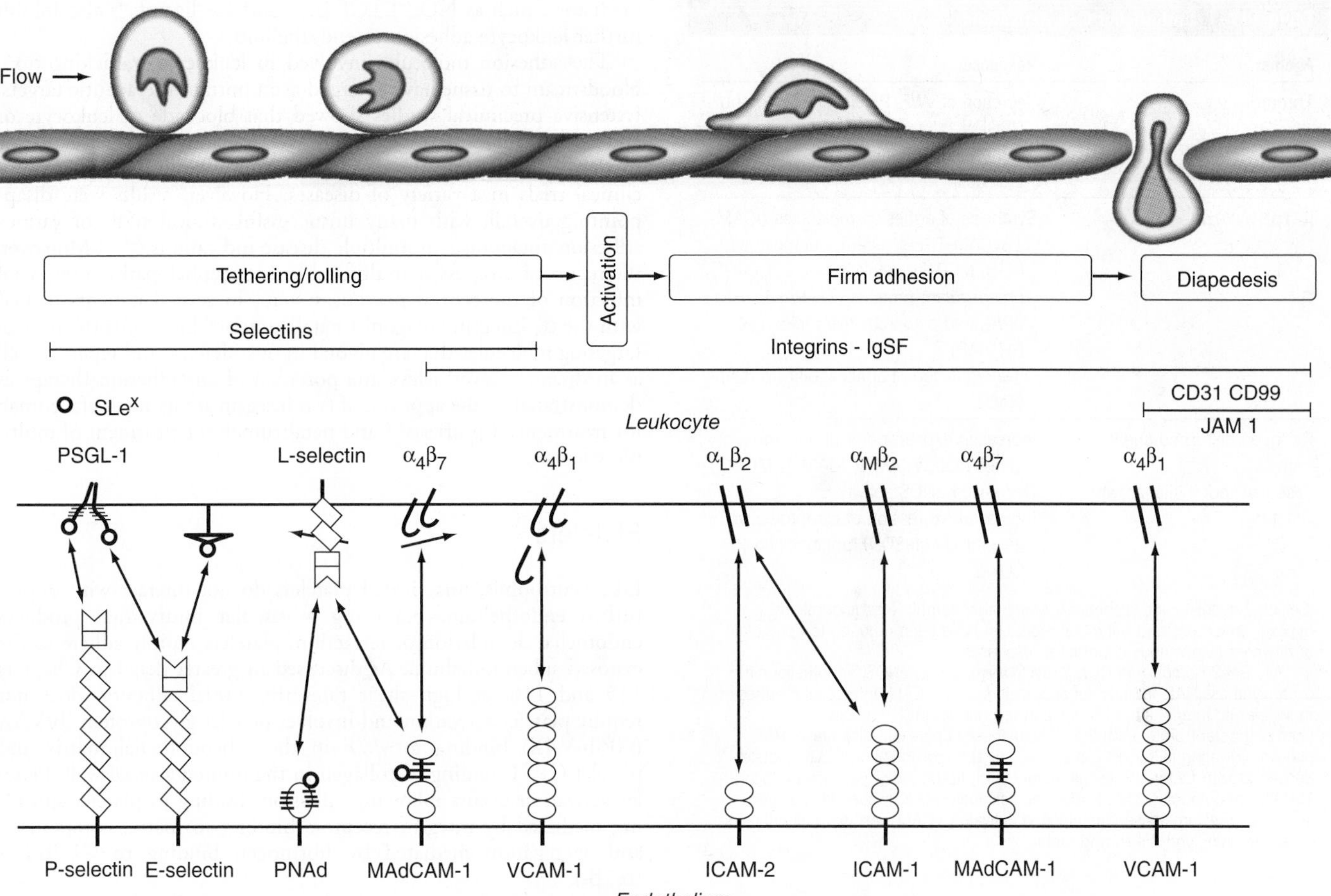

Figure 117–3 Adhesion cascade. Under conditions of flow, leukocytes first tether to endothelial ligands and then roll along the vessel wall. Tethering is mediated predominantly by interaction of P-selectin and L-selectin with their cognate glycoconjugate ligands. P-selectin binds to sialyl Lewis X (SLe^x) and sulfate residues expressed on P-selectin glycoprotein ligand 1 (PSGL-1). L-selectin binds to an uncharacterized ligand(s) on inflamed endothelium and to sulfated SLe^x-like moieties on peripheral node addressin (PNAd) and mucosal addressin cell adhesion molecule 1 (MAdCAM-1) on high endothelial venules. E-selectin, $\alpha_4\beta_1$ (very late antigen 4 [VLA-4]), and $\alpha_4\beta_7$ stabilize rolling initiated by P-selectin and L-selectin. E-selectin recognizes SLe^x on PSGL-1 and other glycoproteins or glycolipids. Following tethering and rolling, leukocyte integrin receptors are activated, most often by chemoattractants (e.g., chemokines) via G protein-coupled receptors. After activation, integrin receptors engage endothelial immunoglobulin gene superfamily ligands to promote firm adhesion. Leukocyte $\alpha_L\beta_2$ (leukocyte function antigen 1 [LFA-1]) binds to intercellular adhesion molecules ICAM-1 and ICAM-2, $\alpha_M\beta_2$ (macrophage 1 [Mac-1]) to ICAM-1, $\alpha_4\beta_1$ (VLA-4) to vascular cell adhesion molecule 1 (VCAM-1), and $\alpha_4\beta_7$ to MAdCAM-1. The adherent leukocyte then migrates across endothelium to interendothelial junctions, where it diapedeses between endothelial cells via leukocyte integrin receptors and their endothelial immunoglobulin gene superfamily ligands as well as endothelial junctional proteins such as CD31, CD99, and junctional adhesion molecule 1 (JAM-1).

tissue- or organ-specific functions. To maintain immune surveillance of tissue, lymphocytes recirculate between blood and lymphatics, gaining entrance to the latter at the high endothelial venule of post-capillary venules in lymphoid tissue.

Intravital microscopic studies have established a sequence of events involved in leukocyte emigration at extravascular sites of inflammation. Under conditions of flow, leukocytes first tether to and then roll along the endothelium of postcapillary venules adjacent to the site of inflammation. Some of the rolling leukocytes are activated and adhere firmly. The adherent leukocytes migrate along the endothelial surface and diapedese between endothelial junctions to enter the extravascular tissue. These steps in emigration tethering, rolling, activation, firm adhesion, and diapedesis also are involved in lymphocyte emigration at high endothelial venules. They result from the interaction of distinct leukocyte and endothelial receptors in an adhesion cascade (Fig. 117–3; see Chapter 16).[223,224] Rolling is observed only under flow conditions and is the consequence of shear forces acting on the leukocyte and adhesive interactions between selectin receptors and their glycoconjugate counterstructures.[225] It is initiated primarily by activation of the endothelium by extravascular stimuli such as bacterial-derived products or by endogenous mediators produced by the endothelium or cells in tissue. Early on, rolling is mediated by endothelial P-selectin, which is rapidly translocated from Weibel-Palade bodies to the luminal surface, and L-selectin on leukocyte microvilli. E-selectin is involved only at later time points, as it is not constitutively expressed by endothelium but rather is induced over hours by de novo synthesis.

In order for leukocytes to circulate freely, their integrin receptors must be minimally adhesive, but they also must be able to increase binding rapidly at sites of inflammation. Once tethered to endothelium by selectin interactions, leukocyte integrin receptors are activated by endothelial membrane-expressed platelet-activating factor, endothelial membrane-bound chemokines, or locally secreted chemoattractants. Activation of leukocyte integrins involves changes in receptor affinity or affinity-independent receptor clustering,[226] which promotes firm adhesion to endothelial ligands, which are members of the immunoglobulin gene superfamily (IgSF). These IgSF ligands are constitutively expressed (ICAM-1, ICAM-2), further upregulated (ICAM-1), or induced (VCAM-1) by inflammatory mediators (Table 117–1). Although these activation-dependent increases in leukocyte integrin binding to endothelial IgSF ligands are necessary for shear-resistant firm adhesion, subsequent leukocyte migration over the endothelium requires reversible adhesion due to cyclic modulation of receptor avidity.[227]

Table 117–1 Endothelial Cell Activation[a]

Agonist	Response
Thrombin	Secretion of vWF, P-selectin, TFPI, and PDGF Synthesis of PAF, IL-8, IL-6, and E-selectin
IL-1β, TNF-α, LPS	Synthesis of adhesion molecules (ICAM-1, VCAM-1, E-selectin), chemokines (IL-8, MCP-1), cytokines (IL-6, CD40), procoagulant proteins (TF, PAI-1, tPA, uPA), and cytoprotective molecules (A1, IAP) Downregulation of anticoagulant proteins (TM)
Reduced/disturbed shear stress	Increased expression of proinflammatory genes (e.g., VCAM-1, ICAM-1, MCP-1)
Vascular endothelial growth factor	Decreased eNOS activity Increased expression of cytoprotective genes (A1, MnSOD), angiopoietin 2, COX-2

[a]Selected agonists and responses. Many other stimuli (e.g., lipoproteins, hypoxia, ,microbes and microbial products) have been reported to upregulate or downregulate various endothelial responses.

A1, Bcl-2 homologue; COX-2, cyclooxygenase 2; eNOS, endothelial nitric oxide synthase; IAP, inhibitor of apoptosis protein; ICAM, intercellular adhesion molecule; IL, interleukin; LPS, lipopolysaccharide; MCP, monocyte chemoattractant protein; MnSOD, manganese superoxide dismutase; PAF, platelet-activating factor; PAI, plasminogen activator inhibitor; PDGF, platelet-derived growth factor; TF, tissue factor; TFPI, tissue factor pathway inhibitor; TM, thrombomodulin; TNF, tumor necrosis factor; tPA, tissue plasminogen activator; uPA, urokinase plasminogen activator; VCAM, vascular cell adhesion molecule; vWF, von Willebrand factor.

There are several caveats regarding the current multistep model of initial selectin-mediated rolling and subsequent integrin-mediated firm adhesion.[228] First, selectin-mediated rolling is not a prerequisite for emigration under conditions of reduced flow, as might occur at sites of inflammation.[229] Second, the model was developed from observations in the systemic microcirculation, where leukocyte emigration occurs in postcapillary venules under relatively low shear forces. However, selectins do not appear to play a major role in neutrophil emigration in the pulmonary microcirculation, where emigration occurs predominantly in capillaries,[230] or in the liver microvasculature, where leukocytes emigrate primarily in sinusoids.[231] Third, under some conditions leukocytes are able to tether and roll via receptors other than selectins and α_4 integrins (e.g., CD44[232] or VAP-1[233]). Finally, several other adhesion pathways have been implicated in leukocyte adhesion to endothelium in vitro, and their roles in the adhesion cascade in vivo remain to be defined.[228]

Once adherent, leukocytes migrate upon the endothelial luminal surface. Upon encountering an intercellular junction, some leukocytes diapedese between endothelial cells, enter extravascular tissue, and then migrate to the site of inflammatory or immune reaction.[234,235] This process of transendothelial migration uses leukocyte integrin interactions with endothelial IgSF ligands[236] and several junctional proteins, including PECAM-1 (CD31)[237] JAM-1,[238] and CD99.[239] Diapedesis involves signaling by the leukocyte to the endothelial cell that triggers opening of endothelial cell junctions.[240] Although leukocyte migration is primarily paracellular (i.e., through endothelial cell–cell junctions), under certain circumstances leukocytes may emigrate by a transcellular pathway.[241]

Leukocyte recruitment is terminated by several mechanisms. E-selectin and P-selectin are removed from the endothelial cell surface by endocytosis,[242] whereas L-selectin is cleaved from leukocytes by a membrane protease.[243] Decay of cytokine, chemokine, or chemoattractant generation leads to gradual resolution of endothelial adhesion molecule expression and integrin activation. Locally expressed mediators, such as NO,[244] TGF-β,[245] and Fas ligand,[246] also inhibit further leukocyte adhesion to endothelium.

The adhesion molecules involved in leukocyte trafficking from bloodstream to tissue have emerged as important therapeutic targets. Extensive preclinical studies showed that blockade of leukocyte or endothelial adhesion molecules was efficacious in diverse disease models,[247] prompting the development of adhesion antagonists for clinical trials in a variety of diseases. However, results were disappointing overall, with many unsuccessful clinical trials of various adhesion antagonists in multiple disease indications.[248,249] Moreover, the report of progressive multifocal leukoencephalopathy, a rare viral infection of the central nervous system, in several patients treated with the α_4-integrin antagonist natalizumab[250] highlights the risks of targeting molecules that are pivotal in host defense and repair as well as in disease. Nevertheless, the potential of antiadhesion therapy is demonstrated by the approval of two integrin antagonists: efalizumab for treatment of psoriasis[251] and natalizumab for treatment of multiple sclerosis.[252]

Platelets

Like neutrophils, unactivated platelets do not interact with unperturbed endothelium. Following a vascular injury that produces endothelial denudation or retraction, platelets rapidly adhere to the exposed subendothelium. As discussed in greater detail in Chapters 115 and 116, at high shear rates this initial adhesion does not require platelet activation and involves platelet glycoprotein Ib/V/IX (GPIb-V-IX) binding to vWF in the subendothelial matrix and platelet GPVI binding to collagen in the injured arterial wall. Platelet activation occurs following adhesion, leading to platelet spreading mediated by integrin receptors binding to matrix components and aggregation mediated by fibrinogen binding to GPIIb/IIIa ($\alpha_{IIb}\beta_3$).

Evidence indicates that platelets can bind directly to activated endothelium in vivo via endothelial P-selectin[253] and PECAM-1[254] and to roll on venular endothelium via interaction of platelet GPIbα and endothelial P-selectin.[255] Platelets have been shown to bind to high endothelial venules in vivo via platelet P-selectin.[256] In vitro platelets can adhere to intact endothelium via a platelet GPIIb/IIIa-dependent bridging mechanism involving platelet-bound adhesive proteins and the endothelial cell receptors ICAM-1, $\alpha_V\beta_3$ integrin, and GPIbα.[257] Platelet adhesion to intact endothelium via these various pathways may contribute to thrombus formation in the circulation and may provide a link between thrombosis and inflammation in diseases such as atherosclerosis.[258] Platelet–endothelial interactions also may contribute to the pathogenesis of thrombotic thrombocytopenic purpura. Normally, ultralarge vWF remains attached to endothelium via P-selectin until it is cleaved by the plasma metalloproteinase ADAMTS-13. Failure of this mechanism in thrombotic thrombocytopenic purpura due to deficiency of ADAMTS-13 may lead to spontaneous platelet adhesion to endothelium and microvascular thrombosis.[259]

Red Blood Cells

Plasmodium falciparum-infected and sickled red blood cells interact significantly with endothelium, and these adhesive interactions are thought to play an important role in the pathogenesis of human diseases.

Among the human malarial parasites, only *Plasmodium falciparum* modifies the surface of the parasitized red blood cells so that asexual parasites and gametocytes are able to adhere to the vascular endothelium.[260,261] Binding of trophozoite- and schizont-infected red blood cells to endothelium not only allows the parasite to escape destruction in the spleen, but it also may contribute to the pathogenesis of cerebral malaria.[261,262] Multiple endothelial adhesion receptors have been implicated in mediating cytoadherence of infected red blood cells, including P-selectin, ICAM-1, VCAM-1, and CD36.[263]

Binding of young sickled red blood cells to postcapillary endothelium with secondary trapping of poorly deformable, often irreversibly sickled cells is thought to be an important pathogenic factor in vasoocclusive events.[264] Several interactions between sickle red cell receptors and endothelial ligands have been described, including $\alpha_4\beta_1$/VCAM-1[265]; $\alpha_4\beta_1$/Lutheran blood group (basal cell adhesion molecule)[266]; and ICAM-4/$\alpha_V\beta_3$.[267] The adhesive proteins thrombospondin and vWF promote adhesion by serving as bridging factors between various sickle red cell and endothelial adhesion molecules. In addition to direct adhesion to endothelium, sickle red cell binding to adherent leukocytes has been proposed as a mechanism for sickle cell vascular occlusion.[268] As with leukocyte adhesion to endothelium in inflammatory and immune disease, drugs targeting sickle red cell adhesive interactions with endothelial cells or leukocytes may prove useful in preventing or treating vasoocclusive crises.

Endothelial Cell Activation and Dysfunction

Although once viewed as a passive barrier between blood and tissue, the endothelium now is evident to be a dynamic and heterogeneous organ that responds to diverse stimuli, ranging from coagulation proteins and cytokines to hemodynamic forces and growth factors. Activation of endothelial cells induces a complex proinflammatory and prothrombotic phenotype as well as expression of certain cytoprotective genes (see Table 117–1).[269,270] Multiple transcription factors, particularly nuclear factor-κB[271] and early growth response 1,[272] regulate these responses.[269] Endothelial activation undoubtedly is an important event in host defense and repair, but it also may contribute to the pathogenesis of diverse diseases, ranging from sepsis[273] to atherosclerosis.[274]

Endothelial dysfunction is characterized by a reduction in the bioavailability of vasodilators, particularly NO, leading to impairment of endothelium-dependent vasodilation, or by an increase in endothelium-derived contracting factors.[275] Endothelial dysfunction is prominent in atherosclerosis but also has been described in diabetes, preeclampsia, hypertension, uremia, and other diseases. In a broader sense, endothelial dysfunction encompasses proinflammatory and procoagulant changes as well as apoptotic cell death.[206,276,277]

A number of noninvasive approaches for assessing endothelial function in vascular diseases have been developed. Endothelial vasodilatory responses can be evaluated by high-resolution ultrasound measurement of flow-mediated vasodilation or by plethysmography of changes in forearm blood flow during reactive hyperemia.[278] Endothelial activation can be assessed in plasma by circulating markers such as soluble endothelial adhesion molecules (e.g., sVCAM-1, sICAM-1, sE-selectin) and endothelial coagulation proteins (e.g., vWF and thrombomodulin)[279] or endothelial microparticles.[280] Circulating endothelial cells reflect significant vascular damage or cell death.[281]

SUGGESTED READINGS

Aird WC: Spatial and temporal dynamics of the endothelium. J Thromb Haemost 3:1392, 2005.

Carmeliet P: Blood vessels and nerves: Common signals, pathways and diseases. Nat Rev Genet 4:710, 2003.

Conway EM, Collen D, Carmeliet P: Molecular mechanisms of blood vessel growth. Cardiovasc Res 49:507, 2001.

Coultas L, Chawengsaksophak K, Rossant J: Endothelial cells and VEGF in vascular development. Nature 438:937, 2005.

De Palma M, Naldini L: Role of haematopoietic cells and endothelial progenitors in tumour angiogenesis. Biochim Biophys Acta 1766:159, 2006.

Harrison DG, Widder J, Grumbach I, Chen W, Weber M, Searles C: Endothelial mechanotransduction, nitric oxide and vascular inflammation. J Intern Med 259:351, 2006.

Hebbel RP, Yamada O, Moldow CF, Jacob HS, White JG, Eaton JW: Abnormal adherence of sickle erythrocytes to cultured vascular endothelium: Possible mechanism for microvascular occlusion in sickle cell disease. J Clin Invest 65:154, 1980.

Kerbel R, Folkman J: Clinical translation of angiogenesis inhibitors. Nat Rev Cancer 2:727, 2002.

Lapidot T, Dar A, Kollet O: How do stem cells find their way home? Blood 106:1901, 2005.

Luster AD, Alon R, von Andrian UH: Immune cell migration in inflammation: Present and future therapeutic targets. Nat Immunol 6:1182, 2005.

Mehta D, Malik AB: Signaling mechanisms regulating endothelial permeability. Physiol Rev 86:279, 2006.

Minami T, Aird WC: Endothelial cell gene regulation. Trends Cardiovasc Med 15:174, 2005.

Petri B, Bixel MG: Molecular events during leukocyte diapedesis. FEBS J 273:4399, 2006.

Pober JS, Min W: Endothelial cell dysfunction, injury and death. Handb Exp Pharmacol 135, 2006.

Rafii S, Lyden D, Benezra R, Hattori K, Heissig B: Vascular and haematopoietic stem cells: Novel targets for anti-angiogenesis therapy? Nat Rev Cancer 2:826, 2002.

Rak J, Milsom C, May L, Klement P, Yu J: Tissue factor in cancer and angiogenesis: The molecular link between genetic tumor progression, tumor neovascularization, and cancer coagulopathy. Semin Thromb Hemost 32:54–70, 2006.

Schofield L, Grau GE: Immunological processes in malaria pathogenesis. Nat Rev Immunol 5:722, 2005.

Shih T, Lindley C: Bevacizumab: An angiogenesis inhibitor for the treatment of solid malignancies. Clin Ther 28:1779, 2006.

Yin T, Li L: The stem cell niches in bone. J Clin Invest 116:1195, 2006.

Yonekawa K, Harlan JM: Targeting leukocyte integrins in human diseases. J Leukoc Biol 77:129, 2005.

REFERENCES

For complete list of references log onto www.expertconsult.com

CHAPTER 118

MOLECULAR BASIS OF BLOOD COAGULATION

Bruce Furie and Barbara C. Furie

Blood coagulation is a host defense system that maintains the integrity of the high-pressure closed circulatory system. After tissue injury, alterations in the capillary bed and laceration of venules and arterioles lead to extravasation of blood into soft tissues or external bleeding. To prevent excessive blood loss, the hemostatic system, which includes platelets, endothelial cells, and plasma coagulation proteins, is called into play. Immediately after tissue injury, a platelet plug is formed through the processes of platelet adhesion and aggregation. Concurrently, blood coagulation stabilizes the platelet plug with a fibrin clot.[1] A series of interdependent enzyme-mediated reactions translates the molecular signals that initiate blood coagulation into a major biologic event, the formation of the fibrin clot. Models of the initiation of blood coagulation by tissue factor emphasize that clotting is a nonlinear process, with a critical threshold of tissue factor activity necessary to generate thrombin.[2,3]

In vitro the generation of thrombin and the formation of a fibrin clot propagate through two separate pathways, the intrinsic pathway and the extrinsic pathway.[4,5] To generate a clot via the intrinsic pathway in a test tube, components intrinsic to whole blood are required. The contact system is activated by surface contact to generate a clot via the intrinsic pathway (Table 118–1). The intrinsic pathway of blood coagulation includes protein cofactors and enzymes (Fig.118–1). This pathway is initiated by activation of factor XII by kallikrein on negatively charged surfaces, including glass in vitro. High-molecular-weight kininogen facilitates this activation. The enzyme form of factor XII, factor XIIa, catalyzes the conversion of factor XI, a proenzyme, to its active enzyme form, factor XIa. In the presence of Ca^{2+}, factor XIa activates the proenzyme factor IX to its enzyme form, factor IXa. Factor IXa binds to the cofactor factor VIIIa bound on membrane surfaces in the presence of calcium ions to generate a complex with enzymatic activity known as "tenase," a nickname for the enzymatic activity that acts on factor X. This tenase complex converts the proenzyme factor X to its enzyme form, factor Xa. In a parallel series of interactions, factor Xa binds to the cofactor factor Va bound on membrane surfaces in the presence of calcium ions to generate a complex with enzymatic activity known as *prothrombinase.* This complex converts the proenzyme prothrombin to its enzyme form, thrombin. Thrombin acts on fibrinogen to generate the fibrin monomer, which rapidly polymerizes to form the fibrin clot. During clinical laboratory analysis of blood clotting, the intrinsic pathway of blood coagulation is evaluated by using the activated partial thromboplastin time. Clotting of plasma is initiated by the addition of negatively charged particles such as kaolin.

The extrinsic pathway of blood coagulation also includes protein cofactors and enzymes (see Fig. 118–1). This pathway is initiated by the formation of a complex between tissue factor on cell surfaces or microparticles and factor VIIa. Although the mechanism by which a small amount of factor VII is converted to factor VIIa in the absence of ongoing blood clotting is unknown, plasma contains factor VIIa at levels of 0.5 to 8.4 ng/mL.[6] When tissue factor is in contact with plasma following vascular injury, this factor VIIa complexes with tissue factor to form an enzyme complex that activates factor X to factor Xa. In turn, factor Xa can feed back to convert more factor VII to factor VIIa,[7] thus accelerating the rate of activation of the extrinsic pathway. Factor VIIa/tissue factor complex, like the tenase complex, converts factor X to its active form, factor Xa, which binds to the cofactor factor V bound on membrane surfaces in the presence of calcium ions to generate the prothrombinase complex. This complex converts prothrombin to thrombin, which converts fibrinogen to fibrin to generate the fibrin clot. During laboratory analysis of blood clotting, the extrinsic pathway of blood coagulation is evaluated using the prothrombin time. Clotting of plasma is initiated by the addition of exogenous tissue factor.

This scheme of blood clotting (see Fig. 118–1) remains invaluable for understanding clot formation in vitro and specifically for laboratory monitoring of anticoagulation therapy for, and diagnosis of, coagulation disorders. Yet the physiologic pathways relevant to blood coagulation in vivo are clearly different. A scheme of blood coagulation in vivo must consider the following salient features. First, because patients with hereditary factor XII, prekallikrein, or high-molecular-weight kininogen deficiency have a markedly prolonged partial thromboplastin time but no bleeding phenotype, these proteins are not required to maintain hemostasis in vivo and should not be included in an in vivo model of blood clotting.[8–10] Second, there is a P-selectin–dependent pathway of blood coagulation.[11] Tissue factor, a normal constituent of the surface of nonvascular cells and of stimulated monocytes and endothelial cells, is present in circulating blood, and bloodborne tissue factor is present in the developing thrombus.[12] Circulating microparticles carrying tissue factor and P-selectin glycoprotein ligand 1 (PSGL-1) accumulate in the region of vessel wall injury due to interaction of microparticle PSGL-1 and platelet P-selectin.[13,14] This tissue factor then initiates fibrin formation. Third, the tissue factor/factor VIIa complex activates not only factor X but factor IX as well, suggesting a central role for factors VIII and IX in coagulation initiated by the tissue factor pathway.[15] Fourth, factor XI deficiency is not invariably associated with a significant bleeding phenotype; as such, the position and prominence of factor IX in the blood coagulation cascade remain uncertain. Fifth, although deficiency of factor XII is not associated with a hemostatic defect, it appears to be protective from thrombosis.[16] Figure 118–2 shows a model of blood coagulation and the pathway of sequential reactions that might lead to clot formation in vivo.[17] The key to initiation of blood coagulation and thrombin generation is tissue factor. Exposure of cell surfaces expressing active tissue factor to the plasma proteins in blood leads to binding of factor VIIa to tissue factor. Tissue factor on some membrane surfaces, including microparticles and certain cells, may be inactive (encrypted). Thiol isomerases may be important for regulating the activity of tissue factor by formation of a disulfide bond on the surface of the protein.[18] Tissue factor complexed to the activated form of factor VII, factor VIIa, activates factors IX and X.[19] The protease responsible for initial activation of factor VII is unknown, but once clotting is activated, several proteases farther down the pathway can activate factor VII. Factors Xa and VIIa both catalyze activation of factor VII, so a potential mechanism for acceleration of factor VII activation exists.[20] Furthermore, both thrombin and factor XIa in the presence of negatively charged surfaces catalyze activation of factor XI.[21] Once factor XIa is generated, an additional mechanism augments activation of factor IX. Factor IXa in complex with factor VIIIa on membrane surfaces activates factor X. Factor Xa in complex with factor Va on membrane surfaces activates prothrombin. Thrombin cleaves fibrinogen, yielding monomeric fibrin, which then polymerizes to form the fibrin clot.

The blood coagulation cascade proceeds on membrane surfaces, although the source of these membranes remains uncertain. Only

Table 118–1 Properties of the Genes, mRNAs, and Gene Products of the Components of the Blood Coagulation Cascade

	Molecular Weight	Gene (kb)	Chromosome	mRNA	Exons (kb)	Plasma Concentration (μg/mL)	Function
Prothrombin	72,000	21	11p11–q12	2.1	14	100	Protease zymogen
Factor X	56,000	22	13q34	1.5	8	10	Protease zymogen
Factor IX	56,000	34	q26–27.3	2.8	8	5	Protease zymogen
Factor VII	50,000	13	13q34	2.4	8	0.5	Protease zymogen
Factor VIII	330,000	185	q28	9.0	26	0.1	Cofactor
Factor V	330,000	7.0	1q21–25	7.0	25	10	Cofactor
Factor XI	160,000	23	15		5		Protease zymogen
Factor XII	80,000	12	5	2.4	14	30	Protease zymogen
Fibrinogen	340,000					3,000	Structural
Aα Chain	64,000		4q26–q28	5			
Bβ Chain	56,000		4q26–q28	8			
γ Chain	47,000		4q26–q28	9			
von Willebrand factor	225,000 n[a]	175	12pter–p12	8.5	52	10	Adhesion
Tissue factor	45,000	12	1pter–p12	2.1	6	0.1	Cofactor/initiator
Factor XIII	320,000					60	Fibrin stabilization

[a]n, number of subunits, where the subunit M_r is 225,000.

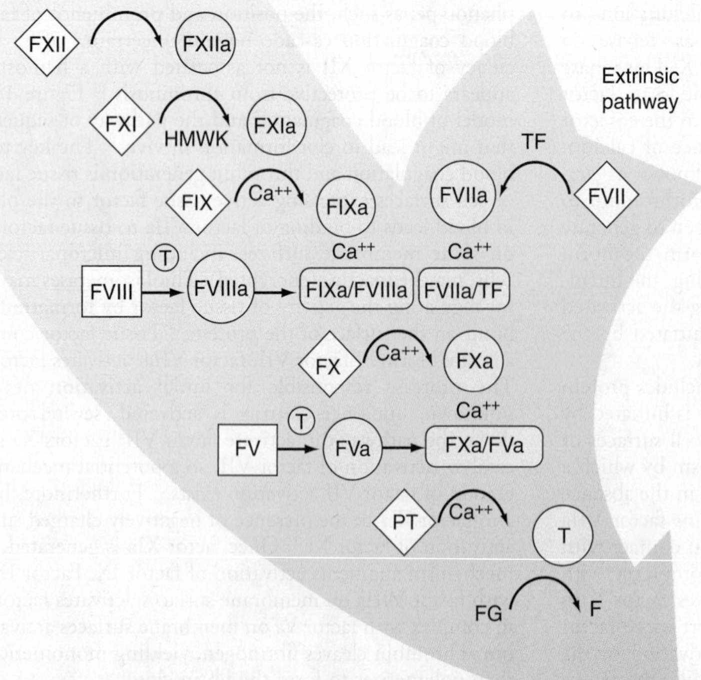

Figure 118–1 Blood coagulation cascade. Glycoprotein components of the intrinsic pathway include factors XII, XI, IX, VIII, X, and V, prothrombin, and fibrinogen. Glycoprotein components of the extrinsic pathway, initiated by the action of tissue factor located on cell surfaces, include factors VII, X, and V, prothrombin, and fibrinogen. Cascade reactions culminate in the conversion of fibrinogen to fibrin and the formation of a fibrin clot. Certain reactions, including activation of factor X and prothrombin, take place on membrane surfaces. Diamonds represent proenzymes; squares represent procofactors; circles represent enzymes and cofactors; shaded rectangles represent macromolecular complexes on membrane surfaces. F, fibrin; FG, fibrinogen; HMWK, high-molecular-weight kininogen; PT, prothrombin; T, thrombin; TF, tissue factor. *(Modified from Furie and Furie.[307])*

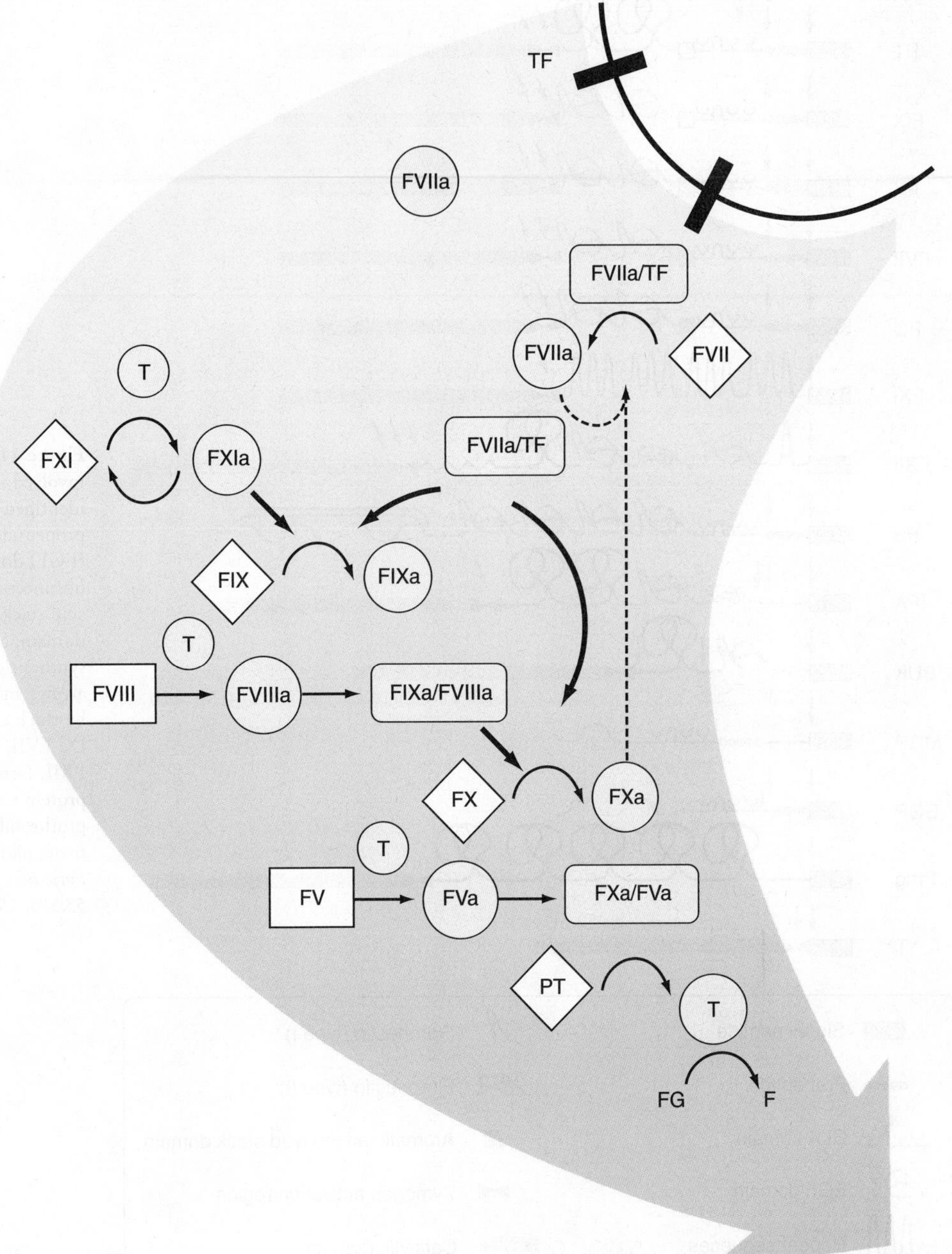

Figure 118–2 Physiologic pathways of blood coagulation. Blood coagulation is initiated by tissue factor (TF) expressed on cell surfaces. When plasma comes in contact with tissue factor, factor VIIa in plasma binds to this receptor. The factor VIIa/tissue factor complex activates both factor IX and factor X. The proteolytic activation of factor VII to VIIa, factor XI to XIa, factor VIII to VIIIa, and factor V to Va through feedback mechanisms (e.g., thrombin [T] or factor XIa [FXIa]) greatly accelerates the rate of blood clotting. The process culminates in the generation of fibrin and its polymerization to form a fibrin clot. *(From Furie B, Furie BC: The molecular basis of blood coagulation. Cell 53:505, 1988.)*

the membrane surfaces of stimulated cells can support the reactions involved in blood clotting. Phosphatidylserine, a critical component of the cell membrane that is required for assembly of blood clotting proteins on membrane surfaces, is exposed on the external membrane surface following cell activation. Phosphatidylserine is asymmetrically distributed on the phospholipid bilayer of the plasma member. An enzyme known as phospholipid scramblase catalyzes the calcium-dependent redistribution and phosphatidylserine exposure to the outer leaflet.[22–24] Tissue factor is an integral membrane protein constitutively expressed on the surface of nonvascular cells,[25–27] on the surface of monocytes and endothelial cells following cell stimulation with certain agonists, and present on leukocyte-derived microparticles circulating in the blood.[13,14,28] This protein binds to factors VII and VIIa, generating the tissue factor/factor VIIa complex on membrane surfaces that activates factor X.[29] In another example of enzyme assembly on membrane surfaces, factors IXa and VIIIa both bind to anionic phospholipid membranes.[30,31] It is envisioned that these two proteins skate about on the membrane, collide, and form the tenase complex, factor IXa/factor VIIIa. This complex has the enzymatic activity to convert factor X, also bound to the cell membrane, to factor Xa. Similarly, factors Xa and Va bind to anionic phospholipid membranes.[32] These two proteins also skate about on the membrane, collide, and form the "prothrombinase" complex, factor Xa/factor Va.[33] This complex has the enzymatic activity to convert prothrombin, also bound to the cell membrane, to thrombin, which is released from the cell surface. Although it has been suggested that individual phospholipids might be allosteric effectors of protein assembly on membrane surfaces,[34,35] a two-dimensional membrane bilayer surface with multisite features of participating phospholipid head groups appears critical.[36] In vivo, platelet membranes, endothelial membranes, or microparticle membranes may contribute to the critical surface for blood clotting. Activated (but not resting) platelets express a factor VIIIa-binding site.[37] During platelet activation in vitro, microparticles are released from the plate-

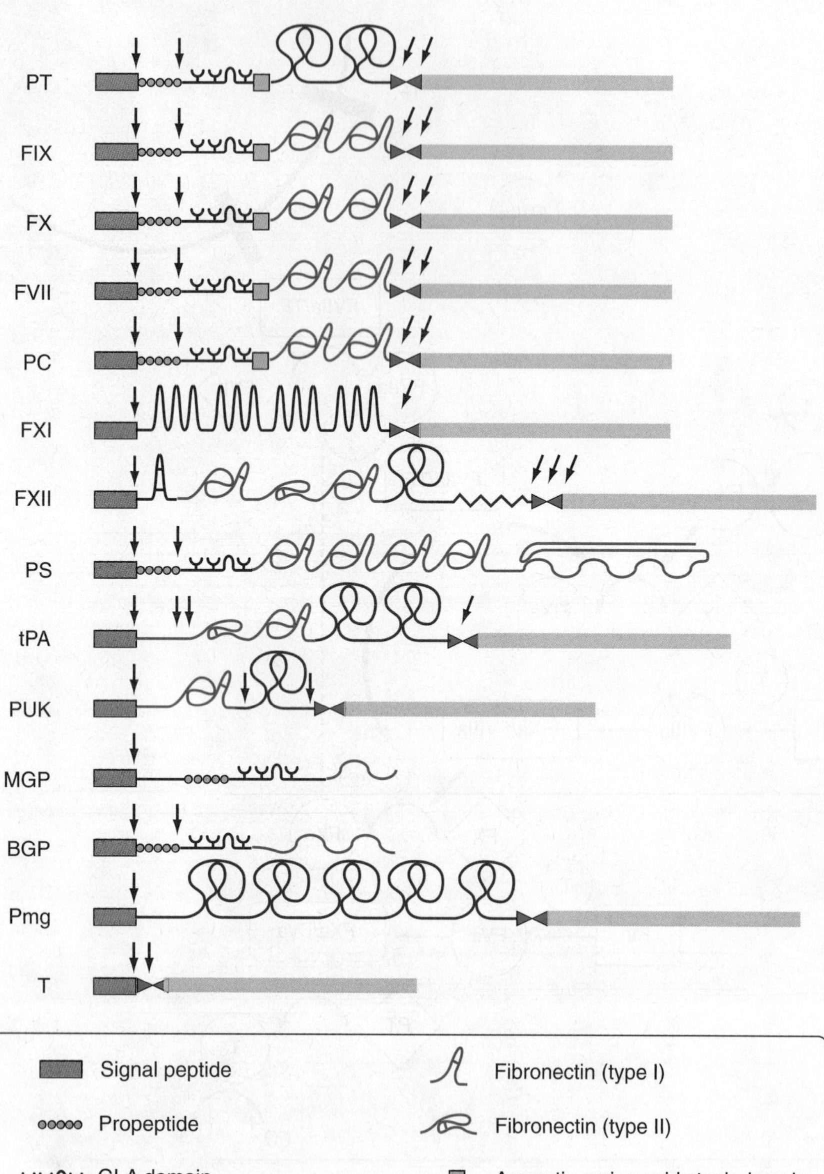

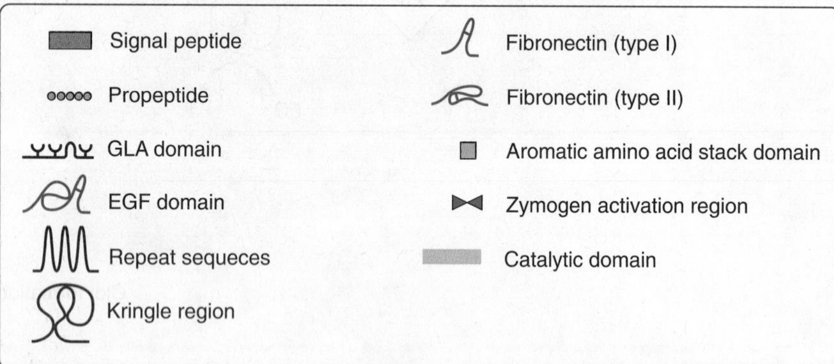

Figure 118–3 Structural domains of the proteins involved in hemostasis and related proteins. Domains, identified in the key, include signal peptide, propeptide, Gla domain, epidermal growth factor (EGF) domain, repeat sequences, kringle region, fibronectin (types I and II) domains, aromatic amino acid stack, zymogen activation region, and catalytic domain. Sites of proteolytic cleavage associated with synthesis of mature protein are indicated by thin arrows and those associated with zymogen activation by thick arrows. BGP, bone Gla protein; FIX, factor IX; FVII, factor VII; FX, factor X; FXI, factor XI; FXII, factor XII; MGP, matrix Gla protein; PC, protein C; Pmg, plasminogen; PS, protein S; PT, prothrombin; PUK, prourokinase; T, trypsin; tPA, tissue plasminogen activator. *(Modified from Furie B, Furie BC: The molecular basis of blood coagulation. Cell 53:505, 1988.)*

let membrane that are especially rich in receptors for factors VIIIa and Va.[38]

STRUCTURE OF THE BLOOD COAGULATION PROTEINS

Domain Structure

Each of the blood coagulation proteins contains multiple functional units, derived from common ancestral genes (Fig. 118–3). As a rule these functional units, or domains, are encoded by individual exons. Although the domains are not structurally identical, they have sufficient homology in structure to suggest homology of function as well. These domains are responsible for directing protein trafficking and posttranslational processing during biosynthesis and for membrane-binding properties, protein complex formation, and enzyme function of the mature protein. In factor IX, for example, these domains are independently folded but give evidence of significant interdomain interaction.[39]

Signal Peptide

The nascent chains of secreted proteins contain a short domain that permits translocation of the growing polypeptide chain into the endoplasmic reticulum. This domain is dominated by hydrophobic amino acids and usually is approximately 15 to 30 residues in length. The blood coagulation proteins found in the plasma initially are synthesized with a signal peptide, which is cleaved within the endoplasmic reticulum by the signal peptidase.

Propeptide/γ-Carboxyglutamic Acid-Rich Domain

The vitamin K–dependent proteins contain a propeptide domain between the signal peptide and the γ-carboxyglutamic acid-rich N-terminal region. This propeptide, 18 residues long in factor IX,[40,41] contains a γ-carboxylation recognition site that directs γ-carboxylation of the vitamin K–dependent proteins after synthesis[42] and is sufficient to carboxylate glutamic acid residues regardless of their sequence context.[43] Adjacent to the carboxylation recognition site is the γ-carboxyglutamic acid-rich region of these proteins. Glutamic acid residues within this region serve as substrates for the vitamin K–dependent γ-carboxylase. After carboxylation, the propeptide is cleaved from the mature protein in a late posttranslational processing step. A single exon in the vitamin K–dependent proteins encodes the propeptide (including the γ-carboxylation recognition site) and the γ-carboxyglutamic acid-rich region of approximately 40 residues. The γ-carboxyglutamic acid (Gla) domain of the vitamin K–dependent proteins contains 10 to 12 γ-carboxyglutamic acid residues and is critical to the Ca^{2+}-binding properties of these proteins. This domain is responsible for promoting the calcium-dependent interaction of these proteins with membrane surfaces, a characteristic essential for the function of these proteins.

The three-dimensional structure of the γ-carboxyglutamic acid-rich region in bovine prothrombin fragment 1 is disordered in the absence of Ca^{2+}.[44] In the presence of Ca^{2+} the Gla domain assumes a unique structure.[45] Of the 10 γ-carboxyglutamic acid residues, four residues on one side and two residues on the other define a carboxylate surface that chelates five Ca^{2+} organized in a linear cluster that extends from one side of the molecule to the other (Fig. 118–4).

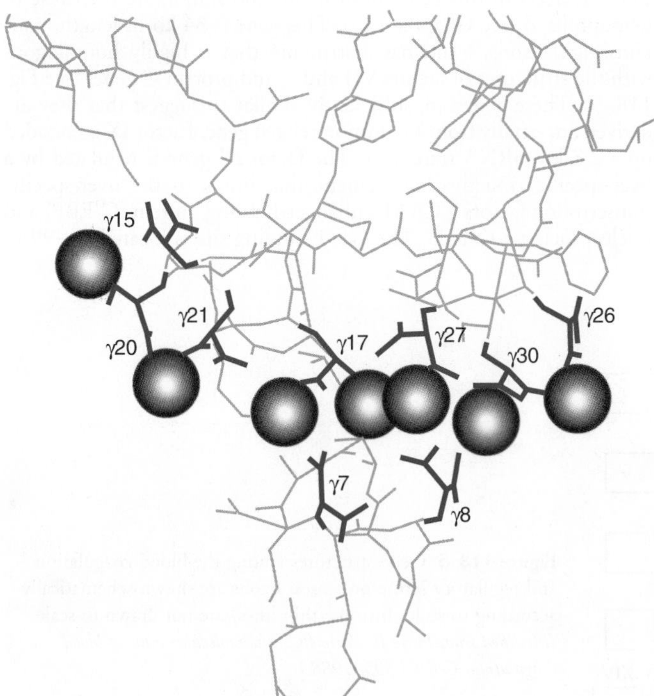

Figure 118–4 Three-dimensional structure of the γ-carboxyglutamic acid-rich region of prothrombin. This region is responsible for metal binding and membrane-protein interaction. *(Modified from Soriano-Garcia M, Padmanabhan K, de Vos AM, Tulinsky A: The Ca^{2+} ion and membrane binding structure of the Gla domain of Ca-prothrombin fragment 1. Biochemistry 31:2554, 1992.)*

The NH_2-terminal alanine loops back to form an ion pair with Gla17, Gla21, and Gla27. With the exception of Gla6, all the γ-carboxyglutamic acid residues are critical for prothrombin function.[46] The mechanism by which this region promotes interaction of the protein with membrane surfaces involves the formation of this unique fold and the expression of a membrane-binding site. The Gla domains of factors VII, X, and IX show marked three-dimensional structural homology in their calcium-stabilized conformer compared to the Gla domain of prothrombin.[47–51]

Epidermal Growth Factor Domain

The epidermal growth factor (EGF)-like domain is a common motif found in many proteins, including some of the proteins involved in blood coagulation. In the blood clotting proteins it is highly homologous with the EGF precursor. This domain, approximately 43 to 50 amino acid residues in length, contains three disulfide bonds arranged in a characteristic covalent structure. Although the EGF domain in some proteins mediates their interaction with an EGF or EGF-like receptor on cell surfaces, the EGF domains on the blood clotting proteins participate in protein complex formation. A calcium-binding site, present in some of the EGF domains of the vitamin K–dependent proteins, is defined by carboxylate groups on aspartic acid.[52] The structures of the EGF domains of factors IX and X, determined by nuclear magnetic resonance spectroscopy, demonstrate marked homology with the three-dimensional structure of EGF.[53,54] Factors IX, X, and VII contain two adjacent EGF domains (as does protein C, whereas protein S has four EGF domains). Factor XII contains two nonadjacent EGF domains, whereas tissue plasminogen activator (tPA) and prourokinase each has a single EGF domain. This domain appears to be critical for protein complex formation.[55]

Kringle Domain

Another common motif in proteins is the kringle domain. This region, with a characteristic covalent structure defined by a pattern of three disulfide bonds, is approximately 100 amino acid residues in length. The three-dimensional structure of the prothrombin kringle reveals an oblate ellipsoid, with folding defined by close contacts between the sulfur atoms of two of the disulfide bridges.[44] Internal structures are well conserved among kringles from various proteins, but molecular surface differences relate to differences in function. The kringle domains play a role in protein complex formation. In prothrombin, the second kringle domain interacts with factor Va in the prothrombinase complex.[56] Among the proteins involved in hemostasis, kringles are found in prothrombin,[57] factor XII,[58] plasminogen,[59] prourokinase,[60] and tPA.[61]

Catalytic Domain

A catalytic domain that is highly homologous with the structure of trypsin and chymotrypsin is common to all blood clotting enzymes. This protease domain includes a site for conversion of an inactive proenzyme to an active enzyme via cleavage of peptide bonds, a regulatory process known as *zymogen activation by limited proteolysis.* Furthermore, this domain contains the enzymatic machinery for cleavage of peptide bonds, the specific recognition site for protein substrates, and the site for interaction with specific protein inhibitors that regulate enzymatic activity. The blood clotting proteases are serine proteases, a class of enzymes with a common mechanism of enzymatic action that requires the catalytic triad of serine, aspartic acid, and histidine within the active site. The catalytic domain of the blood clotting proteases has an active site and an internal core nearly identical to that of trypsin.[62] The molecular surfaces surrounding the enzyme active site are responsible for defining the extended substrate-binding site of the enzyme. Solution of the crystal structure of human α-thrombin has emphasized the structural homology between thrombin and other well-characterized serine proteases.[63] Two patches of positively charged amino acids close to the C-terminal B-chain helix form the presumed heparin-binding site and a secondary fibrinogen-binding site.[64] Interaction of the A and B chains is stabilized by charged residues. A deep canyon-like active site cleft probably contributes significantly to the narrow substrate specificity of thrombin.[63,64]

Other Domains

Other motifs that appear within the proteins involved in hemostasis include the aromatic amino acid stack domain, the apple domains observed in factor XI, and the fibronectin type I and type II domains. The functions of these domains are unknown.

Components of the Intrinsic and Extrinsic Pathways

Factor XII

The factor XII gene, located on chromosome 5, contains 14 exons and 13 introns (Fig. 118–5).[58] Exon I encodes the signal peptide, exon II encodes a segment with no structural homology with other proteins, exons III and IV code for a region homologous with the type II fibronectin structure, exons V and VII each encodes EGF domains, exon VI encodes a fibronectin finger domain that intervenes between the EGF domains, and exons VIII and IX each encodes a kringle domain. The trypsin-like catalytic domain, including the activation region, is encoded by the remaining exons X to XIV. The gene organization of the catalytic domains parallels that of urokinase, factor XI, and tPA. The factor XII mRNA is 2.4 kb in length.[58,65] The mature plasma form of factor XII is composed of 596 amino acid residues in a single polypeptide chain.[58,65]

Factor XII, also known as *Hageman factor,* is the first component of the intrinsic pathway. As such, it is a component of the contact phase of activation of blood coagulation observed in vitro. This protein does not appear to have a physiologic role in hemostasis in vivo, as patients lacking this protein do not have a bleeding disorder. Indeed, the propositus, John Hageman, died of a pulmonary embolism following a fall. The protein circulates in the blood as a single-chain proenzyme of 80,000 molecular weight.[66,67] Factor XII is a glycoprotein, with carbohydrate attached to Asn230 and Asn414. Other glycosylation sites include Thr280, 286, 309, 310, and 318 and Ser289. The surface-binding properties of factor XII, specifically enhancement of the rate of factor XII activation by negatively charged surfaces, may be mediated by the positively charged amino acid sequence His-Lys-Tyr-Lys, a structure common to factor XII and kininogen.[68] The factor XII concentration in plasma is approximately 30 μg/mL. Factor XII has a plasma half-life of 2 days.[69]

Factor XI

The gene for factor XI, an intrinsic pathway component, contains 15 exons and 14 intervening sequences (see Fig. 118–5).[70] Exon I encodes a 5′ untranslated sequence, whereas exon 2 encodes a signal peptide. Four repeat sequences are each encoded by two exons: repeat 1 by exons III and IV, repeat 2 by exons V and VI, repeat 3 by exons VII and VIII, and repeat 4 by exons IX and X. The four apple domains play a role in protein recognition. High–molecular-weight kininogen has binding sites on the apple 1, 2, and 4 domains. Factor IX binds to the apple 2 and 3 domains. Factor XIIa binds to the apple 4 domain. The trypsin-like domain, responsible for the proteolytic function of the enzyme form of the zymogen, is encoded by exons XII to XV. Factor XI has a molecular weight of 160,000[71] and is composed of two identical chains bound together by disulfide bonds.[72] Factor XI circulates in the blood as a disulfide-lined homodimer at a concentration of 5 μg/mL. It has a biologic half-life of approximately 3 days.[73]

The crystal structure of human factor XI at 2.9 Å reveals the four apple domains in a structure resembling a flat saucer.[74] A cavity in the center of the structure is lined with basic and aromatic amino acids. The protease domain has a structure typical of serine proteases. The apple domains form a circular platform around the base of the protease domain.

Factor IX

Factor IX plays a critical role in blood coagulation (see Chapter 124). Its gene, adjacent to the factor VIII gene, is located on the X chromosome. Defects in this gene, both major and minor, are the cause of hemophilia B (see Chapter 125). This gene is 34 kb in length, contains eight exons,[75] and has a structure that is highly homologous with the structures of factors VII and X and protein C genes (see Fig. 118–5). These genes are sufficiently similar to suggest that they are derived ancestrally from a common related gene. Factor IX is encoded on a 2.8-kb mRNA transcript. The factor IX gene is regulated by a liver-specific *cis*-activating element that binds to the liver-specific transcription factors CCAAT enhancer-binding protein (C/EBP) and nuclear factor 1 (NF-1). The NF-1 binding site is located at −99 to

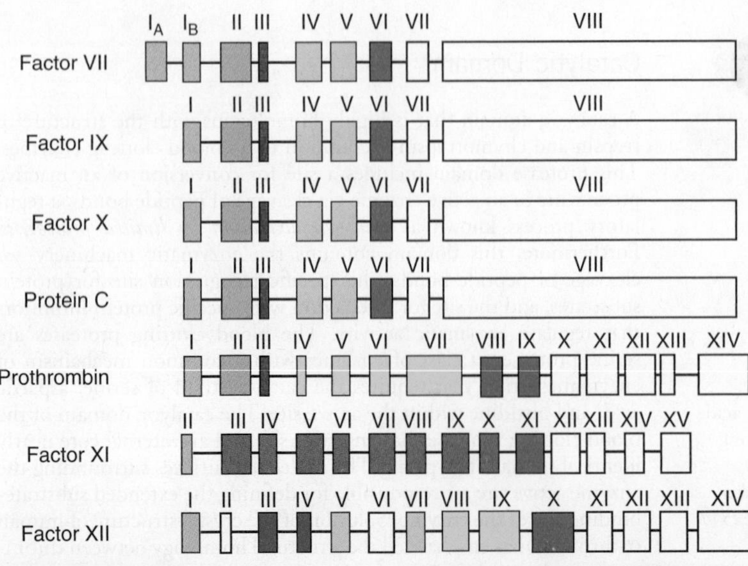

Figure 118–5 Gene structures among the blood coagulation and regulatory serine proteases. Exons are shown schematically according to scale. Introns (thin lines) are not drawn to scale. *(Modified from Furie B, Furie BC: The molecular basis of blood coagulation. Cell 53:505, 1988.)*

−76 upstream of the transcriptional start site.[76] The EBP-binding site is located close to the transcription initiation site. An androgen-responsive promoter element in the factor IX gene explains the curious phenotype of factor IX Leyden (see Chapter 124).[77]

The mature protein, with a molecular weight of 56,000, requires vitamin K for its synthesis and contains 12 γ-carboxyglutamic acid residues. The fully carboxylated form of the protein binds to calcium ions and to membrane surfaces in the presence of calcium ions. Factor IX contains metal-binding sites, defined by γ-carboxyglutamic acid,[78] and another class of metal-binding site that is a component of the EGF domain.[79,80] The site within the EGF domain is defined in part by Asp64, a residue that is partially β-hydroxylated. Factor IX is a glycoprotein containing N- and O-linked sugars. Factors IX and IXa bind to phospholipid membranes composed of phosphatidylserine-phosphatidylcholine.[31,81] This interaction requires both Ca^{2+} and fully carboxylated factor IX.[81] The x-ray structure of porcine factor IXa in the absence of calcium demonstrates the relationship of the two EGF domains and the serine protease domain; however, the Gla domain is partially disordered and not defined.[82] The nuclear magnetic resonance-derived structure of human factor IX Gla domain in the presence of calcium supports, as a first approximation, a model of the Gla domain based upon that of prothrombin.[49,83] The crystal structures of the Gla domain confirm the similarity of this domain in all of the vitamin K–dependent proteins.[50,51]

Expression of phospholipid-binding properties involves two metal-dependent conformational transitions.[81] The calcium-stabilized conformer expresses a phospholipid-binding site that is located at the N-terminus of the protein.[84] Factors IX and IXa bind to activated platelets but not to resting platelets.[85,86] However, there is no evidence for a protein-based receptor for factor IX on the platelet surface. Factor IXa, but not factor IX, binds to factor VIIIa on the surface of activated platelets. The factor VIIIa-binding site includes regions of the second EGF domain and the serine protease domain.[87] The endothelial cell-binding site of factor IX resides in the Gla domain.[88] Collagen on the surface of endothelial cells defines this factor IX-binding site.[89,90] However, the biologic role of this site remains uncertain. The factor IX concentration in plasma is approximately5 μg/mL. This protein has a plasma half-life of approximately 24 hours.[91] As with other proteins of this molecular size, it partitions between the intravascular and extravascular spaces. A comprehensive review of the structure of the factor IX gene and the protein it encodes is given in Chapter 124.

Factor VIII

Factor VIII is a critical cofactor required for normal blood clotting (see Chapter 123). Defects in the factor VIII gene that lead to a deficiency in factor VIII are the cause of hemophilia A. The factor VIII gene is 186 kb in length and is divided into 26 exons (see Fig. 123–1).[92,93] As such, it is one of the largest genes known. Located on the X chromosome, it is near the locus of the factor IX gene. Factor VIII is synthesized as a single polypeptide chain, including a 19-residue signal peptide; in its mature form it contains 2332 amino acid residues.[92,93] Although this protein is synthesized by many cell types, the liver is a major site of synthesis.[94] The glycosylated protein A is estimated to have a molecular weight of 330,000. The protein sequence of factor VIII demonstrates marked sequence homology with factor V, another protein cofactor.[95] Factor VIII circulates in the blood as a heterodimer composed of two polypeptide chains derived from the original single chain. These two chains, including one of relative molecular weight (M_r) 80,000 and one of M_r varying between 90,000 and 200,000, are derived from the COOH-terminus and the NH_2-terminus of the single-chain precursor, respectively. Their interaction is Ca^{2+} dependent. A region of the C2 domain defines the membrane-binding properties of factor VIII and the site of interaction with von Willebrand factor (vWF).[96] The A1 domain interacts with the A3 domain, thus linking the heavy and light chains.[97] Although membranes including phosphatidyl-L-serine are required for factor VIII interaction, phosphatidylethanolamine enhances membrane binding.[98,99] The orientation of factor VIII bound to phospholipid vesicles has been determined by electron microcroscopy.[100] In its circulating form, factor VIII is inactive or minimally active as a cofactor in blood coagulation. It circulates in the blood at very low concentration (100 ng/mL) bound to vWF. Its plasma half-life is approximately 8 to 12 hours.[101] Factor VIII is converted into its active cofactor form by the proteolytic cleavage of two or more peptide bonds within the protein by thrombin. The structure and function of factor VIII are described in detail in Chapter 123.

Factor X

The factor X gene, located on the long arm of chromosome 13 adjacent to the factor VII gene, is composed of eight exons and is 22 kb in length (see Fig. 118–5).[102] The organization of this gene is identical to that of the factor IX gene. Exon I encodes the signal peptide, exon II the propeptide/γ-carboxyglutamic acid-rich domain, exon III the short aromatic amino acid stack domain, exons IV and V the two EGF domains, exon VI the activation region, and exons VII and VIII the catalytic domain. The 5′ end of the factor X gene is linked to the 3′ end of the factor VII gene.[103] The liver-specific promoter element FXP1-binding site was located −63 to −42 bp upstream of the factor X gene, whereas other promoter elements, FXP2 and FXP3, span −215 to −149 and −457 to −351, respectively.[103] After transcription, the factor X mRNA of approximately 1.5 kb includes a short 3′ untranslated region following the stop codon.[104,105] The polyadenylation signal is located within the 3′ end of the coding sequence. Factor X, with a molecular weight of 56,000, is synthesized as a single polypeptide chain.[102,105] However, factor X as isolated from plasma is composed of two polypeptide chains, a heavy chain with a molecular weight of 38,000[106–108] and a light chain with a molecular weight of 18,000.[109,110] These chains are linked by a single disulfide bond. The Arg-Lys-Arg sequence at residues 139 to 141 in the single polypeptide chain appears very susceptible to intracellular or extracellular proteolysis, yielding the predominant two-chain form.[102,105] The light chain of factor X includes 11 γ-carboxyglutamic acid residues at positions 6, 7, 14, 16, 19, 20, 25, 26, 29, 32, and 39 in the human protein. A single β-hydroxyaspartic acid residue is located in the first EGF domain at residue 63. Bovine factor X contains both asparagine-linked carbohydrate at Asn36 and threonine-linked carbohydrate at Thr300.[111] Like prothrombin, the asparagine-linked sugars contain NeuAca263Galβ163(NeuAca266)GlcNAc in the outer chain. The two EGF domains are important for binding to the cofactor, factor Va. The second EGF domain can support factor Va binding but at reduced affinity,[87] suggesting a role for the first EGF domain in this interaction as well.[112]

Factor X is a calcium-binding protein that interacts with membrane surfaces in the presence of calcium. It contains both low-affinity and high-affinity metal-binding sites,[113] occupancy of which leads to conformational changes and expression of membrane-binding properties.[114] Like the other vitamin K–dependent proteins, factor X binds preferentially to acidic phospholipid surfaces.[115,116] Bound factor X is an extrinsic membrane protein in that no component of it is embedded within the membrane. The three-dimensional structure of bovine factor X lacking the Gla domain has been determined by x-ray crystallography and demonstrates marked structural homology with trypsin and the other serine proteases involved in blood coagulation.[117,118] The N-terminus of the Gla domain of factor X shows little stable structure in the absence of Ca^{2+}.[119] However, the structure of the Gla domain of factor X determined when bound to factor X binding protein from a snake venom indicates marked structural homology with other Gla domains.[48] Furthermore, the Gla domain of factor X in the presence of Mg^{2+} assumes a novel conformation, distinct from that in the presence of Ca^{2+}.[120] The Gla domain linked to the first EGF domain shows little interaction between the two domains, but the orientation of these domains is altered by the presence of calcium ions.[121]

The plasma concentration of factor X is maintained at approximately 10 μg/mL. Factor X has a half-life in plasma of approximately 36 hours.[91]

Factor VII

The factor VII gene is 13 kb in length and is located on the long arm of chromosome 13, immediately adjacent to the factor X gene.[122,123] The coding region is found on nine separate exons (see Fig. 118–5). Preprofactor VII is synthesized via two alternative forms. In one form, incorporating exon IB encoding for the signal peptide factor VII arises from a gene whose gene organization is identical to that of the factor IX gene. In a second form, exon IA directs the coding of the signal peptide instead of exon IB. In this form, preprofactor VII has a polypeptide extension of the NH_2-terminus that elongates the signal peptide/propeptide from 38 to 60 residues. Exon II encodes the propeptide and γ-carboxyglutamic acid-rich domain, and exon III encodes the short aromatic amino acid stack domain, a segment common to all vitamin K–dependent proteins. Exons IV and V each encodes one of the EGF domains. The catalytic domain is coded by exons VI to VIII, with the activation peptide encoded within exon VI. The mRNA for factor VII is approximately 2.4 kb in length,[124] with a 3′ untranslated region 1.0 kb in length and a poly(A) tail located after the stop codon.

Factor VII is a component of the extrinsic pathway of blood coagulation. It forms a complex with tissue factor to generate an enzyme complex that activates factor X. Human factor VII, with a molecular weight of 50,000, circulates in plasma as a single-chain zymogen containing 406 amino acid residues.[124] The NH_2-terminal domain includes 11 γ-carboxyglutamic acid residues at positions 6, 7, 14, 16, 19, 20, 25, 26, 29, 34, and 35 in bovine factor VII.[125] Site-specific mutagenesis of some residues in the Gla domain leads to markedly enhanced membrane binding.[126] Asp63 is partially β-hydroxylated. Factor VII is a glycoprotein that contains 13% carbohydrate. The structure of the complex of the active site-inhibited factor VIIa and extracellular domain of tissue factor has been determined by x-ray crystallography.[47] Salient general features of this complex include extensive "embracing" of extended conformations of one protein by the other. This interaction involves multiple domains and multiple contact sites within each domain. The structure of the calcium-stabilized Gla domain is homologous to that of prothrombin and factor IX.

In contrast to other proenzymes involved in blood coagulation, factor VII circulates in the blood in two forms: the inactive zymogen factor VII and the enzymatic active factor VIIa.[6] Factor VII is a zymogen, with no enzymatic activity prior to cleavage.[127] The concentration of factor VIIa is low but sufficient to generate significant factor X-activating activity when the factor VIIa forms a complex with newly exposed tissue factor. The factor Xa formed can activate factor VII to factor VIIa, increasing the amount of factor VIIa available during tissue injury. This model would allow significant amplification of thrombin formation via the extrinsic pathway.

Factor V

Factor V is a plasma glycoprotein with a molecular weight of 330,000. This protein is a critical cofactor that in its activated form facilitates activation of prothrombin by factor Xa. Factor V is a single-chain protein that circulates in the blood in a precursor, inactive cofactor form. The factor V gene, located on chromosome 1 at 1q21–25, encodes a 7-kb mRNA, which itself encodes a prefactor V including a 28-amino–acid-residue signal peptide and a mature protein composed of 2196 amino acid residues.[128,129] The gene contains 25 exons that range in size from 72 to 2820 bp[130] and resembles the factor VIII gene in organization. The heavy-chain region is composed of two domains with notable structural homology, termed the *A domain.* The light-chain region is composed of another A domain and two homologous C domains. The heavy-chain region and light-chain region are joined by a connecting region known as the *B domain.* The A1-A2-B-A3-C1-C2 domain structure is also present in factor VIII.[92] The conversion of factor V into the procoagulant factor Va is a stepwise process related to cleavages adjacent to Arg709, Arg1018, and Arg1545 by either thrombin or factor Xa.[131,132] A single site adjacent to Arg1545 in human factor V is critical for generation of biologically active factor Va.[131] Factor Va is inactivated by cleavage of peptide bonds adjacent to Arg306, Arg506, and Arg679 by activated protein C.[133] Ca^{2+} plays a role in the stabilization of the heavy chain and light chain of factor V.[134] Disruption of this Ca^{2+} binding site by mutagenesis leads to a destabilized factor Va following thrombin activation of factor V, presumably through dissociation of the heavy and light chains.[135] Protein S and phospholipid membranes are critical for this reaction.[136]

Although the liver appears to be the primary site of synthesis of factor V, megakaryocytes also synthesize this protein. In addition to its presence in plasma, factor V is a component of the α granules in megakaryocytes and subsequently in platelets[137] and is secreted on platelet stimulation with specific agonists. Factors V and Va bind to two classes of binding sites on the surface of platelets.[138] However, the higher-affinity binding sites interact specifically with factor Va and not with factor V. The plasma concentration of factor V is 10 μg/mL, and its plasma half-life is approximately 12 hours.[139]

Prothrombin

The prothrombin gene is located on chromosome 11.[140] It is 21 kb in length and is composed of 14 exons, each encoding all or part of a functional domain of prothrombin (see Fig. 118–5)[141]: signal peptide (exon I), propeptide/γ-carboxyglutamic acid-rich domain (exon II), aromatic amino acid stack domain (exon III), two kringle domains (exons IV–VII), activation region (exons VIII and IX), and catalytic domain (exons X–XIV). The introns vary considerably in size, from 84 bp for the intron between exons VIII and IX to 9447 bp for that between exons XII and XIII. Although the structure of prothrombin is homologous with those of factors IX, X, and VII and protein C, the prothrombin gene demonstrates only partial homology with the genes of these proteins. Exons I to III are shared by all these proteins, but prothrombin contains exons IV to VII encoding the kringle domains and has a homologous serine protease domain composed of seven exons, in contrast to the two exons found in the factor IX gene family. Prothrombin mRNA is 2.1 kb in length and includes a 5′ untranslated region greater than 150 bp, a 1.8-kb open reading frame, and a 97-bp 3′untranslated region. The prothrombin gene contains a weak promoter before the transcription initiation site and liver-specific enhancer element spanning approximately 900 bases upstream from the transcription initiation site. This site interacts with hepatic nuclear factor 1.[142,143]

Prothrombin is a plasma glycoprotein with a molecular weight of 72,000.[57,144,145] As with all the blood clotting proteins, prothrombin is synthesized with a hydrophobic signal peptide from residues −43 to −19. After translocation to the rough endoplasmic reticulum, the signal peptide is removed by a signal peptidase. The propeptide, containing the γ-carboxylation recognition site,[42] includes residues −18 to −1. During protein synthesis but after γ-carboxylation, this peptide is removed by an intracellular propeptidase. The mature prothrombin that circulates in the plasma is composed of 579 amino acid residues arranged in a single polypeptide chain. The 10 γ-carboxyglutamic acid residues are located in the Gla domain of human prothrombin at residues 6, 7, 14, 16, 19, 20, 25, 26, 29, and 32. Carbohydrate represents approximately 10% of the mass of prothrombin. *N*-Asparagine–linked carbohydrate is attached to Asn78, Asn100, and Asn373 in bovine prothrombin,[146] and human prothrombin likely contains carbohydrate at the homologous amino acids. Complex asparagine-linked oligosaccharides include NeuAca2 63Galβ163(NeuAca266)GlcNAc. The short aromatic amino acid stack domain has a significant α-helical structure and serves to link the Gla domain to two kringle domains,[45] which are similar to structures found in factor XII, plasminogen, and tPA and are defined structurally by the pattern of disulfide bonds. These domains are important for protein complex formation with factor Va. The remainder of prothrombin, accounting for approximately half the protein structure, represents the catalytic domain. This region includes the activation domain that is critical for conversion of zymogen into the active enzyme and the trypsin-like region that possesses protease activity. Prothrombin has no coagulant activity in its zymogen form and must be converted to thrombin in order to participate in blood coagulation.

The metal-binding properties of prothrombin are conferred by γ-carboxyglutamic acid residues.[147] Abnormal (des-γ-carboxy) prothrombin, lacking γ-carboxyglutamic acid, does not bind to Ca^{2+} and does not interact with membrane surfaces in the presence of calcium.[147,148] Prothrombin binds Ca^{2+} and other metal ions via two classes of metal-binding sites[149–152] and, on metal binding, undergoes conformational changes leading to expression of membrane-binding properties.[114,153,154] Concomitantly, neoantigens are exposed on the metal-stabilized conformers of prothrombin.[155–158] Prothrombin is an extrinsic membrane-binding protein. In the presence of calcium ions, a surface of the prothrombin–metal complex interacts with phospholipid vesicles; a marked preference for acidic phospholipids, specifically phosphatidylserine, has been demonstrated. The N-terminal third of the protein contains the ω loop, and within it the hydrophobic patch;[45] this region is buried within the membrane.[159] Salient features of a model of prothrombin–membrane interaction include the presence of an appropriately charged pocket for the phosphoserine of phosphatidylserine in the Gla domain, electrostatic interaction of the carboxyl group of the serine head group with the γ-carboxyglutamic acid-calcium network of the Gla domain, formation of salt bridges between the positively charged arginine and lysine side chains with the phosphate oxygens, and alignment of the fatty acid tail of phosphatidylserine with the hydrophobic patch of the Gla domain (Fig. 118–6).[160]

The plasma concentration of prothrombin is approximately 100 μg/mL.[161,162] The plasma half-life of prothrombin is approximately 3 days.[91,163]

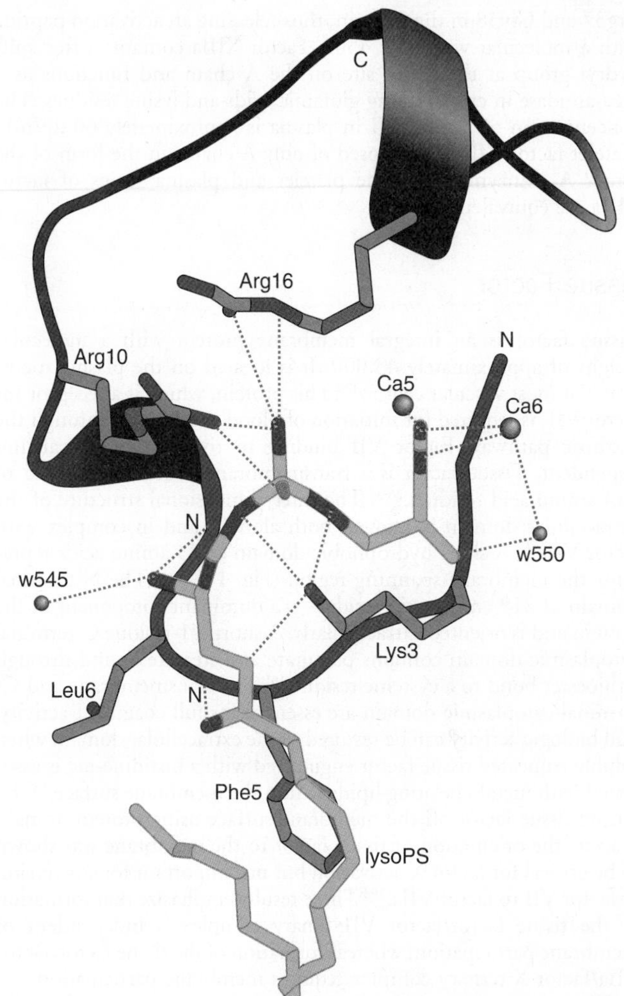

Figure 118–6 Interaction of phosphoserine head group of phospholipid with prothrombin. The hydrogen bonds and salt bridges between atoms in lysophosphatidylserine and the prothrombin-calcium ion complex are indicated as dashed lines (gray). The side chains of Lys3, Phe5, Leu6, Arg10, and Arg16, bound Ca^{2+} ions 5 and 6, and the backbone amide nitrogens of Leu6 and Gla7, N, are labeled. The lysophosphatidylserine (lysoPS) is pink. The phosphate oxygens and carbonyl oxygens labeled red. The Gla domain of prothrombin is black.

Fibrinogen

Fibrinogen is the most abundant plasma protein involved in blood coagulation. At a plasma concentration of 2 to 3 mg/mL, it represents approximately 2% of the total plasma proteins. In addition, platelets contain fibrinogen within their α granules. Variant forms likely arise via posttranslational modifications or protein degradation. Fibrinogen, unique among the blood clotting proteins, is encoded by three separate genes, each of which encodes one of the three subunits. These three genes, located on chromosome 4, are clustered on a 50-kb region.[164] The fibrinogen genes are organized with the α-chain gene 10 kb upstream of the γ-chain gene, which in turn is 13 kb upstream of the β-chain gene. The α-, γ-, and β-chain genes contain nine, five, and eight exons, respectively. The regulation of these genes is coordinated at the transcriptional level by the synchronous production of three separate mRNA species.[165]

Fibrinogen is a structural protein that circulates in the plasma in a functionally inert precursor form. Its conversion to fibrin leads to polymerization of fibrin and to formation of a fibrin clot. Human fibrinogen has a molecular weight of approximately 340,000. It is composed of three pairs of polypeptide chains: two Aα chains, two Bβ chains, and two γ chains.[166] The α, β, and γ chains demonstrate significant structural homology within their amino acid sequences, suggesting their evolutionary origin from a common ancestral gene.[167–169] The Aα chain has a molecular weight of 63,500 and contains 610 amino acid residues. The Bβ-chain has a molecular weight of 56,000 and contains 461 amino acid residues. The γ-chain has a molecular weight of 47,000 and contains 411 amino acid residues. The Aα, Bβ, and γ chains are covalently linked through disulfide bonds. The disulfide bonds near the N-terminal regions of these polypeptide chains link the three chains to each other; they also link the two Aα chains together and the two γ-chains together. This region is known as the *disulfide knot.* Electron micrographs of fibrinogen show a trinodular molecule.[170] X-ray crystal structures of fibrinogen provide insight into the mechanism by which fibrin self-assembles.[171,172] Crystal structures of fragment D consist of a coiled-coil region and two homologous globular regions.[173] Crystal structures of the N-terminal fragment E region show marked symmetry of design.[174] The crystal structure of the C-terminal fragment of the γ chain reveals a mechanism for electrostatic steering that guides the alignment of the fibrin monomers during polymerization.[175] The plasma half-life of fibrinogen is approximately 3 to 5 days.[176]

Factor XIII

Factor XIII is a zymogen of a cysteine transglutaminase that circulates in the blood. It is composed of two peptide subunits, the A chain (M_r 75,000) and the B chain (M_r 80,000).[177] Factor XIII has a molecular weight of 320,000. It is a tetrameric structure with two A chains and two B chains held together noncovalently. After binding to Ca^{2+},[178] factor XIII ($\alpha_2\beta_2$) is activated to its enzyme form factor XIIIa ($\alpha_2\beta_2$) by thrombin through cleavage of the bond between

Arg37 and Gly38 in the A chain, thus releasing an activation peptide with a molecular weight of 4500. Factor XIIIa contains a free sulfhydryl group at the active site on the A chain and functions as a transamidase in cross-linking glutamic acids and lysine residues. The concentration of factor XIII in plasma is approximately 60 μg/mL. Platelet factor XIII is composed of only A chains in the form of the dimer A_2. Enzymatically, the platelet and plasma forms of factor XIIIa are equivalent.

Tissue Factor

Tissue factor is an integral membrane protein with a molecular weight of approximately 43,000. It is located on the plasma membrane of most vascular cells.[25,179] This protein, which is a receptor for factor VII, is required for initiation of blood coagulation through the extrinsic pathway. Factor VII binding to tissue factor is calcium dependent. Tissue factor is a transmembrane protein composed of 263 amino acid residues.[26,27] The three-dimensional structure of the extracellular domain is known, both alone[180] and in complex with factor VIIa.[47] A short hydrophobic domain of 23 amino acids represents the membrane-spanning region (Fig. 118–7). The N-terminal domain of 219 amino acid residues is a dominant component of the protein and is oriented extracellularly. A short, 21-residue C-terminal cytoplasmic domain contains palmitate and stearate bound through a thioester bond to a cysteine residue.[181] The transmembrane and C-terminal cytoplasmic domain are essential for full coagulant activity. Full biologic activity can be restored to the extracellular domain when soluble truncated tissue factor engineered with a histidine-tag is associated with metal-chelating lipids within the membrane surface.[182] By raising tissue factor off the membrane surface using protein domain spacers, the orientation of tissue factor to the membrane was shown to be critical for factor X activation but not important for conversion of factor VII to factor VIIa.[183] These results emphasize that formation of the tissue factor/factor VII binary complex is independent of membrane participation, whereas formation of the tissue factor/factor VIIa/factor X ternary complex requires membrane participation.

Tissue factor is expressed constitutively in most nonvascular cells. In monocytes and endothelial cells, expression of tissue factor is associated with cell stimulation.[184–186] Tissue factor in blood accumulates in the developing thrombus[12] and is delivered to the thrombus via microparticles in a mechanism that is P-selectin and PSGL-1 dependent.[13] The tissue factor gene is 12.4 kb in length and is composed of six exons.[187]

von Willebrand Factor

vWF is a multimeric glycoprotein that is present in the plasma, within the α granules of platelets, and in the Weibel-Palade bodies of endothelial cells (see Chapter 128). The gene for vWF is located on chromosome 12 and is approximately 176 kb in length.[188] The gene includes 52 exons that encode a signal peptide, a large propolypeptide (M_r 80,000), and the mature vWF monomer (M_r 225,000).[189] A 9-kb mRNA encodes a precursor form of the protein, synthesized as a single polypeptide chain containing 2813 amino acid residues.[189–192] Pro-vWF undergoes posttranslational modification involving initial formation of dimers, which undergo multimerization via a process that is dependent on the presence of the intact propeptide.[193,194] The high-molecular-weight vWF multimers vary in size up to approximately 10 million, with the largest forms displaying the most potent biologic activity.

Crystal structures of domains of vWF have provided insight into the organization of the protein. The structure of the A3 domain complexed to antibody indicates the location of the collagen-binding site.[195] Site-specific mutagenesis allowed mapping of this region.[196] The N-terminus of glycoprotein Ibα wraps around the A1 domain of vWF, providing two contact interfaces.[197] Gain-of-function mutations in vWF, as in type IIB von Willebrand disease, show the structural correlates of increased affinity between glycoprotein Ibα and vWF.[198]

Two critical biologic roles are fulfilled by vWF. First, it can mediate the adhesion of platelets to the injured vascular wall. Adhesion occurs through simultaneous binding of vWF to its receptor glycoprotein Ib on platelet surfaces and to collagen in the subendothelium. In addition to being constitutively secreted from endothelial cells, vWF is stored in the Weibel-Palade bodies of endothelial cells and released on stimulation of granule release.[199] As a plasma carrier protein, vWF binds noncovalently to and stabilizes factor VIII and circulates in the blood as a factor VIII/vWF complex. Factor VIII binds stoichiometrically to the vWF subunit.[200] Under physiologic conditions, however, most of the factor VIII-binding sites on mature vWF are unoccupied.

SYNTHESIS OF BLOOD COAGULATION PROTEINS

Biosynthesis of Vitamin K–Dependent Blood Clotting Proteins

Four of the plasma proteins involved in blood coagulation—prothrombin, and factors IX, X, and VII—require vitamin K for their synthesis. These proteins contain between 10 and 12 residues of γ-carboxyglutamic acid[201,202] within the first 45 residues of their NH_2-termini (Fig. 118–8). They represent a unique class of calcium-binding proteins that assemble on membrane surfaces in the presence of Ca^{2+}. These proteins are synthesized in a precursor form, which includes a typical signal peptide and a propeptide that intervenes between the signal sequence and the mature NH_2-terminus of the protein. Following translocation through the rough endoplasmic reticulum, specific glutamic acid residues in the prozymogen are selectively γ-carboxylated.

Vitamin K–dependent carboxylation is catalyzed by a membrane-bound γ-carboxylase located in the endoplasmic reticulum. In the presence of reduced vitamin K, molecular oxygen, carbon dioxide,

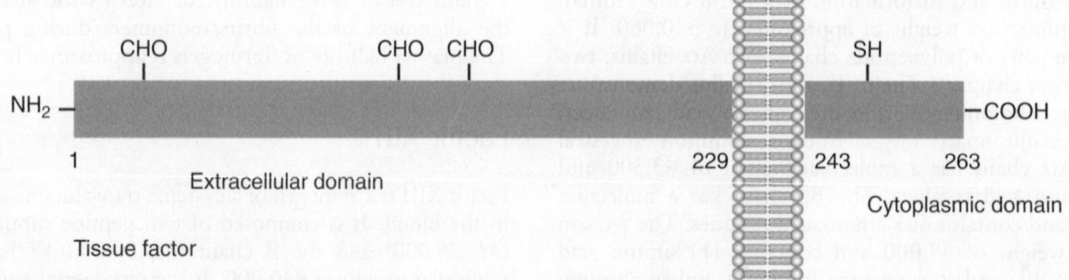

Figure 118–7 Structure of tissue factor. The extracellular domain extends from residues 1 to 229. This region contains three potential glycosylation sites (CHO). A short transmembrane domain is rich in hydrophobic amino acids. The cytoplasmic domain, extending from residues 243 to 263, contains a free sulfhydryl (SH) group, which undergoes esterification to palmitate or stearate.

Residue number	5 10 15 20 25 30 35 40
Human prothrombin	A N T - F L γ γ V R K G N L γ R γ C V γ γ T C S Y γ γ A F γ A L γ S S T A T D V F W A
Human factor IX	Y N S G K L γ γ F V Q G N L γ R γ C M γ γ K C S F γ γ A R γ V F γ N T γ K T T γ F W K
Human factor X	A N S - F L γ γ M K K G H L γ R γ C M γ γ T C S Y γ γ A R γ V F γ D S D K T N γ F W N
Human factor VII	A N A - F L γ γ L R P G S L γ R γ C K γ γ Q C S F γ γ A R γ I F D A γ R T K L F W I
Human protein C	A N S - F L γ γ L R H G S L γ R γ C I γ γ I C D F γ γ A K γ I F N V D D T L A F W S
Human protein S	A N S - L L γ γ T K Q G N L γ R γ C I γ γ L C N K γ γ A R γ V F γ N D P γ T D Y F Y P

Figure 118–8 γ-Carboxyglutamic acid-rich domains of the vitamin K–dependent proteins. A one-letter amino acid code is used (γ denotes γ-carboxyglutamic acid). Sequences have been aligned to maximize sequence homology.

	-24						-18								-10									-1	+1
Factor IX							Thr	Val	Phe	Leu	Asp	His	Glu	Asn	Ala	Asn	Lys	ile	Leu	Asn	Arg	Pro	Lys	Arg	Tyr
Prothrombin	Ser	Leu	Val	His	Ser	Gin	His	Val	Phe	Leu	Ala	Pro	Gln	Gin	Ala	Arg	Ser	Leu	Leu	Gin	Arg	Val	Arg	Arg	Ala
Factor X	Leu	Leu	Leu	Leu	Gly	Glu	Ser	Leu	Phe	Ile	Arg	Arg	Glu	Gin	Ala	Asn	Asn	ile	Leu	Ala	Arg	Val	Thr	Arg	Ala
Protein C	Thr	Pro	Ala	Pro	Leu	Asp	Ser	Val	phe	Ser	Ser	Ser	Glu	Arg	Ala	His	Gin	Val	Leu	Arg	Ile	Arg	Lys	Arg	Ala
Factor VII	Trp	Lys	Pro	Gly	Pro	His	Arg	Val	Phe	Val	Thr	Glu	Glu	Glu	Ala	His	Gly	Val	Leu	His	Arg	Arg	Arg	Arg	Ala
Protein S	Val	Leu	Pro	Val	Leu	Glu	Ala	Asn	Phe	Leu	Ser	Arg	Gin	His	Ala	Ser	Gin	Val	Leu	Ile	Arg	Arg	Arg	Arg	Ala
Bone Gla protein	Ser	Gly	Ala	Glu	Ser	Ser	Lys	Ala	Phe	Val	Ser	Lys	Gin	Glu	Gly	Ser	Glu	Val	Val	Lys	Arg	Pro	Arg	Arg	Tyr

Figure 118–9 Sequence comparison of the propeptide domains of the vitamin K–dependent blood coagulation proteins. Homologous regions of other vitamin K–dependent proteins are aligned. Residues that demonstrate significant sequence homology are boxed and shaded; regions with conservative amino acid substitutions are boxed. *(Modified from Furie B, Furie BC: The molecular basis of blood coagulation. Cell 53:505, 1988.)*

and the protein precursor substrate, specific glutamic acids adjacent to the γ-carboxylation recognition site on the propeptide are converted to the corresponding γ-carboxyglutamic acids. The vitamin K–dependent carboxylase catalyzes both the formation of γ-carboxyglutamic acid from glutamic acid and vitamin K epoxide from vitamin K, which indicates the coupling of these two processes (see Chapter 130).[203] The vitamin K–dependent carboxylase is a single-chain protein with a molecular weight of 94,000 that is composed of a single polypeptide chain of 758 amino acids.[203–206] The carboxylase can be expressed in insect cells otherwise lacking carboxylase activity.[207] The vitamin K–dependent carboxylase includes sulfhydryl groups at the active site.[208] Cysteines critical for carboxylation may include Cys99 and Cys450,[209] although the precise cysteines in the active site remain controversial.[210]

The propeptide within the vitamin K–dependent proteins directs γ-carboxylation. This region demonstrates sequence homology among proteins that contain γ-carboxyglutamic acid (Fig. 118–9),[211,212] an observation that has suggested a role for the propeptide in carboxylation. Site-specific mutagenesis has shown that factor IX species lacking the 18-residue propeptide or containing point mutations at conserved residues −16 or −10 within the propeptide eliminate γ-carboxylation.[42] Analogous studies of prothrombin have demonstrated the importance of amino acids at residues −18, −17, −15, and −10 in the propeptide of prothrombin. Deletion mutants of proprotein C lacking residues in the −17 to −12 portion of the propeptide also are associated with impaired γ-carboxylation.[213] These results demonstrate that the propeptide contains a recognition element, termed the *γ-carboxylation recognition site,* which designates the vitamin K–dependent proteins for γ-carboxylation. This propeptide is required for carboxylation. Furthermore, expression of a cDNA construct in which the propeptide is adjacent to a glutamic acid-rich region of thrombin leads to carboxylation of these glutamic acid residues.[43] Thus, the propeptide is sufficient to support carboxylation, and no other components within the substrate are required, except to improve efficiency of carboxylation.

Peptides containing a complete propeptide sequence and carboxylatable glutamic acid residues are efficiently carboxylated, with a K_m of approximately 3 μM.[214,215] In contrast, peptides without the γ-carboxylation recognition site or with a truncated site are poor substrates for the carboxylase. Glutamic acid, but not aspartic acid, is a substrate for the carboxylase. Based on the predicted structure of the propeptide of factor X, an 18-residue peptide stimulates the carboxylation of the pentapeptide FLEEL (Phe-Leu-Glu-Glu-Leu) by the partially purified carboxylase by approximately eightfold.[216]

The propeptide of prothrombin contains the carboxylation recognition site on its N-terminus and the propeptide cleavage site at the C-terminus. This peptide incorporates a 10-residue amphipathic α helix, from residues −3 to −13.[217] This helix serves as an extension to expose the carboxylation recognition site (Fig. 118–10). In contrast to factor IX, profactor IX cannot be activated to its enzymatically active form and does not bind to acidic membranes even though it is fully carboxylated.[218] The propeptide plays three roles in the synthesis of the vitamin K–dependent proteins: (a) via the γ-carboxylation recognition site, the propeptide signals for carboxylation of adjacent glutamic acid residues; (b) the propeptide inhibits premature zymogen activation and membrane binding during intracellular processing; and (c) the propeptide activates the vitamin K epoxidase activity of the carboxylase.[219]

The propeptide contains a sequence adjacent to the sessile bond that is characteristic of many proproteins and prohormones: Arg-X-Arg/Lys-Arg at residues −4 to −1, where propeptide cleavage occurs between −1 and +1. The propeptidase enzyme responsible for cleavage probably is PACE/furin,[220] a constitutively expressed protease located in the trans-Golgi region that cleaves substrates with adjacent basic amino acid residues. Site-specific mutagenesis of profactor IX has emphasized the importance of Arg−1, the lack of importance of the side chain of residue −3, and the effect of mutation of residue −2 on the efficiency of cleavage.[221]

During synthesis of vitamin K–dependent proteins, the signal peptide contains a recognition element that directs the partially syn-

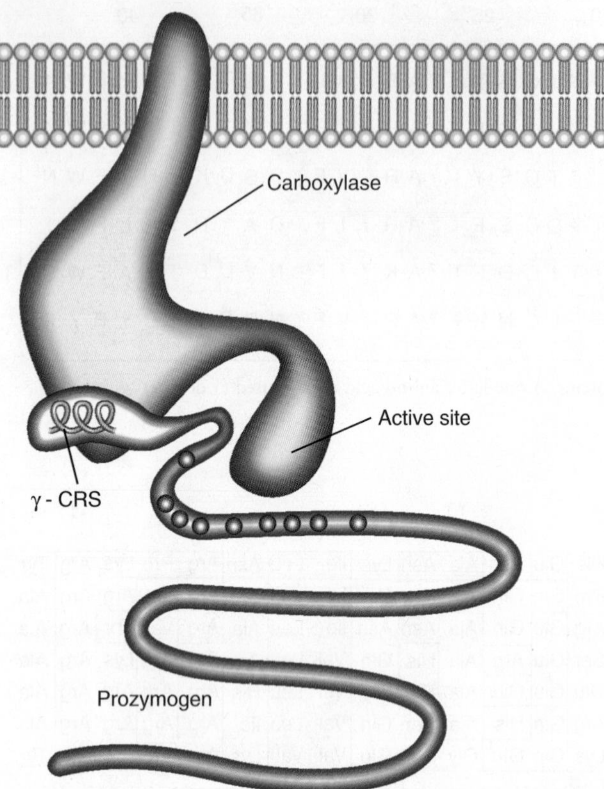

Figure 118–10 Vitamin K–dependent carboxylase. The precursors of the vitamin K–dependent blood clotting proteins, which contain the γ-carboxylation recognition site (γCRS) within the propeptide, bind to carboxylase through this recognition site. Glutamic acids are converted to γ-carboxyglutamic acids by carboxylase in the presence of vitamin K, oxygen, and carbon dioxide. *(Modified from Furie B, Furie BC: The molecular basis of blood coagulation. Cell 53:505, 1988.)*

thesized protein to the endoplasmic reticulum (Fig. 118–11). With cleavage of the signal peptide, the carboxylation recognition site on the propeptide is expressed. The vitamin K–dependent carboxylase is anchored to this region and modifies all the glutamic acids within a given proximity to the recognition site. After carboxylation, the protein is transported to the Golgi apparatus, where the propeptide undergoes cleavage. Final processing of the protein is completed in the Golgi compartment.

Posttranslational β-Hydroxylation

An unusual amino acid, *erythro*-β-hydroxyaspartic acid, is located in the NH_2-terminal EGF domains of protein C[222] and factors IX, X, and VII. *Erythro*-β-hydroxyasparagine also has been identified in protein S.[223] These amino acids are formed by posttranslational hydroxylation of aspartic acid and asparagine. Their function remains unknown, although they may be involved in defining the metal-binding properties of these proteins.

Unlike posttranslational γ-carboxylation, β-hydroxylation of factor IX is not directed by the propeptide, nor does this process require vitamin K or concomitant γ-carboxylation. β-Hydroxylation occurs in domains homologous to the EGF precursor in certain vitamin K–dependent proteins,[223] as well as in proteins outside this family, including the complement proteins Clr and Cls, thrombomodulin, uromodulin, and the low-density lipoprotein recepto.[223–227] A consensus sequence encompassing the β-hydroxylated aspartic acid and asparagine residues within a number of EGF domains has been noted by Stenflo et al.[223]: Cys-X-Asp/Asn-X-X-X-X-Phe/Tyr-X-Cys-X-Cys.

EGF domains that lack the consensus sequence do not contain this posttranslational modification. The hydroxylation is catalyzed by aspartyl β-hydroxylase, an enzyme that requires 2-ketoglutarate and Fe^{2+}.[226] This reaction is blocked by agents that inhibit 2-ketoglutarate–dependent dioxygenases.[228]

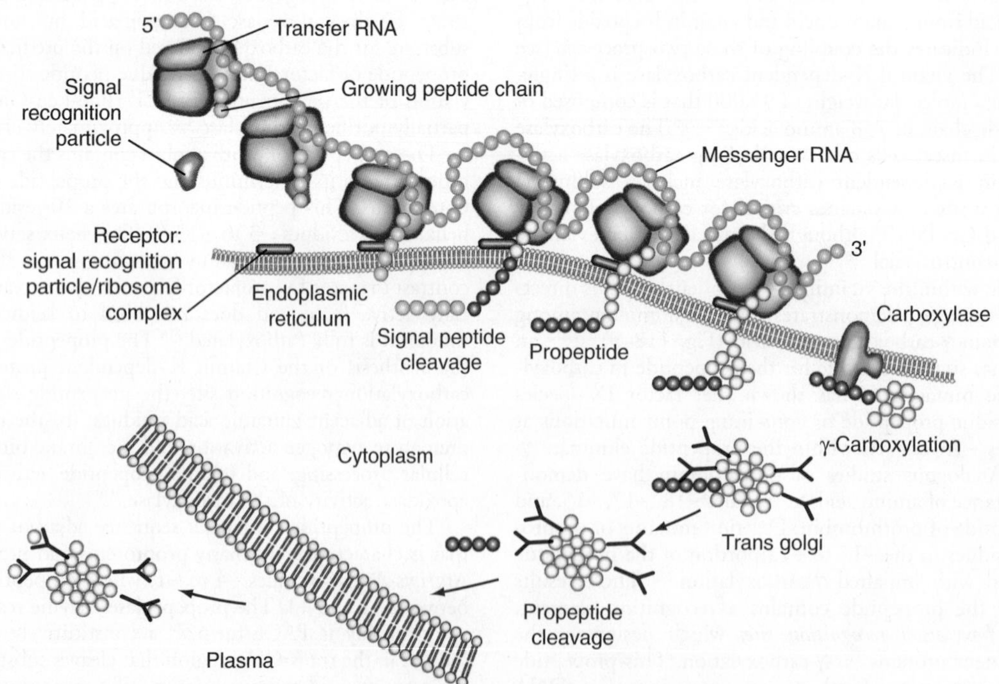

Figure 118–11 Biosynthesis of the vitamin K–dependent blood coagulation proteins. Signal recognition particle binds to the signal peptide, thus directing this complex to the endoplasmic reticulum. Signal peptide directs translocation to the luminal aspect of the endoplasmic reticulum. After signal peptide cleavage by signal peptidase, propeptide is expressed. This region, containing the γ-carboxylation recognition site, binds to the vitamin K–dependent carboxylase. Specific glutamic acids are converted to γ-carboxyglutamic acids by this enzyme. Propeptide is removed in the trans-Golgi region. *(Modified from Furie B, Furie BC: The molecular basis of blood coagulation. Cell 53:505, 1988.)*

Von Willebrand Factor Multimerization

vWF is synthesized as a single polypeptide chain containing a signal peptide, a large propolypeptide (M_r 80,000), and the mature vWF (M_r 225,000). During synthesis, the mature vWF forms a dimer, which multimerizes to the high-molecular-weight, biologically active forms critical for cellular adhesion. Synthesis of vWF takes place in endothelial cells and megakaryocytes. In endothelial cells, vWF is secreted via a constitutive pathway involving mainly dimeric forms. In addition, the regulated pathway involves storage of vWF in Weibel-Palade bodies, within which vWF undergoes multimerization and subsequently cleavage of the propolypeptide. Endothelial cells degranulate under specific stimuli, leading to secretion of vWF. The propolypeptide is required for multimerization[193,194] and is further required for directing vWF to the Weibel-Palade bodies.[229]

ACTIVATION OF BLOOD COAGULATION

Mechanism of Extrinsic Activation

Activation of blood clotting through the tissue factor pathway plays a dominant physiologic role in hemostasis. Tissue factor, a cellular receptor for factors VII and VIIa, is present on most cell surfaces. Expression of tissue factor activity is constitutive on most nonvascular cells and is inducible via de novo synthesis in cells within the blood or on the blood vessel wall. In addition, blood-borne tissue factor circulates in the blood at low concentration. There appear to be two distinct pathways of blood coagulation. In one pathway of hemostasis that follows tissue injury and laceration of blood vessels, nonvascular cells become exposed to blood, leading to contact of nonvascular cell tissue factor with flowing blood. Immediate formation of a complex of tissue factor on the cell surface with factor VIIa from the blood then follows. The formation of this complex initiates the tissue factor pathway, culminating in the generation of thrombin and the formation of a fibrin clot.

An alternate pathway of blood coagulation is P-selectin dependent.[11] This pathway is initiated by vessel wall injury but does not require exposure of flowing blood to tissue factor on nonvascular cells. Rather, tissue factor in the circulating blood, present at very low concentration and possibly inactive, accumulates in the developing thrombus.[12] This tissue factor is present on leukocyte microparticles, along with PSGL-1, and is concentrated on activated platelets within the developing thrombus through platelet P-selectin.[13] The developing thrombus, initiated by endothelial cell damage, contains platelets, tissue factor and fibrin.[1]

Activation of Factor VII

Both pathways involve initiation of fibrin formation via tissue factor. Tissue factor, at a critical concentration, triggers a series of biochemical events in the blood coagulation cascade.

$$\text{Factor VII} \xrightarrow{\text{FVIIa/TF}} \text{Factor VIIa}$$

Through its extracellular domain, tissue factor forms a catalytic complex with factor VIIa in the presence of Ca^{2+}.[29,179] Low amounts (10–100 pM) of factor VIIa are present in normal plasma.[6] With tissue factor as a cofactor, factor VIIa can autocatalyze the activation of factor VII to factor VIIa.[230–232] Deletion of the membrane-anchoring region of tissue factor abolishes autoactivation of factor VII but not cofactor function in the activation of factor X or factor IX.[233] The tissue factor/factor VIIa complex acts on factor IX and factor X, leading to the generation of factor IXa and factor Xa, respectively. Factor Xa is able to feed back to convert more factor VII to factor VIIa, thereby amplifying the initiation of clotting.[7] Activation of factor VII involves cleavage of the Arg152-Ile153 bond, leading to a form of factor VIIa composed of a light chain (M_r 20,000) and a heavy chain (M_r 30,000) linked by a disulfide bond (Fig. 118–12).[20,234,235] This reaction is greatly enhanced by the presence of tissue factor and phospholipid vesicles.[19,236,237] Activation of factor VII is associated with expression of the catalytic triad within the heavy chain, His41, Ser192, and Asn90, common to the active site of all serine proteases. Although the potential for factor Xa-mediated and factor VIIa-mediated amplification of this pathway is apparent, the nature of the protease that generates constitutive factor VIIa in plasma is unknown.

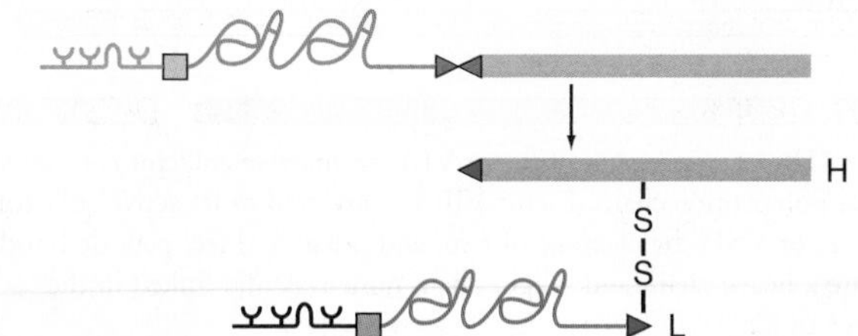

Figure 118–12 Factor VII activation. The zymogen factor VII is composed of a single polypeptide chain. Activation of factor VII to factor VIIa involves cleavage of the bond between Arg152 and Ile153 by factor Xa or factor VIIa. Light (L) chain and heavy (H) chains are linked by a disulfide bond.

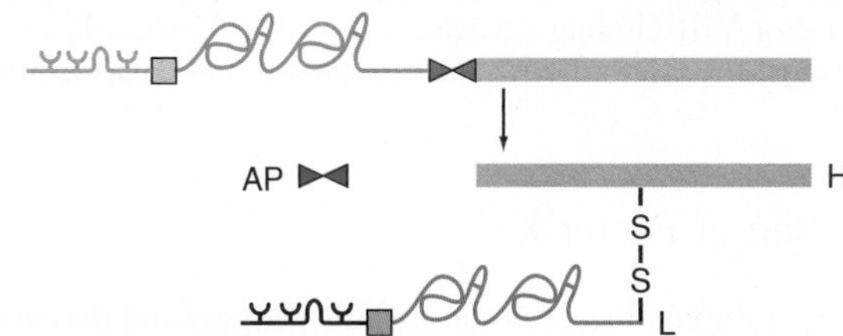

Figure 118–13 Factor IX activation. The zymogen factor IX is composed of a single polypeptide chain. Activation of factor IX to factor IXa involves cleavage of two peptide bonds. Factor IXa contains a light (L) chain and a heavy (H) chain linked by a disulfide bond. An activation peptide (AP) is released during the activation process.

Activation of Factor IX

Activation of factor IX proceeds via the tissue factor pathway in vivo. In vitro (e.g., in the clinical laboratory), the intrinsic pathway is activated via factor XIa:

$$\text{Factor IX} \xrightarrow{\text{TF/factor VIIa or factor XIa}} \text{Factor IXa}$$

Factor IX can be activated through the extrinsic pathway.[15] The factor VIIa/tissue factor complex activates both factor IX and factor X in reactions that require Ca^{2+}. Although the kinetics of factor IX activation by factor XIa and by factor VIIa/tissue factor differ, both enzymes cleave the same peptide bonds and generate the same structural form of factor IXa.

Activation of factor IX by factor XIa, in contrast to the activation of the other vitamin K–dependent blood clotting proteins or the activation of factor IX by factor VIIa tissue factor (which occur on membrane surfaces), takes place in the solution phase. Membrane surfaces, including those of artificial phospholipid vesicles or platelets, do not accelerate the generation of factor IXa. The reaction has an absolute requirement for Ca^{2+}.[238] Factor IX is activated by the cleavage of two internal peptide bonds: the Arg145–Ala146 bond and the Arg180–Val181 bond (Fig. 118–13).[239,240] A factor IXa light chain (M_r 18,000), from residues 1 to 145, and a factor IXa heavy chain (M_r 27,000), from residues 181 to 416, are generated by the proteolytic activation. These chains remain covalently attached through a single disulfide bond. An activation peptide, from residues 146 to 180, is cleaved from factor IX during activation.

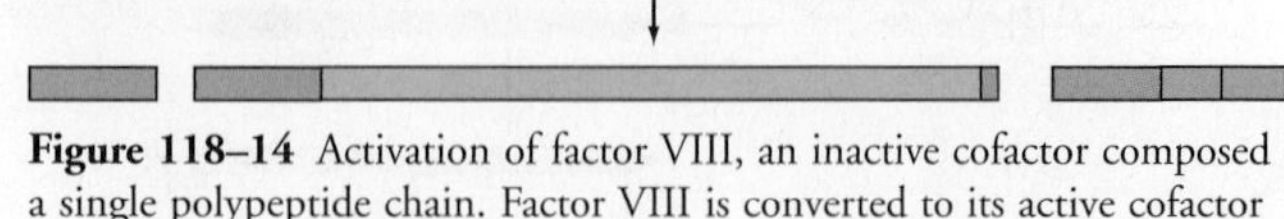

Figure 118–14 Activation of factor VIII, an inactive cofactor composed of a single polypeptide chain. Factor VIII is converted to its active cofactor form, factor VIIIa, by cleavage of two, and possibly three, peptide bonds to generate a heavy chain and a light chain noncovalently linked in the presence of Ca^{2+}.

Like factor IX, factor IXa binds to phospholipid vesicles in the presence of calcium ions and binds to calcium and other metal ions. Activation of factor IX to factor IXa leads to the expression of a factor VIII-binding site and active enzyme site with full coagulant activity. Cleavage of Arg180–Val181 is required for at least partial expression of the factor VIII-binding site; cleavage of Arg145–Ala146 in addition to Arg180–Val181 leads to full enzymatic and cofactor binding activity.

Activation of Factor X

Factor X, at the confluence of the intrinsic pathway and the extrinsic pathway, may be activated by the factor IXa/factor VIIIa complex (tenase complex) or by the factor VIIa/tissue factor complex.

$$\text{Factor X} \xrightarrow{\text{factor IXa/factor VIIIa or factor VIIa/TF}} \text{Factor Xa}$$

The tenase complex, composed of factor IXa and factor VIIIa, requires factor VIII in its active cofactor form (factor VIIIa). Factor VIII expresses either no or minimal cofactor activity but is converted to factor VIIIa by the cleavage of two or possibly three peptide bonds (Fig. 118–14).[241] Factor VIII, a heterodimer composed of a heavy chain that varies in molecular weight from 90,000 to 200,000 and a light chain with a molecular weight of 76,000, is a substrate for thrombin, an enzyme that cleaves at least four peptide bonds within factor VIII. Anion binding site I on thrombin binds to factor VIII.[242] Cleavage of peptide bonds at Arg372–373 and at Arg1686–1689 is required for factor VIII activation.[241] The resulting factor VIIIa contains polypeptide chains of molecular weights 50,000 (derived from the heavy chain), 43,000, and 73,000 (derived from the light chain; see Chapter 123).[243] Factors VIII and VIIIa bind tightly to phospholipid vesicles and to activated platelets.[30,37]

$$\text{factor VIII} \xrightarrow{\text{thrombin}} \text{factor VIIIa}$$

Factor IXa binds to factor VIIIa that is bound to phospholipid membranes and activated platelets. Formation of this enzyme complex is required for activation of factor X on a physiologically relevant time scale.[244] Binding of Na^+ to factor IXa in the tenase complex increases its biologic activity by approximately 12-fold.[245] Similarly, mutation of Glu13 to Ala in factor VIII enhances cofactor interactions with the tenase complex.[246] In the absence of direct structural data, modeling of the tenase complex has suggested multiple interactions between the domains of factor IXa and factor VIIIa.[247] The interface between the second EGF domain and the protease domain of factor IXa contributes to both factor VIII binding and factor X activation.[248]

Alternatively, factor VIIa in complex with tissue factor on cell surfaces can activate factor X on a physiologically relevant time scale. The formation of this complex requires Ca^{2+}.

Factor X, a zymogen with no coagulant activity, is converted to its active enzyme form, factor Xa, by cleavage of a single polypeptide bond between Arg51 and Ile52 in the heavy chain (Fig. 118–15). This cleavage is catalyzed either by the complex of factor IXa and factor VIIIa on membrane surfaces in the presence of Ca^{2+} or by the complex of factor VIIa and tissue factor on membrane surfaces in the presence of Ca^{2+}.[249,250] An activator without physiologic relevance, the coagulant protein of Russell viper venom (RVV) often is used for

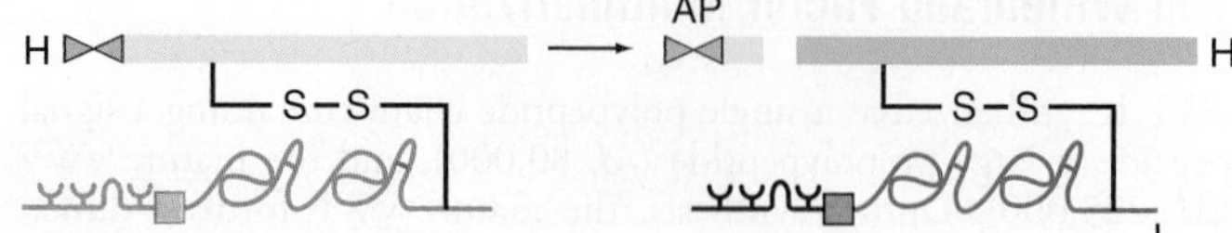

Figure 118–15 Factor X activation. Factor X is composed of two chains, a heavy (H) chain and a light (L) chain, linked by a disulfide bond. Activation of factor X to factor Xa requires cleavage of a single peptide bond on the heavy chain. AP, activation peptide.

clinical laboratory measurements in a test known as the Stypven or RVV time.[251] The activation peptide remains associated with factor Xa[252] but, with the exception of the C-terminal amino acids, does not contribute to the initial formation of a complex with tenase. Although zymogen activation results in a major functional change in the protein, only subtle structural changes in factor X are associated with the development of enzymatic activity.[253] Expression of enzymatic activity involves the catalytic triad common to all serine proteases—His 93, Asp138, and Ser233—in the heavy chain of bovine factor X.

Factor Xa is inhibited by specific plasma protease inhibitors, including antithrombin III and α_2 macroglobulin.[254] These inhibitors probably are scavengers in that they neutralize the potent coagulant activity of any factor Xa that flows past the site of tissue injury. The ternary structure of the antithrombin III/factor Xa/heparin complex reveals that heparin induces an allosteric transition in antithrombin III, thus facilitating the interaction of antithrombin III with the protease domain and active site of factor Xa.[255]

The tissue factor pathway is regulated by a protease inhibitor, tissue factor pathway inhibitor (TFPI).[256–259] The gene for this protein is located on chromosome 2 and includes nine exons.[260,261] This inhibitor, with a molecular weight of 34,000, contains three tandem Kunitz-type protease inhibitor domains.[262] TFPI binds factor Xa directly and inhibits factor VIIa/tissue factor activity in a reaction that appears to involve the formation of a factor Xa/TFPI/factor VIIa/tissue factor complex.[263] Generation of this complex downregulates activity of the tissue factor pathway.

Generation of Thrombin: Assembly of the Prothrombinase Complex

Conversion of prothrombin to thrombin is mediated by the enzyme action of factor Xa and the cofactor factor Va in a complex formed on membrane surfaces. The factor Xa/factor Va complex that is formed on membranes in the presence of Ca^{2+} is known as the "prothrombinase" complex because it serves to act on prothrombin as substrate (Fig. 118–16).

$$\text{prothrombin} \xrightarrow{\text{factor Xa/factor Va}} \text{thrombin}$$

The factor Xa/factor Va/membrane complex has many structural and functional parallels with the factor IXa/factor VIIIa/membrane complex. Factors V and Va are extrinsic membrane-binding proteins. Interaction of these factor V forms with membranes is independent of Ca^{2+} or other metal ions. Factor V binds with high affinity to phospholipid vesicles rich in phosphatidylserine,[264–267] to activated platelets,[138,268] and to microparticles derived from activated platelets.[38,269]

Factor V circulates in the blood as an inactive cofactor or as a cofactor with low intrinsic activity. It is converted to its active cofactor form, factor Va, by the hydrolysis of three peptide bonds, Arg709–Ser710, Arg1018–Thr1019, and Arg1545–Ser1546, by thrombin or factor Xa (Fig. 118–17).[270–273] Anion binding site I on thrombin binds to factor V.[242] These cleavages generate a heavy chain

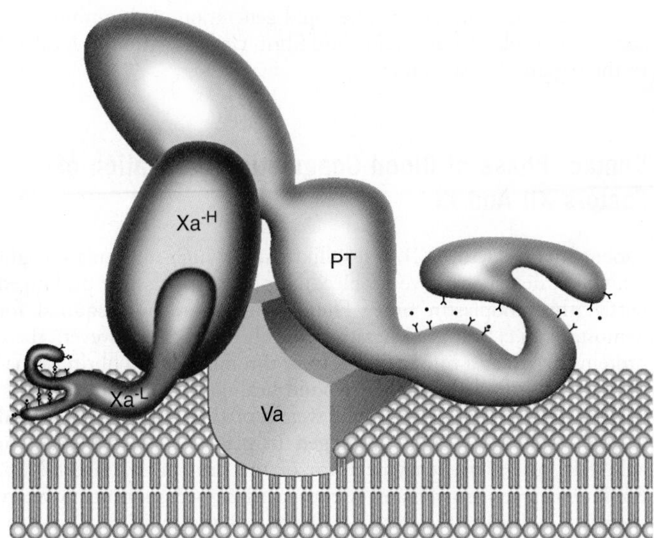

Figure 118–16 Model for the macromolecular complex associated with zymogen activation. A central feature of the proteins involved in blood coagulation is their assembly on membrane surfaces. Interaction of Ca^{2+} with the γ-carboxyglutamic acids on vitamin K–dependent proteins leads to the exposure of a membrane-binding site on these proteins. Assembly of these proteins on membranes in a geometry defined by the protein cofactor facilitates enzyme–substrate interaction. The protein cofactor likely plays an important regulatory role in this complex. Factor Xa, enzyme (L, light chain; H, heavy chain); prothrombin (PT), substrate; factor Va, cofactor; l, Ca^{2+}; U, γ-carboxyglutamic acid; lipid-binding sites in black. *(Modified from Furie B, Furie BC: The molecular basis of blood coagulation. Cell 53:505, 1988.)*

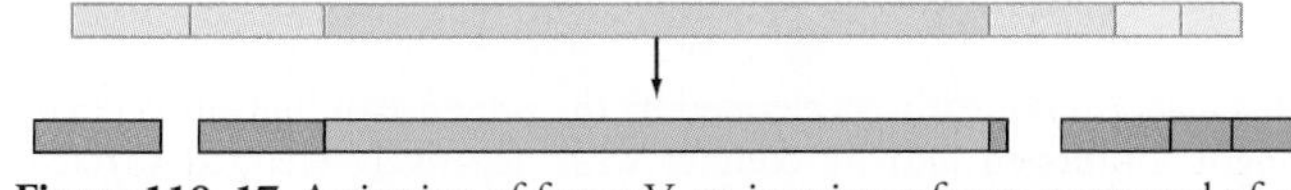

Figure 118–17 Activation of factor V, an inactive cofactor composed of a single polypeptide chain. Factor V is converted to its active cofactor form, factor Va, by the cleavage of two or possibly three peptide bonds to generate a heavy chain and a light chain noncovalently linked in the presence of calcium ions.

(M_r 110,000) and a light chain (M_r 78,000) that are linked noncovalently in the presence of Ca^{2+}. A three-dimensional computational structural model of factor Va has been described.[274]

$$\text{factor V} \xrightarrow{\text{thrombin}} \text{factor Va}$$

In the presence of Ca^{2+}, a complex of factors Xa and Va forms on phospholipid vesicles. Formation of the prothrombinase complex involves three steps: (a) binding of factor Va to membrane surfaces, (b) binding of factor Xa to membrane surfaces, and (c) interaction of membrane-bound factors Va and Xa.[32] Although factor Xa can activate prothrombin directly in the absence of Ca^{2+}, factor Va, and membrane surfaces, the rate of activation is very slow and irrelevant on a physiologic time scale. IN contrast, the rate of prothrombin activation by the prothrombinase complex is approximately 300,000 times as high as the rate of activation by factor Xa.[32]

Although phospholipid vesicles serve as a model system for studying prothrombinase complex formation on platelets, the details of formation of the complex on the two surfaces may vary. Factor Va binds to specific sites on the platelet surface, defining the formation of the prothrombinase complex. Factor Va appears to be the factor Xa receptor on platelets.[275,276] Factor Xa binds to platelets, leading to the expression of prothrombinase activity.[277] Furthermore, factor Va binds to endothelial cells, monocytes, and lymphocytes, facilitating assembly of the prothrombinase complex.[278–281]

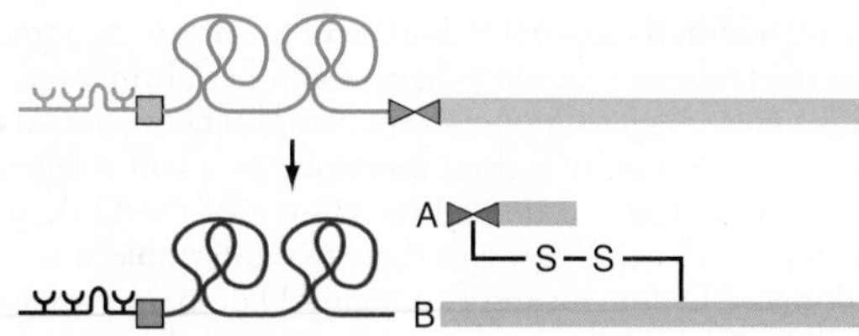

Figure 118–18 Activation of prothrombin, which is composed of a single polypeptide chain. Its activation to thrombin involves cleavage of two or possibly three peptide bonds. Thrombin, the active enzyme, is composed of two chains, the A chain and the B chain, linked by a disulfide bond.

Prothrombin is converted to thrombin by the prothrombinase complex. Although multiple fragments can be generated by the action of prothrombinase on prothrombin, two or possibly three peptide bonds are necessarily cleaved in generating thrombin, a two-chain enzyme with a molecular weight of 38,000 (Fig. 118–18).[282–285] Cleavage of the Arg271–Thr272 or Arg286–Thr287 bond in the presence of plasma proteins yields fragment 1 ≅ 2 (M_r 43,000) or fragment 1 ≅ 2 ≅ 3 (M_r 45,000), respectively, both derived from the NH_2-terminus of human prothrombin.[286,287] With these cleavages, prethrombin 2 (M_r 38,000) or prethrombin 2 with a 13-residue NH_2-terminal extension is generated. Cleavage of the Arg322–IIe323 bond in prothrombin generates meizothrombin and in prethrombin 2 generates both the A chain (M_r 5,000) and the B chain (M_r 32,000) of thrombin, linked by a single disulfide bond. A small peptide, Asp-Tyr-Asp-Tyr-Gln, based on a sequence in the C-terminus of the factor Va heavy chain, inhibits the pathway that generates meizothrombin.[288,289] In contrast to thrombin, meizothrombin has enzymatic activity toward small substrates but does not convert fibrinogen to fibrin.[290] Meizothrombin can be converted to thrombin in the presence of factor Va. The charge relay system, common to the trypsin-like serine proteases, is located at His365, Asp419, and Ser527.

Effector cell protease receptor 1, a receptor for factor X, has a molecular weight of 65,000. It is widely distributed on cells and recognizes a portion of the EGF domain exposed upon zymogen activation of factor X.[291] This receptor is exposed on the platelet surface only upon platelet activation and participates in prothrombinase assembly on cell surfaces.[292]

Thrombin is inhibited by antithrombin III. This inhibition is greatly accelerated by heparin (see Chapter 111).

Conversion of Fibrinogen to Fibrin

$$\text{fibrinogen} \xrightarrow{\text{thrombin}} \text{fibrin} + \text{fibrinopeptide A} + \text{fibrinopeptide B}$$

Fibrinogen circulates as a plasma protein in a biologically inactive form. It is converted to fibrin as a consequence of the cleavage of peptide bonds in both the Aα and the Bβ chain by the enzyme thrombin (Fig. 118–19). Thrombin is specific for the Arg16–Gly17 bond in the Aα chain. Cleavage of this bond releases fibrinopeptide A, a peptide containing 16 amino acid residues from the Aα chain, thereby generating a new amino terminus on the α chain. Thrombin also is specific for the Arg14–Gly15 bond in the Bβ chain, cleavage of which releases fibrinopeptide B, a 14-amino acid peptide, from the Bβ chain, thereby generating a new amino terminus on the β chain. Thus, the covalent structures of fibrinogen and fibrin are identical except for the removal of two fibrinopeptide A and two fibrinopeptide B fragments from fibrinogen.

Upon generation, the fibrin monomer homopolymerizes to form long strands known as *protofibrils* (Fig. 118–20). Both fibrinogen and fibrin are characterized by a trinodal domain structure, with a linear D-E-D domain organization. After removal of the fibrinopeptides, binding sites within the central E domain of the fibrin monomer bind to sites on the D domain of the γ chain of another fibrin monomer.[170] This yields a half-staggered noncovalent complex between two monomeric units.[293] Addition of a third monomer in a half-staggered orientation facilitates the end-on-end interaction of the D domains of two adjacent monomers. Through these two intermolecular interactions, E domain–D domain and D domain–D domain, two-stranded protofibrils are formed. Only after the protofibrils have become sufficiently long is their lateral association—a necessary event in the formation of thick fibrin fibrils—observed.

The polymerized form of fibrin contains fibrin monomers that are noncovalently bound to each other. Thus, the fibrin strands are unstable. Through the action of factor XIIIa, the α and γ chains of adjacent fibrin strands are covalently cross-linked to yield a form of fibrin that is not easily disrupted. Factor XIIIa, a transglutaminase, catalyzes the condensation of lysine residues on one chain and glutamic acid residues on a second chain.[294] Factor XIII, an inactive precursor, is a plasma protein that is converted to its active form, factor XIIIa, by the proteolytic action of thrombin.

Although many details of blood coagulation remain unclear, there has been considerable definition of the structure and function of participating components and of the special role that cell membranes play in complex formation. The rapid generation of thrombin, with concomitant platelet activation and fibrin clot formation, is localized to the region of tissue injury.

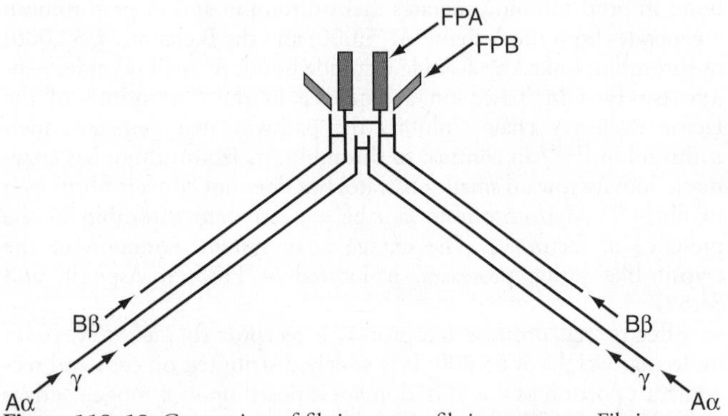

Figure 118–19 Conversion of fibrinogen to fibrin monomer. Fibrinogen is composed of three chains, Aα, Bβ, and γ, arranged as a heterodimer, $A\alpha_2B\beta_2\gamma_2$. The conversion of fibrinogen to fibrin, $\alpha_2\beta_2\gamma_2$, requires cleavage of peptide bonds to release fibrinopeptide A and fibrinopeptide B.

Contact Phase of Blood Coagulation: Activation of Factors XII And XI

Patients with factor XII, prekallikrein, or high-molecular-weight kininogen deficiency have no bleeding phenotype despite prolonged partial thromboplastin time. These proteins are not required for hemostasis (i.e., rapid generation of fibrin clot). However, these proteins may play a role in fibrinolysis, thrombosis, and fibrin formation during inflammation and wound healing.

Prekallikrein, with a molecular weight of 100,000, is partly bound to high-molecular-weight kininogen in plasma. It is converted to kallikrein, the active enzyme form of the protein, by factor XIIa. Kallikrein, a serine protease, is composed of two subunits, a heavy chain of molecular weight 52,000 and a light chain of molecular weight approximately 35,000. The active site resides on the light chain, whereas the heavy chain binds to high-molecular-weight kininogen.[295] In plasma, kallikrein is inactivated by α_2 macroglobulin and by C1 inhibitor.[296,297]

High-molecular-weight kininogen, with a molecular weight of 120,000, is a plasma protein that participates in contact activation. High-molecular-weight kininogen accelerates the rate of surface-dependent activation of factor XII[298] and the rate of prekallikrein activation by activation products derived from factor XIIa.[299]

Factor XII, a zymogen of molecular weight 80,000, is composed of 596 amino acids in its circulating form.[58,65] It is activated to factor XIIa by plasma kallikrein (Fig. 118–21, *A*).[300–302]

$$\text{factor XII} \rightarrow \text{factor XIIa}$$

This reaction is greatly accelerated by the presence of high-molecular-weight kininogen and by contact with negatively charged surfaces such as glass and collagen. Activation of factor XII to generate factor XIIa involves cleavage of the peptide bond between Arg353 and Val354. A heavy chain (M_r 50,000) composed of 353 amino acid residues binds to negatively charged surfaces and is derived from the NH_2-terminus of factor XII. This chain contains the EGF domains, the kringle domain, and the fibronectin type I and type II domains. A light chain (M_r 30,000) composed of 243 amino acid residues

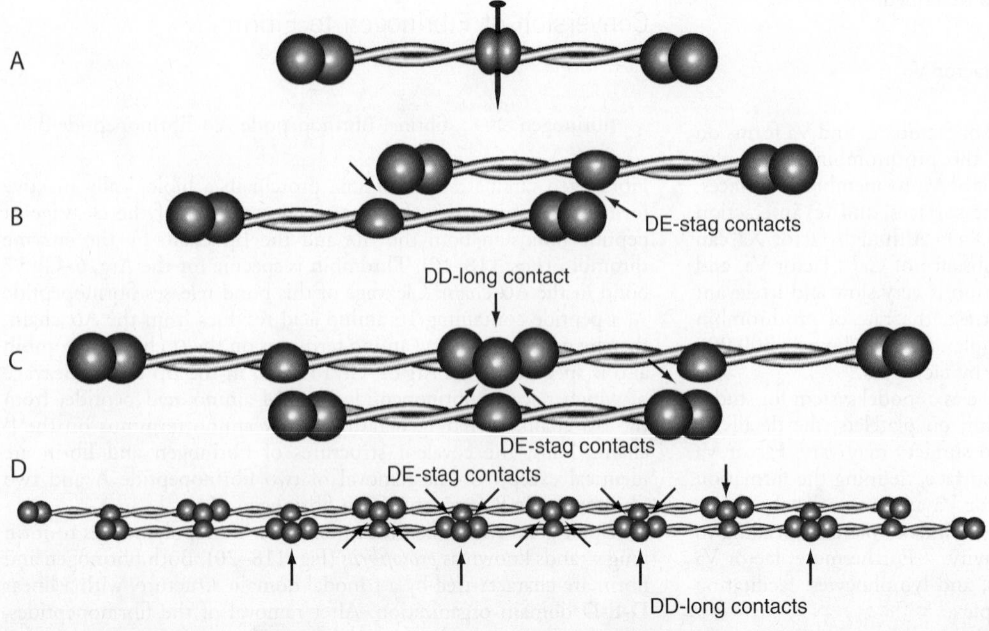

Figure 118–20 Formation of fibrin strands. **A,** Fibrin forms a staggered dimer **(B)**. **C,** Addition of another fibrin monomer end on end yields a trimer. **D,** Continued addition of fibrin monomer generates the fibrin strands.

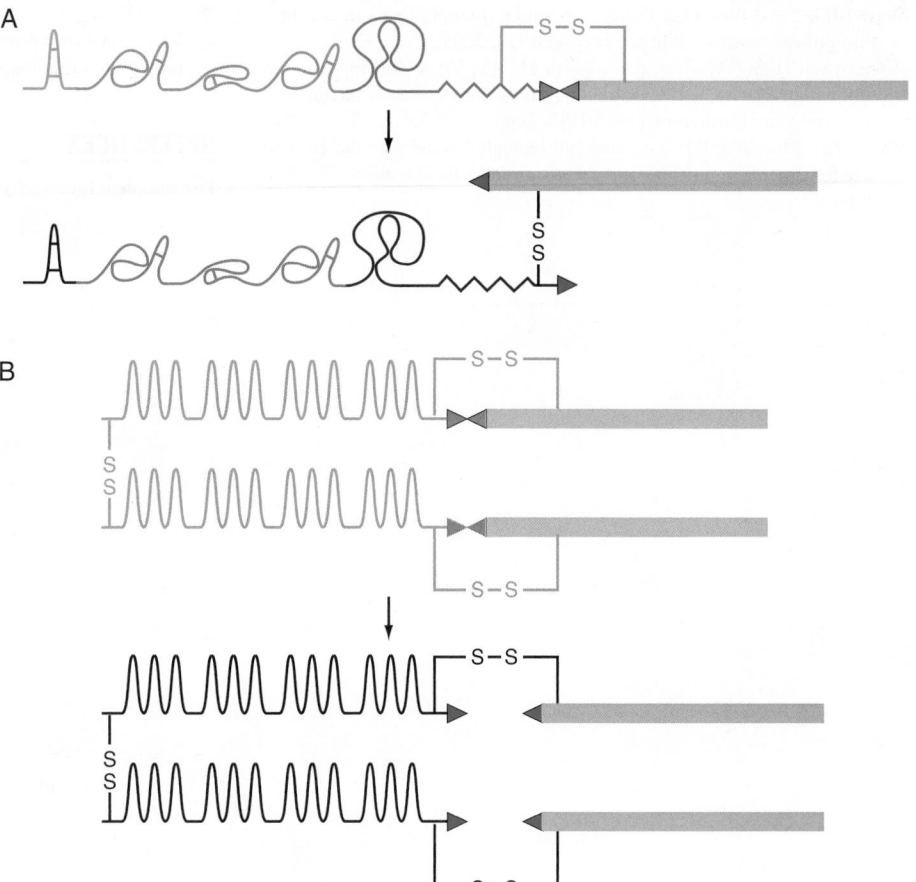

Figure 118–21 Contact phase of blood coagulation. **A,** Factor XII, a zymogen composed of a single polypeptide chain, is converted to its active form, factor XIIa, by cleavage of a single peptide bond. Kallikrein catalyzes this reaction, and the rate of the reaction is greatly accelerated by high-molecular-weight kininogen and by contact with negatively charged surfaces. The light chain of factor XIIa contains the enzyme-active site. **B,** Factor XI, composed of a homodimer formed by two identical subunits, is converted to factor XIa by the enzyme factor XIIa. Each subunit is cleaved to yield a heavy chain and a light chain; the latter contains the enzyme-active site.

contains the catalytic domain, which is common to serine proteases. The catalytic triad includes His393, Asp442, and Ser544. The light chains and heavy chain are linked by disulfide bonds. Factor XIIa functions to convert factor XI to its activated form, factor XIa, and to convert prekallikrein to kallikrein (see Fig. 118–21B).

$$\text{factor XI} \xrightarrow{\text{factor XIIa}} \text{factor XIa}$$

Factor XI is composed of two identical polypeptide chains, each of molecular weight 80,000, connected by a disulfide bond. Factor XI is converted to its enzymatic form, factor XIa, by proteolytic cleavage of the Arg369–Ile370 bond in each chain (see Fig. 118–21, *B).* The heavy chain (M_r 50,000), derived from the amino terminus, and the light chain (M_r 30,000) remain attached through a disulfide bond. Data suggest that thrombin is the physiologically relevant activator of factor XI. The catalytic domain of factor XIa resides on the light chain. The catalytic triad common to all serine proteases includes His44, Asp93, and Ser188.

Factors XI and XIa bind to platelets[303,304] but not to endothelial cells.[305] Whether factor XI–platelet interaction has a physiologic role and whether factor XIa on platelets activates factor IX in the solid phase are uncertain.[306]

SUGGESTED READINGS

Ansong C, Fay PJ: Factor VIII A3 domain residues 1954–1961 represent an A1 domain-interactive site. Biochemistry 44:8850, 2005.

Autin L, Miteva MA, Lee WH, Mertens K, Radtke KP, Villoutreix BO: Molecular models of the procoagulant factor VIIIa-factor IXa complex. J Thromb Haemost 3:2044, 2005.

Bukys MA, Kim PY, Nesheim ME, Kalafatis M: A control switch for prothrombinase: Characterization of a hirudin-like pentapeptide from the COOH-terminus of factor Va heavy chain that regulates the rate and pathway for prothrombin activation. J Biol Chem 281:39194, 2006.

Bukys MA, Orban T, Kim PY, Beck DO, Nesheim ME, Kalafatis M: The structural integrity of anion binding exosite I of thrombin is required and sufficient for timely cleavage and activation of factor V and factor VIII. J Biol Chem 281:18569, 2006.

Chen VM, Ahamed J, Versteeg HH, Berndt MC, Ruf W Hogg PJ: Evidence for activation of tissue factor by an allosteric disulfide bond. Biochemistry 45:12020, 2006.

Fribourg C, Meijer AB, Mertens K: The interface between the EGF2 domain and the protease domain in blood coagulation factor IX contributes to factor VIII binding and factor X activation. Biochemistry 45:10777, 2006.

Johnson DJ, Li W, Adams TE, Huntington JA: Antithrombin-S195A factor Xa-heparin structure reveals the allosteric mechanism of antithrombin activation. EMBO J 25:2029, 2006.

Kastrup CJ, Runyon MK, Shen F, Ismagilov RF: Modular chemical mechanism predicts spatiotemporal dynamics of initiation in the complex network of hemostasis. Proc Natl Acad Sci U S A 103:15747, 2006.

Majumder R, Weinreb G, Lentz BR: Efficient thrombin generation requires molecular phosphatidylserine, not a membrane surface. Biochemistry 44:16998, 2005.

Orban T, Kalafatis M, Gogonea V: Completed three-dimensional model of human coagulation factor va. Molecular dynamics simulations and structural analyses. Biochemistry 44:13082, 2005.

Papagrigoriou E, McEwan PA, Walsh PN, Emsley J: Crystal structure of the factor XI zymogen reveals a pathway for transactivation. Nat Struct Mol Biol 13:557, 2006.

Renne T, Pozgajova M, Gruner S, et al: Defective thrombus formation in mice lacking coagulation factor XII. J Exp Med 202:271, 2005.

Schmidt AE, Stewart JE, Mathur A, Krishnaswamy S, Bajaj SP: Na^+ site in blood coagulation factor IXa: Effect on catalysis and factor VIIIa binding. J Mol Biol 350:78, 2005.

Stone MD, Nelsestuen GL: Efficacy of soluble phospholipids in the prothrombinase reaction. Biochemistry 44:4037, 2005.

Wakabayashi H, Su YC, Ahmad SS, Walsh PN, Fay PJ: A Glu113Ala mutation within a factor VIII Ca^{2+}-binding site enhances cofactor interactions in factor Xase. Biochemistry 44:10298, 2005.

Waters EK, Morrissey JH: Restoring full biological activity to the isolated ectodomain of an integral membrane protein. Biochemistry 45:3769, 2006.

Waters EK, Yegneswaran S, Morrissey JH: Raising the active site of factor VIIa above the membrane surface reduces its procoagulant activity but not factor VII autoactivation. J Biol Chem 281:26062, 2006.

REFERENCES

For complete list of references log onto www.expertconsult.com

CHAPTER 119

MOLECULAR AND CELLULAR BASIS OF FIBRINOLYSIS

H. Roger Lijnen and Désiré Collen

OVERVIEW OF THE FIBRINOLYTIC SYSTEM

The fibrinolytic system in mammalian blood plays an important role in the dissolution of blood clots and in the maintenance of a patent vascular system. The fibrinolytic system (Fig. 119–1) contains an inactive proenzyme, plasminogen, which can be converted to the active enzyme, plasmin, which degrades fibrin into soluble fibrin degradation products. Two immunologically distinct physiologic plasminogen activators have been identified in blood: tissue plasminogen activator (tPA) and urokinase plasminogen activator (uPA). Inhibition of the fibrinolytic system may occur at the level of the plasminogen activators, by specific plasminogen activator inhibitors (plasminogen activator inhibitor 1 [PAI-1] and plasminogen activator inhibitor 2 [PAI-2]), or at the level of plasmin, mainly by α_2 antiplasmin. Some physicochemical properties of the main components of the fibrinolytic system and their gene organization are summarized in Tables 119–1 and 119–2. tPA-mediated plasminogen activation is primarily involved in the dissolution of fibrin in the circulation,[1] whereas uPA binds to the specific cellular receptor for urokinase plasminogen activator (uPAR), resulting in enhanced activation of cell-bound plasminogen. The main role of uPA is induction of pericellular proteolysis during tissue remodeling and repair, macrophage function, ovulation, embryo implantation, and tumor invasion.[2]

Regulation and control of the fibrinolytic system is mediated by specific molecular interactions among its main components and by controlled synthesis and release of plasminogen activators and plasminogen activator inhibitors, primarily from endothelial cells. Disorders of the fibrinolytic system may result from impaired activation (i.e., thrombotic complications) or from excessive activation (i.e., bleeding tendency).

PROTEIN STRUCTURE OF THE MAIN COMPONENTS

The enzymes of the fibrinolytic system are serine proteases; their active site consists of a "catalytic triad" composed of the amino acids serine, aspartic acid, and histidine. This active site is located in the C-terminal serine protease domain, and the N-terminal regions contain one or more functional domains, such as the finger domain (homologous to the fingers in fibronectin), the epidermal growth factor-like domain, and kringle domains. Inhibitors of the fibrinolytic system are grouped into the serpin (serine proteinase inhibitor) superfamily. Serpins have in their C-terminal region a specific reactive site peptide bond that is cleaved by their target enzyme, resulting in release of a peptide from the inhibitor and formation of an inactive enzyme–inhibitor complex (see Table 119–1).

Human plasminogen is a 92-kd, single-chain glycoprotein consisting of 791 amino acids. It contains 24 disulfide bridges and five homologous kringles. All plasminogen activators convert plasminogen to plasmin by cleavage of a single Arg561-Val562 peptide bond. The two-chain plasmin molecule is composed of a heavy chain containing the five kringles (N-terminal part of plasminogen) and a light chain (C-terminal part) containing the catalytic triad, composed of His603, Asp646, and Ser741.[3] Native plasminogen has N-terminal glutamic acid ("Glu-plasminogen") but is easily converted by limited plasmic digestion to modified forms with N-terminal lysine, valine, or methionine, commonly designated "Lys-plasminogen." Plasminogen kringles contain lysine binding sites that mediate the specific binding of plasminogen to fibrin and the interaction of plasmin with α_2 antiplasmin. They play a crucial role in the regulation of fibrinolysis.[4]

tPA is a 70-kd serine protease, originally isolated as a single polypeptide chain of 527 amino acids.[5] However, native tPA contains an N-terminal extension of three amino acids (Gly-Ala-Arg-). tPA is converted by plasmin to a two-chain form by hydrolysis of the Arg275-Ile276 peptide bond. In contrast to the single-chain precursor form of most serine proteases, single-chain tPA is enzymatically active. The N-terminal region of tPA is composed of several domains with homologies to other proteins: a finger domain, including residues 4–50; an epidermal growth factor domain consisting of residues 50–87; and two kringles, including residues 87–176 and 176–262. The region constituted by residues 276–527 represents the serine protease part with the catalytic site, composed of His322, Asp371, and Ser478. These distinct domains in tPA are involved in several functions of the enzyme, including its binding to fibrin, fibrin-specific plasminogen activation, rapid clearance in vivo, and binding to endothelial cell receptors. Binding of tPA to fibrin is mediated by the finger and the second kringle domains.[6] The tPA molecule comprises three potential *N*-glycosylation sites at Asn117, Asn184, and Asn448.

Single-chain urokinase plasminogen activator (sc-uPA) is a 54-kd glycoprotein containing 411 amino acids.[7] On proteolytic cleavage of the Lys158-Ile159 peptide bond, the molecule is converted to the two-chain derivative two-chain urokinase plasminogen activator (tc-uPA). The catalytic triad is located in the C-terminal polypeptide chain and is composed of Asp255, His204, and Ser356. The N-terminal chain contains an epidermal growth factor domain (residues 5–49) and one kringle domain. A low-molecular-mass tc-uPA (33 kd) can be generated with plasmin by hydrolysis of the Lys135-Lys136 peptide bond after previous cleavage of the Lys158-Ile159 bond.

uPAR, the specific cell surface receptor for uPA, is a heterogeneously glycosylated protein of 50 to 60 kd, synthesized as a 313-amino-acid polypeptide, anchored to the plasma membrane by a glycosylphosphatidylinositol (GPI) moiety. The uPAR molecule is composed of three related structural domains. One of the domains, the N-terminal domain, is involved in binding uPA. It binds all forms of uPA containing an intact growth factor domain.[8]

α_2 Antiplasmin is a 70-kd, single-chain glycoprotein containing approximately 13% carbohydrate. The molecule consists of 464 amino acids and contains two disulfide bridges.[9] α_2 Antiplasmin is a serpin with reactive site peptide bond Arg376-Met377. Its concentration in human plasma is approximately 70 μg/mL (approximately 1 μM). α_2 Antiplasmin is synthesized primarily in a plasminogen-binding form that becomes partially converted in circulating blood to an inactive form that lacks a 26-residue peptide from the C-terminal end. The inhibitor is cross-linked to the fibrin α chain when blood is clotted in the presence of calcium ions and factor XIIIa; Gln14 is involved in this cross-linking.[10]

PAI-1 is a 52-kd, single-chain glycoprotein consisting of 379 amino acids. It is a serpin with reactive site peptide bond

Table 119–1 Properties of Main Components of the Fibrinolytic System

Component	M_r	Carbohydrate Content (%)	No. of Amino Acids	Catalytic Triad	Reactive Site	Plasma Concentration (μg/mL)
Plasminogen	92,000	2	791	—	—	200
Plasmin	85,000	2	±715	His603, Asp646, Ser741	—	—
tPA	68,000	7	530 (527)[a]	His322, Asp371, Ser478	—	0.005
uPA	54,000	7	411	His204, Asp255, Ser356	—	0.008
uPAR	55,000				—	—
	60,000	±35	313			—
α_2 Antiplasmin	70,000	13	464	Arg376–Met377	70	
PAI-1	52,000	ND	379	—	Arg346–Met347	0.05
PAI-2	47,000	ND	393	—	Arg358–Thr359	<0.005
TAFI	60,000	23	401		—	5

[a]The numbering of amino acid residues usually is based on the initially determined incorrect value.
ND, not determined; PAI-1, plasminogen activator inhibitor 1; PAI-2, plasminogen activator inhibitor 2; TAFI, thrombin activatable fibrinolysis inhibitor; tPA, tissue plasminogen activator; uPA, urokinase plasminogen activator; uPAR, urokinase plasminogen activator receptor.

Table 119–2 Gene Organization and Chromosome Location of Main Components of the Fibrinolytic System

Component	Symbol	Gene (kb)	mRNA (kb)	Exons	Chromosome
Plasminogen	*PLG*	52.5	2.9	19	6q26–q27
tPA	*PLAT*	32.7	2.7	14	8p12-p11
uPA	*PLAU*	6.4	2.4	11	10q24
uPAR	*PLAUR*	23	1.4	7	19q13.1–q13.2
α_2 Antiplasmin	*PLI*	16	2.2	10	17p13
PAI-1	*PLANH1*	12.2	2.4/3.2	9	7q21.3–q22
PAI-2	*PLANH2*	16.5	1.9	8	18q22.1
TAFI	*CPB*	48	1.8	11	13q14.11

PAI-1, plasminogen activator inhibitor 1; PAI-2, plasminogen activator inhibitor 2; TAFI, thrombin activatable fibrinolysis inhibitor; tPA, tissue plasminogen activator; uPA, urokinase plasminogen activator; uPAR, urokinase plasminogen activator receptor.

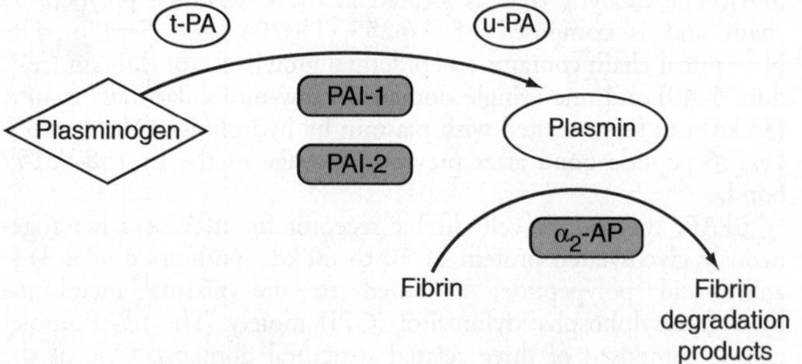

Figure 119–1 Schematic representation of the fibrinolytic system. α_2-AP, α_2 antiplasmin; PAI, plasminogen activator inhibitor; t-PA, tissue plasminogen activator; u-PA, urokinase plasminogen activator.

Arg346-Met347.[11] PAI-1 is stabilized by binding to S-protein or vitronectin.[12]

PAI-2 exists in two different forms with comparable kinetic properties: a 47-kd intracellular nonglycosylated form and a 60-kd secreted glycosylated form.[13] PAI-2 is a serpin[14] containing 393 amino acids with reactive site Arg358-Thr359. The function of intracellular PAI-2 is unclear because its main target enzyme (uPA) occurs extracellularly.

The 60-kd thrombin activatable fibrinolysis inhibitor (TAFI) is a carboxypeptidase B-like enzyme that is primarily produced by the liver and circulates at approximately 75 nM, but the normal variation is wide.[15] The circulating active enzyme has a very short half-life, and only a small fraction of the protein must be activated for normal function. Efficient activation is achieved by the thrombin–thrombomodulin complex.[16]

GENE STRUCTURE OF THE MAIN COMPONENTS

The plasminogen (*PLG*) gene is located on chromosome 6q26–q27, close to the gene for apolipoprotein(a).[17] The 19 exons are separated by 18 introns following the general GT-AG rule. A signal sequence is encoded by the first exon, an activation peptide and each of the five kringles are encoded by two exons, and the remaining six exons code for the intervening sequence and for the protease domain. Several common polymorphisms have been identified, of which the two most common variants observed in all races are *PLGA* and *PLGB*.[18]

The gene for tPA contains 14 exons and is located on chromosome 8, bands p12-p11.[19,20] The intron–exon organization suggests that assembly occurred according to the "exon shuffling" principle, whereby the distinct structural domains are encoded by a single exon or by adjacent exons. An Alu insertion/deletion polymorphism was identified; the homozygous insertion polymorphism is associated with enhanced tPA release under stress conditions.[21]

The uPA gene is located on chromosome 10q24. It contains 11 exons, and the intron–exon organization closely resembles that of the tPA gene.[22] However, some exons are missing in the uPA gene, which accounts for the absence of a finger domain and a second kringle.

The gene for uPAR is located on chromosome 19. It consists of seven exons and six introns, extending over 23 kb.[23,24] Constitutive expression of the uPAR gene is dependent on the −141 to −61 region.

The gene for α_2 antiplasmin is located on chromosome 17p13. It is 16 kb and contains 10 exons.[25] The N-terminal region of the protein, which comprises the fibrin cross-linking site, is encoded by exon IV, whereas both the reactive site and the plasminogen binding site in the C-terminal region are encoded by exon X.

The PAI-1 gene is located on chromosome 7, bands q21.3-q22. It is 12.2 kb and consists of nine exons.[26] As a result of alternative polyadenylation yielding an additional 3′ untranslated region, an mRNA species of 3.2 kb occurs in addition to a region of 2.4 kb. A single 4G/5G polymorphism in the promoter region appears to play an important role in regulation of PAI-1 gene expression, with the 4G allele associated with higher PAI-1 levels.[27]

The gene for PAI-2 is located on chromosome 18q22.1. It spans 16.5 kb and contains eight exons.[28] The gene structure of PAI-2 is different from that of PAI-1 but similar to that of the chicken ovalbumin gene.

The gene for TAFI is located on chromosome 13. It contains 11 exons and spans 48 kb of genomic DNA.[29] Several polymorphisms in the TAFI gene have been claimed to explain the wide normal range of concentrations, but no strong correlations with disease have been established.[30]

MECHANISM OF INHIBITION OF PLASMIN BY α_2 ANTIPLASMIN

α_2 Antiplasmin forms an inactive 1 : 1 stoichiometric complex with plasmin. Inhibition involves two consecutive reactions: a fast, second-order reaction producing a reversible inactive complex, followed by a slower first-order transition resulting in an irreversible inactive complex. The second-order rate constant of inhibition is very high ($2–4 \times 10^7\ M^{-1}\ s^{-1}$), but this high inhibition rate depends on the presence of free lysine binding sites and a free active site in the plasmin molecule and on the availability of a site complementary to the lysine binding site (plasminogen binding site) and of the reactive site peptide bond in the inhibitor. The half-life of plasmin molecules generated at the fibrin surface, which have their lysine binding sites and active site occupied, is two to three orders of magnitude longer than that of free plasmin.[31]

MECHANISM OF ACTION OF TISSUE PLASMINOGEN ACTIVATOR

In the Presence of Fibrin

tPA is a poor enzyme in the absence of fibrin, but the presence of fibrin strikingly enhances the activation rate of plasminogen.[32] Optimal stimulation is only obtained after early plasmin cleavage in the C-terminal Aα chain and the N-terminal Bβ chain of fibrin, yielding fragment X polymer.[33] Kinetic data support a mechanism in which fibrin provides a surface to which tPA and plasminogen adsorb in a sequential and ordered manner, yielding a cyclic ternary complex.[16] Formation of this complex results in enhanced affinity of tPA for plasminogen (K_m 0.16 μM compared with 65 μM without fibrin), yielding up to three orders of magnitude higher catalytic efficiency for plasminogen activation (Fig. 119–2). In agreement with this mechanism, the increase in fibrin stimulation after formation of fibrin X polymers is associated with enhanced binding of tPA and plasminogen, which is mediated in part by C-terminal lysine residues generated by plasmin cleavage. Interaction of these C-terminal lysines with lysine binding sites on tPA and plasminogen may allow improved alignment as well as allosteric changes of the tPA and plasminogen moieties, enhancing the rate of plasminogen activation.[33]

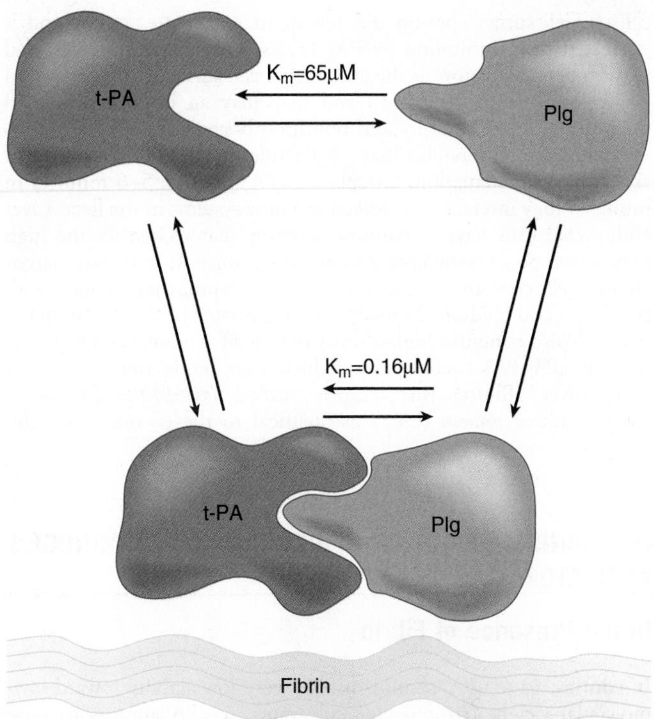

Figure 119–2 Schematic representation of molecular interactions regulating fibrin-specific activation of the fibrinolytic system by tissue plasminogen activator (t-PA). t-PA in circulating plasma in the absence of fibrin has low affinity for its substrate plasminogen (K_m = 65 μM), and no efficient plasminogen activation occurs. t-PA binds specifically to fibrin, and the bimolecular t-PA–fibrin complex has high affinity for plasminogen (K_m = 0.16 μM). Plasminogen binds to the binary t-PA–fibrin complex and is activated to plasmin at the fibrin surface. In loco generated plasmin is protected from rapid inactivation by α_2 antiplasmin. Plg, plasminogen.

Lipoprotein(a) competes with plasminogen for binding to fibrin, suggesting that elevated lipoprotein(a) levels impairs physiologic fibrinolysis.[34]

TAFI inhibits fibrinolysis by downregulating the cofactor functions of partially degraded fibrin. This effect most likely is mediated by removal of newly exposed C-terminal lysine residues that are generated on plasmin cleavage of fibrin.[35]

AT THE CELL SURFACE

A striking analogy exists between the role of fibrin and that of cell surfaces in plasminogen activation.[36] Many cell types bind plasminogen activators and plasminogen, resulting in enhanced plasminogen activation and protection of bound plasmin from inhibition by α_2 antiplasmin.

Most cells bind plasminogen by its lysine binding sites with high capacity but relatively low affinity. Gangliosides as well as a class of membrane proteins with C-terminal lysine residues such as α enolase play an important role in binding of plasminogen to cells.[37] The catalytic efficiency of tPA for activation of cell bound plasminogen is approximately 10-fold higher than in solution, possibly as a result of conversion of the plasminogen conformation to the more readily activatable "Lys-plasminogen-like" structure.[38] Vascular cells have the capacity to regulate pericellular fibrinolysis by modulating the expression of plasminogen receptors; enhanced receptor occupancy results in enhanced plasminogen activation by tPA.[39]

A 40-kd membrane protein (related to annexin II) was proposed as the functional tPA receptor on human umbilical vein endothelial cells.[40] Cell surface–bound tPA retains its enzymatic activity and is protected from inhibition by PAI-1. Assembly of plasminogen and plasminogen activators at the endothelial cell surface provides a focal point for plasmin generation and may play an important role in maintaining blood fluidity and nonthrombogenicity.

Cellular receptors also may play a role in the rapid clearance of tPA from the circulation. Circulating tPA (half-life 5–6 minutes in humans) may interact with several receptor systems in the liver. Liver endothelial cells have a mannose receptor that recognizes the high mannose-type carbohydrate antenna on kringle 1, and liver parenchymal cells contain a calcium-dependent receptor that interacts with the finger and epidermal growth factor domains of tPA.[41] Parenchymal cells also contain a high-affinity receptor for uptake and degradation of tPA–PAI-1 complexes, which also binds free tPA albeit with lower affinity; this receptor, called *low-density lipoprotein receptor-related protein* (LRP), is identical to the α_2-macroglobulin receptor.[42]

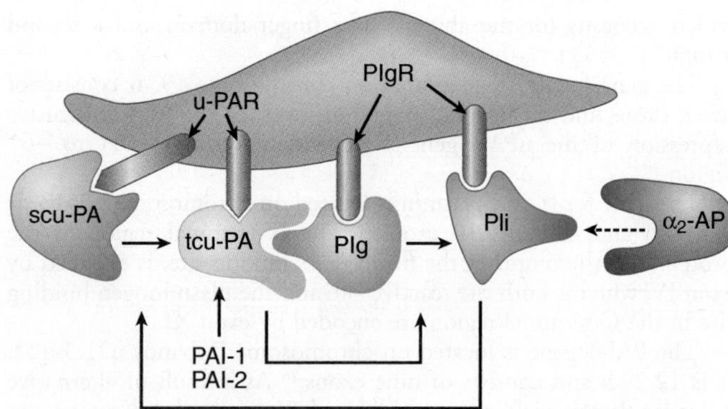

Figure 119–3 Plasminogen activation by urokinase plasminogen activator (u-PA) at the cell surface. The u-PA bound to its cellular receptor (u-PAR) efficiently converts plasminogen (Plg) bound to its cellular receptor (PlgR) to plasmin (Pli), which is protected from rapid inhibition by α_2 antiplasmin (α_2-AP). Plasmin converts u-PAR–bound single-chain urokinase plasminogen activator (scu-PA) to a two-chain derivative (tcu-PA), resulting in enhanced plasminogen activation. Receptor-bound tcu-PA, but not scu-PA, is inhibited by plasminogen activator inhibitor 1 (PAI-1) and plasminogen activator inhibitor 2 (PAI-2).

MECHANISM OF ACTION OF UROKINASE PLASMINOGEN ACTIVATOR

In the Presence of Fibrin

In contrast to tc-uPA, sc-uPA displays very low activity toward low-molecular-weight chromogenic substrates. sc-uPA appears to have some intrinsic plasminogen activating potential, which represents less than 0.5% of the catalytic efficiency of tc-uPA.[43] In plasma in the absence of fibrin, sc-uPA is stable and does not activate plasminogen; in the presence of a fibrin clot, sc-uPA but not tc-uPA induces fibrin-specific clot lysis.[44] sc-uPA is an inefficient activator of plasminogen bound to internal lysine residues on intact fibrin but has a higher activity toward plasminogen bound to newly generated C-terminal lysine residues on partially degraded fibrin. The fibrin specificity of sc-uPA does not require its conversion to tc-uPA but is mediated by enhanced binding of plasminogen to partially digested fibrin.[45]

AT THE CELL SURFACE

The binding of sc-uPA to uPAR on the cell surface was claimed to be crucial for its activity under physiologic conditions. Binding results in strongly enhanced plasmin generation due to effects on activation of plasminogen and on feedback activation of sc-uPA to tc-uPA by generated plasmin. Both effects critically depend on cellular binding of plasminogen. Cell-associated plasmin is protected from rapid inhibition by α_2 antiplasmin, which further favors the activation of receptor-bound sc-uPA. This system can be efficiently inhibited by PAI-1 and PAI-2 (Fig. 119–3). A model based on uPAR-dependent complex formation has been proposed, which would allow initiation of plasminogen activation by the low intrinsic activity of sc-uPA.[46] However, the observation that direct anchorage of uPA to the cell surface (using a GPI-anchored uPA mutant) leads to potentiation of plasmin generation equivalent to that observed in the presence of uPAR suggests that uPAR only functions to localize uPA at the cell surface.[47] In transgenic mice, an uPAR-independent function of uPA has been demonstrated in fibrin clearance and in arterial neointima formation.[48]

MECHANISMS OF INHIBITION OF PLASMINOGEN ACTIVATORS

Multiple mechanisms are involved in the rapid inhibition of tPA in human plasma. PAI-1 is a specific rapid-reacting inhibitor of tPA, which is present at low concentrations in normal plasma but at higher concentrations in many clinical conditions.[49] tPA is inhibited slowly by α_2 antiplasmin, α_1 antitrypsin, and C1 inhibitor. The main mechanism of removal of tPA from the blood, however, is clearance by the liver. In healthy volunteers and in patients with acute myocardial infarction, the initial half-life of tPA is 4 to 6 minutes.[50]

In human plasma, tc-uPA is also slowly inhibited by several proteinase inhibitors, including α_2 macroglobulin, α_1 antitrypsin, antithrombin III, α_2 antiplasmin, and plasminogen activator inhibitor 3 (PAI-3, which is identical to activated protein C inhibitor). More specific and rapid inhibition occurs by PAI-1 and PAI-2. In contrast to tc-uPA, sc-uPA is not inhibited by plasma protease inhibitors. The main mechanism of removal of uPA from the blood is hepatic clearance.[51] In patients with acute myocardial infarction, sc-uPA shows a biphasic disappearance rate with an initial half-life in plasma (after infusion) of approximately 4 minutes.[52]

PAI-1 reacts with single-chain and two-chain tPA and with tc-uPA but not with sc-uPA.[53] PAI-1 inhibits its target proteinases by formation of a 1 : 1 stoichiometric reversible complex, followed by covalent binding between the hydroxyl group of the active site serine residue of the proteinase and the carboxyl group of the P1 residue at the reactive center ("bait region") of the serpin. Highly positively charged regions in tPA (residues 296–304)[54] and in uPA (residues 179–184)[55] are involved in the rapid interaction. A molecular form of intact PAI-1 has been isolated that does not form stable complexes with tPA but is cleaved at the P1-P1′ peptide bond ("substrate PAI-1").[56] Examination of the crystal structure of the cleaved substrate variant using radiographs shows that it has a new β strand (s4A) formed by insertion of the N-terminal portion of the reactive site loop into β-sheet A subsequent to cleavage.[57] Inhibitory PAI-1 may convert not only to latent PAI-1, which can be reactivated, but also to substrate PAI-1, which may be irreversibly degraded by target proteases, including tPA, uPA, and thrombin.[56] PAI activity is very rapidly cleared from the circulation by the liver, with a reported half-life of 7 minutes in rabbit.[58]

PAI-2 inhibits tc-uPA approximately 10-fold slower than PAI-1. PAI-2 efficiently inhibits two-chain tPA and less efficiently inhibits single-chain tPA; it does not inhibit sc-uPA.[53]

MODULATION OF CELL-ASSOCIATED PROTEOLYTIC ACTIVITY BY MATRIX METALLOPROTEINASES

Several regulatory molecular interactions appear to exist between the fibrinolytic and matrix metalloproteinases (MMP) systems, but their exact (patho)physiologic role remains to be elucidated.

MMP-3 (stromelysin 1) specifically cleaves uPA, removing its uPAR binding sequence and resulting in downregulation of cell-associated uPA activity.[59] Several MMPs, including MMP-3, MMP-7, MMP-9, and MMP-12, cleave plasminogen, generating an angiostatin-like fragment containing the receptor-binding domains.[60–62] These MMPs may downregulate cellular fibrinolysis by reducing the amount of activatable cell-bound plasminogen.[63] MMP-3 and MMP-7 also degrade fibrinogen and cross-linked fibrin,[64,65] whereas the catalytic domain of MMP-11 cleaves fibrinogen but not fibrin.[66] The main physiologic inhibitors of the fibrinolytic system, α_2 antiplasmin and PAI-1, are also specifically cleaved by MMP-3, resulting in their neutralization.[67,68]

Inactivation of PAI-1 may be relevant in view of the findings that it plays a role in cell adhesion and migration, independent of its antiproteolytic activity, as a result of high-affinity binding to vitronectin that competes with uPAR-dependent or integrin-dependent binding of cells to the extracellular matrix. Cleavage of PAI-1 by MMP-3 may represent a mechanism decreasing the antiproteolytic activity of PAI-1 and impairing the competitive inhibitory properties on cell adhesion and migration by reducing the binding of cleaved PAI-1 to vitronectin.[68] Plasmin contributes to activation of pro-MMPs secreted by several cell types and thereby may play a role in multiple phenomena requiring extracellular proteolysis, such as atherosclerosis, restenosis after vascular injury, aneurysm formation, and myocardial ischemia.[69]

CONCLUSION

Fibrinolysis is regulated by specific molecular interactions between its main components. Activation of plasminogen by tPA is enhanced in the presence of fibrin or at the endothelial cell surface. uPA binds to the specific cellular receptor uPAR, resulting in enhanced activation of cell-bound plasminogen. Inhibition of fibrinolysis occurs at the level of the plasminogen activators or at the level of plasmin. Assembly of fibrinolytic components at the surface of many cell types by binding to specific receptors provides a mechanism for generation of localized cell-associated proteolytic activity. This may be modulated by interaction with other proteolytic systems, such as MMPs.

SUGGESTED READINGS

Aertgeerts K, De Bondt HL, De Ranter CJ, Declerck PJ: Mechanisms contributing to the conformational and functional flexibility of plasminogen activator inhibitor-1. Nat Struct Biol 2:891, 1995.

Collen D, Lijnen HR: Basic and clinical aspects of fibrinolysis and thrombolysis. Blood 78:3114, 1991.

Collen D: On the regulation and control of fibrinolysis. Thromb Haemost 43:77, 1980.

Declerck PJ, De Mol M, Alessi MC, et al: Purification and characterization of a plasminogen activator inhibitor-1-binding protein from human plasma. Identification as a multimeric form of S protein (vitronectin). J Biol Chem 263:15454, 1988.

Hoylaerts M, Rijken DC, Lijnen HR, Collen D: Kinetics of the activation of plasminogen by human tissue plasminogen activator. Role of fibrin. J Biol Chem 257:2912, 1982.

Madison EL, Goldsmith EJ, Gerard RD, et al: Serpin-resistant mutants of human tissue-type plasminogen activator. Nature 339:721, 1989.

Pannekoek H, Veerman H, Lambers H, et al: Endothelial plasminogen activator inhibitor (PAI): A new member of the serpin gene family. EMBO J 5:2539, 1986.

Pennica D, Holmes WE, Kohr WJ, et al: Cloning and expression of human tissue-type plasminogen activator cDNA in *E. coli.* Nature 301:214, 1983.

Plow EF, Felez J, Miles LA: Cellular regulation of fibrinolysis. Thromb Haemost 66:32, 1991.

Wiman B, Collen D: On the kinetics of the reaction between human antiplasmin and plasmin. Eur J Biochem 84:573, 1978.

REFERENCES

For complete list of references log onto www.expertconsult.com

CHAPTER 120

REGULATORY MECHANISMS IN HEMOSTASIS: NATURAL ANTICOAGULANTS

Björn Dahlbäck and Johan Stenflo

In the absence of an anticoagulant, blood drawn into a test tube clots completely. In the serum that forms, all enzymes participating in coagulation have been activated, and all fibrinogen has been converted to fibrin. In contrast, the coagulation that occurs in vivo after vascular injury is a precisely regulated process.[1–3] This process depends on a delicate balance between coagulation and anticoagulation.[4–6]

INITIATION OF COAGULATION

Blood coagulation is initiated by endothelial cell damage. The damage leads to exposure of the integral membrane glycoprotein tissue factor, which triggers the coagulation process.[1–3,7] Tissue factor is synthesized and expressed by macrophages/monocytes in the adventitia of blood vessels as well as by fibroblasts and keratinocytes in the skin. Healthy endothelial cells that line the luminal side of blood vessels do not express tissue factor activity. However, endothelial cell tissue factor expression can be induced by inflammatory cytokines.

Tissue factor forms a noncovalent complex with activated factor VII that readily cleaves peptidyl substrates and activates factor VII to activated factor VII. Factor VII binds to tissue factor with approximately the same affinity as activated factor VII.[3] Once bound, factor VII is rapidly activated by small amounts of activated factor VII, thrombin, activated factor X, or cellular proteases. The activated factor VII then activates trace amounts of the zymogens factor IX and factor X to the corresponding proteases activated factor IX and activated factor X. Activated factor VII bound to tissue factor is approximately four orders of magnitude more efficient at activating factors IX and X than unbound activated factor VII (Fig. 120–1). This is due to a tissue factor-induced increase in the catalytic constant of activated factor VII and to membrane binding of the substrates factor IX and factor X. Activated factor X leaving the surface of a tissue factor-bearing cell (e.g., a macrophage) is rapidly inactivated by tissue factor pathway inhibitor (TFPI) and by antithrombin, whereas activated factor IX and thrombin are inhibited more slowly. These reactions are often referred to as the *initiation phase of blood coagulation*.[8]

Trace amounts of activated factor IX and thrombin are formed adjacent to platelets bound to subendothelial collagen. The thrombin molecules bind with high affinity to the platelet receptor GP1b and cleave the platelet membrane protein protease-activated receptor 1 (PAR1). Cleavage of PAR1 promotes exocytosis of the platelet granules, which results in exposure of phosphatidylserine-rich cell membranes and release of coagulation components, including factor V/activated factor V and fibrinogen. The phosphatidylserine-containing membranes interact with vitamin K-dependent coagulation factors (factor VII, factor IX, factor X, and prothrombin; Fig. 120–1). Any unactivated factor V released from the platelets is activated by thrombin. These steps are referred to as the *amplification phase* of blood coagulation.[8] Phospholipid-bound protein complexes are formed on the platelet membrane between the cofactors activated factor VIII and activated factor V, and their respective proteases, that is, activated factor IX and activated factor X. Much larger amounts of thrombin are formed than in the initiation phase.[3,9] The process, termed the *propagation phase,* culminates with thrombin-mediated cleavage of fibrinogen, which converts it to fibrin that is deposited at the site of injury.

The tissue factor molecule consists of an N-terminal, extracellular part with two immunoglobulin-like domains.[10,11] There is one disulfide bond in the N-terminal domain and one in the C-terminal domain. The latter bond is adjacent to the cell membrane and is exposed to solvent.[11] The transmembrane region of tissue factor is followed by a short intracellular cytoplasmic tail that has a single Cys residue that is acetylated by stearic or palmitic acid.

Two populations of tissue factor are present on the surface of macrophages. In addition to the active structure that forms an enzymatically active complex with activated factor VII/factor VII there is a second form of tissue factor referred to as *latent* or *cryptic.* Activated factor VII in complex with latent tissue factor cleaves peptidyl bonds but activates factor VII very slowly.[12] The activity of tissue factor appears to be regulated by the conformation of the tissue factor domain that is adjacent to the cell membrane, as revealed by the state of oxidation of the disulfide bond that links Cys186 and Cys209. This disulfide bond is oxidized in the active form and reduced in the latent/cryptic form. The reduction/oxidation state of the disulfide bond appears to be regulated by the extracellular pool of protein disulfide isomerase.[13]

Tissue factor is involved in intracellular signaling.[14] Activated factor X in the ternary activated factor VII–tissue factor–activated factor X complex activates the protease-activated receptors PAR1 and PAR2, which mediate intracellular signaling leading to production of inflammatory cytokines. The in vivo importance of PAR activation at this level compared to activation that is mediated by thrombin remains to be elucidated.

PROCOAGULATION AND ANTICOAGULATION

The coagulation system is balanced in two principally different manners. The protein C anticoagulant system can be regarded as an anticoagulant counterpart of the coagulation system. It is triggered by thrombin, which activates the regulatory protein, protein C, to activated protein C (APC), a serine protease that degrades activated factor V and activated factor VIII by limited proteolysis. In addition there are the two protease inhibitors TFPI, a Kunitz-type inhibitor, and antithrombin, a member of the serine protease inhibitor family (serpins).

Tissue Factor Pathway Inhibitor

The prime inhibitor of activated factor VII is the 46-kd TFPI.[4,15] TFPI is produced by microvascular endothelial cells as well as by monocytes/macrophages.[16] A fraction of TFPI in blood plasma circulates in complex with low-density lipoprotein and high-density lipoprotein. TFPI bound to lipoproteins has less anticoagulant effect than the free form. Also, a fraction of TFPI is noncovalently associated with endothelial cell glycosaminoglycans and can be released by heparin.

TFPI contains three Kunitz-type domains and a C-terminal region that is rich in cationic amino acid residues. There are two alternatively spliced forms of the inhibitor, TFPIα and TFPIβ.[17] The TFPIβ form lacks the Kunitz-3 domain and the region that is C-terminal of this domain in TFPIα. Instead, another C-terminal domain mediates

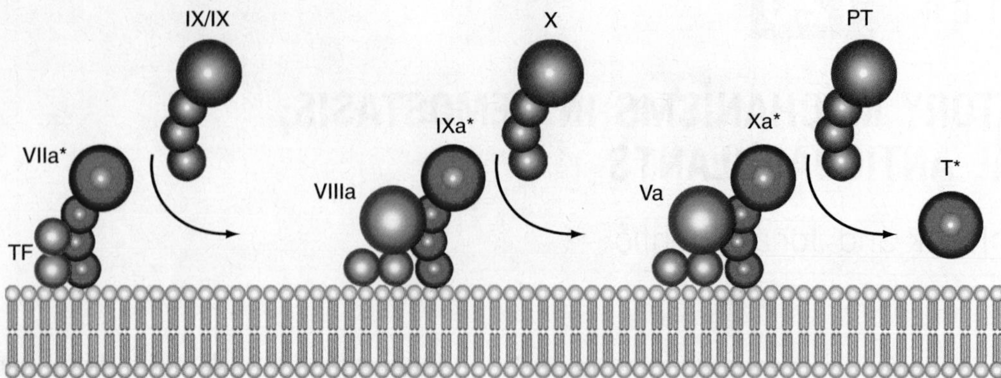

Figure 120–1 Schematic representation of the initiation and propagation of blood coagulation. Blood coagulation is initiated by the exposure of tissue factor (TF) to circulating blood. Factor VII/activated factor VII (VIIa) binds to tissue factor and activates either factor IX (IX) or factor X (X). The activated factor IX (IXa) and activated factor X (Xa) form membrane-bound complexes with their respective cofactor, activated factor VIII (VIIIa) and activated factor V (Va), which activate factor X and prothrombin (PT), respectively. Thrombin is efficiently generated from prothrombin by the activated factor X/activated factor V complex. Thrombin has multiple functions. It activates platelets and several coagulation factors, such as factor VIII, factor V, factor XI, and factor XIII. In addition it converts fibrinogen to fibrin, which constitutes the blood clot.

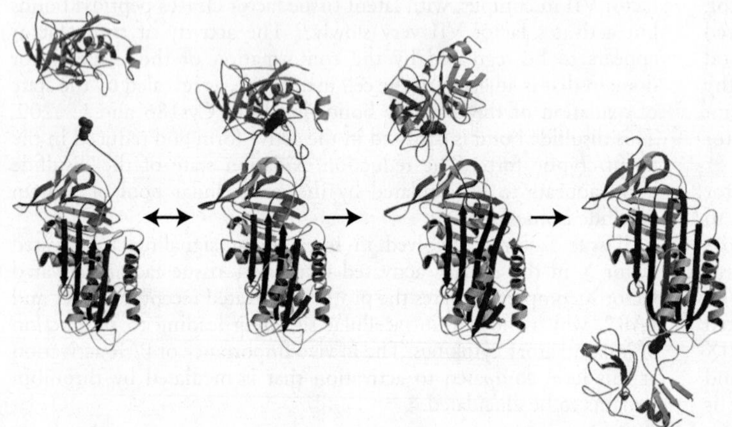

Figure 120–2 Complex formation between a serpin and an enzyme. Inactivation of trypsin by antitrypsin is shown. The mechanism of inhibition is the same for thrombin inhibition by antithrombin (AT). To the left are shown the serpin with the major β-sheet A in blue and the reactive center loop with the scissile bond residue in red. The second section shows the formation of a Michaelis complex between the inhibitor and the enzyme, which results in the formation of a covalent complex between inhibitor and enzyme. The third section shows the complex with the cleaved reactive center loop. The final event is insertion of loop 4 (red) with linked enzyme into the β-sheet A with concomitant denaturation and inactivation of the enzyme (section 4). *(Modified from Huntington JA: Shape-shifting serpins—Advantages of a mobile mechanism. Trends Biochem Sci 31:427, 2006.)*

noncovalent interaction with cellular glycosylphosphatidylinositol. TFPIβ appears to account for most of the tissue factor-activated factor VII inhibitory activity. It is more heavily glycosylated than TFPIα, particularly with respect to sialic acid.

Inhibition of activated factor VII by TFPI can proceed via two pathways. Activated factor X that has been activated by, for example, tissue factor-activated factor VII, is bound to and inhibited by TFPI. In the next step, TFPI-activated factor X complex binds activated factor VII–tissue factor, forming an inactive quaternary complex. Inhibition also can take place by interaction of the activated factor VII–tissue factor-activated factor X complex with TFPI. The tissue factor-activated factor VII complex binds to the Kunitz-1 domain, whereas activated factor X binds to the Kunitz-2 domain of TFPI. The C-terminal cationic residues mediate binding to cell surface heparinoids. These cationic residues are also required for binding to heparin. Thus, heparin treatment releases TFPI from the cell surface. Heparin also seems to form a template for the interaction between activated factor X and TFPI. The tissue factor–activated factor VII complex is cleared from the circulation within a few minutes.[18] Protein S has been shown to have a stimulatory effect on the inhibition of activated factor X by tissue factor.

TFPI-2, a homologue of TFPI, also inhibits tissue factor-activated factor VII.[19] It is expressed in umbilical vein endothelial cells, placenta, and liver. Whether it is involved in the regulation of blood coagulation is unknown.

Serpins

The serine protease inhibitors (serpins) compose a large group of homologous proteins that inhibit trypsin, thrombin, and numerous other serine proteases.[20] The most important serpins in blood coagulation are antithrombin and heparin cofactor II. Antithrombin inhibits activated factor IX, activated factor X, and thrombin, whereas heparin cofactor II inhibits only thrombin. The mechanism of inactivation of a serine protease is the same for all members of the family and can be described as a suicide substrate inhibition mechanism.[20–23]

Serpin-mediated enzyme inhibition is initiated by protease cleavage of the reactive site loop of the inhibitor and formation of an acyl intermediate between the active site of the enzyme and the carboxyl group at the site of cleavage (Fig. 120–2). Once this covalent bond is formed, en route to cleavage of the peptide bond, the reactive site loop with attached enzyme is promptly translocated to the opposite pole of the inhibitor by means of insertion of the reactive site loop as strand 4 into β-sheet A of the serpin.[24,25] This process leads to distortion of the active site of the enzyme and its immediate inactivation. The rate of translocation and hence denaturation of the target enzyme is critical to the process.

The importance of specific regions of antithrombin is illustrated by the functional defects associated with mutations in loops 3 and 5, loops that are adjacent to the inserted loop. These mutations lead to a reduced rate of insertion of the cleaved loop with attached enzyme into β-sheet A. As a result, the acyl intermediate that links enzyme and inhibitor is cleaved with subsequent release of the active enzyme from the cleaved inhibitor.[26]

The rate of inactivation of thrombin by antithrombin in solution is relatively slow. This is due to partial incorporation of the reactive center loop into β-sheet A (see Fig. 120–2).[27] Binding of antithrombin and thrombin to heparin brings the target molecules in proximity and activates antithrombin by removing the partially inserted reactive center loop from β-sheet A. The thrombin–antithrombin complex that is formed has lower affinity for heparin and for endothelial cell glucosaminoglycans (GAGs) than does free antithrombin. It dissociates from the GAGs and is subsequently rapidly removed from the circulation by mononuclear cells ($t_{1/2}$ <5 minutes).[18,22] Heparin, a heterogeneous and negatively charged GAG, is found in mast cell granules, but it is not a normal constituent of blood.[28] Endogenous GAGs are bound to endothelial cells both on the luminal and the abluminal side, although most is bound on the abluminal side. It is estimated that approximately 10% of the endothelial cell GAGs can catalyze complex formation between thrombin and antithrombin.

In heparin obtained from porcine intestines, only a small fraction is active as an anticoagulant. In modern preparations of heparin that are intended for therapeutic use in clinical medicine, the fraction that is active as an anticoagulant has been enriched. Unlike heparin-catalyzed inactivation of thrombin by antithrombin, inactivation of activated factor X does not depend on bridging of activated factor X and antithrombin to heparin but results solely from a heparin-induced conformational change in antithrombin that makes it more reactive with activated factor X.[27] Modern preparations of heparin for clinical use often consist of low–molecular-weight heparin that particularly catalyzes inactivation of activated factor X by antithrombin.

Antithrombin deficiency increases the risk for venous thrombosis (see Chapter 134).[29] It is found in approximately 1 : 3000 persons in the general population and in 1% to 3% of patients with venous thrombosis.[30] Although heparin cofactor II is a specific thrombin inhibiting serpin, its function in vivo is unknown. A few patients with deficiency of the inhibitor have been identified, but no symptoms have been associated with this deficiency.[31]

PROTEIN C SYSTEM

The protein C system exerts its anticoagulant effect by regulating the activities of activated factor VIII and activated factor V, which are cofactors in the tenase and prothrombinase complexes, respectively.[5,32,33] The severe thrombotic disease purpura fulminans, which affects homozygous protein C-deficient individuals in the neonatal period, shows the vital importance of this anticoagulant system. Multiple proteins are involved at different points of the protein C pathway, for example, those that participate in activation of protein C, those supporting the proteolytic activity of APC, and those that inhibit APC (Table 120–1 and Fig. 120–3). Protein C, the key component of the system, is a vitamin K-dependent zymogen of a serine protease that is efficiently activated on the surface of endothelial cells by thrombin bound to thrombomodulin.[33] APC cleaves a limited number of peptide bonds in activated factor V and activated factor VIII, thus providing specific and efficient inhibition of the coagulation pathway. Protein S and the intact form of factor V stimulate the activity of APC. Protein S is sufficient for inactivation of activated factor V, whereas regulation of activated factor VIII requires the synergistic APC cofactor function of both protein S and factor V.[32] In human plasma, protein S is present in two forms: 30% to 40% is free; the rest is bound to C4b-binding protein (C4BP), a regulator of the classical complement pathway. Only free protein S functions as APC cofactor.[34–36] Three protease inhibitors, protein C inhibitor, α_1 antitrypsin, and α_2 macroglobulin, inhibit APC activity in human plasma. However, the half-life (approximately 20 minutes) of APC in circulation is relatively long as the inhibition of APC is slow.[34] The protein C pathway has been found to have anti-inflammatory and antiapoptotic effects.[33,37–39] Moreover, APC has been launched as therapy for patients with severe septic shock and multiple organ failure, resulting in improved survival.[33,37,40–42]

IMPORTANCE OF ENDOTHELIUM IN INITIATION OF THE PROTEIN C PATHWAY

Protein C is a multidomain molecule composed of a γ-carboxyglutamic acid residue (Gla)-rich domain, two epidermal growth factor (EGF)-like domains, a short activation peptide, and the serine protease domain.[34,43] Thrombin is the physiologic activator of protein C, but without its cofactor thrombomodulin it is very inefficient in activating protein C. The high affinity binding of thrombin to thrombomodulin results in greater than 1000-fold amplification of the rate of protein C activation. Thrombomodulin not only functions as an efficient cofactor to thrombin in the activation of protein C but also inhibits the procoagulant properties of thrombin. Thus, thrombomodulin transforms thrombin from a procoagulant to an anticoagulant enzyme. A membrane protein on endothelial cells, endothelial protein C receptor (EPCR), provides another 20-fold stimulation of the thrombin/thrombomodulin-mediated activation of protein C in vivo.[44] The stimulatory effect of EPCR depends on interaction between the Gla domain of protein C and EPCR, which helps orient

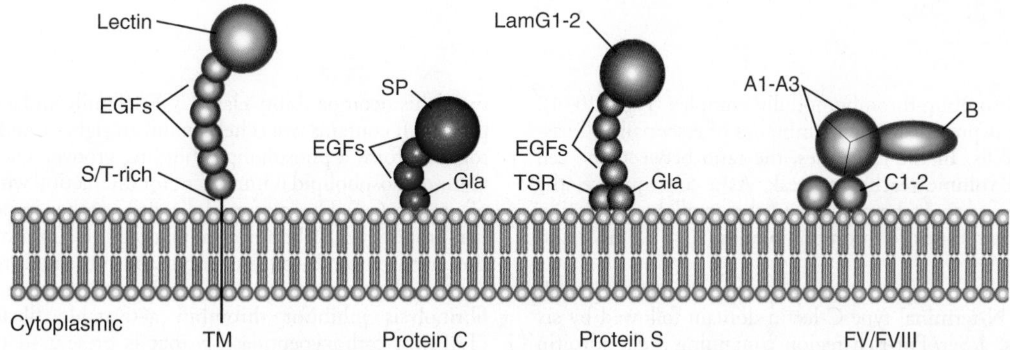

Figure 120–3 Schematic representation of several components of the protein C system. Many multidomain proteins are involved in the protein C system. The domain organization of thrombomodulin (TM), protein C, protein S, and factor V/factor VIII (FV/FVIII) is shown. The following domains are found in the proteins: epidermal growth factor-like domain (EGF); serine/threonine-rich domain of thrombomodulin (S/T-rich), which carries a chondroitin sulfate side chain; serine protease domain (SP); vitamin K-dependent γ-carboxyglutamic acid-rich domain (Gla), which binds calcium and negatively charged phospholipid membranes; and A, B, and C domains of factor V/factor VIII, which attain similar molecular arrangement. During activation of factor V and factor VIII, the B domains are cleaved off and dissociate from the active molecules. TSR, thrombin-sensitive region.

Table 120–1 Components of the Protein C Anticoagulant Pathway

Protein (Amino Acids)	Molecular Mass (kd)	Subunits (Amino Acids)	Domains	Special Functions
Protein C (417)	62	Light chain (155) Heavy chain (262)	Gla, 2 EGFs AP and SP	Zymogen to APC; anticoagulant, antiinflammatory, and antiapoptotic protease, which cleaves factor V/activated factor V and activated factor VIII and PAR1
Protein S (635)	75	Single chain	Gla, TSR, 4 EGFs, SHBG (2 LamG domains)	Cofactor to APC; cofactor to tissue factor pathway inhibitor; binds C4b-binding protein; binds to apoptotic cells; stimulates phagocytosis
Thrombomodulin (554)	75	Single chain	Lectin, hydrophobic, 6 EGFs, S/T-rich, transmembrane, cytoplasmic tail	In membrane of all endothelium; cofactor to thrombin in activation of protein C and thrombin activatable fibrinolysis inhibitor; antiinflammatory
Endothelial protein C receptor (221)	50	Single chain	MHC/CD1	In membrane of endothelium; binds Gla domain of protein C; stimulates protein C activation by thrombin–thrombomodulin and PAR1 cleavage by APC
Factor V (2196)	330	Single chain	A1, A2, B, A3, C1, C3	Precursor to procoagulant activated factor V and to anticoagulant APC; cofactor in activated factor VIII degradation
Factor VIII (2332)	330	Heavy chain (1313) Light chain (684)	A1, A2, B, A3, C1, C3	Precursor to procoagulant activated factor VIII; cofactor in the tenase complex
C4b-binding protein (4078)	570	7 α chains (549) 1 β chain (235)	8 CCPs 3 CCPs	α Chains are cofactors to factor I, an enzyme regulating the complement system; β chain binds to protein S
Protein C inhibitor (387)	60	Single chain	Serpin	Inhibitor of APC and other proteases; stimulated by heparin
α_1 Antitrypsin (394)	60	Single chain	Serpin	Inhibitor of APC and other proteases

The total numbers of amino acids in the mature proteins are given in parenthesis. The molecular masses are approximate and include posttranslational modifications such as carbohydrate side chains. Factor VIII is synthesized as single chain but processed to two chains with heterogeneity of heavy chains; the number of amino acids refers to the longest heavy chain of factor VIII. References to different proteins and their properties are given in the text; some of the information is derived from protein databases available on the Internet. http://www.ncbi.nlm.nih.gov/; http://www.expasy.org/

APC, activated protein C; EGF, epidermal growth factor; Gla, γ-carboxyglutamic acid; PAR, protease-activated receptor 1; S/T-rich, serine/threonine-rich; TSR, thrombin-sensitive region.

protein C to the thrombin–thrombomodulin complex (Fig. 120–4). Thrombomodulin is present in the membranes of essentially all vascular endothelial cells. In the capillaries, the ratio between the cell surface and blood volume reaches its peak. As a consequence, the high concentration of thrombomodulin in the capillary circulation ensures that thrombin binds to thrombomodulin ($K_d = 0.5$ nM) and activates protein C.[33,45,46]

Thrombomodulin is a type I membrane protein containing multiple domains: an N-terminal type C lectin domain followed by six EGF-like domains, a Ser/Thr-rich region containing a chondroitin sulfate side chain, a transmembrane section, and a short cytoplasmic tail (see Fig. 120–3).[33,45,46] Thrombin binds to EGF-5 and EGF-6, whereas EGF-4 interacts with a positively charged cluster in the serine protease domain of protein C.[33,45,47–51] EPCR binds the Gla domain of protein C, which makes protein C accessible to the activating thrombin–thrombomodulin complex.[33,44] EPCR is a member of the major histocompatibility class 1/CD1 family and a type I membrane protein. It contains two α helices and an eight-stranded β sheet, which together form a phospholipid-binding groove. The ability of EPCR to bind phospholipid is important for interaction with the Gla domain of protein C.[52] Thrombomodulin has another important anticoagulant property as its chondroitin sulfate side chain stimulates the inhibition of thrombin by antithrombin and protein C inhibitor.[33]

The thrombin–thrombomodulin complex can also activate the fibrinolysis inhibitor thrombin activatable fibrinolysis inhibitor (TAFI), a carboxypeptidase B that is present in plasma. Activated TAFI removes C-terminal lysine residues from fibrin. Because these lysines constitute a binding site for plasminogen during its activation by tissue plasminogen activator, TAFI inhibits fibrinolysis.[45,53] TAFI also inhibits anaphylatoxins C3a and C5a, suggesting that activation of TAFI by thrombin–thrombomodulin has antiinflammatory consequences.

ACTIVATED PROTEIN C INHIBITS COAGULATION THROUGH CLEAVAGE OF ACTIVATED FACTOR V AND ACTIVATED FACTOR VIII

Factors V and VIII share the domain structure A1-A2-B-A3-C1-C2, with the A domains arranged in a triangular pattern (see Fig. 120–3).[32,54] Activation of factors V and VIII by thrombin releases the carbohydrate-rich B domains from the activated factor V and activated factor VIII which are thus composed of the A1-A2-A3-C1-C2 domains. The high-affinity binding sites for the enzymes activated factor IX and activated factor X are located in the A2 and A3 domains of activated factor VIII and activated factor V, respectively.[55–60] In both activated factor VIII and activated factor V, the C2 domains contain the major sites for phospholipid binding, with some contributions from the C1 domains.[61–64] Molecular models of the A domains of activated factor V and activated factor VIII have been created based on their homology with ceruloplasmin.[65–70] Moreover, three-dimensional structures of APC-cleaved bovine-activated factor V (lacking the A2 domain) and of the C2 domains of both activated factor V and activated factor VIII have been determined.[71–73] The structure of the C1 domain of factor VIII has been predicted by homology and a model of phospholipid-bound activated factor VIII created.[67] These three-dimensional structures, together with experimental results, have made possible the creation of models of both the tenase and the prothrombinase complexes; models that improve our understanding of the molecular interactions involved in two of the important enzymatic reactions of blood coagulation.[59,60]

In human activated factor V, three sites are cleaved by APC: at positions Arg306, Arg506, and Arg679 (Fig. 120–5).[32,54] Cleavage at Arg506 results in partial loss of activated factor X cofactor activity and is kinetically favored over cleavage at Arg306.[32,74–77] Arg306 cleavage results in complete loss of activated factor V activity due to dissociation of the A2 fragments.[78] Regulation of activity of the tenase complex by APC encompasses cleavage of human activated factor VIII at Arg336 and Arg562.[58,79] This reaction is more complex than the degradation of activated factor V because, in addition to protein S, the nonactivated form of factor V serves as an APC cofactor.[32,80,81] In vivo, the concentration of factor VIII is much lower than that of factor V. The complicated task of regulating the highly efficient tenase complex in the presence of a large molar excess of the competing APC substrate factor V/activated factor V may explain the requirement for two APC cofactors.[32,58,79] To serve as an APC cofactor in the regulation of activated factor VIII in the tenase complex, factor V must be cleaved at Arg506 by APC.[32,81,82]

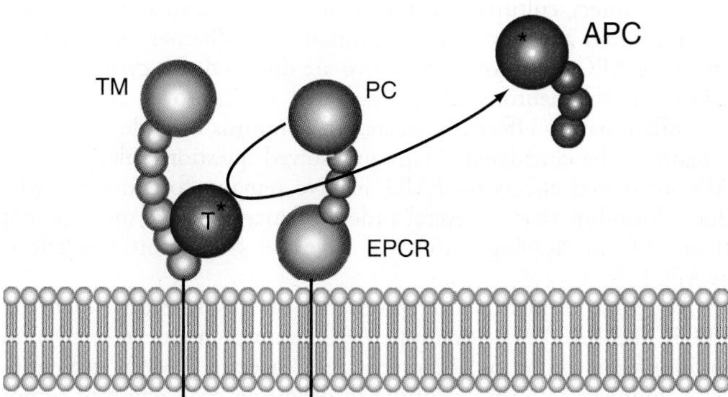

Figure 120–4 Schematic model of the molecular interactions involved in activation of protein C (PC). Thrombin binds to thrombomodulin (TM) with high affinity and efficiently activates protein C. The endothelial protein C receptor (EPCR) interacts with the γ-carboxyglutamic acid (Gla) domain of protein C and helps orient protein C to the thrombin–thrombomodulin complex. The activated protein C (APC) dissociates and leaves room for a new protein C molecule to be activated.

MULTIPLE FUNCTIONS OF VITAMIN K-DEPENDENT PROTEIN S

Protein S consists of an N-terminal Gla domain, a thrombin-sensitive region, four EGF-like domains, and two laminin G-type domains (see Fig. 120–3).[34,35,43] The Gla domain of protein S binds negatively charged phospholipid membranes, and protein S and APC form a membrane-bound complex (Fig. 120–6) that cleaves factor V/activated factor V and activated factor VIII. Several parts of protein S are important for its interaction with APC, including the Gla domain, the thrombin-sensitive region, and the EGF-1 and EGF-2 domains.[34,35,83] During degradation of activated factor VIII, the two laminin G-type domains play a role in the synergistic APC cofactor activity of protein S with factor V.[34,35,84]

Protein S has anticoagulant activity that is independent of APC. According to one hypothesis, direct binding of protein S to activated factor X and activated factor V inhibits the prothrombinase complex.[85,86] Protein S can also function as a cofactor to TFPI in regulation of the tissue factor pathway.[87]

The interaction between protein S and the complement regulatory protein C4BP in human plasma suggests that protein S plays a role in control of the complement system.[34–36] C4BP has an octopus-like structure, with seven identical α chains and a single β chain (see Fig. 120–6).[36] Each α chain can bind a C4b (activated complement protein C4) molecule and convert it into a substrate for factor I, a complement regulatory enzyme in blood. Thus, C4BP is an important regulator of the classical complement pathway. The binding site for protein S is located in the β chain of C4BP.[36,88] In protein S, the interaction site for C4BP is located in the two LamG domains.[89,90] During apoptosis, negatively charged phospholipid is exposed on the surface of cells to which protein S binds. The bound protein S is important for phagocytosis of the apoptotic cell. The molecular mechanisms are unclear but presumably involve an interaction between protein S and the receptors on the surface of the phagocytes.[91,92] In contrast to free protein S, binding of the protein S–C4BP complex to the apoptotic cell surface has been found to inhibit the phagocytic process, suggesting that C4BP blocks the site on protein

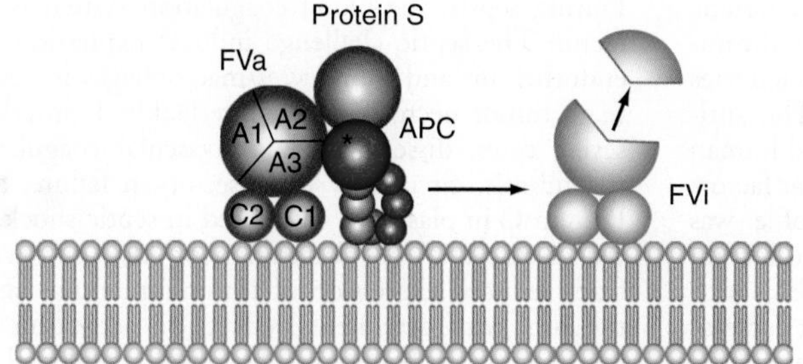

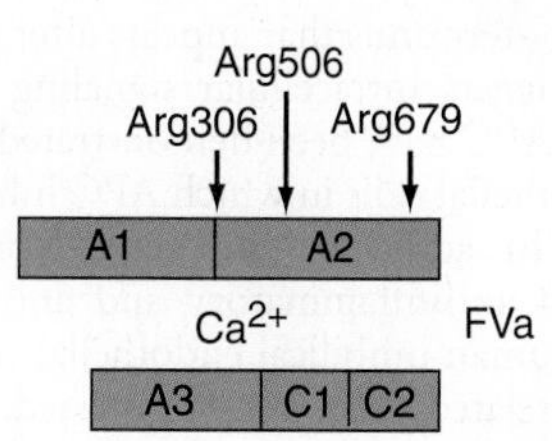

Figure 120–5 Schematic model of the degradation of factor Va (FVa) by activated protein C (APC). Degradation of activated factor V by APC in the presence of protein S, which serves as an APC cofactor. APC cleaves factor V at three sites, Arg306, Arg506 and Arg679, which results in dissociation of degradation fragments from the activated factor V molecule and loss of activated factor V activity.

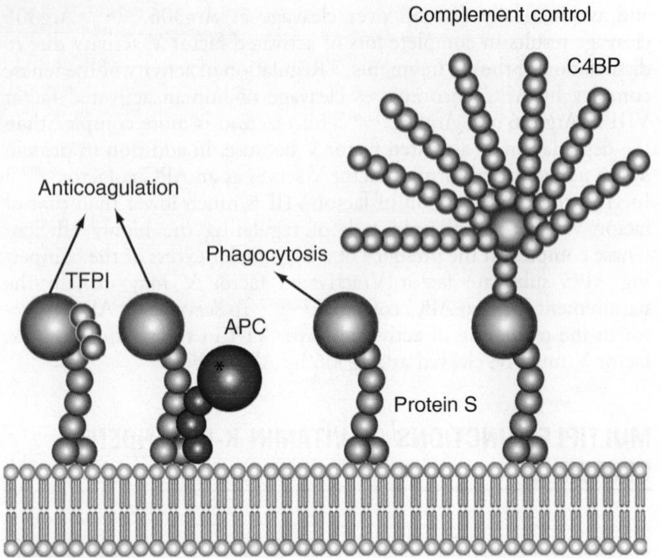

Figure 120–6 Multiple functions of protein S. Protein S binds to negatively charged phosphatidylserine, which is exposed on the surface of cells in certain situations, such as during apoptosis. Protein S has important anticoagulant functions, being a cofactor to both activated protein C (APC) and tissue factor pathway inhibitor (TFPI). Both the free and the C4b-binding protein (C4BP) bound forms of protein S interact with the membrane surface via the γ-carboxyglutamic acid (Gla) domain. The octopus-like shape of C4BP is illustrated with six long α chains and a short β chain that interacts with protein S. This provides the potential for local regulation of both coagulation and the complement (e.g., on apoptotic cells). In addition, the bound protein S stimulates phagocytosis of apoptotic cells.[92]

S interacting with the surface receptors.[93] Binding of protein S and protein S–C4BP complexes to the surface of apoptotic cells may be important for local control of coagulation and complement pathways.

ANTIINFLAMMATORY AND ANTIAPOPTOTIC EFFECTS OF THE PROTEIN C PATHWAY

Several of the proteins of the protein C pathway exert biologic effects other than those strictly referred to as anticoagulant. For example, the lectin domain of thrombomodulin has antiinflammatory effects due to downregulation of nuclear factor-κB and mitogen-activated protein kinase pathways.[46,94] Thrombomodulin also decreases leukocyte adhesion and extravasation, effects that also have been associated with protein C.[94,95] Antiinflammatory and antiapoptotic effects of APC have been demonstrated both in vivo and in vitro. These effects depend on the presence of EPCR and are due to APC-mediated cleavage of PAR1 (Fig. 120–7).[33,37–39,44] PAR1 is a G-coupled protein belonging to the large group of receptors with seven transmembrane spanning regions. PAR1 is primarily known to be cleaved by thrombin, and the novel N-terminus that appears after proteolysis activates the receptor and triggers intracellular signaling events.[96] The antiapoptotic effects of APC have been demonstrated in cultured human umbilical vein endothelial cells in which APC inhibits nuclear factor-κB activation.[38,97] In addition, the gene expression profile was switched toward an antiinflammatory and antiapoptotic direction after treatment of human umbilical endothelial cells (HUVEC) with APC and apoptosis-related genes were suppressed. Genes that decrease proinflammatory signaling pathways and those that are antiapoptotic were instead upregulated. In another study, human APC was shown to inhibit staurosporine-induced apoptosis in the EAhy926 cell line.[98]

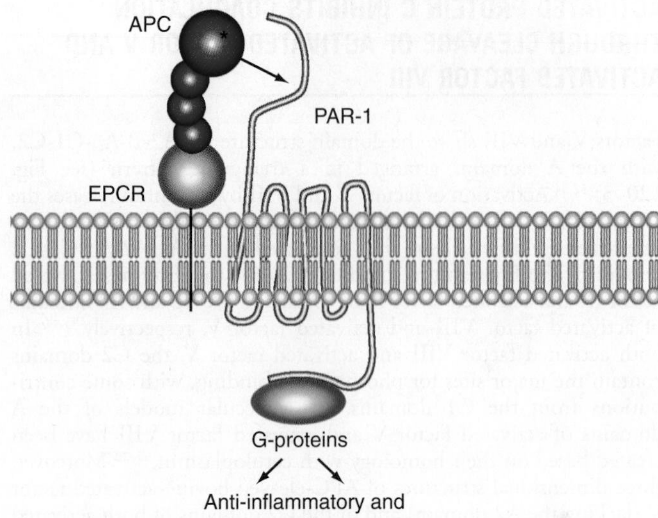

Figure 120–7 Activated protein C (APC) bound to endothelial protein C receptor (EPCR) activates protease-activated receptor 1 (PAR-1). The γ-carboxyglutamic acid (Gla) domain of APC binds to EPCR, which helps orient the active site of APC (marked with asterisk) toward a sensitive peptide bond in PAR-1. PAR-1 spans the membrane seven times, and the cytoplasmic portion of PAR-1 interacts with G proteins. Cleavage of PAR-1 by APC creates a novel N-terminus, which binds and autoactivates the PAR-1 molecule. Intracellular G proteins that are bound to PAR-1 are stimulated and generate the antiinflammatory and antiapoptotic responses of APC.

In a stroke model in mice, APC was shown to be neuroprotective and to protect cultured cortical neurons.[99–101] Similar effects were observed after administration of protein S.[102] Whether the beneficial effects of APC and protein S in vivo are due to direct cytoprotective effects on the neurons or are mediated by improved blood flow, antiinflammatory effects, or decreased apoptosis of endothelial cells remains to be elucidated. Many unresolved questions related to the APC-mediated effects on PAR1 in vivo remain, for example, why does thrombin that is several orders of magnitude[103] more potent than APC in cleaving PAR1 not have the same protective effects as APC?[104]

Not all antiinflammatory properties of APC are dependent on EPCR and PAR1. For example, APC inhibits monocyte activation by interferon γ, phorbol 12-myristate 13-acetate (PMA), and endotoxin-induced pathways resulting in decreased production of tumor necrosis factor α and interleukin 1, selective prevention of downregulation of certain membrane receptors (CD11b, CD14, and CD18), and decreased cell surface exposure of tissue factor.[103,105] APC is also found to stabilize monocyte chemoattractant protein 1 mRNA, a chemokine that is controlled by activation of nuclear factor-κB.[106]

SEVERE SEPSIS AND THE PROTEIN C PATHWAY

During sepsis, the blood coagulation system is activated by tissue factor. The septic challenge induces expression of tissue factor on endothelium and monocytes/macrophages in response to cytokines (e.g., tumor necrosis factor, interleukin 1, interleukin 6).[37,107,108] In severe cases, disseminated intravascular coagulation, microvascular thrombosis, circulatory collapse, organ failure, and shock develop. Protein C in plasma is consumed in septic shock, which can worsen the disease if the concentration of APC decreases. This can result from reduced expression of thrombomodulin and EPCR on endothelium, with detrimental effects on activation of protein C. In a sepsis model in baboons, infusion of a sublethal dose of *Escherichia coli* resulted in more severe disease if APC activity or protein C activation was inhibited.[37,109] Likewise, inhibition of binding of protein C or APC to EPCR exacerbated the septic response to *E. coli* infusion.[110,111] The role of protein S is illustrated by the aggravated effects of sublethal *E. coli* infusion that follow inhibition of protein S by either monoclonal antibodies or C4BP (the latter binds free protein S).[112,113] Beneficial effects of APC infusion were demonstrated in the sepsis model in baboons. The observed prevention of shock and disseminated intravascular coagulation may depend not only on the anticoagulant activity of APC but also on the antiinflammatory effects.[114] APC has also been attempted for treatment of sepsis in humans. In the PROWESS study (1690 patients with severe sepsis), recombinant APC (drotrecogin alfa [Xigris]) resulted in a 19.4% reduction in the relative risk of death and an absolute reduction of 6.1% (30.8% mortality at 28 days in the placebo group vs 24.7% with APC).[41] Further evidence for the efficacy of APC in the treatment of severe sepsis was obtained in the open-label trial ENHANCE.[115] However, in the more recent ADDRESS study of patients with severe sepsis and low risk of death (defined by an Acute Physiology and Chronic Health Evaluation [APACHE I]) score <25 or single-organ failure), no beneficial treatment effects were observed, which argues against the use of APC in such patients.[116] Thus, it appears that APC treatment is efficient in patients with very severe sepsis (APACHE score >25 or multiple-organ failure) when protein C and APC reach very low levels, whereas no beneficial effects of treatment are seen for milder forms of sepsis. The critical factor for the therapeutic effect of APC may be the endogenous level of APC, suggesting that methods for determining the generation of APC in vivo, such as measuring APC directly[117] or indirectly as APC–protein C inhibitor complexes,[118] may have a role in deciding which patients will benefit from treatment with APC.

PROTEIN C PATHWAY AND VENOUS THROMBOSIS

The severe microvascular thrombotic disease of the neonatal period affects individuals with complete inherited protein C deficiency. This disorder demonstrates that the protein C system is vitally important for keeping the blood fluid. In the general population, the prevalence of defective protein C alleles is approximately 1 : 600; thus, complete deficiency affects approximately 1 : 200,000 to 1 : 300,000 newborn babies.[6] The lifelong imbalance between procoagulant and anticoagulant pathways in individuals with heterozygous protein C deficiency is associated with an approximately fivefold increased risk of venous thrombosis (see Chapter 134). Similar thrombosis risk affects patients with heterozygous protein S deficiency; together the two defects account for at most 5% to 10 % of patients with venous thrombosis in western societies (see Chapter 134). Higher prevalences have been reported from Japanese and Chinese studies.[119] The most common genetic risk factor for venous thrombosis in Caucasians is the Arg506 to Gln mutation (factor V Leiden), which causes the condition known as APC resistance. The mutation is found in 20% to 40% of thrombosis patients.[5,6,120,121] The procoagulant activity of factor V is not affected by the mutation, whereas two reactions of the anticoagulant protein C system are affected. Activated factor V Leiden cannot be cleaved at position 506 by APC because of the mutation, but cleavage at the other sites Arg306 and Arg679 are unaffected. In addition, degradation of activated factor VIII is affected by the factor V Leiden mutation because cleavage at Arg506 in factor V is important for the anticoagulant activity of factor V.[32] The relative importance of these two defective reactions, that is, degradation of activated factor V and activated factor VIII, for expression of the prothrombotic phenotype is not known.

The factor V Leiden mutation is found only in individuals with Caucasian background; it is absent or very rare in Asians, Australian Aboriginals, and black Africans. This is explained by the fact that the mutation only occurred once in human history; thus, factor V Leiden is the result of a founder effect, and the mutation is approximately 20,000 to 25,000 years old.[122] With few exceptions, the prevalence of factor V Leiden in European populations exhibit a north to south gradient, with the highest prevalence (10%–15%) in the north and lowest prevalence (approximately 2%) in the south. In United States, the prevalence is approximately 5% in the north and somewhat lower in the south due to differences in ethnic background in the population.[6,121] The relative risk of thrombosis in heterozygous individuals is increased approximately fivefold, whereas homozygotes carry a 50-fold increased risk (see Chapter 134). The factor V Leiden mutation is not a risk factor for arterial thrombosis. Women with factor V Leiden have reduced risk for bleeding after delivery, which may offer a major survival benefit in human history.[120] Moreover, factor V Leiden is suggested to be a positive survival factor in sepsis of either man or mice.[123–125] Thus, the factor V Leiden allele has provided a survival advantage during evolution, which explains its high prevalence in certain populations.

Acknowledgment

We thank Dr. James A. Huntington for Figure 120–2.

SUGGESTED READINGS

Abraham E, Laterre PF, Garg R, et al: Drotrecogin alfa (activated) for adults with severe sepsis and a low risk of death. N Engl J Med 353:1332, 2005.

Ahamed J, Versteeg HH, Kerver M, et al: Disulfide isomerization switches tissue factor from coagulation to cell signaling. Proc Natl Acad Sci U S A 103:13932, 2006.

Autin L, Miteva MA, Lee WH, Mertens K, Radtke KP, Villoutreix BO: Molecular models of the procoagulant factor VIIIa-factor IXa complex. J Thromb Haemost 3:2044, 2005.

Autin L, Steen M, Dahlback B, Villoutreix BO: Proposed structural models of the prothrombinase (FXa-FVa) complex. Proteins 63:440, 2006.

Dahlback B: Blood coagulation and its regulation by anticoagulant pathways: genetic pathogenesis of bleeding and thrombotic diseases. J Intern Med 257:209, 2005.

Dahlback B, Villoutreix BO: Regulation of blood coagulation by the protein C anticoagulant pathway: novel insights into structure-function relationships and molecular recognition. Arterioscler Thromb Vasc Biol 25:1311, 2005.

Hackeng TM, Sere KM, Tans G, Rosing J: Protein S stimulates inhibition of the tissue factor pathway by tissue factor pathway inhibitor. Proc Natl Acad Sci U S A 103:3106, 2006.

Hansson K, Stenflo J: Post-translational modifications in proteins involved in blood coagulation. J Thromb Haemost 3:2633, 2005.

Huntington JA: Shape-shifting serpins–advantages of a mobile mechanism. Trends Biochem Sci 31:427, 2006.

Lane DA, Philippou H, Huntington JA: Directing thrombin. Blood 106:2605, 2005.

Ludeman MJ, Kataoka H, Srinivasan Y, Esmon N, Esmon CT, Coughlin SR: PAR1 cleavage and signaling in response to activated protein C and thrombin. J Biol Chem 280:13122, 2005.

Lwaleed BA, Bass PS: Tissue factor pathway inhibitor: structure, biology and involvement in disease. J Pathol 208:327, 2006.

Mann KG, Brummel-Ziedins K, Orfeo T, Butenas S: Models of blood coagulation. Blood Cells Mol Dis 36:108, 2006.

Monroe DM, Hoffman M: What does it take to make the prefact clot? Arterioscler Thromb Vasc Biol 26:41, 2006.

Piro O, Broze GJ Jr: Comparison of cell-surface TFPIalpha and beta. J Thromb Haemost 3:2677, 2005.

Saller F, Villoutreix BO, Amelot A, et al: The gamma-carboxyglutamic acid domain of anticoagulant protein S is involved in activated protein C cofactor activity, independently of phospholipid binding. Blood 105:122, 2005.

Vincent JL, Bernard GR, Beale R, et al: Drotrecogin alfa (activated) treatment in severe sepsis from the global open-label trial ENHANCE: further evidence for survival and safety and implications for early treatment. Crit Care Med 33:2266, 2005.

REFERENCES

For complete list of references log onto www.expertconsult.com

CHAPTER 121

CLINICAL EVALUATION OF HEMORRHAGIC DISORDERS: THE BLEEDING HISTORY AND DIFFERENTIAL DIAGNOSIS OF PURPURA

Barry S. Coller and Paul I. Schneiderman

The initial evaluation of patients with hemorrhagic problems involves obtaining a detailed history of bleeding symptoms and analyzing any current hemorrhagic lesions, which most often occur on the skin. This chapter focuses on the bleeding history and the differential diagnosis of purpuric skin lesions that may reflect an underlying hemorrhagic or nonhemorrhagic disorder.

THE BLEEDING HISTORY

General Principles

The bleeding history forms the basis of the diagnosis and therapy of hemorrhagic disorders. In order to maximize its value, several basic principles of eliciting and interpreting this information deserve emphasis.

1. Many normal, healthy people consider their bleeding and bruising excessive. For example, using standardized, self-administered questionnaires, Miller et al.[1] found that 23% of the normal population had "positive" bleeding histories, and Wahlberg et al.[2] reported that a remarkable 65% of healthy women and 35% of healthy men answered "yes" to the question: "Do you suffer from a bleeding disorder?" (Table 121–1).[2] Similarly, Plug et al.[3] found that 61% of normal females reported having gum bleeding, 44% reported having nosebleeds, 17% reported having bruising, and 9% reported having prolonged bleeding from small wounds.

2. Patients with profound coagulation disorders invariably have dramatically abnormal bleeding histories, although surprisingly they may not volunteer the information unless specifically questioned.

3. Patients with mild to moderate abnormalities may not have excessive bleeding symptoms or may not recognize subtle symptoms as abnormal, even though they are at risk for developing excessive bleeding if exposed to severe hemostatic challenges. In the study by Miller et al.,[1] 35% of patients with heterozygous von Willebrand disease had negative bleeding histories, and in the study by Wahlberg et al.[2] approximately 54% of the men and 38% of the women with either von Willebrand disease or a platelet function defect failed to identify themselves as suffering from a bleeding disorder (see Table 121–1).

Identifying the group of patients with milder defects and distinguishing them from the normal population require considerable skill and experience and cannot be done with certainty. In fact, given the low frequency of hemorrhagic disorders in the population and the high false-positive rate in the normal population, the task is formidable. For example, if one uses the values of 65% and 100% for the sensitivity of the bleeding history and 77% for its specificity derived from the studies of Miller et al.[1] and Castaman et al.[4] and assumes a prevalence of ten patients with von Willebrand disease in a population of 1000,[5] the predictive accuracy of a positive history is a dismal 3% to 4%. Thus, in a population of 1000 people, either seven or 10 patients with von Willebrand disease with positive histories (65% or 100% of 10) would need to be differentiated from the 228 normal individuals with positive histories (23% of 990) (see Chapter 129).

4. A search for objective confirmation of subjective symptoms provides important information in assessing the severity of the patient's disorder. This is especially important in obtaining a bleeding history because some patients are extremely sensitive to even minor hemorrhagic problems, whereas other patients ignore major problems. Specific objective indicators are discussed with each group of symptoms, but overall indicators include the following: (a) visits to physicians for bleeding problems, along with any laboratory data obtained; (b) need for transfusion of whole blood, packed red blood cells, plasma, platelets, or coagulation factor concentrates; and (c) history of documented anemia and/or physician-prescribed iron therapy.

5. A medication history is incomplete without specific questions concerning aspirin, herbal remedies, dietary supplements, or medications available without prescription that may affect coagulation or platelet function because patients may not recognize these agents as medications. Similarly, it is important to inquire about vitamin tablets that may contain vitamin K in patients taking oral anticoagulants. Hormone replacement therapy and birth controls pills can affect hemostasis.[6,7]

6. Although self-administered questionnaires with yes or no answers facilitate data collection and statistical analysis,[1,2,8,9] obtaining the maximal amount of useful information requires a dialogue between patient and physician. This allows the physician a chance to assess whether the patient truly understands what is being asked, to refine the questions in response to the initial answers, and to follow up on potentially important data that are revealed only as the discussion proceeds.

7. A constellation of hemorrhagic symptoms, rather than any single symptom, is most helpful in suggesting the etiology of the disorder. Thus, spontaneous hemarthroses and muscle hemorrhages are highly suggestive of severe hemophilia, whereas epistaxis, gingival bleeding, and menorrhagia are more commonly found in patients with thrombocytopenia, platelet disorders, or von Willebrand disease (see Chapters 125 and 129).

8. Excessive bruising and bleeding may be a manifestation of diseases of the blood vessel rather than diseases of coagulation or platelets. In patients with impressive bleeding histories but no abnormalities in coagulation or platelets, a high index of suspicion is needed for hereditary hemorrhagic telangiectasia (HHT), Cushing disease, scurvy, Ehlers-Danlos syndrome, and other systemic disorders. In patients whose hemorrhagic symptoms are confined to the skin, consideration must be given to a wide range of dermatologic disorders.

9. The diagnostic value of any single hemorrhagic symptom varies according to the disorder. In studies of hemophilia carriers[10] and of patients with von Willebrand disease or platelet function abnormalities,[2] the individual questions were ranked on the basis of their ability to discriminate between patients and normals. The results from the hemophilia carrier study are given in Table 121–2, and the results of other studies are detailed later in the chapter. Because the patterns of hemorrhage differ with different hemorrhagic disorders, the diagnostic value of any given question will differ as well. For example, a positive response to the question about long bleeding after tooth extractions had a higher sensitivity in the study of patients with von Willebrand disease and platelet disorders[2] (see Table 121–1) than in the study of hemophilia carriers (see Table 121–2).[10]

10. A dietary history is important in patients taking oral anticoagulants because intake of vitamin K will affect the response to medication (see Chapters 130 and 135). In order to maintain a con-

Table 121–1 Results of Self-Administered Questionnaire for Diagnosis of Hemorrhagic Disorders[a]

	Males		Females	
Question	*Normals (n = 23)*	*Patients[b] (n = 24)*	*Normals (n = 20)*	*Patients[b] (n = 21)*
Do you suffer from a bleeding disorder?	35	46	65	62
Bleeding from the gums?	52	67	50	67
Long bleeding after tooth extraction?	4	21	10	24
Skin bleeding?	0	13	15	10
Long bleeding from small wounds?	13	25	10	10
Tendency to bruises?	22	25	55	62
Spontaneous bruises?	0	4	40	48
Nose bleeding?	57	63	85	57
Blood coughed up or vomited?	9	13	5	10
Metrorrhagia?	—	—	55	42
Muscle bleeding?	4	13	15	0
Blood in the urine?	0	8	10	10
Joint bleeding?	0	0	0	10
Blood in the stool?	13	8	5	10
Treated with vitamin K?	0	4	10	19
Treated with plasma or blood transfusion?	0	4	0	0

[a]Values are percent of normal patients and percent of patients with von Willebrand disease, platelet abnormalities, or antithrombin III deficiency answering "yes" to indicated questions. Subjects were given a choice of "yes," "no," and "don't know." The percentage answering "no" and "don't know" varied considerably from question to question.

[b]The patient group consisted of 16 persons with von Willebrand disease, 27 with a variety of qualitative platelet abnormalities, including aspirin-like defects (n = 9), isolated abnormal collagen-induced aggregation (n = 12), and isolated abnormal arachidonic acid-induced aggregation (n = 6), and 2 with antithrombin III deficiency.

Adapted from Wahlberg T, Blomback M, Hall P, Axelsson G: Application of indicators, predictors and diagnostic indices in coagulation disorders. I. Evaluation of self-administered questionnaire with binary questions. Method Inf Med 19:193, 1980.

Table 121–2 Discriminant Capacity of Questions in Distinguishing Between Normal Persons and Hemophilia Carriers

Question	Sensitivity[a] (%)	Specificity[b] (%)	Difference between Carriers and Noncarriers (*P* Value)
Tendency to bruises?	50	77	<0.025
Metrorrhagia?	44	81	<0.025
Abnormal bleeding at delivery?	38	97	<0.005
Abnormal bleeding at operation?	35	92	<0.005
Tendency to nose bleeding?	32	87	<0.05
Long bleeding after tooth extraction?	15	98	NS
Blood in the urine?	11	98	NS
Long bleeding from small wounds?	8	96	NS
Blood in the stool?	3	100	NS

[a]Percentage of positive responses among carriers.

[b]Percentage of negative responses among normals.

From Wahlberg T: Carriers and noncarriers of haemophilia A II. Evaluation of bleeding symptoms registered by a self-administered questionnaire with binary (no/yes) questions. Thromb Res 25:415, 1982.

stant level of anticoagulation, the dietary intake of vitamin K must remain constant.[11] The absolute amount of vitamin K intake is less important, so it is reasonable to permit the patient free choice of diet with the proviso that, once selected, it remain reasonably constant.[12] If the patient wishes to change diets, it is important to monitor the level of anticoagulation more carefully. Patients should be instructed that food additives, such as fish oils, may contain vitamin K. Patients who are not taking food by mouth are at particularly high risk for developing vitamin K deficiency, especially if they are also taking broad-spectrum antibiotics because the latter decrease the vitamin K contribution from bacteria in the gastrointestinal tract (see Chapter 130).[13,14] The combination of decreased oral intake and antibiotic therapy is quite common in patients with bowel disorders during the preoperative and early postoperative periods. Because vitamin K is required on a daily basis despite its fat solubility, significant depression of coagulation factors can occur within several days and lead to excessive operative and/or postoperative bleeding.

11. Potentially confounding pharmacologic and medical influences must be considered in evaluating the history. For example, pregnancy, use of birth control pills, and hormone replacement therapy can variably increase von Willebrand factor levels in some patients with mild to moderate forms of the disease.[6,7,15] Thus, because von Willebrand factor levels decrease soon after parturition, the risk of bleeding actually may increase after delivery and remain high for several weeks thereafter. Similarly, because the stress of surgery or pregnancy can lead to thrombocytopenia in type 2B von Willebrand diseases, bleeding may be especially severe at those times.[16–18]

12. Assessing excessive bleeding in the newborn is especially difficult. For example, some neonates with Glanzmann thrombasthenia

have only minimal symptoms at birth, and the symptoms of von Willebrand disease may be masked by an increase in von Willebrand factor as a result of the stress involved in the delivery. Similarly, a significant number of hemophilic neonates do not have hemorrhagic symptoms in the first weeks of life. Large cephalhematomas may be due to birth trauma, but if they continue to progress after delivery, hemophilia or a vitamin K-dependent factor deficiency should be considered. Delayed bleeding from the umbilical stump should raise the possibility of factor XIII deficiency or a fibrinogen abnormality (quantitative or qualitative).

13. Hemostatic competence during previous severe hemostatic challenges provides particularly valuable data. Thus, a mild bleeding diathesis may not become clinically manifest until the patient experiences a major hemostatic challenge. As a result, it is more difficult to exclude the presence of a mild defect in patients who have not had a significant hemostatic challenge.

Documenting the History

Table 121–3 contains a bleeding history form. It is designed to be filled out by the physician during discussions with the patient. Use of such a form ensures that the major symptoms are elicited and recorded in a standardized manner. The form itself is made a part of the patient's permanent record. Other bleeding history reporting forms have been developed, and their relative value is discussed here, along with general scales of bleeding severity, after considering each of the bleeding symptoms in more detail.[9,19–22]

Evaluating Individual Bleeding Symptoms

Epistaxis

Bleeding from the nose is one of the most common manifestations of platelet disorders and von Willebrand disease. It also is the most common symptom of HHT. At the same time, a large fraction of the normal population has experienced one or more nosebleeds. Thus, when a group of normal subjects was presented with the question, "Nose bleeding?" on a self-administered questionnaire, 57% of the men and 85% of the women answered "yes" (see Table 121–1). To obtain more meaningful data, it is important to inquire about the frequency of nosebleeds and whether the nose bleeding occurs spontaneously or only with trauma. The latter may not always be appreciated because some individuals habitually and subconsciously traumatize their mucous membranes when they use their fingers to remove crusted secretions from their nose. If the bleeding is confined to a single nostril, it more likely is due to a localized vascular abnormality than to a systemic coagulopathy. In northern locales, nosebleed with nonhematologic etiologies is more likely to occur in the dry winter months, especially with use of forced air heating systems that dry out the mucous membranes. It is important to ascertain the effects of aging on epistaxis because many individuals with no discernible abnormalities have childhood epistaxis that disappears after puberty, whereas patients with HHT usually suffer increasingly severe epistaxis with increasing age. Therefore, the age of onset of epistaxis in HHT may provide prognostic information. The length of time for the bleeding to stop gives valuable insight into the severity of the episodes. Objective information can be obtained by inquiring as to whether the epistaxis was severe enough to require evaluation by a physician, and, if so, whether packing, cautery, or transfusions were considered necessary to control the bleeding.

Gingival Hemorrhage

Bleeding from the gums is another common symptom of platelet disorders and von Willebrand disease. It often is the first sign of hemostatic compromise in patients who develop thrombocytopenia after chemotherapy. Interestingly, patients with long-standing hemorrhagic disorders may not recognize that their gingival bleeding is excessive because they assume that everyone bleeds from their gums on a daily basis. In fact, occasional, but not perennial, gum bleeding is very common among the normal population, with 52% of normal males and 50% of normal females answering "yes" to the question, "Bleeding from the gums?" in the study by Wahlberg et al.[2] Therefore, it is important to establish the frequency with which the patient's gum bleeding occurs and whether the bleeding is spontaneous, as the vast majority of normal persons will experience gum bleeding only after the trauma of tooth brushing. If spontaneous gum bleeding occurs during the night, patients may notice blood-tinged stains on their pillowcase. Daily gum bleeding with tooth brushing may or may not be abnormal, depending on whether the patient has gingival disease and whether a hard-bristle or soft-bristle tooth brush is used. Because routine tooth scaling to remove plaque performed by dental hygienists is a significant hemostatic challenge, it is useful to inquire whether the patient was told that he or she bled excessively after this procedure. Finally, some patients have oral mucous membrane bleeding in the form of blood blisters as another manifestation of a hemorrhagic diathesis, most commonly due to severe thrombocytopenia. Such blisters have a predilection to form on the inner surface of the cheek at sites that are traumatized by the teeth.

Skin Hemorrhage

Petechial lesions characteristically appear as crops or showers of lesions in dependent portions of the vasculature. However, the integrity of the microvasculature depends on a variety of vascular and extravascular factors. Therefore, it is not surprising that patients with similar platelet or coagulation disorders show considerable variability in the appearance of petechial lesions. For example, when infants cry, they increase the pressure in the veins draining the face, and in some patients with platelet disorders such as Glanzmann thrombasthenia this may be sufficient provocation to bring out petechial lesions.

Bruising is one of the most difficult symptoms to evaluate because patients vary greatly in their recognition and response to the symptom. Thus, patients who always bruise excessively, even without trauma, may assume that this is normal because they have experienced it all their lives, whereas normal individuals who bruise only rarely may become very concerned about a single large bruise associated with trauma. Bruising is more common in women than in men. For example, 22% of normal men and 55% of normal women responded affirmatively to the question, "Tendency to bruises?," and none of the normal men but 40% of the normal women indicated that they had "spontaneous bruises." Therefore, it is necessary to define better the nature of the bruising so as to determine whether the bruising is part of a hemorrhagic diathesis.

The dermatologic literature recognizes the female easy bruising syndrome (purpura simplex) as one in which women have excessive bruising in relationship to their menstrual cycle, although the time in the cycle when the bruising is excessive varies among women.[23] This diagnosis should be entertained only after excluding other etiologies. Variations in von Willebrand factor levels have been reported during the menstrual cycle, presumably reflecting the effects of estrogen, and this is one potential contributing cause (reviewed by Kujovich[24]). However, not all studies found cyclical variations and not all studies found the same patterns during the menstrual cycle.[24] If there are no underlying hematologic or nonhematologic causes,[25] it is appropriate to reassure the patient that she is unlikely to be at risk of excessive hemorrhage, even with more severe hemostatic challenges such as surgery. It is inappropriate, however, to tell the patient that there is nothing wrong with her, because this can be misinterpreted to suggest that the physician thinks she inappropriately sought medical attention for a trivial matter. These patients clearly do have an abnormality that can be quite frightening, even though at present the molecular basis of the defect has not been identified biochemically.

It is important to try to establish whether the patient's hemorrhagic response is excessive when measured against the inciting

Table 121–3 Form for Documentation of Bleeding History

1. Epistaxis
   A. Ages when affected
   B. Frequency
   C. Spontaneous
   D. Left, right, or both nostrils
   E. Seasonal correlation
   F. Time to stop
   G. Required
      1. Packing
      2. Cautery
      3. Transfusions

Comments:

2. Gingival hemorrhage
   A. Frequency
   B. Spontaneous
   C. With tooth brushing
   D. With dental scaling

Comments:

3. Skin hemorrhage
   A. Petechiae
   B. Bruises
      1. Frequency
      2. Relationship to menses
      3. Spontaneous
      4. Exposed sites
         a. Arms
         b. Legs
      5. Unexposed sites
         a. Trunk
         b. Back
      6. Size
      7. Knots in center
      8. Painful
      9. Color
      10. Time to resolution
      11. Number currently

Comments:

4. Tooth extractions—ages at extractions
   A. Deciduous
   B. Permanent
      Molar
      Other
   C. Duration of bleeding
      1. Packing
      2. Resuturing
      3. Transfusion
   D. Bleeding from injection of anesthetic

Comments:

5. Bleeding from minor cuts
   A. Blade or electric razor
   B. Approximate time to stop
   C. Requires
      1. Direct pressure
      2. Tissue paper

6. Bleeding from major trauma
   A. Knife wound
   B. Motor vehicle accident
   C. Need for
      1. Sutures
      2. Transfusions

Comments:

7. Hemoptysis
   A. Spontaneous
   B. Associated with respiratory infection?

Comments:

8. Hematemesis
   A. Spontaneous
   B. Known increase in portal pressure
   C. Associated with vomiting
      1. Beginning of episode
      2. End of episode

Comments:

9. Hematuria
   A. Frequency
   B. Gross or microscopic
   C. Related to urinary infection
   D. Duration
   E. Required
      1. Cystoscopy
      2. Transfusion

Comments:

10. Hematochezia
   A. Frequency
   B. Duration
   C. Known hemorrhoids

Comments:

11. Melena
   A. Frequency
   B. Duration
   C. Known ulcer disease
   D. Required
      1. Transfusion
      2. Surgery
   E. Documented by tests for occult blood

Comments:

12. Central nervous system bleeding
   A. Hemorrhagic stroke
   B. Documentation
      1. Computed tomography
      2. Magnetic resonance imaging

Comments:

13. Venipuncture site bleeding

Comments:

14. Ophthalmologic bleeding
   A. Subconjunctival hemorrhage
   B. Retinal hemorrhage
   C. Retrobulbar hemorrhage

Comments:

15. Menstrual bleeding
   A. Frequency
   B. Duration in days
      1. Heavy flow
      2. Total flow
   C. Comparison to sisters or friends
   D. Required
      1. Transfusion
      2. Iron therapy
      3. Birth control pills
      4. Dilatation and curettage
      5. Endometrial ablation
      6. Hysterectomy
   E. Known fibroid tumor
   F. Ovarian bleeding

Comments:

16. Pregnancy and delivery bleeding
   A. Pregnancies
   B. Spontaneous abortions (indicate month of gestation)
   C. Induced abortions
   D. Estimated blood loss
   E. Anemia documented
   F. Required
      1. Transfusion
      2. Dilatation and curettage
      3. Hysterectomy
      4. Iron therapy

Comments:

17. Hemarthroses
   A. Joints
      1. Elbow
      2. Knee
      3. Ankle
      4. Wrist
      5. Shoulder
      6. Other
   B. Frequency
   C. Required
      1. Transfusion
      2. Aspiration

Comments:

18. Surgical procedures
   A. Procedure
   B. Date
   C. Excess bleeding
   D. Required
      1. Whole blood
      2. Plasma
      3. Platelets
      4. Coagulation factor concentrate
   E. Reoperation
   F. Wound healing

Comments:

19. Bleeding at circumcision or from umbilical stump

Comments:

20. Telangiectasias
   A. Mucous membranes
   B. Skin
   C. Gastrointestinal tract

Comments:

21. Connective tissue
   B. Skin hyperextensibility
   C. Changes in body fat distribution

Comments:

22. Wound healing

Comments:

23. Medications
   A. Iron
   B. Birth control pills
   C. Aspirin or other antiplatelet medications

Comments:

24. Family history of bleeding

Comments:

25. Immunization history

Comments:

trauma. Thus, spontaneous bruising is most likely to be pathologic, and the patient should be asked specifically whether bruises appear even without any recognized antecedent trauma. Unfortunately, patients vary significantly in appreciating when they have been traumatized. For example, mothers of children who are old enough to be physically active, but still young enough to be held in the mother's arms, may be so focused on other matters that they do not realize that they are being repeatedly kicked. Similarly, normal toddlers and youngsters who are physically active commonly have bruises on their legs and arms.

The location of a bruise may offer indirect evidence of its relationship to trauma. The vast majority of traumatic events occur on exposed sites on the arms and legs. Therefore, if the patient suffers repeated bruises on unexposed sites on the trunk or back, these are more likely to be either spontaneous or in response to minimal trauma. The size of the bruise may also give some indication of the extent of bruising. It is best to provide patients with some size standards that they can relate to, such as "dime-sized," "silver-dollar-sized," or "as large as your palm." When assessing bruise size, it is important to remember that bruises often spread during the resolution phase. With severe bruises there may be hemorrhage into the bruise, resulting in very dark discoloration and the appearance of a raised "knot" in the center of the bruise; such bruises tend to be particularly painful.

The color of the bruise may also be significant. Fresh bruises associated with hemorrhagic phenomena tend to be dark purple, so-called "black-and-blue marks"; they evolve into shades of yellow-green as they resolve. By contrast, patients with senile purpura or Cushing syndrome commonly have bruises that are much redder in appearance. Since easy bruising may be the presenting symptom of Cushing syndrome, it is important to have a high index of suspicion for this disorder in younger patients whose bruises simulate the appearance of senile purpura. Another color variant worth distinguishing is the jet black central area and violaceous-erythematous surrounding area characteristic of warfarin-induced skin necrosis. This thrombotic disorder has a predilection for fatty tissues such as the breasts; it can be mistaken for a hemorrhagic abnormality because of the bruise-like quality of the lesion and the association with oral anticoagulant use.

Bruises usually take 10 days to 2 weeks to resolve, depending on the extent of the bruise. When patients indicate that their bruises take months to resolve or that they have required casting of a limb in order for the bruising to stop, consideration should be given to the poorly understood entity of psychogenic purpura.[26–29]

Tooth Extractions

Bleeding in response to tooth extraction can provide extremely important information. The hemostatic challenge varies, however, with the type of tooth removed; molar extractions are usually the severest tests of hemostasis. Objective information can be obtained about the duration and extent of bleeding by asking about the need to reconsult the dentist for packing, suturing, or even transfusion of blood products. A deep injection given to achieve anesthesia of the lower jaw by nerve block is a particularly dangerous hemostatic challenge since hemorrhage from such an injection may extend down into the neck and compromise the airway.

Bleeding from Minor Cuts

In our society, shaving nicks are the most common minor cuts suffered, and patients with platelet disorders or von Willebrand disease usually bleed excessively from them. If a patient uses an electric razor or a depilatory, it is worthwhile asking whether a razor blade was ever used and, if so, why the switch was made. Although it is difficult to obtain objective information about bleeding after razor nicks, it may be helpful to ask whether the patient delays leaving home in the morning because of persistent oozing from these wounds or whether they leave home with small pieces of tissue paper still attached to their bleeding wounds. It is also useful to instruct the patients that direct pressure for 5 minutes is usually much more effective than tissue paper, since rebleeding is very common when the latter is removed. Patients with purpura secondary to amyloidosis may paradoxically choose to switch from an electric razor to a blade razor because the pressure of the electric razor causes more purpura than razor nicks.

Bleeding from Major Trauma

In the absence of previous surgery, the extent of bleeding in response to major trauma furnishes the most reliable information about future hemostatic risk. In order to assess the appropriateness of the bleeding, the details of the injury must be determined. The need for sutures and transfusions provides objective information. Excessive bleeding due to thrombocytopenia or platelet dysfunction tends to occur immediately, whereas excessive bleeding due to coagulation abnormalities may be delayed. It is especially important to know whether aspirin or other antiplatelet agents were taken after the trauma to alleviate pain.

Hemoptysis

Hemoptysis is virtually never the presenting symptom of a bleeding disorder and is rare even with serious bleeding disorders. Thus, a comprehensive search for an anatomic abnormality or an underlying infectious or neoplastic disease is required, even if the patient has a systemic coagulopathy. Patients with bleeding diatheses may, however, have blood-tinged sputum in association with acute respiratory tract infections. Occasionally, a patient with an upper respiratory tract infection associated with a postnasal drip may also complain of hemoptysis, even though the true source of blood is in the upper airway.

Hematemesis

As with hemoptysis, hematemesis is virtually never the presenting symptom of a hemostatic disorder, and thus a search for an anatomic basis is mandatory. Hemostatic defects may, however, contribute significantly to gastrointestinal bleeding, as in patients with liver disease and esophageal varices, or patients with gastritis secondary to aspirin ingestion.

Hematuria

Urinary tract bleeding is also virtually never the first symptom of a hemostatic disorder and thus a full investigation to define an anatomic defect is required. Hemostatic defects may, however, exacerbate hematuria caused by other disorders; thus, patients with urinary tract infections that might ordinarily produce microscopic hematuria may instead develop gross hematuria. Normal subjects may also develop gross hematuria with urinary tract infections. Since women are much more likely to contract such infections, it may explain why none of the normal men but 10% of the normal women complained of blood in their urine in the study by Wahlberg et al. (see Table 121–1).[2] Even among patients with platelet disorders and von Willebrand disease, however, only 8% of the men and 10% of the women complained of hematuria (see Table 121–1).[2]

Hematochezia

Hemorrhoids are the most common cause of hematochezia, but more serious, less common, causes need to be excluded. In the study by Wahlberg et al.,[2] 13% of normal men and 5% of normal women complained of blood in the stool (see Table 121–1). Although a systemic coagulopathy may exacerbate hematochezia, one should not ascribe the bleeding to the coagulopathy itself without extensive evaluation. Von Willebrand disease, platelet abnormalities, and both inherited and acquired forms of angiodysplasia may all be associated with severe recurrent episodes of hematochezia and often the search for discrete bleeding sites is frustrating and inconclusive. Associations between von Willebrand disease and both angiodysplasia and HHT have been reported,[30] but current information does not support a genetic link between von Willebrand factor and any of the recognized genetic forms of HHT.[31,32] It is more likely, therefore, that having von Willebrand disease makes the hemorrhage associated with vascular anomalies more severe, increasing the probability that the patient will come to medical attention.

Melena

It is important to make certain that the patient understands precisely what is meant by the term melena, because many patients will answer "yes" to a question about black stools when, on further questioning, it is clear that their stools are really dark brown. The black rubber tubing of a stethoscope is a good visual prompt for making this clear. Objective evidence of gastrointestinal hemorrhage can be obtained by explicitly asking whether the patient's stool ever tested positive for occult blood and whether the patient ever underwent endoscopy. As with the other sources of gastrointestinal bleeding, melena is virtually never the presenting symptom of an inherited hemostatic defect. Recurrent episodes of melena may occur, however, in patients with serious hemorrhagic abnormalities or angiodysplasia, and on occasion can even be lethal. Objective data on fecal occult blood tests, previous hospitalizations, the results of endoscopic studies, and the need for blood replacement should also be obtained.

Central Nervous System Bleeding

Severe thrombocytopenia (<5,000–10,000 platelets/μl) is associated with increased risk of central nervous system hemorrhage, including both diffuse petechial lesions and gross hemorrhagic strokes. The latter may occur spontaneously or after just minimal head trauma. It is of interest that spontaneous central nervous system hemorrhage is exceedingly rare in Glanzmann thrombasthenia.[33]

Venipuncture Site Bleeding

Patients with diffuse intravascular coagulation, hyperfibrinolysis, thrombocytopenia, or qualitative platelet disorders characteristically bleed for a long time after venipunctures, whereas patients with coagulation disorders do not. Delayed bleeding, however, may occur in the latter group. Virtually all of the prolonged venipuncture bleeding can be prevented, or at least minimized, by applying direct pressure to the venipuncture site for at least five minutes and then observing the uncovered site for at least one minute for evidence of continual bleeding.

Ophthalmologic Bleeding

Subconjunctival hemorrhages are associated with both platelet and coagulation abnormalities. Activities that increase venous pressure, such as uncontrollable crying in infants, or prolonged Valsalva movements or strangulation, may, however, be sufficient to elicit conjunctival hemorrhages in otherwise normal individuals. These maneuvers will also exacerbate the hemorrhages in patients with hemostatic disorders. Severe thrombocytopenia may also lead to retinal hemorrhage. Many other disorders that are not associated with hemostatic defects can, however, also lead to retinal hemorrhages as a result of damage to the vasculature, including multiple myeloma, retinal vein thrombosis, diabetes, sickle cell anemia, some forms of age-related macular degeneration, and leukemic leukostasis. Orbital hemorrhage is more commonly associated with hemophilia than platelet disorders.

Menses and Ovarian Bleeding

Menorrhagia is defined as loss of more than 80 ml of blood per cycle.[34,35] Assessing the severity of menstrual flow based on the patient's subjective estimation or the number of sanitary napkins or tampons used is generally unreliable because women vary greatly in their perception of excessive bleeding and their hygienic practices.[36] It is usually more helpful to establish the number of days of heavy flow and the total number of days for an average menstrual period; if the former is greater than 3 and/or the latter is greater than 6 or 7, it is likely that the menstrual bleeding is excessive. It may also help to ascertain whether the bleeding is heavy enough to require especially large sanitary napkins or to require curtailment of ordinary activities. Pictorial charts may help quantify blood loss.[35] Objective data include whether a physician 1) prescribed birth control pills to control the bleeding, 2) told the patient she was anemic, 3) prescribed iron, 4) performed a dilatation and curettage (D&C) to assess the bleeding, 5) was forced by circumstances to perform an emergency hysterectomy to secure hemostasis, and/or 6) performed an elective hysterectomy or endometrial ablation as preventive measures. When menorrhagia is confirmed by direct measurement of menstrual blood loss and no gynecologic cause is identified, a search for a hemostatic defect is indicated. In fact, the frequency of von Willebrand disease in patients with menorrhagia has been estimated as 5–20% (reviewed by Kujovich[24]).

Ovarian bleeding at the time of ovulation may be excessive in patients with platelet abnormalities, particularly Glanzmann thrombasthenia. It may result in severe abdominal pain, especially if blood is released into the peritoneal cavity, and may cause damage to the ovary. Repeated events can lead to reduced fertility.[37]

Pregnancy and Delivery

A detailed history of bleeding with each pregnancy should be obtained, including objective data regarding the need for transfusions, dilatation and curettage, iron therapy, and/or hysterectomy. It is useful to specifically ask if the patient's doctor commented on her bleeding being excessive at delivery, even if none of the objective criteria were met. A history of recurrent spontaneous abortion may be part of the antiphospholipid antibody syndrome, which may include lupus-like anticoagulants, anticardiolipin antibodies, and/or false-positive serologic tests for syphilis (see Chapter 133). The suspicion of this syndrome should be even greater if recurrent spontaneous abortions occur after the first trimester. Recurrent spontaneous abortions also have been reported in association with abnormalities of fibrinogen[38] and factor XIII,[39] presumably due to abnormal stability of placental attachment.

Hemarthroses

Joint bleeding is the hallmark of the hemophilias and is extremely rare in all other hemostatic defects except severe von Willebrand disease. Because joint bleeding usually is not associated with discoloration, patients may not appreciate that their symptoms are caused by hemorrhage. Therefore, it is important to inquire specifically about pain, swelling, and limitation of motion rather than merely asking about bleeding into the joints. Pain is the most sensitive indicator and may be the only manifestation.

Surgical Procedures

The details of each surgical procedure should be recorded, including any statements made by the surgeon about the extent of bleeding. In general, the onset of excessive bleeding postoperatively due to coagulation abnormalities may be delayed for hours to approximately 1 day, whereas excessive bleeding due to platelet disorders or thrombocytopenia usually manifests as diffuse oozing intraoperatively or immediately postoperatively. Emphasis should be placed on ascertaining whether any blood products were administered. Specific questioning about tonsillectomy (which is a severe hemostatic challenge because of the large raw surface produced) and appendectomy may be required because some patients forget about these operations, especially if they were performed many years before. It is helpful to ask how long the patient was hospitalized with each operation because delayed discharge may have been due to excessive bleeding. The hospital records should be secured because they may contain important clinical and laboratory data that the patient never knew or forgot.

Circumcision and Umbilical Stump Bleeding

Congenital bleeding disorders, particularly the hemophilias, may cause excessive bleeding at circumcision as their first manifestation. Delayed bleeding from the umbilical stump or after circumcision is said to be particularly suggestive of factor XIII deficiency,[40] but factor VIII or factor IX deficiency also can produce delayed bleeding.

Telangiectasias

Patients may manifest a wide range of telangiectatic lesions, ranging from pinpoint erythematous dots that blanch when compressed to classic cherry angiomata ranging in size up to several centimeters. The vast majority of the otherwise normal population will demonstrate an increase in skin telangiectasias with aging, often associated with the development of papular cherry angiomata. The latter may have a distinctive blue appearance if present in the deeper layers of the skin. Patients with HHT usually have progressively more severe disease as they age. What constitutes the minimal criteria for HHT is not clear; some otherwise normal persons with no clinical manifestations in their early years develop easy bruising in association with skin telangiectasias in their later years. The classic hallmarks of HHT include epistaxis and tongue telangiectasias, but lesions may be present in virtually every organ, manifesting as space-occupying lesions, sources of bleeding, or sources of arteriovenous shunting. On physical examination, the lesions may be much more subtle than the florid examples found in most textbooks. A careful search of the integument is necessary, focusing on the face, chest, shoulders, legs, and under the nails. Lesions are commonly found on the vermilion border of the lips and under the tongue, even when the tip of the tongue is not involved. It is important to distinguish the lesions of HHT from the spider telangiectasias associated with liver disease and pregnancy. The latter have a more splotchy appearance, are concentrated on the shoulders, chest, and face, and have a more serpiginous quality.

Disorders Affecting Connective Tissue

If Ehlers-Danlos syndrome is considered in the differential diagnosis, it is useful to inquire specifically as to whether the patient was "double jointed" as a child or had unusually distensible skin. However, in type IV Ehlers-Danlos syndrome, which is marked by ecchymoses and easy bruisability, joint hypermobility may be confined largely to the fingers, and the skin, although thin and translucent, may be only mildly hyperextensible.[41] More obvious abnormalities, such as lens dislocations, should be apparent. Questions regarding common skin manifestations of Cushing syndrome should be posed, including rounded faces, purple striae, truncal obesity, and fat deposition in the back of the neck. Old photographs of the patient may be extremely helpful in deciding whether facial changes are new. The medication history should provide information on whether the patient is taking glucocorticosteroids.

Wound Healing

Although abnormal wound healing is not a common problem in patients with hemostatic disorders, defects have been reported in association with factor XIII deficiency and fibrinogen abnormalities. Patients with Ehlers-Danlos syndrome and Cushing disease and those taking glucocorticosteroids are likely to have had abnormal wound healing.

Medications

The dose of each prescription and nonprescription drug taken by the patient should be recorded. Specific questions should cover aspirin and other antiplatelet agents, birth control pills, vitamins, herbal remedies, and dietary supplements because these drugs may not be appreciated as medications by the patient. Iron therapy in the past should be noted because it may provide information on previous episodes of anemia due to blood loss.

Family History of Bleeding

A pedigree going back at least one or two generations should be recorded, with emphasis on hemorrhagic and/or thrombotic manifestations for each member. A specific question regarding parental consanguinity should be included because patients may not realize that this is important information. Details about the cause of death for each deceased individual should be obtained.

Immunization History

Because patients with hemostatic disorders may need blood products, it is important to know whether the patient previously was vaccinated against hepatitis B. Vaccination should be considered for all those who have not been vaccinated or whose immunity has decreased below the recommended threshold.

Standardized Questionnaires and Hemorrhage Assessment Instruments

Questionnaires

Rodeghiero et al.[19] developed a physician-administered questionnaire encompassing a range of questions very similar to those included in Table 121–3, with instructions on how to determine when a symptom should be recorded as trivial. In general, the average and most severe manifestations of each symptom are recorded. They also developed a bleeding score to reflect the severity of each symptom. They used the results from 84 symptomatic patients with type 1 von Willebrand disease, 42 type 1 von Willebrand disease obligate carriers who had not sought medical attention, and 215 age- and sex-matched controls to validate the original bleeding score. The symptomatic patients and obligate carriers had similar values for factor VIII (44% and 42%), von Willebrand factor antigen (27% and 27%), and ristocetin cofactor activity (19% and 19%), indicating their biochemical equivalence. The authors analyzed the usefulness of the bleeding history for diagnosing type 1 von Willebrand disease based on both the number and intensity of the bleeding symptoms. Of a possible 10 bleeding symptoms for females and eight for males, fewer than 1% of the controls reported having three hemorrhagic symptoms, 7% reported having two symptoms, and 77% reported having none. In contrast, only 12% of affected patients had no symptoms, 27% had one, 19% had two, 23% had three, and 20% had four or more symptoms. The obligate carriers had results similar to those of the patients, indicating that they suffered similar bleeding symptoms, reinforcing that individuals vary considerably in whether they seek medical attention for hemorrhagic symptoms of equivalent severity. Using a cutoff of three

Table 121–4 Comparison of Different Clinical Criteria for Diagnosis of von Willebrand Disease Developed by Rodeghiero et al.[19]

Criteria	Sensitivity (%)	Specificity (%)
1. Qualitative (>2 symptoms)	50.0	99.5
2. Quantitative (score >3 in males or >5 in females)	64.2	99.1
3. Mixed: criteria 1 and 2	45.2	100
4. Mixed: criterion 1 or 2	69.1	98.6
5. CART model	80.1	91.6

CART, classification and regression tree analysis.

From Rodeghiero F, Castaman G, Tosetto A, et al: The discriminant power of bleeding history for the diagnosis of type 1 von Willebrand disease: An international, multicenter study. J Thromb Haemost 3:2619, 2005.

or more hemorrhagic symptoms, the sensitivity and specificity for diagnosing the obligate carriers were 50.0% and 99.5% (Table 121–4); a cutoff of two or more symptoms would have produced 76.1% sensitivity and 92.1% specificity.

The intensity of the bleeding symptoms, as reflected in the bleeding history scores, correlated with the presence of von Willebrand disease, whether in the affected patient group or the obligatory carrier group (Table 121–4). The diagnostic likelihood ratios differed among the symptoms, with the highest ratios for the questions about cutaneous hemorrhage and excess bleeding with surgery, tooth extraction, or childbirth (Table 121–5). The absence of bleeding with certain provocations may also provided very valuable information. Thus, the absence of bleeding after tooth extractions made it very unlikely that the individual had von Willebrand disease (negative diagnostic likelihood ratio 0.29). The authors found variable increases in sensitivity and specificity when combining both the number and severity of symptoms (see Table 121–4). Application of classification and regression tree analysis (CART) improved the diagnostic sensitivity but decreased the specificity. Classification and regression tree analysis suggested that an efficient strategy for diagnosing or excluding von Willebrand disease consisted of first asking if the individual had undergone tooth extraction. For those who had not or who did not have excess bleeding after tooth extraction, a subsequent negative response to a question about cutaneous bleeding would exclude von Willebrand disease with reasonable probability. In patients with either excess bleeding after tooth extraction or cutaneous bleeding, further laboratory evaluation for von Willebrand disease would be appropriate.

This bleeding history questionnaire subsequently was administered to 712 subjects from 144 families with von Willebrand disease and analyzed with a modified bleeding symptom score (Table 121–6).[20] Three or more hemorrhagic symptoms were present in 79% of index cases and 57% of affected family members. The median bleeding scores for 195 controls, 295 unaffected family members, 273 affected family members, and 144 index cases were −1, 0, 4, and 9, respectively. Figure 121–1A shows the bleeding scores, Fig. 121–1B the odds ratios for individual symptoms, and Fig. 121–1C the correlations of bleeding symptoms with levels of von Willebrand factor antigen, factor VIII, and ristocetin cofactor activity. There was an inverse correlation between bleeding score and each of these laboratory tests. Of note, the mucocutaneous bleeding score, obtained by summing the scores for spontaneous bleeding symptoms, was similar to ristocetin cofactor activity and von Willebrand factor antigen levels in predicting bleeding after tooth extraction but superior to factor VIII values. The mucocutaneous bleeding score was superior to all of the laboratory values in predicting surgical bleeding. The authors concluded that bleeding after minor wounds and cutaneous bleeding were most valuable diagnostically, whereas postpartum hemorrhage, gastrointestinal bleeding, and oral bleeding did not discriminate patients from unaffected family members (Fig. 121–1B).

The data in this study[20] are similar to those in the initial report by Rodeghiero et al.,[19] with the notable exception of postpartum hemorrhage, which was a useful discriminator in the first study but not in the second study. They also identified symptom clusters, including epistaxis with postsurgical or oral bleeding, and cutaneous bleeding with menorrhagia in affected patients. Finally, they noted that index cases had more severe symptoms than did affected family members, despite similar von Willebrand factor laboratory values, suggesting that the index cases may have additional factors compromising their hemostasis. Support for the presence of prohemorrhagic factors in the families was deduced from the slightly elevated bleeding scores in the unaffected family members relative to normal controls (see Fig. 121–1A). Most recently, thus group has applied a Bayesian approach to the diagnosis of type 1 von Willebrand disease, integrating the bleeding score with the von Willebrand factor level and the family history.[8]

Sramek et al.[9] created a self-administered bleeding history questionnaire and analyzed its usefulness in two separate situations: (a) discriminating between individuals referred to a hematologist for evaluation who did and did not have a bleeding disorder, and (b) identifying whether individuals with no known bleeding disorder did or did not have a bleeding disorder. To achieve these goals, they sent questionnaires to 222 patients with a proven bleeding disorder, 134

Table 121–5 Diagnostic Values of Bleeding Scores[a] for Hemorrhagic Symptoms in the Questionnaire Developed by Rodeghiero et al.[19] When Applied to Obligatory Carriers of Type 1 von Willebrand Disease and Healthy Controls

Symptoms	Score 0	Score 1	Score 2	Score 3	Diagnostic Likelihood Ratio
Menorrhagia					
Obligatory carriers	5	4	7	5	4.3
Affected	11	6	9	7	
Controls	101	3	9	8	
Surgical Bleeding					
Obligatory carriers	11	3	6	3	19.1
Affected	26	0	9	7	
Controls	170	2	1	1	
Tooth Extraction Bleeding					
Obligatory carriers	7	5	16	0	13.2
Affected	13	8	24	1	
Controls	171	3	7	0	
Epistaxis					
Obligatory carriers	17	14	11	0	5.1
Affected	38	32	9	3	
Controls	192	20	3	0	
Cutaneous Bleeding					
Obligatory carriers	11	20	9	2	19.1
Affected	25	35	19	2	
Controls	207	8	0	0	
Bleeding from Wounds					
Obligatory carriers	21	17	2	2	10.2
Affected	45	31	3	5	
Controls	205	9	0	1	
Postpartum Bleeding					
Obligatory carriers	7	3	3	1	13.3
Affected	9	6	3	5	
Controls	102	1	2	0	

The bleeding score values for obligatory carriers differed from those of controls for each symptom (all $P < 0.001$) but not from those of affected patients (all $P \geq 0.10$). For each symptom, the number of individuals from each group with the indicated score values is indicated, along with the diagnostic likelihood ratio of the question for differentiating obligatory carriers and affected patients from controls.

[a]Score varies from 0 for no symptom or trivial severity to 3 for severe hemorrhage.

From Rodeghiero F, Castaman G, Tosetto A, et al: The discriminant power of bleeding history for the diagnosis of type 1 von Willebrand disease: An international, multicenter study. J Thromb Haemost 3:2619, 2005.

Table 121–6 Bleeding Symptoms Score Developed by Tosetto et al.[20]

	Score					
Symptom	*−1*	*0*	*1*	*2*	*3*	*4*
Epistaxis	—	No or trivial (<5 min)	>5 or >10 min	Consultation only	Packing or cauterization or antifibrinolytic	Blood transfusion or replacement therapy or desmopressin
Cutaneous	—	No or trivial (<1 cm)	>1 cm and no trauma	Consultation only		
Bleeding from minor wounds	—	No or trivial (<5 min)	>5 or >5 min	Consultation only	Surgical hemostasis	Blood transfusion or replacement therapy or desmopressin
Oral cavity	—	No	Referred at least one	Consultation only	Surgical hemostasis or antifibrinolytic	Blood transfusion or replacement therapy or desmopressin
Gastrointestinal bleeding	—	No	Associated with ulcer, portal hypertension, hemorrhoids, angiodysplasia	Spontaneous	Surgical hemostasis, blood transfusion, replacement therapy, desmopressin, antifibrinolytic	
Tooth extraction	No bleeding in at least two extractions	None done or no bleeding in one extraction	Referred in <25% of all procedures	Referred in >25% of all procedures, no intervention	Resuturing or packing	Blood transfusion or replacement therapy or desmopressin
Surgery	No bleeding in at least two surgeries	None done or no bleeding in one surgery	Referred in <25% of all surgeries	Referred in >25% of all procedures, no intervention	Surgical hemostasis or antifibrinolytic	Blood transfusion or replacement therapy or desmopressin
Menorrhagia	—	No	Consultation only	Antifibrinolytics, pill use	Dilatation and curettage, iron therapy	Blood transfusion or replacement therapy or desmopressin or hysterectomy
Postpartum hemorrhage	No bleeding in at least two deliveries	No deliveries or no bleeding in one delivery	Consultation only	Dilatation and curettage, iron therapy, antifibrinolytics	Blood transfusion or replacement therapy or desmopressin	Hysterectomy
Muscle hematomas	—	Never	Posttrauma, no therapy	Spontaneous, no therapy	Spontaneous or traumatic, requiring desmopressin or replacement therapy	Spontaneous or traumatic, requiring surgical intervention or blood transfusion
Hemarthrosis	—	Never	Posttrauma, no therapy	Spontaneous, no therapy	Spontaneous or traumatic, requiring desmopressin or replacement therapy	Spontaneous or traumatic, requiring surgical intervention or blood transfusion
Central nervous system bleeding	—	Never	—	—	Subdural, any intervention	Intracerebral, any intervention

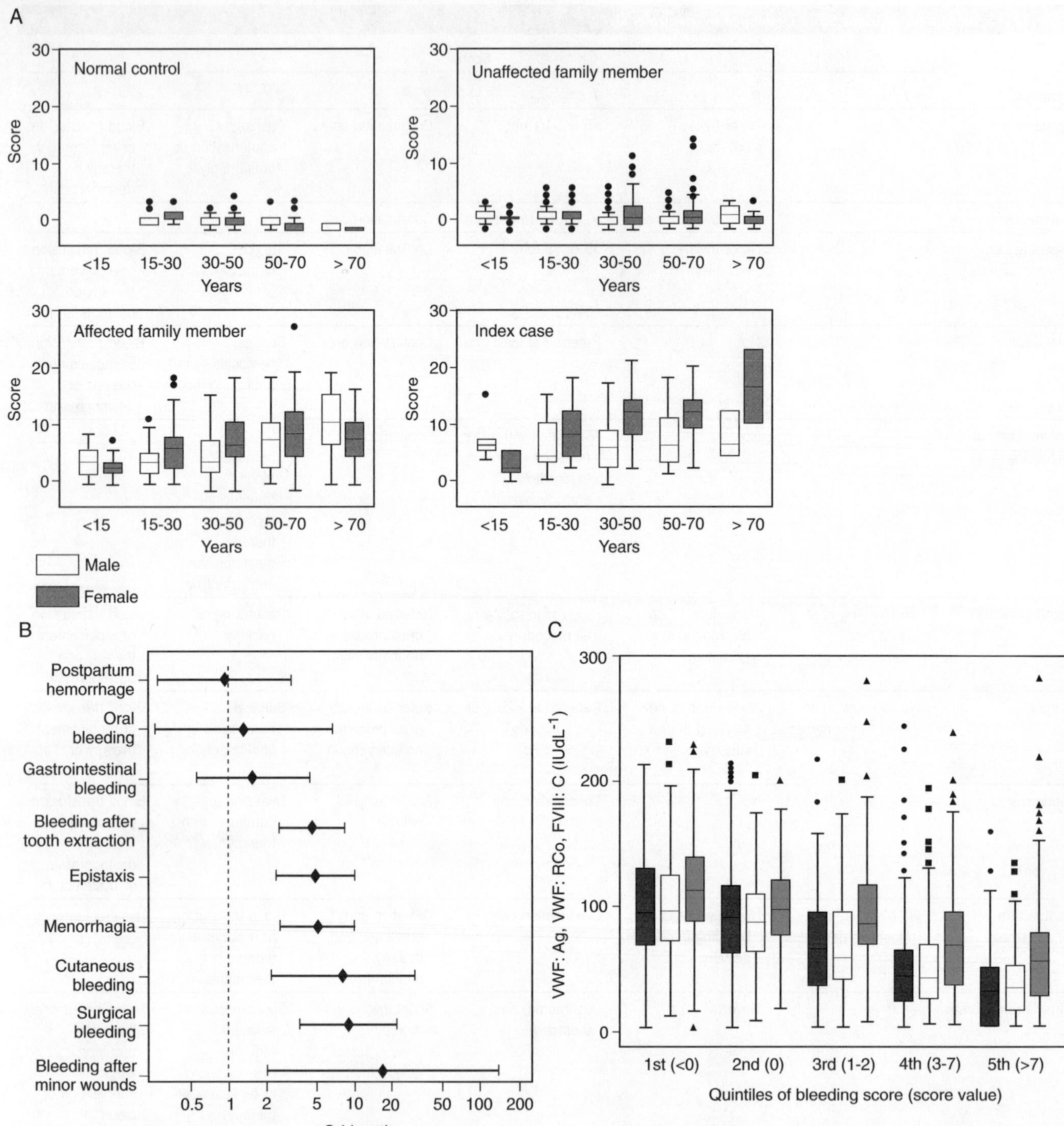

Figure 121–1 Application of a standardized bleeding history assessment questionnaire for diagnosing von Willebrand disease in 195 controls, 295 unaffected family members, 273 affected family members, and 144 index cases.[20] **A,** Bleeding score and age in families with von Willebrand disease and in normal controls. For each category, the boxes represent the 50% of subjects centered around the median. Age is presented on the X-axis. **B,** Association between bleeding symptoms and type 1 von Willebrand disease in the enrolled families in an age-adjusted logistic model. Index cases were excluded from the analysis. A bleeding symptom was considered in the model for a symptom-specific score >1. For each bleeding symptom, the graph reports the logistic estimate and its 95% confidence interval. **C,** Association between bleeding score and levels of von Willebrand factor antigen (VWF:Ag; dark gray boxes), factor VIII coagulant activity (F VIII:C; white boxes), and ristocetin cofactor activity (VWF:RCO, light gray boxes). For each quintile of bleeding score, the boxes span from the 25th to the 75th percentile. Center line represents the median value. *(From Tosetto A, Rodeghiero F, Castaman G, et al: A quantitative analysis of bleeding symptoms in type 1 von Willebrand disease: Results from a multicenter European study (MCMDM-1 VWD). J Thromb Haemost 4:766, 2006.)*[8]

patients referred for evaluation of a bleeding disorder who were found to have no bleeding disorder, and 341 healthy volunteers. Questionnaires were analyzed for both the number and severity of different symptoms. Of note, 70% of the patients with mild von Willebrand disease, 95% of the patients with platelet dysfunction, and 75% of the patients referred for evaluation who were determined to not have a bleeding disorder were women. The questions with the highest univariate positive likelihood ratios (LR+) for distinguishing individuals referred to a hematologist who did, from those who did not, have a bleeding disorder were profuse bleeding with tonsillectomy/adenoidectomy (10.1), muscle bleeding (3.4), joint bleeding (2.5), family member with bleeding disorder (2.4), and profuse bleeding after surgery (2.1). The questions with the lowest negative likelihood ratio (LR–), and thus the best negative predictive values, were profuse bleeding with tooth extraction (0.3) and family member with established bleeding disorder (0.5). The questions with the highest odds ratios (LR+/LR–) by both univariate (shown) and multivariate (not shown) analysis were those about profuse bleeding with tonsillectomy/adenoidectomy (16.2), profuse bleeding with tooth extraction (6.7), and family member with bleeding disorder (5.0). Despite the apparent value of some of these questions, when the overall data were analyzed by receiver operating characteristic curves, the bleeding history was judged to have only minimal discriminatory power for separating referred individuals with, from those without, bleeding disorders. Adding data on the severity of the bleeding symptoms did not improve the test performance meaningfully.

When the bleeding questionnaires of individuals with bleeding disorders were compared to those of healthy controls to simulate the value of the questionnaire as a screening instrument prior to surgery or other invasive procedures, the questions with the highest positive likelihood ratios were those regarding family members with bleeding disorders (34.9), profuse bleeding from small wounds (27.2), profuse bleeding with tonsillectomy/adenoidectomy (16.9), and having a family member with bleeding symptoms (12.9). The questions with the lowest likelihood ratios, and thus the greatest negative predictive values, were those regarding profuse bleeding with tooth extraction (0.2), profuse menstruation (0.3), easy bruising (0.4), and profuse bleeding after surgery (0.4). The questions with the highest odds ratios were those related to family member with a bleeding disorder (97.5), profuse bleeding with small wounds (67.2), and profuse bleeding with tooth extraction (39.4). Receiver operating characteristic curve analysis indicated that the bleeding history had high discriminatory power in separating those with and without a bleeding disorder, either without or with information on the severity of bleeding.

Questions that were weak discriminators in both of the comparisons were those related to profuse bleeding at delivery, hematuria, and hematochezia. The authors noted the differences between their findings and those of Wahlberg[8] with regard to the discriminating value of questions related to dental and surgical bleeding and the presence of a family member with a bleeding disorder and ascribed them to the possible use of prophylactic interventions and the choice of the control population (nonaffected relatives) in the study by Wahlberg.

The bleeding history questionnaire developed by Sramek et al.[9] subsequently was applied to the analysis of bleeding in 274 carriers of hemophilia and 245 noncarrier family members.[3] Carriers were more likely than noncarriers to have (a) required treatment after tooth extraction (relative risk [RR] 23.2), tonsillectomy/adenoidectomy (RR 9.9), or other surgery (RR 2.3); (b) had prolonged bleeding (>5 minutes) from small wounds (RR 2.2) or with nosebleeds (>10 minutes; RR 4.5); or (c) had prolonged (>3 hours) bleeding after tooth extraction (RR 2.3), tonsillectomy/adenoidectomy (RR 1.8), or surgery (RR 2.6). When the results from all participants were analyzed as a function of clotting factor level (0–40, 41–60, and >60 IU/mL), similar increases in bleeding symptoms were observed in individuals with clotting levels less than 40 IU/mL and those with levels between 40 and 60 IU/mL, relative to individuals with levels greater than 60 IU/mL, demonstrating an increased likelihood of symptoms even in those in the 40 to 60 IU/mL group.

Nosek-Cenkowska et al.[22] administered a bleeding history questionnaire to 251 children and their parents prior to tonsillectomy or adenoidectomy and then excluded the results from the 21 patients who had laboratory or clinical evidence of a bleeding disorder. The remaining group was considered to be normal and compared to a group of 31 patients with platelet disorders or von Willebrand disease. The questions that best discriminated between the normals and the patients were those regarding easy bruising (24% vs 67%), bruising every other week (36% vs 68%), bruises confined to areas of trauma (61% vs 39%), bruises affecting more than one part of the body (5% vs 39%), presence of large bruises (>2 inches) at least several times per year (4% vs 30%), hematoma under a bruise (3% vs 22%), nosebleeds (39% vs 69%), nosebleeds at least once per week (3% vs 23%), prolonged nosebleeds (>20 minutes; 4% vs 47%), and relatives with bleeding disorders (44% vs 68%).

Hemorrhage Assessment Instruments

A number of scales of bleeding severity have been developed to standardize reporting of (a) efficacy of prohemostatic agents, (b) surgical or resuscitative interventions, (c) hemostatic impact of an underlying disease, or (d) toxicity of anticoagulants, antiplatelet agents, or chemotherapeutic agents (reviewed by Koreth et al.,[21] Table 121–7). These scales can be characterized by their intraobserver and interobserver consistency (reliability), correlation with a meaningful outcome (validity), sensitivity, and objectivity. Because bleeding manifestations vary considerably depending on the nature of the defect, the scales may differ in usefulness depending on the hemostatic mechanism affected. In general, scales used to quantify bleeding in bone marrow transplantation and/or cancer therapy use broad categories and subjective criteria. They are used primarily to assess the toxicity of treatments and thus are geared to adverse event reporting rather than the delivery of medical care. Bleeding scales used to assess the severity of bleeding associated with immune thrombocytopenia focus on mucocutaneous hemorrhage because this is the most common bleeding manifestation and thus the most valuable for assessing the effect of new therapies. Similarly, multiple scales have

Table 121–7 Scales Used to Assess Clinical Hemorrhage

Primary Use	Scales
1. Bone marrow transplantation toxicity Cancer chemotherapy toxicity	Nevo et al.[403,404]; Miller et al.[405]; Tornebohm et al.[406]; Gmur et al.[407]; Rebulla et al.[408]; National Cancer Institute [Common Terminology Criteria for Adverse Events (CTCAE) 2.0 and 3.0][409]
2. Immune thrombocytopenia	Buchanan and Holtkamp[410]; Buchanan and Adix[411]; Medeiros and Buchanan[412]; Banchette et al.[413]; Lacey and Penner[414]; Bolton-Maggs and Moon[415]
3. von Willebrand disease	ISTH Provisional Consensus[416]; Hospital for Sick Children[416]; Rodeghiero et al.[19]; Tosetto et al.[20]
4. Hemophilia and other coagulation disorders	Multiple Clinical Trials Scales (reviewed in Koreth et al.[21]); World Federation of Hemophilia[417]; Manco-Johnson et al.[418]
5. Hemorrhagic effects of anticoagulants, antiplatelet agents, and fibrinolytic agents	Multiple Clinical Trials Scales (reviewed in Koreth et al.[21]); Salzman et al.[419]; Landefeld et al.[42-44]; Graafsma et al.[420]

Adapted from Koreth R, Weinert C, Weisdorf DJ, Key NS: Measurement of bleeding severity: A critical review. Transfusion 44:605, 2004.

been used to assess the efficacy of different therapies in hemophilia and other coagulation defects; these have focused on joint hemorrhage because it is the most common manifestation of bleeding in hemophilia. Many other scales have been used to assess the hemorrhagic effects of anticoagulants, antiplatelet agents, and fibrinolytic agents used in treating cardiovascular diseases. The Landefeld bleeding severity index, which combines objective evidence of blood loss (by combining data on blood replacement therapy and decreases in hematocrits) and subjective assessment of severity, has been applied in a large number of studies.[42–44] Few attempts have been made to assess the clinical usefulness of these scales or to compare them to each another. However, in one study of hemorrhage associated with percutaneous coronary intervention, the Global Use of Strategies To Open Occluded Coronary Arteries (GUSTO) scale was found to correlate better with clinical outcome than the laboratory-based Thrombolysis In Myocardial Infarction (TIMI) scale.[45] A scale that captures minor bleeding episodes has also been proposed as being more meaningful for assessing long-term antiplatelet therapy.[46] There has been disagreement about whether hemorrhagic toxicity should be evaluated separately from the efficacy of the cardiovascular intervention or combined with it to establish a single composite endpoint. To date, no validated instruments equate the medical significance of hemorrhagic toxicity with efficacy, and because such assessments are intrinsically subjective, broad agreement by either physicians or patients on how to equate them is unlikely. Thus, at present, it appears best to maintain the separation so that efficacy and toxicity can be judged independently.

Summary

Obtaining the details of the bleeding history requires insight into the mechanisms and manifestations of the different hemorrhagic disorders as well as an appreciation of the patient's perceptions of symptoms. Whenever possible, objective data should be obtained to provide a more comprehensive and credible picture. Although obtaining a complete bleeding history may seem tedious, it is well worth the effort because the patient's previous responses to hemostatic challenges are much better predictors of the patient's likelihood of bleeding excessively than are the patient's routine laboratory values. In fact, in one study, routine screening assays of coagulation and platelets failed to detect any clinically significant abnormalities in more than 100 preoperative patients with normal bleeding histories.[47] Although the clinical value of routine laboratory tests for screening for coagulation abnormalities remains uncertain despite many studies of the topic, there is strong consensus on the central role of the bleeding history in evaluating hemostatic risk.[48]

DIFFERENTIAL DIAGNOSIS OF HEMORRHAGIC DERMATOLOGIC LESIONS

Skin hemorrhage is defined as the indiscriminate extravasation of blood cells out of the vasculature and into the skin, subcutaneous tissue, or both. The amount of blood leaking from the vessel determines the size of the lesion, with minute amounts producing pinpoint red lesions less than 2 mm in size (petechiae), and larger amounts producing purpuric lesions (2 mm to 1 cm) or frank ecchymoses (>1 cm).[23] Despite these precise definitions, conventional usage often groups purpuric lesions and ecchymoses under the term *purpura,* and the general group of disorders that produce such lesions is often referred to as *the purpuras.* All these lesions can be readily differentiated from simple erythema and telangiectasias, in which the blood remains confined within the vasculature, because these latter lesions will blanch if direct pressure is applied to them. This can be easily demonstrated using a glass slide. True purpura may demonstrate partial blanching with direct pressure, but a nonblanchable component will remain. The color of the lesion depends on the size and location of the hemorrhage as well as the time since the extravasation occurred. Initially, superficial lesions are bright red or deep red, and deeper lesions have more of a purple appearance. With time, the lesions evolve into deep purple, brown, orange, or blue-green discolorations.

The general mechanisms by which extravasation of blood from the vasculature can occur is depicted schematically in Fig. 121–2. The integrity of the blood vessel depends on (a) the competence of the hemostatic system in combating the basal level of ongoing vas-

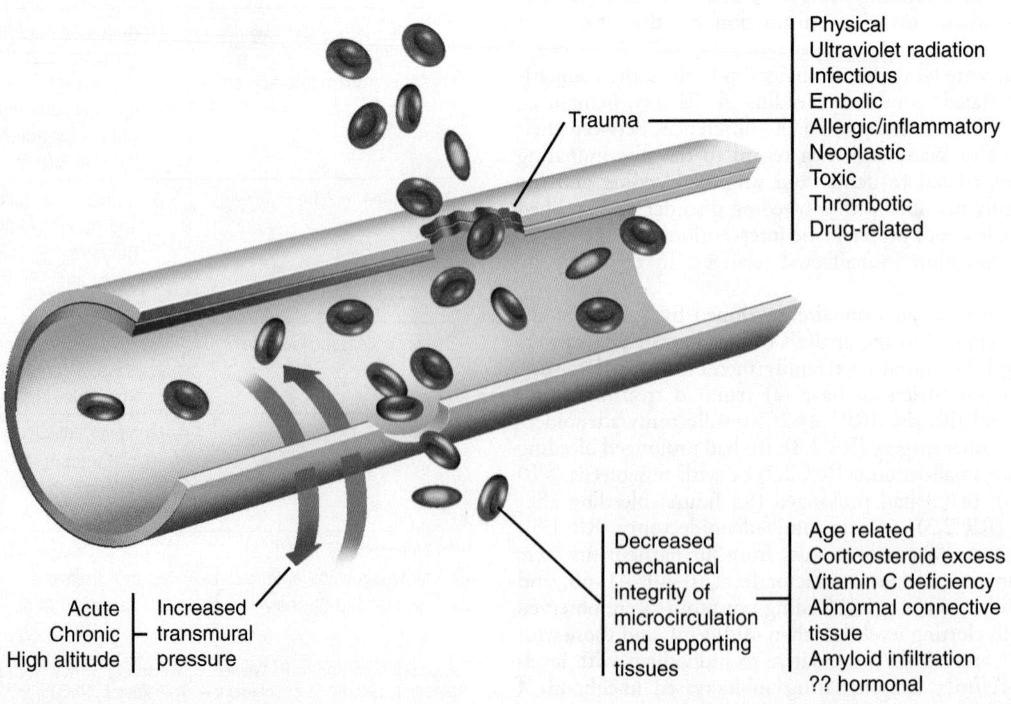

Figure 121–2 Mechanisms of nonpalpable purpura.

Table 121–8 Differential Diagnosis of Purpura

True Purpura

I. Hemostatic Defects
- A. Platelet abnormalities
  - 1. Quantitative
  - 2. Qualitative
- B. Coagulation abnormalities

II. Nonhemostatic Defects—Vascular Purpura
- A. Nonpalpable purpura
  - 1. Increased transmural pressure gradient
    - a. Acute (Valsalva, coughing, vomiting, high altitude, weight lifting)
    - b. Chronic—Venous stasis
  - 2. Decreased mechanical integrity of microcirculation and supporting tissues
    - a. Age related (infancy and actinic purpura)
    - b. Glucocorticoid excess—Cushing syndrome and glucocorticoid therapy
    - c. Vitamin C deficiency (scurvy)
    - d. Abnormal connective tissue—Ehlers-Danlos syndrome
    - e. Amyloid infiltration of blood vessels[a]
    - f. Colloid milium
    - g. ?Hormonal—Female easy bruising syndrome (purpura simplex)
    - h. Lorenzo's oil
    - i. MELAS syndrome
  - 3. Trauma to blood vessels
    - a. Physical
      - 1) Injuries
      - 2) Child abuse
      - 3) Factitial purpura
    - b. Ultraviolet Radiation
      - 1) Purpuric sunburn
      - 2) Solar purpura
    - c. Infectious
      - 1) Bacterial[a]
      - 2) Rickettsial
      - 3) Fungal[a]
      - 4) Viral
      - 5) Parasitic
    - d. Embolic
      - 1) Infectious organisms[a]
      - 2) Atheroemboli (cholesterol crystal emboli)
      - 3) Fat emboli
    - e. Allergic and/or inflammatory
      - 1) Serum sickness
      - 2) Pigmented purpuric eruptions
      - 3) Pyoderma gangrenosum
      - 4) Contact dermatitis
      - 5) Familial Mediterranean fever
    - f. Neoplastic[a]
    - g. Metabolic
      - 1) Erythropoietic porphyria
      - 2) Calciphylaxis
    - h. Immunoglobulin related (hyperglobulinemic purpura of Waldenström and light-chain vasculitis)
    - i. Drug related[a]
    - j. Thrombotic
      - 1) Disseminated intravascular coagulation
      - 2) Warfarin (coumarin)-induced skin necrosis
      - 3) Protein C or protein S deficiency, factor V Leiden, prothrombin G20201A
      - 4) Purpura fulminans
      - 5) Paroxysmal nocturnal hemoglobinuria[a]
      - 6) Antiphospholipid antibody syndrome
      - 7) Hemangioma with thrombocytopenia and consumptive coagulopathy (Kasabach-Merritt syndrome)
  - 4. Unknown cause—Psychogenic purpura
- B. Palpable purpura
  - 1. Cutaneous vasculitis
    - a. Systemic vasculitides[b]
    - b. Paraneoplastic vasculitis
    - c. Henoch-Schönlein purpura
    - d. Acute hemorrhagic edema of infancy
    - e. Livedoid vasculitis
    - f. Idiopathic
    - g. Urticarial
  - 2. Cryoglobulinemia
  - 3. Cryofibrinogenemia
  - 4. Primary cutaneous diseases

Nonpurpuric Disorders Simulating Purpura

I. Disorders with telangiectasias
- A. Cherry angiomas
- B. Hereditary hemorrhagic telangiectasia
- C. Chronic actinic telangiectasia
- D. Scleroderma
- E. CREST syndrome
- F. Ataxia-telangiectasia
- G. Chronic liver disease
- H. Pregnancy-related telangiectasia

II. Kaposi sarcoma and other vascular sarcomas[c]

III. Fabry disease

IV. Neonatal extramedullary hematopoiesis

V. Angioma serpiginosum

[a]May also have a palpable purpuric component.
[b]May also have a nonpalpable purpuric component.
[c]May also have a purpuric component, either nonpalpable or palpable.
CREST, calcinosis cutis, Raynaud syndrome, esophageal motility disorder, sclerodactyly, telangiectasia; MELAS, mitochondrial myopathy, encephalopathy, lactic acidosis, stroke-like episodes.

cular trauma, (b) the integrity of the blood vessel itself and its surrounding tissues, and (c) the transmural pressure gradient tending to drive blood out of the vessel. Even if all these systems are functioning normally, however, serious trauma of diverse etiologies may be sufficient to cause hemorrhagic extravasation.

A classification of disorders producing skin hemorrhage is given in Table 121–8.[23,49] It is organized primarily according to etiology, but a division is made between lesions that are palpable and those that are not palpable because palpability can be readily determined at the bedside and therefore has important practical significance in developing a differential diagnosis. Although the specific mechanism(s) producing palpability is poorly understood, one hypothesis is that a lesion becomes palpable when a generalized increase in vascular permeability secondary to an inflammatory process results in marked extravasation of plasma proteins with the development of extravascular coagulation leading to fibrin deposition. Support for such a mechanism comes from studies showing that the palpable induration accompanying delayed hypersensitivity reactions can be diminished by administration of oral anticoagulants.[50] Alternatively, palpability may be secondary to extensive cellular infiltration, as in certain inflammatory or malignant disorders.

Purpuric lesions secondary to hemostatic defects, including thrombocytopenia and abnormal platelet function, were described in the section. Evaluating Individual Bleeding Symphoms.

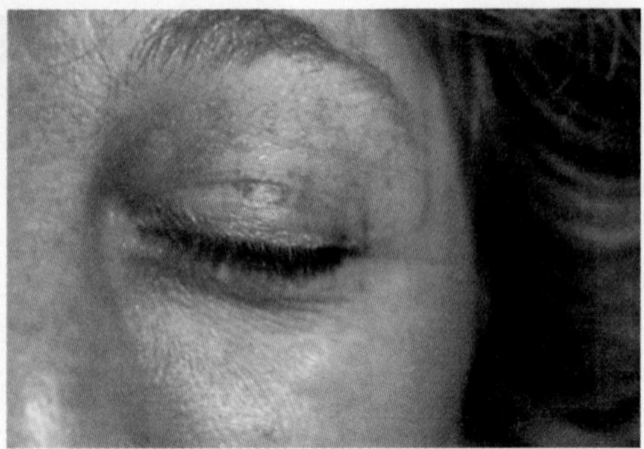

Figure 121–3 Valsalva petechiae.

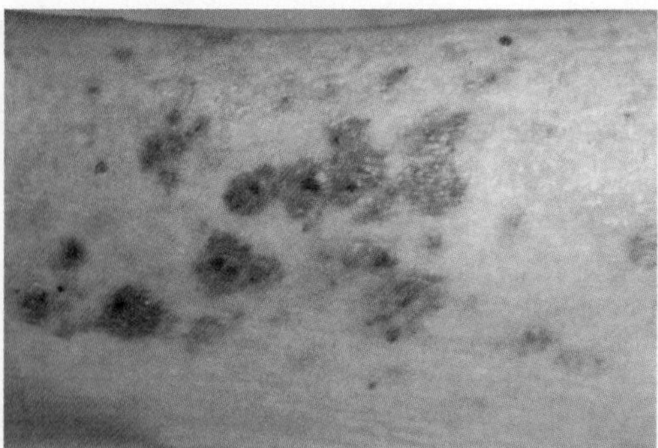

Figure 121–4 Stasis purpura (palpable).

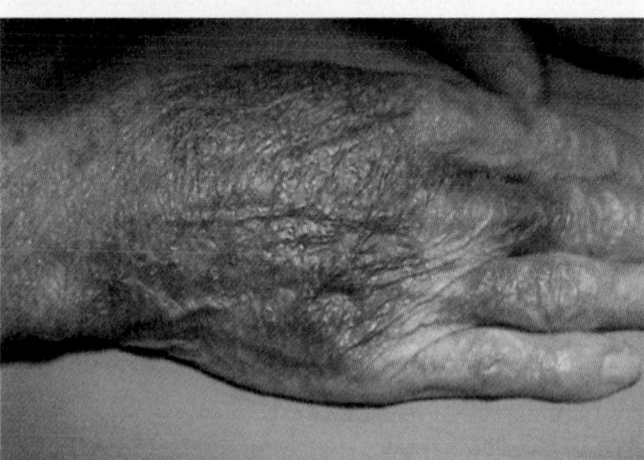

Figure 121–5 Actinic purpura.

Nonpalpable Purpura

Increased Transmural Pressure

Acute

The clinical picture of minute petechiae of the face (especially the eyelids; Fig. 121–3), neck, and upper chest may be seen after prolonged Valsalva maneuvers, crying, coughing, vomiting, childbirth, weight lifting, generalized seizures, vigorous exercise, thoracoabdominal compression, child abuse, bungee jumping, or spirometry.[51–54] A similar syndrome can be found in newborns with umbilical cord strangulation. For the child being evaluated for abuse, the presence of petechiae with or without bruising may indicate an increased likelihood of nonaccidental injury.[55] Lesions on the lower extremities, especially in the elderly, may be due to acute venous stasis from venous insufficiency, compression of the inferior vena cava (as occurs with an aortic aneurysm), or wearing of tight clothing or stockings. Occasionally, such dependent purpura may be palpable (Fig. 121–4), even in the absence of microscopic inflammation.

Purpura may accompany an increase in transmural pressure due to reduced extravascular pressure rather than increased intravascular pressure. Thus, suction purpura may result from application and/or careless removal of electrocardiographic leads, "cupping" devices used during religious rituals, rubber suction cups on toys, sitting in the bathtub,[56] or gas masks; kissing accompanied by suction also may leave its mark.[57] Cutaneous petechiae have been described in mountain climbers ascending higher than 3,800 m above sea level,[58] and petechiae and hemorrhagic bullae have been observed in the external auditory canals of pilots who fly at high altitudes.[59]

Chronic

As a result of humans assuming an upright posture, venous pressure is greater in the lower than the upper extremities. This increased pressure makes the lower extremities more vulnerable to loss of vascular integrity. Thus, the first signs of petechiae due to hemostatic defects commonly, but not universally, appear at the ankles. Moreover, other common cutaneous disorders, such as drug rashes, contact dermatitis,[60] and sunburn, often progress to become petechial and purpuric over the lower extremities. Chronic venous stasis of the lower extremities, due either to venous valvular incompetence or chronic use of tight-fitting garments, exacerbates this phenomenon and can convert subclinical insults of diverse etiologies into frank purpura. Thus, recurrent episodes of extravasation of red blood cells lead to the development of purpuric and yellow brown macules, the latter due to the persistent presence of hemosiderin.

Decreased Mechanical Integrity of Microcirculation and Supporting Tissues

Age Related (Infancy and Actinic Purpura)

Approximately one fourth of normal infants younger than 1 year have some petechiae,[61] and this may reflect vascular incompetence.

At the other end of the age spectrum, chronic solar damage and decreased collagen, elastin, and ground substance due to advanced age may result in the development of characteristic red to purple purpuric patches on the extensor surfaces of the forearms and hands (actinic purpura; Fig. 121–5). The skin accompanying actinic purpura is particularly thin and lacks elasticity, making it especially susceptible to tears induced by shearing forces.[62] Owing to the decreased healing capacity that accompanies aging, the purpuric changes may take months to resolve. Interestingly, the syndromes of premature aging, such as progeria, Werner syndrome, and acrogeria, all may give rise to acral purpuric changes identical to those of purpura in the elderly.[58]

Glucocorticoid Excess (Cushing Syndrome and Glucocorticoid Therapy)

The patches of purpura in Cushing syndrome are classically described as appearing on the extensor surfaces of the forearms, but they may appear on both the flexor and extensor aspects of both the upper and lower extremities. As with actinic purpura, the lesions have a very characteristic bright red appearance, and the skin is fragile.[23] Shearing stress is often the immediate cause of the purpura, and the patches may last for weeks to months. Use of potent fluorinated topical glucocorticosteroids, either with or without occlusive dressings, may result in cutaneous atrophy and purpura.[63] Glucocorticosteroids administered parenterally, orally, or by inhalation may produce similar changes. Microscopy reveals loss of dermal connective tissue with thinning of the epidermis.

Vitamin C Deficiency (Scurvy)

Follicular keratosis, petechiae, and perifollicular purpura with entrapped corkscrew hairs of the arms, legs, back, and buttocks are the characteristic findings of vitamin C deficiency (Fig. 121–6). After 2 to 3 months of inadequate vitamin C intake, swelling, pain, and purpura develop, followed by larger ecchymoses and hemorrhagic

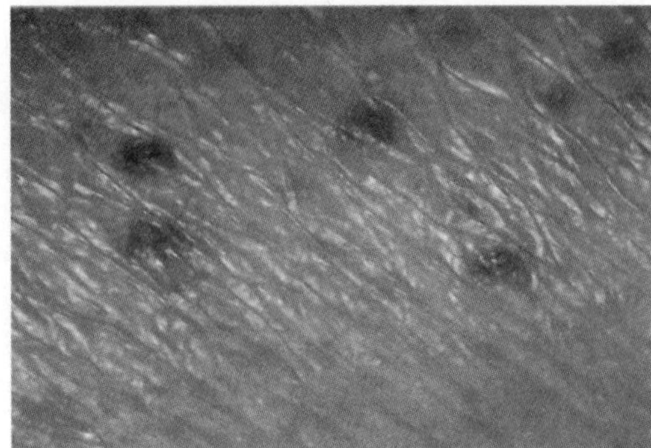

Figure 121–6 Scurvy.

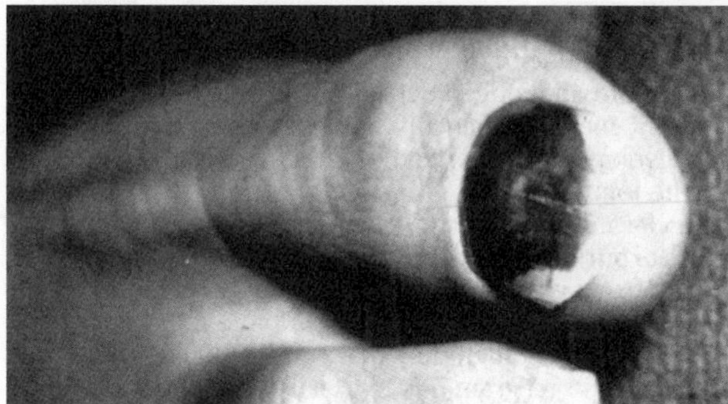

Figure 121–7 "Tennis toe": subungual hemorrhage.

ulcers on the legs and mucous membranes.[64,65] Hemorrhagic gingivitis or stomatitis may occur. Conjunctivitis, myalgias, arthralgias, and bone pain result from localized hemorrhage. Subsequently, woody edema and hyperpigmentation of the legs remain as sequelae of chronic ascorbate deficiency.[66] Scurvy has been reported in the setting of liver transplantation.[67] The prevalence of vitamin C deficiency in hospitalized patients may be as high as 16%.[68]

Abnormal Connective Tissue—Ehlers-Danlos Syndrome

Easy bruising is one of the most prominent features of Ehlers-Danlos syndrome type IV, which is most commonly caused by a defect in the gene for type III collagen. However, bruising also may be seen in the other types. Milder forms of Ehlers-Danlos syndrome that do not meet the diagnostic criteria for the more classic forms have been described, and mild to moderate bruising may be seen in these patients.[69] When evaluating patients for this heterogenous group of connective tissue disorders, it is important to assess the elasticity of the skin, the extensibility of the joints, and the presence of associated abnormalities such as high-arched palate and pectus excavatum. Patients with type IV Ehlers-Danlos syndrome may manifest only joint hyperextensibility of the fingers and modest skin elasticity despite having ecchymoses and easy bruising; However, the skin is thin and translucent.[41] Arterial rupture and intestinal perforations are serious complications of this form of Ehlers-Danlos syndrome.[41] Patients with Marfan or Noonan syndrome also may have mild bleeding tendencies and increased capillary fragility.

Amyloid Infiltration of Blood Vessels

Mucocutaneous manifestations may be prominent in primary systemic amyloidosis associated with plasma cell dyscrasias.[70] Histologic examination demonstrates extensive infiltration of blood vessel walls with amyloid, resulting in increased vascular fragility. As a result, minimal trauma can produce hemorrhagic lesions ("pinch purpura"), and petechiae occur readily with increased transmural pressure (e.g., after Valsalva maneuver or proctoscopy), especially when the amyloid infiltrates the blood vessels in the eyelids and face (postproctoscopic periorbital purpura). A variety of cutaneous lesions can occur in patients with primary systemic amyloidosis, including brown- to tan-colored translucent papules, plaques, nodules, and bullae; these all may become hemorrhagic, either spontaneously or after minimal trauma. An enlarged scalloped tongue with peripheral indentations secondary to pressure from the adjacent teeth is frequently seen. Alopecia and nail changes are less common skin manifestations.

Colloid Milium

Colloid milium is a cutaneous disorder seen in patients with chronic ultraviolet light exposure. It is characterized clinically by translucent yellow papules and plaques and histologically by deposition of upper dermal amorphous eosinophilic material (similar in appearance to amyloid). Lesions of colloid milium may become purpuric after minimal trauma.[71]

?Hormonal—Female Easy Bruising Syndrome (Purpura Simplex)

The female predominance and the frequent association with phases of the menstrual cycle suggest that the female easy bruising syndrome (purpura simplex) is due to hormonal effects on the blood vessel and/or its surrounding tissues.[23] Antibody-mediated platelet dysfunction has been implicated in some patients.[25] Concomitant use of aspirin or other nonsteroidal antiinflammatory drugs may inhibit platelet function and contribute to the severity of the symptoms. Patients complain of frequent purpuric and ecchymotic lesions with minimal trauma. Patients with this entity usually are not at increased risk for hemorrhage from more severe hemostatic challenges such as surgery, but other potentially more serious hemostatic defects must be excluded.

Lorenzo's Oil

Purpura from a defect in vessel wall function has been seen in a patient receiving Lorenzo's oil (glycerol trioleate and glycerol trierucate).[72]

MELAS Syndrome

MELAS (mitochondrial myopathy, encephalopathy, lactic acidosis, stroke-like episodes) syndrome encompasses a group of disorders characterized by one or more enzymatic defects of aerobic metabolism that lead to morphologic changes of mitochondria in multiple organs. Recurrent crops of purpuric macules of the palms and soles have been described in association with MELAS syndrome.[73]

Trauma to Blood Vessels

Physical

Any form of injury, if severe enough, can damage blood vessels sufficiently to cause skin hemorrhage. Thus, it is important to know in detail the extent of the injury before deciding whether the skin hemorrhage is consistent with the magnitude of the trauma.[51] Traumatic lesions usually have well-defined margins. Depending on the etiology (e.g., occupational, accidental, recreational), the pattern may be annular or circumferential (e.g., paintball[74] or baseball injury), linear or loop shaped (e.g., child beating), or subungual (e.g., running shoe injury; Fig. 121–7). The lesions associated with child abuse often include both cutaneous purpura and petechiae of the genitalia, as well as the bulbar and palpebral conjunctivae, the latter reflecting strangulation, smothering, or both.[75,76] Patients with factitial, or self-

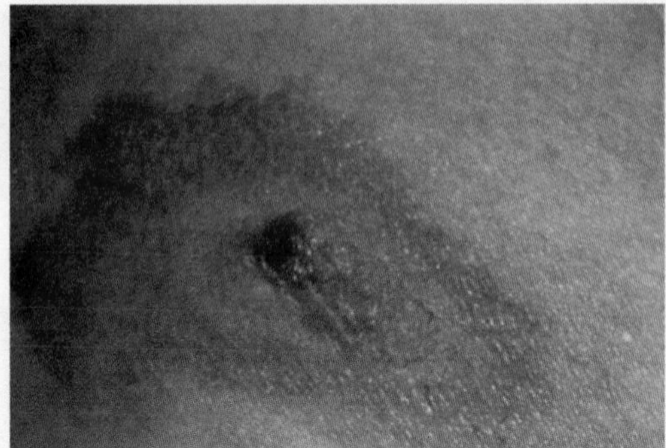

Figure 121–8 Ecthyma gangrenosum.

inflicted, purpura usually have medium- to large-sized lesions on the lower extremities, but other sites may be involved as well. They characteristically express indifference to the bruises. Crush injury may result in petechiae of the face, neck, and chest, sparing the skin of the central chest ("brassier sign").[77] Treatment of cutaneous vascular anomalies with a 585-nm pulsed dye laser can result in purpura.[78,79]

Ultraviolet Radiation

Acute severe sunburn can have a petechial component if the damage is sufficiently extensive. Petechial eruptions on the legs and trunk have been described after just brief exposures to natural sunlight (solar purpura).[80,81] Neonates with hyperbilirubinemia after transfusion may develop transient purpuric patches at sites of maximal exposure to blue light phototherapy, perhaps related to an interaction between the light and circulating porphyrins.[82]

Infectious

Bacterial, viral, fungal, rickettsial, protozoal, and parasitic infections all may produce purpura as a primary clinical manifestation.[83,84] In one study of children with fever and petechiae, approximately 10% had bacterial sepsis and approximately 50% had viral upper respiratory tract infections.[85] The pathogenesis of infectious purpura often is complex and may include direct vascular invasion by the organism, diffuse intravascular coagulation, immune complex vasculitis, Schwartzman-like phenomenon, septic emboli, and/or direct toxic effects on the vasculature. Although characteristic patterns of purpura have been described for the different agents, overlap between the patterns is common.

Gram-negative sepsis with *Pseudomonas* species, *Klebsiella* species, or *Escherichia coli* produces characteristic lesions of ecthyma gangrenosum, which begin as plaque-like areas of edema and erythema with subsequent nodule formation surmounted by irregular purpura (Fig. 121–8). The central area of purpura often is bullous and surrounded by concentric areas of normal skin and a thin band of erythema. Erosions and ulceration may occur. Lesions may be single or multiple, and the palms and soles occasionally may be involved. The differential diagnosis of ecthyma gangrenosum includes fungal sepsis due to *Candida* species, drug eruptions, cryoglobulinemia, Sweet syndrome, pyoderma gangrenosum, necrotizing vasculitis, polyarteritis nodosa, hyperviscosity syndrome, and leukemic infiltrates.[86]

Meningococcemia initially produces erythematous papules, but these soon evolve into stellate purple to slate-gray purpuric lesions (Fig. 121–9). Approximately 5% to 10% of children with fever and petechiae have meningococcemia.[85,87] One useful differentiating finding is that children with purpura confined to the distribution of the superior vena cava are much less likely to have meningococcemia than are those with more generalized purpura.[88] The combination of purulent meningitis and petechiae strongly suggests that *Neisseria meningitides* is the etiologic agent.[89] Acrocyanosis and symmetric peripheral gangrene may ensue and are thought to be due to disseminated intravascular coagulation (DIC). The purpura of meningococcemia may be due to direct vascular invasion by the organism or an

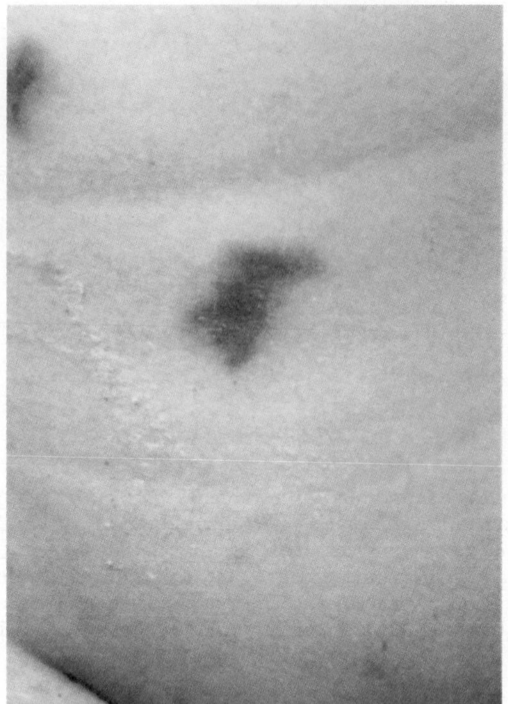

Figure 121–9 Meningococcemia.

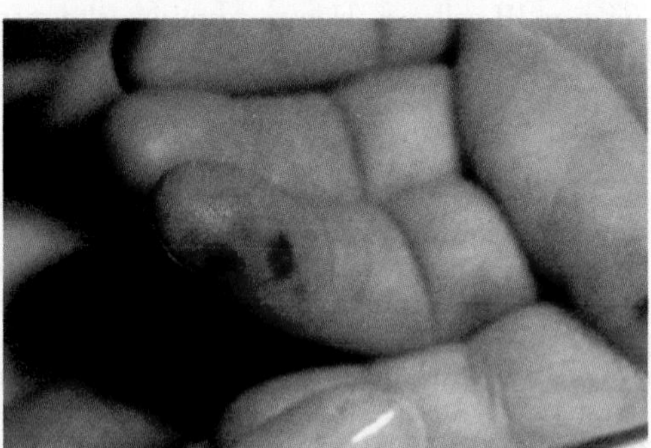

Figure 121–10 Acute bacterial endocarditis.

endotoxin-induced Shwartzman reaction. Microvascular thrombosis is a common pathologic finding, and the importance of thrombosis in the pathophysiology is reinforced by the observation that, in small clinical series, administration of antithrombin III concentrates,[90] recombinant tissue plasminogen activator,[91] or protein C[92,93] improved outcome. In chronic intermittent meningococcemia, an immune complex dermatitis may develop, characterized by hemorrhagic papulovesicles over the joints.

The classic rash of scarlet fever characteristically features linear purpuric lines in the skin folds (Pastia lines). Streptococcal pharyngitis has been reported to produce perioral, neck, and truncal petechiae in a small percentage of patients.

Bacterial sepsis, including acute and subacute bacterial endocarditis due to gram-positive or gram-negative organisms, may cause purpuric macules, papules, hemorrhagic bullae, erosions, and/or ulcers (Fig. 121–10). Some patients with endocarditis have antineutrophil cytoplasmic antibodies (ANCA), one of the manifestations of vasculitis, thus blurring the distinction between primary vasculitis and sepsis.[94]

Widespread ecchymoses and ischemic infarction of the skin are characteristic findings in purpura fulminans, which most commonly is associated with streptococcal, staphylococcal, pneumococcal, and meningococcal bacteremia but also may be caused by other bacteria,

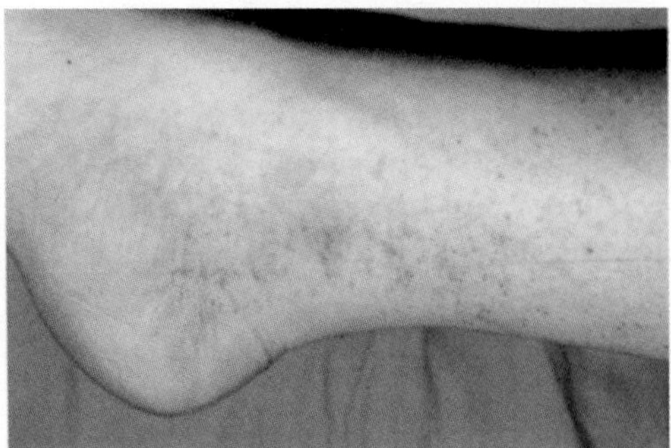

Figure 121–11 Rocky Mountain spotted fever.

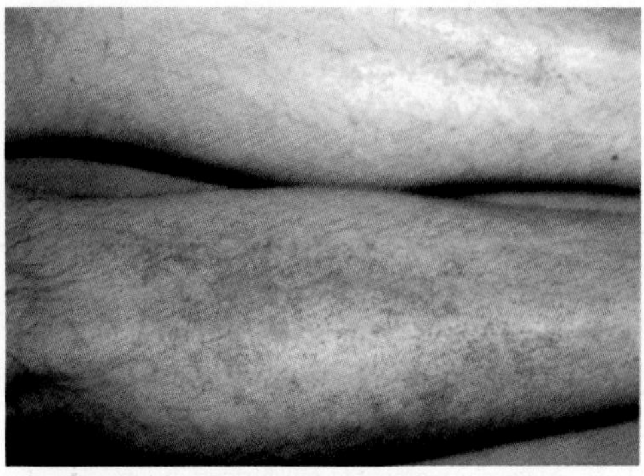

Figure 121–12 Schamberg pigmented purpuric eruption.

viruses, and fungi. The first manifestations of pneumococcal sepsis in asplenic patients may be facial petechiae and purpura, accompanied by acral cyanosis or livedo reticularis.[95] Whipple disease caused by *Tropheryma whipplei* presents rarely with nonthrombocytopenic, nonpalpable purpura.[96]

Splinter hemorrhages of the nails occur in subacute bacterial endocarditis, but they also can be seen in normal individuals following trauma or in patients with trichinosis, peptic ulceration, hypertension, malignancies, severe rheumatoid arthritis, and a number of dermatologic conditions. Thus, the specificity of splinter hemorrhages as a sign of endocarditis is limited.[97,98]

Rickettsial infections, including Rocky Mountain spotted fever (Fig. 121–11) and epidemic typhus, typically produce an array of cutaneous changes ranging from urticarial macules to petechiae, ecchymoses, and areas of hemorrhagic necrosis. Although the characteristic lesion of Lyme borreliosis is a nonpurpuric annular expanding plaque (erythema migrans), the central aspect of this lesion may contain a purpuric macule, papule, or hemorrhagic bulla.

Patients with either disseminated fungal infections (e.g., cryptococcosis, zygomycosis, candidemia, alternariosis, histoplasmosis, aspergillosis)[99,100] or locally invasive fungal diseases (e.g., mucormycosis) may have necrosis, purpura, and/or petechiae early in the course of the illness.[101] Viral infections may have primary purpuric eruptions as their presenting manifestations. Human parvovirus B19 infection has been described as causing a petechial or confluent purpuric rash on the buttocks, axilla, and/or chest,[102] a generalized petechial and purpuric eruption,[103,104] or petechiae limited to the genital area[105] or perioral region and chin (acropetechial syndrome).[106] Palatal petechiae may accompany the exanthem.[107]

One characteristic pattern of infectious purpura is papular purpuric gloves and socks syndrome. This disorder of adolescents and young adults is characterized by well-demarcated symmetric pruritic or painful acral edema and erythema, confluent petechial/purpuric papules and plaques of the hands and feet, oral erythema and erosions, swelling of the lips and tongue, and angular or erosive cheilitis. The inner thighs, inguinal region, buttocks, elbows, and knees may be involved. Systemic manifestations include fever, fatigue, myalgias, anorexia, lymphadenopathy, and arthralgias. The disorder is seen most commonly in association with infections caused by parvovirus B19 but also may be seen with measles virus,[108] cytomegalovirus, Coxsackie B6, rubella, human herpes virus 6, or human herpes virus 7.[109–113]

Patients with virus-associated hemophagocytic syndrome may present with petechiae and purpura.[114] Hanta virus-associated hemorrhagic fever with renal syndrome is transmitted to humans by wild rodents. Signs include fever, acute renal failure, headache, vomiting, and prostration associated with mucocutaneous petechiae, ecchymoses, facial flushing, periorbital edema, and conjunctival and palatal petechiae.[115]

Purpura may be the initial manifestation of parasitic infections, especially in the immunocompromised host. Migration of filariform larvae of *Strongyloides stercoralis* typically produces rapidly progressive abdominal thumbprint linear and reticulated purpura on a background of petechiae; the periumbilical region usually is most severely affected.[116–118] The disorder frequently is fatal. Disseminated *Pneumocystis jiroveci* infections in patients with AIDS may demonstrate purpuric papules and nodules that resemble the lesions of Kaposi sarcoma (see Kaposi Sarcoma and Other Vascular Sarcomas).[119]

Embolic

Atheroemboli with prominent cholesterol crystals, usually originating from atherosclerotic lesions in the aorta, produce a constellation of cutaneous findings, including acral petechiae and purpura, livedo reticularis, nodules, unilateral peripheral ulcers, and bilateral cyanosis and gangrene.[120] Distal pulses are present, and occasionally the emboli are seen in the retinal circulation as refractile interruptions in the column of arterial blood. The syndrome is seen most frequently in older men on anticoagulation or after vascular repair procedures. A high predilection for the pancreas makes elevated serum amylase levels a common accompanying laboratory finding.

Fat embolism may occur 2 to 3 days after severe external trauma or following liposuction. Initial findings include petechiae of the skin folds of the neck and axillae, upper extremities, chest, and/or conjunctivae. The full syndrome consists of hyperthermia, respiratory distress, retinal fat emboli, neurologic symptoms, and pulmonary infiltrates.[121] Emboli from left atrial myxomas may cause acral purpura; necrosis, livedo reticularis, or red papules; splinter hemorrhages; palpable purpura; claudication; peripheral cyanosis; leg ulcers; and/or Raynaud phenomenon.[122] Septic emboli from pseudoaneurysms following percutaneous transluminal coronary angioplasty due to *Staphylococcus aureus* have produced a syndrome of palpable purpura, petechiae, and livedo reticularis.[123]

Allergic and/or Inflammatory

In serum sickness, morbilliform or urticarial eruptions are the most common manifestations. Linear or serpiginous bands of erythema along the sides of the hands and feet may be seen at the margins of the palmar or plantar surfaces.[102] In patients who are thrombocytopenic, purpura usually appears within these linear bands. The eruption often heralds onset of the syndrome. Immunologic evaluation of biopsy material often demonstrates immunoglobulin and complement deposits.

The pigmented purpuric eruptions,[119,124–127] including Schamberg disease, Majocchi disease, and others, are a poorly understood group of disorders characterized by petechiae and purpura on a background of light to dark brown or orange hyperpigmentation (Figs. 121–12 to 121–14). Telangiectasias may or may not be present. Scaling, lichenification, and atrophy are seen occasionally. These eruptions characteristically involve the lower extremities but also may be seen on the arms or trunk; occasionally they are found on the palms and soles.[128] They are not associated with any systemic manifestations. Systemically administered medications (e.g., hydrochlorothiazide, diltiazem, pseudoephedrine, glipizide, and acetaminophen) have been implicated as the cause in some patients,[129,130] as have chronic dental infections.[131] Histologically, extravasation of red blood cells,

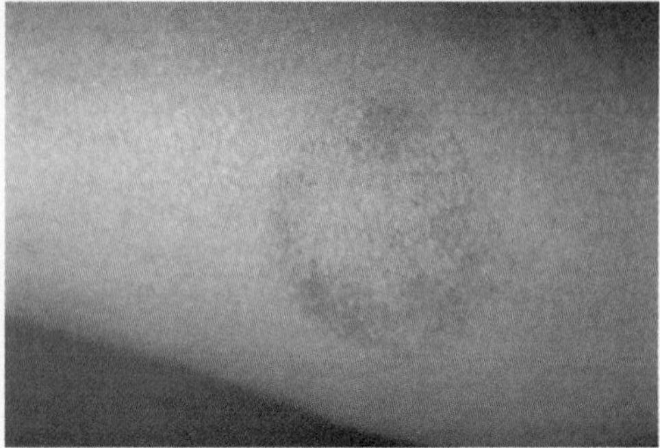

Figure 121–13 Majocchi pigmented purpuric eruption.

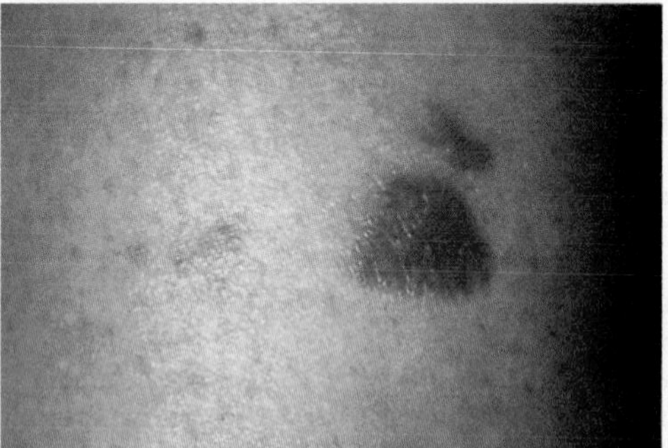

Figure 121–14 Lichen aureus.

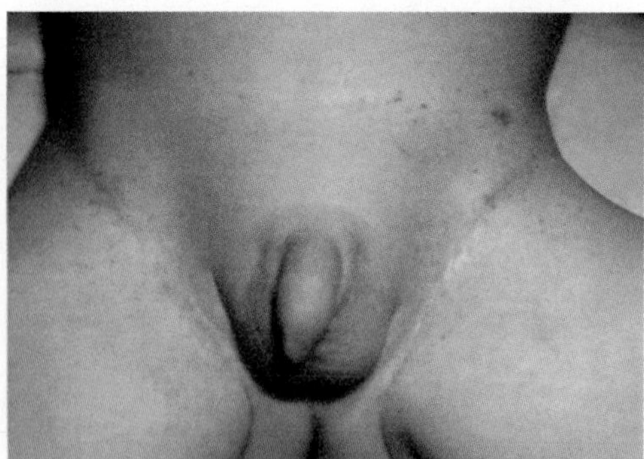

Figure 121–15 Letterer-Siwe disease (Langerhans cell histiocytosis).

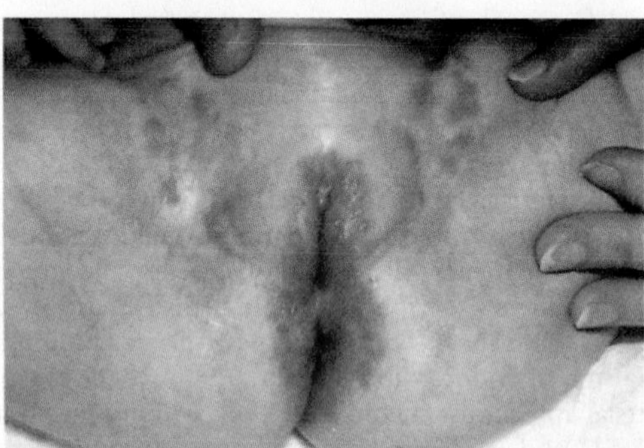

Figure 121–16 Histiocytosis X.

hemosiderin deposits within macrophages, and a perivascular lymphohistiocytic infiltrate with endothelial cell swelling are seen. The pathogenesis of these disorders is not established, but suggested mechanisms include increased capillary fragility with rupture of capillaries in the papillary dermis, aneurysmal dilation of the microvasculature, and abnormal cellular immune responses to an unknown antigen.[132] Involved skin contains activated helper T cells and keratinocytes that stain positive for antigenic markers associated with receptors for effector immune cells.[133] Cutaneous T-cell lymphoma can produce lesions simulating those found with the pigmented purpuric eruptions.[134] Other disorders that must be included in the differential diagnosis are purpuric clothing dermatitis, sensitivity to food additives, lichen nitidus,[135] and hyperglobulinemic purpura of Waldenström.

Pyoderma gangrenosum is a destructive, necrotizing ulceration of the skin presenting as a nodule, pustule, or hemorrhagic bulla. Lesions occur on the calves, thighs, buttocks, and face. Lesions heal with atrophic and cribriform scars. Pyoderma gangrenosum may occur in association with inflammatory bowel disease, rheumatoid arthritis, other polyarthritic and vasculitic syndromes, blood dyscrasias, leukemia, lymphoma, and multiple myeloma. A superficial hemorrhagic bullous form occurs with acute leukemia or other myeloproliferative disorders.

Allergic or irritant contact dermatitis to clothing, rubber, woolen garments, elastic, benzoyl peroxide, dyes, balsam of Peru,[136] eutectic mixture of local anesthetics (EMLA),[137] or detergent whiteners may result in purpuric eruptions that simulate the pigmented purpuric eruptions.[138]

Familial Mediterranean fever is a recessively inherited autoinflammatory disease associated with mutations in the MEFV gene, which codes for the protein pyrin.[139] Petechial or palpable purpuric lesions on the face, trunk, and extremities have been described in a minority of children with familial Mediterranean fever; the lesions usually resolve spontaneously.[140] True vasculitis has been frequently observed in patients with familial Mediterranean fever.[141,142] The protracted febrile myalgia syndrome of familial Mediterranean fever consists of fever, severe paralyzing myalgias, abdominal pain, diarrhea, arthritis and arthralgias, and transient palpable purpuric eruptions mimicking Henoch-Schönlein purpura.[143,144]

Intraabdominal inflammatory diseases such as acute pancreatitis, ruptured ectopic pregnancy, and perforated duodenal ulcer may result in periumbilical purpura (Cullen sign). Similarly, purpura of the flanks (Grey Turner sign) may be an indicator of retroperitoneal hemorrhage. In Langerhans cell histiocytosis, purpuric papules are observed in the seborrheic areas of the scalp, flexures, and groin in children and may be generalized in adults.[145,146]

Neoplastic

Infiltration of the skin in the Langerhans cell histiocytosis group of disorders, including Letterer-Siwe disease and histiocytosis X, can result in the development of a petechial and purpuric papular and crusted dermatitis of the seborrheic areas of the scalp, flexures, and groin (Figs. 121–15 and 121–16). This disorder most commonly affects children but has been reported in adults as a generalized dermatitis.[145,146] Cutaneous T-cell lymphoma may produce cutaneous lesions similar to those seen in the pigmented purpuric eruptions.[147] Similarly, skin infiltrations in patients with leukemias, lymphomas, and plasma cell disorders can produce red to purple papules that simulate purpura.[148] T-cell prolymphocytic leukemia characteristically demonstrates facial edema, purpura, and lesional symmetry.[149] Adult T-cell leukemia may demonstrate purpura at sites of the malignant infiltrate.[150] Patients with hemophagocytic lymphohistiocytosis, a disorder of cytokine dysfunction and uncontrolled activation of T lymphocytes and histiocytes, demonstrate facial erythema and edema, purpura, and morbilliform eruptions.[151]

Metabolic

Patients with erythropoietic protoporphyria may develop purpuric lesions of the dorsum of the hands in areas of edema and erythema after ultraviolet light exposure. Damage to endothelial cells has been postulated as the mechanism of extravasation of red blood cells.[152]

Calciphylaxis is a syndrome consisting of vascular and subcutaneous calcification in patients with secondary hyperparathyroidism due to end-stage renal failure.[153] Livedoid hemorrhagic necrosis may be observed in these patients. Subcutaneous and vascular calcifications

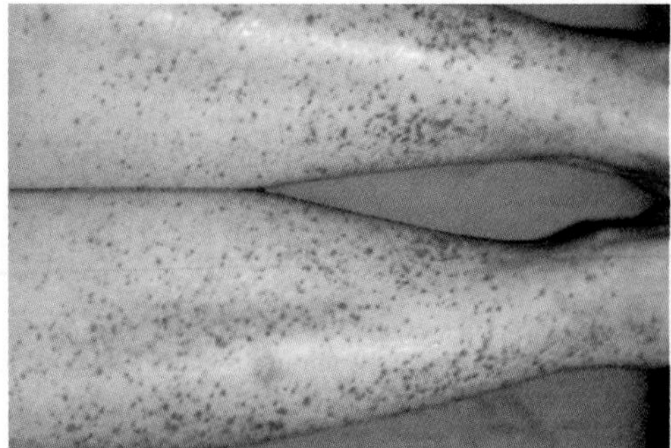

Figure 121–17 Waldenström hyperglobulinemic purpura.

may follow calcium gluconate infusions or may accompany chronic hypercalcemia. They may result in cutaneous necrosis and hemorrhage, typically in a speckled or vascular pattern.

Relapsing showers of petechiae on the trunk and extremities are observed in infants with ethylmalonic aciduria, a metabolic disorder associated with acral cyanosis, chronic diarrhea, and progressive central nervous system dysfunction.[154,155]

Patients with primary hyperoxalosis (deficiency of hepatic alanine-glyoxylate transaminase) may develop a syndrome of necrotizing livedo reticularis, renal failure, and cardiomyopathy.[156]

Immunoglobulin-related (Hyperglobulinemic Purpura of Waldenström and Light Chain Vasculopathy)

Macular or slightly raised discrete or confluent purpuric lesions with hemosiderin staining are the classic cutaneous findings of benign hyperglobulinemic purpura of Waldenström (Fig. 121–17), a syndrome that occurs most often on the legs of women aged 20 to 40 years.[126,157] Palpable purpura is rare. Precipitating factors include increased hydrostatic pressure, hyperviscosity, and low temperatures.[158,159] The polyclonal increase in globulins (mostly IgG1) can be associated with Sjögren syndrome,[160] systemic lupus erythematosus, polymyositis, rheumatoid arthritis, myeloma, thymoma, sarcoid, or multiple sclerosis. Because patients may have recurrent crops of purpuric lesions, pigmented purpuric eruptions must be excluded. Histologically, acute inflammatory cells, red blood cells, and arteriolar necrosis predominate. Elevated serum levels of IgG, IgA, and IgM may be observed.[161] Circulating immunoglobulin-containing complexes may be present.[162] Many patients have antibodies to Ro/SSA,[163] and children born to women with hyperglobulinemic purpura of Waldenström have been reported to develop congenital heart block.[164]

A vasculopathy due to deposition of λ light-chain crystals can produce nonpalpable purpura, hemorrhagic vesicles, ischemic necrosis of the extremities, and rapidly progressive renal failure.[165] Intravascular λ light chains can be observed on direct immunofluorescence of skin, and monoclonal λ light chains are present in the serum.

Drug Related

Petechial and purpuric reactions can be observed after administration of a variety of drugs, including aspirin, alclofenac, allopurinol, atropine, belladonna, bismuth, carbamazepine, carbimazole, carbromal, chloral hydrate, chlordiazepoxide, cimetidine, desipramine, disopyramide, doxepin, fenbufen, gefitinib (epidermal growth factor receptor inhibitor),[166] gold salts, indomethacin, iodides, isoniazid, meclofenamate sodium, mefenamic acid, menthol, mercury, morphine, naproxen, nitrofurantoin, penicillamine, penicillin, phenacetin, phenytoin, piperazine, piroxicam, pyrazolone derivatives, quinine, quinidine, sulfonamides, sulindac, thiouracils, and tolmetin.[167] Topical application of EMLA cream has been reported to result in purpura at the site of application.[168] The mechanism for at least some of these reactions is presumed to be allergic hypersensitivity.

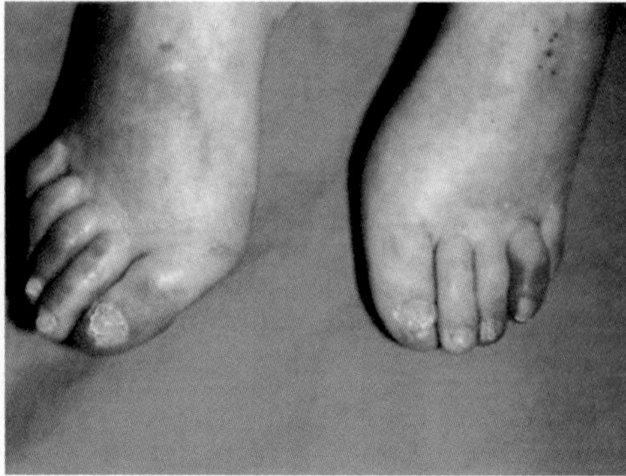

Figure 121–18 Acral cyanosis in disseminated intravascular coagulation.

Thrombotic

Disseminated Intravascular Coagulation. DIC may result from a variety of different insults, many of which have the common denominator of producing hypotension (see Chapter 132). The etiologies of DIC include sepsis, severe trauma, malignancy, obstetric conditions, vascular malformations, toxins, immune-mediated disorders, and shock, cardiac arrest, and heat stroke.[169] Because endothelial cells are active metabolically, hypotension can produce widespread ischemia and endothelial cell damage. The damage can expose subendothelial surfaces, which in turn can initiate an uncontrolled thrombotic response that ultimately selectively depletes coagulation factors and platelets. Alternative mechanisms for initiating the process involve the effects of endotoxin and other mediators, such as interleukin (IL)-1 and tumor necrosis factor, on endothelial cell and monocyte procoagulant activity. This is achieved, at least in part, by induction of tissue factor expression, increased synthesis of tissue plasminogen activator inhibitor, and decreased production of both thrombomodulin and tissue plasminogen activator. Abnormalities of the protein C anticoagulant pathway also are present.[170] Severe deficiency of von Willebrand factor-cleaving protease (ADAMTS13) has been reported in patients with sepsis-induced DIC and may contribute to the renal failure found in association with DIC.[171]

Given the potential for both thrombotic and hemorrhagic manifestations, the diverse skin manifestations are not surprising. The most common skin findings of DIC are acral cyanosis (Fig. 121–18) and variable petechial, purpuric, and ecchymotic lesions (Fig. 121–19). The competence of the fibrinolytic system to digest deposited fibrin determines the extent of tissue compromise. In the most severe cases, acral hemorrhagic gangrene can occur.[83] The presence of peripheral gangrene may be an important consideration in the often difficult decision to use heparin for treatment of the syndrome. The clinical and laboratory differential diagnosis of DIC includes thrombotic thrombocytopenic purpura, chronic DIC (Trousseau syndrome), fulminant hepatic failure, and the HELLP (hemolysis, elevated liver enzymes, and low platelet count) syndrome.[169]

Warfarin-Induced Skin Necrosis. Skin necrosis affects 0.01% to 0.1% of all patients receiving warfarin (Coumarin) and can appear anytime from day 2 to day 14 (usually days 3–6) of therapy.[172,173] Patients who are deficient in protein C appear to be at high risk because the disorder is thought to be due to a temporary imbalance between the procoagulant and anticoagulant vitamin K factors.[174–177] Warfarin-induced skin necrosis begins suddenly as painful erythematous patches (Fig. 121–20) that become edematous and indurated and rapidly progress to irregularly hemorrhagic and necrotic plaques, nodules, and bullae. Eventually large tumid indurations and infarcts occur with eschar formation and sloughing (Fig. 121–21).[178,179] The syndrome is more common in women than in men. The lesions often develop in the skin overlying fatty areas, such as the buttocks, thighs, and breasts. In men, involvement of the penis has been reported.[172] Lesions may be symmetric and widely distributed; occasionally they

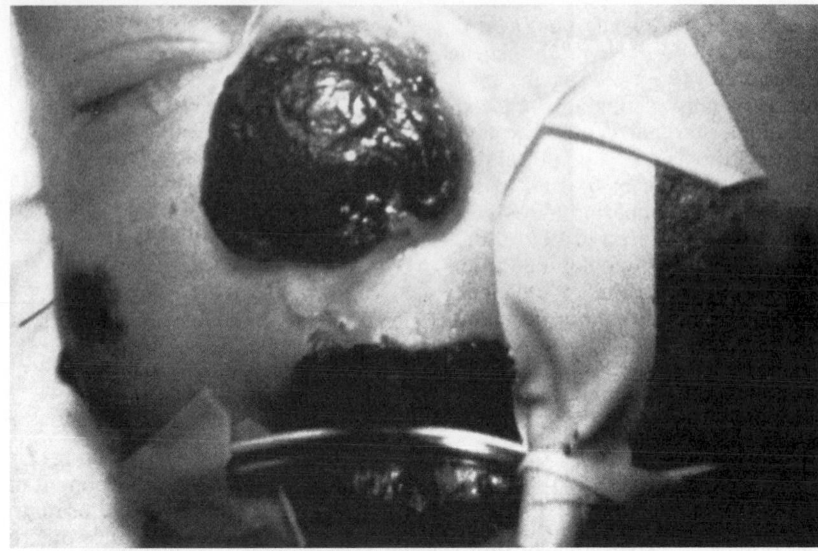

Figure 121–19 Lesion in disseminated intravascular coagulation.

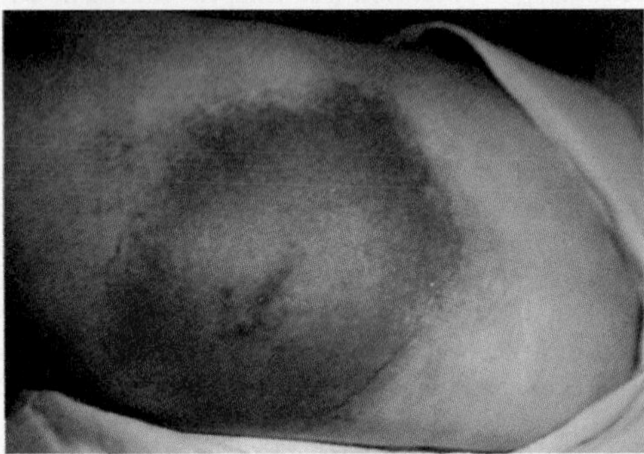

Figure 121–20 Warfarin-induced skin necrosis.

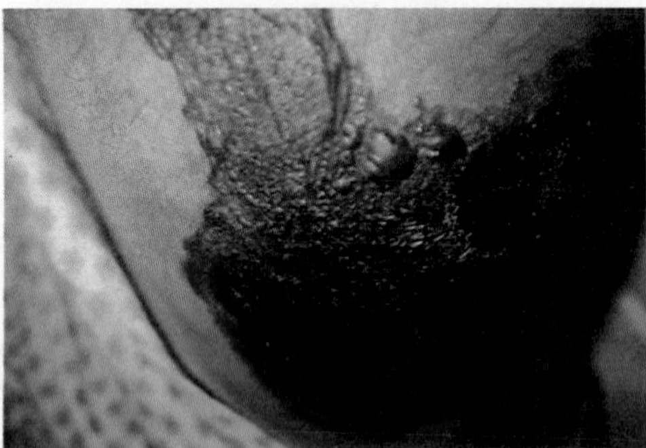

Figure 121–21 Warfarin-induced skin necrosis.

are severe enough to require surgical intervention.[180,181] Histologically, fibrin and platelet thrombi are observed in the dermal and subcutaneous vasculature. In one study, tumor necrosis factor was identified in the lesions, and endothelial cell adhesion molecules were upregulated.[182] The lesions of warfarin-induced skin necrosis can be differentiated from hemorrhagic lesions due to excessive warfarin administration by the presence of the nearly black eschar in the center of the necrotic zone and by histologic examination. Ancillary differentiating points in favor of warfarin-induced skin necrosis include predilection for the female gender, absence of an excessively prolonged prothrombin time, and temporal relationship to the start of warfarin therapy.

Protein C or Protein S Deficiency, Factor V Leiden, Prothrombin G20201A. Homozygous protein C deficiency[183,184] and compound heterozygosity for protein C deficiency[185] have been reported to produce diffuse purpuric and ecchymotic skin lesions suggestive of chronic DIC and purpura fulminans (see Purpura Fulminans).[177,186,187] Widespread venous thrombosis usually accompanies the skin lesions, and central nervous system thrombosis and blindness can occur. The skin lesions and venous thrombosis respond rapidly to therapy with plasma. Long-term therapy may require careful introduction of oral anticoagulants.[188] Replacement therapy with protein C concentrate has been successful.[189,190] Cutaneous necrosis similar to that observed with warfarin-induced skin necrosis has been reported in association with acquired protein C deficiency due to liver disease, malabsorption, antibiotic administration, or autoantibodies to protein C.[191] Infants with homozygous protein S deficiency or resistance to activated protein C due to homozygous factor V Leiden have demonstrated neonatal recurrent purpura fulminans.[192,193] An association between purpura fulminans and combined prothrombotic abnormalities (prothrombin G20201A, factor V Leiden, inherited or acquired protein S deficiency) has been reported in a number of patients, raising the possibility that one or more of these mutations predisposes individuals to infection-related purpura fulminans (see Purpura Fulminans).[194–196] Varicella infection can be accompanied by transient development of autoantibodies to protein S, protein C, or other coagulation proteins, but the development of such antibodies is not predictive of purpura fulminans.[197,198]

Purpura Fulminans. Purpura fulminans is the term given to the most profound cutaneous manifestation of DIC. It is characterized by fever, hypotension, and progression from acral erythema and edema to petechiae, purpura and localized ecchymoses, and ultimately massive, widespread ecchymoses[199,200] and hemorrhagic bullae with progression to infarction of the skin (Fig. 121–22).[201] Widespread arterial and venous thrombosis often accompanies these manifestations. Clinically, purpura fulminans mimics catastrophic antiphospholipid antibody syndrome.[202] Purpura fulminans is associated with a high mortality rate (>50%). It is triggered most commonly by infection with *N. meningitides, Streptococcus pneumoniae,* or *Haemophilus influenzae* in adults or children[203] but may be initiated by any of the infectious agents discussed in Infectious Trauma to Blood Vessels.[83,204] *Staphylococcus aureus*-associated purpura fulminans has been described.[205] The pathogenesis of purpura fulminans is postulated to include a Schwartzman reaction precipitated by endotoxin in gram-negative infections and exotoxin in gram-positive infections mediated by tumor necrosis factor α and IL-1, resulting in consumption of the anticoagulant proteins C and S and antithrombin III.

Patients with sepsis-induced purpura fulminans characteristically have very low levels of protein C.[206] Postvaricella purpura fulminans

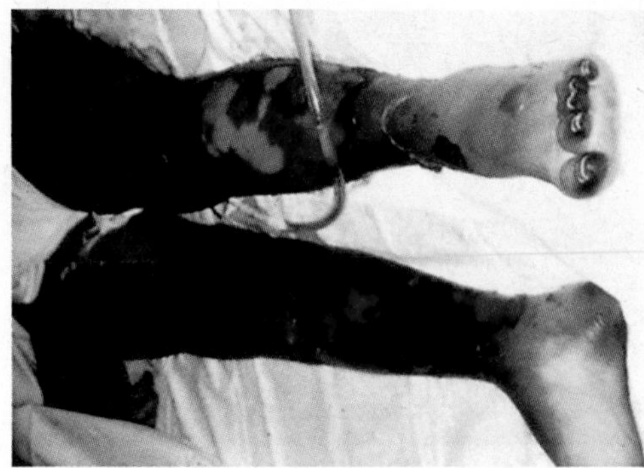

Figure 121–22 Purpura fulminans following herpes zoster.

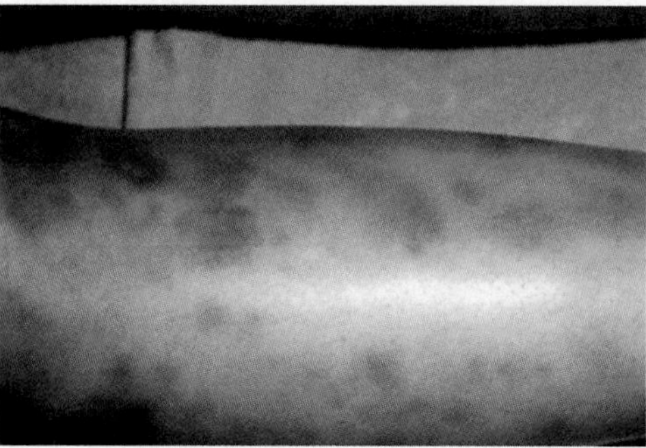

Figure 121–23 Psychogenic purpura.

is associated with acute transient deficiencies of protein C, protein S, or antithrombin III.[207] Anti-protein S antibodies may be transiently present.[208]

Purpura fulminans may occur without antecedent infections.[209] Homozygous protein S, protein C deficiency, or factor V Leiden can produce essentially the same pattern in the neonate,[187] and heterozygous, doubly heterozygous, or acquired abnormalities in these proteins, as well as the prothrombin G20210A mutation, may predispose individuals to develop infection-related purpura fulminans (see Protein C or Protein S Deficiency, Factor V Leiden, Prothrombin G20201A).[194–196] An association between hereditary angioedema, the factor V Leiden mutation, and purpura fulminans has been proposed.[210] Clinically, the syndrome of purpura fulminans most often begins as skin discomfort, followed by erythema, edema, and petechiae. Thereafter painful symmetric purple-gray papules and plaques surrounded by an advancing red border develop. Finally, massive widespread ecchymoses, symmetric, hemorrhagic necrosis, and bulla formation of the arms and legs, abdomen, thighs, and buttocks are seen.[199,200] Head and neck involvement is uncommon, and mucous membranes usually are spared. Ultimately the lesions may progress to gangrene, often with autoamputation of the digits. Associated symptoms and signs include prostration, fever, and edema of the extremities; death is not uncommon. In children, purpura fulminans most commonly follows bacterial infections with the meningococcus, pneumococcus, or group A β-hemolytic streptococcus, or viral infections with varicella or upper respiratory viruses.[211] Treatment with fresh frozen plasma may dramatically improve prognosis.[212] Successful adjunctive treatment of acute infectious purpura fulminans in children and adults with activated protein C has been described.[213,214]

Histopathology reveals hemorrhagic necrosis of the dermis with thromboses of the capillaries and small blood vessels. Fibrinoid necrosis of vessel walls and perivascular granulocytic infiltrates have been described.

The differential diagnosis includes thrombotic thrombocytopenic purpura, allergic or septic vasculitis, postinfectious thrombocytopenia, homozygous protein C or S deficiency, warfarin-induced necrosis, antiphospholipid antibody syndrome, paroxysmal nocturnal hemoglobinuria, and dermal hemorrhage.

Paroxysmal Nocturnal Hemoglobinuria. Occasional patients with paroxysmal nocturnal hemoglobinuria (see Chapter 30) may develop erythematous patches with dusky centers that enlarge to form painful plaques of erythema with central necrosis.[215–217] Hemorrhagic bullae, ulcerations, petechiae, ecchymoses, palpable purpura, and eschar formation may develop. Histologically, intravascular thrombi are seen in the absence of vasculitis.

Antiphospholipid Antibody Syndrome. The antiphospholipid antibody syndrome (see Chapter 131), whose cardinal manifestations are a tendency to thrombosis, thrombocytopenia, and fetal wastage,[218] is often associated with cutaneous manifestations. They are highly variable and may include purpura, ecchymoses, widespread cutaneous necrosis with thrombi within the microvasculature (similar to that seen in purpura fulminans), livedo reticularis, peripheral ischemia and gangrene, leg ulcers, pyoderma gangrenosum-like lesions, dermographism, acrocyanosis, Raynaud phenomenon, urticaria, diffuse alopecia, porcelain white scars, painful skin nodules, subungual splinter hemorrhages, pterygium unguium, and acral red to purple macules.[219,220] A subset of microangiopathic antiphospholipid syndrome may include thrombotic thrombocytopenic purpura, HELLP syndrome, and catastrophic antiphospholipid syndrome (Asherson syndrome).[221,222]

The antibody profile of patients with antiphospholipid antibody syndrome includes IgG and IgM antibodies directed against β_2-glycoprotein I, IgM antibodies to factor VII/activated factor VII, and lupus anticoagulant-type antibodies.[223]

Hemangioma with Thrombocytopenia and Consumptive Coagulopathy (Kasabach-Merritt Syndrome). The Kasabach-Merritt syndrome is defined by the presence of a reddish or purple mass in a neonate or young infant in association with widespread ecchymoses, thrombocytopenia, and a "localized" consumptive coagulopathy.[224] The large mass is a vascular lesion (kaposiform hemangioendothelioma or tufted angioma) in which platelets deposit and coagulation is initiated.[224] Management of such lesions requires stabilization of hemostasis and removal or ablation of the lesion.[224]

Unknown Causes—Psychogenic Purpura

Psychogenic purpura is the term given to a poorly understood disorder characterized by severe recurrent erythema, swelling, pain, and ecchymoses. It affects women much more commonly than men (Fig. 121–23).[26–29,225,226] Patients usually experience pain before or at the time the bruise appears, and the bruising often is so extensive that the patient loses use of the limb during the healing process. In the most severe cases, the patient becomes bedridden. Attempts to identify the etiology have been unsuccessful. Some studies have implicated allergic reactions to blood cells or DNA.[26,28,29,227–230] Localized neurogenic release of fibrinolytic activity in the skin also has been proposed as a mechanism linking the psychological and dermal components of the syndrome.[231] Psychological profiles of patients with this disorder have demonstrated widespread abnormalities,[26,232] raising the possibility of self-inflicted trauma, a view supported by the healing that usually accompanies casting. Whether this is the cause in all cases is far from certain, so it is best to continue to classify the etiology as unknown.

Palpable Purpura

Cutaneous Vasculitides

Patients with lupus erythematosus, dermatomyositis, scleroderma, rheumatoid arthritis,[233] and Sjögren syndrome,[234,235] as well as patients with systemic large and small vessel vasculitis (including urticarial or hypocomplementemic vasculitis,[236] polyarteritis nodosa,[237] micro-

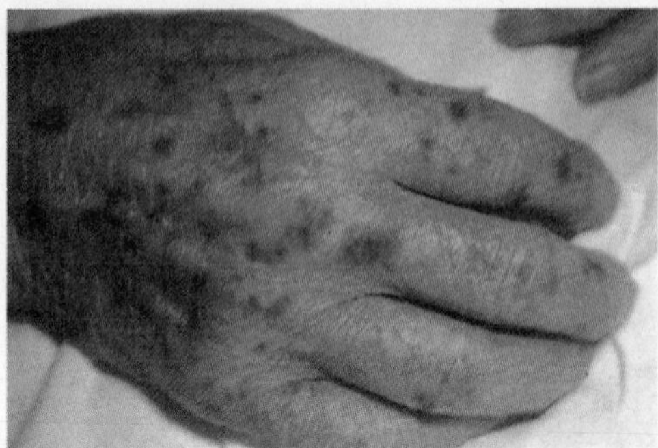

Figure 121–24 Rheumatoid vasculitis.

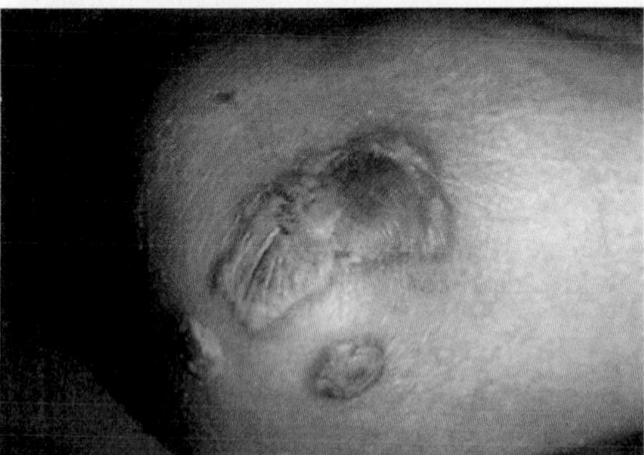

Figure 121–25 Wegener granulomatosis.

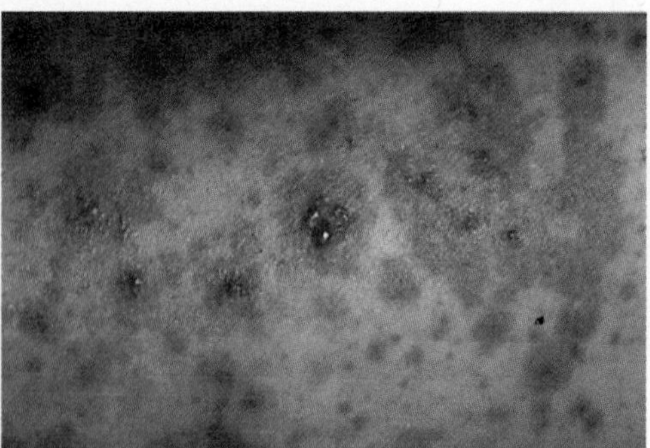

Figure 121–26 Henoch-Schönlein purpura.

scopic polyangiitis,[238–240] Wegener granulomatosis,[241] Behçet disease, Churg-Strauss angiitis,[242] rheumatoid vasculitis, relapsing polychondritis, or undefined vasculitis[243]) may have an array of vasculitic purpuric lesions, including petechiae, papules (palpable purpura), ecchymoses, hemorrhagic bullae, splinter hemorrhages, and periungual hemorrhages (Figs. 121–24 and 121–25).[162,244–254] In microscopic polyangiitis, purpuric skin lesions are present in 15% to 50% of patients.[240] In Sjögren syndrome, approximately 25% of patients have vasculitis with palpable purpura.[234] Nonpurpuric cutaneous lesions may be present, including ulcers, subcutaneous nodules, livedo reticularis, erythema of the face and hands, erythematous plaques, telangiectasias,[255] oral ulcers, and facial edema.[240] Early in the evolution of vasculitis, immune complexes, histamine, thrombin, IL-1, interferon γ, and substance P activate endothelial cells, resulting in release of plasminogen activators and development of urticarial lesions. Late in the process, activated neutrophils release tumor necrosis factor α, proteases, and oxygen free radicals, leading to perturbations of endothelial cells, decreased fibrinolytic activity, microvascular thrombosis, and tissue hypoxia and ischemia, which become manifest as palpable purpura.[256]

Drugs,[257] alcohol,[258] immunoadsorption therapy,[259] and infections are common causes of small vessel (hypersensitivity) vasculitis.[260] Clinical findings include palpable purpura, joint symptoms, and systemic and cutaneous vasculitis. Bacterial infections with staphylococci, streptococci, *Mycobacterium leprae, Mycobacterium tuberculosis,* and others are often associated with vasculitic lesions.[261,262] Subacute bacterial endocarditis due to *Streptococcus viridans* or other organisms may be associated with circulating immune complexes that produce cutaneous and/or systemic leukocytoclastic vasculitis. These syndromes may be accompanied by the development of cytoplasmic antineutrophil cytoplasmic antibodies (cANCA) in association with antiproteinase-3 antibodies.[94,263] Viruses associated with vasculitis include HIV, hepatitis B, hepatitis C, and parvovirus. Hepatitis B is strongly associated with polyarteritis nodosa.[264] Parvovirus has been reported in association with polyarteritis nodosa, Wegener granulomatosis, and Henoch-Schönlein purpura.[265] The tetrad of necrotizing vasculitis, chronic hepatitis C infection, hypocomplementemia, and cryoglobulinemia is a late manifestation of hepatitis C infection.[266]

α_1-Antitrypsin deficiency has been described in association with manifestations of systemic vasculitis, including cutaneous involvement resembling that observed in microscopic polyarteritis, Wegener granulomatosis, and Henoch-Schönlein purpura.[267,268]

Paraneoplastic vasculitis is a syndrome of petechiae, palpable purpura, urticaria, maculopapular lesions, leg ulcers, and/or erythema multiforme seen in association with a number of different solid tumors, hairy cell leukemia, and other lymphoproliferative or myeloproliferative disorders.[269–274] An increased prevalence of solid tumors and lymphoid malignancies has been reported in patients with ANCA-positive vasculitis.[275] In some cases, the cutaneous lesions precede the diagnosis of the malignancy or signal recurrence of the malignancy.

Henoch-Schönlein purpura is the most common leukocytoclastic vasculitis of young children between the ages of 2 and 10 years,[276–278] with a peak age of onset between 4 and 7 years.[279] Adults also are affected, sometimes in association with an underlying malignancy,[280–282] most commonly leukemia and cancer of the lung and prostate.

Palpable purpuric lesions, abdominal pain, and arthritis of the knees and ankles occur together and are the most common findings. However, other organs, including the testicle,[283] may be involved as well. Acute and chronic renal disease is an important associated finding and is more common in adults.[284,285] Adults may have a more severe clinical syndrome compared with children.[284,286,287] There is an increased incidence in males[288,289] and a seasonal increase during the winter months. Many precipitating factors have been implicated, including infections[290] such as streptococcal pharyngitis,[291] staphylococcal sepsis,[292] meningococcal disease,[293] *Bartonella henselae,*[294,295] *Haemophilus parainfluenza*, parvovirus B19,[296] and hepatitis A. In children with Henoch-Schönlein purpura who develop nephritis, mesangial deposition of nephritis-associated plasmin receptor (a group A streptococcal antigen) has been observed.[297] *Helicobacter pylori* has been implicated in the gastrointestinal manifestations of the disease.[298]

Environmental chemicals and toxins, insect bites, physical trauma, familial Mediterranean fever, and malignancies all have been anecdotally reported to be associated with Henoch-Schönlein purpura.[280,299–301]

Genetic predisposition to, or protection from, development of Henoch-Schönlein purpura has been linked to specific major histocompatibility and complement loci.[302–305] Familial cases of Henoch-Schönlein purpura have been described,[306] and inducible nitric oxide synthase polymorphisms have been associated with susceptibility to Henoch-Schönlein purpura.[307]

Clinical presentations of Henoch-Schönlein purpura include explosive onset over the legs and buttocks of urticarial papules and plaques, with or without purpura (Fig. 121–26), palpable purpura, or hemorrhagic vesicles or bullae.[308–310] Larger stellate, reticulate, and necrotic lesions may occur (Fig. 121–27). Often a striking accentuation of palpable purpura demarcated at, and below, the sock line is seen.[311] Occasionally, ecchymotic lesions resembling child abuse are present, but the lesions of Henoch-Schönlein purpura usually are strikingly symmetric. Such lesions are predominantly seen on the arms, hands, and/or face.

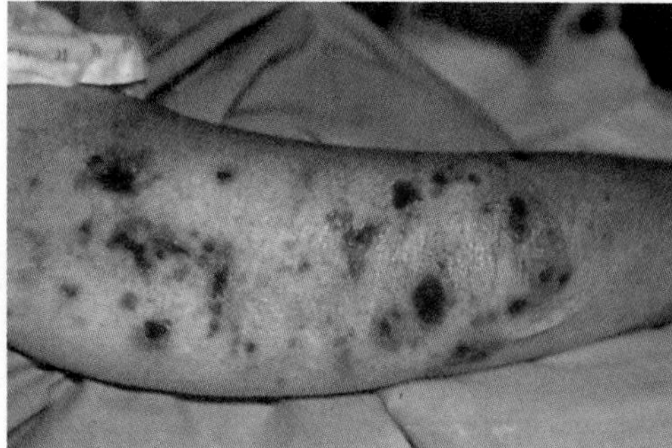

Figure 121–27 Leukocytoclastic vasculitis.

Henoch-Schönlein purpura is thought to be an immune complex disease, with 50% of patients producing IgA rheumatoid factor.[312] IgA-containing immune complexes, including IgA ANCA,[313,314] are detectable in many patients, especially during the early phases of the syndrome.[312,315,316] IgA antiendothelial cell antibodies have been identified in the acute stage of Henoch-Schönlein purpura and may directly activate endothelial cells to produce IL-8.[317] Elevated levels of IgA anticardiolipin antibodies have been reported in children[318] and adults.[319] IgA molecules of some patients with Henoch-Schönlein purpura have been reported to be deficient in sialic acid, an abnormality that may enhance their tendency to aggregate and form macromolecular complexes.[288] The following have all been reported in patients with Henoch-Schönlein purpura: increased levels of von Willebrand factor, an indicator of endothelial cell damage; increased vascular endothelial growth factor; increased intracellular adhesion molecule 1 and vascular cell adhesion molecule 1[320]; attenuated vascular endothelium-dependent relaxation[321]; increased levels of tumor necrosis factor α, leptin, and nitrite[322]; increased plasma levels of matrix metalloproteinase 9[323]; hypocomplementemia[324]; decreased levels of factor XIII[325] (which may be used to support the diagnosis[326]); elevated levels of markers of hypercoagulability[327]; increased numbers of transforming growth factor (TGF)-β–secreting T cells[318]; increased levels of IL-6 associated with thrombocytosis[328]; and increased urinary excretion of tumor necrosis factor α, interleukin 1β, and leukotriene E_4.[329–331] Elevated levels of IL-5 and eosinophilic cationic protein, as well as specific polymorphisms of vascular endothelial growth factor and paired box gene 2 (PAX2), may be associated with development of nephritis.[332–334] Prolonged rash, proteinuria greater than 1g/day, hypertension, and renal impairment at presentation all are unfavorable prognostic indicators.[335–337]

There is no standard therapy for Henoch-Schönlein purpura or the associated IgA renal disease,[338] but there have been numerous conflicting anecdotal reports and nonrandomized retrospective analyses of therapy with systemic glucocorticoids,[339,340] immunosuppressive agents, intravenous γ globulin,[341] and plasmapheresis.[342]

Acute hemorrhagic edema of infancy may mimic Henoch-Schönlein purpura. However, it occurs only in children between the ages of 4 months and 2 years, and its manifestations are exclusively cutaneous. It is characterized by sudden onset of fever, tender iris-like or medallion-like large purpuric cutaneous lesions, and peripheral edema.[343–345] Occasionally reticulate purpura, tender necrotic lesions of the ears, and/or urticaria are observed. The lesions occur on the cheeks, eyelids, ears, extremities, and genitalia and must be differentiated from the cutaneous findings of child abuse, Sweet syndrome, Kawasaki disease, septic emboli, drug eruption, meningococcemia, and hemorrhagic erythema multiforme.

Approximately 10% of adults with leukocytoclastic vasculitis have been reported to demonstrate livedoid superficial plaques, with multifocal areas of hemorrhage or necrosis and reticulate margins connecting adjacent lesions.[346] The blood vessels in these lesions contain deposits of IgA and C3. Smooth-margined purpuric papules with uniform hemorrhage may show IgA but more frequently demonstrate IgG or IgM vascular deposits.

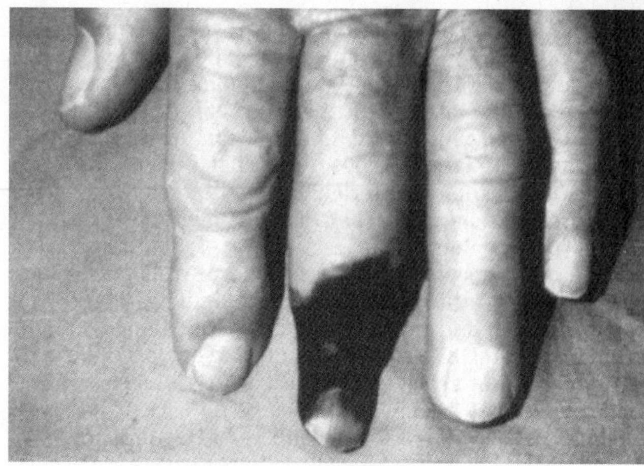

Figure 121–28 Cryoglobulinemia.

Recurrent cutaneous eosinophilic necrotizing vasculitis is characterized by papular, purpuric, and necrotic cutaneous lesions of the legs and feet. Angioedema and arthralgias are common.[347,348] Cutaneous leukocytoclastic vasculitis has been associated with sarcoidosis.[349]

Exercise-induced purpura is a recurrent form of leukocytoclastic vasculitis occurring in marathon runners and long-distance walkers (usually women) in whom erythematous, urticarial, and/or purpuric plaques appear on the lower legs above the malleoli.[350,351] These itching, burning, or painful plaques spare the region compressed by socks. This syndrome also has been called "golfer's vasculitis."[352]

Cryoglobulinemia

Cryoglobulins are cold-precipitable proteins found in plasma or serum. Single component cryoglobulins may be IgG, IgM, or IgA.[353] These cryoproteins may be idiopathic in origin or may occur with Waldenström macroglobulinemia, myeloma, lymphoma, benign paraproteinemias, or visceral leishmaniasis.[322] Mixed cryoglobulins usually are composed of a rheumatoid factor IgM complexed with a monoclonal or polyclonal IgG. Less frequently, IgG or IgA antibodies have anti-IgG activity. Mixed cryoglobulins may be seen as an idiopathic phenomenon or in association with a wide variety of subacute and chronic disorders, most particularly infection with hepatitis C virus (HCV). In fact, it has been reported that 80% to 90% of patients with mixed cryoglobulinemia are positive for anti-HCV antibodies.[354] The immune complexes are commonly composed of HCV and anti-HCV, along with either an IgA or IgM rheumatoid factor.[355,356] T_H1 cytokines have been implicated in the clinical presentation of patients with HCV-induced cryoglobulinemia.[357,358] The clinical triad of purpura, weakness, and arthralgias is characteristic of mixed cryoglobulinemia. Clinical lesions of cryoglobulinemia include the intermittent appearance of acral hemorrhagic necrosis (Fig. 121–28), palpable purpura, livedo reticularis, subungual hemorrhage (Fig. 121–29), urticaria, leg ulcerations, Raynaud phenomenon, and erythema multiforme-like lesions.[162,359–363] Monoclonal cryoglobulins may crystallize and result in livedo reticularis with purpuric necrosis, destructive arthropathy, and malignant hypertension.[364] Rituximab[365] and the combination of prednisolone and the Japanese immunosuppressive reagent mizoribine[366] have been reported to be effective therapy in select groups of patients.

Cryofibrinogenemia

Cryofibrinogenemia indicates the presence in the blood of an abnormal cold-precipitable protein indistinguishable from fibrinogen or fibrin. Essential (primary) cryofibrinogenemia occurs in association

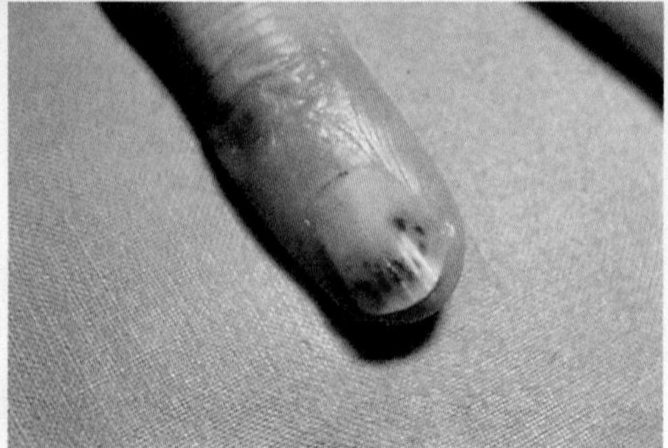

Figure 121–29 Subungual hemorrhage due to cryoglobulins.

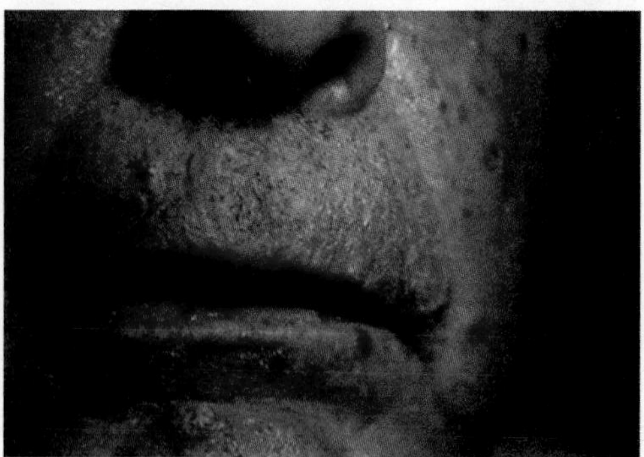

Figure 121–30 Hereditary hemorrhagic telangiectasia.

with DIC. Secondary cryofibrinogenemia may occur with neoplastic, thromboembolic, or infectious disorders. Cutaneous manifestations include sensitivity to cold, purpura, hematoma, livedo reticularis, cyanosis, ulcerations, erythema, urticaria, gangrene, acral blisters, and Raynaud phenomenon.[367–369] The lesions are most commonly observed on the acral areas, including the distal extremities, buttocks, nose, and ears.

Primary Cutaneous Diseases

Allergic contact dermatitis to poison ivy, allergic hypersensitivity to drugs, acne vulgaris, insect bites (especially blackfly bites), dermatitis herpetiformis, pityriasis rosea, and other primary cutaneous disorders may present with purpuric papules and vesicles mimicking septic and vasculitic lesions.[370,371]

NONPURPURIC DISORDERS SIMULATING PURPURA

Disorders With Telangiectasias

Cherry Angiomas

Cherry angiomas are the common papular, brightly erythematous lesions seen on the trunk and extremities of middle-aged and older men and women. They are produced by capillary loop aneurysms.[372] The lesions progress with age and may produce easy bruising because they have an increased tendency to bleed with trauma. On occasion, the lesions have a striking black appearance, mimicking malignant melanoma. Pinpoint or smaller cherry angiomas may be present in large numbers and may mimic petechiae. They may increase the risk of developing purpura in patients taking warfarin.

Hereditary Hemorrhagic Telangiectasia

HHT, also known as Osler-Weber-Rendu syndrome, is an autosomal dominant disorder with an estimated frequency of at least 1 : 8000–50,000, manifested by widespread dermal, mucosal, and visceral telangiectasias.[373–376] One form of the disorder, characterized by a high frequency of symptomatic pulmonary arteriovenous malformations and cerebral abscesses, has been identified as being due to abnormalities in the endothelial protein endoglin (ENG; HHT1).[375] This protein, whose gene is on the long arm of chromosome 9, mediates the response of endothelial cells to members of the TGF-β family.[377] A number of mutations involve the production of truncated forms of the receptor, opening up the possibility of a dominant negative mechanism to explain the autosomal dominant inheritance pattern.[378] A second form of the disease has been linked to the activin receptor-like kinase 1 gene (ACVRL1; ALK-1; HHT2) on chromosome 12, which is also a cell surface receptor for the TGF-β superfamily of ligands.[377,379,380] Dominant negative effects of mutations of ACVRL1 have been identified in zebrafish vascular development.[381] The TGF-β activated kinase 1 (TAK1) may be one of the important downstream molecules mediating the effects of TGF-β on vascular development, as mouse embryos deficient in TAK1 develop vascular lesions akin to those observed in HHT.[382] Other forms of the disease have been linked to loci on chromosome 5q (HHT3), chromosome 7p14 (HHT4), and a region of chromosome 3 containing the TGF-βII receptor.[379,383] An association between juvenile polyposis and HHT has been reported in patients with mutations in SMAD4 (MADH4), a protein in the TGF-β activation pathway.

The pathophysiology of the disorder has been studied by computer reconstruction of cutaneous telangiectasias based on serial sections.[372] Focal dilation of postcapillary venules is followed by connections to dilated arterioles, initially through capillaries, and later directly. Perivascular mononuclear cell infiltrates also are observed. The vessels of HHT show a discontinuous endothelium and an incomplete smooth muscle cell layer. The surrounding stroma lacks elastin. Thus, the bleeding tendencies are thought to be due to mechanical fragility of the abnormal vessels.

Clinically, venous lakes and papular, punctate, mat-like, and linear telangiectasias appear on all areas of the skin and mucous membranes, with a predominance of lesions on and under the tongue and on the face, lips (Fig. 121–30), perioral region, nasal mucosa, fingertips, toes, and trunk.[384] Recurrent epistaxis is a nearly universal finding in patients with this disorder; symptoms almost always worsen with age. Thus, the severity of the disorder often can be gauged by the age at which the nosebleeds begin, with the most severely affected patients developing recurrent epistaxis during childhood. Cutaneous changes usually begin at puberty and progress throughout life. Bleeding can occur in virtually every organ, with gastrointestinal, oral, and urogenital sites most common. In the gastrointestinal tract, the stomach and duodenum are more common sites of bleeding than is the colon. Hepatic and splenic arteriovenous shunts, as well as intracranial, aortic, and splenic aneurysms, may occur. Pulmonary arteriovenous fistulae are associated with oxygen desaturation, hemoptysis, hemothorax, brain abscess, and cerebral ischemia due to paradoxical emboli. Cirrhosis of the liver has been reported in some families.

Therapy for HHT remains problematic, consisting of laser treatment for cutaneous lesions; split-thickness skin grafting, embolization of arteriovenous communications, or hormonal therapy (estrogen or estrogens plus progesterone) for epistaxis; pulmonary resection or embolization for pulmonary arteriovenous malformations; and hormonal therapy and laser coagulation for gastrointestinal lesions.[373,385,386] The nasal vasculature pattern may help to predict the response to laser therapy versus septodermaplasty.[387] Resurfacing the nasomaxillary cavity with radial forearm fasciocutaneous free flaps has been reported to be effective in patients with refractory epistaxis.[388] The antifibrinolytic agents ε-aminocaproic acid and tranexamic acid have been reported to be beneficial in controlling hemorrhage[389,390] but negative results with antifibrinolytic therapy also have been reported.[391,392] Improvement in lesions has been reported in cases using an antagonist to vascular endothelial growth factor,[393] and sirolimus and aspirin.[394]

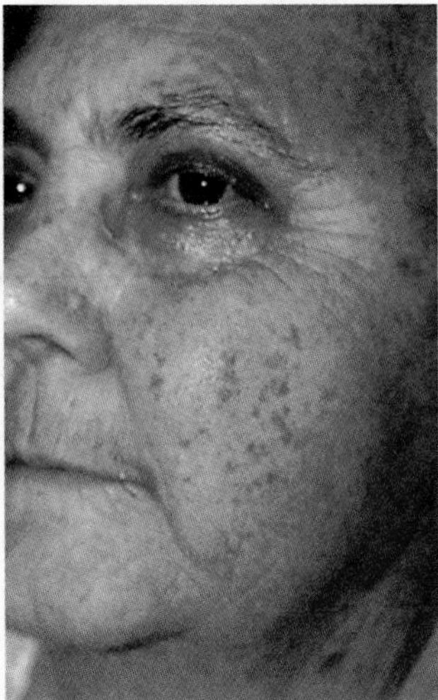

Figure 121–31 Telangiectatic mats.

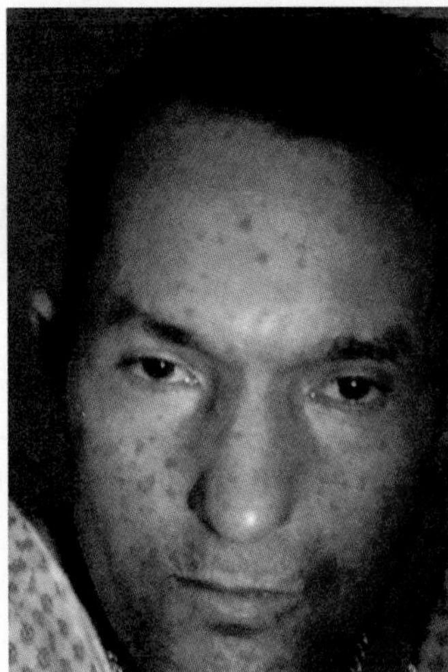

Figure 121–32 CREST syndrome.

Chronic Actinic Telangiectasias, Scleroderma, CREST Syndrome, Ataxia Telangiectasia, Chronic Liver Disease, and Pregnancy-Related Telangiectasias

Telangiectasias from chronic actinic damage (Fig. 121–31), and telangiectatic mats seen in scleroderma and CREST (calcinosis cutis, Raynaud syndrome, esophageal motility disorder, sclerodactyly, telangiectasia) syndrome (Fig. 121–32) may be easily confused with purpura as well as the lesions of vascular nevi and HHT. Angiokeratoma corporis diffusum, ataxia telangiectasia, and spider telangiectasias associated with chronic liver disease also must be differentiated. One point of differentiation is that spider telangiectasias have a central, prominent, easily blanchable feeding vessel with several smaller telangiectasias emanating from the central vessel. Spider telangiectasias seen in patients with chronic liver disease are distributed from the head to the nipple line and correlate with the risk of bleeding from esophageal varices.[395]

KAPOSI SARCOMA AND OTHER VASCULAR SARCOMAS

The epidemic form of Kaposi sarcoma found among some patients infected with HIV is easily confused with purpuric (Fig. 121–33) and ecchymotic (Fig. 121–34) lesions as well as some of the pigmented purpuric eruptions (Fig. 121–35).[396] Oral lesions of epidemic Kaposi sarcoma also may mimic petechiae and purpura (Fig. 121–36). Similarly, angiosarcoma may present as a purple to brown plaque resembling purpura (Fig. 121–37).

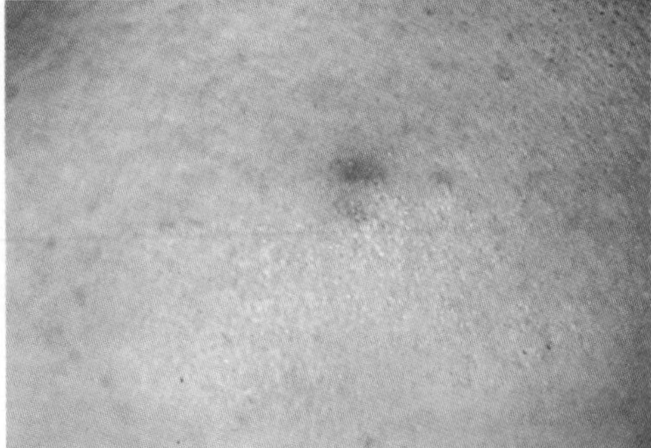

Figure 121–33 Kaposi sarcoma (AIDS).

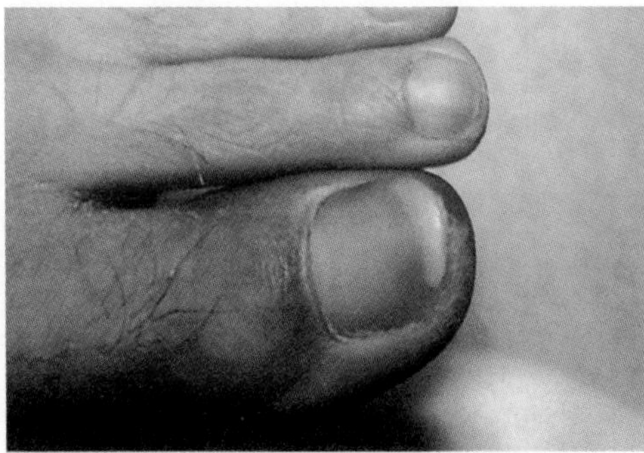

Figure 121–34 Kaposi sarcoma (AIDS).

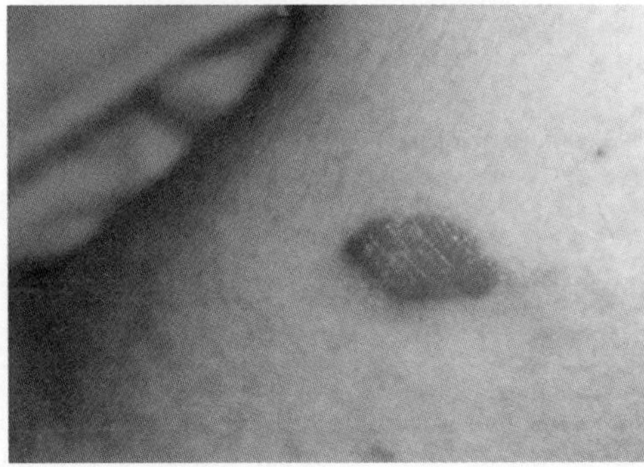

Figure 121–35 Kaposi sarcoma (AIDS).

FABRY DISEASE

Fabry disease (angiokeratoma corporis diffusum) is an X-linked inherited disorder of glycolipid metabolism with deficiency of the enzyme α-galactosidase A.[397] Accumulation of glycolipid throughout the body leads to cutaneous, renal, ophthalmologic, cardiac, and central nervous system manifestations. Angiokeratoma corporis diffusum lesions are pinpoint to 4-mm deep red, blue, or black macules or papules (Fig. 121–38). These nonblanchable lesions are distributed over the trunk, extremities, and genitalia. In mild cases, lesions are localized to the thighs, scrotum, or periumbilical region. Grouping of lesions may occur. Superficial corneal dystrophy and varicosities of the bulbar conjunctivum are commonly seen (Fig. 121–39). Replacement therapy with recombinant human α-galactosidase A is available.[397]

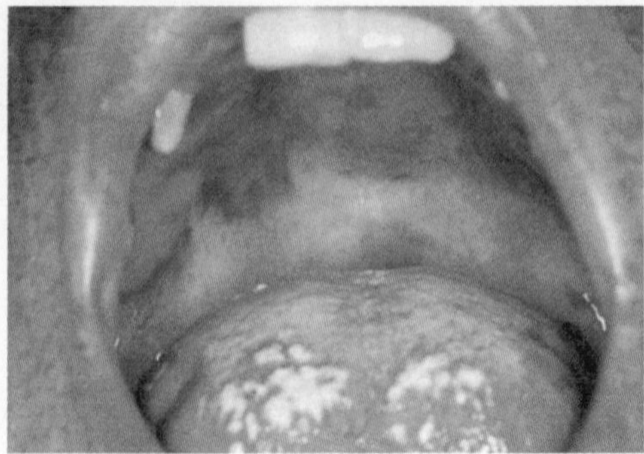

Figure 121–36 Kaposi sarcoma (AIDS).

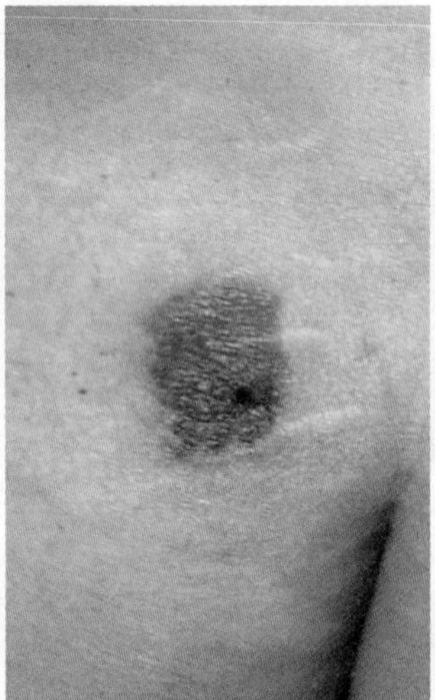

Figure 121–37 Angiosarcoma.

NEONATAL EXTRAMEDULLARY HEMATOPOIESIS (BLUEBERRY MUFFIN BABY)

Infants with congenital infections with toxoplasmosis, rubella, cytomegalovirus, Coxsackie B2 virus, or parvovirus B19, Rh incompatibility, hereditary spherocytosis, or twin transfusion syndrome may have dark red, blue, or blue-gray macules and/or papules at birth or within the first 48 hours of life.[398,399] The lesions contain sites of extramedullary hematopoiesis and are found most commonly on the scalp, neck, and trunk but may be widely distributed. The lesions fade into tan- or copper-colored macules by 8 weeks of age. Infants born with neuroblastoma, rhabdomyosarcoma, leukemia, or Langerhans cell histiocytosis[400] may present with lesions that have a similar appearance.

ANGIOMA SERPIGINOSUM

Angioma serpiginosum is a livedoid vascular nevoid lesion showing pinpoint vascular ectasias on a background of erythema.[23,401,402] The lesion blanches partially with pressure and is not petechial. Capillary microscopy demonstrates punctate dilated capillaries. Lesions usually are seen on the legs and buttocks of women but may occur anywhere; they commonly expand during childhood and regress with age.

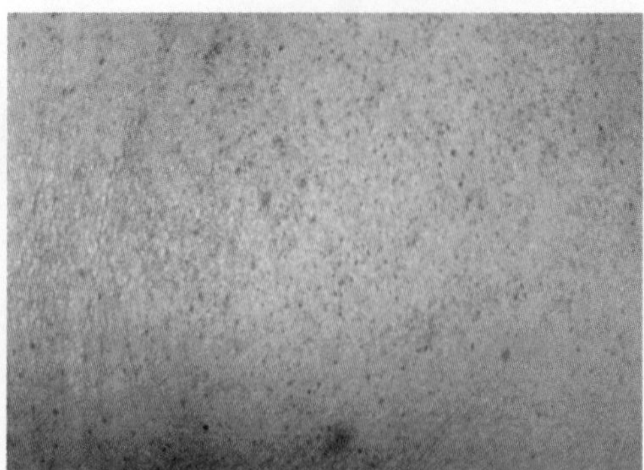

Figure 121–38 Fabry disease.

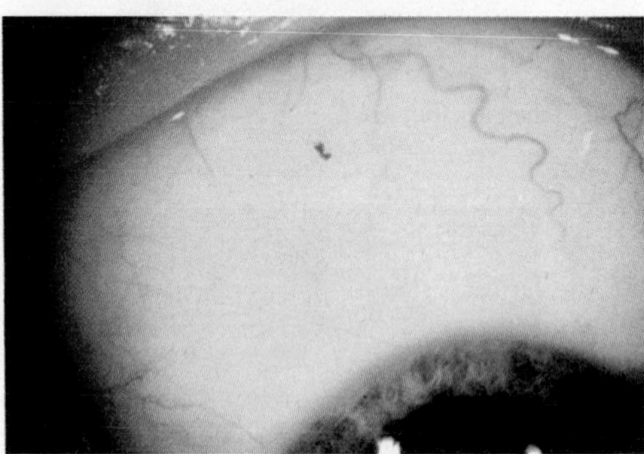

Figure 121–39 Fabry disease.

SUGGESTED READINGS

Castaman G, Rodeghiero F, Tosetto A, et al: Hemorrhagic symptoms and bleeding risk in obligatory carriers of type 3 von Willebrand disease: An international, multicenter study. J Thromb Haemost 4:2164, 2006.

Franchini M: Onset of severe refractory thrombocytopenia following surgery in a patient with type 2B von Willebrand disease—A case report. Hematology 11:127, 2006.

George JN, Caen JP, Nurden AT: Glanzmann's thrombasthenia: The spectrum of clinical disease. Blood 75:1383, 1990.

Hatuel H, Buffet M, Mateus C, Calmus Y, Carlotti A, Dupin N: Scurvy in liver transplant patients. J Am Acad Dermatol 55:154, 2006.

Hengge UR, Ruzicka T, Schwartz RA, Cork MJ: Adverse effects of topical glucocorticosteroids. J Am Acad Dermatol 54:1, 2006.

James AH: Von Willebrand disease. Obstet Gynecol Surv 61:136, 2006.

Nayak K, Spencer N, Shenoy M, Rubithon J, Coad N, Logan S: How useful is the presence of petechiae in distinguishing non-accidental from accidental injury? Child Abuse Negl 30:549, 2006.

Plug I, Mauser-Bunschoten EP, Brocker-Vriends AH, et al: Bleeding in carriers of hemophilia. Blood 108:52, 2006.

Rao SV, O'Grady K, Pieper KS, et al: A comparison of the clinical impact of bleeding measured by two different classifications among patients with acute coronary syndromes. J Am Coll Cardiol 47:809, 2006.

Tosetto A, Rodeghiero F, Castaman G, et al: A quantitative analysis of bleeding symptoms in type 1 von Willebrand disease: Results from a multicenter European study (MCMDM-1 VWD). J Thromb Haemost 4:766, 2006.

REFERENCES

For complete list of references log onto www.expertconsult.com

CHAPTER 122

LABORATORY EVALUATION OF HEMOSTATIC AND THROMBOTIC DISORDERS

Alvin H. Schmaier

The clinical laboratory evaluation is an integral part of the diagnosis and management of patients with hemostatic/thrombotic disorders. A clinical hematologist when challenged by patients with hemostatic/thrombotic disorders is as good as the laboratory that serves him or her for diagnosis and management. This chapter provides a critical practical approach to the diagnosis and management of bleeding and clotting disorders. The chapter discusses how clinicians use the clinical coagulation laboratory for management of patients with hemostatic and thrombotic disorders. The latter activity is a new use of laboratory resources for what until the present era has mostly been a diagnostic facility.

Physiologic hemostasis is the sum of protein (coagulation, fibrinolytic, and anticoagulation) and cellular (platelets, endothelial cells, and leukocytes) elements working in concert to staunch the bleeding at sites of vascular injury without occlusive thrombosis. The coagulation system leads to thrombin formation. The role of the fibrinolytic system is to lyse clot formed by thrombin. The role of the anticoagulation system is to regulate all the enzymes of the coagulation and fibrinolytic systems so that no excess clotting or bleeding occurs. The sum of these elements leads to the hemostatic plug (Fig. 122–1). Thus, the present approach to patients with bleeding disorders is to evaluate the hemostatic, fibrinolytic, and anticoagulation proteins and platelet number and function that contribute to this process. For decades the proteins of the hemostatic system have been referred to as the "coagulation cascade" based on the waterfall hypothesis of Ratnoff and Davies[1] and MacFarland,[2] who almost simultaneously reported a sequence of proteolytic reactions starting with factor XII (Hageman factor) activation and ending with formed thrombin proteolyzing fibrinogen to form a clot. However, at the onset, this hypothesis for physiologic hemostasis was untenable because it was known that factor XII deficiency is not associated with bleeding.[3] By the mid-1970s, the cofactors for factor XII activation (prekallikrein and high-molecular-weight kininogen) were identified, and deficiencies of these proteins also were not associated with a bleeding state.[4–6] In 1977, Osterud and Rappaport[7] recognized that factor VIIa is able to activate factor IX to factor IXa. Later, Broze et al.[8] recognized that the kinetics of tissue factor pathway inhibitor were such that, under physiologic circumstances, the factor VIIa/tissue factor complex cannot directly activate factor X but must go through factor IX activation. If this is the case, how does factor XI, whose deficiency is associated with bleeding, become activated independent of factor XIIa? In 1991, Gailani and Broze[9] showed that formed thrombin cycles back to activate factor XI, resulting in amplification of activation of thrombin formation. Presently, physiologic hemostasis is believed to be an interacting system initiated by factor VIIa and tissue factor activation and amplification of several zymogens that become serine proteases (Fig. 122–2; see Chapter 118). Although this has become a cohesive hypothesis for physiologic coagulation activation, clinical laboratory testing of the proteins of coagulation is not based on this current understanding—it follows the Ratnoff and Davies hypothesis.

The clinical laboratory assays used to examine the proteins of the coagulation system are based on the original surface-activated coagulation cascade hypothesis.[1,2] Although these tests do not represent physiologic hemostasis, they still are useful for diagnosis of defects in coagulation proteins and potential bleeding disorders. Thus, the clinician must understand the distinction between physiologic coagulation, fibrinolysis, and anticoagulation and the diagnostic tests that are used to measure these systems. The first part of this chapter describes the assays used to measure bleeding disorders. Understanding these assays is a practical approach to recognizing a potential bleeding abnormality in a patient. The second part of this chapter provides an overview of an approach to the laboratory diagnosis of thrombosis risk and discusses use of the clinical coagulation laboratory for monitoring activated coagulation states.

When faced with a bleeding patient, the hematologist must use an analytic diagnostic approach to determine its etiology. Most recognized bleeding states are caused by one of three defects: a defect or deficiency in a plasma protein, a defect in platelet number or function, or a defect in platelet–vessel wall interactions (i.e., an abnormality in the adhesive interactions between platelets and the vessel wall), as in defects associated with the presence or function of von Willebrand factor.

When approaching the diagnosis of a coagulation protein defect in a patient, understanding the mechanism is paramount. Any coagulation protein defect can be a true protein deficiency, an abnormal protein that cannot participate in its physiologic function(s), or an inhibitor to the active site of the protein or one that induces enhanced clearance of the protein. In general, inhibitors to a coagulation protein are immunoglobulins, although abnormal production of endogenous heparin, fibronectin, or cryoglobulins has been reported as the source of acquired inhibitors to coagulation proteins.[10] An abnormal coagulation protein can result from missense, deletion, or translocations of its DNA. Last, enhanced clearance of coagulation proteins usually occurs as a result of an antibody–protein complex that is recognized as foreign and thus removed from the circulation.[11] The resultant increased clearance of the protein results in a deficiency of the protein. Thus, clinical laboratory testing, when available, should focus on measuring the presence of the protein by antigen and its functionality by a variety of assays in order to recognize all of these mechanistic possibilities.

In general, hemarthrosis and spontaneous soft-tissue and intramuscular hemorrhage characterize defects of plasma protein, such as hemophilia A and B (factors VIII and IX deficiency). Soft-tissue petechiae, purpura, or ecchymosis characterizes von Willebrand disease or platelet number or functional disorders. However, distinguishing the potential mechanism for bleeding can be difficult. History and physical examination are important components of the hemostatic workup (see Chapter 121) but are inadequate for specific diagnosis of bleeding or clotting disorders. Thus, the clinical laboratory is essential for definitive diagnosis of a bleeding disorder in patients.

CLINICAL SCREENING ASSAYS IN HEMOSTATIC TESTING TO DETECT COAGULATION PROTEIN DEFECTS

In the practice of clinical hemostasis, there are no good global assays for measuring physiologic tissue factor-initiated hemostasis. The three assays most commonly used to examine the coagulation system are (a) the activated partial thromboplastin time (aPTT) induced by surface (contact) activation of the system, (b) the prothrombin time (PT) induced by the addition of excess tissue factor, and (c) the thrombin clotting time (TCT). In the aPTT assay, surface or contact

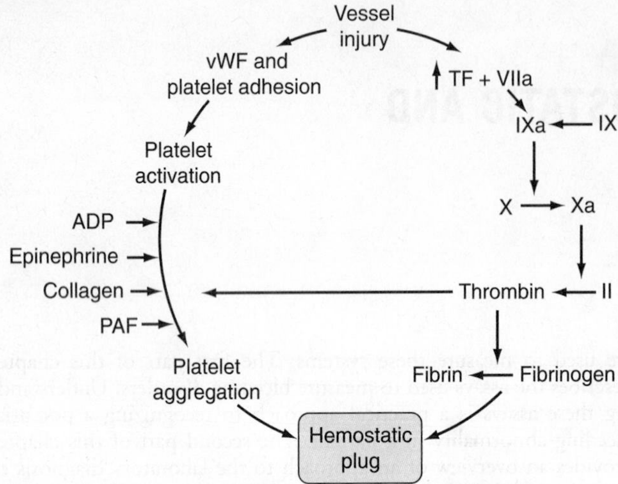

Figure 122–1 Schematic diagram of hemostasis. When a vessel is injured, platelets adhere to the injury site via von Willebrand factor (vWF). Upon adherence, the platelets are activated and release their granule contents. Released adenosine diphosphate (ADP) and exposed collagen recruit more platelets to the injury site. Simultaneously at the site of injury, tissue factor (TF) is upregulated and with activated factor VII activates factor IX to activated factor IX and, sequentially, factor X to activated factor X and prothrombin to thrombin. Thrombin stimulates more platelets, enhancing the platelet plug. Thrombin also proteolyzes fibrinogen to form fibrin monomer, which then polymerizes into a fibrin clot. These events occur on or about the activated platelet surface. PAF, platelet-activating factor. (Adapted from Schmaier AH, Thornburg C, Pipe, S: Coagulation and fibrinolysis. In Henry's Clinical Diagnosis and Management by Laboratory Network. Eds McPherson and Pincus. 21st Edition Elsevier, Philadelphia, PA, 2007, pp 729–745.

activation of the coagulation system occurs because factor XII associates with negatively charged substances in the reagent such that the protein actually stretches to allow expression of its active site, autoactivating factor XII to initiate a cascade of proteolytic reactions seen in the coagulation system.[12–14] These phenomena are the basis of the Ratnoff and Davies hypothesis for activation of the coagulation system. This test measures more proteins (factor XII, prekallikrein, high-molecular-weight kininogen) than those necessary for physiologic hemostasis. In the PT assay, addition of excess tissue factor creates an unphysiologic change in the normal stoichiometric relationship of coagulation factors, thereby allowing factor VIIa to overcome the inhibitory effect of tissue factor pathway inhibitor and favoring direct activation of factor X to factor Xa without the usual physiologic requirement to proceed through factor IX activation. In the TCT assay, exogenous thrombin is added to examine the integrity of its major substrate fibrinogen.

When all three assays are performed simultaneously on a sample of plasma, the results indicate almost all of the diagnostic categories for a bleeding state. It is most useful when performing diagnostic evaluations to perform a complete evaluation of the patient at one time rather than a series of piecemeal studies. Patient conditions usually are dynamic, so piecemeal evaluations often miss evolving clinical states. The three screening tests are performed as follows:

1. *Activated partial thromboplastin time (aPTT).* To perform this common coagulation assay, equal parts of a negatively charged surface and phospholipid mixture and patient plasma are incubated for more than 5 minutes. Calcium chloride 30 mM is added to recalcify citrated plasma, and the time required for clot formation is measured. The aPTT assay assesses the coagulation proteins of the so-called intrinsic system and the common pathways (Fig. 122–3).[15]
2. *Prothrombin time (PT).* To perform this assay, tissue thromboplastin (animal derived or recombinant human tissue factor) and phospholipids and patient plasma are incubated for more than 5 minutes. The plasma then is recalcified by the addition of $CaCl_2$ 30 mM, and the time required for clot formation is measured. The PT assay assesses the coagulation proteins of the so-called extrinsic system and the common pathway (see Fig. 122–3).[16] The sensitivity of the assay is based on likeness of the tissue factor to human tissue factor used in the assay (see Interpretation of Screening Tests of the Coagulation System).
3. *Thrombin clotting time (TCT).* To perform this assay, purified thrombin is added to plasma to determine the time for clot formation. It is a direct measure of the conversion of fibrinogen

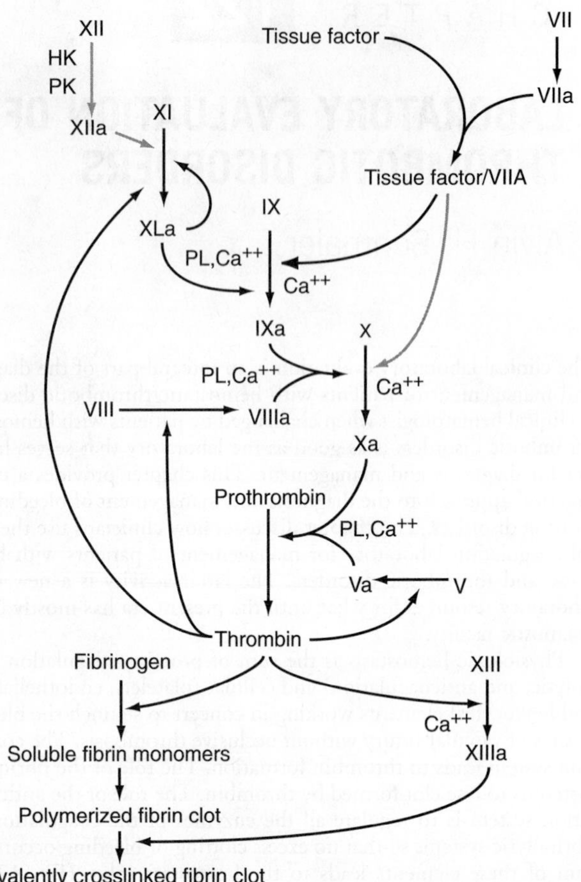

Figure 122–2 Schematic diagram of physiologic hemostasis. Formation of the tissue factor-activated factor VII complex (TF/VIIa) results in factor IX activation to activated factor IX (IXa). TF/VIIa does *not* normally directly activate factor X. Formed activated factor IX activates factor X to activated factor X (Xa) in the presence of activated factor VIII (VIIIa), which must have been formed from some prior thrombin activation of factor VIII). Activated factor X in the presence of activated factor V (Va) activates prothrombin to thrombin (IIa). Thrombin proteolyzes fibrinogen to form a fibrin clot. If more thrombin is needed, thrombin can activate factor XI to activated factor XI (XIa), which then activates more factor IX to activated factor IXa, which makes more activated factor X and thrombin. If more thrombin-induced clot formation is needed, thrombin also activates carboxypeptidase U to form a thrombin activatable fibrinolysis inhibitor (TAFIa) that inhibits fibrinolysis. Factor XI also can be activated by activated factor XII, which is formed secondarily by the constitutive activation of prekallikrein (PK) in the presence of high-molecular-weight kininogen (HK) by the endothelial cell enzyme prolylcarboxypeptidase. These latter mechanisms are *not* constitutive for physiologic hemostasis. However, in nonphysiologic states such as sepsis, clot formation in the intravascular compartment, or cardiopulmonary bypass, activated factor XII can activate factor XI to initiate hemostasis with thrombin formation. This latter mechanism is the basis of the activated partial thromboplastin time, a major screening test for hemostatic disorders. (Adapted from Schmaier AH, Thornburg C, Pipe, S: Coagulation and fibrinolysis. In Henry's Clinical Diagnosis and Management by Laboratory Network. Eds McPherson and Pincus. 21st Edition Elsevier, Philadelphia, PA, 2007, pp 729–745.

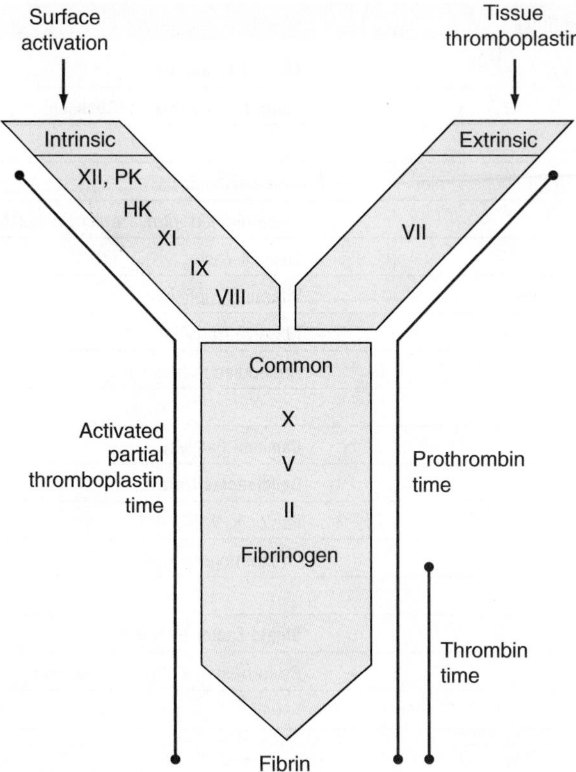

Figure 122–3 Organization of the coagulation system based on current screening assays. The intrinsic coagulation system consists of the proteins factors XII, XI, IX, and VIII and prekallikrein (PK) and high-molecular-weight kininogen (HK). The extrinsic coagulation system consists of tissue factor and factor VII. The common pathway of the coagulation system consists of factors X, V, and II and fibrinogen (I). The activated partial thromboplastin time requires the presence of every protein except tissue factor and factor VII. The prothrombin time (PT) requires tissue factor, factors VII, X, V, and II, and fibrinogen. The thrombin clotting time only tests the integrity of fibrinogen. (Adapted from Schmaier AH, Thornburg C, Pipe, S: Coagulation and fibrinolysis. In Henry's Clinical Diagnosis and Management by Laboratory Network. Eds McPherson and Pincus. 21st Edition Elsevier, Philadelphia, PA, 2007, pp 729–745.

to fibrin (see Fig. 122–3). When performing this assay, it is essential to use the minimal amount of α thrombin (3000 U/mg specific activity) that will reproducibly "clot" fibrinogen, usually 4 to 6 U/mL, aiming for approximately 20 seconds with pooled normal plasma to achieve maximal sensitivity for a clinically useful assay.[17,18] This assay is distinguished from the clottable fibrinogen assay (Clauss assay) by the amount of thrombin used (≈50 U/mL in the Clauss assay).[17,19]

The results of these assays allows the 40-year-old cascade hypothesis to guide the clinician to a practical differential diagnosis of what protein(s) may be affected based on the results of the screening tests. In the coagulation cascade hypothesis, coagulation proteins are classified as members of the intrinsic system, the extrinsic system, or the common pathway (see Fig. 122–3).

All coagulation assays examine the rate of clot formation. In these assays, a sequence of proteolytic reactions take place, leading to thrombin formation and its proteolysis of fibrinogen. Proteolysis of fibrinogen results in clot formation with precipitation of soluble proteins that are detected by either increased impedance or turbidity or decreased optical clarity, based on the instrumentation used to measure the result. Any defect along the pathway to clot formation will give an abnormal result. Furthermore, because a series of reactions must occur to result in the final clot formation, any substance (e.g., inhibitory antibodies, heparinoids, anticoagulants) that interferes with the assay downstream from a specific factor's activity will lead to an abnormal result. For example, a potent inhibitor to factor VIII will give an abnormal factor XI or IX coagulant assay. A deficient or abnormal fibrinogen will affect the results of the aPTT and PT assays even though the levels of all the coagulation factors are normal.

INTERPRETATION OF SCREENING TESTS OF THE COAGULATION SYSTEM

When diagnosing potential bleeding disorders, the coagulation cascade hypothesis and its grouping of coagulation proteins are used to interpret the screening tests for coagulation proteins for various deficiencies or abnormalities in the coagulation proteins (see Fig. 122–3).

The in vitro event of factor XII autoactivating in the aPTT assay initiates the sequence of reactions of the coagulation cascade.[1,2] The aPTT assay measures all the proteins of the so-called intrinsic coagulation protein system (factor XII, prekallikrein, high-molecular-weight kininogen, factor XI, factor IX, and factor VIII) and the proteins of the so-called common pathway (factors X, V, II, and fibrinogen). It is important to realize that coagulation proteins decrease to different levels before the various screening assays show an abnormality. For example, most commercial aPTT reagents detect a decrease in factor VIII when the protein level decreases to 35% to 45% of normal (i.e., 0.35–0.45 U/mL). Alternatively, factor XII and high-molecular-weight kininogen at levels of 10% to 15% of normal will only just begin to show abnormalities on the aPTT assay.[20,21] Similarly, factor VII levels below 35% to 40% will begin to be detected on the PT assay. The sensitivity of the screening tests in detecting specific abnormalities varies with the factor being tested, the commercial reagent used in the assay, and equipment platform for measurement. Ideally, each clinical laboratory should know the level of decrease for each coagulation factor that is detected by an abnormal aPTT or PT by their current equipment and reagents being used.[22]

The PT assay measures the so-called extrinsic protein coagulation pathway of coagulation, which consists of activated factor VII (factor VIIa) and the proteins of the common pathway (factors X, V, II, and fibrinogen).[16] The PT assay also is used as a monitor for patients taking warfarin.[23,24] In this capacity, its result reporting has been modified so that it can be interpreted universally. Because of the plethora of commercially available PT reagents and instruments for assay, it is impossible for physicians to know normal values for the PT from any given laboratory. A convention called the internationalized normalized ratio (INR) was developed to standardize the reporting of PT for patients taking warfarin.[23] INR = (patient's PT/mean laboratory control PT)^{ISI}, where ISI (international sensitivity index) for a reagent is a measure of the responsiveness of a given thromboplastin to reduction of the vitamin K-dependent coagulation factors. The reliability of PT becomes less with increasing ISI of the thromboplastin as the therapeutic range for PT diminishes.[24] It is provided by each manufacturer based on the degree of variation of the thromboplastin from the World Health Organization (WHO) reference thromboplastin that has an arbitrarily assigned value of 1, as determined by z, the logarithm of a PT per second determined with the WHO standard, and x, the logarithm of PT in seconds determined with the test preparation, according to the equation $z = a_1 + b_1x$, where $b_1 = m +$ square root of $m^2 + 1$ and $a_1 = z - b_1x$ (see Pollar[24] for meaning of m in these equations). Manufacturer determination of ISI requires a minimum of 20 normal donors and 60 samples of patients stable on warfarin therapy with INRs between 1.5 to 5.0.[24] The higher the ISI, the less sensitive the thromboplastin. Human recombinant thromboplastin gives an ISI value of approximately 1.0. In practice, the term INR has become common parlance to describe all PT changes from normal. In reality, it should be used only to characterize the degree of PT prolongation of a plasma sample from a patient on warfarin.

Table 122–1 Laboratory Evaluation of Abnormalities of Coagulation Protein: aPTT and PT Screening Tests

Long aPTT, Normal PT	Long PT, Normal aPTT	Long aPTT and PT
Associated with Bleeding	Factor VII (rare)	**Think Medical States (Common)**
Factor VIII (male only)		
Factor IX (male only)	Slight defects[b] in factors X, II, and V and dysfibrinogenemias	Anticoagulants
Factor XI		Disseminated intravascular coagulation
Antibodies to factor VIII		Liver disease
Amyloid adsorbed factor IX		Vitamin K deficiency
		Massive transfusion
Not Associated with Bleeding		Antibodies to factor V
Factor XII	**Single Factor Deficient**	
Prekallikrein	Perform specific inhibitor assay	**Common Pathway**
High-molecular-weight kininogen		**Deficiencies (rare)**
Lupus anticoagulant		Factor X, V, II
Single Factor Deficient		Dysfibrinogenemias
Perform specific inhibitor assay		
		Single Factor Deficient
		Perform specific inhibitor assays
Multiple Factors Deficient		
Pan inhibitors,[a] e.g., lupus anticoagulant, immunoglobulin		**Multiple Factors Deficient** Pan inhibitors

[a]Pan inhibitors: General description of a nonspecific inhibitor that can be an immunoglobulin (e.g., lupus anticoagulant, myeloma protein) or natural substance (heparin, fibronectin, amyloid) that binds coagulation proteins and interferes with their function.

[b]Occurs with more sensitive PT reagents, international sensitivity index ≈ 1.0.

aPTT, activated partial thromboplastin time; PT, prothrombin time.

Table 122–2 Clinical Peculiarities of Coagulation Protein Screening Tests

Long aPTT, normal or long PT, *no bleeding*	Normal aPTT, PT, *with bleeding*
Long APTT only	
Factor XII deficiency	Factor XIII deficiency or inhibitor
Prekallikrein deficiency	α_2-Antiplasmin deficiency or defect
High-molecular-weight kininogen	Plasminogen activator inhibitor deficiency or defect
Lupus anticoagulant	α_1-Antitrypsin Pittsburgh defect
Long aPTT and PT	
Dysfibrinogenemia with fibrinopeptide B release defect	
Lupus anticoagulant	

aPTT, activated partial thromboplastin time; PT, prothrombin time.

TCT only measures the ability of exogenous thrombin to proteolyze (clot) fibrinogen. It only assesses fibrinopeptide A and B release from fibrinogen and fibrin polymerization. Prolonged TCTs as indicated by values outside the 95% confidence interval for the time to clot of a population of 20 or more normals suggest reduced fibrinogen levels or abnormal fibrinogen function.

Knowing what each test measures, the following approach can be used to evaluate bleeding risk in patients who have prolonged values in one or more of these assays (Table 122–1). For example, if a patient has an isolated prolonged aPTT, determination of the patient's risk to bleed begins with the addition of historical information (see Chapter 121). If isolated prolongation of the aPTT is associated with bleeding, then the differential diagnosis in decreasing likelihood of frequency is factor VIII, factor IX, or factor XI deficiency. Factor VIII and IX deficiencies are sex linked and usually are seen only in males; factor XI deficiency is autosomal recessive and is seen in males and females (see Chapters 123 to 126 for a full discussion). If the aPTT alone is prolonged and the patient has no history of bleeding, the most common cause is a lupus anticoagulant (see Chapter 131). The specific proteins of the so-called intrinsic coagulation system associated with a prolonged aPTT but no bleeding history in decreasing frequency are factor XII, prekallikrein, and high-molecular-weight kininogen deficiency (Table 122–2). All of these defects are autosomal recessive and rare. Knowing about these latter three proteins is essential to evaluating a prolonged aPTT, even though the patient is not at bleeding risk. It also is important to recognize these protein defects so that patients do not undergo unnecessary plasma replacement therapy. Information indicates that factor XII contributes to the extent of thrombosis independent of hemostasis.[25] Factor XII activation contributes to the extent of clot formation of induced arterial thrombus by fibrin, platelets, or other material that function as negatively charged surfaced for autoactivation.[25–27]

Individuals can have acquired disorders that inhibit specific coagulation factors and increase their risk for bleeding. The clinical laboratory phenotype of these patients depends on the protein to which the coagulation protein inhibitor is directed. The most common severe acquired coagulation protein inhibitor is a spontaneous antibody inhibitor to factor VIII that is seen in both males and females (see Chapter 131). Patients with the disorder present with bleeding and a long aPTT. Characteristically, this inhibitor is seen in elderly patients, patients with B-cell malignancies, patients with connective tissue disorders such as systemic lupus erythematosus, and women postpartum. Patients are managed acutely with replacement therapy (high-dose factor VIII, activated vitamin K-dependent coagulation factor concentrates, or recombinant factor VIIa), but long-term management may require immunosuppression with cyclophosphamide (Cytoxan) and prednisone and/or rituximab.[28,29] Management decisions in these patients are influenced by the severity of bleeding and the height of the titer of the inhibitor to factor VIII as determined by the Bethesda assay.[30–32]

Alternatively, an isolated PT prolongation associated with bleeding usually indicates factor VII deficiency (see Chapter 127). Patients usually have partial VII defects as a true deficiency is incompatible with life.[33] At times, defects in some common pathway proteins (fibrinogen and factors II, V, and X) may first appear as an isolated PT prolongation; if severe, these latter protein defects will yield prolonged PT and aPTT results. The reason for the former is that certain more sensitive PT reagents first detect the defect before the aPTT. Recombinant tissue factor-based PT reagents with an ISI value approaching "I" constitute these more sensitive PT reagents.[24]

In general, defects in the common pathway proteins (fibrinogen, and factors II, V, and X) usually result in a prolonged PT and aPTT. When confronted with laboratory results of prolonged PT and aPTT, the hematologist should first not consider the specific proteins mentioned but rather should address the differential diagnosis for medical states such as anticoagulation therapy, disseminated intravascular coagulation (DIC), liver disease, vitamin K deficiency, and massive transfusion.[34,35] These general medical conditions are the most common causes of abnormal results in the two screening tests. Anticoagulation, unless the patient is faking medical illness, and massive transfusion are excluded by history.[36] Vitamin K deficiency is rare except in patients who are receiving warfarin therapy, are nutritionally depleted alcoholics, are having IV replacement without vitamins, have bacterial overgrowth in the gastrointestinal tract as result of antibiotic therapy, or, very rarely, have defects in transport proteins or enzymes for metabolism (see Chapter 130). Liver disease has several mechanisms that contribute to prolonged aPTT and PT. Prekallikrein, factor VII, and factor V are the first proteins to be decreased in liver disease. Abnormal fibrinogens often are produced in liver disease.[37] TCT detects defects in fibrinopeptide A and B release as well as polymerization defects. The reptilase time uses a snake venom enzyme to "clot" fibrinogen by liberating only fibrinopeptide A.[38] An abnormal TCT with a normal reptilase time indicates a fibrinopeptide B release defect, an abnormality that gives very long aPTT and PT values but is not associated with bleeding (see Table 122–2).[18] The reptilase time also will not be altered by the presence of heparin and can be used to determine if long aPTT and TCT are due to heparin.[36]

In addition to these general medical conditions, acquired disorders can present with the clinical laboratory phenotype of a long PT and aPTT. Acquired deficiencies or inhibitors are also seen in a number of medical conditions. Systemic amyloidosis is associated with decreases in plasma factor X or IX as a result of adsorption of the coagulation proteins onto the amyloid protein.[39] In the former condition, PT and aPTT may be affected; in the latter, only aPTT is affected. Hypergammaglobulinemic states seen with multiple myeloma or Waldenström macroglobulinemia (immunoglobulin M) can be associated with pan inhibitors to coagulation protein function.[40] Dysfibrinogenemias are common in these patients because fibrinogen binds immunoglobulin.[18] These phenomena are recognized by performing specific factor assays against the one or more proteins affected at multiple dilutions of the patient's plasma. In general, as the factor assay is performed at lower dilutions (e.g., 50%, 25% and 10% of normal plasma), the degree of inhibition of the coagulation factor reduces, suggesting that as the plasma is diluted, the effect of the inhibitor is lost. This coagulation test pattern is characteristic of a specific inhibitor to a coagulation protein.

Another acquired inhibitor that influences coagulation protein reactions is the lupus anticoagulant (see Chapter 131). This inhibitor represents antibodies directed to epitopes of proteins bound to certain phospholipids.[41] Lupus anticoagulants variably interfere with aPTT and PT. Detection of the degree of interference depends on the nature of the commercial reagent. Characteristically, a lupus anticoagulant will have a greater effect on a coagulation assay as the reagents, not protein, in the assay are diluted out.[42] For example, the degree of prolongation of PT or aPTT in a plasma sample will be greater at 1 : 50 dilution and 1 : 500 dilution of the assay reagent in a patient with a lupus anticoagulant than in a patient with a specific inhibitor to a coagulation protein.[42,43] In the latter case, the inhibitor level will change only when the patient's plasma, not the reagent for the assay, is diluted. Specific criteria have been developed to recognize lupus anticoagulants.[41,44,45] In general, assays that have some dilution of the coagulation reagent (dilute PT or tissue thromboplastin inhibition assay, dilute aPTT, dilute Russell viper venom time, or kaolin clotting time) are useful but are not specifically diagnostic for the condition.[41,43,44] Correction of the defect with excess phospholipids or platelet membranes is an additional characteristic of the disorder noted on clot-based assays.[41,46] However, no clot-based assay is diagnostic for lupus anticoagulants. All criteria also emphasize that the diagnosis is one of exclusion.[41,46]

FACTOR-SPECIFIC COAGULATION PROTEIN TESTING

All specific coagulation factor assays of the intrinsic system (XII, prekallikrein, high-molecular-weight kininogen, factors XI, IX, and VIII) are measured on one-stage assays using aPTT as its assay platform.[47,48] These assays became readily available because of accessibility of specific factor-deficient plasma. For example, a factor VIII assay uses a mixture of aPTT reagent, factor VIII-deficient plasma, and patient (test sample) plasma. After incubation for more than 5 minutes, the time to clot is initiated by recalcification with calcium chloride. All coagulation factors of the extrinsic system and common pathway (factors VII, X, V, and II) are measured in assays using PT as its platform.[47,48] For example, a factor X assay is a mixture of PT reagent that contains tissue factor (thromboplastin), factor X-deficient plasma, and patient (test sample) plasma. After incubation for more than 5 minutes, the time to clot is initiated by addition of calcium chloride. The amount of factor present in a given patient sample is determined by comparing the patient sample against a standard curve made with 10% to 100% normal plasma using the factor-deficient plasma and PT reagent.

Coagulation-based assays are sensitive and specific. They are simpler to perform than antigen assays for each of the coagulation proteins. Additional assays such as TCT and reptilase time specifically examine the integrity of fibrinogen.[17,38] Coagulation-based assays examine the function of the protein, antigen assays establish its presence, and, combined, these assays may detect protein with reduced function. Such a situation commonly arises when examining fibrinogen. The most useful means for determining the presence of an abnormal fibrinogen (dysfibrinogenemia) is to measure clottable fibrinogen and fibrinogen antigen on the same sample.[18,49] If fibrinogen clottability is less than 90% the amount of fibrinogen antigen, the protein produced probably is functionally abnormal.[37,49]

In addition to clot-based assays, the modern coagulation laboratory performs antigen assays for various proteins, which is important in the diagnosis of abnormal proteins.[49] Chromogenic assays also are used to measure certain enzymes (factor VIII, factor Xa, thrombin, plasmin, activated protein C) and various plasma protease inhibitors (antithrombin, α_2 antiplasmin, C1 inhibitor). The ability to neutralize the enzymatic activity of factor Xa or thrombin is a useful way to assay for the plasma level of anticoagulants, such as heparin, low molecular weight heparins, or for heparinizing which inhibit factor Xa or hirudin, argatroban a biualirudin which inhibit thrombin.[50]

PRACTICAL APPROACH TO THE BLEEDING PATIENT WITH A COAGULATION PROTEIN DEFECT

Patients with abnormal results on coagulation assays can be evaluated by the differential diagnosis of an isolated aPTT abnormality, PT abnormality, or both. When presented with a prolonged coagulation assay, the differential diagnosis often is between a true deficiency and an inhibitor to a specific coagulation protein. Two approaches can be used to obtain a specific diagnosis.

A common practice when approaching the problem of determining specific coagulation factor defects begins with a mixing test of patient and normal plasma. Mixing studies based on PT or aPTT are interpreted based on the fact that a 50% level of any coagulation factor alone gives normal PT and aPTT values. Both of these screening assays have hyperbolic curves, that is, a decrease in any one factor does not lead to a linear prolongation of either of the two assays. At 50% levels of any coagulation factor, global clotting assays will fall in the normal range.[51] Only with values less than 50% of specific factors will PT and aPTT begin to prolong. The sensitivity of PT and aPTT to prolongation with lowering of clotting factors varies depending on the factor and the reagent made by the manufacturer.[22] Thus, if patient plasma is mixed 1:1 with normal plasma, PT or aPTT should be normal if no factor is present in the patient plasma. If the mixture does not correct to normal, something in the patient plasma may be interfering with function of the protein in normal plasma.

Because screening assays for inhibitors are not standardized, a mixing study is a weak assay fraught with misinterpretation and, in many ways, is a much less attractive initial approach. Almost no studies provide evidence-based laboratory procedures for inhibitor screening assays. Some approaches to the use of mixing studies were developed for testing for lupus anticoagulants, which have their own peculiar aspects.[43–46] Critical issues in performing mixing studies is the ratio of patient plasma to normal plasma (1:1 to 4:1), the time of incubation from mixing to assay (immediate to 2 hours), and the assays used for measuring results (PT, aPTT). One critical investigation examined the sensitivity and specificity of mixing studies for assessing factor deficiencies and anticoagulants.[52] Patient and normal plasma were incubated at 37°C for 1 hour before assay in a ratio of 1:1 or 4:1 patient to normal plasma. On an aPTT mix of 1:1 with percent correction of 70% to 75% calculated using a specific formula (see reference for formula), the sensitivity and specificity in recognizing a factor deficiency or anticoagulant were 100% and 33% or 33% and 100%, respectively. When the percent correction was 50% calculated from a ratio of 4:1 patient to normal in the plasma mix for the aPTT, the sensitivity and specificity in recognizing a factor deficiency or anticoagulant improved to 88% and 100% or 100% and 88%, respectively.[52] Likewise, on a PT mix of 1:1 with a percent correction of 70% to 75% calculated using a specific formula (see reference for formula), the sensitivity and specificity in recognizing a factor deficiency or anticoagulant were 95% and 50% or 50% and 95%, respectively. When the percent correction was greater than 40% calculated from a ratio of 4:1 patient to normal in the plasma mix for the PT, the sensitivity and specificity in recognizing a factor deficiency or anticoagulant improved to 96% and 100% or 100% and 96%, respectively.[52] Further studies showed that assay after an immediate mix versus 1-hour incubation at 37°C had lower sensitivity and specificity. These investigations show the variability of mixing studies test performance and their "usefulness" in translating their information into meaningful diagnostic data. Once the presence of an inhibitor is determined, factors assays must be performed to isolate the specific protein to which the inhibitor is directed. Furthermore, specific inhibitor studies are needed to confirm the diagnostic impression and determine titer.

As a second initial approach to diagnosis of a specific coagulation protein defect, the specific defect of a prolonged coagulation assay can be obtained by performing all relevant coagulation factor assays indicated by the abnormal PT and aPTT. If any one test value is decreased, then a specific coagulation factor inhibitor assay for that factor can be performed. One can argue that an excess number of specific assays is being performed, but in most developed clinical institutions, these assays are automated and can be performed more efficiently in batch fashion than piecemeal with sequential ordering. The value of such an approach is the shortened time to a specific factor diagnosis. If more than one factor is found to be low using such an approach, then efforts are made to determine the global reason for the result. Finding a single factor decrease by any initial approach requires more effort to perform the specific assays and determine if there are inhibitors to that factor. One general approach to a specific inhibitor study can be performed by mixing various ratios of patient plasma to normal plasma (e.g., 1:1, 2:1, 4:1, 1:2, 1:4), incubating the samples for 2 hours at 37°C, and then assaying the level of the specific factor in the mixture.[53] Simultaneously, the patient plasma and normal plasma used in the mixing study are incubated under the same conditions. At the time of assay, the percent activities of the specific factor under study in the normal plasma, patient plasma, and each of the mixtures are obtained. If the *observed value* at any given ratio of patient plasma to control plasma is less than the calculated *expected value* of mixing the two plasmas in the various ratios (e.g., 1:1, 2:1, 1:2, etc.), then one can conclude that an inhibitor present in patient plasma transferred to the normal plasma sample. For example, if there is 100% activity (1 U/mL) of the factor being studied in an undiluted sample, a 1:1 dilution of normal plasma with factor-deficient plasma should give an activity level of approximately 50%. If the same normal plasma was incubated 1:1 with patient plasma and the activity was 32%, one should conclude that something in the patient plasma transferred and inhibited the factor's activity in normal plasma, which is the definition of an inhibitor. This approach is a general, nonquantitative method for assessing a coagulation factor inhibitor. A specifically quantitative method for determining inhibitors to any coagulation factor can be developed for all coagulation factors using a modification of specific inhibitor assays used to characterize factor VIII inhibitors.[30–32] This approach is preferred because it standardizes assay performance and method for reporting inhibitor assay results. Given the vagaries of general mixing studies for inhibitors, my approach has been to determine if a single coagulation factor is affected when the screening tests are abnormal and then determine if there is a specific inhibitor to the activity of that factor using a standardized approach to a specific factor inhibitor assay.[30–32]

SCREENING TESTS USED TO RECOGNIZE PATIENTS WITH DISORDERS OF PLATELET NUMBER OR FUNCTION

Recognition of platelet function disorders is critical to any hemostatic evaluation (see Chapters 129, 141, and 142). Knowing the platelet count is essential because thrombocytopenia alone may increase bleeding risk. Obtaining a detailed medication history from patients is important in order to realize the mechanism of action of each medication and its possible influence on assays for platelet function. It is clinically not useful to document abnormal platelet function in a patient taking interfering medication. Screening tests for platelet function testing have been developed; each has advantages as well as disadvantages. The screening tests for platelets are as follows:

1. *Platelet count.* This assay measures the number of platelets in 1 μL of blood. It is used to exclude a quantitative platelet defect as the cause of a bleeding disorder. Causes of thrombocytopenia are discussed in Chapters 32 and 138 to 140.
2. *Bleeding time.* To perform this assay, the forearm is pierced, and the time until bleeding stops is measured. Specific devices have been manufactured to perform this assay, which assesses platelet number or function. The bleeding time is a very qualitative assay influenced by technique, skin characteristics, and platelet count.[54] It should only be performed by experienced technologists. In general, it should not be performed on any patient with a platelet count less than 100,000/μL because a low platelet count alone can lead to prolongation of the bleeding time. The bleeding time assay is not a good predictor of surgical bleeding.[55,56] It is seldom useful when performed on a hospitalized patient. However, in the outpatient setting for an individual who has a bleeding history and is not taking any medications, an abnormal bleeding time may provide useful information. It can predict whether more costly von Wille-

brand factor studies and platelet aggregation and secretion studies will be useful for the diagnosis of a bleeding state. If thrombocytopenia is not present, the differential diagnosis of the long bleeding time includes von Willebrand disease and platelet function defects. Patients with Ehlers-Danlos syndrome, osteogenesis imperfecta, and scurvy may have variable prolongation of bleeding times that are not necessarily due to platelet dysfunction.[57–59]

3. *High-shear platelet function analyzers.* Several automated platelet function analyzers have come into use as screening tests for platelet function abnormalities, replacing the bleeding time as a diagnostic assay. Each method is unique to and should be evaluated against the wide range of congenital and acquired platelet function disorders before it is accepted as a screening assay. One product, the platelet function analyzer PFA-100 (Siemens, Deerfield, IL), has been best evaluated and is most widely used.[60,61] In citrated whole blood, the PFA-100 measures the "closure time" required for platelets to adhere to agonist-coated membranes and aggregate under high sheer stress (5000–6000 s^{-1}). It is a novel technology and not analogous to the bleeding time or light transmission platelet aggregometry. Two cartridges are available: collagen–ADP and collagen–epinephrine-coated membranes. Platelet function is measured as a function of the time needed to occlude the aperture, termed "closure time." Abnormal closure times are longer than the mean values of laboratory-specific values for normals. Each laboratory that uses this technology must determine its own normal values because of influences of different collection tubes and anticoagulant concentrations. Test results can only be interpreted as normal or abnormal. The assay does not make a specific diagnosis (e.g., von Willebrand disease). The PFA-100 may be useful to screen for individuals with von Willebrand disease, Glanzmann thrombasthenia, and Bernard-Soulier syndrome but may be less sensitive to primary platelet secretion defects and storage pool disorders.[62–66] Any abnormality detected by the PFA-100 requires specific testing for von Willebrand disease and platelet function disorders for diagnosis.

INTERPRETATION OF SCREENING TESTS OF PLATELET FUNCTION

Abnormalities on one or more of the screening tests in a patient with a normal platelet count usually suggests von Willebrand disease or a defect in platelet function. Of note, von Willebrand disease or platelet function defects leading to bleeding can be present even with one or both of the screening assays is normal. At present, no screening assay can exclude the diagnosis of von Willebrand disease or a platelet function defect. If the clinical history is compelling but the screening tests are normal, more definitive von Willebrand factor or platelet function testing is needed. Likewise, if a screening test for platelet function abnormalities is abnormal, the consulting physician has the onus to diagnose or exclude von Willebrand disease or a platelet function defect. Thus, once medication or nonprescription drug use is excluded, more sophisticated, specifically diagnostic studies for von Willebrand disease and a platelet function defect are needed for most patients requiring invasive procedures. In general, one of 10 patients in this diagnostic category have a platelet function defect. The majority of individuals fall into the category of von Willebrand disease. Von Willebrand disease is discussed in Chapters 128 and 129. Its diagnosis is made by abnormal studies of von Willebrand antigen, von Willebrand factor activity (ristocetin cofactor assay and/or collagen binding assay), and von Willebrand factor multimers. Some patients with von Willebrand disease also have a reduced factor VIII assay, presenting with a long aPTT. Certain subtypes of patients with von Willebrand disease (type IIB or platelet-type) have a lower threshold to agglutinate and aggregate to ristocetin (0.3–0.6 mg/mL) in platelet-rich plasma; normal individuals do not respond to this concentration of ristocetin. However, all normals respond to 1.0 mg/mL and higher concentrations of ristocetin added to platelet-rich plasma.

In addition to evaluation for von Willebrand disease, individuals with an abnormal bleeding time or PFA-100 result may require evaluation with platelet aggregation studies. Two forms of platelet aggregation studies are available: light transmission aggregometry in platelet-rich plasma and impedance aggregometry in platelet-rich plasma or whole blood. Light transmission aggregometry in platelet-rich plasma is the gold standard of platelet function testing[67]; impedance aggregometry is less well characterized.[68] Whole-blood impedance aggregometry to some extent is a screening study as well. When performed in conjunction with platelet secretion, either of ATP or serotonin, light transmission aggregometry can be diagnostic of several well-characterized platelet function defects and can characterize defects in others (see Chapters 141 and 142). The procedures for light transmission aggregometry have been reviewed.[69–71] Because of the wide variability in how light transmission aggregometry is performed in clinical laboratories, efforts are being made to develop minimal standards for the performance of platelet function testing in clinical laboratories.[72,73] In light transmission aggregometry, the absence of platelet aggregation in response to physiologic platelet agonists is indicative of Glanzmann thrombasthenia (defects in integrin $\alpha_{IIb}\beta_3$), whereas absent agglutination/aggregation in response to ristocetin suggests Bernard-Soulier syndrome (defects in glycoproteins Ib, IX, and V) or von Willebrand disease. Platelet storage pool disorders can be diagnosed if platelet light transmission aggregometry is performed simultaneously with studies that include measurement of proteins within or released from platelet α or dense granules or measurement of granule membrane proteins (e.g., P-selectin) that become surface expressed after cell activation. Platelet activation defects, such as that induced by aspirin, can be diagnosed as well using this combination of techniques (see Chapters 141 and 142). Finally, with appropriate monoclonal antibodies, flow cytometry can be useful in measuring the surface expression of platelet glycoproteins and the activation state of the cell.[74]

BLEEDING DISORDERS NOT RECOGNIZED BY SCREENING TESTS FOR COAGULATION PROTEINS OR PLATELETS

A few rare bleeding disorders are not recognized by routine blood coagulation and platelet screening tests (see Table 122–2). These entities include, in order of frequency, factor XIII defects, α_2-antiplasmin defects, plasminogen activator inhibitor 1 defects, and α_1-antitrypsin Pittsburgh. Factor XIII deficiency can be congenital or acquired, especially after isoniazid therapy.[75] α_2-Antiplasmin defects and plasminogen activator inhibitor 1 defects produce hyperfibrinolytic states as a result of reduced inhibition of plasmin and tissue plasminogen activator or urokinase, respectively.[76,77] α_2-Antiplasmin deficiency can be acquired in acute leukemia or other activated coagulation states.[78] Deficiency or abnormal forms of plasminogen activator inhibitor 1 also are associated with a bleeding state.[77] α_1-Antitrypsin Pittsburgh is an exceedingly rare bleeding disorder caused by a mutation in antitrypsin that results in potent thrombin inhibition, preventing clot formation.[79]

OTHER ACTIVITIES FOR HEMOSTASIS LABORATORIES

Thrombosis Evaluation

In addition to the diagnosis of bleeding disorders, the hemostasis laboratory is important in the evaluation of prothrombotic states (see Chapter 134). Evaluation of prothrombotic states serves the patient in many ways. In individuals with idiopathic thrombosis, recognition of a specific molecular or protein defect may be important in determining the duration of anticoagulant therapy. Certain prothrombotic states (e.g., antithrombin, protein C, and protein S deficiencies, antiphospholipid antibody syndrome) may confer higher risk for recurrence and thus suggest long-term anticoagulation after the first event. Recognition of less severe prothrombotic states (e.g., factor V Leiden and prothrombin 20210 polymorphisms, functional defects in fibrinogen and plasminogen) do not in themselves confer high risk for thrombosis but when conjoined with another risk factor may confer higher risk. Knowing this information helps patients engage in risk modification activity (e.g., stop taking oral contraceptives). Finally, 18% of patients without a family history of thrombosis and 30% to 40% of patients with a family history may have an identifiable molecular or protein risk factor for venous thrombosis.[80] This information helps many patients deal with anticoagulant management issues after they present with idiopathic thrombosis.

Monitoring Acute Hemostatic and Thrombotic Conditions

In addition to the diagnosis of hemostatic and thrombotic disorders, the coagulation laboratory has the function of monitoring patient therapy. Patients receiving unfractionated heparin (UFH) and warfarin are monitored by aPTT and PT, respectively. New monitoring roles are being established for these facilities. This section is divided into two parts: monitoring of anticoagulation therapy and measurement of activated coagulation.

Anticoagulation monitoring is an increasingly larger activity of hemostasis laboratories. In addition to UFH and warfarin monitoring using clot-based assays, low-molecular-weight heparin monitoring is an important activity in the hospitalized patient. This monitoring is especially important in patients who are obese, in those who have renal function compromise, and in patients prior to elective surgery.[81] Anti-factor Xa assays for monitoring low-molecular-weight heparins can be developed against each agent using the WHO's low-molecular-weight heparin for the standard curve.[50] Similarly, there is interest in developing clinical assays in addition to the aPTT for monitoring direct thrombin inhibitors, such as argatroban hirudin or bivalirudin as antifactor IIa chromogenic assays.[50]

Monitoring of activated coagulation states and their amelioration with treatment is another activity of the specialized hemostatic laboratory. The classic activated coagulation state is DIC (see Chapter 132). DIC is a clinicopathologic state associated with tissue destruction as a result of infectious, traumatic, obstetrical, malignant, and connective tissue disorders. The two forms of clinical presentation are an *acute* form that is a hyperfibrinolytic state and a *subacute* form that is more indolent. In the acute form, aPTT and PT are elevated, and the fibrinogen and platelet count are low. In the subacute form, aPTT, PT, and platelet may be normal or slightly, low and fibrinogen can be normal or even elevated. Finding a prolonged PT and aPTT with a reduced fibrinogen and platelet count usually indicates DIC in the hospitalized patient until proven otherwise.[82] This clinical laboratory phenotype of DIC most probably results from a secondary hyperfibrinolytic state and is the form of DIC most commonly recognized. The biochemical diagnosis of DIC then is simplified to finding evidence of simultaneous thrombin and plasmin formation. The D-dimer is a plasmin-proteolyzed fragment of insoluble, cross-linked fibrin.[83,84] It is a confirmatory assay for DIC in the appropriate clinical condition. Insoluble fibrin results from thrombin cleavage of soluble fibrinogen and cross-linking of fibrin by thrombin/activated factor XIII. Presently, a scoring system to aid in the diagnosis of DIC is available.[85] D-Dimer elevation characterizes DIC but is not specific for it. It is positive in patients in postoperative states, with resolving hematomas, and after large-vessel or pulmonary thrombosis. A positive D-dimer also has become an adjunct to the clinical diagnosis of pulmonary embolism.[86] Heparin-induced thrombocytopenia is another coagulation laboratory activation state. Laboratory diagnosis and monitoring the effectiveness of therapy for heparin-induced thrombocytopenia is discussed in detail in Chapter 140.

SUGGESTED READINGS

Chen X, Wang J, Paszti Z, Wang F, et al: Ordered adsorption of coagulation protein factor XII on negatively charged polymer surfaces probed by sum frequency generation vibrational spectroscopy. Anal Bioanal Chem 388:65, 2007.

Field JJ, Fenske TS, Blinder MA: Rituximab for the treatment of patients with very high-titre acquired factor VIII inhibitors refractory to conventional chemotherapy. Haemophilia 13:46, 2007.

Hayward CPM, Harrison P, Cattaneo M, Ortel TL, Rai AK: Platelet function analyzer (PFA)-100 closure time in the evaluation of platelet disorders and-platelet function. J Thromb Haemost 4:312, 2006.

Jennings LK, White MM: Platelet aggregation. In Michelson AD (ed.): Platelets, 2nd ed. Amsterdam, Elsevier, 2007, p 495.

Kannemeier C, Shibamiya A, Nakazawa F, et al: Extracellular RNA constitutes a natural procoagulant cofactor in blood coagulation. Proc Natl Acad Sci U S A 104:6388, 2007.

Kearon C, Ginsberg JS, Douketis J, et al: Canadian Pulmonary Embolism Diagnosis Study (CANPEDS) Group: An evaluation of D-dimer in the diagnosis of pulmonary embolism: A randomized trial. Ann Intern Med 144:812, 2006.

Michelson AD, Linder MD, Barnard MR, Furman MI, Frelinger AL III: Flow cytometry. In Michelson AD (ed.): Platelets, 2nd ed. Amsterdam, Elsevier, 2007, p 545.

Moffat KA, Ledford-Kraemer MR, Nichols WL, Hayward CP: Variability in clinical laboratory practice in testing for disorders of platelet function: Results of two surveys of the North American Specialized Coagulation Laboratory Association. Thromb Haemost 93:549, 2005.

O'Donnell MJ, Kearon C, Johnson J, et al: Preoperative anticoagulation activity after bridging low-molecular-weight heparin for temporary interruption of warfarin. Ann Intern Med 146:184, 2007.

Renne T, Pozagajova M, Gruner S, et al: Defective thrombus formation in mice lacking coagulation factor XII. J Exp Med 202:271, 2005.

Smith SA, Mutch NJ, Baskar D, Rohloff P, Docampo R, Morrissey JH: Polyphosphates modulates blood coagulation and fibrinolysis. Proc Natl Acad Sci U S A 103:903, 2006.

Zhou L, Schmaier AH: Platelet aggregation testing in platelet-rich plasma: Description of procedures with the aim to develop standards in the field. Am J Clin Pathol 123:172, 2005.

REFERENCES

For complete list of references log onto www.expertconsult.com

CHAPTER 123

STRUCTURE, BIOLOGY, AND GENETICS OF FACTOR VIII

Geoffrey Kemball-Cook, John H. McVey, and Edward GD Tuddenham

Factor VIII is a key cofactor in blood coagulation. Absence of functional factor VIII in plasma results in the serious bleeding disorder hemophilia A, which affects approximately one in 10,000 live births (see Chapter 125). Although hemophilia A has been regarded as a good candidate for gene therapy, traditional treatment of hemophilia consists of factor VIII replacement using plasma-derived or recombinant factor VIII products. Developments in factor VIII biochemistry have improved our understanding of how factor VIII interacts with other macromolecules in the performance of its normal procoagulant (clotting) function and how naturally occurring mutations result in the spectrum of clinical phenotypes found in hemophilia A (see box on Plasma Protein Factor VIII).

FACTOR VIII STRUCTURE AND FUNCTION

For successful normal human hemostasis, both tissue factor/activated factor VII-dependent initiation of clotting and factor VIII-dependent amplification of this initial response are absolutely required. Initiation of blood coagulation generates small quantities of activated factor IX and factor X. However the factor VIII-dependent mechanism catalyzes conversion of factor X to factor Xa far more efficiently, thus dramatically amplifying the events triggered by the tissue factor-dependent pathway.[1] This factor VIII-dependent amplification is indispensable for maintaining hemostasis, as shown by the fact that absence of circulating functionally active factor VIII causes the coagulation disorder hemophilia A.

Coagulation is a complex network of interactions (see Chapter 118). Factor VIII is proteolytically activated in the early stages of clotting to activated factor VIII. It is released from its plasma carrier protein, von Willebrand factor (vWF), and then complexes with and functions as a cofactor for the serine protease factor IXa. The membrane-bound complex (the so-called *tenase complex*) activates factor X to factor Xa.[2] Factor Xa thus produced can participate in a similar complex ("prothrombinase") with activated factor V for proteolytic conversion of prothrombin into thrombin, the key enzyme of the coagulation cascade that generates insoluble fibrin from soluble fibrinogen. It is possible that the procoagulant membrane surface on which the tenase complex assembles is provided by activated platelets,[3] although this has not been proven. Although detailed understanding of the assembly and function of these membrane-associated complexes is lacking, it is clear that a major role of the membrane surface is to concentrate components of the tenase and prothrombinase complexes, limit their diffusion to two dimensions, and provide the optimal spatial orientation of the components. For the factor VIII-dependent complex, this results in a large increase in factor Xa generation resulting from lowering the Michaelis constant (K_m) for factor X[2,4] and increase in the catalytic constant of the reaction (k_{cat}).[5]

Factor VIII Structure

Factor VIII is a large plasma protein with a predicted molecular mass of approximately 270 kd in the absence of additional posttranslational glycosylation. Inspection of the predicted linear amino acid sequence of the factor VIII molecule (mature sequence 2332 amino acid residues after removal of the signal peptide) demonstrates a clear domain organization consisting of three homologous A domains, two homologous C domains, and the unique large B domain, together with three short highly acidic sequences *a1, a2,* and *a3.* These sequences are arranged in the order (N-terminus to C-terminus) A1-*a1*-A2-*a2*-B-*a3*-A3-C1-C2 (Fig. 123–1).[6,7] Much evidence from a large range of proteins of known structure strongly indicates that such homologous domains fold independently from each other and thus are structurally distinct. This domain structure is similar to that of the homologous factor V,[8] except that factor V lacks the three short acidic peptides. The A domains have approximately 40% identity with each other and with the A domains of factor V, as well as with the three-A-domain proteins ceruloplasmin (Cp) and hephaestin. The C domains are homologous to several proteins, including the lipid-binding lectin discoidin I. The C domains also exhibit 40% identity to the C domains of factor V. The B domains of factors VIII and V do not show any sequence conservation with each other or with any other known protein.[9] However, they show strong similarities in two other respects: overall size and high density of N-linked glycosylation.

These sequence data provide clear indications that factors VIII and V are derived from a common ancestor, which itself was derived from a three-A-domain progenitor for all four related A-domain proteins.[10,11]

Prior to secretion into plasma, factor VIII is proteolytically processed within the cell to a series of metal ion-linked heterodimers produced by cleavage at the B-*a3* junction and by a number of additional cleavages within the B domain.[12] These cleavages generate the heavy chain composed of A1 (1-336: mature protein numbering), *a1* (337-372), A2 (373-719), and *a2* (720-740) with variable lengths of B (741-1648), and the light chain composed of *a3* (1649-1689), A3 (1690-2019), C1 (2020-2172), and C2 (2173-2332). Thus, circulating factor VIII in vivo consists of a heavy chain of variable molecular mass (e.g., from 90 kd, when only the A1-A2 domains are present, to 220 kd when the full-length B domain is present) and a light chain of 76 kd.[13]

Much is known from genetic and biochemical approaches. However, in order to relate further information about structure–function relationships in factor VIII and to interpret mutations, information on the three-dimensional structure of the protein is required. X-ray crystallography can give the highest resolution but requires large amounts of pure protein and successful crystallization of the target protein. Nuclear magnetic resonance also is high resolution, requires smaller amounts of protein, and does not require crystallization, but the factor VIII molecule is too large for this technique. However, these techniques can be applied to individual domains of factor VIII.

Electron microscopy either of individual protein molecules or of ordered arrays can provide medium-resolution structural information. Finally, homology modeling can be used to predict the structure of a domain or group of domains based on an existing high-resolution structure for a related protein.

Election microscopy studies at very low resolution led to characterization of the size and shape of factor VIII molecules in solution.[14,15] A globular core of approximately 12-nm diameter with a rod-like protrusion, suggested to be the B domain, up to 50 nm long, was defined. Fluorescence energy transfer studies also suggested close association of light chain and heavy chain.[16]

Plasma Protein Factor VIII

The plasma protein factor VIII is essential for rapid blood clotting. The absence of functional factor VIII is the cause of the bleeding disorder hemophilia A, which affects one in 5,000 male births.

Homology modeling was used in an attempt to generate useful models for part of the factor VIII molecule. Homology modeling required the availability of high-resolution structures for proteins or domains homologous to all or part of the factor VIII molecule. The first model, based on the crystal structure of the protein nitrite reductase, which has three domains rather distantly related to the factor VIII A domains, suggested a "triangular" structure for these domains in factor VIII.[17] Shortly afterward, a crystal structure of the related protein human Cp was produced.[18] This was used as the basis for construction of an improved A-domain homology model confirming the triangular layout and providing a revised arrangement for the

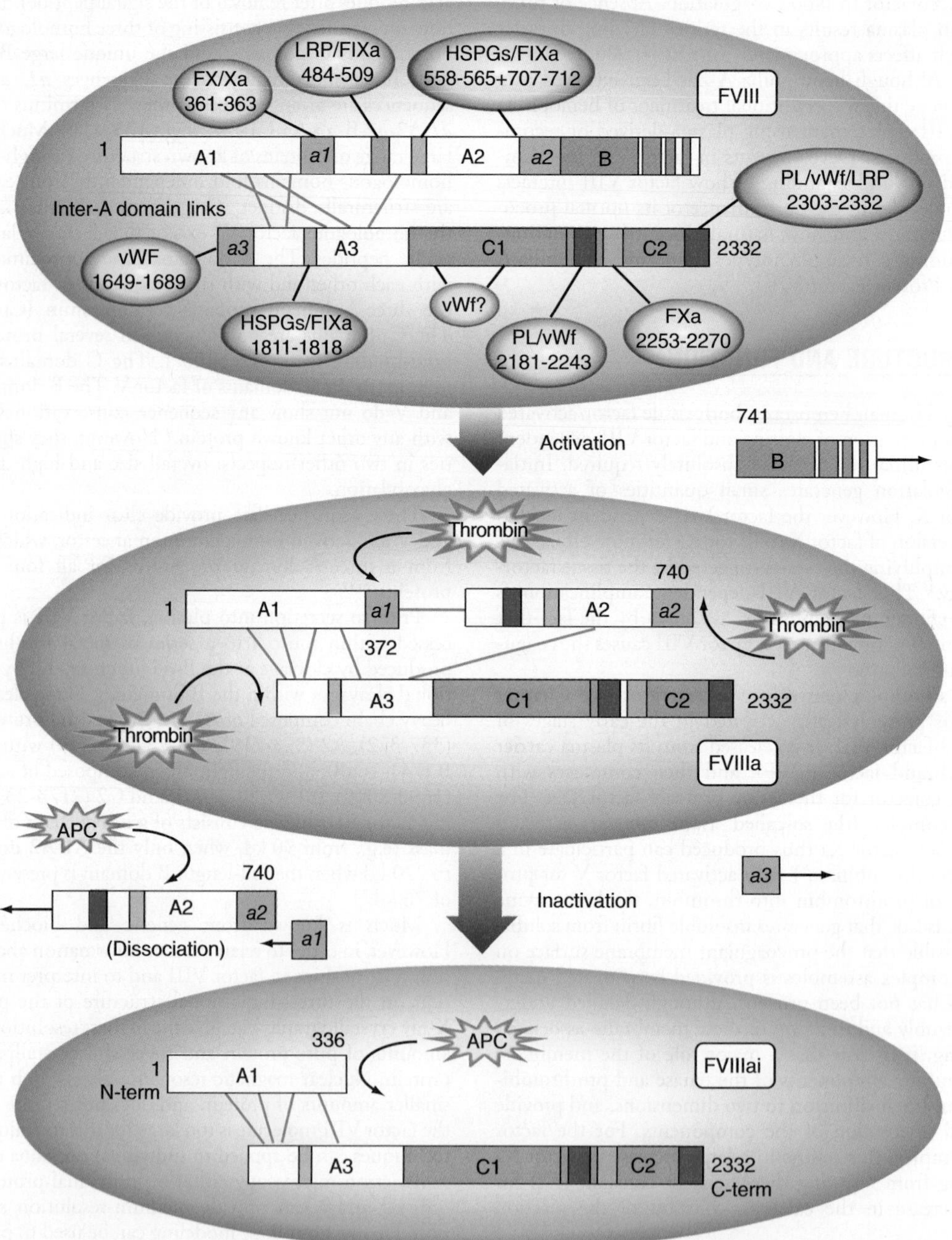

Figure 123–1 Factor VIII domain structure and functional regions, proteolytic activation by thrombin, and subsequent inactivation by subunit dissociation or activated protein C cleavage. Prior to activation, factor VIII circulates as a two-chain noncovalently linked heterodimer held together by electrostatic and hydrophobic interaction between the A domains. The regions of factor VIII involved in binding various macromolecules are indicated. Activation of factor VIII by cleavages at positions 372, 740, and 1689 releases the B domain and acidic peptide *a3*, generating the factor VIIIa heterotrimer. Here the A2 subunit is weakly associated with the stable A1/A3-C1-C2 heterodimer through electrostatic interactions. Following activation, inactivation of factor VIIIa proceeds either by spontaneous dissociation of the A2 domain or by proteolytic cleavage by APC after residues 336 and 562 in A1 and A2, respectively. LRP, low-density lipoprotein receptor-related protein; PL, phospholipid; vWf, von Willebrand factor.

orientation of the subdomains, together with more reliable detail of the structure.[19] This model, together with the growing online database of hemophilic mutations,[20] was used to investigate structure–function in factor VIII as well as for direct experimental studies with recombinant factor VIII variants.

Electron microscopic studies of arrays of factor VIII molecules adhering to a phospholipid monolayer defined the overall shape of the factor VIII molecule at low resolution and provided information on factor VIII–phospholipid interaction.[21] Contemporaneously, a high-resolution crystal structure for the factor VIII C2 domain was derived, obtained with highly purified recombinant C2 domain. Although preliminary homology models had been constructed previously for the factor VIII C domains,[22] this was the first high-quality structural information available for either C domain. For the first time, hemophilic mutations could be unambiguously studied at high resolution in part of the factor VIII molecule; in addition, a plausible mechanism for the interaction of factor VIII with a membrane via the C2 domain was derived.[23]

Because the C1 and C2 domains of factor VIII are closely related by homology, a homology model for the factor VIII C1 domain was generated that facilitated analysis of factor VIII functions.[24] In further studies, the C1 and C2 structures were combined with refined electron microscopic array data to produce a five-domain factor VIII structure (A1-A2-A3-C1-C2) bound to a phospholipid membrane.[25] This factor VIII model satisfied a large number of detailed biochemical and biophysical criteria and thus was used for a number of detailed studies of both naturally occurring hemophilic variants and in vitro mutagenesis. A draft molecular model for the factor VIIIa-IXa complex on the phospholipid membrane was produced by manually docking the factor VIII model with the crystal structure of factor IXa.[13] This model for the complex is consistent with many existing data, including defined binding sequences on both proteins. This basic tenase model was adopted for various mutation/mutagenesis studies.[26,27] Since the release of this model, a crystal structure for part of the related factor Va molecule lacking the A2 domain has been reported.[28] In addition, detailed combined modeling/docking methods have generated further hypothetical models of tenase that can be used to test hypotheses of function.[29] Most recently two groups have solved the crystal structure of B-domainless human factor VIII, confirming the predicted triangular arrangement of the three A domains, associated with tow C domains suggested to interact side-by-side with phospholipid membranes following activation.[29a,29b] The availability of these structures facilitates both close analysis of hemophilia-causing mutations together with the design of altered factor VIII molecules with greater stability or potency.

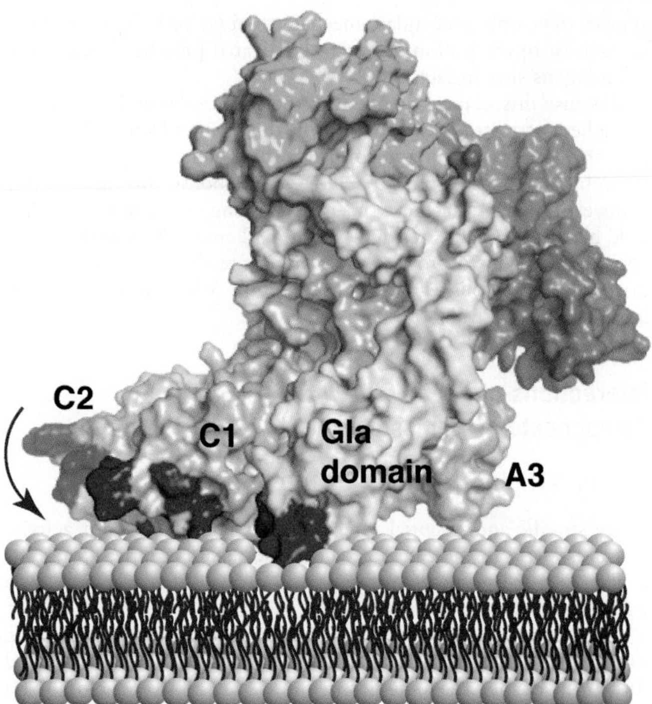

Figure 123–2 Model of the factor IXa-factor VIIIa complex. The complex of factor VIIIa (heavy chain [dark grey] and light chain [light grey and grey]) and factor IXa (heavy chain [orange] and light chain [yellow] includes four putative membrane binding sites: the bases of C1 and C2 domain, the A3 domain loop of factor VIII and the Gla domain of factor IXa [blue]. Possible interactions of the factor IXa-factor VIIIa complex with phospholipid membrane surfaces are illustrated.[29a]

Mechanisms of Factor VIII Action

Activation of Factor VIII

Factor VIII circulates in plasma as an inactive pro-cofactor and must be activated to factor VIIIa by specific proteolytic cleavages for full activity. After initiation of coagulation, factor VIII is activated by two major physiologic activators: factor Xa and thrombin. The cleavages resulting in factor VIII activation by thrombin and factor Xa have been defined.[30] Both proteases cleave the factor VIII molecule after Arg372 (between *a1* and A2), after Arg740 (between *a2* and B) within heavy chain, and after Arg1689 (between *a3* and A3) within light chain, yielding noncovalently linked A1-*a1*, A2-*a2*, and A3-C1-C2 fragments, which remain associated as heterotrimeric factor VIIIa (see Fig. 123–1). The short acidic *a3* peptide is lost. Because the *a3* region bears an important vWF-binding site, removal of *a3* by cleavage at Arg1689 promotes release of factor VIIIa from vWF and a substantial increase in factor VIIIa affinity for platelets.[31] In addition, cleavage at Arg1689 is required for generation of the maximal cofactor activity of factor VIIIa.[32]

Removal of *a3* leads to a 10-fold decrease in the association rate constant and a 160-fold increase in the dissociation rate constant of interaction of factor VIIIa with vWF in comparison with nonactivated factor VIII[33] and a 1600-fold decrease in factor VIIIa affinity for vWF, enabling factor VIIIa to bind to a membrane surface and to factor IXa during assembly of the tenase complex. The A1 and A3 domains retain a metal ion-mediated interaction, and this relatively stable A1/A3-C1-C2 dimer is more weakly associated with the separate A2 domain through electrostatic interactions. The role of individual metal ions and amino acids in the association for factor VIII domains has been extensively studied.[26,34,35]

Information on the factor VIII sites responsible for binding of these activators is available. An important factor Xa-binding site was localized to C2 residues 2253-2270[36] and a site responsible for thrombin-catalyzed cleavage at Arg1689 in the light chain assigned to the C2 domain of factor VIII.[37] Residues 361-363 in the acidic peptide *a1* have been implicated in binding factor Xa during activation of factor VIII.[38] In addition, sites in A1 and A2 are associated with cleavage at Arg740.[39]

Inactivation of Factor VIII

Clotting in response to injury must be rapid but also localized in both place and time, because uncontrolled thrombin generation would risk intravascular thrombosis. Thus, factor VIIIa activity is degraded by two separate processes, resulting in an inactivated cofactor often referred to as *factor VIIIai* (see Fig. 123–1).

First, spontaneous dissociation of the A2 domain from the factor VIIIa heterotrimer in the absence of any further cleavage of factor VIIIa results in loss of factor VIIIa procoagulant function, and hemophilic mutations at the A2 interdomain interface display more rapid dissociation. This mechanism appears to be the primary cause of the rapid downregulation of tenase activity in vivo.[40] Second, specific proteolytic cleavage by activated protein C after Arg336 and Arg562 effectively destroys the procoagulant modulation of factor VIIIa of the factor IXa active site in the tenase complex.[41] However, this appears to be only a secondary mechanism of factor VIIIa control,[42,43] in contrast to the profound effect of activated protein C cleavage at homologous sites in factor Va.

Because dissociation of A2 from the noncovalently linked factor VIIIa heterotrimer appears to limit the duration of factor VIII action in vivo, one strategy for maximizing the potency of administered recombinant factor VIII is to delay or even abolish this dissociation. A novel approach to achieve this goal is to engineer a novel disulfide link between cysteine residues in the A2 and A3 domains. This approach has shown promise in laboratory testing.[44,45] Although A2 dissociation is abolished, the mutant factor VIII molecules can be inactivated by activated protein C.

Interactions of Factor VIII with Components of Hemostasis

Factor VIII Interactions in the Tenase Complex

Three specific and essential interactions enable the cofactor activity of factor VIIIa in the assembled intrinsic tenase complex: with the enzyme factor IXa, the substrate factor X, and the membrane upon which the tenase complex assembles.

The factor VIIIa light chain bears an important factor IXa binding site ($K_d \approx 15$ nM) within A3 domain residues 1811-1818,[46,47] and this largely enables the high-affinity interaction between factors VIIIa and IXa, although the sequence is not involved in modulation of the factor IXa active site. The exact region of factor IXa involved is not clear; however, the site is included within the factor IXa light chain formed of its γ-glutamyl carboxylic acid (Gla)-epidermal growth factor 1 (EGF1)-EGF2 domains. In addition, cleavage of the factor IX zymogen is required, and the Ca^{2+} binding site in the EGF1 domain and EGF1-EGF2 salt bridge must be intact.[48,49] An interaction with the N-terminal Gla domain of factor IXa was suggested.[50]

The A2 domain also interacts with factor IXa directly through residues 330-338 in the factor IXa protease domain.[51,52] Although the affinity of factor IXa for isolated A2 is low ($K_d \approx 300$ nM), this interaction enables the cofactor activity of factor VIIIa, as interaction of the A2 domain with the factor IXa protease domain amplifies its enzymatic activity.[53] The A2 domain contains three amino acid sequences that are involved in interaction with factor IXa (see Fig. 123–1): 558-565,[54] 707-712,[55-57] and 484-509.[58] The 558-565 sequence has been modeled as an extended interface with the factor IXa protease domain helix.[52] In addition, a full FVIII-FIXa clocked structure using crystal structures of B-domainless FVIII and porcine FIXa has been constructed (Ngo et al, 2008).

The functionally important A2 sites that affect factor IXa enzymatic activity apparently are exposed only upon cleavage within the factor VIIIa heavy chain at Arg372, by either factor Xa or thrombin.[59] Recruitment of the light chain and A2 sites with factor IXa stabilizes factor VIIIa within the tenase complex, where factor IXa serves as a bridge linking the A2 subunit and A1/A3-C1-C2 heterodimer[60]; this delays spontaneous inactivation of factor VIIIa heterotrimer due to dissociation of A2.[40,61] The effect of the cleavages at Arg372 in the heavy chain and Arg1689 within the light chain on the assembly of the functional tenase complex has been studied by fluorescence anisotropy with active site-labeled factor IXa.[32,59,62] The anisotropy increase induced by a factor VIII molecule with cleaved light chain (HC/A3-C1-C2) was significantly higher than that observed for factor VIII with intact light chain (HC/LC) and comparable to that for factor VIIIa.[32] That anisotropy change correlates with modulation of the factor IXa active site by factor VIII suggested that removal of the acidic sequence *a3* following cleavage at Arg1689 is required for optimal interaction of factor VIIIa with factor IXa. These studies also indicated that maximal stimulation of the factor IXa active site by factor VIIIa requires cleavage between A1 and A2 at Arg372 in addition to removal of *a3*.[53,59] Addition of factor X led to a further marked increase in anisotropy, suggesting that factor X also contributes to optimal orientation of the factor IXa active site in the assembled tenase complex.[53]

Limited information defines the factor VIII site(s) involved in interaction with the factor X, the zymogen substrate of the tenase complex. One site has been localized to *a1* (residues 337-372) based on the ability of the corresponding synthetic peptide to inhibit factor X binding to the isolated A1 domain and also on chemical cross-linking of this peptide with factor X.[63] This factor X interactive site subsequently was narrowed down to *a1* residues 349-372.[64] The *a1* peptide facilitates substrate binding into the complex, as cleavage of factor VIIIa by activated protein C (releasing the *a1* fragment) and mutation of acidic residues in the sequence 361-363 both raised the K_m for factor X.[65,66]

The factor VIII heavy chain does not appear to contribute to factor VIII membrane binding. The factor VIII light chain is important for interaction with phospholipids[67] and is entirely responsible for their interaction at high affinity. Activation of factor VIII to factor VIIIa by thrombin increases this affinity.[31] A conformational change occurs within the C2 domain associated with factor VIIIa release from vWF after loss of the *a3* peptide, resulting in a 10-fold increase in its affinity for phospholipid membranes.[31] The plasma concentration of factor VIII is approximately 1 nM, so decrease of the K_d for factor VIIIa–phospholipid interactions to a comparable nanomolar level (0.4–1.1 nM)[31] suggests that conditions favorable for factor VIIIa association with membranes may result after factor VIII activation at the site of coagulation.

Studies with synthetic factor VIII peptides suggested that the major factor VIII light chain sequence involved in phospholipid binding is located within the C2 domain at residues 2303-2332, as peptides encompassing this region inhibited factor VIII–phospholipid binding.[68,69] Binding localization to the C2 region 2181-2243 of various antibodies that prevent factor VIII–phospholipid interaction suggested it should contain factor VIII residues critical for interaction with phospholipid.[70] The 1.5-Å x-ray structure of the human factor VIII C2 domain further implicated this factor VIII region in phospholipid binding, as analysis of the structure suggested that three hydrophobic projections or "feet" formed by the side chains of Met2199/Phe2200, Val2223, and Leu 2251/Leu2252 might penetrate into the hydrophobic interior of the membrane bilayer.[23,71]

Interaction of factor VIII requires phospholipid surfaces with negatively charged head groups (e.g., phosphatidylserine). Thus, four basic residues were postulated to stabilize factor VIII–phospholipid binding by electrostatic interaction with such head groups (Arg2215, Arg2220, Lys2227, and Lys2249) because they lie close to the "feet."[25] Further direct analysis of factor VIII–phospholipid binding by electron crystallography permitted the resolution of five functional domains of factor VIII (A1, A2, A3, C1, and C2) on a phospholipid surface and strongly supported the contribution of these three loops, together with a fourth, Trp2313-His2315, in forming the phospholipid-interacting region.[25] Thus, two of the first three loops lie in the implicated 2181-2243 sequence and the fourth loop within the implicated 2303-2332 sequence. Predictions based on the x-ray structure of C2 and electron crystallographic studies of factor VIII were supported by alanine mutagenesis of the residues composing the hydrophobic "feet" Met2199/Phe2200 and Leu 2251/Leu2252, which strongly reduced the affinity of factor VIII for phospholipid.[72] In parallel with this effect on factor VIII–phospholipid binding, these mutations reduced factor VIII affinity for vWF, indicating that these two residues are important contributors to factor VIII–vWF interaction. Interestingly, the recent crystal structures of B-domainless FVIII suggest that both C1 an C2 contribute hydrophobic residues to phospholipid interaction in a side-by-side fashion (Ngo et al, 2008).

Interactions with von Willebrand Factor

von Willebrand factor is a large multimeric plasma protein composed of identical subunits of 220 kd (see Chapter 128). In the circulation, factor VIII molecules interact via the factor VIII light chain with vWF in a tight noncovalent complex with K_d of approximately 0.4 nM.[33,73] This complex is required for maintaining the normal factor VIII level in plasma. Binding to vWF reduces premature assembly of the tenase complex prior to factor VIII activation and prevents factor VIII inactivation by activated protein C, factor IXa, and factor Xa. Deficiency of vWF leads to a secondary deficiency of factor VIII[74,75] due to a lack of its protection from proteases and faster clearance from the circulation.

The factor VIII light chain contains at least two regions directly involved in binding to vWF (see Fig. 123–1): the acidic sequence *a3* (residues 1649-1689) preceding the A3 domain,[33,76] and one or more sequences within the C1 and C2 domains. Synthetic peptide studies had suggested that the sequence 2303-2332 in C2 was involved in both vWF and phospholipid binding,[33,68] and this was supported by the finding that the purified 2303-2324 peptide assumed an amphipathic helical conformation, in free solution, with affinity for phospholipid membranes.[69] However, x-ray crystallography of the C2 domain showed unambiguously that the 2303-2332 sequence lies largely within the domain core,[23] so such a helical structure is very unlikely, although individual residues within the sequence still could be important.

Involvement of the C1 domain in addition to C2 was demonstrated by the fact that vWF binding was affected by mutation of three C1 residues (Tyr2105, Arg2116, and Ser2119) in hemophilia A patients[77] and that Arg2150 in C1 also is associated with vWF interaction.[78–80] In addition, isolated C1-C2 fragment was shown to interact much more tightly with vWF than does the isolated C2 domain.[81] This finding suggests that vWF interaction is mediated by contributions from the *a3* peptide, C1, and C2, oriented to form a combined surface for interaction with either vWF or the phospholipid surface.[25] Although the heavy chain does not appear to interact directly with vWF, it is required for maximal affinity of factor VIII–vWF interaction, as affinity of the whole factor VIII molecule for vWF is 10-fold higher than for isolated light chain.[33]

Loss of the acidic *a3* peptide following factor VIII activation by thrombin promotes factor VIIIa dissociation from vWF, as *a3* is also suggested to be required for maintaining the C2 conformation optimal for vWF binding. A conformational change within the C2 domain upon removal of *a3* was indicated by a reduction in affinity of thrombin-cleaved light chain, compared to intact LC, for an anti-C2 monoclonal antibody NMC-VIII/5 that is conformationally sensitive.[33] Additional evidence for this conformational change was obtained using another antibody with a discontinuous epitope composed of two portions of the C2 domain, residues 2227-2241 and 2259-2279.[82] This antibody binding to these spatially close but distinct regions of C2 may account for its ability to "lock" the C2 conformation, thus preventing conformational changes within C2 induced by removal of *a3*. Affinity of factor VIIIa for vWF in the presence of the conformation-specific antibody (K_d 36 nM)[83] was 20-fold higher than in its absence (K_d 640 nM).[33] This confirms that after factor VIII activation by thrombin, the C2 domain undergoes a conformational change that is required for complete release of factor VIIIa from vWF.

Biosynthesis and Metabolism of Factor VIII

Factor VIII Biosynthesis and Processing

Expression profile analysis suggests expression in a variety of different tissues, with the highest levels of factor VIII mRNA detected in the liver and kidney.[84] Further evidence from liver transplantation in humans and dogs demonstrating restoration of normal levels of factor VIII in subjects with hemophilia A suggested the liver was the major site of synthesis. However, the cell type within the liver responsible for factor VIII synthesis is unclear. Synthesis of factor VIII has been attributed to hepatocytes, sinusoidal endothelial cells, and Kupffer cells. However, more recent data suggest the major cell type responsible for factor VIII synthesis are the liver sinusoidal endothelial cells, as these cells secrete active factor VIII when maintained in vitro,[85] and after transplantation in vivo these endothelial cells corrected the phenotype of hemophilia A mice.[86,87]

Much insight into the biosynthesis of factor VIII has come from analysis of expression in heterologous cell types with the purpose of producing recombinant factor VIII for therapeutic purposes.[88] In addition, characterization of the molecular defects responsible for the autosomal recessive bleeding disorder associated with combined deficiency of factors V and VIII revealed the importance of intracellular trafficking in the biosynthesis of factor VIII.[89]

The B domain of factor VIII can be deleted without loss of factor VIII procoagulant activity.[90] Expression cassettes encoding B-domain–deleted recombinant factor VIII resulted in significantly higher levels of mRNA over equivalent full-length recombinant factor VIII expression cassettes, resulting in higher levels of recombinant factor VIII protein synthesis. However, the levels of recombinant factor VIII secreted into the media did not increase proportionately, suggesting intracellular interactions were limiting efficient secretion.[91,92] Recombinant factor VIII is cotranslationally translocated into the lumen of the endoplasmic reticulum (ER) where it folds and assembles into tertiary structures. These reactions are facilitated by enzymes and molecular chaperones that interact with folding intermediates of recombinant factor VIII.

As the nascent protein chain enters the ER lumen, the sequence is scanned for asparagine residues in the consensus Asn-X-Ser/Thr motif, and preassembled core glycans are covalently added. Sequential trimming of two glucose residues allows the peptide to associate with the ER chaperones calnexin and calreticulin,[93] which associate with other luminal factors including members of the protein disulfide isomerase family. This most probably creates a protected environment that allows correct folding and formation of appropriate disulfide bonds. Release from calnexin/calreticulin is followed by cleavage of the innermost glucose residue from the N-glycan core. The structure of the released peptide is checked and a terminal glucose residue is added back onto the N-glycan core of polypeptides that have not folded correctly, allowing it to reassociate with the calnexin/calreticulin system in an attempt to acquire the native conformation. Another important protein chaperone in recombinant factor VIII expression is immunoglobulin heavy-chain binding protein BiP (GRP78 [78-kd glucose-regulated protein]).[94–96] BiP has an ATPase domain and interacts with recombinant factor VIII through an 11-residue hydrophobic β sheet that occurs within the homologous type 1 copper ion binding site in the A1 domain of factor VIII. Mutation of amino acid residue Phe309 within the β sheet to serine increased secretion of recombinant factor VIII several-fold and reduced the ATP requirement, suggesting that BiP plays a role in copper ion binding to recombinant factor VIII.[97]

A significant amount of recombinant factor VIII within the ER never transits to the Golgi compartment due to a failure to fold correctly. Improperly folded recombinant factor VIII proteins are targeted for ER-associated degradation by translocation back across the ER membrane to the cytosol where proteosomal degradation takes place.

If after release from chaperones recombinant factor VIII has folded correctly, then it will exit the ER. Studies of the molecular defect responsible for combined deficiency of factor V and factor VIII revealed that mutations lay in the genes encoding two proteins: either LMAN1 (also known as ERGIC 53) or MCFD2.[98–102] LMAN1 and MCFD2 form a stable complex that serves as a cargo receptor for efficient transport of factor V and factor VIII from the ER to the Golgi via COPII-coated vesicles.[103] The B domain of factor VIII appears to be the primary determinant of LMAN1-MCFD2 binding, most probably through mannose residues in the heavily glycosylated B domain as LMAN1 contains a carbohydrate recognition domain that binds mannose residues. MCFD2 contains two calcium ion-binding EF hands and interacts with LMAN1 in a calcium ion-dependent manner. MCFD2 is important in the efficient recruitment of factor VIII to LMAN1 and therefore ensures efficient ER export. The overall biosynthetic process in the ER and Golgi is shown in Fig. 123–3.

In the Golgi apparatus, factor VIII is further posttranslationally modified by proteolytic cleavage within the B domain at positions 1313 and 1648, modification of the *N*-linked oligosaccharides to

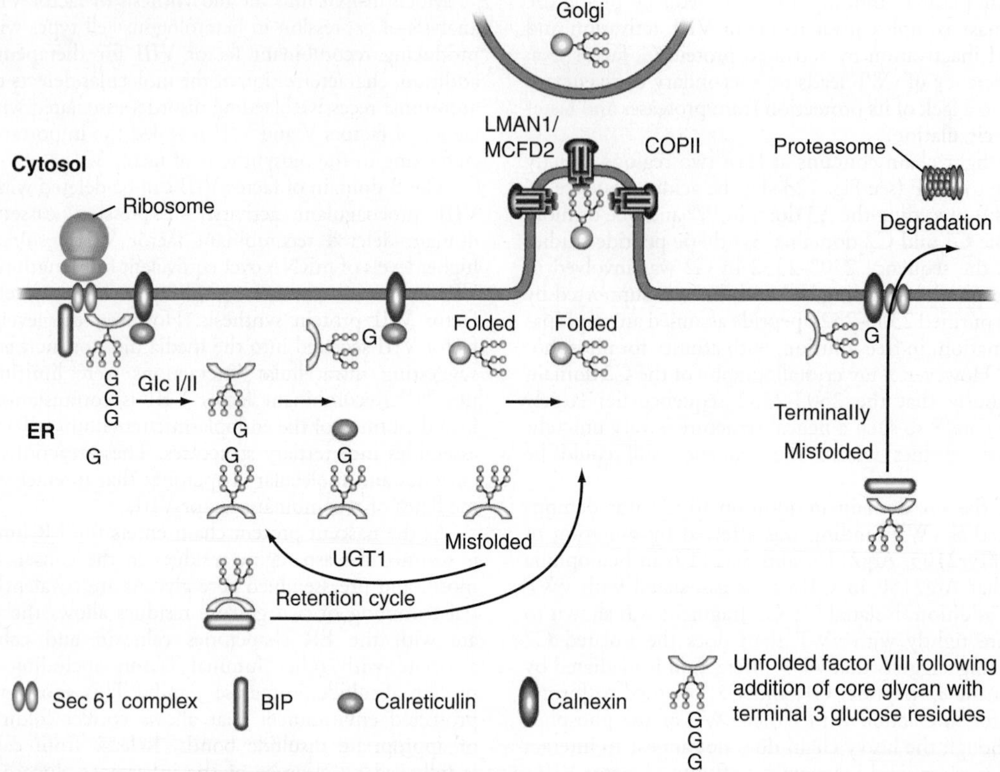

Figure 123–3 Biosynthesis of factor VIII. The proposed pathway of translation and trafficking through the endoplasmic reticulum (ER) to the Golgi compartment is indicated. Newly synthesized factor VIII is cotranslationally modified by addition of N-linked core glycans in the ER. Newly synthesized factor VIII associates with chaperones (calnexin, calreticulin, and immunoglobulin heavy-chain binding protein [BiP]) and their accessory proteins that aid the folding of the protein into its native conformation. Quality control mechanisms ensure misfolded protein is not transported from the ER but is retained to allow further refolding attempts. Terminally misfolded protein is transported to the cytosol for degradation by the proteasome. Correctly folded factor VIII is recruited to COPII vesicles by MCFD2 and LMAN1 for efficient transport to the Golgi.

complex types, addition of *O*-linked carbohydrate, and sulfation of six tyrosine residues.[104]

Low-Density Lipoprotein Receptor-Related Protein and Factor VIII Clearance

Factor VIII turnover in plasma and the mechanisms responsible are relatively poorly characterized. A key role in factor VIII catabolism has been found for low-density lipoprotein (LDL) receptor-related protein (LRP),[105–107] a broad-specificity hepatic clearance receptor.[108] The wide spectrum of plasma ligands for LRP includes blood clotting and fibrinolytic proteins such as factor Xa,[109,110] factor IXa,[111] tissue factor pathway inhibitor, the thrombin–antithrombin complex, plus plasminogen activators and their complexes with plasminogen activator inhibitor.[108]

LRP is one member of the LDL receptor family of structurally related endocytic receptors, in humans also containing LDL, very-low-density lipoprotein (VLDL), gp330/megalin, and apolipoprotein E receptor 2.[108,112] Mature LRP is a noncovalently linked heterodimer made up of a 515-kd extracellular ligand binding subunit and an 85-kd transmembrane/cytoplasmic subunit. Ligand binding to LRP occurs via the cysteine-rich LDL receptor class A (LDLRA) repeats featuring a highly conserved patch of negatively charged amino acid side chains that interact with positively charged ligand residues.

The involvement of LRP in factor VIII catabolism and clearance rests on the findings that (a) factor VIII is able to bind to purified LRP, (b) factor VIII is efficiently internalized and degraded by LRP-expressing cell lines, and (c) factor VIII plasma half-life in a mouse model could be prolonged threefold by blocking LRP with its classical antagonist, the 39-kd receptor-associated protein.[106,113] At least two separate factor VIII regions are involved in LRP interaction: one within the light-chain C2 domain[105] and the other one within heavy-chain A2 domain mapped to the 484-509 sequence.[106] This A2 site is inaccessible unless factor VIII is proteolytically activated to factor VIIIa,[114] probably serving to maintain plasma factor VIII levels during normal circulation. The C2 site of factor VIII has not been finely mapped but likely shares vWF-binding residues, as an anti-C2 monoclonal antibody that inhibits LRP–factor VIII binding also inhibits its binding to vWF.[105,115]

Taken together, these findings suggest that, in the normal circulation, where factor VIII will be complexed with vWF, only the A2 LRP-binding site would be exposed and thus mediate factor VIII clearance. This hypothesis was supported experimentally by showing that catabolism by LRP-expressing cells, both of the isolated A2 domain and of factor VIII from its complex with vWF, showed similar kinetics.[116]

The importance of the C2 site for LRP-mediated factor VIII clearance derives from comparison of factor VIII catabolism by LRP-expressing cells in the presence and absence of vWF. Purified isolated factor VIII in which the C2 site is exposed was internalized and degraded twice as efficiently as factor VIII complexed with vWF.[106] The C2 site may be similarly exposed in vivo in patients with severe von Willebrand disease who have no circulating plasma vWF. In such patients, infused factor VIII had a half-life three times shorter than either normal subjects[117–119] or hemophilia A patients, who also have normal plasma vWF levels.[120] The role of LRP in accelerated clearance of factor VIII in the absence of vWF is consistent with studies in vWF-deficient mice. Preadministration of receptor-associated protein inhibited clearance of factor VIII.[75,107]

Proteolytic activation to factor VIIIa also leads to exposure of the C2 site upon dissociation of factor VIII from vWF. Thus, exposure of both A2 and C2 LRP-binding sites in factor VIIIa (A1/A2/A3-

C1-C2) may be important for LRP-mediated regulation of factor VIIIa levels at the site of vascular injury.[121] Factor VIIIa is an unstable heterotrimer owing to rapid dissociation of A2 from the A1/A3-C1-C2 fragments,[122] so the fact that both isolated A2 domain[116] and the A3-C1-C2 cleaved light chain of factor VIII[121] can be efficiently cleared by LRP-expressing cells suggests the existence of an LRP-mediated pathway for clearance of both constituents of activated factor VIII in vivo, enabled via the A2 and C2 LRP-binding sites. Because two other protein components related to the tenase complex, factor Xa and factor IXa, also are LRP ligands,[109,111] LRP may have a role in regulation of tenase activity at the site of coagulation by reducing the levels of factor IXa, for which factor VIIIa serves as a cofactor, and the product of tenase, factor Xa, capable of activating factor VIII.

A mechanism for "preconcentrating" factor VIII near the cell surface has been suggested, as actual factor VIII–LRP interaction has an affinity only of K_d 60 to 116 nM.[105,106] LRP-mediated endocytosis is facilitated for many LRP ligands by cell surface heparan sulfate proteoglycans, which are a major glycoprotein component of the extracellular matrix. LRP-mediated clearance of factor VIII from its complex with vWF is promoted by heparan sulfate proteoglycans.[116] Simultaneous blocking of both LRP and heparan sulfate proteoglycans confirmed a synergistic effect in factor VIII clearance, as a more significant prolongation of factor VIII half-life was seen in mice (5.5-fold) than with blocking of LRP alone (3.3-fold). The heparan sulfate proteoglycan-binding site in factor VIII has been localized within A2 domain residues 558-565,[116] which also bind factor IXa. Use of a factor V/factor VIII chimeric molecule also suggested that another factor IXa-binding site in factor VIII A3, residues 1811-1818, binds significantly to heparan sulfate proteoglycans.[123] Thus, the catabolic pathway of factor VIII may involve initial binding of factor VIII/vWF complex to heparan sulfate proteoglycans, which concentrate the complex on the cell surface and present it to LRP, followed by LRP-mediated catabolism of factor VIII.

FACTOR VIII GENETICS AND GENOMICS

Factor VIII Genomics

The human factor VIII gene *F8* is located on the X chromosome at band q28 and consists of 26 exons spanning 186,933 base pairs (bp)[124] (reference genomic sequence GI 67083285, reverse complement 498-187430 bp). The exons range in size from 69 bp (exon 5) to 3106 bp (exon 14); the vast majority are between 69 and 250 bp in length. The 25 introns vary considerably in size, ranging from 207 bp (intron 17) to 32,849 bp (intron 22). The encoded mRNA is 9030 nucleotides in length (reference mRNA sequence GI 10518504), including a 171-nucleotide 5′ untranslated region and a 1803-nucleotide 3′ untranslated region. The 7053-nucleotide sequence encoding the 2351-amino-acid primary translation product is split across all 26 exons. Exon 1 encodes the 19-amino-acid secretory leader and the first 29 amino acids of the A1 domain. The remainder of the A1 domain is encoded by exons 2-8, the A2 domain is encoded primarily by exons 9-13, with a short segment and the acidic sequence *a2* encoded on the large exon 14 that primarily encodes the B domain. The most 3′ segment of exon 14 encodes *a3* and the start of A3, with the remainder of A3 encoded by exons 15-19. The C1 and C2 domains are encoded by exons 20-23 and 24-26, respectively.

Intron 22 of the *F8* gene contains three additional transcribed genes: *F8A, F8B,* and *H2AFB1*. These genes are contained within a 9.5-kb segment of intron 22 known as *int22h-1* that is present as multiple copies (*int22h*-2 and *int22h*-3) approximately 400 kb telomeric of *F8*. *F8A*, a gene devoid of introns, is transcribed in the opposite direction to *F8* on the complementary strand.[125] It is abundantly transcribed in a wide variety of tissues, and the 40-kd protein is associated with huntingtin (Htt), the aberrant protein in Huntington disease, and therefore is also known as Htt-associated protein 40 (HAP40).[126] It acts as an adaptor protein linking Htt with the GTPase Rab5, a key regulator of endocytosis.[127] *F8B* is transcribed in the same direction as *F8* and uses a unique 5′ exon spliced to exons 23-26 of *F8*. It encodes a putative protein, with eight novel amino acids followed by the C2 domain of factor VIII. Its function is unknown. No *F8B* gene is known to exist in mice, as only one copy of the *int22h* interval is present extragenic to *F8*. However, overexpression of a transgene encoding F8B produced multiple eye defects in transgenic mice.[128] The *H2AFB1* gene is transcribed in the opposite direction to F8 and encodes a member of the histone H2A B1 family.

The 1.2 kb of 5′ flanking region of the *F8* gene that includes most of the 5′ untranslated region contains numerous transcription factor binding sites. Functional analysis of a series of 5′ deletion constructs linked to a luciferase reporter gene following transient transfection of liver-derived cell lines showed that most of the upstream sequence was dispensable for liver-specific expression.[129,130] A fragment of 215 bp containing 109 bp of 5′ flanking sequence and 106 bp of 5′ untranslated sequence contained all the necessary elements for maximal expression. This fragment contains binding sites for the transcription factors C/EBP, nuclear factor-κB (NF-κB) and HNF1 and mutation analysis demonstrated a key role for HNF1 in transcriptional regulation. Factor VIII is known to increase under conditions that induce the acute phase response. Functional deletion/mutation analysis has shown this requires the NF-κB and C/EBP binding sites located in the 5′ untranslated region.[131]

Biochemical evidence, molecular cloning data, and comparative sequence analysis support the existence of all components of the coagulation network in jawed vertebrates and suggest that it evolved before the divergence of teleosts more than 430 million years ago.[10,11] The *F8* gene has been cloned and sequenced in a variety of vertebrates, ranging from mammals to birds and bony fish (teleosts). Comparative analysis of the gene organization in *Fugu rubripes* (Japanese puffer fish) and *Danio rerio* (zebrafish) with the human gene indicates an identical genomic organization with conservation of the exon–intron boundaries, with the exception of exon 14, which is much smaller due to a reduction in the size of the B domain. The introns in *Fugu F8* gene are condensed, with sizes ranging from 69 to 461 bp, accounting for the considerably smaller size (9.2 kbp vs 186.9 kbp) of the *Fugu* ortholog. Expansion of the human *F8* is due, in part, to the presence of repetitive elements within introns in the human *F8* gene that are not present in the *Fugu F8* gene. Approximately 70% of the human *F8* gene (129 kbp) consists of repetitive elements such as SINES (65), LINES (102), LTRs (50) and other DNA (21) elements. None of these repeat elements are found in the coding sequences; however, two are located in the 3′ untranslated region.

Hemophilia A

Genetic Disorders

Hemophilia A is an X-linked single gene bleeding disorder resulting from mutations in or close to the *F8* gene, which leads to loss of the circulating plasma coagulation protein factor VIII or production of a defective variant. The factor VIII protein was first purified 25 years ago.[132] Cloning of the *F8* gene was accomplished soon after[124] and was followed by descriptions of the mutations in many patients with hemophilia A.[133–135]

F8 gene defects associated with hemophilia A can be divided into two classes: (a) large gene rearrangements, insertions, and deletions, and (b) small mutations affecting only a small number of nucleotides. All types of defects may result in severe disease, but the single most clinically important defect is a recurrent large gene rearrangement (an "inversion") involving *F8* intron 22, which results in approximately 45% to 50% of *all* severe disease cases of hemophilia A worldwide.

The worldwide online hemophilia A mutation database[20] (http://europium.csc.mrc.ac.uk) lists more than 2800 individual reports of *F8* variants, including all insertion/deletions and single-base DNA replacements. In some cases, assessment of the severity of disease associated with a mutation casts light on the functional aspects of

Table 123–1 Summary of Mutation Data Available from Analysis of 2853 Individual Reports in the Online Hemophilia A Database[20]

Hemophilia A Mutations	Unique Reports	Reported Clinical Severity: Severe (%)	Moderate (%)	Mild (%)	Variable (%)	Reported Inhibitor Status: Positive (%)	Negative (%)
Total Unique Mutations	1221	718 (67)	123 (11)	212 (20)	23 (2)	171 (19)	727 (81)
Unique Single-Base Variants	809	369 (52)	105 (15)	206 (29)	23 (3)	78 (13)	513 (87)
Missense	583	204 (40)	92 (18)	187 (37)	23 (5)	44 (10)	391 (90)
Stop	131	112 (97)	4 (3)	0 (0)	0 (0)	31 (31)	69 (69)
Splice	95	53 (66)	9 (11)	19 (23)	0 (0)	3 (5)	53 (95)
Unique Insertions	80	67 (91)	5 (7)	2 (3)	0 (0)	16 (26)	46 (74)
Small (<50 bp)	75	63 (92)	5 (7)	1 (1)	0 (0)	15 (25)	45 (75)
Large (>50 bp)	5	4 (80)	0 (0)	1 (20)	0 (0)	1 (50)	1 (50)
Unique Deletions	332	282 (95)	13 (4)	4 (1)	0 (0)	77 (31)	168 (69)
Small (<50 bp)	197	157 (93)	9 (5)	4 (2)	0 (0)	31 (22)	113 (78)
Large (>50 bp)	135	125 (97)	4 (3)	0 (0)	0 (0)	46 (46)	55 (55)

The distribution of these mutations among severe, moderate, and mild disease, and relation to inhibitor status where known, are given. Human factor VIII gene *(F8)* inversions invariably result in severe disease but are not included in the database because of their high redundancy. Inversions are responsible for approximately 45% of all severe disease.

Hemophilia A database[20] from http://europium.csc.mrc.ac.uk.

Online Hemophilia A Database

The worldwide online hemophilia A mutation database (http://europium.csc.mrc.ac.uk) lists more than 2800 individual reports of *F8* variants, whether directly submitted to the database or derived from published reports.

factor VIII protein. Inversions are omitted from the database because they are almost entirely identical both genetically and phenotypically and therefore are highly redundant. A summary of mutations listed in the online database is given in Table 123–1 (see box on Online Hemophilia A Database).

Gross Genetic Changes

A mutation hotspot specific to hemophilia A is the recurrent rearrangement responsible for 50% of all severe cases in which homologous recombination of a sequence within intron 22 of the *F8* gene and two extragenic and telomeric copies of the sequence results in an inversion that disrupts the *F8* gene.[136,137]

Inversions (IVS 22 and IVS 1)

Half of all severe hemophilia A is caused by spontaneous homologous recombination resulting in inversion of the *F8* gene (Fig. 123–4). Two types of inversion involving a sequence in intron 22 and either the proximal (*int22h-2*) or the distal (*int22h-3*) of two extragenic copies of this sequence were thought to be responsible for the two forms of inversion observed in hemophilia A patients.[138] However, genomic sequence data following the completion of the DNA sequence of the human X chromosome[139] indicate that recombination leading to inversion can occur only between intron 22 and distal copies of the sequence.[140] Recombination between intron 22 and the proximal copies of the sequence would be predicted to lead to duplication and deletion because they are in the same orientation to each other. The new sequence information also revealed that *int22h-2* and *int22h-3* form the arms of a large palindrome. Therefore it has been suggested that recombination occurs between the arms of the palindrome, creating alleles where either the *int22h-2* or the *int22h-3*

Inversions and Severe Hemophilia

Half of all cases of severe hemophilia A worldwide are caused by spontaneous homologous recombination resulting in inversion of part of the *F8* gene.

occupies the proximal position, thus explaining the observed rearrangements[141,142] (see box on Inversions and Severe Hemophilia).

A second inversion found in 5% of severe hemophilia A cases involves a 1-kb sequence in intron 1 (*int1h-1*) and a repeated copy (*int1h-2*) 140 kb telomeric of the *F8* gene between the *C6.1A* and *VBP1* genes. The inversion results in the production of two chimeric mRNAs that compose either exon 1 of the *F8* gene and exons 2-6 of the *VBP1* gene or exons of the *C6.1A* gene and exons 2-26 of the *F8* gene. The inversion causes severe hemophilia A because the coding sequence for factor VIII (exons 2-26) is downstream of the translation stop codon of the *C6.1A* gene.[143,144]

Large Insertions and Deletions

Approximately 5% of patients with hemophilia A have large deletions (>50 base pairs). The online mutation database[20] (http://europium.csc.mrc.ac.uk) lists 137 individual deletions of varying size scattered throughout the *F8* gene. Few of the deletions have been mapped at the nucleotide level. Deletions usually are associated with a severe bleeding phenotype, although four cases are reported to be associated with a moderate bleeding phenotype. The observed clinical phenotype most probably is due to in-frame joining of the exons flanking the deletion during mRNA processing.

Insertions of large elements in the *F8* gene are a rare cause of hemophilia A; only five such events have been reported.[20] Two involve insertion of LINE repetitive elements, which are members of the class of transposable elements, also known as interspersed repeats, that are the largest single component of mammalian genomes. LINEs mobilize by an ancient reverse transcription mechanism shared with the group II introns of mitochondria and eubacteria.[145] Two of the other insertions described in the *F8* gene involve Alu repeat elements, members of the SINE family of short interspersed nucleotide elements that lack the ability to retrotranspose autonomously but can coopt LINE machinery for their replication.

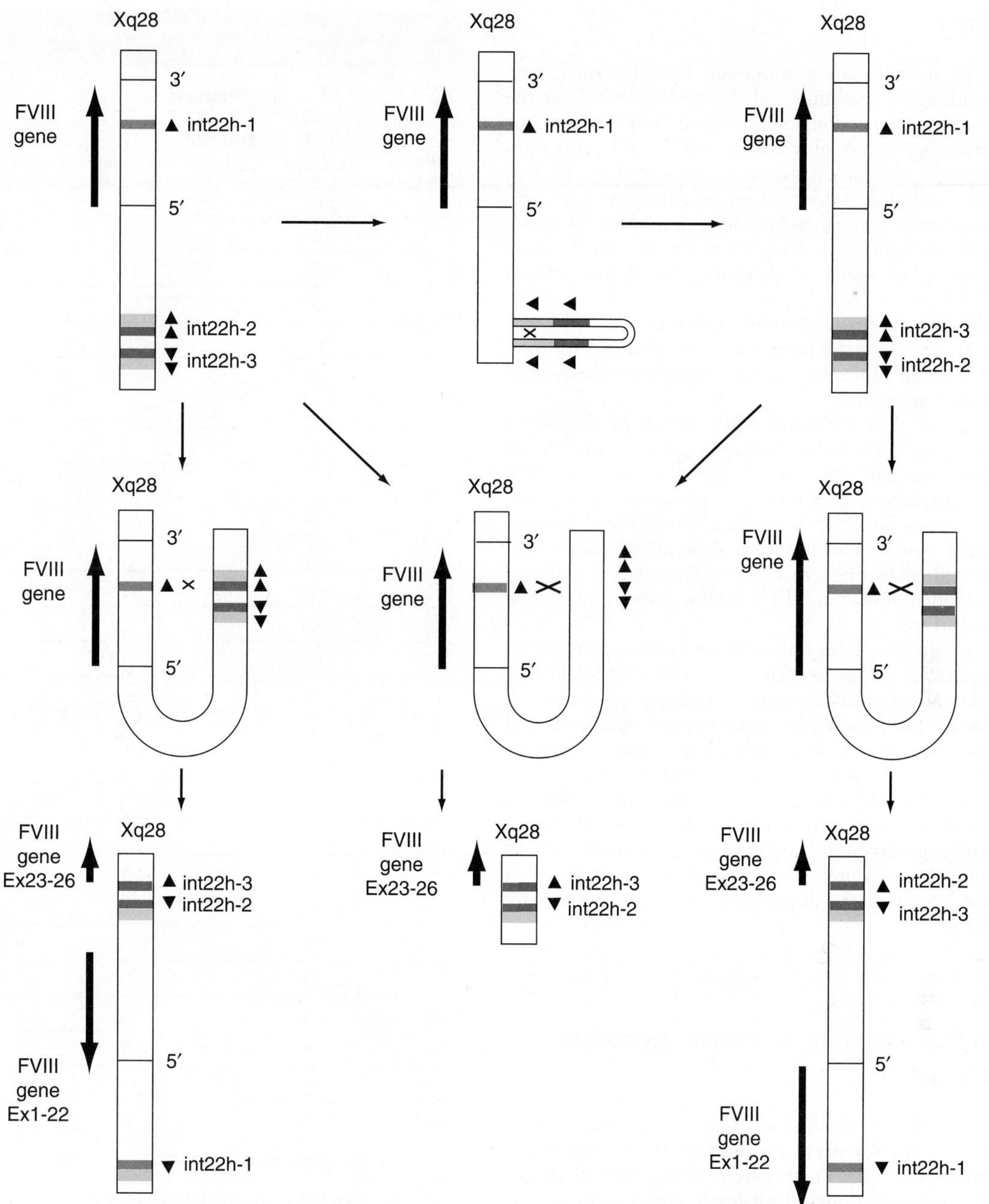

Figure 123–4 Inversions in Xq28 causing hemophilia A. Proposed mechanism causing polymorphic inversion and recombination between *int22h* repeats leading to inversion of the *F8* gene. The *F8* gene is indicated by the large arrow. Inversions disrupting the *F8* gene result from recombination between *int22h-1* region (in intron 22 of the *F8* gene) and either *int22h-2* or *int22h-3*, which lie 400 kb distal to *F8*. The three copies of the *int22h* sequence are indicated by the red, purple, and green boxes, and their orientation relative to the intron 22 copy is indicated by the arrowhead. The distal copies (*int22h-2* and *int22h-3*) are in opposite orientation to each other and are flanked by a large imperfect palindrome, indicated by blue boxes. Proposed recombination between the arms of the palindrome would generate alleles where either the *int22h-2* or the *int22h-3* is most telomeric and in the opposite orientation to *int22h-1*. The consequences of the recombination between the *int22h-1* and either *int22h-3* or *int22h-2* in the distal position leading to inversion are indicated to the left and right of the figure, respectively. The consequence of the recombination between the *int22h-1* and either *int22h-2* or *int22h-3* (indicated by the checkered colors) in the proximal position, leading to deletion rather than inversion, is indicated in the center of the figure.

Other Rearrangements

Two examples of duplication of parts of the *F8* gene causing hemophilia A have been described. In one case, a 23-kb sequence in intron 22 is duplicated and inserted between exons 23 and 24 in one of the maternal *F8* genes. This was presumed to be unstable and led to deletion of 39 kb of DNA including exons 23-25, thus causing hemophilia A in the patient' son.[146] The other duplication, of exon 13 was identified in a cohort of northern Italian patients in which it was found to be responsible for mild hemophilia A in 32% of subjects from the area.[147,148] The duplication is associated with a mild bleeding phenotype because exon skipping of one of the duplicated exons during mRNA processing leads to production of a wild-type factor VIII mRNA. More recently, a complex genetic rearrangement consisting of a 15.5-kb deletion/16-bp insertion located 0.6 kb from a 28.1-kb deletion/263-kb insertion at Xq28 has been described in a patient with hemophilia A. Although this arrangement affects the copy number of several genes, with deletion of part of the *F8* gene and the *FUNDC2* gene and duplication of the *FAM11A*, *HSFX1*, *MAGEA9*, and *MAGEA11* genes, the patient exhibits no clinically detectable phenotype other than hemophilia A.[149]

Small Mutations

This category of disease-causing mutations includes single-base replacements resulting in an amino acid change ("missense") or the introduction of a new stop codon ("nonsense" or "stop"). Occasionally, such a base change occurs at or near an mRNA splice junction, resulting in skipped exons or premature truncation of the protein ("splice" variants). Included in this category are small insertion/deletion events, commonly defined as involving less than 50 bases, and frequently involving a single base. These defects usually cause frameshifts in the DNA sequence, generating novel stop codons downstream.

In general these mutations result from small-scale errors of DNA replication that are not successfully repaired. The spectrum of clinical severity and presence of inhibitors depends strongly on the type of small mutation and its location.

As of 2007, more than 1800 individual reports of single-base substitutions are given in the online hemophilia A database.[20] Some are recurrent, but more than 800 *unique* single-base variants are listed as being causative of disease. Even for a large protein of 2332 amino acids, this is an extraordinarily rich database of functional disorder in a single protein. Annotations in the database include factor VIII clotting activity and circulating factor VIII antigen (factor VIII:Ag) levels, clinical severity, antifactor VIII inhibitor status, and journal reference for each report.

To date, the unique single-base substitution variants are made up of 583 unique missense mutations that result in an amino acid substitution, 131 unique stop mutations, and 90 unique splice variants. The distribution of these mutations among severe, moderate, and mild disease, and relation to inhibitor status where known, are given in Table 123–1. Table 123–2 lists the distribution of the mutations by *F8* exon. Exon 14 is approximately 10 times larger than the average size of the other exons, so it has a much higher burden of causative mutations generally, although missense mutations actually are relatively poorly represented when normalized per kilobase of coding sequence, reflecting the dispensability of the B domain for functional activity.

Table 123–2 Summary of the Distribution of Mutations in the Online Hemophilia A Database[20] by *F8* Exon

	Point Mutations			Deletions		
***F8* Exon**	***Missense***	***Nonsense (Stop)***	***Splicing***	***Small***	***Large***	***Insertions***
1	15	2	4	2	NA	1
2	10	1	5	8	NA	4
3	25	0	6	5	NA	0
4	35	7	4	1	NA	1
5	13	1	10	4	NA	1
6	11	2	6	4	NA	2
7	38	5	4	8	NA	1
8	27	6	1	8	NA	1
9	27	3	5	7	NA	3
10	10	3	3	5	NA	0
11	36	1	4	2	NA	1
12	20	5	4	2	NA	1
13	32	3	2	7	NA	3
14	43	52	6	77	NA	39
15	19	2	3	4	NA	0
16	26	7	2	7	NA	0
17	28	3	2	6	NA	5
18	34	5	1	5	NA	4
19	16	1	8	4	NA	4
20	8	1	0	2	NA	2
21	9	5	1	0	NA	1
22	19	5	4	3	NA	1
23	30	1	4	7	NA	0
24	13	5	4	3	NA	2
25	13	2	2	7	NA	3
26	26	3	0	9	NA	0
TOTAL	583	131	95	197	135	80

Total unique single-base (point) mutations: 824. Total unique mutations of all types: 1236.

F8, human factor VIII gene; NA, not applicable.

Single-Base Substitutions: Missense, Nonsense, and Splice Mutations

Table 123–1 shows the stratification of unique single-base substitution mutations by clinical severity and antifactor VIII inhibitor status. Missense mutations and splice variants are associated with all disease severities, unlike stop mutations, which result almost exclusively in severe disease as usually no protein circulates.

In approximately 590 single-base substitution cases of reported known inhibitor status, 78 (13%) are reported as inhibitor positive. Most of these are associated with severe disease, indicating a likely role for regular replacement therapy in the development of an antibody response. Stop mutations result in a higher proportion of cases with positive inhibitor status (31/100 [31%]) in comparison to the missense mutation group in which only 10% (44/435) are inhibitor positive. Only three of 56 cases report the presence of an inhibitor in the splice variant group, an unexplained low incidence.

For stop mutations, a skewed pattern of inhibitor development in relation to exon number is seen. Of 30 unique stop mutations associated with the generation of antifactor VIII antibodies in vivo, none are found in exons 1-7 and only four in the first 13 exons. The reasons are unknown, although various hypotheses have been formulated for this distribution of inhibitor-positive cases (see Chapter 126).[150,151]

Many single-base mutations occur numerous times in different populations; 32 unique mutations have been reported independently on 10 occasions or more, with six of those reported independently over 25 times. Enhanced predisposition to replication errors at the local chromatin level clearly is involved, whether caused by the CpG dinucleotide "hotspot" effect (i.e., CG→TG), by specific sequence motifs, or by other local factors.

Within these groups with an identical mutation, the variabilities of clinical phenotype and factor VIII activity level are notable. For example, the mutation Arg1997→Trp has been reported 34 times in unrelated families, with factor VIII activity varying from less than 1% to 5% of normal plasma values, and clinical severity varying from severe to mild. This variability suggests that besides the defined disorder in the *F8* gene, additional factors must be controlling factor VIII activity. Other genes do affect factor VIII levels. Detailed studies of a small number of families with the rare clotting disorder of combined factor V–factor VIII deficiency have demonstrated that mutations in at least two genes coding for proteins involved in glycoprotein trafficking in the ER and Golgi apparatus result in reductions in the secreted levels of both factor V and factor VIII. Other causes of variation are undefined.

With a three-dimensional structure for factor VIII or its domains, structural rationales for defects in function can be attempted. The many missense mutations in the database can be a fertile area for correlating factor VIII function with protein structure and explaining how these small changes in protein sequence result in clinical disease.

Knowing circulating factor VIII antigen levels as well as factor VIII activity levels is necessary in order to make interpretations about factor VIII function in plasma or about the ability of a variant molecule to be secreted. A plasma activity of 5% of normal associated with a hemophilic missense mutation might result from either a molecule that is present at a normal 100% antigen level but is dysfunctional (i.e., cross-reactive material [CRM]-positive) or a poorly secreted or unstable yet functionally normal molecule that circulates at the 5% level (i.e., CRM-negative).

The abolition of existing cysteine residues known to be involved in disulfide bridge formation is associated with low levels or an absence of factor VIII molecules in the plasma of patients. von Willebrand factor interaction is impacted by mutations in the *a3* peptide at Tyr1680 and in the C1 residues Tyr2105, Arg2116, Ser2119, and Arg2150, either directly or indirectly. In all these cases, the effect is a reduction of circulating levels of factor VIII protein, which appears otherwise functionally normal, and mild to moderate hemophilia usually results.

In some cases, antigen values are normal, whereas activity values are grossly reduced or undetectable. This finding indicates that, in these patients, hemophilia is caused by generation of a functionally inactive molecule that circulates normally. This small class of missense mutations gives strong clues as to which amino acids or regions are crucial for functional interactions in this molecule, and structure–function relationships have been suggested by several groups based on CRM-positive mutations.[19,152–155]

Because factor VIII can express its procoagulant function only after specific proteolytic cleavages, modifications of the relevant proteolytic sites (e.g., Arg372→Cys/His, Ser373→Pro/Leu, Arg1689→Cys) would severely reduce or even abolish this activity. In fact, these mutations all result in normal circulating factor VIII protein levels with functional activity of 12% or below. Arg1689→His has a milder effect on function, with a mean activity value of 23% from seven reports.

Alternatively, modifying interactions with one of the functionally important ligands of factor VIII (e.g., factor IXa, factor X, phospholipid membrane) by mutation would reduce functional activity. In the case of factor IXa binding, two mutations associated with very low factor VIII activity and normal antigen levels are N-glycosylation variants. Ile566→Thr leads to a new glycosylation site at Asn564, at a factor IXa binding site. Met1772→Thr predicts a new N-glycosylation at Asn1770, also close to a factor IXa binding region. These novel glycosylations appear to hinder the functional association of the two proteins.

Because factor VIIIa instability is mediated by the dissociation of the A2 domain from the A1 and A3 domains, for other variants, amino acid changes impacting the stability of the proteolytically activated heterotrimeric factor VIIIa itself, via the interdomain interfaces, might reduce functional integrity sufficiently to cause clinical disease. Examples have been experimentally confirmed.[156,157]

Approximately one third of all hemophilic missense mutations cause the clinical phenotype by generating a dysfunctional molecule that circulates normally in plasma. The remaining mutations are associated with defective factor VIII secretion or stability.

Small Deletions and Insertions

The mutation database lists both *F8* deletions and the less common insertions. Together they can be termed "indels." *F8* indels have been divided into large and small. In general, large indels involve stretches of hundreds or many thousands of DNA bases, whereas most small indels result from deletion or insertion of a single base.

The database lists 296 individual small deletion reports (defined as smaller than 50 bases deleted), comprising 197 unique small deletions of which approximately 50% are of single bases. Small deletion reports outnumber those of large deletions by 2:1. Overall inhibitor development is lower than expected at 22% of all unique cases, compared to values of approximately 30% for insertion frameshifts and nonsense point mutations.

A small but significant number of small deletion variants occur with high frequency in unrelated families across the world, as seen with some small insertions. Almost all of these multiple reports are of deletions of a single adenine base (A) in a consecutive run of As. For example, there are more than 50 separate reports of an A deletion in a run of nine As at codons 1191-1194, which also is a "hot spot" for single-base insertions. Most patients with this mutation are severely affected, so it is a highly significant cause of disease.

Small deletions are found throughout the factor VIII sequence and generally cause frameshifts followed by chain termination as a result of generation of novel termination signals and a truncated protein product. Almost all are associated with severe disease. However, as also found with small insertions, there are a small number of moderate or mild cases, often associated with "A runs" with predicted truncated protein product. It is postulated that some low-level miscopying in this region results in generation of small amounts of mRNA with the correct wild-type sequence, allowing synthesis of sufficient functional protein to moderate the clinical phenotype.

In a small number of rare in-frame deletions, a multiple of three bases is deleted. Most of these occurrences are predicted to result in deletion of a single amino acid. Some are associated with detectable factor VIII activity and protein, indicating that the deletion has been accommodated in the protein structure. Deletions of two or four amino acids are associated with severe disease.

Insertion events causing hemophilia are much less frequent overall than are deletions (see Table 123–1). An additional difference in the mutation spectrum between the two types of indel events is that large insertions are extremely rare events, unlike large deletions. Of the 144 individual insertion reports in the hemophilia A database, only five feature more than a few bases in total. The dominant group of small insertions are composed of just 75 unique insertion events, the vast majority of which are less than 10 bp in length. Insertions of an additional adenine base at the site of a run of adenines accounts for most of the repetitious reports, for example, more than 27 separate unrelated cases of insertion of an A into a run of eight As at codons 1439-1441, and another 14 cases of insertion of A into a run of nine As at codons 1191-1194. Runs of As in the *F8* cDNA are relatively common, and these insertions, and small deletions at the same loci, are thought to result from uncorrected DNA polymerase slippage during replication.

The vast majority of insertions cause frameshifts and result in severe hemophilia (see Table 123–1). However, similar to the situation with small deletions, a small number of "A-run" insertion cases are associated with low but measurable factor VIII activity levels and only moderate clinical severity. This situation probably is the result of a small percentage of normal mRNA molecules being produced by "corrective" slippage errors on the mutant template during transcription.

Promoter Mutations

Mutations in the 5′ flanking sequence of the *F8* gene responsible for hemophilia A are extremely rare. Only two sequence variants in this region have been identified, both associated with mild bleeding phenotypes. One patient was asymptomatic until age 53 years, when he suffered abdominal bleeding while undergoing anticoagulation therapy for heart insufficiency. The other patient had no spontaneous bleeding into joints and muscles but suffered bleeding complications only after surgery.[158] The functional consequences of these mutations are not fully characterized.

Clinical Aspects

Inhibitors and Gene Deletions

The presence of a severe gene lesion preventing factor VIII expression is strongly associated with the development of alloantibodies to factor VIII introduced via replacement therapy. The most severe gene lesions affecting *F8* are large deletions, and patients with this genotype very frequently develop inhibitors. Of 98 patients with deletions larger than 50 bp, 44 had inhibitors (45%). This is a higher percentage than for any other class of gene lesion[151] but still not a predictable event, perhaps because intravenous infusion is a weak route to immunization in the absence of adjuvant, and the infused material will bind to its natural carrier vWF, which is present at normal levels in the circulation of the recipient.

Carrier Detection and Antenatal Diagnosis

For every affected male with an X-linked recessive disorder in the population there are approximately two carriers of the disease. However, the number of putative carriers related to a case likely is at least double that figure and often much higher, although the prior risk of being a carrier decreases with genetic distance from the proband. In practice this works out to approximately five females requesting carrier determination for every affected male in a static population.

Prior to the era of widespread gene sequencing, the first step in carrier detection was to estimate the ratio of plasma factor VIII activity to vWF antigen. The mean for noncarrier females is a ratio of 1.0, whereas the mean for carriers of hemophilia A is 0.5. There is wide individual variation in this ratio due to random X inactivation, but performing this phenotypic test still is clinically useful and important because a proportion of carrier females have sufficiently low factor VIII levels to be classified as bleeding carriers, with the phenotype of mild hemophilia. Rarely as a result of processes that interfere with X inactivation of the mutation-bearing allele, girls with severe hemophilia are born. Another potentially confusing factor in the interpretation of factor VIII : vWF ratios is the presence of a von Willebrand disease allele segregating in the same kindred as one affected by hemophilia A (Fig. 123–5).

The next step in carrier status determination uses linkage markers; a highly informative set located within *F8* is available.[159] Combination of the dinucleotide repeat polymorphisms in introns 13 and 22 with single nucleotide polymorphisms in introns 18 and 22 gives heterozygosity and therefore useful information in approximately 90% of carriers in most populations from diverse ethnic groups. Therefore, linkage analysis is uninformative for approximately 10% of families. It now is common practice to perform direct mutation detection by sequencing to track the disease allele in hemophilia A families. Other reasons for using this approach are that issues of paternity are circumvented, intermediate family members are not required to conclusively demonstrate linkage, and the mutation itself can provide useful information about clinical phenotype when it is not known from the affected relative. If the potential carrier herself is the only available member of the kindred and if she is heterozygous for a known or plausible novel mutation in her *F8* gene, her status is at once resolved (see Fig. 123–5). In approximately 2% of cases of severe and moderate hemophilia A, no mutation can be found in the coding regions usually sequenced. Linkage then is the only method available for carrier determination.

Antenatal diagnosis is offered to carriers of hemophilia A based on direct mutation analysis or on linkage analysis if the mutation is not known from DNA extracted from a chorionic villus sample taken at approximately 12 weeks of gestation. Before then, determining whether the conceptus is male or female is possible by noninvasive testing of maternal blood Y chromosome DNA at approximately 10 weeks. If the conceptus is female, then chorionic villus sampling with its risk of pregnancy loss (≈1% in experienced centers) is not needed. Preimplantation diagnosis of hemophilia has been successfully demonstrated with selection of embryos for transfer that are not affected.[160]

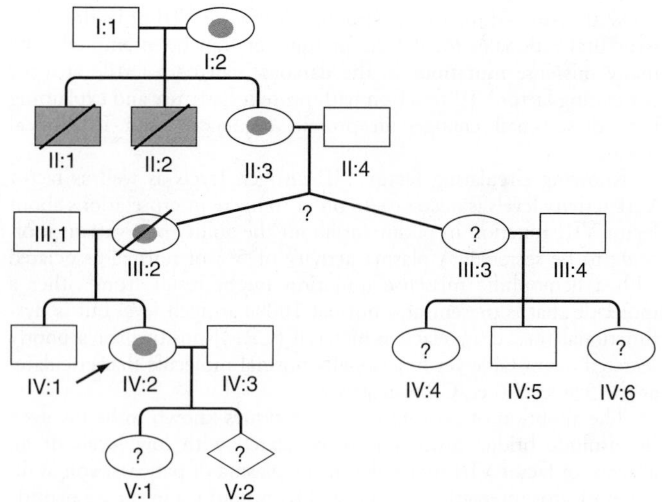

Figure 123–5 Sequencing the *F8* gene to correct diagnosis in a hemophilia A carrier. The proband (IV:2, arrow) was recalled for reevaluation of her original diagnosis of mild von Willebrand disease. Review of her family tree and phenotypic data (two antecedent males died of bleeding; factor VIII activity 33 IU/mL; von Willebrand factor antigen 63 IU/mL) suggested that she had been misclassified and that she might be a hemophilia A carrier. Sequencing of her *F8* gene showed her to be heterozygous for Arg372→Cys, a known cause of moderately severe hemophilia A. Although pregnant and carrying a male conceptus (according to Y chromosome analysis of maternal blood), she elected to continue the pregnancy and to be managed at delivery with appropriate precautions for the possibility of an affected infant. Because it now is clear that her mother was an obligate carrier, the surviving twin sister (III:3) almost certainly is a carrier (they were said to be identical), and her two daughters (IV:4 and IV:6) also are putative carriers as is the proband's daughter (V:1). Of note, both male relatives died of bleeding at a young age, and no DNA was available from them. Hence, sequencing of the putative carrier's *F8* gene was the only option for resolution of both the diagnosis and the inheritance in this family. The question mark indicates status is unconfirmed.

SUGGESTED READINGS

Bagnall RD, Giannelli F, Green PM: Polymorphism and hemophilia A causing inversions in distal Xq28: A complex picture. J Thromb Haemost 3:2598, 2005.

Eaton D, Rodriguez H, Vehar GA: Proteolytic processing of human factor VIII. Correlation of specific cleavages by thrombin, factor Xa, and activated protein C with activation and inactivation of factor VIII coagulant activity. Biochemistry 25:505, 1986.

Fay PJ, Jenkins PV: Mutating factor VIII: Lessons from structure to function. Blood Rev 19:15, 2005.

Gale AJ, Radtke KP, Cunningham MA, et al: Intrinsic stability and functional properties of disulfide bond-stabilized coagulation factor VIIIa variants. J Thromb Haemost 4:1315, 2006.

Gitschier J, Wood WI, Goralka TM, et al: Characterization of the human factor VIII gene. Nature 312:326, 1984.

Kemball-Cook G: The Haemophilia A Mutation Database. http://europium.csc.mrc.ac.uk 1 June 2008.

Lenting PJ, Van Mourik JA, Mertens K: The life cycle of coagulation factor VIII in view of its structure and function. Blood 92:3983, 1998.

Mann KG: Biochemistry and physiology of blood coagulation. Thromb Haemost 82:165, 1999.

Miao HZ, Sirachainan N, Palmer L, et al: Bioengineering of coagulation factor VIII for improved secretion. Blood 103:3412, 2004.

Nathwani AC, Davidoff AM, Tuddenham EG: Prospects for gene therapy of haemophilia. Haemophilia 10:309, 2004.

Naylor J, Brinke A, Hassock S, et al: Characteristic mRNA abnormality found in half the patients with severe haemophilia A is due to large DNA inversions. Hum Mol Genet 2:1773, 1993.

Naylor JA, Buck D, Green P, et al: Investigation of the factor VIII intron 22 repeated region (int22h) and the associated inversion junctions. Hum Mol Genet 4:1217, 1995.

Ngo JC, Huang M, Roth DA, Furie BC and Furie B: Crystal structure of human factor VIII: implications for the formation of the factor IXa-factor VIII complex. Structure 16:597, 2008.

Pratt KP, Shen BW, Takeshima K, et al: Structure of the C2 domain of human factor VIII at 1.5 A resolution. Nature 402:439, 1999.

Ross MT, Bentley DR: More on: Polymorphism and hemophilia A causing inversions in distal Xq28: A complex picture. J Thromb Haemost 3:2600, 2005.

Saenko EL, Ananyeva NM, Tuddenham EG, et al: Factor VIII—Novel insights into form and function. Br J Haematol 119:323, 2002.

Shen BW, Spiegel PC, Chang CH, Huh JW, Lee JS, Kim J, Kim YH and Stoddard BL: The tertiary structure and domain organisation of coagulation factor VIII. Blood 111:1240, 2008.

Toole JJ, Knopf JL, Wozney JM, et al: Molecular cloning of a cDNA encoding human antihaemophilic factor. Nature 312:342, 1984.

Zhang B, Ginsburg D: Familial multiple coagulation factor deficiencies: New biologic insight from rare genetic bleeding disorders. J Thromb Haemost 2:1564, 2004.

Zhang B, McGee B, Yamaoka JS, et al: Combined deficiency of factor V and factor VIII is due to mutations in either LMAN1 or MCFD2. Blood 107:1903, 2006.

REFERENCES

For complete list of references log onto www.expertconsult.com

CHAPTER 124

BIOCHEMISTRY OF FACTOR IX AND MOLECULAR BIOLOGY OF HEMOPHILIA B

David A. Roth, Steven J. Freedman, and Bruce Furie

Factor IX is a plasma protein with a molecular weight of 56,000. Synthesis of factor IX by the liver requires vitamin K. Factor IX participates in an intermediate phase of the blood coagulation pathway (see Chapter 118). Activated factor XI (factor XIa) or activated factor VII (factor VIIa) complexed with tissue factor can activate factor IX. In complex with factor VIIIa on membrane surfaces, activated factor IX (factor IXa) then activates factor X. The critical importance of factor IX is emphasized by the phenotype of hemophilia B, a hereditary disease characterized by factor IX deficiency.

In 1952, factor IX was discovered to be distinct from factor VIII by the observation that the clotting time corrected after mixing the plasmas from two unrelated patients with hemophilia.[1,2] Hemophilia B, or Christmas disease, is an X-linked disorder defined by a hereditary decrease in factor IX activity. The molecular defect leading to factor IX deficiency in the index patient has been shown to be a point mutation, with a substitution of Cys206 to serine in the catalytic domain.[3] Hemophilia B accounts for approximately 12% of the total cases of hemophilia. The disease is variable in phenotype, and the degree of bleeding severity usually correlates with the level of factor IX activity present in the patient's plasma. As anticipated from the variable phenotypes of hemophilia B and the similarity of phenotypes within each particular family, hemophilia B is caused by a variety of genetic defects. It is estimated that one third of cases of hemophilia B arise from spontaneous mutations.

GENE STRUCTURE AND REGULATION

The factor IX gene is located on the tip of the long arm of chromosome X at Xq27.1,[4] close to the factor VIII gene. The gene is 34 kb in size and was derived ancestrally from a precursor of the prothrombin gene, like other genes encoding vitamin K-dependent proteins.[5] The factor IX gene contains eight exons (Fig. 124–1), which range in size between 25 and 1935 nucleotides, and seven introns, which range in size from 188 to 9473 nucleotides. The messenger RNA (mRNA) comprises a 205-base pair (bp) 5′ untranslated region, a 1383-bp preprofactor IX region that encodes for a 461-amino-acid precursor protein, and a 1392-bp 3′ untranslated region.[6–8] Exons I, II, and III encode the prepro leader sequence, the γ-carboxyglutamic acid (Gla) domain, and the aromatic amino acid stack domain. Exons IV and V encode the two consecutive epidermal growth factor (EGF)-like domains. Exons VI, VII, and VIII encode the activation peptide and the serine protease catalytic domain.

Regulation of the factor IX gene is mediated by elements in the 5′ untranslated region, intron sequences, and the 3′ untranslated region. The 5′ proximal region extending to −270 contains the minimal promoter sequence required for maximal factor IX expression.[9,10] Multiple promoters exist within this region, including a CAAT box at −238 and a TATA box at −181.[11,12] A transcription start site has been defined at approximately −176.[9] Multiple negative regulatory elements (silencers) that suppress gene expression exist upstream of −416. One such silencer consists of a promoter (−766 to −417) oriented in the reverse direction of the factor IX promoter activity.[12] Experiments using transgenic mice indicate that the introns of factor IX are required for its expression in vivo.[13] Furthermore, expression vectors that include the first intron of the factor IX gene produce sevenfold to ninefold higher levels of mRNA than vectors lacking this sequence.[14] The 3′ untranslated region contains polyadenylation signal sequences that are important in normal gene expression. A 653-bp deletion of this region has been found in a mild form of hemophilia B.[15]

Factor IX levels increase with age.[16] Longitudinal analysis of human factor IX gene expression patterns in transgenic mice identified two *cis*-acting elements that control age-dependent levels of circulating factor IX.[17] AE5′ (age-regulatory element in the 5′ end) resides between −770 and −802 of the 5′ untranslated region and is responsible for age-stable expression of the human factor IX gene. The other element, AE3′, is found in the middle of the 3′ untranslated region and causes age-associated increases in factor IX, most likely by stabilizing factor IX mRNA.

Factor IX Leyden is a form of hemophilia B characterized by a severe bleeding disorder during childhood; factor IX activity and antigen levels are less than 1%.[18] With the onset of puberty or with the administration of androgen therapy,[19] factor IX levels rise to 30% to 60% of normal, and the hemophilia phenotype disappears (Fig. 124–2). In normal individuals, factor IX levels increase modestly after puberty.[20] Analysis of factor IX genes from patients with various pedigrees with the factor IX Leyden phenotype demonstrated 11 unique point mutations clustered in a region between nucleotides −40 to +20.[11] A transgenic mouse with a mutation at +13 in the factor IX promoter shows age-dependent, male-specific expression of factor IX, mimicking the factor IX Leyden phenotype.[21] Several transcription factors that bind within or immediately upstream of the factor IX Leyden promoter region have been identified.[11,22,23] For example, CCAAT/enhancer-binding protein binds between +1 and +18,[22] and hepatic nuclear factor 4 binds between −19 and −27.[24,25] CCAAT/enhancer-binding protein α and Ets factor GA-binding protein (GABPα/β) bind between −195 and −220, which lies upstream of the Leyden promoter region.[26] Binding of these two transcription factors enhances transactivation of the factor IX gene by two proline- and acidic-amino-acid-rich (PAR) proteins, D-site-binding protein and hepatic leukemia factor.[26,27] Studies have also demonstrated transcriptional activation of the factor IX gene after cotransfection of hepatocytes with the androgen receptor and the CCAAT/enhancer binding protein, and androgen receptor binding to the proximal factor IX promoter was disrupted by mutation at nucleotide −26.[28] Levels of many of these transcription factors rise at different time points during development. Thus, they may play an important role in the developmental expression of the factor IX gene through wild-type and factor IX Leyden promoters.

SYNTHESIS OF FACTOR IX

Factor IX is synthesized in the hepatocyte as a precursor protein. It then undergoes a series of intracellular posttranslational modifications and is secreted as a zymogen (Fig. 124–3). The coding sequence of the factor IX gene encodes two peptides that are removed prior to secretion of the mature factor IX into the blood: a 28-residue signal peptide that directs the nascent peptide chain to the endoplasmic reticulum and an 18-residue propeptide between the signal peptide and the mature amino terminus of factor IX.[8] The signal peptide is cleaved cotranslationally by the signal peptidase. The propeptide contains the γ-carboxylation recognition site that directs

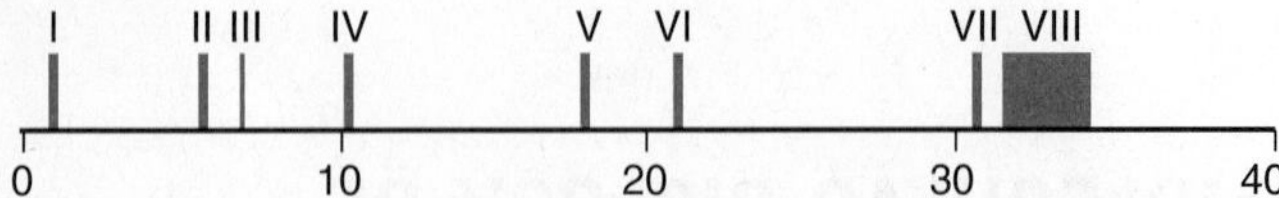

Figure 124–1 Structure of the factor IX gene and encoded factor IX domains. The factor IX gene includes eight exons and seven introns. Exons 1 to 8 are represented as solid bars and designated with roman numerals I to VIII.

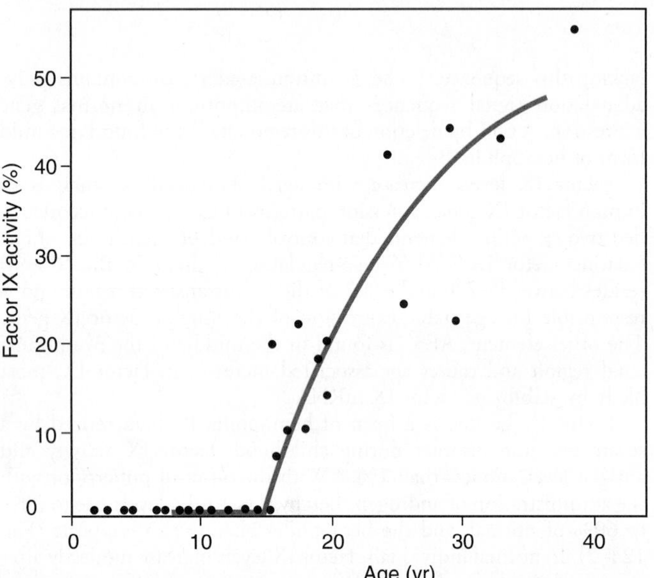

Figure 124–2 Factor IX Leyden. Changes in the plasma factor IX level as a function of age. (From Briet E, Bertina RM, van Tilburg NH, Veltkamp JJ: Hemophilia B Leyden: A sex-linked hereditary disorder that improves after puberty. N Engl J Med 306:788, 1982.)

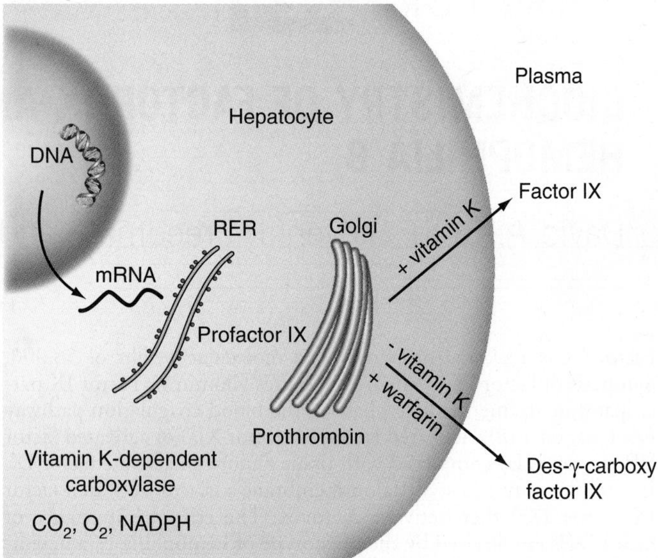

Figure 124–3 Biosynthesis of factor IX. Factor IX is synthesized in the liver in a precursor form. The signal peptide is responsible for translocation of the nascent peptide chain to the endoplasmic reticulum. Profactor IX undergoes posttranslational processing, including γ carboxylation, glycosylation, β hydroxylation, disulfide bond formation, and propeptide cleavage. γ Carboxylation requires molecular oxygen, reduced vitamin K, and carbon dioxide in the presence of the vitamin K-dependent γ carboxylase.

γ carboxylation of the adjacent glutamic acid residues in the Gla domain of mature factor IX.[29] This recognition element is defined by amino acids −18, −17, −16, −14, and −10 toward the amino terminus of this region.[30] The vitamin K-dependent carboxylase binds to the γ-carboxylation recognition site within the propeptide.[29–32] The carboxylation reaction, catalyzed by the carboxylase, requires a reduced form of vitamin K (vitamin KH_2), molecular oxygen, carbon dioxide, and the factor IX precursor uncarboxylated profactor IX, which contains glutamic acid residues.[33] The carboxylase is an enzyme with a molecular weight of 94,000 that is sufficient to carboxylate a precursor substrate in the presence of the necessary cofactors.[34–37] The carboxylase is a membrane protein, and its catalytic activity resides on the luminal side of the rough endoplasmic reticulum.[38,39] Multiple glutamic acids are carboxylated within a single precursor upon interaction with the carboxylase.[40] The Gla residues bind calcium, and this in turn facilitates membrane binding by factor IX and factor IXa.

Aspartic acid 64 within the first EGF-like domain undergoes β hydroxylation in the rough endoplasmic reticulum. From the cDNA sequences of factor IX,[7,8] factor X,[41] protein C,[42,43] protein S,[44] and factor VII,[45] it is apparent that specific aspartic acid residues in precursor forms of these proteins undergo β hydroxylation posttranslationally. Stenflo et al.[46] suggest that a consensus sequence consisting of Cys-X-Asp/Asn-X-X-X-Phe/Tyr-X-Cys-X-Cys signals this event. Factor IX contains approximately 0.4 moles of β-hydroxyaspartic acid per mole of factor IX.[47,48] This modified amino acid is formed from aspartic acid by a posttranslational process catalyzed by the α-ketoglutarate–dependent dioxygenase[49] aspartyl β-hydroxylase.[50,51] Mutants lacking Asp64 have decreased calcium binding, which suggests that β-hydroxyaspartic acid is involved in calcium binding. However, detailed studies using nuclear magnetic resonance spectroscopy failed to show a significant difference in calcium binding between β-hydroxylated and non–β-hydroxylated factor IX peptides.[52] Furthermore, recombinant factor IX expressed in the presence of dipyridyl, *o*-phenanthroline, or pyridine 2,4-dicarboxylate, which are inhibitors of 2-ketoglutarate–dependent dioxygenases, retains full activity.[53] These data are consistent with the hypothesis that Asp64 is required for full functional activity, but β hydroxylation is not.

Bovine and human factor IX are glycoproteins that contain approximately 17% carbohydrate by weight. The first EGF-like domain is glycosylated at two *O*-linked glycosylation sites. Xyl α(1 → 3) Gluβ1 → *O*-Ser and Xyl α(1 → 3) Xyl α(1 → 3) Glcβ1 → *O*-Ser saccharides are glycosidically linked to Ser53.[54] A tetrasaccharide NeuAc α(2 → 6) Gal β(1 → 4) GluNAc β(1 → 3) Fucα1 → *O*-Ser is linked to Ser61.[55–57] A putative UDP-glucose:protein *O*-glucosyltransferase that makes *O*-glucose modifications in EGF repeats has been identified.[58] A second heavily glycosylated portion of factor IX is the activation peptide (Ala146-Arg180). It is glycosylated at two *N*-linked and two *O*-linked glycosylation sites.[59] Asn157 and Asn167 are fully glycosylated. Thr159 and Thr169 are partially glycosylated. Additional posttranslation modifications including sulfation of Tyr155 and phosphorylation of Ser158 have been identified. Although these modifications on factor IX have no effect on specific coagulant activity, tyrosine sulfation may influence in vivo recovery of factor IX.[60]

Profactor IX, including the propeptide and factor IX sequence, undergoes carboxylation in the endoplasmic reticulum. Profactor IX, even in its fully carboxylated form and in contradistinction to factor IX, is not capable of binding to membrane surfaces.[61] Presumably this property prevents factor IX from being retained inside the cell, where high levels of calcium ions within the endoplasmic reticulum could support factor IX–membrane interaction. Profactor IX undergoes additional posttranslational processing, including disulfide bond formation and glycosylation, characteristic of other secreted plasma proteins. The propeptide is cleaved as a late processing event.[8,62,63] Furin or a furin-like converting enzyme cleaves peptide bonds at a site adjacent to the sequence RXRR, where X can be any amino acid and R is arginine.[64] Bristol et al.[65] used site-directed mutagenesis to define a hierarchy of the efficiency of cleavage given different paired amino acids at the P1 and P2 positions: Lys-Arg > Arg-Arg > Thr-Arg > Arg-Lys > Lys-Lys >> Lys-Thr. γ Carboxylation precedes propeptide cleavage.[65]

The carboxyl terminus of factor IX contributes to intracellular factor IX stability and cellular secretion. Mutant factor IX with substitutions in amino acids 403 to 415 are degraded and secreted only at low levels when expressed in a hepatoma cell line.[66] Addition of proteosome inhibitors to this system leads to increased intracellular mutant factor IX concentrations and recovery of factor IX secretion.[66] Consistent with these observations, naturally occurring mutations in the carboxyl terminus of factor IX lead to hemophilia B with severely depressed factor IX protein levels in the plasma.[67]

STRUCTURE OF FACTOR IX

Human factor IX is a single-chain glycoprotein composed of 415 amino acids (Fig. 124–4).[7,8,68] It has a molecular weight of 56,000.[69,70] Factor IXa is composed of a light chain of molecular weight 18,000 and a heavy chain of molecular weight 28,000.[71] The structure of porcine factor IX has been determined by x-ray crystallography in the absence of calcium ions.[72] The protein resembles a tulip in which the amino terminal Gla domain represents the bulb, the two EGF domains represent the stalk, and the catalytic domain represents the flower (Fig. 124–5).

PROPEPTIDE

The propeptide directs γ carboxylation of profactor IX and then is cleaved to yield factor IX. The propeptide includes an amphipathic α helix with a hydrophobic face and a hydrophilic face.[73] The carboxylation recognition site is located proximal to this helix. This recognition site binds the amino-terminal third of the carboxylase.[74,75] Curiously, the propeptide also interacts with a region of the carboxylase having sequence homology to itself. This region of the carboxylase between residues 495 and 513 has been named the "internal propeptide."[74,76,77] Mutations in the propeptide have been documented as the cause of some forms of hemophilia B. Diuguid et al.[62] determined the size of the propeptide of factor IX by analysis of a mutant factor IX, factor IX Cambridge. This mutant has an 18-residue amino-terminal extension due to mutation of Arg–1 to a serine, precluding propeptide cleavage by the propeptidase furin. Concurrently, Bentley et al.[63] evaluated factor IX Oxford 3, a mutant factor IX in which Arg–4 is mutated to glutamine; this mutation also prevents propeptide cleavage. Similar mutations have been described, each characterized by the complete absence of factor IX activity and the presence of the 18-residue propeptide extension.[78–81] Of the several proteins studied,[62,78,82,83] there is a partial defect in γ carboxylation of factor IX. Because of the failure of propeptide cleavage, these profactor IX mutants cannot bind to phospholipid vesicles, nor can they be activated by factor XIa. In fact, the propeptide prevents binding of profactor IX to membranes even if profactor IX is fully carboxylated.[61] These data and the marked sequence homology of this domain in Gla-containing proteins led to the proposal that the propeptide participates in γ carboxylation.[84] Using site-specific mutagenesis and a heterologous mammalian expression system, Jorgensen et al.[29] and Rabiet et al.[48] demonstrated that factor IX lacking the 18-residue propeptide was not carboxylated in vivo. Similarly, point mutations at −16 (Phe → Ala) or −10 (Ala → Glu), both positions highly conserved in the propeptides of the vitamin K-dependent proteins, inhibited γ carboxylation. These results demonstrated that the propeptide contains a recognition element, designated the γ-carboxylation recognition site, that signals γ carboxylation of vitamin K-dependent proteins during hepatic biosynthesis. The propeptide is sufficient to direct γ carboxylation when engineered immediately amino terminal to an unrelated glutamic acid-rich region of prothrombin.[85]

γ-Carboxyglutamic Acid Domain

The amino-terminal Gla domain of human factor IX includes 12 Gla residues, located at positions 7, 8, 15, 17, 20, 21, 26, 27, 30, 33, 36, and 40.[86,87] The Gla domain defines some of the critical calcium-binding sites of the protein and is required for the interaction of factor IX with membrane surfaces in the presence of calcium ions.[88] At present, naturally occurring mutations have been described for nine of the 12 Gla residues. Patients with these mutations have moderate to severe hemophilia, an observation emphasizing the functional importance of these residues.[67] In contrast, factor IX, which lacks Gla36 and Gla40, Gla residues that are not found in other vitamin K-dependent blood coagulation proteins, maintains full function.[89,90] In the absence of calcium, the Gla domain consists of three well-defined structural elements linked by a flexible polypeptide backbone.[90] The three structural elements are a short amino-terminal ω loop (residues 6–9), a hexapeptide loop formed by a disulfide bridge between cysteines 18 and 23, and a carboxyl-terminal α helix (residues 37–46). The hexapeptide loop is essential for factor IX function, as evidenced by the fact that factor IX Zutphen (Cys18 → Arg) cannot form the Ca^{2+}-dependent conformation and results in severe hemophilia.[91] When bound with calcium, the Gla domain folds in a manner that exposes the ω-loop–containing hydrophobic residues Leu6 and Phe9 on the surface. This region forms at least part of the phospholipid-binding site in factor IX (see Membrane-Binding Properties below).[92,93] The Gla domain also interacts directly with the light chain of factor VIII.[94]

EPIDERMAL GROWTH FACTOR-LIKE DOMAINS

Two consecutive EGF-like domains bridge the amino-terminal Gla domain/aromatic amino acid stack and the carboxyl-terminal serine protease domain in factor IXa. The EGF domains are approximately 50 amino acids long and have three conserved disulfide bonds. The three-dimensional structures of these domains closely resemble that of other EGF domains and contain two antiparallel β sheets.[72,95,96] The carboxyl-terminal end of the first EGF domain fills a hydrophobic pocket at the amino-terminal end of the second EGF domain.[97] Only the first of the two EGF domains binds calcium ions and provides one of two high-affinity calcium-binding sites outside of the Gla domain.[96] The other high-affinity calcium-binding site resides in the serine protease domain.[98] The importance of this calcium-binding site for factor IX function is illustrated by mutations of Asp47 and Asp64 (factor IX Alabama) that disrupt calcium binding and cause hemophilia B.[99–102] Engineered mutations of Asp64 have widespread effects on factor IXa function, including assembly into the tenase complex and enzymatic activity for its substrate factor X.[103]

Analysis of EGF peptides and mutants helps to define the function of these domains in factor IX and factor IXa. The isolated first EGF domain inhibits factor Xa generation by intact factor IXa in the presence or absence of factor VIIIa, and it can be directly cross-linked to Gla domainless factor X.[104,105] Alanine scanning mutagenesis of the second EGF domain shows that residues 102 to 108 bind factor X.[106] Data using EGF chimeras, deletions, and point mutants indicate that the first EGF domain directly interacts with tissue factor in the factor VIIa/tissue factor complex.[107,108] Mutation of Gly48 → Arg in factor IX Tainan and factor IX Malmo are poorly activated by factor VIIa/tissue factor.[109] Substitution of Arg94 in the second EGF domain with a serine, a naturally occurring hemophilia B defect, introduces an *O*-linked carbohydrate that attenuates factor IX activation by both factor XIa and the factor VIIa/tissue factor complex.[110] Alanine scanning mutagenesis of the second EGF domain shows that residues 89 to 93 are involved in factor VIIIa binding. In contrast, studies with factor IX chimeras in which the first EGF domain is replaced with the first EGF domain of other coagulation proteins suggest that this region does not interact with factor VIIIa.[111,112] However, Asp64 mutations in factor IX affect binding to the factor VIII light chain.[113] Thus, both EGF domains are involved in protein–protein

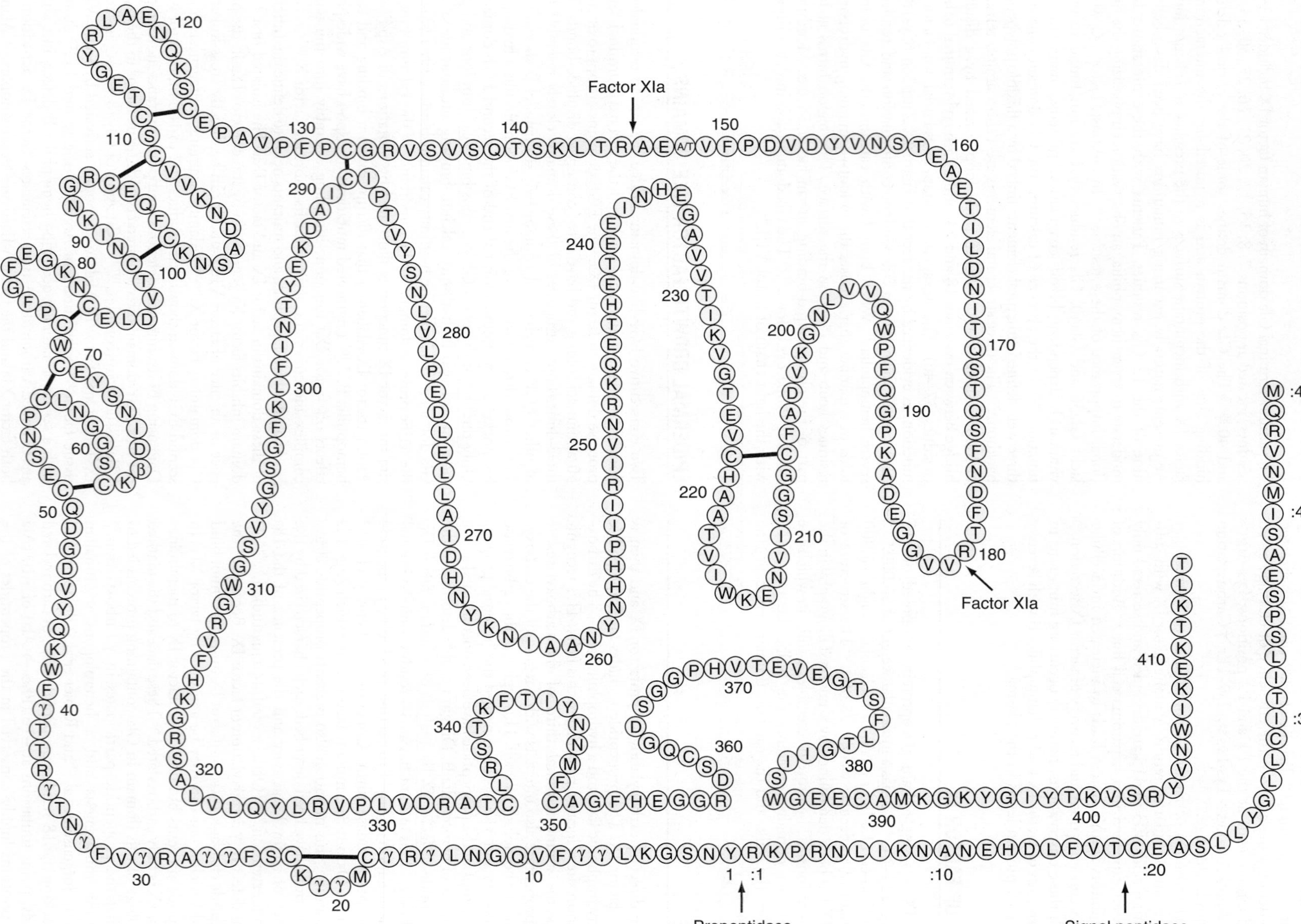

Figure 124–4 Amino acid sequence of factor IX. The preprofactor IX sequence includes the signal peptide, propeptide, γ-carboxyglutamic acid domain, aromatic amino acid stack domain, two EGF domains, and the serine protease domain. Amino acids are designated by the one-letter code. β, β-hydroxyaspartic acid; γ, γ-carboxyglutamic acid; EGF, epidermal growth factor.

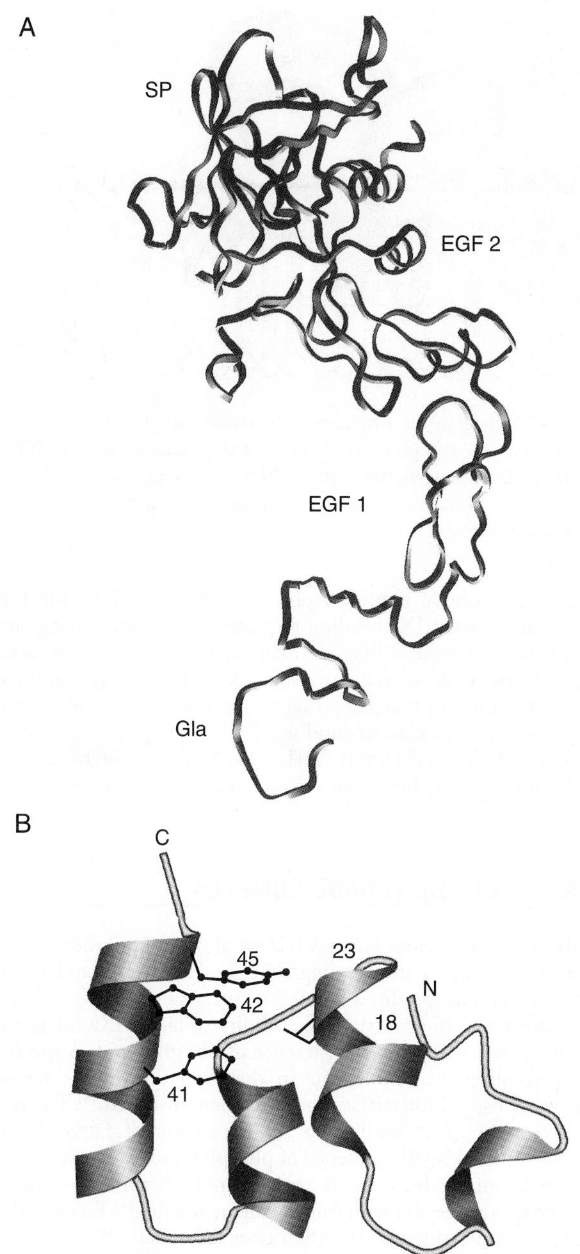

Figure 124–5 A, Ribbon model of the three-dimensional structure of factor IXaβ as determined by x-ray crystallography. **B,** Ribbon model of glutamic acid-containing region as determined by nuclear magnetic resonance. The cysteines of the hexapeptide disulfide loop, residues 18 and 23, are labeled by residue number, and the disulfide bond is indicated. The side chains of the conserved aromatic residues of the aromatic amino acid stack domain are displayed and labeled by residue number. EGF 1, first epidermal growth factor-like region; EGF 2, second epidermal growth factor-like region; Gla, γ-carboxy glutamic acid-containing region; NMR, nuclear magnetic resonance; SP, serine protease-containing region.

interactions that contribute to factor IX activation and factor IXa function.

SERINE PROTEASE DOMAIN

The carboxyl-terminal portion of factor IX demonstrates marked sequence homology with zymogens of serine proteases, such as trypsin and chymotrypsin. This region is 235 amino acids long and contains, in latent form, the enzyme active site of factor IXa. The mechanism of factor IX activation involves limited proteolysis through cleavage of two peptide bonds that release the activation peptide between residues Ala146 and Arg180. Consequently, the serine protease domain is within the heavy chain of factor IXa. The enzyme active site is common to all serine proteases and contains the enzymatic machinery for the hydrolysis of peptide bonds. The classic catalytic triad is composed of factor IXa residues His221, Asp269, and Ser365. An extended substrate-binding site surrounds the active site and defines the high substrate specificity of factor IXa for protein substrates.[114]

CALCIUM-BINDING PROPERTIES

Factor IX binds to metal ions. As with the other vitamin K-dependent proteins, there are two classes of metal-binding sites: high affinity and low affinity.[114,115] Occupation of these two classes of metal-binding sites leads to two sequential conformational changes in these proteins.[116,117] The first conformational change can be induced by calcium, magnesium, and many other divalent cations. The second conformational change is induced only by calcium ions. Fab fragments of conformation-specific antibodies, directed against factor IX after it has undergone the conformational transition that is calcium ion selective, block the binding of factor IX to phospholipid vesicles and the activation of factor IX by factor XIa. These findings suggest that the conformer achieved only in the presence of calcium is necessary for expression of a phospholipid-binding site and for binding of factor IX by factor XIa.[117]

The binding of calcium to the Gla domain involves formation of an internal calcium-binding pocket formed by the amino-terminal nine Gla residues. The binding results in the formation of a calcium-carboxylate network with an exposed amino-terminal hydrophobic loop.[92,93] The crystal structure of the factor IX Gla domain shows that six calcium ions are coordinated by Gla residues. However, it is possible that other calcium ions bind to low-affinity sites not detectable by x-ray crystallography. The binding of calcium to the first EGF-like domain is mediated by a consensus sequence including Asp47, Asp49, Gln50, Asp64, and Tyr69. Asp47, Gln50, and Asp64 residues interact directly with calcium.[97,99,104] Astermark et al.[118] demonstrated that the individual Gla and EGF domains bind calcium ions, but the intact Gla–EGF domain unit binds calcium ions with even higher affinity. Another high-affinity calcium-binding site in the heavy chain of factor IX involving residues 235, 237, 240, and 245 has been described.[98]

MEMBRANE-BINDING PROPERTIES

The interaction of factor IX and factor IXa with phospholipid membranes has been studied using phospholipid vesicles.[101] Factor IX affinity for phosphatidylcholine-phosphatidylserine membranes is independent of the phosphatidylserine concentration above 20% to 30%.[119] K_d of approximately 1 to 2 μM has been measured. Factor IX binds to vesicles in the presence of Ca^{2+} but not in the presence of Mg^{2+} or ethylenediaminetetraacetic acid (EDTA). Furthermore, des-γ-carboxy factor IX does not interact with phospholipid vesicles, even in the presence of Ca^{2+}. These results emphasize the importance of the Gla domain in defining phospholipid-binding properties. Several lines of experimental evidence indicate that the amino-terminal region of the Gla domain is the phospholipid-binding site (Fig. 124–6). First, Leu6 and Phe9 form a hydrophobic surface patch as demonstrated in the human factor IX Gla domain solution and crystal structures.[92,93] Second, these residues can be directly cross-linked to phospholipids.[120] Third, the Mg^{2+}-coordinated Gla domain, which does not bind phospholipid membranes, lacks a well-ordered hydrophobic surface patch.[120] Fourth, this patch is part of the epitope for an antifactor IX antibody that inhibits phospholipid binding.[93] Finally, and most convincingly, the homologous region in the prothrombin : Ca^{2+}: phosphoplipid ternary complex crystal structure directly interacts with phospholipid membranes.[121] Other structural

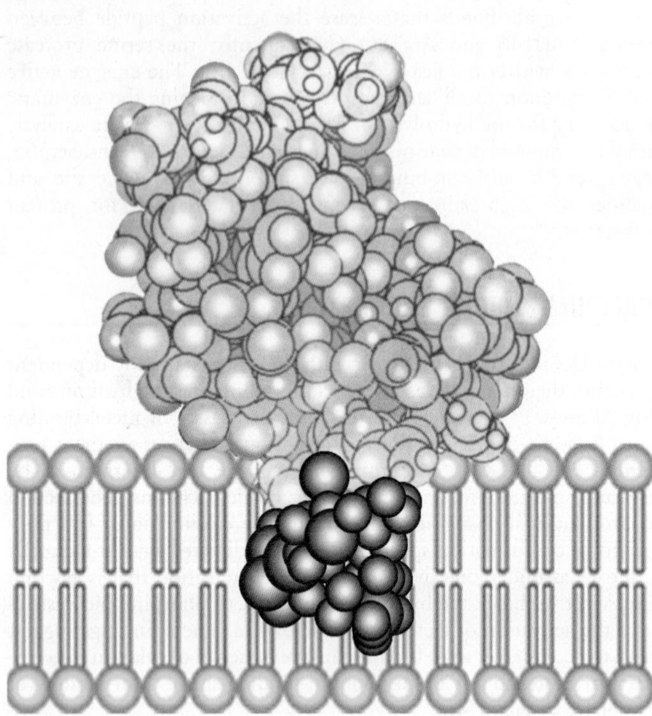

Figure 124–6 Model of the interaction of factor IX and phospholipid membrane. The hydrophobic residues (black) that form the hydrophobic patch in the phospholipid-binding site of factor IX are buried in the phospholipid bilayer. The phosphatidylserine binds specifically through electrostatic interactions with amino acid side chains of the γ-carboxyglutamic acid (Gla) domain.

similarities between factor IX and prothrombin interactions with phospholipid membranes may be present.

Factors IX and factor IXa bind to bovine aortic endothelial cells and compete for the same site.[122–124] K_d binding constants ranging between 127 pM and 7.4 nM have been reported. Factor IXa binding to endothelial cells is greater in the presence of both factor VIII and factor X.[125] Interaction of factor IX with endothelial cells is inhibited by a Gla peptide corresponding to residues 1 to 42 of factor IX.[126] K_i for this interaction is approximately 0.05 μM. A chimeric protein in which the Gla domain of protein C is replaced with that of factor IX is able to bind endothelial cells.[127] These results suggest that the endothelial binding site resides within the Gla domain. More specifically, factor VII can be converted to a protein that binds endothelial cells if Gla domain residues 3 to 11 are replaced with those of factor IX.[128] However, Gla peptides corresponding to residues 1 to 14 and 1 to 24 do not compete with intact factor IX for binding to endothelial cells.[129] Because purified natural variants of factor IX with mutations within the hydrophobic stack domain or the first EGF-like domain do not compete effectively with wild-type factor IX for binding to endothelial cells, the functional integrity of the Gla domain in the interaction with endothelial cells depends on these regions.[130] Interestingly, factor IX can bind to collagen IV with K_d of 6.8 nM, which approximates the binding affinity of factor IX to endothelial cells.[124] In this study, mutant factor IX containing Lys5 → Ala or Val10 → Lys could not compete with wild-type factor IX binding to collagen IV. Further support for collagen IV as the endothelial cell-binding site is provided by data by Gui et al.,[131] who showed that factor IX binds to endothelial cell collagen IV surfaces in vivo.

Activated platelets, but not resting platelets, bind factors IX and IXa.[132,133] Factor IX and factor IXa have some common binding sites on activated platelets. There are 250 to 300 sites per platelet for factor IX and 500 to 600 sites per platelet for factor IXa. The interaction of factor IXa with platelets is mediated at least in part by the Gla domain.[134] A synthetic peptide from residues 4 to 11 in the Gla domain inhibits factor IXa binding to platelets.[135] Studies using chimeras in which the second EGF domain of factor IX/IXa is replaced with the second EGF domain of factor X or factor VII exhibited decreased binding to platelets, suggesting that the second EGF domain plays a role in platelet binding.[136,137] In the presence of saturating concentrations of factors VIIIa and X, the K_d of factor IXa (0.5 nM) binding is five times lower than that of factor IX alone.[138,139]

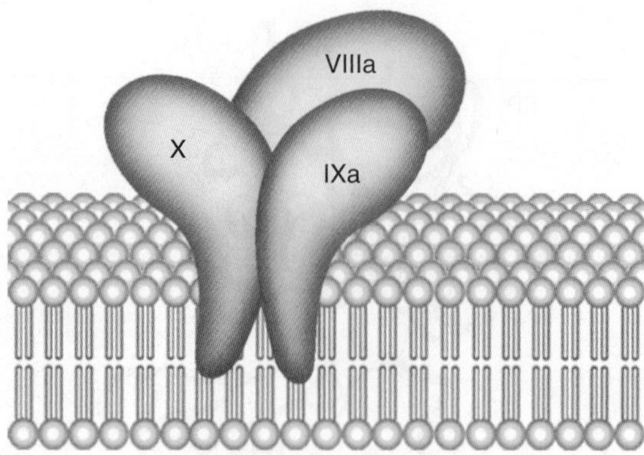

Figure 124–7 Model of the structure of the tenase complex. The tenase complex (the enzyme complex capable of activating factor X to factor Xa) includes factor IXa as enzyme and factor VIIIa as cofactor bound to the membrane surface. The substrate factor X interacts with factor IXa, factor VIIIa, and the membrane.

FORMATION OF THE TENASE COMPLEX

Assembly of factor IXa and factor VIIIa on phospholipid membranes constitutes the tenase complex (Fig. 124–7). Factor IXa and factor VIIIa interact on phospholipid membrane surfaces with a K_d of 2 nM at a 1 : 1 molar stoichiometry.[140] The affinity of factor IXa for factor VIIIa is increased 10-fold in the presence of phospholipid. A specific role for phosphatidylethanolamine in the formation of the tenase complex on phospholipid surfaces has been demonstrated.[141] The rate of bond cleavage (k_{cat}) leading to the formation of factor Xa is increased 1500-fold by the presence of phospholipid.[142] Activation of factor IX to factor IXa leads to the expression of a factor VIII-binding site and active enzyme site with full coagulant activity.[143] Factor VIIIa binds more tightly to factor IXa than does factor VIII.[140] A conformational change in the factor IXa active site is induced by factor VIIIa, thus providing a structural basis for enhancement of factor IXa activity upon cofactor binding.[144]

Factor IX domains are involved in protein–protein interactions that facilitate tenase complex formation. The affinity of a naturally occurring factor IX mutant (Gly12 → Arg) for factor VIIIa is 172-fold less than that for wild-type factor IX, suggesting a role for the Gla domain in formation of the tenase complex.[145] Both EGF domains of factor IXa interact with factor X, and the second EGF domain interacts with factor VIIIa. Helix 330 in the protease domain of factor IXa interacts with residues 558 to 565 in the A2 subunit of factor VIIIa.[146]

ACTIVATION OF FACTOR IX BY THE INTRINSIC PATHWAY

Factor IX is a proenzyme with no catalytic activity. It is activated to factor IXa, formally known as factor IXaβ, by factor XIa in the presence of calcium, or by factor VIIa/tissue factor in a reaction that occurs on a membrane surface and in the presence of calcium (Fig. 124–8). The kinetics of factor IX activation by factor VIIa/tissue

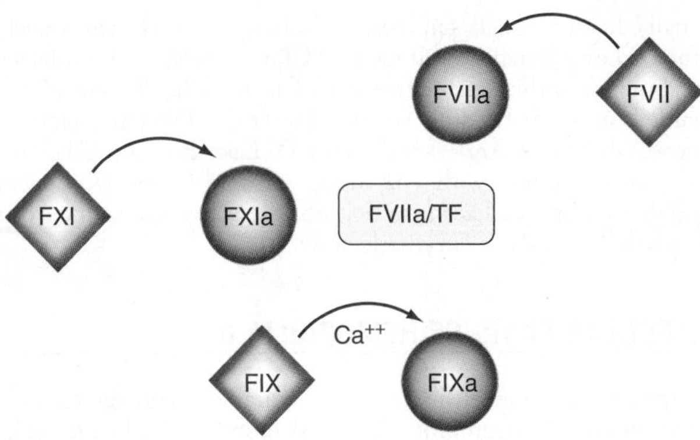

Figure 124–8 Pathways of factor IX activation. Factor IX is activated independently by either factor XIa or factor VIIa/tissue factor. Factor XIa can activate factor IX in the absence of membrane surfaces, but calcium ions are required. The complex of factor VIIa and tissue factor on membrane surfaces in the presence of calcium ions also converts factor IX to its active enzyme form.

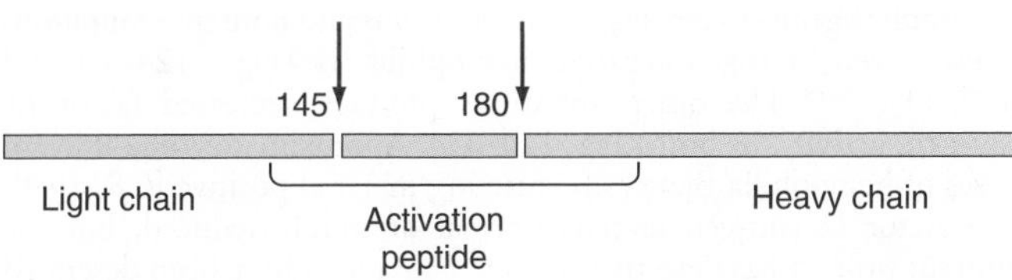

Figure 124–9 Activation of factor IX by limited proteolysis. The zymogen factor IX has no enzymatic activity. Upon cleavage of the peptide bonds adjacent to Arg145and Arg180, enzymatically active factor IXa is generated. Cleavage of these peptide bonds is associated with expression of enzyme activity and a factor VIIIa binding site.

factor and factor XIa are comparable. In contrast to the other vitamin K-dependent blood clotting proteins, membrane surfaces, including phospholipid vesicles or cell surfaces, do not enhance factor IX activation by factor XIa. When factor IX is activated by factor XIa, two peptide bonds are cleaved: one bond located at Arg145-Ala146 and the other bond at Arg180-Val181 (Fig. 124–9).[147] With release of the internal carbohydrate-rich activation fragment (M_r 11,000) from residues 146 to 180, the factor IXa light chain (M_r 17,000) and heavy chain (M_r 28,000) remain bound by a single disulfide bond (see Fig. 124–4). The enzyme active site is located on the heavy chain. Cleavage of factor IX appears to occur via a processive mechanism in which both cleavages are made by factor XIa before factor IXa is produced.[148] The protease from Russell viper venom activates factor IX to factor IXaα by cleaving only the Arg180-Val181 bond.[71]

Factor IX Chapel Hill (Arg145 → His), the first factor IX mutation to be defined at the molecular level, is the prototype of a genetic defect in which activation of a zymogen is impaired due to the mutation of an arginine preceding a sessile bond.[138] It has minimal coagulant activity.[100] Factors IX Chicago-2 (Arg145 → His)[139] and factor IX Albuquerque (Arg145 → Cys)[149] have mutations at the same site. In both of these mutations, loss of the arginine at position 145 precludes cleavage of the sessile bond separating the factor IX light chain from the activation peptide. Failure to cleave this bond, but normal cleavage of the Arg180-Val181 bond, produces factor IXaα, which activates factor X very slowly. The active site of factor IXa is formed, however, as demonstrated by its ability to cleave synthetic substrates normally.[150] Cleavage of the Arg145-Ala146 bond exposes a binding site for factor VIIIa. Conversely, factor IXα, an intermediate with a cleaved Arg145-Ala146 bond but a noncleaved Arg180-Val181 bond, binds factor VIII normally but cannot generate factor Xa from factor X.[151] Factor IX mutants at position 180 include factor IX Hilo (Arg180 → Gln), factor IX Milano (Arg180 → Gln), factor IX Deventer (Arg180 → Trp), and factor IX Nagoya (Arg180 → Trp), all of which result in hemophilia Bm, a type of hemophilia in which the patient's mutant factor IX causes a marked prolongation of the ox brain prothrombin time. This phenotype results because factor IX Bm variants are more effective inhibitors of the factor VIIa/tissue factor complex-induced activation of factor X than is wild-type factor IX.[152,153] Factor IX Novara (Val181 → Phe)[153] and factor IX Tokyo (Val182 → Ala)[154] also result in the hemophilia Bm phenotype, whereas factor IX Kashihara (Val182 → Phe) results in hemophilia B.[155,156]

Activation of factor IX by factor XIa is highly metal selective, with optimal activation only in the presence of Ca^{2+} and suboptimal activation in the presence of Sr^{2+}.[103,157] K_m for activation of factor IX by factor XIa without calcium is 18 μM, and k_{cat} is 2.4 min^{-1}. In the presence of calcium, K_m is decreased to 2 μM, and k_{cat} is increased to 10.4 min^{-1}.[158,159] Although the proteolytic activity of factor XIa is present on the light chain, the heavy chain of factor XIa is responsible for Ca^{2+}-dependent acceleration of factor IX activation.[159,160] The region of the factor XIa heavy chain that interacts with factor IX has been localized to residues 134 to 172 in the heavy chain of factor XI.[161] Interestingly, conformation-dependent, Ca^{2+}-specific antifactor IX antibodies, which inhibit phospholipid binding, also inhibit factor IX activation by factor XIa.[116] Based on this observation, it was proposed that the phospholipid-binding site and factor XIa-binding site on factor IX overlap. In support of this hypothesis is the finding that if the factor IX Gla domain, which binds Ca^{2+} and phospholipid, is either decarboxylated or replaced with the factor VII Gla domain in factor IX, then activation by factor XIa is attenuated.[162] Unexpectedly, the isolated Gla domain (residues 1–47), which binds phospholipid and is recognized by conformation-dependent, Ca^{2+}-specific antifactor IX antibodies, did not inhibit factor XIa activation of factor IX.[163] Therefore, the Gla domain is necessary but not sufficient for factor XIa binding. As such, other data implicate a role for the neighboring EGF domain. For example, activation of factor IX New London (Pro50 → Glu) by factor XIa is abnormally slow.[164] Also, a monoclonal antibody directed against the first EGF domain of factor IX inhibits its activation by factor XIa.[165]

ACTIVATION OF FACTOR IX BY THE EXTRINSIC PATHWAY

Factor IX is also activated by factor VIIa and tissue factor (see Fig. 124–8).[142,166] This reaction, which is dependent on calcium ions, is characterized by K_m of 0.3 μM.[167,168] The k_{cat} for this reaction is between 13 and 68 min^{-1}.[167,168] Structure–function studies indicate that both of the factor IX EGF domains may be involved in binding the factor VIIa/tissue factor complex. The relative importance of factor IX activation by factor XIa or the factor VIIa/tissue factor complex was evaluated by measuring the level of the factor IX activation peptide in patients with factor VII and XI deficiencies.[169] A significant reduction in the baseline levels of the factor IX activation peptide was noted in patients with factor VII deficiency but not in patients with factor XI deficiency compared with normal controls. Furthermore, administration of recombinant factor VIIa to patients deficient in factor VII resulted in significant elevations of the factor IX activation peptide.[170] Almus et al.[171] evaluated activation of factors IX and X by the factor VIIa/tissue factor complex in an umbilical vein model. In this system, activation of factors IX and X occurs at the same rate. These studies, along with the observation that patients with factor XI deficiency have variable bleeding, suggest that the factor VIIa/tissue factor complex initiates blood clotting. A revised model for blood coagulation was proposed whereby the factor VIIa/tissue factor complex initiates blood clotting and thrombin activation of factor XI maintains it.[172]

ENZYMATIC ACTIVITY OF FACTOR IXa

Activation of factor X by factor IXa has been evaluated under multiple experimental conditions. Calcium by itself accelerates factor IXa activation of factor X, but it has a more important role in allowing for formation of the tenase complex on membrane surfaces. The presence of both factor VIIIa and Factor IXa on membrane surfaces greatly accelerates activation of factor X, whereas the presence of only one of these cofactors alone has a minimal effect.[173,174] The k_{cat} for factor X activation by factor IXa in the presence of factor VIIIa but without phospholipid vesicles is 0.058 min^{-1}. The same reaction without factor VIIIa but with phospholipid vesicles has k_{cat} of 0.095 min^{-1}, whereas in the presence of factor VIIIa and phospholipid vesicles the reaction is greatly accelerated, with k_{cat} of 1740 min^{-1}.[132] Activation of factor X by factor IXa is also supported by activated platelets and endothelials cells. The k_{cat} for factor X activation on activated platelets is 1240 min^{-1}, which is very close to the k_{cat} for factor X activation in the presence of phospholipid vesicles. The rate of activation of factor X on endothelial cells is approximately one sixth the rate on activated platelets.[175]

Physiologic inhibitors of factor IXa circulate in plasma. Factor IXa is inhibited by antithrombin III, which forms a 1 : 1 stoichiometric complex with factor IXa as well as other activated coagulation factors. This reaction is accelerated approximately 1000-fold by the addition of heparin.[176–179] Some factor IX Bm variants with mutations at the amino terminus of the heavy chain or within the catalytic domain are unable to bind antithrombin III.[153] Protease nexin 2, an amyloid β-protein precursor containing a Kunitz-type protease inhibitor domain, is an even more potent inhibitor of factor IXa than is antithrombin III.[180,181] However, it is present in plasma at only picomolar concentrations. Nonetheless, the protease nexin 2 is an α-granule component of platelets and may achieve physiologically significant concentrations in areas of platelet degranulation.[182]

Mutations within the catalytic domain of factor IX also decrease enzymatic activity. A mutation of Ile397 → Thr has been recognized in many hemophilia B families, including factor IX Vancouver,[183] factor IX Long Beach,[184] and factor IX Los Angeles.[185] This defect is near, but not within, the active site of factor IXa. It may alter the extended substrate-binding site for factor X. Likewise, factor IX Angers (Gly396 → Arg)[186] and factor IX Lake Elsinore (Ala390 → Val)[187] also interfere with enzymatic activity. Factor IX Bergamo (Pro368 → Thr) is adjacent to Ser365, the active site serine, so not unexpectedly it ablates enzymatic activity.[153]

MOLECULAR BASIS OF HEMOPHILIA B

An updated comprehensive list of naturally occurring factor IX mutations causing hemophilia B can be found in the Hemophilia B Mutation Database (version 13; www.kcl.ac.uk/ip/petergreen/haemBdatabase.html). This list is compiled from 2891 patient entries and includes various types of mutations, including 91 gross deletions or insertions, 211 short deletions and insertions, one triple mutation, 34 double mutations, and the remainder single mutations. Of note, this database overrepresents mutations causing a more severe bleeding phenotype, and certain mutations are overrepresented due to a founder effect, whereas double mutants are underrepresented due to incomplete gene sequencing. Gross deletions and nonsense mutations cause severe, antigen-negative hemophilia B (Figs. 124–10 and 124–11).[188,189] The other mutations produce decreased factor IX antigen, activity, or both (Fig. 124–11). Approximately one third of cases of hemophilia B are cross-reacting material positive [CRM(+)]; the factor IX antigen level is normal or mildly reduced, but the mutant protein has defective activity. Mutations have been described

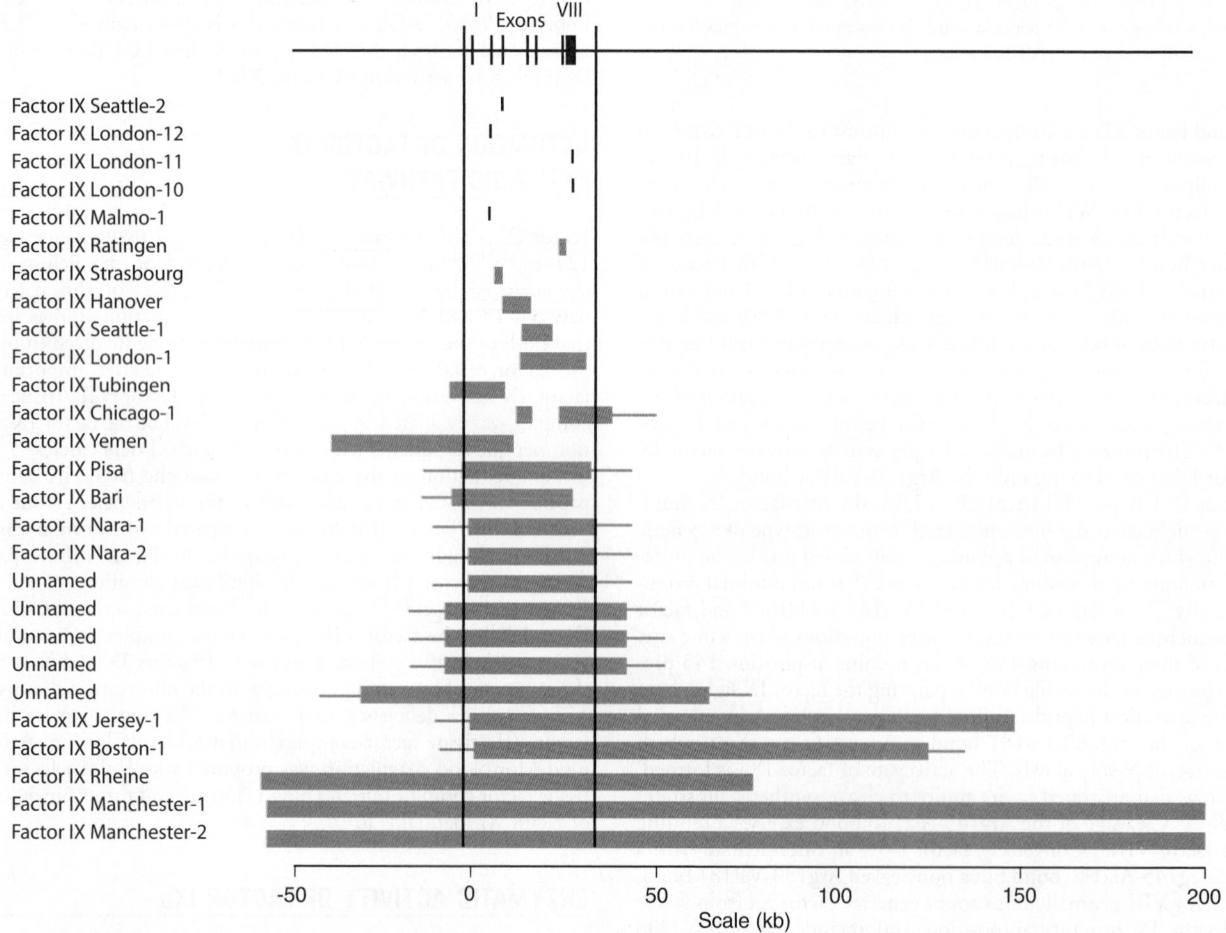

Figure 124–10 Factor IX gene deletions as a cause of hemophilia B. Almost 150 deletions are reported in the hemophilia B mutation database, of which a representative set is illustrated here. Deleted portions of factor IX gene are indicated by light blue rectangles; an uncertain extent of deletion is indicated by blue lines. The factor IX gene (exons 1–8) is shown in black.

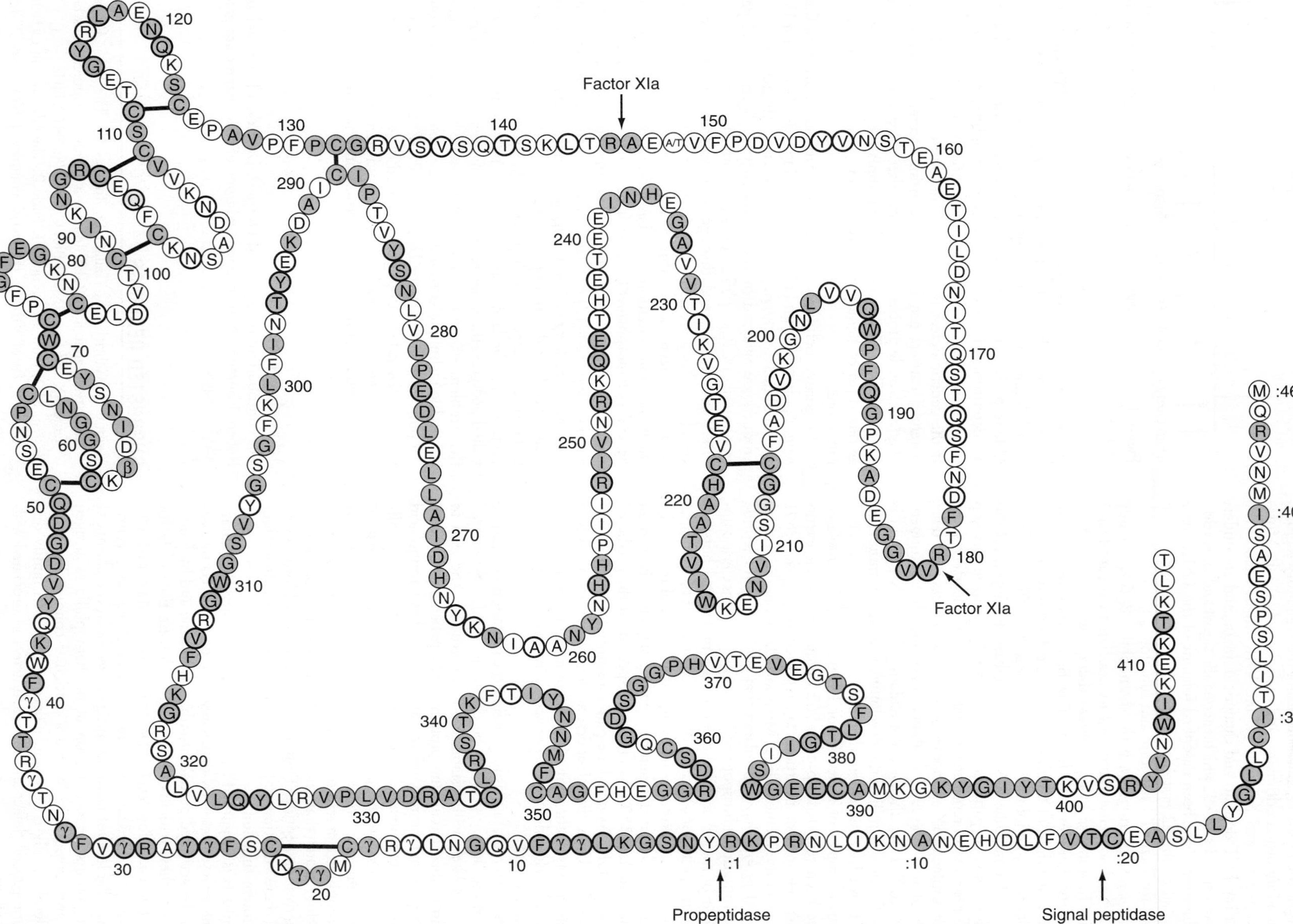

Figure 124–11 Point mutations in the factor IX amino acid DNA sequence as a cause of hemophilia B. Missense mutations are designated by red shading and nonsense/frameshift mutations are designated by a black bold circle. Amino acids are designated by the one-letter code. β, β-hydroxyaspartic acid; γ, γ carboxyglutamic acid.

in all regions of the factor IX gene, including the regulatory regions, the exon-encoding protein domains, and even the poly A tail. Mutations are overrepresented in exons IV and VIII, which encode the calcium-binding EGF domain and catalytic domain, and are underrepresented in exons I and VI, which encode the signal and activation peptides. Mutations have been described for nine of the 12 Gla residues and for all of the 22 cysteines, emphasizing the importance of these residues for factor IX structure and function.

Mutations causing antigen-negative hemophilia B (i.e., mainly gross deletions and nonsense mutations) are associated with antifactor IX antibodies in response to replacement therapy with factor IX.[188] In a series of 62 families with hemophilia B, a family member in approximately one third of families exhibiting deletions or nonsense mutations developed an inhibitor.[190] Slightly less than 2% of patients reported in the Hemophilia B Mutation Database developed inhibitors. Therefore, not all patients without factor IX antigen develop inhibitors in response to replacement therapy.[191,192] Conversely, some patients with antifactor IX antibodies do not possess gross gene deletions.[80,193] In at least one case, antibodies developed in an antigen-positive patient.[193] Thus, the lack of circulating factor IX protein is not the only factor controlling the development of an immunologic response to factor IX replacement therapy.

Numerous examples of repeat factor IX mutations in unrelated families have been reported. To date, 962 unique molecular events and 91 gross deletions or insertions are reported among the 2891 patient entries in the Hemophilia B Mutation Database; the rest are repeats. Several groups have postulated that the CpG dinucleotide sequence is a mutational hotspot.[194–196] The CpG sequence is a component of four of the six arginine codons. As a mutational hotspot, it may represent an important cause of the development of spontaneous point mutations. Furthermore, using a mathematical model, the 20 CpG dinucleotides in the factor IX coding sequence showed an observed mutation rate 150 times the rate expected for the predicted transition rate.[197] Of 51 single base-pair substitutions found in one study, 27 were at CpG dinucleotides, which represents a 38-fold excess for mutations at these sites.[198] In another study, point mutations at CpG dinucleotides were estimated to be increased by 77-fold over the expected rate.[199]

In patients with mutant plasma proteins, the mutation of arginine to another amino acid appears to be common. Insofar as internal point mutations likely will destabilize protein structure and lead to markedly diminished circulating protein levels, patients preselected for circulating mutant protein antigen are likely to have amino acid substitutions on the protein surface. Proteases of the trypsin family use arginines located on the protein surface to hydrolyze adjacent bonds during protein processing and zymogen activation. For instance, hemophilia Bm results from mutation of Arg180 to a variety of other amino acids that prevent carboxyl-terminal cleavage to release the activation peptide. Thus, given the functional importance of arginines, these mutations appear to lead to phenotypically obvious defects in protein function.

Hemophilia B is diagnosed by the finding of isolated, hereditary factor IX deficiency. Factor IX deficiency may be observed by prolongation of the activated partial thromboplastin time and by failure of plasma from these patients to correct the clotting time of factor IX-deficient plasma. A low level of factor IX activity combined with a lifelong history of bleeding or a family history of bleeding secures the diagnosis. The level of factor IX antigen present in the plasma of each patient permits characterization of the hemophilia as antigen negative or antigen positive. Within a particular cohort, the factor IX activity level usually is constant, reflecting that each family displays the same genetic defect and that each defect is associated with a particular phenotype.

The bleeding disorder associated with moderate or severe hemophilia B and the sex-linked nature of the disorder make genetic counseling for affected persons and potential carriers an important issue. Carrier analysis has been performed by differentiating between factor IX activity and factor IX antigen levels. However, this method at best is only 80% effective, partially because of the preponderance of mutations yielding markedly diminished factor IX antigen and

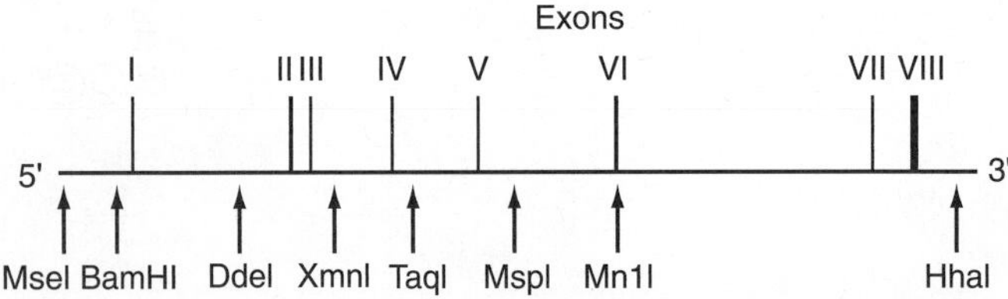

Figure 124–12 Restriction fragment length polymorphisms in the factor IX gene.

partially because of "lyonization," which causes differential levels of inactivation of the X chromosome carrying the mutant gene.[200]

With knowledge of the sequence of the factor IX gene, it is possible to probe for the precise genetic defect among potential carriers. To determine whether a person is a hemophilia B carrier, genomic DNA is isolated from the potential carrier and key family members. If the genetic defect for a particular cohort is known, the DNA of potential carriers can be screened using stringent hybridization to oligonucleotide probes to detect whether these individuals carry that genetic defect. This method is compromised by the fact that as many as one third of hemophilia cases in any generation arise from new mutations.

Of greater usefulness for diagnosing carriers is restriction fragment length polymorphism linkage analysis (Fig. 124–12). Factor IX genes are amplified by polymerase chain reaction (PCR), and the PCR products are analyzed by restriction enzyme digestion and gel electrophoresis. PCR amplification allows prenatal diagnosis using fetal DNA samples obtained through amniocentesis or chorionic villus sampling. Cosegregation of a specific polymorphism that creates a restriction enzyme site within or adjacent to the factor IX gene and the hemophilic mutation is used as indirect evidence for carrier state. Several polymorphisms have been described within and adjacent to the factor IX gene, and they are informative in more than 90% of families (Fig. 124–12).[201] Ethnic variation in the frequency of polymorphisms makes restriction fragment length polymorphism analysis more useful for determining carrier state in some populations (e.g., Caucasians) compared with others (e.g., Asians).[202,203] Other limitations include the lack of an informative polymorphism for any individual pedigree, the absence of key family members for analysis, and the problem of genetic recombination. Perhaps a more generally applicable technique is conformation-sensitive gel electrophoresis.[204] Amplification of the factor IX gene by PCR, followed by conformation-sensitive gel electrophoresis, and DNA sequencing or restriction enzyme digestion should facilitate rapid identification of a hemophilia B mutation in suspected carriers and their fetuses.

Acknowledgments
The contributions of Dr. David Diuguid, Dr. Steven Limentani and Dr. Robert Flaumenhaft to previous editions of this chapter are gratefully acknowledged.

SUGGESTED READINGS

Aktimur A, Gabriel MA, Gailani D, Toomey JR: The factor IX gamma-carboxyglutamic acid (Gla) domain is involved in interactions between factor IX and factor XIa. J Biol Chem 278:7981, 2003.

Blostein MD, Furie BC, Rajotte I, Furie B: The Gla domain of factor IXa binds to factor VIIIa in the tenase complex. J Biol Chem 278:31297, 2003.

Chang YJ, Wu HL, Hamaguchi N, et al: Identification of functionally important residues of the epidermal growth factor-2 domain of factor IX by alanine-scanning mutagenesis. Residues Asn(89)-Gly(93) are critical for binding factor VIIIa. J Biol Chem 277:25393, 2002.

Gui T, Lin HF, Jin DY, et al: Circulating and binding characteristics of wild-type factor IX and certain Gla domain mutants in vivo. Blood 100:153, 2002.

Huang M, Furie BC, Furie B: Crystal structure of the calcium-stabilized human Factor IX Gla domain bound to a conformation-specific anti-Factor IX antibody. J Biol Chem 279:14338, 2004.

Huang M, Rigby AC, Morelli X, et al: Structural basis of membrane binding by Gla domains of vitamin K-dependent proteins. Nat Struct Biol 10:751, 2003.

Lin PJ, Jin DY, Tie JK, et al: The putative vitamin K-dependent gamma-glutamyl carboxylase internal propeptide appears to be the propeptide binding site. J Biol Chem 277:28584, 2002.

Persson KE, Villoutreix BO, Thamlitz AM, et al: The N-terminal epidermal growth factor-like domain of coagulation factor IX: Probing its functions in the activation of factor IX and factor X with a monoclonal antibody. J Biol Chem 277:35616, 2002.

Shao L, Luo Y, Moloney DJ, Haltiwanger R: O-glycosylation of EGF repeats: Identification and initial characterization of a UDP-glucose: Protein O-glucosyltransferase. Glycobiology 12:763, 2002.

Wilkinson FH, Ahmad SS, Walsh PN: The factor IXa second epidermal growth factor (EGF2) domain mediates platelet binding and assembly of the factor X activating complex. J Biol Chem 277:5734, 2002.

Zhong D, Bajaj MS, Schmidt AE, Bajaj SP: The N-terminal epidermal growth factor-like domain in factor IX and factor X represents an important recognition motif for binding to tissue factor. J Biol Chem 277:3622, 2002.

REFERENCES

For complete list of references log onto www.expertconsult.com

CHAPTER 125

CLINICAL ASPECTS AND THERAPY FOR HEMOPHILIA

Margaret V. Ragni, Craig M. Kessler, and Jay Nelson Lozier

[I]f the first son of a woman is circumcised and he dies and the second son is circumcised and he dies, you must not circumcise the third son. . . . Additionally, the sons of the woman's sister should not be circumcised but the sons of her brother can be circumcised.

The Talmud (Yebamot 64b)

The existence of a sex-linked hereditary coagulopathy was first recognized and the disorder first described in the Talmud in the fifth century. This entity eventually was labeled "haemorrhaphilia" (love of bleeding) in 1828.[1] By means of early crude assays developed at the end of the nineteenth century, the clotting times of plasma from persons with hemophilia were found to be greatly prolonged compared with the clotting times in nonbleeders.[2] Mixing two sources of hemophilic plasma sometimes corrected the abnormality in vitro.[3] By 1947, the defect in hemophilia had been attributed to a single deficient plasma protein, which was required for platelet utilization and thromboplastin generation.[4,5] Shortly thereafter, the recognition by Pavlovsky[6] that the plasma of some hemophilic patients could correct the in vitro or in vivo defects of other patients having a clinically identical bleeding disorder led to recognition of the existence of multiple types of hemophilia. The clinical entity related to the protein defect described by Brinkhous[4] and Quick[5] was termed *hemophilia A* and was shown to be related to deficiency of factor VIII (antihemophilic factor or antihemophilic globulin). The other type was termed *hemophilia B* and was shown to result from factor IX deficiency (antihemophilic factor B, plasma thromboplastin component, or Christmas factor, named after a patient with factor IX deficiency).[7,8] These two types of hemophilia are similar clinically and have identical hereditary patterns (sex-linked recessive).

The pathophysiology of hemophilia A and hemophilia B is based on the insufficient generation of thrombin by the factor IXa/factor VIIIa complex through the intrinsic pathway of the coagulation cascade. Formation of the tissue factor/factor VIIa complex is the initiating event in mammalian hemostasis and is triggered immediately after vascular injury, when factor VII in plasma interacts with tissue factor in the membranes of cells that are extrinsic to the vasculature. The fact that factor IX, not factor X, is the preferred substrate for the tissue factor/factor VIIa complex indicates that the intrinsic and extrinsic pathways of blood coagulation are not as distinct as initially proposed in the "waterfall" or "cascade" models of the 1960's.[9–14] A scant amount of thrombin is generated, enough to activate platelets and to cleave factor VIII from its pro-cofactor form to yield its active cofactor form (see Chapter 123). In turn, the factor IXa/VIIIa "tenase" complex assembles on membrane surfaces to activate factor X. Deficiencies of either factor VIII or IX lead to ineffective hemostasis due to inadequate thrombin generation.

EPIDEMIOLOGY

Accurate estimates of the incidence and prevalence of hemophilia depend on the reliable diagnosis and differentiation of hemophilia A and B from von Willebrand disease and other, less common congenital bleeding disorders. Hemophilia A and hemophilia B are clinically identical and must be distinguished from von Willebrand disease, which is due to decreased von Willebrand factor (vWF) activity.[15] Hemophilia A is four to six times more common than hemophilia B,[16–31] and mutations that cause hemophilia occur throughout the genes for factor VIII[32] and factor IX.[33] Based on worldwide surveys of patients with hemophilia, the annual incidence of hemophilia A has been estimated at approximately 1 : 5000 male births (Table 125–1).[16–28,31,34] The incidence of hemophilia B is estimated at approximately 1 : 30,000 male births.[30]

The prevalence of hemophilia indicates the number of patients alive with the disease at a given point in time. Hemophilia A and hemophilia B are observed in all ethnic and racial groups. Although some studies suggest a lower prevalence in the Chinese population and a higher prevalence among Caucasians,[35,36] the demographics of hemophilia mirror the general population (Table 125–2).[37]

The prevalence of hemophilia varies with age. The peak prevalence occurs in the second or third decade of life,[16–28] likely due to underdiagnosis or delayed diagnosis of mild hemophilia in young individuals[38,39] and excess mortality in older individuals with severe disease. As the overall fitness of patients with hemophilia improves with advances in therapy[40] and as the rate of detection of mild cases increases, a corresponding overall increase in both the true and the observed prevalence of hemophilia is likely.[41] In the developing world, the diagnostic rate is much lower, even that for severe disease.[31] The epidemic of acquired immunodeficiency syndrome (AIDS), although devastating to infected persons, has been predicted to have a transitory and relatively modest effect on the future prevalence of hemophilia.[36,42,43] Carrier testing and prenatal diagnosis (see box on Carrier Detection and Prenatal Diagnosis in Hemophilia) have not had a great impact on the incidence of hemophilia, because a substantial number of cases are the result of unanticipated new mutations. Furthermore, not all known female carriers undergo prenatal diagnostic testing, and most pregnant carriers diagnosed with a hemophilic fetus do not opt for pregnancy termination.[22,23,28,44,45]

The hemophilias are more common than autosomal recessive bleeding disorders because disease manifests in the first male to inherit a defective factor VIII or factor IX allele, unlike recessive diseases, which require inheritance of two defective alleles and may have an incidence of 1 : 500,000 to 1 : 2,000,000.[46] Consanguinity is not a typical feature of families in which hemophilia occurs, in contrast with autosomal recessive bleeding disorders.[46] Hemophilic females are exceedingly rare because the 50% factor levels typical of carriers protect against bleeding so that most carriers are asymptomatic. However, among hemophilic females doubly heterozygous for the disease who inherit the affected gene from a carrier mother and an affected father, postpartum bleeding is common.[47] Some female carriers may be affected as a result of unequal inactivation (lyonization) of factor VIII or factor IX alleles, hemizygosity for all or part of the X chromosome, or other mechanisms.

Three degrees of clinical severity correspond to the level of plasma coagulant factor activity. Persons with factor VIII or factor IX levels less than 1% of normal have severe hemophilia characterized by frequent spontaneous bleeding into joints and soft tissues as well as prolonged bleeding with trauma or surgery. Patients with 1% to 5% of normal levels have a moderate course characterized by occasional spontaneous bleeding and excessive bleeding with surgery or trauma. Levels greater than 5% of normal seem to protect against spontaneous bleeding, although excessive bleeding with surgery or trauma occurs.

Table 125–1 Prevalence, Incidence, and Severity of Hemophilia in Various Countries

	Hemophilia A			Hemophilia B		
Population	***Prevalence (per 100,000 Males)***	***Annual Incidence (per 10,000 Males)***	***Severe Disease (% of Cases)***	***Prevalence (per 100,000 Males)***	***Annual Incidence (per 10,000 Males)***	***Severe Disease (% of Cases)***
United States	20.6	—	60%	5.3	—	44%
Sweden	10.7–11.1	1.4	30%–40%	2.6–3.2	0.3	28%–32%
Greece	10.7–12	1.9	38%–58%	1.6–2.0	0.4	52%–60%
Spain	5.7	—	—	0.9	—	—
United Kingdom[a]	9.5–15.7	—	44%–61%	1.0–2.8	0.4	52%–60%
Finland	5.4	0.7	63%	3.2	—	19%
Netherlands[b]	14.5	—	(40%)	2.6	—	(40%)
Italy[a]	8.2	—	65%	1.5	—	70%
Canada	11.6	—	34%	2.7	—	24%
Japan	6.5	—	—	1.4	—	—
India[c]	2.4	—	45%	0.6	—	—

[a]Severe disease is defined as coagulant factor activity levels <1% of normal, except in the United Kingdom and Italy, where severe disease includes coagulant factor activity levels <2% of normal.
[b]Percent severe disease reported for the Netherlands is the overall average for hemophilia A and B combined.
[c]Figures for India do not reflect an estimated 43% underreporting of cases.
Data from references 16–28, 31, 34.

Table 125–2 Prevalence of Hemophilia in Various Racial Groups in the United States[a]

Combined Prevalence of Hemophilia A and B in Various Racial Groups

Racial Group	Prevalence (Cases/100,000 Males)
White	13.4
African American	12.3
Hispanic American	11.4

Racial Distribution of Patients with Hemophilia A and B

Group	Hemophilia A	Hemophilia B
White	71.7%	69.6%
African American	12.6%	17.2%
Hispanic American	7.8%	4.7%
Other/unknown	7.9%	8.4%

[a]The prevalence for each group is derived by dividing the number of cases of hemophilia A and B by the total number of males in a six-state region (Colorado, Georgia, Louisiana, Massachusetts, New York, and Oklahoma) from 1993 to 1994. The distribution of hemophilia A and B in various groups is derived from the number of cases of hemophilia A or B in each group divided by the total number of cases of hemophilia A and B.
Data from Soucie JM, Evatt B, Jackson D: Occurrence of hemophilia in the United States. The Hemophilia Surveillance System Project Investigators. Am J Hematol 59:288–294, 1998.

In patients with severe or moderate disease, the disorder is readily diagnosed because of spontaneous bleeding and joint disease, but mild hemophilia is substantially underdiagnosed. The proportion of hemophilia A patients with severe disease differs among series, ranging from 30% to 80% of cases, with 60% in the largest series (see Table 125–1). The proportion of cases that are severe is lower in hemophilia B, ranging from 20% to 45%.[16–28] Hemophilia treatment/referral centers may be more likely to diagnose mild and moderate disease that might otherwise be missed in a community hospital where subtle bleeding abnormalities cannot be analyzed with sophisticated laboratory testing.

GENETIC ASPECTS

Hemophilia A demonstrates sex-linked inheritance, by virtue of the location of the factor VIII gene on the long arm of the X chromosome (Xq28).[48] The factor IX gene also is located on the long arm of the X chromosome, at Xq27.[49] Accordingly, males bearing a defective allele on their single X chromosome are affected with hemophilia, the severity of which is determined by the particular mutation. Hemophilic males do not transmit the gene to their sons except under extraordinary circumstances,[50] but all of their daughters are obligate carriers for hemophilia. The diagnosis of mild hemophilia may be significantly delayed in females, even in those with a family bleeding history.[38] Although female carriers usually are not affected, they can become symptomatic with hemophilia via a number of mechanisms.[51]

Carriers with a defective allele on one X chromosome and a normal allele on the other X chromosome may undergo X chromosome inactivation, or *lyonization* (described by Mary Lyon), which results in unequal inactivation of alleles so that the defective (hemophilic) allele is expressed in preference to the normal allele. The lyonization process may be the result of random X-chromosome inactivation[52–54] or may be nonrandom in some cases (i.e., a distinct tendency for inactivation of the normal X allele is seen in all females from the same kindred).[55] Females who have hemophilia due to this process are said to be *lyonized carriers.* The phenotype in the lyonized carrier is no more severe than in the hemophilic male in such families, because any expression from the normal allele in such carriers will ameliorate the hemophilia phenotype. Accordingly, symptomatic lyonized carriers are seen only in hemophilic kindreds in which the male phenotype is symptomatic.

Other mechanisms for female hemophilia include homozygosity for the defective factor VIII allele and hemizygosity for the defective gene. Homozygosity may occur as the result of mating between a hemophilic male and a female carrier. This mechanism may be inferred if multiple hemophilic sons are born to a hemophilic woman, which has been confirmed in one case through detailed genetic analysis of the kindred.[56] Hemizygosity for the X chromosome may occur in females who have the 45,XO (Turner syndrome) karyotype limited to cells that synthesize factor VIII or

Carrier Detection and Prenatal Diagnosis in Hemophilia

Carrier testing and prenatal diagnosis can be offered to women who are related to obligate carrier females or males with hemophilia and who are interested in childbearing. It also may be important to other members of the family to ascertain the mechanism of mutation of the factor VIII or factor IX genes. For instance, germline mutation in a maternal grandfather has different implications for maternal aunts of a patient with hemophilia than does germline mutation in the mother of the patient. This analysis is especially pertinent in de novo cases of hemophilia.

Prenatal diagnosis may be useful even when pregnancy termination is not acceptable based on moral or ethical grounds. For instance, a prenatal diagnosis of hemophilia may be an indication for cesarean section and perinatal factor replacement and may allow more time for psychological preparation of the parents before delivery. Conversely, ruling out hemophilia as soon as possible is advantageous to parents of a normal child.

Accuracy rates greater than 90% for carrier detection and 95% for prenatal diagnosis have been achieved in laboratories having special expertise in blood coagulation testing using assays for factor VIII, factor IX, and von Willebrand factor. Sampling of fetal blood for factor activity cannot be performed before approximately 16 weeks of gestation, however, and procoagulant proteins in amniotic fluid may give spurious coagulant activity on coagulation factor assays. Furthermore, maternal factor IX (but not factor VIII) is found in amniotic fluid, which may contaminate fetal blood samples, making prenatal diagnosis of hemophilia B more difficult than diagnosis of hemophilia A. Phenotypic diagnosis of carriers may be misleading in females with extreme inactivation of the X chromosome with the abnormal factor VIII or factor IX allele. Analysis of factor VIII levels in potential carriers must take into account the age of the woman as well as ABO blood type, which affects the normal range of factor VIII and von Willebrand factor levels. Despite these limitations, phenotypic analysis still is useful as an adjunct to genotypic analysis and may be the only option when key family members are not available for genetic analysis.

Genotypic analysis requires either that the specific gene defect be known or that the carrier be heterozygous for at least one DNA polymorphism within, or closely linked to, the gene in question. DNA from the affected male must be available for analysis if the genetic defect is not known in advance. Prenatal diagnosis by genotypic analysis has advantages over phenotypic analysis. Results are not affected by X inactivation, blood type, or factor levels. Because less material is needed for genetic analysis, the test can be performed during the first trimester (e.g., chorionic villus sampling at 12 weeks of gestation).

When a carrier is heterozygous for a restriction fragment length polymorphism and the DNA of the hemophilic male is available for analysis, it is possible to determine which restriction fragment length polymorphism is associated with the gene defect. Fetal DNA can be characterized for the presence of the restriction fragment length polymorphism to determine whether or not an allele associated with the defective gene has been inherited. The analysis of fetal DNA is a probabilistic venture because of a (small) chance of recombination between the marker site and the actual gene defect. Accordingly, the best markers for analysis are within the gene (and therefore less likely to be subject to recombination with the defect) or very close to the gene of interest. When the specific gene defect is known, the analysis becomes deterministic.

Polymerase chain reaction amplification of DNA and denaturing gradient gel electrophoresis analysis may facilitate rapid screening of mutations in the known coding sequence for factor VIII. However, this analysis does not account for intervening sequences, which compose the vast majority of the gene. If the known male with hemophilia A is not available for analysis or if informative polymorphisms are not observed in the carrier female, analysis of the fetal DNA for the common intron 22 inversions, responsible for almost half of all severe cases of hemophilia A, may be useful.

IX (somatic mosaicism)[51,57] or in all cells as a consequence of a germline event (Turner syndrome).[58]

One report documents a female carrier who inherited an affected factor VIII allele from her mother (an unaffected carrier) and an X isochromosome from her nonhemophilic father. In this case, expression of factor VIII from the isochromosome was defective, and the daughter displayed severe hemophilia A.[59] In another case, a structurally abnormal X chromosome deleted at the tip (Xq27) distal to a normal factor IX gene resulted in inactivation of that chromosome, and expression from the other X chromosome revealed a defective factor IX gene for which the affected female was a carrier. As a consequence, she demonstrated severe hemophilia B.[60]

Evaluation of "hemophilia" in a female should begin with testing for von Willebrand disease as well as autosomal recessive coagulation factor deficiencies associated with a bleeding phenotype. In hemophilic females, karyotyping is necessary not only to rule out Turner syndrome but also to rule out a male (46,XY) karyotype associated with testicular feminization, which has been described in hemophilia A.[61,62]

No single mutation is responsible for hemophilia, in contrast with cystic fibrosis, sickle cell anemia, and Duchenne muscular dystrophy, which are caused by either one or a limited number of mutations. Hundreds of point mutations, deletions, and inversions that cause hemophilia have been described throughout the factor VIII and factor IX genes (see Chapters 123 and 124).[30,63]

An inversion of the factor VIII gene accounts for approximately 40% of cases of severe hemophilia A. Because of the presence of a transcribed gene (*F8A*) within intron 22 of the factor VIII gene[64] and at least two nontranscribed copies of the *F8A* gene lying telomeric to the factor VIII gene, homologous recombination can occur during spermiogenesis.[65] With this mechanism, the first 22 exons of the factor VIII gene are inverted with respect to the last four exons, resulting in a defective truncated factor VIII transcript that lacks functional factor VIII. This inversion may occur with either of the extragenic copies of *F8A* and can be detected and differentiated by restriction fragment length polymorphism analysis on Southern blot preparations.[66] A similar mechanism has been described in dogs with hemophilia A but not in mice, perhaps because dogs have multiple copies of the *F8A* gene and mice have only the single copy in intron 22.[67–69] Because of the high incidence of the intron 22 inversion in patients with severe hemophilia A, testing for this rearrangement should be the first step in carrier and prenatal testing, before sequence analysis of the large factor VIII cDNA/gene. In humans, the inversion usually is the result of a recombination event during spermiogenesis in the maternal grandfather of the person who represents the index case.[70]

Careful analysis of factor IX gene mutation patterns in Caucasian,[71] Asian,[72] Hispanic,[73] and Amerindian[74] populations indicates that hemophilia B results from similar endogenous processes (e.g., deamination of CpG dinucleotides) rather than from environmental mutagens. Although no single common gene defect causes hemophilia B, haplotype analysis indicates that point mutations derived from three "founder" patients account for approximately 25% of all cases of hemophilia B in North America.[75]

ETIOLOGY AND PATHOGENESIS

The hallmark of hemophilia is bleeding into joints (hemarthrosis), which is painful and leads to chronic inflammation and joint destruction similar to those seen in rheumatoid arthritis. Abnormal bleeding originates from the subsynovial venous plexus underlying the joint capsule, where a lack of thromboplastic activity has been demonstrated.[76] The high degree of factor Xa inhibitory activity conveyed by the tissue factor pathway inhibitor synthesized by human synovial cells also may predispose hemophilic joints to bleeding,[77] which may explain the impressive hemostatic response after intravenous administration of recombinant factor VIIa for acute hemarthroses in patients with factor VIII inhibitors.[78,79]

Untreated, inadequately treated, or recurrent joint bleeds result in chronic synovial and intraarticular pathology produced by the toxic effects of hemosiderin and release of proteolytic enzymes (e.g., elastase, collagenase) from the cellular blood components. As synovial iron from recurrent bleeding accumulates, the c-*myc* and *mdm*-2 oncogenes are induced, resulting in synovial cell proliferation.[80,81] Synovial hypertrophy, hemosiderin deposition, fibrosis, and damage to cartilage progress until subchondral bone cyst formation becomes apparent radiographically. Abnormal mechanical forces of weight bearing on these joints exacerbate the damage, which ultimately results in permanent deformities with subluxation, misalignment, loss of mobility, occasional ankylosis, and unequal extremity lengths. Once hemophilic arthropathy compromises one joint, destruction may be precipitated in another joint as a result of unusual and increased stresses placed on it to compensate for the dysfunction of the damaged joint.

Radiologically and clinically, hemophilic arthropathy evolves through five stages (Fig. 125–1). Stage 1 consists of intraarticular and periarticular swelling due to acute bleeding. The joint structure appears normal. Stage 2 is associated with loss of bone density around the joint and epiphyseal hypertrophy secondary to chronic synovial inflammation. Stage 3 is characterized by progression of the epiphyseal hypertrophy with widening of the intercondylar notch. The articular cartilage surfaces are not affected until stage 4, when secondary joint space narrowing becomes apparent. Stage 5 is characterized by advanced cartilage erosion, loss of joint space, joint fusion, and development of fibrosis of the joint capsule.

Because radiographic and clinical examinations frequently underestimate the extent of joint disease, new approaches to evaluation are being introduced.[82] Magnetic resonance imaging (MRI)[83,84] permits better discrimination of changes in the cartilage, synovium, and joint space and earlier detection of synovial hypertrophy than possible by physical examination or radiography (Fig. 125–2).

CLINICAL PRESENTATION

The clinical presentations of patients with hemophilia A and with hemophilia B are indistinguishable. Hemophilia, especially severe disease with less than 1% of normal factor activity, is readily diagnosed, especially in patients with a family history of hemophilia. The diagnosis of hemophilia usually is made on the basis of unusual bleeding symptoms early in life, and the age at first bleeding episode varies with the severity of disease. Infants with severe disease typically present with their first bleeding between 12 and 18 months (despite undetectable factor VIII or factor IX activity). The first manifestations of disease in mild hemophilia may be seen at age 2 to 5 years.[14,39,85] Severe hemophilia most often manifests as easy bruising. Mild to moderate disease more often is associated with bleeding after trauma or dental procedures.[14] Spontaneous hemarthroses occur in individuals with severe disease but are rare before age 9 months, when weight bearing and walking begin.[14]

Coinheritance of "prothrombotic" genes such as factor V Leiden or prothrombin A20210 may mitigate the severity of bleeding, if not arthropathy, in patients with severe hemophilia A.[86,87] These mutations or protein C deficiency may delay the onset of clinically significant bleeding associated with severe hemophilia A[88] or render a more moderate phenotype, as demonstrated in a hemophilia mouse model heterozygous or homozygous for factor V Leiden.[89] In contrast, the occurrence of combined coagulation factor deficiencies (e.g., type 1 von Willebrand disease with hemophilia) may render the phenotype more severe.[90]

That the trauma of childbirth does not cause intracranial hemorrhage more often than it does is remarkable, although some infants may be born with hemophilia A as a result of de novo mutation and die of intracranial hemorrhage at birth undiagnosed. A study of the modes of delivery and prenatal complications in 117 moderately or severely affected infants (those with hemophilia A and B) shows that the risk of serious bleeding in conjunction with normal vaginal delivery is small (<3.8%).[91–93] Vacuum extraction is a major risk factor for subgaleal or cephalic hematomas, and cesarean section does not eliminate the risk of intracranial hemorrhage. In addition, forceps deliveries and prolonged labor increase the risk of intracranial bleeds (Fig. 125–3).[94] Use of fetal scalp electrodes and fetal blood sampling for intrapartum monitoring of affected neonates does not appear to cause bleeding complications.[95]

It is often assumed that excessive bleeding with circumcision is usual for hemophilic infants. In fact, such bleeding occurs in less than half of severely affected infants after circumcision.[85] Of note, those who bleed are circumcised several days later than those who do not bleed. Thus, failure to bleed excessively with circumcision does not rule out hemophilia.

Although the individual with severe hemophilia may bleed from any anatomic site after negligible or unnoticed trauma, intraarticular and intramuscular bleeds are the most common clinical symptoms of severe and moderate hemophilia, yet they rarely occur before the child begins to ambulate. In fact, the most common *presenting* manifestations of hemophilia A and B in one series of patients were soft-tissue bleeds in 41%, bleeding associated with intramuscular injections and surgery in 16%, and oral bleeding from tongue or lip biting in 11%,[96] 14% of which were severe enough to require transfusion of packed red blood cells.

Soft-tissue hemorrhages advance along tissue planes, and blood loss may be extensive and even life threatening because the bleeding is not confined to a closed space (e.g., the joint capsule) as in hemarthrosis. Intracranial hemorrhage was the leading cause of death before the AIDS epidemic and remains the most common hemorrhagic cause of death. Hematuria and gastrointestinal tract bleeding are common. Retroperitoneal bleeding (Fig. 125–4), although uncommon, may occur spontaneously, with extension downward along the psoas muscle through the inguinal canal into the thigh or dissection upward along the vertebral muscles even as far as the neck.

Isolated hemorrhage into a closed space such as the forearm may lead to a compartment syndrome, which is characterized by severe pain with compromise of nerve function and blood flow. Without factor replacement and surgical decompression, compartment hemorrhage may lead to permanent neuropathy, tissue necrosis, or even loss of limb. Compartment syndromes of the forearm may be caused even by venipuncture at the antecubital fossa, and patients should be alert for this uncommon but devastating complication of phlebotomy.

The extreme examples of soft-tissue hemorrhage, which are common in severe hemophilia A, are less common in moderate or mild disease. Moderate or mild disease may not be detected until adulthood (e.g., during dental extraction), when unexplained bleeding, such asa hematoma initially regarded as a recurrent "pulled muscle," prompts evaluation. Routine preoperative laboratory tests may reveal a prolonged activated partial thromboplastin time (aPTT) that triggers further testing, leading to a diagnosis of hemophilia. Some patients with mild disease serve in the military or engage in other hazardous pursuits, only to have hemophilia diagnosed later in life.

Intraarticular bleeding becomes problematic usually between the ages of 2 and 3 years. It occurs most prominently in the knees, followed by the elbows and ankles. Bleeding into the shoulders, hips, and wrists is less common, although trauma may precipitate bleeding in any joint. Bilateral involvement may occur but is uncommon.[97]

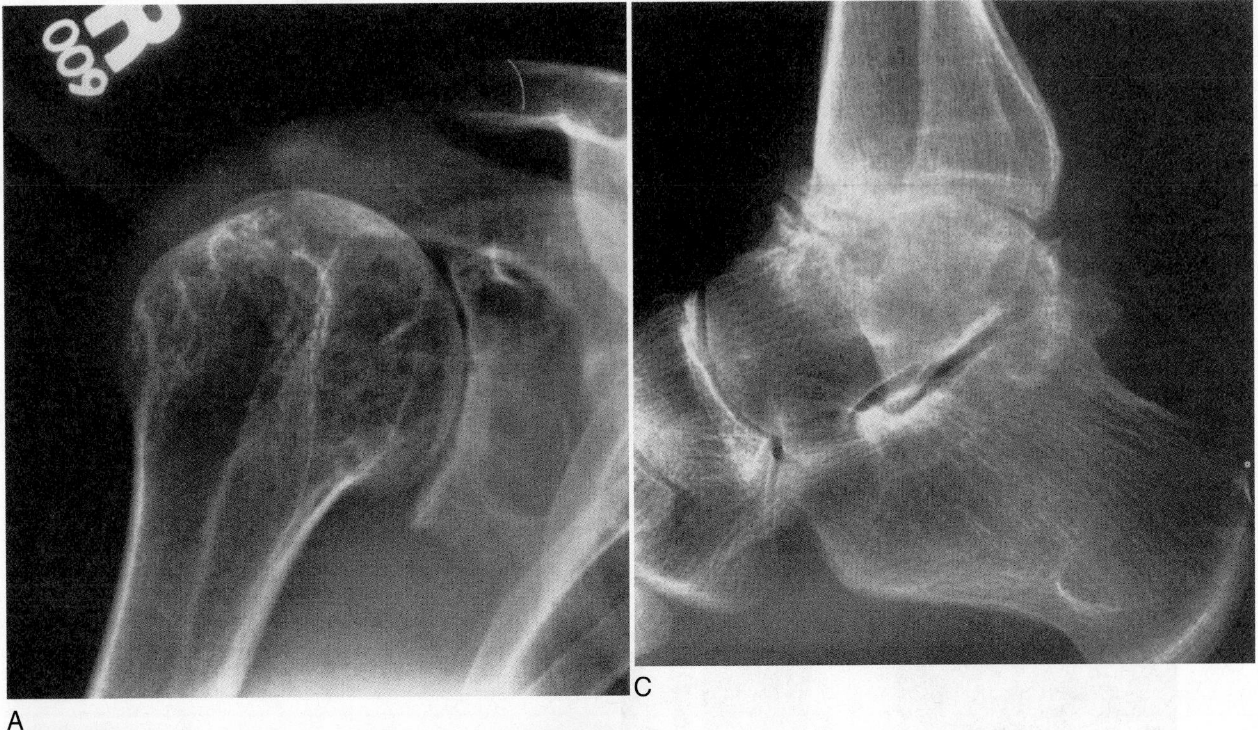

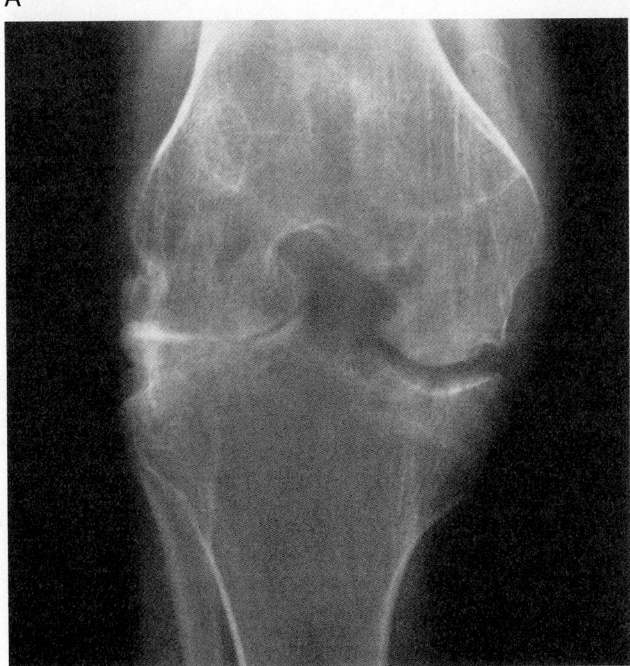

Figure 125–1 Radiographic changes associated with hemophilic arthropathy. **A,** Radiograph of the shoulder showing multiple subchondral cysts in the head of the humerus, an early finding in hemophilic arthropathy. The glenohumeral joint space is fairly well preserved, and range of motion is normal. **B,** Widening of the intercondylar notch and near fusion of the femur and medial tibial condyle in the knee joint affected by hemophilic arthropathy. **C,** Narrowing and fusion of the tibiotalar joint in the ankle.

In acute hemarthroses, a tingling or burning sensation often precedes the onset of intense pain and swelling. Joint mobility is compromised by pain and stiffness, and the joint is maintained in a flexed position. In most cases, replacement of the deficient clotting factor gradually reverses the pain, and once the bloody joint effusion resorbs, joint range of motion and function are regained.

Chronic hemophilic arthropathy often is painful with weight bearing and normal use, but frequently the pain is related to the arthritic changes in the joint. Pain may disappear or subside once the joint becomes ankylosed. Muscle atrophy around the joints may lead to further instability, loss of use, valgus deformities, and increased bleeding due to loss of cushioning around the joint and uncoordinated function among muscle groups. Individuals with factor VIII and factor IX levels greater than 20% of normal rarely develop hemophilic arthropathy, even if they had experienced previous bleeds, as reported in 6% to 20%.[98]

Socioeconomic and other health issues may affect the severity and degree of disability associated with hemophilic joint disease. Obesity, which is not uncommon in individuals with hemophilia, significantly worsens joint range of motion.[99] Whether higher body mass index in hemophilic men occurs because of immobilization, sedentary lifestyles, or inability to work due to recurrent bleeds is a major focus of current hemophilia care. In addition, the place of care may influence outcomes: those who receive care outside a hemophilia treatment center have significantly lower quality of life and shorter lifespans than those who receive care from experienced, knowledgeable staff at a hemophilia center.[40]

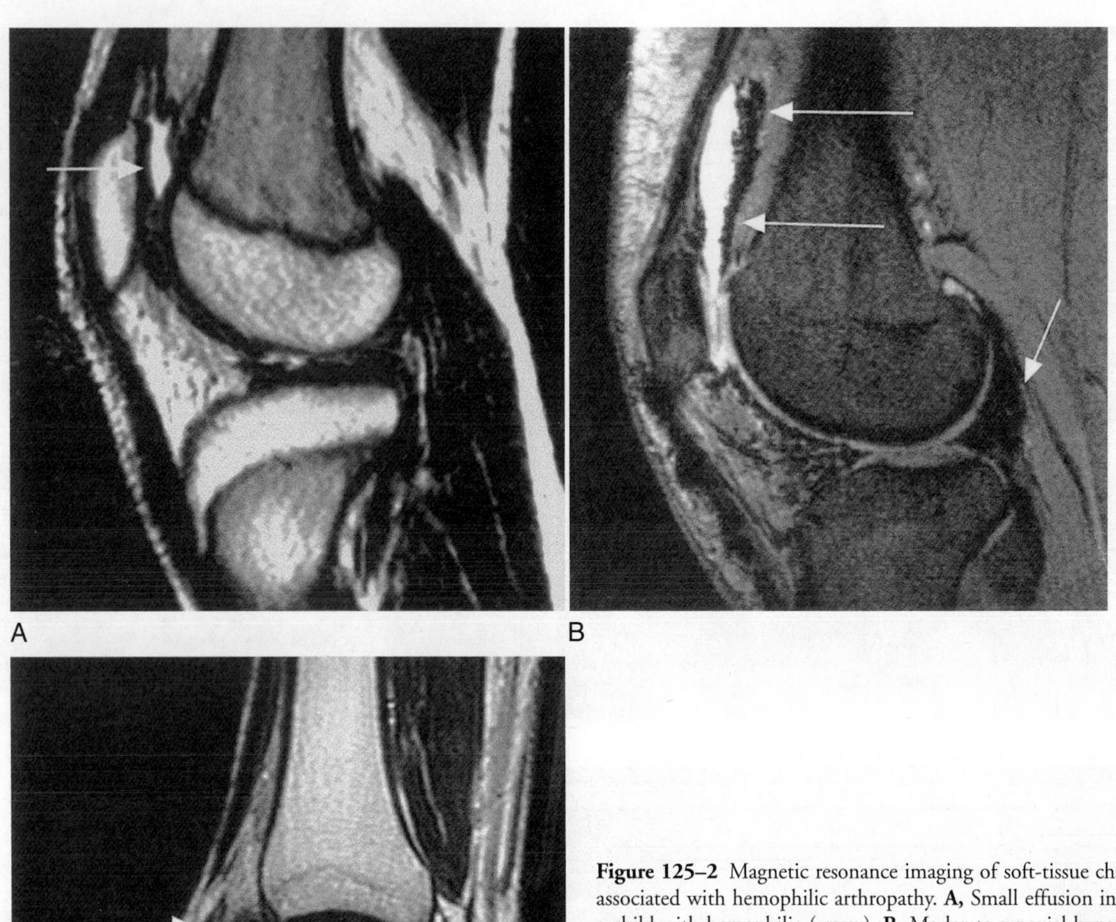

Figure 125–2 Magnetic resonance imaging of soft-tissue changes associated with hemophilic arthropathy. **A,** Small effusion in the knee of a child with hemophilia (arrow). **B,** Moderate synovial hyperplasia in the knee of an adult with hemophilia (arrows). **C,** Small effusion in the ankle of an adult with hemophilia (arrow). (From Nuss R, Kilcoyne RE [eds.]: The MRI Atlas of Hemophilic Arthropathy. New York, Professional Publishing Group, 2002.)

LABORATORY EVALUATION

The severity, frequency, and location of bleeding in patients with hemophilia are determined by the plasma concentration of factor VIII or factor IX. Typically, the same degree of severity exists within families, and little fluctuation of coagulation factor levels occurs within an individual over time. Exceptions include Heckathorn syndrome,[100] in which factor VIII levels vary within affected family members; moderate or mild hemophilia A, in which factor VIII levels vary as acute-phase reactants with exercise and inflammation; and the unusual hemophilia B variant factor IX Leyden,[101] in which reduced factor IX levels progressively rise after puberty, eventually approaching the normal range (3%–4% increase per year through adolescence). This rise has been attributed to the effects of androgenic steroids on the mutated promoter region of the factor IX gene in affected patients.[102,103]

Factor VIII and factor IX levels are assayed against a normal pooled plasma standard, which is designated as 100% activity, equivalent to that of 1 U/mL of factor VIII or factor IX. The normal range of factor VIII and factor IX levels varies between 50% and 150%, although increases in either factor are associated with pregnancy and aging. Use of estrogen-containing contraceptives and replacement therapies produce substantially higher rises in factor VIII than in factor IX. In the normal healthy premature and term neonate, factor IX (but not factor VIII) levels typically are 20% to 50% of normal and rise to nearly normal adult levels within 6 months. This situation is attributed to hepatic immaturity at birth. In congenital factor VIII or factor IX deficiencies, persons with undetectable activity (<0.01 U/mL) will experience the most severe and frequent spontaneous bleeding complications, whereas those with higher levels will manifest moderate (with 2%–5% of normal activity) or mild (>5% of normal activity) symptomatology.

The whole blood clotting time, results of the prothrombin consumption test, and aPTT are abnormal in hemophilia A and B because of intrinsic pathway coagulation protein deficiencies. Various other laboratory techniques are available for specific determination of factor VIII and factor IX activities. The one-stage assay based on aPTT is most commonly used because of its reproducibility, simplicity, and low cost. In Europe, use of a chromogenic assay is advocated for determination of factor VIII levels and has been

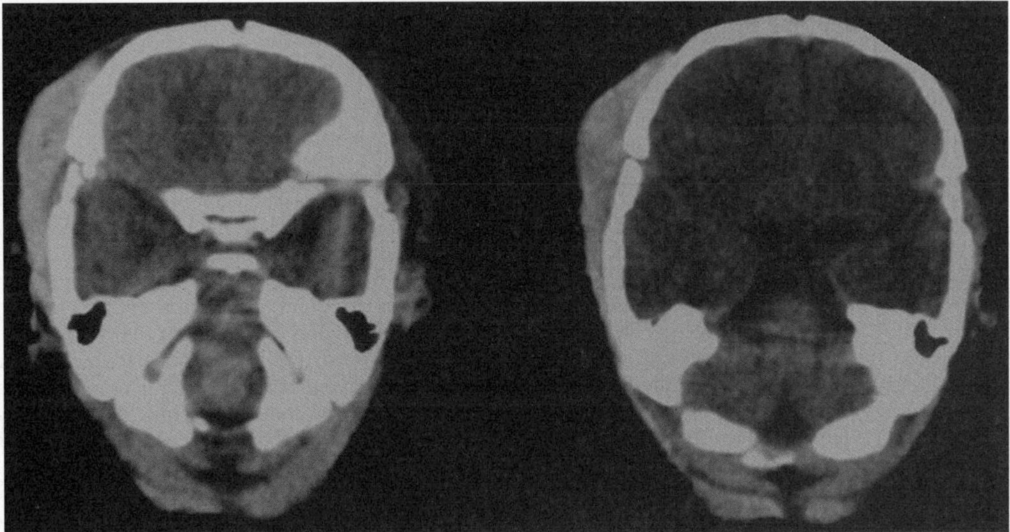

Figure 125–3 Subgaleal bleed in 2-day old male infant with severe hemophilia A. Computed tomographic scan shows a large right subgaleal hematoma. The infant was born by spontaneous vaginal delivery, without assistance of forceps or vacuum, with Apgar scores of 8 and 10. The presentation was breech, and delivery was difficult. He developed edema of the right eye and right face and hemoglobin 6.4 gm% in the first day of life. He received two units of blood and factor VIII concentrate. At age 4 months he developed an inhibitor, anti-factor VIII 50 Bethesda units, as had two older affected siblings before him.

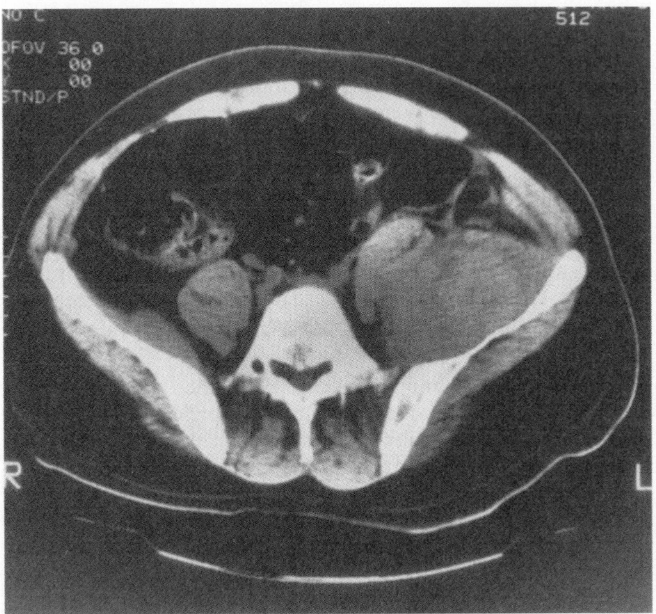

Figure 125–4 Retroperitoneal hemorrhage involving the iliopsoas muscle of the left iliac fossa in a patient with hemophilia A and a high-titer inhibitor.

adopted by the European Pharmacopoeia and the International Society on Thrombosis and Haemostasis,[104] but this assay is much less commonly used in the United States. Factor VIII assays performed by chromogenic techniques and by the aPTT method in patients receiving recombinant factor VIII concentrates (particularly B domain-deleted products) give consistently different results. Values determined by the chromogenic substrate method are approximately twice as high as those determined by the one-stage aPTT method.[104,105] The laboratory discrepancy is based on the relative amount of phospholipid in the activating reagent for the one-stage assay compared with the chromogenic assay, as well as modifications to the activation time in the chromogenic assay as performed in some laboratories.

The wide variety of aPTT reagents, standards, assay methods, and laboratories used to perform current one-stage and chromogenic assays[106] complicates both the pharmacokinetics and dosing of factor concentrates. For these reasons, use of product-specific standards in place of plasma standards has been recommended, with better agreement on product recoveries, for example, with B-domain–deleted factor VIII, which differs in structure and half-life from full-length factor VIII.[107] Adopting product standards for such assays may improve patient care by providing more accurate factor levels and avoiding breakthrough bleeds.[108] An alternate assay, the thrombin generation assay, measures peak thrombin generation, total thrombin generated, and $t_{1/2}$ max (time to half maximum) thrombin generation.[109,110] Because the thrombin generation assay provides absolute values and requires no standards, it may provide more accurate postinfusion values as well as better detection of low factor levels.[110] Preliminary data from study of a more global assay that incorporates clot formation and fibrinolysis may provide better risk assessment than provided by standard clotting time assays.[111]

Hemophilia A usually can be differentiated from von Willebrand disease in the laboratory by the presence of normal or increased vWF antigen and ristocetin cofactor activity.[112] Of note, the rare von Willebrand 2N variant, in which the vWF protein does not bind factor VIII, may be phenotypically identical to severe hemophilia A except for its autosomally transmitted inheritance pattern.[113,114] Specialized assays for measuring the factor VIII-vWF protein-binding characteristics and genetic testing for the specific point mutations involved are necessary to diagnose this entity. Bleeding times or closure times, which are prolonged in von Willebrand disease, are normal in persons with hemophilia. However, prolonged bleeding times have been documented in patients with hemophilia A and B in the absence of abnormal platelet aggregation assays or following the surreptitious use of aspirin or nonsteroidal antiinflammatory drugs (NSAIDs) in several series of patients.[115,116] Although there is no obvious explanation for this phenomenon, bleeding times tend to be more prolonged when the Simplate device is used and correlate with severity of bleeding events, platelet IgG levels, circulating immune complexes, and vascular injury. The effects of concurrent hepatitis or human immunodeficiency virus (HIV) infection have not been evaluated.

Most individuals with severe factor VIII or factor IX deficiency (<1% activity) have undetectable levels of the corresponding factor antigen when assayed against a specific antibody: they are designated cross-reactive material-negative [CRM(−)]. In contrast, moderately and mildly affected patients may have normal or slightly reduced levels of antigen [CRM(+)].[117] The clinical significance of CRM(−) versus CRM(+) status remains unclear; however, it has been conjectured that CRM(−) persons are more likely than those who are CRM(+) to develop alloantibodies directed against their specific clotting protein defect.[118] A special subset of CRM(+) hemophilia B, hemophilia B_M, is associated with an abnormal factor IX protein that prolongs the prothrombin time when an ox or bovine (rather than human) brain source of thromboplastin is used. This product of point mutations in the factor IX gene possesses decreased coagulation function and acts as a competitive inhibitor of factor VIIa.[119,120]

Although the presence of an inhibitor to factor VIII or factor IX is clinically suspected when a bleeding episode fails to respond to an adequate dose of factor concentrate, laboratory confirmation is critical to the diagnosis and subsequent treatment strategy. For alloantibody inhibitors (associated with congenital defect) or autoantibody inhibitors (associated with previously normal coagulation), if the initial aPTT is prolonged, aPTT determination should be repeated after incubation of the patient's plasma with normal plasma at 37°C for 1 to 2 hours. If the prolonged aPTT does not correct, the presence of an inhibitor should be evaluated through specific clotting factor assays performed in multiple dilutions and subsequently quantified according to the Bethesda method (see Chapter 126). The clotting factor against which the inhibitor is directed will remain persistently and equally deficient at all dilutions, whereas the apparent activity of other factors will increase as the inhibitor is diluted out.[121,122] Increasing dilutions of the patient's plasma are incubated with an equal volume of normal plasma (standardized to contain 1 U/mL) for 2 hours at 37°C until a residual factor activity level falls within 25% to 75% of the control mixture of normal plasma and buffer. A standard curve is estab-lished, which defines 1 Bethesda unit (BU) as a measure of the inhibitor potency that results in 50% neutralization of factor VIII or factor IX activity in the pooled normal plasma.[123] The Nijmegen modification of the Bethesda method, which eliminates the pH-dependent variation of factor VIII activity in the incubation mixtures of the Bethesda assay and uses immunodepleted factor VIII-deficient plasma, increases the specificity of the assay in the very low range of factor VIII antibody inhibitor titers. This assay usually is reserved for research protocols because titers of the clinically relevant inhibitors typically are greater than 5 to 10 BU.[124] By convention, a titer greater than 0.6 BU is considered positive for the presence of an inhibitor. Inhibitors present at less than 5 BU are termed low-titer inhibitors and usually are not associated with anamnestic responses when sources of the specific clotting factor protein are administered. Inhibitors present at greater than 10 BU are defined as high-titer inhibitors and often are associated with anamnestic responses. The most sensitive means for detecting an inhibitor antibody is measurement of a decrease in the recovery and half-life of factor VIII in vivo.

DIFFERENTIAL DIAGNOSIS

Considerations in the differential diagnosis of hemophilia include congenital bleeding disorders such as von Willebrand disease, platelet disorders (e.g., Glanzmann thrombasthenia), and deficiency of various other coagulation factors such as factor V, VII, X, or XI or fibrinogen.[44] In addition are autoimmune syndromes in which antibodies to factor VIII may spontaneously develop, leading to "acquired hemophilia."[125]

The diagnosis of hemophilia is made on the basis of family history, bleeding symptoms, and findings on physical examination and laboratory evaluation. The hallmarks of severe hemophilia include prolonged bleeding with surgical procedures, trauma, or dental extraction, as well as hemarthroses and spontaneous bleeding into soft tissues. The last of these conditions distinguishes severe hemophilia A from von Willebrand disease and platelet disorders, in which soft-tissue hemorrhage and hemarthropathy are uncommon (except in severe, type 3 von Willebrand disease). In addition, a family history indicating autosomal dominant transmission is characteristic of von Willebrand disease rather than hemophilia, which has a sex-linked recessive pattern of inheritance. Family history may be unrevealing in de novo presentations of hemophilia.

Severe hemophilia A is not clinically distinguishable from severe hemophilia B by either historical features (bleeding symptoms) or findings on physical examination; the two must be distinguished by specific assays for factor VIII and factor IX. Accurate diagnosis of hemophilia A and hemophilia B is critical for appropriate clinical management. Autosomally inherited disorders of coagulation factors V, VII, X, and XI and fibrinogen also must be diagnosed by specific coagulation factor assays.[46]

Mild hemophilia A may be difficult to distinguish from von Willebrand disease because factor VIII levels tend to be depressed in the latter, and prolongation of the bleeding time (characteristic of von Willebrand disease but not hemophilia) is not reliably present. Specific assays for vWF and analysis of the vWF multimeric pattern by gel electrophoresis may distinguish the two disorders. Repeat testing is sometimes required to make a definitive diagnosis in the case of von Willebrand disease, especially mild (type 1) forms of the disease (see Chapters 128 and 129).

TREATMENT

Factor Replacement Therapy

The key to treatment of bleeding in hemophilia is replacement of the missing coagulation protein to achieve hemostasis. The dose and choice of product are influenced by the severity of disease, the site and severity of the bleeding, and the clinical scenario. The patient's weight, inhibitor antibody status, and treatment history (especially with respect to exposure to bloodborne pathogens) also are important. The annual cost of factor replacement therapy for an adult receiving weekly treatments may range from $20,000 to $100,000, and the cost for patients with inhibitors may be greater, particularly for those undergoing immune tolerance induction protocols. Therefore, patients are best managed in a comprehensive hemophilia center, where multispecialty expertise and ancillary support services for diagnosis, therapy, and management are in place. The comprehensive hemophilia center also serves as a resource for patients with related bleeding disorders such as von Willebrand disease. Replacement therapy involves educating the patient and his or her family in self-infusion techniques, the cornerstone of home-based treatment.

Guidelines for replacement therapy have been determined empirically over many years; however, the minimal doses of clotting factor replacement for adequate hemostasis have not been established (Tables 125–3, 125–4, 125–5, and 125–6). Typically, hemostasis for minor bleeding can be achieved at plasma factor levels of 25% to 30% of normal (0.25–0.30 U/mL), whereas severe bleeding requires at least 50% of normal activity. Surgical procedures and life-threatening bleeding require targets of 75% to 100% of normal activity. For factor VIII replacement, each unit of factor VIII per kilogram of body weight is assumed to raise the plasma level by 2% (0.02 U/mL). Thus, injection of 1750 U of factor VIII will provide for an incremental rise of 50% (0.5 U/mL) of normal (1750 U/70 kg × 0.02 U/mL), which then declines according to the pharmacokinetics associated with factor VIII. This calculation estimates the peak level, and in critical bleeding situations common practice involves doubling the initial dose to ensure that the trough level after one half-life exceeds the desired value. Because factor VIII has a half-life of 8 to 12 hours, repeat dosing at least two or three times daily is required to maintain the desired factor VIII level. One half of the initial dose is given every half-life (i.e., every 8–12 hours) to maintain the desired factor VIII level.

Similar calculations can be made for dosing factor IX concentrates. Factor IX demonstrates a volume of distribution approximately twice that of factor VIII because of equilibration with the extravascular extracellular fluid compartment (in which factor VIII does not exchange) and a half-life of approximately 24 hours. One unit of factor IX administered per kilogram of body weight results in a 1% (0.01 U/mL) increment in the circulating factor IX level in plasma. Thus, 3500 U of factor IX provides an incremental rise of 50% of normal (0.5 U/mL; 3500 U/70 kg × 0.01 U/mL). For low-purity, low specific activity factor IX preparations, it is best to aim for a maximum level of 50% of normal to avoid the thrombotic complications that have occurred with these preparations. This is not a problem with the highly purified, high specific activity factor IX preparations.

A recovery rate 20% lower than expected has been observed in approximately 30% of patients who receive recombinant factor IX. This finding may have implications for therapy for acute bleeding, so patients should undergo a baseline pharmacokinetic study with the factor IX preparation of choice. The initial dose is adjusted accordingly, as are subsequent maintenance doses of factor IX, which are given every 18 to 24 hours.[118] For replacement therapy for hemophilia A or B, subsequent dosing is adjusted on the basis of measured factor levels. The duration of treatment is determined by the rapidity of pain relief and recovery of range of motion of an affected joint or resolution of a hematoma. For major surgery, replacement therapy usually is continued for at least 10 to 14 days to allow for efficient wound healing and scar formation. This is consistent with data showing that impaired coagulation delays wound healing in hemophilia B mice related to greater iron deposition that is thought to induce angiogenesis in wound sites.[126] This emphasizes the importance of factor replacement in achieving early and rapid hemostasis as well as wound healing after trauma or surgery.

Intermittent bolus infusions of factor concentrates have been used successfully for treatment and prophylaxis for many years. However, pharmacokinetics may vary between products and patients, and the wide fluctuations in factor levels during therapy may make management difficult (see box on Choice of Factor Concentrate). Continuous infusion protocols have been developed, which reduce factor use, facilitate laboratory monitoring of factor levels (because laboratory values reflect a steady state rather than a peak or a trough), and decrease the overall cost of therapy. This approach has been associated with excellent hemostasis and safety and has been used with factor VIII, factor IX, porcine factor VIII, recombinant human factor VIIa, and activated prothrombin complex concentrates for therapy for patients with inhibitors. Some studies note a 30% to 75% decrease in the use of concentrate with continuous infusions administered in the surgical setting and report a progressive decrease in the plasma clearance of coagulation factors.[122,138,139] Most high-purity preparations maintain more than 80% of initial activity 3 to 7 days after reconstitution.[140] A typical continuous infusion protocol begins with a bolus designed to achieve 100% of normal levels followed by an infusion of 2 U/kg/hour. The results of factor VIII or factor IX assays obtained thereafter are used to guide changes in the infusion regimen. Typically, if the measured factor level is low, the infusion rate can be increased or a small bolus given to bring the levels up to the desired value. Addition of small amounts of heparin (1–5 U/mL of infusion

Table 125–3 Guidelines for Replacement Dosing with Factor VIII and Factor IX

	Desired Plasma Level (% of Normal)		Initial Dose (IU/kg body weight)		
Type of Lesion	***Factor VIII***	***Factor IX***	***Factor VIII***	***Factor IX***	**Duration of Therapy (Days)**
Mild (often spontaneous) hemarthrosis	30%	20%–30%	15	20–30	q8–12h over 1–2 days for factor VIII q12–24h over 1–2 days for factor IX (often only one dose required)
Superficial hematoma					
Oropharyngeal or dental					
Severe epistaxis					
Persistent hematuria					
Major central nervous system trauma or hemorrhage; lumbar puncture or epidural anesthesia	80%–100%	80%–100%	>50	50	q8–12h over at least 10–14 days for factor VIII q12h over at least 10–14 days for factor IX
Surgery					High-purity products are recommended to avoid thrombotic complications
Retroperitoneal hemorrhage					
Dental extraction with nerve block					Continuous infusion with high-purity products recommended to avoid peak and trough level fluctuations and to save on overall use of factor concentrate
Severe gastrointestinal bleeding					

Table 125–4 Factor VIII Concentrates Available in the United States

Category	Manufacturer	Method Viral Depletion/Inactivation	Specific Activity (IU/mg)
Recombinant Factor VIII Products			
Advate	Baxter	Immunoaffinity chromatography/solvent detergent (TNBP/polysorbate 80)[a]	4000–10,000
Helixate FS	ZLB Behring	Immunoaffinity chromatography/solvent detergent (TNBP/polysorbate 80)	4000
Kogenate FS	ZLB Behring	Immunoaffinity chromatography/solvent detergent (TNBP/polysorbate 80)	4000
Recombinate	Baxter	Immunoaffinity chromatography	4000
ReFacto	Wyeth	Immunoaffinity chromatography/solvent detergent (TNBP/Triton X-100)	9110–13,700[b]
Plasma-Derived Factor VIII Products			
Hemophil M	Baxter	Immunoaffinity chromatography/solvent detergent (TNBP/octoxynol 9)[a]	2–20
Monarc-M	Baxter	Immunoaffinity chromatography/solvent detergent (TNBP/octoxynol 9)[a]	2–20
Monoclate P	ZLB Behring	Immunoaffinity chromatography/pasteurization (60°C, 10 hours)	5–10
Plasma-Derived Factor VIII Products Containing von Willebrand Factor			
Alphanate	Grifols	Affinity chromatography/solvent detergent (TNBP/polysorbate 80)/dry heat (80°C, 72 hours)	8–30
Humate-P	ZLB Behring	Pasteurization (60°C, 10 hours)	1–2
Koate-DVI	Talecris	Solvent detergent (TNBP/polysorbate 80)/dry heat (80°C, 72 hours)	9–22
Porcine Factor VIII Products			
Hyate:C	Ipsen (Wales)	None	>50

[a]TNBP is tri (*n*-butyl) phosphate.
[b]Measured by ReFacto standard using chromogenic assay.

Table 125–5 Factor IX Concentrates Available in the United States

Category Manufacturer Method Viral Depletion/Inactivation	Specific Activity (IU/mg)
Recombinant Factor IX Products	
BeneFix Wyeth affinity chromatography/viral filtration	200–360
Plasma-Derived Factor IX Products	
AlphaNine SD Grifols dual-affinity chromatography/solvent detergent (TNBP/polysorbate 80)/[a] nanofiltration 229 ± 23	
Mononine ZLB Behring immunoaffinity chromatography/sodium thiocyanate/ultrafiltration	>160
Plasma-Derived Prothrombin Complex Concentrates	
Bebulin VH Baxter (Vienna) vapor heat (60°C, 10 hours, 190 mbar plus 80°C, 1 hour, 375 mbar)	2.0
Profilnne Grifols solvent/detergent (TNBP/polysorbate 80)	4.5
Proplex-T Baxter dry heat (60°C, 144 hours)	>0.8
Plasma-Derived Activated Prothrombin Complex Concentrates	
FEIBA VH Baxter (Vienna) vapor heat (60°C, 10 hours, 190 mbar plus 80°C, 1 hour, 375 mbar)	0.8

[a]TNBP is tri (*n*-butyl) phosphate.

Table 125–6 Factor VIIa Concentrates Available in the United States

Category Manufacturer Method Viral Depletion/Inactivation	Specific Activity (IU/mg)
Recombinant Factor VIIa Products	
NovoSeven Novo Nordisk affinity chromatography/viral filtration/solvent detergent (TNBP/polysorbate 80)	—

[a]TNBP is tri (*n*-butyl) phosphate.

solution) may reduce the incidence of local thrombophlebitis at the venous access site.

The pharmacokinetics of factor products are different in children than in adults: children have lower factor VIII recovery and shorter half-life.[141] Recovery appears to be highly correlated with body surface area, whereas half-life is strongly correlated with vWF levels. These findings suggest the need for pharmacokinetics studies in children to assure the adequacy of prophylaxis and the treatment regimen, especially before surgery.[141] Use of ideal weight for height, age, and gender also has been advocated to assist dosing in obese children and adults.[142]

Benefits and Risks of Use of Factor Preparations

Bloodborne Pathogens

Until the availability of recombinant factor VIII products in the late 1980s and recombinant factor IX in the late 1990s, patients with hemophilia received thousands of units of concentrates derived from plasma obtained from tens of thousands of donors. Patients who received these products prior to 1985, when viral inactivation procedures were introduced, were infected by various transfusion-transmitted infectious agents, including HIV, hepatitis A virus (HAV), hepatitis B virus (HBV), hepatitis C virus (HCV), hepatitis G virus, and parvovirus B19. Virtually all patients who received plasma-derived concentrates before 1985 have been infected with

Choice of Factor Concentrate

The choice of factor concentrate is based on safety, as there is no difference in efficacy among the preparations, whether recombinant or plasma derived. Since implementation of viral attenuation methods in the manufacture of these products, no seroconversions to HIV, HBV, or HCV with any plasma-derived product have been reported. Because there remains the possibility of transmission of HIV-1, HIV-2, hepatitis B or C virus, nonlipid-enveloped viruses, hepatitis A virus, and parvovirus B19 despite viral inactivation and viral filtration methods, recombinant factor VIII and factor IX concentrates are recommended as first-line treatment of all individuals with hemophilia, regardless of HIV or HCV serostatus (see Bloodborne Pathogens). If plasma-derived products are used, high-purity products are preferred over lesser-purity products. For example, plasma-derived coagulation factor IX is recommended over plasma-derived prothrombin complex concentrates or their activated prothrombin complex concentrates because of potential thromboembolic risk with the latter product. Recombinant products also are preferred in prophylaxis regimens.

Among the 15% to 25% of affected patients who develop inhibitors, those with high-titer antibodies may require immune tolerance induction to neutralize the inhibitor; once eradicated, factor VIII can be used effectively to achieve hemostasis (see Chapter 126). Until tolerance is achieved, however, hemostasis in inhibitor patients is achieved with recombinant factor VIIa, activated prothrombin complex concentrates, or porcine factor VIII concentrates. The latter are generally less effective than recombinant factor VIII or IX concentrates are in noninhibitor patients, which is not surprising given that the former agents fall short of the normal thrombin-generating activity possible with the latter agents.[127] A prospective crossover comparison study of recombinant factor VIIa and activated prothrombin complex concentrate factor VIII inhibitor bypass activity for treatment of hemarthroses in subjects with high-responding factor VIII or IX inhibitors found neither agent to be superior.[128] Porcine factor VIII is effective, however, only in patients with low antiporcine factor VIII titers. As might be expected, titers of antiporcine factor VIII typically rise a few days after its administration, but there may be an important window of opportunity to achieve hemostasis with this agent, for example, in surgery, prior to development of an anamnestic response. The high rate of endogenous porcine parvovirus in swine has been a problem for production of plasma-derived porcine factor VIII products, and a recombinant product is under development. Prophylaxis in inhibitor patients may be effective with use of several different agents, including factor VIII inhibitor bypass activity and recombinant factor VIIa.[129] Immune tolerance induction, which neutralizes factor VIII inhibitors, is generally performed with recombinant factor VIII, although plasma-derived vWF concentrate has shown superior efficacy in some patients.[130,131] Immunosuppression with cyclosporine,[132] mycophenolate,[133] and rituximab[134,135] have shown efficacy as single agents in tolerance induction, although only in small studies. Preliminary results with rituximab indicate tolerance can be maintained for 12 or more months, potentially providing the opportunity for treatment with factor VIII during elective surgery. A phase II clinical trial of rituximab in inhibitor patients through the NHLBI Transfusion Medicine Hemostasis Clinical Trials Network (TMH-CTN) should help determine the efficacy, safety, and durability of this modality. Inhibitor formation is a T-cell–dependent immune response, suggesting the potential usefulness of a dendritic cell vaccine approach. In the hemophilia A murine model, factor VIII-pulsed dendritic cells have led to successful tolerance induction and prevented an anamnestic response on rechallenge with factor VIII.[136,137]

All replacement therapy options should be discussed with the patient or the family. Patient preferences must be given serious consideration because extensive scientific data are not always available to determine the "best" treatment and because of the wide variation in cost among the clotting factor concentrates. Regardless of product choice, elective major surgery should be approached with great caution and performed in a major hemophilia treatment center with expertise in hemophilia management and with a wide range of products available should one prove ineffective.

HCV, with 60% genotype 1, the predominant phenotype of United States donors. The HCV genotype 1 is characterized by a poorer response to interferon-ribavirin antiviral therapy and more frequent progression to hepatic failure.[143] HCV infection is characterized by asymptomatic hepatic transaminasemia, which may be either intermittent or persistent. Spontaneous clearance may occur in up to 20% of infected patients, primarily in those with hepatitis B coinfection acquired before age 2 years and those with HCV coinfection since 1983.[144] Progression to liver failure occurs in approximately 10% to 20% of HCV-seropositive patients with 20 to 25 years of exposure, and hepatitis C liver disease is the leading cause of morbidity and mortality in this population.[145,146] Among those coinfected with HIV, there is persistent HCV replication, high HCV RNA viral load, advanced fibrosis, and more rapid liver disease progression, with a 3.7-fold increased relative risk of end-stage liver disease.[145] Risk factors for liver disease progression in hemophilia include age at HCV exposure, hepatitis B surface antigenemia, HIV coinfection, and alcohol use. This latter risk factor underscores the importance of avoiding or minimizing alcohol use in this group.

Liver biopsy, the standard for determining the extent of liver damage and degree of fibrosis, is not commonly performed in patients with hemophilia.[147] Although percutaneous liver biopsy has been complicated by bleeding,[148] the less invasive transjugular liver biopsy, which accesses the liver via the jugular vein, appears to be safe in patients with hemophilia when performed under factor coverage.[147,149]

Treatment with interferon-ribavirin antiviral therapy leads to durable viral suppression in fewer than 50% of patients, just as in nonhemophilic subjects. However, among those with HIV–HCV coinfection, significantly fewer respond (≤20%), and hepatotoxicity is not uncommon.[145,150] Therapy, if successful, may not only prevent liver disease progression but also development of hepatocellular carcinoma,[151,152] which is associated with chronic HCV and HBV infections.

For patients with HIV–HCV coinfection there is increasing evidence that HIV antiviral therapy, or highly active antiretroviral therapy (HAART), reduces the severity of liver disease progression,[153] presumably related to HIV viral load reduction. For those who develop end-stage liver disease, liver transplantation is becoming the standard of care for coinfected individuals just as for HIV-negative/HCV-positive individuals,[150] although not all centers perform the procedure, and some assign lower priority to those with HIV infection. Even if accepted onto a waiting list, coinfected patients are more likely to die preoperatively of severe bacterial sepsis and multiorgan failure.[154] Recognition of the signs and symptoms of end-stage liver disease and early referral to hepatologists and transplant surgeons are essential for optimal care. Yet, coinfected patients may not receive standard HIV or HCV antiviral therapy or be referred to a hepatologist. If patients do receive a donor organ, which cures the hemophilia,[155–157] hepatitis C is difficult to eradicate because it recurs in all HCV-positive liver transplant recipients,[153] underscoring the need for better hepatitis C treatment.

The risks of horizontal transmission of HCV from the infected hemophiliac to his sexual partner or subsequent vertical transmission of HCV to the unborn fetus appear to be minimal (<3%), unless the patient and the pregnant female are coinfected with HIV. In that case, vertical HIV transmission is more likely than is HCV infection,[158] although the risk of HIV transmission to sexual partners is greatly reduced by HAART and the absence of a detectable HIV viral RNA.

Hepatitis B is a problem of the past for patients with hemophilia as a result of testing of plasma donors for hepatitis B surface antigen and routine administration of recombinant hepatitis B vaccine shortly after birth. HBV titers from prior vaccination may disappear with the progression of AIDS; in these patients, vaccination should be repeated. Of the HBV-seropositive patients who were exposed to the virus in concentrates administered before 1985, approximately 5% are chronic carriers of hepatitis B surface antigen. In these patients, development of progressive hepatic failure or hepatocellular carcinoma is more likely, and they are susceptible to coinfection with the hepatitis D virus ("deltavirus"), which accelerates liver failure.

Although HAV transmission is not considered an important bloodborne pathogen, HAV seroconversions have been detected in hemophiliacs who received high-purity concentrates treated with solvent detergent.[159] HAV in plasma pools containing one or more transiently viremic donors are not susceptible to currently available viral inactivation processes because HAV is a nonenveloped virus. Thus, manufacturers of plasma-derived concentrates now screen prospective donors and donor pools by polymerase chain reaction testing for viral nucleic acids to minimize the risk of transmission of HAV (as well as HIV-1 and HIV-2, HBV, and HCV). The HAV vaccine series is recommended for all seronegative hemophilic children older than 2 years and is effective by both the intramuscular and subcutaneous routes.[160] The immune response to the vaccine of HIV-seropositive patients should be checked because booster doses may be needed.

Hepatitis E is not transmitted through plasma-derived concentrates. This is in contrast to hepatitis G virus, a human flavivirus distantly related to HCV. Approximately 15% to 25% of hemophiliacs who received nonviral attenuated concentrates are seropositive for hepatitis G virus, compared with 3% of healthy blood donors.[161] Hepatitis G virus appears to be susceptible to the same viral inactivation processes used for HCV and other lipid-enveloped viruses and should not be a substantial threat to hemophiliacs.

Human parvovirus B19, a single-stranded DNA virus, is associated with fifth disease (erythema infectiosum) in children, transient aplastic anemia in patients with chronic hemolytic diseases, and chronic bone marrow aplasia in patients with AIDS. Through transplacental transmission, B19 parvovirus can induce hydrops fetalis and fetal loss. Because infection is ubiquitous and frequently asymptomatic in healthy adults, viremia often is undetected. The prevalence of B19 viremia in normal blood donor populations ranges up to 1 : 1000,[162] ensuring that most large plasma pools used to make factor concentrates are contaminated with virus. The seroprevalence of hemophiliacs treated repeatedly with plasma-derived concentrates approaches 80% even in those who have received only viral-attenuated products deemed safe from HCV and HIV.[163,164] This is considerably higher than observed in age-matched control groups (approximately 40% seroprevalence). Previous exposure to B19 parvovirus is not affected by age, type or severity of hemophilia, HIV status, $CD4^+$ lymphocyte counts, or purity of the plasma-derived concentrate.[165] Although a few anecdotes describe pure red cell aplasia or pancytopenia, the long-term consequences of parvovirus infection in hemophilia are not established. To date, parvovirus B19, a nonlipid-enveloped virus, has been resistant to inactivation by all available heating and solvent-detergent techniques, used alone or in combination, in the manufacture of concentrates.[166] Adjunctive nanofiltration steps have been implemented for additional viral depletion. Of concern to many physicians who care for patients with hemophilia is the fact that parvovirus B19 is representative of other nonlipid-enveloped viral pathogens (known or unknown) that might contaminate plasma-derived concentrates. These compelling considerations have served as the rationale for administering only recombinant factor VIII or factor IX to parvovirus B19-seronegative patients, previously untreated hemophiliacs, or pregnant carriers. The viruses responsible for West Nile fever and severe acute respiratory syndrome are lipid-enveloped and should be excluded from the plasma-derived concentrates by currently available viral attenuation processes. Furthermore, donor screening procedures and specific virus testing likely will help exclude these pathogens from plasma-derived products.

Other agents potentially transmissible through plasma-derived transfusion include SEN virus, TT virus, both of which cause hepatitis; human herpesvirus 8; simian foamy virus; coronavirus of the severe respiratory syndrome, and prion variant Creutzfeldt-Jakob, which causes the human form of bovine spongiform encephalopathy.[167]

The causative agent of the progressive dementia and spongiform encephalopathy characteristic of Creutzfeldt-Jakob disease (CJD) has been considered infectious since the mid 1960s; however, its transmissibility through the transfusion of blood or blood components remains controversial. Because it cannot be detected in asymptomatic donors, is resistant to chemical and physical inactivation, and does not induce antibodies in carriers, which could be a marker of exposure, CJD prions remain a theoretical threat to individuals using plasma-derived concentrates. CJD is not known to be transmitted to humans by blood components, and no CJD-related deaths are known or reported in hemophilia or other heavily transfused populations.[168] The possibility of bloodborne transmission, however, has not been completely excluded because of its decades-long incubation period prior to symptomatic disease.

A variant form of CJD (vCJD) that causes a neurologic disorder similar to bovine spongiform encephalopathy, a prion disease of cattle, has been recognized in nonhemophilic individuals in the United Kingdom. Between 1995 and 2006, 200 individuals worldwide developed vCJD, including three individuals in the United States who acquired vCJD through blood cell transfusion outside the United States.[169] vCJD has not been transmitted through plasma-derived clotting factor,[168] although it remains a potential risk. The Food and Drug Administration has evaluated the potential for transmission of vCJD by plasma-derived factor VIII concentrates from subclinically infected donors that might be inadvertently included in source plasma. The conclusion was that all U.S.-licensed products probably achieve a 4 $\log_{10}$ reduction of vCJD during manufacture (www.fda.gov/ohrms/dockets/ac/06/briefing/2006-4271B1-01.pdf). The clearance of prions from factor VIII products is hindered because factor VIII is purified from cryoprecipitate, and current manufacturing processes do not inactivate or destroy prions. Prion clearance is entirely the result of partitioning away from intermediates and final product during manufacture and is not as robust as viral clearance measures capable of 10 $\log_{10}$ reduction, for instance. Based on these data, the risk of vCJD transmission via plasma-derived clotting factor concentrates is estimated to range from 1 : 9.4 billion per person-year, based on episodic treatment, to 1 : 15,000 per person-year, based on daily treatment.[170] The risk, although low, has contributed to patient preference for recombinant products only and for elimination of animal proteins from the manufacturing process to the greatest extent possible. Monitoring and surveillance for CJD and vCJD in individuals receiving blood products and clotting factor concentrates continues.[170]

Noninfectious Complications of Replacement Therapy

Other than infectious complications, clotting factor concentrates produce few clinically significant adverse reactions. Transfusion-associated anaphylaxis is rare, although anaphylaxis to factor IX concentrates in persons with severe hemophilia B in close association with the development of a factor IX inhibitor has been reported.[171] Genetic analysis reveals complete deletion or rearrangements of the factor IX gene in most affected patients. Induction of immune tolerance to factor IX has not been generally successful, and these patients may be predisposed to developing nephrotic syndrome.[172] Any plasma-derived or recombinant factor IX concentrate is capable of producing such a complication; treatment of bleeding events with recombinant human factor VIIa is the only effective alternative. Urticarial reactions and low-grade fevers can be treated with antihistamines and acetaminophen.

Thrombotic Complications of Replacement Therapy

Thrombotic complications with use of factor VIII concentrates have not been commonly reported. However, low-purity factor IX complex concentrates have been associated with occurrence of thrombotic complications when infused repeatedly in large amounts. Similar complications have been reported with administration of the activated factor IX complex concentrates used in inhibitor patients. Disseminated intravascular coagulation, deep vein thrombosis, pulmonary embolism, and fatal or life-threatening acute myocardial infarction in young men and boys have been described.[173–175] The introduction of high-purity plasma-derived and recombinant factor IX preparations has virtually eliminated this thrombogenicity, and in vivo studies show little or no rise in the surrogate markers of coagulation activation (e.g., fibrinopeptide A, prothrombin fragment 1.2). Thrombotic events have been reported with use of recombinant factor VIIa,[176,177] including local phlebitis if the drug is administered in small peripheral veins.[178]

Adjunctive Therapeutic Measures

In most persons with mild or moderate hemophilia A, the expense of replacement therapy can be reduced and exposure to bloodborne pathogens eliminated through administration of desmopressin (desamino-8-arginine vasopressin [DDAVP]), a pharmacologic analogue of the hormone 8-arginine vasopressin. DDAVP usually is administered intravenously or intranasally as a spray, with subsequent rise in factor VIII coagulant activity adequate to achieve hemostasis for surgical procedures or symptomatic bleeding. Peak factor VIII activity two to five times baseline level typically is observed within 30 minutes after intravenous infusion of DDAVP (0.3 μg/kg of body weight) and within 60 minutes after intranasal delivery 150 μg per nostril of metered spray: one puff in one nostril for those <50 kg and one puff in each nostril for those ≥50 kg). Because of the variability in individual response, potential candidates for this form of treatment should be tested in advance of its use to provide hemostasis. Dosing can be repeated at 8- to12-hour intervals; however, a progressive tachyphylaxis frequently occurs, making DDAVP less useful for long-term hemostatic support in the postoperative period. Furthermore, the antidiuretic effects of the drug may produce water intoxication and severe hyponatremia, particularly if free water intake is not restricted. Seizure activity is uncommon but has been reported, predominantly in small children and the elderly, but it may occur at any age. Monitoring of fluids and serum sodium levels should minimize these risks. Virtually all patients experience transient facial flushing; mild headaches and minimally decreased blood pressure occasionally are noted. DDAVP should be used cautiously in elderly men with risk factors for coronary or cerebral arterial thrombosis because of an apparent increased risk for angina pectoris, myocardial infarction, or stroke after administration. This may be due to DDAVP-mediated release of supranormal vWF protein multimers from endothelial cells, which promote platelet adhesion in conditions of high shear stress. DDAVP also stimulates the release of tissue plasminogen activator from endothelial cells, potentially producing fibrinolysis at the site of hemostasis. Therefore, for treatment or prevention of mucosal surface bleeding (e.g., dental, gastrointestinal, or vaginal [in carriers]), antifibrinolytic agents should be added immediately before administration of DDAVP and continued for 5 to 7 days thereafter. Similarly, adjunctive administration of antifibrinolytic agents, such as ε-aminocaproic acid or tranexamic acid, in combination with clotting factor concentrates enhances control of bleeding during and after dental surgery in patients with hemophilia A. Use of these agents should be reserved for patients with hemophilia B who are receiving high-purity factor IX preparations because any thrombotic tendency induced by low-purity materials may be exacerbated by inhibition of fibrinolysis.

Experience with use of fibrin sealants in patients with hemophilia both as a hemostatic agent and as a promoter of wound healing is growing. Fibrin sealant has reduced blood loss and requirements for factor replacement therapy in major and minor surgical procedures, including circumcisions and dental procedures.[179] Fibrin sealants also have been used successfully to limit hemorrhage from the cavities remaining after percutaneous evacuation of hemophilic pseudotumors (see box on Pseudotumors in Hemophilia).[180–182]

Pseudotumors in Hemophilia

Hemophilic pseudotumors are large encapsulated hematomas that represent progressive cystic swelling from persistent bleeding and incomplete resorption. This serious complication is evident in approximately 1% to 2% of severely affected patients, usually adults. The pseudotumor is composed of clot and necrotic tissue.

Three types of pseudotumors predominate in hemophilia. The most common type arises from repeated hemorrhage and inadequate clot resorption and usually is confined within fascial and muscle planes. Radiologically they appear as simple cysts; infrequently, they expand to involve adjacent structures or erode through the skin layers. The second type involves large muscle groups, such as the gluteus maximus and iliopsoas. These lesions are especially problematic because they may gradually enlarge, develop a fibrous capsule, and eventually destroy adjacent underlying structures by pressure necrosis. Skeletal fractures and bony deformities produced by cortical erosion may result. The third and rarest type of pseudotumor arises from within bone itself, often secondary to subperiosteal bleeding. This lesion typically is observed in the long bones of the lower extremities and pelvis but has been reported to occur within the calcaneus, cranium, and mandible (Fig. 125–5). As the periosteum expands, it is stripped and raised, leading to displacement and erosion of adjacent muscle and bone. Most such pseudotumors arise in adults and occur in proximal skeletal structures; distal lesions occur more frequently in children before skeletal maturity and are associated with a better prognosis.

Pseudotumors are best diagnosed by computed tomographic scanning, magnetic resonance imaging, ultrasonography, and vascular injection studies. Although the presence of one or more progressively enlarging pelvic or skeletal masses in a hemophiliac is consistent with the diagnosis of a pseudotumor, the lesions may resemble osteomyelitis, metastatic neoplasms, Ewing sarcoma, primary osteosarcomas, tuberculosis abscesses, aneurysmal bone cysts, giant cell tumors, or plasmacytomas. Chondrosarcomas and liposarcomas have occurred in such patients. Preoperative biopsy is contraindicated because catastrophic complications, including life-threatening bleeding and infection, are common. Distal pseudotumors respond well to conservative treatment consisting of aggressive clotting factor replacement and cast immobilization. Because conservative treatment has not been nearly as successful for lesions of the proximal musculoskeleton and because complete regression is rare,[180] this approach is reserved primarily for inhibitor patients with high-titer inhibitors. High- and low-intensity radiotherapy regimens have been successful in eradicating pseudotumors in the long bones and may offer an alternative conservative approach.[181] Surgical extirpation is the most effective therapy for pseudotumors and is the treatment of choice when it can be performed in major hemophilia centers. Nevertheless, the operative mortality rate approaches 20%.[182] Depending on the size and location of the pseudotumor, percutaneous evacuation of the cavity and subsequent introduction of fibrin sealant or cancellous bone may be considered.

Orthopedic and Musculoskeletal Bleeding

Occasionally, repetitive bleeding occurs in a single joint despite intensive prophylactic factor replacement therapy and physiotherapy. The synovitis and pain in this "target joint" warrant definitive treatment to prevent progressive degeneration. Prophylaxis (see box on Prophylaxis: The Joint Outcome Study), that is, the infusion of factor concentrate two or three times weekly, may prevent bleeds by maintaining a level of at least 0.01 U/mL, sufficient to prevent spontaneous bleeding. New data support the concept that prophylaxis prevents recurrent bleeds and ongoing joint damage, which may prevent long-term adverse joint outcomes, if initiated early enough.[183] However, if prophylaxis is started after joint damage has occurred (i.e., "secondary prophylaxis"), cartilage destruction may continue, as evidenced radiographically.[184] Because prophylaxis may be difficult to maintain in young children due to complicated venous access and the need for a dedicated individual to perform the infusion, some families have opted for surgery despite the risks and lack of evidence-based data supporting this approach. Among the surgical procedures for chronic hemophilic arthropathy, arthroscopic synovectomy is considered for some children in whom joint damage is increasing and prophylaxis is unsuccessful or impractical, or for adults who prefer not to undergo a major surgical procedure. By contrast, open synovectomy usually is performed in adults with long-standing joint pain and disability.

Standard scoring systems for hemophilic arthropathy, including the Arnold-Hilgartner scale,[97] which measures single joint pathology, and the Pettersson score,[185] which measures multiple joint pathology radiologically, now are used together with MRI,[186] which provides for earlier detection of synovial hypertrophy than possible by physical examination or radiography. MRI is increasingly used in clinical hemophilia management and in prospective outcome studies. Open surgical or arthroscopic synovectomy may reduce the frequency of hemarthroses and reduce pain by removing inflamed tissue and most of the blood vessels in the joint. Synovectomy should not be performed with the sole intent of improving joint mobility, because loss of motion in the affected joint often occurs after surgery. Arthroscopic surgery is increasingly being used to control recurrent bleeds and slow progression of joint disease.[187] In this procedure, thickened synovium is removed, reducing the number and frequency of joint hemorrhages but not the relentless radiographic deterioration.[188] In those with advanced arthropathy, improvement may be transient. The optimal time to perform this procedure is unknown.

An alternative approach, nonoperative synovectomy ("synoviorthesis" or "radionuclide synovectomy"), involves injection of a radioisotope (usually phosphorus-32) into the joint space. The procedure may be appropriate for selected patients to ablate inflamed synovial tissue or for inhibitor patients in whom control of bleeding often is problematic. Although radionuclide synovectomy results in better preservation of range of motion than is obtained with operative synovectomy,[189] it may not eliminate hemarthroses as effectively as opera-

Prophylaxis: The Joint Outcome Study

Prophylaxis, the three to four times weekly infusion of factor to prevent hemorrhages, is considered optimal therapy and is recommended for children as soon as recurrent bleeds in joints occur. A number of studies have demonstrated that, if begun early, when patients are 1 to 4 years old, prophylaxis decreases spontaneous bleeds, arthropathy, joint scores, radiologic abnormalities, and surgical intervention.[207,208] The success of prophylaxis is based on administering factor VIII or factor IX concentrates 25 to 40 U/kg three times weekly for hemophilia A and twice weekly for hemophilia B to achieve factor levels of 1% to 2%, essentially converting a patient with severe disease into one with mild or moderate disease, essentially eliminating *spontaneous* bleeds. Outcomes are correlated with both the intensity of treatment and the level of compliance[209,210] and translate into decreased absence from school or work, fewer bleeds and days spent in the hospital, increased personal and professional productivity, improved overall performance status, and a healthier self-image.[209] Although "prophylactic" treatment was long thought to be more effective than "episodic" or "on-demand" treatment in terms of long-term joint outcomes,[209] no comparison of these modalities were available and this conjecture remained unproven until the "Joint Outcome Study."

A multicenter, prospective randomized trial, the Joint Outcome Study for the first time confirmed that prophylaxis reduces or prevents acute joint bleeds as well as clinical joint damage and is superior to episodic on-demand treatment.[211] Studying a group of 65 children with hemophilia A, the investigators randomized half (n = 32) to receive factor VIII prophylaxis every other day at a dose of 25 U/kg and half (n = 33) to receive intensive episodic treatment in three or more infusions totaling greater than 80 U/kg factor VIII concentrate at the time of each joint bleed. Subjects between the ages of 12 and 30 months were enrolled and were followed to age 6 years. At baseline, each child was required to have two or fewer hemorrhages into any one joint with normal roentgenogram and magnetic resonance MR) imaging studies. Compared with patients receiving episodic treatment, those receiving prophylaxis had 10-fold fewer bleeds per year (0.47 vs 4.9 per year, $P < 0.01$. Moreover, those receiving prophylaxis also had lower joint scores (4.7 vs 8.6, $P < 0.01$). Not unexpectedly, prophylaxis requires a significantly greater total amount of factor and is more costly than episodic treatment: patients receiving prophylaxis used 3.5-fold more factor per year than did those receiving episodic treatment ($P < 0.001$). Thus, this clinical trial for the first time demonstrated the efficacy of prophylaxis, including both acute and intermediate-term benefits. Longer followup is needed to establish long-term clinical and structural joint improvement as defined clinically, radiographically, and by magnetic resonance imaging.

A study of 60 hemophilic children has shown that prophylaxis does prevent long-term radiographic evidence of arthopathy.[212] Furthermore, a case-control study of 100 children with hemophilia A (60 with inhibitors and 40 noninhibitor controls) provides preliminary yet compelling evidence that early initiation of prophylaxis also protects against inhibitor development.[213] No study has provided evidence that prophylaxis, when started early in childhood, increases the incidence of inhibitor antibody formation.

Factor concentrate expense is substantially greater with prophylaxis. Cost may be substantially reduced if the factor is administered by continuous infusion and dosing is based on measured pharmacokinetics.[214,215] In addition to cost, children receiving prophylaxis may develop infectious and thrombotic complications of CVADs,[216,217] which are commonly placed to facilitate access (see Complications of Factor Replacement Therapy). These potential risks may dissuade some families from initiating prophylaxis.[218]

"Primary prophylaxis" (i.e., prophylaxis initiated prior to joint damage and/or recurrent hemarthroses in a target joint) is the preferred "preventive" approach. "Secondary prophylaxis" (i.e., prophylaxis initiated after onset of significant joint damage) may be beneficial in patients reluctant to begin primary prophylaxis. However, it should be recognized that although stabilization of articular function and joint scores may occur over time, reversal of joint damage or radiographic deterioration of previously damaged joints may not be possible.[184]

tive synovectomy. Of considerable concern is the finding that radionuclide synovectomy has been complicated by the occurrence of acute lymphoblastic leukemia in two hemophilic children within 1 year of the procedure.[190,191] Because leukemia rarely, if ever, occurs in hemophilia,[192] longer surveillance will be required before the long-term safety of this procedure is established.

Orthotics may play an important role in management of joint disease, and orthotic intervention can serve as an interim measure before definitive reconstructive surgery. The goal of orthotic intervention is to transform a subluxed, flexed joint into a functional stiff limb rather than a functional articulation. Ankle guards and arch supports are useful in patients with ankle arthropathy and can assist in maintaining and improving gait and weight bearing. Shoe lifts can equalize the lengths of the lower extremities. Otherwise, orthotics are applied most commonly to the knees and occasionally to the elbows. Dynamic braces equipped with adjustable hinges to correct extension deformities of joints with successive, painless manipulations have supplanted traditional plaster casting of the joint with serial extension wedging, which requires anesthesia, is painful, and does not permit active muscle contraction.[193] These methods do not address subluxation deformities; however, promising results have been reported with the Ilizarov apparatus, which applies significant skeletally mediated forces simultaneously in both the subluxation and the extension planes.[193,194]

Pain and deformity that limit mobility, quality of life, and performance status are indications for joint reconstruction. Arthroplasty with prosthetic joint replacement has been performed to restore function in knees, hips, elbows, and shoulders.[195] Improvements in durability and design of joint prostheses allow their use in younger patients, in whom knee prostheses may remain intact for more than 15 years. Prosthetic loosening is observed in hip replacements within 6 to 10 years after surgery and is due to increased stresses on the joint, probably from weight bearing and abnormal torque produced by the ipsilateral or contralateral knee.[196] Staged surgical procedures or multiple joint procedures in a single operative session performed in patients with hemophilia should be considered because the costs of rehabilitation and clotting factor replacement are considerably lower using this approach.[197] An evaluation of orthopedic surgery in HIV-infected hemophiliacs with an absolute CD4 count of 200/μL or less suggests that arthroplasty increases the risk of infection 10-fold, particularly staphylococcal prosthetic joint infection, chronic osteomyelitis, and sepsis.[198] Although not a universal experience,[199] this finding suggests that surgical intervention should be based on the overall balance of risks and potential benefits.

Arthrodesis (surgical fixation) is reserved for painful joints with greatly compromised mobility. Fixation is most commonly performed on the ankle by interposition of autologous iliac crest bone, which fuses the juxtaposed bone surfaces. Fixation of bones into a single, well-aligned unit can be facilitated with intramedullary nails or external fixators; however, pin site infections may occur in up to 10% of patients. Arthroscopic ankle arthrodesis has been developed using demineralized bone matrix–bone marrow slurry as a graft substitute. Although this approach has not yet been widely applied for hemophilic arthropathy, it has the potential to obviate open surgery and reduce the need for factor replacement.[200] Ankle fusion allows patients good mobility in normal shoes because the joints of the feet and toes are less commonly affected by bleeds, and the pain and frequency of hemarthroses are markedly diminished. Supramalleolar varus osteotomy may be a useful alternative in hemophilic arthropathy with secondary valgus deformity.[201]

Intramuscular Hematoma

Approximately 30% of bleeding episodes in persons with hemophilia occur in muscles. Although most intramuscular hematomas are trivial and resolve spontaneously, some produce significant morbidity and, depending on their location and size, can lead to death. Intramuscular bleeds occur less commonly than hemarthroses and usually are not life threatening. The most serious hematomas occur in the iliopsoas muscle or retroperitoneal space, where bleeding can be profuse. These lesions can mimic hip hemarthroses and appendicitis. Large hematomas can produce fever, neutrophilia, ecchymoses, hyperbilirubinemia, and elevated lactate dehydrogenase levels. They may be painful and may impair the sensory and motor function of adjacent nerves, which they entrap and compress. Occasionally, flexion contractures involving muscles innervated by these nerves develop (e.g., in the hip). Muscle bleeds are precipitated by incidental trauma in severe hemophilia and by more significant degrees of trauma in moderate or mild disease (e.g., contact sport injuries). Iatrogenic hematomas may form in association with intramuscular injections of medications (e.g., vaccines) and can be prevented by administering replacement clotting factor beforehand. All significant muscle bleeds should be treated aggressively to raise the factor level above 50% of normal.

Mucous Membrane Bleeding

Although fatal gastrointestinal tract bleeding was a greater problem before the introduction of factor concentrates, significant hemorrhage occurs in 13% of adult patients with hemophilia.[202] Gastric mucosal bleeding has become more common in recent years with the increased use of NSAIDs for treatment of painful hemophilic hemarthropathy. NSAIDs have supplanted aspirin as the major cause of this complication. In patients with hemophilia, aspirin in any form should be avoided altogether and NSAIDs prescribed judiciously for limited time periods under strict medical supervision.

Hemorrhagic complications of portal hypertension in long-term survivors of viral hepatitis have occurred more commonly as hemophilia patients have lived longer. Massive, life-threatening melena and hematemesis can result from esophageal varices in patients with hemophilia complicated by portal hypertension. Sclerotherapy at the site of bleeding varices has been successful for treatment of gastrointestinal bleeding, as has the transjugular intravenous portal vein–systemic shunt procedure for decompression of varices, and probably is safer than aggressive open surgical procedures. In selected patients, orthotopic liver transplantation offers another option for treatment of symptomatic portal hypertension complicating terminal liver failure. This approach has the additional advantage of providing a cure of the underlying hemophilia by restoring normal coagulant factor synthesis.[155–157] Gastrointestinal blood loss in a patient with hemophilia demands an exhaustive evaluation for anatomic lesions, as in any other patient.

Bleeding from the mucous membranes of the nose and mouth is common in hemophilia. Posttraumatic tongue bleeding must be treated aggressively to prevent progressive airway obstruction, which can develop rapidly. In infants, the frenulum is a frequent site of bleeding, and as the hemophilic child grows older, the loss of deciduous teeth and the eruption of secondary dentition can be complicated by prolonged bleeding. Fortunately, these episodes usually respond well to antifibrinolytic agents (e.g., ε-aminocaproic acid, tranexamic acid) or fibrin sealants without factor replacement. Factor replacement may be required for more difficult cases. For major dental surgery, particularly those necessitating nerve blocks, factor replacement to achieve 15% to 25% of normal activity should prevent bleeding into the tissue planes of the neck, which can lead to respiratory embarrassment. In mild hemophilia, intranasal or subcutaneous/intravenous DDAVP is an excellent choice, with or without antifibrinolytics or fibrin sealants. Spontaneous epistaxis is relatively uncommon without an anatomic lesion or trauma. Nevertheless, it may necessitate factor replacement, packing, cauterization, or fibrinolytic therapy. Urologic bleeding is common in patients with hemophilia[203–206] and usually is spontaneous, episodic, and painless. In addition to factor replacement, fluid intake should be increased. If bleeding is protracted and severe, a short course of steroids may be helpful. If the hematuria is caused by nephrolithiasis, extracorporeal shock lithotripsy can be performed safely under coverage of factor replacement.

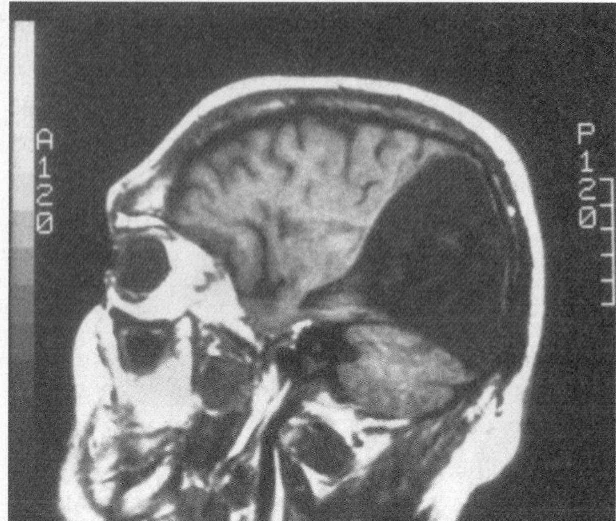

Figure 125–5 Massive pseudotumor resulting from repeated intracranial hemorrhage in a patient with hemophilia.

Complications of Factor Replacement Therapy

With the virtual elimination of pathogen risk through the introduction of recombinant factors and the chemical and physical inactivation of plasma-derived and recombinant clotting factor products, the major complications of hemophilia are spontaneous life-threatening and disabling central nervous system (CNS) bleeds, inhibitor formation, and central venous access device (CVAD) infection. Currently, individuals exposed to HIV and HCV through infusion of blood products represent approximately bout 40% and 80% of adults with hemophilia, whereas those younger than 20 years remain free of HIV or HCV.[145] With the introduction of HAART, HIV infection is a chronic treatable disease, with a life expectancy in patients with hemophilia similar to that before the HIV epidemic (Fig. 125–5).[35,36,43,219] Among patients with hepatitis C, fibrosis and cirrhosis may occur in 20% or more of patients and up to twofold or more higher among those who are HIV positive. Several large prospective studies, including the HHH (Impact of HIV on Hepatitis C Infection in Hemophilia A), will determine the incidence of fibrosis and end-stage liver disease, comparing HIV-negative with HIV-positive subjects. Hepatitis C remains the major cause of morbidity and the leading cause of death among individuals with hemophilia.[135] Nearly all patients with HIV infection are coinfected with HCV, and HIV upregulates cytokines that increase liver fibrosis and progression to end-stage liver disease. Among coinfected patients with end-stage liver disease, liver transplantation, which effects phenotypic cure of hemophilia, now is considered safe and effective.[150]

CNS bleeding, including intracranial hemorrhage[220] (see Fig. 125–3) and soft-tissue hemorrhage in or around vital areas such as the airway or internal organs, is particularly life threatening in patients with hemophilia. The estimated lifetime risk of intracranial hemorrhage, based on clinical presentation, has been reported to be 2% to 8%. After HCV and HIV infections, intracranial hemorrhage constitutes the third leading cause of death among individuals with hemophilia.[145,221] Clinically, early signs of CNS bleeding may include headache, nausea and vomiting, and increased sleepiness, which, if missed, may delay treatment and worsen outcome. Psychomotor retardation, cerebral palsy, and/or seizures may occur in a substantial proportion of patients; the most common inciting event is trauma, including birth trauma.[222] In a longitudinal study of children with hemophilia, in whom the prevalence of intracranial hemorrhage was assessed by both clinical surveys and radiologic imaging (head MRI), the combined rate of symptomatic and silent intracranial hemorrhage was 12%.[223] However, this figure may underestimate the true frequency, as a significant fraction of cases of intracranial hemorrhage diagnosed by MRI are clinically silent[223] (see box on Intracranial Hemorrhage in Hemophilia).

Intracranial Hemorrhage in Hemophilia

Intracranial hemorrhage is the third leading cause of death in patients with hemophilia, after hepatitis C and HIV infection.[145,221] This complication develops in 10% of patients with severe hemophilia, with a mortality rate greater than 30%. Survivors have a significant incidence of psychoneurologic sequelae, including mental retardation, seizure disorders, and motor dysfunction. Because even minimal trauma to the head may precipitate severe hemorrhage and serious intracranial pathology, aggressive treatment with clotting factor concentrates should be initiated immediately to achieve 100% levels of factor VIII or IX, *even if there is only a clinical suspicion of bleeding.* Replacement therapy should precede any diagnostic procedures because less than 5% of acute head injuries in hemophiliacs are accompanied by early abnormalities on computed tomographic scan.[220] When intracranial injury is demonstrated on computed tomographic scans, neurologic deficits, vomiting, or altered mental status is apparent on physical examination. Neurosurgical intervention may be necessary but carries high risks despite maintenance of adequate hemostasis with clotting factor concentrates.

Intracranial hemorrhage in the neonate is invariably preceded by mild to moderate head injury. The risk of serious bleeding associated with vaginal delivery is small, but vacuum extraction has been associated with subgaleal bleeds (Fig. 125–3) and should be avoided when delivering offspring of known hemophilia carriers. In hemophilic adults, CNS bleeding may arise in individuals with hepatitis C and end-stage liver disease associated with portal hypertension and thrombocytopenia or in those with HIV-associated immune thrombocytopenia. However, the latter is responsive to HAART. The risk of CNS bleeding in patients with hemophilia increases when the platelet count falls below 50,000/μL, likely in association with factor VIII or IX deficiency. For this reason, regular (every other day) treatment with factor is recommended to prevent CNS bleeding.[240]

Factor VIII inhibitors alloantibodies directed at infused factor VIII or, less commonly, factor IX are the major noninfectious complication of factor replacement. These IgG antibodies typically occur after a median of nine factor exposures and at a median age of 2 years.[224] They are more common in patients with severe disease and in Caucasians, although the prevalence is twofold higher among African Americans with hemophilia.[224] Inhibitor formation has been linked to genetic factors, including large deletion phenotypes, African American race, and familial occurrence. However, the nonconcordance of inhibitor formation in brother studies suggests that nongenetic factors play an important role. Several small studies have reported that the earlier[225] and the more intense[213,226,227] the exposure to factor VIII, the greater the likelihood of inhibitor development in patients with hemophilia A. These findings will require prospective studies for confirmation. Because inhibitor patients are difficult to treat, they have greater associated morbidity and a somewhat shorter life expectancy than do noninhibitor patients.[228]

CVADs are widely used in children with hemophilia for factor infusion to prevent joint bleeding (prophylaxis) and for induction of immune tolerance. Yet, despite the potential benefits of these devices, their use is complicated by CVAD infection, which accounts for significant cost, morbidity, hospitalization, sepsis, and sepsis-related deaths. From 30% to 40% of patients receiving prophylaxis may develop CVAD infection,[216] with an incidence of 0.66 per 1000 CVAD days.[229] The rate of CVAD infection appears to be related to the frequency of access, with twice as many infections occurring in patients undergoing daily tolerance induction versus prophylaxis three to four times per week.[216,229,230] Increasing evidence suggests that small clots propagated in CVADs by frequent factor infusion serve as a nidus for surface bacteria and propagate CVAD infection.[231] An alternative to standard ports for venous access in children with hemophilia is use of arteriovenous fistulae. In a 3-year study of 27 hemophilia patients, half of whom had inhibitors, proximal forearm fistulae were well tolerated, although thrombosis occurred in one and inadequate AVF maturation occurred in five with inhibitors.[232] Whether arteriovenous fistula placement will prove to be a practical alternative approach to venous access is not known.

Hemophilia as a chronic disease has been recognized to affect the physical and cognitive growth of affected children independent of HIV serologic status. Data from the United States indicate that a significant proportion (approximately 25%) of hemophilic children 6 to 18 years old exhibit below-normal performance in motor skills, lower-than-expected academic performance (measured by IQ scores), and more behavioral and emotional problems than expected, as reported by parents.[233] The presence of HIV and the absolute CD4+ counts were not related to neuropsychological performance at baseline. Causality has not been established, but the potential contributions of minimal head trauma with clinically silent bleeding and the effects of hemophilia on the emotional well-being of the family cannot be overlooked.

The major cause of death in individuals with hemophilia is liver disease, followed by HIV disease and CNS bleeding.[145,219] Only rarely do individuals with hemophilia or hemophilic carriers develop or succumb to myocardial infarction or stroke.[219,234] Of note, only approximately 20% of the expected number of deaths from cardiovascular disease occur, suggesting a protective effect of hemophilia A.[41,228]

Prognosis

Before the widespread use of replacement therapy, the prognosis for patients with severe hemophilia was poor and their quality of life greatly diminished. The outlook improved dramatically in the modern era of hemophilia treatment, beginning in the 1960s with the development of cryoprecipitate,[235] factor VIII concentrates[236] (for hemophilia A), and prothrombin complex concentrates[237] (for hemophilia B). It then became possible to achieve high levels of factor VIII or factor IX without volume overload, which limits plasma therapy. This advance permitted effective therapy for life-threatening soft tissue bleeding, which requires high doses of factor VIII or factor IX for prolonged periods. Furthermore, the convenience of factor concentrates made home therapy of hemarthroses practicable. Use of lyophilized factor concentrates administered at home saved many patients from the delays, expense, and inconvenience of hospital- or clinic-based treatment with cryoprecipitate or plasma. The availability of factor concentrates facilitated prophylactic therapy, which has been shown to virtually eliminate bleeding episodes and actually prevent joint deterioration, especially when started early in life (i.e., at age 1–2 years)[207] (see box on Prophylaxis: The Joint Outcome Study[184,208–212,218]).

Many large studies documented the dramatic gains in life expectancy of patients with hemophilia during the era of replacement therapy. The life expectancy of patients with severe hemophilia, which had remained relatively constant from the nineteenth century to the 1960s, has risen from 11 years (or less) for severely affected patients up to 50 or 60 years by the early 1980s in reported series.[16,18,22–26,35,238,239] Significant progress has been evident even in patients with mild or moderate disease, for whom life expectancy is closer to that for the normal population in the pretreatment era (Fig. 125–6).

With the efficacy of prophylaxis in reducing the frequency of joint hemorrhage demonstrated in a randomized clinical trial[183] (see box on Prophylaxis: The Joint Outcome Study), primary prophylaxis is expected to become a more acceptable approach to treatment. Accordingly, chronic orthopedic disability resulting from progressive hemophilic arthropathy and the associated social and economic consequences should become less common. Results of a study of U.S. boys 6 to 12 years old with factor VIII levels less than 2% of normal indicate that those on prophylactic treatment regimens had higher total academic achievement and mathematical scores than those receiving "on demand" treatment.[241] The superior academic performance was associated with less absenteeism, which was correlated with less frequent bleeding episodes per year (6 vs 25) and better scores on the Physical Summary aspect of the Child Health Questionnaire (48.4 vs 41.3). These findings make a case for prophylactic treatment as a method by which children with hemophilia can reach their full academic and physical potential.

Significant impairment of physical stature and sexual maturation has been observed in HIV-infected boys with hemophilia compared with uninfected boys or population norms.[242] The discrepancy between total serum testosterone levels (compared with age-adjusted levels in HIV-uninfected boys) and observed physical changes arises as a result of HIV infection and the impact on the immune and endocrine systems; thus, the effects are potentially reversible with HAART.

The combined morbidity and mortality associated with hemophilia and its treatment constitute a powerful argument for prophylactic treatment, development of safer concentrates, elimination of inhibitor antibodies when they occur, and gene therapy, which currently is the only prospect (other than liver transplantation) for the cure of hemophilia.

Gene Therapy

Gene therapy or, more correctly, gene transfer can be defined as the clinical delivery of gene constructs whose expression compensates for a missing protein.

Hemophilia has attracted a great deal of attention from investigators interested in gene therapy for several reasons: (a) the complementary DNAs (cDNAs) have been cloned,[243,244] (b) fully functional factor VIII and factor IX may be produced in various cell types if the correct posttranslational modifications are made and the protein is delivered to the circulation, and (c) the amount of factor VIII or factor IX required to improve the bleeding phenotype can be as little as 1% of normal plasma levels. There may be some margin for error with regard to overexpression due to regulation of factor VIII/factor IX enzyme activity by anticoagulant proteins C and S and antithrombin III. Although elevated factor VIII or factor IX levels may be risk factors for thrombotic diseases,[245,246] it seems unlikely that prolonged superphysiologic levels of factor VIII or factor IX would ensue from current gene transfer technology. Factor VIII and factor IX knockout mice[247–250] and spontaneous hemophilia A and B dog colonies[67,68,251–253] have facilitated preclinical gene therapy development. It also has proved possible to detect epitope-tagged human factor VIII[254] or normal human factor IX[255–258] in normal rhesus monkeys after gene transfer with various vectors, which permits testing of gene transfer vectors in nonhuman primates.

Skin fibroblasts or keratinocytes, readily obtained and easily transduced by gene transfer vectors, may be reintroduced to the patient for delivery of the secreted protein to the bloodstream. Therapeutic levels of factor IX or factor VIII have been achieved in rodents using this approach.[259–264] A recurring problem is the lack of sustained expression of factor VIII or factor IX, which may be due to cell-mediated immunity or promoter shutdown in implanted cells.[265] Factor VIII-transfected skin fibroblasts reimplanted in the omentum of hemophilia A subjects in a phase I trial achieved levels that were only marginally therapeutic and were not sustained.[266]

Gene transfer to muscle cells can be performed ex vivo or in vivo, although the latter approach is more practical because of the lack of suitable human muscle cell lines that can be used in immune-competent humans.

The most successful application of in vivo gene therapy has been gene transfer with adeno-associated virus (AAV) vectors. AAV vectors can transfer only DNA with a total length of less than 4.5 kilobases, which is sufficient for factor IX gene transfer but not for factor VIII gene transfer. In vivo preclinical studies with AAV vectors in hemo-

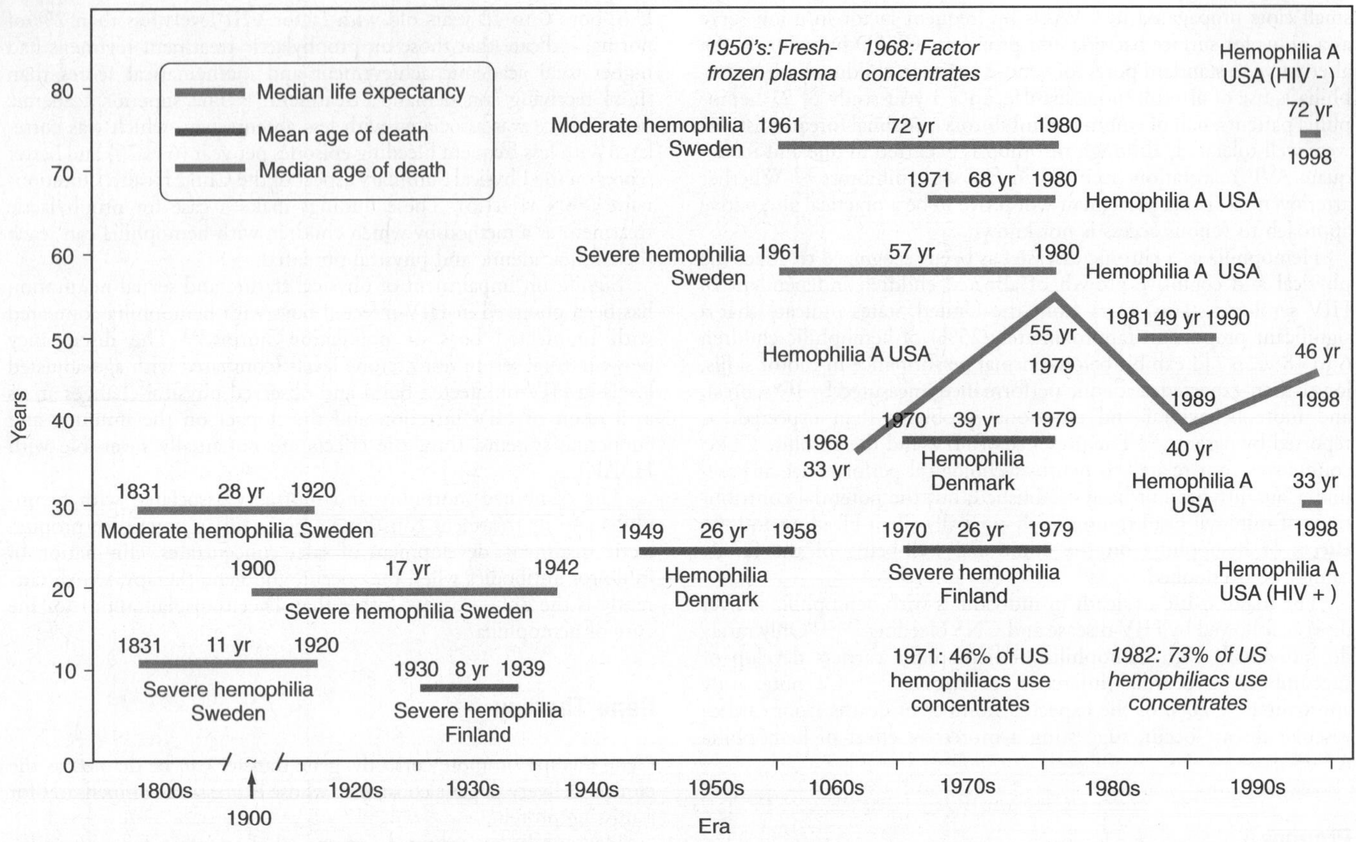

Figure 125–6 Effect of therapy with plasma and plasma-derived factor concentrates on the prognosis of hemophilia. The natural history of hemophilia in the era before the advent of effective therapy is documented in the Scandinavian data from the nineteenth and early twentieth centuries. Progress is seen beginning in the 1950s and 1960s with the introduction of plasma, cryoprecipitate, and factor concentrates. The effect of human immunodeficiency virus (HIV) infection on life expectancy in the 1980s is especially pronounced in the United States, where nearly all patients with severe hemophilia received concentrates made from pooled contaminated plasma. The subsequent elimination of HIV and hepatitis virus from factor concentrates has permitted their use, with minimal risk for viral infection. The median age at death for patients with hemophilia in the United States has risen, from a local nadir of 40 years in 1989 to 46 years as of 1998. The dramatic effect of HIV infection is apparent when the data for HIV-seropositive and HIV-seronegative patients in the United States are compared.

philia B knockout mice and hemophilia B dogs have shown that clinically relevant levels of factor IX in the plasma can be achieved for sustained periods using this approach.[267–274] A key problem directly related to the use of muscle as a target for gene transfer has been poor delivery of recombinant factor IX from muscle into plasma because of binding of factor IX by type IV collagen.[275] Clinical trials of AAV factor IX gene transfer in vivo targeting muscle have demonstrated therapeutically significant plasma factor IX levels (approximately 1% of normal) at doses of 2×10^{11} vector genomes per kilogram of body weight.[276] Although the trial was an open label study and a placebo effect cannot be excluded, patients did report a lower frequency of joint bleeds.[266] Fortunately, there were no inhibitors or other safety issues in these subjects.[277] However, long-term followup of these patients and two subsequent groups receiving threefold and ninefold higher vector doses, although not associated with toxicity or inhibitor formation, showed no improvement from the initial results.[278] Levels greater than 1% are unlikely to be achieved with higher doses because the volume and number of intramuscular injections become impractical.

Hepatocytes, which synthesize plasma proteins including factors VIII and IX as well as albumin, may be transduced by various vectors. As with muscle cells, hepatocytes are not easily propagated ex vivo, but in vivo gene transfer has been accomplished in animals using adenovirus, AAV, and retrovirus vectors. Adenovirus vectors are capable of high-efficiency factor VIII or IX gene transfer to hepatocytes in vivo in mice,[279–291] monkeys,[254,256,257] and hemophilic dogs,[292–296] although this is limited by the lack of integration of the vector DNA into the target cell DNA and gradual loss of gene expression. Adenovirus vector proteins may be toxic by inducing the cytokine cascade,[297] which may be immediately toxic to the recipient, by removing transduced cells by cell-mediated immunity, and by inducing the formation of antibodies to the expressed gene.[256,293,294,298] Based on the observation that removal of adenovirus genes may permit longer periods of gene expression and reduced immune response,[298] gutted adenoviral vectors (most of the adenovirus genes deleted) have been tested for hemophilia gene therapy[284,287,299–301] but are limited by problems in large-scale production. Clinical use of adenovirus vectors also is limited by the common presence of neutralizing antibodies in the population and the likelihood of ubsequent anamnestic response with repeated administration of the vector.[302]

AAV-mediated factor VIII gene transfer to liver has been performed in animals[303–305] but because of size constraints of vector DNA packaging, AAV gene transfer to liver has focused primarily on factor IX. In vivo gene transfer of factor IX by intravenous, portal vein, or hepatic artery injection of AAV vectors has resulted in expression of factor IX in mice,[306–314] dogs,[307,315,316] and nonhuman primates.[258] However, although transient therapeutic levels of factor IX (>10% of normal) were achieved in hemophilia B patients for up to several weeks,[317] levels were not sustained, coincident with immune-mediated elimination of vector-transduced hepatocytes as evidenced by asymptomatic liver transaminase elevation and T-cell reactivity to AAV capsid proteins.[278,317] Vector shedding in the semen was detected in several subjects but was asymptomatic and transient[318] and was not predicted in animals.[319] Thus, even if reasonably safe, repeated administration of AAV-factor IX vector is hampered by the humoral immunity to vector capsid proteins.

Although long-term expression of clotting factor and phenotypic correction of hemophilia A and B have been accomplished in animal models of hemophilia by retroviral vector given systemically,[320] in bone marrow stromal cells, epidermis, or rapidly dividing hepatoycytes,[321] and by AAV vector in skeletal muscle[278] and in mature hepatocytes,[317] long-lasting expression has not been accomplished in humans.[278,317,320] Some of the new gene transfer approaches being developed in murine hemophilia models include assessment of transient cytotoxic suppression of the acute humoral response to AAV-mediated gene transfer, induction of immune tolerance to factor IX by hepatic gene transfer,[322] factor VIII-targeted expression in megakaryocytes,[323] and endothelial targeted factor VIII expression by a sleeping beauty transposon.[324] Gene therapy in hemophilia will become practicable when the emerging issues of vector safety, vector immune response, and inhibitor antibody formation are eliminated and optimal levels of transgene expression are determined. Differing approaches to gene transfer likely will be needed in hemophilia (e.g., hepatocyte-directed gene transfer might be avoided in patients with underlying liver disease).

Interest continues in the development of factor VIII and factor IX products with lower immunogenicity, longer duration, and greater efficacy. A number of potential new products are in the pipeline, including substituted or mutated factor VIII A2, C2 immunogenic epitopes to reduce inhibitor formation[325] and pegylated factor VIII molecules of longer duration.[326] There Progress is being made with regulation of protein expression (when gene transfer becomes a reality), including use of silencing mRNA that allows for transcription correction or enhanced functional factor IX production.[327]

Acknowledgment
The opinions expressed in this chapter do not constitute U.S. government policy.

SUGGESTED READINGS

Astermark J, Donfield SM, DiMichele DM, et al: A randomized comparison of bypassing agents in hemophilia complicated by an inhibitor: The FEIB Novoseven Comparative (FENOC) Study. Blood 109:546, 2007.
Among the first randomized trials to compare bypassing agents with activated factor VIIa in inhibitor treatment.

Blajchman MA, Vamvakas EC: The continuing risk of transfusion-transmitted infections. N Engl J Med 355:1303, 2006.
Up-to-date summary and discussion of the current risks of transmissible agent risk of plasma.

High KA: Gene transfer for hemophilia: can therapeutic efficacy in large animals be safely translated to patients? J Thromb Haemost 3:1682, 2005.
Excellent review of current state of the art and the difficulties in predicting human immune response from animal models.

Kulkarni R: Perinatal management of newborns with hemophilia. Br J Haematol 112:264, 2001.
Outstanding review of the problems and approach to management of infants with hemophilia.

Lorenzo JI, Lopez A, Altisent C, Anzar JA: Incidence of factor VIII inhibitors in severe haemophilia: The importance of patient age. Br J Haematol 113:600, 2001.
Careful detailed analysis of time to development of inhibitors and factor usage in hemophilia.

Loveland KA, Stehbens J, Contant C, et al: Hemophilia growth and development study: Baseline neurodevelopmental findings. J Pediatr Psychol 19:223, 1994.
Important study assessing the impact of hemophilia and its complications on neurologic development.

Lusher JM, Arkin S, Abildgaard CF, Schwarz RS: Recombinant factor VIII for the treatment of previously untreated patients with hemophilia A. Safety, efficacy, and development of inhibitors. N Engl J Med 328:453, 1993.
Landmark study defining the safety and efficacy of recombinant factor concentrate in hemophilia A.

Mannucci PM, Tuddenheim EGD: Medical progress: the hemophilias: From royal genes to gene therapy. N Engl J Med 344:1773, 2001.
Outstanding and thorough review of the clinical, laboratory, treatment, and management of the hemophilic patient.

Manco-Johnson MJ, Abshitre TC, Shapiro AD, et al. Prophylaxis versus episodic treatment to prevent joint disease in boys with severe hemophilia. N Engl J Med 357:535, 2007.
First randomized clinical trial establishing the efficacy and safety of primary prophylaxis in the prevention of joint bleeding in children with hemophilia.

Naylor JA, Nicholson P, Goodeve A, et al: A novel DNA inversion causing severe hemophilia A. Blood 87:3255, 1996.
Landmark paper describing the intron 22 inversion mutation that underlies nearly half of cases with severe hemophilia A.

Nelson MD Jr, Maeder MA, Usner D, et al: Prevalence and incidence of intracranial haemorrhage in a population of children with haemophilia: The Hemophilia Growth and Development Study. Haemophilia 5:306, 1999.
Important study assessing the problem of intracranial hemorrhage and impact on growth and development in children with hemophilia.

Pipe WE: The promise and challenges of bioengineered recombinant clotting factors. J Thromb Haemost 3:1692, 2005.
Cogent review of new concepts in bioengineering factor molecules with longer half-life and greater efficacy.

Ragni MV: Impact of human immunodeficiency virus (HIV) on progression to end-stage liver disease in individuals with hemophilia and hepatitis C. J Infect Dis 183:1112, 2001.
Current understanding of the impact of HIV on progression of end-stage liver disease in individuals with hemophilia.

Soucie JM, Muss R, Evatt B, et al: Mortality among males with hemophilia: relations with source of medical care. The Hemophilia Surveillance Project Investigators. Blood 96:437, 2000.
Evidence-based description of the negative impact on hemophilia life expectancy of receiving care outside hemophilia treatment centers.

Triemstra M, Rosendaal FR, Smit C, et al: Mortality in patients with hemophilia. Changes in a Dutch population from 1986 to 1992 and 1973 to 1986. Ann Intern Med 123:823, 1995.
Summary of impact of HIV and HCV on hemophilia mortality in the last 30 years.

Valentino LA, Ewenstein B, Navickis RJ, Wilkes MM: Central venous access devices in hemophilia: A meta-analysis. Haemophilia 10:134, 2004.
Meta-analysis of central venous access device infection in hemophilia.

Wiedel J: Arthroscopic synovectomy: State of the art. Haemophilia 8:372, 2002.
State-of-the-art paper defining the role, indications, and outcomes of arthroscopic synovectomy in hemophilia.

REFERENCES

For complete list of references log onto www.expertconsult.com

CHAPTER 126

INHIBITORS IN HEMOPHILIA A AND B

Ara Metjian and Barbara A. Konkle

Patients with factor VIII deficiency (hemophilia A) or factor IX deficiency (hemophilia B) are at risk for developing neutralizing antibodies after receiving factor replacement therapy. Patients with severe factor VIII deficiency (<1%) are particularly at risk. With the availability of plasma-derived and recombinant replacement products safe from transmission of known infectious agents, the development of inhibitors has become the major complication of hemophilia treatment.

Inhibitor formation in hemophilia was first reported in 1941.[1] A 44-year-old man with classic hemophilia had been treated numerous times with blood products, and his coagulation time subsequently became refractory to transfusions. The authors realized that transfusion may have caused this heretofore unknown complication and suggested that coagulation times should be checked after administration of blood products to monitor for the phenomenon. This report soon was followed by numerous cases[2–5] reporting the development of a substance that counteracted infused blood product components. The nature of the inhibitor was shown to be an IgG antibody of the IgG4 subclass.[6]

HEMOPHILIA A

Epidemiology

The formation of inhibitors is more common in hemophilia A than in hemophilia B.[7] In hemophilia A, the severe phenotype most often is due to a null mutation, which is less common in hemophilia B. Null mutations result in a complete absence of the protein product and are more likely to predispose to inhibitor formation. Second, factor IX shares significant homology with the other vitamin K-dependent clotting factors, possibly protecting against inhibitor development.[8] Finally, it is hypothesized that because factor IX is a smaller and more abundant protein than factor VIII, enough protein may cross the placenta to induce tolerance in the developing fetus.[8]

Patients with severe hemophilia are at highest risk for inhibitor formation. Among those with hemophilia A, approximately 30% of patients with severe disease will develop an inhibitor versus 3% of those with moderate hemophilia and 0.3% with mild hemophilia.[9] Inhibitor formation occurs early after initiation of replacement therapy. Data from prospective clinical trials of recombinant factor VIII reveal that inhibitor development typically arises within a median of 8 to 10 exposure days, but a wide range is not uncommon.[10] The risk of inhibitor development decreases with more days of treatment and is extremely uncommon after 150 exposure days. For patients with mild or moderate disease, inhibitors are reported to develop after periods of intense replacement, during times of surgery or other "inflammatory states."[9]

Both genetic and environmental factors place individuals at risk for inhibitor development (Table 126–1). Family history of inhibitor formation, race, and underlying mutation resulting in the hemophilia are important genetic risk factors. Among many studies, the Malmö International Brother Study, which examined the genetics of monozygotic and dizygotic twins and of brother pairs, found an inhibitor rate that was higher than could be explained by chance alone. Having a first-degree relative with an inhibitor raised the risk of inhibitor development threefold, resulting in an approximately 50% chance of inhibitor development compared to a baseline 15% risk.[11,12]

Patient race as a risk factor was first noted in studies examining the prevalence of inhibitors.[13] In the prospective recombinant factor VIII trials, African Americans were observed to have twice the rate of inhibitor formation compared to Caucasians. In a retrospective survey, Latinos were observed to have a trend toward a higher prevalence rate. Although no definitive genetic cause has been identified, this observation implicates a broad genetic mechanism in inhibitor formation.[14,15]

The type of mutation is an important factor in inhibitor formation.[8] Three general categories of mutations in factor VIII place a patient at "high risk" for inhibitor formation: (a) inversions of intron 22, (b) large deletions affecting more than one domain, and (c) nonsense mutations involving the light chain.[7] These mutations either eliminate circulating factor VIII or alter exposed areas on factor VIII to make exogenously administered factor VIII appear "foreign."[16] The "low-risk" mutations consist of small deletions/insertions, missense mutations, and splice site mutations. It has been postulated that these mutations, although significant enough to diminish the coagulant activity of factor VIII, even to undetectable levels by our current clinical assays, allow generation of enough endogenous factor VIII such that tolerance can be achieved.[7]

Despite the strong genetic influences that underlie inhibitor formation, there exist clinical observations of an environmental pressure for the creation or inhibition of inhibitors. First, the Malmö International Brother Study cohort contains discordant monozygotic twins (i.e., identical twin brothers with the same mutations) of which only one brother developed an inhibitor.[17] Second, among the high-risk mutations, only 30% to 35% of patients with hemophilia and the intron 22 inversion form inhibitors. Even with multidomain deletions, the highest estimated risk approaches 75%,[18] implying other patients with the same mutation are somehow protected against inhibitor formation.

Age at first treatment has been evaluated as a risk factor for inhibitor development, and a relationship with earlier exposure to factor VIII-containing products and the development of inhibitors has been observed.[19–22] This is in contrast to a case-control study that observed an initial trend toward an increase in inhibitor formation in children who were treated at a younger age. However, when the severity of the genetic mutation was factored into the analysis, it ceased to be statistically significant. In fact, there appeared to be a protective effect against the formation of inhibitors when children were started on prophylaxis early in life.[23]

The method of factor VIII infusion in provoking an alloimmune response is another matter of speculation. Administration of factor VIII via continuous infusion has the advantage of requiring less factor replacement and avoiding the peaks and troughs seen with bolus intravenous administration.[24] However, intense replacement of factor VIII, especially in the form of a continuous infusion, has been observed to provoke the generation of inhibitors in patients who are otherwise considered to be at low risk.[25,26] This usually is seen in patients with mild hemophilia A who are undergoing surgery. These patients have less historical exposure to factor concentrate, which could place them at higher risk for inhibitor development when exposed to concentrate.[27]

Table 126–1 Risk Factors for Inhibitor Formation

Established Risk Factors	Possible[a]
Type (hemophilia A > hemophilia B)	Age at first exposure
Severity (severe > mild/moderate)	Type of factor concentrate (plasma-derived vs recombinant factor VIII)
Underlying mutation (e.g., intron 22)	Method of infusion (continuous vs bolus)
Race (African/Latino > Caucasian)	Prophylaxis vs on-demand
Family history	

aConflicting results reported in the literature.

The most controversial "environmental" factor is the type of factor VIII concentrate used, low-/intermediate-purity plasma-derived factor VIII versus high-purity plasma-derived factor VIII or recombinant factor VIII, in inhibitor formation. For more than 15 years, the debate on whether recombinant factor VIII leads to a higher inhibitor incidence remained largely unresolved.[28,29] This originated with the prospective trials of first-generation recombinant factor VIII in previously untreated patients. Part of the trial design consisted of frequent monitoring for inhibitor formation at least every 3 months.[30,31] In the Kogenate trial, the total incidence of any inhibitor formation in patients with severe hemophilia A was 29.2% within a median of 9 exposure days.[32] A similar inhibitor incidence rate of 31.5% was found in a prospective trial of Recombinate.[33] Thus, compared to historical values and older retrospective studies that used low-/intermediate-purity plasma-derived factor VIII with reported rates of approximately 10%,[34] recombinant factor VIII appeared to be more immunogenic.

A number of factors likely account for this observation. The recombinant factor VIII trials of previously untreated patients were the first large prospective clinical trials of hemophilia treatment, so their comparison to anecdotal or retrospective case reports and case series is largely untenable.[30–33] The trials of previously untreated patient were also the first to monitor routinely for the development of inhibitors prospectively. Prior to this study, historical references tested for inhibitors only when clinically indicated, and even then testing was performed twice yearly at most. Prospective monitoring of patients receiving high-purity plasma-derived factor VIII revealed a similar inhibitor rate.[35] Continued analysis of the recombinant factor VIII trials results showed that almost half (11/23) of the inhibitors in the Kogenate trial were transient in nature, decreasing the prevalence of inhibitors upon extended observation.[32] A similar pattern was observed in the Recombinate trial, in which alloantibodies disappeared in 14 of 22 study subjects who had developed an inhibitor, even with continued treatment, reducing the prevalence rate to 11.1%.[33] The older studies likely missed these ephemeral inhibitors.

Potential causes of increased immunogenicity of factor VIII products include neoantigen formation during manufacturing and, among other variables, the absence of von Willebrand factor (VWF), which is present in low-/intermediate-purity plasma-derived factor replacements.[21,36] New factor VIII concentrates can be immunogenic, as in the case of a double virus inactivated factor VIII product that was used in Belgium[37] and two new plasma-derived factor VIII products that were used in the Netherlands and Belgium.[38,39] However, when currently available factor VIII products were given to previously treated patients, the rate of inhibitor formation has been low, confirming low immunogenicity in this setting.[40]

The role of VWF in the factor concentrate is under study. Compared to historical controls using VWF-containing concentrates, lower response rates of immune tolerance have been reported with use of recombinant factor VIII than with use of VWF-containing plasma-derived factor VIII.[41] Goudemand et al.[21] reported a 2.5- to 3-fold increased risk for inhibitor generation when recombinant factor VIII was used. A possible mechanism is that VWF protects factor VIII from endocytosis by dendritic cells and subsequent presentation to factor VIII-specific T cells.[42]

Pathobiology

Circulating antigens initially are taken up by antigen-presenting cells.[43] These proteins undergo proteolysis, and the digested peptides are placed upon major histocompatibility (MHC) II molecules for presentation to CD4+ T cells. Interactions between antigen-presenting cells and CD4+ T cells include binding between MHC II and the T-cell receptor and costimulatory molecules. The costimulation allows for activation and differentiation into T_H1 or T_H2 cells. T_H2 cells secrete interleukin (IL)-4, IL-5, and IL-10, which promote the synthesis of noncomplement binding immunoglobulins, namely IgG4.[43]

Once the appropriate B cells have been stimulated, the expressed immunoglobulin is secreted, and further changes in the B-cell genome and evolution enhance its binding and eventually its inhibitory characteristics. The ultimate production of a polyclonal antibody response leads to disruption of factor VIII function on numerous levels.[44] These phenomena have provided an in vivo revelation of the structure, function, and biochemical impact of factor VIII inhibitors.

The role of MHC II alleles in factor VIII inhibitor formation has been investigated. There are some weak associations, with some MHC class I/II alleles being "risk" alleles.[45,46] T-cell involvement in inhibitor formation is evidenced by the presence of isotype switching and somatic hypermutation of the B cells, both of which are T cell dependent.[47] There exists within the factor VIII molecule several epitopes against which CD4+ T cells react strongly.[48–50]

Factor VIII exists as a heterodimer, with a heavy chain containing the A1, A2, and B domains connected with a light chain containing the A3, C1, and C2 domains (Fig. 126–1). Short intervening acidic regions (*a1*, *a2*, and *a3*) aid in binding to factor X and serve as important sites for proteolysis by thrombin and factor Xa.[51] By serving as a cofactor for factor IX in the "Xase" complex, it aids in the conversion of factor X to its active form, factor Xa, which along with factor V on a phospholipid bilayer cleaves prothrombin to form thrombin, which in turn amplifies the coagulation cascade (see Chapter 123).[52]

Normally when factor VIII is secreted, it is noncovalently bound to vWF via the light chain, particularly through interactions with *a3* and the C2 domain.[53] Upon thrombin activation, factor VIIIa dissociates from VWF and via the C2 domain, which is no longer bound by VWF, binds to phosphatidylserine on the platelet membrane.[54] Inhibitors interrupt this process through a number of different mechanisms (see Fig. 126–1): by preventing factor VIII interaction with VWF, thereby significantly decreasing its half-life; by slowing the release of factor VIIIa from VWF after thrombin activation, increasing the time for inactivation prior to association with the Xase complex; and by preventing C2 domains from binding with phospholipids.[55–59]

Other mechanisms of inhibition rely upon antibodies that recognize the Arg484-Ile508 epitope in the A2 domain, which is responsible for binding with the protease domain of factor IXa.[60] Interference at this site interrupts the cofactor activity with factor IXa, inhibiting Xase function.[61] When bound by inhibitors, the A3 domain, which contains a binding site for factor IX, prevents factor VIII from binding to factor IX, inhibiting the Xase complex.[62–64]

Although inhibitors that react with the acidic regions and the A1 and C1 domains are reported,[65–67] they usually constitute the minority of the polyclonal immune response in hemophilia A. Patients treated with plasma-derived factor VIII tend to have antibodies directed against the light chain and the C2 domain, whereas patients treated with recombinant factor VIII have antibodies targeting the A2 domain.[68] One other mechanism of inhibition is an alloantibody that catalyzes proteolysis of factor VIII.[69–71]

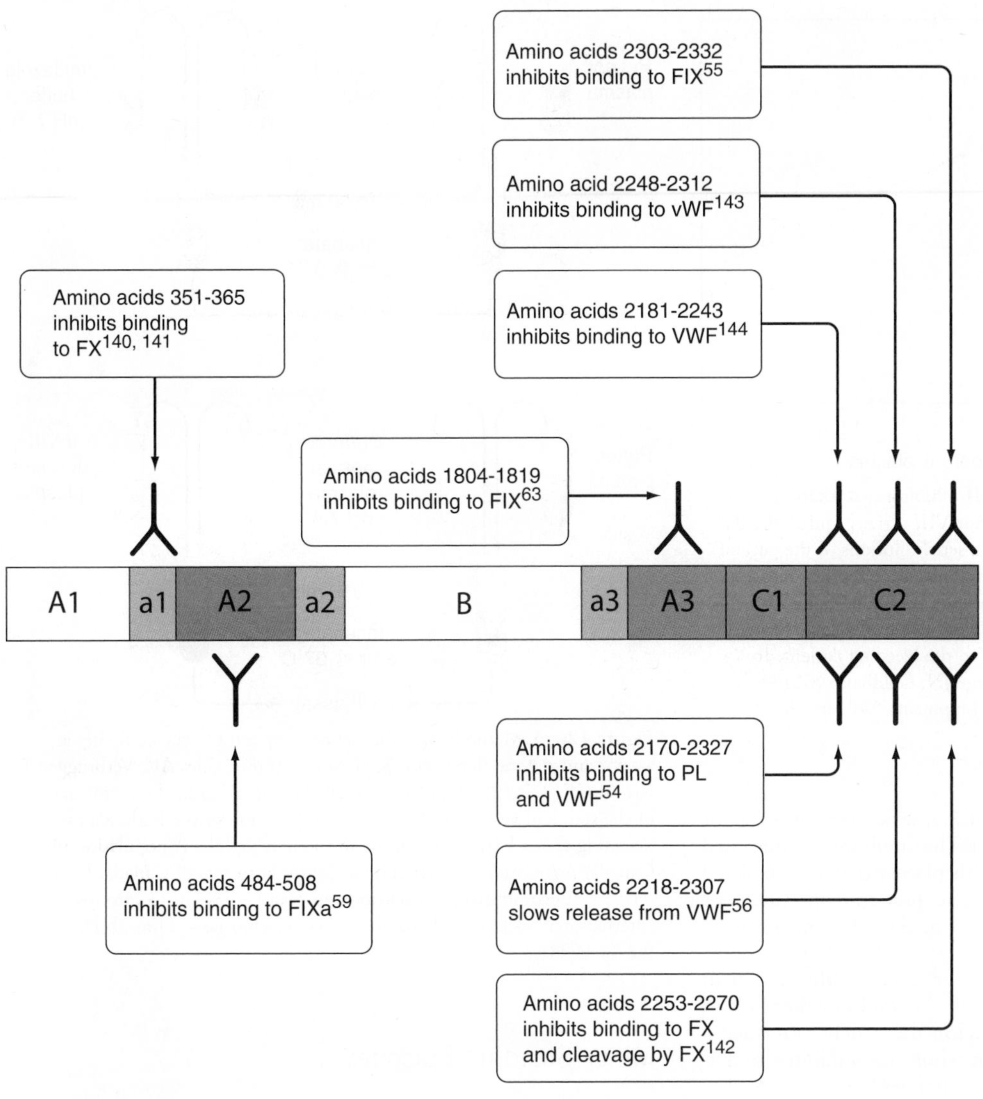

Figure 126–1 Factor VIII domains and binding site by amino acid location and effect on factor VIII. Intensity of color reflects the frequency of inhibitors to the epitope.[140–144] FIX, factor IX; FIXa, activated factor IX; FX, factor X; PL, phospholipid; VWF, von Willebrand factor.

Clinical Manifestations

In patients with severe hemophilia, acquiring an inhibitor does not initially increase the frequency of bleeding. However, as treatment options are less effective in preventing and treating bleeding, these patients are more likely to develop damaged joints that bleed more frequently.[72] Inadequate treatment of joint bleeds may result in progressive severe arthropathy with resultant disability. General health status and quality of life of these patients are reduced compared to those without inhibitors.[73] They have more hospital visits and absences from school or work, and they are more likely to need assistive devices such as a wheelchair or crutches.[74] In the past, development of an inhibitor increased the mortality risk, but with current therapy the mortality rate is nearly identical to the rate in patients without an inhibitor.[75]

In patients with mild to moderate hemophilia, development of an inhibitor usually occurs after a period of intense factor replacement.[9,26] The clinical indication that a patient with mild to moderate hemophilia has developed an inhibitor is the patient's failure to respond to factor replacement or his or her lack of appropriate recovery after factor VIII infusion. Even worse, a patient with mild disease may convert to a severe phenotype and present with spontaneous bleeding, reminiscent of severe hemophilia, when the inhibitor cross-reacts with endogenous factor VIII, reducing the patient's factor VIII activity to less than 1%.[76]

Any person with hemophilia, regardless of severity, who is undergoing treatment and fails to respond should be promptly evaluated for the development of an inhibitor. Any change in clinical responsiveness should be investigated for the development of an inhibitor.[77–79] Testing a patient for the presence of an inhibitor prior to any major surgical procedure is recommended.

Laboratory Diagnosis

In 1975 the Bethesda assay was devised as a simple and reproducible method for determining antibody titer. It is based on the ability of patient plasma to inactivate factor VIII in normal plasma. The result is expressed in Bethesda units (BU).[80] Patient plasma is serially diluted in normal plasma, incubated for 2 hours at 37°C, and residual factor VIII activity measured using a one-stage assay. One BU correlates to a patient factor VIII activity of 50%. A standard curve is generated, and the patient's plasma is diluted until factor VIII activity is between 25% and 75%, the linear portion of the standard curve. The inhibitor units are read from the graph and multiplied by the dilution factor to determine the number of BU in the undiluted plasma (Fig. 126–2).

In order to improve the specificity and reliability of the Bethesda assay, two groups developed the Nijmegen modification to the Bethesda assay.[81] The Bethesda assay can produce false-positives results, usually evidenced as low-titer inhibitors due to decreased factor VIII activity as pH increased and protein concentration decreased. The Nijmegen modification made two important changes to the Bethesda assay. (a) The normal plasma and control mixture

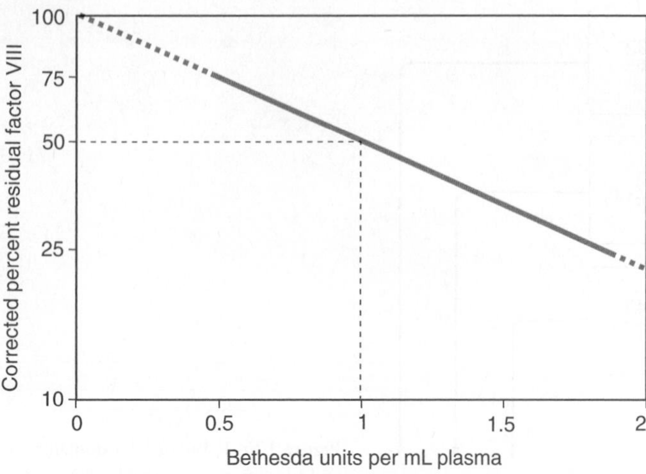

Figure 126–2 Bethesda assay for factor VIII inhibitor quantitation. Relationship between corrected residual factor VIII activity and Bethesda titer is shown. If the result is less than 25%, serial dilutions of the patient's plasma are tested until the result is between 25% and 75%. The result is multiplied by the dilution to assign the Bethesda titer. One Bethesda unit is defined by a corrected residual factor VIII of 50% in the assay (dotted line). (From Konkle BA: Clinical approach to the bleeding patient. In Colman RW, Marder VJ, Clowes AW, George JN, Goldhaver SZ [eds.]: Hemostasis and Thrombosis. Philadelphia, Lippincott, Williams & Wilkins, 2006, p 1147.)

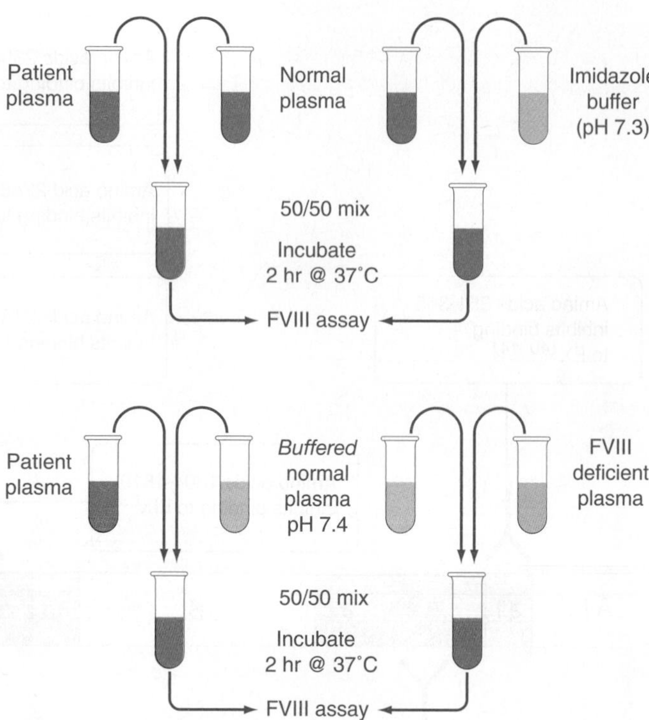

Figure 126–3 Methodologic differences between the classic Bethesda assay[80] and the modified Nijmegen assay.[81] (From Giles AR, Verbruggen B, Rivard GE, Teitel J, Walker I: A detailed comparison of the performance of the standard versus the Nijmegen modification of the Bethesda assay in detecting factor VIII:C inhibitors in the haemophilia A population of Canada. Association of Hemophilia Centre Directors of Canada. Factor VIII/IX Subcommittee of Scientific and Standardization Committee of International Society on Thrombosis and Haemostasis. Thromb Haemost 9:872, 1998.)

were buffered with imidazole to a pH of 7.4, which prevented factor VIII:C inactivation at higher pH. (b) The imidazole buffer used in the control mixture was replaced with plasma that was depleted of factor VIII in order to have similar protein concentrations (Fig. 126–3). This is the recommended method for diagnosis of inhibitors.[82]

Based upon the results of the inhibitor assay, a value less than 5 BU is considered a low-titer inhibitor. If the inhibitor titer fails to rise despite repeated challenges with factor, the patient is termed a low responder. In contrast, a patient in whom the inhibitor titer is greater than 5 BU is considered a high responder.[83]

Pharmacokinetics studies should be performed in patients who show clinical behavior of inhibitor formation but have a negative inhibitor assay.[77,79] Although a distinct minority of the inhibitor repertoire, not all antibodies that are raised against factor VIII interfere with its coagulant function. These inhibitors shorten the half-life of infused factor VIII and are suspected only when factor VIII recovery or half-life is shortened.[44]

Monitoring for inhibitor development in previously untreated patients is of paramount importance, especially when starting treatment or prophylaxis because inhibitor development occurs early in the course of treatment.[30–32] Guidelines recommend screening previously untreated patients every fifth exposure day up to the 20th exposure day, and then every 3 months up until the 150th exposure day.[77,79] Repeat testing should be performed before any invasive procedure or elective operation.[77,79] If porcine factor VIII is available, antiporcine antibody titers can be tested to determine the feasibility of this treatment option.[84]

Treatment

The standard of care dictates that patients with hemophilia receive comprehensive and routine therapy at a hemophilia treatment center having specialized care and experience in the treatment of individuals with severe bleeding disorders. In cases requiring emergency treatment or surgery, patients should be transferred to the hemophilia treatment center after their condition has been stabilized (see box on Treatment of Bleeding in a Patient with Factor VIII Deficiency and an Inhibitor).

Minor Bleeding Episodes

In low responding patients with a known inhibitor titer, larger doses of factor VIII can be given to overcome the inhibitor and provide therapeutic levels of factor VIII. Optimally, the titer is *less than* 5 BU. Equation 126–1 approximates the dose necessary to overcome a low titer:

Loading Dose =
2 (Body Weight)[(80)(100 − Hematocrit)/100] (B.U.)

However, after this loading dose, factor levels must be determined to ensure that therapeutic levels are sustained.[85] Treatment should be maintained ideally with continuous infusion. If bolus dosing is used, the treatment interval will need to be shortened. With both approaches, factor levels must be followed closely.

In high responding patients who have inhibitor titers that have decreased to *less than* 10 BU, factor VIII replacement therapy should be avoided. This attempt to avoid an anamnestic response is made for two reasons. If immune tolerance therapy is possible, keeping the titer low will increase the chances for success. More importantly, a low titer will allow for use of factor VIII therapy in bleeds that are life or limb threatening. Controversy exists whether anamnesis occurs with activated prothrombin complex concentrates, which contain a small amount of factor VIII.[10,77–79]

For patients with mild to moderate hemophilia and an inhibitor, treatment with desmopressin (desamino-8-arginine vasopressin [DDAVP]) is an alternative. These patients should undergo DDAVP testing in advance to gauge their response. DDAVP can be used prior to minor procedures and in cases of mild bleeding.[86]

Treatment of Bleeding in a Patient with Factor VIII Deficiency and an Inhibitor

Low Titer, Low Responder

Mild Bleeding

- Local and conservative measures, such as rest, ice, compression, and elevation
- If the patient is known to respond to DDAVP (i.e., mild hemophilia A), 0.3 μg/kg IV or 300 μg intranasal (150 μg for patients <50 kg), for minor bleeding or treatment before minor surgery
- Antifibrinolytic therapy (ε-aminocaproic acid or tranexamic acid) for mucosal bleeding
- Factor VIII dosing to raise the level to 50%
- Recombinant factor VIIa, 90–120 μg/kg, followed by 90 μg/kg every 2–3 hours
- Activated prothrombin complex concentrates, 50–100 U/kg, with maximum daily dose of 200 U/kg
- Concurrent treatment with antifibrinolytics is discouraged

Life- or Limb-Threatening Bleeding

- Factor VIII dosing to maintain factor VIII activity levels at 100%
- Recombinant factor VIIa, 90–120 μg/kg, followed by 90 μg/kg every 2–3 hours
- Activated prothrombin complex concentrates, 50–100 U/kg, with maximum daily dose of 200 U/kg
- Concurrent treatment with antifibrinolytics is discouraged

Low Titer, High Responder

Mild Bleeding

- Local and conservative measures, such as rest, ice, compression, and elevation
- If the patient is known to respond to DDAVP (i.e., mild hemophilia A), 0.3 μg/kg IV or 300 μg untranasal (150 μg for patients <50 kg), for minor bleeding or treatment before minor surgery
- Antifibrinolytic therapy (ε-aminocaproic acid or tranexamic acid) for mucosal bleeding
- Recombinant factor VIIa, 90–120 μg/kg, followed by 90 μg/kg every 2–3 hours
- Activated prothrombin complex concentrates, 50–100 U/kg, with maximum daily dose of 200 U/kg
- May induce anamnesis

Life- or Limb-Threatening Bleeding

- Factor VIII in high doses to maintain levels of 100 U/mL
- Frequent monitoring for an anamnestic response, usually within 5–7 days
- After the anamnestic response develops:
    - Recombinant factor VIIa, 90–120 μg/kg, followed by 90 μg/kg every 2 hours
    - Activated prothrombin complex concentrates, 50–100 U/kg, with maximum daily dose of 200 U/kg

High Titer, High Responder

Mild Bleeding

- Local and conservative measures, such as rest, ice, compression, and elevation
- If the patient is known to respond to DDAVP (i.e., mild hemophilia A), 0.3 μg/kg IV or 300 μg/kg intranasal (150 μg/kg for patients <50 kg), for minor bleeding or treatment before minor surgery
- Antifibrinolytic therapy (κ-aminocaproic acid or tranexamic acid) for mucosal bleeding
- Recombinant factor VIIa, 90–120 μg/kg, followed by 90 μg/kg every 2–3 hours
- Activated prothrombin complex concentrates, 50–100 U/kg, with maximum daily dose of 200 U/kg
- Concurrent treatment with antifibrinolytics is discouraged

Life- or Limb-Threatening Bleeding

- If available, immunoadsorption can be attempted to rapidly lower the inhibitor titer so as to allow use of factor VIII
- Recombinant factor VIIa, 90–120 μg/kg, followed by 90 μg/kg every 2 hours
- Activated prothrombin complex concentrates, 50–100 U/kg, with maximum daily dose of 200 U/kg

Severe Bleeding Episodes

For patients who have an inhibitor titer less than 5 BU, use of factor VIII therapy should be considered if factor VIII levels can be monitored closely. This likely provides the most effective therapy if adequate factor VIII levels can be maintained. Patients should be monitored closely for anamnesis, which should be expected in patients with a history of a high-titer inhibitor, because switching to a bypassing agent will be needed.

In the case of a severe bleed or a life-threatening emergency, an immediate assay of the patient's inhibitor titer should be determined but should not delay initial treatment. For patients with a known and persistently high-titer antibody, prompt treatment should consist of therapy with a bypass agent, either an activated prothrombin complex concentrates or factor VIIa.[78,79]

Surgery

Surgery in patients with hemophilia, especially those who have an inhibitor, requires the involvement of an entire facility experienced in the preoperative and postoperative care of such patients.[87] However, treatment recommendations for surgical procedures are similar to those for hemorrhage. In a patient who is a low responder, adequate hemostasis can be achieved with higher doses of factor VIII. For the high responding patient, use of activated prothrombin complex concentrates or recombinant factor VIIa has been shown to be effective in the postoperative setting.[88–90]

Prothrombin Complex Concentrates

Prothrombin complex concentrates originally were used for treatment of hemophilia B. Their use evolved to encompass hemophilia A with inhibitors because of their thrombogenic properties. Prepared from large volumes of plasma, prothrombin complex concentrates contain the vitamin K-dependent clotting factors prothrombin, factor VII, factor IX, and factor X.[91] Heparin or antithrombin is added to some preparations to limit coagulation during the manufacturing process and administration. All prothrombin complex concentrate products undergo a viral inactivation process. In comparison to placebo, a prothrombin complex concentrate was effective in controlling approximately 50% of bleeding episodes in patients with inhibitors compared to 25% for product containing albumin alone.[92]

Activated Prothrombin Complex Concentrates

Activated prothrombin complex concentrates are prothrombin complex concentrates that undergo partial "activation" during the manufacturing process. Although results comparing prothrombin complex concentrates to activated prothrombin complex concentrates have not been definitive,[93,94] activated prothrombin complex concentrates may be more effective treatment and are more commonly used to treat bleeding in patients with FVIII inhibitors.[72,85,91,95]

Clinical studies have shown that activated prothrombin complex concentrates are effective in treating bleeding in 81% to 93% of joint bleeds.[96,97] Use of activated prothrombin complex concentrates has allowed for surgery in inhibitor patients and has been reported to be effective.[97] A review of surgical cases of patients with an inhibitor and an activated prothrombin complex concentrate showed adequate hemostatic control without any adverse outcomes.[88]

During an acute bleed, activated prothrombin complex concentrates are administered at 50–100 U/kg, every 6 to 12 hours based upon the clinical severity, with the maximum daily dose capped at 200 U/kg.[78] This broader time frame allows for use at home for treatment of acute bleeds, as well as prophylaxis. A study compared an activated prothrombin complex concentrate (factor eight inhibitor bypassing activity [FEIBA, Baxter], 85 IU/kg) with one to two doses of recombinant factor VIIa (NovoSeven [Novo Nordisk Health Care AG] ≈105 μg/kg) for response at 6 hours to treatment of joint bleeding. Although both products showed 80% to 90% efficacy at some time point, equivalency was not shown due to differences in rating by a substantial proportion of patients.[98]

Use of activated prothrombin complex concentrates is hampered by the lack of a laboratory test to measure efficacy, the possibility of anamnesis with the amounts of factor VIII present in the product, and the risk of thrombotic events. The risk of thrombosis is increased with dosing that varies from the recommended dosage and in patients with increased risk for thrombotic events (elderly, coronary artery disease).[77,78]

Recombinant Factor VIIa

Factor VIIa was purified from plasma and first used to treat a patient with an inhibitor in 1983.[99] Later it was produced by recombinant technology and found to be effective for treatment of bleeding and in allowing surgery. A randomized dose finding trial found recombinant factor VIIa to be effective in 71% of joint and muscle bleeds within two to three doses, given every 2 to 3 hours.[100] Likewise, a prospective randomized dose finding study in surgery found that although 35 μg/kg of recombinant factor VIIa was effective for minor procedures, 90 μg/kg was statistically superior in achieving adequate hemostasis during major surgical procedures, with an efficacy rate of 83% to 100%.[101] However, use of recombinant factor VIIa is limited by the lack of effective laboratory monitoring, very short half-life (≈2 hours) requiring frequent administration, potential for thrombotic events, and expense.[85]

For serious hemorrhages or for surgery, an initial dose of 90 μg/kg is recommended. Some experts advise an initial dose of 120 μg/kg, followed by the 90 μg/kg dose.[102] With serious bleeds or after surgery, current recommendations are to continue with dosing every 2 hours for 1 to 2 days and then to start tapering to every 3 hours for another 2 days, followed by every 4 to 6 hours for days 5 to 14, depending on the type of surgery.[103] Although continuous infusion is an option to decrease cost and avoid prolonged troughs, it still is being investigated as a viable alternative to 2-hour dosing.

Combining Bypass Agents

For bleeding that is unresponsive to treatment with an activated prothrombin complex concentrate or recombinant factor VIIa alone, use of both products in an alternating regimen has been reported.[104,105] This combination is not recommended by the product manufacturers. Laboratory tests document increased coagulation activation. Given the risk of thrombosis, this regimen should be considered only under extreme, emergent conditions.

Fibrinolytic Inhibitors

ε-Aminocaproic or tranexamic acid has a long safety record and is commonly used as a treatment alone or in combination with factor replacement for mucosal bleeding or dental procedures. Fibrinolytic inhibitors are routinely used with factor for orthopedic surgery.[106]

For children, ε-aminocaproic acid is administered at 50 to 100 mg/kg/dose every 6 hours. If used prior to a procedure, the first dose should be given 4 hours before the start of the procedure. In adults, a loading dose of 4 to 5 g is given initially, followed by 1 g/hour for 8 hours or until bleeding is controlled. Fibrinolytic inhibitors should not be used when activated prothrombin complex concentrates are used, and care must be used in the case of urogenital bleeding. These agents are considered safe for use with recombinant factor VIIa.[77]

Immune Tolerance Therapy

The ultimate therapy for a patient with hemophilia and an inhibitor is induction of immune tolerance. The goal of this procedure is eradication of the inhibitor. Successful immune induction therapy enables use of factor VIII replacement therapy for both acute bleeding and prophylaxis to prevent joint arthropathy.

The first episode of immune tolerance arose from an emergency situation in 1974 when a child with a high-titer inhibitor (>500 BU) required immediate treatment.[107] The clinical decision was made to treat the child with high doses of factor VIII and a prothrombin complex concentrate, which controlled the child's hemorrhage. A serendipitous finding was that the child's inhibitor titer fell to almost 40 BU. This marked the first episode where high-dose factor VIII led to a decrease in inhibitor titer and ushered in the "Bonn protocol," which uses high doses of factor VIII (100 IU/kg) given twice daily.[108,109] Activated prothrombin complex concentrates are administered based on the bleeding tendency of the patient. This regimen is followed until the inhibitor has disappeared, sometimes as long as 3 years.[107,110]

The Malmö protocol also developed out of the need for emergent elimination of an inhibitor in a patient with hemophilia B who required urgent orthopedic surgery.[111] Unique among other immune tolerance regimens, the Malmö protocol uses a number of immunomodulatory therapies to lower the inhibitor level. Among them is serial use of a *Staphylococcal aureus* protein A column to adsorb out the inhibitory immunoglobulin(s) until the inhibitor titer is less than 10 BU. This regimen is coupled with administration of intravenous immunoglobulin,[112] which is thought to exert antiidiotypic effects. Cyclophosphamide is given to prevent or attenuate the formation of new antibodies. Like the Bonn protocol, high doses of factor VIII are given so that the inhibitors are neutralized and therapeutic levels are maintained.[113,114]

In contrast to the other immune tolerance protocols that use higher doses of factor VIII as part of the regimen, a low-dose regime has been used with success. In 1981, the van Creveld clinic, which cares for a majority of the patients with hemophilia with inhibitors in the Netherlands, adopted a protocol of immune tolerance using low-dose factor VIII infusions, starting at 25 IU/kg every other day, a 16- to 24-fold less dose than the other high-dose immune tolerance protocols used. These studies found that low-dose factor VIII was very effective in inducing immune tolerance, without the need for immunoadsorption, immunosuppression, or lengthy treatment courses.[115–117]

Several retrospective immune tolerance registries have been established.[118–126] Although several key facets remain in disagreement with each other, most registries have found that the most consistent predictors of success were (a) beginning immune tolerance therapy when the inhibitor titer is as low as possible (ideally <10 BU), and (b) lower historical peak antibody titers.[122]

Uncertainty remains regarding the optimal total dose of factor VIII, the age at which to start immune tolerance therapy, the interval time between development of the inhibitor and start of immune tolerance therapy, the use of immunosuppressives, and especially the type of factor replacement used in immune tolerance therapy. Use of low-/intermediate-purity factor concentrate containing vWF may be more efficacious than use of recombinant factor VIII.[36,127,128] These questions currently are being addressed in a multinational immune tolerance trial comparing two different dosing regimens that allows investigators choice of treatment with a recombinant or a vWF-containing factor VIII product.[129]

HEMOPHILIA B

The development of inhibitors in hemophilia B follows the same general principles as in hemophilia A. Inhibitory antibodies arise after treatment with infused factor IX-containing products, and this phenomenon was observed very soon after hemophilia B was differentiated from hemophilia A.[130] However, several distinct differences in the epidemiology and treatment of hemophilia B deserve special mention. These differences include the lower incidence and prevalence of inhibitors in hemophilia B, the risk of anaphylaxis to infused factor IX-containing concentrates, the lower success rate of immune tolerance therapy, and the risk of nephrosis associated with immune tolerance therapy.[131]

Epidemiology

Overall, the incidence of inhibitors in severe hemophilia B is much less than that of severe hemophilia A (≈3% vs ≈30%).[132] A very-low-risk mutation for inhibitor development is one with a single amino acid substitution and is considered to have a risk of almost 0%, whereas an unknown genotype generally is assigned a risk of approximately 3%.[133] The risk of inhibitor development approaches 20% with more significant mutations such as frameshift mutations, premature stop codons, and splice site mutations.[133] Patients with hemophilia B who are at highest risk for development of inhibitors have a severe phenotype as a result of large gene deletions or another significant aberration of the gene product, such as nonsense mutations. Although these significant mutations affect only a fraction of the hemophilia B population, they account for approximately 50% of the inhibitor population.[133]

Diagnosis

Similar to hemophilia A, an inhibitor should be suspected in hemophilia B when a patient ceases to respond to conventional treatment. Given the possibility of anaphylaxis that may occur during the initial treatment episodes, patients with high-risk mutations must be regularly screened for the generation of inhibitors. The laboratory diagnosis for inhibitors in hemophilia B involves a modification of the Bethesda assay, in which factor IX-deficient plasma is used instead of factor VIII-deficient plasma.[77]

Treatment

Treatment of hemophilia B in patients with inhibitors mirrors that of hemophilia A, ranging from use of conservative local measures to infusion of bypassing agents. Both activated prothrombin complex concentrates and factor VIIa are useful for treatment of bleeding and for control of hemorrhage after surgery.[77] However, because activated prothrombin complex concentrates contain significant amounts of factor IX, recombinant factor VIIa is more commonly used.

A major complication is the development of anaphylaxis upon the initial receipt of factor IX concentrates. Although only an estimated 35 cases have been reported, given the paucity of hemophilia B patients with inhibitors, these cases nevertheless represent a significant complication.[131,134–136] Because these severe reactions occur only after initiation of treatment, they have been observed exclusively in children (median age 12 months), occurring at a median of 11 exposure days. The development of anaphylaxis also has been noted to occur at the same time as the appearance of an inhibitor. The major risk factor for developing an anaphylactic reaction is the presence of a null mutation, leading to an absence of circulating factor IX.[137]

Although experience with anaphylaxis occurring in response to factor replacement is limited by the relative scarcity of its occurrence, some general practice recommendations have been posed. For newly diagnosed hemophilia B patients, especially those with high-risk mutations, the initial treatments should be conducted in a medical facility with resuscitation equipment available.[131] Immune tolerance is generally ineffective in these patients, although tolerance to factor IX has been reported with progressively increasing doses of factor IX administered with hydrocortisone.[136]

Unlike hemophilia A, immune tolerance therapy in hemophilia B has a much lower rate of success.[131] This is further complicated by the risk of developing nephrotic syndrome during immune tolerance therapy, especially in patients who had an allergic reaction to factor IX replacement. The limited data available suggest that this syndrome is not due to immune complex deposition and is not responsive to corticosteroids.[138,139] The development of nephrosis should be monitored by frequent urinalysis during immune tolerance therapy. Should nephrosis occur, factor IX doses should be reduced or discontinued.[139]

SUGGESTED READINGS

Ananyeva NM, Lacroix-Desmazes S, Hauser CA, et al: Inhibitors in hemophilia A: Mechanisms of inhibition, management and perspectives. Blood Coagul Fibrinolysis 15:109, 2004.

Astermark J: Why do inhibitors develop? Principles of and factors influencing the risk for inhibitor development in haemophilia. Haemophilia 12(Suppl 3):52, 2006.

Astermark J: Treatment of the bleeding inhibitor patient. Semin Thromb Hemost 29:77, 2003.

DiMichele DM: Immune tolerance: A synopsis of the international experience. Haemophilia 4:568, 1998.

Hay CR, Brown S, Collins PW, et al: The diagnosis and management of factor VIII and IX inhibitors: A guideline from the United Kingdom Haemophilia Centre Doctors Organisation. Br J Haematol 133:591, 2006.

Ingerslev J: Hemophilia. Strategies for the treatment of inhibitor patients. Haematologica 85(10 Suppl):15, 2000.

Key NS: Inhibitors in congenital coagulation disorders. Br J Haematol 127:379, 2004.

Ludlam C: Identifying and managing inhibitor patients requiring orthopaedic surgery—The multidisciplinary team approach. Haemophilia 11(Suppl 1):7, 2005.

Lusher JM: Hemophilia treatment. Factor VIII inhibitors with recombinant products: Prospective clinical trials. Haematologica 85(10 Suppl):2, 2000.

Oldenburg J, Schroder J, Brackmann HH, et al: Environmental and genetic factors influencing inhibitor development. Semin Hematol 41(1 Suppl 1):82, 2004.

Scandella D: New characteristics of anti-factor VIII inhibitor antibody epitopes and unusual immune responses to factor VIII. Semin Thromb Hemost 28:291, 2002.

Scharrer I, Bray GL, Neutzling O: Incidence of inhibitors in haemophilia A patients—A review of recent studies of recombinant and plasma-derived factor VIII concentrates. Haemophilia 5:145, 1999.

Schwaab R, Brackmann HH, Meyer C, et al: Haemophilia A: Mutation type determines risk of inhibitor formation. Thromb Haemost 74:1402, 1995.

White GC 2nd, Kempton CL, Grimsley A, et al: Cellular immune responses in hemophilia: Why do inhibitors develop in some, but not all hemophiliacs? J Thromb Haemost 3:1676, 2005.

Wight J, Paisley S, Knight C: Immune tolerance induction in patients with haemophilia A with inhibitors: A systematic review. Haemophilia 9:436, 2003.

REFERENCES

For complete list of references log onto www.expertconsult.com

CHAPTER 127

RARE COAGULATION FACTOR DEFICIENCIES

David Gailani and Anne T. Neff

Inherited deficiencies of blood clotting proteins distinct from those involved in hemophilia A and B are rare, and the clinical presentations, diagnostic options and treatments differ from those for deficiencies of factor VIII (see Chapters 123 and 125) and factor IX (see Chapters 124 and 125). The rare disorders include deficiencies of fibrinogen; the plasma protease zymogens prothrombin, factors VII, X, XI, and XII, and prekallikrein; the cofactors factor V and high-molecular-weight kininogen; and the transaminase factor XIII. Reactions involving these proteins are shown in Fig. 127–1. Conversion of soluble fibrinogen to fibrin at a wound site is triggered by binding of factor VIIa to tissue factor (Fig. 127–1, *A*).[1–3] The factor VIIa/tissue factor complex converts factor X to Xa, which then converts prothrombin to thrombin in the presence of factor Va. Mice lacking prothrombin, factor VII, factor X, or factor V die in utero or soon after birth,[4] consistent with the rarity of these deficiencies in humans. Thrombin has many functions, including conversion of fibrinogen to fibrin through limited proteolysis (Fig. 127–2). Factor IX is also activated by factor VIIa/tissue factor and, with factor VIIIa, sustains thrombin generation by activating factor X.[1–3] Factor IX activation by factor XIa is required in some situations.[5] In the model shown in Fig. 127–1, *B,* which serves as the basis for the prothrombin time and partial thromboplastin time (PTT) assays, factor XI activation requires factor XII, prekallikrein, and high-molecular-weight kininogen, the contact factors.[6] However, deficiency of a contact factor does not result in abnormal bleeding, and other mechanisms likely exist for factor XI activation. For example, thrombin can activate factor XI (Fig. 127–1, *A*).[7] Finally, factor XIII is activated by thrombin and cross-links fibrin monomers to complete the process of fibrin formation.[8] The number from the Online Mendelian Inheritance in Man (OMIM) database for each congenital deficiency is given in the section title, and each section references Web sites that compile and regularly update lists of mutations that cause factor deficiencies.

Most coagulation protein disorders are recessive traits, with severe deficiency occurring in one in 500,000 to 2,000,000 individuals. This implies a carrier frequency of approximately 1 : 1000,[9] which is 10-fold higher than the frequency of mutant alleles causing factor VIII deficiency (≈1 : 10,000). Therefore, these disorders are rare because they are recessive traits and not because of low allele frequencies. As with any recessive trait, incidences are higher in areas where consanguineous marriages are common. Overall, the rare factor deficiencies represent approximately 3% to 5% of all coagulation factor deficiencies.[10] An international database for these disorders (www.rbdd.org) has been established for the purpose of collecting clinical, genetic, and therapeutic information to facilitate development of evidenced-based diagnostic and treatment recommendations.[10]

FIBRINOGEN DEFICIENCY (OMIM 202400)

The fibrous nature of a blood clot has been recognized for centuries.[11] The plasma precursor of the fibrin component of the clot, fibrinogen, was first purified in the late nineteenth century.[11] Fibrinogen and fibrin are designated factors I and Ia, respectively, by the committee that established the nomenclature system currently used for coagulation proteins.[12] In 1947, fibrinogen was identified as a major component of cryoprecipitate, the preparation commonly used in the United States to treat fibrinogen deficiency.[13] Congenital absence of fibrinogen (*afibrinogenemia*) was first described in 1920[9] and has an estimated incidence of 1 : 1–2,000,000.[14] Partial deficiency of fibrinogen is called *hypofibrinogenemia.* Afibrinogenemia and hypofibrinogenemia traditionally have been considered separate disorders, however, it now is clear that they represent the homozygous and heterozygous states, respectively, for mutations affecting plasma fibrinogen concentration.

Fibrinogen is a 340,000 molecular weight plasma glycoprotein composed of two heterotrimers, each containing an Aα, Bβ, and γ chain (see Fig. 127–2).[15] The protein is synthesized in hepatocytes,[16] and the three chains are encoded by separate genes within a 50-kb region on chromosome 4.[17] Fibrinogen in platelet α granules is taken up from the plasma by a glycoprotein IIb/IIIa–dependent mechanism.[18] Thrombin converts fibrinogen to fibrin monomer through proteolysis, removing fibrinopeptides A and B from the N-termini of the Aα and Bβ chains, respectively (Fig. 127–2).[15,19] Fibrinogen also binds to glycoprotein IIb/IIIa, facilitating platelet aggregation.[20]

Afibrinogenemia is an autosomal recessive disorder caused by homozygosity or compound heterozygosity for mutations in the fibrinogen genes, with the Aα gene most often affected.[21] Afibrinogenemic patients have undetectable or nearly undetectable levels of fibrinogen (<10 mg/dL; normal 150–400 mg/dL) by activity-based clotting assays and by measurement of immunoreactive fibrinogen. Hypofibrinogenemia is associated with partial deficiency of fibrinogen due to heterozygosity for a mutation. Since the first report of a causative mutation in 1999,[22] more than 70 abnormalities have been described in the fibrinogen genes of afibrinogenemic/hypofibrinogenemic patients (www.geht.org/databaseang/fibrinogen).[21,23] Most are deletions, frameshifts, splice site mutations, or nonsense mutations. A relatively small number of missense mutations that are clustered in the C-termini of the Bβ and γ chains in the D domain (see Fig. 127–2) interfere with protein secretion. Missense mutations such as Glyγ284Arg (Fibrinogen Brescia)[24] and Argγ375Trp (Fibrinogen Aguadilla)[25] cause hypofibrinogenemia with accumulation of fibrinogen in hepatocytes, leading to hepatic dysfunction and cirrhosis (endoplasmic reticulum storage disease).

Acquired hypofibrinogenemia is common in disseminated intravascular coagulation and primary fibrinolysis. Fibrinogen levels typically are normal or increased in liver disease but may be low (<100 mg/dL) in cirrhosis with hepatic failure or with fulminant hepatic necrosis.[26] A severely depressed fibrinogen level due to hepatic insufficiency indicates a poor prognosis.[27] Patients receiving L-asparaginase for hematologic malignancies may develop severe hypofibrinogenemia (<20 mg/dL),[28] with normal or only slightly reduced levels of other coagulation factors.

Hemorrhagic symptoms in fibrinogen deficiency are most significant when the plasma level is less than 50 mg/dl.[29,30] Most afibrinogenemic patients have bleeding from the umbilical cord and from mucosal surfaces.[29,31,32] Bleeding from the skin, gastrointestinal tract, and genitourinary tract are common, as is menorrhagia.[33–35] Hemarthroses (54%) and muscle hematomas (72%) were frequent in one series.[29] However, hemarthrosis-related arthropathy appears to be less pronounced than in hemophilia. Intracranial bleeding is a frequent

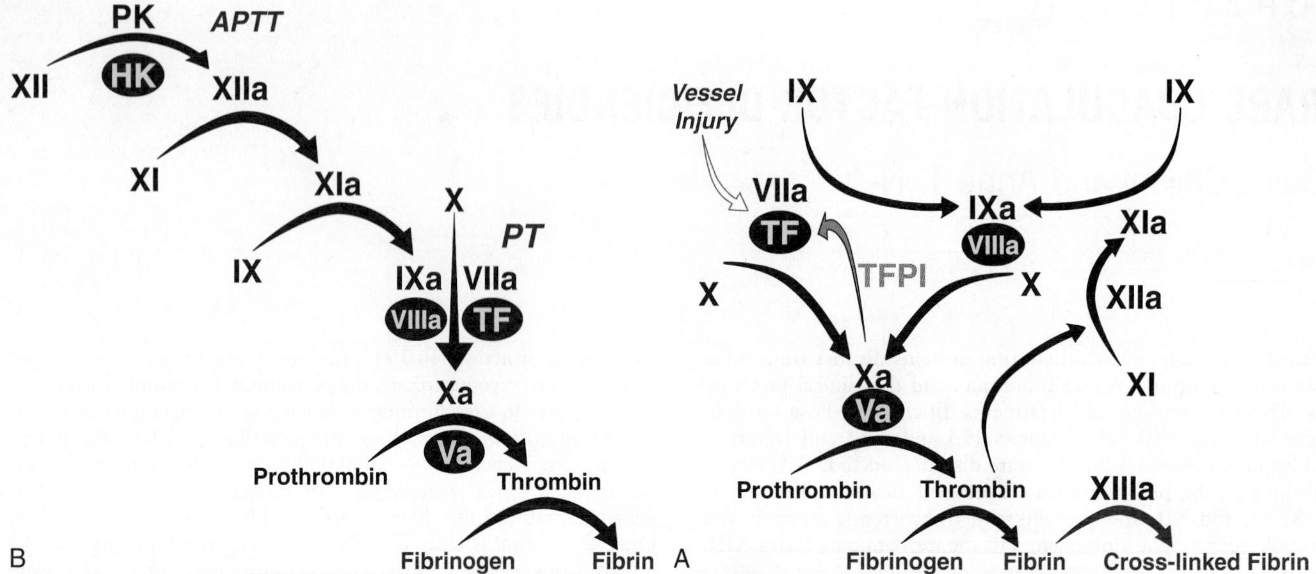

Figure 127–1 Models of plasma coagulation. Unactivated factors are indicated by a Roman numeral, and activated factors by Roman numerals followed by a lower case "a." Enzymes are indicated by black lettering and cofactors by yellow lettering in black ovals. Black arrows indicate reactions involving factor activation, blue arrow indicates fibrin cross-linking by factor XIIIa, and red arrow indicates the factor Xa–dependent inhibition of the factor VIIa/tissue factor (TF) complex by tissue factor pathway inhibitor (TFPI). **A,** Model of TF-initiated hemostasis. See introduction for a description of the events leading to formation of a fibrin clot. **B,** Cascade/waterfall model of hemostasis. This model serves as the basis for the prothrombin time and activated partial thromboplastin time (PTT) assays. In the prothrombin time assay, a reagent containing TF is added to plasma, and the factor VIIa/TF complex induces clot formation through activation of factor X. In the PTT assay, a reagent containing a negatively charged substance initiates clot formation through activation of factor XII (contact activation; see Fig. 127–3 for details). HK, high-molecular-weight-kininogen; PK, plasma prekallikrein.

cause of death in these patients.[32–35] Spontaneous rupture of the spleen has been reported.[36] Hypofibrinogenemic patients usually are asymptomatic but may have excessive bleeding with trauma or surgery, particularly if the fibrinogen level is less than 50 mg/dL. Some mutations causing hypofibrinogenemia result in liver insufficiency due to accumulation of fibrinogen in the endoplasmic reticulum of hepatocytes,[24,25] similar to the syndrome associated with α_1-antityrpsin deficiency.[37]

The incidence of spontaneous abortions is high in afibrinogenemic and hypofibrinogenemic woman.[29,38–40] Fibrinogen-deficient mice also have difficulty sustaining pregnancies,[41] confirming the importance of the maternal protein to fetal viability. Prepartum and postpartum bleeding are relatively common,[39,40] and intraabdominal bleeding from ruptured corpus luteal cysts have been reported. Arterial and venous thrombotic events have been described in afibrinogenemic patients.[42] Although some cases are associated with other risk factors for thromboembolism or with administration of replacement therapy, in most instances no risk factor was identifiable. Fibrinogen and fibrin have been shown to downregulate thrombin activity, providing a possible explanation for these events.[43,44] Alternatively, some thrombotic episodes could occur in patients with dysfibrinogenemia or hypodysfibrinogenemia who have been mistakenly diagnosed as afibrinogenemic.

Plasma assays measuring time to fibrin clot formation, such as the prothrombin time, PTT, and thrombin time, will be infinitely prolonged in afibrinogenemia. The template bleeding time and platelet aggregation studies often are abnormal.[34,45] Fibrinogen is absent, but other coagulation factor levels are normal. The von Clauss method is the most commonly used technique for measuring fibrinogen in clinical laboratories.[46] It is based on determining the time to clot formation after addition of thrombin to plasma. This assay is not reliable at very low fibrinogen levels (<10 mg/dL) and may give falsely low readings with fibrin variants that polymerize slowly (dysfibrinogenemia) or if substances that interfere with fibrin polymerization (paraproteins, high levels of fibrin degradation products) are present. Therefore, it is important to demonstrate the absence of immunoreactive fibrinogen to confirm the diagnosis of afibrinogenemia.[47] In hypofibrinogenemia, functional and antigenic fibrinogen levels are proportionately decreased. A disproportionately lower functional level suggests the diagnosis of dysfibrinogenemia. The prothrombin time and PTT are relatively insensitive to fibrinogen and may not be prolonged in mild to moderate hypofibrinogenemia. The thrombin time is more sensitive in these situations. Afibrinogenemic patients have low erythrocyte sedimentation rates and develop little induration in skin tests for delayed hypersensitivity because of the absence of fibrin deposition.[48]

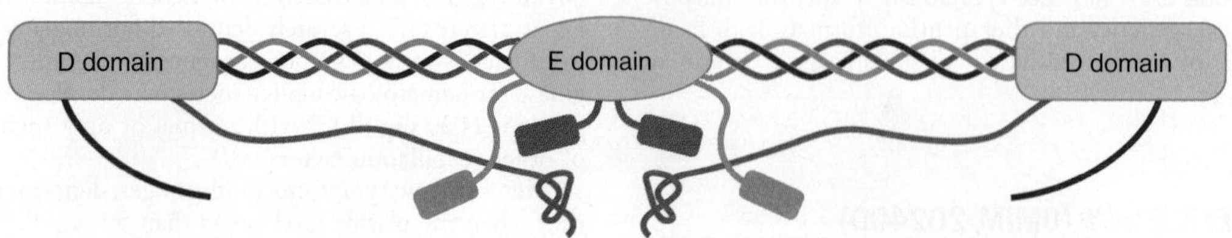

Figure 127–2 Model of human fibrinogen. Each half of the molecule contains an Aα (blue), Bβ (red), and γ (green) chain. The amino-termini of the six chains that compose the whole molecule are linked by disulfide bonds in the central E domain. The carboxy-terminal regions of the polypeptides form two nodular D domains at the extremes of the molecule. Fibrinopeptides A (blue boxes) and B (red boxes) reside in the E domain and are removed by the proteolytic activity of thrombin during conversion of fibrinogen to fibrin. (Adapted from Mosesson MW: Fibrinogen and fibrin structure and functions. J Thromb Haematol 3:1894, 2005, with permission.)

Afibrinogenemic and hypofibrinogenemic patients can be treated with cryoprecipitate, fresh frozen plasma, or fibrinogen concentrate, depending on availability. In the United States, cryoprecipitate is used most frequently. A 30- to 50-mL unit contains approximately 300 mg of fibrinogen. Fibrinogen has an extravascular distribution of approximately 30%, and an afibrinogenemic adult with an estimated 3-L plasma volume will require 12 units of cryoprecipitate to achieve a plasma level of 100 mg/dL. Recommendations regarding target levels for treating bleeding range from 30–50 mg/dL[30] to 100 mg/dL.[40] The following are guidelines for treating afibrinogenemia from the United Kingdom Haemophilia Centre Doctors Organization.[40] For significant bleeding, the plasma fibrinogen level should be increased to 100 mg/dL until hemostasis is achieved and then maintained above 50 mg/dL until wound healing is complete. A similar strategy is recommended for managing surgery patients. The half-life of transfused fibrinogen is 3 to 5 days,[49] and every-other-day treatment usually is adequate to maintain levels in the absence of consumption. Infusions may need to be more frequent in certain clinical settings, and close monitoring of fibrinogen levels is recommended to facilitate dosing. Data are insufficient to base recommendations for primary prophylaxis to prevent bleeding. However, secondary prophylaxis is reasonable to prevent recurrent intracranial hemorrhage, with trough levels kept above 50 mg/dL.

Administration of regular infusions of fibrinogen is recommended to maintain pregnancies in afibrinogenemic woman and to reduce the incidence of postpartum hemorrhage.[50,51] Therapy should be initiated as early as possible because fetal loss in the first trimester is frequent. Fetal loss has occurred in some patients with fibrinogen levels above 50 mg/dL; therefore, it is recommended that levels be kept above 100 mg/dL through the duration of the pregnancy.

Antifibrinolytic therapy with ε-aminocaproic acid may be an effective replacement for blood products for some mucosal bleeding and for dental extractions (see box on Antifibrinolytic Therapy for Congenital Factor Deficiencies). However, this therapy is associated with an increased risk for thrombotic events and must be used cautiously in patients with a history of thrombosis, pregnancy, surgery, or immobilization. Fibrin glues also may be useful for tooth extraction, and estrogen/progesterone therapy may be helpful for controlling menorrhagia.[52]

Antifibrinolytic Therapy in Congenital Factor Deficiencies

The antifibrinolytic agents ε-aminocaproic acid and tranexamic acid are effective adjuncts to factor replacement in many situations when treating bleeding disorders and may be useful alternatives to replacement therapy for mild bleeding or minor procedures. These drugs inhibit clot dissolution by blocking plasminogen activation and plasmin activity. They are particularly valuable when bleeding involves tissues with high fibrinolytic activity, such as the oral cavity, and have been useful for treating menorrhagia, limiting blood loss at surgery, controlling epistaxis, and reducing some forms of gastrointestinal bleeding. A typical loading dose of ε-aminocaproic acid is 50 to 100 mg/kg, followed by 2 to 4 g every 6 hours. If bleeding subsequently occurs, the dose can be increased to a maximum of 24 g in 24 hours. ε-Aminocaproic acid is available in oral and intravenous formulations, and identical dosing can be used for either preparation due to excellent bioavailability. For dental extraction in patients with factor VIII or IX deficiency, many hemophilia centers use a single 50% to 100% loading dose of clotting factor concentrate, followed by 7 days of ε-aminocaproic acid as the sole prophylaxis. It is reasonable to extrapolate this approach to patients with some of the rare bleeding disorders. Patients with factor XI deficiency do well with antifibrinolytic agents alone for tooth extractions. Dental procedures such as scaling or root canal can be performed safely using ε-aminocaproic acid mouthwash prepared from the intravenous formulation three to four times daily with or without systemic antifibrinolytic therapy.

Prolonged therapy with antifibrinolytic agents must be used with caution in patients who are not mobile, who have a history of thromboembolic events, or who have significant urogenital bleeding because of an increased risk for thrombus formation. These drugs interfere with urokinase-mediated fibrinolytic activity in the genitourinary tract and can cause renal outflow obstruction by thrombotic occlusion of the ureter. Concomitant use of antifibrinolytic agents with activated prothrombin complex concentrates or, possibly, recombinant factor VIIa may result in a particularly high risk for thrombus formation. Patients may develop nausea or vertigo with high doses of ε-aminocaproic doses and, rarely, rhabdomyolysis.

DYSFIBRINOGENEMIA (OMIM 134820 Aα CHAIN, 134830 Bβ CHAIN, AND 134850 γ CHAIN)

In *dysfibrinogenemia,* structural variants of fibrinogen circulate in the plasma. These abnormal proteins are designated by the city of origin of the patient in whom they are identified, with additional Roman numerals if more than one variant is found in a city. Cases in which the dysfunctional protein is present at low levels in plasma are referred to as *hypodysfibrinogenemia.* The first family with dysfibrinogenemia (fibrinogen Paris I, 15-amino-acid insertion after Gln350 in the γ chain)[53] was described in 1964.[54] The actual incidence for congenital dysfibrinogenemia is not known because the majority of patients appear to be asymptomatic, and most probably do not come to medical attention. Although a rare cause of excessive bleeding, it has been estimated that 0.8% of patients with a history of venous thromboembolism have dysfibrinogenemia.[55]

Congenital dysfibrinogenemia and hypodysfibrinogenemia are predominantly autosomal dominant disorders caused by a missense mutation in one of the fibrinogen genes, although some insertions and deletions have been identified.[9] More than 100 mutations associated with dysfibrinogenemia (www.geht.org/databaseang/fibrinogen/) have been identified in approximately 300 families. The types of functional defects most often reported are largely determined by the clinical assays available for assessing fibrin formation and likely do not represent the full spectrum of mutations that can cause fibrinogen dysfunction. Variants that are easily detected by conventional clinical assays primarily have defects in fibrinopeptide release (e.g., Fibrinogens Bicêtre [AαArg16His] and Metz [AαArg16Cys]; see Fig. 127–2)[56] or polymerize slowly (e.g., Fibrinogen Caracas II [AαSer434Asn]).[57] Fibrinogens Bicêtre and Metz cumulatively have been reported more than 70 times, likely reflecting the ease with which these variants are detected by functional fibrinogen assays found in most clinical laboratories and their relatively high frequency.

Thrombotic events have been reported in numerous patients with dysfibrinogenemia.[55,58] A subcommittee of the International Society on Thrombosis and Haemostasis concluded that a significant relationship exists between certain fibrinogen variants and venous thrombosis.[55] Thrombosis-associated mutations tend to cluster at the C-terminus of the Aα chain and near the thrombin cleavage site on the Bβ chain[58]; however the mechanisms by which these variants cause thromboembolism are not well understood. Abnormalities in fibrin polymerization,[59] cross-linking,[59,60] clot structure,[61,62] and susceptibility to fibrinolysis[60,62,63] have been described. The "Dusart syndrome"[62] associated with fibrinogen Paris V (AαArg554Cys)[64] has been identified in several apparently unrelated families (Fibrinogens Chapel Hill III and Nashville).[64,65] In one family, this mutation was associated with multiple cases of venous thromboembolism and sudden death in teenagers and young adults.[65]

A group of mutations in the C-terminus of the fibrinogen Aα chain is associated with autosomal dominant hereditary amyloidosis in which the amyloid deposits contain fragments of the variant fibrinogens.[16,66–68] The kidneys are primarily affected, but wider visceral and nerve involvement may occur with time.[66–68] Renal grafts subsequently become involved with amyloid,[16,66] and liver transplantation may be a better option for treating this condition.[16,69,70] The allele frequency for one responsible mutation, the AαGlu526Val variant, is relatively common and may account for 5% of patients with apparent sporadic amyloid.[68]

Acquired dysfibrinogenemia is most frequently diagnosed in liver disease, with up to 80% to 90% of patients with cirrhosis or liver failure showing some degree of fibrinogen dysfunction.[71,72] Increased sialic acid content leading to an enhanced negative charge likely is responsible for the impairment in fibrin polymeirzation.[73] Homocysteine-induced modifications of fibrinogen have been proposed to contribute to the hypercoagulable state associated with elevated plasma levels of homocysteine.[74] The monoclonal antibody in patients with multiple myeloma can interfere nonspecifically with fibrin polymerization in tests such as the thrombin time[75] but usually do not cause abnormal hemostasis. Acquired dysfibrinogenemia also has been associated with malignancies,[76,77] bone marrow transplantation,[78] and rarely with medications such as mithramycin.[79]

The majority of patients with dysfibrinogenemia (55%–60%) are not symptomatic, and the condition is identified by an abnormal result on a coagulation screening assay.[55] Approximately 25% of patients have abnormal bleeding, and 20% have thrombotic episodes.[55] Correlation between functional abnormalities and clinical symptoms is difficult in many cases. The relatively common AαArg16His and AαArg16Cys variants have been observed in asymptomatic individuals as well as in patients with bleeding or thrombotic events.[9] Epistaxis, easy bruising, and menorrhagia are relatively common.[75,80] Many bleeding episodes are mild, but significant events, including soft-tissue hematomas, hemarthroses, postoperative hemorrhage, and bleeding during pregnancy and postpartum, have been observed.[75,80] Abnormalities with wound healing and spontaneous abortions have been reported.[80] Thrombosis primarily involves the venous circulation (deep vein thrombosis, pulmonary embolism, thrombophlebitis), although some arterial events or combinations of venous and arterial thrombosis have been reported.[55] Approximately one fourth of patients with thrombotic symptoms also experience excessive bleeding.

Most cases of dysfibrinogenemia present as abnormalities on routine coagulation screening tests such as the prothrombin time and PTT. The thrombin time is considered the primary screening test for dysfibrinogenemia, although its sensitivity is not established.[80] The test involves measuring the time to clot formation in citrated plasma after addition of a standard amount of thrombin. The specificity of the thrombin time is relatively poor because a low level of fibrinogen, the presence of heparin, elevated fibrin degradation products, and high levels of some paraproteins may affect the result. The reptilase time has been used as an alternative screen for dysfibrinogenemia and is useful in combination with the thrombin time.[75] The assay involves inducing clot formation with an enzyme from the venom of *Bothrops jararaca* or *Bothrops atrox* that cleaves fibrinopeptide A from fibrinogen and is not sensitive to heparin. Plasma concentration of clottable fibrinogen as determined by the von Clauss method may be low in some types of dysfibrinogenemia. Levels of immunoreactive fibrinogen usually are normal but are decreased in some cases (e.g., hypodysfibrinogenemia). With some variants, fibrin degradation products may be elevated using certain assays because the variant fibrinogen is not incorporated into a clot. This may lead to the false impression that disseminated intravascular coagulation is present.

Given that most dysfibrinogenemic patients are asymptomatic and that symptoms correlate poorly with abnormalities in coagulation assays, generalized recommendations for treating dysfibrinogenemia are not possible. Therapy must be individualized, and most patients will not require treatment. The patient's personal and family histories are useful for guiding therapy. Active bleeding can be treated with replacement therapy as described for afibrinogenemia, and replacement may be indicated in some patients prior to invasive procedures with a high risk of bleeding.

In general, patients with thrombosis and dysfibrinogenemia should be treated similarly to other patients with hypercoagulable conditions. No data are available on which to formulate recommendations regarding duration of therapy. The past history, family history, coexisting conditions, and the nature (idiopathic, pregnancy, postsurgery) and seriousness of the thrombotic event all must be taken into consideration. As with any thrombotic event, the risk of bleeding associated with prolonged therapy must be considered. Recurrent spontaneous abortions have been associated with dysfibrinogenemia in several families, and some pregnancies have been carried to term under replacement therapy with cryoprecipitate.[29]

PROTHROMBIN DEFICIENCY (OMIM 176930)

More than a century ago, Morawitz proposed that an insoluble fibrin clot is formed from fibrinogen through the activity of *fibrin ferment* or thrombin.[11,81] Thrombin was generated from a precursor, prothrombin, by thrombokinase (probably factor Xa). Prothrombin and thrombin are designated factors II and IIa.[12] Total prothrombin deficiency probably is not compatible with life, as absence of the protein has not been observed in humans and prothrombin null mice die in utero or shortly after birth.[4] Congenital partial prothrombin deficiency (*hypoprothrombinemia*) and abnormal circulating prothrombin (*dysprothrombinemia*) affect an estimated 1:2,000,000 persons (Table 127–1).[14] Prothrombin deficiency is relatively common in Puerto Rico, accounting for 6% of non–von Willebrand disease congenital bleeding disorders seen at the University of Puerto Rico Hemophilia Center. The estimated carrier frequency is 1:700 in the Puerto Rican population.[82]

Prothrombin is a 72,000 molecular weight protein that is converted to thrombin by factor Xa in complex with factor Va on phospholipid surfaces (see Fig. 127–1, *A*).[1,2] Thrombin is a pivotal protease in hemostasis, with multiple procoagulant activities including cleavage of fibrinopeptides A and B from fibrinogen to form fibrin (see Fig. 127–2), activation of factors V, VIII, XI, and XIII, and cleavage of protease activated receptors.[83] Thrombin also downregulates fibrinolysis by activating the metalloproteinase thrombin activatable fibrinolysis inhibitor,[84] forms a complex with thrombomodulin to downregulate coagulation through the activation of protein C,[85] and has cytokine and growth factor-like properties.

Prothrombin deficiency is an autosomal recessive disorder manifested as hypoprothrombinemia (reduced activity and antigen; cross-reactive material negative deficiency [CRM−]), dysprothrombinemia (reduced activity with normal to moderately reduced antigen; cross-reactive material positive deficiency [CRM+]), or a combination of both. Plasma prothrombin activity typically is approximately 1% to 10% of normal in hypoprothrombinemia and 1% to 20% in dysprothrombinemia. Heterozygotes for either condition have approximately 50% normal activity and are not symptomatic. More than 50 prothrombin gene mutations have been described (www.med.unc.edu/isth/; www.hgmd.org).[86] In dysprothrombinemia, missense mutations cause defects in prothrombin conversion to thrombin (e.g., prothrombin Puerto Rico I [Arg457Gln][82] and Madrid [Arg271Cys][87]) or result in functionally defective thrombin (e.g., prothrombin Tokushima [Arg418Trp][88]).

Prothrombin deficiency can be inherited in combination with deficiencies of other vitamin K–dependent proteins (see Combined Deficiency of Vitamin K–Dependent Proteins below). Acquired prothrombin deficiency occurs with warfarin therapy, poisoning with rodenticides such as brodifacoum, with vitamin K deficiency or liver disease, and in disseminated intravascular coagulation. Cephalosporins, particularly those with *N*-methyl-thiotetrazole side chains, can decrease prothrombin levels.[89] Antiprothrombin antibodies are common antiphospholipid antibodies in patients with lupus anticoagulants or the antiphospholipid antibody syndrome.[90] More rarely, patients with lupus anticoagulants or systemic lupus erythematosus have antibodies that enhance prothrombin clearance, causing true deficiency.[91,92] Formation of neutralizing antibodies after replacement therapy in congenital prothrombin deficiency has not been reported.

Prothrombin gene mutations are associated with variable levels of activity (1%–50% of normal) that may correlate poorly with clinical

Table 127–1 Properties of Plasma Coagulation Factors and Characteristics of Deficiency States

Protein	Incidence of Severe Congenital Deficiency	Inheritance Pattern	Sources for Proteins in Blood	Other Names for Deficiency States	Bleeding Diathesis	Null Mouse phenotype
Fibrinogen	≈1:1–2 × 10⁶	Autosomal recessive or dominant	Liver		Mild to severe	Severe bleeding, reduced fertility
Prothrombin	≈1:2 × 10⁶	Autosomal recessive	Liver		Mild to severe	Lethal in utero or perinatal
Factor V	≈1:1 × 10⁶	Autosomal recessive	Liver, megakaryocytes?	Parahemophilia	Mild to moderately severe	Lethal in utero or perinatal
Factor VII	≈1:5 × 10⁵	Autosomal recessive	Liver	Serum prothrombin conversion accelerator deficiency	Mild to severe	Lethal in utero or perinatal
Factor X	≈1:1 × 10⁶	Autosomal recessive	Liver	Stuart-Prower factor deficiency	Mild to severe	Lethal in utero or perinatal
Factor XI	≈1:1 × 10⁶	Autosomal recessive or dominant	Liver	Hemophilia C, plasma thromboplastin antecedent deficiency	Asymptomatic to moderate	No bleeding diathesis, protected from thrombosis
Factor XII	Unknown	Autosomal recessive	Liver	Hageman trait	None	No bleeding diathesis, protected from thrombosis
Prekallikrein	Unknown	Autosomal recessive	Liver	Fletcher trait	None	Not available
High-molecular-weight kininogen	Unknown	Autosomal recessive	Liver	Flaujeac trait, Williams trait, Fitzgerald trait	None	No bleeding diathesis
Factor XIII	1:1–5 × 10⁶	Autosomal recessive	A chain: liver, platelets, monocytes B chain: liver	Fibrin stabilizing factor deficiency	Moderate to severe	Bleeding diathesis, reduced fertility

symptoms. Life-threatening bleeding occurred in a patient with 8% normal activity, whereas patients with 2% activity were asymptomatic.[93,94] The bleeding diathesis can present at circumcision in neonates; it also can present as easy bruising, epistaxis, or menorrhagia, or with trauma or surgery. Muscle hematomas and hemarthroses were the most frequent manifestations in a series of patients.[35] Central nervous system hemorrhage was reported in 8% of prothrombin-deficient patients in one registry and in 20% of patients with less than 1% normal activity.[33]

In the prothrombin time and PTT assays, prothrombin is converted to thrombin by factor Xa in complex with factor Va on phospholipids vesicles (see Fig. 127–1, *B*), and severe prothrombin deficiency prolongs both test results. Some prothrombin time and PTT reagents are relatively insensitive to reductions in prothrombin level, and mild deficiencies may be missed. The diagnosis is confirmed and the degree of deficiency established by a modified prothrombin time assay using prothrombin-deficient plasma. Prothrombin deficiency must be distinguished from deficiencies of fibrinogen, factor V, or factor X, which are also associated with a prolonged prothrombin time and PTT.

Prothrombin complex concentrates approved for use in factor IX deficiency contain variable amounts of prothrombin and factors VII and X (Table 127–2) and are the preferred product for treating prothrombin deficiency, although they are not approved for this use by the Food and Drug Administration. Prothrombin complex concentrates are derived from human plasma and undergo viral inactivation to enhance safety. The prothrombin activity in these concentrates is comparable to or higher than the factor IX activity. Hemostatic levels of prothrombin are estimated to be approximately 30% of normal, and 20 to 30 factor IX units/kg of prothrombin complex concentrate produces plasma prothrombin levels of 20% to 30%.[95] The half-life of prothrombin is approximately 3 days, and dosing every 2 to 3 days maintains adequate levels until healing is complete.[14] Use of prothrombin complex concentrates has been associated with thrombotic events, and it is recommended that levels of factors VII, IX, and X be kept below 150% to minimize this risk.[14] Dental procedures or minor hemorrhage may respond to antifibrinolytic therapy with ε-aminocaproic acid.[35] Prothrombin deficiency also can be treated with fresh frozen plasma for bleeding episodes or surgical intervention (15–20 mL/kg loading dose followed by 3 mL/kg/day). Due to the long half-life, additional doses may not be required in all situations. Cryoprecipitate is not a source of prothrombin, and plasma prothrombin levels do not increase after infusion or inhalation of desmopressin (L-desamino-8-D-arginine vasopressin [DDAVP]). These agents should not be used to treat prothrombin deficiency.

FACTOR V DEFICIENCY (OMIM 227400)

In 1943, Quick reported that aged plasma clotted more slowly than fresh plasma in a prothrombin time assay and proposed that a *labile factor* distinct from prothrombin was required for normal coagulation.[96] At the same time, Owren noted that a patient with a lifelong bleeding problem appeared to lack a factor normally found in plasma that does not adsorb onto aluminum hydroxide, in contrast to prothrombin.[97] It subsequently was determined that Owren's patient was deficient in the labile factor described by Quick, which now is called *factor V.* Congenital deficiency of factor V has been estimated to occur in 1:1,000,000 persons (see Table 127–1).[98,99]

Factor V is the 330,000 molecular weight precursor of factor Va, which facilitates prothrombin activation by factor Xa on phospho-

Table 127–2 Treatment Considerations for Rare Coagulation Factor Deficiencies

Protein	Plasma Half-Life (hours)	Blood Sources	Concentrate Available	Level for Major Surgery	Dosing Frequency (hours)	Minimum for Hemostasis	Other Considerations
Fibrinogen	72–120	Cryoprecipitate plasma	Available, but not in the United States	100 mg/dL	q24–48h	30–50 mg/dL	Level of 100 mg/dL is recommended in pregnancy
Prothrombin	60–100	Plasma	Prothrombin complex concentrate	30%	q2–3days	≈5%	
Factor V	12–14	Plasma, platelets	No	25%	q12–24h	≈10%	Platelets may be used if factor V inhibitor is present
Factor VII	3–4	Plasma	Recombinant factor VIIa, prothrombin complex concentrate	15%–25%	q2–3h for factor VIIa q4–6h for fresh frozen plaza	5%–10%	Frequent infusion of plasma due to short half-life can cause volume overload
Factor X	20–40	Plasma	Prothrombin complex concentrate	25%–40%	q24h	≈10%	Deficiency in amyloidosis will respond poorly to replacement therapy
Factor XI	45	Plasma	Hemoleven®, LFB, Les Ulis, France, received orphan-designation from FDA, November 2007	30%–45%	q1–2days	15%	Limit plasma exposure to prevent inhibitor development
Factor XII	60	Plasma	No	Not required	None	0	No bleeding diathesis
Prekallikrein	Unknown	Plasma	No	Not required	None	0	No bleeding diathesis
High-molecular-weight kininogen	170	Plasma	No	Not required	None	0	No bleeding diathesis
Factor XIII	240–336 (10–14 days)	Plasma, cryoprecipitate	Available in the United States as part of a protocol	20%–50%	q5–6weeks for prophylaxis qweek for pregnancy, surgery	1%–2%	Plasma levels may need to be maintained above 10% to sustain pregnancy

lipid surfaces (see Fig. 127–1, *A*).[1,2] Most factor V (80%) is in plasma; the remainder is stored in a partially proteolyzed form in platelet α granules.[99,100] In humans, platelet factor V is primarily of plasma origin.[101] Severe factor V deficiency is an autosomal recessive trait. Approximately 40 factor V gene mutations associated with factor V deficiency have been described (www.med.unc.edu/isth/; www.hgmd.org).[99] Two thirds result in premature termination of protein synthesis, and most are unique to specific families,[99,102] although Tyr1702Cys has been identified several times in the Italian population.[103] No large gene deletions have been found, and most patients have some detectable factor V antigen in plasma. Studies of factor V missense mutations indicate that most abnormal polypeptides are degraded within the cell, resulting in low factor V antigen in plasma (CRM− deficiency). The only well characterized CRM+ factor V mutation is factor V New Brunswick [Ala221Val],[104] which interferes with stability of factor Va.

Patients with low plasma factor V also have low platelet factor V. A few patients with disproportionately low platelet factor V compared to plasma activity have been identified. Factor V Quebec is an autosomal dominant bleeding disorder with low platelet factor V levels and normal plasma factor V.[105] Proteolytic degradation of multiple α granules proteins in this syndrome is possibly due to deficiency or abnormality of the protein multimerin.[106] Factor V New York is associated with defective platelet factor V not related to generalized proteolysis of platelet proteins.[107] The underlying mutations in factor V Quebec and factor V New York are not known. Combined deficiency of factor V and factor VIII may be caused by mutations in proteins required for secretion of both proteins (see Combined Factor V and Factor VIII Deficiency below).

Acquired factor V deficiency occurs in liver disease and disseminated intravascular coagulation. Factor V inhibitors may occur with antibodies to thrombin in patients exposed to topical bovine thrombin or human thrombin in fibrin sealants or glues.[108] Most patients with these inhibitors are asymptomatic, but some have significant bleeding. Factor V inhibitors have been observed in deficient patients treated with plasma, in otherwise normal individuals, in patients with malignancies and autoimmune disease, after treatment with aminoglycosides, and in association with systemic amyloidosis.[108,109]

Bleeding in patients with severe factor V deficiency (1%–10% of normal levels) varies considerably.[99] Although significant bleeding occurs, the frequency tends to be less than in severe factor VIII or factor IX deficiency. Common presenting findings include bruising, epistaxis, prolonged bleeding from lacerations, and soft-tissue hemorrhage.[98] Hemarthroses are less common than in hemophilia, and debilitating arthropathy is not common.[98] Bleeding into the central nervous system has been reported.[99] Heavy menses and postpartum hemorrhage are common in severe factor V deficiency.[110] Trauma, surgery, and dental extraction are associated with a high risk of bleeding in untreated patients. Bleeding with surgery involving the urogenital tract, nose, or mouth may be particularly problematic because of high fibrinolytic activity in these tissues. Mild (heterozygous) factor V deficiency (25%–60% of normal factor level) usually is not associated with excessive bleeding,[14] although approximately 10% of patients are symptomatic.

An association between factor V deficiency and thromboembolism has been observed.[42,111] In some cases, factor V deficiency may simply have not been sufficient to prevent thrombosis. With the exception of deficiencies of prothrombin and factor X, thrombosis has been reported with all coagulation factor deficiencies.[42] However, the situation with factor V is more complex. Factor V deficiency can occur in patients with the procoagulant polymorphism factor V Arg506Gln (factor V Leiden).[99,111,112] If Arg506Gln and a mutation causing deficiency occur on opposite alleles (*in trans*), most factor V in blood is factor V Leiden, resulting in a significantly increased risk of thrombosis (pseudohomozygous activated protein C resistance).[111,112] Alternatively, Arg506Gln may occur on the same allele as a null mutation (*in cis*), and the prothrombotic effect of Arg506Gln is masked.[113] These patients may have a bleeding tendency.

Factor V is required for normal prothrombin activation by factor Xa (see Fig. 127–1, *B*), and factor V deficiency causes prolongation of both the prothrombin time and the PTT. The diagnosis and severity are established by a modified prothrombin time using factor V–deficient plasma. In some cases of severe factor V deficiency, the template bleeding time also is prolonged, perhaps related to low levels of factor V in platelet α granules.[114] Patients with factor V deficiency should also be tested for factor VIII deficiency so that combined deficiency is not missed.

Managing factor V deficiency is challenging because factor V concentrate is not commercially available (see Table 127–2). Mucosal bleeding from the nose and mouth may respond to ε-aminocaproic acid, and superficial lacerations often respond to local pressure. Administration of fresh frozen plasma is the preferred treatment for serious bleeding or in preparation for surgery. The minimal factor V level for hemostasis is approximately 10% to 20%,[33] although some patients in this range have bleeding symptoms. A plasma level of at least 25% is recommended for major surgery.[115,116] Estimates of the factor V plasma half-life vary widely, but 12 to 14 hours should be assumed for replacement purposes. Infusion of a loading dose of fresh frozen plasma (20 mL/kg over 3–4 hours) prior to surgery and then 5 to 10 mL/kg every 12 hours usually is adequate. Infusions should be continued for 7 to 10 days to maintain adequate hemostasis. Factor V–deficient women can have significant bleeding with childbirth and should be treated in a similar manner.[117,118] Care must be taken to avoid fluid overload from large volumes of fresh frozen plasma, especially in older patients. Plasma exchange has been successful in a few factor V–deficient patients requiring surgery.[119] Although the defect caused by factor V deficiency hypothetically would render therapy with recombinant factor VIIa relatively ineffective, a single case of successful use of this agent in a patient with severe factor V deficiency requiring surgery has been reported.[120]

Platelets are a source of factor V and may be particularly useful in patients with factor V inhibitors, as platelet factor V either may be protected from inhibition or differ in structure from plasma factor V sufficiently to not cross-react with the antibody.[121] However, platelet transfusions are not routinely recommended for treating factor V–deficient patients because of concern for developing antiplatelet alloantibodies. Cryoprecipitate is not a source of factor V, and plasma levels do not respond to administration of DDAVP.[122]

FACTOR VII DEFICIENCY (OMIM 227500)

Factor VII deficiency was first reported in 1951 by Alexander et al.[123] and was called *serum prothrombin conversion accelerator deficiency*. Factor VII deficiency is the most common of the nonhemophilic coagulation deficiencies (see Table 127–1), with an estimated prevalence of 1:500,000 for the severe form (activity <2% of normal).[95]

Factor VII is the 50,000 molecular weight precursor of the protease factor VIIa.[1,2] Factor VII/VIIa binds to tissue factor to initiate coagulation through activation of factors X and IX (see Fig. 127–1, *A*).[1–3] Mice lacking factor VII develop normally in utero but succumb to bleeding at birth.[4] An infant born with complete absence of factor VII died at 12 days with intracerebral hemorrhage[124]; however, another child survived with replacement therapy.[125] Thus, low levels of factor VII activity appear necessary to sustain life. Factor VII deficiency is considered an autosomal recessive trait, although observations of symptomatic heterozygotes call this into question.[33,126]

More than 100 factor VII gene mutations have been found in factor VII–deficient patients, with CRM+ missense mutations predominating (http://www.med.unc.edu/isth/; http://193.60.222.13/). Ala244Val accounts for 84% of abnormal factor VII alleles in 88 unrelated Iranian-Jewish and Moroccan-Jewish patients.[127] Arg304Gln may have originated more than once.[128] Mutations such as Ala294Val[129] appear to result from a founder effect. Some factor VII variants demonstrate variable activity in the prothrombin time assay, depending on the species of origin (e.g., rabbit or human) of the tissue factor used. The name "factor VII Padua" has been applied to these variants, and several cases are associated with a missense mutation (Arg304Gln) in the tissue factor binding site.[130,131] Factor VII deficiency has been reported in conjunction with abnormalities of bilirubin metabolism, mental retardation, microcephaly, epicanthus, cleft palate, and persistent patent ductus arteriosus.[132] It also has been seen in cases of trisomy 8,[133] and a chromosome 13 q34 deletion causes loss of the factor VII and factor X genes. The latter condition may be associated with carotid body tumors and other malformations.[132] Inherited factor VII deficiency may occur in combination with deficiencies of other vitamin K–dependent proteins (see Combined Deficiency of Vitamin K–Dependent Proteins below).

Reduced levels of factor VII occur with warfarin therapy, liver disease, biliary tract disease, vitamin K deficiency, and cephalosporin therapy.[134] In these situations, other vitamin K–dependent factors usually are decreased, although the effect on factor VII often is the greatest. Inhibitors of factor VII have been reported in deficient patients after replacement therapy.[135]

The clinical spectrum of bleeding in factor VII deficiency is broad. Significant bleeding is greatest with severe deficiency, and patients with levels less than 1% may have a syndrome similar to hemophilia, with spontaneous joint and soft-tissue bleeding leading to hemarthrosis-related arthropathy.[136,137] Central nervous system hemorrhage is common (4%–17%).[33,138,139] Patients with factor VII activity 5% of normal or greater tend to have milder symptoms, such as epistaxis, menorrhagia, and bruising. Although little bleeding occurs in patients with levels of 10% to 15%, some describe significant bleeding that occurs either spontaneously or in response to challenges.[140] In one report, 36% of heterozygotes (factor VII activity 21%–69%) reported bleeding problems, mostly involving skin and mucous membranes.[33] Excessive bleeding often complicates dental extraction and surgery on the oropharynx or urogenital tract in untreated patients. Abdominal surgery and hysterectomy are associated with fewer problems, likely related to varying levels of fibrinolytic activity in different tissues. Postpartum bleeding is not common in factor VII–deficient women.[136,141]

Thrombosis associated with factor VII deficiency has been reported.[142] The database of the International Factor VII Deficiency Study Group contained nine thromboembolic events among 514 entries in 2002.[143] Failure to bind tissue factor pathway inhibitor (see Fig. 127–1, *A*), the natural inhibitor of factor VIIa/tissue factor, has been proposed as an etiology, although a mutation operating by this mechanism has not been identified. Some patients may have factor VII Padua, and apparent low activity may be an artifact of the thromboplastin reagent used.

In the prothrombin time assay, factor VII/VIIa binds to tissue factor in the thromboplastin reagent. The factor VIIa/tissue factor complex then activates factor X (see Fig. 127–1, *B*). In severe factor VII deficiency the prothrombin time is prolonged, but the PTT is normal. The diagnosis is confirmed and the factor level determined by a modified prothrombin time assay using factor VII–deficient plasma. With some very sensitive thromboplastin reagents, the prothrombin time may be prolonged, with factor VII levels at the lower end of the normal range. When assessing patients for factor VII deficiency, the source of the tissue factor must be considered, as factor VII Padua-type variants interact poorly with reagents containing rabbit tissue factor.[131]

A major consideration when treating factor VII–deficient patients is the short 3- to 4-hour plasma half-life of the protein. Factor replacement can be accomplished with a variety of products (see Table 127–2). Recombinant factor VIIa is approved for use in congenital factor VII deficiency. The recommended dose is 15 to 30 μg/kg body weight every 2 to 6 hours, with the frequency adjusted to the clinical situation. Hemarthroses often respond to single infusions, whereas prophylaxis for invasive procedures may require treating every 2 to 3 hours. Bleeding can be treated with infusions every 4 to 6 hours until hemostasis is achieved.[144] Fresh frozen plasma is widely used for factor VII deficiency, but limited information on efficacy is available. The plasma factor VII level required for surgery is not formally established, but levels of 15% to 25% usually are adequate, and most bleeding episodes respond to infusions every 6 to 12 hours despite the short plasma half-life of factor VII. Use of frequent doses of fresh frozen plasma may result in volume overload. Prothrombin complex concentrates contain variable amounts of factor VII and have been used to treat factor VII deficiency. However, these products are not favored because they contain other vitamin K–dependent factors that are thrombogenic at high concentrations.[14,145] Cryoprecipitate is not a source of factor VII, and plasma levels do not respond to administration of DDAVP.

Not all bleeding in factor VII–deficient patients requires replacement. Minor injuries may be controlled with local measures, and fibrinolytic inhibitors such as ε-aminocaproic acid may be effective as single agents for minor bleeding, dental procedures, or other procedures involving mucous membranes. Fibrin glues may be effective in some situations.[95]

FACTOR X DEFICIENCY (OMIM 227600)

Factor X deficiency was described in two patients in the 1950s.[146,147] The missing plasma factor was called *Stuart-Prower factor* after the two index cases and subsequently was designated *factor X.* Patient Stuart originally was thought to have factor VII deficiency, but mixing of his plasma with factor VII–deficient plasma corrected the abnormalities in clotting assays.[146] Patient Prower had a bleeding tendency and multiple coagulation assay abnormalities, including a prolonged thromboplastin generation test and prothrombin time.[147] Prevalence rates for symptomatic factor X deficiency are thought to be approximately 1 : 1,000,000 (see Table 127–1).[148,149]

Factor X is a 58,000 molecular weight protein that is the precursor of factor Xa.[1,2] Factor X may be activated by the factor VIIa/tissue factor complex or by the factor IXa/factor VIIIa complex (see Fig. 127–1, *A*).[1–3] Factor Xa converts prothrombin to thrombin in the presence of factor Va, phospholipid, and calcium ions; it also catalyzes conversion of factor V to factor Va.

Congenital factor X deficiency is an autosomal recessive trait, with severely affected persons having activity levels less than 1%. Rarely, heterozygotes bleed abnormally.[33] Factor X–deficient mice die in utero or shortly after birth from hemorrhage,[4] and most patients with severe factor X deficiency probably have traces of plasma factor X. Most (75%) of the approximately 60 known mutations identified in the factor X gene are missense mutations, and many are CRM+ variants (www.med.unc.edu/isth/; www.hgmd.org). Mutations affecting the catalytic activity of factor Xa or its interactions with prothrombin or factor V (e.g., Gly381Asp)[150] cause abnormalities in both the prothrombin time and PTT. Mutations that preferentially interfere with activation of factor X by factor VIIa/tissue factor, such as Gla14Lys (Factor X Vorarlberg),[151] preferentially prolong the prothrombin time, whereas Thr318Met (factor X Roma)[152] interferes with interactions with factor IXa, preferentially prolonging the PTT. Factor X deficiency can be inherited with deficiencies of other vitamin K–dependent proteins (see Combined Deficiency of Vitamin K–Dependent Proteins below).

Acquired factor X deficiency occurs with warfarin therapy, vitamin K deficiency, liver disease and disseminated intravascular coagulation, all of which cause concomitant decreases of other coagulation factor levels. Factor X deficiency has been reported with malignancy,[153] infections,[154] and medication.[155] There are rare reports of acquired factor X inhibitors,[156] some after exposure to topical thrombin.[157] Amyloidosis has been implicated in acquired factor X deficiency,[158,159] occurring in 8.7% of patients with AL amyloidosis in one study[160] but rarely in secondary (AA) amyloidosis.[161] Factor X binds to amyloid fibrils, greatly reducing the plasma half-life of the protein.[159] Distinguishing this type of factor X deficiency from the inherited disorder is based on the clinical setting and poor clinical response to infusion of factor X–containing products in the amyloidosis patients.

Bleeding in factor X deficiency is severe and occurs earlier in life in patients with the lowest plasma levels.[149] Factor X–deficient patients bleed more severely than do patients with other rare congenital coagulopathies.[162] The most frequent symptom is epistaxis (72%), but soft-tissue hematomas and menorrhagia are common.[149] Hemarthrosis, hematuria, postoperative bleeding, central nervous system hemorrhage, and gastrointestinal bleeding occur in severe deficiency, and umbilical stump bleeding in newborns is common (28%). Mildly affected persons (factor X activity >15%) may have increased bruising or bleeding with trauma. Most heterozygotes are asymptomatic. However, one third may have excessive bleeding from mucous membranes or after invasive procedures.[33]

As the first protein in the common pathway (see Fig. 127–1, *B*), factor X deficiency typically prolongs the prothrombin time and PTT and must be distinguished from deficiencies of fibrinogen, prothrombin, and factor V, which are associated with similar test results. Definitive diagnosis and determination of severity are established by a modified prothrombin time or PTT assay using factor X–deficient plasma. Some factor X variants preferentially prolong either the prothrombin time or the PTT. Distinguishing congenital factor X deficiency from acquired deficiency associated with amyloidosis cannot be determined in the coagulation laboratory because assays that are dependent on factor X will correct after mixing with normal plasma in both conditions. The findings of a serum M protein, signs of amyloidosis, and histologic confirmation of amyloid in tissues point toward AL amyloidosis. A poor response to factor X infusion in the absence of an inhibitor distinguishes the two conditions.

Factor X–deficient patients are treated with fresh frozen plasma[163] or prothrombin complex concentrate[164,165] for most bleeding episodes (see Table 127–2). A level of 10% to 15% usually is sufficient for hemarthroses and soft-tissue bleeding. The half-life of factor X is approximately 20 to 40 hours,[166] and levels of 10% to 20% are easily obtained with fresh frozen plasma. Recommended fresh frozen plasma doses are 20 mL/kg initially and 3 to 6 mL/kg every 24 hours to keep trough activity levels at 10% to 20%.[95] Higher factor X levels may be required for severe bleeding or surgery, and accumulation of factor X in plasma can be achieved by increasing the transfusion frequency to every 12 hours. Prothrombin complex concentrates contain approximately 1 unit of factor X per unit of factor IX, and doses of 20 to 30 units/kg daily or every other day have been suggested for major surgery.[14,35] Risk of thromboembolism and disseminated intravascular coagulation is a concern when using prothrombin complex concentrates, and it is recommended that plasma factor X levels not exceed 50% of normal, unless absolutely required.[14,164,165] Minor bleeding episodes can be treated with local measures and/or ε-aminocaproic acid. Cryoprecipitate lacks factor X, and DDAVP infusion has no effect and should not be used.

Patients with acquired factor X deficiency and amyloidosis usually are unresponsive to administration of products containing factor X. Treatment has been based on chemotherapy,[166] splenectomy,[167] plasma exchange,[168] prothrombin complex concentrates,[169] and activated factor VIIa.[170]

FACTOR XI DEFICIENCY (OMIM 264900)

In 1953, Rosenthal et al.[171] described three members of a family with abnormal hemostasis, prolonged time to clot formation in a glass tube, and normal prothrombin times. In mixing studies, patient plasma shortened the clotting times of factor VIII–deficient or factor IX–deficient plasma. Unlike the X-linked hemophilias, the new disorder, sometimes referred to as *hemophilia C*, was transmitted as an autosomal trait.[172] The missing factor was called *plasma thromboplastin antecedent* and subsequently factor XI. Early estimates placed the incidence of factor XI deficiency at 1 : 1,000,000.[173] However, other studies suggest an incidence as high as 1%,if symptomatic cases with mild deficiency are included (see Table 127–1).[174,175] Severe factor XI deficiency is common in persons of Ashkenazi Jewish decent, with an incidence of 1 : 450.[176]

Factor XI, the precursor of the 160,000 molecular weight protease factor XIa, is a dimer of two identical polypeptides.[1,2] This structure is unique among coagulation proteases and has implications for inheritance patterns in factor XI deficiency. In the PTT assay, factor XI is activated by factor XIIa (see Fig. 127–1, *B*). However, in vivo factor XI is likely to be activated by factor XII–independent processes as well, because factor XII deficiency does not cause abnormal bleeding.[6] Factor XI may be activated by thrombin, factor XIIa, or factor XIa,[7] and factor XIa activates factor IX (see Fig. 127–1, *A*).[1–3]

The carrier (heterozygous) frequency for factor XI deficiency in Ashkenazi Jews is 5% to 11%, and severe deficiency (<15% of normal) occurs in 0.1% to 0.3%.[5] Early observations of factor XI–deficient parents passing severe deficiency to their children suggested an autosomal dominant or incompletely recessive mode of inheritance.[172,177] It is likely that the unaffected parent in many cases was an asymptomatic carrier, and it is the current opinion that factor XI deficiency in the Jewish population is an autosomal recessive disorder.[176,178] Asakai et al.[179] identified three factor XI gene mutations, two of which account for more than 90% of abnormal factor XI alleles in Jews.[178,180] Glu117Stop codes for a truncated protein, and homozygotes lack plasma factor XI antigen and activity.[179] Phe283Leu causes a partial defect in dimer formation with retention of monomerie protein within the cell of origin.[181] Phe283Leu homozygotes have plasma factor XI activity and antigen levels of 10%,[5] and the plasma protein is dimeric.[181] Compound heterozygotes for Glu117Stop and Phe283Leu have activity of approximately 3%, and heterozygotes have activities of approximately 50% to 60%.[5]

More than 100 mutations in the human factor XI gene have been identified (www.med.unc.edu/isth/; www.hgmd.org; www.FactorXI.org). Cys38Arg has an allele frequency of approximately 0.5% in French Basques,[175] and Cys128Stop[174] accounts for approximately 10% of mutant factor XI alleles in Great Britain.[173] In most cases, plasma factor XI activity and antigen are comparably reduced (CRM− deficiency).[182–184] A classification scheme with three categories has been proposed for CRM− deficiency.[185] The first category contains mutations that prevent factor synthesis (e.g., Glu117Stop), whereas the second contains mutations that interfere with dimer formation (e.g., Phe283Leu). Inheritance in both categories likely follows an autosomal recessive pattern, as mutant polypeptide would not interfere with the product of the normal allele in a heterozygote. The third category includes mutations that block secretion but do not prevent dimerization (e.g., Gly400Val).[185,186] In heterozygotes, mutant polypeptides form dimers with wild-type factor XI, trapping the normal protein in the cell (dominant negative effect). This mechanism may account for families in which severe to moderate factor XI deficiency appears to be a dominant trait. CRM+ factor XI mutations are rare and usually involve catalytic defects (e.g., Gly555Glu).[187] Factor XI Ser248Asn has activity similar to normal factor XI in the PTT assay but binds poorly to platelets,[188] possibly explaining the bleeding disorder associated with the mutation.

Factor XI levels decrease in liver disease and disseminated intravascular coagulation but are not affected by vitamin K deficiency or warfarin therapy. Mild factor XI deficiency is common in patients with Noonan syndrome[189] and the carbohydrate-deficient glycoprotein syndrome, a group of genetic disorders involving multiple organ systems caused by defects in glycosylation of secretory glycoproteins.[190] Antibody inhibitors to factor XI are a relatively common consequence of replacement therapy in factor XI–deficient patients, with up to one third of homozygotes for the Glu117Stop mutation developing inhibitors, often after a single exposure to plasma.[178,191]

Significant bleeding in severe factor XI deficiency is triggered by trauma or surgery.[177,178,192] Spontaneous soft-tissue bleeding or bruising is uncommon.[177,182,184] Bleeding may start at the time of injury or be delayed several hours, and oozing from wounds such as tooth extraction sites may persist for hours to days. Bleeding correlates relatively poorly with plasma factor XI levels.[182,184] Patients with severe deficiency may not bleed excessively, even during surgery without treatment,[5] whereas patients with milder deficiency (15%–50% of normal) may have abnormal hemostasis.[182,184,192] A patient may exhibit different bleeding tendencies over time.[177,184] A study of severe factor XI deficiency clarified this situation by showing that both factor XI level and site of injury influence bleeding.[5] Injury to tissue with high fibrinolytic activity, such as the oral cavity or urinary tract, is associated with excessive bleeding in two thirds of cases, regardless of genotype. Bleeding with surgery or injury at other locations is less frequent but is more common in patients with the lowest factor XI levels.[5,193,194] Thus, homozygotes for Phe283Leu experienced less bleeding than did homozygotes for Glu117Stop or compound heterozygotes.

The association between abnormal hemostasis and mild factor XI deficiency is controversial. Some studies demonstrated minimal bleeding with procedures including tooth extraction, tonsillectomy, nasal surgery, and urologic surgery,[5,195] others found poor correlation between factor XI levels and bleeding,[193,196] and some suggest it is difficult to distinguish severe from mild deficiency based on bleeding tendency.[184,195] Using a logistic regression model, Brenner et al.[193] assessed bleeding in 45 families with factor XI deficiency and determined the odds ratios for bleeding were 13.0 and 2.6 for homozygotes and heterozygotes, respectively. Thus, mild factor XI deficiency may be a mild risk factor for bleeding, but with a significantly smaller risk than for severe deficiency.

In the PTT assay, factor XI is bound to the contact surface through high-molecular-weight kininogen and is activated by factor XIIa (see Figs. 127–1, *B*, and 127–3). Factor XIa then activates factor IX. Therefore, factor XI deficiency prolongs the PTT. Diagnosis and severity are established by a modified PTT using factor XI–deficient plasma. The PTT may be normal in heterozygotes.

Planning perioperative therapy is a challenge in factor XI–deficient patients (see box on Treating Factor XI–Deficient Patients). Factor XI concentrates are available in some countries. Replacement therapy with fresh frozen plasma is used most often in the United States (see Table 127–2). Cryoprecipitate does not contain factor XI, and factor XI levels do not respond to DDAVP. The half-life of factor XI from fresh frozen plasma is approximately 45 hours. When deciding which patients require replacement therapy, it is important to consider the type of hemostatic challenge anticipated. In patients with severe deficiency, most major surgery or procedures involving tissues with high fibrinolytic activity (oropharynx or urinary tract) should be covered with fresh frozen plasma to keep plasma levels at approximately 45% for 10 to 14 days.[197] In the past, it has been recommended that surgery at other sites be treated with replacement to achieve a target of approximately 30% for 5 to 7 days. However, a current retrospective analysis has confirmed that for certain procedures such as circumcision, orthopedic surgery, and appendectomy, the risk of bleeding is low, and replacement therapy can be withheld, unless bleeding occurs.[194] Similar "on-demand" recommendations have been made for treating women during and after labor, which usually is not associated with excessive bleeding.[184,196] Dental procedures, such as tooth extraction, and minor surgical procedures should be covered with antifibrinolytic therapy and in most cases do not require replacement therapy.[198] Patients with factor XI levels greater than 40% do not require replacement therapy for surgery.[195]

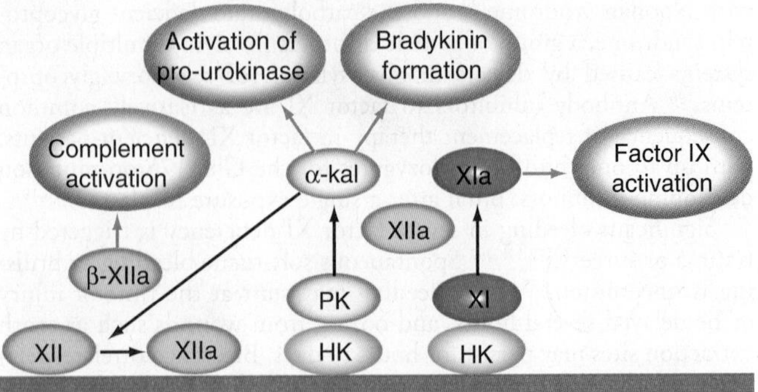

Figure 127–3 Contact activation reactions. Contact activation is initiated by activation of factor XII (XII) to α-factor XIIa (XIIa) when plasma is exposed to a negatively charged surface. Factor XIIa converts prekallikrein (PK) to the active protease α-kallikrein, and α-kallikrein reciprocally activates additional factor XII, amplifying the contact process. Factor XIIa initiates coagulation in the activated partial thromboplastin time assay through conversion of factor XI (XI) to factor XIa (XIa). Note that both PK and factor XI require high-molecular-weight kininogen (HK) to bind properly to the negatively charged surface. The products of the contact activation process can contribute to activation of several host defense mechanisms, at least in vitro. Factor XIa promotes thrombin generation and fibrin clot formation through activation of factor IX. A fragment of α-factor XIIa (β-XIIa—Hageman factor fragment) can initiate the complement cascade through activation of C1. α-Kallikrein cleaves HK to liberate the nanopeptide bradykinin, which has important effects on inflammation and on regulation of local blood flow. α-Kallikrein also can convert prourokinase to the plasminogen activator urokinase, initiating fibrinolysis. Large black arrows indicate the main reactions of contact activation that require the negatively charged surface. Gray arrows indicate subsequent effects on host defense mechanisms that are not surface dependent.

Factor XI concentrates have shown efficacy in factor XI–deficient patients[199,200] but have not been available in the United States. In November 2007, the plasma factor XI concentrate Hemoleven® (LSB, Les Ulis, France) was granted orphan-designation by the Food and Drug Administration. The use of these concentrates has been associated with evidence of intravascular coagulation and thromboembolic events,[201,202] particularly in elderly patients with cardiovascular disease receiving doses greater than 30 U/kg. Current concentrates contain antithrombin and heparin to reduce the procoagulant nature of the product. Factor XI–deficient patients with inhibitors usually do not have an increased bleeding tendency. Activated prothrombin complex concentrates and recombinant factor VIIa both have been used successfully for major surgery in patients with inhibitors.[203,204]

DEFICIENCIES OF THE CONTACT FACTORS: FACTOR XII, PREKALLIKREIN, AND HIGH-MOLECULAR-WEIGHT KININOGEN

Factor XII, prekallikrein, and high-molecular-weight kininogen along with factor XI are involved in the "contact phase" that initiates coagulation in the PTT (see Figs. 127–1, *B,* and 127–3). Patients with deficiency of these proteins have prolonged PTTs but do not have abnormal bleeding, even with major surgery.[6] Therefore, either these proteins do not participate in hemostasis, or redundant mechanisms compensate for their absence. No specific therapy is required to prepare deficient patients for invasive procedures. It is clinically important to distinguish factor XII, prekallikrein, and high-molecular-weight kininogen deficiency from deficiencies of factors VIII, IX, or XI, which also prolong the PTT but cause abnormal hemostasis.

Treating Factor XI–Deficient Patients

When preparing patients with severe factor XI deficiency (plasma level <15%) for an invasive procedure, it is important to remember that (a) a negative bleeding history does not indicate low risk with subsequent procedures, (b) certain procedures are associated with low bleeding risk, and (c) patients with very low factor XI levels (<1%) may develop neutralizing inhibitors when exposed to factor XI. These observations have led to refinements in treatment recommendations that limit exposure to factor XI. Antiplatelet drugs should be stopped 1 week before surgery. Dental extraction can be managed with antifibrinolytic drugs alone (tranexamic acid 1 g qid or ε-aminocaproic acid 4–6 g qid), starting 12 hours before the procedure and continuing for 7 days. Surgery on the oropharynx, nasopharynx, or urinary tract should be treated with fresh frozen plasma for 10 to 14 days, as more than half of patients will bleed if not treated. A similar strategy is appropriate for neurosurgery, head and neck surgery, and cardiothoracic procedures. Antifibrinolytic therapy is a useful adjunct to replacement for surgery on the oropharynx or nasopharynx. Fresh frozen plasma infusion is not necessary prior to circumcision, orthopedic surgery, or appendectomy, as the incidence of excessive bleeding is less than 5%. If bleeding subsequently occurs, fresh frozen plasma should be administered. For vaginal delivery, replacement may be withheld unless bleeding occurs. A similar approach may be acceptable for cesarean section, although data are limited. It is not clear if epidural anesthesia is safe in the absence of factor coverage, and replacement therapy should be used. Patients with factor XI levels greater than 40% do not require replacement, and a history of excessive bleeding in these individuals suggests the presence of other hemostatic abnormalities. Replacement therapy to reach appropriate target levels may be required for factor XI levels of 15% to 40%, depending on the procedure. Aspirin or clopidogrel can be used in factor XI–deficient patients with myocardial infarction or other manifestations of atherosclerosis. Atrial fibrillation or venous thromboembolism should be treated with warfarin, with the goal of not allowing the international normalized ratio to exceed 2.5.

Factor XII Deficiency (OMIM 234000)

In 1955, Ratnoff and Colopy[205] described three asymptomatic individuals with a novel abnormality of surface-induced coagulation. The missing plasma component was called *Hageman factor* after the index case[206] and later was designated *factor XII.* The incidence of severe factor XII deficiency is not known. Many deficient persons go undiagnosed due to the absence of a phenotype. Moderate to severe factor XII deficiency was reported in 1.5% to 3.0% of healthy blood donors. This unexpectedly high prevalence may be related to antibodies to factor XII or antiphospholipid antibodies that interfere with factor XII activity assays.[207,208]

Factor XIIa is an 80,000 molecular weight protease that activates factor XI and prekallikrein during the contact phase of the PTT.[1,2] A 46C/T polymorphism in the 5′-untranslated region of the factor XII gene strongly influences plasma levels, with the 46T allele associated with lower plasma factor XII compared to 46C.[209] The frequency of 46T is high (73%) in East Asians (compared to 20% in Caucasians), who have lower factor XII levels than other ethnic groups. Factor XII activity and antigen usually are reduced in parallel in deficient individuals, and circulating dysfunctional variants are rare.[210] A small number of factor XII gene mutations have been identified (www.hgmd.org), most residing in the protease domain.[211] Factor XII deficiency is not associated with spontaneous or excessive posttraumatic bleeding, and most cases are identified by the incidental finding of a prolonged PTT. There is controversy regarding an association between factor XII deficiency and thrombosis[212] or recurrent abortion.[213] Although studies indicate no increased risk for thrombosis,[214,215] results from the SMILE (Study of myocardial infarction—Leiden) project demonstrated an inverse relationship between factor XII levels and risk of myocardial infarction.[212] In contrast, factor XII–deficient mice are relatively protected from developing pathologic thrombi.[216] An association between factor XII deficiency and thrombosis in humans remains uncertain.

Factor XII undergoes autoactivation when exposed to the contact surface in the PTT. Factor XIIa activates factor XI and prekallikrein, with α-kallikrein reciprocally activating additional factor XII (see Fig. 127–3). In severe factor XII deficiency, the PTT is very prolonged. Definitive diagnosis is established by a modified PTT using factor XII–deficient plasma. Antiphospholipid antibodies may disproportionately affect measurement of factor XII by PTT-based assays.[217] In addition, factor XII antibodies have been detected in up to half of plasmas with antiphospholipid antibodies[207,208] and may account for many or most cases of presumed mild factor XII deficiency.

Prekallikrein Deficiency (OMIM 229000)

In 1965, Hathaway et al.[218] reported on members of a family with long plasma clotting times that corrected on prolonged incubation with glass. The family had no history of bleeding. The missing plasma component, initially called *Fletcher factor* after the index cases, subsequently was shown to be prekallikrien.[219] Severe prekallikrein deficiency apparently is a rare disorder. However, many mild cases may be missed because 2% to 5% of normal plasma prekallikrein activity is sufficient to bring some PTT assays into the normal range.

Prekallikrein is the 95,000 molecular weight precursor of the kininogenase α-kallikrein. Prekallikrein deficiency is an autosomal trait, presenting in the homozygous or compound heterozygous forms with plasma levels less than 1%. CRM+ prekallikrein variants account for about half of cases and are common in Caucasian and Japanese patients; most black patients are CRM–.[6] Few prekallikrein gene mutations have been identified (www.hgmd.org). Partial prekallikrein deficiency (10%–50%) may be seen in patients with severe high-molecular-weight kininogen deficiency,[220] likely due to increased catabolism or clearance, because prekallikrein circulates as a complex with high-molecular-weight kininogen. Severe prekallikrein deficiency presents as an incidental prolongation of the PTT in a person without a history of excessive bleeding. Although thrombotic events have been described with prekallikrein deficiency, whether the deficiency contributes to thrombosis is unclear.

In the PTT assay, prekallikrein is converted to α-kallikrein by factor XIIa, which reciprocally activates factor XII (see Figs. 127–1B and 127–3). Severe prekallikrein deficiency causes a prolonged PTT, and the diagnosis is confirmed by a modified PTT using prekallikrein-deficient plasma. The prolonged PTT in prekallikrein deficiency may be shortened by prolonged incubation with the contact reagent, which allows factor XII sufficient time to activate by prekallikrein-independent mechanisms. This distinguishes prekallikrein deficiency from other deficiencies associated with a prolonged PTT, which do not correct with prolonged incubation. Some PTT reagents use the contact activator ellagic acid, which is relatively insensitive to prekallikrein deficiency and may fail to detect some patients with prekallikrein deficiency.

High-Molecular-Weight Kininogen Deficiency (OMIM 228960)

In 1974, Schiffman and Lee[221] reported that a plasma factor distinct from prekallikrein was required for factor XI activation by factor XIIa. In 1975, three asymptomatic patients from three separate families with in vitro abnormalities of coagulation, fibrinolysis, and kinin generation were described who appeared to lack the unknown factor. The condition, originally named for the affected families (Fitzgerald trait, Williams trait, and Flaujeac trait),[6,220] subsequently was determined to be due to high-molecular-weight kininogen deficiency. The disorder appears to be very rare.

High–molecular-weight kininogen is a 110,000 molecular weight glycoprotein that contains the vasoactive peptide bradykinin.[222,223] Prekallikrein and factor XI circulate in plasma as complexes with high-molecular-weight kininogen. Low-molecular-weight kininogen and high–molecular-weight kininogen are alternatively spliced products of a single gene; however, low–molecular-weight kininogen does not play a role in coagulation in vitro. High-molecular-weight kininogen deficiency is an autosomal recessive trait. Depending on the genetic abnormality (www.hgmd.org), patients may have isolated high-molecular-weight kininogen deficiency or combined high-molecular-weight kininogen and low-molecular-weight kininogen deficiency.[6] Patients with high-molecular-weight kininogen deficiency usually are identified by the incidental finding of a prolonged PTT and do not have excessive bleeding.

In the PTT assay, high-molecular-weight kininogen facilitates binding of prekallikrein and factor XI to the contact surface, enhancing their activation by factor XIIa (see Fig. 127–1B and 127–3). Severe high-molecular-weight kininogen deficiency is characterized by a very prolonged PTT, and definitive diagnosis is established by modified PTT using high-molecular-weight kininogen–deficient plasma. Partial prekallikrein deficiency is common in severe high-molecular-weight kininogen deficiency, likely due to increased catabolism of prekallikrein when it is not in complex with high-molecular-weight kininogen.[220]

FACTOR XIII DEFICIENCY (OMIM 134570 [A SUBUNIT] AND 134580 [B SUBUNIT])

In 1944, Robbins[224] demonstrated that fibrin formed from purified components was soluble in weak acid, whereas fibrin formed in the presence of serum or plasma was not. He proposed that a *fibrin stabilizing factor* was present in plasma, and that its deficiency would cause excessive bleeding. This idea was confirmed in 1960, when Duckert et al.[225] described the first patient with deficiency of fibrin stabilizing factor, which subsequently was designated *factor XIII.* The incidence of symptomatic factor XIII deficiency is estimated to be 1 : 1–5,000,000 (see Table 127–1).[226]

Plasma factor XIII is a 330,000 molecular weight tetramer composed of two catalytic "A" subunits and two carrier "B" subunits.[8,227] About half of factor XIII in blood is in platelets, with a small amount in monocytes. Platelet and monocyte factor XIII consist only of A subunits. Factor XIII is converted to the transglutaminase factor XIIIa by thrombin and catalyzes formation of γ-glutamyl-ε-lysyl bonds between fibrin monomers (see Fig. 127–1, *A*), resulting in a fibrin meshwork that is insoluble in mild acids and urea. Factor XIIIa also cross-links fibrin to plasma, extracellular matrix, and cytoskeleton proteins, facilitating clot adherence to an injury site. Congenital factor XIII deficiency is an autosomal recessive trait. In type I deficiency, A and B subunits are reduced, whereas in type II deficiency A subunits are reduced and in type III deficiency B subunits are reduced.[228] Deficiency usually is caused by mutations in the A subunit.[35] B subunit mutations are rare (www.med.unc.edu/isth/; www.hgmd.org). The incidence of factor XIII mutations probably is higher than the incidence of the bleeding diathesis, as hemorrhage and screening test abnormalities occur almost exclusively with severely decreased plasma activity (<1%–2%). For some mutations, a founder effect is likely. For example, Leu660Pro in the A subunit is relatively prevalent in Palestinian Arabs.[229] The molecular heterogeneity of factor XIII deficiency may explain variability in bleeding, with mutations in specific areas of the molecule affecting certain functions.

Plasma factor XIII levels are low in disseminated intravascular coagulation. Significant deficiency is rare in liver disease and may indicate a poor prognosis. Acquired deficiency has been seen in inflammatory disorders, including Henoch-Schönlein purpura,[230] and inflammatory bowel disease.[231] Factor XIII neutralizing antibodies rarely occur in deficient patients as a consequence of factor replacement but have been observed in collagen vascular disorders such as systemic lupus erythematosus[232] and with therapy with isoniazid, penicillin, procainamide, and phenytoin.[233]

Newborns with factor XIII deficiency frequently bleed from the umbilical stump.[234–236] Ecchymoses, soft-tissue hematomas, and prolonged bleeding with trauma are common, and recurrent soft-tissue bleeding may lead to formation of hemorrhagic cysts (pseudotumors).[234,235] Hemarthroses is less frequent than in factor VIII or IX deficiency. Bleeding often is delayed 12 to 36 hours postinjury[225] but may be immediate. Bleeding at the time of invasive procedures may be minimal, but delayed hemorrhage often occurs. Intracranial hemorrhage is more frequent in factor XIII deficiency than in other inherited coagulation disorder; its incidence of 25%[235–237] justifies prophylactic factor XIII replacement. Delayed wound healing has been observed in deficient patients, possibly related to a defect in angiogenesis.[238] Recurrent spontaneous abortions occur with most pregnancies in untreated factor XIII–deficient women,[239] possibly due to abnormal formation of the cytotrophoblastic shell and poor attachment of the placenta to the uterus.[240]

The prothrombin time and PTT measure time to fibrin clot formation; they do not assess clot stability. Therefore, results of these assays are normal in factor XIII–deficient patients. Clots in factor XIII–deficient plasma are soluble in 5 M urea or 1% monochloroacetic acid, whereas normal clots are stable for at least 24 hours.[241] Solubility in 5 M urea (urea clot stability assay) is the most frequently used clinical assay for screening for factor XIII deficiency or inhibitors. Clots from plasma lacking α_2 antiplasmin also may show increased solubility in this assay[242] and can be identified with specific assays. Specific assays measuring factor XIIIa activity are available but have yet to achieve widespread clinical use.[241]

The plasma half-life of factor XIII is 10 to 14 days,[243] and hemostasis can be achieved in most situations by maintaining levels above approximately 5%, thus facilitating prophylactic replacement therapy to prevent intracranial bleeding. Factor XIII concentrate (Fibrogammin) is available in the United States only as part of a company-sponsored study (see Table 127–2),[244,245] A regimen of 10 to 20 U/kg every 5 to 6 weeks is sufficient for normal hemostasis. Single doses of 10 to 20 U/kg have been used successfully for treatment of poor wound healing. If concentrate is not available, fresh frozen plasma (1–2 units every 4–6 weeks) or cryoprecipitate (1 unit/10–20 kg body weight every 3–4 weeks) can be used. Limited information is available to guide the use of replacement therapy during surgery or major bleeding. Factor XIII concentrate (50–75 U/kg) has been recommended for these situations.[245] Adequate hemostasis has been achieved during intracranial surgery by administering concentrate to achieve a level of 50% during surgery and then maintaining the level above 20% for the first few postoperative weeks before returning to prophylactic dosing.[246] Factor XIII levels higher than those achieved with prophylactic dosing are also required to prevent fetal loss during pregnancy.[38,247] In pregnancy, factor XIII replacement should be started early, preferably before gestational week 5, as decidual bleeding from implantation will occur without replacement. The optimal plasma factor XIII concentration in pregnancy is not clear, but at least 10% of normal is recommended.[247] This can be achieved by infusing 250 units of concentrate every 7 days through week 22 of gestation and 500 units per week for the remainder of pregnancy, with a bolus of 1000 units during labor.[247]

CONGENITAL DEFICIENCIES INVOLVING MULTIPLE COAGULATION FACTORS

Cases of congenital deficiencies of more than one coagulation factor have been described. Some likely represent chance coinheritance of distinct factor deficiency states, but several represent familial syndromes (Table 127–3). Such syndromes likely are caused by abnormalities in intracellular processing of factors (e.g., type 1 deficiency) or alterations in the structure/activity of multiple factors (e.g., type 3 deficiency). Remember that common nonspecific inhibitors such as lupus anticoagulants interfere with coagulation assays and can lead to erroneous interpretations when they suggest multiple factor deficiencies (see box on Laboratory Testing in Rare Coagulation Factor Deficiencies). Similarly, potent inhibitors directed at a single coagulation factor (e.g., factor VIII) occasionally may interfere with assays for other factors. Two familial multiple factor deficiency states, combined factor V and VIII deficiency (type 1) and deficiency of vitamin K–dependent factors (type 3), are well characterized.

Combined Factor V and Factor VIII Deficiency (OMIM 227300)

Combined factor V and factor VIII deficiency was first recognized in 1954.[248] The familial form is an autosomal recessive trait caused by mutations (www.med.unc.edu/isth/) in either the LMAN1 (mannose binding lectin, formerly ERGIC-53) or MCFD2 (multiple combined factor deficiency protein) gene.[249,250] These proteins form a complex required for transport of factors V and VIII from the endoplasmic reticulum to the Golgi apparatus.[251] Although very rare, the allele frequency is high (≈1%) in Tunisian Jews originating from a community on the island of Djerba.[252]

Deficiency of either LMAN1 or MCFD2 causes a partial defect in factor V and VIII secretion, lowering plasma levels to approximately 5% to 30%. The mutation in Tunisian Jews is a T to C transition at a donor splice site in intron 9 of the LMAN1 gene.[252] A history of consanguinity, cosegregation of the factor deficiencies, and similar reductions in factor V and VIII favor the familial disorder. Homozygotes or compound heterozygotes bleed primarily after trauma, and epistaxis, gingival bleeding, easy bruising, and menorrhagia are common.[253,254] Nontrauma-related hemarthrosis may occur in 20% of patients, but bleeding from the gastrointestinal

Table 127–3 Combined Familial Deficiency States

Type	Deficient Factors	OMIM Designation	Reference	Underlying Cause
1	V, VIII	227300	249, 250	Mutations in LMAN1 or MCFD2
2	VIII, IX	134510	266	Unknown
3	II, VII, IX, X, protein C, protein S	277450 (γ-glutamyl carboxylase) 608547 (vitamin K oxidoreductase)	259, 260, 262	Mutations in γ-glutamyl carboxylase or vitamin K oxidoreductase
4	VII, VIII	134430	266	Unknown
5	VIII, IX, XI	134520	267	Unknown
6	IX, XI	134540	267	Unknown

OMIM, Online Mendelian Inheritance in Man.

Laboratory Testing in Rare Coagulation Factor Deficiencies

When considering one of these diagnoses, remember that (a) acquired conditions causing multiple factor deficiencies are far more common than is congenital deficiency of a single factor, and (b) common nonspecific coagulation inhibitors such as lupus anticoagulants and heparin can interfere with coagulation assays. Unexplained prolongation of the prothrombin time or partial thromboplastin time (PTT) should be evaluated in a qualified laboratory. A mixing study with normal plasma is recommended as an initial step to determine if the abnormality is related to a factor deficiency or an inhibitor. The mixing study should be done with and without incubation (1–2 hours), as some inhibitors show a time-dependent pattern of inhibition. Slight prolongation of the prothrombin time or PTT can be difficult to evaluate with a mixing study, and we frequently test for lupus anticoagulants in these cases prior to specific assays for coagulation factors. Ideally, samples should be collected by venipuncture and not from central lines or ports, because contamination of samples with heparin may distort results. Many laboratories use the thrombin time assay to screen samples for possible heparin contamination. Tests for hepatic function (albumin) or injury (transaminases) facilitate interpretation. If a vitamin K–dependent protein (prothrombin or factor VII, IX, or X) is low, a level for factor V and at least one other vitamin K–dependent factor should be determined. If levels of multiple vitamin K–dependent factors are low and factor V is normal, a process affecting vitamin K is likely. If factor V also is low, liver disease or disseminated intravascular coagulation should be considered. Distinguishing disseminated intravascular coagulation from liver disease can be difficult, because standard tests may be abnormal in both conditions. Measuring factor V and factor VIII levels can be useful in this situation, because both factors usually are low in disseminated intravascular coagulation, whereas the factor VIII level often is normal or elevated in liver disease.

Patients with factor XI, XII, prekallikrein, or high-molecular-weight kininogen deficiency may require anticoagulation for thromboembolism or other indications. However, the PTT cannot be used for monitoring therapy with unfractionated heparin or thrombin inhibitors such as lepirudin and argatroban. Measuring heparin with a factor Xa-based chromogenic assay or by protamine titration can be done but requires a sophisticated laboratory. Alternatively, low-molecular-weight heparin, which usually does not require monitoring, may be used. Specific tests for direct thrombin inhibitors have been developed, some based on modifications of the thrombin time assay.

tract or intracranial hemorrhage is less common. Postpartum hemorrhage occurs in most affected women, and invasive procedures including dental extraction usually are accompanied by excessive bleeding without replacement therapy. In one study, approximately 13% of heterozygotes reported excessive bleeding; however, there was no correlation between symptoms and factor levels.[253] The disorder is associated with a prolonged prothrombin time and PTT (see Fig. 127–1, *B*). Isolated factor V deficiency also gives this pattern, so it is recommended that factor VIII levels be measured in patients with factor V deficiency so that combined deficiency is not overlooked.

Patients with mucosal bleeding and menorrhagia may respond to antifibrinolytic therapy. For more significant bleeding, surgical procedures, or tooth extraction, a combination of fresh frozen plasma and factor VIII concentrate should be used. DDAVP can raise factor VIII[253] but not factor V levels.[255] Trough levels of approximately 50% for both proteins have been recommended for surgery. Plasma exchange to raise factor V levels has been suggested to avoid volume overload from large volumes of fresh frozen plasma.[255]

Combined Deficiency of Vitamin K–Dependent Proteins (OMIM 277450 and 608547)

In 1979, Chung et al.[256] described a newborn girl with a prolonged prothrombin time and PTT, low levels of prothrombin and factors VII, IX, and X and no evidence of liver disease or malabsorption. She had a partial response to large doses of vitamin K. In subsequent cases, low protein C and protein S levels also were noted[257,258] in association with mutations in the γ-glutamyl carboxylase gene.[259,260] The condition is a rare autosomal recessive trait.[261]

Prothrombin, factors VII, IX, and X, proteins C and S, and some bone proteins require γ-carboxylation of glutamic acid residues in the N-terminal Gla domain (see Chapter 130).[1,2] γ-Carboxylation is mediated by γ-glutamyl carboxylase, which uses reduced vitamin K as a cofactor. γ-Carboxylation results in formation of vitamin K 2,3-epoxide, which must be reduced by vitamin K oxidoreductase to replenish the pool of vitamin K. Mutations in the γ-glutamyl carboxylase gene (e.g., Arg394Leu; www.hgmd.org) or vitamin K oxidoreductase gene (e.g., Arg98Trp) can impair this process and result in low levels of all vitamin K–dependent proteins.[260,262] The factors are reduced to 10% to 50% of normal, resulting in a variable bleeding tendency that may be severe. Some patients have skeletal abnormalities, possibly related to reduced function of vitamin K–dependent bone proteins.[263] Low levels of vitamin K–dependent proteins are also seen in patients receiving warfarin, in poisoning with rodenticides such as brodifacoum, and in vitamin K deficiency. The levels of these proteins are low in liver failure, in conjunction with other proteins synthesized in the liver.

The low levels of prothrombin and factors VII, IX, and X cause prolongation of the prothrombin time and PTT. Protein C and S levels also are reduced. The abnormalities correct upon mixing with normal plasma. Failure to correct suggests that a nonspecific inhibitor such as a lupus anticoagulant is interfering with the assay. Patients with deficiencies of vitamin K–dependent proteins should be evaluated for liver disease and for exposure to warfarin or rodenticides containing vitamin K antagonists such as brodifacoum. Due to their long half-lives, these agents can be identified by toxicology screens long after ingestion. Some patients have adequate clinical response to vitamin K but require unusually high doses. Non-responders or responders with significant bleeding episodes can be treated with fresh frozen plasma or prothrombin complex concentrate.[261,264,265]

SUGGESTED READINGS

Asselta R, Tenchini ML, Duga S: Inherited defects of coagulation factor V: The hemorrhagic side. J Thromb Haemost 4:26, 2006.

Asselta R, Duga S, Tenchini ML: The molecular basis of quantitative fibrinogen disorders. J Thromb Haemost 4:2115, 2006.

Darghouth D, Hallgren KW, Shtofman RL, et al: Compound heterozygosity of novel missense mutations in the gamma-glutamyl-carboxylase gene causes hereditary combined vitamin K-dependent coagulation factor deficiency. Blood 108:1925, 2006.

Davie EW, Kulman JD: An overview of the structure and function of thrombin. Semin Thromb Hemost Suppl 1:3, 2006.

Doggen CJ, Rosendaal FR, Meijers JC: Levels of intrinsic coagulation factors and the risk of myocardial infarction among men. Opposite and synergistic effects of factors XI and XII. Blood 108:4045, 2006.

Girolami A, Ruzzon E, Tezza F, et al: Arterial and venous thrombosis in rare congenital bleeding disorders: A critical review. Haemophilia 12:345, 2006.

Girolami A, Ruzzon E, Tezza F, et al: Congenital combined defects of factor VII: A critical review. Acta Haematol 117:51, 2007.

Hedner U: Mechanism of action of recombinant activated factor VII: An update. Semin Hematol 43(1 Suppl 1):S105, 2006.

Herrman FH, Auerswald G, Ruiz-Saez A, et al: Factor X deficiency: Clinical manifestations of 102 subjects from Europe and Latin America with mutations in the factor 10 gene. Haemophilia 12:479, 2006.

Inbal A, Dardik R: Role of coagulation factor XIII (FXIII) in angiogenesis and tissue repair. Pathophysiol Haemost Thromb 35:162, 2006.

Kawasaki K, Komura H, Nakahara Y, et al: Factor XIII in Henoch-Schonlein purpura with isolated gastrointestinal symptoms. Pediatr Int 48:413. 2006.

Lee CA, Chi C, Pavord SR, et al: UK Haemophilia Centre Doctors' Organization: The obstetric and gynaecological management of women with inherited bleeding disorders—Review with guidelines produced by a taskforce of UK Haemophilia Centre Doctors' Organization. Haemophilia 12:301, 2006.

Mitchell M, Mountford R, Butler R, et al: Spectrum of factor XI (F11) mutations in the UK population—116 index cases and 140 mutations. Hum Mutat 27:829, 2006.

Moen JL, Lord ST: Afibrinogenemia and dysfibrinogenemia. In Colman RW, Marder VJ, Clowes AW, George JN, Goldhaber SZ (eds.): Hemostasis and Thrombosis: Basic Principles and Practice, 5th ed. Philadelphia, Lippincott, Williams & Wilkins, p 939, 2006.

Perdekamp MT, Rubenstein DA, Jesty J, et al: Platelet factor V supports hemostasis in a patient with an acquired factor V inhibitor, as shown by prothrombinase and tenase assays. Blood Coagul Fibrinolysis 17:593, 2006.

Peyvandi F, Haertel S, Knaub S, Mannucci PM: Incidence of bleeding symptoms in 100 patients with inherited afibrinogenemia or hypofibrinogenemia. J Thromb Haemost 4:1634, 2006.

Peyvandi F, Jayandharan G, Chandy M, et al: Genetic diagnosis of haemophilia and other inherited bleeding disorders. Haemophilia 12(Suppl 3): 82, 2006.

Pollak ES, Russell TT, Ptashkin B, et al: Asymptomatic factor VII deficiency in African Americans. Am J Clin Pathol 126:128, 2006.

Roberts H, Escobar M: Inherited disorders of prothrombin conversion. In Colman RW, Marder V, Clowes A, George JN, Goldhaber SZ (eds.): Hemostasis and Thrombosis: Basic Principles and Clinical Practice, 5th ed. Philadelphia, Lippincott Williams & Wilkins, 2006, p 923.

Rubbia-Brandt L, Neerman-Arbez M, Rougemont AL, Male PJ, Spahr L: Fibrinogen gamma375 arg>trp mutation (fibrinogen aguadilla) causes hereditary hypofibrinogenemia, hepatic endoplasmic reticulum storage disease and cirrhosis. Am J Surg Pathol 30:906, 2006.

Salomon O, Steinberg DM, Seligsohn U: Variable bleeding manifestations characterize different types of surgery in patients with severe factor XI deficiency enabling parsimonious use of replacement. Haemophilia 12:490, 2006.

Sauls DL, Lockhart E, Warren ME, Lenkowski A, Wilhelm SE, Hoffman M: Modification of fibrinogen by homocysteine thiolactone increases resistance to fibrinolysis: A potential mechanism of the thrombotic tendency in hyperhomocysteinemia. Biochemistry 45:2480, 2006.

Vellinga S, Steel E, Vangenechten I, et al: Successful pregnancy in a patient with factor V deficiency: Case report and review of the literature. Thromb Haemost 95:896, 2006.

Wong AYK, Hewitt J, Clarke B, et al: Severe prothrombin deficiency caused by prothrombin-Edmonton (R-4Q) combined with a previously undetected deletion. J Thromb Haemost 4:2623, 2006.

REFERENCES

For complete list of references log onto www.expertconsult.com

CHAPTER 128

STRUCTURE, BIOLOGY, AND GENETICS OF VON WILLEBRAND FACTOR

David Ginsburg and Denisa D. Wagner

The adhesive glycoprotein von Willebrand factor (VWF) was named after Dr. Erich von Willebrand, who described in 1926 a new bleeding disorder[1] distinct from hemophilia. von Willebrand disease (VWD) was later recognized to be caused by qualitative or quantitative defects in VWF.[2] VWF circulates in plasma at concentrations of 5 to 10 μg/mL. Some of the molecules are complexed with factor VIII, protecting factor VIII against degradation. VWF is synthesized by only two cell types: endothelial cells and megakaryocytes.[3,4] Besides plasma, VWF is found in platelets, endothelial cells, and the basement membrane of blood vessels.[5] All these pools of VWF contribute to the protein's main function: to promote attachment of platelets to areas of vessel injury. To optimize the availability of VWF at the site of injury, a highly active form of the protein is stored in secretory granules of platelets and endothelial cells. When these cells sense tissue injury (eg, by contact with thrombin), they instantly mobilize the stored protein. The released VWF binds to glycoprotein Ib (GPIb) on the platelet surface and to components of the basement membrane, forming a bridge that can withstand the high sheer stress of blood flow. VWF is necessary for this initial attachment step of platelets to the injured area.[6] Together with other adhesive proteins, such as fibrinogen, fibronectin, and thrombospondin, VWF interacts with glycoprotein IIb (GPIIb)/IIIa on activated platelets and contributes to platelet spreading and aggregation. VWF is a large protein composed of many subunits held together covalently by disulfide bonds. In this way, the protein acquires multiple binding sites for platelets and the basement membrane, which may strengthen its interactions during hemostasis. The ultra-large forms of VWF assembled within the endothelial cell are processed to smaller forms in circulating plasma through the action of a recently identified plasma protease, ADAMTS13.[7–9] Deficiency of this protease is now known to be the cause of thrombotic thrombocytopenic purpura (TTP) (see Chapter 139). This is presumably because of the abnormally enhanced adhesive function of unprocessed ultra-large VWF multimers. In contrast, qualitative or quantitative deficiency of VWF adhesive function results in the common bleeding disorder, VWD (see Chapter 129).

THE VON WILLEBRAND FACTOR GENE

The full-length VWF complementary DNA (cDNA) sequence predicts a protein of 309,000 molecular weight (2813 amino acids).[10–13] In addition, the location of *N*- and *O*-linked glycosylation sites within the mature VWF subunit have been determined by direct protein analysis.[14] Comparison of the cDNA and primary amino acid sequences identified a large propeptide (741 amino acids) preceding the mature VWF subunit sequence. This propeptide is identical to a previously observed immunologic activity in plasma called VWF antigen II. This propeptide plays an important role in VWF multimer assembly and processing but has no known function after secretion. The *VWF* gene is located on the short arm of human chromosome 12[10,12] and a partial, nonfunctional duplication (pseudogene) is on human chromosome 22.[15] The structures of the unusually large *VWF* gene and pseudogene are shown schematically in Fig. 128–1.[16,17] The gene is composed of 52 exons spanning a total of 178 kb of the human genome. It is similar in size to the factor VIII gene (see Chapter 123) and more than 100 times larger than the gene for β-globin (see Chapter 33). The *VWF* gene accounts for approximately 0.1% of human chromosome 12. The *VWF* pseudogene duplicates the middle portion of the gene from exons 23 to 34, including the intervening sequences. The pseudogene is approximately 97% homologous to the authentic gene and is only present in humans.[17]

Analysis of the VWF amino acid sequence identifies a pattern of homologous repeated segments, designated by the letters A through D in Fig. 128–1. This pattern suggests that the *VWF* gene arose by a complex series of partial gene duplications. The expression of the *VWF* gene is tightly regulated and restricted exclusively to endothelial cells and megakaryocytes.[18] For this reason, VWF is frequently used as a primary histochemical marker to identify cells of endothelial cell origin. A 734-base pair DNA fragment extending from approximately 500 base pairs upstream of the transcription start site into the first intron confers endothelial cell-specific *VWF* gene expression in vitro[19] and directs gene expression to a subpopulation of endothelial cells in transgenic mice.[20] However, as in the case of β-globin, another highly tissue-specific regulated gene (see Chapter 27), critical transcription regulatory sequences located a great distance from the 5′ end of the *VWF* gene may be required for the high-level expression observed in a wide range of endothelial cells in vivo.

Comparison of the *VWF* DNA sequence to that of other known genes identifies potential relationship to a number of other adhesive proteins. A superfamily of proteins sharing sequence similarity with VWF A domains contains a number of proteins associated with the extracellular matrix, hemostasis, or cell adhesion. The crystal structure of the VWF A1 and A3 domains have been solved[21,22] and are remarkably similar to the structure for the homologous I domain of the integrin α2/β1.[23] The structure of the VWF A1 domain in complex with GPIbα demonstrates that the latter platelet receptor wraps around one side of the A1 domain, providing two areas of contact bridged by charged interactions. These findings may explain the effect of mutations in type 2B VWD and provide a model for activation of the VWF molecule.[24]

Exons of *VWF* range in size from 40 base pairs to 1.4 kb for exon 28, one of the larger known single exons. This latter exon encompasses most of the A1 and A2 homologous repeats, a region containing several important VWF functional domains, as well as most human mutations associated with type 2A and 2B VWD.

DOMAIN STRUCTURE

VWF exists as a series of multimers varying in molecular weight between 0.5 (dimer) and 20 million (multimer). Electron microscopic observations of VWF molecules reveals that they are filamentous and contain subunits arranged in a head-to-head and tail-to-tail configuration.[25,26] The building block of multimers is a dimer, held together by disulfide bonds located near the carboxyl-terminal end of each subunit. The dimers are joined to each other by disulfide bonds located near the *N*-terminal end of the mature subunit.[27,28] The mature subunit has a mass of approximately 270 kd and contains 18.7% carbohydrate.[14] *N*- and *O*-linked carbohydrates are found clustered at both ends of the subunit. All 169 cysteine residues (8.2% of the amino acid content) are involved in interchain or intrachain disulfide bonds.[29] Two Arg-Gly-Asp (RGD) sequences are found in pro-VWF. The one in the mature VWF subunit is part of the binding site for the platelet integrin receptor, GPIIb/IIIa (see Fig. 128–1).

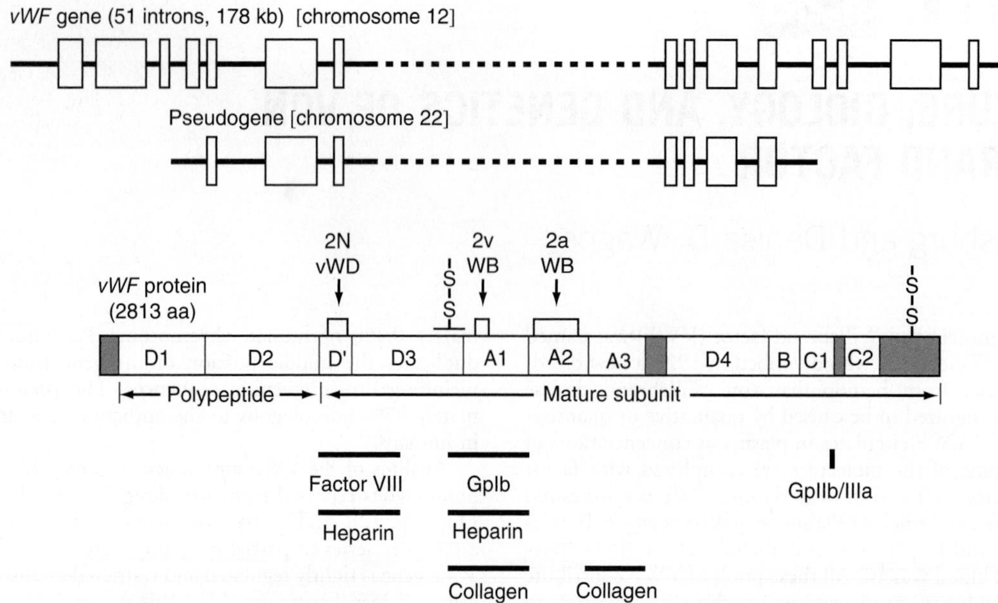

Figure 128–1 The structure of the *VWF* gene and protein. The structures of the *VWF* gene and pseudogene are indicated schematically at the top of the figure. The corresponding protein is also depicted, including the homologous repeat domain structure. The localization within VWF of point mutations associated with VWD variants are also indicated. AA, amino acids; VWD, von Willebrand disease; VWF, von Willebrand factor. *(Adapted from Ginsburg D, Bowie EJW: Molecular genetics of von Willebrand disease. Blood 79:2507, 1992.)*

The significance of the other RGD sequence located on the propeptide is unknown.

Several functional domains in VWF have been identified on the VWF subunit (see Fig. 128–1).[30] Two collagen-binding sites have been mapped to the mature VWF subunit and potentially a third to the propeptide. However, studies of recombinant VWF suggest that the major physiologically active binding site for fibrillar collagen lies within the A3 domain.[31,32] VWF also has at least two binding sites for heparin and may interact with heparin-like molecules in the basement membrane. The factor VIII–binding domain is located in the *N*-terminal portion of the VWF subunit[33] and interacts with the *N*-terminal portion of the factor VIII light chain.[34,35] VWF also has affinity for two platelet receptors. VWF binding to GPIb plays a pivotal role in the early events of hemostasis, leading to the attachment of platelets to the area of injury.[6] Several potential, short-binding sequences for GPIb on VWF have been identified, all localized to a large disulfide loop contained within the VWF A1 repeat (see Fig. 128–1).[36,37] The binding region of VWF to GPIIb/IIIa on activated platelets is located in the carboxyl-terminal portion of the mature subunit. This recognition site can be specifically inhibited by the Arg-Gly-Asp sequence contained within peptides and is, therefore, likely to include the Arg-Gly-Asp-Ser sequence. VWF (with other adhesive proteins, such as fibrinogen and fibronectin) may compete for binding to this glycoprotein. In vivo studies in knock-out mice demonstrate that all three of these adhesive ligands (VWF, fibrinogen, and fibronectin) contribute to platelet adhesion in thrombus formation following vascular injury.[38] Finally, the VWF A2 domain contains the cleavage site for the plasma protease ADAMTS13, which reduces VWF multimer size and biologic activity.

BIOSYNTHESIS

The processing steps leading to the formation of mature VWF multimers have been studied chiefly in endothelial cells,[39] but evaluation of megakaryocyte biosynthesis indicates an identical pattern of synthesis (Fig. 128–2).[4] VWF is first synthesized as a pro-VWF monomer.[40–42] Co-translationally, high-mannose carbohydrate is added to the polypeptide chain. There are 13 potential *N*-linked

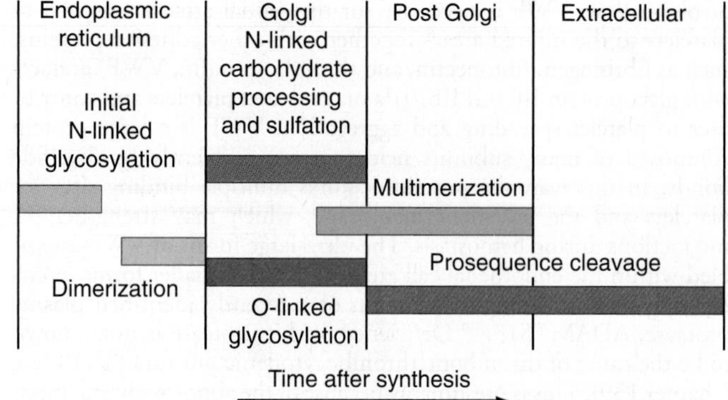

Figure 128–2 Map of processing steps in the biosynthesis of VWF. Interchain disulfide bonds are formed in two steps (dimerization and multimerization, pink). The propeptide is cleaved late in VWF processing (prosequence cleavage, red). VWF, von Willebrand factor. *(Adapted from Handin RI, Wagner DD: Molecular and cellular biology of von Willebrand factor. Prog Hematol 9:233, 1989.)*

glycosylation sites on mature VWF and 4 on the propeptide. Although residing within the endoplasmic reticulum, the carboxyl-termini of the pro-VWF subunits are linked together by an unknown number of disulfide bonds.[43] Only dimeric molecules are transported to the Golgi apparatus, where their processing continues.

In the Golgi apparatus, common modifications, including the addition of *O*-linked carbohydrate, high-mannose carbohydrate processing, and sulfation, take place (see Fig. 128–2). In addition, a unique processing event includes the multimerization of dimers by disulfide bond formation. VWF is the only protein known that has disulfide bonds formed late in protein synthesis, as disulfide bonds are usually formed in the endoplasmic reticulum. The latter process is catalyzed by the enzyme disulfide isomerase. The contents of the last compartment of the Golgi apparatus (*trans*-Golgi), and the post-Golgi secretory vesicles are slightly acidic. It is likely that multimerization occurs in these acidic compartments because this process can be completely inhibited by culturing cells in the presence of a weak base[44] that increases the pH of acidic cellular compartments. The VWF propeptide plays an active role in the interdimer disulfide bond formation. When prepro-*VWF* cDNA is expressed in a monkey kidney cell line or other cells that normally do not synthesize VWF, these cells are capable of supporting VWF multimerization. By contrast, if pre-*VWF* cDNA (with the cDNA coding for the propeptide deleted) is expressed in these cells, only dimeric molecules are synthesized and secreted.[45,46] In in vitro multimerization experiments, pro-VWF dimers spontaneously form larger multimers, whereas VWF mature dimers remain dimeric. The in vitro multimerization is promoted by a slightly acidic environment (optimal pH is ~5.8) and will not occur at a neutral or basic pH.[47] Under these acidic pH conditions, the propeptide may catalyze disulfide bond formation among the mature VWF subunits. The propeptide contains sequences similar to those found at the active site of protein disulfide isomerase. These are cysteines separated by two amino acids that readily interchange with disulfide bonds in the substrate. When an additional amino acid was inserted between the cysteines of the propeptide by site-specific mutagenesis, the VWF expressed did not form multimers.[48] During the biosynthesis of VWF multimers, the propeptide self-associates, but it is not known whether this association is linked to noncovalent multimer assembly that likely precedes the interchain disulfide bond formation.[49]

The propeptide cleavage is one of the final processing steps in the biosynthesis of VWF. Similar to other prosequences, the VWF propeptide is cleaved adjacent to two basic amino acids, Lys-Arg at residues −2 and −1. An Arg at −4 position from the cleavage site is also part of the cleavage recognition sequence, providing evidence that an enzyme with furin-like specificity is responsible for the intracellular prosequence cleavage.[50] Multimerization and propeptide cleavage are separate events. Site-specific mutagenesis of the cleavage site inhibits propeptide cleavage, but the expressed protein has a normal multimeric composition.[51] Propeptide cleavage and multimerization occur after sulfation in the *trans*-Golgi network but prior to formation of the Weibel-Palade body.[52]

Although VWF processing is chiefly intracellular, some modifications to the protein occurs after secretion. Cleavage of the propeptide, which begins in the *trans*-Golgi compartment, may continue extracellularly.[53] The largest VWF multimers found in plasma are smaller than those found in endothelial cells.[54] A plasma protease,[55,56] ADAMTS13,[7–9] specifically cleaves VWF in the circulation between Tyr 842 and Met 843 in the VWF A2 domain,[57] resulting in reduction of unusually large multimers to smaller species. Mutant VWF in group II type 2A VWD exhibits increased susceptibility to cleavage by this protease,[58] the apparent mechanism for loss of large VWF multimers in this disorder. In addition, genetic or acquired deficiency of this protease activity is responsible for most cases of TTP (see Chapter 139). Mice engineered to be genetically deficient in ADAMTS13 exhibit enhanced platelet adhesion and thrombus formation on injured blood vessels, suggesting that ADAMTS13 functions as a natural antithrombotic by regulating VWF multimer structure.[59,60]

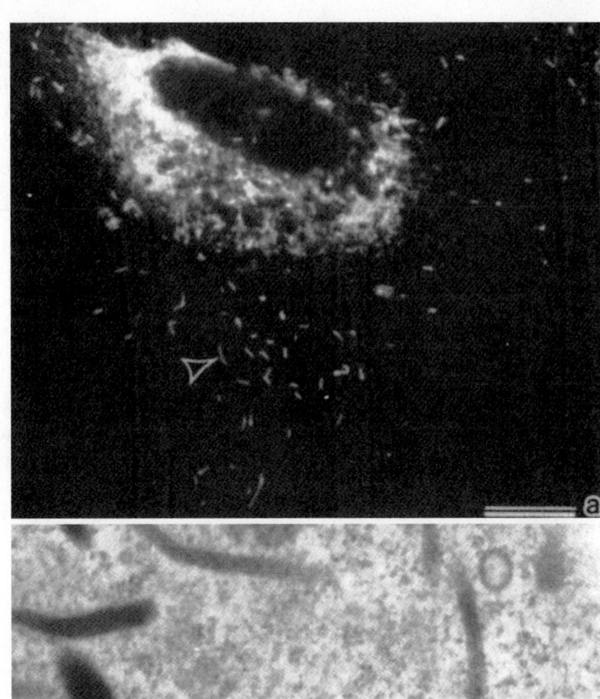

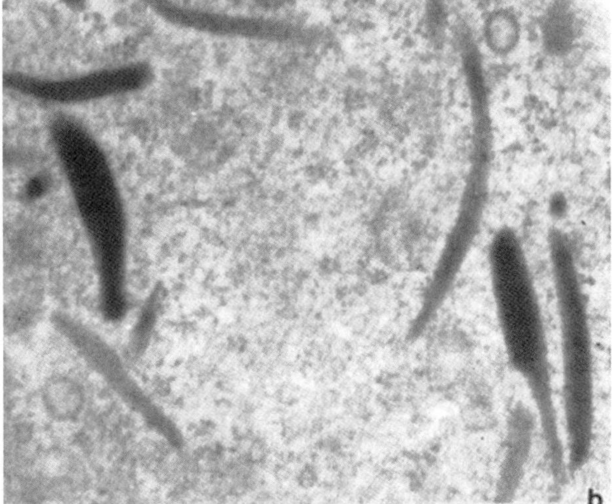

Figure 128–3 Weibel-Palade bodies of endothelial cells. **A,** Immunofluorescence staining of a human umbilical vein endothelial cell with anti-VWF antiserum. VWF is present in the perinuclear region, where it is synthesized and in the Weibel-Palade bodies (*arrowhead*) throughout the cytoplasm. Bar = 10 μm. (**B**) Electron micrograph of Weibel-Palade bodies of the same origin. Bar = 0.5 μm. VWF, von Willebrand factor.

VON WILLEBRAND FACTOR STORAGE AND SECRETION

VWF is the only known adhesive protein that is stored and undergoes regulated secretion from cells other than platelets.[39] Both the platelet pool and the endothelial pool of VWF are important physiologically, as demonstrated by crossed bone marrow transplantation experiments between normal and VWD pigs.[61,62] In platelets, VWF is present in the α-granules with many other stored proteins. Only a few secreted proteins, including angiopoietin-2, tissue plasminogen activator (tPA) and interleukin (IL)-8 have been shown to be costored in the Weibel-Palade bodies of endothelial cells, along with VWF and the VWF propeptide.[63,64] In both organelles, the stored VWF molecules appear to form tubular structures, 150 Å in diameter.[65,66] These tubules are absent in the α-granules of pigs with VWD.[67] A transmembrane glycoprotein of the α-granule, P-selectin, is a component of the Weibel-Palade body membrane. Like VWF, the biosynthesis of this protein is restricted to endothelial cells and to megakaryocytes. When expressed on the plasma membrane, P-selectin promotes the adhesion of monocytes, neutrophils, and some other subsets of leukocytes.[68,69] Weibel-Palade bodies originate from the Golgi apparatus. They are up to 4 μm long and 0.1 μm thick (Fig. 128–3) and are found in endothelial cells of virtually all blood vessels types. There is, however, variation in the number of Weibel-Palade bodies per cell in endothelium of different origin.[70]

Fully processed VWF is secreted from cultured endothelial cells by one of two pathways. The constitutive pathway is directly coupled to VWF synthesis and occurs without stimulation. The regulated pathway, involving VWF stored in Weibel-Palade bodies, is initiated by the action of secretagogues. Another important difference between the two pathways is the biologic activity of the VWF secreted. Although mostly small multimers are secreted constitutively, only the largest, biologically most potent multimers are stored in Weibel-Palade bodies (Fig. 128–4).[71,72] It is not known whether the large multimers are selected for storage or whether the conditions found in the Weibel-Palade body promote multimer assembly. The VWF stored in platelet α-granules is also enriched in large multimers.[73] All the N-terminal D domains (D1–D3) appear to be necessary for VWF storage. Deletions of these individual domains lead to constitutive secretion of the expressed protein.[74,75] Although the propolypeptide remains in the Weibel-Palade bodies noncovalently associated with the mature subunit,[52] cleavage of the prosequence has to occur for efficient formation of the storage granules.[76] Although the VWF propeptide is required for VWF multimerization, as well as VWF storage in the Weibel-Palade body, these functions can be dissociated, and VWF multimerization is not required for storage.[77] The biologic function of the two secretory pathways may be different. The largest multimers released from Weibel-Palade bodies at the time of vascular injury may act to attach platelets to the injured endothelium and the vessel wall. Some of the released large VWF molecules remain associated with the endothelial membrane,[72] where their highly adhesive interaction with circulating platelets is regulated by ADAMTS13 proteolysis.[59,60,78] Circulating VWF may also self-associate on the endothelial surface to facilitate platelet adhesion.[79] Binding of VWF to the GPIb receptor of platelets and the integrin-type receptors, such as the GPIIb/IIIa complex on platelets and the vitronectin receptor on endothelial cells, is enhanced by the presence of large numbers of binding sites on VWF multimers. The exceptional adhesive activity of ultralarge VWF multimers may be regulated by its sequestration in storage organelles, with rapid local release at the site of vascular injury.

Secretagogues for VWF that may be of physiologic importance include thrombin,[80] fibrin,[81] histamine,[82] the terminal complement proteins C5b-9,[83] and several bioactive lipids such as sphingosine-1 phosphate.[84] The release of Weibel-Palade bodies appears to be coupled to Ca^{2+} influx. Thrombin activity as a secretagogue is related to its proteolytic activity and the cleavage of a specific receptor.[80,85] Interaction with a cellular receptor is a likely mechanism for fibrin release of VWF. A specific N-terminal fragment of the fibrin β-chain appears to interact with the endothelium.[86] Histamine-induced release can be blocked by histamine H_1-receptor antagonists.[82] Desamino-8-arginine vasopressin (DDAVP) administration results in VWF release from endothelial cells and a two- to threefold increase in plasma levels of VWF and factor VIII, the basis for use of this agent as a key treatment modality for VWD and mild hemophilia (see Chapters 125 and 129). DDAVP appears to induce VWF secretion by binding to the vasopressin V2 receptor, which is expressed on microvascular endothelial cells.[87] The regulation of Weibel-Palade body exocytosis is important for many biologic processes, and the cellular machinery involved is only beginning to be understood.[88]

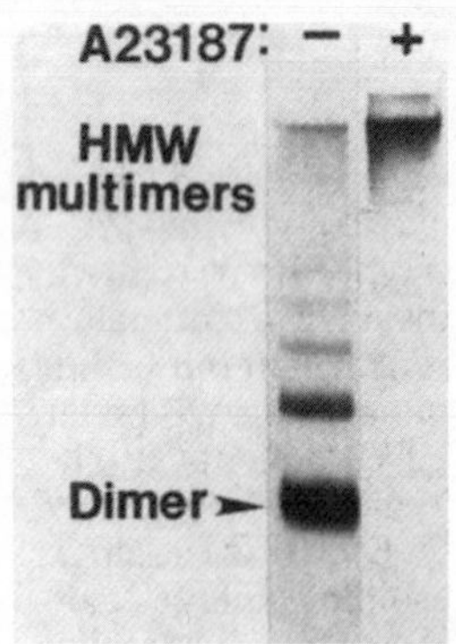

Figure 128–4 Multimeric composition of VWF secreted by endothelial cells in culture. Human umbilical vein endothelial cells were metabolically labeled with 35S-methionine and the constitutively secreted protein (–), which, released during a 10-minute treatment with the secretagogue A23187(+), were purified and analyzed nonreduced on an agarose gel. The autoradiograph of the gel is shown. The protein secreted constitutively is composed predominantly of small multimers, whereas the VWF secreted from Weibel-Palade bodies is only of high molecular weight (HMW multimers). VWF, von Willebrand factor. *(Adapted from Sporn LA, Marder VJ, Wagner DD: Inducible secretion of large, biologically potent von Willebrand factor multimers. Cell 46:185, 1986.)*

VON WILLEBRAND DISEASE

Molecular Genetics

With the availability of *VWF* cDNA and genomic sequences, a molecular genetic approach to the characterization of VWD became possible. Southern blot analysis identified large gene deletions as the molecular basis for VWD in a small subset of patients with severe, or type 3, disease.[2,15] With the advent of the polymerase chain reaction (PCR), extensive direct DNA sequence analysis has been conducted on material from patients with a variety of VWD variants, using platelets as a source for *VWF* messenger RNA (mRNA) or by direct analysis of genomic DNA. A large number of human mutations have been cataloged (Fig. 128–5).[2,89] A database of known *VWF* mutations and polymorphisms is maintained by the VWF Scientific and Standardization Committee of the International Society of Thrombosis and Haemostasis.[90] Molecular genetic analysis has shed important light on the molecular pathogenesis of VWD and promises to improve diagnosis. For some VWD variants, mutations have been

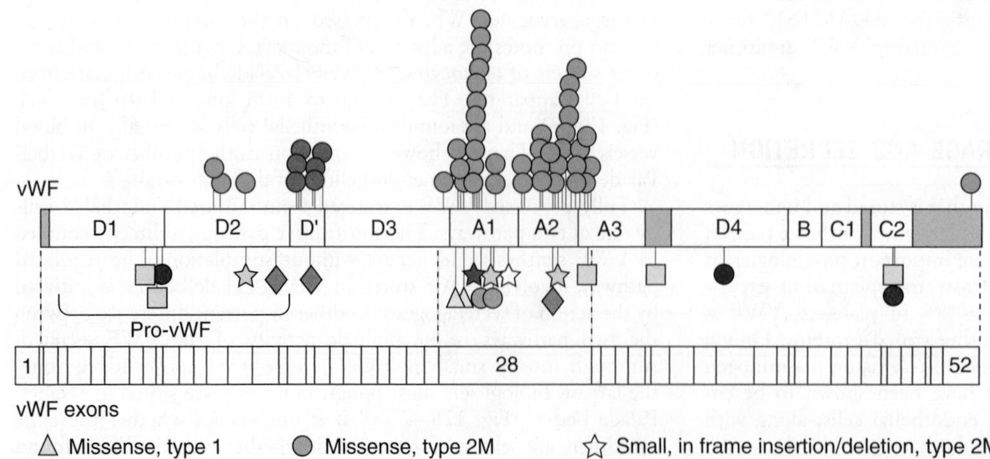

Figure 128–5 VWD mutations. The location of all point mutations and small, in-frame insertions and deletions reported to the VWD database[90] as of 1997 are shown schematically here within the VWF domain structure. The relative positions of each of the 52 VWF exons are shown below. VWD, von Willebrand disease; VWF, von Willebrand factor. *(From Nichols WC, Ginsburg D: von Willebrand disease. Medicine 76:1, 1997.)*

identified in most patients studied, and precise diagnosis and classification by DNA screening may soon become practical.

VWD can be divided into two general categories: those variants caused by a pure quantitative deficiency and those caused by a qualitative structural or functional abnormality within the VWF protein. Total disruption of gene function by deletion of a segment of the gene or a nonsense mutation (abrupt termination of the protein by insertion of a stop codon into the coding sequence) results in quantitative VWF abnormalities. Conversely, most qualitative variants are a result of mutations resulting in single amino acid substitutions that interfere with protein structure or function. The current classification scheme for VWD is based on an improved understanding of molecular pathogenesis.[91,92]

Types 1 and 3 von Willebrand Disease

Quantitative VWF abnormalities can be either mild or pronounced. Patients with type 3 (severe VWD) suffer from a profound bleeding disorder (see Chapter 129) with very little or no detectable plasma or platelet VWF. Type 3 VWD is a relatively rare disease, with an incidence of approximately 1 : 1 million.[93] By contrast, type 1 is the most common form of VWD, accounting for 70% to 80% of cases; it is associated with a mild to moderate quantitative decrease in VWF (levels in the range of 20% to 50% of normal). Type 3 VWD appears to result from the inheritance of a dysfunctional *VWF* gene from both parents. Gene deletions varying from 2.3 kb to more than 180 kb have been identified in several patients and may be associated with an increased risk for developing VWF inhibitor antibodies.[2] Several other defects resulting in complete loss of VWF function have been identified in patients with type 3 VWD, including nondeletion defects resulting in loss of mRNA expression,[94] as well as specific nonsense mutations or frameshift mutations resulting in disruption of the VWF protein coding sequence (see Fig. 128–5).[2]

Until recently, only a limited number of point mutations responsible for type 1 and 3 VWD had been identified, compared with the large number of mutations reported for the less common qualitative VWD variants described in the following section (see Fig. 128–5). This is caused, at least in part, by the complexity of screening all 52 exons of the *VWF* gene in a patient with type 1 or 3 VWD. In contrast, for many of the qualitative variants, the observed clustering of mutations focuses the search to a limited region of *VWF*. Several mutations resulting in truncation or disruption of the VWF protein coding sequence have been identified in patients with type 3 VWD. A particularly common frameshift mutation in exon 18, because of the deletion of a single cytosine, accounts for approximately 50% of type 3 VWD alleles in Sweden and has also been shown to be the molecular defect in the original patient reported by von Willebrand.[95] The resulting frameshift produces a stable mRNA encoding a truncated protein that is rapidly degraded in the cell.[96] This mutation is also common in the German population[97] but not in the United States.[96]

In the most straightforward model, type 1 VWD would simply represent the heterozygous form of type 3 VWD. However, there is some controversy on this point.[98] Type 3 VWD has classically been defined as "recessive" in inheritance and parents, who are obligate carriers for the defect and are often completely asymptomatic with normal laboratory numbers. However, in other cases, parents are affected with classic type 1 VWD. In addition, the reported prevalence of type 1 VWD (~1% of the population[99,100]) would predict a much higher frequency of type 3 VWD (1 : 40,000) than is observed (1 : 1 million). This discrepancy may be explained in part by over diagnosis of type 1 VWD in patients with only mildly decreased plasma VWF levels near the lower limit observed in the general population.[92,101]

The spectrum of mutations known to be responsible for type 1 VWD has recently been markedly expanded through two large studies, one in Europe[102] and the other in Canada.[103] These reports include more than 200 index cases, with VWF gene mutations identified in 60% to 70% of the patients analyzed. In the European study,[102] approximately one-third of the cases could be reclassified as a type 2 variant, with mutations detected in 95% of this subgroup. For the remaining "true" type 1 VWD families, mutations were only identified in 55%. In both reports, patients with lower VWF levels were more likely to carry VWF gene mutations. Previous studies have suggested that a subset of type 1 VWD mutations may produce a mutant VWF subunit that interferes in a dominant-negative way with the normal allele, accounting for the autosomal dominant inheritance and resulting in particularly reduced VWF levels. Mutations at cysteine residues in the D3 domain of VWF have been identified in several patients with moderately severe VWD. Expression of recombinant VWF carrying one of these mutations (Cys1149Arg) resulted in a mutant protein that was retained within the endoplasmic reticulum, potentially acted in a dominant negative manner when co-transfected with wild-type VWF.[104]

The observations that ~80% of reported mutations in type 3 VWD are predicted to lead to null alleles, whereas only 11% of type 1 VWD mutations are predicted to be null[102] suggests that the penetrance of clinical bleeding in patients heterozygous for a null mutation may in general be much lower than the corresponding penetrance in patients heterozygous for a VWF amino acid substitution. This hypothesis could explain the apparent recessive inheritance of type 3 VWD, as well as the high frequency of missense mutations identified in symptomatic type 1 VWD patients. The underlying mechanisms for VWD in the 30% to 50% of mild type 1 patients in whom no VWF gene mutation is detected remain unknown. Some of these patients may have regulatory mutations in distant parts of the VWF gene not covered by current sequence analysis. The possibility of locus heterogeneity (ie, defects in other genes giving rise to a disorder clinically indistinguishable from VWD) has also been proposed. Consistent with this idea, studies of an animal model of type 1 VWD in the mouse identified a mutation in a glycosyltransferase gene (*B4galnt2*) that results in reductions of plasma VWF levels of up to 20-fold.[105] Although comparable effects for non-*VWF* genes in human VWD have not yet been demonstrated, other genetic factors are known to significantly modify human VWF levels, including ABO blood group (see Chapter 129). The effects of such modifying genes are likely to determine the penetrance of symptomatic type 1 VWD, particularly in patients with "milder" type 1 VWD mutations. In addition, the combined effects of several modifier genes could conceivably account for type 1 VWD in a subset of patients with two normal *VWF* gene alleles. Consistent with this idea, inheritance of type 1 VWD in some families does not clearly track with the VWF gene.[2,102,103] Recently, a subset of type 1 VWD has been identified, which results from accelerated clearance of VWF from plasma.[106] Although the four reported families all carry VWF gene missense mutations, the accelerated clearance in other patients could result from mutations in components of the protein clearance machinery or in genes responsible for VWF posttranslational modification.

Type 2A von Willebrand Disease

Type 2A VWD is the most common qualitative abnormality of VWF and is associated with selective loss of large and intermediate-sized VWF multimers (see Chapter 129). Direct sequence analysis from platelet mRNA and genomic DNA has identified a panel of mutations within *VWF* exon 28, accounting for most of patients with type 2A VWD.[2,89] Nearly all of these mutations are clustered within the VWF A2 repeat (see Figs. 128–1 and 128–5). One particular mutation (Arg1597Trp) accounts for approximately one-third of type 2A VWD cases around the world. In vitro analysis of recombinant VWF containing type 2A VWD mutations suggests that two distinct mechanisms contribute to the pathogenesis of this disorder (Fig. 128–6).[107] In the first group, the single amino acid substitution results in a defect in VWF intracellular processing, with retention of the abnormal VWF in the endoplasmic reticulum. In the second group, VWF synthesis and processing in vitro is normal, and the loss of multimers is caused by increased sensitivity to proteolysis in plasma by ADAMTS13 at a site within the type 2A VWD mutation cluster in

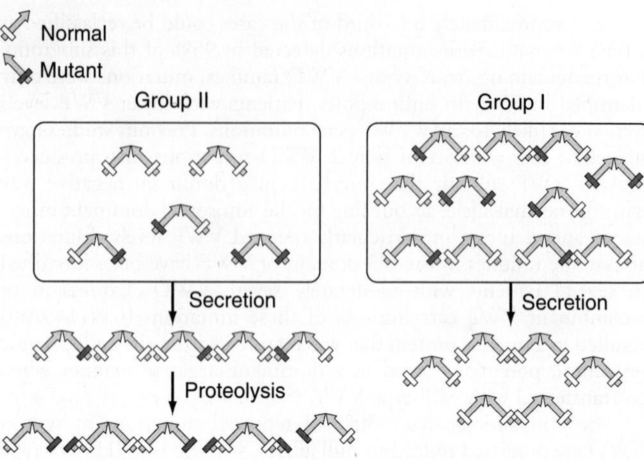

Figure 128–6 Two mechanisms for the molecular pathogenesis of type 2A VWD. Each VWF monomer is indicated as a gray arrow with the normal sequence indicated by white boxes and mutant sequence by black boxes. Within the cell, mixed dimers are formed, as well as homodimers of mutant and wild-type monomers. In group II, full-size multimers are assembled and proteolyzed after secretion. In group I, mutant subunits are held up in the endoplasmic reticulum; only homomultimers of normal subunits are secreted, predominantly of small size, VWD, von Willebrand disease; VWF, von Willebrand factor.

the VWF A2 domain (Tyr 1605-Met 1606).[7–9,57] Recombinant VWF carrying type 2A mutations shows increased sensitivity,[58] and recombinant VWF deleted for the A2 domain is resistant to cleavage by this protease.[108]

Type 2B von Willebrand Disease

Type 2B VWD is also characterized by the loss of large VWF multimers but through a unique mechanism, distinct from those described earlier for type 2A VWD. A panel of mutations has been identified in type 2B VWD patients, all located within a short stretch of the VWF A1 domain (see Fig. 128–5). Four of these mutations, clustered within a 35-amino acid segment of the 2813-amino acid *VWF* coding sequence, account for more than 90% of type 2B VWD patients studied.[2,89] Therefore, screening for this panel of mutations could provide precise and rapid DNA diagnosis for this disorder.

These observations also identify a critical region of VWF involved in binding to the platelet GPIb receptor. Each of these single amino acid substitutions is thought to result in a unique *gain of function*, leading to spontaneous binding of VWF to platelets. Under normal conditions, plasma VWF is inert in its interaction toward platelets until it encounters an exposed subendothelial surface. Binding of VWF to collagen or other ligands within the vessel wall at sites of vascular injury presumably results in a secondary conformational change, which then facilitates binding to the GPIb platelet receptor. In type 2B VWD, the mutant VWF is capable of spontaneously binding to GPIb in the absence of subendothelial contact. Analysis of recombinant VWF demonstrates very similar increases in VWF binding to platelets for each of six distinct type 2B VWD mutations, supporting the hypothesis that the VWF GPIb binding domain can adopt either a discrete "on" or "off" conformation.[109] The large multimers appear to have the highest affinity for GPIb (presumably because of multivalency) and are rapidly cleared from plasma, along with the bound platelets, resulting in the characteristic loss of large multimers, as well as thrombocytopenia.

Type 2N von Willebrand Disease

Type 2N is a unique variant of VWD that has important implications for the differential diagnosis of hemophilia and provides an instructive example of genetic locus heterogeneity. Rare cases of "autosomal" hemophilia have been reported in the past, in which deficiencies in factor VIII activity were inherited in an apparently autosomal manner. Biochemical analysis in several families identified a defect residing within the patient's plasma VWF, interfering with its ability to bind and stabilize factor VIII.[110,111] This variant is called type 2N,[91] although it is sometimes referred to as VWD Normandy, after the province of origin of one of the first patients.[112]

DNA sequence analysis in type 2N VWD has identified several mutations, mostly clustered in a region at the N-terminus of VWF previously shown to be important for factor VIII binding (see Figs. 128–1 and 128–5).[2,30,89] One of these mutations, Arg854Gln, appears to be particularly common.[113] Although usually silent in the heterozygote, homozygosity or compound heterozygosity for a type 2N *VWF* allele can result in clinically significant factor VIII deficiency. Therefore, type 2N VWD should be considered in the differential diagnosis of hemophilia A, particularly in a female patient or in the context of other features suggesting an autosomal pattern of inheritance.[112] Most type 2N VWD mutations result in only mild to moderate reductions in plasma factor VIII. However, at least one mutation (Glu787Lys) is associated with factor VIII levels as low as 1%, when co-inherited with a type 3 VWD allele.[114] This latter observation suggests that a diagnosis of type 2N VWD should also be considered in patients with more profound reductions in factor VIII level.

Prenatal Diagnosis

With the advent of molecular tools for the analysis of VWD, prenatal diagnosis has become possible and has been applied in a few cases. Given the generally mild clinical manifestations of most VWD variants, prenatal diagnosis is generally not indicated. However, in the case of type 3 or severe VWD, the indications for prenatal diagnosis are similar to those of severe hemophilia. For those VWD variants for which the mutation is known, direct analysis of chorionic villus samples or amniotic fluid can be performed rapidly by polymerase chain reaction and can be expected to provide a highly accurate, specific, and rapid diagnosis. For VWD families in which the specific mutation is unknown, genetic linkage analysis can be performed using a large panel of highly informative DNA sequence polymorphisms (http://www.shef.ac.uk/vwf/index.html). One particularly useful polymorphism is a highly variable TCTA repeat in intron 40, which has been reported to have more than 100 distinct alleles. Although all cases of type 3 VWD analyzed to date appear to be linked to defects within the *VWF* gene, the possibility of locus heterogeneity (ie, involvement of other genes outside of *VWF*) should be considered when performing this kind of analysis.

SUGGESTED READINGS

Chauhan AK, Motto DG, Lamb CB et al: The metalloprotease ADAMTS13 is a natural anti-thrombotic. J Exp Med 2006;203:767.

Goodeve A, Eikenboom J, Castaman G, et al: Phenotype and genotype of a cohort of families historically diagnosed with type 1 von Willebrand disease in the European study, Molecular and Clinical Markers for the Diagnosis and Management of Type 1 von Willebrand Disease (MCMDM-1VWD). Blood 2007;109:112.

Huizinga EG, Tsuji S, Romijn RA, et al: Structures of glycoprotein Ib alpha and its complex with von Willebrand factor A1 domain. Science 2002;297:1176.

James PD, Notley C, Hegadorn C, et al: The mutational spectrum of type 1 von Willebrand disease: Results from a Canadian cohort study. Blood 2007;109:145.

Lyons SE, Bruck ME, Bowie EJW, Ginsburg D: Impaired intracellular transport produced by a subset of type IIA von Willebrand disease mutations. J Biol Chem 1992;267:4424.

Mayadas TN, Wagner DD: Vicinal cysteines in the prosequence play a role in von Willebrand factor multimer assembly. Proc Natl Acad Sci U S A 1992;89:3531.

Mohlke KL, Purkayastha AA, Westrick RJ, et al: MVWF, a dominant modifier of murine von Willebrand factor, results from altered lineage-specific expression of a glycosyltransferase. Cell 1999;96:111.

Motto DG, Chauhan AK, Zhu G, et al: Shigatoxin triggers thrombotic thrombocytopenic purpura in genetically susceptible ADAMTS13-deficient mice. J Clin Invest 2005;115:2752.

The University of Sheffield. ISTH SSC VWF Database. http://www.shef.ac.uk/vwf/index.html. Accessed June 11, 2007.

Tsai HM, Sussman II, Ginsburg D, et al: Proteolytic cleavage of recombinant type 2A von Willebrand factor mutants R834W and R834Q: Inhibition by doxycycline and by monoclonal antibody VP-1. Blood 1997; 89:1954.

von Willebrand EA: Hereditär Pseudohemofili. Finska Läkarsällskapetes Handl 1926;67:7. [Hereditary pseudohaemophilia. Haemophilia 1999;5:223].

Weibel ER, Palade GE: New cytoplasmic components in arterial endothelia. J Biol Chem 1964;23:101.

REFERENCES

For complete list of references log onto www.expertconsult.com

CHAPTER 129

VON WILLEBRAND DISEASE: CLINICAL ASPECTS AND THERAPY

Gilbert C. White, II and J. Evan Sadler

von Willebrand disease (VWD) is an inherited hemorrhagic disorder caused by a deficiency or dysfunction of von Willebrand factor (VWF), a large adhesive glycoprotein found in plasma, platelets, and endothelial cells. As a result, the interaction of platelets with the vessel wall is defective, and primary hemostasis is impaired.

VWD was first reported in 1926 by Erik von Willebrand,[1] who described a 5-year-old Finnish girl from the Åland Islands with a bleeding disorder that could be distinguished from classic hemophilia by an autosomal pattern of inheritance, mucocutaneous hemorrhage rather than joint and soft tissue hemorrhage, a prolonged bleeding time, and normal clot retraction. Of 66 family members, 23 had a similar hemorrhagic diathesis. Two years later, George Minot[2] reported a similar bleeding disorder in five patients and described the intermittent nature of the bleeding. von Willebrand originally attributed the bleeding defect in his patients to either a platelet defect or abnormal capillaries.[1] In 1953, three independent groups reported deficiency of factor VIII in VWD,[3–5] and in 1957, Nilsson and coworkers[6] showed that the infusion of fraction I-0 from normal human plasma led to a greater-than-expected increase in factor VIII levels in patients with VWD, suggesting that the defect might be found in the plasma. More importantly, the infusion of fraction I-0 from hemophilic plasma also led to a greater-than-expected increase in factor VIII, indicating that the plasma component was something other than factor VIII.[7]

The abnormal interaction between platelets and the vessel wall in VWD was first demonstrated in 1960 by Borchgrevink[8] and was confirmed by numerous workers.[9,10] The next major discovery was the observation by Zimmerman and colleagues[11] that an antigen associated with factor VIII was decreased in patients with VWD. This antigen is now known as VWF and is a protein distinct from factor VIII. The in vitro measurement of VWF activity was facilitated by the observation by Howard and Firkin[12] that ristocetin, an antibiotic isolated from the actinomycete species *Nocardia lutea*, induced agglutination of platelets in the presence of VWF. The primary structure of VWF was determined in 1985, when the complementary DNA (cDNA) for VWF was independently cloned and sequenced by four groups.[13–16] Recent analysis has identified the *VWF* gene mutation in the families from the Åland islands first studied by von Willebrand.[17]

PREVALENCE

The apparent prevalence of VWD depends on how patients are ascertained and on the criteria for diagnosis. Patients with severe mucocutaneous bleeding and very low or dysfunctional VWF are easily diagnosed but also are relatively uncommon. The more typical patient with bleeding and only modest quantitative VWF deficiency is a diagnostic challenge. Based on the number of persons from specific geographic regions who are evaluated for bleeding in hematology clinics, VWD affects 35 to 100 per million (0.0035%–0.01%), which is comparable to the prevalence of hemophilia A.[18] Population screening discovers more potential patients but with a risk of increased diagnostic uncertainty. For example, screening of schoolchildren for bleeding symptoms and VWF defects has suggested that the prevalence of VWD is 0.82% to 1.6%.[19] However, few patients so identified have medically significant bleeding, and their families rarely exhibit cosegregation of low VWF levels with either bleeding or *VWF* genotype.[20] The prevalence of heterozygosity for null *VWF* alleles also can be estimated from the prevalence of severe (recessive) VWD type 3, which affects between 0.55 to 6 per million people. Taking these values as estimates for q^2, heterozygosity for nonfunctional *VWF* alleles ($2pq$) would affect 1480 to 3580 persons per million.[18] A comparison of this number with estimates of prevalence based on bleeding symptoms suggests that less than 10% of these heterozygotes will have medically significant bleeding.

GENETICS

The *VWF* gene is on human chromosome 12,[13,14] and VWD usually exhibits an autosomal pattern of codominant inheritance: One mutant *VWF* allele may cause disease (although penetrance and expressivity can be variable), and two mutant alleles usually cause more severe disease. Some less common variants exhibit recessive inheritance, so that only homozygotes or compound heterozygotes have symptoms. Recent studies suggest that autosomal recessive VWD may be more common than previously recognized. Several families with type 2A (some formerly designated type IIC)[21,22] and type 1 VWD[23] appear to fit this pattern. In addition, the VWF protein is multimeric, which provides opportunities for mutant VWF subunits to disrupt the assembly, secretion, or function of associated normal subunits. In such cases, a single mutant *VWF* allele may cause exceptionally severe, dominant disease. von Willebrand disease illustrates some limitations of the terms *dominant* and *recessive* for the description of genetic disease. Nevertheless, these terms usually are satisfactory in practice.

Modifiers unlinked to the *VWF* locus also influence plasma VWF levels and may cooperate with *VWF* mutations to affect the severity of bleeding symptoms. For example, blood type O is overrepresented among patients diagnosed with VWD type 1, probably because the mean VWF level for persons with blood type O is at least 25% lower than for those with other ABO blood types (Table 129–1).[24] The basis for this relationship is not fully understood. However, some *N*-linked oligosaccharides on VWF bear ABO blood group determinants, and the absence of A or B antigens appears to slightly decrease the circulatory half-life of VWF.[25,26]

ABO blood type accounts for approximately 30% of the observed heritable variation in plasma VWF level,[27] suggesting that additional modifying loci remain to be identified. Studies in mice suggest that several other changes in protein glycosylation could affect VWF levels by a mechanism analogous to that proposed for ABO blood type. In the RIIIS/J mouse, ectopic expression of the *N*-acetylglucosaminyltransferase (*Galgt2*) gene in endothelial cells causes abnormal glycosylation of VWF and leads to its rapid clearance from plasma.[28] These mice have VWF levels substantially lower than strains with normal *Galgt2* expression. Similarly, mice deficient in ST3Gal-IV sialyltransferase have a bleeding disorder associated with reduced levels of VWF, probably because of the increased hepatic clearance of VWF bearing oligosaccharides that lack certain sialic acid residues.[29]

Table 129–1 Influence of ABO Blood Group on VWF : Ag in Blood Donors

ABO Type	n	VWF:Ag Geometric Mean	VWF:Ag Geometric Mean ±2 SD
O	456	74.8	35.6–157.0
A	340	105.9	48.0–233.9
B	196	116.9	56.8–241.0
AB	109	123.3	63.8–238.2

Entries for VWF : Ag are in IU/dL. For unselected blood donors, the range of values for VWF : Ag ± 2 SD was 45–203 IU/dL (Montgomery RR, personal communication). All groups are significantly different in pair-wise comparisons except for B vs. AB. VWF : Ag, von Willebrand factor antigen immunoassay; SD, serologically detectable. Adapted from reference 24.

Table 129–2 Common Laboratory Tests in von Willebrand Disease

Property Assessed	Test Name or Method (Abbreviation)
Screening Tests	
VWF-platelet GPIb binding	Ristocetin cofactor activity (VWF : RCo)
VWF-collagen binding	VWF binding to immobilized collagen (VWF : CB)
VWF protein concentration	Immunoassay (VWF : Ag)
Factor VIII stabilization in vivo	Factor VIII coagulation assay (FVIII : C)
Specialized Tests	
VWF-platelet GPIb binding	Ristocetin-induced platelet aggregation (RIPA)
VWF multimer distribution and structure	Multimer gel electrophoresis
VWF-factor VIII binding	Factor VIII binding to immobilized VWF (VWF : FVIIIB)

GPIb, glycoprotein Ib; VWF, von Willebrand factor; Nomenclature for VWF and its activities is according to reference 228.

LABORATORY TESTING

A typical screening laboratory evaluation for VWD includes assays of plasma VWF mediated platelet function, VWF antigen level, and factor VIII level. In most laboratories, measurement of VWF-mediated platelet function consists of platelet binding activity, but it is increasingly apparent that collagen-binding activity should also be measured. Depending on the clinical situation, additional specialized tests may be indicated to assess the structure and distribution of VWF multimers or factor VIII binding activity (Table 129–2). Assays of platelet VWF antigen, activity, or multimer structure may be useful in selected patients.[30]

A similar unit definition is used for all quantitative assays of plasma VWF: The concentration in suitably pooled normal plasma is defined as 1 IU/mL, and 95% of values obtained in healthy populations lie between approximately 50 and 200 IU/dL. In general, laboratories should calibrate all of their assays with respect to the current World Health Organization (WHO) VWF reference plasma standard.

von Willebrand Factor Platelet-Binding Activity

When added to a suspension of platelets in plasma that contains VWF, ristocetin promotes the binding of VWF to platelet membrane glycoprotein Ib (GPIb), which causes platelet agglutination at a rate that depends on the concentration of VWF and ristocetin.[12] Ristocetin dimerizes in solution with a dissociation constant of approximately 1 mg/mL. Ristocetin dimers bind VWF at multiple proline-rich sites and also bind to platelets, which alters the affinity of VWF binding to platelet GPIb by a mechanism that has not been fully elucidated.[31]

Two main assay designs are used. Ristocetin cofactor activity (VWF : RCo) is measured by adding a fixed concentration of ristocetin to a suspension of formalin or paraformaldehyde-fixed platelets in a sample of patient plasma, and agglutination is assessed macroscopically or in an aggregometer.[32–34] The initial rate of agglutination varies directly with the concentration of VWF, which is determined by comparison to results obtained with dilutions of a calibrated plasma standard. Automated methods to measure VWF : RCo have been developed that appear to have similar characteristics to conventional aggregometric methods.[35] Regardless of methodology, VWF : RCo assays are somewhat imprecise and insensitive. In laboratory surveys, the coefficient of variation typically is 30% or greater and is even higher when the plasma level of VWF : RCo is less than 15 IU/dL.[36,37] Assay variations employing purified platelet GPIb in an enzyme-linked immunosorbent assay (ELISA) method have been described that are more sensitive and reproducible but are not widely available at this time.[38]

Ristocetin-induced platelet aggregation (RIPA) is the second major ristocetin-dependent assay of VWF activity. RIPA is measured by adding increasing concentrations of ristocetin to platelet-rich plasma and assessing the rate and extent of platelet aggregation by aggregometry. In samples from healthy persons, RIPA is absent or very weak at 0.3 to 0.5 mg/mL ristocetin and brisk at greater than 1.2 mg/mL ristocetin. Because RIPA uses the patient's own platelets, it gives abnormal results if the platelet count is low or if platelet GPIb is defective. For example, Bernard–Soulier syndrome[39] is caused by congenital deficiency of platelet GPIb (see Chapter 141), and in this condition RIPA is absent, but VWF : RCo (performed with exogenous platelets) is normal. RIPA also is relatively insensitive at low concentrations of VWF. The major use of RIPA is to distinguish between qualitative defects of VWF that are associated with decreased affinity for GPIb (type 2A, some type 2M) or increased affinity for GPIb at low concentrations of ristocetin (type 2B).[40] Because RIPA can only be performed with fresh platelet-rich plasma, the test requires scheduling with a specialized laboratory capable of performing platelet aggregometry.

The venom of *Bothrops jararaca* and closely related snakes contains a protein named botrocetin[41] that binds tightly to the A1 domain of VWF and promotes binding to platelet GPIb, possibly by forming a ternary complex.[42] When added to a suspension of platelets, botrocetin causes platelet aggregation or agglutination in a VWF-dependent manner similar to that observed with ristocetin, although botrocetin and ristocetin interact with different sequences of the VWF molecule.[43] These properties have been exploited to devise an assay of *botrocetin-cofactor activity* that has been used mainly in a research setting.

von Willebrand Factor Collagen-Binding Activity

Another function of VWF is binding to collagen because VWF mediates the interaction of platelets with collagen. This function depends on multimer size and on the properties of the major collagen-binding site in VWF domain A3. Collagen-binding activity (VWF : CB) may be measured by an ELISA-style method in which a preparation of fibrillar collagen is immobilized in microtiter wells. Patient plasma is added, and bound VWF is detected immunologically.[44] The behavior of the assay depends critically on the kind of collagen used.[45] In general, decreased VWF : CB correlates with decreased VWF concentration, decreased high molecular weight multimers, or (rarely) specific defects in collagen binding.

von Willebrand Factor Antigen

Immunoassays for VWF antigen (VWF:Ag) are performed by ELISA or newer automated methods, or, sometimes, by quantitative immunoelectrophoresis (Laurell assay).[46,47] The results with Laurell assays may be dominated by the smallest VWF multimers, which migrate faster on electrophoresis. Consequently, the Laurell method may overestimate the concentration of VWF:Ag in VWD type 2A.

Factor VIII Activity

Factor VIII circulates in a complex with VWF, and factor VIII levels usually are roughly proportional to VWF levels. Factor VIII coagulant activity is usually measured by a one-stage clotting assay using human factor VIII-deficient plasma as substrate.[48] Factor VIII levels also are reduced in patients with hemophilia A, factor VIII inhibitors, and sometimes in disseminated intravascular coagulation (see Chapters 125, 126, 132).

von Willebrand Factor Multimers

In normal human plasma, VWF is present as a series of multimers composed of dimers of 300-kd VWF subunits. Multimers range in size from dimers of 600 kd to species of more than 20,000 kd in increments of 600 kd (Fig. 129–1), and the largest multimers are most effective at mediating platelet adhesion.[49] The VWF multimers are analyzed by sodium dodecyl sulfate (SDS)-agarose gel electrophoresis and immunodetection of VWF.[50,51] The ability of the method to discriminate among certain VWD subtypes depends strongly on the technique used.

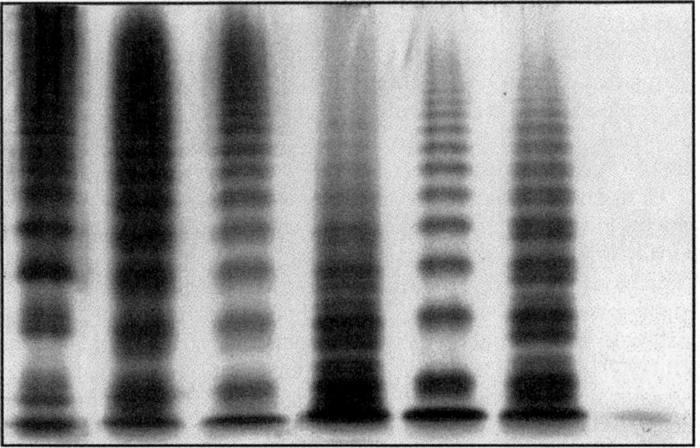

Figure 129–1 von Willebrand factor (VWF) multimer patterns. Samples were electrophoresed on a 1.2% agarose gel and VWF was visualized by binding ^{125}I-labeled anti-VWF antibody followed by autoradiography. Platelet lysate (Plt) contains larger multimers than are present in normal plasma (NP). Platelet multimers contain only intact VWF subunits and have no smaller satellite bands under the major bands, whereas plasma multimers show some evidence of degradation. Plasma samples were analyzed for patients with von Willebrand disease (VWD) types 1, 2A, 2B, and 3 as indicated. The type 2A sample in lane 4 is from a patient with enhanced sensitivity to proteolysis typical of mutations in VWF domain A2. The type 2A sample in lane 5 is from a patient with impaired multimer assembly typical of mutations in the VWF propeptide. *(Image provided courtesy of Marlies Ledford.)*

Factor VIII Binding

Abnormal binding of factor VIII to VWF may be caused by mutations in the factor VIII binding site on VWF, and such defects occur in VWD type 2N.[52,53] Distinguishing VWD type 2N from mild hemophilia A may require a direct assessment of factor VIII-VWF binding (VWF:FVIIIB), which usually is performed in an ELISA-style assay. For example, plasma samples are added to microtiter wells coated with antibody to VWF. Endogenous factor VIII (if any) is removed from the bound VWF by washing with high ionic strength buffer. After incubation with a fixed concentration of pure factor VIII, the amount of bound factor VIII is determined enzymatically, and the amount of immobilized VWF in the same sample is determined immunochemically. Defects in factor VIII-VWF binding are identified by a decreased slope of the regression line of factor VIII versus VWF, compared with the result obtained using a VWF standard.[54,55] An autosomal pattern of inheritance is a strong clue of VWD type 2N as opposed to hemophilia.

Other Tests

VWF-mediated platelet function may be assessed by measurement of the bleeding time, an in-vivo general test of platelet-vessel wall interactions (see Chapter 122).[56] The bleeding time usually is performed using a modification of the technique described by Ivy and coworkers.[57] Standardized incisions are made on the volar aspect of the forearm, keeping venous pressure at 40 mm Hg with a blood pressure cuff. Blood from the incisions is blotted to filter paper every 30 seconds, and the bleeding time is the time required for bleeding to stop.

Although the bleeding time has been a traditional measurement of VWF-mediated platelet function, a prolonged bleeding time is not specific for defects in VWF. The bleeding time procedure is difficult to standardize and results are critically dependent on the experience of the person performing the test. Differences in mean bleeding time can be demonstrated between sufficiently large groups of healthy controls and patients with VWD. However, the broad range of normal values and extreme lack of reproducibility makes the bleeding time very difficult to interpret for most patients.[58]

A platelet function analysis (PFA-100) has been developed as an automated in-vitro test of platelet function. The PFA-100 test involves passing citrated whole blood through a perforated membrane that is coated with collagen plus adenosine diphosphate (ADP) or collagen plus epinephrine. The aperture becomes occluded by a platelet plug, and the time required (the closure time) is prolonged by defects in platelet function or VWF. The closure time is sensitive to many other variables, including hematocrit and leukocyte count; and the distribution of closure times in healthy controls is broad. Nevertheless, the PFA-100 closure time appears to be more sensitive and reproducible than the bleeding time, and has replaced the bleeding time as a test for platelet-dependent hemostasis at some centers (see Chapter 122). Like the bleeding time, PFA-100 closure times do not correlate with surgical blood loss,[59] and the role of PFA-100 testing for the diagnosis of VWD or the assessment of bleeding risk remains uncertain.[60,61]

CLASSIFICATION AND MOLECULAR DEFECTS

Many mutations have similar effects on VWF structure and function, which permits a simpler classification of VWD-based mainly on pathophysiologic mechanism. Three major VWD types are designated: Type 1 refers to partial quantitative deficiency of VWF; type 2 includes qualitative defects of VWF; and type 3 refers to virtually complete absence of VWF (Table 129–3).[62] von Willebrand disease type 2 is further divided into four subtypes that have distinct mechanisms and clinical features. There is a good correlation between VWD type 2 subtypes and the location of causative *VWF* gene mutations. A database of *VWF* gene mutations and polymorphisms[63,64] is

Table 129–3 Classification of von Willebrand Disease

Type	Description
1	Partial quantitative deficiency of VWF
2	Qualitative deficiency of VWF
2A	Decreased platelet-dependent VWF function with selective deficiency of high-molecular-weight multimers
2B	Increased affinity for platelet GPIb
2M	Decreased platelet-dependent VWF function with high-molecular-weight multimers present
2N	Markedly decreased binding of factor VIII to VWF
3	Complete deficiency of VWF

GPIb, glycoprotein Ib; VWF, von Willebrand factor.

Table 129–4 Correspondence of von Willebrand Disease Classification and Previous Nomenclature

VWD Type	Previous Type	References
1	I	
	IA	86
	I-1, I-2, I-3	76
	I-platelet normal	30
	I-platelet low	30
	Vicenza*	66, 67
2A	IIA	50
	IIA-1, IIA-2, IIA-3	69
	I-platelet discordant	30
	IB	86
	IIC	87
	IID	88
	IIE	89
	IIF	90
	IIG	91
	IIH	92
	II-I	93
2B	IIB	40
	I New York	101
	Malmö	102
2M	B	106
	IC	107
	ID	108
2N	Normandy	52, 53
3	III	

*Whether von Willebrand disease (VWD) Vicenza is best considered VWD type 1 or type 2M is controversial. The most recent classification places it under VWD type 1.[62]

maintained at the University of Sheffield and can be accessed at http://www.shef.ac.uk/vwf/index.html.

von Willebrand Disease Type 1

von Willebrand disease type 1 is characterized by partial quantitative deficiency of VWF, and bleeding risk is attributed to decreased amount of VWF with normal function. The values for VWF:Ag typically fall between less than 10 IU/dL and 50 IU/dL (or 2 standard deviations [SD] below the normal mean). Values for VWF functional assays and factor VIII are decreased concordantly. In practice, a common rule of thumb is to require the value of VWF:RCo, for example, to be greater than 70% of the value for VWF:Ag, although this criterion may not be reliable, especially when the VWF:Ag level is low (eg, VWF:Ag < 40 IU/dL).[65] The distribution of plasma VWF multimer is normal. Specifically, the proportion of high molecular weight multimers is not decreased; whether to include patients with exceptionally large VWF multimers (eg, VWD Vicenza[66,67]) is controversial. von Willebrand disease type 1 is the most commonly diagnosed variant of VWD, accounting for 60% to 80% of cases.

von Willebrand disease type 1 usually is transmitted dominantly with variable penetrance. In general, the lower the VWF level, the more likely that both the VWF level and the associated bleeding phenotype will be penetrant. Apparently recessive inheritance of partial quantitative VWF deficiency does occur with a relatively low frequency, usually through the acquisition of a null allele from one parent and a hypofunctional allele from the other parent.[23,68] The occurrence of more severe bleeding symptoms in such compound heterozygous patients may explain the phenotypic variability observed in certain families.

A few patients with VWD type 1 are heterozygous for null alleles that produce undetectable or greatly reduced amounts of messenger RNA (mRNA) for VWF.[69–71] However, most patients with particularly severe forms of VWD type 1 appear to have missense mutations that interfere with the VWF secretion or promote the rapid clearance of VWF from the circulation. Such patients usually have VWF levels <20 IU/dL.[23,72,73] Examples have been reported in Canada[74] and Italy[75] of highly penetrant VWD type 1 mutations that occur in an extended *VWF* haplotype, consistent with descent from one founder in each population.

Although the diagnosis of VWD type 1 depends on testing of plasma VWF, examination of platelet VWF reveals additional heterogeneity (Table 129–4). Some patients have concordant decreases of both plasma and platelet VWF. This group was described previously as type I-1[76] or type I-platelet low[30] and proposed to be caused by defective VWF synthesis. Other patients have low plasma VWF and normal platelet VWF. This phenotype, termed type I-2[76] or type I-platelet normal,[30] was proposed to be caused by impaired release from cellular stores, although increased clearance from plasma would be an alternative mechanism. An additional variant in which plasma VWF is normal and platelet VWF multimers are reduced was termed type I-3.[76] Interestingly, VWF-mediated platelet function in patients with VWD type I-platelet normal was normal or nearly normal, suggesting that platelet VWF content may correlate inversely with bleeding tendency.[30,77] Patients with normal platelet VWF also appeared to have a better response to 1-desamino-8-D-arginine vasopressin (DDAVP; desmopressin).[30]

Despite the straightforward definition of VWD type 1, some patients present a difficult diagnostic challenge. Those with exceptionally low values of VWF are relatively easy to diagnose. Very low VWF levels (eg, 10 to 30 IU/dL) and significant bleeding symptoms usually cosegregate within a family as dominant traits, and linkage analysis or DNA sequencing often supports the existence of an intragenic VWF mutation.[78,79] These mutations can have dominant negative effects. For example, different single amino acid substitutions in the VWF D3 domain may cause VWD type 1 by reducing the secretion[80] or intravascular survival[67] of VWF multimers.

In contrast to patients with very low VWF levels, subjects with VWF levels just below the normal range often do not fit comfortably into a diagnosis of VWD type 1. The population distribution of VWF levels is very broad, and mild mucocutaneous bleeding symptoms are common (see Chapter 121). As a consequence, chance association of low VWF and bleeding also is common.[81] In such cases, it is common to find that bleeding symptoms and low VWF levels do not cosegregate, or that low VWF levels are not associated with specific VWF alleles within a family.[20,78,79,82,83] Furthermore, the bleeding risk conferred by a VWF level just below the normal range is not known precisely but probably is modest. For example, the relative risk for menorrhagia, given a low VWF level, appears to be approximately 3.9.[81] The limited ability of low VWF to predict bleeding also is illustrated by a longitudinal study of children diagnosed with VWD through population screening. Among 1218 school children in Italy, 9 new cases of VWD were identified based on a low VWF and bleeding symptoms plus a family history of bleeding and at least 1 relative with low VWF.[19] However, in these families there was no concordance between low VWF levels and bleeding symptoms, and none of the new cases had medically significant bleeding during 13 years of follow-up.[20] The modest bleeding risk and lack of heritability suggest that a low VWF level could be treated as a modest risk factor for bleeding, without necessitating the diagnosis of a genetic disorder.

von Willebrand Disease Type 2

von Willebrand disease type 2 is characterized by qualitative abnormalities of VWF. Patients may have normal levels of VWF : Ag, but the protein is dysfunctional. These variants account for 7% to 30% of cases. Four subtypes are currently recognized. The distribution among the subtypes varies among centers. For example, in France patients with VWD type 2 were partitioned as follows: type 2A equaled 30%, type 2B equaled 28%, type 2M (or unclassified) equaled 8%, and type 2N equaled 34%.[84] In contrast, the distribution in Bonn, Germany, was type 2A equaled 74%, type 2B equaled 10%, type 2M equaled 13%, and type 2N equaled 3.5%.[51]

Von Willebrand disease type 2A refers to qualitative variants of VWD in which platelet-VWF interactions are markedly decreased because hemostatically effective large VWF multimers are absent. The VWF : Ag may be normal or decreased. The VWF : RCo is decreased disproportionately. A VWF : RCo/VWF : Ag ratio of less than 0.7 may be used as criterion of abnormal function,[85] although VWF : RCo may be extremely low in VWD type 2A. On multimer gels, the high-molecular-weight and intermediate multimers are absent or markedly decreased. Satellite multimer bands may or may not be normal. Patients previously classified as II-1, II-2, and II-3,[76] I-platelet discordant,[30] IIA,[50] IB,[86] IIC,[87] IID,[88] IIE,[89] IIF,[90] IIG,[91] IIH,[92] and II-I[93] are included under VWD type 2A (see Table 129–4).

At least two distinct mechanisms cause VWD type 2A: (1) abnormal assembly and secretion of large VWF multimers; and (2) increased susceptibility of VWF to proteolysis in the circulation. The two mechanisms may be distinguished by examining platelet VWF, which lacks large multimers if assembly is abnormal but has a normal multimer pattern if the VWF has increased susceptibility to proteolysis. The mutations that cause VWD type 2A by interfering with multimer assembly can act at any of several steps in the biosynthetic process, and the location of these mutations often can be inferred from the appearance of the VWF multimers. For example, mutations in the propeptide D1 and D2 domains (Fig. 129–2) interfere with multimerization in the Golgi apparatus and cause a recessive variant originally named *type IIC* that exhibits an exceptionally clean multimer pattern characterized by the absence of prominent satellite bands (see Fig. 129–1).[87,94,95] Mutations in the D3 domain that interfere with multimerization have also been identified in patients with the dominant variant originally named *type IIE* (see Fig. 129–2), with an indistinct or "smeary" multimer pattern.[89,96] Mutations in the cystine knot (CK) domain prevent dimerization in the endoplasmic reticulum and cause a dominantly inherited variant originally named *type IID* (see Fig. 129–2), which exhibits a characteristic single satellite band between the major bands consistent with some multimers having an odd number rather than the normal even number of subunits.[88,97]

Some mutations within the A2 domain render VWF more susceptible to proteolytic digestion by the metalloprotease ADAMTS13, probably by destabilizing the domain structure and facilitating exposure of the bond to be cleaved. Other mutations within domain A2 or adjacent domains have more extreme effects on structure and cause VWD type 2A at least partly by impairing multimer assembly.[98–100] Mutations in domain A2 frequently appear to be responsible for most cases of the variant originally named *type IIA* (see Fig. 129–2).

Although VWD type 2A mutations throughout the VWF subunit interfere with distinct steps of multimer assembly that correlate with

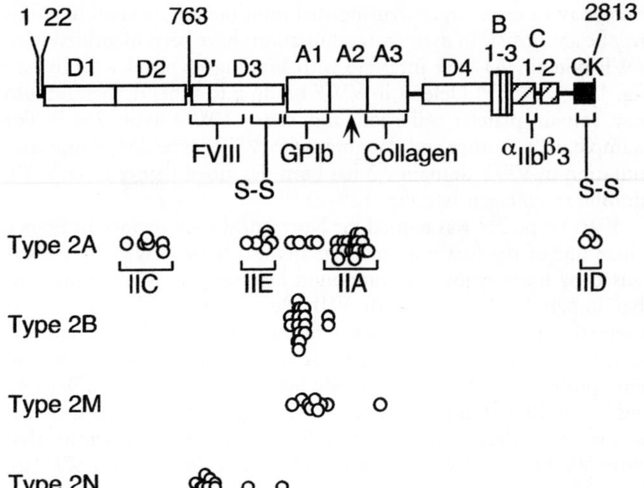

Figure 129–2 von Willebrand factor mutations in von Willebrand disease (VWD) type 2. Amino acid residues of prepro-VWF are indicated by codon number. The signal peptide comprises residues 1–22, the propeptide contains residues 23–763, and the mature subunit contains residues 764–2813. Conserved structural domains (A, B, C, D, and CK) are labeled. Multimers are linked together by disulfide bonds (S-S) located in the D3 and CK domains. Binding sites are indicated for factor VIII (FVIII), platelet GPIb (GPIb), collagen, and platelet integrin αIIbβ3. The metalloprotease ADAMTS13 cleaves the Tyr^{1605}-Met^{1606} bond in domain A2 (*arrow*). *Circles* indicate the position of mutations that cause the VWD types indicated at the left. For VWD type 2A, the *lettered brackets* show the location of mutations that correspond to variants with characteristic multimer patterns as discussed in the text, including type 2A, caused by increased sensitivity to proteolysis (IIA) or by defective multimer assembly because of mutations in the propeptide (IIC), the D3 domain (IIE), or the cystine knot (CK) domain (IID).

distinct satellite band patterns on multimer gels, or spare the process of multimer assembly and instead promote intravascular degradation of VWF, ultimately they all appear to promote bleeding through a shared mechanism, by reducing the concentration of large VWF multimers and thereby impairing platelet binding to VWF at sites of vascular injury.

VWD type 2B is caused by a qualitative abnormality of VWF in which there is increased platelet-VWF interaction because of an increased affinity of VWF for its platelet receptor, GPIb. Patients previously diagnosed with VWD types IIB,[40] I-New York,[101] and Malmö[102] are included in this category (see Table 129–4). The hallmark of type 2B VWD is brisk RIPA at low concentrations of ristocetin (0.3–0.5 mg/mL) that do not induce platelet aggregation in normal platelet-rich plasma. In the most common form of type 2B VWD, high-molecular-weight multimers are absent from plasma (see Fig. 129–1) but are present in platelets. A full range of normal multimer sizes is synthesized, but the largest multimers bind spontaneously to platelets and are cleared rapidly[103] because of the increased affinity of VWF for platelet GPIb.[40] Patients with type 2B VWD often have mild thrombocytopenia.

The mutations that cause VWD type 2B are within or adjacent to the Cys1272-Cys1458 disulfide loop in the A1 domain of VWF (see Fig. 129–2).[63,96,104] The A1 domain binds directly to a site near the N-terminus of platelet GPIb, and type 2B mutations appear to stabilize the bound conformation.[105]

VWD type 2M (*M* for *multimer*) refers to qualitative variants in which decreased platelet-dependent VWF function is not caused by the absence of high-molecular-weight multimers, but instead is caused by mutations that interfere with VWF binding to platelets or subendothelium.[62] Previous VWD types B,[106] IC,[107] and ID[108] are grouped in this category (see Table 129–4). Assays of VWF activity are decreased disproportionately relative to levels of VWF : Ag and factor VIII. The VWF multimer distribution is typically normal, and there may be even larger-than-normal multimers. The satellite bands may be abnormal. In many cases, mutations have been identified with VWF domain A1 that interfere with binding to platelet GPIb (see Fig. 129–2).[63,96,104] Defects in VWF binding to subendothelium also may impair platelet adhesion and cause VWD type 2M.[62] For example, in a mother and daughter with VWD type 2M, a missense mutation in VWF domain A3 has been described that reduces VWF binding to collagen (see Fig. 129–2).[109]

VWD type 2N was named for Normandy, the province in France where one of the first reported patients was born. VWD type 2N is caused by homozygous or compound heterozygous *VWF* mutations that impair binding to factor VIII. Because the VWF-factor VIII interaction is necessary for normal factor VIII survival in the circulation, VWD type 2N masquerades as an autosomal recessive form of hemophilia A.[52,53] Patients typically have normal levels of VWF : Ag and VWF : RCo, but reduced factor VIII and VWF : FVIIIB is absent or markedly decreased.[54,55] With few exceptions, mutations that cause VWD type 2N occur in the D′ or D3 domain of VWF (see Fig. 129–2).[55,63]

von Willebrand Disease Type 3

VWD type 3 is characterized by complete or nearly complete deficiency of VWF and accounts for less than 5% of patients with VWD. This recessive, severe form of VWD is the result of homozygosity or compound heterozygosity for *VWF* alleles that produce little or no protein. The prevalence of VWD type 3 is approximately 0.5 per million for many European countries,[110] approximately 1.4 per million for North America,[111] approximately 3 per million for Sweden,[110] and up to 6 per million for populations in which consanguinity is prevalent, such as Iran.[18,112] In most cases, VWF : RCo and VWF : Ag are undetectable and factor VIII levels are less than 10 IU/dL. Multimeric analysis of plasma from patients with VWD type 3 disease shows essentially no multimers because of the marked reduction in VWF. The gene defects associated with VWD type 3 usually are nonsense mutations or frameshifts because of small insertions or deletions; large deletions, splice-site mutations and missense mutations are less common. The mutations are distributed throughout the *VWF* gene and most are unique to the family in which they were first identified.[63,113,114]

APPROACH TO DIAGNOSIS

If the diagnosis of VWD is suspected, VWF : Ag, VWF : RCo, factor VIII and platelet count may be used as screening tests, in addition to other testing that may be considered, such as a prothrombin time and activated partial thromboplastin time (see Chapter 122). In some patients with VWD, the level of factor VIII may be decreased sufficiently to prolong the activated partial thromboplastin time. Thrombocytopenia may cause bleeding similar to that observed in VWD, although the platelet count also may be low in VWD type 2B. The bleeding time and PFA-100 closure time have been recommended as screening tests in the diagnosis of VWD, but as discussed in a preceding section (Laboratory Testing, Other Tests), they are not specific and have very limited predictive power to exclude or support the diagnosis.[58,60,61,115]

Normal values in screening assays, including a normal VWF : RCo/VWF : Ag ratio (eg, >0.7), exclude medically significant VWD with a few caveats discussed under Issues in Diagnosis and Classification. A decreased but detectable level of VWF, with proportionate decrease in factor VIII and no evidence of qualitative VWF defect, suggests a diagnosis of VWD type 1. Disproportionate decreases in VWF : RCo or VWF : CB, with ratios of VWF : RCo/VWF : Ag or VWF : CB/VWF : Ag (eg, less than 0.7,[65,85,109]) suggest a diagnosis of VWD type 2A, 2B, or 2M, and merit further specialized testing for discrimination.

The absence of high-molecular-weight VWF multimers excludes VWD type 2M[62] and narrows the possibilities to type 2A and type 2B. Sometimes the multimer pattern is so characteristic of a specific VWD type 2A mechanism[51,96,104] that VWD type 2B also can be excluded, but in most cases, RIPA is necessary. Markedly impaired RIPA is typical of VWD type 2A, and increased RIPA at low ristocetin concentrations is required to diagnose VWD type 2B.[50]

If high-molecular-weight multimers are present but the VWF : RCo or VWF : CB is disproportionately decreased, then the most likely diagnosis is VWD type 2M.[65,104] However, some VWD type 2B mutations do not markedly alter the VWF multimer distribution,[101,102] and RIPA may be necessary to distinguish VWD type 2M from these uncommon forms of VWD type 2B.

In the evaluation of patients for possible VWD type 2M, VWF : RCo and VWF : CB could be considered complementary because each assesses a different binding function. In practice, however, most centers have chosen one or the other as a measure of VWF functional activity, which means that certain VWD type 2M defects may be overlooked. The VWF : CB does not detect mutations that specifically impair binding to platelet GPIb. Conversely, VWF : RCo would be normal in patients with isolated collagen-binding defects, although only one such family has been reported so far.[109] The prevalence of collagen-binding defects in VWD type 2M may be low but will not be known until more experience is obtained with the VWF : CB assay.

A normal level of VWF, a decreased level of factor VIII, and evidence against X-linked inheritance suggest a diagnosis of VWD type 2N, although assays of factor VIII-VWF binding (VWF : FVIIIB) may be necessary to exclude hemophilia A.[55] In VWD type 2N, the ratio FVIII : C/VWF : Ag generally is less than 0.5. Patients with *VWF* gene mutations that severely impair factor VIII binding had FVIII : C levels of 8.4 ± 5.2 IU/dL, and those with less severe binding defects had FVIII : C levels of 21.8 ± 9.8.[54] VWF : FVIIIB results for patients with VWD type 2N are typically less than 0.1 and the results for heterozygous carriers cluster around 0.5, where the result for normal standard VWF is defined to be 1.0.[54]

The absence of detectable VWF is characteristic of VWD type 3. In most cases, the factor VIII level also is below 10 IU/dL.[112,116,117] A small subset of patients with VWD type 3 has higher factor VIII levels of 12 to 32 IU/dL. In contrast to other patients with VWD type 3, some of those with relatively high baseline values for factor VIII may have a clinically useful increase in factor VIII level after treatment with desmopressin.[118]

ISSUES IN DIAGNOSIS AND CLASSIFICATION

von Willebrand Disease Type 1 or Low von Willebrand Factor

The diagnosis of VWD type 1 is easy if the level of VWF is very low, but it becomes problematic as the level of VWF approaches the lower end of the normal population distribution. For example, VWF levels less than 30 IU/dL have been associated with recurrent and medically significant bleeding, a clearly dominant pattern of inheritance, and mutations in the *VWF* gene.[30,75,78,79,80] For patients with such dominant, symptomatic, and relatively severe VWF deficiency, the diagnosis of VWD type 1 is likely to be useful for counseling them about their bleeding risk and facilitating appropriate treatment.

In contrast, VWF levels near the lower end of the normal distribution usually are not associated with significant bleeding, tend not to be heritable, often do not cosegregate with any bleeding symptoms that may occur, and do not show consistent linkage to the *VWF* locus.[20,78,79,82,83] Many factors contribute to this uncertainty. Increases in VWF are associated with pregnancy, hyperthyroidism, renal failure, and the stress of exercise, fainting, inflammation, trauma, or surgery.[119–124] Levels of VWF also vary during the menstrual cycle in women,[125] although there are significant discrepancies among studies concerning the timing of minimum and maximal levels. Consequently, test results for persons having moderately low VWF levels may be intermittently normal or abnormal.[82,126] In addition, a modestly low VWF level confers only a modestly increased risk of minor bleeding that rarely requires medical treatment or a change in lifestyle. For example, the relative risk of menorrhagia was estimated to be approximately 3.9 for women with VWF levels of approximately 30 to 50 IU/dL.[81] Rather than labeling them with the diagnosis of VWD type 1, patients with VWF levels in this range could be informed that they have "low VWF," which is a modest risk factor for minor bleeding. Conversely, serious bleeding symptoms associated with only moderately low levels of VWF should prompt investigation for a disorder other than VWD.

von Willebrand Disease Type 1 or Type 2

Similar concerns apply to distinguishing between VWD type 1 and VWD type 2, or among the VWD type 2 variants. Very abnormal VWF phenotypes are easy to recognize, but subtle defects can be difficult to characterize. As a general rule, however, the closer the laboratory phenotype approximates that of VWD type 1, the more likely the clinical course will be as well. For example, patients with the VWD type 2N mutation R816W have low levels of factor VIII (<10 IU/dL) and a poor response to desmopressin, whereas patients with the VWD type 2N mutation R854Q tend to have higher levels of factor VIII (20–40 IU/dL) and a clinically useful response to desmopressin.[127] Differentiating VWD type 1 from VWD type 2M can be particularly difficult because the distinction depends on the VWF:RCo/VWF:Ag ratio, and VWF:RCo assays are notoriously imprecise. VWF:RCo/VWF:Ag ratios of <0.6 or <0.7 have been proposed for the diagnosis of VWD type 2M, but a recent clinical study observed that satisfactory discrimination from VWD type 1 required a VWF:RCo/VWF:Ag ratio <0.4.[65] Therefore, diagnoses based on the VWF:RCo/VWF:Ag ratio may require repeated testing or confirmation by other methods.

Influence of ABO Blood Type

Because VWF plasma level varies with ABO blood type, some laboratories employ different normal ranges for different ABO blood types,[24] but the value of this refinement for VWD diagnosis is uncertain. Also, the risk of bleeding associated with a particular VWF level does not appear to depend on ABO blood type.[128] Consequently, the use of ABO-adjusted reference ranges for VWF parameters may not significantly increase the precision of VWD diagnosis.

Mixed von Willebrand Disease Phenotypes

Mutations may disrupt the function of *VWF* alleles in many distinct ways, and, therefore, compound heterozygosity can sometimes produce VWD phenotypes that combine features of several VWD subtypes. For example, inheritance of a factor VIII binding defect from one parent and a hypofunctional allele from another can produce a mixed phenotype of VWD type 2N and VWD type 1. Such interactions may contribute to the variability in laboratory findings and symptoms observed in certain families.[23] In favorable cases, such combined defects may be deciphered by genetic and phenotype studies of the patient's relatives.

DIFFERENTIAL DIAGNOSIS

Bleeding symptoms in VWD include those characteristic of platelet dysfunction and sometimes of factor VIII deficiency. Consequently, the differential diagnosis includes other defects of platelets and blood clotting, both congenital and acquired. Such disorders usually can be identified readily, but some can pose special problems.

Hemophilia A

Factor VIII deficiency occurs in both VWD and hemophilia A (see Chapter 125), and a patient with hemophilia who ingests aspirin, or who has another cause for platelet dysfunction, can have a combination of bleeding symptoms that resembles VWD type 3. Hemophilia A and VWD can be distinguished by appropriate laboratory testing (see Chapters 122 and 125). VWF:Ag and VWF:RCo are normal in hemophilia and absent in VWD type 3. However, factor VIII is selectively low in both hemophilia A and VWD type 2N. Without a clear pattern of X-linked recessive inheritance to support hemophilia A, or autosomal recessive inheritance to support VWD type 2N, distinguishing between these diagnoses may require testing of factor VIII binding to patient VWF (VWF:FVIIIB). The VWF:FVIIIB is normal in hemophilia A and markedly decreased in VWD type 2N. In a screening study of 177 patients previously diagnosed with hemophilia A, 5 were found instead to have VWD type 2N.[129]

Thrombocytopenia

Thrombocytopenia associated with VWD type 2B may be discovered incidentally during a medical evaluation for other reasons and may be exacerbated by pregnancy,[130–133] surgery,[134] or other physiologic stress. Platelet counts less than 20,000 cells/μL may occur under these conditions. This finding sometimes has led to the erroneous diagnosis of autoimmune thrombocytopenia, resulting in unnecessary treatment with corticosteroids, intravenous immunoglobulins, and splenectomy.[130–136] VWD type 2B also may present as neonatal thrombocytopenia.[137,138]

Platelet-Type Pseudo-von Willebrand Disease

Platelet-type pseudo-VWD was first described by Miller and Castella[139] and Weiss and coworkers[140] as a hemorrhagic disorder caused by gain-of-function defects in the platelet receptor for VWF (see Chapter 141). Phenotypically, patients with platelet-type pseudo-VWD are similar to patients with VWD type 2B. Multimeric analysis shows the absence of high-molecular-weight multimers and factor VIII, VWF:RCo, and VWF:Ag are variably reduced. RIPA is enhanced in response to low concentrations of ristocetin (0.3–0.5 mg/mL), and mild thrombocytopenia is commonly present. However, in contrast to VWD type 2B, in which the abnormality is in the VWF, the defect in platelet-type pseudo-VWD is in platelet GPIb. The mutant GPIb binds VWF with increased affinity, and the deficiency of high-molecular-weight VWF multimers is thought to occur as a consequence of increased binding to platelets. Platelet-type pseudo-VWD can be distinguished from VWD type 2B by suitable mixing experiments. In platelet-type pseudo-VWD, the addition of normal human VWF to a patient's platelet-rich plasma induces platelet aggregation, whereas in VWD type 2B it does not.[141] The converse test also can be useful: In VWD type 2B the VWF in patient plasma binds to formalin-fixed platelets at low concentrations of ristocetin, whereas in platelet-type pseudo-VWD it does not.[142]

Platelet-type pseudo-VWD is caused by missense mutations in the VWF binding site located in the N-terminal end of the platelet GPIb α-chain; the substitutions Gly233Val and Val239Met have been reported in different families.[143–145] When VWF binds GPIbα, conformational changes occur in both proteins, and the crystallographic structures of the bound and free proteins suggest that the mutations that cause platelet-type pseudo-VWD increase the affinity of binding by stabilizing the bound conformation of GPIbα.[105]

Acquired von Willebrand Syndrome

Deficiency of VWF may occur as an acquired condition, in which case it is referred to as *acquired von Willebrand syndrome* (AvWS).

The laboratory findings in AvWS are similar to those in VWD, with decreased values for VWF:Ag, VWF:RCo, and factor VIII. The VWF multimer pattern often shows a decrease in large multimers compatible with a diagnosis of VWD type 2A, but the multimer distribution also may be normal.[146,147]

AvWS usually appears to be caused by one of three mechanisms involving VWF: autoimmune clearance, fluid shear stress-induced proteolysis, or increased binding to platelets or other cells. Immune mechanisms are thought to explain AvWS that occurs in association with lymphoproliferative disorders, monoclonal gammopathy of unknown significance, systemic lupus erythematosus, autoimmune hypothyroidism, other autoimmune diseases, and some cancers. Antibodies to VWF have been found only in less than 20% of such patients, suggesting that current methods for antibody detection are too insensitive, or that AvWS associated with these conditions may not always have an immunologic basis.

Some cardiovascular conditions expose the blood to increased fluid shear stress and thereby appear to increase the proteolytic cleavage of VWF, probably by the metalloprotease ADAMTS13, which causes the loss of large VWF multimers and may cause AvWS. For example, AvWS has been reported in patients with aortic stenosis, mitral valve prolapse, pulmonary hypertension, ventricular septal defect, and patent ductus arteriosus. The AvWS resolves or improves on surgical correction of the vascular defect or pharmacologic treatment of pulmonary hypertension.[146–151]

AvWS may result from increased binding of VWF platelets in patients with thrombocytosis caused by myeloproliferative disorders, such as essential thrombocythemia, polycythemia vera, and chronic myelogenous leukemia or by reactive thrombocytosis after splenectomy. There is an inverse relationship between platelet count and the proportion of high-molecular-weight VWF multimers, and measures to reduce the platelet count can restore a normal multimer distribution and normal hemostatic function.[152–154] Binding of VWF to the surface of malignant lymphocytes or other tumor cells also has been reported to cause AvWS. In some cases, increased VWF binding may be a consequence of the abnormal expression of GPIb or other VWF binding proteins on the cell surface.[146,147]

A few other conditions may cause AvWS. Mildly decreased VWF levels may occur in hypothyroidism by nonimmune mechanisms and are corrected with appropriate thyroid hormone therapy.[155] Case reports have described AvWS in patients receiving valproic acid, ciprofloxacin, griseofulvin, or hydroxyethyl starch.[146,147]

Recognizing AvWS is important because treatment of associated predisposing conditions may improve the hemostatic defect. If correction of the underlying disorder is not possible, then several strategies may be tried to control bleeding. Despite the fact that most AvWS is caused by rapid clearance of VWF, treatment with desmopressin reportedly is effective in approximately one-third of patients. As is true of VWD, a test dose of desmopressin appears to predict future responses in AvWS. Factor VIII-VWF concentrates were effective in a similar fraction of cases.[146] The likelihood of response to desmopressin or factor VIII-VWF concentrates appears to be greatest for AvWS associated with autoimmune clearance. Approximately one-third of patients with immune-mediated AvWS also respond well to high-dose intravenous immunoglobulin, although a good response seems to be less likely for patients with IgM monoclonal gammopathy.[156] If these interventions are ineffective, then plasmapheresis or extracorporeal immunoadsorption may be considered.[146]

In contrast to the relatively good outcome in immune-mediated disease, AvWS associated with either high fluid shear stress or increased binding to platelets does not usually respond well to desmopressin, factor VIII-VWF concentrates, or intravenous immunoglobulin.[146] However, AvWS in the setting of cancer, particularly Wilms tumor,[147] may be quite responsive to desmopressin and also have good responses to factor VIII-VWF concentrates.[146]

CLINICAL MANIFESTATIONS

Bleeding Symptoms

Depending on the subtype, bleeding in VWD may have features of bleeding because of platelet dysfunction or factor VIII deficiency, and VWD type 3 combines these hemostatic defects. Bruising, recurrent severe nosebleeds, oral cavity bleeding, and menorrhagia are characteristic of platelet adhesion defects, whereas joint and deep tissue bleeding are more likely to be caused by factor VIII deficiency (see Chapter 121). A recent study summarized bleeding episodes in 385 patients with VWD type 3, 182 of whom were women.[112] The reported symptoms included gastrointestinal bleeding in 20%, hemarthrosis in 37%, postoperative bleeding in 41%, muscle hematoma in 52%, menorrhagia in 69%, oral cavity bleeding in 70%, and severe nosebleeds in 77%. Compared with these figures for VWD type 3, patients with hemophilia A had approximately twice the frequency of bleeding into joints and muscles and a similar frequency of postoperative bleeding but rarely had bleeding from mucosal surfaces. Pregnancies in VWD type 3 were not associated with excessive bleeding and did not require prophylactic replacement therapy prior to delivery. However, postpartum bleeding that delayed discharge from the hospital or required blood transfusion occurred in 15% of pregnancies. Menorrhagia requiring medical treatment, causing iron deficiency, or requiring transfusion of blood or plasma occurred in at least two-thirds of women with VWD type 3.[112,157] In addition to menorrhagia, women may experience midcycle pain with ovulation and significant bleeding into the corpus luteum, which rarely may cause life-threatening hemoperitoneum.[158,159]

Patients with other types of VWD may experience some or all of the symptoms associated with VWD type 3, depending on the severity of VWF dysfunction and on whether the defect affects mainly platelet adhesion, factor VIII level, or both. Women with VWD are more frequently symptomatic than are men, mainly because of the hemostatic challenges of the menstrual cycle and childbirth. Including all VWD types, women account for approximately two-thirds of patients.[82,158]

Standardized bleeding questionnaires have been developed and tested retrospectively on patients with VWD type 1 (see Chapter 121).[160,161] The most common symptoms were bleeding after tooth extraction, nosebleeds, menorrhagia, bleeding into the skin, postoperative bleeding, and bleeding from minor wounds. At least one bleeding symptom was reported by 98% of index cases, 89% of affected relatives, 32% of unaffected relatives, and 12% of healthy controls. Such questionnaires may be useful in deciding whether a patient's bleeding symptoms merit laboratory testing for VWD.

Other Disorders Associated With von Willebrand Disease

Many conditions that affect hemostasis, directly or indirectly, can interact with VWD and exacerbate bleeding symptoms, which contributes to the phenotypic heterogeneity of VWD. For example, recurrent bleeding from gastrointestinal angiodysplasia is relatively common in AvWS and in VWD types 2 and 3.[162–164] Similarly, VWD may be associated with bleeding at various sites in hereditary hemorrhagic telangiectasia[165] and Ehlers-Danlos syndrome.[166,167]

THERAPY

The aim of therapy in VWD is to correct abnormalities of VWF-dependent platelet function and blood coagulation, as necessary, usually by raising plasma levels of VWF and factor VIII. In contrast to hemophilia, which frequently is associated with severe spontaneous bleeding, few patients with VWD require chronic prophylactic treatment to prevent bleeding. The major indications for treatment in

VWD are to stop bleeding episodes and to prevent surgical or postpartum bleeding. As a general rule, mucosal bleeding responds to correction of the platelet adhesion defect by raising the level of hemostatically effective, large VWF multimers,[168–170] whereas surgical and soft tissue bleeding respond to correction of the blood clotting defect by raising the level of factor VIII.[171,172] Recommendations for specific clinical situations are summarized in Table 129–5.

Patients with VWD can have venous thrombosis, particularly when receiving treatment with factor VIII-VWF concentrates,[173,174] and should receive prophylactic antithrombotic therapy when indicated by other aspects of the clinical situation.

DESMOPRESSIN

The synthetic vasopressin analog, 1-desamino-8-D-arginine vasopressin (desmopressin) lacks the pressor activity of vasopressin (antidiuretic hormone [ADH]) and was developed initially for the treatment of diabetes insipidus. When given at much higher doses to normal volunteers or to persons with mild hemophilia A or VWD, desmopressin was found to induce a rapid increase in plasma levels of VWF and factor VIII, with peak levels achieved approximately 30 minutes after intravenous administration.[119,175] Desmopressin promotes the secretion of VWF from storage sites in endothelium. One study has demonstrated the loss of VWF staining of capillary endothelial cells after desmopressin administration.[176] The rapid changes in factor VIII and VWF levels coincide, suggesting that factor VIII is released from cells in which both proteins are stored together, although the identity of these cells is unknown at present.

Bleeding and Surgery in von Willebrand Disease

Desmopressin (DDAVP; Aventis, Ferring) is available in an injectable or a nasal spray formulation. The injectable preparation (4 μg/mL) usually is administered intravenously and maximal responses are obtained with a dose of 0.3 μg/kg. The total dose is diluted in normal saline (eg, 50 mL) and infused over 30 minutes. Healthy controls and patients with type 1 VWD or mild hemophilia A usually obtain a reproducible twofold to fivefold increase in VWF and factor VIII within 30 minutes after the end of the infusion.[175] Subcutaneous administration produces similar peak levels of factor VIII and VWF but with a delay of 1.5 to 2 hours.[175,177] For subcutaneous administration, 0.3 μg/kg of injectable desmopressin is administered at less than 1.5 mL/site, and a single treatment may require three or four subcutaneous injections.

Because of its decreased bioavailability, approximately 10-fold more intranasal desmopressin must be given to achieve a useful hemostatic response. Two intranasal preparations are available. One is a dilute solution (100 μg/mL) used for patients with diabetes insipidus that cannot be used to treat VWD. The other is a concentrated preparation (Stimate, 1.5 mg/mL) specifically formulated for self-treatment of bleeding in hemophilia A and VWD. The spray pump delivers 0.1 mL (150 μg), and the usual dose is two sprays (one per nostril) for a total of 300 μg. Patients weighing less than 50 kg may use a single spray. Maximal levels of factor VIII and VWF are reached in approximately 1.5 hours, and usually are less than those achieved with optimal intravenous dosing and similar to those reached after an intravenous dose of 0.2 μg/kg.[175,177,178]

For all routes of administration, the half-life of the stimulated increase in factor VIII and VWF is approximately 5 to 8 hours in most patients.[175,177] Therefore, a dose interval of 24 hours is usually sufficient. Patients with VWD type 1 caused by rapid clearance of VWF, or VWD type 2A caused by intravascular proteolysis of VWF may have very brief responses to desmopressin. A dose interval of 12 hours may be required in such patients, or desmopressin may simply be ineffective. The individual response to desmopressin is reproducible, and an elective test dose (see box on Performing a Desmopressin Test Dose) is advisable to characterize the response to desmopressin before depending on it for hemostasis.

Tachyphylaxis to desmopressin is common but does not always impair its hemostatic effect. The levels of factor VIII and VWF after the second dose are approximately 30% less than after the first dose, and responses to subsequent doses tend to be similar.[179] Because some patients (≈20%) fail to sustain effective responses after the initial dose,[179] desmopressin alone should not be relied on for hemostasis over several days unless the patient's pattern of response is known to be satisfactory. In practice, one can follow factor levels and switch to coverage with factor VIII-VWF concentrates if necessary.

Common immediate side effects of intravenous desmopressin include transient headache, facial flushing, and mild hypotension with compensatory tachycardia. These symptoms generally abate with a reduction in the dose or the rate of infusion. Among patients using intranasal desmopressin, headache, and flushing occurred with approximately 3% of doses; nausea, vomiting, dizziness, abdominal cramping, and peripheral edema were reported infrequently (in total, 0.14% of doses).[180]

Desmopressin has potent antidiuretic activity and can cause hyponatremia and seizures if free water intake is not restricted appropriately. This complication appears to be a particular concern for infants and young children but may occur at any age. The risk of hyponatremia is increased for patients who receive repeated intravenous doses of desmopressin and intravenous hydration[181] but has occurred after a single intranasal dose of desmopressin followed by excessive oral fluid intake.[182] Patients using intranasal desmopressin should be instructed about the importance of restricting water intake and the significance of symptoms that may be associated with hyponatremia. For patients receiving intravenous desmopressin, monitoring of water intake, body weight, and serum electrolytes should be considered for children or for persons of any age given intravenous fluids or repeated doses of desmopressin.

Performing a Desmopressin Test Dose

Desmopressin 0.3 μg/kg in 50 to 100 mL of normal saline is infused intravenously over 30 minutes with monitoring of vital signs and for side effects of flushing or headache. Levels of factor VIII, VWF:RCo (or VWF:CB), and optionally VWF:Ag are checked 1 hour and 4 hours, respectively, after the start of the infusion. Bleeding time need not be measured because it does not correlate with clinical efficacy. The values for factor VIII and VWF at 1 hour indicate the maximum response. The values at 4 hours permit calculation of the half-life of the endogenous factors and, therefore, predict the duration of an effective response. In most patients the half-life of the increased factor VIII and VWF is 5 to 8 hours.[175,177] The subset of patients with VWD type 1 who have normal platelet VWF content often exhibit an exaggerated peak increase (up to 20-fold) of both VWF and factor VIII but with a very short half-life of approximately 1 hour, adequate for oral surgery but possibly not for major surgery.[183] Patients with VWD type 2N exhibit dissociation between a normal VWF response and a brief and often insufficient factor VIII response.[22,127] Patients with VWD type 2A may have a satisfactory factor VIII response but a small or very brief VWF:RCo response.[103,184] Comparison of peak VWF:RCo and VWF:Ag values can help to discriminate between qualitative and quantitative VWF defects when the distinction is unclear from assays before treatment.

Peak factor VIII and VWF:RCo values of 40 to 60 IU/dL may be sufficient for minor surgery including dental extractions. Peak values of greater than 100 IU/dL are satisfactory for major surgery if the trough level can be maintained above approximately 50 IU/dL with a dose interval of 12 or 24 hours, depending on the duration of response based on the test dose.

Performing a Desmopressin Test Dose

Desmopressin 0.3 μg/kg in 50 to 100 mL of normal saline is infused intravenously over more than 30 minutes with monitoring of vital signs and for side effects of flushing or headache. Levels of factor VIII, VWF:RCo (or VWF:CB), and optionally VWF:Ag are checked 1 hour and 4 hours, respectively, after the start of the infusion. Bleeding time need not be measured because it does not correlate with clinical efficacy. The values for factor VIII and VWF at 1 hour indicate the maximum response. The values at 4 hours permit calculation of the half-life of the endogenous factors and, therefore, predict the duration of an effective response. In most patients the half-life of the increased factor VIII and VWF is 5 to 8 hours.[175,177] The subset of patients with VWD type 1 who have normal platelet VWF content often exhibit an exaggerated peak increase (up to 20-fold) of both VWF and factor VIII but with a very short half-life of approximately 1 hour, adequate for oral surgery but possibly not for major surgery.[183] Patients with VWD type 2N exhibit dissociation between a normal VWF response and a brief and often insufficient factor VIII response.[22,127] Patients with VWD type 2A may have a satisfactory factor VIII response but a small or very brief VWF:RCo response.[103,184] Comparison of peak VWF:RCo and VWF:Ag values can help to discriminate between qualitative and quantitative VWF defects when the distinction is unclear from assays before treatment.

Peak factor VIII and VWF:RCo values of 40 to 60 IU/dL may be sufficient for minor surgery including dental extractions. Peak values of greater than 100 IU/dL are satisfactory for major surgery if the trough level can be maintained above approximately 50 IU/dL with a dose interval of 12 or 24 hours, depending on the duration of response based on the test dose.

Myocardial infarction, stroke, and venous thromboembolism have been reported rarely in association with desmopressin use in adults. In clinical trials evaluating desmopressin to reduce blood loss during surgery, the incidence of thrombosis was similar in the treated and untreated groups.[185] Therefore, the risk of thrombosis appears to be small, but desmopressin should not be used in patients with significant coronary or cerebrovascular atherosclerosis.

Desmopressin is effective for most patients with VWD type 1, who make reduced amounts of a functionally normal VWF molecule.[175] The subset of VWD type 1 characterized by normal levels of platelet VWF (VWD type 1 platelet normal) appears to be caused by accelerated clearance of VWF from the blood, and these patients often have exaggerated responses to desmopressin that are of relatively short duration but are hemostatically effective.[183]

Desmopressin usually is not effective in patients with VWD type 2 or type 3. In VWD type 2A, the VWF secreted in response to desmopressin usually has markedly abnormal function and good hemostatic responses are uncommon.[103] Desmopressin causes acute, reversible thrombocytopenia in VWD type 2B[186] (and in platelet-type pseudo-VWD[187]), and usually does not correct the hemostatic defect.[103,186,188] Therefore, many consider desmopressin to be contraindicated in VWD type 2B, although good responses have been reported for a few patients.[138,189–192] Published experience in VWD type 2M is limited, but the properties of the mutant VWF suggest that desmopressin should be ineffective. Aside from patients with the mutation R854Q, which causes a relatively mild factor VIII binding defect, desmopressin usually does not effectively increase the level of factor VIII in VWD type 2N.[22,127] With a few exceptions,[118] desmopressin does not change VWF or factor VIII levels in VWD type 3.[103] The relatively rare patients with VWD type 2 or type 3 who respond satisfactorily can be identified with a test dose of desmopressin.

Plasma Products

Fresh-frozen plasma is too dilute for the specific treatment of VWD in most cases. Cryoprecipitate is prepared from frozen plasma by thawing at 4°C (39.2°F). The precipitate that forms is collected by centrifugation and refrozen. When thawed, cryoprecipitate from 1 unit of blood donation can be dissolved in 10 mL of saline for intravenous administration. One unit of cryoprecipitate contains approximately 100 U of factor VIII and VWF, and 200 to 250 mg of fibrinogen, representing a 10-fold concentration relative to plasma. Cryoprecipitate is not generally subjected to virus inactivation treatments and, therefore, may transmit certain infections. For this reason, virucidally treated factor VIII-VWF concentrates are preferred for therapy of VWD in countries where they are available (Table 129–5). Most of the clinical experience using such concentrates is with Humate-P (Aventis)[193] or Alphanate (Alpha Therapeutic Corp.),[194] but published results suggest that other factor VIII-VWF concentrates may be similarly effective.[195] The manufacturing process for all of these concentrates reduces the average size of the VWF multimers,[196] which could impair their adhesive function, but this has not proved to be a significant problem in practice. Most factor VIII-VWF concentrates are standardized only for factor VIII content, so that initial dosing must be based on factor VIII levels. They also differ substantially from each other in VWF content, and the VWF levels obtained during therapy must be determined by laboratory testing. Humate-P is labeled with both factor VIII and VWF:RCo

Table 129–5 Treatment with Factor VIII-VWF Concentrate

Bleeding	Initial Dose and Frequency	Target
Major surgery or bleeding	50 IU/kg daily	Trough level of VIII:C > 50 IU/dL until healing is satisfactory, typically 5–10 days
Minor surgery	40 IU/kg daily or every other day	Trough level of VIII:C > 30 IU/dL until healing is satisfactory, typically 2–4 days
Dental extractions	30 IU/kg one dose	VIII:C > 30 IU/dL for >12 hours
Minor bleeding	25 IU/kg daily	Trough level of VIII:C > 30 IU/dL until bleeding stops, typically 2–4 days
Delivery and postpartum	50 IU/kg daily starting the day of delivery	Trough level of VIII:C > 50 IU/dL until healing is satisfactory, typically 3–4 days postpartum

Initial doses of factor VIII-von Willebrand factor (VWF) concentrate have been calculated for adults with von Willebrand disease (VWD) type 3, or with VWD type 2 variants and completely dysfunctional endogenous VWF. Doses may be increased ≈ 20% for children younger than age 18 years to compensate for their relatively increased plasma volume.[194] For patients with some VWF that is normally functional (VWD type 1) or partially functional (mild type 2 variants), doses should be decreased based on the factor levels present before treatment. For concentrates labeled with VWF:RCo content, dosing may be based on VWF:RCo instead of factor VIII. Trough levels of factor VIII and VWF:RCo should be monitored at least daily. If necessary, reduced doses may be given at shorter dose intervals to decrease the range of peak and trough factor levels. If concentrates are not available locally and the risk of infection is judged to be acceptable, cryoprecipitate may be substituted assuming that one unit of cryoprecipitate contains 100 IU of factor VIII and VWF. If the patient is known to be responsive, desmopressin starting 1 hour before surgery may be substituted for factor VIII-VWF concentrates. If desmopressin is used to cover major surgery, peak and trough factor levels should be monitored and concentrates should be available in case the response to desmopressin becomes inadequate.

Primary or adjunctive therapy with antifibrinolytics, the role of platelet transfusions, and the approach to VWF inhibitors are discussed in the text.

Adapted from reference 229.

content, and initial dosing can be based on VWF level if desired.[193]

Factor VIII and VWF levels fall at different rates in patients with VWD who are treated with factor VIII-VWF concentrates,[194] and this phenomenon has important consequences when treatment is prolonged. The VWF:Ag declines with a half-time of approximately 13 hours; VWF:RCo declines more quickly with a half-time of approximately 7 hours because proteolysis in vivo converts the largest multimers into less active smaller forms more quickly than the VWF:Ag is cleared from circulation. Factor VIII levels decline slowly with an apparent half-time of approximately 24 hours that reflects both normal catabolism and stabilization of endogenously synthesized factor VIII through binding to the transfused VWF. Therefore, if dosing is adjusted to maintain the VWF:RCo level at 50 to 100 IU/dL, the factor VIII level can increase to several hundred IU/dL after a few days, which may confer a significant risk of thrombosis.[173,174,194] Excessive factor VIII levels can be avoided by laboratory monitoring and changing the concentrate dose accordingly.

Unnecessarily high factor VIII levels also could be avoided by switching to a pure VWF concentrate and relying on endogenous synthesis to maintain the factor VIII level. Such a high-purity VWF concentrate prepared from human plasma has been used successfully in Europe[197] (VWF-VHP, Biotransfusion) but is not available in the United States. Recombinant human VWF has been prepared and tested in animal models[198] but is not available for clinical use.

Pure factor VIII, plasma-derived or recombinant, is not appropriate for routine use in VWD. These preparations do not contain significant amounts of VWF and cannot correct quantitative or qualitative deficiencies of VWF. Also, when given to patients with VWD type 3 or VWD type 2N, the infused factor VIII is cleared rapidly with a half-life of less than 2 hours because there is no endogenous functional VWF to bind and stabilize it in the circulation.[199,200]

Platelets

The platelet VWF pool normally accounts for approximately 15% of total blood VWF,[201] and both plasma and platelet VWF contribute to hemostasis.[202] The transfusion of a normal platelet pheresis unit (4 to 5 × 10^{11} platelets) partially corrects the bleeding time of adult patients with VWD type 3, and appears to reduce the amount of cryoprecipitate necessary to fully correct the bleeding time.[203,204] Platelet transfusion could be considered for patients with VWD in whom therapy with factor VIII-VWF complex does not control serious bleeding.

Antifibrinolytic Agents

The fibrinolytic inhibitors ε-aminocaproic acid and tranexamic acid can be used in conjunction with desmopressin or factor VIII-VWF concentrates, and can be given orally or intravenously.[205] Systemic administration of either drug appears particularly effective for bleeding in the oral cavity.[206,207] Bleeding after oral surgery also was decreased by using mouth rinses containing tranexamic acid to supplement other systemic therapy.[208] Systemic antifibrinolytic agents are contraindicated in patients with bleeding in the upper urinary tract, where the formation of a stable clot may cause obstruction. Antifibrinolytics are contraindicated in patients with active thromboembolic disease and should be used with caution in patients with a history of thromboembolism.

Menstrual Cycle Bleeding

Midcycle bleeding from a hemorrhagic corpus luteum may be prevented by the use of combined oral contraceptives.[159] Menorrhagia in VWD, including VWD type 3, has been controlled with combined oral contraceptives, although the reported response rate varies among surveys from 24%[209] to 73%.[157] Estrogens at high doses can raise the plasma level of factor VIII and VWF, but current oral contraceptives do not contain sufficient estrogen and their efficacy probably depends instead on hormone-induced changes in the endometrium.

Menorrhagia also can be treated with tranexamic acid 1 g every 6 hours for 5 days,[210] or with a single dose of 4 g a day for 3 to 5 days, started at the onset of bleeding.[211] Although ε-aminocaproic acid has not been tested specifically in VWD, it has been effective for menorrhagia in otherwise healthy women at doses of 5 g three times daily for 5 days,[212] or 3 g every 6 hours for 3 to 5 days.[213] Occasional side effects include nausea, diarrhea, and orthostatic hypotension.

Desmopressin has been evaluated for the treatment of menorrhagia in two small randomized placebo-controlled trials including 22 women with VWD[214] or 20 women with unexplained prolonged bleeding times.[215] Each study reported a trend in favor of desmopressin for the reduction of menstrual bleeding, but the difference was not statistically significant. A larger open-label trial in 90 women (most with VWD) reported shortened or decreased bleeding in 88% of treated menstrual cycles.[180]

Pregnancy, Labor, and Delivery

Excessive bleeding during pregnancy is uncommon in VWD, and replacement therapy is rarely needed, even for patients with VWD type 3. Fertility is not impaired, and the rate of spontaneous abortion does not appear to be increased.[112,157] However, bleeding at delivery and postpartum may occur if the factor VIII and VWF levels are sufficiently low. Factor VIII and VWF levels normally begin to increase by the second trimester, increase approximately twofold by the end of the third trimester,[216] and decrease to baseline within a week after delivery. For patients with VWD, factor VIII and VWF levels below approximately 50 IU/dL are associated with increased risk of peripartum hemorrhage.[217] Whether factor VIII or VWF correlates best with bleeding risk has not been determined conclusively.[217,218] Severe peripartum hemorrhage has occurred in VWD patients with isolated decreases in VWF:RCo (VWD type 2A)[219] or factor VIII (VWD type 2N),[53,220] suggesting that both factors are relevant. Factor VIII and VWF levels should be checked antepartum and, if necessary, factor VIII-VWF concentrate given to increase the levels to greater than 50 IU/dL at delivery.[217] Administration of concentrate may reverse the thrombocytopenia as well as the bleeding tendency associated with VWD type 2B at delivery.[133] If factor levels are greater than 50 IU/dL, epidural anesthesia has been used without complications.[217,221] Complete evacuation and effective uterine contraction after delivery are important to prevent bleeding.[218]

In the postpartum period, desmopressin or factor VIII-VWF concentrate should be used to maintain levels greater than 50 IU/dL for 3 to 4 days.[112,217,218] Delayed bleeding may occur 2 to 3 weeks after delivery, and patients should be instructed about this risk. If hemorrhage occurs despite prophylaxis, full replacement therapy should be given using desmopressin or factor VIII-VWF concentrate as appropriate, and antifibrinolytics may be useful adjunctive treatment.

Alloantibody Inhibitors of von Willebrand Factor

Inhibitors to VWF in patients with VWD are uncommon and occur exclusively in patients with VWD type 3 who have been transfused repeatedly with plasma, cryoprecipitate, or factor VIII-VWF concentrates. Inhibitors have been identified by patient screening or physician surveys in 2.6% to 9.5% of patients with VWD type 3, although selection bias makes it difficult to know the true incidence.[112,222] Patients with large deletions of the VWF gene may be at higher risk for the development of inhibitors,[222] and a familial tendency to inhibitor formation has been noted.[223] The presence of a VWF inhibitor is suggested by the failure to respond clinically to replacement therapy, by decreased recovery of infused VWF, and by lack of correction of abnormal VWF-dependent platelet function tests. The presence of an antibody inhibitor can be confirmed by demonstrating that patient plasma, serum or purified immunoglobulin inhibits RIPA of normal platelet-rich plasma. The inhibitors that have been characterized so far have been IgG alloantibodies and all but one were clearly polyclonal.[222] The antibodies typically inhibit the function of factor VIII-VWF complex (as in plasma) but not that of pure factor VIII, suggesting that inhibition of factor VIII-VWF is caused by steric hindrance.[223]

When transfused with a product containing VWF, patients with VWF inhibitors commonly experience serious allergic reactions with back pain, abdominal pain, and hypotension, and they may have life-threatening anaphylactic reactions.[112,170] These adverse consequences can be avoided by the use of recombinant factor VIII preparations that are free of VWF. Although the infused factor VIII is cleared rapidly, factor VIII levels of 40 to 60 IU/dL can be achieved by intravenous infusion of 700 to 900 U/kg/day, given continuously or by bolus infusion every 4 hours, and this approach has controlled bleeding after abdominal surgery or cesarian section.[224,225] Recombinant factor VIIa (NovoSeven) also has been used effectively for surgical or postpartum bleeding by continuous infusion (≈ 20 μg/kg/hour) or bolus infusion (≈ 90 μg/kg every 4 hours).[225–227]

SUGGESTED READINGS

Eikenboom J, Van Marion V, Putter H, et al: Linkage analysis in families diagnosed with type 1 von Willebrand disease in the European study, molecular and clinical markers for the diagnosis and management of type 1 VWD. J Thromb Haemost 4:774, 2006.

Goodeve A, Eikenboom J, Castaman G, et al: Phenotype and genotype of a cohort of families historically diagnosed with type 1 von Willebrand disease in the European Study, Molecular and Clinical Markers for the Diagnosis and Management of Type 1 von Willebrand Disease (MCMDM-1VWD). Blood 109:112, 2007.

Hayes TE, Brandt JT, Chandler WL, et al: External peer review quality assurance testing in von Willebrand disease: the recent experience of the United States College of American Pathologists proficiency testing program. Semin Thromb Hemost 32:499, 2006.

James PD, Notley C, Hegadorn C, et al: Association of Hemophilia Clinic Directors of Canada. Challenges in defining Type 2M von Willebrand disease: Results from a Canadian cohort study. J Thromb Haemost 5:1914–22, 2007.

James PD, Notley C, Hegadorn C, et al: The mutational spectrum of type 1 von Willebrand disease: Results from a Canadian cohort study. Blood 109:145, 2007.

James PD, Paterson AD, Notley C, et al: Genetic linkage and association analysis in type 1 von Willebrand disease: results from the Canadian Type 1 VWD Study. J Thromb Haemost 4:783, 2006.

Kitchen S, Jennings I, Woods TA, et al: Laboratory tests for measurement of von Willebrand factor show poor agreement among different centers: Results from the United Kingdom National External Quality Assessment Scheme for Blood Coagulation. Semin Thromb Hemost 32:492, 2006.

Rodeghiero F, Castaman G, Tosetto A, et al: The discriminant power of bleeding history for the diagnosis of type 1 von Willebrand disease: An international, multicenter study. J Thromb Haemost 3:2619, 2005.

Sadler JE, Budde U, Eikenboom JC, et al: Update on the pathophysiology and classification of von Willebrand disease: A report of the Subcommittee on von Willebrand Factor. J Thromb Haemost 4: 2103, 2006.

Tosetto A, Rodeghiero F, Castaman G, et al: A quantitative analysis of bleeding symptoms in type 1 von Willebrand disease: Results from a multicenter European study (MCMDM-1 VWD). J Thromb Haemost 4:766, 2006.

REFERENCES

For complete list of references log onto www.expertconsult.com

CHAPTER 130

VITAMIN K: METABOLISM AND DISORDERS

Barbara C. Furie and Bruce Furie

INTRODUCTION

Vitamin K plays a critical role in the posttranslational modification of the blood coagulation proteins, factors VII, IX, and X, and prothrombin, and of the plasma regulatory proteins, proteins C and S. Vitamin K serves as a cofactor for an enzymatic reaction that converts glutamic acid residues in the NH_2-termini of these proteins into γ-carboxyglutamic acid (Gla) residues (Fig. 130–1).[1,2] There are three well-defined classes of Gla-containing proteins that have been isolated and extensively characterized: (1) the mammalian Gla-domain containing, vitamin K-dependent blood clotting and regulatory proteins; (2) γ-carboxyglutamic acid-containing proteins of vertebrate mineralized tissue, including osteocalcin and matrix Gla protein; and (3) conotoxins of the marine snail, *Conus*. A new class of transmembrane Gla-domain containing proteins has been identified in vertebrates and ascidians, marine invertebrates, by interrogation of gene data bases and complementary DNA (cDNA) cloning.[3–5] These proteins may suggest a role for vitamin K-dependent proteins in signal transduction.

Gla acid residues confer essential metal-binding properties on the vitamin K-dependent proteins of blood coagulation.[6] If γ-carboxylation is impaired either as a result of vitamin K deficiency or through pharmacologic intervention, the newly synthesized vitamin K-dependent proteins are secreted into the blood in their des-γ-carboxy or "abnormal" forms. The des-γ-carboxylated proteins cannot bind Ca^{2+}, and the physiologically important metal ion-mediated binding to phospholipid vesicles or cell membranes does not occur.[7,8] Because many critical enzymatic reactions of blood coagulation proceed on membrane surfaces, coagulation and its regulation are impaired. Therefore, vitamin K metabolism is essential to normal hemostatic and antithrombotic mechanisms. Indeed, inhibition of vitamin K action is the primary mechanism of oral anticoagulant therapy (see Chapter 137).

THE VITAMIN K CYCLE

In its role as a cofactor for the vitamin K-dependent carboxylase, vitamin K participates in a series of linked enzyme reactions that result in the generation of γ-carboxyglutamic acid and the regeneration of active cofactor. This series of reactions is known as the *vitamin K cycle* (Fig. 130–2). In addition to the enzyme, the reduced form of vitamin K and a glutamic acid-containing polypeptide substrate, the reactions require carbon dioxide and molecular oxygen. In the first reaction in the cycle (see Fig. 130–2), a hydrogen ion, H^+, is abstracted from the γ-carbon of the glutamyl residue and a carboxyl group is added.[9] Concomitantly, the cofactor, vitamin K, is converted from the reduced to the epoxide form.[10] The enzyme, the vitamin K-dependent carboxylase, catalyzes both carboxylation and epoxidation.[11]

THE VITAMIN K-DEPENDENT CARBOXYLASE

The vitamin K-dependent carboxylase is a single polypeptide chain of 758 amino acids.[12–15] The enzyme is found in vertebrates and invertebrates, including Drosophila,[16,17] cone snail *Conus*,[18–20] *Ciona intestinalis* (sea squirt, an *urochordates*)[3] and *Halocynthia roretzi* (a tunicate).[21] Although vertebrates and molluscs diverged on the evolutionary tree more than 500 million years ago, the vitamin K-dependent carboxylase and its gene are highly conserved.[22,23] Mice lacking the gene for the vitamin K-dependent carboxylase demonstrate a partial developmental block with only 50% of null animals surviving to term.[24] Those animals that survive to term die uniformly at birth of massive intra-abdominal hemorrhage. These data indicate that there is no redundant pathway for carboxylation of glutamic acid.[24]

The vitamin K-dependent carboxylase is an integral membrane protein that binds directly to the γ-carboxylation recognition site on the precursor forms of the vitamin K-dependent proteins.[25] The enzyme is located in both the endoplasmic reticulum and the Golgi apparatus.[26,27] However, carboxylation is an efficient process such that carboxylation of protein substrates is completed in the endoplasmic reticulum.[28] The presence of carboxylase in the Golgi apparatus is likely caused by the recycling of the membrane-bound enzyme between the endoplasmic reticulum and the Golgi apparatus.

The active site responsible for glutamate binding is located in the N-terminal one-third of the protein.[29] The complementary site on the carboxylase that binds the propeptide carboxylation recognition site also resides in part in the N-terminal one-third of the protein,[30] the C-terminal one-third of the protein[31] or perhaps both.[32] Regions around residues 234, 406, and 513 have been implicated in propeptide-binding site whereas regions around residue 359 have been implicated in catalysis.[33] The vitamin K epoxidase activity of the protein requires a C-terminal region of this enzyme for this activity.[34]

MECHANISM OF ACTION OF VITAMIN K

The most attractive hypothesis has been that an active oxygenated species of vitamin K abstracts a hydrogen from the γ-carbon of glutamic acid, with subsequent collapse of the activated vitamin K species to vitamin K epoxide and the addition of carbon dioxide to the γ-carbon of glutamic acid.[35] In support of this hypothesis, oxygen and vitamin KH_2-dependent exchange of tritium from tritiated water to the γ-carbon of a glutamic acid in a carboxylase substrate at low carbon dioxide concentrations have been taken as evidence of a carbanion mechanism.[36] Based on a nonenzymatic model, a *base strength amplification mechanism* has been proposed to explain the conversion of vitamin KH_2 into an oxygenated intermediate of sufficient basicity to abstract a hydrogen from the γ-carbon of a glutamyl residue in a carboxylase substrate.[37–39] Recent advances have been made that help resolve the conundrum of how the carboxylase active site might generate a vitamin K species of sufficient basicity. Although a vitamin K-dependent γ-glutamyl carboxylase cysteine or histidine residue was suspected of serving as the enzyme active site residue that deprotonates vitamin K,[11,40–45] more recent studies have eliminated these residues from consideration for this role.[46,47] The enzyme active site base that deprotonates vitamin K has been identified as Lys218 based on evidence that the active site base is an amine, evolutionary comparison of vitamin K-dependent carboxylases, mutagenesis studies, and chemical rescue experiments.[46,48]

The base amplification mechanism for vitamin K activation suggests that epoxidation of vitamin KH_2 by the vitamin K-

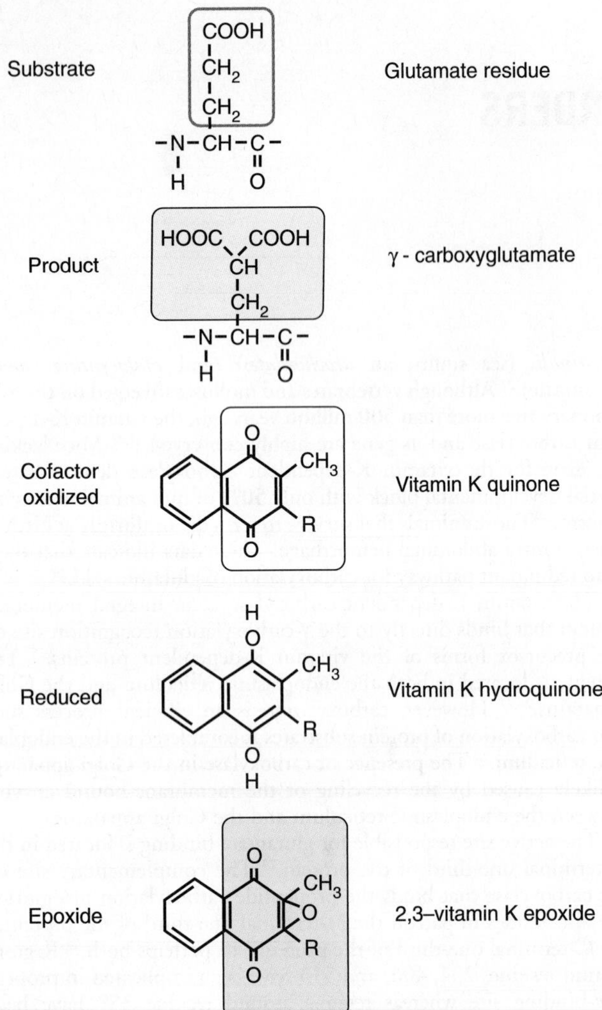

Figure 130–1 Reactants in the vitamin K-dependent carboxylation pathway.

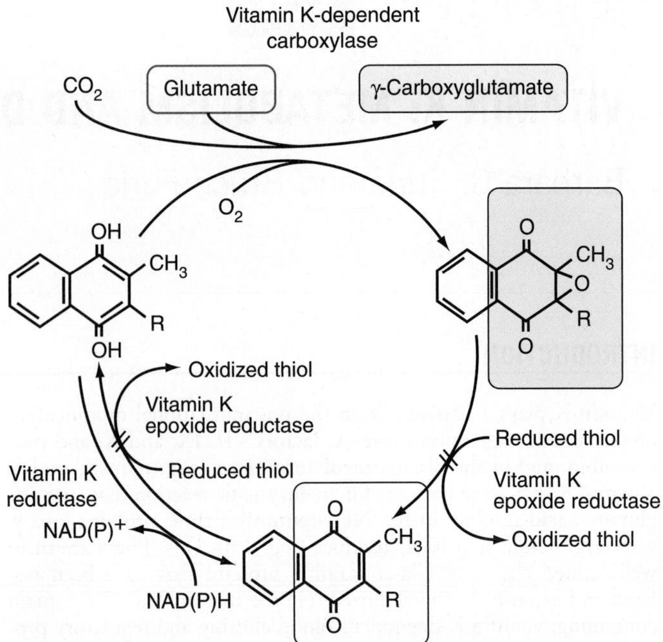

Figure 130–2 The vitamin K cycle. Reduced vitamin K, the hydroquinone form, is a cofactor for the conversion of glutamate to γ-carboxyglutamate by the vitamin K-dependent carboxylase, also known as the vitamin K epoxidase. Concomitant with conversion of glutamate to γ-carboxyglutamate, the hydroquinone is converted to 2,3-vitamin K epoxide. The epoxide can be converted to vitamin K quinone by the vitamin K epoxide reductase. Vitamin K quinone can be reduced by two pathways to the vitamin K hydroquinone, completing the cycle.

dependent carboxylase can occur in the absence of formation of γ-carboxyglutamic acid but that carboxylation cannot occur in the absence of epoxidation. However in the absence of propeptide and glutamate-containing substrate, the carboxylase lacks vitamin K epoxidase activity. When these substrates are added to the enzyme, vitamin K epoxidase activity is upregulated.[49] These results were originally interpreted to indicate that the propeptide and glutamate-containing substrate induced a conformational change in the vitamin K-dependent carboxylase that exposed a free cysteine at the catalytic site for vitamin K epoxidation.[50] In light of the observation that Lys218 is the critical active site base, an alternate hypothesis is that binding of the propeptide and glutamate substrate modify the active site environment, changing the equilibrium between the protonated state of the lysine side chain, favored at physiologic pH, and the unprotonated state required for its action as a general base.[48]

As epoxidation occurs concomitant with carboxylation and because vitamin K either from dietary sources or gut flora is in the quinone form, tissues in which γ-carboxylation takes place must have a mechanism for generating the reduced form of vitamin K. Vitamin K epoxide reductase, a dithiol-requiring enzyme, reduces vitamin K epoxide to the vitamin K quinone (see Fig. 130–2). Two enzymatic activities, including the epoxide reductase, have been identified that convert vitamin K quinone to the biologically active hydroquinone (see Fig. 130–2). The epoxide reductase activity resides in the endoplasmic reticulum. Originally thought to be part of an enzyme complex,[51,52] current evidence suggests the vitamin K epoxide reductase, capable of reducing vitamin K epoxide to vitamin K and vitamin K to the reduced form of the vitamin, is a single gene product.[53–55] However the vitamin K epoxide reductase must be recycled to its reduced form to perform another round of vitamin K reduction. Protein disulfide isomerase, an endoplasmic reticulum enzyme involved in dithiol redox exchange, has been linked to the vitamin K cycle in the endoplasmic reticulum and may be responsible for reduction of the vitamin K epoxide reductase.[56] Because both activities of the vitamin K epoxide reductase are inhibited by warfarin, an additional enzyme must be responsible for reducing vitamin K to its active cofactor form when the vitamin is given to reverse anticoagulation with warfarin.[53]

NATURE OF THE SUBSTRATE

Although many tissues contain the enzymes to carry out γ-carboxylation and the reactions of the vitamin K cycle, the primary site of synthesis of the vitamin K-dependent proteins of the blood is the liver. These proteins are synthesized with both a signal sequence and a propeptide. The canonical leader sequences provide the signal that indicates that the protein is to be secreted and thus allows the growing polypeptide chain to be translocated to the rough endoplasmic reticulum. All sequences of the propeptides of the vitamin K-dependent proteins are highly homologous and unique to this class of proteins.[57] These propeptides serve as recognition signals that designate these proteins as substrates for the vitamin K-dependent carboxylase.[58] The γ-carboxylation recognition site resides on the N-terminus of the propeptide. It is extended by a 10-residue amphipathic α-helix.[59] The propeptide of the precursor forms of the vitamin K-dependent proteins serves three functions: (1) to direct γ-carboxylation by the γ-carboxylase,[58] (2) to inhibit binding of the carboxylated precursor proteins to membranes,[60] and (3) to upregulate vitamin K epoxidase activity of the carboxylase.[49]

VITAMIN K

Forms and Distribution

The vitamin K family of chemical compounds has many members. Vitamin K_1 (2-methyl-3-phytyl-1,4-naphthoquinone) is the major form of the vitamin found in plants. Animal tissue and bacteria produce menaquinones, a series of vitamin K forms similar in structure to vitamin K_1 but with varying lengths of unsaturated polyprenyl groups at the 3 position.

Nutritional Sources

Vitamin K is an essential fat-soluble vitamin. The diet is the primary source of vitamin K in humans. Leafy green vegetables, in particular, are a good source of vitamin K_1,[61] although vitamin K_1 is widely distributed in the normal human diet. A contribution to adequate vitamin K intake in humans may be provided by the vitamin K_2 synthesized by intestinal bacteria.[62] The daily dietary requirement for the vitamin has been estimated to be 100 to 200 (μ) μg/day.[63]

Physiology

Vitamin K is absorbed in the ileum. The presence of bile salts and normal fat absorption are required for effective uptake. The storage pool of vitamin K is modest. In the absence of a dietary source of the vitamin, this storage pool can be exhausted within 1 week in an otherwise normal person. Such a deficiency does not generally lead to clinical manifestations, as the vitamin K synthesized by gut flora is available to provide suboptimal but adequate synthesis of vitamin K-dependent proteins.

VITAMIN K DISORDERS

Hemorrhagic Disease of the Newborn

Hemorrhagic disease of the newborn, because of vitamin K deficiency, develops during the first week of life, usually between days 2 and 7 (see Chapter 133).[61–66] Clinical manifestations include bleeding in the skin or from mucosal surfaces, circumcision, or venipuncture sites.[67] Rarely, internal bleeding, including retroperitoneal or intracranial hemorrhage, is the primary manifestation of hemorrhagic disease of the newborn. These ominous complications are the rationale for the use of vitamin K prophylaxis in neonates.

Almost all neonates are vitamin K deficient, presumably as a result of deficient vitamin K nutriture in the pregnant mother during the third trimester and because of the lack of colonization of the colon by bacteria that produce vitamin K in the neonate.[68] However, this deficiency is further aggravated in some patients by inadequate dietary intake of vitamin K. This disorder is more prevalent in breast-fed babies, as human milk, in contrast to cow's milk, contains only 15 μg/L of vitamin K.[67,69]

Neonates with hemorrhagic disease of the newborn have a prolonged prothrombin time and partial thromboplastin time (PTT). However, it is critical to distinguish whether the prolongation of these times is a manifestation of the deficiency of the vitamin K-dependent proteins because of vitamin K deficiency or to decreased synthetic capacity of the liver in newborns. Elevation of the abnormal (des-γ-carboxy) prothrombin (PIVKA-II) antigen level is indicative of vitamin K deficiency, as this form of prothrombin appears only when post-translational modification is impaired but not when protein synthesis is impaired.[68] Administration of vitamin K (100 μg) corrects the deficiency state and usually does not need to be repeated in the otherwise healthy infant.

Prophylactic vitamin K has been in use for in-hospital births for the past 45 years. Vitamin K (100 μg to 1 mg) is administered intramuscularly to the newborn immediately after birth. At these doses, vitamin K administration carries little morbidity and can prevent hemorrhagic disease of the newborn. Some of these vitamin K protocols are under revision[70] and have been updated.[71]

ACQUIRED VITAMIN K DEFICIENCY

Dietary Deficiency States and Antibiotics

The requirement for vitamin K is sufficiently low relative to the vitamin K content of a normal diet that clinically significant vitamin K deficiency does not occur as a result of inadequate dietary intake. Although sensitive markers of vitamin K deficiency, such as abnormal (des-γ-carboxy) prothrombin antigen,[72] indicate that diet truly depleted of vitamin K can lead to mild vitamin K deficiency, no evidence shows that an inadequate diet alone can have clinical manifestations. Bacteria in the large intestine produce functional forms of vitamin K. In the absence of dietary vitamin K, small amounts of vitamin K in the large intestine are absorbed passively and prevent severe vitamin K deficiency. In patients medicated with antibiotics that destroy the intestinal flora, this vitamin K source is eliminated. Thus, a common setting of vitamin K deficiency is the case of a patient with inadequate or minimal dietary intake treated simultaneously with antibiotics (Fig. 130–3). This form of vitamin K deficiency occurs within 1 to 3 weeks, after depletion of body stores of vitamin K.[73]

Malabsorption syndromes are commonly associated with vitamin K deficiency. Defects in the enterohepatic circulation because of biliary disease interfere with absorption of fat-soluble vitamins in the ileum. Primary biliary cirrhosis,[74] cholestatic hepatitis, and other causes of cholestasis can lead to impaired absorption of vitamin K.

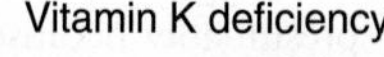

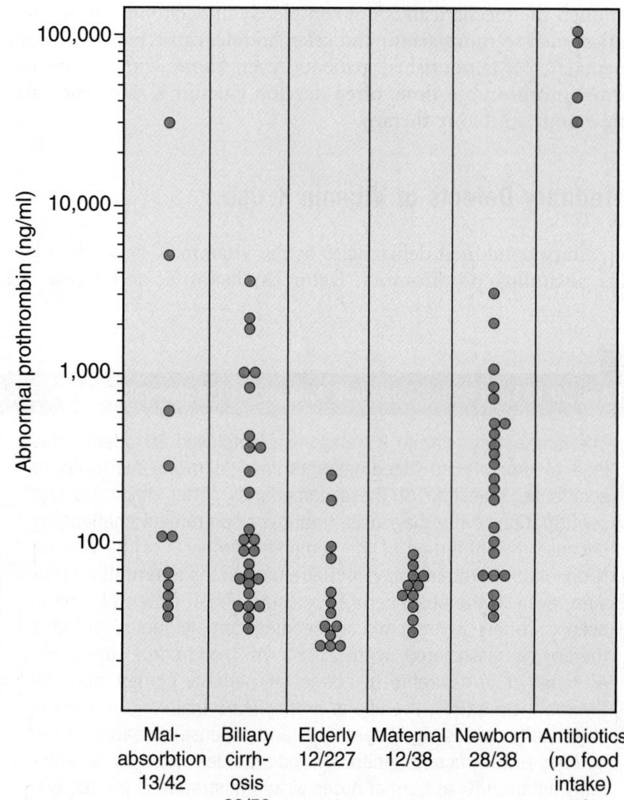

Figure 130–3 Abnormal (des-carboxy) prothrombin antigen as a marker for vitamin K deficiency. Normal subjects have no detectable abnormal prothrombin. Vitamin K deficiency arises as a result of disorders of absorption, including mild abnormalities in otherwise normal elderly subjects, or because of impaired intake.

Furthermore, intestinal malabsorption, as in sprue or regional enteritis, impairs vitamin K use. Older adults also have evidence of mild vitamin K deficiency, presumably because of intestinal malabsorption.[75]

Vitamin K Antagonists

Drugs that inhibit the reuse of vitamin K lead to a buildup of vitamin K epoxide at the expense of vitamin K hydroquinone. Warfarin and related vitamin K antagonists, whether ingested accidentally, factitiously, or as an overdose of oral anticoagulant therapy, lead to a deficiency of the vitamin K-dependent proteins, prolongation of the prothrombin time and PTT, and clinical bleeding manifestations.[76–78] Although such patients are not vitamin K deficient, the clinical and laboratory manifestations because of vitamin K antagonists are identical to those of vitamin K deficiency. Factitious warfarin ingestion may be seen as a component of a major psychiatric disturbance. Despite repeated denials of use of such medications by suspect patients, this diagnosis must be considered in all patients with *acquired* deficiency of all the vitamin K-dependent proteins. Measurement of serum warfarin level can confirm such suspicions. With the introduction of second-generation rodenticides that inhibit vitamin K action, including brodifacoum, cases of factitious ingestion and accidental poisonings have been increasingly reported.[79–87] These long-acting poisons, now widely available (eg, d-Con; see box on Reversal of Long-Acting Vitamin K Antagonists ["Superwarfarins"]), can lead to prolongation of the prothrombin time for more than 1 year after a single dose; fatalities have been reported.[88] Chemically distinct from warfarin, these compounds are not detected in serum warfarin assays. Specific serum assays have been developed.[89,90]

Other drugs cause a vitamin K deficiency-like state as well and respond to vitamin K therapy. Excessive doses of aspirin cause hypoprothrombinemia,[91] presumably because of oxidation of vitamin K. Although the mechanism is not completely understood, certain antibiotics, such as moxalactam and cefamandole, cause hypoprothrombinemia.[92–95] Malnourished patients, even those with an initially normal prothrombin time, often develop vitamin K deficiency after intravenous antibiotic therapy.[96]

Hereditary Defects of Vitamin K Use

Hereditary combined deficiencies of the vitamin K-dependent proteins, including prothrombin, factor IX, factor X, and factor VII, have been recognized for some time, although the molecular bases for the phenotype in these kindred was unknown.[97–101] Mutations in the vitamin K-dependent carboxylase and in the vitamin K epoxide reductase have been established as causes of hereditary deficiencies in the vitamin K-dependent proteins in a number of kindred. Defects in the absorption and transport of vitamin K might also be anticipated to manifest with this clinical presentation.

In kindred where hereditary combined deficiency of vitamin K-dependent proteins is caused by abnormalities in the vitamin K-dependent carboxylase point mutations in the enzyme are most often responsible. Arg394 6Leu, Trp501 6Ser, Arg485 6Pro, Trp157 6Arg, Thr591 6Lys and His404 6Pro mutations have all been linked to this disorder.[102–106] In addition a splice site mutation in carboxylase has been identified.[105] Some cases have been responsive to high daily doses of vitamin K.[101,103,107] Other cases have been resistant to vitamin K therapy, which emphasizes the heterogeneity of this disorder.

Mutations in the vitamin K epoxide reductase are causative for combined deficiency of vitamin K-dependent proteins of blood coagulation[55,106,108] and for warfarin resistance (see Chapter 137).[55,109–111] Hereditary combined deficiency of vitamin K-dependent proteins has also been shown to result from an Arg98 6Trp mutation in the vitamin K epoxide reductase.[55]

Mutations in the propeptide of factor IX render otherwise normal patients sensitive to warfarin.[112]

Therapy for Vitamin K Deficiency

Vitamin K deficiency is treated by the administration of vitamin K_1. The preferred route of administration depends on the urgency for correcting the bleeding tendency and on the risk of inducing local hematoma formation. If the bleeding is severe or life-threatening, fresh frozen plasma should be administered. Because of the risk of transmission of viral infection, the use of blood products must be weighed carefully, although this risk has been greatly reduced in recent years. (See box on Therapy for Vitamin K Deficiency.)

Reversal of Long-acting Vitamin K Antagonists ("Superwarfarins")

The long-acting vitamin K antagonists employed as rodenticides lead to pronounced bleeding syndromes following factitious or accidental ingestion of these compounds. After diagnosis and confirmation of the diagnosis, treatment can remain challenging because the inhibition of the complete synthesis of the vitamin K-dependent proteins may continue for months after initial exposure, even in the absence of reexposure. Fresh frozen plasma is used routinely to treat major bleeding complications, but this therapy is associated with a risk of blood-borne infection. Although it is desirable to correct or partially correct the prothrombin time (PT), the use of prophylactic fresh frozen plasma chronically carries significant risks and expense. Because of the potency of the second-generation rodenticides and their fat solubility, vitamin K_1 at normal doses of administration is ineffective. However, daily doses of 100 to 150 mg of vitamin K_1 administered orally have been effective in normalizing the PT. Over time, the dose of vitamin K_1 needed to correct the PT can be adjusted downward, so that only the required amounts of vitamin K are employed.

Therapy for Vitamin K Deficiency

The approach to the treatment of vitamin K deficiency depends on the clinical setting and the severity of bleeding. Except in the face of serious internal bleeding, reversal of the vitamin K deficiency by the administration of vitamin K is generally adequate. If the prothrombin time (PT) is significantly prolonged to indicate that a bleeding complication may be induced by intramuscular injection, that route of administration of vitamin K_1 (phytonadione [AquaMEPHYTON]) should be avoided. Because the delivery of vitamin K by the subcutaneous route is variable, intravenous vitamin K_1 (phytonadione [AquaMEPHYTON], 10–15 mg) is the recommended approach, as it ensures rapid delivery. However, intravenous vitamin K_1 does require monitoring, because of early reports of severe allergic reactions with the intravenous route of administration; care must be given to initiate rapid reversal of an untoward reaction. With vitamin K, the PT should return toward the normal range within 12 hours and should have corrected within 24 to 48 hours. Serious bleeding complications attributed to vitamin K deficiency, such as intracranial bleeding, must be reversed immediately. Despite the rapid action of vitamin K, administration of vitamin K should be preceded by the infusion of fresh frozen plasma. This blood component contains all the vitamin K-dependent blood-clotting proteins. In sufficient quantities, fresh frozen plasma can correct, or nearly correct, the PT, as well as the bleeding tendency.

Patients with vitamin K deficiency without bleeding manifestations can be treated with oral vitamin K or, as in patients with chronic vitamin K deficiency secondary to malabsorption syndromes, with subcutaneous vitamin K.

SUGGESTED READINGS

Berkner KL: The vitamin K-dependent carboxylase. Annu Rev Nutr 25:127, 2005. This reviews vitamin K–dependent carboxylation of glutamic acids in target proteins. The emphasis is on structure function relationships in the carboxylase and on its enzymatic mechanism.

Furie B, Bouchard BA, Furie BC: Vitamin K-dependent synthesis of γ-carboxyglutamic acid. Blood 93:1798, 1999. This is a broad review of the vitamin K cycle, action of the carboxylase and mammalian vitamin K-dependent proteins.

Li T, Chang CY, Jin PJ, et al: Identification of the gene for vitamin K epoxide reductase. Nature 457:541, 2004. This paper describes the discovery of the gene for the vitamin K epoxide reductase based on a positional cloning strategy using information derived from warfarin resistant rats and humans with hereditary deficiency of vitamin K-dependent proteins.

Rishavy MA, Pudota BN, Hallgren KW, et al: A new model for vitamin K-dependent carboxylation: The catalytic base that deprotonates vitamin K hydroquinone is not Cys but an activated amine. Proc Natl Acad Sci U S A 101:13732, 2004. This paper demonstrates convincingly that in spite of a wealth of literature that implicates a cysteine as the active site base in the carboxylase the key residue is an amino acid bearing an amine side chain.

Rishavy MA, Hallgren KW, Yakubenko AV, et al: Bronsted analysis reveals Lys218 as the carboxylase active site base that deprontonates vitamin K hydroquinone to initiate vitamin K-dependent protein carboxylation. Biochemistry 45:13239, 2006. This paper establishes that the active site base responsible for deprotonation of vitamin K is Lys218 and provides the basis for reinterpretation and integration of a large body of previously existing data.

Rost SA, Fregin V, Ivaskevicius E, et al: Mutations in VKORC1 cause warfarin resistance and multiple coagulation factor deficiency type 2. Nature 427:537, 2004. This paper identifies the vitamin K epoxide reductase gene based on linkage information from two heritable human diseases: combined deficiency of vitamin K–dependent blood clotting proteins and resistance to warfarin.

Stafford DW: The vitamin K cycle. J Thromb Haemost 3:1873, 2005. This review provides a pithy account of the vitamin K cycle and the nature and action of the carboxylase and the epoxide reductase.

REFERENCES

For complete list of references log onto www.expertconsult.com

CHAPTER 131

LUPUS ANTICOAGULANT AND ACQUIRED INHIBITORS OF BLOOD COAGULATION

Donald I. Feinstein

Spontaneously acquired inhibitors of blood coagulation, also known as circulating anticoagulants, are pathologic macromolecules in blood that directly inhibit blood clotting proteins or reactions involving blood clotting. Most have been characterized as antibodies. These inhibitors arise secondary to transfusion of plasma or recombinant replacement proteins in patients with hereditary bleeding disorders (see Chapter 126) or arise de novo in patients with previously normal hemostatic mechanisms. This chapter will include discussion of the lupus anticoagulant and spontaneously acquired inhibitors of blood coagulation proteins. Inhibitors are usually recognized in the laboratory by prolonged coagulation tests that are subsequently found to be uncorrected by the addition of normal plasma. They may be clinically silent or may be associated with a history of excessive bleeding or paradoxically by thrombosis (see box on Diagnostic Approach to Inhibitors)

LUPUS ANTICOAGULANT AND ANTI PHOSPHOLIPID ANTIBODIES

General Considerations

The lupus anticoagulant is an antibody that prolongs phospholipid-dependent coagulation tests in vitro. It was given this name in 1972 because clear proof of its site of action was lacking, and because the anticoagulant had been recognized in patients with systemic lupus erythematosus (SLE).[1] It is a misnomer because the lupus anticoagulant is more frequently encountered in patients without lupus[1,2] and is associated with thrombosis rather than with bleeding.[1,2] Immunoglobulins reacting with other hemostatic factors, such as von Willebrand factor (VWF),[3] factor VIII,[4] factor IX, and factor XI, inhibitors of thrombin and fibrin polymerization, and factor XIII[5] have also been described in patients with SLE, but they are rare compared with the lupus anticoagulant.

Patients with the lupus anticoagulant who do not have established SLE fall into several different categories: (1) patients with "lupus-like" chronic autoimmune disorders but without findings that fit the criteria for the diagnosis of SLE;[6,7] (2) patients with other chronic systemic autoimmune disorders; (3) patients presenting with a venous or arterial thrombotic event for which no underlying cause may be apparent;[8–13] (4) patients receiving certain drugs, including procainamide[14] and phenothiazines[15] (a high prevalence of the lupus anticoagulant and a positive antinuclear antibody test are observed in psychotic patients receiving long-term chlorpromazine therapy);[15] other drugs or biologics that can induce the lupus anticoagulant include hydralazine, quinidine, and possibly α-interferon; (5) patients with a recent acute viral infection,[16] in whom the antibody is usually transient; (6) patients with human immunodeficiency virus infection;[17,18] (7) women with recurrent fetal wastage;[6,15,16,19–28] (8) occasionally in older patients with malignancies[28a] and (9) patients seeking medical attention for a variety of disorders in whom the lupus anticoagulant is discovered as an incidental finding, usually discovered because of a prolonged partial thromboplastin time (PTT) performed as a routine preoperative evaluation.

The lupus anticoagulant, and related antibodies, anticardiolipin antibody (a CL antibody) and anti-beta$_2$-glycoprotein I antibody (β_2-GPI) are antiphospholipid antibodies that are associated with the antiphospholipid antibody syndrome (APS). Criteria for the diagnosis of the antiphospholipid syndrome have been proposed and validated.[29,30] Recently, these criteria were updated.[31] The updated criteria require one or more clinical episodes of arterial, venous, or small vessel thrombosis and/or increased pregnancy morbidity plus the presence of the lupus anticoagulant, anticardiolipin antibody in medium or high titer (ie, >40 GPL or MPL units or >99th percentile, on two or more occasions, at least 12 weeks apart, measured by a standardized enzyme-linked immunoabsorbent assay [ELISA]) (Table 131–1). The syndrome may be primary when not associated with SLE and secondary when it occurs in association with SLE.[29–34]

The prevalence of lupus anticoagulant in patients with SLE in which the PTT was used for its detection is approximately 10%.[1] In other studies using various screening tests, it varied from 11% to 30%.[35] Using the kaolin clotting time—a test with increased sensitivity for detecting low-titer lupus anticoagulants because it contains no added exogenous phospholipid—evidence of inhibitor activity can be demonstrated in the plasma of 30% to 50% of randomly selected patients with SLE.[36] The percentage approximates the 42% to 44% incidence of the frequency of anticardiolipin antibodies in patients with SLE,[37] although in most other studies it varies from 17% to 39%.[35]

The prevalence of positive tests for lupus anticoagulant and anticardiolipin antibody in a normal population has been reported in several studies.[38–40] Because of the non-Gaussian distribution of anticardiolipin antibody levels in normal subjects, the cut-off points between normal and abnormal results is difficult to determine.[32,40] One study reported IgG and IgM anticardiolipin antibodies in approximately 5% of normal individuals, although only 2% had persistently elevated levels on repeat testing.[40] Shi and colleagues detected anticardiolipin antibodies in 6% of normal blood donors, respectively, and detected lupus anticoagulant activity by kaolin clotting time in 4%.[38] The prevalence of anticardiolipin antibody appears to increase with age.[35]

The prevalences of elevated levels of IgG and IgM anticardiolipin antibody in healthy pregnant women were 2% to 3% and 4%, respectively.[41–43] Most of these were low titer; only 0.2% were high titer. In other studies, the incidence of anticardiolipin antibodies in pregnant individuals ranged from 1% to 2% and lupus anticoagulant 1% to 4%.[35]

Properties, Epitope Specificity, Mechanism of Action, and Relationship of the Lupus Anticoagulant to Anticardiolipin Antibodies and Anti-β_2 Glycoprotein I Antibodies

Lupus anticoagulants and anticardiolipin antibodies are immunoglobulins that were originally thought to react only with phospholipid. However, it is now well established that these antibodies react directly with epitopes on β_2-GPI[44,45] or prothrombin,[46,47] that subsequently bind to anionic phospholipid.[46] Anticardiolipin antibodies are low-affinity monovalent antibodies to β_2-GPI when in solution, and the monovalent complexes bind weakly to anionic

Diagnostic Approach to Inhibitors

The approach to patients with abnormal coagulation tests should initially include a complete history regarding excessive bleeding, particularly as it relates to hemostatic challenges and thrombotic problems—venous or arterial. Initial laboratory studies should include a repeat of the abnormal coagulation test on a mixture of the patient's plasma and normal plasma. Correction of the abnormal test indicates a deficiency state, whereas poor correction indicates the presence of an inhibitor.

Approach to Inhibitors Associated with Bleeding

Patients who present with an acquired bleeding disorder and in whom an inhibitor is demonstrated most often have antibodies to a specific clotting factor. Subsequent laboratory evaluation should attempt to demonstrate the specific coagulation factor to which the antibody is directed and to determine the specificity of the antibody. The former is done using a specific assay for the coagulation factor suspected of being affected, and the latter is done using a specific assay for the coagulation factor of a mixture of various dilutions of patient's plasma (antibody) and normal plasma (antigen) over time. If the inhibitor is specific for a single clotting factor, procoagulant activity of that coagulation factor is neutralized over time, whereas other clothing factors assays are unaffected. For example, if an acquired inhibitor of factor VIII is suspected and the factor VIII assay is low, a factor VIII assay of a mixture of the patient's plasma and normal plasma should demonstrate a progressive decrease in factor VIII activity from immediately after the mixture was made to 1 to 2 hours later. By contrast, if factor IX and XI assays were done on the same mixture, factors IX and XI would be unaffected.

Rarely, a spontaneously acquired autoantibody reacts with a non-coagulant epitope of a specific hemostatic factor (eg, prothrombin in the lupus anticoagulant-hypoprothrombinemia syndrome) or a specific clotting factor is adsorbed to cellular surfaces (eg, VWF) or to amyloid (eg, factor X). In these patients, the addition of normal plasma to the patient's plasma results in correction of the abnormality. In these patients, the in-vivo half-life of the affected hemostatic factor is shortened significantly because of rapid clearance of the antigen-antibody complex or by adsorption of the clotting factor to a pathologic surface.

Spontaneously acquired heparin-like anticoagulants differ from the aforementioned inhibitors in that they are not immunoglobulins, and they do not specifically affect one specific clotting factor. These anticoagulants are easily recognized because their major effect is on the thrombin time, but the reptilase time is normal.

Approach to Inhibitors Not Associated with Excessive Bleeding

If the patient has a history of thrombotic disease or repeated episodes of fetal loss, he or she should be evaluated for the presence of a lupus anticoagulant and elevated levels of anticardiolipin and anti–β_2-GPI antibodies. Most commonly, patients with the former have a prolonged PTT and a normal or slightly prolonged prothrombin time. However, on occasion, the prothrombin time may be more prolonged than usual, particularly when using recombinant human tissue factor (Innovin) even in the absence of an associated prothrombin deficiency. If the patient is suspected of having a lupus anticoagulant, several relatively simple tests can be used to confirm the diagnosis. For sensitivity, the kaolin clotting time, the dilute Russell's viper venom time test, the dilute prothrombin time, or the Staclot lupus anticoagulant test are excellent tests with very good sensitivity. Some believe that more than one test should be done if a lupus anticoagulant is suspected, and a single test is negative. Correction of a prolonged clotting time by the addition of phospholipid is specific for the lupus anticoagulant. In the presence of a lupus anticoagulant with a prolonged PTT, specific intrinsic clotting factor assays are frequently low but increase with increasing dilution of test plasma. For example, assays for factor IX would be 5%; factor XI, 9%; and factor XII, 10%; and all would progressively increase with increasing dilution of the test plasma. In some cases, the factor XI or XII assay is more affected than the other assays. The lupus anticoagulant may affect all the specific assays, in contrast to an antibody to a specific clotting factor, for which a single assay shows irreversible inactivation of that clotting factor. In the latter case, dilution would not result in an increase in the level of that clotting factor.

phospholipids. However, when the antigen density is high, bivalent complexes are formed that have a high affinity for phospholipid surfaces.[48–50] The fact that β_2-GPI antibodies are polyclonal reacting with different epitopes on the β_2-GPI molecule and the increased affinity of the divalent antigen-antibody complexes for phospholipid surfaces explains why some anticardiolipin antibodies have anticoagulant activity and some do not.[50] This anticoagulant activity correlates best with the incidence of thrombosis,[51] and a subset of lupus anticoagulants caused by anti–β_2-GPI antibodies with specificity for an epitope on domain I.[52] In some patients the anticardiolipin antibody will react with immobilized cardiolipin in vitro but not prolong phospholipid-dependent coagulation tests. Similarly, some of the antiprothrombin antibodies can prolong coagulation tests and some will not.[50]

Anticardiolipin antibodies are usually IgG or IgM immunoglobulins. In some patients, for example, those in whom it arises secondary to long-term chlorpromazine therapy, it is IgM;[15] in other patients, it is IgG,[2] and in still others, it may be an IgG and IgM.[2] In addition, anticardiolipin antibodies can also be IgA but are usually associated with IgG and/or IgM isotype, and are highly prevalent in African Americans with SLE.[53]

The anti–β_2-GPI and antiprothrombin antibodies responsible for the lupus anticoagulant effect react in coagulation assay systems containing anionic phospholipids. Reducing the phospholipid component of clotting mixtures amplifies the effect of the inhibitor. The most sensitive tests for detecting the lupus anticoagulant contain only limited amounts of procoagulant phospholipid: a sensitive or dilute activated partial thromboplastin time,[54,55] the kaolin clotting time,[36] the silica clotting time,[56,57] the dilute Russell's viper venom time, the prothrombin time performed with very dilute tissue factor, the dilute prothrombin time (formerly called the tissue thromboplastin inhibition test), and the Taipan snake venom time.[58] Adding liposomes containing phosphatidylserine,[59] rabbit brain phospholipid,[60] freeze-thawed platelets[61,62] or hexagonal phospholipids[63,64] markedly shortens the prolonged PTT of plasma containing the lupus anticoagulant and is used as a confirmatory test to increase specificity for presence of a lupus anticoagulant when there is a prolonged clotting test.

Patients with antiphospholipid antibodies also frequently have evidence of anticardiolipin antibodies. These antibodies were first recognized in association with a biologic false-positive test for syphilis,[2,65] a test in which cardiolipin is the antigen. This reaction is β_2-GPI dependent, and it results from the increased binding of antigen-antibody complexes containing β_2-GPI and cardiolipin. Anticardiolipin antibody assays are measured by an ELISA using cardiolipin.[66] Bovine serum is added to block nonspecific antibody binding and to provide a source of β_2-GPI.[67] Assay results are usually reported as MPL units for IgM anticardiolipin antibody or GPL units for IgG anticardiolipin antibody. Because of assay variability, a lack of standardization of the assay and a non-Gaussian distribution in normal people, the distinction between normal and abnormal values are not clear. Although the assay is not standardized, most laboratories discriminate between normal and abnormal as 20 GPL (IgG) or MPL (IgM) units, with the cutoff values in different laboratories varying from greater than 10 GPL or MPL units[54] to 20.[68] However, in the updated Consensus Statement[31] the cutoff value has been increased to 40 GPL or MPL units. IgA anticardiolin antibodies are

Table 131–1 Updated International Consensus Statement on Classification Criteria for Definite Antiphospholipid Syndrome

Antiphospholipid antibody syndrome (APS) is present if at least one of the clinical criteria and one of the laboratory criteria that follow are met:

Clinical Criteria

1. Vascular thrombosis
   One or more clinical episodes of arterial, venous, or small vessel thrombosis, in any tissue or organ. Thrombosis must be confirmed by objective validated criteria (ie, unequivocal findings of appropriate imaging studies or histopathology). For histopathologic confirmation, thrombosis should be present without significant evidence of inflammation in the vessel wall.
2. Pregnancy morbidity
   One or more unexplained deaths of a morphologically normal fetus at or beyond the 10th week of gestation, with normal fetal morphology documented by ultrasound or by direct examination of the fetus, or
   One or more premature births of a morphologically normal neonate before the 34th week of gestation because of: (i) eclampsia or severe pre-eclampsia defined according to standard definitions, or (ii) recognized features of placental insufficiency, or
   Three or more unexplained consecutive spontaneous abortions before the 10th week of gestation, with maternal anatomic or hormonal abnormalities and paternal and maternal chromosomal causes excluded.

Laboratory Criteria

Lupus anticoagulant (LA) present in plasma, on two or more occasions at least 12 weeks apart, detected according to the guidelines of the International Society on Thrombosis and Haemostasis (see Table 2 in Miyakis S, Lockshin MD, Atsumi T, et al.).

Anticardiolipin (aCL) antibody of IgG and/or IgM isotype in serum or plasma, present in medium or high titer (ie, >40 GPL or MPL units, or > the 99th percentile), on two or more occasions, at least 12 weeks apart, measured by a standardized enzyme-linked immunosorbent assay (ELISA).[67]

Anti–β_2-glycoprotein I antibody of IgG and/or IgM isotype in serum or plasma (in titer > the 99th percentile), present on two or more occasions, at least 12 weeks apart, measured by a standardized ELISA, according to recommended procedures.[69,71]

Classification of APS should be avoided if less than 12 weeks or more than 5 years separate the positive antiphospholipid antibody (aPL) test and the clinical test and the clinical manifestation. Coexisting inherited or acquired factors for thrombosis are not reasons for excluding patients. A thrombotic episode in the past could be considered as a clinical criterion, provided that thrombosis is proved by appropriate diagnostic means and that no alternative diagnosis or cause of thrombosis is found. Superficial venous thrombosis is not included in the clinical criteria. Generally accepted features of placental insufficiency include: (i) abnormal or nonreassuring fetal surveillance test(s); eg, a nonreactive nonstress test, suggestive of fetal hypoxemia; (ii) abnormal Doppler flow velocimetry waveform analysis suggestive of fetal hypoxemia, eg, absent end-diastolic flow in the umbilical artery; (iii) oligohydramnios, eg, an amniotic fluid index of 5 cm or less; or (iv) a postnatal birth weight less than the 10th percentile for the gestational age.

Adapted from Miyakis S, Lockshin MD, Atsumi T, et al: International consensus statement on an update of the classification criteria for definite antiphospholipid syndrome (APS). Thromb Haemost 4:295, 2006.

Table 131–2 Detection of Antiphospholipid Antibodies

Lupus Anti Coagulant Antibodies

Prolongation of at least one phospholipid-dependent coagulation assay with the use of platelet-poor plasma (dilute prothrombin time, activated partial thromboplastin time (PTT), dilute activated PTT, colloidal-silica clotting time, dilute Russell's viper venom time, and kaolin clotting time).

Failure to correct the prolonged coagulation time on one of the above phospholipid-dependent tests by mixing the patient's plasma with normal platelet-poor plasma.

Confirmation by shortening or correction of the prolonged coagulation time after the addition of excess phospholipid or platelets that have been frozen or thawed.

Exclusion of the other coagulation with the use of specific factor assays if the confirmatory test is negative or if a specific factor inhibitor is suspected.

Anticardiolipin Antibodies

Enzyme-linked immunosorbent assay performed with cardiolipin-coated plates in the presence of *bovine* serum β_2-glycoprotein I. IgG and/or IgM in medium or high titer (ie, >40 GPL or MPL units or >99th percentile) on two or more occasions at least 12 weeks apart measured by a standardized enzyme-linked immunosorbent assay (ELISA).[67]

Anti-β_2-Glycoprotein I Antibodies

Enzyme-linked immunoadsorbent assay using *human* β_2-Glycoprotein I. IgG and or IgM titers >99th percentile on two or more occasions at least 12 weeks apart measured by a standardized ELISA.[69,71]

From Brandt JT, Tiplett DA, Arving B, et al: Criteria for the diagnosis of lupus anticoagulants: An update on behalf of the subcommittee on Lupus Anticoagulant/Antiphospholipid Antibody of the Scientific and Substandisation Committee of the ISTH. Thromb Haemost 74(4):1185, 1995.

usually associated with increased IgM and IgG isotypes in patients with APS (Table 131–2). However, occasionally it might be the only anticardiolipin antibody that is elevated.

The recent update of the International Consensus Statement on the diagnosis of APS also included increased IgG and IgM anti–β_2-GPI antibodies[31] (see Table 131–2). These antibodies are measured by an ELISA.[69] However, although increased levels of these antibodies are independent risk factors for thrombosis[70,71] and pregnancy complications,[72,73] measurement of these antibodies also suffer from lack of standardization and lack of agreement in cutoff values. However, the Committee recommended that the cutoff value be greater than the 99th percentile of controls.[31] In 3% to 10% of patients with APS, the anti–β_2-GPI antibody might be the only one that is positive.[74]

Antiprothrombin antibodies detected by ELISA include those against prothrombin alone and those against the prothrombin-phosphatidylserine complex. The extensive review by Galli and coworkers[70] failed to find an association with these antibodies and thrombosis. However, in one study the antiphosphatidylserine prothrombin complex antibodies had a very high correlation with the presence of the lupus anticoagulant and thrombotic complications in patients with SLE.[75]

Although most patients with elevated levels of anticardiolipin antibodies also test positive for lupus anticoagulant activity, considerable data support lupus anticoagulant activity and anticardiolipin antibodies as distinct subgroups of antibodies that can be separated by affinity or physicochemical methods and have different antigenic specificities.[76,77] Antibodies to β_2-GPI can be further separated into those that have anticoagulant activity and those that do not.[78,79] Lupus anticoagulants and anticardiolipin antibodies occur concurrently in only approximately 50% to 75% of patients, and a patient may have no anticoagulant activity simultaneously with a markedly elevated anticardiolipin antibody titer by ELISA, and vice versa. Patients who are being evaluated for possible APS must have tests for lupus anticoagulant activity based on a clotting assay and anticardiolipin antibody activity by ELISA.

The mechanism by which the different antiphospholipid antibodies interfere with coagulation in vitro is not clear. However, phospholipid participates in coagulation at several steps: as a component of the prothrombinase complex, as a cofactor for factor VIIIa and factor IXa in the tenase complex, and as a cofactor for activation of factor X by factor VIIa in complex with tissue factor. The lupus anticoagulant may impede each of these reactions of blood coagulation, and it can inhibit the binding of factor X and prothrombin to negatively charged surfaces.[36,80] Because β_2-GPI and prothrombin also bind tightly to phospholipid, it is possible that antibodies directed to epitopes on β_2-GPI and prothrombin could also interfere with phospholipid-dependent clotting reactions, particularly the tenase and prothrombinase complexes, accounting for the anticoagulant effect in vitro.

Mechanism of Hypoprothrombinemia in the Hypoprothrombinemia-Lupus Anticoagulant Syndrome

A small subset of patients with the lupus anticoagulant also have a selective deficiency of prothrombin. The plasma of these patients does not contain an antibody that neutralizes prothrombin activity,[81] and the plasma prothrombin antigen is decreased to the same extent as prothrombin activity.[82] Bajaj and colleagues[83] demonstrated that the plasma from patients with the hypoprothrombinemia-lupus anticoagulant syndrome contains antibodies that bind prothrombin without neutralizing its in-vitro coagulant activity. The decreased concentration of plasma prothrombin in patients with this syndrome results from the rapid removal of the prothrombin-prothrombin antibody complexes. Altered mobility of prothrombin antigen on crossed immunoelectrophoresis, indicative of the presence of plasma prothrombin antigen-antibody complexes, has been demonstrated in 66% to 75% of patients with the lupus anticoagulant in whom plasma prothrombin activity was not substantially decreased.[84] It is probable that the latter antibodies have less affinity for prothrombin than the antibodies found in patients with a very low prothrombin level, and that the prothrombin deficiency stems from rapid clearance of the antigen-antibody complexes.

Laboratory Evaluation

The results of screening coagulation tests usually found in patients with the lupus anticoagulant include a prolonged PTT, which is prolonged when the patient's plasma is mixed with equal parts of normal plasma (see box on Diagnostic Approach to Inhibitors). The prothrombin time is minimally to moderately prolonged (0.5 to 3 seconds), and occasionally, it is normal. However, the prothrombin time is prolonged more than normal plasma when diluted tissue factor is used, as in the dilute prothrombin time test.[85] The thrombin time is normal. The sensitivity of the PTT for lupus anticoagulant detection varies with different commercial reagents used for the test,[86,87] probably reflecting, at least in part, variation in the phospholipid composition of these reagents. Some commercial PTT reagents have been created to be very sensitive to the presence of lupus anticoagulants. The prevention of platelet activation in plasma samples is crucial because procoagulant phospholipid, in the patient plasma or in the normal plasma used for mixing studies, may neutralize weak lupus coagulant activity.[54,56,88,89] It is recommended that test plasmas and normal plasma be initially centrifuged at 2000 g for 10 minutes, followed by centrifugation at 10 to 15,000 g for 10 minutes or filtered through 0.22 μm screens to remove platelets before freezing. A normal dilute thrombin time assures that the plasma does not contain heparin.

Confirmation of the Diagnosis

The pattern of the lupus anticoagulant manifestations in coagulation testing is often indistinguishable from that of an anticoagulant directed against any one of the several clotting factors that influence the result of the PTT, but not the prothrombin time. Therefore, further tests are needed to confirm that the prolonged PTT of a mixture of the patient's plasma and normal plasma results from the lupus anticoagulant (see Table 131–2 and box on Methods for Establishing the Presence of a Lupus Anticoagulant). It is particularly important to rule out a factor VIII inhibitor, which, in contrast to the lupus anticoagulant, is associated with serious bleeding.

Methods for Establishing the Presence of a Lupus Anticoagulant

1. Platelets and platelet debris must be removed from the patient's plasma and the normal plasma used for mixed studies before any testing is carried out.
2. A screening test with very high sensitivity (eg, kaolin clotting time, dilute activated PTT, dilute Russell's viper venom time test, colloidal-silica clotting time, and dilute prothrombin time) should be used.
3. The clotting time of a mixture of test and normal plasma should be significantly longer than that of the normal plasma mixed with various non-lupus anticoagulant plasmas.
4. To increase specificity, there should be a relative correction of the defect by the addition of lysed washed platelets, phospholipid liposomes containing phosphatidylserine, or hexagonal-phase phospholipids.
5. Testing must be repeated 12 weeks apart to establish the presence of a persistent abnormality.

Various tests have been devised to increase the sensitivity to lupus anticoagulants, including examination of clotting time in systems containing reduced phospholipid, such as the kaolin clotting time,[36] the silica clotting time,[90] the dilute Russell's venom time test,[91] a modified PTT that uses polybrene to neutralize heparin and hexagonal phospholipids to correct the lupus anticoagulant effect (Staclot-LA),[54] the Taipan snake venom time,[92] and the dilute prothrombin time. The latter's sensitivity and specificity have been improved with the use of recombinant tissue factor.[93] The sensitivity and specificity of the tests vary in different reports.[54] However, there is evidence that to maximize the number of patients with lupus anticoagulants identified, more than one test should be done.[54,55] Because studies show that the lupus anticoagulant activity is the most important risk factor for thromboembolic events, it is most important to identify those patients at risk.[94,51]

Lupus anticoagulant tests should include a heparin neutralizer, or the dilute thrombin time should be done to rule out the presence of heparin. In addition, if the patient is on oral anticoagulants with an international normalized ratio (INR) greater than 3.5, the patient's plasma sample should be diluted 1:2 with normal plasma before the test is done.

Mixing studies are important in distinguishing factor deficiencies from inhibitors. One study provides evidence that β_2-GPI–dependent antibodies prolong the dilute Russell's venom time test more than the kaolin clotting time, and the prothrombin-dependent antibodies prolong the kaolin clotting time to a greater extent than the dilute Russell's venom time.[95,96]

Tests based on the observation that excess phospholipid substantially shortens the prolonged PTT of lupus anticoagulant plasma are important as a means of differentiating the lupus anticoagulant from other inhibitors. The excess phospholipid is added as freeze-thawed platelets,[62] liposomes containing phosphatidylserine,[59] platelet-derived microvesicles,[97] rabbit brain phospholipid,[60] or hexagonal phase phospholipids.[64] Correction of prolonged clotting times by excess phospholipid significantly increases specificity, and false-positive results are encountered only for heparinized patients or extremely high-titer inhibitors to other clotting factors. However, no positive results are obtained from patients with other low-titer clotting factor inhibitors, congenital factor deficiencies, hepatic insufficiency, or in patients receiving warfarin therapy. The correction of a prolonged clotting time by phospholipid is almost always confirmatory for the presence of a lupus anticoagulant.

Another novel test for the detection of lupus anticoagulants uses two different snake venoms, one that depends on the presence of phospholipid and one that does not.[98] The ecarin time is phospholipid independent, whereas the textarin time is phospholipid-dependent. In the presence of the lupus anticoagulant the ecarin time is unaffected, but the textarin time is prolonged. Because textarin also requires factor V for prothrombin activation and ecarin does not, this test may give false-positive results in patients with factor V inhibitors.

One diagnostic approach that is helpful in ruling out other types of coagulation factor inhibitors is to perform specific one-stage clotting factor assays based on the PTT. Low values for several clotting factors and increasing values for each clotting factor with increasing dilution of the test plasma in the assay system are commonly observed test patterns. Inhibitors affecting more than one clotting factor using the PTT are usually lupus anticoagulants. In contrast, in patients with acquired factor VIII inhibitors, the factor VIII levels are lower than one sees with lupus anticoagulants and the factor VIII level does not increase with plasma dilution. The inhibitor is not neutralized by a high concentration of phospholipid. Occasionally, the factor XI and XII assays may be more affected than the other intrinsic assays, and an occasional patient will have a factor XII inhibitor associated with a lupus anticoagulant.[99] Several reviews of laboratory testing for lupus anticoagulants have been published.[54,55,100]

Laboratory Recognition of the Hypoprothrombinemia-Lupus Anticoagulant Syndrome

Although minimal to moderate prolongation of the prothrombin time, up to approximately 3 seconds beyond a control value, can be accounted for by the lupus anticoagulant, the finding of a substantially prolonged prothrombin time represents presumptive evidence of an associated specific prothrombin deficiency. Unlike the specific clotting factors assayed in modified PTT test systems, the specific clotting factors affecting the prothrombin time—factor VII, factor X, and factor V—are assayed in clotting systems that are affected only by rare, high-titer lupus anticoagulants. Therefore, the finding of a low value in a prothrombin assay may be taken as evidence of an associated prothrombin deficiency. If, however, further evidence is desired, three additional findings may be demonstrated: (1) a mixture of equal parts of the patient's plasma and normal plasma gives the expected value calculated from the mean of the levels in individual plasmas; (2) prothrombin activity and prothrombin antigen are concordantly decreased; or (3) prothrombin has abnormal mobility on crossed immunoelectrophoresis.[84,101]

CLINICAL RELATIONSHIPS OF LUPUS ANTICOAGULANT AND ANTICARDIOLIPIN ANTIBODIES: PRIMARY AND SECONDARY ANTIPHOSPHOLIPID SYNDROME

Lupus anticoagulant and anticardiolipin antibodies are associated with thrombosis or fetal wastage with or without autoimmune disorders. This clinical entity is known as the *antiphospholipid syndrome*[102,103] (see Table 131–1).[29,31] The primary antiphospholipid syndrome is defined as venous or arterial thrombotic disease, or both, or as recurrent fetal wastage associated with elevated levels of antiphospholipid antibodies in the absence of any definite autoimmune disease.[29,31] These patients do not demonstrate any other clinical or serologic evidence of autoimmune disease, except for occasional low-titer (<1 : 160) antinuclear antibodies. In contrast, the secondary antiphospholipid syndrome is associated with SLE and related disorders. Some patients have some evidence of a systemic autoimmune disorder but demonstrate insufficient criteria to make the diagnosis of SLE (overlap syndrome). Primary antiphospholipid syndrome rarely progresses to SLE. In one report of 128 patients with primary antiphospholipid syndrome followed for an average of 9 years only 8% developed SLE, and the presence of a positive Coombs test was a significant predictor of progression.[104] However, the recent Consensus Statement advises against using the term *secondary*, but this is controversial.[105] In addition, the Consensus Conference recognized that there are other clinical manifestations that can occur in antiphospholipid syndrome in the absence of the specific classification criteria. Such clinical manifestations include cardiac manifestations (valve disease, coronary artery disease, and ventricular dysfunction), neurologic manifestations (transient ischemic attack, stroke, dementia, cognitive dysfunction, transmyelopathy, seizures, and migraines), shin manifestations (livedo reticularis and other rare lesions), renal manifestations (thrombotic microvascular angiopathy), and thrombocytopenia.[31]

An occasional patient with high-titer anticardiolipin antibodies and/or a lupus anticoagulant can present with fulminant disease with multiorgan system involvement (eg, lung, kidney, or brain), hypertension, and microvascular and macrovascular thrombosis. This clinical presentation is known as the catastrophic antiphospholipid syndrome.[106,107] Because these patients have a high mortality rate, they require aggressive treatment.

Most patients who test positive for the lupus anticoagulant have elevated levels of anticardiolipin antibody. However, although the correlation between the two is significant, many patients showing positivity for lupus anticoagulant activity do not have elevated levels of anticardiolipin antibody or other antiphospholipid antibodies, and vice versa.[108–110]

Because anticardiolipin antibody levels can fluctuate significantly,[111] a negative test for the lupus anticoagulant and anticardiolipin antibody does not completely rule out the presence of antiphospholipid syndrome. This is particularly true during an acute thrombotic episode, when antibody titers may transiently decline to normal.[112]

Several studies[22,113] suggest that when tests for the lupus anticoagulant and anticardiolipin antibodies are performed at two separate time intervals (6 to 16 weeks), a statistically significant association can be shown between persistently positive tests and prior thromboembolic events and fetal loss. The strength of the association is much reduced when transiently positive patients are included. It is strongly recommended that repeat testing be done 12 weeks apart. In children, particularly, the antibody may persist for many months and then spontaneously disappear. These studies also showed that a combination of tests for detecting lupus anticoagulant activity is superior to a single test.

A false-positive Venereal Disease Research Laboratory test in low-titer (1 : 4 to 1 : 8) can be demonstrated in less than or equal to 30% of patients with the lupus anticoagulant or anticardiolipin antibodies. These cross-reacting antibodies differ from reagin, the antibody responsible for the Wasserman reaction in patients with syphilis and usually do not require the presence of β_2-GPI for their detection. The detergent, Tween 20, can be used in the anticardiolipin antibody assay to distinguish β_2-GPI–dependent and –independent antibodies.[114] These β_2-GPI–independent antibodies are true antiphospholipid antibodies and are frequently seen in patients with infection and usually are not associated with thrombosis.

Relationship of Lupus Anticoagulant and Anticardiolipin Antibodies to Other Antibodies

In some subjects with lupus anticoagulant, anticardiolipin antibody and/or anti–β_2-GPI antibodies that react to other anionic phospholipids, such as phosphatidylserine, phosphatidylinositol, and phosphatidic acid, have been demonstrated.[110] In some patients with lupus anticoagulant or anticardiolipin antibody, antibodies to neutral phospholipids (phosphatidylethanolamine or phosphatidylcholine) have been demonstrated.[115] Sugi and colleagues[116] have demonstrated that autoantibodies to phosphatidylethanolamine recognize a kininogen-phosphatidylethanolamine complex. Smimov and colleagues[117] have shown that inhibition of activated protein C is antibody- and phosphatidylethanolamine-dependent. However, the significance of these antibodies in the absence of the lupus anticoagulant or anticardiolipin antibodies is unknown.

Correlation between Clinical Findings and Antiphospholipid Antibodies

Bleeding

Most patients with the lupus anticoagulant do not have a bleeding phenotype. Patients with the lupus anticoagulant have undergone needle biopsy of the kidney and the severe hemostatic challenges of major surgery,[2,8] including prostatectomy[2] and open heart surgery,[2] without excessive postoperative bleeding.

Nevertheless, patients with the lupus inhibitor may have clinically significant bleeding. In all but a few, the bleeding can be attributed to some abnormality other than the lupus inhibitor, such as depressed prothrombin activity. The combination of the lupus anticoagulant and a prothrombin coagulant activity below approximately 20% of normal has resulted in severe and even fatal bleeding. In other patients, thrombocytopenia, alone or in combination with moderate prothrombin deficiency, accounted for the bleeding tendency. The hemorrhagic manifestations may also be related to severe uremia.

Evaluation of the risk of abnormal bleeding in patients with the lupus anticoagulant includes establishing the presence or absence of prothrombin deficiency, thrombocytopenia, or uremia. Occasionally a patient may have only a prolonged bleeding time associated with excessive bleeding.[118] In the absence of these coexisting risk factors, abnormal bleeding is minimal even after trauma or surgery.[8,32] In summary, most patients with the isolated finding of lupus anticoagulant do not experience abnormal bleeding. On rare occasions, excessive postoperative bleeding has been attributed to the lupus anticoagulant.[119,120]

Thrombosis

Since the initial observation of Bowie and colleagues in 1963, it has become clear that thrombosis is a major concern in patients with the lupus anticoagulant. The reported incidence has varied from 17% to 71%, averaging approximately 30% to 40%.[6,8,37,121–123] In patients with an elevated level of anticardiolipin antibody, a high incidence (~40%) of thrombotic disease has been reported.[37,102,124] Of unselected patients with antiphospholipid antibody, 1% to 2.5% per year will develop thromboembolism,[123,125] and 10% to 25% of patients with deep venous thrombosis will be found to have antiphospholipid antibodies.[126] However, in a prospective population based study of 66,140 in Norway,[127] elevated anticardiolipin antibody levels were not a risk factor for predicting an initial venous thrombosis. Thrombosis is more frequent as the level of anticardiolipin antibody increases, and medium and high titers (>40 GPL and/or MPL units) are more frequently associated with thrombotic events. Although some investigators believe that elevated levels of IgG or IgA isotypes are more common than IgM in patients with thrombotic complications,[111,128] this has not been clearly established. The lupus anticoagulant or increased levels of anticardiolipin antibody must be persistently present on more than one occasion at least 12 weeks apart because the incidence of thrombotic complications is almost the same in patients with transiently positive tests as in patients with negative tests at two different time intervals.[21,22,113] The persistent presence of elevated levels of anticardiolipin antibody has been shown to be associated with indices of in-vivo coagulation activation. In a study of patients with SLE[129] who were persistently anticardiolipin antibody–positive versus patients who were transiently positive or persistently negative, anticardiolipin antibody–positive patients had a higher mean level of F1+2 and fibrinopeptide A than patients who were transiently positive, persistently negative, or on warfarin therapy. The differences remained significant even if patients with prior thromboembolism were excluded from the analysis. These results suggest that the presence of persistently elevated levels of anticardiolipin antibody in SLE patients is associated with an ongoing prothrombotic state. Studies suggest that the presence of lupus anticoagulants was more strongly associated with venous and arterial thrombosis than the presence of anticardiolipin antibody.[51,94,130,131] Galli and colleagues[96] have suggestive evidence that β_2-GPI antibodies that prolong the dilute Russell's viper venom time test more than the kaolin clotting time (*dilute Russell's viper venom time test phenotype*) are associated with a higher incidence of thrombosis than the prothrombin-dependent antibodies, which prolong the kaolin clotting time more than the dilute Russell's viper venom time test (*kaolin clotting time phenotype*). However, because of different commercial and noncommercial dilute Russell's viper venom time test assays, these results are difficult to reproduce in all laboratories.[132] Direct immunoassays (ELISA) for human β_2-GPI (rather than bovine β_2-GPI in the anticardiolipin assay) are also strongly associated with thrombosis and are commercially available. However, any one of these tests may be positive in patients with antiphospholipid syndrome. Studies by Galli and coworkers[51,93,123] strongly suggest that lupus anticoagulant activity is the strongest risk factor for thromboembolic events-independent of the type and site of thrombosis, the presence of SLE, and the laboratory methods used to detect them.[123] Anticardiolipin and β_2-GPI antibodies were not as strong a risk factor.

Thrombosis may be venous or arterial,[102] with events occurring nearly equally in the arterial and venous circulation[51,123,133,134] in some studies, whereas in other studies the incidence of venous thrombosis (70%) is greater than the incidence of arterial thrombosis.[95,135] Venous thrombosis is usually manifested as deep venous thrombosis of the lower extremities with or without pulmonary emboli. Unusual sites of venous thrombosis, such as hepatic veins, portal vein, inferior vena cava, mesenteric veins, renal veins, cerebral venous sinuses, retinal veins, and upper extremity veins, have been reported.[102,136,137] Arterial thrombosis is usually manifested as stroke[32,102,138] or transient ischemic attacks.[139] Nonbacterial mitral and aortic endocardial valve lesions, with or without SLE, accompanied by thromboembolic transient ischemic attacks and strokes have also been reported.[140] Some studies have suggested that stroke is most commonly an embolic event originating from cardiac vascular lesions.[141,142] In one study, 75% of patients with recurrent cerebral ischemic events had vascular thickening or vegetations found on transesophageal echocardiography.[141,142] In another study, 20% of patients admitted to a cardiology department for severe valvular heart disease had antiphospholipid antibodies.[143] Thromboembolic events were more common in the antiphospholipid antibody group. Livedo reticularis alone is common at presentation (~20%) and occasionally may be associated with cerebrovascular disease (Sneddon's syndrome). Other neurologic manifestations include epilepsy, migraine, chorea, and transverse myelitis. The association of antiphospholipid antibodies and coronary artery disease is controversial. Hamsten and colleagues[144] reported that young survivors of myocardial infarction had a high incidence of anticardiolipin antibody, and those patients with a persistently elevated anticardiolipin antibody had a higher incidence of recurrent events. Similar findings were reported in another prospective study of 133 patients who had a significant number of subsequent events compared with matched control subjects.[145] In contrast, other studies did not find elevated anticardiolipin antibody or subsequent events in patients with an acute myocardial infarction.[146,147] However, in the report from the Euro-Phospholipid Project,[136] which included the study of 1000 patients with primary or secondary antiphospholipid syndrome, 2.8% of patients presented with acute myocardial infarction and, during the evolution of the disorders, a total of 8.2% had developed a myocardial infarction or angina. Patients admitted for peripheral vascular surgical procedures also have a high incidence of phospholipid antibodies.[148]

Thromboembolic pulmonary hypertension with or without SLE can occur in association with the lupus anticoagulant or elevated levels of anticardiolipin antibody, or both.[102,149,150] Other thrombotic manifestations reported include: gangrene of extremities and digits, multi-infarct dementia, retinal arterial and venous thrombosis, renal arterial and venous thrombosis, adrenal infarction and insufficiency, mesenteric ischemia and infarction, vascular necrosis of bone, cerebral venous thrombosis, leg ulcers, and cutaneous necrosis.[136] Patients can develop an acute or subacute microangiopathy and microvascular thrombosis with progressive loss of organ function and can be associated with a fragmentation type hemolytic anemia and thrombocytopenia (catastrophic antiphospholipid syndrome).[106] It is clear from the Euro-phospholipid Project Group who have accumulated data on 1000 patients with antiphospholipid syndrome that patients with this syndrome may have a variety of clinical manifestations that involve any organ.[136]

Although thrombosis is supposedly not associated with the lupus anticoagulant or anticardiolipin antibody induced by infection or drugs, there have been several reports of human immunodeficiency virus- or drug-associated thrombosis.[8,151] In a report of the treatment of patients with melanoma with immunotherapy, 5 of 12 patients receiving interferon-α had lupus anticoagulants and anticardiolipin antibodies within 4 to 28 days, and deep vein thrombosis developed in 4 of these 5 patients.[152] In patients with infections, anticardiolipin antibodies bind cardiolipin directly and usually do not require the presence of β_2-GPI,[32,152] except for those patients with leprosy who have β_2-GPI and prothrombin-dependent antibodies.[153,154] Despite this fact, patients with leprosy do not have an increased incidence of thrombosis.[153,154]

Patients who are persistently positive for the lupus anticoagulant or who have persistently elevated levels of anticardiolipin antibody and suffer a thromboembolic event have a recurrence rate of approximately 50% within 2 years.[133,134,155,156] Recurrences tend to occur in most of the patients on the same side of the circulation as the initial event—venous recurrences after an initial venous event and arterial recurrences after an initial arterial event.[133]

Fetal Loss, Thrombocytopenia, Hemolytic Anemias, and Other Associations

Another major clinical manifestation associated with the lupus anticoagulant or anticardiolipin antibody is fetal loss.[6,21,22,26–28,102,121,128,157] Fetal wastage may occur at any time during pregnancy.[26,27,68,102] Fetal wastage in antiphospholipid syndrome is defined as (1) any patient with three or more unexplained consecutive spontaneous abortions before the 10th week of gestation (pre-embryonic and embryonic period); (2) any patient with one or more unexplained deaths of morphologically normal fetuses at or after the 10th week of gestation; (3) one or more premature births of morphologically normal neonates before the 34th week of gestation; or (4) intrauterine growth retardation and premature birth (see Table 131–1).[31] Any patient with such a history should be tested for the lupus anticoagulant and anticardiolipin antibody. A recent study showed that increased pregnancy loss was associated with the presence of the lupus anticoagulant and elevated levels of antihuman anti–β_2-GPI antibodies, whereas it was not associated with the lupus anticoagulant and increased levels of anticardiolipin antibodies in the absence of anti–β_2-GPI antibodies.[158] Fifty percent of pregnancy losses in patients with antiphospholipid syndrome occur beyond the 10th week of pregnancy in contrast to pregnancy losses in patients without antiphospholipid syndrome, where most losses occur before the 10th week of gestation.[68] This syndrome occurs in patients with or without SLE. Thrombosis of placental vessels and placental infarction are thought to be one of the mechanisms by which fetal loss occurs.[159,102] The high incidence of thrombotic disease in these patients lends further support to this hypothesis. There is also evidence that antiphospholipid antibodies may impair trophoblastic invasion and cause embryonic loss or uteroplacental insufficiency and fetal loss.[157] The Euro Project Group identified a significantly increased incidence of preeclampsia, eclampsia, and abruptio placentae in patients with antiphospholipid syndrome.[136]

Thrombocytopenia is a frequent finding in patients with the lupus anticoagulant or anticardiolipin antibody and is seen in 30% to 50% of the patients.[157,160] Patients with SLE or related autoimmune disorders have an even higher incidence of thrombocytopenia and leukopenia.[136,161] The incidence of antiphospholipid antibodies is increased (~30%–40%) in patients with idiopathic autoimmune thrombocytopenic purpura.[157,162]

Coombs-positive hemolytic anemia has also been associated with lupus anticoagulants and/or anticardiolipin antibodies in patients with or without SLE[163,164] and occurred in approximately 10% of patients reported from the Euro-Phospholipid Project Group.[136]

CATASTROPHIC ANTIPHOSPHOLIPID ANTIBODY SYNDROME

A few patients with antiphospholipid syndrome present with an acute syndrome characterized by multiple vascular occlusions, usually affecting small vessels in several organ systems occurring over a relatively short period of time (days to weeks) and resulting in a 50% mortality.[106,107] Reviews describing the clinical characteristics of more than 230 patients with this disorder have been published.[165,166] Forty percent of the patients had SLE, 40% primary antiphospholipid syndrome, and 6% had lupus-like disease. Previous clinical findings of antiphospholipid syndrome were present in approximately 50% of the patients, most commonly venous thromboembolic disease, recurrent fetal loss, or thrombocytopenia. The most common factors that seemed to precipitate the acute syndrome were infection, trauma or invasive procedures, warfarin withdrawal, SLE flare, or the presence of a malignancy. The initial presentation was usually complex with multiorgan involvement because of thromboembolic microangiopathy. The most common systems involved were cardiorespiratory, central nervous system, and renal. Pulmonary involvement was usually caused by acute respiratory distress syndrome with or without pulmonary emboli and occasionally alveolar hemorrhage. Cardiac involvement was usually manifested as congestive heart failure with or without acute myocardial infarction or valvular lesions. The major central nervous system manifestation was ischemic stroke. Deep venous thrombosis, acute peripheral arterial occlusive disease, and skin involvement were relatively common. Manifestations of systemic inflammatory response syndrome was also common. Less common complications include hypoadrenalism because of adrenal venous occlusion and bone marrow necrosis.[106]

Laboratory findings, other than positive tests for antiphospholipid antibodies, included thrombocytopenia (60%), autoimmune hemolytic anemia (33%), and evidence of disseminated intravascular coagulation (20%). Fragmented red cells were seen in 9%.

The mortality of this large group of patients was approximately 50% with the most common cause of death being cardiac or pulmonary related. The only therapy that seemed to be of benefit was anticoagulation and corticosteroids, whereas plasmapheresis, and intravenous gammaglobulin seemed to be less effective.[106,165,166] Aggressive supportive therapy such as dialysis, mechanical ventilation, treatment of infection, and so on were important. If the patient recovered, continued anticoagulation was important. Two-thirds of patients who survive the initial catastrophic event remain symptom free, whereas approximately 25% develop noncatastrophic clinical manifestations of antiphospholipid syndrome.[166]

PATHOPHYSIOLOGIC MECHANISM(S) OF THROMBOSIS

The nature of the association between thrombosis and antiphospholipid antibodies, such as the lupus anticoagulant and anticardiolipin antibody, is uncertain. Because many people with antiphospholipid antibodies never experience thrombosis, it is not clear whether antiphospholipid antibodies are direct causative factors for thrombosis, or whether they represent secondary consequences of thrombosis with no direct pathophysiologic role. Because many of these antibodies perturb hemostasis in vitro, it has been assumed that they also directly affect the hemostatic system in vivo, so the prothrombotic-antithrombotic equilibrium is perturbed enough that it becomes unbalanced, favoring thrombosis or placental ischemia. There is evidence substantiating this in patients with SLE and elevated anticardiolipin antibodies, in whom elevated levels of fibrinopeptide A and the prothrombin fragment F1+2 have been demonstrated.[129,167] In contrast, in the study by Ferro and coworkers,[167] F1+2 was elevated in patients with SLE who were lupus anticoagulant-positive, but patients who were positive only for anticardiolipin antibody did not have elevated levels of F1+2. In other studies of patients who were lupus anticoagulant positive, the mean level of thrombin-antithrombin complexes was higher than it was in control subjects.[99,168]

Antiphospholipid Antibodies as Direct Causative Factors for Thrombosis

There are experimental animal models that suggest that antiphospholipid antibodies directly cause thrombosis and pregnancy loss. The antiphospholipid syndrome has been produced in normal mice by passive transfer of human immunoglobulin with anticardiolipin activity[169] or by active immunization with a human monoclonal anticardiolipin antibody[170]or with β_2-GPI.[171,172] Pregnant mice that were passively[169] or actively immunized with anticardiolipin antibody IgG had increased fetal loss.[169,173] In another experimental model,[174] mice injected with purified anticardiolipin antibody from patients with antiphospholipid syndrome followed by a "pinch" injury to their femoral vein had significantly larger thrombi that persisted for a longer period of time than in appropriate control animals. A monoclonal human anticardiolipin antibody generated from a patient with the antiphospholipid syndrome caused thrombosis in mice.[175] All of these experimental models strongly suggest that antiphospholipid antibodies have a direct pathophysiologic role in thrombosis. Human anticardiolipin antibodies accelerated atherosclerosis in an low-density lipoprotein (LDL)-receptor null mouse.[176]

Mechanism of Thrombosis

The various pathophysiologic mechanisms possibly causing thrombosis have been recently extensively reviewed by Giannakopoulos and coworkers.[177] Antiphospholipid antibodies could directly contribute to thrombosis by altering platelet activity, procoagulant or anticoagulant pathways, or vascular endothelial function. Several considerations support a possible role for platelet activation in the pathogenesis of antiphospholipid antibody–associated thrombosis.[177] First, many subjects with antiphospholipid antibody–associated thrombosis have some degree of thrombocytopenia,[8,10,121] presumably immune in origin. Second, there is an association between antiphospholipid antibodies and antiplatelet antibodies.[160,161] Antiphospholipid antibodies may directly cross-react with platelets.[178,179] The third consideration is the occurrence of arterial, as well as venous, thrombotic episodes. Platelet activation is thought to play a role in the pathogenesis of arterial thrombotic disease, whereas other causes of increased thrombotic risk, such as deficiencies of antithrombin, protein C, protein S, or factor V Leiden, predispose primarily to increased venous thrombotic risk. Increased levels of a urinary metabolite of thromboxane A_2 have been demonstrated in patients with antiphospholipid antibodies.[180] However, in contrast, another study showed that although antiphospholipid antibodies could bind to circulating platelets, no evidence of measurable platelet activation was found.[178] Fourth, serum or purified IgG from subjects with antiphospholipid antibodies inhibits the release of the platelet inhibitor, prostacyclin, from vascular segments or cultured vascular endothelial cells.[181–183] This finding suggests that in some subjects with antiphospholipid antibodies, impaired prostacyclin release might lead to excessive platelet activity, resulting in thrombosis. Platelets from subjects with antiphospholipid antibody–associated thrombosis are more resistant to in-vitro inhibition by the inhibitory prostaglandin E_1, than are normal platelets. However, except for one study,[184] the correlation between in-vitro inhibition of prostacyclin release and thrombosis in subjects with antiphospholipid antibodies has been poor.[183] Shi and colleagues[185] showed that purified IgG from patients with lupus anticoagulants and anticardiolipin antibodies bound to thrombin-activated, but not resting, platelets, and antibody binding did not produce any evidence of platelet activation. There is little evidence that lupus anticoagulants or anticardiolipin antibodies directly cause platelet activation. However, Arvieux and colleagues[186] showed that murine monoclonal antibodies to β_2-GPI with lupus anticoagulant activity could activate platelets when there were subthreshold concentrations of epinephrine or adenosine diphosphate in the presence of β_2-GPI. Subsequent platelet activation was shown to depend on binding to the platelet Fc receptor, similar to the pathophysiologic process occurring in heparin-induced thrombocytopenia. As an extension of the latter hypothesis, Arnout[50] has suggested that the deposition of immune complexes (containing β_2-GPI or prothrombin) on partially activated platelets induces further cell activation by a yet to be identified signal transduction mechanism leading to full platelet activation, microvesicle generation, the formation of platelet-leukocyte aggregates, and the provision of a large anionic phospholipid surface that could generate increased thrombin.[50] The increased concentration of prothrombin on the phospholipid surface can result in the generation of excess thrombin at sites of injury.[187]

Between 30% and 70% of sera from patients with antiphospholipid antibodies contains endothelial cell-reactive antibodies.[188] Some of these antibodies bind to β_2-GPI on the endothelial cell surface and result in endothelial cell activation.[189,190] There is evidence that β_2-GPI binds with high affinity to annexin V or antibodies directly bind to annexin A_2 independent of β_2-GPI on the endothelial cell surface.[191,192] These antibodies might cause thrombosis by directly damaging endothelial cells; by impairing endothelial, antiplatelet, anticoagulant, or fibrinolytic activities; or by bringing about procoagulant changes in endothelial function, such as expression of tissue factor.[193,194] Antiphospholipid antibody–containing sera from patients with systemic lupus and thrombosis induced a small, but significant, increase of endothelial cell tissue factor activity. When added in combination with a low dose of tumor necrosis factor, a synergistic enhancement of tissue factor activity was found.[190] These antiphospholipid antibody–containing sera led to enhanced thrombosis formation in an in-vitro thrombosis model. In contrast, non–antiphospholipid antibody–containing sera from patients with systemic lupus did not generate tissue factor activity, nor did the sera produce enhanced thrombus formation.[194] Antiphospholipid antibodies stimulate tissue factor expression by human monocytes.[195,196] Simantov and coworkers[190] showed that purified IgG from lupus patients with elevated anticardiolipin antibody and antiphospholipid syndrome causes increased monocyte adhesion when reacted with endothelial cells in vitro. Monocyte adhesion depended on the presence of β_2-GPI. These data strongly suggest that anticardiolipin antibody is capable of binding to and activating vascular endothelial cells.

All of the experimental evidence at the present time suggests that anti-β_2 GPI-β_2 GPI antigen-antibody complexes binding to platelet or endothelial receptors as insufficient in themselves to activate platelets and/or endothelial cells and require a primary stimulus.[177]

Annexin V is a potent anticoagulant protein that has a high affinity for phospholipid and competes with activated coagulation factors for binding to phospholipid surfaces.[191] Thus annexin V forms a protective anticoagulant shield on endothelial cells and when disrupted by anti-β_2 GPI antibodies can result in accelerated coagulation reactions.[197] IgG fractions from patients with antiphospholipid syndrome reduce the quantity of annexin V on cultured endothelial cells and trophoblasts and accelerate the coagulation reactions of plasma clotting factors expressed on these cells.[198]

Several abnormalities of natural anticoagulant pathways have also been reported in patients with antiphospholipid antibody–associated thrombosis.[177] In one study, thrombomodulin antibodies were found in 30% of patients with the lupus anticoagulant, in 10% of patients with unexplained thromboembolism, and in 10% of control subjects.[199] However, in another study, inhibition of thrombomodulin activity was found in only 2 of 46 patients with lupus anticoagulants.[200] In that same study, plasma from 24 of 33 patients with thrombosis showed significant inhibition of activated protein C, whereas plasma from 13 patients with thrombosis showed no inhibition. In other studies,[17,18,201] serum and purified IgG impaired activation of protein C by thrombin complexed to the endothelial cofactor, thrombomodulin,[202] and impaired the phospholipid-dependent anticoagulant action of activated protein C and its cofactor, protein S.[17] In addition, murine monoclonal anti–β_2-GPI antibodies in the presence of β_2-GPI are able to inhibit protein C anticoagulant activity in vitro.[203] Reduced plasma levels of free protein S have also been observed in subjects with antiphospholipid antibody-associated thrombosis.[151,181,204] In another study, purified IgG from seven patients with antiphospholipid antibodies reacted with the disaccharide present in the heparin-heparan pentasaccharide that binds antithrombin III, and these antibodies inhibited formation of thrombin-antithrombin complexes.[205]

It appears that plasma from some patients with antiphospholipid antibodies inhibits several natural anticoagulant pathways, and whether this inhibition stems from other antibodies has not yet been established. Although several abnormalities of the natural anticoagulant pathway have been demonstrated in patients with antiphospholipid antibodies, a close correlation between abnormalities of these pathways and thrombosis in patients with antiphospholipid antibodies has not been consistently demonstrated. A defect in natural anticoagulant pathways could not, by itself, explain the presence of arterial thromboembolism.

Because anticardiolipin antibodies are antibodies directed against β_2-GPI,[76,77] it suggests that possibly the antihemostatic effect is caused by inhibition of β_2-GPI function. Although patients with severe β_2-GPI deficiency do not have thromboembolic disease,[206] the presence of anti-β_2-GPI antibodies is associated with lupus anticoagulant activity, anticardiolipin antibodies, and thromboembolic complications in patients with systemic lupus.[207]

Impaired fibrinolysis may contribute to thrombosis in patients with antiphospholipid antibodies.[208,209] However, active systemic lupus[209,210] is independently associated with impaired fibrinolysis.[211] More recent studies of patients with antiphospholipid antibody–associated thrombosis without lupus have failed to document impaired fibrinolysis in vivo[212] or any effect of plasma-containing antiphospholipid antibodies on in-vitro endothelial secretion of tissue plasminogen activator or plasminogen activator inhibitor-1.[213] However, interference with annexin A2 function could result in impaired fibrinolysis because annexin A2 allows tissue plasminogen activator and plasminogen to bind on the endothelial cell surface.[177,192,214]

Harkko and colleagues[215] found that apolipoprotein E-deficient mice who had active atherogenesis developed high titers of autoantibodies to epitopes of oxidized LDL and to cardiolipin, and that sera or anticardiolipin antibody-IgG from patients with antiphospholipid syndrome bind to oxidized cardiolipin but does not bind to reduced cardiolipin. Antiphospholipid antibodies are directed at neo-epitopes of oxidized lipoproteins. It had been previously shown by Vaarla and colleagues[216] that binding of anticardiolipin antibody to solid-phase cardiolipin was inhibited by oxidized LDL, but not by native LDL, suggesting cross-reactivity between antiphospholipid antibodies and antibodies to oxidized LDL. Other data suggest that antiphospholipid antibodies may be pathogenic in the formation of atherosclerotic lesions and result in increased atheroma development.[217]

Although it has been proposed that fetal loss and/or growth retardation is probably also caused by placental vascular thrombosis and/or insufficiency, not all placentas show thrombosis[218] and not all patients with antiphospholipid antibodies suffer fetal loss. The passive administration of polyclonal or monoclonal antibodies from patients with antiphospholipid syndrome and healthy controls to pregnant mice does lead to adverse pregnancy outcomes. Moreover, this phenomenon appears to require complement activation.[219,220] In many patients with second or third trimester fetal loss or growth retardation, placental vascular thrombosis can be demonstrated. In addition, it has been shown that patients with β_2-GPI–dependent lupus anticoagulant activity displayed increased annexin V resistance in an in-vitro assay suggesting that anti–β_2-GPI antibodies compete with annexin V for anionic phospholipids, and thus promote thrombosis by interfering with annexin V's anticoagulant activity.[221] However, in many patients with fetal loss no placental vascular thrombosis can be found. In addition, there is evidence that trophoblast function can be disrupted because anti–β_2-GPI antibodies can inhibit trophoblast gonadotropin secretion and invasiveness in vitro.[222] Thus, there may be more than one mechanism whereby antiphospholipid antibodies may effect placental function.

THERAPY FOR PATIENTS WITH LUPUS ANTICOAGULANT AND/OR OTHER ANTIPHOSPHOLIPID ANTIBODIES

The lupus anticoagulant usually persists in the untreated adult patient. However, it frequently disappears spontaneously when it occurs in children in whom the anticoagulant develops after a viral infection and may be transient in adult patients without systemic lupus, thromboembolic disorders, or fetal loss.

When the lupus anticoagulant or elevated levels of antiphospholipid antibodies, or both, are found in patients with underlying autoimmune disease, treatment of the underlying disease with immunosuppressive therapy may result in reduction or disappearance of the antibody.[65,81] When the anticoagulant is found in association with severe prothrombin deficiency or severe thrombocytopenia (<20,000 cells/µL), treatment with corticosteroids is indicated (see preferred treatment box on Therapy for Patients with Lupus Anticoagulant or Increased Levels of Anticardiolipin or Antihuman β_2-GPI). There has been one case report of a patient with a lupus anticoagulant and hypoprothrombinemia who was resistant to corticosteroids but was responsive to intravenous gammaglobulin.[223] However, when the lupus anticoagulant or anticardiolipin antibody is discovered as an isolated finding, not associated with thrombosis or fetal loss, treatment is not indicated. Although aspirin may be effective in primary prevention of arterial thrombosis and may be effective in some patients with antiphospholipid antibodies and recurrent fetal loss, it did not show efficacy in preventing venous thrombosis and pulmonary embolism in the Physician's Health Study.[126] If low-dose aspirin is prescribed for prophylaxis, the patient should be educated about efficacy and its side effects. It is important to educate patients about the symptoms of venous thrombosis and its prophylaxis, and the symptoms of pulmonary embolism, heart attack, stroke, and in women-fetal loss. Any factors predisposing the patient to thrombosis, such as medication containing estrogen, should be discontinued. Smoking cessation should be pursued, and hypertension, hyperlipidemia, and diabetes should be aggressively treated.

Therapy for thrombosis associated with the lupus anticoagulant or elevated levels of anticardiolipin antibodies should be guided by the knowledge that recurrence is common.[126,133,134,156] In one study, patients who had discontinued oral anticoagulation had a 50% probability of recurrence in 2 years and a 78% recurrence in 8 years.[224] Similar results have been published by others with a recurrence rate of 10% to 30% per year.[123,133,134,155] Three prospective studies reported that there was an increased risk of recurrence that varied from 10% to 67% per year.[225–229] However, in many of these studies the patients did not fulfill the consensus definition of antiphospholipid syndrome.[31] In most reports the incidence of recurrence is highest in the first 6 months after discontinuing anticoagulant therapy.[225,229] Venous recurrence usually occurs in patients who have an initial venous event, whereas arterial recurrences usually occur in patients who sustain an initial arterial event.[133] Although it was initially thought that prevention of venous recurrence required high-intensity warfarin with a target INR of 3.5,[230] evidence has been accumulating from recent studies that standard intensity warfarin (INR 2 to 3) can almost completely abrogate recurrence of venous thromboembolic disease.[231,232] The pooled data from these two studies revealed no difference in recurrent thrombosis between moderate-intensity warfarin (INR 2 to 3) and high-intensity (INR 3 to 4), nor was there a greater bleeding risk.[231,232] However, it should be noted the recurrent venous events in the moderate-intensity warfarin groups were lower than expected and that patients with recurrent venous thromboembolic disease were excluded.[233–236] As the data from several studies

Therapy for Patients with the Lupus Anticoagulant or an Increased Level of Anticardiolipin Antibodies

The lupus anticoagulant persists in most untreated adults. Often it disappears spontaneously when it occurs in children in whom the anticoagulant is acquired after a viral infection, and it may be transient in adult patients without SLE, thromboembolic disorders, or fetal loss.

When the lupus anticoagulant, increased levels of anticardiolipin antibodies, or anti–β_2-GPI antibodies are found in patients with underlying autoimmune disease, treatment of the underlying disease with immunosuppressive therapy may result in reduction or disappearance of the antibody. When the lupus anticoagulant is found in association with severe prothrombin deficiency or severe thrombocytopenia (<20,000 cells/μL), treatment with adrenal corticosteroids is indicated. If the patient is actively bleeding with severe hypoprothrombinemia, adjunctive therapy with intravenous immunoglobulin (IVIg) can be given, whereas if the patient has active bleeding with only severe thrombocytopenia anti-D (if Rh+) or IVIg can be given. However, when the lupus anticoagulant, increased levels of anticardiolipin, or anti–β_2-GPI antibodies are discovered as an isolated finding and not associated with thrombosis or fetal loss, treatment is not indicated except for possibly prophylactic low-dose aspirin and/or hydroxychloroquine plus aggressive treatment of comorbid conditions such as smoking, diabetes mellitus, dyslipidemia, hypertension, and so on.

Therapy for thrombosis associated with the lupus anticoagulant or significant levels of anticardiolipin or β_2-GPI antibodies should be guided by the knowledge that recurrence is common. The site of the first event (arterial or venous) tends to predict the site of subsequent events. It is recommended that patients with acute venous thromboembolic events receive low-molecular-weight heparin subcutaneously in the usual therapeutic doses, or alternatively, intravenous unfractionated heparin in the usual therapeutic doses to achieve a plasma heparin level of 0.3 to 0.7 units using a factor Xa inhibition assay. Long-term anticoagulation with warfarin can be started simultaneously with a dose to maintain the INR between 2 and 3 using a thromboplastin insensitive to the lupus anticoagulant. If recurrent venous events occur at a therapeutic INR, then the patient should be treated with either therapeutic low-molecular-weight heparin, or alternatively, to continue with warfarin with an INR of 2.5 to 3.5.

Long-term anticoagulants are also probably efficacious in secondary prevention of arterial thrombosis depending on the vascular bed involved. In patients with ischemic coronary artery disease the target INR should be 2.5 to 3.5 or, alternatively, 2 to 3 along with low-dose aspirin (81 mg/day). If coronary ischemic events recur at an INR of 2.5 to 3.5, then low-dose aspirin (81 mg/day) can be added. In patients with cerebrovascular ischemic events aspirin alone (325 mg/day) or warfarin alone (INR of 2 to 3) are reasonable alternatives. In addition, comorbid conditions such as dyslipidemia, hypertension, diabetes, and smoking should be aggressively treated.

Because of the increased recurrence of thrombotic disease antihemostatic therapy should be continued for life, except when they occur exclusively in pregnancy. Because of the efficacy of antihemostatic therapy in preventing recurrent thrombosis, the use or corticosteroids and other immunosuppressive agents to suppress antibody production is usually not necessary in the absence of SLE. However, in patients with refractory SLE and severe manifestation of APS hematopoietic stem cell transplantation should be considered.

A pregnant patient—with or without SLE—with the lupus anticoagulant and/or a significant level of anticardiolipin or anti–β_2-GPI antibodies associated with a history of fetal wastage (see Table 123–1) should be treated with low-dose aspirin 81 mg/day plus prophylactic doses of low-molecular-weight heparin 4000 to 5000 anti-Xa units subcutaneously once every 24 hours. If fetal loss recurs on this regimen, a therapeutic dose of low-molecular-weight heparin should be tried. A pregnant patient with or without SLE with a previous thrombotic event usually is already receiving oral anticoagulants. At the time of diagnosis of pregnancy, the oral anticoagulant should be immediately replaced with low-molecular-weight heparin in full therapeutic doses (adjusted to periodically determine serum anti-Xa levels with low-molecular-weight heparin standard). Oral anticoagulants can be resumed in the postpartum period for 4 to 6 weeks.

For the patient, with or without SLE, who becomes pregnant for the first time and who has not had a prior thromboembolic event or fetal wastage, no treatment is indicated. However, the patient should be educated regarding the possibility of increased risk of fetal loss or thrombosis, the potential side effects of therapy, and the contradictory results from uncontrolled and controlled trials. After full disclosure—if the patient desires treatment—she should be given prophylactic doses of low-molecular-weight heparin and/or low-dose aspirin.

If an asymptomatic patient with persistently present antiphospholipid antibodies requires a major surgical procedure, prophylactic low-molecular-weight heparin and intermittent pneumatic compression should be used.

The patient who presents with catastrophic APS should receive anticoagulant therapy with an intravenous bolus of 80 units/kg of unfractionated heparin, followed by a continuous intravenous infusion of 18 units/kg/h or alternatively, therapeutic doses of low-molecular-weight heparin (if renal function is normal). Simultaneously, the patient should be given a pulse of high-dose methylprednisolone, 2 g intravenously daily for 3 days. If the patient's condition stabilizes within the first 24 hours, rituximab, 375 mg/m^2 should then be administered. Although plasmapheresis and/or IVIg may be helpful in some cases, these therapeutic maneuvers may interfere or make heparin and rituximab administration difficult. Because it appears that anticoagulation is much more efficacious than plasmapheresis and IVIg in this syndrome, then these therapeutic modalities could be reserved for recurrent adverse events.

---

noted above have demonstrated that patients with antiphospholipid syndrome have a high risk for recurrent venous thromboembolic disease after anticoagulation is discontinued, many feel that anticoagulation should be continued indefinitely.[225,229] The American College of Chest Physicians recommends treatment for 12 months and consideration of indefinite therapy after an initial event.[229,237] Because of the efficacy of warfarin therapy in preventing recurrences, the use of corticosteroids and other immunosuppressive agents to suppress antibody production in the absence of autoimmune disease is not recommended.

Monitoring anticoagulant therapy may be difficult in patients with lupus anticoagulants and a prolonged PTT. It is mandatory when using unfractionated heparin to monitor therapy using a specific heparin assay, such as the one dependent on factor Xa inhibition (therapeutic range, 0.3 to 0.7). In most instances, it is preferable to use low-molecular-weight heparin in therapeutic doses, which usually eliminates the need for monitoring. When using warfarin, the optimal INR for patients with lupus anticoagulants is controversial,[133,134,238,239] because patients with lupus anticoagulants may have a variably prolonged prothrombin time,[238,240] and various thromboplastins have a different sensitivity in the presence of a lupus anticoagulant.[238] Therefore, it is possible that in various studies of therapy in patients with lupus anticoagulants that the degree of anticoagulation is overestimated, and the target INR of 3.0 noted earlier might be an overestimate because of the presence of the lupus anticoagulant. This hypothesis is substantiated by the report by Moll and Ortel,[238] in which the prothrombin time done by the prothrombin-proconvertin test and a chromogenic factor X level correlated well with established therapeutic ranges. The prolongation of the prothrombin time in some patients with the lupus anticoagulant is prolonged by some tissue thromboplastins, particularly recombinant tissue factor, but not the other tissue factor reagents.[241,242] A tissue factor reagent that is known to be insensitive to the effect of the lupus anticoagulant can be used. However, it is important that the specific international sensitivity index of the specific thromboplastin is used in the calculation of the INR.[241] If an insensitive tissue factor cannot be found, then a chromogenic factor X assay with a target therapeutic range of 10% to 40% (which is equal to an INR of 2 to 3) can be used. Alternatively, low-molecular-weight heparin can be used. Rarely, patients may continue to have recurrent venous thromboembolic events despite INR values in the therapeutic range. These patients can be treated with long-term low-molecular-weight heparin, warfarin with a target INR of 3.0, or aspirin in addition to warfarin.[243]

The treatment of patients with arterial thrombotic disease is less clear than in patients with venous disease. Although the recent trials with venous disease also enrolled patients with arterial thrombotic disease, there were too few patients to come to any definite conclusion.[231,232] However, in both trials there was a low recurrence rate in patients assigned to moderate-intensity warfarin (INR 2–3), and the recurrence rate was no different than with high-intensity warfarin. However, it should be noted that the patients in these two trials were patients who suffered an initial thrombotic event and excluded patients with recurrent vascular events. Thus, it is probably premature to conclude that warfarin alone with a target INR of 2 to 3 is adequate to prevent arterial thrombosis. However, it has been shown in well-controlled trials in patients with coronary artery disease that secondary prevention is effective with high-intensity warfarin (INR 2.8 to 4.8)[244–246] or moderate-intensity warfarin (INR 2.0 to 2.5) plus low-dose aspirin (75 mg).[247] In the latter study,[247] aspirin and warfarin (INR 2.2) was shown to be equivalent to high-intensity warfarin (INR 3.5) and was superior to aspirin alone. In contrast, in the antiphospholipid and stroke study (Antiphospholipid Antibodies and Stroke Study Group [APASS]),[248] aspirin alone was equivalent to warfarin (INR 1.4 to 2.8). Considering the successful trials using warfarin alone in secondary prevention in patients with coronary artery disease with a reduction in the INR to 2.5 to 3.5,[249,250] it would also be reasonable to use warfarin alone (without aspirin) with a target INR of 3.0. Thus, the treatment of arterial thrombosis in patients with associated antiphospholipid antibodies remain controversial.[225,229,231,232] However, it appears from the above studies that aspirin alone, aspirin plus moderate-intensity warfarin (INR 2–3), or moderate-intensity warfarin alone (INR 2.5–3.5) are reasonable alternatives after an initial arterial ischemic event depending on the arterial bed involved. In addition, recently it has been shown that in patients with systemic lupus with or without antiphospholipid antibodies that treatment with chloroquine and hydroxychloroquine reduced the incidence of thrombosis and prolonged survival, particularly in patients with a previous history of thrombosis and/or the presence of antiphospholipid antibodies.[251] Moreover, hydroxychloroquine has been shown to inhibit platelet activation in the presence of antiphospholipid antibodies.[252]

The optimum treatment of patients with recurrent arterial events is yet to be determined and requires either more intensive or alternative antihemostatic treatment. In addition, comorbid conditions such as diabetes, smoking, dyslipidemia, and hypertension, must be aggressively treated.

Recently it has been reported that several patients with refractory SLE with secondary antiphospholipid syndrome were treated with autologous hematopoietic stem cell transplantation with excellent results.[253] There was no treatment-related mortality, and the majority of patients remained thrombosis free without anticoagulant therapy.

A pregnant patient with or without SLE with the lupus anticoagulant or elevated levels of anticardiolipin antibody associated with a history of recurrent fetal wastage should be treated. However, the precise regimen to be followed has not been clearly established. Lubbe and colleagues[254] described a successful pregnancy outcome in a patient with the lupus anticoagulant and fetal wastage who was treated with prednisone and low-dose aspirin. Subsequently, the same regimen led to successful pregnancy outcomes in 10 of 16 pregnancies in 12 patients, some of whom had SLE.[255] Other investigators, using a similar regimen in patients without SLE, also reported a decrease in fetal wastage in a significant number of patients.[256] In a study by Silveira and associates,[256] prednisone and low-dose aspirin given to 11 patients with recurrent fetal wastage (32 previous fetal losses and 5 live-born infants) resulted in 100% live-born infants (12 pregnancies and 12 live-born infants), and no significant adverse effects to mother or infants. The levels of anticardiolipin antibody decreased in most patients. Lockshin and colleagues[257] have cast significant doubt regarding the efficacy of aspirin with or without corticosteroids in high-risk patients with high-titer anticardiolipin antibodies. In 11 pregnancies receiving corticosteroids and low-dose aspirin, there were 9 fetal losses, whereas in 10 pregnancies receiving aspirin alone or no therapy, there were 5 fetal losses. However, in a large, randomized trial in 202 patients with autoantibodies (lupus anticoagulant, anticardiolipin antibody, antinuclear antibody, anti-DNA, or antilymphocytic IgM) and unexplained loss of at least 2 fetuses, corticosteroids plus low-dose aspirin resulted in 65% viable infants, compared with 57% in the placebo group.[258] Despite these variable results with corticosteroids with or without aspirin, the formidable toxicity of corticosteroids, including hypertension, preeclampsia, gestational diabetes, and premature labor and delivery, and the lack of such toxicity with other regimens, resulted in the deletion of corticosteroids as part of the therapeutic armamentarium. However, in an occasional patient with active SLE, corticosteroids may be necessary to suppress the underlying disease.

Wallenberg and Rotmans[259] used low-dose aspirin and dipyridamole in 37 patients with obstetric histories similar to those with antiphospholipid antibodies, with a 93% success rate. Unfortunately, these patients were not systematically examined for the presence of antiphospholipid antibodies. Likewise, Elder and colleagues[159] reported similar success using low-dose aspirin alone in 42 patients, of whom 16 had SLE (13 with antiphospholipid antibodies). One other randomized double-blind trial in patients with three or more miscarriages and the presence of antiphospholipid antibodies compared low-dose aspirin 75 mg/day to placebo.[260] In this small trial of 40 patients, 85% of the placebo group and 80% of the aspirin group were delivered of live infants.

In another small, randomized trial,[261] 50 patients with at least three consecutive episodes of spontaneous pregnancy loss and positive antiphospholipid antibody were assigned low-dose aspirin alone or low-dose aspirin plus heparin with increasing doses throughout pregnancy to achieve a PTT between 1.2 and 1.5. Viable infants were delivered by 11 of 25 (44%) women receiving aspirin alone, whereas 20 of 25 women (80%) receiving aspirin plus heparin delivered viable fetuses. In another randomized trial[262] in patients with persistently positive antiphospholipid antibodies and three or more fetal losses, low-dose aspirin (75 mg) plus unfractionated heparin (5000 units twice daily) resulted in live births in 32 of 45 (71%) pregnancies, compared with 19 of 45 (42%) live births in patients receiving low-dose aspirin alone. In contrast, in a randomized trial, 98 patients with persistently positive antiphospholipid antibodies and recurrent fetal loss were assigned low-dose aspirin alone or low-dose aspirin plus 5000 units of low-molecular-weight heparin daily.[263] There was no difference in live births between the two groups with 72% fetal survival with aspirin alone versus 78% with aspirin plus heparin. This well controlled and randomized study contrasts to a large meta-analysis of several controlled trials of therapy for pregnancy loss associated with antiphospholipid antibodies, (excluding the randomized trial noted earlier).[264] Ten trials fulfilled their inclusion criteria (627 patients). Three trials of aspirin alone showed no reduction in pregnancy loss. Heparin (in prophylactic to intermediate doses) combined with aspirin resulted in a significant reduction in fetal loss compared with aspirin alone. Prednisone and aspirin resulted in a significant increase in prematurity but no significant reduction in pregnancy loss.

Rosove and colleagues[265] reported 14 successful outcomes in 15 pregnancies in 14 patients (5 with lupus) using adjusted full-dose heparin therapy throughout pregnancy. None of the patients was treated with aspirin, and only one patient received a short course of corticosteroids for a lupus flare. Ruffatti and coworkers[266] reported 100% fetal survival in 53 patients treated with heparin alone.

Different therapeutic regimens in controlled and uncontrolled clinical trials have resulted in a decrease in fetal loss. Some trials are difficult to evaluate because the cutoff levels between normal and abnormal for anticardiolipin antibodies were lower (<20 GPL units) than the cutoff values in other studies (>20 GPL units).[68] This is obviously a reflection of the lack of standardization of the anticardiolipin assay. Despite this problem, the most efficacious regimens appear to be low- or intermediate-dose heparin plus low-dose aspirin, or adjusted-dose heparin without aspirin. Although the trials in pregnant patients with antiphospholipid antibodies used unfractionated heparin, it has been clearly shown that low-molecular-weight heparin (4000 to 5000 anti-Xa units subcutaneously every 24 hours) is safe, efficacious, and easy to use in pregnancy. Unlike unfractionated heparin, it does not cause clinically significant osteoporosis. Whether it can be used alone (without aspirin) in prophylactic doses remains to be determined in clinical trials. The only other issue regarding low-molecular-weight heparin is its use just before delivery, which may complicate the timing of epidural analgesia. However, this can be obviated by a planned delivery or switching to unfractionated heparin before delivery. The use of aspirin alone remains controversial, despite its demonstrated efficacy in some of the trials. Regimens containing corticosteroids appear in most studies to cause significant adverse events (hypertension, diabetes, and preterm labor and delivery).

Whether asymptomatic patients with antiphospholipid antibodies who desire pregnancy should be treated prophylactically is not clear. Low-titer anticardiolipin antibody occurs in up to 2% to 4% of healthy young women and high-titer antibody in approximately 0.2%.[43] Young women with antiphospholipid antibodies who wish to become pregnant may be referred for consultation. If the patient does have a high titer of IgG anticardiolipin antibody, the risk of fetal loss approximates 25%, whereas the risk of fetal loss in patients without antiphospholipid antibodies is approximately 13%. The patient should be educated regarding these data, the possibility of fetal loss, the potential side effects of therapy, and the lack of controlled trials in these patients. Because low-dose aspirin was demonstrated to be efficacious in a well-controlled clinical trial without significant side effects, its use would probably do no harm.

Treatment of Catastrophic Antiphospholipid Antibody Syndrome

In the extensive reviews of patients with catastrophic antiphospholipid syndrome, various therapeutic interventions were analyzed.[107,108,165,166] Because most patients received more than one intervention, the analysis was difficult. Recovery occurred in 62% of patients treated with anticoagulation versus 23% in those who were not.[107] The use of steroids, cyclophosphamide, plasmapheresis, or intravenous gammaglobulin did not seem to affect outcome. However, considering the various combinations, recovery occurred in 64% of patients treated with anticoagulants and steroids and only in 38% of those who were not. Other combinations did not significantly affect outcome. However, intravenous gammaglobulin or plasma exchange with fresh frozen plasma have shown some efficacy in some cases.[166] In addition, rituximab has occasionally been added to corticosteroids with positive results.[229,267,268]

An analysis of the long-term outcome of patients with catastrophic antiphospholipid syndrome that were originally reported[107] and survived the initial event revealed that 66% had no recurrence while on long-term anticoagulants, whereas 26% developed further thromboembolic events.[269] Twenty-five percent of the latter patients died from the event. Five percent of the patients died of multiorgan failure and 2% of other causes.

SPONTANEOUSLY ACQUIRED INHIBITORS OF FACTOR VIII (ACQUIRED HEMOPHILIA A)

Clinical Setting

Virtually all inhibitors of factor VIII are recognized because of their neutralization of factor VIII activity. Most occur in five clinical situations: alloantibodies in hemophilia A; postpartum; in association with various immunologic disorders; in association with various malignancies; and in older patients without any associated disorder. The last four clinical situations occur with an estimated incidence of 0.2 to $1.48/1 \times 10^6$ persons/year.[270–273]

In 1981, Green and Lechner[271] surveyed 215 patients with factor VIII inhibitors in an effort to gather demographic information regarding spontaneously arising inhibitors to factor VIII. The gender incidence was approximately equal, and almost 60% of the patients were older than 60 years of age. No associated disease was found in 50% of patients, but rheumatoid arthritis, SLE, drug reactions, dermatologic disorders, and different types of malignancies (solid tumors and lymphoproliferative malignancies) were each seen in 8% to 15% of the total group. In 13.5% of cases, the disorder occurred during the postpartum period. These associations have been corroborated by other reports.[272,273] Overall mortality was 22%. Approximately 38% showed eventual spontaneous disappearance of the inhibitor. The spontaneous remission rate was confirmed by Lottenberg and colleagues,[270] who reported that among 16 patients receiving no immunosuppressive therapy, 5 had spontaneous remissions.

Factor VIII Inhibitors Occurring in Patients with Immunologic Disorders, in Patients with Cancer and in Patients without Underlying Disease

Immune disorders associated with factor VIII inhibitors include rheumatoid arthritis,[274,275] SLE, and other systemic autoimmune diseases,[274–276] penicillin or other drug reactions,[1] bronchial asthma,[274,275] inflammatory bowel disease,[275] erythema multiforme,[275] dermatitis herpetiformis,[275] graft-versus-host disease,[114] and interferon-α therapy.[277,278] Occasionally, factor VIII inhibitors are associated with monoclonal gammopathies. More than 40 cases with various types of cancers have been reported.[279] Solid tumors were found in 25 patients, and 16 had hematologic malignancies.[279]

Factor VIII Inhibitors Occurring Postpartum

Factor VIII inhibitors can occur during the postpartum period,[274–276,280–283] and rarely during pregnancy.[284] Most often, the inhibitor occurs after the birth of the first or second child. Although a bleeding tendency may become evident immediately or after a prolonged interval, there is usually a 2- to 5-month delay before the diagnosis is made. The course in these patients is variable, but the inhibitor disappears spontaneously in many patients after 12 to 18 months.[280–282] In a review of 51 patients with postpartum inhibitors, the survival rate was 97% at 2 years, and Kaplan-Meier analysis revealed a probability of complete remission of almost 100%.[114] The median time to complete remission was 11 months, an interval shortened with immunosuppressive drugs.

In patients who became pregnant again after the occurrence of a postpartum factor VIII inhibitor,[281,285] only a rare patient who had achieved a remission have had a recurrence.[283,286] The cause of these postpartum inhibitors is unknown.

Properties of Spontaneously Acquired Factor VIII Inhibitors

With rare exceptions, factor VIII inhibitors are IgG antibodies. Some of these inhibitors have restricted heterogeneity because some possess κ or λ light chains.[1,275,287–292] These inhibitors frequently contain mixtures of heavy chain subclasses. Hultin and coworkers[290] found that hemophilic and nonhemophilic inhibitors contain mixtures of IgG_1 and IgG_4 subclasses. The high incidence of factor VIII inhibitors containing a subpopulation of IgG_4 is significant because this subclass constitutes less than 5% of plasma IgG. The inhibitors are specific for factor VIII activity, and most do not interfere with the activities of VWF within the factor VIII-VWF complex. The VWF antigen and function are normal in patients with these inhibitors. Factor VIII inhibitors do not participate in complement fixation.[275,276] They show species specificity in vitro and in vivo in that human factor VIII is generally neutralized to a greater extent than is bovine or porcine factor VIII. Infusion of bovine or porcine factor VIII into a patient with an inhibitor often raises the factor VIII level.[293]

The kinetics of the reaction between factor VIII and most hemophilic inhibitors is first order with respect to factor VIII and to inhibitor (type I).[294] The inhibitor can be completely neutralized by excess factor VIII.[294] A time dependence of the neutralization of factor VIII sometimes requires 1 to 2 hours to reach equilibrium at low inhibitor concentrations.[294] Neutralization occasionally takes place in an initial rapid phase, followed by a very slow second phase.[295,296] By contrast, inhibitors arising in most nonhemophiliac patients frequently differ in their reaction kinetics from inhibitors arising in hemophiliac patients.[296,297] A linear relationship between the inhibitor concentration and the amount of factor VIII inactivated is observed with hemophilia inhibitors (type I), but not with most spontaneous inhibitors (type II). Most spontaneous inhibitors do not totally inactivate factor VIII in vitro. Although most factor VIII inhibitor patients have no factor VIII in the plasma, the occasional patient exhibits some plasma factor VIII activity.[276,297,298]

Epitope Specificity of Factor VIII Antibodies

The antigenic regions on the factor VIII molecule to which factor VIII inhibitors bind have been identified.[137,299–301] The epitopes to which alloantibodies or autoantibodies are directed are limited to certain areas of the factor VIII light or heavy chains[300,301] and interfere with factor VIII interaction with factor IX, factor X, VWF, or phospholipid.[300,301] The factor VIII molecule consists of two series of repeated homologous domains and a single B domain arranged in the following order: A1-A2-B-A3-C1-C2. Small regions rich in acidic amino acids are located between A1 and A2 (called a1), A2 and B (a2), and B and A3 (a3).[301] The heavy chain consists of A1-a1-A2-a2-B and the light chain consists of a3-A3-C1-C2.[301] The A and C domains are required for functional activity, whereas the B domain is not. A variety of immunologic techniques have been used to characterize the parts of the factor VIII molecule to which antibodies bind. These include immunoblot analysis after sodium dodecyl sulfate-polyacrylamide gel electrophoresis of purified factor VIII, immunoprecipitation assays using recombinant polypeptide fragments of factor VIII, the effects of inhibitory antibodies on functional hybrid recombinant human-porcine factor VIII peptides, enzyme-linked immunosorbent assay techniques that measure antibody binding to intact recombinant or plasma-derived factor VIII, and the use of monoclonal anti-factor VIII antibodies derived from the plasma of inhibitor patients.[300,301] The A2, A3, and C2 domains and the light chain are most immunogenic, whereas the A1 and B domains are poorly or nonimmunogenic.[300] Anti-A2 and -C2 antibodies are present in approximately 68% of plasmas tested by immunoprecipitation assays using recombinant polypeptide fragments of factor VIII.[302] Less commonly, antibodies to the different acidic regions (a_1, a_2, a_3) are also found.[302,303] The antibody or combinations of antibodies that inhibit factor VIII activity predominantly consist of those directed toward A2, A3, C2, and a3 epitopes because of the ability of polypeptides containing those epitopes to completely neutralize inhibitor activity.[300,301] Anti-C2 antibodies interfere with factor VIII function by blocking the binding of factor VIII to phospholipid or VWF[300–303] or slowing the release of VWF from factor VIII.[300,301] These antibodies interfere with the assembly of the tenase complex. Anti-A2 and anti-A3 antibodies prevent factor VIIIa interaction with factor IXa or Xa, and interfere with the function of the tenase complex.[300–303] On occasion, antibodies are generated to the a1 residues between A1 and A2, which prevents binding of factor X to factor VIII,[300,301] or more commonly anti-a3 antibodies, which interfere with the binding of VWF to factor VIII.[301]

Antibody patterns in hemophilic patients differ from those in autoantibody patients.[304] C2 antibodies were the only antibodies found in 48% of autoantibody patients, whereas this pattern occurred in only one of 34 hemophiliacs.[304] Sixty-two percent of autoantibody patterns were directed to a single epitope, in contrast to only 17% of hemophiliac patterns. Fewer autoantibody patients contained anti-A2 and anti-A3 antibodies, and the occurrence of A2 plus C2 antibodies was also less common. Hemophiliacs treated with plasma-derived factor VIII or recombinant factor VIII have equally complex patterns, but they differ in epitope specificity from one another.[304] The relative amounts of antibody to the A2 and C2 domains can vary over time, and neither level is always correlated with the other inhibitor level.[304,305]

Recognition, Identification, and Quantitation of Factor VIII Inhibitors

The presence of a factor VIII inhibitor should be suspected whenever a patient with no prior bleeding history presents with spontaneous massive bruising or with large, unexplained hematomas. For unknown reasons, patients with spontaneously acquired factor VIII inhibitors have a more severe bleeding diathesis than hemophilia A patients with inhibitors with very severe skin, mucous membrane, and soft tissue bleeding. In contrast to hemophilia A patients with inhibitors, hemarthroses are rare. Some patients will present with no or minor bleeding (see box on Diagnostic Approach to Inhibitors).[273] The PTT is prolonged, whereas the prothrombin time and thrombin time are normal. The PTT of a mixture of the patient's plasma and normal plasma is also prolonged, although inactivation of factor VIII may require preincubation for 1 to 2 hours.[40,41] Confirmation that an inhibitor acts specifically with factor VIII requires incubating the patient's plasma diluted with an equal volume of normal plasma and performing assays of factors VIII, IX, XI, and XII at 0, 60, and 120 minutes. If the inhibitor is specific for factor VIII, only factor VIII decreases over time. A technique that uses the PTT rather than a factor VIII assay detects weak inhibitors of less than 0.4 Bethesda units.[306,307] Because heparin can also prolong the PTT, it is important to exclude the presence of heparin in the sample by performing a dilute thrombin time. In addition, because the lupus anticoagulant can also present with a prolonged PTT and can also be associated with the presence of a specific factor VIII inhibitor, it is important to exclude its presence by a dilute Russell viper venom time and its correction with exogenous phospholipid.

Quantitative inhibitor measurements are important in the emergency management of hemorrhage and for evaluation of long-term therapy. A standard unit of measurement, termed the *Bethesda unit,*[308] is best suited for the measurement of inhibitors arising in hemophiliacs, but the complexity of reaction kinetics and variations in antibody affinities for factor VIII, particularly in nonhemophilic inhibitors with high residual factor VIII, limit standardization. The reason for the high residual factor VIII is not clear but Nogami[309] reported that immune complexes of autoantibody and factor VIII prevented the inactivation of factor VIII by activated protein C. The presence of factor VIII in the antigen-antibody complexes prevented its binding to phospholipid membranes where it forms the tenase complex. Despite significant residual factor VIII levels in vitro, the patient has severe bleeding. Because of the high residual factor VIII, it may be difficult to determine the inhibitor titer in nonhemophilic patients with spontaneously acquired inhibitors. The results of the Bethesda assay underestimate the actual in vivo level of human factor VIII autoantibodies. Assay results are less valuable in guiding therapy than they are in hemophiliac patients with inhibitors. There is little correlation between the factor VIII level, titer of inhibitor, and degree of prolongation of the partial thromboplastin time with bleeding complications nor is the inhibitor titer at presentation useful for predicting the severity of bleeding. Frequently, more factor VIII must be given to obtain hemostatic levels in patients with autoantibodies to factor VIII. In the United Kingdom, the New Oxford method is used to quantitate factor VIII inhibitors,[310] with 1 Bethesda unit equaling approximately 1.21 times 1 New Oxford unit. The Bethesda assay does not ensure pH control during the incubation period, and this may result in nonantibody-mediated inactivation of factor VIII. In 1995, the Nijmegen modification of the Bethesda assay was introduced wherein the substrate plasma used in the test and control plasma is buffered to 7.4, and factor VIII-deficient plasma is substituted for imidazole buffer in the control sample.[311] Because some factor VIII-immunodepleted plasma lacks VWF, the results of the modified assay may give lower inhibitor titers compared with assay results when the factor VIII-deficient plasma in the control sample contained VWF.[312] These results were probably a result of the lack of the stabilizing effect of VWF resulting in a decrease in factor VIII level when incubated with the normal pooled plasma.[312] Recent studies suggest that 4% bovine serum albumin could be substituted for the factor VIII-deficient plasma in the control mixture without loss of specificity.[313]

Therapy of Patients with Factor VIII Inhibitors

The major objectives in the treatment of these patients are twofold: (1) the treatment of acute bleeding episodes, and (2) the elimination of the autoantibody to factor VIII (see box on Management of Spontaneously Acquired Factor VIII Inhibitors). When a patient with an inhibitor hemorrhages, conservative measures, including immobilization, compression, and possibly ε-aminocaproic acid, should be considered. The use of intramuscular injections or the use of aspirin-containing compounds is contraindicated. If the patient's bleeding is mild to moderate and the inhibitor titer is low (<3 Bethesda units) then desmopressin acetate (DDAVP) can be tried, and has been helpful in some cases.

The indication for the use of factor VIII concentrates or factor VIII bypassing agents is serious active bleeding. If the patient is not actively bleeding, transfusion is not indicated. Unlike inhibitors associated with hemophilia A, most spontaneously acquired inhibitors are usually not inducible when the patient is exposed to factor VIII. When the patient is bleeding, highly purified human factor VIII, or recombinant factor VIII is indicated in low titer inhibitor patients.

An important parameter in determining the amount of factor VIII to be infused is the titer of the inhibitor. If the titer is low (<5 Bethesda units), a large dose of human factor VIII sufficient to neutralize all the circulating inhibitor and provide enough excess factor VIII to achieve a plasma factor VIII of greater than 0.3 units/mL can be given. This can be achieved usually with the rapid infusion of human factor VIII (100 to 150 units/kg) followed by a continuous infusion of 10 units/kg/h. Alternatively, a large amount of human factor VIII can be given every 1 to 4 hours, giving 40 units of factor VIII/kg plus an additional 20 units/kg per Bethesda unit. When the inhibitor titer is slightly elevated (5–10 Bethesda units), the antibody level can be lowered by plasmapheresis or, alternatively, by one of several methods of immunoadsoprtion.[314,315] This can be followed by a bolus infusion (150–250 units/kg) followed by a continuous infusion of human factor VIII.

When factor VIII replacement is used, factor VIII levels must be assayed frequently to monitor the plasma factor VIII level achieved in vivo, particularly after the infusion of a factor VIII concentrate. The infused factor VIII may be efficacious in vivo before it is inactivated.

In the past porcine factor VIII has been used effectively in these patients because most autoantibodies have much less inhibitor activity against porcine factor VIII.[293,316,317] However, porcine factor VIII is no longer commercially available but a recombinant porcine concentrate is undergoing clinical trial.[318]

Management of Spontaneously Acquired Factor VIII Inhibitors

Conservative Measures

When a patient with an inhibitor has a hemorrhage, conservative hemostatic measures should be taken to complement whatever other therapy is used. These measures include immobilization, application of cold compresses, local application of hemostatic agents, and, on occasion, administration of ε-aminocaproic acid. The patient should not receive intramuscular injections, unnecessary venipunctures, aspirin-containing compounds, or nonsteroidal antiinflammatory drugs. If the patient has a low inhibitor level (<3 Bethesda units) then desmopressin (DDAVP) 0.3 µg/kg can be given immediately.

Selection of a Blood Product

For patients who are actively bleeding, therapeutic options include treatment with human plasma-derived or recombinant factor VIII concentrates, activated prothrombin complex concentrates, and recombinant factor VIIa. If the patient is not actively bleeding, transfusion is unnecessary. Unlike inhibitors associated with hemophilia A, most spontaneously acquired inhibitors do not increase in titer after exposure to factor VIII. This consideration should not impede transfusion therapy. If the titer is low (<5 Bethesda units), a large dose of factor VIII sufficient to neutralize all of the circulating inhibitor and provide enough excess factor VIII to achieve a plasma factor VIII of greater than or equal to 0.3 units/mL (30%) can be given. This usually can be achieved by giving a rapid infusion of giving 100 to 150 units/kg of human factor VIII concentrate followed by a continuous infusion of 10 units/kg/h. Alternatively, a large amount of human factor VIII can be given every 1 to 4 hours, giving 40 units of factor VIII/kg and an additional 20 units/kg for each Bethesda unit. If a patient has a moderately high inhibitor level of 5 to 10 Bethesda units, the inhibitor level may be lowered by approximately 50% to 65% by a 1.5-volume plasmapheresis or by using one of several methods of extracorporeal immunoadsorption. After apheresis or immunoadsorption, the patient is initially given human factor VIII (150 to 250 units/kg), followed by a continuous infusion in the dose noted previously. If plasmapheresis cannot be done promptly or if the patient has a very high titer inhibitor, it is impossible to achieve hemostatic levels of factor VIII, except by bypassing the site of inhibitor action with activated prothrombin complex concentrate (factor VIII inhibitor bypassing activity [FEIBA]) with a dose of 75 to 100 units/kg every 12 hours or recombinant factor VIIa at a dose of 90 µg/kg every 2 hours until the bleeding ceases followed by decreasing intervals of the administration of either concentrate. If factor VIII inhibitor titers are not readily available, then freeze plasma to be subsequently sent to a reference laboratory and infuse activated prothrombin complex concentrate or factor VIIa.

Immunosuppression of the Inhibitor

The long-term goal in the management of these patients should be aimed at immunosuppression of the autoantibody production. Although many immunosuppressive regimens have proved efficacious, we now initiate therapy with rituximab 375 mg/m^2 intravenously followed by weekly doses for a total of 4 weeks, immunosuppressive therapy with dexamethasone (Decadron) 40 mg/day, days 1 to 4, followed by prednisone 1mg/kg starting on day 5. Cyclophosphamide (2 mg/kg/day orally) is initiated concurrently with rituximab and dexamethasone. Inhibitor titers are determined every 1 to 2 weeks. This regimen is continued for 4 weeks. If a significant decrease in titer occurs (>50% reduction), the regimen is continued for 4 more weeks. If the preceding regimen is unsuccessful, the patient is placed on azathioprine (2 mg/kg), and serial inhibitor titers are performed. If no significant response occurs in 8 weeks, the regimen is discontinued, and cyclosporine or interferon-α therapy is tried.

If human factor VIII is ineffective, or the inhibitor level is too high, an attempt may be made to bypass the need for factor VIII by giving a prothrombin complex concentrate or recombinant factor VIIa. The prothrombin complex concentrates exhibit a procoagulant activity that bypasses the factor VIII-dependent clotting reactions. Two types of prothrombin complex concentrate have been used in the treatment of patients with factor VIII inhibitors: regular inactivated intermediate-purity prothrombin complex concentrates (eg, Bebulin VH [Baxter]); and activated concentrates, so-called anti-inhibitor coagulant complex. Both types of concentrates contain various amounts of activated factors VII, IX, and X and phospholipids, and should be distinguished from the highly purified factor IX concentrates used in the treatment of hemophilia B. The activated concentrates (FEIBA-VH [Baxter]) contain a greater amount of the factor VIII bypassing material and are specifically designed for patients with factor VIII inhibitors. Both types of concentrates have proved efficacious in hemophiliacs with inhibitors in controlled clinical trials,[319–321] but today the activated concentrates are the ones used to treat patients with inhibitors. The doses are arbitrary, but the usual initial dose of FEIBA is 75 to 100 units/kg. In a French multicenter retrospective survey of the use of FEIBA in 60 patients with factor VIII or IX inhibitors (6 of whom had spontaneously acquired inhibitors) with 433 bleeding episodes or surgical procedures, efficacy was good to excellent in 81.3% of the episodes.[322] Adverse effects were seen in only 5 of 433 episodes (12%), but an anamnestic response occurred in 17 of 54 evaluable patients (31.5%). A retrospective study of 34 patients with spontaneously acquired factor VIII inhibitors revealed a complete response rate of 86% with a dose of FEIBA of 75 units/kg every 8 to 12 hours with a median number of doses of 10 to control a severe bleed.[323] The authors emphasize that a dose of 200 units/kg/24-hour period should not be exceeded because of an increased incidence of thromboembolism.

Purified components of the prothrombin complex have been used to treat hemorrhages in patients with inhibitors. A highly purified concentrate containing factor VIIa achieved good hemostasis[324] and, subsequently, a recombinant preparation of human factor VIIa has shown significant efficacy in patients with inhibitors.[325,326] This product is designed to generate thrombin only at sites of vascular injury. In a survey of more than 240 patients, 18 of whom were patients with spontaneously acquired factor VIII autoantibodies, the recombinant factor VIIa was used successfully for critical bleeds or for surgery.[327] Dosage and interval of dosing are still being evaluated, but factor VIIa therapy is initiated with doses of 90 μg/kg, and this dose is repeated every 2 to 3 hours (half-life is 2.9 hours) for one to two times for spontaneous bleeds and every 2 to 3 hours for 48 hours for surgical procedures, followed by tapering doses over several days. Efficacy has been reported in approximately 90% of patients with spontaneous bleeds and in approximately 80% of patients undergoing surgical procedures. Treatment is not influenced by the inhibitor titer, and no specific assay reflects clinical efficacy. Antibodies to factor VII do not occur except in factor VII-deficient patients.[328] The safety profile has been excellent, and thrombotic events are rare. Continuous infusion has been evaluated and proved efficacious in some studies,[329,330] but not in others.[331]

In a recent comparison of FEIBA with recombinant factor VIIa in hemophilia patients with inhibitors with joint bleeds, both treatments were efficacious in 80% to 90% of patients.[332] However, both products did not meet statistical equivalence at the majority of time that patients were examined.

Long-term goals in the management of these patients should be aimed at immunosuppression of the autoantibody production. Assessment of immunosuppressive therapy is difficult because inhibitors occasionally disappear spontaneously, particularly in patients with postpartum inhibitors and patients with drug-induced inhibitors.[271] In patients with underlying disorders, such as systemic autoimmune disorders or cancer, treatment of the underlying disease may result in disappearance of the inhibitor. Many patients respond to corticosteroids alone; in one report of 16 patients receiving only steroids,[333] 7 were complete responders, 4 were partial responders, and 5 were nonresponders. The time to response averaged approximately 16 days. In their 1981 survey, Green and Lechner[271] found that inhibitors disappeared in 22 of 41 steroid-treated patients. In a prospective, multicenter, controlled clinical trial, antibody disappeared in 10 of 30 patients treated with prednisone alone (1 mg/kg) in the first 3 weeks, and in 3 of 4 other patients randomized to continue prednisone after the first 3 weeks of prednisone therapy.[334] In patients resistant to steroids, the use of cytotoxic agents, particularly cyclophosphamide alone or in combination with corticosteroids, can be efficacious. Antibody disappeared in three of six patients randomized to oral cyclophosphamide and prednisone after the patients were resistant to prednisone alone in the first 3 weeks. Eight patients did not respond. In this trial, the titer of antibody was significantly lower in responders than in nonresponders, and most responses occurred within 6 weeks of starting therapy.

The use of factor VIII concentrate infusion before immunosuppressive therapy was first proposed by Green.[335] The hypothesis proposed that the factor VIII concentrate infusion stimulates the abnormal clone of immune cells responsible for autoantibody synthesis and results in a greater cytotoxic effect by the immunosuppressive therapy. A combination of cyclophosphamide, vincristine, and prednisone every 3 weeks, preceded by an infusion of factor VIII concentrate (50 to 100 units/kg), resulted in complete disappearance of the inhibitor in 11 of 12 patients.[336] The responses occurred rapidly, usually within only two or three courses, and remissions in all patients were durable over 2 to 5 years. The same group reported similar response rates with a similar chemotherapeutic regimen without the infusion of human factor VIII.[337] Others have reported similar results with various combinations of prednisone, cyclophosphamide, and vincristine. The initial inhibitor titer may be an important prognostic factor in the treatment of these patients.

In one report, nine consecutive patients with a spontaneously acquired factor VIII autoantibody were treated with oral cyclophosphamide (100 to 200 mg/day) and prednisone (50 to 80 mg/day) until the inhibitor titer reached zero, followed by slowly decreasing doses.[338] All patients achieved a complete remission, with a median time of 3 weeks to resolution of all bleeding symptoms and a median time to undetectable factor VIII inhibitor of 12 weeks (range, 3 to 37 weeks). Two patients had a relapse as the immunosuppressive drugs were tapered, but the patients reattained a complete response with reinstitution of therapy. Initial titers of factor VIII inhibitor levels ranged from 2.5 to 1040 units (mean = 174), and the patients with higher inhibitor titers required a longer duration of therapy. However, in a more recent uncontrolled trial patients with spontaneously acquired factor VIII inhibitors from the United Kingdom,[273] prednisone alone (1 mg/kg) was compared to prednisone and oral cyclophosphamide (1–2 mg/kg), and there was no difference in remission rate (76% versus 78%) nor the time to remission (49 days vs. 39 days). In contrast a meta-analysis of 249 patients from 20 publications, none of which were controlled studies, found that 70% achieved remission with steroids alone and 89% with the combination of steroids and cyclophosphamide without any advantage in survival.[339] The results of these studies, along with the results of the prospective clinical trial reported by Green and associates,[334] strongly suggest but do not prove that the initial immunosuppressive treatment of choice is oral prednisone and cyclophosphamide; a preliminary dose of human factor VIII is unnecessary.

Immunosuppressive therapy should be continued as long as the inhibitor titer is decreasing because patients with high inhibitor titers respond more slowly than patients with low inhibitor titers. Patients with inhibitors who have high residual factor VIII levels in vitro (0.04 to 0.34 units/mL) respond well.[298]

If prednisone and/or cyclophosphamide are ineffective, then azathioprine in doses of 100 to 200 mg/day (or 2 mg/kg/day) has also proved effective; Green and Lechner[271] found 19 of 28 patients to respond completely. Söhngen and colleagues[340] reported five patients who responded to a combination of corticosteroids and azathioprine within 6 weeks of initiating therapy. Sallah[341] reported the use of 2-chlorodeoxyadenosine in six patients refractory to other immunosuppressive regimens. The dose used was 0.1 mg/kg/day for 7 days by continuous infusion; five patients received a single course, and one patient received two courses of therapy. All six of the patients had a significant decrease in inhibitor titer with the median time to reach nadir being 137 days. Although no patient attained a complete remission with a zero inhibitor titer, all of them had a significant increase in factor VIII level and no further bleeding. There have also been cases reported in which cyclosporine[342,343] or interferon-α[344] resulted in a complete response.

Any response to immunosuppressive therapy generally occurs within 6 to 12 weeks. If the titer has not decreased significantly in that period, therapy should be discontinued. Although most patients who obtain a complete response do not relapse, an occasional patient relapses early at the time of tapering or withdrawal of immunosuppressive therapy, and some patients relapse several months later.[273]

Spontaneously acquired factor VIII inhibitors respond to high-dose intravenous IgG.[345] In a prospective, multicenter study of high-dose intravenous IgG, 19 patients received 1 g/kg for 2 days or 400 mg/kg for 5 days, followed by periodic maintenance doses.[346] A rapid decline in inhibitor titer occurred in 3 to 4 days in two patients, and a gradual decline occurred in four other patients, with nadirs occurring several weeks to many months after starting therapy. Concurrent therapy with prednisone could have contributed to the response in two patients. The response rate was estimated to be between 25% and 37.5%. In another report[347] seven patients were treated with intravenous IgG 0.4 gm/kg/day × 5 days, plus prednisone 1 mg/kg/day for 14 days followed by tapering of the dose. Four patients had a complete response by day 21. In a more recent report where 31 patients received intravenous IgG in addition to immunosuppressive therapy, there was no evidence of additional efficacy of intravenous IgG in patients receiving prednisone or prednisone and cyclophosphamide.[273] The mechanism by which patients with inhibitors respond to intravenous IgG is unknown. However, IgG may have a short- and long-term immunosuppressive effect.[348,349] Anti-idiotypic antibodies are present in the IgG preparations;[350–352] the emergence of anti-idiotypic antibodies may be the explanation for the occasional spontaneous remission and some instances of remission induced by immunosuppressive agents.[351]

During the past few years, the administration of anti CD-20 monoclonal antibody, rituximab, has been used in the treatment of various autoimmune disorders including spontaneously acquired factor VIII inhibitors.[353,354] Up to this time more than 50 patients with spontaneously acquired factor VIII inhibitors have been reported who have received rituximab.[355,356] Treatment with rituximab resulted in an overall rate of complete remission of approximately 75% to 80% with no difference on whether the patients had or had not received immunosuppressive drugs previously or concomitantly. The median time to complete remission was approximately 8 weeks, but some were as short as 1 to 2 weeks.[355,356] In comparison to 44 patients treated with prednisone and cyclophosphamide reported in the literature, the complete remission rate was 84% with a median time to complete remission of approximately 6 weeks.[355] Two-thirds of patients who received rituximab remained in complete remission after 2 years as compared to 94% who received prednisone/cyclophosphamide. Most patients received 4 weekly doses of rituximab, and it was less efficacious in patients with higher antibody levels[355,357] or they took longer to respond.[356]

In light of the above data, rituximab is efficacious but less so than the efficacy of prednisone and cyclophosphamide. Suggested regimens include prednisone and cyclophosphamide alone or rituximab with prednisone and cyclophosphamide.

The great majority of patients (~75%–80%) eventually attain complete remission, and approximately 20% relapsed on withdrawal of immunosuppressive therapy.[273] Thus, these patients frequently require repeat or alternative immunosuppressive therapy.

ACQUIRED INHIBITORS OF VON WILLEBRAND FACTOR

Patients with von Willebrand disease may acquire inhibitors after plasma transfusion. Usually this occurs in patients with type 3 von Willebrand disease. An acquired syndrome similar to hereditary von Willebrand disease with onset later in life has been described.[358] More than 260 cases of the acquired syndrome have been reported, several reviews have been published,[359–362] and an international registry has been established.[363] The acquired syndrome occurs in patients with systemic autoimmune disease, B-cell lymphoproliferative disorders, myeloproliferative diseases, cardiovascular disorders, Wilms tumor, hypothyroidism, and a variety of other associations.[363] The most common associations are with lymphoproliferative and myeloproliferative disorders.[363] The clinical course in these patients is extremely variable from the new onset of mild bruising and mucous membrane bleeding to severe life-threatening bleeding.

Laboratory studies in these patients are extremely variable. Screening studies of hemostasis may show a prolonged bleeding time, an abnormal platelet function analysis (PFA)-100 test, or a prolonged PTT. Analysis of VWF usually reveals low ristocetin cofactor activity or collagen binding activity, low to normal VWF antigen level, and low to normal factor VIII activity. There is frequently an increased ratio of VWF antigen to ristocetin cofactor activity and, in approximately two-thirds of the cases, high-molecular-weight multimers are missing, as in type 2 von Willebrand disease,[364–368] and in one-third the multimers are proportionally decreased as in type 1 von Willebrand disease.[364] In a few patients, their plasma could be demonstrated to impair ristocetin cofactor activity of normal plasma.[360,364–370] In some, IgG antibodies could be demonstrated by a competitive ELISA assay.[371] In contrast, in most of the patients, inhibitor activity cannot usually be demonstrated by incubating the patient's plasma with normal plasma and measuring VWF activity, VWF antigen, or factor VIII.[360,364–370,372] Although factor VIII activity levels may be low, in only a rare case can inhibitor activity against factor VIII be demonstrated.[373] The bleeding time is variable and may be normal, similar to the variable bleeding times in patients with hereditary von Willebrand disease.

Because acquired von Willebrand disease is associated with a variety of different disorders and is characterized by variable clinical and laboratory features, many different pathophysiologic mechanisms leading to low VWF levels exist. Some patients develop IgG antibodies that can impair VWF activity,[360,364–368,370] whereas in other cases the antibody does not impair VWF activity but probably binds to a nonactive site on the molecule resulting in rapid clearance of the protein from the circulation.[369,374–376] In other patients, selective adsorption of VWF by tumor cells was demonstrated.[377–380] In two cases, the mechanism of adsorption was caused by aberrant expression of the glycoprotein Ib receptor on the surface of the tumor cell.[380,381] In a case of Waldenström macroglobulinemia, selective adsorption of VWF by monomeric IgM on the lymphocyte surface was demonstrated, but there was no impairment of VWF activity by the monoclonal IgM in plasma.[377]

In patients with myeloproliferative disorders, the mechanism is thought to be caused by increased adsorption of high-molecular-weight multimers by platelets or increased proteolysis of high-molecular-weight multimers.[363,382] Other mechanisms that have been implicated as a cause of the syndrome include decreased synthesis of VWF in hypothyroidism,[383] adsorption of VWF by hyaluronic acid in patients with Wilms tumor,[384] and increased proteolysis by ADAMTS 13 of high-molecular-weight multimers because of high plasma shear rates in the area of the cardiac defect in patients with congenital heart disease or aortic stenosis.[363,385] When these various underlying disorders are abrogated by appropriate therapy, the acquired syndrome disappears.

In addition, acquired von Willebrand syndrome has occasionally been described in association with the use of certain drugs, in other systemic disorders, and in a few cases where the patient had no underlying disease and was not taking any medications.[363]

Because there are a variety of pathophysiologic mechanisms that can cause acquired von Willebrand disease, many different therapeutic approaches have been tried with varying success. Frequently, successful treatment of the underlying disease or discontinuation of a drug results in disappearance of the syndrome. In patients with lymphoproliferative disorders or systemic autoimmune disease who are bleeding, attempts can be made to increase VWF with administration of DDAVP, cryoprecipitate, or VWF concentrate. The latter (eg, Humate-P, Alphanate, or Koate-HP) may result in a transient and blunted increase in VWF activity, VWF antigen, and factor VIII, such that effective hemostasis can be achieved.[363] Moreover, a bolus infusion followed by a continuous infusion of VWF concentrate may be more efficacious than periodic bolus infusion in the presence of an inhibitor.[386] Whenever administering DDAVP or transfusing VWF, efficacy should be measured by serial VWF and factor VIII assays. There are reports of patients with acute bleeding who failed to respond to DDAVP and VWF concentrate but responded to recombinant factor VIIa.[387,388] Several patients have been reported who responded to intravenous Ig (400 mg/kg × 5 days or 1 gm/kg × 2 days).[366,389–392] Although the response may be transient, in a few patients the response may last 2 to 3 weeks. After recurrence, repeat administration may result in repeated responses.[363,393] The patients who appear to respond to intravenous Ig are those patients with a demonstrable inhibitor in vitro and/or an associated IgG monoclonal gammopathy.[393] In patients in whom the syndrome is thought to be antibody mediated, it is conceptually possible that they respond to immunosuppressive therapy with or without the addition of rituximab, as has been reported in patients with autoantibodies to factor VIII.

ACQUIRED INHIBITORS OF FACTOR V

Rarely, factor V inhibitors occur in patients with hereditary factor V deficiency after transfusion.[394] However, most factor V inhibitors occur spontaneously in older, previously healthy patients in the absence of a common underlying disease.[394–402] The most common association seen in approximately two-thirds of the cases is a surgical procedure preceding the development of the inhibitor.[401] Other significant associations include blood transfusion, antibiotics, and malignant diseases.[401,402] Many of the cases that followed surgery were associated with the use of topical bovine thrombin or fibrin glue. Both of these substances contain a large amount of bovine thrombin and small amounts of bovine factor V. This can result in the production of antibovine thrombin antibodies or antibovine factor V antibodies that cross-react with human thrombin and factor V.[403,404] Bleeding is usually secondary to cross reactive antihuman factor V antibodies rather than to the antithrombin antibodies. Despite the various associations with factor V antibodies, in approximately 20% of cases, no associations can be identified,[401] and in these patients, true autoantibodies to factor V presumably are present.

The degree of clinical bleeding in these patients varies, in contrast to the uniformly severe bleeding in patients with factor VIII inhibitors. This extreme variability, from no clinical sequelae to fatal hemorrhage, can possibly be explained by the accessibility of platelet factor V to the antibody.[399,400] Studies by Nesheim and associates[399] on a patient with a factor V inhibitor suggest that platelet factor V is relatively protected from an antifactor V antibody in whole blood, even though plasma factor V is completely neutralized. Platelet factor V may play a key role in maintaining hemostatic competency in the presence of a factor V inhibitor. This hypothesis is supported by the efficacy of platelet concentrates in a factor V inhibitor patient.[397] Fresh frozen plasma failed to effect hemostasis, but on four separate occasions, effective hemostasis was achieved with platelet transfusions. Two other patients responded to platelet transfusions, but others were not responsive. In one recent report,[405] the amount of functional factor V was low in plasma and platelets, but the amount of factor V antigen was normal. It was subsequently shown that this was a result of the presence of factor V antigen-antibody complexes in plasma and the α granules of platelets. The course of the factor V inhibitor is short lived in most patients, disappearing within 10 weeks. Removal of the antibody by plasmapheresis or immunoadsorption resulted in decreased bleeding in some patients.[401] In one report, the administration of intravenous IgG in a patient with cross-reactive antibodies to bovine and human factor V resulted in rapid elimination of the human antibody without any effect on the titer of bovine antibody concomitant with abrogation of the hemorrhagic disorders.[403] Two other cases have been reported with a rapid response to intravenous Ig.[406] Whether steroids or other immunosuppressive agents influence the natural history of the inhibitors is unclear. The inhibitor may disappear with immunosuppressive therapy,[397] including one case with rituximab,[407] or it may disappear spontaneously without specific therapy.[394–396]

With rare exceptions the factor V inhibitors are polyclonal IgG or polyclonal IgM and IgG antibodies.[398,401,408] One study of 12 patients with factor V inhibitors showed that the IgG autoantibodies and the bovine protein-induced IgG alloantibodies immunoprecipitated the factor Va light chain, and in 9 cases the C2 domain.[408] Five of the antibodies inhibited binding of factor V to phospholipids, presumably interfering with the assembly of the prothrombinase complex.[408] Only the IgG antibodies in patients with excessive bleeding inhibited factor V in a prothrombinase assay.

The laboratory identification of a factor V inhibitor is based on coagulation assays. PTT and prothrombin time are prolonged, and normal plasma fails to correct these assays. These findings in the presence of a normal thrombin time should strongly suggest the presence of a factor V inhibitor although similar findings may also be seen in a few patients with the lupus anticoagulant.[394,398] In those patients who develop a factor V inhibitor after the use of topical thrombin, a prolonged thrombin time is a clue to the diagnosis, particularly when it is associated with a history of recent surgery. The demonstration that a mixture of the patient's plasma and normal plasma specifically lacks factor V clotting activity is required for a definitive diagnosis. The antibody can be quantitated by using an assay similar to the Bethesda assay used for the quantitation of factor VIII inhibitors.

A few patients with factor V antibodies have been reported with thrombotic manifestations rather than bleeding.[409–412] Two of the four cases had an autoimmune process in which lupus-like anticoagulant activity associated with anticardiolipin antibodies was present.[410,411,128] The third case was associated with Sjögren syndrome.[412] In three of four of these patients clotting times were prolonged, and the procoagulant function of factor V was also affected, but the patients did not have any bleeding manifestations. In the one patient, clotting times were not prolonged, but the antibody interfered with the interaction of activated protein C and factor V.[409]

ACQUIRED INHIBITORS OF FACTORS VII, IX, AND X AND PROTHROMBIN

Although prothrombin antibodies are common in patients with a lupus anticoagulant, most of the patients do not have hypoprothrombinemia (see box on Methods for Establishing the Presence of a Lupus Anticoagulant). However, in an occasional patient, the prothrombin level may be sufficiently depressed (<30%) to cause excessive bleeding. In these patients the antibody does not inactivate prothrombin activity in vitro but binds to a nonactive site on the molecule at the carboxy-terminal latent thrombin segment.[413] Consequently, the prothrombin antigen-antibody complex is rapidly cleared from the circulation, and the in-vitro laboratory findings are more consistent with a deficiency of prothrombin rather than an inhibitor of prothrombin activity (ie, the addition of normal plasma to patient plasma results in correction of the prolonged clotting time). Whether this antibody is similar to the prothrombin antibody associated with lupus anticoagulant activity (66% to 75% of patients with lupus anticoagulant) but without significant prothrombin deficiency is not clear.[100,131] It is conceptually possible that these antibodies are the same and that the rare instances of prothrombin deficiency associated with lupus anticoagulants stems from an excess of antibody or, alternatively, increased affinity of the antibodies for prothrombin, causing very rapid prothrombin antigen clearance and inadequate hepatic synthesis to compensate for the rapid clearance.

Another prothrombin antibody directed at an epitope at the amino terminal end of the prothrombin molecule has been described in a patient without an associated lupus anticoagulant. This antibody also did not neutralize prothrombin activity in vitro and resulted in an acquired prothrombin "deficiency" state.[413] Another patient with a prothrombin antibody without a lupus anticoagulant was recently described in a patient with lymphoma in whom the antibody disappeared after treatment of the lymphoma.[414]

Several patients have been reported whose plasma contained an antibody that reacted with thrombin.[415–421] Many of these patients bleed, but some are asymptomatic. The most common cause of spontaneously acquired inhibitors to thrombin are antibodies that develop in patients exposed to bovine topical thrombin or fibrin glue preparations during surgical procedures.[403,421–426] Thirty-five percent to 50% of these patients exposed to such preparations develop antibodies to bovine thrombin and/or bovine factor Va[403,423–426] that can cross-react with their human counterparts. Other patients appeared to spontaneously develop autoantibodies to thrombin,[415–420] and some of these patients also had systemic autoimmune disorders.[418–420] Coagulation tests in these patients are distinguished by a prolonged thrombin time that does not correct on mixing with normal plasma or protamine, and the reptilase time is normal. The PTT and prothrombin times are prolonged. In contrast, a rare patient may develop a thrombin inhibitor affecting the anticoagulant function of thrombin, causing thrombosis rather than bleeding.[427,428]

Five patients in whom IgG autoantibodies to factor VII developed had a prolonged prothrombin time but a normal PTT.[429–431] Weisdorf and coworkers[432] described a patient with severe aplastic anemia who had acquired factor VII deficiency. A factor VII-binding immunoglobulin in the patient's plasma bound to factor VII, resulting in rapid clearance of the immune complex. In one patient the inhibitor was characterized as an IgG antibody that bound to the light chain of factor VIIa within or near the Gla domain and inhibited the activity of the tissue factor-factor VIIa complex.[431] There also have been several patients with hereditary factor VII deficiency who have become alloimmunized after being treated with recombinant factor VIIa.[328]

Spontaneously acquired factor IX inhibitors are extremely rare.[433–437] The clinical setting in which these inhibitors occur is similar to that associated with the development of factor VIII inhibitors. Three were associated with SLE and two with the postpartum state. Those that have been characterized are polyclonal IgG antibodies. Treatment is similar to patients with factor VIII inhibitors using factor IX concentrates, activated prothrombin complex concentrates, and recombinant factor VIIa. Most seem to disappear within 1 to 7 months of onset, but whether immunosuppressive therapy alters the natural history is unknown.

Three documented patients with a factor X inhibitor have been reported.[438,439] These patients were elderly without underlying disease who had the sudden onset of a bleeding diathesis. In two of three cases, the inhibitor was characterized as IgG antibodies and disappeared spontaneously without specific therapy.

ACQUIRED INHIBITORS OF FACTORS XI AND XII

Inhibitors directed against factors XI or XII have been reported.[440–447] Some were detected in patients with hereditary factor XI deficiency after transfusions, whereas most occurred spontaneously in patients with SLE. Many of the latter patients also had low factor XII levels. When the latter are studied with dilution, phospholipid or platelet neutralization, and dilute Russell's viper venom time tests, the diagnosis of a lupus anticoagulant becomes evident. Zucker and colleagues[443] studied several patients on long-term chlorpromazine therapy in whom asymptomatic IgM inhibitors of the intrinsic phase of blood coagulation developed. The inhibitor resulted in decreased measurements of all the plasma clotting factors in the intrinsic pathway and was shown to interfere with the coagulant activity of contact product. Some of these patients also had antibodies to various components of the contact system, including high and low-molecular-weight kininogens and factor XII.[447] Except for those with hereditary factor XI deficiency, none of the patients in whom inhibitors to the contact system developed has had excessive bleeding.

ACQUIRED INHIBITORS THAT AFFECT FIBRIN STABILIZATION, FIBRINOGEN, OR FIBRIN POLYMERIZATION

The terminal phase of blood coagulation is characterized by the cleavage of fibrinopeptides A and B from fibrinogen, polymerization of fibrin monomers, and the covalent cross-linking of the α-and γ-chains of fibrin by factor XIIIa. Spontaneously acquired inhibitors of each of these reactions have been described.

Inhibitors of fibrinogen have been reported in patients with hereditary afibrinogenemia after transfusion.[448,449] Marciniak and Greenwood[449] reported a patient in whom a polyclonal IgG antibody developed that caused a delay in the release of fibrinopeptide A from normal fibrinogen reacting with thrombin, which retarded the onset of clot formation. This patient had a prolonged PTT, prothrombin time, thrombin time, and reptilase time. The isolated inhibitor prolonged the thrombin time of normal plasma.

A high incidence of prolonged plasma thrombin time has been observed in patients with SLE. Galanakis and coworkers[450] found that two such patients had monoclonal antibodies that reacted with different parts of fibrin and fibrinogen, delaying fibrin polymerization. Autoantibodies that inhibit fibrin monomer polymerization have developed in some patients.[451,452]

Although a variety of abnormalities of hemostasis are associated with monoclonal gammopathies,[453] isolated M proteins can interfere with the conversion of fibrinogen to fibrin monomer or with the aggregation of fibrin monomers into polymers.[453–455] Coleman and associates[455] provided indirect evidence that at least some M proteins act as antibodies because Fab fragments of IgG monoclonal proteins were more inhibiting than intact protein, the isolated chains, or the Fc fragments.

Spontaneous inhibitors of fibrin stabilization can lead to severe hemorrhagic complications, some fatal.[275,456] Of the approximate 32 reported patients, several developed the inhibitor while taking isoniazid or procainamide.[5] Three other patients had SLE.[5] Non–cross-linked fibrin clots can result from neutralization of factor XIII by (1) inhibition of activation of factor XIIIa; (2) inhibition of the transamidation function of factor XIIIa; or (3) interference with the cross-linking sites on the fibrinogen substrate. Therefore, a classification scheme for the various types of factor XIII inhibitors was based on the step of the reaction sequence that is inhibited. Type I inhibitors are directed against the activation of the factor XIII zymogen but do not interfere with transamidase activity.[457] Type II inhibitors impair the transamidase activity of factor XIIIa.[5] Type III inhibitors complex with the fibrin substrate and prevent its binding by factor XIIIa. A fourth type of inhibitor was reported in which the antibody inhibits factor XIII activity by binding to the fibrin-binding site on factor XIIIa.[458] This inhibitor was characterized as an IgG antibody and disappeared with immunosuppressive therapy. Another type of IgG antibody bound the inactive and thrombin-activated factor XIII but had much greater affinity for the activated zymogen and was specific for the A subunit of factor XIII.[5] Most of the inhibitors of fibrin stabilization are IgG antibodies and usually disappear with immunosuppressive therapy or cessation of the associated drug.[5] One patient responded to rituximab.[459] Acute bleeding can sometimes be controlled by transfusion of factor XIII concentrate or cryoprecipitate.[5]

HEPARIN-LIKE ANTICOAGULANTS

The development of spontaneously acquired heparin-like anticoagulants has been reported in patients with neoplasms or those undergoing suramin therapy for the treatment of adrenocortical carcinoma.[460–465]

Reports of heparin-like anticoagulants associated with neoplastic disorders[460,461,463–466] include cases of plasma cell malignancies and a severe hemorrhagic disorder.[460,463] Coagulation studies are characterized by a prolonged thrombin time that can be corrected by the addition of protamine sulfate, toluidine blue, or heparinase to the patient's plasma. All these inhibitors possess biochemical and physicochemical properties of glycosaminoglycans. One patient treated intravenously with protamine sulfate showed an improvement in his laboratory study results, as well as decreased bleeding.[463]

A complex coagulopathy was reported in three women receiving suramin for adrenocortical carcinoma.[464] The severe hepatocellular dysfunction that developed accounted for some of the coagulopathy. Each patient acquired a potent inhibitor to the thrombin time, which increased markedly during exacerbations of hepatic injury. Anticoagulant activity was eliminated in vitro by a combination of heparitinase and chondroitinase ABC, suggesting that the activity was mediated by heparan sulfate and dermatan sulfate. Because suramin inhibits enzymes that normally degrade glycosaminoglycans, hepatic injury was hypothesized to cause the release of glycosaminoglycans, which then accumulate because of failure of degradation.

SUGGESTED READINGS

Feinstein DI, Rapaport S: Acquired inhibitors of blood coagulation. Prog Hemost Thromb 1:75, 1972.

Feinstein D: Lupus anticoagulant, anticardiolipin antibodies, fetal loss, and systemic lupus erythematosus. Blood 80:859, 1992.

Giannakopoulos B, Passam F, Rahgozar S, et al: Current concepts on the pathogenesis of the antiphospholipid syndrome. Blood 109(2):422, 2007.

Lim W, Crowther MA, Eikelboom JW: Management of antiphospholipid antibody syndrome. JAMA, 295(9):1050, 2006.

Miyakis S, Lockshin MD, Atsumi T, et al: International consensus statement on an update of the classification criteria for definite antiphospholipid syndrome (APS). Thromb Haemost 4:295, 2006.

Sailer T, Zoghlami C, Kurz C, et al: Anti-β2-glycoprotein I antibodies are associated with pregnancy loss in women with the lupus anticoagulant. Thromb Haemost 95:796, 2006.

Shapiro SS, Thiagarajan P: Lupus anticoagulants. Prog Hemost Thromb 6:263, 1982.

Shapiro SS: The lupus anticoagulant/antiphospholipid syndrome. Annu Rev Med 47:533, 1996.

REFERENCES

For complete list of references log onto www.expertconsult.com

CHAPTER 132

DISSEMINATED INTRAVASCULAR COAGULATION

Howard A. Liebman and Ilene C. Weitz

Disseminated intravascular coagulation, frequently designated by its acronym DIC, is a pathologic syndrome arising from a heterogeneous group of medical disorders (Table 132–1). It is characterized by laboratory evidence of consumption and proteolytic degradation of hemostatic components. The clinical expression varies and may be manifested by laboratory abnormalities alone or in combination with hemorrhagic and thrombotic complications. Because of the variable clinical manifestations and heterogeneity of primary disorders associated with the development of DIC, the syndrome has been characterized under a number of designations, including *defibrination syndromes*, *consumptive coagulopathies*, or *consumptive thrombohemorrhagic disorders*.[1–12] Significant controversies exist in regard to the pathophysiology, diagnosis, and treatment of DIC. However, certain generally accepted clinical and laboratory observations regarding this syndrome can provide a model to assist the clinician in the diagnosis and therapy of these patients.

GENERAL PATHOGENESIS

Central to the pathogenesis of DIC is the unregulated and excessive generation of thrombin. This results in the consumption of coagulation factors that are the natural substrates of this protease, such as fibrinogen, factor V, and factor VIII. Thrombin, acting as a ligand, binds to thrombin receptors on platelets and endothelial cells[13,14] and is a potent agonist inducing platelet activation and aggregation.[15] Thrombin also induces endothelial cell release of tissue plasminogen activator (tPA).[16] In the presence of the newly formed fibrin monomer,[17] plasmin is formed from plasminogen. This results in an aggressive secondary fibrinolysis. Therefore, the clinical and laboratory manifestations of DIC result from generation of these two proteases, thrombin and plasmin. The generation of excess amounts of thrombin with relatively reduced expression of plasmin may result in large-vessel thrombosis or microvascular fibrin deposition leading to organ dysfunction and ischemic necrosis. Excessive thrombin generation with a vigorous secondary fibrinolysis may result in increased consumption of hemostatic components and bleeding. The bleeding and thrombotic manifestations of DIC are well documented in autopsy studies.[9,18–20]

INITIATION OF PHYSIOLOGIC AND PATHOLOGIC

Thrombin Generation

The physiologic formation of the hemostatic plug requires the localized and limited generation of thrombin at the site of vessel injury. DIC results from a failure of the mechanisms that limit the regulation of blood clotting and thrombin generation. This site-specific generation of thrombin is accomplished by a combination of regulatory mechanisms (Fig. 132–1). Tissue factor (TF) is expressed at the site of vessel injury. This is followed by the sequential proteolytic conversion of proenzymes to enzymes by a mechanism that involves the formation of macromolecular complexes of enzymes and cofactors on specific receptors on membrane surfaces.[21–25] The excessive generation of thrombin is limited by several natural inhibitory mechanisms. TF pathway inhibitor modulates the local effects of TF-factor VIIa expression.[26,27] The protease inhibitors, antithrombin and heparin cofactor II are bound to endothelial- and subendothelial-associated proteoglycans.[28,29] When bound to these endothelial-associated, heparin-like molecules, they become potent inhibitors of factor IXa, factor Xa, and thrombin. Thrombomodulin, a thrombin-specific receptor present on the surface of endothelial cells, binds thrombin and modifies its substrate specificity. Thrombin bound to thrombomodulin can no longer act as a procoagulant enzyme[30,31] and becomes the activator of protein C.[32] The resulting activated protein C, along with its cofactor, protein S, degrades factors Va and VIIIa, destroying their procoagulant activity.[33] The fibrin-platelet hemostatic plug is limited by a highly regulated fibrinolytic system. Plasmin, the mediator of fibrinolysis, is produced by the proteolysis of plasminogen by tPA. Plasmin rapidly degrades newly formed fibrin, reducing the size of the clot and initiating events that lead to vascular repair. DIC arises from an overwhelming of these regulatory mechanisms that leads to excessive generation of thrombin and a failure of the normal inhibitory pathways to prevent the systemic effects of the enzyme.

Although many disorders are associated with the development of DIC, initiation most often involves a common pathway (see Fig. 132–1). Initiation of DIC usually involves one or two mechanisms: mechanical tissue injury and endothelial and/or monocyte-macrophage activation and injury. Primary to both initiating pathways is the exposure of blood to excessive amounts of TF. Mechanical injury of organs rich in TF, such as brain or placenta, may result in fulminant consumption, as observed in gunshot wounds to the brain[34] or abruptio placentae.[35] A variation of tissue injury is observed in patients with malignancy-associated DIC. Malignant tissues disrupt the normal vascular hemostatic regulatory mechanisms and expose blood to tumor-associated procoagulant activity. Malignant tissues have been shown to express TF activity,[36–38] and some tumors have been shown to produce a cysteine protease capable of directly activating factor X.[36] Recent studies have shown an association between oncogenic transformation and the increased expression of tissue factor in the cancer cells.[37,38] An extreme example of malignancy-associated DIC is observed in patients with acute promyelocytic leukemia. The coagulopathy persists while the TF-rich leukemic blasts are present in blood and bone marrow.[39,40] The down-regulation of TF expression in the leukemic blasts by all-*trans*-retinoic acid, resulting in the correction of the coagulopathy, is an excellent demonstration of the importance of TF in the initiation of DIC in this disease.[41,42] Studies using sepsis or endotoxin models of DIC have clearly demonstrated the primary role of TF.[43–44] These studies have shown that the contact-phase proteins of the classic intrinsic pathway are not directly linked to the initiation of DIC and have only an ancillary role in the coagulopathy of sepsis.[45]

The intricate interactions between inflammation and coagulation have been elucidated using the model of bacterial endotoxin. Sepsis triggers a series of reactions that enhance cytokine expression and release. Levels of tumor necrosis factor (TNF), and interleukins (IL)-1, IL-6, and IL-8 are increased in response to endotoxin exposure. These cytokines, in turn, promote TF expression and thrombin generation, as well as suppression of fibrinolysis, tipping the balance in favor of the procoagulant state.[46–48] Endotoxin stimulates monocyte production of TNF. Levels of TNF increase quite early in sepsis, simultaneously with activation of coagulation. However, studies using inhibitory monoclonal antibodies to TNF show that activation

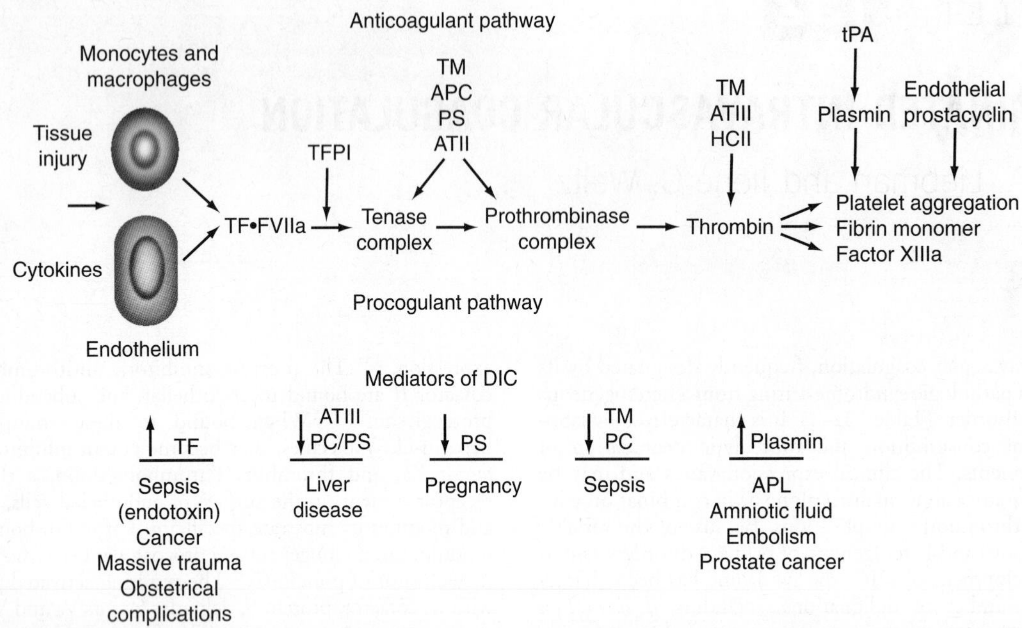

Figure 132–1 Regulatory pathways of hemostasis and pathophysiology of DIC. APC, activated protein C; APL, acute promyelocytic leukemia; ATIII, antithrombin III; HCII, heparin cofactor II; prothrombinase complex, membrane complex of factors Xa and Va and prothrombin; PS, protein S; tenase complex, membrane complex of factors IXa, VIIIa, and X; TF, tissue factor; TF · FVIIa, tissue factor–factor VIIa complex; TFPI, TF pathway inhibitor; TM, thrombomodulin; tPA, tissue plasminogen activator.

Table 132–1 Underlying Conditions Associated With Disseminated Intravascular Coagulation

Acute and Subacute
Infection
Gram-negative bacteria
Encapsulated gram-positive bacteria
Viruses (eg, varicella)
Obstetric complications
Abruptio placentae
Amniotic fluid embolism
Sepsis
Saline-induced abortion
Malignancies
Leukemia, lymphoma
Tissue injury
Burns
Heat stroke
Chronic
Malignancies
Solid tumors
Obstetric complications
Dead fetus syndrome
Localized intravascular coagulation
Aortic aneurysm
Hemangiomas (Kasabach-Merritt syndrome)
Advanced liver disease
LeVeen shunt
Fatty liver of pregnancy

of coagulation is not inhibited by abolishing TNF activity.[49] In contrast, IL-6 has a central role in endotoxin-induced activation of coagulation because the activation could be abolished by using inhibitory monoclonal antibodies to IL-6.[50]

Resting endothelium and monocytes do not express TF.[51] Endothelial cells activated by cytokines, such as IL-1, IL-6, and TNF, or injured by endotoxin express TF activity in vitro.[52,53] Viruses and other pathogens capable of infecting endothelium are also capable of inducing increased TF expression.[54] Subsequently, TF-factor VIIa and thrombin can activate monocyte and endothelial protease-activated receptors, inducing expression of IL-6/IL-8.[55,56] Clinical studies have found elevated levels of IL-6 and IL-8 in patients with recurrent venous thrombosis, suggesting a role for these cytokines in amplifying thrombin generation.[57,58] IL-8, in conjunction with monocyte chemotactic factor, upregulates endothelial leukocyte adhesion molecules.[59,60] In murine models, blockade of leukocyte/platelet adhesion molecules combined with anticoagulants provided superior protection against the development of DIC.[61] In these circumstances, even without mechanical injury or cell death, blood is exposed to a potent procoagulant surface. The coagulation inhibitors antithrombin III, heparin cofactor II, and thrombomodulin, although highly effective in regulating the localized generation of thrombin, are overwhelmed in DIC by the more potent systemic generation of thrombin and its precursor enzymes.

The endotoxin model of sepsis-induced DIC reveals significant effects on the anticoagulant and fibrinolytic system. In addition to enhanced endothelial procoagulant activity, there is a suppression of endothelial anticoagulant properties as reflected in decreased thrombomodulin expression.[44,55,62] Levels of protein C decrease significantly in patients with sepsis-induced DIC.[63,64] Therefore, the combination of low plasma levels of protein C and decreased endothelial expression of thrombomodulin necessary for protein C activation result in a significant depression of this important antithrombotic mechanism. The physiologic importance of this protein C anticoagulant pathway is further demonstrated by the inherited deficiencies of protein C or protein S, which are associated with microvascular thrombosis and intravascular consumption, as observed in purpura fulminans of the newborn or warfarin necrosis in deficient adults.[65–68] Endotoxin has also been shown to increase plasminogen activator inhibitor synthesis and secretion, resulting in suppression of tPA-mediated activation of fibrinolysis.[69,70] In addition, thrombin-activated platelets release large amounts of plasminogen activator inhibitor-1.[70]

Antithrombin levels decrease as a result of binding to the excess thrombin generated. Significant acquired deficiencies of antithrombin are rare but can be observed in cases of overwhelming acute DIC or cases complicated by significant hepatic dysfunction.[10,71–75] Antithrombin levels of less than 60% have been associated with an extremely high mortality rate.[74] The use of antithrombin and activated protein C concentrates has been associated with a decrease in the coagulopathy associated with severe sepsis. In vitro, antithrombin blocks the stimulatory effects of lipopolysaccharide on cultured endothelial cells and peripheral blood monocytes.[75] Induction of IL-6 and TF by lipopolysaccharide can also be blocked by antithrombin in a dose-dependent manner, independent of direct thrombin inhibition.[76] The infusion of activated protein C appears to protect against endotoxin-induced upregulation of TNF expression.[48,77] In clinical studies of patients with severe sepsis, activated protein C infusion was associated with a decrease in D-dimers and IL-6.[48] The impact of tissue factor pathway inhibitor (TFPI) in DIC associated with sepsis remains unclear. Increased, decreased, and normal levels of TFPI have been reported.[57,77]

Monocytes and neutrophils play an important ancillary role in the initiation of DIC. Monocytes activated by endotoxin or antibody-antigen complexes can express TF activity and assemble the prothrombinase complex on their membranes.[78,79] Activated monocytes also secrete the inflammatory cytokines, interleukin-1 and TNF,[80,81] which modulate endothelial procoagulant activity.[53,54]

Activated platelets expressing P-selectin also induce monocyte TF expression. Platelet-activating factor, another monocyte-derived cytokine, induces additional platelet activation and aggregation[82] and increases vascular permeability.[83] Activated neutrophils release a number of cellular enzymes that can injure endothelium and degrade subendothelial matrix.[84] Neutrophil elastase has been shown to degrade and inactivate a number of coagulation proteins and inhibitors, including factor V, factor VIII, antithrombin III, TFPI and plasminogen activator inhibitor.[85–89]

The variable clinical expressions of DIC result from this complex interaction of thrombin, plasmin, proteolytic inhibitors, platelets, endothelium, monocytes, and neutrophils. The underlying disorders that initiate DIC, such as sepsis, malignancy, or mechanical tissue injury, may trigger different hemostatic and cellular pathways for thrombin and plasmin generation, resulting in a clinical pathologic process that favors thrombosis or consumption with bleeding. The intensity and duration of hemostatic activation can result in a fulminant (acute), subacute, or chronic presentation. Fulminant DIC is usually characterized by coagulation factor consumption and bleeding. The chronic forms of DIC are more frequently characterized by thrombotic manifestations. However, in a significant number of cases, there are few or no clinical manifestations of DIC exclusive of the abnormal laboratory findings. Morbidity and mortality in these patients predominantly result from the underlying disease, and no specific treatment for the DIC is indicated.[90–93]

DIAGNOSIS OF DIC: CLINICAL AND LABORATORY FINDINGS

Clinical Features

The clinical manifestations of DIC are frequently obscured by the clinical features associated with the primary initiating illness (see Table 132–1). There is considerable variation in the frequency of specific clinical findings described in different case series, which probably reflects differences in the underlying primary disorders reported in each study.[7,9,10,91,92] Many of the clinical findings ascribed to DIC in early case series, such as adult respiratory distress syndrome (ARDS) or acute tubular necrosis, are probably a direct result of the primary illness, shock, and hypoperfusion. Their onset frequently has no direct relationship to the initiation of DIC and may precede its appearance. However, the microvascular thrombosis associated with DIC may aggravate multiorgan dysfunction, and less frequent pathologic features, such as pulmonary hemorrhage and renal cortical necrosis may be directly linked to the development of DIC.[7,9,10,18,20,91]

Bleeding is the predominant clinical manifestation observed in DIC and is reported in 70% to 90% of patients.[7,9,10,91,92] Cutaneous, gastrointestinal, genitourinary, and pulmonary bleeding, along with bleeding at surgical sites, are the most frequently reported. However, in earlier case series, the definition of DIC was based primarily on laboratory studies that clearly defined a patient population with severe consumption of hemostatic components, including fibrinogen and platelets. Studies that use laboratory criteria of DIC based primarily on markers of thrombin generation find many more cases of DIC without clinical evidence of bleeding than previously reported.[93,94,95]

Overt thromboembolic manifestations have been less frequently observed in DIC and have been reported in 10% to 40% of patients.[7,9,10,91,92] In patients with cancer, laboratory evidence of thrombin generation is frequently present without evidence of severe coagulation factor or platelet consumption.[94–100] However, activation of coagulation pathways in the patient with cancer usually results in thromboembolic manifestations.[98–100]

Table 132–2 Laboratory Diagnostic Studies for Disseminated Intravascular Coagulation

Laboratory Markers of Thrombin Generation
D-dimer
Protamine paracoagulation assay for fibrin monomer
Ethanol gel assay for fibrin monomer
Fibrinopeptide A
Prothrombin fragment 1.2
Thrombin–antithrombin complex
Screening assays for factor and platelet consumption
Prothrombin time
Partial thromboplastin time
Thrombin time
Quantitative fibrinogen
Platelet count
Ancillary tests
Fibrin/fibrinogen degradation products
Euglobulin or dilute whole-blood clot lysis
Antithrombin-III level
α_2-Antiplasmin level
Factor V level

Laboratory Features

Laboratory studies used in the diagnosis and evaluation of patients with DIC can be characterized as tests of thrombin and plasmin generation and screening tests for hemostatic function that delineate the severity of coagulation factor consumption (Table 132–2). Although abnormalities in the screening assays, such as the prothrombin time (PT), partial thromboplastin time (PTT), or platelet count may provide important corroborative evidence of hemostatic component consumption, the diagnosis of DIC should not be made without at least one positive test indicative of excessive thrombin generation. The two most readily available studies that document the excess activity of thrombin are immunoassays for D-dimers and the protamine paracoagulation assay for fibrin monomer.[96,101–106] D-dimers are the proteolytic by-products of plasmin degradation of cross-linked fibrin monomers. In contrast, to the older assays for fibrin/ fibrinogen degradation products (FDP), which do not distinguish between the plasmin degradation by-product of fibrin or fibrinogen, the formation of D-dimers requires prior formation of fibrin monomer, which is cross-linked by factor XIIIa. The formation of fibrin monomer and the generation of factor XIIIa from its zymogen require thrombin. When using the D-dimer assay as the only laboratory marker of thrombin generation, caution must be exercised in interpreting abnormal results in patients who have had recent surgery, bleeding into tissues, cirrhotic liver disease, or renal failure. In each of these clinical circumstances, D-dimers can be moderately elevated without DIC. Therefore, patients with D-dimer levels less than 2000 ng/mL should not be diagnosed as having DIC unless there is other corroborating evidence.[93,101,102,104]

The protamine paracoagulation test detects the presence of excess soluble fibrin monomer, which is associated with fibrinogen in plasma. The presence of fibrin monomer documents prior action of thrombin on fibrinogen. This assay can be particularly helpful in clinical circumstances when there may be other disorders that could contribute to elevations in D-dimers. However, the assay is difficult and is most reliable when the laboratory has extensive experience performing this assay. Additional assays of thrombin generation that have been used in the evaluation of patients with DIC include the ethanol gel assay for fibrin monomer,[105] immunoassays for fibrinopeptide A,[106] thrombin-antithrombin complexes,[107] and prothrombin fragment 1 · 2.[108] However, the routine clinical use of these assays is limited by their cost and complexity for simple and rapid laboratory screening. In addition, the latter three immunoassays have an excessive degree of sensitivity to thrombin generation, and positive results may not reflect clinically significant DIC.

Laboratory studies that delineate the severity of hemostatic component consumption in the patient with DIC include quantitative platelet counts and screening assays for plasma coagulation function. The screening tests include the PT, PTT, and thrombin time. Prolongations of the PT, PTT, and thrombin time assays result from the combined primary and secondary consumption of coagulation factors. Plasmin generated by secondary fibrinolysis results in the proteolytic degradation of factors, including fibrinogen and factors V, VIII, and XII. The intermediate plasmin degradation products of fibrin inhibit fibrin polymerization, which further contributes to the prolongations observed in these assays.[109] The results from these screening assays provide the information necessary for appropriate decisions regarding replacement treatment. These screening tests direct the clinician toward a diagnosis of acute DIC.

In five case studies of acute DIC, combining more than 900 patients, the most frequent laboratory abnormalities reported, in decreasing order of frequency, were thrombocytopenia, elevated fibrin degradation products, prolonged PT, prolonged thrombin time, prolonged PTT, and a low fibrinogen.[7,9,10,91,92] Although deficiencies of nearly every coagulation factor have been reported, acquired deficiencies of factor V and fibrinogen are the most frequently observed in patients with acute DIC. A fibrinogen less than 100 mg/dL, in the absence of severe liver disease, is invariably associated with acute DIC, usually associated with bleeding manifestations, and denotes a poor prognosis.[7,9,10]

In chronic DIC syndromes, the degree of clotting protein consumption may be limited and can be balanced by hepatic synthesis of coagulation factors, resulting in only minor abnormalities in the screening assays. Platelet counts may be at low normal levels and fibrinogen levels can be normal because hepatic synthesis of fibrinogen can be significantly upregulated by inflammatory cytokines.[110] In these circumstances, the presence of high levels of the markers of thrombin generation, in the appropriate clinical settings, may be sufficient to make the diagnosis of DIC.

Despite the presence of a significant secondary fibrinolysis, screening assays for increased fibrinolysis, such as the dilute whole-blood clot lysis test or euglobulin clot lysis test, usually give normal results in patients with DIC.[7,10] However, the use of these screening assays should be considered in clinical circumstances, such as DIC in association with severe liver disease,[111] in acute promyelocytic leukemia,[112,113] heat stroke,[114] amniotic fluid embolism,[115] or metastatic prostate carcinoma.[116] The clinician should be aware that there can be false-positive studies if these screening tests are performed in patients with fibrinogens less than 100 mg/dL.

The presence of thrombocytopenia, the most frequent laboratory abnormality observed in patients with DIC, should always direct the clinician to a review of the peripheral blood film. Fragmented red blood cells, although reported in patients with DIC, rarely constitute greater than 10% of the red cells.[10] However, in some cases of chronic DIC with elevated D-dimers but normal coagulation screening assay results, the presence of fragmented red cells may provide supportive evidence. In contrast, disorders, such as acute leukemia, sepsis, and thrombotic thrombocytopenic purpura can result in significant thrombocytopenia and a markedly abnormal blood film without laboratory evidence of DIC.

The diagnosis of DIC should never be made based solely on laboratory abnormalities but must include consideration for the underlying primary initiating illness and the patient's clinical presentation. Several scoring systems combining clinical and laboratory data have been devised to assist in the diagnosis and determination of prognosis of patients with DIC.[117,118,119,120] Proposed in 2001, the International Society of Thrombosist Haemostory (ISTH) scoring system uses a combination of risk assessment and simple, widely available coagulations assays. The scoring system appears to be both sensitive (93%) and specific (98%) in diagnosing patients with overt and nonovert DIC (Table 132–3).[117,118,120,121] The algorithm is similar to that used by the Japanese Ministry of Health Working group (JMHW).[119] Correlation with the Acute Physiology and Chronic Health Evaluation II (APACHE II), logistic organ dysfunction (LOD), and Sequential Organ Failure Assessment (SOFA) score have validated the usefulness of the ITSH scoring system.[122] The ISTH scoring system for DIC is only valid if the patient has a clinical syndrome that would lead to DIC.[117,118,120,122] A scoring system proposed by the Japanese Association of Acute Medicine (JAAM) expands on the JMHW by incorporating criteria for the systemic inflammatory response syndrome (SIRS), as well as the rate of decrease of the platelet count.[119] A recent prospective comparison of the algorithms used in the three scoring systems, the JAAM demonstrated a higher sensitivity rate (97%), but the specificity is unclear.[119,123] The prospective use of the ISTH scoring system is particularly useful in predicting 28-day mortality.[118,120,123] This may lead to earlier intervention and perhaps improvement in mortality.

Differential Diagnosis of Disseminated Intravascular Coagulation

A number of clinical disorders not associated with DIC can result in an acquired bleeding diathesis and significant laboratory hemostatic laboratory abnormalities. Thrombocytopenia can result from primary bone marrow failure; an infiltrative marrow process, such as leukemia; endothelial-mediated platelet activation, such as in vasculitis or thrombotic thrombocytopenic purpura; or immunologic destruction. A difficult clinical problem occurs in the patient with sepsis.[124,125] Sepsis without DIC can be associated with a variable degree of thrombocytopenia; however, sepsis with platelet counts less than 50,000 is most often associated with DIC.[124,125]

A rare syndrome of primary fibrinolysis occurs with the independent generation of plasmin without concomitant thrombin generation.[126–130] Such patients can have low fibrinogen, and elevated fibrin degradation products. In addition, patients with liver disease and primary fibrinolysis with portal hypertension may have thrombocytopenia secondary to splenic sequestration. Therefore, the differential diagnosis in these patients may prove difficult. In these patients, the dilute whole-blood clot lysis and euglobulin clot lysis tests are significantly shortened, and the protamine paracoagulation assay is negative for fibrin monomer. Despite significantly elevated fibrin degradation products, the D-dimer assay results are normal or only minimally elevated.[130]

CLINICAL PRESENTATIONS

Acute and Subacute DIC

Infection

Bacterial sepsis is a common cause of acute DIC. Thrombin generation results from bacterial or endotoxin-associated endothelial cell perturbation and monocyte activation, leading to enhanced TF activity and inflammatory cytokine secretion.[22,43,44,53,54,62] Gram-negative

Table 132–3 ISTH Scoring System for Disseminated Intravascular Coagulation

Overt DIC			
Risk assessment: Does the patient have an underlying disorder known to be associated with DIC (see Table 132–1)? Score =			
Yes = 2; No = 1			
If yes proceed. If no, do not use the algorithm. Order global coagulation test—platelet count, PT, fibrinogen soluble fibrin monomers of fibrin degradation products.			
Score global coagulation test results as follows:			
Platelet count	>100 × 10⁹/L = 0 <100 × 10⁹/L = 1 <50 × 10⁹/L = 2		Score =
Fibrin related marker	No increase = 0 Moderate increase = 2 Strong increase = 3		Score =
Prolongation of prothrombin time	<3 seconds = 0 >3 seconds <6 seconds = 1 >6 seconds = 2		Score =
Fibrinogen level	>1.0 gram/L = 0 <1.0 gram/L = 1		Score =
Calculate score: total score = 5. If ≥5, compatible with overt DIC: Repeat scoring daily.			
If <5, suggestive of nonovert DIC: Repeat in 1 to 2 days.			
Nonovert DIC			
1. Risk assessment: Does the patient have an underlying condition associated with DIC (see Table 132–1)? Score =			
Yes = 2; No = 0			
If yes, proceed. If no, do not use the algorithm.			
Major Criteria			
Platelet count	>100 × 10⁹/L = 0 <100 × 10⁹/L = 1	+ increasing count = −1 stable count = 0 decreasing count = 1	Score =
PT prolongation	<3 seconds = 0 >3 seconds = 1	+ increasing value = 1 stable value = 0 decreasing value = −1	Score =
Soluble fibrin or FDP	Normal = 0 Raised = 1	+ increasing value = 1 stable value = 0 decreasing value = −1	Score =
Specific Criteria			
Antithrombin		Normal = −1 Low = 1	Score =
Protein C		Normal = −1 Low = 1	Score =
TAT-complexes		Normal = −1 High = −1	Score =
4. Calculate score: Total score =			

DIC, disseminated intravascular coagulation; FDP, fibrin/fibrinogen degradation products; PT, prothrombin time; TAT, thrombin-antithrombin.
From reference 117.

organisms are more commonly associated with sepsis and DIC, although cases are associated with gram-positive sepsis.[124,125] Infection with viruses, such as varicella, rubella, rubeola, and influenza, along with intracellular pathogens, such as *Mycobacterium tuberculosis*, can also lead to DIC through enhanced endothelial and monocyte TF activity.[131–135] Fungal infections and malaria have similarly been complicated by DIC.[136–138]

There is a wide range of clinical manifestations of sepsis-associated DIC. Many cases are characterized by laboratory changes without bleeding or clinical evidence of microthrombus formation. Examples of clinical entities at the other end of the spectrum include Waterhouse-Friderichsen syndrome and purpura fulminans. The Waterhouse-Friderichsen syndrome is rare and is most often seen in association with fulminant meningococcal sepsis.[139,140] It is characterized by widespread intravascular fibrin deposition and platelet thrombi that lead to microvascular obstruction of vital organs, along with hemorrhagic necrosis of the adrenal glands. The latter leads to significant, often irreversible shock associated with a high mortality rate. Virtually any gram-negative organism can cause DIC. The gram-positive bacterial infections associated with DIC often involve encapsulated organisms, such as pneumococci. The overwhelming infection observed in those with diminished circulatory clearance because of functional or anatomic asplenia is frequently implicated.[141] Clostridial species are also associated with severe DIC because of septic abortion, which carries a very high mortality rate.[142,143]

Purpura Fulminans

Purpura fulminans is a rare, severe skin disorder associated with DIC that primarily affects children and infants. Extensive areas of skin develop blue-black hemorrhagic necrosis, and biopsy typically reveals small-vessel microthrombi and vasculitis. Distribution of necrotic areas typically depends on the clinical setting. Patients are acutely ill with fever and hemorrhage from multiple sites, are hypotensive, and manifest typical laboratory signs of DIC.[144,145] The pathogenesis of purpura fulminans is unknown, but histologic findings have been likened to the animal model of consumptive coagulopathy, the local Shwartzman reaction.[144] It has also been suggested that the development of purpura fulminans in meningococcemia may result from acquired defects in the protein C pathway because similar lesions are seen in two other protein C deficiency states, namely, neonatal purpura fulminans and warfarin-induced skin necrosis.[145–148]

Purpura fulminans occurs in three clinical settings.[148] In acute sepsis-associated or secondary purpura fulminans, the initial presentation is one of overwhelming infection that is most commonly meningococcemia but has been reported with many other gram-positive and gram-negative organisms.[147,149,150] Patients are hypotensive with reduced peripheral perfusion contributing to skin necrosis on distal extremities; alternatively, skin necrosis can occur in a patchy distribution.[150–158] Idiopathic purpura fulminans can manifest within 10 days of an antecedent illness, most commonly scarlet fever and varicella in children. Most skin lesions are localized to the breasts or lower half of the body. Third, purpura fulminans can be seen in association with homozygous protein C deficiency in affected neonates, in whom massive intravascular thrombosis and abdominal wall gangrene can also develop.[65–68,155] Acquired inhibitors of the protein C pathway can also be associated with this presentation.[156] Patients with warfarin-induced skin necrosis may present with a similar but usually less severe form of purpura fulminans and warrant consideration of protein C or protein S deficiency.[72,157,158] The mortality rate has recently been significantly reduced in purpura fulminans, largely because of more widespread use of therapeutic heparinization in these patients and aggressive transfusion support factor replacement.[145,146,159]

Obstetric Complications

Pregnancy predisposes patients to DIC through the generation of a hypercoagulable state manifested by increased levels of most coagulation factors along with reduced fibrinolytic activity because of decreased tPA production and increased plasmin activator inhibitor levels.[160,161] Overt clinical DIC manifestations occur when these baseline conditions are complemented by the occurrence of any of a number of acute obstetric complications that lead to the release of TF or endothelial cell perturbation, followed by consumption of clotting factors and enhanced fibrinolysis.

The manifestations of DIC associated with obstetric complications are varied, with different grades of severity noted depending on the degree of hypofibrinogenemia and depletion of other clotting factors seen in each case. Because of this variation and baseline pregnancy-associated coagulation abnormalities, it is prudent to consider serial assessment of coagulation parameters when DIC is suspected to detect progressive alterations over time. Similarly, the coagulopathy may be localized to the uterus or disseminated through the blood.

Abruptio placentae, or placental detachment, has a wide range of clinical presentations—from incidental detection on pathologic examination of the placenta, to vaginal bleeding, to pronounced DIC with accompanying shock, bleeding, severe abdominal pain because of uterine contractions, and fetal death.[161,162] The exact causes of placental abruption, outside of trauma, and the subsequent processes leading to DIC remain unclear. Placenta is rich in TF activity, which likely is an important component of the DIC pathophysiologic process.[160,161] Hypofibrinogenemia has been documented in 38% of abruptio placentae cases, which implies that potentially serious and life-threatening DIC is present in a significant number of patients.[32]

Amniotic fluid embolism is a rare, usually fatal catastrophe occurring in 1 in 8000 to 1 in 80,000 deliveries. Amniotic fluid is introduced into the circulation of multiparous, postmature women with large-for-date fetuses and in those undergoing long and vigorous labor after induction.[161–165] DIC is triggered by amniotic fluid TF and an activator of factor X.[161–165] The extensive occlusion of the pulmonary arteries that causes sudden dyspnea, cor pulmonale, shock, and seizures is a result of blockage with fetal debris and meconium. This, in turn, enhances local platelet-fibrin thrombus formation. There can be secondary fibrinolysis, further contributing to defibrillation and bleeding. This is followed after a latent period of up to 3 hours by severe bleeding in 37% of cases.[166] The mortality rate associated with this condition, primarily caused by respiratory failure, is greater than 80%.[164] As with abruptio placentae, the pathogenetic mechanism for the clinical manifestations is unclear. Because of the rapid course of this complication and its infrequency, specific treatment modalities, such as heparin and fibrinolysis inhibitors have not been adequately assessed but may be considered in individual cases. Red cell and coagulation factor replacement therapy warrants consideration in patients with active bleeding, along with pulmonary and hemodynamic support.

Sepsis during pregnancy is often caused by gram-negative bacteria and *Clostridium* species, with the patient being particularly susceptible to DIC under these circumstances. Septic abortions are often associated with severe DIC, accompanied by endotoxin-mediated shock and a high mortality rate.[166] Virtually any organism can be associated with septic abortion. In addition, saline-induced abortion during the second trimester without sepsis also has a clear association with hypofibrinogenemia, thrombocytopenia, and increased fibrin degradation products.[167,168]

Malignancies

Cancer can be associated with acute or chronic DIC, depending primarily on the type of cancer. Malignancy-associated chronic DIC associated with solid tumors is reviewed later in the chapter, whereas acute DIC associated with leukemia is discussed here. DIC has been associated with acute myelocytic and lymphocytic leukemia, chronic myeloid and myelomonocytic leukemia, hairy cell leukemia, and angioimmunoblastic lymphadenopathy.[169–180] Among these diagnostic entities, acute promyelocytic leukemia is most commonly associated with life-threatening hemorrhage secondary to DIC and other hemostatic abnormalities.

The pathogenesis of DIC associated with acute promyelocytic leukemia has remained controversial; consequently, the optimal therapeutic approach associated with this condition remains unclear. Leukemic cells from patients with acute promyelocytic leukemia have been found to harbor TF, a factor X-activating protease, and to produce IL-1.[169–171,176,181,182] Increased levels of prothrombin fragment 1·2 and thrombin-antithrombin III complexes have also been described in these patients and document the excessive generation of thrombin in this leukemia.[183]

Investigators have also provided evidence for primary fibrinogenolysis as a contributing factor associated with serious bleeding seen in patients with acute promyelocytic leukemia. In this respect, urokinase-type plasminogen activator and tPA have been found in acute promyelocytic leukemia cells along with reduced plasma activity of plasminogen activator inhibitor and reduced α_2-antiplasmin plasma levels.[109,184–193] It is likely that DIC and primary fibrinogenolysis contribute to bleeding in the patient with acute promyelocytic leukemia.

Although bleeding predominates in acute promyelocytic leukemia, thromboembolic complications have been noted in up to 5% of patients and 15% to 25% of autopsy results.[192–195] One study suggested that acute promyelocytic leukemia cells from a patient with coagulopathy did not, in fact, have procoagulant activity, but rather were capable of elaborating IL-1 that induced endothelial TF activity when mixed with endothelial cells.[190]

Acute promyelocytic leukemia-associated bleeding as a result of DIC is further exacerbated by thrombocytopenia because of marrow suppression. Once treatment is initiated, subclinical DIC often becomes clinically apparent because of chemotherapy-induced acute promyelocytic leukemia cell lysis.[195] The incidence of coagulopathy- and hemorrhage-related mortality associated with acute promyelocytic leukemia-has significantly decreased since the introduction of the differentiating agent all-*trans*-retinoic acid into induction regimens, with bleeding frequently abating within 48 hours of treatment initiation.[38,195]

Tissue Injury, Burns, and Heat Stroke

Extensive trauma and burns are often associated with localized and disseminated intravascular coagulation. This is particularly true if there is a component of head injury associated with multiple trauma because brain parenchyma is rich in TF. In this respect, laboratory-based "DIC scores" have been shown to have prognostic value in patients with head injury.[196–197] Studies have demonstrated a high mortality rate when head injuries are accompanied by bleeding and laboratory evidence of DIC, along with a correlation between time to treatment after trauma and the development and extent of DIC.[197–199]

Extensive exposure of circulating blood to TF is probably the most prevalent causative factor in trauma-associated DIC. Other possible contributions to this clinical picture may relate to dilutional coagulopathy caused by blood loss or replacement with crystalloid solutions and packed red cells alone; ischemic or trauma-associated hepatic dysfunction with reduced clotting factor and natural inhibitor synthesis; and ARDS.

Massive trauma is often accompanied by ARDS, to which hypotension followed by aggressive fluid replacement contribute. Obstruction of the pulmonary circulation secondary to multiple thrombi may also contribute to ARDS.[200,201] One study noted that among 30 patients with ARDS, 7 had evidence of additional thrombotic microangiopathy in the skin and kidneys, whereas an additional 12 had thrombocytopenia, and 4 had pulmonary vessel fibrin deposition on postmortem examination.[201]

Serious trauma cases involving multiple fractures, usually (but not always) can lead to fat embolism within the first 48 hours.[202,203] This is associated with respiratory distress and neurologic impairment secondary to marrow fat emboli from associated fractures. If the pulmonary picture is complicated by ARDS, laboratory evidence of DIC may also be present because of endothelial perturbation, TF expression, and inhibition of fibrinolysis.[203]

Burns can be associated with DIC through release into the circulation of TF from damaged tissues expressing TF, often with associated hypovolemic shock and infection, which occur later in the clinical course. In addition to DIC, significant local consumption of clotting factors has also been associated with burns.[204]

DIC and primary fibrinogenolysis have been demonstrated in association with heat stroke, a syndrome defined as a body temperature greater than 42° C (107.6°F) caused by collapse of thermoregulatory mechanisms.[205,206] Pathophysiologic mechanisms associated with the disorder include TF expression from damaged tissues and endothelial cell perturbation.[207] Extensive fibrin deposition with subsequent increased release of plasminogen activators and secondary fibrinolysis has been associated with the generalized bleeding and multiorgan failure accompanying fatal cases of heat stroke.[208]

CHRONIC DIC

Malignancies

The association between solid tumors and thrombotic and bleeding symptoms was initially described by Trousseau in 1865. *Trousseau syndrome* refers to spontaneous recurrent or migratory venous thrombosis or arterial emboli because of nonbacterial thrombotic endocarditis, or both, occurring in the setting of malignancy.[209] There is a spectrum of thrombohemorrhagic diagnostic entities seen in association with solid tumors, including low-grade DIC, venous thromboembolic disease, primary fibrinogenolysis, microangiopathic hemolytic anemia, and nonthrombotic valvular endocarditis.[210] These different disorders can present singly or multiply at any location and with any degree of acuteness or chronicity.

DIC associated with solid tumors demonstrates pathophysiologic mechanisms similar to those of the DIC seen with acute promyelocytic leukemia. These include TF secreted by tumor cells and activated monocytes.[211] A factor X-activating cysteine protease has been described in human carcinoma tissue.[36,37] Tumor cells or media conditioned by these cells induce platelet aggregation in vitro and in vivo.[212]

In a retrospective study of 1117 patients with solid tumors, a clinical and laboratory diagnosis of DIC could be made in 76 (6.8%) patients.[214] In multivariate analysis, older patients, male patients, patients with advanced-stage tumors, and patients with breast cancer were statistically more likely to develop DIC.[214] Chronic DIC is classically associated with thrombosis. Among the many studies done in the area of thrombosis and bleeding in association with solid tumors, one group documented deep venous thrombosis in 113 of 182 (62%) patients with cancer. Ninety-six of the 182 (53%) manifested migratory thrombophlebitis; 41 (23%) demonstrated nonbacterial thrombotic endocarditis, a disorder classically associated with mucin-producing carcinomas; and 75 (41%) had bleeding manifestations.[215]

Classic laboratory findings associated with chronic DIC and solid tumors include thrombocytopenia and circulating fibrin degradation products. Hypofibrinogenemia also occurs but is less common. Microangiopathic hemolytic anemia may occur in the absence of other DIC laboratory abnormalities, usually in association with disseminated mucin-secreting adenocarcinoma. Laboratory manifestations of increased thrombin generation are seen in patients with solid tumors and may not be accompanied by clinical thrombosis or bleeding.

Primary fibrinogenolysis is primarily seen in patients with prostate cancer and acute promyelocytic leukemia. These tumors are capable of producing activators of plasminogen and thrombin.[115,216] Biopsy of prostate tumors is sometimes accompanied by prolonged postoperative bleeding as a result of this phenomenon, and hemorrhagic manifestations can dominate the clinical picture.[217]

Dead Fetus Syndrome

The dead fetus syndrome occurs several weeks after intrauterine fetal death and can be accompanied by DIC.[218,219] The clinical syndrome is usually one of insidious-onset DIC mediated by TF from the placenta or dead fetus entering the maternal circulation over the ensuing days, eventually causing bleeding. Serial laboratory monitoring of the mother after diagnosis of intrauterine fetal death is warranted to detect possible progressive coagulopathy; in this event, immediate evacuation of uterine contents is indicated.

Localized Intravascular Coagulation

Aortic Aneurysm

Extensive aortic aneurysms have been associated with significant laboratory abnormalities and bleeding secondary to platelet and fibrinogen consumption.[220] These complications are characteristically associated with extensions and enlargements of the dissecting aneurysm, which are often accompanied by sudden onset of severe pain. In one series of patients with aortic aneurysms, 40% had chronically elevated levels of fibrin split products, with 4% showing evidence of significant bleeding and laboratory findings of DIC.[220]

Hemangiomas

Kasabach and Merritt were the first to report localized intravascular coagulation in association with hemangiomas.[221] These are usually benign tumors seen mostly in infants and children that typically enlarge over time. They are associated with consumption of platelets and fibrinogen as demonstrated by radiolabeling studies showing intravascular clotting and excessive fibrinogenolysis (the latter caused by tPA release from abnormal endothelium of tumor vessels).[222–225] Microangiopathic hemolytic anemia has also been observed in this setting along with laboratory evidence of DIC.[225,226] Clinical DIC and emboli to other organs, however, usually are not seen in association with hemangiomas. Severe bleeding is normally noted only after surgery or other invasive procedures associated with the hemangioma.[226]

Liver Disease and DIC

Patients with advanced liver disease are prone to a plethora of hemostatic and thrombotic derangements that are often very difficult to classify and successfully manage. Alterations in hepatic synthesis and hepatic and renal clearance of activated coagulation, fibrinolytic, and natural inhibitor proteins, along with the thrombocytopenia and the deranged hemodynamics typically seen in this patient population, collectively contribute to the difficulties encountered.

In those with advanced or acute, severe liver disease, the clinician may expect to find decreased hepatic synthesis of most coagulation proteins, protein C, protein S, antithrombin III, and plasminogen, along with α_2-antiplasmin. The liver also demonstrates defective clearance of activated clotting proteins.[227,228] Portal hypertension leads to splenomegaly with enhanced platelet sequestration and thrombocytopenia.

Given these circumstances, the issue of whether DIC is directly associated with liver disease, as opposed to the observation that these patients may simply be more sensitive to DIC, is an unsettled one. Experimental observations suggest the existence of an association[229–235] or support the hypothesis that these hemostatic derangements may stem from disorders other than DIC.[236–239]

As is the case with the pregnancy-associated disorders, the diagnosis of DIC in patients with liver disease and generalized bleeding not caused by a local source is most readily appreciated by following serial hemostatic parameters and noting a significant reduction in these values over a short period of time. If available, tests reflecting thrombin generation, such as the protamine paracoagulation assay, the prothrombin fragment 1·2 or thrombin-antithrombin III complex levels, along with D-dimer levels, can also contribute to establishing the diagnosis.

Disseminated intravascular coagulation is also seen after the placement of peritoneovenous (LeVeen) shunts for complications associated with massive ascites. The incidence is variously quoted in different studies as ranging from 3% to 91%, and may depend on whether the primary disease is peritoneal or hepatic in origin.[240–246] Ascitic fluid possesses TF activity in association with monocytes and thrombin activity, which likely contribute to the DIC.[244,246] Clamping the shunt is the only effective treatment in severe cases because heparin and antithrombin III concentrates have not proved efficacious.[245]

Fatty liver of pregnancy has also been associated with DIC on the basis of labor-induced protein factor and platelet consumption in the presence of decreased synthesis of the clotting factors and natural inhibitors.[247] The clinical and laboratory features have been attributed to low plasma antithrombin III levels, and patients have responded to antithrombin III concentrate.[248]

TREATMENT OF DIC

General Measures and Replacement Therapy

Given the heterogeneity of the underlying disorders with which DIC is associated, the difficulties often encountered with determining the extent of consumption of clotting factors and fibrinogenolysis in each case, and the relative lack of well-controlled studies of treatment of homogeneous subgroups with DIC, many aspects of treatment of DIC are controversial. Part of the problem resides with the fact that studies are very difficult to perform in view of the variety of pathophysiologic triggers and clinical presentations associated with DIC. DIC is one disorder in which management has to be individualized, with careful attention to variables, such as the initiating illness and the presence of bleeding or thrombosis.

The cornerstones of management of DIC include aggressive basic support measures, paying close attention to circulatory volume status, gas exchange, and electrolyte balance, along with prompt, vigorous treatment of the underlying cause of the DIC. This includes, for example, intravenous antibiotics for gram-negative septicemia, prompt uterine evacuation for abruptio placentae, and restoration of hemodynamic stability for hypovolemic shock. The other management components of the disorder include determining whether replacement of depleted platelets or clotting factors is necessary and whether attempted abrogation of the DIC with heparin or natural inhibitors should be considered.

The idea that blood replacement therapy may be "fueling the fire" of DIC has never been proved (see box on Replacement Therapy for DIC). Transfusion of platelets, cryoprecipitate, and fresh frozen plasma should be reserved for those with clear laboratory evidence of DIC and bleeding or a pending invasive procedure. It is typically most effective in those with very low platelet and fibrinogen levels in whom DIC is self-limited or concluded.

Patients with head injury-associated brain tissue destruction are particularly prone to acute, limited defibrination (hypofibrinogenemia, elevated levels of serum fibrinogen-related or fibrin-related split products, and low levels of factors V and VIII or platelets), in which laboratory abnormalities often return toward normal within hours.[31] These patients benefit from rapid, optimal correction of hemostatic deficiencies to minimize the neurologic consequences of intracranial bleeding, whereas heparin therapy to prevent ongoing intravascular coagulation is not helpful because of the associated intracranial bleeding risk.

Platelets should ideally be maintained at more than 20 to 30 × 10^9/L in a bleeding patient, whereas those who are undergoing procedures or who have concurrent functional impairment or significant blood loss should have higher counts. Cryoprecipitate should be given to maintain plasma fibrinogen greater than 100 mg/dL, whereas fresh frozen plasma is indicated to correct a prolonged PT and PTT in appropriate clinical circumstances. To determine the efficacy of transfusion, platelet and fibrinogen levels should be checked 30 to 60 minutes after the transfusion and every 6 hours after that. Replacement therapy may be required every 8 hours while the underlying cause of the DIC is being addressed. Transfusions can be discontinued when the coagulation parameters are almost or fully normalized and symptoms have abated. If laboratory parameters fail to improve with transfusions because of DIC-associated bleeding, a concurrent heparin infusion may warrant consideration.

The Role of Heparin in DIC Management

Heparin should be considered in the management of DIC if (1) a patient has strong clinical and laboratory evidence of DIC and thromboembolic manifestations predominate (eg, purpura fulminans, dead fetus syndrome before induction, aortic aneurysm before

Replacement Therapy for DIC

The symptoms and abnormal laboratory findings associated with DIC are most readily addressed through the prompt recognition and treatment of the underlying disorder. Until the underlying cause can be definitively managed, blood product replacement therapy warrants consideration in the patient with significant bleeding or a planned procedure and coagulation parameters compatible with DIC. Replacement folate and vitamin K therapy also warrant consideration in any patient with prolonged DIC.

Platelet transfusions should be considered to maintain the count greater than 20 to 30 × 10^9/L in a bleeding patient, although aiming for higher values if concurrent functional impairment is present, a procedure is planned, or blood loss is significant. DIC-associated thrombocytopenia does not usually reach levels of 20 × 10^9/L, without concurrent contributing factors, such as sepsis. One unit of donor platelets is expected to contain at least 5.5 × 10^9 platelets and increases the count 6 to 8 × 10^9/L, assuming normal splenic pooling. The platelet count should be repeated 10 to 60 minutes after the first transfusion to confirm the expected increment, and every 6 hours after that. Poor postplatelet transfusion increments are often seen in consumptive thrombocytopenia, making transfusion support difficult under these circumstances.

Cryoprecipitate administration is considered in a symptomatic patient to maintain plasma fibrinogen more than 100 mg/dL. The fibrinogen content of each cryoprecipitate unit varies from 100 to 250 mg, depending on variable storage volumes and pooling methods. From 1 to 4 units/10 kg can be given, with the postinfusion increment checked 30 to 60 minutes later and followed by repeat determinations every 6 hours.[249]

Fresh frozen plasma is given if significant DIC-associated bleeding is accompanied by a prolonged PT and PTT. The aim is to reduce the PT, with the target in each case dependent on the nature and extent of bleeding, the presence and extent of coexisting hemostatic defects, and whether a procedure is planned and its attendant bleeding risk. This is accomplished by administration of 10 to 15 mL/kg of plasma.[249] Each milliliter of plasma contains 0.7 to 1 unit of activity of each clotting factor and 1 to 2 mg of fibrinogen, so an alternative formula to 10 to 15 mL/kg incorporates estimated plasma volume, desired factor level increment, and the half-life of the factor being replaced into the equation. The PT and PTT should be checked every 6 hours and plasma given as needed based on the patient's clinical response. Depending on clinical circumstances, bleeding patients with DIC given plasma transfusions can exhibit poor clinical and laboratory responses, particularly if advanced liver disease with coexistent diminished clotting factor synthesis and altered hemodynamics complicate the picture.

surgery); or (2) intensive blood replacement therapy fails to alleviate excessive bleeding and increase the level of coagulation proteins. These circumstances notwithstanding, it is important to consider that heparin is less likely to lead to clinical improvement in DIC once it is established and ongoing, which is usually the case by the time it is diagnosed. Heparin is also capable of exacerbating DIC-associated bleeding in these populations and should be used very cautiously. For these reasons, heparin usually has a limited role, if any, in acute DIC.

In chronic DIC associated with solid tumors, the dead fetus syndrome, or hemangiomas, continuous heparin infusion without a loading bolus can be given with blood products if the clinical picture warrants treatment (eg, deteriorating coagulation parameters in dead fetus syndrome, thrombosis, or before chemotherapy). Patients with solid tumors can be given long-term, adjusted-dose subcutaneous unfractionated heparin or low-molecular-weight heparin rather than

Heparin in the Management of DIC

The circumstances under which a trial of heparin should be considered in the management of a patient with clinical and laboratory evidence of DIC are outlined in the text. In general, if the clinical setting is more compatible with chronic DIC (eg, secondary to solid tumor), the picture is more likely to be complicated by thromboembolic phenomena rather than bleeding, which necessitates consideration of heparin therapy.

If an initial heparin bolus is indicated, one nomogram suggests 80 units/kg intravenously can be given, followed by an 18 units/kg/h infusion.[250] Heparin has variable sensitivity to different thromboplastin reagents incorporated in individual laboratory PTT assays. Therefore, any laboratory nomogram used in heparin dosing needs to have its dosing recommendations based on the therapeutic range for the local PTT reagent tailored to corresponding heparin levels of 0.2 to 0.4 units/mL by protamine titration or anti-factor Xa levels of 0.3 to 0.7 units/mL. If no bolus is indicated, patients can be started on an 18 units/kg/h infusion. The PTT, heparin level, or anti-factor Xa level should be checked 6 hours after the start of therapy, and dosage adjustments made accordingly.[250]

For long-term outpatient therapy (eg, for solid tumor-associated chronic DIC), it is also possible to achieve therapeutic heparin levels through subcutaneous injection, with its anticoagulant effect occurring 1 hour later and peak levels after 3 hours. Typically, 35,000 units are given daily, divided into two doses 12 hours apart, with a PTT drawn 6 hours after a dose, and subsequent dosage adjustments made based on the result. Serial heparin or anti-factor Xa levels may be preferable for monitoring if the baseline PTT is prolonged. If an initial rapid effect is desired, a 5000 unit intravenous heparin bolus can be given before the initial subcutaneous dose. Efficacy of heparin treatment can be monitored by changes in D-dimer, fibrinogen, and platelet levels.

Early evidence suggests a potential role for low-molecular-weight heparin in the prevention and management of DIC in association with acute promyelocytic leukemia and Trousseau syndrome.[251,252,253] In this case, low-molecular-weight heparin may be administered subcutaneously in prophylactic doses, enoxaparin 30 mg every 12 hours, or therapeutically at 1 mg/kg every 12 hours, dalteparin doses are 5000 units daily or 200 units/kg every 24 hours, or tinzaparin 75 units/kg to 175 units/kg daily.

oral anticoagulants, which are ineffective in this circumstance (see box on Heparin in the Management of DIC).[251,252] Because the baseline PTT is often prolonged in these patients, the antithrombotic effect of heparin may be monitored by serial heparin or anti-factor Xa levels.

The role of heparin in the treatment of the complex coagulopathy associated with acute promyelocytic leukemia remains controversial.[253–256] Supportive care aimed at maintaining the platelet count above 50,000 and replacing fibrinogen is critical in preventing bleeding complications. Because of the rapid improvement of the DIC in patients receiving all-*trans*-retinoic acid as part of the induction therapy, the role heparin has in acute promyelocytic leukemia is likely to be limited to patients with overt thrombotic complications.[41,42,195] Similarly, the use of heparin in DIC associated with advanced liver disease remains unclear.[257–259] It is contraindicated in abruptio placentae because of bleeding complications associated with delivery and hysterectomy, if these are carried out, and controlled trials have not been done in acute DIC associated with septic abortion.

The role of heparin in management of aortic aneurysms depends on whether the patient is a surgical candidate. Although a nonsurgical patient with only laboratory evidence of DIC does not need heparin, it is prudent to obtain a DIC screen on any patient with an aortic aneurysm in whom surgery is contemplated to avoid serious intraoperative and postoperative bleeding. Preoperative correction of any hemostatic defects with replacement therapy and continuous heparin infusion is in order.[260] These maneuvers should also be considered in patients with bleeding aortic aneurysms. Those with evidence of an aneurysmal leak associated with factor consumption require transfusion of platelets and cryoprecipitate and emergency surgery, and they should not receive heparin.

The use of low-molecular-weight heparins in prophylaxis and treatment of DIC has recently been described in several case reports.[252,253] Although no control trials have yet been reported, these early reports suggest that low-molecular-weight heparins may be as efficacious as adjusted-dose heparin, providing reproducible anticoagulation with less frequent dosing. In one study, six patients with acute promyelocytic leukemia received enoxaparin from the day of admission until presenting skin and mucous membrane bleeding resolved, and the coagulation values returned to normal (11 to 23 days). Three had laboratory evidence of DIC on presentation, and significant bleeding complications developed in two patients while on low-molecular-weight heparin, and in a third, bleeding occurred 3 days after its discontinuation.[253]

Antithrombin and Protein C Concentrates

Antithrombin concentrate has been used in the management of subsets of patients with DIC on the premise that systemic consumptive coagulopathies often lead to a relative plasma deficiency of natural inhibitors, such as antithrombin, that contributes to a procoagulant state. Antithrombin deficiency would also be expected to decrease the effect of any therapeutic heparin used to treat DIC, and so antithrombin concentrates warrant consideration in any heparinized patient with DIC, particularly if heparin resistance is encountered.

Exogenous antithrombin neutralizes thrombin generated in DIC and potentially ameliorates thrombosis, particularly if there is hepatic insufficiency with its associated decrease in antithrombin synthesis. In this respect, antithrombin shortens the duration of DIC in some patients with fatty liver of pregnancy, and its use should be considered in this setting.[261] Except for hepatic insufficiency, other studies have shown improved hemostatic function in most patients with DIC given antithrombin, but no effect on mortality.[262,263] A phase III randomized placebo-controlled trial of antithrombin concentrate failed to demonstrate any statistically significant benefit in survival at any point during the study period.[261]

Activated protein C has been given to animals in concert with infusion of *Escherichia coli* with the subsequent prevention of DIC and gram-negative septicemia.[264] Conversely, when these infusions were supplemented with anti-protein C antibody, inhibition of protein C led to enhanced *E. coli*-associated lethality. Additional studies suggested activated protein C concentrates ameliorated DIC in a rabbit model, with less bleeding than was associated with heparin.[265] This was confirmed in humans in a prospective, double-blind study comparing the safety and efficacy of activated protein C and unfractionated heparin in the treatment of DIC.[266] The death rate at 28 days was significantly reduced in the activated protein C arm.[266,267] Studies of protein C concentrate replacement in infants with purpura fulminans because of severe protein C deficiency and in infants, children, and adults with meningococcemia appear promising.[268–270] A phase III, randomized placebo-controlled trial of activated protein C concentrate was performed in patients with severe sepsis and demonstrated a statistically significant reduction in absolute risk of death of 6.1% and a relative risk reduction of 19.4%.[271] The benefit was seen early and maintained throughout the study period. The risk reduction was independent of the baseline protein C level. Analysis of IL-6 and D-dimer levels showed statistically significant decreases in the activated protein C compared with controls. Bleeding complications were described but were manageable in the antithrombin and activated protein C trials. Activated protein C concentrate has been approved for clinical use in patients with severe sepsis. A case series of pediatric patients with meningococcemia and DIC managed with plasma or whole-blood exchange led to survival of seven of eight patients, with no associated bleeding or cardiovascular complications during the procedure.[271] A prospective, randomized study should be performed to see if activated protein C concentrate can substitute for plasma exchange in the management of meningococcal sepsis.

Fibrinolysis Inhibitors

Under most circumstances, patients with DIC should not be treated with fibrinolytic inhibitors. These agents act by blocking the secondary fibrinogenolysis that accompanies DIC to various extents and may prevent tissue perfusion.[272–275]

The DIC setting in which fibrinolytic inhibitors may warrant consideration includes (1) when intense primary fibrinogenolysis can be demonstrated in association with disease states, such as acute promyelocytic leukemia,[115] Kasabach-Merritt syndrome,[276,277] prostate cancer; and (2) when the patient is bleeding profusely and is not responding to replacement therapy. In the latter case, factor degradation products may be contributing to bleeding, and the use of fibrinolytic agents should be considered only after the continuously bleeding patient has received replacement therapy for depleted hemostatic factors, and intravenous heparin infusions ε-aminocaproic acid or tranexamic acid may be useful in these cases in concert with heparin for the coexisting DIC.[278–281]

An approach to treatment of Kasabach-Merritt syndrome entails administering a fibrinolytic inhibitor alone or in combination with cryoprecipitate.[115,276] The result has been tumor shrinkage and correction of hemostatic defects through induction of thrombosis within the tumor.

SUGGESTED READINGS

Angstwurn MWA, Dempfle CE, Spannagi M: New disseminated intravascular coagulation score: A useful too to predict mortality in comparison with Acute Physiology and Chronic Health Evaluation II and Logistic Organ Dysfunction scores. Crit Care Med 34(2):314, 2006.

Aoki N, Matsuda T, Saito H, et al: A comparative double-blind randomized trial of activated protein C and unfractionated heparin in the treatment of disseminated intravascular coagulation. Int J Hematol 75(5):540, 2002.

Bakhtiari K, Meijers JCM, de Jonge E, Levi M, Prospective validation of the International Society of Thrombosis and Haemostasis scoring system for disseminated intravascular coagulation. Crit Care Med 32(12):2416, 2004.

Boccaccio C, Sabatino G, Medico E, et al. The *MET* oncogene drives a genetic programme linking cancer to haemostasis. Nature 434:396, 2005.

Esmon CT: Role of coagulation inhibitors in inflammation. Thromb Haemost 83(1):51, 2001.

Gando S, Iba T, Euguchi Y, et al: A multicenter, prospective validation of disseminated intravascular coagulation diagnostic criteria for critically ill patients: Comparing current criteria. Crit Care Med 34(3): 625, 2006.

Levi M: Disseminated intravascular coagulation: What's new? Crit Care Clin 21:449, 2005.

Marin V, Montero-Julian FA, Gres S, et al: The IL-6 soluble IL-6R autocrine loop of endothelial activation as an intermediate between acute and chronic inflammation: An experimental model involving thrombin. J Immunol 167(6):3435, 2001.

Norman KE, Cotter MJ, Stewart JB, et al: Combined anticoagulant and antiselectin treatments prevent lethal intravascular coagulation. Blood 101(3):921, 2003.

Sallah S, Wan J, Nguyen N, et al: Disseminated intravascular coagulation in solid tumors: Clinical and pathologic study. Thromb Haemost 86:828, 2001.

Souter PJ, Thomas S, Hubbard A, et al: Antithrombin inhibits lipopolysaccharide-induced tissue factor and interleukin-6 production by mononuclear cells, human umbilical vein endothelial cells and whole blood. Crit Care Med 29(1):134, 2001.

Taylor FBJ, Toh CH, Hoots WK, Wada H, Levi M: Toward definition, clinical and laboratory criteria and a scoring system for disseminated intravascular coagulation. Thromb Haemost 86:1327, 2001.

van Aken BE, Reitsma PH, Rosendaal FR: Interleukin 8 and venous thrombosis: Evidence for a role of inflammation in thrombosis. Br J Haematol 116(1):173, 2002.

Woodside KJ, Hunter GC, Disseminated intravascular coagulation scoring systems in the critically ill. Crit Care Med 34(3):899, 2006.

Yu JL, May L, Lhotak V, et al: Oncogenic events regulate tissue factor expression in colorectal cancer cells: implications for tumor progression and angiogenesis. Blood 105:1734, 2005.

REFERENCES

For complete list of references log onto www.expertconsult.com

CHAPTER 133

DISORDERS OF COAGULATION IN THE NEONATE

Cameron Trenor, III and Ellis J. Neufeld

Neonates experience rapid physiologic changes after birth, some of which impact the hemostatic system. Evaluation of disorders of coagulation in the neonate requires an understanding of the evolution of physiologic normal values for age, the congenital disorders that present in early life, and the clinical settings common in neonatology that affect hemostasis and thrombosis risks. The rapid evolution of the blood coagulation system after birth leads to a dynamic group of age-dependent reference ranges in factors that should be considered physiologically normal. Developmental hemostasis is the term applied to the evolution of the hemostatic and fibrinolytic systems through infancy and childhood.

DEVELOPMENTAL HEMOSTASIS

The hemostatic system evolves throughout childhood and most rapidly during the neonatal period. Changing plasma concentrations of proteins involved in blood coagulation lead to a dynamic group of reference ranges for preterm and term infants. Although discrepant from adult values, these reference ranges are neither "abnormal" nor pathologic. The relative rarity of hemorrhagic or thrombotic complications in this population argues that the neonatal coagulation system is physiologically replete.

Laboratory Evaluation

Laboratory evaluation of thrombosis or bleeding in a neonate requires recognition that reference ranges for healthy newborns are age-dependent and differ from adult values. The concept of developmental hemostasis was pioneered by Maureen Andrew, and her seminal papers describing reference ranges for healthy premature and full-term neonates are still widely referenced.[1,2] However, recent data suggest that reference ranges for coagulation assays in infants vary with analyzer and reagents systems used.[3] As current instrumentation for coagulation testing has evolved since age-specific normal ranges were defined, reference laboratories should develop their own age-related reference ranges specific for their own testing systems. Neonatal samples should be drawn by experienced staff, ideally from free-flowing veins. Samples are processed in 1 mL tubes containing 0.1 mL of 3.2% buffered sodium citrate, aiming for a final ratio of one part citrate to nine parts blood.

The prothrombin time, expressed in seconds, is usually similar between full-term neonates and adults despite relative deficiencies of vitamin K-dependent coagulation factors.[2] However, premature infants and cord blood samples exhibit a prolonged prothrombin time[1,4] compared to adults. Activated partial thromboplastin time (PTT) is prolonged in newborns, attributed to relative deficiencies in contact factors.[5] Thrombin time is similar to adult values when measured in the presence of calcium to compensate for the unique fetal form of fibrinogen with increased sialic acid content.[6] The template bleeding time is reportedly preserved in neonates, but this is an unreliable technique in neonatology and is not recommended for bleeding evaluations.

Blood Coagulation Proteins

The synthesis of fetal and neonatal coagulation proteins begins at approximately 10 weeks of gestation, and plasma concentrations of these proteins increase with gestational age. Maternal coagulation proteins cannot cross the placenta.[7] However, the impact of maternal drug use on fetal vitamin K-dependent coagulation protein synthesis has been described, with warfarin, phenytoin, barbiturates, and antibiotics as examples.

The study of coagulation factors in neonates is confounded by a dynamic group of age-dependent reference ranges. Physiologic ranges for coagulation factors in healthy newborns having received intramuscular vitamin K after delivery have been established and are shown in Table 133–1. Plasma levels of fibrinogen and factors V, VIII, and XIII are present at adult levels at birth. Levels of von Willebrand factor (vWF), particularly high-molecular-weight multimers, are higher than adult levels from birth until 3 months of age,[8] in part because of maternal estrogen and despite adult levels of the vWF processing enzyme, ADAMTS-13.[9] Vitamin K-dependent factors (prothrombin and factors VII, IX, and X) are present at significantly lower levels than in adults, as are the four contact factors (factor XI, factor XII, prekallikrein, and high molecular weight kininogen). Both the contact factors and the vitamin K-dependent factors approach adult levels by approximately 6 months of age.

Regulation of Thrombin

Direct thrombin inhibition occurs via α_2-macroglobulin, antithrombin, and heparin cofactor II. Unlike in adults, α_2-macroglobulin is the dominant thrombin inhibitor in neonates, with twice the plasma concentration and thrombin binding of antithrombin.[10] Thrombin inhibition through heparin cofactor II is catalyzed by a fetal proteoglycan anticoagulant produced by the placenta and found in both maternal and fetal circulation.[11,12]

Inhibition of thrombin generation is also accomplished by upstream inhibition of the clotting proteins in the prothrombinase and *tenase* complexes (see Chapter 118). Thus, protein C, its cofactor protein S, and tissue factor pathway inhibitor (TFPI) serve as they do in adults. Circulating levels of proteins S and C are substantially lower than adult levels, requiring 6 to 12 months respectively to reach adult levels. Despite lower total protein S, free protein S levels are preserved because of low levels of C4b-binding protein in newborn plasma. The interaction of protein S with activated protein C in neonatal plasma may be limited by elevated levels of α_2-macroglobulin.[13] Free TFPI levels are lower than in adults, despite total TFPI levels being similar in neonatal and adult plasma.[14]

Thrombin regulation in neonatal plasma is similar to the plasma from therapeutically anticoagulated adults.[15] The amount of thrombin generated in neonates is proportional to available prothrombin concentrations,[16] whereas the rate of thrombin generation is dependent on other procoagulant protein concentrations. The capacity of neonatal fibrin clots to bind thrombin is lower than in adults because of lower plasma prothrombin levels.[17] This observation implies that

Table 133–1 Reference Values (Ranges) for Common Coagulation Tests and Blood Coagulation Protein Levels by Age, Comparing Two Comprehensive Prospective Studies with Different Methodologies†

	Day 1		Day 3 (ref 3) vs. Day 5 (ref 2)		1 month–1 year		Adult (measured)	
	Ref 3	Ref 2	Ref 3	Ref 2	Ref 3	Ref 2	Ref 3	Ref 2
Prothrombin time (sec)	15.6 (14.4–16.4)	13 (11.6–14.4)	14.9 (13.5–16.4)	12.4 (10.5–13.9)	13.1 (11.5–15.3)	12.3 (10.7–13.9)	13 (11.5–14.5)	12 (11–14)
PTT (sec)	38.7 (34.3–44.8)	42.9 (31.3–54.5)	36.3 (29.5–42.2)	42.6 (25.4–59.8)	39.3 (35.1–46.3)	35.5 (28.1–42.9)	33.2 (28.6–38.2)	33 (27–40)
Thrombin time (sec)	N/A	23.5 (19–28.3)	N/A	23.1 (18–29.2)	17.1 (16.3–17.6)	24.3 (19.4–29.2)	16.6 (16.2–17.2)	N/A
Fibrinogen (mg/dL)	280 (192–374)	283 (225–341)	330 (283–401)	312 (237–387)	242 (82–383)	251 (150–387)	310 (190–430)	278 (156–400)
Prothrombin (%)	54 (41–69)	48 (37–59)	62 (50–73)	63 (48–78)	90 (62–103)	88 (60–116)	110 (78–138)	108 (70–146)
Factor V (%)	81 (64–103)	72 (54–90)	122 (92–154)	95 (70–120)	113 (94–14)	91 (55–127)	118 (78–152)	106 (62–150)
Factor VII (%)	70 (52–88)	66 (47–85)	86 (67–107)	89 (62–116)	128 (83–160)	87 (47–127)	129 (61–199)	105 (67–143)
Factor VIII (%)	182 (105–329)	100 (61–139)	159 (83–274)	88 (55–121)	94 (54–145)	73 (53–109)	160 (52–290)	99 (50–149)
Factor IX (%)	48 (35–56)	53 (34–72)	72 (44–97)	53 (34–72)	71 (43–121)	86 (36–139)	130 (59–254)	109 (55–163)
Factor X (%)	55 (46–67)	40 (26–54)	60 (46–75)	49 (34–64)	95 (77–122)	78 (38–118)	124 (96–171)	106 (70–152)
Factor XI (%)	30 (7–41)	38 (24–52)	57 (24–79)	55 (39–71)	89 (62–125)	86 (49–134)	112 (67–196)	97 (67–127)
Factor XII (%)	58 (43–80)	53 (33–73)	53 (14–80)	47 (29–65)	79 (20–135)	77 (39–115)	115 (35–207)	108 (52–164)
Antithrombin III (%)	76 (58–90)	63 (51–75)	74 (60–89)	67 (54–80)	109 (72–134)	104 (84–124)	96 (66–124)	100 (74–126)
Protein C activity (%)	36 (24–44)	35 (26–44)	44 (28–54)	42 (31–53)	71 (31–112)	59 (37–81)	104 (74–164)	96 (64–128)
Protein S activity (%)	36 (28–47)	36 (24–48)	49 (33–67)	50 (36–64)	102 (29–162)	87 (55–119)	75 (54–103)	81 (60–113)
D-dimer (μg/mL)	1.47 (0.41–2.47)	N/A	1.34 (0.58–2.74)	N/A	0.22 (0.11–0.42)	N/A	0.18 (0.05–0.42)	N/A

N/A, not available; PTT, partial thromboplastin time; Ref 2, Andrew et al; Ref 3, Monagle et al.
†Adapted from Monagle et al and Andrew et al (range inferred from published statistical documentation).

decreased plasma prothrombin levels may suppress thrombus propagation in neonates when compared to adults.

In sum, this implies relatively increased thrombus stability in healthy newborns that is normalized under physiologic stress.

The Fibrinolytic System

Although some components of the neonatal fibrinolytic system are distinct from adult proteins, their clinical relevance is probably minimal. The fibrinolytic system functions to control thrombus size by influencing clot lysis through the actions of plasminogen. Fetal plasminogen circulates at substantially lower levels than in adults yet has increased receptor affinity because of a relative increase in mannose and sialic acid side chains.[18] Whereas a healthy neonate has decreased plasmin-generating potential than an adult,[19] the stress of illness can increase depressed baseline levels of tissue plasminogen activator (tPA) up to eightfold. Neonates with severe plasminogen deficiency have only a minimal increased risk of thrombosis, and most of their clinical findings result from poor extravascular fibrinolysis.[20] The major plasmin inhibitors are found at near adult levels in the neonate.

Platelets

Neonatal platelet count and mean platelet volume are similar to adult values. Thrombocytopenia is common in neonates. Thrombocytosis is rare in neonates but is associated with prematurity and occurs 4 to 6 weeks after delivery. This correlates with evidence of increased megakaryocytopoiesis in the third trimester.[21]

Platelet function is altered at birth. Platelets are activated to a degree during the birth process, hypothesized to be a result of temperature change, hypoxia, acidosis, adrenergic stimulation, and amniotic fluid exposure. In contrast, platelet adhesion and aggregation may be inhibited by the transient perinatal release of nitric oxide.[22] Consistent with this, both bleeding times[23] and platelet function analyzer (PFA)-100 closure times are shorter in neonates than adults, perhaps mediated by increased neonatal high multimeric vWF.[24] If available, PFA-100 is preferred to bleeding time for testing platelet-related hemostasis. The bleeding time is inconsistent in neonates, and this test is to be discouraged in nearly every clinical circumstance. The PFA-100 is not a perfect surrogate for clotting status in vivo so that mild defects in platelet function might provide false negative results.[25] As a practical matter, it is not often clinically necessary to diagnose mild congenital platelet disorders in the neonate because severe neonatal bleeding is rare with mild defects.

The Vessel Wall

Animal models and in-vitro systems provide evidence that young blood vessels possess greater antithrombotic potential than adult vessels. In both rabbit venous and aortic models, increased heparin sulfate glycosaminoglycans are associated with increased antithrombin-mediated anticoagulant activity in rabbit pups compared to adults.[26,27] Circulating levels of endothelial cell adhesion markers vary with age, implying that expression or secretion of these proteins from the vessel wall may be dynamic in neonates.[28]

NEONATAL HEMORRHAGIC DISORDERS

Significant bleeding in neonates should prompt a hemostasis evaluation. In sick infants, acquired factor deficiencies or thrombocytopenia are frequently to blame, but rare congenital factor deficiencies often present with neonatal bleeding. Attention to maternal contributing factors (eg, infection, thrombocytopenia, drugs) is critical when evaluating neonates. Initial empirical therapy consists of platelet and/or factor supplementation, often while diagnostic studies are underway.

Evaluation of the Bleeding Neonate

Neonatal, peripartum, maternal, and family histories are each important in the evaluation of a newborn with hemorrhagic complications. Documentation of vitamin K administration in the delivery room should be confirmed. Maternal factors that can directly lead to neonatal thrombocytopenia include infection, immune thrombocytopenia, or drugs. Maternal vitamin K deficiency or drugs impairing vitamin K metabolism can lead to severe deficiencies of vitamin K-dependent blood coagulation proteins at birth. On physical examination, the location and characteristics of bleeding (eg, procedural, mucosal, cutaneous, intraventricular), whether diffuse or localized and the general appearance of the baby as sick or well will help predict the underlying etiology of hemorrhage. Ill-appearing newborns are prone to disseminated intravascular coagulation or liver disease as reasons for acquired factor deficiencies. These disorders tend to present with diffuse bleeding. Well-appearing newborns are more likely to have localized bleeding or ecchymoses because of thrombocytopenia from a transplacental antibody, vitamin K deficiency, or a rare inherited factor deficiency.

Laboratory evaluation of the hemorrhage in newborns should include sepsis evaluation, platelet count, prothrombin time, PTT, thrombin time, fibrinogen, and if other causes are not identified, consideration of a PFA-100. In male infants with a positive family history of hemophilia or strong clinical suspicion, factors VIII and IX should be measured regardless of a PTT prolongation. Deficiencies of factor XIII, α_2-antiplasmin or plasminogen activator inhibitor-1 will not be detected by standard screening, and specific testing should be obtained if suspected. Further evaluation of this laboratory screening approach is summarized in Fig. 133–1, modified from Blanchette and Rand.[29]

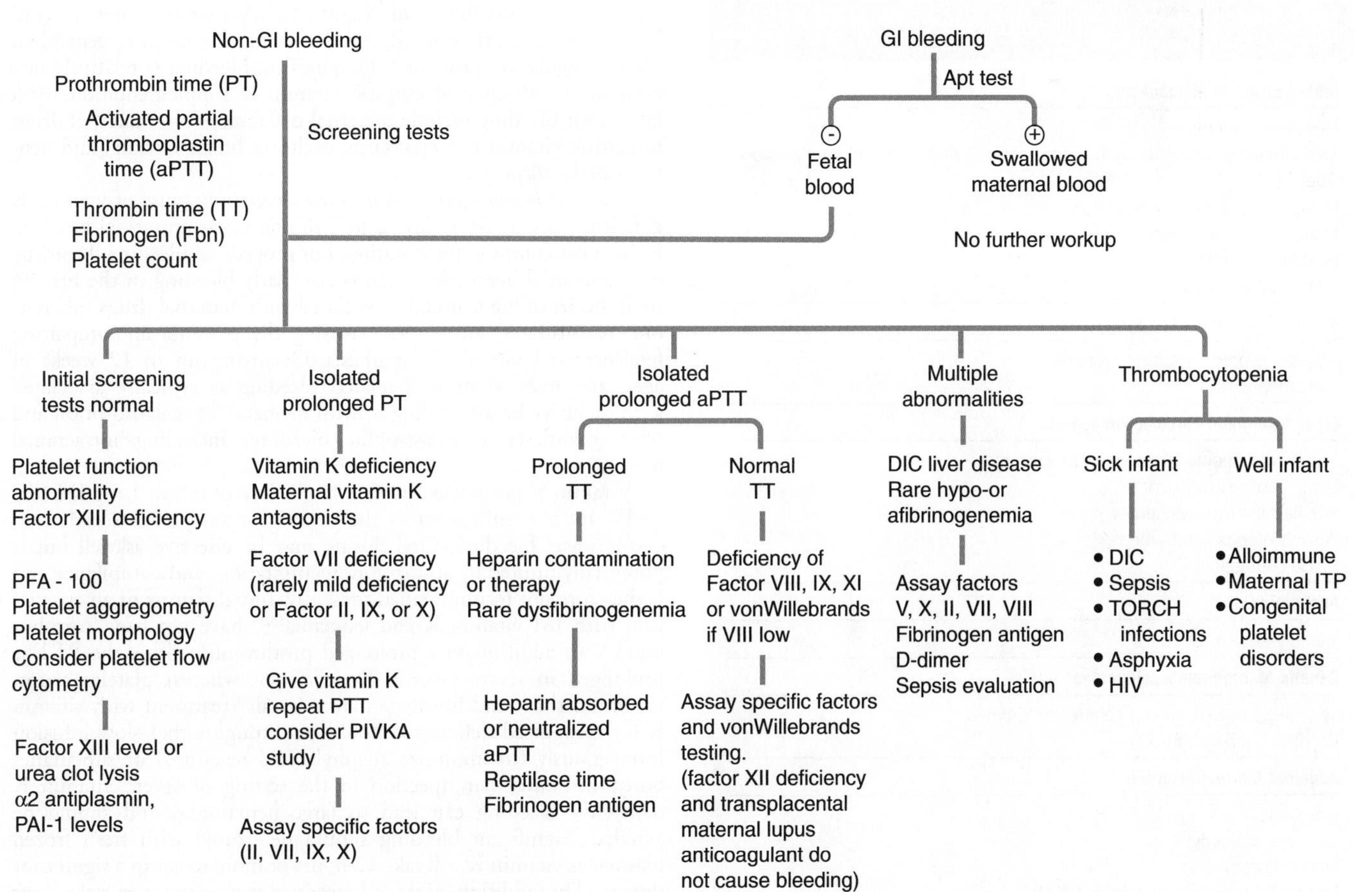

Figure 133–1 Diagnostic approach to the bleeding neonate.

Neonatal Thrombocytopenia

The following factors are important to consider when evaluating neonatal thrombocytopenia: congenital or acquired, sick or well, maternal antibody or drug, and platelet size. Platelet number and size in healthy neonates is equivalent to adults and thrombocytopenia is defined as less than 150,000 cells/μL. Significant thrombocytopenia (less than 50,000 cells/μL) in neonates rarely manifests with bleeding, particularly in the absence of maternal antiplatelet antibodies.[30] In the absence of maternal thrombocytopenia, fewer than 1% of healthy newborns have thrombocytopenia,[30] compared to more than 20% of newborns requiring intensive care.[31]

The majority of causes of neonatal thrombocytopenia involve increased platelet destruction. In well-appearing newborns, thrombocytopenia is usually an immune-mediated phenomenon related to maternal transplacental IgG antibodies or drugs (eg, quinine, hydralazine, thiazides, tolbutamide). In sick newborns, platelet destruction is often related to infection, disseminated intravascular coagulation, extracorporeal membrane oxygenation (ECMO), thrombosis, or mechanical ventilation performed for hyaline membrane disease. Significant localized thrombosis in large vessels can also lead to thrombocytopenia, as can specific recognizable syndromes including renal vein thrombosis, necrotizing enterocolitis, or vascular anomalies (Kasabach-Merritt syndrome).

Platelet production is impaired after significant hypoxic-ischemic injury, perhaps because fetal megakaryocytes are particularly sensitive to hypoxia. Newborns from pregnancies complicated by intrauterine growth restriction or pregnancy-induced hypertension frequently have transient mild to moderate thrombocytopenia. Other causes of decreased platelet production in neonates include rare primary congenital platelet or marrow disorders and infiltrative disorders. These are summarized in Table 133–2.

Table 133–2 Syndromic, Genetic, and Acquired Etiologies of Neonatal Thrombocytopenia

Inborn Errors of Metabolism
Isovaleric acidemia
Methylmalonic acidemia (with acute acidosis) and cobalamin metabolic defects
Holocarboxylase deficiency
Mitochondrial disorders
Pearson syndrome
Kearns-Sayer syndrome
Genetic Marrow Failure Syndromes
Amegakaryocytic thrombocytopenia
Fanconi anemia
Other Syndromic Thrombocytopenias
Thrombocytopenia-absent radius syndrome
Paris-Trousseau syndrome
X-linked thrombocytopenias
Wiskott-Aldrich syndrome
GATA-1 mutations
Aneuploidy
Trisomy 21, 13, or 18
Genetic Macrothrombocytopenias
May-Hegglin, Sebastian, Fechtner syndromes
Bernard Soulier syndrome
Acquired Marrow Disorders
Oncologic
Neonatal leukemia
Neuroblastoma
Histiocytic Lymphohistiocytosis (HLH)

Platelet Abnormalities

Qualitative platelet disorders are only rarely associated with overt neonatal bleeding. Clinical suspicion should be aroused in patients with clinical bleeding in the setting of normal coagulation screening and platelet counts. Bleeding may include mucocutaneous sites, heelsticks for capillary blood sampling, cephalohematoma, umbilical stump bleeding, or postprocedural bleeding. Neonatal presentation usually involves only the most severe genetic disorders of platelet function, because of defects of platelet fibrinogen receptor, integrin glycoproteins IIb and IIIa, (Glanzmann thrombasthenia), and von Willebrand receptor glycoprotein Ib (Bernard-Soulier syndrome) (see Chapter 141). Maternal medications may affect platelet function, most notably aspirin, although low-dose aspirin does not appear to significantly alter neonatal platelet function.[32] Neonatal medications may also affect platelet function. Common offenders include nitric oxide, prostaglandin E2, indomethacin, and aspirin. Suspected platelet disorders should be evaluated by platelet morphology and direct platelet aggregation studies after initial screening by PFA-100. Additional flow cytometry for specific surface glycoproteins or electron microscopy studies for granule morphology by an expert consultant should be considered. Evaluation of the bleeding time is rarely more helpful than clinical assessment and direct tests on blood. Treatment with platelet infusion is standard if bleeding is present. The potential risk of allosensitization from normal platelets in congenital deficiencies of platelet surface antigens must be weighed against the severity of bleeding when functional defects are suspected.

Vitamin K Deficiency Bleeding

Vitamin K is a necessary cofactor for γ-glutamyl carboxylase, the enzyme required for posttranslational carboxylation of prothrombin, factors VII, IX, and X, and proteins C, S, and Z. Many newborns are significantly deficient in vitamin K, whether measured in cord blood[33] or indirectly through activity levels of vitamin K-dependent blood coagulation proteins.[34] Despite this, bleeding is relatively rare even in the absence of empiric vitamin K supplementation. Risk factors for bleeding include maternal malabsorption, maternal drugs impairing vitamin K metabolism, exclusive breast-feeding, and neonatal malabsorption.

Classical *hemorrhagic disease of the newborn* because of vitamin K deficiency occurs from days 2 to 7 of life. Gastrointestinal bleeding is the most common presentation, but procedural bleeding, bruising, or intracranial hemorrhage can occur. Early bleeding in the first 24 to 48 hours of life is usually associated with maternal drugs (phenytoin, barbiturates, antibiotics) crossing the placenta and impairing fetal/neonatal vitamin K synthesis. Occurring up to 12 weeks of age, late onset vitamin K-related bleeding is typically associated with exclusive breast-feeding or with neonatal fat malabsorption and often manifests as catastrophic bleeding, including intracranial hemorrhage.

Vitamin K prophylaxis with a single dose of 0.5 to 1 mg IM (SC or IV are also sufficient) in the delivery room prevents early and classic onset bleeding. Oral dosing may be effective as well but is potentially limited by absorption, regurgitation, and compliance and is therefore not recommended presently. Initial reports of an association with IM vitamin K and leukemia[35,36] have not been corroborated.[37] In addition to a prolonged prothrombin time, the PTT is prolonged in severe vitamin K deficiency, whereas platelet count, thrombin time, and fibrinogen are normal. Treatment with vitamin K for recognized deficiency should be through either slow infusion intravenously (to minimize anaphylactoid reactions) or subcutaneously. Intramuscular injection in the setting of severe vitamin K deficiency bleeding can lead to large hematomas and should be avoided. Significant bleeding should be treated with fresh frozen plasma, as vitamin K will take 12 hours or more to act to a significant degree. The addition of blood product concentrates enriched for vitamin K-dependent proteins (prothrombin complex concentrates) should be reserved for life-threatening bleeding, given concerns about precipitating thrombosis.[38]

Inherited Coagulation Disorders

Prolonged PTT

Hemophilia is the most common inherited coagulation disorder, as discussed in detail in Chapter 125. Evaluation for factor VIII, IX, and XI deficiencies should be undertaken immediately in any neonate with an isolated prolonged PTT and bleeding or positive family history. Male newborns with a positive (maternal) family history of hemophilia should be evaluated prior to intramuscular injections, including vitamin K. Typically, newborns with hemophilia and bleeding are well-appearing. Male infants far outnumber females, given the location of both factor VIII and factor IX genes on the X chromosome. However, severe factor VIII or factor IX deficiency can, albeit rarely, present in females. Factor XI deficiency is an autosomal recessive disorder, so female newborns with bleeding and isolated prolonged PTT should also be tested. Evaluation of hemophilia carrier status in mothers of unknown status (eg, single prior affected child or positive history in maternal grandmother) can be performed genetically, as factor levels in carriers range widely and overlap with normal levels. Most bleeding episodes in newborn males occur after circumcision or occasionally umbilical stump separation, although intracranial hemorrhage is reported in approximately 3.5% of hemophiliac newborns,[39] and cephalhematomas are common. Joint bleeding is very rare in the neonatal period. For patients with known or suspected hemophilia or severe deficiencies of factors VII, X, or XIII, screening for intracranial bleeding should be considered. Although head ultrasound is often used for screening, head computed tomography (CT) is more sensitive than ultrasound for small parafalcine bleeds, which can also occur in a small percentage of normal infants with no sequelae.

Isolated Prolonged Prothrombin Time

Inherited factor VII deficiency is a rare, autosomal recessive condition with a strong gene dosage effect. Neonatal bleeding can occur in severe cases (ie, homozygosity or compound heterozygosity for two mutations in the factor VII gene). Factor VII deficiency is rarely reported to be associated with microcephaly or midline defects because of loss of adjacent genes in disruptions on chromosome 13q. Additionally, factor VII deficiency is found in combined factor defects associated with abnormalities of the vitamin K pathways. Replacement with fresh frozen plasma or recombinant factor VIIa at very low doses is used to correct the deficiency.

Prolonged Prothrombin Time and PTT

The association of bleeding with prolongation of both the prothrombin time and PTT in a healthy newborn may indicate vitamin K deficiency or congenital deficiencies of prothrombin, factors V or X, and also rare combined deficiencies. More commonly, combined prothrombin time and PTT prolongation occurs in sick newborns with disseminated intravascular coagulation (DIC) pathophysiology or severe perturbed liver synthetic function. Any of these factor deficiencies may present with postprocedure, umbilical stump, intracranial, or gastrointestinal bleeding.

Combined factor deficiencies are rare but must be considered when laboratory evaluation or clinical course are confusing. Autosomal recessive mutations in the LMAN1 (ERGIC-53) or MCFD2 result in combined factor V and VIII deficiency,[40] because of defective intracellular processing of both factors. Mutations in γ-glutamyl carboxylase are associated with inherited combined deficiencies of all vitamin K-dependent proteins.[41] Factor VII deficiency has rarely been reported in combination with factors V, VIII, IX, X, XI, and protein C defects, as reviewed by Girolami.[42]

Factor XIII

Factor XIII is a transpeptidase that crosslinks fibrin strands and is required for clot stability. Severe factor XIII deficiency may present with neonatal bleeding and is not detected by screening prothrombin time, PTT, or thrombin-time assays. Specific factor XIII levels or urea clot solubility testing are used for diagnosis, and treatment is replacement with factor XIII concentrate or by cryoprecipitate. Intracranial bleeding in a child with no other risk factors should prompt a search for factor XIII deficiency.

Other Inherited Deficiencies Associated with Neonatal Bleeding

Von Willebrand disease (vWD) is the most common inherited bleeding diathesis and is discussed in Chapter 129. vWD has been associated with neonatal bleeding, although very rarely, and generally with severe subtypes. The largest case series of 55 newborns with vWD reports no bleeding complications,[43] although individual cases of scalp hematomas and bleeding after vitamin K injection or umbilical stump detachment are reported. Acquired forms of vWD also occur rarely and may complicate obstetric management of afflicted patients and affect their newborns. Family history of vWD, especially type 2 (dominant, qualitative defects), should prompt vWD evaluation in the neonate prior to circumcision, and possibly before intramuscular injections. There is possible association of vWD and acute idiopathic pulmonary hemorrhage.[44] Children with new diagnoses of type 3 vWD should be genetically tested for mutations predisposing for inhibitory alloantibody formation prior to aggressive replacement with exogenous vWF.[45] Treatment in neonates for prophylaxis or bleeding is with plasma-based factor VIII:vWF concentrates that contain von Willebrand factor (e.g., Humate-P or Alphanate), dosed initially at 40 to 60 ristocetin cofactor units/kg.

Afibrinogenemia can be associated with neonatal bleeding. Severe deficiency of fibrinogen is rare and can manifest as bleeding in soft tissue, after circumcision, or after umbilical stump detachment. Diagnosis is evident by standard fibrinogen assays, and treatment involves replacement with cryoprecipitate or, if available, fibrinogen concentrate.

Even complete deficiencies of the contact factors, high-molecular-weight kininogen, prekallikrein, and factor XII, are not associated with bleeding phenotypes. Autosomal recessive deficiencies of the fibrinolytic proteins α_2-antiplasmin[46] and plasminogen activator inhibitor-1[47] have been associated with case reports of pediatric bleeding, but no cases are reported in the neonatal period.

Liver Disease

Coagulopathy and bleeding because of inadequate hepatic synthetic function is not unique to neonates. Liver disease in neonates may be caused by viral hepatitis, parenteral nutrition, cholestasis, hypoxic injury, or metabolic disease. Rare disorders presenting with liver failure in neonates include hereditary tyrosinemia, neonatal hemochromatosis, and hemophagocytic lymphohistiocytosis.

Because of synthetic deficiencies of multiple coagulation proteins, laboratory workup typically reveals prolonged prothrombin time and PTT. Platelet count may be depressed, especially if hypersplenism is present, and platelet dysfunction is often present. Hypofibrinogenemia is a late effect of liver disease and elevated fibrin degradation products and D-dimer occur because of delayed hepatic clearance.

Diagnostically, measurement of factors V, VII, and VIII can help distinguish liver disease, vitamin K deficiency, and consumptive coagulopathy (eg, DIC or large vascular malformations). Factors V and VIII are not vitamin K-dependent, are made by the liver and multiple cell types respectively, and have neonatal concentrations similar to adult levels. Deficiency of all three implies consumption, whereas decreased levels of factors V and VII with normal factor VIII is consistent with liver disease.

Treatment should include factor replacement with fresh frozen plasma or cryoprecipitate and platelet transfusion. Patients with biliary atresia or other cholestatic liver failure syndromes may also benefit from parenteral administration of vitamin K. Successful therapy is predicated on treatment of the underlying cause of liver disease.

Intraventricular Hemorrhage

Intraventricular hemorrhage carries significant morbidity and mortality in the newborn period. With improvements in neonatal care, the incidence of intraventricular hemorrhage is decreasing despite its association with prematurity. The etiology of intraventricular hemorrhage is multifactorial but includes prematurity of cerebral vasculature and ischemia-reperfusion injury related to ventilatory support, blood pressure lability, or extracorporeal membrane oxygenation. The role of coagulopathy or thrombocytopenia is unclear. One study reports hypofibrinogenemia, thrombocytopenia, or prolonged clotting time in 11 of 15 neonates with intraventricular hemorrhage whereas only in 5 of 35 control newborns.[48] Hemorrhage after thrombosis may explain some cases (especially in full-term infants), with factor V Leiden heterozygosity identified in 18% of neonates with grade 2 to 4 intraventricular hemorrhage compared to 3% of controls.[49] Multiple trials have analyzed antenatal vitamin K administration, indomethacin, antithrombin, fresh frozen plasma, factor XIII, tranexamic acid, or ethamsylate for prevention of intraventricular hemorrhage. Studies to date have drawn mixed conclusions or lack long-term developmental outcomes, thus preventing a consensus recommendation. Cerebellar hemorrhage should raise suspicion for an organic acidemias, such as methylmalonic, propionic, or isovaleric acidemia.

Extracorporeal Membrane Oxygenation

Extracorporeal membrane oxygenation is occasionally used in neonates with severe persistent pulmonary hypertension or in conjunction with cardiac surgery for patients with severe cardiomyopathy. The extracorporeal membrane oxygenation pump, oxygenation membrane, and large-bore catheters in the patients all pose thrombotic risk, whereas the requirement for long-term high-dose systemic anticoagulation can pose a severe bleeding risk in sick neonates. Protocols that strike a balance between too little and too much anticoagulation have been worked out empirically over the last 20 years, following activated clotting time assays. With extracorporeal membrane oxygenation anticoagulation, prothrombin time and PTT assessments of coagulation status may give results that do not correlate with activated clotting time assays. Complicating this, there is evidence that heparin dose is prognostic of extracorporeal membrane oxygenation survival independent of the activated clotting time, implying that an activated clotting time of 180 to 220 seconds may not represent adequate anticoagulation.[50] Further, prolonged use of extracorporeal membrane oxygenation reliably causes a state of depleted clotting factors and high levels of fibrin degradation products. However, this depletion does not mean patients are adequately anticoagulated. The laboratory hallmark of this state is a very prolonged PTT or moderately long activated clotting time and high D-dimers, at very low heparin doses (compared to those used at initiation of extracorporeal membrane oxygenation). In neonates with thrombosis or specific high-risk situations, daily fresh frozen plasma infusion is sometimes used as a source of plasminogen and anticoagulant proteins. Data supporting specific regimens for this purpose are lacking.

Respiratory Distress Syndrome

Respiratory distress syndrome (RDS), also known as hyaline membrane disease, is an acute pulmonary process common in premature neonates. Part of the pathophysiology of RDS includes hyaline membrane formation and fibrin deposition through diffuse areas of atelectasis. Although increasing thrombin generation and decreased antithrombin levels correlate with the severity of RDS, therapeutic interventions addressing the coagulation system have been inconclusive. Studies using plasmin[51] or plasminogen[52] demonstrated a survival benefit; heparin is controversial, and antithrombin supplementation may lead to increased mortality.[53] Further clinical studies are needed to address possible benefits of antithrombotic or thrombolytic therapies in RDS. The generation of thrombin and deposition of fibrin leads to a laboratory profile consistent with mild DIC or thrombosis. Low fibrinogen and elevated D-dimer are present in RDS and may mask the laboratory evaluation of thromboembolic disease. Doppler ultrasound should be relied on for diagnosis of deep venous thrombosis or suspected pulmonary embolism. Unexpected increase in ventilatory support should raise suspicion for pulmonary embolism in this population.

NEONATAL THROMBOEMBOLIC DISORDERS

Thrombosis in neonates is uncommon, but more than half of pediatric thromboembolic events occur in the neonatal period. The incidence of neonatal thromboembolic events is increasing because of improved neonatal survival and an increased use of thrombogenic surfaces (eg, catheters, extracorporeal membrane oxygenation circuits) for advanced neonatal care. Approximately 80% of neonatal thrombi are associated with indwelling catheters. However, rare severe congenital thrombophilias present in the newborn period and deserve special consideration in this population. Positive family history or prior miscarriages may indicate a hereditary thrombophilia. Heparin remains the mainstay of therapy, but newer agents have been successfully employed in special circumstances, such as heparin-induced thrombocytopenia.

Incidence

Current estimates of the incidence of neonatal thrombosis are provided by three international registries with different inclusion criteria. German, Dutch, and Canadian registries have independently reported the incidence of neonatal thromboembolic events at 15 to 51 events per 10,000 patients.[54–56] Two-thirds of thromboembolic events were venous, and 80% were either catheter-associated or followed a severe illness.[57] Arterial thromboembolic events in neonates usually involve either stroke or emboli to limbs from catheter-associated thrombi.

Acquired Thrombophilia

Indwelling Catheters

Central venous and arterial access is required for the advanced care provided in modern neonatology. The most common acquired thrombotic risk factor in neonates is the presence of an indwelling vascular catheter. Awareness of the prothrombotic biases of catheter location, size, material, duration of placement, and type of fluid delivered is important in this population. Symptomatic venous thrombosis presents with swelling, discoloration, and temperature decrease of an affected limb. Loss of catheter patency, evidence of collateral circulation and/or unexplained thrombocytopenia should raise clinical suspicion for thrombosis. Importantly, prospective imaging prior to indwelling central access catheter removal find high rates of asymptomatic thrombi (up to 86%)[55] with an unknown potential for long-term morbidity. Treatment often begins with removal of the catheter, although consideration of anticoagulation prior to catheter removal is warranted, especially in infants with right to left intracardiac or intrapulmonary shunting. Small catheter-mediated thrombi may resolve without specific therapy.[58] Larger thrombi or those in locations associated with greater morbidity (eg, sinovenous, renal, portal) may warrant short courses of heparin or thrombolytic agents. Platelets should never be administered through arterial catheters because of the potential risk of embolisms.

Disseminated Intravascular Coagulation

Neonates are susceptible to DIC because of immature anticoagulant and fibrinolytic pathways. Most cases of neonatal DIC are associated with tissue ischemia and acidosis secondary to sepsis, low output cardiac failure, perinatal asphyxia, severe respiratory distress syndrome, or necrotizing enterocolitis.[59] Other causes of consumption coagulopathy include large vascular anomalies (the nidus for consumption being the abnormal vascular endothelium of the lesion), severe liver disease, massive hemolysis, or hereditary thrombophilia. DIC may present with hemorrhage and/or thrombosis. Laboratory evaluation reveals prolonged prothrombin time, PTT and thrombin clotting time, decreased fibrinogen, thrombocytopenia, and increased D-dimer and fibrin split products. Sepsis-induced DIC in premature infants may be predicted by elevation of serum interleukin (IL)-6 and IL-10 without elevation of regulated on activation, normal T-cell expressed and secreted (RANTES).[60] Definitive therapy for DIC requires identification and reversal of the trigger for coagulation activation. Treatment of bleeding or prophylaxis for procedures is provided by infusion of fresh frozen plasma, platelets (if bleeding is severe) and, if needed for hypofibrinogenemia, cryoprecipitate. A reasonable target range for bleeding in neonatal DIC is to maintain fibrinogen greater than 100 mg/dL, platelets greater than 50,000 cells/μL, and a prothrombin time that is only modestly elevated. Heparin should be given in thrombotic DIC with antithrombin repletion by concentrate when indicated and attention to the high risk of bleeding complications. Animal models have demonstrated reversal of DIC and improved mortality with replacement of antithrombin, activated protein C, tissue factor pathway inhibitor, and tPA,[61,62] but confirmatory studies in neonates have not been performed to date.

Congenital Thrombophilia

Healthy newborns with spontaneous thrombi are rare, and this presentation should prompt an evaluation for congenital thrombophilia. Heterozygosity at a single thrombophilia locus is generally insufficient to promote neonatal thrombus formation without an additional inciting event (eg, central access catheter placement). However, rare homozygous and compound heterozygous mutations in multiple genes can present with thrombophilia in the neonatal period. Congenital thrombophilia should be considered in patients with spontaneous or extensive thrombosis, ischemic skin lesions or purpura fulminans or a family history of purpura fulminans.[63] It is difficult to promptly distinguish acquired deficiencies from heterozygous inherited deficiencies, so thrombophilia evaluations other than for homozygous states should be deferred from the acute setting. Amongst the several known causes of congenital thrombophilia, only homozygous or compound heterozygous protein C and/or protein S deficiencies are clearly sufficient for neonatal thrombosis. However, antithrombin deficiency, mutations in the prothrombin gene (G20210A), factor V Leiden, elevated lipoprotein (a), and maternal anticardiolipin or lupus anticoagulant have all been associated with thrombosis in neonates.

Specific Neonatal Thrombotic Syndromes

Renal Vein Thrombosis

The renal vein is one of the most common sites of neonatal thrombotic events. Renal vein thrombosis is more common in males[54] and in the left renal vein, although 28% to 44% occur bilaterally.[64,65] Renal vein thrombosis presents with hematuria, thrombocytopenia, and a palpable abdominal mass and may include proteinuria, edema, hypertension, renal failure, anuria, adrenal hemorrhage, or anemia. Diagnosis is reliably confirmed by Doppler ultrasound. Renal vein thrombosis is associated with prematurity, umbilical venous catheters, diabetic mothers, asphyxia, and infections. Factor V Leiden and prothrombin mutation G20210A and elevated lipoprotein(a) have also been found in association with renal vein thrombosis. However, these are very common traits, and it would be inaccurate to say they are proven to be causal, despite the associations.[64,66] Although no clear treatment guidelines exist, supportive care is reasonable for unilateral renal vein thrombosis. Treatment with heparin, either unfractionated or low-molecular-weight, and fibrinolytics are considered for renal insufficiency or involvement of bilateral renal veins or the inferior vena cava. Neonates with renal vein thrombosis should be followed closely for persistent hypertension and chronic renal insufficiency.[67]

Portal Vein Thrombosis

The true incidence of portal vein thrombotic events is unknown but is at least 36 cases per 10,000 neonatal intensive care unit admissions.[68] Prospective ultrasonography revealed 43% of neonates with umbilical venous catheters harbor a clinically silent portal venous thrombus.[58] Most cases are asymptomatic and are identified incidentally by abdominal ultrasound. Major risk factors for occurrence are umbilical venous catheter placement and severe illness; correlation with inherited thrombophilias is controversial.[68,69] The long-term complications of portal venous thrombi are lobar atrophy and portal hypertension with associated gastrointestinal bleeding. These complications are distinctly associated with ectopic umbilical venous catheter placement (below or in the liver) or with occlusive thrombi concurrent with ultrasonographic liver parenchymal changes. Neonates with umbilical venous catheters should be monitored with ultrasound and catheter removal and/or anticoagulation should be considered for portal venous thrombosis.

Purpura Fulminans

Purpura fulminans is a catastrophic presentation of disseminated purpuric lesions, often associated with bullae and necrosis. The histopathology of these lesions reveals diffuse cutaneous microthrombi with surrounding hemorrhage. Diffuse thrombosis including stroke, retinal infarcts, arterial infarction with gangrene, and disseminated intravascular coagulation is often associated with purpura fulminans. Neonatal presentation is associated with severe protein C,[70] antithrombin or protein S[71] deficiency, either acquired in sepsis or inherited as homozygous or compound heterozygous conditions. Some infants with severe protein C deficiency do not develop thrombosis until adulthood,[72] implying that additional factors influence neonatal presentation. Treatment with heparin and replacement with protein C concentrate or fresh frozen plasma is indicated, and successful long-term anticoagulation has been reported.[73]

Arterial Ischemic Stroke

Perinatal arterial ischemic stroke is an important cause of cerebral palsy, epilepsy, and cognitive impairment. Perinatal arterial ischemic stroke is predominantly diagnosed in full-term neonates[74] and has a prevalence of 20 cases per 100,000 live births.[75] In the neonatal period, perinatal arterial ischemic stroke often presents with focal or generalized seizure, although pathologic hand preference before 1 year of age is most common if the stroke was asymptomatic in the newborn period.[76] Ischemic injury is usually detected by magnetic resonance imaging (MRI) or magnetic resonance angiography, and unilateral lesions favor the left hemisphere.[75] It is now accepted that perinatal arterial ischemic stroke risk factors differ from those of older infants and children, as maternal and placental factors are probably often involved, and some events even occur in utero.[77] The most common acquired risk factors for perinatal arterial ischemic stroke are perinatal asphyxia, fetal distress, chorioamnionitis or other infections, preeclampsia, congenital heart disease, and dehydration. The contribution of congenital thrombophilia to perinatal arterial ischemic stroke risk in unclear, although the transient presence of maternal anticardiolipin antibodies may be common.[76] The majority of perinatal ischemic strokes have no detectable hypercoagulable states on subsequent analysis. One possible explanation is embolic arterial occlusion from placental thrombi through the umbilical vein and across the physiological right to left shunts of the fetus and neonate. Evaluation of placental pathology is important because demonstration of placental thrombi or abruption may indicate maternal prothrombotic states. Furthermore, if placental thrombi can be proven histologically, the recurrence risk for infants is especially low. No controlled trials have been performed to date involving anticoagulation in perinatal arterial ischemic stroke, and such studies are needed. One current guideline suggests 10 to 14 days of therapeutic heparin (unfractionated or low-molecular-weight heparin [LMWH]) for perinatal stroke.[78] Because of a low risk of recurrence, long-term anticoagulation or antiplatelets agents are not routinely recommended. Long-term developmental outcomes depend on stroke size, with poorer outcomes for large strokes, especially those involving Broca and Wernicke areas, the internal capsule, and basal ganglia.[79] Cerebral palsy is particularly associated with delayed presentation of symptoms[79] and quantified diffusion restriction of descending corticospinal tracts on MRI.[80]

Sinovenous Thrombosis

The Canadian Pediatric Ischemic Stroke Registry identified 0.67 cases of cerebral venous sinus thrombosis per 100,000 children, with 43% occurring in the neonatal period.[81] Risk factors for neonatal sinovenous thrombosis include perinatal asphyxia, dehydration, infection, congenital heart disease, and severe illness, with ECMO now recognized as a specific risk factor.[82,83] The frequencies of congenital thrombophilias are estimated at 20% to 40% of neonates with venous sinus thrombosis, with factor V Leiden and methyltetrahydrofolate reductase C677T mutation occurring most commonly.[82,83] The latter is so common in the general population that it is not believed to be causally related to thrombosis. In contrast to purpura fulminans, no cases of congenital deficiencies of protein C, protein S or antithrombin have been reported. Clinical presentation ranges from silent or subtle to diffuse neurologic changes, seizures, and intraventricular hemorrhage. Up to 31% of full-term neonates with intraventricular hemorrhage are found to have associated venous sinus thrombosis.[84] This suggests a different pathophysiology than intraventricular hemorrhage in premature infants. Diagnosis in neonates is frequently made by transcranial Doppler ultrasound. However, MRI with magnetic resonance venogram is the most sensitive diagnostic technique.[81] The Canadian Pediatric Ischemic Stroke Registry reports that 42% of neonatal sinovenous thrombi have associated cerebral parenchymal infarcts, and 83% of these are hemorrhagic infarcts.[81] Treatment recommendations for neonatal venous sinus thrombosis are not standardized, aside from treatment of underlying conditions, when relevant (eg, infection, congenital heart disease, dehydration). The high rate of associated hemorrhage increases the risk of treatment with heparin, either unfractionated or LMWH, so treatment plans should be individualized. In older patients, punctate hemorrhage behind a cerebral venous infarct is not an absolute contraindication to anticoagulation, but studies in neonates are lacking. Nevertheless, in the Canadian registry, 36% of neonates were treated with heparin, unfractionated or LMWH, most for 3 months, and no cases of death or neurologic compromise from hemorrhage were reported.[81] Overall outcomes from the Canadian registry reveal neurologic impairment in up to two-thirds of cases and approximately 2% mortality.[82] Associated parenchymal infarction is associated with prolonged neurologic deficits.

Principles of Therapy

As with other age groups, therapeutic modalities available to neonates include supportive care, anticoagulation, thrombolytic agents, and surgical thrombectomy. The British Haemostasis and Thrombosis Task Force has proposed guidelines for the management of neonatal thrombosis.[63] Supportive therapy is recommended for clinically silent thrombi, including catheter-mediated events. As soon as practical, catheters associated with thrombi should be removed, and all documented thrombi should be followed closely with serial imaging.

Anticoagulation with unfractionated or LMWH is described in neonates and is the mainstay of anticoagulant therapy. Oral vitamin K antagonists are not recommended in the acute settings for management of neonatal thrombosis. Anticoagulation with heparin in neonates often requires supplementation of physiologically low levels of antithrombin with concentrate or fresh frozen plasma, especially for

Treatment of Neonatal Thrombosis

Unfractionated Heparin
Bolus: 75 unites/kg UFH over 10 minutes
Maintenance: 28 units/kg/h, therapeutic goal = 0.3–0.7 U/ml
Prophylaxis: 10 U/kg/h
Follow platelet count q2d to detect 2–5% chance of HIT

Enoxaparin
1.5 mg/kg SC q12h (with normal renal function)
Check anti-Factor Xa level by peripheral venipuncture 4–6 hours after 2nd or 3rd dose therapeutic goal 0.5–1 U/ml (goal 0.4–0.6 U/ml if concurrent thrombocytopenia or other bleeding risk factor)
Hold for 12 hours prior to minor procedures, 24 h prior to major procedures
Follow platelet count q2d to detect 2–5% chance of HIT

Prophylaxis with Enoxaparin
0.75 mg/kg SC q12h
If checked, anti-Factor Xa level 4–6 hours after 2nd or 3rd dose should be <0.4 U/ml
Hold for 12 hours prior to procedures

Purpura Fulminans
Concurrent unfractionated heparin (as above); goal = 0.3–0.7 U/ml and replacement with FFP or protein C concentrate.
FFP: 15 ml/kg BID until specific diagnosis is clear
Protein C concentrate for severe protein C deficienty
Load with 100–120 U/kg, then 60–80 U/kg q6h × 3 doses (goal protein C activity 100%). Once therapeutic anticoagulation is achieved, maintenance therapy with 45–60 U/kg q6–12h (goal protein C activity >25%)

Antithrombin III Repletion
Antithrombin III (functional) should be maintained at >35% of normal levels for effective heparin-based anticoagulation
Dose in International Units = (desired – current ATIII*) × weight (kg)

*expressed as % normal level based on functional ATIII level.

tPA Thrombolysis in Neonatal Thrombosis

Concurrent Heparin (Unfractionated Heparin or Enoxaparin) Should Be Considered at Prophylactic Dosing

- Non-life or limb-threatening thrombi:
  - 0.05 mg/kg h × 2 h
  - If no improvement 0.1 mg/kg/h × 6 hours
  - Discontinue after 8 hours
- Life or limb-threatening thrombi:
  - 0.1 mg/kg/h for up to 6 hours
  - If no response, consider increase by 0.1 mg/kg/h increments to max 0.5 mg/kg/h
  - Maintain fibrinogen >150 mg/dL
  - Reversal of severe bleeding with aminocaproic acid at 100 mg/kg IV q6h

Recommended Dosing for Transfusion in Neonatal Hemorrhage

PRBCs: 10–15 cc/kg single donor PRBCs infused over 4 hours
Platelets*: 10 ml/kg raises platelet count by 75 K (goal >50 K if bleeding, >20 K if not)
FFP: 10 ml/kg raises factor levels 0.1–0.2 U/ml; 15 ml/kg BID for purpura fulminans
Cryoprecipitate: 0.15 U/kg raises fibrinogen about 100 mg/dL (goal >150 mg/dL if bleeding, >50 mg/dL if not bleeding)
Von Willebrand Factor: 40–69 "ristocetin cofactor units"/kg of plasma-derived FVIII/VWF preparations
Factor VIII: for hemophilia A—50 U/kg load, then 25 U/kg q12h. Recombinant factor preferred.
Factor IX: for hemophilia B—80–100 U/kg daily. Recombinant factor preferred.
Factor VIIa: for severe factor VII deficiency—20–30 mcg/kg q6–12h

*Volume limits transfusion of platelets by the "unit" in small neonates. Practices vary—follow institutional guidelines for volume dosing or volume reduction.

apparent heparin resistance. The starting doses for heparin (unfractionated and LMW) are outlined in the Treatment of Neonatal Thrombosis box. Management of heparin anticoagulation in neonates requires special consideration for physiologically low antithrombin levels and prolonged PTT. Antithrombin should be corrected in laboratory evaluation of anti-Xa levels. Therapeutic anticoagulation is defined by therapeutic anti-Xa levels (0.3–0.7 units/mL for unfractionated heparin and 0.5–1 units/mL for LMWH). Unfractionated heparin dosing may also be adjusted according to the PTT that correlates to anti-Xa levels of 0.3 to 0.7 units/mL. Three LMWHs have been studied in neonates,[85] and the most experience lies with enoxaparin. Prophylactic heparin administration is recommended for umbilical arterial lines (0.5 units/h) and for cardiac catheterization (bolus 100–150 units/kg with catheter insertion, repeat for prolonged procedures).

The antibodies that cause heparin-induced thrombocytopenia (HIT) are found in neonates with an estimated incidence as high as 1.5%,[86] particularly in patients following cardiac surgery. Overt HIT with thrombosis is apparently much more rare, although it has been observed in neonates and can be life-threatening. Mothers with HIT can passively transfer this antibody to their fetus. Diagnostic criteria for HIT include platelet count decrease by more than 50%, timing 5 to 10 days after heparin initiation (neonates cannot exhibit an anamnestic response) and new thrombosis with a positive HIT antibody. Treatment includes cessation of heparin therapy and anticoagulation with argatroban or lepirudin. Data supporting use of these agents is sparse in neonates but is reviewed by Risch and colleagues.[87] Fondaparinux might be a reasonable option in selected cases, but experience in neonates is limited.

Guidelines for thrombolytic management of neonatal thrombi have been reported by the British Haemostasis and Thrombosis Task Force[63] and the Perinatal and Pediatric Subcommittee of the International Society of Thrombosis and Haemostasis.[88] Both groups agree that thrombolysis should be considered for extensive thrombosis, organ dysfunction, limb-threatening ischemia, and low-dose thrombolysis for catheter-occluding thrombi. Tissue plasminogen activator is the most studied thrombolytic reagent in pediatric patients. Transfusion support for hypofibrinogenemia and thrombocytopenia should be provided to minimize bleeding risk. Contraindications for thrombolytic therapy include active bleeding and major surgery or bleeding within 10 days, whereas relative cautions include severe asphyxia within 7 days, seizures within 48 hours, sepsis or prematurity of less than 32 weeks of gestation. When required, heparin given concomitantly with tPA should be given at prophylactic dosing (0.75 mg/kg every 12 hours for LMWH or 10 units/kg/h for unfractionated heparin). Surgical thrombectomy is reserved for organ, limb, or life-threatening thrombi when tPA is impractical or predicted to be ineffective or too slow.

SELECTED READINGS

Monagle P, Barnes C, Ignjatovic V, et al: Developmental haemostasis. Impact for clinical haemostasis laboratories. Thromb Haemost 95:362, 2006.

Andrew M, Paes B, Milner R, et al: Development of the human coagulation system in the full-term infant. Blood 70:165, 1987.

Reverdiau-Moalic P, Delahousse B, Body G, Bardos P, Leroy J, Gruel Y: Evolution of blood coagulation activators and inhibitors in the healthy human fetus. Blood 88:900, 1996.

REFERENCES

For complete list of references log onto www.expertconsult.com

CHAPTER 134

HYPERCOAGULABLE STATES

Kenneth A. Bauer

INTRODUCTION

Improved understanding of the molecular basis of the coagulation mechanism coupled with clinical investigation has facilitated the identification of hemostatic risk factors in substantial numbers of patients presenting with venous thrombosis. Persons with a tendency to thrombosis are defined as having thrombophilia, and the term *inherited thrombophilia* is applied to persons with genetic defects that predispose them to the development of venous thromboembolism.

This chapter describes the hereditary thrombotic disorders or primary hypercoagulable states (Table 134–1), as well as some of the major acquired or secondary hypercoagulable states (malignancy, nephrotic syndrome, paroxysmal nocturnal hemoglobinuria [PNH], hyperviscosity syndromes, drug-induced thrombosis, and antiphospholipid antibody syndrome).

CLINICAL APPROACH

Differential Diagnosis

A clinically useful approach to patients with an active thrombotic process is to categorize the underlying disorder as either a primary or an acquired hypercoagulable state. Thus, one group of patients will have features that suggest the presence of an inherited thrombotic disorder or a primary hypercoagulable state (see Table 134–1). Such disorders result from mutations in single genes encoding a plasma protein component of one of the major natural anticoagulant mechanisms. The anticoagulant systems most frequently involved in the inherited hypercoagulable states include antithrombin III in the heparan sulfate-antithrombin III mechanism and protein C, protein S, and factor V Leiden in the protein C anticoagulant pathway (Fig. 134–1). An elevation in the plasma prothrombin level in association with a G to A transversion at position 20210 in the 3′-untranslated region of the prothrombin gene also is a risk factor for venous thrombosis.

A second group of patients have an acquired or secondary hypercoagulable state. The underlying disorder may be any of a heterogeneous group of disorders characterized by an increased risk for the development of thrombotic complications compared with that in the general population (Table 134–2).

The inherited thrombotic disorders (see Table 134–1) have been associated almost exclusively with *venous thrombosis*. Hereditary deficiencies of antithrombin III, protein C, or protein S will be found in less than 10% of unselected individuals presenting with venous thromboembolism (Table 134–3). Resistance to activated protein C because of the factor V Leiden mutation and the prothrombin G20210A mutation are more prevalent defects that can also be found in significant numbers of persons with first episodes of idiopathic venous thrombosis older than age 50 in the absence of a positive family history.[1–3]

A significant percentage of women with thrombosis in association with oral contraceptive use or pregnancy will have an inherited disorder, especially the factor V Leiden[4,5] and prothrombin G20210A mutations.[6] Hereditary thrombophilia has also been identified as a risk factor in patients with venous thrombosis in uncommon sites such as the portal, hepatic, mesenteric, axillary, and cerebral veins. The presence of indwelling venous catheters however, is the most common risk factor today for upper extremity venous thrombosis, and this complication generally does not warrant evaluation of the patient for an underlying hypercoagulable state.

Although classification of patients as having either a hereditary or an acquired disorder is useful in directing the laboratory evaluation for hypercoagulability, thrombosis frequently results from the interplay of genetic and acquired factors. Patients with hereditary defects are at lifelong risk of developing thrombosis, and stimuli such as pregnancy, estrogen use, or surgery trigger thrombotic episodes in perhaps 50% of affected persons. Also, defects in more than one coagulation protein can be identified in some patients who have experienced venous thrombosis, reflecting the high background frequency in the general population of abnormalities such as factor V Leiden[2] and the prothrombin G20210A mutation.[8] Such patients have a more severe thrombotic tendency than those with a single identifiable mutation.[9–15] Thus, thrombosis can be viewed as a multigene disorder in which susceptible persons will have one or more genetic mutations, with clinical events occurring when they are exposed to exogenous prothrombotic stimuli (Fig. 134–2).[16] In many cases, however, the inciting precipitant to thrombosis is not reported by the patient and presumably is subclinical.

History and Physical Examination

In the evaluation of patients with a recent or remote history of thrombosis, historical details should be obtained regarding the age of onset, location of prior thrombotic lesions, and results of objective diagnostic studies documenting thrombosis. Such diagnostic studies are critical, because the clinical diagnosis of deep vein thrombosis, in particular, is notoriously inaccurate (see Chapter 135). The patient should be carefully questioned about circumstances proximate to the time of thrombosis that might have precipitated the event. Possible inciting factors include surgical procedures, trauma, pregnancy, immobility, and estrogen administration. Women should be carefully questioned regarding prior use of oral contraceptives or hormone replacement therapy and obstetric history. An increased risk of recurrent fetal loss is associated with the presence of lupus anticoagulants or antiphospholipid antibodies, as well as with the hereditary thrombotic disorders.[17–21] A family history is particularly important because a well-documented history of venous thrombosis in one or more first-degree relatives strongly suggests the presence of a hereditary defect. The initial manifestation of a malignancy can be a thrombotic event, so inquiry should be made regarding the presence of constitutional symptoms (eg, diminished appetite, weight loss, fatigue), pain, hematochezia, hemoptysis, or hematuria. It also should be ascertained whether the patient has an underlying disease, such as cancer, collagen-vascular disease, a myeloproliferative disorder, atherosclerotic disease, or nephrotic syndrome, or takes synthetic or natural estrogens, or drugs that can induce lupus anticoagulants, such as hydralazine, procainamide, or phenothiazines. Recurrent thrombosis despite therapeutic anticoagulation with oral anticoagulants is common in patients with an occult neoplasm or an established diagnosis of cancer.

In the physical examination, special attention should be directed to the vascular system, extremities to look for signs of superficial or

Table 134–1 Differential Diagnosis of the Patient Presenting with Thrombosis or Thrombotic Diathesis

Inherited (Primary) Hypercoagulable States
- Activated protein C resistance caused by factor V Leiden Mutation
- Prothrombin gene mutation (G to A transition at position 20210 in the 3′-untranslated region)
- Antithrombin III deficiency
- Protein C deficiency
- Protein S deficiency
- Dysfibrinogenemias (rare)

Acquired (Secondary) Hypercoagulable States

In association with physiologic or thrombogenic stimuli
- Pregnancy (especially the postpartum period)
- Estrogen use (oral contraceptives, hormone replacement therapy)
- Immobilization
- Trauma
- Postoperative state

Advancing age

Obesity

Prolonged air travel

Lupus anticoagulant or antiphospholipid antibody syndrome

In association with other clinical disorders (see Table 134–2)

Mixed/Unknown
- Activated protein C resistance in the absence of factor V Leiden
- Elevated factor VIII level
- Elevated factor XI level
- Elevated factor IX level
- Elevated thrombin activatable fibrinolysis inhibitor (TAFI) level
- Decreased free tissue factor pathway inhibitor (TFPI) level
- Decreased plasma fibrinolytic activity

deep vein thrombosis, chest, heart, abdominal organs, and skin to detect skin necrosis or livedo reticularis. Because venous thromboembolism may be the first manifestation of an underlying malignancy, rectal examination and stool testing for occult blood should be done, and women should undergo a pelvic examination.

The hereditary thrombotic disorders include deficiencies of antithrombin III, protein C, or protein S; the factor V Leiden and prothrombin G20210A mutations; and rarely, dysfibrinogenemias. The most common sites of thrombosis in such patients are the deep leg veins, iliac veins, and pulmonary arteries. Thrombosis in mesenteric, portal, and cerebral veins as well as superficial thrombophlebitis has been described in patients with these disorders. Typical precipitating

Table 134–2 Acquired Conditions and Disorders Associated with Hypercoagulable States

Systemic lupus erythematosus in association with the presence of a lupus anticoagulant or antiphospholipid antibodies

Malignancy
- Disease-related: includes migratory superficial thrombophlebitis (Trousseau syndrome), nonbacterial thrombotic endocarditis, thrombosis associated with chronic DIC, thrombotic microangiopathy
- Treatment-related: associated with the administration of various chemotherapeutic agents (L-asparaginase, mitomycin, some adjuvant chemotherapeutic agents for treatment of breast cancer, thalidomide or lenalidomide in conjunction with high doses of dexamethasone

Infusion of prothrombin complex concentrates

Nephrotic syndrome

Heparin-induced thrombocytopenia

Myeloproliferative disorders

Paroxysmal nocturnal hemoglobinuria

DIC, disseminated intravascular coagulopathy

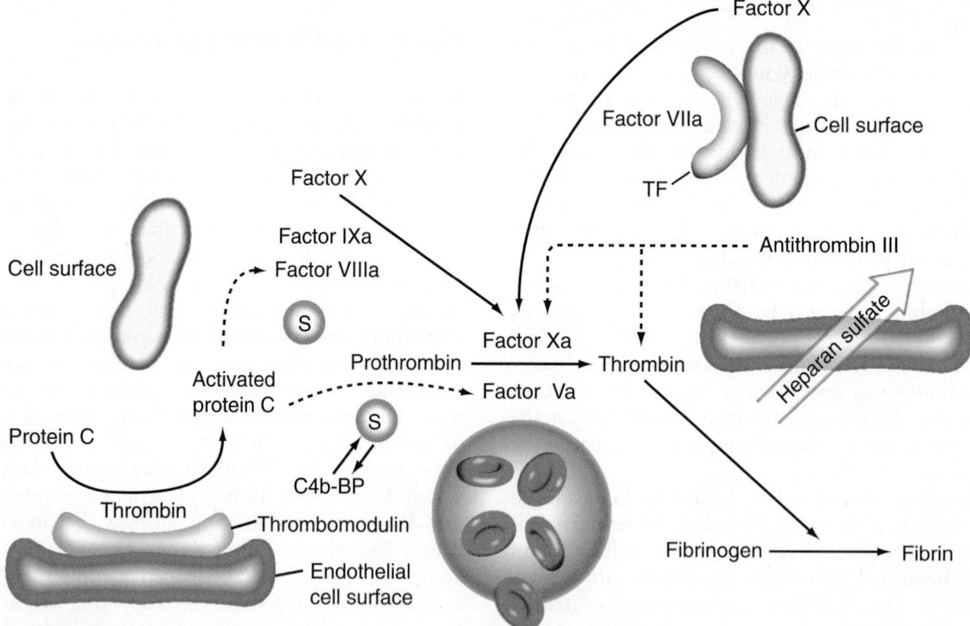

Figure 134–1 A SCHEMATIC DIAGRAM OF THE PATHWAYS THAT GENERATE FACTOR XA AND THROMBIN, AND THE NATURAL ANTICOAGULANT MECHANISMS THAT REGULATE THE ACTIVITY OF THESE ENZYMES. Factor X can be activated by factor VIIa-tissue factor (TF) complex or the factor IXa-VIIIa-activated cell surface complex. Factor Xa binds to the factor Va on activated platelets and mediates the conversion of prothrombin to thrombin under physiologic conditions. Thrombin is then able to act upon fibrinogen to form a fibrin clot. Thrombin and factor Xa are inactivated by antithrombin III bound to heparan sulfate molecules associated with the vascular endothelium, resulting in the formation of factor Xa-antithrombin III and thrombin-antithrombin III complexes. Protein C is activated by thrombin bound to the endothelial cell receptor thrombomodulin. Once activated, protein C functions as a potent anticoagulant by inactivating factors VIIIa and Va. Protein S enhances the binding of activated protein C to phospholipid-containing membranes and is able to accelerate the inactivation of factors VIIIa and Va by this enzyme. The complement component, C4b-binding protein (C4b-BP), forms complexes with protein S, which neutralizes its ability to serve as a cofactor for activated protein C in inactivating factors VIIIa and Va.

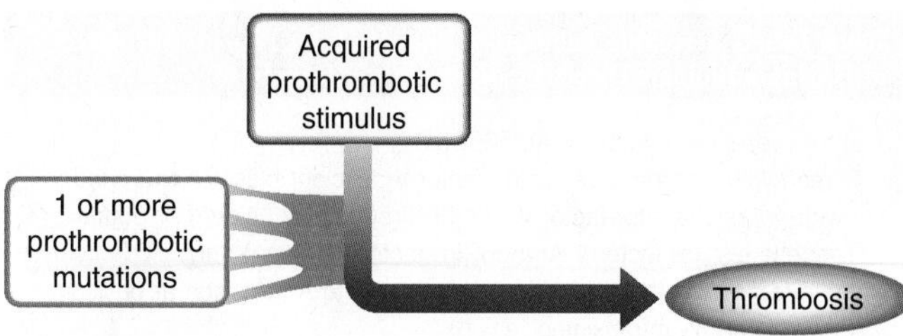

Figure 134–2 Venous thrombosis can be viewed as a multigene disorder in which susceptible persons will have one or more genetic mutations. Clinical events often occur when they are exposed to exogenous prothrombotic stimuli. *(Modified from Schafer AI: Hypercoagulable states: Molecular genetics to clinical practice. Lancet 344: 1739, 1994, with permission. © by the Lancet, Ltd.)*

Table 134–3 Prevalence of Defects in Patients with Venous Thrombosis

Defect	Prevalence
Activated protein C resistance (factor V Leiden)	12–40%[a]
Prothrombin gene mutation (G to A transition at position 20210 in the 3′-untranslated region)	6–18%[a]
Deficiencies of antithrombin III, protein C, protein S	5–15%
Antiphospholipid antibody syndrome	5–10%

[a]Prevalence restricted to white populations.

factors for thrombosis in such patients are the postoperative state, immobilization, trauma, pregnancy, oral contraceptive use, and advancing age.

Patients with thrombosis should be questioned regarding their ethnic background. The factor V Leiden and prothrombin G20210A mutations are not found in aboriginal African, Native American, or Asian populations.[22,23] The two mutations arose approximately 30,000 years ago in whites in Europe.[24,25] The carrier frequency of the factor V Leiden in the U.S. population with African, Native American, or Asian ancestry is 1.23%, 1.25%, and 0.45%, respectively.[26]

Laboratory Evaluation

Routine Tests

The initial laboratory evaluation for patients with thrombosis should include a complete blood count, review of the peripheral blood smear, and serum chemistries including liver and renal function tests, and urinalysis.

Elevations in the hematocrit, white blood cell count, or platelet count should lead to consideration of polycythemia vera and essential thrombocythemia in the differential diagnosis. These myeloproliferative disorders predispose patients to venous as well as arterial thrombotic events, particularly when the hematocrit or platelet count is not controlled by therapy. In addition, secondary polycythemia or secondary thrombocytosis may provide a clue to an underlying occult neoplasm that may itself be the predisposing factor to thrombosis. Leukopenia and thrombocytopenia often are found in PNH, a hematologic disorder characterized by chronic intravascular hemolysis with episodes of gross hematuria and a unique constellation of thrombotic complications. These occur almost exclusively in the abdominal venous network, including the mesenteric, hepatic, portal, splenic, and renal veins, and the cerebral venous circulation. The development of thrombosis and thrombocytopenia concurrent with heparin administration should always prompt consideration of the diagnosis of heparin-induced thrombocytopenia.

If the blood smear shows evidence of red-cell fragmentation or schistocytes, the differential diagnosis includes disseminated intravascular coagulation (see Chapter 132) and the thrombotic microangiopathies (thrombotic thrombocytopenic purpura/hemolytic-uremic syndrome). Although bleeding is the most common coagulation problem in disseminated intravascular coagulation, patients with malignancy can have a low-grade consumptive coagulopathy leading to the development of venous or arterial thrombosis. The latter can result from emboli arising from fibrin vegetations on the mitral or aortic valves (ie, nonbacterial thrombotic endocarditis). A leukoerythroblastic picture with nucleated red blood cells or immature white cells on the peripheral smear should suggest the possibility of bone marrow involvement by tumor.

Patients with Budd-Chiari syndrome, which occurs when there is obstruction of the hepatic venous circulation, have ascites and hepatomegaly along with abnormal liver function tests. The nephrotic syndrome is characterized by large amounts of protein in the urine, hypoalbuminemia, and hyperlipidemia. Renal vein thrombosis can complicate the clinical course in up to one-third of such patients, but patients with nephrotic syndrome are prone as well to venous thrombosis in sites such as leg veins and pulmonary arteries.

Patients with thrombosis should routinely undergo baseline coagulation tests, including prothrombin time and partial thromboplastin time (PTT). For the latter test, use of a reagent sensitive to the presence of lupus anticoagulants will provide an initial screen for this acquired abnormality. If the PTT is normal, the use of additional specialized clotting assays such as the dilute Russell viper venom time, kaolin clotting time, and the tissue thromboplastin inhibition test, may facilitate making this diagnosis in patients suspected on clinical grounds of having a lupus anticoagulant (see Chapter 131). Some, but not all, individuals with lupus anticoagulants have elevated titers of cardiolipin or β_2-glycoprotein-I antibodies. Patients with abnormal test results should be periodically reevaluated, because lupus anticoagulants or elevated cardiolipin antibody levels are considered to be risk factors for thrombosis only if the abnormalities persist over several months.

In patients who present with idiopathic venous thromboembolism, the available data do not support an extensive search (eg, computed tomography scans of the chest, abdomen, and pelvis) for occult malignancy. It is however important to pursue symptoms or findings on physical examination that suggest an underlying malignancy and to ensure that age-appropriate screening tests have been performed (ie, mammography, colonoscopy).

Tests for Specific Biologic Risk Factors

Based on the history and physical examination, a decision must be made as to whether testing should be performed to identify specific biologic risk factors predisposing to thrombosis. Clinical judgement must be exercised with regard to the scope of the evaluation as well as the optimal time for its performance. The decision as to which tests should be ordered is determined partly by the type of thrombotic event (Table 134–4). Hereditary deficiencies of antithrombin III, protein C, and protein S, and the factor V Leiden mutation and the prothrombin G20210A mutations are risk factors for venous thrombosis. Although there are reports of an association with arterial thrombosis in select populations, such as children and young women with myocardial infarction, it is generally not recommended to test for these defects in most such patients. The presence of a lupus anticoagulant is a risk factor for venous as well as arterial thrombosis. Therefore, performance of these tests is warranted in the latter group of patients, particularly when other factors predisposing to arterial thrombosis are absent.

Additional factors will guide the extent of the laboratory evaluation. Clinical features that increase the likelihood of identifying individuals with deficiencies of antithrombin III, protein C, and protein

Table 134–4 Sites of Thrombosis According to Coagulation Defect

Abnormality	Arterial	Venous
Factor V Leiden	–	+
Prothrombin gene mutation	–	+
Antithrombin III deficiency	–	+
Protein C deficiency	–	+
Protein S deficiency	–	+
Lupus anticoagulant	+	+

S include an initial venous thrombotic event younger than the age of 50 years, recurrent thrombosis, and positive family history.[27] These features also increase the chances of identifying individuals with factor V Leiden and the prothrombin gene mutation, although these genetic defects also can frequently be identified in older individuals with an initial episode of deep venous thrombosis who do not have acquired risk factors or a positive family history. Screening for all of these defects and lupus anticoagulant/antiphospholipid antibodies also is warranted in patients with thrombosis in unusual vascular beds (eg, mesenteric vein thrombosis, cerebral venous thrombosis).

Some clinical features have been associated with individual hereditary thrombotic disorders. Approximately one-third of individuals who sustain the rare complication of warfarin-induced skin necrosis will prove to have protein C deficiency; however, this syndrome has also been reported in patients with protein S deficiency[28] and factor V Leiden.[29] In newborn infants, the development of skin necrosis and visceral thrombosis (eg, neonatal purpura fulminans) indicates a likely diagnosis of severe hereditary protein C deficiency, although cases have been reported in association with homozygous protein S deficiency as well. Both conditions require emergent therapy if major morbidity or mortality are to be averted. Although the presence of resistance to heparin's anticoagulant effect, as measured by the PTT, often leads to consideration of antithrombin III deficiency, congenital antithrombin III deficiency is infrequently diagnosed in such individuals.

Table 134–5 gives a list of tests useful in screening patients suspected of having a biologic defect predisposing to thrombosis. Coagulation assays with high sensitivity and specificity for the factor V Leiden mutation are available and are based on the resistance of the mutant factor Va molecule to inactivation by activated protein C. Positive results are confirmed by genetic testing of DNA obtained from peripheral blood mononuclear cells. Initial testing for the factor V Leiden mutation can also be done genetically; testing for the prothrombin G20210A mutation must be done genetically. The best screening tests for deficiencies of antithrombin III, protein C, and protein S are functional assays that detect both quantitative and qualitative defects. Immunologic assays detect only quantitative deficiencies of these proteins. For antithrombin III, convenient functional assays are available that measure the heparin cofactor activity of the molecule. Among protein C assays, coagulation assays provide a more complete evaluation of the functional activity of the molecule than is possible with amidolytic assays. However, coagulation assays for protein C as well as protein S can give falsely low values if the factor V Leiden mutation is present,[30] and reliable application of these assays requires initial assessment as to whether this mutation is present. To screen for a dysfibrinogenemia, the thrombin time is recommended along with measurements of plasma fibrinogen by clotting and immunologic assay.

Timing of Laboratory Testing

An important consideration in the laboratory evaluation of patients with a suspected deficiency of antithrombin III, protein C, or protein S is the timing of testing. Erroneous diagnoses can be made because of the influence of acute thrombosis, comorbid illness, or anticoagulant therapy on the levels of these plasma proteins. Table 134–6 provides a list of some of the common causes of acquired deficiencies of antithrombin III, protein C, or protein S.

Acute thrombosis by itself can result in transiently reduced levels of antithrombin III and, occasionally, protein C and protein S. Heparin therapy can be associated with up to a 30% decline in plasma antithrombin III levels over several days, whereas warfarin produces a marked drop in the functional activity of protein C and protein S and a lesser decline in immunologic levels. Warfarin has also been shown to rarely elevate antithrombin III levels significantly, sometimes into the normal range, in patients with a hereditary deficiency of this inhibitor. For these reasons, it is optimal to test for

Table 134–5 Screening Laboratory Evaluation for Patients Suspected of Having a Biologic Defect Predisposing to Thrombosis

Test for presence of factor V Arg506Gln
- Screen with clotting assay using factor V-deficient plasma[a] and confirm with genetic test for factor V Arg506Gln (factor V Leiden) or obtain genetic test for factor V Arg506Gln (factor V Leiden) only

Genetic test for prothrombin gene mutation (G to A transition at position 20210 in the 3′-untranslated region)

Functional assay of antithrombin III (heparin-cofactor assay)[a]

Functional assays of protein C[a]

Functional assay of protein S/immunological assays of total and free protein S[a]

Screen for dysfibrinogenemias (immunologic and functional assays of fibrinogen, thrombin time)[a]

Clotting assay for lupus anticoagulant[a]/serologic tests for antiphospholipid antibodies

[a]Coagulation assays are performed on platelet-poor plasma obtained from blood samples drawn into a solution containing 3.8% (wt/vol) sodium citrate. The ratio of anticoagulant to blood is 0.1:0.9 (vol/vol). In the absence of an accompanying clinical history for the patient, determination of the prothrombin time will help to exclude the ingestion of warfarin, which will affect the measurements of protein C and protein S. Determination of the thrombin time as well as the PTT will help to exclude the administration of heparin.

PTT, partial thromboplastin time.

Table 134–6 Causes of Acquired Deficiencies in Antithrombin III, Protein C, or Protein S

Antithrombin III	Protein C	Protein S
Neonatal period	Neonatal period	Neonatal period
Pregnancy		Pregnancy
Liver disease	Liver disease	Liver disease
DIC[a]	DIC[a]	DIC
Nephrotic syndrome	Chemotherapy (CMF)	
Major surgery		Inflammatory states
Acute thrombosis	Acute Thrombosis	Acute thrombosis
Treatment with:		
Heparin	Warfarin	Warfarin
L-asparaginase	L-asparaginase	L-asparaginase
Estrogens		Estrogens

CMF, cyclophosphamide, methotrexate, 5-fluorouracil; DIC, disseminated intravascular coagulation.

these deficiency states at least 2 weeks after the patient has completed the initial course of oral anticoagulant therapy following a thrombotic event. If, however, levels of antithrombin III, protein C, or protein S are obtained on acute presentation and are well within the normal range, these findings will effectively exclude the diagnosis of these deficiency states. The finding of a low level during this period will need to be confirmed by repeat testing after anticoagulation is discontinued.

The investigation of first-degree family members is useful to document the hereditary nature of the deficiency. Confirmation of a deficiency state in first-degree family members is particularly helpful diagnostically in patients in whom the risks of recurrent thrombosis are too great to temporarily discontinue anticoagulation. In such patients, a diagnosis of protein C or protein S deficiency can be confirmed by carrying out testing after warfarin has been discontinued for 2 weeks under the cover of heparin or low-molecular-weight heparin at therapeutic doses.

Other Coagulation Abnormalities

Elevations in the levels of several coagulation factors, including factor VIII,[31–33] factor XI,[34] factor IX,[35] thrombin activatable fibrinolysis inhibitor,[36] and decreased levels of free tissue factor pathway inhibitor[37] and plasma fibrinolytic activity[38] have been implicated as risk factors for a first episode of venous thrombosis. The molecular basis for these abnormalities has not been elucidated. For factor VIII, high plasma activity levels cannot be attributed to overt inflammation because patients with levels greater than 150% did not have elevations in acute phase reactants such as C-reactive protein, fibrinogen, and erythrocyte sedimentation rate.[39] Austrian investigators found that the probability of recurrent venous thrombosis at 2 years in persons with factor VIII levels greater than 234% of normal (the 90th percentile of the values for the study sample) was 37% compared with 5% in patients with levels less than 120% of normal. This observation has not however been corroborated by other groups.[40,41]

In the absence of the factor V Leiden mutation, a significantly increased risk for venous thrombosis is associated with a reduced sensitivity to activated protein C, as measured by a clotting assay that does not mix patient's plasma with factor V-deficient plasma.[42] However, this risk is lower than in carriers of the factor V Leiden mutation. This increased risk remains after adjustment for elevated levels of factor VIII and oral contraceptive use, both of which are known to lead to a reduced response to activated protein C.

Many other hemostatic gene polymorphisms have been investigated and suggested to be risk factors for venous and arterial thrombosis; most of these associations have not been substantiated by subsequent studies.[43–46]

There have been reports of thrombosis in association with abnormalities in other coagulation or fibrinolytic system proteins. These include heparin cofactor II deficiency, plasminogen deficiency (either hypo- or dysplasminogenemias), factor XII deficiency, and elevations in plasminogen activator inhibitor type 1 (PAI-1). Causal associations between these abnormalities and an increased risk of thrombosis have not been clearly defined, however.

INHERITED HYPERCOAGULABLE DISORDERS

Antithrombin III Deficiency

In 1965, Egeberg[47] described a Norwegian family in which certain members who had a history of thrombosis had plasma concentrations of antithrombin III that were 40% to 50% of normal. Subsequently, other investigators described additional families with a similar constellation of clinical and laboratory abnormalities.[48,49]

Antithrombin III deficiency is inherited in an autosomal dominant fashion and thus affects both sexes equally. Two major types of inherited antithrombin III deficiency have been delineated (Table 134–7). The type I deficiency state is a result of reduced synthesis of biologically normal protease inhibitor molecules.[50] In these cases, the antigenic and functional activity of antithrombin III in the blood is reduced in parallel. The molecular basis of this disorder is either a deletion of a major segment of the antithrombin III gene or, more commonly, the occurrence of small deletions/insertions, or single base substitutions. These mutations will introduce a frameshift, a direct termination codon, a change in messenger RNA (mRNA) processing, or unstable translation products. The antithrombin III mutation database includes more than 100 distinct mutations in patients with a type I deficiency.[51] The second type of antithrombin III deficiency is produced by a discrete molecular defect within the protease inhibitor (type II). The plasma levels of antithrombin III are greatly reduced as judged by functional activity, whereas antithrombin III immunologic activity is essentially normal.

Table 134–7 Assay Measurements in Heterozygous Antithrombin (ATIII) Deficiency

Types	Antigen	Activity: Heparin Cofactor	Activity: Progressive ATIII
I	Low	Low	Low
II			
Active site defect	Normal	Low	Low
Heparin-binding site defect	Normal	Low	Normal

The prevalence of type I antithrombin III deficiency in the adult population is approximately 1 : 2000.[52,53] Studies of healthy blood donors employing functional assays that measure heparin cofactor activity have found that the prevalence of antithrombin III deficiency in the general population is 1 : 250 to 1 : 500;[54,55] a substantial number, however, have a type II defect with mutations at the heparin-binding site that are associated with a lower risk of thrombosis.[53] The best single screening test for the disorder is the antithrombin III-heparin cofactor assay that measures factor Xa inhibition.

The thrombotic risk associated with antithrombin III deficiency depends on population selection. In older reviews of antithrombin III deficiency including families with a high penetrance of thrombosis, more than 50% of affected patients experience venous thrombotic episodes.[56,57] The initial clinical manifestations occur apparently spontaneously in approximately 42% of subjects but are related to pregnancy, parturition, oral contraceptive ingestion, surgery, or trauma in the remaining 58% of patients.[56] The most common sites of disease are the deep veins of the leg and the mesenteric veins. Recurrent thrombotic episodes occur in approximately 60% of affected persons, and clinical signs of pulmonary embolism are evident in 40%.[56] Although cases have been reported in which antithrombin III-deficient infants sustained cerebral venous thrombosis,[58–60] thrombotic episodes are rare in affected children before puberty. After puberty, thrombotic events occur with some frequency and the risk of thrombosis increases substantially with advancing age.[56] First-degree relatives of symptomatic individuals with antithrombin III deficiency have an 8- to 10-fold increased risk of thrombosis over that in noncarriers.[61,62] In the Leiden Thrombophilia Study, a case-control study of 474 consecutive patients following an initial episode of deep vein thrombosis,[63] the prevalence of antithrombin III deficiency was only 1.1%, and the odds ratio for thrombosis was only 5.0.[64]

The first family with type II antithrombin III deficiency was described in 1974.[65] Many families with this type of deficiency state have been reported, and they have been further subcategorized on the basis of two different functional assays of antithrombin III activity. The first is the antithrombin III-heparin cofactor assay, which measures the ability of heparin to bind to lysyl residues on the inhibitor and catalyze the neutralization of coagulation enzymes such as thrombin and factor Xa. This assay, based on factor Xa inhibition, is currently the most widely used functional antithrombin III assay. The second test is the progressive antithrombin III activity assay, which quantitates the capacity of this inhibitor to neutralize the enzymatic activity of thrombin in the absence of heparin.

Heparin cofactor II is another protein in human plasma that exhibits heparin cofactor activity.[66,67] In contrast to antithrombin III, this inhibitor does not inhibit factor Xa or other serine proteases and requires concentrations of heparin of at least 1 unit/mL in the reaction mixture to function as an efficient inhibitor of thrombin; it therefore probably plays a minimal role when heparin is used clinically as an anticoagulant.[67] Because some functional antithrombin III assays employ heparin concentrations greater than 1 unit/mL, an assay based on factor Xa inhibition is more specific than one based on thrombin inhibition to identify patients with congenital antithrombin III deficiency.[68] Heparin cofactor II can also interact with another glycosaminoglycan, dermatan sulfate, and this binding dramatically accelerates the neutralization of thrombin by this inhibitor. Several patients have been described with inherited deficiencies of heparin cofactor II and thrombotic phenomena,[69,70] but the causal relationship is uncertain.[71]

Many mutant antithrombin III molecules have been identified with reductions in heparin cofactor activity without a concordant reduction in progressive antithrombin III activity.[51] These variants generally have mutations at a heparin-binding site at the N-terminal end of the molecule. Variants with decreased activity in both antithrombin functional assays generally have mutations near the Arg393-Ser394 site at the C-terminal end of the molecule. Another type of mutation has been described at the C-terminal end of the antithrombin III molecule between amino acids 402 and 429. These type II variants are termed *pleiotropic* because they exhibit multiple functional defects.[72] Mutations at positions 402 to 407 can lead to the presence of trace amounts of an electrophoretically and functionally abnormal antithrombin III molecule.[72] The similarity of characteristics of these mutations indicates that the region of residues 402 to 407 is important for the maintenance of normal plasma levels of antithrombin III antigen.[73]

A case-control study of 1,018 Spanish patients with venous thromboembolism recently reported that the antithrombin A348S mutation was present in 1.7% and 0.2% of cases and controls, respectively.[74] Presence of the mutant allele was associated with an adjusted odds ratio of 9.75 (95% confidence interval [CI], 2.2–42.5) for venous thrombosis. This mutation did not decrease antithrombin III antigen or anti-factor Xa activity in a heparin cofactor assay, and it only slightly reduced anti-thrombin activity. As only six cases were identified as having antithrombin III deficiency by anti-factor Xa activity assay, this antithrombin variant represented the primary cause of antithrombin III deficiency in this population.

The risk of thrombosis is substantially less in heterozygous patients with type II defects at the heparin-binding site as compared to the thrombin-binding site.[75] Persons with plasma antithrombin III-heparin cofactor activity measurements of approximately 50% and normal progressive antithrombin III activity (ie, heparin binding site defects) have infrequent thrombotic episodes.[76,77] Several of these cases came to clinical attention when severe venous or arterial thrombosis, or both, accompanied by plasma antithrombin III-heparin cofactor levels below 10%, developed in young children of these heterozygous subjects.[78,79] There often was a history of parental consanguinity, and these children were homozygous for an antithrombin molecular defect. In contrast with this subgroup of patients, heterozygous type II patients with both diminished progressive antithrombin III activity and antithrombin III-heparin cofactor activity (ie, thrombin-binding site defects) sustain venous thromboembolism as often as type I patients do.

The mean concentration of antithrombin III in normal pooled plasma is approximately 140 μg/mL. Most laboratories report a normal range between 75% and 120% of normal pooled plasma for antithrombin III-heparin cofactor determinations, and a somewhat wider range for immunoassay results.

Healthy newborns have approximately one-half the normal adult concentration of antithrombin III;[80] levels gradually reach those in adults by 6 months of age.[81] The levels may be considerably lower in infants born after 30 to 36 weeks of gestation[81] and are even further reduced in infants with respiratory distress, necrotizing enterocolitis, sepsis, or disseminated intravascular coagulation (DIC). Thromboembolic events are rare in children with hereditary antithrombin III deficiency. In the absence of heparin, antithrombin III contributes approximately 80% of the thrombin-neutralizing capacity of normal adult plasma. The levels of a second thrombin inhibitor, α_2-macroglobulin, are higher during the first two decades of life than in adults, which may lessen the risk of thromboembolic complications in antithrombin III-deficient patients during childhood.[82]

A variety of pathophysiologic conditions can reduce the concentration of antithrombin III in the blood (see Table 134–6). Acute thrombosis infrequently lowers antithrombin III levels substantially, but DIC usually reduces the level of this inhibitor. Lowered antithrombin III concentrations occur in patients with liver disease as a result of decreased protein synthesis. Decreased antithrombin III levels are also observed in individuals with the nephrotic syndrome as a consequence of urinary excretion.[83] Furthermore, modest reductions in plasma antithrombin III concentration are found in users of oral contraceptives as well as in women receiving hormone replacement therapy.[56,84] The levels of antithrombin III do not change substantially during normal pregnancy but may decrease significantly in women with pregnancy-induced hypertension, preeclampsia, or eclampsia. Infusions of L-asparaginase can substantially lower the plasma concentration of this inhibitor. In addition, the administration of heparin decreases plasma antithrombin III levels,[85] presumably on the basis of accelerated in-vivo clearance. Evaluation of plasma samples from patients during a period of heparinization can therefore potentially lead to an erroneous diagnosis of antithrombin III deficiency.

Owing to the number of clinical disorders that can be associated with reductions in the plasma concentration of antithrombin III, definitive diagnosis of the hereditary deficiency state is often difficult. Although an antithrombin III level in the normal range usually is sufficient to exclude the disorder, low levels should be confirmed by obtaining another sample at a subsequent time point. This determination is ideally performed when the patient is no longer receiving oral anticoagulants, because these medications have occasionally been reported to increase plasma antithrombin III concentrations into the normal range in patients with the hereditary deficiency state.[48] Confirmation of the hereditary nature of the disorder requires the investigation of other family members. Diagnosis of other affected family members also allows for appropriate counseling regarding the need for prophylaxis against venous thrombosis.

Protein C Deficiency

In 1981, Griffin and colleagues[86] described the first kindred in which several persons had plasma levels of protein C antigen of approximately 50% of normal and a history of recurrent thrombotic events. Subsequently, others[87–89] reported families with heterozygous protein C deficiency.

Heterozygous protein C deficiency is inherited in an autosomal dominant fashion; a more severe form of protein C deficiency is an autosomal recessive disorder. The phenotype of patients with heterozygous protein C deficiency is similar to that of persons with hereditary antithrombin III deficiency. In severely affected families, approximately 75% of protein C-deficient individuals experienced one or more thrombotic events. The initial episode occurs apparently spontaneously in approximately 70% of those experiencing such events. The remaining 30% have typical associated risk factors, such as pregnancy, parturition, contraceptive pill use, surgery, or trauma, at the time they develop acute thrombotic events. Patients are infrequently symptomatic until their early 20s, but increasing numbers experience thrombotic events by the time that they reach the age of 50 years.

The most common sites of disease are the deep veins of the legs, the iliofemoral veins, and the mesenteric veins. Approximately 63%

of affected patients develop recurrent venous thrombosis, and approximately 40% exhibit signs of pulmonary embolism.[90] Superficial thrombophlebitis of veins in the lower extremity as well as cerebral venous thrombosis can occur in protein C-deficient patients.[87] There have been reports of nonhemorrhagic arterial stroke in young adults with hereditary protein C deficiency, but a causal relationship is uncertain.

The prevalence of protein C deficiency in outpatients presenting with an initial episode of venous thromboembolism ranges from 0.5% to 4%.[27,64,91] In earlier reports of more selected patient populations, protein C deficiency was more frequently identified, ranging from 2% to 9%. Initial estimates placed the prevalence of protein C deficiency between 1 : 16,000 and 1 : 32,000 within the general population, based on the assumption that protein C was an autosomal dominant disorder with high penetrance and that at least one-half of the individuals with the deficiency would demonstrate symptomatic thrombosis. However, it was difficult to reconcile this figure with the infrequent history of thrombosis in parents of infants presenting with purpura fulminans, which is caused by the homozygous or doubly heterozygous form of protein C deficiency. This disparity led to studies of healthy blood donors, which found a much higher prevalence of heterozygosity for protein C deficiency than was previously estimated, ranging from 1 : 200 to 1 : 500.[92,93]

The risk of thrombosis initially attributed to protein C deficiency was subject to selection bias, being overestimated from familial reports. Data from the Leiden Thrombophilia Study indicate that heterozygous protein C deficiency is associated with about a sevenfold increased risk for an initial episode of deep vein thrombosis over that in normal persons.[64] Among Italian patients, protein C deficiency is associated with a similar sevenfold increase in venous thrombotic risk.[61] In asymptomatic carriers of protein C deficiency, the incidence of thrombosis is fairly low at 0.4 to 1.0% annually.[94]

Two major subtypes of heterozygous protein C deficiency have been delineated using immunologic and functional assays (Table 134–8). The type I deficiency state is the most common form and is characterized by a reduction in both the immunologic and biologic activity of plasma protein C to approximately 50% of normal. Studies of the genetic defects in patients with protein C deficiency have led to the identification of 195 different mutations.[95] In persons with a type I deficiency, missense and nonsense mutations are most common. Other types of mutations resulting in type I protein C deficiency include promoter mutations, splice-site abnormalities, in-frame deletions, frameshift deletions, in-frame insertions, and frameshift insertions. In families with a type II deficiency state, affected persons have normal protein C levels on immunologic examination yet possess lowered functional levels of the zymogen. Point mutations in the protein C gene result in the presence of dysfunctional protein C molecules in the affected patient's plasma.

Warfarin-induced skin necrosis has been associated with the presence of heterozygous protein C deficiency.[96,97] This syndrome typically occurs during the first several days of warfarin therapy, often in association with the administration of large loading doses of the medication. The skin lesions occur on the extremities, breasts, and trunk, as well as the penis, and extend over a period of hours from an initial central erythematous macule. If protein C is not rapidly administered, the affected cutaneous areas become edematous, develop central purpuric zones, and ultimately become necrotic. Biopsies demonstrate fibrin thrombi within cutaneous vessels with interstitial hemorrhage. The dermal manifestations of warfarin-induced skin necrosis are clinically and pathologically similar to those seen in infants with purpura fulminans because of severe protein C deficiency.

The pathogenesis of warfarin-induced skin necrosis is attributable to the emergence of a transient hypercoagulable state. The initiation of the drug at standard doses leads to a decrease in protein C anticoagulant activity levels to approximately 50% of normal within 1 day.[98] Although factor VII activity measurements follow a pattern similar to that of protein C, the levels of the other vitamin K-dependent factors decline at slower rates, consistent with their longer half-lives (Fig. 134–3). During this period, it therefore appears that the drug's suppressive effect on protein C has a greater influence on the hemostatic mechanism than that caused by its reduction in factor VII. These effects are augmented when greater than 10 mg of warfarin daily is administered to initiate oral anticoagulation or if the patient has an underlying hereditary deficiency of protein C. Only approximately one-third of patients with warfarin-induced skin necrosis, however, have an inherited deficiency of protein C, and this complication is only infrequently reported in individuals with the heterozygous deficiency state. This syndrome has also been reported in association with an acquired functional deficiency of protein C.[99]

A rare disorder exists in which newborns develop a syndrome described as *purpura fulminans* and exhibit laboratory evidence of DIC in association with protein C antigen levels less than 1% of normal.[100–102] In some instances, there was a history of consanguinity in the family, making it highly likely that the affected infants were homozygous for the deficiency state.[101,102] These newborns can also be double heterozygotes, as was demonstrated in a Chinese patient who had a 5-nucleotide deletion in one protein C allele and a missense mutation in the other.[103] The heterozygous parents of these infants only infrequently had thromboses, in contrast to patients with thrombotic histories and a hereditary partial deficiency of protein C. There have also been a number of reported cases of older patients with homozygous or doubly heterozygous protein C deficiency who do not present with lesions resembling purpura fulminans. These individuals generally had protein C levels less than 20% of normal in the absence of oral anticoagulant therapy, and their clinical presentation was similar to that of severely affected persons from thrombophilic kindreds with the heterozygous deficiency state.[104,105] Genotyping of such homozygous individuals identified several missense mutations in the protein C gene; the variant protein C molecules produced by these individuals are either synthesized at a decreased rate or rapidly cleared from the circulation. The parents of these patients and infants with purpura fulminans have a type I deficiency state.

The nature of the molecular defect in the protein C gene per se does not explain the marked phenotypical variability in heterozygous type I protein C deficiency. A mutation common among symptomatic Dutch patients has also been found in an asymptomatic Swedish parent[106] of a doubly heterozygous child.[107] Also 4 of the 11 mutations observed in homozygotes, whose parents frequently are asymptomatic, have been found in symptomatic heterozygotes.[108] As in other inherited thrombotic disorders, the variable penetrance of thrombosis in heterozygous protein C deficiency reflects a complex interaction with other modulating factors.

A variety of immunologic and functional techniques have been developed to measure protein C levels in plasma samples. Enzyme-linked immunosorbent assays are commonly used to determine protein C antigen levels. Functional assays initially used either thrombin or the thrombin-thrombomodulin complex to activate protein C. Enzymatic activity is then assessed using either a chromogenic substrate or by measuring its anticoagulant activity in a clotting assay.[98] The development of simpler functional assays was facilitated by the observation that the venom of the Southern copperhead snake (*Agkistrodon contortrix*) activates protein C in plasma. After activation of protein C by this venom, the enzyme's amidolytic activity can be

Table 134–8 Assay Measurements in Heterozygous Protein C Deficiency

Activity			
Types	**Antigen**	**Amidolytic**	**Coagulant**
I	Low	Low	Low
II	Normal	Low	Low
	Normal	Normal	Low

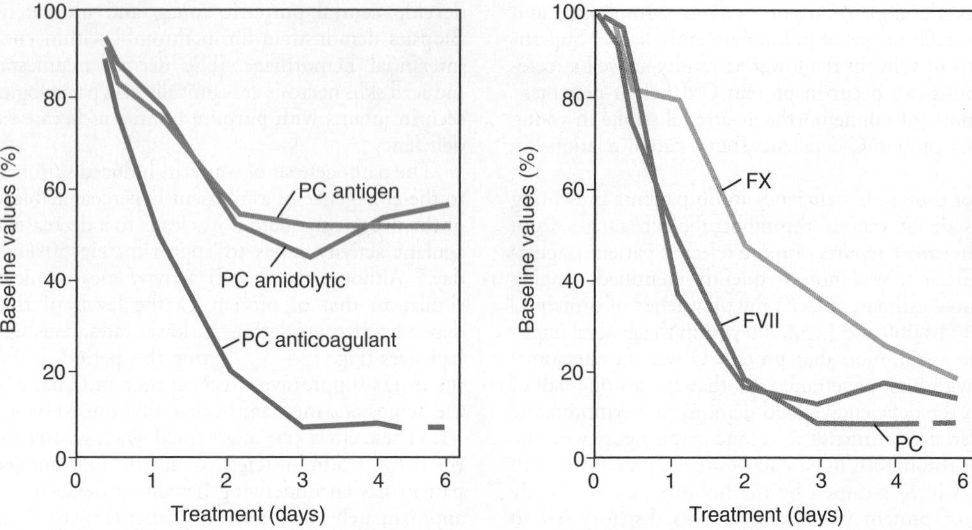

Figure 134–3 Mean levels of protein C (PC) anticoagulant activity, PC amidolytic activity, and PC antigen (left graph), and of PC anticoagulant activity and factor VII activity and factor X activity (right graph), following the initiation of warfarin therapy in patients with deep venous thrombosis. Patients were maintained on heparin infusions, and 10 mg of warfarin were administered for the first three days. Dosages were subsequently adjusted on the basis of the prothrombin time. Measurements are expressed as percentages of prewarfarin levels. *(From D'Angelo SV, Comp PC, Esmon CT, D'Angelo A: Relationship between protein C antigen and anticoagulant activity during oral anticoagulation and in selected disease states. J Clin Invest 77:416, 1986, with permission).*

measured using a suitable chromogenic substrate, or its anticoagulant activity can be measured in a clotting assay.

Functional assays using amidolytic and clotting endpoints may give useful information about the nature of the molecular defect in patients with type II protein C deficiency. Several persons have been described with normal protein C antigen measurements who have substantial reductions in protein C anticoagulant activity, but normal or near normal amidolytic activity.[98] These defects potentially reflect a reduced ability of activated protein C to interact with platelet membranes or with its substrates such as factor V and factor VIII. Thus, the protein C anticoagulant activity assay should have greater sensitivity than the amidolytic assay in screening for molecular defects resulting in type II protein C deficiency. Most clinical laboratories, however, prefer to use a chromogenic assay for initial screening, because it is technically easier to perform and has a smaller coefficient of variation than that of the clotting assay. "Global" coagulation assays also have been developed to screen for any major abnormality in the entire protein C pathway (eg, protein C deficiency, protein S deficiency, the factor V Leiden mutation).[109] The usefulness of these assays has been limited, however, by a poor sensitivity for protein S deficiency.

Protein C normally circulates in human plasma at an average concentration of 4 μg/mL. The levels of protein C antigen in healthy adults are log-normal distributed, with 95% of the values ranging from 70% to 140%.[92] There is no significant gender dependence, but mean protein C concentrations increase by approximately 4% per decade. The relatively wide normal range of protein C measurements in the general population occasionally makes it difficult to identify a given person as having heterozygous protein C deficiency. If medical and pharmacological causes of low levels are excluded, patients with a protein C value of less than 55% of normal are very likely to have the genetic abnormality, whereas levels from 55% to 65% are consistent with either a deficiency state or the lower end of the normal distribution.[92] To document the presence of protein C deficiency with confidence, it is therefore useful to obtain repeat laboratory determinations as well as to perform family studies to identify an autosomal dominant inheritance pattern.

Protein C levels in newborns are 20% to 40% of normal adult levels.[110] Preterm infants have even lower levels, and babies with significant perinatal thrombosis can have levels suggestive of the homozygous deficiency state. Acquired protein C deficiency (see Table 134–6) occurs in liver disease, severe infection and septic shock, DIC, adult respiratory distress syndrome, the postoperative state,[110] breast cancer patients receiving cyclophosphamide, methotrexate, and 5-fluorouracil,[111] and in association with L-asparaginase. A particularly severe form of acquired protein C deficiency has been described in association with purpura fulminans and DIC in patients with acute viral or bacterial infections, in particular meningococcemia.[112] In contrast to antithrombin III, the antigenic concentrations of vitamin K-dependent plasma proteins, including protein C, often are elevated in patients with the nephrotic syndrome.[113]

Warfarin therapy reduces functional[98] and, to a lesser extent, immunologic measurements of protein C,[86,114] making it difficult to diagnose heterozygous protein C deficiency in this setting. Research laboratories have used a reduced ratio of protein C antigen to prothrombin or factor X antigen to identify patients with a type I deficiency state.[86,114] This approach, however, can be used only in persons in a stable phase of oral anticoagulation, and the diagnostic criteria for the disorder vary with the intensity of warfarin therapy.[114] Therefore, evaluation in patients suspected of having the deficiency state should be delayed until after oral anticoagulation has been discontinued for at least 2 weeks, and family studies should also be performed. If warfarin cannot be discontinued because of the severity of the thrombotic diathesis, such patients can be studied while receiving unfractionated or low-molecular-weight heparin therapy, which does not alter plasma protein C levels.

An acquired inhibitor of protein C has been documented in an Australian patient.[115] This patient had a bleeding diathesis for several years, with the development of purpura fulminans before his death. An autopsy showed arterial and venous thrombi in many organs. Laboratory evaluation demonstrated the presence of chronic DIC. The immunoglobulin G (IgG) fraction of the patient's plasma completely inhibited the functional anticoagulant activity of activated protein C.

Protein S Deficiency

In 1984, members from several kindreds who exhibited reduced levels of protein S were described who had a striking history of recurrent venous thrombotic disease.[116,117] Subsequently, many additional families with this disorder have been reported.

Heterozygous protein S deficiency is inherited in an autosomal dominant fashion, with a reported frequency of approximately 10% in families with inherited thrombophlia.[61] However, the prevalence is less (between 1% and 7%) among consecutive outpatients with deep vein thrombosis.[27,64] Protein S deficiency generally is considered to confer a risk of thrombosis similar to that in protein C deficiency, although the association has been complicated by considerable phenotypical variability. A more severe form of protein S deficiency is an autosomal recessive disorder.

The clinical presentation of patients with heterozygous protein S deficiency is similar to that outlined for deficiencies of antithrombin III and protein C. Of 71 protein S-deficient members from 12 Dutch pedigrees,[118] 74%, 72%, and 38% of the individuals sustained deep vein thrombosis, superficial thrombophlebitis, and pulmonary emboli, respectively. The mean age of the first thrombotic event was 28 years, with a range of 15 and 68 years; 56% of the episodes were apparently were spontaneous, and the remainder were precipitated by an identifiable factor. Thrombosis also has been reported in the axillary, mesenteric, and cerebral veins. Although there have been case reports of young patients with arterial thrombosis and protein S deficiency, current data do not support an association between hereditary protein S deficiency and an increased risk of arterial thrombosis.[119]

Under normal conditions, approximately 60% of the total protein S antigen in plasma is complexed to a complement component, C4b-binding protein. Only the free 40% is functionally active as a cofactor in mediating the anticoagulant effects of activated protein C. This observation has led to the development of methods for measuring total[117] and free protein S antigen.[120] Total protein S antigen can be reliably measured by enzyme-linked immunosorbent assay techniques following dilution of plasma samples to allow dissociation of the protein S-C4b-binding protein complexes. After removal of protein S-C4b-binding protein complexes from plasma by polyethylene glycol precipitation,[120] free protein S can be quantitated by immunoassay of the supernatant fractions. It is also possible to measure free protein S specifically by a monoclonal antibody-based immunoenzymatic assay that uses antibodies specific for the free form.[121] Functional assay methods are based on the ability of protein S to serve as a cofactor for the anticoagulant effect of activated protein C. Some of the original coagulation assays developed to measure the functional activity of plasma protein S were later found to be sensitive to abnormalities associated with resistance to activated protein C (factor V Leiden),[122] which has led to the development of more accurate assays.[123]

Three types of protein S deficiency states can be identified on the basis of measurements of total and free antigen as well as functional activity (Table 134–9). Type I deficiency is associated with approximately 50% of the normal total protein S antigen level,[117] and decrements in free protein S antigen and protein S functional activity to less than approximately 40% of normal.[120] Another type of hereditary deficiency (type II) has been described in which the functional activity of protein S is decreased, but with normal total and free antigen levels. A type III deficiency state is characterized phenotypically by a decreased concentration of free and functional plasma protein S, but a normal level of total protein S antigen.

The analysis of mutations in patients with protein S deficiency was complicated by the presence of a protein S pseudogene.[124] Mutations, however, were subsequently identified in approximately 70% of thrombophilic families with protein S deficiency using mutation screening strategies.[125] Type I deficiency most often is secondary to missense mutations, base pair insertions or deletions, premature stop codons, or mutations affecting a splice site. There have been a few cases of large deletions of the gene. Of the more than 130 different mutations documented in patients with various types of protein S deficiency, only 7 different nucleotide substitutions have been identified with a type II deficiency.[126] Several of these mutations are located in the N-terminal end of the protein S molecule, which includes the domains that interact with activated protein C.

The biologic basis of type III protein S deficiency state is uncertain. Furthermore, the coexistence of the type I and type III deficiencies has been reported in some protein S-deficient families, which has led to the proposal that the two types of protein S deficiency are phenotypical variants of the same genotype and are not the product of distinct genetic mutations.[127] In a followup analysis of one large family with a high prevalence of both type I and type III deficiencies, total protein S antigen, but not free protein S antigen levels, were shown to directly correlate with age.[128] These findings were independent of gender and also seen in non-deficient family members. A single point mutation in the protein S gene was responsible for the quantitative type I deficiency, but the type III phenotype was actually caused by an age-dependent free protein S deficiency; with increasing age, the relative concentrations of free protein S to total protein S decreased. However, a Dutch cohort study of first-degree family members with protein S deficiency found that affected relatives of probands with type I deficiency were at increased risk for venous thromboembolism, whereas affected relatives of probands with type III deficiency were not.[119]

Young patients with recurrent venous thromboembolic disease associated with doubly heterozygous or homozygous protein S deficiency have been identified.[116] The parents of the patients were asymptomatic and had laboratory studies consistent with type I protein S deficiency. Neonatal purpura fulminans has been described in association with homozygous protein S deficiency.[129,130]

The average concentration of total protein S antigen in normal adults is 23 μg/mL, but there is considerable overlap between "low normals" and individuals with heterozygous protein S deficiency. Levels increase with advancing age and are lower and more variable in females than males. These factors have confounded the reliable estimation of the prevalence of heterozygous protein S deficiency in the normal population as well the relative risk for thrombosis conferred by the disorder.[64] Thus, it is difficult to make the diagnosis of heterozygous protein S deficiency by performing only a single assay; repeat sampling and family studies usually are required to establish the diagnosis firmly.

Acquired protein S deficiency occurs during pregnancy[131] and in association with the use of oral contraceptives.[132] Reduced protein S levels also have been noted in patients with DIC and acute thromboembolic disease.[133] C4b-binding protein is an acute phase protein, and the decline in protein S activity in the latter two conditions as well as in other inflammatory disorders is attributable to a shift of the protein to the complexed, inactive form.[133] The levels of total and especially free protein S are significantly reduced in men with human immunodeficiency virus infection.[134] Total protein S antigen measurements are generally increased in patients with the nephrotic syndrome,[113] although functional assays give reduced values. This is caused in part by the loss of free protein S in the urine and by elevations in C4b-binding protein levels. Total and free protein S antigen levels are moderately decreased in liver disease[133] and in association with L-asparaginase chemotherapy. An acquired severe deficiency of protein S also has been reported in association with cutaneous necrosis.[135] Several studies have noted an association between antiphospholipid antibodies and acquired protein S deficiency, especially in severe cases of varicella complicated by purpura fulminans.[136]

Interpretation of protein S measurements in patients receiving oral anticoagulants is complicated inasmuch as the antigenic and functional levels of the protein drop substantially with vitamin K antagonists. In stably anticoagulated patients, research investigators used reductions in the ratio of total protein S antigen to prothrombin antigen to infer a diagnosis of type I protein S deficiency; the strategy employed was similar to that described for the diagnosis of protein C deficiency.[117]

TABLE 134–9 Assay Measurements in Heterozygous Protein S Deficiency

Types	Protein S Total Antigen	Protein S Free Antigen	Protein S Activity
I (classic)	Low	Low	Low
II	Normal	Normal	Low
III	Normal	Low	Low

Total protein S antigen values in healthy newborns at term are 15% to 30% of normal, whereas C4b-binding protein is markedly reduced to less than 20%. Thus, the free form of the protein predominates in this setting, and functional levels are only slightly reduced compared with those in normal adults.[137]

Activated Protein C Resistance and the Factor V Leiden Mutation

In 1993, Dahlbäck[138] identified a novel mechanism for familial thrombophilia: the plasmas of persons with unexplained personal and familial histories of venous thromboembolism exhibited a poor response to activated protein C (APC) in a PTT assay. The observations of Dahlbäck facilitated the development of a PTT-based assay to screen for APC resistance, which demonstrated the abnormality in 33% of Swedish patients referred for evaluation of venous thrombosis.[139] Precipitating factors for thrombosis, such as pregnancy and the use of oral contraceptives, were identified in 60% of the patients. Family studies revealed that relatives with APC resistance had a significantly higher frequency of thrombosis than that in relatives without the defect. In a U.S. referral population of patients younger than age 50 years with unexplained venous thromboembolic disease, approximately 50% were found to have APC resistance.[140] Investigators in Italy and Austria confirmed that APC resistance was a frequent laboratory abnormality in patients with unexplained venous thrombosis.[122,141]

Major contributions to our understanding of the molecular basis and clinical relevance of APC resistance were made by Dutch investigators from Leiden. In 1987, they initiated the Leiden Thrombophilia Study, a large case-control study to investigate risk factors for first episodes of venous thrombosis in the general population of The Netherlands. The rationale for undertaking this study was, in part, to define the true risk of venous thrombosis associated with protein C deficiency. There was a seeming paradox in that referred patients from families with protein C deficiency had a high frequency of venous thrombosis, but the deficiency state is present in 1:200 to 1:500 healthy blood donors. The selection criteria for accruing subjects into these studies turns out to be a major factor underlying this difference.

Following the initial observations of Dahlbäck, patients entering the Leiden Thrombophilia Study were screened for APC resistance after the completion of anticoagulant therapy.[1] Entry criteria were a first episode of deep venous thrombosis in outpatients younger than 70 years and confirmation of the diagnosis by objective evaluation. Patients with malignancy were excluded. Each thrombosis patient was assigned a healthy age- and gender-matched control. APC resistance was found in 21% of thrombosis patients and 5% of controls. Patients with APC resistance were calculated to have a sevenfold increased relative risk of venous thrombosis over that in controls. This corresponds to an incidence for an initial episode of deep venous thrombosis among carriers in the general Dutch population of approximately 0.06 episodes per 100 person-years (Table 134–10). A lower frequency of APC resistance in this study compared with that in studies of referral populations is attributable to different selection criteria for the thrombosis cohorts.

It subsequently was shown that a defect in factor V involving the mutation of arginine 506 to glutamine (Arg506Gln or factor V Leiden) is most often the cause of APC resistance.[142] This is the site at which APC cleaves factor Va, and this sequence alteration makes the mutant factor Va molecule biochemically resistant to inactivation by the activated protein C.[142,143] The Arg506Gln substitution was found to be the cause of APC resistance in about 90% of Dutch patients with APC resistance in the PTT assay,[142] and the mutation was found in 2% to 4% of healthy Dutch controls. Most patients with APC resistance are heterozygous for the factor V Leiden mutation, but a number of homozygous patients with heightened APC resistance in PTT assays have been identified.[142,144] Homozygotes are at higher thrombotic risk than that noted for heterozygotes (see Table 134–10),[145] as are patients with heterozygous resistance to APC combined with mutations in the genes for protein C, antithrombin III, and probably protein S.[10,13,146] The genes for factor V and antithrombin III both are located on the long arm of chromosome 1, thereby allowing for coinheritance of the factor V Leiden mutation and an antithrombin III mutation within all affected members of a family. This situation is expected to lead to an even more severe thrombotic diathesis.[13]

Table 134–10 The Leiden Thrombophilia Study Data: Relative and Absolute Risks of an Initial Episode of Deep Venous Thrombosis in the General Population Because of Common Risk Factors

Factors	Risk	Incidence*	Reference
Normal	–	0.008	
Prothrombin gene mutation	2.8 × ↑	0.022	(3)
Oral contraceptives	4 × ↑	0.03	(212)
Factor V Leiden heterozygotes	7 × ↑	0.057	(1)
Oral contraceptives + Factor V Leiden	35 × ↑	0.285	(212)
Factor V Leiden Homozygotes	80 × ↑	0.5–1	(145)

*Episodes per 100 person-years.

The U.S. Physicians' Health Study also has provided valuable data regarding factor V Leiden as a risk factor for venous as well as arterial thrombosis. In a retrospective case-control study of 14,916 healthy men older than age 40 years with a mean followup period of 8.6 years, heterozygosity for the factor V Leiden mutation was identified in 12% of patients with a first episode of deep vein thrombosis or pulmonary embolism and in 6% of controls.[2] The relative risk of venous thromboembolism was increased 3.5-fold in those persons with no other concomitant risk factors but was reduced to 1.7-fold in those with preexistent cancer or recent surgery. This study also showed that elderly patients with venous thrombosis frequently have the mutation.[2] Among men older than 60 years with initial episodes of venous thrombosis and no identifiable triggering factors, 26% were heterozygotes for factor V Leiden.

A cohort study of more than 9000 randomly selected adults in Denmark found that the simultaneous presence of smoking, obesity (body mass index greater than 30 kg/m^2), older age (older than 60 years), and the factor V Leiden mutation resulted in absolute 10-year venous thromboembolism rates of 10% in heterozygotes and 51% in homozygotes.[147]

A prospective cohort study determined the incidence of venous thromboembolism in asymptomatic carriers of the factor V Leiden mutation identified through family studies of symptomatic probands. Nine events occurred in 1564 observation-years resulting in an annual incidence of 0.58%. It was concluded that the absolute annual incidence of venous thromboembolism in asymptomatic carriers of the mutation is low.[148]

A number of studies have examined whether factor V Leiden, a prevalent abnormality in white populations, leads to an increased risk for arterial thrombotic events. There are no convincing data that other thrombophilic states such as deficiencies of antithrombin III, protein C, and protein S confer an increased risk of arterial thrombosis, but evaluation of these associations is complicated by the relative infrequency of these defects. In a cohort of men older than age 40 years in which there was a low prevalence of smoking, the U.S. Physicians' Health Study did not find an association between the factor V Leiden mutation and myocardial infarction or stroke.[2] In a younger cohort of Italian patients with myocardial infarction occurring younger than age 45 years, an increased incidence of the factor V Leiden mutation relative to that in controls also was not found.[149] Furthermore, a report of 36 French homozygous patients with the mutation did not identify a tendency for the development of arterial thrombosis.[150]

Data from a case-control study, however, suggest that heterozygosity for factor V Leiden is a risk factor for a myocardial infarction in young women (18 to 44 years old), but only in the presence of other cardiac risk factors.[151] The presence of the factor V Leiden mutation was associated with a 2.4-fold increased risk of myocardial infarction after adjustment for age (9.5% of patients with myocardial infarction, compared with 4.1% in controls). The risk of myocardial infarction associated with factor V Leiden was observed only among current cigarette smokers, in whom the mutation conferred a threefold increased risk. Compared with women who did not smoke and did not carry the factor V Leiden mutation, women who smoked and carried the mutation had a 30-fold increased risk of myocardial infarction. Although other cardiac risk factors such as older age, obesity, hypercholesterolemia, hypertension, diabetes, family history of ischemic heart disease, and postmenopausal status that is surgically induced were associated with cardiac events, the use of low-dose oral contraceptives was not. Data from this cohort indicate that the prothrombin gene mutation is also a risk factor for myocardial infarction, but only in current cigarette smokers.[152]

Obstetric complications, such as severe preeclampsia, abruptio placentae, fetal growth retardation, and stillbirth, are associated with intervillous or spiral artery thrombosis and consequent placental insufficiency. Factor V Leiden as well as other hereditary thrombophilias is associated with an approximate tripling of the risk of late fetal loss.[17,21] An increased incidence of factor V Leiden, as well as other thrombophilias, also was reported in women in association with other obstetric complications;[153] associations with preeclampsia and intrauterine growth restriction/retardation have, however, not been corroborated.[154,155]

The prevalence of heterozygosity for the factor V Leiden mutation in whites, including European, Jewish, Israeli Arab, and Indian populations, ranges between 1% and 8.5%. The mutation apparently is not present in African blacks or in Chinese, Japanese, or Native American populations.[22] In Europe, the mutation has been found to be more prevalent in northern countries such as Sweden than in southern countries such as Spain and Italy. Using dimorphic sites in the factor V gene to do haplotype analysis, data have been provided supporting the existence of a founder effect among whites of differing ethnic background.[24] It also was estimated that the mutation originated approximately 30,000 years ago, which came after the evolutionary divergence of white, African, and Asian populations.

Two mutations at the Arg306 residue in factor V, the second APC cleavage site in the activated cofactor, have been described in patients with a history of thrombosis. These mutations involve substitutions of Arg306 with threonine (factor V Cambridge)[156] or glycine (in Hong Kong Chinese).[157] The latter mutation, however, evidently has no clinical relevance because it is not associated with APC resistance, and the mutation is as common in healthy Chinese blood donors as in patients with thrombosis (4.5% and 4.7%, respectively).[158] The factor V Cambridge mutation is extremely rare among whites with venous thromboembolic disease.

Cosegregation of heterozygous APC resistance caused by the factor V Leiden mutation and type I factor V deficiency has been reported in some patients.[159,160] The plasma of these individuals manifests severe APC resistance in PTT assays, as found in patients homozygous factor V Leiden patients (ie, the patients with such cosegregation are pseudo-homozygous). These patients were seemingly more thrombosis-prone than were heterozygous relatives with factor V Leiden alone, suggesting that their clinical phenotype is similar to homozygous factor V Leiden patients.

Several polymorphisms are present in the factor V gene.[161,162] An extended factor V gene haplotype (HR2) containing the R2 polymorphism (His1299Arg) is associated with mild APC resistance and occurs with increased frequency in heterozygous patients with the factor V Leiden mutation with the lowest APC resistance ratios.[162] Although one case-control study found that the R2 allele was a risk factor for venous thromboembolism with an odds ratio of 2.0 after excluding subjects with genetic defects such as factor V Leiden,[163] another case-control study found no significant increase in risk.[164]

The initial observations of Dahlbäck[138] facilitated the development of a PTT-based assay that serves as a screening test for APC resistance. The PTT assay is performed in the presence or absence of a standardized amount of APC, and the two clotting times are converted to an APC ratio. Results can be interpreted by comparing the ratio with the normal range, or by normalizing it to the APC resistance ratio obtained using normal pooled plasma. Although this first generation APC resistance assay was conceptually quite simple and easy to perform in a coagulation laboratory, it required careful standardization and determination of the normal range in at least 50 controls. The level of APC, the PTT reagent, and the instrumentation used for clot detection affected the performance characteristics of the assay. Some assays using this format, therefore, had inadequate sensitivity and specificity for the factor V Leiden mutation. Also, patients receiving anticoagulants or with an abnormal PTT caused by other coagulation defects could not be evaluated with this assay, and the test was not validated in patients with acute thrombosis or in pregnant women.

The discovery that factor V Leiden is the dominant genetic defect responsible for APC resistance facilitated the development of second-generation coagulation tests. With proper standardization, this assay is characterized by nearly 100% sensitivity and 100% specificity for the mutation. For these tests, patient plasma is diluted in a sufficient volume of factor V-deficient plasma, and then a PTT-based assay is performed. This modification also permits the evaluation of plasmas of patients receiving anticoagulants or with abnormal PTT results caused by coagulation factor deficiencies other than factor V.

The fact that the dominant mutation underlying APC resistance is factor V Leiden makes it attractive to diagnose this defect by analyzing genomic DNA in peripheral blood mononuclear cells. This can be readily accomplished by amplifying a DNA fragment containing the factor V mutation site by polymerase chain reaction and analyzing the cleavage products on ethidium bromide-stained agarose gels after restriction enzyme digestion with MnlI.[142] The substitution of an A for a G at nucleotide 1691 in the factor V cDNA (CGA to CAA) results in the Arg506Gln mutation and the loss of a MnlI cleavage site. Other diagnostic approaches include hybridization with allele-specific oligonucleotide probes.

Some patients with APC resistance without the factor V Leiden mutation can be identified using the first generation PTT-based assay. The Leiden Thrombophilia Study demonstrated that this abnormality is a significant independent risk factor for an initial venous thrombotic event.[42] Performance of this assay is not recommended, however, as part of the routine laboratory evaluation, because the commercially available APC resistance assays using undiluted plasma do not replicate the performance characteristics of the assay used in the Leiden Thrombophilia Study, and the clinical implications of this type of APC resistance are uncertain.

Prothrombin Gene Mutation

In 1996, investigators from Leiden reported that a G to A substitution at nucleotide 20210 in the 3′-untranslated region of the prothrombin gene is associated with elevated plasma prothrombin levels and an increased risk of venous thrombosis.[3] This mutation, which was discovered by sequencing the prothrombin gene of selected patients with venous thrombosis, is located at the last position of the 3′-untranslated region at the cleavage site for polyadenylation of prothrombin mRNA. The prothrombin 20210A mutation changes the position of the 3′-cleavage/polyadenylation reaction in prothrombin mRNA, thereby leading to increased prothrombin biosynthesis by the liver.[165] This finding is in contrast to previous data that the mutation changes mRNA stability by increasing mRNA 3′-end formation.[166]

Investigation of a referral population with a personal and family history of venous thrombosis demonstrated that 18% had the mutation in the 3′-untranslated region of the prothrombin gene, whereas it was present in only 1 of 100 healthy controls.[3] Among these thrombosis patients, 40% also carried the factor V Leiden mutation, again emphasizing the current view of venous thrombosis as a multigene disorder.

In the Leiden Thrombophilia Study, 6.2% of venous thrombosis patients and 2.3% of healthy matched controls had the prothrombin gene mutation.[3] This mutation independently confers a 2.8-fold increased risk of venous thrombosis (see Table 134–10) and the effect is operative in both genders and all age groups. Among heterozygotes with the prothrombin gene mutation, 87% of thrombosis patients and controls in the study had prothrombin activity levels that were greater than 1.15 units/mL, whereas only 23% of those with a normal prothrombin genotype were elevated to this degree.

In subsequent studies, the prothrombin G20210A mutation was found at significantly higher frequency in patients with venous thrombosis than healthy controls.[167,168] As with the factor V Leiden mutation, the risk of venous thrombosis among carriers of the prothrombin mutation is substantially increased by the use of oral contraceptives.[6] Large population studies have shown that the prevalence of the mutation is approximately 2% in the general white population, albeit with significant geographic variation. Among southern Europeans the prevalence was approximately 3%, but it was only very rarely identified in individuals of Asian or African descent.

Polymerase chain reaction methods are used to detect the prothrombin G20210A mutation in genomic DNA[3] and methods are available to detect both the prothrombin G20210A mutation and factor V Leiden in the same reaction. Although plasma prothrombin activity and antigen levels are significantly higher in individuals with the prothrombin G20210A mutation, concentrations cannot be used to screen for the defect due to significant overlap with values in the normal population.[3]

Dysfibrinogenemias

Qualitative abnormalities of fibrinogen are inherited in an autosomal dominant manner. The dysfibrinogenemias are a heterogeneous group of disorders that may be asymptomatic or manifest with a bleeding diathesis or recurrent venous or arterial thromboembolism (see Chapter 127). A small number of variant fibrinogens have been reported to be associated with thrombotic complications. These defects can be detected with thrombin and reptilase times, which often are prolonged. Functional fibrinogen measurements usually are substantially lower than antigenic measurements in the plasmas of affected patients. An occasional patient with a dysfibrinogemia may have a prolonged prothrombin time or PTT, and the inability of some abnormal fibrinogens to clot completely in vitro can result in false-positive results in fibrin(ogen) degradation product tests.

The functional and biochemical defects of a number of abnormal fibrinogens associated with thromboembolic disease have been characterized (see Chapter 127).[169,170] The conversion of fibrinogen to fibrin by thrombin results in the proteolytic cleavage of fibrinopeptides A and B from the molecule. Defects in the release of these two peptides or abnormalities in fibrin polymerization have been reported. Such functional defects do not, however, offer a ready explanation for the thrombotic diathesis seen in these subjects. Abnormalities in the binding of thrombin to fibrin also have been found in some dysfibrinogenemias.[171,172] In one of these kindreds, three homozygous siblings with a Bβ chain substitution of Ala by Thr at position 68 had a severe clinical phenotype sustaining both arterial and venous thrombosis at a young age.[171] Decreased binding of thrombin by this mutant fibrinogen has been suggested to lead to the presence of excessive thrombin in the circulation and the occurrence of thrombosis. Other fibrinogen mutants have been shown to cause abnormal fibrin polymerization. Some of the abnormal fibrinogens have been evaluated for their ability to resist or promote fibrinolysis on incorporation into a fibrin clot. The fibrin formed from fibrinogen *Chapel Hill III* has been demonstrated to be abnormally resistant to lysis by plasmin.[173] Plasminogen activation is decreased in the presence of the fibrin formed from fibrinogen Dusart, despite normal tissue-type plasminogen activator binding to the substrate.[174] These abnormalities have the potential for decreasing fibrinolytic activity in vivo, which results in a familial thrombotic diathesis in biochemically affected persons.

Inherited Abnormalities of Fibrinolysis

Although investigators have identified a few individuals with inherited abnormalities of the fibrinolytic mechanism and recurrent venous thromboembolism, the clinical association is considerably less striking than that in many kindreds with deficiencies of antithrombin III, protein C, or protein S, or with the factor V Leiden mutation and the prothrombin gene mutation. Dysplasminogenemia or hypoplasminogenemia has been reported in a number of individuals with thromboembolic disease; the first case of an abnormal plasminogen was identified in Japan.[175] The propositus had a history of recurrent thrombosis, and family studies demonstrated that the biochemical abnormality followed an autosomal dominant inheritance pattern. Despite the hereditary nature of the defect, none of the other biochemically affected members of the kindred had experienced a thrombotic event. Other Japanese pedigrees without thrombosis have since been described with the same biochemical defect; the gene frequency of this variant in the Japanese population was 0.018.[176] Population studies in the United States have not uncovered any cases of this dysplasminogenemia. The non-Japanese cases of dysplasminogenemias and hypoplasminogenemias also have been characterized by the absence of thrombotic episodes in biochemically affected family members other than the propositi.

Severe type 1 plasminogen deficiency is associated with a rare chronic inflammatory disease of the mucous membranes. The disorder is characterized by the presence of fibrin-rich pseudomembranous lesions and the most common clinical manifestations are ligneous conjunctivitis (80%) and ligneous gingivitis (34%). Less common sites of involvement are the vagina, respiratory tract, ears, and gastrointestinal tract.[177] Patients with this disorder have been found to be homozygous or compound heterozygous for a number of different mutations in the plasminogen gene.[177] Although this disorder occasionally can be life-threatening, venous and thrombosis was not observed among these patients. A severely affected infant with ligneous conjunctivitis has been treated successfully with a purified plasminogen concentrate,[178] but this product is not commercially available.

There were reports documenting the existence of thrombophilic families in association with impaired fibrinolysis.[179,180] Reevaluation of several of these families demonstrated the presence of hereditary protein S deficiency and no association between elevations in PAI-1 activity and a history of thrombosis.[181,182]

Immunochemical methods for the measurement of tissue-type plasminogen activator and functional assays for its inhibitors have been applied to the study of patients with documented venous thromboembolism. These studies suggested that defective synthesis or release of tissue-type plasminogen activator, as well as increased levels of PAI-1, may be important pathogenetic factors in as many as one-third of these individuals.[183–185] Subsequent studies however have not found a relationship between impaired fibrinolytic activity and venous thromboembolism.[186,187]

Factor XII Deficiency

Factor XII is the zymogen of a serine protease that initiates the contact activation reactions and intrinsic blood coagulation in vitro but probably plays no physiologic role in hemostasis in vivo. Persons with severe factor XII deficiency (factor XII activity less than 1% of normal) have markedly prolonged PTTs but do not exhibit a bleeding disorder. The absence of a hemostatic defect in patients with a severe deficiency of factor XII, prekallikrein, or high-molecular-weight-kininogen indicates that these factors are not required for in-vivo hemostasis. A number of cases of venous thromboembolism or myocardial infarction in factor XII-deficient patients,[188] including the initial patient described with the abnormality,[189] have been reported, however.

A literature review of 121 patients with factor XII deficiency found an 8% incidence of thromboembolism, including several myocardial infarctions in relatively young persons.[188] Interpretation of such data is difficult, because such complications are likely to be reported in the literature, whereas the asymptomatic patient with factor XII deficiency may go unrecognized. This problem has led some groups to perform cross-sectional analyses of thromboembolic events in larger numbers of unselected families with factor XII deficiency.[190,191] In Swiss families with factor XII deficiency, 2 of 18 homozygous or doubly heterozygous patients had sustained deep vein thrombosis, although each occurred at a time when other predisposing thrombotic risk factors were present.[190] Among heterozygotes with factor XII deficiency, only 1 of 45 had a possible history of venous thrombosis. These investigators concluded that heterozygous factor XII deficiency does not constitute a major thrombotic risk factor, whereas a severe deficiency may predispose some affected persons to venous thrombosis. Other groups of investigators have found a 10% to 20% incidence of thrombotic episodes in heterozygotes.[191,192] Thus, it remains uncertain whether an increased thrombotic risk is associated with factor XII deficiency.

Hyperhomocysteinemia

Homocysteine is a sulfur-containing amino acid that is formed from methionine (Fig. 134–4). It is converted back to methionine by one of two remethylation pathways or undergoes transsulfuration to cysteine. In remethylation catalyzed by the enzyme methionine synthase, homocysteine acquires a methyl group from 5-methyltetrahydrofolate and vitamin B_{12} (cobalamin) acts as a cofactor. In a secondary pathway, betaine is the methyl donor in a reaction catalyzed by betaine-homocysteine methyltransferase. In transsulfuration, homocysteine condenses with serine to form cystathionine in a reaction catalyzed by cystathionine-β-synthase followed by hydrolysis by the enzyme γ-cystathionase to cysteine and α-ketobutyrate. Vitamin B_6 (pyridoxine) is a cofactor in both of these reactions. The normal plasma homocysteine concentration is 5 to 16 μM.

Homocystinuria is a rare autosomal recessive inborn error of metabolism presenting in childhood. The most frequent cause is homozygous cystathionine-β-synthase deficiency, which has a frequency in the general population of approximately 1:250,000. As a result of impaired intracellular metabolism of homocysteine, increased amounts of the amino acid accumulate in the blood and are excreted in the urine. Children with homocystinuria exhibit premature atherosclerosis and venous thromboembolism, along with mental retardation, ectopic lenses, and skeletal abnormalities. A small number of cases are caused by homozygous defects encoding 5,10-methylenetetrahydrofolate reductase (MTHFR), and persons so affected are similarly afflicted with premature vascular disease and thrombosis along with neurologic problems. The mechanisms by which hyperhomocysteinemia act as an atherogenic and thrombogenic risk factor have been only partially elucidated.[193,194]

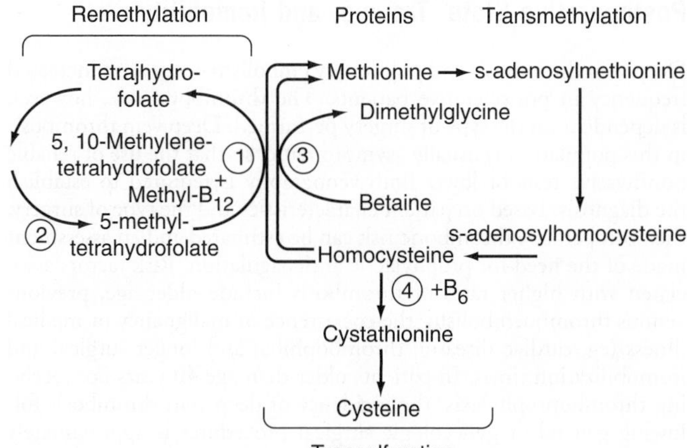

Figure 134–4 Intracellular metabolism of homocysteine occurs through remethylation to methionine or transsulfuration to cysteine. Numbered circles indicate the enzymes involved: 1, methionine synthase; 2, methylenetetrahydrofolate reductase (MTHFR); 3, betaine-homocysteine methyltransferase; 4, cystathionine beta-synthase. *(From De Stefano V, Finazzi G, Mannucci PM: Inherited thrombophilia: Pathogenesis, clinical syndromes, and management. Blood 87:3531, 1996, with permission).*

During the last two decades, mild or moderate hyperhomocysteinemia was identified as a seemingly independent risk factor for venous and arterial thrombotic events.[195–197] Mild (16–24 μmol/L) or moderate (25–100 μmol/L) hyperhomocysteinemia results from genetic and acquired abnormalities. Although heterozygous cystathionine-β-synthase deficiency is found in only approximately 0.3% of the general population, a MTHFR variant with an alanine to valine substitution at amino acid 677 is common[198] and can be present in 1.4 to 15% of the population, depending on their origin.[197] This mutation causes thermolability of MTHFR and a 50% reduction in its specific activity. The most common causes of acquired hyperhomocysteinemia are deficiencies of vitamin B_{12}, folate, or vitamin B_6, which are cofactors in homocysteine metabolism. There is a strong inverse correlation between hyperhomocysteinemia and folate levels and, to a lesser extent, with vitamin B_{12} and B_6 concentrations. Elderly patients frequently have elevated plasma homocysteine concentrations even in the absence of vitamin deficiencies, as do patients with renal failure. Cigarette smoking is also associated with acquired hyperhomocysteinemia.

Although patients with homocystinuria because of cystathionine-β-synthase deficiency have levels greater than 100 μmol/L, individuals with heterozygous defects in this gene or inadequate vitamin B_6 levels may have normal or only slightly elevated levels of fasting homocysteine. The discrimination of such patients from normal individuals can be improved by demonstrating an abnormal increase in plasma homocysteine 4 hours after an oral methionine load. Defects in the remethylation pathway because of MTHFR gene defects or inadequate folate or vitamin B_{12} levels tend to cause elevated homocysteine levels under fasting conditions. The prevalence of hyperhomocysteinemia is almost twice as high when based on homocysteine measurements performed after methionine loading as when based on fasting levels.

As folic acid, vitamin B_6, and vitamin B_{12} supplementation can decrease plasma homocysteine levels, it was hypothesized that treatment with these supplements would reduce the risk of arterial and venous thrombosis. Large randomized placebo-controlled clinical trials, however, reported that clinical outcomes are not improved by providing supplements of these vitamins to patients with histories of ischemic stroke,[199] myocardial infarction,[200] vascular disease,[201] or venous thrombosis.[202]

Because there are currently no data that persons with mild hyperhomocysteinemia and a history of venous or arterial thrombosis should be managed any differently than those with normal homocysteine levels, there is no longer justification for routinely obtaining homocysteine levels in such patients. In addition, results from the Leiden MEGA study indicate that presence of homozygosity for the MTHFR C677T polymorphism, which mildly increases homocysteine levels, is not associated with an increased risk for venous thrombosis.[203] These testing for this polymorphism should not be performed. It should furthermore be noted that the prevalence of hyperhomocysteinemia in the U.S. population has declined since the wheat supply was fortified with folic acid in the late 1990s. Although there were previous reports that hyperhomocysteinemia significantly increased the risk for a first venous thrombotic event in patients with the factor V Leiden mutation,[204] a recent publication found no additive or multiplicative interaction between these abnormalities for the risk of venous thrombosis.[205]

ACQUIRED THROMBOTIC DISORDERS

Pregnancy, Oral Contraceptives, and Hormone Replacement Therapy

Pregnancy is associated with an approximately sixfold increased risk of venous thromboembolism. Although the incidence of deep vein thrombosis and pulmonary embolism has been estimated to be as high as 1%, the true incidence is unknown because of difficulties in performing screening radiologic studies in pregnant women. Although relatively rare, pulmonary embolism causes 12 deaths per 1 million pregnancies in the state of Massachusetts and is estimated to account for 12% of fatalities during pregnancy.[206]

The puerperium, defined as the 6-week period following delivery, is associated with a higher rate of thrombosis than that associated with pregnancy itself. Risk factors for thrombosis in pregnancy include increasing age, Cesarean delivery, prolonged immobilization, obesity, and previous thromboembolism. Coexistent thrombophilia represents a major risk factor.[207] Factor V Leiden and the G20210A prothrombin gene mutation individually are associated with an increased risk of venous thromboembolism during pregnancy and the puerperium, and the risk among women with both mutations is disproportionately higher than that among women with only one mutation.[208]

Thrombosis during pregnancy and the puerperium is attributable to pregnancy-induced alterations in hemostasis as well as venous stasis in the lower extremities caused by the gravid uterus. Trauma to the pelvic veins during vaginal delivery or tissue injury during Cesarian section also contributes to the hypercoagulable state. Compression of the left iliac vein by the crossing right iliac artery is a local, mechanical factor that is believed to underlie the threefold higher incidence of deep vein thrombosis in the left leg compared to the right.

Marked changes in the coagulation mechanism occur during pregnancy. Increased levels of markers of coagulation system activation can be detected in the systemic circulation by the end of the first trimester. The elevations in thrombin generation probably arise from the uteroplacental circulation because the placenta is rich in tissue factor. The vasculature of the placenta is unique from other tissues in that it is lined by chorionic villi that are covered by trophoblast tissue, rather than endothelium, which is in direct contact with maternal blood.

The levels of most procoagulant factors increase during pregnancy, with fibrinogen increasing markedly from a normal level of 250 to 400 mg/dL to 600 mg/dL in late pregnancy. Among the natural anticoagulant proteins, there is a significant decline in the level of free and total protein S in the second trimester.[131] At the same time, fibrinolytic system activity declines progressively during pregnancy. Platelet activation and increased platelet turnover also probably occur during pregnancy; mild thrombocytopenia, possibly as a result of increased consumption, occurs in 8.3% of healthy women at term.[209] The net effect of these hemostatic changes is to promote blood coagulation so as to provide adequate hemostasis at the time of placental separation. The altered levels of hemostatic proteins return to normal within 4 weeks after delivery. Fibrinolytic activity rapidly returns to nonpregnant levels within hours after placental separation.

Oral contraceptive use is associated with an increased risk of venous and arterial thrombosis.[4] The risk of venous thrombosis is related to the estrogen dose, and most oral contraceptives prescribed in the United States contain less than 50 μg of ethinylestradiol in combination with a progestational agent (ie, combined oral contraceptives). The use of low dose-estrogen preparations containing older progestational agents (levonorgestrel, lynoestrenol, and norethisterone), however, still confers approximately a fourfold increased risk of venous thromboembolism, compared with that in nonusers (see Table 134–10). The risk of myocardial infarction and stroke is less. Oral contraceptives affect lipid profiles by lowering low-density lipoprotein cholesterol and raising high-density lipoprotein cholesterol levels. Unexpectedly, newer progestogens (desogestrel, gestodene, and norgestimate) with less deleterious effects on lipid profiles are associated with a higher risk of venous thromboembolism than that noted for the previous generation of combined oral contraceptives.[210,211] This risk is particularly high among carriers of the factor V Leiden mutation[212,213] and women with a family history of thrombosis. It is not yet known whether oral contraceptives containing the newer progestogens are associated with any increase in risk of myocardial infarction, which is a rare event in young women.

The mechanism by which oral contraceptives are prothrombotic is complex and uncertain. Prothrombotic effects include modest increases in the levels of procoagulant factors (factor VII, factor VIII, factor X, prothrombin, fibrinogen) and decreases in the levels of anticoagulant proteins (antithrombin III, protein S). The development of *acquired* APC resistance has been demonstrated, by means of a thrombin generation assay, in women taking oral contraceptives. Although the molecular basis for this phenomenon is unknown, it provides a plausible explanation for the greatly increased thrombotic risk among oral contraceptive users who are carriers of the factor V Leiden mutation.[4]

Although the thrombogenicity of oral contraceptives was recognized shortly after their introduction in the 1960s, convincing evidence that the lower estrogen dose used for hormone replacement therapy leads to an increased risk of venous thromboembolism was conclusively reported only in 1996. The estrogens commonly prescribed for hormone replacement are chemically different than those in oral contraceptives and are considered to have substantially lower biologic potency. Venous thrombotic risk associated with hormone replacement therapy is increased two- to fourfold, an effect similar in magnitude to that noted for oral contraceptives. The use of hormone replacement therapy, however, leads to a considerably larger number of excess cases of thrombosis, as a result of an overall age-related increase in the incidence of thrombosis. Carriers of the factor V Leiden mutation receiving hormone replacement therapy have a significantly increased risk of venous thromboembolism.[214,215] Data from the Heart and Estrogen Replacement Study (HERS) and the Estrogen Replacement and Atherosclerosis Trial indicate that heterozygous carriers of factor V Leiden on hormone replacement therapy had an odds ratio that was 14.1-fold higher for venous thromboembolism, as compared to noncarriers receiving placebo.[215]

Raloxifene, a selective estrogen receptor modulator that has antiestrogenic effects on breast and endometrial tissue but estrogenic effects on bone, lipid metabolism, and coagulation, is also associated with an increased risk of venous thromboembolic disease.[216]

Postoperative State, Trauma, and Immobility

Deep vein thrombosis and pulmonary embolism occur with increased frequency in postoperative patients. The thrombotic risk, however, is dependent on the type of surgery performed. Deep vein thrombosis in this population is usually asymptomatic, so that the use of reliable noninvasive tests or lower limb venography is required to establish the diagnosis. Based on patient characteristics and the type of surgery, the postoperative thrombotic risk can be estimated and an assessment made of the need for prophylactic anticoagulation. Risk factors associated with higher rates of thrombosis include older age, previous venous thromboembolism, the coexistence of malignancy or medical illness (eg, cardiac disease), thrombophilia, and longer surgical and immobilization times. In patients older than age 40 years not receiving thromboprophylaxis, the incidence of deep vein thrombosis following general or gynecologic surgical procedures is approximately 20% to 25%, and clinically significant pulmonary embolism occurs in 1% to 2% of these patients. For urologic surgery, the incidence of deep vein thrombosis ranges from 10% for transurethral procedures to up to 40% for radical prostatectomies. Orthopedic procedures on the hip and lower extremities are among the most thrombogenic surgical procedures. In the absence of prophylaxis, the risk of deep vein thrombosis following total knee replacement is 45% to 70%, and fatal pulmonary embolism has been reported to occur in 1% to 3% of patients undergoing hip surgery. The increased thrombotic risk is not confined to the immediate postoperative period and continues for several weeks.

Deep vein thrombosis and pulmonary embolism also are commonly encountered following major trauma. A study of patients admitted to a Canadian regional trauma unit demonstrated that 58% of patients had lower extremity deep vein thrombosis, which usually was asymptomatic.[217] Risk factors for thrombosis in this setting were older age, the need for surgery or blood transfusions, and the presence of lower extremity fractures or spinal cord injury. Pulmonary embolism occurs in 2% to 22% of trauma patients, and is the third most common cause of death in those who survive the first 24 hours.[218]

The mechanism of activation of the coagulation system following surgery or trauma has not been elucidated, but the exposure of tissue factor from injured tissue or activated monocytes is the most likely pathway for increased thrombin generation in these settings. In postoperative patients, the occurrence of thrombosis is also influenced by fibrinolytic system activity. Minor alterations in a number of hemostatic parameters have been reported in postoperative patients, including elevated levels of fibrinogen and von Willebrand factor and decreased levels of antithrombin III and protein C. Decreased venous blood flow in the lower extremities also contributes to postoperative hypercoagulability. In hip replacement surgery, the femoral vein in the operated leg may kink, thereby stimulating proximal venous thrombosis in the absence of preexistent calf vein thrombosis.

Venous stasis can be a precipitating cause of venous thromboembolism, particularly in hospitalized patients. An increased risk for venous thromboembolism also has been observed with prolonged air travel, particularly when the distance is greater than approximately 3000 miles.[219–221] Venous stasis secondary to immobilization is likely the major mechanism underlying this risk, which is increased in the presence of other predisposing thrombotic risk factors.[222,223]

Malignancy

The incidence of clinical thromboembolic disease in the cancer population has been estimated to be as high as 11%.[224] Autopsy series have described even higher rates of thrombosis for certain tumor types. One autopsy study found a 30% incidence of thrombosis in patients who died of pancreatic cancer and more than 50% in patients with tumors in the body or tail of the pancreas. Other tumor types commonly associated with thromboembolic complications are carcinomas of the gastrointestinal tract, ovary, prostate, and lung.

Patients with malignancy also have a higher rate of postoperative venous thrombotic complications than the general population, with an incidence of approximately 40%. Careful attention should therefore be paid to prophylaxis of deep vein thrombosis in such patients undergoing major abdominal or pelvic surgical procedures.

In some instances thrombosis manifests itself before the diagnosis of an underlying malignancy. Prandoni[225] investigated 250 consecutive patients with symptomatic deep vein thrombosis that was objectively documented by venogram. Cancer was identified at the time of diagnosis of the thrombotic event in 3.3% of patients with idiopathic venous thrombosis (ie, those with no other known risk factors), but no cases were found in patients with secondary venous thrombosis (those with documented additional risk factors such as prolonged immobilization, leg trauma, or hereditary thrombotic disorder). During a 2-year followup period, cancer was diagnosed in 7.6% of the patients with idiopathic venous thrombosis and in 1.9% of the patients with secondary venous thrombosis. The incidence of cancer was considerably higher in patients with recurrent idiopathic venous thrombosis.

The probability of detecting an occult neoplasm in patients with a documented thrombotic event also was evaluated by Monreal and colleagues,[226,227] who found a malignant lesion in 22.6% of patients with idiopathic deep vein thrombosis in contrast to 6.1% of patients with secondary thrombosis and in 11.5% patients with pulmonary embolism. The higher incidence of cancer reported by these investigators probably is because of a more aggressive diagnostic approach, which included chest radiography, upper gastrointestinal endoscopy, abdominal ultrasound study, and computed tomography scan.

Nonbacterial thrombotic endocarditis, characterized by sterile vegetations composed of platelets and fibrin on heart valves, is highly associated with malignant disorders. In autopsy series, cancer was found in as many as 75% of cases of nonbacterial thrombotic endocarditis. The majority of cases of nonbacterial thrombotic endocarditis occur in patients with adenocarcinomas, and its incidence among lung cancer patients may run as high as 7%. Laboratory evidence for DIC is often present. The aortic and mitral valves are most commonly affected. The diagnosis of nonbacterial thrombotic endocarditis can be difficult to make ante mortem, because less than 50% of patients have audible cardiac murmurs, and small lesions may not be identified by echocardiography.

The major clinical manifestations of nonbacterial thrombotic endocarditis are caused by systemic emboli from the vegetations on the heart valve(s) rather than from valvular dysfunction itself. Common sites of embolization include the spleen, kidney, and extremities, with the most significant morbidity arising from emboli to the central nervous system and coronary arteries. Nonbacterial thrombotic endocarditis should be considered in all cancer patients who develop an acute stroke syndrome, as well as in others who have cerebral embolism with an unknown etiology.

DIC is the cardinal coagulopathy associated with malignancy and results from generalized activation of the coagulation system. Malignancy is the third most common cause of DIC after infection and trauma and accounts for 7% of cases. DIC is a common coagulopathic complication in cancer patients and has been reported in as many as 15% of patients with malignancy. DIC occurs in virtually all patients with acute promyelocytic leukemia. The leukemic promyelocytes contain procoagulants that can trigger DIC, as well as fibrinolytic activators. The cell lysis that results from conventional chemotherapy releases these enzymes and can exacerbate the coagulopathy. Other disease entities, particularly sepsis, which in itself may be responsible or may contribute to the development of DIC in cancer patients, should be ruled out.

Various patterns of DIC are seen in association with malignancy. Acute forms of DIC are rare and usually present with minor bleeding from mucosal or cutaneous surfaces or extensive life-threatening hemorrhage involving visceral sites. Laboratory evaluation demonstrates prolongation of the prothrombin time, PTT, thrombin time, and reptilase time; decreased fibrinogen concentration; thrombocytopenia; and elevated levels of fibrin degradation products. More common in cancer patients are chronic forms of DIC. Many patients with chronic DIC are asymptomatic, and laboratory data often show modest reductions in fibrinogen and platelet count, elevated fibrin degradation products, and minimal changes in the prothrombin time or PTT. Others may have more obvious evidence of platelet, fibrinogen, and coagulation factor consumption. These latter patients often demonstrate hypercoagulability and can manifest deep vein thrombosis, Trousseau syndrome (ie, migratory superficial phlebitis involving the upper or lower extremities), or nonbacterial thrombotic endocarditis.

Thrombotic microangiopathy is the descriptive term for a syndrome characterized by hemolytic anemia, thrombocytopenia, pathognomonic microvascular thrombotic lesions, and the involvement of various specific organs (see Chapter 139). Depending on the differences in organ involvement, thrombotic microangiopathy is commonly called *thrombotic thrombocytopenic purpura* or *hemolytic uremic syndrome*. Severe thrombotic microangiopathy associated with thrombocytopenia may occur in as many as 5.7% of patients with metastatic carcinomas, most frequently with gastric, breast, or lung primary sites. Despite the classical manifestations of a Coombs-negative hemolytic anemia and severe thrombocytopenia, patients usually present with neurologic abnormalities, including headache, confusion or paresis, and occasionally signs of DIC. Renal failure is an uncommon feature of carcinoma-associated thrombotic microangiopathy. The goal of treatment of malignancy-related thrombotic microangiopathy is to decrease the tumor burden, because other treatment modalities, such as corticosteroids, plasma exchange or plasma infusion, result in only moderate and transient clinical improvement.

Probably contributing to the thrombotic tendency in cancer patients are clinical factors such as vascular stasis because of obstruction of blood flow by the tumor or patient immobility, hepatic involvement and dysfunction, sepsis, advanced age, other comorbid conditions, and certain antineoplastic agents. Thus, the exact details of the mechanisms underlying coagulation activation in malignancy remain uncertain, and a complex interaction of several of the above mechanisms, as well as others yet to be identified, may be responsible.

Nephrotic Syndrome

The nephrotic syndrome results from a variety of pathologic processes that cause excessive kidney glomerular leakage of plasma proteins into the urine. It is clinically characterized by edema, proteinuria, hypoalbuminemia, and hyperlipidemia. Thrombosis is a major cause of morbidity in patients with the nephrotic syndrome; the renal veins are the most commonly affected sites.[228] Renal vein thrombosis occurs in approximately 35% of cases, but the incidence varies considerably based on the underlying renal pathology and on the severity and duration of the proteinuria. The incidence of thrombosis in other sites is approximately 20%.[228,229] In adults, deep vein thrombosis and pulmonary embolism are the most common thrombotic complications. Arterial thrombosis is seemingly more common in children with nephrotic syndrome, resulting in stroke, mesenteric infarction, or limb ischemia.

Alterations in many blood coagulation parameters have been reported in patients with the nephrotic syndrome, although some abnormalities are inconsistently reported, of relatively minor magnitude, and poorly correlated with thrombotic events. The variability in findings is attributable to the complex nature of the nephrotic syndrome itself and the resultant marked stimulation of hepatic protein biosynthesis.

Among the natural anticoagulant proteins, plasma antithrombin III levels often are decreased, owing at least in part to urinary excretion. The antigenic levels of protein C and protein S generally are increased.[113] Plasma levels of several components of the coagulation cascade—factors XII, XI, and X—are reported to be decreased as a result of urinary excretion, whereas factors XIII, X, VIII, VII, and V characteristically are elevated in these patients. Some data suggest that platelet hyperreactivity, increased whole blood viscosity, and abnormal fibrin clot architecture related to hypofibrinolysis may contribute to the thrombotic diathesis in the nephrotic syndrome.

Hemolytic Anemias

PNH is a rare acquired clonal disorder of bone marrow stem cells. Patients generally manifest chronic intravascular hemolysis, with episodes of gross hemoglobinuria accompanied by leukopenia and thrombocytopenia. Many have a prior history of aplastic anemia. Despite the presence of thrombocytopenia, thrombosis is more commonly encountered than bleeding. Indeed, thrombosis can be a presenting feature of PNH, as well as an important cause of morbidity and mortality in this disorder. A diagnosis of PNH should be suspected in patients with a negative family history of thrombosis but with evidence of pancytopenia, an elevated reticulocyte count, or results of iron studies consistent with iron deficiency.

A unique feature of PNH is the predilection for thrombosis to occur in the intraabdominal venous network (mesenteric, hepatic, portal, splenic, and renal veins) and cerebral vessels, as opposed to deep vein thrombosis or pulmonary embolism. Arterial events such as myocardial infarction, stroke, and aortic thrombosis have rarely been reported. Acute thrombotic episodes should be treated with heparin or low-molecular-weight heparin. Fibrinolytic agents have been used successfully to treat acute intraabdominal venous thrombosis. Long-term oral anticoagulation should be considered in patients with thrombosis in association with PNH.

The abnormality of PNH erythrocytes that leads to hemolysis is their increased sensitivity to complement-mediated lysis. Deficiencies of a number of membrane proteins have been observed in PNH, including acetylcholinesterase, leukocyte alkaline phosphatase, *decay accelerating factor*, CD59 (membrane inhibitor of reactive lysis) antigen, homologous restriction factor, CD58, 5′-ectonucleotidase, CD16, urokinase-type plasminogen activator, and CD14 antigen. These proteins all are attached to the cells by a glycosylphosphatidylinositol anchor, and PNH appears to be the consequence of somatic mutations in the X-linked PIG-A (phosphatidylinositol glycan class A) gene, which participates in an early step in glycosylphosphatidylinositol anchor synthesis. Several of the membrane abnormalities involve proteins that modulate complement function, and the absence of CD59 antigen on erythrocytes appears to be the most critical defect. Granulocytes and platelets, like red cells, show increased sensitivity to complement-mediated lysis. Shed circulating platelet microparticles in PNH result in the dissemination of procoagulant phospholipids in the blood flow, possibly contributing to the thrombotic tendency in these patients. Although it has been suggested that the membrane abnormalities in PNH may lead to increased platelet activation by complement, there is not currently an adequate explanation for the thrombotic tendency in this disease. There is no apparent association between hemolytic and thrombotic episodes, nor does the onset of thrombosis correlate with the duration or degree of hemolysis.

Thrombosis is also a serious complication in patients with other types of hemolytic anemias, including sickle cell disease and thalassemia. In sickle cell disease, increased blood viscosity because of sickled erythrocytes contributes to microvascular occlusion. Asymptomatic patients with sickle cell disease also exhibit ongoing platelet activation, thrombin generation, and, fibrinolysis that increases during episodes of pain. These changes have been noted to be predictive of frequency of pain and interval to next pain episode, thereby implicating thrombogenic activity in the development of sickle cell pain crises. There is evidence for endothelial activation and increased numbers of circulating microvascular endothelial cells (CD36+) overexpressing intercellular adhesion molecule 1, vascular cell adhesion molecule 1, E-selectin, P-selectin, and tissue factor in patients with sickle cell disease.[230] Although much of the morbidity in sickle cell disease is a result of tissue ischemia and infarction (sickle cell crisis) caused by sickle cell occlusion of the microvasculature, both children and adults with sickle cell disease also have an increased risk of thrombosis of large blood vessels.

As standards of care for thalassemic patients have improved in recent years, resulting in an almost doubling of life expectancy, previously undescribed complications of the disease are being recognized, particularly thromboembolic complications.[231] These include cerebral thrombosis, deep vein thrombosis, pulmonary embolism, and recurrent arterial occlusions. Venous thrombosis develops following splenectomy in some patients with thrombocytosis. Associated with these clinical thromboembolic complications, profound hemostatic abnormalities have been observed in patients with β-thalassemia major, β-thalassemia intermedia and hemoglobin H disease.[231]

Hyperviscosity

Thrombosis can be a manifestation of diseases associated with hyperviscosity. Hyperviscosity of the blood may be caused by increased plasma viscosity, an increased number of red or white blood cells, or decreased deformability of cells.

Increased plasma viscosity can result from hypergammaglobulinemia or hyperfibrinogenemia. Hypergammaglobulinemia associated with the hyperviscosity syndrome is most commonly encountered in patients with Waldenström's macroglobulinemia or multiple myeloma. Presenting manifestations of the hyperviscosity syndrome include bleeding because of platelet dysfunction, visual disturbances, and neurologic defects. Thrombosis in hypergammaglobulinemic states is attributable to abnormal rheology.

Hyperviscosity plays an important role in the pathogenesis of thrombosis in polycythemia vera, which is a major complication of this disorder. Patients with elevated hematocrits have increased whole blood viscosity, and this abnormality has been inversely correlated with cerebral blood flow. Acquired qualitative platelet defects also have been implicated in the pathogenesis of the hemostatic defects in polycythemia vera. Common thrombotic complications in this disorder include cerebrovascular accidents, myocardial infarction, peripheral arterial occlusion, deep vein thrombosis, pulmonary embolism, and portal and hepatic vein thrombosis (Budd-Chiari syndrome).

In the myeloid and monocytic leukemias, the presence of very elevated white blood counts (generally greater than 100,000 cells/mm^3) can increase the viscosity in the microcirculation, which can play a role in the pathogenesis of thrombosis. Small vessels in the lungs, brain, and less commonly, other organs may be obstructed by large numbers of immature leukocytes.

In sickle cell disease, the increase in blood viscosity secondary to sickling of erythrocytes may contribute to the occlusion of small blood vessels. Enhanced adhesion of sickle erythrocytes to vascular endothelium, along with increased coagulation and platelet activation, promotes vascular occlusion.

Drug-Induced Thrombosis

The contribution of cancer therapies to the development of thrombotic events can be difficult to evaluate, because the neoplasm itself and other risk factors predispose cancer patients to thromboembolic complications.

Thrombotic events have been reported with induction chemotherapy regimens for acute lymphoblastic leukemia (ALL) that include L-asparaginase. Intracranial thrombosis with hemorrhage is observed most frequently, but deep venous thrombosis and pulmonary embolism can also occur. The incidence of thrombotic complications in children receiving L-asparaginase as part of induction chemotherapy for ALL is approximately 1%. Generalized bleeding episodes have only rarely been observed.

The inhibition of protein synthesis by L-asparaginase causes deficiencies of numerous plasma proteins, including albumin, thyroxine-binding globulin, and various coagulation proteins. Decreased levels of prothrombin, factors V, VII, VIII, IX, X, XI, fibrinogen, antithrombin III, protein C, protein S, and plasminogen have all been described secondary to L-asparaginase chemotherapy. Decreased levels of procoagulant factors lead to prolongation of the prothrombin time, PTT, and thrombin time. These coagulation abnormalities resolve within 1 to 2 weeks after cessation of the drug.

It is difficult to assess the role of the substantial reductions in the levels of natural anticoagulant proteins such as antithrombin III, protein C and protein S in the pathogenesis of the thrombotic events. Both procoagulant and anticoagulant protein synthesis in the liver are decreased by L-asparaginase, leading to uncertainty about whether there is an alteration in the balance of the opposing forces of the hemostatic mechanism. In one study of children with ALL receiving L-asparaginase, prednisone, and vincristine, no correlation was found between protein C, protein S, or antithrombin III levels and the presence or absence of thrombosis.[232] Other clinical factors may contribute to the pathogenesis of thrombotic complications that are observed in these patients, including immobility and concurrent sepsis.

Women with breast cancer receiving certain chemotherapy regimens are at increased risk for developing thrombosis. The availability of large numbers of patients receiving standard adjuvant chemotherapy programs as well as appropriate matched, untreated control populations has facilitated studies of this association. One study found a 5% incidence of symptomatic venous thrombosis among patients with stage II breast cancer treated with chemotherapy regimens that included cyclophosphamide, methotrexate, and 5-fluorouracil (CMF).[233] All of the thrombotic events occurred while the patients were receiving chemotherapy. In the post-treatment followup period, no clinically evident thromboses were observed. Goodnough[234] reported a 17.6% incidence of thrombosis in a series of patients with metastatic breast cancer receiving chemotherapy, with pulmonary embolism or deep vein thrombosis accounting for a majority of the thrombotic events. Levine[235] randomized 205 patients receiving adjuvant chemotherapy for stage II breast cancer to either a 12-week or a 36-week course of chemotherapy after primary surgical treatment. During the first 12 weeks of chemotherapy, there were similar numbers of thrombotic events; however, during the following 24 weeks, there were 5 additional thrombotic events in the 36-week treatment group, whereas no further thromboses were seen in the 12-week treatment group who had already completed therapy. Thus, 6.8% of the patients had a thromboembolic event while on chemotherapy, but no further thrombotic events were detected during the postchemotherapy followup period of more than 2400 patient-months. No relationships were found in this study between the development of thrombosis and estrogen or progesterone receptor status, age, number of involved lymph nodes, or subsequent tumor recurrence.

The association of arterial thrombosis and cancer therapy was shown in studies by Wall[236] and Saphner.[237] The Cancer and Acute Leukemia Group B study[236] found a 1.3% incidence of arterial thrombosis, either peripheral arterial or cerebrovascular, in 1014 patients during treatment for stage II or III breast cancer on two separate chemotherapy protocols. All except one of the thrombotic events occurred while patients were receiving chemotherapy. In the study by Saphner,[237] which included 2352 patients, a significant increase in arterial thrombosis was found in premenopausal women who received combined chemohormonal therapy, whereas no higher risk for arterial thrombosis was seen in postmenopausal women receiving tamoxifen either alone or in combination with chemotherapy. In both studies, arterial thrombotic events tended to occur early in the course of treatment.

The pathophysiologic basis for the thrombogenicity of chemotherapy in breast cancer patients is not well understood. In a prospective study of patients receiving adjuvant chemotherapy for breast cancer, no alterations in antithrombin III levels were detected. Rogers[111] found a statistically significant decrease in protein C and protein S levels during CMF chemotherapy. Some of these patients had decrements in protein C and S levels that fell below the range of values seen in hereditary thrombotic disorders. Decreases in factor VII and fibrinogen levels also were reported. None of the patients in this small study, however, had clinically evident thrombosis. Other investigators have observed significant declines in protein C concentration during CMF chemotherapy, which returned to baseline values after the completion of therapy.[238] Possible explanations for these chemotherapy-induced abnormalities include impairment of vitamin K metabolism, inhibition of DNA/RNA synthesis leading to a decrease in protein synthesis by the liver, and initiation of intravascular coagulation.

Hormonal therapies, such as estrogen therapy for prostate carcinoma, have clearly been linked to an increased incidence of thromboembolic disease. In the Veterans Administration Cooperative Urologic Research Group's studies of estrogen therapy in patients with prostate cancer, death rates from cardiovascular events were higher in those on 5 mg of diethylstilbestrol daily than in those on a 1 mg daily dose.[239] The antitumor effect of these two dosages was similar.

The use of tamoxifen, an antiestrogen with some proestrogenic activity for the prevention and treatment of breast cancer, is associated with an increased risk of venous thromboembolic events.[240,241] The factor V Leiden and prothrombin G20210A mutations are not associated with thrombosis in women on tamoxifen.[242,243]

For the treatment of multiple myeloma, thalidomide or lenalidomide, particularly when given in protocols that include high doses of dexamethasone, is associated with a high incidence of venous thromboembolism.[244]

Lupus Anticoagulants and the Antiphospholipid Syndrome

A diagnosis of antiphospholipid antibody syndrome requires an initial thrombotic event in association with a persistent lupus anticoagulant and/or persistently elevated levels of cardiolipin (IgG or IgM) or β_2-glycoprotein I antibodies (see Chapter 131). Clinical manifestations include venous or arterial thrombosis and recurrent fetal loss. Thrombocytopenia and livedo reticularis may also be found in patients with the syndrome. Antiphospholipid antibody syndrome frequently occurs in patients with systemic lupus erythematosus but also occurs in patients with cancer and with some infections and with the administration of certain drugs. Lupus anticoagulants result from the presence of immunoglobulins, which bind to phospholipids and plasma proteins (β_2-glycoprotein 1, prothrombin) and prolong phospholipid-dependent clotting assays in vitro (see Chapter 131). Persons with lupus anticoagulants do not suffer from a bleeding diathesis unless other hemostatic defects are present (eg, severe thrombocytopenia, prothrombin deficiency). Paradoxically, a persistent lupus anticoagulant and/or a high level of cardiolipin or β_2-glycoprotein-I antibodies identifies thrombotic patients at substantially increased risk for recurrence. However, asymptomatic patients with transient lupus anticoagulants in association with infections or drugs may not be at increased risk for thrombosis.

The management of acute venous thromboembolism in patients with lupus anticoagulants is similar to that in other patients without this laboratory abnormality. The initial treatment of patients with a prolonged PTT at baseline, however, is complicated by the fact that the PTT cannot reliably be used to monitor unfractionated heparin dosage unless proper in-vitro calibration studies are done by adding known amounts of heparin into plasma samples and measuring the response of the PTT. Thus, it is preferable to monitor anticoagulant therapy in these individuals by performing plasma heparin measurements using factor Xa and a suitable chromogenic substrate. These problems are obviated by the use of low-molecular-weight heparin, which does not require coagulation monitoring. The presence of lupus anticoagulants also can interfere with heparin monitoring during cardiac surgery.

Warfarin is effective in preventing recurrent thrombosis, although retrospective studies indicated that an international normalized ratio (INR) greater than 3 is required.[245,246] Randomized clinicals trial in patients with the antiphospholipid antibody syndrome have shown that an INR of 2 to 3 is as effective as an INR of 3 to 4 in preventing recurrent venous thrombosis.[247,248]

The clinical heterogeneity of the individual populations in which lupus anticoagulants develop makes it difficult to generalize regarding their long-term antithrombotic management. Persons in whom transient lupus anticoagulants develop in association with infections do not experience thromboembolic episodes, and it is unclear whether drug-associated lupus anticoagulants are associated with thrombosis. Thus, the presence of persistent lupus anticoagulant or a high-titer antiphospholipid antibody, or both, in an asymptomatic subject with no prior thrombotic history is not an indication for anticoagulant or antiplatelet medications. Inasmuch as it is not currently possible to determine reliably the risk of thrombosis in an asymptomatic individual with these laboratory abnormalities, however, all such individuals should receive appropriate prophylaxis in conjunction with major surgical procedures, prolonged immobilization, pregnancy, and the postpartum period, unless there is a strong contraindication to such treatment. Corticosteroids can normalize clotting assay times or reduce antiphospholipid antibody titers in persons with lupus anticoagulants. These and other immunosuppressive medications have not been proved to prevent recurrent thrombosis, however.

MANAGEMENT

Acute Thrombosis

The acute management of venous thrombosis or pulmonary embolism in patients with biologic risk factors for thrombosis generally is not different from that in other individuals. Massive acute venous thrombosis and pulmonary embolism are strong indications for thrombolytic therapy. The usual treatment consists of unfractionated heparin or low-molecular-weight heparin followed by long-term anticoagulation with warfarin (or other vitamin K-antagonists). Warfarin can be started within the first 24 hours. Heparin or low-molecular-weight heparin is continued for at least 5 days or until the prothrombin time is in the therapeutic range, namely, until an INR of 2.0 to 3.0 is achieved. Special considerations may apply to selected patients with antithrombin III deficiency and hereditary protein C deficiency. The principles of anticoagulation are described in further detail in Chapter 137.

Antithrombin III Deficiency

Persons with antithrombin III deficiency can usually be managed successfully with low-molecular-weight heparin or intravenous heparin, although in some situations, higher than usual doses are required to achieve adequate anticoagulation. In antithrombin III-deficient individuals receiving heparin for the treatment of acute thrombosis, the adjunctive role of antithrombin concentrate purified from human plasma is not clearly defined because controlled trials have not been performed. Antithrombin III concentrate has been used safely and effectively in patients with antithrombin deficiency and acute venous thrombosis. It is recommended in those patients who have unusually severe thrombosis, have difficulty achieving adequate anticoagulation, or experience recurrent thrombosis despite adequate anticoagulation. It can also be used for antithrombotic prophylaxis in antithrombin III-deficient patients in whom anticoagulation is contraindicated. The use of antithrombin concentrate as adjunctive therapy or as an alternative to heparin, however, has not been studied in a controlled trial.[249]

Antithrombin concentrate is prepared from pooled normal human plasma. The manufacturing processes used to prepare antithrombin concentrate result in a product that is greater than 95% pure; this process inactivates the hepatitis B virus and human immunodeficiency virus-I. It is preferable to administer antithrombin concentrate rather than fresh frozen plasma. A human antithrombin concentrate has also been produced from the milk of transgenic goats using recombinant DNA technology[250] and is commercially available in Europe.

The infusion of 50 units of plasma-derived antithrombin concentrate per kilogram of body weight (1 unit is defined as the amount of antithrombin in 1 mL of pooled normal human plasma) usually will increase the plasma antithrombin III level to approximately 120% in a congenitally deficient individual with a baseline level of 50%. Plasma levels should be monitored to ensure that they remain above 80%. The administration of 60% of the initial dose at 24-hour intervals is recommended to maintain inhibitor levels in the normal range.[251] Recovery of plasma-derived antithrombin concentrate in vivo in patients with antithrombin deficiency is 1.4% to 2.7% per unit per kilogram of body weight. Recovery is lower in patients with acute thrombotic events and those receiving heparin therapy. The biologic half-life approximates 2.8 to 4.8 days.

Oral anticoagulants are highly effective in the management of patients with antithrombin III deficiency. Warfarin should be continued indefinitely in patients with recurrent venous thrombosis. Asymptomatic antithrombin III-deficient persons from thrombophilic kindreds are not generally given prophylactic anticoagulation unless they are exposed to situations that predispose them to the development of thrombosis (eg, prolonged immobilization, surgery, pregnancy).

Protein C Deficiency

Hereditary protein C deficiency can rarely be associated with warfarin-induced skin necrosis because of the induction of a transient hypercoagulable state by warfarin. Despite this risk, routine measurement of plasma protein C concentrations in all individuals with thrombosis before the initiation of oral anticoagulants is not recommended. This conclusion is based on three observations: the infrequent occurrence of warfarin-induced skin necrosis even among patients with hereditary protein C deficiency; the frequency of asymptomatic hereditary protein C deficiency in the general population (1:200 to 1:500); and the diagnostic difficulty in making a rapid and definitive laboratory diagnosis of the deficiency state.

Conversely, oral anticoagulation in a patient who is known or likely to be protein C deficient should be started under the cover of full heparinization. The dose of warfarin should be increased gradually, starting from a relatively low level (eg, 2 mg for the first 3 days and then in increasing amounts of 2 to 3 mg/day until therapeutic anticoagulation is achieved). Patients with heterozygous protein C deficiency and a history of warfarin-induced skin necrosis have been successfully retreated with oral anticoagulants. Administration of protein C, in the form of either fresh frozen plasma or protein C concentrate derived, can provide protection against recurrent skin necrosis until a stable level of anticoagulation is achieved. A highly purified protein C concentrate derived from human plasma is commercially available.

Long-Term Therapy to Prevent Recurrent Venous Thromboembolism

After initial heparinization, standard therapy for patients with deep venous thrombosis or pulmonary embolism typically includes anticoagulation with warfarin for 3 to 12 months at a target INR of between 2 and 3; this regimen results in more than a 90% reduction in recurrence risk. In patients presenting with a first episode of symptomatic venous thromboembolism, Prandoni[252] found the cumulative incidence of recurrent venous thrombosis after the cessation of anticoagulant therapy to be 24.8% at 5 years and 30.3% at 8 years. Other investigators have confirmed that this risk is approximately 5% to 15% per year for the first several years after a first or even a second episode of unprovoked venous thrombosis.

Recurrences are less common when the initial event is associated with a transient risk factor (eg, surgery, trauma, pregnancy). Despite the relatively high recurrence risk in patients with a first episode of unprovoked venous thrombosis, anticoagulation with warfarin has not proved to have sufficient benefit, compared with the bleeding risk, to support long-term prophylaxis for all patients at substantial recurrence risk. For example, one controlled trial evaluated the efficacy of long-term warfarin therapy (INR 2 to 2.85) for 6 months or indefinitely in 227 patients with a second venous thrombotic episode, but not specifically inherited thrombophilia.[253] Long-term warfarin was highly effective in preventing recurrences as compared with 6 months of therapy (2.6% vs. 21% over 4 years). This benefit was partially counterbalanced by a trend toward an increased incidence of major hemorrhage (8.6% vs. 2.3%), and there was no difference in mortality rate between the two groups.

Owing to the relatively high frequency of the factor V Leiden mutation in patients with a first episode of venous thromboembolism, there is a substantial amount of data on the risk of recurrence. Although two groups initially reported that patients with factor V Leiden who had a first venous thrombotic event were more than twice as likely to have a recurrent episode than those without the mutation,[204,254] several other groups have not found that heterozygosity for this defect or the prothrombin G20210A mutation confers a higher recurrence risk.[14,40,255–257] Thus, the consensus view is that neither of these defects alone is predictive of recurrence, and several studies have argued against the use of long-term warfarin therapy after a first thromboembolic episode in these patient populations. As an example, the recurrence rate after discontinuation of oral anticoagulant therapy was assessed in 62 patients with factor V Leiden.[258] None of the patients had a recurrent event while taking warfarin. The median time to recurrence after stopping warfarin was 9 years; the period was shorter (3.5 years) among patients who suffered an idiopathic rather than precipitated first event. It was estimated that, even in the latter group, death from hemorrhage would probably exceed the number of fatal pulmonary emboli prevented with chronic warfarin therapy. A decision analysis model concerning the value of extended anticoagulation in patients with factor V Leiden who had a first deep vein thrombosis concluded that the number of major induced hemorrhages would exceed the number of clinical pulmonary emboli that would be prevented, and that extension of oral anticoagulation beyond 1 year would not produce clinical benefit.[259] There is no increase in mortality among patients with the factor V Leiden mutation,[260] further supporting the argument that the mortality risk of chronic warfarin therapy at a target INR of 2 to 3 in the average thrombophilic patient may exceed the potential benefit.

The recurrence risk appears to be significantly higher in the small subset of patients who are heterozygous for both mutations, homozygous for factor V Leiden, or have another thrombophilic defect.[10–15]

The presence of antiphospholipid antibody syndrome[246] or cancer[261,262] are also important risk factors for recurrence. A randomized clinical trial of patients with venous thromboembolism in the setting of active cancer demonstrated that chronic low-molecular-weight heparin leads to a significantly lower recurrence rate than that with standard therapy (low-molecular-weight heparin for 5–7 days followed by warfarin at a target INR between 2 and 3).[263]

Owing to the relatively low frequency of antithrombin, protein C, or protein S deficiency in unselected cohorts with an initial episode of venous thromboembolism, randomized clinical trials have included too few patients with these deficiencies to draw firm conclusions. A literature review and retrospective cohort study suggested that they have a high annual incidence of recurrent venous thromboembolism during the years immediately following a first episode and that this incidence declines thereafter.[264] The application of decision analysis to this problem indicates that optimal anticoagulant treatment duration will vary depending on the type of initial event (spontaneous or secondary; deep vein thrombosis or pulmonary embolism), patient age, and time passed since the initial thromboembolic episode.[265] Of interest, retrospective studies are unable to demonstrate an increase in mortality in patients with antithrombin III[266] or protein C deficiency.

For the individual patient, the decision to continue anticoagulation indefinitely requires estimation of the quantitative risk of recurrent thrombosis, including fatal pulmonary embolism, and major bleeding, including fatal bleeding over time. Patient compliance has a major impact on the success of therapy, and patient preferences must be factored into the decision. Many clinicians with experience managing these disorders recommend indefinite anticoagulation for patients with heterozygous antithrombin III deficiency. Some also recommend such an approach for patients with heterozygous deficiencies of protein C and protein S.

In summary, the decision whether to undertake extended or indefinite anticoagulation must be tailored to the individual patient based on several factors (Table 134–11). Commonly cited criteria for indefinite anticoagulation include the following:

Two or more spontaneous venous thrombotic events that are separated by a relatively short period of time (less than 2 years)

One spontaneous thrombosis in the case of antithrombin III deficiency, the antiphospholipid antibody syndrome, and active cancer

A single unprovoked venous thrombotic event in the presence of more than one genetic abnormality (eg, combined heterozygosity

Table 134–11 Long-Term Management of Patients with Venous Thromboembolism

Risk Classification	Management
High-Risk	Indefinite anticoagulation
2 or more spontaneous events for all high-risk patients	
1 spontaneous life-threatening thrombosis	
1 spontaneous thrombosis at unusual sites (mesenteric or cerebral venous)	
1 spontaneous thrombosis in association with the antiphospholipid antibody syndrome, active cancer, antithrombin III deficiency, or more than one genetic or allelic abnormality	
Moderate-Risk	Vigorous prophylaxis in
1 thrombosis with a known provocative stimulus	High-risk settings in asymptomatic patients

for the factor V Leiden mutation and the prothrombin G20210A mutation)

A single spontaneous pulmonary thromboembolic event that is massive or submassive

One spontaneous thrombosis at an unusual site (eg, mesenteric, portal, or cerebral veins)

Management of Pregnancy

The management of pregnancy in women with a history of thrombosis or hereditary thrombotic disorders poses special problems. The incidence of thrombotic complications during pregnancy and the postpartum period appears to be greater in women with antithrombin III deficiency than in those with deficiencies of protein C or protein S.[267] During pregnancy, adjusted-dose unfractionated heparin or low-molecular-weight heparin administered by the subcutaneous route is the anticoagulant of choice, because its efficacy and safety for the fetus are established. Low-molecular-weight heparin is an attractive alternative to unfractionated heparin in these women because of its better bioavailability and longer half-life. There is a low risk of venous thromboembolism antepartum without prophylactic anticoagulation in women with a history of thrombotic episodes[268] in association with transient risk factors; the risk appears to be higher in women with the factor V Leiden mutation. Treatment, however, should be administered during the postpartum period. Affected women with antithrombin III deficiency with or without previous thrombotic events probably should receive treatment. Treatment for asymptomatic women with other hereditary thrombotic disorders should be considered on an individual basis, but asymptomatic women with heterozygosity for factor V Leiden or the prothrombin G20210A mutation are at low risk and generally will not require prophylactic anticoagulation.

The dose and duration of heparin or low-molecular-weight heparin therapy in pregnancy are uncertain, because appropriately designed clinical trials have not been performed. Women considered to be at high risk should receive therapeutic doses by subcutaneous injection every 12 hours for the duration of pregnancy. The dose of unfractionated heparin should be adjusted to maintain the 6-hour postinjection PTT at 1.5 times the control value. In women considered to be at intermediate risk, lower doses of heparin (5000 to 10,000 units subcutaneously every 12 hours), or low-molecular-weight heparin can be started during the second or third trimester and continued for approximately 6 weeks into the postpartum period. Low-risk patients can be observed closely throughout the pregnancy.

In women who are planning pregnancy while receiving long-term oral anticoagulant therapy, several approaches can be taken to minimize the risk of both thrombotic complications and warfarin embryopathy. One is to stop warfarin and commence subcutaneous heparin or low-molecular-weight heparin therapy. This approach potentially exposes the patient to many months of heparin therapy while she is trying to conceive. Alternatively, warfarin therapy could be continued with the performance of pregnancy tests on a frequent basis. As soon as pregnancy is diagnosed and before the sixth week of gestation, oral anticoagulants must be discontinued and heparin therapy initiated. The risk of warfarin embryopathy appears to be quite small during the first 6 weeks of pregnancy.

Management of Warfarin-Induced Skin Necrosis and Neonatal Purpura Fulminans

As warfarin-induced skin necrosis is a rare complication, therapy has been guided primarily by knowledge regarding its pathogenesis. The diagnosis should be suspected in individuals with painful, red skin lesions developing within a few days after the initiation of the drug, and immediate intervention is required to prevent rapid progression and reduce complications. Therapy should consist of immediate discontinuation of warfarin, administration of vitamin K, and infusion of heparin at therapeutic doses. Lesions have been reported to progress despite adequate anticoagulation with heparin.

In persons with hereditary protein C deficiency, the administration of a source of protein C should be considered. This measure also may be appropriate in other patients with warfarin-induced skin necrosis, because they invariably have reduced plasma levels of functional protein C when the skin lesions first appear. Fresh frozen plasma has been used, but improved results can be expected with the administration of a highly purified protein C concentrate, which facilitates the rapid and complete normalization of plasma protein C levels.

The management of neonatal purpura fulminans in association with homozygous or doubly heterozygous protein C deficiency is more complicated, and heparin therapy has not been shown to be effective. The administration of a source of protein C appears to be critical in the initial treatment for these patients. Fresh frozen plasma has been used with success in affected infants. However, the half-life of protein C in the circulation is only approximately 6 to 16 hours, and the administration of plasma on a frequent basis is limited by the development of hyperproteinemia or hypertension, loss of venous access, and the potential for exposure to infectious viral agents. Protein C concentrate is efficacious in treating neonatal purpura fulminans.[269] Warfarin has been administered to these infants without the redevelopment of skin necrosis during the phased withdrawal of fresh frozen plasma infusions, and this medication has been used chronically to control the thrombotic diathesis. Successful liver transplantation was performed in a child with liver failure and homozygous protein C deficiency, which resulted in normalization of the plasma protein C level and resolution of the thrombotic diathesis.[270]

SUGGESTED READINGS

Abramson N, Costatino JP, Garber JE, et al: Effect of factor V Leiden and prothrombin G20210→A mutations on thromboembolic risk in the national surgical adjuvant breast and bowel project breast cancer prevention trial. J Natl Cancer Inst 98:904, 2006.

Bayston T, Lane D: Antithrombin mutation database. Department of Haematology, Imperial College Faculty of Medicine, Charing Cross Hospital Campus, Hammersmith, London. http://www1.imperial.ac.uk/medicine/about/divisions/is/haemo/coag/antithrombin/ 2007.

Bennett CL, Angelotta C, Yarnold PR, et al: Thalidomide- and lenalidomide-associated thromboembolism among patients with cancer. JAMA 296:2558, 2006.

Bezemer ID, Doggen CJ, Vos HL, et al: No association between the common MTHFR 677C→T polymorphism and venous thrombosis: Results from the MEGA Study. Arch Intern Med 167:497, 2007.

Bønaa KH, Njølstad I, Ueland PM, et al: Homocysteine lowering and cardiovascular events after acute myocardial infarction. N Eng J Med 354:1578, 2006.

Corral J, Hernandez-Espinosa D, Soria JM, et al: Antithrombin Cambridge II (A384S): an underestimated genetic risk factor for venous thrombosis. Blood 109:4258, 2007.

Corral J, González-Conejero R, Soria JM, et al: A nonsense polymorphism in the protein Z-dependent protease inhibitor increases the risk for venous thrombosis. Blood 108:177, 2006.

Cuzick J, Forbes JF, Sestak I, et al: Long-term results of tamoxifen prophylaxis for breast cancer—96-month follow-up of the randomized IBIS-I trial. J Natl Cancer Inst 99:272, 2007.

den Heijer M, Willems HP, Blom HJ, et al: Homocysteine lowering by B vitamins and the secondary prevention of deep vein thrombosis and pulmonary embolism: A randomized, placebo-controlled, double-blind trial. Blood 109:139, 2007.

D'Ursi P, Marino F, Caprera A, et al: ProCMD: A database and 3D web resource for protein C mutants. BMC Bioinformatics 8(Suppl 1):S11, 2007.

Investigators THOPEH: Homocysteine lowering with folic acid and B vitamins in vascular disease. N Engl J Med 354:1567, 2006.

Keijzer MB, Borm GF, Blom HJ, et al: No interaction between factor V Leiden and hyperhomocysteinemia or MTHFR C677T genotype in venous thrombosis. Results of a meta-analysis of published studies and a large case-control study. Thromb Haemost 97:32, 2007.

Schreijer AJ, Cannegieter SC, Meijers JC, et al: Activation of coagulation system during air travel: A crossover study. Lancet 367:832, 2006.

Shrivastava S, Ridker PM, Glynn RJ, et al: D-dimer, factor VIII coagulant activity, low-intensity warfarin and the risk of recurrent venous thromboembolism. J Thromb Haemost 4:1208, 2006.

Tefs K, Gueorguieva M, Klammt J, et al: Molecular and clinical spectrum of type I plasminogen deficiency: A series of 50 patients. Blood 108:3021, 2006.

REFERENCES

For complete list of references log onto www.expertconsult.com

antithrombin and proteins C and S, the factor V Leiden and prothrombin G20210A mutations, hyperhomocysteinuria, and the presence of antiphospholipid antibodies. Hypercoagulable states are the subject of Chapter 134.

NATURAL HISTORY OF VENOUS THROMBOEMBOLISM

Most thrombi are asymptomatic and confined to the intramuscular veins of the calf. These calf vein thrombi often undergo spontaneous lysis and rarely, if ever, produce long-term sequelae.[21] By contrast, complete lysis of proximal vein thrombosis is uncommon even when heparin treatment is given.[22]

The symptoms and signs of venous thromboembolism are caused by obstruction to venous outflow, inflammation of the vessel wall or perivascular tissues, or embolization of thrombus into the pulmonary circulation. Asymptomatic pulmonary embolism is detected by perfusion lung scanning in approximately 50% of patients with documented proximal vein thrombosis.[23] Most clinically significant and fatal pulmonary emboli probably arise from thrombi in the proximal veins of the legs. Although pulmonary embolism also may complicate calf vein thrombosis, these emboli tend to be smaller in size, and pulmonary embolism occurs less commonly than in patients with proximal vein thrombosis.[23] Asymptomatic venous thrombosis is found in 70% of patients who present with confirmed pulmonary embolism.[24] These thrombi usually are large and involve the proximal veins.

Extensive venous thrombosis causes venous valvular damage, which leads to the postphlebitic syndrome.[25] Patients with a previous history of venous thrombosis are at increased risk of further episodes of venous thrombosis, particularly when patients are exposed to high-risk situations.[26]

PROGNOSIS WITH VENOUS THROMBOSIS

Untreated or inadequately treated venous thrombosis is associated with a high complication rate, which can be decreased markedly by adequate anticoagulant therapy. Approximately 20% of untreated silent calf vein thrombi and 20% to 30% of untreated symptomatic calf vein thrombi extend into the popliteal vein. When extension occurs and is untreated, it is associated with a 40% to 50% risk of clinically detectable pulmonary embolism.[21] Patients with proximal vein thrombosis who receive inadequate treatment[27] have a 47% frequency of recurrent venous thromboembolism over 3 months, and patients with symptomatic calf vein thrombosis who receive a 5-day course of intermittent intravenous unfractionated heparin without continuing oral anticoagulants have a recurrence rate greater than 20% over the next 3 months.[28]

By contrast, clinically detectable recurrence occurs in less than 2% of patients with proximal vein thrombosis during the initial period of unfractionated heparin therapy[23] if an adequate anticoagulant response is achieved, and the recurrence rate during the subsequent 3 months of treatment with oral anticoagulants or moderate doses of subcutaneous unfractionated heparin is 2% to 4%.[27,29,30] After 3 months of anticoagulant therapy, the recurrence rate is 5% to 10% in the subsequent year.[27,29,30] Patients whose first episode of venous thrombosis was idiopathic and those who have ongoing risk factors, such as prolonged immobilization or cancer, have a higher risk of recurrence.

The significance of asymptomatic calf deep vein thrombosis discovered incidentally by screening venography after orthopedic surgery is unclear although the risk of clinical sequelae from these thrombi is low.[31] As a result, if adequate perioperative deep vein thrombosis prophylaxis is given, it probably is not necessary to perform screening tests for deep vein thrombosis in asymptomatic patients at the time of hospital discharge.

POSTPHLEBITIC SYNDROME

The postphlebitic syndrome is caused by venous hypertension, usually resulting from valve destruction. Valve destruction results in malfunction of the muscular pump mechanism, which leads to increased pressure in the deep calf veins during ambulation. The high pressure ultimately renders the perforating veins of the calf incompetent, so that blood flow is directed from the deep veins into the superficial venous system during muscular contraction. This leads to edema and impaired viability of subcutaneous tissues and, in its most severe form, to venous ulceration. Outflow obstruction initially may be bypassed by the development of collateral veins, but with time, the veins distal to the obstruction become dilated and their valves become incompetent.

In patients whose thrombosis extends into the iliofemoral veins, the leg swelling at initial presentation may not resolve entirely. This is in contrast to patients with less extensive proximal vein thrombosis, where the swelling may subside after initial treatment but recur months or years later. Other symptoms and signs of the postphlebitic syndrome may be delayed for 5 to 10 years after the initial thrombotic event. These symptoms include pain in the calf that is relieved with rest and leg elevation, pigmentation and induration around the ankle and lower one-third of the calf, and ulceration, which usually occurs in the region of the medial malleolus.

Patients with extensive thrombosis involving the iliofemoral vein frequently have greater disability and may even have venous claudication, which is characterized by incapacitating, bursting pain with exercise.[32] This complication rarely occurs in patients with thrombosis involving the more distal veins.

The frequency with which postphlebitic syndrome occurs after venous thromboembolism is controversial. Prandoni and colleagues[33] demonstrated that 29% of patients with acute deep vein thrombosis will develop the syndrome after 8 years of followup; however, other investigators have found a much lower rate.[34] The development of ipsilateral recurrent thrombosis was associated with a large increase in risk for the development of postphlebitic syndrome.

Whether therapy for acute venous thrombosis reduces the long-term risk of postphlebitic syndrome is unclear. In practical terms, therapy that reduces thrombus extension or prevents the development of profound outflow obstruction from the limb is likely to reduce the long-term risk of postphlebitic syndrome. In addition, the use of below-knee graduated compression stockings has been shown to reduce the risk of postphlebitic syndrome in patients with deep vein thrombosis.[35]

DIAGNOSIS OF VENOUS THROMBOSIS

The approach to the diagnosis of venous thrombosis has changed radically over the past 2 decades. It is now accepted that the clinical diagnosis of venous thrombosis is unreliable and that objective tests are necessary to confirm the diagnosis.

In symptomatic patients, venous ultrasonography has a sensitivity and specificity for detection of proximal (femoral or popliteal vein) deep vein thrombosis of more than 95%.[36] However, ultrasonography is insensitive for detection of calf vein thrombosis and of any deep vein thrombosis occurring after orthopedic surgery.[37] Ultrasound examination can be repeated 7 days after the initial study to increase its sensitivity for detection of clinically important calf vein thrombosis and to improve the safety of diagnostic strategies that do not include venography in patients with suspected calf vein thrombosis. This strategy will detect the 10% to 30% of calf vein thrombi that extend proximally. If examination findings remain negative after 7 days, the risk of clinically important proximal extension is negligible, and it is safe to withhold antithrombotic treatment.[38–41]

CLINICAL DIAGNOSIS

Although clinical diagnosis is unreliable, careful documentation of clinical symptoms and signs is helpful in ruling out venous thrombosis when an alternative cause is identified. The conditions that most frequently mimic venous thrombosis are a ruptured Baker cyst, cellulitis, sciatica, muscle or tendon tear, muscle cramp, muscle hematoma, external venous compression, superficial thrombophlebitis, and the postphlebitic syndrome. In assessing patients for suspected venous thrombosis, patients can be reliably classified into high-, intermediate-, and low-probability groups based on their clinical manifestations and the presence or absence of risk factors such as recent immobilization, hospitalization within the past 6 months, or malignancy.[42] In one series, patients with the classic symptoms and signs of deep vein thrombosis such as localized pain, tenderness, swelling, and discoloration, and who had at least one risk factor had an 85% probability of venous thrombosis, whereas those with atypical symptoms and no risk factors had only a 5% probability of venous thrombosis. These low- and high-pretest probabilities can be combined with the results of objective noninvasive tests to make clinical decisions (Fig. 135–1). A low clinical pretest probability and a negative result on noninvasive testing can be used to exclude a diagnosis of venous thrombosis and obviate further testing, whereas a high clinical pretest probability and a negative noninvasive test result should prompt further investigation with venography.

In approximately 70% of patients referred for clinically suspected venous thrombosis, the diagnosis will be excluded by objective tests.[38,39] Of the 30% who have venous thrombosis, approximately 85% will have proximal vein thrombosis, and the remainder will have thrombosis confined to the calf.[38,39]

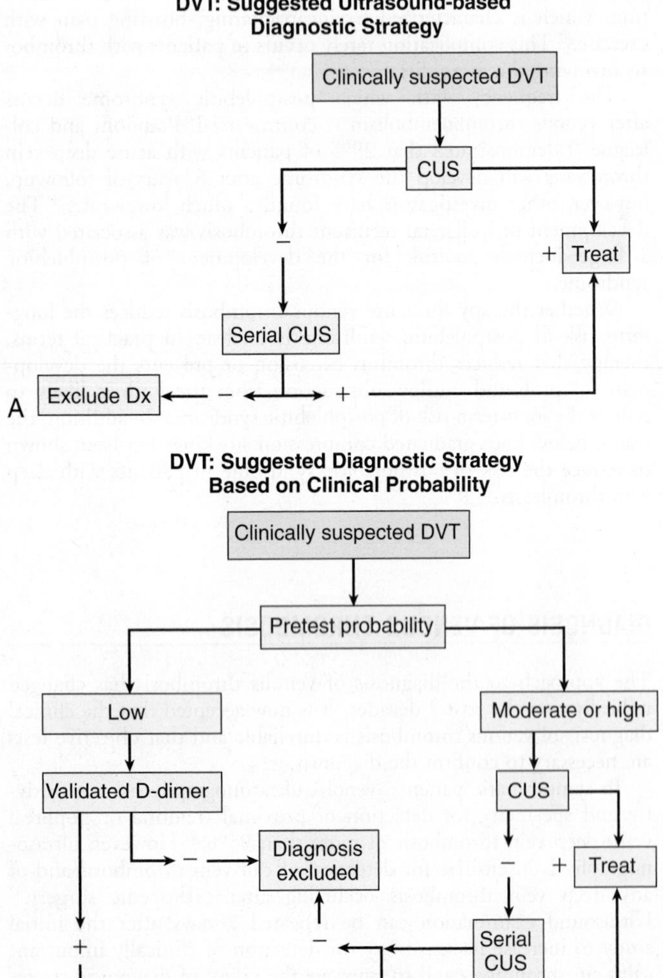

Figure 135–1 Diagnostic algorithms for the management of patients with suspected deep vein thrombosis (DVT). **(A)** Ultrasound examination-based strategy. **(B)** Clinical probability-based strategy. CUS, compression ultrasound.

OBJECTIVE DIAGNOSTIC TESTS

Both invasive and noninvasive tests are useful for the diagnosis of venous thrombosis. Venography is the only invasive test of proven value; the noninvasive test that has been most widely studied is venous ultrasonography. Unlike venography, ultrasonography lacks sensitivity for detection of calf vein thrombosis.

Venography

Venography remains the reference standard for the diagnosis of venous thrombosis.[43] It is technically difficult, and its proper execution and interpretation require considerable experience. Venography may produce superficial phlebitis and can cause deep vein thrombosis,[43] but with good technique, ascending venography outlines the entire deep venous system of the lower extremities, including the calf and iliac veins.

Venous Ultrasonography

Venous ultrasonography is performed using a high-resolution real-time scanner equipped with a 5-MHz electronically focused linear array transducer. The common femoral vein and femoral artery are first located in the groin, with the patient in a supine position. The superficial femoral vein is then examined along its course. Next, the popliteal vein is located and examined down to the level of its trifurcation into the peroneal and tibial veins. At each of these locations, the vein being examined is compressed gently but firmly with the transducer probe, and the results are observed on the monitor. Hard copies from freeze-frame images of both stages of the procedure are obtained and serve as a permanent record.

Venous ultrasonography is very accurate for the detection of proximal vein thrombosis in symptomatic patients but relatively insensitive for detection of calf vein thrombosis. If the field of examination is extended to the distal popliteal vein and the proximal deep calf veins, venous ultrasonography detects approximately 50% of calf vein thrombi in symptomatic patients.[44,45] Although there are reports that ultrasound examination of the calf can detect thrombi reliably, most such reports have not used venography as their reference standard. Furthermore, whether the value of this test is maintained when it moves from highly specialized vascular laboratories into community ultrasonography laboratories is unknown. A potential limitation of venous ultrasonography is its inability to visualize the iliac veins and the segment of the superficial femoral vein within the femoral canal. This is not a serious limitation, because isolated thrombi within the femoral canal or the iliac vein are rare.[46] Furthermore, the obstruction produced by iliac vein thrombi often limits the compressibility of the common femoral vein segment and hence will be detected indirectly.

D-Dimer Assays

D-dimer assays use mono- or polyspecific antibodies against D-dimer to provide quantitative or qualitative data on the concentration of D-dimer in whole blood or plasma. D-dimer is a product of fibrin lysis and is increased in patients with acute venous thromboembolism. However, the test is nonspecific because the level of D-dimer also is increased in a variety of conditions including malignancies and infections. Therefore, the D-dimer assay is most useful as a tool to rule out suspected deep vein thrombosis.[47,48]

D-dimer assays have two principal limitations: (1) A positive test is nonspecific and should not be used as the sole criterion for diagnosis of venous thrombosis; and (2) numerous test kits are available that have different sensitivities for deep vein thrombosis. Thus, D-dimer results are not interchangeable between kits. This has led to significant confusion regarding the use of D-dimer assays, and this confusion is exacerbated by the fact that the use of an insensitive D-dimer assay to rule out venous thrombosis could result in omission of required diagnostic testing, placing patients at risk for pulmonary embolism and death.

The optimal setting for use of a D-dimer assay is in the assessment of patients with a low clinical pretest probability of deep vein thrombosis. The combination of a low pretest probability (determined using a validated scoring system) and a negative result on a validated D-dimer assay essentially rules out the diagnosis of acute deep vein thrombosis, obviating the need for additional testing. Some D-dimer kits have been studied in patients with low and moderate pretest probabilities of deep vein thrombosis and have been shown to reliably exclude deep vein thrombosis in both patient groups.[49,50] Evaluation of the levels of D-dimer may be of particular value in patients with suspected recurrent venous thrombosis, and it may assist in decision making about optimal duration of anticoagulation.[51]

DIAGNOSTIC STRATEGIES

Diagnostic algorithms for the noninvasive diagnosis of clinically suspected venous thrombosis are presented in Fig. 135–1. If ultrasonography is not immediately available, patients can receive a therapeutic dose of low molecular weight heparin and return for diagnostic testing on the subsequent day. Patients with a high pretest likelihood of deep vein thrombosis and negative findings on ultrasound examination require an additional diagnostic test; either venography or serial ultrasonography (with two repeat tests, the first on day 3 to 5 and the second on day 7 to 14) must be performed.

PULMONARY EMBOLISM

Clinical Manifestations

In most instances, pulmonary embolism is clinically silent. Dyspnea is the most frequently reported symptom.[52,53] Chest pain is common and typically pleuritic in nature but may be substernal and compressing. Hemoptysis is a less frequent feature of pulmonary embolism.[24,52,53]

The physical signs of pulmonary embolism are nonspecific. Syncope usually is associated with massive pulmonary embolism and is caused by a reduction in cardiac output. This in turn results in hypotension and transient impairment of cerebral blood flow.

Although 70% of patients with pulmonary embolism have venographic evidence of thrombosis at presentation, less than 20% of these patients have leg symptoms.[24] Massive pulmonary embolism causes tachypnea, tachycardia, cyanosis, and hypotension. In these patients, cardiac examination may reveal a right ventricular heave, a loud pulmonary second sound, and a gallop rhythm. Physical examination of the chest may be normal, or nonspecific abnormalities may be detected. Patients with pulmonary infarction or atelectasis may have reduced movement of the affected portion of the chest. There may be signs of pulmonary consolidation or atelectasis, a pleural friction rub, crackles, or a pleural effusion, and a low-grade fever may be present.

Differential Diagnosis

The differential diagnosis of dyspnea and pleuritic chest pain, in addition to pulmonary embolism, includes pneumonia, pleurisy, chest wall pain from trauma, pericarditis, atelectasis, pneumothorax, acute bronchitis, acute bronchiolitis and acute bronchial obstruction as a result of mucous plugging or bronchoconstriction.

Diagnosis

The clinical diagnosis of pulmonary embolism is as unreliable as the diagnosis of venous thrombosis. Consequently, objective tests are necessary. The chest radiograph is not specific for pulmonary embolism and usually does not show any diagnostic abnormality. Nevertheless, it is useful in excluding other causes for the presenting symptoms (eg, pneumothorax) and is essential for interpreting the lung scan findings. Like the chest radiograph, the electrocardiogram frequently is normal or shows nonspecific abnormalities. However, in the appropriate clinical setting, electrocardiograph evidence of right ventricular strain is strongly suggestive of pulmonary embolism. Similarly, elevated levels of cardiac troponin frequently are seen in patients with massive pulmonary embolism as a result of right ventricular strain and associated myocardial ischemia.[54]

Diagnostic Tests for Pulmonary Embolism

Pulmonary Angiography

Pulmonary angiography is the reference standard for establishing the presence or absence of pulmonary embolism. Selective angiography and magnification views improve resolution and reduce the risk of the procedure. When pulmonary angiography is adequately performed, a negative result excludes the diagnosis of pulmonary embolism. Unless the tertiary pulmonary arteries are visualized in a patient with a small perfusion defect, however, the diagnosis of pulmonary embolism cannot be excluded.[55]

Arrhythmias, cardiac perforation, cardiac arrest, and hypersensitivity reactions to contrast material occur in 3% to 4% of patients undergoing pulmonary angiography.[56] Patients with a history of allergy to radiopaque dye should not undergo pulmonary angiography.

Ventilation-Perfusion Lung Scan

The lung scan consists of a perfusion and a ventilation component. For the perfusion component, particles of isotopically labeled microaggregates of human albumin are injected intravenously and become trapped in the pulmonary capillary bed. Their distribution reflects lung blood flow and is recorded with an external photoscanner. A normal perfusion scan excludes pulmonary embolism, but an abnormal perfusion scan is nonspecific.[24,53,57]

Ventilation lung scanning is performed using either radioactive gases or aerosols that are inhaled and exhaled by the patient while a gamma camera records the distribution of radioactivity within the alveolar gas exchange units. The purpose of ventilation imaging is to improve the specificity of perfusion scanning for the diagnosis of pulmonary embolism. A high-probability ventilation-perfusion scan (in which a segmental or greater area is ventilated but not perfused) has a positive predictive value for pulmonary embolism of more than 90%, obviating the need for angiography.

Helical Computed Tomography Scanning

Helical or spiral computed tomography (CT) scanning of the chest has emerged as a preferred test for the diagnosis of pulmonary embolism. This test is relatively insensitive, particularly for detection of emboli that lodge in the peripheral pulmonary vasculature. However, when performed in experienced clinical centers with use of validated scanning protocols, helical CT scanning is a useful tool to rule out pulmonary embolism in patients with compatible clinical symptoms.

For example, in one study where patients with suspected pulmonary embolism were evaluated with single-detector helical CT scanning and those with negative or inconclusive findings on CT scanning underwent ultrasonographic evaluation of their legs on the day of presentation and on days 4 and 7 after scanning, 124 of 510 enrolled patients had pulmonary embolism.[58] In 130 patients, an alternate diagnosis for their chest symptoms was found with the CT scan, 10 patients either could not have a CT performed or had a uninterpretable scan, and 248 patients had normal scans. Two of these 248 patients had proximal deep vein thrombosis on their initial ultrasound study, and all other patients had normal findings on serial ultrasound examinations. This and other similar studies suggest that if used correctly, helical CT scanning is a useful test in patients with suspected pulmonary embolism. In fact, systematic reviews suggest that a correctly done spiral CT effectively rules out pulmonary embolism in patients suspected to be at low or moderate risk of this complication.[59]

Diagnostic Strategy

Patients with large perfusion defects (involving one or more segments, or more extensive defects) and a ventilation-perfusion mismatch have a 90% probability of pulmonary embolism. Similarly, patients with a normal perfusion scan have less than a 2% probability of having pulmonary embolism, excluding the diagnosis. However, most patients who have ventilation-perfusion scanning performed will have neither of these findings; rather, they will have either matched defects or small perfusion defects.[24,53,57] Patients with these findings require further investigation with either pulmonary angiography or objective tests for venous thrombosis. A patient with suspected pulmonary embolism, an indeterminate ventilation-perfusion scan, and positive findings on leg ultrasound examination can be assumed to have pulmonary embolism. A patient with suspected pulmonary embolism, an indeterminate ventilation-perfusion scan, and a negative result on leg ultrasound examination requires additional testing, because the thrombus may have completely embolized to the lungs.[24,53]

A diagnostic algorithm for the management of clinically suspected pulmonary embolism is shown in Fig. 135–2. After a history and physical examination, electrocardiograph , and chest radiography, all patients with suspected pulmonary embolism should undergo helical CT scanning or ventilation-perfusion lung scanning. A negative result on perfusion lung scan, or a negative helical CT, rules out clinically significant pulmonary embolism, and anticoagulant therapy can be withheld. If the perfusion scan demonstrates one or more segmental (or larger) defects and ventilation to these regions is normal, or if an intraluminal filling defect is seen on helical CT, a diagnosis of pulmonary embolism is made. Although a ventilation-perfusion mismatch supports a diagnosis of pulmonary embolism, a ventilation-perfusion "match" does not exclude pulmonary embolism, and further objective testing is required in these patients. Similarly, the diagnosis of pulmonary embolism cannot be excluded in patients with small perfusion defects (one or more subsegmental defects) or those with indeterminate lung scan findings (in which the perfusion defects correspond with abnormalities on the chest radiograph). In these patients, venous ultrasonography should be performed. If deep vein thrombosis is documented, a diagnosis of pulmonary embolism can be assumed, and anticoagulant therapy should be started, thereby obviating the need for pulmonary investigations.

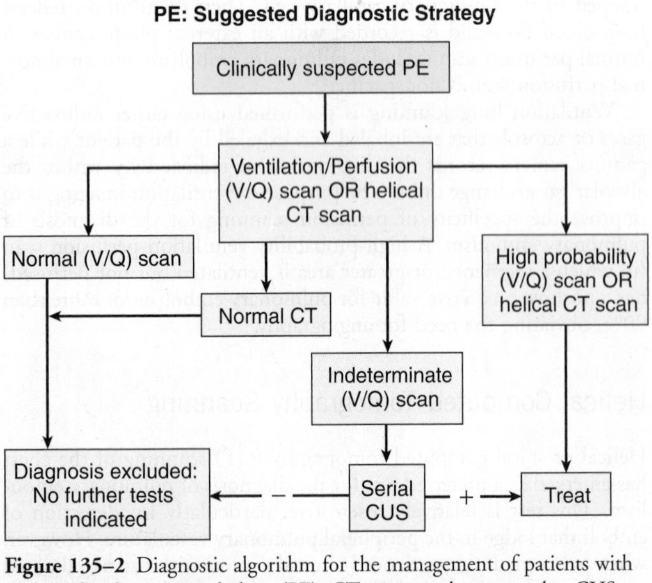

However, if results on these tests are negative, additional objective investigations (including, perhaps, pulmonary angiography) are required in patients with a high clinical suspicion. For those with a lower pretest probability of pulmonary embolism, an alternative strategy is to withhold anticoagulants and to perform serial noninvasive tests to detect ongoing venous thrombosis. In patients with a low or low-to-moderate pretest probability of pulmonary embolism, a D-dimer test may prove useful. If the D-dimer assay result is negative, further testing could be avoided, whereas if it is positive (increasing the likelihood of acute thrombosis), further testing is warranted.[60,61]

PE: Suggested Diagnostic Strategy

Figure 135–2 Diagnostic algorithm for the management of patients with suspected pulmonary embolism (PE). CT, computed tomography; CUS, ultrasound compression.

MANAGEMENT OF PATIENTS WITH SUSPECTED RECURRENT VENOUS THROMBOEMBOLISM AND POSTPHLEBITIC SYNDROME

A majority of patients with a history of venous thrombosis who develop new onset leg pain do not have recurrent deep vein thrombosis when investigated with the appropriate diagnostic tests. Some of these patients have the postphlebitic syndrome; in others, the pain is unrelated to venous thrombosis.[62] Misdiagnosis of postphlebitic syndrome as acute deep vein thrombosis has immediate consequences for patients, because many such patients will be treated with life-long warfarin. In these patients, who in fact did not experience recurrent thrombosis, this treatment is unneeded, costly, and associated with significant risk.

DIAGNOSIS OF ACUTE RECURRENT VENOUS THROMBOSIS

The diagnosis of acute recurrent venous thrombosis is difficult to make, because the clinical manifestations of recurrence are nonspecific. In addition, all of the validated diagnostic tests for acute venous thrombosis have limitations in this setting, because the venous occlusion produced by the initial episode of venous thrombosis makes it difficult to identify new abnormalities.

The most appropriate diagnostic strategy for suspected recurrent venous thrombosis has yet to be determined. The patient's history may be helpful in determining the likelihood of recurrent thrombosis. Leg pain with ambulation and leg swelling that is relieved with overnight rest is typical of the postphlebitic syndrome. New, clinically significant and persistent leg swelling, particularly if the symptoms do not abate overnight, is consistent with recurrent thrombosis and should prompt diagnostic evaluation. It may also be useful to obtain a measurement of the international normalized ratio (INR) at the time of presentation, and to assess the INR measurements in recent weeks. Warfarin is a very effective antithrombotic; thus, the risk of recurrent thrombosis in therapeutically anticoagulated patients irrespective of their symptoms is very low. Nevertheless, recurrent thrombosis despite therapeutic anticoagulation occasionally is seen in patients with cancer or those with antiphospholipid antibodies.

Many patients with a history of venous thrombosis will have a heightened level of concern about the risk of recurrent thrombosis. This heightened concern will lead these patients to seek testing for recurrent thrombosis even with incompatible symptoms. Such patients require careful clinical and radiologic evaluation. If there is no evidence of acute recurrence, they may require counseling and significant education about their condition.

The best test for recurrent thrombosis is the demonstration of a new thrombus in a previously unaffected venous segment. Thus, lack of compressibility on ultrasonography or an intraluminal filling defect on venography is diagnostic of recurrent thrombus, if the lesion involves an area that was previously documented to be free of thrombus. Similarly, a normal venogram rules out recurrence, and normal findings on ultrasound examination rule out proximal thrombus. A normal result on ultrasound study does not rule out calf vein thrombosis, and requires that additional testing with serial ultrasonography be performed if this is suspected. Other findings, such as lack of compressibility of the veins or an intraluminal filling defect with flow seen on Doppler ultrasound studies, are not sufficiently reliable to either confirm or rule out acute thrombosis. In these cases, serial testing (to detect extension) may be useful.

D-dimer–based testing strategies are very attractive in patients with suspected recurrence, because they may obviate the need for additional diagnostic testing. Until such strategies are carefully studied, however, they should not be used in these patients.

Magnetic resonance imaging may be of use in some patients with suspected recurrence as it appears that selected magnetic resonance protocols may be able to reliable classify the age of the thrombus.

DIAGNOSIS OF THE POSTPHLEBITIC SYNDROME

The clinical spectrum of the postphlebitic syndrome varies from a course that may mimic acute venous thrombosis to one of persistent leg pain that is worse at the end of the day and is associated with dependent edema, stasis pigmentation, and, in its most severe form, skin ulceration.[63] Rarely, patients may complain of venous claudication on walking.[64] When symptoms are acute or subacute in onset, a diagnosis of postphlebitic syndrome should be considered only after recurrent venous thrombosis has been excluded by objective tests. There is no single definitive diagnostic test for the postphlebitic syndrome, but a history of objectively documented deep vein thrombosis, appropriate clinical findings, and evidence of venous reflux or outflow obstruction on venous ultrasonography constitute sufficient evidence to make this diagnosis.

Other causes of recurrent leg pain or swelling include recurrent muscle strain, internal derangement of the knee or hip, recurrent cellulitis, extrinsic compression of the vein, lumbosacral disk disease, sciatic pain, and factitious causes of leg pain and swelling.

PROPHYLAXIS OF VENOUS THROMBOEMBOLISM

Pulmonary embolism is a common preventable cause of death in hospitalized patients.[65] Hospitalized patients can be classified as at low, moderate, or high risk for developing venous thromboembolism. Effective prophylaxis is cost-effective and is available for most high-risk groups.[66]

Low-Dose Unfractionated Heparin

Low doses of unfractionated heparin prevent thrombosis by catalyzing the inhibition of thrombin, factor Xa, and the other serine proteases by antithrombin. Unfractionated heparin is usually given subcutaneously at a dose of 5000 units 2 hours before surgery and continued postoperatively at a dose of 5000 units every 8 to 12 hours. Low-dose unfractionated heparin prophylaxis does not require laboratory monitoring and is simple and convenient to administer. It is the method of choice for moderate risk general surgical and medical patients, and it reduces the risk of venous thromboembolism by 50% to 70%.[65,67–69] When used in these doses, unfractionated heparin is both highly effective and associated with only a small increase in the risk of bleeding. Although low-dose unfractionated heparin is effective in patients undergoing elective hip surgery and reduces the incidence of venous thrombosis by approximately 40%, it is less effective than other current prophylactic strategies and thus should not be used as the sole form of prophylaxis in such patients. Low-dose unfractionated heparin has not been shown to be effective in patients with hip fractures or those undergoing major knee surgery. In addition, use of subcutaneous heparin may be associated with heparin induced thrombocytopenia, particularly in the postoperative period.

Intermittent Pneumatic Compression

Intermittent pneumatic compression of the legs enhances blood flow in the deep veins and increases blood fibrinolytic activity.[65] Although there are few methodologically rigorous studies that support the effectiveness of intermittent pneumatic compression for venous thrombosis prophylaxis, this modality is virtually free of clinically important side effects and is particularly useful in patients who have a high risk of bleeding. It also is frequently used, albeit with little supporting evidence, during the operative procedure in patients undergoing extended-duration surgery and in patients after trauma. Intermittent compression is the prophylactic measure of choice in selected patients undergoing neurosurgical procedures;[70] however, most of these patients should eventually receive low molecular weight heparin as well.[71]

Graduated Compression Stockings

Graduated compression stockings also reduce venous stasis in the legs and are effective for preventing postoperative venous thrombosis in low- and moderate-risk general surgical patients[68] and in medical or surgical patients with neurologic disorders, including paralysis of the lower limbs.[70] In surgical patients, the combination of graduated compression stockings and low-dose unfractionated heparin is significantly more effective than low-dose unfractionated heparin alone.[72,73] Use of graduated compression stockings alone, however, constitutes inadequate prophylaxis in patients undergoing surgery associated with a very high risk of thromboembolism.[74] Graduated compression stockings are inexpensive and should be considered for use in all high-risk surgical patients, even if other forms of prophylaxis are used.

Oral Anticoagulants

When administered in doses that prolong the prothrombin time to an INR of 2.0, oral anticoagulants effectively prevent postoperative venous thromboembolism in patients in all risk categories.[65,69] Oral anticoagulants can be given preoperatively, at the time of surgery, or in the early postoperative period. When these agents are started at the time of surgery or in the early postoperative period, the anticoagulant effect is not achieved until the third or fourth postoperative day. Nevertheless, when used in this fashion, oral anticoagulants are effective in very high-risk patient groups, including patients with hip fractures.[75] Prophylaxis with oral anticoagulants is relatively inconvenient, however, because careful laboratory monitoring is necessary.

Low-Molecular-Weight Heparins and Fondaparinux

When used in prophylactic doses, once or twice daily, low-molecular-weight heparin is an effective and safe agent for prophylaxis in the following high-risk groups: patients undergoing elective hip surgery, those with hip fractures, patients undergoing major general surgery or major knee surgery, those with spinal injury, and those who have sustained a stroke. Low-molecular-weight heparin is more effective than standard low-dose unfractionated heparin in general surgical patients, patients undergoing elective hip surgery, and patients with stroke or spinal injury. In addition, low-molecular-weight heparin also has been shown to be more effective than warfarin in patients undergoing hip or major knee surgery, better than adjusted-dose unfractionated heparin in preventing proximal vein thrombosis after elective hip surgery, and superior to dextran or aspirin after hip surgery.[76] Recently, concern about the coadministration of epidural anesthesia or analgesia and low-molecular-weight heparins has led to recommendations against the coincident use of these modalities. Recent evidence suggests that once-daily low-molecular-weight heparin may be safer than twice-daily low-molecular-weight heparin, allowing coincident use.[77]

Low-molecular-weight heparins produce their anticoagulant effect by preferentially catalyzing the inactivation of factor Xa by antithrombin. This effect is produced by a *pentasaccharide based on* a conserved sequence in the heparin molecule. The pentasaccharide moiety, fondaparinux, has been synthesized chemically and has been studied for the prevention and treatment of venous thromboembolism. Fondaparinux has been shown to be superior to low-molecular-weight heparin for the prevention of venous thrombosis after high-risk orthopedic surgery and is the only agent to demonstrate clear efficacy in patients undergoing surgical repair of a fractured hip. Extended use of fondaparinux in this patient population significantly reduces the risk of clinical venous thromboembolism over an extended followup period.[78] Fondaparinux has also been shown in clinical trials to be as effective and safe as unfractionated intravenous heparin for the treatment of acute symptomatic pulmonary embolism,[79] as effective and safe as twice-daily low-molecular-weight heparin for the treatment of deep vein thrombosis[80] and as effective as therapeutic dose enoxaparin in patients with unstable coronary syndromes. In this latter study fondaparinux was also safer than enoxaparin.

Choice of Prophylaxis in Different Patient Groups

General Surgical and Medical Patients

Early ambulation should be encouraged, and use of graduated compression stockings should be considered for all general surgical and medical patients. Moderate-risk patients should be given prophylaxis with low-dose unfractionated heparin. If anticoagulants are contraindicated because of an unusually high risk of bleeding, intermittent pneumatic compression should be used. Patients at very high risk, such as those with recent venous thrombosis, should receive low-molecular-weight heparin, oral anticoagulants, or adjusted-dose unfractionated heparin.

Hip Surgery

Low-molecular-weight heparin, oral anticoagulants, fondaparinux, or adjusted-dose unfractionated heparin are all effective in preventing venous thrombosis in patients undergoing hip surgery. In direct comparisons, fixed-dose low-molecular-weight heparin was more effective than warfarin in preventing thrombosis and was better than adjusted-dose unfractionated heparin in preventing proximal vein thrombosis. Fondaparinux is more effective than low-molecular-weight heparin. Extended duration anticoagulation is now recommended by consensus conferences for such patients; as a result extended prophylaxis after hospital discharge should be considered in all such patients.

Major Knee Surgery

Low-molecular-weight heparin or fondaparinux is the prophylactic agent of choice in patients undergoing major knee surgery. Early mobilization should be encouraged. Extended duration anticoagulation is now recommended by consensus conferences for such patients; as a result extended prophylaxis after hospital discharge should be considered in all such patients.

Genitourinary Surgery, Neurosurgery, and Ocular Surgery

In patients undergoing genitourinary surgery, neurosurgery, or ocular surgery, intermittent pneumatic compression, with or without the use of static graduated compression stockings, is effective and does not increase the risk of bleeding. Selected patients undergoing neurosurgery should receive low-molecular-weight heparin. Some patients undergoing surgery for urogenital cancer are at very high risk of venous thrombosis; there is increasing enthusiasm for prolonging prophylaxis after hospital discharge in such patients particularly if they are discharged from the hospital early in their postoperative course.

Stroke and Spinal Injury

Low-molecular-weight heparin is more effective than low-dose standard unfractionated heparin in patients who have suffered stroke or spinal injury and is the prophylactic method of choice for prevention of venous thrombosis. Extended prophylaxis with warfarin (target INR 2.0 to 3.0) should be used in patients who remain at high risk for venous thrombosis because of paralysis. Whether such prophylaxis should be continued after hospital discharge is unknown; in most centers, prophylaxis is discontinued at the time of discharge.

Trauma

Most trauma patients should receive low-molecular-weight heparin prophylaxis. In patients deemed to be at very high risk of bleeding, intermittent compression can be used until the bleeding risk has declined. Routine interruption of the inferior vena cava with a filter device has never been studied and will be associated with an increased risk of subsequent venous thrombosis.

Extending Prophylaxis after Hospital Discharge

Venographic studies suggest that approximately 1 of 5 (20%) patients undergoing elective orthopedic surgery who receive standard antithrombotic prophylaxis will have asymptomatic deep vein thrombosis found by venography at the time of hospital discharge. However, in the 3 months after hospital discharge, symptomatic nonfatal venous thromboembolism occurs in only approximately 1 of 42 (2.4%) patients, and fatal pulmonary embolism occurs in approximately 1 of 1250 (0.08%) patients.[81] Thus, treatment with a short, 5- to 10-day course of anticoagulant therapy after hip or knee arthroplasty is associated with a low risk for the development of subsequent clinically important symptomatic venous thromboembolism. Nevertheless, some authorities advocate extended-duration anticoagulation after hospital discharge. This treatment is designed to further reduce this low risk by providing additional prophylaxis during the period when patients are returning to a normal level of mobility.

A variety of treatment strategies have been used for extended prophylaxis, including use of aspirin, low-molecular-weight heparin, warfarin, and fondaparinux. Each of these strategies has been shown to reduce the risk of both venographic and clinically apparent deep vein thrombosis, suggesting that extended duration anticoagulation should be considered in all patients undergoing very high-risk surgery. Extended duration prophylaxis may be particularly important in patients who are discharged soon after surgery, at which time they have markedly reduced mobility.

To further refine post-discharge prophylaxis, it would be helpful to identify high-risk patient groups. This approach would allow therapy to be administered to those most in need, rather than exposing all patients to the costs, bleeding risk, and inconvenience of 3 to 4 weeks of anticoagulant therapy. For example, it may be reasonable to limit extended duration anticoagulation to high-risk patients, such as those with limited postoperative mobility, patients with a noncemented hip prosthesis who are non–weight-bearing, those with previous venous thromboembolism or morbid obesity, and those with cancer. This approach has not been tested in prospective clinical trials.

TREATMENT OF VENOUS THROMBOEMBOLISM

The objectives of treatment for venous thromboembolism are to prevent death from pulmonary embolism, to reduce morbidity from the acute event, to minimize postphlebitic symptoms, and to prevent chronic thromboembolic pulmonary hypertension. All of these goals can be achieved with adequate anticoagulant therapy.

PREVENTING DEATH CAUSED BY PULMONARY EMBOLISM

Anticoagulants are effective in reducing mortality from pulmonary embolism.[82] However, some patients have relative or absolute contraindications to anticoagulant therapy. Such patients can be broadly divided into two groups. The first group consists of patients with a transient risk factor for bleeding, such as surgery for resection of a bowel tumor or active ulcer disease. Although not formally studied in randomized trials, insertion of a temporary vena cava filter, followed by its removal and subsequent therapeutic anticoagulation when the bleeding risk is diminished, should be considered for such patients. This strategy reduces the initial risk of bleeding while eliminating the long-term increase in the risk of deep vein thrombosis associated with permanent caval interruption.

The second group of patients consists of those with a persistent, major risk factor for bleeding; because the mortality rate for major bleeding occurring during therapeutic anticoagulation is approximately 20%, such patients should be considered for insertion of a permanent vena cava filter. This procedure is associated with a significant risk of immediate worsening of leg symptoms because of blockage of the inferior vena cava by thrombus and a long-term increase in the risk of recurrent deep vein thrombosis.

Thrombolytic therapy with streptokinase, urokinase, or tPA is more effective than unfractionated heparin alone in correcting the angiographic defects produced by pulmonary embolism[82] and may be better than unfractionated heparin in preventing death in patients with massive pulmonary embolism associated with shock.[83,84] Based on these findings, thrombolytic therapy is the treatment of choice for patients with massive pulmonary embolism, or in those with underlying cardiac or pulmonary disease, in whom even a small or moderate-sized embolus may be life-threatening.

Thromboendarterectomy is effective in selected cases of chronic thromboembolic pulmonary hypertension with proximal pulmonary arterial obstruction.[85] Urgent pulmonary embolectomy is usually reserved for patients with a saddle embolism lodged in the main pulmonary artery or for those with massive embolism whose blood pressure cannot be maintained despite thrombolytic therapy and vasopressor agents.[82] Although this procedure can be successfully performed by experienced surgical teams, in inexperienced hands it is associated with high complication and mortality rates. Patients with repeated episodes of pulmonary embolism and significant chronic pulmonary hypertension with right ventricular compromise should be carefully anticoagulated and monitored. If pulmonary pressures do not decrease, they should be evaluated for surgical fitness. If deemed necessary, surgery should be carried out in expert centers, within which the likelihood of success of the procedure is high.[85]

ANTICOAGULANT THERAPY TO REDUCE MORBIDITY FROM THE ACUTE EVENT

The first principle of treatment for acute venous thrombosis is to deliver effective doses of a parenteral anticoagulant as soon as the diagnosis is confirmed (or, if testing is delayed and the clinical likelihood of disease is moderate or high, before confirmation of the diagnosis). The second principle is that the initial anticoagulant should be a fast-acting parenteral drug, because currently available oral anticoagulants have a delayed onset of action. Third, patients should receive a full course of therapeutic-dose anticoagulants because use of subtherapeutic drug doses are associated with a high risk of recurrent thrombosis.

Traditionally, patients with acute venous thrombosis were admitted to the hospital and given intravenous unfractionated heparin, administered to achieve a therapeutic partial thromboplastin time (PTT). Warfarin was then started, and the heparin continued until the INR was more than 2.0. This treatment strategy remains a practice standard. However, recent work has confirmed that the vast majority of patients with acute venous thrombosis are safely and effectively managed as outpatients with therapeutic doses of low-molecular-weight heparin and warfarin.

Treatment should consist of weight-adjusted, once- or twice-daily subcutaneous low-molecular-weight heparin. Monitoring of the anticoagulant effect of the low-molecular-weight heparin is not required. If anticoagulant-related complications develop, or if the patient is at extremes of weight (less than 40 kg or greater than 100 kg), or has severe renal insufficiency, then the anticoagulant effect of the low-molecular-weight heparin can be assessed using an antifactor Xa assay. The target factor Xa assay target is 0.5 to 1.0 unit/mL measured 4 hours after a subcutaneous injection using a twice-daily dosing schedule. Low-molecular-weight heparin does not have a predictable effect on the PTT; thus, this test cannot be used for monitoring low-molecular-weight heparin. Warfarin should be initiated on the same day as the institution of unfractionated heparin. The low-molecular-weight heparin should be continued for at least 4 days and until the INR has been between 2.0 and 3.0 on two consecutive days.

Patients with comorbid conditions that preclude outpatient treatment, those with significantly symptomatic pulmonary embolism, or those in whom thromboembolism develops during hospitalization should receive either unfractionated heparin or low-molecular-weight heparin in the hospital.[86] Prospective randomized trials have compared the safety and effectiveness of unfractionated heparin given by either continuous intravenous infusion, intermittent intravenous injection, or subcutaneous injection. Although continuous intravenous unfractionated heparin infusion produces less bleeding than occurs with intermittent intravenous injections, unfractionated heparin delivery by intermittent subcutaneous injections appears to be as safe and efficacious as continuous intravenous unfractionated heparin infusion in the treatment of venous thrombosis.[82,87]

Unfractionated heparin has a half-life that varies considerably among different people.[88] After a single intravenous injection, there is an initial rapid disappearance owing to a saturable clearance mechanism, followed by a more gradual linear clearance,[89] with a mean heparin half-life of approximately 60 minutes. Whereas intravenous unfractionated heparin produces an immediate anticoagulant effect, peak heparin levels are not achieved until 3 hours after subcutaneous injection, but the levels will remain therapeutic for up to 12 hours, depending on the dose.

Unfractionated heparin therapy can be monitored using the activated clotting time and the PTT, or by heparin assays that measure the ability of heparin to accelerate the inactivation of factor Xa or thrombin. It is important to give adequate doses of unfractionated heparin at initial presentation because the risk of recurrent venous thromboembolism probably is increased if insufficient doses are given. Accordingly, the PTT should be maintained above a level equivalent to a heparin level of 0.3 unit/mL as determined by measuring the antifactor Xa activity. For most currently used PTT reagents, this is equivalent to a PTT ratio of 1.8 times the control value. Thus, the recommended therapeutic range is a PTT ratio of 1.8 to 2.5.[90] Higher unfractionated heparin doses may be associated with an increase in the risk of bleeding.[89]

In the past, heparin was administered for a period of 7 to 10 days, and oral anticoagulants were started after 3 to 5 days and overlapped with heparin for 4 to 5 days. The period of overlap is necessary because the antithrombotic effects of oral anticoagulants are delayed and because the initial increase in the INR is attributable to a decrease in the level of factor VII, which has a short half-life, and not to reductions in the levels of prothrombin and factor X, which have longer half-lives and therefore must be reduced to produce therapeutic anticoagulation.[91,92] Two studies have demonstrated that 9 to 10 days of unfractionated heparin therapy are no better than a 4- to 5-day course of unfractionated heparin with overlapping warfarin.[93] Because neither study included many patients with major pulmonary embolism or extensive iliofemoral vein thrombosis, it would be prudent to use heparin for at least 7 days in these patients.

Recent evidence suggests that unfractionated heparin can be used without laboratory monitoring, similar to low-molecular-weight heparin; in a study of more than 700 patients, unfractionated heparin was administered using a fixed, weight adjusted dose without PTT monitoring. The risk of bleeding and recurrent thrombosis was found to be similar to that seen in patients treated with twice daily dalteparin or enoxaparin.[94]

After an initial course of heparin therapy, patients with venous thromboembolism require continuing anticoagulant therapy for several months to prevent recurrence.[27,28] Both therapeutic doses of subcutaneous heparin or low-molecular-weight heparin and oral anticoagulants are effective for this indication. Some patients will require long-term anticoagulation: patients with multiple previous episodes of venous thrombosis; those with a persistent, major risk factor for venous thrombosis; and those in whom the consequences of recurrence would be dire. Other patients, particularly those with an episode of venous thrombosis that occurred in the absence of a clear cause should receive a minimum of 6 months of therapeutic anticoagulation.

Fondaparinux is as effective as low-molecular-weight heparin in patients with acute deep vein thrombosis or pulmonary embolism.

PREVENTING MORBIDITY FROM THE POSTPHLEBITIC SYNDROME

The postphlebitic syndrome is a major cause of morbidity. The risk of postphlebitic syndrome in patients with symptomatic deep vein thrombosis may be as high as 29% after 8 years if the definition of this syndrome includes symptoms such as occasional leg pain or swelling.[33] The ability of thrombolytic therapy to prevent the postphlebitic syndrome has been evaluated to a limited extent. Streptokinase treatment produces complete lysis of acute venous thrombi in 30% to 40% of cases and causes partial lysis in an additional 30%.[82] By contrast, complete lysis of venous thrombi occurs in less than 10% of patients given unfractionated heparin. It is estimated that thrombolysis occurs 3.7 times more often in patients who receive streptokinase than in those given unfractionated heparin, but major bleeding occurs 2.9 times more frequently with streptokinase. Although five randomized studies have reported that the frequency of the postphlebitic syndrome is significantly higher in patients who receive unfractionated heparin than in those given streptokinase,[82] one trial[95] reported that patients given streptokinase and those given unfractionated heparin had similar manifestations of the postphlebitic state after 5 years of followup. Two studies reported that the incidence of the postphlebitic syndrome was reduced by the early use of graduated compression stockings, a finding disputed by another study.[82] In view of their low cost and lack of toxicity, most experts recommend that patients with persistent leg swelling after deep vein thrombosis wear compression stockings.

Catheter-directed lysis of deep vein thrombosis is widely practiced in the United States. Using a variety of techniques, with the usual lytic agent being tPA, rapid and near complete resolution of thrombus can be demonstrated in many patients. Unfortunately, neither the immediate or long-term benefit of such expensive and potentially toxic therapy has been demonstrated in controlled clinical trials. In particular, there is no good quality evidence of improved venous valvular function after catheter-directed lysis.

PREVENTION OF LATE EFFECTS OF PULMONARY EMBOLISM

Clinically significant pulmonary hypertension is an uncommon complication of pulmonary embolism. In randomized trials comparing unfractionated heparin with either streptokinase or urokinase for the treatment of acute pulmonary embolism, thrombolytic therapy produced greater improvement in lung scan-detected perfusion defects than that obtained with unfractionated heparin during the first week. However, there were no apparent differences in the lung scan findings at 2 weeks, 3 months, and 1 year.[96] Subsequent long-term followup in small subgroups of patients indicated that pulmonary capillary blood volume and both pulmonary vascular resistance and functional status were significantly better in patients who received fibrinolytic therapy than in those given unfractionated heparin.[82] As a result, thrombolysis is reserved in most centers for patients with massive pulmonary embolism causing cardiovascular collapse.

Moser and colleagues[85] have reported their experience with surgical pulmonary endarterectomy in carefully selected patients with chronic thromboembolic pulmonary hypertension. Most patients with obstruction of the proximal pulmonary arteries show impressive improvement after endarterectomy. These investigators stress the importance of careful patient selection and expert perioperative management.

SIDE EFFECTS, COST, AND CLINICAL USEFULNESS OF THROMBOLYTIC THERAPY

Bleeding occurs more frequently with thrombolytic therapy than with unfractionated heparin.[82,97] The risk of hemorrhage increases with the duration of thrombolytic infusion and usually occurs at a site of previous surgery or trauma. Intracranial hemorrhage occurs in approximately 1% of patients at risk, approximately twice as frequently as with unfractionated heparin treatment.

PRACTICAL RECOMMENDATIONS

A majority of patients with proximal deep vein thrombosis, calf vein thrombosis, and minimally symptomatic pulmonary embolism should receive outpatient low-molecular-weight heparin. Selected patients may be admitted for intravenous unfractionated heparin although there is no evidence that this therapy is superior to low-molecular-weight heparin in any clinical setting.

Warfarin should be started at the same time as for initiation of the heparin, considering patient age and gender in selecting a warfarin dose. An initial dose of 5 to 10` mg can be given to most individuals, and initial doses less than 5` mg should be used for elderly patients. Women generally require lower warfarin doses than men. The duration of warfarin therapy is variable. Patients with a persistent, major risk factor for recurrence, such as malignancy, should receive warfarin for as long as the risk factor persists. Those with a secondary thrombosis (such as after orthopedic surgery) who have returned to normal mobility may need warfarin for as little as 6 weeks, although a 3-month treatment period probably is preferable. Patients with idiopathic deep vein thrombosis (ie, those without a clear precipitant) should receive a minimum of 6 months, although consideration may be given for longer duration of therapy. The optimal duration of warfarin therapy for these patients is unknown and some of these patients receive indefinite anticoagulant therapy. Two potential tests that may prove of value are compression ultrasonography when anticoagulant discontinuation is being considered, and D-dimer assays. A persistent intraluminal filling defect seen on ultrasonography and/or a persistently positive D-dimer may predict recurrent thrombosis and mandate extended duration anticoagulant therapy.

A large randomized trial has suggested that patients with venous thrombosis in the setting of ongoing or recently treated cancer have a lower risk of recurrent thrombosis when given extended-duration low-molecular-weight heparin than when given warfarin.[98] This treatment should probably be considered in all patients with acute venous thrombosis occurring in the setting of cancer.

The dose of unfractionated heparin should be adjusted to maintain the PTT at 1.8 to 2.5 times control. To monitor unfractionated heparin given by continuous intravenous infusion, the PTT should be measured 6 hours after the bolus dose so that it reflects the anticoagulant effects of the infusion. If twice-daily subcutaneous unfractionated heparin is given, a mid-interval PTT should be measured 6 hours after the injection.

The INR is used to monitor oral anticoagulant therapy, and the dose of warfarin should be adjusted to achieve an INR of 2.0 to 3.0. Heparin can be discontinued when the INR has been therapeutic for 2 successive days.

VENOUS THROMBOSIS IN UNUSUAL SITES

Subclavian or Axillary Vein Thrombosis

Although thrombosis of the subclavian or axillary veins most frequently occurs as a complication of a chronic indwelling catheter, it also may occur as a consequence of local malignancy and is a well-documented complication of mastectomy and radiation therapy.[99] Subclavian vein thrombosis is particularly common in children with indwelling central venous catheters; this complication develops in up to 20% of children who have catheters placed for cancer chemotherapy or parenteral nutrition. In adults, the cause of subclavian or axillary vein thrombosis is frequently uncertain, and idiopathic subclavian or axillary vein thrombosis often occurs in young patients preceded by repetitive, strenuous activity that involves the affected arm. Occasionally, subclavian or axillary vein thrombosis can occur in patients with activated protein C resistance or congenital deficiency of antithrombin, protein C, or protein S, or in patients with antiphospholipid antibodies. Finally, thrombosis of the axillary or subclavian vein or the superior vena cava is a rare complication of perivenous endocardial pacing using an implantable system.[100,101] Upper extremity deep vein thrombosis is associated with pulmonary embolism, a complication seen frequently in children with catheter-related thrombosis. In adults, however, such emboli are predominately small and minimally symptomatic.

Patients with subclavian or axillary thrombosis usually experience pain in the axilla and edema and cyanosis of the arm. If thrombosis extends into the superior vena cava, edema and cyanosis of the face, neck, and upper extremities may develop. Dilated superficial veins on the chest and arms may appear after a number of days. Occasionally, asymptomatic thrombosis of the internal jugular vein accompanies subclavian vein thrombosis. The definitive diagnosis is made with venography, although venous ultrasonography is frequently used as the first-line diagnostic test. Patients with a negative ultrasound and a high clinical suspicion for upper extremity thrombosis should undergo venography.

Subclavian or axillary vein thrombosis usually is treated with anticoagulants. Thrombolytic therapy also is effective and should be considered, because it is estimated that greater than two-thirds of the patients with subclavian vein thrombosis will have persistent symptoms in the affected arm. Subclavian vein stenosis that persists after thrombolytic therapy may predispose to recurrence and may limit the benefits of thrombolysis.[102] In some settings, stenting of subclavian vein stenosis after venous thrombosis may reduce symptoms, particularly in patients requiring dialysis in whom outflow obstruction from the arm may cause major morbidity.

Mesenteric Vein Thrombosis

Mesenteric vein thrombosis is uncommon. This disorder occurs most commonly in the sixth and seventh decades of life and affects segments of the small bowel, leading to hemorrhagic infarction rather than gangrene. Bowel infarction often produces bloody ascites, and adhesions frequently develop between the involved bowel and the omentum. Many of the affected patients have associated disorders, such as thrombosis at other sites, inflammatory bowel disease, recent abdominal surgery, malignant disease, and portal hypertension. Mesenteric vein thrombosis also may complicate hypercoagulable states (such as antithrombin, protein C, or protein S deficiencies), polycythemia vera, or the use of oral contraceptives, and it also has been reported in late pregnancy. In approximately 20% of cases, no underlying cause is found. The clinical manifestations of mesenteric vein thrombosis include intermittent abdominal pain, abdominal distention in the later stages of the disorder, vomiting, diarrhea, and melena. Although the diagnosis often is difficult to make, blood-stained ascitic fluid on abdominal paracentesis and hemorrhagic bowel infarcts at peritoneoscopy are characteristic findings. Management includes supportive care and surgical resection followed by anticoagulant therapy. The mortality rate is approximately 20%, and recurrence is seen in up to 20% of cases.

Renal Vein Thrombosis

Renal vein thrombosis can occur as a complication of the nephrotic syndrome, possibly because antithrombin is lost in the urine, and is commonly seen in association with membranous glomerulonephritis. Patients may be asymptomatic, may present with mild symptoms of abdominal or back pain, or may have severe flank pain and tenderness. Pulmonary embolism has been described as a relatively common complication of renal vein thrombosis. With anticoagulant therapy there is a gradual improvement in renal function tests, although patients may suffer from long-standing proteinuria. Thrombolytic therapy has been used successfully in a small number of patients with renal vein thrombosis.

Cerebral Vein Thrombosis

Spontaneous venous thrombosis of the cerebral veins is an uncommon manifestation of thrombophilia. Patients may present with signs and symptoms of raised intracerebral pressure: headache, nausea, vomiting. Many patients with spontaneous cerebral vein thrombosis will be found to have a hypercoagulable state (see Chapter 134).[103] A relationship among cerebral vein thrombosis, oral contraceptive use, and the prothrombin gene 20210A mutation has been described.[183] Patients with cerebral vein thrombosis should be given therapeutic doses of heparin followed by warfarin and monitored for development of symptomatic intracerebral hemorrhage.[104]

SUGGESTED READINGS

Kearon C, Ginsberg JS, Anderson DR, et al: SOFAST Investigators: Comparison of 1 month with 3 months of anticoagulation for a first episode of venous thromboembolism associated with a transient risk factor. J Thromb Haemost 2:743, 2004.

Prandoni P, Lensing AW, Prins MH, et al: Below-knee elastic compression stockings to prevent the post-thrombotic syndrome: A randomized, controlled trial. Ann Intern Med 141:249, 2004.

Ridker PM, Goldhaber SZ, Danielson E, et al: Long-term, low-intensity warfarin therapy for the prevention of recurrent venous thromboembolism. N Engl J Med 348:1425, 2003.

Van Strijen MJ, De Monye W, Schiereck J, et al: Single-detector helical computed tomography as the primary diagnostic test in suspected pulmonary embolism: A multicenter clinical management study of 510 patients. Ann Intern Med 138:307, 2003.

REFERENCES

For complete list of references log onto www.expertconsult.com

CHAPTER 136

ARTERIAL THROMBOEMBOLISM

Elizabeth F. Krakow, Jeffrey S. Ginsberg, and Mark A. Crowther

INTRODUCTION

Arterial thrombosis usually occurs as a complication of atherosclerosis. Atherosclerosis is the most common underlying cause of coronary heart disease, cerebrovascular disease, and peripheral arterial disease and as such is the single most common cause of mortality and morbidity in Western populations. Arterial narrowing caused by atherosclerosis limits blood flow and causes ischemic symptoms when the oxygen requirements are increased by exercise. For example, angina pectoris occurs when the coronary arteries cannot supply sufficient blood flow to meet the demands of the myocardium. Similarly, intermittent claudication reflects ischemia of the leg muscles as a result of an imbalance between arterial blood supply and the demands of the exercising muscles, whereas intestinal angina typically occurs after a large meal when the blood supply to the gut is insufficient to meet the requirements.

Tissue infarction occurs when the arterial supply is completely occluded for a critical period of time. Arterial occlusion usually is the result of the rupture or fissuring of an atherosclerotic plaque, which exposes thrombogenic material and triggers the formation of a platelet-fibrin thrombus.

PATHOGENESIS OF ATHEROSCLEROSIS

The term *atherosclerosis* was introduced by Marchand, who recognized the association of fatty degeneration and vessel stiffening.[1] Atherosclerosis affects medium and large-sized arteries and is characterized by patchy intramural thickening of the subintima that encroaches on the arterial lumen and eventually leads to vascular obstruction. The earliest lesion of atherosclerosis is the fatty streak, which is caused by an accumulation of lipid-laden foam cells in the intimal layer of the artery. With time, the fatty streak evolves into a fibrous plaque, the hallmark of established atherosclerosis.

Atherosclerotic lesions are composed of three major components. The first is a cellular component with increased numbers of intimal smooth muscle cells and an accumulation of macrophages. The second component is the connective tissue matrix, large amounts of which are produced by the proliferating smooth muscle cells, and extracellular lipid. The third component is lipid that accumulates within the smooth muscle cells and the macrophages, thereby converting them into foam cells. Thus, the development of atherosclerotic lesions involves proliferation of smooth muscle cells, synthesis of connective tissue matrix, and accumulation of macrophages and lipid.

Over the years, two main hypotheses have been proposed to explain the pathogenesis of the atherosclerotic process: the lipid hypothesis[2,3] and the chronic endothelial injury hypothesis.[4] Experimentally, atherosclerosis can be produced by cholesterol feeding or by chronic endothelial injury.

The Lipid Hypothesis

The lipid hypothesis postulates that with increased levels of low-density lipoproteins (LDLs), lipid accumulates in smooth muscle cells and macrophages as the LDL penetrates the arterial wall. LDL is oxidized in the presence of endothelial cells. In its oxidized form, LDL becomes more atherogenic. Thus, oxidized LDL causes endothelial damage[5] and is chemotactic for monocyte-macrophages. Monocytes first adhere to the altered endothelium by interacting with surface adhesion molecules (eg, vascular cell adhesion molecule 1 [VCAM-1]), and then migrate through the endothelium and basement membrane by elaborating hydrolases that degrade connective tissue matrix (matrix metalloproteinases). As these cells accumulate, they take up lipid and are converted to foam cells. Macrophages bind intra-intimal LDL through a family of novel receptors, known as scavenger receptors, which recognize LDL only after it has been oxidized. Oxidation affects both lipid and apoprotein moieties of the LDL molecule; the lecithin component of LDL phospholipid undergoes conversion to lysolecithin, which is chemotactic for monocytes.[6] In addition, uptake of oxidized LDL renders the macrophages less mobile, thereby promoting the accumulation of these lipid-laden cells in the intima (Fig. 136–1).

An experimental model of atherosclerosis has been developed in monkeys fed a diet rich in cholesterol.[2] Within 2 weeks of induction of hypercholesterolemia, monocytes become attached to the surface of the arterial endothelium, migrate into the subendothelium, and accumulate lipid, which gives them the appearance of foam cells. Proliferating smooth muscle cells then emerge, and they also accumulate lipid. As the fibrous plaque enlarges, the endothelial cells retract, exposing the subendothelium to the blood and triggering the formation of platelet-fibrin thrombi. The release of platelet-derived growth factor leads to further smooth muscle proliferation, as described in the response-to-injury hypothesis. Support for the important role of oxidized LDL in atherogenesis comes from several sources. Administration of antioxidants to hyperlipidemic rabbits inhibits the formation of fatty streaks. Oxidized LDL can be extracted from human lesions, and many humans have circulating antibodies that are specific for epitopes of oxidized LDL.[6]

The Chronic Endothelial Injury Hypothesis

The response-to-injury hypothesis was proposed by Russell Ross.[4,7] It postulates that endothelial injury results in loss of endothelium, adhesion of platelets to subendothelium, aggregation of platelets, release of platelet-derived growth factors and elaboration of chemotactic factors that attract leukocytes, which in turn release other growth factors. The growth factors induce replication and migration of smooth muscle cells into the intima and result in the formation of a fibrous plaque. The smooth muscle cells synthesize and secrete connective tissue matrix containing collagen, proteoglycans, and elastic fibers, which contributes to the mass of the lesion. Plaque fissure or rupture may trigger the formation of a platelet-fibrin plug, which is then incorporated into the lesion. With repeated injury there is further intimal proliferation and progressive narrowing of the lumen.

The earliest stages of atherosclerosis are mediated by the inflammatory cascade. This cascade is initiated as the response to the injury caused by turbulent blood flow in the setting of an unfavorable serum lipid profile. Animals fed an atherogenic diet rapidly overexpress VCAM-1. VCAM-1 expression on endothelial surfaces is an early and necessary step in the pathogenesis of atherosclerosis.[8] VCAM-1

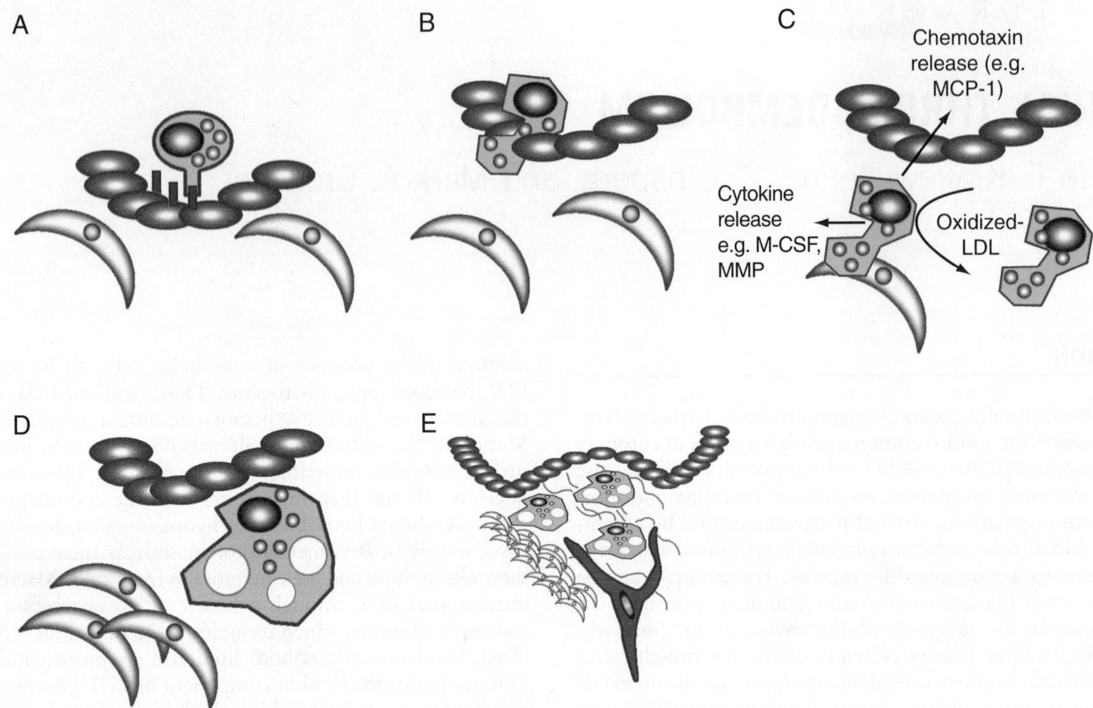

Figure 136–1. Atherosclerosis is initiated when adhesive proteins are expressed by the endothelium, causing leukocytes to adhere to the endothelium (Panel A). Leukocytes then cross the endothelial barrier (B). Monocytes within the subendothelial space "orchestrate" the development of atherosclerosis through cytokine release (C). The first clinically apparent lesion is the accumulation of foam cells (D). The clinically important lesion is characterized by intimal narrowing, many foam cells, neovascularization and flow-limiting stenosis (E). LDL, low density lipoprotein. MCP-1, monocyte chemoattractant protein 1; M-CSF, monocyte-colony stimulating factor; MMP, matrix metalloproteinase. *(Adapted with permission from Crowther M, Pathogenesis of atherosclerosis. Hematology Am Soc Hematol Educ Program 436, 2005.)*

expression increases recruitment of monocytes and T-cells to sites of endothelial injury. Subsequently, monocyte chemoattractant protein 1 (MCP-1) and other chemokines (eg, leukotactin-1[9,10]) released by leukocytes and stimulated monocytes magnify the inflammatory cascade by recruiting additional leukocytes, activating leukocytes in the media, and causing proliferation and migration of smooth muscle cells. The smooth muscle cells in turn elaborate a monocyte chemotactic factor and synthesize connective tissue matrix. Locally-elaborated monocyte-colony stimulating factor causes monocyte proliferation, and local activation of monocytes leads to both cytokine-mediated progression of atherosclerosis and oxidation of LDL. Oxidized LDL is cytotoxic to cultured endothelial cells.

The molecular mechanisms by which oxidized LDL may cause or perpetuate endothelial injury, attract monocytes, stimulate smooth muscle growth and promote arterial thrombosis are now being elucidated. Specifically, oxidation of LDL upregulates genes involved in the inflammatory cascade, such as a ligand in the tumor necrosis factor receptor superfamily 14 (LIGHT). LIGHT may in turn promote further lipid accumulation by upregulating a scavenger receptor and enhance macrophage expression of tissue factor and plasminogen activator inhibitor 1, creating a prothrombotic cell phenotype.[11] Through these molecular pathways, the lipid hypothesis and the endothelial injury hypothesis are closely linked.

Once initiated, many mediators of inflammation have been described to influence mitogenesis, intracellular matrix proliferation, angiogenesis, foam cell development and thrombosis. For example, CD40 ligand (CD40L) elaborated within the plaque increases the local expression of tissue factor, and thus, presumably, increases the likelihood of thrombosis. Anti-CD40L abrogates evolution of established atherosclerotic lesions in animal models.[12] Inflammatory mediators expressed by smooth muscle cells within the atherosclerotic plaque include, but are not limited to, interleukin (IL)-1β, tumor necrosis factor α and β, IL-6, monocyte-colony stimulating factor, MCP-1, IL-18, and CD40L.

Functional and Structural Consequences of Early Lesions

With the development of atherosclerosis, there is impaired regulation of vascular tone. This is caused in part by decreased production of endothelial-derived nitric oxide. The impaired release of nitric oxide is associated with increased vascular tone and may be associated with increased platelet activation and intimal proliferation.[13]

Atherosclerotic lesions can develop in the absence of endothelial denudation and without the involvement of platelet-derived growth factors.[2] Thus, smooth muscle hyperplasia occurs in hypertension without associated endothelial cell loss[14–17] and persists long after platelet interaction with the vessel wall has ceased.[18–20] Cells other than platelets produce growth factors,[7] including macrophages,[21] endothelial cells,[22] and arterial smooth muscle cells,[23] and these may contribute to the growth of the atherosclerotic plaque.[4] In this context, local synthesis of platelet-derived growth factor has been demonstrated in human atherosclerotic plaques.[24]

Growth of the Atherosclerotic Plaque

The atherosclerotic plaque grows slowly over a period of years and can produce severe stenosis or even total vascular occlusion. The mature plaque consists of a fibrous cap composed of collagen, a lipid core containing intracellular and extracellular lipid, and areas of calcification. Lipid-rich plaques are prone to spontaneous fissuring or rupture when exposed to high shear stress at sites of stenosis and arterial branching. Two forms of plaque injury are recognized: superficial and deep. Superficial injury produces areas of focal endothelial denudation that can enlarge and lead to the formation of mural or even occlusive thrombi. Plaques that are capped with superficial collagen fibers separated by large number of lipid-filled macrophages predispose to superficial injury.[25,26]

Deep intimal injury is characterized by a split or tear that extends from the luminal surface of a plaque deep down into the plaque substance. This type of injury, which tends to occur in plaques that contain a large lipid-rich pool, exposes blood to the highly thrombogenic contents of the plaque. In particular tissue factor is elaborated within the plaque, a process exacerbated by local expression of CD40L, and leads to intraluminal and extraluminal thrombosis. Intraluminal thrombi become incorporated into, and increase the size of, the atherosclerotic plaque, whereas extraluminal thrombi can be partly or completely occlusive.[27]

Angiogenesis within the Plaque

Angiogenic signaling and proliferation of microvessels within the plaque is incompletely understood. Plaque hemorrhage is likely attributable to bleeding from fragile microvessels that proliferate within the plaque itself, presumably in response to local angiogenic stimuli. Kockx and colleagues proposed that intraplaque microhemorrhage may initiate platelet and erythrocyte deposition, lead to iron deposition, activate macrophages, and contribute to foam cell formation.[28] Support for this hypothesis lies in the finding that intraplaque microvessels are an independent predictor of plaque rupture.[29] The potential importance of angiogenesis in the development of atherosclerosis is found in experiments demonstrating that thalidomide reduced atherosclerotic lesion development in a placebo-controlled trial in atherosclerosis-prone mice.[30] However, thalidomide and its analogs have pleiotropic effects, including anti-inflammatory and matrix stabilizing effects. For example, in early pilot studies in humans with chronic heart failure, it is unlikely that the prompt improvement in ejection fraction was caused by the anti-angiogenic properties of thalidomide.[31]

Anti-Atherogenic Pathways

Understanding of the pathogenesis of atherosclerosis on the molecular level will lead to new therapeutic targets. For example, peroxisome proliferator-activated receptors (PPARs)[32] have numerous potential anti-atherogenic activities. PPAR-α can inhibit adhesion molecules including VCAM-1, increase endothelial nitric oxide release, reduce foam cell formation, and reduce uptake of glycated LDL and triglyceride-rich remnant lipoproteins. PPAR-γ is expressed on endothelial cells, smooth muscle cells, macrophages, and T-cells in the atherosclerotic lesion. The functions attributed to this receptor include:[1] increased nitric oxide synthesis and release,[2] decreased recruitment of T cells,[3] reduced angiogenesis,[4] inhibition of smooth muscle cell migration,[5] decreased smooth muscle cell expression of matrix degrading enzymes,[6] decreased macrophage-dependent expression of matrix metalloproteinase 9 and osteopontin,[7] enhanced release of the IL-1 receptor antagonist, and[8] enhanced reverse cholesterol transport. The thiazolidinedione oral hypoglycemic medications (commonly called *glitazones*) are PPAR-γ agonists. They might also activate PPAR-α. Glitazones reduce serum C-reactive protein (CRP), matrix metalloproteinase 9, and tumor necrosis factor-a in humans.[33,34] PPAR agonists might prove effective in treating atherosclerosis in nondiabetic patients.[35]

PATHOGENESIS OF ARTERIAL THROMBOSIS

Arterial thrombi form under conditions of high blood flow and are composed mainly of platelet aggregates held together by fibrin strands. Thrombosis is initiated by rupture of the atherosclerotic plaque, which exposes thrombogenic material in the subendothelium to the blood.[27,36] If the thrombus is nonocclusive and blood flow remains rapid, the thrombi may organize and become incorporated into the atherosclerotic plaque.[36] With more marked arterial narrowing, shear rates increase and promote more extensive platelet and fibrin deposition, which can result in the formation of an occlusive thrombus.

Thrombogenic Factors

Thrombosis occurs when the balance between thrombogenic factors and protective mechanisms is perturbed. The protective mechanisms include the nonthrombogenic properties of intact endothelial cells, fluid-phase antiproteases, and the dissolution of fibrin by the fibrinolytic system. Thrombogenic stimuli include injury or loss of endothelial cells and activation of platelets and blood coagulation.

Nonthrombogenic Properties of Endothelial Cells

The fluidity of blood *in vivo* is enhanced by the thromboresistant properties of intact vascular endothelium and is threatened by damage to the vessel wall.[37] Endothelial cell-surface glycosaminoglycans and thrombomodulin are potent inhibitors of coagulation. Vessel wall generation of prostacyclin and nitric oxide limits platelet aggregation. Finally, plasminogen activators limit fibrin deposition.[38]

Damage to the Vessel Wall

Thrombogenesis is promoted by loss of endothelium, which may be caused by direct physical damage such as occurs with angioplasty, hemodynamic stress, use of tobacco products, high blood cholesterol levels, or enzymes released from platelets and leukocytes.[7] The shedding of endothelial cells exposes the subendothelium to platelets and blood coagulation proteins. Platelets that adhere to the subendothelium undergo a shape change, aggregate, and secrete their granular contents, thereby recruiting more platelets. At physiologic shear rates, platelet adhesion to subendothelial collagen is mediated by von Willebrand factor, glycoprotein VI, and glycoprotein Ib on the platelet surface[39] as well as to subendothelial components.

Although endothelial cell loss represents the most severe form of vascular damage, more subtle injury may also promote thrombogenesis. Thus, endothelial cells exposed to endotoxin, cytokines such as IL-1 and tumor necrosis factor, thrombin, hypoxia, or increased shear stress synthesize tissue factor and internalize thrombomodulin, thereby promoting coagulation. In addition, these perturbed cells also produce plasminogen activator inhibitor type 1, which impairs fibrinolysis, and acquire receptors to which leukocytes and platelets adhere.[38] Finally, the altered endothelial cells synthesize factors that regulate local blood flow. These include vasoconstrictors known as *endothelins*, as well as vasodilators such as prostacyclin and nitric oxide.[13,38]

Platelet Activation

Platelets adhering to collagen undergo a shape change, secrete their granular contents, and aggregate. In addition to collagen, a variety of other agonists, including thrombin, epinephrine, and thromboxane A_2 (TXA_2), also promote platelet aggregation.[40] Whereas all of these agents stimulate the synthesis of TXA_2, collagen, thrombin, and TXA_2 also induce the release of adenosine diphosphate from platelet granules, which amplifies the aggregation process. In addition to these pathways, thrombin-induced platelet aggregation occurs through a third mechanism that may involve the activation of platelet calpain.[41]

Activated platelets contribute to chronic lesional development. They secrete vascular endothelial growth factor, its relative vascular endothelial growth factor-C, and fibroblast growth factor, which might promote or sustain neoangiogenesis within the plaque.[42] They also elaborate tumor growth factor β and platelet-derived growth factors. These two mitogenic cytokines act at the site of the thrombus to promote the development of atherosclerotic lesions.

Virtually all agonists that induce platelet aggregation act through a common pathway that involves the increase in ionized calcium within the platelet cytoplasm either by mobilization of calcium from the dense tubular system or by increased transport across the membrane. This in turn results in the functional expression of the platelet glycoprotein GPIIb/IIIa, which serves as a receptor for fibrinogen and other Arg-Gly-Asp–containing adhesive proteins such as fibronectin, von Willebrand factor, and thrombospondin.[41] Binding of fibrinogen to GPIIb/IIIa is essential for platelet aggregation because fibrinogen bridges the platelets together.

An increase in platelet cyclic adenosine monophosphate levels reduces the calcium-mobilizing effect of all agonists. Prostacyclin produced by endothelial cells inhibits platelet aggregation by activating platelet adenylate cyclase, thereby elevating cyclic adenosine monophosphate levels.[43]

Activation of Coagulation

Damage to the vessel wall activates the blood coagulation pathway by exposing blood to tissue factor or collagen in the subendothelial matrix, thus activating platelets. Thrombin formed as a result of these processes then serves to convert fibrinogen to fibrin, which stabilizes the platelet aggregates.

EPIDEMIOLOGY AND PREVENTION OF ATHEROSCLEROSIS

The most effective means of preventing arterial thrombosis is to prevent atherosclerosis. The proven risk factors for atherosclerosis are abnormal lipids, hypertension, cigarette smoking, obesity, physical inactivity, diabetes, age, family history, and male gender. The first five of these risk factors are potentially reversible, and there is evidence that their reversal reduces the complications of atherosclerosis. At least 90% of the risk for myocardial infarction is attributable to modifiable risk factors.[44] In general, compliance with recommendations for lifestyle modification is poor.

Cholesterol and Lipids

The plasma level of cholesterol is determined by genetic factors, by the type and amount of fat in the diet, and by other factors such as obesity, physical activity, and disease states. Based on the results of animal studies, epidemiologic data, and interventional studies, there is good evidence for an association between hypercholesterolemia and atherosclerosis.

Of the three major classes of lipoproteins, very-low-density lipoproteins, LDL, and high-density lipoproteins (HDLs), LDL contain 60% to 70% of the total serum cholesterol and are the most atherogenic. In contrast, the levels of HDL are inversely correlated with the risk of coronary heart disease.

The association between serum cholesterol levels and the risk of coronary heart disease is continuously graded.[45,46] Familial hypercholesterolemia, a disorder caused by an absent or defective LDL receptor, causes premature coronary heart disease.[47,48] In the heterozygous form of this disorder, which occurs in 1 in 500 in the population, the total cholesterol concentration is usually in excess of 300 mg/dL. Approximately 5% of all patients who present with acute myocardial infarction younger than the age of 60 years have heterozygous familial hypercholesterolemia. The homozygous form of familial hypercholesterolemia occurs in approximately 1 in 1 million individuals and presents with cholesterol levels ranging from 600 to 1,000 mg/dL. Patients usually develop severe coronary heart disease younger than the age of 20 years.

Reduced levels of HDL cholesterol are associated with an increased risk of coronary heart disease. The main causes of reduced HDL cholesterol include cigarette smoking, obesity, physical inactivity, androgenic and related steroids (including anabolic steroids), beta-blocking agents, hypertriglyceridemia, and genetic factors. In contrast, weight reduction, exercise, and some medications elevate HDL cholesterol levels.

Both the cholesterol level and the prevalence of coronary heart disease are influenced by environmental factors, including diet. Thus, individuals who immigrate from countries where the prevalence of coronary heart disease and the serum cholesterol levels are low to a country with a high prevalence of coronary heart disease will often have increases in both serum cholesterol levels and rates of coronary heart disease.

The evidence that decreasing serum cholesterol levels with cholesterol-lowering drugs or dietary modification slows and even reverses the progression of coronary atherosclerosis[49–52] and reduces coronary events[53] comes from many randomized trials.[49,53–55] Lowering the serum cholesterol level with diet or drug therapy also slows the progression of angiographically documented coronary atherosclerosis in patients with arterial bypass grafts.[49] Modifying several risk factors, such as lowering the serum cholesterol level, the blood pressure, and the levels of LDL cholesterol and cessation of smoking, reduces the risk of ischemic heart disease.[56,57] Individuals with several risk factors benefit most from these measures (see box on Clinical Controversy).[58]

Despite the enthusiasm for a lower target LDL to prevent cardiovascular events (including coronary death), the effect of statins on overall mortality is debated. A large meta-analysis of standard-dose statin therapy found a 12% relative reduction in all-cause mortality that was driven by the reduction in coronary deaths; there was no significant reduction in other vascular causes of death or in noncardiovascular mortality.[68] Despite the apparent safety of most statins, intensive statin therapy has not lowered all-cause mortality.[60–63] In recent trials, overall mortality was essentially the same in standard and intensive therapy arms. Although these trials involved 27,548 patients, even in aggregate they may be underpowered to detect a difference in this endpoint.[59] Although one trial showed a trend toward more noncardiovascular deaths associated with intensive therapy,[60] in pooled analyses, it does not appear that intensive therapy increases the risk of noncardiovascular death over standard-dose therapy.[59]

Another specific modifiable risk factor for atherosclerosis has recently emerged. Trans fats are unsaturated fats with at least one double bond in the *trans* configuration. Industrially-produced trans fats are found in partially hydrogenated vegetable oils common in baked goods, margarines, and other manufactured food products. As

Clinical Controversy

How low should cholesterol levels for secondary prevention of cardiovascular events be reduced? Meta-analysis[59] has confirmed that aggressive lowering of the serum cholesterol level in patients with stable coronary artery disease[60,61] or recent acute coronary syndrome or myocardial infarction[62,63] results in a rapid decrease in the risk of subsequent ischemic cardiac complications, the need for surgical revascularization, stroke, and coronary death rates. This effect occurs even in patients with minimal risk factors, (such as hypertensive patients older than 65 years but without evidence of coronary heart disease), and whose LDL cholesterol level falls within the normal range (2.6–3.4 mmol/L, 100–130 mg/dL).[64] Clinical trials have demonstrated that each incremental reduction of LDL achieved with hydroxymethylglutaryl-coenzyme A reductase inhibitors (*statins*) leads to an incremental reduction of cardiovascular events, across LDL levels.[60–66] Target LDL values for secondary prevention have been revised accordingly: Although a target of less than 100 mg/dL (2.6 mmol/L) is mandated, treating to less than 70 mg/dL (1.8 mmo/L) is considered reasonable.[67]

compared with an equal number of calories from saturated or *cis*-unsaturated fatty acids, trans fats increase LDL, decrease HDL, increase lipoprotein(a) levels, and reduce LDL particle size. In prospective studies, the relation between trans fats and coronary events has been even greater than predicted from these deleterious effects on the lipid profile. In randomized controlled trials, trans fats were shown to promote inflammation and induce endothelial cell dysfunction. In meta-analyses, a 2% increase in trans fat consumption was associated with greater than 20% increase in incident coronary heart disease. In individual epidemiologic studies, they have been linked to sudden cardiac death. It has been estimated that 6% to 22% of cardiac events could be averted if intake of trans fats were broadly reduced.[69] Many countries are now regulating the elimination of trans fats from commercial products.

Tobacco

Cigarette smoking increases the risk of coronary heart disease, peripheral arterial disease, cerebrovascular disease, and graft occlusion after reconstructive arterial surgery. It is particularly hazardous in those with a poor cardiovascular risk profile and in women taking estrogens, and there is a dose relationship between the risk of coronary heart disease and the number of cigarettes smoked daily.[70] Within 1 year of abstinence, those who stop smoking have only half the risk of those who continue to smoke, regardless of how long they smoked. After 15 years of abstinence, their risk of dying from coronary heart disease is similar to that of persons who have never smoked.[71] Smoking cessation also reduces mortality after coronary artery bypass graft surgery, reduces morbidity and mortality in patients with peripheral vascular disease, and decreases mortality after myocardial infarction.[72]

Although the mechanism by which smoking increases the risk of atherosclerosis is uncertain, there are several possibilities. Cigarette smoking decreases the levels of HDL, increases LDL cholesterol, and, by raising levels of carbon monoxide, leads to hypoxia, thereby perturbing the anticoagulant properties of the endothelium. In addition, smoking increases platelet reactivity and, by elevating the plasma fibrinogen and the hematocrit, also increases blood viscosity.

Hypertension

Hypertension is a risk factor for stroke, myocardial infarction, and cardiac and renal failure.[73] Beginning at 115/75 mm Hg, cardiovascular disease risk doubles for each increment of 20/10 mm Hg.[74] Treatment of hypertension reduces the incidence of stroke and lowers overall mortality, but there is less convincing evidence that it affects coronary events.[75] Thus, pooled analysis of all studies examining the effects of lowering the blood pressure shows a 10% risk reduction for mortality and a 40% risk reduction for stroke. However, there is only an 8% risk reduction for fatal and nonfatal myocardial infarction, a difference that is not statistically significant.

Diabetes

Patients with diabetes have twice the risk of incident myocardial infarction and stroke as the general population.[76] Asymptomatic patients with diabetes may have the same atherosclerotic burden as nondiabetic persons with symptomatic coronary artery disease.[77] Persons with diabetes and no prior history of myocardial infarction have as high a risk of myocardial infarction and of fatal myocardial infarction as nondiabetic patients who previously suffered a myocardial infarction.[78] Therefore, national guidelines for cholesterol and hypertension management recommend the same treatment targets for diabetic patients without known cardiovascular disease as for patients with established cardiovascular disease.[74,79–81]

The mechanisms by which insulin resistance and hyperglycemia promote atherosclerosis and endothelial dysfunction are complex.[82] For example, hyperglycemia induces procoagulant proteins and inhibits fibrinolysis. Advanced glycation end products produce reactive oxygen species and increase oxidative stress by activating nicotinamide adenine dinucleotide phosphate oxidase through specific receptors. Reactive oxygen species stimulate expression of procoagulant and proinflammatory genes, leading to apoptosis of endothelial cells and decreased endothelial cell proliferation. Advanced glycation end products also modify extracellular matrix proteins, resulting in decreased vessel elasticity. Intermolecular cross-linking by advanced glycation end products impairs the function of endothelial proteins. Endothelial cells express specific receptors, which in turn promote inflammation through activation of NF-κB and through interactions with macrophages in the vessel wall. These macrophages become foam cells and contribute to progression of the atherosclerotic lesion.

Physical Inactivity

Individuals who exercise regularly have less cumulative disability[83] and a lower incidence of myocardial infarction and death,[84–92] but it is uncertain whether the association is causal or whether it merely reflects the fact that healthier individuals are more likely to exercise. In patients who have recovered from an acute myocardial infarction, exercise produces approximately 20% reduction in the risk of recurrent infarction or death.[93,94] Regular exercise may exert these protective effects by increasing the levels of HDL cholesterol and lowering the blood pressure.[95,96]

Obesity

Although some observational studies[97] have suggested that obesity is an independent risk factor for coronary heart disease, this has not been a universal finding. Obesity is linked to the development of insulin resistance, type 2 diabetes, hypertension, obstructive sleep apnea, and dyslipidemia.[98] Whether obesity confers a substantial risk of cardiovascular events independent of these risk factors is debated. Even among patients with established coronary artery disease, it has been difficult to show an independent effect of obesity on mortality.[99] However, weight loss ameliorates the risk factors cited and is currently considered an important therapeutic goal.

Emerging Risk Factors

Evidence is increasing that a variety of additional risk factors for atherosclerotic disease exist.

Inflammation

Given the importance of the inflammatory cascade in the pathogenesis of atherosclerosis, clinical interest has focused on the development of markers of risk attributable to inflammation. Predominant among these is C reactive protein (CRP). CRP is a pentraxin that is central to the human innate immune response.[100] CRP is predominantly produced by the liver as an acute phase reactant. Arterial smooth muscle cells can express CRP in response to inflammatory cytokines.[101] Whether CRP is causally related to atherogenesis is controversial. Even experimental work reached differing conclusions about whether a direct association between CRP and the pathogenesis of atherosclerosis exists. For example, Danenberg and colleagues evaluated the proinflammatory and prothrombotic effects of CRP on monocytes and endothelial cells in vivo by subjecting wild-type mice, which do not express CRP, and human CRP-transgenic mice to models of arterial injury. In one model, complete thrombotic occlusion of the femoral artery at 28 days was seen in 17% of wild-type mice compared with 75% of CRP-transgenic mice.[102] However, Hirschfield and colleagues found transgenic expression of CRP in mice prone to atherosclerosis had no effect on the development, progression, or severity of spontaneous atherosclerosis.[103]

Regardless of whether it has any pathogenic role in atherosclerosis, in humans CRP is a mild-to-moderate biomarker of atherosclerotic complications.[104–108] Many large, prospective, primary prevention studies have shown that highly-sensitive CRP measurement is an independent predictor of stroke,[109] peripheral arterial disease,[108] acute myocardial infarction, and cardiovascular death even after adjustment for traditional cardiac risk factors such as serum LDL or the composite Framingham risk score.[110–116] Studies in populations experiencing stable angina or acute coronary syndromes,[104,117–119] undergoing elective or acute percutaneous[120–122] or surgical[123] coronary revascularization, or who have established coronary artery disease[124] have reached similar conclusions.

Whether the success of statin therapy is attributable only to its LDL-lowering effects, or whether it is also attributable to antiinflammatory effects, is unknown.[125,126] Outcome trials designed to evaluate this question have found that lowering CRP is at least as important as lowering LDL and that patients with the lowest levels of LDL but elevated levels of CRP carry a substantial risk for atherosclerotic progression (as measured by intravascular ultrasound[127]) and for cardiac events[128] compared with patients with the lowest levels of both LDL and CRP (see box on Who Should Be Screened with CRP?). Other clinical evidence that systemic inflammation contributes to the progression of atherosclerosis comes from the increased rate of cardiac events in patients with connective tissue diseases, such as systemic lupus erythematosus[131] or rheumatoid arthritis.[132,133]

Lipoprotein(a)

Lipoprotein(a) [Lp(a)] is composed of a lipoprotein attached to apolipoprotein B-100. Its physiologic role is not known but it might mediate transport of oxidized LDL. Elevated levels of Lp(a) have also emerged as a potential risk factor for atherosclerosis.[134–137] However, the data are inconsistent,[138] and it is unclear that focusing on Lp(a) over and above LDL has any therapeutic benefit[139] even if the two molecules are under separate metabolic control. Genetically determined elevation of Lp(a) may play a larger role in young patients with premature atherosclerosis.[135,140] Interest in this biochemical abnormality is heightened by the observation that niacin therapy reduces Lp(a) levels. There are limited data showing that niacin reduces the risk of atherothrombotic complications in the setting of secondary prevention,[141] but niacin has not been adequately evaluated for primary prevention.

Homocysteine

Congenital or acquired hyperhomocysteinemia is associated with an increase in the risk of both arterial and venous thromboembolism.[142,143] Genetic studies of polymorphisms in the methylenetetrahydrofolate reductase gene corroborate results from observational studies linking hyperhomocysteinemia to stroke.[144] In most cases, homocysteine levels may be reduced with the administration of folic acid or vitamins B_6 or B_{12}.[145,146] Although one randomized, placebo-controlled trial suggested that aggressive lowering of homocysteine levels reduces the risk of stenosis after percutaneous coronary interventions,[147] other studies have not found this association[148] or even found increased rates of in-stent restenosis.[149] Three large randomized controlled trials focused on secondary prevention found no benefit to lowering homocysteine levels. High-dose folate therapy showed no ability to prevent ischemic stroke in the Vitamin Therapy for Prevention of Stroke trial,[150] and two studies actually demonstrated possible harm.[151,152] In the Norwegian Vitamin Trial, although B_6, folate, B_{12}, or all three effectively lowered homocysteine levels by 27%, the group taking B_6 alone or folate and B_{12} alone suffered roughly the same rate of stroke and myocardial infarction as the placebo group, although the group randomized to combination therapy had an absolute increase in stroke or myocardial infarction of approximately 5% over the placebo and other treatment arms when followed for 3 years.[151] The Heart Outcomes Prevention Evaluation II found a protective effect on stroke (possibly because of uncorrected statistical testing of multiple endpoints), no effect on myocardial infarction or cardiovascular death, and a slight increase in hospitalization for unstable angina.[152] The role of hyperhomocysteinemia in atherosclerosis is debated; it is not thought to be directly responsible for initiating or propagating whatever processes confer an increased risk of arterial thromboses to such patients.[153]

Who Should Be Screened with CRP?

At present, guidelines from the American Heart Association/Centers for Disease Control recommend against screening the entire adult population with CRP. The guidelines endorse measurement of CRP at the discretion of the physician, particularly in persons deemed an intermediate risk by the Framingham criteria, where the finding of an elevated CRP might prompt further intensification of therapy. However, low-risk individuals are unlikely to be reclassified as high-risk based solely on elevation of the CRP, although high-risk persons and patients with established atherosclerotic disease should be treated intensively regardless of the CRP value.[129,130] Serial monitoring of the CRP or treating to particular CRP targets has not been evaluated.

Impaired Endothelial Progenitor Cell Production or Function

Early endothelial cell dysfunction is manifested by impaired nitric oxide production and poor vascular responses to vasodilators. These changes predict progression of atherosclerosis and confer an increased risk of cardiac events.[154,155] Endothelial injury manifests as changes at the luminal surface of the cell and eventually apoptosis occurs. In this way, a functional and presumably reversible impairment progresses to permanent structural damage.[156] As in other organs, repair of these lesions and regeneration of a healthy endothelium might depend on stem cell proliferation and local engraftment.

Endothelial progenitor cells (EPCs) are derived from the bone marrow (Fig. 136–2) and circulate throughout adult life.[157,158] Preliminary evidence for this phenomenon came from two observations. In canines, bone-marrow derived cells were shown to "endothelialize" Dacron grafts rendered impervious to capillary ingrowth.[158] In humans, endothelial cells from male heart transplant recipients were observed to have engrafted in the blood vessels in female donor hearts.[159] EPCs are thought to serve two roles: endothelialization and neovascularization. A putative hematopoietic/angiopoietic stem cell that gives rise to EPCs has been postulated. Other sources for circulating EPCs have been postulated as well. These include myeloid cells (which can be coaxed to differentiate into endothelial cells *in vitro*), mature endothelial cells that have shed from the vessel wall, and tissue stem cells in the myocardium. Agreement on the cell markers that define an EPC and the most accurate methods of quantifying EPC number and biologic functionality is lacking.[156,160,161] Like T-cells, EPCs may be a heterogeneous population of closely related cells with highly specialized functions.

Decreased numbers and decreased proliferative potential of circulating EPCs predict cardiovascular events.[162–164] These relationships hold true even after adjustment for traditional cardiac risk factors.[164] Three possible explanations exist: Poor EPC mobilization and engraftment may be a primary mechanism of atherosclerosis; it may be caused by the same underlying etiology as atherosclerosis (eg, impaired nitric oxide synthesis); or it may be an epiphenomenon. These competing hypotheses do not detract from the potential usefulness of EPCs as a biomarker of cardiovascular risk.

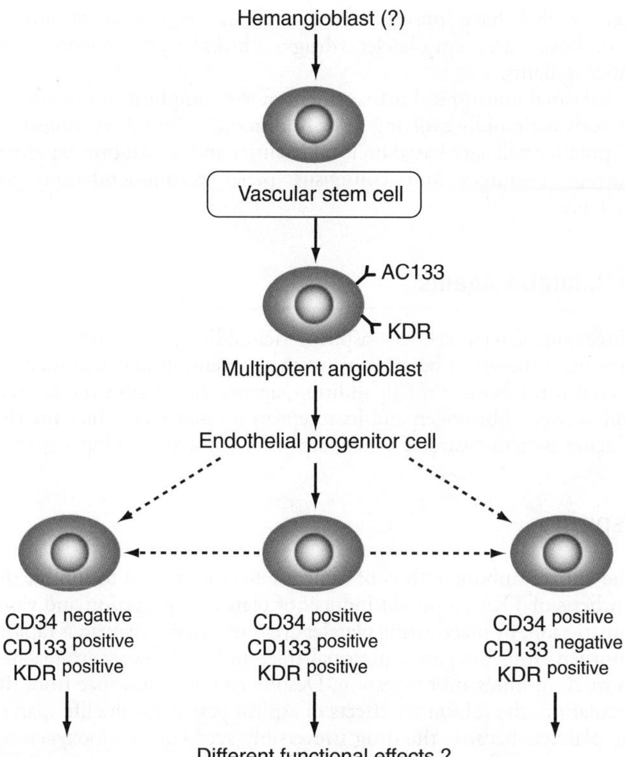

Figure 136–2. Endothelial progenitor cells are putatively derived from the hemangioblast, circulate in peripheral blood, and have the potential to differentiate into mature endothelial cells. The surface markers CD34, KDR (VEGFR2), and CD133 define circulating endothelial progenitor cells. Different subpopulations display different functional activities concerning angiogenesis and endothelial cell repair. The CD34 negative, CD133 and VEGFR2 positive EPC subpopulation may be a precursor of the CD34/CD133 positive EPC population and preferably homes to sites of ischemia. *(Adapted with permission from Werner N, Nickenig G. Clinical and therapeutical implications of EPC biology in atherosclerosis. J Cell MolMed Apr-Jun;10(2):318, 2006.)*

Many modifiable factors influence circulating EPC levels and function. These include physical activity,[165] smoking,[166] estrogen,[167] and inflammation.[168] The capacity of EPCs to differentiate may influence recovery following acute myocardial infarction.[169] Early studies have explored pharmacologic approaches to increase circulating EPCs,[170] stents impregnated with "EPC-capturing" antibodies or peptides[171,172] or seeded with EPCs themselves,[173,174] vascular endothelial growth factor gene transfer,[175] and autotransplantation.[176–179] Sources of autologous EPCs include peripheral blood[176,178] and bone marrow.[177–179] Different cell preparations yield differing amounts of EPCs, hematopoietic cells, and mesenchymal cells. The EPCs may be expanded by culture *ex vivo*.[176,178] The timing of transplant in relation to myocardial infarction varies among studies. Intracoronary infusion of marrow[176,180–182] and peripheral blood[176,183] presumed to contain functional EPCs is feasible in the early period after acute myocardial infarction. Similar studies have been performed in patients with chronic myocardial ischemia.[178,183–185] Granulocyte colony-stimulating factor has occasionally been used for progenitor cell mobilization.[183,185] Most of these early trials assessed surrogate endpoints, such as change in left ventricular ejection fraction or myocardial perfusion. Follow-up has been short. The improvements have been modest at best and inconsistent. Only one randomized study detected a clinical benefit.[179]

Four classes of drugs already known to benefit patients at risk for cardiovascular events may increase circulating EPCs. Angiotensin II accelerates EPC senescence such that their proliferation is impaired, but valsartan (an angiotensin I receptor blocker) attenuates this process.[186,187] In small studies in humans, olmesartan, irbesartan, and ramipril increased the number of circulating EPCs.[188,189] Ramipril (an angiotensin-converting enzyme inhibitor) was also shown to increase their functional activity.[189] Preclinical data suggest that hydroxymethylglutaryl coenzyme A reductase inhibitors can also augment circulating EPCs.[190–193] Erythropoietin can mobilize EPCs,[194–196] but it might have deleterious cardiovascular effects for other reasons, such as increasing blood viscosity and blood pressure, particularly in patients who are not anemic. Whether elevation of circulating EPCs persists with chronic pharmacologic treatments and whether achieving a given level of circulating EPCs can be considered a surrogate marker for decreasing clinical events—and hence an important therapeutic target—has not been validated.

Nonsteroidal Anti-inflammatory Drugs

Cyclooxygenases (COX) 1 and 2 form prostaglandins from arachidonic acid. Prostaglandins are lipid mediators of pain, fever, inflammation, vasodilation, smooth muscle function, and gastric mucus secretion. Nonsteroidal anti-inflammatory drugs (NSAIDs) inhibit prostaglandin synthesis by inhibiting COX enzymes. Traditional NSAIDs inhibit both COX isoforms reversibly, whereas aspirin inhibits both irreversibly. The original but oversimplified "COX-2 hypothesis" stated that the prostaglandins formed by constitutively-expressed COX-1 have a homeostatic role, whereas those formed by inducible COX-2 are primarily responsible for inflammation. Available NSAIDs have a spectrum of COX-2:COX-1 selectivity: Indomethacin, ibuprofen, and naproxen are essentially nonselective; celecoxib and diclofenac have similar but only moderate COX-2 selectivity; rofecoxib and valdecoxib are more COX-2 specific; whereas lumiracoxib is the most COX-2 specific.[197] COX-2 selectivity can be lost at high drug concentrations.[197] Relative selectivity may also be affected by polymorphisms of the COX-1 and COX-2 genes themselves and of the enzymes involved in NSAID metabolism.[198]

It was proposed that selective COX-2 inhibitors would be as effective as traditional NSAIDs with a lower incidence of gastrointestinal ulceration and bleeding. However, the biology of COX-1 and COX-2 predicts that selective COX-2 inhibition could promote cardiovascular events. Mature platelets express only COX-1, which is responsible for TXA_2 production. COX-2 selective inhibitors substantially impair vascular biosynthesis of prostaglandin I_2 (prostacyclin) without impairing platelet production of TXA_2.[199,200] Normally, prostaglandin I_2 opposes various mediators of platelet aggregation, vasoconstriction and attendant blood pressure elevation, and atherogenesis—including TXA_2. In animal models, unopposed TXA_2 effects accelerate initiation and progression of atherosclerosis.[201,202] Indeed, several clinical trials designed to address the gastrointestinal safety,[203–205] colorectal adenoma prevention,[206,207] and analgesia in the immediate post–coronary bypass period[208,209] detected a higher incidence of myocardial infarction among patients allocated to COX-2 inhibitors versus placebo or nonselective NSAIDs. This risk appeared not only among populations considered at high risk of myocardial infarction[208,209] but also among those whose baseline risk of myocardial infarction was probably intermediate[203] or low.[206] Duration of exposure seems to increase the risk of cardiovascular endpoints, in line with the hypothesis that selective COX-2 inhibition promotes atherogenesis. Meta-analysis suggests the overall risk for myocardial infarction in chronic users of COX-2 inhibitors is approximately twofold compared to placebo (corresponding to an excess of 1 to 4 myocardial infarctions in 1000 person-years).[210] Accordingly, rofecoxib and valdecoxib have been withdrawn from the market. The incidence of serious vascular events seems similar between COX-2 inhibitors and traditional NSAIDs (ibuprofen and diclofenac—although one caveat in interpreting these results is that diclofenac has relatively more COX-2 selectivity).[210] It is unknown whether the risk associated with the high doses of traditional NSAIDs employed as comparators in the COX-2 inhibitor trials may overrepresent the risk associated with more moderate doses (see box on Do All NSAIDs Increase the Risk of Cardiac Events?).

Do All NSAIDS Increase the Risk of Cardiac Events?

Whether certain traditional NSAIDs may not impact cardiovascular risk, or may even be cardioprotective, is a matter of debate. For example, in small, short-term studies, flurbiprofen was effective in reducing reinfarction and the need for secondary revascularization after a first myocardial infarction[211] and indobufen reduced cardioembolic events.[212] High-dose naproxen does not appear to carry the same cardiovascular risks as other NSAIDs.[210] To account for this finding, it has been suggested that the long half-life of naproxen (14 hours) compared to other NSAIDs might promote more sustained inhibition of platelet aggregation. However, whether naproxen offers cardioprotection compared to aspirin has not been prospectively evaluated, and early experiments indicate that aspirin is probably the better choice for two reasons. First, naproxen's pharmacodynamic effect is strictly tied to its systemic bioavailability, so missing one or two doses allows prompt recovery of platelet COX-1 activity within 24 hours. Second, naproxen inhibits prostacyclin production to a substantial degree whereas aspirin does not,[213] raising the possibility that long-term use of naproxen could be atherogenic.

Finally, the interaction between NSAIDs and aspirin remains far from clear. *In vitro* and human studies suggest that ibuprofen negates the beneficial antiplatelet effects of aspirin.[214–216] Such a negative interaction was not found to hold for rofecoxib or diclofenac.[216] Studies examining clinical outcomes of combined NSAID-aspirin therapy have been conflicting.[217–219] This is likely caused by differences in study design, difficulty accounting for nonprescription use of these medications, and difficulty in estimating adherence to therapy. A very large case-control study sought to overcome these limitations. The authors concluded that there in no increased risk of myocardial infarction among patients simultaneously taking aspirin and ibuprofen chronically, compared with those taking aspirin alone.[219]

At this time, sufficient evidence does not exist to recommend concurrent use of aspirin to mitigate cardiovascular effects of long-term NSAID use. Similarly, some patients choose long-term COX-2 specific NSAID therapy over nonselective NSAIDs for noncardiovascular indications, either to minimize gastrointestinal effects or because anecdotally occasional patients may experience superior analgesia with COX-2 inhibitors. In this instance, some clinicians prescribe concurrent low-dose aspirin therapy. However, it is crucial to realize that low-dose aspirin negates the gastrointestinal benefits of the COX-2 inhibitor[204] and that this approach has not been prospectively evaluated with a cardiovascular endpoint.

Other Risk Factors

Impaired fibrinolysis has been linked to atherosclerotic vascular disease in some but not all studies. Antiphospholipid antibodies are clearly associated with premature arterial thromboembolism and may be associated with accelerated atherosclerosis. Both thoracic radiation therapy and heart transplantation are associated with accelerated atherosclerosis and ischemic cardiac syndromes.

NONINVASIVE TREATMENT OF ARTERIAL THROMBOEMBOLISM

Treatment of atherosclerosis and its thromboembolic complications includes interventional procedures such as endarterectomy, embolectomy, arterial bypass surgery, and angioplasty with or without stenting, as well as medical management. The three forms of medical therapy that have proven effective in the treatment of arterial thrombosis are antiplatelet drugs, thrombolytic agents, and anticoagulants.

Optimal nonsurgical management of the complications of atherosclerosis is a rapidly evolving field. Additionally, "standard" nonsurgical practice will vary based on local facilities and health care expertise. Current resources and consensus panel recommendations are available.[67,220–223]

Antiplatelet Agents

Three antiplatelet agents—aspirin, ticlopidine, and clopidogrel—have been shown to be effective in the prevention and treatment of arterial thrombosis.[224,225] In addition, agents that inhibit the interaction between fibrinogen and its receptors on platelets reduce the risk of acute ischemic cardiac syndromes after coronary angioplasty.[226]

Aspirin

The antithrombotic effects of aspirin reflect its ability to inhibit the synthesis of TXA_2, a potent inducer of platelet aggregation and vasoconstriction, by inactivating platelet cyclooxygenase. Aspirin is rapidly absorbed from the gastrointestinal tract and peak levels are reached 15 to 20 minutes after ingestion. Despite its rapid clearance from the circulation, the inhibitory effects of aspirin persist for the life span of the platelets because the drug irreversibly acetylates cyclooxygenase. A dose as small as 80 mg of aspirin per day is sufficient to inhibit TXA_2 synthesis. Aspirin therapy is inexpensive, widely available, and largely nontoxic; thus it should be used in all patients with evidence of atherosclerotic disease unless a specific contraindication exists.

The side effects of aspirin are primarily gastrointestinal, and gastrointestinal hemorrhage can occur in some patients. These complications are dose-related and are reduced if enteric-coated aspirin is used. Aspirin is contraindicated in patients with active peptic ulcer disease or aspirin-induced asthma, and it should be discontinued if gastrointestinal side effects are severe.

In most randomized studies, patients with a history of active peptic ulcer disease were excluded, and the beneficial effects of aspirin occurred without hemorrhagic complications.[227] However, in a U.S. Physicians Study the use of aspirin was associated with an increased incidence of cerebral hemorrhage, a finding not observed in symptomatic patients treated with aspirin to prevent the complications of atherosclerosis.[227,228]

Dipyridamole

Dipyridamole interferes with platelet function by inhibiting adenosine deaminase and phosphodiesterase, causing accumulation of adenosine, adenine dinucleotides, and cyclic adenosine monophosphate. It also causes vasodilation. In studies in which aspirin alone was compared with the combination of aspirin and dipyridamole for cardiovascular events, no additional benefit was observed from the addition of dipyridamole.[227,229] However, two trials showed that the combination of aspirin and dipyridamole is somewhat more effective than aspirin alone for patients who suffer transient ischemic attacks or minor ischemic strokes.[230,231] Like aspirin, dipyridamole also augments the antithrombotic effect of oral anticoagulants in patients with mechanical prosthetic valves.[232]

Ticlopidine and Clopidogrel

Ticlopidine and clopidogrel are thienopyridine derivatives that inhibit adenosine diphosphate-dependent platelet aggregation by antagonizing the $P2Y_{12}$ adenosine diphosphate receptor. They are metabolized by the liver, producing active metabolites. Because the production of intermediate active metabolites is required, the inhibitory effects of ticlopidine and clopidogrel on platelet function are delayed after administration.

Ticlopidine is more effective than aspirin in reducing stroke in patients with transient cerebral ischemia or minor stroke. Ticlopidine is also effective in 1) reducing the risk of the combined outcome of stroke, myocardial infarction, or vascular death in patients with thromboembolic stroke, 2) decreasing vascular death and myocardial infarction in patients with unstable angina, 3) reducing acute occlusion of coronary bypass grafts, and 4) improving walking distance and decreasing vascular complications in patients with peripheral vascular disease.[224]

The most common side effects of ticlopidine are diarrhea and skin rash; the most serious complications are neutropenia and thrombotic thrombocytopenic purpura. Nevertheless, ticlopidine should be considered in place of aspirin in patients who are allergic to or intolerant of aspirin, or who have had a vascular event despite the use of aspirin.

Clopidogrel and ticlopidine are more effective than aspirin for the prevention of ischemic stroke, myocardial infarction, or vascular death in patients at high risk of these complications.[225] Compared to ticlopidine, clopidogrel poses a much lower risk for the development of neutropenia or thrombotic thrombocytopenic purpura.

Combined use of aspirin and clopidogrel is of established benefit in the acute setting, especially to maintain patency of intraluminal arterial stents. Long-term combined use of aspirin and clopidogrel in patients with established coronary artery disease may marginally reduce the risk of recurrent arterial thrombosis.[233] Whether the added cost of clopidogrel is worth this marginal benefit is unclear. Furthermore, the same trial studied combined use of aspirin and clopidogrel for primary prevention in patients with a high risk for atherothrombotic events but no known coronary artery disease and found both cardiovascular death and all-cause mortality were increased in the primary prevention group.[233] Caution must be exercised in interpreting these results as they are derived from subgroup analysis. Combined treatment can be considered for many patients with established atherosclerosis (especially for those patients who recently suffered myocardial infarction, who have unstable angina, or have undergone percutaneous coronary intervention), but it is not currently advocated for primary prevention, even in high-risk patients. At what time point the risk-benefit balance in patients who had indications for using clopidogrel in an acute setting, for secondary prevention, approaches the increased risk seen in patients who have no such indications is unknown.

Platelet Glycoprotein IIb/IIIa Blockade

Blockade of the platelet fibrinogen receptor (glycoprotein IIb/IIIa [GPIIb/IIIa]) using humanized monoclonal antibodies (abciximab) or small molecule inhibitors (eptifibatide, tirofiban) reduces the risk of clinically significant ischemic events in patients undergoing coronary angioplasty. Large studies have demonstrated that GPIIb/IIIa antagonists reduce the risk of death, myocardial infarction, or urgent coronary artery bypass grafting in the first 30 days after percutaneous coronary intervention in patients with acute or chronic coronary syndromes. The absolute risk reduction for death or myocardial infarction at 30 days is on the order of 3%.[234–242] Demonstration that GPIIb/IIIa antagonists reduce the risk of ischemic events after percutaneous coronary intervention led to their use in other settings.

In ST-elevation myocardial infarction, there is a need for reperfusion strategies that improve on the outcomes of fibrinolytic therapy. Fibrinolytic therapy may achieve adequate epicardial blood flow, but distal plaque embolization may nonetheless compromise myocardial reperfusion. Early dose-finding trials found that adding a GPIIb/IIIa inhibitor to full-dose fibrinolytic therapy may be beneficial,[243,244] but in at least one such trial, the enthusiasm for this approach was tempered by increased bleeding.[245] Likewise, large trials of high-dose and low-dose fibrinolytic therapy combined with GPIIb/IIIa inhibition have not found clear reductions in long-term mortality and the risk of major bleeding persists.[246,247]

In non–ST-elevation myocardial infarction and unstable angina, GPIIb/IIIa antagonists have a larger role. In patients not scheduled for percutaneous coronary intervention (PCI), trials involving greater than 31,000 patients have demonstrated an absolute risk reduction of death or myocardial infarction of approximately 1% at 30 days after the index event.[248] Platelet fibrinogen receptor blockade is now a standard component of the treatment of refractory acute coronary syndromes while awaiting resolution or definitive therapy.

Abciximab produces an immediate and profound inhibition of platelet activity that persists for 6 to 12 hours after termination of its infusion. Administration of abciximab is associated with an increase in the risk of hemorrhage, although this risk can be moderated with the judicious use of heparin and careful patient selection. Eptifibatide and tirofiban have shorter half-lives, and platelet function normalizes within 4 to 8 hours of termination of the infusion. Drug-induced thrombocytopenia is more common with abciximab than with the small molecule inhibitors, but severe thrombocytopenia is rare (0.9%–1.6%), usually transient, and generally responds to platelet transfusions. A thrombogenic syndrome analogous to heparin-induced thrombocytopenia has not been observed.

Thrombolytic Therapy

Thrombolytic therapy is useful in the treatment of arterial thrombosis because rapid clot lysis and restoration of blood flow prevent permanent tissue damage. More than 80% of patients with acute myocardial infarction have thrombotic occlusion of the infarct-related coronary artery, and thrombolytic agents produce rapid lysis of these thrombi in 50% to 75% of cases.[220] Tissue plasminogen activator (tPA) is more effective than streptokinase in achieving early coronary lysis, but both agents improve left ventricular function and reduce mortality.[249] Thus, streptokinase and tPA decrease mortality by approximately 25% when used without adjunctive aspirin or intravenous heparin, and reduce mortality by 40% to 50% when either agent is combined with aspirin.[53,250] In the Global Utilization of Streptokinase and t-PA for Occluded Coronary Arteries-I (GUSTO-I) study, an accelerated tPA regimen combined with high-dose intravenous heparin produced a 14% greater reduction in mortality than streptokinase. This difference was most evident in patients treated within 4 hours of onset of symptoms. Unfractionated heparin or low-molecular-weight heparin is usually advised in conjunction with the so-called "fibrin-specific" fibrinolytics (reteplase, alteplase, tenecteplase). Recent American College of Chest Physicians guidelines emphasize the importance of using unfractionated heparin in conjunction with the non–fibrin-specific streptokinase as well.[220]

Following successful thrombolysis there is a 10% to 20% reocclusion rate and a 3% to 4% reinfarction rate.[250] Aspirin reduces the incidence of reinfarction.[220,251] Reocclusion is less common with streptokinase than with tPA. The traditional explanation is that streptokinase induces extensive plasma proteolysis and release of fibrinogen degradation products. However, at pharmacologic doses used for acute myocardial infarction, all thrombolytic agents cause a high degree of systemic fibrinolysis and hence systemic anticoagulation. Direct thrombin inhibitors, such as bivalirudin (Hirulog) and hirudin, are more effective than heparin at preventing reocclusion after coronary thrombolysis. However, large-scale clinical trials have been disappointing.[251–253]

Recent developments in thrombolytic medications have focused both on improving efficacy and increasing the convenience of thrombolytic therapy. Thus, agents that can be administered by rapid intravenous bolus, oftentimes outside the hospital setting, have recently been the focus of research studies. In general, these agents are either not, or only marginally, more effective than traditional thrombolytic medications, but are more convenient to use.

Anticoagulants

Heparin

The role of anticoagulant therapy in the treatment of arterial thrombosis is controversial.[254,255] When used alone, heparin is effective in the short-term treatment of unstable angina,[254] but a rebound effect is seen when the drug is stopped.[256] Aspirin appears to prevent the cluster of ischemic events that occur when heparin is discontinued. There is some suggestion that the addition of heparin to aspirin improves the short-term outcome in patients with unstable angina, but it is uncertain whether this effect is sustained. Moderate doses of heparin (12,500 units subcutaneously every 12 hours) also reduce the incidence of mural thrombosis detected by two-dimensional echocardiography, which is a particular problem in patients with anterior infarction.

Heparin prevents early reocclusion of the infarct-related artery after successful thrombolysis with tPA. However, a meta-analysis has suggested that routine administration of heparin to patients with acute myocardial infarction is not indicated.[257] Heparin therapy reduced mortality by 6% (95% confidence intervals: 0%–10%), and the rate of reinfarction by 1.3%. However, heparin was associated with a clinically important increase in the risk of major hemorrhage that outweighed its observed benefit. A more recent meta-analysis could not detect a beneficial effect of heparin on reinfarction or death in patients treated with thrombolysis. A trend toward bleeding complications with heparin was noted. However, there are limitations among the studies of patients receiving thrombolytics for acute myocardial infarction. These limitations include a serious lack of power to detect even a modest benefit of heparin and lack of routine aspirin prescription.[258]

Low-Molecular-Weight Heparin

In patients with ST-elevation myocardial infarction, the most recent meta-analysis concluded that at 30 days, subcutaneous low-molecular-weight heparin given for 4 to 8 days after thrombolysis reduces reinfarction by approximately one-quarter and death by approximately 10% compared with placebo and, when directly compared with heparin, low-molecular-weight heparin reduces reinfarction by almost one-half.[258] Whether the various low-molecular-weight heparins differ in efficacy from one another in terms of clinical endpoints is not known. Reviparin compared to placebo showed a slight benefit on reinfarction and mortality in patients with ST-elevation myocardial infarction.[259]

In patients with unstable angina or non–ST-elevation myocardial infarction, the benefit of low-molecular-weight heparin over heparin is not clear. Both had a similar risk of mortality, recurrent angina, and major bleeding, but low-molecular-weight heparin decreased the risk of myocardial infarction.[260]

There is limited experience with intravenous low-molecular-weight heparin during percutaneous intervention, but one meta-analysis suggests that employed without monitoring of the anticoagulant effect, it may be comparable to heparin and may even carry a lower risk of hemorrhage.[261]

Fondaparinux

Fondaparinux is a synthetic pentasaccharide that binds antithrombin and catalyzes its inhibition of factor Xa.

The Sixth Organization to Assess Strategies in Acute Ischemic Syndromes (OASIS-6) trial studied patients presenting with ST-elevation myocardial infarction.[262] Patients underwent PCI or thrombolysis. In subjects without a clear indication for anticoagulation, fondaparinux was compared to placebo or heparin. Subjects with a clear indication for anticoagulation (ie, those destined for primary PCI or receiving so-called fibrin-specific thrombolytics) were randomized to fondaparinux or heparin. There was no benefit to adjunctive therapy with fondaparinux in patients undergoing primary PCI. However, in those receiving thrombolytics or no reperfusion therapy at all, fondaparinux yielded an absolute risk reduction of approximately 1.5% in the incidence of reinfarction or death, whether compared to placebo or to heparin.

OASIS-5 studied patients presenting with acute coronary syndromes (unstable angina or non–ST-elevation myocardial infarction).[263] Fondaparinux was not inferior to enoxaparin in the early postinfarction period in terms of death, progression to myocardial infarction, or refractory ischemia. Fondaparinux led to an absolute reduction in mortality of 0.7% up to 180 days after the index event. In both OASIS-5 and OASIS-6, fondaparinux was associated with less major bleeding compared to heparin or low-molecular-weight heparin. The reduction in major bleeding has been postulated to contribute to the observed mortality difference. Whether it results from an intrinsic property of the drugs, or whether the commonly employed doses of heparin and low molecular weight heparin are in fact too high, is a matter for debate. Fondaparinux is also attractive because it is administered in a fixed dose (2.5 mg daily) without monitoring in patients with creatinine clearance as low as 30 mL/min.

Warfarin

Oral anticoagulants are effective for the treatment of arterial thrombosis. Two studies have shown that oral anticoagulants are effective for long-term treatment of patients with myocardial infarction, an observation confirmed in a meta-analysis.[264–266] This meta-analysis also confirmed that low-dose warfarin (1 or 3 mg) combined with 80 mg of aspirin per day does not provide benefit beyond that achieved with 160 mg of aspirin/day.[267] Therapeutic doses of warfarin are not commonly administered for primary or secondary prophylaxis of myocardial infarction because of the inconvenience associated with international normalized ratio (INR) monitoring.

Direct Thrombin Inhibitors

The role of bivalirudin and other direct thrombin inhibitors, which have been licensed in some jurisdictions for the treatment of acute coronary syndromes, is currently evolving.[268] To date, there does not appear to be any benefit to using direct thrombin inhibitors in lieu of heparin for acute coronary syndromes. Also, direct thrombin inhibitors have not been evaluated for this indication in the era of aggressive antiplatelet therapy with clopidogrel, aspirin, and GPIIb/IIIa inhibitors. For patients undergoing percutaneous coronary intervention, bivalirudin may be safer than heparin because of reduced bleeding.[269]

Atrial Fibrillation

Patients with nonvalvular atrial fibrillation have an increased risk of stroke, which occurs at a frequency of 5% per year.[270–274] The risk of stroke is similar for persistent and paroxysmal atrial fibrillation. The risk of stroke increases with age,[275,276] and is increased by a number of associated cardiac disorders, including a history of myocardial infarction, angina, heart failure, and previous thromboembolic event, and the presence of left atrial dilation, left ventricular dysfunction, mitral calcification, or hypertension. In such patients, warfarin (INR 2.0–3.0) produces a 60% to 80% reduction in the risk of stroke, with only a modest increase in bleeding complications.[270–274] Therefore, warfarin (target INR 2.0–3.0) should be administered to all patients with persistent or paroxysmal nonvalvular atrial fibrillation who do not have a contraindication to anticoagulant therapy. This recommendation applies particularly to those patients with nonvalvular atrial fibrillation who have an additional risk factor for stroke,[277] such as hypertension, impaired left ventricular function and/or congestive heart failure, diabetes, previous cerebral ischemia or systemic embolization. In these patients, warfarin therapy (target INR 2.0–3.0) is more effective than either fixed low-dose warfarin,[278] aspirin,[278] or aspirin and clopidogrel in combination.[279] Aspirin should be used in patients with nonvalvular atrial fibrillation who are at high risk for stroke when warfarin is contraindicated. Low-risk patients (ie, those who are younger than 65 years old and without a history of cerebral ischemia, diabetes, hypertension, left ventricular dysfunction, or structural heart defects) should receive aspirin, 325 mg/day. Such patients who are between 65 and 75 years of age should receive either aspirin or warfarin. Several scoring systems to stratify the risk of stroke in atrial fibrillation patients have been developed.[277]

Mechanical and Bioprosthetic Valves

Patients with prosthetic heart valves have an increased risk of systemic embolism, which most often manifests as a stroke. The embolic risk is greater with mechanical than with bioprosthetic valves, with prosthetic mitral rather than aortic valves, and when there is associated atrial fibrillation.[232] For patients with tissue prosthetic valves who are in sinus rhythm, the risk of embolism is largely confined to the first 3 months after valve insertion, whereas patients with mechanical prosthetic valves have a lifelong risk of systemic embolism. The general consensus is that patients with tissue valves but no other risk factors for thrombosis should receive warfarin for 3 months after valve placement, with a goal INR of 2.0 to 3.0, followed by lifelong low-dose aspirin.[232,280]

Randomized trials in patients with mechanical prosthetic valves have shown that warfarin is effective in reducing the risk of systemic embolism, even when given at a lower intensity than that used in the past.[281,282] Current American College of Chest Physician recommendations are for a target INR of 2.5 (range 2.0–3.0) with a St. Jude Medical bileaflet valve in the aortic position, a target INR of 3.0 (range 2.5–3.5) with a tilting disk or bileaflet valve in the mitral position, and a target INR of 3.0 (range 2.5–3.5) in combination with low-dose aspirin for patients with caged ball or caged disk valves in either position.[232] Current American College of Cardiology/American Heart Association recommendations are to increase the target INR to the 2.5 to 3.5 range for patients with mechanical aortic valves who have additional risk factors for thromboembolism (atrial fibrillation, left ventricular dysfunction, prior thromboembolism, or a hypercoagulable condition). The American College of Cardiology/American Heart Association also strongly recommends adding low-dose aspirin to warfarin in all patients with risk factors for thromboembolism, unless aspirin is contraindicated for reasons such as gastrointestinal bleeding.[280]

SUGGESTED READINGS

Cannon CP, Steinberg BA, Murphy SA, Mega JL, Braunwald E: Meta-analysis of cardiovascular outcomes trials comparing intensive versus moderate statin therapy. J Am Coll Cardiol 48(3):438, 2006.

Fries S, Grosser T: The cardiovascular pharmacology of COX-2 inhibition. Hematology Am Soc Hematol Educ Program 445, 2005.

Harrington RA, Becker RC, Ezekowitz M, et al: Antithrombotic therapy for coronary artery disease: The Seventh ACCP Conference on Antithrombotic and Thrombolytic Therapy. Chest 126(3 Suppl):513S, 2004.

Kim JA, Montagnani M, Koh KK, Quon MJ: Reciprocal relationships between insulin resistance and endothelial dysfunction: Molecular and pathophysiological mechanisms. Circulation 113(15):1888, 2006.

Menon V, Harrington RA, Hochman JS, et al: Thrombolysis and adjunctive therapy in acute myocardial infarction: The Seventh ACCP Conference on Antithrombotic and Thrombolytic Therapy. Chest 126(3 Suppl):549S, 2004.

Pi-Sunyer FX: The obesity epidemic: Pathophysiology and consequences of obesity. Obes Res 10(Suppl 2):97S, 2002.

Ross R: The pathogenesis of atherosclerosis: A perspective for the 1990s. Nature 362(6423):801, 1993.

Smith SC Jr, Allen J, Blair SN, et al: AHA/ACC guidelines for secondary prevention for patients with coronary and other atherosclerotic vascular disease: 2006 update: Endorsed by the National Heart, Lung, and Blood Institute. Circulation 113(19):2363, 2006.

Werner N, Nickenig G: Clinical and therapeutical implications of EPC biology in atherosclerosis. J Cell Mol Med 10(2):318, 2006.

Yusuf S, Hawken S, Ounpuu S, et al: Effect of potentially modifiable risk factors associated with myocardial infarction in 52 countries (the INTERHEART study): Case-control study. Lancet 364(9438):937, 2004.

REFERENCES

For complete list of references log onto www.expertconsult.com

CHAPTER 137

ANTITHROMBOTIC DRUGS

Jeffrey I. Weitz

Arterial and venous thromboses are major causes of morbidity and mortality. Arterial thrombosis is the most common cause of acute myocardial infarction, ischemic stroke and limb gangrene, whereas deep vein thrombosis leads to pulmonary embolism, which can be fatal, and to the postphlebitic syndrome. Most arterial thrombi are superimposed on disrupted atherosclerotic plaque because plaque rupture exposes thrombogenic material in the plaque core to the blood. This material then triggers platelet aggregation and fibrin formation, which results in the generation of a platelet-rich thrombus that can temporarily or permanently occlude blood flow.[1] In contrast to arterial thrombi, venous thrombi rarely form at sites of obvious vascular disruption. Although they can develop after surgical trauma to veins, or secondary to indwelling venous catheters, venous thrombi usually originate in the valve cusps of the deep veins of the calf or in the muscular sinuses,[2] where they are triggered by stasis. Sluggish blood flow in these veins reduces the oxygen supply to the avascular valve cusps.[3] Endothelial cells lining these valve cusps become activated and express adhesion molecules on their surface. Tissue factor-bearing leukocytes and microparticles adhere to these activated cells and induce coagulation.[4] Local thrombus formation is exacerbated by reduced clearance of activated clotting factors as a result of impaired blood flow. If the calf vein thrombi extend into more proximal veins of the leg, thrombus fragments can dislodge, travel to the lungs, and produce a pulmonary embolism.[5]

Arterial and venous thrombi are composed of platelets and fibrin, but the proportions differ. Arterial thrombi are rich in platelets because of the high shear in the injured arteries. In contrast, venous thrombi, which form under low-shear conditions, contain relatively few platelets and are predominantly composed of fibrin and trapped red cells.[6] Because of the predominance of platelets, arterial thrombi appear white, whereas venous thrombi are red in color, reflecting the trapped red cells.

Antithrombotic drugs are used for prevention and treatment of thrombosis. Targeting the components of thrombi, these agents include (a) antiplatelet drugs, which inhibit platelets; (b) anticoagulants, which attenuate coagulation; and (c) fibrinolytic agents, which induce fibrin degradation (Fig. 137–1). With the predominance of platelets in arterial thrombi, strategies to inhibit or treat arterial thrombosis focus mainly on antiplatelet agents, although, in the acute setting, they often include anticoagulants and fibrinolytic agents. Anticoagulants are the mainstay of prevention and treatment of venous thromboembolism because fibrin is the predominant component of venous thrombi. Antiplatelet drugs are less effective than anticoagulants in this setting because of the limited platelet content of venous thrombi. Fibrinolytic therapy is used in selected patients with venous thromboembolism. For example, patients with massive or submassive pulmonary embolism can benefit from systemic or catheter-directed fibrinolytic therapy. Catheter-directed fibrinolytic therapy also can be used as an adjunct to anticoagulants for treatment of certain patients with extensive iliofemoral vein thrombosis.[7]

ANTIPLATELET DRUGS

Role of Platelets in Arterial Thrombosis

In healthy vasculature, circulating platelets are maintained in an inactive state by nitric oxide (NO) and prostacyclin released by endothelial cells lining the blood vessels. In addition, endothelial cells also express ADPase on their surface which degrades ADP released from activated platelets. When the vessel wall is damaged, release of these substances is impaired and the subendothelial matrix is exposed.[8] Platelets adhere to exposed collagen, von Willebrand factor, and fibronectin via receptors constitutively expressed on the platelet surface. Adherent platelets undergo a change in shape, secrete ADP from their dense granules, and synthesize and release thromboxane A_2. Released ADP and thromboxane A_2, which are platelet agonists, activate ambient platelets and recruit them to the site of vascular injury.

Disruption of the vessel wall also exposes tissue factor-expressing cells to the blood. Tissue factor initiates coagulation. Activated platelets potentiate coagulation by binding clotting factors and may support the assembly of activation complexes that enhance thrombin generation. In addition to converting fibrinogen to fibrin, thrombin also serves as a potent platelet agonist and recruits more platelets to the site of vascular injury.

When platelets are activated, GPIIb/IIIa, the most abundant receptor on the platelet surface, undergoes a conformational change that enables it to ligate fibrinogen. Divalent fibrinogen molecules bridge adjacent platelets together to form platelet aggregates. Fibrin strands, generated through the action of thrombin, then weave these aggregates together to form a platelet/fibrin mesh.

Antiplatelet drugs target various steps in this process (Fig. 137–2). The commonly used drugs include aspirin, thienopyridines (clopidogrel and ticlopidine), dipyridamole, and GPIIb/IIIa antagonists.

Aspirin

The most widely used antiplatelet agent worldwide is aspirin. As an inexpensive and effective antiplatelet drug, aspirin serves as the foundation of most antiplatelet strategies.

Mechanism of Action

Aspirin produces its antithrombotic effect by irreversibly acetylating and inhibiting platelet cyclooxygenase (COX)-1 (Fig. 137–2), a critical enzyme in the biosynthesis of thromboxane A_2. At high doses (approximately 1 g/day), aspirin also inhibits COX-2, an inducible COX isoform found in endothelial cells and inflammatory cells.[8,9] In endothelial cells, COX-2 initiates the synthesis of prostacyclin, a potent vasodilator and inhibitor of platelet aggregation.

COX-2 inhibitors were developed to block the production of inflammatory prostaglandins without affecting platelet function. The

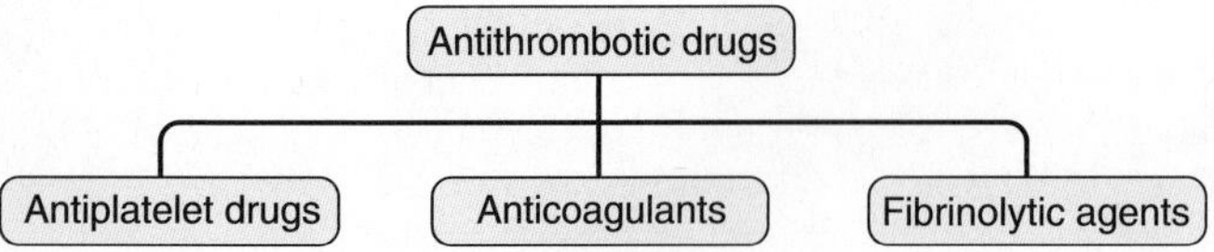

Figure 137–1 Classification of antithrombotic drugs.

various COX-2 inhibitors differ in their selectivity for COX-2 relative to COX-1. By blocking prostacyclin synthesis without concomitant inhibition of thromboxane A_2 production, highly selective inhibitors of COX-2 increase the risk of cardiovascular events. Thus, long-term rofecoxib therapy increases the risk of myocardial infarction three- to fivefold,[10,11] a finding that led to the withdrawal of this drug from the market.

Indications

Aspirin is widely used for secondary prevention of cardiovascular events in patients with coronary artery disease, cerebrovascular disease, or peripheral vascular disease. Compared with placebo, aspirin produces a 25% reduction in the risk of cardiovascular death, myocardial infarction or stroke in these patients.[12] Aspirin also is used for primary prevention in patients whose estimated annual risk of myocardial infarction is in excess of 1%, a point where its benefits are likely to outweigh harms.[13] This includes patients older than 40 with two or more major risk factors for cardiovascular disease, or those older than 50 with one or more such risk factor.[9] Aspirin is equally effective in men and women. In men, aspirin mainly reduces the risk of myocardial infarction, whereas in women aspirin lowers the risk of stroke.[14]

Dosages

Aspirin is usually administered at doses of 75 to 325 mg once daily. There is no evidence that higher doses of aspirin are more effective than lower doses, and some analyses suggest reduced efficacy with higher doses.[9] Because the side effects of aspirin are dose-related, daily aspirin doses of 75 to 150 mg are recommended for most indications. When rapid platelet inhibition is required, an initial aspirin dose of at least 160 mg should be given.[9]

Side Effects

Most common side effects are gastrointestinal and range from dyspepsia to erosive gastritis or peptic ulcers with bleeding and perforation.[9] These side effects are, at least to some extent, dose-related. Use of enteric-coated or buffered aspirin in place of plain aspirin does not eliminate the risk of gastrointestinal side effects. The overall risk of major bleeding with aspirin ranges from 1% to 3% per year.[9,15] The risk of bleeding is increased when aspirin is given in conjunction with anticoagulants, such as warfarin. When dual therapy is used, low-dose aspirin should be given (75–100 mg daily). Eradication of *Helicobacter pylori* infection and administration of proton pump inhibitors may reduce the risk of aspirin-induced gastrointestinal bleeding in patients with peptic ulcer disease.

Aspirin should not be administered to patients with a history of aspirin allergy characterized by bronchospasm. This problem occurs in approximately 0.3% of the general population, but is more common in those with chronic urticaria or asthma, particularly in subjects with coexisting nasal polyps or chronic rhinitis.[16] Hepatic and renal toxicity are observed with aspirin overdose.

Aspirin Resistance

The term *aspirin resistance* has been used to describe both clinical and laboratory phenomena.[17] Clinical aspirin resistance is defined as the failure of aspirin to protect patients from ischemic vascular events. This is not a helpful definition because it is made after the event occurs. Furthermore, it is not realistic to expect aspirin, which only blocks thromboxane A_2-induced platelet activation, to prevent all vascular events.

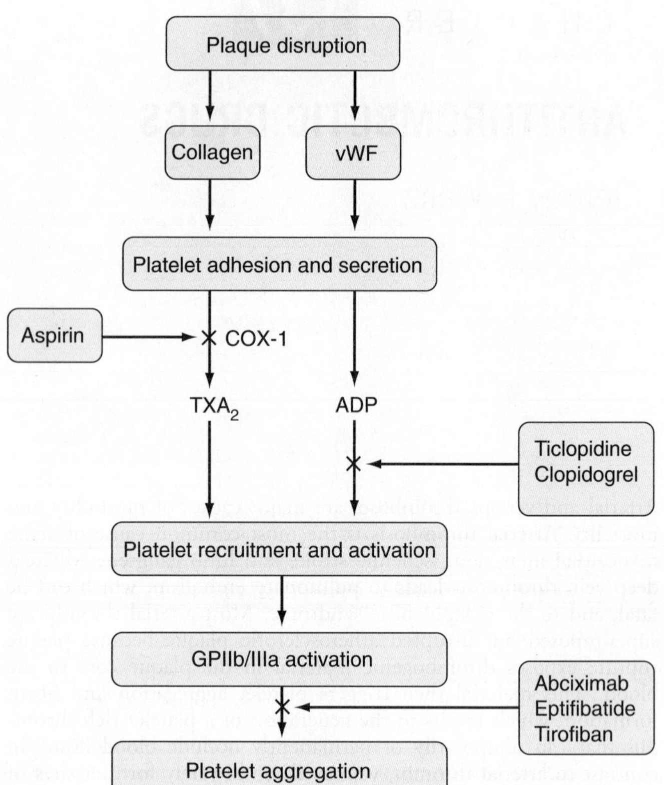

Figure 137–2 Site of action of antiplatelet drugs. Aspirin inhibits thromboxane A_2 (TXA_2) synthesis by irreversibly acetylating cyclooxygenase-1 (COX-1). Reduced TXA_2 release attenuates platelet activation and recruitment to the site of vascular injury. Ticlopidine and clopidogrel irreversibly block $P2Y_{12}$, a key ADP receptor on the platelet surface. Therefore, these agents also attenuate platelet recruitment. Abciximab, eptifibatide, and tirofiban inhibit the final common pathway of platelet aggregation by blocking fibrinogen binding to activated glycoprotein (GP) IIb/IIIa.

Aspirin resistance also has been described biochemically as failure of the drug to produce its expected inhibitory effects on tests of platelet function, such as thromboxane A_2 synthesis[18] or arachidonic acid-induced platelet aggregation.[19] However, the tests of platelet function used for diagnosis of biochemical aspirin resistance have not been well standardized.[17] Furthermore, there is no definitive evidence that these tests identify patients at risk of recurrent vascular events, or that resistance can be reversed either by giving higher doses of aspirin or by adding other antiplatelet drugs.[17] Until this information is available, testing for aspirin resistance remains a research tool.

Thienopyridines

The thienopyridines include ticlopidine (Ticlid) and clopidogrel (Plavix), drugs that target $P2Y_{12}$, a key ADP receptor on platelets.

Mechanism of Action

The thienopyridines are structurally related drugs that selectively inhibit ADP-induced platelet aggregation by irreversibly blocking $P2Y_{12}$ (Fig. 137–2). Ticlopidine and clopidogrel are both prodrugs that must be metabolized by the hepatic cytochrome P450 (CYP) enzyme system to become biologically active. Consequently, when given in usual doses, their onset of action is delayed for several days.[20]

Indications

Like aspirin, ticlopidine is effective at reducing the risk of cardiovascular death, myocardial infarction, and stroke in patients with atherosclerotic disease.[21] Because of its delayed onset of action, ticlopidine is not recommended in patients with acute myocardial infarction. Ticlopidine was used routinely as an adjunct to aspirin after coronary artery stenting and as an aspirin substitute in those intolerant to aspirin.[20] Because clopidogrel is more potent than ticlopidine and has a better safety profile, clopidogrel has replaced ticlopidine.[20]

When compared with aspirin in patients with recent ischemic stroke, myocardial infarction or peripheral arterial disease, clopidogrel reduced the risk of cardiovascular death, myocardial infarction, and stroke by 8.7%.[22] Therefore, clopidogrel is more effective than aspirin but also is more expensive. In some patients, clopidogrel and aspirin are combined to capitalize on their capacity to block complementary pathways of platelet activation. For example, the combination of aspirin plus clopidogrel is recommended for at least 4 weeks after implantation of a bare metal stent in a coronary artery and longer in those with a drug-eluting stent.[20] Recent concerns about late in-stent thrombosis with drug-eluting stents have led some experts to recommend long-term use of clopidogrel plus aspirin for this indication.[23,24]

The combination of clopidogrel and aspirin also is effective in patients with unstable angina. Thus, in 12,562 such patients, the risk of cardiovascular death, myocardial infarction or stroke was 9.3% in those randomized to the combination of clopidogrel and aspirin and 11.4% in those given aspirin alone. This 20% relative risk reduction with combination therapy was highly statistically significant.[25] However, combining clopidogrel with aspirin increases the risk of major bleeding to approximately 2% per year. This bleeding risk persists even if the daily dose of aspirin is 100 mg or less.[26] Therefore, the combination of clopidogrel and aspirin should only be used when there is a clear benefit. For example, this combination has not proven to be superior to clopidogrel alone in patients with acute ischemic stroke,[27] or to aspirin alone for primary prevention in those at risk for cardiovascular events.[28]

Dosing

Ticlopidine is given twice daily at a dose of 250 mg. The more potent clopidogrel is given once daily at a dose of 75 mg.[20] Because its onset of action is delayed for several days, loading doses of clopidogrel are given when rapid ADP receptor blockade is desired. For example, patients undergoing coronary stenting are often given a loading dose of 300 mg, which effects inhibition of ADP-induced platelet aggregation in approximately 6 hours. Loading doses of 600 or 900 mg produce an even more rapid effect.[20]

Side Effects

The most common side effects of ticlopidine are gastrointestinal. More serious are the hematologic side effects, which include neutropenia, thrombocytopenia, and thrombotic thrombocytopenic purpura. These side effects usually occur within the first few months of starting treatment. Therefore, blood counts must be carefully monitoring when initiating therapy with ticlopidine. Gastrointestinal and hematologic side effects are rare with clopidogrel.[20]

Thienopyridine Resistance

There is subject variability in the capacity of the thienopyridines to inhibit ADP-induced platelet aggregation.[29] This variability reflects, at least in part, genetic polymorphisms in the CYP isoenzymes involved in the metabolic activation of the drugs. For example, subjects with the *CYP2C19*2* allele exhibit decreased responsiveness to clopidogrel as do those with reduced CYP3A4 activity.[30,31] These findings raise the possibility that pharmacogenomic profiling may help identify clopidogrel-resistant patients. Point-of-care devices that assess the extent of platelet inhibition may also help to identify these patients.[32] It is currently unknown, however, whether patients with biochemical evidence of clopidogrel resistance have a poorer outcome and whether administration of higher doses of clopidogrel to these patients overcomes this problem.

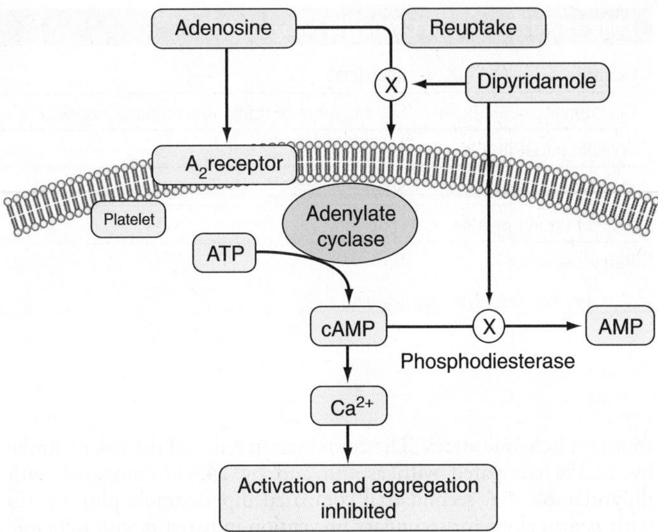

Figure 137–3 Mechanism of action of dipyridamole. Dipyridamole increases levels of cAMP in platelets by (**A**) blocking the reuptake of adenosine and (**B**) inhibiting phosphodiesterase-mediated cAMP degradation. By promoting calcium uptake, cAMP reduces intracellular levels of calcium. This, in turn, inhibits platelet activation and aggregation.

Dipyridamole

A relatively weak antiplatelet agent on its own,[20] an extended release formulation of dipyridamole combined with low-dose aspirin, a preparation known as Aggrenox, is used for prevention of stroke in patients with transient ischemic attacks.[33]

Mechanism of Action

By inhibiting phosphodiesterase, dipyridamole blocks the breakdown of cAMP. Increased levels of cAMP reduce intracellular calcium and inhibit platelet activation. Dipyridamole also blocks the uptake of adenosine by platelets and other cells. This produces a further increase in local cAMP levels because the platelet adenosine A_2 receptor is coupled to adenylate cyclase (Fig. 137–3).

Dosing

Aggrenox is given twice daily. Each capsule contains 200 mg of extended release dipyridamole and 25 mg of aspirin.[33]

Side Effects

Because dipyridamole has vasodilatory effects, it must be used with caution in patients with coronary artery disease. Gastrointestinal complaints, headache, facial flushing, dizziness, and hypotension also can occur. These symptoms often subside with continued use of the drug.[33]

Indications

Dipyridamole plus aspirin was compared with aspirin or dipyridamole alone, or with placebo, in patients with an ischemic stroke or

Table 137–1 Features of GPIIb/IIIa Antagonists

Feature	Abciximab	Eptifibatide	Tirofiban
Description	Fab fragment of humanized mouse monoclonal antibody	Cyclical KGD-containing heptapeptide	Nonpeptidic RGD mimetic
Specific for GPIIb/IIIa	No	Yes	Yes
Plasma half-life	Short (minutes)	Long (2.5 hours)	Long (2.0 hours)
Platelet-bound half-life	Long (days)	Short (seconds)	Short (seconds)
Renal clearance	No	Yes	Yes

KGD, Lys–Gly–Asp; RGD, Arg–Gly–Asp.

transient ischemic attack. The combination reduced the risk of stroke by 22.1% compared with aspirin and by 24.4% compared with dipyridamole.[34] A second trial compared dipyridamole plus aspirin with aspirin alone for secondary prevention in patients with ischemic stroke. Vascular death, stroke, or myocardial infarction occurred in 13% of patients given combination therapy and in 16% of those treated with aspirin alone.[35] On the basis of these data, Aggrenox is often used for stroke prevention. However, because of its vasodilatory effects and the paucity of data supporting the use of dipyridamole in patients with symptomatic coronary artery disease, Aggrenox should not be used for stroke prevention in such patients.

GPIIb/IIIa Receptor Antagonists

As a class, parenteral GPIIb/IIIa receptor antagonists have an established niche in patients with acute coronary syndromes. The three agents in this class are abciximab (ReoPro), eptifibatide (Integrilin), and tirofiban (Aggrestat).

Mechanism of Action

A member of the integrin family of adhesion receptors, GPIIb/IIIa, is found on the surface of platelets and megakaryocytes.[36] With approximately 80,000 copies per platelet, GPIIb/IIIa is the most abundant receptor. Consisting of a noncovalently linked heterodimer, GPIIb/IIIa is inactive on resting platelets. When platelets are activated, inside–outside signal transduction pathways trigger a conformational activation of the receptor. Once activated, GPIIb/IIIa binds adhesive molecules, such as fibrinogen and, under high-shear conditions, von Willebrand factor. Binding is mediated by the Arg–Gly–Asp (RGD) sequences found on the α chains of fibrinogen and on von Willebrand factor, and by the Lys–Gly–Asp (KGD) sequence located within a unique dodecapeptide domain on the γ chains of fibrinogen. Once bound, fibrinogen and/or von Willebrand factor bridge adjacent platelets together to induce platelet aggregation.[36]

Although abciximab, eptifibatide, and tirofiban all target the GPIIb/IIIa receptor, they are structurally and pharmacologically distinct (Table 137–1). Abciximab is a Fab fragment of a humanized murine monoclonal antibody directed against the activated form of GPIIb/IIIa.[37] Abciximab binds to the activated receptor with high affinity and blocks the binding of adhesive molecules. In contrast to abciximab, eptifibatide and tirofiban are synthetic small molecules.[37] Eptifibatide is a cyclic heptapeptide that binds GPIIb/IIIa because it incorporates the KGD motif, whereas tirofiban is a nonpeptidic tyrosine derivative that acts as an RGD mimetic. Abciximab has a long half-life and can be detected on the surface of platelets for up to 2 weeks. Eptifibatide and tirofiban have shorter half-lives.[37]

In addition to targeting the GPIIb/IIIa receptor, abciximab also inhibits the closely related $a_v\beta_3$ receptor, which binds vitronectin, and $a_M\beta_2$, a leukocyte integrin. In contrast, eptifibatide and tirofiban are specific for GPIIb/IIIa. Inhibition of $a_v\beta_3$ and $a_M\beta_2$ may endow abciximab with antiinflammatory and/or antiproliferative properties that extend beyond platelet inhibition.[37]

Dosing

All of the GPIIb/IIIa antagonists are given as an intravenous bolus followed by an infusion. Because they are cleared by the kidneys, the doses of eptifibatide and tirofiban must be reduced in patients with renal insufficiency.[37]

Side Effects

In addition to bleeding, thrombocytopenia is the most serious complication. Thrombocytopenia is immune-mediated and is caused by antibodies directed against neoantigens on GPIIb/IIIa that are exposed upon antagonist binding.[38] With abciximab, thrombocytopenia occurs in up to 5% of patients, and is severe in approximately 1% of these individuals. Thrombocytopenia is less common with the other two agents, occurring in approximately 1% of patients.

Indications

Abciximab and eptifibatide are used in patients undergoing percutaneous coronary interventions, particularly those with acute myocardial infarction.[39] Tirofiban is used in high-risk patients with unstable angina. Eptifibatide also can be used for this indication.[40]

New Antiplatelet Agents

Thienopyridines that produce more predictable suppression of ADP-induced platelet aggregation are under investigation.[41,42] Direct acting reversible $P2Y_{12}$ antagonists also have been developed. These agents can be given orally or parenterally and have a rapid onset of action because they are not prodrugs.[42] Finally, orally active inhibitors of the type 1 protease-activated receptor (PAR-1), the major thrombin receptor on platelets, also are entering clinical trials.

ANTICOAGULANTS

There are both parenteral and oral anticoagulants. Currently avail-able parenteral anticoagulants include heparin, low-molecular-weight heparin (LMWH) and fondaparinux, a synthetic pentasaccharide. The only available oral anticoagulants are the vitamin K antagonists, of which warfarin is the agent most often used in North America.

Parenteral Anticoagulants

Heparin

A sulfated polysaccharide, heparin is isolated from mammalian tissues rich in mast cells. Most commercial heparin is derived from porcine intestinal mucosa and is a polymer of alternating D-glucuronic acid and *N*-acetyl-D-glucosamine residues.[43]

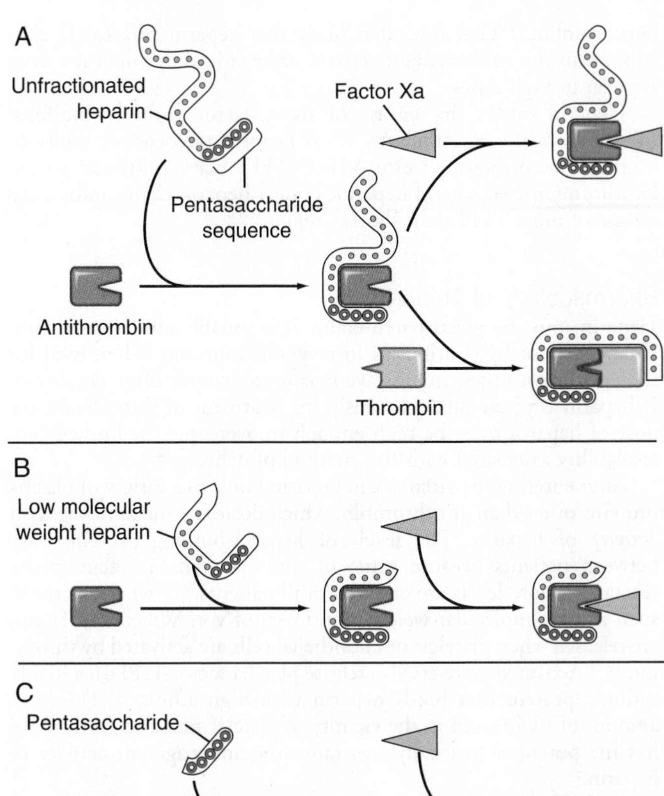

Figure 137–4 Mechanism of action of heparin, low-molecular-weight heparin, and fondaparinux, a synthetic pentasaccharide. (**A**) Heparin binds to antithrombin via its pentasaccharide sequence. This induces a conformational change in the reactive center loop of antithrombin that accelerates its interaction with factor Xa. To potentiate thrombin inhibition, heparin must simultaneously bind to antithrombin and thrombin. Only heparin chains composed of at least 18 saccharide units, which corresponds to a molecular weight of 5400, are of sufficient length to perform this bridging function. With a mean molecular weight of 15,000, all of the heparin chains are long enough to do this. (**B**) Low-molecular-weight heparin (LMWH) has greater capacity to potentiate factor Xa inhibition by antithrombin than thrombin because, with a mean molecular weight of 4500 to 5000, at least half of the LMWH chains are too short to bridge antithrombin to thrombin. (**C**) The pentasaccharide only accelerates factor Xa inhibition by antithrombin because the pentasaccharide is too short to bridge antithrombin to thrombin.

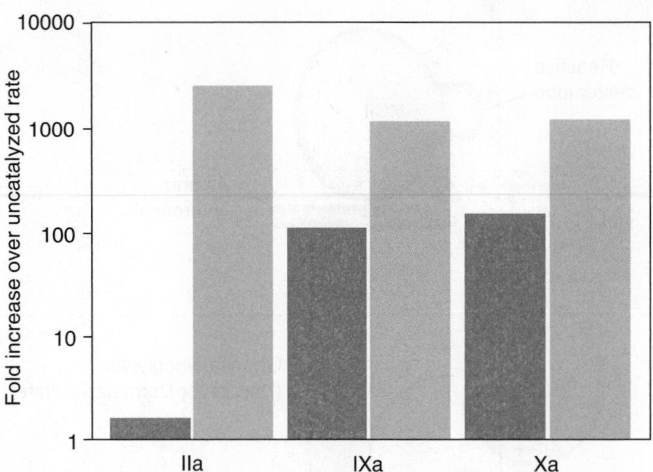

Figure 137–5 Comparison of the stimulatory effects of pentasaccharide and unfractionated heparin on catalysis of antithrombin-mediated inhibition of thrombin (IIa), factor IXa (IXa), and factor Xa (Xa). Second-order rate constants of inhibition of IIa, IXa, or Xa by antithrombin, measured in the presence of heparin (open bars) or fondaparinux (closed bars) were divided by those determined in the absence of glycosaminoglycan and are plotted as fold increase over the uncatalyzed rate of inhibition (reprinted with permission from Wiebe EM, Stafford AR, Fredenburgh JC, et al: Mechanism of catalysis of inhibition of factor IXa by antithrombin in the presence of heparin or pentasaccharide. J Biol Chem 278(37):35767, 2003.

Mechanism of Action

Heparin acts as an anticoagulant by activating antithrombin and accelerating the rate at which antithrombin inhibits enzymes involved in blood coagulation, particularly thrombin and factor Xa.[44] Antithrombin, the obligatory plasma cofactor for heparin,[44] is a 58,000 molecular weight single-chain polypeptide that is a member of the serine protease inhibitor (serpin) superfamily. Synthesized in the liver and circulating in plasma at a concentration of 2.6 μM, antithrombin acts as a suicide substrate for its target enzymes.

To activate antithrombin, heparin binds to the serpin via a unique pentasaccharide sequence that is found on one-third of the chains of commercial heparin (Fig. 137–4). The remainder of the heparin chains that lack this pentasaccharide sequence have little or no anticoagulant activity.[45] Once bound to antithrombin, heparin induces a conformational change in the reactive center loop of antithrombin that renders it more readily accessible to its target proteases. This conformational change enhances the rate at which antithrombin inhibits factor Xa by at least two orders of magnitude, but has little effect on the rate of thrombin inhibition by antithrombin.[46] To catalyze thrombin inhibition, heparin serves as a template that binds antithrombin and thrombin simultaneously.[47] Formation of this ternary complex brings the enzyme in close apposition to the inhibitor, thereby promoting the formation of a stable covalent thrombin–antithrombin complex.[47,48]

Only pentasaccharide-containing heparin chains composed of at least 18 saccharide units (which correspond to a molecular weight of 5400) are of sufficient length to bridge thrombin and antithrombin together.[49] With a mean molecular weight of 15,000, and a range of 5000 to 30,000, almost all of the chains of unfractionated heparin are long enough to effect this bridging function.[44] Consequently, by definition, heparin has equal capacity to promote the inhibition of thrombin and factor Xa by antithrombin and is assigned an anti–factor Xa to anti–factor IIa (thrombin) ratio of 1 : 1.[44]

Although current dogma states that heparin catalysis of factor Xa inhibition by antithrombin is mediated solely by the conformational changes evoked by pentasaccharide binding to antithrombin, recent studies have challenged this concept. Thus, in the presence of calcium, a heparin-binding site on factor Xa is exposed.[50,51] By binding simultaneously to this site on factor Xa and to antithrombin, longer pentasaccharide-containing heparin chains accelerate the rate of factor Xa inhibition by antithrombin more than shorter chains. The same is true for heparin catalysis of factor IXa inhibition by antithrombin.[52,53] Thus, maximum enhancement in the rate of factor Xa or factor IXa inhibition by antithrombin requires heparin chains that are of sufficient length to bridge the enzymes to antithrombin (Fig. 137–5).

In addition to activating antithrombin, heparin also can catalyze heparin cofactor II. This 66,000 molecular weight serpin, which is found in plasma at a concentration of 1.2 M, is a specific inhibitor of thrombin.[54] Two features account for the specificity of heparin cofactor II. First, the reactive site of heparin cofactor II contains the sequence Leu444–Ser445, a peptide bond that is not readily susceptible to cleavage by coagulation proteases other than thrombin.[55] Second, heparin cofactor II possesses a unique anionic sequence at its N-terminal. In its unactivated state, this sequence forms an intramolecular bond with the positively charged glycosaminoglycan-binding site located on the body of heparin cofactor II. When heparin or dermatan sulfate, a glycosaminoglycan that interacts only with

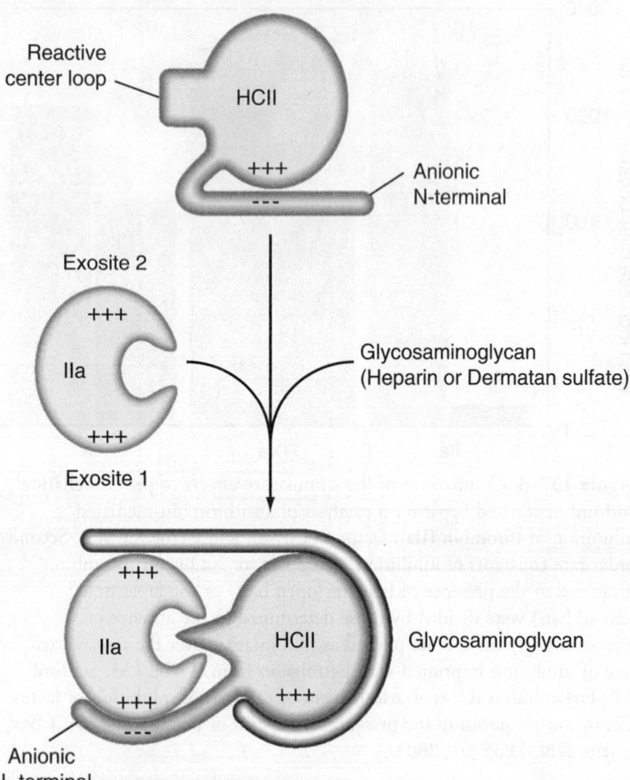

Figure 137–6 Catalysis of heparin cofactor II (HCII) by glycosaminoglycans. In its inactivated form, the acidic N-terminal tail of HCII is tethered to the positively charged glycosaminoglycan-binding site on the body of the serpin. The binding of heparin or dermatan sulfate to this binding site displaces the N-terminal tail, thereby facilitating the interaction of this anionic domain with exosite 1 on thrombin. Glycosaminoglycan binding also evokes a conformational change in the reactive center loop of HCII that contributes to the formation of the HCII–thrombin complex. Longer heparin chains not only bind to HCII, but also bind to the heparin-binding domain on thrombin, so-called exosite 2. Heparin-mediated bridging of HCII to thrombin enhances the rate of inhibition. Consequently, longer heparin chains that contain at least 26 saccharide units promote thrombin inhibition by HCII to a greater extent than shorter chains. Unlike heparin, dermatan sulfate does not need to bind to thrombin for maximal enhancement in the rate of thrombin inhibition because shorter dermatan sulfate fragments are just as active as longer ones.

heparin cofactor II, binds to heparin cofactor II, this N-terminal sequence is displaced, which enables its tethering to a positively charged domain on thrombin, exosite 1.[56–59] This tethering interaction occurs only with thrombin and facilitates thrombin inhibition by heparin cofactor II (Fig. 137–6).

Maximum catalysis of heparin cofactor II by heparin requires heparin chains composed of at least 26 saccharide units, which corresponds to a molecular weight of 7800.[60,61] Longer heparin chains activate heparin cofactor II to a greater extent than shorter chains because the longer chains are of sufficient length to not only bind to heparin cofactor II, but to also bind to thrombin to form a ternary complex.[62] Formation of this complex brings thrombin and heparin cofactor II into close apposition.

The interaction of heparin with heparin cofactor II is not mediated by the antithrombin-binding pentasaccharide sequence.[63] Because heparin lacks a specific heparin cofactor II-binding domain, heparin's affinity for heparin cofactor II is lower than that for antithrombin. Consequently, 10-fold higher heparin concentrations are needed to accelerate thrombin inhibition by heparin cofactor II in plasma than are necessary to enhance thrombin's inactivation by antithrombin.[64] Therefore, it is likely that heparin cofactor II contributes to the anticoagulant activity of heparin only when the drug is given in high doses.

Heparin causes the release of tissue factor pathway inhibitor (TFPI) from the endothelium.[65,66] A factor Xa-dependent inhibitor of tissue factor-bound factor VIIa,[67] TFPI may contribute to the antithrombotic activity of heparin. Longer heparin chains induce the release of more TFPI than shorter chains.[65,66]

Pharmacology of Heparin

Heparin must be given parenterally. It is usually administered subcutaneously or by continuous intravenous infusion. When used for therapeutic purposes, the intravenous route is most often employed. If heparin is given subcutaneously for treatment of thrombosis, the dose of heparin must be high enough to overcome the limited bioavailability associated with this method of delivery.[44]

After entering the circulation, heparin binds to a variety of plasma proteins other than antithrombin, which decreases the anticoagulant activity of heparin. The levels of heparin-binding proteins vary between patients because some of these proteins are acute-phase reactants whose levels are elevated in ill patients,[68,69] whereas others, such as high-molecular-weight multimers of von Willebrand factor, are released when platelets or endothelial cells are activated by thrombin.[70,71] Activated platelets also release platelet factor 4 (PF4), a highly cationic protein that binds heparin with high affinity.[72] The large amount of PF4 found in the vicinity of platelet-rich arterial thrombi has the potential to locally neutralize the anticoagulant activity of heparin.[73]

Because the levels of heparin-binding proteins are so variable between patients, the anticoagulant response to fixed or weight-adjusted doses of heparin is unpredictable. Consequently, coagulation monitoring is essential to ensure that a therapeutic response is obtained when heparin is administered for treatment purposes.

Heparin is cleared through a combination of a rapid saturable and a much slower first-order mechanism.[74–76] The saturable phase of heparin clearance is thought to be due to binding to endothelial cell receptors[77,78] and macrophages.[79] Bound heparin is internalized and depolymerized.[80,81] The slower nonsaturable mechanism of clearance is largely renal. At therapeutic doses, a large proportion of heparin is cleared through the rapid saturable, dose-dependent mechanism. The complex kinetics of clearance make the anticoagulant response to heparin nonlinear at therapeutic doses, with both the intensity and duration of effect rising disproportionately with increasing dose. Thus, the apparent biological half-life of heparin increases from approximately 30 minutes after an intravenous bolus of 25 U/kg, to 60 minutes with an intravenous bolus of 100 U/kg, to 150 minutes with a bolus of 400 U/kg.[74–76]

Monitoring

Heparin therapy can be monitored using the activated partial thromboplastin time (aPTT) or anti–factor Xa level. Although the aPTT is the test most often employed for this purpose, there are problems with this assay. aPTT reagents vary in their sensitivity to heparin, and the type of instrumentation used for testing can influence the results.[82] Consequently, laboratories must establish a therapeutic aPTT range with each reagent–instrument combination by measuring the aPTT and anti–factor Xa level in plasma samples collected from heparin-treated patients. For most of the aPTT reagents and instruments in current use, therapeutic heparin levels are achieved with a two- to threefold prolongation of the aPTT.[83]

Anti–factor Xa levels also can be used to monitor heparin therapy. With this test, therapeutic heparin levels range from 0.3 to 0.7 units/mL. Although this test is gaining in popularity, anti–factor Xa assays have yet to be standardized, and results can vary widely between laboratories.

Up to 25% of heparin-treated patients with venous thromboembolism require more than 35,000 units/day to achieve a therapeutic aPTT. These patients are considered heparin resistant.[84] It is useful to measure anti–factor Xa levels in these patients because many will have a therapeutic anti–factor Xa level despite a subtherapeutic aPTT. This dissociation in test results occurs because elevated plasma levels of fibrinogen and factor VIII, both of which are acute-phase proteins, shorten the aPTT but have no effect on anti–factor Xa levels.[85] Heparin therapy in patients who exhibit this phenomenon is best monitored using anti–factor Xa levels instead of the aPTT.[84] Patients with congenital or acquired antithrombin deficiency and those with unusually high levels of heparin-binding proteins often require very high doses of heparin to achieve a therapeutic aPTT or anti–factor Xa level. If there is good correlation between the aPTT and the anti–factor Xa levels, either test can be used to monitor heparin therapy.

Dosing

For prophylaxis, heparin is usually given in fixed doses of 5000 units subcutaneously two or three times daily. With these low doses, coagulation monitoring is unnecessary.[86] In contrast, monitoring is essential when heparin is given in therapeutic doses because a subtherapeutic anticoagulant response has been associated with a higher risk of recurrent thrombosis.[87–90] Fixed-dose or weight-based heparin nomograms are used to standardize heparin dosing and to shorten the time required to achieve a therapeutic anticoagulant response. At least two heparin nomograms have been validated in patients with venous thromboembolism and reduce the time required to achieve a therapeutic aPTT.[91,92] Weight-adjusted heparin nomograms also have been evaluated in patients with acute coronary syndromes.[93,94]

A recent study indicates that unmonitored twice daily subcutaneous heparin is as effective and safe as once-daily low-molecular-weight heparin for initial treatment of venous thromboembolism. High doses of heparin were used; treatment was started with a dose of 333 units/kg followed by 250 units/kg twice daily thereafter.[95] Based on these findings, unmonitored high-dose subcutaneous heparin is a viable treatment option in patients with renal insufficiency where low-molecular-weight heparin or fondaparinux is problematic.

Limitations of Heparin

Heparin has pharmacokinetic and biophysical limitations (Table 137–2). The pharmacokinetic limitations reflect heparin's propensity to bind in a pentasaccharide-independent fashion to cells and plasma proteins. Heparin binding to cells explains its dose-dependent clearance, whereas binding to plasma proteins results in a variable anticoagulant response and can lead to heparin resistance.

The biophysical limitations of heparin reflect the inability of the heparin-antithrombin complex to (a) inhibit factor Xa when it is incorporated into the prothrombinase complex,[96,97] the complex that converts prothrombin to thrombin, and (b) to inhibit thrombin bound to fibrin.[98,99] Consequently, factor Xa bound to activated platelets within platelet-rich thrombi has the potential to generate thrombin, even in the face of heparin.[100] Once this thrombin binds to fibrin, it too is protected from inhibition by the heparin–antithrombin complex.[98,99] Clot-associated thrombin can then trigger thrombus growth by locally activating platelets and amplifying its own generation through feedback activation of factors V, VIII, and XI.[101–103] Further compounding the problem is the potential for heparin neutralization by the high concentrations of PF4 released from activated platelets within the platelet-rich thrombus.[73]

Table 137–2 Pharmacokinetic and Biophysical Limitations of Heparin

Limitations	Mechanism
Poor bioavailability at low doses	Limited absorption of long heparin chains
Dose-dependent clearance	Binds to endothelial cells
Variable anticoagulant response	Binds to plasma proteins whose levels vary from patient to patient
Reduced activity in the vicinity of platelet-limited activity against factor Xa incorporated in the prothrombinase complex and thrombin bound to fibrin	Neutralized by platelet factor 4–released rich thrombi from activated platelets Reduced capacity of heparin-antithrombin complex to inhibit factor Xa bound to activated platelets and thrombin bound to fibrin

Side Effects

The most common side effect of heparin is bleeding. Other complications include thrombocytopenia, osteoporosis, and elevated levels of transaminases.

Bleeding

The risk of heparin-induced bleeding increases with higher heparin doses. Concomitant administration of drugs that affect hemostasis, such as antiplatelet or fibrinolytic agents, increases the risk of bleeding, as does recent surgery or trauma.[104] Heparin-treated patients with serious bleeding can be given protamine sulfate to neutralize the heparin. Protamine sulfate, a mixture of basic polypeptides isolated from salmon sperm, binds heparin with high affinity, and the resultant protamine–heparin complexes are then cleared. Typically, 1 mg of protamine sulfate, administered intravenously, neutralizes 100 units of heparin. Anaphylactoid reactions to protamine sulfate can occur, and drug administration by slow intravenous infusion is recommended to reduce the risk of these problems.[105,106]

Thrombocytopenia

Heparin can cause thrombocytopenia. Heparin-induced thrombocytopenia (HIT) is an antibody-mediated process that is triggered by antibodies directed against neoantigens on PF4 that are exposed when heparin binds to this protein.[107] These antibodies, which usually are of the IgG class, bind simultaneously to the heparin-PF4 complex and to platelet Fc receptors. Such binding activates the platelets and generates platelet microparticles. Circulating microparticles are prothrombotic because they express anionic phospholipids on their surface and can bind clotting factors, thereby promoting thrombin generation.[108]

The features of HIT are illustrated in Table 137–3. Typically, HIT occurs 5 to 14 days after initiation of heparin therapy, but it can manifest earlier if the patient has received heparin within the past 3 months.[109] It is rare for the platelet count to fall below 100,000/μL in patients with HIT, and even a 50% decrease in the platelet count from the pretreatment value should raise the suspicion of HIT in those receiving heparin.[107] HIT is more common in surgical patients

Table 137–3 Features of Heparin-Induced Thrombocytopenia

Features	Details
Thrombocytopenia	Platelet count of 100,000/μL or less or a decrease in platelet count of 50% or more
Timing	Platelet count falls 5–10 days after starting heparin
Type of heparin	More common with unfractionated heparin than low-molecular-weight heparin
Type of patient	More common in surgical patients than medical patients. More common in women than in men
Thrombosis	Venous thrombosis more common than arterial thrombosis

Management of Heparin-Induced Thrombocytopenia

- Stop all heparin
- Give an alternative anticoagulant, such as lepirudin, argatroban, bivalirudin, danaparoid or fondaparinux
- Do not give platelet transfusions
- Do not give warfarin until the platelet count returns to its baseline level. If warfarin was administered, give vitamin K to restore the INR to normal
- Evaluate for thrombosis, particularly deep vein thrombosis

than in medical patients and, like many autoimmune disorders, occurs more frequently in females than in males.[110]

HIT can be associated with thrombosis, either arterial or venous. Venous thrombosis, which manifests as deep vein thrombosis and/or pulmonary embolism, is more common than arterial thrombosis. Arterial thrombosis can manifest as ischemic stroke or acute myocardial infarction. Rarely, platelet-rich thrombi in the distal aorta or iliac arteries can cause critical limb ischemia.[107]

The diagnosis of HIT is established using enzyme-linked assays to detect antibodies against heparin–PF4 complexes or with platelet activation assays. Enzyme-linked assays are sensitive but can be positive in the absence of any clinical evidence of HIT.[107] The most specific diagnostic test is the serotonin release assay. This test is performed by quantifying serotonin release when washed platelets loaded with labeled serotonin are exposed to patient serum in the absence or presence of varying concentrations of heparin. If the patient serum contains the HIT antibody, heparin addition induces platelet activation and subsequent serotonin release.[107]

Management of HIT is outlined in the box below. Heparin should be stopped in patients with suspected or documented HIT, and an alternative anticoagulant should be administered to prevent or treat thrombosis.[107,111] The agents most often used for this indication are parenteral direct thrombin inhibitors, such as lepirudin, argatroban or bivalirudin, or factor Xa inhibitors, such as fondaparinux or danaparoid.

Patients with HIT, particularly those with associated thrombosis, often have evidence of increased thrombin generation that can lead to consumption of protein C. If these patients are given warfarin without a concomitant parenteral anticoagulant to suppress thrombin generation, the further decrease in protein C levels induced by warfarin can trigger skin necrosis.[112,113] To avoid this problem, patients with HIT should be treated with a direct thrombin inhibitor or fondaparinux until the platelet count returns to normal levels. At this point, low-dose warfarin therapy can be introduced, and the thrombin inhibitor or fondaparinux can be discontinued when the anticoagulant response to warfarin has been therapeutic for at least 2 days.[107]

Osteoporosis

Treatment with therapeutic doses of heparin for over a month can cause a reduction in bone density. This complication has been reported in up to 30% of patients given long-term heparin therapy,[114–117] and symptomatic vertebral fractures occur in 2% to 3% of these individuals.

Studies in vitro[118] and in laboratory animals[119–121] have provided insights into the pathogenesis of heparin-induced osteoporosis. These investigations suggest that heparin causes bone resorption both by decreasing bone formation and by enhancing bone resorption. Thus, heparin affects the activity of both osteoblasts and osteoclasts.

Elevated Levels of Transaminases

Therapeutic doses of heparin frequently cause modest elevation in the serum levels of hepatic transaminases, without a concomitant increase in the level of bilirubin.[122,123] The levels of transaminases rapidly return to normal when the drug is stopped. The mechanism responsible for this phenomenon is unknown.

Advantages of Low-Molecular-Weight Heparin over Heparin

Advantage	*Consequence*
Better bioavailability and longer half-life after subcutaneous injection	Can be given subcutaneously once or twice daily for both prophylaxis and treatment
Dose-independent clearance	Simplified dosing
Predictable anticoagulant response	Coagulation monitoring is unnecessary in most patients
Lower risk of heparin-induced thrombocytopenia	Safer than heparin for short or long-term administration
Lower risk of osteoporosis	Safer than heparin for extended administration

Low-Molecular-Weight Heparin

Consisting of smaller fragments of heparin, low-molecular-weight heparin is prepared from unfractionated heparin by controlled enzymatic or chemical depolymerization. The mean molecular weight of low-molecular-weight heparin is approximately 5000, one-third the mean molecular weight of unfractionated heparin.[124] Low-molecular-weight heparin has advantages over heparin and has replaced heparin for most indications.

Mechanism of Action

Like heparin, low-molecular-weight heparin exerts its anticoagulant activity by activating antithrombin. With a mean molecular weight of 5000, which corresponds to approximately 17 saccharide units, at least half of the pentasaccharide-containing chains of low-molecular-weight heparin are too short to bridge thrombin to antithrombin (Fig. 137–4). However, these chains retain the capacity to accelerate factor Xa inhibition by antithrombin because this activity is largely the result of the conformational changes in antithrombin evoked by pentasaccharide binding. Consequently, low-molecular-weight heparin catalyzes factor Xa inhibition by antithrombin more than thrombin inhibition.[125] Depending on their unique molecular weight distributions, low-molecular-weight heparin preparations have anti–factor Xa to anti–factor IIa ratios ranging from 2:1 to 4:1.

Pharmacology

Although usually given subcutaneously, low-molecular-weight heparin also can be administered intravenously if a rapid anticoagulant response is needed. Low-molecular-weight heparin has pharmacokinetic advantages over heparin.[124,125] These advantages reflect the fact that shorter heparin chains bind less avidly to endothelial cells, macrophages, and heparin-binding plasma proteins.[126–128] Reduced binding to endothelial cells and macrophages eliminates the rapid, dose-dependent, and saturable mechanism of clearance that is a characteristic of unfractionated heparin. Instead, the clearance of low-molecular-weight heparin is dose-independent and its plasma half-life is longer.[85,86] Based on measurement of anti–factor Xa levels, low-molecular-weight heparin has a plasma half-life of approximately 4 hours. Low-molecular-weight heparin is cleared almost exclusively by the kidneys and the drug can accumulate in patients with renal insufficiency.[124,125]

Low-molecular-weight heparin exhibits approximately 90% bioavailability after subcutaneous injection.[124,125] Because low-molecular-weight heparin binds less avidly to heparin-binding proteins in plasma than heparin, low-molecular-weight heparin produces a more predictable dose response and resistance to low-molecular-weight heparin is rare. With a longer half-life and more predictable anticoagulant response, low-molecular-weight heparin can be given subcutaneously once or twice daily without coagulation monitoring, even when the drug is given in treatment doses.[124] These properties render low-molecular-weight heparin more convenient than unfractionated heparin. Capitalizing on this feature, studies in patients with venous thromboembolism have shown that home treatment with low-molecular-weight heparin is as effective and safe as in-hospital treatment with continuous intravenous infusions of heparin.[129–131] Out-patient treatment with low-molecular-weight heparin streamlines care, reduces health care costs, and increases patient satisfaction.

Monitoring

In the majority of patients, low-molecular-weight heparin does not require coagulation monitoring. If monitoring is necessary, anti–factor Xa levels must be measured because most low-molecular-weight heparin preparations have little effect on the aPTT. Therapeutic anti–factor Xa levels with low-molecular-weight heparin range from 0.5 to 1.2 units/mL when measured 3 to 4 hours after drug administration. When low-molecular-weight heparin is given in prophylactic doses, peak anti–factor Xa levels of 0.2 to 0.5 units/mL are desirable.[132]

Indications for low-molecular-weight heparin monitoring include renal insufficiency and obesity. Low-molecular-weight heparin monitoring in patients with a creatinine clearance of 50 mL/minute or less is advisable to ensure that there is no drug accumulation. Although weight-adjusted low-molecular-weight heparin dosing appears to produce therapeutic anti–factor Xa levels in patients who are overweight, this approach has not been extensively evaluated in those with morbid obesity. It may also be advisable to monitor the anticoagulant activity of low-molecular-weight heparin during pregnancy because dose requirements can change, particularly in the third trimester.[132] Monitoring also is important in high-risk settings, such as in patients with mechanical heart valves who are given low-molecular-weight heparin for prevention of valve thrombosis.

Dosing

The doses of low-molecular-weight heparin recommended for prophylaxis or treatment vary depending on the low-molecular-weight heparin preparation. For prophylaxis, once-daily subcutaneous doses of 4000 to 5000 units are often used, whereas doses of 2500 to 3000 units are given when the drug is administered twice daily. For treatment of venous thromboembolism, a dose of 150 to 200 units/kg is given if the drug is administered once daily. If a twice-daily regimen is employed, a dose of 100 units/kg is given. In patients with unstable angina, low-molecular-weight heparin is given subcutaneously on a twice-daily basis at a dose of 100 to 120 units/kg.[124]

Side Effects

The major complication of low-molecular-weight heparin is bleeding. Recent meta-analyses suggest that the risk of major bleeding may be lower with low-molecular-weight heparin than with unfractionated heparin.[133,134] HIT and osteoporosis are less common with low-molecular-weight heparin than with unfractionated heparin.[124]

Bleeding

Like the situation with heparin, bleeding with low-molecular-weight heparin is common in patients receiving concomitant therapy with antiplatelet or fibrinolytic drugs. Recent surgery, trauma, or underlying hemostatic defects also increase the risk of bleeding with low-molecular-weight heparin.[104]

Although protamine sulfate can be used as an antidote for low-molecular-weight heparin, protamine sulfate incompletely neutralizes the anticoagulant activity of low-molecular-weight heparin because it only binds the longer chains of low-molecular-weight heparin.[135] Because longer chains are responsible for catalysis of thrombin inhibition by antithrombin, protamine sulfate completely reverses the antithrombin activity of low-molecular-weight heparin. In contrast, protamine sulfate only partially reverses the anti–factor Xa activity of low-molecular-weight heparin because the shorter pentasaccharide-containing chains of low-molecular-weight heparin do not bind to protamine sulfate. Consequently, patients at high risk for bleeding may be more safely treated with continuous intravenous unfractionated heparin than with subcutaneous low-molecular-weight heparin. In addition to the potential for complete reversal with protamine sulfate, the short half-life of intravenous heparin also is an advantage if major bleeding occurs.

Thrombocytopenia

The risk of HIT is approximately fivefold lower with low-molecular-weight heparin than with heparin.[136,137] Low-molecular-weight heparin binds less avidly to platelets and causes less PF4 release. Furthermore, with lower affinity for PF4 than heparin, low-molecular-weight heparin is less likely to induce the conformational changes in PF4 that trigger the formation of HIT antibodies.

Low-molecular-weight heparin should not be used to treat HIT patients[107,111] because most HIT antibodies exhibit cross reactivity with low-molecular-weight heparin.[138,139] This in vitro cross reactivity is not simply a laboratory phenomenon because there are case reports of thrombosis when HIT patients are treated with low-molecular-weight heparin.

Osteoporosis

The risk of osteoporosis is lower with long-term low-molecular-weight heparin than with heparin.[140] For extended treatment, therefore, low-molecular-weight heparin is a better choice than heparin because of the lower risk of both osteoporosis and HIT.

Fondaparinux

A synthetic analog of the antithrombin-binding pentasaccharide sequence, fondaparinux differs from low-molecular-weight heparin in several ways (Table 137–4). Fondaparinux is licensed for (a) thromboprophylaxis in medical, general surgical and high-risk orthopedic patients, and (b) as an alternative to heparin or low-molecular-weight heparin for initial treatment of patients with established venous thromboembolism. In some countries, fondaparinux also is approved for treatment of patients with acute coronary syndromes.

Table 137–4 Comparison of Low-Molecular-Weight Heparin and Fondaparinux

Features	LMWH	Fondaparinux
Molecular weight	4500–5000	1728
Catalysis of factor Xa inhibition	Yes	Yes
Catalysis of thrombin inhibition	Yes	No
Bioavailability after subcutaneous administration (%)	90	100
Plasma half-life (hours)	4	17
Renal excretion	Yes	Yes
Induces release of tissue factor pathway inhibitor	Yes	No
Neutralized by protamine sulfate	Partially	No

LMWH, low-molecular-weight heparin.

Mechanism of Action

As a synthetic analog of the antithrombin-binding pentasaccharide sequence found in heparin and low-molecular-weight heparin, fondaparinux has a molecular weight of 1728. Fondaparinux binds only to antithrombin (Fig. 137–4) and is too short to bridge thrombin to antithrombin. Consequently, fondaparinux catalyzes factor Xa inhibition by antithrombin and does not enhance the rate of thrombin inhibition.[141]

Pharmacology of Fondaparinux

Fondaparinux exhibits complete bioavailability after subcutaneous injection. With no binding to endothelial cells or plasma proteins, the clearance of fondaparinux is dose independent and its plasma half-life is approximately 17 hours.[142] The drug is given subcutaneously once daily. Because fondaparinux is cleared unchanged via the kidneys, it is contraindicated in patients with a creatinine clearance less than 30 mL/minute and it should be used with caution in those with a creatinine clearance less than 50 mL/minute.[141]

Fondaparinux produces a predictable anticoagulant response after administration in fixed doses because it does not bind to plasma proteins. The drug is given at a dose of 2.5 mg once daily for prevention of venous thromboembolism. For initial treatment of established venous thromboembolism, fondaparinux is given at a dose of 7.5 mg once daily. The dose can be reduced to 5 mg once daily for those weighing less than 50 kg and increased to 10 mg for those more than 100 kg. When given in these doses, fondaparinux is as effective as heparin or low-molecular-weight heparin for initial treatment of patients with deep vein thrombosis or pulmonary embolism and is associated with similar rates of bleeding.[143,144]

Fondaparinux is used at a dose of 2.5 mg once daily in patients with acute coronary syndromes. When this prophylactic dose of fondaparinux was compared with treatment doses of enoxaparin in patients with non-ST-segment elevation acute coronary syndromes, there was no difference in the rate of cardiovascular death, myocardial infarction, or stroke at 9 days.[145] However, the rate of major bleeding was 50% lower with fondaparinux than with enoxaparin, a low-molecular-weight heparin preparation—a difference that likely reflects the fact that the dose of fondaparinux was lower than that of enoxaparin. In acute coronary syndrome patients who require percutaneous coronary interventions, there is a risk of catheter thrombosis with fondaparinux unless adjunctive heparin is given.[146]

Side Effects

Fondaparinux does not cause HIT and, in contrast to low-molecular-weight heparin, there is no cross reactivity of fondaparinux with HIT antibodies. Fondaparinux can induce the formation of HIT antibodies to the same extent as low-molecular-weight heparin, however.[147] In contrast to heparin or low-molecular-weight heparin, fondaparinux is too short to cluster PF4 tetramers together, which is a prerequisite for HIT antibody binding.[148] This phenomenon not only explains why HIT antibodies do not cross-react with fondaparinux, but also explains why fondaparinux does not cause HIT despite the fact that it induces the formation of HIT antibodies. Fondaparinux has been successfully used for HIT treatment.[149] However, large clinical trials supporting the use of fondaparinux for this indication are lacking.

The major side effect of fondaparinux is bleeding. There is no antidote for fondaparinux. Protamine sulfate has no effect on the anticoagulant activity of fondaparinux because it fails to bind to the drug. Recombinant activated factor VII reverses the anticoagulant effects of fondaparinux in volunteers,[150] but it is unknown whether this agent will control fondaparinux-induced bleeding.

Parenteral Direct Thrombin Inhibitors

Heparin and low-molecular-weight heparin are indirect inhibitors of thrombin because their activity is mediated by antithrombin. In contrast, direct thrombin inhibitors do not require a plasma cofactor; instead, these agents bind directly to thrombin and block its interaction with its substrates. Approved parenteral direct thrombin inhibitors include lepirudin (Refludan), argatroban (Novastan), and bivalirudin (Angiomax) (Table 137–5). Lepirudin and argatroban are licensed for treatment of patients with HIT, whereas bivalirudin is approved as an alternative to heparin in patients undergoing percutaneous coronary interventions, including those with HIT.[151]

Table 137–5 Comparison of the Properties of Hirudin, Bivalirudin, and Argatroban

	Hirudin	Bivalirudin	Argatroban
Molecular mass	7000	1980	527
Site(s) of interaction with thrombin	Active site and exosite 1	Active site and exosite 1	Active site
Renal clearance	Yes	No	No
Hepatic metabolism	No	No	Yes
Plasma half-life (minute)	60	25	45

Lepirudin

A recombinant form of hirudin, lepirudin is a bivalent direct thrombin inhibitor that interacts with both the active site and exosite 1, the substrate-binding site, on thrombin.[151] For rapid anticoagulation, lepirudin is given by continuous intravenous infusion, but the drug can be given subcutaneously for thromboprophylaxis. Lepirudin has a plasma half-life of 60 minutes after intravenous infusion and is cleared by the kidneys. Consequently, lepirudin accumulates in patients with renal insufficiency.[152] A high proportion of lepirudin-treated patients develop antibodies against the drug.[153] Although these antibodies rarely cause problems, in a small subset of patients they can delay lepirudin clearance and prolong its anticoagulant activity. Serious bleeding has been reported in some of these patients.[153]

Lepirudin is usually monitored using the aPTT and the dose is adjusted to maintain a aPTT that is 1.5 to 2.5 times the control. The aPTT is not an ideal test for monitoring lepirudin therapy because the clotting time plateaus with higher drug concentrations. Although the ecarin clotting time provides a better index of lepirudin dose than does the aPTT, the ecarin clotting time has yet to be standardized.

Argatroban

A univalent inhibitor that targets the active site of thrombin, argatroban is metabolized in the liver.[151] Consequently, this drug must be used with caution in patients with hepatic insufficiency. Argatroban is not cleared via the kidneys so this drug is safer than lepirudin for HIT patients with renal insufficiency.

Argatroban is administered by continuous intravenous infusion and has a plasma half-life of approximately 45 minutes. The aPTT is used to monitor its anticoagulant effect and the dose is adjusted to achieve a aPTT 1.5 to 3 times the baseline value, but not to exceed 100 seconds. Argatroban also prolongs the international normalized ratio (INR), a feature that can complicate the transitioning of patients from argatroban to warfarin.[154] This problem can be circumvented by using the levels of factor X to monitor warfarin in place of the INR. Alternatively, the argatroban infusion can be stopped for 2 to 3 hours prior to INR determination.

Bivalirudin

A synthetic 20-amino acid analog of hirudin, bivalirudin is a divalent thrombin inhibitor.[151] Thus, the N-terminal portion of bivalirudin interacts with the active site of thrombin, whereas its C-terminal tail binds to exosite 1, the substrate-binding domain on thrombin. Bivalirudin has a plasma half-life of 25 minutes, the shortest half-life of all the parenteral direct thrombin inhibitors.[151] Bivalirudin is degraded by peptidases and is partially excreted via the kidneys. When given in high doses in the cardiac catheterization laboratory, the anticoagulant activity of bivalirudin is monitored using the activated clotting time. With lower doses, its activity can be assessed using the aPTT.

Studies comparing bivalirudin with heparin suggest that bivalirudin produces less bleeding.[155,156] This feature plus its short half-life make bivalirudin an attractive alternative to heparin in patients undergoing percutaneous coronary interventions,[157] and it is licensed for this indication. Bivalirudin also is approved for management of HIT patients who require percutaneous coronary interventions.[158]

ORAL ANTICOAGULANTS

Current oral anticoagulant practice dates back almost 60 years to when the vitamin K antagonists were discovered as a result of investigations into the cause of hemorrhagic disease in cattle. Characterized by a decrease in prothrombin levels, this disorder is caused by ingestion of hay containing spoiled sweet clover. Hydroxycoumarin, which was isolated from bacterial contaminants in the hay, interferes with vitamin K metabolism, thereby causing a syndrome similar to vitamin K deficiency. A variety of coumarin derivatives are available. The agent most widely used in North America is warfarin.

Warfarin

A water-soluble vitamin K antagonist, warfarin was initially developed as a rodenticide. Like other vitamin K antagonists, warfarin interferes with the synthesis of the vitamin K-dependent clotting proteins, which include prothrombin and factors VII, IX, and X. The synthesis of the vitamin K-dependent anticoagulant proteins, proteins C and S, also is reduced by vitamin K antagonists.

Mechanism of Action

All of the vitamin K-dependent clotting factors possess glutamic acid residues at their N-termini. A posttranslational modification adds a carboxyl group to the γ-carbon of these residues to generate γ-carboxyglutamic acid.[159] This modification is essential for expression of the activity of these clotting factors because it permits their calcium-dependent binding to negatively charged phospholipid surfaces.[160,161] The γ-carboxylation process is catalyzed by a vitamin K-dependent carboxylase. Thus, vitamin K from the diet is reduced to vitamin K hydroquinone by vitamin K reductase (Fig. 137–7). Vitamin K hydroquinone serves as a cofactor for the carboxylase enzyme, which in the presence of carbon dioxide replaces the hydrogen on the γ-carbon of glutamic acid residues with a carboxyl group. During this process, vitamin K hydroquinone is oxidized to vitamin K epoxide, which is then reduced to vitamin K by vitamin K epoxide reductase.[162]

Warfarin inhibits vitamin K epoxide reductase (VKOR), thereby blocking the γ-carboxylation process.[162,163] This results in the synthesis of vitamin K-dependent clotting proteins that are only partially γ-carboxylated.[164] Warfarin acts as an anticoagulant because these partially γ-carboxylated proteins have reduced or absent biological activity. The onset of action of warfarin is delayed until the newly synthesized clotting factors with reduced activity gradually replace their fully active counterparts.

The antithrombotic effect of warfarin depends on a reduction in the functional levels of factor X and prothrombin, clotting factors that have half-lives of 24 and 72 hours, respectively.[165] Because of the delay in achieving an antithrombotic effect, initial treatment with warfarin is supported by concomitant administration of a rapidly acting parenteral anticoagulant, such as heparin, low-molecular-weight heparin, or fondaparinux, in patients with established thrombosis or at high risk for thrombosis.[126]

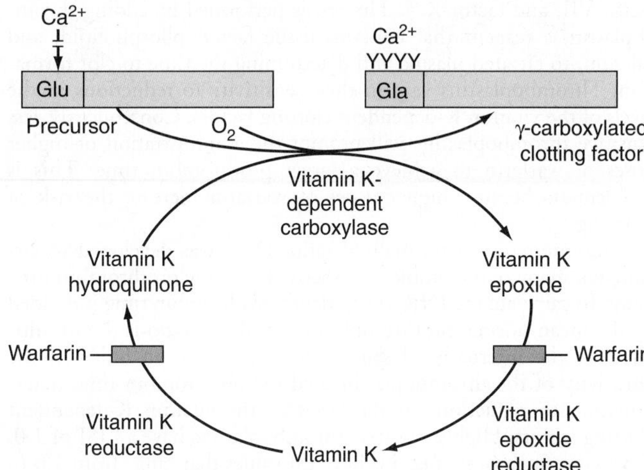

Figure 137–7 The vitamin K cycle and its inhibition by warfarin. Dietary vitamin K is reduced by vitamin K reductase to generate vitamin K hydroquinone. Vitamin K hydroquinone serves as a cofactor for the vitamin K-dependent carboxylase that converts glutamic acid residues at the N-termini of the vitamin K-dependent precursors to γ-carboxyglutamic acid residues, thereby creating the so-called Gla-domain. By binding calcium, the Gla-domain is critical for the interaction of the vitamin K-dependent clotting factors with negatively charged phospholipid membranes. During vitamin K-dependent carboxylation, vitamin K is oxidized to vitamin K epoxide. Vitamin K epoxide is then converted to vitamin K by vitamin K epoxide reductase. Vitamin K antagonists, such as warfarin, interfere with this cycle by inhibiting vitamin K epoxide reductase and vitamin K reductase. Of these two enzymes, vitamin K epoxide reductase is more readily blocked by vitamin K antagonists than vitamin K reductase. Consequently, supplemental vitamin K can overcome the inhibitory effects of vitamin K antagonists.

Pharmacology

Warfarin is a racemic mixture of *R* and *S* isomers. Of these, the *S* isomer is more active. Warfarin is rapidly and almost completely absorbed from the gastrointestinal tract. Levels of warfarin in the blood peak approximately 90 minutes after drug administration.[165] Racemic warfarin has a plasma half-life of 36 to 42 hours, and more than 97% of circulating warfarin is bound to albumin. It is only the small fraction of unbound warfarin that is biologically active.[165]

Warfarin accumulates in the liver, where the two isomers are metabolized via distinct pathways. Oxidative metabolism of the *S* isomer is effected by CYP2C9. Two relatively common variants, *CYP2C9*2* and *CYP2C9*3*, have reduced activity. Patients with these variants require lower maintenance doses of warfarin. Polymorphisms in *VKORC1* also can influence the anticoagulant response to warfarin.[166,167] These findings have prompted a recommendation that patients starting on warfarin should be tested for these polymorphisms and that this information should be incorporated into their warfarin-dosing algorithms. Whether this approach will increase the efficacy and/or safety of warfarin therapy is unproven.

In addition to genetic factors, the anticoagulant effect of warfarin is influenced by diet, drugs, and various disease states. Fluctuations in dietary vitamin K intake affect the activity of warfarin. A wide variety of drugs can alter absorption, clearance, or metabolism of warfarin.[165] Because of the variability in the anticoagulant response to warfarin, coagulation monitoring is essential to ensure that a therapeutic response is obtained.

Monitoring

Warfarin therapy is most often monitored using the prothrombin time, a test that is sensitive to reductions in the levels of prothrombin, factor VII, and factor X.[165] The test is performed by adding thromboplastin, a reagent that contains tissue factor, phospholipid, and calcium, to citrated plasma and determining the time to clot formation. Thromboplastins vary in their sensitivity to reductions in the levels of the vitamin K-dependent clotting factors. Consequently, less sensitive thromboplastins will prompt the administration of higher doses of warfarin to achieve a target prothrombin time. This is problematic because higher doses of warfarin increase the risk of bleeding.

The international normalized ratio (INR) was developed to circumvent many of the problems associated with the prothrombin time assay. To calculate the INR, the patient's prothrombin time is divided by the mean normal prothrombin time and this ratio is then multiplied by the international sensitivity index (ISI), an index of the sensitivity of the thromboplastin used for prothrombin time determination to reductions in the levels of the vitamin K-dependent clotting factors. Highly sensitive thromboplastins have an ISI of 1.0. Most current thromboplastins have ISI values that range from 1.0 to 1.4.[165]

Although the INR has helped standardize anticoagulant practice, problems persist. The precision of INR determination varies depending on reagent–instrumentation combinations. This leads to variability in the INR results. Also complicating INR determination is unreliable reporting of the ISI by thromboplastin manufacturers.[165] Furthermore, every laboratory must establish the mean normal prothrombin time with each new batch of thromboplastin reagent. To accomplish this, the prothrombin time must be measured in fresh plasma samples from at least 20 healthy volunteers using the same instrumentation that is used for patient samples.[165]

For most indications, warfarin is administered in doses that produce a target INR of 2.0 to 3.0. An exception is patients with mechanical heart valves where a target INR of 2.5 to 3.5 is recommended.[165] Vitamin K antagonists have a narrow therapeutic window. Thus, studies in atrial fibrillation demonstrate an increased risk of cardioembolic stroke when the INR falls below 1.7 and an increase in bleeding with INR values greater than 4.5.[168] Likewise, a study in patients receiving long-term warfarin therapy for unprovoked venous thromboembolism demonstrated a higher rate of recurrent venous thromboembolism when the warfarin dose was adjusted to achieve a target INR of 1.5 to 1.9 than with a target INR of 2.0 to 3.0. Rates of major bleeding were similar.[169]

Dosing

Warfarin is usually started at a dose of 5 to 10 mg. The dose is then titrated to achieve the desired target INR. Because of its delayed onset of action, patients with established thrombosis or those at high risk for thrombosis are given concomitant treatment with a rapidly acting parenteral anticoagulant, such as heparin, low-molecular-weight heparin, or fondaparinux. Initial prolongation of the INR reflects reduction in the functional levels of factor VII. Consequently, concomitant treatment with the parenteral anticoagulant should be continued until the INR has been therapeutic for at least 2 consecutive days. A minimum 5-day course of parenteral anticoagulation is recommended to ensure that the levels of prothrombin have been reduced into the therapeutic range with warfarin.[165]

Because warfarin has a narrow therapeutic window, frequent coagulation monitoring is essential to ensure that a therapeutic anticoagulant response is obtained. Even patients with stable warfarin dose requirements should have their INR determined every 2 to 4 weeks. More frequent monitoring is necessary when new medications are introduced because so many drugs enhance or reduce the anticoagulant effects of warfarin.

Side Effects

Like all anticoagulants, the major side effect of warfarin is bleeding. A rare complication is skin necrosis. Warfarin crosses the placenta and can cause fetal abnormalities. Consequently, warfarin is contraindicated during pregnancy.

Bleeding

At least half of the bleeding complications with warfarin occur when the INR exceeds the therapeutic range. Bleeding complications may be mild, such as epistaxis or hematuria, or more severe, such as retroperitoneal or gastrointestinal bleeding. Life-threatening intracranial bleeding also can occur.[165]

To minimize the risk of bleeding, the INR should be maintained in the therapeutic range. In asymptomatic patients whose INR is between 3.5 and 4.5, warfarin should be withheld until the INR returns to the therapeutic range. If the INR is greater than 4.5, a therapeutic INR can be achieved more rapidly by administration of low doses of sublingual vitamin K.[170,171] A sublingual vitamin K dose of 1 mg usually is adequate for patients with an INR between 4.9 and 9, whereas 2 to 3 mg can be used for those with an INR greater than 9. Higher doses of vitamin K can be administered if more rapid reversal of the INR is required or if the INR is excessively high.

Patients with serious bleeding need more aggressive treatment. These patients should be given 10 mg of vitamin K by slow intravenous infusion. Additional vitamin K should be given until the INR is in the normal range. Treatment with vitamin K should be supplemented with fresh frozen plasma as a source of the vitamin K-dependent clotting proteins. For life-threatening bleeds, or if patients cannot tolerate the volume load, recombinant factor VIIa or prothrombin complex concentrates can be used.

Warfarin-treated patients who experience bleeding when their INR is in the therapeutic range require investigation into the cause of the bleeding. Those with gastrointestinal bleeding often have underlying peptic ulcer disease or a tumor. Similarly, investigation of hematuria or uterine bleeding in patients with a therapeutic INR may unmask a tumor of the genitourinary tract.

Skin Necrosis

A rare complication of warfarin, skin necrosis usually is seen 2 to 5 days after initiation of therapy. Well-demarcated erythematous lesions form on the thighs, buttocks, breasts, or toes. Typically, the center of the lesion becomes progressively necrotic. Examination of skin biopsies taken from the border of these lesions reveals thrombi in the microvasculature.

Warfarin-induced skin necrosis is seen in patients with congenital or acquired deficiencies of protein C or protein S.[172,173] Initiation of warfarin therapy in these patients produces a precipitous fall in plasma levels of proteins C or S, thereby eliminating this important anticoagulant pathway before warfarin exerts an antithrombotic effect through lowering of the functional levels of factor X and prothrombin. The resultant procoagulant state triggers thrombosis. Why the thrombosis is localized to the microvasculature of fatty tissues is unclear.

Treatment involves discontinuation of warfarin and reversal with vitamin K, if needed. An alternative anticoagulant, such as heparin or low-molecular-weight heparin, should be given in patients with thrombosis. Protein C concentrates or recombinant activated protein C can be given to protein C-deficient patients to accelerate healing of the skin lesions; fresh frozen plasma may be of value for those with protein S deficiency. Occasionally, skin grafting is necessary when there is extensive skin loss.

Because of the potential for skin necrosis, patients with known protein C or protein S deficiency require overlapping treatment with a parenteral anticoagulant when initiating warfarin therapy. Warfarin should be started in low doses in these patients and the parenteral anticoagulant should be continued until the INR is therapeutic for at least 2 to 3 consecutive days.

Pregnancy

Warfarin crosses the placenta and can cause fetal abnormalities or bleeding. The fetal abnormalities include a characteristic embryopathy, which consists of nasal hypoplasia and stippled epiphyses. The risk of embryopathy is highest if warfarin is given in the first trimester of pregnancy.[174] Central nervous system abnormalities also can occur with exposure to coumarins at any time during pregnancy. Finally, maternal administration of warfarin produces an anticoagulant effect in the fetus that can cause bleeding. This is of particular concern at delivery when trauma to the head during passage through the birth canal can lead to intracranial bleeding. Because of these potential problems, warfarin is contraindicated in pregnancy. Instead, heparin, low-molecular-weight heparin, or fondaparinux can be given during pregnancy for prevention or treatment of thrombosis.

Warfarin does not pass into the breast milk. Consequently, warfarin can safely be administered to nursing mothers.[174]

Special Problems

Patients with a lupus anticoagulant or those who need urgent or elective surgery present special challenges. Although observational studies suggested that patients with thrombosis complicating the antiphospholipid antibody syndrome required higher-intensity warfarin regimens to prevent recurrent thromboembolic events, two recent randomized trial demonstrated that targeting an INR of 2.0 to 3.0 is as effective as higher-intensity treatment and produces less bleeding.[175,176] Monitoring warfarin therapy can be problematic in patients with antiphospholipid antibody syndrome if the lupus anticoagulant prolongs the baseline INR.

If patients receiving long-term warfarin treatment require an elective invasive procedure, warfarin can be stopped 5 days prior to the procedure to allow the INR to return to normal levels. Those at high risk for recurrent thrombosis can be bridged with once- or twice-daily subcutaneous injections of low-molecular-weight heparin when the INR falls below 2.0. The last dose of low-molecular-weight heparin should be given 12 to 24 hours prior to the procedure, depending on whether low-molecular-weight heparin is administered twice or once daily, respectively. After the procedure, treatment with warfarin can be restarted.

New Oral Anticoagulants

New oral anticoagulants that target thrombin or factor Xa are under development.[177] These drugs have a rapid onset of action and have half-lives that permit once- or twice-daily administration. Designed to produce a predictable level of anticoagulation, these new oral agents can be given in fixed doses without coagulation monitoring. Therefore, these drugs will be more convenient to administer than warfarin. The results of ongoing phase II and III clinical trials will determine the role of these new oral anticoagulants in the prevention and treatment of thrombosis.

FIBRINOLYTIC DRUGS

Role of Fibrinolytic Therapy

Used to degrade thrombi, fibrinolytic drugs can be administered systemically or they can be delivered via catheters directly into the substance of the thrombus. Systemic delivery is used for treatment of acute myocardial infarction, acute ischemic stroke and most cases of massive pulmonary embolism. The goal of therapy is to produce rapid thrombus dissolution, thereby restoring antegrade blood flow. In the coronary circulation, restoration of blood flow reduces morbidity and mortality by limiting myocardial damage, whereas in the cerebral circulation, rapid thrombus dissolution decreases the neuronal death and brain infarction that produce irreversible brain injury. For patients with massive pulmonary embolism, the goal of fibrinolytic therapy is to restore pulmonary artery perfusion.

Peripheral arterial thrombi and thrombi in the proximal deep veins of the leg are most often treated using a catheter-directed approach. Catheters with multiple side holes can be utilized to deliver fibrinolytic drugs. In some cases, intravascular devices that fragment and extract the thrombus are used to hasten treatment. Although these devices can be used alone, they are often used in conjunction with fibrinolytic agents.

Mechanism of Action

Currently approved fibrinolytic agents include streptokinase, acylated plasminogen streptokinase activator complex (anistreplase), urokinase, recombinant tissue-type plasminogen activator (rt-PA) (Alteplase; Activase), and two recombinant derivatives of rt-PA, tenecteplase (TNKase) and reteplase (Retaplase). All of these agents act by converting the proenzyme, plasminogen, to plasmin, the active enzyme (Fig. 137–8). Plasmin then degrades the fibrin matrix of thrombi, thereby producing soluble fibrin degradation products.[178]

Endogenous fibrinolysis is regulated at two levels. Plasminogen activator inhibitors, particularly the type 1 form, known as PAI-1,[179] prevent excessive plasminogen activation by regulating the activity of t-PA and urokinase-type plasminogen activator (u-PA). Once plasmin is generated, it is regulated by plasmin inhibitors, the most important of which is α_2-antiplasmin. The plasma concentration of plasminogen is twofold higher than that of α_2-antiplasmin. Consequently, with pharmacological doses of plasminogen activators, the concentration of plasmin that is generated can exceed that of α_2-antiplasmin.[180] In addition to degrading fibrin, unregulated plasmin also can degrade fibrinogen and other clotting factors. This process, which is known as the systemic lytic state, reduces the hemostatic potential of the blood and increases the risk of bleeding.

The endogenous fibrinolytic system is geared to localize plasmin generation to the fibrin surface. Both plasminogen and *t*-PA bind to fibrin to form a ternary complex that promotes efficient plasminogen activation.[181–183] In contrast to free plasmin, plasmin generated on the fibrin surface is relatively protected from inactivation by α_2-antiplasmin, a feature that promotes fibrin dissolution.[184,185] Furthermore, C-terminal lysine residues exposed as plasmin degrades fibrin serve as binding sites for additional plasminogen and t-PA molecules. This creates a positive feedback that enhances plasmin generation. When used pharmacologically, the various plasminogen activators capitalize on these mechanisms to a lesser or greater extent.

There are two pools of plasminogen: circulating plasminogen and fibrin-bound plasminogen (Fig. 137–9). Plasminogen activators that preferentially activate fibrin-bound plasminogen are considered fibrin-specific. In contrast, nonspecific plasminogen activators do not

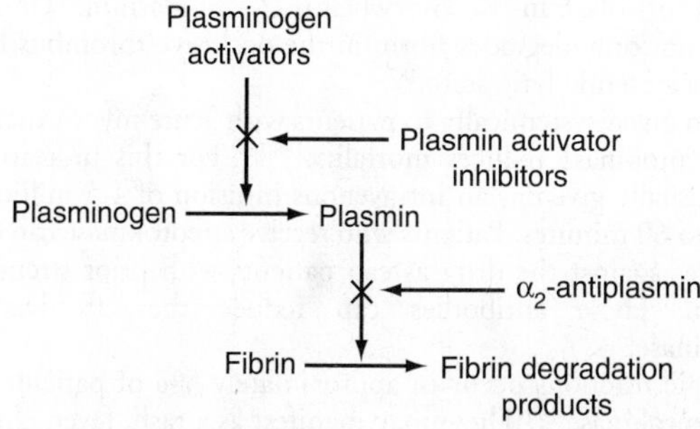

Figure 137–8 Fibrinolytic system and its regulation. Plasminogen activators convert plasminogen to plasmin. Plasmin then degrades fibrin into soluble fibrin degradation products. The system is regulated at two levels. Type 1 plasminogen activator inhibitor (PAI-1) regulates the plasminogen activators, whereas α_2-antiplasmin serves as the major inhibitor of plasmin.

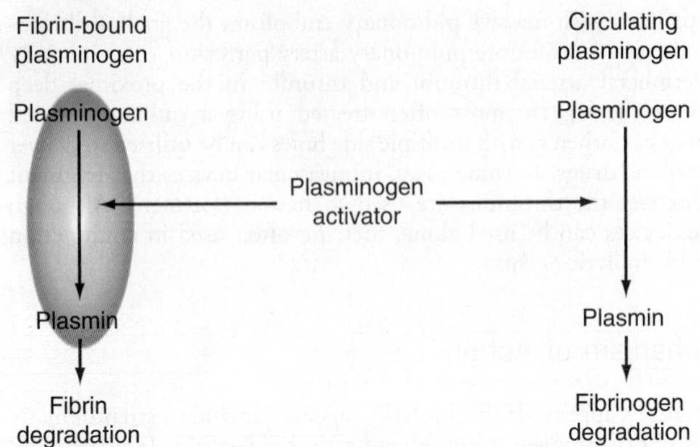

Figure 137–9 Consequences of activation of fibrin-bound or circulating plasminogen. The fibrin specificity of plasminogen activators reflects their capacity to distinguish between fibrin-bound and circulating plasminogen. This, in turn, reflects their affinity for fibrin. Plasminogen activators with high affinity for fibrin preferentially activate fibrin-bound plasminogen. This results in the generation of plasmin on the fibrin surface. Fibrin-bound plasmin, which is protected from inactivation by α_2-antiplasmin, degrades fibrin to yield soluble fibrin degradation products. In contrast, plasminogen activators with little or no affinity for fibrin do not distinguish between fibrin-bound and circulating plasminogen. Activation of circulating plasminogen results in systemic plasminemia and subsequent degradation of fibrinogen and other clotting factors.

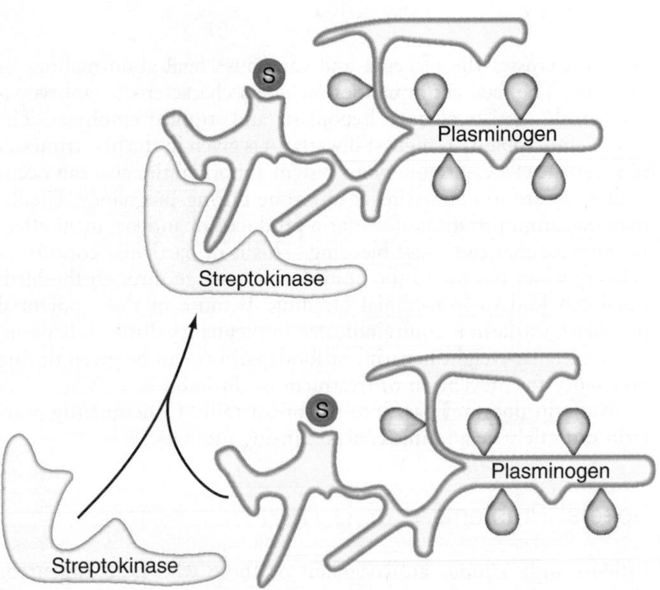

Figure 137–10 Mechanism of action of streptokinase. Streptokinase binds to plasminogen and induces a conformational change in plasminogen that exposes its active site. The streptokinase/plasmin(ogen) complex then serves as the activator of additional plasminogen molecules.

discriminate between fibrin-bound and circulating plasminogen. Activation of circulating plasminogen results in the generation of unopposed plasmin that can trigger the systemic lytic state. Alteplase and its derivatives are fibrin-specific plasminogen activators, whereas streptokinase, anistreplase, and urokinase are nonspecific agents.

Streptokinase

Unlike other plasminogen activators, streptokinase is not an enzyme and does not directly convert plasminogen to plasmin. Instead, streptokinase forms a 1 : 1 stoichiometric complex with plasminogen. Formation of this complex induces a conformational change in plasminogen that exposes its active site (Fig. 137–10). This conformationally altered plasminogen then converts additional plasminogen molecules to plasmin.[186]

Streptokinase has no affinity for fibrin and the streptokinase–plasminogen complex activates both free and fibrin-bound plasminogen. Activation of circulating plasminogen generates sufficient amounts of plasmin to overwhelm α_2-antiplasmin. Unopposed plasmin not only degrades fibrin in the occlusive thrombus but also induces a systemic lytic state.[187]

When given systemically to patients with acute myocardial infarction, streptokinase reduces mortality.[188,189] For this indication, the drug is usually given as an intravenous infusion of 1.5 million units over 30 to 60 minutes. Patients who receive streptokinase can develop antibodies against the drug as can patients with prior streptococcal injection. These antibodies can reduce the effectiveness of streptokinase.

Allergic reactions occur in approximately 5% of patients treated with streptokinase.[190] These may manifest as a rash, fever, chills, and rigors. Although anaphylactic reactions can occur, these are rare. Transient hypotension is common with streptokinase and has been attributed to plasmin-mediated release of bradykinin from kallikrein.[191] The hypotension usually responds to leg elevation and administration of intravenous fluids and low doses of vasopressors, such as dopamine or norepinephrine.[192]

Anistreplase

To generate this drug, streptokinase is combined with equimolar amounts of Lys-plasminogen, a plasmin-cleaved form of plasminogen with a lysine residue at its N-terminal. The active site of Lys-plasminogen that is exposed on combination with streptokinase is then masked with an anisoyl group. After intravenous infusion, the anisoyl group is slowly removed by deacylation, giving the complex a half-life of approximately 100 minutes. This allows drug administration via a single bolus infusion.

Although it is more convenient to administer, anistreplase offers few mechanistic advantages over streptokinase. Like streptokinase, anistreplase does not distinguish between fibrin-bound and circulating plasminogen. Consequently, it too produces a systemic lytic state. Likewise, allergic reactions and hypotension are just as frequent with anistreplase as they are with streptokinase.[193]

When anistreplase was compared with ateplase in patients with acute myocardial infarction, reperfusion was obtained more rapidly with alteplase than with anistreplase.[194] Improved reperfusion was associated with a trend toward better clinical outcomes and reduced mortality with alteplase. These results and the high cost of anistreplase have dampened the enthusiasm for its use.

Urokinase

Derived from cultured fetal kidney cells, urokinase is a two-chain serine protease with a molecular weight of 34,000.[195] Urokinase directly converts plasminogen to plasmin by cleaving the Arg560–Val561 bond. Unlike streptokinase, urokinase is not immunogenic and allergic reactions are rare. Urokinase produces a systemic lytic state because it does not discriminate between fibrin-bound and circulating plasminogen.

Despite many years of use, urokinase has never been systemically evaluated for coronary fibrinolysis. Instead, urokinase is often employed for catheter-directed lysis of thrombi in the deep veins or the peripheral arteries. Because of recent production problems, the availability of urokinase is limited.

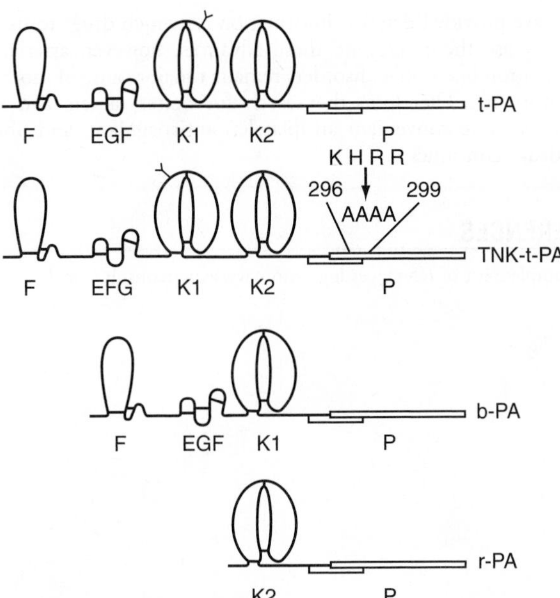

Figure 137–11 Domain structures of alteplase (*t*-PA), tenecteplase (TNK-*t*-PA), desmoteplase (b-PA), and reteplase (r-PA). The finger (F), epidermal growth factor (EGF), first and second kringles (K1 and K2, respectively), and protease (P) domains are illustrated. The glycosylation site (Y) on K1 has been repositioned in tenecteplase to endow it with a longer half-life. In addition, a tetra-alanine substitution in the protease domain renders tenecteplase resistant to PAI-1 inhibition. Desmoteplase differs from alteplase and teneteplase in that it lacks a K2 domain. Reteplase is a truncated variant that lacks the F, EGF, and K1 domains.

Alteplase

A recombinant form of single-chain t-PA, Alteplase has a molecular weight of 68,000.[196] Alteplase is rapidly converted into its two-chain form by plasmin. Although single- and two-chain forms of t-PA have equivalent activity in the presence of fibrin, in its absence, single-chain t-PA has 10-fold lower activity.[197,198]

Alteplase consists of five discrete domains (Fig. 137–11). The N-terminal A-chain of two-chain Alteplase contains four of these domains; residues 4 through 50 make up the finger domain, a region that resembles the finger domain of fibronectin, resides 50 through 87 are homologous with epidermal growth factor, whereas residues 92 through 173 and 180 through 261, which have homology to the kringle domains of plasminogen, are designated as the first and second kringle, respectively. The fifth Alteplase domain is the protease domain; it is located on the C-terminal B-chain of two-chain Alteplase.

The interaction of Alteplase with fibrin is mediated by the finger domain, and to a lesser extent, by the second kringle domain.[199,200] The affinity of Alteplase for fibrin is considerably higher than that for fibrinogen.[200] Consequently, the catalytic efficiency of plasminogen activation by Alteplase is two to three orders of magnitude higher in the presence of fibrin than in the presence of fibrinogen. This phenomenon helps to localize plasmin generation to the fibrin surface.

Although Alteplase preferentially activates plasminogen in the presence of fibrin, Alteplase is not as fibrin-selective as was first predicted. Its fibrin specificity is limited because like fibrin, the fibrin fragments (DD)E, the major soluble degradation product of cross-linked fibrin,[201] binds Alteplase and plasminogen with high affinity.[200] Consequently, (DD)E is as potent as fibrin as a stimulator of plasminogen activation by Alteplase. Whereas plasmin generated on the fibrin surface results in thrombolysis, plasmin generated on the surface of circulating (DD)E degrades fibrinogen.[202] Fibrinogenolysis results in the accumulation of fragment X, a high molecular weight clottable fibrinogen degradation product. Incorporation of fragment X into hemostatic plugs formed at sites of vascular injury renders them susceptible to lysis.[203–205] This phenomenon may contribute to Alteplase-induced bleeding.

A trial comparing Alteplase with streptokinase for treatment of patients with acute myocardial infarction demonstrated significantly lower mortality with Alteplase than with streptokinase,[206] although the absolute difference was small. The greatest benefit was seen in patients less than 75 years of age with anterior myocardial infarction who presented less than 6 hours after symptom onset.

For treatment of acute myocardial infarction or acute ischemic stroke, Alteplase is given as an intravenous infusion over 60 to 90 minutes. The total dose of Alteplase usually ranges from 90 to 100 mg. Allergic reactions and hypotension are rare and Alteplase is not immunogenic.[190]

Tenecteplase

A genetically engineered variant of t-PA, tenecteplase was designed to have a longer half-life than t-PA and to be resistant to inactivation by PAI-1.[207] To prolong its half-life, a new glycosylation site was added to the first kringle domain (Fig. 137–11). Because addition of this extra carbohydrate side chain reduced fibrin affinity, the existing glycosylation site on the first kringle domain was removed. To render the molecule resistant to inhibition by PAI-1, a tetra-alanine substitution was introduced at residues 296–299 in the protease domain, the region responsible for the interaction of t-PA with PAI-1.[207–209]

Tenecteplase is more fibrin-specific than t-PA. Although both agents bind to fibrin with similar affinity, the affinity of tenecteplase for (DD)E is significantly lower than that of t-PA.[210] Consequently, (DD)E does not stimulate systemic plasminogen activation by tenecteplase to the same extent as t-PA. As a result, tenecteplase produces less fibrinogenolysis than t-PA.

For coronary fibrinolysis, tenecteplase is given as a single intravenous bolus. In a large phase III trial that enrolled more than 16,000 patients, the 30-day mortality rate with single bolus tenecteplase was similar to that with accelerated dose t-PA.[211] Although rates of intracranial hemorrhage also were similar with both treatments, patients given tenecteplase had fewer noncerebral bleeds and a reduced need for blood transfusions than those treated with t-PA.[211] The improved safety profile of tenecteplase likely reflects its enhanced fibrin specificity.

Reteplase

A recombinant *t*-PA derivative, reteplase is a single-chain variant that lacks the finger, epidermal growth factor, and first kringle domains (Fig. 137–11). This truncated derivative has a molecular weight of 39,000.[212] Reteplase binds fibrin more weakly than t-PA because it lacks the finger domain.[213] Because it is produced in *Escherichia coli*, reteplase is not glycosylated. This endows it with a plasma half-life longer than that of t-PA. Consequently, reteplase is given as two intravenous boluses, which are separated by 30 minutes.[214] Clinical trials have demonstrated that reteplase is at least as effective as streptokinase for treatment of acute myocardial infarction,[214] but the agent is not superior to t-PA.[215]

New Fibrinolytic Agents

Several new drugs are under investigation. These include desmoteplase (Fig. 137–11), a recombinant form of the full-length plasminogen activator isolated from the saliva of the vampire bat,[216,217] and alfimeprase, a truncated form of fibrolase, an enzyme isolated from the venom of the southern copperhead snake.[218] Desmoteplase, which is more fibrin-specific than t-PA,[200,219,220] is being investigated for the treatment of acute ischemic stroke. With a potential for enhanced safety, desmoteplase may extend the window for treatment beyond 3 hours. An ongoing phase III clinical trial is exploring this possibility.

Alfimeprase is a metalloproteinase that degrades fibrin and fibrinogen in a plasmin-independent fashion.[218] In the circulation, alfimeprase is inhibited by α_2-macroglobulin.[179] Therefore, the drug must be delivery to the thrombus via a catheter. Once localized on the thrombus, alfimeprase produces rapid fibrin degradation.

Arterial and venous thrombosis reflect a complex interplay among the vessel wall, platelets, the coagulation system, and the fibrinolytic pathways. Activation of coagulation also triggers inflammatory pathways that may contribute to thrombogenesis. A better understanding of the biochemistry of blood coagulation and advances in structure-based drug design have identified new targets and resulted in the development of novel antithrombotic drugs. Well-designed clinical trials have provided detailed information on which drugs to use and when to use them. Despite these advances, however, arterial and venous thromboembolic disorders remain a major cause of morbidity and mortality. Therefore, the search for better targets and more potent or more convenient antiplatelet, anticoagulant, and fibrinolytic drugs continues.

REFERENCES

For complete list of references log onto www.expertconsult.com

CHAPTER 138

IMMUNE THROMBOCYTOPENIC PURPURA, NEONATAL ALLOIMMUNE THROMBOCYTOPENIA, AND POSTTRANSFUSION PURPURA

James Bussel and Douglas B. Cines

IMMUNE THROMBOCYTOPENIC PURPURA

Introduction

Immune thrombocytopenic purpura (ITP) is the most common cause of acquired severe thrombocytopenia. ITP has been estimated to affect approximately 1 in 10,000 in the general population, about half of whom are children, and to account for 0.18% of hospital admissions (reviewed in reference 1). The clinical presentation varies from severe thrombocytopenia and bleeding to the discovery of mild asymptomatic thrombocytopenia during evaluation of another illness or during routine annual checkup.[2] ITP can occur as an isolated condition or it may accompany other systemic disorders, requiring separate or integrated management. ITP in pregnant women has more limited therapeutic options and is infrequently complicated by severe neonatal thrombocytopenia. ITP is caused by autoreactive antibodies that bind to platelets and shorten their lifespan. Substantial strides have been made toward understanding the pathophysiology of ITP, including the role of persistent infection in certain cases and the understanding that platelet production may be impaired. Important new treatment modalities, each with their own efficacy, side effects, tolerability, and cost, have been introduced. Practice guidelines were developed in the United States in 1996[3] and the United Kingdom in 2003,[4] but require updating. The intent of this chapter is to review the clinical features of ITP, consider new developments in diagnosis and in management, and provide the practitioner with our view of how these are best incorporated into patient care. The discussion of ITP in adults and children is separated to emphasize the issues pertinent to each population, but general concerns common to both are covered in the section on adults.

Immune Thrombocytopenic Purpura in Adults

Presentation

It had long been thought that in adults, ITP occurs most commonly in women during the second and third decades of life.[5] Recent surveillance studies indicate that ITP may actually be more common in older individuals of both sexes in some settings.[6,7] Patients may come to medical attention with platelet counts between 10,000 and 20,000/μL because they develop petechiae, purpura or ecchymoses, and/or epistaxis over the course of several days. Those with platelet counts between 30,000 and 50,000/μL often give a history of easy bruising. Patients with platelet counts below 10,000/μL are more likely to have widespread cutaneous bruising accompanied by bleeding from mucosal sites, including epistaxis, gingival bleeding, hematuria, menorrhagia or, less commonly, melena. Rarely, the presentation is intracranial hemorrhage or significant bleeding at other internal sites. Platelet counts above 50,000/μL are likely to be discovered incidentally.[8] Most patients are otherwise in their usual state of health, although chronic fatigue, inability to focus, and similar protean complaints are not uncommon.[9] Few adults give a history of a viral illness in the preceding weeks. A few show evidence of another systemic disorder associated with immune thrombocytopenia. However, the typical patient is well with the exception of bleeding and possibly fatigue.

Differential Diagnosis

ITP is the most common cause of severe thrombocytopenia in otherwise healthy young adults. ITP remains a diagnosis of exclusion.[3,4] Other disorders that need to be considered are divided into those that cause isolated thrombocytopenia and those usually associated with additional hematologic abnormalities. The former include inherited thrombocytopenia (Chapter 32), drug-induced thrombocytopenia (Chapter 140), and secondary immune thrombocytopenias (see below), including HIV and hepatitis C infection (Chapter 158). During pregnancy, the differential diagnosis also includes gestational thrombocytopenia, preeclampsia and HELLP, and less commonly other disorders. Other causes of thrombocytopenia are generally evident from the initial presentation (Chapter 121). Among elderly adults, the major additional consideration is myelodysplasia in which thrombocytopenia can precede other manifestations by months to years.[10] Myelodysplasia with a relatively normal-appearing bone marrow and refractory ITP can be virtually indistinguishable on presentation. Thrombocytopenia with additional hematologic abnormalities has multiple causes, including hypersplenism, leukemia, aplastic anemia, and the thrombotic thrombocytopenic purpura/hemolytic uremic syndrome (TTP/HUS) or disseminated intravascular coagulation (DIC), among others (Chapters 139 and 140).

Initial Evaluation

The physical examination reveals only signs of bleeding, typically petechiae and purpura unless there are comorbid conditions. Splenomegaly or lymphadenopathy suggests another diagnosis or an underlying illness with secondary thrombocytopenia. The blood counts are normal except for the platelet count unless there has been significant bleeding, in which case normocytic or, if chronic bleeding has led to iron deficiency, microcytic anemia may be seen. Thrombocytopenia determined by automated analyzer must be confirmed by examination of the peripheral blood smear to exclude pseudothrombocytopenia (see below) and hematologic conditions that affect multiple cell lines (Fig. 138–1). Platelet size is increased in many patients; however, the mean platelet volume determined by automated counter is inaccurate at very low platelet counts and platelets consistently approaching the size of erythrocytes are more typical of hereditary macrothrombocytopenias. Conversely, unusually small platelets are associated with Wiskott–Aldrich syndrome. Schistocytes should suggest TTP, HUS, or DIC (Chapters 132 and 139) and

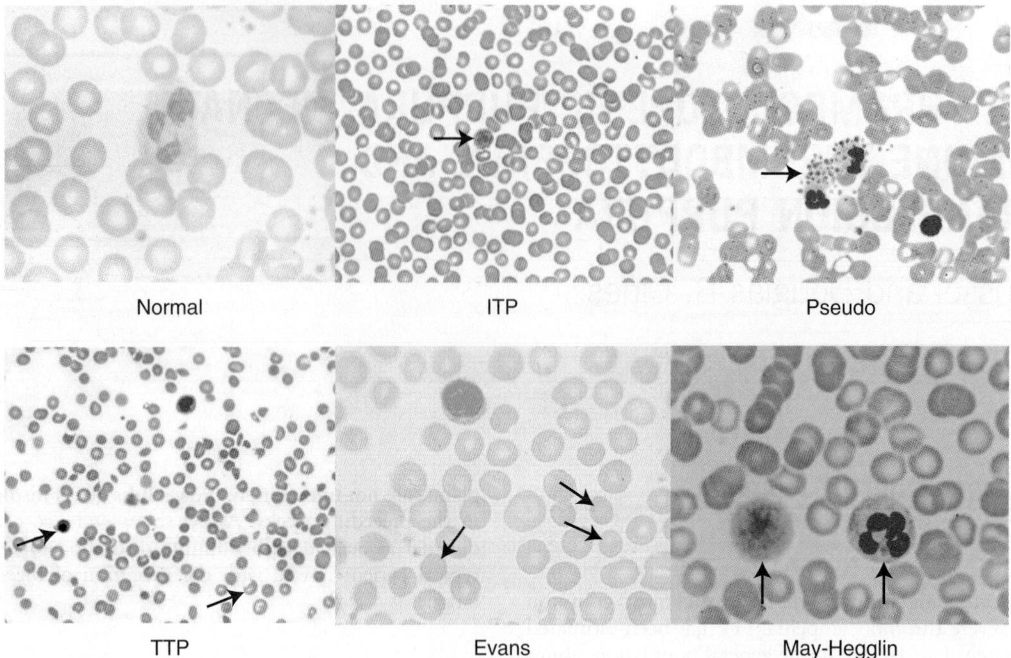

Figure 138–1 Peripheral blood smear in immune thrombocytopenic purpura (ITP) and other conditions. Normal: Blood smear from healthy individual showing normal number and size distribution of platelets. ITP: Blood smear confirms low platelets count and shows a megathrombocyte (arrow) but no other abnormalities. Pseudo: Pseudothrombocytopenia. Blood smear shows platelet clumping and rosetting around leukocyte (arrow). TTP: Thrombotic thrombocytopenia purpura. Arrows point to a schistocyte and a nucleated red blood cell. Evans: Evans syndrome refers to concurrent ITP and autoimmune hemolytic anemia as suggested by spherocytes (arrows). May-Hegglin: Inherited thrombocytopenia characterized by giant platelets and leukocyte inclusion bodies (arrows).

polychromasia with spherocytes might indicate Evans syndrome (see below).

No additional diagnostic studies are required to make a diagnosis of ITP in the typical cases. Testing for platelet antibodies is not recommended. The marrow, if performed, reveals normal erythroid and myeloid development, normal to increased numbers of megakaryocytes, and no marked dysplastic features such as megakaryocyte clumping or bare nuclei. Even when the presentation is typical, bone marrow aspiration and biopsy are probably indicated in older individuals.[3] The initial history, course, and response to therapy provide important diagnostic clues,[3] including those suggesting secondary ITP. Serological evaluation for HIV and/or hepatitis C infection is indicated in at-risk populations because of the potential adverse effect of prolonged corticosteroid usage on viral replication and the utility of antiviral therapy in treating the accompanying thrombocytopenia.[11] Quantification of immunoglobulins and immunoelectrophoresis may be appropriate in the elderly, those with hepatosplenomegaly or lymphadenopathy, and in patients with a history of recurrent infections. Both hypothyroidism and hyperthyroidism are common. The role of testing for antiphospholipid antibodies (APLA) is uncertain. Testing for a lupus anticoagulant should be performed if there is a history of a thromboembolic event, recurrent miscarriages, a prolonged aPTT or other suggestion of a systemic autoimmune disease. APLA are common[12] but do not affect response to ITP-directed therapy.[13,14] On the other hand, there is divergence in the literature as to the risk of thrombosis in patients with APLA during or after recovery.[13,14]

The role of testing for infection with *Helicobacter pylori* or the empiric use of antibiotics on presentation remains controversial because the outcome of this approach has been highly variable (reviewed in reference 15). Patients are often asymptomatic, in which case the best way to establish the diagnosis is by using ^{13}C-breath urea or the stool antigen tests rather than serology; false positive serology has been reported after treatment with IVIG. Antibiotic therapy is least likely to be effective in patients with severe ITP of long-standing duration.[16]

Pseudothrombocytopenia

Pseudothrombocytopenia is an in vitro artifact of automated cell counting that occurs with a frequency of between 1 in 1000 and 1 in 10,000 blood specimens collected in EDTA.[17] The phenomenon involves platelet agglutination by autoantibodies that bind to a conformer of the platelet glycoprotein IIb-IIIa complex induced by low concentrations of ionized calcium only attained in vitro. The diagnosis is suspected when platelet clumping is observed on a blood smear made from EDTA-anticoagulated blood.[17] The diagnosis is confirmed by demonstrating that the platelet count is substantially higher when measured in citrated or heparinized blood, or in blood obtained without an anticoagulant and analyzed by blood smear. Platelet clumping occurs at body temperature, distinguishing it from cold agglutinins, although the two may coexist. Falsely low platelet counts may also occur when giant platelets are excluded from automated analysis. The blood smear of all patients with ITP must be analyzed to confirm the automated platelet count before therapy is initiated or changed.

Pathogenesis and Laboratory Diagnosis

Eluates from ITP platelets contain autoantibodies to platelet glycoproteins IIb/IIIa (integrin αIIbβ3), Ib/IX, and Ia/IIa (integrin $\alpha2\beta1$), among other determinants (see references 18 and 19 for review). It is common to find antibodies to multiple platelet antigens.[20] Detecting antibodies in platelet eluates is estimated to have a sensitivity of between 49% and 66%, a specificity of 79% to 92% and a positive predictive value of 78% to 92%.[21,22] However, interlaboratory agreement is only 55% to 67%, and detection of circulating antibody is less useful and reproducible. A negative test does not exclude the diagnosis of ITP.[21,23] The sensitivity and specificity for using these tests to distinguish ITP from thrombocytopenia associated with myelodysplasia, systemic lupus, chronic hepatitis, and other conditions have not been determined in a systematic way. Therefore, ITP remains a clinical diagnosis made by excluding other diseases and it is still premature to rely on platelet antibody tests to confirm or to exclude the diagnosis.[3] The most reliable diagnostic criterion continues to be a response to "ITP specific" therapies, especially IVIG and IV anti-D.

Platelet life span is reduced in almost all patients[24,25] because of accelerated clearance of antibody-coated platelets by Fcγ receptors expressed on tissue macrophages. In most patients, an increased percentage of young, large (>20 fL) or reticulated platelets is seen suggesting an attempt to compensate by increasing platelet production.[26] However, in up to two-thirds of patients, platelet production is impaired[27,28] because nascent antibody-coated platelets are destroyed or damaged by intramedullary macrophages,[29] autoantibodies impede megakaryocyte differentiation and platelet release,[30–32] and/or because cytotoxic $CD8^+$ T cells damage megakaryocytes. Thrombopoietin levels are normal or minimally elevated in contrast to the marked elevations seen in hypomegakaryocytic disorders.[33] Although most identified autoantibodies bind to glycoproteins that serve important hemostatic functions, only a few patients note easy bruising at platelet counts above 50,000/μL as a result of antibody-induced storage pool deficiency or other qualitative defects.[34] In rare cases, platelet autoantibodies cause an acquired thrombasthenia or Bernard–Soulier-like disorder.[35,36]

Initial Treatment of Adults With Immune Thrombocytopenic Purpura

Management is predicated on the platelet count and severity of bleeding (Panel 1; top panel).[37] The primary short-term goal is to provide the minimal therapy needed to attain a hemostatic platelet count (>20,000–30,000/μL) and then to temporize until the disease improves or remits.[38] Because few adults with ITP remit spontaneously soon after diagnosis (reviewed in reference 39), treatment is indicated for the typical patient who presents with platelet counts lower than 20,000 to 30,000/μL, especially those over the age of 60 or with a previous history or ongoing bleeding, who are at greatest risk for life-threatening hemorrhage.[40] Treatment may be required at higher presenting platelet counts in patients with medical conditions that predispose to bleeding, in need of surgery, on mandated antiplatelet agents or anticoagulation, or who are at high risk of trauma owing to employment or difficulty in self-care as a result of physical, mental, or emotional disturbance, among other reasons.[37] In the absence of hemorrhage or other medical emergency, such as concurrent trauma or surgery, or another issue as indicated above, treatment is generally initiated with prednisone 1 to 2 mg/kg/day. IV anti-D (especially at a dose of 75 μg/kg) is a suitable alternative in Rh(D)-positive individuals with a negative direct antiglobulin test (DAT) and is less toxic, but considerably more expensive (Fig. 138–2B).[41] Approximately 50% of patients show sustained improvement with repeated infusions.[42] Intravenous immunoglobulin (IVIG; 1 g/kg for 1–2 days) should be used with IV methylprednisolone (30 mg/kg up to 1 g) when platelet counts remain below 5000/μL despite several days of corticosteroids or when bleeding is more widespread (see below). Others advocate basing initial therapy on the severity of bleeding.[43] Recent studies indicate that initiating therapy with one to four 4-day courses of high-dose dexamethasone may lead to sustained hemostatic responses in approximately 50% of patients.[44,45] Therapy is generally not required at platelet counts above 30,000/μL in the absence of bleeding or predisposing comorbid conditions.[3,37]

Glucocorticoids impair the clearance of antibody-coated platelets by tissue macrophages,[46] inhibit antibody production[47] and/or may increase platelet production,[29] possibly by inhibiting phagocytosis of platelets by bone marrow macrophages. Petechiae and purpura may resolve before the platelet count rises through a direct effect on vascular integrity and because newly formed platelets are preferentially recruited to sites of bleeding. Sixty to 90% of patients respond to prednisone depending on the intensity and duration of treatment,[3,48] most within 3 to 4 weeks[49,50] by which time considerable toxicity is usually evident. Although there is little consensus on the appropriate duration of therapy,[3] our opinion is that there is no compelling evidence that prolonging treatment further will alter the natural history and that it will clearly increase toxicity. Alternative forms of management should be sought if the platelet count does not increase sufficiently or falls below hemostatic levels during tapering rather than resuming prednisone or increasing the dose. Long-term remission rates of 9% to 32% are reported with prednisone alone.[3,48–50] Therefore, it is likely that most patients, including initial responders, will require additional forms of treatment.

Emergent Treatment

Consideration should be given to hospitalizing all patients who present with platelet counts lower than 10,000 to 20,000/μL until a beneficial effect of treatment can be documented, unless the patient is known to have shown a good response previously to a specific agent. Emergency treatment is indicated for internal or profound mucocutaneous bleeding (Fig. 138–2A) (reviewed in reference 37). General measures to reduce the bleeding risk should be instituted, including avoidance of drugs that interfere with platelet and hemostatic function, control of blood pressure, measures to minimize the risk of trauma, and treatments that have beneficial local effects on bleeding, for example, Amicar for epistaxis and oral bleeding and progesterone for vaginal bleeding. Treatment is initiated with IVIG (1 g/kg/day for 1–3 consecutive days) or IV anti-D (75 μg/kg) and intravenous methylprednisolone (1–2 g/day for 1–3 consecutive days) unless the platelet exceeds 30,000 to 50,000/μL sooner.[3,51,52] Platelet transfusions are indicated for life-threatening bleeding and are often surprisingly effective,[53] especially when given continuously after an initial bolus and preceded by other therapies, such as IVIG.[54] Multimodality therapy with corticosteroids, IVIG and/or anti-D and/or vincristine has recently been shown to be effective in patients with poor outcomes to individual agents.[55] Splenectomy is reserved for the rare patient who fails to respond and requires immediate additional treatment, for example, prior to emergency craniotomy for intracranial hemorrhage. A bone marrow documenting a normal-appearing marrow with active megakaryocytopoiesis should be performed if there is any question regarding the diagnosis. Experience with plasmapheresis is limited (reviewed in reference 56). Recombinant factor VIIa can be administered if bleeding remains uncontrolled while awaiting a response to treatment; dosing is not well established, but a minimum of 40 U/kg has been used successfully in patients with thrombocytopenia of diverse etiologies.[57]

Management of First Relapse—Medical Therapy and Splenectomy

Prednisone is generally tapered over 1 to 4 months, at which time most adults relapse. For those who do not respond or fail to sustain a response (platelet count <30,000–50,000/μL) (Fig. 138–2C), either splenectomy (Fig. 138–2E) or medical therapy (Fig. 138–2D) can be pursued. Prolonged reliance on corticosteroids to maintain a hemostatic platelet count should be avoided whenever possible. A trial of steroid-sparing agents or alternatives to steroids (see below) should be implemented. More patients and physicians are waiting for at least 6 to 12 months before proceeding to splenectomy even in the face of persistent thrombocytopenia. The argument for medical therapy is based on recent evidence that a substantial fraction of patients treated repetitively with anti-D or with a course of dexamethasone or rituximab (see below) can postpone or avoid splenectomy.[58] The decision to defer or proceed with splenectomy is predicated on disease severity, side effects of therapy, desired level of physical activity, travel (eg, exposure to malaria and poor access to medical care), compliance, and, importantly, patient and physician preference.

Response to splenectomy cannot be predicted from results of prior treatment, though patients totally refractory to several prior

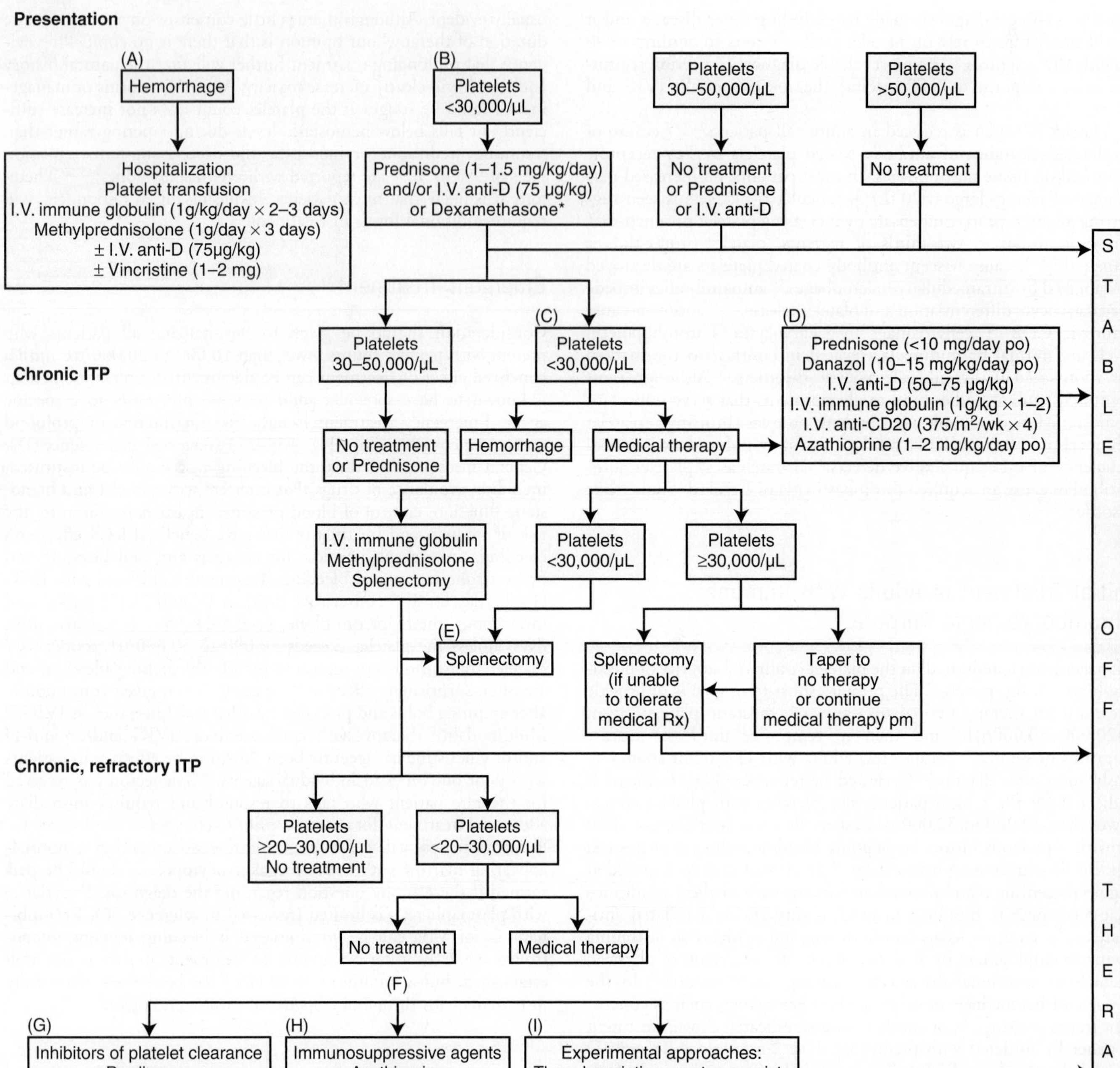

Figure 138–2 Treatment algorithm for management of adult-onset ITP. Letters refer to specific aspects of management cited in text. *Presentation.* Some advocate the use of 20,000/μL as a guideline for therapy. The decision to treat patients with platelet counts lower than 50,000/μL is based in part on evidence of bleeding, a history of bleeding, comorbid risk factors, life-style and tolerance of therapy. There is no consensus as to duration of steroid therapy. The use of anti-D as initial therapy is appropriate only for Rh$^+$, DAT$^-$ individuals who are not markedly anemic or hemolyzing. *Chronic ITP.* The goal of medical therapy is to attain a hemostatic platelet count, generally greater than 20,000 to 30,000/μL. The threshold for treatment depends on comorbid risk factors for bleeding and risk of trauma. Higher platelet counts may be appropriate for surgery or after trauma. Medications can be used individually but combinations of azathioprine and danazol (or corticosteroids) may provide added benefit and allow lower doses to be utilized. IVIG and anti-D is generally reserved for severe thrombocytopenia unresponsive to oral agents. The decision to proceed to splenectomy depends on intensity of therapy required, tolerance to side effects, risk of surgery and patient preference. IVIG and/or methylprednisolone may help to increase the platelet count immediately prior to splenectomy. Laparoscopic and open splenectomy have comparable outcomes. *Chronic, refractory ITP.* The decision to treat patients who have platelet counts lower than 20,000 to 30,000/μL after splenectomy involves an assessment of the risk of hemorrhage versus the side effects of each form of therapy (see text). *Accessory splenectomy is reserved for those who have had a durable remission from splenectomy. **Drugs are often used in combination (e.g. azathioprine and danazol). Patients receiving protracted courses of corticosteroids should be monitored for osteopenia and cataracts. Modified from the New England Journal of Medicine 364:995, 2002.

approaches to management fair less well. IVIG, anti-D, and/or pulse doses of corticosteroids are used to boost the platelet count above 50,000/μL preoperatively. Prophylactic platelet transfusions are discouraged as bleeding is rare even in the face of severe thrombocytopenia and the platelet count typically rises rapidly once the splenic artery is ligated. Approximately 85% attain a stable hemostatic response initially (reviewed in reference 59), of whom approximately 20% relapse within 5 to 10 years.[38,59] The short- and long-term outcomes of laparoscopic and conventional transabdominal approaches are comparable[60] and the former hastens recovery. Splenic irradiation is less effective and is reserved for the elderly and others in whom splenectomy is indicated but hazardous.[61] The major known risks of splenectomy are overwhelming bacterial sepsis and reduced ability to control certain infections such as malaria and babesiosis. Sepsis occurs in less than 1% of otherwise healthy adults with uncomplicated ITP managed appropriately.[62] Immunization with polyvalent pneumococcal, *Haemophilus influenzae* type B, and quadrivalent meningococcal polysaccharide vaccines, depending on age and immunization history, should be given at least 2 weeks prior to splenectomy.[63,64] Our experience is that immunizations can be given successfully 6 or more weeks postoperatively in those receiving immunosuppression, that is, rituximab or azathioprine prior to splenectomy. Evidence is lacking to suggest any benefit of prophylactic antibiotics in otherwise healthy adults or even in children more than 5 years of age. Pneumococcal vaccination should be readministered at 5- to 10-year intervals; the conjugated vaccine, effective in infants under the age of 2 when Pneumovax is not, can be tried in patients not responding to Pneumovax. Any febrile illness demands careful evaluation and IV antibiotics should be instituted immediately at the onset of a systemic illness with fever higher than 101°F even when a specific bacterial etiology is not evident.

Chronic Immune Thrombocytopenic Purpura: Splenectomy Failures

As many as 50% of adults require therapy after splenectomy (Fig. 138–2F).[3] Response to splenectomy is lower in elderly patients, and probably in those with Evans syndrome or secondary immune thrombocytopenias. The incidence of major hemorrhage in patients failing splenectomy is in the range of 2% to 3% per year in referral practices.[38,72] The initial approach to patients with bleeding or severe thrombocytopenia after splenectomy is generally the same as at presentation: the diagnosis should be reevaluated, alternative reasons for thrombocytopenia and bleeding must be excluded, measures to limit bleeding instituted, and treatment with corticosteroids and/or IVIG reinstituted depending on the severity. IV anti-D is the one treatment that is much less effective after splenectomy.[73] Once the platelet count has increased to a safe level, steroids are tapered. An occasional patient can be managed with alternate-day corticosteroids or sufficiently low daily doses of prednisone (5–10 mg) to permit long-term use, but most will require one or more of the treatments described below (Fig. 138–2E). Osteoporosis and cataracts should be monitored on a regular basis and prophylactic measures instituted to mitigate accelerated bone loss in patients continuing to be maintained on corticosteroids.

The goal of therapy for those who fail or relapse after splenectomy may differ from the initial presentation because fewer patients attain a durable unmaintained remission. In guidelines issued by the American Society of Hematology and by others, a platelet count of 30,000/μL is recommended as a surrogate endpoint.[37,48] However, some experts recommend using a platelet count as low as 10,000 to 20,000/μL in the absence of bleeding.[39] Treatment must be individualized as the tolerance for severe thrombocytopenia varies considerably and somewhat unpredictably, and unnecessary or prolonged steroid treatment increases mortality due to infection.[74] The risk of bleeding is influenced by the patient's age, bleeding history, and comorbid conditions,[40] which must be balanced against an individualized estimate of potential complications of each treatment modality. Elderly patients are more likely to bleed and to be exposed to medications that impair platelet function, but also are more likely to suffer debilitating side effects of therapy. Therefore, no treatment paradigm is applicable to all patients and intangibles such as level of physical activity, other medical conditions, tolerance to the side effects of therapy, and life expectations must be taken into consideration (Fig. 138–2F).

Place of Splenectomy in the Management of Adults with Immune Thrombocytopenic Purpura

For more than 50 years, splenectomy has been the treatment of choice for adults with ITP whose platelet counts have fallen after a course of prednisone, generally given at a dose of 1 to 1.5 mg/kg/day. The initial response to splenectomy exceeds 70% and most responding patients remain in clinical remission indefinitely (reviewed in reference 65). The efficacy and safety of laparoscopic splenectomy further enhanced patient acceptance. However, concerns about overwhelming sepsis postsplenectomy remain and recent studies have raised questions about pulmonary hypertension, atherosclerosis and thromboembolic complications, albeit generally in patients undergoing the procedure for other indications. The development of new drugs to treat ITP and the use of the internet have combined to increase patient concerns about undergoing surgery to remove a "normal" organ. However, until recently, there has been no indication that any treatment favorably alters the natural history of ITP, permitting splenectomy to be deferred without unacceptable medication-related toxicity.

Studies by Cooper et al using repeated injections of IV anti-D,[42] a study by George et al comparing repeated infusions of IV anti-D to prednisone,[66] a single course of rituximab (reviewed in reference 67), and three recent studies using short courses of dexamethasone as initial treatment[44,45,68] suggest that one-third to 50% of patients may attain hemostatic platelet counts without additional therapy and without splenectomy. Follow-up is short and it is now clear that some initial responders to rituximab relapse at later times.[69] Moreover, not all patients can tolerate the effects of dexamethasone on mood, rituximab may alter the T- and B-cell repertoire even after peripheral B-cell numbers have returned to normal, and rare cases of severe intravascular hemolysis and disseminated intravascular coagulation have occurred in patients who tolerated an initial course of anti-D.[70,71] Moreover, a platelet count that is generally adequate for hemostasis (>30,000/μL) may be unsuitable for patients with an active lifestyle, comorbid risk factors for bleeding, or settings where use of drugs that interfere with platelet function are deemed mandatory. Lastly, the treatment landscape may be altered soon by the introduction of thrombopoietin receptor agonists. Therefore, the proper timing of splenectomy has become a matter of considerable discussion between patients and their hematologists and the verdict is by no means "in."

Accessory Spleens

Residual splenic tissue is identified using either radionucleotide, MR imaging or CT scan. Response rates to removing an accessory spleen vary considerably (see reference 75 for review), but success appears more likely if the duration of initial response to splenectomy exceeded 2 years (Fig. 138–2G).[75]

Agents That Impair Platelet Clearance

Most postsplenectomy patients require maintenance doses of corticosteroids that are intolerable in order to maintain adequate platelet counts. Although the options for treatment are discussed below as if each is to be used as a single agent, benefits are often at least additive when agents are used in combination and the toxicity is reduced because lower doses may suffice (Fig. 138–2G).

Intravenous Immunoglobulin

Approximately 85% of adults respond to IVIG given by intermittent intravenous infusion at a dose of 1 g/kg/day for 2 consecutive days with an increase in platelet count to higher than 50,000/μL and in approximately 65% the peak platelet count exceeds 100,000/μL,[76] although the response rate may be lower in patients failing splenectomy. Single infusions are repeated as needed every 7 to 28 days. IVIG impairs the clearance of IgG-coated platelets,[77] perhaps indirectly by activating the inhibitory receptor FcRγIIb.[78]

There is no evidence that commercial preparations of IVIG differ in efficacy but they may differ in toxicity in certain subpopulations, for example, IgA content in the rare patient with IgA deficiency and anti-IgA antibodies and high osmolarity due to sucrose in elderly, diabetic patients at risk for renal failure. Toxicity is generally mild and self-limited. However, many patients complain of postinfusion headaches that, in a few, are unusually severe because of aseptic meningitis.[79] Positive antiglobulin tests after infusion due to isohemagglutinins are common but are typically short-lived and overt hemolytic anemia is very rare.[80] Other side effects in order of frequency include thrombosis,[81] pulmonary or renal failure,[82] and anaphylactoid reactions in IgA-deficient patients with IgE anti-IgA antibodies (in whom IgA-depleted preparations should be used).[83,84] Antiviral antibodies[85] can be passively acquired but there are no documented cases of HIV, hepatitis A, B, or C, HTLV1, or parvovirus transmission with currently available preparations. The major limitations of IVIG are the need for frequent infusion, availability, duration, and severity of postinfusion headaches, time of infusion, and cost. Approximately one-third of patients who respond initially ultimately may become refractory.[86] The major indications for IVIG are (a) treatment of hemorrhagic emergencies; (b) preparation for splenectomy or other surgical procedures in patients intolerant of or resistant to corticosteroids who are Rh- or have a positive direct antiglobulin test, precluding the use of anti-D; (c) to defer splenectomy in debilitated adults; (d) during pregnancy when potentially teratogenic drugs must be avoided; and (e) chronic management of patients who are either refractory to other modalities or who are awaiting response to slower-acting agents.

Anti-D

The response rate of Rh(D)+ individuals given IV anti-D at a dose of 75 μg/kg intravenously is comparable to IVIG.[41,87] Treatment takes approximately 5 minutes, is less expensive than IVIG, the product is not currently in short supply, and the systemic side effects of the latter are avoided. The most common toxicity of anti-D is hemolytic anemia. The mean decrease in hemoglobin is 1 to 2.0 g/dL, which may be accompanied by chills and nausea notwithstanding premedication with acetaminophen, antihistamines, and steroids, or, in less than 1% of cases, by intravascular hemolysis (IVH).[70] Disseminated intravascular coagulation, renal failure, and even death has been reported in a few patients with IVH.[71] Anti-D should probably be avoided in patients with ongoing hemolysis or positive direct antiglobulin tests not attributable to prior anti-D treatment, and in those with comorbidities such as cirrhosis or renal insufficiency that may predispose to these serious complications of IVH. Other limitations of anti-D treatment include its inapplicability to Rh(D)– individuals and very limited efficacy postsplenectomy. The indications for use of anti-D are essentially the same as for IVIG. However, anti-D appears to work through a different mechanism than IVIG, that is, by blocking FcγRIIA and/or FcγRIIIA,[88] suggesting the two agents may provide additive benefits in urgent situations. Anti-D has been especially useful in HIV-positive individuals and those needing chronic treatment, in whom it is desirable to avoid long-term use of corticosteroids and splenectomy.[89]

Danazol

Approximately 20% to 40% of pre- and postsplenectomized patients respond to the attenuated androgen, danazol, at a dose of 10 to 15 mg/kg/day for 4 to 6 months (Fig. 138–2-D, G).[90,91] However, danazol is generally less effective in refractory patients.[92,93] Part of the variation in reported response is due to differences in the duration of treatment,[90] because some individuals require up to 6 months for a benefit to be seen. Danazol impairs macrophage-mediated clearance of antibody-coated platelets initially[94] and may inhibit antibody production with prolonged use.[90,95] The major indications for danazol are to defer splenectomy and as a corticosteroid-sparing drug. Most patients require continued treatment at low daily doses to maintain remission.[96] Danazol shares with other androgens the potential to increase cholesterol, and to cause masculinization, mood and menstrual changes, and hepatic injury, including cholestatic hepatitis, peliosis hepatis,[97] and neoplasia.[98] We have found the combination of danazol and azathioprine (see below) to be more effective than either drug alone, using IV steroids and IVIG as supplements until a stable response is seen.[37]

Agents that Impair Antibody Production

Rituximab

Rituximab is being used more frequently as second-line therapy before as well as after splenectomy. Rituximab is a chimeric anti-CD20 monoclonal antibody that depletes B cells. When given at a dose of 375 mg/m^2 once weekly for 4 weeks, durable complete responses lasting at least 1 year are seen in 25% to 40% of patients, whereas others may attain relatively brief partial responses lasting weeks to months.[99–101] Response rates are not influenced by splenectomy status. However, in one study, 40% of 47 patients in CR at 1 year relapsed by year 5.[69] Patients with a durable initial complete response often respond to a second course if they relapse (reviewed in reference 102) but the duration is rarely longer than the initial response. Complete responses to a single dose have been reported in children.[103] The mechanism of response continues to defy simple categorization. An early-response phase, possibly due to macrophage inhibition by opsonized B-cells, and a late response phase, presumably resulting from inhibition of antibody synthesis and other B-cell functions, are both seen.[104] Recent work suggests that depletion of B cells removes an important source of stimulation for autoreactive T cells.[69] To date, patients with ITP have experienced few side effects other than transient serum sickness in children[104] provided that appropriate premedication is used and that the initial infusion rate is slow and increased gradually. Reactivation of hepatitis B in carriers has been seen and there have been a few cases of progressive multifocal leukoencephalopathy in patients with systemic lupus who were receiving additional immunosuppressants at the time they were treated with rituximab. As of now, no long-term clinical sequelae of immunosuppression have been demonstrated in the approximately 700,000 patients treated for a variety of indications although there is evidence for prolonged perturbation in the B-cell and T-cell repertoire in patients treated for other autoimmune disorders.[105]

Azathioprine

Twenty to 40% of patients respond to azathioprine (1–3 mg/kg/day as tolerated to maintain an absolute neutrophil count of approximately 1500/μL) depending on intensity and duration of treatment.[106–108] As with all modalities, responses are less frequent in refractory patients. The median time to response in one study was 4 months, and maximal benefit was not attained in some until 7 to 8 months. Complete responses tend to be durable and, on occasion, persist after treatment is discontinued. Serious side effects are rare and predominantly limited to reversible elevations of serum transaminases; some patients experience diarrhea, nausea, and depression that can be avoided by ingestion at bedtime.

Cyclophosphamide

Comparable response rates have been reported using cyclophosphamide as a single agent (1–2 mg/kg/day titrated based on the neutrophil count or 1–2 courses given intravenously at a dose of 1–1.5 g/m^2 every 3 weeks).[108,109] Cyclophosphamide can cause alopecia, hemorrhagic cystitis, and bladder fibrosis and should be used cautiously in younger patients because of its potential to cause infertility and leukemia. The combination of cyclophosphamide, prednisone, and other agents, for example, vinca alkaloids, may be effective in some refractory patients with acceptable toxicity and lasting efficacy.[110]

Other Immunosuppressants

Patients have been treated successfully with cyclosporine[111,112] or mycophenolate mofetil.[113] The former has been effective but its toxicity would appear to preclude long-term use if other modalities were available. The latter is best used as part of a combination approach. Other patients have been treated by incubating their plasma with columns coated with staphylococcal protein A, but this approach has been largely discontinued because of toxicity and lack of efficacy.

Additional Approaches

Dapsone (75 mg qd)[114] is effective in some patients, presumably by impeding macrophage function as a result of oxidant-mediated hemolysis; screening for G6PD deficiency may be advisable in males prior to use. Response rates in refractory patients are low.[115] Vinca alkaloids bind avidly to platelets and are released slowly into the plasma, which allows antibody-coated platelets to target the drug to tissue macrophages, inhibiting phagocytosis.[94,116] Vincristine (0.03 mg/kg or 1–1.5 mg/m^2; not to exceed 2 mg) and vinblastine (4–6 mg/m^2; not to exceed 10 mg) can be administered either by IV push or by slow infusion.[117] The response rate to either drug is approximately 10% in patients with chronic refractory ITP when used as a single agent and sustained complete remissions are uncommon.[118] Treatment generally has to be given every 2 to 4 weeks for an indefinite period and patients often become refractory or treatment has to be stopped because of neurologic toxicity. Vinca alkaloids are most effective when used as part of combination treatment.

Chronic Refractory Immune Thrombocytopenic Purpura

Approximately 20% of patients either do not respond to these approaches, relapse when the medications are stopped, or are unable to tolerate them (Fig. 138–2H). At this point, there must be a reassessment as to whether any therapy is needed, as some patients tolerate low platelet counts without bleeding.[39] However, the mortality rate from bleeding ranges from 2.2% for those younger than 40 years of age to more than 40% in those older than 60 in this subpopulation.[72,119] Therefore, almost all refractory patients with platelet counts lower than 20,000 to 30,000/μL will ultimately require treatment. The use of experimental approaches is to be considered in this setting.

High-dose immunosuppression followed by autologous bone marrow or peripheral stem cell transplantation has been used by several groups in this setting (Fig. 138–2I). In the largest reported series, 6 of 14 patients developed a complete or partial remission; however, some of the 6 suffered other complications.[120] Studies using a humanized monoclonal antibody to the T-cell costimulatory molecule CD154[121] have shown success even in previously refractory patients but its use has been discontinued because of the advent of thromboembolic complications.

Investigational trials using thrombopoietin-receptor agonists have shown great success in most patients, even those with severe disease. Dose-dependent increases in platelet counts have been reported in the majority of even refractory patients with few serious side effects.[122–124] In one study of AMG531, patients maintained their platelet counts for more than 2 years with weekly treatment with good drug tolerance and minimal toxicity. With more protracted usage, reticulin fibrosis has been seen in a small number of patients, which resolved on discontinuation of the agent; it is not yet known if this is a class effect. A high response rate has also been seen in two randomized, placebo-controlled studies of eltrombopag given for 6 weeks.[125] If these agents continue to show high response rates without serious unforeseen toxicities, it is anticipated that they will be incorporated into the management of patients at many stages of the disease and have the potential to be especially useful in refractory patients.

SECONDARY THROMBOCYTOPENIAS

Introduction

Secondary immune thrombocytopenias comprise as many as 40% to 50% of cases of ITP in some series.[126,127] The reason for the increased recognition of secondary ITP is not apparent other than the spread of HIV-1 and hepatitis C infections and increasingly effective therapy for chronic lymphoid malignancies (Chapters 83). This incidence needs to be considered in determining which patients with ITP should be investigated for an underlying disorder and whether to treat a patient with a systemic illness for presumed ITP when other causes of thrombocytopenia may coexist.

Systemic Lupus Erythematosus

An estimated one-third of patients with SLE develop thrombocytopenia sometime during their illness, although not all require treatment.[128–130] Thrombocytopenia may precede the diagnosis of SLE by months to years, but this occurs in only 2% to 5% of patients with classic ITP.[5,131,132] Therefore, serologic evaluation should be restricted to those with additional clinical or laboratory evidence consistent with lupus[3] rather than an isolated positive ANA.[132]

The pathogenesis of thrombocytopenia in SLE is multifactorial. Antibodies to platelet glycoproteins, like those seen in ITP, to DNA,[133,134] to phospholipids and phospholipid-binding proteins[135–137] to CD40 ligand,[138] to thrombopoietin[139] and immune complexes of diverse composition[140,141] have been identified, but bear an inconstant relationship to thrombocytopenia. When severe thrombocytopenia is part of a systemic relapse, platelet deposition may occur in vessels involved by inflammation,[142] as part of the hemophagocytic syndrome or a systemic thrombotic microangiopathy, in which cases ITP-directed approaches are often ineffective. The distinction may be difficult.[143] Evidence of marrow damage not found in ITP has been reported,[139] but amegakaryocytic thrombocytopenia is rare.[144]

The significance of thrombocytopenia depends on the clinical context. Thrombocytopenia has been associated with increased disease activity and mortality in some but not in all studies.[130,145] However, the clinical course of thrombocytopenia in the absence of other disease manifestations is similar to primary ITP,[128,146] whereas severe thrombocytopenia that develops during a systemic exacerbation of vasculitis may carry a poorer prognosis.[128,129,147] Treatment decisions should be predicated on the extent to which thrombocytopenia per se is the predominant reason for treatment and the likelihood that systemic vasculitis will necessitate treatment in the future.

Because patients with persistent SLE often experience repeated episodes of thrombocytopenia, treatment should only be used when there is a risk of bleeding in order to avoid excessive use of corticosteroids or other medications in these heavily treated patients. Patients with severe thrombocytopenia and no evidence of active SLE should be treated as if they had primary ITP, in which case the initial response to corticosteroids, danazol, IVIG, and immunosuppression is comparable.[130,148–151] There is less published experience with other medical approaches although rituximab has activity in SLE and the thrombopoietic agents may be useful in the future. The role of splenectomy remains controversial. Variation in the response rates reflects differences in disease severity.[152,153] Reliance on splenectomy should be tempered by the knowledge that patients may often require corticosteroids or immunosuppressants to control the underlying disease. In our opinion splenectomy is indicated when thrombocytopenia is severe and persistent, is the predominant reason for treatment, when other tolerable options are ineffective, and when the SLE is otherwise well controlled.[154] Profound thrombocytopenia occurring during the course of a systemic exacerbation of SLE requires control of the underlying disease.[155]

Common Variable Immunodeficiency and IgA Deficiency

ITP occurs with increased frequency in patients with common variable immunodeficiency (CVID) and other forms of immunodeficiency. Approximately 10% of patients with CVID develop ITP and a similar proportion autoimmune hemolysis. Conversely, approximately 1% of adults with otherwise typical ITP meet criteria for CVID.[156] The average age at diagnosis was 28 years in one large series.[157] CVID should be suspected in patients with even mild recurrent infections and allergies, as should IgA deficiency. A higher than expected incidence of mutations in the transmembrane activator and calcium modulator and cyclophilin ligand [CAML] interactor (TACI) have been reported in patients with CVID with ITP and Evans syndrome.[158] Splenectomy and immunosuppressive agents should be avoided to the extent possible and treatment with IVIG is preferable. IgA deficiency also occurs in at least 1% of ITP patients although anti-IgA antibodies are rare.

Lymphoproliferative Disorders

Chronic Lymphocytic Leukemia

Thrombocytopenia caused by marrow and splenic infiltration is a common feature of advanced CLL; these patients have a mean survival of about 19 months. By contrast, ITP occurs in more than 10% patients with CLL,[159] may precede the diagnosis of CLL or develop at any stage and does not necessarily confer a poor prognosis.[160–162] The diagnosis of ITP becomes progressively more difficult as the CLL progresses. ITP should be suspected in early-stage disease when the bone marrow contains "adequate" numbers of megakaryocytes or in advanced stages when the severity of thrombocytopenia is disproportionate to the extent of marrow infiltration or splenomegaly. The concurrent development of autoimmune hemolytic anemia may suggest the diagnosis as well.[161] Several cases have been associated with the use of fludarabine.[163] When ITP is difficult to diagnose, a course of therapy with IVIG may be indicated for therapeutic and diagnostic purposes, although most patients with CLL and immune thrombocytopenia respond to corticosteroids or splenectomy.[160–162] Rituximab has been useful to inhibit both B-cell proliferation and antibody production, although additional agents are necessary to treat the CLL itself. IVIG prophylaxis (400 mg/kg/month) should be considered in patients postsplenectomy and in those with a history of infection or who require chronic immunosuppressive therapy.

Hodgkin Disease and Non-Hodgkin Lymphomas

ITP occurs in up to 1% of patients with Hodgkin disease. The clinical course of approximately 50 patients has been reported.[164–166] In three-quarters of these, ITP was diagnosed an average of 52 months (1 month–22 years) after the Hodgkin disease was diagnosed,[167] whereas it was discovered at the time of splenectomy for ITP in a few.[5] In the rest, ITP preceded the diagnosis of Hodgkin disease, although in some the interval was so long as to place the association in doubt.[167–169] In approximately one-third of the reported cases, ITP heralded a recurrence.[164,166,167,170,171] Most patients without evidence of recurrent Hodgkin disease responded to corticosteroids,[167,171] splenectomy,[170] and/or azathioprine,[171] whereas chemotherapy treatment of the underlying disease was effective in others.[161]

The association between immune thrombocytopenia and non-Hodgkin lymphoma appears almost coincidental[164,170,172–174]; however, autoimmune hemolysis occurs in some patients as well. In most cases, thrombocytopenia proved difficult to manage unless the underlying malignancy responded to chemotherapy.

Leukemia of Large Granular Lymphocytes

The term LGL leukemia is applied to two disorders distinguished by the phenotype of the clonally expanded cell population.[175] In more than 90%, there is a clonal expansion of $CD3^+CD16^+$ T cells (T-LGL) and the natural history is typically one of stability or slow progression. In the remaining patients, the LGL cells express an NK phenotype ($CD3^-CD16^+CD57^+$), the disorder is more aggressive, and severe thrombocytopenia caused by marrow replacement and splenic infiltration may develop over months.[175] Most patients with T-LGL present with recurrent infections secondary to neutropenia. Five to 20% develop thrombocytopenia, which is generally mild and secondary to splenomegaly. An occasional patient presents with severe thrombocytopenia and the clinical picture of ITP.[176] The diagnosis should be suspected when thrombocytopenia is accompanied by neutropenia, arthralgia, splenomegaly, and/or a positive test for rheumatoid factor, similar to Felty syndrome. On occasion, the number of LGL cells is only slightly increased,[175] making it hard to distinguish from severe ITP in which an increase in $CD56^+D3^-$ cells[177] may also be observed.[178] Insufficient patients have been reported to determine whether the response to treatment in T-LGL differs from that of primary ITP.

Posttransplantation

Persistent thrombocytopenia develops in 3% to 5% of recipients of allogeneic bone marrow and solid organ transplants as a result of allo- or autoimmune or nonimmune causes, including partial reconstitution, graft versus host disease, CMV infection, venoocclusive disease, sepsis, and microangiopathic processes, among others.[179–181] Alloimmune thrombocytopenia may result from residual host B-cell reactivity against donor platelets.[182] Autoimmune thrombocytopenia, which has also been reported after autologous bone marrow or peripheral blood stem cell transplantation, is presumed to result from immune dysregulation or, rarely, donation by patients with compensated ITP.[183,184] Thrombocytopenia is often mild and transient, but in others is persistent, severe, and occasionally refractory and fatal. In the latter cases, patients do not respond to typical ITP therapies and careful exploration for infections and GVHD is warranted. In general, the treatment options are the same as those for primary ITP including, on occasion, splenectomy and retransplantation, but response rates are low (reviewed in reference 180). Thrombopoietic agents may prove useful in the future.

Miscellaneous Disorders

An increased incidence of immune thrombocytopenia is reported in patients with autoimmune thyroid disease.[185,186] Also, mild thrombocytopenia may be caused by hypersplenism that responds slowly to control of the hyperthyroid state.[185] The incidence of hypothyroidism also appears to be increased in ITP patients. In patients with sarcoidosis, immune platelet destruction may be superimposed on thrombocytopenia caused by splenic and marrow infiltration with granulomas.[187,188] ITP is also reported in association with myasthenia gravis,[189] multiple sclerosis,[1] and in patients with a variety of benign and malignant neoplasms, most of whom respond to conventional treatment for ITP.[174,190,191] Evans syndrome is the combination of autoimmune hemolysis and ITP. Response rates to medical therapy and splenectomy are lower than in primary ITP, especially in children. Severe ITP and other cytopenias also occur in patients with autoimmune lymphoproliferative syndrome caused by mutations in the Fas gene, Fas, caspase-8, or caspase-10; the disorder may present in adults and occasionally without marked lymphadenopathy (reviewed in reference 192).

IMMUNE THROMBOCYTOPENIC PURPURA IN CHILDHOOD

Introduction

The child with ITP differs from adults with ITP with respect to the differential diagnosis, the higher frequency of earlier spontaneous remission, and the greater reluctance to proceed to splenectomy. Potential long-term effects of treatment require careful consideration in a population with a greater-than-50-year life expectancy. There is as yet no pathophysiological explanation that explains the differences in ITP between these two age groups.

Presentation

Children with acute ITP typically present with the sudden onset of petechiae and purpura and platelet counts lower than 20,000 to 30,000/μL. The relationship between the bleeding risk and platelet count appears to be similar to that found in adults. Intracranial hemorrhage (ICH) has been reported in approximately 0.1% to 1% of children.[193] This may be higher than the incidence in adults and may occur earlier in the course. Both sexes up to teen age are affected with equal frequency. The peak incidence of ITP occurs between the ages of 3 and 5 but it may occur at any age after 2 to 3 months.[194] Many children have a history of nonspecific viral infection or vaccination with live virus[195] in the week(s) prior to developing symptoms. However, causality is hard to prove. The parents and pediatrician are often more concerned than the child, who usually feels well. As in adults, the physical examination is notable only for signs of bleeding, absence of hepatomegaly or lymphadenopathy, and a normal uvula and radial rays; minimal splenomegaly is detectable in less than 10% of children. The CBC should be within normal limits for age with the exception of the platelet count; if anemia is due to chronic bleeding, microcytosis and hypochromia may be present. The white blood cell differential, which normally has more lymphocytes than neutrophils in children less than 4 to 5 years of age,[194] is also expected to be normal, although some young, activated cells may be seen on smear.

Evaluation

To experienced pediatric hematologists, this constellation of findings (ie, an otherwise healthy child with the apparent rapid onset of isolated thrombocytopenia and a physical examination notable only for bleeding) is sufficient to make a diagnosis of ITP, which is by far the most common (>95%) cause of isolated, especially severe, thrombocytopenia in childhood. No additional testing, including a bone marrow, is required if the presentation is typical irrespective of choice of therapy.[3,196,197] Red blood cell typing for the presence of the Rh(D) antigen, a reticulocyte count, and direct antiglobulin test is appropriate if use of anti-D is contemplated.[3,196,197] Cooperative childhood cancer study group trials, which included thousands of children with leukemia, demonstrated that none presented with isolated thrombocytopenia, an otherwise normal blood count and smear, and the absence of hepatosplenomegaly or lymphadenopathy.[193,198] Moreover, although some pediatricians are more comfortable if a bone marrow examination is performed prior to treatment with corticosteroids, in a study of more than 100 thrombocytopenic children with a classical presentation of ITP, only one child was found to have another diagnosis (aplastic anemia, not leukemia).[197] Finally, as in adults, a substantial response to IVIG or anti-D is diagnostic of ITP.[199] Additional testing should be performed, e.g., HIV, only if the appropriate signs, symptoms, or history are present.[200]

Differential Diagnosis

Once thrombocytopenia is documented, three questions arise: (a) Is the thrombocytopenia isolated? (b) If isolated, is it immune? and (c) If immune, is it primary? Additional diagnoses must be considered if other cytopenias or abnormalities on physical examination are present.

1. Severe anemia, even if there has been significant epistaxis or metromenorrhea, should lead to an investigation of alternative diagnoses, for example, aplastic anemia and dysplastic marrow disorders occasionally characterized by an elevated MCV (>90 in preteens), microangiopathic hemolytic disorders (Chapter 139) and Evans syndrome (see above). Orthopedic abnormalities are common in children with Fanconi anemia (thumbs) and with Thrombocytopenia and Absent Radius syndrome (TAR) syndrome. Neutropenia may be caused by an associated neutrophil antibody (analogous to anemia in Evans syndrome) or a sign of an underlying marrow disorder.
2. In a healthy child with an otherwise normal CBC and no abnormalities other than bleeding manifestations on physical examination, the next consideration is to exclude other nonimmune inherited disorders that account for 2% to 10% of the children presenting with isolated thrombocytopenia.[201] A bone marrow examination will not usually help to differentiate ITP from these syndromes. The diagnosis of a familial disorder may be difficult for many reasons. Affected family members may be asymptomatic or the disorder may be inherited in an autosomal recessive manner. Commonly, an inherited cause of thrombocytopenia is suspected only after the child has failed to respond to treatment for ITP. Fortunately, most children with inherited thrombocytopenias have mild to moderate thrombocytopenia (20,000–100,000/μL) and do not have symptoms or require treatment other than prior to surgery or when the platelet count is further decreased by infection. Small platelets should raise a suspicion of Wiscott–Aldrich syndrome, the XLT form may present with thrombocytopenia alone. The Bernard–Soulier syndrome should be suspected if there is moderate thrombocytopenia and giant platelets, as should the group of MHY9-RD macrothrombocytopenias, such as May–Hegglin, which are characterized by mutations in the heavy chain of nonmuscle myosin (Chapter 32). Non-TAR, congenital amegakaryocytic thrombocytopenia may be indistinguishable from ITP on presentation. The diagnosis is often first considered in a child less than 1 to 3 years of age when thrombocytopenia only responds to platelet transfusions. Testing for a c-mpl mutation will identify most patients, although bone marrow biopsy remains the definitive diagnostic test.
3. Underlying disorders associated with ITP should be excluded. HIV as a cause of ITP in childhood is usually the result of in utero transmission; effective antiretroviral therapy almost always suppresses clinical manifestations in the infant. Hepatitis C and *H pylori* need to be considered, as in adults, although there is far less information in this age group. SLE (with or without antiphospholipid syndrome) may develop in 2% to 5% of female adolescents

who present with ITP. Testing for antinuclear antibodies should only be performed if suggestive symptoms or laboratory findings are present. Humoral immunodeficiency is found in 1% to 2% of children with ITP, most commonly due to CVI or IgA deficiency. Almost 10% of ITP patients were IgG_2 deficient in one study[157]; the incidence may be sufficient to warrant measuring immunoglobulin and subclass levels and/or documenting response to polyvalent pneumococcal vaccine prior to splenectomy.[202] Immunoglobulin measurements may also be indicated in children who are to receive IVIG.[203] Autoimmune lymphoproliferative syndrome is characterized by marked hepatosplenomegaly and/or lymphadenopathy beginning in childhood[192,204]; autoimmune hemolysis is common. Most cases have an abnormality in CD95 (Fas), resulting in persistence of autoreactive T cells that fail to undergo timely programmed cell death.

Management at Presentation

Which children with acute ITP should be treated and which treatment should be used remain controversial.[3,196,205,206] Treatment is intended to prevent ICH and to improve quality of life. However, the incidence of ICH is too low[207] to perform a controlled study of treatment. The risk of ICH is higher in children with platelet counts lower than 10,000/μL,[208] those presenting with extensive "wet" purpura or additional sites of bleeding, with coexisting coagulopathies, or with a history of significant head trauma. However, as ICH can occur in the absence of bleeding at other sites, our approach is to treat all children with platelet counts below 15,000 to 20,000/μL. It should be emphasized that no trial has demonstrated a reduction in ICH with treatment, and other experienced pediatric hematologists use more (or less) restrictive criteria. At least 80% of affected children recover spontaneously, approximately half within the first 2 months.[209,210] Chronicity is more likely to develop in teenagers, and in children with SLE or Evans syndrome. However, children of any age can develop chronic ITP even with an otherwise typical presentation, and there is as yet no evidence that the natural history of childhood ITP is altered by early treatment.[211]

Prednisone (2–4 mg/kg/day),[212] IV or oral methylprednisolone (30 mg/kg/day for 3 days),[213] IVIG (1 g/kg/day for 2 days)[214] and IV anti-D (75 μg/kg)[73,87] shorten the duration of severe thrombocytopenia compared with observation alone. IVIG increased the platelet count by an average of 54,000/μL within the first 24 hours in one study.[199] The combination of IVIG and corticosteroids may be synergistic. Platelet transfusions should be reserved for ongoing or imminent, (e.g., post head trauma), major hemorrhage.[53] We recommend that all children with acute ITP, platelet counts lower than 20,000/μL, and wet purpura, hematuria, hematochezia, or metromenorrhagia, be treated with a combination of IVIG (1 g/kg/day) and intravenous methylprednisolone (30 mg/kg/day), both for 1 to 3 days, with the goal of increasing the platelet count to exceed 30,000/μL and cessation of bleeding. If bleeding continues and the platelet count does not increase, adding IV anti-D (75 μg/kg in an Rh+, DAT− patient) and/or vincristine (0.03 mg/kg) is almost always effective. The diagnosis of ITP should be reconsidered if a child fails to respond to therapy, in which case a bone marrow should be performed or repeated.[55]

Management of Acute Immune Thrombocytopenic Purpura After the First Week

The goal of treatment is to maintain a platelet count higher than 20,000 to 30,000/μL with a minimum of toxicity, allowing normal or near normal activity until further improvement occurs spontaneously. Drugs that impair platelet function, such as aspirin, nonsteroidal antiinflammatory agents, and glycerol guaiacolate, should be avoided. Guidelines must be set for physical activity. Our policy is to interdict only high-contact sports such as football, lacrosse, and hockey at platelet counts lower than 30,000/μL, but not to restrict other physical activities, including basketball, soccer, track, swimming, bicycling, baseball, and tennis, although such decisions need to be individualized.[37]

Primary reliance may be placed upon prednisone because it is relatively inexpensive, given orally, and toxicity is not intolerable as long as treatment duration is limited. The dose is usually tapered over 2 to 6 weeks, although there is no evidence in favor of any specific duration. If prednisone is continued, an attempt should be made to administer it on alternate days to minimize toxicity, especially osteoporosis, the most significant, long-term side effect of corticosteroids in children. The utility of high-dose dexamethasone in children with chronic ITP has been disappointing.[211]

We recommend IVIG[217] or IV anti-D (Winrho-SD)[73] either as initial treatment or for children who require more than 0.1 to 0.2 mg/kg/day of prednisone as continued treatment. Both IVIG and anti-D are generally administered on an "as needed" basis rather than at fixed intervals. Treatment may be continued for at least 12 months if a response is seen, as spontaneous improvement may be delayed. In general, few children will require splenectomy. Treatment with rituximab[104,218] or, less commonly, azathioprine[219] may be used on occasion to defer splenectomy. Although short-term treatment results may mimic those seen in adults, the long-term outcome is not known. Evidence of special toxicity is not present, but some clinicians give IVIG to young children treated with rituximab to avoid potential hypogammaglobulinemia.[220] Danazol is reserved for peri- and postpubertal ITP because of its effect on bone age.

The advantage of IVIG in managing children includes the high response rate and lack of serious long-term toxicity.[199,206] The disadvantages are that IVIG must be infused over hours, depending upon the platelet count, postinfusion headaches are common and often marked, and the cost is high.[217] In contrast to adults, few pediatric patients become refractory even with prolonged treatment. There is no evidence that any of the commercially available products differ in clinical effectiveness. Anti-D appears to be equally safe as and comparably effective to IVIG in Rh+ patients who have not undergone splenectomy[73] and infusion is complete within minutes. Whether early treatment with IVIG or anti-D will alter the incidence of chronic ITP remains to be determined. Children have been treated with each modality for years without evidence of cumulative toxicity.

Chronic Immune Thrombocytopenic Purpura in Children: Management After 6 to 12 Months

Durable clinical remission occurs in 70% to 90% of children with typical ITP after splenectomy.[221] Laparoscopic splenectomy has less long-term impact on physical activity and child-bearing than an open procedure. Yet, pediatric hematologists delay recommending splenectomy for at least 1 year after diagnosis for two reasons. First, children who have platelet counts higher than 20,000 to 30,000/μL and are asymptomatic can be followed safely with little or no treatment. Virtually all children can be managed with IVIG or anti-D if the platelet count falls below 20,000 to 30,000/μL; low doses of prednisone (<0.2 mg/kg/qod) can be added, as needed. Our experience and those of others is that the platelet count often improves over time, although on occasion a previously stable patient will develop thrombocytopenia and menorrhagia at puberty. Second, the risk of postsplenectomy sepsis may be as high as 2% over 10 years in children. Indeed, there have been deaths reported from postsplenectomy sepsis as well as from bleeding in this age group. The risk appears to be reduced substantially by administering pneumococcal, H Flu B, and meningococcal vaccines in conjunction with prophylactic antibiotics, which is the current standard of care. How often to revaccinate and the value of prophylactic antibiotics in this setting remain unsettled. We currently recommend that Pneumovax be readministered every 5 to 10 years, but do not readminister H Flu B vaccine unless a specific risk is identified. Meningococcal vaccine is typically

Initial Management of Immune Thrombocytopenic Purpura in Childhood

It is well known that children with newly diagnosed immune thrombocytopenic purpura (ITP) often improve on their own, with or without treatment. A recent study suggests that the rate of spontaneous improvement may be as high as 90% by 1 year, with half of the children showing improvement within 2 months.[215] This high rate of spontaneous improvement has led to the evolution of two distinct schools of thought regarding the approach to the initial management of children who present with acute ITP.

Proponents of one school believe that if patients are likely to get better on their own, little is to be gained by intervention until at least 3 to 6 months has passed from diagnosis. Even then therapy is not indicated unless the platelet count is very low and there is significant bleeding, as the prognosis for eventual improvement or resolution is still good. The rationale is that intracranial hemorrhage (ICH) is a very rare event, that all therapies have toxicities, and the entire process of providing treatment, including doctor's visits and obtaining blood counts, generates more distress than benefit.

In contrast, advocates of the other school believe that it is appropriate to provide treatment to a child if the platelet count is very low, that is, less than 15,000 to 20,000/μL, in order to minimize the risk of bleeding. This approach takes into account parental anxiety regarding low counts, risk of nonfatal but serious bleeding in addition to ICH, and the need to restrict physical activities until the count improves.

Observational studies are underway that may provide insight into this controversy, but an unequivocal answer may remain elusive because too many unmeasurable variables contribute to the risk of bleeding, especially when the incidence of severe bleeding is low. In the absence of such information, one clear change in medical practice has been that the cutoff platelet count for intervention even among "treaters" has decreased from 30,000–50,000/μL to 10,000–20,000/μL in children with no bleeding or only scattered petechiae or minimal bruising. Also, there is more emphasis on basing treatment decisions on the extent of bleeding, although there is neither precision nor uniformity in approach among even the most experienced pediatric hematologists.

Even in settings where there is reasonable consensus that treatment is indicated, considerable variation remains in practice patterns. Some assume that in the most severely affected patients,[216] any of the most effective treatments (IVIG 1 g/kg, IV anti-D 75 μg/kg, and very high-dose corticosteroids), each of which have their own kinetics, cost and toxicity profile, can be used supplemented by platelet transfusions as needed. Recent data indicate that the combination of IVIG (1 g/kg), IV methylprednisolone (30 mg/kg), IV anti-D (75 μg/kg), and/or vincristine (0.03 mg/kg) is often effective when single agents are not.[55]

Whatever criteria for instituting treatment are used and whatever treatment is instituted, the most important clinical message is the need to monitor the patient very closely for new signs of bleeding and the readiness to provide additional treatment within 12 to 72 hours if there is no response to the first agent chosen. Additional studies of acute ITP in children are needed to predict risk of bleeding and chronicity that would permit more rational intervention in a disorder that is generally benign but that is rarely occasioned by catastrophic bleeding complications or by severe thrombocytopenia lasting for years.

(re)administered prior to starting college. Intravenous antibiotics should be initiated urgently for children with a fever higher than 102°F. Most pediatric hematologists prefer waiting until a child has reached 5 years of age before recommending splenectomy because of the frequency of infection and high fevers in this population, although there is insufficient data on the risk of sepsis after the age of 2 to make firm recommendations in difficult-to-manage patients. In younger children, it may be wise to document protective titers of antibody to the most common serotypes of pneumococcus prior to splenectomy. No other long-term health risks have been identified in children who have been splenectomized for ITP to date although this has received little study and pulmonary hypertension has been reported after splenectomy, primarily to treat or as a result of hemolytic disorders.

Among the few children refractory to splenectomy, alternate diagnoses should be reinvestigated. Few children have significant bleeding problems even if they remain thrombocytopenic, an observation that must be borne in mind when recommending potentially toxic forms of treatment for platelet counts higher than 20,000/μL. The rare, symptomatic, refractory pediatric patient should be approached in the same manner as the comparable adult, although the potential side effects of various drugs may differ depending on the age of the child. The efficacy of treatment in this setting is entirely anecdotal.

IMMUNE THROMBOCYTOPENIC PURPURA DURING PREGNANCY

Diagnosis

The incidence of ITP is reported to be 1 to 2 per 1000 deliveries.[222] Proper management involves not only careful attention to the mother but also an awareness of the incidence and consequences of neonatal thrombocytopenia caused by transplacental passage of maternal autoantibodies. This includes the risks and benefits to the fetus of maternal therapy, invasive monitoring, and surgical delivery. Comprehensive reviews of the differential diagnosis and management of thrombocytopenia in pregnancy have been published.[223,224]

The most common condition confused with ITP is gestational thrombocytopenia, which occurs in 4% to 8% of pregnancies. Gestational thrombocytopenia is likely when an otherwise healthy woman with a previously documented normal platelet count develops mild thrombocytopenia (>70,000–100,000/μL) in the third trimester of an uncomplicated pregnancy.[225] Severe maternal or neonatal thrombocytopenia is rare and there is no indication for additional diagnostic or therapeutic interventions other than following the maternal platelet count until term when epidural anesthesia becomes an issue (see below). Because gestational thrombocytopenia and ITP are both diagnoses of exclusion, it may be difficult to make the distinction in an asymptomatic woman with no previous platelet count who presents with moderate to severe thrombocytopenia earlier in pregnancy.[226,227] Although the incidence of gestational thrombocytopenia far exceeds all other causes combined, previously healthy women can present for the first time during gestation with ITP, early preeclampsia, type IIb von Willebrand disease, a microangiopathic disorder, or hereditary thrombocytopenia.

Therapy of Immune Thrombocytopenic Purpura in Pregnancy

Most women are managed through pregnancy without major difficulty, although a severe exacerbation may occur on occasion. The only contraindication to pregnancy is the (inadvertent) use of cytotoxic drugs with teratogenic potential during the first trimester. Pregnancy does not alter the threshold for maternal treatment in ITP, as platelet counts higher than 20,000 to 30,000/μL are adequate for otherwise uncomplicated pregnancy until term.[3] Prednisone has been the mainstay of therapy and appears to pose little risk to the human fetus owing to placental metabolism.[228] However, protracted use of prednisone is associated with a higher rate of premature labor and pregnancy-induced hypertension[227] and may exacerbate gestational diabetes. For these reasons, refractory patients and those requiring more than 20 mg of prednisone daily are generally managed with IVIG. Laparoscopic splenectomy has been performed successfully during the second trimester,[229] but is rarely needed and should be avoided unless absolutely necessary. There is limited experience with azathioprine for ITP, although it has been used to suppress renal transplant rejection without evidence of teratogenicity.[228] We have reported on the treatment of eight women with anti-D (1–7 courses) without evidence of fetal hydrops by ultrasound or of neonatal anemia or jaundice in the seven Rh+ neonates.[230] Rituximab can be detected in serum for 3 to 6 months after completion of treatment and in theory can be transported across the placenta and cause B-cell depletion in the fetus. Other drugs, for example, vinca alkaloids, should also be avoided if at all possible.

The major therapeutic challenge generally comes at delivery. Maternal platelet counts greater than 50,000/μL suffice for cesarean section[227,231] and this level is a useful goal as term approaches when emergent obstetrical indications are more common. Cesarean sections have been performed safely at lower platelet counts when necessary.[226] Anesthesiologists require higher platelet counts for epidural anesthesia, although studies to support any minimal threshold are lacking.[226] Severe bleeding after vaginal delivery is uncommon even at very low platelet counts.[226,227] A second major goal of management is to prevent neonatal ICH. However, there is no noninvasive means to identify neonates at risk, and the best approach to managing delivery remains unsettled.[232] The risk of neonatal thrombocytopenia lower than 50,000/μL is estimated to be 9% to 15%, the incidence of platelet counts below 20,000/μL is approximately 5%,[226] and the risk of ICH is below 1%.[231] Antenatal ICH is extremely rare,[226] arguing against maternal treatment of the fetus (in contrast to alloimmune thrombocytopenia) except for very special cases, for example, the mother's previous child was born with an ICH or a platelet count lower than 10,000/μL.

The risk of severe neonatal thrombocytopenia appears to be substantially greater if a previous fetus has been severely affected[226,233] and perhaps if the mother is more severely affected.[226,234] Otherwise, there is at best a weak correlation between fetal and maternal platelet counts.[222,226,227,235,236] Severely thrombocytopenic neonates have been born to mothers with normal platelet counts,[237] including those who responded to splenectomy, corticosteroids, or IVIG.[238]

There is no noninvasive means to predict the fetal platelet count. Although prenatal platelet counts can be measured by fetal scalp or percutaneous umbilical blood sampling (PUBS), neither is in widespread use. Too often fetal scalp sampling platelet counts are falsely low because of clumping, which leads to unnecessary emergency cesarean sections, and the risk of hemorrhage after PUBS exceeds that of ICH even in skilled hands. Although there is no direct evidence that cesarean section prevents ICH in ITP,[231] we consider the procedure if severe neonatal thrombocytopenia is documented or expected[3,239] or if there is a difficult delivery. Neonatal platelet counts often fall transiently in the first few days postpartum, possibly related to the maturation of the reticuloendothelial cell system. Treatment with IVIG and steroids is indicated at platelet counts lower than 30,000/μL in view of the vulnerability of neonates to ICH. A head sonogram, CT, and/or MRI should be obtained as soon as possible after birth to exclude ICH. Emergent management of the neonate with platelet transfusions and IVIG with or without corticosteroids[240] should be instituted if there is any suspicion of bleeding, even in the absence of overt neurologic impairment or documented hemorrhage until ICH can be excluded on radiologic grounds. Close monitoring should continue until a normal platelet count is documented.

Neonatal Alloimmune Thrombocytopenia

Clinical Presentation

Alloimmune thrombocytopenia (AIT) is the platelet analog of hemolytic disease of the newborn, although there are important differences in natural history and management. AIT is identified clinically in approximately 1 in 5000 term pregnancies (approximately 800–4000 cases per year in the United States),[241,242] accounting for as many as 50% of the cases of severe neonatal thrombocytopenia.[241,243] Large screening studies have documented that AIT actually occurs as often as 1 in 1000 deliveries based on both systematically performed neonatal platelet counts and screening of HPA-1a negative families.[244–246] Neonates with moderate thrombocytopenia are now being identified more often as a result of greater awareness and the wider availability of recently developed serologic techniques. However, in contrast to hemolytic disease of the newborn, routine screening is still not performed.[241,247] Typically, the diagnosis is suspected when bleeding and severe thrombocytopenia occur unexpectedly in a neonate born after an otherwise uneventful pregnancy. A platelet count lower than 50,000/μL, unknown etiology of the thrombocytopenia, and possibly a family history of transient neonatal thrombocytopenia point to the diagnosis of AIT.[245] ICH is common (10%–20%) and is fatal in 1% to 5% of cases.[241,248] Hydrocephalus or porencephaly due to ICH in utero occurs in up to 10% of severely thrombocytopenic fetuses.[248–251] Thrombocytopenia typically persists for up to 3 weeks.[243]

Pathogenesis

AIT is caused by the transplacental passage of maternal alloantibodies against platelet antigens shared by the father and fetus. Shed fetal platelet antigens can pass into the maternal circulation by the end of the first trimester,[252] by which time the placenta has developed the capacity to transport maternal IgG antibodies to the fetus. Serologic diagnosis involves demonstrating parental platelet antigen incompatibility and antiplatelet antibody in maternal serum of matching specificity. Diverse biallelic antigen systems have been implicated. Most cases identified in non-Asian populations occur in homozygous HPA-1b (Pl(A2)/Pl(A2)) mothers.[241] Most neonates are severely affected as are the few cases attributable to alloantibodies against other determinants on platelet glycoprotein IIIa, for example, anti-HPA-1b[253] and anti-HPA-4 (Yuk(a)/Pen) in Asian populations[254] and glycoprotein IIb, for example, anti-HPA-3a (Bak(a)/Lek) and anti-HPA-9(Max).[255] Br(a)/Br(b) incompatibility, which accounts for 15% to 20% of the cases of AIT in Europe,[241,256] is generally milder and is more likely to occur during subsequent pregnancies, presumably because platelets express fewer copies of the glycoprotein Ia/IIa complex on which the HPA-5 alleles are located. Too few cases of AIT due to antibodies to other antigens[257–259] have been reported to estimate the severity or prevalence because a severe clinical presentation is the usual reason to initiate an investigation. There is debate regarding the frequency of Gov (HPA-15a and 15b) incompatibility as a cause of AIT. ABO- and HLA antibodies rarely, if ever, cause AIT. Additional alloantibodies with novel specificities will likely be identified in the future. These advances place additional demands on referral laboratories to acquire and maintain the appropriate roster of typed controls, reference sera, and DNA-based techniques for haplotyping.

Neonatal thrombocytopenia develops in 1% to 6% of women who are homozygous for the HPA-1b allele and carry an HPA-1a fetus.[241,242] Production of anti-HPA-1a antibodies occurs almost exclusively in women who carry the HLA haplotype DRB30101 also known as Dw52a[260–263]; the incidence of AIT in this subpopulation exceeds 25%,[242] a relative risk 10- to 100-fold above HPA-1b/1b women with other HLA haplotypes. Genetic restriction in the development of anti-HPA-5a antibodies may exist as well.[264] These genetic linkages have important implications in managing relatives of affected women. Because fetal blood sampling may induce sensitization, it is our policy to test previously unsensitized HPA-1b/1b, DRB30101 positive women for circulating anti-HPA-1a antibodies monthly, and at 36 to 38 weeks if the child's father is HPA-1a positive. A PUBS is performed only if antibodies are detected. Amniocentesis is performed for fetal platelet typing if the father is unavailable, uncertain, or a heterozygote.

Management of the Affected Child

The index case can be devastating and typically occurs without warning. ICH is identified in approximately 10% of neonates during the peripartum period, making immediate diagnosis and treatment mandatory. A normal maternal platelet count should be documented, although AIT can occur coincidentally with ITP or other causes of maternal thrombocytopenia, especially gestational.[265] A neonate born with a platelet count lower than 50,000/μL should be presumed to have AIT even if there is evidence of another etiology such as bacterial sepsis, disseminated intravascular coagulation, congenital viral (herpes, CMV, varicella, rubella) or toxoplasma infection. AIT should also be considered in any neonate with parenchymal ICH. If AIT is suspected, treatment followed by testing should be initiated.

The urgency of treatment should be governed by the likelihood of ICH and the severity of the thrombocytopenia. If the ultrasound or CT is normal and there is no clinical evidence of ICH, transfusion of random donor platelets, which has been shown to be effective in most cases of neonatal AIT in two recent studies, should also be started.[266,267] IVIG should also be started[241,268,269] although responses can take 1 to 3 days. Therefore, corticosteroids may provide added benefit but should not be used as the sole modality.[241,270] If ICH has occurred, then random donor platelets should be given immediately, and repeated as needed to maintain the count higher than 50,000 to 100,000 along with IVIG (with or without corticosteroids) while antigen-negative, often maternal, platelets are procured.[271] Although in theory maternal platelets should be washed to remove circulating alloantibody and resuspended in AB-positive plasma, in actual practice they can be administered safely after centrifugation alone. The platelets should be irradiated to lessen the risk of graft-versus-host disease.[272] A rise in the platelet count should be verified. Serologic studies of the parents should be performed to confirm the diagnosis because of the implications for subsequent pregnancies and the possible need for genetic counseling of other family members. Maternal antibodies that react with paternal platelets are not detected in up to 15% of otherwise typical cases.[241]

Management of Subsequent Pregnancies

An aggressive approach is warranted, especially in cases of HPA-1a incompatibility[273] for several reasons: (a) Severe thrombocytopenia recurs in more than 99% of subsequent pregnancies. (b) Most will be more severely affected than their previously affected sibling. (c) Severe fetal thrombocytopenia occurs early, with 40% of fetuses having platelet counts lower than 20,000/μL by 24 weeks. (d) Neither the presence nor the absence of alloantibody in the mother nor a change in antibody titer predicts the fetal platelet count.[242,274] (e) At least one-half of ICH occurs antenatally and, therefore, would not be prevented by elective cesarean section at term. (f) When treatment is withheld, fetal platelet counts often fall rapidly or remain very low during gestation.[275] (g) Effective antenatal treatment is available.[275,276]

Antenatal management has changed over the past several years as newer studies have enabled better informed therapeutic decisions to be made. Two approaches to antenatal management of thrombocytopenic fetuses have been studied. The more aggressive approach, pursued primarily in several European centers, involves weekly transfusion of maternal or antigen-matched platelets in utero starting as early as 20 to 26 weeks' gestation.[275,277] Each procedure carries a risk of fetal exsanguination and side effects from transfusion[278] and the long-term outcomes reflect the high risk to the fetus of repeated procedures. More recent studies have added to the concerns regarding fetal blood sampling.[279,280] In the United States, initially IVIG (1 g/kg/week) was administered weekly to the mother once it was clear that she was carrying an HPA-1a-positive fetus and thrombocytopenia was documented or could be assumed based on paternal homozygosity.[273,275,281–284] One randomized study clarified that IVIG alone at 1 g/kg/week was not sufficient if there had been an antenatal ICH or if the pretreatment fetal count was lower than 10,000 to 20,000/μL. Therefore a second dose of 1 gm/kg/week has been explored, as has the addition of prednisone (0.5–1 mg/kg/day).

We currently initiate therapy at 12 weeks of gestation with IVIG at a dose of 2 g/kg/week if an antenatal ICH occurred during a prior pregnancy. Otherwise IVIG either at 1 to 2 g/kg/week or at 1 g/kg/week together with 0.5 mg/kg/day of prednisone can be started at 20 to 26 weeks of gestation without fetal blood sampling. Whether to sample at 32 to 34 weeks of gestation in order to augment treatment for persisting fetal thrombocytopenia, continue treatment until term without sampling, or increase treatment without sampling at 32 weeks remains unsettled. Avoiding the initial fetal sampling has sufficed to provide good control of the fetal platelet count while substantially minimizing the number of invasive procedures.[285] Long-term outcome studies suggest that antenatal treatment does not result in residual complications for the fetus and may even preserve immunologic and neurologic development.[286,287]

POSTTRANSFUSION PURPURA

Clinical Presentation

Posttransfusion purpura (PTP) is an uncommon (1/7000 transfusions),[288] acquired thrombocytopenia that develops approximately 1 week after blood transfusion. The typical patient is a multiparous, middle-aged or elderly female who presents with the acute onset of bleeding due to severe thrombocytopenia a mean of 6 to 8 days (range 1–14 days) after receiving a blood product containing platelet material.[289] Almost all other affected patients have a history of prior transfusion, making PTP exceptionally rare in males and in previously untransfused nulliparous females.[247,290] In such cases, the onset may be delayed.[291] Subclinical cases have been reported,[292,293] but the incidence of asymptomatic, milder forms is unknown. PTP after bone marrow[294] or solid organ transplantation[295] has been described. On rare occasions, thrombocytopenia develops within hours after transfusion of a blood product containing alloantibodies to recipient platelets.[296,297]

Pathogenesis

The pathogenesis of PTP remains unclear. Alloantibodies are found in essentially all patients. However, the enigma is whether the alloantibodies are responsible for destroying autologous platelets, which appear to lack the relevant antigen. Any proposed explanation must also account for the low incidence in genetically susceptible individuals exposed to products known to contain the provoking antigen, the absence to date of the PTP syndrome in women whose pregnancies are complicated by AIT due to alloantibodies with same apparent specificity, the prolonged duration of the thrombocytopenia, the occasional failure to respond to transfusion of "antigen-negative" platelets,[298] and the fact that the syndrome may not recur after inadvertent or deliberate reexposure to antigen-mismatched products.[247,292,299] Indeed, in at least one instance, reinfusion of plasma obtained during the period of severe thrombocytopenia did not reproduce the syndrome.[300]

Sera from more than 90% of patients with PTP contain antibodies to the Pl(A1) antigen (HPA-1a), which is expressed on the platelets of 97% to 98% of the Caucasian population. In the remaining cases, antibodies to the Pl(A2) (HPA-1b) allele,[289] other epitopes on platelet glycoproteins IIb-IIIa or, less commonly, other platelet antigens are responsible. Although only anti-HLA antibodies were detected in several patients, their role is unclear.[289,301] Another unanswered question is why PTP is a rare disorder. On the basis of the prevalence of HPA-1b homozygosity, it would be expected that anti-HPA-1a antibodies would develop in 1% to 3% of all recipients of random donor transfusions. The lower-than-expected frequency may result in part from genetic restriction on antibody production. PTP and NAIT are both closely linked to HLA B8 and DRB30101.[242,260,263] Yet, only single instances of PTP occurring in sisters[302] or in a woman with a history of AIT have been reported.[303] Three theories to explain the clinical features of PTP have been proposed.

It was initially suggested that the alloantibodies cause complement-dependent lysis of donor platelets, releasing antigen–antibody complexes that bind to HPA-1a-negative host platelets via Fcγ receptors, perpetuating the destructive process.[300] Antigen-independent platelet destruction could explain why transfusing HPA-1a negative platelets may be ineffective as well as the failure to detect autoantibodies. Platelet eluates collected as long as 100 days after the acute episode may contain immunoglobulin with anti-HPA-1a reactivity[304,305] that also binds to autologous and other HPA-1 negative platelets.[304] However, it has not been proven that these sera or eluates contain immune complexes composed of HPA-1a and anti-HPA-1a, or that they volley between rapidly destroyed platelets and their replacements for several weeks without themselves being cleared from the circulation.

An interrelated hypothesis is that the immune complexes bind to HPA-1a-negative platelets through the antigen, followed by the formation of immune complexes in situ. Only during an anamnestic response would sufficient alloantibody and donor antigen be present coincidentally to initiate PTP. PTP plasma has been reported to contain HPA-1a antigen, both soluble and in the form of microparticles,[306,307] capable of binding to antigen-negative platelets in vitro.[308] It is estimated that binding of less than 5% of the amount of soluble HPA-1a antigen potentially present in a single unit of blood may suffice to destroy all circulating platelets.[309,310] The remaining antigen–antibody complexes could perpetuate sensitization of the markedly reduced number of residual platelets left after the initial round of destruction.[309] Although measurable amounts of HPA-1a antigen have been detected in PTP plasma during the acute syndrome,[309,310] it remains to be proven that HPA-1 antigen complexed with anti-HPA-1a antibody is present on host platelets in vivo.

A more compelling case can be made for the hypothesis that a subset of anti-HPA-1a antibodies cross-react with undefined determinants on HPA-1b platelets.[311] Although the HPA-1a and 1b antigens differ at a single amino acid, it is likely that the conformation of the gpIIb-IIIa complex diverges sufficiently that only a small proportion of anti-HPA-1a antibodies cross-react with host protein or that autoantibodies directed at entirely different epitopes are generated.[312] Sera and platelet eluates from some individuals with PTP have been found to contain immunoglobulin with anti-HPA-1a reactivity that also bind to autologous platelets and platelets lacking gpIIb-IIIa.[313,314] The hypothesis that a subset of antibodies cross-reacts with autologous platelets would be consistent with (a) the infrequent occurrence of overt PTP in HPA-1 negative patients (re)exposed to blood products containing the antigen; (b) the absence of PTP in HPA-1a negative mothers with AIT; (c) the prolonged course in the absence of treatment; and (d) the presence of anti-HPA-1a reactivity in eluates from autologous platelets and those congenitally lacking gpIIIa.

Diagnosis

PTP should be suspected in any patient, especially older multiparous or previously transfused women, who develop severe thrombocytopenia approximately 1 week after transfusion. Suspicion is heightened if the patient's plasma lyses platelets from random normal donors, because there are few other conditions (eg, quinidine and heparin-associated purpura) in which this occurs. Treatment must be initiated immediately based on clinical criteria, because it may take several days before the results of confirmatory tests become available. The sine qua non of diagnosis is the demonstration of platelet-specific alloantibodies to determinants that are not present on the patient's own platelets determined by genotyping.[315] Alloantibodies to HPA-1a/1b and HPA-5/5b are readily detected using a commercial ELISA but may be missed if the patient has received multiple platelet transfusions.[316] Detection of antibodies to other, less common antigens requires co-ordination with a reference center.

Treatment

The clinical course of untreated patients is typically prolonged. In one series, bleeding lasted a mean of 10.2 days.[289] It took a mean of 14.6 days until the platelet count exceeded 50,000/μL (range 3–90), and 19.5 days until it exceeded 100,000/μL (range 3–130). Thrombocytopenia can persist for 60 to 120 days[292] and fatality rates approach 10%.[247,298,317] Therefore, intervention must be initiated once the disorder is suspected clinically. The treatment of choice is intravenous immunoglobulin (IVIG) 1 g/kg/day for 2 days; a second course may be required.[318] More than 90% of patients respond, generally beginning within 2 to 3 days.[289,318] Corticosteroids have an adjunctive role, if any. A response to splenectomy in a refractory patient has been reported.[319] Thrombocytopenia may recur within days of stopping treatment; relapses are generally milder and more easily managed than was the initial episode.[289,310] The role of prophylactic platelet transfusions in patients with profound thrombocytopenia but non–life-threatening bleeding is unclear. Sera from affected patients often contain antibodies to many HLA determinants, making provision of antigen-matched platelets problematic. Administration of random donor platelets is commonly associated with moderate to severe transfusion reactions, including bronchospasm and hypotension, rarely succeeds in raising the platelet count, and theoretically may perpetuate the disease.[300,318,320,321] Even when antigen-matched platelets can be procured in time, they may or may not suffer the same fate as the patient's own "antigen-negative" cells (reviewed in reference 322).

Anti-HPA-1a antibodies may persist for more than a year[323] and PTP may recur.[292,299,324] Although reexposure to blood products containing the relevant antigen does not invariably provoke PTP,[300,310] antigen-matched or autologous blood products should be used whenever possible.[289] It is unknown whether washing or using frozen and thawed red cells removes sufficient antigen to prevent recurrence.[324,325] The increased use of leukodepletion may have contributed to the apparent decreased incidence of PTP.[288] There is no data as to the risk of PTP developing in unaffected multiparous or in previously transfused siblings who share HLA haplotypes. The risk of women with pregnancies complicated by NAIT developing PTP is sufficiently low that only awareness and close monitoring of platelet counts after transfusion appears warranted.

SUGGESTED READINGS

Burrows RF, Kelton JG: Fetal thrombocytopenia and its relation to maternal thrombocytopenia. N Engl J Med 329:1463, 1993.

Bussel JB, Kuter DJ, George JN, et al: AMG 531, a thrombopoiesis-stimulating protein, for chronic ITP. N Engl J Med 355(16):1672, 2006.

Cines DB, Bussel JB: How I treat idiopathic thrombocytopenic purpura (ITP). Blood 106(7):2244, 2005.

Cohen YC, Djulbegovic B, Shamai-Lubovitz O, et al: The bleeding risk and natural history of idiopathic thrombocytopenic purpura in patients with persistent low platelet counts. Arch Intern Med 160:1630, 2000.

Cooper N, Stasi R, Cunningham-Rundles S, et al: The efficacy and safety of B-cell depletion with anti-CD20 monoclonal antibody in adults with chronic immune thrombocytopenic purpura. Br J Haematol 125(2):232, 2004.

Diz-Kucukkaya R, Hacihanefioglu A, Yeneri M, et al: Antiphospholipid antibodies and antiphospholipid syndrome in patients presenting with immune thrombocytopenic purpura: A prospective cohort study. Blood 98:1760, 2001.

Gaines AR: Disseminated intravascular coagulation associated with acute hemoglobinemia or hemoglobinuria following Rho(D) immune globulin intravenous administration for immune thrombocytopenic purpura. Blood 106(5):1532, 2005.

George JN, Woolf SH, Raskob GE, et al: Idiopathic thrombocytopenic purpura: A practice guideline developed by explicit methods for the American Society of Hematology. Blood 88:3, 1996.

Gernsheimer T, Stratton J, Ballem PJ, et al: Mechanisms of response to treatment in autoimmune thrombocytopenic purpura. N Engl J Med 320:974, 1989.

Houwerzijl EJ, Blom NR, van der Want JJL, et al: Ultrastructural study shows morphological features of apoptosis and para-apoptosis in megakaryocytes from patients with idiopathic thrombocytopenic purpura. Blood 103:500, 2003.

Kojouri K, Vesely SK, Terrell DR, et al: Splenectomy for adult patients with idiopathic thrombocytopenic purpura: A systematic review to assess long-term platelet count responses, prediction of response, and surgical complications. Blood 104(9):2623, 2004.

Mazzucconi MG, Fazi P, Bernasconi S, et al: Therapy with high-dose dexamethasone (HD-DXM) in previously untreated patients affected by idiopathic thrombocytopenic purpura: A GIMEMA experience. Blood 109:1401, 2007.

McCrae KR, Samuels P, Schreiber AD: Pregnancy-associated thrombocytopenia: Pathogenesis and management. Blood 80:2697, 1992.

McMillan R, Durette C: Long-term outcomes in adults with chronic ITP after splenectomy failure. Blood 104(4):956, 2004.

Newman GC, Novoa MV, Fodero EM, et al: A dose of 75 mg/kg/d of IV anti-D increases the platelet count more rapidly and for a longer period of time that does 50 mg/kg/d in adults with immune thrombocytopenic purpura (ITP). Br J Haematol 112:1076, 2001.

Portiejle JEA, Westendorp RGJ, Kluin-Nelemans HC, et al: Morbidity and mortality in adults with idiopathic thrombocytopenic purpura. Blood 97:2549, 2001.

Provan D, Newland A, Bolton-Maggs P, et al: Guidelines for the investigation and management of idiopathic thrombocytopenic purpura in adults, children and in pregnancy. Br J Haematol 120:574, 2003.

Rajan SK, Espina BM, Liebman HA: Hepatitis C virus-related thrombocytopenia: Clinical and laboratory characteristics compared with chronic immune thrombocytopenic purpura. Br J Haematol 129(6):818, 2005.

Siragam V, Crow AR, Brinc D, et al: Intravenous immunoglobulin ameliorates ITP via activating Fc gamma receptors on dendritic cells. Nat Med 12(6):688, 2006.

REFERENCES

For complete list of references log onto www.expertconsult.com

CHAPTER 139

THROMBOTIC THROMBOCYTOPENIC PURPURA AND THE HEMOLYTIC UREMIC SYNDROME

Keith R. McCrae, J. Evan Sadler, and Douglas B. Cines

INTRODUCTION

In 1925, Moschowitz described a 16-year-old girl who died of a previously undescribed illness characterized by microangiopathic hemolytic anemia, petechiae, hemiparesis, and fever.[1] Postmortem examination revealed numerous hyaline thrombi, most prevalent in the terminal arterioles and capillaries of the heart and kidneys. In 1936, four similar cases were reported by Baehr et al, who proposed that the hyaline thrombi were secondary to agglutinated platelets,[2] and in 1947 Singer suggested that the term *thrombotic thrombocytopenic purpura* be used to describe this disorder.[3] In 1955 Gasser used the term *hemolytic uremic syndrome* (HUS) to describe a related syndrome that consisted of Coombs-negative hemolytic anemia, thrombocytopenia, and renal failure.[4] When considered together, these disorders are referred to as thrombotic microangiopathies, based on their shared features of microangiopathic hemolytic anemia, thrombocytopenia, and microvascular thrombotic lesions.[5–7]

The clinical and pathologic features of TTP and HUS often overlap.[6,8–10] However, these disorders appear to have a different pathogenesis as demonstrated by the high incidence of severe deficiency of the von Willebrand factor (VWF)-cleaving protease ADAMTS13 in patients with clinically diagnosed TTP, but not HUS.[11–13] Similarly, deficiency of complement regulatory proteins, particularly factor H or membrane cofactor protein, appears to be a unique characteristic of some familial and sporadic cases of HUS.[14–16] Moreover, although TTP and HUS affect many of the same organ systems, the frequency with which they do so differs, and the histopathologic features of the lesions of TTP and HUS are also distinct.[17] Finally, plasma exchange is a highly effective therapy for idiopathic TTP[10,18–21] but is usually ineffective for sporadic HUS or *Escherichia coli* verotoxin-associated HUS.[21,22] Based on these considerations, a better understanding of these disorders may be facilitated by continuing to distinguish them, while recognizing that extensive overlap in clinical features may prevent an unambiguous diagnosis of TTP or HUS in some patients. The measurement of ADAMTS13 levels is still not standardized among laboratories, and its utility in diagnosing or distinguishing between these disorders remains uncertain.[10,23–25] Given the growing number of clinical situations that may be associated with thrombotic microangiopathies, a simplified classification scheme that provides a practical framework for classifying these syndromes has been proposed (Table 139–1).[21]

GENETIC ASSOCIATIONS AND FAMILIAL THROMBOTIC MICROANGIOPATHY

Over the last 5 years an abundance of information concerning the genetics and pathogenesis of thrombotic microangiopathies has emerged. These data are considered in two primary categories—the role of complement regulatory factor deficiencies in the hemolytic uremic syndrome, and that of VWF cleaving protease (ADAMTS13) deficiency in TTP.

Complement Regulatory Factor Deficiencies in Familial Hemolytic Uremic Syndrome

The term *HUS* is generally used to encompass several diverse disorders discussed in detail below. By far the most common is the epidemic, or "typical" form of HUS that is associated with diarrhea caused by verotoxin-producing *E coli* (VTEC). VTEC-associated HUS accounts for at least 95% of all cases in children[7,26] and most nonsporadic cases in adults. The remaining "atypical" forms of HUS often exhibit autosomal dominant or recessive inheritance,[27] and have been associated with deficiencies in proteins that regulate the alternative pathway of complement activation.[28–30]

Diagnosis and Pathophysiology

Loss of function mutations in complement regulatory proteins, factor H (FH), factor I (FI) and membrane complement protein (MCP, CD46) have been identified in approximately 15% to 30%, 5% to 12%, and 10% to 13% of patients with atypical HUS, respectively.[31–33] Antibodies to FH have been identified in a few affected children.[34] Deletion of factor H-related molecules 1 and 3 (FHR1 and FHR3)[35] also has been described. Conversely, gain of function mutations in complement factor B[36] and complement factor C3[37] have been reported.

Factor H acts in concert with plasma cofactor I[14,38] and the transmembrane cofactor protein MCP[15] to downregulate C3b-mediated amplification of the alternative complement pathway by promoting the decay of C3bBb, the alternative pathway C3 convertase, and by cleaving and inactivating C3b.[16] HUS-associated mutations in FH cluster primarily in the C-terminal region, leading to impaired binding to cell-surface or subendothelial C3b, whereas binding to fluid phase C3b is preserved.[39,40] Thus, plasma levels of C3 are only reduced in 30% to 50% of affected patients at diagnosis.[41] A Web site for genotypic, phenotypic, and structural information on FH, FI, and MCP mutations has been developed (http://FH-HUS.org/).[42,43]

The mechanism(s) by which complement activation leads to the clinical manifestations of HUS remains uncertain. Moreover, approximately one-half of patients with familial HUS have not had mutations identified in complement regulatory proteins, implicating other pathways in pathogenesis.

Clinical Course

Inherited HUS associated with deficiency of complement regulatory proteins typically runs a chronic relapsing course, often complicated by hypertension and renal insufficiency.[14,44,45] Exacerbations may be preceded by infection, but occasionally are associated with pregnancy or seemingly incidental events. Penetrance is approximately 60% in families with heterozygous mutations in FH; thus HUS may occur in siblings with identical genetic abnormalities at different times, or not at all.[46] The prognosis of patients with FH and IF deficiencies is especially poor, with a high rate of recurrence and progression to end-stage renal disease or death approaching 70% in the former, whereas MCP deficiency carries a better prognosis.[31] Aggressive treat-

Table 139–1 Proposed Classification Scheme for Thrombotic Microangiopathies

Category	Clinical Features*	Mechanism	Treatment
Idiopathic TTP	Coombs negative, without DIC or other conditions† associated with secondary TTP. Severe renal failure is uncommon.	Autoimmune ADAMTS13 deficiency in a majority of patients	>80% respond to plasma exchange. May benefit from immunosuppression.
Secondary TTP	Associated conditions include cancer, infection, hematopoietic stem cell transplantation, chemotherapy, specific drugs such as cyclosporine, quinine, ticlopidine.	Mechanisms are mostly unknown. ADAMTS13 deficiency is uncommon.	With occasional exceptions, responses to plasma exchange are unlikely. Treatment and prognosis are dictated by the specific associated conditions.
Verotoxin-associated HUS (usually accompanied by diarrhea; D+ HUS)	Acute renal failure, often oliguric, preceded by bloody diarrhea	Endothelial damage by Shiga toxin-producing *Escherichia coli.* ADAMTS13 deficiency is extremely rare.	Usually self-limited though extensive support required. No demonstrated efficacy of plasma exchange.
Atypical HUS	Acute renal failure, often oliguric, without a preceding diarrheal illness.	Complement regulatory protein deficiencies in at least 50% of patients; ADAMTS13 deficiency is extremely rare.	No demonstrated efficacy of plasma exchange, except possibly for factor H deficiency.

*Clinical features listed are in addition to microangiopathic hemolytic anemia and thrombocytopenia.
†Conditions associated with autoimmune ADAMTS13 deficiency and idiopathic TTP include certain autoimmune disorders, pregnancy, and ticlopidine.

ment with plasma exchange[45] or plasma infusions of 15 to 20 mL/kg weekly or biweekly[47,48] may slow the progression of renal failure in some patients. However, the evidence that plasma-based therapy or immunosuppression affects the clinical course in most patients is limited.

Affected patients have a high risk of recurrence after renal allografting[31,49,50] and HUS has been reported in related donors after surgery. Factor H is a soluble blood protein made in the liver. Therefore Factor H deficiency is not corrected by renal allografting, and HUS often recurs in the transplanted kidney, especially living-related donors.[27,28] One patient appears to have been cured by combined kidney and liver transplantation.[51] HUS recurs rarely in renal allografts of patients with MCP deficiency, suggesting that local expression of MCP is protective.[15,32]

ADAMTS13 Deficiency in Familial Thrombotic Thrombocytopenic Purpura

Schulman[52] and Upshaw[53] described a distinct form of autosomal recessive TTP, referred to as Upshaw–Schulman syndrome. Patients often have neonatal jaundice without maternal blood type incompatibility, and experience repeated episodes of thrombotic microangiopathy during early childhood.[54–57] Exacerbations often occur in association with minor respiratory infections, tonsillitis, sinusitis, otitis media, surgery, or routine vaccinations.[52,53,58,59] A substantial fraction of patients, perhaps one-half, are asymptomatic until early adulthood.[55] Affected women may present with thrombotic microangiopathy during pregnancy. Rare asymptomatic males have been identified in their fourth or fifth decade of life.[55]

The patients frequently present with microangiopathic hemolytic anemia, severe thrombocytopenia and neurologic defects that may range from mild alterations in mental status or visual disturbances to paralysis, seizures, or coma. Renal involvement causes proteinuria and hematuria, with granular and red cell casts. In contrast to familial HUS, serum creatinine usually is only modestly elevated, although patients may occasionally have severe acute renal insufficiency and some develop chronic renal failure requiring dialysis.[56,57] Symptomatic gastrointestinal involvement appears to be rare but may include abdominal pain, nausea, and vomiting.[60] One patient was reported to reproducibly develop pulmonary infiltrates during relapses.[61] These clinical and laboratory abnormalities resolve promptly with plasma replacement, and patients usually can be maintained symptom-free by small transfusions of plasma, typically 5 to 20 mL/kg every 2 to 3 weeks,[54] although some patients require larger volumes of plasma.[56]

The defect in Upshaw–Schulman syndrome was first linked to VWF by Moake,[62] who found "unusually large" VWF multimers in the plasma of patients with chronic relapsing TTP. He proposed that the patients lacked a plasma protease or reductase that normally cleaves "unusually large" VWF multimers, and that the abnormal multimers then cause uncontrolled intravascular platelet aggregation, thrombosis, and tissue infarction. Subsequently, a plasma metalloprotease was discovered that degrades VWF multimers by cleaving the Tyr (1605) Met (1606) bond in the VWF subunit,[63,64] and patients with Upshaw–Schulman syndrome were shown to lack this enzyme,[58] supporting Moake's model for the pathogenesis of VWF-dependent thrombotic microangiopathy.

The VWF protease was purified from plasma, cloned, and found to be a member of the ADAMTS family of metalloproteases, where "ADAMTS" stands for "a disintegrin-like and metalloprotease (reprolysin type) with thrombospondin type 1 motif" (Fig. 139–1). Simultaneously, genome-wide linkage analysis showed that Upshaw–Schulman syndrome is caused by mutations in the *ADAMTS13* gene on chromosome 9q34.[65] Like other members of the family, ADAMTS13 has a metalloprotease domain followed by a disintegrin domain, a thrombospondin-1 repeat, and a cysteine-rich and spacer domain characteristic of the family. These domains are followed by seven additional thrombospondin-1 repeats and two CUB domains. Several of the structural domains distal to the metalloprotease domain participate in the recognition of VWF.[66]

ADAMTS13 is synthesized mainly in the liver by hepatic stellate cells but also in vascular endothelial cells[67] and renal glomerular podocytes.[68] Small amounts of functional ADAMTS13 are present in platelets.[69]

Deletion, splice site, frameshift, and missense mutations that cause Upshaw–Schulman syndrome have been found in almost all structural domains of ADAMTS13, and there is no obvious hot spot for such mutations. Expression studies have shown that the missense mutations almost always prevent the secretion of ADAMTS13 protein, although some also impair catalytic activity.[66,70,71]

ACQUIRED THROMBOTIC MICROANGIOPATHIES

Idiopathic Thrombotic Thrombocytopenic Purpura

Clinical Manifestations

The classic pentad of symptoms that comprise the syndrome of TTP include microangiopathic hemolytic anemia (MAHA), thrombocytopenia, neurologic symptoms, fever, and renal dysfunction.[10,72–77] In

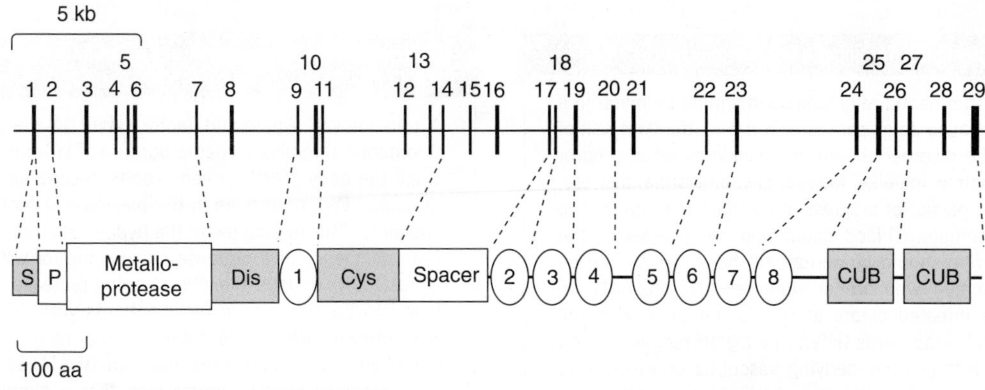

Figure 139–1 Structure of ADAMTS13. The *ADAMTS13* gene contains 29 exons and spans 37 kb on chromosome 9q34. Dashed lines show the relationship between the gene structure and domains of the ADAMTS13 protein. The ADAMTS13 precursor contains 1427 amino acid residues and includes a signal peptide (S), propeptide (P), metalloprotease, disintegrin domain (Dis), thrombospondin type 1 repeats (numbered 1–8), cysteine-rich domain (Cys), spacer domain, and CUB domains. Adapted with permission from Zheng X, Chung D, Takayama TK, et al: Structure of von Willebrand factor-cleaving protease (ADAMTS13), a metalloprotease involved in thrombotic thrombocytopenic purpura. J Biol Chem 276:41059, 2001.

earlier studies, approximately 75% of patients presented with a triad of MAHA, neurologic symptoms, and thrombocytopenic purpura[75,76]; however earlier recognition of TTP[78] and the established therapeutic efficacy of plasma exchange had led to a gradual appreciation that MAHA and thrombocytopenia alone in the absence of an obvious precipitating condition are sufficient diagnostic criteria for diagnosis of TTP.[6,23] Indeed, the evolution of this diagnostic approach has led to a sevenfold increase in the use of plasma exchange for TTP.[23,79]

TTP occurs with an estimated annual incidence of 3.7 to 11 cases per million,[80,81] is more common in females (female/male ratio of 3 : 2),[75,76,82,83] and has a peak incidence in the fourth decade.[75,76,83] Other risk factors appear to include African ancestry[80,84] and obesity.[84,85] Ten to 40% of patients complain of an upper respiratory tract infection or flu-like syndrome in the weeks preceding the diagnosis. Occasional patients present with malaise, fatigue, fever, or other nonspecific symptoms of days' to weeks' duration that are unresponsive to antibiotics or symptomatic management. The diagnosis of TTP may be overlooked until these prodromal symptoms become unrelenting or neurologic dysfunction develops. Neurologic symptoms ranging from headache and confusion to somnolence, seizures, aphasia, or coma often dominate the clinical picture in TTP[75–78,86] and may fluctuate in severity, a characteristic attributed to the repetitive formation and dissolution of microthrombi in the cerebral microvasculature.[87,88] Thrombocytopenia may be severe, with platelet counts below 20,000/μL, and mucocutaneous bleeding is common.[75–77,86] The prothrombin time, partial thromboplastin time, and fibrinogen levels are usually normal or only mildly perturbed; mild elevations in fibrinogen degradation products occur in 50% of patients[89] although more sensitive assays, such as those for prothrombin fragment 1+2, thrombin–antithrombin and plasmin–antiplasmin complexes often demonstrate subtle activation of coagulation and fibrinolytic pathways.[90] Evidence of renal involvement may include hematuria, proteinuria, granular or red cell casts, and mild azotemia, though anuria and renal failure are uncommon presenting features.

MAHA, resulting from fragmentation of red blood cells in the microvasculature[89,90] is a sine qua non of this disorder. The presence of schistocytes on the peripheral blood smear is the most characteristic laboratory finding of thrombotic microangiopathy (Fig. 139–2), although these may not be apparent in rare patients at the onset of their disease.[91,92] The markedly elevated levels of plasma lactate dehydrogenase (LDH) that are typically seen in patients with TTP, once believed to result primarily from hemolysis, also reflect a contribution from tissue ischemia.[93] Nucleated red blood cells are present in many patients, and their number may be disproportionately increased in comparison to the degree of reticulocytosis.[75] With rare exceptions, the direct antiglobulin test is negative.[76] Other less common symptoms may include abdominal pain and respiratory distress. The differential diagnosis of TTP is broad.[23,77] Although a severe deficiency (<5%) of ADAMTS13 is consistent with a diagnosis of TTP, it is not diagnostic. Similarly, TTP cannot be excluded by a normal or only moderately decreased level of ADAMTS13.[94]

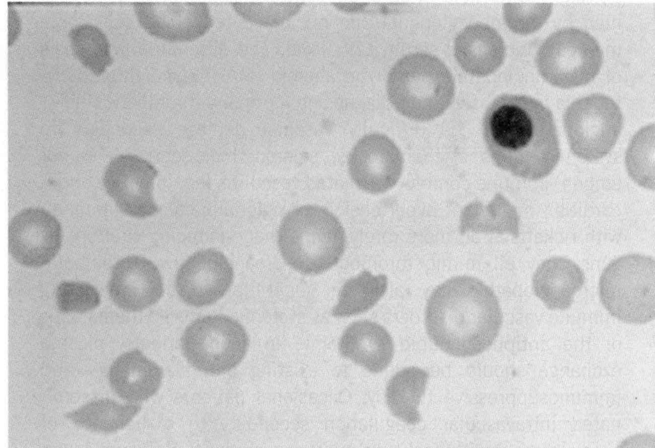

Figure 139–2 This peripheral blood film was obtained from a 28-year-old woman who presented with fever, epistaxis, and altered mental status. Note the absence of platelets and the presence of a nucleated erythrocyte and schistocytes (*arrows*), consistent with a microangiopathic process.

Pathogenesis

The cloning and biochemical characterization of ADAMTS13 has provided new insight into its role in the pathogenesis of TTP,[95,96] and facilitated the development of a model for how VWF and ADAMTS13 regulate platelet adhesion.[97] Endothelial cells secrete "unusually large" VWF multimers that may remain adherent to the cell surface and promote platelet attachment, or enter the circulation and promote intravascular platelet aggregation. Under high shear, vWF multimers elongate along the endothelium and promote platelet adhesion as well as susceptibility to vWF enzymatic cleavage.[64] ADAMTS13 regulates the activity of vWF by cleaving the most hemostatically active high-molecular-weight multimers; failure of this feedback mechanism may lead to the microvascular thrombosis, tissue ischemia, and infarction that are characteristic of TTP. However, many questions yet remain concerning the pathogenesis of this disorder.[21,98] For example, the factors that trigger sporadic episodes of TTP remain undefined. Although endothelial damage or

Approach to the Patient with Thrombotic Microangiopathy

The diagnosis of thrombotic microangiopathy must be made in a timely manner because delay carries with it the attendant risk of sudden death. The disorder should be considered when prodromal symptoms such as malaise, fatigue, gastrointestinal distress, or low-grade fever persist or progress in the face of symptomatic therapy, and a complete blood count and an analysis of the peripheral blood film should be performed. Suspicion should be heightened in women who are or were recently pregnant, in patients who are infected or are at risk for infection with the human immunodeficiency virus (HIV), in allograft recipients, and in those with a history of underlying vasculitis or exposed to specific drugs described in the text. Patients with early, idiopathic TTP frequently present without the classic triad or pentad of signs and symptoms. Thus, a provisional diagnosis of a primary thrombotic microangiopathy should be made, and plasma-based therapy instituted, in any patient with microangiopathic hemolytic anemia and thrombocytopenia, unless an alternative cause is evident. We consider an average of one or more schistocytes per high-power field to be of concern, especially when accompanied by thrombocytopenia and nucleated red blood cells, or a markedly increased serum LDH level. The differential diagnosis of microangiopathic hemolytic anemia (MAHA) and thrombocytopenia is extensive, and diagnosing a primary thrombotic microangiopathy can be difficult. Vascular damage secondary to systemic lupus erythematosus, scleroderma, septic or tumor emboli, immune complex-mediated vasculitis (eg, infective endocarditis), malignant hypertension, cryoglobulinemia, or infection with rickettsial or, more rarely, hemorrhage-inducing viral organisms, may all mimic thrombotic microangiopathy. Thrombotic microangiopathy may also be superimposed on preexisting immune vascular disorders such as systemic lupus erythematosus or the antiphospholipid syndrome; in such patients, plasma exchange should be added to existing antiinflammatory and immunosuppressive therapy. Occasional patients with disseminated intravascular coagulation secondary to malignancy or sepsis present with occlusive microangiopathy of sufficient severity to be confused with primary thrombotic microangiopathy. In the setting of renal transplantation, a biopsy may be required to distinguish thrombotic microangiopathy from allograft rejection or recurrence of a preexisting renal vascular disorder. Occasional patients with thrombotic microangiopathy may present with acute pancreatitis, acute respiratory distress syndrome, memory and personality changes, or other poorly defined neurologic symptoms that themselves have a broad differential diagnosis. Again, the finding of MAHA and thrombocytopenia provides important clues to the underlying problem and the urgent need for intervention with plasma-based therapy.

ADAMTS13 in the Management of Thrombotic Thrombocytopenic Purpura

A role for von Willebrand factor (vWF) in the pathogenesis of thrombotic thrombocytopenic purpura (TTP) has been suspected since the early 1980s, when reports describing the presence of ultralarge vWF multimers in the plasma of affected patients first appeared. This finding led to the hypothesis that TTP might result from deficiency of a protease responsible for vWF cleavage, and almost 20 years later the vWF-cleaving protease was isolated and found to be deficient in most patients with TTP. This protease was subsequently cloned, found to be a member of the ADAMTS metalloprotease family, and denoted ADAMTS13. This tremendous progress raised expectations that a simple and accurate diagnostic test would soon be available for the diagnosis of TTP. However, the utility of ADAMTS13 testing remains undefined, due in part to issues such as a lack of assay standardization and different inclusion criteria in studies that have assessed the relevance of ADAMTS13 measurements. Despite these obstacles, areas where this assay may or may not be useful have begun to emerge. *First*, ADAMTS13 measurements may be useful but are not sensitive for the diagnosis of TTP and specificity depends on the clinical setting. The incidence of severe ADAMTS13 deficiency (defined as <5% activity) has been reported to be as low as 33% in some series of patients with apparently idiopathic thrombotic microangiopathy. However, for patients with thrombotic microangiopathy, severe ADAMTS13 deficiency is very specific for idiopathic TTP, but may also occur, uncommonly, in other disorders such as sepsis-induced DIC or severe liver failure. Thus, although a severe ADAMTS13 deficiency is consistent with TTP, it is not diagnostic in the absence of other clinical information. Moreover, normal or moderately reduced ADAMTS13 levels (20%–40%) do not exclude TTP. *Second*, there is insufficient evidence at present to demonstrate a clear relationship between the levels of ADAMTS13 and/or anti-ADAMTS13 antibodies in acute TTP with short-term outcomes. Though two prospective studies suggest a higher first remission rate in patients with severe deficiencies of ADAMTS13, these findings require validation in larger, prospective studies. There is also no evidence that real-time monitoring of ADAMTS13 or anti-ADAMTS13 antibodies during initial treatment improves outcomes; both the diagnosis and initial management of TTP should be based on clinical and laboratory parameters, such as the platelet count and LDH. *Third*, patients with severe deficiencies of ADAMTS13, or detectable levels of anti-ADAMTS13 antibodies obtained either at diagnosis or during initial remission, are at markedly increased risk for subsequent TTP relapse, which may occur in 30% to 55% of patients with TTP. Thus, patients in this category might be considered for additional immunosuppressive therapy with anti-CD20 or other agents during remission, although the benefit of such intervention on long-term outcomes remains uncertain.

activation has been suggested as one such factor, exactly what may initiate such insults is uncertain. Moreover, some patients develop TTP despite normal levels of circulating ADAMTS13, whereas patients with congenital deficiencies of ADAMTS13 may not develop TTP until adulthood, and sometimes not at all.[55] The latter observations emphasize that factors other than ADAMTS13 deficiency contribute to the development of TTP, and suggest that ADAMTS13 deficiency should be considered an important risk factor, though perhaps not always a sufficient cause of this syndrome. This concept has been borne out in studies of ADAMTS13-deficient mice; the risk of developing a TTP-like syndrome depends strongly on the genetic background, and in some mice ADAMTS13 deficiency causes disease only after exposure to agents like Shigatoxin that induce endothelial cell dysfunction.[99]

Pathology

The prototypic vascular lesions of TTP are characterized by platelet-rich thrombi within or beneath a damaged endothelium.[54] Involved microvascular endothelial cells are swollen and in some cases detached. The subendothelium contains hyaline material that is relatively poor in fibrin but consists instead largely of von Willebrand factor (VWF) and platelet remnants.[17,100] In contrast, the lesions of HUS are rich in fibrin and contain comparatively little VWF.[17] Involved vessel walls characteristically display a paucity of mononuclear leukocytes; fibrinoid necrosis, aneurysm formation, and other evidence of vasculitis are absent in primary or idiopathic cases. Medium- and large-sized arteries show less extensive involvement and the venous system

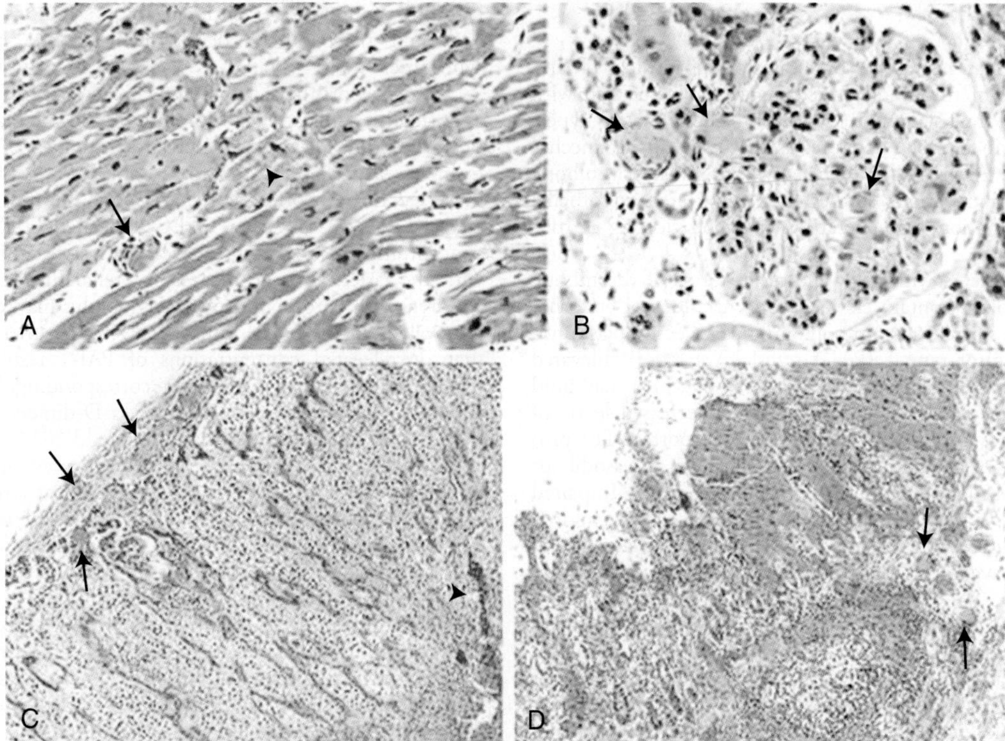

Figure 139–3 Tissue specimens obtained at autopsy from a patient with abnormalities characteristic of TTP. A specimen from the heart (*Panel A*) shows multiple intramyocardial microthrombi (*arrow*), hemorrhage, and early ischemic changes, with scattered foci of contraction-band necrosis (*arrowhead*). A specimen from the kidney (*Panel B*) shows characteristic microthrombi in an afferent arteriole, the glomerular hilum, and glomerular capillaries (*arrows*), with vascular congestion and parenchymal hemorrhage in the surrounding interstitium. A tissue specimen from the adrenal gland (*Panel C*) shows characteristic subcapsular microthrombi (*arrows*), with congestion of cortical arterioles and medullary parenchymal hemorrhage (*arrowhead*). A specimen from the cecum (*Panel D*) shows submucosal microthrombi (*arrows*) and hemorrhagic mucosal ulceration and necrosis. Microthrombi were also present in the pancreas, thyroid gland, and other organs. Photographs and interpretation by Patrick Stangeby. (Reproduced from George JN: Thrombotic thrombocytopenic purpura. N Engl J Med 354:1927, 2006, with permission).

is typically spared. The most commonly affected organs include the brain, pancreas, heart, and adrenal glands.[17,75] Involvement of other sites such as the kidney, spleen, gingiva, bone marrow, and skin (Fig. 139–3) may occur as well.[17,86] A characteristic pathologic lesion involving adjacent areas of vascular dilatation and constriction accompanied by segmental hyaline change may occur in the placenta of pregnant patients with TTP.[101]

von Willebrand Factor and ADAMTS13

Shortly after the congenital absence of ADAMTS13 was discovered to cause familial TTP, almost all patients with nonfamilial, idiopathic TTP were found to have acquired absence of ADAMTS13 activity, usually associated with autoantibody IgG inhibitors of the protease.[12,102] These initial findings have been confirmed repeatedly, although the prevalence of ADAMTS13 deficiency in TTP has not always been as high. Some of this variation may reflect the inclusion or exclusion of patients with acute renal failure or other preexisting conditions. For example, one study found ADAMTS13 deficiency in 18 of 48 adults with idiopathic thrombotic microangiopathy unselected for renal function,[84] whereas another study reported ADAMTS13 deficiency in 22 of 22 patients without acute anuric renal failure.[103] Conversely, acquired severe ADAMTS13 deficiency is extremely rare in patients without thrombotic microangiopathy,[13] with the possible exception of sepsis. For example, a retrospective study of 109 patients with sepsis-induced DIC found ADAMTS13 levels lower than 5% in 17 of them (16%).[104] Severe liver failure is another setting in which rare patients may have severe ADAMTS13 deficiency. Modest decreases in plasma ADAMTS13 activity have been reported in newborns and among adults with cirrhosis, chronic renal insufficiency, pregnancy, connective tissue diseases, and various inflammatory conditions, but the mean ADAMTS13 levels in all of these groups were higher than 40% and none of the patients had levels lower than 6%.[105,106] Therefore, severe ADAMTS13 deficiency (<5%) appears to be quite specific for TTP, although its sensitivity depends on how patients are identified and whether they have other conditions that may predispose to thrombotic microangiopathy.[13,107]

Antibodies against ADAMTS13 have been demonstrated in 59% to 100% of patients with acquired severe ADAMTS13 deficiency.[12,84,102,103,108,109] This variability probably reflects the relative insensitivity of certain assays for detecting inhibitors.[110] In addition, some IgG and IgM antibodies may cause ADAMTS13 deficiency by promoting its clearance from the circulation without inhibiting activity.[111]

Plasma exchange is effective for patients with or without inhibitors, and clinical responses frequently occur despite the persistence of both the inhibitor and severe ADAMTS13 deficiency, although patients with high-titer inhibitors may respond more slowly and relapse more often.[55,103,112] Both congenital and acquired ADAMTS13 deficiency are characterized by unpredictable periods of stability between relapses, which probably reflects a role of stress in exacerbating the disease by activating or damaging endothelium, increasing the release of unusually large VWF multimers, and triggering microvascular platelet thrombosis. An interaction between ADAMTS13 deficiency and stress would account for the frequent occurrence of thrombotic microangiopathy in association with pregnancy, surgery, infections, and various other inflammatory conditions that raise VWF levels.

Other Mechanisms

ADAMTS13 levels are normal in some cases of idiopathic TTP, and in almost all cases of thrombotic microangiopathy associated with stem cell or organ transplantation, cancer, infections, severe hypertension, and certain drugs. Therefore, as discussed above, mechanisms other than ADAMTS13 deficiency can cause thrombotic microangiopathy, and various studies have implicated endothelial injury, platelet activation, and alterations in blood clotting as contributory factors.

Plasma from patients with TTP and other forms of thrombotic microangiopathy often contain elevated concentrations of endothelial-derived proteins such as thrombomodulin, P-selectin, plasminogen activator inhibitor type 1 (PAI-1), and VWF.[88,113,114] Elevated levels of endothelial cell microparticles,[115] some of which may bind vWF[116] and induce platelet aggregation,[117] and decreased levels of tissue factor pathway inhibitor[118] have also been reported. The production and stability of endothelial cell prostacyclin, a vasodilator and inhibitor of platelet activation, may be decreased.[119,120] Impaired renal generation of prostacyclin has been observed in children with *Escherichia coli*-associated HUS.[121] However, treatment of patients with intravenous prostacyclin has met with inconsistent responses.[122–124]

Antiplatelet and endothelial cell antibodies of diverse specificity have been identified in TTP, and may bind preferentially to microvascular endothelial cells.[125,126] Some antiendothelial cell antibodies recognize CD36[125,127] and might inhibit the binding of thrombospondin-like domains in ADAMTS13 to microvascular endothelium.[18] However, the pathophysiological significance of these antibodies has not been established.

Plasma from patients with idiopathic and human immunodeficiency virus (HIV)-associated TTP and sporadic HUS, but not *E coli* verotoxin-associated HUS, induce apoptosis of dermal microvascular, renal and cerebral, but not pulmonary or hepatic endothelial cells. Apoptosis involves the induction of Fas (CD95)[128,129] and upregulation of caspases 1 and 3, and is inhibited by overexpression of Bcl-X_L or the Bcl-2 homolog A1.[130] DNA array analysis suggests that the resistance of pulmonary endothelial cells to apoptosis induced by TTP plasma may reflect increased expression of survival factors such as the TRAIL antagonist osteoprotegerin and vascular endothelial cell growth factors and their receptors.[131] Ticlopidine and plasma from patients with ticlopidine-associated TTP also induced apoptosis of microvascular endothelial cells in vitro, possibly related to altered interactions of endothelial cells with the extracellular matrix.[132]

In addition to alterations in endothelial cell function, TTP plasma may promote platelet aggregation directly.[133] Platelet microparticles have been detected in essentially all patients with thrombotic microangiopathy, their number correlating inversely with the platelet count and their disappearance with clinical improvement.[134] Circulating endothelial microparticles may directly bind vWF, and aggregate platelets through a vWF-dependent pathway.[135] Though several additional platelet-activating moieties have been identified,[136–139] their role in the pathogenesis of TTP has not been defined. Indeed, recent thought concerning the pathogenesis of TTP has evolved toward a model in which platelet aggregation occurs primarily in response to high-molecular-weight vWF multimers bound to the surface of stimulated endothelial cells and not appropriately cleaved in the absence of ADAMTS13, rather than on spontaneous aggregation of platelets in plasma.[140]

Some reports suggest a role for increased procoagulant activity in the pathogenesis of thrombotic microangiopathy. Acquired deficiencies of proteins C and S have been described in some patients.[141,142] Analysis of a small case series suggested that the prevalence of Factor V Leiden was increased in patients with TTP and normal ADAMTS13 activity,[143] though this was not observed in a larger study.[144] In patients with verotoxin-producing *E coli* infection (see section on Verotoxin-Associated Thrombotic Microangiopathy), evidence for activation of the coagulation system, as documented through the measurement of prothrombin fragment 1+2 and thrombin–antithrombin complexes,[145,146] closely follows the onset of bloody diarrhea and precedes the development of the hemolytic uremic syndrome.[145]

Several reports have focused on characterization of the fibrinolytic abnormalities in patients with thrombotic microangiopathies, particularly HUS. Plasminogen activator activity was reportedly absent from vessels occluded by microthrombi.[147] Plasma levels of PAI-1 are increased in both primary[90,148] and bone marrow transplant-associated TTP,[149] as well as in VTEC-associated HUS.[141,150–152] Plasma concentrations of PAI-1 may have prognostic significance in children with the latter, and the recovery of renal function in a cohort of children with thrombotic microangiopathy may correlate with the removal of PAI-1 by peritoneal dialysis.[152] Others, however, argue that the elevated concentrations of PAI-1 result primarily from renal insufficiency,[153,154] and that corresponding increases in t-PA, t-PA:PA1-1 complexes and fibrinogen D-dimers suggest that fibrinolysis is stimulated rather than impaired.[153,155]

Vasoregulators such as endothelin[156] may also contribute to microvascular constriction and increased shear stress in thrombotic microangiopathy, particularly within the renal vasculature. Nitric oxide metabolites may be involved in the generation of lipid peroxides, superoxide anions, peroxynitrite and hydroxyl radicals, though increased production of nitric oxide diminished renal injury in a rat model of thrombotic microangiopathy.[157] Nitric oxide depletion as a result of binding to free hemoglobin has been postulated to mediate vasoconstriction in patients with TTP.[158] Products of activated leukocytes, such as elastase and cathepsin G may also contribute to tissue damage.[159]

Therapy

The mortality rate of TTP exceeds 90% without therapy. Through the mid-1970s, splenectomy remained the only modality with more than an anecdotal response rate.[76] Since that time, there has been a dramatic reversal of this prognosis with the advent of plasma-based therapy, such that long-term survival now approaches 80%.[6,20,160,161] Moreover, with the appreciation that TTP may in many cases be an immune-mediated disorder, the use of immune-based approaches is expanding.

Plasma Therapy

Anecdotal responses to whole blood infusion were reported after Moschowitz's initial description of TTP, in which he noted that a colleague had seen four similar patients who recovered promptly after transfusion of whole blood.[1] Yet the remarkable benefit of plasma therapy was not appreciated until 1976, when Bukowski et al reported a 50% survival rate in 16 patients with thrombotic microangiopathy treated by exchange transfusion.[162] The next year, Byrnes and Khurana reported that the active component in whole blood was contained in plasma, an observation that led to the widespread use of plasma infusion.[163] The same year, Bukowski et al[164] demonstrated the efficacy of plasma exchange, which suggested that the response rate might be improved by removing a toxic substance from patient plasma.

The results of a prospective trial reported in 1991 appeared to resolve the long-debated issue of the relative efficacy of plasma exchange versus infusion in favor of the former. At 6 months, complete remissions were seen in 78% of patients treated with exchange versus 31% in those treated with plasma infusion.[165] This study did not resolve the question of whether removal of a disease-inciting agent or replacement of a missing factor accounted for the superior response observed with plasma exchange, particularly because patients in the exchange arm received a threefold greater volume of plasma. Indeed, a retrospective study demonstrated no significant difference in outcome in patients with acquired TTP who received equal volumes of plasma by exchange or infusion.[166] However, the current model for the pathogenesis of acquired idiopathic TTP suggests that plasma exchange is superior because it both removes an IgG inhibitor of ADAMTS13 and replaces the deficient protein, and the benefit of plasma exchange over infusion has also been suggested by a recent systematic review.[167] In contrast, plasma infusion may be sufficient for patients with a genetic cause of ADAMTS13 deficiency, or perhaps acquired deficiency due to a low-titer inhibitor.[164,168] From a practical perspective, large volumes of plasma are more easily administered by plasma exchange, and unless a genetic deficiency of ADAMTS13 has been documented, plasma infusion should be reserved for situations in which exchange is not immediately available.[169] It is worth noting that plasma exchange is highly effective even in patients who do not have a severe deficiency of ADAMTS13,[84] suggesting that this modality may have additional therapeutic mechanisms. This observation highlights the belief that monitoring of ADAMTS13 and/or anti-ADAMTS13 levels during plasma therapy for acute TTP does not improve outcomes (see box on ADAMTS13 in the Management of Thrombotic Thrombocytopenic Purpura).

Plasma exchange is generally initiated with the goal of exchanging 1 to 1.5 plasma volumes (40–60 mL/kg) daily although the optimal regimen has not been determined.[20,23] Patients begun on a regimen of 1 plasma volume daily may be increased to 1.5, or in some cases, 2 plasma volumes daily if their initial response is poor. Neurologic improvement occurs most rapidly, often within hours to days.[78] The serum LDH level typically falls by 50% within 3 days in responders, and the platelet count begins to rise in a mean of 5 days, although normalization may take several weeks.[78] Impaired renal function is generally the last to improve. Several prognostic factors at the time of presentation have been suggested through multivariate analysis, including an age greater than 40 years, hemoglobin less than 9.0 g/dL, and the presence of a fever greater than 38.5°C.[170]

Fresh frozen plasma remains the most commonly used replacement product. An advantage to the use of cryosupernatant, which is depleted of von Willebrand factor, was suggested by a retrospective study in which 50% of patients seemingly refractory to exchange with FFP responded to subsequent exchange with cryosupernatant (cryopoor plasma, CPP).[165] However, a small prospective study found no difference in outcomes between patients treated with these products as initial therapy.[171] These findings are consistent with a recent study in which similar concentrations and stability of ADAMTS13 during storage at 1 to 5°C were observed in CPP and fresh frozen plasma.[172] Experience with solvent-detergent treated plasma has been increasing, and in a recent pilot study this product appeared to have similar efficacy as standard fresh frozen plasma with a lowered incidence of allergic/urticarial and citrate reactions; an increased risk of thrombosis was not observed.[173] Solvent-detergent treated plasma contains ADAMTS13 at concentrations approximately 20% below those observed in fresh-frozen plasma.[174]

Daily plasma exchange should be continued until neurologic symptoms have resolved and both a normal serum LDH and platelet count have been maintained for at least 2 to 3 days[10,20,23,72,175]; a shorter duration of therapy risks immediate and occasionally fatal relapse. Approximately 85% to 90% of patients will show a clinical and laboratory response to plasma exchange within 3 weeks, most often within 10 days (mean 15.8; range 3–36 days).[165] However, at least 30% of patients experience one or more relapses, the exact frequency depending on the definition used; recurrence within 30 days of discontinuing plasma exchange is considered exacerbation of existing disease.[6] The decision to switch from FFP to cryosupernatant or to introduce another form of therapy remains a matter of clinical judgment but has historically not been considered until the patient has received a minimum of 10 to 14 days of daily exchange with FFP, unless extraordinary circumstances intervene. There is little data to support an approach of either abrupt discontinuation of plasma exchange after remission is achieved or "tapering" the frequency of therapy; thus, this decision must be empiric. The benefit of using other modalities with plasma exchange in the treatment of TTP is unproven, although the addition of rituximab and other agents has been proposed based on anecdotal results from small studies.[176–179]

Contemporary studies have highlighted the complications of plasma exchange therapy. Complication rates may approach 30%, mostly related to central venous catheter insertion or infection.[180–182] Thrombosis has also been reported, and some, but not all reports have suggested a higher incidence when solvent-detergent (S/D) treated plasma, which contains reduced amounts of protein S, is used as a replacement fluid.[183,184]

Corticosteroids

Corticosteroids are often used as part of initial therapy or in those who fail to show a brisk response to plasma-based therapy.[6] Corticosteroids are of little benefit on their own[87,160] and retrospective studies do not provide compelling evidence that they improve the response to plasma exchange.[160] However, the antiinflammatory and immunosuppressive effects of corticosteroids make them attractive adjunctive therapy for autoimmune idiopathic TTP and they have been recommended for routine use for patients receiving plasma exchange.[20]

Splenectomy

Before the introduction of plasma therapy, splenectomy was considered first-line treatment for TTP, inducing remission in up to 50% of patients when used in conjunction with other agents.[160] In the plasma exchange era splenectomy has generally been reserved for refractory patients, with variable response rates.[43,119,120] Recent reports demonstrate that laparoscopic splenectomy may be safely performed in TTP patients with minimal morbidity,[185] and that excellent responses occur in some refractory patients.[121,122] Some series suggest that splenectomy induces an enhanced response to plasma exchange in patients initially refractory.[78,87] Splenectomy during hematologic remission may reduce the incidence of relapses in patients with chronic relapsing TTP.[186] Therefore, splenectomy may be considered in patients refractory to large-volume plasma exchange or immunosuppression (see below). Plasma exchange should be continued after surgery and until the thrombotic microangiopathy remits.

Other Modalities

The response rate to *antiplatelet agents* such as aspirin, dipyridamole, sulfinpyrazone, or ticlopidine as single agents approximates 10%,[87,160] essentially indistinguishable from the natural history of thrombotic microangiopathy. Antiplatelet agents have not been convincingly shown to increase the response to plasma exchange[6,165,187,188] and may promote bleeding in the setting of severe thrombocytopenia and invasive procedures.[6,189] Hence, their use as first-line therapy cannot be recommended, though a potential role in preventing relapse has been reported.[190] The use of *intravenous immunoglobulin* is predicated on a report that IgG from healthy individuals inhibits the capacity of TTP plasma to agglutinate platelets in vitro,[191] a finding that has not been reproduced. Most reports supporting the efficacy of intravenous immunoglobulin[192] are compromised by the delay in the initiation of treatment or concomitant administration of other agents, and others have failed to demonstrate responses to intravenous immunoglobulin after failure of plasma exchange. A recent study described a response to the combination of plasma exchange and intravenous immunoglobulin in a patient who was refractory to plasma exchange alone.[179] There are anecdotal reports of favorable responses to *vincristine*[87,160,193–195] as well as other immunosuppressive therapies such as azathioprine, cyclophosphamide, cyclosporine, and staphylococcal protein A immunoadsorption.[196,197]

With numerous reports documenting its efficacy[92,198–200] the anti-CD20 monoclonal antibody, rituximab, has been used with increasing frequency in TTP.[201] The bulk of rituximab use has been in patients refractory to plasma exchange, in whom it has been used alone[202] or in conjunction with additional plasma exchange.[177,178,203] In some individuals, rituximab has been employed in the treatment of one or more relapses.[204,205] Rituximab administration has been associated with a decrease in the level of inhibitory ADAMTS13 IgG antibodies,[202,203,206] which has led to its use in patients with TTP in remission in whom decreasing levels of ADAMTS13 activity with recurrence of inhibitors has been noted during follow-up.[207] However, there have been no prospective, randomized trials of rituximab in

Transfusion Therapy in Thrombotic Microangiopathy

Patients with TTP often develop symptomatic anemia because of bleeding and partially compensated hemolytic anemia. Packed red blood cells can be transfused safely in this setting. In elderly patients and in those with an impaired cardiovascular system, it may be prudent to provide an additional margin of safety when choosing a threshold for transfusion. In contrast, platelet transfusions are relatively contraindicated in TTP. Though no controlled studies have addressed this issue, there are several published reports of patients under treatment for TTP whose clinical situation deteriorated markedly within 1 to 24 hours of receiving allogeneic platelets; the authors are aware of similar experiences. Clinical deterioration after platelet transfusion can also occur in patients with HUS, as well as VTEC-associated and drug-induced thrombotic microangiopathies. Postmortem examination of such patients has revealed widespread microthrombi involving the brain, heart, lung, kidney, and multiple other organs. Many of these appeared "fresh," in that they showed no evidence of overgrowth by proliferative endothelial cells. Sudden death has also been reported on rare occasions in patients who responded to plasma therapy with a rapid rise in the platelet count. Thus, we consider platelet transfusions to be relatively contraindicated in patients with TMA in the absence of overt major bleeding or a comparable hemostatic challenge.

either primary or relapsed TTP, and thus its efficacy and optimal application in TTP remain uncertain. A randomized, prospective trial of plasma exchange alone compared to plasma exchange and rituximab is under development through the NIH-sponsored Transfusion Medicine and Hemostasis Clinical Trials Network.[208]

Cyclosporine is another immunotherapy that has been used anecdotally in TTP, with studies showing promise both in reducing the incidence of relapse,[209] and treating early relapse.[210] Responses correlate with improvements in ADAMTS13 activity and decreases in anti-ADAMTS13 antibody titer.[211] As with rituximab, the role of cyclosporine in the treatment of TTP remains uncertain because of the paucity of information derived from prospective, randomized trials.[212] Anecdotal success with mycophenolate mofetil has also been reported.[213]

The use of low-dose aspirin (81 mg daily) commenced on platelet recovery (platelet count >50,000/µL) has been recommended by some, particularly in patients who experience a rapid rise in the platelet count.[20,87] Folate supplementation and administration of the hepatitis B vaccine should be considered routine components of supportive care.[20] Platelet transfusion is relatively contraindicated in patients with TTP.

THE HEMOLYTIC UREMIC SYNDROME

The hemolytic uremic syndrome is considered as two primary syndromes that differ in cause and outcome, though each of these may have several variations (Table 139–1).

Verotoxin-Associated Thrombotic Microangiopathy

Epidemiology

This variant of thrombotic microangiopathy has been referred to as "typical," "epidemic," "childhood," diarrheal D+, verotoxin *E coli*-associated (VTEC), and Shiga-like toxin (Stx)-related HUS. The incidence is highest in children below the age of 5 years,[214] but the disorder can occur at any age.[7,214–217] In one epidemiologic study conducted in the United States, the median age of patients with D+ HUS was 4 years; 55% of patients were less than 5 years of age, 33% between 5 and 17 years, 6% between 18 and 44 years, and 6% older than 45 years of age.[218] The pathogenesis, and in particular its association with verotoxin-producing *E coli*,[26] has been established; these organisms account for 80% to 86% of HUS in the United States and Europe.[216] The major reservoir of verotoxin-producing *E coli* is domestic cattle; approximately 2% to 3% harbor enteropathic *E coli* in their gastrointestinal tract at the time of slaughter,[219] and meat becomes contaminated with *E coli* during processing. The organism has also been isolated from deer, sheep, goats, horses, dogs, birds, and flies.[214] Outbreaks are most often associated with ingestion of inadequately cooked ground beef,[214,218,220] though contamination of poultry, cheese, fruits, and vegetables has also been reported. Other cases have been attributed to ingestion of contaminated water[221] or unpasteurized apple cider or milk.[222] The incidence of Stx-HUS may be increasing as a result of developments in food production methods.[219] Meat is now more likely to be prepared from hundreds or thousands of grain-fed cows. Industrial farming also generates large quantities of potentially contaminated manure that periodically enters streams where it can contaminate feed and uncooked vegetables.[219] Carriage may be asymptomatic[223] and fecal–oral transmission may contribute to spread in settings such as day care centers[224] and nursing homes,[225] whereas aerosolization in barns has been implicated in outbreaks at fairs. Petting zoos have also been a source of pathogenic *E coli*.[226]

The relationship of Stx-producing organisms to human disease was first recognized in 1983 based on the identification of *E coli* strain O157:H7 as the probable cause of two outbreaks of hemorrhagic gastroenteritis.[227] VTEC were implicated in the development of HUS after the organisms were detected in stools from 11 of 15 Canadian children with HUS.[228] Subsequent studies demonstrated an association between HUS and additional verotoxin-producing strains of *E coli*,[218,229] of which more than 100 have now been identified.[148,152] In one outbreak, toxigenic *E coli* were detected in 68% of children with HUS; 46% of cases were due to *E coli* O157:H7, 25% to *E coli* O26, and the rest due to other serogroups.[230,231] VTEC are also associated with sporadic, nonepidemic cases of HUS,[214,220,232] although molecular subtyping may be required for documentation.[233] The disease occurs more frequently during summer and autumn in temperate climates,[26] with approximately 50% of cases occurring between June and September.[216] In addition to *E coli*, infection by Shigatoxin-producing *Shigella dysenteriae* serotype 1 is associated with HUS in developing countries, particularly in Asia and Africa, though *S dysenteriae* is a very uncommon cause of HUS in industrialized countries.[217] The mortality of *S dysenteriae*-associated HUS is significantly higher than that of *E coli*-associated disease despite a similar pathogenesis.[216] Cases resulting from verotoxin-producing *Citrobacter freundii* have also been reported.[230]

Clinical Manifestations

Stx-induced HUS occurs most commonly after *E coli* O157:H7-induced gastroenteritis,[234,235] with rare cases reported after infection of the urinary tract or skin, or infection with non-*E coli* organisms.[216,217,230,236,237] The disease begins with the sudden onset of abdominal pain and watery diarrhea a mean of 3.7 (range 2–12) days after toxin exposure.[151,238,232] Abdominal pain may be severe and precede the onset of diarrhea. This presentation, particularly in the absence of fever, may be difficult to differentiate from inflammatory bowel disease, appendicitis, ischemic colitis, or intussusception. Bloody diarrhea generally ensues on the second day accompanied in some cases by nausea and vomiting,[7,218,238] though up to one-third of patients do not report blood in the stool.[239] Fever is typically absent or mild. Colonoscopy reveals edematous colonic mucosa, with occasional ulceration and pseudomembrane formation. Thumbprinting in the distal ascending and proximal transverse colon, suggesting an ischemic colitis, may be seen on barium enema and is attributed to exotoxin-induced thrombi in the microvasculature of the bowel wall.[7,232]

It is estimated that *E coli*-associated hemorrhagic gastroenteritis is complicated by HUS in 8% to 18% of sporadic cases, and more than

20% in certain epidemic outbreaks.[7,240] Young children and the elderly are at greatest risk,[238] perhaps due in part to slower clearance of the organism from the gastrointestinal tract. HUS typically develops 1 to 3 days after the onset of bloody diarrhea, with oliguria or other evidence of renal impairment[7,216,218,241]; 50% of patients require dialysis, at least temporarily.[235] The severity of MAHA varies considerably, but many affected individuals require red cell transfusions.[238] Thrombocytopenia is common, with a median platelet count of 30,000/μL in one study,[218] but may be mild or absent in up to 30% of cases at presentation. Twenty-five percent of patients develop neurologic manifestations, which may include irritability and somnolence, and less commonly, confusion, paresis, and seizures.[7,218,242]

The disease should be suspected in a patient who presents with the characteristic clinical manifestations after an episode of bloody diarrhea, although the prototypic history of a preceding hemorrhagic gastroenteritis may be absent in up to 30% of cases.[7,218,238,243] Stool cultures are positive in approximately 50% of those whose diagnosis is confirmed serologically.[218,235] *E coli* O157:H7 ferment sorbitol slowly, appearing as colorless overnight colonies on sorbitol–MacConkey agar; sorbitol-negative cultures may be characterized further using commercially available O157:H7-specific antisera.[218,244] Methods to detect Stx or their structural genes[232] improve diagnostic sensitivity, and a point-of-care card that detects *E coli* O157:H7 by immunodiffusion has been developed.[245]

The risk of developing HUS when Stx is associated with non-O157:H7 species of *E coli* varies.[246,231] A fourfold or greater rise in antibody titer to either Stx or O157 lipopolysaccharide confirms the diagnosis.[232] Serologic assays are more sensitive than stool cultures and may remain positive for up to 8 weeks.[218,247] Algorithms developed to diagnose Stx-HUS have recently been developed.[248]

Pathology

Renal biopsy, though rarely required for diagnosis in endemic areas, suggests that endothelial damage is central to the pathogenesis of Stx-HUS. Involved glomeruli show widening of the subendothelial space, which is filled with cellular debris and fibrin (Fig. 139–3). Concurrent thickening of the capillary wall results in a "double contour" appearance.[249] In some specimens, infiltration of glomeruli by monocytes and, to a lesser extent, neutrophils has been observed, perhaps as a result of elevated urinary levels of monocyte chemoattractant protein-1 and interleukin 8.[250] Glomerular capillary endothelial cells are swollen and occasionally detached, leading to obliteration of the capillary lumens.[251] Thrombi in glomerular capillaries may be sparse,[120] though thrombotic occlusion of afferent arterioles may be present. Glomerular involvement with sparing of larger arterioles and arteries is generally associated with a better prognosis.[252] In older children and adults (who primarily develop sporadic, D^- HUS), involvement of arterioles and interlobular arteries, with relative sparing of glomeruli, is observed more commonly. Lesions are characterized by edema and myointimal proliferation, necrosis of the vascular wall, and patchy renal cortical necrosis. Glomeruli exhibit ischemic changes, characterized by collapse, retraction, and wrinkling of the capillary loops. This pattern is associated with a poor prognosis and a high incidence of chronic renal insufficiency.[252]

Toxins

Enteropathic *E coli* are generally noninvasive. These organisms create a tight zone of attachment to the intestinal wall through the actions of intimin, and express several other virulence factors that enhance their proliferation locally.[22,253,254] Their capacity to cause HUS is attributed to two 70-kd bacterial exotoxins[255] named verotoxins for their cytotoxicity against African green monkey kidney (Vero) cells. The toxins are transported across the intestinal epithelium through specific para- and intercellular mechanisms[256] and then circulate, most likely by binding with low affinity to the surface of neutrophils, before being transferred to receptors expressed on glomerular endothelial cells that are upregulated by proinflammatory cytokines (see below).[257,258] Verotoxins also bind to platelets, red cells, and activated monocytes; however, the majority of transport appears to result from neutrophil binding because toxin incubated with whole blood binds preferentially to the latter.[217,257]

Verotoxin-1 is homologous to a Shigella toxin[214,255] and is therefore generally referred to as Shiga-like toxin 1 (SLT-1 or Stx1). Most strains of pathogenic *E coli* produce a second toxin, Stx2, which is 30-fold more potent[259] and associated with a higher risk of developing HUS.[260] The toxins are carried on a lysogenic bacteriophage that is capable of infecting other strains of *E coli*. The intact, 70-kd Stx holotoxins consist of a 32-kd A subunit and five 7.7-kd B receptor-binding subunits.[259] The toxin binds to terminal Gala1-4Galb (galabiose) residues primarily on globosyltriaosylceramide (Gb_3; also known as CD77 and the human blood group P(k) antigen)[261] that are highly expressed on capillary endothelium in the glomerulus and brain; the expression of these receptors is upregulated by TNF released as a consequence of toxin-induced leukocyte activation.[262] Receptor-bound holotoxin is internalized[263] and transported in a retrograde manner to the endoplasmic reticulum and then to the nucleus.[262,264] The A subunit is proteolyzed to a 27-kd A1 subunit that binds the 60s ribosomal subunit and cleaves adenosine from ribosomal RNA and RNA-free chromatin and DNA.[265] This prevents elongation factor 1-dependent binding of aminoacyl tRNA, which inhibits protein synthesis and leads to caspase-mediated endothelial cell apoptosis.[266] Signal transduction through cross-linked B-unit–CD77 complexes may also contribute to its cytotoxicity.[256,267] Recently, additional virulence factors, such as cytolethal distending toxin, which may interfere with the endothelial cell cycle, have been described, though their specific role in disease pathogenesis has yet to be fully defined.[268]

Pathophysiology

HUS is caused by endothelial cell damage initiated by Shiga toxins and the inflammatory cytokines they induce. The subytpe and amount of Stx, as well as other virulence factors, contribute to risk.[269] Stx promotes bacterial adhesion to the intestinal epithelium and stimulates a local inflammatory response that recruits neutrophils and monocytes, leading to toxic and ischemic intestinal inury. Stx translocates across the epithelium where it binds to and activates leukocytes, and is then transported via leukocytes to target organs such as the kidney. There, Stx upregulates expression of high-affinity Gb3 receptors on renal capillary endothelium, mesangial and tubular epithelial cells.[270] Increased expression of Gb3 on glomerular microvascular and cerebral endothelium compared with other vascular beds[271] contributes to their heightened sensitivity to apoptosis, cytotoxicity, upregulation of integrins, and procoagulant activity.[271,272] The predilection of children to develop HUS may relate to the higher levels of Gb_3 expression compared with adults.[271] *E coli* lipopolysaccharide and Stx also stimulate leukocyte and intrarenal expression of diverse proinflammatory cytokines including IL-1, -6 and -8, MCP-1, interleukin-1β, and interferon-γ that exacerbate toxin- and leukocyte-induced endothelial dysfunction.[270,273,274] Interactions between endothelial cell fractalkine and mononuclear leukocytes expressing the fractalkine receptor, CX3R1, may play a particularly important role in the renal damage characteristic of HUS.[275] Stx also acts in concert with lipopolysaccharide to trigger a procoagulant state early in the course of the disease that involves platelet activation,[276,277] expression of tissue factor, release of unusually large von Willebrand factor multimers,[278] and elaboration of plasminogen activator-1,[145] promoting thrombosis at sites of damaged endothelium.

Management

Stx-associated HUS is the most common cause of acute renal failure in children[26,243] and its management has been recently reviewed.[248,279]

Patients with acute bloody diarrhea, especially in the absence of fever, and those with very painful diarrhea should be considered to have *E coli* O157:H7 infection and be admitted for hydration and infection control.[248,280] Aggressive hydration has been shown to be nephroprotective,[281] though careful attention to fluid and electrolyte status is essential.[282] Although approximately 60% of children require dialysis initially, the disorder is typically self-limited and mortality has been reduced to 3% to 5%[283] with appropriate supportive care[266,218] with death usually due to severe involvement of the central nervous system, intestine or myocardium.[283] Renal insufficiency generally resolves within 2 to 3 weeks, although some patients have prolonged anuria, requiring several months before return to normal, and renal recovery after up to 40 months of dialysis has been reported.[284] Though angiotensin converting enzyme inhibitors (ACEI) may diminish renal blood flow in acute HUS, they may have a renoprotective effect in patients with persistent proteinuria following the disease.[281] Despite a favorable short-term outcome, many children with Stx-associated HUS develop chronic renal insufficiency over time.[285] In one report of 29 patients with "typical" childhood HUS followed for 15 to 28 years, 7 developed chronic renal failure and 12 developed hypertension, proteinuria, or reduced glomerular filtration rate, whereas only 10 showed no residual abnormalities.[252] Thus, approximately 50% to 60% of patients have complete recovery with long-term preservation of renal function.[283,286] Long-term outcome is worse in those presenting with prolonged anuria,[287] an elevated leukocyte count,[288] elevated levels of prothrombin fragment 1+2, tissue type plasminogen activator and plasminogen activator 1[145] and older age.[22,225,289] There is also a correlation between the extent of histological damage on presentation and eventual outcome; virtually all patients with cortical necrosis are left with significant chronic renal disease.[252] Proteinuria persisting for more than 1 year after the initial episode of thrombotic microangiopathy is likewise associated with progressive renal disease.[243,283]

In randomized trials, neither plasma infusion nor exchange has been of benefit in children or adults with Stx-associated HUS.[20,286,290] A trial of pheresis is indicated only in the adult with episodic HUS that cannot be distinguished from TTP on presentation.[6] Corticosteroids, heparin, urokinase, aspirin, and dipyridamole have been ineffective.[216] A silicon dioxide particle covalently linked to a trisaccharide, designed to bind toxin in the intestine and block systemic effects, has not shown benefit in clinical trials.[291] Antimotility agents and narcotics delay clearance of *E coli* and toxin from the GI tract and may increase the risk of progression to thrombotic microangiopathy.[292,293] Nonsteroidal antiinflammatory agents may reduce renal blood flow. Most experts believe that antibiotics increase the risk of progression to HUS by lysing bacteria, releasing Stx and inducing bacteriophages on which *stx* genes are expressed,[248,294] though this was not confirmed in a recent metanalysis.[295]

Sporadic (D^-) Hemolytic Uremic Syndrome

"Sporadic" HUS is a form of systemic thrombotic microangiopathy in which renal failure developing in the absence of an obvious precipitating factor is the predominant feature. This disorder may be referred to as the "adult" or "atypical" HUS, but also accounts for up to 10% of cases in the pediatric population. Sporadic HUS is not associated with a prodrome of bloody diarrhea and therefore is also referred to as D^- or $VTEC^-$ HUS to contrast with HUS associated with verotoxin-producing *E coli* or other bacteria.[28] However, D^+ cases do occur in adults, often in epidemics associated with a contaminated food source.[219] "Sporadic" cases occurring in more than one family member[296] may follow an autosomal recessive or dominant pattern, and many are associated with a mutation in complement regulatory proteins (vide supra).[14,38,200] The course of thrombotic microangiopathy that complicates bone marrow transplantation, immunosuppressive medication, pregnancy, and chemotherapy most closely resembles that of D^- HUS.[28] Although D^- HUS is significantly less common than TTP, the fact that up to 16% of patients in large TTP series have required dialysis demonstrates that these disorders can be indistinguishable on clinical gounds.[6,10,23,297]

Patients with sporadic HUS often experience a prodrome suggestive of an upper respiratory tract infection or nonspecific symptoms of malaise and fatigue, but severe abdominal pain and bloody diarrhea as observed in D^+ HUS is notably absent. Neurologic manifestations are typically less common and severe than in TTP and are less likely to dominate the clinical course.[298] MAHA is universal, and the reticulocyte count and LDH concentration are elevated,[299] but severe thrombocytopenia is less common than in TTP.[299,300] Sporadic HUS does not display the seasonal variability characteristic of verotoxin-associated HUS.[26] Renal involvement is more severe than in TTP, with up to 60% of patients requiring dialysis.[301]

Because of its rarity, lack of clear diagnostic criteria, and the inclusion of patients with HUS in series consisting primarily of patients with TTP, the responsiveness of patients with atypical HUS to therapy is ill defined. This disorder is also frequently grouped with pregnancy, cancer, and chemotherapy-associated thrombotic microangiopathies that may have similar clinical presentations but different natural histories. Nevertheless, overt sporadic HUS is associated with a poor prognosis, especially in the elderly and those with severe renal dysfunction.[299] The mortality rate approaches 25%, and 50% of surviving patients develop chronic renal insufficiency.[26,216,217,285,302] Responses to plasma exchange have been reported, but their frequency is difficult to assess.[302,303] Likewise, it is not clear whether this disorder responds to the above-mentioned ancillary agents appropriate for use in TTP. Nevertheless, and despite a lack of definitive evidence that plasma exchange prevents the progression of sporadic HUS to chronic renal insufficiency, a trial of plasma exchange is appropriate in patients able to undergo the procedure safely.[6,20,302,303] Recurrences during pregnancy have been reported.[304,305] Renal transplantation is associated with a high risk of recurrence.[49,50] Guidelines for transplantation have been published (http://espn.cardiff.ac.uk/hus_guideline_2005.pdf).

Cyclosporine A–Associated and Posttransplantation Thrombotic Microangiopathy

Thrombotic microangiopathies occur most commonly in three transplant-related settings: (a) in association with the use of cyclosporine A (CyA), (b) as recurrent disease after transplantation for a thrombotic microangiopathy-related disorder, and (c) after bone marrow transplantation.

Cyclosporine:

Cyclosporine A is the most common cause of drug-induced thrombotic microangiopathy.[306] Thrombotic microangiopathy occurs in 1% to 5% of renal transplant recipients,[307–312] as well as in occasional solid organ recipients (reviewed in reference 308) treated with CyA or FK506. CyA-induced thrombotic microangiopathy typically develops insidiously with progressive, otherwise unexplained renal insufficiency.[307] MAHA or thrombocytopenia develops in only half the patients and is usually mild.[307,310] The appearance of the glomerular capillary and arteriolar thrombotic lesions is similar to de novo cases of thrombotic microangiopathy.[313] The distinction of CyA-induced thrombotic microangiopathy from acute tubular necrosis or rejection can often be made only by biopsy, and not in every case can an unequivocal distinction be established.[314] Broad alloantibody reactivity[307] and coinfection with cytomegalovirus[311] may predispose to CyA-associated thrombotic microangiopathy.

CyA is cytotoxic to cultured endothelial cells at concentrations similar to the peak plasma levels and tissue concentrations achieved in vivo.[315] CyA acts synergistically with IL-1α, IL-1β, and TNF-α to induce endothelial cell tissue factor expression[316] and inhibit thrombomodulin activity.[317] CyA also enhances the secretion of thromboxane by cultured endothelial cells[315] and inhibits the production or activity of a putative plasma prostacyclin stimulating factor.[318] Plasma levels of VWF[319] and endothelin-1[320] are elevated during episodes of nephrotoxicity, consistent with endothelial cell injury. CyA also enhances platelet aggregation and thromboxane release.[321]

CyA-induced thrombotic microangiopathy often responds to a reduction of the dose or temporary discontinuation of CyA. The prognosis is generally good, although some patients develop permanent renal failure.[306] In many patients, CyA can be reintroduced at a lower dose[307,322]; in others, FK 506 has been substituted successfully,[323] although the latter may also precipitate thrombotic microangiopathy.[324] The utility of plasma exchange is uncertain.

Renal Transplantation:

Approximately 50% of patients with idiopathic HUS develop end-stage renal insufficiency, thus becoming candidates for renal transplantation. Thrombotic microangiopathy can recur in the transplanted kidney, even in the absence of CyA. The reported frequency of this complication varies widely,[325–327] with the lowest incidence (approximately 10%) in young children with a history of Stx-associated HUS.[328–330] The incidence approaches 50% in older children and adults with atypical presentations in whom a familial etiology is likely.[328–330] Recurrence rates are lower in those with a longer duration between the initial episode of HUS and transplantation, and perhaps in those who have had bilateral nephrectomy.[330] A careful, multigenerational history must be taken to exclude the possibility of familial thrombotic microangiopathy when a living related donation is being considered.[200,329,330] The management of HUS associated with deficiencies in complement regulatory proteins is discussed above.

Bone Marrow Transplantation:

Thrombotic microangiopathy occurs in approximately 6% of patients who undergo allogeneic marrow transplantation; the incidence is estimated to be 0.1% to 1% after autologous marrow or stem cell transplantation.[83,331–337] The incidence is difficult to determine and diagnostic criteria are somewhat arbitrary as schistocytes and thrombocytopenia are nearly universal findings after bone marrow transplantation,[333,338] and the differential diagnosis of fever, renal failure, and neurologic complications is extensive. Indeed the utility of considering thrombotic microangiopathy to be a specific disorder in this setting has been questioned.[339] The clinical manifestations typically begin months after transplantation.[335,340] The pathophysiology is assumed to reflect systemic endothelial cell injury from a variety of causes. VWF protease activity may fall after transplantation,[341] but severe deficiency as occurs in TTP is uncommon (reviewed in references 308 and 342). Risk factors include use of an unrelated or mismatched donor,[336–338] total body irradiation as part of the pretransplant conditioning regime,[343] CyA or FK506 posttransplant,[331,333,344] systemic cytomegalovirus or other infection, older age,[336] female gender,[335] and graft-versus-host disease.[334,336,339,342,344] Systemic microangiopathy is rare,[339] but an intestinal biopsy may be needed to distinguish thrombotic microangiopathy from GVH in patients with refractory diarrhea.[345]

Withdrawal or substitution of another immunosuppressive for cyclosporine, if possible, and aggressive therapy with plasma exchange is often considered.[335,346] Discontinuing CyA may worsen underlying GVH and the benefit of plasma exchange has not been established; plasma exchange has also been associated with transfusion-related acute lung injury.[49] Alternative causes should be sought and aggressive treatment of infection and graft-versus-host disease be employed first in all but the most overt cases.[337] It is difficult to establish the prognosis because of variable inclusion criteria. Although patients may show an initial response to plasma therapy, the effectiveness of exchange has not been established and mortality exceeds 50%, often due to complications of graft-versus-host disease or opportunistic infection.[83,308,336,337,339,342] Defibrotide has been used with reported success in a few cases.[347]

Cancer and Chemotherapy-Associated Thrombotic Microangiopathy

Thrombotic microangiopathies may terminate the course of some patients with disseminated malignant neoplasms and large tumor burdens, most commonly adenocarcinoma of the gastrointestinal tract, breast, and lung.[77,348,349] Patients generally present with the abrupt onset of moderate to severe MAHA and thrombocytopenia. Renal insufficiency and neurologic dysfunction occur less commonly than in idiopathic or chemotherapy-induced thrombotic microangiopathy,[350,351] and may result from concurrent metabolic disturbances, central nervous system metastases, or hemorrhage.

The pathogenesis of cancer-associated thrombotic microangiopathy remains poorly understood.[77] Laboratory evidence of disseminated intravascular coagulation (DIC) is found in 25% to 80% of patients based on findings of elevated fibrin split products[348,350,352] or more sensitive measures of fibrinogen turnover.[77,348,350] However, the observation that thrombotic microangiopathy occurs in only 5% of patients with disseminated malignancy and DIC[349] suggests that additional factors, such as microvascular occlusion or intimal proliferation induced by tumor emboli within the pulmonary vasculature,[350,353,354] or formation of an incompletely endothelialized tumor vasculature that predisposes to platelet adhesion, must be involved. Severe deficiency of ADAMTS13 is not typical.[355] Survival is generally measured in weeks. The only effective therapy is reduction of the tumor burden, a goal that is often not attainable. A role for plasma exchange has not been established.

Specific cancer chemotherapeutic agents have also been implicated in the development of thrombotic microangiopathy.[351,356] Many patients were receiving therapy for an adenocarcinoma at the time thrombotic microangiopathy developed,[357,358] making the risk attributable to the neoplasm versus the therapy difficult to determine.[349,357,359,360] However, unlike cancer-associated thrombotic microangiopathy, most patients with chemotherapy-associated thrombotic microangiopathy do not carry a large tumor burden, and some may be in remission.[77,353] Mitomycin-C, a known nephrotoxin[357] is the most commonly reported cause, though other agents, including gemcitabine, *cis*-platininum, bleomycin, docetaxel, 5-fluourouracil, deoxycoformycin, carboplatin, and interferon-α, either alone or in combination, have been implicated.[77,308,358–362] Most patients who develop thrombotic microangiopathy due to mitomycin-C do so after having received a cumulative dose in excess of 60 mg,[357] but the syndrome has been reported after minimal exposure.[359] Most (77%) cases occur within 4 months of the last exposure to chemotherapy, and it is uncommon for cases to develop beyond 1 year.

Patients with chemotherapy-associated thrombotic microangiopathy generally present with moderate to severe MAHA, thrombocytopenia, and renal insufficiency (median creatinine value of 4.2 mg/dL).[349,357] Approximately 15% to 20% develop neurologic dysfunction, which may include confusion, headache, and seizures. A unique feature in some series is noncardiogenic pulmonary edema in more than 50% of patients.[358] Pulmonary function may deteriorate rapidly after red blood cell or platelet transfusion,[357] which should be used with caution.

Chemotherapy-associated thrombotic microangiopathy is presumed to result from direct toxicity to the endothelium. Mitomycin inhibits the production of prostacyclin by umbilical vein endothelium, and the infusion of mitomycin-C into the rat kidney induces histological changes similar to those of chemotherapy-induced thrombotic microangiopathy.[363] ADAMST13 levels are not severely depressed.[84] Chemotherapy-induced thrombotic microangiopathy confers a grave prognosis. Fewer than 20% of affected patients respond to plasma exchange and corticosteroids, and more than 50% die within 2 months.[349,353,357,364] Anecdotal responses to immunophoresis with staphylococcal protein A columns have been reported in approximately 50% of patients, typically those with no clinically evident tumor, though these reports require confirmation.[357,365,366]

Miscellaneous, Drug-Associated Thrombotic Microangiopathy

In addition to chemotherapeutic agents, thrombotic microangiopathy has been associated uncommonly with more than 50 drugs, including penicillins,[77] ciprofloxacin[367] and clarithromycin,[368] histamine H_2-receptor antagonists,[369] the norplant contraceptive,[370] and thienopyridines,[371–373] among others.[77,374] Interestingly, the mechanisms by which each of these agents induce the thrombotic microangiopathy may differ, as may the natural history and response to therapy. Although mitomycin C, gemcitabine, and cyclosporine appear to induce TMA in a cumulative dose-dependent manner, quinidine[375] and thienopyridines (ticlopidine and clopidogrel) induce thrombotic microangiopathy through either idiosyncratic, immune-mediated mechanisms or acute endothelial toxicity.[371,374,376]

An association of quinine with thrombotic microangiopathy was first reported by Gottschall et al in 1991, who described the course of three patients with a syndrome resembling idiopathic HUS.[377] Patients generally present with severe MAHA, platelet counts lower than 50,000/μL and renal insufficiency, usually requiring dialysis.[375] Neurologic dysfunction occurs in a minority of patients, but can be severe; granulocytopenia and lymphopenia have been reported.[378] In earlier reports, the prognosis was favorable once quinine was withdrawn and plasma exchange instituted.[375] However, in a recent series, 17 of 225 patients with HUS had quinine-associated thrombotic microangiopathy; 4 of these died, and 7 survivors were left with chronic renal failure.[379] Although this disorder occurs most commonly after the ingestion of quinine tablets, cases have been reported after exposure to quinine in beverages such as tonic water, and the syndrome may recur rapidly upon reexposure.[379,380] The pathogenesis may involve idiosyncratic, quinine-dependent antibodies reactive with platelet glycoproteins IIb/IIIa and Ib/IX and related antigens on endothelial cells and neutrophils[375,377,378,381] that promote neutrophil aggregation and binding to endothelial cells in a drug-dependent manner.[375,378,381]

The thienopyridines ticlopidine and clopidogrel are another common cause of drug-induced TTP. TTP occurs in a higher percentage of patients exposed to ticlopidine, with an incidence ranging from 1:600 to 1:4814 patient exposures[373,376,382,383] in contrast to an estimated incidence of 4 per 1,000,000[384] to 1 per 8,500 to 26,000[385] exposures in patients taking clopidogrel.[372] No cases of clopidogrel-associated TTP were encountered in the CAPRIE and CURE studies, each of which enrolled more than 6200 patients.[376] Despite the low frequency of cases in patients treated with clopidogrel, the fact that this drug is the second most commonly prescribed drug in the United States renders it the most commonly reported drug associated with TTP in the FDA's MedWatch database, accounting for more than 30% of all drug-associated TTP cases. Interestingly, the pathogenesis and natural history of TTP associated with ticlopidine and clopidogrel may differ in many cases.[371] Reductions in ADAMTS13 activity below 15% occur in 85% of patients with ticlopidine-exposed patients, but in only 15% of patients with clopidogrel-associated TTP. These reductions reflect the development of anti-ADAMTS13 antibodies.[112] TTP generally develops within 2 to 12 weeks of starting the drug,[376] and responds relatively quickly to plasma exchange, which reduces mortality and should be initiated promptly on diagnosis.[386] Spontaneous relapses may occur in these patients.[371,373] In contrast, 90% of patients exposed to clopidogrel, but only 10% of patients exposed to ticlopidine, develop a syndrome characterized primarily by microangiopathic hemolytic anemia and renal insufficiency, without severe thrombocytopenia[371,387]; these individuals have normal levels of ADAMTS13, usually develop disease within the first 2 weeks of drug treatment, and may require several weeks of plasma exchange to achieve remission. Whether plasma exchange actually improves the clinical outcome is uncertain.[371] Spontaneous relapses are uncommon in these individuals.[372,376,385,386]

HIV-Associated Thrombotic Microangiopathy

An association between HIV infection and thrombotic microangiopathy has been recognized since 1984.[388–390] The incidence of HIV infection in patients with thrombotic microangiopathy varies from 15% to 50% in endemic areas.[389–391] The presentation of HIV-associated thrombotic microangiopathy and TTP in non–HIV-infected individuals are similar,[77,78,391,392] although some patients with HIV present with acute renal failure.[393] Thrombotic microangiopathy may occur at any time during the course of HIV infection, but is rare in patients with hemophilia.[394] Diagnosis may be difficult because fever, anemia,[395] thrombocytopenia,[396,397] nephropathy, neurologic dysfunction, and elevated LDH levels secondary to lymphoma, drug reactions or pulmonary infection with *Pneumocystis carinii* occur commonly in this population.[391] The pathogenesis of HIV-associated thrombotic microangiopathy is not well understood. It has been suggested that the function of the microvascular endothelium is disrupted by opportunistic organisms or infection with HIV, drugs such as fluconazole[398] or valacyclovir,[187] and alterations in plasma cytokines.[391] ADAMTS13 deficiency in the presence or absence of inhibitory antibodies has been reported[399,400] and may be associated with high D-dimer levels.[401] HIV-associated thrombotic microangiopathy responds to plasma exchange, and responses to antiretroviral therapy have been reported.[78,391] The role of splenectomy is less well studied.[78] The long-term prognosis is dependent on the severity of the underlying syndrome.[7,402] Prior to the introduction of effective antiretroviral therapy, many patients had advanced AIDS on presentation and died within 1 to 2 years of their underlying disease, but survival has improved in patients treated with aggressive plasma therapy, antiretrovirals, and other supportive measures.[7,78,391]

Pregnancy-Associated Thrombotic Microangiopathy

The differential diagnosis of MAHA associated with gestation is complex.[20,403–405] Thrombotic microangiopathy may be difficult if not impossible to distinguish from other causes of MAHA unique to pregnancy, such as preeclampsia, the syndrome of hemolysis-elevated liver function tests and thrombocytopenia (HELLP) and acute fatty liver associated with DIC.[403,406] The severity of the renal and neurologic abnormalities and the time during gestation at which the signs and symptoms of thrombotic microangiopathy first appear may provide clues needed to prevent critical delays in therapy.[20,403,404]

Approximately 10% of cases of idiopathic TTP occur in association with pregnancy.[75,305,407] In one series, 40 of 45 cases of TTP were diagnosed antepartum. Among those diagnosed during pregnancy, the mean gestational age at the onset of symptoms was 23.5 weeks in one series,[408] although overall TTP is more common in the third trimester or immediately postpartum.[305,406] In the absence of appropriate therapy, maternal and fetal mortality approach 90%. There is no evidence that uterine evacuation leads to resolution.[403,404,409,410] ADAMST13 levels fall progressively during pregnancy but severe deficiency (<5%) is seen only in women with TTP.[305] The prognosis has improved dramatically since the advent of plasma exchange, and continuing pregnancy does not impair response.[407,408] Many patients carry to term successfully, although the overall risk of fetal loss remains significant.[411]

Patients with chronic, relapsing TTP are likely to recur during subsequent pregnancies.[304,407] Anecdotal evidence suggests that prophylactic treatment with antiplatelet agents or corticosteroids may reduce the frequency and severity of relapse.[407] Other patients have been managed with periodic transfusion of plasma or plasma fractions, but more intensive treatment may be needed during pregancy.[304]

Sporadic HUS also occurs in association with pregnancy and has previously been termed malignant nephrosclerosis, irreversible postpartum renal failure, or postpartum intravascular coagulation.[403] The disorder primarily affects primiparas who present with MAHA, thrombocytopenia, renal insufficiency and hypertension beginning a minimum of 48 hours after an otherwise normal pregnancy. Neurologic symptoms are less frequent and severe.[404] In one series, the mean time to onset of symptoms was 26.6 days after delivery,[408] a finding that helps to distinguish HUS from other causes of pregnancy-associated MAHA and thrombocytopenia such as preeclampsia and HELLP. Occasional patients with familial thrombotic microangiopathy display clinical manifestations for the first time during pregnancy, and occasional cases associated with VTEC infection have occurred intrapartum.[20,412,413] The prognosis of pregnancy-associated HUS remains relatively poor. The mortality rate formerly approached 50% and an additional 10% to 15% were left with chronic renal insufficiency.[414] Responses to plasma exchange or infusion have been reported, though their frequency is uncertain. Uterine evacuation does not lead to remission, and fetal outcome depends on successful treatment of the mother.[404]

FUTURE DIRECTIONS

The syndromes of thrombotic microangiopathy are uncommon, though the associated morbidity and mortality are significant. Despite dramatic progress in understanding the genetic and molecular basis of these disorders, important aspects of their pathogenesis, for example the factors that incite these disorders in specific individuals, remain poorly understood. Nevertheless, a disorder universally fatal 30 years ago has a far better prognosis today, and we are beginning to understand the reasons why therapy previously considered empiric is efficacious. As our understanding of the genetics, biochemistry, and immunology of these disorders evolves, it is likely that improved approaches to treatment will follow as well. We look forward to better definition of the role of ADAMTS13 protease and antibody levels in diagnosing, guiding therapy for, and predicting relapse of TTP, as well as to a better understanding of the risk of pregnancy in women with a history of thrombotic microangiopathy. The application of new and specific immunosuppressive approaches may also lead to improved outcomes and prevention of relapse.

SUGGESTED READINGS

George JN: How I treat patients with thrombotic thrombocytopenic purpura-hemolytic uremic syndrome. Blood 96:1223, 2000.

George JN: Thrombotic thrombocytopenic purpura. New Engl J Med 354:1927, 2006.

Furlan M, Robles R, Galbusera M, et al: von Willebrand factor-cleaving protease in thrombotic thrombocytopenic purpura and the hemolytic-uremic syndrome. N Engl J Med 339:1578, 1998.

Tsai H-M, Lian ECY. Antibodies to von Willebrand factor-cleaving protease in acute thrombotic thrombocytopenic purpura. N Engl J Med 339:1585, 1998.

Caprioli J, Noris M, Brioschi S, et al: Genetics of HUS: the impact of MCP, CFH, and IF mutations on clinical presentation, response to treatment, and outcome. Blood 108:1267, 2006.

Zimmerhackl LB, Besbas N, Jungraithmayr T, et al: Epidemiology, clinical presentation, and pathophysiology of atypical and recurrent hemolytic uremic syndrome. Semin Thromb Hemost 32:113, 2006.

Levy GG, Nichols WC, Lian EC, et al: Mutations in a member of the ADAMTS gene family cause thrombotic thrombocytopenic purpura. Nature 413:488, 2001.

Ridolfi RL, Bell WR: Thrombotic thrombocytopenia purpura: Report of 25 cases and a review of the literature. Medicine 60:413, 1981.

Amarosi EL, Ultmann JE: Thrombotic thrombocytopenic purpura. Report of 16 cases and review of the literature. Medicine 45:139, 1966.

Mannucci PM, Peyvandi F: TTP and ADAMTS13: When is testing appropriate? Hematology (Am Soc Hematol Educ Program) 79, 2007.

Rock GA, Shumak KH, Buskard NA, et al: Comparison of plasma exchange with plasma infusion in the treatment of thrombotic thrombocytopenic purpura. N Engl J Med 325:393, 1991.

Fakhouri F, Vernant JP, Veyradier JP, et al: Efficiency of curative and prophylactic treatment with rituximab in ADAMTS13-deficient thrombotic thrombocytopenic purpura: a study of 11 cases. Blood 106:1932, 2005.

Amirlak I, Amirlak B: Haemolytic uremic syndrome: an overview. Nephrology 11:213, 2006.

Tarr PI, Gordon CA, Chandler WL: Shiga-toxin-producing *Escherichia coli* and haemolytic uraemic syndrome. Lancet 365:1073, 2005.

Gagnadoux MF, Habib R, Gubler MC, et al: Long-term (15–25 years) outcome of childhood hemolytic-uremic syndrome. Clin Neph 46:39, 1996.

Repetto HA: Long-term course and mechanisms of progression of renal disease in hemolytic uremic syndrome. Kidney Int Suppl 97:S102, 2005.

Karch H, Friedrich AW, Gerber A, et al: New aspects in the pathogenesis of the enteropathic hemolytic uremic syndrome. Sem Thromb Hemost 32:105, 2006.

George JN: The association of pregnancy with thrombotic thrombocytopenic purpura-hemolytic uremic syndrome. Current Opinion in Hematology 10:339, 2003.

Qu L, Kiss JE: Thrombotic microangiopathy in transplantation and malignancy. Seminars in Thrombosis and Haemostasis 31:691, 2005.

Bren A, Pajek J, Greco K, et al: Follow-up of kidney graft recipients with cyclosporine-associated hemolytic-uremic syndrome and thrombotic microangiopathy. Transplant Proc 37:1889, 2005.

Batts ED, Lazarus HM: Diagnosis and treatment of transplantation-associated thrombotic microangiopathy: real progress or are we still waiting? Bone Marrow Transplant 40:709, 2007.

Bennett CL, Kim B, Zakarija A, et al: Two mechanistic pathways for thienopyridine-associated thrombotic thrombocytopenic purpura: a report from the SERF-TTP Research Group and the RADAR Project. J Am Coll Cardiol 50:1138, 2007.

Zakarija A, Bennett C: Drug-induced thrombotic microangiopathy. Sem Thromb Hemost 31:681, 2005.

McCrae KR: Thrombocytopenia in pregnancy: differential diagnosis, pathogenesis and management. Blood Rev 17:7, 2003.

Veyradier A, Obert B, Houllier A, et al: Specific von Willebrand factor-cleaving protease in thrombotic microangiopathies: a study of 111 cases. Blood 98:1765, 2001.

Vesely SK, George JN, Lammle B, et al: ADAMTS13 activity in thrombotic thrombocytopenic purpura-hemolytic uremic syndrome: relation to presenting features and clinical outcomes in a prospective cohort of 142 patients. Blood 102:60, 2003.

Zheng XL, Kaufman RM, Goodnough LT, et al: Effect of plasma exchange on plasma ADAMTS13 metalloprotease activity, inhibitor level, and clinical outcome in patients with idiopathic and nonidiopathic thrombotic thrombocytopenic purpura. Blood 103:4043, 2004.

REFERENCES

For complete list of references log onto www.expertconsult.com

CHAPTER 140

THROMBOCYTOPENIA DUE TO PLATELET DESTRUCTION AND HYPERSPLENISM

Theodore E. Warkentin

Thrombocytopenia is defined as a platelet count below the lower limit of the normal range (approximately 150 × 10^9/L). Sometimes, an expanded definition of thrombocytopenia is appropriate. For example, an abrupt drop in the platelet count can signify the onset of a platelet-destructive process such as heparin-induced thrombocytopenia (HIT)[1] or bacteremia, even if the platelet count remains above 150 × 10^9/L.

In the clinical evaluation of the thrombocytopenic patient, three questions must be asked. First, could the patient have pseudothrombocytopenia? Second, what is the most likely explanation for the thrombocytopenia? And third, what are the likely risks posed by the causative disorder and the severity of the thrombocytopenia? For example, very severe thrombocytopenia caused by drug-dependent antibodies or platelet-reactive autoantibodies often is associated with bleeding. By contrast, thrombocytopenia caused by heparin-dependent antibodies or attributable to disseminated intravascular coagulation (DIC) secondary to adenocarcinoma is strongly associated with thrombosis. Often, the underlying cause of the thrombocytopenia (eg, bacteremia, cancer, cirrhosis), rather than the thrombocytopenia itself, poses the greater risk.

Thrombocytopenia can be caused by any of four general mechanisms: (a) platelet underproduction, (b) increased platelet destruction, (c) platelet sequestration, and (d) hemodilution. Platelet underproduction usually occurs with underproduction of other blood cell lines and usually is characterized by pancytopenia. Thrombocytopenia caused by increased platelet destruction develops when the rate of platelet destruction surpasses the ability of the bone marrow to produce platelets. Platelet destruction may be caused by immune or nonimmune mechanisms (Table 140–1). Thrombocytopenia due to platelet sequestration is caused by redistribution of platelets from the circulation into an enlarged splenic vascular bed. Hemodilution is characterized by a decrease in the number of platelets, as well as red and white cells, caused by the administration of colloids, crystalloids, or platelet-poor blood products. In pregnant women, the differential diagnosis must be expanded to include causes unique to these patients (Table 140–2).

APPROACH TO THE THROMBOCYTOPENIC PATIENT

History and Physical Examination

Certain information should be ascertained, including (a) the location and severity of bleeding (if any); (b) the temporal profile of the hemostatic defect (acute, chronic, or relapsing); (c) presence of symptoms of a secondary illness, such as a neoplasm, infection, or an autoimmune disorder such as systemic lupus erythematosus (SLE); (d) a history of recent medication use, alcohol ingestion, or transfusion; (e) presence of risk factors for certain infections, particularly human immunodeficiency virus (HIV) infection and viral hepatitis; and (f) family history of thrombocytopenia (see Chapter 121).

During the physical examination, evidence of hemostatic impairment should be sought, as well as secondary causes for thrombocytopenia. The signs of platelet bleeding include petechiae and purpura (see Chapter 121). Petechiae typically occur in the dependent regions of the body or on traumatized areas. Spontaneous mucous membrane bleeding (wet purpura), epistaxis, and gastrointestinal bleeding indicate more serious hemostatic defects. Although petechiae are common in patients whose platelet count is less than 10 to 20 × 10^9/L, most patients whose platelet count is greater than 50 × 10^9/L do not exhibit any signs of hemostatic impairment. The physical examination may identify an explanation for the thrombocytopenia. For example, enlarged lymph nodes can indicate a viral infection, such as infectious mononucleosis or HIV infection, or a neoplastic lymphoproliferative disorder. An enlarged spleen suggests hypersplenism.

Laboratory Evaluation

The laboratory tests used for the evaluation of a patient with thrombocytopenia are summarized in Table 140–3 (also see Chapter 122). The blood film is examined to exclude pseudothrombocytopenia, which is characterized by in vitro platelet clumping. This phenomenon, which occurs in approximately 1/1000 blood samples examined, is most often caused by naturally occurring, platelet glycoprotein complex GPIIb/IIIa (integrin $\alpha_{IIb}\beta_3$)-reactive autoantibodies that produce aggregation of platelets in the presence of the calcium-chelating anticoagulant ethylenediamine tetra-acetic acid (EDTA).[2,3] The platelet aggregates are not counted by the electronic particle counter, so the automated platelet count appears falsely low. The correct platelet count usually can be determined by collecting the blood into sodium citrate or heparin anticoagulants or performing a count on nonanticoagulated finger prick samples; maintaining the blood sample at 37°C also will reduce platelet clumping in many instances.[3] EDTA-dependent pseudothrombocytopenia has no pathologic significance, other than potentially placing a patient in jeopardy for inappropriate treatment for thrombocytopenia that does not exist. A much less common (1/10,000 blood samples) antibody-mediated pseudothrombocytopenic disorder is platelet satellitism, in which rosette-like clusters of platelets are seen around neutrophils.[4] This entity is produced by immunoglobulin G (IgG) antibodies that recognize EDTA-induced cryptic epitopes on both platelet GPIIb/IIIa and neutrophil FcγIII receptors.

The bone marrow examination can be helpful in assessing platelet production, particularly if megakaryocytes are reduced in number or abnormal in appearance. Examination of the bone marrow can be diagnostic in a few disorders (eg, leukemia, metastatic tumor, Gaucher disease, megaloblastic anemia).

Elevated platelet-associated IgG (PAIgG) is observed in patients with either immune or nonimmune thrombocytopenia; therefore, these assays are not useful diagnostically. There is evidence that glycoprotein-specific platelet antibody assays, such as the monoclonal antibody immobilization of platelet antigens (MAIPA) assay or antigen capture enzyme (ACE) immunoassay, are relatively specific for detection of autoimmune thrombocytopenic disorders.[5] Chapter 138 discusses these disorders in more detail.

In patients in whom the mechanism of chronic thrombocytopenia is unclear, an indium 111 (^{111}In)-labeled autologous platelet survival study can be helpful. Three patterns can be seen: (a) a normal platelet survival and recovery (underproduction); (b) a marked reduction in the platelet life span (increased destruction); and (c) a reduced recovery but a normal or near-normal life span (sequestration). ^{111}In-labeled platelets also can be used to image accessory splenic tissue in patients with idiopathic thrombocytopenic purpura (ITP) in whom

Table 140–1 Mechanisms of Platelet Destruction

Type of Thrombocytopenia	Specific Example(s)
Immune-Mediated	
Autoantibody-mediated platelet destruction by reticuloendothelial system (RES)	Primary and secondary idiopathic (immune) thrombocytopenic purpura*
Alloantibody-mediated platelet destruction by RES	Neonatal alloimmune thrombocytopenia*; posttransfusion purpura*; passive alloimmune thrombocytopenia; alloimmune platelet transfusion refractoriness*
Drug-dependent, antibody-mediated platelet destruction by RES	Drug-induced immune thrombocytopenic purpura (eg, quinine) (see Table 140–6)
Platelet activation by binding of immunoglobulin G (IgG) Fc of drug-dependent IgG to platelet FcγIIa receptors	Heparin-induced thrombocytopenia
Non–Immune-Mediated	
Platelet activation by thrombin or proinflammatory cytokines	Disseminated intravascular coagulation (DIC)*; septicemia/systemic inflammatory response syndromes
Platelet destruction via ingestion by macrophages (hemophagocytosis)	Infections, certain malignant lymphoproliferative disorders
Platelet destruction through platelet interactions with altered von Willebrand factor (vWF)†	Thrombotic thrombocytopenic purpura*; hemolytic uremic syndrome*
Platelet losses on artificial surfaces	Cardiopulmonary bypass surgery*; use of intravascular catheters
Decreased platelet survival associated with cardiovascular diseases	Congenital and acquired heart disease; cardiomyopathy; pulmonary embolism

*See other relevant chapters for a discussion of thrombocytopenia in these disorders.

†Although platelet destruction is not directly caused by antibodies, immune mechanisms can explain altered vWF (eg, autoimmune clearance of vWF-cleaving metalloprotease).

Table 140–2 Differential Diagnosis of Thrombocytopenia in Pregnancy

Incidental thrombocytopenia of pregnancy (gestational thrombocytopenia)
Preeclampsia/eclampsia*
Disseminated intravascular coagulation (DIC) secondary to:
Abruptio placentae
Endometritis
Amniotic fluid embolism
Retained fetus
Preeclampsia/eclampsia*
Peripartum/postpartum thrombotic microangiopathy
Thrombotic thrombocytopenic purpura
Hemolytic uremic syndrome

*Preeclampsia/eclampsia usually is not associated with overt DIC.

splenectomy fails to effect a cure or in whom postsplenectomy relapse occurs.

Therapy

The bleeding risk for thrombocytopenic patients can be reduced by avoiding drugs that impair hemostasis (eg, alcohol, antiplatelet agents, anticoagulants) and invasive procedures (intramuscular injections). If drug-induced thrombocytopenia is suspected, as many medications as possible should be stopped. Life-threatening bleeding episodes should be treated with platelet transfusions, regardless of the mechanism of the thrombocytopenia.

The underlying cause and anticipated natural history of the thrombocytopenic disorder influence the decision whether to transfuse platelets for prophylaxis against bleeding. As a general rule, patients with chronic thrombocytopenic disorders characterized by increased platelet destruction (eg, chronic ITP) or chronic underproduction (eg, aplastic anemia, myelodysplasia) can tolerate long periods of severe thrombocytopenia without major bleeding. In addition, a prophylactic transfusion can trigger alloimmunization against human leukocyte antigen (HLA) or platelet antigens, thereby jeopardizing future therapeutic platelet transfusions. Therefore, prophylactic platelet transfusions are seldom indicated for these patients. When such patients have a transient but major hemostatic risk such as trauma or certain surgeries, however, the platelet count should be maintained above 50×10^9/L. Invasive procedures such as thoracentesis, paracentesis, and liver biopsy usually are not associated with excess bleeding if the platelet count is greater than 50×10^9/L.[6]

Prophylactic platelet transfusions should not be given to patients with HIT, thrombotic thrombocytopenic purpura, or hemolytic uremic syndrome, because they could exacerbate platelet-mediated thrombotic complications.

ANATOMY AND PHYSIOLOGY

The Spleen: Anatomy and Function

The spleen is a small, well-perfused organ receiving about 5% of the cardiac output.[7] Its anatomy is uniquely suited for its function; the progressive branching of the splenic artery into the trabecular and then central arteries helps separate the plasma from the cellular elements (see Chapter 163). The central arteries arise perpendicularly from the trabecular arteries and skim off the plasma layer from the cells. Soluble antigens in the plasma are delivered to the white pulp, where phagocytic cells process the antigens and initiate antibody production.

The cell-rich hemoconcentrated fraction of the blood is delivered to the red pulp. A small percentage of this blood flows directly to the splenic veins (the closed system), but most moves into the splenic cords (the open system). Here the cellular elements percolate through a meshwork of reticulum fibers, reticuloendothelial cells, and supporting cells, to reach the splenic sinuses. The cells enter the sinuses by passing through narrow fenestrations in the basement membrane of the endothelial cells lining the sinuses. The blood exits through the splenic vein into the portal system. Because the veins in the portal system lack valves, any increase in portal pressure is transmitted to the splenic microcirculation.

The spleen has a number of important roles. It is the largest lymphoid organ in the body and plays a pivotal role in host defense by

Table 140–3 Laboratory Tests Used to Investigate a Patient With Thrombocytopenia

Test	Rationale
Common Tests	
Complete blood count (CBC)	Isolated thrombocytopenia usually is caused by platelet destruction, whereas involvement of all cell lines suggests underproduction or sequestration
Examination of the blood film	Pseudothrombocytopenia (platelet clumps) Toxic changes and granulocyte "left shift" suggest septicemia Atypical lymphocytes suggest viral infection Red cell fragments suggest TTP or HUS Parasites (eg, in malaria) White cell inclusions suggest hereditary macrothrombocytopenia
Blood cultures	Bacteremia, fungemia
Antinuclear antibody test	Systemic lupus erythematosus
Direct antiglobulin test	Exclude immune hemolysis accompanying ITP (Evans syndrome)
Coagulation assays	
Activated partial thromboplastin time (APTT), prothrombin time (INR), thrombin time, fibrinogen, D-dimer assay	Disseminated intravascular coagulation (DIC)
Lupus anticoagulant assay (nonspecific inhibitor), anticardiolipin and anti-β_2-glycoprotein I assays	Antiphospholipid antibody syndrome
Serum protein electrophoresis; IgG, IgM, IgA levels	ITP associated with lymphoproliferative disorder (monoclonal); hypersplenism associated with chronic hepatitis (polyclonal)
HIV serologic studies	HIV-associated thrombocytopenia
Bone marrow aspiration, biopsy	Assess megakaryocyte numbers and morphology; exclude primary marrow disorder
Specialized Tests	
Glycoprotein-specific platelet antibody assays (eg, MAIPA)	Relatively specific assay for primary and secondary ITP
Drug-dependent increase in platelet-associated IgG	Specific assay for drug-induced immune thrombocytopenia
Drug-dependent platelet activation (eg, platelet serotonin release assay) and/or Platelet factor 4/heparin (or polyanion) ELISA	Heparin-induced thrombocytopenia
Radionuclide platelet lifespan study with imaging (eg, ^{111}In platelet survival study)	Define the mechanism of thrombocytopenia; identify an "accessory" spleen postsplenectomy

ELISA, enzyme-linked immunosorbent assay; HIV, human immunodeficiency virus; HUS, hemolytic uremic syndrome; IgG, immunoglobulin G; INR, international normalized ratio; ITP, idiopathic (immune) thrombocytopenic purpura; MAIPA, monoclonal antibody immobilization of platelet antigens; TTP, thrombotic thrombocytopenic purpura.

clearing microorganisms and antibody-coated cells. The spleen also is important for antibody synthesis, especially against soluble antigens. The filtering function of the spleen includes (a) culling (removal of damaged or senescent cells and bacteria), (b) pitting (removal of red cell inclusions and parasites), and (c) remodeling (reticulocyte sequestration and maturation). The spleen also acts as a (d) large reservoir for platelets (accommodating about one-third of the platelet mass in normal individuals).[7] By contrast, the human spleen contains less than 2% of the total red blood cell mass, although in some animals (dogs and cats), the spleen is a much more important red cell reservoir.

Physiologic Platelet Sequestration

Radiolabeled platelet studies have shown that approximately 30% of the total platelet mass exists as a freely exchangeable pool in the spleen.[7] Because the normal platelet life span is 9 to 10 days, a platelet spends approximately a third of its life, or 3 days, within the spleen. In patients with hypersplenism, as many as 90% of platelets can be found in the spleen.

After the labeled platelets are injected, accumulation is apparent in both the liver and the spleen.[8] An initial, irreversible phase of hepatic uptake occurs. This equilibrates during the first 5 minutes and may reflect hepatic clearance of platelets damaged in the labeling procedure. Simultaneously, there is a slow rise in activity over the spleen that peaks in about 20 minutes. Splenic platelet uptake is thus dependent on input (spleen blood flow) and output (clearance).

The splenic platelet pool size can be decreased and the platelet count increased with intravenous infusions of epinephrine in normal persons and in patients with splenomegaly.[7] By contrast, isoprenaline increases the pool size.[9] Splenic blood flow increases with increasing spleen size, although perfusion (flow per unit of tissue volume) falls.[10] Blood flow can be increased in some inflammatory disorders (eg, SLE) without an increase in spleen size. A marked increase or decrease in splenic perfusion alters the proportion of platelets within the spleen.

The most important determinant of the splenic platelet pool is the spleen size.[10] The measurement of spleen size can thus be helpful in predicting the degree of thrombocytopenia expected from excess platelet pooling in the spleen. For example, if the splenic platelet pool is 90% (ie, 10% outside the spleen), the platelet count will be reduced by a factor of 7 (because normally 70% of platelets lie outside the spleen). Consequently, and as a general rule, even if the spleen is massively enlarged, very severe thrombocytopenia ($<20 \times 10^9$/L) is virtually never seen. On the other hand, mild thrombocytopenia may be explained by mild splenomegaly that may not be detectible on physical examination but demonstrable by imaging studies.

PATHOLOGIC PLATELET SEQUESTRATION: HYPERSPLENISM

Definition

Hypersplenism is a syndrome characterized by splenomegaly and any or all of the following cytopenias: anemia, leukopenia, or thrombocytopenia. Implicit in the definition is that the cytopenias will correct following splenectomy. Although splenomegaly is almost always present in hypersplenism, many patients with splenomegaly do not have hypersplenism. The hypersplenism usually is the result of an identifiable pathologic process, but rarely, the cause of the splenomegaly remains elusive, and the hypersplenism is termed *primary.*

Pathogenesis

A list of the disorders producing splenomegaly and hypersplenism is presented in Table 140–4. An increase in the size of the spleen can be caused by several mechanisms. An increase in the workload of the spleen can be due to immunologic stress (infection, inflammation, or an autoimmune disorder) or to increased red cell removal (red cell membrane disorders, hemoglobinopathies). Portal hypertension also will increase the size of the spleen, producing congestive splenomegaly. Benign and malignant infiltrative disorders also can increase splenic size (infiltrative splenomegaly) and cause hypersplenism. Some of these disorders produce thrombocytopenia by more than just hypersplenism (eg, marrow replacement by tumor, immune-mediated platelet clearance). Thus, the demonstration of an enlarged spleen does not necessarily mean that the cytopenias are caused solely by hypersplenism.

The thrombocytopenia of hypersplenism is caused primarily by increased splenic platelet pooling.[7,10] A massively enlarged spleen can hold greater than 90% of the total platelet mass. In the absence of altered platelet production, the total body platelet mass usually is normal and the platelet life span is near normal.[7] Usually, the splenic transit time remains normal (approximately 10 minutes), but the absolute number of platelets retained within the enlarged spleen is increased. All of these platelets remain part of the exchangeable pool. In hypersplenism, the thrombocytopenia is moderately severe (platelet counts of 50×10^9/L to 150×10^9/L). Severe thrombocytopenia (less than 20×10^9/L) suggests another diagnosis. Therefore, it is unusual for patients with hypersplenism to have evidence of hemostatic impairment attributable to thrombocytopenia, or to need specific interventions to raise the platelet count. Plasma volume expansion occurs in hypersplenism, but hemodilution plays a relatively minor role in the thrombocytopenia. In some patients, impaired hepatic production of thrombopoietin may contribute to severe thrombocytopenia that cannot be explained solely by hypersplenism in advanced liver disease.[11]

The neutropenia of hypersplenism is caused by an increase in the marginated granulocyte pool, a portion of which is located in the spleen. The neutropenia of hypersplenism usually is asymptomatic.

Diagnosis

Thrombocytopenia is likely to be caused by hypersplenism when (a) splenomegaly is present, (b) the thrombocytopenia is mild to moderate in severity, (c) moderately reduced neutrophil and low-normal hemoglobin levels are found, and (d) no or minimal evidence for impaired hematopoiesis is observed on bone marrow examination. Ultrasonography, computed tomography (CT), and radionuclide imaging are of comparable sensitivity in documenting splenomegaly,[12] and an imaging study should be performed when suspected splenomegaly is not evident on physical examination. The mean platelet volume (MPV) often is slightly decreased in hypersplenism, but this finding is not sufficiently specific to be diagnostically useful. An ^{111}In-labeled platelet survival study can be diagnostic of hypersplenism, demonstrating reduced platelet recovery and a normal platelet life span. Determining the cause of the splenomegaly usually is the most important issue.

Therapy

Several maneuvers can improve or correct the cytopenias attributable to hypersplenism, including total or partial[13] splenectomy, partial splenic embolization,[14] and, in patients with congestive splenomegaly, surgical or transjugular intrahepatic portosystemic shunting.[15] Cytopenias secondary to hypersplenism, and thrombocytopenia in particular, are almost never sufficiently severe to justify treatment, however. Consequently, the decision to perform one of these interventions usually depends on other considerations. For example, splenectomy should be considered for relief of pain or early satiety

Table 140–4 Differential Diagnosis of Splenomegaly and Hypersplenism

Infections
Acute
Viral (viral hepatitis, infectious mononucleosis, cytomegalovirus infection)
Bacterial (septicemia, salmonellosis, brucellosis, splenic abscess)
Parasite (toxoplasmosis)
Subacute and chronic
Subacute bacterial endocarditis
Tuberculosis
Malaria
Kala-azar
Fungal disease
Inflammation
Felty's syndrome
Systemic lupus erythematosus
Serum sickness
Rheumatic fever
Sarcoidosis
Congestive Splenomegaly
Intrahepatic
Cirrhosis
Extrahepatic
Portal vein obstruction
Splenic vein obstruction
Hepatic vein occlusion (Budd-Chiari syndrome)
Chronic passive congestion
Heart failure
Hematologic Disorders
Red cell disorders: hemolytic anemias, thalassemia, sickle cell disorders
Neoplasia
Malignant
Myeloproliferative disorders
Myeloid metaplasia
Polycythemia rubra vera
Essential thrombocythemia
Chronic leukemia
Chronic myeloid leukemia
Chronic lymphocytic leukemia
Hairy cell leukemia
Lymphoma
Acute leukemia
Malignant histiocytosis
Benign
Hamartoma
Hemangioma
Lymphangioma
Fibroma
Storage Diseases
Gaucher disease
Niemann-Pick disease
Miscellaneous
Amyloidosis
Cysts

associated with massive splenomegaly (eg, in myelo- or lymphoproliferative disorders), or for splenomegaly of unknown origin (for investigation of possible splenic lymphoma[16]).

Short-term complications from splenectomy include infections, bleeding, and thromboembolism. The major long-term risk associated with splenectomy is overwhelming septicemia; this risk can be reduced by vaccination. All patients should be vaccinated against pneumococci, meningococci, and *Haemophilus*, preferably at least 2 weeks before splenectomy.[17] Splenectomy for congestive hypersplenism in the setting of portal hypertension carries high morbidity and mortality rates[18]; consequently, splenectomy is performed only after careful consideration. Splenectomy also is associated with high morbidity (50%) and mortality (10%–15%) rates in myeloid metaplasia and does not alter the natural history of this disorder. Thus, splenectomy usually is performed for palliation of intractable symptoms.

Splenectomy in Gaucher disease usually corrects the cytopenias, relieves abdominal discomfort, and in children improves growth. Partial rather than total splenectomy has been used in an attempt to avoid shifting the deposition of glucocerebroside from spleen to bones. Often, however, recurrence of splenomegaly and hypersplenism results after partial splenectomy. Enzyme replacement therapy can reduce the morbidity from hypersplenism (see Chapter 53).

DRUG-INDUCED THROMBOCYTOPENIC SYNDROMES

Many drugs can cause thrombocytopenia. Some drugs (eg, anticancer chemotherapeutic agents, valproic acid[19]) cause dose-dependent thrombocytopenia, generally through myelosuppressive mechanisms. An important disorder encountered by hematologists is unexpected thrombocytopenia caused by immunologic (idiosyncratic) mechanisms. The frequency of these reactions varies considerably among drugs, and ranges from very rare (less than 1/10,000), for commonly used drugs such as acetaminophen, aspirin, quinine/quinidine, and trimethoprim-sulfamethoxazole,[20] to common (1%–5%), for other drugs such as gold[21] and unfractionated heparin.[1,22–25]

Immunologic drug-induced thrombocytopenia can occur by different mechanisms (Fig. 140–1).[26] For example, thrombocytopenia can result when the Fab terminus of the pathogenic IgG binds to a complex composed of drug (or drug metabolite) and a platelet mem-

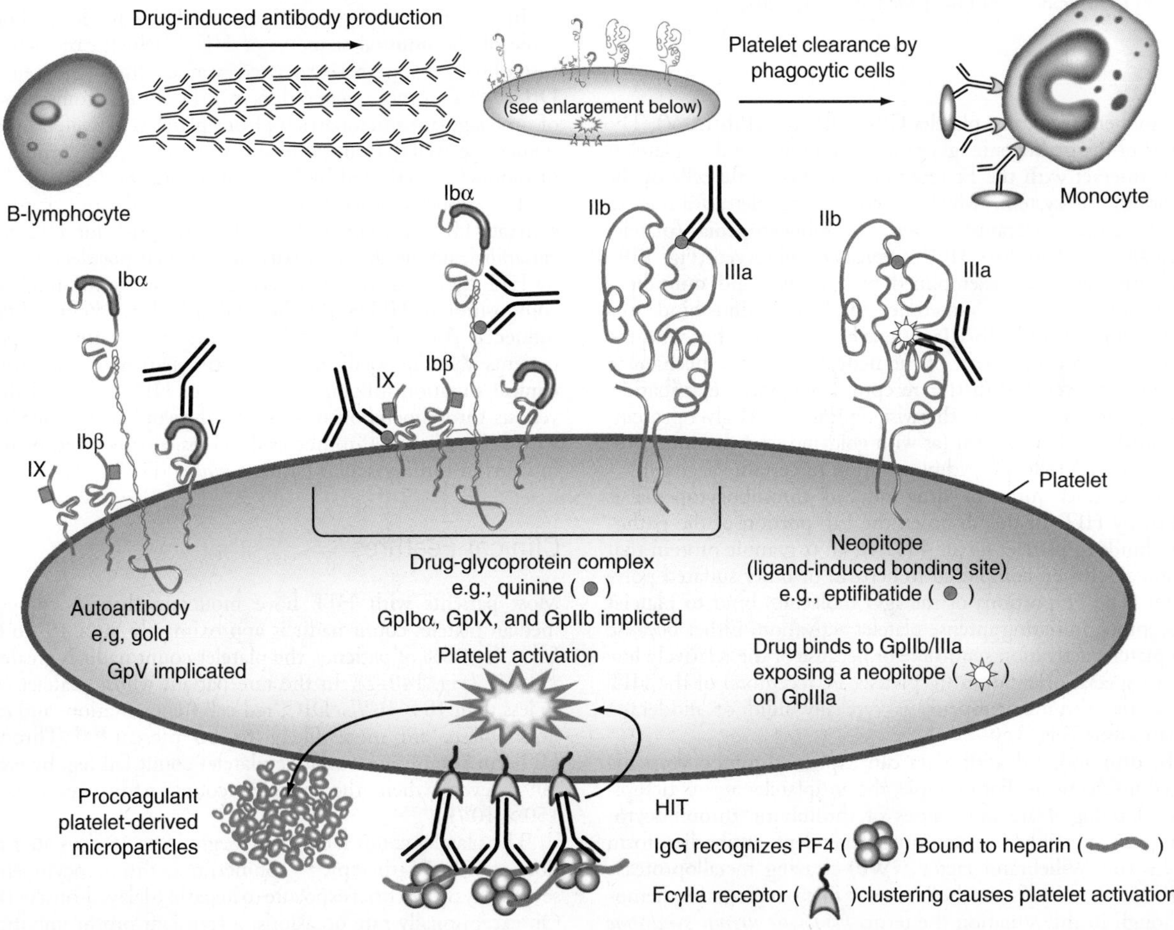

Figure 140–1 Mechanisms of drug-induced immune thrombocytopenia. Four immune thrombocytopenic syndromes are illustrated. On the bottom of the schematic platelet, heparin-induced thrombocytopenia (HIT) is illustrated, indicating that IgG antibodies bind to complexes of platelet factor 4 (PF4) and heparin, with the Fc regions of the antibodies binding to the platelet FcγIIa receptors, resulting in platelet activation (including generation of procoagulant, platelet-derived microparticles). On the top of the schematic platelet, three mechanisms are illustrated that lead to increased platelet clearance by phagocytic cells. From left to right, these are: autoantibody-induced immune thrombocytopenia (eg, gold-induced antiglycoprotein V [GPV] antibodies); drug-dependent antibodies reactive against drug (or drug metabolite)/platelet glycoprotein complex(es) (eg, quinine-induced thrombocytopenia, in which drug-dependent antibodies against GPIbα, GPIX, and GPIIb have been implicated, resulting in an antibody/drug/glycoprotein ternary complex); and antibodies against neoepitope(s) formed in the presence of a drug (eg, eptifibatide-induced immune thrombocytopenia caused by formation of ligand-induced binding site elsewhere on the GPIIb/IIIa complex following eptifibatide binding). Note that preexisting (naturally occurring) antibodies can explain abrupt-onset thrombocytopenia in a patient receiving eptifibatide for the first time.

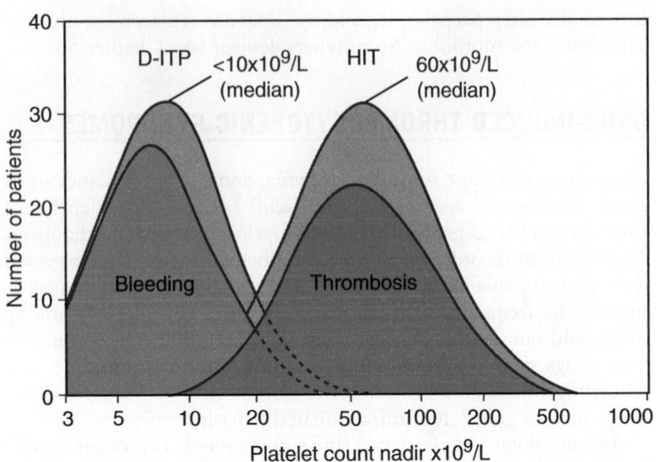

Figure 140–2 Severity of thrombocytopenia in drug-induced immune thrombocytopenia: a comparison of HIT versus other drug-induced immune thrombocytopenic disorders (D-ITP). Whereas D-ITP is strongly associated with petechiae and purpura, HIT is strongly associated with thrombosis. Note: the heights of the D-ITP and HIT curves are not drawn to scale, as HIT is more common than all D-ITP disorders combined. From: Warkentin TE: Drug-induced immune-mediated thrombocytopenia-from purpura to thrombosis. N Engl J Med 356:891, 2007.

brane component (typically, platelet GPIIb/IIIa or GPIb/IX/V). The Fc portions of the pathogenic IgG molecules do not bind to platelets but rather interact with the Fc receptors on phagocytic cells of the reticuloendothelial system, which ingest the platelets, leading to accelerated platelet clearance. Severe thrombocytopenia (platelet counts usually less than 20×10^9/L) typically is observed (Fig. 140–2).[26] This mechanism is exemplified by quinine- and quinidine-induced thrombocytopenia. Sometimes, the Fab terminus binds to a neoepitope on platelet GPIIb/IIIa induced by the drug, but with the drug itself not comprising part of the neoepitope. This mechanism is exemplified by the GPIIb/IIIa receptor antagonist, eptifibatide. Rarely, some drugs may cause otherwise typical platelet glycoprotein-reactive autoantibodies to form (as with gold-induced thrombocytopenia or acute ITP following administration of certain vaccines).

Another distinct form of drug-induced thrombocytopenia is exemplified by HIT. In this disorder, the Fab portion of the pathogenic IgG binds to platelet factor 4 (PF4), an α-granule protein that is immunogenic when complexed to heparin or other sulfated polysaccharides. The Fc portions of the IgG molecules bind to platelet FcγIIa receptors, initiating intense platelet activation. Either because HIT is a platelet activation syndrome or because of the relatively low numbers or special orientation (to platelet Fc receptors) of the HIT antibodies, the thrombocytopenia is typically mild or moderate, rather than severe (Fig. 140–2).

Finally, drug-induced antibodies can explain thrombocytopenia by unusual mechanisms. For example, the antiplatelet agents ticlopidine and clopidogrel are rare causes of thrombotic thrombocytopenic purpura, possibly because drug-dependent antibodies form against the von Willebrand factor (vWF)-cleaving metalloprotease ADAMTS13. Quinine is another cause of microangiopathic hemolysis, although in this situation the terms *hemolytic uremic syndrome* and *DIC* are often used, reflecting the prominent renal failure and/or coagulation abnormalities observed in some affected patients.

Heparin-Induced Thrombocytopenia

Heparin is the most important cause of immune-mediated drug-induced thrombocytopenia for several reasons. First, heparin is a widely used anticoagulant (see Chapter 137). Second, HIT is relatively common, occurring in approximately 1% to 5% of postoperative patients, and 0.5% to 1% of medical patients who receive unfractionated heparin derived from porcine intestine for 7 to 14 days.[1,22–25] The risk of HIT is somewhat higher in women (odds ratio, 1.5–2.0).[25] Finally, HIT paradoxically can cause life- or limb-threatening venous or arterial thrombosis.[22,27,28]

Pathogenesis

Heparin binds reversibly and saturably to platelets and can weakly activate platelets in vitro. In general, the direct platelet-activating effects of heparin, as well as its immunogenicity, are proportional to its size and degree of sulfation; consequently, low-molecular-weight heparin (LMWH) is less likely to cause HIT than is unfractionated heparin.[22–25]

HIT is caused by heparin-dependent IgG that activates platelets via their FcγIIa receptors.[29] The HIT antigens reside on large multimolecular complexes formed between (cationic) PF4—a member of the C-X-C subfamily of chemokines—and (anionic) heparin.[30–32] Although heparin-treated patients can form IgM and IgA heparin-dependent antibodies, these are unlikely to cause HIT.[33] A unique laboratory characteristic of HIT is that high heparin concentrations (10–100 U/mL) inhibit platelet activation by the pathogenic IgG[34]; this laboratory feature is exploited in diagnostic testing for HIT (see the later section "Diagnosis").

In vivo thrombin generation contributes to the pathogenesis of some of the unusual sequelae of HIT,[28] which can include venous thrombosis,[22] warfarin-associated venous limb gangrene,[35–37] and DIC.[38–40] Thrombin generation in HIT results from the generation of procoagulant microparticles from platelets activated by HIT antibodies,[41] as well as from expression of tissue factor by endothelial cells or monocytes activated by HIT antibodies (Fig. 140–3).[28,31,42]

Thrombocytopenia develops in only a minority of patients who generate HIT antibodies.[1,22–24,33] Differing risk for HIT may reflect variability among different patients for their platelets to be activated by HIT IgG,[43] as well as differing levels and immunoglobulin class composition of HIT antibodies.[33] Poorly defined clinical factors also influence risk of HIT, which occurs more often in postsurgery patients than in medical or obstetric patients.[25] Additionally, the clinical situation influences the type of HIT-associated thrombosis: venous thromboembolism typically develops in orthopedic patients with HIT, whereas thrombosis develops equally often in arteries and in veins in cardiovascular patients with HIT.[24]

Clinical Features

Most patients with HIT have moderate thrombocytopenia: The median platelet count nadir is approximately 50×10^9 to 60×10^9/L[24,44]; for 90% of patients, the platelet count nadir is greater than 20 $\times 10^9$/L (Fig. 140–2). In the rare patient whose platelet count falls to less than 10×10^9/L, DIC, red cell fragmentation, and circulating normoblasts are more likely to be present.[39,40] Thrombosis in HIT can complicate a relative platelet count fall (eg, by greater than 50%) even when the platelet count nadir never falls below 150×10^9/L).[1,23,38]

The platelet count fall usually begins 5 to 10 days after the initiation of heparin therapy.[22,45] Sometimes, thrombocytopenia begins several days *after* a brief exposure to heparin (delayed-onset HIT).[27,38–40] On exceptionally rare occasions, a transient prothrombotic disorder that resembles HIT clinically and serologically occurs without apparent preceding heparin exposure ("spontaneous HIT").[46] HIT is highly prothrombotic: In at least 50% of patients, a thrombosis develops in association with HIT.[1,22–26,45] Both venous (deep vein thrombosis, pulmonary embolism) and arterial (especially aortic and iliofemoral arterial thrombosis, cerebrovascular accidents, myocardial infarctions) thrombi occur. Other complications include painful dermal erythema or necrosis at the sites of subcutaneous heparin injection[47] and acute inflammatory[38] or transient memory disturbances[38] following heparin bolus injections to sensitized persons.

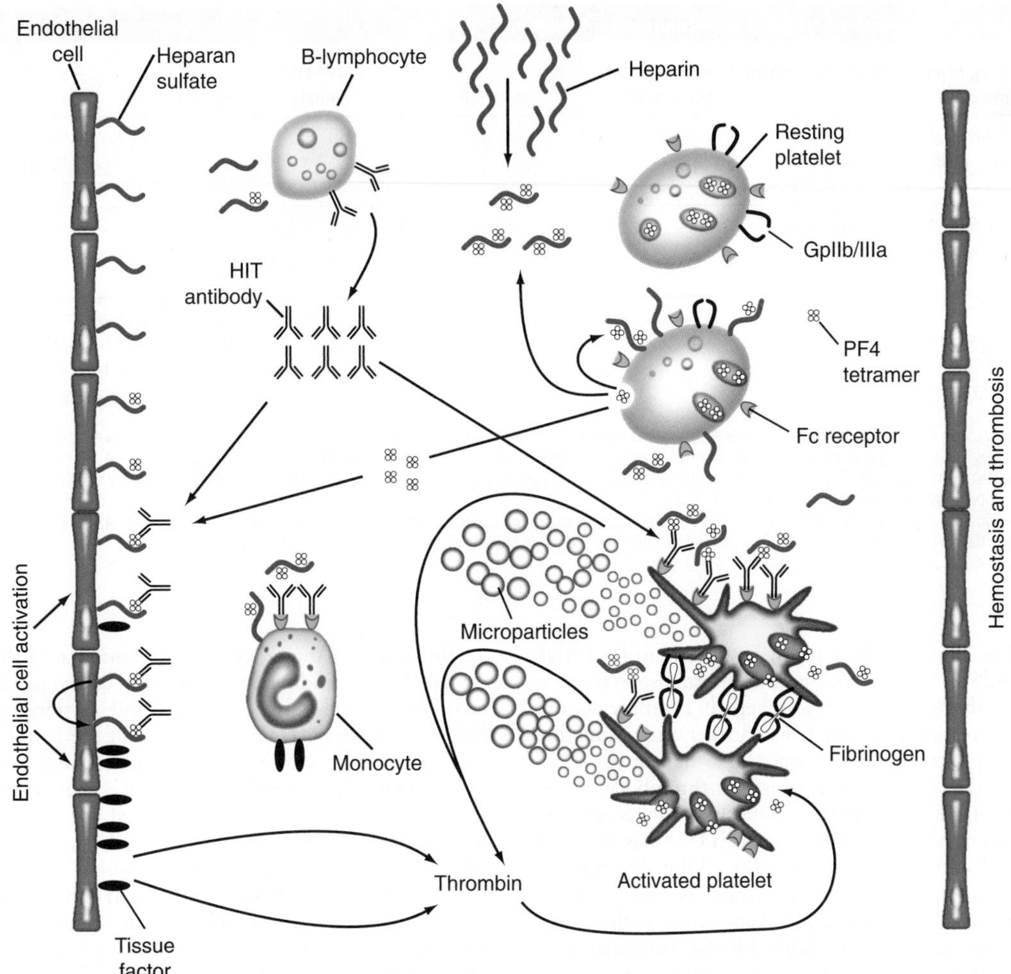

Figure 140–3 Pathogenesis of heparin-induced thrombocytopenia (HIT). Heparin produces mild platelet activation, resulting in release of platelet factor 4 (PF4) from platelet α-granules and the formation of immunogenic PF4-heparin complexes. B lymphocytes generate IgG immunoglobulins that recognize the PF4-heparin complexes; the Fc "tails" of the IgG bind to platelet FcγIIa receptors, resulting in Fc receptor clustering and consequent "strong" platelet activation. Platelet-derived microparticles are generated that accelerate thrombin generation. The HIT antibodies also recognize PF4 bound to endothelial heparan sulfate, leading to immunoinjury that causes endothelial activation. Recent evidence suggests that HIT antibodies also activate monocytes. The greatly increased thrombin generation observed in HIT helps to explain its association with venous and arterial thrombosis, as well as some of its unusual clinical features (eg, warfarin-induced venous limb gangrene, decompensated disseminated intravascular coagulation [DIC]), and also provides a rationale for treatments that control thrombin (eg, with direct thrombin inhibitors). (Reprinted with permission from Greinacher A, Warkentin TE: Treatment of heparin-induced thrombocytopenia: An overview. In Warkentin TE, Greinacher A [eds.]: Heparin-Induced Thrombocytopenia, 4th ed. New York, Informa Healthcare USA, 2007, p 287.)

Unexplained hypotension or abdominal pain in a patient with HIT suggests bilateral adrenal hemorrhagic infarction, which can lead to acute adrenal failure; this hemorrhagic necrosis results from adrenal vein thrombosis.[48]

Diagnosis

Assays for HIT antibodies can be classified as platelet "activation" and PF4-polyanion "antigen" assays.[49,50] Activation assays that utilize washed platelets (eg, platelet carbon 14 (^{14}C) labeled-serotonin release assay) are quite sensitive and specific for detecting clinically significant HIT antibodies.[1,22,23,33,44,50] Important quality control maneuvers include the selection of platelet donors whose platelets respond well to Fc receptor stimulation, as well as the inclusion of negative and positive HIT sera of variable reactivity to ascertain that the test platelets can identify weaker HIT sera.[43] A characteristic activation profile is produced by HIT serum: increased platelet activation at low heparin concentrations (0.05–0.3 U/mL), but background platelet activation at high heparin concentrations (10–100 U/mL).[43,50]

Two enzyme-linked immunosorbent assays (ELISAs) are commercially available for detecting antibodies that recognize PF4 bound either to heparin or to the polyanion, polyvinyl sulfonate.[49,50] These assays are very sensitive for detecting HIT antibodies but are more likely than washed platelet activation assays to detect clinically insignificant anti-PF4/heparin antibodies.[33] Thus, results of laboratory tests must be interpreted in the clinical context—that is, HIT is a clinicopathologic syndrome.[49,50] Activation and antigen assays are not 100% concordant, and there are advantages for reference laboratories to be able to perform both types of assay.[33] In general, serum or plasma from patients with clinical HIT have strongly positive assay results, whereas clinically insignificant antibodies give weaker results.[33,49,50]

Management

All heparin should be discontinued in patients strongly suspected to have HIT, including heparin "flushes" of intravascular catheters (with

Table 140–5 Treatment Schedules for Lepirudin, Bivalirudin, and Argatroban

Anticoagulant	Dosing Protocol for HIT-Associated Thrombosis*	Anticoagulant Monitoring†	Metabolism	Half-Life (minute)	Comment
Lepirudin	±Bolus: 0.4 mg/kg; initial infusion rate: 0.05–0.10 mg/kg/hour‡[52,56]	1.5–2.5 × baseline aPTT	Renal	80	Approved dosing regimen is too high; risk of anaphylaxis, especially on reexposure; minor prolongation of INR (compare to "Argatroban")
Bivalirudin	No bolus; initial infusion rate: 0.15–0.20 mg/kg/hour	1.5–2.5 × baseline aPTT	Enzymatic (80%); renal (20%)	25	Small but favorable experience for treating HIT; minor prolongation of INR (compare to "Argatroban")
Argatroban	No bolus: initial infusion rate: 2 μg/kg/minute	1.5–3.0 × baseline aPTT	Hepatobiliary	40–50	Initial dose 0.5 μg/kg/minute in hepatic insufficiency**; moderate or marked prolongation of INR, which complicates warfarin anticoagulation

*The initial lepirudin infusion rate range is substantially less than that indicated in the package insert (0.15 mg/kg/hour), as there is emerging evidence that the approved dosing regimen is too high. Some experts routinely avoid the bolus except for life- or limb-threatening thrombosis.
†Generally, the patient's baseline aPTT should be used for calculating target range, when appropriate; otherwise, the mean laboratory normal range can be used.
‡Major dose reduction in renal insufficiency is required.
**Reduced initial dosing (eg, 0.5–1.0 μg/kg/min) is also appropriate in patients in intensive care units, with cardiac failure, or postcardiac surgery.
aPTT, activated partial thromboplastin time; HIT, heparin-induced thrombocytopenia; INR, international normalized ratio.

substitution of saline flushes). Of note, there appears to be a high risk (approximately 25%–50%) for subsequent thrombosis in patients with serologically confirmed HIT in whom heparin is simply discontinued.[27,44,51] It is increasingly accepted that further anticoagulation is indicated in most patients strongly suspected as having "isolated" HIT[28,52]—that is, HIT recognized because of thrombocytopenia rather than because of HIT-associated thrombosis.[24] The recognition of thrombin generation in the pathogenesis of HIT[28,35] has provided a rationale for use of anticoagulant agents that inhibit thrombin or its generation. Currently, three such anticoagulants—recombinant hirudin (lepirudin), bivalirudin, and argatroban—are available in the United States for treatment of HIT (Table 140–5). (Danaparoid is an anticoagulant "heparinoid" with predominant antifactor Xa activity that is effective for treating HIT[52–54]; however, danaparoid was discontinued in the United States in April 2002, but it remains available in Canada, the European Union, Australia, New Zealand, and Japan.)

The recombinant hirudin derivative lepirudin (Refludan) is a 65-amino-acid polypeptide that inactivates thrombin by forming a tight, noncovalent 1 : 1 complex with it. Lepirudin is approved for the treatment of HIT-associated thrombosis in the European Union, the United States, and elsewhere.[55] Hirudin is renally excreted, and the drug must be avoided (or the dosage substantially reduced) in patients with renal failure. With normal renal function, the half-life is about 80 minutes. Anticoagulant monitoring is performed using the activated partial thromboplastin time (target aPTT, 1.5 to 2.5 times the baseline aPTT). In the treatment of HIT-associated thrombosis, lepirudin reduced a composite end point (encompassing new thrombosis, limb amputation, and all-cause mortality) from 47.8% (in historical controls) to 21.3%.[55] The end point of new thrombosis was reduced from 27.2% to 10.1%.[55] Major bleeding complications were seen in about 20% of patients (compared with 7.1% in controls), which has resulted in recommendations to administer initial doses lower than that recommended in the package insert, even in patients with normal renal function.[52,56] In patients with isolated HIT (an "off-label" indication), lepirudin given in "prophylactic" doses (0.1 mg/kg/hour given intravenously without an initial bolus, and adjusted to an aPTT of 1.5 to 2.0 times baseline) resulted in new thrombosis in 2.7% of patients and in 9.0% of patients with the combined end point.[57] Similarly low rates of thrombosis have also been observed in postmarketing studies of patients given lepirudin for isolated HIT. Recently, fatal anaphylactic reactions following administration of an intravenous bolus have been reported, with a frequency as high as 1/400 patients following reexposure.[58] The risk of anaphylaxis is another reason to avoid bolus dosing in most clinical situations.[52]

Bivalirudin (Angiomax) is a 20-amino-acid thrombin inhibitor modeled after hirudin that is composed of two peptide fragments that recognize the thrombin active site and its fibrinogen-binding sites, linked by a tetraglycine spacer. Its half-life is only about one-third that of lepirudin (25 vs 80 minutes), and only minor dose adjustments are needed in renal insufficiency because bivalirudin undergoes enzymatic metabolism. It is approved for anticoagulation during percutaneous coronary interventions (PCIs), including for patients in whom heparin is contraindicated because of HIT.[59] Its short half-life and predominant enzymatic (nonorgan) elimination are reasons why it is a major option for intraoperative anticoagulation for cardiac surgery, when heparin is contraindicated because of acute or recent HIT.[52,60] Experience using bivalirudin "off-label" to treat HIT outside the setting of PCI is limited.[59,60] Anaphylaxis has not been reported.

Argatroban (marketed without a trademark in the United States; Novastan, Argatra, and Arganova outside the United States) is a small-molecule (527-Da) direct thrombin inhibitor that undergoes predominant hepatobiliary excretion and is therefore suitable for use without dose adjustment in patients with renal failure (the dose is reduced by three-quarters in patients with hepatic insufficiency).[61–63] Argatroban is approved in the United States for both treatment and prevention of thrombosis in HIT. It is given in the same dosage for both indications (usual starting infusion rate of 2 μg/kg/minute without initial bolus). Argatroban (in substantially higher doses) is also approved for anticoagulation during PCI in patients with previous or acute HIT. Its half-life is 40 to 50 minutes. Argatroban prolongs the INR more than lepirudin and bivalirudin, and a higher-than-usual target INR during warfarin cotherapy (which depends on the thromboplastin reagent used to measure the INR) can be expected (see Caveats in next section).[63] Argatroban reduced the frequency of a composite end point (new thrombosis, limb amputation, and all-cause mortality) from 56.5% (in historical controls) to 43.8% and 41.5% in two studies of patients with HIT complicated by thrombosis; new thrombosis event rates were reduced from 34.8% to 19.4% and 13.1%, respectively.[61,62] In patients with isolated HIT, argatroban reduced the rate of new thrombosis from 15.0% to 6.9%, and the combined event rate of new thrombosis, limb amputation, and all-cause mortality from 38.8% to 25.6%.[61]

Caveats in Treatment of Heparin-Induced Thrombocytopenia

Warfarin and other vitamin K antagonists (coumarins) should not be used during the acute thrombocytopenic phase of HIT.[26,28,35–37,52] A particularly high-risk situation is HIT associated with deep vein thrombosis, especially if there is overt (decompensated) DIC. This is because deep vein thrombosis in a patient with HIT treated with warfarin can progress to venous limb gangrene.[35–37] The laboratory marker of this unusual syndrome is a high INR (generally, greater than 4.0), which corresponds to the combination of a marked reduction of protein C together with persisting thrombin generation (as shown by elevated thrombin–antithrombin complex levels) during warfarin therapy.[35] However, although warfarin (in theory) should be safe in a patient whose thrombin generation is controlled (eg, using a thrombin inhibitor), it is important nevertheless to delay warfarin until substantial resolution of thrombocytopenia has occurred (to more than 150 × 10^9/L).[52] This is because warfarin-induced prolongation of the aPTT can result in underdosing of the direct thrombin inhibitor,[37] and because stopping the direct thrombin inhibitor before resolution of the HIT during warfarin overlap can lead to limb loss due to fulminant venous limb gangrene.[36,37]

Using sensitive assays for HIT antibodies, LMWH reacts similarly to standard, unfractionated heparin in vitro. Furthermore, because LMWH can lead to worsening of clinical HIT, these agents should not be used to treat HIT.[52] Fondaparinux (Arixtra) is a novel anticoagulant with exclusive antifactor Xa activity based on its strong resemblance to the antithrombin-binding "pentasaccharide" sequence within heparin (see Chapter 137). Fondaparinux use has been associated with formation of anti-PF4/heparin antibodies at a frequency similar to that of LMWH; however, unlike the situation with LMWH, the antibodies do not interact with PF4/fondaparinux.[64] Fondaparinux may prove to be an effective anticoagulant in patients with acute HIT, although to date, experience in patients with serologically confirmed HIT is minimal, and important questions regarding appropriate dosing for HIT are unresolved.[28,52]

Although primary treatment for HIT should include an anticoagulant that inhibits thrombin or reduces thrombin generation, certain treatment adjuncts can be used in certain situations. These include surgical thromboembolectomy, high-dose intravenous immunoglobulin (VIG), antiplatelet drugs such as aspirin, and plasmapheresis.

These several caveats, along with recommendations for management of patients with suspected HIT, are summarized in the box on Diagnosis and Treatment of Heparin-Induced Thrombocytopenia.

Prevention

Platelet monitoring in patients receiving heparin should reflect the overall risk of HIT (ie, the preparation, the dose, and the clinical situation).[49,52] At least alternate-day platelet count monitoring should be considered in patients at relatively high risk for developing HIT (eg, postoperative orthopedic and cardiovascular patients receiving prophylactic-dose unfractionated heparin). Monitoring at least two or three times a week should be considered for patients at moderate risk for developing HIT (eg, medical patients receiving unfractionated heparin, postoperative patients receiving unfractionated heparin "flushes" or LMWH). The frequency of HIT is low with LMWH,[22–25] particularly in medical patients or during pregnancy, and routine platelet count monitoring may not be required in such settings.[49,52] In addition, HIT only rarely begins 14 or more days after initiation of a course of heparin, so routine monitoring beyond this period may not be required.

Anticoagulation and Previous Heparin-Induced Thrombocytopenia

HIT antibodies are transient and usually are undetectable several weeks or a few months after an episode of HIT.[45] Thus, if HIT antibodies are not detectable, it is appropriate to use heparin for a brief indication in those situations in which an alternative anticoagulant has drawbacks (eg, heart surgery).[45,52,65] Heparin should be avoided preoperatively (eg, argatroban[66] or bivalirudin[59] can be used for heart catheterization). Patients requiring urgent heart surgery during acute or recent HIT (with antibodies still detectable) have been successfully anticoagulated with alternate anticoagulant approaches (eg, bivalirudin, lepirudin[67] or heparin plus an antiplatelet agent such as epoprostenol[68] or tirofiban[65]), but each of these approaches has certain disadvantages. For example, lepirudin in high doses for cardiac surgery requires monitoring with the ecarin clotting time (not widely available), and patients can develop severe bleeding if renal failure occurs; epoprostenol causes hypotension, and there is limited experience in cardiac surgery using this approach. Bivalirudin shows the greatest promise for use in cardiac surgery, but special surgical and anesthesiologic maneuvers are required (as bivalirudin undergoes proteolysis, thus posing risk of thrombosis within stagnant blood).[52]

A diagnostic and therapeutic approach to HIT, beginning with the "4 T's,"[69] is shown in the accompanying box.

DRUG-INDUCED IMMUNE THROMBOCYTOPENIA

A large number of drugs can cause a syndrome that mimics acute ITP (Table 140–6).[20,21,26,70–103] Typically, severe thrombocytopenia (platelet count usually less than 20 × 10^9/L) (Fig. 140–2), together with petechiae and purpura, develops usually within weeks, but occasionally much longer after initiation of therapy with the responsible drug. Drug-induced immune thrombocytopenia is much less common than HIT. For example, a relatively "common" cause of this syndrome is trimethoprim-sulfamethoxazole (*co*-trimoxazole), even though it occurs in only approximately 1/25,000 patients who receive this drug combination.[20] Important exceptions to these generalizations occur with immune thrombocytopenia that results from GPIIb/IIIa receptor antagonists; these reactions are relatively common (affecting about 0.5%–1% of patients) and usually occur within hours of first use, as a result of preexisting, naturally occurring antibodies.[82–95] Another exception is carbimazole-induced thrombocytopenia, in which mild thrombocytopenia is explained by the presence of the platelet glycoprotein target (platelet endothelial cell adhesion molecule-1 [PECAM-1]) in relatively small quantities on the platelet surface.[99] Besides the atypical immune-mediated syndromes of HIT and GPIIb/IIIa antagonist thrombocytopenia, the most common drugs in absolute terms that are implicated as causing severe immune thrombocytopenia are quinine (outpatients) and vancomycin (inpatients).[79]

Pathogenesis

Drug-dependent binding of the Fab component of IgG to platelet glycoproteins leads to platelet destruction. This occurs because the IgG-sensitized platelets are recognized by the Fc receptors of phagocytic cells. For quinine- and quinidine-induced immune thrombocytopenia, both the GPIIb/IIIa and GPIb/IX/V complexes have been implicated as targets for the drug-dependent IgG (see Fig. 140–1). By contrast, for sulfa antibiotic- and naproxen-induced immune thrombocytopenia, the GPIIb/IIIa complex is predominantly involved.[76,104] Sometimes, drug metabolites rather than the parent drug form the antigen.[80] A trimolecular complex is formed among IgG Fab, the drug (or metabolite), and the platelet glycoprotein. In contrast with HIT, platelet Fc receptors are not involved. Drug-dependent IgG binding is remarkably heterogeneous with respect to binding affinity, number of binding sites per platelet, and the range of drug concentrations required. A recent study of quinine-induced immune thrombocytopenia identified two different types of antibodies: quinine-dependent antibodies that bind to platelets in the presence of drug, and quinine-specific antibodies that reacted with quinine-conjugated albumin. The pathophysiologic implications of this latter group of antibodies remains unclear.

Diagnosis and Treatment of Heparin-induced Thrombocytopenia

Heparin-induced thrombocytopenia (HIT) should be clinically suspected when thrombocytopenia occurs during (or soon after) heparin therapy that has a temporal profile consistent with immune sensitization to heparin. Four relevant questions-the "4 T's"-should be asked[69]:

Thrombocytopenia: Does the patient have thrombocytopenia? A greater than 50% fall in the platelet count can indicate HIT even if the platelet count has not fallen to below 150×10^9/L). (*Note*: Very severe thrombocytopenia, such as with platelet count below 10×10^9/L, is only very rarely caused by HIT.[26])

Timing: Is the timing of the platelet count fall consistent with immune sensitization? In HIT, platelets usually fall 5 to 10 days after starting a course of heparin (first day of heparin is day zero); a more rapid fall in the platelet count can occur if the patient is already sensitized from an exposure to heparin within the past 100 days.

Thrombosis: Has thrombosis or other sequelae of HIT occurred? (*Note*: Besides venous and arterial thrombosis, patients with HIT can develop skin lesions at heparin injection sites, or systemic inflammatory or cardiorespiratory reactions that begin 5 to 30 minutes after an intravenous heparin bolus).

Other: Are other explanations for thrombocytopenia present? HIT is relatively less likely when compelling clinical evidence exists for another cause for the thrombocytopenia, such as positive blood cultures.

Steps in Management of Clinically Suspected Heparin-Induced Thrombocytopenia

1. Confirm that thrombocytopenia is present (repeat CBC), test for DIC, and test for HIT antibodies.
2. Assess clinically and radiologically for thrombosis (eg, duplex ultrasound for lower-limb deep vein thrombosis).
3. Stop all heparin (including heparin "flushes" and, possibly, use of heparin-coated intravascular catheters [catheters in situ for several days may not have significant residual heparin).
4. Initiate alternative anticoagulation, generally in therapeutic doses (options: lepirudin, argatroban, bivalirudin,* danaparoid,*† fondaparinux [?]‡), if HIT is strongly suspected.
5. Although initial treatment decisions are made on clinical grounds, results of testing for HIT antibodies can influence subsequent treatment, including the decision to resume heparin if HIT has been ruled out using one or more sensitive assays for HIT antibodies.

Caveats

- Do not give low-molecular-weight heparin to treat HIT.
- Do not give warfarin or other coumarin anticoagulants until the platelet count has substantially recovered (to greater than 150×10^9/L), and administer only in low initial doses (warfarin, 5 mg or less) and with a minimum 5-day overlap with a parenteral anticoagulant.
- Do give vitamin K (e.g. 5–10 mg IV over 30–60 min) if HIT is diagnosed after warfarin has already been given, so as to reduce risk of coumarin necrosis and to avoid underdosing of direct thrombin inhibitor because of aPTT prolongation by warfarin.
- Do not give prophylactic platelet transfusions (unless the patient is bleeding).

*Not approved for treatment of HIT in the United States (except, in the case of bivalirudin, for anticoagulation during PCI).

†Withdrawn from US market, but is available in numerous other countries.

‡Theoretically, fondaparinux should be effective for HIT, but only anecdotal use has been reported, and appropriate dosing for acute HIT is unresolved.

Clinical Features

Patients with drug-induced immune thrombocytopenia typically present with petechiae, purpura, and severe thrombocytopenia (platelet count often less than 20×10^9/L). Sometimes systemic symptoms such as fever and chills occur in patients with abrupt-onset thrombocytopenia. Usually, the thrombocytopenia becomes clinically apparent 1 to 2 weeks after initiation of the drug,[79] but the thrombocytopenia can begin even after a patient has been taking a drug for several years. Usually the platelet count begins to rise within a few days of discontinuing the implicated drug, but occasionally several weeks are required for recovery, possibly because of generation of drug-independent IgG (platelet autoantibodies).[105]

Rarely, distinct drug-dependent IgG molecules destroy red and/or white cells in addition to platelets. For example, both platelet- and leukocyte-reactive quinidine-dependent IgG molecules have been detected in a patient with quinidine-induced bicytopenia.[106] Sometimes, the immune process is directed against a pluripotent hematopoietic stem cell, resulting in pancytopenia accompanied by marrow aplasia or hypoplasia (eg, gold-, carbamazepine-, or quinidine-induced pancytopenia). A bone marrow biopsy should be performed in patients with suspected drug-induced bicytopenia or pancytopenia, because a hypoplastic marrow can indicate the serious complication of drug-induced aplastic anemia.

Diagnosis

A high index of clinical suspicion often is required to make the diagnosis. Quinine is widely available—as an ingredient in tonic water, for example, or as an additive to street drugs. Demonstration of drug-dependent binding of IgG to platelets in vitro is important in diagnosis. Labeled immunoglobulin-specific probes (eg, phase II assays) or glycoprotein capture techniques (phase III assays) can be used (see Table 140–6).

There are certain caveats in diagnostic testing. First, metabolites rather than parent drug must sometimes be used to detect the IgG.[80] Second, wash buffer in these assays may require the inclusion of the target drug (or metabolite). Third, even despite these maneuvers, the sensitivity of in vitro assays is relatively low, and the diagnosis of drug-induced immune thrombocytopenia often must be made on clinical grounds alone. Sometimes, the diagnosis is confirmed by inadvertent or deliberate reexposure to the suspected drug. However, deliberate drug rechallenge often is not performed because of its risk.

Management

As many drugs as possible should be discontinued in patients with suspected drug-induced immune thrombocytopenia. If further drug treatment is necessary, an alternate, immunologically non–cross-reactive substitute should be used. Spontaneous improvement in the platelet count usually begins within a few days of discontinuing the offending drug, although in some cases, complete recovery may take 2 weeks or longer. Platelet transfusions should be given to patients with life-threatening bleeding. High-dose IVIG, 1 g/kg given over 6 to 8 hours for 2 consecutive days, could be helpful in some situations. Corticosteroids appear to be relatively ineffective for treatment of drug-induced immune thrombocytopenia.[107]

GOLD-INDUCED THROMBOCYTOPENIA

Gold-induced immune thrombocytopenia occurs in as many as 1% to 3% of treated patients.[21] A genetic predisposition is suggested by the association with HLA-DR3, which is found in approximately 85% of affected patients.[21] The thrombocytopenia typically occurs during the first 20 weeks of therapy, before 1000 mg of gold has been given. Rarely, the thrombocytopenia begins much later, sometimes

Table 140–6 Drug-Induced Immune Thrombocytopenia

Drug	Platelet Count <20 × 10^9/L	Drug Rechallenge	Drug-Dependent In Vitro Testing*
Quinine/Quinidine Group			
Quinine[20,73,74]	Y	Y	Y[I,II,III]
Quinidine[20]	Y	Y	Y[I,II,III]
Gold Salts[21,75]			
Gold sodium thiomalate	Y	Y	Y[II,III]
Auronofin (oral gold)	Y	Y	Y[II]
Aurothioglucose	Y		
Antimicrobials			
Antimony-containing			
Stibophen	Y	Y	Y[I]
Sodium stibogluconate		Y	
Cephalosporins			
Cefamandole	Y		Y[II]
Cefotetan	Y		Y[II]
Ceftazidime[76]	Y		Y[III]
Ceftizoxime[76]			Y[III]
Ceftriaxone[77]			
Cephalothin	Y	Y	Y[I]
Ciprofloxacin			
Clarithromycin	Y	Y	
Fluconazole	Y		
Fusidic acid	Y	Y	Y[II,III]
Gentamicin	Y	Y	Y[I]
Nalidixic acid	Y	Y	
Penicillins			
Amoxicillin[76]			Y[III]
Ampicillin	Y		Y[II]
Apalcillin	Y		
Methicillin	Y	Y	Y[I]
Mezlocillin	Y		Y[I]
Penicillin	Y		Y[II]
Piperacillin	Y	Y	
Pentamidine	Y		Y[II,III]
Rifampin[76]	Y	Y	Y[I,II,III]
Sulfa antibiotics			
Sulfamethoxazole[20]	Y		Y[I,II,III]
Sulfamethoxypyridazine	Y		
Sulfisoxazole	Y		Y[I,II,III]
Suramin	Y		Y[I]
Teicloplanin[78]	Y		Y[II,III]
Vancomycin[79]	Y	Y	Y[II,III]
Antiinflammatory Drugs			
Acetaminophen[76,80]	Y	Y	Y[I,III]
Salicylates[20]			
Acetylsalicylic acid	Y	Y	Y[I]
Diflunisal	Y		Y[I]
Mesalamine[81]	Y	Y	
Sodium *para*-aminosalicylic acid	Y	Y	Y[I]
Sulfasalazine	Y	Y	
Other nonsteroidal antiinflammatory drugs			
Diclofenac	Y	Y	Y[I]
Fenoprofen	Y		
Ibuprofen[76]	Y		Y[II,III]
Indomethacin	Y		
Meclofenamate	Y	Y	
Mefenamic acid	Y		Y[I,II]
Naproxen[76,80]	Y		Y[III]
Oxaprozin[76]			Y[III]
Oxyphenbutazone	Y		
Phenylbutazone			Y[II]
Piroxicam	Y		
Sulindac			Y[I]
Tolmetin	Y	Y	

Table 140–6 Drug-Induced Immune Thrombocytopenia—cont'd

Drug	Platelet Count <20 × 10⁹/L	Drug Rechallenge	Drug-Dependent In Vitro Testing*
Cardiac and Antihypertensive Drugs			
Positive inotropic drugs			
Digitoxin		Y	Y[I]
Digoxin		Y	Y[I]
Antiarrhythmic drugs			
Amiodarone	Y	Y	
Procainamide	Y	Y	Y[I]
Quinidine (see above)			
β-Blockers			
Alprenolol	Y	Y	
Oxprenolol	Y	Y	
Other antihypertensive drugs			
Captopril	Y		
Diazoxide		Y	
α-Methyldopa	Y	Y	Y[I]
Diuretics			
Acetazolamide	Y		Y[I]
Chlorothiazide	Y	Y	Y[I]
Chlorthalidone			Y[I]
Furosemide	Y	Y	Y[I]
Hydrochlorothiazide	Y	Y	Y[I]
Spironolactone	Y		Y[I]
Antiplatelet Agents			
GPIIb/IIIa receptor antagonists			
Intravenous agents			
Abciximab[82–88]	Y		Y[II,III]
Eptifibatide[89–91]	Y		Y[II,III]
Tirofiban[90,92]	Y		Y[II,III]
Oral agents (investigational)			
Orbofiban[93]	Y		Y[II,III]
Roxifiban[94,95]	Y		Y[III]
Xemilofiban[93]	Y		Y[II,III]
ADP Receptor Blockers			
Ticlopidine			Y[II]
Benzodiazepines			
Diazepam	Y	Y	Y[I,II]
Antiepileptic Drugs			
Carbamazepine[76]	Y	Y	Y[I,II,III]
Phenytoin	Y		Y[I]
Valproic acid	Y	Y	
Histamine H_2 Receptor Antagonists			
Cimetidine	Y	Y	Y[II]
Ranitidine			Y[I,II]
Sulfonylurea Drugs[20]			
Chlorpropamide	Y		
Glibenclamide (glyburide)	Y		
Iodinated Contrast Agents			
Diatrizoate	Y	Y	
Iocetamic acid	Y		
Iopanoic acid	Y	Y	Y[I]
Sodium ipodate	Y	Y	Y[I]
Retinoids			
Isotretinoin	Y	Y	
Etretinate			
Antihistamines			
Antazoline	Y	Y	Y[I]
Chlorpheniramine	Y	Y	Y[I]

Table 140–6 Drug-Induced Immune Thrombocytopenia—cont'd

Drug	Platelet Count <20 × 10⁹/L	Drug Rechallenge	Drug-Dependent In Vitro Testing*
Illicit Drugs			
Cocaine	Y	Y	
Heroin	Y	Y	
Quinine contaminant ("filler")	Y		Y[I,II]
Antidepressants			
Tricyclic antidepressants			
Amitriptyline	Y	Y	
Desipramine			Y[I]
Doxepin	Y		
Imipramine			Y[I]
Tetracyclic antidepressants			
Mianserin	Y	Y	Y[I]
Mirtazapine[96]	Y		Y[II,III]
Antineoplastic Drugs			
Actinomycin D	Y	Y	
Aminoglutethimide	Y	Y	
Oxaliplatin[97]			
Tamoxifen		Y	Y[I]
Miscellaneous Drugs and Foods			
Atorvastatin[98]	Y	Y	
Carbimazole[99]			[YII,III]
Danazol	Y	Y	
Deferoxamine		Y	
Efalizumab[100]	Y		
Jui (Chinese herbal medicine)[101]	Y		
Levamisole		Y	
Levodopa[102]	Y		
Lidocaine	Y	Y	Y[I]
Morphine	Y		Y[I]
Papaverine	Y	Y	Y[II]
Tahini (pulped sesame seeds)[103]	Y	Y	

ADP, adenosine diphosphate.

even several months after discontinuation of the gold. Although the onset of thrombocytopenia typically is abrupt, regular platelet count monitoring is important, because an early diagnosis can be made in some patients. The thrombocytopenia often persists for several months despite discontinuation of the gold, probably because of gold-induced autoimmune thrombocytopenia (drug-independent autoantibodies against GPV have been implicated) (see Fig. 140–1).[75] Although most patients will eventually respond to corticosteroids, immediate albeit generally transient correction of severe thrombocytopenia usually can be achieved with high-dose IVIG. Some patients with persisting thrombocytopenia benefit from splenectomy or use of gold-chelating agents (dimercaprol, *N*-acetylcysteine).

DRUG-INDUCED AUTOIMMUNE THROMBOCYTOPENIA

Certain drugs besides gold have been reported to initiate autoimmune thrombocytopenia (eg, levodopa,[102] procainamide[108]). Because the pathogenic antibodies are by definition drug independent, however, it is difficult to establish causation. The mumps–measles–rubella vaccine can cause a severe but generally self-limited thrombocytopenia that is clinically and serologically indistinguishable from childhood acute ITP.[109]

DRUG-INDUCED IMMUNE THROMBOCYTOPENIA OF RAPID ONSET

Rapid onset of thrombocytopenia (within hours) can occur if a patient with preexisting drug-dependent antibodies is (re)exposed to the drug. This situation is relatively common in HIT (about 25% of patients identified),[45] because repeated treatment with heparin is common, and heparin use itself can result in the complication (HIT-associated thrombosis) that might lead to further use of heparin. However, because HIT antibodies are transient, rapid-onset HIT occurs in patients with recent heparin exposures, usually within the past 100 days.[45] By contrast, repeated episodes of quinine-induced thrombocytopenia of abrupt onset can be many months or even years apart, because these antibodies persist for much longer in the circulation. Thrombocytopenia of rapid onset is commonly seen with GPIIb/IIIa receptor antagonists (see next section).

THROMBOCYTOPENIA DUE TO GPIIB/IIIA RECEPTOR ANTAGONISTS

Several thrombocytopenic syndromes have been reported with use of GPIIb/IIIa receptor antagonists (abciximab, eptifibatide, tirofiban) administered briefly by the intravenous route during PCIs such as angioplasty or stenting: (a) rapid-onset thrombocytopenia, within a few hours of drug administration (in 0.4%–2% of patients)[82,83,89,94]; (b) rapid-onset pseudothrombocytopenia (in approximately 1%–2%)[84]; and (c) delayed-onset thrombocytopenia, beginning 5 to 7 days after drug administration (rare).[85,86] In patients who have received continuous dosing with an oral GPIIb/IIIa antagonist (one of the investigational agents roxifiban, orbofiban, and xemilofiban), thrombocytopenia has developed beginning either within hours or a few days of initial dosing, or during the second or third week of therapy.[93–95] The frequency of rapid-onset thrombocytopenia is higher among patients who receive a second course, especially if it follows the initial exposure by only a few weeks.[87] Thrombocytopenia typically is severe (median platelet count nadir, about 5×10^9/L to 10×10^9/L), but clinical effects vary dramatically, ranging from absence of petechiae or other signs of bleeding (in 50% of patients) to fatal hemorrhage (in less than 5%).[90,93] Some patients develop anaphylactoid reactions accompanying the abrupt platelet count declines.[82] Some investigators have proposed that the antibodies may cause thrombosis in some patients.[91,92]

These syndromes are caused by at least two mechanisms. First, antibodies of IgG (and possibly IgM[87]) class can bind to neoepitopes on the GPIIb/IIIa complex generated by these drugs (or their metabolites)—that is, ligand-induced binding sites (see Fig. 140–1).[90,93,95] Up to 5% of humans and nonhuman primates have naturally occurring IgG antibodies that will bind to GPIIb/IIIa receptors in the presence of drug,[93,110] which could explain why rapid-onset thrombocytopenia occurs so often with these agents. A second mechanism is applicable to abciximab (ReoPro), a chimeric Fab fragment comprised of murine GPIIb/IIIa-reactive sequences and human framework sequences). Interestingly, although a high frequency of normal persons (74%) have antibodies that recognize platelets coated with abciximab, these "normal" antibodies were shown to differ from those detected in patients in whom thrombocytopenia developed after a second exposure to abciximab[87]: whereas the pathogenic antibodies recognized murine sequences within abciximab, the "normal" (nonpathogenic) antibodies were specific for the carboxyl terminus (C terminus) (papain cleavage site) of Fab fragments prepared from normal human IgG.[87] Drug-dependent antibodies also can be generated beginning about a week following a brief intravenous exposure. The antibodies differ among patients with respect to the precise neoepitopes recognized and display variable degrees of cross-reactivity among the different GPIIb/IIIa receptor antagonists ("fibans")[90]; this explains why a repeat treatment course with another GPIIb/IIIa receptor antagonist may not necessarily produce a repeat thrombocytopenic episode.[88]

Some naturally occurring antibodies bind to GPIIb/IIIa only in the presence of low calcium concentrations, thus explaining pseudothrombocytopenia—falsely low platelet count estimates due to ex vivo aggregation of platelets collected into anticoagulants, especially EDTA.[84] The rare syndrome of delayed-onset thrombocytopenia following brief intravenous exposure might result from high-titer GPIIb/IIIa-reactive antibodies that bind even in the absence of the drug.

Platelet transfusions are indicated in bleeding patients, although their efficacy has not been established. Platelet transfusions are most likely to be effective in the treatment of abciximab-induced thrombocytopenia, because its highly avid binding to GPIIb/IIIa means that little free plasma abciximab can bind to the transfused platelets (cf. the reversible GPIIb/IIIa receptor antagonists eptifibatide and tirofiban). Platelet transfusions are not indicated in pseudothrombocytopenia, which underscores the importance of reviewing the blood film when apparent thrombocytopenia is recognized after treatment with one of these agents.

Various in vitro assays utilizing flow cytometry[87,90,110] or ELISA[87,90,95] have been developed recently to detect these antibodies. Because some pathogenic antibodies are naturally occurring, it is theoretically possible to identify patients at high risk for rapid-onset thrombocytopenia in elective situations (see box on Approach to Patients With Thrombocytopenia Following Percutaneous Coronary Interventions).

Approach to Patients with Thrombocytopenia Following Percutaneous Coronary Interventions

Four diagnoses should be considered in patients who develop thrombocytopenia within minutes or a few hours following percutaneous coronary interventions (PCIs) utilizing one or more of the following pharmacologic agents: (a) heparin, (b) platelet glycoprotein GPIIb/IIIa inhibitor (eg, abciximab, eptifibatide, tirofiban), or (c) iodinated contrast agent.

- **GPIIb/IIIa inhibitor-induced pseudothrombocytopenia.** The patient has no symptoms or signs of bleeding, and platelet aggregates are seen in the blood film. The platelet count is falsely reported as low by the automated particle counter, which fails to count aggregated platelets. No treatment is required.
- **GPIIb/IIIa inhibitor-induced thrombocytopenia.** The platelet count falls abruptly, often to profoundly reduced levels (typical nadir, 5 to 20×10^9/L). Hemostatic impairment is variable, ranging from no petechiae to fatal hemorrhages; occasionally, patients develop anaphylactoid reactions. Treatment involves stopping all platelet antagonists and anticoagulants and giving platelets if the patient has signs of bleeding. Prophylactic platelet transfusions also can be considered if the platelet count is very low (less than 10×10^9/L). Testing for drug-dependent antibodies can be accomplished using flow cytometry or enzyme-linked immunosorbent assay (ELISA).
- **Rapid-onset heparin-induced thrombocytopenia.** In patients who have preexisting HIT antibodies because of recent heparin exposure (generally, within the past 100 days), rapid-onset HIT can occur when heparin is given during PCI. This is much less common than GPIIb/IIIa inhibitor-induced thrombocytopenia or pseudothrombocytopenia, so presumptive treatment of HIT with a nonheparin anticoagulant is rarely indicated in this situation.
- **Radiocontrast-induced immune thrombocytopenic purpura.** Very rarely, patients who have previously received iodinated contrast can develop abrupt-onset, severe thrombocytopenia following exposure to contrast during PCI. Platelet transfusions (with or without high-dose intravenous immunoglobulin [IVIG]) are appropriate for a bleeding patient.

MISCELLANEOUS DRUG-INDUCED THROMBOCYTOPENIC SYNDROMES

Drug-Induced Thrombotic Microangiopathy

Several drugs can trigger a syndrome of thrombocytopenia, fragmentation hemolysis, and renal failure known as drug-induced hemolytic uremic syndrome (see Chapter 139). This syndrome has been established for quinine, in which multiple quinine-dependent antibodies reactive against platelets, red cells, leukocytes, and endothelial cells have been reported.[111] Treatment is with plasmapheresis, as for more typical thrombotic thrombocytopenic purpura (TTP). Typically, affected patients recover, although some require short-term hemodialysis. Although a similar syndrome may be caused by mitomycin, cyclosporine, and penicillamine, it should be noted that many patients who receive these drugs have underlying illness (gastric adenocarcinoma, bone marrow transplantation,[112] and collagen vascular disease, respectively) that are themselves associated with hemolytic uremic syndrome These patients generally are much less responsive to plasma exchange than others with idiopathic TTP. TTP rarely can be caused by drugs[113] such as ticlopidine,[114] clopidogrel,[115] and simvastatin. Autoantibodies against vWF-cleaving metalloproteinase have been identified in ticlopidine-induced TTP.[114]

Drug-Induced Disseminated Intravascular Coagulation

On rare occasions, quinine causes severe thrombocytopenia accompanied by marked coagulation abnormalities indicative of DIC.[116,117] This syndrome overlaps that of quinine-induced thrombotic microangiopathy, and the explanation for why some patients have more prominent coagulopathy is unknown. Although all patients with HIT have biochemical evidence of increased thrombin generation, only about 10% to 20% evince overt DIC.

Nonidiosyncratic Drug-Induced Thrombocytopenia

Most antineoplastic drugs produce a dose-dependent pancytopenia caused by injury to hematopoietic cells, including megakaryocytes and their progenitor cells. Typically, the platelet count nadir occurs at a predictable period following treatment and then quickly recovers. Unexpectedly severe or prolonged thrombocytopenia in patients receiving chemotherapy should suggest alternate explanations for the thrombocytopenia (eg, idiosyncratic thrombocytopenia caused by another drug).

Mild to moderate thrombocytopenia develops in approximately 20% of patients who take valproic acid (an antiepileptic agent); bleeding symptoms are uncommon.[19] The mechanism of thrombocytopenia in this setting is unknown, but the condition appears to be nonidiosyncratic, because the risk of thrombocytopenia correlates strongly with serum concentrations of valproic acid metabolite.[19] Amrinone is another agent that can cause generally mild, dose-dependent thrombocytopenia.[118]

Rapid Nonimmune Drug-Induced Thrombocytopenia

Some drugs produce rapid but generally mild and transient drops in the platelet count. These drugs include heparin,[28] protamine, bleomycin, hematin, ristocetin (no longer clinically used), desmopressin (particularly in patients with type 2B von Willebrand disease), and porcine factor VIII. The mechanism(s) for thrombocytopenia in these syndromes are obscure. Sometimes, however, acute thrombocytopenia is IgG-mediated: for example, we have observed that some rapid-onset thrombocytopenic reactions to heparin—particularly when accompanied by systemic inflammatory symptoms and signs—are attributable to IgG-mediated HIT in patients who were recently sensitized to heparin.[38,45]

Drug Hypersensitivity Reactions

Mild to moderate thrombocytopenia is sometimes observed in patients with systemic drug hypersensitivity reactions.[119,120] Comorbid clinical features can include generalized rashes, fever, cholestasis, and leukopenia. Allopurinol, isoniazid, sulfasalazine, and phenothiazine drugs, among others, have been implicated in these reactions.

Thrombocytopenia Secondary to Biologic Response Modifiers

Use of purified or recombinant biologic response modifiers such as interferon,[121,122] interleukin-2,[123] and certain colony-stimulating factors has resulted in severe, reversible thrombocytopenia in some patients. Antilymphocyte globulins also can produce severe thrombocytopenia.[124]

OTHER CAUSES OF DESTRUCTIVE THROMBOCYTOPENIA

Incidental Thrombocytopenia of Pregnancy

Maternal thrombocytopenia occurs in 4% to 8% of pregnancies.[125–128] Most affected women are healthy and have no history of thrombocytopenia, and their thrombocytopenia is incidentally detected by routine blood testing. The cause of the mild reduction in platelet count (usually 75×10^9/L to 150×10^9/L) is unknown. This condition is benign, without an increased risk for maternal bleeding or neonatal thrombocytopenia. Accordingly, no special maneuvers are indicated in these women, and the route of delivery should be determined by obstetric indications (see Chapter 138).

Preeclampsia/Eclampsia

Preeclampsia is characterized by the onset of hypertension and proteinuria during pregnancy, especially in a primigravida near term. Preeclampsia complicates approximately 5% of pregnancies, and the frequency is higher in black women. Thrombocytopenia occurs in about 20% of preeclamptic patients, and in almost half of patients with eclampsia.[126,128] In addition, some patients have evidence for a platelet function defect.[129] A subset of patients with preeclampsia have microangiopathic *h*emolysis, *e*levated *l*iver enzymes, and *l*ow *p*latelets, widely known as the HELLP syndrome.[130] This condition usually indicates severe preeclampsia and may be associated with a higher risk of maternal and fetal complications.[130,131] Repeated clinical and laboratory assessment of these patients is important, because this syndrome can mimic other life-threatening complications of pregnancy, such as overt DIC, TTP, septicemia, and acute fatty liver of pregnancy.

Increased platelet destruction is the mechanism for the thrombocytopenia in preeclampsia. However, activation of the coagulation system is relatively modest,[132] suggesting that thrombin generation may not be a major factor to explain the thrombocytopenia. Endothelial dysfunction (impaired nitric oxide synthesis) is another potential explanation for increased platelet turnover in preeclampsia.[133]

Pharmacologic control of hypertension and rapid delivery are the treatments for preeclampsia and will usually result in resolution of the thrombocytopenia within a few days. Because of the associated platelet function defects, some physicians recommend demonstrating a normal bleeding time in moderately thrombocytopenic patients before epidural anesthesia is performed in this group of patients. Some physicians, however, consider epidural anesthesia to be relatively safe, even in patients with moderate thrombocytopenia.[134] In those patients in whom delivery is not an option (ie, premature fetus), treatment with bed rest and aggressive antihypertensive therapy has been reported to result in an improved platelet count. However, the clinical course is markedly variable, and some patients develop life-threatening organ failure. Plasmapheresis has been used in some patients, especially if there is evidence of thrombotic microangiopathy and organ dysfunction.[135] Plasma exchange would seem appropriate in such a patient whose clinical picture has features that overlap with those of TTP.

Infection

Infection is a common cause of thrombocytopenia, occurring in approximately 50% to 75% of patients with bacteremia or fungemia, and in almost all patients with septic shock or DIC.[136] Even when caused by bacteremia, the thrombocytopenia generally is mild to moderate in severity and usually is not accompanied by significant coagulation abnormalities or bleeding. The likelihood of laboratory evidence for DIC increases as the platelet count falls to less than 50 $\times 10^9$/L, however. The mechanisms for thrombocytopenia in septicemia in the absence of DIC are uncertain but could include chemokine-induced macrophage ingestion of platelets (hemophagocytosis[137]) and direct activation of platelets by endogenous mediators of inflam-

Table 140–7 Mechanisms for Thrombocytopenia Complicating Infections

Mechanism for Thrombocytopenia	Selected Example(s)*
Increased Platelet Destruction	
Disseminated intravascular coagulation	Meningococcemia
Hemophagocytosis	Septicemia, Epstein–Barr virus infection
Platelet-reactive autoantibodies (acute)	Varicella, subacute bacterial endocarditis (rare)
Platelet-reactive autoantibodies (chronic)	HIV infection
Hemolytic uremic syndrome	Verocytotoxin-producing *Escherichia coli*, *Shigella*, HIV infection
Antibodies against platelet-adsorbed microbial antigens	Malaria
Hypersplenism	
Acute	Disseminated *Mycobacterium avium* infection in HIV infection
Chronic	Viral chronic active hepatitis, malaria
Decreased Platelet Production	
Replacement of marrow by granulomas	Ehrlichiosis, tuberculosis
Infection of megakaryocytes	HIV infection
Transient virus-induced aplasia	Parvovirus B19 infection (erythroblastopenia predominates)
Multiple Mechanisms	
Platelet destruction plus hypersplenism	Recurrent malaria
Increased platelet destruction, decreased platelet production, hypersplenism	Chronic HIV infection

*References can be found in Hoffman R, Benz EJ Jr, Shattil SJ, et al (eds.): Hematology: Basic Principles and Practice, 3rd ed. New York, Churchill Livingstone, 2000.

mation (eg, platelet-activating factor)[138] or certain microbial products.[139,140] In rare situations, platelet-reactive autoantibodies are implicated.[141] Various explanations for thrombocytopenia in different types of infection are listed in Table 140–7.

Unexplained thrombocytopenia in a hospitalized patient warrants studies to exclude infection, such as blood cultures. Prompt recognition and treatment of the infection constitute the most important therapy, as platelet count recovery tends to parallel the resolution of the infection. Prophylactic platelet transfusions are generally not required unless the platelet count falls to less than 10×10^9/L, or unless comorbid clinical features increase the likelihood of serious bleeding (eg, concomitant coagulopathy, an invasive procedure, uremic platelet dysfunction). The use of heparin for patients with septic shock and DIC is controversial (Chapter 132). However, heparin may benefit a subset of patients with clinical evidence of DIC and microvascular thrombosis (eg, acral tissue ischemia or necrosis) and is recommended for use in these patients. The possibility of acquired protein C deficiency complicating acute DIC also should be considered in septic patients with purpura fulminans, such as that secondary to meningococcemia, because treatment with vitamin K, plasma, and possibly recombinant activated protein C[142] could be beneficial.

Thrombocytopenia in patients infected with HIV poses a special diagnostic problem, because there are many potential explanations for the thrombocytopenia, which often coexist (see Chapter 158).[143,144] These include immune platelet destruction, impaired platelet production secondary to HIV infection of megakaryocytes, drug-induced myelosuppression (commonly implicated drugs include zidovudine, ganciclovir, and trimethoprim-sulfamethoxazole), HIV-associated thrombotic microangiopathy, hypersplenism, and marrow infiltration by tumor or opportunistic infections. Platelet kinetic studies have shown a complex interaction of decreased platelet production, increased platelet destruction, and splenic platelet sequestration.[145] Immune mechanisms for platelet destruction include antibodies that cross-react with GPIIb/IIIa complexes ("molecular mimicry")[146,147] and immune complexes containing IgM antiidiotype antibodies (which could explain the paradox of high levels of platelet-associated IgG and IgM with low serum levels of platelet-reactive antibodies).[148] Anti-HIV chemotherapy (eg, zidovudine, HAART) often raises the platelet count in patients with HIV-associated thrombocytopenia. Most patients with HIV-associated thrombocytopenia respond to conventional treatments for ITP, including corticosteroids, splenectomy, IVIG, and, particularly, anti-D.[143,149,150]

Systemic Lupus Erythematosus

Immune-mediated thrombocytopenia, which occurs in as many as 25% of patients with SLE,[151] is associated a twofold increased risk of organ-damage events in this patient population.[152] Many different types of platelet-IgG interactions are described (eg, antiglycoprotein,[153,154] anti-antiglycolipid,[155] β_2-glycoprotein I-containing immune complexes[156]). In addition, antithrombopoietin, anti-c-Mpl (thrombopoietin receptor), and anti-CD40 ligand autoantibodies have been reported.[154,157–159] Multiple causes for thrombocytopenia-increased platelet destruction, hypersplenism, even impaired platelet production related to antibody-induced megakaryocytic hypoplasia[157,158]—are reported. The predominant explanation for thrombocytopenia in SLE remains unknown.

Several thrombocytopenic syndromes are seen in patients with SLE. For many patients, the thrombocytopenia is chronic, resembling ITP, and is the predominant clinical manifestation of the lupus.[151] Often, these patients have a prolonged bleeding time despite mild thrombocytopenia.[160] Some thrombocytopenic patients with SLE have antiphospholipid antibodies and are at increased risk for thrombotic rather than bleeding complications (see Chapter 131). Acute, severe thrombocytopenia can be a prominent feature in patients with a severe multisystem exacerbation of lupus.[151] Rarely, patients with SLE develop an illness that closely resembles TTP or hemolytic uremic syndrome; these patients should be treated with plasma exchange.[161,162] Thrombocytopenia as a feature of SLE-associated, viral-induced macrophage activation syndrome has been reported.[163,164]

Treatment of the thrombocytopenia of SLE is similar to that of ITP (see Chapter 138). Corticosteroids constitute the first line of therapy, but many patients do not respond or require high doses. Additionally, patients with SLE may be at relatively higher risk for avascular necrosis of the femoral head. High-dose IVIG may be useful in a bleeding patient to transiently increase the platelet count.[165] Before resorting to splenectomy, one could try danazol (an attenuated androgen), in doses of 200 to 800 mg/day.[166,167] Higher doses can cause hepatitis. Typically, several weeks are required before a benefit is seen. Splenectomy probably is as effective in achieving platelet count remission in SLE as in ITP.[167,168] Patients with refractory thrombocytopenia sometimes benefit from more aggressive therapies, such as with azathioprine, intermittent-pulse cyclophosphamide, plasmapheresis synchronized with pulse cyclophosphamide,[169] cyclosporine,[170,171] or, possibly, rituximab (anti-CD20 chimeric monoclonal antibody).[172]

Antiphospholipid Syndrome

The antiphospholipid syndrome (Chapter 131) is characterized by occurrence of one or more clinical events (venous or arterial thrombosis, recurrent miscarriages, thrombocytopenia) associated with IgG, IgM, or IgA antibodies that recognize a complex of one or more protein cofactors (eg, β_2-glycoprotein I, annexin V, prothrombin, protein C, protein S) bound to negatively charged phospholipid.[173–175] Many patients (30%–50%) with this syndrome have thrombocytopenia,[176–178] which is typically mild and intermittent; approximately 15% have autoimmune hemolysis. The antiphospholipid syndrome should be considered in patients who develop idiopathic lower-limb or abdominal vein (mesenteric, renal, adrenal) thrombosis, cerebral venous (dural sinus) thrombosis, cardiac valvulitis, nonatheromatous arterial thrombosis (especially thrombotic stroke in a patient younger than 50 years of age), dermal microvascular thrombosis (acrocyanosis, digital ulceration or gangrene, livedo reticularis), or acute multiorgan failure associated with DIC and/or widespread thrombosis of the microvasculature ("catastrophic antiphospholipid syndrome").[173–180]

The mechanism of the prothrombotic tendency in patients with antiphospholipid syndrome remains elusive, but interference with endothelial cell function, impaired fibrinolysis,[181,182] antibody-mediated platelet activation, formation of endothelial microparticles,[183] interference with thrombin,[184] and factor Xa[185] degradation by antithrombin, disturbance in the protein C anticoagulant pathway[186] or anticoagulant activity of β_2-glycoprotein I all have been described.[187] Disruption of the antithrombotic annexin V antithrombotic "shield" by antiphospholipid antibodies has been proposed to explain pregnancy losses through placental vascular thrombosis.[188] There is evidence that thrombocytopenia in patients with antiphospholipid syndrome is associated with platelet glycoprotein-reactive autoantibodies.[189]

Antiphospholipid antibodies are detected by either of two methods: (a) solid-phase ELISA with purified phospholipids (usually cardiolipin) as target antigens or (b) a "functional" assay for so-called lupus anticoagulant activity, shown by demonstrating inhibition of certain phospholipid-dependent coagulation assays, such as the aPTT or the Russell viper venom time.[173] Although antiphospholipid antibodies frequently are detected in patients with SLE, they also can be found in patients with other autoimmune disorders, malignancy, or infections, or as a complication of certain drugs (eg, procainamide). Often no associated condition is identified ("primary" antiphospholipid syndrome). Antiphospholipid antibodies of low titer are sometimes found in normal persons, particularly the elderly, or during normal pregnancy. Autoantibody "cluster" studies show that anticardiolipin, lupus anticoagulant, and anti–double-stranded DNA antibodies occur together more often than with other SLE-associated autoantibodies (eg, anti-Sm, anti-Ro, anti-RNP).[190]

There are intriguing parallels between the antiphospholipid syndrome and HIT[191]: in both disorders, the antibodies are directed at a protein target (β_2-glycoprotein I and PF4, respectively) bound to a negatively charged species (anionic phospholipid and heparin, respectively). For both, high-titer IgG antibodies that result in a positive "functional" test result (lupus anticoagulant activity and HIT-IgG-induced platelet activation, respectively) are most likely to be associated with clinical disease.[192] Both disorders are characterized by the paradox of thrombocytopenia associated with increased risk for venous and arterial thrombosis.

To help physicians diagnose the antiphospholipid syndrome, clinical and laboratory criteria have been developed,[193,194] with recent revisions.[195,196] The laboratory criteria include the presence of anticardiolipin, anti-β_2-glycoprotein I, or lupus anticoagulant antibodies (moderate- to high-titer IgG or IgM) on two or more occasions at least 12 weeks apart. The major clinical criteria are thrombosis and complications of pregnancy. Thrombosis can involve large arteries or veins, or small vessels within any organ. The complications of pregnancy include one or more unexplained deaths of normal fetus(es) after week 10 of gestation or premature births (before 34 weeks), or greater than three spontaneous abortions before week 10 of gestation.

Specific treatment for the thrombocytopenia usually is not required. For many patients, long-term anticoagulant or antiplatelet therapy, or both, are needed to prevent recurrent thromboses. For those patients with recurring pregnancy losses and antiphospholipid antibodies, randomized trials have documented the benefit of low-dose aspirin combined with either low-dose unfractionated heparin[197] or LMWH.[198,199]

Malignancy

Thrombocytopenia complicating malignant disorders most frequently results from antineoplastic treatment or marrow replacement by tumor. However, certain thrombocytopenic syndromes have been associated with malignancy, including autoimmune thrombocytopenia, DIC, and thrombotic microangiopathy.

Immune thrombocytopenia attributable to platelet glycoprotein-reactive autoantibodies can complicate neoplastic lymphoproliferative diseases such as Hodgkin disease, non-Hodgkin lymphoma, chronic lymphocytic leukemia, and multiple myeloma.[200,201] Sometimes the thrombocytopenia responds to treatment of the neoplasm, although in some patients (particularly those with Hodgkin disease), the thrombocytopenia is indistinguishable from ITP and is not related to the activity of the lymphoma.

DIC occurs in certain malignancies, particularly adenocarcinomas of the pancreas, stomach, lung, colon, breast, and prostate.[202–204] Some patients present with venous or, less commonly, arterial thrombosis as the first clinical manifestation of their malignancy. In these patients, the presence of thrombocytopenia is an important clue that should prompt investigations for DIC, such as measurement of fibrinogen or fibrin D-dimer levels. In our experience, the platelet count typically rises to normal or even elevated levels during heparin therapy, as heparin ameliorates the DIC process; however, recurrent thrombocytopenia and thrombosis can recur within hours of discontinuing the heparin therapy.[204,205] Cancer patients with DIC and deep vein thrombosis also are at increased risk for warfarin-associated venous limb gangrene.[204,205] The role of various tumor-associated procoagulant substances—such as "cancer procoagulant' (a 68-kd cysteine proteinase that activates factor X independently of tissue factor/factor VIIa[206]) and cancer-associated tissue factor (which is expressed on tumor cells,[207] as well as circulating microparticles,[208–210]) —suggest pathophysiologic parallels with microthrombosis in HIT, as both cancer-associated DIC and acute HIT are risk factors for phlegmasia cerulean dolens and venous limb gangrene during anticoagulation with warfarin. Thus, cancer patients with DIC should receive heparin (especially, LMWH) rather than warfarin anticoagulation (see box on Diagnostic Considerations in the Patient with Limb Ischemia and Thrombocytopenia). DIC with hemorrhagic manifestations is characteristically seen in some patients with prostate adenocarcinoma, and in many patients with acute promyelocytic leukemia. It is crucial to recognize promyelocytic leukemia, because treatment with all-*trans*-retinoic acid produces differentiation of the malignant cells, thereby rapidly reducing the life-threatening bleeding risks attributable to hyperfibrinolysis in this disorder.[211]

A destructive thrombocytopenic disorder that resembles hemolytic uremic syndrome or TTP has been described in patients with advanced cancer.[212] In some patients, mitomycin treatment may have contributed to the microangiopathy. DIC usually is not present. Some patients respond transiently to plasmapheresis, but for many, response to any therapy is poor.

Diagnostic Considerations in the Patient with Limb Ischemia and Thrombocytopenia

Concurrence of limb ischemia/necrosis and thrombocytopenia suggests one of several hematologic emergencies:

- **Heparin-induced thrombocytopenia (HIT).** Occlusion of large lower-limb arteries by platelet-rich "white clots" is characteristic of heparin-induced thrombocytopenia. The major clue is an otherwise unexplained platelet count fall that begins 5 or more days after initiation of heparin. Urgent thromboembolectomy may be limb sparing. Sensitive assays for HIT antibodies give strong positive results. See also subsequent entry for warfarin.
- **Adenocarcinoma-associated disseminated intravascular coagulation.** Severe venous or arterial thrombosis can develop in patients with metastatic adenocarcinoma who have disseminated intravascular coagulation (DIC), especially within hours after stopping heparin. A clinical clue is an otherwise unexplained rise in platelet count that occurred during initial heparin therapy. See also entry for warfarin.
- **Warfarin-induced phlegmasia cerulea dolens/venous limb gangrene.** Coumarin anticoagulants such as warfarin can lead to venous ischemia (phlegmasia cerulea dolens) or venous limb gangrene in patients with DIC caused by HIT or adenocarcinoma. Limb loss can occur even though the limb pulses are palpable.
- **Sepsis-associated microvascular thrombosis.** Acquired natural anticoagulant failure (eg, antithrombin or protein C depletion) can complicate DIC associated with sepsis, leading to acral limb ischemia or necrosis.
- **Septic embolism.** Rarely, infective endocarditis or aneurysmal thrombosis leads to the constellation of thrombocytopenia with infection and acute limb ischemia.
- **Antiphospholipid syndrome.** Autoimmune thrombocytopenia and hypercoagulability can interact to produce acute limb ischemia and thrombocytopenia in a patient with antiphospholipid syndrome.

Macrophage Activation (Hemophagocytic) Syndrome

The macrophage activation (or hemophagocytic) syndrome comprises a heterogeneous group of disorders characterized by variable cytopenias and morphologic evidence of macrophage phagocytosis of red cells, granulocytes, and platelets; hyperferritinemia, hypercytokinemia, and sepsis-like features are characteristic, with potential for evolution to fatal multiple organ failure.[213,214] Some adult patients have an aggressive disease characterized by high fever, weight loss, prominent hepatosplenomegaly, severe pancytopenia, elevated liver enzymes, and often a terminal infection. Both T- and B-cell lymphomas can explain such a dramatic syndrome.[215,216] However, similar patients with fulminant illness have been described following otherwise unremarkable bacterial or viral infections (particularly those due to the Epstein–Barr virus[217]). In children also, the high mortality rate associated with hemophagocytic lymphohistiocytosis warrants aggressive treatment, including antineoplastic chemotherapy and bone marrow transplantation.[218] Nonneoplastic but nonetheless severe hemophagocytosis can be seen in patients with certain infections (eg, babesiosis,[219] ehrlichiosis,[220] HIV infection[221,222]), as well as in patients with rheumatologic disorders (SLE,[163,164,223] Still disease,[224] ankylosing spondylitis[225]). Laboratory indicators of macrophage activation syndrome include markedly elevated ferritin, soluble CD163 and CD25 levels, and morphologic evidence of hemophagocytosis.[213,214] Treatment should be directed at the underlying illness. Early administration of high-dose gammaglobulin appears to benefit some patients with nonneoplastic macrophage activation syndrome.[226]

Solid Organ and Bone Marrow Transplantation

Thrombocytopenia commonly occurs during episodes of solid organ allograft rejection.[227] It is possible that platelet activation and deposition in the transplanted organ vasculature contribute to the rejection process. Antirejection therapies also can cause thrombocytopenia through increased platelet destruction (antilymphocyte globulin[228]) or marrow suppression (azathioprine[228]). Posttransplantation hemolytic uremic syndrome develops in approximately 5% of renal transplant recipients[229,230] and in even fewer recipients of liver or heart transplants.[230] Although cyclosporine sometimes is implicated in hemolytic uremic syndrome, it usually can be safely resumed following recovery.[231]

Early, severe thrombocytopenia caused by marrow-ablative therapy invariably accompanies bone marrow transplantation (BMT). Platelet count recovery to greater than 50×10^9/L is more rapid (16 vs 35 days) in patients receiving autologous mobilized peripheral blood progenitor cells than in those undergoing autologous BMT.[231] Severe persistent thrombocytopenia despite recovery of red and white cells is relatively common following marrow or peripheral blood transplantation[232]; autoimmune thrombocytopenia has been implicated in some patients.[233] Late-onset thrombocytopenia following BMT that responds to corticosteroids, IVIG, and splenectomy also has been attributed to autoimmune thrombocytopenia. Rarely, transplantation-associated alloimmune thrombocytopenia can be caused by donor–recipient incompatibility involving platelet-specific alloantigens such as Pl^{A1} or Br^{a}.[234]

A syndrome of thrombocytopenia, red cell fragmentation, and renal impairment can occur in as many as 10% of patients undergoing BMT, usually beginning 3 to 12 months following transplantation (BMT-associated thrombotic microangiopathy).[112,235,236] The pathogenesis remains obscure; reduced ADAMTS13 levels have not been implicated.[237,238] The hematologic abnormalities can be mild and remit spontaneously, although patients often have residual azotemia and hypertension. More severely affected patients usually do not benefit from plasmapheresis.[239] The syndrome has a poor overall prognosis, and many patients will die irrespective of any intervention.

Cardiopulmonary Bypass Surgery

Excess bleeding is an important problem in patients who undergo heart surgery utilizing cardiopulmonary bypass.[240] Many of these patients receive blood transfusions, and approximately 5% require reoperation for postoperative bleeding.

Thrombocytopenia and transient platelet dysfunction (Chapter 142) are observed in virtually every patient. Typically, the platelet count falls by 35% to 65%, primarily as a result of hemodilution, but also because of bleeding and losses within the extracorporeal perfusion device. The bleeding time rises markedly during heart surgery (to greater than 30 minutes) but usually improves to less than 15 minutes shortly after surgery, and to normal several hours later. By contrast, the thrombocytopenia persists for 3 to 4 days, followed by recovery of the platelet count to values exceeding the preoperative baseline.

The pathogenesis and clinical significance of the hemostatic defect in these patients remain uncertain, but the explanation probably is multifactorial. Studies have described transient, *intrinsic* defects in platelet function.[241] These defects include decreased in vitro platelet aggregation, decreased platelet surface membrane proteins,[242] selective depletion of platelet α-granules,[241] and evidence of in vivo platelet activation[243] and platelet vesiculation.[243] The platelet dysfunction in heart surgery also is attributable to an *extrinsic* platelet defect resulting from thrombin inhibition by the high doses of heparin.[244] Furthermore, an important role for hyperfibrinolysis in the pathogenesis of bleeding is shown by elevated D-dimer levels in bleeding patients,[245] as well as the efficacy of antifibrinolytic agents[246] in the prevention and treatment of heart surgery-associated bleeding. Other factors in some patients include residual heparin effect following bypass (including heparin rebound[247]) and preoperative use of aspirin. Treatment of platelet dysfunction after cardiopulmonary bypass is discussed in Chapter 142.

THROMBOCYTOPENIA ASSOCIATED WITH CARDIOVASCULAR DISEASE

Congenital Cyanotic Heart Disease

Thrombocytopenia caused by a decrease in platelet life span occurs in some patients with severe cyanotic congenital heart disease and is approximately related to the severity of the polycythemia. Bleeding occurs in a few patients and can be related to platelet function defects, coagulopathy, or hyperfibrinolysis. Reducing the hematocrit by phlebotomy sometimes helps to correct the hemostatic defects.

Valvular Heart Disease

Increased platelet turnover is common in valvular heart disease, and some patients have mild thrombocytopenia. The pathogenesis of the platelet consumption is not well understood, but the defect could be related to increased platelet–vWF interactions at high shear.[248,249] Indeed, high-molecular-weight multimers of vWF are reduced in some of these patients, which explains why bleeding from gastrointestinal angiodysplasia in patients with aortic stenosis typically resolves following aortic valve replacement.[250,251] Thrombocytopenia secondary to consumptive coagulopathy can be seen in intracardiac thrombosis associated with valvular heart disease.[140,252]

Pulmonary Vascular Disorders

Disorders characterized by pulmonary hypertension can be accompanied by thrombocytopenia, the pathogenesis of which is poorly defined. Thrombocytopenia can occur in association with pulmonary embolism,[205,253,254] possibly as a result of DIC. When evaluating such a patient, the clinician should inquire about current or recent heparin exposure, because HIT and pulmonary embolism are strongly associated.[22,44]

SUGGESTED READINGS

Arepally GM, Ortel TL: Clinical practice. Heparin-induced thrombocytopenia. N Engl J Med 355:809, 2006.

Aster RH, Curtis BR, Bougie DW, et al: Thrombocytopenia associated with the use of GPIIb/IIIa inhibitors: Position paper of the ISTH working group on thrombocytopenia and GPIIb/IIIa inhibitors. J Thromb Haemost 4:678, 2006.

Bougie DW, Wilker PR, Aster RH: Patients with quinine-induced immune thrombocytopenia have both "drug-dependent" and "drug-specific" antibodies. Blood 108:922, 2006.

Brighton TA, Evans S, Castaldi PA, et al: Prospective evaluation of the clinical usefulness of an antigen-specific assay (MAIPA) in idiopathic thrombocytopenic purpura and other immune thrombocytopenias. Blood 88:194, 1996.

Emmenegger U, Frey U, Reimers A, et al: Hyperferritinemia as indicator for intravenous gammaglobulin treatment in reactive macrophage activation syndromes. Am J Hematol 68:4, 2001.

Francois B, Trimoreau F, Vignon P, et al: Thrombocytopenia in the sepsis syndrome: Role of hemophagocytosis and macrophage colony-stimulating factor. Am J Med 103:114, 1980.

Kitchens CS: Thrombocytopenia due to acute venous thromboembolism and its role in expanding the differential diagnosis of heparin-induced thrombocytopenia. Am J Hematol 76:69, 2004

Levine JS, Branch DW, Rauch J: The antiphospholipid syndrome. N Engl J Med 346:752, 2002.

Lo GK, Juhl D, Warkentin TE, et al: Evaluation of pretest clinical score (4 T's) for the diagnosis of heparin-induced thrombocytopenia in two clinical settings. J Thromb Haemost 4:759, 2004.

Lubenow N, Eichler P, Lietz T, et al: Lepirudin in patients with heparin-induced thrombocytopenia-results of the third prospective study (HAT-3) and a combined analysis of HAT-1, HAT-2, and HAT-3. J Thromb Haemost 3:2428, 2005.

Miyakis MS, Lockshin MD, Atsumi T, et al: International consensus statement on an update of the classification criteria for definite antiphospholipid syndrome J Thromb Haemost 4:295, 2006.

Tesselaar ME, Romijn FP, van der Linden IK, et al: Microparticle-associated tissue factor activity: A link between cancer and thrombosis? J Thromb Haemost 5:520, 2007.

Tinmouth AT, Semple E, Shehata N, Branch DR: Platelet immunopathology and therapy: A Canadian Blood Services Research and Development Symposium. Transfus Med Rev 20:294, 2006.

Von Drygalski A, Curtis BR, Bougie DW, et al: Vancomycin induced immune thrombocytopenia. N Engl J Med 356:904, 2007.

Warkentin TE: Drug-induced immune-mediated thrombocytopenia-from purpura to thrombosis. N Engl J Med 356:891, 2007.

Warkentin TE: Venous limb gangrene during warfarin treatment of cancer-associated deep venous thrombosis. Ann Intern Med 135:589, 2001.

Warkentin TE, Elavathil LJ, Hayward CPM, et al: The pathogenesis of venous limb gangrene associated with heparin-induced thrombocytopenia. Ann Intern Med 127:804, 1997.

Warkentin TE, Greinacher A, Koster A, Lincoff AM: Treatment and prevention of heparin-induced thrombocytopenia: ACCP evidence-based clinical practice guidelines (8th edition). Chest 2008; in press.

Warkentin TE, Kelton JG: Delayed-onset heparin-induced thrombocytopenia and thrombosis. Ann Intern Med 135:502, 2001.

Warkentin TE, Kelton JG: Temporal aspects of heparin-induced thrombocytopenia. N Engl J Med 344:1286, 2001.

Warkentin TE, Levine MN, Hirsh J, et al: Heparin-induced thrombocytopenia in patients treated with low-molecular-weight heparin or unfractionated heparin. N Engl J Med 332:1330, 1995.

REFERENCES

For complete list of references log onto www.expertconsult.com

CHAPTER 141

HEREDITARY DISORDERS OF PLATELET FUNCTION

Joel S. Bennett

A prolonged bleeding time in a patient with a normal platelet count suggests the presence of von Willebrand disease or a disorder of platelet function. von Willebrand disease is discussed in Chapter 129, and acquired disorders of platelet function are discussed in Chapter 142. Hereditary disorders of platelet function disorders are considered in this chapter. For discussion purposes, these disorders can be classified into disorders of platelet adhesion, aggregation, secretion, or procoagulant activity according to the predominant aspect of platelet function affected.

DISORDERS OF PLATELET ADHESION

Bernard-Soulier Syndrome (Glycoprotein Ib/IX/V Deficiency)

Described in 1948 by Bernard and Soulier, the Bernard-Soulier syndrome is a rare platelet function disorder characterized by a prolonged bleeding time, large platelets, and thrombocytopenia.[1] Patients with the Bernard-Soulier syndrome bleed because their platelets cannot adhere to von Willebrand factor (VWF), a consequence of deficiency or dysfunction of the platelet glycoprotein (GP) Ib/IX/V (GPIb-IX-V) complex.[2–4]

Biology and Molecular Aspects of the Disorder

Following disruption of the vascular endothelium, circulating platelets adhere to exposed subendothelial connective tissue. In addition to connective tissue components such as collagen, fibronectin, and laminin, at the high shear rates present in arterioles and the microcirculation, platelet adhesion requires the presence of VWF.[5,6] VWF is an elongated multimeric glycoprotein, each monomer of which contains two sequence motifs that interact with platelets (see Chapter 128).[7] One motif located in the A1 domain of VWF enables subendothelial VWF to interact transiently with the GPIb-IX-V complex on unactivated platelets, thereby causing platelets to translocate (or roll) along the exposed subendothelial surface. The second motif, located in the C1 domain, mediates the stable interaction of VWF with the integrin αIIbβ3 (GPIIb-IIIa) on activated platelets.[8] Although VWF is also a component of plasma, soluble VWF does not bind spontaneously to GPIb-IX-V.[9] What prevents the spontaneous binding of soluble VWF to platelets is uncertain. However, exposing soluble VWF to the antibiotic ristocetin or the snake venom protein botrocetin in vitro enables it to bind to GPIb-IX-V.[10,11] Whether there are physiologic correlates for ristocetin and botrocetin is unclear. One possibility is that the A1 domain of subendothelial VWF, but not soluble VWF, is in a conformation that allows it to bind to GPIb-IX-V.[12] A second possibility is that shear stress changes the conformation of the A1 domain, GPIb-IX-V, or both, allowing spontaneous VWF binding to GPIb-IX-V.[13]

GPIb-IX-V, the protein complex affected in Bernard-Soulier platelets, is a noncovalent heterotrimer consisting of the heavily glycosylated 165,000 mol wt protein GPIb,[14] the 20,000 mol wt protein GPIX[15] and the 82,000 mol wt protein GPV.[16] There are approximately 25,000 copies of GPIb and GPIX on the platelet surface but only half as many copies of GPV, suggesting that individual GPIb-IX-V complexes contain two copies of GPIb, two copies of GPIX, and one copy of GPV. Whether GPIb-IX-V is also expressed by endothelial cells remains an area of controversy.[17–19] GPIb itself is a disulfide-linked heterodimer containing a 143,000 mol wt α subunit (GPIbα) and a 22,000 mol wt β subunit (GPIbβ).[20] GPIbα can be cleaved by trypsin or a calcium-dependent platelet protease into a soluble 135,000 mol wt heavily glycosylated amino (N)–terminal fragment named glycocalicin and a membrane-embedded 25,000 mol wt carboxyl (C)–terminal remnant that remains disulfide-linked to GPIbβ and associated with GPIX.[21] The N-terminal portion of glycocalicin contains binding sites for VWF and thrombin. Its C-terminal portion consists of a variable number of tandem 13 residue mucin-like repeats to which multiple O-linked, sialic acid–rich hexasaccharides are appended.[22,23] GPIbα extends into the platelet cytoplasm where residues 567 to 571 in its cytoplasmic tail bind to the C-terminus of filamin A (actin-binding protein),[24,25] thereby linking it to the platelet cytoskeleton[26] and where residues 580 to 590 and 605 to 610 bind to the adaptor protein 14–3-3 linking it to platelet signaling pathways.[27–29] The cytoplasmic portions of GPIbβ and GPIX are acylated with palmitic acid through thioester linkages at free cysteine residues.[30] This modification may stabilize the interaction of these subunits with the membrane lipid bilayer or with other membrane proteins. In addition, the cytoplasmic portion of GPIbβ can be phosphorylated at Ser166 by cyclic AMP-dependent protein kinase A,[31] a reaction that inhibits collagen-induced platelet actin polymerization.[32] The role of GPV in GPIb-IX-V function is unclear. Although GPV can be cleaved by thrombin,[33] this is not required for VWF binding to GPIbα. GPV cleavage also does not activate platelets,[34] and it is controversial whether it has a role in regulating the ability of thrombin to activate platelets.[35–38]

The N-terminal portion of GPIbα, as well as GPIbβ, GPIX, and GPV, contain leucine rich repeats (LRRs) with the consensus sequence L-L--N-L--LPPGLL-G---L-.[16,39] LRR were first detected in the plasma protein leucine rich α_2 glycoprotein and have been detected in an increasing number of proteins.[39] GPIbα contains eight LRR (seven were predicted from sequence information),[9] whereas GPIbβ and GPIX contain one each and GPV contains fifteen. The amino acids flanking the LRR are also conserved.[39] A crystal structure for the VWF A1 domain bound to residues 1 to 290 of GPIbα revealed that LRR 1 and five to eight of GPIbα bound tightly to the A1 domain, largely as a result of long-range electrostatic attraction.[9] Moreover, conformational changes in a flexible loop located near the carboxyl terminus of the GPIbα fragment, termed the *β-switch*[9] or *R-loop*,[40] and the site of several gain-of-function mutations responsible for platelet-type von Willebrand disease,[9] may be needed for VWF binding to GPIbα. The function of the LRR in GPIbβ, GPIX, and GPV is unknown; but they do not function as *leucine-zippers* and are not located in regions known to be involved in intermolecular associations.

Studies of GPIb-IX-V biosynthesis using Chinese hamster ovary cells indicate that although small amounts of GPIbα can be detected on the surface of cells expressing GPIbα and GPIbβ, GPIbα expression is much more efficient when the cells coexpress GPIbα, GPIbβ, and GPIX.[41] Moreover, GPIbβ is the subunit that links GPIbα to GPIX.[42] Thus, mutations that result in the deficient expression of any one of the components of GPIb-IX-V can produce the Bernard-

Soulier syndrome. Conversely, GPV is not required for GPIb-IX-V expression, and the basis for its absence from Bernard-Soulier platelets is unknown.[43]

Etiology and Pathogenesis

The effects of GPIb-IX-V deficiency are not limited to the inability of affected platelets to adhere to VWF. Most Bernard-Soulier platelets are large when observed on peripheral blood smears.[16] However, there is contradictory evidence about the size of these platelets in the circulation. It has been reported that circulating Bernard-Soulier platelets are of normal size,[44] but have increased membrane, perhaps located in the surface-connected open-canalicular system and extruded when platelets spread during the preparation of a blood smear.[45] Others have found that circulating Bernard-Soulier platelets have an increased volume,[46] a more spherical shape,[46] and a more deformable membrane than normal platelets.[47] The molecular basis for the large size of Bernard-Soulier platelets is unknown. However, amelioration of macrothrombocytopenia in a murine Bernard-Soulier model via expression of an IL4-GPIbα fusion protein suggests that the absence of the GPIbα cytoplasmic domain contributes to this abnormality.[48] Although the serum prothrombin time has been reported to be shortened in the Bernard-Soulier syndrome[49] and collagen-induced platelet procoagulant activity and Factor XI binding to be absent,[50] prothrombin consumption, measured by a two-stage assay, is normal[51]; and the expression of platelet factor 3[51] and prothrombinase activity by Bernard-Soulier platelets is increased.[52] An unexplained decrease in thrombin-, trypsin-, and thromboxane-stimulated phospholipase C activity has also been reported.[53] GPIb-IX is a target for some drug-dependent antiplatelet antibodies induced by quinidine and quinine[54]; and as would be expected, these antibodies fail to bind to Bernard-Soulier platelets.[55]

Genetic Aspects

The Bernard-Soulier syndrome is an autosomal recessive disorder.[16] In most instances, GPIb-IX-V is not present on the surface of Bernard-Soulier platelets; but in a few cases, 7% to 47% residual GPIb or GPIb-IX has been detected.[56] When it has been possible to study heterozygotes, many, but not all, have had platelets that are larger than normal and a GPIb content intermediate between normals and affected individuals.[57,58] Consistent with the rarity of the syndrome, consanguinity has often been present in affected families.

The gene for each component of the GPIb-IX-V complex has been localized and characterized. The *GPIbα* gene is located on chromosome 17p12-ter, the *GPIbβ* gene on chromosome 22q11.2, the *GPIX* gene on chromosome 3q21, and the *GPV* gene on chromosome 3q29.[16] Each gene has a compact *intron-depleted* structure, such that the genes for GPIbα, GPIbβ, and GPV contain two exons and the gene for GPV contains three.[59] The open reading frame and 3′ untranslated region of each is encoded by a single exon except for the *GPIbβ* gene where its single intron is inserted into the codon for the fourth residue of its signal peptide.[60] The genes are also similar in that their 5′ flanking regions contain potential binding sites for GATA, Ets, and Sp-1 transcription factors like other genes expressed by megakaryocytes.[61–63] In addition, polymorphic variation in the region surrounding the translation initiation site of GPIbα seems to be a determinant of the level of GPIb-IX-V expression.[64]

At least 47 different mutations responsible for the Bernard-Soulier syndrome have been identified: 18 involving the gene for GPIbα, 18 involving the gene for GPIbβ, and 11 involving the gene for GPIX. Most mutations have been missense mutations or nucleotide deletions and insertions resulting in frameshifts and premature stop codons. However, several unique mutations have been identified: deletion of the entire GPIbβ locus on chromosome 22q11.2, occasionally in the setting of the velocardiofacial syndrome;[65] a C to G transversion in the GATA binding site of the GPIbβ promoter resulting in decreased GPIbβ gene transcription[66]; and an Ala140Thr substitution in the transmembrane domain of GPIX.[67] The latter is noteworthy because it suggests that transmembrane domain interactions are involved in efficient GPIb-IX-V expression and is consistent with the impaired GPIb-IX expression observed when the transmembrane domain of GPIbβ was mutated in vitro.[68] It is also noteworthy that eleven mutations have been reported multiple times, suggesting that there may be *hot spots* for mutation in the *GPIbα, GPIbβ*, and *GPIX* genes.

Clinical Presentation

The Bernard-Soulier syndrome presents in infancy or childhood with bleeding characteristic of defective platelet function: ecchymoses, epistaxis, and gingival bleeding.[16] Later manifestations include menorrhagia and postpartum, gastrointestinal, and posttraumatic hemorrhage. Hemarthroses and expanding hematomas are unusual. Although the severity of hemorrhage among affected individuals is variable, bleeding can require frequent transfusion and suppression of menses. In a review of 59 cases, there were 10 deaths.[69] In some patients the severity of hemorrhage inexplicably declined over the course of the disease.[69]

Laboratory Findings

The bleeding time in patients with the Bernard-Soulier syndrome is markedly prolonged to greater than 20 minutes.[16] Platelet counts may vary within kindreds and in a given patient. Most patients are thrombocytopenic to some degree and patients with platelet counts less than 20,000/μl have been reported.[70] Platelets seen on stained peripheral blood smears are large with 30% to 80% having a mean diameter greater than 3.5 μm.[57] Occasional platelets are as large as 20 to 30 μm in diameter. Erythrocytes and white blood cells are normal and distinctive abnormalities have not been observed in marrow megakaryocytes by light microscopy,[71] but abnormalities in the demarcation membrane system have been observed by electron microscopy.[72] The laboratory tests that distinguish Bernard-Soulier from normal platelets are the failure of Bernard-Soulier platelets to agglutinate in the presence of ristocetin and decreased or absent agglutination after exposure to botrocetin.[16] In contrast to von Willebrand disease, these abnormalities cannot be corrected by the addition of normal plasma. Absent ristocetin-induced agglutination and normal platelet aggregation can be reproduced in the whole blood aggregometer, obviating the difficulty of preparing platelet-rich plasma containing a sufficient number of Bernard-Soulier platelets for conventional aggregometry.[73] Aggregation of Bernard-Soulier platelets induced by agonists such as adenosine diphosphate (ADP), collagen, and epinephrine is normal (Fig. 141–1).[16] However, the rate of thrombin-stimulated aggregation has been reported to be reduced.[74] Although a defect in prothrombin consumption, manifested by a short serum prothrombin time, has been reported, expression of platelet factor 3 activity by Bernard-Soulier platelets is normal or increased.[51]

Differential Diagnosis

There are several conditions associated with large platelets and thrombocytopenia (macrothrombocytopenia, Table 141–1) that can be readily differentiated from the Bernard-Soulier syndrome because Bernard-Soulier platelets fail to agglutinate in the presence of ristocetin.[75]

Macrothrombocytopenia is characteristic of patients with mutations in the *MYH9* gene located on chromosome 22q12.3-q13.2 that encodes the nonmuscle myosin heavy chain IIA (NMMHC-IIA).[76,77] Although classically segregated into four separate autosomal dominant inherited syndromes (the May-Hegglin anomaly and the Sebastian, Fechtner, and Epstein syndromes) based on the presence or absence of Döhle body-like leukocyte inclusions, hereditary nephritis, cataracts, and sensorineural deafness, detailed evaluation of families

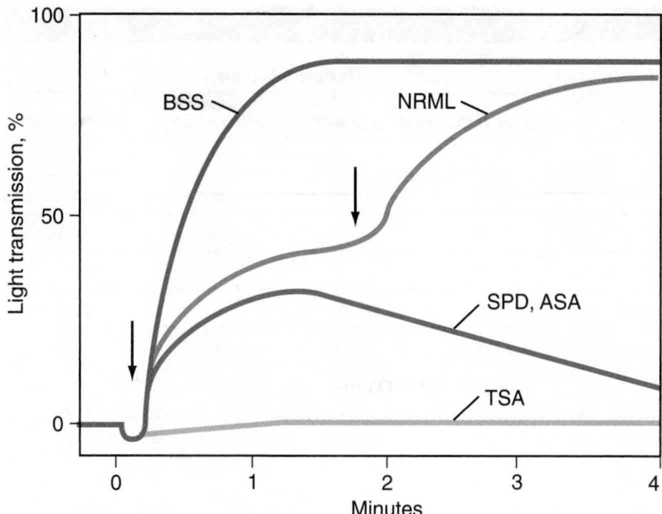

Figure 141–1 Platelet aggregation in response to adenosine diphosphate (ADP). Following the addition of ADP to a stirred aliquot of platelet-rich plasma in an aggregometer, there is a brief decrease in light transmission, indicated by the solid arrow, because of platelet shape change. When normal (**NRML**) or Bernard-Soulier platelets (**BSS**) are examined, shape change is followed by either a single continuous wave of aggregation at high ADP concentrations or two waves of aggregation at lower ADP concentrations. The hatched arrow at the inflection point between the first and second waves of aggregation is the point at which platelet secretion occurs. δ-Storage pool deficient platelets (**SPD**) generally undergo only a first wave of aggregation and the aggregates may dissociate. Aspirin-treated platelets (**ASA**) only undergo first wave aggregation when stimulated by ADP. Thrombasthenic platelets (**TSA**) undergo shape change, but do not aggregate regardless of the platelet agonist.

Table 141–1 Causes of Inherited Macrothrombocytopenia

Bernard-Soulier syndrome
MHY9-related disorders
May-Hegglin anomaly
Sebastian syndrome
Fechtner syndrome
Epstein syndrome
Gray platelet syndrome
Montreal platelet syndrome
Mediterranean macrothrombocytopenia
Mediterranean stomatocytosis/macrothrombocytenia
GATA1 mutations
Sialyl-Lewis-S antigen deficiency
Paris-Trousseau syndrome
Platelet-type von Willebrand disease

in whom *MYH9* mutations have been identified has revealed a heterogeneous distribution of symptoms within individual families and has not revealed genotype-phenotype correlations.[78] For example, cataracts, hearing loss, and abnormal renal function has be detected in family members affected by the May-Hegglin anomaly, but this syndrome was initially defined by the absence of these symptoms. Thus, it seems appropriate to consider these syndromes as a single entity whose variability results from the variable expression of *MHY9* mutations and whose common feature is macrothrombocytopenia. In general, the function of platelets affected by *MHY9* mutations is normal[79–81]; if hemorrhage occurs, it is usually caused by thrombocytopenia.[82] However, in some patients said to have the Fechtner and Epstein syndromes, abnormal platelet aggregation and secretion have been described.[83,84]

The pathogenesis of *MHY9*-related disorders is currently unclear. Most cells express multiple myosin II isoforms; but platelets only express NMMHC-IIA, perhaps accounting for the commonality of macrothrombocytopenia. Cytoskeletal proteins are involved in the biogenesis of platelets from megakaryocyte proplatelets, but exactly how they participate in the release of platelets from proplatelets is still poorly understood.[85,86] Nonetheless, altered cytoskeletal organization has been observed in platelets from patients with *MYH9* mutations,[87] implying that perturbed cytoskeletal dynamics is responsible for the macrothrombocytopenia. Whether perturbed cytoskeletal dynamics results from deficient myosin ATPase activity,[88] haploinsufficiency caused by protein instability,[89,90] or a dominant-negative effect on NMMHC-IIA assembly seems to vary according to the particular MHY9 mutation.[91] The Döhle body-like inclusions in the leukocytes of patients with the May-Hegglin anomaly and the Sebastian and Fechtner syndromes observed on stained blood smears are composed of aggregates of NMMHC-IIA and ribosomes.[92] However, it is important to note that even in the absence of visible Döhle body-like inclusions, NMMHC-IIA aggregates may be detected in leukocytes by immunostaining.[78,93] Thus, *MHY9*-related disorders must always be considered in the differential diagnosis of macrothrombocytopenia.

Large platelets and thrombocytopenia also occur in the Gray Platelet syndrome, a disorder resulting from platelet α granules deficiency.[94] In contrast to Bernard-Soulier platelets, these platelets are pale gray on Wright-stained blood smears and agglutinate normally in the presence of ristocetin.[95] In the autosomal dominant Montreal platelet syndrome, giant platelets, thrombocytopenia, and a prolonged bleeding time are associated with spontaneous platelet aggregation at pH 7.4 and normal agonist-induced platelet aggregation.[96] So-called Mediterranean macrothrombocytopenia refers to putative differences in platelet count and platelet size among Europeans of Northern and Mediterranean origin;[97] in Italy, this may be caused by heterozygosity for the Bernard-Soulier syndrome.[98] Conversely, Mediterranean stomatocytosis/macrothrombocytenia, the rare combination of stomatocytic hemolysis and macrothrombocytopenia, has been reported to result from excess plant sterols in the blood and to be caused by mutations in the *ABCG5* and *ABCG8* genes linked to phytosterolemia.[99] Sex-linked macrothrombocytopenia has been described in patients with specific mutations of the GATA-1 transcription factor[100–102] and macrothrombocytopenia with dystrophic megakaryocytes and neutrophils lacking sialyl Lewis S antigen has been described in an infant who died at age 37 months because of hemorrhage.[103] In the Paris-Trousseau syndrome,[104] a component of the Jacobsen syndrome,[105] deletion of the long arm of chromosome 11 at q23.3 results in mild thrombocytopenia, subpopulations of large platelets and platelets containing giant α granules, and the expansion of immature megakaryocyte progenitors.[106] The syndrome is thought to be caused by loss of *FLI1*, a gene located on the deleted portion of chromosome 11, whose product is a transcription factor that acts synergistically with GATA-1 to mediate the transcription of megakaryocytic-specific genes.[107,108] In the context of the Jacobsen syndrome, the Paris-Trousseau syndrome is accompanied by facial dysmorphism; ophthalmic, digital, and cardiac abnormalities; and variable psychomotor retardation.[105] There are also anecdotal reports of thrombocytopenia and giant platelets, often associated with a mild bleeding diathesis, but lacking the features of either Bernard-Soulier syndrome or the *MHY9* disorders.[109,110] In two of these reports, macrothrombocytopenia was associated with the presence of large platelet granules whose origin was uncertain.[111,112]

Acquired Bernard-Soulier-like disorders can be differentiated from the congenital Bernard-Soulier syndrome by history. Antibodies to GPIb occur in some patients with idiopathic thrombocytopenic purpura,[113] but it has not been possible to determine if the antibodies

Table 141–2 Treatment of Inherited Disorders of Platelet Function

Disorder	Defect in Platelet Function	Structural Defect	Treatment Options			
			Platelet Transfusion	*DDAVP*	*Corticosteroids*	*Recomb. VIIa*
BSS	Adhesion	GPIb-IX deficiency	Y	?	N	Y
GT	Aggregation	GPIIb-IIIa deficiency	Y	N	N	Y
Gray platelet syndrome	Secretion	α granule deficiency	Y	?	NIA	NIA
Storage pool disease	Secretion	δ granule deficiency	Y	Y	?	Y
Primary secretion defects	Secretion	Defective signal transduction	Y	Y	?	NIA
Scott syndrome	Procoagulant activity	Decreased exposure of anionic phospholipids	Y	N	N	NIA

?, may be effective in some cases; BSS, Bernard-Soulier syndrome; DDAVP, desmopressin; GT, Glanzmann thrombasthenia; N, no; NI, no information available; Y, yes.

themselves are responsible for bleeding because of concomitant thrombocytopenia. Two patients with myelodysplasia and an acquired Bernard-Soulier–like syndrome have been reported.[114,115] A patient has also been reported with a lymphoproliferative disorder and clinical bleeding; the patient had a prolonged bleeding time, normal platelet count and platelet morphology, and a circulating IgG antibody that inhibited ristocetin-induced platelet agglutination but was directed against an unidentified 210,000 mol wt platelet protein.[116] In *Platelet-Type von Willebrand disease*, mutations within the VWF binding domain of GPIbα induce spontaneous VWF binding to GPIbα and the clinical picture of Type IIB von Willebrand disease.[9,117,118]

Therapy

Treatment of hemorrhage in patients with the Bernard-Soulier syndrome usually requires platelet transfusion (Table 141–2). Hormonal control of menses has been effective in managing menorrhagia.[119] Splenectomy has been attempted to increase the platelet count[120] but has resulted in only transient increases and has not ameliorated the platelet function defect. Corticosteroids are not beneficial in this disorder. Desmopressin acetate (DDAVP) has been reported to shorten the bleeding time in some, but not all, affected individuals in whom it has been administered,[121–124] but its efficacy in patients with hemorrhage is unclear. Conversely, a number of anecdotal reports suggest that recombinant VIIa may be effective in the treatment of hemorrhage in Bernard-Soulier syndrome patients, but the degree of effectiveness has varied[125–129] Lastly, two sisters with the Bernard-Soulier syndrome and histories of significant bleeding were successfully treated by hematopoietic stem-cell transplantation.[130]

Platelet Collagen Receptors

Collagen plays an essential role in platelet function as a substrate for platelet adhesion, a binding site for VWF in the extracellular matrix, and an agonist for platelet aggregation and secretion. Although several platelet membrane proteins interact with collagen (including GPIIb,[131] GPIV,[132] a 65,000 mol wt protein that binds to type 1 collagen,[133] a 47,000 mol wt protein[134] and a 68,000/72,000 mol wt doublet[135] that bind to type III collagen, and a protein with a mol wt of 85,000 to 90,000[136]) only GPVI[137] and the integrin α2β1[138,139] are physiologic platelet receptors for collagen.

GPVI

GPVI, a 62,000 mol wt member of the immunoglobulin gene superfamily,[140,141] is associated with the γ chain of the Fc receptor in the plasma membrane of human platelets.[142] Exposure of normal platelets, but not GPVI-deficient platelets, to collagen or collagen-like peptides results in the tyrosine phosphorylation of the Fc receptor γ chain and the proteins SLP-76, Syk, Lyn, LAT, and phospholipase Cγ2, followed by platelet aggregation.[143,144] Murine platelets lacking either the Fc receptor γ chain or Syk are unable to respond to collagen[145] and the interaction of GPVI-deficient human platelets with either immobilized and soluble collagen is markedly impaired.

There are eight reports of patients whose platelet specifically lacked GPVI,[146] three of which concern patients with congenital GPVI deficiencies.[147–149] These patients had mild bleeding diatheses[147–149] and platelets that failed to aggregate following stimulation with collagen despite the presence of normal amounts of α2β1. However, the platelets of two retained some ability to adhere to collagen-coated surfaces.[148,149] A fourth patient has been reported with a more severe bleeding disorder that included epistaxis requiring transfusion, severe bleeding after trauma, and significant postpartum hemorrhage.[150] The platelets of this patient expressed GPVI and the FcR γ chain, but aggregated poorly in response to collagen, convulxin, and collagen-related peptide (CRP), as well as to heparin-induced thrombocytopenia antibodies, implying a defect in collagen-induced signaling downstream of the FcR γ chain. GPVI deficiency as been reported in conjunction with the gray platelet syndrome.[151] Four patients have been described, whose plasma contained autoantibodies against GPVI that inhibited collagen-induced platelet function,[152–155] as well as two patients, one with myelodysplasia and a second with chronic lymphocytic leukemia, whose platelets did not respond to collagen or convulxin but contained GPVI by flow cytometry.[156]

α2β1

α2β1 (GPIa-IIa, VLA-2) is a widely expressed integrin that binds with high affinity to type I collagen, as well as to collagen types II to V and to laminins 1 and 5, depending on the cellular context.[157] Besides platelets, α2β1 is present on endothelial cells, fibroblasts, epithelial cells, Schwann cells, and activated T cells.[158] α2β1 is one of nine integrins whose α subunit contains a 200 residue I-domain that is largely, if not exclusively, responsible for ligand binding.[159] The relative contributions of α2β1 and GPVI to collagen-initiated platelet function remains unclear. Current data suggest a model in which platelet tethering initiated by platelet GPIb-IX-V binding to collagen-bound VWF enables GPVI to bind to collagen and generate *outside-in* signals. In turn, these signals increase the affinity of α2β1 for collagen, resulting in platelet adhesion to collagen that is sufficiently firm to resist the shear stress of flowing blood.[139,160,161]

In support of a role for α2β1 in mediating physiologic platelet responses, several patients have been reported with platelets lacking α2β1 and failing to interact normally with collagen. Two patients were investigated because of the presence of a bleeding diathesis.

Platelets from the first contained approximately 15% to 25% of the normal amount of α2, failed to aggregate in response to collagen, and failed to adhere to collagen under both static and flow conditions.[162,163] Platelets from the second lacked α2 as well as the α granule protein thrombospondin, failed to aggregate in response to low concentrations of collagen, and adhered to, but did not spread on, collagen-coated surfaces.[164] Two families were also investigated because of autosomal dominant thrombocytopenia and mild cutaneous bleeding.[165] Platelets of affected family members expressed 38% to 63% of the normal amount of α2β1 and adhered poorly to collagen-coated surfaces, whereas collagen-induced platelet aggregation was either normal or only slightly perturbed.

There are also inherited differences in the density of α2β1 on the platelet surface that result from polymorphisms in the coding and promoter regions of the α2 gene.[166–168] In vitro studies suggest a positive correlation between α2β1 expression and platelet adhesion to type I and type III collagen.[169] In addition some, but not all, epidemiologic studies have suggested that increased α2β1 expression is a risk factor for myocardial infarction and stroke in younger individuals and for diabetic retinopathy in patients with type II diabetes mellitus.[170–176]

DISORDERS OF PLATELET AGGREGATION

Glanzmann Thrombasthenia (Glycoprotein IIb-IIIa Deficiency)

Originally described by Glanzmann in 1918,[177] thrombasthenia is a rare bleeding disorder characterized by a prolonged bleeding time, a normal platelet count, and absent macroscopic platelet aggregation.[178] Platelets from affected individuals are unable to aggregate because of a deficiency or dysfunction of the platelet membrane GPIIb-IIIa complex.[179]

Biology and Molecular Aspects of the Disorder

The formation of a hemostatically effective platelet plug requires platelet aggregation.[180] In contrast to platelet adhesion, platelet aggregation is an active metabolic process, requiring platelet stimulation by agonists such as thrombin, collagen, and ADP and exposure of a binding site for fibrinogen or VWF on the GPIIb-IIIa complex.[181–183] Fibrinogen or VWF bound to GPIIb-IIIa crosslinks adjacent platelets into an occlusive plug. The GPIIb-IIIa complex, also known as αIIbβ3, is a member of the integrin family of adhesion receptors[184] and like other members of this family, resides on the cell surface in an equilibrium between inactive (low affinity) and active (high affinity) conformations.[185] Platelet stimulation shifts GPIIb-IIIa to its active conformation, enabling it to bind ligands and mediate platelet aggregation.[185] Platelet stimulation also enables the interaction of the GPIIb-IIIa cytoplasmic tails with submembranous actin filaments via intermediary cytoskeletal proteins such as talin and α-actinin, thereby providing a mechanism for transmitting the force of cytoskeletal contraction to the fibrin clot resulting in clot retraction.[186,187]

GPIIb-IIIa is a calcium-dependent heterodimer and dissociates into GPIIb and GPIIIa monomers in the presence of calcium chelators.[188] By electron microscopy, the heterodimer appears as a 12 × 8 nm globular head with two 18 nm stalks extending from one side.[189] When incorporated into phospholipid vesicles, the globular head extends approximately 20 nm above the vesicle surface with the tips of the tails inserted into the phospholipid.[190]

GPIIb has an unreduced mol wt of 136,000 and dissociates into a 125,000 mol wt heavy chain (GPIIbα) and 23,000 mol wt light chain (GPIIbβ) following disulfide bond reduction.[188] GPIIbα binding to GPIIIa is responsible for heterodimer formation,[191] whereas GPIIbβ anchors GPIIb in the platelet membrane.[192] GPIIb is synthesized as single chain precursor (pro-GPIIb) in the rough endoplasmic reticulum (ER)[192] where it associates with GPIIIa. The resulting heterodimer is then transported to the Golgi complex where pro-GPIIb is cleaved into heavy and light chains.[193] In contrast to GPIIb, GPIIIa is a single chain protein containing 56 cysteine residues and 28 disulfide bonds;[194] its apparent mol wt of 90,000 on unreduced sodium dodecyl phosplate (SDS) gels increases to 110,000 following disulfide bond reduction.[188] The disulfide bonds in GPIIIa are concentrated in three regions of the extracellular portion of the molecule: a cysteine-rich, protease-resistant amino terminus (residues 1–62), a protease-sensitive central region (residues 101–422), and a disulfide-rich, protease-resistant core (residues 423–622).[195] In addition, there is a long-range disulfide bond between cysteine residues 5 and 435 that results in a large protease-sensitive loop.[196]

In the absence of heterodimer formation, GPIIb and GPIIIa monomers are retained in the ER and are eventually degraded.[197] The factors responsible for the retention of uncomplexed monomers are unknown. However, it is clear from studies of various thrombasthenic mutants that the formation of GPIIb-IIIa heterodimers alone is not sufficient to guarantee egress of GPIIb-IIIa from the ER.[197,198]

Platelets also express a second GPIIIa (β3)-containing integrin, the vitronectin receptor (αvβ3), whose αv subunit is highly homologous to GPIIb.[199] There are 50- to 500-fold fewer copies of αvβ3 than GPIIb-IIIa on platelets.[200,201] Moreover, GPIIb-IIIa expression is restricted to cells of the megakaryocytic lineage,[202] whereas αvβ3 is expressed by a variety of cells including endothelial cells, smooth muscle cells, and osteoclasts.[203] The extracellular portions of αvβ3 and GPIIb-IIIa have been crystallized and their structures solved.[204,205] The structures reveal that the amino terminus of αv and GPIIb fold into a β-propeller, as had been predicted.[206] The β-propeller is followed by *thigh* and two *calf* domains with a flexible *genu* between the thigh and first calf domains. The GPIIIa head consists of a βA domain whose fold resembles that of integrin α subunit *I-domains* and contains a metal ion binding or MIDAS motif. The interface between the β-propeller and the βA domain is the site at which αv and GPIIb interact with the β3 and resembles the interface between the Gα and Gβ subunits of G proteins. The remainder of the extracellular portion of GPIIIa consists of plexin semaphorin integrin (PSI) domain, four tandem epideimal growth factor (EGF) repeats, and a relatively unique carboxyl-terminal βTD domain. In the crystal structure of αvβ3, the molecule is severely bent because of the flexibility of the αv and GPIIIa stalks. Thus, it has been proposed that when αvβ3 (and by analogy GPIIb-IIIa) is activated, the molecule straightens to resemble the molecules visualized by electron microscopy.[189,204,207]

Etiology and Pathogenesis

There are approximately 80,000 copies of GPIIb-IIIa on the surface of unstimulated platelets.[208] Glanzmann thrombasthenia results when platelets lack sufficient numbers of functional GPIIb-IIIa complexes to support platelet aggregation.[179] However, the platelets of obligate thrombasthenic heterozygotes aggregate normally, indicating that 50% of the normal amount of GPIIb-IIIa is at least sufficient to support platelet aggregation.[209]

GPIIb-IIIa deficiency is responsible for additional abnormalities of platelet function. Thrombasthenic platelets do not spread normally on the subendothelial matrix, an aspect of platelet adhesion that is mediated by GPIIb-IIIa binding to fibronectin and VWF.[210] The amount of fibrinogen in the α granules of thrombasthenic platelets is decreased to absent.[178] Because human megakaryocytes do not synthesize fibrinogen,[211] α granule fibrinogen is derived from plasma by a GPIIb-IIIa-mediated endocytic process.[212–215] Thus, the absence of functional GPIIb-IIIa on thrombasthenic platelets accounts for their deficit in α granule fibrinogen. Several biochemical reactions in platelets that require the presence of GPIIb-IIIa are impaired in thrombasthenic platelets. For example, the tyrosine phosphorylation of multiple platelet proteins, including proteins with molecular weights of 140,000 and 50,000 to 68,000, depends on ligand binding to GPIIb-IIIa; and the tyrosine phosphorylation of proteins such as pp125FAK as well as proteins with molecular weights of 95,000 to 97,000 requires platelet aggregation.[216] Calpain, a calcium-dependent thiol protease, is activated when stirred normal platelets are stimulated by thrombin, but not when thrombasthenic platelets are treated in a similar manner.[217] The redistribution of several proteins, including spectrin, talin, vinculin, pp60(src), and p62(yes), to a detergent-insoluble platelet cytoskeleton follows thrombin-stimulated platelet aggregation; but it does not occur when thrombasthenic platelets are treated in this way.[218] The kinetics of calcium exchange in unstimulated thrombasthenic platelets is inexplicably decreased[219] because it is unclear what role, if any, GPIIb-IIIa plays in calcium transport.[220,221] Clot retraction in blood containing thrombasthenic platelets is either absent or reduced,[178] a finding consistent with the ability of GPIIb-IIIa to link the fibrin clot to the platelet cytoskeleton.[186]

Aspects of platelet function that do not depend on GPIIb-IIIa are normal in thrombasthenia. Thrombasthenic platelets interact normally with collagen fibrils[222] and undergo secretion when stimulated by "strong agonists" such as thrombin.[223] Incubation of thrombasthenic platelets with ristocetin induces VWF binding to GPIb-IX-V[10] and thrombasthenic platelets adhere to VWF in the subendothelium.[210] Thrombasthenic platelets also express normal amounts of procoagulant activity following lysis.[52] However, agonist-stimulated prothrombinase activity varies and is influenced by the nature of platelet agonist.[52,224]

Table 141–3 Mutations That Impair GPIIb-IIIa Function

Mutation	Affected Subunit	Reference
Tyr143His	GPIIb	242
Arg-Thr insertion into the Cys146-Cys167 loop	GPIIb	257
Arg995Gln	GPIIb	258
Cys560Arg	GPIIIa	255
Arg214Gln	GPIIIa	247
Ser752Pro	GPIIIa	250–252
Asp119Tyr	GPIIIa	243
Val193Met	GPIIIa	244
Arg214Trp	GPIIIa	245, 246
Ser123Pro	GPIIIa	253
Cys560Phe	GPIIIa	254
Cys560Arg	GPIIIa	255
Cys579Ser	GPIIIa	254
Arg724Stop	GPIIIa	256

Genetic Aspects

The genes for GPIIb and GPIIIa are located on the long arm of chromosome 17 at q21→23[225] with the GPIIb gene a minimum distance of 365 kb downstream from the GPIIIa gene.[226] The GPIIb gene (*ITGA2B*) spans approximately 18 kb, is located in a region that contains at least 7 complete and 3 incomplete Alu repeats, and consists of 30 exons ranging in size from 46 bp to 220 bp.[227] Like the genes for other proteins expressed in megakaryocytes, its 5′ flanking region lacks TATA or CAAT boxes. Instead it contains a linear array of regulatory elements that includes two motifs recognized by the GATA-1 transcription factor and its cofactor FOG;[228,229] sequences flanking each GATA-1 binding site that are recognized by Fli-1 and perhaps other members of the Ets family of transcription factors;[230–233] and an Sp1-binding silencer element located between the GATA-1 sites.[234] In addition, regions located 2.5 to 7.1 kb upstream and 2.2 to 7.4 kb downstream from the GPIIb gene are necessary for consistent high level gene expression.[235] The gene for GPIIIa (*ITGB3*) spans 63 kb and contains 15 exons.[236,237] Like the GPIIb gene, the 5′ flanking region of the GPIIIa gene lacks TATA or CAAT boxes.[238] Specific regulatory motifs that control GPIIIa gene expression in megakaryocytes have not been identified. Although the organization of exons in many genes reflects the distribution of functional domains in the protein they encode, this does not appear to be true for either the GPIIb or the GPIIIa gene.

Glanzmann thrombasthenia is an autosomal recessive disorder with clusters of disease in populations where consanguinity is common and has been subclassified into three types based on the amount of GPIIb-IIIa present per platelet and the presence or absence of α granule fibrinogen and clot retraction.[178] In type I, platelets contain less than 5% of the normal amount of GPIIb-IIIa and clot retraction and α granule fibrinogen are absent. In type II, platelets contain 10% to 20% of the normal amount of GPIIb-IIIa, clot retraction is decreased, and α granule fibrinogen is present. In *variant* thrombasthenia, the platelet content of GPIIb-IIIa equals 50% of normal, indicating that the GPIIb-IIIa abnormality is qualitative, rather than quantitative.

Expression of GPIIb-IIIa on the platelet surface requires the formation of correctly folded GPIIb-IIIa heterodimers in the ER of megakaryocytes.[239] Thus, a mutation in the gene for either GPIIb or GPIIIa can impair GPIIb-IIIa expression and produce thrombasthenia, observations confirmed in murine models of GPIIb-IIIa deficiency.[240,241] At least 126 unique mutations responsible for thrombasthenia have been identified in the genes for GPIIb and GPIIIa, 68 in *ITGA2B*, and 58 in *ITGB3*. Many mutations are listed in a Glanzmann thrombasthenia database that can be queried at http://sinaicentral.mssm.edu/intranet/research/glanzmann/menu. The mutations are a mix of missense mutations (52%), nonsense mutations (14%), nucleotide deletions and insertions (28%), and alternative splicing (6%). Most mutations result in Type I and Type II thrombasthenia, but several have resulted in *variant thrombasthenia* where the GPIIb-IIIa abnormality is qualitative rather than quantitative (Table 141–3). Five such mutations (Tyr143His in GPIIb[242] and Asp119Tyr,[243] Val193Met,[244] Arg214Trp,[245,246] and Arg214Gln[247] in GPIIIa) are located in regions of GPIIb-IIIa that have been implicated in ligand binding and may perturb GPIIb-IIIa function by preventing its interaction with fibrinogen or VWF.[248,249] A sixth mutation, a Ser752Pro substitution in the cytoplasmic tail of GPIIIa, inexplicably prevents GPIIb-IIIa activation by cellular agonists.[250–252] A seventh mutation in GPIIIa, Ser123Pro, did not impair GPIIb-IIIa expression or agonist-induced ligand binding but was associated with absent ADP- and collagen-induced platelet aggregation.[253] In addition, three mutations involving cysteine residues located at the third and fourth EGF domains of GPIIIa (Cys560Phe,[254] Cys560Arg,[255] and Cys579Ser[254]) resulted in type II thrombasthenia and also induced constitutive ligand binding activity in the residual GPIIb-IIIa.

Four nonvariant mutations in GPIIb and GPIIIa are also noteworthy. In the first, the codon for Arg724 in GPIIIa is converted to a stop codon, resulting the synthesis of a truncated molecule lacking 39 carboxyl-terminal amino acids and the assembly of GPIIb-IIIa heterodimers that are unable to transduce inside-out and outside-in signals.[256] In the second, the insertion of two amino acids (arginine and threonine) into the Cys146-Cys167 loop of GPIIb results in an inactive thrombasthenic variant,[257] attesting to the importance of this region of GPIIb in ligand binding. In the third, an Arg995Gln mutation in the conserved GFFKR motif of the GPIIb cytoplasmic tail resulted in *poor*, but not absent, platelet aggregation,[258] in contrast to the constitutive GPIIb-IIIa activation predicted from disruption of a activation-constraining cytoplasmic clamp.[259] In the fourth, a Cys560Arg mutation in GPIIIa locked GPIIb-IIIa in a high-affinity conformation but produced a thrombasthenic-phenotype, perhaps because the low number of constitutively active GPIIb-IIIa complexes expressed on the platelet surface were insufficient to support platelet aggregation.[255]

Clinical Presentation

The clinical manifestations of thrombasthenia in a large cohort of patients have been described in detail.[178] Thrombasthenia typically presents with mucocutaneous bleeding during the neonatal period or infancy, occasionally with bleeding following circumcision. Spontaneous petechiae are uncommon and bleeding generally results from conditions that would cause bleeding in an otherwise normal individual. Next to purpura, epistaxis is the most frequent type of bleeding, especially during childhood. Gingival bleeding, often related to poor dental hygiene, and menorrhagia are frequent. Bleeding at menarche may be severe and require transfusion. Similarly, parturition represents a severe hemorrhagic risk. Other hemorrhagic manifestations include gastrointestinal bleeding and hematuria, but hemarthroses and deep hematomas are unusual. Serious bleeding may follow trauma or surgery in patients not transfused with normal platelets. However, the severity of hemorrhage in thrombasthenia is unpredictable, even within single kindreds, and does not correlate with the extent of GPIIb-IIIa deficiency. Thus, one sibling may experience life-threatening bleeding requiring frequent transfusion, whereas another suffers only mild bruising and epistaxis. The apparent decline in the clinical severity of thrombasthenia with age is likely caused by a decrease in the incidence of conditions such as epistaxis with aging.

Laboratory Findings

Platelet counts and platelet morphology on peripheral blood smears are normal. The bleeding time of affected individuals is markedly prolonged.[222] A diagnosis of thrombasthenia is usually suspected after platelet aggregometry reveals absent agonist-stimulated platelet aggregation (see Fig. 141–1). Platelet secretion induced by strong agonists such as thrombin is normal, but secretion in response to weak agonists such ADP and epinephrine does not occur. Coagulation tests, such as the prothrombin time and the partial thromboplastin time, are normal in thrombasthenia, whereas clot retraction in the presence of thrombasthenic platelets is absent or reduced.

Differential Diagnosis

A history of lifelong bleeding, a prolonged bleeding time, and absent platelet aggregation are diagnostic of thrombasthenia and differentiate it from other disorders of platelet adhesion and secretion. Instances of acquired thrombasthenia have been reported and can be differentiated from congenital thrombasthenia by history. Although autoantibodies against GPIIb-IIIa have been detected frequently in patients with idiopathic thrombocytopenic purpura,[260,261] autoantibodies that induce a thrombasthenic-like state are unusual.[262–265] A patient with multiple myeloma has been reported whose $IgG_1\kappa$ paraprotein was directed against GPIIIa and inhibited GPIIb-IIIa function.[266] Congenital afibrinogenemia may be associated with a prolonged bleeding time and decreased in vitro platelet aggregation caused by the absence of sufficient fibrinogen to support normal platelet aggregation.[267]

Patients have also been reported who presented with a thrombasthenia-like phenotype, but whose GPIIb-IIIa abnormality is unclear. In one patient with variant thrombasthenia, GPIIb-IIIa was present but dissociated abnormally in the presence of low concentrations of EDTA.[268] The platelets of a second patient with a mild thrombasthenia-like illness aggregated poorly in response to ADP and other agonists and had a deficit in the surface pool, but not the internal pool, of GPIIb-IIIa.[269] Similarly, the platelets of a third reported patient contained a normal amount of GPIIb-IIIa but here unable to aggregate in response to the usual platelet agonists.[270] In the LAD-III/LAD-1/variant syndrome, patients manifest mucocutaneous bleeding and absent platelet aggregation, despite normal or nearly normal GPIIb/IIIa expression.[271–273] Concurrently, they suffer from recurrent and severe bacterial infections caused by defective leukocyte integrin function, implying that the syndrome results from a general defect in integrin activation. In some affected kindreds, defective expression of the Rap-1 activator CalDAG-GEFI has been detected in platelets and leukocytes.[273,274] Moreover, disruption of the gene for CalDAG-GEFI in mice reproduces many of the features of the syndrome.[275] Thus, because Rap-1 has been implicated in the activation of both platelet and leukocyte integrins, it is likely that at least in some patients, CalDAG-GEFI deficiency is the abnormality responsible for the syndrome.

Therapy

The mainstay of treatment of bleeding in thrombasthenia is transfusion of normal platelets (see Table 141–2). Because bleeding is a life-long problem, use of HLA-matched platelets should be considered to lessen the chance of refractoriness to transfusion due to platelet alloimmunization. In rare instances thrombasthenic patients develop antibodies against normal GPIIb and GPIIIa following transfusion, potentially limiting the effectiveness of transfused platelets.[276,277] Protein A Sepharose immunoadsorption has been reported to restore the efficacy of transfused platelets in this situation.[278] Oral contraceptives have been useful in controlling menorrhagia. Regular dental care is essential in minimizing gingival bleeding. Fibrinolytic inhibitors such as epsilon aminocaproic acid or tranexamic acid, in addition to platelet transfusions, may help control bleeding after dental extractions. Corticosteroids are not efficacious in managing bleeding in thrombasthenic patients.[222] Although DDAVP has been reported to shorten the bleeding time in a patient with thrombasthenia and to have a beneficial effect during minor dental surgery,[121] this is the only report of an effect of DDAVP in thrombasthenia.[279] Recombinant factor VIIa has been found to be efficacious for the treatment of bleeding episodes and for obtaining surgical hemostasis in thrombasthenic patients, particularly in patients who have developed alloantibodies from prior platelet transfusions.[280–282] Lastly, the thrombasthenia of five affected individuals has been corrected by bone marrow transplantation.[283–286]

DISORDERS OF PLATELET SECRETION

Platelets contain four types of granules: dense granules containing ADP, adenosine triphosphate (ATP), calcium, serotonin, and pyrophosphate; α granules containing a variety of proteins, some derived from the plasma, others synthesized by the megakaryocyte; lysosomes containing acid hydrolases; and microperoxisomes containing a peroxidase activity. Following platelet activation, the contents of these granules are extruded in an exocytic process known as *platelet secretion*.[287] Inherited disorders of platelet secretion result from a deficiency of one or more of the types of platelet granules or from abnormalities in the platelet secretory mechanism. Secretion disorders are a frequent cause of mild to moderate bleeding manifested by easy bruising, menorrhagia, and excessive postoperative and postpartum blood loss. In one group of 145 patients presenting with such symptoms, 18% were found to have a deficiency of platelet granules, 19% to have an abnormality in the platelet secretory mechanism, and 36% to have von Willebrand disease.[288] No explanation for the bleeding diathesis could be found in 27% of the patients. Patients with platelet secretion disorders usually have a prolonged bleeding time, absence of the second wave of platelet aggregation when platelets are stimulated by ADP and epinephrine, and decreased aggregation when platelets are stimulated by collagen. These disorders must be differentiated from the acquired abnormalities of platelet secretion induced by drugs such as aspirin or systemic diseases such as uremia and multiple myeloma (see Chapter 142) and from the various types of von Willebrand disease (see Chapter 129).

DISORDERS OF SECRETION CAUSED BY ABNORMALITIES OF PLATELET α GRANULES

The Gray Platelet Syndrome (α Granule Deficiency)

The gray platelet syndrome, described by Raccuglia in 1971,[94] is a rare disorder that results from the specific absence of morphologically recognizable α granules in the platelets of affected individuals.

Biology and Molecular Aspects of the Disorder

Normal platelets contain approximately 50 spherical or elongated structures termed α *granules* that contain a variety of proteins, some of which are specific or relatively specific for platelets and others that are also found in plasma.[289] The former include platelet factor 4 (PF4) , β-thromboglobulin (βTG), platelet-derived growth factor, and thrombospondin and the latter include fibrinogen, VWF, albumin, coagulation factor V, IgG, fibronectin, and a number of protease inhibitors.[290] The platelet-specific proteins and several of the plasma proteins such as VWF[291] are synthesized by megakaryocytes, whereas others reach the α granules via endocytosis of circulating protein.[292] The α granule membrane contains many of the same proteins present in the platelet plasma membrane (GPIIb-IIIa[293] and GPIb-IX-V)[294] and others specific for α granules (P-selectin[295,296] and osteonectin).[297] Each can be translocated to the platelet surface following platelet activation.

Etiology and Pathogenesis

Electron micrographs of megakaryocytes and platelets from patients with the gray platelet syndrome reveal absence of normal α granules[298] and the presence of vacuoles and small α granule precursors containing material that stains for VWF and fibrinogen.[299] The other types of platelet granules are present in normal numbers. The outer membranes of the vacuoles and small α granule precursors contain P-selectin and GPIIb-IIIa which can be translocated to the platelet surface after thrombin stimulation.[293,300] These observations indicate that α granules are present in gray platelets and suggest that the abnormality responsible for the gray platelet syndrome is an inability to target proteins to these structures.[301] The inability to package and retain PF4, βTG, and platelet-derived growth factor in α granules would account for the elevated plasma concentrations of PF4 and βTG and the bone marrow fibrosis observed in patients with the syndrome.[302] The abnormality responsible for the gray platelet syndromes appears to be restricted to megakaryocytes because electron micrographs of endothelial cells from affected patients reveal typical Weibel-Palade bodies suggesting that these cells are capable of packing VWF normally.[303] A report of three children with the gray platelet syndrome whose neutrophils also had a gray appearance caused by a decrease in secondary granules suggests that the abnormality responsible for the gray platelet syndrome could also affect other blood cell lines.[304] However, in another report of five affected individuals, neutrophil granularity was normal,[305] suggesting that either the gray platelet syndrome is heterogenous or that the three reported children suffer from a unique familial hypogranular neutrophil and platelet disorder. With regard to the former possibility, two macrothrombocytopenic disorders resembling the gray platelet syndrome have been described. In the White platelet syndrome, autosomal dominant macrothrombocytopenia was associated with mild to moderate bleeding, defective platelet aggregation, incomplete α granule formation, and 30% or more gray-appearing platelets on blood smears.[306] In the Medich giant platelet disorder, macrothrombocytopenia was associated with a marked decrease in platelet α granules. In contrast to classic gray platelets, empty vacuoles without granule contents were not present in the platelet cytoplasm but were replaced by membranous inclusions resembling cigars or scrolls.[307]

Clinical Presentation and Laboratory Findings

Patients with the gray platelet syndrome present with a lifelong history of mild to moderate mucocutaneous bleeding,[308] but one patient developed subgaleal and epidural hematomas following head trauma.[309] Patients also exhibit variably prolonged bleeding times, moderate thrombocytopenia, reticulin fibrosis of the bone marrow, and large platelets whose gray appearance on a Wright-stained blood smear gives the name to the disorder.[94,95] Platelet counts vary from 25,000 to 150,000/μl, but generally range between 60,000 and 100,000/μl. Studies of platelet aggregation have produced variable results. Aggregation induced by ADP, epinephrine, arachidonic acid, and the calcium ionophore A23187 has generally been normal or nearly normal,[310] but collagen-induced aggregation has been reported to be decreased to absent in some, but not all, cases, perhaps due to an associated deficiency of GPVI.[95,151,309] Responses to thrombin have also been variable, with reports of decreased aggregation and secretion in response to low thrombin concentrations,[95,310–312] impaired increments in intracellular calcium[313] and decreased generation of inositol-1,4,5-triphosphate.[314] Gray platelets agglutinate normally when exposed to ristocetin and the content of their dense granules is normal.[315] As expected, the PF4, βTG, fibrinogen, VWF, factor V, fibronectin, and thrombospondin content of gray platelet α granules is markedly decreased. Surprisingly, gray platelets contain substantial quantities of albumin and IgG,[316] proteins normally present in α granules. The PF4 and βTG concentrations in the plasma of affected individuals are normal or elevated.[95,310]

Genetic Aspects

Genetic analysis of families with the gray platelet syndrome support the possibility that platelet α granule deficiency may be a heterogenous disorder. Falik-Zaccai and colleagues reported 59 cases of the gray platelet syndrome.[308] Although the presence of the disorder in males and females in the same family suggested that it is an autosomal disease, its mode of inheritance remains uncertain. For example, a family has been reported in which the gray platelet syndrome was inherited in an X-linked fashion and associated with an Arg216Gln mutation in the *GATA1* gene.[317] A disorder resembling the gray platelet syndrome is present in the Wistar Furth strain of rat and is inherited as an autosomal recessive.[318] Hematopoietic zinc finger (*HZF*) null mice also have features resembling the gray platelet syndrome, but sequence analysis of the *HZF* gene and studies of *HZF* protein expression in five gray platelet syndrome patients from three different families did not identify abnormalities in this gene.[319]

Therapy

Treatment of severe bleeding episodes may require the transfusion of normal platelets (see Table 141–2). DDAVP was found to shorten the bleeding time in one patient and was used as successful prophylaxis for a dental extraction.[320]

The Quebec Platelet Disorder (Factor V Quebec)

Two unrelated families with an autosomal dominant bleeding disorder of moderate severity have been identified in Quebec.[321–323] Their disorder is characterized by mild thrombocytopenia, defective epinephrine-induced platelet aggregation, a decrease in the amount of multiple α granule proteins, and bleeding unresponsive to platelet transfusion, but controlled by fibrinolytic inhibitors. The disorder in the index family was initially attributed to a decrease in platelet factor V, hence the name Factor V Quebec.[324] In contrast to the gray platelet syndrome, the α granules in platelets of the Quebec platelet disorder appear to be morphologically normal.[322] However, the amount of α granule proteins, including factor V, multimerin, fibrinogen, VWF, fibronectin, osteonectin, and thrombospondin, is decreased and many are substantially degraded.[322] Further, analysis of α granule proteolytic activity revealed that the ectopic expression of urokinase-type plasminogen activator in α granules is responsible for the biochemical and clinical features of the disorder.[325,326] The basis for the ectopic expression of urokinase-type plasminogen activator is unknown.[327] A patient with a longstanding bleeding disorder has also been reported with platelets containing a reduced amount of α granule factor V but no evidence of ectopic α granule proteolytic activity, indicating that some other process was responsible for the reduction in α granule factor V.[328]

DISORDERS OF SECRETION DUE TO DEFICIENCY OF PLATELET DENSE GRANULES

Dense Granule Deficiency (δ-Storage Pool Disease)

Biology and Molecular Aspects of the Disorder

Normal platelets contain three to six 200 to 300 nm dense or δ granules that serve as intracellular storage sites for ADP, ATP, calcium, pyrophosphate, and serotonin.[329] Because of their high calcium content, δ granules can be visualized in electron micrographs of unfixed, unstained platelet whole mounts.[329] They can also be visualized by electron microscopy of thin sections of fixed platelets after staining with uranyl ions (uranaffin reaction) and by fluorescence microscopy after staining platelets with mepacrine (quinacrine).[329] The δ granule membrane contains a 40,000 mol wt protein named granulophysin (CD63) that is translocated to the platelet surface following platelet activation[330] and corresponds to the melanoma-associated antigen ME491, the lysosomal membrane protein-1 (LIMP-1), and the lysosomal membrane-associated protein-3 (LIMP-3).[331] The δ granule membrane also contains P-selectin, GPIb, and GPIIb-IIIa.[332] δ Granules undergo exocytosis coincident with the second wave of platelet aggregation (see Fig. 141–1).[333] ADP secreted from δ granules is thought to be involved in propagation of the primary platelet response;[334,335] the function of the other δ granule contents is presently unknown.

Platelet δ granules are related to a group of lysosome-related granules including melanosomes, neutrophil azurophilic granules, the lytic granules of cytotoxic T lymphocytes and natural killer cells, basophilic granules in basophils and mast cells, and class II major histocompatibility complex compartments in antigen-presenting cells.[331,336] The biogenesis of δ granules in megakaryocytes is poorly understood. However, δ-storage pool deficiency occurs in tyrosinase-positive albinism in humans[331]; pigment dilution syndromes in mice and rats[331]; and as part of a Chediak-Higashi–like syndrome in cattle, cats, mink, foxes and killer whales,[337] implying that that the biogenesis of dense granules, melanosomes, and lysosomes is related. How dense granules accumulate ATP and ADP is also unknown. One candidate for mediating ATP and ADP accumulation is MRP4 (multidrug resistance protein 4, ABCC4), a nucleotide transport pump, because it colocalizes with dense granules by immunofluorescence microscopy and its distribution is altered in dense granule-deficient platelets.[338] A second candidate is the gene *Slc35d3*, a nucleotide sugar transporter, that was identified in a strain of hypopigmented ashen mice (a model of the human Griscelli syndrome[339]) that independently developed platelet dense granule deficiency.[340]

Normal platelets contain two pools of adenine nucleotides that exchange slowly, if at all.[341] One pool is a metabolic nongranule pool in which the ratio of ATP : ADP content is 8 : 1 to 10 : 1. The second pool is present in the δ granules and contains 65% of the platelet adenine nucleotides with an ATP : ADP ratio of 2 : 3. Thus, in normal platelets, the whole platelet ATP : ADP ratio is less than 2.5. Conversely, serotonin is not synthesized by megakaryocytes, but it is taken up from the plasma and stored in the δ granules where it is protected from platelet monoamine oxidase.[342]

Etiology and Pathogenesis

δ-Storage pool disease is a heterogeneous group of disorders with δ granule deficiency as the common feature. The disorder can be subdivided into deficiency states associated with albinism and those in otherwise normal individuals.[343] δ-Storage pool disease has been reported in some patients with the Wiskott-Aldrich syndrome/X-linked thrombocytopenia,[344,345] the syndrome of thrombocytopenia with absent radii,[346] Ehlers-Danlos syndrome,[347] and osteogenesis imperfecta.[348] When δ-storage pool disease is associated with albinism, as in the Hermansky-Pudlak syndrome (HPS) (oculocutaneous tyrosinase-positive albinism, platelet dense granule deficiency, ceroid-like inclusions in cells of the reticuloendothelial system, progressive pulmonary fibrosis, and granulomatous colitis)[331] and the Chediak-Higashi syndrome (CHS) (partial oculocutaneous albinism, frequent pyogenic infections, and giant lysosomal granules in cells of hematologic and non-hematologic origin),[337] there is a quantitative deficiency of δ granules. In the platelets of nonalbinos, however, the number of uranaffin- and mepacrine-positive granules is normal to only slightly decreased, suggesting an inability to package the δ granule contents.[349,350] The platelet content of granulophysin also parallels the apparent number of δ granules in storage pool–deficient patients, being low in patients with the HPS and CHS, but normal in nonalbinos.[351] In some nonalbino patients, the δ granule abnormality is also associated with a variable deficiency of α granules (αδ-storage pool disease).[352,353] Although the content of lysosomal acid hydrolases in platelets from patients with δ-storage pool disease is normal, thrombin-induced acid hydrolase secretion may be impaired in severely affected individuals, an abnormality that can be corrected by the addition of ADP in vitro.[335] The ability of δ-storage pool–deficient platelets to form thrombi on the subendothelium has been studied ex vivo under various conditions of shear.[210] Thrombus dimensions are reduced in proportion to the magnitude of the dense granule deficit and are reduced even further when αδ-storage pool disease platelets are examined, suggesting that δ and α granule contents either potentiate thrombus growth on the subendothelium or help to stabilize thrombi in the presence of high shear stress.

Clinical and Laboratory Findings

Patients with δ-storage pool disease have a mild to moderate bleeding diathesis characteristic of patients with platelet secretion defects. Platelet counts and morphology are usually normal and bleeding times are usually prolonged.[288] Further, the volume of blood emerging from bleeding time wounds is increased over normal, particularly at early time points,[354] suggesting that δ granule contents may be involved in the contraction that follows vascular transection. The quantity of thromboxane B_2, a metabolite of thromboxane A_2, in the collected blood is also decreased, especially in patients with αδ-storage pool disease, a finding consistent the impaired agonist-induced prostaglandin and thromboxane synthesis often detected in these platelets.[355] Aggregometer tracings of δ-storage pool–deficient platelets stimulated by weak agonists such as ADP and epinephrine usually lack a second wave of aggregation (see Fig. 141–1).[356] Responses to low concentrations of collagen are also diminished to absent, but responses to high collagen concentrations may be normal or nearly normal.[357] Although this pattern of aggregation is typical for δ-storage pool disease, patients have been reported with normal aggregation studies.[288] The steady-state serotonin content of δ-storage pool–deficient platelets is decreased even though the rate of uptake of serotonin is normal,[341] because without storage sites, the serotonin either leaks out of the platelet or is metabolized by platelet monoamine oxidase. In δ-storage pool deficiency, the dense granule pool of ADP no longer contributes to the whole platelet content of ADP and the ATP : ADP ratio of δ-storage pool–deficient platelets is 3.0 or greater. This alteration in ATP : ADP ratio is extremely helpful in the diagnosis of δ-storage pool deficiency, especially when the typical aggregation abnormalities are absent.[288] Flow cytometry of mepa-

Table 141–4 Hermansky-Pudlak Syndrome Subtypes[360,361]

Human Subtype	Mouse Mutation	Affected Gene	Protein Complex	Reference
HPS-1	Pale ear	*HSP1*	BLOC-3	360–362, 367, 368
HPS-2	Pearl	*AP3B1*	AP-3	372, 374, 375
HPS-3	Cocoa	*HPS3*	BLOC-2	377, 378
HPS-4	Light ear	*HPS4*	BLOC-3	371
HPS-5	Ruby eye-2	*HPS5*	BLOC-2	379, 380
HPS-6	Ruby eye	*HPS6*	BLOC-2	380, 381
HPS-7	Sandy	*DTNBP1*	BLOC-1	383
HPS-8	Reduced Pigmentation	*BLOC1S3*	BLOC-1	386

crine-labeled platelets may be a rapid method to detect δ-storage pool–deficient platelets,[358,359] but its sensitivity compared to measurement of the ATP : ADP ratio has not been tested.

Genetic Aspects

HPS and CHS are inherited as autosomal recessive disorders.[331,337] There are eight known human HPS genes and fifteen genetically distinct strains of mice have phenotypes similar to human HPS.[360,361] Moreover, eight of the mutant mouse genes are orthologs of the human HPS genes (Table 141–4). HPS-1, the HPS prototype, although rare in the general population, occurs with a frequency of 1 in 1800 in northwest Puerto Rico.[362,363] It is also one of the most common causes of oculocutaneous albinism in Japanese.[364] Besides δ-storage pool disease and tyrosinase-positive albinism, patients with HPS-1 suffer from decreased visual acuity, nystagmus, granulomatous colitis, and usually fatal pulmonary fibrosis.[365,366] HPS-1 results from mutations in a gene located on human chromosome 10q23.1–23.3 that encodes an 80,000 mol wt protein and corresponds to the gene responsible for the mouse mutant *pale ear*.[362,367,368] HPS-1 in Puerto Rico results from a 16-bp duplication in exon 15 of *HPS-1*[369] and at least 22 additional mutations have been identified in non-Puerto Ricans.[361] The HPS-1 protein is one component of a cytosolic and membrane-bound complex (BLOC-3, biogenesis of lysosome-related organelles complex 3) that also contains the 77,000 mol wt protein that is mutated in HPS-4.[360] Thus, the HPS-1 and HPS-4 proteins participate in the same step in vesicle development, and the phenotypes of patients with HPS-1 and HPS-4 are similar.[370] The gene mutated in HPS-4 corresponds to the gene involved in the mouse mutant *light ear*.[371] HPS-2 results from mutations in *ADTB3A*, the gene encoding the β3A subunit of the adaptor complex AP-3; mutations in this gene are also responsible for the mouse mutant *pearl*.[372] The AP-3 complex contains four subunits (δ, β3A, μ3A, and σ3), interacts with clathrin, and is thought to recruit cargo proteins to newly formed vesicles.[373] Patients with HPS-2 have phenotypes ranging from mild to severe and are distinguished from other HPS mutants by the presence of neutropenia and recurrent childhood infections.[372,374,375] HPS-3, a relatively mild form of HPS,[376] is the human homologue of the mouse mutant *cocoa*.[377] HPS-3 results from mutation of a gene located on human chromosome 3q24 encoding a 113,700 mol wt protein of unknown function.[378] HPS-5 results from mutation of a gene located on chromosome 11p14 and has been identified in five patients who manifested hypopigmentation and platelet storage pool disease without colitis or pulmonary fibrosis.[379] HPS-6, detected in a single patient from Belgium[380] and 20 individuals from an extended Israeli Bedouin family,[381] produces a phenotype similar to HPS-5 and results from mutation of the HPS6 gene located on chromosome 10q24.1-q25.1.[381] HPS-5 and HPS-6 correspond to the mouse mutants *ruby-eye 2* and *ruby-eye*, respectively.[380] Like HPS 1 and 4, the similarity of the phenotypes of HPS3, HPS5, and HPS6 suggest the responsible genes act within the same pathway. In support of this suggestion, biochemical studies indicate that HPS3, HPS5, and HPS6 interact to form a multisubunit complex called BLOC-2.[382] HPS-7, identified in a Portuguese woman with mild HPS, results from a mutation in the gene for dysbindin, mutation of which is also responsible for the mouse mutant *sandy*.[383] Dysbindin is a component of the BLOC-1 complex that also contains the proteins pallidin, muted, and cappuccino, each of which is associated with a variant of murine HPS.[384,385] HPS-8 was identified in a large consanguineous Pakistani family that presented with incomplete oculocutaneous albinism and platelet storage pool disease and was found to be caused by a frameshift mutation in the gene *BLOC1S3*, another component of the BLOC-1 complex.[386] Although the function of BLOC-1, BLOC-2, BLOC-3, and AP-3 in the biogenesis of platelet δ granules is not known, BLOC-1 and AP-3 have been shown to physically associate and to facilitate the trafficking of melanosomal membrane protein tyrosinase-related protein 1.[387] Similarly, BLOC-1 has been found to associate with BLOC-2 where it participates in a cargo transport pathway from early endosomes to melanosomes.[387,388]

CHS results from mutations in the gene *CHS1* (*LYST*) located on human chromosome 1q42–q43.[389,390] *CHS1* is the ortholog of the murine *bg* gene, mutation of which is responsible for the beige mouse.[390] *CHS1* encodes a 430,000 mol wt cytosolic protein whose role in normal lysosome development is unknown.[337] There appears to be a genotype–phenotype correlation between various *CHS1* mutations and the clinical course of CHS.[391–393] Thus, mutations that prevent the synthesis of the full-length CHS1 protein are associated with a severe childhood form of CHS that usually progresses to a fatal accelerated lymphoproliferative phase, often following infection with Epstein-Barr virus. Missense mutations, however, have been associated with a milder clinical course with less frequent infections and survival into adolescence and adulthood, but are associated with progressive neurologic deficits.

Therapy

Bleeding in patients with δ-storage pool disease can be controlled by the transfusion of normal platelets (see Table 141–2). However, this is seldom necessary because the potential risks of platelet transfusion far outweigh the benefits when bleeding is not life-threatening. Moreover, other methods to readily improve hemostasis without the risks of transfusion are available. Bleeding has been controlled by the administration of cryoprecipitate[394] or DDAVP.[395] The latter avoids the transfusion of blood products and should be regarded as the initial therapy of choice. DDAVP is a vasopressin analogue whose pressor effects (V_1 vasopressin receptors) are substantially less than its antidiuretic effects (V_2 vasopressin receptors). Infusion of the drug releases large multimers of VWF and tissue plasminogen activator from tissue stores.[279] The released VWF accounts for the beneficial effect of the drug on the bleeding time in some forms of von Willebrand disease. The precise mechanism of its ability to shorten the bleeding time in patients with platelet function disorders is uncertain. Nonetheless, in several series of patients with platelet disorders, shortening of the bleeding time in response to DDAVP occurred in 43% to 100% of patients.[395–397] This variability in response rate indicates that if DDAVP is to be used for surgical prophylaxis, a bleeding time must be obtained after the DDAVP infusion to insure that the patient has responded.

In a single unconfirmed study, prednisone at doses of 20 to 50 mg for 3 to 4 days was used to improve hemostasis in patients with inherited platelet disorders.[398] Shortening of the bleeding time was seen within 3 days and persisted for up to 3 to 7 days after the prednisone was stopped. However, prednisone was ineffective in shortening the bleeding time in patients with thrombasthenia[222] or in normal individuals given aspirin.[399] There are also reports suggesting that recombinant VIIa can be effective in managing bleeding in patients with storage pool disease.[126,400]

HPS, in particular the HPS-1 and HPS-4, is associated with progressive pulmonary fibrosis that is generally fatal by the fourth to sixth decades of life.[401] The pathogenesis of the fibrosis is uncertain, but it may result from the disruption of type II pneumocytes by ceroid, resulting in inflammation, cytokine production, and fibroblast proliferation.[401] The drug pirfenidone, an antifibrotic agent, has been reported to slow the progression of pulmonary fibrosis in patients with HPS.[402] One patient with HPS and pulmonary fibrosis was treated successfully by bilateral lung transplantation.[403]

Bone marrow transplantation has been effective in reversing the immunologic and hemostatic manifestations of CHS,[404] but surviving patients later develop neurologic deficits.[337]

DISORDERS OF SECRETION DUE TO AN ABNORMAL SECRETORY MECHANISM

In this uncommon group of disorders, platelet function resembles that of individuals who have been given platelet inhibitory drugs such as aspirin (see Fig. 141–1). Thus, there is marked impairment of aggregation and secretion in response to weak platelet agonists such as ADP, epinephrine, and low concentrations of collagen, whereas responses to stronger agonists such as higher concentrations of collagen may be normal or near normal. Bleeding times of patients with this type of secretion defect are usually prolonged. However, when the bleeding time is normal or only slightly prolonged, it may become markedly prolonged 2 hours after the ingestion of three aspirin tablets.[405]

Etiology and Pathogenesis

Stimulated platelets secrete the contents of their cytoplasmic granules by a process that involves granule convergence at the center of the platelet, fusion of the granule membranes with the membranes of the surface-connected open canalicular system, and extrusion of the granule contents into the platelet's external milieu.[287] This process requires coupling agonist receptors on the platelet surface to the effector systems responsible for platelet secretion and is discussed in detail in Chapter 116.

The disorders of platelet secretion discussed in this section represent a heterogeneous collection of abnormalities in stimulus-response coupling. In many instances, the evidence linking the reported biochemical abnormalities to defective platelet secretion is not definitive. Patients have been reported with platelets displaying abnormalities in arachidonic acid metabolism including impaired coupling of the thromboxane A_2 (TxA_2) receptor and phospholipase C,[406] as well as deficiencies of cyclooxygenase[407–412] and thromboxane synthetase.[413,414] Diminished platelet responsiveness to endogenous and exogenous TxA_2 has been attributed to abnormalities of platelet TxA_2 receptors.[415–417] An Arg 60 Leu mutation in the first cytoplasmic loop of the TxA_2 receptor, detected in five Japanese patients, impairs TxA_2-stimulated inositol-1,4,5-triphosphate formation, calcium mobilization, and phosphatidic acid formation without affecting TxA_2-binding.[418] Impaired platelet responsiveness to the calcium ionophores A23187[416,419,420] and ionomycin[421] has been reported, as has impaired GPIIb-IIIa activation and pleckstrin phosphorylation following platelet stimulation by multiple agonists caused by a mutation in the transcription factor CBFA2 that results in decreased expression of protein kinase C-θ.[422,423] A patient whose platelets responded poorly to ADP, epinephrine, collagen, thrombin, the TxA2 analogue U46619, and platelet-activating factor was found to have decreased platelet membrane GTPase activity caused by decreased expression of the gene for Gαq,[424,425] a phenotype that reproduces that of the Gαq-deficient mouse.[426] Another patient with a mild inherited bleeding disorder associated with abnormal platelet aggregation and secretion, reduced generation of inositol 1,4,5 trisphosphate, and reduced intracellular calcium mobilization was found to have a platelet-specific defect in phospholipase C-β2.[427,428] Several patients have been reported with platelets responding poorly to ADP because of defects in the Gαi-coupled ADP receptor $P2Y_{12}$.[429–435] A patient with a lifelong bleeding diathesis and platelets that responded poorly or not all to weak agonists was found to have reduced expression of the Gα subunit $G\alpha_{i1}$.[436] In addition, there are reports of patients whose platelets respond poorly to epinephrine[437–439] and to platelet-activating factor.[439,440] In one group of eleven patients with impaired platelet responses to low concentrations of collagen, eight were noted to have abnormal responses to other weak agonists, such as ADP, epinephrine, TxA_2, and the prostaglandin endoperoxide analogue U44169, but normal responses to strong agonists such as thrombin and high concentrations of collagen.[441] This suggests a defect in coupling weak agonist stimulation to secretion, rather than a defect in the secretory machinery itself. In the remaining patients, responses to strong agonists were abnormal and the platelets were unable to synthesize TxA_2.

Genetic Aspects

Most reports have been of individual patients so that determination of the mode of inheritance has not been possible. When families were studied, the mode of inheritance appeared to be autosomal dominant in some cases[409,411,414,415,437] and autosomal recessive in others.[442]

Therapy

The approach to therapy in patients with these disorders is identical to that described above for patients with disorders of platelet secretion due to deficiency of platelet dense granules (see Table 141–2).

DISORDERS OF PLATELET PROCOAGULANT ACTIVITY

The plasma membrane of activated platelets provides a surface for the assembly of the *tenase* and *prothrombinase* complexes that activate coagulation factor X and prothrombin, respectively (see Chapter 118). This procoagulant activity was previously termed *platelet factor 3*. Although there remains uncertainty whether specific membrane structures serve as receptors for this activity, it is clearly associated with a calcium-induced exposure of anionic phospholipids on the platelet surface.[443] The phospholipid composition of the platelet plasma membrane, like that of other cells, is asymmetric with phosphatidylcholine and sphingomyelin localized predominantly in the outer membrane leaflet and phosphatidylserine and phosphatidylethanolamine concentrated in the inner leaflet. This asymmetry is established by at least two enzymatic activities: *flippase*, an ATP-dependent aminophospholipid translocase[444,445] that directs the inward transporter of lipids and *floppase*, an ATP-requiring transporter encoded by the gene *ABCC1*, that directs the transport of choline- and amino-phospholipids to the outer leaflet.[443] Following an agonist-stimulated rise in intraplatelet Ca,$^{2+}$ membrane asymmetry is lost with exposure of anionic phospholipids on the platelet surface,[446] as well as on platelet membrane vesicles or microparticles,[447] events that may or may not be related.[448] A similar response to increased intracellular calcium has been detected in erythrocytes[449] and lymphocytes.[450] The rapid Ca^{2+}-induced movement of phospholipids between membrane leaflets may be mediated by a membrane-associated phospholipid *scramblase,* the precise identity of which remains unresolved.[451] One such candidate scramblase may be a proline-rich 37,000 mol wt type II membrane protein that is a member of a four-gene family[452] expressed by erythrocytes and platelets as well as a variety of hematologic and nonhematologic tissues and cell lines.[453] Although the redistribution of membrane phospholipids that accompanies apoptosis also requires scramblase activity, the development of platelet procoagulant activity and apoptotic membrane changes appear to operate through different pathways.[454]

Isolated deficiency of platelet procoagulant activity is exceedingly rare. In addition to the one well-studied patient after whom the disorder was named (Scott syndrome),[455] three additional patients have been reported.[224,456] A recessive disorder identical to the Scott syndrome has also been reported in a pedigree of German shepherd dogs.[457] The initial patient presented with a history of a spontaneous retroperitoneal hematoma and bleeding after surgery and dental procedures.[455] Although prothrombin and partial thromboplastin times, bleeding times, and platelet function studies were normal, serum prothrombin times were short and the patient's platelets were unable to express normal procoagulant activity. Although the patient's platelets secreted normal quantities of factor Va activity, they expressed only 20% to 25% of the normal number of factor Xa binding sites.[458] In addition, factor X activation by factor IXa and factor VIIIa was impaired, suggesting a concomitant deficiency of factor IXa and/or factor VIIIa binding sites.[459] When stimulated with the combination of thrombin and collagen, there was decreased exposure of anionic phospholipids on the platelet surface and decreased membrane vesiculation.[460–462] Similarly, there was decreased membrane vesiculation and procoagulant activity when the patient's erythrocytes were treated with the ionophore A23187.[449] Although membrane-associated phospholipid scramblase activity in the patient's platelets, erythrocytes, and lymphocytes was impaired, Ca^{2+} induced function of the isolated scramblase incorporated into proteoliposomes was indistinguishable from normal[451] and normal amounts of scramblase mRNA and protein were present in Scott syndrome lymphocytes.[463] This suggests that a reaction affecting scramblase function may be responsible for the syndrome. In support of this suggestion, decreased store-operated (capacitative) Ca^{2+} entry has been detected in a French patient.[464,465] Conversely, store-operated Ca^{2+} entry was unaffected in two unrelated patients,[466] whereas partial restoration of platelet procoagulant activity by valinomycin suggested a defect in the Gardos channel, a Ca^{2+} dependent K^+ channel.[467]

SUGGESTED READINGS

Arthur JF, Dunkley S, Andrews RK: Platelet glycoprotein VI-related clinical defects. Br J Haematol 139:363, 2007.

Bergmeier W, Goerge T, Wang HW, et al: Mice lacking the signaling molecule CalDAG-GEFI represent a model for leukocyte adhesion deficiency type III: J Clin Invest 117:1699, 2007.

Chintala S, Tan J, Gautam R, et al: The Slc35d3, gene, encoding an orphan nucleotide sugar transporter, regulates platelet-dense granules. Blood 109:1533, 2007.

De Candia E, Pecci A, Ciabattoni G, et al: Defective platelet responsiveness to thrombin and protease-activated receptors agonists in a novel case of gray platelet syndrome: Correlation between the platelet defect and the alpha-granule content in the patient and four relatives. J Thromb Haemost 5:551, 2007.

Dunkley S, Arthur JF, Evans S, Gardiner EE, Shen Y, Andrews RK: A familial platelet function disorder associated with abnormal signalling through the glycoprotein VI pathway. Br J Haematol 137:569, 2007.

Hacihanefioglu A, Tarkun P, Gonullu E: Use of recombinant factor VIIa in the management and prophylaxis of bleeding episodes in two patients with Bernard-Soulier syndrome. Thromb Res 120:455, 2007.

Kuijpers TW, van Bruggen R, Kamerbeek N, et al: Natural history and early diagnosis of LAD-1/variant syndrome. Blood 109:3529, 2007.

Pasvolsky R, Feigelson SW, Kilic SS, et al: A LAD-III syndrome is associated with defective expression of the Rap-1, activator CalDAG-GEFI in lymphocytes, neutrophils, and platelets. J Exp Med 204:1571, 2007.

Setty SR, Tenza D, Truschel ST, et al: BLOC-1, is required for cargo-specific sorting from vacuolar early endosomes toward lysosome-related organelles. Mol Biol Cell 18:768, 2007.

Tubman VN, Levine JE, Campagna DR, et al: X-linked gray platelet syndrome due to a GATA1, Arg216Gln mutation. Blood 109:3297, 2007.

Westbroek W, Adams D, Huizing M, et al: Cellular defects in Chediak-Higashi syndrome correlate with the molecular genotype and clinical phenotype. J Invest Dermatol 127:2674, 2007.

White JG, Keel S, Reyes M, Burris SM: Alpha-delta platelet storage pool deficiency in three generations. Platelets 18:1, 2007.

REFERENCES

For complete list of references log onto www.expertconsult.com

CHAPTER 142

ACQUIRED DISORDERS OF PLATELET FUNCTION

José A. López and Evelyn Lockhart

The acquired disorders of platelet function are among the most common of hematological abnormalities, a reflection of the sensitivities of platelets to external and internal perturbations. The clinical challenge in evaluating acquired disorders of platelet function is to determine whether observed derangements in platelet function pose a threat to the patient. Although platelet function can be altered to predispose to either hemostatic or thrombotic disorders, this chapter deals primarily, but not exclusively, with platelet disorders that may compromise hemostasis. We attempt also to guide the clinician in trying to determine the clinical importance of these disorders, but the marked variations in bleeding risks associated with any particular disorder of platelet function make this a difficult task. Bleeding in patients with acquired platelet dysfunction is likely to occur less frequently and predictably than in those affected by severe inherited platelet disorders such as Bernard-Soulier or Glanzmann thrombasthenia (see Chapter 141) and may manifest itself only in the setting of trauma or surgery or in the presence of additional hemostatic defects.

The laboratory evaluation of these patients may illuminate these disorders (see Chapter 122) but offer little concrete guidance in management. Acquired platelet defects (Table 142-1) often exhibit abnormal laboratory test results, such as a prolonged closure time on a platelet function analyzer or abnormal aggregation. Historically, the bleeding time has been used to evaluate bleeding risk in patients with jaundice or uremia; but it measures hemostasis only in one vascular bed (the skin) and bears inherent interoperator variability. These platelet assays are useful as a research tool; however, defects as quantified by laboratory tests, including the bleeding time, do not correlate precisely with risk for bleeding, and thus are not predictive of bleeding in these patients. Additionally, some acquired platelet disorders manifest with thrombosis, a risk that currently has no effective screening test. Lastly, tests that depend on assessing the functions of platelets ex vivo do not assess the contributions of labile substances from the endothelium (see Chapter 117) and occasionally (as in platelet aggregometry) lack the component of flow, a key factor with in vivo platelet function.

INTRINSIC DISORDERS OF PLATELET FUNCTION

Chronic Myeloproliferative Disorders

Clinical Features and Epidemiology

The myeloproliferative disorders (MPDs) include polycythemia rubra vera (PV), essential thrombocythemia (ET), and myelofibrosis with myeloid metaplasia. All three disorders are characterized by bone marrow hypercellularity, atypical megakaryocytic hyperplasia, and megakaryocyte clustering. Each chronic MPD is clonal, with the molecular lesion involving a hematopoietic stem cell. Thus, even when the phenotype is dominated by excessive proliferation of erythrocytes, such as in PV, the platelets are also products of the abnormal clone. Recent work from several laboratories has defined an important causative mutation in the disorder as producing a single, relatively conserved amino acid change (V617F) in the signaling protein JAK2.[1–5] This gain-of-function mutation is not present in the germ line but is acquired in hematopoietic stem cells, increasing the sensitivity of hematopoietic precursors to stimulation by erythropoietin and thrombopoietin, accounting for the increased red cell and platelets counts observed in the MPDs. It is estimated that this mutation can be found in 95% of patients afflicted with polycythemia vera and in 50% to 60% of those with essential thrombocythemia or idiopathic myelofibrosis (see Chapters 68, 70, 71).[6]

The MPDs all can display various degrees of leukocytosis or thrombocytosis; PV is often characterized by a marked elevation in the hematocrit. Particularly in PV and ET, thrombosis or bleeding account for a high percentage of the associated morbidity of the disorders, with thrombosis being the most frequent consequence. Thrombosis in PV and ET varies in location, with reports of arterial, venous, and microcirculatory locations; generally, arterial thrombosis is the most common.[7] Microcirculatory disturbances such as erythromelalgia, a syndrome of erythema and burning pain, are more frequently seen with ET, and result from platelet-rich arteriolar microthrombi that can lead to ischemia and gangrene. Bleeding in both PV and ET is primarily mucocutaneous. Some bleeding episodes can be in part attributed to thrombosis, such as variceal bleeding resulting from thrombosis-induced portal hypertension.[8] However, bleeding tendencies in these patients can be worsened by the use of aspirin as medical intervention for their thrombotic risks.

Polycythemia rubra vera in particular has been well studied in a large, prospective clinical study with respect to the risks of this disorder for hemorrhage and thrombosis. In the recently completed European Collaboration on Low-dose Aspirin in Polycythemia study, 633 (38.4%) of the 1638 patients enrolled had a history of thrombotic events. Of these cases, approximately three-quarters were arterial and one-quarter were venous. Of the former, ischemic stroke and transient ischemic attacks accounted for most events. The mean followup duration was 2.7 ± 1.3 years (range, 0–5.3 years). During this time, 122 patients (7.4%) experienced nonfatal thrombosis, of which 87 cases were arterial and 50 were venous. Of the 164 patients who died during the study, thrombosis accounted for 41% of the deaths and bleeding for only 7%. In this study, the biggest predictors of thrombotic risk were age older than 60 years and prior history of thrombosis. Risk was also increased in patients with diabetes mellitus or congestive heart failure and in smokers.

The rates of thrombotic and hemorrhagic complications in essential thrombocythemia have been studied in 21 retrospective cohort trials, reviewed by Barbui and colleagues.[9] At the time of diagnosis, the rates of thrombosis ranged from 9% to 84% in these trials, whereas rates of hemorrhage ranged from 3.9% to 63%. As in patients with PV, age older than 60 and a history of prior thrombosis predict the risk for recurrent thrombosis.[10]

The Pathogenesis of Bleeding and Thrombosis

Several intrinsic platelet function defects have been associated with the MPDs, but their clinical importance is uncertain. These may result, at least in part, from an increased sensitivity of the platelets to activation, a potential consequence of the JAK2 gain-of-function mutation. For example, a recent study demonstrated an increased risk for thrombosis in patients with chronic MPD when the mutant kinase could be detected in platelets alone or in platelets and

Table 142–1 Acquired Disorders of Platelet Function

Intrinsic disorders
Chronic myeloproliferative disorders
Leukemias and myelodysplastic syndromes
Paroxysmal nocturnal hemoglobinuria
Extrinsic disorders
Drugs that affect platelet function (see Table 142–2)
Foods and food additives:
ω3-fatty acids, vitamin E, ethanol, Chinese black tree fungus, garlic extract (ajoene)
Chronic renal failure
Cardiopulmonary bypass
Antiplatelet antibodies
Dysproteinemias
Disseminated intravascular coagulation
Hypothermia
Miscellaneous disorders

granulocytes.[11] Likewise, a study of patients with essential thrombocythemia demonstrated that the presence of the JAK2 mutation in platelets correlated with increased platelet expression of tissue factor and P-selectin, decreased expression of CD41and CD42b, and increased quantities of platelet-neutrophil aggregates, all indicators of a hyperreactive platelet phenotype.[12] However, the precise relationship of the JAK2 mutation to platelet function and thrombotic risk remain to determined.

The bleeding time is prolonged in few patients, and significant bleeding complications can occur in patients with normal bleeding times. Elevation of the platelet count per se correlates poorly with the risk for hemorrhage or thrombosis in some studies, but spontaneous bleeding is rare in patients with platelet counts of less than 1,000,000/μL. Very high platelet counts, more than 1.5×10^6 platelets/μL, have been associated with an acquired form of von Willebrand disease, in which the largest multimers of von Willebrand factor (vWF) are deficient, presumably because many are adsorbed by the binding sites on the elevated numbers of platelets.[13–16]

One situation clearly associated with an increased risk for excessive bleeding, particularly with surgery, is the increased whole blood viscosity and high hematocrit in patients with uncontrolled polycythemia vera.[17] Leukocytosis has also recently been identified as a risk factor for thrombosis in PV, as it is in ET.[18,19]

The platelets of patients with MPDs can show various morphologic abnormalities, including size and shape variability as well as decreased numbers of secretory granules. Platelet survival may be decreased in ET. The most common platelet abnormality is decreased aggregation and secretion in response to agonists, particularly epinephrine, adenosine diphosphate (ADP), and collagen. These abnormalities are not merely caused by the high platelet count, because patients with reactive thrombocytosis have functionally normal platelets.[20] In what may appear to be a paradox, some patients demonstrate spontaneous in vitro platelet aggregation in platelet-rich plasma. The significance of this is unknown because it is also occasionally seen in normal individuals. Decreased platelet aggregation or secretion and decreased procoagulant activity may be caused by the following: (a) decreased agonist-induced release of arachidonic acid from membrane phospholipids; (b) decreased conversion of arachidonic acid to prostaglandin endoperoxides or lipoxygenase products; (c) decreased platelet responsiveness to thromboxane A_2 (TXA_2); (d) decreased dense-granule or α granule contents; or (e) decreased α_2-adrenergic receptors. Specific platelet membrane abnormalities have also been reported, including deficiencies of glycoproteins Ib and IX, causing an acquired form of the Bernard-Soulier syndrome[21]; a deficiency of receptors for prostaglandin D_2[22]; a deficiency in the number of c-*MPL* receptors[23]; and an increased number of Fc receptors.[24] Because MPDs are clonal in origin, the platelet abnormalities may develop from a clone of abnormal megakaryocytes.[25] Alternatively, such findings may result from platelet hyperreactivity and previous activation.[12]

It is important to emphasize several features about the platelet function defects reported in MPDs. First, no defect has consistently predicted a risk for bleeding or thrombosis. Second, no defect is unique to, and therefore predictive of, a particular MPD. Third, their relative frequency has varied widely in different reported series. Therefore, the clinical importance of the described abnormalities of platelet function in MPDs is unknown. It is unlikely that any of these abnormalities of platelet function has a major clinical role in myeloproliferative diseases, given that the major complication associated with these disorders is thrombosis rather than bleeding and the observation that bleeding is most commonly seen with platelet counts greater than 1.5×10^6/μL.[13–15] Nevertheless, the recent elucidation of the gain-of-function JAK2 mutation as an important molecular cause of the MPDs suggests that platelet hyperfunction contributes to the increased risk of thrombosis associated with these disorders.

Management

Two large studies have established age and history of a prior thrombosis as important risk factors for thrombosis in PV.[26,27] In 1986 the Polycythemia Vera Study Group published guidelines recommending that all patients with PV be phlebotomized to keep the hematocrit less than 45%. Those at low risk for thrombosis (age younger than 60 years and no history of prior thrombosis) generally required no further therapy. In patients at higher risk, cytoreduction was recommended. Current recommendations for therapy still largely follow these guidelines, but new treatments are available for cytoreduction.[28] Hydroxyurea, with or without aspirin, has been shown effective in reducing the risk of thrombosis in patients with essential thrombocythemia.[29] Younger patients can be treated with α-interferon, because they tolerate this therapy better than older patients. Even in those receiving cytoreductive therapy, thrombosis remains a serious complication, a fact that served as the rationale for the European Collaboration on Low-dose Aspirin in Polycythemia study. Aspirin therapy in PV had not been in routine use, except for the treatment of digital ischemia,[30] because of its perceived association with hemorrhagic complications, a perception based on the early cessation of an aspirin trial by the Polycythemia Vera Study Group.[31] The European Collaboration on Low-dose Aspirin in Polycythemia study was a multicenter study conducted in Europe that examined both the natural history of PV and the antithrombotic effect of low-dose (100 mg/d) aspirin. Aspirin lowered the incidence of nonfatal myocardial infarction and stroke by approximately 60% and reduced both overall mortality and cardiovascular mortality by 46% and 59%, respectively. Patients with PV should therefore be treated with low-dose aspirin unless there is a clear contraindication to its use.[32]

In patients with low-risk essential thrombocythemia and moderate platelet counts, platelet-lowering therapy is unnecessary, given the low risk for thrombosis and bleeding.[5] Reduction of the platelet count with hydroxyurea should be considered in patients with other risk factors for cardiovascular disease and in patients otherwise at high risk: those with a prior history of thrombosis, age older than 60 years, and with platelet counts of greater than 1.5×10^6/mL. A recent study compared hydroxyurea plus aspirin with anagrelide plus aspirin for the prevention of the thrombotic complications of essential thrombocythemia.[33] Anagrelide is a drug originally developed as a platelet inhibitor, but it was found to lower platelet counts by inhibiting the proliferation and differentiation of megakaryocytes.[34–36] Anagrelide is much more expensive than hydroxyurea. Both regimens achieved good long-term control of platelet counts, but patients in the anagrelide group were much more likely to suffer both thrombotic and hemorrhagic complications, and to progress to myelofibrosis. Inexplicably, those in the anagrelide group experienced more venous thrombosis. There was no significant difference in death rate between the two groups. This study reinforces the recommendation of hydroxyurea with aspirin as first-line therapy for high-risk patients, on the basis of efficacy, safety, and cost.

LEUKEMIAS AND MYELODYSPLASTIC SYNDROMES

Bleeding in patients with the leukemias and myelodysplastic syndrome is almost always caused by thrombocytopenia, but abnormalities of platelet function have been described. In acute myelogenous leukemia and its variants, platelets may be larger than normal, abnormally shaped, and have a marked variation in the number of granules. Abnormal platelet structure and function have been described, especially associated with acute megakaryoblastic leukemia (FAB M7),[37,38] with one study describing three patients with decreased aggregation to collagen, ADP, epinephrine, and the thromboxane analogue U46619, along with a decreased platelet serotonin content.[37] Platelet abnormalities can also be seen in the myelodysplastic syndromes, with defective aggregation and glass bead retention described, associated most commonly with hypolobulated megakaryocytes and the 5q⁻ syndrome.[39] Abnormal platelet function has also been described in association with B-cell malignancies: with hairy cell leukemia, which can persist after splenectomy,[40] and with chronic lymphocytic leukemia,[41] in which the patient's platelets showed dramatically reduced responses to glycoprotein VI agonists collagen and convulxin.

Paroxysmal Nocturnal Hemoglobinuria

Paroxysmal nocturnal hemoglobinuria (PNH) is another clonal disorder that involves all blood cells. The hematopoietic stems cells and their progeny are defective in the synthesis of the glycosylphosphatidylinositol attachments required for some membrane proteins, leading to a defect in all glycosylphosphatidylinositol-linked proteins on blood cells,[42] including platelets.[43] Thromboembolism is a leading cause of mortality in PNH, affecting at least half of these patients and preferentially targeting the hepatic veins.[44] Several mechanisms have been proposed to explain this association, but it is unclear that the platelets have an important role.[45] The platelet function abnormalities described in PNH range from hypersensitivity to agonists to dysfunction. One study showed platelets to be hypersensitive to epinephrine, ADP, and collagen, as judged by their abilities to aggregate and to release ^{14}C serotonin.[46] The release of total nucleotides was also markedly increased over normal with all aggregating agents. By contrast, another study examining platelets from PNH patients showed them to be profoundly hyporeactive, as measured by defective clot formation, adhesion, and aggregation.[47] However, this was interpreted as being a consequence of chronic overstimulation of the platelets while in the circulation.

Platelet activation and increased platelet microparticle formation have also been demonstrated in patients with paroxysmal nocturnal hemoglobinuria.[48,49] Nevertheless, a strong correlation exists between thromboembolic disease and the number of circulating abnormal neutrophil clones.[50] It is likely that the level of abnormal granulocyte clones reflect the number of abnormal platelet clones.[51] Warfarin prophylaxis in patients with high numbers of abnormal clones significantly reduces the thrombotic risk and carries minimal bleeding risk in nonthrombocytopenic patients. A recent open-label study of eculizumab, a humanized monoclonal antibody against human complement C5 that prevents assembly on the cell surface of the membrane-attack complex, demonstrated a greater than 10-fold reduction in thromboembolic events in treated patients as compared with untreated patients.[52] Eculizumab effectively reduced thrombotic episodes, even in those taking antithrombotic medications, and reduced the rates of both arterial and venous thromboses. These encouraging results may signal a new era of therapy for PNH patients, because eculizumab has also been shown to decrease transfusion requirements, reduce fatigue, and improve general well being.[53]

Table 142–2 Drug-Induced Platelet Dysfunction

Mechanism: Known
Inhibition of GPIIb/IIIa-fibrinogen Interaction
Abciximab, eptifibatide, oral $\alpha_{IIb}\beta_3$ inhibitors, fibrinolytic agents
Inhibition of ADP Receptors
Ticlopidine, clopidogrel
Stimulation of Adenyl Cyclase
Epoprostenol, iloprost, beraprost
Stimulation of Guanyl Cyclase
Nitrites, nitroprusside
Inhibition of Phosphodiesterase
Methyl xanthines (theophylline), dipyridamole, sildenafil and related drugs
Inhibition of Thromboxane Pathway
Aspirin, nonsteroidal antiinflammatory drugs, moxalactam, losartan
Inhibition of Calcium Flux
Verapamil, calcium channel blockers (nifedipine, diltiazem)
Inhibition of Serotonin Uptake
Tricyclic antidepressants, fluoxetine
Mechanism: Unknown
Antibiotics
β-Lactam antibiotics, penicillins, nitrofurantoin
Plasma Expanders
Dextran, hydroxyl ethyl starch
Anesthetics
Dibucaine, procaine, cocaine, halothane
Phenothiazines
Chlorpromazine, promethazine, trifluoperazine
Oncologic Drugs
Mithramycin, daunorubicin, BCNU
Immunosuppressive Drugs
FK 506, cyclosporin, mycophenolic acid
Radiographic Contrast Agents
Renographin-76, Renovist II, Conray 60
Antihistamines
Diphenhydramine, chlorpheniramine
Miscellaneous
Clofibrate, hydroxychloroquine

ADP, adenosine diphosphate; BCNU, bis-chloroethyl-nitrosourea.

EXTRINSIC PLATELET DISORDERS

Drugs That Affect Platelet Function

Numerous drugs affect platelet function (Table 142-2). For several, inhibition of platelet function is their intended effect (Fig. 142-1); for most, platelet dysfunction is an unintended and undesired side effect. Antiplatelet agents are discussed more fully in Chapter 137. For all these drugs, their effects on platelet function are defined by an abnormality of platelet aggregation or of the bleeding time, but

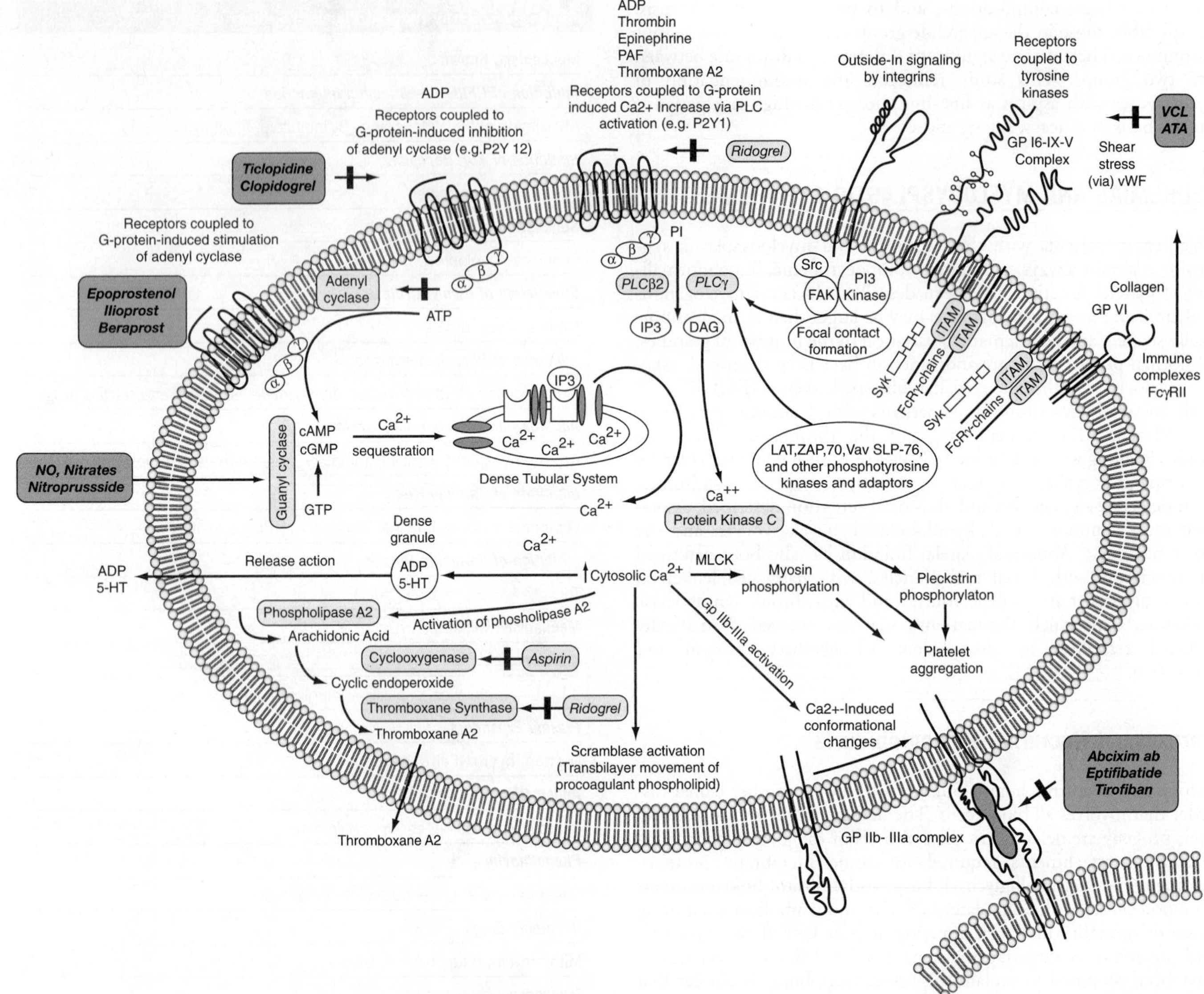

Figure 142–1 Mechanism of inhibition of platelet function by various drugs. Some of the drugs shown, such as Ridogrel, VCL, and ATA, are not now used clinically. ADP, adenosine diphosphate; ATA, aurin tricarboxylic acid; ATP, adenosine triphosphate; cAMP, cyclic adenosine monophosphate; cGMP, cyclic guanyl monophosphate; DAG, diacylglycerol; GP, glycoprotein; GTP, guanyl triphosphate; 5-HT, serotonin (5-hydroxytryptamine); IP3, inositol triphosphate; ITAM, immunoreceptor tyrosine-based activation motif; MLCK, myosin light chain kinase; NO, nitric oxide; PAF, platelet activating factor; PI, phosphatidylinositol; PLA2, phospholipase A2; TXA_2, thromboxane A_2; VCL, rA1 domain of von Willebrand factor; vWF, von Willebrand factor.

their contribution to a risk of excessive bleeding is definitively established only for aspirin, clopidogrel, ticlopidine, and the inhibitors of $\alpha_{IIb}\beta_3$ function.

Aspirin

Aspirin has been in routine use worldwide for more than 100 years and is still by far the most common agent associated with platelet dysfunction.[54] The primary mechanism by which aspirin impairs hemostasis is through irreversible acetylation of the enzyme cyclooxygenase (COX)-1, an early enzyme in the synthetic pathway that leads to the formation of the potent platelet agonist, TXA_2. Because platelets have no nuclei and therefore retain only a limited capacity to synthesize new proteins, a single small dose of aspirin (40–100 mg) or as little as 10 mg taken daily for one week can completely inhibit TXA_2 production and therefore impair the function of a cohort of platelets for their circulating life span. Aspirin also acetylates the isoform of cyclooxygenase present in endothelial cells, COX-2; COX-2 acetylation blocks synthesis of prostacyclin, a strong inhibitor of platelet function.[55] However, COX-2 is markedly less sensitive than COX-1 inhibition by aspirin,[54] and endothelial cells, unlike platelets, are able to synthesize new enzymes quite rapidly.[56]

Platelets exposed to aspirin either in vivo or in vitro predictably demonstrate impaired aggregation to epinephrine, ADP, arachidonic acid, and low concentrations of collagen and thrombin,[57] a result of defective TXA_2 production. These agonists have therefore been defined as *weak* agonists, requiring that TXA_2 diffuse out of the platelet, bind its platelet membrane receptors, and reinforce aggregation by promoting α and dense granule secretion. Aspirin-treated platelets stimulated with these agonists demonstrate only a primary, reversible wave of aggregation without granule secretion. Stronger agonists (high concentrations of thrombin and collagen) do not require TXA_2 synthesis to cause platelet secretion and irreversible aggregation, which probably accounts for the observation that hemostasis in healthy aspirin-treated subjects is usually normal.

Aspirin also prolongs the bleeding time but less consistently than it induces the platelet aggregation abnormality. Early studies demonstrated that the mean template bleeding time of a group of normal subjects was significantly increased 2 hours after ingestion of two to three aspirin tablets (650–975 mg).[58,59] Prolongation of the bleeding time can be demonstrated as long as 4 days after a single dose of aspirin[60] when new, normally functioning platelets replace a sufficient fraction of the aspirin-inhibited cohort. Despite its effect on the mean bleeding times, aspirin prolongs the bleeding time above the normal range in only about one half of normal subjects.[58,59] Smaller single doses of aspirin (150–160 mg) that consistently cause abnormal platelet aggregation do not prolong the bleeding time; daily ingestion of 30 mg of aspirin (but not 10mg) usually does.[61]

The bleeding time is reputed to be the most direct test of platelet function because it is performed directly on the patient and because it correlates with the platelet count in select patients.[62] However, the bleeding time did not predict bleeding in one study of patients taking aspirin for rheumatic disease who were undergoing gastric endoscopic biopsy[63] or in uremic patients undergoing renal biopsy.[64] These data emphasize that the bleeding time cannot be automatically accepted as an accurate representation of systemic hemostasis.[65]

Aspirin most dramatically prolongs the bleeding times in patients with other hemostatic defects. For example, one study of patients with severe hemophilia, who often already have slightly prolonged bleeding times,[66] showed that 5 of 11 patients treated with two to three aspirin tablets experienced sustained hemorrhage from the bleeding time incisions,[67] requiring transfusion with plasma or factor VIII. Patients with mild hemophilia appeared to be at less risk from aspirin ingestion; in none of 16 patients was the bleeding time prolonged longer than values in the normal control group.[67] Small doses of aspirin also cause a greater than normal prolongation of the bleeding time in patients with chronic renal failure and have been associated with reports of major bleeding.[68] The combination of ethanol and aspirin has a synergistic effect on increasing the bleeding times in normal subjects.[69]

Clinical Importance of the Aspirin-Induced Defect in Platelet Function

In contrast to the antithrombotic effect of aspirin, which appears unrelated to the dose above small threshold doses, gastrointestinal mucosal toxicity is dose related.[70] The mechanism of mucosal injury appears to be separate from the effect on hemostasis, involving ionic trapping of aspirin within gut mucosal cells[71] and diminished synthesis of protective gut prostaglandins.[72,73] The inhibitory effect of even a single dose of aspirin on gastric prostaglandin synthesis is prolonged, with one study showing that gastric COX activity was still suppressed by 57% 72 hours after a single 325-mg dose of aspirin.[74]

Bleeding can originate from both discrete ulcers and diffuse mucosal damage and is more common from the upper gastrointestinal tract. The risk of bleeding is increased even with doses of aspirin as low as 10 to 30 mg/day;[75] the protective effect of resistant coatings is unproved.[76] Recently, a nitric oxide-donating form of aspirin (NCX-4016) has been shown to enhance the cardioprotective effect of aspirin while sparing the gastrointestinal tract.[77]

The gastrointestinal risk of aspirin is enhanced in the elderly (older than 65) and in those with concomitant medical conditions such as cardiovascular disease, as well as in those taking certain other medications, such as other nonsteroidal antiinflammatory agents.[76] Aspirin seems to also delay the healing of gastric ulcers, possibly because it interferes with the release of growth factors such as endostatin and vascular endothelial growth factor from platelets.[78]

The clinical importance of the antithrombotic effect of aspirin was clearly demonstrated in a study of 22,071 physicians who received either 325 mg of aspirin every other day or placebo over the course of 5 years.[79] Those receiving aspirin had a 44% decreased incidence of myocardial infarction. Aspirin treatment was also associated with a small but significant increase in mucocutaneous bleeding as evidenced by easy bruising, hematemesis, melena, epistaxis, as well as an increased incidence of blood transfusion. Because even lower doses have been shown to be effective in preventing thrombosis, it is likely that the risk of bleeding can be reduced further while maintaining an antithrombotic effect.

The likelihood that aspirin will cause bleeding is increased in the presence of other hemostatic defects. The risk of bleeding is increased if aspirin is given simultaneously with warfarin in high-intensity anticoagulation regimens (international normalized ratio 3.0–4.5), but the occurrence of major hemorrhagic events may not be increased.[80] Similarly, aspirin may unmask mild hereditary disorders of platelet function.[81] For example, patients with mild von Willebrand disease often have a normal bleeding time that becomes markedly increased with aspirin therapy.[81] Conversely, aspirin given during treatment of acute coronary syndromes in combination with fibrinolytic and other antithrombotic agents does not appear to increase the incidence of major bleeding episodes,[82,83] with the exception of its combination with clopidogrel, which is associated with a slight increase in bleeding complications over treatment with aspirin alone.[84]

Several studies have addressed the risk of postoperative hemorrhage in patients taking aspirin. The results, as may be expected with a very mild hemostatic defect, are inconsistent. Some studies report increased blood loss in patients taking aspirin who undergo cardiac surgery, but others do not.[85] Increased chest tube blood loss in aspirin-treated patients was not associated with worse clinical outcomes, such as a need for reoperation or greater numbers of units of blood transfused.[68,86]

In studies of patients undergoing elective total hip replacement by a single surgeon, aspirin treatment (1.2–3.6 g/day) was begun the day before surgery and continued for 7 days.[87] The blood loss was 20% greater in the treated group in one study, but this was considered clinically unimportant and required no additional care.[87] A study of 200 patients undergoing general or gynecologic surgery also suggested that there was greater surgical blood loss in patients who had taken aspirin.[88] The surgeon and the anesthesiologist observed "greater than expected bleeding" in 12 of 55 patients who had taken aspirin and had abnormal results on platelet aggregation studies, compared with 7 of 97 patients who had not taken aspirin and had normal aggregation studies. The other 48 patients in this study either claimed they had not taken aspirin but were found to have abnormal platelet aggregation—a frequent occurrence in many studies caused by habitual and forgotten aspirin use (33 patients)—or had taken aspirin but their platelet aggregations were normal (15 patients). Of these 48 patients 8 were believed to have excessive bleeding at surgery. Although the results were interpreted as demonstrating increased surgical bleeding following aspirin treatment, it is important to note that "greater than expected bleeding" also occurred in the control patients. This observation is inevitable in all subjective evaluations of bleeding, either surgical or medical. The observer always expects and hopes for a normal hemostatic response, but the range of "normal" bleeding is great, and patients with more bleeding are often viewed with concern.

Recent evidence suggests that aspirin may in fact be beneficial in the perioperative period. There is a well-recognized syndrome of platelet dysfunction following cardiopulmonary bypass (see also section on cardiopulmonary bypass), and until recently aspirin administration has been believed to be contraindicated.[89] However, a recent observational study noted that patients receiving aspirin within 4 hours of cardiopulmonary bypass had markedly improved outcomes, with improvements in virtually every parameter of bypass-related morbidity, including, unexpectedly, the incidence of bleeding.[90] The benefit of aspirin in this study has been attributed to modulation of the proinflammatory properties of platelets[89] but may also involve benefits unrelated to aspirin's effect on platelets. Aspirin was also noted to positively influence the outcome of microsurgery, a benefit ascribed to decreased thrombosis at the sites of microsurgical anastomoses and to decreased TXA_2-mediated vasoconstriction downstream of these sites.[91]

Thus, aspirin appears to have a small effect on increasing surgical bleeding, which can be significant. The risk is not increased, however, with minimally invasive trauma such as spinal or epidural anesthesia.[92,93] In other cases aspirin therapy may actually positively influence the outcome of surgery.[90,91] These data on aspirin represent well the clinical paradigm for acquired disorders of platelet function: they are common; the defect is usually mild; normal individuals vary in their sensitivities to aspirin; platelet aggregation and the bleeding time are subject to technical vagaries; the risk for increased bleeding in the individual subject who is otherwise healthy is minimal and unpredictable; but a definite risk for increased bleeding with aspirin can be demonstrated when large groups of healthy subjects are analyzed or when individuals are studied who have concomitant pathologic (eg, hemophilia) or physiologic (eg, childbirth) conditions that predispose them to hemorrhage.

Other Nonsteroidal Antiinflammatory Drugs

In addition to aspirin, many other drugs used for their antiinflammatory and analgesic properties can cause platelet dysfunction.[85] As with aspirin, their mechanism of action appears to be the inhibition of the activity of COX-1; but in contrast to aspirin, these agents only temporarily affect COX-1 function, inhibiting the enzyme only as long as the active drug circulates. Among these agents, therefore, only drugs such as piroxicam, which has a plasma half-life of more than 2 days,[94] affect platelets for more than a few hours. As with aspirin, the most sensitive indication of impaired platelet function is the inhibition of in vitro platelet aggregation and secretion. These agents prolong the bleeding time minimally and transiently or not at all, consistent with the bleeding time being a less sensitive measure of the aspirin-induced defect.[85] The platelet function analyzer–100 more reliably detects the defect manifested as a prolonged clotting time with the collagen/epinephrine cartridge.[95]

Reports of bleeding correlate with the effects of these agents on platelet function, suggesting that they increase the risk for excessive bleeding less than aspirin. As with aspirin, they may increase the bleeding times in patients with severe hemophilia; but in two studies, therapeutic doses of ibuprofen had no effect on the bleeding time in 19 of 20 patients with hemophilia.[96] Therefore, the clinical approach to patients taking any drug that can inhibit COX-1 should be similar, but the reversibility of the effect of nonaspirin antiinflammatory drugs provides an added margin of safety when these agents are used. The additional risk for bleeding with surgery should be negligible, but a prudent course would be to discontinue these drugs the day before a procedure. Analgesics such as acetaminophen and sodium or choline salicylate do not inhibit platelet function and have no adverse effects on hemostasis.[96]

Recently, a class of drugs with greater selectivity for COX-2 than for COX-1 has entered clinical use, the coxibs. These drugs were developed for the treatment of patients with chronic pain or chronic inflammatory disorders to diminish the risk of gastrointestinal bleeding and ulceration.[97] Although these drugs have little affect on platelet function because they do not inhibit COX-1, nevertheless they have as a group been associated with an increased risk of cardiovascular events, including thrombosis.[98] Although COX-2 is involved in promoting inflammatory states, which are associated with thrombosis, a major consequence of its inhibition is to diminish endothelial synthesis of prostacyclin I_2, a major component of the platelet inhibitory functions of healthy endothelium.[98]

Adenosine Diphosphate Receptor Antagonists

The thienopyridines ticlopidine, clopidogrel, and prasugrel inhibit ADP-mediated platelet activation and aggregation.[99] ADP-induced platelet activation involves a rise in free cytoplasmic Ca^{2+} because of influx from the extracellular fluid and mobilization from internal stores, and a drop in intracellular cyclic adenosine monophosphate (cAMP) coupled to inhibition of adenylyl cyclase. ADP receptors can be divided into two groups: the G-protein-coupled receptors, termed *P2Y,* and the inotropic receptors, *P2X.* Platelets contain two P2Y receptors, $P2Y_1$ and $P2Y_{12}$, complexed to the heterotrimeric G proteins, G_q and G_{i2}, respectively. ADP binding to $P2Y_1$ is necessary for platelet aggregation but is not sufficient. Rather, $P2Y_1$ is responsible for ADP-induced platelet shape change, and its engagement by ADP triggers a transient aggregatory response. $P2Y_{12}$, coupled to inhibition of adenylyl cyclase, mediates the amplification of the aggregation response and increases thrombus stability.[100]

The thienopyridine derivatives covalently modify the $P2Y_{12}$ receptor, preventing receptor-coupled inhibition of adenylyl cyclase activity. These drugs have no effects on arachidonic acid metabolism and hence act synergistically with aspirin to inhibit platelet function. The thienopyridines are all prodrugs of similar structures that produce active metabolites that bind irreversibly to $P2Y_{12}$, inhibiting ADP-mediated aggregation for up to 10 days after withdrawal of the drug, paralleling the platelet life span.[101] Because most platelet agonists require ADP for their full activity, the thienopyridines inhibit platelet activation by all agonists except strong agonists at high concentrations.[102] They have a further hypothetical advantage over aspirin in that they inhibit shear-induced platelet aggregation.[103]

The thienopyridines are administered orally, with fewer gastrointestinal side effects if taken with meals. All thienopyridines must be metabolized in the liver to their active forms. At lower doses, the full pharmacologic effect requires 3 to 5 days for ticlopidine and 4 to 7 days for clopidogrel. A doubling of the bleeding time can be observed after 3 to 7 days of treatment. When a rapid therapeutic effect is desired, therapy can be initiated with a loading dose, 500 mg for ticlopidine, and 300 to 600 mg for clopidogrel. At these doses, clopidogrel significantly impairs platelet function within 90 minutes of administration.[104,105]

Ticlopidine was the first thienopyridine for which clinical benefit was demonstrated in patients presenting with a wide range of cardiovascular diseases, including stroke, myocardial infarction, and the thrombotic complications of peripheral arterial disease.[106] Ticlopidine use, however, is limited by its slow onset of action and frequent side effects, which force discontinuation of the drug in 20% of patients. The most common side effects are diarrhea, nausea, and skin rash, but neutropenia and thrombotic thrombocytopenic purpura are the most severe, with estimated incidences of about 3.3% and 0.02%, respectively.[106]

Clopidogrel has an excellent side-effect profile, is well tolerated even at high doses (600 mg/day), and has largely replaced ticlopidine in the United States. More importantly, the incidence of thrombotic thrombocytopenic purpura is 100-fold less than with ticlopidine and is comparable to that of the general population, with about one case per 4 million patients treated.[107] No cases of clopidogrel-associated severe neutropenia have been reported, and the Clopidogrel versus Aspirin in Patients at Risk of Ischemic Events trial showed that there is no need for routine complete blood counts in patients taking clopidogrel.[108]

Prasugrel, an investigational drug, appears to be converted to its active form much more efficiently than does clopidogrel.[109]

Overall, the rates of bleeding complications of the thienopyridines are similar to those seen with aspirin, with the combination of aspirin and clopidogrel being associated with higher postoperative bleeding after coronary artery bypass grafting than with either drug alone.[110]

Platelet $\alpha_{IIb}\beta_3$ Antagonists

In the past decade, a new class of agents targeted at the major platelet integrin, $\alpha_{IIb}\beta_3$, has emerged for use in the treatment of acute coronary syndromes[111]; these agents are intended to produce a transient effect akin to the defect in Glanzmann thrombasthenia, but there are important differences between the drug effect and the disease.

Three intravenous $\alpha_{IIb}\beta_3$ antagonists are currently in use, having been evaluated in tens of thousands of patients presenting with various forms of cardiovascular disease. Although these agents share many similarities in their pharmacodynamics and therapeutic effects, they also have a number of clinically important pharmacokinetic differences.

Abciximab

The first $\alpha_{IIb}\beta_3$ inhibitor approved for clinical use, abciximab (ReoPro), is a human-murine chimeric Fab fragment of a monoclonal antibody that targets the β_3 subunit of $\alpha_{IIb}\beta_3$ and therefore also reacts with another integrin that shares the β_3 subunit, $\alpha_V\beta_3$. Although $\alpha_{IIb}\beta_3$ expression is restricted to megakaryocytes and platelets, $\alpha_V\beta_3$ is expressed on platelets, at low levels, and in cells of the vascular wall, including endothelial cells and fibroblasts.[112] The clinical relevance of this cross-reactivity is unclear.

Intravenous administration of a standard 0.25 mg/kg bolus of abciximab blocks approximately 80% of surface $\alpha_{IIb}\beta_3$ and inhibits platelet aggregation to a similar extent, although the extent of inhibition is variable.[111] This level of blockade increases the bleeding time only mildly.[54] The bleeding time is only markedly prolonged when receptor blockade exceeds 90%. Following the bolus dose, abciximab is infused at 0.125 g/kg/min for 12 hours. Several trials have established this as a clinically effective regimen.[111]

Free plasma levels of abciximab drop rapidly after its administration, with an initial half-life of approximately 30 minutes and most of the drug remaining bound to platelets. This explains why patients with thrombocytosis may require larger weight-adjusted doses of abciximab to attain a therapeutic antiplatelet effect.[113] Conversely, platelet inhibition is more profound in patients with lower platelet counts treated with the usual dose of abciximab.

Abciximab is not excreted in the urine and is probably metabolized by the reticuloendothelial system at the time platelets (with bound abciximab) are cleared from the circulation. Although a daily platelet turnover rate of 10% would predict that no abciximab would be detected in blood after 10 days of its administration, platelet-bound abciximab has been observed up to 3 weeks following its initial administration, suggesting platelet-to-platelet redistribution of the drug or release of new platelets from megakaryocytes that had previously bound the drug. Several in vitro and in vivo studies confirm abciximab's ability to exchange from one platelet to another.[114]

Because of the low plasma levels of unbound abciximab, the drug's inhibitory effect can be rapidly reversed by platelet transfusion; and hemostasis should be normal when the concentration of infused platelets exceeds 50,000/μL, as it is in normal individuals. However, because of abciximab's ability to redistribute to the newly transfused platelets, the platelet-bound abciximab may produce a gradual inhibitory effect on the infused platelets[114]; and in severe or refractory bleeding it may be necessary to infuse a very large dose of platelets, sufficient to leave 50% of $\alpha_{IIb}\beta_3$ receptors free, a number shown to be sufficient for normal hemostasis in studies of Glanzmann thrombasthenia heterozygotes. Without platelet transfusions, platelet aggregation generally returns to baseline levels within 12 to 24 hours after discontinuing abciximab.

Eptifibatide

Eptifibatide (Integrilin) is a cyclic heptapeptide based on the KGD (Lys-Gly-Asp) sequence found in barbourin, a platelet-inhibitory disintegrin from the venom of the Southeastern Pigmy rattlesnake, *Sistrurus miliarius barbouri.*[115] Barbourin differs from other integrin-binding proteins with the Arg-Gly-Asp (RGD) canonical sequence in that the arginine is conservatively substituted by lysine, a change that renders the protein a specific inhibitor of $\alpha_{IIb}\beta_3$.[115] Eptifibatide incorporates the KGD sequence within a cyclic seven-member peptide of high potency.

Eptifibatide differs pharmacokinetically from abciximab in several important ways.[111] For example, unlike abciximab, intravenous eptifibatide infusion produces high levels of unbound drug. Platelet transfusions therefore are not a good method for acutely reversing eptifibatide's antiplatelet effect, because the newly transfused platelets are rapidly inhibited. However, its short plasma half-life of approximately 2.5 hours allows for rapid clearance of eptifibatide and the reversal of its antiplatelet effect when administration is discontinued. Platelet aggregation has been shown to return to normal in approximately 4 hours, with the bleeding time normalizing within 1 hour.[111]

Tirofiban

Tirofiban (Aggrastat) is a peptidomimetic agent based on the RGD sequence, with a pharmacokinetic profile similar to that of eptifibatide.[111] Tirofiban antagonizes $\alpha_{IIb}\beta_3$ and does not cross-react with $\alpha_V\beta_3$.[116,117] As with eptifibatide, the maximum antiplatelet effect is seen at concentrations that leave a high concentration of unbound drug in the plasma.[111] Therefore, platelet transfusions are not commonly effective in reversing tirofiban's antiplatelet effect. However, its half-life is even shorter than that of eptifibatide (approximately 2 hours), and its anti-platelet effect is reversed rapidly after discontinuation of infusion.

The data thus far indicate that the main therapeutic benefit of $\alpha_{IIb}\beta_3$ antagonists is obtained in patients undergoing percutaneous coronary intervention (PCI), regardless of whether it is elective or for the treatment of an acute coronary syndrome.[118] As a class, the $\alpha_{IIb}\beta_3$ antagonists have been demonstrated to be beneficial in patients undergoing PCI, with an overall relative risk reduction in the composite of death, myocardial infarction, or urgent target vessel revascularization of 30% to 50% at 30 days ($P < 0.01$).[119,120] Whether the three drugs in current use are significantly different in their clinical efficacy in patients undergoing PCI is a matter of controversy. However, the data thus far indicate that the three drugs are probably similar in the long-term (<6 months after PCI) in the reduction of death, myocardial infarction, and the need for urgent target-vessel revascularization.[121]

Limitations and Adverse Effects of the $\alpha_{IIb}\beta_3$ Antagonists

Bleeding

Millions of patients have been treated with intravenous $\alpha_{IIb}\beta_3$ antagonists in various clinical scenarios, and the data are compelling that these drugs have a very good safety profile.[118] Importantly, none is associated with an increased risk of intracranial hemorrhage.[122]

Thrombocytopenia

Up to 1% of patients receiving abciximab may develop profound thrombocytopenia (platelet count <20,000/μL).[123] A decrease in the platelet count is appreciable within the first hours after administration. It is therefore essential that a platelet count be obtained 2 to 4 hours after initiating treatment. Most patients with severe thrombocytopenia respond well to platelet transfusions and their platelet counts usually recover within 5 days but may take more than one week to do so. Because patients receiving abciximab frequently also receive heparin, heparin-induced thrombocytopenia must be excluded. Ethylenediaminetetraacetic acid–dependent pseudothrombocytopenia should also be considered and ruled out by examination of a blood smear for the presence of platelet aggregates.

Many patients require readministration of abciximab, raising the possibility that antibodies against the drug will complicate therapy. The safety of readministration was studied systematically in the ReoPro Readministration Registry.[123] The study found that abciximab readministration has a high clinical success rate and is not associated with hypersensitivity reactions, excessive bleeding, or death, and the incidence of thrombocytopenia is no greater than that seen in patients receiving abciximab for the first time. However, thrombocytopenia tended to be profound, relatively refractory to platelet infusion, and more often delayed. It is therefore recommended that clinicians obtain a second platelet count 24 hours after the readministration of abciximab and that they maintain a high index of suspicion for the delayed development of abciximab-induced thrombocytopenia.

Antibiotics

Antibiotics can also affect platelet function.[85] Those most commonly affecting platelet function are the penicillins and cephalosporins, which share a β-lactam ring structure. Some of these produce predictable dose- and duration-related effects on the bleeding time.[124–126] Because the effect on bleeding time is seen only in patients who are receiving large parenteral doses of antibiotics, this is a potential problem only for hospitalized patients. In a study of 74 hospitalized patients with a consistently prolonged bleeding time, the likely cause was penicillin in 39 patients (30 patients were receiving penicillin G, more than 15,000,000 U/day, and 9 were receiving ampicillin, 6 to 8 g/day) and aspirin or related drugs in 7 patients.[126]

The structural properties that cause some, but not all, penicillins and cephalosporins to affect platelet function are unknown. The side chain structure alters the antibacterial and pharmacologic properties of the penicillins and cephalosporins and may also determine their effects on platelet function. It is postulated that the antibiotic associates with the platelet plasma membrane by a lipophilic mechanism, perturbing multiple receptor-agonist interactions and/or stimulus-response coupling.[127] The characteristic laboratory observation is the occurrence of a prolonged bleeding time and abnormal platelet aggregation after several days of high-dose parenteral therapy.[125,126] These abnormalities usually do not subside until several days after the antibiotic is discontinued.

The frequency of clinically important bleeding in patients taking β-lactam antibiotics is low and is not predicted by a prolonged bleeding time, and the causal relation to antibiotic treatment is unproved.[128] For each report implicating an antibiotic as a cause of hemorrhage, many more patients receive the same antibiotics in large doses without bleeding complications.[128]

In conclusion, antibiotic-induced platelet dysfunction appears to have little clinical importance, and the potential effect on platelet function should not be considered in the decision to use any antibiotic in any clinical situation. An exception to this conclusion may be moxalactam. The frequency of clinically important hemorrhagic complications with moxalactam appears to be greater than with other antibiotics.[128] This drug has been demonstrated to produce a dose-dependent inhibition of ADP- and collagen-induced platelet aggregation, and to result in defective TXA_2 generation,[129] which suggests that it acts on the thromboxane synthesis pathway, much as aspirin does. Furthermore, unlike most other β-lactam antibiotics, moxalactam contains a methylthiotetrazole-leaving group that has been implicated in the inhibition of synthesis of vitamin K-dependent coagulation factors.[130] Therefore, moxalactam-induced bleeding may be caused by the combination of deficiencies in vitamin K-dependent coagulation factors and impaired platelet function.

Nitrofurantoin, an antibiotic structurally unrelated to the β-lactam antibiotics, may mildly prolong the bleeding time and impair platelet aggregation at blood concentrations higher than 20 μM.[131] Nitrofurantoin is not known to cause clinical bleeding.

Other Drugs

Drugs That Increase Platelet Cyclic Nucleotide Concentration

Elevation of the platelet concentration of cAMP by any mechanism inhibits platelet function and is a major mechanism of action of the thienopyridines, discussed earlier in adenosine diphosphate receptor antagonists section. Prostacyclin and its analogues increase cAMP synthesis by the stimulation of adenylyl cyclase, and they have been studied as antithrombotic substitutes for heparin in cardiopulmonary bypass surgery and hemodialysis.[132] Prostacyclin is one of the most potent endogenous inhibitors of platelet functions but has not been shown to be more effective than aspirin in clinical trials, and its clinical use is limited by its vasodilatory side effects. Prostacyclin-like agents that have been used include epoprostenol (the synthetic salt of prostacyclin), treprostinil, inhalational prostacyclin (iloprost), and an orally active stable analogue (beraprost). In spite of the potent inhibition of platelet aggregation by prostacyclin in vitro, the effects on the bleeding time are minimal and inconsistent.

Cilostazol is a cyclic nucleotide phosphodiesterase inhibitor with both platelet inhibitory and vasodilatory effects; its current clinical use for peripheral vascular disease in the United States was preceded by its use in Japan and other Asian countries. In addition to its selective inhibition of phosphodiesterase (one of the major cAMP hydrolyzing enzymes in platelets), cilostazol also inhibits adenine nucleotide uptake, a property not seen in other phosphodiesterase inhibitors that further enhances its antiplatelet activity.[133]

Dipyridamole has several biologic effects, including phosphodiesterase inhibition, targeting the PDE5 isoform that degrades cyclic guanosine monophosphate (cGMP).[134] It also enhances the release, and prevents the breakdown, of prostaglandin prostacyclin I_2.[135] Primarily used for prevention of stroke, its usefulness was demonstrated by a meta-analysis of recent randomized trials showing that the combination of dipyridamole, particularly the modified release form, and aspirin was more efficacious than aspirin alone in secondary prevention of vascular events after transient ischemic attacks or stroke.[136] Dipyridamole has been associated with a significantly increased risk of gastrointestinal bleeding when used either as a single agent or in combination with aspirin.[137]

Recently, inhibitors of PDE5 have become popular in the treatment of erectile dysfunction.[138] PDE5 is expressed in platelets and its inhibition results in increases in the level of platelet cGMP, an effect similar to the effect of the well-known inhibitor of platelet function, nitric oxide. One study examined the activation response of platelets drawn from patients taking sildenafil (Viagra) when stimulated with either ADP or low-dose thrombin. The results showed significantly reduced activation to ADP in sildenafil-treated platelets, suggesting that the drug impairs selected pathways of platelet function in vivo. Several reports of sildenafil-associated bleeding have appeared, including epistaxis,[139,140] hemorrhoidal bleeding,[141] spontaneous intracranial hemorrhage,[142] and acute variceal bleeding.[143]

Anticoagulants

Although heparin is best known for its anticoagulant effect and its adverse effect in causing thrombocytopenia and paradoxical thrombosis (see Chapter 137), it has the potential to affect platelet function. Heparin can bind to the platelet surface,[144] cause platelet aggregation and secretion,[145] and impair vWF-dependent platelet function.[146] Heparin can also increase the bleeding time.[147] Whether these phenomena are related to the bleeding complications of heparin use is unknown. The prolonged bleeding time is probably caused by heparin's inhibition of thrombin generation, analogous to the slight but significant increase in bleeding times in patients with hemophilia.[66]

Paradoxically, heparin has also been shown to be capable of inducing the association of vWF with the GPIb complex.[148] Whether this is restricted to certain individuals or occurs only at certain heparin doses is unclear, but it raises the possibility that this mechanism may contribute to heparin-induced thrombosis.

Fibrinolytic Agents

Bleeding during therapy with plasminogen activators is predominantly caused by the effects of hypofibrinogenemia and increased fibrin(ogen) degradation products on fibrin clot formation, usually combined with a structural lesion in the blood vessel wall (see Chapter 137). In addition, pharmacologic doses of streptokinase, urokinase, and tissue plasminogen activator may impair platelet function through several potential mechanisms, all related to excessive production of plasmin.[149] First, very high levels of fibrin(ogen) degradation products coupled with very low levels of fibrinogen may impair platelet aggregation. Second, the binding of plasminogen to the platelet surface may facilitate its conversion to the proteolytic enzyme, plasmin, by plasminogen activator.[150] On the platelet surface, plasmin can degrade GPIb (thereby impairing the interaction of the platelet with vWF[151]) and fibrinogen (thereby dispersing platelet aggregates).[152] Third, plasmin can inhibit platelet aggregation by blocking the release of arachidonic acid from platelet membranes, limiting thromboxane production.[153] The clinical importance of these observations is unknown.

In addition to depressing platelet function, plasmin has been shown to directly activate platelets,[154–157] an effect that has been postulated to account for reocclusion after tissue plasminogen activator treatment for myocardial infarction.[158] The mechanism involves cleavage of protease-activated receptors, in particular PAR4.[159]

Plasma Expanders

Dextrans are partially hydrolyzed branched polysaccharides of glucose. Of the two preparations in clinical use, one has an average molecular size of 70,000 to 75,000 (often termed *dextran 70*) and one has an average molecular size of 40,000 (termed *dextran 40* or *low-molecular-weight dextran*). Both preparations are effective plasma expanders and can affect platelet function, but there are data suggesting that the high-molecular-weight molecules have a greater effect on hemostasis.[160] Dextran infusion also impairs platelet aggregation and platelet procoagulant activity and can cause a modest reduction in plasma vWF concentration. However, dextran has no effect on platelet function when added directly to platelet-rich plasma in vitro.[161] Because of these effects on platelet function, dextran has been used as an antithrombotic agent, and its efficacy in preventing fatal postoperative pulmonary emboli appears to be equivalent to that of subcutaneous heparin.[162] This therapeutic effect is achieved without any increased risk for bleeding, as demonstrated in a large double-blind trial comparing dextran with placebo during general surgery.[163]

Hydroxyethyl starch, known as *hetastarch,* is a synthetic glucose polymer with an average molecular weight of 450,000 (range, 10,000–1,000,000) that is also used for plasma expansion. Hetastarch use has been associated (albeit inconsistently) with abnormal platelet function, and this appears to be more evident with use of the higher molecular weight forms.[164] Like dextran, it can prolong the bleeding time, particularly if administered in doses of greater than 20 mL/kg of a 6% solution, and predispose to bleeding if administered simultaneously with heparin or is used in a patient with a preexisting hemostatic defect.[165]

Cardiovascular Drugs

Administration of nitroglycerin, isosorbide dinitrate, or nitroprusside can decrease platelet aggregation and secretion in vitro; but the effects in vivo are minimal and inconsistently observed.[85] The mechanism of platelet inhibition appears to involve the production of nitric oxide from the drug, with concomitant increases in platelet cAMP and, more markedly, cGMP.[166] α-Adrenergic receptor blockers such as propranolol, metoprolol, nebivolol, and pindolol have also been shown to inhibit platelet aggregation, apparently through mechanisms independent of α-adrenoreceptor blockade.[167,168] Several of these agents have been shown to blunt platelet aggregatory responses to ADP and collagen[169] and decrease platelet TXA_2 production in response to agonists.[167] Blunting of serotonin uptake by platelets and inhibition of the response to serotonin have also been demonstrated.[170] Numerous reports also exist on antiplatelet effects of the calcium channel blockers nifedipine, verapamil, and diltiazem. These studies have demonstrated inhibition of platelet aggregation in vitro when high concentrations (micromolar) of the drug were used with washed platelets.[152] This effect is seen primarily with epinephrine as the agonist, and it does not appear to be related to inhibition of calcium ion flux. The proposed mechanisms of action include inhibition of epinephrine binding to α_2-adrenergic receptors, inhibition of the platelet response to TXA_2, and inhibition of serotonin-induced aggregation. In therapeutic doses, the calcium channel blockers do not prolong the bleeding time. Quinidine, an antiarrhythmic drug, can act as an antagonist of platelet α_2-adrenergic receptors at high concentrations. In a single report, a patient taking 800 mg of quinidine and 650 mg of aspirin daily developed melena and generalized petechiae with a normal platelet count and a bleeding time of longer than 35 minutes.[171] Subsequent studies on two normal volunteers showed that quinidine caused a mild increase in the bleeding time that was apparently potentiated by aspirin.

Psychotropic Agents

Platelets from patients taking tricyclic antidepressant drugs (imipramine, amitriptyline, nortriptyline) or phenothiazines (chlorpromazine, promethazine, trifluoperazine) may have impaired in vitro aggregation and secretion responses to ADP, epinephrine, and collagen; but this effect is not associated with an increased risk for bleeding.[85] Numerous reports have also appeared on the antiplatelet effects of the widely used selective serotonin reuptake inhibitors (paroxetine, sertraline, fluoxetine), which may block the only means of platelet serotonin uptake for storage;[172,173] the effect of the drug in decreasing platelet serotonin levels has been documented.[174,175] Prolonged bleeding time,[176] excessive bruising,[177] and defective platelet aggregation have all been noted in patients taking fluoxetine.[178] Additionally, patients taking serotonin reuptake inhibitors exhibit a higher incidence of gastrointestinal bleeding, with concomitant nonsteroidal antiinflammatory drug use increasing the bleeding risk beyond the sum of the individual effects of the two drugs.[179] Further evidence of the antiplatelet effects of serotonin reuptake inhibitors, especially those that bind the serotonin transporter with high affinity, is the reduction in risk for myocardial infarction seen in patients taking these drugs when compared to patients taking other antidepressants or no drugs at all.

Cocaine

Cocaine accounts for more drug-related visits to emergency departments in the United States than any other drug except alcohol. Its use is associated with a large increase in the incidence of myocardial infarction in individuals who are otherwise at low risk, and it has been hypothesized that platelet aggregation contributes substantially to this risk.[180] In vitro, however, cocaine has been shown to inhibit platelet aggregation to several agonists and to be capable of dissociating preformed aggregates.[181]

Oncologic Drugs

Administration of mithramycin has been associated with decreased platelet aggregation, increased bleeding time, and mucocutaneous bleeding.[182] Daunorubicin and bis-chloroethyl-nitrosourea can each inhibit platelet aggregation and secretion when added to platelet-rich plasma, but there has been no suggestion of clinically important bleeding caused by defective platelet function in patients receiving the drug.[85]

Statins

The statins, inhibitors of the key enzyme in cholesterol synthesis, 3-hydroxy-3-methylglutaryl coenzyme A reductase, are widely used in the therapy of hypercholesterolemia.[183] These agents, which include lovastatin, pravastatin, simvastatin, fluvastatin, atorvastatin, and cerivastatin, decrease the risks for cardiovascular death and complications through a variety of mechanisms, including reductions in the rate of thrombosis. Among these effects are decreases in platelet reactivity, brought about by the beneficial effects on vascular thrombogenicity, with increased production of endothelial nitric oxide and prostacyclin, and by directly decreasing platelet reactivity.[184] Membrane cholesterol content, which is lowered by the statins, has been correlated with platelet reactivity,[185,186] with recent evidence demonstrating that the content of cholesterol in these membranes correlates with localization of important membrane adhesive and agonist receptors within membrane microdomains known as rafts.[187] Statins, in addition to lowering plasma and membrane cholesterol levels, also reduce the activity of stimulatory signaling pathways that employ such signaling molecules as the small GTP-binding proteins Ras, Rho, and Rac, which require posttranslational prenylation to be targeted to cell membranes. Statins inhibit protein prenylation.[188] No bleeding complications have been associated with statin use, but a substudy of the Platelet Receptor in Ischemic Syndrome Management (PRISM) trial showed that their sudden withdrawal in the setting of acute coronary events (known coronary artery disease and chest pain within the previous 24 hours) was associated with an increased cardiac risk compared with that seen in patients who continued to receive statins (relative risk, 2.93) or who had never received statins.[189] This increase in cardiac events was partially attributed to increased platelet reactivity, mediated through direct and indirect mechanisms.

Miscellaneous Drugs

Clofibrate, another lipid-lowering drug, diminishes platelet responsiveness to ADP, collagen, and epinephrine when given to patients with type II hyperbetalipoproteinemia and can diminish the responsiveness of normal platelets to ADP and epinephrine in vitro.[85] Ketanserin, which has been studied for its potential to prevent atherosclerotic complications, decreases platelet aggregation in response to serotonin. Antihistamines and some radiographic contrast agents can also impair platelet aggregation. The mechanism of action of these agents is unknown.[85] The commonly used antihypertensive drug losartan, an angiotensin II receptor antagonist, interacts with the TXA_2 receptor and inhibits thromboxane-dependent platelet adhesion and aggregation.[190]

Foods and Food Additives

Certain foods and food additives can have important effects on platelet function, particularly when consumed in large quantities. In a classic study published in 1979, Dyerberg and Bang[191] reported that Greenland Eskimos on traditional diets had markedly prolonged bleeding times compared with gender- and age-matched Danish control subjects (mean 8.1 min versus 4.8 min), and they correlated this finding with an impaired secondary wave of platelet aggregation to ADP and collagen and high plasma levels of ω-3 fatty acids. The proposed mechanisms by which ω-3 fatty acids (eicosapentaenoic acid, C20:5ω-3; and docosahexaenoic acid, C22:6ω-3) interfere with platelet function is through their competition with arachidonic acid for the 2-acyl position of membrane phospholipids, or access to COX-1.[192,193] The action of platelet cyclooxygenase on the ω-3 fatty acids not only reduces TXA_2 synthesis to platelet agonist stimulation through competition with the substrate arachidonic acid, it also leads to the production of inhibitory eicosanoids. The latter mechanism was substantiated in the original study of Eskimos by the demonstration that administration of aspirin decreased the bleeding time in all subjects tested but not to *normal* levels.[191] Additionally, ω-3 fatty acids may increase the production of antiaggregatory prostaglandins from cells of the vascular wall.[191]

Ethanol, one of the most commonly and excessively ingested substances in the world, acts synergistically with aspirin to prolong the bleeding time.[69] In addition, ethanol acts cooperatively with agents that block binding of fibrinogen to GPIIb/IIIa in reducing platelet aggregation to several agonists; this effect is not solely caused by effects on TXA2 generation.[194] One study found that ethanol was capable of inhibiting collagen-induced platelet aggregation, secretion, arachidonate mobilization, and TXA_2 formation but did not inhibit platelet adhesion to deendothelialized rabbit aortae.[195]

Other food components or additives may affect platelet function and have been suspected of increasing the risk for minor bleeding. Easy bruising noted after eating Chinese food has been attributed to an effect on platelets by a substance in black tree fungus.[196] A component of onion extract can inhibit platelet arachidonic acid metabolism.[197] Ajoene, a component of garlic, is an inhibitor of fibrinogen binding to platelets and platelet aggregation.[198] Extracts from frequently consumed spices—cumin, turmeric, and clove—can decrease platelet thromboxane production and inhibit platelet aggregation.[199]

It can be concluded that platelets are sensitive to an enormous variety of therapeutic and dietary compounds.[85] However, an increased risk for clinically important bleeding has been demonstrated only for aspirin and agents specifically designed to inhibit platelet function. Reports of increased bleeding with all other agents must be viewed with caution. Despite this qualification, it would be prudent for the clinician to have a thorough understanding of the antiplatelet effects of drugs prescribed and to always consider the potential impacts of drug- or diet-induced platelet dysfunction, particularly in patients with coexisting hemostatic defects (see later in Patients on Anti-platelet Drugs Awaiting Surgery).

CHRONIC RENAL FAILURE

Clinical Features

The recognition of severe hemorrhage as a distinct complication of renal failure is generally attributed to Reisman's description in 1907 of two patients with Bright disease who had severe and generalized bleeding.[200] Reisman proposed that the cause was "a toxin analogous to the hemorrhagins of snake venom." However, the bleeding in Reisman's patients could have been attributed to any of a number of other associated conditions.[200] Others observed a "tendency to hemorrhage" in patients with chronic glomerulonephritis in the predialysis era, and the descriptions of epistaxis and menometrorrhagia[201] suggest a primary platelet abnormality. However, in the era before dialysis, death in patients with chronic renal failure occurred primarily from hyperkalemia and pulmonary edema.[202] After dialysis treatment became established, the major causes of death became infection and the underlying cause of the renal failure. Hemorrhage caused 6 of 100 deaths in one series, but additional factors could have contributed in each case.[202] The current prognosis for patients with end-stage renal disease is excellent, with a significant proportion surviving past 10 years and some reported to survive up to three decades on hemodialysis.[203] Bleeding problems were not mentioned in this discussion, and bleeding was not considered in reviews published in the past 25 years on the clinical course and management of patients with chronic renal failure. However, bleeding and thrombosis in patients with chronic uremia continue to be discussed.[204]

A more objective indication of the rarity of a significant bleeding diathesis in patients with renal failure is the extensive experience with percutaneous renal biopsy. In a study of 1000 consecutive percutaneous renal biopsies performed at the Mayo Clinic, 69 patients had hematuria, which cleared in 50 patients within 2 days.[64] Hypertension was a more significant factor than the bleeding time in predicting the occurrence of complications.[64] Another study of 183 consecutively performed renal biopsies reported three episodes of hemorrhage that required surgical intervention; all were the results of needle lacerations of the kidney or spleen.[205] In an analysis of 5120 renal biopsies performed at 15 institutions, there were no deaths, and the severe bleeding complications appeared to be related to anomalous vessels, heparin anticoagulation, or the presence of amyloid in the kidney.[206] The reports with other invasive procedures in patients with chronic renal disease are few, but they suggest that bleeding complications are rare after abdominal surgery, liver and bone marrow biopsies, and tooth extractions.[207]

By contrast, gastrointestinal tract hemorrhage is a common complication and frequent cause of death in patients with acute renal failure, and patients with chronic renal failure account for a significant proportion of patients undergoing endoscopy for upper gastrointestinal bleeding.[208] Experimental data suggest that chronic uremia renders the gastric mucosa susceptible to acid injury.[209] More than 90% of patients with renal failure and gastrointestinal bleeding have an anatomic diagnosis at endoscopy: Angiodysplasia is most common, with *peptic* lesions (gastric or duodenal ulcer, erosive esophagitis, gastritis, or duodenitis) also common.[208] Rectal ulcers can also cause sudden, massive lower gastrointestinal hemorrhage.

These observations suggest that serious, spontaneous hemorrhage is uncommon in patients with chronic renal failure. Nevertheless, platelet dysfunction is believed to constitute the primary hemostatic abnormality in uremia.[210] Descriptions of bleeding in uremia have often focused on the laboratory phenomena of abnormal platelet aggregation or a prolonged bleeding time, rather than actual hemorrhagic episodes in patients.[204] As with the drug-induced disorders of platelet function discussed earlier in drugs that affect platelet function section, abnormal platelet function in uremia is far more common than clinically important bleeding. Furthermore, laboratory evaluation of platelet function may not be a good predictor of the risk of hemorrhage.

Tests of Hemostasis and Platelet Function in Uremia

Platelet aggregation studies are frequently abnormal in uremic patients, but the occurrence abnormalities do not appear to correlate with the severity of the renal failure or the occurrence of bleeding.[211] The bleeding time may also be prolonged in uremia and does not necessarily correlate with the severity of the renal failure.[211] Furthermore, controversy exists as to whether the bleeding time is a useful predictor of risk for clinically important bleeding.[65,212] One study found no difference in bleeding complications whether or not a bleeding time was performed before renal biopsy.[213]

Anemia, which does correlate with the severity of renal failure, is an independent cause of a prolonged bleeding time.[214–217] The relation of the hematocrit to the bleeding time was first discerned by Duke, in 1910, who found that the bleeding time in thrombocytopenic patients was corrected by transfusion of fresh whole blood, but when thrombocytopenia recurred, the bleeding time was not as prolonged in the presence of a higher hematocrit. Furthermore, it has been noted that bleeding times can be prolonged with severe anemia caused by vitamin B_{12} or iron deficiency and can be corrected when the anemia is corrected with red blood cell transfusions.[214] Therefore, severely anemic patients with chronic renal failure would be expected to have prolonged bleeding times. The relation of the bleeding time to hematocrit in these patients has been confirmed by correction of the bleeding time with the transfusion of washed red blood cells and by treatment with erythropoietin.[216,218] There was a suggestion in these reports that bleeding symptoms also improved with the correction of the anemia. It is believed that anemia is associated with an increased bleeding time because of the demonstrated tendency of red blood cells to displace the less dense platelets to the periphery of the cylindrical blood vessel, where the platelets are able to surveil the vascular wall for defects.[219]

In contrast to the studies of platelet function performed to understand the possible increased risk for bleeding in patients with chronic renal failure, coagulation and fibrinolytic activities have been investigated to understand the increased risk for thrombotic complications, a major cause of mortality.[204] Although the data are inconsistent, markers of ongoing coagulation are often seen in patients with uremia, suggesting the presence of a prothrombotic state.[204,220]

Pathogenesis of Abnormal Platelet Function in Uremia

Even though the anemia of renal failure appears to be the major cause of the prolonged bleeding time, there is also evidence of abnormal platelet function. Platelet aggregation abnormalities persist when the hematocrit is normalized by red blood cell transfusion[215,216] or erythropoietin treatment.[221] The defects appear to result from intrinsic defects of the platelets and from substances in the plasma capable of inhibiting the function of normal platelets. Deficiencies in the number of GPIb complexes in uremic platelets have been reported, the number inversely correlating with the creatinine level.[222] Consistent with this finding, another study demonstrated that defective ristocetin-induced platelet aggregation of uremic platelet-rich plasma was not corrected by resuspending the platelets in normal platelet-poor plasma. Likewise, uremic platelets suspended in normal plasma were defective in their adhesion to deendothelialized rabbit vessels at a high shear rate, a test of the competency of the interaction between GPIb and vWF.[223] Conversely, the same study demonstrated that plasma factors also influence platelet function by showing that normal platelets suspended in uremic plasma acquire an adhesion defect that is possibly related to an abnormality of the interaction of vWF with the subendothelium. This led to the suggestion that vWF may be abnormal in uremia. Two studies have demonstrated normal to elevated vWF antigen and activity (measured as ristocetin cofactor activity) in uremic patients, but with decreased levels of the largest and most hemostatically active multimers,[224,225] reflected in one study as a decreased ratio of activity to antigen level compared with normal subjects.[224] Taken together, the various studies consistently indicate that the first step of platelet adhesion at sites of vessel wall injury is defective, a defect that could reach clinical significance if coupled with other defects of platelet function.

The platelets of uremic patients frequently exhibit reduced fibrinogen binding, aggregation, and secretion in response to a wide variety of agonists. This abnormality may be retained by the platelets after their separation from uremic plasma, and in some experiments uremic plasma has induced these defects in normal platelets. Uremic platelets may also exhibit a reduction in several of the biochemical responses necessary for aggregation and secretion, including the rise in cytoplasmic free calcium levels, release of arachidonic acid from membrane phospholipids, conversion of arachidonic acid to TXA_2, and dense-granule and α-granule secretion. Abnormal cytoskeletal assembly and deficient tyrosine phosphorylation have also been noted in uremic platelets, abnormalities only partially corrected by dialysis.[226]

The accumulation of dialyzable platelet-inhibitory substances in the plasma of uremic patients has long been recognized. The ability of uremic plasma to inhibit platelet function was demonstrated by Horowitz and colleagues,[227] who showed reduced ADP-induced platelet aggregation and a prolonged Stypven clotting time, a measure of platelet procoagulant activity. This activity, previously called *platelet factor 3,* is vital to the support of blood coagulation on the platelet surface and requires externalization of the anionic phospholipid phosphatidylserine. One uremic substance described by Horowitz and coworkers with platelet inhibitory properties is guanidinosuccinic acid,[228] which accumulates in uremic plasma as an alternative byproduct of L-arginine metabolism,[212] a consequence of the inhibitory effect of high urea levels on enzymes of the urea cycle. Like L-arginine, guanidinosuccinic acid is a precursor of nitric oxide, production of which is increased in endothelial cells and platelets in uremic patients and experimental animals.[212] Consistent with an important role for nitric oxide in uremia, infusion of the nitric oxide synthesis inhibitor monomethyl L-arginine reduced the bleeding time in uremic rats.[229] Suppression of nitric oxide production appears to correlate with the benefit of conjugated estrogens in improving the bleeding time in uremia.[230] Increased expression of vascular prostacyclin has also been described in uremic rats, a factor that would further depress in vivo platelet function.[231]

Dialysis itself may be associated with alterations in platelet function. For example, hemodialysis may cause transient increases in the bleeding time and reduced responsiveness to platelet agonists in vitro,[232] and chronic hemodialysis and peritoneal dialysis are associated with an increase in *reticulated* platelets, suggesting accelerated platelet turnover.[233] Of the two forms of dialysis, hemodialysis appears to have the greatest effect on platelet function, with one study noting abnormal cytoskeletal assembly and defective tyrosine phosphorylation to thrombin stimulation in the platelets of patients on hemodialysis, parameters that returned almost to normal with the institution of ambulatory peritoneal dialysis.[226] The cause of the defect associated with hemodialysis is likely to be the chronic low-level platelet activation associated with the procedure. In particular, polymerization and depolymerization of actin, release of granules and exposure of granule proteins on the platelet surface, and shedding of membrane proteins are all effects likely to render the platelets relatively refractory to subsequent activation.

As would be expected, platelets from uremic patients may be unusually sensitive to medicines that decrease platelet function. Aspirin has been reported to be more effective in prolonging the bleeding time in uremic patients than in control subjects, and this effect may occur by mechanisms other than the irreversible inhibition of COX-1 function. Similarly, β-lactam antibiotics that prolong the bleeding time may have a greater effect in uremic patients and may increase the occurrence of bleeding, particularly if renal clearance of the antibiotic is reduced.[85,217]

Mild thrombocytopenia has been reported in cases of chronic renal failure, in which setting it is probably caused by a combination of diminished marrow production and diminished platelet survival.[217] However, a platelet count of less than 100,000/μL should alert the physician to the possibility of thrombocytopenia caused by a systemic disease, such as multiple myeloma, systemic vasculitis, the hemolytic-uremic syndrome, preeclampsia, renal allograft rejection, or an adverse reaction to a drug such as heparin.

Erythropoietin deficiency can also contribute to the hemostatic defect of uremia. Consistent with this, defective tyrosine phosphorylation in uremic endothelial cells is restored when erythropoietin is added (see Uremic Bleeding section).[234]

CARDIOPULMONARY BYPASS

Clinical and Laboratory Features

Although cardiopulmonary bypass is accompanied by decreased plasma levels of coagulation factors and increased fibrinolytic activity, abnormal platelet function is a prominent observation in these patients. A fall in the platelet count and platelet dysfunction are seen in most patients undergoing bypass surgery with either a bubble or a membrane oxygenator.[235] A prolonged bleeding time (longer than expected for the degree of thrombocytopenia), decreased platelet aggregation, decreased platelet agglutination in response to ristocetin, and a decreased concentration of α-granule or dense granule contents are typically found in patients following bypass surgery.[235] Despite these abnormalities, excessive bleeding is uncommon, occurring in only approximately 5% of patients. Bleeding, usually manifesting as excessive chest tube blood loss (defined as >100 mL/h), has multiple causes: surgical complications, excessive protamine dose, and possibly also platelet function abnormalities.[236–240]

Recently, several surgeries have taken advantage of deep hypothermia circulatory arrest, especially those involving the thoracic aorta and congenital heart abnormalities. Neurological dysfunction is associated with this procedure and is believed to be at least partially caused by platelet microaggregates formed in response to the low temperature.

Pathogenesis of the Platelet Disorder

As with hemodialysis, the platelet defect caused by cardiopulmonary bypass is most likely caused by the effects of platelet activation and fragmentation within the extracorporeal circulation. The severity of the platelet abnormalities thus correlates with the duration of the bypass procedure.[241,242] Following uncomplicated surgery, platelet function returns to normal in 1 hour[241]; however, a much longer time may be required in some patients,[243] and the platelet count typically does not return to normal for several days.[240] Thrombocytopenia is caused by hemodilution, accumulation of platelets within the bypass circuit, and, to a lesser extent, sequestration of damaged platelets in the liver. Platelet dysfunction following bypass may be caused by reversible adhesion and aggregation of platelets to fibrinogen adsorbed from plasma onto the bypass circuit material; mechanical trauma and shear stress; cardiotomy suction; trace concentrations of circulating thrombin and ADP; complement activation; hypothermia; blood conservation devices; bypass priming solutions; and, with bubble oxygenators, exposure of platelets to the blood–air interface.[85] Cardiopulmonary bypass also consistently causes the appearance of platelet fragments, or membrane *microparticles,* evidence that the platelet surface membrane is subjected to severe mechanical stress and activation during the procedure.[242] These data indicate that a considerable amount of platelet aggregation occurs during cardiopulmonary bypass, simultaneously producing deleterious effects from substances released from the platelets and the new adhesive molecules exposed on their surfaces, and rendering the platelets relatively refractory to subsequent activation stimuli.

Another surgical cause of platelet dysfunction relates to the use of deep hypothermic circulatory arrest in some surgeries. This procedure involves cooling the vital organs to temperatures between 15°C and 22°C (59°F and 71.6°F) for the purpose of neuroprotection during complex surgeries of the aortic arch or intracerebral aneurysms.[244] During the period of deepest hypothermia, the circulation is stopped, making for bloodless surgical fields. Complications of deep hypothermic circulatory arrest include coagulopathy and neurological sequelae, with evidence that the latter problem may involve hypothermic activation of platelets and formation of microaggregates.[245]

Management

A study on the use of aspirin in patients undergoing coronary artery bypass grafting indicates that earlier practices of avoiding platelet inhibitors may in fact lead to increased morbidity of all types, ranging from death to ischemic complications involving the heart, the gut, and the kidneys.[90] Patients who received aspirin within 48 hours of their surgery reduced their risk of dying by one-third and their risk of nonischemic complications involving the heart, kidneys, and gastrointestinal tract by approximately two fifths. In the same study, it was noted that the patients who received either platelets or antifibrinolytic therapy as prophylaxis against postoperative bleeding were at increased risk for adverse complications and death. Thus, except in the setting of acute hemorrhage with evidence of platelet dysfunction, platelet transfusion should be avoided. Likewise, it is perhaps best to treat patients with aspirin soon after bypass surgery to decrease the incidence of deleterious effects. In addition to the known benefit of aspirin in preventing graft occlusion in patients undergoing coronary artery bypass grafting, the evidence would appear to warrant early institution of aspirin therapy in patients who have undergone cardiopulmonary bypass for other reasons and in whom aspirin therapy is not otherwise contraindicated.

When postoperative blood loss is greater than anticipated, it can be treated with DDAVP after cessation of bypass, but most clinical trials have not demonstrated a beneficial effect of this agent.[246,247] In these studies, a benefit of DDAVP seemed more apparent in patients undergoing more complex cardiac surgical procedures. Potential risks of DDAVP include hyponatremia, hypotension, and thrombosis.[246]

Attempts have been made to prevent platelet activation during bypass surgery in humans and experimental animals by infusion of prostaglandin E_1 or prostacyclin. By increasing the platelet concentration of cAMP and reducing platelet responsiveness, these agents partially prevent the occurrences of thrombocytopenia and platelet function abnormalities.[248] However, the hypotensive properties of these agents limit their usefulness. Antifibrinolytics (tranexamic acid, ε-aminocaproic acid, aprotinin) have been shown to be effective in reducing the loss of blood following cardiopulmonary bypass.[249] Aprotinin has been studied for its potential to protect platelets from activation by thrombin, plasmin, and other proteases generated during cardiopulmonary bypass. At high doses, aprotinin appears better than either ε-aminocaproic acid or desmopressin at reducing postoperative blood loss and is at least as good as tranexamic acid.[250] However, aprotinin has recently been reported to be associated with increases in late mortality and renal toxicity after cardiopulmonary bypass. Because the methodologies of these studies have clear limitations, continued use has been approved after review by the Food and Drug Administration, albeit limited to coronary artery bypass grafting and with cautions for greater postoperative vigilance.

In the management of the neurological sequelae of deep hypothermic circulatory arrest, evidence exists that treatment with the $\alpha_{IIb}\beta_3$ inhibitors eptifibatide or tirofiban may improve outcomes by preventing microvascular occlusion.[245]

ANTI-PLATELET ANTIBODIES

Immunoglobulins bind platelets nonspecifically and specifically and have the potential in both instances of interfering with platelet functions. In several pathologic conditions, including idiopathic thrombocytopenic purpura (ITP), systemic lupus erythematosus (SLE), and platelet alloimmunization, the antibodies lead to accelerated platelet destruction and thrombocytopenia. Generally, the surviving platelets, known as *stress platelets* display enhanced function.[251] Indeed, bleeding times in ITP may be shorter than expected for the degree of thrombocytopenia. Sometimes, however, the hemorrhagic tendency is greater than expected from the drop in platelet count or persists when the platelet count has recovered, signaling that the bound antibody may be perturbing platelet function. Immune thrombocytopenia is common; significantly impaired hemostasis caused primarily by antibody-mediated platelet dysfunction is not. In one study, 3 of 49 patients with ITP, whose platelet counts had recovered after therapy with either corticosteroids or splenectomy, continued to display elevated bleeding times and persistence of mucocutaneous hemorrhage.[252]

Clinical and Laboratory Features

In some patients with ITP or SLE, platelet dysfunction may be suspected because mucocutaneous bleeding symptoms occur at a platelet count that is usually sufficient for normal hemostasis (>50,000/μL), and the bleeding time may be longer than expected for the degree of thrombocytopenia. Patients with antiplatelet antibodies may exhibit defective platelet function in vitro, even if they do not have prolonged bleeding times or clinical symptoms of excessive bleeding—a situation similar to that described for the effects of aspirin ingestion and renal disease. For example, in two studies, 13 of 19 patients with ITP demonstrated impaired platelet aggregation to ADP, epinephrine, or collagen.[253,254] In two other studies, 22 of 35 patients with SLE were found to have decreased platelet aggregation in response to these agonists.[255,256] These platelet function abnormalities appeared to be antibody-mediated, because IgG purified from the plasma or eluted from the platelets of some of the patients inhibited the aggregation of normal platelets.

Platelet antibodies may impair several aspects of platelet function. The most frequently observed abnormality is absence of platelet aggregation in response to low concentrations of collagen, and absence of the second wave of irreversible aggregation in response to ADP or epinephrine. This pattern is identical to the abnormalities caused by aspirin, described earlier. In ITP and SLE, the abnormal aggregation may be related to the decreased platelet content of dense- and α-granule contents or to an activation defect manifested by diminished conversion of arachidonic acid to TXA_2.

Pathogenesis

Impairment of platelet function by autoantibodies or alloantibodies usually involves interference with the functions of the target antigens. For example, alloantibodies (eg, anti-Pl^{A1}) and autoantibodies have been described that interfere with the functions of $\alpha_{IIb}\beta_3$, sometimes causing a syndrome similar to Glanzmann thrombasthenia.[257–261] These antibody-associated thrombopathies can be severe. Interference with $\alpha_{IIb}\beta_3$ function perhaps is to be expected, given that $\alpha_{IIb}\beta_3$ is the most common protein antigen on the platelet surface and the most common target of autoantibodies.[262] Impairment of GPIb functions has also been described, in one case producing a syndrome of severe refractory thrombocytopenia and a functional defect closely resembling that seen in Bernard-Soulier syndrome.[263] An interesting aspect of antibodies against GPIb is the potential that they may be associated with more severe thrombocytopenia than when other antigens are targeted[264]; this finding is consistent with the observation that anti-GPIb antisera inhibited megakaryopoiesis in vitro[265] and with the finding that monoclonal GPIb antibodies inhibited in vitro proplatelet formation.[266] Autoantibodies have also been described that interfere with platelet collagen-binding function, targeting GPIa (integrin α_2),[267,268] GPIV,[268] and GPVI.[269,270] The latter glycoprotein was in fact identified as an important receptor for collagen based on the functional impairment in collagen response caused by patient antisera.[269,271]

Other antibodies have been described that can activate platelets. Of particular interest is the report of a patient who presented with immune thrombocytopenia and an antibody against CD9 (a member of the tetraspanin protein family) whose antibody could activate normal platelets.[272] After remission with recovery of the platelet count, the patient relapsed, this time with an antibody against the platelet Fc receptor, FcγRIIA. The latter antibody blocked the ability of the first antibody to activate platelets, confirming that activation involved stimulation of the Fc receptor. Platelets that have been activated and induced to secrete, but have not been incorporated into aggregates, are expected to be refractory to platelet agonists and deficient in secretory granule contents, essentially leading to an acquired storage pool deficiency, which has also been described in association with autoantibodies.[273]

DISSEMINATED INTRAVASCULAR COAGULATION

Disseminated intravascular coagulation (see Chapter 132) is sometimes associated with acquired storage pool disease, believed to result from repeated stimulation leading to what are graphically termed *exhausted platelets*.[274] It has also been suggested that the elevated fibrin(ogen) degradation products and low fibrinogen levels that occur in patients with disseminated intravascular coagulation may inhibit platelet function. Although purified fibrin(ogen) degradation products can impair platelet aggregation in vitro, the concentrations required to do this are unlikely to be found in vivo.[275] Another feature of disseminated intravascular coagulation, hypofibrinogenemia, is unlikely to contribute to a defect in platelet aggregation, except in extreme cases, as fibrinogen concentration in plasma exceeds by at least 10-fold the quantity needed to saturate fibrinogen receptors on platelets.[276]

DYSPROTEINEMIAS

Clinical Features

Although thrombotic complications are not uncommonly seen in dysproteinemias (and attributed to hyperviscosity), bleeding complications have likewise been attributed to excessive paraproteins acting through several pathophysiologic mechanisms. Platelet dysfunction is observed in approximately one-third of patients with IgA myeloma or Waldenström macroglobulinemia, in 15% of patients with IgG myeloma, and occasionally in patients with benign monoclonal gammopathy.[277] Additional hemostatic problems in these patients can be caused by the hyperviscosity syndrome,[278] a heparin-like coagulation inhibitor,[279] or complications of amyloidosis (eg, acquired factor X deficiency[280] or fibrinolysis[281]). Patients may have markedly abnormal results on laboratory tests (eg, the thrombin time) with no evidence of clinical bleeding.[277]

Pathogenesis

Abnormalities of platelet function correlate with the concentration of the plasma paraprotein. Myeloma proteins can inhibit all platelet functions—aggregation, secretion, procoagulant activity, and clot retraction—and normal platelets can acquire these defects when incubated with the purified monoclonal immunoglobulin.[282] In some cases, specific interactions of the monoclonal protein have been described. One IgA myeloma protein inhibited the ability of a suspension of aortic connective tissue to aggregate normal platelets.[283] The bleeding time and bleeding symptoms of the patient from whom this paraprotein was isolated were corrected when the IgA myeloma protein was removed by plasmapheresis. One patient suffered a fatal hemorrhage from an IgG1κ paraprotein that bound GPIIIa (β_3 integrin) and inhibited platelet aggregation.[284] A number of reports have described acquired von Willebrand disease in patients with myeloma, benign monoclonal gammopathy, or chronic lymphocytic leukemia.[285] In some patients, the plasma concentration of vWF was decreased, in others the larger multimers were deficient. The myeloma protein may interact with vWF and accelerate its clearance from plasma or interfere with its binding to platelet GPIb.

Management

Because bleeding appears to be correlated to high plasma paraprotein concentrations,[286] plasmapheresis should be performed expeditiously to reduce the paraprotein; effectiveness of this therapy can be evaluated by amelioration of bleeding symptoms. Chemotherapy for the underlying plasma cell neoplasm should be begun to effect a longer-lasting reduction of the paraprotein. DDAVP infusion, with or without plasmapheresis, may be transiently effective in patients with acquired von Willebrand disease.[285]

COMMENTS ON THE MANAGEMENT OF SELECTED BLEEDING DISORDERS

Liver Disease

The bleeding diathesis observed with fulminant or end-stage liver disease is multifactorial, with contributing causes such as thrombocytopenia, anemia, deficiencies in liver-synthesized coagulation factors, and excessive fibrinolysis well-described.[287,288] Chronic liver disease and hepatic cirrhosis of various causes have been reported to prolong the bleeding time and cause other platelet function abnormalities that may be related to a decrease in GPIb.[289] Although some studies have shown an association between prolonged bleeding time and gastrointestinal hemorrhage in cirrhotic patients,[290] other studies showed that the bleeding time and platelet aggregation abnormalities correlated best with the degree of thrombocytopenia,[291] suggesting that no specific platelet function defect exists in liver disease. However, this latter study did not evaluate patients by the severity of liver disease. One study found an aspirin-like defect in patients with severe liver disease, with defective aggregation and TXB_2 production.[292] Interestingly, one study of cirrhotic patients with hepatocellular carcinoma showed that platelets sampled from the portal circulation showed significantly decreased and delayed collagen aggregation as compared to samples from the systemic circulation.[293] In addition to portal hypertension and esophageal varices, this finding may point to localized vascular bed factors (including increased prostacyclin I_2) which may contribute specifically to variceal bleeding.

Patients on Antiplatelet Drugs Awaiting Surgery

Hematologists are often consulted to assess the risk of bleeding and to advise on the management of patients taking antiplatelet drugs and those who are scheduled for surgery and other invasive procedures. The decision to discontinue antiplatelet therapy is arbitrary, and there are no empirical guidelines. It is a common practice to discontinue antiplatelet therapy even for minor surgery. However, serious adverse events have been reported in association with preoperative interruption of antithrombotic treatments. Therefore, the risk of intraoperative or postoperative bleeding should be carefully weighed against the dangers of precipitating a thrombotic event.

The risk of bleeding in patients taking aspirin is minimal. Nevertheless, when a relatively healthy patient who is taking aspirin is scheduled for an invasive procedure, aspirin should ideally be discontinued for at least 5 days. This period of time is sufficient for replacement of approximately one-half of the aspirin-exposed platelets with new platelets that were not exposed to aspirin, resulting in a sufficient number (eg, approximately 100,000/μL) to affect hemostasis during any surgical procedure. However, because aspirin use is so common and because the drug is present in hundreds of pharmaceutical products, it may not be feasible to discontinue aspirin and wait 5 days for a procedure in some patients. Significant excessive bleeding caused by aspirin is rare, and any serious bleeding that does occur during an operative procedure is likely caused by a surgically correctible lesion. If severe hemorrhage caused by deficient platelet function is suspected, a platelet transfusion would be promptly effective, but this will only rarely be indicated. Aspirin use does not appear to be a reason to delay necessary surgery except in patients in whom the nature of the surgical procedure requires the absolute minimum risk for excessive bleeding (eg, some plastic-surgical, neurosurgical, or ophthalmologic procedures). The use of prophylactic platelet transfusions in this clinical setting is discouraged.

The thienopyridines, ticlopidine and clopidogrel, when used as a single agent, have a safety profile for bleeding similar to that of aspirin, but the data are less extensive. These two drugs undergo biotransformation in vivo to active metabolites that covalently modify the ADP receptor $P2Y_{12}$. The full antiplatelet effect of ticlopidine in vivo requires 3 to 5 days of oral administration, whereas an antiplatelet effect of clopidogrel is apparent within 2 hours of administration. Because, like aspirin, platelet inhibition with these agents is irreversible, it would be prudent to wait 5 days off the drug before surgery.

Because the thienopyridines have been found to be synergistic with aspirin in their effects on platelet function, their use in combination with aspirin has become standard therapy after stent placement and for the treatment of acute coronary syndromes. The bleeding risk is increased in patients receiving both medications. In the case of a patient presenting for emergency surgery, prophylactic platelet transfusion should still be avoided, and platelet transfusion should be considered only in the setting of severe or refractory hemorrhage.

Uremic Bleeding

Prolonged bleeding times and abnormal platelet aggregation are common in uremic patients, but they do not always predict an increased risk for hemorrhage or constitute an indication for transfusion or therapeutic intervention. If a patient with abnormal platelet function and a long bleeding time requires an invasive procedure, such as a kidney or lung biopsy or a laparotomy, and there is no history to suggest an increased risk for bleeding, it may be less risky to carry out the procedure without specific treatment to correct the platelet defect than to delay and attempt to normalize a laboratory value.

When therapy is indicated, the best strategy to improve hemostasis is to perform dialysis. Dialysis improves platelet function and normalizes the prolonged bleeding time in uremia and diminishes the risk for bleeding. For example, intensive dialysis decreases the occurrence of acute gastrointestinal bleeding, a major cause of morbidity and mortality in patients with acute renal failure. Peritoneal dialysis and hemodialysis are equally effective, but evidence of in vivo platelet activation is only seen in patients treated with hemodialysis.

If bleeding does complicate a procedure, the cause is most likely structural and should be managed as it would be in patients without renal failure. Similarly, patients with chronic renal failure who present with hemorrhage should by evaluated as are other bleeding patients; uremia should not be assumed to be the cause of bleeding.

Several treatment modalities, apart from intensive dialysis, may improve the bleeding time, and anecdotal observations suggest that they may also improve hemostasis. However, these modalities have not been uniformly effective, and prospective studies have not been performed. Therefore, therapy for bleeding in a patient with chronic renal failure should take into consideration the severity of bleeding, the anticipated severity of the hemostatic risk from surgery or trauma, and the risks of the therapy.

Infusion of DDAVP (L-deamino-8-D-arginine vasopressin, desmopressin) has been used in the management of bleeding in uremia and avoids the risk associated with the infusion of blood products. An intravenous or subcutaneous dose of 0.3 mg/kg administered over 15 to 30 minutes shortens the bleeding time in 50% to 75% of uremic patients. This correction occurs within 30 to 60 minutes and lasts for up to 4 hours, correlating with increases in the overall plasma concentration of vWF and in the fraction of vWF made up of higher-molecular-weight multimers. DDAVP has been reported to be effective in preventing surgical bleeding in uremic patients, but controlled trials of its efficacy are lacking. Another unresolved issue is whether uremic patients as a whole experience excessive surgical bleeding. DDAVP has less pressor effect than natural vasopressin, and side effects are uncommon but may include facial flushing, mild tachycardia, water retention, hyponatremia severe enough to cause seizures, arterial thrombosis, and memory loss. DDAVP stimulates the release of vWF from endothelial cells, which may account for its therapeutic effect, but other mechanisms may be involved, including a direct priming effect on the platelets.

Increasing the hematocrit, either by red blood cell transfusion or by treatment with recombinant human erythropoietin, is associated with a correction of the bleeding time and possibly reduced tendency to bleed. The mechanism by which anemia prolongs the bleeding time in uremia is unknown but may relate to the absence of the normal effect of axial streaming of erythrocytes in the center of the bloodstream that forces the platelets toward the edge of the blood vessel and thereby facilitates their ability to detect disruptions of the endothelium.[219] It has also been proposed that erythrocytes facilitate activation of platelets by releasing ADP, a contribution diminished by anemia.[294] The benefits of increasing the hematocrit by transfusion must be weighed against the risk of infection associated with transfusion of blood products.

Conjugated estrogens have also been reported to shorten prolonged bleeding times in uremic patients and to correct the bleeding diathesis.[295] Even a single 50-mg dose of oral conjugated estrogen (Premarin) may be effective. In support of this, conjugated estrogens have been shown to shorten the prolonged bleeding time in uremic rats.[296] The correction of the bleeding time in this model was abolished by the nitric oxide precursor L-arginine, and administration of estrogens to uremic rats decreases the expression of nitric oxide synthase. These findings suggest that the estrogen effect on hemostasis in uremia might be mediated by changes in the nitric oxide synthetic pathway.

Some studies have reported that cryoprecipitate infusions shorten the bleeding time in patients with uremia, but others have not; it is unlikely that the benefit justifies the risk.

SUGGESTED READINGS

Barbui T, Finazzi G: Therapy for polycythemia vera and essential thrombocythemia is driven by the cardiovascular risk. Semin Thromb Hemost 33:321, 2007.

Carobbio A, Finazzi G, Guerini V, et al: Leukocytosis is a risk factor for thrombosis in essential thrombocythemia: Interaction with treatment, standard risk factors, and Jak2 mutation status. Blood 109:2310, 2007.

Falanga A, Marchetti M, Vignoli A, et al: V617F JAK-2 mutation in patients with essential thrombocythemia: Relation to platelet, granulocyte, and plasma hemostatic and inflammatory molecules. Exp Hematol 35:702, 2007.

Fontana P, Reny JL: New antiplatelet strategies in atherothrombosis and their indications. Eur J Vasc Endovasc Surg 34:10, 2007.

Hillmen P, Muus P, Duhrsen U, et al: Effect of the complement inhibitor eculizumab on thromboembolism in patients with paroxysmal nocturnal hemoglobinuria. Blood 110:4123, 2007.

Strand V: Are COX-2 inhibitors preferable to non-selective non-steroidal anti-inflammatory drugs in patients with risk of cardiovascular events taking low-dose aspirin? Lancet 370:2138, 2007.

Sugidachi A, Ogawa T, Kurihara A, et al: The greater in vivo antiplatelet effects of prasugrel as compared to clopidogrel reflect more efficient generation of its active metabolite with similar antiplatelet activity to that of clopidogrel's active metabolite. J Thromb Haemost 5:1545, 2007.

Toyama K, Karasawa M, Yamane A, et al: JAK2-V617F mutation analysis of granulocytes and platelets from patients with chronic myeloproliferative disorders: Advantage of studying platelets. Br J Haematol 139:64, 2007.

REFERENCES

For complete list of references log onto www.expertconsult.com

PART IX

TRANSFUSION MEDICINE

CHAPTER 143

HUMAN BLOOD GROUP ANTIGENS AND ANTIBODIES

Marion E. Reid and Connie M. Westhoff

INTRODUCTION

An important clinical concern in transfusion medicine occurs when a patient requiring transfusion is found to have unexpected blood group antibodies. Although these antibodies can be characterized in terms of specificity, immunoglobulin class, and in vitro characteristics, no fool-proof method exists to predict the clinical significance. The potential for adverse effects of transfusion should be assessed by correlating the serological information with clinical experiences reported in the literature and with the patient's medical history. For example, a patient who has not been exposed to red blood cells (RBCs) by transfusion or pregnancy is unlikely to have a clinically significant alloantibody.

ERYTHROCYTE BLOOD GROUP ANTIGENS

Erythrocyte blood group antigens are polymorphic, inherited, carbohydrate, or protein structures located on the surface of the RBC membrane. There are 29 different blood group systems, with more than 250 associated blood group antigens (Table 143–1). The protein antigens are primarily located on integral transmembrane proteins, but a few are on glycosylphosphatidylinositol (GPI)-linked proteins. Some antigens are carbohydrates attached to proteins or lipids, some require a combination of a specific portion of protein and carbohydrate, and a few antigens are carried on proteins that are adsorbed from the plasma. Many proteins carrying blood group antigens reside in the erythrocyte membrane as complexes with other proteins,[1] and many components carrying blood group antigens have been assigned cluster of differentiation numbers.

Recognition of a blood group antigen begins with discovery of an antibody. When an individual whose RBCs lack an antigen is exposed to RBCs that possess the antigen, he or she may mount an immune response and produce antibodies that react with the antigen. Depending on the characteristics of the antibody and the number and topology of antigens in the RBC membrane, the interaction between antibody and antigen may result in sensitization, agglutination, or hemolysis when complement is activated. In blood group testing, most assays are designed to result in agglutination and clumping of the RBCs is the detectable endpoint.[2] The ability to detect and identify blood group antigens and antibodies has contributed significantly to current safe supportive blood transfusion practice, to the appropriate management of pregnancies at-risk for hemolytic disease of the newborn (HDN), and to management of organ transplantation.

Terminology

Some blood group systems bear the family surname in which the antibody was first discovered (Kell, Kidd, Duffy, etc.), with abbreviations to indicate alleles (K/k, Jk^a/Jk^b, and Fy^a/Fy^b etc.). Others were given letter designations (A, B, D, M, N, etc.). A committee for terminology of RBC surface antigens, organized by the International Society for Blood Transfusion, works to standardize terminology of new blood group antigens.[3]

MOLECULAR BASIS OF BLOOD GROUP ANTIGENS AND PHENOTYPES

Most genes encoding blood group antigens have been cloned and sequenced,[4] and the molecular basis of most blood group antigens has been determined.[5,6] Details concerning the alleles associated with blood group antigens and phenotypes can be obtained from the following Web site: www.ncbi.nlm.nih.gov/projects/mhc/xslcgi.fcgi?cmd=bgmut/home. Knowledge of the gene has allowed determination or predictions regarding the structure and function of the components carrying blood group antigens as well as an appreciation of diseases associated with loss of expression of some blood groups, such as null phenotypes (Table 143–2). Knowledge of the gene has made it possible to perform DNA analyses to type multiply transfused patients, determine gene dosage (zygosity), and perform noninvasive fetal typing not possible by classical hemagglutination. Table 143–3 lists examples of DNA-based assays useful in the transfusion medicine.

Blood Group Antibodies

The common causes of immunization against blood group antigens are transfusion, pregnancy and occasionally transplantation or practices such as sharing needles. In addition, microbes encountered by way of the digestive tract and other mucosal surfaces regularly (eg, anti-A, -B, -P, $-P^k$) or sometimes (eg, anti-M, -P1, $-Le^a$, $-Le^b$) result in production of so-called naturally occurring antibodies. These antibody specificities are the most common antibodies present in children and nontransfused male patients.

Antibodies recognizing antigens in the ABO blood group system are by far the most clinically significant. Others occur in the following approximate order, from the most to the least commonly encountered in transfusion practice: anti-D, anti-K, anti-E, anti-c, anti-Fy^a, anti-C, anti-Jk^a, anti-S, and anti-Jk^b. Other clinically significant antibodies occur with an incidence of less than 1% of immunized patients.[7,8]

Antibodies considered clinically insignificant unless the antibody reacts in tests performed strictly at 37°C (98.6°F) include those to A1, P1, M, N, Lu^a, Le^a, Le^b, and Sd^a antigens. A few antibodies that react at 37°C (98.6°F) by the indirect antiglobuin test (IAT) but are usually clinically insignificant include those of the Knops and Ch/Rg systems. Table 143–4 summarizes the immunoglobulin class and clinical significance associated with some alloantibodies. A brief clinical and technical description of most blood group antibodies can be found in reviews.[9–11]

Compatibility testing (patient's serum against donor's RBCs) still uses techniques that were described more than 100 years ago for direct agglutination, and more than 50 years ago for indirect agglutination. The hemagglutination technique is simple; is inexpensive; does not require sophisticated equipment; and, when done correctly, is sensitive and specific in terms of clinical relevance.

Blood group IgM antibodies to carbohydrate antigens (eg, in ABO, P1, Le, H and P systems) often agglutinate antigen-positive RBCs suspended in a saline medium (direct agglutination). Most

Table 143–1 Blood Group Systems

ISBT System Name (Number)	Gene Name HGNC (ISBT)	Chromosome Location	Predicted Topology (Number of amino acids AA)	Component Name (CD number)	Associated Blood Group Antigens (Null phenotype)
ABO (001)	*ABO*	9q34.2	Glycosyltransferases Type II (354 AA)	Carbohydrate	A, B, A, B, A1
MNS (002)	*GYPA (MN)* *GYPB (Ss)*	4q31.21	Type I (131 AA) (72 AA)	GPA (CD235a) GPB (CD235b)	M, N, S, s, U, Vw + 40 more (En(a–); U–; M^kM^k)
P (003)	*P1*	22q11.2-qter	Galactosyltransferase	Carbohydrate	P1
Rh (004)	*RHD* *RHCE*	1p36.11	Multipass: 12 spans (417 AA)	RhD (CD240D) RhCE (CD240CE)	D, C, E, c, e, G, V, Rh17 + 42 more (Rh_{null})
Lutheran (005)	*LU*	19q13.32	Type I IgSF (597 AA) (557 AA)	Lutheran glycoprotein B-CAM (CD239)	Lu^a, Lu^b, Lu3, Lu4, Au^a, Au^b + 13 more (Recessive Lu[a–b–])
Kell (006)	*KEL*	7q34	Type II (732 AA)	Kell glycoprotein (CD258)	K, k, Kp^a, Kp^b, Ku, Js^a, Js^b + 21 more (K_0 or K_{null})
Lewis (007)	*FUT3(LE)*	19p13.3	Fucosyltransferase Type II (361 AA)	Carbohydrate Adsorbed from plasma	Le^a, Le^b, Le^{ab}, Le^{bh}, ALe^b, BLe^b (Le[a–b–])
Duffy (008)	*DARC (FY)*	1q23.2	Multipass: 7 spans (338 AA)	Fy glycoprotein (CD234)	Fy^a, Fy^b, Fy3, Fy4, Fy5, Fy6 (Fy[a–b–])
Kidd (009)	*SLC14A1(JK)*	18q12.3	Multipass: 10 spans (389 AA)	Kidd glycoprotein	Jk^a, Jk^b, Jk3 (Jk[a–b–])
Diego (010)	*SLC4A1 (DI)*	17q21.31	Multipass: 14 spans (911 AA)	Band 3, AE1 (CD233)	Di^a, Di^b, Wr^a, Wr^b, Wd^a, Rb^a + 15 more
Yt (011)	*ACHE (YT)*	7q22	GPI-linked (557 AA)	Acetyl-cholinesterase	Yt^a, Yt^b
Xg (012)	*MIC2 (XG1)*	Xp22.33	Type I (180 AA) (163 AA)	Xg^a glycoprotein CD99	Xg^a
Scianna (013)	*ERMAP(SC)*	1p34.2	Type I (475 AA)	*ERMAP*	Sc1, Sc2, Sc3, Rd + 3 more (Sc: –1,–2,–3)
Dombrock (014)	*ART4 (DO)*	12p12.3	GPI-linked (314 AA)	Do glycoprotein; ART 4 (CD297)	Do^a, Do^b, Gy^a, Hy, Jo^a (Gy[a–])
Colton (015*)*	AQP1 (CO)	7p14	Multipass: 6 spans (269 AA)	*Aquaporin*	Co^a, Co^b, Co3 (Co[a–b–])
Landsteiner-Wiener (016)	ICAM4 (LW)	19p13.2	Type I IgSF (241 AA)	LW glycoprotein (ICAM-4) (CD242)	LW^a, LW^{ab}, LW^b (LW[a–b–])
Chido/ Rodgers (017)	*C4A, C4B (CH/RG)*	6p21.32	Adsorbed from plasma	C4A; C4B	CH1, CH2, Rg1 + 6 more
Hh (018)	*FUT1(H)*	19q13.33	Fucosyltransferase Type II (365 AA)	Carbohydrate (CD173)	H (Bombay or Oh)
Kx (019)	*XK (XK)*	Xp21.1	Multipass: 10 spans (444 AA)	XK glycoprotein	Kx (McLeod)
Gerbich (020)	*GYPC (GE)*	2q14.3	Type I (128 AA) (107 AA)	GPC (CD236) GPD	Ge2, Ge3, Ge4 + 5 more (Leach phenotype)
Cromer (021)	*CD55 (CROM)*	1q32.2	GPI-linked (347 AA)	DAF (CD55)	Cr^a, Tc^a, Tc^b, Tc^c, Dr^a, Es^a, IFC + 8 more
Knops (022)	*CR1(KN)*	1q32.2	Type I (1998 AA)	CR1 (CD35)	Kn^a, Kn^b, McC^a, Sl^a, Yk^a + 4 more
Indian (023)	*CD44 (IN)*	11p13	Type I (341 AA)	Hermes antigen (CD44)	In^a, In^b + 2 more
Ok (024)	*BSG (OK)*	19p13.3	Type I IgSF (248 AA)	Neurothelin, basigin (CD147)	Ok^a
RAPH (025)	*MER2*	11p15.5	Not known	Not defined	MER2 (Raph–)
JMH (026)	*SEMA-L (JMH)*	15q24.1	GPI-linked (656 AA)	H-Sema-L, Semaphorin 7A (CD108)	JMH + 4 more
I (027)	*IGNT*	6p24.2	*N*-Acetylglucosaminyltransferase type II (400 AA)	Carbohydrate	I (I– or i adult)
Globoside(028)	*3GALT3* or *βGalNAcT1*	3q26.1	*N*-acetylgalactosaminyltransferase type II (331 AA)	Carbohydrate (Gb_4, globoside)	P (P–)
GIL (029)	*AQP3(GIL)*	9p13.3	Multipass: 6 spans (292 AA)	AQP3	GIL (GIL–)

IgSF, immunoglobulin super family; ISGN, International Society for Gene Nomenclature; type I, Protein with a single pass through the RBC lipid bilayer with its amino terminus to the outside of the cell; type II = Protein with a single pass through the RBC lipid bilayer with its amino terminus to the inside of the cell.

Table 143–2 Blood Groups, Function and Disease Association

Function	System Name	Present in Other Tissue	Null Phenotype	Disease Association
Structure				
Interacts with protein 4.1 and p55	Gerbich	Fetal liver, renal endothelium	Leach	Hereditary elliptocytosis, hemolytic anemia; decreased protein 4.1 and p55 *Plasmodium falciparum*[96]
Structure and Transport				
Anion transport	Diego	Granulocytes, kidney: intercalated cells of distal and collecting tubules	1 case: transfusion dependent	Southeast Asian ovalocytosis, hereditary spherocytosis, renal tubular acidosis
Transport; possible neurotransmitter	Kx	Fetal liver, adult skeletal muscle, brain, pancreas, heart	McLeod	Acanthocytosis, muscular dystrophy, hemolytic anemia; McLeod syndrome sometimes associated with CGD
Possible structural function	Rh	No	Rh_{null}	Hemolytic anemia; hereditary stomatocytosis–Rh_{null} syndrome; reduced expression and mosaicism; hematological malignancies
Ammonia Transport	RhAG	Homologs in kidney, brain, gut, gallbladder, liver, etc.		
Urea transport	Kidd	Vasa recta endothelium Renal medulla	Jk(a–b–)	Impaired urea transport, urine concentrating defect
Water transport	Colton	Kidney, liver, gall bladder, eye, capillary endothelium	Co(a–b–)	Urine concentrating defect
Glycerol/water/urea transport	GIL		GIL-negative	
Receptor and adhesion molecules				
Chemokine/*Plasmodium vivax* receptor	Duffy	Endothelial and epithelial cells, Purkinje cells, colon, lung, spleen, thyroid, thymus, kidney	Fy(a–b–): Resistance to *P. vivax*	Receptor for *P. vivax*
Binds hyaluronic acid, mediates adhesion of leukocytes	Indian	Wide tissue distribution	1 case: congenital dyserythropoietic anemia	
Binds laminin	Lutheran	Fetal liver, placenta, arterial walls, BM epithelium	Lu(a–b–) recessive type	Increased expression possibly involved in vasoocclusion in sickle cell disease[83]
Ligand for integrins	Landsteiner-Wiener		LW_{null} also Rh_{null}	Depressed in pregnancy and in some malignant diseases
Possible adhesion	Ok	All cells tested		
Adhesion molecules	Xg	Fibroblasts, fetal liver, spleen, thymus, adrenal, adult BM		
Adhesion molecule. Function in RBCs not known	JMH			Absent from PNH III RBCs
Possible adhesion	Scianna		Sc:–1,–2,–3	See reference 79
Enzymes				
Cleaves big endothelin 3 to ET-3 (a potent vasoconstrictor)	Kell	Bone marrow, fetal liver, testes, brain, lymphoid tissue, heart	K_{null} (K_0)	
Enzymatic (AChE)	Yt	Granulocytes, innervated tissue, including brain and muscle		Absent from PNH III RBCs
Enzymatic (ART4)	Dombrock		Gy(a–)	Absent from PNH III RBCs
Complement				
Part of the complement cascade	Chido/Rodgers	Plasma	C4: deficient RBCs predispose for SLE	Certain phenotypes increased susceptibility to autoimmune conditions and infections
Complement regulation; binds C3b; disassembles C3/C5 convertase	Cromer	Vascular endothelium, Epithelia GI, GU, CNS. Soluble form in plasma and urine	*Inab*	Absent from PNH III RBCs; Dr^a is the receptor for uropathogenic *Escherichia coli*
Complement regulation; binds C3B and C4b; mediates phagocytosis	Knops	Blood cells, glomerular podocytes, follicular dendritic cells	No case reported	Antigens depressed in certain autoimmune and malignant conditions

Table 143–2 Blood Groups, Function and Disease Association—cont'd

Function	System Name	Present in Other Tissue	Null Phenotype	Disease Association
Other				
	ABO	Epithelial cells, secretions, ectoderm, and endoderm	Group O	Altered expression in some hematological disorders: leukemia
	H	Broad distribution soluble: all fluids except CSF in secretors	Bombay (O_h)	Decreased in some tumour cells; increased in hematopoietic stress
	Lewis	Blood cells, GI, skeletal muscle, kidney, adrenal	Le(a–b–)	Increased expression in fucosidosis
Glycosylation	I	Broad tissue distribution	i	Cataracts in Asians
	GLOB	Blood cells; soluble form in cyst fluid	P^k and p	Receptor *E. coli* and Parvovirus B19
Carrier of negative charge on sialic acid; complement regulation; receptor for microbes	MNS		$M^k M^k$ lack GPA and GPB En(a–) lack GPA S–s–U: lack GPB	Decreased *P. falciparum* invasion; may be receptor for *E. coli*

CGD, chronic granulomatous disease; CNS, central nervous system; GI, gastrointestinal; GL, glycolipid; GP, glycoprotein; GU, genitourinary; IgSF = immunoglobulin super family; PNH, paroxysmal nocturnal hemoglobinuria; RBC, red blood cell; BM = bone marrow.

Table 143–3 Uses of DNA-Based Assays in the Clinical Laboratory

Type patients who have been recently transfused
Identify a fetus at risk for hemolytic disease of the newborn
Type RBCs coated with immunoglobulin
Type patients with AIHA to select antigen-negative RBCs for absorption of autoantibodies when searching for underlying alloantibodies
Type donors, including mass screening for antigen-negative donors, when appropriate antisera are not readily available
Type donors for antibody screening cells and identification panels
Determine which phenotypically antigen-negative patients can receive antigen-positive RBCs without being immunized
Type patients who have an antigen that is expressed weakly on RBCs
Identify partial D
Resolve blood group A, B, and Rh discrepancies
Determine *RHD* zygosity

AIHA, autoimmune hemolytic anemia; RBC, red blood cell.

other antigens (eg, in Rh, Kell, Duffy, and Kidd systems) are proteins and are detected by the antiglobulin test, which detects IgG antibodies and/or complement on the RBCs. The *indirect* antiglobulin test (IAT) is used to detect RBCs sensitized in vitro, such as antibody detection and identification, antigen typing, and crossmatching. The *direct* antiglobulin test (DAT) is used to detect RBCs sensitized in vivo such as alloantibodies in transfusion reactions or HDN, and autoantibodies in warm autoimmune hemolytic anemia or cold hemagglutinin disease.

Compatibility Procedures and Location of Antigen-Negative Blood

In most countries, a blood sample from a prospective recipient is tested for ABO, D, and detection of unexpected (ie, other than anti-A and anti-B) blood group antibodies. Blood typing problems should be resolved and when antibodies are detected they should be identified. Once a patient is actively immunized to an RBC antigen and produces a clinically significant alloantibody, the patient is considered immunized for life and should be transfused with antigen-negative RBCs, even if the antibody is no longer detectable. Patients with passively acquired antibody (eg, neonates, recipients of plasma and platelet products, Rh immune globulin, intravenous immune globulin) must be transfused with antigen-negative RBCs only while the passive antibody is present. Knowing the specificity of an antibody helps establish whether it is likely to be clinically significant and determine the approach necessary to provide an adequate supply of compatible blood. Selection of blood for transfusion to patients with blood group alloantibodies is the joint responsibility of staff at the hospital and donor blood center. The transfusion service staff are a vital conduit for communication between the patient's physician and/or consultant hematologist and the donor center staff to determine the predicted immediate and on-going transfusion needs of the patient and to ensure that antigen-negative blood is available for the patient as appropriate. To some extent selection of antigen-negative blood depends on the urgency of the transfusion.

Transfusion management of patients who require chronic transfusion therapy, in particular patients with sickle cell anemia, has been the subject of much debate.[12,13] Some programs attempt to prevent alloimmunization by prophylactic transfusion of blood that is antigen-matched for D, C, E, and K or for many additional antigens (Table 143–5). There is no consensus at present as to the best approach, but the goal is to provide blood that will survive maximally.

It is important not to delay surgery or transfusion unnecessarily by attempting to obtain antigen-negative RBCs for patients with antibodies that are not clinically significant. Also, in hemolytic anemia caused by warm-reactive autoantibodies, compatibility may be difficult to demonstrate. In this scenario, the important issue is to be sure that there are no clinically significant alloantibodies underlying the warm reactive autoantibodies (see box on "Laboratory Methods for Detecting Blood Group Antigens and Antibodies").

Disease Association

The absence of some blood group antigens and their carrier molecules can result in disease. For example, an absence of the Rh proteins causes stomatocytosis and compensated hemolytic anemia (Rh_{null} syn-

Table 143–4 Characteristics of Some Blood Group Alloantibodies (the Antibodies Are Listed in Approximate Order of Clinical Significance)

			Clinical	
Antibody specificity	**IgM (Direct)**	**IgG (Indirect)**	***Transfusion Reaction***	***HDN***
ABO	Most	Some	Immediate; mild to severe	Common; mild to moderate
H in Bombay	Most	Some	Immediate; mild to severe	Mild to severe
Rh	Some	Most	Immediate/delayed; mild to severe	Common; mild to severe
Kell	Some	Most	Immediate/delayed; mild to severe	Sometimes; mild to severe
Kidd	Few	Most	Immediate/delayed; mild to severe	Rare; mild
Duffy	Rare	Most	Immediate/delayed; mild to severe	Rare; mild
S	Some	Most	Delayed/mild	Rare; mild to severe
s	Rare	Most	Delayed/mild; immediate/delayed;	Rare; mild to severe
U	Rare	Most	Mild to severe	Rare; severe
PP1P^k	Most*	Most*	Mild to severe	Mild to severe**
Vel	Most*	Most*	Mild to moderate	Mild to severe
Diego	Some	Most	Delayed; none to severe	Mild to severe
Colton	Rare	Most	Delayed; mild	Rare; mild to severe
Lutheran	Some	Most	Delayed	Rare; mild
Dombrock	Rare	Most	Immediate/delayed; mild to severe	Rare; mild
M	Some	Most	Delayed (rare)	Rare; mild
N	Most	Rare	None	None
LW	Rare	Most	Delayed; none to mild	Rare; mild
Yt^a	Rare	Most	Delayed (rare); none to mild	None
Ch/Rg	Rare	Most	Anaphylactic (3)	None
JMH	Rare	Most	Delayed (rare in genetic variants); none to mild	None
P1	Most	Rare	None (rare)	None
Le^a	Most	Few	Immediate (rare)	None
Le^b	Most	Few	None	None
I	Most	Rare	None None to mild in I-adults	None
Knops	Rare	Most	None	None
Xg^a	Rare	Most	None	None

HDN, hemolytic disease of the newborn.
*Most examples of these antibodies are both IgM and IgG.
**Seldom hemolysis of fetal cells but high incidence of recurrent spontaneous abortions.

Table 143–5 Approaches to Supplying RBC Products to Sickle Cell or Other Transfusion-Dependent Patients

Provide antigen-negative blood after the patient has made the corresponding alloantibody
Provide phenotype-matched blood after the patient makes the first antibody
Provide blood matched for D, C, E, and K antigens
Provide blood matched for D, C, E, c, e, K, Fy^a, Fy^b, Jk^a, and Jk^b antigens
Provide completely phenotyped RBC products including antigens such as U, Js^b, and hr^B

RBC, red blood cell.

drome), whereas an absence of Xk protein causes the McLeod syndrome. RBCs and white blood cells from patients with leukocyte adhesion deficiency II (also known as congenital disorder of glycosylation type II) lack antigens that depend on fucose. Thus, the RBCs have the Bombay, Le(a–b–) phenotype and the white blood cells lack sialy-Le^x, which explains the high white blood cell count and infections in these patients.[14,15] Hemagglutination is a simple test that can be used to diagnose these three syndromes.

In patients with paroxysmal nocturnal hemoglobinuria, a proportion of the RBCs will lack antigens carried on GPI-linked proteins. Other associations between blood group antigens and diseases are summarized in Table 143–2. Diseases associated with antibodies to blood group antigens include hemolytic disease of the newborn, warm autoimmune hemolytic anemia, cold hemagglutinin disease, and paroxysmal cold hemoglobinuria. Hemagglutination is a valuable aid in diagnosis of these conditions.

Blood Group Systems

Presented here is a brief description of the most clinically relevant blood group systems in approximate order of clinical significance. Information about these and other blood group systems is given in Table 143–1, Table 143–2, and Table 143–4. For further information and prevalence of blood group antigens in different populations, the interested reader is referred to specialized texts such as *Human*

Laboratory Methods for Detecting Blood Group Antigens and Antibodies

Manual or gel-column methods based on agglutination of red blood cells (RBCs) are still the most common serologic assays performed in transfusion medicine laboratories. Automated assays based on agglutination, and automated solid-phase adherence assays are primarily used in large centers.

The serologic behavior of RBC antibodies primarily reflects the immunoglobulin isotype, but is also influenced by the target antigen copy number. Most antibodies to carbohydrate antigens such as those in the ABO, Lewis, and P blood group systems are naturally occurring and are of the IgM isotype. These multivalent antibodies optimally bind and directly agglutinate to RBCs at temperatures less than 37°C (98.6°F). In contrast, antibodies occurring following immunization to protein antigens such as those in the Rh, Kell, Kidd, and Duffy blood group systems are of the IgG isotype. These bivalent antibodies optimally bind to, but do not directly agglutinate, RBCs at 37°C (98.6°F). The addition of an antiglobulin reagent (ie, rabbit antihuman IgG; Coombs serum) is required to induce RBC agglutination.

Blood Group Typing

ABO

Commercially available human polyclonal and mouse monoclonal anti-A and anti-B are used to determine the ABO type of patient and donor, and these reagents directly agglutinate RBCs at room temperature. To confirm a patient's ABO type, the serum is tested for the presence of the corresponding agglutinins by testing with commercially available group A and group B RBCs. In both cases, hemagglutination is macroscopically visible, and an antiglobulin reagent is not required.

Rh

Patient and donor RBCs are routinely tested for the presence of the D antigen in the Rh system. Reagents containing monoclonal anti-D that directly agglutinate D-positive RBCs (designated Rh positive) suspended in saline at room temperature are commonly used for patient testing. Testing for expression of a weak D antigen on RBCs is required for donor units.

Identification of Serum Alloantibodies or Autoantibodies

Most alloantibodies in patient sera are of the IgG isotype and do not directly agglutinate antigen-positive RBCs. Thus, the most common assay used to detect these antibodies is the indirect antiglobulin test (IAT), formerly known as the indirect Coombs test. In this assay (*antibody screening*), patient serum is incubated at 37°C (98.6°F) with commercially available reagent RBCs of known antigen type. After incubation unbound antibodies are removed from the RBCs by washing with saline; and an antiglobulin reagent containing either rabbit antihuman IgG, or a mixture of rabbit antihuman IgG and murine monoclonal antihuman complement, is added. If the RBCs are agglutinated, this indicates the presence of an alloantibody, an autoantibody, or both. The distinction between alloantibody and autoantibody and the determination of the specificity of the alloantibody are determined by testing the serum against a panel of different

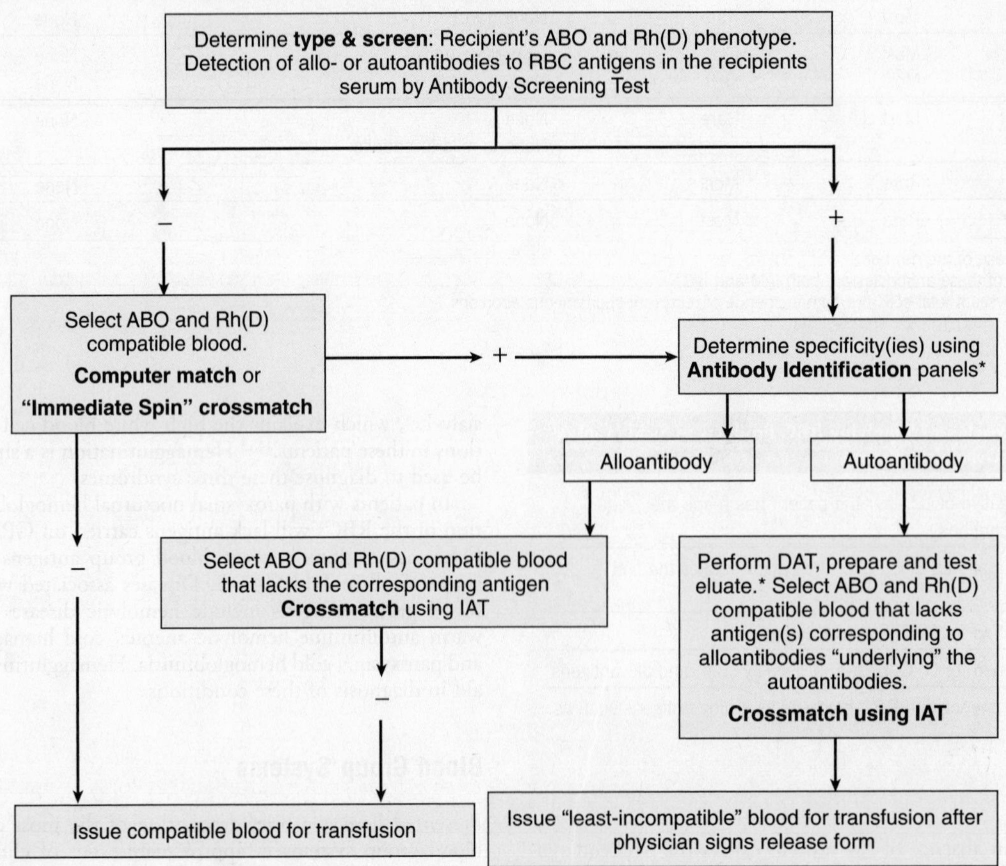

Laboratory Methods for Detecting Blood Group Antigens and Antibodies—cont'd

reagent RBCs (usually 10) varying in antigen phenotype (*antibody identification*). Agglutination of all panel cells suggests the presence of an antibody to a high prevalence antigen or of an autoantibody; differential reactivity suggests the presence of an alloantibody or antibodies to a specific RBC antigen.

The IAT is also used to crossmatch donor blood for transfusion. Patient serum is tested against RBCs from a donor with a compatible ABO and D (not necessarily identical) antigen type. A positive reaction indicates the probable presence of an alloantibody in the recipient directed against a donor RBC antigen. The specificity of this alloantibody can be determined by testing panel cells as discussed above.

Detection of RBC Coated in Vivo With Immunoglobulin and Complement (DAT)

The direct antiglobulin test (DAT), formerly known as the direct Coombs' test, detects the presence of antibody or complement (or both) on the surface of RBCs. This technique is used in the analysis of delayed hemolytic transfusion reactions, testing for hemolytic disease of the newborn, and the evaluation of patients with suspected autoimmune hemolytic anemia. Patient RBCs obtained in ethylenediaminetetraacetic acid (EDTA) are washed with saline and then incubated with a commercially available antiglobulin reagent containing either anti-human IgG or a mixture of anti-human IgG and anti-human complement. The test is positive if agglutination is seen after the addition of the antiglobulin reagent. Antiglobulin reagents containing anti-IgM or anti-IgA are available in specialized centers to detect coating of RBCs *in vivo* by antibodies of these isotypes.

Blood Groups, The Blood Group Antigen FactsBook, and AABB *Technical Manual.*[2,5,6]

Carbohydrate Blood Groups

ABO and Hh

The ABO blood group system is by far the most clinically significant, because of the presence of naturally occurring IgM antibodies (and sometimes IgG). The original observation by Landsteiner that certain human erythrocyte suspensions were agglutinated other human sera, led to the recognition of ABO polymorphism. This initial observation is still the cornerstone of modern transfusion practice more than a century later.

Antigens and Their Synthesis

ABH antigens occur on glycoproteins and glycolipids and are synthesized in a stepwise fashion by glycosyltransferases that sequentially add specific monosaccharides in specific linkages to a growing oligosaccharide precursor chain (reviewed in Clausen and Hakomori[16]). The terminal sugar determines antigen specificity (Fig. 143–1). The precursor substrate for A and B antigens is the H antigen, the terminal sugar of which is fucose added by fucosyltransferases encoded by the *FUT1* gene. The A and B transferase enzymes differ only by the nature of the monosaccharide added to the chain. *N*-acetyl-D-galactosamine is added by A-transferase, and D-galactose by B-transferase. In clinical practice, four ABO phenotypes (A, B, O, and AB) are discriminated. In addition, two common variations of group A, A_1, and A_2, can be distinguished. The differences between A_1 and A_2 phenotypes are both quantitative and qualitative. The A_1 transferase is more efficient in converting H to A antigen (approximately 5 times more A sites per RBC on A_1 RBCs than on A_2 RBCs) and in addition has the capacity to make the A_1 antigen the repetitive A epitope.[17] Quantitatively normal ABH expression also requires the branching of carbohydrate chains, which is performed by the blood group I enzyme, a 6-β-*N*-acetylglucosaminyltransferase.

Some H antigen precursor remains on A and B RBCs in this order: $A_2 > B > A_2B > A_1 > A_1B$. In addition to expression on cells of ectodermal and mesodermal origin (eg, RBC), some individuals also express ABH antigens in cells of endodermal origin (eg, secretions and plasma). This is caused by the activity of another fucosyltransferase (Secretor or Se transferase), encoded by *FUT2*, which has similar properties but different tissue expression compared to *FUT1* (H transferase). Approximately 20% of the population are nonsecretors and lack FUT2 activity.[18]

Inherited and Acquired ABH Variants

In addition to the main ABO blood types, there are many other inherited phenotypes, which have a weaker expression of the specified antigen, eg, A_3, A_x, A_{el}, B_3, B(A), and cisAB.[6,19] This can cause problems in determining the ABO blood group; but for patients needing immediate transfusion, the selection of O red cells and AB plasma products are an option. In blood donors, if weak expression of A or B antigens is not detected, the major risk is if the red cells are transfused to a patient whose antibodies may cause accelerated destruction of the transfused cells.

Rare *Bombay* phenotype RBCs (first reported in Bombay, India) lack H antigen, and consequently, A and B antigens. Other variants with weak H expression on RBCs, with or without H in secretions, also occur (para-Bombay) and have been reviewed by Oriol.[18]

Acquired B antigen results from the action of bacterial deacetylase, an enzyme that can remove an acetyl group from the A-terminal sugar, *N*-acetylgalactosamine. Galactosamine is similar to galactose, the B-specific terminal residue, and anti-B reagents can crossreact with the deacetylated structure.[20] Acquired B can occur in individuals suffering from gram-negative infections of gastrointestinal origin or carcinoma. The clinical significance is that AB blood may be transfused, sometimes with fatal outcome.[21] Other polyagglutinable states exist (eg, T, Tn, Tk) that are detected by naturally occurring antibodies found in the serum of most people, which can be identified by a panel of lectins.

A or B antigen expression can weaken in patients with acute leukemia or stress hematopoiesis. Chromosomal deletions or lesions that involve the *ABO* locus can result in the loss of transferase expression in the leukemic cell population. A decrease in A or B antigen expression, when found without a hematological disorder, can be prognostic of a pre-leukemic state.

Genes

The *ABO* gene was cloned in 1990 following purification of A transferase.[22,23] There are only four amino acid differences between A and B transferases in the catalytic domain, two of which (Leu266Met and Gly268Ala) are primarily responsible for the substrate specificity.[24] The group O phenotype results from mutations in A or B alleles that cause a loss of glycosyltransferase activity. The most common group O (O_1) results from a single nucleotide deletion near the 5′ end of

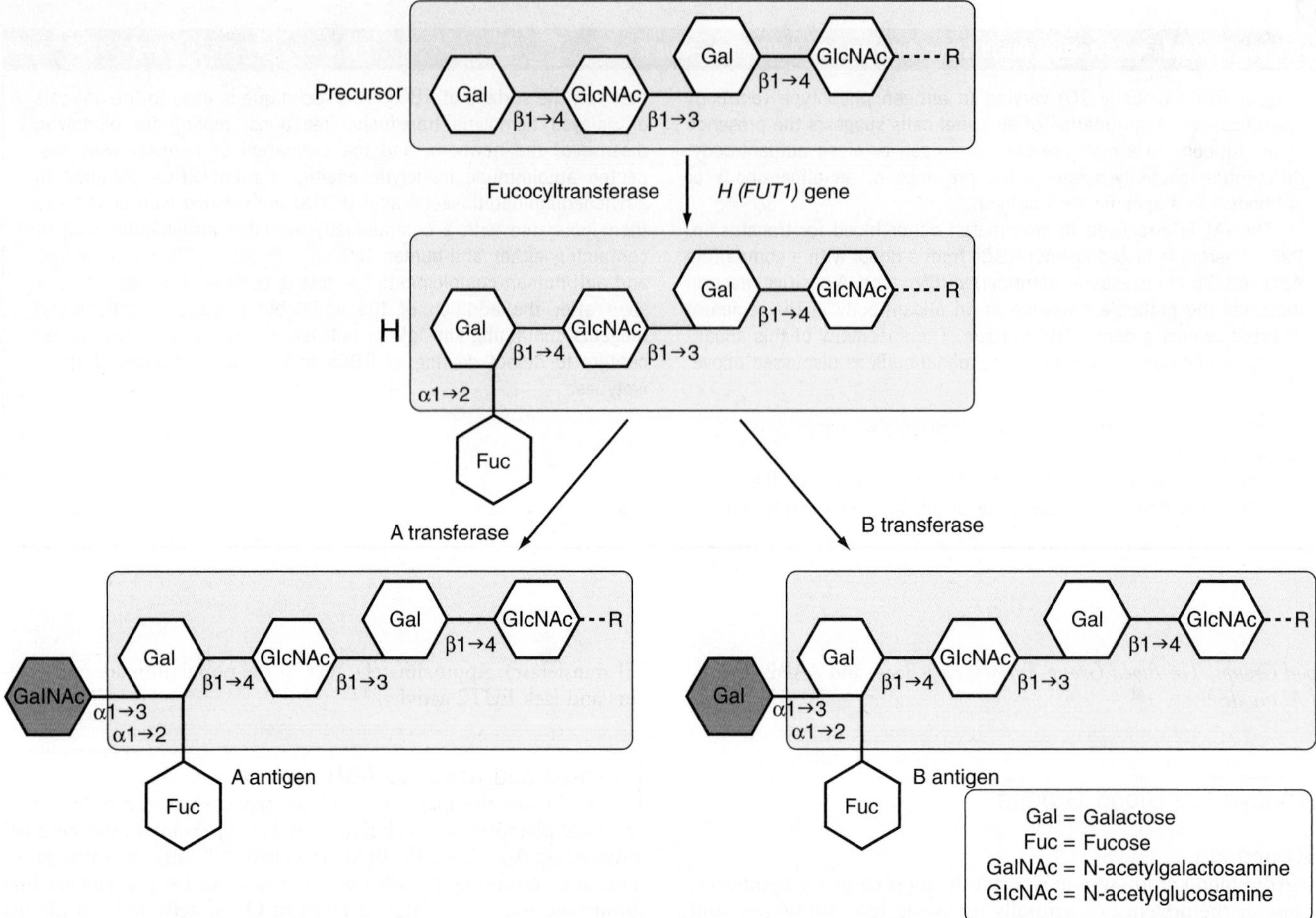

Figure 143–1 Biochemical structures of ABH antigens. Schematic representation of the terminal portions of the carbohydrate structures carrying the H, A, and B antigens on red blood cells.

the gene that causes a frameshift and early termination with no active enzyme production.[25] The *ABO* gene has seven exons and A or B subgroups (with few exceptions) result from a variety of mutations in exon 7 that cause alterations in the catalytic domain of the glycosyltransferase.[26] The rare B(A) and *cis*-AB phenotypes express both A and B from a single allele caused by variant glycosyltransferases that have a combination of A- and B-specific residues. Numerous common and rare *ABO* alleles have been reported and current information is available on the blood group antigen gene mutation database Web site (www.ncbi.nlm.nih.gov/projects/mhc/xslcgi.fcgi?cmd=bgmut/home). In addition to single-point mutations, recombination and gene conversion events between common alleles can result in hybrids with unexpected transferase activity. This makes genomic typing of ABO difficult.[27]

The fucosyltransferase enzymes required for H synthesis are encoded by two closely linked genes on chromosome 19, *FUT1* (or *H*) and *FUT2* (or *Se* for *secretor)* with differential substrate and expression in tissues.[18] Homozygosity for defective *FUT2* alleles is responsible for the nonsecretor phenotype in which A, B, and/or H antigen are not present in secretions. Individuals homozygous for null alleles at both the *FUT1* and *FUT2* loci have the Bombay phenotype.[28,29]

Transplantation

As tissue antigens, ABH are important in solid organ transplantation. Recipient antibodies react with antigens on the transplanted organ and complement activation at the surface of endothelial cells can result in rapid destruction and hyperacute rejection.[30] However, successful transplantation across ABO barriers is possible, particularly with blood group A_2 to O, and with current immunosuppressive and pretreatment regiments including removal of ABO antibodies.[31] Allogeneic bone marrow transplantations are routinely performed irrespective of ABO compatibility, but occasionally initial hemolysis or pure red cell anemia can result because of persisting anti-A or anti-B titers in the recipient.

ABO Antibodies

Anti-A and anti-B are found in the sera of individuals who lack the corresponding antigens. They are produced in response to environmental stimulants, such as bacteria, and have therefore been termed *naturally occurring* antibodies.[32] These antibodies are produced after birth, reaching a peak at 5 to 10 years of age, and declining with increasing age. The antibodies are mostly IgM and can activate complement, which, in conjunction with the high density of ABO antigen sites on RBCs, are responsible for the severe, life-threatening transfusion reactions that may result following ABO-incompatible transfusions. In contrast, HDN caused by ABO antibodies is usually mild because, (a) placental transfer is limited to the fraction of IgG anti-A and anti-B found in maternal serum, (b) ABH antigens are not fully developed on fetal RBCs because of lack of fully branched carbohydrate chains, and (c) tissue ABH antigens provide additional targets for the antibodies. ABO HDN is most often seen in non–group O infants of non-white group O mothers.

Platelets have intrinsic A, B, and H antigens, and thus ABO incompatibility can compromise the outcome in platelet transfusions.[33] However, platelets from donors with an A_2 phenotype lack both A and H antigens. Approximately 20% of group A platelets would be from A_2 donors and would be appropriate for *universal* use.

Platelets from A_2 donors may also be a superior product for patients undergoing A/O major mismatch allogeneic progenitor cell transplantation.[34]

Potent anti-H (along with anti-A and anti-B) found in O_h (Bombay) or para-Bombay nonsecretors will destroy transfused RBCs of any ABO group, so these individuals must be transfused only with blood of the Bombay phenotype. In contrast, anti-H in non-Bombay individuals including those with low expression of H antigen, notably A_1B and A_1, is usually IgM, reacts only at lower temperatures and is, therefore, clinically insignificant.[6]

Other Carbohydrate Blood Group Systems

In addition to the ABO and H blood group systems, several other antigens of carbohydrate nature are known. As for all glycoconjugate structures, sequential enzymatic action is required to build the antigenic epitopes and the genetic background of all these involves different glycosyltransferase loci.

The *null* p, P_2^k and P_1^k phenotypes are of clinical interest because of potent naturally occurring antibodies that are present in plasma of individuals whose RBCs lack the glycolipid-based antigens $P1/P/P^k$, P1/P or P, respectively. In analogy with the ABO blood group system, antibodies of IgM and IgG class (anti-$PP1P^k$, anti-P1P, or anti-P) are made against the missing antigens. Although the incidence of the null phenotypes is only 5 to 10 per million, they have attracted considerable interest because of their relationship to disease and as receptors for pathogens.

Women with p and P^k phenotypes suffer a high incidence of spontaneous abortion, a phenomenon most likely caused by attack of the placenta by anti-P. Anti-P and anti-P^k cause hemolytic transfusion reactions if antigen-positive blood is transfused. Transient auto–anti-P, produced following a viral infection, causes paroxysmal cold hemoglobinuria and lysis of P-positive RBC. P antigen (also known as globoside) is the cellular receptor for parvo-B19 virus that causes *Erythema infectiosum* (fifth disease) in children, sometimes complicated by severe aplastic anemia caused by lysis of early erythroid precursors. P-fimbriated *Escherichia coli* express both P- and P^k-binding molecules at the tips of their pili, a finding with implications for uropathogenicity. Individuals lacking P, or P^k and P, appear naturally resistant to these bacterial and viral infections. In contrast to anti-P and anti-P^k, it should be noted that anti-P1 is a cold-reactive agglutinin that seldom has clinical importance.[35]

Lewis antigens are fucosylated glycolipids synthesized by nonerythroid cells, circulate in plasma, and are passively adsorbed onto RBC.[36] Antibodies to Lewis can be made by people homozygous for nonfunctional 4-α-fucosyltransferases encoded by the FUT3 gene. The Le^a and Le^b antigens are not antithetical and in clinical practice only Le(a–b–) people make anti-Le^a or anti-Le^b. These antibodies are of IgM class and seldom cause any clinical problems.[6]

The i and I antigens are nonterminal epitopes on linear and branched carbohydrate structures, respectively, carrying ABH antigens in their terminal ends. During the first years of life, linear chains are modified into branched chains, resulting in the appearance of I antigens.[37] The i phenotype is rare among adults but is the normal state on RBCs from fetuses and infants. The gene encoding the I-branching β-1,6-*N*-acetylglucosaminyltransferase (IGnT) has three alternative forms of exon 1 with common exons 2 and 3. Mutations in exon 2 or exon 3 silence IGnT and give rise to the form of the i phenotype that is associated with cataracts in Asians.[38,39] Mutations in exon 1C (IGnTC or IGnT3) silence the gene in erythrocytes, but not in other tissues, and lead to the i phenotype without cataracts.[40]

Alloanti-I made by a person with the rare i adult phenotype can be clinically significant and cause destruction of transfused I+ RBCs. The sera of all people contain auto-anti-I that is clinically benign and reactive only at or below room temperature. In contrast, cold hemagglutinin disease is characterized by a high titer of complement-fixing monoclonal anti-I, which cause in vivo hemolysis and hemolytic anemia. The titer and thermal range of anti-I is often increased following infection with *Mycoplasma pneumoniae*. If transfusion cannot be avoided, donor RBCs should be transfused through a blood warmer.[41]

Table 143–6 The Incidence of the Principal Rh Haplotypes

Fisher-Race Haplotype	Modified Weiner Haplotype	Incidence (%)		
		White	*African Black*	*Asian*
Rh-positive				
DCe	R_1	42	17	70
DcE	R_2	14	11	21
Dce	R_0	4	44	3
DCE	R_Z	<0.01	<0.01	1
Rh-negative				
ce	r	37	26	3
Ce	r′	2	2	2
cE	r″	1	<0.01	<0.01
CE	r^y	<0.01	<0.01	<0.01

Protein Blood Groups

Rh and LW Blood Group Systems

The Rh system is second only to the ABO system in importance in transfusion medicine. This is because Rh antigens, especially D, are highly immunogenic. Thus, in most countries, blood for transfusion is tested and labeled with the D antigen type (Rh-positive or Rh-negative); and D–recipients are transfused with D–RBC products.

Three systems for naming Rh antigens have been used. Two are shown in Table 143–6, which indicates the incidence of the common Rh haplotypes present in different ethnic groups. The Fisher-Race nomenclature was based on the premise that there were three closely linked genes (D, C/c, and E/e), whereas the Wiener nomenclature (Rh-Hr) was based on his belief that a single gene encoded one *agglutinogen* that carried the factors D, C/c, and E/e. Although neither theory was correct (there are two genes; *RHD* and *RHCE*, correctly proposed by Tippett[42]), for written communication the Fisher-Race designation (CDE) is often preferred, and for spoken communication a modified version of Wiener's nomenclature is preferred. Use of uppercase *R* indicates that D antigen is present and use of a lowercase *r* (or *little r*) indicates that it is absent. The C or c and E or e antigens carried with D are represented by subscripts: 1 for Ce (R_1), 2 for cE (R_2), 0 for ce (R_0), and Z for CE (R_z). The presence of these antigens without D are represented by superscript: *prime* for Ce (r′), *double-prime* for cE (r″), and *y* for CE (r^y). This terminology allows one to convey the common Rh antigens present (the phenotype) with a single term.

The third system uses numerical designations to more accurately represent the serologic data, to be free of genetic interpretation, and to be computer friendly. This numerical nomenclature, with a few exceptions (Rh17, Rh32, Rh33), is not widely used in the clinical laboratory.

Genes, Proteins, Antigens, and Phenotypes

The Rh proteins are designated RhD (encoded by *RHD*), which carries the D antigen, and RhCE (encoded by *RHCE*), which carries the CE antigens (either ce, cE, Ce, or CE). RhD differs from the various forms of RhCE by 32 to 35 amino acids (Fig. 143–2), and both are covalently linked to fatty acids (palmitate) in the lipid bilayer of the RBC. RhD and RhCE form a complex in the RBC membrane with the RhAG (Rh-associated glycoprotein). Other proteins present in the Rh-complex are CD47 (an integrin-associated protein), LW, glycophorin B, and possibly band 3 (the anion exchanger).[43]

The D-negative (Rh-negative) phenotype is prevalent in whites (15%–17%), less common in African descent (3%–5%), and rare in Asians (<0.1%). The absence of D in Europeans is primarily caused by a deletion of the *RHD* gene. Rare D-negative whites and Asians carry a *RHD* gene that is silenced because of a variety of molecular events. D-negative African blacks have *RHD* genes that either contain a 37-bp duplication that results in a premature stop codon, a hybrid *RHD-CE-D*, or *RHD* deletion.[6] This is important when designing PCR-based methods to predict the D status.

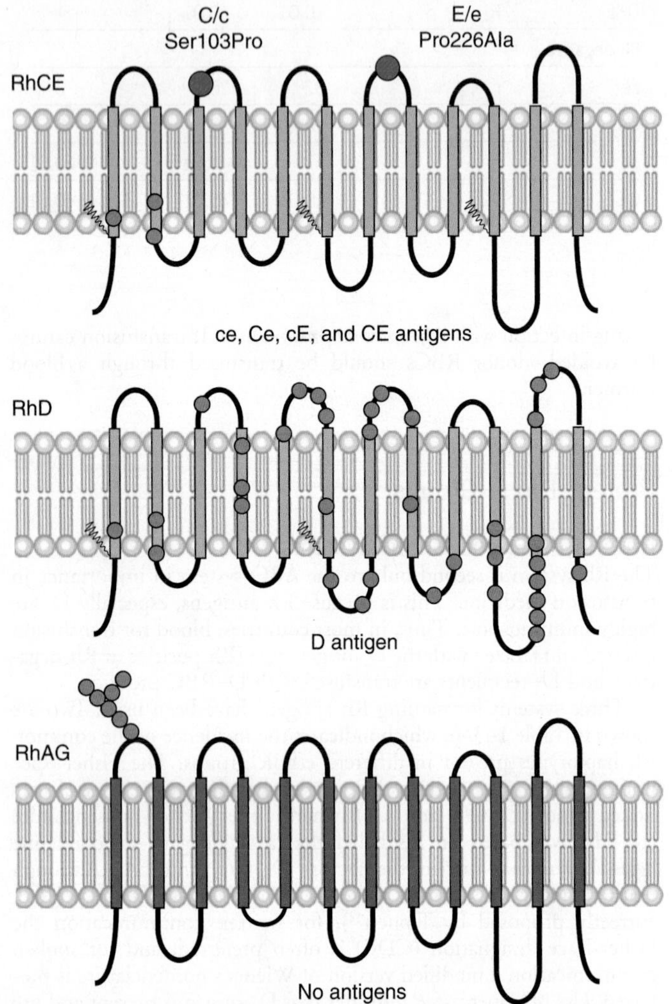

Figure 143–2 Model of Rh proteins RhCE, RhD, and RhAG. The Rh proteins are predicted to have a similar membrane topology. The amino acid differences between RhD and RhCE are shown as **open circles**. Positions 103 and 226, which are critical for C/c and E/e expression, respectively, are indicated as **black circles**.

RBCs with weak D (formerly known as D[u]) require the IAT for detection and are caused by amino acid changes predicted to be in the intracellular or transmembrane regions of RhD (Fig. 143–3).[44] Most individuals with a weak D phenotype can safely receive D-positive blood and do not make anti-D.[45]

Partial D antigens (D categories or D mosaics) result from a single point mutation in *RHD* resulting in amino acid changes, which are predicted to be extracellular (see Fig. 143–3), or by replacement of *RHD* nucleotides or exons by the equivalent of part of *RHCE*. RBCs with a partial D antigen may have a strong or weak expression of the D antigen. Because patients with partial D antigens can make anti-D to the D epitopes they lack, they ideally should receive D-negative blood. In practice most type as D-positive and are recognized only after they make anti-D. Future implementation of *RHD* genotyping will help distinguish partial D.[46]

Several phenotypes, including D - -, Dc- and DC[w]-, have an enhanced expression of D antigen and no or variant CE antigens. They are caused by replacement of portions of *RHCE* by *RHD*. The RhD sequences in RhCE along with a normal RhD explain the enhanced D and account for the lack, or reduced expression, of CE antigens. Immunized people with these CE depleted phenotypes make anti-Rh17.

C and c antigens differ by four amino acids, but only residue Ser103Pro is predicted to be extracellular. E and e differ by one amino acid, Pro226Ala (see Fig. 143–2). The RhD and various combinations of RhCE proteins (ce, Ce, cE, and CE) depicted in Figure 143–2 are typical for most white transfusion recipients. However, Rh proteins in other ethnic groups often have additional polymorphisms, and this fact often complicates transfusion in patients with sickle cell disease. For example, the RBCs of more than 30% of blacks are VS+ because of a Leu245Val and Gly336Cys substitution in Rhce, and expression of these antigens is associated with variant expression of e. Many other amino acid changes in Rhce, as well as in RhD, are associated with production of Rh antibodies in patients with sickle cell disease.[5,46–48]

The Rh_{null} phenotype is rare and occurs on two genetic backgrounds; the *regulator* type caused by mutations in *RHAG*, which encodes Rh-associated glycoprotein, and the *amorph* type caused by mutations in *RHCE* on a deleted *RHD* background. Rh_{null} RBCs are stomatocytic, fragile, and the patients have anemia, suggesting that the Rh proteins have an important structural role in the erythrocyte membrane.[49]

Antibodies

Most Rh antibodies are IgG and do not activate complement. As a result, primarily extravascular hemolysis, rather than intravascular hemolysis, occurs in transfusion reactions involving Rh antibodies. Rh antibodies are almost always caused by red cell immunization from pregnancy or transfusion, and usually persist for many years.

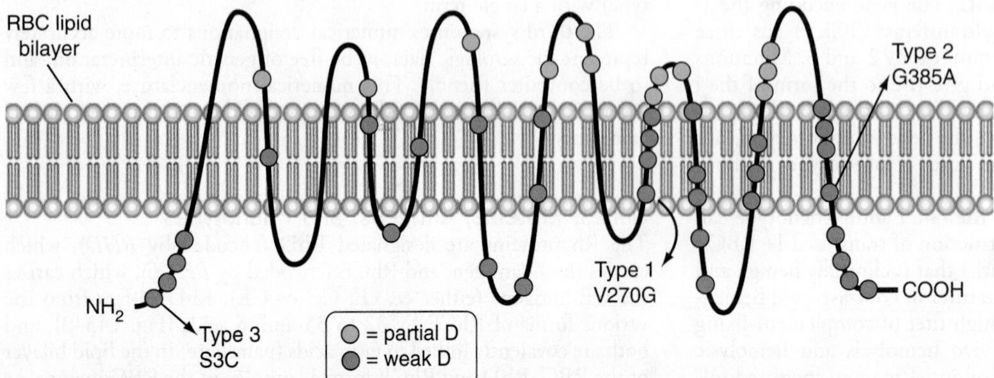

Figure 143–3 Model of weak D and partial D. The predicted location of the amino acid mutations responsible for weak D phenotypes is shown as **black circles**. Type 1, 2, and 3 (shown at the three **arrows**) are found in approximately 90% of weak D phenotypes. The location of amino acid residues responsible for partial D phenotypes is shown as **open circles**.

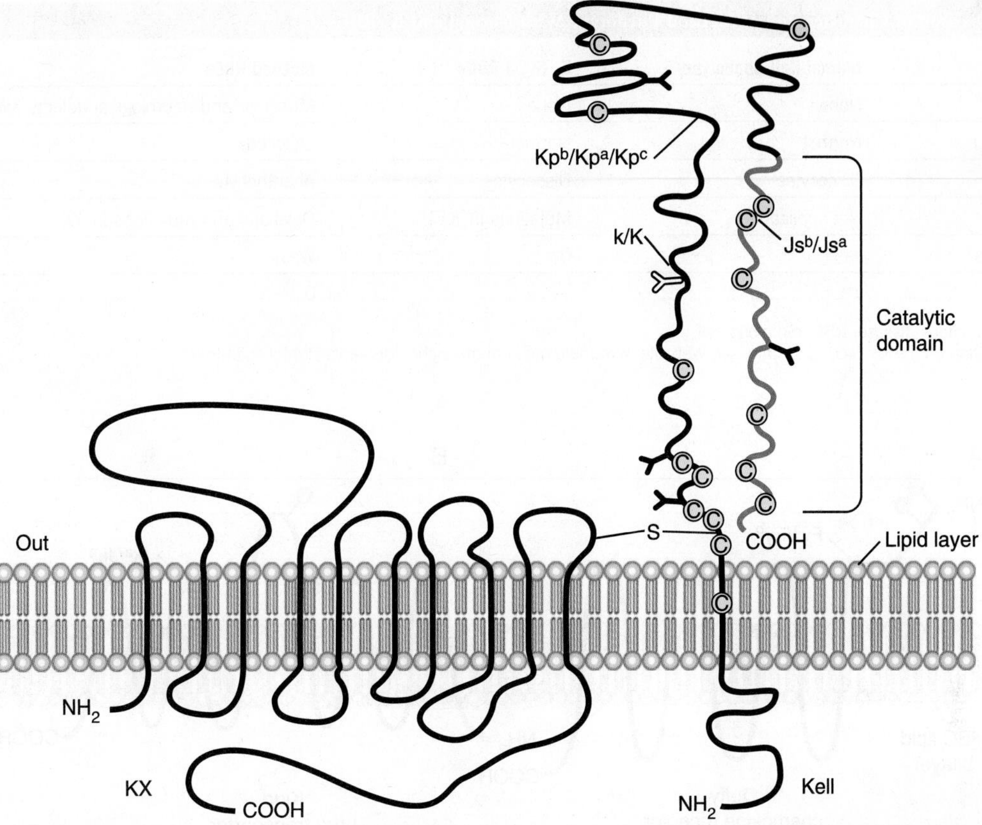

Figure 143–4 Model of Kell and Kx proteins. Kell is a single-pass protein, but Kx is predicted to span the red blood cell membrane 10 times. In the RBC, Kell and Kx are linked by a disulfide bond, shown as **S**, and the locations of the more common Kell antigens are indicated. The N-glycosylation sites are shown as **Y**. The **hollow Y** represents the N-glycosylation site that is not present on the K (K1) protein.

Anti-D can cause severe transfusion reactions and HDN, but the incidence of anti-D has decreased with the prophylactic use of Rh immune globulin. Most Rh antibodies should be considered as having the potential to be clinical significant for HDN and transfusion reactions. If serum antibody levels fall below detectable levels, subsequent exposure to the antigen characteristically produces a rapid secondary immune response.

Autoantibodies to high-prevalence Rh antigens often occur in the sera of patients with warm autoimmune hemolytic anemia as well as in some cases of drug-induced autoimmune hemolytic anemia.[50]

LW Blood Group System

Rh and LW are independent blood group systems but have a phenotypic relationship: In adults, D-positive RBCs have a stronger expression of LW antigen than D-negative RBCs, and anti-LW can be confused with anti-D. Transient loss of LW antigens from RBCs has been described in pregnancy and patients with diseases, particularly Hodgkin disease, lymphoma, leukemia, sarcoma, and other forms of malignancy. Loss of LW antigens is usually associated with the production of antibodies that appear to be alloanti-LW.[51]

Kell and Kx Systems

The Kell protein is highly folded through multiple intrachain disulfide bonds and in the RBC membrane Kell is covalently linked to XK protein (Fig. 143–4). Twenty-seven of the Kell antigens result from a single amino acid substitution in the Kell protein.[52] The K antigen is remarkably immunogenic for only differing from wild-type (k) by one amino acid, and it appears that loss of an N-glycan exposes the peptide, thereby rendering it immunogenic.

Weak expression of Kell antigens can be inherited, or acquired and transient. Inherited weak expression occurs with the K_{mod} phenotype, the McLeod phenotype, when Kp^a is in *cis*, or with the Leach and Gerbich types of Ge-negative phenotypes.[53] Transient depression of Kell system antigens occurs in autoimmune hemolytic anemia, with microbial infections, and in two cases of idiopathic thrombocytopenia purpura.[6] The lack of Kell antigens (the K_0 or K_{null} phenotype) is caused by several different gene defects.[54]

HDN caused by anti-K can result in severe neonatal anemia. Maternal antibody titers and amniotic bilirubin levels are not good predictors of the severity of the disease. Kell antigens are expressed early during erythropoiesis and anti-K has been shown to suppress erythropoiesis in vitro.[55,56] This may explain the low level of bilirubin observed, in the face of neonatal anemia. Other unusual consequences of Kell antibodies include risk of fetal thrombocytopenia and neutropenia.[57,58]

McLeod Syndrome

This rare syndrome is associated with the loss of expression of Kx protein caused by mutations and deletions in the *XK* gene.[59,60] The syndrome, manifest only in males, may be underdiagnosed. The characteristics, which often develop only after the fourth decade of life, are summarized in Table 143–7. Few patients with chronic granulomatous disease also have the McLeod phenotype because of X-chromosome deletions encompassing both genes. Carrier females have two populations of RBCs (one of the McLeod phenotype and one of normal phenotype).

Duffy Blood Group System

The Duffy (FY) glycoprotein (Fig. 143–5) is a promiscuous chemokine receptor found on RBCs and on endothelial cells in the kidney and brain that binds a family of chemotactic and proinflammatory peptides from the CXC (IL-8, MGSA) and the CC (RANTES, MCP-1, MIP-1) classes. The physiological role of FY is unclear, but on RBCs the receptor may allow RBCs to act as scavengers for excess

Table 143–7 Comparison of Characteristics of McLeod Phenotype With Normal and K_0 RBCs

Characteristics	Normal Kell phenotype	K_0 (K_{null}) RBCs	McLeod RBCs
Pathology	None	None	Muscular and neurological defects (with and without CGD)
Creatine kinase level	Normal	Normal	Elevated
Morphology	Discocytes	Discocytes	Acanthocytes
Gene defect	Not applicable	Mutations in *KEL*	Deletions and mutations in *XK*
Kell system antigens	++++	0	Weak
Kx antigen	+	++	0

CGD, chronic granulomatous disease; RBC, red blood cell.
For more information on the McLeod syndrome, see Web site: www.nefo.med.uni-muenchen.de/~adanek/McLeod.html/.

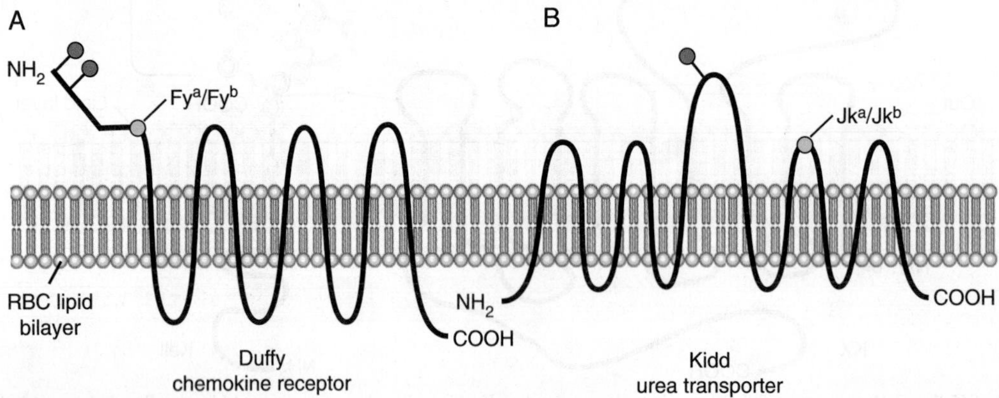

Figure 143–5 Model of Duffy (FY) and Kidd (JK) proteins. **A.** The Duffy glycoprotein is homologous to chemokine receptors and is predicted to have a seven-transmembrane domain structure. The location of the Fy^a/Fy^b polymorphism is shown as an **open circle**, and the glycosylation sites as a **ball and stick**. **B.** Predicted 10-transmembrane domain structure of the Kidd/urea transporter. The location of the polymorphism responsible for the Kidd antigens is shown as an **open circle** and the site for the N-glycan (**ball and stick**) are indicated.

chemokines. FY is also a receptor to which *Plasmodium vivax* merozoites can bind to invade RBC and cause malaria.[61]

Antigens. The Fy^a and Fy^b antigens differ by a single amino acid (Gly42Asp) located on the N-terminal extracellular domain of the FY glycoprotein and is responsible for the common Fy(a+b–), Fy(a–b+), and Fy(a+b+) phenotypes. The null Fy(a–b–) phenotype is rare in most ethnic groups but is common in people of African and Arabian origins. The null phenotype most often results from a mutation in the promoter region of *FYB* that disrupts a binding site for the erythroid transcription factor GATA-1 and results in loss of FY on RBCs.[62] Because the erythroid promoter controls expression only in erythroid cells, FY expression in other tissues is unaffected. All African blacks with a mutated GATA box to date have been shown to carry *FYB* and therefore Fy^b is expressed on nonerythroid tissues. This explains why Fy(a–b–) individuals make anti-Fy^a but not anti-Fy^b. Fy(a–b–) caused by a mutated GATA box on an *FYA* allele has been found in Papua New Guinea, another malaria-endemic region.[63]

Antibodies. FY antigens are much less immunogenic than K; and most antibodies are IgG, subclass IgG1, and arise from stimulation by transfusion. Anti-Fy^b is much less common than anti-Fy^a and the antibodies can cause delayed hemolytic transfusion reactions (DHTR) and rarely HDN. Anti-Fy3 is made by extremely rare Fy(a–b–) individuals who lack FY protein on all cells.

Kidd Blood Group System

The JK blood group molecule (see Fig. 143–5) was implicated in urea transport when RBCs lacking all JK antigens were shown to resist lysis in 2 M urea.[64] The gene encoding a human urea transporter, *HUT11*, was cloned and the protein was shown to express antigens in the Kidd system.[65,66] The JK/HUT11 protein in RBCs and kidney medulla is a constitutive urea transporter. Failure to express Kidd does not result in an overt clinical syndrome; the only observed manifestation is a reduced capacity to concentrate urine.[67]

Antigens. The Jk^a and Jk^b antigens differ by a single amino acid (Asp280Asn)[68] and are responsible for the common Jk(a+b–), Jk(a–b+) and Jk(a+b+) phenotypes. The Jk(a–b–) or Jk_{null} phenotype is rare but occurs with greater incidence in Polynesians, Asians, and Finns. The silent alleles in Polynesians/Asians have splice-site or missense mutations that abolish expression of Jk^b, and large deletions and premature stop codons in *JKA* alleles have been found in rare white Jk_{null} pedigrees.[6]

Antibodies. Neither anti-Jk^a nor anti-Jk^b is common, but JK antibodies are responsible for at least one-third of cases of delayed DHTRs.[41] The antibodies often drop to undetectable levels, or react only with cells that are homozygous for the antigen, and escape detection in the sensitized patient's serum prior to transfusion. JK antibodies only rarely cause HDN; and if they do, typically, it is not severe. Anti-Jk3, sometimes referred to as anti-Jk^{ab}, is produced by Jk(a–b–) individuals and reacts with Jk(a+) and Jk(b+) RBCs and rare donor components must be located for transfusion.

MNS System

M and N antigens are carried on alternative forms of glycophorin A (GPA), whereas S and s antigens are carried on alternative forms of glycophorin B (GPB). M/N and S/s are homologous proteins encoded by adjacent genes, and therefore, show linkage disequilibrium in inheritance of the antigens. The MNS system is highly polymorphic and most of the 46 antigens are the result of amino acid substitutions or rearrangements between *GYPA* and *GYPB*.[69] Persons who are S-s-, usually blacks, may lack the high incidence antigen, U, caused by a deletion of *GYPB* or express U weakly due to an altered form of *GYPB*.[69,70]

Antibodies. Anti-S, -s, and -U are usually IgG and can be clinically significant antibodies. Anti-M and anti-N are usually naturally occurring, reactive at room temperature or below, and often clinically insignificant. Anti-En^a is an umbrella term for immune antibodies that react with determinants on GPA.

Other Protein Antigens. Antibodies to antigens in these systems are less common than those described earlier in this chapter. Information regarding their general clinical significance is summarized it Table 143–4.

The Lutheran System

Lutheran (LU), along with *Secretor*, provided the first example of autosomal linkage in humans, the first example of autosomal crossing over, and the first indication that crossing over in humans is more common in females than in males.[71,72] The Lutheran system consists of four antithetical pairs of antigens and 10 independent high-prevalence antigens.

Antibodies. Antibodies in this system are rarely encountered because the antigens are not highly immunogenic. They are usually IgG and give characteristic agglutinates surrounded by unagglutinated RBCs. They can cause mild transfusion reactions but do not typically cause HDN. Anti-LU3 is found in the serum of immunized people of the rare recessive LU(a–b–) phenotype, and the antibody is usually IgG and may cause a delayed transfusion reaction or HDN. Blood with the LU(a–b–) phenotype should be used for transfusion of patients with these antibodies.

Diego System

The Diego blood group antigens are on Band 3, the red cell anion exchanger (AE1), and the N-glycan on AE1 carries most red cell A, B, H, I, and i blood group activity. The Di^b antigen has a prevalence of greater than 99.9%. The Di^a antigen is rare in most populations, with the exception of South American Indians where Di^a occurs in 54%, and approximately 12% of Native Americans are Di(a+).[73]

Antibodies. Diego antibodies are usually IgG and do not bind complement. These antibodies have caused transfusion reactions (usually delayed) and HDN.

Yt Blood Group System

The Yt system was named in 1956 when and antibody was found in the serum of patient whose last name was Cartwright. Yt^a occurs with a prevalence of more than 99% in random blood samples; and Yt^b is found with a prevalence of approximately 8%, with the exception of Israelis where it has a prevalence of 20% or higher.[74]

Antibodies. Yt antibodies usually are IgG and do not bind complement. These antibodies have caused delayed transfusion reactions, but not HDN.

Xg Blood Group System

Xg glycoprotein has 48% identity with CD99 glycoprotein, which has been implicated in cell-to-cell adhesion events, activates a caspase-independent apoptosis pathway in T cells, and is expressed on human RBCs as well as all other human tissue tested.[75,76,77] The gene encoding Xg^a is not subject to X-inactivation caused by the expression of a duplicate gene, *MIC2*, located telomeric and in the pseudoautosomal region of the X chromosome. The difference between Xg(a+) and Xg(a–) is the level of Xg^a antigen on the RBC. The prevalence of Xg^a differs in males (65.6%) and females (88.7%), and there is a phenotypic association between the expression of Xg^a and CD99.[5]

Antibodies. Anti-Xg^a is usually IgG and may bind complement. Some anti-Xg^a are apparently naturally occurring. These antibodies have not caused transfusion reactions or HDN.[5]

Scianna Blood Group System

The Scianna antigens are expressed by the red cell adhesion protein, erythrocyte membrane-associated protein.[78,79] Sc1 is a high-prevalence antigen (prevalence ≈99.9%), and Sc2 is a low-prevalence antigen (1%).

Antibodies. Scianna antibodies are usually IgG and some bind complement. These antibodies have not caused transfusion reactions; and although they have caused cord RBCs to be positive in the DAT, they have not caused HDN. Several examples of autoanti-Sc1 have been reported, some reactive in tests using patient serum but not plasma. Autoanti-Sc3-like antibodies have been described in one patient with lymphoma and in one patient with Hodgkin disease whose RBCs had suppressed Sc antigens.[80]

Dombrock Blood Group System

Dombrock antigens are carried on a GPI-linked glycoprotein that is a member of the mono-ADP-ribosyltransferase family (ART4), but Do has no demonstrable enzyme activity on the RBC. The Dombrock blood group system consists of two antithetical antigens, Do^a and Do^b, and three antigens of high prevalence; Gregory (Gy^a), Holley (Hy), and Joseph, (Jo^a). The Gy(a–) phenotype is the null of the system.

Antibodies. Do^a and Do^b antigens are poor immunogens, and anti-Do^a and anti-Do^b are rarely found as single specificities. Antibodies in the Do system are usually IgG and do not bind complement. These antibodies have caused delayed transfusion reactions and a positive DAT, but no clinical HDN.[9]

Colton Blood Group System

The Colton antigens are carried on aquaporin-1 (AQP-1), the first water channel protein characterized in mammals, and is also found in the kidney.[81] The function of AQP-1 in RBCs may be to rehydrate rapidly after shrinking in the hypertonic environment of the renal medulla.[82] Co^a has a prevalence of 99.9%, its antithetical antigen Co^b has a prevalence of 10%, and Co3 is present on all RBCs except those of the very rare Co(a–b–) null phenotype. Apparently healthy propositi with the Co(a–b–) phenotype and AQP-1 deficiency have RBCs with an 80% reduction in the ability to transport water.[83] The residual water transport in these RBCs may be through another member of the water channel protein family, AQP-3, which transports water, glycerol, and urea, and carries the blood group antigen GIL.[84]

Antibodies. Antibodies in the Colton system are usually IgG and some bind complement. The antibodies have caused delayed transfusion reactions and HDN.[9]

Gerbich Blood Group System

The Gerbich system antigens are carried on glycophorin C (GPC) and glycophorin D. There are three high-prevalence antigens (Ge2, Ge3, and Ge4) and five low-prevalence antigens. The two glycoproteins are products of the *GYPC* gene. The gene consists of four exons and the smaller glycophorin D is generated by the use of an alternative translation initiation site. There are three different molecular bases for the Gerbich null phenotype.[85]

Antibodies. The antibodies may be immune or naturally occurring. Most are IgG and some of these bind complement; some antibodies may be IgM. Although some antibodies have caused delayed transfusion reactions, others have been benign. Clinical HDN has not been reported, but the antibodies have been eluted from cord RBCs that tested positive on DAT. Clinically significant auto–anti-Ge have been reported. Because Ge-negative donors are rare, it is important to test siblings of Ge-negative patients for compatibility, and to urge such patients to donate blood for long-term storage.[9] Antibodies to low-prevalence antigens in the Ge blood group system are rare, and RBCs from almost all random donors are compatible; there is no difficulty in finding blood for transfusion of patients with these antibodies.

Cromer Blood Group System

The Cromer antigens are carried on decay accelerating factor (DAF, CD55), a complement control protein attached to the RBC membrane through GPI-linkage. Cromer is a system of two sets of antithetical antigens, Tc^a/Tc^b/Tc^c and WES^a/WES^b, eleven high-prevalence antigens, and three low-prevalence antigens. The Cr(a–) phenotype is the least rare of the negative phenotypes, and with the exception of one Spanish-American woman, all people with Cr(a–) RBCs are black. Most of the other phenotypes are exceedingly rare.

Antibodies. Antibodies in the Cromer system are usually IgG and do not bind complement. The antibodies have caused mild delayed transfusion reactions but not HDN. When a patient's antibody is directed at a high-prevalence antigen, it is important to test siblings in the quest for compatible blood and to urge the patient to donate blood for long-term storage when clinical status permits.

Knops Blood Group System

The Knops blood group antigens are carried on complement receptor 1 (CR1). Kn^a, Sl^a, and McC^a, antigens are fairly common and have a similar prevalence (>90%) in different populations; however, Sl^a is present on RBCs of 98% of whites, but on only 60% of blacks. Typing for Knops system antigens can be challenging because of the low level of expression on the RBCs, as some disease processes cause CR1 deficiency can lead to false-negative results. RBC CR1 is important in the processing of immune complexes, binding them for transport to the liver and spleen for removal from the circulation. The CR1 copy number per RBC (and thus antigen strength) is reduced in Systemic lupus erythematous (SLE), cold hemagglutinin disease, paroxysmal nocturnal hemoglobinurin (PNH), hemolytic anemia, insulin-dependent diabetes mellitus, AIDS, some malignant tumors, and any condition associated with increased clearance of immune complexes. CR1, and the Sl^a antigen in particular, may act as a receptor for the malarial parasite *Plasmodium falciparum*, and thus, the Sl(a–) phenotype may provide selective advantage.[86]

Antibodies. Antibodies in the Knops system are usually IgG and they do not bind complement. The antibodies do not cause transfusion reactions or HDN, and once identified, they can be ignored for clinical purposes. Identification may be complicated by the fluctuation of antigen expression on RBCs. Anti-Kn^a is the most common antibody in whites, and anti-Sl^a is the most common in African Americans.[19]

Indian Blood Group System

The antigens of the Indian system are carried on CD44.[87] CD44 has a diverse range of biologic functions involving cell–cell and cell–matrix interactions in cells other than RBCs.[87] It is an adhesion molecule in lymphocytes, monocytes, and some tumor cells. CD44 binds to hyaluronate and other components of the extracellular matrix and is also involved in immune stimulation as well as signaling between cells.[88] In^b is a common antigen, and In^a is rare in white persons but has a prevalence of 4% in Indians, 10% in Iranians, and nearly 12% in Arabs.

Antibodies. Antibodies in the Indian system are usually IgG and do not bind complement. Some antibodies may directly agglutinate RBCs, but the reactivity is greatly enhanced by the IAT. These antibodies have caused decreased RBC survival and a positive DAT in the neonate but not HDN. A severe, delayed, hemolytic transfusion reaction caused by anti-In^b has been reported.[89]

Ok Blood Group System

The Ok antigen is carried on CD147, whose function on RBCs is unknown. CD147 on tumor cells is thought to bind an unknown ligand on fibroblasts, which stimulates their production of collagenase and other extracellular matrix metalloproteinases, thus enhancing tumor cell invasion and metastasis.[90] In studies with CD147 knockout mice, RBCs were apparently not compromised. CD147 may be involved in the function of the blood-brain barrier[91] and lymphocyte inactivation.[92] The eight known Ok(a–) probands are Japanese.

Antibodies. The original example of anti-Ok^a is IgG and does not bind complement. This antibody caused reduced red cell survival but not HDN. Only one other example of human anti-Ok^a is known.

RAPH Blood Group System

The MER2 antigen in the RAPH blood group system was originally defined by monoclonal antibodies (1D12, 2F7). It is carried on CD151 (tetraspanin). All three people (two probands) with anti-MER2 had renal failure requiring dialysis, skin lesions, neurosensory deafness, and nail dystrophy.[93,94] Of English blood donors 92% are MER2-positive, and 8% are MER2-negative. The antigen strength varies among different RBC samples.

Antibodies. The three examples of human anti-MER2 (anti-RAPH) are IgG and two of the three antibodies bind complement. These antibodies have not caused HDN or transfusion reactions; indeed, two siblings with the antibody have received numerous crossmatch-incompatible RBC transfusions without problems. The three antibody producers were Indian Jews.[93]

Antigens Adsorbed From Plasma

Chido/Rodgers Blood Group System

Although the Ch and Rg antigens are readily detected on RBCs, they are located on the fourth component of complement (C4), which becomes bound to RBCs from the plasma. In complement activation through the classical pathway, C4 becomes bound to the RBC membrane and undergoes further cleavage; ultimately, a tryptic fragment, C4d, remains on the RBC. This C4d glycoprotein carries the Ch/Rg blood group antigens. The antigens are stable in stored serum or plasma, and the phenotypes of this system are most accurately defined in plasma by hemagglutination inhibition tests.

Antibodies. Antibodies in the Ch/Rg system are usually IgG and do not activate complement and are considered benign and nebulous. There can be considerable variation in the reaction strength obtained with different RBC samples. Although these antibodies do not generally cause transfusion reactions, they have caused anaphylactic reactions.[95] The antibodies have not caused HDN.

FINAL COMMENTS

Over the last decade, as information was gained about the genes encoding the membrane components carrying blood group antigens, it has been possible to determine the function of many of the components, understand the basis of disease associations, and develop DNA-based assays with clinical usefulness. Despite the rapid growth of knowledge about blood groups, the simple hemagglutination test remains the principle assay for blood grouping and compatibility testing; it also is valuable in aiding in diagnosis. For example, it is used as part of the investigation of hemolytic disease of the newborn, warm autoimmune hemolytic anemia, cold hemagglutinin disease, paroxysmal hemoglobinuria, and paroxysmal nocturnal hemoglobinuria, and it can be used to directly diagnose rare conditions such as the Rh syndrome (by testing and showing that they lack D, C, E, c and e antigens), the McLeod Syndrome (by testing RBCs with anti-Kx and showing they lack Kx antigen), and leukocyte deficiency syndrome II (LADII) (by testing RBCs and showing they lack A, B, H, Le^a and Le^b antigens). DNA-based genotyping assays are an invaluable adjunct to classic hemagglutination but are unlikely to completely replace this simple, effective technique.

SUGGESTED READINGS

Brecher M (ed.): Technical Manual, 15th ed. Bethesda, MD, American Association of Blood Banks, 2005.

Daniels G: Human Blood Groups, 2nd ed. Oxford, Blackwell Science, 2002.

Daniels GL, Fletcher A, Garratty G, et al: Blood Group Terminology 2004. Vox Sang 87:316, 2004.

Issitt PD, Anstee DJ: Applied Blood Group Serology, 4th ed. Durham NC, Montgomery Scientific Publications, 1998.

Lee S, Russo D, Redman CM: The Kell Blood Group System: Kell and XK Membrane Proteins. Semin Hematol 37:113, 2000.

Lögdberg L, Reid ME, Lamont RE, et al: Human Blood Group Genes 2004: Chromosomal Locations and Cloning Strategies. Transfus Med Rev 19:45, 2005.

Mollison PL, Engelfriet CP, Contreras M: Blood Transfusion in Clinical Medicine, 10th ed. Oxford, Blackwell Science, 1997.

Ness PM: To Match or Not To Match: The Question for Chronically Transfused Patients With Sickle Cell Anemia. Transfusion 34:558, 1994.

Noizat-Pirenne F, Lee K, Le Pennec P-Y, et al: Rare RHCE Phenotypes in Black Individuals of Afro-Caribbean Origin: Identification and Transfusion Safety. Blood 100:4223, 2002.

Olsson ML, Chester MA: Polymorphism and Recombination Events at The Locus *ABO*: A Major Challenge for Genomic ABO Blood Grouping Strategies. Transfus Med 11:295, 2001.

Petz LD, Garratty G: Acquired Immune Hemolytic Anemias, 2nd ed. New York, Churchill Livingstone, 2003.

Reid ME, Lomas-Francis C: Blood Group Antigen FactsBook, 2nd ed. San Diego, Academic Press, 2004.

Reid ME, Lomas-Francis C: Blood Group Antigens & Antibodies: A Guide to Clinical Relevance & Technical Tips. New York, Star Bright Books, 2007.

Reid ME, Øyen R, Marsh WL: Summary of the Clinical Significance of Blood Group Alloantibodies. Semin Hematol 37:197, 2000.

Wagner FF, Gassner C, Müller TH, et al: Molecular Basis of Weak Phenotypes D. Blood 93:385, 1999.

Westhoff CM: The Structure and Function of the Rh Antigen Complex. Semin Hematol 44:42, 2007.

Westhoff CM: Molecular Testing for Transfusion Medicine. Curr Opin Hematol 13:471.

REFERENCES

For complete list of references log onto www.expertconsult.com

CHAPTER 144

HUMAN PLATELET ANTIGENS

Thomas J. Kunicki and Diane J. Nugent

PLATELET MEMBRANE GLYCOPROTEINS

Among the variety of glycoproteins (GPs) on the human platelet surface, there are several that contribute to the immunogenic makeup of the platelet (Table 144–1). Foremost among these are the integrins, which serve important roles in platelet function as receptors for protein components of the extracellular matrix, such as collagen, and/or bind to plasma glycoproteins, such as fibrinogen or von Willebrand factor (VWF). Other immunogenic glycoprotein receptors are unique to the megakaryocyte/platelet lineage, such as the GP Ib-IX-V complex.

INTEGRINS

The integrins are membrane GP heterodimers, each consisting of noncovalently associated α and β subunits.[1] The specificity of an integrin is dictated in large part by the identity of its α subunit, even though ligand binding per se may occur with a significant portion of the β subunit. The number of possible $\alpha\beta$ combinations is apparently limited, however, and selective pairing in humans between several α and β subunits has led to the discovery of more than 24 different integrins. These ubiquitous receptors mediate a wide range of cell adhesion events that are important to every fundamental area of human biology, including embryonal development, immunocompetence, wound healing, and hemostasis. Two platelet membrane receptors that figure prominently in the antigenic profile of platelets, the cohesion receptor $\alpha_{IIb}\beta_3$ and the collagen receptor $\alpha_2\beta_1$, belong to the integrin receptor family.

THE PLATELET COHESION RECEPTOR, INTEGRIN $\alpha_{IIb}\beta_3$

The numerically predominant platelet integrin $\alpha_{IIb}\beta_3$ (initially designated GP IIb-IIIa) mediates the common cohesive pathway that results from platelet activation in vivo, that is, platelet aggregation supported by the binding of adhesive proteins, such as fibrinogen and VWF. The α subunit of this integrin, α_{IIb}, is synthesized exclusively by megakaryocytes. Consequently, $\alpha_{IIb}\beta_3$ is a unique marker for platelets or cell lines with a megakaryocytic phenotype. Glanzmann thrombasthenia (GT) is an inherited disorder of platelet function characterized by an inability of platelets to bind fibrinogen and undergo agonist-induced aggregation.[2] The molecular defect in this disease involves either a quantitative or a qualitative abnormality of $\alpha_{IIb}\beta_3$.

THE PLATELET COLLAGEN RECEPTOR, INTEGRIN $\alpha_2\beta_1$

Another integrin that contributes significantly to platelet function is the collagen receptor $\alpha_2\beta_1$ (GPIa-IIa). A high affinity interaction of platelet $\alpha_2\beta_1$ with collagen anchors the platelet more firmly to the matrix, permitting the formation of an activated, procoagulant platelet monolayer.[3] Platelet adhesion in flowing blood mediated by $\alpha_2\beta_1$ is supported by several collagen types, including types I, III, IV, and VI, and the rate of platelet monolayer formation is directly proportional to the platelet $\alpha_2\beta_1$ density.[4] Signal transduction is mediated by both $\alpha_2\beta_1$ and the platelet-specific collagen receptor, GPVI, facilitating and likely accelerating platelet activation and leading to aggregate formation.[5,6] Unlike α_{IIb}, the α_2 subunit is a single chain molecule and, like several other integrin α subunits, contains an additional 129 amino acid segment known as the *I-domain.*[1] Inherited platelet deficiencies of the α_2 subunit have been described, and patients with these deficiencies exhibit chronic mucocutaneous bleeding and prolonged bleeding times.[7,8] The expression of $\alpha_2\beta_1$ on platelets differs markedly between normal subjects and depends on the inheritance of at least three haplotypes of the α_2 gene.[4]

Regulation of $\alpha_2\beta_1$ expression could certainly modulate the antigenicity of this membrane receptor. It is also possible that similar factors influence expression of other platelet integrins, including $\alpha_{IIb}\beta_3$, but the extent to which that occurs remains to be determined. Two other integrins, the fibronectin receptor $\alpha_5\beta_1$[9] and the laminin receptor $\alpha_6\beta_1$,[10] are expressed by platelets, but neither has yet been shown to contribute significantly to platelet immunogenicity.

THE RECEPTOR COMPLEX GLYCOPROTEIN Ib-IX-V

The pattern of membrane GPs existing as functional complexes is repeated in the case of the nonintegrin adhesion receptor complex Ib-IX-V. The functional complex is actually a heptamer composed of one molecule of GPV associated with two molecules of each of three other gene products, GPIbα, GPbβ, and GPX .[11] With blood flow conditions ranging from low to high shear, the initial *transient* arrest of platelets on collagen requires VWF acting as a bridge between collagen and the GPIb complex.[12] The VWF binding site on the complex is located within the amino-terminal domain of GPIbα.[13] The Bernard-Soulier syndrome (BSS) is an inherited disorder of platelet function characterized by defective platelet adhesion to subendothelium and a quantitative or qualitative defect in the Ib-IX-V complex caused by mutations in genes encoding the GPIbα or the GPIX components.[2]

PLATELET GLYCOLIPIDS

Glycolipids play an important role in the structural and functional characteristics of the platelet membrane, as is true of all cell types. Less is known about platelet glycolipid structure and immunogenicity, compared to our knowledge of the platelet GPs. Several immunogenic glycolipid components of the membrane have been identified (Table 144–2).[14] The predominant glycolipid on human platelets is lactosyl ceramide, representing 64% of the neutral glycolipids. Other neutral glycolipids include trihexosyl ceramide, glycosyl ceramide, and globoside. The principal fatty acids associated with these neutral glycolipids are behenic acid (22 : 0), arachidic acid (20 : 0), and lignoceric acid (24 : 0). Ganglioside I (identified as hematoside or GM3) represents 92% of the acidic glycolipids, ganglioside II represents 5% of the platelet acidic glycolipid composition.

Table 144–1 Functional Properties of Selected Membrane Glycoprotein Complexes

GP	Alternate Names	Receptor Function	Protein Ligands
Ib-IX-V	GPIb complex	Adhesion	VWF
$\alpha_{IIb}\beta_3$	GPIIb-IIIa, CD41/CD61	Adhesion Cohesion	Fibrinogen Fibrinogen Fibronectin Vitronectin VWF
$\alpha_2\beta_1$	GPIa-IIa, VLA-2, CD49b/CD29	Adhesion	Collagen
$\alpha_5\beta_1$	GPIc-IIa, VLA-5, CD49e/CD29	Adhesion	Fibronectin
$\alpha_6\beta_1$	GPIc′-IIa, VLA-6, CD49f/CD29	Adhesion	Laminin

CD, cell differentiation (antigen); GP, glycoprotein; VLA, very late activation (antigen); VWF, von Willebrand factor.

Table 144–2 Glycolipid Antigens of Platelets

Cardiolipin
Lactosylceramide
Glycosphingolipids
Acidic: Sulfatides/gangliosides Monogalactosyl sulfatide (16/6 idiotype)
Neutral: Globotriaosyl ceramide Globotetraosyl ceramide

ALLOANTIGENS

The proliferation of serologically defined alloantigens on platelet GPs has led to the development of a consensus nomenclature, in which each of the alloantigens is prefixed as *human platelet antigen* (HPA-).[15] These designations as well as the alternate (original) names are given in Table 144–3. The HPA- nomenclature does not take into consideration linkage between many of these polymorphisms. Particularly in the case of integrin β_3, they are distributed among a limited number of major haplotypes. Two clinically significant syndromes are the direct result of sensitization to platelet-specific alloantigens: neonatal alloimmune thrombocytopenia and posttransfusion purpura.

NEONATAL ALLOIMMUNE THROMBOCYTOPENIA AND POSTTRANSFUSION PURPURA

Neonatal Alloimmune Thrombocytopenia Purpura

Neonatal alloimmune thrombocytopenia purpura (NATP) is caused by maternal sensitization to paternal alloantigens on fetal platelets (Table 144–4). A correct diagnosis of NATP must first eliminate other causes of thrombocytopenia that may occur during pregnancy. When severe, NATP may result in intracerebral hemorrhage leading to hydrocephalus and fetal death. Fetal hydrocephalus, unexplained fetal thrombocytopenia with or without anemia, or recurrent miscarriages should be considered as indicators of possible NATP.[16] Multiparous women with a history of at least one incident of NATP should be monitored carefully for subsequent episodes. Postnatal management involves transfusion of compatible platelets, and washed maternal platelets are often used. Antenatal management is controversial but can include a combination of maternal intravenous gamma globulin administration, intrauterine platelet transfusions, and corticosteroid therapy, with simultaneous close monitoring of fetal platelet counts throughout the pregnancy.[16]

The biologic diagnosis is normally made by genotyping of maternal and paternal platelet alloantigens and a serologic search for antibodies in maternal plasma or serum that react with paternal platelets.

It is intriguing that only a fraction of those mothers negative for the platelet antigen in question deliver infants affected with NATP. For example, in Western populations, responsiveness to HPA-1a is most commonly the cause of NATP, yet the frequency of homozygous HPA-1b mothers in the general white population is 2%, and estimates of the incidence of NATP are no greater than 0.05%. A key to understanding this discrepancy lies in the finding that responsiveness to HPA-1a shows an human leukocyte antigen (HLA) restriction.[17] Individuals who are homozygous for Pro_{33} (homozygous HPA-1b) and responsive to the predominant HPA-1a antigen are almost exclusively HLA DRB3*0101[17] or DQB1*02.[18] In the case of DRB3*0101, the calculated risk factor is 141, a risk level equivalent to that of the hallmark of HLA-restriction in autoimmune disease, ankylosing spondylitis and HLA B27.[19] In contrast, responsiveness of homozygous HPA-1a individuals to the HPA-1b allele is not linked to HLA.[19,20] T cells are the likely candidates for providing HLA-restriction in this case, and Maslanka and colleagues[19] provided evidence that in one case of NATP, T cells that share CDR3 (CD) R3 motifs are stimulated by peptides that contain the same Leu_{33} polymorphism that is recognized by anti-HPA-1a alloantibodies.

In five cases of alloimmunization against the less frequent antigen, HPA-6b, there was a clear association between responsiveness and the major histocompatibility complex haplotype DRB1*1501, DQA1*0102, DQB1*0602.[21] This alloimmunization likely involves different HLA class II molecules than those involved in immunization against HPA-1a.

Responsiveness to HPA-1a is not the sole cause of NATP. In a large study of 348 cases of clinically suspected NATP,[22] 78% of serologically confirmed cases were caused by anti-HPA-1a and 19% anti-HPA-5b. All other specificities accounted for no more than 5% of cases. In reports from other laboratories, the association of NATP with other alloantigens, such as HPA-3a, HPA-3b, HPA-1b, or HPA-2b, has been noted but is rare.[23] Obviously, differences in allelic gene frequencies between different racial or ethnic populations have an important affect on the frequency of responsiveness to a particular alloantigen. Table 144–5 summarizes some known variation in allelic gene frequencies between different world populations.[24–31] Thus, in the Japanese population, anti-HPA-1a has never been shown to be involved in NATP, and antibodies specific for HPA-4b play a dominant clinical role.[32] This is probably because the gene frequency for the HPA-1b allele among the Japanese (0.02) is much lower than that found in Western populations (0.15). Conversely, the gene frequency of the HPA-4b allele in Japan (0.0083) is higher than that observed in Western populations (<0.001).

Posttransfusion Purpura

Posttransfusion purpura (PTP) is a rare transfusion reaction that follows 7 to 10 days after an immunogenic blood (platelet) transfusion (see Table 144–4). It most often affects previously nontransfused, multiparous women. As with NATP, there is an increased risk to develop PTP among HLA-DR3–positive individuals, and HPA-1a is the antigen most often implicated (in European white populations).[33,34] High-titered antibodies against HPA-1a are usually detected in the patient's serum. Several cases of PTP associated with antibodies specific for HPA-5a have been reported,[35,36] and antibodies specific for HPA-15a have also been documented.[37] The paradox of PTP is that, although the recipient's platelets do not express the immunogen (typically, HPA-1a), the offending antibodies bind to

Table 144–3 Molecular Genetics of Human Platelet Alloantigens*

Antigen	Synonym	Glycoprotein Location	Nucleotide Substitution	Amino Acid Substitution	Study
HPA-1a	Zw^a, Pl^{A1}	Integrin β_3	T_{196}	Leu^{33}	Newman et al.[40]
HPA-1b	Zw^b, Pl^{A2}		C_{196}	Pro^{33}	
HPA-2a	Ko^b	GPIbα	C_{524}	Thr^{145}	Kuijpers et al.[47]
HPA-2b	Ko^a, Sib^a		T_{524}	Met^{145}	
HPA-3a	Bak^a, Lek^a	Integrin α_{IIb}	T_{2622}	Ile^{843}	Lyman et al.[48]
HPA-3b	Bak^b		G_{2622}	Ser^{843}	
HPA-4a	Yuk^b, Pen^a	Integrin β_3	G_{526}	Arg^{143}	Wang et al.[49]
HPA-4b	Yuk^a, Pen^b		A_{526}	Gln^{143}	
HPA-5a	Br^b, Zav^b	Integrin α_2	G_{1648}	Glu^{505}	Santoso et al.[51]
HPA-5b	Br^a, Zav^a, Hc^a		A_{1648}	Lys^{505}	
HPA-6W	Ca^a, Tu^a	Integrin β_3	A_{1564} G_{1564}	Gln^{489} Arg^{489}	Wang et al.[55]
HPA-7W	Mo^a	Integrin β_3	G_{1317} C_{1317}	Ala^{407} Pro^{407}	Keijpers et al.[57]
HPA-8W	Sr^a	Integrin β_3	T_{2004} C_{2004}	Cys^{636} Arg^{636}	Santoso et al.[56]
HPA-9W	Max^a	Integrin α_{IIb}	A_{2603} G_{2603}	Met^{837} Val^{837}	Noris et al.[58]
HPA-10W	La^a	Integrin β_3	A_{281} G_{281}	Gln^{62} Arg^{62}	Peyruchaud.[59]
HPA-11W	Gro^a	Integrin β_3	A_{1996} G_{1996}	His^{633} Arg^{633}	Simsek et al.[60]
HPA-12W	Iy^a	GPIbβ	A_{141} G_{141}	Glu^{15} Gly^{15}	Sachs et al.[61]
HPA-13W	Sit^a	Integrin α_2	T_{2531} C_{2531}	Met^{799} Thr^{799}	Santoso et al.[62]
HPA-14W	Oe^a	Integrin β_3	$\Delta AAG_{(1929-31)}$ $AAG_{(1929-31)}$	ΔLys^{611} Lys^{611}	Santoso et al.[63]
HPA-15a	Gov^b	CD109	C_{2108}	Ser^{703}	Schuh et al.[66]
HPA-15b	Gov^a		A_{2108}	Try^{703}	
HPA-16W	Duv^a	Integrin β_3	T_{517} C_{517}	Ile^{140} Thr^{140}	Jallu et al.[153]
	Va^a	Integrin β_3			Kekomaki et al.[67]
	Pe^a	GPIbα			Kekomaki et al.[154]

*Adapted from Santoso S, Kiefel V: Human platelet alloantigens. Wien Klin Wochenschr 113:806, 2001.

and can be eluted from the recipient's platelets. An interesting theory is that, in cases of PTP, a transient loss of tolerance for the immunogen (most often integrin $\alpha_{IIb}\beta_3$) results in autoantibody production.[38] This theory is supported by the finding that recombinant antibodies derived from PTP patients during the acute stage resemble autoantibodies, with a low degree of somatic mutation,[38] and PTP does not reoccur if incompatible platelets are readministered.[39] In this scenario, the allospecific antibodies detected after the acute phase of PTP may not completely explain the pathophysiology of the disorder.

MOLECULAR GENETICS OF PLATELET ALLOANTIGENS

By convention, the designation HPA has been assigned to alloantigen systems in which the precise polymorphism that accounts for the serologic difference between alleles has been identified. Of the sixteen HPA systems defined to date (see Table 144–3), nine are expressed by the integrin β_3 subunit (HPA-1, HPA-4, HPA-6, HPA-7, HPA-8, HPA-10, HPA-11, HPA-14, and HPA-16); two are localized on the integrin α_{IIb} subunit (HPA-3 and HPA-9); two are found on the integrin α_2 subunit (HPA-5 and HPA-13); one is expressed by the GP Ibα (HPA-2); one, by GPIbβ (HPA-12); and the last is located on CD109 (HPA-15).

Table 144–4 Alloimmune Thrombocytopenias

Neonatal Alloimmune Thrombocytopenia
Incidence is 1 per 3000 in a retrospective study and 1 per 2200 births in one prospective study.
Maternal antibodies are produced against paternal antigens on fetal platelets.
Similar to erythroblastosis fetalis, except that 50% of cases occur during first pregnancy.
Most frequently implicated antigens are HPA-1a and HPA-5$_\alpha$ (United States/Europe).
In the case of responsiveness to HPA-1a, there is a high-risk association with HLA DRB3*0101 or DQB1*02.
In the case of responsiveness to HPA-6b, there is an increased association with HLA DRB1*1501, DQA1*0102, or DQB1*0602.
Posttransfusion Purpura
Nearly all reported patients have been women previously sensitized by pregnancy or transfusion (<5% were men).
Thrombocytopenia usually occurs 1 week after transfusion.
Homozygous HPA-1b individuals account for most (>60%) cases.
High-risk association with HLA DRB3*0101 or DQB1*02.
Enigmatically, the recipient's antigen-negative platelets are destroyed by autologous antibody.

HLA, human leukocyte antigen; HPA, human platelet antigen.

HPA-1

The HPA-1 alloantigen system is defined by the Leu[33]/Pro[33] polymorphism that is enclosed within a small 13 amino acid loop formed by the pairing of Cys[26] with Cys[38].[40] This region of the molecule is held proximal to the distal cysteine-rich region in the middle of β_3 by a long-range disulfide bond linking Cys[5] and Cys[435].[41] The importance of three-dimensional structure imposed by the Cys[26]-Cys[38] disulfide bond constraint to expression of the HPA-1 determinants is evidenced by the fact that linear peptides corresponding to the β_3(26–38) sequence are not antigenic[42] and the antigens are not lost following denaturation of β_3 in ionic detergents. However, they are immediately destroyed on subsequent disulfide bond reduction. The complex structure of the β_3 molecule and the sensitivity of the determinants to this structure is the likely explanation for observed heterogeneity in binding properties of anti-HPA-1a alloantibodies.[43] Although all alloantibodies would bind to the denatured molecule or to recombinant amino-terminal segments of the molecule expressed in *Escherichia coli*,[44] a subset of antibodies appear to require presentation of the antigenic loop within a more native environment, such as the nondenatured molecule.[43] Anti–HPA-1a antibodies inhibit clot retraction and platelet aggregation, in the latter case presumably because they block the binding of fibrinogen.[45]

An R93Q mutation in β_3 can also attenuate antibody binding to the HPA-1a epitope,[46] either through conformational changes in the amino terminal region of the β_3 molecule or through an attenuation of the immune processing of that epitope.

Other cells that express β_3, as the beta subunit of the vitronectin receptor, including endothelial cells, fibroblasts, and smooth muscle cells, also express HPA-1 epitopes. This could contribute to the complexity of the clinical symptoms in alloimmune-mediated thrombocytopenia. At this time, little, if anything, is known about the involvement of tissues other than platelets in these conditions.

HPA-2

Two previously described polymorphisms of the Ib-IX-V complex, termed *Ko* and *Sib*, are now known to be reflections of two linked polymorphisms, one of which defines the diallelic system, HPA-2.[47]

Table 144–5 Gene Frequencies of the Major Alloantigenic Alleles in Various World Populations

HPA-	Western	Japanese	Amerindian	Black	Korea	African-American	Finnish	Thai
1a	0.85	0.998	>0.993	0.885	0.995		0.86	>0.998
1b	0.15	0.002	<0.007	0.115	0.005		0.14	<0.002
2a	0.93		0.058	0.852		0.82	0.91	0.917
2b	0.07		0.042	0.148		0.18	0.09	0.083
3a	0.61						0.59	0.37
3b	0.39						0.41	0.63
4a	>0.99	0.989						0.991
4b	<0.01	0.011						0.009
5a	0.89					0.79	0.95	0.973
5b	0.11					0.21	0.05	0.027

In the GP Ibα sequence, a Thr/Met polymorphism at residue 145, is associated with HPA-2a and HPA-2b epitopes, respectively.

HPA-3

The HPA-3 system is associated with an Ile^{843}/Ser^{843} polymorphism of α_{IIb}.[48]

HPA-4

Another diallelic human alloantigen system known as *Pen* (or *Yuk*) is found on β_3 and is associated with an Arg^{185}/Gln^{186} polymorphism.[49] Given the proximity of the Pen polymorphism to the RGD binding domain (residues 109–171) of β_3, it is not surprising that anti–HPA-4a antibodies completely inhibit aggregation of HPA-4a homozygous platelets.[45]

Other cells that express β_3 as the β subunit of the vitronectin receptor, including endothelial cells, fibroblasts, and smooth muscle cells, also express HPA-1 and HPA-4 epitopes.[50] This could contribute to the complexity of the clinical symptoms in patients with alloimmune-mediated thrombocytopenia. At this time, little, if anything, is known about the involvement of tissues other than platelets in these conditions.

HPA-5

The HPA-5 system is located on the integrin subunit α_2.[51] The detection of this system was facilitated by the development of a highly sensitive murine monoclonal antibody-based monoclonal antibody immobilization of platelet antigen assay.[52] Like the preceding alloantigenic systems, the HPA-5 system is diallelic. Roughly 1000 to 2000 copies of α_2 are present on the surface of normal platelets, and each α_2 molecule expresses a single HPA-5 epitope.[53] The integrin α_2 is distributed on a wide variety of cells, but nothing is currently known about the antigenicity of the HPA-5 determinants on receptors expressed by cell types other than platelets.

The density of the $\alpha_2\beta_1$ integrin is known to correlate with the α_2 SNP C807T. However, in a study of 79 HPA-5(a/a) mothers giving birth to HPA-5(a/b) offspring, Panzer and colleagues[54] determined that there was no increased risk of maternal-fetal HPA-5 incompatibility among mothers whose genotype is 807T.

HPA-6

This system, originally defined by the alloantigens Ca^a or Tu^a, is created by the β_3 Arg^{489}/Gln^{489} polymorphism resulting from a G/A substitution at base 1564.[55]

HPA-7 and HPA-8

The alloantigen Mo^a has been localized to β_3.[56,57] The alloantigen Sr^a is classified as a private alloantigen, because it appears to be inherited within a single family or family group but not expressed by the general population. The unique feature of the HPA-8 polymorphism is that it is associated with an Arg^{636}/Cys^{636} substitution and thereby results in an additional unpaired cysteine residue.[56] Since its initial characterization, it has been accepted that all cysteine residues in β_3 are involved in disulfide bridges. Despite the addition of this new sulfhydryl group, the Arg^{636}-containing β_3 subunit still associates with α_{IIb} and contributes to an expressed $\alpha_{IIb}\beta_3$ complex without apparent impairment of function.

The alloantigen system HPA-7 results from a C to G substitution at bp 1267 of β_3 resulting in replacement of Pro^{407} by Ala^{407}.[57] Mo^a is a low-frequency alloantigen and has been detected in only 1 of 450 random donors outside of the initial family of the propositus.

HPA-9

The HPA-9 system, originally named for the alloantigen Max^a, is the second system to be localized to the integrin α_{IIb} subunit. It is defined by the Val^{837}, Met^{837} polymorphism.[58]

HPA-10

This system, initially named *La*, is defined by the β_3 Arg^{62}/Gln^{62} polymorphism.[59]

HPA-11

The private antigen Gro^a is defined by integrin β_3 residue His^{633} (A_{1996}).[60] The corresponding Gro^b allele is defined by the substitution Arg^{633} (G_{1996}).

HPA-12

On GPIbβ, the Glu^{15}/Gly^{15} (A_{141}/G_{141}) dimorphism creates the ly^a and ly^b alleles, respectively.[61] Ly^a (HPA-12a) has been found in 1 of 300 unrelated German donors.

HPA-13

The Sit(a) alloantigen, identified in a single severe case of NATP and present in 1 in 400 German subjects, is defined by integrin α_2 mutation C2531T.[62] This mutation results in a Thr^{799} Ø Met^{799} substitution and results in a modest decrease in platelet response to collagen in vitro.

HPA-14

One case of NATP has been attributed to antibodies specific for Oe^a, and none of 600 unrelated blood donors was found to carry this antigen. Deletion of the $\beta3$ residue $Lysine^{611}$ is the cause of the expression of Oe^a,[63] and this isoform is in linkage disequilibrium with HPA-1b.

HPA-15

The HPA-15 alloantigenic polymorphism, Gov, is uniquely expressed by a different protein receptor. Kelton and colleagues[64] initially described the Gov system that is now known to be carried by the 175 kd glycosyl phosphatidylinositol-anchored GP CD109. Alloantibodies defining each of two alleles (Gov^a/Gov^b) were detected in two patients who had received multiple platelet transfusions[64] and, more recently, three patients who had developed NATP.[65] An A2108C single nucleotide polymorphism of the CD109 gene, resulting in a Tyr^{703} Ø Ser^{703} substitution, defines the Gov alloantigen system.[66]

ADDITIONAL ALLOANTIGENS

One additional private antigen, Va^a, is associated with the integrin $\alpha_{IIb}\beta_3$, but it has not been determined which subunit bears the determinants.[67] Lastly, the alloantigen Pe^a is expressed by GPIba.[68]

ISOANTIGENS

Isoantibodies are produced against an epitope that is expressed by all normal individuals and is not polymorphic. In the area of human platelet immunology, a classic example of isoimmunization can and does occur when a patient with an inherited deficiency of a membrane GP has been subjected to multiple platelet transfusions to correct a bleeding diathesis. Such inherited disorders are GT and BSS, wherein the individual either lacks or expresses an altered form of $\alpha_{IIb}\beta_3$ in the case of GT or Ib-IX-V in the case of BSS. Isoantibodies developed by transfused patients do not distinguish any of the allelic forms of the GPs (eg, HPA-3 or HPA-1 alloantigens on $\alpha_{IIb}\beta_3$) but react with the platelets of all normal persons tested. Because the propositus does not express the platelet GP that carries the epitope in question, these antibodies do not bind to their own platelets.

ISOANTIBODIES IN GLANZMANN THROMBASTHENIA

Several cases have been documented in which GT patients have produced antibodies specific for α_{IIb}, β_3, or the $\alpha_{IIb}\beta_3$ complex. Recently, we defined an idiotype (OG) that is associated at high frequency with isoantibodies specific for integrin subunit β_3 generated by GT patients.[69,70] Patient OG suffered from persistent, often serious bleeding episodes as a result of both his GT phenotype and the fact that he had generated a very high-titered IgG isoantibody inhibitor of platelet cohesion.[70] The study of the OG idiotype presented an excellent opportunity to compare and contrast disease-related $\alpha_{IIb}\beta_3$ inhibitors of human origin with other natural or synthetic inhibitors of this integrin receptor. Rabbit polyclonal anti-OG idiotype binds to IgG specific for $\alpha_{IIb}\beta_3$ obtained from eleven nonrelated GT patients, including an unrelated patient ES, studied extensively by Coller and colleagues,[71] who had developed isoantibodies of very similar specificity. Conversely, anti-OG does not recognize $\alpha_{IIb}\beta_3$-specific antibodies produced by other unrelated GT patients, who had developed isoantibodies with specificities distinct from that of the OG isoantibody. Moreover, anti-OG does not recognize $\alpha_{IIb}\beta_3$-specific antibodies developed by any patients with idiopathic thrombocytopenic purpura (ITP) or six representative patients with alloimmune thrombocytopenias; and anti-OG never binds to IgG from any of several nonimmunized control individuals.

Anti-OG binds to selected protein ligands of $\alpha_{IIb}\beta_3$, namely, fibrinogen, vitronectin, and VWF, but not to other known protein ligands, such as fibronectin or type I collagen. The epitope or epitopes recognized by anti-OG on these three adhesive proteins are either very similar or identical, because each protein can inhibit the binding of anti-OG to any of the others. The epitope on fibrinogen recognized by anti-OG resides in the β_3 chain and is likely contained within the first 42 amino acids from the amino-terminus.[72] Because OG IgG inhibits fibrinogen binding to $\alpha_{IIb}\beta_3$, the specificity of the OG idiotype defines a novel binding motif for the integrin $\alpha_{IIb}\beta_3$ that is shared by fibrinogen, vitronectin, and VWF but distinct from previously described RGD-containing sites on the fibrinogen α_{IIb} chain or the fibrinogen β_3 chain carboxyl-terminal decapeptide site. Moskowitz and colleagues[72] have employed specific proteolytic forms of fibrinogen to confirm that the epitope recognized by anti-OG is located within Bβ(1–42). This represents an excellent example of molecular mimicry in which an antigen-selected IgG inhibitor of $\alpha_{IIb}\beta_3$ function shares a novel recognition sequence common to three physiologic protein ligands of that receptor.

ISOANTIBODIES IN BERNARD-SOULIER SYNDROME

Because BSS is less frequently encountered than GT, it follows that isoantibodies produced in conjunction with this syndrome are also less frequently encountered. In the only clear-cut case of such an isoantibody,[73] the isolated IgG impaired both normal platelet adhesion to subendothelial elements and in vitro aggregation in response to ristocetin and bovine factor VIII.

CD36

The frequency of platelet CD36 (GPIV) deficiency, which occurs most often in Asians and blacks, is approximately 4%; and a subset of these individuals is at risk for immunization against CD36.[74] In five cases of neonatal thrombocytopenia, isoantibodies reactive with CD36 were identified in the mothers of the affected infants. Two black mothers were homozygous for a T1264G substitution in the CD36 gene, and a European white mother was homozygous for a novel deletion of exons 1 through 3. These findings and the results of prior reports indicate that isoimmunization against CD36 can cause neonatal isoimmune thrombocytopenia, refractoriness to platelet transfusions, and PTP.[74]

AUTOANTIGENS

Autoimmune (or idiopathic) thrombocytopenia purpura (AITP or ITP) is the most frequently encountered form of immune thrombocytopenia.[75] This disorder can be classified as acute or chronic on the basis of the duration of the thrombocytopenia, the chronic form persisting longer than 6 to 12 months (see Chapter 131). The acute, self-limiting form occurs predominantly in children, often after a viral illness or immunization, and affects boys and girls with equal frequency. The chronic form is mainly an adult illness and affects twice as many women as men. Life-threatening bleeding occurs in up to 1% percent of patients with ITP. The reason that some patients sustain severe hemorrhagic complications and others do not remains unexplained; but because of differences seen in the clinical expression of chronic and acute ITP, it has been theorized that the mechanisms of disease for each form are probably different.

It had been hoped that the antigenic targets in acute and chronic forms of ITP might be different so that antigen identity might one day be used as an early indicator of clinical outcome. Subsequent studies have shed more light on this issue and have demonstrated that autoantibody specificity in chronic versus acute ITP is quite similar, particularly in children.[76,77] Nonetheless, a distinction between antigen specificity and an acute versus chronic course in cases of ITP may yet be found in the early stages of the autoimmune response. Clearly, prospective studies aimed at answering this question are still warranted.

Although most autoantibodies apparently induce thrombocytopenia, few induce platelet dysfunction without an increase in platelet clearance (see Chapter 131).[78,79] The proportion of the two types of autoantibody, that which leads to platelet clearance and that which blocks platelet function, may be an important factor controlling the unpredictable clinical severity of ITP.

GLYCOPROTEINS AS AUTOANTIGENS

Integrin $\alpha_{IIb}\beta_3$

The integrin $\alpha_{IIb}\beta_3$ was the first platelet membrane component to be identified as a dominant antigen in patients with chronic ITP,[80] and subsequent studies from several laboratories have confirmed the important contribution of this receptor to the autoantigenic makeup of the human platelet.[75]

Integrin Subunit β_3

Attempts to further localize autoepitopes on either integrin subunit have been more successful with regard to β_3. Early on, Kekomaki and colleagues[81] defined a prominent autoantigenic region as the 33 kd chymotryptic fragment of β_3 located within the cysteine-rich region of β_3, which was bound by both plasma autoantibodies and autoantibody eluted from patients' platelets. Fujisawa and colleagues[82] subsequently determined that plasma autoantibodies in 5 of 13 patients with chronic ITP was bound to peptides representing β_3 residues 721 to 744 or 742 to 762, namely, the carboxy-terminal region of β_3 that is presumed to be located in the cytoplasm of the platelet. Their role in the pathogenesis of immune thrombocytopenia is clouded by the fact that this portion of the β_3 molecule is located within the cytoplasm, not on the surface, of the resting platelet.

However, internal autoantigens are the hallmark of many immune-mediated diseases, such as polymyositis and systemic lupus erythematosus.[83] As with these diseases, one can postulate that the autoantigen is primarily internal, but at some point is expressed on the surface of the platelet surface, perhaps with activation or senescence, at which time the autoantibody can bind and remove the cell from circulation.

The report by Fujisawa[84] is one of many suggesting that autoantibodies to $\alpha_{IIb}\beta_3$ can bind to cryptic epitopes or neoantigens that are expressed with platelet activation or senescence. Platelets normally accumulate IgG on the membrane surface as they age or become activated over 7 to 10 days, and then they are cleared by reticuloendothelial cells in the spleen.[85] Using Fab′2 fraction of IgG it has been shown that normal individuals have autoantibodies in their sera that specifically bind to senescent antigens on red blood cells and platelets to mediate clearance of spent or dysfunctional cells.[86,87] The role of these naturally occurring autoantibodies in pathologic immune destruction of cells is unclear. Animal studies suggest that the initial binding of the pathogenic antiplatelet autoantibody may trigger the expression of senescent or cryptic antigens on the platelet membrane, resulting in a second wave of immunoglobulin binding and clearance by naturally occurring autoantibodies.[88]

More recently, additional autoantigenic epitopes have been identified on the β_3 subunit. Nardi and colleagues[89] identified the peptide β_3^{49-66} as a site that is bound by most affinity-purified antibodies isolated from serum immune complexes of immunologic thrombocytopenic patents infected with human immunodeficiency virus type 1. This is not a peptide that is bound by serum IgG antibodies from control subjects or patients with the classic form of ITP.

Identification of autoimmune epitopes has been aided by the development of the phage-display peptide library. Bowditch and colleagues[90] used a filamentous phage library that displays random linear hexapeptides to identify peptide sequences recognized by AITP autoantibodies. Plasma antibody eluates from patients were used to select for phage-displaying autoantibody-reactive peptides. They identified anti-$\alpha_{IIb}\beta_3$ antibody-specific phage encoding the hexapeptide sequences Arg-Glu-Lys-Ala-Lys-Trp (REKAKW), Pro-Val-Val-Trp-Lys-Asn (PVVWKN), and Arg-Glu-Leu-Leu-Lys-Met (RELLKM). Each phage showed saturable dose-dependent binding to immobilized autoantibody, and binding could be blocked with purified $\alpha_{IIb}\beta_3$. The binding of plasma autoantibody to the phage encoding REKAKW could be blocked with a synthetic peptide derived from the β_3 cytoplasmic tail; however, the PVVWKN was not. Using sequential overlapping peptides from the β_3 cytoplasmic region, an epitope was localized to the sequence Arg-Ala-Arg-Ala-Lys-Trp (β_3 734–739).

Integrin Subunit α_{IIb}

Autoantibodies reactive with α_{IIb} were identified in two patients with chronic ITP[91,92]; and in one patient, the antibody was subsequently shown to react with a chymotryptic, 65 kd, COOH-terminal fragment of the α_{IIb} heavy chain.[92] Ethylenediaminetetraacetic acid (EDTA)–dependent autoantibodies represent a special category that are absorbed by autologous platelets when whole blood is drawn in EDTA. In one such case of EDTA-dependent *pseudothrombocytopenia*, an IgM antibody was shown to bind to α_{IIb} by immunoblot assay and crossed immunoelectrophoresis.[93]

Further work by Gevorkian and associates[94] used phage display to map an autoepitope on α_{IIb}. A filamentous phage library was employed that displays random peptides, 11 amino acids in length flanked on each side by a cysteine, to identify peptide sequences recognized by an antiplatelet autoantibody known to block fibrinogen binding to $\alpha_{IIb}\beta_3$. Phage from individual colonies, after the fourth round of purification, were tested for binding to the autoantibody. A phage expressing the sequence CTGRVPLGFEDLC exhibited saturable dose-dependent binding to immobilized autoantibody. This binding could be blocked with purified $\alpha_{IIb}\beta_3$ and α_{IIb} but not by β_3. The peptide amino acid sequence has partial identity with amino acids 4 through 10 and with amino acids 31 through 35 on α_{IIb}. This work suggests that the autoantibody binds to a combinatorial epitope within the first 35 amino acids of α_{IIb}.

Autoantigenic epitopes may be conformational and dependent on the tertiary configuration of the molecule. Given the fluid nature of the platelet membrane and the remarkable metamorphosis that occurs with activation and adhesion, it is not surprising that conformational antigenic sites would come and go. In fact, Shadle and associates[95] describe a neoantigen on α_{IIb}, which is only revealed following the normal binding of fibrinogen to its receptor, the $\alpha_{IIb}\beta_3$ complex. Serum autoantibodies have been described that demonstrate increased binding to platelets in the presence of calcium chelators, such as EDTA, heparin, or other drugs.[93] Some autoantibody binding may be directed to neoantigens and thus is enhanced after changes in membrane GPs induced by agents such as EDTA or heparin.

Human Monoclonal Autoantibodies

How large is the autoepitope repertoire on a given GP antigen? The answer to this important question affects on the feasibility of developing therapeutic and diagnostic measures based on epitope specificity. Since the autoantibodies that react with a given epitope are likely to share idiotypes, one can approach this question from two angles, analyzing the epitope repertoire, the idiotype repertoire, or both. Two studies have addressed the extent of the autoantigen repertoire on $\alpha_{IIb}\beta_3$ by analyzing the competitive binding between human autoantibodies and murine monoclonal antibodies.[96,97] However, the limited number of studies that have used this approach have generated conflicting results, and there remain insufficient data to judge the size of the autoepitope repertoire on $\alpha_{IIb}\beta_3$. Additional analyses aimed at epitope localization will be necessary, and perhaps novel approaches will expedite this task. One such novel approach is the development of human monoclonal autoantibodies specific for $\alpha_{IIb}\beta_3$ and other platelet GPs.

Human monoclonal antibodies are an alternative tool in the search for GP epitopes that are autoimmunogenic in humans. The first human monoclonal antibody against a platelet GP was developed by Nugent and associates,[83] derived from an ITP individual producing an antibody against β_3. This human monoclonal antibody detects a neoantigen associated with β_3 that is expressed only on stored or thrombin-activated platelets. A number of human monoclonal autoantibodies specific for the heavy chain of GPIb were generated from the lymphocytes of an ITP patient with serum autoantibody specific for Ib.[98] The heavy chain variable region genes of four of these antibodies have been sequenced and found to be markedly homologous to human immunoglobulin, germ-line, heavy-chain variable region genes.[98] Another human monoclonal autoantibody was produced that is specific for the heavy chain of α_{IIb}.[84] The epitope recognized by this antibody (2E7) has been identified as a contiguous amino acid sequence with residues 231 to 238 with an immunodominant tryptophan residue at position 235.[99] This was the first time that the precise epitope on α_{IIb} or β_3 recognized by a human antibody had been identified.

The $\alpha_{IIb}\beta_3$ molecule is a member of the greater family of adhesion molecules or integrins, and α_{IIb} has significant homology with other integrin α chains. A comparison of the 220 to 238 sequence of α_{IIb} and seven other integrin α subunits revealed significant homology between α_{IIb} and other α integrin chains, yet 2E7 did not bind to the other cell types that express these related integrin family members, such as endothelial cells, lymphocytes, monocytes, or neutrophils. In the highly homologous region spanning residues 234 through 238, α_{IIb} differs from the other α chains only in position 235 (TrpØLeu). Ironically, this tryptophan plays a critical role in determining the immunogenic epitope recognized by 2E7.

From the foregoing analysis, it is clear that further studies are required to determine the extent to which the production of human autoantibodies to platelet GPs is clonally restricted. Given a selected number of idiotypes (Ids) related to autoimmunity to $\alpha_{IIb}\beta_3$, one could potentially use the antiidiotype (anti-Id) to modulate immunization to $\alpha_{IIb}\beta_3$. Along these lines, it has been reported that intravenous immunoglobulin, which is routinely used to reverse acute thrombocytopenia in patients with ITP, may contain anti-Id directed to idiotypes of autoantibody but not alloantibodies that recognize $\alpha_{IIb}\beta_3$.[100] Nugent and colleagues[101] have defined a DM idiotype that is characteristic of human autoantibodies that are specific for the Ib heavy chain. Their study clearly suggests that the repertoire of idiotypes expressed by human autoantibodies specific for membrane GPs, such as those of the human platelet, will be narrowly defined and thus amenable to study.

The production of human monoclonal autoantibodies or recombinant Fab fragments from patients with immune thrombocytopenia provides researchers with specific antibody probes to map target antigens. Human monoclonal antibodies have an advantage over serum antibodies in that they are monoclonal and circumvent problems associated with using a polyclonal serum where many different, low-titer autoantibodies can be found with reactivity against a variety of epitopes.

GPIb Complex

Autoantibodies to components of the GPIb complex are also frequently encountered in adult chronic ITP. He and associates[102] have made progress in the localization of selected autoantigenic epitopes on the GP Ib molecule. Epitopes were most frequently found on a recombinant fragment of Ibα corresponding to residues 240 through 485 and next most often on a fragment representing residues 1 through 247. In the case of those antibodies reactive with the former sequence, further epitope mapping identified the dominant determinant as the nine amino acid sequence TKEQTTFPP (residues 333–341).[102] In some cases in which autoantibody to Ib-IX was detected, the clinical presentation proved to be particularly severe and refractory to therapy.[101] One case of *pseudo–Bernard-Soulier syndrome* (dysfunction of the Ib-IX-V receptor complex) was reported to be caused by an autoantibody to Ib.[103] Finally, in the subset of childhood ITP cases associated with varicella-zoster infection, the GP V component of this receptor was found to be the dominant target of serum autoantibodies that do not cross-react with viral antigens.[104] At the same time, in another group of children with this disease, it was found that serum antibodies specific for viral antigens can cross-react with normal platelet antigens and may thus contribute to platelet clearance.[105]

Unlike the $\alpha_{IIb}\beta_3$ complex, autoantibodies directed against GPIb are almost universally associated with pathologic immune destruction of platelets. Thus far, no one has described naturally occurring antibodies reacting with GPIb in either resting or activated platelets. Although only 15% to 30% of AITP patients have autoantibodies that bind to GPIb, there is no background binding of antibodies in normal plasma, so the characterization of this antigen is much more straightforward. Furthermore, using antiidiotypic reagents, it appears that the repertoire of idiotypes expressed by anti-GPIb antibodies from patients with AITP is very narrowly defined.[101] In this study, affinity purified antiplatelet GPIb antibody from patient DM who produced a very high titer anti-GPIb autoantibody was used to immunize rabbits and mice for the production of rabbit polyclonal and murine monoclonal anti-DM idiotypic antibodies. These reagents were highly specific for the DM idiotype and could be used to screen a large number of serum samples from normal individuals and patients with AITP. Furthermore, the rabbit polyclonal and certain of the murine monoclonal antibodies block binding of the immunizing antibody, DM, to platelets or purified GPIb. Approximately 95% of AITP serum samples from patients who are positive for the DM idiotype contained anti-GPIb autoantibody (P < 0.00001).

The GPIbα heavy chain is a large molecule and contains Leucine-rich repeats and a region in the middle of the GP that is heavily glycosylated. The NH2-terminal region of GPIb is responsible for binding to von Willebrand antigen, mediating platelet adhesion. Theoretically, there could be a variety of antigenic sites on this molecule; but in the studies examining frequency of DM idiotype positive, anti-GPIb autoantibodies, only 12% to 15% of the anti-GPIb plasmas was negative for DM idiotypic antibodies. Half of these were from patients who had developed drug-dependent antibodies, which bound to the GPIb-IX complex, particularly those associated with the ingestion of quinine or quinidine. These results suggest that the DM idiotype is tightly associated with autoantibodies against GPIb in patients with AITP; and, although DM is not the only autoepitope on GPIb, it is certainly present as one of the anti-GPIb antibodies in the serum of most patients with autoantibodies to this complex.

The DM autoantigen has been mapped to the heavy chain of the GPIb complex. Following trypsin treatment of affinity purified GPIb complex, the DM autoantibody specifically recognizes a site on the 40 to 45 kd fragment of the GPIbα molecule, the same region where von Willebrand protein binds to mediate platelet adhesion. Ongoing research to identify the sequence of the DM autoepitope will provide a critical piece of information which is currently lacking in AITP, namely what role do these GP sequences play in antigen selection of certain pathologic autoantibody idiotypes.

GPV

In the mid-1980s, when screening for antigen specific autoantibodies became available, many researchers hoped that the patterns of target antigen reactivity might be predictive of the clinical course of AITP, that is, acute versus chronic. In fact, an initial report looking at eight children with acute AITP using immunoblot technique failed to demonstrate anti-β_3 antibody even though this was the dominant antigenic target recognized by autoantibodies from patients with chronic AITP.[106] This was followed by a report from the same laboratory[107] demonstrating serum antibody reactivity to GPV in four pediatric patients with thrombocytopenia associated with varicella (chickenpox) infection. GPV is a thrombin-sensitive, 85 kd GP of unknown function on the platelet surface. There was no evidence of immune complexes in these patients or varicella antigens adsorbed to the surface of their platelets. Because all of the children with varicella-related AITP and acute childhood form of AITP achieved resolution of thrombocytopenia within 6 months, there was some hope that GPV reactivity would be a marker for mild disease and these patients could escape aggressive immunosuppressive therapy.

Integrin $\alpha_2\beta_1$

Platelet integrin $\alpha_2\beta_1$ is an important collagen receptor on the platelet membrane. Although present in a much lower concentration than $\alpha_{IIb}\beta_3$ or the GPIb complex, this receptor has also been shown to be a target autoantigen in 10% to 20% of chronic AITP patients.[108] Moreover, serum IgG autoantibodies specific for integrin subunit α_2 were identified in a unique case of autoimmune platelet dysfunction after myasthenia gravis.[108] This autoantibody inhibited aggregation of normal platelets induced by collagen or wheat germ agglutinin. This was the first case wherein autoantibodies to α_2 were associated with a chronic hemorrhagic disorder.

Efforts to map the specific epitope on this receptor have been unsuccessful even though several groups have suggested that the binding of these antibodies, because they impair function, might be near the binding site of collagen. Deckmyn and associates describe a plasma autoantibody directed against a protein comigrating with α_2 and recognized by the patient's antibody when affinity-purified $\alpha_2\beta_1$ was used as antigen.[108] The $\alpha_2\beta_1$ complex was immunoprecipitated from a platelet lysate by the patient's plasma, and purified platelet specific IgGs from this patient inhibited aggregation of normal platelets induced by collagen or by wheat germ agglutinin. Dromigny and associates[109] described a 48-year-old woman in whom they found increased bleeding times, impaired collagen-induced platelet aggregation, and the presence of autoantibodies directed against $\alpha_2\beta_1$ and the GPIb complex.

CHAPTER 145

HUMAN LEUKOCYTE ANTIGEN AND HUMAN NEUTROPHIL ANTIGEN SYSTEMS

Ena Wang, Sharon Adams, David F. Stroncek, and Francesco M. Marincola

This chapter reviews human leukocyte antigen (HLA) and human neutrophil antigen (HNA) systems. A general background of the structure, function, and nomenclature of both systems and their relevance in clinical hematology is presented. Analysis of HLA gene products is applied in clinical settings (a) to select compatible donor-recipient pairs for transplantation, (b) to select HLA-compatible single donor platelet products for thrombocytopenic patients refractory to standard transfusion of random pooled platelets, (c) to screen for genetic factors that may contribute to the prevalence of diseases, and (d) for forensic purposes in which the identity of individuals may contribute to solving legal disputes or criminal investigations. In addition, we discuss new applications that have broadened the relevance of HLA in the area of immune pathology. Human leukocyte antigen phenotypes determine the suitability of patients for epitope-specific immunization. Tetrameric HLA/epitope complexes (tHLA) allow enumeration of antigen-specific T-cell responses. Furthermore, molecular identification of T-cell epitopes associated with distinct diseases and characterization of the communication between immune effector cells through HLA/HLA ligand interactions extend the relevance of HLA to biologic fields. These biologic fields encompass natural killer (NK) and cytotoxic T-cell function, antigen recognition in the context of infection, autoimmunity, graft-versus-neoplasia (GVN) effect, and autologous cancer rejection. Finally, the recognition that polymorphism extends to other protein families relevant to immune pathology including cytokines, their receptors, and killer cell inhibitory receptors has broadened the significance of immunogenetics beyond HLA. Thus, this chapter emphasizes the importance of viewing human pathology through the kaleidoscopic complexity of human polymorphism.

GENETICS, STRUCTURE, AND FUNCTION OF HLA MOLECULES

Human leukocyte antigen embrace a family of genes clustered in the short arm of chromosome 6 as the human version of the major histocompatibility complex (MHC), initially identified in mice as responsible for graft rejection between genetically unrelated strains (transplantation antigens).[1] Credit for the description of the human MHC goes to three individuals. In 1952, Jean Dausset observed that serum of individuals who had received several transfusions contained hemoagglutinins specific for donor's leukocytes. In 1958, Rose Payne noted that the only requirement for the development of hemoagglutinins against leukocytes was a history of previous transfusion or pregnancy and concluded that these antibodies were directed against antigens on the surface of circulating leukocytes. This conclusion was concomitantly and independently confirmed by Jon van Rood, who observed that multiple pregnancies immunize mothers against leukocytes leaked from the fetus into the mother's circulation. Based on these discoveries, the term *human leukocyte antigen* was subsequently adopted.[2] It should be clarified, however, that this historical name is misleading. Neither is HLA molecule expression limited to leukocytes nor do they display, in natural conditions, antigenic behavior. In fact, several are expressed by most somatic cells; and, rather than being antigens, they chaperon protein bioproducts to the cell surface for recognition by T cells. There is, however, some substance to the name, because HLA, by virtue of being densely packed on the cell surface, are exposed to recognition in a foreign environment such as allotransplantation or xenoinfusion performed to induce anti-HLA antibodies as diagnostic reagents.

ORGANIZATION OF THE HLA GENES

Human leukocyte antigen genes comprise a string of coding sequences that regulate the expression of molecules with similar but not identical function. Residing in a region that spans approximately 4000 kb of the short arm of chromosome 6 (Figure 145–1),[3] HLA contains several genes and pseudogenes characterized by sequence homology and functional similarity. Of them, 47 are officially recognized by the World Health Organization nomenclature committee[4] and include classic HLA class I and class II genes associated with antigen processing such as *PSMB8* and *PSMB9* (proteasomal units) or *TAP1* and *TAP2* associated with peptide transport. Both HLA and HLA-associated genes can be physically grouped into three subregions according to chromosomal location. In centromeric to telomeric direction, the first is HLA class II region comprising the α and β chains of HLA-DR, -DQ, -DP, -DM, and -DO as well as *TAP* and *PSMB.* Sandwiched between the class II and class I region, class III region encodes for functionally unrelated genes such as complement components, heat shock proteins, and tumor necrosis factor. The reason for their genetic link to the HLA complex is unknown, but their immunologic function seems more than coincidental. The class I region is most telomeric and includes HLA-A, -B and -Cw loci, the nonclassic HLA-E, -F, and -G loci and several pseudogenes.

General terminology separates HLA genes into classic and nonclassic. Classic HLA genes have been well characterized and are clearly associated with presentation of antigen to immune cells. They are further subdivided into class I (HLA-A, -B, -C) and class II (HLA-DR, -DQ, and -DP). In general, HLA class I and II genes have very similar structure and function.[5,6] They contain six to eight exons coding for functionally distinct domains (Figure 145–2). The first exon encodes a leader sequence; the following exons (exons 2–4) are highly polymorphic and encode extracellular domains responsible for peptide binding and T-cell antigen receptor (TCR) engagement. Because they are exposed on the cell surface, these domains are also responsible for alloreactivity. The last exons encode a conserved transmembrane and small intracellular domains whose function is unclear.

Only the heavy chain of HLA class I is encoded in the MHC region. Genes encoding HLA-A, -B, and -C contain three exons coding for α_1, α_2, and α_3 extracytoplasmic domains, one transmembrane, and three cytoplasmic domains (Figure 145–3). The associated class I light chain, β_2-microglobulin, is encoded on chromosome 15.[7] By contrast, the HLA class II molecule is composed of a heterodimer of an α and a β chain encoded in the MHC region. Although the genetics are different, the protein product is structurally similar to HLA class I, with two helices resulting in the antigen presenting part of the molecule (Figure 145–4).

All DR molecules use DRA for α chains but can use alleles coded by DRB1, DRB3, DRB4, or DRB5 for β chains. DP, DQ, DM, and DO molecules are the product of *DPA1* and *DPB1, DQA1* and *DQB1, DMA* and *DMB,* and *DOA* and *DOB* genes, respectively.

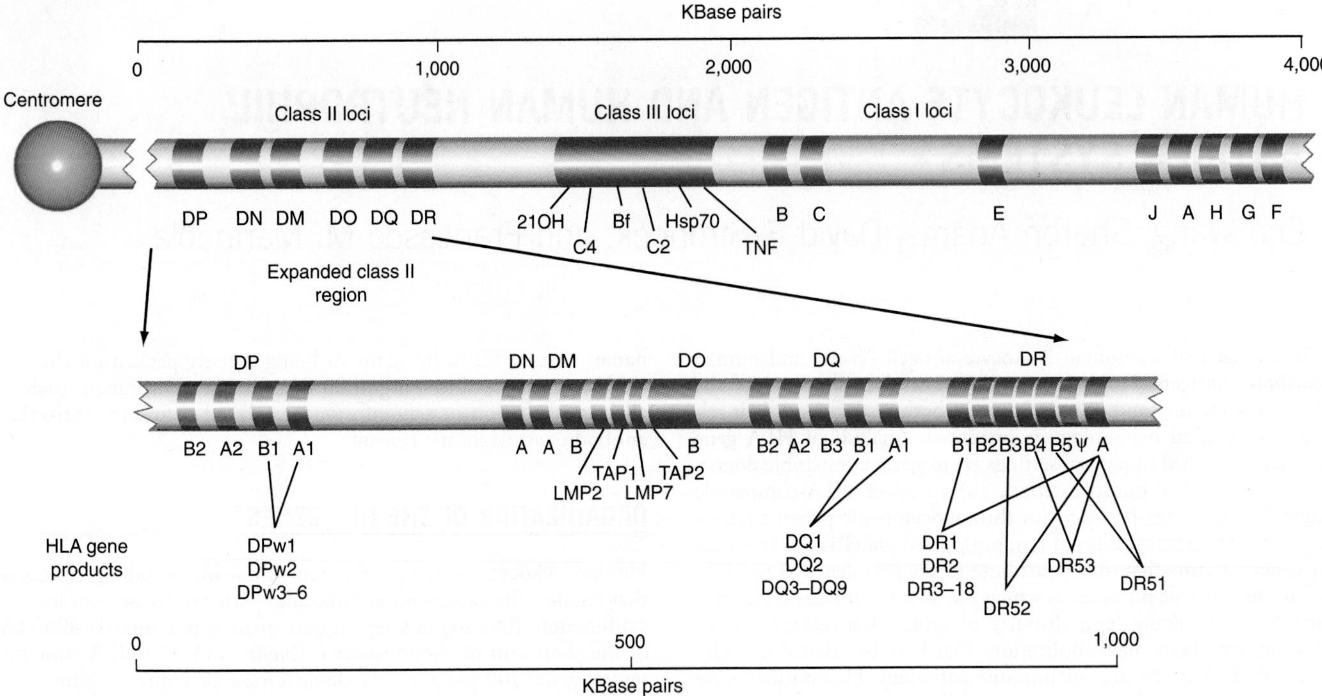

Figure 145–1 Physical map of the HLA genetic complex, illustrating the clusters of genes according to the class of encoded gene products. The symbol ψ represents four DRB pseudogenes, designated 7, 8, and 9. Other pseudogenes are shown in gray. HLA, human leukocyte antigen.

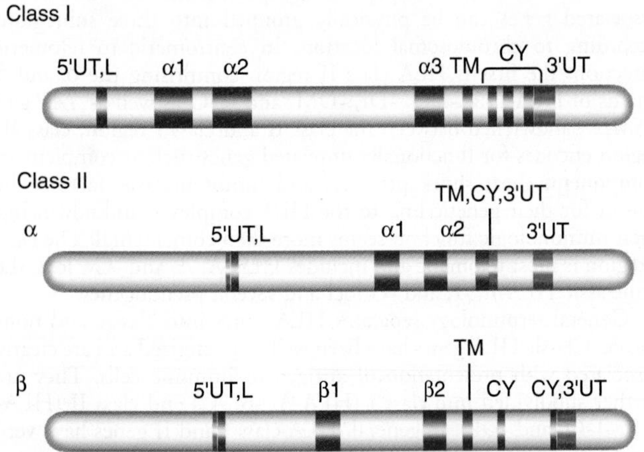

Figure 145–2 Organization of class I and II MHC genes. 5′ UT and 3′ UT, untranslated regions in the 5′ and 3′ ends of the gene; α, β, exons encoding extracellular domains; CY, exon encoding cytoplasmic tail; L, leader sequence; TM, transmembrane exon. (From Germain RN, Malissen B: Analysis of the expression and function of class-II major histocompatibility complex-encoded molecules by DNA-mediated gene transfer. Annu Rev Immunol 4:281, 1986.)

Human leukocyte antigen DRB1 locus is expressed in all HLA haplotypes (the set of HLA alleles derived from the same parental chromosome and therefore genetically linked). However, only one other HLA DR locus is present in each individual chromosome. Thus, each haplotype can have either DRB5 (DR1 haplotype); DRB3, -B4, or -B5 loci (DR2 haplotype); DRB4 locus (DR4 and DR7 haplotype); or none (DR8 and DR10 haplotype).[3]

INHERITANCE AND LINKAGE DISEQUILIBRIUM

Because of their proximity within a short chromosomal distance, HLA genes are inherited en bloc from each parent unless a recombi-

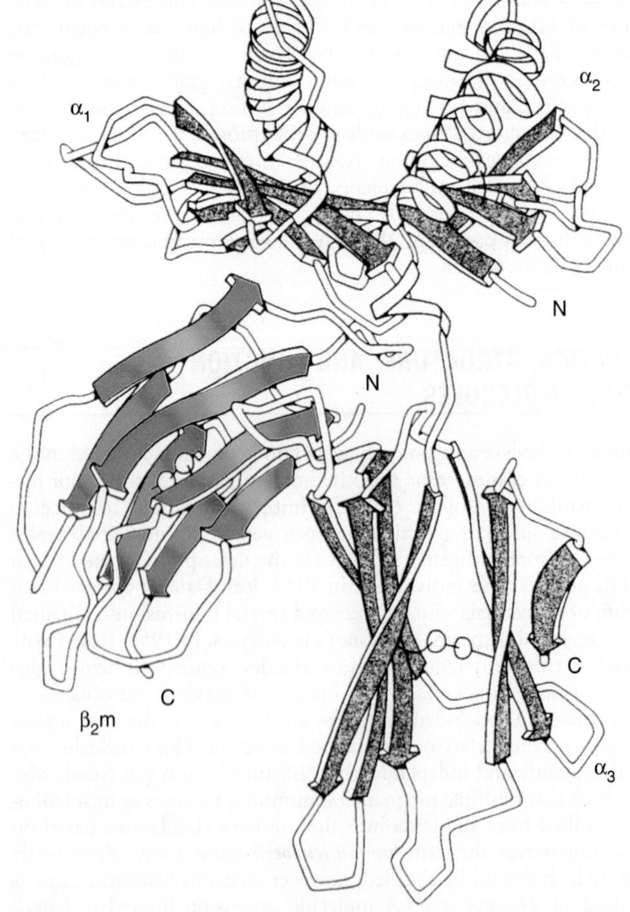

Figure 145–3 Three-dimensional configuration of HLA-A2, modeled from x-ray crystallographic studies. HLA, human leukocyte antigen. (From Bjorkman PJ, Saper MA, Samraoui B, et al: Structure of the human class I histocompatibility antigen, HLA-A2. Nature 329:506, 1987.)

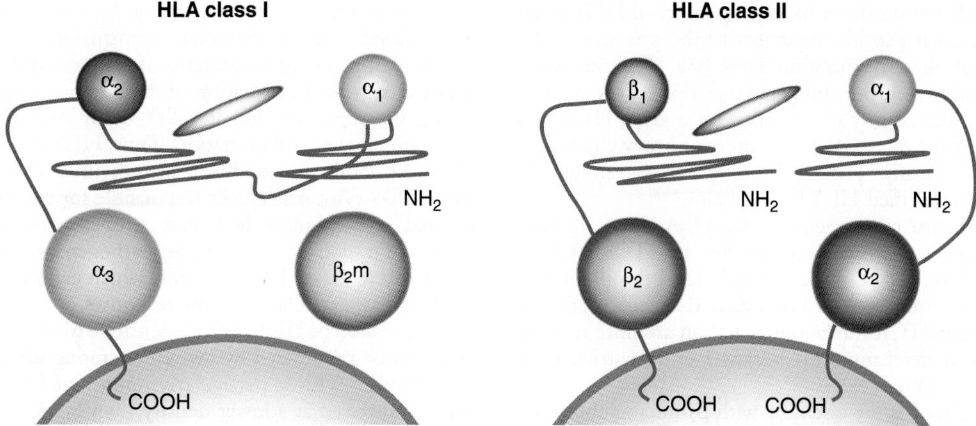

Figure 145–4 Schematic diagram of HLA class I and class II molecules pointing to their structural similarity. In both HLA classes, two immunoglobulin-type domains reside close to the cell membrane (α_3 and β_2 m for class I and α_2 and β_2 for class II). The other two domains project toward the extracellular milieu with α-helices (α_1 and α_2 for class I and α_1 and β_1 for class II) and a platform of parallel β-sheets that form a peptide binding groove. HLA, human leukocyte antigen.

nant event occurs. Thus, each HLA haplotype behaves as a unit and is transmitted through generations according to mendelian principles. Because there are four possible genotypes (two from each parent), the probability of genotypic identity between two siblings is 25%. Most HLA phenotypically identical siblings are also HLA genotypically identical, because the genetic pool of derivation is restricted to the parents. In 2% of cases, recombinant HLA haplotypes (a set of genes derived partially from two chromosomes through recombination) deviate from this rule.

The occurrence of HLA haplotypes within a population with a frequency higher than expected from the prevalence of individual alleles is called *linkage disequilibrium.* In large populations gene frequencies achieve equilibrium within a few generations unless selective pressure influences individuals' survival and mating capacity (Hardy-Weinberg principle). In equilibrium, gene prevalence is maintained based solely on its frequency. Thus, assuming that there were 18, 36, and 8 alleles for the HLA-A, -B, and -C loci, respectively (number of alleles known when this example was described[2]), theoretically 18 × 36 × 8 = 5184 HLA class I allelic combinations or haplotypes would be possible. Adding HLA class II genes to the calculation yields an astronomical number, making unlikely the identification of two HLA-matched individuals. However, individual alleles occur with different frequency, and an allele that occurs with high frequency is predominant in a given population, such as HLA-A2 in whites and A24 or A11 in Asians.[8] Because predominant alleles come with the related haplotype, most theoretical permutations never occur, and the chances of identifying matched individuals are much higher than theoretically possible.

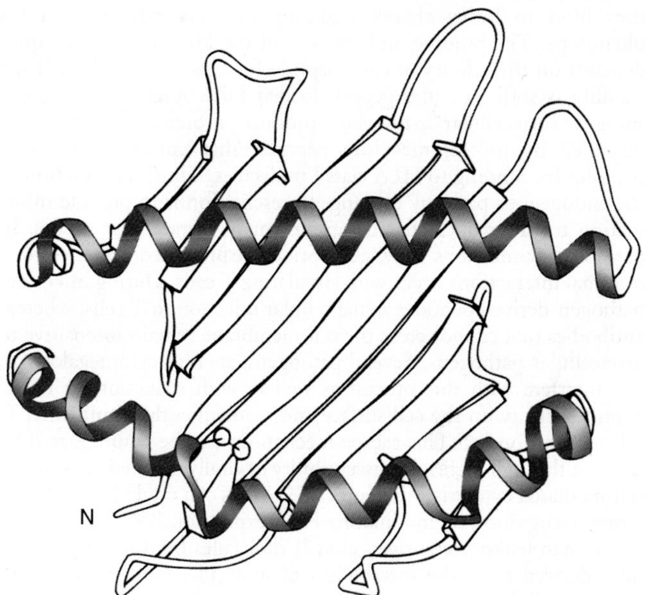

Figure 145–5 Scheme of the peptide groove of an HLA class I molecule, formed by the α_1 and α_2 domains at the side and the β-sheets at the bottom. The view is looking down on the vertically oriented molecule: the T-cell receptor point of view. HLA, human leukocyte antigen. (From Bjorkman PJ, Saper MA, Samraoui B, et al: Structure of the human class I histocompatibility antigen, HLA-A2. Nature 329:506, 1987.)

STRUCTURE OF THE HLA CLASS I AND II

The structure of HLA molecules and their relationship with their natural ligand, the TCR, has been well characterized by crystallography.[9–11] Human leukocyte antigen molecules are heterodimer glycoproteins belonging to the immunoglobulin super family with common features (see Figure 145–4). This includes two α-helical domains protruding toward the extracellular milieu. Between them lies a flat surface formed by β-sheet structures that contributes to the formation of a groove accommodating peptides generated from intracellular (HLA class I) or extracellular proteins (HLA-class II) (Figure 145–5). The helixes/peptide complex is exposed for TCR recognition. Because HLA polymorphism is clustered within the α-helixes and β-sheets domains, peptides display variable affinity for distinct HLA alleles.[12,13] It has been proposed that a given peptide can bind to closely related alleles, and HLA superfamilies with similar binding characteristics have been described.[14–16] However, peptide binding to related but distinct HLA alleles is associated with conformational dissimilarity caused by differential interaction with variant residues in the binding groove.[17] The TCR interaction with HLA required for productive engagement spans a surface including the peptide and portions of the α and β helix.[11,18–20] This double requirement of interaction between TCR and HLA/peptide complex represents the structural basis for HLA restriction. Degenerate and promiscuous TCR recognition of peptides presented by distinct HLA alleles within the same superfamily has also been described.[21] Although this concept holds in general, several exceptions can be expected because single amino acid variants in the HLA molecule may disallow binding of a peptide[22] or may not be permissive to TCR engagement.[23,24]

The binding affinity of a given peptide for a HLA allele can be predicted through algorithms that compile available information to identify amino acid residues that fit distinct pockets of the HLA groove.[12,25] Several algorithms implement this information with experimental testing based on the refolding capability of HLA heavy chains exposed to known peptide sequences in the presence of β_2-microglobulin and/or their dissociation rates (see Web site www.bimas.dcrt.nih.gov or www.uni-tuebingen.de/uni/kxi). This is based on the principle that the affinity of a peptide for a given HLA promotes that stability of the noncovalent assembly of heavy chain with β_2-microglobulin.[12,26] Finally, peptide binding can be shown by direct elutriation from purified HLA heavy chains.[13,27]

Beyond the *interactive* component of the HLA molecule with TCR, other domains act as coreceptors for the TCR. CD8+ cytotoxic T cells bind to the α_3 domain of HLA class I through CD8, whereas CD4+ T cells interact with HLA class II-specific domains. Although the coreceptor/TCR interaction is not an absolute requirement in most cases, it determines HLA class I or II restriction of individual T cells.[28]

Specific to HLA class I is the assembly with β_2-microglobulin on stabilization in the presence of high-affinity peptides derived from the cleavage of intracellular proteins (endogenous pathway of antigen presentation).[29] Most peptides derive from degradation of self-protein in the cytosol by proteasomes (PSMB) and other proteases.[30] Soluble peptides (9–10 amino acids long) are then chaperoned into the endosomal compartment by transporter molecules associated with antigen processing (TAP1 and TAP2). Within this compartment, they bind to heavy chains according to each individual's HLA phenotype. The binding and stability of the HLA/peptide complex depends on the affinity of each peptide for a particular allele. If the stability is sufficient, the peptide-loaded HLA migrates to the cell surface. Intracellular pathogens produce proteins that are also degraded by proteasomes into peptides that compete with self-peptides for binding to HLA class I molecules. Thus, the function of the endogenous pathway of antigen presentation is to provide information to the extracellular compartment of intracellular events. In physiologic conditions, only self-peptides are presented, and therefore, minimal interactions occur with circulating T cells. During infection, pathogen-derived peptides signal cellular infection to T cells, whereas antibodies that cannot cross the cell membrane remain insensitive to intracellular pathogens. Several pathogens, such as cytomegalovirus, can interfere with this process as well as with reduction of HLA/peptide density on the cell surface and, consequently, diminished T-cell recognition.[31,32] This escape mechanism can be counteracted by the host through increased susceptibility of virally infected cells to NK cell-mediated cytolysis.[33] Reciprocally, viruses can evade NK cells and escape recognition by modulating HLA expression.[34–36]

Human leukocyte antigen class II molecules bind to longer peptides derived from the metabolism of molecules endocytosed from the extracellular compartment (exogenous pathway of antigen presentation).[29] This is a specialized process used by *professional* antigen-presenting cells such as macrophages and dendritic cells. Human leukocyte antigen class II molecules are assembled within the endosomal compartment where they are composed of a heterotrimer. This includes the α and β chains plus a short invariant chain that stabilizes the molecule by occupying its groove while chaperoning its migration to the endosomal compartment where exogenous antigen is processed. Upon uptake, the exogenous antigen undergoes limited proteolysis in the membrane-bound acidic endosomal compartment (MHC class II peptide-loading compartment, MIIC). Upon entering the MIIC, the pre-HLA class II complex is degraded and antigenic peptides are loaded with the help of the nonclassic HLA-DM molecule.[37]

EXPRESSION OF HLA MOLECULES

There are genetic and structural differences between the two classes of HLA alleles. The most striking difference is functional, because HLA class I molecules are expressed by most nucleated cells with the exception of germinal cells, whereas HLA class II molecules are expressed mainly by specialized antigen presenting cells.[38,39] Human leukocyte antigen class I molecules are also expressed by platelets.[40] They are responsible for refractoriness after multiple transfusions[41–44] and sufficiently, though minimally, by reticulocytes to be targets of alloantibodies during hemolytic transfusion reactions.[45] Human leukocyte antigen class II proteins are expressed constitutively by cells associated with the initiation of the immune response such as monocytes, macrophages, and B cells[46] or by immune cells activated by cytokines during inflammation. Thus, HLA class I molecules instruct the host about the condition of individual cells as potential targets for CD8+ cytotoxic T cells responsible for clearing the organisms of altered cells. Human leukocyte antigen class II molecules initiate immune responses by taking up pathogen components and presenting them to CD4+ helper T cells, which can in turn initiate humoral and facilitate cellular immune responses.

Expression of HLA alleles is sensitive to environmental conditions and can be modulated by cytokines among which interferons play a major role.[47] This is particularly important for HLA-B and -C normally expressed at a lower density than HLA-A but which are more sensitive to cytokine induction.[48,49] In addition, HLA class II molecules can be expressed by most cells following cytokine stimulation.[50,51] Thus, the ability of cells to present antigen in association with HLA is strongly influenced by the surrounding environment. This might explain why chronic inflammation induced by alloreactions during graft-versus-host disease (GVHD) may facilitate the presentation of tumor-specific antigens by tumor cells with consequent development of GVN effect. In addition, it might explain how systemic administration of proinflammatory cytokines such as intereleukin-2 may stimulate immune responses by increasing the antigen-presenting ability of cells within the tumor microenvironment.[52]

HLA POLYMORPHISM AND ITS CLINICAL SIGNIFICANCE

A striking characteristic of the HLA system is its extreme polymorphism.[53] By chance, most individuals are heterozygote and, therefore, carry two different alleles for each HLA gene that, being codominant, are equally expressed on the cell surface. Because everybody carries three HLA class I (-A, -B, and -C) and three HLA class II (-DR, -DQ, and -DP) genes, most individuals (with the exception of homozygotes) express six different HLA class I and six different HLA class II molecules on the surface of their cells. This has important functional implications, because HLA polymorphism is clustered in domains of the HLA molecule associated the peptide-binding and interaction with the TCR. Thus, most individuals have a broad repertoire of molecules capable of presenting different pathogen components to immune cells. Therefore, it is believed that HLA polymorphism improves the chances of a given species of surviving infection.[54] This paradigm is difficult to demonstrate in human pathologic conditions in which the natural history of infectious diseases rarely correlates with HLA phenotype. An exception is the strong association between HLA-B*5701 and lack of progression to acquired immunodeficiency syndrome of individuals infected with HIV.[55] Associations have been observed between HLA phenotype and predisposition for nasopharyngeal carcinoma.[56,57] This is of particular interest because nasopharyngeal carcinoma is a virally induced cancer against which T cells can mediate immune surveillance. Human leukocyte antigen associations have also been described with less consistency for other virally driven tumors, such as cervical carcinoma,[58] or immunogenic tumors, such as melanoma.[59,60]

The difficulty in demonstrating conclusive associations between infectious disease and HLA in humans could be caused by the successful implementation of antigen presentation through a broad repertoire of HLA genes, which could compensate for each other in limitations in antigen presentation. Chickens carry a single MHC locus and their susceptibility to infection appears to be clearly related to MHC. For instance, Kaufman has shown that chickens carrying a particular Bf (the only MHC class I gene in chickens) allele are fully protected from Rouse virus–induced sarcomas, because this allele (B-f12) can bind several antigenic peptides from its proteins. On the contrary chickens homozygous for B-f4 are killed by the same infection, since this allele cannot bind peptides from sarcoma virus proteins.[54]

HLA polymorphism is the basis of alloimmunization, because most individuals are likely to have different HLA molecules on the surface of their cells. Hundreds of HLA alleles have been identified through high-resolution typing, making the chances of two individuals having identical HLA phenotypes extremely low. Thus, partial mismatches are commonly accepted in transplantation cases, which are at the root of hyperacute, acute, and chronic rejections. Hyperacute rejection is caused by preformed antibodies against donor HLA alleles in patients presensitized by multiple transfusions.[61] Acute and chronic rejection result from a combination of humoral and cellular immune reactivity toward HLA alleles of the donor.[62,63] In addition to allosensitization, HLA alleles can mediate GVHD, whereby hematopoietic cells derived from the grafted tissue recognize and reject the host tissues. They do this by identifying polymorphisms of intracellular proteins of the host (minor histocompatibility antigens) presented in association with donor/recipient matched HLA alleles.

NONCLASSIC MHC AND MHC CLASS I CHAIN-RELATED MOLECULES

Besides the three ubiquitously expressed highly polymorphic *classic* HLA class I molecules, humans encode three relatively conserved *nonclassic,* selectively expressed (HLA-E, -F, and -G) MHC class I genes (also known as MHC-Ib). These evolved at different rates in primates reflecting differential involvement in the modulation of immune responses.[4,64,65] In addition, these molecules are characterized by unique patterns of transcription, protein structure, and immunologic function.[66]

The MHC class I–related chain genes (*MICA* and *MICB*) are located within the MHC region and are characterized by high polymorphism (more than 50 alleles so far identified).[67] The molecules encoded by these genes do not appear to bind peptides or associate with β_2 microglobulin. Their polymorphic variants are not concentrated around the peptide binding groove, yet they seem to have functional significance, because most mutations are nonsynonymous, suggesting selective pressure as a driving force. Their tissue distribution is restricted to epithelial and endothelial cells and fibroblasts. It appears that *MIC* genes modulate the function of NK and CD8+ T cells by binding the NKG2D stimulating receptor.[68] Also, *MIC* has been implicated in transplant rejection because alloantibodies against them are often found in transplant recipients that may exert complement mediated cytotoxicity against endothelial cells from the graft.

Other *unusual* MHC-like molecules are present in the genome and have disparate functions, including presentation of lipid antigens (CD1), transport of immunoglobulins (Fc receptor), and regulation of iron metabolism (hemochromatosis gene product).[69] Contrary to classic MHC class I genes that are constitutively expressed, nonclassic MHC and *MIC* gene expression is dependent on stimulation by proinflammatory cytokines.[70] In addition, two nonclassic MHC class II proteins (HLA-DM and HLA-DO) have been described that function as mediators of peptide exchange by stabilizing empty MHC class II molecules.[37] Finally, it is possible that several nonclassic MHC molecules whose function is to present peptides to lymphocytes may be present throughout the genome. Because of their limited polymorphism, however, these genes may have evolved to serve specialized presentation functions.[71]

Characterized by low polymorphism, the regulation of HLA-G expression follows a nonclassic behavior. *Aberrant* cytokine-responsive regulatory sequences[72–74] may be responsible for its predominant expression by trophoblasts that do not express other HLA proteins.[75] It may also account for its low levels in a variety of human tissues.[76] Lack of responsiveness to common immunostimulatory pathways (NFκB, interferon-γ, or CIITA) is most pronounced in HLA-G cells and is shared by other nonclassic MHC such as HLA-E.[77] Also, HLA-G is expressed in a variety of cancers.[72] It is hard to know what the relevance of HLA-G expression is, because it can occur in various membrane-bound or soluble isoforms with distinct functional characteristics.[72] Functional isoforms that include the α-1 and α-2 domains bind and present peptides from cytoplasmic proteins.[78] Because of the minimal polymorphism, however, the repertoire of peptides presented is likely to be limited, suggesting that peptide binding is necessary to stabilize the molecule rather than being involved in antigen presentation.

Functionally, HLA-G is thought to modulate the function of NK cells through interactions with their inhibitory receptors.[79] In addition, the HLA-G leader sequence contains a peptide that can bind and stabilize the expression of HLA-E, which, in turn, inhibits NK cells.[80] Because the HLA-G-derived leader peptide has the strongest affinity for HLA-E (among all HLA class I molecules), it is likely that HLA-G is a powerful direct and indirect inhibitor of NK cells, reducing the risk of cardiac rejection[81] or inducing immune escape of cancer cells.[72] Although much has been published about the immunoregulatory role of HLA-G, its true function remains mysterious, principally because of discordant findings reported by various groups.[73] With the goal of achieving consensus, a workshop was recently organized to standardize methods of analysis of HLA-G.[66]

HLA-E is minimally polymorphic,[4] binds hydrophobic peptides from other HLA class I leader sequences, and interacts with CD94/NKG2 lectin-like receptors present predominately on NK and partially on CD8+ T cells.[82–85] The peptide binding is highly specific and stabilizes the HLA-E protein, allowing its migration to the cell surface. Thus, surface density of HLA-E is an indirect reflection of the number of HLA class I alleles expressed by a cell.[86] The interaction of HLA-E with CD94/NKG2 protects HLA-E expressing cells from killing. Cells damaged by viral infection or neoplastic degeneration may lose HLA class I expression. As a backup mechanism of protection, reduced HLA class I expression results in decreased expression of HLA-E, leading to vulnerability to NK cells.[87] Some viruses express mimic peptides that bind and stabilize HLA-E so that, although classic MHC molecules are downregulated, HLA-E expression is maintained, allowing the pathogen to simultaneously escape CD8+ T and NK cell killing.[88]

The function of HLA-F remains enigmatic. Its transcriptional regulation is closest to classic HLA molecules in that it can be induced by NFκB, interferon regulatory factor-1, and class II trans-activator.[89] However, contrary to classic HLA molecules, HLA-F is predominantly empty, mostly intracellular, with a restricted pattern of expression.[90] Its tissue distribution appears to be limited to B cells, and therefore it is mostly found in lymphatic organs.[90] Structural studies suggest that HLA-F is a peptide-binding molecule and may reach the cell surface under favorable conditions when a suitable peptide is present.[91] Once on the cell surface, HLA-F may interact with the effector cell receptors IL-T2 and IL-T4, as suggested by HLA-F tetrameric complexes binding studies.[91] Thus, it is possible that in specific yet unknown conditions, HLA-F may modulate the function of immune effector cells similarly to HLA-E and HLA-G.

NON-HLA POLYMORPHISM AND ITS CLINICAL SIGNIFICANCE

Although this chapter is dedicated to HLA, it would be incomplete without mentioning the increasingly recognized polymorphisms of other immune modulators. The significance of non-HLA polymorphism is evidenced by the development of GVHD in the presence of HLA identical matching among relatives. As recently summarized,[92] three general areas of polymorphism are being investigated: NK cell receptor genes, minor histocompatibility antigens, and cytokines. Over the last decade, much progress has been made in identifying the mechanisms of action of NK cells. A major breakthrough was made in the discovery of HLA class I–specific inhibitory receptors as well as on the role that they play in the regulation of NK function with consequent effects on the eradication of hematologic malignancies, prevention of graft rejection, or induction of GVHD.[93] NK cells recognize HLA molecules via killer immunoglobulin-like inhibitory receptors (KIR). The regulation of NK cell function by KIR receptors is further discussed in Chapter 13. KIRs are glycoproteins encoded

Table 145–1 HLA Class-I Alleles Recognized by Different KIRs

KIR	HLA Class I Allele	Amino Acid Sequence Motif
P58.1 (KIR2DL1)	HLA-Cw2, Cw4, Cw5, Cw6	*Asn 77, Lys 80*
P58.2 (KIR2DL2/3)	HLA-Cw1, Cw3, Cw7, Cw8	*Ser 77, Asn 80*
P70 (KIR3DL1)	HLA-Bw4 public specificity	*Aa 77–83*
P140 (KIR3DL2)	HLA-A3, A11	
(KIR2DL4)	HLA-G	

HLA, human leukocyte antigen; KIR, killer immunoglobulin-like receptor.

by at least 17 different genes located on chromosome 19q13.4.[94] All human KIR genes derive from a gene encoding three immunoglobulin (Ig)-like domains (D0, D1, and D2) and a long cytoplasmic tail. However, the KIRs genes are diverse and may encode either two or three Ig-like domains and either a long or short cytoplasmic tail (Table 145–1). The long cytoplasmic tails contain one or two immunoreceptor tyrosine-based inhibition motifs.[95] Although KIR molecules with long cytoplasmic tails inhibit NK cytotoxicity, those with short tails do not. The names given to KIR genes are based on the molecule that they encode. The first digit corresponds to the number of Ig-like domains in the molecule and a *D* denotes *domain.* The D is followed by either an *L* for *long* cytoplasmic tail or *S* for *short* cytoplasmic tail or *p* for a *pseudogene.* The last digit indicates the number of the KIR gene.[96]

Expression of KIR in individual NK cells is complex because NK cells may express several members of the KIR family. The number of KIR genes in each haplotype varies among individuals. The most common haplotype is known as group A, which is made up of 6 genes (2DL1, 2DL2 or 2DL3, 3DL1, 3DL2, 2DS4, and 2DL4). Various KIR genes can recognize different HLA-A, -B and -C molecules. Human leukocyte antigen-C antigens can be divided into two groups based on polymorphisms at amino acid positions 77 and 80 of their class I heavy chains. One group has asparagine (asn) at position 77 and lysine (lys) at 80 and the other has serine (ser) at 77 and asn at 80. Some KIRs recognize HLA-C antigens with asn 77 and lys 80, whereas other KIRs recognize HLA-C antigens with ser 77 and lys 80. The polymorphism at position 80 is most important. Another group of KIR reacts with HLA-B antigens that carry specific combinations of amino acids at positions 77 and 83 of the heavy chain that form HLA-Bw4. Because a single KIR can interact with multiple HLA class I alleles, KIR recognition of HLA class I molecules is degenerate. Another NK inhibitory receptor (CD94-NKG2A) recognizes the nonclassical HLA-E molecule. In addition, each of the KIR genes are extensively polymorphic.

Because the genes for KIR, HLA, and CD94-NKG2A are located in separate chromosomes, they segregate independently and, consequently, individuals can carry genes for KIR for which there is no correspondent HLA ligand.[97] Because HLA-E is expressed in all individuals, NK cells that bear the CD94-NKG2A receptor are not alloreactive. Because the specificity of KIR for their ligands is broad and each individual carries several KIRs, it is likely that in most cases all NK cells of a given person express at least one KIR that is specific for a self-HLA class I allele. Thus, in autologous settings, NK cells kill only aberrant cells that have lost HLA class I expression. By contrast, NK cells can kill allogeneic cells that do not express HLA class I alleles recognized by their KIR. Thus, by knowing the KIR repertoire of a given transplant recipient and the HLA type of the donor, it would theoretically be possible to predict the likelihood of an NK-mediated alloreaction. Importantly, it appears that *alloreactive* NK cells undergo proliferation on exposure to the stimulatory cells and, therefore, can preferentially expand in the presence of allogeneic tissue. NK cells also express activating receptors that are responsible for their lytic activity. Although the identity of the ligands for these receptors has not been identified, it is possible that they are expressed primarily by activated or proliferating cells. It is therefore possible that during the inflammatory process induced in allogeneic conditions, normal cells can become activated by cytokines and express ligands, which are responsible for NK activation in the absence of HLA class I molecules reactive with the inhibitory receptors.[93] The relevance of KIR in transplantation has been well studied in the context of haploidentical hematopoietic transplantation. In this case, several combinations are possible: NK cells from the graft express KIRs that do not interact with the donor's HLA (graft-versus-host alloreactivity). It seems that the presence of graft-versus-host reactive NK cells associated with incompatibilities between donor and recipient (especially HLA-Cw families) has favorable effects in the outcome of acute myeloid leukemia.[98] Alternatively, a good match may be present between graft NK and host HLA as well as between host NK and graft HLA. In such a case, no alloreactivity occurs. Finally, the graft's HLA type may be unsuitable for the host's NK repertoire and the host's reactivity may lead to graft rejection. Alloreactive grafted NK cells seem to prevent GVHD while inducing GVN.[93]

Like HLA, KIR genes are polymorphic, and their variability is clustered in positions likely to affect the overall structure of the molecule. The relevance of KIR gene polymorphism in the outcome of bone marrow transplantation (BMT) is unclear. It appears that the risk of GVHD is highest in the context of unrelated BMT when the recipient KIR genotype is *included* in the donor KIR genotype.[99] These results show that compatibility between KIR genotypes themselves may influence the outcome of BMT.

The minor histocompatibility antigens (mHags) are represented by polymorphic molecules whose peptides containing variant sequences are presented by HLA alleles. They have been shown to be targets of cytotoxic T cells, which can lyse leukemia cells.[100,98] In addition, some mHags are selectively expressed by neoplastic cells.[101] At present, little is known about the identity of mHag epitopes in the context of various HLA types and their significance in the development of GVHD and GVN.

Cytokines are another large family of molecules associated with antigen recognition, graft rejection, and GVHD. Their polymorphism is becoming an important area of investigation in the context of transplantation, autoimmunity, and cancer.[102] Polymorphic sites reside in regulatory regions so that genetic variants are associated with high or low production of a given cytokine rather than differences in its function. A Web site compiles information about cytokine polymorphism (www.bris.ac.uk/Depts/PathAndMicro/services/GAI/cytokine4.htm). Although no consensus has been achieved yet, several studies have shown associations between various cytokine genotypes and propensity toward disease and transplant outcome. These studies have been summarized elsewhere.[92,103] A strong association was recently noted between a low interleukin-10 producer genotype and a tendency to develop melanoma and prostate cancer.[104,105]

HLA NOMENCLATURE

The history of the HLA system nomenclature was summarized by Sir Walter Bodmer who, together with Ruggiero Ceppellini, was primarily involved in its development.[106] It began as HL-A, for *human leukocyte locus A.* With the recognition that HLA molecules are encoded by more than one locus, the A came to stand for *antigen* and a locus designation was added after HLA (ie, HLA-A, -B, -C, -D, etc.).[2] From then on, the World Health Organization has updated the nomenclature regularly, the last being in December 2004 after the 14th International Histocompatibility Workshop (Table 145–2).[4] At present two systems are used. An immunologically defined nomenclature is based on the identification of HLA antigens on the surface of leukocytes. Therefore, HLA phenotypes described by immunologic methods are conventionally called *HLA antigens.*[107] The second system is based on the molecular identification of nucleotide sequences in genomic DNA, and results are conventionally referred to as HLA-alleles. Because molecular typing has higher resolution, it has gained increasing popularity.

IMMUNOLOGICALLY DEFINED HLA NOMENCLATURE

Immunologically defined nomenclature follows this rule: HLA separated by a hyphen from a capital letter identifying the locus encoding distinct HLA class I (-A, -B, -C) or class II (-DR, -DQ, -DP) antigens. The letter is followed by a number that identifies a serologic family of alleles sharing epitopes recognized by alloantibodies or alloreactive cytotoxic T cells. With improved understanding of the molecular genetics of the HLA region, various appendages have been removed from the HLA nomenclature. For instance, the letter *w* was used to indicate a provisional assignment, and this has been discontinued, but it is occasionally added to HLA-C antigen nomenclature to distinguish it from complement genes; DP and DW also maintained this letter to reinforce the dependency of their immune identification predominantly through cellular techniques. Finally, HLA-Bw4 and -Bw6 retain the *w* to emphasize that the public epitopes are shared by several HLA-B and some HLA-antigens. More recently, a bridge between immunologic and molecular nomenclature has been proposed whereby HLA antigens that encompass a single gene product can be assigned a two-digit numeric extension corresponding to the molecular nomenclature for that allele.[108]

SEQUENCE-DEFINED ALLELIC NOMENCLATURE

The Tenth International Histocompatibility Workshop recommended in 1987 a sequence-based nomenclature[108] to describe alleles not distinguishable by immunologic methods. Since then, the number of HLA alleles has rapidly increased. A total of 422 new alleles were named since the previous report in 2003, and as of December 2004,[4] 349 designations were given to HLA-A, 627 to -B, and 182 to -Cw alleles (1180 named HLA class I alleles). Assignments for HLA class II included 394 HLA-DRB1, 61 -DQB1, and 116 -DPB1 alleles. Other designations are summarized in Table 145–2. Human leukocyte antigen designates molecules belonging to the human MHC followed by the locus (-A, -B, etc). Alleles are then identified after an asterisk (*). A four-digit number is used in which the first two digits refer to the original serologic family (eg, HLA-A2 serologically would be HLA-A*02). The last two digits designate alleles sequentially identified within that family. Often numbers are missing because an original assignment was revoked (eg, this is why there is no HLA-A*2401). When silent mutations are identified (variation in nucleotide sequence that does not translate into changes in amino acid sequence), the name of the allele remains identical, but another two digits are added to designate a variant that has no functional significance. New sequences are submitted to EMBL (www.ebi.ac.uk/Submissions/index.html), GeneBank (www.ncbi.nlm.nih.gov/Genbank/index.html), or DDBJ (http://www.ddbj.nig.ac.jp/sub-e.html).

Requirements for new allele naming were described by Marsh and associates.[4] The World Health Organization committee also made recommendations about naming alleles with aberrant expression such as HLA-G isoforms and KIR. Some alleles are identifiable at the genomic level but are not translated into protein (pseudo genes). These are indicated by the addition of an N (for null) following the numerical designation of the allele. Mutations inducing a reduction of expression are marked by *L* (*low expression*). An *S* denotes alleles expressed as soluble *secreted* molecules, such as HLA-B*4402010S characterized by an intronic variant that disallows the expression of the trans-membrane domain of the HLA molecule and is, therefore, only in soluble form. Differential splicing of HLA-G leads to production of membrane-bound and soluble forms, which are respectively denoted by a lower-case *m* or *s* before HLA. Limited cytoplasmic expression is denoted by C and aberrant expression by A. Finally, KIR polymorphism will be classified by a new system that is in preparation.[4,97,109] A nomenclature system for cytokine polymorphism has not yet been developed.[110]

HLA TYPING IN CLINICAL HEMATOLOGY AND DETERMINATION OF COMPATIBILITY HLA TYPING

Originally, HLA typing was done primarily in support of transplantation or transfusion needs with the purpose of identifying histocompatibility through the best match between donor and recipient. Allosensitization of recipients previously exposed to heterologous cell products is tested by identifying alloreactive antibodies in serum and cross-match procedures are performed to grade compatibility of candidate donor-recipient pairs. In addition, HLA testing has been applied to identify links between a given disease and the genetic make-up of its carriers.[111] Strong associations are exemplified by birdshot uveitis (a disease occurring exclusively in HLA-A29 individuals),[112] type I diabetes and other autoimmune diseases,[113–115] or long-term survival of HIV infected individuals.[55] These studies evaluated the role that genetic background may have contributed over environmental factors.[111,116] Human leukocyte antigen associations are thought to be caused by the differential ability of distinct alleles to present immunogenic epitopes[112,113] or by the close linkage to the HLA class III region where potent immunomodulators such as tumor necrosis factor α are located.[117] It has also been suggested that HLA associations may be predictors of immune responsiveness of cancer to immune therapy.[60] However, such associations have remained quite difficult to reproduce.[118] Human leukocyte antigen typing is requested for enrollment of patients into and interpretation of immunization protocols,[24] because specific HLA/epitope combinations require high-resolution typing.[22,119]

Serologic testing takes advantage of fetomaternal sensitization. In mammals, the progeny carries a full haplotype of paternal origin, and pregnant women may develop antibodies against the paternal haplotype. Maternal serum samples are collected at term and characterized by testing their ability to kill HLA-bearing repository cell lines of known phenotype in the presence of complement (complement-dependent cytotoxicity [CDC]).[120] Then CDC is used for HLA typing by exposing circulating cells expressing HLA class I (most cells) and class II (predominantly B cells) antigens from the individual (to be typed to previously characterized sera or monoclonal antibodies).[121] Conversely, already typed repository cell lines are used in CDC to identify alloantibodies in sera of sensitized individuals. The fraction of cell lines killed by the sera roughly grades the intensity of allosensitization or panel reactive antibody (PRA) reactivity. Some antibodies activate complement and kill with poor efficiency, known as the *cytotoxicity negative absorption positive (CYNAP) phenomenon.*[122] As judged by cytotoxicity testing, CYNAP may underestimate allosensitization. By modifying CDC with the addition of antihuman antibodies suitable for complement activation, CYNAP can be circumvented (augmented CDC). In this case, however, relatively innocuous antibodies can cause overestimation of clinically relevant allosensitization.[123] Other methods identify alloantibodies, including immobilization of HLA molecules on solid surface to capture soluble antibodies[124–126] and flow cytometry using a spectrum of microbeads loaded with known HLA alleles.[127,128] An interlaboratory comparison of serum screening for HLA antibody determination suggested that enzyme-linked immunosorbent assay and flow cytometry yield higher PRA activity values compared with CDC or augmented CDC.[125] However, the study suggested a lack of consistency among participant laboratories, leaving unsolved the question of which method most accurately defines clinically relevant allosensitization and a panel of various methods may be most informative.[72]

Complement-dependent cytotoxicity is declining in interest in the United States because most laboratories are switching to easier-to-handle and higher resolution molecular methods. However, immunologic methods remain valuable to characterize functional aspects of HLA because molecular methods cannot define whether an HLA allele is expressed nor, at least until recently,[129] grade allosensitization. Thus, it is likely that immunologic methods will continue to complement molecular methods in the future.[129]

The usefulness of conventional serologic typing has been limited by the availability of allele-specific sera. Most importantly, as anti-

Table 145–2 Name of Genes in the HLA Region Considered by the WHO Nomenclature Committee[4]

Name	Previous Equivalents	Molecular Characteristics	# of Alleles (July 2004)
HLA-A	–	Class I α-chain	349
HLA-B	–	Class I α-chain	627
HLA-B	–	Class I α-chain	182
HLA-E	E, '6.2'	Associated with class I 6.2-kB Hind III fragment	5
HLA-F	F, '5.4'	Associated with class I 5.4-kB Hind III fragment	2
HLA-G	G, '6.0'	Associated with class I 6.0-kB Hind III fragment	15
HLA-H	H, AR, '12.4', HLA-54	Pseudogene association with class I 5.4-kB Hind III fragment	
HLA-J	cda 12, HLA-59	Pseudogene association with class I 5.9-kB Hind III fragment	
HLA-K	HLA-70	Pseudogene association with class I 7.0-kB Hind III fragment	
HLA-L	HLA-92	Pseudogene association with class I 9.2-kB Hind III fragment	
HLA-N	HLA-30	Pseudogene association with class I 1.7-kB Hind III fragment	
HLA-S	HLA-17	Pseudogene association with class I 3.0-kB Hind III fragment	
HLA-X	–	Class I gene fragment	
HLA-Z	HLA-Z1	Class I gene fragment located in HLA class II region	
HLA-DRA	DRα	DR α chain	3
HLA-DRB1	DRβI, DR1B	DR $β_1$ determining specificity for DR1, DR2, DR3, etc.	394
HLA-DRB2	DRβII2	Pseudogene with DRβ-like sequence	1
HLA-DRB3	DRβIII, DR3B	DR β3 determining DR52, Dw24, w25, –26 specificity	41
HLA-DRB4	DRβIV, DR4B	DR β4 determining DR53 specificity	13
HLA-DRB5	DRβV, DR5B	DR β5 determining DR52, Dw24, w25, –26 specificity	18
HLA-DRB6	DRBX, DRBσ	Pseudogene found in DR1, DR2, and DR10 haplotypes	3
HLA-DRB7	DRBψ1	Pseudogene found in DR4, DR7, and DR9 haplotypes	2
HLA-DRB8	DRBψ2	Pseudogene found in DR4, DR7, and DR9 haplotypes	1
HLA-DRB9	M 4.2 β exon	Pseudogene isolated fragment	1
HLA-DQA1	DQα1, DQ1A	DQ α chain as expressed	28
HLA-DQB1	DQβ1, DQ1B	DQ β chain as expressed	61
HLA-DQA2	DXα, DQ2A	DQ α–related chain, not known to be expressed	
HLA-DQB2	DXβ, DQ2B	DQ β–related chain, not known to be expressed	
HLA-DQB3	DVβ, DQB3	DQ β–related chain, not known to be expressed	
HLA-DOA	DNA, DZα, DOα	DO α chain	8
HLA-DOB	DOβ	DO β chain	9
HLA-DMA	RING 6	DM α chain	4
HLA-DMB	RING 7	DM β chain	7
HLA-DPA1	DPα1, DP1A	DP α chain as expressed	22
HLA-DPB1	DPβ1, DP1B	DQ β chain as expressed	116
HLA-DPA2	DPα2, DP2A	DP α chain–related pseudogene	
HLA-DPA3	DPA 3	DP α chain–related pseudogene	
HLA-DPB2	DPβ2, DP2B	DP β chain–related pseudogene	
TAP1	ABCB2, RING4	ABC (ATP-binding cassette) transporter	7
TAP2	ABCB3, RING 11	ABC (ATP-binding cassette) transporter	4
PSMB9	LMP2, RING 12	Proteasome-related sequence	
PSMB8	LMP7, RING 10	Proteasome-related sequence	
MICA	PERB 11.1	Class I chain–related gene	57
MICB	PERB 11.2	Class I chain–related gene 18	
MICC	PERB 11.3	Class I chain–related gene	
MICD	PERB 11.4	Class I chain–related gene	
MICE	PERB 11.5	Class I chain–related gene	

HLA, human leukocyte antigen; WHO, World Health Organization.

bodies identify structural differences on the surface of HLA molecules, variants caused by nucleotide polymorphism in nonexposed areas such as the peptide binding groove of the HLA heavy chain are not detectable. However, these differences are of functional significance because they determine the specificity and affinity of peptide binding[130,131] and T-cell recognition of self and allogeneic target cells.[23,132] DNA-based typing directly determines the sequence,[133] and its resolution is limited only by the number of allele-specific probes used to identify an ever growing number of alleles (see Web site www.anthonynolan.com/HIG/index.htm). Various polymerase chain reaction (PCR)-based methods have been described among which sequence-specific primer[133,134] and sequence-specific oligonucleotide probe[135,136]–based methods are the most universally used. The rich nature of HLA has led to proportionally increasing complexity of the assays used to cover all possible alleles. As a consequence, accurate HLA typing for donor and recipient matching in transplantation has become increasingly complex and burdensome. In addition, because of the important role that HLA molecules play in antigen presentation and the stringency of the relationship between epitope and associated HLA allele, high-resolution typing is increasingly requested for appropriate enrollment of patients into immunization protocols aimed at the enhancement of T-cell responses.[137] Therefore, high-resolution HLA typing is increasingly in demand in clinical and experimental settings.

Although oligonucleotide-based methods could theoretically discriminate any known polymorphic site, they have two major limitations. First, they require a specific PCR reaction for each allele investigated. Because each individual has only two alleles for each locus, a disproportionately large number of PCR reactions must be performed to cover all possible polymorphisms to identify the two borne by the individual tested. Because both methods are based on specific interactions with known oligonucleotide sequences unique to a particular allele, they cannot identify unknown polymorphisms unless the variation occurs within the region spanned by one of the oligos used in the assay. Because of these limitations, interest is growing for definitive typing methods that yield conclusive information about the identity of the alleles typed. The most comprehensive method is sequence-based typing. Unfortunately, its use has been limited by cost of equipment and reagents and by the high level of expertise and time required for the interpretation of each typing. More recently, high-throughput, robotic, sequence-based typing has been developed that allows sequencing of hundreds of genomic fragments each day.[138–140] However, even sequence-based typing has some technical limitations. Some combinations of HLA class I and class II alleles result in ambiguous allele combinations that require additional testing for resolution.[141] Finally, new methods based on high-density array technology are being developed that may allow extensive typing of known and unknown polymorphisms on microchips.[142,143]

High-resolution methods yield high-resolution information of an individual's HLA type. However, the wealth of information is counterbalanced by increased difficulty in identifying suitable HLA alleles during donor-recipient pairing or accrual into immunization protocols restricted to specific HLA-epitope combinations. Thus, at present, clinicians are faced with the daunting task of applying high-resolution typing results of unclear relevance to clinical settings.[144]

TESTING FOR ALLOSENSITIZATION AND DETERMINATION OF COMPATIBLE RECIPIENT/DONOR PAIRS

Any cell containing product transfused or transplanted between different individuals should be compatible in an ideal situation. Yet, in most cases, histocompatibility is not prospectively sought. Thus, patients with multiple exposures to blood products often become reactive to various antigens, including HLA. Transplant candidates often develop prior alloreactivity following transfusion of platelet concentrates contaminated with leukocytes, even though the incidence of allosensitization is much less because of leukodepletion of blood products. Alloreactivity must be documented before transplantation, because alloreactive patients can still undergo transplantation, provided that the donor has no mismatched HLA antigens reacting with the patient's antibodies. Patients who have received repeated platelet transfusions may become allosensitized and, consequently, refractory to further transfusions unless HLA-compatible platelets are used. Obviously, the best compatibility consists of identical matching. It is often impossible to identify a perfectly matched unrelated donor, particularly in the case of rare HLA types, Thus, other strategies are adopted to identify the best possible match or *compatible mismatch.* Selection of unrelated donor-recipient pairs is carried out through typing with serologic, cellular, and molecular methods.[145] The chances of identifying compatible donors based on full or partial HLA matching have become increasingly low with the increasing resolution of the typing methods.[144] To broaden compatibility, matching criteria of donor-recipient pairs are based on shared public epitopes assigned to cross-reacting groups (CREGs)[146] or shared amino acid polymorphisms defined through sequence information (Table 145–3).[147] The preexistence of alloantibodies restricts the identification of compatible donors even further. Highly sensitized recipients with PRA activity exceeding 85% of tested specificities (generally between 30 and 60) represent a particularly challenging group.[148] An alternative approach to the exclusion of alloreactive determinants is the inclusion of *acceptable* antigen mismatches expressed in a panel of cells that give negative reactions with the recipient sera,[149] which extends the repertoire of possible donors. All these are fundamental tools for the identification of nonrelated, not fully matched donor-recipient pairs. Unfortunately, even these compromises often fail to identify a suitable match.

Duquesnoy[148] recently described a molecularly based algorithm to identify histocompatible pairs called HLAMatchmaker. This method focuses on the structural basis of HLA class I polymorphism so that compatible HLA mismatches can be identified without extensive serum screening. This algorithm is based on the principle that short amino acid sequences (triplets) characterizing polymorphic sites of the HLA molecules are critical components of allosensitizing epitopes. Such amino acids reside in the α helices and β loops of the heavy chain. Because each HLA molecule expresses a characteristic string of these determinants, it is possible to characterize each molecule according to the linear sequence of amino acid triplets present on its surface. Based on the reasonable assumption that none of the triplets present in the HLA repertoire of the recipient is self-immunogenic, it is possible through a process of *electronic recombination* to identify donors with HLA alleles different from the recipient's but containing exclusively shared triplets. These HLA alleles will be compatible, because they do not contain any epitope absent in the recipient.

In theory, a large number of triplets could occur if polymorphisms were randomly distributed. However, most HLA molecules span conserved domains and only a total of 142 different polymorphic triplets designate serologically defined HLA-A, -B, and -C antigens.[148] Triplet polymorphism can occur in 30 locations on HLA-A, 27 in HLA-B, and 19 in HLA-C chains. Because the HLAMatchmaker algorithm includes interlocus comparison, it is possible to accumulate the information into a single database. Among the 142 polymorphic triplets, 29 are polymorphic for one class I locus but monomorphic for another class I locus. Such polymorphic triplets cannot be immunogenic because they are always present on the patient's own HLA antigens, whereas the remaining 113 triplets have immunogenic potential. With this algorithm, it is possible to significantly broaden the number of *molecularly matched* HLA alleles and significantly increase the chances of identifying a compatible donor, particularly in those cases in which the recipient has a rare HLA phenotype. In addition, HLAMatchmaker considers triplets that are present in the panel cells that give negative reactions with the recipient's serum. These negative panel cells can be expected to share antigens with the patient's, but other HLA antigens may be present and contain mismatched triplets apparently not immunogenic for that patient. Such triplets are therefore acceptable and can be added to the algorithm for the identification of possible donors. Thus, HLAMatchmaker

Table 145–3 Population Frequencies of Major Cross Reactive or Determinants Present on HLA-A and -B Gene Products

Major Cross-Reactive Group	Public Epitope	Associated Private Epitopes	Approximate Epitope Frequency (%)*
1C	1p	A1, 3, 9 (23, 24), 11, 29, 30, 31, 36, 80	79
	10p	A10 (25, 26, 34, 43, 66), 11, 28 (68, 69), 32, 33, 74	
2C	28p	A2, 28 (68, 69), 9, 17	70
	9p	A2, 28 (68, 69), 9 (23, 24)	
	17p	A2, B17 (57, 58)	
5C	5p	B5 (51, 52), 18, 35, 53, 78	50
	21p	B5 (51, 52), 15 (62, 63, 75, 76, 77), 17 (57, 58), 21 (49, 50), 35, 53, 70 (71, 72), 73, 74, 78	
7C	7p	B7, 8, 41, 42, 48, 81	54
	22p	B7, 22 (54, 55, 56), 27, 42, 46	
	27p	B7, 13, 27, 40 (60, 61), 47	
8C	8p	B8, 14 (64, 65), 16 (38, 39), 18	38
12C	12p	B12 (44, 45), 13, 21 (49, 50), 40 (60, 61), 41	44
Bw4	Bw4	B13, 27, 37, 38, 47, 49, 51, 52, 53, 57, 58, 59, 63, 77, A24, 25, 32	79
Bw6	Bw6	B7, 8, 18, 35, 39, 41, 42, 45, 46, 48, 50, 54, 55, 56, 60, 61, 62, 64, 65, 67, 71, 72, 73, 75, 76, 78, 81	87

HLA, human leukocyte antigen.
*North American white populations of European origin.

assesses HLA compatibility at a molecular level by determining whether or not a triplet in a given position of a mismatched HLA antigen is also found in the same position in any of the recipient's own HLA-A, HLA-B, and HLA-C molecules. A shared triplet in the same position on a mismatched HLA antigen cannot elicit a specific antibody response in that patient. This hypothesis needs future testing, because this strategy might represent a revolutionary tool for the identification of potential donors. Preliminary verification of the algorithm in a series of high PRA renal patients suggested that this is a proper strategy at least in highly sensitized renal transplantation candidates waiting for unrelated donors.[150] HLAMatchmaker is also effective at selecting an optimal HLA-typed platelet component for alloimmunized thrombocytopenic patients.[151]

A new version of HLAMatchmaker considers so-called eplets and is based on the structural definitions of functional epitopes on well-characterized protein antigens that have been complexed with antibody.[152] Eplets represent amino acid residue configurations within a 3 to 3.5 Angstrom radius of each polymorphic residue on the HLA molecular surface. Many eplets correspond to triplets but eplets represents a more complete repertoire of structurally defined epitopes.

THE HLA MOLECULES AS ANTIGENS AND HLA ALLOIMMUNIZATION

By no means are HLA molecules antigenic in physiologic condition (with the exception of maternofetal alloimmunizaton). However, because of their high density on the surface of cells, they can become highly immunogenic in the nonphysiologic event in which cells from different individuals are exposed to another person's immune system. The mechanism or mechanisms leading to allosensitization are believed to follow two pathways. The first pathway mimics the one followed during most immune reactions in which antigen is up taken by antigen-presenting cells and presented to autologous lymphocytes (indirect pathway). In this case the donor's HLA molecules are processed into peptides through the exogenous pathway of antigen presentation and presented to autologous T cells as linear peptides.[153,154] This pathway is believed to be responsible for the development of alloantibodies as well as T-helper cell responses, but its role in the development of cytotoxic T cell responses remains unclear. Because this pathway depends on the presentation of donor HLA molecules by recipient HLA alleles, it may explain why the humoral response to HLA class I allodeterminants correlates with the HLA phenotype of the responder.[155] The indirect pathway of HLA allorecognition has been associated with allograft rejection.[156] Because the function of HLA molecules is to present antigenic determinants to T cells, it could be easily envisioned how minor changes in their structure could be misinterpreted as antigenic epitopes. Intact HLA molecules residing on the surface of donor cells are a perfect target for T-cell–mediated allorecognition (direct pathway) either through the direct cytotoxic effect of T cells against target cells or by the activation of helper T cells, through HLA class II engagement, which leads to stimulation of antibody-mediated immune responses.[157]

Humoral responses mediated most frequently by IgM are predominant in the sensitization to infrequent allogeneic exposure, because they require smaller amounts of antigenic material. T-cell responses become more manifest in the context of transplantation in which the persistence of the allogeneic stimulus allows the expansion and sustenance of alloreactive cytotoxic T cells. Antibodies and TCR have different requirements for their engagement, which means epitopes recognized by T cells and antibodies are different. Antibodies require interaction with a small structure, including a limited number of amino acids; thus, any sequence combination on the surface of an HLA allele not present in the individual exposed to the alloreaction may represent an epitope. T cells have much lower binding affinity for their ligand and require a complete interaction with the peptide as well as the α and β helices of the HLA class I heavy chain.[11] Although several B-cell epitopes recognized by antibodies can be identified in a given HLA molecule, generally the whole HLA molecule is necessary for T-cell–dependent allorecognition. Definition and topographic mapping of epitopes defined by serologic or cellular methods has revealed distinct regions of hypervariability in the α-1 and α-2 domains of the class I heavy chains and in the α-1 and β-1 domains of class II molecules.[158] Two types of antibody-defined epitopes can be identified according to their frequency among HLA alleles. Private epitopes are almost but not totally unique for a single serologically defined HLA antigen and are used for typing. These epitopes are generally shared by all molecular alleles present in that given family, and fine differences among alleles within a general family cannot be distinguished by antibodies. Public epitopes are more widely distributed and cluster distinct serologic families into groups. These epitopes bear an immunodominant character. Immune sera that identify public epitopes have been considered predictive of major CREGs with the idea that alloreactivity among patients belonging to the same CREG may be less likely (Table 145–3). The predictive value of CREGs in transplant outcome or platelet transfusion results, however, remains to be demonstrated.

Not all subjects who have been exposed to alloantigens develop alloantibodies, and in fact exposure to low doses of donor-specific HLA antigens through donor transfusion may have a beneficial effect on graft survival.[159] Obviously, the degree of compatibility in the context of allosensitization may vary according to the degree of mismatch between donor and recipient. In addition, alloantibodies are one aspect of alloreaction that does not take into account cellular responses. These have been more difficult to document, although they are likely to play an important role in the context of acute transplant rejection. Several hypotheses have been discussed about the reason or reasons for the capriciousness of allosensitization, including the presence of regulatory immune responses or cytokine-mediated immunosuppression. Currently, the mechanism modulating the quality and quantity of alloimmunity remains elusive; and different aspects of this algorithm are discussed ad hoc in this chapter, with particular attention to molecularly defined algorithms for the prediction of histocompatibility.[129,148,160,161]

Clearly, HLA matching is beneficial in patients undergoing renal transplantation. An analysis of more than 150,000 recipients receiving transplants in different centers participating in the Collaborative Transplant Study showed that a complete mismatch (6 HLA-A+B+DR) had a 17% lower survival expectation than no mismatch ($P < 0.0001$).[162] Matching was particularly beneficial in patients with highly reactive preformed alloantibodies. The same study suggested that high-resolution matching based on molecular typing improved graft survival. Similar results were observed in cases of cardiac transplantation in which HLA matching yielded significantly better results ($P < 0.0001$). This is particularly important because donor hearts are currently not allocated according to HLA match in most centers. In cases of liver transplantation, HLA matching was not beneficial.[163]

Donor-specific hyporesponsiveness has been particularly well documented in the context of renal allotransplantation and may limit the need for immunosuppression. A recent randomized study suggested that pretransplant donor transfusions improved the survival of cadaver kidney grafts in patients receiving modern immunosuppressive regimens, but the mechanism remains unclear.[164,165] Although most centers currently do not implement deliberate blood transfusions, the usefulness of this approach needs to be investigated further.

Approximately 5% to 10% of platelet transfusions are given to patients who have been previously exposed to HLA class I expressing heterologous cells and are reactive to HLA antigens. Such patients are refractory to random-donor platelets and must be given HLA-matched or *semi-matched* plateletpheresis components.[41–44] However, a provision of HLA-matched platelets does not always improve platelet recovery and survival. Possibly, the ineffective platelet transfusion is in part caused by unrecognized HLA mismatches between the donor and recipient resulting from the low-resolution methods used for typing, and higher resolution methods have been advocated. It is currently controversial whether or not molecularly based HLA typing confers an advantage over serologic typing, and this principle was recently questioned in the context of hematopoietic cell transplantation.[166,167]

HLA AS A FUNCTIONAL MEDIATOR OF GRAFT-VERSUS-HOST DISEASE AND/OR GRAFT-VERSUS-NEOPLASIA EFFECT

Allogeneic or syngeneic bone marrow transplantation is used predominately for the treatment of hematologic malignancies[168–170] and other hematologic disorders such as aplastic anemia,[171] thalassemia,[172] or myelodysplastic syndrome.[173] This strategy can induce long-term disease-free survival in chronic myelogenous leukemia patients.[168,169] The objective of bone marrow transplantation in cases of malignancy is to cure the patient by eradication of the neoplastic cells with myeloablative chemotherapy followed by restoration of hematopoiesis through the transplantation of normal hematopoietic stem cells derived from HLA-compatible normal donors. This strategy is characterized by the insurgence of an immune reaction toward the host's normal cells (GVHD),[174–176] which is often associated and preferentially targets neoplastic cells (GVN effect).[177–184] Both the GVHD and the GVN effect occur in the presence of a full HLA match; thus, the HLA molecules are not targets of allosensitization themselves but present polymorphic molecules expressed by the recipient's cells recognized by the grafted immune cells.

GRAFT-VERSUS-HOST DISEASE

Graft-versus-host disease represents the alloimmune reaction of donor lymphocytes against normal cells of the recipient. Graft-versus-host disease occurs predominantly in association with hematopoietic progenitor cell transplantation (HPCT) compared to other types of transplants because the hematopoietic transplant is enriched of immune cells. Myeloablative therapy is generally administered before transplantation and, as a consequence, in most cases prevents graft rejection. Graft-versus-host disease is a major complication of HPCT, and a fine balance between GVHD and graft rejection is maintained by modulating the level of posttransplantation immunosuppression.[184] In addition, other major disturbances associated with HPCT such as overwhelming infection, leukemia or tumor relapse, and other regimen-related morbidities are strongly influenced by the treatment of GVHD. With the advent of nonmyeloablative HPCT for the treatment of nonhematologic diseases such as solid tumors, GVHD has reached a predominant role because of its close association with GVN effect.

T-cell depletion has been advocated for the prevention of GVHD by decreasing the probability of cellular and humoral alloresponses.[185,186] This strategy decreases the occurrence of GVHD but is associated with an increased risk of graft rejection and tumor or leukemia relapse.[184] In fact, Weiden and colleagues[187] observed that survivors of severe acute GVHD had a significantly lower incidence of tumor relapse compared with patients who did not experience GVHD. This association appeared mandatory and it was believed that the beneficial GVN reaction was inseparable from GVHD.

The risk of GVHD increases with genetic distancing between donor and recipient. Thus, recipients of transplants from HLA-identical twins have a lesser chance of developing GVHD than recipients of transplants from HLA-unrelated donors and from donors with only a partial HLA match.[188,189] Interestingly, however, although the genetic closeness between donor and recipient appears to decrease the risk of GVHD, it also decreases the therapeutic benefit, with increased chances of tumor relapse.

GRAFT-VERSUS-NEOPLASIA EFFECT

It was originally observed that a beneficial collateral effect of GVHD was the rejection of neoplastic cells by the donor immune system in the context of hematologic malignancies (graft-versus-leukemia effect).[177] It was rapidly recognized that the graft-versus-leukemia effect could play a powerful therapeutic role in the treatment of refractory malignant disorders, including some solid tumors (graft-versus-tumor effect).[181] Because the biology and clinical principles underlining the two effects are likely similar, for simplicity, in this chapter we coin a unifying term: *graft-versus-neoplasia effect.* Indeed, there is a perception that the GVN reaction is the most potent form of tumor immunotherapy currently in clinical use. Its mechanism of action is still poorly understood. T cells definitely play a fundamental role in the initiation and maintenance of the alloreaction toward neoplastic cells.[190] A sevenfold increase in the chance of relapse was noted in patients with chronic myelogenous leukemia who received a T-cell–depleted BMT as compared with a subset of patients who had received a T-cell–repleted BMT but did not develop GVHD.[185,186] This result suggested that GVHD is a biologic entity different from GVN effect. In addition, on leukemia relapse, administration of donor lymphocyte infusion could re-induce clinical remission.[191] Finally, leukemia-specific CD8+ T cells have been identified in circulating lymphocytes at the time of leukemia regression.[192] NK cells play an additional role in mediating this phenomenon, and clinical data suggest that mismatch of NK receptor and ligands during allogeneic BMT can be used to enhance the GVN effect.[93,193] Appreciation of the GVN effect has led to the development of nonmyeloablative stem cell transplants designed to immunosuppress the host to a level sufficient to permit engraftment of the donor immune cells to generate GVN without inducing the serious complications associated with myeloablation.[184] The GVN effect has gained popularity in the last decade to the point that allogeneic-based immunotherapeutic approaches have been advocated for several nonhematologic malignancies.[184] The rationale is largely based on the assumption that the immune cell repertoire capable of recognizing cancer cells in the allogeneic context is broader than in the autologous system. Donor T cells can target not only tumor-specific antigens but also allelic variants of these antigens; mHag; and, in the case of HLA-mismatched transplants, HLA antigens disparate from the donor expressed by the tumor cells.[194–196] Although there are several theories about how GVN effect occurs, it remains unclear why allo-T cells have a better chance of targeting tumor cells in an allogeneic context as compared with the natural insurgence of antitumor immunity described for several solid tumors.

HLA AND T-CELL–DIRECTED IMMUNIZATION

The last decade has witnessed remarkable progress in the identification and mapping of T-cell epitopes for various infectious diseases and cancer. In particular, progress was made in mapping HLA associated epitopes for HIV, cytomegalovirus, and Epstein-Barr virus.[197–200] In addition, the molecular identification of tumor-associated antigens has yielded a large number of epitopes that could be used to immunize against neoplasia.[201] A comprehensive discussion of these topics is beyond the scope of this chapter, but we address a few points framing the relevance of HLA in the context of T-cell–directed immunization.

The identification of T-cell epitopes led to two major areas of clinical investigation. The first is active-specific immunization to prevent or treat ongoing infections or cancer. The second is the harvest and in vitro expansion of immunization-induced T cells for adoptive transfer. In general, active immunization has proved successful in inducing epitope-specific T cells easily detectable among circulating lymphocytes.[119,202–204] However, often the immunization-induced enhancement of T-cell function is not associated with clinical improvement. Although the reason for the clinical ineffectiveness of immunization-induced T cells is unclear, it has been postulated that they may be quantitatively[203] or qualitatively[205] inadequate for eradicating disease. Therefore, a second strategy is being pursued whereby the number of antigen-specific T cells is amplified in vitro for autologous or donor-derived adoptive transfer. This second strategy has met some promising success in the context of ganciclovir-resistant cytomegalovirus infection,[206] Epstein-Barr virus–induced posttransplantation lymphoproliferative disorders,[207] and metastatic melanoma.[208]

Whether delivered as a primary form of therapy or to prime in vivo T cells for further ex vivo expansion, epitope-specific vaccination encounters the major limitation of a stringent requirement for HLA allelic association. Although superfamilies of HLA alleles may share epitopes,[14,15] in practical terms, clinically relevant HLA/epitope associations are restricted to few peptide/allele combinations for a given protein.[22] Patients considered for enrollment in immunization protocols are best served by high-resolution HLA typing to exclude subtypes with unproven immunogenic potential for a given epitope. To bypass the stringent HLA requirements demanded by epitope-specific vaccination, whole-antigen delivery is suggested. This is based on the assumption that the epitope repertoire of a protein can be adjusted to distinct HLA phenotypes by a cellular process of *self-selection* naturally coupling peptides to HLA according to binding affinity. Although theoretically indisputable, in practice the truth of this assumption depends on the efficiency with which individual molecules are processed and presented in association with distinct HLA alleles. Even in these settings, high-resolution typing is desirable because it allows accurate interpretation of immunization results by allowing a comparison between the detailed genetic makeup of the individual receiving the vaccine and his or her antigen-specific immune response. It is likely that in the future HLA laboratories will receive increasing demands for high-resolution, definitive typing for appropriate patient enrollment and for subsequent interpretation of immune responses.

MONITORING IMMUNE RESPONSES WITH TETRAMERIC HLA-PEPTIDE COMPLEXES

A growing understanding of the molecular immunology of T-cell interactions with HLA/epitope complexes in the context of infectious disease, virally induced malignancies, and spontaneous tumors as well as interest in their treatment with T-cell–directed vaccines has generated more attention on issue of using accurate methods to quantify ex vivo the extent of antigen-specific immune responses.[209] The most commonly used assays available for the enumeration of antigen-specific T cells include tHLA; intracellular fluorescence-activated cell sorter staining for cytokine expression on cognate stimulation; detection of cytokine release by enzyme-linked immunospot assay; and quantitative real-time PCR, recently reviewed by Keilholz and associates.[210] Tetrameric HLA/peptide complexes are complexes of four HLA molecules combined with a specific peptide and bound to a fluorochrome (Figure 145–6). These complexes bind to complementary TCR and identify antigen-specific T cells,[211] measuring cellular responses against specific epitopes with sensitivity as low as 1 in 5000 CD8+ T cells. To synthesize tHLA molecules, soluble HLA heavy chain containing a biotinylation site and recombinant β_2-microglobulin are synthesized and purified. They are then refolded in the presence of the specific epitope and the monomer is isolated by gel filtration and is biotinylated. Fluorescent streptavidin is added to induce tetramerization. An aliquot of tetramers is added to the peripheral blood mononuclear cells together with other antibodies for a more detailed characterization of antigen-specific T cells.[205] Analysis is performed using a flow cytometer. Because of the specificity of vaccines, the patient's HLA type and specific peptide must be identified and synthesized to provide the adequate tetramer. Pentameric HLA/peptide complexes have recently become available and in some laboratories have replaced the use of tHLA.

Analysis of tHLA offers many potential advantages over other T-cells assays. This method is quantitative and enables an estimation of the avidity between TCR and peptide-loaded HLA class I molecules. Tetrameric HLA/peptide complexes staining does not kill the labeled cells, allowing sorting of subpopulations by flow cytometry for additional analysis or expansion for adoptive transfer. With tHLA specific T cells can be analyzed from blood samples without the prerequisite of in vitro culture and all specific cytotoxic T lymphocytes are detected, regardless of their functional status.[203,205,212]

HLA Summary

The relevance of HLA in clinical pathology has broadened from its role as a predictor of allosensitization to a mediator of GVHD and GVN. The understanding of action mechanisms in various nonclassic HLA genes as well as KIR has opened a new field. The study examining the function of the innate immune response in the context of transplantation and other immunopathologies is a result of this.

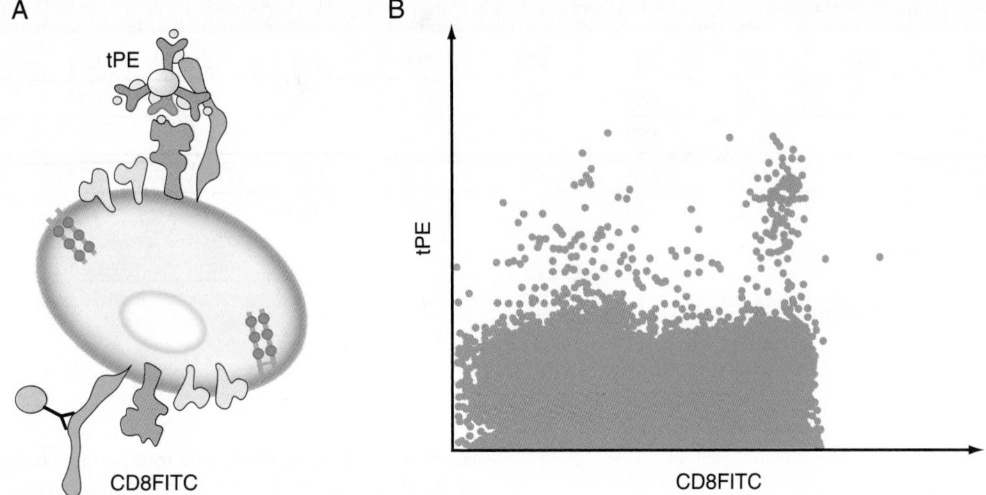

Figure 145–6 Schematic representation of the mechanism of binding of tetrameric peptide/human leukocyte antigen complexes (tHLA) to antigen-specific T cells. **A**, Binding of tHLA to T-cell receptor (TCR). The tHLA consists of four HLA/peptide complexes identical to the ones recognized by the T cell on the surface of live cells. Each HLA molecule is modified to contain one biotin molecule that serves as a bridge for binding to tetravalent streptavidin molecules fluorescently labeled. **B**, Actual FAC analysis result of CD8+, tHLA-positive T cells. (Modified from Monsurro V, Nargosen D: Immunotracking of specific cancer vaccine CD8+ lymphocytes. ASHI Q 26:100, 2003.)

Together with HLA, immunogenetics is rapidly growing, driven by the realization that polymorphism is the hallmark of human immunopathology as its spans mHag, KIR, cytokines, and their receptors. Each of these is interwoven in an intricate array of interdependent functions that cannot be discounted. Modern methods should be able to adopt high-throughput systems for the parallel assessment of all these variables when addressing the genetic makeup of an individual in correlation with the natural or therapeutic history of his or her disease. The comparison of donor and recipient protein profiling and cytokine polymorphism may offer insights into the rejection mechanism when matched-donor grafts are used. Finally, the increased use of T-cell–directed immunization is driving renewed interest in high-resolution typing of HLA molecules to allow a more accurate interpretation of clinical and immunologic results.

HUMAN NEUTROPHIL ANTIGENS AND THEIR CLINICAL SIGNIFICANCE

Lalezari and colleagues described the first granulocyte antigens. These antigens were designated *N* for neutrophil. Each antigen system was described alphabetically and each allele was described numerically in order of discovery. They identified NA1 in 1966 and its allele, NA2, in 1972.[213,214] In 1971, Lalezari and coworkers described another granulocyte antigen, NB1.[215] Reports of several other granulocyte antigens followed.

A new nomenclature was established in 1998 by the International Society of Blood Transfusion Working Party (Table 145–4).[216] In this nomenclature, antigen systems are referred to as *human neutrophil antigens,* or HNA. The antigen systems—that is, the polymorphic forms of the immunogenic proteins—are indicated by integers, and specific antigens within each system are designated alphabetically by date of publication. Alleles of the coding genes are named according to the Guidelines for Human Gene Nomenclature. Neutrophil antigens NA1 and NA2 became HNA-1a and HNA-1b in the new nomenclature and NB1 became HNA-2a.

Neutrophil antigens were first characterized using clinically important allo- and autoantibodies. Most often, neutrophil-specific alloantibodies are directed toward antigens in the HNA-1 or HNA-2 systems. The availability of many different alloantibodies and monoclonal antibodies to HNA-1 and HNA-2 antigens has allowed the characterization of these antigen systems. In addition, three other antigens systems have been partially characterized, HNA-3, HNA-4, and HNA-5. The serology, biochemistry, molecular biology, and clinical significance of these antigens are reviewed here.

Table 145–4 ISBT Nomenclature

Antigen System	Antigens	Location	Former Name	Alleles
HNA-1	HNA-1a	FcγRIIIb	NA1	FCGR3B*1
	HNA-1b	FcγRIIIb	NA2	*FCGR3B*2*
	HNA-1c	FcγRIIIb	SH	*FCGR3B*3*
HNA-2	HNA-2a	CD177 (NB1 gp)	NB1	*CD177*1*
HNA-3	HNA-3a	70–95 kD gp	5b	Not defined
HNA-4	HNA-4a	CD11b (CR3)	Mart[a]	CD11B*1
HNA-5	HNA-5a	CD11a (LFA-1)	Onda	*CD11A*1*

CR3, C3bi receptor; gp, glycoprotein; HNA, human neutrophil antigen; ISBT, International Society of Blood Transfusion; LFA-1, leukocyte function antigen-1.

THE HNA-1 ANTIGEN SYSTEM

Expression of HNA-1 Antigens

Human neutrophil antigens -1 antigens are expressed only on neutrophils. HNA-1 antigens are located on the low-affinity Fc-γ receptor IIIb (FcγRIIIb), CD16.[217–220] FcγRIIIb, HNA-1a, HNA-1b, and HNA-1c antigens are expressed on all segmented neutrophils, approximately one-half of neutrophilic metamyelocytes, and approximately 10% of neutrophilic myelocytes.[221] Neutrophil expression of FcγRIIIb and HNA-1 antigens are diminished by the treatment of neutrophils with stimulants such as complement component C5a and chemotaxin F-met-leu-phe or granulocyte colony-stimulating factor (G-CSF). Soluble FcγRIIIb is present in plasma and it has the same HNA-1 polymorphisms found on neutrophils. FcγRIIIb released from granulocytes is the source of the soluble FcγRIIIb and HNA-1 antigens.[222]

Table 145–5 Nucleotide Differences Among the Genes Encoding the HNA-1a, HNA-1b, and HNA-1c Antigens of FcγRIIIb Base Pair Position

Gene	141	147	227	266	277	349	473	505	559	641	733
FCGR3B*1	AGG	CTC	A**A**C	GCT	GAC	**G**TC	GAC	CAC	GTT	TCT	TGA†
FCGR3B*2	AG**C**	CT**T**	AGC	GCT	**A**AC	ATC	GAC	CAC	GTT	TCT	TGA†
FCGR3B*3	AG**C**	CT**T**	AGC	G**A**T	**A**AC	ATC	GAC	CAC	GTT	TCT	TGA†
FCGR3A	AGG	CTC	AGC	GCT	GAC	ATC	G**G**C	**T**AC	**T**TT	T**T**T	**C**GA

HNA, human neutrophil antigen.
*N-Glycosylation site.
†Stop codon.
Note: Differences among genes are in bold.

Biochemistry

FcγRIIIb is a glycoprotein with 233 amino acids and is glycosylphosphatidylinositol (GPI) anchored.[217–220] Its molecular weight is 50 to 80 kD, and the glycoprotein has *N*-linked carbohydrate side chains. Human neutrophil antigen–1a form of FcγRIIIb is 50 to 65 kD, the HNA-1b form of FcγRIIIb is 65 to 80 kD, and the heterozygous form is 50 to 80 kD. Differences in *N*-glycosylation account for the differences in molecular mass.

Molecular Biology

FcγRIIIb and the HNA-1 antigens are encoded by the *FCGR3B* gene located on chromosome 1q23–24 within a cluster of two families of FcγR genes, *FCGR2* and *FCGR3.* The *FCGR3* family is made up of *FCGR3A* and *FCGR3B. FCGR3B* is highly homologous to *FCGR3A,* which encodes FcγRIIIa. Only four nucleotides differ between *FCGR3B* and *FCGR3A* (Table 145–5). The most important difference between the two genes is a C to T change at 733 in *FCGR3B* that creates a stop codon. As a result, *FCGR3A* has 21 more amino acids than *FCGR3B* and *FCGR3A* is a transmembrane rather than GPI-anchored glycoprotein. FcγRIIIa is not recognized by antibodies specific to HNA-1 antigens, but the similarities between *FCGR3A* and *FCGR3B* complicate genotyping of HNA-1 alleles.

HNA-1a, -1b, and -1c Polymorphisms

The neutrophil-specific HNA-1 antigen system is made up of the three alleles, HNA-1a, -1b, and -1c.[223] The antigens are also known as NA1, NA2, and SH (see Table 145–4). The gene frequencies of the three alleles vary widely among different racial groups. Among whites, the frequency of the gene encoding HNA-1a, *FCGR3B*1,* is between 0.30 and 0.37 and the frequency of the gene encoding HNA-1b, *FCGR3B*2,* is from 0.63 to 0.70.[224–228] In Japanese and Chinese populations, the *FCGR3B*1* gene frequency is from 0.60 to 0.66 and the *FCGR3B*2* gene frequency is from 0.30 to 0.33.[224,226–228,217,219–221] The gene frequency of the gene encoding HNA-1c, *FCGR3B*3,* also varies among racial groups. *FCGR3B*3* is expressed by neutrophils in 4% to 5% of whites and 25% to 38% of African Americans.[229]

The *FCGR3B*1* gene differs from the *FCGR3B*2* gene by only five nucleotides in the coding region, at positions 141, 147, 227, 277, and 349 (see Table 145–5).[217–220] Four of the nucleotide changes result in changes in amino acid sequence between the HNA-1a and HNA-1b forms of the glycoprotein. The fifth polymorphism at 147 is silent. The glycosylation pattern of the protein differs between the two antigens because of two nucleotide changes at bases 227 and 277. HNA-1b form has six *N*-linked glycosylation sites and HNA-1a form has four glycosylation sites.

The gene encoding the HNA-1c form of FcγRIIIb, *FCGR3B*3,* is identical to *FCGR3B*2* except for a C to A substitution at nucleotide 266 resulting in an alanine to aspartate change at amino acid 78 of FcγRIIIb (see Table 145–5).[223] In many cases, *FCGR3B*3* exists on the same chromosome with a second or duplicate *FCGR3B* gene.[230,223] One group has found that in Danish people, *FCGR3B*3* always exists as a duplicate gene in association with *FCGR3B*1.*[231] However, in other populations duplicate *FCGR3B*3* genes were associated with both *FCGR3B*1* and *FCGR3B*2.*

Several other sequence variations in *FCGR3B* have been described.[226] These chimeric alleles have single-base substitutions involving one of the five single nucleotide polymorphisms that distinguish *FCGR3B*1* and *FCGR3B*2. FCGR3B* alleles that more closely resembled *FCGR3B*2* were found more often in African Americans than in whites or Japanese.[226]

FCγRIIIB Deficiency

Blood cells from patients with paroxysmal nocturnal hemoglobinuria lack the GPI-linked glycoproteins and their granulocytes express reduced amounts of FcγRIIIb and the HNA-1 antigens.[220] Genetic deficiencies of granulocyte FcγRIIIb and HNA-1 antigens have also been reported. With inherited deficiency of FcγRIIIb, the *FCGR3B* gene is deleted along with an adjacent gene, *FCGR2C.*[232,225] Among white subjects the incidence of individuals homozygous for *FCGR3B* deletion is about 0.1%.[233,234] However, among Africans and African Americans the incidence is much higher; in one study, 3 of 126 Africans were found to be *FCGR3B* deficient[229] and in another 1 of 53 were found to be *FCGR3B* deficient.[226]

Function of HNA-1 Antigens

The low-affinity Fc-γ receptors link humoral immunity to cellular immune function; specifically, FcγRs on effector cells recognize cytotoxic IgG molecules and immune complexes containing IgG molecules. Polymorphisms in FcγRIIIb affect neutrophil function. Neutrophils that are homozygous for HNA-1b have a lower affinity for IgG3 than granulocytes homozygous for HNA-1a.[235] Neutrophils from people who are homozygous for HNA-1b phagocytize erythrocytes sensitized with IgG1 and IgG3 anti-Rh monoclonal antibodies and bacteria opsonized with IgG1 at a lower level than granulocytes homozygous for HNA-1a.[236,237]

Clinical Relevance of FCγRIIIB Deficiency

Despite the important role of FcγRIIIb in neutrophil function, deletion of the entire *FcγRIIIB* gene does not cause major clinical problems, and most people with FcγRIIIb deficiency are healthy. However, too few patients have been studied to identify a slight increase in susceptibility to infection or autoimmune disease due to FcγRIIIb deficiency. In a study of 21 people with FcγRIIIb deficiency, 2 were found to have autoimmune thyroiditis and 4 had multiple episodes of bacterial infections.[232] Other smaller studies and case reports have found that despite their FcγRIIIb deficiency, all individuals, except for the one person with systemic lupus erythematosus, were healthy, had no circulating immune complexes, and showed no increased susceptibility to infections.

FCGR3B Polymorphisms and Disease Associations

Several studies suggest that *FCGR3B* polymorphisms affect the incidence and outcomes of some autoimmune and inflammatory diseases, but the results seem contradictory. Children with chronic immune thrombocytopenia purpura are more likely to be *FCGR3B*1* homozygous than control subjects,[238] but Spanish patients with systemic lupus erythematosus are more likely to be *FCGR3B*2* homozygous.[239] Myasthenia gravis is more severe in *FCGR3B*1* homozygous patients,[240] but multiple sclerosis is more benign in *FCGR3B*1* homozygous patients.[241] Patients with chronic granulomatous disease who are *FCGR3B*1* homozygous are less likely to develop major gastrointestinal or genitourinary tract infectious complications than heterozygous and *FCGR3B*2* homozygous chronic granulomatous patients.[242] Because *FCGR3B* is clustered with FCGR3A and FCGR3B on chromosome 1q22, it is possible that some of these findings may be caused in part by linkage disequilibrium among Fc receptors.

THE HNA-2 ANTIGEN SYSTEM

Human neutrophil antigen–2 system has one well-described allele, HNA-2a. It was previously known as NB1.[215] Monoclonal antibodies specific to HNA-2a have been clustered as CD177.

Expression of HNA-2a

HNA-2a is neutrophil-specific antigen. It is expressed only on neutrophils, neutrophilic metamyelocytes, and myelocytes.[221,243] HNA-2a is unique in that it is expressed on subpopulations of neutrophils. The mean size of the HNA-2a-positive subpopulation of neutrophils is 45% to 65%.[244–246] The expression of HNA-2a is greater on neutrophils from women than men.[246,247] The size of the HNA-2a positive subpopulation of neutrophils from women is approximately 60%, compared with approximately 50% for men. The expression of HNA-2a falls with age in women but remains constant in men.[246] Neutrophil expression of HNA-2a is greater in pregnant women than in healthy female blood donors.[247] The surface expression of HNA-2a is slightly upregulated by treatment with the chemotactic peptide F-met-leu-phe.[244] The administration of G-CSF to healthy subjects for several days increases the proportion of neutrophils expressing HNA-2a to near 90%.[248]

NB1 Glycoprotein Biochemistry

The glycoprotein carrying HNA-2a, NB1 glycoprotein, is located on neutrophil plasma membranes and secondary granules[244,249] and is linked to the plasma membrane via a GPI anchor.[244] Although some GPI-anchored proteins are shed by F-met-leu-phe treated neutrophils, NB1 glycoprotein is not, nor is soluble NB1 glycoprotein present in plasma.[244] The molecular weight of NB1 glycoprotein is 58 to 64 kD and it contains *N*-linked carbohydrate side chains.[244,249]

Molecular Biology

The gene encoding NB1 glycoprotein, *CD177,* is located on chromosome 19q13.31 and its coding region consists of 1311 bp that code for a protein of 416 and a signal peptide of 21 amino acids.[250,251] The predicted protein has two cysteine-rich domains, three potential *N*-linked glycosylation sites, and a potential ω-site for attachment of the GPI anchor.[250] This gene belongs to the *Ly-6* snake toxin superfamily. Other genes in this family include urokinase type plasminogen activator receptor (uPAR) (CD87) and decay accelerating factor (CD59).

Two different groups sequenced *CD177* independently. One group sequenced it as the gene encoding HNA-2a and called the gene *NB1,*[250] and the other group sequenced it as a gene overexpressed in granulocytes from people with polycythemia rubra vera and called the gene *PRV-1.*[252] The *NB1* and *PRV-1* alleles differ at only 4 bp.[250] Bettinotti and colleagues[253] used Human Genomic Project databases to characterize the structure of the *PRV-1* and *NB1* genes. They described the intron and exon structure of *NB1,* but they found only one gene homologous to both *PRV-1* and *NB1,* suggesting that they are alleles of the same gene that they called *CD177.* In addition, they found a pseudogene homologous to exons 4 through 9 of *CD177.*[253]

Polymorphisms

HNA-2a is expressed on neutrophils by approximately 97% of whites, 95% of blacks, and 89% to 99% of Japanese.[246,254,255] HNA-2a has been reported to have an allele, NB2; but the product of this gene cannot be reliably identified with alloantisera, and no monoclonal antibody specific for NB2 has been identified.[256]

Human neutrophil antigen–2a negative neutrophil phenotype is caused by a *CD177* transcription defect.[257] HNA-2a genes from two women with HNA-2a-negative neutrophils who produced HNA-2a-specific alloantibodies have been studied, and *CD177* cDNA sequences were present in both women.[257] However, all neutrophil CD177mRNA contained accessory sequences that were considered to be introns. Human neutrophil antigen 2a–negative phenotype was the result of different off-frame insertions at the RNA level, resulting in NB1 gp deficiency in neutrophils.[257]

Role of NB1 Glycoprotein in Neutrophil Function

The role of *CD177* in neutrophil function is unknown. In some studies HNA-2a may have a role in the adhesion of neutrophils to endothelial cells.[258] Upregulation of HNA-2a after F-met-leu-phe stimulation, HNA-2a internalization on antibody cross-linking, and activation of the respiratory burst after binding of HNA-2a antibodies to HNA-2a-bearing neutrophils suggest a possible role as receptor molecule.[259]

Clinical Relevance of HNA-2 Antigens

The rare women who produce HNA-2a–specific alloantibodies and who lack NB1 glycoprotein are healthy. The expression of HNA-2a is reduced on neutrophils from people with paroxysmal nocturnal hemoglobinuria and chronic myelogenous leukemia.[243] It is unknown whether the lack of expression of HNA-2a on neutrophils from patients with paroxysmal nocturnal hemoglobinuria or chronic myelogenous leukemia has any clinical significance. *CD177* mRNA is overexpressed by neutrophils from patients with polycythemia rubra vera and essential thrombocytosis.[252,260] Some groups are using quantitative real-time PCR to measure neutrophil *CD177* mRNA levels to assist with the diagnosis of polycythemia rubra vera and essential thrombocytosis. Patients with essential thrombocytosis and increased CD177 mRNA levels have been reported to have increased risk of thrombocytosis and bleeding.[261] Patients with polycythemia rubra vera and essential thrombocytosis have been found to have gain of function mutations in the gene encoding Janus kinase-2 (JAK2)[262–266] and the increased expression of CD177 mRNA in neutrophils from these patients may be secondary to the JAK2 mutation.

HNA-3 ANTIGEN SYSTEM

Human neutrophil antigen–3 antigen system has one antigen, HNA-3a, that was previously known as 5b. HNA-3a is expressed by neutrophils, lymphocytes, platelets, endothelial cells, kidney, spleen, and placental cells. HNA-3a has a gene frequency of 0.66 and is located on a 70 to 95 kD neutrophil glycoprotein.[267] The gene encoding HNA-3a has not yet been cloned, and the nature and function of the 70 to 95 kD gp is unknown. Although the biologic role for this system has not been established, several cases of transfusion-related acute lung injury (TRALI) have been associated with transfusion of plasma containing anti-5b.[268,269]

HNA-4 AND HNA-5 ANTIGEN SYSTEMS

Human neutrophil antigen–4 and HNA-5 antigens are located in the β_2 integrins. Each antigen system contains only a single antigen, HNA-4a and HNA-5a, respectively. Human neutrophil antigen–4a antigen was previously known as Mart(a). HNA-4a was defined by an antibody in the sera of three nontransfused multiparous blood donors. The antigen was shown to have autosomal dominant inheritance and has a phenotype frequency of 99.1% in white subjects. HNA-4a has been located on the αM chain (CD11b) of the C3bi receptor (CR3) and is caused by a single nucleotide substitution of G to A at position 302.[270] The substitution would be predicted to result in an Arg to His polymorphism at amino acid 61. The significance of the antibody is unknown and none of the infants of the three multiparous women with anti-HNA-4a showed evidence of neonatal alloimmune neutropenia.

A second polymorphism of the β_2 integrins, HNA-5a, was first described as Ond(a). A chronically transfused man with aplastic anemia became alloimmunized to HNA-5a. HNA-5a was found to be expressed on the αL integrin unit, leukocyte function antigen-1 (LFA-1) (CD11a), and is caused by a G to C single nucleotide substitution at position 2446. This change predicts an amino acid change of Arg to Thr at amino acid 766.[270]

CLINICAL SIGNIFICANCE OF ANTIBODIES TO NEUTROPHIL ANTIGENS

Alloimmune Neonatal Neutropenia

During pregnancy, mothers can become alloimmunized to neutrophil antigens. Maternal IgG directed to neutrophils can cross the placenta and destroy the neonate's neutrophils. Maternal alloimmunization to neutrophil antigens can occur in utero and affect the first child. Most neonates experience isolated neutropenia, but the cytopenias are self-limiting and resolve as the antibody is cleared. The alloimmunized mothers produce and carry the antibodies; but the antibodies do not react with the mother's blood cells or tissues, and they have normal neutrophil counts. Antibodies to neutrophil-specific antigens HNA-1a, HNA-1b, and HNA-2a most commonly cause neonatal alloimmune neutropenia (Table 145–6).[267,271] Antibodies to HNA-1c and HNA-3a rarely cause alloimmune neonatal neutropenia. Mothers with FcγRIIIb deficiency have produced FcγRIIIb-specific antibodies that caused neonatal neutropenia.[234,267,271]

Newborns with alloimmune neutropenia are usually asymptomatic. Most often, the neutropenia is detected in the first week of life when the neonate becomes febrile or develops an infection and a neutrophil count is done. Typically, the counts are 0.100 to 0.200 × 10^9/L. Some neonates have normal neutrophil counts the first day of life, but they become neutropenic on their second day.[271] White blood cell count, platelet count, and hemoglobin are usually normal; but eosinophilia or monocytosis may be present. If a bone marrow biopsy is performed, it often shows normal numbers of erythroid progenitors and megakaryocytes with hyperplasia of myeloid progenitors.

Table 145–6 Specificities of Antibodies in Alloimmune Neonatal Neutropenia

Antigen	N = 18[271,251]	N = 48[267,253]
HNA-1a	28%	10%
HNA-1b	22%	8%
FcγRIIIb	0%	8%
HNA-2a	11%	2%
HNA-3a	0%	2%
Unknown	0%	15%
HLA class I[271,251]	11%	54%
Negative	28%	38%

HLA, human leukocyte antigen; HNA, human neutrophil antigen.

The clinical course is quite variable. An occasional infant is asymptomatic, but almost all affected children have an infection. The most common infections are umbilicus infections, skin infections, abscesses, and respiratory tract infections. Less commonly, infants experience otitis media, urinary tract infections, and gastroenteritis. Serious infections such as sepsis, pneumonia, and meningitis can occur. The duration of the neutropenia may be as short as a few days or as long as 28 weeks.[271] The mean duration of neutropenia is about 11 weeks.[271]

For an asymptomatic child, no immediate treatment may be required. Prompt and aggressive antibiotic treatment of children with fevers or other signs of infections is indicated. Intravenous immunoglobulin has a limited role in the treatment of neonatal alloimmune neutropenia. Approximately half the patients treated have a transient increase in count lasting only a few days. The use of G-CSF to treat alloimmune neutropenia has also had mixed results. The administration of G-CSF elevates the neutrophil count in some but not all neonates.[271]

AUTOIMMUNE NEUTROPENIA OF CHILDHOOD

Autoimmune neutropenia has been well described in children.[272–275] Typically, the onset of the autoimmune neutropenia of children begins at 8 months of age, but children between 1 and 36 months of age can be affected. Most studies found that neutrophil counts recover spontaneously by the age of 5 years, with a median of 13 to 20 months of neutropenia.[272–275]

In most cases, children presented with severe neutropenia, having neutrophil counts less than 0.5 × 10^9/L. Monocytosis has been reported to occur in up to 38% of patients. Bone marrow biopsies in affected patients usually show normal to hypercellular marrow with a decreased number of mature granulocytes. Febrile episodes and infections, including bacterial skin infections, otitis media, respiratory tract infections, and urinary tract infections, are common. Life-threatening complications are rare.

Antibodies to neutrophils can be detected in up to 98% of affected patients. If an antibody specificity is identified, the antibodies are almost always specific to epitopes located on FcγRIIIb. The antibodies are directed to HNA-1a in 10% to 46% of patients, to HNA-1b in 2% to 3% of patients, and rarely to FcγRIIIb epitopes expressed by granulocytes from all donors.[273,274]

Autoimmune neutropenia has been treated with corticosteroids, intravenous immunoglobulin, and G-CSF. Approximately half the patients responded to intravenous immunoglobulin, but neutrophil counts remained elevated for only 1 week.[273] Almost all the patients responded to G-CSF and 75% to corticosteroids, and neutrophil counts remained elevated as long as the drugs were given.

TRANSFUSION REACTIONS

Antibodies to neutrophil and HLA antigens can cause febrile nonhemolytic transfusion reactions and TRALI. Prior to the widespread transfusion of leukocyte-reduced blood components, approximately 0.5% of transfusions were associated with febrile nonhemolytic transfusion reactions, and leukocyte antibodies are a common cause of these reactions. These febrile reactions are caused by the interaction of leukocyte antibodies in the transfusion recipient with leukocytes contained in the transfused blood components. These reactions can be prevented by the use of components that have been filtered to remove leukocytes.

A more serious type of transfusion reaction associated with leukocyte antibodies is the acute noncardiac pulmonary edema, or TRALI. This entity is characterized by acute respiratory distress that usually occurs within 4 hours after a transfusion. These reactions are characterized by dyspnea, hypoxia, and bilateral pulmonary infiltrates on chest radiograph without cardiomegaly or pulmonary vascular congestion. The mortality rate associated with TRALI is approximately 5%.[276] Of patients with TRALI, 80% have rapid resolution of pulmonary infiltrates and return of arterial blood gas values to normal within 96 hours after the initial respiratory insult. However, pulmonary infiltrates have persisted for at least 7 days after the transfusion reaction in 17% of TRALI patients.

Transfusion-related acute lung injury has been associated with both neutrophil and HLA antibodies. Antibodies reported in these reactions include HNA-1a, HNA-1b, HNA-2a, HNA-3a, and HLA class I and II antibodies. Most these cases involve the passive transfusion of the offending antibody in donor plasma, as contrasted with the reactivity of the recipient's antibody with donor leukocytes to cause febrile nonhemolytic reactions. Retrospective studies involving antibodies to HNA-3a have implicated blood components from single donors with anti-HNA-3a in several TRALI cases.[269]

GRANULOCYTE TRANSFUSIONS

Granulocyte transfusion recipients sometimes produce antibodies specific to HNA-1a, HNA-1b, and HNA-2a. The transfusion of granulocytes to patients with these antibodies can result in febrile transfusion reactions and pulmonary transfusion reactions.[277] Hematopoietic progenitor cell transplant recipients who produce HNA-2a antibodies as a result of granulocyte transfusions have experienced marrow graft failure.[278]

NEUTROPHIL ANTIGENS SUMMARY

Two neutrophil antigen systems, HNA-1 and HNA-2, have been well described, and three others, HNA-3, HNA-4, and HNA-5, have been described in part. HNA-1 antigens are located on FcγRIIIb, and antibodies to these antigens are frequently implicated in autoimmune and alloimmune neutropenia. HNA-2a is located on NB1 glycoprotein, and antibodies to HNA-2a are found in patients with alloimmune and autoimmune neutropenia. The gene expressing this protein is overexpressed by neutrophils in patients with polycythemia rubra vera. Antibodies to HNA-3a are rare; but relative to other neutrophil antibodies, may be more frequently associated with cases of TRALI. The significance, if any, of HNA-4a and HNA-5a antibodies is uncertain.

SUGGESTED READINGS

Braun WE: Update in kidney transplantation: Increasing clinical success, expanding waiting lists. Cleve Clin J Med 69:501, 2002.

Bux J, Jung KD, Kauth T, Mueller-Eckhardt C: Serological and clinical aspects of granulocyte antibodies leading to alloimmune neonatal neutropenia. Transfus Med 2:143, 1992.

Bux J, Behrens G, Jaeger G, Welte K: Diagnosis and clinical course of autoimmune neutropenia in infancy: Analysis of 240 cases. Blood 91:181, 1998.

Childs R, Srinivasan R: Advances in allogeneic stem cell transplantation: Directing graft-versus-leukemia at solid tumors. Cancer J Sci Am 8:2, 2002.

Daser A, Michinson H, Michinson A, Muller B: Non-classical-MHC genetics of immunological disease in man and mouse: The key role of pro-inflammatory cytokine genes. Cytokine 8:593, 1996.

Dawkins RL, Degli-Esposti MP, Abraham LJ, et al: Conservation versus polymorphism of the MHC in relation to transplantation, immune responses and autoimmune disease. In Klein J, Klein D (eds.): Molecular Evolution of the Major Histocompatibility Complex. Berlin, Springer-Verlag, 1991, p 391.

De Haas M, Kleijer M, van Zwieten R, et al: Neutrophil FcγRIIIb deficiency, nature, and clinical consequences: A study of 21 individuals from 14 families. Blood 86:2403, 1995.

Duquesnoy RJ, Marrari M: HLA matchmaker: A molecularly based algorithm for histocompatibility determination. II. Verification of the algorithm and determination of the relative immunogenicity of amino acid triplet-defined epitopes. Hum Immunol 63:353, 2002.

Hennecke J, Wiley DC: T cell-receptor-MHC interactions up close. Cell 104:1, 2001.

Kim CJ, Parkinson DR, Marincola FM: Immunodominance across the HLA polymorphism: Implications for cancer immunotherapy. J Immunother 21:1, 1997.

Kissel K, Santoso S, Hofmann C, et al: Molecular basis of the neutrophil glycoprotein NB1 (CD177) involved in the pathogenesis of immune neutropenias and transfusion reactions. Eur J Immunol 31:1301, 2001.

Matzinger P: An innate sense of danger. Semin Immunol 10:399, 1998.

Opelz G, Vanrenterghem Y, Kirste G, et al: Prospective evaluation of pretransplant blood transfusion in cadaver kidney recipients. Transplantation 63:964, 1997.

Opelz G, Wujciak T, Dohler B, et al: HLA compatibility and organ transplant survival: Collaborative transplant study. Rev Immunogenet 1:334, 1999.

Parker KC, Bednarek MA, Coligan JE: Scheme for ranking potential HLA-A2 binding peptides based on independent binding of individual peptide side-chains. J Immunol 152:163, 1994.

Petersdorf EW, Hansen JA, Martin PJ, et al: Major-histocompatibility-complex class I alleles and antigens in hematopoietic-cell transplantation. N Engl J Med 345:1794, 2001.

Petz LD, Garratty G, Calhoun L, et al: Selecting donors of platelets for refractory patients on the basis of HLA antibody specificity. Transfusion 40:1446, 2000.

Stroncek DF, Skubitz KM, McCullough J: Biochemical nature of the neutrophil-specific antigen NB1. Blood 75:744, 1990.

Velardi A, Ruggeri L, Moretta A, Moretta L: NK cells: a lesson from mismatched hematopoietic transplantation. Trends Immunol 23:438, 2002.

REFERENCES

For complete list of references log onto www.expertconsult.com

CHAPTER 146

PRINCIPLES OF RED BLOOD CELL TRANSFUSION

Melissa M. Cushing and Paul M. Ness

The clinical practice of transfusion medicine has evolved substantially in the past century. Several critical advances have spurred progress since the discovery of the ABO system just over 100 years ago. The description of Rh and the introduction of a safe and effective anticoagulant-preservative solution (suggested by Loutit and Mollison[1]) allowed for the preservation of blood products. Another important landmark was the development of the antiglobulin test by Coombs,[2] which permitted the detection of antibodies in recipient plasma that did not produce direct agglutination in the test tube but might be capable of causing in vivo red blood cell destruction.

It was not until the mid-1960s, however, with the introduction of plastic blood packs by Walter and Murphy,[3] that the era of component therapy began. This innovation, combined with the ability to store blood for extended periods, revolutionized transfusion practice. Today, approximately 15 million units of blood are transfused each year in the United States.

RED BLOOD CELL PRESERVATION AND STORAGE

The first key to the storage of blood for later transfusion is a stable, minimally toxic anticoagulant with preservative properties. During the early 1900s, it was recognized that citrate met these criteria.[4] Although slightly more toxic than heparin, if given rapidly and in large amounts, citrate has preservative action that heparin lacks. Citrate has the added advantage of not causing systemic anticoagulation in the recipient.

The other factor essential for long-term storage is a mechanism to maintain cell viability and function. Fresh transfused red blood cells have a good survival rate in the recipient's circulation, with a destruction rate approximately equal to that of the recipient's own cells: 1% per day.[5] The arbitrary standard used for stored red blood cells requires 75% to remain in the circulation for 24 hours.

Adenosine Triphosphate Levels

Adenosine triphosphate (ATP) levels appear to be a major determinant of red blood cell viability.[6] The drop in cellular ATP levels during storage has been correlated with increased cell rigidity and with loss of membrane lipid, leading to decreased red blood cell life span.[7] For this reason, most efforts to extend red blood cell storage have focused on ways to maintain intracellular ATP levels. First, dextrose was introduced into the citrate solution (citrate-phosphate-dextrose [CPD]: 21 days), to which adenine was added (CPDA-1: 35 days). Three additive solutions containing additional dextrose and adenine (Nutricel, or AS-3) or dextrose and adenine plus mannitol (Adsol, or AS-1) and (Optisol, or AS-5) allow extension of the maximum storage time to 42 days (Table 146–1).

2,3-Diphosphoglycerate Levels

Stored red blood cells must also maintain their capacity to deliver oxygen. It was not until 1967 that the central role of 2,3-diphosphoglycerate (2,3-DPG) in releasing oxygen from oxyhemoglobin was recognized.[8,9] Attention was then focused on ways to maintain high levels of 2,3-DPG in stored blood cells. The first anticoagulant introduced on a large scale, acid citrate-dextrose, was ineffective because of its low initial pH; however, the subsequently developed CPD, with its higher initial pH and slower fall in pH, was superior. CPDA-1 and additive solutions have not further improved 2,3-DPG maintenance. Although 2,3-DPG depletion of stored red blood cells is known to decrease oxygen delivery, the clinical significance of this finding is unclear. 2,3-DPG levels in stored blood cells are rapidly regenerated in vivo, rising to greater than 50% of normal within several hours and to normal within 24 hours.[10] Although a patient with normal cardiac status should be able to compensate by increasing cardiac output to maintain normal oxygen delivery until 2,3-DPG levels are regenerated, an improvement in 2,3-DPG preservation in stored red blood cells is still desirable.

By-Products of Red Blood Cell Storage With Potentially Adverse Effects

Infusion of large volumes of blood with citrate anticoagulant over a short period may cause plasma citrate levels to reach the toxic range. The primary concern is the cardiovascular effects of hypocalcemia caused by chelation of calcium by citrate. The risk of citrate toxicity is exacerbated by liver dysfunction or liver immaturity. Despite these theoretical considerations, there is little documented evidence of clinical citrate toxicity, and the problem can usually be prevented by slower infusion. If large amounts of blood have to be infused over a very short period, administration of calcium gluconate can be considered, but whether the benefits justify the risk is controversial.[11]

Another issue with prolonged storage is the excess potassium in the red blood cell supernatant that could potentially cause cardiac arrhythmias. At a storage temperature of 4°C, the red blood cell sodium-potassium pump is essentially nonfunctional, and intra- and extracellular levels gradually equilibrate. In addition, hemolysis results in increased potassium in the supernatant. However, because the total volume of plasma in red blood cell concentrates is low (approximately 70 mL), the total potassium burden is only approximately 5.5 mEq at product expiration. Practically speaking, the potassium load is rarely a clinical problem except in the setting of preexisting hyperkalemia and renal failure. In this situation, fresher units of red blood cells or washed red blood cells can be used.

Microaggregates consisting of platelets, leukocytes, and fibrin form during blood storage. Although studies have shown that pulmonary dysfunction after massive transfusion may be significantly diminished by the use of a microaggregate filter of pore size 20 to 40 μm,[12] other studies have not confirmed microaggregates as the cause of hypoxia.[13] Because microaggregate filters have been found to slow the infusion rate, their use is not uniformly recommended in cases of trauma. The growing use of prestorage, leukoreduced blood has reduced the importance of this issue. Since their introduction in the 1960s, plastic blood bags used for storing red blood cells have been made from polyvinylchloride containing the lipophilic plasticizer di(2-ethyl)phthalate (DEHP), which confers pliability. The safety of DEHP has been questioned for years owing to its tendency to leach from the bag and to be present at levels of 50 to 70 mg/L in stored red blood cells.[14] Numerous studies in animal models have addressed the toxicity of the substance and are summarized in a comprehensive review.[15,16] The situation is complicated by a significant stabilizing effect of DEHP on the red blood cell membrane, with red blood cells stored in various containers that lack DEHP having unacceptable recovery at the end of the storage period. This decreased recovery has been shown to be due to increased hemolysis and increased osmotic fragility.[17]

Storage Length of Red Blood Cells

During storage, RBCs undergo a series of biochemical and biomechanical changes that reduce their survival and function. In addition, accumulation of biological by-products during RBC storage may be harmful to recipients of blood transfusions. Increasing numbers of studies have raised concern that prolonged RBC storage adversely affects clinical outcomes.[18] One recent study reported an association between red cell storage length and adverse outcome in cardiac surgery patients.[19] Multivariate analysis in another recent study, also looking at cardiac surgery patients, showed no effect of storage time on survival or ICU stay.[20] A large, prospective, randomized clinical trial would be helpful in determining the true clinical significance of the effect of red cell storage duration on patient outcomes.

RED BLOOD CELL COMPONENTS

Modern transfusion medicine practice is aimed at providing the specific component of the blood required, rather than whole blood: red cells for oxygen-carrying capacity, plasma for coagulation proteins, and platelets for microvascular bleeding. The component therapy approach allows for optimal use of a limited community resource (Table 146–2). Today, the clinician wishing to increase the patient's oxygen-carrying capacity is more likely to be using a red blood cell concentrate than whole blood, although there may still be situations in which whole blood, if available, is appropriate. For particular clinical applications, several modifications can be made to red blood cell products to render them leukocyte or plasma depleted. Red blood cells can also be frozen for long-term storage.

Table 146–1 Biochemical Changes in Stored Red Blood Cells

Variable	CPDA-1 *Fresh*	CPDA-1 *35 Days*	Adsol *35 Days*
In vivo survival (at 24 hours) (%)	100	<71.0	<88.0
pH	<7.5	<6.7	<6.7
ATP (% initial)	100	<45.0	<76.0
2,3-DPG (% initial)	100	<10.0	<10.0
Plasma K^+ (mEq/L)	5.1	<78.5	<49.0

Data from Zuck TF, Bensinger TA, Peck CC, et al: The in vivo survival of red cells stored in modified CPD with adenine: Report of a multi-institutional cooperative effort. Transfusion 17:34, 1977; and Moore GL, Peck CC, Sohmer RR, Zuck TF: Some properties of blood stored in anticoagulant CPDA-1 solution: A brief summary. Transfusion 21:135, 1981.

Whole Blood

A unit of whole blood is collected in CPDA-1 anticoagulant, giving it a shelf-life of 35 days and a volume of approximately 510 mL (450 mL of blood plus 63 mL of CPDA-1). Within 24 hours of collection, the platelets,[21] as well as the granulocytes, are dysfunctional, and several plasma coagulation factors have fallen to suboptimal levels.[22]

Whole blood has the advantage of correcting simultaneous deficits in oxygen-carrying capacity and blood volume. Therefore, whole blood is indicated in the management of trauma or in surgical cases involving extensive blood loss. In this setting, whole blood has two distinct advantages: (a) it provides colloid osmotic pressure and some coagulation factors not supplied by crystalloid solutions and (b) it does not expose the recipient to red blood cells and plasma from different donors.

The goal of using whole blood for all cases of concomitant red blood cell and volume deficit is difficult to achieve in practice. Most indications for whole blood transfusion are now well managed exclusively with blood component therapy, but the use of fresh whole blood has persisted in military settings.[23] In the civilian setting, the simultaneous need for volume and oxygen-carrying capacity can usually be met by combining red cells with crystalloid or colloid solutions. In some cases of trauma and cardiovascular surgery, platelet transfusion may be indicated to combat microvascular bleeding from dilutional thrombocytopenia or bypass-associated platelet dysfunction. The transfusion of platelets usually supplies the equivalent of several units of relatively fresh plasma so that there is often no reason for further donor exposure by the administration of frozen plasma.

Red Blood Cell Concentrates

Red blood cell concentrates are obtained from whole blood after removal of most of the plasma for the production of frozen plasma or platelets, or both. At most blood centers, the red blood cells are then mixed with 100 mL of an additive nutrient solution that extends the storage period to 42 days and results in flow properties similar to those of whole blood.[24]

Table 146–2 Red Blood Cell Components: Characteristics and Indications

Component	Characteristics	Indications
Whole blood	High volume; good flow	Combined red cell/volume deficit (massive hemorrhage; exchange transfusion)
Red blood cells	Lower volume Higher hematocrit	Red cell deficit
Leukocyte-reduced red blood cells	Good flow in AS-1	Prevention of febrile reactions Reduction of alloimmunization Reduction of immunomodulatory effects
Washed red blood cells	Plasma depletion Must use within 24 hours	Prevention of severe allergic reactions Prevention of anaphylaxis in IgA deficiency
Frozen red blood cells	Long-term storage Plasma and leukocyte depletion Must use within 24 hours of thawing	Rare donor unit storage Autologous storage for postponed surgery

Red blood cell concentrates are the product of choice for the correction of an isolated defect in oxygen-carrying capacity, as in cases of chronic anemia. In addition, red blood cells rather than whole blood are used for the emergent transfusion of patients of unknown ABO type. Concentrated type O red blood cells are transfused after the plasma containing isohemagglutinins is removed to prevent potential hemolysis of the recipient's red blood cells.

Leukocyte-Reduced Red Blood Cells

Leukocyte-reduced red blood cells (LRRCs) can be prepared by a variety of methods, resulting in differing degrees of white blood cell removal. Early techniques of preparation involved centrifugation or washing with saline, whereby the buffy coat was repeatedly removed. Currently, the most widely used method of leukoreduction is filtration, which can be performed either in the laboratory or at the bedside. The various filters on the market result in greater than 99% leukocyte reduction while depleting less than 10% of the red blood cells.[25] Blood bags with in-line filters, which allow prestorage leukoreduction, are now more commonly used and have been shown to decrease febrile nonhemolytic transfusion reactions compared to bedside leukoreduction filters.[26]

The major indication for the use of LRRCs has been the prevention of the nonhemolytic febrile transfusion reaction, the most common adverse effect of transfusion, particularly in multiply transfused patients or multiparous females. Traditionally, these reactions are believed to be mediated by antibodies directed against leukocyte antigens,[27] but whether lymphocyte HLA antigens or granulocyte-specific antigens are the major targets has remained a subject of controversy. Depletion of leukocytes to less than 5×10^8 has been shown to prevent, or at least ameliorate, such reactions in most patients.[28] Increasing evidence has accumulated suggesting that cytokines play a role in causing these reactions.[29] Because cytokines may be released from leukocytes during storage, prestorage leukoreduction procedures have become the preferred mode of leukoreduction.

A second important indication for LRRCs is the prevention of alloimmunization to HLA antigens that can adversely affect posttransfusion platelet increments, such as in cancer patients undergoing chemotherapy. This approach will be effective only if platelets for transfusion can also be white blood cell depleted. According to current AABB standards, the total leukocyte number must be less than 5×10^6 when intended for this purpose. With the introduction of third-generation leukoreduction filters for both red blood cells and platelets, this goal is achievable. A multicenter study known as TRAP showed that the use of leukoreduction filters for platelet products significantly decreased the rate of alloimmunization but did not totally eliminate the problem.[30] Leukoreduction has also been studied for its ability to prevent transfusion-mediated immunosuppression, which is of particular concern in the postoperative period. Data collected to date suggest that this practice may be of value.[31] Indeed, even simple removal of the buffy coat from red blood cells (which is a routine procedure during component preparation in Europe) may provide a sufficient degree of leukoreduction.[32] Because component preparation in the United States does not include a buffy coat removal step and because soluble white blood cell fragments may be capable of mediating immunomodulation, a prestorage leukoreduction method would be required to abrogate this adverse effect in transfusion recipients in the United States. However, despite numerous studies looking for cancer recurrence or increases in infections, the data remain contradictory.[33]

Washed Red Blood Cells

Red blood cells are washed, using isotonic saline solutions, by either automated or manual techniques. Automated techniques are more efficient, but there is always some degree of red blood cell loss with each wash cycle. When the washing is performed in an open system, the resulting product must be transfused within 24 hours because of concerns over potential bacterial contamination.

The primary aim of washing is to remove plasma proteins, although some leukocytes and platelets are removed simultaneously. The major indication for washed red blood cells is the prevention of severe allergic transfusion reactions, thought to be mediated by recipient antibodies (most likely IgE) to donor plasma proteins. Washing is recommended when reactions are recurrent and severe, even in the face of antihistamine administration. In IgA-deficient patients who have preformed antibody to IgA, IgA-containing plasma can actually cause anaphylaxis.[34] Multiple cell washes may be required to remove the contaminating plasma protein.[35]

Another setting in which washed cells have been advocated is paroxysmal nocturnal hemoglobinuria. However, one study has suggested that these patients do not require washed cells and this indication for washed cells has become less popular in recent times.[36]

Irradiated Red Blood Cells

Red blood cells are irradiated with a minimum dose of 25 Gy. Red cells expire 28 days after irradiation or the original expiration date, whichever is sooner. A method is used to ensure that irradiation has occurred with each batch. The primary aim of irradiating is to prevent the frequently fatal risk of transfusion-associated graft-versus-host disease (TA-GVHD). Graft-versus-host disease can occur after the transfusion of immunologically competent donor lymphocytes, usually to an immuno-incompetent recipient. Irradiation is performed to inactivate immunocompetent lymphocytes. Some indications for irradiated products include neonates, patients with hematologic malignancies, stem cell transplant recipients, and patients with congenital immune deficiencies. There is still much debate among experts regarding which additional patient populations may be at risk for TA-GVHD. It has been suggested that a policy of universal blood component irradiation could prevent TA-GVHD in patients with currently unsuspected risks, including advanced age.[37]

Frozen Red Blood Cells

Red blood cells can be frozen (with glycerol used as a cryoprotective agent) and stored in liquid nitrogen or mechanical freezers. The required concentration of glycerol depends on the rate and the temperature of freezing.[38,39] The freezing process destroys other blood constituents, except for a small percentage of immunocompetent lymphocytes. Red blood cells are prepared for transfusion by thawing and washing away the glycerol using a series of progressively less hypertonic saline solutions, allowing glycerol to diffuse gradually from the cells to prevent hemolysis. The cells are resuspended in isotonic saline solution containing glucose. The extensive washing removes approximately 99.9% of the plasma as well as cellular debris.

Red blood cells can be stored in the frozen state for at least 10 years with good viability. After thawing and washing, storage is typically limited to 24 hours because of the open system. Frozen cells have been shown to maintain prefreezing ATP and 2,3-DPG levels. To maintain these factors at high levels, the standard is to freeze within 6 days of collection. When it is necessary to freeze older units, rejuvenation with a solution containing pyruvate, glucose, phosphate, and adenine has provided excellent results.[40] The major indication for frozen red blood cells is the stockpiling of rare donor units for patients who have developed alloantibodies. Some patients with rare phenotypes can make autologous donations that can be frozen for later use. Cells from autologous donors can be frozen if more units are required than can be collected in the 42-day liquid storage period or if surgery is postponed. Because of the high cost and cumbersome nature of freeze–thaw procedures, other uses of frozen red blood cells are somewhat difficult to justify.

APPROPRIATE TRANSFUSION PRACTICE IN VARIOUS CLINICAL SETTINGS

The response to red blood cell transfusion varies from patient to patient. In the absence of increased red blood cell destruction or sequestration, 1 unit of red blood cells can be expected to increase the hemoglobin level by 1 g/dL or the hematocrit level by approximately 3%. This rise is usually not measurable until approximately 24 hours after transfusion, when the plasma volume has had time to return to normal. On the basis of a half-life of approximately 57.7 days for donor red blood cells, Mollison and associates[5] calculated that an average-sized adult requires 24 mL of red blood cells per day to maintain a given hematocrit level, assuming no red blood cell production. Patients with red cell aplasia require approximately 2 units of red blood cells every 2 weeks.

Several factors can adversely affect the survival of transfused red blood cells. Hemolysis, caused by either immune red blood cell damage or mechanical trauma, shortens the survival of transfused cells, much as it shortens the survival of the patient's own cells. Hypersplenism can lead to initial sequestration as well as increased destruction of red blood cells. Continued blood loss is another obvious cause of suboptimal response to transfusion. It should also be emphasized that transfusion suppresses erythropoiesis, so that the net result of transfusion may be less than expected if transfusions are administered on a chronic basis.

Chronic Anemia

As a rule, signs and symptoms attributable to anemia are unlikely to develop at a hemoglobin level of greater than 7 or 8 g/dL. When the anemia is of gradual onset, the body's compensatory mechanisms for maintaining oxygen delivery to the tissues come into play. Both cardiac output and intracellular 2,3-DPG increase, and thus, oxygen unloads at a lower oxygen saturation of hemoglobin. When chronic anemia is due to red blood cell destruction, the healthy bone marrow responds by increasing production up to sixfold.

Red blood cell transfusion is always symptomatic and supportive rather than definitive therapy for anemia. Transfusion should be used only when there is no definitive treatment for the underlying cause, or when the severity of the anemia and the clinical manifestations in the patient make it impossible to wait for the effects of the treatment to be realized.

Generalizations about whether or when to transfuse red blood cells, and how many, are difficult to make and are usually inappropriate. The clinical impact of anemia varies, depending on its pathogenesis, rate of onset, the presence or absence of accompanying hypovolemia, and, most importantly, the individual patient. The hemoglobin level at which a given individual manifests the signs and symptoms of anemia relates, in part, to underlying health status, cardiorespiratory reserve, and activity level.

Perioperative Period

Many generalizations have been made about the appropriate transfusion management of acute blood loss, often with little hard data to support the arguments. One rule of thumb is that blood loss of 10% or less of total blood volume requires no replacement therapy at all; loss of up to 20% can be replaced exclusively with crystalloid solutions; and loss of greater than 25% generally requires red blood cell transfusion to restore oxygen-carrying capacity, along with crystalloid and sometimes colloid solutions to restore intravascular volume to maintain perfusion. For years, the figure of 10 g/dL of hemoglobin had been used as the gold standard for the red blood cell transfusion trigger during the perioperative period, but 7 g/dL is now more commonly used.[41,42]

In the aftermath of transfusion-transmitted human immunodeficiency virus, however, this approach is no longer justified. Each case must be evaluated individually on the basis of clinical signs and symptoms, rather than on the basis of laboratory values. If the cardiovascular system is healthy and the degree of hypoperfusion is not significant, good tissue oxygenation can be maintained at much lower hemoglobin levels. A National Institutes of Health consensus conference suggested that many surgical patients do not need transfusion unless the hemoglobin level falls to less than 7 g/dL.[41] Reexamination of these issues has laid to rest the long-held belief that these lower hemoglobin levels interfere with wound healing or automatically make general anesthesia a risk.

Given that red blood cell transfusion should be tailored to individual needs, the question arises as to whether there is any readily available, objective measurement that can be used to determine how low the hemoglobin level can safely be allowed to fall before red blood cell transfusion is initiated. Several studies of acute normovolemic anemia in rats,[43] dogs,[44] and baboons[45,46] have focused on the whole-body oxygen extraction ratio as an indicator of when to transfuse. These studies make the seemingly valid assumption that the heart is the major organ at risk. With progressive hemodilution, healthy animals with normal coronary arteries were able to maintain normal levels of oxygen consumption through a moderate increase in cardiac output, an increase in coronary blood flow, and a linear increase in the extraction ratio up to 50%. As the hematocrit level fell to less than 10%, however, oxygen consumption began to fall off and the animals were no longer able to increase the extraction ratio enough to compensate for the low oxygen blood tension. An extraction ratio of 50% was found to represent the critical point at which the myocardium converted from aerobic to anaerobic metabolism, reflected in net lactate production. At this point, metabolic acidosis set in, resulting in hemodynamic instability. In a subsequent study, investigators compared the response to acute normovolemic anemia in healthy dogs to the response in dogs with critical coronary stenosis and found that both groups converted to anaerobic metabolism and went into congestive heart failure at an extraction ratio greater than 50%, but that an extraction ratio greater than 50% occurred at a hematocrit level of 17.0% in the dogs with critical stenosis, compared with a hematocrit level of 8.6% in the healthy group.[47] On the basis of these studies, it seems reasonable to extrapolate to humans and to suggest that the extraction ratio, if it were readily obtainable from standard hemodynamic monitoring devices, could be used to help assess transfusion need and that an extraction ratio of 50% might be a useful red blood cell transfusion trigger, because it appears to be a valid indicator of marginal myocardial oxygen reserve in both healthy persons and individuals with coronary artery disease. A limited number of studies have addressed the usefulness of the extraction ratio as a transfusion trigger in humans. One study monitored the oxygen extraction ratio in patients undergoing CABG and found that an extraction ratio of 45% or more could act as a safe transfusion trigger and allow a reduction in allogeneic blood transfusion.[48]

Clinical studies within the last 10 years make this issue even more confusing. Physicians have used a hemoglobin value of 10 g/dL for many years as a convenient transfusion trigger. A recent randomized controlled trial compared a liberal transfusion strategy with hemoglobin maintained at 10 to 12 with a restrictive hemoglobin value of 7 to 8 for critically ill patients. The study showed that patients with the lower hemoglobin values did better than the patients who underwent transfusion with the liberal indication.[49] On the other hand, a retrospective analysis of a large cohort of elderly patients with acute myocardial infarction showed that patients with a hematocrit level less than 33% who subsequently underwent transfusion had a lower mortality rate when measured at 30 days.[50]

The possibility of immunomodulation by allogeneic transfusions in humans was first suggested more than 30 years ago when improved renal allograft survival was reported in pretransplant transfusion recipients.[51] A potential link between allogeneic transfusion and an increased rate of cancer recurrence and postoperative infection was first raised in the 1980s, and numerous retrospective and prospective observational studies supporting these contentions have been reported in the literature since that time. These studies, as well as reports from investigations with opposing data, have been analyzed in numerous reviews on the topic.[52–55] Studies in experimental animals have also yielded contradictory results. Research using animal models and human subjects on the specific immunomodulatory effects of transfusion has consistently pointed to depression of cell-mediated immunity, although the specific defects seen have varied.[56,57] The mediators of these immunomodulatory effects appear to be leukocytes present in cellular blood components, including whole blood and red blood cells.[53] Several well-designed, prospective, randomized controlled trials have been conducted comparing transfusion with leukoreduced blood components or autologous blood to transfusion with unmodified allogeneic blood components. On the basis of previous reports and the apparent pathogenesis of the immunomodulation, it was predicted that the recipients of leukoreduced blood or autologous blood would have a significantly lower risk of immunomodulation. However, the results of these studies have also varied, and controversy continues.[58]

In the debate concerning leukoreduction, some experts believe that the medical benefit has been demonstrated for many recipients and suggest that the technology be applied universally because the only downside is cost.[58] In the absence of data suggesting universal benefit,[59] however, others argue that the technology should be applied selectively to patients who will clearly benefit. Although it is generally agreed that leukoreduced red blood cells will lower the risk of febrile, nonhemolytic transfusion reactions, lower the risk of cell-associated viral infections, such as cytomegalovirus, and reduce the risk of alloimmunization, it is not clear whether patients without specific indications will benefit. A large randomized study showed no benefits to patients without specific indications in a short-term analysis.[60] The long-term benefits of universal leukoreduction and the ability of a universal program to avoid transfusion errors are promoted by some experts.[61] Several randomized controlled clinical studies of leukoreduced red blood cells in cardiac surgery have demonstrated decreased mortality in recipients of leukoreduced blood components; perhaps these studies will become the tipping point to universal leukoreduction in the United States.[62–64]

Red Blood Cell Transfusion in Neonates

In neonates, as is often the case with adult patients, it is convenient to consider periodic, small-volume transfusion separately from massive transfusion situations. The trigger for transfusion and the optimal type of component are very different in the two settings. The potential adverse effects may be quite distinct, particularly in infants.

Low-volume red blood cell transfusion is rarely indicated in full-term infants unless acute blood loss has occurred at birth or an intrauterine situation has led to prenatal anemia. In contrast, premature infants are frequent recipients of these transfusions. In the intensive care setting, the premature infant is subjected to frequent blood sampling, and iatrogenic anemia may necessitate transfusion. Anemia of prematurity is also a well-recognized entity, with premature infants having a slightly lower Hb value at birth. In addition, the postnatal decline in Hb occurs earlier and is more pronounced in premature infants.[65] The mechanism for anemia of prematurity appears to involve a relatively lower output of erythropoietin in response to a given degree of anemia.[66] This phenomenon is attributed in part to the fact that the liver, rather than the kidney, is the major site of erythropoietin production in these infants.[67] Although some practitioners have considered this degree of anemia to be physiologic, the benign nature of this condition remains controversial.

Another debate among neonatologists concerns the triggers for red blood cell transfusion, as in what clinical signs and symptoms are valid reflections of poor tissue oxygenation. Congestive heart failure and severe pulmonary disease are generally accepted indications for transfusion, but recurrent apnea, tachypnea, tachycardia, and failure to thrive are also used as transfusion triggers.[65,68] In recent times, the rate of transfusion and the donor exposure rate of premature infants have consistently declined. These changes, however, reflect improvements in patient care (eg, microtesting methods resulting in less iatrogenic blood loss; the use of surfactant resulting in decreases in respiratory distress) and the use of a single unit to supply one infant over a longer period rather than being attributable to changes in the transfusion trigger. The prolonged use of single units has become possible with the advent of the sterile docking technology, which preserves the full shelf-life of the unit of red blood cells, as well as with the accumulating solid evidence that fresh blood is not necessary for low-volume transfusions in neonates, because supernatant potassium and decreased pH are not of concern in this setting.[62,65] Two recent studies have provided additional information about the relative risks and benefits of using restrictive rather than more liberal criteria for very low birth weight infants. One study showed that a liberal transfusion practice resulted in more infants receiving transfusion but conferred little evidence of benefit.[69] The other study showed a lower risk of apnea and major brain injury for the liberal transfusion arm of the study.[70] Therefore, the safest transfusion trigger in the preterm infant still remains unclear and further studies are indicated. Finally, several trials of erythropoietin therapy in premature infants have been undertaken.[71] The administration of relatively high-dose erythropoietin has been shown to raise hemoglobin levels and reticulocyte counts in healthy premature infants, but the effect in sicker neonates is unclear. Although transfusion exposure was decreased, the significance of this observation is diminished, given the promise of new strategies for limiting transfusions and donor exposure. Therefore, the high cost of erythropoietin treatment and the increased risk of retinopathy associated with erythropoietin treatment may not be justified in this patient population.[72,73]

In the case of massive transfusion, the situation differs, with marked increases in transfusion in recent years in full-term as well as premature infants. Despite the decline in Rh hemolytic disease of the newborn, this disease remains a prominent indication for exchange transfusion. The two triggers for exchange are (a) rapidly rising levels of unconjugated bilirubin that may lead to kernicterus and permanent central nervous system damage and (b) congestive heart failure secondary to severe anemia. Exchange transfusion is especially beneficial in cases of hemolytic disease of the newborn because it clears the bilirubin and the offending antibody from the circulation and removes antibody-coated red blood cells before lysis, while providing a source of red blood cells lacking the offending antigen. A two-blood-volume exchange is commonly performed by using a fresh unit of blood concentrated to a final hematocrit level of approximately 50%. In cases of hyperbilirubinemia resulting from other causes (eg, that associated with liver immaturity in premature infants), phototherapy is the treatment of choice because its effects are usually more sustained, and exchange transfusion is used only for cases of marked elevations.[74] Extracorporeal membrane oxygenation and open-heart surgery are two other situations in which the neonate may be exposed to large volumes of allogeneic red blood cells. The extracorporeal membrane oxygenation circuit requires a prime with red blood cells, as do many of the types of extracorporeal circuits used for cardiopulmonary bypass.[74]

Although accumulating evidence supports the safety of using red blood cell units of any age and with any preservative solution for low-volume transfusions in neonates, the same transfusion policies may not apply to massive transfusion. Newborn physiology is unique in several ways that may have implications for massive transfusion therapy. The newborn does not handle metabolites in a mature fashion. Renal immaturity may lead to problems in clearing potassium or acid from stored red blood cells, and the immature liver may not catabolize citrate efficiently. These problems are accentuated and protracted in the premature infant. To address the concern about potassium load, fresh (<5 days old) or washed red blood cells are often used, although the necessity of this practice is actively debated.[75,76] Fresh blood may also be preferred because of its higher 2,3-DPG levels and better red blood cell integrity. The citrate problem is probably best handled by using slow infusion rates, because the use of bicarbonate or calcium replacement to counteract the acid load or calcium-chelating effects of citrate is controversial. Finally, the use of red blood cells stored in the newer preservative solutions (CPDA-1, Adsol, Nutricel, Opitsol) is avoided by some authorities because of the risk of renal damage and renal stones due to adenine metabolites. In addition, the potential toxicity of the various additives is of concern, as is a significant depletion of plasma proteins associated with transfusion of units with additive solutions.[77,78] If CPD red blood cells are not available, the additive solution can be removed and the cells washed. Red blood cells preserved in additive solutions also have a lower hematocrit, which must be taken into account in making calculations for exchange transfusion.[74]

The humoral and cellular immune systems of the neonate are also immature; again, the problem is accentuated in the premature infant with two implications for transfusion therapy. There is a small but real risk of transfusion-induced graft-versus-host disease in premature infants receiving red blood cell transfusions[79] and in the fetus undergoing intrauterine transfusion.[80] Irradiation of red blood cells should be performed in both settings. Another risk of transfusion in low birth weight (<1500 g) premature infants is the development of clinical cytomegalovirus (CMV) infection in infants of cytomegalovirus-seronegative mothers.[81] CMV safe blood, either CMV seronegative or leukoreduced, should be provided to these infants.[82]

ALTERNATIVES TO ALLOGENEIC RED CELL TRANSFUSIONS

There are many alternatives to standard allogeneic red cell transfusions for a patient requiring elective surgery (Table 146–3). Alternatives include banking autologous units before the surgery, acute normovolemic hemodilution, pharmacologic therapies (ie, erythropoietin or fibrinolysis inhibitors), perioperative salvage, virally inactivated donor red cells, or blood substitutes. All options have their own unique benefits and drawbacks. In cases where an emergency transfusion is needed, the first three options would not be available, as they all require significant planning. Only virally inactivated components and red cell substitutes (both of which are still works in progress) would be available for unanticipated transfusion needs.

Autologous Blood Transfusion

Advantages of Autologous Blood Transfusion

The substitution of autologous blood components for those collected from other (allogeneic) donors eliminates transfusion-transmitted diseases such as hepatitis and acquired immunodeficiency syndrome. Immunologic complications related to the transfusion of foreign cells, including hemolysis and febrile reactions to white blood cells, are also prevented. Other advantages, though possible, are less clearly established. For example, erythropoiesis may be sufficiently stimulated in the repeatedly bled autologous donor to hasten recovery from postoperative anemia.[83] Intraoperatively salvaged red blood cells are spared the acquired membrane defects ("storage lesion") and 2,3-diphosphoglycerate deficiency of refrigerated allogeneic cells.[84] Some investigators believe that allogeneic blood transfusions may contribute to immunosuppression in the recipient[85] and therefore to an increased risk of cancer dissemination[86] whereas autologous blood should not. However, a randomized trial of autologous versus allogeneic blood transfusion in patients with colon cancer was unable to detect any differences in prognosis, thereby disputing the contribution to immunosuppression by allogeneic blood.[87]

An important drawback to these techniques is their increased expense, in contrast to the simpler allogeneic transfusions they replace.[88] In addition, the availability of autologous components may result in their use in situations where transfusion might not have otherwise been considered.[89] Patients with suboptimal compensatory erythropoiesis and donation-induced anemia at the time of surgery are also more likely to be given transfusions.

Some patients and their families ask for directed blood donations, hoping to select blood donors that are known to them and presumably have less risk. This practice has not been shown to have any medical benefit, may cause reduced or delayed blood availability, and should not be considered a worthwhile transfusion alternative.

Preoperative Autologous Blood Collection

The typical volunteer allogeneic blood donor is allowed to give 1 unit of blood no more than once every 8 weeks, to prevent iron deficiency. However, provided that bone marrow erythropoiesis can be stimulated and satisfactory iron supplies maintained, blood can be collected as frequently as once a week from an autologous donor.[90] Although the shelf-life of refrigerated red blood cells is limited to 42 days, frozen storage for up to 10 years is possible at less than −65°C, using glycerol as a cryopreservative.

From a cardiovascular standpoint, phlebotomy is well tolerated by a variety of seemingly high-risk donors, including the elderly,[91] children,[92] pregnant women,[93] and patients with coronary artery disease.[94] By contrast, anemia frequently develops during the donation interval and limits the number of autologous units that can be collected. In addition to marginal iron stores, erythropoietin levels often do not increase during the donation interval, probably because the hematocrit level of most donors is not allowed to fall to less than 30%.[95] This situation may be improved by the administration to autologous donors of the recombinant growth hormone erythropoietin.[96] Common indications for autologous blood donation are listed in Table 146–4. The use of preoperatively donated autologous blood

Table 146–3 Alternatives to Standard Allogeneic Transfusions

Hemodilution
Intraoperative autologous transfusion
Perioperative blood salvage
Lower transfusion trigger
Pharmacologic therapies
Viral inactivation
Red Cell Substitutes

Table 146–4 Common Indications for Autologous Blood Techniques

Surgical/Obstetric Procedures	Preoperative Donations	Perioperative Salvage
Intraabdominal vascular procedures	Yes	Yes*
Open heart surgery	Yes	Yes*
Total hip replacement	Yes	Yes†
Total knee replacement	Yes	Yes‡
Scoliosis repairs	Yes*	Yes
Radical prostatectomy	Yes	Yes§
Placenta previa	Yes	No*
Multiple gestations	Yes	No*

*The safety of blood containing amniotic fluid has not been conclusively established.

†The need for postoperative salvage has not been conclusively established.

‡Intraoperative salvage is unnecessary when a tourniquet technique is used; postoperative salvage may be of value when procedure is performed without cement.

§The risk of cancer spread after transfusion of intraoperatively salvaged blood has not been established.

Adapted from Kruskall MS: On measuring the success of an autologous blood donation program [editorial]. Transfusion 31:481, 1991.

Table 146–5 Autologous Blood Salvage Systems*

Characteristics of Collected Blood							
System	*Hardware*	*Software*	*Hematocrit*	*Free Hemoglobin*	*Platelet Count*	*Coagulation Factors*	*Fibrin Degradation Products*
Collection without washing	Rigid plastic container	Plastic bag	Low (25%)	Very high (200 mg%)	Low (100,000/mm³)	Low (35%–75%)	High (300 mg%)
Collection followed by washing	Integral or separate blood cell processor	Disposable plastic bowl and tubing	High (60%)	Low (<50 mg%)	Very low (10,000/mm³)	Absent (0%)	Absent (0%)

*Typical results of laboratory tests are shown. Transfusion of large volumes of salvaged blood results in similar alterations in these tests in the recipient. Data from Noon GP: Intraoperative autotransfusion. Surgery 84:719, 1978; and Silva R, Moore EE, Bar-Or D, et al: The risk: benefit ratio of autotransfusion-comparison to banked blood in a canine model. J Trauma 24:557, 1984.

has also been reported for a variety of other surgical procedures, including radical prostatectomy; hysterectomies and other gynecologic procedures; colorectal, biliary, and gastric surgery; and neurosurgery.[97]

Autologous blood has been safely collected from women during pregnancy for use during childbirth. Nevertheless, the transfusion rate at delivery is quite low (<2.5% in many institutions)[98] and most autologous donations are unused. Long-term (frozen) storage of autologous red blood cells in the absence of a planned transfusion episode is largely ineffective and expensive.

Intraoperative Blood Salvage

Interest in salvaging blood shed at surgery has been stimulated by the introduction of automated instruments for autologous blood salvage over the past 30 years. Systems for blood collection without processing are usually modifications of disposable suction devices (Table 146–5). Blood is collected under low vacuum pressure into a plastic bag seated within a hard outer canister. An anticoagulant such as citrate can be added. As soon as the bag is full, or within 4 hours of the start of collection (to prevent bacterial overgrowth), the contents of the bag are reinfused into the patient by gravity without any washing or further processing, except passage through a standard blood filter.

Alternatively, the contents in the bag can be washed to remove free hemoglobin, surgical irrigant solutions, and other debris. Although this step is theoretically attractive and increasingly popular, its necessity before reinfusion of shed blood has not been established.[99] Instruments that include both a reservoir for collecting salvaged blood and a centrifugal washer have been developed. Large aliquots (>500 mL) can be fully washed in as little as 3 minutes. As a result of this speed, autologous blood salvage has become practical in situations in which blood loss may be extremely rapid, such as trauma or liver transplantation.

The hematocrit level of unwashed blood is typically low because of dilution from irrigating surgical fluids and some degree of mechanical hemolysis. Free hemoglobin levels are sometimes greater than 1000 mg% in unwashed blood, and hemoglobinemia and hemoglobinuria may occur after the transfusion, although renal sequelae are surprisingly low.[99] Despite this evidence of red blood cell injury, the survival rate of ^{51}Cr-labeled salvaged cells is normal in most patients studied.[100]

Transfusion of salvaged blood has resulted in coagulation abnormalities, including hypofibrinogenemia, prolonged prothrombin time and partial thromboplastin time, elevated fibrin degradation products, and thrombocytopenia.[101] These coagulation abnormalities most likely reflect the characteristics of the salvaged blood itself, which, after exposure to serosal surfaces, becomes deficient in coagulation factors and platelets and, in the case of unwashed blood, has high levels of fibrin degradation products (see Table 146–4).[102]

Fat, fibrin, bone fragments, and microaggregates often contaminate salvaged autologous blood. However, infusion of unwashed blood has not been proved harmful in either animals or humans, possibly because routine blood filters remove most particulate material.[103] Other contaminants, such as heparin, topical antibiotics, hemostatic agents, and biologic substances such as tissue enzymes, can be at least partially removed by washing.[104,105] Complete removal of bacteria is also not possible, even when the salvaged blood is washed with antibiotics. Thus, collection of blood from a contaminated site (eg, with intestinal contents) is usually considered to be contraindicated. Tumor cells have also been found in blood salvaged during cancer operations and many practitioners consider cancer another contraindication.[105]

Approximately one-half the blood lost during surgery can be salvaged. The rest is usually irretrievably absorbed in drapes and sponges or damaged during collection. The use of salvaged autologous blood has been associated with a 50% reduction in allogeneic blood use in orthopedic procedures such as spinal surgery[106] and hip replacement[107] and is also effective in vascular surgical procedures such as aortic reconstruction.[108] Autologous salvage has been a useful adjunct in the treatment of some Jehovah's Witnesses, whose literal acceptance of the Bible includes abstention from routine allogeneic blood transfusions.[109]

Both the canister systems and red blood cell processors used to collect intraoperative autologous blood can also be employed to collect postoperative blood drainage, such as that from the mediastinum after open heart surgery,[110] from the knee or hip after orthopedic procedures,[111] or from the peritoneal cavity after hepatic injury.[112] Because blood salvaged from a serosal cavity has little residual fibrinogen and platelets, clotting is not a problem, and the addition of anticoagulants is usually unnecessary.[113] Shed mediastinal blood after open-heart surgery contains high levels of cardiac muscle enzymes, especially creatine kinase, as well as lactate dehydrogenase from hemolyzed red blood cells.[114,115] Therefore, reinfusion of shed blood results in elevated levels of both enzymes, which can confound the diagnosis of myocardial infarction in the postoperative period.[116,117] Reinfusion of shed mediastinal blood has been shown to reduce the need for allogeneic transfusions.[118]

Hemodilution

The collection of autologous blood during surgery for later reinfusion at the end of the procedure was first suggested in open-heart operations, in which it was hoped that a supply of platelets undamaged by exposure to the membrane oxygenator might reduce the incidence of coagulopathies.[119] Hemodilution itself reduces red blood cell loss: a patient with a hematocrit level of 45% and 2 L blood loss during surgery loses roughly 900 mL of red blood cells, but one with a hematocrit level of 20% from hemodilution loses only 400 mL of red blood cells. Hemodilution is probably less expensive to accomplish than preoperative autologous blood donation and may be the only option available when surgery is performed in other than elective settings.[120] Proponents claim that the induced anemia may even be beneficial to the patient, in that oxygen delivery at a hematocrit level of 30% is enhanced by an increased cardiac output resulting from the decreased blood viscosity.[121]

Reductions in allogeneic blood needs have been reported after marked intraoperative hemodilution (after the hematocrit is lowered by 50%).[122] More modest hemodilution (eg, removal of 2 U of blood at the beginning of surgery) is also beneficial, according to some investigators.[123,124] but not others.[125,126] Furthermore, one group has provided evidence that hemodilution may jeopardize patients at risk of ischemic myocardial injury. More research is needed to establish the safety and ideal protocols for this form of blood conservation. The availability of blood substitutes may facilitate augmented hemodilution for some patients who are expected to have large volumes of blood loss or who refuse blood transfusions.

BLOOD SUBSTITUTES

The search for blood substitutes began when our early scientific ancestors tested alternatives to human blood, including animal blood, milk, and wine. Modern research into the use of animal blood includes the work by Amberson et al, who reported the successful use of a bovine hemosylate for exchange transfusions in cats and dogs.[127] Further work revealed that human and bovine hemosylates caused renal dysfunction in human recipients. The suspected cause of this nephrotoxicity was the stromal lipid component of the RBC membrane.[128,129] The logical next step in the search for the ideal substitute was the development of stroma-free hemoglobin (hemoglobin tetramer). Unfortunately, in 1978 Savitsky et al demonstrated renal dysfunction, hypertension, and abdominal pain using stroma-free hemoglobin (Hb) in healthy volunteers.[130] It was hypothesized that these adverse events were due to the instability of the hemoglobin tetramer. Since then, efforts have been made to produce stabilized products with desirable oxygen off-loading characteristics and extended intravascular retention times.

Today, the US blood supply is safe and has sufficient capacity to meet most patient needs. There is room for considerable improvement, however, in supply levels and risk reduction. The gap between a shrinking donor pool (owing to willingness and/or ability) and increasing transfusion requirements of an aging population continues to narrow. The threat of new and emerging infections results in the vulnerability of human-derived oxygen carriers. Recent battles against West Nile virus and variant Creutzfeldt–Jakob disease underscore the risk of a tainted blood supply and depletion of transfusion resources. Theoretically, the ideal red cell substitute would solve both of these issues (Table 146–6). There have been many attempts to develop red cell substitutes in the past, but no product has been able to fulfill all of the above criteria or meet the Food and Drug Administration's requirements of purity, potency, and safety.

Table 146–6 The Ideal Red Cell Substitute

Delivers oxygen (and maybe enhances delivery)
Does not transmit disease
Does not have immunosuppressive effects
Available in abundant supply
Universally compatible (no need to type and crossmatch)
Prolonged shelf-life and stable at a range of temperatures
Similar in vivo half-life to the red blood cell
Available at a reasonable cost
Easy to administer
Able to access all areas of the human body (including ischemic tissue)
Effective on room air or ambient conditions

TYPES OF RED CELL SUBSTITUTES

It is important to differentiate between "blood substitutes" and red cell substitutes. Red cell substitutes are oxygen carriers and do not replace all components and functions of blood, for example, coagulation factors and white blood cells. There are three categories of oxygen carriers that show promise as red blood cell substitutes: perfluorocarbons, hemoglobin-based oxygen carriers (HBOC), and engineered red blood cells.

Perfluorocarbons

Perfluorocarbons (PFC) are chemically and biologically inert artificial fluorinated organic fluids that are immiscible in water and have a high solubility for oxygen. The amount of dissolved oxygen in PFC is directly related to the ambient oxygen tension—unlike Hb; gas molecules are not chemically bound to PFC, but are absorbed and released by simple diffusion.[131] Oxygent (Alliance Corp, San Diego, CA) is a second-generation concentrated PFC emulsion based on perflubron (perfluorooctyl bromide; $C_8F_{17}Br$) with a shelf-life of up to 2 years. It requires oxygen inhalation by the patient, as the oxygen delivery capacity is less than 30% of normal blood. A large European multicenter phase III study has shown that Oxygent in conjunction with acute normovolemic hemodilution (ANH) reduced the need for RBC transfusion in 492 patients undergoing major noncardiac surgery.[132] However, a phase III trial studying Oxygent in patients undergoing cardiopulmonary bypass was terminated in the United States because of a possible increase in stroke rates in the Oxygent treatment arm. Although some PFC are still being investigated, there are no major trials ongoing in the United States. Perftoran, a perfluorocarbon approved for clinical use in Russia and Mexico, has been shown to be safe in a study of cardiac surgery patients who received Perftoran along with acute normovolemic hemodilution. The patients who received Perftoran had higher arterial oxygen levels and received less allogeneic transfusions than the patients who just underwent hemodilution.[133]

Hemoglobin-Based Oxygen Carriers

The stroma of the red cell causes many of the problems in allogeneic human red cell transfusions. The red cell membrane ultimately fails and limits the shelf-life. The red cell membrane also contains the antigens that limit compatibility. Unfortunately, initial efforts to develop HBOC that focused on unmodified Hb failed—unmodified tetramers naturally dissociate into dimers outside of the RBC. This unmodified tetrameric Hb is associated with renal toxicities, gastrointestinal effects, and vasoconstriction.

The HBOC currently in clinical development are stroma-free and engineered to produce desirable oxygen dissociation characteristics as well as an adequate in vivo half-life with minimal toxicities. Stroma-free Hb has a very high oxygen affinity compared with native Hb in an RBC because of a lack of 2,3-diphosphoglycerate (DPG). Furthermore, the Hb tetramer is such a small molecule that the kidney rapidly removes it.

Four different methods have been suggested to avoid toxicities: stabilization, polymerization, conjugation, and Hb vesicles. Hb can be stabilized using an alpha-chain cross-linker (Diaspirin Cross-Linked Hb); this approach was pursued by Baxter Healthcare (Deerfield, IL). The second approach, polymerization, involves intermolecular cross-linking of tetramers to increase intravascular retention time. Polymerization with agents such as glutaraldehyde not only increases the molecular size of the molecule but also increases Hb concentration and decreases oncotic pressure. This approach is being pursued by Northfield Laboratories (Evanston, IL). Conjugation involves the binding of a larger molecule, such as polyethylene glycol or dextran, potentially allowing the Hb-conjugate to remain in the vasculature longer due to its increased size. Conjugation is being attempted by Sangart (San Diego, CA). A drawback of conjugation is an increased viscosity compared to normal blood.[134] The final approach, Hb vesicles, uses liposome-encapsulated Hb to mimic the actual red blood cell. The Hb molecule is inserted into a lipid membrane derived from natural lecithins or synthetic phospholipids. These products have an effective oxygen delivery system, high Hb concentration and should be stable during storage with a plasma half-life of 4 to 20 hours without risk of renal toxicity; however, they have a tendency toward methemoglobin formation. Although Hb vesicles appear to be an attractive option, there are no clinical trials with these products at the current time.

HBOC can be prepared from different Hb sources. Human Hb probably would not alleviate supply concerns, because the amount of outdated human blood is likely to be inadequate to make large supplies of HBOC. Bovine Hb has been used as a source of Hb because of its naturally low oxygen affinity and its ability to be directly polymerized (to avoid renal excretion) without prior manipulation. Bovine Hb has a molecular structure similar to human Hb but has enhanced oxygen unloading in ischemic tissue. Unlike human Hb, which is regulated by 2,3-DPG, the affinity of bovine Hb is partially regulated by serum chloride ions.[135] Although this product removes the constraint of using human donated red blood cells, there are uncertainties about using bovine Hb because of its potential to transmit disease (eg, bovine spongiform encephalopathy) and its potential immunogenicity. Biopure Corp (Cambridge, MA) has pursued the commercial development of a bovine HBOC.

Researchers have explored two options for recombinant sources of Hb. There is a hybrid Hb product which is a synthetic heme bound to recombinant human serum albumin. This product has a similar p50 to human red blood cell Hb and has an intravascular circulation time of greater than 36 hours in rats.[136] The second alternative, which was pursued by Somatogen, is completely recombinant Hb molecules. These products are either developed in microorganisms (*Escherichia coli*, yeast) or in transgenic plants or animals. A first-generation product developed in *E coli* was discontinued because of vasoconstrictive effects in animals. Harvesting of the human Hb and purification techniques still require major improvement, and scaling up research methods to make an adequate supply of clinical material will be a significant hurdle. At the current time, recombinant Hb is still within preclinical development.

HBOC are a work in progress, but several shortcomings have emerged across the class. Although molecular size has increased to the point where it is not immediately removed by the kidney, the molecules are still seen as foreign in the recipient and quickly cleared by the reticuloendothelial system. The plasma half-life is generally 24 hours or less, thus unlikely to have a role in patients with chronic anemia. In addition, free Hb is a scavenger of nitric oxide (NO); because NO plays a key role in vasomotor control, specifically vasodilation, its removal by Hb results in a vasoconstrictive effect leading to hypertension (systemic and pulmonary).

Three HBOC products remain in advanced clinical development (Fig. 146–1): Hemopure (Biopure Corp, Cambridge, MA), Hemospan (Sangart, San Diego, CA), and Polyheme (Northfield Laboratories, Evanston, IL). All three products have recently faced significant challenges in proving their safety and efficacy in late phase clinical trials.[137]

Engineered Red Blood Cells

Owing to the difficulty of finding compatible red blood cells in patients who become alloimmunized as a result of frequent transfusions, there have been efforts to create universal donor red blood cells. Two approaches have been proposed to attain this goal. Covalent binding of polyethylene glycol masks red cell antigens. Alternatively, red cell antigens can be enzymatically removed by exoglycosidase treatment, which has only been partially successful thus far. The strategy of an engineered red blood cell, though still in its infancy, does not address concerns such as limited supply, storage limitations, and disease transmission.

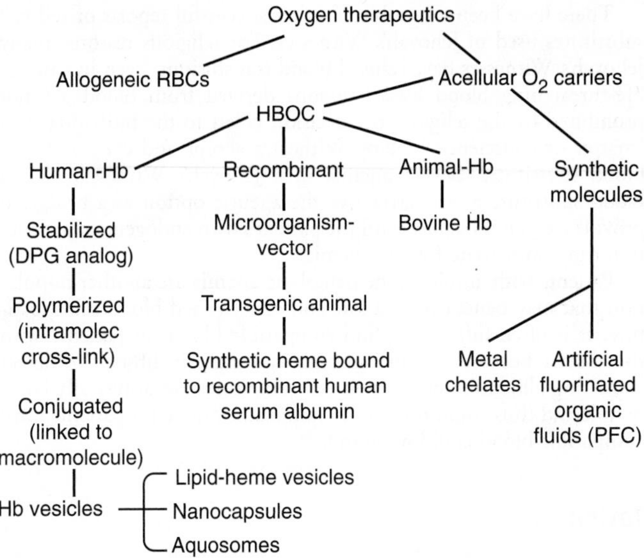

Figure 146–1 Three HBOC products remain in advanced clinical development: Hemopure (Biopure Corporation, Cambridge, MA), Hemospan (Sangart, San Diego, CA), and Polyheme (Northfield Laboratories, Evanston, IL).

Potential Clinical Applications

Red blood cell substitutes have many potential applications. One of the most compelling would be use for resuscitation during military and civilian traumas. In developing a specific plan to avoid the consequences of blood unavailability after national disasters involving large-scale injuries, blood substitutes could play a key role as an immediate treatment option. In addition to these acute emergency situations, there is a wide range of less urgent applications where oxygen carriers might provide a viable solution to difficult situations, including augmenting perioperative hemodilution, transfusion of patients who refuse human blood components because of religious beliefs, transfusion of patients with rare blood types or antibodies to high incidence antigens, organ preservation for transplant surgery, and transfusion in patients with autoimmune hemolytic anemia in whom it is difficult to detect underlying antibodies.

One of the most promising roles for red cell substitutes is to avoid transfusion of donor red cells, especially when compatible red blood cells are not available. Other roles include use as a volume expander or resuscitative fluid, as well as clinical situations where tissue oxygenation is needed but the tissues do not have access to red blood cells. An example of this attractive potential indication for the use of red blood cell substitutes is to target tissue ischemia, with specific focus on vital organs. Another application that has been studied in both preclinical and clinical studies is the use of red cell substitutes to increase tumor Po_2 levels to enhance sensitivity to radiation and chemotherapy.[138,139] Finally, preclinical studies using red cell substitutes to preserve tissues and prolong the storage time of an organ prior to transplantation have been conducted.[140]

Patients with hemoglobinopathies comprise a unique population that might receive added benefits from red cell substitutes versus donor red cells. These patients tend to be chronically transfused and also seem to be at a higher risk for becoming alloimmunized per unit transfused compared to the general population.[141] The universal compatibility of red cell substitutes would be ideal to protect these patients from further alloimmunization and the risks of delayed hemolytic transfusion reactions. In addition, the availability of blood for sickle cell patients requiring phenotyped RBCs would be improved. Red cell substitutes could be useful as urgent therapy for acute chest syndrome or other emergency vasoocclusive events until compatible blood is found.

There have been a number of other successful reports of red cell substitutes used in Jehovah's Witnesses. For religious reasons, many Jehovah's Witnesses have refused blood transfusions, even in cases of life-threatening blood loss. Fractions derived from blood are not prohibited by the religion; the decision is left to the individual as a "matter of conscience." Many Witnesses accept and even seek out blood substitutes. Severe anemia in a Jehovah's Witness makes a blood substitute a very attractive therapeutic option as a bridge to provide oxygen transport until the patient's own endogenous production can compensate for the anemia.

Patients with autoimmune hemolytic anemia are another population that may benefit from a safe and effective red blood cell substitute. It is often difficult to find compatible blood for patients with this disease because the autoantibody can make it difficult to detect coexisting alloantibodies.[142] Red cell substitutes are universally compatible and thus could become an important bridge for patients until compatible blood could be found.[143]

Toxicities

The safety of red cell substitutes remains a serious concern. Although cross-linking and polymerizing Hb subunits have reduced the incidence of nephrotoxicity, problems with vasoconstriction and pressor effects have not been completely eliminated. Vasoconstrictive responses, including increased systemic and pulmonary arterial pressures, are thought to result from the binding of nitric oxide to Hb. Hb interaction and scavenging of nitric oxide is also thought to play a role in some gastrointestinal effects of the products, such as dysphagia.[144]

The complications of red cell substitutes in septic patients are not known. Cell-free Hb substances may support bacterial virulence by offering a ready supply of iron, thus sustaining bacterial replication and inhibiting neutrophil function.[145] Although animal data has been suggestive of a potential clinical problem, clinical trials to date have not established this risk.

The immunogenicity of HBOC is still being studied. Because the modified human hemoglobins have been chemically changed it may be possible for them to trigger an immune response in humans. Bovine Hb has an even greater chance of causing immunogenicity in humans, because of its substantial differences from the protein structure of human Hb. To date, no serious immune or allergic responses have been reported, but most patients have only had single-incident exposures to these products, usually over short periods of time. Animal studies by manufacturers have not demonstrated a problem.

The Future of Red Cell Substitutes

Proving the benefit of red cell substitutes in clinical trials has not been easy for a number of reasons. First, in order to reduce use of donor red blood cells, we must prove that the risks presented by HBOC or PFC are not greater than those of blood transfusions. This fact has not yet been established. Second, without specific transfusion triggers or guidelines, it is difficult to establish whether a transfusion has actually been avoided. Finally, the goal of reducing transfusion-related expenses may not be achievable because HBOC are likely to initially be very expensive.

Red cell substitutes have a promising value proposition for transfusion services—increase the availability of blood components and remove donor and contamination safety risks. Existing products suffer from critical shortcomings (in vivo half-life) that make them more suitable for short-term gaps (eg, acute blood loss, ischemia, bridge until compatible red cells become available) than long-term solutions. Substitutes not based on human blood introduce potentially more complex safety hurdles, such as immunogenicity and fear of prion contamination in bovine-derived products.

SUGGESTED READINGS

Ansell J, Parrilla N, King M, et al: Survival of autotransfused red blood cells recovered from the surgical field during cardiovascular operations. J Thorac Cardiovasc Surg 84:387, 1982.

Blajchman MA: Transfusion immunomodulation or TRIM: What does it mean clinically? Hematology 10(Suppl 1):208, 2005.

Dzik WH, Anderson JC, O'Neill EM, et al: A prospective, randomized clinical trial of universal WBC reduction. Transfusion 42:1114, 2002.

Goodnough LT, Rudnick S, Price TH, et al: Increased preoperative collection of autologous blood with recombinant human erythropoietin: A controlled trial. N Engl J Med 321:1163, 1989.

Hebert PC, Wells G, Blajchman MA, et al: A multicenter, randomized controlled clinical trial of transfusion requirements in critical care. N Engl J Med 340:409, 1999.

King KE, Ness PM: Treatment of Autoimmune Hemolytic Anemia. Semin Hematol 42:131, 2005.

Klein HG: Transfusion-associated graft-versus-host disease: Less fresh blood and more gray (Gy) for an aging population. Transfusion 46:878, 2006.

Meryman HT, Hornblower M: A method for freezing and washing red blood cells using high glycerol concentration. Transfusion 12:145, 1972.

Ness PM, Bourke DL, Walsh PC: A randomized trial of perioperative hemodilution versus transfusion of preoperatively deposited autologous blood in elective surgery. Transfusion 32:226, 1992.

NIH Consensus Conference: Perioperative red blood cell transfusion. JAMA 260:2700, 1988.

Paglino JC, Pomper GJ, Fisch GS, et al.: Reduction of febrile but not allergic reactions to RBCs and platelets after conversion to universal prestorage leukoreduction. Transfusion 44(1):16, 2004.

Ress PM, Cushing MM: Oxygen therapeutics: Pursuit of an alternative to the donor red blood cell. Arch Pathol Lab Med 131:734, 2007.

Schmidt H, Mortensen PE, Folsgarrd SL, Jensen EA: Autotransfusion after coronary artery bypass grafting halves the number of patients needing blood transfusion. Ann Thorac Surg 61:1177, 1996.

Sehgal LR, Sebala LP, Takagi I, Curran RD, et al: Evaluation of oxygen extraction ratio as a physiologic transfusion trigger in coronary artery bypass graft surgery patients. Transfusion 41(5):591, 2001.

Tinmouth A, Fergusson D, Yee IC, Hebert PC: Clinical consequences of red cell storage in the critically ill. Transfusion 46:2014, 2006.

TRAP Study Group: Leukocytic reduction and ultraviolet B irradiation of platelets to prevent alloimmunization and refractoriness to platelet transfusions. N Engl J Med 337:1861, 1997.

Vamvakas EC: Pneumonia as a complication of blood product transfusion in the critically ill: Transfusion-related immunomodulation (TRIM). Crit Care Med 343:S151, 2006.

Vyas GN, Holmdahl L, Perkins HA, Fudenberg HH: Serologic specificity of human anti-IgA and its significance in transfusion. Blood 34:573, 1969.

REFERENCES

For complete list of references log onto www.expertconsult.com

CHAPTER 147

PRINCIPLES OF PLATELET TRANSFUSION THERAPY

Aleksandar Babic and Richard M. Kaufman

PLATELET COLLECTION AND MANUFACTURING

Platelet products are either prepared from whole blood donations (platelet concentrates), or are collected by apheresis (single donor platelets, SDPs). In the United States, whole blood-derived platelet concentrates are made using the platelet-rich plasma (PRP) method. First, a whole blood unit is separated by gentle centrifugation (slow spin) into red cells and PRP. The PRP is then centrifuged a second time (hard spin) to isolate one platelet concentrate plus one unit of plasma. Each platelet concentrate contains approximately 5.5×10^{10} platelets suspended in a plasma volume of approximately 50 mL. In Europe and Canada, the alternate buffy coat method is used to produce platelet concentrates. Platelets are stored at room temperature under continuous gentle agitation for up to 5 days. (Seven-day platelet storage is permissible under certain conditions, discussed in Infections Risks.) To prepare an adult dose of platelets for transfusion, four to six platelet concentrates are pooled together.

Apheresis platelet units are collected from a single platelet donor by continuous flow centrifugation using an automated device. A high volume of whole blood is processed through the machine, and the platelets are retained in a sterile collection bag. By AABB standards, an apheresis platelet unit should contain a minimum of 3×10^6 platelets,[1] a dose that is approximately equivalent to six pooled platelet concentrates. Current devices actually allow many different combinations of blood products to be collected during a single apheresis donation, such as a unit of platelets plus a unit of RBCs. Apheresis platelet units generally contain less than 1×10^6 white blood cells per unit; thus they meet the current AABB definition for leukoreduced blood products ($<5 \times 10^6$ WBCs/unit).[1] Although apheresis platelets cost more to produce than whole blood derived platelet concentrates, they have become increasingly popular. In the United States in 2004, approximately 1.4 million therapeutic doses of platelets were provided as apheresis platelets, and only 256,000 doses were administered as whole blood-derived platelet concentrates.[2,3]

Apheresis platelets provide some (limited) advantages over whole blood-derived platelet concentrates. Radiolabeling studies indicate that apheresis platelets circulate longer in vivo than pooled concentrates,[4] most likely reflecting gentler handling and less platelet activation during collection. Recipients of apheresis platelets are exposed to fewer donors per transfusion (one donor versus six as with a pool of platelet concentrates), so in principle apheresis platelets should pose a lower risk of viral transmission than whole blood-derived platelets. However, given that the per unit transfusion-transmission risks for HIV and Hepatitis C Virus have been cut to approximately 1 in 2,000,000,[5] the actual safety advantage of apheresis platelets over whole blood-derived platelets is small. Data from surveillance culture studies do suggest that apheresis platelets may be less likely than platelet concentrates to become contaminated with bacteria.[6] At one time, it was predicted that apheresis platelets would be less likely than pooled concentrates to provoke platelet alloimmunization, by virtue of exposing recipients to fewer unique donor HLA antigens. This hypothesis was not confirmed empirically, however.[7,8] Although they express surface HLA class I antigens, platelets appear to be rather poor immunogens. HLA alloimmunization to platelets primarily appears to be triggered by contaminating white blood cells within a platelet unit. Thus, alloimmunization is not platelet dose-dependent, and simply providing leukoreduced platelet units prevents most cases of immune-mediated platelet refractoriness.[8]

PROPHYLACTIC PLATELET TRANSFUSION

Today, the vast majority of platelet units are transfused prophylactically, to prevent bleeding in nonbleeding patients rather than to treat active bleeding.[9] Prior to 1960, platelet transfusions were not widely available, and death from hemorrhage was common among patients with leukemia who received chemotherapy. In 1962, Gaydos and colleagues published a seminal study demonstrating a relationship between platelet count and likelihood of bleeding.[10] After this study was published, prophylactic platelet transfusion rapidly became standard practice. Of note, no specific platelet transfusion trigger was suggested by the authors based on their data. Regardless, a platelet count of 20,000/μL was widely adopted as the standard prophylactic platelet transfusion trigger.

Later studies suggested that a lower transfusion trigger would be as effective as a trigger of 20,000/μL. Slichter and Harker, for instance, performed red cell radiolabeling studies in thrombocytopenic patients who were not receiving platelet transfusions. They demonstrated that only patients with platelet counts below 5000/μL had significantly elevated fecal red cell loss.[11] Years later, several clinical studies directly challenged the 20,000/μL trigger. Platelet transfusion triggers of 10,000/μL versus 20,000/μL were compared directly in three randomized prospective studies of patients with acute leukemia.[12–14] All of these studies, as well as large nonrandomized prospective trials,[15,16] demonstrated no increased risk of bleeding when a trigger of 10,000/μL is used. Notably, all of these trials included provisions for transfusing thrombocytopenic patients at platelet counts above 10,000/μL if associated risk factors for bleeding (eg, fever) were present. Although few studies have directly examined prophylactic platelet transfusion in the specific setting of hematopoietic stem cell transplantation (HSCT), the 10,000/μL trigger has been widely applied to the HSCT patient population, and it appears to be safe.[17,18] Clinical factors are usually more important determinants of bleeding risk than the platelet count alone. Approximately two-thirds of bleeding events post-HSCT occur in patients with platelet counts above 20,000/μL.[19,20]

Prophylactic Platelets for Invasive Bedside Procedures

At present, there are no large randomized trials evaluating the need for platelet prophylaxis prior to invasive bedside procedures such as lumbar puncture. However, there exist retrospective data providing reassurance that moderate thrombocytopenia does not pose a serious risk for performing such procedures. Howard et al[21] reviewed the records of 956 consecutive pediatric patients with newly diagnosed acute lymphoblastic leukemia who underwent lumbar puncture. No serious hemorrhagic complications were observed following 5223 lumbar punctures, including 170 procedures that were done when the platelet count was 11,000 to 20,000/μL. The authors concluded that prophylactic platelet transfusion was unnecessary in patients with platelet counts above 10,000/μL. Lumbar punctures were performed in only 29 patients with platelet counts of 10,000/μL or less, making it difficult to assess the risk of bleeding in patients with very low platelet counts. A similar, albeit much smaller retrospective study examined the same issue in adult patients with acute leukemia.[22] No hemorrhagic complications were observed following 195 lumbar punctures, including 35 that were done with a platelet count of 20,000 to 30,000/μL. Finally, for other common bedside procedures such as central venous catheter placement, platelet counts of 20,000 to 30,000/μL are generally considered to be adequate, although again data from prospective studies are unavailable.

Prophylactic Platelets for Major Surgical Procedures

There are currently no data from randomized trials addressing the question of what constitutes an adequate platelet count prior to surgery. Retrospective studies, though, suggest that patients with platelet counts of 50,000/μL or higher are not at excess bleeding risk during surgery. Bishop and colleagues[23] reported a series of 95 patients with acute leukemia who underwent 130 surgical procedures with platelet counts of less than 50,000/μL. Intraoperative blood loss exceeded 500 mL in only 7% of cases. No relationship was seen between the preoperative platelet count and surgical blood loss. These data suggest that prophylactic platelet transfusions need not be administered prior to surgery when the preoperative platelet count is at least 50,000/μL. This rule-of-thumb is thought to apply to most types of surgery (cardiac, orthopedic, etc.). For a few types of surgeries though, requiring a higher platelet count (70,000–100,000/μL) is traditional, although no published data currently exist either to support or refute this approach. These settings include neurosurgery, retinal surgeries, and other procedures where the risk is not that the patient may exsanguinate, but rather that even a minor bleed might cause clinically significant damage in a vulnerable vital structure such as the brain.

Prophylactic Platelet Dosing

Lowering the standard prophylactic platelet transfusion trigger from 20,000/μL to 10,000/μL is believed to have helped conserve the limited supply of platelets in the United States. A complementary approach to lowering the transfusion trigger is altering the dose of prophylactic platelets administered. There are currently thought to be two distinct clearance mechanisms for platelets. Most platelets undergo senescence after circulating in the peripheral blood for 8 to 10 days. But there is also evidence for a second clearance route, in which there is a fixed daily loss of platelets that occurs independent of platelet age. Platelets exiting the circulation via this second route are postulated to function in maintaining vascular integrity.[24] This small fixed daily platelet requirement has been estimated to be 7.1×10^9 platelets/L/day. In principal, a low dose of platelets could be used to meet this daily requirement. Mathematical modeling has suggested that using a low dose (eg, pools of three whole blood-derived platelets versus the current six) would save approximately 22% of prophylactic platelets over time.[25] On the other hand, higher prophylactic platelet doses would be predicted to reduce the total number of transfusion events.[26,27] Randomized trials are now underway that are designed to empirically determine the optimal dosing strategy for prophylactic platelets.[28–30]

THERAPEUTIC PLATELET TRANSFUSION

A small number of studies published in the 1970s and early 1980s suggested the idea of using a purely therapeutic platelet transfusion strategy—transfusing platelets only to treat active bleeding, rather than administering prophylactic platelets in thrombocytopenic patients.[31–33] This concept was revived recently by Wandt and colleagues,[16] who reported a series of 140 hematopoietic stem cell transplants in which no prophylactic platelets were given to clinically stable patients, regardless of platelet count, unless the patient had WHO grade II or higher bleeding. Patients deemed to be clinically unstable (defined as fever >38.5°C, infection or known coagulation factor disorder) were given prophylactic platelet transfusions for platelets less than 10,000/μL. No WHO grade III or IV bleeding was observed. Grade II bleeding was seen in 26 transplants (19%). No clinically relevant bleeding was seen in the remaining 114/140 patients (81%). The first 60 patients in this study were compared to 60 historical controls who were transfused with prophylactic platelets for a platelet count of less than 10,000/μL. The total number of platelets transfused was only 111 in the therapeutic group compared to 237 in the historical control group. Thus the therapeutic strategy was quite effective in this study.

ADVERSE EFFECTS OF PLATELET TRANSFUSION

Infectious Risks

Platelets are associated with the same range of infectious pathogens as any other blood component, but septic transfusion reactions, caused by bacterially contaminated units, comprise a unique risk of platelet transfusion. Over time, improvements in donor screening virtually eliminated the risk of transfusion transmission of hepatitis B virus, hepatitis C virus, and HIV. The risk of septic transfusion reactions remained fairly constant over this same time period, so eventually platelet bacterial contamination became, by default, the most frequent infectious risk of transfusion. Unlike other blood components, which are stored either refrigerated or frozen, platelets are stored at room temperature. The reason is that if platelets are refrigerated prior to transfusion, they are cleared rapidly from the recipient's circulation.[34] Although room temperature storage allows transfused platelets to circulate in vivo, it has the downside of promoting bacterial growth. Because of this risk, platelet storage is ordinarily limited to only 5 days, making platelet inventory management extremely challenging.

In the 1990s, numerous studies demonstrated that contaminating bacteria, usually representing skin flora from the donor, could be cultured out of approximately 1/3,000 platelet units.[35] Clinically apparent septic transfusion reactions were thought to occur following approximately 1/25,000 platelet transfusions, although there is considerable uncertainty around this point estimate.[35] In 2002, an open letter calling for immediate action to reduce the risk of platelet bacterial contamination[36] led to the proposal of AABB standard 5.1.5.1. The standard states:

> *5.1.5.1 The blood bank or transfusion service shall have methods to limit and detect bacterial contamination in all platelet components. Standard 5.6.2 applies [skin disinfection].*[37]

How this standard is being met varies by facility. Many blood collection centers have begun routinely culturing platelet units using an automated culture system. The BacT/ALERT system (Bio-Merieux), used by many centers, works by continuously monitoring for bacterial production of CO_2 within culture bottles. Platelet units are sampled on the day after collection. The samples are cultured for a period of time, typically 24 hours, and if the cultures fail to produce abnormal levels of CO_2, the product is released into inventory. Overall, culture-based bacterial screening appears to have decreased, but not eliminated, the risk of septic reactions. Reducing the risk even further may ultimately require alternative approaches, such as pathogen reduction.[38–41] Nonculture methods such as pH and glucose testing (using a dipstick or automated analyzer) and Gram staining are employed by some facilities; however, the sensitivity and specificity of these nonculture methods is demonstrably inferior to culture-based methods.[42,43] Rapid, point-of-issue tests that could be used to verify the sterility of a platelet unit just before release are under development. It is hoped that that some of the costs associated with testing for platelet bacterial contamination will be offset by the benefits of being able to extend platelet storage beyond the 5-day limit.

The FDA has approved the use of 7-day-old platelets in the context of a large surveillance study (PASSPORT)[44,45]; the quality of even older platelet units is being evaluated.

A number of alternate approaches to the problem of bacterial contamination have been proposed. These include freezing platelets using a cryopreservative such as DMSO or trehalose[46,47] and refrigerating platelets after glycosylation.[48–50] Pathogen inactivation systems, utilizing photosensitive dyes/UV light, can provide up to 6 logs of killing of spiked virus or bacteria within a unit of platelets or red cells.[51–56] One such system has been licensed for use in Europe. At this time, however, no pathogen inactivation system is licensed for use in the United States.

Allergic and Febrile Nonhemolytic Transfusion Reactions

The typical RBC unit contains approximately 20 mL of plasma. Platelet units contain far more plasma, approximately 200 mL on average. There are multiple potential adverse effects associated with this large plasma content. First, allergic transfusion reactions are frequently associated with platelet transfusion. Allergic reactions to platelet transfusions occur when the recipient has a preexisting allergy to a plasma protein component. Allergic reactions can range from mild, uncomplicated urticarial reactions to full-blown anaphylaxis. Febrile nonhemolytic reactions, defined as a rise in temperature of more than 1°C, may also be seen following platelet transfusion. In a provocative study, Heddle and colleagues demonstrated that it is in fact the plasma component of platelet units, rather than the cellular component, that causes most such reactions.[57] Cytokines that accumulate during product storage have been implicated.

ABO and Hemolytic Reactions to Platelets

Whenever possible, platelet units are assigned so as to match the donor plasma with recipient red cell type. For example, a type A patient would ordinarily receive type A or AB platelets, which do not contain anti-A antibody. When platelet inventories are constrained, however, it is a frequent practice to provide ABO-incompatible platelets: for example, type A patient can receive type O platelets, containing anti-A. The passive transfusion of donor anti-A or anti-B to a patient rarely results in a clinically apparent reaction. Occasionally, however, hemolysis may be observed. Most often, this occurs with units from type O donors, who occasionally have high titer anti-A, anti-B and/or anti-A,B antibody. In a typical type O adult, the titer of circulating anti-A is on the order of 1 : 128-1-256. Some donors, for unclear reasons, have anti-A titers of 1 : 10,000 or higher. Recipients of products from donors with high-titer anti-A (and less frequently, anti-B) rarely do have clinically apparent hemolysis, and a small number of fatalities have been reported.[58] This is considered to be a low-risk event, but may be on the rise in the United States because of the increased number of single-donor apheresis platelet units used.[59] One strategy to deal with this issue is to measure the anti-A/B titer on all platelet donors; components exceeding a threshold titer are assigned to type-specific recipients. An alternate strategy is to gently reduce the load of plasma in a platelet unit prior to transfusing the unit to a non–ABO-identical recipient.

Transfusion-Related Acute Lung Injury

Transfusion-related acute lung injury (TRALI), an acute respiratory distress reaction associated with the transfusion of any plasma-containing blood component, deserves mention. Although TRALI can be seen with any blood component, it most commonly follows transfusion of plasma or platelet units. RBCs are a much less common cause of TRALI. It is hypothesized that higher volumes of plasma provide higher loads of TRALI-precipitating anti-HLA or antineutrophil antibody, making plasma and platelets higher-risk components for TRALI. Irrespective of the type of blood component causing TRALI, the diagnosis of TRALI remains one of exclusion, and treatment is supportive.

Rh(D) Sensitization

The Rh(D) antigen is the most immunogenic red cell protein antigen. More than 80% of individuals who are Rh(D) negative will form an anti-D antibody following a single Rh(D)-positive RBC transfusion.[44] Anti-D antibodies are associated with both hemolytic transfusion reactions as well as hemolytic disease of the fetus and newborn. For this reason, it is standard practice to provide Rh(D)-negative individuals exclusively with Rh(D)-negative RBC units. Platelet units contain a small number of contaminating RBCs. In the case of platelet concentrates, approximately 0.3 to 0.5 mL RBCs may be present. Current apheresis platelets contain far fewer RBCs—approximately 0.0002 to 0.0007 mL per unit.[60] Ordinarily, Rh(D)-negative platelet units are given to Rh(D)-negative recipients. However, inventory constraints frequently force blood banks to provide Rh(D)-positive platelet products to Rh(D)-negative recipients. Transfusion of such units is associated with a low but nonzero risk of sensitization and formation of anti-D. Anti-D antibody formation can be prevented by administering Rh immune globulin, as is done to prevent fetomaternal Rh sensitization in Rh(D)-negative mothers of Rh(D)-positive children. The risk of sensitization is especially low among Rh(D)-negative immunocompromised patients transfused with Rh(D)-positive platelets, for example, HSCT patients.[61] In this setting, the value of RhIg prophylaxis appears to be marginal.

PLATELET REFRACTORINESS

Causes of Refractoriness to Platelet Transfusion

Platelet refractoriness is defined as an inappropriately low platelet increment following repeated platelet transfusions. It can be caused by nonimmune and/or immune factors (Table 147–1). The most commonly reported nonimmune causes of platelet refractoriness include fever, sepsis, bleeding, splenomegaly, and disseminated intravascular coagulation.[62] In a subset of cases, platelet refractoriness is immune-mediated. Platelets express HLA class I antigens, ABO antigens,[63] and several platelet-specific antigens. Any of these molecules may potentially serve as an immune stimulus in a transfusion recipient. Antibodies directed against HLA molecules are responsible for most cases of immune-mediated platelet refractoriness, whereas antibodies to the human platelet antigens (anti-HPA antibodies) are less frequently implicated.[8]

Diagnosis of Platelet Refractoriness

Because less than half of all platelet-refractory patients have demonstrable anti-HLA or antiplatelet antibodies,[64,65] evaluation of both an immediate response to platelet transfusion and an 18- to 24-hour posttransfusion platelet survival is needed to help establish the cause of platelet refractoriness. Platelet counts obtained from 10 minutes to 1 hour after transfusion that repeatedly fail to demonstrate a corrected count increment (CCI) of more than 5000/μL usually indicate immune-mediated platelet refractoriness.[66] If the 10-minute to 1-hour posttransfusion platelet count shows a reasonable increment but the platelet count falls back to baseline by 18 to 24 hours, a nonimmune mechanism of refractoriness may be presumed (Table 147–1). In cases of suspected immune-mediated refractoriness, HLA antibody screening (panel reactive antibody or PRA) provides valuable supporting evidence that allosensitization has occurred.[67,68] A patient with a PRA greater than 70% may be considered to be "severely immunized,"[69] and a good candidate for HLA-matched platelets (below).

Table 147–1 Causes of Refractoriness to Platelet Transfusion

Nonimmune
Fever
Sepsis
Drug-associated
Active bleeding
Splenomegaly
Disseminated intravascular coagulation
Venoocclusive disease
Immune
Anti-HLA antibodies
Anti-HPA antibodies
ABO mismatch
Drug-dependent antibodies

Table 147–2 Management of the Platelet-Refractory Patient

Obtain 10-minute to 1-hour posttransfusion platelet count on two occasions.
If there is an appropriate increment in platelet count after a single platelet transfusion, continue to transfuse random platelets and treat nonimmune factors associated with decreased platelet survival such as sepsis, DIC; discontinue offending drugs, etc.
If the 10-minute to 1-hour posttransfusion platelet counts demonstrate no platelet increment (or only a marginal increment) obtain patient's HLA type and also screen the patient for presence of anti-HLA antibodies (Panel Reactive Antibody test, PRA).
While awaiting HLA antigen typing and antibody screening results, consider transfusion of "fresh" (<3 days old) ABO-matched platelets.
If PRA shows less than 20% reactivity, continue with "fresh" ABO matched random platelets.
If PRA shows more than 20% reactivity, obtain anti-HLA antibody specificity. Use recipient's HLA typing information to locate grade A or B matched platelet units for transfusion. Avoid transfusion of platelets containing antigens against which the recipient has antibodies. Consider recruiting recipient's family for platelet donation.
Transfusion of crossmatch-compatible platelets is an option if there is a poor response to grade A or B matched platelets and/or if recipient has antibodies to platelet-specific antigens.
All HLA-matched or crossmatched platelet units must be irradiated prior to transfusion to prevent transfusion-associated graft-versus-host disease.

Table 147–3 Traditional Platelet Selection Guidelines for Refractoriness Due To Alloimmunization

ABO antigens are expressed on platelets. Consider transfusion of ABO-matched platelets while awaiting recipient's HLA type and antibody specificity.
Platelet matching for recipient's HLA-A and HLA-B antigens is important.
Platelet matching for recipient's HLA-C antigens is not essential.
Determine the antigen specificity of recipient's antiplatelet antibodies and try to transfuse antigen-negative platelets.
Some HLA antigens may be weakly expressed on platelets. Consider giving platelets mismatched for those antigens (eg, HLA-B12 and its splits B44,B45)
If HLA-matched platelets are unavailable, consider transfusion of platelets mismatched for HLA antigens that are serologically cross-reactive with recipient's HLA antigens.
If platelets mismatched for serologically cross-reactive antigens are not effective, matching for HLA associated antigen systems such as Bw4/Bw6 may be helpful.[94]

Detection of Anti-HLA Antibodies

Several assays are available to detect presence of anti-HLA class I antibodies in serum of alloimmunized patients. One of the most commonly used tests is the National Institutes of Health lymphocytotoxicity assay (LCTA).[70] The results of LCTA correlate well with the response to platelet transfusion.[18,71] However, this assay will not detect anti-HLA antibodies that do not activate complement.[72] The anti-HLA antibodies can also be detected using HLA-specific solid-phase enzyme-linked immunosorbent assay,[73] glycoprotein-specific monoclonal antibody-specific immobilization of platelet antigens,[72] or flow cytometric detection of antibody binding to beads coated with purified HLA antigens.[74] This flow cytometry-based methodology has significantly improved sensitivity over LCTA[75] and, similarly to solid-phase assays, it can detect both complement-fixing and non–complement-fixing antibodies.[74] All our patients with suspected platelet refractoriness due to alloimmunization are evaluated for presence of anti-HLA antibodies using flow cytometry-based assays.

Detection of Antiplatelet Antibodies

Most commonly used methods for detection of anti-HPA antibodies are solid-phase assays utilizing purified platelet antigens for detection of antibody specificity. However, extensive testing for anti-HPA antibodies is not widely accepted as a critical step in the workup of platelet refractory patients, mostly because of conflicting data on significance of these antibodies in platelet refractoriness.[8,76,77]

Prevention of Alloimmunization

Although they express HLA class I antigens, platelets themselves are fairly weak immunogens. It has been shown that contaminating leukocytes in platelet products are primarily responsible for stimulating HLA antibody formation in platelet transfusion recipients.[8,78–80] Thus, removing white cells from blood products (leukoreduction) is an essential means of preventing alloimmunization and subsequent platelet refractoriness. The definitive study showing this was the Trial to Reduce Alloimmunization to Platelets (TRAP study),[8] which compared alloimmunization rates in 530 newly diagnosed AML patients randomized to receive either unmodified, pooled platelet concentrates (control); filtered, pooled platelet concentrates (F-PC); filtered single-donor apheresis platelets (F-AP); or UV-B-irradiated pooled platelet concentrates (UVB-PC). Anti-HLA antibodies were detected in 45% of controls, compared with 17% to 21% of patients receiving modified platelets. 13% of control group patients became platelet-refractory, versus only 3% in the F-PC group, 4% in the F-AP group, and 5% in the UVB-PC group.

Management of the Platelet-Refractory Patient

When platelet refractoriness has been demonstrated, several strategies may facilitate achieving therapeutic platelet increments in vivo (Table 147–2). A trial of ABO-matched, fresh (1–2 days old) platelets may be helpful.[81,82] In cases of immune-mediated refractoriness, a trial of HLA-matched platelets,[67,83–85] antigen-negative platelets,[86] or cross-matched platelets[87–89] should be considered. The basic principles for selection of HLA-matched platelets are outlined in Table 147–3. In

Table 147–4 Grades of HLA-Matched Platelets

Match Grade	Description
A	4-antigen match (Donor and recipient match at both HLA-A and -B loci)
B1U	1 antigen unknown or blank (eg, Donor is: A2, –; B5, 27)
B1X	1 cross-reactive group*
B2UX	1 antigen blank and 1 cross-reactive*
C	1 mismatched antigen present
D	2 or more mismatched antigens present
R	Random

*The clusters of HLA antigens that share antigenic epitopes can be classified into cross-reactive antigen groups (CREG). Antibodies recognizing one HLA molecule within the group cross-react with other members of the same group.

Adapted from Brecher ME (ed.): Technical Manual, 15th ed. Bethesda, MD, AABB, 2005.

most cases, alloimmune refractory patients will show some degree of response to HLA-matched platelets.[90] Because of the high degree of polymorphism of the HLA loci, it is often not possible to find perfect HLA-A and -B locus matches, leading to the use of platelets mismatched at one or more loci (Table 147–4). In general, transfusion of grade A or BU matched platelets can result in an increase in platelet count that is superior to platelet increment obtained using either crossmatched platelets or platelets with different degrees of HLA mismatching (BX, C, or D).[83] Examples of different categories of matches are provided in Fig. 147–1. An additional step that may help in finding compatible platelets is flow cytometric detection of anti-HLA antibody specificity using single HLA antigen-coated beads.[91] This information can be used to find donors that may be HLA mismatched with the recipient but whose platelets lack the antigens to which the patient has specific antibodies.[86] Furthermore, family members may be considered as platelet donors in addition to the available pool of HLA-matched volunteer donors. As an alternative to HLA antigen matching, patients may benefit from receiving donor platelets that are crossmatch compatible with the patient's serum.[92] The major benefit of crossmatching is a potentially larger pool of donors that would have been excluded by strict HLA antigen matching. Also, platelet crossmatching may be helpful in cases of refractoriness due to antibodies directed against platelet-specific antigens.

The most challenging cases are those rare instances involving immune-refractory patients who are actively bleeding, and HLA-matched platelets or crossmatched platelets are either ineffective or unavailable. In such cases, patients are typically transfused with repeated doses of random HLA-incompatible platelets during hemorrhagic episodes. The efficacy of this practice is unclear. Data from an animal model system suggest that limited benefits might be obtained in alloimmune-refractory patients transfused with a large number of pooled random donor platelets because of a transient decrease in the alloantibody titer.[93]

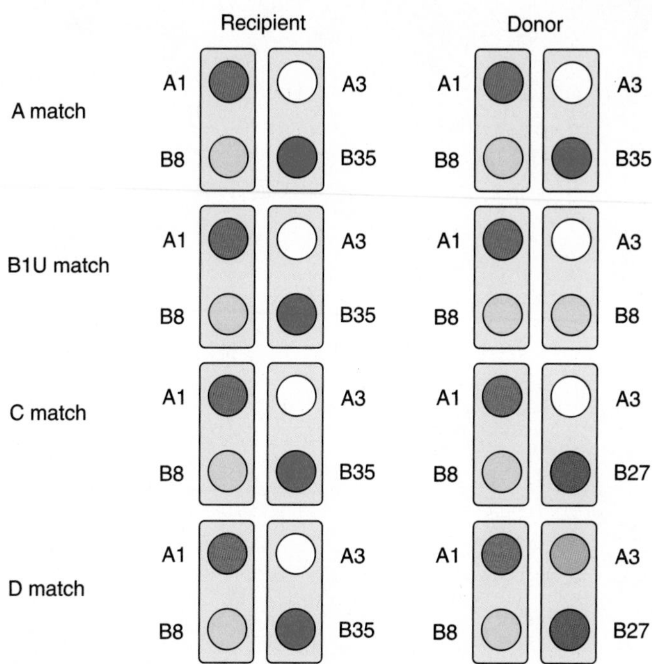

Figure 147–1 Examples of donor/recipient pairs on the basis of HLA match.

SUGGESTED READINGS

Bishop JF, Schiffer CA, Aisner J, Matthews JP, Wiernik PH: Surgery in acute leukemia: A review of 167 operations in thrombocytopenic patients. Am J Hematol 26:147, 1987.

Cid J, Lozano M, Fernandez-Aviles F, et al: Anti-D alloimmunization after D-mismatched allogeneic hematopoietic stem cell transplantation in patients with hematologic diseases. Transfusion 46:169, 2006.

Daly PA, Schiffer CA, Aisner J, Wiernik PH: Platelet transfusion therapy. One-hour posttransfusion increments are valuable in predicting the need for HLA-matched preparations. JAMA 243:435, 1980.

Fang CT, Chambers LA, Kennedy J, et al: Detection of bacterial contamination in apheresis platelet products: American Red Cross experience, 2004. Transfusion 45:1845, 2005.

Hanson SR, Slichter SJ: Platelet kinetics in patients with bone marrow hypoplasia: Evidence for a fixed platelet requirement. Blood 66:1105, 1985.

Hillyer CD, Josephson CD, Blajchman MA, Vostal JG, Epstein JS, Goodman JL: Bacterial contamination of blood components: Risks, strategies, and regulation: Joint ASH and AABB educational session in transfusion medicine. Hematol Am Soc Hematol Educ Program 575, 2003.

Hoffmeister KM, Felbinger TW, Falet H, et al: The clearance mechanism of chilled blood platelets. Cell 112:87, 2003.

Howard SC, Gajjar A, Ribeiro RC, et al: Safety of lumbar puncture for children with acute lymphoblastic leukemia and thrombocytopenia. JAMA 284:2222, 2000.

Rebulla P, Finazzi G, Marangoni F, et al, for the Gruppo Italiano Malattie Ematologiche Maligne dell'Adulto: The threshold for prophylactic platelet transfusions in adults with acute myeloid leukemia. N Engl J Med 337:1870, 1997.

Slichter SJ: Background, rationale, and design of a clinical trial to assess the effects of platelet dose on bleeding risk in thrombocytopenic patients. J Clin Apher 21:78, 2006.

The Trial to Reduce Alloimmunization to Platelets Study Group: Leukocyte reduction and ultraviolet B irradiation of platelets to prevent alloimmunization and refractoriness to platelet transfusions. N Engl J Med 337:1861, 1997.

Wandt H, Schaefer-Eckart K, Frank M, Birkmann J, Wilhelm M: A therapeutic platelet transfusion strategy is safe and feasible in patients after autologous peripheral blood stem cell transplantation. Bone Marrow Transplant 37:387, 2006.

REFERENCES

For complete list of references log onto www.expertconsult.com

CHAPTER 148

PRINCIPLES OF NEUTROPHIL (GRANULOCYTE) TRANSFUSIONS

Ronald G. Strauss

Current cytapheresis technology permits collection of large numbers of several types of blood leukocytes from healthy donors or patients—who often are stimulated with recombinant cytokines—to be used for transfusion and transplantation or for further processing (eg, ex vivo expansion and genetic manipulation) and storage. Neutrophils (PMNs) are granulocytic leukocytes that are collected and issued as a standard blood component (granulocytes, pheresis). This chapter analyzes the use of granulocyte (ie, neutrophil) transfusions (GTX) as an adjunct to antimicrobial drugs in the treatment and prevention of progressive infections in patients with neutropenia or PMN dysfunction.

Life-threatening infections with bacteria, yeast, and fungus continue to be a consequence of severe neutropenia ($<0.5 \times 10^9$/L blood PMNs) and disorders of PMN dysfunction. The most frequent situation seen today is neutropenic fever and infection with yeast or fungus after intense chemotherapy for hematologic malignancies or in conjunction with hematopoietic progenitor cell transplantation. Neutropenic infections cause considerable morbidity, occasionally are fatal, and add considerable cost to the management of these patients.

Previous attempts to prevent infections in severely neutropenic patients by transfusing PMN concentrates (ie, prophylactic GTX) achieved only questionable success. Although rates of certain infections were significantly reduced by prophylactic GTX, many adverse effects, such as pulmonary infiltrates and cytomegalovirus infections, were reported, and GTX were expensive. Similarly, use of therapeutic GTX to resolve existing infections has not gained lasting acceptance, despite many reports documenting significant benefit.[1] This lack of enthusiasm for GTX can be explained by the continuing development of new and very effective antimicrobial drugs to prevent and treat infections and by the availability of recombinant hematopoietic growth factors and peripheral blood hematopoietic progenitor cell (PBHPC) transfusions—both of which hasten patient recovery from myelotoxic therapy and shorten the period of risk for neutropenic infections. The lack of familiarity of some oncology and transplant physicians with the markedly improved modern PMN concentrates available for transfusion today may limit use of GTX.

Historically, PMN concentrates were collected for transfusion from unstimulated donors or those stimulated only with corticosteroids and contained woefully inadequate numbers of PMNs.[1] Currently, very large numbers of PMNs can be collected from normal donors using granulocyte-colony stimulating factor (G-CSF) plus corticosteroid marrow stimulation followed by large-volume leukapheresis, during which several liters of donor blood are processed.[2] In this chapter, the historic and modern experiences with GTX is reviewed and the current technology of PMN collection is discussed.

THERAPEUTIC GRANULOCYTE TRANSFUSIONS IN NEUTROPENIC PATIENTS' HISTORICAL EXPERIENCE

In the third edition of this book, 34 papers were reviewed that reported the therapeutic use of GTX—collected before the advent of G-CSF donor stimulation—in severely neutropenic patients ($<5 \times 10^9$/L blood PMNs). Data were tabulated (Table 148–1) according to the index infection that prompted GTX therapy. Patients were counted only once (eg, patients with septicemia were listed only in the septicemia group, even if they had another infection, such as pneumonia). As an exception, all patients with invasive fungal infections were counted together because it was impossible to accurately separate sepsis, pneumonia, sinusitis, and so forth into distinct categories. All patients given GTX for a designated type of infection were enumerated in the "Treated" column. The treated patients, those for whom the actual course and mortality of the index infection could be clearly documented, were enumerated again in the "Evaluable" column. GTX therapy was considered successful if so stated by the author. Combining data from multiple reports of varying experimental design is of limited value for drawing conclusions, and it was done simply to document the breadth of historic reported experience.

To obtain more definitive information regarding efficacy of historic GTX (ie, collected without G-CSF), the seven controlled studies were analyzed in more detail.[3–9] In these seven studies, the response of infected neutropenic patients to treatment with GTX plus antibiotics (study group) was compared with that of comparable patients given antibiotics alone and evaluated concurrently (control group). The design, size, and results of these seven studies are presented in Tables 148–2 and 148–3. Three of the seven studies reported a significant overall benefit for GTX.[6–8] In two additional studies,[3,5] overall success was not demonstrated for GTX, but certain subgroups of patients were found to benefit significantly. Some measure of success for GTX was evident in five of the seven controlled studies. However, this success was counterbalanced by four studies that were negative in some respect—two totally[4,9] and two partially negative.[3,5]

An explanation of these inconsistent results is evident on critical analysis of the adequacy of GTX support (see Table 148–3). Patients in the three successful trials received relatively high doses of PMNs (generally $\geq 1.7 \times 10^{10}$/day).[6–8] Donors were selected to be erythrocyte and leukocyte compatible. By contrast, the four controlled studies yielding negative results can legitimately be criticized. Two of the four studies with negative conclusions used PMNs collected by filtration leukapheresis for some patients.[3,5] It is now known that such PMNs are defective, and they are no longer transfused. In the negative studies using PMNs collected by centrifugation leukapheresis,[4,5,9] the dose was extremely low (0.41 to 0.56×10^{10} per concentrate). As another factor, investigators in two of the four negative studies[3,9] made no provision for the possibility of leukocyte alloimmunization, as donors were selected solely on the basis of erythrocyte compatibility. Finally, control subjects responded reasonably well to antibiotics alone in three of the four negative studies,[3,5,9] suggesting that some patients fared so well with conventional treatment that they had no apparent need for additional therapeutic modalities.

These impressions from the seven controlled GTX trials have been analyzed by formal meta-analysis,[10] and conclusions were that the dose of PMNs transfused and the survival rate of the nontransfused control subjects were primarily responsible for the differing success rates of the historical studies. In clinical settings in which the survival rate of nontransfused control subjects was low, study subjects benefitted from receiving adequate doses of GTX—prompting the authors to suggest that severely neutropenic patients with life-threatening infections be considered for GTX given in adequate doses.[10]

MODERN EXPERIENCE

Fungal and yeast infections occur frequently in patients with severe neutropenia or PMN dysfunction, and these infections pose a major challenge to the efficacy of modern therapeutic GTX. Recipients of hematopoietic progenitor cell transplants—particularly marrow transplant patients—often become severely neutropenic, exhibit PMN dysfunction, and manifest defective cellular and humoral immunity for months after transplantation. Altered immunity is particularly profound when marrow is T-lymphocyte depleted to diminish graft-versus-host disease. Hence, all types of infection pose a threat, with fungal and yeast infections being major problems.[11,12] In a series of 1186 marrow transplant patients, 10% developed a non-candidal fungal infection, with only 17% of infected patients surviving.[11] When the marrow graft is depleted of T lymphocytes, the rate of infection is increased two- to sevenfold above that occurring with standard bone marrow transplantation.[12]

Data are insufficient to determine the proper role of GTX in treating fungal infections. Historic case reports,[13–15] experimental studies in animals,[16,17] and experience in treating patients with chronic granulomatous disease[18] have supported the efficacy of GTX in fungal infections. In contrast, a large clinical study reported that GTX, collected in the pre G-CSF era, were of no benefit in treating fungal and yeast infections in 87 bone marrow transplant patients, 50 of whom received GTX.[19] Unfortunately, this study was a retrospective review with several shortcomings and must be interpreted cautiously.

At this time, no randomized clinical trials of therapeutic GTX collected after G-CSF donor stimulation have been reported to establish the efficacy or potential toxicity of modern GTX. However, 10 case reports and uncontrolled studies will be reviewed.[13,20–28] Clark and colleagues[13] and Catalano and coworkers[21] each reported single patients (Table 148–4) with aplastic anemia undergoing progenitor cell transplantation with fungus infections that responded favorably to strikingly different doses of PMNs. Similarly, Ozsahin and associates[22] and Bielorai and colleagues[23] each reported single patients (see Table 148–4) with chronic granulomatous disease and fungal infections that responded favorably to GTX during the transplantation period. Bielorai and coworkers[24] reported a single patient (see Table 148–4) with acute leukemia and sepsis with progressive, antibiotic-resistant bacteria whose infection cleared slowly with GTX. It is impossible, in these single reports of very complicated patients, to firmly ascribe the good outcome to the GTX.

Hester and colleagues[20] transfused 15 patients with hematologic malignancies and infections (Table 148–5). PMNs were collected from donors stimulated only with G-CSF and selected without regard for leukocyte compatibility. Although GTX were successful in most patients, it was not possible to distinguish responses of fungus versus yeast infections. Lee and associates[28] transfused 25 patients with hematologic malignancies (see Table 148–5), many of whom were infected with multiple organisms. PMNs were colleted from donors stimulated with G-CSF alone (66% of donors), G-CSF plus dexamethasone (25% of donors), or dexamethasone alone (8% of donors). Of patients with sepsis, 50% (2 of 4) responded favorably, and 38% (8 of 21) of patients with progressive localized infections responded favorably.

Grigg and associates[25] transfused 11 patients (see Table 148–5). Eight patients had hematologic malignancies and progressive infections—five of the eight undergoing progenitor cell transplantation and three receiving chemotherapy. Three additional patients who were undergoing progenitor cell transplantation had stable fungus infections. PMNs were collected from donors stimulated only with G-CSF and selected without regard for leukocyte compatibility. Success was excellent for bacterial and stable fungus infections,

Table 148–1 Infectious Problems in Neutropenic Patients Treated With Historic Granulocyte Transfusions in 34 Studies

Type of Infection	Treated	Evaluable	Success Rate (%)
Bacterial septicemia	298	206	127/206 (62)
Sepsis organism unspecified	132	39	18/39 (46)
Invasive fungus and yeast	83	77	28/77 (36)
Pneumonia	120	11	7/11 (64)
Localized infections	143	47	39/47 (83)
Fever etiology unknown	184	85	64/85 (75)

Table 148–2 Results of Seven Controlled Studies Evaluating Historical Therapeutic Granulocyte Transfusions in Neutropenic Patients

		Study Group		Control Group	
Investigators	**Success**	***N***	***Survival (%)***	***N***	***Survival (%)***
Higby et al[7]	Yes	17	76	19	26
Volger and Winton[8]	Yes	17	59	13	15
Herzig et al[6]	Yes	13	75	14	36
Alavi et al[3]	Partial	12	82	19	62
Graw et al[5]	Partial	39	46	37	30
Winston et al[9]	No	48	63	47	72
Fortuny et al[4]	No	17	78	22	80

Table 148–3 Design of Seven Controlled Studies Evaluating Historical Therapeutic Granulocyte Transfusions in Neutropenic Patients

Investigators	Randomized?	Collection Method	Dose ($\times 10^{10}$)	Schedule	HLA*	WBC*
Higby et al[7]	Yes	Filtration	2.2	Daily	No	Yes
Vogler and Winton[8]	Yes	Centrifugation	2.7	Daily	Yes	Yes
Herzig et al[6]	Yes	Filtration Centrifugation	1.7 0.4	Daily Daily	No No	Yes Yes
Alavi et al[3]	Yes	Filtration	5.9	Daily	No	No
Graw et al[5]	No	Filtration Centrifugation	2.0 0.6	Daily Daily	No No	Yes Yes
Winston et al[9]	Yes	Centrifugation	0.5	Daily	No	No
Fortuny et al[4]	No	Centrifugation	0.4	Daily	No	Yes

*Donors selected to be compatible with recipient either by HLA typing (A and B loci matched, at least in part) or by leukocyte cross-matching.

Table 148–4 Case Reports of Modern Therapeutic Granulocyte Transfusions Using PMNs Collected From Granulocyte-Colony Stimulating Factor–Stimulated Donors in Neutropenic Patients

Investigators	PMNs × 10¹⁰ per Each GTX	Stimulation	Leukapheresis	Outcomes
Clarke et al[13]	5.3*	G-CSF 5–10 μg/kg	Dextran 10 L processed	One patient with fungus recovered
Catalano et al[21]	1.9	G-CSF 300 μg/dose	Not described	One patient with fungus recovered
Ozsahin et al[22]	3.1	G-CSF 5 μg/kg	Hetastarch 5–7 L processed	One patient with fungus recovered
Bielorai et al[23]	7.0*	G-CSF 5 μg/kg	Not described	One patient with fungus recovered
Bielorai et al[24]	4.8–6.8	Not described	Not described	One patient with vancomycin-resistant *Enterococcus* recovered

G-CSF, granulocyte-colony stimulating factor; GTX, granulocyte transfusions.
*Assumptions made as PMN dose expressed × 10¹⁰ unclear in these reports. Dose calculated that would be given to a 70-kg recipient for Clarke et al, and Bielorai et al.

Table 148–5 Groups of Neutropenic Patients Treated With Modern Therapeutic Granulocyte Transfusions Using PMNs Collected From Granulocyte-Colony Stimulating Factor–Stimulated Donors

Investigators	PMNs × 10¹⁰ per Each GTX	Stimulation	Leukapheresis	Outcomes
Hester et al[20]	4.1	G-CSF 5 μg/kg	Pentastarch 7 L processed	60% (9 of 15) Success with fungus (11 patients) and yeast (4 patients)
Grigg et al[25]	5.9*	G-CSF 10 μg/kg	Dextran 10 L processed	100% (3 of 3) Success with bacterial infection 0% (0 of 5) Success with progressive fungus 67% (2 of 3) success with stable fungus
Peters et al[26]	3.5*	G-CSF 5 μg/kg -or- Prednisolone	Hetastarch 6.4 L processed	82% (14 of 17) Success with bacterial infection 54% (7 of 13) Success with fungal infection
Price et al[27]	8.2	G-CSF 600 μg/kg -plus- Dexamethasone 8 mg	Hetastarch 10 L processed	100% (4 of 4) Success with bacterial infection 0% (0 of 8) Success with invasive fungus 57% (4 of 7) Success with yeast infection
Lee et al[28]	5.1–10.6	G-CSF 5 μg/kg -and/or- Dexamethasone 3 mg/m²	Pentastarch 6–10 L processed	40% (10 of 25) Success with multiple-organism infections

G-CSF, granulocyte-colony stimulating factor; GTX, granulocyte transfusions.
*Assumptions made as PMN dose expressed ×10¹⁰ unclear in these reports. PMN dose calculated using values for range of leukocytes collected, percentage of collected cells being myeloid and volume of units collected (Grigg et al). Dose calculated that would be given to a 70-kg recipient for Peters et al.

but was quite poor for progressive fungus infections with organ dysfunction—a troubling pattern reported by others.[27]

Peters and colleagues[26] transfused 30 patients (see Table 148–5) with hematologic disorders—18 undergoing progenitor cell transplantation. PMNs were collected from donors stimulated with G-CSF or prednisolone and selected without regard for leukocyte compatibility. The exact PMN dose transfused is uncertain because values from 0.9×10^{10} to 14.4×10^{10} can be calculated from data reported, and it was impossible to distinguish the success of GTX from G-CSF versus prednisolone-stimulated donors. However, the outcome of bacterial infections appeared to be superior to that of fungus infections.

Price and coworkers[27] transfused 19 patients (see Table 148–5) with hematologic malignancies, 16 of whom had received progenitor cell transplants and 3 who were pretransplantation recipients. PMNs were collected from donors stimulated with G-CSF and dexamethasone. Although donors were selected without regard for leukocyte compatibility, recipients were documented not to exhibit evidence of leukocyte alloimmunization at study entry. Bacterial infections responded well and yeast infections responded modestly. Despite very high PMN doses, success for invasive fungus infections was dismal.

No firm conclusions can be drawn from these somewhat anecdotal reports of modern therapeutic GTX for several reasons: (a) no concurrent control subjects were included (ie, randomly assigned to receive no GTX or GTX from donors stimulated only with corticosteroids); (b) the number of patients reported was quite small; and (c) PMN collection methods were variable, with a broad range of PMN doses transfused. On the basis of these preliminary findings, bacterial infections appeared to respond well to modern GTX, relatively mild fungus and yeast infections responded modestly well, whereas serious fungus infections with tissue damage resisted even the large doses of PMNs transfused with modern GTX.[25–27] The precise role of modern therapeutic GTX, collected from donors stimulated with G-CSF plus corticosteroids, in the management of infected, neutropenic, oncology/transplant patients awaits definition by randomized clinical trials.

EXPERIENCE IN INFANTS AND CHILDREN

Most patients with congenital disorders of PMN dysfunction have adequate numbers of blood PMNs, but they are susceptible to serious infections because their PMNs fail to kill pathogenic microorganisms. Patients with severe forms of PMN dysfunction are relatively rare, and no randomized clinical trials have been reported to establish the efficacy of therapeutic GTX in their management. Firm recommendations about the use of GTX to treat patients cannot be made. However, several patients with chronic granulomatous disease, complicated by progressive life-threatening fungal infections, have been reported to benefit.[29–37] Because of the possibility of alloimmunization to leukocyte and red blood cell antigens plus the risk of transfusion-transmitted infections, therapeutic GTX are recommended only for progressive infections that cannot be controlled with antimicrobial drugs. Because of lifetime problems with infections, prophylactic GTX are impractical.

Neonates (infants within the first month of life) are another group of patients who may suffer life-threatening bacterial infections caused, at least in part, by PMN dysfunction and neutropenia. Neutropenia must be viewed differently in neonates than in older patients, as in the latter, GTX are considered usually when the blood PMN count falls to less than 0.5×10^9/L. By contrast, because normal neonates exhibit a physiologic neutrophilia, absolute blood PMN counts as high as 3.0×10^9/L (ie, relative neutropenia) might prompt consideration of GTX in neonates.[38] The mechanism of neutropenia cannot always be identified, but in some infants, a marked decrease in the marrow PMN storage pool can be demonstrated. For example, these forms (metamyelocytes and segmented PMNs) account for 26% to 65% of all nucleated cells in normal marrow, but in some neonates with sepsis, this value will be less than 10% of nucleated marrow cells.

Six controlled trials[39–44] have assessed the role of GTX in treating neonatal infections. Although four of the six[39–42] found a significant benefit for GTX, the controlled studies, when assessed by meta-analysis, were insufficiently homogeneous to permit clear recommendations regarding the efficacy of GTX.[10] The dose of PMNs transfused was identified as the primary reason for disagreements between studies. When leukapheresis PMN concentrates were transfused, GTX were beneficial. When buffy coats were transfused, GTX were not beneficial.[10] The role of therapeutic GTX for neonatal infections is unclear at present and, because they are transfused only rarely at this time, they will not be discussed further. However, the possible roles of immunoglobulin and cytokine therapies for neonatal sepsis will be discussed later.

PROPHYLACTIC GRANULOCYTE TRANSFUSIONS IN NEUTROPENIC PATIENTS

Based on historic reports, prophylactic GTX were of marginal value. In 12 reports,[45–56] benefits were few, whereas risks and expenses were substantial. However, some measure of success was found in 7[45–51] of 12 studies; the remaining 5 studies failed to show a benefit for prophylactic GTX.[52–56] In none of these five negative studies were large numbers of PMNs obtained from matched donors and transfused daily. In a situation analogous to that for the negative therapeutic GTX trials, the failure of prophylactic GTX might be explained, at least in part, by inadequate transfusions.

The role of modern prophylactic GTX (ie, from G-CSF stimulated donors) has not been established by definitive clinical trials. However, two factors suggest possible success (a) because of the rapid recovery from myeloablation, hastened by peripheral blood hematopoietic progenitor (PBHPC) transfusions and treatment of patients with recombinant growth factors, the period of severe neutropenia may be as short as 1 week; and (b) this relatively brief period of severe neutropenia might literally be eliminated by transfusing large doses of PMNs collected from donors stimulated with G-CSF plus corticosteroids. A few studies have begun to explore this possibility (Table 148–6).

Bensinger and colleagues[57] transfused seven allogeneic marrow recipients with PMNs collected from their HLA-identical or syngeneic marrow donors after G-CSF stimulation. Because donors experienced leukapheresis on consecutive days, collection techniques were quite variable in terms of quantities of hydroxyethyl starch infused and liters of donor blood processed, and the number of PMNs collected varied from 0.3 to 14.4 × 10.[10] Recipients received an average of 7.6 GTX while awaiting marrow recovery, and recipients were given 5 µg/kg G-CSF daily to maintain a mean blood PMN count of 0.95×10^9/L measured 24 hours posttransfusion. The goals of this study were to evaluate the feasibility and safety of collecting and transfusing PMNs from G-CSF stimulated donors; patient outcomes were not reported.

Adkins and associates[58] transfused 10 allogeneic marrow recipients with PMNs collected from their HLA-matched sibling marrow donors (see Table 148–6). Leukapheresis was performed on days 1,

Author's Approach to Therapeutic GTX

Indicated for severe bacterial, yeast, or fungal infection in a neutropenic patient (<0.5×10^9 neutrophils (PMN)/µL blood) when the infection progresses despite optimal antimicrobial therapy.

Collect PMNs (4 to 8×10^{10}) from allogeneic blood donors, as follows:

1. Stimulate neutrophilia by giving the donor 300 to 480 µg of G-CSF subcutaneously 12 hours before beginning leukapheresis, with or without 8 mg dexamethasone orally 12 hours before beginning leukapheresis.
2. Process 10 L of donor blood using a continuous-flow blood separator with citrated hydroxyethyl starch solution infused throughout the collection.

Transfuse one granulocyte concentrate (4 to 8×10^{10} PMNs) daily until bone marrow recovery (blood PMNs > 1.0×10^9/L without GTX) or clinical resolution of infection.

Table 148–6 Modern Prophylactic Granulocyte Transfusion Studies Using PMNs Collected From Granulocyte-Colony Stimulating Factor–Stimulated Donors in Hematopoietic Progenitor Cell Transplant Recipients

Investigator	PMNs × 10^{10} Per Each GTX	Stimulation	Leukapheresis	Outcomes
Bensinger et al[57]	4.2	G-CSF 3.5–6 µg/kg	Variable	Not reported
Adkins et al[58]	4.1 (day 1) 5.1 (day 3) 6.1 (day 5)	G-CSF 5 µg/kg × 5 days posttransplant	Hetastarch 7 L processed Days 1, 3, and 5	60% (6 of 10) afebrile 40% (4 of 10) febrile 3 culture positive
Adkins et al[59]	5.6 (day 2) 7.0 (day 4) 8.5 (day 6) 9.9 (day 8)	G-CSF 10 µg/kg	Hetastarch 7 L processed Days 2, 4, 6, and 8	Reduction of fever and antibiotics if no leukocyte antibodies

G-CSF, granulocyte-colony stimulating factor; GTX, granulocyte transfusions.

3, and 5 posttransplant, and GTX were infused. Recipients were given 7.5 μg/kg G-CSF every 12 hours until blood PMNs were greater than or equal to 1.5×10^9/L. Recipient blood PMNs were maintained at greater than 1.5×10^9/L throughout the 5 days of posttransplant GTX. By comparison, a historic group of control recipients treated with G-CSF, but no GTX, exhibited mean blood PMN counts less than 0.5×10^9/L posttransplant. Prophylactic GTX seemed promising in this setting and, perhaps, would have been even more effective (ie, higher recipient blood PMN counts and fewer infections) if given daily. In another study, Adkins and coworkers[59] transfused 23 autologous PBHPC recipients with PMNs collected from first-degree relative donors (see Table 148–6). Leukapheresis was performed on posttransplant days 2, 4, 6, and 8, and GTX were infused. Recipients were given 5 μg/kg G-CSF daily until the blood PMN count was greater than or equal to 1.5×10^9/L. Recipients were studied for the effects of lymphocytotoxic antibodies (ie, leukocyte alloimmunization) on GTX effectiveness. The 15 recipients who did not exhibit lymphocytotoxic antibodies during the 10-day study period experienced a mean of 4.1 febrile days and required 7.3 days of antibiotics. Values for the eight recipients with lymphocytotoxic antibodies were less desirable—6.3 febrile days and 10.5 days of antibiotics. Rates of documented infections were not reported.

No firm conclusions can be drawn from these reports of modern prophylactic GTX because no nontransfused control subjects were included; few patients were studied; and most patients were given GTX every other day, rather than daily—possibly providing a less than optimal dose of PMNs. Modern prophylactic GTX appear promising, but their efficacy, potential adverse effects, and economic analysis await definition by randomized clinical trials.

ALTERNATIVE OR ADDITIVE MEASURES TO GRANULOCYTE TRANSFUSIONS

Patients with severe neutropenia, particularly those undergoing chemotherapy or hematopoietic progenitor cell transplantation, exhibit a variety of abnormalities in multiple body defense mechanisms, not all of which can be corrected by GTX. Consequently, infections that occur in these patients do not always respond to GTX, and a number of additional therapies have been evaluated. Two that appear to hold promise are the use of recombinant myeloid growth factors (ie, cytokines) and intravenous immunoglobulin (IVIG).

Recombinant myeloid growth factors such as G-CSF and granulocyte–macrophage colony-stimulating factor (GM-CSF) are glycoprotein cytokines that enhance the production, differentiation, and function of myeloid cells.[60] As recently reviewed,[61] studies of cytokine production in neonates have yielded conflicting results, with investigators reporting values that are higher than, equal to, or lower than adult values. Generally, the dysregulation of expression and production of hematopoietic cytokines in neonates contributes to quantitative and qualitative myeloid abnormalities that lead to decreased availability and function of blood PMNs.[61] Several trials of G-CSF and GM-CSF, used to prevent and to treat neonatal sepsis, have been reported.[61] Although most studies have shown some benefit, such as improved production and function of PMNs, reduction in the incidence of infections and/or mortality has not been convincingly shown.[61]

In older children and adult patients, G-CSF and GM-CSF have been used to accelerate marrow recovery after chemotherapy and to successfully diminish the rate of acquired infections and the need for prolonged hospitalization.[60] In contrast to success in preventing neutropenic infections, the role of G-CSF and GM-CSF in treating already established infections is not as firmly documented. Regardless of solid evidence, these growth factors frequently are given to patients with neutropenia and severe infections, and it seems reasonable to consider adding therapeutic GTX when severe bacterial, yeast, or fungal infections are progressing in neutropenic patients, despite the use of appropriate antibiotics plus recombinant cytokines.

Collection and Transfusion of Neutrophil Concentrates

To ensure adequate numbers and quality of PMNs for transfusion, PMNs must be collected from stimulated donors by automated leukapheresis using an erythrocyte sedimenting agent, such as hydroxyethyl starch.[2] A major limitation of GTX efficacy has been the inability to transfuse adequate numbers of perfectly functioning PMNs. Under the stress of a severe bacterial infection, the marrow of an otherwise healthy adult will produce between 10^{11} and 10^{12} PMNs in 24 hours. Granulocyte concentrates collected from healthy donors who are not stimulated with corticosteroids or G-CSF will contain between 0.2 and 0.8×10^{10} PMNs—approximately 1% of a healthy marrow's output. Hence, donor stimulation is mandatory to achieve even a hope of a reasonable PMN dose per GTX.

Donor stimulation with properly timed corticosteroids (≥24 hours before leukapheresis) will increase the yield to approximately 2×10^{10} PMNs.[67] Stimulation with G-CSF, alone or in combination with corticosteroids, will produce higher but variable PMN yields; yields with prophylactic GTX were of marginal value Yields of 4 to 8×10^{10} PMNs are achieved regularly, and posttransfusion blood PMN counts frequently increase to 1 to 3×10^9/L, with PMNs detected in the recipient's bloodstream for several hours after GTX. Currently, PMN donors are optimally stimulated using 300 to 480 μg G-CSF given subcutaneously, plus 8 mg dexamethasone taken orally approximately 12 hours before beginning leukapheresis.[68] A recent report suggested that adrenal corticosteroids might cause posterior subcapsular cataracts in PMN donors.[69] Although this report must be confirmed by study of larger numbers of PMN donors, it seems logical to include this cautionary information in donor consent forms or to stimulate PMN donors using only G-CSF until the issue is resolved.

Each institution must assess local needs. If, despite optimal antimicrobial and other supportive therapy, neutropenic patients suffer significant morbidity or mortality from infections, GTX should be considered. Once therapeutic transfusions have been prescribed, they must be given effectively (≥2×10^{10} PMNs per dose with corticosteroid stimulation, ≥4×10^{10} PMNs per dose with G-CSF, and never <1×10^{10} PMNs per dose). Transfusions are continued until the infection has resolved or until blood PMNs have risen above 1.0×10^9/L. It seems logical that patients with evidence of alloimmunization (platelet refractoriness, leukocyte antibodies, repeated febrile transfusion reactions, or posttransfusion pulmonary infiltrates) should receive GTX collected from donors selected to be leukocyte compatible by HLA matching and/or leukocyte crossmatching. However, it has not been clearly shown that attempts to improve leukocyte antigen compatibility do, in fact, increase the success of GTX in alloimmunized patients—particularly when modern GTX from G-CSF-stimulated donors are transfused. Granulocyte concentrates should be transfused as soon as possible after collection because PMN functions begin to deteriorate rapidly. Some delay between collection and transfusion is inevitable, and granulocyte concentrates are usually stored briefly at 22°C, with little or no agitation. It is highly desirable to transfuse granulocyte concentrates within 6 hours of collection; they should not be given if more than 24 hours old.

The use of IVIG, to prevent or to treat neonatal sepsis, has appeal because this therapy may correct abnormalities of humoral immunity and neutrophil function. In studies of experimental infections, IVIG proved beneficial by increasing opsonic activity and by improving PMN kinetics.[62,63] Although the precise role of IVIG in the management of human infants is controversial, this therapy has been given (with mixed results) to prevent and to treat infections. Most prophylactic studies evaluating IVIG to prevent infections have documented few positive effects, but a few have reported true benefit.[64,65] In contrast, several therapeutic studies reported benefit from adding IVIG to antibiotics during the treatment of neonatal infections.[66] However, the data remain insufficient to justify the routine use of IVIG as standard therapy to prevent and/or treat infections in preterm infants.

SUGGESTED READINGS

Adkins DR, Goodnough LT, Shenoy S, et al: Effect of leukocyte compatibility on neutrophil increment after transfusion of granulocyte colony-stimulating factor-mobilized prophylactic granulocyte transfusions and on clinical outcomes after stem cell transplantation. Blood 95:3605, 2000.

Bielorai B, Neumann Y, Avigad I, et al: Successful treatment of vancomycin-resistant *Enterococcus* sepsis in a neutropenic patient with G-CSF-mobilized granulocyte transfusions. Med Pediatr Oncol 34:221, 2000.

Bielorai B, Toren A, Wolach B, et al: Successful treatment of invasive aspergillosis in chronic granulomatous disease by granulocyte transfusions followed by peripheral blood stem cell transplantation. Bone Marrow Transplant 26:1025, 2000.

Ghodsi Z, Strauss RG: Cataracts in neutrophil donors stimulated with adrenal corticosteroids. Transfusion 41:1464, 2001.

Lee J-J, Chung I-J, Park M-R, et al: Clinical efficacy of granulocyte transfusion therapy in patients with neutropenia-related infections. Leukemia 15:203, 2001.

Liles WC, Rodger E, Dale DC: Combined administration of G-CSF and dexamethasone for the mobilization of granulocytes in normal donors: Optimization of dosing. Transfusion 40:642, 2000.

Parravicini E, van de Ven C, Anderson L, Cairo MS: Myeloid hematopoietic growth factors and their role in prevention and/or treatment of neonatal sepsis. Trans Med Rev 16:11–24, 2002.

Price TH, Bowden RA, Boeckh M, et al: Phase I/II trial of neutrophil transfusions from donors stimulated with G-CSF and dexamethasone for treatment of patients with infections in hematopoietic stem cell transplantation. Blood 95:3302, 2000.

REFERENCES

For complete list of references log onto www.expertconsult.com

CHAPTER 149

TRANSFUSION OF PLASMA DERIVATIVES: FRESH-FROZEN PLASMA, CRYOPRECIPITATE, ALBUMIN, AND IMMUNOGLOBULINS

Cassandra D. Josephson and Christopher D. Hillyer

Plasma and its derivatives are valuable resources, but cost, risk of infectious disease transmission, although rare, and other adverse effects mandate their appropriate use. Plasma can be separated from packed red blood cells (pRBC) through centrifugation of whole blood at the time of collection or can be collected by apheresis as a single product or as a byproduct of platelet or red blood cell apheresis. Plasma can be processed into derivatives through cold ethanol fractionation (method of Cohn).[1] In this chapter, the features and uses of fresh-frozen plasma (FFP), F24 plasma (F24), cryoprecipitate, albumin, and intravenous (IVIG) and intramuscular immunoglobulin are discussed. The use of plasma-derived clotting factor concentrates as therapy for specific congenital clotting factor deficiencies is discussed in Chapter 150.

FROZEN PLASMA

Plasma is the acellular, fluid compartment of blood and it consists of 90% water, 7% protein and colloids, and 2% to 3% nutrients, crystalloids, hormones, and vitamins. The protein fraction contains the soluble clotting factors: fibrinogen, factor XIII, von Willebrand Factor (vWF), factor VIII primarily bound to its carrier protein vWF, and the vitamin K-dependent coagulation factors II, VII, IX, and X. Clotting proteins are the constituents for which transfusion of plasma is most often required.

Plasma frozen at −18°C or colder within 6 hours of donation can be labeled as FFP. This product may be stored up to 1 year before use, at which time it is thawed over 20 to 30 minutes. The activities of the labile coagulation factors (V and VIII) decrease after thawing, but remain adequate for at least 24 hours. A second type of frozen plasma, the most commonly used in the United States, is F24 plasma. To be labeled as F24 plasma, it must be frozen at −18°C or colder within 24 hours of collection. FFP and F24 are considered to be equivalent products for most patient populations. The difference between the historic data on FFP compared to F24 is a reduction in the following factors: fibrinogen 12%, FV 15%, FVIII 23%, and FXI 7%.[2] However, because factor VIII is an acute phase reactant, its levels are quickly replenished in recipients without hemophilia A. Therefore, FFP and F24 use may be interchangeable for patients without factor VIII deficiency.[3] A third type of frozen plasma is termed *cryosupernatant* or *cryoreduced-plasma* (CRP). The Food and Drug Administration (FDA) has recently licensed this component as "Plasma, Cryoprecipitate Reduced"—notice that it is devoid of its cryoprecipitate fraction, formed when FFP is thawed at 4°C.[19] The cryosupernatant component is then refrozen at −18°C or colder. A fourth frozen product, solvent detergent-treated plasma, is no longer commercially available because of the manufacturer's loss of licensure in April 2002. Plasma that is not immediately frozen as FFP or F24 becomes "liquid plasma" (stored at 1 to 6°C) or "source plasma" (stored at −18°C or colder). These products are used for the preparation of plasma derivatives: albumin, clotting factor concentrates, and immunoglobulin preparations.

INDICATIONS

The indications for the use of FFP and F24, the clinical conditions for which FFP and F24 administration is not indicated, and investigational uses are listed in Table 149–1. Audits of transfusion practices have consistently demonstrated that frozen plasma use is inappropriately high.[4,5] Specifically, FFP and F24 should not be used (a) to reconstitute "whole blood" by coadministration with red blood cells (RBCs); (b) as a simple volume expander; or (c) as a source of nutrients. Appropriate uses are described in detail in the following sections.

Liver Disease and Transplantations

Patients with severe liver disease may have low levels of the vitamin K-dependent clotting factors (II, VII, IX, and X) (see Chapter 124). These patients develop a prolonged prothrombin time (PT) and partial thromboplastin time (PTT). In addition, the thrombin time (TT) may be prolonged, fibrin split products may be elevated, and in later stages the fibrinogen level may decrease. Hemorrhage, most often secondary to an anatomic lesion, may be complicated by the coagulopathy resulting from these abnormalities.

Infusions of FFP and F24 are indicated during bleeding if the coagulation test results are abnormal. In the absence of anatomic lesions, bleeding does not usually occur until the PT is greater than 16 to 18 seconds or the PTT is greater than 55 to 60 seconds. Frozen plasma products are not recommended prophylactically before a surgical challenge or liver biopsy unless these values are exceeded.[6] In fact, the PT and PTT are poor predictors of surgical bleeding, and mild abnormalities in these coagulation tests may be impossible to correct—even with infusion of large quantities of plasma.[7,8] Orthotopic liver transplantation complicated by preexisting severe liver disease, lack of clotting factor synthesis during the anhepatic stage, massive pRBC transfusion, and disseminated intravascular coagulation (DIC) may require large volumes of FFP.[9] Transfusion should be guided by clinical assessment of bleeding, coagulation test results, and thromboelastographic changes.[10,11]

Massive Transfusion

The administration of FFP and F24 to patients receiving large quantities of pRBC (>1 blood volume in 24 hours in an adult) is often recommended because of a dilutional coagulopathy arising from blood replacement with pRBC and crystalloid solutions, both of which lack coagulation factors. Dilutional thrombocytopenia, another potential result of massive transfusion, may complicate the coagulopathy in these patients.[12]

In general, FFP and F24 transfusions are of little value in nonbleeding patients who have received less than 6 to 10 units of pRBC. In some patients, however, shock associated with DIC and dilutional

Table 149–1 Administration of Fresh-Frozen Plasma and F24 Plasma

Indicated
Multiple acquired coagulation factor deficiency[9–19]
Liver disease
Massive transfusion
Disseminated intravascular coagulation
Rapid reversal of warfarin effect
Plasma infusion or exchange for thrombotic thrombocytic purpura, hemolytic uremic syndrome, syndrome of hemolysis, elevated liver enzymes, and low platelets or Refsum's disease[20–23]
Congenital coagulation defects (see Chapter 126)[a]
C1-esterase inhibitor deficiency[a]—acute episodes and prophylaxis of angioedema
Investigational
Meningococcal sepsis[104]
Acute renal failure in the context of multiorgan failure[105]
Not Indicated
Immunodeficiency
Burns
Wound healing
Reconstitution of packed red blood cells
Volume expansion
Source of nutrients

[a]Fresh-frozen plasma is used in the absence of specific factor concentrate.

coagulopathy may occur, necessitating use of frozen plasma products.[11] Although several studies have demonstrated the ineffectiveness of routine FFP infusions in patients receiving more than 10 units of pRBC within 24 hours, many physicians still choose to transfuse FFP in the face of continued bleeding. Ketchem et al has shown that early use of plasma and platelets in trauma patients undergoing massive transfusion appears to decrease the incidence of coagulopathy in those patients.[13] However, it is far more effective to use FFP to replace depleted clotting factors reflected by abnormal laboratory tests than to use predetermined formulations (eg, 1 unit of FFP for every 5 units of pRBC transfused).[14]

Disseminated Intravascular Coagulation

Disseminated intravascular coagulation may be secondary to sepsis, liver disease, hypotension, surgery-associated hypoperfusion, trauma, obstetric complications, leukemia (usually promyelocytic), or underlying malignancy (see Chapter 131). Successful treatment of the underlying cause is paramount. Patients with DIC and bleeding should be given frozen plasma products in amounts sufficient to correct or ameliorate the hemorrhagic diathesis. However, in patients with severe liver disease, bleeding, and DIC, FFP infusions often fail to normalize the PT and PTT.[15]

Rapid Reversal of Warfarin Effect

Warfarin inhibits the hepatic synthesis of vitamin K-dependent clotting factors (II, VII, IX, and X) by blocking the recovery of the form of vitamin K that is active in the carboxylation of these proteins (see Chapter 129). Warfarin therapy induces functional deficiencies of these factors, which correct within 48 hours after the discontinuation of warfarin if diet and vitamin K absorption are normal. Vitamin K administration corrects the coagulopathy in 12 to 18 hours.[16] In patients anticoagulated with warfarin who have active bleeding, require emergency surgery, or have serious trauma, the deficient clotting factors can be immediately provided by prothrombin complex concentrates (PCC), or frozen plasma product transfusion. PCC should be chosen as first-line therapy, especially if volume overload is a concern. FFP is recommended as standard of care if PCCs are unavailable.[17,18] To replenish the vitamin K-dependent coagulation factors such that adequate hemostasis (normalized PT) is established, a large volume of frozen plasma may be required. Markris et al has demonstrated that FFP contains insufficient amounts of vitamin K-dependent factors to reverse the effects of warfarin completely.[18] In patients without bleeding but with significantly prolonged PTs, the potential danger of significant hemorrhage is often overemphasized and must be weighed against the risks of plasma infusion when PCCs are not available.[19] In addition, some case reports appear to support the "off label" use of recombinant FVIIa for warfarin reversal in the context of head trauma; controlled trials have not been executed as yet.[156]

Thrombotic Thrombocytopenic Purpura and Hemolytic Uremic Syndrome

In patients with thrombotic thrombocytopenic purpura (TTP), FFP/F24 as simple transfusion or in plasma exchange is the treatment of choice because plasma contains the needed vWF-cleaving protease. Plasmapheresis is preferred in most patients, including those at risk for fluid overload, such as those with renal or cardiac impairment (see Chapter 138). Plasmapheresis is most effective in those patients who have an autoantibody, acquired TTP. This is due to the removal of a patient's plasma containing the inhibitor coupled with the addition of donor plasma containing the functional vWF-cleaving protease.[20,21] The FDA has approved the use of CRP for refractory TTP, defined as those who are unresponsive to standard therapy with FFP. Some authorities advocate the use of CRP as a first-line therapy for TTP, an off-label use of the component. However, in 2001 The North American TTP Group published a multicenter prospective randomized trial comparing exchange transfusion with FFP to CRP for the initial treatment of TTP. They demonstrated that survival was the same in both study groups and established equal efficacy between FFP and CRP for the initial therapy in TTP.[22,23]

Standard therapy involves daily plasmapheresis with FFP/F24 or CRP replacing 1.0 to 1.5 plasma volumes. Treatment should be initiated immediately or at least within 24 hours of diagnosis.[24] The total number of treatments is based on the patients' clinical response, but the average number of exchanges to achieve remission are approximately.[25]

DOSAGE

One unit of FFP or F24 derived from a unit of whole blood contains 200 to 280 mL. When plasma is collected by apheresis, as much as 800 mL can be obtained from one individual (jumbo plasma units). On average, there is 0.7 to 1 unit/mL of activity of each coagulation factor per milliliter of FFP and 1 to 2 mg/mL of fibrinogen. The appropriate dose of FFP may be estimated from the plasma volume, the desired increment of factor activity, and the expected half-life of the factor being replaced. Alternatively, the plasma dosage may be estimated as 8 to 10 mL/kg, and ideally should be ordered as the number of milliliters to be infused.[26] In critically ill patients higher doses of FFP should be considered, 30 mL/kg.[27] The frequency of administration depends on the clinical response to the infusion and the normalization of laboratory parameters.

COMPATIBILITY AND SIDE EFFECTS

Frozen plasma is screened for unexpected RBC antibodies at the time of collection and should be ABO-type compatible for transfusion. Tests for serologic compatibility, major and/or minor crossmatching, are not performed before administration. Alloimmunization to RBC antigens may occur with FFP transfusion, but this is rare.[28]

A Case of Transfusion-Related Acute Lung Injury

A 30-year-old woman with precursor B-cell ALL in DIC presents with respiratory distress, severe hypoxemia, hypotension, and fever 2 hours after receiving 2 units of FFP. The patient's hypotension does not respond well to intravenous fluids. On physical exam she has rales and decreased breath sounds. No murmur is auscultated and no jugular venous distention is observed. Her chest x-ray reveals bilateral pulmonary infiltrates.

Transfusion-related acute lung injury (TRALI) is a clinical diagnosis. The exact pathophysiology of TRALI has not been clearly established. Clinicians should be keenly aware of the transfusion reaction and especially how it relates to plasma product administration. Reporting these types of cases to the medical director of the blood bank at the institution is imperative to help with the understanding of this type of transfusion reaction and prevention of the reaction in the patient or other patients in the future. Please see the transfusion reaction chapter for more details about TRALI.

Fever, chills, and allergic reactions may occur and are treated symptomatically. Occasionally, severe allergic reactions with symptoms of bronchoconstriction or noncardiogenic pulmonary edema are seen. Some of these cases are thought to be due to HLA antibodies present in donor plasma that react with recipient leukocytes. The phenomenon has been termed transfusion-related acute lung injury (TRALI). TRALI is now reportedly the leading cause of mortality related to transfusion, and may be underdiagnosed because it can occur in the context of extremely ill patients.[29,30]

Anaphylactic reactions may occur after infusion of plasma (containing IgA) into patients with complete IgA deficiency and antibodies to IgA.[31] For such patients, it is possible to obtain IgA-deficient plasma from donors in the national registry.

Transmission of infectious disease by frozen plasma products has been significantly reduced, but the risk is not yet completely eliminated. Frozen plasma is not thought to transmit the cell-associated cytomegalovirus.[32]

CRYOPRECIPITATE

Cryoprecipitate is prepared from 1 unit of FFP thawed at 4°C. The precipitate is then refrozen in 10 to 15 mL of plasma and stored at −18°C or colder for 1 year. Cryoprecipitate contains 80 to 100 units of factor VIII, 100 to 250 mg of fibrinogen, and 50 to 60 mg of fibronectin. Initially the plasma also contains 40% to 70% of vWF. Anti-A and anti-B antibodies may also be present, but in small amounts.

For clinical purposes, cryoprecipitate should be considered the blood product most rich in factor VIII, vWF, XIII, fibrinogen, and fibronectin—the plasma proteins with the highest molecular weights. Cryoprecipitate is used predominately to treat bleeding associated with fibrinogen and factor XIII deficiency states.[33] It is rarely used to treat vWF and factor VIII deficiencies. Congenital deficiencies of these factors and their treatments are discussed in Chapters 122, 124, 126, 117, 128, 32, and 150.

Indications

The indicated, investigational, and nonindicated clinical conditions for administration of cryoprecipitate are listed in Table 149–2. Specific indications and inappropriate uses are discussed subsequently.

Table 149–2 Administration of Cryoprecipitate

Indicated
Fibrinogen deficiency
Massive transfusion[35]
Reversal of thrombolytic therapy[154,155]
Congenital afibrinogenemia
Dysfibrinogenemia[34]
Factor XIII deficiency[a]
Fibrin glue[41–44]
Renal stone removal[106]
Possibly Indicated
Some patients with hemophilia A or von Willebrand disease[39]
Uremic bleeding
Investigational
Wound healing (as a source of fibronectin)[107]
Premature rupture of membranes[45]
Not Indicated
Sepsis (postoperative)

[a]Cryoprecipitate is used in the absence of specific factor concentrate. This product is not FDA-approved in the United States.

Fibrinogen Deficiency

Fibrinogen deficiency is the primary indication for cryoprecipitate transfusion. The deficiency may present in the form of congenital afibrinogenemia (rare) or dysfibrinogenemia, severe liver disease, DIC, or during massive transfusion.[34–38] These patients often have concomitant decreases in clotting factor levels and require the coadministration of frozen plasma products. It is important to obtain fibrinogen measurements because levels less than 100 mg/dL cause prolongation of the PT and PTT, despite adequate clotting factor replacement. Very low levels of fibrinogen occur during liver transplantation, where transfusion support with cryoprecipitate is vital.[9,19]

Von Willebrand Disease

Von Willebrand factor (vWf), required for platelet binding to damaged vascular endothelium, is low, absent, or dysfunctional in von Willebrand disease (vWD). DDAVP (desmopressin acetate [1-deamino, 8-D-arginine], vasopressin) remains the treatment of choice in type I vWD. However, in DDAVP nonresponders who have type I vWD or in those individuals not eligible for DDAVP with types II and III vWD, therapy with plasma-derived vWF-containing concentrates is the treatment of choice. As a last resort, if vWF-containing concentrates are unavailable and severe bleeding is occurring, cryoprecipitate may be administered. However, recent advances in clotting factor concentrates and viral inactivation methods may make the use of "wet" cryoprecipitate to treat vWD obsolete.[39,40]

Fibrin Glue and Sealants

Fibrin glue results from the mixture of a fibrinogen source (from FFP, platelet-rich plasma, or heterologous [90%] or, more recently, autologous cryoprecipitate) with bovine thrombin. The enhanced local hemostasis achieved by fibrin glue is through the action of thrombin on fibrinogen. As adjunct therapy, this product has been used successfully in cardiac surgery to control multiple small blood leaks as a result of adhesions, and to reduce blood loss and the factor concentrate requirement in patients with von Willebrand disease undergoing various surgical procedures.[41] Autologous and heterologous fibrin clot preparations have been used in meniscal tear repair,[42] in establishing patency of anastomosis in vasovasostomy,[43] in the treatment of postoperative neonatal chylothorax, and midtrimester premature rupture of membranes.[44,45] The infectious risks (eg, human immunodeficiency virus [HIV] and hepatitis) associated with the use of heterologous fibrin glue are eliminated by replacement with the autologous source. Production of fibrin glue is a non-FDA-approved preparation, but it has been widely used in Europe for more than 20 years. There are recently FDA-approved alternatives to fibrin glue termed *fibrin sealants*. They may have some advantages—such as standardization of production—over locally made fibrin glue, but are much more expensive.[46] Other complications related to bovine thrombin (anaphylaxis, formation of antibodies to factor V) or related to the activation of coagulation have been reported with fibrin glue and fibrin sealants.[47]

Uremic Bleeding

Abnormal bleeding is a common complication of uremia and is primarily due to platelet dysfunction and defective interaction with endothelium. Use of cryoprecipitate as a source of vWF has been speculated to correct the platelet dysfunction. However, cryoprecipitate has been shown not to affect platelet aggregation in vitro, but does shorten the bleeding time. In 1980, a single study published in the *New England Journal of Medicine* led to the widespread, but temporary, use of cryoprecipitate for the treatment of uremic bleeding.[48] Since that time, variable response reports have been published.[49] Therefore, cryoprecipitate may be beneficial in the management of uremic bleeding.

Dosage

The dosage of cryoprecipitate is calculated on the basis of the amount of fibrinogen present in 1 unit of cryoprecipitate, the plasma volume, and the desired increment. The difficulty in determining the correct amount to administer is due primarily to variability in the fibrinogen content of cryoprecipitate, secondary to variable storage volume and pooling methods used. The goal of therapy should be to maintain the measured fibrinogen at greater than 100 mL/dL. This can usually be accomplished by the transfusion of 2 to 4 units/10 kg if the fibrinogen content of the concentrate is low and by 1 to 2 units/10 kg if the fibrinogen content is high. For these doses, the expected increment in fibrinogen should be approximately 60 to 100 mg/dL. Dosing frequency should be determined based on clinical and laboratory response.

Compatibility and Side Effects

Cryoprecipitate can contain anti-A and/or anti-B antibodies and, as such, the American Association of Blood Banks (AABB) Standards recommends ABO compatibility for cryoprecipitate transfusions.[50] However, because of the small amounts of these isohemagglutinins in each unit, "out of ABO group" cryoprecipitate is sometimes administered when "in ABO group" cryoprecipitate is unavailable. As with FFP/F24, compatibility testing is not required and because cryoprecipitate does not contain red blood cells, Rh matching is unnecessary. The risks of fevers, chills, allergic reactions, and infectious disease transmission are similar to those of frozen plasma products.

ALBUMIN

Albumin, an important plasma protein, contributes primarily to the maintenance of plasma colloid oncotic pressure. It is clinically available in three forms: a 5% solution in saline; a 25% solution in distilled water; and purified protein fraction (PPF), which is 5% total protein (88% albumin and 12% globulins). These products are heat treated and unable to transmit viruses. The high cost, periodic shortages, and lack of efficacy in some clinical situations have led to increased scrutiny over the appropriate use of this important plasma derivative.[51,52] In many clinical situations, the use of albumin remains controversial and is the subject of continued debate. Many authorities believe that albumin is extensively overused. Listed in Table 149–3 are our preferences for indications, possible indications, investigational uses, and clinical situations in which administration is contraindicated. Under common usages, the table contains clinical situations in which albumin is frequently used.

Table 149–3 Administration of Albumin

Indicated
After large-volume paracentesis[62–64]
Nephrotic syndrome resistant to potent diuretics[66]
Ovarian hyperstimulation syndrome[68–70]
Volume/fluid replacement in plasmapheresis[109]
Possibly Indicated
Adult respiratory distress syndrome
Cardiopulmonary bypass pump priming[56]
Fluid resuscitation in shock/sepsis/burns[57]
Neonatal kernicterus
To reduce enteral feeding intolerance[110]
Not Indicated
Correction of measured hypoalbuminemia or hypoproteinemia
Nutritional deficiency, total parenteral nutrition[111]
Preeclampsia[112]
Red blood cell suspension
Simple volume expansion (surgery, burns)[57]
Wound healing
Investigational
Cadaveric renal transplantation[113]
Cerebral ischemia[114]
Stroke[115]
Common Usages
Serum albumin <20 g/dL
Nephrotic syndrome, proteinuria, and hypoalbuminemia
Labile pulmonary, cardiovascular status
Cardiopulmonary bypass, pump priming
Extensive burns
Plasma exchange
Hypotension
Liver disease, hypoalbuminemia, diuresis
Protein-losing enteropathy, hypoalbuminemia
Resuscitation
Intraoperative fluid requirement exceeding 5 to 6 L in adults
Premature infant undergoing major surgery

Indications

A decrease in measured plasma albumin is found in many situations and is often not a clinically significant concern. Mild edema due to hypoalbuminemia does not require albumin therapy. However, inadequate synthesis, as seen in severe liver disease and severe malnutrition, or excessive loss, as seen in nephrotic syndrome and protein-losing enteropathy, can lead to significant hypoalbuminemia with intravascular volume depletion, anasarca, ascites, and pleural effusions. Historically, albumin has had a broader use (ie, nutritional support, correction of hypoalbuminemia, volume replacement), but recent studies support its benefit in fewer situations, including nephrotic syndrome resistant to potent diuretic therapy, after large-volume paracentesis, and in ovarian hyperstimulation syndrome (OHSS).[53,54]

The indications and inappropriate uses of albumin are described in detail in the following sections.

Intravascular Volume Expansion

Albumin provides the most (80%) of plasma colloid oncotic pressure. Infused albumin provides colloid oncotic pressure; however, 50% of the infused protein is lost to the extravascular fluid compartment within 4 hours. Crystalloid may also provide volume expansion and is more quickly redistributed into total body fluids. Studies investigating the use of albumin in various situations including volume expansion during and after surgery,[55] as priming solution in cardiopulmonary bypass,[56] or in maintaining colloid oncotic pressure,[57] found no clinical benefit compared with controls. In 1998, the Cochrane Injuries Group performed a systematic review of randomized control trials in albumin treatment of critically ill patients and concluded that there was no evidence that albumin reduces mortality in patients with hypovolemia, burns, or hypoalbuminemia. In fact, they suggested that albumin may increase mortality. On the basis of their findings, the group recommended that hypoalbuminemia be eliminated from the list of indications and called for a large randomized trial to assess the effect of albumin on mortality.[58] Critics of the meta-analysis sharply disagreed with the Injuries Group findings and have extensively disputed each study's individual and cumulative conclusions.[59] At this time albumin therapy cannot be recommended for simple volume expansion or for the maintenance of albumin levels or colloid oncotic pressure. This conclusion is not definitive and *it will not be definitive* until a large, randomized control trial on albumin administration in critically ill patients is performed. Currently, the Australia and New Zealand Intensive Care Society in conjunction with the Institute for International Health of the University of Sydney are embarking on such a study.[60]

Cirrhosis

The use of albumin in cirrhotic patients dates to before 1950. In this setting, albumin is recommended for temporary improvement in hyponatremia, spontaneous bacterial peritonitis, or prevention of the complications associated with paracentesis, including volume shifts and hyponatremia.[61] Several studies demonstrated that after large-volume paracentesis, hyponatremia and renal insufficiency were improved with albumin infusion compared with other volume-expanding agents.[62–64]

Nephrotic Syndrome

Albumin has been used to increase colloid oncotic pressure with the intention of increasing diuresis. This use is currently limited to patients in whom diuretic therapy is poorly tolerated or ineffective or in those with massive ascites or anasarca.[65,66]

Ovarian Hyperstimulation Syndrome

Ovarian hyperstimulation syndrome is characterized by ovarian enlargement and increased capillary permeability that results in ascites and renal impairment with fluid and electrolyte imbalance.[67] This potentially lethal syndrome is associated with exogenously administered gonadotrophins for the induction of ovulation in women undergoing reproductive procedures. Several vasoactive substances, including an unidentified factor released by the hyperstimulated ovary, have been implicated in the pathogenesis of OHSS. In high-risk patients, the use of prophylactic IV human albumin at the time of oocyte retrieval has been shown to decrease significantly the incidence and severity of OHSS,[68–70] although the pregnancy rate may be less than that associated with embryo cryopreservation.[71] Furthermore, a meta-analysis by Aboulghar et al in 2002 demonstrated that albumin administration was effective in the prevention of severe OHSS.[72] However, it is unknown if therapeutic albumin treatment for women with a diagnosis of severe OHSS is effective. It is postulated that albumin exerts its beneficial effect through binding and inactivating the OHSS-associated factor.

Dose

The volume and speed of administration should be determined by the patient's volume status, condition, and response to the product. Albumin 5% is oncotically equivalent to normal human plasma. Albumin 25% provides less infusion volume per amount of albumin and is usually administered to patients with a tenuous volume status.

Compatibility and Side Effects

Albumin is a plasma derivative used widely and associated with rare adverse reactions. Still, allergic reactions, including urticaria, may be encountered. Volume overload may occur with excessive doses, and a decrease in ionized calcium is, at least, a theoretical possibility. Albumin is an excellent growth medium for bacteria, and bacterial contamination can lead to febrile and more serious reactions. Albumin lots are tested for contaminants and pyrogens before shipment. Transmission of infectious diseases is no longer a concern.

INTRAVENOUS IMMUNOGLOBULIN

Intravenous immunoglobulin is prepared by fractionation of large pools of human plasma. There are numerous preparations available in the United States and throughout the world. Each preparation is slightly different and has theoretical advantages and disadvantages and specific licensed indications. Ideally, IVIG should contain each IgG subclass; retain Fc receptor activity; have a normal half-life; demonstrate virus neutralization, opsonization, and intracellular killing; and have antibacterial capsular polysaccharide antibody. Furthermore, vasoactive impurities should be absent, and no transmissible infectious agents should be present.[73]

Indications

Indications, possible indications, and investigational uses of IVIG are listed in Table 149–4.

Primary Immunodeficiency Syndromes

Primary congenital immunodeficiency syndromes have been treated with intramuscular immunoglobulin for the past 30 years. The use of intramuscular immunoglobulin has certain disadvantages: delayed absorption, delivery of inadequate amounts due to small muscle mass, and pain at the injection site. IVIG overcomes these disadvantages, and used prophylactically in patients with primary immunodeficiency[74] has been demonstrated to reduce the number of febrile and infectious episodes as well as improve survival rate.[75] IVIG use in IgG subclass deficiencies is also beneficial.[76]

Chronic Lymphocytic Leukemia

Chronic lymphocytic leukemia (CLL) may be associated with hypogammaglobulinemia and complications of repeated bacterial infections (see Chapter 79). IVIG decreases the incidence and severity of bacterial infections in CLL patients with hypogammaglobulinemia and has become accepted prophylactic therapy.[77,78]

Table 149–4 Administration of Intravenous Immunoglobulins

Indicated
Primary immunodeficiency syndromes
Common variable immunodeficiency
X-linked agammaglobulinemia
Severe combined immunodeficiency
Ataxia-telangiectasia
Wiskott–Aldrich syndrome
IgG subclass deficiency[76]
Cytomegalovirus-interstitial pneumonia after bone marrow transplantation[79]
Chronic inflammatory demyelinating polyneuropathy[121]
Chronic lymphocytic leukemia[77]
Guillain–Barré syndrome[123,124]
Idiopathic thrombocytopenic purpura (refractory)[83-88]
Inflammatory myopathies (refractory, dermatomyositis, and polymyositis)[108,128,129]
Mucocutaneous lymph node syndrome[91]
Pediatric HIV infection[82]
Parvovirus infection
Possibly Indicated
Antiphospholipid syndrome in pregnancy[118]
Autoimmune hemolytic anemia (warm type unresponsive to prednisone)[119]
Factor VIII inhibitors (refractory)[151]
Graves ophthalmopathy[132]
Immune neutropenia[126]
Multiple myeloma (stable disease, high risk for infections)[1331]
Myasthenia gravis (refractory, acute severe decompensation)[133]
Pemphigus[152]
Systemic lupus erythematosus (refractory, severe, active)[148]
Thrombocytopenia refractory to platelet transfusion[149]
Vasculitis (refractory to standard therapy)[150]
Investigational
Acquired von Willebrand disease[116]
Amyotrophic lateral sclerosis[117]
Burn patients[120]
Chronic fatigue syndrome[122]
Fetomaternal alloimmune thrombocytopenia[136]
Graft-versus-host disease[81]
Human immunodeficiency virus infection[125]
Immune-mediated aplastic anemia[77]
Inflammatory bowel disease[77]
Intractable childhood epilepsy[130]
Multiple sclerosis[134]
Neonatal hemolytic disease[137,138]
Neonatal sepsis[135]
Prevention of nosocomial postoperative infections[139,140]
Prophylaxis in transplant recipients against cytomegalovirus infection[141]
Recurrent unexplained spontaneous abortions[142,143]
Rheumatoid arthritis[144]
Solid organ transplantation[145–147]

Bone Marrow Transplantation

The use of prophylactic IVIG or cytomegalovirus (CMV)–IVIG in CMV-negative bone marrow transplant recipients during the first 100 days posttransplant has been demonstrated to reduce the incidence of symptomatic CMV-associated disease, including CMV interstitial pneumonia, in some trials.[78] Because of the high cost of this treatment and the increasing use of prophylactic ganciclovir, IVIG is currently not indicated for the prophylaxis of CMV infections in bone marrow transplant recipients. In established CMV-interstitial pneumonia, IVIG in combination with ganciclovir has been shown to reduce the mortality rate and has become the recommended treatment modality.[80] Its role in preventing severe graft-versus-host disease is unclear. Prolonged IVIG therapy during GVHD prevention may suppress humoral immunity recovery.[79,81]

Pediatric Human Immunodeficiency Virus Infection

The defects in humoral and cellular immunity observed in children with HIV infection predispose them to life-threatening bacterial infections. Studies have shown that the administration of IVIG to HIV-infected children can reduce the incidence and severity of bacterial infections as well as the frequency of hospitalization.[82] Prevention of maternal–fetal transmission of HIV infection through the use of hyperimmune HIV-IVIG is being investigated.

Idiopathic Thrombocytopenic Purpura

The use of IVIG represents a major advance in the treatment of acute and chronic idiopathic thrombocytopenic purpura (ITP) (see Chapter 132). IVIG significantly raises the platelet count within 5 days in adults with chronic ITP and in children with acute ITP.[7,83,84] The mechanism of action of IVIG in ITP is unknown, but most clinicians believe that Fc receptor blockade decreases the removal of antibody-coated platelets. Other proposed mechanisms include suppressed antiplatelet antibody synthesis, increased antiviral immunity, and blockage by antiidiotypic antibodies. In general, IVIG induces responses in most patients within 1 to 2 days. Responses are of variable duration and are rarely sustained, although maintenance therapy may be of some value. IVIG may be effective in chronic ITP refractory to corticosteroids or splenectomy[85,86]; may show greater efficacy in conjunction with corticosteroids[87]; and has been demonstrated to be superior to oral corticosteroids in children with acute ITP.[88]

Although IVIG has shown equal efficacy with corticosteroids in pediatric acute ITP and in 75% of adults with chronic ITP, because of the transient responses and high cost, its use is justified only in clinical situations requiring rapid elevation of platelet count or if standard therapy has failed. IVIG is, therefore, indicated in acute bleeding episodes or before urgent surgery, including splenectomy; in patients at high risk of intracranial hemorrhage; and in those in whom corticosteroids are contraindicated or ineffective. IVIG has also been used to treat ITP during pregnancy, postinfectious thrombocytopenia, ITP associated with HIV infection, and neonatal thrombocytopenia. Intravenous anti-D immune globulin has demonstrated efficacy in Rh-positive, nonsplenectomized individuals with ITP. It has been suggested that the mechanism of action may involve a shift in the immune-mediated destruction from platelets to the antibody-coated RBCs.[89]

Mucocutaneous Lymph Node Syndrome

The mucocutaneous lymph node syndrome (Kawasaki disease) has been treated with aspirin with or without concomitant IVIG administration.[90] Coronary artery aneurysm, a serious complication of this disease, was significantly reduced in the IVIG-treated group.[91] However, in a multicenter retrospective survey of all children treated with Kawasaki disease, persistent or recrudescent fever after their first course of IVIG was associated with a statistically significant risk of treatment failure. Furthermore, IVIG retreatment in those patients with persistent fever after IVIG treatment failure was approximately 60%. A call was made for a randomized trial to assess the efficacy of this practice.[92] With regard to the pathogenesis of Kawasaki disease, decreased peripheral blood lymphocyte apoptosis has been demonstrated. Therefore, the effect of IVIG in Kawasaki disease has been postulated to partially reverse inhibited lymphocyte apoptosis.[93]

Dosage

Patients with primary immunodeficiency syndromes and IgG levels less than 200 mg/dL are candidates for immunoglobulin replacement. Most patients require 100 to 200 mg/kg IV every 3 to 4 weeks to achieve adequate IgG levels (usually >800 mg/dL) and protection against infection. Initially, serial IgG level determination may allow the physician to individualize the dose and schedule. These are affected by the recovery, half-life, redistribution, and catabolism of IVIG, which vary from product to product and patient to patient. Patients with ITP are usually treated with 400 mg/kg daily for 5 days or 1000 mg/kg daily for 2 days (see Chapter 132). Repeat single doses (400 mg/kg) have been used intermittently in some patients (particularly children) to maintain platelet counts greater than 50,000/μL. Kawasaki disease is treated with higher doses ranging from 1800 mg/kg to 2000 mg/kg as a single dose.[90,91,94]

Compatibility and Side Effects

Infusions of IVIG should be started slowly and patients should be closely monitored. If the initial rate (0.5 mL/kg/hour) is well tolerated, the rate can be increased gradually, but not more than eightfold. Fever, headache, nausea, vomiting, fatigue, backache, leg cramps, urticaria, flushing, elevation of blood pressure, and thrombophlebitis may be seen. IgA-deficient patients may have IgG anti-IgA antibodies, which can cause anaphylactic reactions.[94] This complication is rare and may be avoided by using products with a lower concentration of IgA.[95] Aggregated IgG may produce chills, nausea, flushing, chest tightness, and wheezing. Rarely, IVIG preparations contain IgG anti-A and/or anti-B RBC antibodies that can produce hemolysis[96] or interfere with serologic evaluations, including RBC compatibility testing.[97] IVIG treatment will produce a positive direct antiglobulin test (DAT), rendering the DAT test result unhelpful with regard to potential red blood cell autoantibody interpretation. Serum sickness can occur. Improved manufacturing processes currently in place render IVIG free of envelope and nonenvelope viruses.[98] Nevertheless, hepatitis C virus transmission has been reported in certain patient populations.[99,100] High-dose IVIG therapy has been associated with reversible, acute renal failure[101] and aseptic meningitis.[102]

HYPERIMMUNE AND INTRAMUSCULAR IMMUNOGLOBULINS

Hyperimmune immunoglobulin is prepared from large pools of plasma known to contain elevated antibody titers against specific infectious agents. The intramuscular and hyperimmune immunoglobulins[73] are listed in Table 149–5.

Antithymocyte globulin (ATG) is a purified concentrated γ-globulin made from hyperimmune serum of horses immunized with human T lymphocytes. ATG is used in renal transplant patients as an adjunct therapy in the treatment of graft rejection.[102] It is also used in patients with aplastic anemia who are not candidates for bone marrow transplantation (see Chapter 25).[103]

Hyperimmune immunoglobulin is used to prevent the development of specific clinical disease or alter its symptomatology. CMV Ig is indicated in all kidney and liver transplant recipients who are seronegative for CMV and who receive the respective organ from a seropositive donor and in bone marrow transplant patients with CMV interstitial pneumonia.[79] Hepatitis B immunoglobulin is used to provide passive immunity to hepatitis B virus associated with needlestick exposure or sexual contact with HBsAg-positive individuals.

Rh immunoglobulin is used when fetal Rh(D)-positive RBCs may have entered the maternal circulation of an Rh(D)-negative mother. This means that Rh(D) immunoglobulin is given to Rh(D)-negative mothers after abortion or amniocentesis, as well as before delivery and again postpartum if the child proves to be Rh(D) positive.[153] The therapeutic effect is thought to be caused by antibody feedback with T-cell suppression of the B-cell clone responsible for the formation of anti-Rh antibody. Rh immunoglobulin can also be given to prevent immunization in Rh(D)-negative individuals given Rh(D)-positive components, such as platelets. Transfusion of Rh(D)-positive RBCs to Rh(D)-negative recipients is occasionally necessary, and prevention of immunization is not possible unless IV Rh immunoglobulin is made available by the manufacturers. Rh immunoglobulin has also been used to treat ITP.[89]

Experimentally, immunoglobulin has also been administered by oral, intrathecal, and aerosolized routes. Oral administration has been tried with some success in the prevention of rotavirus infection and necrotizing enterocolitis in premature infants, in the treatment of *Cryptosporidia*-associated diarrhea, and in the prevention of viral gastroenteritis after bone marrow transplant. Intrathecal administration has been tried in the treatment of viral encephalitis and tetanus, aerosolized administration in infections with respiratory syncytial virus.

Table 149–5 Hyperimmune and Intramuscular Immunoglobulins

Antithymocyte globulin
Cytomegalovirus immunoglobulin
Hepatitis B immunoglobulin
Rabies immunoglobulin
Rh(D) immunoglobulin
Tetanus immunoglobulin
Vaccinia immunoglobulin
Varicella-zoster immunoglobulin
Western equine encephalitis immunoglobulin

SUGGESTED READINGS

Blood Products Advisory Committee: 80th Meeting. Department of Health and Human Services, Food and Drug Administration, Center for Biologics Evaluation and Research. July 22, 2004. (Available at www.fed.gov/ohrms/dockets/ac/04/transcripts/2004-405t1.doc).

British Society of Haematology: Guidelines on the diagnosis and management of thrombotic microangiopathic haemolytic anaemias. Br J Haematol 120:556, 2004.

Buchanan GR, Journeycake JM, Adix L: Severe chronic idiopathic thrombocytopenic purpura during childhood: Definition, management, and prognosis. Sem Thromb Haemost 29:595, 2003.

Cardigan R, Lawrie AS, Mackie IJ, et al: The quality of fresh-frozen plasma produced from whole blood stored at 4°C overnight. Transfusion 45:1342, 2005.

Cherin P, Pelletier S, Teixeira A, et al: Results and long-term follow-up of intravenous immunoglobulin infusions in chronic, refractory polymyositis: An open study with thirty-five adult patients. Arthritis Rheum 46:467, 2002.

Ketchem L, Hess JR, Hiippala S: Indications for early fresh frozen plasma, cryoprecipitate, and platelet transfusion in trauma. J Trauma 60:S51, 2006.

MacLennan S, Hamilton PJ: Management of massive blood loss: A template guide. Br J Anaesth 85:387, 2000.

Newburger JW, Takahashi M, Gerber MA, et al: Diagnosis, treatment, and long-term management of Kawasaki disease: A statement for health professionals from the Committee on Rheumatic Fever, Endocarditis, and Kawasaki Disease, Council on Cardiovascular Disease in the Young, American Heart Association. Pediatrics 114:1708, 2004.

Pantanowitz L, Kruskall M, Uhl L: Cryoprecipitate patterns of use. Am J Clin Pathol 119:874, 2003.

Roberts I: Albumin and hypovolemia: Time to move on and generate new evidence. Lancet 259:72, 2002.

REFERENCES

For complete list of references log onto www.expertconsult.com

CHAPTER 150

PREPARATION OF PLASMA-DERIVED AND RECOMBINANT HUMAN PLASMA PROTEINS

William N. Drohan and David B. Clark

The development of large-scale methods for the preparation of human plasma proteins began more than 60 years ago. In 1940, after the outbreak of World War II, a meeting was called to discuss the urgent request of the United States Armed Forces for 300,000 units of human whole blood or plasma for transfusion, which at that time seemed an impossibly large amount.[1] Dr. Edwin J. Cohn of the Harvard Medical School was approached to determine whether animal plasma could be made safe for human use. Cohn drew together a task force of investigators and developed a method for the fractionation of bovine plasma based on differential precipitation of various plasma proteins by appropriate combinations of ethanol concentration, pH, low temperature, ionic strength, and protein concentration. Within a short time, highly purified preparations of bovine serum albumin were available for clinical trials. Although there were no immediate reactions, the frequency of severe delayed reactions made it obvious that these preparations were unsuitable for clinical use. Meanwhile, Cohn had arranged with the American Red Cross to provide his laboratory with a supply of human plasma, and the ethanol method was quickly adapted for human plasma fractionation. Although albumin was the only product distributed during the war, the remaining plasma fractions were carefully preserved, and other preparations, including fibrinogen and immunoglobulins, were soon developed.

Since World War II, major improvements have occurred in the preparation of human plasma proteins. The ethanol process has been supplemented by more selective purification techniques to produce a wide variety of products of high purity. Genetic engineering technology has allowed recombinant human plasma proteins to be produced in tissue culture systems and transgenic animals. Most important, the safety of plasma products has been increased significantly by the development of improved methods for the inactivation and removal of viruses, as well as for the screening and testing of donors and donations. Transfusion-transmitted diseases and the safety of blood and plasma products are described in detail in Chapter 154. Today, methods for inactivation or removal of viruses and other pathogens that might be present in the starting materials are integral parts of all manufacturing processes. This chapter describes current methods and future directions for the preparation of plasma-derived and recombinant human plasma proteins for clinical use, mainly for products available in the United States.

FRESH FROZEN PLASMA

Plasma from a single donor that has been separated from the red cells, placed in a freezer within 8 hours after phlebotomy and stored at 18°C or less meets the criteria for labeling as Fresh Frozen Plasma (FFP).[2] Clinical indications for the administration of FFP are described in Chapter 149. FFP has a very low risk of infectious disease transmission[3]; however, its viral safety depends entirely on donor selection and blood screening techniques. One method is currently being used to increase the safety of plasma for transfusion. Fresh Frozen Plasma, Donor Retested[4] is FFP that is held in quarantine for a minimum of 112 days after collection, through the "window" period during which a donor can be infectious but not test positive in the screening tests. Once the donor from whom it was collected has been retested and found negative in all tests, the plasma may be released for use. A similar method is used by most manufacturers to quarantine plasma for fractionation until a donor again tests negative at a subsequent donation.[5]

PLASMA FRACTIONATION

Plasma for fractionation is derived from two sources, either directly by plasmapheresis, termed Source Plasma, or as a by-product of whole blood donation, termed Recovered Plasma. Source and recovered plasma differ slightly in protein and lipid content, and fractionation parameters may be adjusted slightly to accommodate those differences, but in general, either type may be used interchangeably. The plasma is usually shipped frozen as individual units from local blood or plasma collection centers to a central processing plant. At the plant, sufficient units to produce typically 2000- to 3000-L pools are thawed slowly to produce a cryoprecipitate, a cold-insoluble fraction that contains significant amounts of factor VIII, von Willebrand factor (vWF), which is usually in a complex with FVIII, fibrinogen, fibronectin, and factor XIII along with a number of other proteins present in smaller quantities.[6] The cryoprecipitate is usually removed by centrifugation. The supernatant may be treated with a chromatographic media to remove the factor IX complex and antithrombin III before it is processed by the ethanol method to obtain immunoglobulins, albumin, and other products.

Cohn's Method[7] is still the basis for most of the large-scale plasma fractionation today in the United States and much of the world. Other manufacturers use a modified ethanol precipitation method developed by Kistler and Nitschmann,[8] whereas others use newer chromatographic methods.[9,10] In the Cohn method, the ethanol concentration is increased in steps from 8% to 40% at specific combinations of pH, ionic strength, protein concentration, and cold temperature to precipitate several fractions.

The first precipitate, fraction I, contains factor VIII, fibrinogen, and other poorly soluble proteins, many of which are also removed by cryoprecipitation. Fractions II and III are precipitated together and contain the immunoglobulins that are further purified in a separate process. Because many of the fraction I proteins are removed in the cryoprecipitate, some manufacturers do not produce a separate fraction I. Instead they collect a combined fraction I+II+III. Fraction IV is often produced in two subfractions. Fraction IV-1 contains the vitamin K-dependent clotting factors, antithrombin and α_1-antitrypsin. Fraction IV-4 contains transferrin, haptoglobin, and some of the albumin, whereas fraction V is almost pure albumin.[11] The overall scheme of plasma fractionation is shown in the box.

IMMUNE GLOBULINS AND HYPERIMMUNE GLOBULINS

Since the early 1950s, immune globulin products have been prepared from Cohn fraction II + III by the method developed by Oncley.[18] Oncley's method uses additional ethanol precipitations to remove lipoproteins, IgA, IgM, and other plasma proteins, leaving fraction II, which contains purified IgG.[11] The overall ethanol method is often referred to as Cohn–Oncley fractionation. Immune Globulin is prepared from the plasma of unselected normal donors, whereas hyperimmune globulins are prepared from the plasma of donors with high

ALBUMIN AND PLASMA PROTEIN FRACTION

Albumin remains one of the major products of human plasma fractionation. During the 60 years since the initial use of human serum albumin in treating the casualties at Pearl Harbor, literally tons of albumin have been isolated and millions of units have been infused.[12] Albumin, having the highest solubility and the lowest isoelectric point of all the major plasma proteins, remains in solution until the pH is adjusted to 4.8 in the presence of 40% ethanol at −5°C when the bulk of the albumin is finally precipitated in fraction V.[13] After the removal of ethanol and salts, sodium acetyltryptophanate and sodium caprylate are added as stabilizers, and the albumin is sterile-filtered and bottled. The vials are then heated for 10 hours at 60°C to inactivate any remaining blood-borne viruses. This pasteurization method was the first significant viral inactivation process developed for a plasma product.[14]

Three albumin products are manufactured in the United States: Albumin (Human) 25% solution, Albumin (Human) 5% solution, and Plasma Protein Fraction (Human). To be designated Albumin, more than 96% of the protein content must be albumin. Plasma Protein Fraction (PPF), also usually a 5% solution, is an albumin product of lower purity obtained by coprecipitating fraction IV-4 with fraction V.[15] The total protein in PPF must be 83% or more albumin, with 17% or less globulins, and 1% or less γ-globulin. PPF is more economical to produce than albumin,[16] but the rapid infusion of PPF has been associated with hypotensive episodes.[17] Clinical indications for the use of Albumin and PPF are described in Chapter 149. Albumin (Human) is also sometimes used as a stabilizer in the formulation of other highly purified plasma and recombinant products.

antibody titers against specific antigens (eg, rho(D), hepatitis B, rabies, and tetanus). These donors may be identified during convalescent periods after infection or transfusion, or they may be specifically immunized to produce the desired antibodies. Immune Globulin products and indications are described in Chapter 149.

Intravenous Immune Globulin Concentrates

The original immune globulin concentrates, originally termed Immune Serum Globulin and currently Immune Globulin (Human), were administered by the intramuscular route, with the associated problems of limited injectable volume, poor bioavailability, and discomfort at the injection site.[19] Intravenous injection of immune globulin causes serious clinical reactions, attributed to complement-activating aggregates in these products.[20]

To overcome these limitations, Immune Globulin Intravenous (Human) (IGIV) products have been developed using a variety of methods to remove or inactivate anticomplementary aggregates. Processing and formulation techniques have been improved, and conditions have been identified, to permit these products to be prepared as either freeze-dried or liquid concentrates.[21] Today most intramuscular Immune Globulin usage is limited to hyperimmune products. Immune Globulin products tend to be self-protecting from viral transmission because of the large pools of antibodies they contain.[22] However, postinfusion viral infections have occurred. As a result, all manufacturers have incorporated viral inactivation or removal steps in the production of IGIV.[23]

The development of IGIV has permitted the administration of much higher doses, with a subsequent expansion in immunoglobulin therapy. In addition to providing passive immune protection, IGIV has been found to modulate the immune response to autoimmune diseases such as idiopathic thrombocytopenic purpura.

Subcutaneous Immune Globulin Concentrates

The first patient treated for primary immune deficiency was actually given subcutaneous injections of immunoglobulins.[24] However, as described above, intramuscular and later intravenous injections became the preferred methods. Recently one manufacturer has developed an immune globulin concentrate for subcutaneous injection, termed Immune Globulin Subcutaneous (Human).[25] It is a 16% solution administered using an infusion pump. The product is intended for patients who have problems with intravenous infusion.

COAGULATION FACTOR CONCENTRATES

The distinction between hemophilia A and B was unknown in the mid-1800s when it was first shown that the transfusion of whole blood could be used to curtail bleeding in patients with hemophilia.[26,27] By 1940, bleeding episodes were being routinely treated with plasma. However, large amounts of plasma were needed, and this method of therapy could not provide normal levels of coagulation factors without producing hypervolemia.[28] The development of more highly purified plasma-derived coagulation factor concentrates and more recently of recombinant concentrates has resulted in dramatic increases in life expectancy and quality of life for patients with hemophilia.

The major issues in the preparation and use of coagulation factor concentrates are viral safety and purity. The benefit of viral safety is obvious; with the exception of cryoprecipitate, all concentrates are now subjected to some form of treatment for the inactivation or removal of viruses that might be present in the input plasma. Purity, as it affects product efficacy and adverse reactions, is discussed below for both factor VIII and factor IX products. The purity of factor IX concentrates has definitely been shown to be important; however, the situation for factor VIII products is less clear. The development of improved coagulation factor concentrates continues to be a major focus of research.

See Chapter 151 for a detailed discussion of indications and use of coagulation factor concentrates.

FACTOR VIII CONCENTRATES

Factor VIII concentrates, generically termed Antihemophilic Factor (Human) (AHF), for the treatment of hemophilia A have evolved from cryoprecipitates to very-high-purity plasma-derived products to recombinant products. The various AHF concentrates available in the United States are shown in Table 150–1.

Cryoprecipitate

In 1959, Pool and Robinson[29] reported that when frozen plasma is thawed slowly, a residual "cryoprecipitate" results that contains most of the factor VIII activity of the original plasma. By 1965, single-donor cryoprecipitate with factor VIII concentrations 5 to 30 times that of plasma became widely available for use in the treatment of hemophilia A.[30] Single-donor cryoprecipitate is still available from many blood banks but carries a risk of viral transmission. However, large-scale cryoprecipitation is the first step in most procedures for the preparation of plasma derivatives containing high concentrations of its constituent proteins. Cryoprecipitate contains approximately one-half of the factor VIII/vWF complex and one-third of the fibrinogen and factor XIII in whole plasma.[31]

Intermediate- and High-Purity Antihemophilic Factor Concentrates

Product purity is generally measured by specific activity, the activity of the protein of interest, such as factor VIII, divided by the total

Table 150–1 Antihemophilic Factor Concentrates Marketed in the United States

Antihemophilic Factor Methods	Manufacturer	Product Name	Specific Activity†	Production Methods	Virus Inactivation/Removal
Antihemophilic Factor (Human)	Baxter	Hemofil M	2–20 2000‡	Cryoprecipitation, cold-acid precipitation, IAC, IEC	S/D (TNBP/octoxynol 9), purification steps, lyophilization
	Grifols	Alphanate	5–30§ 140‡	Cryoprecipitation, salt precipitation, PEG precipitation, AC	S/D (TNBP/polysorbate 80), dry heat (80°C, 72 hours), purification steps, lyophilization
	Talecris	Koate-DVI	9–22§ 50‡	Cryoprecipitation, $Al(OH)_3$ adsorption, PEG precipitation, glycine precipitation, SEC	S/D (TNBP/polysorbate 80), dry heat (80°C, 72 hours), purification steps
	CSL Behring	Monoclate-P	4–10 >3000‡	Cryoprecipitation, cold precipitation, $Al(OH)_3$ adsorption, IAC, AC	Pasteurization (60°C, 10 hours), purification steps
Antihemophilic Factor/von Willebrand Factor Complex (Human)	CSL Behring	Humate-P	1–2§ 40‡	Cryoprecipitation, $Al(OH)_3$ adsorption, glycine precipitation	Pasteurization (60°C, 10 hours), purification steps
Antihemophilic Factor (Recombinant)	Baxter	Recombinate	2–20 >4000‡	CHO Cell culture, IAC, IEC	Purification steps
	Baxter	Advate	4000–10,000	CHO Cell culture, IAC, IEC	S/D (TNBP/polysorbate 80, octoxynol 9)
	Bayer	Kogenate FS¶	4000‡	BHK Cell culture, IEC, IAC, IMAC	S/D (TNBP/polysorbate 80), purification steps
	Wyeth	ReFacto	9000–13,000	CHO Cell culture, IEC, IAC, HC, SEC	S/D (TNBP/octoxynol 9), purification steps

AC, affinity chromatography; BHK, baby hamster kidney cells; CHO, Chinese hamster ovary cells; HC, hydrophobic chromatography; IAC, immunoaffinity chromatography; IEC, ion-exchange chromatography; IMAC, immobilized metal affinity chromatography; PEG, polyethylene glycol; S/D, solvent/detergent; SEC, size exclusion chromatography; TNBP, tri-*n*-butyl phosphate.

*These concentrates were marketed in the United States in 2006. Data were obtained from manufacturers, distributors, and available literature.

†Factor VIII U/mg of protein.

‡Before addition of human albumin.

§Also contains active von Willebrand Factor. Humate-P is the only AHF product with a licensed indication for von Willebrand disease treatment.

¶Also distributed by ZLB Behring as Helixate FS.

mass of protein in the product. The activity of most plasma proteins is measured in units, where one unit is defined as the activity in one milliliter of normal human plasma. If the product is assayed against an international reference standard, the activity is expressed in International Units (IUs). There is no consensus for classification of concentrate purity. Berntorp[32] suggests intermediate purity as having specific activities of 1 to 50 IU/mg and high purity as having specific activities of 50 to 200 IU/mg. The specific activity of plasma is on the order of 0.01 IU/mg and that of cryoprecipitate is approximately 0.3 IU/mg.[33] Many of the highly purified products contain human albumin as a stabilizer, which adds additional protein and thus lowers the apparent specific activity. To describe the effective purity of such products, the specific activity is often given in the absence of the added albumin. Table 150–1 shows both values, where applicable.

After the discovery of cryoprecipitation, the development of intermediate-purity AHF concentrates was the next significant advance in the treatment of hemophilia A. Cryoprecipitate was used as the starting material, and a variety of methods were developed to remove fibrinogen, immunoglobulins, and other proteins. Fibrinogen can be removed at specific conditions of temperature and pH or by precipitation with glycine or polyethylene glycol. Aluminum hydroxide can be used to adsorb and remove the vitamin K-dependent clotting factors II, VII, IX, and X.[34] Intermediate-purity concentrates are enriched approximately 3000-fold over plasma. Until effective methods were developed for viral inactivation following the AIDS crisis of the early 1980s, patients receiving these concentrates were exposed to all of the blood-borne viruses in the donor population. It is not surprising that frequently treated patients uniformly became infected with hepatitis[35] and, later, often HIV.[36]

Intermediate-purity AHF concentrates were the mainstay of hemophilia A treatment until the development of high-purity concentrates in the late 1980s. They are still available, their chief advantage being lower cost. As described below, some intermediate-purity concentrates are also used as a source of von Willebrand factor. More recently, various ion-exchange and gel-filtration techniques were added to the precipitation methods to produce high-purity concentrates with specific activities of 50 to 200 IU/mg of protein.[37,38] However, even though these concentrates are highly purified in comparison with the intermediate-purity concentrates, significant amounts of high-molecular-weight proteins such as fibrinogen, fibronectin, and vWF tend to fractionate with factor VIII and remain in the preparations. The only high-purity concentrates currently available in the United States are the immunoaffinity-purified concentrates discussed next.

Product purity has always been an issue with AHF concentrates. The initial improvement from plasma to cryoprecipitate to intermediate-purity concentrates primarily affected infusion volume and convenience. In the early years of the AIDS crisis, some researchers wondered if the frequent exposure to the impurities in AHF concentrates depressed the immune system of hemophiliacs and made them more susceptible to adventitious diseases. As more became known about AIDS, that idea was discarded,[39] but it did provide some of the impetus for development of higher purity products. The current focus is the effect of purity on inhibitor development. Inhibitors are antibodies produced against factor VIII because the immune system sees the protein as a foreign molecule. A number of studies have been done to look at the effect of purity on inhibitor development, but the results are still controversial.[40–42]

Antihemophilic Factor Concentrates Purified by Immunoaffinity Chromatography

The next major advance in the preparation of AHF concentrates was the use of murine monoclonal antibodies (mAbs) immobilized on a chromatographic column for the purification of factor VIII by immunoaffinity chromatography. Two different methods were developed that both start with factor VIII concentrates partially purified by conventional means.[43,44] One procedure uses an mAb that binds to the vWF portion of the factor VIII–vWF complex; the other uses an mAb that binds directly to factor VIII. In both processes, the columns are loaded with the low-purity intermediate product, washed extensively to remove unwanted proteins, and then eluted, respectively, by separation of factor VIII from the vWF–mAb complex or directly from the mAb itself. Both processes use a final chromatography step to remove the harsh elution solutions as well as any mAb that might have leached off the column. These processes produce factor VIII that is essentially pure prior to the addition of albumin as a stabilizer. Both processes include several steps that inactivate or remove viruses.

Recombinant Antihemophilic Factor Concentrates

One of the remarkable early accomplishments of molecular biology was the elucidation of the structure of factor VIII, its molecular cloning, and the successful production of recombinant human factor VIII. Because proper posttranslational processing is essential to factor VIII functionality, the products are produced in mammalian cells, either baby hamster kidney (BHK) cells or Chinese hamster ovary (CHO) cells. The CHO cells used to produce Recombinate also coexpress recombinant vWF, which helps to stabilize the FVIII and substantially increase its recovery from the culture medium. The recombinant factor VIII is purified by various combinations of immunoaffinity chromatography, ion-exchange chromatography, and gel filtration.[45] The final products contain minimal or no recombinant vWF and only trace quantities of mouse immunoglobulin, hamster protein, and cellular DNA. The second-generation product ReFacto consists of a shortened FVIII molecule with the central portion of the B-domain deleted. This produces a molecule with full activity but that is more stable during processing. The recombinant products have been shown to be safe, effective, and well-tolerated and to perform similarly to plasma-derived factor VIII in a number of clinical studies.[46]

Recombinant products have the advantage that they are nominally free from contamination with human viruses. However, some contain human or bovine components in their cell culture medium, some are purified by immunoaffinity chromatography using mAbs grown in cell culture, several are stabilized with human albumin (pasteurized) in the final product and all are produced in mammalian cells that potentially harbor unrecognized viruses in their genome. Thus there exists the theoretical possibility of virus transmission. To further minimize any possible viral risk, the three second-generation products, ReFacto, Kogenate FS, and Advate are treated with a solvent and detergent mixture that inactivates all lipid-enveloped viruses. The products are formulated without albumin or other human- or animal-derived compounds, using sugars, amino acids, and polysorbate 80 as stabilizers, with no reduction in the 2-year shelf life. ReFacto and Kogenate FS employ only human-derived compounds in their cell culture systems, and Advate employs no human- or animal-derived compounds in the cell culture systems used to produce either the product or the mAb used for purification.

FACTOR IX CONCENTRATES

Two types of plasma-derived factor IX concentrates are available today: Factor IX Complex, which contains significant amounts of the other vitamin K-dependent clotting factors, and Coagulation Factor IX (Human), a preparation substantially free of these other proteins. A recombinant product, Coagulation Factor IX (Recombinant) is also available. The factor IX concentrates available in the United States are shown in Table 150–2.

Factor IX Complex Concentrates

The vitamin K-dependent clotting factors, because of their similar structures, tend to copurify by most of the methods used to isolate them from plasma. Thus, the original factor IX products for treatment of hemophilia B were mixtures of the vitamin K-dependent

Table 150–2 Factor IX Concentrates and Related Products Marketed in the United States*

Product Type	Manufacturer/ Distributor	Product Name	Specific Activity†	Purification Methods	Virus Inactivation/ Removal Methods
Factor IX Complex	Baxter	Bebulin VH	2	IEC	Vapor heating: 60°C for 10 hours at 190 mbar, then 80°C for 1 hour at 375 mbar
	Grifols	Profilnine SD	4	IEC	S/D (TNBP/polysorbate 80), purification steps
Coagulation Factor IX (Human)	Grifols	AlphaNine SD	>150	IEC, barium citrate precipitation, AC, nanofiltration	S/D (TNBP/polysorbate 80), nanofiltration, purification steps
	CSL Behring	Mononine	>190	IEC, IAC, HIC	Sodium thiocyanate, ultrafiltration, purification steps
Coagulation Factor IX (Recombinant)	Wyeth	BeneFix	>200	CHO cell culture, IEC, IAC, IMAC, nanofiltration	Nanofiltration
Anti-Inhibitor Coagulant Complex	Baxter	FEIBA VH	NA	IEC, surface activation	Vapor heating (60°C for 10 hours at 190 mbar, then 80°C for 1 hour at 370 mbar
Coagulation Factor VIIa (Recombinant)	Novo Nordisk	NovoSeven	NA	BHK cell culture, IEC, IAC	Detergent treatment, purification steps

AC, affinity chromatography; BHK, baby hamster kidney cells; CHO, Chinese hamster ovary cells; HIC, hydrophobic interaction chromatography; IAC, immunoaffinity chromatography; IEC, ion-exchange chromatography; IMAC, immobilized metal affinity chromatography; NA, not available or not applicable; S/D, solvent/detergent; TNBP, tri-*n*-butyl phosphate.

*These concentrates were marketed in the United States in 2006. Data were obtained from manufacturers, distributors, and available literature.

†Factor IX U/mg of protein.

proteins including factor II (prothrombin), factor VII, factor IX, factor X, protein C, and protein S. Because the protein in highest concentration in these products is prothrombin, they have also been identified as prothrombin complex concentrates; however, Factor IX Complex is the generic name in the United States.

The first factor IX-rich concentrate used for the treatment of hemophilia B was developed in France more than 40 years ago.[47] It was produced by the adsorption of the plasma vitamin K-dependent clotting factors with tricalcium phosphate and was successfully used to treat hemophilia B for a number of years. The original production process had a number of disadvantages and was eventually discontinued.[48] However, this method led to the development of several other processes based on tricalcium phosphate adsorption.[49] Factor IX Complex produced by these methods contains approximately equal amounts of factor II, VII, IX, and X activity units.

The next major development in the production of Factor IX Complex concentrates was the introduction of ion-exchange chromatography.[50] This represented one of the first major uses of chromatography in plasma fractionation. As shown in the box, the vitamin K-dependent clotting factors can be captured from cryoprecipitate-poor plasma by adsorption onto diethylaminoethyl (DEAE)–cellulose or DEAE–Sephadex, and the supernatant plasma can then be further fractionated by the Cohn–Oncley method for the production of immune globulins, albumin, and other products. The eluate from the DEAE resin may be further purified by additional precipitation or adsorption steps.[51] Such processes give 100-fold or more purification of factors II, IX, and X. Factor VII does not bind to DEAE under the conditions in plasma, however, and is present in only very low concentrations in concentrates prepared by these methods.

Coagulation Factor IX Concentrates

With the widespread use of Factor IX Complex, it soon became apparent that serious thromboembolic episodes and acute myocardial infarction were major complications of its infusion, especially when used in large quantities for extended periods, such as for surgical procedures or in patients with liver disease.[52,53] The cause of the thrombogenicity has not been conclusively determined. It may be due to the presence of activated clotting factors,[54,55] contaminating phospholipids,[56] or the result of an overload of factors II and X.[57,58]

On the basis of these hypotheses, methods have been developed for the preparation of second-generation factor IX concentrates that are more highly purified and essentially free of the other vitamin K-dependent clotting factors. These have been designated Coagulation Factor IX (Human). Coagulation Factor IX concentrates are manufactured from factor IX complex by additional purification steps. Of the two products available in the United States, one is prepared by immunoaffinity chromatography using an mAb to factor IX.[59] The other is purified by heparin affinity chromatography.[60] Both methods also include viral inactivation steps. These preparations have been proven to be largely nonthrombogenic in clinical use.[61,62]

Recombinant Factor IX Concentrates

A recombinant coagulation factor IX has also been developed. It is produced in cell culture by CHO cells that also coexpress a protease that enhances the ability of the cells to remove the amino-terminal propeptide. The cell culture product is purified with several chromatography steps and treated to remove viruses.[63] The product was developed with the aim of essentially eliminating any risk of viral transmission, including elimination of blood or plasma proteins from the cell culture medium and the final product formulation, avoidance of monoclonal antibodies in the purification process, and use of a nanofiltration step in the purification process to remove any viruses that might be present.[64] The final product has been shown to be structurally and functionally similar to plasma-derived factor IX.[65] However, it gives a lower recovery when infused into patients, probably because of differences in posttranslational glycosylation.[66]

OTHER COAGULATION FACTOR CONCENTRATES

As described in Chapter 151, one of the major complications in the treatment of hemophilia patients is the development of inhibitors, antibodies directed against factor VIII or factor IX. Low-titer inhibitors can usually be saturated by administering large amounts of factor VIII or factor IX. This is not an effective therapy for higher-titer inhibitors because of the large amount of factor concentrate required. However, high-titer inhibitors may be treated by immune tolerance induction therapy in which higher than usual doses of FVIII or FIX are given regularly over an extended period of time.[67] Another widely used method of treatment for patients with high-titer inhibitors is administration of either Factor IX Complex or an activated factor IX complex termed Anti-Inhibitor Coagulant Complex to "bypass" the factor VIII step in the coagulation cascade.[68]

Although the bypass mechanism is not completely understood, one hypothesis is that activated clotting factors such as factor VIIa and FXa are involved.[69,70] This has led to the development of recombinant activated factor VII (rFVIIa) for the treatment of both hemophilia A and B patients with inhibitors.[71] Recombinant factor VIIa is produced in tissue culture in BHK cells and then purified by ion-exchange and immunoaffinity chromatography.[72] The molecule is spontaneously activated during the final ion-exchange chromatography steps.[73] Factor VIIa is currently the most widely used option for inhibitor treatment,[74] especially for patients who have never been exposed to plasma-derived products. However, one issue in the use of the factor IX complexes and factor VIIa is a risk of thromboembolic complications.[75]

Another interesting approach for treating hemophilia A patients with high-titer inhibitors had been the use of a porcine factor VIII concentrate. Porcine factor VIII is efficacious in controlling hemostasis and is less readily inactivated by some human factor VIII inhibitors.[76] However, the manufacturer has discontinued the product because of the difficulty of obtaining parvovirus-free porcine plasma. They are reportedly developing a recombinant porcine FVIII concentrate to replace the discontinued plasma-derived product.[77]

von Willebrand disease (vWD), caused by missing or abnormal von Willebrand factor (vWF), is the most commonly inherited coagulation disorder.[78] There are several types of vWD, many of which can be treated with the drug desmopressin. However, a number of vWD patients do not respond to desmopressin but can be treated by replacement therapy with plasma-derived vWF. In the past, such patients were treated with plasma or, more effectively, with cryoprecipitate.[79] Cryoprecipitate has a population of vWF multimers similar to that of normal plasma; however, it is not treated for viral inactivation and therefore carries a risk of infection. More recently patients have been treated with several intermediate-purity viral-inactivated AHF concentrates that contain significant amounts of vWF.[79] Humate-P has been licensed in the United States for treatment of vWD and therefore is labeled with its vWF content.[79,80] Alphanate and Koate-DVI also contain significant amounts of vWF and have been used for treatment of vWD.[79]

A recombinant human activated protein C, generic name Drotrecogin alfa (activated), is available for treatment of severe sepsis. A protein C zymogen is produced in a human kidney cell line and purified by chromatography, including an ion-exchange step operated in a pseudo-affinity mode. The zymogen is activated with bovine thrombin. The final product has an identical amino acid sequence as plasma protein C but a slightly different glycosylation pattern.[81,82] The efficacy of activated protein C in treatment of sepsis is controversial.[83,84]

FIBRIN SEALANTS

Fibrin sealants, or fibrin glues, are topical hemostatic agents that have been used in a variety of surgical situations for their hemostatic and adhesive properties.[85] The preparations consist of two components derived from human plasma that are mixed together immediately prior to use. The first component, derived from cryoprecipitate,

Table 150–3 Additional Plasma Derivative Concentrates Marketed in the United States

Product Type	Manufacturer/Distributor	Product Name	Purification Methods	Virus Inactivation/Removal Methods
Fibrin Sealant	Baxter	Tisseel VH	Fibrinogen component: cryoprecipitation Thrombin component: IEC, calcium chloride incubation	Both components: Vapor heating (60°C for 10 hours at 190 mbar, then 80°C for 1 hour at 370 mbar), lyophilization, purification steps
	OMRIX/Johnson & Johnson	Crosseal	Fibrinogen component: cryoprecipitation, $Al(OH)_3$ adsorption, ultrafiltration Thrombin component: IEC, nanofiltration	Fibrinogen component: S/D (TNBP/octoxynol 9) Pasteurization (60°C, 10 hours) Thrombin component: S/D (TNBP/octoxynol 9), nanofiltration
Alpha$_1$-Proteinase Inhibitor (Human)	Baxter	Aralast	Cohn fractionation, PEG precipitation, $ZnCl_2$ precipitation, IEC	S/D (TNBP/polysorbate 80), nanofiltration
	Talecris	Prolastin	Cohn fractionation, PEG precipitation, IEC	Pasteurization (60°C, 10 hours) Purification steps
	ZLB Behring	Zemaira	Cohn fractionation, NA	Pasteurization (60°C, 10 hours), ultrafiltration
Antithrombin III (Human)	Talecris	Thrombate III	Ethanol fractionation, dual AC	Pasteurization (60°C, 10 hours)

AC, affinity chromatography; IEC, ion-exchange chromatography; NA, not available; PEG, polyethylene glycol; S/D, solvent/detergent; TNBP, tri-*n*-butyl phosphate.
*These concentrates were marketed in the United States in 2006. Data were obtained from manufacturers, distributors, and available literature.

contains fibrinogen, along with factor XIII, and other plasma proteins.[86] Both also contain added plasmin inhibitors to delay clot lysis. Tisseel contains aprotinin, derived from bovine plasma, whereas Crosseal contains tranexamic acid.[85] The second component is human plasma-derived thrombin purified from cryo-poor plasma. Both products are treated for viral inactivation. Bovine thrombin was used for many years; however, research suggests that it may be responsible for many postsurgical hemostatic problems.[87,88] The fibrin sealant products available in the United States are shown in Table 150–3.

Because commercial fibrin sealants have only been available in the United States for a few years, a variety of methods had been used previously to prepare fibrin sealant for use in the treatment of individual patients. These "homemade" preparations are usually made with single-donor or autologous cryoprecipitate plus bovine thrombin. Some surgeons still advocate their use because of cost considerations, especially with autologous cryoprecipitate for which there is no risk of disease transmission. However, the methods are somewhat cumbersome, and the concentration of fibrinogen in the preparations, and thus their performance, is highly variable.[89,90]

PLASMA PROTEINASE INHIBITORS

The proteinase inhibitors that are present in human plasma play critical roles in the regulation of the proteolytic cascades of the coagulation, fibrinolytic, complement, and kinin systems. Most of these inhibitors have similar amino acid and structural properties and are members of a superfamily of proteins designated serpins (serine proteinase inhibitors).[91,92] Hereditary deficiencies in α_1-antitrypsin and antithrombin III can cause specific disease states, and inhibitor concentrates have been developed. The plasma proteinase inhibitor concentrates available in the United States are shown in Table 150–3.

Alpha$_1$-Proteinase Inhibitor

Alpha$_1$-Proteinase Inhibitor (Human) (API), also known as α_1-antitrypsin, was the first of the serpins to be isolated and characterized.[93] Although the protein was originally named for its antitrypsin activity, its primary physiologic function appears to be the inhibition of neutrophil elastase in the lung. Patients with hereditary deficiencies of this inhibitor develop pulmonary emphysema and liver disease.[94] In the most common form of API deficiency, mutant API protein accumulates in the liver, where it is produced, causing neonatal hepatitis, cirrhosis, and hepatocellular carcinoma.[95] This mechanism, in which mutant serpin proteins form polymers that accumulate in hepatocytes, has recently been recognized as a general characteristic of the serpins resulting in diseases called the serpinopathies.[96]

API therapy is indicated for chronic treatment of individuals with hereditary deficiency. Until recently API was an orphan drug with only one supplier and subject to chronic shortages.[97] The licensure of two more products in 2002 and 2003 has helped to ease the shortages, however, only a limited amount is ultimately available from plasma. One issue is the inefficiency of intravenous administration. It is estimated that only approximately 2% of the infused API ends up in the lung. Studies suggest that aerosol delivery of API directly into the lungs by inhalation would be efficacious and could replace intravenous administration because of its lower cost and greater convenience.[98] API is also a good candidate for recombinant production.[99]

Antithrombin III

Antithrombin III (Human) (ATIII) plays a critical role in the regulation of hemostasis as the major physiologic inhibitor of thrombin and factor Xa. Heterozygous hereditary deficiency of ATIII has been linked to an increased tendency to thrombosis. Acquired deficiencies have also been reported in women taking oral contraceptives and as a consequence of pregnancy, surgery, cirrhosis, and hepatic malignancies.[100]

The affinity of ATIII for heparin, essential for the pharmacologic effect of the drug, has also been employed as a means of purifying ATIII. Use of immobilized heparin as an affinity adsorbent for ATIII is the key step in large-scale preparation of ATIII concentrates for clinical use.[101] Thrombate III, the only product currently on the US market is purified by heparin affinity chromatography from Cohn fraction IV-1,[102] but, as shown in the box, ATIII may also be isolated from cryosupernatant or Cohn fraction I supernatant. Although heparin-based adsorbents are not specific for ATIII, other plasma proteins are bound less tightly and may be washed off with medium ionic strength buffers prior to the elution of ATIII with a high ionic strength buffer. Additional purification steps produce concentrates that contain more than 95% ATIII.[101] ATryn, a recombinant ATIII, was recently licensed in Europe and is the first recombinant human plasma protein produced in transgenic animals to be approved anywhere.[103]

FUTURE DIRECTIONS

New Plasma-Derived Concentrates

A number of additional plasma protein concentrates that are not currently available in the United States are available in Europe and other parts of the world. These include concentrates of protein C,[104] von Willebrand factor,[105] factor VII,[106] factor XI,[107] factor XIII,[108] and C_1-esterase inhibitor.[109] There are also several other proteins in plasma that would be potentially useful as therapeutic products. These include butyrylcholinesterase for reversal of succinylcholine-induced apnea[110] and treatment of cocaine overdose.[111] Other coagulation factors and inhibitors, such as factors X[112] and XII[113] and protein S,[114] may also be candidates for use in treatment of congenital and acquired deficiencies. However, the prevalence of these disorders is small, so they would be true orphan drugs. There are also potential improvements that can be made to current plasma-derived concentrates. In addition to enhanced purification and viral clearance methods, products can be made more user-friendly. For instance, alternate delivery systems could replace intravenous administration of coagulation factors by subcutaneous injection.[115] As described above, several studies have looked at aerosol delivery of Alpha-1 Proteinase Inhibitor.[98] Fibrin Sealant products are being developed consisting of precoated resorbable bandages.[116]

Recombinant Plasma Protein Concentrates

Almost all plasma proteins licensed for human use have been cloned and expressed in a biologically active form in animal cells, and several have been developed into licensed products, as described above. The main advantages of recombinantly produced plasma proteins include freedom from human viruses and a potentially unlimited supply. Several recombinant products that are currently being developed will be produced in transgenic animals, including antithrombin III (already available in Europe)[103] and alpha-1 proteinase inhibitor.[99,117] Transgenic cows, goats, pigs, and sheep can produce large quantities of human proteins, typically 1 to 10 g/L in milk, whereas animal tissue culture systems routinely produce substantially less protein, typically 10 to 100 mg/L.[117]

Recombinant proteins can also be produced in modified forms that may give them advantageous new properties such as increased potency, longer half-life, or varied specificity.[118,119] One product already available is B-domain deleted factor VIII described above.

SUGGESTED READINGS

General Overviews of Plasma Products

Farrugia A, Robert P: Plasma protein therapies: Current and future perspectives. Best Pract Res Clin Haematol 19:243, 2006.

Mertens K: The future of plasma derivatives. Transfus Clin Biol 8:303, 2001.

Production Method for Plasma Products

Buchacher A, Iberer G: Purification of intravenous immunoglobulin G from human plasma—aspects of yield and virus safety. Biotechnol J 1:148, 2006.

Burnouf T, Radosevich M: Affinity chromatography in the industrial purification of plasma proteins for therapeutic use. J Biochem Biophys Methods 49:575, 2001.

Johnston A, Adcock W: The use of chromatography to manufacture purer and safer plasma products. Biotechnol Genet Eng Rev 17:37, 2000.

Vandersande J: Current approaches to the preparation of plasma fractions. Biotechnology 19:165, 1991.

van Oss CJ: On the mechanism of the cold ethanol precipitation method of plasma protein fractionation. J Protein Chem 8:661, 1989.

Production of Recombinant Plasma Products

Larrick JW, Thomas DW: Producing proteins in transgenic plants and animals. Curr Opin Biotechnol 12:411, 2001.

Pipe SW: The promise and challenges of bioengineered recombinant clotting factors. J Thromb Haemost 3:1692, 2005.

Saenko EL, Ananyeva NM, Shima M, et al: The future of recombinant coagulation factors. J Thromb Haemost 1:922, 2003.

Safety of Plasma Products

Cai K, Gierman TM, Hotta J, et al: Ensuring the biologic safety of plasma-derived therapeutic proteins: Detection, inactivation, and removal of pathogens. BioDrugs 19:79, 2005.

MacLennan S, Barbara JA: Risks and side effects of therapy with plasma and plasma fractions. Best Pract Res Clin Haematol 19:169, 2006.

Schlesinger KW, Ragni MV: Safety of the new generation recombinant factor concentrates. Expert Opin Drug Saf 1:213, 2002.

Safety of Plasma Products in Regard to Prion Transmission

Burdick MD, Pifat DY, Petteway SR Jr, Cai K: Clearance of prions during plasma protein manufacture. Transfus Med Rev 20:57, 2006.

Dolan G: Clinical implications of emerging pathogens in haemophilia: The variant Creutzfeldt-Jakob disease experience. Haemophilia 12(Suppl 1):16, 2006; Discussion 26.

Ludlam CA, Turner ML: Managing the risk of transmission of variant Creutzfeldt Jakob disease by blood products. Br J Haematol 132:13, 2006.

History of Plasma Product Production

Menache D: Coagulation factor IX concentrate: Historical perspective. Haemophilia 1(Suppl 3):7, 1995.

Owen WG: Big piece, little piece or: Yes, factor VIII is a protein. J Thromb Haemost 3:1905, 2005.

Palmer JW: The evolution of large-scale human plasma fractionation in the United States. In Sgouris JR, Rene A (eds.): Proceedings of the Workshop on Albumin. Washington, DC, US Government Printing Office, 1976, p 255.

Starr D: Blood: An epic history of medicine and commerce. London, Warner, 1999.

REFERENCES

For complete list of references log onto www.expertconsult.com

CHAPTER 151

TRANSFUSION THERAPY FOR COAGULATION FACTOR DEFICIENCIES

Catherine S. Manno and Peter J. Larson

This chapter covers products available to treat deficiencies of plasma coagulation proteins. The development of blood component therapy, and subsequently protein concentrates that are enriched in particular coagulation factors and other proteins, made possible the effective treatment of bleeding episodes in patients with hemophilia and other diatheses. In the 1940s, a collaborative effort funded by the US government was undertaken among protein scientists with the goal of rapidly developing a method to isolate albumin from human plasma to provide a lyophilized intravascular volume expander for use in the military. As part of this effort, Dr. Edwin Cohn developed an ethanol fractionation procedure that was amenable to large-scale manufacture.[1] Building on the foundation of the Cohn fractionation procedure (see Chapter 143), the first coagulation factor concentrates were developed in the mid-1960s and provided a safer and more effective treatment for patients with the X-linked coagulation deficiencies, hemophilia A and B. Given the limited human plasma resource as a raw material for production of all but a few coagulation protein concentrates, manufacturers of human plasma-based products attempt to derive the maximum yield from each pool of plasma. Manufacturers of plasma-derived products strive to maximize the therapeutic potential of pooled human plasma by deriving more products from these processes.

Development of recombinant products has been fueled by concerns of infectious disease transmission through the human plasma resource. Currently licensed products are produced in mammalian cell culture to optimize necessary posttranslational modifications required for biologic activity. These recombinant expression processes are complicated and expensive. Transgenic recombinant technology is currently being explored as a way to decrease or eliminate reliance on the human plasma resource and the technically rigorous production of recombinant proteins using mammalian cell culture methods.

HEMOPHILIA A AND B

The hemophilias are X-linked disorders caused by deficiencies of either factor VIII (hemophilia A, or classic hemophilia) or factor IX (hemophilia B, or Christmas disease). The genes for these coagulation factors are located in close proximity on the long arm of the X chromosome. Hemophilia A affects 1 in 10,000 males, whereas hemophilia B affects 1 in 30,000. This difference in incidence is roughly correlated with the size of the genes, and more than 30% of cases arise from spontaneous mutations.

The major morbidity of the severe hemophilias A or B is arthropathy, developing over the course of years in untreated or undertreated adults as a result of recurrent spontaneous joint bleeding. The major cause of hemorrhagic mortality is bleeding into critical closed spaces (eg, intracranial or retroperitoneal).[2] Central nervous system (CNS) bleeding occurs in 3% to 14% of patients, and mortality from CNS hemorrhage ranges from 20% to 50%[3–5] with neurologic sequelae (including seizures, motor impairment, or mental retardation) observed in 40% to 50% of survivors.[3] CNS bleeding episodes occur predominantly in patients with severe disease (<1% factor level).[3] A more detailed discussion of the hemophilias and the molecular biology of factors VIII and IX can be found in Chapters 114 through 117.

TRANSFUSION THERAPY OF HEMOPHILIA A AND B

History of Transfusion for Hemophilia

Transfusion was first proposed by Schönlein and his student Hopf in 1832 as a treatment for "bleeders" who were suffering from exsanguinating hemorrhage, and these two were likely the first to have used the term *Haemophilie* to describe the disease.[6,7] The first effective transfusion-based intervention for hemophilia is credited to Samuel Lane who, in 1840, infused 10 to 12 ounces of fresh human blood into a 12-year-old boy with postoperative hemorrhage following eye surgery for correction of a squint.[8] Subsequently, a variety of interventions employing the infusion of human and animal blood and blood derivatives were utilized in the therapy of hemorrhage in patients with congenital bleeding diatheses (Table 151–1). Citrated plasma was first employed in 1923 for the treatment of hemophilia by Feissly to overcome a major ABO incompatibility in a father-to-son transfusion.[9] Development of modern blood banking in the 1930s and expansion of transfusion during and after World War II allowed for more widespread use of whole blood and subsequently frozen plasma in the treatment of hemophilia. Because of limited availability, the use of whole blood and components of whole blood for the treatment of hemophilia and other diseases was initially confined to larger metropolitan areas. In addition, volume constraints with the infusion of whole blood and plasma made the achievement of high plasma levels of coagulation factors (>5%) difficult.[10]

The advent of modern transfusion therapy for hemophilia came with the observation that the cold-insoluble precipitate remaining following thawing of frozen plasma at 4°C contains high concentrations of factor VIII.[11] Application of this procedure to the separation of components of whole blood[12] allowed for the production of a low-volume blood product known as "cryoprecipitate." Cryoprecipitate derived from a single whole blood collection contains approximately 125 U of factor VIII and quickly replaced frozen plasma as the therapy of choice for the treatment of bleeding episodes in hemophilia A in the 1960s. The availability of cryoprecipitate made the treatment of bleeding episodes by patients in their homes, rather than at a hospital, a reality. In addition, the development of quantitative assays for factor VIII[13] and for factor IX[14] meant that the two diseases could now be distinguished and effects of transfusion therapy on circulating levels of factors could be more accurately assessed.

Prior to the discovery of plasma cryoprecipitate, significant advances had been made in the fractionation of plasma utilizing ethanol,[1] glycine,[15] polyethylene glycol,[16] a combination of glycine and polyethylene glycol,[17] and calcium or barium[18–20] to precipitate plasma proteins. These techniques, in conjunction with cold precipitation of frozen plasma, laid the groundwork that resulted in the production of the first factor VIII and factor IX concentrates for clinical use.[17,19] These concentrates could be lyophilized and stored at temperatures up to 4°C with extended stability. Infusion of factor concentrates resulted in high circulating levels of factor VIII and factor IX without the complication of volume overload and paved the way for intensive infusion therapy for serious and life-threatening bleeding complications such as intracranial, retroperitoneal, and retropharyngeal hemorrhages and major surgery. Because they were produced from large pools of single plasma donations (>1000), initial concentrates were nearly universally contaminated with viral patho-

Table 151–1 Development of Transfusion Therapy for Hemophilia

Year	Development
1832	Schönlein proposes transfusion for exsanguination[7]
1840	Lane transfuses whole blood to stop postoperative bleeding in hemophilia[8]
1905	Weil reports use of human serum to treat hemophilia[89]
1911	Addis fractionates plasma by acid method[90]
1923	Feissly uses citrated plasma in ABO-mismatched father-to-son transfusion for hemophilia[9]
1930s–1940s	Development of modern blood banking. Availability of whole blood and frozen plasma for therapy (allows levels of approximately 5%)
1946	Cohn develops ethanol fractionation of plasma[1]
1949	Graham uses FFP in canine hemophilia model[91]
1945–1960	Fractionation of plasmas with AHF activity
1952	Biggs distinguishes hemophilia B from hemophilia A[14]
1953	Graham, Langdell, and Brinkhous develop quantitative assays to measure AHF[13,92]
1958	Barium precipitation of plasma to enrich for factor IX[18,93]
1963	Wagner uses glycine precipitation to partially purify factor VIII
1964	Pool develops clinically useful cryoprecipitate for factor VIII deficiency (allows levels of >20%)[12]
1966	Johnson uses polyethylene glycol (PEG) to partially purify factor VIII[16]
1967	Brinkhous develops glycine and PEG method to produce large-scale high potency factor VIII product (allows levels of 100%)[17]
1965–1970	Home infusion therapy
1969	Hoag produces large-scale prothrombin complex concentrate for factor IX deficiency[19]
1970s	Hepatitis B surface antigen assay is developed
1978–1985	HIV contaminates blood supply and factor concentrates
1979–1986	Heat treatment of factor concentrates reduces transmission of hepatitis B and HIV[23,24]
1985	Assay for HIV is licensed
1982	Immunoaffinity method of purification for factor VIII[94,95]
1986	Solvent/detergent method of treating infusible protein solutions to inactivate enveloped viruses[96,97]
1992–1993	First recombinant factor VIII concentrates are licensed[30,98]
1998	Recombinant factor IX concentrate is licensed[99]

gens such as hepatitis B and non-A non-B hepatitis (hepatitis C).[21] Initial attempts to attenuate viral transmission using pasteurization and dry heat, instituted by manufacturers in the late 1970s and early 1980s,[22,23] were found to limit the transmission of hepatitis B. Eventually these techniques were found to inactivate the human immunodeficiency virus (HIV).[24–26] Before the widespread application of these techniques, however, the majority of patients with severe hemophilia treated with concentrates between 1978 and 1985 were infected with HIV and HCV. This tragic consequence of infusion therapy helped fuel the development of modern strategies to reduce the risk of viral transmission by products derived from human plasma. These strategies include (a) careful screening of potential donors for risk factors leading to infection with transfusion-transmissible infections, (b) more vigilant surveillance of the blood donor base for the appearance of new pathogens, (c) development and implementation of testing specific for markers of infectious agents, (d) purification strategies that reduce viral load in final products, and (e) physical and chemical viral inactivation methods to treat infusible products. Finally, development and refinement in techniques of molecular biology in the 1970s and 1980s resulted in the cloning of the genes for many plasma proteins, including factor VIII and factor IX.[27–29] Within the next decade, the production and licensure of biologically active recombinant factor VIII and factor IX products had become a reality.[30–33] Concentrates of these recombinant products have been shown to be effective and have not been associated with the transmission of pathogens. Further development of recombinant products centers on the removal of all human and animal proteins in the production and formulation of products to further reduce the risk of their inadvertent contamination with emerging pathogens, such as variant prions,[34,35] and newly discovered agents, such as hepatitis G virus and TTV.[36,37] In addition, episodic supply constraints incurred in the manufacture of recombinant proteins in mammalian cell culture systems resulting in supply shortages of recombinant factor VIII[38] have led to greater interest in transgenic production of human plasma proteins compared to mammalian cell culture. With transgenic systems, raw material from which the protein of interest is purified (milk, plant tissue) can be produced in abundance.

Attenuation of Pathogens in Blood-Derived and Other Biologic Products

The development of factor VIII and factor IX concentrates in the 1960s improved the life expectancy of patients with hemophilia from approximately 11 years (prior to effective transfusion therapy) to nearly normal.[39] Experience with these first-generation concentrates, however, showed that they invariably transmitted the viral agents responsible for hepatitis B and hepatitis C,[21] which are associated with chronic hepatitis with attendant morbidity and mortality, including cirrhosis and hepatocellular carcinoma. Although efforts were being directed at methods to attenuate these known hepatitis viruses during the late 1970s and early 1980s, HIV contaminated the human blood supply. More than 70% of patients in many countries and 30% to 40% of hemophilia patients worldwide were infected with HIV.[40–43] The devastating effects of both HIV and chronic hepatitis in the hemophilia patient population provided a major impetus for the improvement in viral safety of all infusible products derived from human and, in the case of porcine factor VIII, animal blood. More recently, concern about the prion agents responsible for transmissible spongiform encephalopathies such as CJD, variant CJD, and bovine spongiform encephalopathy, as well as newly identified viral agents in the blood supply,[36,37] have reinforced the need for continued surveillance and further refinements in the production of products for the treatment of hemophilia. This attention has also been focused on recombinant products, because nearly all currently licensed products use added human or animal protein in fermentation or as stabilizers during purification or formulation. Table 151–2 lists agents that are potential contaminants of human plasma. Other viruses such as cytomegalovirus and HTLV-1 are transmissible primarily by cellular blood products.

Although ideal, the absolute removal of infectious agents in transfusable products may be unattainable and in fact may be unnecessary, because the primary goal is to make them noninfectious. Practically, this can be accomplished by reducing the levels of the contaminating agent below the level of infectivity. The most relevant agents, viruses and prions, are small and therefore difficult to separate from protein components of plasma. Some pathogens are resistant to currently employed methods of inactivation. In addition, as exemplified by HIV and prions, new agents may periodically emerge in the human population by crossing species barriers. Unless detected rapidly, newly emerging agents have the potential for global dissemination, especially if they are transmitted by transfusion of contaminated blood products. Despite these limitations, the safety of infusible products derived from human or animal sources (which includes

Table 151–2 Viruses Implicated in Transfusion of Plasma-Derived Products

Virus	Nucleic Acid	Human Disease	Known Transmission by Blood	Lipid Enveloped	Size (nm)	Reduction/Inactivation
HIV	RNA	Yes (AIDS)	Yes	Yes	100–120	S/D
HBV	DNA	Yes (acute and chronic hepatitis)	Yes	Yes	40–45	S/D
HCV	RNA	Yes (acute and chronic hepatitis)	Yes	Yes	40–60	S/D
Parvo B19	DNA	Yes (Fifth disease, transient erythroblastopenia of childhood, chronic anemia in immunocompromised patients)	Yes	No	18–20	Incompletely by heat; nanofiltration
HAV	RNA	Yes	Yes	No	25–30	Incompletely by heat
Hepatitis G	RNA	No	Yes	Yes		?S/D
TTV	DNA	No	Yes	No		?S/D
HHV-8	DNA	Kaposi sarcoma	Unknown			
SEN V	DNA			No		
TSE (prion)	peptide	Yes (Jakob-Creutzfeld disease)	Unknown	N/A	250 kd	Unknown

Data from Teitel J: Transmissible agents and the safety of coagulation factor concentrates. World Federation of Hemophilia: Facts and Figures 7:1, 1999; and Allain JP: Emerging viruses in blood transfusion. Vox Sang 78(Suppl 2):243, 2000.

cultured mammalian cells expressing recombinant protein) can be optimized by reducing the initial viral load in the source material (human plasma, culture medium, or transgenic material). With human plasma, this is accomplished by screening to limit potentially infected donors, by removal and inactivation of infectious agents, and by prospective surveillance of all products and recipients of products that potentially may become contaminated.

Current discussions in the medical, health economic, and patient communities center around achieving an appropriate balance between safety and costs given that plasma-derived products on the market today are extremely safe with regard to pathogen transmission.[44]

Infusion Regimens and Dosing for Hemophilia

The mainstay of therapy for hemophilia involves the treatment of bleeding episodes with the infusion of products capable of replacing the missing factor VIII or IX. This so-called on-demand therapy is effective in staunching hemorrhage, but not before tissue damage has occurred. Bleeding is especially destructive in the synovium, where a vicious cycle develops in which the initial bleed results in a proliferative inflammatory response and hypertrophy of synovial tissues that then become more susceptible to further trauma and bleeding. The result in the short term is repeated bleeds into the same joint, referred to as a "target joint," and eventually chronic joint destruction or hemophilic arthropathy. Chronic arthropathy often requires surgical intervention, including synovectomy, debridement, joint replacement, or even joint fusion.

With the availability of factor concentrates that allowed for the attainment of high plasma levels of factor VIII or IX, prophylactic therapy became possible. This approach was pioneered by Swedish treaters who have demonstrated that the use of prophylactic regimens,[45] wherein trough factor levels are maintained at greater than 1% of normal, reduces the incidence of arthropathy and CNS hemorrhage.[44] Greater availability of virally safe factor concentrates has allowed for the initiation of prophylactic regimens in early childhood. This "primary" form of prophylaxis has become the standard of care in developed countries. Prophylaxis is not universally practiced, however, owing to the high cost of factor concentrates, the requirement for frequent intravenous infusion, and the need for placement of central venous catheters in some patients, especially small children, to obtain intravenous access. Use of central catheters is attended by the risks of catheter-induced septic and thrombotic complications.

Dosing regimens for the treatment of bleeding episodes in hemophilia and for prophylactic regimens have evolved paralleling the availability of high-concentration pathogen-safe replacement products. Although no universal regimen for treatment has been established, certain trends prevail. In general, for non–life-threatening bleeding episodes, the goal of therapy is to achieve a plasma factor VIII or IX level of between 30% and 100%. For life-threatening bleeds or prophylaxis for surgical procedures, the goal is a level of 100% to be maintained by repeated bolus infusions or continuous infusion for a duration of 10 to 14 days or longer, depending on the severity of the bleed or surgical intervention.

The majority of prophylaxis regimens aim at achieving a trough factor level of approximately 1%. For hemophilia A, this is usually accomplished by dosing two or three times a week. Prophylactic regimens can be "primary," instituted in young children to prevent bleeding episodes, especially hemarthroses that result in chronic arthropathy, or "secondary," in which limited or prolonged periods of prophylactic therapy are instituted following a serious bleed or the development of repeated bleeding into a single joint (target joint). To prevent the development of a target joint and chronic arthropathy, many hemophilia treatment centers have recently adopted a regimen of two, three, or more infusions following a hemarthrosis. Specific dosing regimens for bleeding episodes have been developed by treaters and treatment centers. Although slight variations in indications and target plasma levels of factor VIII and factor IX between treatment centers exist, representative dosing regimens are similar and are presented in Table 151–3.[46–48]

TREATMENT OF HEMOPHILIA

Products Available for Treatment of Factor VIII Deficiency

Products available for the treatment of bleeding episodes or prophylaxis against bleeding in patients with hemophilia A include DDAVP, a vasoactive peptide that stimulates release of stored factor VIII, and infusible products containing exogenous factor VIII protein. These may be blood components, concentrates purified from blood plasma, or concentrates containing recombinant factor VIII protein.

Table 151–3 Dosing Regimens for Bleeding and Prophylaxis in Hemophilia

Site	Factor Level	Dose Hemophilia A	Dose Hemophilia B	Duration of Treatment	Comments
Joint	30%–70%	15–35 U/kg	30–70 U/kg	1–3 days	Splinting temporary splinting, no weight bearing
Life threatening (eg, intracranial, retropharyngeal, retroperitoneal)	80%–100%	40–50 U/kg	80–100 U/kg	10–14 days	Antifibrinolytic therapy with retropharyngeal bleeds
Soft tissue	30%–50%	15–25 U/kg	30–50 U/kg	2–5 days	Higher levels can be used for compartment syndrome
Surgery	80%–100%	40–50 U/kg	80–100 U/kg	10–14 (or shorter for minor procedures)	Significant blood loss can occur into large muscles of the lower extremity and the iliopsoas
Oral	20%–50%	10–25 U/kg	20–50 U/kg	1–2	Antifibrinolytic therapy
Gastrointestinal*	30%–100%	15–50 U/kg	30–100 U/kg	2–3	Should be evaluated for source
Genitourinary†	30%–50%	15–25 U/kg	30–50 U/kg	1–2	Avoid antifibrinolytic therapy
Prophylaxis‡	50%	25 U/kg	50 U/kg	qod or 3×/week	Steroids may be useful

*Depending on severity.
†Painless spontaneous hematuria often requires no treatment other than fluid intake. Persistence requires treatment and evaluation.
‡Use of a schedule of 25 U/kg qod and a dose of 40 U/kg with an interval of 2 days between the next dose may increase compliance by decreasing infusions to three per week.
Data from DiMichele,[46] Lusher,[47] and Mannucci.[48]

1-Deamino 8-D Arginine Vasopressin

The preferred product for treatment of patients with mild or moderate hemophilia A is the synthetic octapeptide DDAVP (1-deamino 8-D arginine vasopressin), a vasopressin analog. DDAVP causes a release of factor VIII (and von Willebrand factor) from endothelial cells, raising plasma factor VIII by approximately threefold (range, 2- to 12-fold) in patients with hemophilia in whom the disease is caused by decreased production or secretion of a functional protein or a protein that has decreased activity. To be effective, DDAVP relies on a partial quantitative deficiency of factor VIII; thus, patients with severe hemophilia will not benefit from its use if the causative mutation results in no synthesis, secretion, or a protein with no activity. The response to DDAVP in an individual patient is typically reproducible, and an effective response must be documented prior to its routine use or as prophylaxis for bleeding in surgical procedures. Intravenous and intranasal preparations are available. The intravenous product has been used in a subcutaneous route of administration. The intranasal preparation more easily allows a patient to administer the compound on an as-needed basis in a home therapy regimen. The phenomenon of tachyphylaxis, the decreased effectiveness of repeated doses of the compound, occurs after several, typically three, consecutive doses.

Injectable DDAVP (ZLB Behring) is available in 4 μg/mL or 15 μg/mL preparations. The recommended dose is 0.3 μg/kg, mixed in 30 mL normal saline, infused intravenously slowly over 30 minutes. This dose can be repeated after 12 to 24 hours. DDAVP nasal spray Stimate® (ZLB Behring) is available in a metered-dose pump that delivers 0.1 mL (150 μg) per activation (spray). The dose is one activation for patients less than 50 kg and two activations in separate nostrils for those more than 50 kg. Generally, only three consecutive doses of DDAVP should be used unless otherwise advised by an experienced hemophilia treater. Because DDAVP is a vasopressin analog, there is a risk of fluid retention with its use. Changes in fluid balance can result in hyponatremia and seizures, especially when DDAVP is used in individuals on nonfluid-restricted or salt-restricted diets (eg, the elderly or very young or surgical patients undergoing fluid replacement with solutions with concentrations <0.9% sodium). Caution is advised with the use of DDAVP in patients at risk for arterial thrombosis, as there have been reports of myocardial infarction and cerebral thrombosis with its use.[49] DDAVP is not recommended for children younger than 2 years of age.

1-DEAMINO 8-D ARGININE VASOPRESSIN (DDAVP) TRIAL

1. Collect citrated plasma from the patient immediately before DDAVP infusion for testing with the postinfusion blood specimen.
2. Administer DDAVP intravenously (0.3 μg/1 kg).
3. Wait approximately 30 minutes postinfusion, carefully observing the patient for possible adverse side effects (increased blood pressure, facial flushing, rarely surgeries).
4. Collect post-DDAVP infusion specimen in sodium citrate.
5. Measure the pre- and post-DDAVP FVIII : C and VWF : Ag levels to confirm a therapeutic response.

Factor VIII Concentrates

In developed countries, the current standard of care for the treatment and prevention of bleeding episodes in patients with severe hemophilia A, and in patients with mild or moderate disease who do not respond to DDAVP, is the infusion of recombinant human factor VIII. Recovery of recombinant factor VIII ranges from 1.5 to 2.5%/IU/kg so that dosing assumes a rise in plasma factor VIII activity of 2% for every 1 IU/kg infused. Available concentrates are optimized to enhance viral clearance during purification and undergo one or more viral inactivation steps during manufacture. Plasma-derived FVIII concentrates, treated with multiple purification and viral inactivation steps, are also available and have an excellent recent record of safety.

Intermediate- and High-Purity Plasma-Derived Concentrates

Intermediate-purity plasma-derived concentrates are prepared from cryoprecipitated plasma or fresh frozen plasma, from which factor VIII is further purified using precipitation, gel permeation, ion exchange, or affinity chromatography, often in combination. Specific factor VIII coagulant activity in these products ranges from 2 to more than 100 IU/mg of protein, and many of the methods used also copurify significant amounts of von Willebrand factor, making them useful for the treatment of some patients with von Willebrand disease (see later discussion on treatment of von Willebrand disease). More highly purified plasma-derived concentrates are produced using heparin ligand or immunoaffinity purification methods and have specific activities ranging from 140 to greater than 3000 IU/mg. To stabilize the factor VIII molecule, the majority of these products are formulated by adding human albumin prior to lyophilization.

Highly purified recombinant factor VIII concentrates have been licensed in North America, Europe, and Japan since the early 1990s. These are either full-length or B-domain deleted molecules (the B-domain is not required for activity in coagulation) that are expressed in mammalian cell culture (Chinese hamster ovary or baby hamster kidney cell lines) and are purified using immunoaffinity techniques. The development of these recombinant products was fueled primarily by concerns regarding safety of the human blood donor pool and the viral epidemics that occurred within the hemophilia population with the use of early plasma-derived products. As with highly purified plasma-derived factor VIII concentrates, the first-generation recombinant products are formulated with added albumin as a stabilizer. Newer products (Kogenate FS, Bayer, Advate, Baxter Biosciences Refacto, Wyeth) have been developed that stabilize the factor VIII molecule with nonprotein excipients.[50–52] Recombinant production methods that do not rely on the human plasma resource theoretically should provide for unlimited supply.

Plasma/Cryoprecipitate

In communities where virally inactivated factor VIII concentrates are not available, cryoprecipitate provides an effective alternative to therapy with concentrates for hemophilia A and VWD patients. Cryoprecipitate is a small-volume product (10–15 mL) enriched in factor VIII, von Willebrand factor, fibrinogen, fibronectin, and factor XIII. Dosing can be calculated assuming approximately 80 to 150 IU of factor VIII per bag of cryoprecipitate (derived from a 450-mL single whole blood donor collection unit). Thus, a typical 1750-IU dose (50% correction for a 70-kg patient) would require between 10 and 21 bags or units. The limitations of cryoprecipitate therapy are (a) lack of a viral inactivation step in manufacture of the component and (b) lack of convenience, because multiple units must be pooled into a large volume (approximately 70–100 mL) for infusion. Fresh frozen plasma and whole blood provide less desirable alternatives because adequate therapy with both of these products suffers from the limitations described for cryoprecipitate, and their use often results in intravascular volume overload. Solvent detergent (SD)-treated fresh frozen plasma product is available in some countries. ABO group-specific SD plasma is prepared by solvent detergent treatment (TNBP and Triton X100) of a pool of up to 2500 donors. Following removal of the solvent and detergent components, 200-mL aliquots are refrozen for infusion.

Products Available for Treatment of Factor IX Deficiency

Factor IX Concentrates

As with replacement therapy for factor VIII deficiency, intermediate- and high-purity products derived from plasma for the treatment of factor IX deficiency are available, as well as a single recombinant factor IX product. All of these concentrates also undergo at least one viral inactivation or exclusion step in manufacture. The volume of distribution of factor IX is approximately twice the plasma volume. This can be explained in part by the affinity of factor IX for type IV collagen present in the extracellular matrix.[53] Recovery of factor IX following infusion is therefore approximately 1%/IU/kg. The recovery observed with recombinant factor IX is approximately 20% lower than that observed with plasma-derived factor IX.[54] This is likely due to differences in posttranslational modifications between recombinant factor IX and plasma-derived factor IX.

Intermediate purity factor IX products are generally purified from plasma using anion-exchange chromatography or calcium or barium precipitate adsorption. These methods select for proteins that contain highly negatively charged epitopes. The vitamin K-dependent coagulation factors, by virtue of their gamma-carboxyglutamic acid (gla) rich domains, are such proteins; thus, these techniques copurify varying amounts of the other vitamin K-dependent coagulation factors, factor VII, factor X, and prothrombin with factor IX. Hence, the products are referred to as "prothrombin complex concentrates" (or PCCs). The levels of vitamin K proteins in these products vary and can be obtained from the manufacturer. In addition, the PCCs are contaminated with trace amounts of activated forms of vitamin K-dependent factors. The presence of these *activated* factors is the likely explanation for thromboses that have occurred with the use of these intermediate-purity products, typically in the setting of postoperative immobility or hepatic dysfunction.[55] To minimize the risk of thrombosis with the use of PCCs, it is advisable to achieve a peak factor IX level no higher than 50%.[56] Some clinicians add small amounts of heparin to infusions of these products to prevent thrombosis, and some manufacturers have formulated PCCs with heparin or antithrombin III.

High-purity factor IX products are produced from plasma using techniques of ligand affinity or immunoaffinity chromatography and typically have specific activities greater than 150 IU/mg. Two single high-purity recombinant factor IX products have been licensed in the U.S. (Alphanine, Grifols; Mononine, ZLB Behring) Thrombotic complications have not been reported with these high-purity products.

In communities where factor IX concentrates are not available, plasma may provide a means of replacing factor IX in hemophilia B patients during bleeding episodes. Each unit of fresh frozen plasma (FFP) derived from a 450-mL whole blood collection contains approximately 200 IU of factor IX. Replacement to therapeutic levels of factor IX with FFP is difficult because of the complication of volume overload. In some areas, solvent-detergent plasma provides a virally inactivated alternative to FFP.

Other Useful Adjuncts for Treatment of Bleeding in Hemophilia A and B

The antifibrinolytic agents tranexamic acid and ε-aminocaproic acid (EACA) are sometimes used in conjunction with clotting factor replacement therapy or DDAVP in the treatment of bleeding that occurs with hemophilia and other bleeding disorders. These agents interact with the lysine-binding site of plasminogen and enhance its activation. The more important effect of lysine analogs is that their occupancy of this site inhibits binding of the zymogen, plasminogen, to fibrin, which is necessary for full fibrinolytic activity. Antifibrinolytics are useful in the setting of mucosal bleeding and may substantially reduce the need for clotting factor concentrates in the setting of oral mucosal bleeding with tooth extractions. These agents are administered preoperatively and continued postoperatively until wound healing occurs. Although tranexamic acid is more potent, it is less readily absorbed when given orally. Tranexamic acid is administered at 25 mg/kg orally or 10 mg/kg intravenously preoperatively, and therapy can be continued postoperatively using oral rinses with a 5% solution. EACA is used at a dose of 100 mg/kg preoperatively followed by 100 mg/kg every 6 hours either orally or intravenously (maximum dose 24 g/day). Dosing of EACA should be reduced in patients with renal insufficiency.

INHIBITORS OF FACTOR VIII AND FACTOR IX

A major complication in the treatment of patients with hemophilia is the development of inhibitory antibodies against the infused factors that interfere with factor activity. Rarely, antibodies may develop that do not affect activity but increase clearance of factor VIII or factor IX. The incidence of factor VIII inhibitors is approximately 30%, and inhibitors typically develop within the first 20 exposures to replacement therapy.[57,58] Well-designed prospective studies of the use of recombinant factor VIII in previously untreated patients revealed that many of these inhibitors are low titer and transient in nature.[31,32] Patients with low-titer, transient inhibitors can be managed with increased doses of factor VIII. Inhibitors to factor IX occur less frequently, with an estimated incidence of approximately 1% to 3%.[59] Patients with factor IX antibodies may have anaphylactic reactions when treated with high-purity products.[60,61]

Patients with high-titer inhibitors to either factor VIII or factor IX do not usually achieve hemostasis following factor replacement and thus present a treatment challenge. Treatment of patients who develop inhibitors involves two approaches: (a) acute treatment of bleeding episodes and (b) immune tolerance induction therapy, whereby the patient is treated frequently (often daily) with factor VIII or factor IX in an effort to suppress the production of inhibitors by the immune system (similar to allergic desensitization therapy).

Treatment of acute bleeding episodes can be accomplished by two methods. For patients with low-titer inhibitors (<5 Bethesda units [BU], a laboratory measurement of inhibitor activity), hemostasis can be accomplished with large doses of factor VIII or factor IX (eg, as high as 200 IU/kg given at frequent intervals) in an effort to neutralize or "override" the circulating inhibitor. A neutralization approach is usually ineffective for patients with high-titer inhibitors (>5–10 BU), and is also expensive because of the large amounts of factor required. These patients and patients with low-titer inhibitors who fail to respond to override therapy can be treated using products that act to "bypass" the inhibitor. The only current bypass agents include activated prothrombin complex concentrates (FEIBA, Baxter Bioscience) (aPCC), which contain factors VII, X, and prothrombin in addition to factor IX that enhance production of thrombin generation by activating the coagulation pathway at points farther down than the factor VIIIa/factor IXa step. FEIBA is used as first-line treatment of bleeding episodes in patients with inhibitors by some treaters, despite the fact that the concentrate is derived from human plasma.

Recombinant activated factor VII (rFVIIa) (NovoSeven, Novo Nordisk) product was licensed in Europe and the United States with an indication for use as a bypass agent in the treatment of inhibitors in patients with hemophilia A and hemophilia B. This product has the advantage of being the only recombinant product available for the treatment of bleeding episodes in patients with inhibitors. The dose of rFVIIa is 90 μg/kg. Recombinant factor VIIa is administered every 2 hours, compared with every 8 to 12 hours for PCCs or activated PCCs. Thrombosis has also been reported with the use of rFVIIa[62,63] and PCCs.

Despite the success achieved with immune tolerance induction regimens (80%–90%),[64] "bypass" agents will still be needed in patients undergoing tolerization, because an interval potentially as long as 2 to 3 years exists between the time that induction is initiated and the inhibitor is suppressed. Bleeding episodes that occur prior to achievement of tolerance will usually require treatment with one or other of the bypassing agents.

Treatment of Life-Threatening Bleeding Episodes in Patients With Inhibitors Against Factor VIII or Factor IX

Concentrates

1. Factor VIII containing concentrates in high doses (as high as 150–200 IU/kg) if inhibitor titer is low (<5–10 BU) or if neutralization can be demonstrated with high doses. High-dose continuous infusion of factor VIII (~10 IU/kg/hour) following a high dose bolus may be useful.
2. Recombinant factor VIIa. Dose is 90 μg/kg (or a dose up to 320 μg/kg) administered every 2 hours. Risk of thrombosis exists with this product.
3. Activated PCCs at a dose of 50 to 75 IU/kg every 8 to 12 hours. Risk of thrombosis exists with this product.

Immunomodulation

1. Antibody depletion
   a. Plasmapheresis
   b. Extracorporeal immunoadsorption of plasma (staph protein A column therapy and other methods)
2. Suppression of antibody production
   a. High-dose steroids (equivalent of prednisone 80 mg/day)
   b. Cyclophosphamide (10–15 mg/kg load and 2–3 mg/kg/day)
   c. Intravenous immunoglobulin (1 g/kg daily for 2 days)
   d. More aggressive regimens that may include vincristine, azathioprine, cyclosporine, or interferon-γ

Conservative Measures

1. Immobilization
2. Compression
3. Local application of hemostatic agents
4. Antifibrinolytics
5. Avoid venipunctures, intramuscular injections, arterial puncture, or lumbar punctures
6. Avoid use of medications that inhibit platelet function
7. DDAVP may be effective in some patients with low titer inhibitors

Treatment of life-threatening bleeds in the context of a high-titer inhibitor represents a significant challenge. The infusion of non-factor VIII concentrates, when the inhibitor titer precludes the use of factor VIII, is less effective than treatment with factor VIII concentrates and is difficult to monitor, because plasma factor VIII levels are of no value. Adjunctive therapies are frequently employed in this setting to lower the titer of the antibody to allow for treatment of the patient with factor VIII concentrates. Aggressive regimens are employed in which circulating antibodies are depleted using plasmapheresis or staphylococcal protein A immunoadsorption, and reduction of antibody production is attempted using immunomodulatory agents such as steroids, cyclophosphamide, and intravenous infusion of gamma globulin (IgG).[65–68] These strategies for acutely reducing antibody titers are also employed by some hemophilia treaters at the outset of immune tolerance induction.

VON WILLEBRAND DISEASE

Von Willebrand disease (VWD) is an autosomal dominant bleeding disorder first described by Erik von Willebrand in 1926, who named this bleeding diathesis "pseudohemophilia." Von Willebrand disease is relatively common, with a prevalence of up to 2% of the general population.[69] The penetrance and severity of the disease vary depending on the type of VWD (type 1, 2, or 3), the specific mutation, the number of affected genes, the patient's blood type, and numerous drug, hormonal, and stress-related parameters. These factors, particularly the subtype of VWD and the patient's response to DDAVP, influence the recommended treatment for acute bleeding episodes or for prophylaxis against bleeding.

Although the disease had been described in the 1920s, and the primary defect had earlier been attributed to either platelets or the vessel wall. An understanding of the missing protein in VWD and its relationship to factor VIII was not appreciated until the 1950s. Correction of the defect with transfusion of plasma, but not with platelet concentrates alone, defined the disease as one involving a missing plasma protein factor (von Willebrand factor [VWF]) not a platelet or vessel wall defect.[70] A correlation between VWD and factor VIII activity had previously been observed, the observation that a plasma fraction from patients lacking factor VIII (hemophilia A) could correct the defect in VWD, in addition to the autosomal inheritance pattern, which helped further differentiate hemophilia A from VWD.[70] A more detailed discussion of clinical features and pathophysiology of VWD and the molecular biology of VWF can be found in Chapters 120 and 121.

TRANSFUSION THERAPY FOR VON WILLEBRAND DISEASE

The specific treatment for VWD varies with the bleeding symptoms and signs and with the subtype of VWD. Treatment is guided further by laboratory results indicating the potential success of increasing VWF with DDAVP, and the clinical experience with a particular patient and his or her natural biological family members who have VWD. When possible, attempts should be made to treat the patient without exposing him or her to plasma-derived products.

Non–Protein-Based Treatment

DDAVP is a synthetic octapeptide homolog of vasopressin that results in the release of stored VWF from Weibel Palade bodies of the endothelium (see section on treatment of hemophilia A). DDAVP is often effective for type 1 disease and may be useful in certain patients with type 2 disease. It is not appropriate for use in patients with type 3 disease in whom no stores of VWF exist. Prior to the use of DDAVP, a DDAVP trial should be conducted to document its efficacy in an individual patient. The trial is performed as described for hemophilia A. The phenomenon of tachyphylaxis is also observed when DDAVP is used to treat VWD. For bleeding that does not respond to DDAVP or in patients in whom a poor response is observed with DDAVP, other modalities (typically protein-based) must be employed.

As described for hemophilia A, the antifibrinolytic agent ε-aminocaproic acid or tranexamic acid are often administered in the setting of dental surgery to inhibit fibrinolysis. Care should be taken when these agents are administered in patients with a predisposition to thrombosis.

Estrogens upregulate VWF synthesis and may be useful especially in women. Therapy with estrogens should also help ameliorate menorrhagia in affected symptomatic patients.

Plasma-Protein-Based Therapy

Factor VIII Concentrates

Some intermediate-purity factor VIII concentrates are manufactured from plasma using methods that copurify significant amounts of VWF. Many of the products listed in Table 151–4 contain VWF, but only Humate-P (ZLB Behring) is currently licensed for the treatment of VWD. Alphanate (Grifols USA) has been studied in clinical trials to support an indication for VWD, and others, including Koate-DVI (Talecris Biotherapeutics), have been tested in vitro and in vivo for their potential use in therapy for VWD.[71–73] The multimeric pattern of VWF in these concentrates varies, and no product has the pattern of multimers that is present in normal plasma.[72] Because many of these products are effective clinically, the importance of these differences in multimer pattern remains to be determined.

Table 151–4 Other Coagulation Deficiencies

Factor	Incidence	Inheritance	Chromosome	Half-Life	Target Plasma Level	Treatment Product*
I (fibrinogen)	1–2/10^6		4	2–4 days	50–100 mg/dL	Concentrates
Afibrinogen		AR				Cryoprecipitate
Hypofibrinogen		AR or AD				
Dysfibrinogen		AR or AD				
II (prothrombin)	<1/10^6	AD	11	3 days	30%	PCCs Plasma
V	1/10^6	AR	1	36 hours	25%	Plasma
VII	2/10^6	AR	13	3–6 hours	25%	rFVIIa Concentrates PCCs Plasma
X	2/10^6	AR	13	40 hours	10%–25%	PCCs Plasma
XI		AR or AD	4	80 hours	20%–40%	Concentrates Plasma
XIII	<1/10^6	AR	1.6	9 days	5%	Concentrates Cryoprecipitate Plasma

AD, autosomal dominant; AR, autosomal recessive; PCC, prothrombin complex concentrates.
*Products are listed in order of viral safety.
Data from Cohen AJ, Kessler CM: Treatment of inherited coagulation disorders. Am J Med 99:675, 1995.

von Willebrand Factor Concentrates (Plasma-Derived and Recombinant)

Several chromatography-purified plasma-derived concentrates enriched in VWF have been studied by manufacturers in Europe.[74,75] Preliminary reports suggest that these are amenable to viral inactivation steps and may be effective both in vitro and in vivo.[72] To date, none of these have been developed as widely licensed products. Recombinant VWF has been successfully isolated from a number of expression systems and partially characterized, but a recombinant product for the treatment of patients has not yet been developed clinically.

Cryoprecipitate

Cryoprecipitate had been the mainstay of plasma-based therapy for bleeding in patients with VWD until the availability of virally inactivated intermediate-purity factor VIII concentrates with preserved functional VWF protein. These factor VIII concentrates are the products of choice for the treatment of bleeding in patients with types 1 and 2 VWD who are unresponsive to DDAVP, and for bleeding in patients with type 3 VWD. Owing to the small potential for viral contamination of cryoprecipitate, manufacture of which does not include steps to inactivate viral pathogens, cryoprecipitate is currently indicated only when virally safe concentrates containing VWF are unavailable.

ACQUIRED FACTOR VIII AND VON WILLEBRAND FACTOR DEFICIENCY

Antibodies that inhibit the activity of factor VIII can develop in previously normal patients. Most of these patients have no underlying disease; however, factor VIII antibodies can arise in the setting of autoimmune disorders or in the postpartum period. Although approximately one-third of inhibitors will disappear spontaneously, the mortality rate among affected patients is significant.

Acquired VWD is a rare autoimmune disorder that can occur in association with other autoimmune disorders or lymphoproliferative disease. Antibody may interact with the epitopes on VWF required for its normal activity or result in increased clearance of antibody–VWF complexes.

Treatment

Therapy for those patients with relatively high inhibitor titers (>5 BU) includes bypassing agents (FEIBA or rFVIIa) to stop bleeding and immunosuppression to reduce inhibitor levels. Plasmapheresis or immunoadsorption can be employed to reduce the circulating levels of inhibitors. Immunosuppressive agents and intravenous immunoglobulin (IgG) are useful adjuncts to abrogate production o the autoantibody. DDAVP can also be effective in some patients with low-titer inhibitors. Unlike inhibitors that develop with hemophilia A, exposure to factor VIII usually does not result in increased antibody titers.[76] Conservative measures to control hemorrhage should also be used in conjunction with the above, including immobilization and compression, topical or local hemostatic agents, and antifibrinolytic therapy. The use of venipunctures, intramuscular injections, and drugs with platelet inhibitory activity should be minimized or avoided.

OTHER COAGULATION PROTEIN DEFICIENCIES

Approximately 15% of inherited bleeding disorders are caused by deficiencies of coagulation factors other than factor VIII, factor IX, or VWF. Inherited deficiencies of fibrinogen and factors II, V, VII, X, XI, and XIII may result in bleeding, requiring treatment. The genes for these factors are not located on the X chromosome; thus two gene defects are typically required for symptomatic disease. Consanguinity is frequent in affected kindreds. Characteristics of these deficiencies are presented in Table 151–2. Hereditary deficiencies of factor XII, pre-kallikrein, and high-molecular-weight kininogen have not been described to result in bleeding diatheses.

The mainstays of therapy for these disorders are cryoprecipitate (for fibrinogen and factor XIII deficiencies) and plasma. In some countries, concentrates enriched in the missing protein have been available. A solvent-detergent treated pooled plasma product is also available in some regions. Pooled solvent-detergent treated plasma has the advantage over fresh frozen plasma in that it is virally inactivated but has the drawback of exposing the patient to a large number of donors (2500) with each dose.

Fibrinogen Deficiency

Bleeding disorders can result from low to absent levels of fibrinogen (hypofibrinogenemia or afibrinogenemia) or a protein with abnormal function (dysfibrinogenemia). The inheritance pattern for the former is autosomal recessive and for the latter is autosomal dominant. Dysfibrinogenemias can result in bleeding or hypercoagulability. The gene for fibrinogen is located on chromosome 4. Because fibrinogen is required for the formation of a fibrin clot, it is surprising that afibrinogenemic patients survive gestation and birth. Diagnosis is made when patients present with bleeding from the umbilical stump, intracranial hemorrhage, or mucosal bleeding. Hemarthroses can occur but are less common than observed with the hemophilias. Wound healing may be delayed. Increased incidence of fetal wastage in patients with afibrinogenemia and hypofibrinogenemia is observed, and term gestation is rarely achieved without replacement of fibrinogen.[77–79] Because the substrate for clot formation, fibrinogen, is missing or deficient, the prothrombin time (PT), activated partial thromboplastin time (aPTT), thrombin clotting time (TCT), and coagulation assays that have fibrin formation as their end points are all prolonged. Replacement of fibrinogen is accomplished with cryoprecipitate, with a goal of achieving a plasma level between 50 and 100 mg/dL and at least 60 mg/dL for maintenance of pregnancy.[79] Each bag of cryoprecipitate contains approximately 200 to 300 mg of fibrinogen. The biologic half-life of fibrinogen is between 2 and 4 days. Virally inactivated fibrinogen concentrates are available in Europe, China, and Japan (Japan Green Cross, Aventis, LFB). Adverse reactions to treatment include the development of fibrinogen antibodies, allergic reactions, and, paradoxically, thrombosis.

Prothrombin Deficiency

Congenital prothrombin deficiency is a rare autosomal recessive disorder estimated to be present at a rate of 0.5 cases per million. Disease has been described with both homozygous and heterozygous defects (including compound heterozygotes). Hemorrhagic symptoms include bruising; intracranial, mucosal, and deep tissue bleeding; and menorrhagia. Hemarthroses are rare. Correlation between bleeding and prothrombin levels is poor. No reports of a prothrombinemia appear in the literature, suggesting that complete lack of the protein is incompatible with normal development. Both the PT and the aPTT time are prolonged, and the thrombin time is normal. Treatment of prothrombin deficiency includes plasma at a dose of 15 to 20 mL/kg followed by 3 mL/kg every 12 to 24 hours to achieve levels of approximately 30%. The half-life of prothrombin is approximately 3 days. Prothrombin complex concentrates contain prothrombin and other vitamin K-dependent factors and can be used to treat prothrombin-deficient patients who are undergoing major surgery or life-threatening bleeds. Caution should be exercised, as these have been associated with thrombosis.

Factor V Deficiency

Inherited deficiency of factor V occurs in fewer than 1 per 1,000,000 people, with an autosomal recessive inheritance pattern (homozygous or compound heterozygous), resulting in factor V levels less than 20%. Symptoms include bleeding from the umbilical stump and mucous membranes, ecchymoses, menorrhagia, postpartum bleeding, and intracranial hemorrhage. Hemarthroses can occur but are less common than with severe hemophilia. No factor V-enriched plasma concentrates are available. Because factor V is in the common pathway of coagulation, both the PT and the aPTT are prolonged. Treatment of bleeding involves the infusion of plasma at 15 to 20 mL/kg with a goal of achieving levels of 20%. The half-life of factor V is approximately 36 hours. Because platelets contain stored factor V, this product has been used to treat bleeding. Platelet infusion may result in the production of platelet-specific antibodies.

Factor VII Deficiency

Factor VII deficiency occurs in approximately 1 in 500,000 people. Severe bleeding occurs with levels below 5%, and symptoms in severely affected patients are similar to those observed with severe hemophilia. Intracranial hemorrhage may occur in up to 16% of cases and in neonates following vaginal delivery. The PT is prolonged, but the aPTT and thrombin time are normal. Prothrombin complex concentrates contain factor VII and may provide a benefit over plasma because they are virally inactivated. As with the use of these products for factor VIII and factor IX inhibitors, thrombosis has been reported. Several plasma-derived factor VII concentrates have been developed and have been used to treat congenital deficiency. Recombinant activated factor VII concentrate is effective in the treatment of bleeding with factor VII deficiency.[80–83] Inhibitors to factor VIIa have developed in patients with congenital factor VII deficiency.[80]

Factor X Deficiency

Congenital deficiency of factor X is a rare condition resulting from homozygous or compound heterozygous defects in the autosomal genes for factor X located on chromosome 13. Bleeding is correlated with factor X levels, and symptoms include epistaxis, menorrhagia, hemarthrosis, intracranial hemorrhage, hematuria, and umbilical cord bleeding. Because factor X is a component of prothrombinase (the first step in the common pathway), diagnosis is suggested by both a prolonged PT and a prolonged aPTT but a normal TCT. Treatment is with plasma products (FFP or solvent-detergent treated plasma) at approximately 10 to 15 mL/kg followed by 5 mL/kg every 24 hours with a goal of plasma factor X activity levels of 20%. No factor X-specific concentrates are available, but PCCs contain variable amounts of factor X. As with the use of PCCs for other indications, the risk of thrombosis is increased.

Factor XI Deficiency

Congenital factor XI deficiency (sometimes called hemophilia C) is an autosomal disorder with a recessive pattern of inheritance and is particularly common in Ashkenazi Jews, in whom two specific mutations account for the approximately 8% prevalence of an abnormal factor XI gene.[81,82] Bleeding symptoms are variable and include postsurgical or traumatic bleeding or heavy menses in women. Spontaneous hemorrhage is not typical of the disorder, and this characteristic distinguishes the disorder from hemophilia A and B. Plasma levels of factor XI do not correlate with bleeding symptoms, as factor levels do in hemophilia A and B. The aPTT is prolonged with factor XI deficiency; PT and thrombin time are normal. Patients with factor XI deficiency are usually treated prior to surgical procedures with a goal of factor XI levels between 30 and 45 U/dL.[81] Plasma (FFP and solvent-detergent treated plasma) provides the mainstay of therapy, and dosing takes into consideration the long half-life of 60 to 80 hours. Although the half-life of factor XI in solvent-detergent plasma is comparable to that of FFP, decreased levels of factor XI in the product (approximately 30%–50%) have been reported.[83] Two virally reduced or inactivated factor XI concentrates have been developed using affinity chromatography or cation-exchange chromatography.[84] These have been demonstrated to be effective, but there have been reports of thromboembolic complications with their use, presumably because of contaminant activated factor IX. Both products are now formulated with antithrombin and heparin, but caution is advised with their use in elderly patients and in patients with preexisting cardiovascular disease. Doses should not exceed 30 U/kg and peak FXI should not exceed 100 U/dL.[85]

Because bleeding occurs in patients with factor IX deficiency more often in settings in which fibrinolysis is more active (oral mucosa, urinary tract), antifibrinolytic agents can be useful adjuncts in the treatment of such bleeding episodes or used as sole agents to prevent bleeding with dental procedures. Fibrin glue can provide a useful adjunct or be used solely in topical bleeding (dental extractions, circumcisions). DDAVP has been reported as useful for the prevention of surgical bleeding in factor XI deficiency.[86] The mode of effect of DDAVP is unclear but is likely due to the coexistence of mild VWF deficiency.

Factor XIII Deficiency

Factor XIII is a transglutaminase that catalyzes the cross-linking of γ-glutamyl and ε-lysyl groups of fibrin monomers, stabilizing the forming clot by decreasing its susceptibility to fibrinolysis. Inherited deficiency of factor XIII is autosomal recessive and results from defects in the genes for the two subunits of factor XIII located on chromosome 1 (B subunit) and chromosome 6 (A subunit). The majority of reported defects involve the A subunit. Umbilical bleeding in homozygotes may be observed at birth. Soft-tissue bleeds, hemarthroses, excessive intracranial bleeding (relative to other coagulation deficiencies), pseudotumors, and bleeding at surgery are observed in affected patients. Surgery is also complicated by poor wound healing. Affected male patients may have oligospermia and female patients may have recurrent miscarriages. Coagulation screening tests (PT, aPTT, and TCT) are normal. Solubility of clots is increased with factor XIII deficiency; thus, the diagnosis can be made by incubating clots in the presence of solubilizing agents such as 5 M urea or 1% to 2% chloroacetic acid. Factor XIII has a long half-life (9–15 days). FFP (2–3 mL/kg) or cryoprecipitate (1 bag/10–20 kg) can be administered to raise levels of factor XIII. Because of the long half-life of factor XIII, FFP and cryoprecipitate can be used on a prophylactic basis (dosing every 3–4 weeks) to prevent intracranial hemorrhage and other bleeding episodes. Two plasma-derived factor XIII concentrates have been developed and may be available in the United States on a limited basis. Dosing with factor XIII concentrate is 10 to 75 IU/kg every 4 to 6 weeks, with lower doses for prophylaxis and higher doses for the treatment of bleeding episodes. A recombinant FXIII-A_2 concentrate was found in phase I testing to be safe and potentially effective for replacement in patients with FXIII deficiency and is currently in clinical trials.[87]

OTHER PLASMA-DERIVED PROTEIN CONCENTRATES

As discussed in Chapter 143, plasma fractionation processes also allow for the isolation of plasma components other than the coagulation proteins. Immunoglobulins are isolated by a variety of techniques from the Cohn fraction II-III. α_1-Antitrypsin and antithrombin are produced from fraction IV. As with other vitamin K-dependent proteins, protein C may be isolated from Cohn fraction II.

Anticoagulant Proteins (Protein C and Antithrombin)

Brief mention should be made of plasma-derived concentrates enriched in protein C and antithrombin III. These products have been used for a variety of indications, but both are licensed for the treatment of congenital deficiencies that result in thrombosis. Protein C concentrate has also been used in the treatment of purpura fulminans with meningococcemia. Antithrombin has been used for the treatment of venoocclusive disease in patients undergoing bone marrow transplantation, heparin resistance in patients undergoing cardiopulmonary bypass, and sepsis. Recent results using a recombinant activated protein C[88] have shown efficacy in the treatment of sepsis, and its utility for other indications is not yet known.

Immunoglobulins

The use of immunoglobulins (both intravenous and hyperimmune products) for a variety of diseases is discussed elsewhere in this book.

α_1-Protease Inhibitor (Antitrypsin)

α_1-Protease inhibitor (or antitrypsin) concentrates (Prolastin, Bayer Healthcare LLC; Aralast, Baxter Biosciences; Zemaira, ZLB-Behring) are available for the prophylactic treatment of people with congenital deficiency of α_1 antitrypsin. α_1 Antitrypsin inhibits neutrophil elastase, which is thought to be responsible for the alveolar damage resulting in emphysema. These replacement products, administered intravenously, are presumed to act to delay the progression of congenital emphysema associated with this protease inhibitor deficiency.

CONCLUSION

Virally safe plasma-derived concentrates have been developed that are enriched in a variety of coagulation and other proteins. Initially, refinements in techniques of plasma fractionation formed the basis for the development of these concentrates as an improvement over the use of blood component therapy (whole blood, plasma, and cryoprecipitate). Plasma-derived protein concentrates were first developed for the treatment of the more common hemophilias A and B. Subsequent refinements were made to reduce, then eliminate, the transmission of viral and other pathogens present in the human plasma pool while increasing product purity. Techniques in molecular biology and heterologous expression of mammalian proteins have allowed for the production of some proteins, most notably factor VIII and factor IX, without reliance on the limited plasma resource. These plasma-derived and recombinant concentrates have supplanted the use of plasma or cryoprecipitate for the treatment of some congenital and acquired deficiencies of soluble plasma factors and have decreased or eliminated the attendant risks of allergic reactions, volume overload, and pathogen transmission. For patients on home infusion regimens, protein concentrates also have the benefit of increasing patient convenience, as infusion volumes are small relative to blood component therapy. Although the development of high-purity, virally safe concentrates to treat other plasma protein deficiencies that are currently treated with blood components is technically feasible, such development is limited by the very small numbers of patients with these disorders. In the future, the development of products produced in transgenic animals holds the promise of producing large quantities of recombinant proteins, thus making available more of these life-saving products for use clinically.

SUGGESTED READINGS

Bernard GR, Vincent JL, Laterre PF, et al: Efficacy and safety of recombinant human activated protein C for severe sepsis. N Engl J Med 344:699, 2001.

Bray GL, Gomperts ED, Courter S, et al: A multicenter study of recombinant factor VIII (recombinate): Safety, efficacy, and inhibitor risk in previously untreated patients with hemophilia A. The Recombinate Study Group. Blood 83:2428, 1994.

Ehrenforth S, Kreutz W, Scharrer I, et al: Incidence of development of factor VIII and factor IX inhibitors in haemophiliacs. Lancet 339:594, 1992.

Horowitz B, Wiebe ME, Lippin A, Stryker MH: Inactivation of viruses in labile blood derivatives. I. Disruption of lipid-enveloped viruses by tri(*n*-butyl)phosphate detergent combinations. Transfusion 25:516, 1985.

Lusher JM, Arkin S, Abildgaard CF, Schwartz RS: Recombinant factor VIII for the treatment of previously untreated patients with hemophilia A: Safety, efficacy, and development of inhibitors. Kogenate Previously Untreated Patient Study Group. N Engl J Med 328:453, 1993.

Nilsson IM, Berntorp E, Zettervall O: Induction of immune tolerance in patients with hemophilia and antibodies to factor VIII by combined treatment with intravenous IgG, cyclophosphamide, and factor VIII. N Engl J Med 318:947, 1988.

Roberts H: The treatment of hemophilia: Past tragedy and future promise. N Engl J Med 321:1188, 1989.

Schwartz RS, Abildgaard C, Aledort L, et al, Group TRFVS: Human recombinant DNA derived antihemophilic (factor VIII) in the treatment of hemophilia A. N Engl J Med 323:1800, 1990.

United Kingdom Haemophilia Centre Doctor's Organization: Guidelines on the selection and use of therapeutic products to treat haemophilia and other hereditary bleeding disorders. Haemophilia 9:1, 2003

White GC, Beebe A, Nielsen B: Recombinant factor IX. Thromb Haemost 78:261, 1997.

REFERENCES

For complete list of references log onto www.expertconsult.com

CHAPTER 152

HEMAPHERESIS AND CELLULAR THERAPY*

Ellen F. Lazarus and Harvey G. Klein

Bloodletting is an ancient therapy, fashionable, albeit unproved, well into the 19th century. About the time that scientific skepticism began to temper the widespread use of therapeutic phlebotomy, a new technique for blood removal, apheresis, appeared in the research laboratory.[1] The term *apheresis*, derived from a Greek verb meaning "to take away or withdraw," was coined to describe removal of one component of blood with return of the remaining components to the donor. Like phlebotomy, apheresis was used first to treat patients but later became more important for collecting blood components for transfusion. Increasingly, apheresis techniques are used to collect cell populations from the peripheral blood of healthy donors and patients for purposes of hematopoietic stem/progenitor cell (HPC) transplantation and immune cell therapies. Annually in the United States, up to 20,000 units of peripheral blood stem cells (PBSC) and therapeutic lymphocytes are collected at hospital and blood center apheresis facilities.[2]

PRINCIPLES OF APHERESIS

The principal objective of apheresis is efficient removal of some circulating blood component, either cells (cytapheresis) or some plasma solute (plasmapheresis). For most disorders, the treatment goal is to deplete the circulating cell or substance directly responsible for the disease process. Apheresis can also mobilize cells and plasma components from tissue depots. For example, lymphocytes may be mobilized from the spleen and lymph nodes of some patients with chronic lymphocytic leukemia, and low-density lipoproteins can be removed from tissue stores in patients with familial hypercholesterolemia. Apheresis also appears to mobilize $CD34^+$ cells from extravascular depots in peripheral blood stem/progenitor cell (PBSC) donors, resulting in collection of more than twice as many $CD34^+$ cells than estimated based on preapheresis peripheral blood cell counts (Fig. 152–1).[3] Apheresis may have other, less obvious effects. Lymphocyte depletion may modify immune responsiveness in some disease states, possibly by disturbing the control mechanisms of cellular immune regulation. Plasmapheresis enhances splenic clearance of immune complexes in certain autoimmune disorders.[4] When therapeutic effect is judged by clinical improvement rather than by efficiency of solute removal, apheresis is more often a helpful adjunct than a form of first-line therapy.

Several mathematic models formulated for different clinical conditions describe the kinetics of apheresis.[5–7] Removal of most blood constituents follows a logarithmic curve (Fig. 152–2). This model assumes that the substance removed is neither synthesized nor degraded substantially during the procedure, remains within the intravascular compartment, and mixes instantaneously and completely with any plasma replacement solution. When the goal of plasmapheresis is to supply a deficient substance, for example, the cleavase ADAMTS13 in the treatment of thrombotic thrombocytopenic purpura, replacement follows logarithmic kinetics similar to those developed for solute removal. From Fig. 152–2, it is evident that removal of 1.5 to 2.0 volumes will reduce an intravascular substance by approximately 80% and that processing larger volumes results in little additional gain.

Specific cell removal with centrifugal automated cell separators depends on the number of cells available, the volume of blood processed, the efficiency of the particular instrument, and the separation characteristics of the different cells. Most commercially available instruments remove platelets and lymphocytes extremely efficiently. Granulocytes and other mononuclear cells, including HPC from peripheral blood, cannot be cleanly separated from other cells by standard centrifugal apheresis equipment (Fig. 152–3). Optimal harvesting of these cells requires special techniques such as stimulating the donor with corticosteroids or cytokines and adding sedimenting agents to enhance cell separation.

TECHNOLOGY AND TECHNIQUES

The plasmapheresis technique that originated in the animal laboratory required manual resuspension of red cells and posed a substantial risk of microbial contamination of the components being reinfused. With the introduction of sterile, disposable, interconnected plastic blood bags, plasmapheresis became relatively safe and easy. However, manual apheresis proved too inefficient and labor-intensive for collecting large component volumes and raised concerns that the separated units of red blood cells might be reinfused accidentally into the wrong donor or patient. The introduction of automated on-line blood cell separators solved these problems.[8,9] Automated apheresis instruments use microprocessor technology to draw and anticoagulate blood, separate components either by centrifugation or by filtration, collect the desired component, and recombine the remaining components for return to the patient or donor.[10,11] The equipment contains disposable plastic software in the blood path and uses anticoagulants containing citrate or combinations of citrate and heparin that do not result in clinical anticoagulation of the patient or donor. Most instruments function well at blood flow rates of 30 to 80 mL/min and can operate from peripheral venous access or from a variety of multilumen central venous catheters. Newer therapeutic apheresis devices are smaller and more automated, allowing for implementation of more safety functions and improved portability.

Because the ideal method for treating disorders mediated by abnormal plasma components is to remove the offending substance selectively, a variety of on-line filtration and column adsorption techniques have been introduced or proposed. Ligands bound to a column matrix may be relatively nonspecific chemical sorbents, such as charcoal or heparin, or specific ligands, such as monoclonal antibodies and recombinant protein antigens. Two such columns are commercially available: one using staphylococcal protein A and the other using dextran sulfate cellulose beads. Staphylococcal protein A has high affinity for the Fc portion of IgG1, IgG2, and IgG4 and for immune complexes containing these IgG subtypes. This column is approved for use in therapeutic apheresis procedures for patients with chronic immune thrombocytopenia and selected adult patients with rheumatoid arthritis. The dextran sulfate cellulose columns selectively remove low-density lipoproteins and have proved effective in managing patients with homozygous hypercholesterolemia who have not responded to diet and cholesterol-lowering drug therapy (Fig. 152–4). Apheresis technology has also been adapted for extracorpo-

Disclaimer: No official support or endorsement of this chapter by the Food and Drug Administration is intended or should be inferred. The views presented herein do not necessarily reflect those of the Food and Drug Administration, the National Institutes of Health, or the Department of Health and Human Services.

Cell type	Blood concentration			Cell content			Apparent volume of distribution	
	Initial	End	% change*	Blood†	Product‡	Fraction§	Liters	No. of blood volumes
CD34 Cells								
25 l	0.077	0.045	−45	3.8	7.9	2.3	25.9	5.3
15 lx 2	0.078	0.039	−50	3.9	8.1	2.3	22.2	5.1

* Percentage change, end vs. iniial

† Estimated initial content in peripheral blood

‡ Total product content

§ Total product content divided by estimated initial content in peripheral blood. l, liters. CD34 cell concentration in 10^9/l, CD34 cell content x 10^8 cells.

Figure 152–1 Twenty healthy mobilized donors underwent either a single large volume leukapheresis procedure of 25 L or two consecutive-day smaller volume procedures of 15 L each. In both study groups, more than twice as many CD34 cells were collected than the estimated total content of these cells in the peripheral blood before apheresis, providing evidence for the existence of a large extravascular pool of PBSC which becomes accessible to collection by leukapheresis. *Modified from Bolan, C.D.* et al, *British Journal of Haematology, 2003, by permission of the authors.*

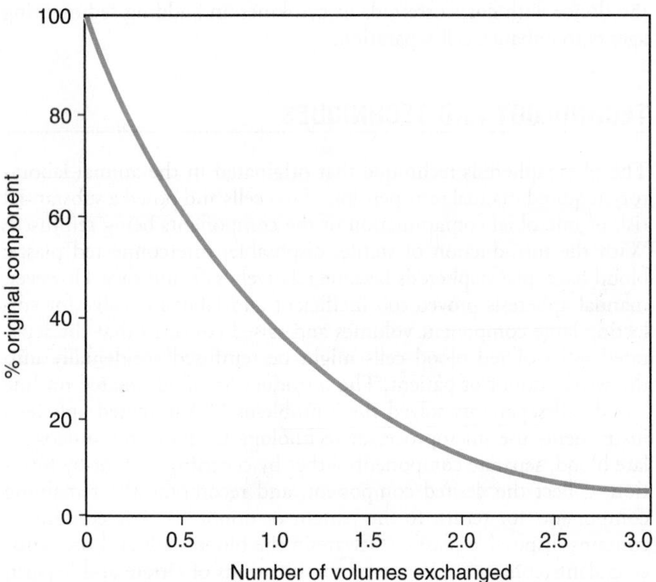

Figure 152–2 Relation between volumes removed by apheresis and percentage of the target component remaining. The relation is valid for blood volumes during red cell exchange or for plasma volumes during plasmapheresis if the target solute remains primarily within the intravascular compartment.

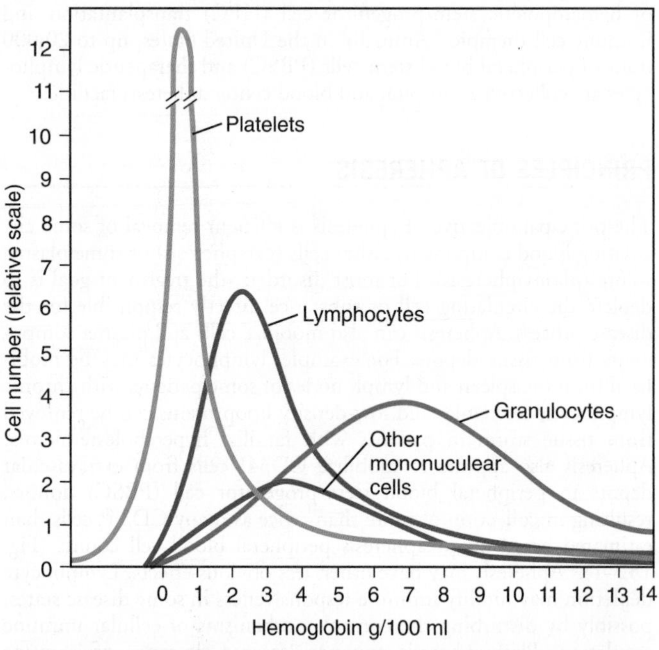

Figure 152–3 Schematic distribution of cells at the collection port of a centrifugal cell separator. The number and percentage of each cell type collected can be varied by adjusting the site of collection along the interface or by changing centrifugal force, blood flow rate, or rate of cell removal.

real phototherapy of patient leukocytes (photopheresis) to treat cutaneous T-cell lymphoma and to modulate the pathologic immune response in graft-versus-host disease, solid organ transplant, and autoimmune diseases (see below).

THERAPEUTIC CYTAPHERESIS

Common indications for therapeutic cell removal are listed in Table 152–1. Most of these procedures entail simple apheresis of the patient's peripheral blood with diversion for discarding the affected red cell, white cell, or platelet fraction. Special apheresis technologies have been approved, such as photopheresis devices, which divert a cell fraction that is photochemically treated in the extracorporeal circuit and returned to the patient's circulation, and apheresis immunoabsorption columns, which selectively remove immunoglobulins in the plasma by binding to a solid matrix.

Erythrocytapheresis

Red cell exchange (erythrocytapheresis) is used most often to manage or prevent the acute vasoocclusive complications of sickle cell disease. Compared with manual exchange transfusion, mechanical cell separators offer the advantages of speed and ease and reduce the risks of rapid blood volume alteration and increased blood viscosity that may occur with simple transfusion. Automated procedures can be performed with all centrifugal instruments and programmed procedures allow accurate prediction of target hemoglobin concentration and percent hemoglobin A (HbA) at the conclusion of the procedure.

Sickle cell anemia occurs in individuals who are homozygous for a single mutation in codon 6 of the β-globin gene, resulting in substitution of a single amino acid. Although the defect appears simple, the pathophysiology of the vasoocclusive crises is complex, involving hemoglobin polymerization, change in cell shape, adhesion to endothelial cells, dysregulated nitric oxide homeostasis, and release of free

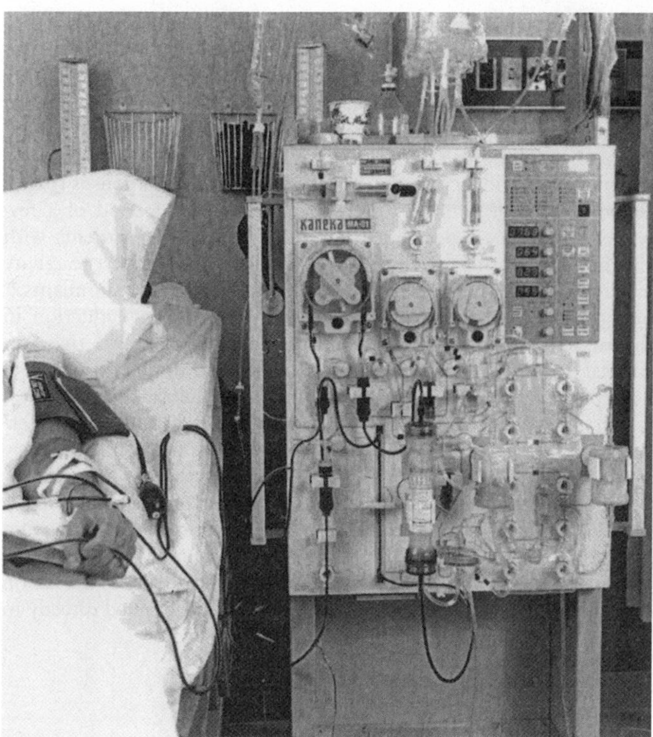

Figure 152–4 Two-stage therapeutic plasmapheresis. Plasma is separated from cells by filtration and then passed through parallel adsorption columns to remove low-density lipoproteins from a patient with homozygous familial hypercholesterolemia.

Table 152–1 Common Indications for Therapeutic Cytapheresis

Erythrocytapheresis
Sickle cell disease
Acute complications
Prophylaxis for recurrent stroke
Frequent severe pain crises
Hyperparasitemia (malaria, babesiosis)
Hemochromatosis
Leukapheresis
Leukemia with hyperleukocytosis syndrome
Cutaneous T-cell lymphoma (photopheresis)
Peripheral blood stem cell collection
Plateletpheresis
Symptomatic thrombocytosis

hemoglobin and inflammatory cytokines[12] Clinical manifestations vary from patient to patient. The rationale behind exchange transfusion involves improving tissue oxygenation, reducing hemolysis, and preventing microvascular sickling by diluting the patient's abnormal red cells, simultaneously correcting anemia and favorably altering whole blood viscosity and rheology. No clinical data support a single optimal level of hemoglobin A (Hb A); however, as few as 30% of transfused cells markedly decrease blood viscosity. At mixtures of 50% or greater, resistance to membrane filterability approaches normal.[13,14] In nonemergency situations, such levels can often be achieved with a simple transfusion regimen. For simple and exchange transfusions, raising the level of Hb A to between 60% and 70% while lowering the level of Hb S to 30% is generally efficacious, although even higher levels of HbA may be required to treat an ongoing crisis.

Clinical indications for exchange transfusion in patients with sickle cell anemia remain controversial, with limited controlled study data available. Simple transfusion has been shown to improve renal concentrating ability and splenic function in young sickle cell patients; exchange transfusion improves exercise tolerance and reverses the periodic oscillations in cutaneous blood flow associated with this disease.[15–17] Such observations have encouraged the use of exchange transfusion for acute complications of sickle cell disease such as acute chest syndrome, priapism, cerebrovascular accident, and hepatic and retinal infarction. Exchange transfusion for sickle cell patients has also been used for prophylaxis during pregnancy and before surgery, although prophylactic transfusion in these settings is controversial. The only randomized trial of transfusion during pregnancy has shown that prophylactic transfusion sufficient to reduce the incidence of painful crises did not reduce other maternal morbidity or perinatal mortality.[18] In a randomized study of sickle cell disease patients undergoing surgery, a conservative simple transfusion regimen (to increase the Hb level to 10 g/dL) was as effective as an aggressive regimen (to lower the Hb S level to <30%) with respect to perioperative non–transfusion-related complications. The patients in the aggressive regimen group received twice as many units of blood, had a proportionally increased red blood cell alloimmunization rate, and had more hemolytic transfusion reactions.[19] The results of this and other studies suggest that if prophylactic preoperative exchange transfusion is used, it should be limited to patients undergoing high-risk procedures in whom simple transfusion could not effectively raise the Hb A level to 70% or higher.

Transfusion prophylaxis is now clearly indicated for children at high risk for stroke. A randomized controlled study demonstrated a risk reduction of 90% in the patients who were maintained at levels of 30% or less Hb S by simple or exchange transfusion.[20] This result confirms earlier experience and indicates that in this group of children with sickle cell anemia, transfusion therapy should begin before the first event and continue indefinitely. Long-term erythrocytapheresis may be preferable for patients at high risk for stroke who have developed iron overload to levels associated with organ damage.[21]

Exchange transfusion, although relatively safe and convenient, carries all the complications of red cell transfusion. Patients are exposed to a large number of donors and are at a small but significant risk of contracting hepatitis and other blood-borne infections. As many as 33% of all patients develop alloantibodies, and life-threatening delayed hemolytic transfusion reactions have been reported.[22,23] In addition, an immunohematologic study of multiply transfused sickle cell patients shows that 85% of heavily transfused patients are alloimmunized to human leukocyte antigens (HLAs), platelet-specific antigens, or both.[24] Most centers avoid inducing nonhemolytic transfusion reactions and HLA alloimmunization by using leukocyte-depleted red cells. Extended red blood cell phenotyping at diagnosis and provision of phenotypically matched blood, when practical, can reduce the risk of red cell alloimmunization and associated hemolytic transfusion reactions. Despite the removal of red cells during exchange, patients remain in positive iron balance, although iron accumulation is slow and chelation is rarely required to prevent transfusional hemosiderosis.[21]

Other indications for red cell exchange are rare. The procedure has been used for patients with overwhelming red cell parasitic infections, such as severe and complicated malaria and babesiosis.[25,26] In these situations, red cell exchange decreases the concentration of circulating parasites and may help sustain life until conventional therapy and natural immunity take effect. Although the efficacy of this therapy has not been evaluated by controlled trials, prospective studies and review of published cases suggest the use of erythrocytapheresis for parasitemia greater than 10% to 15%, or even less in selected patients.[27] Automated red cell removal with volume replacement (isovolemic hemodilution) can be performed rapidly and safely in polycythemic subjects.[28] This maneuver should be reserved for polycythemic patients with an urgent clinical indication to lower the hematocrit (eg, evolving thrombotic stroke) for which standard single-unit manual phlebotomy might be inadvisably slow. Automated double red cell apheresis technology has more recently been used to treat individuals with hereditary hemochromatosis. This procedure removes excess iron more rapidly than manual phlebotomy, and may be more tolerable to patients because of the lower frequency of maintenance procedures required (Fig. 152–5).[29]

Leukapheresis

Therapeutic leukapheresis has been used most successfully to help manage patients with acute leukemia and extremely high white blood cell (WBC) numbers, so-called acute hyperleukocytic leukemia (AHL). When the fractional volume of leukocytes (leukocrit) exceeds 20%, blood viscosity increases and leukocytes can interfere with pulmonary and cerebral blood flow and compete with tissue for oxygen in the microcirculation.[30] Investigations of the expression and function of adhesion receptors in leukemic cells and the role of adhesion molecules in leukocyte-induced acute lung injury in sepsis suggest that the pathophysiology of leukostasis in AHL may also be related to interactions between leukemic blasts and endothelial cells mediated by locally released adhesion molecules.[31] A single leukapheresis procedure generally reduces the WBC count by 20% to 50%, depending on the differing sedimentation characteristics of the specific blast cell population. Ordinarily, leukapheresis is initiated in a patient with acute myeloid leukemia (AML) when the blast count is higher than 100,000/mm^3 or when rapidly rising blast counts are higher than 50,000/mm^3, especially when evidence of central nervous system or pulmonary symptoms appears. The threshold for initiation of leukapheresis in patients with acute lymphocytic leukemia (ALL) is generally higher (WBC count >200,000/mm^3).[32] Other immediate measures for treatment of patients with AHL include infusion of IV fluids, administration of hydroxyurea and allopurinol, and correction of coagulopathy and thrombocytopenia.[31]

Mechanical cytoreduction for managing other leukemic processes has limited value. Although repeated leukapheresis has adequately reduced the WBC count in a series of patients with chronic myeloid leukemia, the median patient survival rate was not significantly different from that of similar patients treated with conventional chemotherapy.[33] Chronic leukapheresis can provide acceptable control of the peripheral WBC count in clinical situations such as pregnancy, when cytotoxic agents may best be avoided, but cytoreduction alone does not appear to alter the course of chronic myeloid leukemia. Some studies of patients with chronic lymphocytic leukemia suggested short-term clinical benefit, but long-term support of patients when the disease is refractory to chemotherapy does not appear to prolong life.[34,35]

Lymphocyte removal by apheresis has also been used to modify immune responsiveness in patients with autoimmune diseases, and to enhance solid organ allograft survival and reverse solid organ graft rejection, but evidence of clinical efficacy in these situations is sparse. Removal of large numbers of lymphocytes over a period of a few weeks can suppress peripheral lymphocyte counts in patients with rheumatoid arthritis for up to 1 year and can alter skin-test reactivity and lymphocyte mitogen responsiveness to a variety of stimulants.[36] Selected patients experience a modest but significant reduction in disease activity; however, the subset of patients who may derive substantial benefit from this therapy is difficult to identify.[37,38] An adsorptive type extracorporeal column of cellulose acetate beads, which selectively adsorb circulating granulocytes and monocytes/macrophages, is undergoing study in patients with inflammatory bowel disease.[39]

Photopheresis is an automated extracorporeal photochemotherapy treatment that involves leukapheresis, extracorporeal photoactivation with a light-sensitizing agent, 8-methoxypsoralen (8-MOP) and ex vivo ultraviolet A irradiation, and reinfusion of the leukocyte fraction (Fig. 152–6). The light-sensitizing agent is often delivered directly to

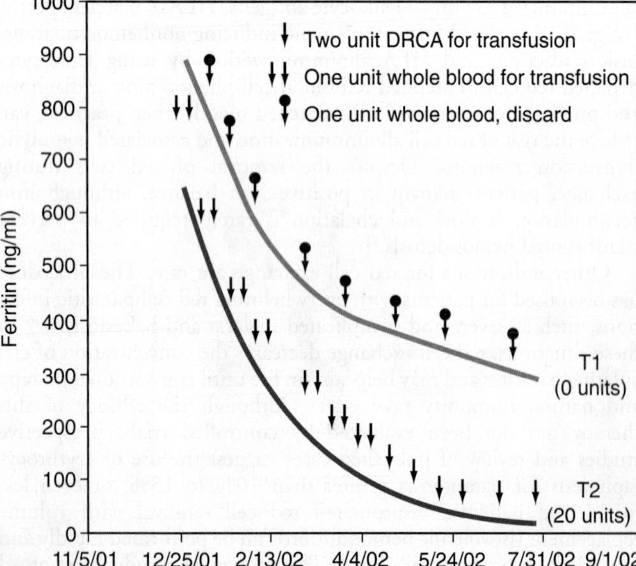

Figure 152–5 One twin was treated with manual phlebotomy (T1), and the other with double red cell apheresis (DRCA) (T2). In the same time period, ferritin levels declined more rapidly and to lower levels in the twin treated with double red cell apheresis. (*Unpublished data from Bolan CD, Leitman SF, with permission of the authors.*)

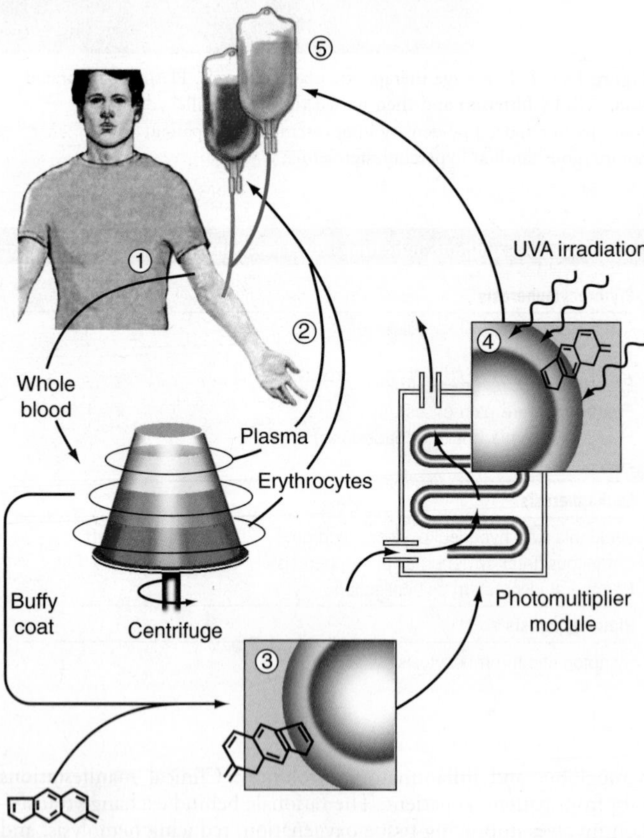

Figure 152–6 Overview of a photopheresis procedure. 1) Vascular access is achieved by placement of a peripheral intravenous line or through a temporary central venous catheter. Whole blood is withdrawn from the patient, mixed with an anticoagulant solution, and pumped to a centrifuge where it is separated into plasma, red cell, and mononuclear cell (buffy coat) fractions by elutriation. 2) Following the collection of each mononuclear cell fraction, the uncollected red cells and plasma are pumped from the plasma/return bag through a blood filter and returned to the patient. 3) The mononuclear cell fractions are mixed with 8-methoxypsoralen and then 4) pumped through a sterile cassette surrounded by UV-A bulbs, resulting in a controlled rate and amount of UV-A exposure. 5) The treated cell fraction is filtered and returned to the patient.

the extracorporeal leukocyte fraction, which may reduce the adverse effects such as nausea and vomiting associated with oral administration. The mechanism of action of photopheresis is unclear, but may involve induction of apoptosis in pathogenic T-lymphocytes and induction of a dendritic cell-mediated cytotoxic T-cell response. This therapy has minimal toxicity and is highly effective in the treatment of patients with advanced cutaneous T-cell lymphoma.[40,41] Other disorders reported to respond to photopheresis therapy include cardiac and other solid organ graft rejection,[42,43] and graft-versus-host disease (GVHD) following bone marrow transplantation in patients who do not respond to standard immunosuppressive therapy.[44,45] Acute adverse effects include skin erythema, low-grade fever, and transient hypotension. Anemia due to incomplete reinfusion of red cells may occur in patients undergoing long-term photopheresis.[41]

Plateletpheresis

Therapeutic plateletpheresis is generally reserved for patients with myeloproliferative disorders and hemorrhage or thrombosis associated with an increase in circulating platelets. Many centers consider using plateletpheresis when the patient's peripheral platelet count is greater than 10^6/mm^3, although no consistent relation between the level of platelet elevation and the occurrence of symptoms has been found, and no generally accepted assay of platelet dysfunction predicts which patients are at risk.[46,47] A single cytapheresis procedure can lower the platelet count by 30% to 50%. Plateletpheresis can have dramatic effects for selected patients such as those with evolving digital gangrene. Attempts to maintain thrombocythemic patients at normal platelet counts by cytapheresis alone have not been successful; more practical long-term chemotherapy should be instituted concurrently. As most patients with thrombocytosis do not develop symptoms, including patients with myeloproliferative disorders, prophylactic plateletpheresis is unwarranted regardless of the platelet count.[47]

THERAPEUTIC PLASMAPHERESIS

Common clinical indications for therapeutic plasmapheresis are outlined in Table 152–2. Most procedures are performed for treatment of immunologic and hematologic disorders. A course of plasmapheresis generally consists of five to seven exchanges of 1 to 1.5 plasma volumes each, either daily or with an interval of 1 to 2 days between procedures, although the course of therapy will vary depending on the specific disease indication and rate and duration of response. Several expert committees have published practice guidelines for using plasmapheresis in a wide variety of disease states.[48–50] Some of the least controversial indications for plasmapheresis are supported by small series of uncontrolled cases that rely on some objective clinical or laboratory measurement of patient improvement.

Table 152–2 Common Indications for Therapeutic Plasmapheresis

Hematologic diseases (including blood cell–specific autoimmune diseases)
Thrombotic thrombocytopenic purpura
Idiopathic thrombocytopenic purpura (immunoabsorption)
Hyperviscosity
Posttransfusion purpura
Cold agglutinin syndrome
Coagulation factor inhibitors
ABO-mismatched marrow transplant (recipient)
Autoimmune diseases
Cryoglobulinemia
Rheumatoid arthritis (immunoadsorption, lymphoplasmapheresis)
Myasthenia gravis
Goodpasture syndrome
Guillain–Barré syndrome
Chronic inflammatory demyelinating polyneuropathy
Metabolic diseases
Homozygous familial hypercholesterolemia (selective adsorption)
Refsum disease
Other
Drug overdose and poisoning

Hematologic Indications

Two of the most common indications for plasmapheresis are treatment of thrombotic thrombocytopenic purpura (TTP) and treatment of clinical syndromes associated with paraproteinemias. Plasma exchange with fresh-frozen plasma (FFP) replacement has been estimated to improve survival rates of patients with TTP from 10% to more than 75%. Comprehensive reviews of the clinical and laboratory evaluation and treatment of patients with suspected TTP, including management with plasma exchange therapy, have been published.[51,52] Treatment usually involves daily single-volume plasma exchange with both frequency and duration of treatment guided by clinical response, increase in platelet count to 100,000/μL or more, and evidence of declining hemolysis as measured by normalization of serum L-lactate dehydrogenase (LDH) and decline in the number of schistocytes on the peripheral blood smear. Despite initial reports of improved response rates in certain patients, recent experience suggests that the use of cryoprecipitate-poor plasma may not be more effective than the use of standard FFP as a specific replacement fluid for plasma exchange in patients with TTP.[53]

The effectiveness of plasma exchange in this setting may derive from removal of antibody to and/or replacement of the von Willebrand factor-cleaving zinc metalloprotease, ADAMTS13.[54–56] However, patients with clinical features of TTP and only moderate ADAMTS13 deficiency or even normal activity may respond to plasma exchange.[57] Plasma exchange for hematopoietic progenitor cell transplant recipients with clinical features of TTP has proved far less efficacious. This syndrome likely differs in pathogenesis from classic TTP.

Small, uncontrolled studies and extensive clinical experience support the use of plasmapheresis as an adjunctive therapy for patients with paraproteinemia and hyperviscosity syndrome, and with some paraproteinemias in the absence of hyperviscosity.[58,59] Comprehensive review articles describing the rationale and treatment schedules for plasmapheresis in patients with a variety of paraproteinemias, including cryoglobulinemia and Waldenström macroglobulinemia, and other hematologic-oncologic indications, have been published.[60,61]

Low-Density Lipoprotein Apheresis and Other Metabolic Disease Indications

Evidence that cutaneous lesions and vascular lesions regress in individuals with familial hypercholesterolemia as low-density lipoprotein levels are controlled by plasmapheresis has encouraged the use of apheresis column absorption procedures in patients with homozygous disease and in poorly controlled heterozygous patients. Low-density lipoprotein apheresis is a procedure for removing apolipoprotein B-containing lipoproteins specifically from the blood by a variety of techniques, including dextran sulfate cellulose adsorption, immunoadsorption, and heparin-induced extracorporeal precipitation. Short-term safety and efficacy have been demonstrated.[62] Patients have now been treated successfully for several years; however, additional experience with this therapy will be required to prove long-term benefit for refractory hypercholesterolemia and coronary artery disease.

Simple plasma exchange may be used in patients with other inherited metabolic diseases, such as Refsum disease.[63] The frequency of

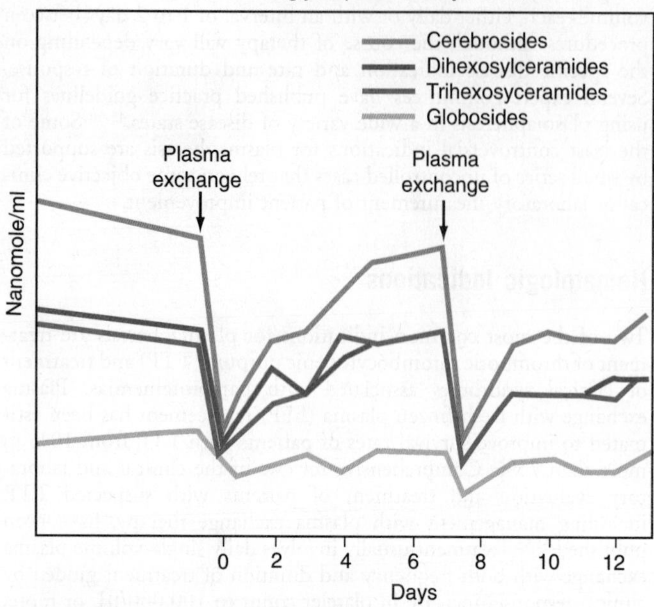

Figure 152–7 Plasma exchange to remove plasma neutral glycolipids in a patient with Fabry disease. The plasma lipid recovery curve appears to be biphasic, reflecting initial reequilibration from tissue stores and subsequent new synthesis of that glycolipid.

exchange depends primarily on total body burden, rate of synthesis, and plasma concentration of the solute to be removed (Fig. 152–7). Less evidence exists to support a role for repeated treatments in these diseases.

Immune Disease Indications and Immunoadsorption Therapies

Plasma exchange appears to have at least a temporary adjunctive role in managing some rheumatic diseases and other immune disorders characterized by circulating autoantibodies. Early success was reported in patients with Goodpasture syndrome, a disorder characterized by a specific pathogenic autoantibody directed against the renal glomerular and pulmonary alveolar basement membrane. Plasmapheresis has demonstrated similar success in myasthenia gravis, pemphigus, and Eaton-Lambert syndrome. Although nonselective plasma exchange has been used in a variety of other rheumatic diseases such as systemic lupus erythematosus and rheumatoid vasculitis, with the exception of treatment of patients with Goodpasture syndrome (in which plasma exchange is considered first-line adjuvant therapy), such use remains unproved and should be reserved for circumstances where a vital organ or life itself is endangered. In some immune disorders, such as immune thrombocytopenic purpura (ITP) and immune inhibitors to coagulation proteins, plasma exchange may be helpful during a catastrophic event, but in general, benefit of nonselective plasma exchange therapy is not established.[64]

Plasma exchange appears to be a useful therapeutic option in renal transplant patients with refractory humoral rejection and also may be used to overcome ABO and HLA incompatibilities between renal transplant patients and their only available donors. Montgomery et al have published several studies showing successful reversal of acute humoral rejection mediated by HLA-specific donor antibody using a combination of plasmapheresis and intravenous immune globulin.[65] They have also demonstrated the use of a conditioning regimen consisting of pretransplant plasmapheresis, immunosuppressive medications, and low-dose CMV immune globulin to effectively reduce donor-specific antibody and isoagglutinin titers, with and without posttransplant splenectomy and anti-CD20 treatment.[66,67]

Another promising indication for plasma exchange is treatment of patients with focal segmental glomerulosclerosis (FSGS), for primary disease refractory to standard immunosuppressive therapy and for treatment of patients with recurrent disease after renal transplantation.[68]

Two immunoadsorption columns have been approved in the United States for removal of autoantibodies to factor VIII or factor IX (Immunosorba staphylococcal protein A–agarose column), and treatment of ITP and rheumatoid arthritis (Prosorba staphylococcal protein A–silica column). Several case series describe the use of immunoadsorption for patients with immune inhibitors to factor VIII or factor IX.[69–71] A phase III, multicenter, sham-controlled randomized study of staphylococcal protein A column immunoadsorption shows a significant increase in clinical response in adult patients with longstanding rheumatoid arthritis.[72] Sparse published evidence exists to support the use of immunoadsorption therapy in patients with chronic ITP refractory to standard medical management.

Plasmapheresis is also an effective first- or second-line therapy in selected patients with certain neurologic disorders. Controlled clinical trials of plasmapheresis have demonstrated efficacy in at least two of the polyradiculoneuropathies.[73,74] However, intravenous immunoglobulin alone may be equally effective in the treatment of severe Guillain–Barré syndrome.[75] A review of published studies of therapeutic plasmapheresis in multiple sclerosis (MS) concludes that plasmapheresis may be an effective therapy in acute or chronic progressive MS when conventional corticosteroid or other immunosuppressive drug therapies have failed.[76] The long-term benefit for patients with chronic progressive MS remains controversial.[77] Anecdotal reports of dramatic responses to plasma exchange in patients with primary autoimmune autonomic failure support the hypothesis that antibodies to ganglionic acetylcholine receptors are the causative agents of the severe nervous system failure characteristic of this disease.[78]

REPLACEMENT FLUIDS FOR PLASMA EXCHANGE

The success of therapeutic apheresis procedures seldom depends on the composition of the replacement solution that is used; the single exception is TTP (discussed in the previous section). With therapeutic plasmapheresis for most other disorders, the primary function of the replacement solution is to maintain intravascular volume. Additional requirements include restoration of important plasma proteins, maintenance of colloid osmotic pressure, maintenance of electrolyte balance, and preservation of trace elements lost during a prolonged course of plasmapheresis procedures. In moderately well-nourished patients, homeostatic mechanisms normally obviate the need for precise plasma replacement, and 5% albumin in normal saline or combinations of albumin and crystalloid are usually sufficient. Commonly used is 60% to 80% replacement by colloid, with the crystalloid component consisting of a combination of normal saline and an anticoagulant. Patients with clinical conditions such as hypotension, hypoalbuminemia, or preexisting coagulopathies should receive solutions prepared specifically to meet their individual requirements. Routine supplementation with calcium, potassium, or immunoglobulins is unnecessary. However, for large-volume apheresis procedures to collect PBSCs, intravenous calcium supplementation is beneficial (discussed in the following section). Because less than 500 mL is removed during most cell collection procedures and therapeutic cell depletions, no volume replacement beyond the anticoagulant and saline priming solution is required.

Problems of decreased availability and high cost of albumin have led some centers to develop protocols for alternatives to plasma-derived volume expanders, such as hydroxyethyl starch (HES), for full or partial volume replacement with plasma exchange.[79] These solutions are generally well tolerated. However, extensive replacement with HES in patients undergoing longer courses of plasmapheresis, especially those with impaired renal function, can result in diffuse tissue accumulation of the larger starch molecules (acquired lysosomal storage).[80]

COMPLICATIONS OF THERAPEUTIC APHERESIS

Automated apheresis is a minimal-risk procedure for normal healthy donors. The current generation of blood cell separators is remarkably reliable and equipped with sensitive detection and alarm systems to alert the operator to potential problems. Nevertheless, serious morbidity and rare deaths have been associated with therapeutic procedures. In most reports, deaths are related to either complications associated with the use of central venous access catheters or to cardiac and respiratory problems in patients who were critically ill before apheresis; in the latter, the contributory role of the apheresis procedure is often questionable. The most common adverse effects of therapeutic apheresis are citrate-induced hypocalcemia, allergic reactions (usually to donor plasma or other blood components), vasovagal reactions, and hypovolemia.[81] If transient paresthesia and mild vasovagal events are excluded, approximately 5% of all therapeutic apheresis procedures have medical complications.[82] The frequency of adverse reactions is influenced by the experience of the operator and the nature of the patient population under treatment.[83]

Expected and predictable effects of therapeutic apheresis include alterations in laboratory parameters due to removal and dilution by replacement fluids. A 5% to 15% decrease in hemoglobin-hematocrit, a 20% to 30% decrease in platelet count, and mild transient increase in leukocyte count are commonly observed.[84] Significantly but transiently abnormal coagulation test results are often observed (recovery generally occurs within 48 hours after a single-volume exchange procedure), as well as clinically insignificant decreased levels of other plasma proteins after serial plasma exchange procedures.[84,85]

The most common adverse effect of both donor and therapeutic apheresis procedures is symptomatic hypocalcemia caused by infusion of calcium-chelating citrate ions in the anticoagulant, and, if used as replacement fluid, anticoagulated donor plasma. It is usually manifested by mild perioral or acral paresthesia, or both, requiring no intervention other than slowing the reinfusion rate. The benefit of oral calcium supplements in this setting is questionable, although the practice is widespread. Hyperventilation may exacerbate the symptoms of hypocalcemia. More severe citrate toxicity is uncommon; signs may range from involuntary carpopedal spasm, nausea, and vomiting, to frank tetany with spasm in other muscle groups, including life-threatening laryngospasm and grand mal seizure.[86] Severe toxicity is most commonly experienced by small patients, particularly women, when the blood flow rate is rapid and the procedure is prolonged beyond a few hours. Symptoms correlate inversely with the level of ionized calcium.[87] Extremely low concentrations of ionized calcium are encountered routinely in therapeutic procedures that process more than 15 L of blood. Acute severe hypocalcemia leading to fatal cardiac arrhythmia has been reported in patients who have undergone apheresis. Controlled infusions of 10% calcium gluconate or calcium chloride are effective in the management of these complications. Because metabolism of citrate occurs predominantly in the liver and kidney, patients with conditions affecting these organs are at increased risk for severe citrate reactions. Studies of therapeutic plasma exchange procedures and of PBSC donations performed with and without calcium gluconate or calcium chloride infusion show the effectiveness of continuous calcium infusion for the prevention of mild to moderate citrate toxicity (Fig. 152–8).[87,88]

In a study of plateletpheresis donors, Bolan et al documented sustained effects of citrate infusion on bone metabolism demonstrated by changes in alkaline phosphatase, osteocalcin, parathyroid hormone, and 1,25-dihydroxyvitamin D levels, suggesting the potential for long-term effects on bone metabolism in these donors.[89] Magnesium, another divalent cation, is also bound by citrate. Despite decreases in serum ionized magnesium levels to 39% below baseline, clinical effects are not typically observed, even during large-volume leukapheresis procedures.[90]

The most severe allergic complications occur when plasma is used as the replacement solution, and this risk increases with repeated exposure.[83] Allergic reactions to ethylene oxide, an agent used in the sterilization of plastic disposable equipment, have been reported.[91] Intravenous diphenhydramine is usually effective in managing allergic reactions; premedication with steroids and precautions against anaphylaxis may be necessary for sensitized individuals. Atypical (hypotension and flushing) and anaphylactic reactions have been reported in patients receiving angiotensin-converting enzyme inhibitors undergoing different apheresis procedures, including immunoadsorption with staphylococcal protein A columns. These medications should be discontinued for at least 24 hours before apheresis.[92]

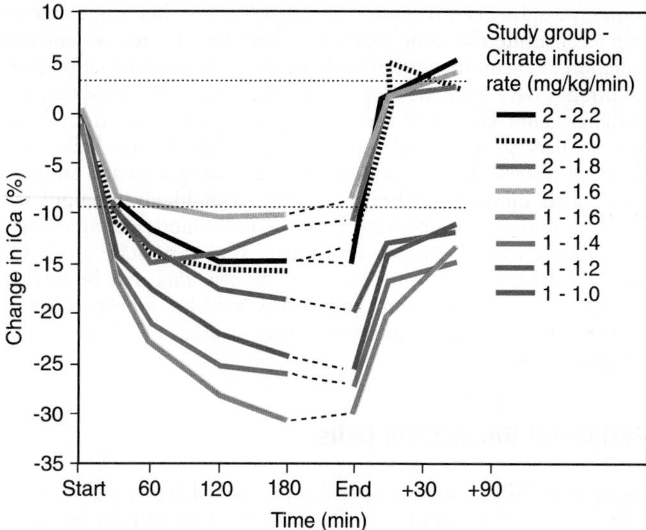

Figure 152–8 Levels of iCa are markedly lower in procedures performed without prophylactic Ca infusion and remain below the reference range 90 minutes after completion of apheresis. Dotted lines indicate upper and lower limits of the reference range. Open symbols represent procedures without prophylactic Ca; solid symbols represent those with Ca infusion. Dashed lines between 180 minutes and end-procedural values (End) reflect varying procedure duration. *(From Bolan CD, Cecco SA, Wesley RA, et al: Transfusion 2002;42:935–946, used by permission).*

Unlike donors undergoing apheresis for donation of red cells, platelets, or plasma, donors undergoing apheresis for collection of therapeutic granulocytes are stimulated with steroids and G-CSF prior to donation. The well-known association of long-term steroid treatment and posterior subcapsular cataracts has not been felt to be relevant in the context of short-term steroid stimulation for donor granulocyte mobilization. However, a small observational study showed that the frequency of posterior subcapsular cataracts was greater in granulocyte donors than in an age-matched plateletpheresis donor control group, suggesting that granulocyte donors may be at increased risk for certain types of cataract formation.[93]

Serious complications indirectly associated with therapeutic apheresis include adverse consequences of vascular access; namely, retroperitoneal or pericardial hemorrhage, pneumo- or hemothorax, thrombosis, nerve damage, and infection. A retrospective review of 381 therapeutic plasma exchange procedures at one institution reported an approximately 1% incidence of severe complications, all of them related to central venous catheters.[94]

CELLULAR THERAPY

Blood cell separators developed for hemapheresis are used increasingly to collect peripheral blood cells for novel forms of cellular therapy. The most common application of apheresis technology for cell therapy indications is the collection of HPC from peripheral blood after administration of recombinant hematopoietic growth factor or chemotherapy, or both, to “mobilize” large numbers of HPC into the circulation. The collected mononuclear cell fraction contains a subset of progenitor cells that, on infusion, can home to and reconstitute the bone marrow in patients who receive ablative radiation or chemotherapy, or both. In the cell-processing laboratory, techniques have been developed for removing T lymphocytes, for purging tumor cells, and for selecting progenitor cells from bone marrow harvests and PBSC collection products. Donor leukocytes obtained from leukapheresis procedures are being used and studied, either with minimal further processing or in highly manipulated forms, as immunotherapy for leukemia, solid tumors, and viral complications of transplantation. Preliminary studies promise a role for autologous HPCs and other mononuclear cells that may be further manipulated in the laboratory and used as "vehicles" for experimental immune therapies in patients with cancer or infectious diseases, and for gene therapies.

Peripheral Blood Stem Cells

Pluripotent HPCs, and quite possibly primordial hematopoietic stem cells capable of reconstituting the bone marrow and the immune system, have long been known to circulate in the peripheral blood.[95] Numerous studies have confirmed the potential for rapid and durable engraftment of PBSCs mobilized into the circulation by hematopoietic growth factors, harvested by large-volume leukapheresis procedures, and subsequently administered to patients with marrow aplasia following high-dose chemotherapy. The concentration of hematopoietic stem cells in the peripheral blood can be increased by the administration of cytokines such as granulocyte colony-stimulating factor (G-CSF) and granulocyte-macrophage colony-stimulating factor (GM-CSF), and by the administration of chemotherapy. CD34$^+$ hematopoietic cell numbers in the peripheral blood generally rise 20- to 40-fold (from 1 to 3 cells/μL to 40 to 70 cells/μL) following administration of G-CSF alone, and they increase 100- to 1000-fold when chemotherapy rebound is enhanced by administration of G-CSF.[96] Efforts to define optimal collection conditions have been limited by the lack of a standardized assay; however, time and level of increase of donor peripheral blood WBC and CD34$^+$ cell counts after administration of mobilizing agents have proved to be useful indicators.[97,98] Hematopoietic colony assays have been used to characterize and quantify stem cells collected by hemapheresis. Colony assays have limited immediate utility because they require a 10- to 14-day incubation period before results are obtained. Assays that use the CD34 antigen as a marker for primitive HPCs can be used to predict the yield of PBSCs collected by leukapheresis and have the advantage of a relatively rapid turnaround time. Despite ongoing problems with interlaboratory standardization, flow cytometric analysis of cells labeled with a fluorochrome-conjugated CD34 antibody are being used increasingly for "real-time" decision making about the timing and adequacy of PBSC collections.

Several clinical scale devices for CD34$^+$ cell enrichment of leukapheresis collections by immunoabsorption or immunomagnetic techniques are available. This "positive selection" of CD34$^+$ hematopoietic cells also results in reduced numbers of cells that do not express the CD34 antigen, such as T lymphocytes. T-cell-reduced products may confer a lower risk of GVHD, and the ability to produce apheresis products enriched for CD34$^+$ cells facilitates graft manipulations for experimental cell therapies such as ex vivo expansion of CD34$^+$ cells. However, some studies suggest a higher incidence of engraftment failure and possibly delayed immune reconstitution in certain patient populations when transplants are performed with highly purified CD34-selected, T cell-depleted products.[99] As yet, no data confirm the clinical benefit of CD34$^+$ cell selection strategies. Please see Chapter 109, Graft Engineering, for a more complete discussion of ex vivo HPC enrichment and T-cell depletion.

Several problems have slowed enthusiastic universal adoption of PBSC transplants for all recipients. Concerns remain regarding the hypothetical long-term effects of exposure of healthy donors to growth factors. The possible risks of donor G-CSF administration and leukapheresis must be weighed against less evidence of benefit of PBSC compared to bone marrow (or against the rapid availability of cord blood) for pediatric recipients.[100] Also, some clinical data suggest the possibility that allogeneic PBSC transplant may result in more frequent chronic graft-versus-host disease in certain patient populations than occurs with bone marrow transplant, without obvious reciprocal benefit with regard to graft-versus-leukemia effect. [Schmitz N et al: Long-term outcome of patients given transplants of mobilized blood or bone marrow: a report from the International Bone Marrow Transplant Registry and the European Group for Blood and Marrow Transplantation. Blood 108(13): 4288, 2006].

Patient Management Issues for Therapeutic Apheresis

Important issues to consider when preparing a patient for therapeutic apheresis, for monitoring the patient during the procedure, and for managing the patient after removal from the apheresis device include:

Preparation

- Volume considerations—Calculate volume to be processed or exchanged; order replacement solutions; assess patient volume status
- Vascular access—Assess need for apheresis line placement. Note that not all large catheters are suitable for apheresis procedures.
- Medications—Evaluate impact of medications (coumadin, platelet inhibitory agents, ACE inhibitors) and indications to suspend certain medications. Albumin-bound medications may be depleted by apheresis.
- Cell counts—Patient may require transfusion for preprocedure anemia or thrombocytopenia
- Electrolytes—Assess risks for citrate toxicity; order calcium replacement solutions if indicated

Procedure

- Volume considerations—Monitor replacement fluids (saline/albumin ratio). Rapid infusion of refrigerated solutions may cause hypothermia.
- Vascular access—Observe for impaired, intermittent, or obstructed flow. Kinked tubing can result in hemolysis.
- Medications—Limitations on blood or citrate flow rate due to symptomatic citrate-induced hypocalcemia may necessitate addition of anticoagulant to the final apheresis product or inclusion of heparin in the anticoagulant regimen.
- Cell counts—Consider impact of very high or low cell counts on device settings and procedure efficiency
- Electrolytes—Continually monitor for adverse citrate effects; bolus or continuous intravenous calcium administration may be required

Postprocedure management:

- Volume considerations—Review net volume balance and consider additional infusion or administration of diuretic if needed
- Vascular access—The decision to remove the apheresis catheter should include the possibility of additional apheresis or procedures; monitor for complications associated with maintenance or removal of venous catheter
- Medications—Determine when to restart medications; consider impact of transiently reduced coagulation factor levels
- Cell counts—Patient may require transfusion for postprocedure thrombocytopenia; monitor cumulative red cell and platelet loss following repeated procedures
- Electrolytes—Assess for imbalance postprocedure, with attention to ionized calcium and magnesium, as indicated by symptoms

For allogeneic donors, the discomfort and inconvenience of multiple-day cytokine administration may be a significant deterrent. Most donors experience some degree of malaise and bone pain, and some donors require hospitalization for more serious adverse reactions to G-CSF administration. Splenic enlargement occurs commonly, and several instances of splenic rupture have been reported.[101] Citrate toxicity is a common complication of PBSC collections; although usually mild and transient, it may be severe and even life threatening in some individuals (see previous section). Venous access requires large-bore multilumen catheters, and these appear particularly susceptible to clotting, especially when patients receive recombinant cytokine stimulation. Hemorrhage, especially in thrombocytopenic patients, is another potentially severe complication of central venous catheter placement. Some patients who have received multiple prior cycles of chemotherapy and a small proportion of normal healthy donors, referred to as "poor mobilizers," fail to respond adequately to mobilization regimens.

Finally, a problem associated with all sources of HPC for transplantation is that the cells may be stored frozen in liquid nitrogen with the cryoprotectant dimethylsulfoxide (DMSO). Cryopreservation is expensive, and rapid infusion of DMSO has been associated with cardiac arrhythmias, hypertension, nausea, and vomiting. Fortunately, DMSO toxicity can be minimized by appropriate premedication, careful attention to infusion rates, and also by washing the thawed product prior to administration, although this strategy does result in measurable loss of progenitor cells. Please see Chapter 108 for a more thorough discussion of practical aspects of HPC mobilization and collection.

Adoptive Immunotherapy

The ability to mobilize and collect large numbers of mononuclear cells, along with the ability to expand these cells ex vivo and in vivo, has led to the development of therapeutic cell products for adoptive immunotherapy of some neoplastic and infectious diseases. Apheresis components collected from nonmobilized donors consist predominantly of mature blood cells, whereas those obtained from growth factor-mobilized donors contain large numbers of HPCs, mature mononuclear cells, and a variety of other cell types. Cell collections that are intended for adoptive immunotherapy may be minimally manipulated after apheresis collection, or they may be enriched for specific cell populations and/or modified ex vivo by addition of small molecules or by insertion of transgenes.

Donor Leukocytes-Lymphocytes for Infusion

Early studies of adoptive immunotherapy involved infusion of unmanipulated donor leukocytes (donor leukocyte-lymphocytes for infusion [DLI] or therapeutic cells [TC]) to chronic myeloid leukemia patients with relapse after bone marrow transplantation to induce a graft-vs-leukemia effect resulting in cytogenetic remission.[103] A retrospective analysis of DLI for relapsed hematologic malignancies after allogeneic bone marrow transplantation documents a 60% complete response rate in chronic myeloid leukemia patients overall, with an even higher response rate in patients with relapsed chronic-phase disease.[104] DLI has also effected complete or partial remission in patients with relapsed multiple myeloma after allogeneic bone marrow transplantation.[105] Newer strategies include administration of DLI after nonmyeloablative conditioning and allogeneic HPC transplant for treatment of several malignant and nonmalignant diseases.

Because small numbers of cells generally suffice, donor cells collected by leukapheresis are often aliquoted and cryopreserved for repeated treatment over a period of months. Response to DLI is often associated with the development of acute and chronic GVHD, although the severity is usually mild to moderate and controlled by immunosuppressive therapy. Another serious complication of DLI is transient or persistent marrow aplasia, which may be attributed to the destruction of residual host hematopoiesis by the infused mononuclear cells before recovery of normal donor hematopoiesis.[106]

Cytotoxic T Lymphocytes and Other Therapeutic Cell Products

Leukapheresis is also used to obtain mononuclear cells that can be manipulated ex vivo using cell selection and cell culture techniques to generate activated or cytotoxic lymphocytes to treat hematologic malignancies and solid tumors. The ability to identify and isolate human tumor antigens by advanced molecular genetic techniques has resulted in the formulation of other extensively manipulated cell products for adoptive immunotherapy of cancer. Some strategies use peptides derived from tumor antigens to sensitize antigen-presenting cells, such as dendritic cells in vitro, which can then be either directly infused as cancer vaccines, or can be used to sensitize tumor infiltrating lymphocytes or unselected peripheral blood lymphocytes ex vivo for reinfusion as specific antitumor effector cells. Techniques to translate these experimental strategies into clinically practicable therapies are under development.

In addition to treatment of neoplastic diseases, highly manipulated donor lymphocyte products are being developed as prophylaxis and therapy for serious infectious diseases, including infectious complications of bone marrow transplantation such as Epstein–Barr virus-associated lymphoproliferative disorders, adenovirus, and cytomegalovirus infection.[107] Early experience shows that adoptive immunotherapies for infection are promising, but the technology is extremely complex and prohibitively expensive at this stage of development. Please see Chapter 111 for a more complete discussion of experimental cell therapies.

Cellular Gene Therapy

Cellular gene therapy is a technique in which a functioning gene is inserted ex vivo into somatic cells to correct an inborn genetic error or to provide some new function to the cell. The gene-modified cells may be purified, concentrated, expanded, or infused without further manipulation. Successful therapy requires gene identification and isolation, efficient insertion and expression in the target cells, and sufficient circulation or engraftment of the corrected cells after infusion into the patient.

The ability to collect large numbers of lymphocytes and HPCs and to expand and manipulate their growth and differentiation in vitro makes these cells logical candidates for cellular gene therapy. Peripheral blood lymphocytes are easily collected with automated cell separation devices, can be expanded in culture systems, and can withstand cryopreservation and thawing with good recovery of viability and function. They can circulate in vivo for months and possibly years after infusion, and may persist even longer at tissue sites. Permanent correction of genetic and acquired defects might be effected by inserting the missing or defective gene into HPCs. HPCs are easily accessible in bone marrow, mobilized peripheral blood by apheresis, and umbilical cord blood. They can be concentrated to high purity using immunologic cell selection techniques, and can be cryopreserved in DMSO and subsequently thawed with good recovery of viability and engraftment potential. Pluripotent cells comprise only 1% to 2% of the total progenitor cell pool, but because of the ability of the pluripotent cells to maintain hematopoiesis for years, correction of even a small number of cells could, in theory, provide a patient with a several-log increase in gene-modified cells within each hematopoietic lineage. Unfortunately, gene transduction of long-lived progenitors has proved extremely inefficient, and risks associated with integration of the vector into the target cell DNA, including reports of ALL-like complications due to retroviral transduction of $CD34^+$ cells, must be addressed before the promise of cellular gene therapy is fulfilled. Please see Chapter 110 for a more complete discussion of gene transfer for hematologic disorders.

SUGGESTED READINGS

Hemapheresis and Cellular Therapy

Bolan CD et al: Prospective evaluation of cell kinetics, yields and donor experiences during a single large-volume apheresis versus two smaller volume consecutive day collections of allogeneic peripheral blood stem cells. B J Haematol 120:801, 2003.

Bolan CD et al: Controlled study of citrate effects and response to i.v. calcium administration during allogeneic peripheral blood progenitor cell donation. Transfusion 42(7):935, 2002.

Burgstaler E: Current instrumentation for apheresis. In McCleod B, Price T, Drew M (eds.): Apheresis: Principles and Practice. Bethesda, MD, AABB Press, 1997, p 85.

George JN, Vesely SK, Terrell DR: The Oklahoma Thrombotic Thrombocytopenic Purpura-Hemolytic Uremic Syndrome (TTP-HUS) Registry: A community perspective of patients with clinically diagnosed TTP-HUS. Semin Hematol 41(1):60, 2004.

Gordon BR, Saal SD: Low-density lipoprotein apheresis using the Liposorber dextran sulfate cellulose system for patients with hypercholesterolemia refractory to medical therapy. J Clin Apheresis 11(3):128, 1996.

Hester JP, McCredie KB, Freireich EJ: Response to chronic leukapheresis procedures and survival of chronic myelogenous leukemia patients. Transfusion 22(4):305, 1982.

Jones HG, Bandarenko N: Management of the therapeutic apheresis patient. In McCleod B, Price T, Weinstein R (eds.): Apheresis: Principles and Practice. Bethesda, MD, AABB Press, 2003, p 253.

Kato GJ, Gladwin MT, Steinberg MH: Deconstructing sickle cell disease: Reappraisal of the role of hemolysis in the development of clinical subphenotypes. Blood Rev 21:37–47, 2007.

Kim HC: Therapeutic pediatric apheresis. J Clin Apheresis 15(1–2):129, 2000.

Lockwood CM et al: Reversal of impaired splenic function in patients with nephritis or vasculitis (or both) by plasma exchange. N Engl J Med 300(10):524, 1979.

McCullough J, Chopek M: Therapeutic plasma exchange. Lab Med 12:745, 1981.

McLeod BC et al: Frequency of immediate adverse effects associated with therapeutic apheresis. Transfusion 39(3):282, 1999.

Montgomery RA et al: Plasmapheresis and intravenous immune globulin provides effective rescue therapy for refractory humoral rejection and allows kidneys to be successfully transplanted into cross-match-positive recipients. Transplantation 70(6):887, 2000.

Pulsipher MA et al: Weighing the risks of G-CSF administration, leukopheresis, and standard marrow harvest: Ethical and safety considerations for normal pediatric hematopoietic cell donors. Pediatr Blood Cancer 46(4):422, 2006.

Randomised trial of plasma exchange, intravenous immunoglobulin, and combined treatments in Guillain-Barre syndrome. Plasma Exchange/Sandoglobulin Guillain-Barre Syndrome Trial Group. Lancet 349(9047):225, 1997.

Szczepiorkowski ZM et al: Guidelines on the use of therapeutic apheresis in clinical practice—Evidence-based approach from the Apheresis Applications Committee of the American Society for Apheresis. J Clin Apheresis 22(000), 2007.

Tsai HM: Current concepts in thrombotic thrombocytopenic purpura. Annu Rev Med 57:419, 2006.

REFERENCES

For complete list of references log onto www.expertconsult.com

CHAPTER 153

TRANSFUSION REACTIONS

Yan Yun Wu, Simon Mantha, and Edward L. Snyder

A *transfusion reaction* can be defined as any untoward reaction that occurs as a consequence of infusion of blood or one of its components. Reactions are considered to be acute when they occur during transfusion or within several hours after the transfusion has been terminated (Table 153–1). Reactions also can be classified as delayed. Delayed hemolytic transfusion reactions, for example, usually occur days after the transfusion. Other types of delayed reactions occur long after the blood has been infused—months or even years—as in the case of some transfusion-transmitted diseases. From 1995 to 2004, there were 665 transfusion related fatalities reported to the FDA.[1] This chapter reviews various types of transfusion reactions.

HEMOLYTIC TRANSFUSION REACTIONS

Hemolytic transfusion reactions are caused by the immune-mediated lysis of transfused red cells. Immune-mediated hemolysis can be divided conveniently into four categories by time of reaction (acute or delayed) and by site of hemolysis (intravascular or extravascular). The four types are acute intravascular, acute extravascular, delayed intravascular, and delayed extravascular reactions (Table 153–2).

ACUTE INTRAVASCULAR HEMOLYTIC TRANSFUSION REACTIONS

Acute reactions occur when incompatible red cells are transfused into a patient who already possesses the corresponding antibody, and a reaction occurs within minutes. Because of naturally occurring ABO antibodies, infusion of ABO-incompatible blood is the most likely cause of a clinically significant acute intravascular hemolytic transfusion reaction.[2] Such a reaction could occur, for example, after transfusion of A red cells into an O recipient who has significant amounts of circulating anti-A. Although the titer and avidity of the antibody affect the extent of the hemolytic reaction, the clinical severity of an ABO-incompatible blood transfusion is greatly influenced by the degree of complement activation and cytokine stimulation. In an ABO-incompatible transfusion reaction, fixation of the C5b-9 complex occurs with release of C3a and C5a (anaphylatoxins 1 and 2, respectively). These low-molecular-weight peptides produce bronchospasm, mast cell degranulation, hypotension (C3a), and pulmonary dysfunction (C5a); the latter is secondary to migration of granulocytes to the pulmonary capillary bed, resulting in V/Q abnormalities.[3] Fixation of the C5b-9 complement membrane attack complex produces pores in the red cell membrane, and the resultant osmotic lysis produces hemoglobinuria and hemoglobinemia.[3,4] The sine qua non of an acute intravascular hemolytic transfusion reaction is the presence of red plasma and red (dark) urine.

It is critical to distinguish, as quickly as possible, hemoglobinuria and hemoglobinemia resulting from an acute hemolytic transfusion reaction from similar signs caused by other causes. Hemoglobinuria can be confused with hematuria from bladder hemorrhage or myoglobinuria. Hemoglobinemia caused by non-immune-mediated lysis can result from mechanical hemolysis from an improperly collected blood sample. The direct antiglobulin test (DAT) usually becomes positive in an immune hemolytic reaction (if tested before all the incompatible red blood cells [RBCs] are destroyed); preparation of an antibody eluate is often necessary to identify the offending antibody. An antibody elution is the removal of antibody from the red cell by various physical or chemical techniques with concentration of the antibody in the eluting solution, which is usually albumin or saline. This antibody-containing solution, the eluate, is then treated as a serum sample and used to identify the offending blood group antibody.

The time lost in making a clinical diagnosis can turn a mild treatable reaction into one that is life-threatening. A full-blown acute intravascular hemolytic transfusion reaction is a true medical emergency. Antibody-coated red cell stroma produced during an immune hemolytic transfusion reaction induces renal vasoconstriction, resulting in acute tubular necrosis.[3,5] Another contributing cause of ischemic renal failure involves the release of free plasma hemoglobin. It has been shown that cell-free hemoglobin binds tightly to nitric oxide. Endothelium-derived relaxing factor, a powerful vasodilator, is composed in part of nitric oxide. By binding to nitric oxide, free plasma hemoglobin blocks relaxing factor and prevents renal vasodilation. This also promotes renal vasoconstriction and renal tubular ischemia, with eventual tubular necrosis.[6] The C3a and C4a generated may cause hypotension and tachycardia and may produce shock. Clinical symptoms include shortness of breath, chest pain, dizziness, and nausea. C3a can also cause bronchospasm, and C5a generation causes further pulmonary dysfunction. Many patients, curiously even anephric patients, often complain of lower back pain.[7] This is believed to be caused by ischemic muscle pain or vasospasm, rather than kidney pain from developing renal failure. In addition to complement components, cytokines and interleukins (ILs) also play a role in the clinical symptom complex associated with acute intravascular hemolytic transfusion reactions. For example, IL-1β, IL-6, and tumor necrosis factor-α (TNF-α) have pyrogenic activity; IL-8 is a neutrophil chemotactic and activating factor. These four cytokines have been generated in in vitro models of intravascular hemolysis and IgG-mediated red cell incompatibility.[8–11] The clinical variability of hemolytic transfusion reactions is likely explained by the relative balance of cytokine production in the transfusion recipient. Factors that increase the circulating levels of proinflammatory cytokines and chemokines result in more severe reactions.[12]

Therapy

Initial therapy consists of immediately stopping the transfusion, maintaining a patent intravenous line, supporting the cardiorespiratory system, and ensuring a brisk diuresis. Increasing renal blood flow is the best way to prevent acute oliguric renal failure. The usual therapeutic maneuver used to induce a diuresis is infusion of 0.9% NaCl or some other suitable crystalloid solution. Crystalloid should be given to maintain a urine output of 100 mL/hour for approximately 24 hours. Diuretics such as furosemide also can be used and are preferred by some to infusion of mannitol to increase intravascular volume.[13,14] Mannitol, if chosen, must be used with caution; if acute tubular necrosis (ATN) occurs before mannitol infusion, pulmonary edema may occur as a result of the acute increase in intravascular volume secondary to fluid expansion. Similarly, excessive crystalloid infusion should be avoided in patients with borderline congestive heart failure. Renal damage must be minimized, however, and increasing renal blood flow helps to prevent anuric renal failure. The mechanisms responsible for the beneficial effect of increased renal blood flow likely include increased clearance of free hemoglobin, resulting in decreased binding of nitric oxide, and a return of more physiologic control of renal vasodilation. Creatinine and blood urea nitrogen (BUN) should be closely monitored; dialysis may be necessary for therapy of acute renal failure. As difficult as ATN therapy is, it is easier to treat a patient in the diuretic phase than in the oliguric phase of ATN. Support of blood pressure and respiration may require the use of vasopressors, bronchodilators, and, when necessary, intubation. High levels of dopamine cause vasoconstriction and should be avoided unless the patient's blood pressure requires high dosage. Disseminated intravascular coagulation (DIC) can occur in severe cases. The prothrombin time, partial thromboplastin time, and fibrinogen level should be closely monitored.

Laboratory Evaluation

Laboratory findings include hemoglobinuria, hemoglobinemia, and a haptoglobin level that is low to 0 mg/dL. During the hemolytic episode, the bilirubin (especially indirect bilirubin) usually increases only to 2 to 3 mg/dL if the patient has normal liver function. Elevations of bilirubin to 20 to 30 mg/dL are not seen in otherwise normal patients, even with florid hemolysis. Very elevated bilirubin levels are seen only in patients with concurrent hepatocellular disease, such as viral hepatitis or hepatic carcinoma. Because of the lysis of red cells, levels of lactate dehydrogenase (LDH) may rise markedly. If the patient shows no signs of vasomotor instability and if hemostatic and renal function is unchanged 24 to 36 hours after the incompatible transfusion, the episode can be considered to be over, with serious sequelae unlikely.

Although ABO-incompatible blood transfusions are the most common cause of an acute intravascular hemolytic transfusion reaction, other complement-fixing antigen–antibody systems, such as the Jk^a (Kidd) or Fy^a (Duffy) blood group systems, can also produce these reactions.[15]

ACUTE EXTRAVASCULAR HEMOLYTIC TRANSFUSION REACTION

In an extravascular hemolytic transfusion reaction, complement is not fixed at all or is fixed only to C3b. In either situation, because of the nature of the antigen–antibody reaction, complement activation with fixation of the C5b-9 complex does not occur. The presence of IgG on the red cell or fixation of complement to C3b results in an extravascular reaction because the antibody-coated cells are cleared by the IgG receptors in the spleen or the C3b receptors in the liver. Red cell lysis does not occur in the intravascular space. Largely as a result of the lack of generation of C3a or C5a, an extravascular hemolytic transfusion reaction does not usually present as a clinical emergency. It is characterized, as are most immune hemolytic transfusion reactions, by development of a positive DAT due to recipient

Workup of an Acute Intravascular Hemolytic Transfusion Reaction

If an acute transfusion reaction occurs:

1. *Stop blood component infusion immediately.*
2. Maintain intravenous access with a suitable crystalloid or colloid solution.
3. Maintain blood pressure, heart rate.
4. Maintain an adequate airway.
5. Give a diuretic or institute fluid diuresis, or both.
6. Obtain blood and urine for transfusion reaction workup.
7. Blood bank workup of suspected transfusion reaction:
   - Check paperwork to ensure correct blood component was transfused to the correct patient.
   - Observe plasma for hemoglobinemia.
   - Perform direct antiglobulin test.
   - Repeat compatibility testing (crossmatch).
   - Repeat other serologic testing as needed (ABO, Rh).
   - Analyze urine for hemoglobinuria.

If intravascular hemolytic reaction is confirmed:

8. Monitor renal status (BUN, creatinine).
9. Monitor coagulation status (prothrombin time, partial thromboplastin time, fibrinogen).
10. Monitor for signs of hemolysis (lactate dehydrogenase, bilirubin, haptoglobin).
11. If sepsis is suspected, culture as appropriate.

Table 153–1 Types of Acute Transfusion Reactions

Reaction Type	Presenting Signs and Symptoms
Acute intravascular hemolytic	Fever, chills, dyspnea, hypotension, tachycardia, flushing, vomiting, back pain, hemoglobinuria, hemoglobinemia, shock
Acute extravascular hemolytic	Fever, indirect hyperbilirubinemia, posttransfusion hematocrit increment lower than expected
Febrile reaction	Fever, chills
Allergic (mild)	Urticaria, pruritus, rash
Anaphylactic	Dyspnea, bronchospasm, hypotension, tachycardia, shock
Hypervolemic	Dyspnea, tachycardia, hypertension, headache, jugular venous distention
Septic	Fever, chills, hypotension, tachycardia, vomiting, shock
Transfusion-related acute lung injury	Dyspnea, decreased oxygen saturation, fever, hypotension

Table 153–2 Hemolytic Transfusion Reactions: Serologic Presentation

Type	Antibody Detectable Initially	Primary Antibody Type	Degree of Complement Binding	Example
Acute intravascular	Yes	IgM	Full (C1–9)	ABO system
Acute extravascular	Yes	IgG	None/partial	Rh system
Delayed intravascular	No	IgG	Full (C1–9)	Kidd system
Delayed extravascular	No	IgG	None/partial	Duffy system

Adapted from Blood Transfusion Therapy: An Audiovisual Program, 2nd ed. Arlington, VA, American Association of Blood Banks, 1991.

red cell alloantibody binding to the circulating donor red cells. Moreover, an increase in indirect bilirubin, an increase in LDH, a decline in hematocrit, a decline in haptoglobin, and an increase in colorless urine urobilinogen occurs; hemoglobinuria and hemoglobinemia, however, are rarely present. The patient typically remains clinically stable; and renal failure, shock, and hemostatic abnormalities, such as DIC, are rarely seen unless the amount of incompatible blood infused is excessive. However, patients often have a low-grade fever, probably from the generation of IL-1 or other proinflammatory cytokines.[12]

The diagnostic test of choice is a DAT with an eluate. The eluate is performed to identify the antibody coating the red cells.[15] The positive DAT result reflects the patient's antibody (or antibodies) coating of the donor red cells. This is not an autoantibody (or antibodies), and the patient's own RBCs are not usually involved in the reaction.

Typically, an acute extravascular hemolytic transfusion reaction requires no special therapeutic intervention. Maintaining a good urine output and monitoring renal and hemostatic function are usually sufficient. The patient characteristically recovers in a few days as the offending donor red cells are cleared from the circulation. The pathogenic alloantibody can often be identified in the patient's serum. These acute transfusion reactions may occur if the patient's preexisting alloantibody was missed by the blood bank during the antibody screening process, if the unit of blood was labeled for the wrong patient, or if the unit was hung in error on the wrong patient.[2]

DELAYED HEMOLYTIC REACTIONS

The pathogenesis of a delayed intravascular transfusion reaction is similar to that described for an acute intravascular hemolytic reaction. However, in the delayed type, the patient develops the antigen–antibody reaction some time (3–10 days) after the transfusion. The process occurs more slowly and is less likely to present as a clinical emergency. Hemoglobinuria and hemoglobinemia can occur but often are less profound and pronounced than with an acute intravascular reaction. This probably is caused by the continual and gradual removal of antibody-coated red cells as the antibody titer rises and by the more gradual generation of C3a and C5a. The same serologic diagnostic and treatment concepts used for an acute intravascular hemolytic reaction apply here. However, the need for acute intervention is much less likely. Initiating a diuresis and monitoring renal and hemostatic function may be sufficient.

Delayed extravascular hemolytic transfusion reactions occur as well. Such antigen–antibody reactions often involve the Rh system. The clinical presentation is similar to that of an acute extravascular reaction: the patient often has no acute clinical symptoms but may present with a fever, a falling hematocrit, and the development of a new DAT. Serologic evaluation of a transfusion reaction in a patient who had a positive pretransfusion antiglobulin test result, caused by autoantibody or medication, may be confusing. Such a workup requires an expert serologist to detect the new alloantibody in the patient's serum and make a diagnosis of a hemolytic transfusion reaction.

FEBRILE NONHEMOLYTIC TRANSFUSION REACTIONS

A febrile nonhemolytic transfusion reaction (FNHTR) is suspected when a temperature rise of 1°C or more occurs during or after transfusion when no other cause can be found. In addition to fever, an FNHTR is often accompanied by shaking chills. Febrile reactions are believed to be largely mediated by cytokines. The cause of cytokine release can be related to antibody–leukocyte or antibody–platelet interactions. These could be due to cytotoxic or agglutinating antibodies in the recipient's plasma reacting against antigens present on transfused donor lymphocytes, granulocytes, or platelets.[16–19] These antibodies often have human leukocyte antigen (HLA) specificity, although they also may be neutrophil- or platelet-specific.[20,21] Conversely, the donor plasma also can contain antibody that can react with the corresponding cellular antigens in the recipient's blood.[22] The febrile reaction is mediated largely by the release of cytokines such as IL-1β, IL-6, and TNF-α from macrophages, monocytes, granulocytes, or lymphocytes.[23] IL-1 (endogenous pyrogen), through prostaglandin PGE_2 synthesis, probably stimulates the thermoregulatory center of the hypothalamus to produce fever. Other mediators such as macrophage inflammatory proteins (MIP-1) may also participate in the febrile response, but this reaction is not mediated through prostaglandin synthesis.[24] CD154 (CD40 ligand) derived from platelets may also be involved in febrile reactions by inducing cyclooxygenase-2 and PGE_2.[25]

These cytokines could be derived from three possible sources in the transfusion setting. The first is synthesis by recipient leukocytes in response to transfusion. The second is production by donor leukocytes after infusion into the recipient. The third mechanism is generation by donor leukocytes in vitro during storage before transfusion.[26] Red cells and units of platelet concentrates have sufficient potential sources of cytokines in the large number (10^7–10^8) of mononuclear leukocytes capable of cytokine synthesis. Studies have shown that generation of cytokines does occur in units of blood during storage and that such generation is directly proportional to the leukocyte count of the unit and the duration of storage.[27–29] Use of third-generation leukocyte reduction filters can lower the incidence of febrile reactions. Judging from reports of persistent febrile reactions despite use of these 3 to 4 $\log_{10}$ leukocyte reduction filters, such filtration needs to occur before storage and before the donor leukocytes begin to generate these proinflammatory cytokines in the blood storage bag. Heddle and colleagues[30] showed that febrile reactions to platelet transfusions were more likely due to proinflammatory cytokines present in the supernatant platelet-poor plasma than to the cellular elements in the platelet concentrates. Proinflammatory cytokines are not removed by bedside blood filters and enter the circulation.[31] Chemokines, such as IL-8 and RANTES, and complement components C3a and C5a are removed to various degrees by some bedside leukoreduction filters.[32,33] Prevention of cytokine generation by prestorage leukoreduction, however, is more efficient and effective than is scavenging of the biologic response modifiers by using bedside filtration technology.

The frequency of febrile reactions for a nonleukoreduced unit has been estimated to be 0.5% per unit transfused.[34,35] Reactions are most commonly seen in recipients who have been exposed to multiple white cell or platelet antigens, such as oncology patients or multiparous women. Oncology patients are at risk as a result of frequent transfusions, multiparous women from multiple exposures during childbirth. Both of these groups of patients can form multiple HLA-, granulocyte-, or platelet-specific antibodies that will react with white cells or platelets on subsequent exposure. Antigen–antibody reactions are capable of stimulating cellular activation with resultant complement fixation, cytokine generation, and activation of other biologic response modifiers.[36,37]

CLINICAL MANIFESTATIONS

Clinically, an FNHTR is characterized by fever and chills occurring shortly after the transfusion has begun.[38] The patient may have nausea and vomiting. Various factors, including rate of infusion of the blood and leukocyte content of the transfused blood (antigen load), may affect the severity of the clinical presentation of the febrile reaction. Febrile reactions also can occur several hours after the transfusion has ended.[17] Although an FNHTR often starts with the patient's complaining of feeling uneasy or "chilly," symptoms may progress from a slight tremor to true rigors. The chills or rigors are a manifestation of heat-conserving cutaneous vasoconstriction and cytokine release and result in muscular heat production.[39] These thermogenic responses, coupled with any effects due to release of IL-1β or other cytokines, may cause the patient's temperature to rise several degrees above pretransfusion levels. Although these reactions are rarely dangerous, the severity often increases as the rate and dose of the infusion increase. Mild reactions are generally more uncomfortable and frightening than life threatening. FNHTRs are usually self-limited, with fever persisting for no more than 8 to 10 hours. Elderly patients with a tenuous cardiovascular status and critically ill patients may develop respiratory complications, hypotension, or shock. Young adults, however, are less likely to become seriously ill even with development of a high fever. As in any transfusion reaction, the onset of fever and chills requires that the transfusion be stopped, the intravenous line kept open with normal saline or a suitable crystalloid, and appropriate samples sent to the blood bank. The patient should be reassured, because anxiety may be extreme.

LABORATORY EVALUATION

The workup of a febrile reaction must be undertaken promptly. Fever may also be the first sign of an acute hemolytic reaction or infusion of a unit of red cells or platelets contaminated with bacteria. The workup consists of ruling out a hemolytic reaction by reconfirming the ABO type of the patient and the donor blood unit, repeat crossmatching to confirm patient-donor compatibility, evaluating the results of the pretransfusion and posttransfusion direct antiglobulin tests, evaluating the serum for hemolysis, and rechecking the accuracy of paperwork.[40–42] The posttransfusion DAT should yield negative findings, because an FNHTR does not involve red cell alloantibody.

As laboratory testing is being completed, the workup should extend beyond the blood bank to include bedside patient evaluation. Because fever and chills also may be caused by drugs or by diseases associated with infection or inflammation, these factors also should be evaluated. Blood cultures of the patient and the blood product, to rule out infusion of a contaminated unit of blood, is becoming more common at many medical centers. The difficulty lies in knowing when to order blood cultures: they are expensive and there is a 3% incidence of positive cultures as a result of contamination during culturing (see the Bacterial Contamination section). Most routine hospital blood banks do not have the expertise or reagents needed to identify specific HLA, platelet, or granulocyte antibodies. Accordingly, the diagnosis of a febrile hemolytic transfusion reaction is usually made without isolating an identifiable antibody. The FNHTR is often a diagnosis of exclusion arrived at after ruling out a hemolytic reaction, a septic transfusion, or other possible causes of fever.

TREATMENT AND PREVENTION

Fever from an FNHTR usually responds to antipyretics, including aspirin, nonsteroidal antiinflammatory drugs (NSAIDs), and acetaminophen. For thrombocytopenic adult patients, acetaminophen (325–650 mg, taken orally) is the antipyretic of choice. Thrombocytopenic patients must avoid aspirin: it further compromises platelet function because of its inhibitory effect on platelet cyclooxygenase, an enzyme involved in the platelet release reaction. Nonthrombocytopenic patients may receive aspirin if its use is not contraindicated for other medical reasons. Many house officers routinely order diphenhydramine for treatment of febrile reactions. This therapy, however, should be reserved for pretreatment or treatment of possible allergic reactions. Unless the patient has a history of allergic reactions or shows signs of an allergic component to an FNHTR, such as flushing, hives, or pruritus, there is no benefit from the use of antihistamines for febrile reactions. Antihistamines produce drowsiness in some patients.

For patients with no history of febrile reactions, routine premedication is unnecessary. Adult patients with severe reactions despite premedication may require more intensive pharmacotherapy, including hydrocortisone sodium succinate (100 mg administered intravenously) given 1 to 2 hours before transfusion. Patients with severe shaking chills can be treated with meperidine (25–50 mg) intramuscularly or subcutaneously, if there are no medical contraindications. Meperidine can stop shaking chills almost immediately.[43] Febrile reactions after granulocyte transfusions and, less frequently, after platelet transfusions can be so severe that hypotension and cardiovascular collapse can occur.

Prevention of febrile reactions when pharmacologic therapy fails relies on the use of leukocyte-depleted blood components. Several leukocyte depletion techniques are available. Centrifugation can remove approximately 70% of the leukocytes in a unit of blood; cell washing or use of frozen deglycerolized red cells can remove up to 95% of contaminating white cells. Older microaggregate blood filters can reduce leukocyte content by approximately 1 to 2 logs (90%–93%).[44–51] Third-generation leukocyte-depletion red cell filters are more useful for preventing febrile reactions.[52–54] They can remove up to 4 logs (99.99%) of white cells, often lowering the level of white cells in a unit of blood from 10^9 to 10^5. They also may be useful for preventing or delaying the onset of HLA alloimmunization.[55,56] Leukocyte depletion platelet filters are also available.[57–63] The results of a multiinstitutional trial to reduce alloimmunization to platelets (TRAP Trial) have shown that reduction of leukocytes by filtration and UV-B irradiation of platelet concentrates were equally effective compared with a control group for preventing alloantibody-mediated refractoriness to platelets during chemotherapy for acute myeloid leukemia.[64]

The degree of usage of leukocyte-depleted blood components is still controversial.[65–67] Data show that a patient who has had one febrile transfusion reaction has a 1 in 8 chance of having another one.[35] Individuals with a history of recurrent severe febrile reactions should have notations made in their blood bank record to ensure future use of leukocyte-reduced components.

Although they clearly are indicated for people with multiple and recurrent febrile reactions, many physicians question whether leukodepleted blood products should be used indiscriminately for all patients.[68,69] The immunomodulatory effects of allogeneic blood transfusions on tumor growth and recurrence and susceptibility to viral infection is poorly understood, and much research has yet to be performed.[70–72] The cost of filtration is often cited as a reason to limit use of leukoreduction technology. Cost considerations, however, are often discounted when a significant threat, imagined or real, to the world's blood supply is posed. Such a threat may be associated with the risk of transmission of variant Creutzfeldt–Jakob disease (vCJD).[73] There is concern that vCJD may be transmitted by eating tissue from cows with bovine spongiform encephalopathy. In a murine model, there are some data that the agent may be present in the blood and can be associated with B cells.[74] Two reports implicate the transmission of vCJD by blood transfusion; studies are continuing. There are discussions about whether all blood should be leukodepleted in an attempt to address this potential risk to the world's blood supply.[73,75] Studies such as these[64,73–75] may begin to influence physicians to use leukoreduction technology for more patients. Such increased use, although improving the safety of the blood supply, can significantly raise the cost of medical care. However, the cost increment may be offset by reducing the potential complications.[76] After universal leukoreduction, the rate of FNHTR decreased significantly compared with nonuniversal leukoreduced blood, although this finding has not been confirmed by all studies.[77,78]

ALLERGIC TRANSFUSION REACTIONS

Allergic transfusion reactions are believed to be most commonly due to infusion of plasma proteins.[79,80] The allergic manifestations produced vary. They include skin erythema with associated mild urticaria and pruritus; a confluent rash, which is intensely pruritic; extensive urticaria; severe vasomotor instability; bronchospasm; and anaphylaxis. A patient who develops hives and a mild allergic reaction during a blood transfusion usually does not progress to a more severe anaphylactic reaction after infusion of additional blood from the same unit. The severity of allergic transfusion reactions is not necessarily dose-related.

The exact nature of the antibodies involved in the various types of allergic reactions is unclear. The mild allergic reactions are usually IgE-mediated, but other immunoglobulins may also be involved; anaphylactic reactions are most often IgE mediated.[7,81] Allergic reactions are believed to be mediated by histamine. Histamine can be released through the Ag–Ab interactions involving antibodies present in recipients against donor antigens or via antibodies passively transferred from donor against recipient antigens. Histamine can also be passively transferred from donors to recipients by transfusion of stored blood components.[82,83] Allergic transfusion reactions are quite common, occurring in approximately 1% of all transfusions.[84,85] Most of these reactions start with pruritus, followed by the development of hives. At this point, the transfusion should be stopped and the patient given 25 to 50 mg of diphenhydramine, if there are no medical contraindications and if the patient had not already been maximally premedicated. After a short interval, the transfusion can be continued, but only if the rash decreases or the hives disappear and the patient feels well and shows no signs of fever, chills, or vasomotor instability. For mild allergic transfusion reactions not associated with any cardiorespiratory problems, such as fever, bronchospasm, dyspnea, hypotension, or tachycardia, it is acceptable to continue the transfusion after the reaction has subsided, because it is not likely to recur. The risk of transfusion-transmitted disease posed by infusion of another unit of blood is greater than the risk posed by continuing a transfusion that has produced only mild urticaria. This is not true, however, if the patient shows signs of systemic toxicity from the transfusion, such as fever hypotension, bronchospasm, or tachycardia.

The treatment of mild allergic reactions involves the use of diphenhydramine or other H1 blocker.[81] Reactions are rarely serious and often do not recur with subsequent transfusions. The pathogenesis is thought to be recipient antibody directed against donor plasma proteins. Most blood banks, however, cannot identify the offending antibody; identification usually requires research laboratory techniques. Accordingly, the diagnosis of an allergic transfusion reaction is a diagnosis of exclusion. Washed red cells can be used to prevent reactions.[46,86] Leukocyte depletion or microaggregate filters are of no value because the plasma protein passes through the filter.

Most patients who have more than one mild allergic reaction should continue to receive routine bank blood and may be premedicated with diphenhydramine or similar agents. Washed cells should not be provided until a second reaction has occurred and generally should be provided only for patients with severe or recurrent reactions. The occurrence of one or two hives or mild pruritus after transfusion is not an indication for the use of washed cells or pharmacotherapy. Anaphylactic reactions, however, can be life threatening and may require intubation and pressor agents. The use of washed cells for patients experiencing these reactions is appropriate. For patients with severe or recurrent reactions, combination of H1 and H2 blockers may be more effective for treatment and premedication, and the addition of steroids may be necessary if not otherwise contraindicated.[81,87]

Although it is convenient to characterize a transfusion reaction as being purely febrile or allergic, in reality there is often a mix of the two symptoms, and the reaction is designated according to the predominant clinical sign.

BACTERIAL CONTAMINATION

Bacterial contamination of stored blood can pose grave risks to the recipient. Bacteria can enter the blood bag during venipuncture as a result of inadequate skin preparation or during component preparation.[88] Some bacteria grow best at room temperature; other (psychrophilic) organisms grow optimally at refrigerated blood bank (1°C to 6°C) temperatures. Gram-negative bacteria, including *Pseudomonas*, *Yersinia*, *Enterobacter*, and *Flavobacterium*, are organisms commonly associated with a contaminated unit of refrigerated blood.[89,90] Platelet concentrates, stored at room temperature, are also known to be subject to bacterial contamination; several reports have described fatal septic transfusion reactions due to platelets containing *Salmonella* or *Staphylococcus*.[91–93] Units of blood that are contaminated need not be obviously discolored, malodorous, or clotted; by simple visual inspection, it is extremely difficult to determine whether a unit is contaminated. However, Kim and coworkers[94] reported that visual inspection, with comparison of the blood bag segmented tubing with that of the blood bag itself, can occasionally identify units likely to be bacterially contaminated.

Individuals who receive a unit of contaminated blood may develop fever, rigors, skin flushing, abdominal cramps, myalgias, DIC, renal failure, cardiovascular collapse, and cardiac arrest. Clinically the patient presents in warm shock. These reactions may be immediate, or there may be a delay of several hours before the symptom complex becomes apparent. Reaction to infusion of a unit of contaminated blood is distinguishable from FNHTR by the former's more severe clinical presentation and is distinguishable from intravascular hemolytic transfusion reaction by the absence of the latter's characteristic hemoglobinuria and hemoglobinemia. Reactions after transfusion of infected units of blood are often attributable to endotoxin produced by gram-negative bacteria. The presence of bacteria alone, however, can also cause many of these symptoms. The symptom complex often is attributable in part to cytokines and interleukins that are generated in the contaminated, in vitro stored blood. These biologic response modifiers produce severe reactions in vivo after transfusion.[27–29,95–97] For example, nitric oxide, produced locally in smooth muscle by the synergistic action of TNF-α, IL-1, and interferon-γ, probably mediates refractory hypotension and vasoplegia associated with septic shock.[96,98]

If, during transfusion, a patient who appeared well suddenly develops rigors and shock, infusion of an infected component should be considered. If on further evaluation this diagnosis is still considered likely, the patient should be treated immediately, because delay significantly contributes to the chance of a fatal outcome. Blood pressure, pulse, respiration, and renal blood flow need to be supported. Blood infusion should be stopped the moment any transfusion reaction is suspected, and appropriate samples should be sent to the blood bank for a DAT and other studies. Cultures of the untransfused blood remaining in the blood bag should be obtained because they may be diagnostic. Broad-spectrum antibiotics should be started immediately if infusion of contaminated blood is suspected and continued until the culture results are reported. These reactions are rare[99] but can be fatal. Use of recombinant IL or cytokine inhibitors is still experimental to be useful clinically.

Because of the decrease in viral transmission by blood transfusion, septic transfusion reactions now account for a significant portion of the transfusion-related mortality in the United States.[100] Data from the BaCon (Bacterial Contamination of Blood) study showed that from 1998 to 2000, the rate of transfusion-transmitted bacteremia was 9.98 per million single-donor platelets, 10.64 per million pooled platelets, and 0.21 per million RBC units; the rate of fatal reactions was 1.94 per million single-donor platelets, 2.22 per million pooled platelets, and 0.13 per million RBC units, respectively.[100] To reduce the risk of bacterial transmission through platelet transfusion, the American Association of Blood Banks has mandated that starting in March 2004 platelet concentrates should be tested for bacterial contamination.[101] There are two bacteria detection systems approved by the US Food and Drug Administration (FDA) to be used for screening of blood components.[102,103] Since the implementation of bacterial testing of platelets, although the risks of septic transfusion reaction have been reduced, they have not been eradicated.

TRANSFUSION-RELATED ACUTE LUNG INJURY (NONCARDIOGENIC PULMONARY EDEMA)

Transfusion-related acute lung injury (TRALI), the third leading cause of transfusion-related death, was thought to be rare in the past, but it is now believed to occur in as many 1 of 5000 to 1120 transfusions.[104–108] With increasing recognition and knowledge of this clinical syndrome, the current view of TRALI is much broader. It may range from mild dyspnea to severe noncardiogenic pulmonary edema, with symptoms including dyspnea, oxygen desaturation, respiratory failure, chills, fever, and hypotension. Most patients require oxygen support, and many may require mechanical ventilation. TRALI may develop within 1 to 6 hours of starting a transfusion, without an elevation in cardiac pressure.[22,104,105,109–113] The chest radiograph may reveal a pulmonary edema pattern (bilateral infiltrates), and there is respiratory insufficiency with a decrease in O_2 saturation, but without development of elevated left-side cardiac pressure. Copious amounts of pulmonary edema fluid are produced, as is characteristic of hypervolemia; however, the noncardiogenic reaction usually follows infusion of volumes of blood too small to produce fluid overload. The postulated pathologic mechanism includes a reaction between donor HLA (class I and II) or white blood cell antibody and recipient leukocytes. Complement and monocyte activation with aggregation of white blood cells also may occur when leukoagglutinins present in the recipient react with leukocytes contained in the infused donor blood,[22,106,107,114–117] As a result of the HLA Ag–Ab reaction, the activated leukocytes generate adhesive molecules on their surface (CD11/CD18). These proteins permit the leukocytes to attach to the cell membrane of the pulmonary endothelial cells and by diapedesis enter the interstitial space between the pulmonary capillaries and the alveolar epithelium. Once they are in the interstitial space, the neutrophils degranulate and release destructive enzymes, which produce a capillary leak, resulting in fluid filling the alveolar air sacs. Pulmonary leukostasis with pulmonary edema occurs as a result of microvascular occlusion and capillary leakage.[118,119] Complement-activated granulocytes also produce toxic oxygen radicals that damage pulmonary endothelial cells, resulting in an increase in pulmonary vascular permeability and further passage of fluid into alveolar spaces. Silliman and associates[120,121] postulated a two-step approach to the pathogenesis of TRALI. After an initial neutrophil activation step, neutrophil-priming lipids, which they believe play a key role in the process, further activate the granulocytes and produce the clinical syndrome.[113,120] Rodent model systems for TRALI have also been described.[122]

Because a definitive diagnosis of TRALI usually requires that cardiac monitoring (Swan–Ganz) catheters be in place, TRALI is difficult to diagnose outside the operating room or intensive care unit. When a patient shows signs of noncardiogenic pulmonary edema, as with all other reactions, the infusion should be stopped. These HLA/neutrophil antigen–antibody reactions may be idiosyncratic and often do not recur. Because of the difficulty in differentiating TRALI from other competing diagnoses such as circulatory overload and the patient's underline pulmonary status, efforts have been made to develop consensus guidelines to diagnose TRALI.[123,124]

To remove leukocyte antigens from units of red cells or platelets, leukocyte reduction filters may be useful; washed red cells are useful for that component as well. Treatment is symptomatic (Table 153–3). Donors who are implicated in moderate to several TRALI reactions should not be maintained as blood donors. In November 2006, the American Association of Blood Banks (AABB) made further recommendations to reduce the risks of TRALI.[125] Even though it is controversial whether multiparous women who are blood donors and blood donors who have been multiply transfused should be used as plasma donors, because their serum may contain high titers of leukoagglutinating antibodies, more and more collection facilities started to limit their use as a source for plasma components.

Table 153–3 Diagnosis of Transfusion-Related Acute Lung Injury

Onset	Within 6 hours of start of transfusion
Frequency	1 : 1000 to 1 : 4500 transfusions (probably underreported)
Signs and symptoms	Decreased O_2 saturation, fever, hypotension, tachypnea, dyspnea, diffuse pulmonary infiltrates, normal cardiac pressures (requires Swan–Ganz catheter), copious amounts of pulmonary edema fluid
Pathogenesis	HLA/granulocyte-specific antibodies (usually of donor origin) reacting with recipient leukocytes. Activates recipient neutrophils; stimulates complement activation; generates CD11/18 on the polymorphonuclear neutrophil surface, resulting in pulmonary capillary adherence and diapedesis and eventual pulmonary capillary leak syndrome. The latter is associated with generation of proteolytic enzymes and toxic O_2 metabolites, which cause endothelial cell damage.
	Neutrophil priming lipids may also play a role.
Diagnosis	Chest radiograph; blood gases; blood for HLA or antineutrophil antibodies
Differential diagnosis	Fluid overload; septic transfusion; anaphylaxis
Treatment	STOP TRANSFUSION; ventilatory support (administer O_2, intubate as needed), support blood pressure, administer steroids; diuretics of *no* value

Data from Levy GJ, Shabot MM, Hart ME, et al: Transfusion-associated noncardiogenic pulmonary edema. Report of a case and a warning regarding treatment. Transfusion 2:278, 1986.

OTHER ADVERSE EFFECTS OF TRANSFUSION

Circulatory Overload (Hypervolemia)

Hypervolemia is a form of transfusion reaction that should be considered in patients who, during a blood infusion, develop sudden severe headache, dyspnea, tachycardia, congestive heart failure, or other signs of fluid overload. Unless the patient is actively hemorrhaging, blood should never be infused rapidly, because the acute expansion of the patient's intravascular volume may exceed the capacity of the cardiovascular system to compensate. Rapidly transfusing a patient who is anemic but who is euvolemic and not actively bleeding produces no benefit and may cause harm. This caveat applies to transfusion of any blood component. Patients with compromised cardiopulmonary status may not tolerate acute blood volume expansion and may develop right- or left-sided heart failure. This is especially true for infants and the elderly. If symptoms occur, the transfusion should be stopped and some form of volume reduction, either diuretics or phlebotomy, instituted. If there is a concern that the patient may not tolerate infusion of a full unit of blood or component within the 4-hour period allotted for infusion of blood components, the blood bank can divide the product into smaller portions, which can be transfused in aliquots. As a general guide, infusions in nonbleeding adults should occur at less than 2 to 3 mL/kg/hour. The rate should be lowered to 1 mL/kg/hour for patients at risk for fluid overload. Diuretics may be given to patients with compromised cardiopulmonary status before transfusion.

The initial stages of transfusion-induced hypervolemia may be difficult to distinguish from hemolytic transfusion reaction as well as from febrile, allergic reactions or TRALI. The absence of hemoglobinuria and hemoglobinemia or the absence of a positive posttransfusion DAT result should serve to distinguish the reaction from one due to immune hemolysis, and the absence of fever, chills, or urticaria from the febrile or allergic types of reactions. The clinical use of laboratory testing such as brain natriuretic peptide (BNP) to aid in the differential diagnosis is currently under active investigation.[126] A normal BNP value suggests TRALI, whereas a high BNP suggests cardiac myocyte stretching from fluid overload.

Anaphylactic Reactions

When plasma containing IgA is transfused to patients with IgG or IgE anti-IgA antibodies, anaphylactic reactions can occur. Similarly, it may also occur in patients with deficiency of other plasma proteins such as haptoglobin.[127] Anaphylactic reactions have also been reported after transfusion of platelets administered through some types of bedside leukoreduction filters.[128] The pathogenesis of this syndrome appeared to be the activation of the contact pathway (prekallikrein converting to kallikrein) induced in plasma by the negatively charged surface of some leukoreduction filters. Kallikrein activation stimulates the conversion of high-molecular-weight kininogen to bradykinin. The bradykinin generated by the negatively charged bedside filter enters the circulation and produces a symptom complex characterized by pain, cutaneous flushing, and hypotension without fever or chills. The syndrome is often much more severe in patients already taking angiotensin-converting enzyme (ACE) inhibitors. ACE is identical to kininase II, which is responsible for degrading bradykinin. Blockage of the kininase II degradation of bradykinin by ACE inhibitors results in a prolonged bradykinin half-life and a reaction that can be very severe. Accordingly, physicians should let the blood bank know of any patients taking ACE inhibitors who require blood transfusion. Prestorage leukoreduction avoids this problem, because the half-life of bradykinin is approximately 15 seconds. Reactions have been reported with platelet as well as red cell transfusions, but most commonly with platelet transfusions administered through a bedside leukoreduction filter, with a negative surface charge. Although these reactions are rare, they can be quite serious.

Transfusion-Associated Graft-Versus-Host Disease

Transfusion-associated graft-versus-host disease (GVHD) occurs when immunologically competent lymphocytes are introduced into an immunoincompetent host who cannot destroy the donor lymphocytes. The immunocompetent donor lymphocytes engraft, recognize the host as foreign, and then attack host tissues. GVHD occurs after allogeneic bone marrow transplantation and less often after transfusion of nonirradiated cellular blood components, especially when the blood donor and recipient share some HLA antigens.[129] There is an increased danger from posttransfusion GVHD, in part because of the frequent failure of physicians to recognize the risk. Another major factor, however, is the propensity of the donor's lymphocytes to produce recipient bone marrow aplasia. In GVHD after bone marrow transplantation, the bone marrow is of donor origin, and bone marrow aplasia does not occur. In posttransfusion GVHD, however, the donor's lymphocytes attack the bone marrow of recipient/host origin, producing aplasia.

Posttransfusion GVHD is fatal in more than 90% of cases, primarily because of aplasia of the recipient's bone marrow.[130–132] It may occur 8 to 10 days after transfusion with a marked pancytopenia as well as multiorgan involvement of GVHD such as skin and liver. The signs and symptoms include nausea, vomiting, anorexia, fever, watery diarrhea, liver function abnormality, and rash. Patients often die of infection and bleeding within 3 to 4 weeks. There is no effective treatment, with the possible exception of stem cell transplantation, if posttransfusion GVHD is recognized early and if a suitable donor can be found in a short time.[133] Reports have shown that haploidentical directed donor units of blood may produce fatal posttransfusion GVHD even in immunocompetent recipients.[134,135] The use of irradiated blood (2500 cGy) is recommended in clinical situations in which posttransfusion GVHD is considered likely, such as when patients receive directed blood transfusions from their relatives. Leukocyte-reduction filters should not be used as prophylaxis against GVHD, because the exact number of leukocytes needed to produce the disease is not known with certainty. Case reports of fatal GVHD in patients who received leukoreduced but not irradiated blood have been published.[136] Several articles have addressed this subject.[137–140] Irradiation of red cells produces a membrane defect, however, which causes slow leakage of potassium and hemoglobin.[141] Accordingly, the FDA ruled that irradiated units of red cells shall have an outdate not to exceed 28 days from the time of irradiation. GVHD continues to be a rare but extremely serious complication of blood transfusion.[131,142,143] Although it is controversial, prophylactic irradiation is usually not indicated for patients with human immunodeficiency virus (HIV) infection.

Posttransfusion Purpura

Posttransfusion purpura (PTP) is a rare and self-limiting thrombocytopenia occurring 5 to 10 days posttransfusion in patients lacking a specific platelet antigen, usually PLA1 (HPA-1a).[144] They often have a history of sensitization with prior transfusions or pregnancies. After resensitization by the transfusion or additional pregnancy, patients developed potent antibodies against the platelet-specific antigen that they are lacking but are present on donor platelets. These platelet antibodies often have a high titer and can fix complement. As a result, the transfused platelets and the patient's own platelets are also destroyed through the adsorption of the antigen on their own platelets. A concurrent autoimmune process may also involve destruction of the recipient's own platelets, as shown in one case report of a positive antiantibody against the patient's own platelets.[145] The thrombocytopenia can be marked with a platelet count below 10,000/μL. The onset is sudden, although self-limited, and usually resolves in 2 weeks. Intravenous immunoglobulin (IVIG) appears to be an effective treatment, although plasma exchange, steroids, and splenectomy can also be useful. Patients with acute bleeding and needing platelet support should receive platelets without the platelet-specific antigen. If random donor platelets are given, patients can develop severe reactions, including allergic reactions. Recurrence of PTP is rare.

Microaggregate Debris and Adult Respiratory Distress Syndrome

Much has been published regarding the use of microaggregate filters for preventing adult respiratory distress syndrome after massive transfusion.[65,146–151] Microaggregate debris consists of dead platelets, granulocytes, and fibrin strands that form in blood during storage.[152–154] It was hypothesized that infusion of blood containing microaggregate debris through standard 170-μm-pore filters resulted in the passage of these 20- to 120-μm microaggregates into the pulmonary vasculature, producing occlusion of the pulmonary capillaries and pulmonary failure. Published studies have shown, however, that microaggregate filters are not required and transfused microaggregates do not appear to influence the onset of adult respiratory distress syndrome.[155,156] This syndrome is most likely, and most often, attributable to concurrent hypotension and sepsis rather than to infusion of microaggregate debris, per se. Improvements in surgical techniques, posttrauma medical care, perfusion technology, and especially treatment of shock and sepsis have contributed more to the decreased incidence of postperfusion respiratory distress syndrome than has use of microaggregate filters.[157]

LEUKOCYTE REDUCTION

There are multiple reasons to leukoreduce units of blood and components. Standards of the American Association of Blood Banks require that to be considered leukoreduced for any indication, the level of leukocytes in the final component must be less than 5×10^6.[158] This value applies to units of RBCs and single-donor apheresis platelets. For platelets prepared from whole blood, the value is less than 8.3×10^5 in all bags. Because the final pooled component also must have less than 5×10^6 leukocytes, this implies that the final pool size should not exceed 6 units. Generally accepted indications for leukocyte reduction include decreasing the incidence of HLA alloimmunization,[55,56,64] decreasing incidence of febrile transfusion reaction, and decreasing cytomegalovirus (CMV) transmission. Other areas include decreasing the incidence of tumor recurrence and improving certain clinical outcomes.[159-161] Leukoreduction is an effective approach to reduce CMV transmission through blood transfusion, and many hospitals now use leukoreduced blood components (CMV safe) to replace CMV serologic negative blood components to prevent CMV transmission, even for allotransplantation patients.[162] As more data are published, the indications for use of leukocyte reduction filters will become clearer. Although a conservative approach to their use for well-established indications would seem most prudent, changes for the indications are always being reviewed.[69,77,163]

HYPOTHERMIA

Hypothermia can occur with rapid infusion of large quantities of refrigerated (1–6°C) blood.[164-166] Data have shown that rapid infusion of blood (1 unit every 5 minutes) may lower the temperature of the sinoatrial node to less than 30°C, at which point ventricular fibrillation may occur.[167] Most transfusions need not be given this rapidly. For routine transfusion, blood does not have to be warmed. Overwarming the blood can cause thermal injury and produce hemolysis, DIC, or shock. Use of warming techniques for some trauma patients may reduce the incidence of coagulopathies associated with major trauma.[168]

If blood is to be warmed, the temperature must be monitored and kept below a level that could cause hemolysis.[158,169] Usually, this is less than 42°C. Heating blood under running hot tap water or heating in a microwave device is unacceptable; microwave devices produce hot spots that can cause hemolysis.[170,171]

ELECTROLYTE TOXICITY

Citrate, a component of the preservative solution used in blood storage, functions as an anticoagulant by chelating calcium and interfering with the coagulation cascade. Rapid transfusion of citrated blood can be associated with a drop in ionized calcium levels.[172-174] Citrate-containing blood products, however, are routinely infused without any problem, because the citrate is rapidly metabolized to bicarbonate. In patients with normal liver function, citrate infusion is very unlikely to produce reactions. Mild to severe citrate toxicity can be seen, however, in individuals undergoing cytapheresis when large volumes of citrated plasma are reinfused.[175,176]

The effects of hypocalcemia range from mild circumoral paresthesias to frank tetany. However, severe citrate toxicity, even with massive transfusion, is very rare. More commonly, the reaction is mild and self-limiting and can be treated by merely slowing the rate of reinfusion.[177] If prolonged QT intervals or signs of tetany are seen, calcium can be administered. Infusion of calcium, however, may be associated with the development of ventricular arrhythmias and cardiac arrest.[178] Calcium should not be infused routinely, even after large-volume blood transfusions. Under no circumstances should calcium be added to a unit of blood, because it would recalcify the unit and cause clots to form in the bag.

Hypomagnesemia, presumably due to chelation of magnesium by citrate, has also been reported. Actual clinical complications of transfusion-induced hypomagnesemia, however, have not been well documented, other than in the cases of cytapheresis.[176,179,180]

Hyperkalemia due to infusion of stored blood is a rare occurrence. Although hyperkalemia is often thought to be a problem in massive transfusion, in reality development of hypokalemia is of greater concern. With storage, leakage of potassium from red cells to the extracellular fluid occurs. However, after infusion, the red cells reverse the biochemical storage lesion by restoring the Na–K ATP membrane pump, and intracellular potassium levels are restored. As the citrate is metabolized to bicarbonate, the blood becomes alkalotic, contributing to hypokalemia.[181-183] In massive transfusion, this may not uncommonly result in the need for administration of potassium. Extracellular potassium increases at the rate of approximately 1 mEq/day during the first few weeks of storage. If this presents a concern for neonates or patients with renal failure, fresher or washed blood can be requested. As there is increased potassium leakage from red cells after exposure to 25 Gy of radiation to prevent posttransfusion GVHD, a maximum 28-day shelf life from the day of irradiation is imposed on this blood component.[158] Ammonia toxicity, previously a concern with stored blood, rarely presents problems.[184]

Risk Groups for Transfusion-Associated Graft-Versus-Host Disease

Risk Well Defined
Congenital T-cell defects (known or suspected)
Immunologic immaturity (fetus or premature infant)
Intrauterine transfusion
Exchange transfusion
Acquired T-cell defects
Bone marrow or peripheral blood stem cell transplant recipients (allogeneic or autologous)
Hodgkin's disease
Haplotype sharing between donor and recipient
Transfusions from blood relatives
HLA-matched platelets

Risks Identified But Not Clearly Defined
Hematologic malignancies (other than Hodgkin's disease)
Solid tumors
Immunologic immaturity or prematurity (in the context of small-volume transfusion)
Certain immunosuppressive agents such as Fludarabine

Risks Not Identified
Acquired immunodeficiency syndrome (AIDS)
Aplastic anemia (except in setting of bone marrow transplantation or immunosuppressive therapy)

PLASTICIZERS

Plasticizers are chemicals used to make the rigid polyvinyl chloride plastic used in blood bags more malleable. The traditional plasticizer is di-2-ethylhexylphthalate (DEHP).[185] There has been some question as to whether DEHP is carcinogenic and whether its breakdown product, monoethylhexylphthalate, may cause problems because of production of peroxisomes, which may be destructive to vital organs.[186-189] Citrate-based[190,191] plasticizer and new-generation blood bags are commercially available. Ironically, DEHP plasticizers may actually serve a useful function in that they appear to stabilize the red cell membrane and also may have a beneficial effect on platelet morphology.[192-194]

HEMOSIDEROSIS

One milliliter of red blood cells contains 1 mg of iron. A unit of blood with 250 mL of red blood cells contains approximately 250 mg of iron, and 4 units of blood contain 1 g of iron, roughly the amount stored in the bone marrow. Men and nonmenstruating women lose only approximately 1 mg iron each day. Continued use of transfusion therapy in individuals with an extravascular type of hemolytic anemia, such as those with thalassemia or sickle cell anemia, in which iron is not lost from the body but is recycled, can thus result in the accumulation of excessive tissue stores of iron. Over long periods, the iron that is stored in parenchymal cells results in death of the cell and eventual organ failure.[195] Transfusion of reticulocyte-rich blood (neocytes) generally has not been found to be of value for decreasing the transfusion requirement in patients with chronic hemolytic anemias.[196]

Iron chelation therapy, such as that with deferoxamine, is now widely used and is often able to maintain patients with chronic hemolytic anemias in negative iron balance.[197,198] The recent approval of an new oral iron chelater Deferasirox provides an alternative mode of iron chelation therapy.[199]

AIR EMBOLI

With replacement of evacuated glass bottles by plastic blood bags, the risk of air embolism from phlebotomy or transfusion virtually disappeared from transfusion practice. Air, however, still may be pumped into patients by the roller pumps contained in various transfusion devices, especially apheresis and intraoperative salvage machines.[200] All such devices currently manufactured, however, contain air in-line sensors. However, any operators using this equipment must be well-trained and remain alert to the potential risk of air embolization at all times while the patient is being treated. Patients who receive air intravenously experience acute cardiopulmonary insufficiency. The air tends to lodge in the right ventricle, preventing blood from entering the pulmonary circulation. Acute cyanosis, pain, cough, shock, and arrhythmia may occur, and death may result unless immediate action is taken. The patient should be placed head down on the left side; this usually displaces the air bubble from the pulmonary valve. Use of central lines may also pose an additional risk of air embolism.

TRANSFUSION REACTIONS FROM THE INFUSION OF HEMATOPOIETIC STEM CELLS

For patients receiving hematopoietic stem cell infusions, transfusion reactions can occur similar to regular blood components. However, certain reactions are unique to the transfusion of hematopoietic stem cells. The most common are the acute reactions associated with infusion of DMSO, a cryopreservative used for freezing hematopoietic stem cells.[201,202] Signs or symptoms of DMSO toxicity range from an unpleasant taste or smell, nausea, vomiting, diarrhea, chills, and hypertension to flushing, hypotension, bronchospasm, pulmonary edema, cardiac arrhythmias, and neurologic symptoms. Antihistamines have been used to prevent and to treat DMSO-related toxicity. In addition, DMSO toxicity is dose related, and it sometimes can be prevented by washing the components before transfusion.

PATHOGEN INACTIVATION

With improvement of donor testing, especially NAT testing, the risk of transfusion-transmitted diseases has decreased dramatically, such as approximately 1 : 1,900,000 for the risk of HIV, 1 : 137,000 for HBV, and 1 : 1,000,000 for HCV.[203] However, the risk is never zero. Moreover, there are emerging pathogens, such as the West Nile virus,[204] that may pose risk to the blood supply. It is expensive and impossible to screen all potential pathogens to protect the blood supply. To improve blood safety, new technologies such as pathogen inactivation have been developed.[205–207] There are several platforms of pathogen inactivation technologies. The principle of most pathogen inactivation is that agents added to blood components modify DNA or RNA templates, making them inaccessible to DNA or RNA polymerase, thus inactivating pathogens, including viruses, bacteria, and parasites; and also inactivating white blood cells. Available pathogen inactivation compounds include alkylating compounds, binary ethyleneimine-like compounds, riboflavin, and methylene blue. There are available systems for pathogen inactivation of RBCs, plasma, and platelets. Preclinical studies and clinical trials including phase III have shown promising results in the efficacy and safety of pathogen inactivation agents.[208,209]

SUGGESTED READINGS

AABB, Association Bulletin #06-07: Transfusion-Related Acute Lung Injury, in AABB PulsePoint. 2006.

ASBMTJ: Guidelines for preventing opportunistic infections among hematopoietic stem cell transplant recipients. Biol Blood Marrow Transplant 6:659, 2000.

Biggerstaff BJ, Petersen LR: Estimated risk of West Nile virus transmission through blood transfusion during an epidemic in Queens, New York City. Transfusion 42:1019, 2002.

Blajchman MA: Immunomodulation and blood transfusion. Am J Ther 9:389, 2002.

Brecher ME: Technical Manual. Bethesda, MD, AABB Press, 2002.

Carey PM, Sacher RA: Transfusion-associated graft versus host disease. In Simon TL, Dzik WH, Snyder EL, et al (eds.): Rossi's Principles of Transfusion Medicine. Philadelphia, Lippincott Williams & Wilkins, 2002, p 852.

Dzik WH: Leukoreduced blood components: Laboratory and clinical aspects. In Simon TL, Dzik WH, Snyder EL, et al (eds.): Rossi's Principles of Transfusion Medicine. Philadelphia, Lippincott, Williams & Wilkins, p 270, 2002.

Fang CT, Chambers LA, Kennedy J, et al: Detection of bacterial contamination in apheresis platelet products: American Red Cross experience, 2004. Transfusion 45:1845, 2005.

Kopko PM, Paglieroni TG, Popovsky MA, et al: TRALI: Correlation of antigen-antibody and monocyte activation in donor-recipient pairs. Transfusion 43:177, 2003.

Leukocyte reduction and ultraviolet B irradiation of platelets to prevent alloimmunization and refractoriness to platelet transfusions. The Trial to Reduce Alloimmunization to Platelets Study Group [comment]. N Engl J Med 337:1861, 1997.

Menitove J: Standards for Blood Banks and Transfusion Services. Bethesda, MD, AABB Press, 2002.

Nichols WG, Price TH, Gooley T, et al: Transfusion-transmitted cytomegalovirus infection after receipt of leukoreduced blood products. Blood. (accessed online January 16, 2003)

Paglino JC, Pomper GJ, Fisch G, et al: Reduction of febrile but not allergic reactions to red cells and platelets following conversion to universal prestorage leukoreduction. Transfusion 4:16, 2004.

Popovsky MA: Guidelines for the Management of Transfusion-Related Acute Lung Injury Developed for the Scientific Section Coordinating Committee. Bethesda, MD, AABB Press, 2003.

Silliman CC, Boshkov LK, Mehdizadehkashi Z, et al: Transfusion-related acute lung injury: Epidemiology and a prospective analysis of etiologic factors. Blood 101:454, 2003.

Stack E, Pomper GJ: Febrile, allergic, and nonimmune transfusion reactions. In Simon TL, Dzik WH, Snyder EL, et al (eds.): Rossi's Principles of Transfusion Medicine. Philadelphia, Lippincott Williams & Wilkins, 2002, p 831.

Wu Y, Snyder EL: Safety of the blood supply: Role of pathogen reduction. Blood Rev 17:111, 2003.

Zhou L, Giacherio D, Cooling L, Davenport RD: Use of B-natriuretic peptide as a diagnostic marker in the differential diagnosis of transfusion-associated circulatory overload [see comment]. Transfusion 45:1056, 2005.

REFERENCES

For complete list of references log onto www.expertconsult.com

CHAPTER 154

TRANSFUSION-TRANSMITTED DISEASES

Jay E. Menitove, Eberhard W. Fiebig, and Michael P. Busch

INTRODUCTION

During the 1980s and 1990s, transfusion medicine specialists focused their attention on reducing the risks of transfusion-transmitted human immunodeficiency virus (HIV) and hepatitis C infections. Currently those risks approximate 1 per 2 million transfusions. By 2003, additional testing prevented transfusion transmission of the West Nile Virus, a viral etiology of an emerging epidemic. Further risk reduction followed introduction of bacterial testing of platelet concentrates in 2004 that reduced the risk of transfusion-associated sepsis from 1 per 5000 to approximately 1 per 100,000. By early 2007, another new test was introduced. This one seeks to lower *Trypanosoma cruzi* transmission rates in the United States from the 1 per 25,000 risk approximated prior to test implementation.

In light of the significant progress achieved to date, this chapter reviews the residual risk from the above-cited adverse infectious complications of transfusion and presents the current knowledge, pathogenesis, and risk-reduction strategies aimed at emerging pathogens threatening the blood supply.

HEPATITIS INFECTION

Hepatitis A

The hepatitis A virus (HAV), a nonenveloped RNA virus in the picornavirus family, is transmitted predominantly through the fecal–oral route. The incubation period averages 28 days (range 15–50 days) and signs or symptoms persist for less than 2 months. Approximately 10% to 15% of infected individuals develop prolonged or relapsing illness, but HAV is self-limited with no chronic carrier state. HAV is the most frequent cause of hepatitis among children under 11 years of age. Risk factors for acquiring infection include close personal contact with infected individuals and injecting drug use. Approximately 45% to 50% of those infected have no identifiable transmission source. The peak viremic period occurs 2 weeks before onset of jaundice or elevation of liver function tests. Transfusion transmission occurs infrequently and corresponds to donation by a recently infected, asymptomatic individual.[1–3] Viremia persists for a median period of 42 days (range up to 59 days) in patients with hepatitis A.[1–3] The virus resists heating at 60°C for 1 hour and is difficult to inactivate by pathogen reduction procedures developed for cellular components (eg, psoralens, and riboflavin) and fresh-frozen plasma (solvent/detergent and methylene blue). Transmission by clotting factor concentrates treated with the solvent/detergent pathogen process occurred in the 1990s and remains low-risk despite the lack of HAV infection among hemophiliac patients treated in the early 2000s.[4,16,170,268]

Hepatitis B

The hepatitis B virus (HBV) is a DNA virus in the Hepadnaviridae family. The infective virion is known as the Dane particle and has surface and core components, HBsAg and HBc antigen, respectively. In addition, within infected hepatocytes nonstructural regulatory proteins, hepatitis B e antigen, polymerase proteins, and viral progeny DNA are produced. Epitopes on the virus surface provide a basis for epidemiologic studies and consist of the HBsAg "a" d/y and w/r determinants. Recombinant vaccines target the "a" determinant of HBsAg and confer protective immunity. During active HBV infection, significant HBsAg overproduction results in the release of self-assembled 22-nm-diameter spheres and tubules in addition to Dane particles.

The average incubation period, defined as the time from infection to liver enzyme elevation and symptomatic hepatitis, is 59 days (range: 5–12 weeks) but may be as long as 6 months. Symptoms, which occur in 30% to 50% of infected persons, include anorexia, nausea, vomiting, jaundice, arthralgias, rashes, vasculitis, and glomerulonephritis. Chronicity, defined as persistent HBsAg and HBV DNA in plasma, follows acute infection in 2% to 10% of adults and 30% to 90% of young children and infants. Approximately 5% of the US population has serologic evidence of prior HBV infection (anti-HBc-reactive), and 0.4% to 0.5% (1–1.3 million) are chronically infected (HBsAg-positive). Between 1987 and 1998, reported cases of acute HBV infection in the United States declined by 76%, in great part because of expanded hepatitis B vaccination programs. Among blood donors, new HBV infections declined from 1.97 per 100,000 person-years to 1.27 between 1998 and 2001.[5]

Viral titers in blood are significantly greater than those present in the semen, vaginal fluid, and saliva. In relative terms, HBV is 100 times more infective than HIV and 10 times more infective than HCV. The predominant mode of transmission in adults and adolescents is through sexual contact. Forty percent have infected partners, 15% are males having sex with other males, injecting drug users account for 14% of cases, and one-third have no identifiable risk.

HBsAg is detectable in blood approximately 4 weeks (30–60 days) after infection. Subsequently, IgM anti-HBc antibodies appear coinciding with symptom onset. High viral titers (10^{10} genomes/mL) present at that time decline subsequently. HBsAg persists transiently in acute infections for up to 4 months (average 63 days). Antibodies against HBsAg (anti-HBs) arise subsequently and protect against reinfection. Anti-HBc identifies chronically infected low-level carriers; some anti-HBc-positive and anti-HBsAg-negative carriers contain circulating HBV DNA.[6] Although anti-HBs confers immunity, sufficient virus remains in the liver to transmit HBV following liver transplant from anti-HBs-positive donors.[7]

Most current HBV transfusion transmission cases are attributable to blood donations by asymptomatic donors during the acute infection phase prior to HBsAg appearance.[8] During this "window period" between infection and routine laboratory detection, HBV replicates relatively slowly with a doubling time of HBV viral load of approximately 2.6 days[8] (see text box below on estimating residual risk of blood screened for TTVs). Other cases are due to HBV mutants not detectable by HBsAg testing.[9] With current routine testing for HBsAg and anti-HBc, the risk for HBV transmission per unit is approximately 1 per 205,000 units.[5] Further risk reduction can be expected from recently implemented high-sensitivity serologic assays for HBsAg detecting approximately 0.1 ng/mL HBsAg compared with an average of 0.3 ng/mL with previous assays, and HBV NAT on either single donation samples or samples from multiple donors in minipools.[10,11] NAT on single donation samples has the potential to reduce the risk of transfusion-transmitted HBV by detecting newly

The Incidence Rate (IR) / Window Period (WP) Model: Estimating Residual Risk of Blood Screened for Transfusion-Transmitted Viruses

Accurate estimates of the risk of transmission of viral infections are important for monitoring and improving blood safety and for helping physicians and patients to make informed decisions about the use of blood products. As a consequence of improved protection of the blood supply from contamination with HIV and HCV, direct methods to estimate risks, such as prospective studies of transfusion recipients or testing of donor samples with sensitive research tests, have become impractical and prohibitively expensive because of the very large sample size required to conduct such studies.[13] Alternative, widely adopted and validated approaches to estimate the risk of viral transmission from blood units screened for HIV and HCV are based on mathematical modeling of the likelihood that a blood donor presents in the so-called window period of infection. The rationale is that in this period screening assays are not yet reactive but infectious virus is present in the bloodstream. The most widely used method is based on the IR/WP model, which estimates the residual risk for the virus in question by multiplying the IR (the rate of new infections in the specific blood donor population per year) by the length of the WP (in fractions of a year).[14] The model assumes that the WP risk is the single most contributing factor to residual risk (minor contributors being variant viral strains escaping detection, immunosilent carriers, and testing errors), that accurate figures for IR and WP are available, and that donors present for blood donation at the same rate during the length of the WP. These assumptions can be reasonably made, and the predictions derived from the model have been remarkably accurate over time. A major advantage of this approach is that it can be easily implemented with existing databases. The IR/WP model and its modifications have been applied worldwide to provide region-specific risk estimates. The model has also been applied to other viruses, including HBV and HTLV, although for various reasons estimates derived for the latter are less reliable.[5,8] Current US risk estimates for HIV, HCV, HBV, and HTLV shown in Table 154–1 are derived from IR/WP model calculations. Figure 154–1 shows the decline in IR, WP length, and resultant residual risk of the three major transfusion-transmitted viruses over time.

infected donors 21 to 29 days earlier than currently licensed HBsAg tests; minipool testing on the other hand offers little or no improvement over current and new investigational HBsAg assays for donor screening.[10,12] The cost and complexity of performing individual donation NAT for HBV, combined with declining HBV incidence and relatively low rate of chronic infection and clinical disease, resulted in minimal adoption of HBV NAT in the United States through 2007 despite licensure of HBV NAT assays by the FDA.[9,12] Subsequently, NAT assay revisions resulted in widespread texting.

Hepatitis C

The hepatitis C virus (HCV) is an RNA virus in the Flaviviridae family that has six genotypes. In the United States, genotypes 1, 2, and 3 cause 75%, 10%, and 10% of infections, respectively, and have similar replication and transmission rates and natural history. Genotype 1 responds less favorably to current treatment than genotypes 2 or 3.

Overall 4.1 million people (1.6% of the US population) have evidence of HCV infection and 3.2 million have ongoing chronic infections. Almost 90% of infected persons born between 1943 and 1972 reported injection drug use, high risk sexual behavior (more than 20 lifetime partners), or transfusion before 1992. Among those born before 1942, 0.9% are infected and more than 60% of those

Table 154–1 Risk of Transfusion-Transmitted Diseases in the United States

Pathogenic Agent	Average Estimated Risk per Unit
Hepatitis A	unknown, presumably <1:1 million
Hepatitis B	1:205,000[a]
Hepatitis C	1:1,935,000[b]
Human Immunodeficiency Virus-1	1:2,135,000[b]
Human T-Lymphotropic Virus-I, II	1:2,993,000
Cytomegalovirus (CMV)	infrequent[c]
Parvovirus B19	unknown, presumably <1:1 million
West Nile & other Arbo Viruses	unknown, presumably <1:1 million
Malaria	1:4,000,000
Babesia	<1:1 million
Chagas disease	~1:25,000 prior to testing
Creutzfeldt–Jakob Disease (CJD), vCJD	4 vCJD cases reported
Bacterial contamination associated with symptomatic sepsis	1:500,000 per red blood cell unit 1:70,000–118,000 per apheresis platelet unit[d]

[a]Estimates for HBV reflect risk projections prior to implementation of blood donor screening with nucleic acid testing (NAT).
[b]Estimates for HIV, HCV indicate risk projections following implementation of NAT for these agents in 1999.
[c]In association with CMV risk-reduced components.
[d]Reference 155.

infected in this age range (approximately 240,000 persons) have a history of prior blood transfusion.[15] Sexual transmission is considered an inefficient mechanism for viral transfer. Vertical transmission occurs in 3% to 7% of infants of mothers with active infections.[15] Among blood donors, 0.07% to 0.09% have confirmed positive test results.[5]

Only 20% to 30% of newly infected persons develop symptoms during the acute infection phase. However, chronic infection develops in 75% to 85% of persons infected after 45 years of age and in 50% to 60% of those infected as children or young adults.[16] Of patients with chronic HCV infection, approximately 25% develop fibrosis that evolves into cirrhosis over an average 20-year interval. Biochemical evidence of liver inflammation occurs in 70% of those infected as adults compared to 10% of those infected as juveniles. The risk of progression to cirrhosis varies from 10% to 20% of those infected as adults to approximately 5% of those infected earlier in life.[16,17] Alcohol consumption increases the risk of progression to cirrhosis. Hepatocellular carcinoma occurs in 1% to 4% per year in those with cirrhosis.

The risk of HCV transmission by transfusion declined following introduction of surrogate markers for non-A, non-B hepatitis in the 1980s (ALT and anti-HBc) and of serologic testing for HCV antibodies in May 1990 (Fig. 154–1). The window period for the first-generation HCV antibody test extended to 6 months, but was reduced to 82 and 70 days with second- and third-generation assays, respectively.[8] Introduction of nucleic acid amplification testing for the HCV viral genome in 1999 reduced the window period to 10 to 25 days.[18] By combining NAT with serologic testing, the resultant risk per unit declined from an estimated 1 per 276,000 units to 1 per 1,935,000 units.[5,19] Of note, the residual risk estimates based on serologic testing alone have been confirmed by NAT screening in that the yield of HCV RNA-positive/HCV antibody-negative donations found among donations (1 per 263,000) was as predicted by the incidence-window period model.[20,21]

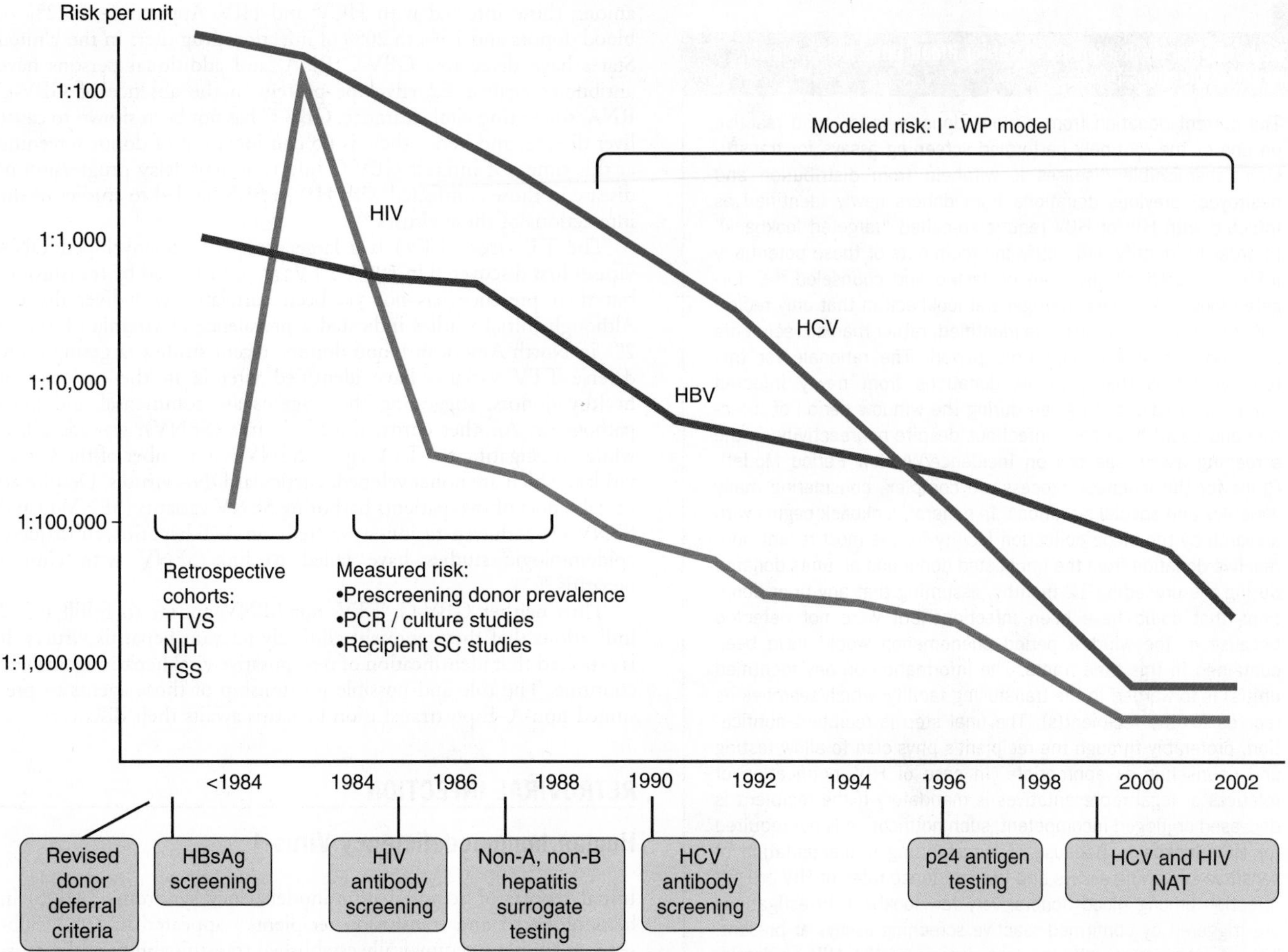

Figure 154–1 HIV, HBV, and HCV transfusion-transmission risks declined significantly during the past two decades. The boxed text below the *x*-axis indicates the major interventions contributing to risk reduction. (Data from Busch MP: Transfusion-transmitted viral infections: Building bridges to transfusion medicine to reduce risks and understand epidemiology and pathogenesis. Transfusion 46(9):1624, 2006.)

Because NAT is labor and resource intensive, HCV NAT feasibility depended on the use of so-called minipools, created by combining aliquots from 16 to 24 donations. Loss of test sensitivity due to sample pooling was tolerable given the rapid increase or burst of HCV viremia prior to antibody seroconversion (estimated doubling time of 10.8 hours in that period) and the high titer of viremia during the 40- to 50-day plateau phase preceding antibody seroconversion.[18] Consequently, NAT-positive donations that test HCV antibody negative contain 5×10^2 to 5×10^9 HCV copies per mL.[21–23] Although minipool NAT has been implemented successfully and with moderate yield in many developed countries,[21] NAT testing is expensive and the cost-effectiveness low.[24,25]

As an alternative to NAT assays, enzyme immunoassays have been developed that detect HCV core antigen in serum or plasma, either as separate tests that are run in parallel with HCV antibody screening assays or as so-called fourth-generation HCV antigen–antibody combination assays.[26,27] Although these tests significantly reduce the preseroconversion window period and are being adopted in developing countries, they have slightly less sensitivity than HCV NAT, approximately 10^5 gEq per mL,[28] and have not been introduced in the United States.

The remarkable advances in safety achieved by HCV NAT greatly reduced transfusion-associated HCV cases. Nonetheless, some newly infected individuals demonstrate fluctuations in HCV RNA, at times below NAT detection levels prior to HCV antibody seroconversion.[29] This possibly explains some of the low residual risk of transfusion-transmitted HCV infection despite the ongoing combination of HCV antibody and NAT testing.

The prolonged interval between infection and HCV clinical sequelae prompted blood bankers to conduct "Lookback" notification of previous recipients of blood donated by donors found HCV antibody positive.[30,31]

Hepatitis D

Originally called the delta agent, this is a defective RNA-containing passenger virus that requires HBV to act as a "helper" for assembly of envelope proteins. Screening for hepatitis B acts synergistically in preventing transfusion-associated hepatitis D cases by identifying donors that are coinfected with hepatitis B and D.[35]

Hepatitis E

The hepatitis E virus (HEV) is an RNA calicivirus associated with fecal-contaminated water supply that usually causes a self-limited illness. Transmission by transfusion had been postulated on the basis of cohort studies in endemic countries that showed a high prevalence of HEV among transfused patients. Recently transfusion transmission of HEV has been established in Japan, which led to the decision to screen blood donations by NAT in high-risk regions.[36] Fortunately, HEV is rare in the United States and most other developed countries and hence screening is not under active consideration.[35]

Lookback: Tracing Recipients of Earlier Blood Units from a Newly Identified Infectious Donor

The current donation from a blood donor who is found reactive on one of the routinely performed screening assays for transfusion-transmissible diseases is withheld from distribution and destroyed; previous donations from donors newly identified as infected with HIV or HCV require so-called "targeted lookback" in order to identify and notify the recipients of these potentially infectious units so they can be tested and counseled.[32,33] Targeted lookback differs from general lookback in that only recipients of "at risk donations" are identified, rather than all recipients of blood during a certain time period. The rationale for this requirement is that previous donations from newly infected donors may have been given during the window period of infection and could have been infectious despite nonreactivity on the screening assay (see box on Incidence/Window Period Model). Rules for the lookback process are complex, considering many variables and special situations. In general, lookback begins with a search by the blood collection facility for the most recent nonreactive donation from the implicated donor and all units donated during the preceding 12 months, assuming that any prior donations that could have been infectious but were not detected because of the window period phenomenon would have been contained in this time frame. The information on any identified unit(s) is forwarded to the transfusing facility, which searches its records for the recipient(s). The final step is recipient notification, preferably through the recipient's physician to allow testing and counseling as appropriate. In case of HIV, notification of relatives or legal representatives is mandatory if the recipient is deceased or judged incompetent, such notification is not required for HCV lookback. Because of longstanding implementation of sensitive screening assays and low incidence rates of HIV or HCV infection among blood donors, very few lookback investigations are triggered by confirmed reactive screening assays at present. This is in contrast with the first decade of the HIV epidemic, when it was not uncommon to perform lookback on prior donations from blood donors who were implicated because of presumed transfusion-associated HIV infection in the recipient. Large-scale targeted retrospective HCV lookback investigations were launched in many countries in the mid- to late 1990s to identify recipients of blood components who were donated by individuals before they were found to be HCV positive through blood donor screening beginning in 1990.[30,31] The efficacy of these programs have been low in general, and their value has been questioned. Recent experience in Canada further demonstrates the very limited value of targeted HCV lookback in the current setting of low disease prevalence and sensitive screening assays.[34] On the other hand it is clear that through this program some recipients could be contacted who would not have otherwise benefited from testing, counseling, adoption of a healthier lifestyle, and antiviral therapy.

Non-A–E Hepatitis

Several observations suggest hepatitis viruses other than those identified as hepatitis A-E viruses cause viral hepatitis. For example, cases of posttransfusion hepatitis occur occasionally despite screening or diagnostic testing for known hepatitis viruses. Similarly, a small but consistent percentage of community-acquired and chronic hepatitis cases test negative for known hepatitis viruses, some cirrhosis cases are classified as "cryptogenic," the etiologic agent for hepatitis-associated aplastic anemia eludes description, and the cause of some cases of acute liver failure remains undefined.[37]

Several candidate agents have been proposed as non-A–E hepatitis viruses.[38] GBV-C (initially also referred to as Hepatitis G Virus [HGV]) is a member of the Flaviviridae family and is transmitted predominantly by the parenteral route. Infection occurs frequently among those infected with HCV and HIV. Approximately 2% of blood donors and 15% to 20% of infection-drug users in the United States have detectable GBV-C RNA, and additional persons have antibodies against E2 envelope protein in the absence of GBV-C RNA, suggesting viral clearance. GBV-C has not been shown to cause liver disease, and hence there is no consideration of donor screening at this time. Of interest GBV-C infection may delay progression of disease in those coinfected with HIV, which has led to studies of the interactions of these viruses.[39]

The TT virus (TTV) is a large group of nonenveloped DNA viruses first discovered in 1997. TTVs are transmitted by transfusion, but their presence has not yet been correlated with liver disease. Although initial studies indicated a prevalence of viremia of 1% to 2% in North American blood donors, recent studies targeting more diverse TTV variants have identified viremia in the majority of healthy donors, suggesting these agents are commensal and nonpathogenic. Another entity, the SEN virus (SENV), was identified while investigating the TTV agent. SENV is a member of the Circoviridae, which are nonenveloped, curricular DNA viruses. Despite an initial report of two patients harboring SENV variants (SENV-D and SENV-H) with transfusion-associated non-A–E hepatitis, subsequent epidemiologic studies have failed to link SENV with clinical hepatitis.[37]

Thus neither GBV-C, TTV, nor SENV appear to fulfill initial indications that they represent clinically relevant hepatitis viruses. It is expected that identification of new putative viral hepatic agents will continue. The role and possible relationship of those agents to presumed non-A–E posttransfusion hepatitis awaits their discovery.

RETROVIRAL INFECTION

Human Immunodeficiency Virus-1

Initial reports of acquired immunodeficiency syndrome (AIDS) in hemophiliacs[40] and transfusion recipients[41] appeared in 1982. Subsequent studies unequivocally established transmissibility of the causative agent (HIV) by untreated coagulation factor concentrates and blood components.[42] According to the Centers for Disease Control and Prevention (CDC) 9706 AIDS cases in the United States were linked to transfusion through December 31, 2005, including 47 adults/adolescents and 3 children who were infected by blood from HIV-seronegative donors since antibody screening was implemented in early 1985.[43] In addition, since the early 1980s, 5712 hemophilic and other patients with coagulation disorders acquired HIV as a result of therapy with plasma derivatives. In hindsight the initial response to this crisis was criticized as perhaps too slow and indecisive.[44] Nevertheless, preventive measures to protect the blood supply were put in place quickly once the threat was fully recognized. Implementation of detailed blood donor history questioning with deferral of high-risk blood donors began in spring of 1983 and antibody testing for HIV in 1985. Almost all new cases after implementation of antibody screening were attributable to blood donations given during the so-called window period of infection (see text box).

Sequential introduction of improved, highly sensitive enzyme immunoassays for detection of HIV antibodies in the early 1990s, addition of testing for HIV-1 (p24) antigen in 1995, and HIV RNA testing on pooled donor samples in 1999 were instrumental in reducing the risk of HIV transmission by transfusion to its current low level (Fig. 154–1, Table 154–1). The risk for manufactured blood products, such as coagulation factor concentrates, albumin and immune globulin preparations, can be expected to be even lower because of additional viral inactivation processes, including heat (pasteurization), physicochemical processes (solvent/detergent treatment), and nanofiltration that have been implemented since the mid-1980s; indeed, no new HIV infections have been attributed to manufactured plasma derivatives since 1990.[45]

Blood centers notify donors found repeatedly reactive in HIV antibody-screening tests with appropriate counseling messages, even if confirmatory or supplemental testing results by Western blot (WB) or immunofluorescence are negative or indeterminate. Donors with positive and persistently indeterminate WB are permanently deferred from giving blood for use in transfusion. Experimental data indicate that very few blood donors with indeterminate results by HIV supplemental tests are infected with HIV,[46] and that low-risk blood donors on occasion may have false-positive supplementary test results.[47] Recipients of prior donations from donors with confirmed positive results are traced through lookback investigations (see text box).

Human Immunodeficiency Virus-2

Human immunodeficiency virus-2, a retrovirus linked more closely to the simian immunodeficiency virus than to HIV-1, was recognized initially in West Africa in the late 1980s. Transmissibility of HIV-2 appears to be lower, the course of infection milder, and the interval between infection and AIDS and disease longer than associated with HIV-1.[48] Sixty-two cases of HIV-2 were reported in the United States as of June 30, 1995, leading to substantial concern over transfusion safety.[49] Antibody testing for HIV-1 detects 60% to 91% of HIV-2-infected persons, whereas HIV-2 antibody test kits detect more than 99%.[50] Blood donor testing for both HIV-1 and HIV-2 antibodies began in 1992. From 1992 through 1998, only three donors with HIV-2 infection were identified in the United States after screening more than 50 million donations, suggesting a very low risk for HIV-2 transmission by transfusion.[51] Almost all cases occur in Africa or have historical links to that region.[52]

HIV-1 Group M Subtype and Group O Infections

The majority of HIV-1 infections are caused by subtypes of group M (main group) viruses. In the United States and Europe almost all HIV-1 infections are caused by subtype B viruses, but worldwide other subtypes dominate locally.[52] Widely used antibody assays for detection of HIV-1 infection are based on subtype B antigens and do not perform as well with non–subtype B viral strains[53] leading to concern that infections with such strains could be missed. Fortunately, HIV-1 NAT assays appear to have good sensitivity to all group M variants, which has tempered this concern. Ongoing surveillance studies have recently been launched to monitor emergence of new HIV variants and the effectiveness of routine HIV test kits for detecting these viruses.[54]

The HIV-1 group O (outlier group) viruses were isolated from patients in Central and West Africa in 1994. These HIV-1 variants share 65% to 70% homology with HIV-1 and 56% with HIV-2. Through 1997, two HIV-1 group O-infected persons were identified in the United States and only rare cases have been reported subsequently in industrialized nations.[52,55] To safeguard against possible false-negative HIV antibody test results in blood donor screening, blood donors are deferred if they were born in, lived in, traveled to and received a blood transfusion, or had risk exposures in HIV-1 group O-endemic African countries.[56]

This deferral policy may be reversed once antibody and NAT assays with established sensitivity to group O viruses are licensed by FDA and implemented.

Human T-Lymphotropic Virus-I and -II

HTLV-I and -II are closely related retroviruses in the oncovirinae group with 60% to 70% sequence homology and shared tropism for T lymphocytes. In contrast to HIV, HTLV is rarely present in cell-free plasma and shows little active replication in infected humans. HTLV is found around the globe, with endemic foci in southern Japan, the Caribbean, certain parts of South America, Africa, the Middle East, and Melanesia.[57] An epidemic of HTLV-II infection has been observed over the past 40 to 50 years among intravenous drug users in the United States, Brazil, and Europe.[58] Transmission of both HTLV-I and -II occurs by parenteral exposures, through sexual contact, and by vertical transmission from mother to child during pregnancy and breast feeding.

Diseases associated with HTLV-I infection include adult T-cell leukemia/lymphoma (ATL), HTLV-associated myelopathy/tropical spastic paraparesis (HAM/TSP), lymphocytic pneumonitis, uveitis, polymyositis, and arthritis.[59] HTLV-II does not appear to cause hematologic malignancy but has been associated with the other conditions attributed to HTLV-I infection, and also has been linked to a higher rate of common infections such as acute bronchitis, pneumonia, and urinary tract infections, suggesting a mild immunosuppressive effect of the virus.[60]

Patients with ATL have HTLV-I provirus integrated into $CD4^+$ flower-like cells.[61] ATL occurs in 2% to 4% of infected persons following a latent period that extends for many decades. The illness is characterized by leukemia, generalized peripheral lymphadenopathy, hepatomegaly, impaired liver function tests, splenomegaly, skin lesions, bone lesions, and hypercalcemia.[62,63] HAM/TSP occurs in approximately 2% of HTLV-I- and HTLV-II-infected individuals. Patients with transfusion-associated HAM/TSP develop neurologic symptoms at a median of 3.3 years after transfusion.[63] This illness is characterized by slowly progressive chronic spastic paraparesis, lower limb weakness, urinary incontinence, impotence, sensory disturbances, low back pain, hyperreflexia, and impaired vibration sense.

Risk factors for HTLV-I and -II infections in blood donors include low educational attainment, accidental needle sticks, previous blood transfusion, seven or more lifetime sex partners, and a sex partner from an HTLV endemic area. Injection drug use or having sex with a drug user associates significantly with HTLV-II but not with HTLV-I infection.[64]

Blood donor screening for HTLV-I antibodies began in 1988, and a more sensitive HTLV-I/II combination assay that detects close to 100% of HTLV-II infections was introduced in 1998.[65] The prevalence of HTLV confirmed positive infectious markers among first-time blood donors decreased approximately 10-fold during the 1990s to 0.01% in 2001 with a similar decline in incidence rates in repeat donors.[1] Consequently, risk projections based on the incidence rate / window period model were lowered to approximately 1 in 3 million blood donations in 2001.[5] Because essentially cell-free components such as plasma and cryoprecipitate do not transmit HTLV and only 30% of infected cellular components result in transmission,[66] the threat of acquiring HTLV infection from screened blood appears to be minimal at this time.

More problematic is the notification of healthy blood donors of possible HTLV infection because of a false-positive result with the screening EIA. This is more likely to occur with HTLV than with HIV or hepatitis infection because of a lack of licensed confirmatory tests for HTLV. In recognition of this deficiency, FDA approved an algorithm that accepts nonreactivity on repeat testing with a second screening EIA from a different manufacturer as evidence that infection is absent.[67] This strategy resolves nearly two-thirds of false-positive screening results but still results in a large number of false notifications and does not address the issue of providing targeted counseling for HTLV-I versus HTLV-II infection. Because blood donors who are notified of possible infection suffer considerable psychosocial stress,[68] development of supplemental tests that meet criteria for licensing is a priority.

HUMAN HERPES VIRUS INFECTIONS

Human herpes viruses (HHV) are enveloped, structurally complex double-stranded DNA viruses that cause common infectious diseases, usually associated with life-long carrier states and the possibility of recurrent reactivation infections. They are classified in 3 subfamilies, alpha-, beta- and gamma-herpesvirinae, of which the latter two contain the herpes viruses that are of greatest concern from a transfusion medicine standpoint. Members of the alpha herpes virus subfamily, herpes simplex viruses, and varicella zoster virus, rarely, if ever cause transfusion-transmitted infections.

Cytomegalovirus (HHV-5)

Cytomegalovirus (CMV), a beta herpes virus, can infect a wide range of cell types, including leukocytes of monocyte-macrophage lineage and their progenitors, of which the former represent the preeminent source of transfusion-transmitted infection.[69] Consequently, cell-depleted blood components (plasma, cryoprecipitate) do not transmit CMV. Primary CMV infection in immunocompetent individuals is usually community-acquired and often asymptomatic or associated with a mild, self-limited infectious mononucleosis syndrome. However, in virtually all cases, latent virus persists permanently in cellular reservoirs, allowing lifelong reactivation infections, or in the setting of transfusion or transplantation, viral transmission via cellular blood products, or transplanted donor organs.

In immunosuppressed patients, CMV infection leads to pneumonitis, hepatitis, gastroenteritis, retinitis, and other inflammatory conditions, often associated with considerable morbidity and mortality. Primary infection in pregnancy does not pose a threat for the woman but is associated with severe fetal malformation syndromes and congenital infections complicated by jaundice, hepatosplenomegaly, microencephaly, and thrombocytopenia. Fetal mortality rates approach 20%.[70] Premature infants (<1200 g birth weight) born to CMV-seronegative women are at particular high risk for symptomatic CMV disease, including hemolytic anemia. Morbidity varies considerably from a few percent to 50% of seronegative infants receiving unscreened, nonleukoreduced blood. CMV-seronegative marrow transplant patients are also strongly susceptible to CMV infection, with approximately 30% of those infected developing symptomatic CMV disease in the past, before institution of routine monitoring for CMV antigenemia and preemptive antiviral therapy.[71] Seronegative renal and liver transplant recipients are also susceptible to symptomatic transfusion-transmitted CMV infections, but the risk associated with receiving seropositive solid organs outweighs that attributed to blood transfusion. CMV-seronegative HIV-infected patients represent another group at risk for transfusion-transmitted primary CMV infection.[72]

On average 50% of US blood donors have antibodies against CMV, thereby indicating prior CMV exposure and potential to transmit the disease via latently infected circulating monocytes.[69] The reported risk of (usually asymptomatic) CMV infection in seronegative immunocompetent patients who receive non–leukocyte-reduced cellular blood components unscreened for presence of CMV antibodies is approximately 1%.[73,74] In contrast, the historical risk of CMV infection in immunocompromised recipients receiving CMV-unscreened, non–leukocyte-reduced blood components has been reported in various studies from 13.5% to 53.3%.[75] Selection of CMV seronegative or leukocyte-reduced blood components for susceptible patient groups have significantly reduced the risk of transfusion-transmitted CMV infection. Neither method is fail-safe in preventing transfusion-associated CMV transmission, however, and "breakthrough" infections have been reported in bone marrow transplant recipients at a rate of 1% to 2% for CMV-seronegative units and 1% to 6% for leukocyte-reduced blood components.[76,77] Whether both methods of creating "CMV-safe" or "risk-reduced" blood components are equivalent in protecting transfusion recipients continues to be a matter of debate.[78–80] At least in the allogeneic bone marrow transplant setting, a recent meta-analysis of available studies comparing both strategies found selection of CMV-seronegative components more effective than leukocyte reduction.[75] This may not translate in a difference in clinical outcomes, though, as implementation of prospective monitoring for CMV antigenemia and preemptive treatment with ganciclovir is preventing all but rare cases of CMV disease nowadays.[77]

In the absence of clear-cut scientific data and interpretation, it has been recommended that each institution review its internal policies for blood use in patients vulnerable to CMV infection.[81,82] Table 154–2 lists patient populations for whom use of CMV "risk-reduced" components, that is, CMV seronegative, leukocyte-reduced or units meeting both criteria, are thought to be beneficial. If leukocyte reduction is chosen as a means to reduce the risk of CMV transmission, components prepared by prestorage-leukocyte reduction should be selected because leukocyte removal by this method is more reliable than bedside filtration.[81,82]

Table 154–2 Patients Benefiting From CMV-Risk-Reduced Blood Components*

- Infants <1200 g with CMV-seronegative mothers
- Seronegative autologous and allogenic (CMV-seronegative donors) progenitor cell transplant recipients
- Seronegative progenitor cell transplant candidates
- Seronegative recipients of seronegative solid organ transplants
- Seronegative pregnant women
- Fetuses receiving intrauterine transfusions
- Immunosuppressed patients receiving granulocyte transfusions
- HIV-seropositive/CMV-seronegative patients

*CMV-risk reduced components include CMV-seronegative and leukocyte-reduced components. From references 69 to 82.

In the future, nucleic acid testing (NAT) for CMV genomic sequences in plasma may offer an approach for additional risk reduction by blood donor screening, as rare blood donors who present with window period infections prior to emergence of CMV antibody may be detected and their donations discarded.[83] Presently, it is not clear, however, if detection of plasma viremia by NAT equates infectivity. Current NAT assays also do not seem to be more effective than serologic screening in detecting latently infected healthy blood donors, as CMV DNA was not reproducibly detected in unequivocally seronegative samples.[84] Most promising appears to be CMV NAT screening of umbilical cord blood transplants as an adjunct to serologic screening.[85]

Another concern is CMV seropositive patients who theoretically remain at risk for second-strain infections. These have been reported in immunocompetent patients, where they appear not to be associated with added morbidity, and in recipients of solid organ transplants, where they do contribute to more severe disease than from reactivation of endogenous virus.[72,81] The source of second-strain infections in the latter setting is frequently the transplanted organ, whereas evidence linking blood transfusions as the source is not available. Furthermore, because reactivation of latent infections is a common occurrence in seropositive immunosuppressed patients, the benefit of providing reduced-risk CMV components for these patients is unproven and generally not recommended.

Ex vivo and observational clinical studies suggest a link between allogeneic leukocytes in blood transfusion and reactivation of latent CMV infection,[86] providing an argument for using leukocyte-reduced blood to decrease infections in immunosuppressed CMV-seropositive patients. Although theoretically compelling, the effectiveness of this approach has not been demonstrated in prospective studies.[87]

Epstein–Barr Virus (HHV-4)

Epstein–Barr virus (EBV), a gamma herpes virus, is the etiologic agent of heterophile antibody-positive infectious mononucleosis and is closely associated with Burkitt lymphoma, nasopharyngeal carcinoma, and posttransplant lymphoproliferative disease (PTLD).[88] Transfusion transmission of the virus is unlikely because more than 90% of the adult population has evidence of previous exposure, and infection is deterred by host virus-specific cytotoxic T lymphocytes, capable of lysing EBV-infected B lymphocytes when viral peptides are expressed on the lymphocyte surface.[89] Rare cases of transfusion-transmitted EBV presenting as infectious mononucleosis have been described in both immunocompetent recipients[90,91] and in immunosuppressed patients following solid organ transplantation.[92] Aggressive EBV-associated lymphoproliferative disorders have been observed in patients with weakened immune system following cord blood stem cell transplantation[93] but have not been documented following transfusion. Because B lymphocytes are the likely source of transfusion-transmitted EBV infection, leukocyte reduction of cellular blood components that efficiently removes B cells is an attractive strategy to prevent infection in transfusion recipients.[94] The validity of this assumption has yet to be validated in controlled clinical trials.

Kaposi Sarcoma Virus (HHV-8)

HHV-8, a gamma herpes virus linked to Kaposi sarcoma, body cavity based lymphoma and Castleman disease has tropism to lymphocytes and monocyte-macrophages, and has been shown to be transmitted by transplantation. The possibility has been raised that transfusions given in the United States have transmitted HHV-8,[95] but definitive evidence is lacking. The seroprevalence of HHV-8 among US blood donors has been reported in regional studies as high as 20% to 25%.[96] However, a recent multicenter study in five representative US regions found a seroprevalence of only 3% to 3.5% and no evidence of viremia.[97] These findings are in agreement with epidemiologic studies that suggest sexual contact is the preferred route of HHV-8 transmission whereas blood-borne transmission appears to be an unlikely event.[98,99] On the other hand there is convincing evidence of HHV-8 transmission by transfusion in sub-Saharan Africa where seroprevalence of HHV-8 among blood donors is 40%, and fresh, nonleukoreduced transfusions are common practice.[100] Similar to what has been established for CMV infection, it can be assumed that leukocyte reduction mitigates the risk of HHV-8 transmission via transfusion, but this has not been demonstrated.

Parvovirus

Human parvovirus B19 is a 19- to 23-nm-diameter nonenveloped, single-stranded DNA virus that is included in the Parvoviridae family along with adeno-associated viruses and newly discovered viruses PARV 4, PARV 5 and bocavirus.[101] Parvovirus B19 causes fifth disease or erythema infectiosum and has been linked with transient aplastic crises in patients with sickle cell anemia, inherited hemolytic diseases, and malaria as a result of severe reticulocytopenia and anemia.[102] Acute infection impairs erythropoiesis for 7 to 10 days and causes complete cessation for 3 to 7 days, resulting in hemoglobin decreases. Arthropathy has been reported in adults and loss of joint range of motion in children with hemophilia.[103] Immunocompromised patients have been reported to suffer prolonged anemia, erythrodermia, hepatitis, myocarditis, and pancytopenia.[104] Although B19 has at least three genotypes, little is known about transmission and pathogenicity of genotypes 2 and 3.[105]

B19 infects only humans.[106] Transmission occurs through the respiratory route most commonly, through the placenta to a fetus in up to 30% of women infected during pregnancy, and through transfusion of blood, blood components, and plasma derivatives. Transmission to immunocompetent patients, and those with hemolytic hemoglobin disorders, rarely results in systemic illness. In contrast, in women infected during weeks 9 to 20 of pregnancy, fetal death occurs in approximately 11% from hydrops fetalis.[108] The overall low incidence of infection in transfused patients results from coinfusion of neutralizing antibodies or because of low viral load, less than 4×10^3 genome equivalents per mL.[105,109] B19 is highly tropic for erythroid progenitor cells gaining access to cells through the blood group P antigen, or globoside, that serves as the virus receptor.[106,107] Following acute infection, viral replication leads to extremely high viremic levels that decline in response to IgM antibody production approximately 9 days following infection.[102] B19 may persist in bone marrow, liver, tonsils, and skin of healthy persons.[101]

B19 infection is ubiquitous, with 50% of high school children demonstrating seropositivity that increases to 90% in older adults.[106,107,110] Persistent infection, including pure red cell aplasia, occurs in those not developing neutralizing antibodies to the viral capsical protein 1 (VP1). In these patients, the virus circulates at high titer, greater than 10^{12} genome copies/mL.[106,107] Patients at risk for persistent infection include those receiving chemotherapy, immunosuppressive drugs, organ transplant recipients, and those with HIV.

Blood and blood-derivative transmission involves donations during the transient 1- to 2-week high-titer viremic period. The prevalence of B19 viremia has been reported as 0.003% to 0.6% in blood and plasma donors.[109] Hence, most blood transfusion recipients are at relatively low risk of exposure whereas recipients of pooled, plasma-derived products involving thousands of donors have a significant risk. In one report, 14% of viremic plasma donors had titers between 10^4 and 10^7 genome equivalents/mL and 1 in 13,000 had titers greater than 10^7.[110] In observational studies, seroconversion occurred among recipients of plasma with high titers, $10^{7.5}$ to $10^{8.5}$ genome copies/mL treated with the solvent/detergent pathogen reduction technique suggesting the presence of anti-B19 antibodies are not protective against large viral loads. (See Pathogen Reduction/Inactivation Methods) Seroconversion did not occur among recipients of plasma with viral titers between $10^{0.5}$ and $10^{3.5}$ genome copies per mL. However, parvovirus transmission has been reported in a recipient of solvent/detergent-treated antihemophilic factor concentrate containing 1.3×10^3 genome equivalents/mL and in a recipient of a dry-heat-treated, 80°C for 72 hours, factor VIII product containing 4×10^3 genome equivalents per mL.[109,111] Solvent/detergent treatment is ineffective in preventing B19 transmission, but freeze-drying and dry-heat treatment (80°C for 72 hours) inactivates more than 4.7 logs B19, which may not be sufficient to prevent transmission.[112]

Currently, plasma derivative manufacturers use "in-process" nucleic acid testing to identify source plasma units with high-titer parvovirus B19, greater than 10^4 genome equivalents/mL. Approximately 1 per 10,000 plasma units are withheld from further processing. Because individual whole-blood donations rarely cause parvovirus infection, testing of single red cell units, platelet or plasma for parvovirus B19 is not under consideration currently. Of note, PARV4 and PARV5, but not human bocavirus, have been detected in pooled plasma derivative samples.[101]

West Nile Virus

The West Nile Virus (WNV) is a mosquito-borne lipid-enveloped RNA virus in the Japanese encephalitis flaviridae complex. Transmitted bird-to-bird by mosquito vectors, human infections occur incidentally. The first cases were identified in the West Nile district of Uganda in 1937. Subsequently, outbreaks occurred in the Middle East, South Africa, and Europe. The first North American cases appeared in New York City in 1999.[124] Starting in July 2000, WNV cases spread to the Mid-Atlantic states. In July 2001, 66 cases were reported in the eastern one-third of the United States. In 2002 the epidemic spread to the Midwest and eastern plains states. Four organ transplant recipients developed WNV infection.[125] In 2003, the epidemic intensified into in Nebraska, Colorado, North and South Dakota, and Wyoming with 9862 cases reported and more than 1000 healthy blood donors testing positive. By 2004, case reports declined in the Northeast but extended westward into Arizona and Southern California. In 2005, more than 2800 cases were reported, with approximately 25% occurring in California, relatively high activity in South Dakota, Nebraska, Louisiana, and Illinois, and low activity in the Northeast. Approximately 400 viremic blood donors were identified. In 2006, more than 4050 cases occurred with WNV activity reported in Washington for the first time and high-frequency reports in Idaho, California, Nebraska, Illinois, Louisiana, and the Dakotas.[126] More than 340 blood donors had positive test results.

WNV viremia appears 1 to 3 days following a bite from an infected mosquito. In contrast to HIV and HCV, peak WNV levels are relatively low, median 3500 copies/mL compared to 10^5 to 10^7 copies for HIV and HCV. In a cohort analysis comparing blood donors with positive WNV RNA tests to presumably uninfected donors, 61% of those with positive tests described symptoms such as headache, eye pain, new rash, or weakness within 21 days of donation

Pathogen Reduction/Inactivation Methods

Expanded blood donor screening coupled with deferral of high-risk donors have greatly reduced the risk of transfusion-transmitted diseases (TTDs) over the last two decades. These passive protective measures, however, cannot ensure complete protection from known TTDs and are of limited utility in safeguarding the blood supply from emerging and currently unknown infectious agents. Pathogen reduction and inactivation methods (PRIMs) promise to add another layer of safety by removing a broad range of pathogenic agents, reducing their capabilities to cause disease, or both.

PRIMs have long been employed in the manufacture of plasma derivatives such as albumin, gammaglobulins, and coagulation factor concentrates.[113] The relative stability of these proteins made it comparatively easy to use heat or chemical processes to inactivate infectious agents in the product without damaging the therapeutic ingredient. The principal limitation of these methods is their relative inefficiency against non-lipid-enveloped viruses such as HAV and parvoviruses. Recently, nanofiltration has become available as another effective approach to remove nonenveloped viruses in the manufacture of plasma derivatives.[114]

More challenging is treatment of blood components containing living cells or labile plasma proteins. Pathogen reduction and inactivation in acellular components poses lesser problems, and several chemical and photochemical principles have been developed.[115] Longest in use is solvent detergent-treated plasma (SDP), which has been available in Europe since the early 1990s and became available in the United States in 1998. Solvent detergent treatment is highly effective against lipid-enveloped viruses, including HIV and HCV, but is relatively ineffective against nonenveloped viruses.[116] In this context, the concern was raised that the pooling process in the manufacture of SDP that combines plasma donations from approximately 2500 individuals could lead to the inadvertent spread of viruses not affected by the treatment. Validating this concern, numerous lots of SDP were recalled in the United States following parvovirus seroconversions in recipients of SDP; rare cases of clinical disease due to parvovirus infection were also reported.[117] Unrelated to considerations regarding infectious disease transmissions, the product was withdrawn from distribution in the United States in 2002 following a series of deaths from excessive bleeding and thrombotic complications associated with use of SDP in patients with severe liver disease and liver transplants. The product is still available outside the United States, however. An alternative PRIM for treatment of plasma is photodynamic treatment in which photosensitive compounds such as methylene blue (MB), psoralens, or riboflavin (vitamin B_2) are added and activated by exposure to UV light. Pathogen inactivation occurs through oxidation (MB) or binding to DNA or RNA in case of psoralens and riboflavin. The photodynamic methods have the advantage of being suitable for single-unit treatment, avoiding the problems with pooling. Some loss of coagulation factor activity and platelets occurs, the significance of which is being studied. MB-treated plasma has been available for years in European countries, and psoralen/UV light plasma is undergoing clinical studies.[118–120] Platelets treated with psoralen/UV light are available for routine clinical practice in Europe and have successfully completed clinical studies prior to product approval in the United States[121]; a riboflavin-based method is in earlier stages of investigation. Adoption of photodynamic principles for pathogen inactivation of red blood cell components is complicated by absorption of long-wave UV light by hemoglobin. Overall pathogen reduction is seen by some transfusion medicine leaders as an important step in mitigating transfusion risk in a era of emergency pathogens.[115]

A unique problem is posed by removal or inactivation of prions, the abnormal cellular protein that has been identified as causative agent of transmissible spongiform encephalopathies, including vCJD. Existing physical or chemical methods are ineffective, and methods that work are too severe to be applied to blood products.[122] Initial hopes that leukocyte reduction would remove prions were not fulfilled, but an experimental, specially designed leukocyte reduction filter may be effective for prion removal as well.[123]

Although there is no dearth of PRIMs for blood components already available or under consideration, remaining questions of efficacy, component function, residual toxicity, and cost have to be answered before these methods will find widespread acceptance in clinical practice. It is expected, however, that newer-generation PRIMs will fulfill the stringent requirements and will provide an added layer of safety to transfusable products in the future.

compared to 20% of those not infected.[127] These findings suggest donor history information is insufficient to prevent transfusion transmission. Testing for antibodies, also, does not prevent transmission because IgM antibodies appear a median of 14 days and IgG antibodies a median of 17 days postinfection. Hence, nucleic acid testing for WNV RNA was selected as the testing strategy. Following intense collaboration among virologists, government officials test manufacturers and blood centers; WNV RNA testing was introduced at the start of the 2003 WNV season. To achieve efficiency, blood donors' samples were tested in minipools containing aliquots from 6 or 16 donors. More than 1000 donors tested positive[128–133] and six transfusion-associated WNV cases occurred during 2003. The implicated donors had low-level viremia that escaped detection in the minipool samples. Subsequently, test performance improved and blood collection agencies implemented strategies in which individual donation rather than minipool testing occurred in areas experiencing proportionally high WNV attack rates. One transfusion-associated case occurred in 2004 and one in 2006.[134] Of the 30 cases reported prior to 2006, all implicated donations tested WNV IgM-antibody negative.[135,136]

In a study involving more than 13 million blood donations between 2003 and 2005, WNV RNA testing performed on individual donation samples detected 22% of WNV-infected donors who tested negative using minipool samples.[137] Of these donations, 5.3% were antibody negative and presumably infectious. In test-positive donors, WNV RNA persisted in 42% for a median of 14 days. On the basis of multiple reports, the median viremic duration approximates 6 days but may persist for up to 104 days.[128–133,138] IgM antibodies appear 7 to 14 days postinfection and correspond to a decrease in RNA levels. IgM antibodies persist for more than 398 days in approximately two-thirds of those infected.

Up to 1% of WNV-infected patients develop neuroinvasive disease manifest by meningitis, encephalitis, or acute flaccid paralysis. Even among those with mild illness, 13 months after diagnosis, 50% WNV-infected patients report that fatigue, memory problems, and extreme weakness occurs, one-third have headaches, one-quarter suffer intention tremors, and 13% have word-finding difficulty.[138] The overall mortality rate in reported cases approximated 3.6% in 2006.

Currently, blood collection agencies conduct WNV RNA on every donation despite questions about the cost-effectiveness, $483,000 per quality-adjusted life-year for year-round minipool testing, compared to target testing based on WNV prevalence and seasonality.[139,140]

BACTERIAL CONTAMINATION

Bacterial contamination of red cell and platelet components ranked among the top three causes of transfusion-related fatalities reported to the FDA, with 85 cases (13% of all reported) in the 1995 to 2004 time period.[141] Bacteria enter blood containers as a result of inadequate skin disinfection at the phlebotomy site, transient asymptomatic bacteremia at the time of blood donation, a break in technique during pooling or sealing, or through disruption of container integrity. Bacterial proliferation occurs more rapidly in platelet concentrates stored for up to 5 days at room temperature than in red cells stored for up to 42 days at refrigerated temperatures.[142,143] Importantly, bacterial contamination represents a well established risk associated with autologous transfusion, because of more permissible acceptance standards of autologous donors and usually long storage times of donated blood units which favors bacterial growth.[144]

The frequency of bacterial contamination in red blood cell units has not been well established but can be expected in the order of at least 1 in 30,000 transfusions, with a prevalence of significant clinical outcomes of 1 in 500,000 transfusions and fatalities at a rate of 1 in 10,000,000. Prior to universal screening of platelet products for bacterial contamination in the US which occurred in March of 2004, the rate of bacterial contamination in allogeneic platelets was estimated at 1 in 1,000 to 3,000 units, the rate of life-threatening septic reactions at least at 1 in 100,000 recipients, and the rate of fatalities at 1 in 500,000.[145,146] Large-scale culturing of platelet component samples since implementation of screening for bacterial contamination demonstrated a lower contamination rates of approximately 1 in 5,000,[147,148] but the previously observed rates for sepsis and fatalities are probably low estimates, related to underreporting.[149] It can be expected that because of interception of screening-positive platelets, current transfusion reaction and fatality rates have improved, although it is clear that contaminated platelets may escape detection with available methods, and breakthrough cases of transfusion-associated sepsis continue to occur.[147,150]

Septic transfusion reactions should be suspected if the following occur within 1 to 4 hours of transfusion: fever greater than 1°C to 2°C from pretransfusion levels, chills and rigors, tachycardia more than 120 beats per minute or an increase of 40 beats per minute, or an increase or fall in systolic blood pressure of greater than 30 mm Hg. Additional signs and symptoms include nausea, vomiting, diarrhea, bleeding, oliguria, or septic shock.[142,145] Septic transfusion reactions may be confused with febrile, nonhemolytic transfusion reactions or may be masked by concurrent antibiotic administration.

Microorganisms isolated from contaminated red cell units include *Serratia liquefaciens*, *Pseudomonas* species, the plant pathogen *Enterobacter agglomerans*, and most important, *Yersinia enterocolitica*. The latter, a gram-negative endotoxin-producing organism is remarkable for its preference to grow at colder temperature in iron-enriched environments. Gram-positive skin saprophytes account for most of the organisms contaminating platelet concentrates, with the remaining attributed to gram-negative organisms associated with occult bacteremia. Most fatal reactions are due to endotoxin reactions associated with gram-negative bacteria. Platelet concentrates contaminated with *Bacillus* species, *Escherichia coli*, *Klebsiella* species, *Staphylococcus aureus* and *S epidermidis*, *Serratia marcescens*, and *Streptococcus* species account for 85% of fatal reactions.[151] The bacterial dose in platelet concentrates leading to morbidity or mortality is not known precisely. Bacterial concentration of 10^8 CFU per mL resulted in fatalities.[152]

Immediate recognition of a septic reaction, followed by prompt discontinuation of the transfusion, and antibiotic administration form the mainstay of therapy. Prevention relies on careful donor selection, and scrupulous adherence to aseptic techniques and precautions from component collection, processing, transport and storage to transfusion at the bedside. Better prevention of bacterial contamination may be achieved by newly introduced skin disinfection solutions and diversion and discard of the first 15–30 mL of collected blood. These methods alone or in combination may reduce the bacterial load in skin fragments trapped in the phlebotomy needle that subsequently enter blood storage containers.[153,154]

In addition to precautionary measures to minimize bacterial contamination of blood products, screening for and interdiction of affected units is now in place for whole blood derived and apheresis platelets. Both culture-based methods and alternative approaches, such as microscopic examination of stained platelet smears, detection of decrease in pH and glucose associated with bacterial growth, and visual assessment for loss of "swirling," which describes the normal shimmering light reflection of platelets bags when viewed against a light source, have been applied to screening. Culture-based methods are more sensitive and reliable than surrogate tests but require time for bacterial growth to occur. Depending on the system used, contamination rates from 1 to 500 bacterial CFU/mL are generally detected 24 hours after inoculation of the culture media.[153] It should be noted, however, that bacteria grow at variable rates.[151] *Staphylococcus epidermidis* grows slowly and *Propionibacterium acnes* requires, on average, 69 hours for detection. Despite excellent sensitivity some slow-growing bacteria, which nevertheless can cause significant reactions, will be missed with the usual approach of platelet release after the first 12 to 24 hours of incubation, if the cultured sample shows no growth. As culturing generally continues until the expiration date of the platelet unit or detection of growth, there is further opportunity to intercept released platelets that have not been transfused or alert physicians about the potential risk of bacterial contamination in cases where the units were already administered.

Non-culture methods for detecting bacteria in platelet units allow rapid testing just before transfusion, that is, at a time point when assessment for bacterial contamination is most relevant and has the greatest chance to identify a significant bacterial concentration. Current tests defect 10^{4-6} CFU/mL, and are used as an adjunct point of care test for platelets tested by bacterial culture. Visual inspection for discoloration or loss of swirling is subjective and performs poorly. Gram staining and multireagent strip testing generally require bacterial contamination levels of at least 10^6 CFU/mL, a threshold that may not reliably detect all platelet units that have the potential to cause septic reactions.[153] In addition, the latter test can be expected to have a 1% false-positive rate, which translates into substantial product wasting. Future nucleic acid-based nonculture methods currently under development promise to be more sensitive and specific, which would make them a more suitable alternative to culture methods.

Prior to the mid-1980s, platelet concentrates were stored for 7 days. Following reports of septic reactions, the shelf-life was reduced to 5 days to decrease the interval during which bacteria could proliferate. Methods for detecting and interdicting contaminated platelets may permit return to a 7-day storage interval, with the benefits of decreasing outdating and increasing availability of this component with limited shelf-life. In the United States, blood suppliers briefly distributed platelets with a 7-day shelf life following enrollment in an FDA-mandated postmarket surveillance (PASSPORT) study that included testing for bacterial contamination by a sensitive culture method.[155] Initial experience suggested that extended platelet storage coupled with bacterial testing substantially decreased platelet loss from outdating, but some platelet products with negative bacterial cultures obtained 24 hours postcollection had bacterial growth when tested 7 days later, leading to discontinuation of 7 day storage.

SPIROCHETE INFECTIONS

Syphilis

No cases of transfusion-associated syphilis (*Treponema pallidum*) infections have been reported in the United States in the past 4 decades. Donor selection changes, uniform serologic testing, lack of spirochete viability in blood stored at refrigerated temperatures, decreases in the rate of primary syphilis, and widespread antibiotic usage either alone or in combination contributed to this successful outcome.[156–159] Currently, most blood collection agencies use an automated test for detecting treponemal antibodies. Approximately 50% of donors with confirmed positive test results, have evidence of a treated syphilis infection.[157] Persistent false-positive reactions occur in patients with hepatitis, mononucleosis, viral pneumonia, chicken pox, measles, immunizations, or pregnancy. Donations with reactive syphilis tests are discarded unless nonreactive in a confirmatory test. Blood centers defer donors with positive confirmatory tests for 1 year and then restore donor eligibility provided the donor underwent adequate syphilis treatment and has a negative non-treponemal serologic test result.[158]

Lyme Disease

The *Borrelia burgdorferi* spirochete causes Lyme disease, the most frequently occurring tick-borne infection in North America and Europe.[160] *Ixodes scapularis*, the black-legged tick, transmits *B burgdorferi* in the northwestern and north-central parts of the United States, and *I pacificus*, the western black-legged tick, transmits the infection along the Pacific coast. The ticks feed predominantly in late spring and early summer during the nymphal stage whose bites are associated predominately with transmission to humans. Deer are not infected; rather they transport and maintain the ticks.

B burgdorferi spirochetemia occurs in 44% of patients with Lyme disease and peaks 7 to 10 days post–tick bite. The spirochete survives routine red cell and frozen plasma storage for up to 45 days and in platelets for 6 days. Transfusion transmission of *B burgdorferi* has been demonstrated in a murine model.[161-164] Despite these observations, no human transfusion-associated cases have been reported. This may reflect the relatively short spirochetemia phase and deferral of donors with fever, headache, malaise, myalgia, arthralgia, Bell Palsy or rash that occurs 3 to 30 days after exposure. Individuals with a history of Lyme disease are accepted as blood donors 12 months following treatment and resolution of symptoms.

Other Tick-Borne Pathogens

The rickettsial agents, human monocytic ehrlichiosis (HME) and human granulocytic anaplasmosis (HGA), formerly human granulocytic ehrlichiosis, are intracellular organisms that survive in stored blood. *Ehrlichia chaffeensis* causes HME and is transmitted to humans through Lone Star tick bites (*Amblyomma americanum*).[161,165] Most cases occur in the south-central and southeastern United States. *Anaplasma phagocytophilum* causes HGA and occurs predominately in the northeastern, upper Midwestern areas of the United States. *I scapularis* or *I pacificus* ticks transmit the organism. Coinfection with the agents of Lyme disease, babesiosis, HGA have occurred. In a murine study, coinfection with *A phagocytophilum* and *B burgdorferi* result in decreased antibody response to the former but not the latter.[166] Symptoms include fever, chills, and headache often associated with thrombocytopenia, leukopenia, and increased liver enzymes.[160] Intracellular aggregates appear in monocytes in the HME and inclusions appear in granulocytes in HGA. Seroprevalence studies in blood donors in Wisconsin and Connecticut report 0.5% to 3.5% seropositivity for *A phagocytophilum* antibodies.[165]

One case of transfusion-associated HE occurred 9 days after an RBC transfusion donated by an asymptomatic donor exposed to deer ticks 2 months previously. The RBCs had been stored for 30 days prior to transfusion.[167] Leukocyte reduction does not completely remove *E chaffeensis*.[168]

In a study involving military recruits in Arkansas who had been exposed to tick bites and unknowingly infected with *E chaffeensis* and *Rickettsia rickettsii*, the agent of Rocky Mountain Spotted Fever (RMSP), no clinical illness occurred in recipients. One possible RMSP seroconversion was reported.[169] A case report of transfusion-associated RMSP involved a donor developing symptoms 3 days postdonation. The recipient developed symptoms 6 days posttransfusion.

Other tick-borne agents implicated in transfusion include Colorado tick fever virus and tick-borne encephalitis virus.

PARASITIC INFECTIONS

Malaria

Four plasmodium species (*P falciparum*, *P vivax*, *P ovale*, and *P malariae*) cause the protozoan disease, malaria. Up to 150 million cases occur worldwide annually, with most occurring in sub-Saharan Africa. Other endemic areas include parts of Asia and Central and South America. Local, mosquito-borne transmission occurred in the United States in 2003 in Palm Beach County, Florida in which seven persons were infected.[170] Of 1,066 imported cases in civilian travelers in 2003, 561 traveled to Africa, 109 to Asia/Western Pacific, 59 to Central America/Caribbean, 21 to South America, and only 6 from Mexico.[171] Transmission occurs through the bite of an infected female Anopheles mosquito and, rarely, transfusion or congenitally. Anopheles mosquitoes generally feed between dawn and dusk thereby limiting the risk to travelers who usually visit malaria areas during daylight hours.

In nonendemic countries, transfusion-associated malaria risk arises from semiimmune blood donors. Such persons are asymptomatic despite high titer antimalaria antibodies and low-level malaria parasitemia. Those donors without malarial immunity who travel to endemic areas and became infected, generally, are symptomatic when they are parasitemic and would not be accepted as blood donors.

Between 1979 and 1986 most malaria cases in the United States occurred among foreign civilians rather than US civilians. Currently, most cases occur in US civilians, reflecting increased travel and reduced immigration. Transfusion-associated malaria cases occur infrequently, approximately once per 4 million transfusions.[172] Through 2003, 95 transfusion-associated malaria episodes or 2.5 per year were reported. *P falciparum* accounted for 36% of the cases, *P malariae* for 28%, *P vivax* for 27%, *P ovale* for 5% with the remainder unknown or mixed species. *P falciparum* cases increased in frequency between 1990 and 2003, accounting for 73% of the cases compared to 24% of the cases between 1970 and 1989.

The incubation period for transfusion-associated malaria ranges between 8 and 90 days. *P falciparum* has the shortest time, mean 17 days (range 8 to 36 days) and *P malariae* the longest, mean 51 days (range 8 to 90 days).[172] Among the cases reported, 94% were associated with RBC or whole blood and 6% with platelets. Foreign-born donors accounted for 60% (64% from Africa). Transmission from fresh frozen plasma has not been reported.

The current strategies for reducing the low risk of transfusion transmission in the United States involve deferral of donors who have traveled to malarious endemic regions during the previous 12 months; who have a history of malaria within the previous 3 years, and who emigrated from a malarial area or revisited that area within the previous 3 years. Some residual risk remains because transfusion transmission of *P falciparum*, *P vivax*, and *P ovale* has been reported 5, 2.5, and 7 years, respectively, after departing malarious areas.[172] In contrast, under the current policy, approximately 1% of US blood donors are deferred because of travel to malarious areas, of which nearly 40% traveled to Mexico, where only 6 of the more than 1000 imported cases originated.

To create a more approximate balance between geographic deferral and actual risk of malaria infection, various strategies are under discussion. These include antibody testing (which identifies the 1.5% to 3% of infected travelers), malaria antigen detection, and nucleic acid testing. The sensitivity of the latter may be insufficient, 0.004 parasites per μL (or 200 parasites per mL whole blood) because a dose of 100 parasites transmits infection.[173]

Babesia

Babesia microti, a piroplasm protozoan, causes the rodent-borne zoonosis babesiosis. The deer or black-legged tick *I scapularis* transmits this organism following 48 hours or more of feeding. In addition, these ticks transmit *B burgdorferi* and ehrlichiosis agents. *Peromyscus leucopus*, or the white footed mouse, serves as the natural reservoir. *B. microti* is the agent most frequently associated with babesiosis, but MO-1, WA-1, CA-1 and B. divergens also cause clinical disease. Infections often go unrecognized.

Parasitemia persists for an average 82 days in asymptomatic patients but chronic carrier states have been identified.[174,175] *Babesia* has been found by polymerase chain reaction in approximately one-half of seropositive blood donors.[176,177] In asplenic patients, intraerythrocyte parasitemic levels can approach 85% resulting in severe, life-threatening anemia.

Endemic areas include coastal and island areas of New England and New York as well as parts of California, Washington, Missouri, Wisconsin, and Minnesota.[165,176,178–180] Seroprevalence in blood donors varies and recently was found in 1.4% of blood donors in endemic areas of Connecticut.[177] At least 70 cases of transfusion-associated Babesia infections have been reported in the endemic and nonendemic regions of the United States. The parasite retains infectivity in red cell components at refrigerated or frozen temperatures and in residual RBCs contained in platelet concentrates stored at room temperature. The intraerythrocytic location of *B microti* favors transfusion transmission of this agent over *B burgdorferi*.[178] Transfusion-acquired cases occur 1 to 9 weeks following transfusion.[181] Based on studies in an endemic region where more than 1% of blood donors are seropositive for *B microti* infection the risk of acquiring *B microti* infection from an RBC transfusion was 1 in 1800 and for platelets 0 in 371.[181] The diagnosis is made by examining blood smears for intraerythrocytic ring forms, maltese cross-like tetrads, antibabesial antidotes and PCR assays for babesial DNA.[175,182] Treatment includes clindamycin or guinine or other antimicrobials. In severe cases, clinicians perform exchange transfusions especially in splenectomized patients.[181]

Currently, no specific strategies exist to prevent transfusion-associated babesia cases. Hence, clinical awareness and prompt antibiotic therapy serve as the primary treatment modalities. Questioning donors about tick exposure or tick bite has a low predictive value[165] and serologic or PCR testing await availability. All prospective blood donors are asked about prior Babesia infections and those answering affirmatively are deferred.

Leishmaniasis

Phlebotomine sand fly bites transmit Leishmania infections to humans. In addition, transplacental, sexual, and transfusion transmission occurs. The promastigote form of the parasite resides in the gastrointestinal tract of sand flies and is injected into humans through a skin bite. In humans, promastigotes are phagocytosed by monocytes and transformed into amastigotes. The latter then reproduce and reside in macrophages and the reticuloendothelial system. Organisms present within monocytes and free amastigotes that are released during refrigerated storage temperatures that transform into promastigotes and remain extracellularly are involved in transfusion transmission. *L tropica* survives also in monocytes contained in frozen red cell preparations and in platelet concentrates stored at room temperature. However, *L tropica* has not been found in cell-free plasma.[183]

At least 10 cases of transfusion-associated leishmaniasis attributed to *L donovani* have been reported in endemic areas, mostly in young children or neonates. A probable case of platelet transfusion-transmitted *L donovani* was reported in India. Several animal model studies demonstrate transmission by blood transfusion.[184,185]

Following reports of *L. tropica*-related viscerotropic leishmaniasis in veterans of the Persian Gulf Operation Desert Storm conflict between August 1990 and December 1992, those serving in this theater of operations were deferred from blood donation for 1 year. The deferral period reflected the development of fever, malaise, abdominal pain, and intermittent diarrhea that occurred up to 7 months following return to the United States. *L tropica* was found in the bone marrow of 7 patients and in the lymph node in one. Intracellular amastigotes were seen in the peripheral blood of the one patient in whom this was studied.[186] Following reports of cutaneous and visceral leishmaniasis in troops involved in the Afghanistan and Iraq wars, a similar 1-year deferral following departure from Iraq was instituted in October 2003.[187] Those with skin infections are deferred permanently. Questions have been raised about extending the deferral period.[188] Desert Storm occurred during a season when sand flies are inactive compared to the much longer exposure time for troops stationed in Afghanistan and Iraq where infections with *L tropica* and *L major* predominate, but where *L donovani* is also present. Asymptomatic infections occur frequently in healthy donors and organisms may circulate in peripheral blood more than 1 year following exposure. Foxhounds infected with Leishmania species have been found in 18 states and 2 Canadian provinces. Transmission occurred only among dogs.[189] The possibility of transmission to humans and the increased number of military personnel returning from Iraq raise concerns of future transfusion transmission.

To date, there are no cases of transfusion-transmitted Leishmaniasis in the United States. The widespread use of leukocyte-reduction filters, may have a beneficial role because these filters reduce both intracellular and extracellular parasite contaminations by 3 to 4 logs.[183,190] Awareness of potential transfusion transmission and surveillance remain important mechanisms for determining the transfusion risk.

Toxoplasmosis

Toxoplasmosis is caused by the intracellular protozoal parasite *Toxoplasma gondii*, whose usual host is the domestic cat. The parasite is transmitted by infected cats or soiled cat litter and by eating raw or undercooked pork, goat, lamb, beef, or wild game. Approximately 20% to 25% of the US population has evidence of infection. Transfusion-associated disease has been described in immunocompromised patients.[191–193]

Chagas Disease

American trypanosomiasis, or Chagas disease, consists of an acute phase that varies from no symptoms to manifestations that may include fever, skin rash, conjunctivitis with palpebral edema, lymphadenopathy, and hepatosplenomegaly. The acute phase usually resolves in 4 to 8 weeks unless severe myocarditis or meningoencephalitis intervenes. The latter is associated with fatal outcomes. Following a latent stage of undetermined duration, the chronic phase occurs in up to 30% to 40% of infected patients, manifesting as cardiac disease, megacolon, or achalasia.[194–197]

The flagellate protozoal parasite *T cruzi* causes Chagas disease. The disorder is widespread in Latin America. Humans become infected when bitten by *T cruzi*-infected insects of the Reduviidae family.[198,199] Once infection occurs, low-level parasitemia usually persists for life; treatment is effective in eradicating the parasite only when rendered during the initial acute stage.[194–201] Vector transmission is unlikely in the United States, but 50,000 to 100,000 infected Latin American immigrants reside in the United States.[194] The organisms remain viable in whole blood stored at refrigerator temperatures for 18 days, for longer than 8 months in citrated blood samples stored at room temperature, and following freezing and thawing. In South America, approximately 13% to 49% of recipients of parasitemic blood become infected. There is concern that additional transfusion-associated Chagas disease cases will occur as immigration increases to the United States from Central and South America.[194–199,202,203]

Risk factors for *T cruzi* infection include birth or residence in endemic regions such as Central America, South America, or Southeastern Mexico; living in dwellings with palm leaf-thatched roofs or mud walls, where vector insects reside; oral intake of contaminated foodstuff; and a history of receiving a blood transfusion in Latin America.[194–198,201,204] Among donors who lived in poor housing or received a blood transfusion in endemic areas, 3% to 4% had *T cruzi* antibodies.[205] One study, conducted in California, found that 1/340 donors had a risk factor for Chagas disease.[206] A large survey conducted from 1994 to 1998 in Los Angeles and Miami among immigrant blood donors from endemic areas observed *T cruzi* seroprevalence rates of 1/7500 and 1/9000, respectively.[202] The risk of transmission of *T cruzi* infection from these donors remains unclear, however, as none of the 18 recipients in the survey who received blood from a seropositive donor, and who were available for testing, had evidence of infection.

Some studies have estimated the transmission rate per infected blood unit to be approximately 18%. A recently reported lookback study involving blood donations in Mexico made prior to determining the donors were *T cruzi* seropositive found four of nine recipients of subsequently determined seropositive whole blood or platelets to be seropositive.[208] Lifelong low-grade parasitemia persist in approximately 50% of those infected and 13% to 63% of those seropositive have been found parasitemic.[196,207]

Since 1987, seven cases of transfusion-associated Chagas disease have been reported in the United States and Canada and symptoms developed 2 to 3 months' posttransfusion.[209–214] In at least six cases, platelets were the implicated component; the unit in the seventh case was not identified. *T cruzi* may separate with platelets or room-temperature storage may favor parasite survival, although *T cruzi* survives 18 to 21 days in refrigerated RBCs.[197] In each of the 6 cases, the implicated donor emigrated from a *T cruzi* endemic region (Bolivia, Mexico, Paraguay, Chile) between 16 to 33 years before the implicated donation. In addition, acute Chagas' disease has been reported in organ transplant recipients.[215,216]

The increasing prevalence of *T cruzi*-infected blood donors, the reports of transfusion-associated cases in the United States, and some autochthonous cases,[217] have triggered efforts to mitigate the risk of transfusion transmitted Chagas disease. Questioning donors about geographic location of birth or extended stay or transfusion in Chagas endemic areas interdicts 75% of donors. However, implementing this approach without a testing protocol has a high degree of nonspecificity causing unnecessary donor deferrals.[197,206,208,218] Leukocyte reduction by filtration decreases *T cruzi* transmission in a mouse model by 50% to 70%.[219]

Serologic testing, under development for many years achieved FDA licensure as a blood donor screening test in December 2006. The approved assay uses a *T cruzi* epimastigote lysate.[220] Another assay based on chimeric recombinant antigens is undergoing clinical trials.[221] These sensitive and specific assays were predicted to remove approximate 600 potentially *T cruzi*-infected blood components annually in the United States. Initial testing results show this 1 per 30,000 donors test positive, but none of more than 50 lookback cases showed serologic evidence of infection. Long-term serologic testing strategies remain under consideration. For example, testing each donor once or twice, recording the results, and retesting only if potential risk exposure occurs. Plasma used for derivative manufacturing undergoes pathogen inactivation procedures that have demonstrated activity against *T cruzi*. Methylene blue and visible illumination reduce *T cruzi* viability in plasma intended for direct transfusion.[222,223]

CLASSIC AND VARIANT CREUTZFELDT–JAKOB DISEASE

Classical Creutzfeldt–Jakob disease (CJD) is a rare, fatal, degenerative neurologic disease with a long asymptomatic latent period that was first described in 1920. The etiologic agent of CJD is thought by most experts to be a prion protein (PrPsc), an abnormal conformation of a normal cellular protein (PrPc) that can induce conformational transformation (recruitment) of additional PrPc to PrPsc, resulting in deposition of insoluble precipitates in neural tissue and progressive dementia.[224,225] CJD is one of a variety of prion diseases of humans that occur spontaneously at a rate of approximately 1 per million throughout the world, or can be transmitted vertically in familial conditions such as Gerstmann Straussler Scheinker syndrome or horizontally through ritualistic cannibalism (Kuru).

There are no reported cases of transmission of classical CJD by blood transfusion. Nevertheless, as a result of the long incubation phase of the disease (as demonstrated from growth hormone transmissions), concern arose in the mid-1990s that CJD transmission could occur from asymptomatic donors to blood transfusion recipients.[226] This theoretical risk led to the establishment of enhanced donor deferral policies (based on iatrogenic exposure or family history of the disease) for potential CJD carriers. Several recent epidemiologic studies have confirmed earlier studies in failing to establish a link between transfusion and transmission of CJD.[227,228] Although still regarded as a theoretical risk, there is an emerging consensus that classical CJD is not transmitted by transfusion.

Like classical CJD, variant (vCJD) is a fatal, degenerative neurologic disease, although it occurs in younger persons and has distinctive clinical, histopathologic, and biochemical features. In contrast to classical CJD, vCJD disease is new, with the first reports from the United Kingdom (UK) occurring in 1996.[229] The etiologic agent of vCJD, a prion, is the same agent that causes bovine spongiform encephalopathy (BSE). The outbreak of vCJD in the United Kingdom followed a massive epidemic of BSE in the 1980s and 90s that was traced to the recycling and processing of material (offal) from dead sheep and cattle into food meal for cattle. After this practice was banned in 1988, the outbreak eventually subsided after reaching a peak in the early 1990s. Transmission of the BSE prions to humans occurred by oral consumption of beef and other cattle products containing reticular endothelial or neural tissue. The number of new vCJD diagnoses in the United Kingdom rose steadily in the first few years after 1995 from 3 to 28 cases annually in 2000 but has decreased since then to 5 cases in 2005 and 3 in 2006. At the end of December 2006, 162 definite or probable cases of vCJD have been reported in the United Kingdom.[230] An additional 36 cases originated elsewhere, mostly in France and several other European countries, but a few cases were identified outside Europe, including 3 cases in the United States and 1 each in Canada, Japan, and Saudi Arabia. Several but not all of the patients in the latter category had spent more than 6 months in the United Kingdom between 1980 and 1996, that is, during the BSE epidemic in Britain. Although it appears that the vCJD outbreak is resolving and has been much smaller than initially feared, concern persists that there could be a second larger wave of the epidemic because of delayed onset of the disease in an affected population that is currently asymptomatic but harbors abnormal prion proteins. This is based in part on observing abnormal prion protein accumulation in random surgical tissue samples in the United Kingdom, which may represent preclinical vCJD disease. In one retrospective study, 3 of 12,674 (approximately 1 in 3500) appendectomy and tonsillectomy specimens from persons aged 20 to 29 showed this finding.[231] Furthermore, a critical polymorphism at codon 129 of the normal prion protein coding for methionine or valine leads to significant variation in the susceptibility to, and incubation period of, human prion diseases.[232] As only 37% of the general British population is homozygous for methionine, and therefore most susceptible, a larger population (52%) of heterozygotes may still be in the latent stage of the disease.

On the basis of findings in animal models which suggested that blood and its components could be infectious via transfusion,[233–235] and the observation that initially all known cases of vCJD could be traced to time spent in the United Kingdom, a policy was adopted in 1999 of indefinite deferral of persons who spent more than 6 months in the United Kingdom from 1980 to 1996.[236] The prediction was that this would reduce the number of donors potentially infected with vCJD by approximately 70% and would result in the deferral of approximately 2.5% of otherwise eligible donors. Following discovery of vCJD cases in continental Europe, the deferral policy was later revised to include donors if they had spent more than 3 months in the United Kingdom or 5 years in Europe since 1980.[236]

As of 2006, four probable cases of transfusion-transmitted vCJD have been reported in the United Kingdom, meaning that they could have developed vCJD independent of transfusion, but this possibility is regarded highly unlikely based on epidemiologic considerations.[228] Three of the four cases were diagnosed 6.5, 7.8, and 9 years after receiving non–leukocyte-reduced red blood cells or a blood component from two different donors who developed clinical symptoms of vCJD 40 and 21 months after donating. In the other case, the recipient of non–leukocyte-reduced red cells had no clinical symptoms of vCJD but showed abnormal prion proteins in lymphoid (but not neural) tissues postmortem and was therefore considered to be in a preclinical stage of the disease. Five years before his death from unrelated causes he had received non–leukocyte-reduced red blood cells from a donor who showed clinical symptoms of vCJD infection 18 months after donating. These four cases represent 6% of the total population of 66 UK recipients who received blood components from 18 different donors subsequently diagnosed with vCJD. No further cases of probable transfusion-transmitted vCJD have been identified in this cohort or anywhere else so far (as of January 2007, 23 of the 66 UK recipients were alive and could still develop clinical disease later on). It is not possible to derive general predictions on vCJD risk associated with blood transfusion from the UK experience but prion transmissibility by transfusion leading to clinical disease cannot be regarded a mere theoretical consideration anymore. As there are no blood donor screening tests for vCJD, development of suitable pathogen reduction or inactivation methods (PRIMs), in case of prevention of prion transmission most likely a filtration-based approach,[123] holds the greatest promise for protection from transfusion-transmitted prion diseases (see box on PRIMs).

POTENTIAL EMERGING INFECTIONS

Simian Foamy Virus and Other Non-Human Primate Retroviruses

The pandemic human retroviruses, HIV-1/2 and HTLV-I/II, were each the result of multiple independent introductions of viruses from nonhuman primates (NHPs). A series of recent findings focused on populations exposed to NHPs has demonstrated that transmission of retroviruses from NHPs to humans is a regular and ongoing phenomenon.[237–246] These results show that three new retroviruses previously undocumented in humans, including the simian foamy viruses (SFVs), HTLV-3, and HTLV-4, have all been identified in persons exposed to NHPs,[240–246] which has raised concern over risks to the safety of the blood supply.

SFVs are of particular concern because these are widespread retroviruses among Old and New World monkeys, apes, and prosimians.[247] SFV infects more than 70% of captive adult NHPs, but does not appear to be associated with disease in any host species.[240,243,246] SFV is genetically diverse and has persisted in primates for more than 30 million years.[248] Humans are susceptible to infection with a variety of SFV subtypes from both monkey and ape species. Persistent cell-associated viremia has been found in infected persons.[240,243] SFV sequences can be consistently amplified from peripheral blood mononuclear cells (PBMNCs), and virus can be readily isolated from these cells.[240,243] SFVs have been found among humans exposed to NHPs in natural settings in Cameroon through hunting, butchering, and keeping wild NHP pets, suggesting that SFV may likely be prevalent among West and Central African populations who frequently hunt, butcher, and consume bushmeat.[241] SFV also has been found in persons occupationally exposed to captive NHPs in primate research facilities and zoos in North America and Europe.[240,243,244] A study of workers exposed to Asian macaques around religious temples in Indonesia reported one infected worker.[245] No disease has been seen in 14 infected primate workers in the United States.[240,243] The limited number of cases and potential selection biases inherent in studying a healthy worker cohort, however, limit the ability to identify potential disease associations in these studies.[240,243]

It is noteworthy that many of the SFV-infected primate workers have donated blood in the United States, and several were retrospectively confirmed to be SFV-infected at the time of their donation.[240,243] A retrospective study of recipients from an SFV-infected blood donor failed to identify evidence of infection in three recipients of red cells (one of whom received leukoreduced units, the other two did not) and one recipient of platelets.[249] Several recent reports by Khan and Kumar[250] and Brooks et al[251] provided direct evidence of SFV transmission by transfusion of whole blood into rhesus monkeys. Evidence of transfusion-transmitted infection included seroconversion, identification of SFV sequences in monkey PBMNCs, and isolation of infectious virus from PBMNCs.

In assessing the potential impact of an emerging infection like SFVs, one must examine person-to-person transmissibility, survival in blood products, measurable frequency in the population, availability of a blood screening test, and evidence of disease in infected individuals. For SVF, lack of documented disease associations and of sensitive and specific serologic assays, has led the US FDA to postpone consideration of deferral or screening of potential donors exposed to NHPs. In contrast, in Canada health authorities have recently recommended deferral from blood transfusion and cell, organ and tissue donation for those individuals who work directly with NHP in institutions such as zoos, public or private biomedical research institutions, and animal sanctuaries. This approach provides additional protection against unrecognized simian viruses other than SFV that may also be infecting these donors.[242,246,252]

Influenza Viruses

Influenza remains a major cause of morbidity and mortality in the United States and worldwide, particularly in the elderly and immunosuppressed populations. In years of high influenza activity, influenza incidence in pediatric populations range from 5% to 9.5% and weekly mortality incidence due to pneumonia and influenza can peak at over 10% of all cause mortality in the United States. The threat of pandemic influenza A has recently gained prominent attention with human cases of highly pathogenic avian influenza A (H5N1) detected in China, Southeast Asia, and more recently in Turkey and Africa.[253]

The threat that influenza poses to the blood supply remains largely unexplored. It has been assumed to be negligible based on the premise that asymptomatic donors will not be viremic and potential donors with symptomatic influenza infection (with or without viremia) will be deferred from donation. However, murine models suggest that viremia is transient and only present early in the disease course,[254] raising the possibility that significant numbers of blood donors harbor influenza viremia during a presymptomatic or asymptomatic phase. A human study of nasal challenge of volunteers with Asian influenza demonstrated viremia within 24 hours of challenge in 4 of 11 subjects, and 4 of 4 subjects tested with the most sensitive assay available at the time.[255] Viremia was cleared prior to the development of symptoms or nasal shedding of virus. During epidemic spread of influenza, a pre-symptomatic viremic phase could result in significant numbers of transmission events. Viremia during the symptomatic phase of influenza is rare,[256–258] and the frequency of viremia during presymptomatic or asymptomatic infection is unknown.

Quantifying the potential threat to the blood supply is particularly crucial in preparation for a predicted global influenza pandemic. A more virulent strain of influenza could result in higher blood viral loads and cause increased morbidity and mortality compared to circulating influenza A and B strains. This is even more relevant when one considers that highly pathogenic avian influenza H5N1 is a systemic disease.[259,260] A recent report suggests that infection with avian influenza among human populations exposed to sick birds may not be uncommon,[261] further underlining the need to study whether influenza A infection is associated with viremia.

If influenza infection resulted in a viremic phase prior to the onset of symptoms, it would have implications for blood safety. Because of their underlying health problems, blood product recipients would be expected to suffer increased morbidity and mortality secondary to influenza A infection compared to healthy donors. If influenza was transmissible by transfusion, testing of the blood supply could become particularly important during pandemic outbreak of highly pathogenic influenza A. Additional product discards (as a result of a positive test) would further endanger blood donation availability and such additional stress on the system would need to be taken into consideration when modeling the effect of a potential pandemic on the blood supply.

Detection of influenza in the blood presents a challenge owing to the lower viral loads found in blood compared to nasopharyngeal secretions. Red blood cell fractions may contain more influenza than plasma or white blood cell fractions because of the hemagglutinin moiety of influenza.[262] Both NAT-based and rapid antigen or neuraminidase detection tests have been developed to detect influenza A and B in recent years. Although NAT tests appear to have higher sensitivity than antigen or neuraminidase activity assays for nasopharyngeal samples, the relative abundance of viral RNA to influenza antigen or neuraminidase in the bloodstream of infected individuals has not been determined. Studies are now in progress to validate NAT and antigen assays for detection of influenza A in blood and to quantify the proportion of blood donors with detectable viremia and antigenemia during periods of high influenza activity.

Dengue

Dengue viruses, transmitted by Aedes mosquitoes, infected at least 96 US travelers in 2005, almost as many as occurred in the previous 5 years. Illness associated with infection ranges from no symptoms to fever, minor or major bleeding, thrombocytopenia, and increased vascular permeability manifest by hemoconcentration and pleural or abdominal effusions. The incubation period varies between 3 and 14 days. The travel destination of those infected included Mexico (44% of cases), Central America (26%), Caribbean (22%), and Asia (8%). No transfusion-associated cases occurred. However, the increased number of cases and reports of transmission by bone marrow transplantation and needle-stick injuries involving symptomatic patients raises the possibility of transfusion transmission by asymptomatic travelers returning from endemic areas.[263–267]

Severe Acute Respiratory Syndrome

A novel enveloped RNA coronavirus infected more than 1800 patients in 17 countries between February and March 2003 causing the Severe Acute Respiratory Syndrome. A two week asymptomatic incubation period fostered virus spread through close person-to-person contact and raised the possibility of blood-borne infection. For this reason blood collection agencies deferred anyone from donating blood for at least 14 days after possible exposure to SARS and those with illness for at least 28 days after recovery.[268,269] The epidemic subsided within months and no transfusion-associated SARS cases occurred.

Lymphocytic Choriomeningitis

Organ transplantation-associated lymphocytic choriomeningitis virus (LCMV) infection occurred in two clusters involving two donors and eight transplant recipients. Seven of the eight recipients died. Transmission of LCMV, a rodent-borne arena-virus occurs through contact with pet rodents, mice, and hamsters. The transplant-related cases represent the first person-to-person transmission other than vertical transmission during pregnancy. Serologic surveys indicate that up to 5% of US adults have evidence of LCMV infection. Viremia has been documented in mice and humans. In light of other pathogen transmission by both organ transplantation and transfusion, for example, West Nile Virus, *T cruzi*, rabies, the future possibility of LCMV transmission by blood transfusion remains a possibility.[270,271]

Rabies

The Rabies virus is not transmitted hematologically. Contact with blood, urine, or feces is not considered an exposure risk. However, an organ donor infected via a bat bite transmitted rabies to the liver and the two kidney recipients.[272] The transmission occurred presumably through exposure to infected neuronal tissue.

CONCLUSION

Progress in testing technologies continues to decrease the residual risk of transmitting known pathogens through transfusion. Additional efforts, such as pathogen reduction and improved donor screening for pathogens, should provide further benefit. The emergence of newly discovered pathogens and wider geographic spread of known pathogens through emigration and commercial globalization, however, will create pressure for additional interventions. Unfortunately, all of these approaches increase costs and conflict with the simultaneous, ongoing interest in controlling medical care costs.

As such, global surveillance and public health measures, not priority issues previously, take on greater significance not only for public health in general but also for reducing the risk of transfusion-transmitted infections.

SUGGESTED READINGS

Brooks JI, Merks HW, Fournier J, et al: Characterization of blood-borne transmission of simian foamy virus. Transfusion 47:162, 2007.

Busch MP, Glynn SA, Stramer SL, et al, for the NHLBI-REDS NAT Study Group: A new strategy for estimating risks of transfusion-transmitted viral infections based on rates of detection of recently infected donors. Transfusion 45:254, 2005.

Busch MP, Caglioti S, Robertson EF, et al: Screening the blood supply for West Nile Virus RNA by nucleic amplification testing. N Engl J Med 353:460, 2005.

Cardo LJ: Leishmania: Risk to the blood supply. Transfusion 46:1641, 2006.

Cervia JS, Sowemimo-Coker SO, Ortolano GA, et al: An overview of prion biology and the role of blood filtration in reducing the risk of transfusion-transmitted variant Creutzfeldt-Jakob disease. Transfus Med Rev 20(3):190, 2006.

Fryer JF, Delwart E, Hecht FM, et al: Frequent detection of the parvovirus, PARV4 and PARV5, in plasma from blood donors and symptomatic individuals. Transfusion; 47:1054, 2007.

Hewitt PE, Llewelyn CA, Mackenzie J, Will RG: Creutzfeldt-Jakob disease and blood transfusion: Results of the UK Transfusion Medicine Epidemiological Review study. Vox Sang 91(3):221, 2006.

Hladik W, Dollard SC, Mermin J, et al: Transmission of human herpesvirus 8 by blood transfusion. N Engl J Med 355(13):1331, 2006.

Hollinger FB: Hepatitis B virus infection and transfusion medicine: science and the occult. Transfusion 48:1001, 2008.

Kitchen AD, Chiodini PL: Malaria and blood transfusion. Vox Sang 90:77, 2006.

Kleinman SH, Kamel HT, et al: Two-year experience with aerobic culturing of apheresis and whole blood-derived platelets. Transfusion 46(10):1787, 2006.

Leiby DA: Babesiosis and blood transfusion: Flying under the radar. Vox Sang 90:157, 2006.

Stramer SL, Glynn SA, Kleinman SH, et al, for the National Heart, Lung, and Blood Institute Nucleic Acid Test Study Group: Detection of HIV-1 and HCV infections among antibody-negative blood donors by nucleic acid amplification testing. N Engl J Med 351:760, 2004.

Tobler LH, Contestable P, Pitina L, et al: Evaluation of a new ELISA for detection of Chagas' antibody in U.S. blood donors. Transfusion 47:90, 2007.

Vamvakas EC: Is white blood cell reduction equivalent to antibody screening in preventing transmission of cytomegalovirus by transfusion? A review of the literature and meta-analysis. Transfus Med Rev 19(3):181, 2005.

REFERENCES

For complete list of references log onto www.expertconsult.com

CHAPTER 155

TRANSFUSION MEDICINE IN HEMATOPOIETIC STEM CELL AND SOLID ORGAN TRANSPLANTATION

Richard M. Kaufman and Jerome Ritz

HEMATOPOIETIC STEM CELL TRANSPLANTATION

The array of hematopoietic stem cell transplantation (HSCT) approaches used to treat patients with malignant or nonmalignant diseases has continued to grow in complexity. In concert, the scope of transfusion medicine has expanded to support the development of novel hematopoietic stem cell therapies. Currently, hematopoietic stem cells are obtained from three sources: bone marrow (BM), mobilized peripheral blood stem cells (PBSCs), and umbilical cord blood (UCB). After harvesting, and before infusion into the patient, stem cell products undergo a variety of manipulations in the laboratory, ranging from simple processing (eg, red blood cell depletion, freezing) to sophisticated graft engineering (eg, T-cell depletion, retroviral transduction). Like conventional blood components, hematopoietic stem cell products are prepared in rigorously controlled environments using good manufacturing practices. Specific details of hematopoietic stem cell mobilization, collection, and processing are discussed elsewhere (see Chapter 146).

The focus of this section is on the unique issues involved with providing optimal transfusion support to the HSCT patient. After myeloablative conditioning and stem cell transplantation, there is a 1- to 4-week period of pancytopenia when patients require multiple RBC and platelet transfusions.[1–3] In general, the criteria for transfusion after HSCT mirror those of other clinical settings, but the magnitude of support required may be great. Frequent platelet transfusions are given to prevent bleeding, and as a result, alloimmunization and platelet refractoriness are important concerns. Switching of ABO blood groups occurs commonly in the allogeneic HSCT patient population, posing unique problems to the blood bank and transfusion service. Because HSCT patients are typically highly immunocompromised, strategies are needed to prevent transfusion-transmitted cytomegalovirus (CMV) disease and transfusion-associated graft-versus-host disease (TA-GVHD).

ENGRAFTMENT AND BLOOD COMPONENT SUPPORT AFTER HEMATOPOIETIC STEM CELL TRANSPLANTATION

The level of transfusion support required by a particular patient after HSCT is dictated largely by the kinetics of engraftment and subsequent hematopoietic reconstitution. A key parameter affecting the engraftment rate is the source of stem cells used (Fig. 155–1). In the 1990s, several randomized trials demonstrated the superiority of PBSC over BM-derived stem cells in terms of faster platelet and neutrophil recovery for patients undergoing autologous HSCT.[4–6] More rapid recovery using PBSC rather than BM was later documented in the allogeneic HSCT setting as well. On average, neutrophil recovery (neutrophil count >0.5 × 10^9/L) occurs 2 to 6 days earlier when PBSC versus BM is used as the source of stem cells. Similarly, platelet recovery (platelet count >20 × 10^9/L) occurs 5 to 8 days earlier after PBSC transplantation than after BMT.[7–11] One reason for the faster engraftment of PBSC products is that the cellular composition of PBSC and BM is very different. PBSC products contain approximately threefold more CD34$^+$ cells and 10-fold more mature T cells than BM products.[7]

There is a strong relationship between the CD34$^+$ cell dose administered and the speed of hematopoietic recovery.[12–17] Faster engraftment rates have translated into decreased blood component usage.[13,14] For example, Haas and colleagues[14] reported that autologous PBSC transplant patients given more than 2.5 × 10^6 CD34$^+$ cells/kg received significantly fewer platelet transfusions than patients receiving less than 2.5 × 10^6 CD34$^+$ cells/kg (median of 4 vs 13 platelet units). In addition to the higher numbers of CD34$^+$ cells in PBSC products, there are multiple qualitative factors that differ between PBSC- and BM-derived stem cells, including cell surface molecule expression, metabolic activity, clonogenicity, and cell cycle status.[18,19] What impact these factors have on engraftment remains incompletely understood.

Several clinical factors may affect the rate of hematopoietic recovery and transfusion requirements after HSCT. Accelerated platelet recovery has been associated with a higher pretransplantation platelet count and receiving a graft from a human leukocyte antigen (HLA)-identical sibling donor. Factors associated with delayed platelet recovery include prior radiation therapy, the presence of fever, hepatic venoocclusive disease, GVHD, and the use of posttransplantation granulocyte colony-stimulating factor (G-CSF) or granulocyte–macrophage colony-stimulating factor (GM-CSF).[24] The use of recombinant human erythropoietin (rHuEPO) has been shown to accelerate RBC recovery and decrease RBC transfusion requirements among allogeneic HSCT patients.[25–28] The particular conditioning regimen that is used also affects hematopoietic recovery. In particular, nonmyeloablative transplantation protocols predictably result in decreased transfusion requirements.[29]

Although PBSC products are the most commonly transplanted source of stem cells currently, the use of UCB transplants for both pediatric and adult recipients has continued to grow at a rapid pace.[20] One reason is that only approximately 30% of patients requiring HSCT have an HLA-matched related donor.[21] Precise HLA matching has been demonstrated to be significantly less important for UCB products versus BM or PBSC. Also, UCB transplants are associated with a lower rate of graft-versus-host disease (GVHD). A primary disadvantage of UCB is the lower CD34$^+$ cell content of these products. The currently accepted minimum cell dose for UCB transplant is 1.7 × 10^5 CD34$^+$ cells/kg or 2.5 × 10^7 nucleated cells/kg, about one order of magnitude lower than the threshold for PBSC or BM transplant.[20] The lower cell content of UCB has been linked to a higher rate of graft failure as well as slower hematopoietic recovery.[22,23] For this reason, UCB transplants using two (or sometimes more) grafts simultaneously are often performed, particularly in adult patients.

The growth in UCB banking has created the (potential) advantage of rapidly available grafts to patients requiring transplantation. The University of Minnesota, for example, has reported that the search for a UCB unit typically takes approximately 1 day, compared with 3 to 4 months for a PBSC or BMT donor.[20] It is possible that the ability to provide UCB grafts quickly will translate into better patient outcomes, but this has not been proven to date. UCB transplantation is a fairly new field, yet considerable efforts have already been made to standardize UCB banking practices. The FDA has driven the concept that all human cellular or tissue-derived therapies, regardless of source, need to fit into an established regulatory framework and must meet the same essential requirements for donor screening and

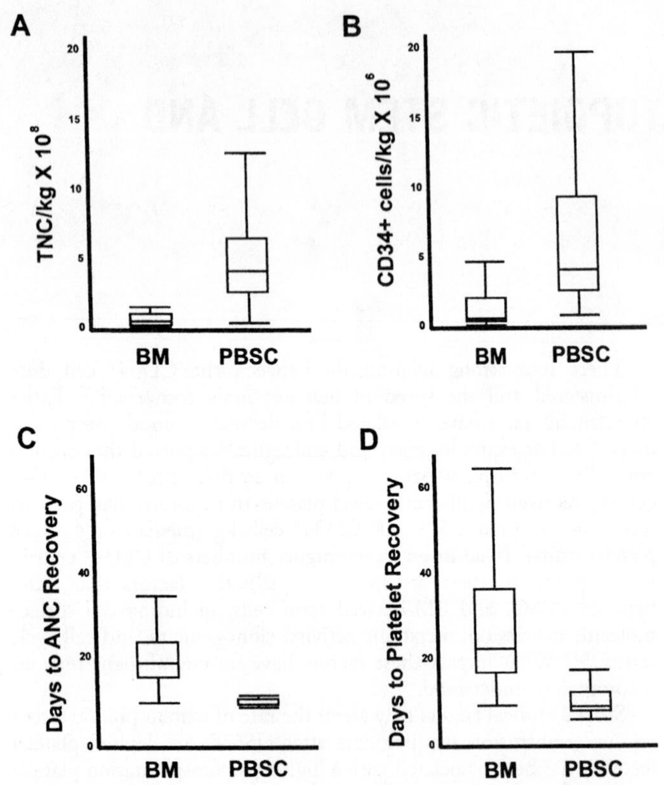

Figure 155–1 Comparison of peripheral blood stem cell (PBSC) products with bone marrow (BM). BM (n = 187) and PBSCs (n = 104) were collected from autologous donors at the Dana-Farber Cancer Institute and Brigham and Women's Hospital from 2000 through 2002. **A,** The total nucleated cell content (TNC/kg recipient weight) was significantly higher in PBSC products (median, 4.2×10^8 nucleated cells/kg) than in BM products (0.5×10^8 nucleated cells/kg). **B,** The $CD34^+$ cell content of PBSC products was also significantly higher compared with BM (median, 4.3×10^6 $CD34^+$ cells/kg versus 0.5×10^6 $CD34^+$ cells/kg). **C,** Reconstitution of neutrophils (absolute neutrophil count $>0.5 \times 10^9$/L) occurred more rapidly in recipients of PBSCs (median, 10 days) compared with BM (median, 18 days). **D,** Similarly, platelet recovery (platelet count $>20 \times 10^9$/L) was more rapid in PBSC recipients (median, 11 days versus 27 days for BM recipients). *(Courtesy of G. Kao, Dana-Farber Cancer Institute, Boston, MA.)*

good tissue practices.[23a] Two US accrediting agencies, the AABB and the Foundation for Accreditation of Cellular Therapy (FACT), have developed standards for collecting, testing, processing, and storing UCB samples, with the intent of ensuring the quality of UCB products provided.[23b]

ABO-INCOMPATIBLE HEMATOPOIETIC STEM CELL TRANSPLANTATION

In approximately 20% of allogeneic HSCT, ABO incompatibility exists between the donor and recipient.[30] ABO incompatibility is classified as major (the recipient has ABO antibody directed against donor RBCs), minor (the donor has ABO antibody directed against recipient RBCs), or both (major–minor). In most cases, the clinical impact of donor–recipient ABO incompatibility on HSCT is minimal. ABO incompatibility does not appear to affect overall patient survival, graft rejection, or GVHD.[31–33] Nevertheless, clinically significant hemolytic complications resulting from ABO incompatibility occasionally do occur.

In major ABO-incompatible HSCT (eg, group A donor → group O recipient), two types of hemolytic complications may be seen.

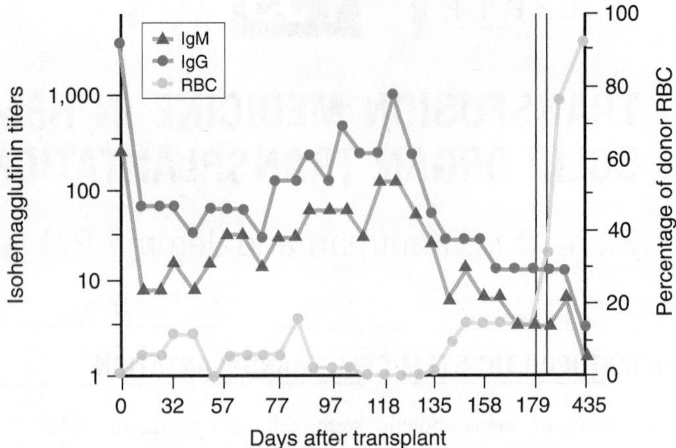

Figure 155–2 Delayed red blood cell (RBC) reconstitution in the recipient of a major ABO-incompatible stem cell transplant. The appearance of mature RBCs corresponded to declining anti-donor isoagglutinin titers. This patient remained RBC transfusion dependent for 12 months after transplantation. *(From Maciej Zaucha J, Mielcarek M, Takatu A, et al: Engraftment of early erythroid progenitors is not delayed after non-myeloablative major ABO-incompatible hematopoietic stem cell transplantation. Br J Haematol 119:740–750, 2002.)*

Immediately on infusion, mature donor RBCs contained within the stem cell product may be destroyed by preformed ABO antibody in the recipient. The usual practice is to reduce the volume of RBCs contaminating major ABO incompatible stem cell products to less than 10 mL. This manipulation effectively eliminates most immediate hemolytic reactions.

The second potential hemolytic complication of major ABO-incompatible HSCT is that recovery of the recipient's RBC counts may be delayed, in some cases dramatically (Fig. 155–2). This condition is a form of pure red cell aplasia (PRCA).[34] PRCA is characterized by peripheral blood reticulocytopenia and the absence of histologically detectable erythroid precursors in the bone marrow of the recipient. Peripheral-blood ABO antibody titers are characteristically elevated. Red cell transfusion dependence may last for several months after the recovery of platelets and granulocytes. Although red cell *reconstitution* is delayed in these cases, red cell *engraftment* is not. Using in vitro colony assays, the presence of early erythroid progenitors can be demonstrated in the bone marrow at the same time after transplantation as myeloid progenitors.[35] Early erythroid progenitors do not express ABO antigens and appear to survive normally in the bone marrow. On undergoing differentiation, the erythroid precursors begin expressing ABO antigens and are targeted by host ABO antibodies. It has been proposed that PRCA associated with major ABO-mismatched HSCT may be more likely to occur in the setting of nonmyeloablative SCT, because host hematopoiesis may be relatively preserved.[36] A higher PRCA rate in nonmyeloablative SCT has not been observed consistently,[35,37] perhaps because of differences in treatment regimens. The optimal therapy for PRCA after major ABO-incompatible HSCT has not been defined. Various treatment modalities used with variable success have included plasma exchange,[30,34] corticosteroids,[38] rHuEPO,[39,40] antithymocyte globulin,[41] donor lymphocyte infusion (DLI),[42] rituximab,[43] and discontinuation of cyclosporine.[36]

Minor ABO-incompatible HSCT (eg, group O donor → group A recipient) has been associated with immediate hemolysis from passively transfused donor ABO antibody and with delayed hemolysis caused by ABO antibodies produced by mature donor lymphocytes contained in the graft. Minor ABO incompatibility does not affect overall rates of graft rejection, GVHD, or patient survival.[31,33] Depletion of donor plasma in the graft generally eliminates the problem of immediate hemolysis caused by passively transfused ABO antibody. The more serious potential problem is the passenger lymphocyte

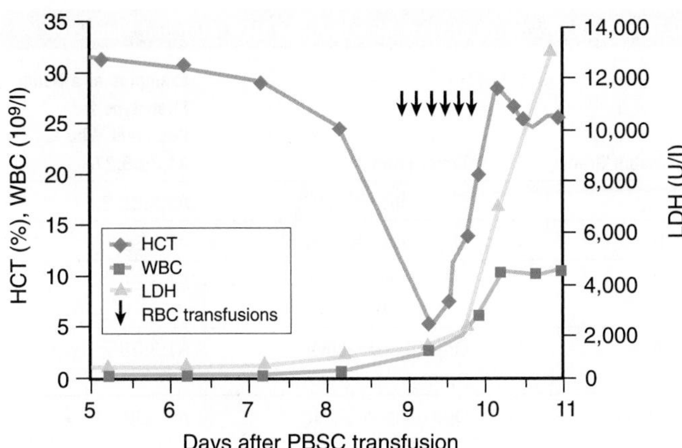

Figure 155–3 Severe hemolysis in the recipient of a minor ABO-incompatible stem cell transplant. Serologic testing revealed that donor-type anti-A isoagglutinins caused the hemolysis. *(From Bolan CD, Childs RW, Procter JL, et al: Massive immune haemolysis after allogeneic peripheral blood stem cell transplantation with minor ABO incompatibility. Br J Haematol 112:787, 2001.)*

Table 155–1 Examples of Transfusion Restrictions After ABO-Incompatible Hematopoietic Stem Cell Transplantation

ABO Type Recipient	ABO Type Donor	Type of Mismatch	Transfusion Restriction Red Blood Cell	Plasma
A	A	None	A or O	A or AB
A	O	Minor	O	A or AB
A	AB	Major	A or O	AB
A	B	Major/minor	O	AB

syndrome, whereby mature donor lymphocytes engraft in the host and produce anti-A or anti-B antibodies that bind to and cause the destruction of circulating host RBCs (Fig. 155–3). This complication typically occurs 1 to 3 weeks after transplantation and is heralded by a positive direct antiglobulin test (DAT) and a fall in hematocrit level. Rarely, hemolysis may be massive.[44] Standard practice is to transfuse group O or donor group RBCs to dilute the recipient red cells and to monitor patients closely for clinical and laboratory evidence of hemolysis. Exchange transfusion has been performed in this setting but is usually unnecessary.

Less is known about ABO incompatibility with respect to UCB transplantation versus PBSC transplantation or BMT. Recent case series, however, suggest that PRCA and other isoagglutinin-mediated potential adverse consequences of ABO-incompatible stem cell transplantation are far less likely to occur with UCB than with the other stem cell sources. Tomonari and colleagues, for example, reported zero cases of PRCA among 21 major and 18 major–minor ABO-mismatched UCB recipients. Zero of 29 recipients of minor ABO-incompatible UCB transplants developed immune hemolysis in their series.[44a] Similarly, Snell and colleagues[44b] reported that 0/14 minor ABO-incompatible UCB recipients developed immune hemolysis, compared with 14/25 contemporaneous patients who developed immune hemolysis after receiving a minor ABO-incompatible PBSC transplant.

The blood bank places specific RBC and plasma restrictions on patients undergoing ABO-incompatible HSCT (Table 155–1). RBCs are selected to be compatible with donor and recipient plasma, and plasma products are selected to be compatible with donor and recipient RBCs. These practices are begun on day 0 of HSCT or earlier if feasible. ABO antigens are widely expressed on endothelial tissues; HSCT recipients therefore may be considered ABO chimeras even after full RBC recovery.

PROPHYLACTIC PLATELET TRANSFUSIONS

Most platelet transfusions administered to cancer patients are given prophylactically rather than to control active bleeding. In the past, a platelet count of 20,000/mm^3 was generally used as a transfusion "trigger."[45,46] Later studies have supported the concept that prophylactic platelet transfusions can safely be provided using even lower platelet thresholds, with associated inventory and cost savings. In an observational study of acute leukemia patients, Gmur and colleagues[47] demonstrated that the platelet transfusion threshold could be set safely at 5,000/mm^3 for patients without fever or bleeding, and at 10,000/mm^3 for patients with such signs. Platelet transfusion triggers of 10,000/mm^3 versus 20,000/mm^3 were compared directly in two randomized, prospective studies of patients with acute leukemia.[48,49] Both of these studies and a third nonrandomized, prospective study[50] demonstrated no increased risk of bleeding when a trigger of 10,000/mm^3 was used. All of these trials included provisions for transfusing thrombocytopenic patients at higher platelet counts if associated risk factors for bleeding (eg, fever) were present. Relatively few studies have directly examined prophylactic platelet transfusion specifically in the setting of HSCT. Nevertheless, the 10,000/mm^3 trigger has been widely applied to the HSCT patient population, and it appears to be safe for patients lacking associated clinical factors (eg, infection, GVHD).[51,52] Frequently, these clinical factors are more important determinants of bleeding risk than the platelet count alone. Approximately two-thirds of bleeding events after HSCT occur in patients with platelet counts above 20,000/mm^3.[24,53]

The widespread use of a 10,000/mm^3 transfusion trigger is believed to have helped conserve the overall platelet supply. A complementary approach that is being studied currently is one of optimizing the dose of prophylactic platelets transfused. Most platelets undergo senescence after circulating for 8 to 10 days. But there is thought to be a second platelet clearance route: a small fixed daily loss of platelets that occurs independent of platelet age. Platelets leaving the circulation via this route (approximately 7.1×10^9 platelets/L/day) are hypothesized to help maintain vascular integrity.[55] In theory, a low dose of prophylactic platelets could meet this daily requirement, and using a low dose (eg, transfusing pools of 3 whole-blood derived platelet concentrates rather than the current 6) might yield considerable component savings over time.[56] A randomized controlled trial designed to empirically determine the optimal prophylactic platelet dose is being performed by the US Transfusion Medicine/Hemostasis Clinical Trials Network.[57] In this study, termed "PLADO" (PLAtelet DOsing), thrombocytopenic patients are randomized to receive either medium- (standard) (2.2×10^{11} platelets/m^2), low- (1.1×10^{11} platelets/m^2), or high-dose prophylactic platelets (4.4×10^{11} platelets/m^2). The primary end point is the percentage of patients with Grade 2 or higher bleeding in each arm. An interesting alternative approach, using therapeutic rather than prophylactic platelet transfusions, is being studied by Wandt and colleagues in Germany.[58]

ALLOIMMUNIZATION AND PLATELET REFRACTORINESS

Because HSCT patients typically receive large numbers of transfusions with cellular blood products, they are at risk to become alloimmunized to HLA antigens. Although graft failure associated with histocompatibility differences between donor and recipient is usually attributed to rejection by host T lymphocytes, host antibodies may also mediate graft failure by complement-mediated cytotoxicity or by antibody-dependent cell-mediated cytotoxicity.[59] To prevent graft failure and platelet refractoriness, it is important to prevent HLA alloimmunization in patients who are possible candidates for HSCT. In particular, blood transfusions from the potential stem cell donor

Table 155–2 Causes of Platelet Refractoriness

Patient Factor	Clinical Effects	Blood Bank
Alloimmunization	Fever	ABO match
Bone marrow transplantation	Sepsis	Platelet storage time
Gender	Splenomegaly	Platelet cross-match
Circulating IVIG	Clinical bleeding	HLA match
Transfusion number	RBC use DIC Neutropenia	

DIC, disseminated intravascular coagulation; HLA, human leukocyte antigen; IVIG, intravenous immunoglobulin G; RBC, red blood cell.

Adapted from Friedberg RC, Donnelly SF, Boyd JC, et al: Clinical and blood bank factors in the management of platelet refractoriness and alloimmunization. Blood 81:3428, 1993.

Table 155–3 Degree of HLA Matching for HLA-Matched Platelets

Match Grade	Description	Examples of a Donor Phenotype for Recipient Who Is A1,3;B8,27
A	Four antigen match	A1,3;B8,27
B	No mismatch present	A1,-;B8,27
B1U	One antigen blank or unknown	A1,3;B8,27
B1X	One cross-reactive group	A1,3;B8,7
B2UX	One antigen blank and one cross-reactive	A1,-;B8,7
C	One mismatched antigen	A1,3;B8,35
D	Two or more antigen mismatched	A1,32;B8,35

Data from Vengelen-Tyler V: Technical Manual, 12th ed. Bethesda, American Association of Blood Banks Press, 1996.

should be avoided because of the risk of sensitizing the patient to HLA and non-HLA antigens.

Platelet refractoriness may be defined as the failure to achieve an adequate platelet increment after two or more platelet transfusions (Table 155–2). A number of nonimmune factors have been linked to platelet refractoriness, including fever, sepsis, disseminated intravascular coagulation (DIC), drugs (eg, amphotericin), bleeding, splenomegaly, hepatic venoocclusive disease, and GVHD. In a subset of cases, platelet refractoriness is caused by alloimmunization. Platelets express HLA class I antigens, relatively low levels of ABO antigens, and several platelet-specific antigens. All of these molecules are potential targets of an immune response. Antibodies directed against HLA molecules are responsible for most cases of immune-mediated platelet refractoriness. Notably, less than half of all platelet-refractory patients have demonstrable antiplatelet or anti-HLA antibodies.[60,61] Platelet counts obtained at 10 minutes to 1 hour posttransfusion that repeatedly fail to demonstrate an adequate corrected count increment (CCI) usually indicate an immune mechanism of platelet destruction.[62] If the 10-minute to 1-hour posttransfusion platelet count shows a reasonable increment, but the platelet count falls back to baseline by 18 to 24 hours, a nonimmune mechanism of refractoriness may be presumed. HLA antibody screening of patients provides a second important line of evidence. A panel reactive antibody (PRA) level of 70% is often used as a threshold for diagnosing alloimmunization.[63]

Although platelets express class I HLA antigens, platelets themselves are poor immunogens. Preclinical studies in mice[64] and rats[65] suggested that white blood cells (WBCs) contaminating platelet products are the cells primarily responsible for stimulating an anti-HLA immune response in platelet transfusion recipients. It was hypothesized that removing WBCs from platelet products could prevent alloimmunization and platelet refractoriness. This was subsequently shown to be true in human studies.[66–69] The definitive study was the multicenter prospective Trial to Reduce Alloimmunization to Platelets (TRAP study),[69] which compared alloimmunization rates in 530 newly diagnosed AML patients randomized to receive unmodified, pooled platelet concentrates (control); filtered, pooled platelet concentrates (F-PC); filtered single-donor apheresis platelets (F-AP); or UV-B-irradiated pooled platelet concentrates (UVB-PC). Anti-HLA antibodies were detected in 45% of controls, compared with 17% to 21% of patients receiving modified platelets. Thirteen percent of control group patients became platelet-refractory, compared with only 3% in the F-PC group, 4% in the F-AP group, and 5% in the UVB-PC group.

Current filtration and apheresis technology can yield blood products with less than 10^6 residual leukocytes. It is standard practice to provide patients requiring long-term blood component support with leukoreduced products. Leukoreduction provides the additional benefit of reducing CMV risk in susceptible patients and of reducing the rates of febrile nonhemolytic transfusion reactions. The benefits in the HSCT patient population are clear; whether prestorage leukoreduced products need to be provided to all patients is controversial.[70–73] Blood suppliers in many European countries and Canada have moved to providing exclusively prestorage leukoreduced products. Suppliers in the United States have made efforts to do the same, although universal prestorage leukoreduction is currently not mandated by the regulatory agencies (eg, US Food and Drug Administration, American Association of Blood Banks) overseeing blood transfusion practices.

Once platelet refractoriness has been demonstrated, several strategies may help in obtaining therapeutic platelet increments in vivo. If refractoriness is nonimmune in nature (eg, sepsis), the underlying cause must be treated. A trial of ABO-matched, fresh (1 to 2 days old) platelets may be helpful.[74] In cases of immune-mediated refractoriness, a trial of HLA-matched platelets or crossmatched platelets may be indicated. Owing to the polymorphism of the HLA loci, it is often not possible to find perfect HLA-A and -B locus matches, leading to the use of platelets mismatched at one or more loci (Table 155–3). Grade A (4 antigens matched) or BU (3 antigens matched/one antigen unknown) matched platelets provide the highest probability of a successful response.

CYTOMEGALOVIRUS INFECTION

CMV is a human herpesvirus (HHV-5) capable of infecting a variety of cell types, including mature WBCs and their progenitors. CMV causes significant morbidity and mortality in immunocompromised patients, including seronegative HSCT recipients. Allogeneic HSCT patients in particular are at risk to develop serious manifestations of CMV disease, which include pneumonitis, gastroenteritis, hepatitis, encephalitis, and retinitis. CMV disease is considerably less common in the autologous transplant setting.[75] When a patient who is CMV-seropositive at baseline undergoes HSCT, CMV disease occurs primarily as a result of reactivation of latent virus.[76] In those cases where the HSCT donor is seropositive and the recipient is seronegative, CMV transmission may occur by means of the stem cell product. When both donor and recipient are seronegative, CMV infection results primarily from the transfusion of infectious blood components.[78,79]

Serologic screening of blood products is currently the most effective means of reducing the risk of transfusion-transmitted CMV. In a randomized study by Miller and coworkers,[77] only 18% of seronegative allogeneic BM recipients who received seronegative blood components developed CMV infection, versus 38% of patients receiving unscreened blood products. No benefit of serologic screening was observed in cases where the donor or recipient was seropositive. As the use of CMV seronegative blood components for seronegative HSCT recipients became adopted widely, CMV infection rates dropped from approximately 23%–37%[77–79] to 1%–4%.[80] The infrequent CMV infections still seen in part represent limitations of the serologic testing methodologies, such as donations made in the preseroconversion window period.[81] A number of sensitive PCR-based methods have been explored to measure CMV viral load in blood donors.[82] The clinical utility of DNA-based screening for CMV is unclear.

Because the seroprevalence of CMV in various communities ranges from 40% to 80%, it is logistically difficult for blood banks to maintain an inventory of CMV seronegative components.[83] As an alternative to serologic screening, leukoreduction of blood components using filtration or other means has been used to render blood products "CMV safe." The AABB defines leukoreduced products as containing less than 5×10^6 WBCs.[81] Using current apheresis and filtration technologies, residual WBC counts of less than 1×10^6 are readily obtainable. In 1977, a study of seronegative heart surgery patients showed that whole blood leukoreduced by centrifugation (58% reduction of leukocytes) resulted in a seroconversion rate of 12.5%, compared with 67% in recipients of nonleukoreduced blood.[84] Since then, a number of studies have demonstrated lower seroconversion rates, with blood products leukoreduced by saline washing, freeze-deglycerolization, and filtration. Filtration of red cells was shown to decrease transfusion-acquired CMV infection in infants,[85] and the use of filtered blood components was shown to decrease CMV seroconversion in patients undergoing treatment for acute leukemia.[81,82] Leukocyte depletion was further reported to be effective for preventing CMV disease in the autologous[86] and allogeneic[87] HSCT settings.

In 1995, Bowden and colleagues[80] reported a large prospective study of 502 seronegative marrow transplant patients randomized to receive seronegative or filtered blood products to test the hypothesis that these methods are equivalent in preventing CMV transmission. In the primary statistical analysis, there were no significant differences in the rates of CMV infection (1.3% vs 2.4%) or CMV disease (0% vs 2.4%) between the seronegative and filtered arms, respectively. The primary analysis excluded patients who seroconverted within the first 21 days of HSCT, based on the premise that they most likely would have been infected with CMV before transplantation. Complicating the interpretation of this study is that a secondary analysis of all patients seroconverting between days 0 and 100 showed a significantly worse outcome for patients in the filtered arm: 2.4% of patients in the filtered arm developed CMV disease, compared with 0% in the seronegative arm. Moreover, five of the six patients in the filtered arm who developed CMV disease progressed to fatal pneumonia. There were no deaths in the seronegative arm. Another confounding factor is that bedside filtration was used, which was subsequently shown to suffer from a relatively high rate of failure.[88] Later methods would be expected to provide better and more consistent leukoreduction. Nevertheless, patients receiving leukoreduced blood showed a low level (2.4%) of CMV infection, which is in keeping with the historical figures of 1% to 4% CMV seroconversion with the use of CMV-seronegative components. The investigators conclude by stating: "We believe that the results of this study justify abandoning the maintenance of dual inventories of seronegative and unscreened blood products. The need to perform serologic screening of blood products of CMV could be eliminated altogether."[80]

Given the previous considerations and the data associating filtered RBC units with an increased risk for CMV infection in HSCT patients,[89] it remains unclear whether leukoreduced products are equivalent to seronegative products for the prevention of CMV transmission. It is certain that leukoreduction is extremely effective in decreasing CMV transmission, and the use of leukoreduced CMV-safe products as a substitute for seronegative products has become an accepted practice standard.[81] Overall, although transfusion-transmitted CMV remains a problem in the HSCT population, the rates seen using seronegative or leukoreduced products are far lower than they have been in the past, in large part because of improvements in surveillance and preemptive therapy.[90]

TRANSFUSION-ASSOCIATED GRAFT-VERSUS-HOST DISEASE

TA-GVHD is a devastating complication of blood transfusion primarily affecting immunocompromised patients, including patients undergoing allogeneic or autologous HSCT. The basic mechanism underlying TA-GVHD is that viable, immunocompetent lymphocytes in a blood product engraft and proliferate in the transfusion recipient. The donor lymphocytes attack host tissues, including skin, liver, intestine, and marrow. Signs and symptoms generally appear 7 to 10 days after transfusion. Patients typically present with fever, rash, elevated liver function test results, and nausea, vomiting, and diarrhea. Severe, refractory pancytopenia often develops as well, in most cases leading to the patient's death. The pancytopenia seen differentiates TA-GVHD from classic GVHD after HSCT. Whereas TA-GVHD involves immune rejection of host marrow cells, the marrow is spared in classic GVHD, because donor and recipient BM are selected to be HLA-compatible. In most cases, TA-GVHD is fatal within 3 to 4 weeks of transfusion, with most patients dying from complications of marrow failure (i.e., bleeding or infection).

TA-GVHD occasionally occurs in completely immunocompetent patients. In these cases, the mechanism is a "one-way" HLA match, in which the transfusion recipient shares an HLA haplotype with a donor who is homozygous for that haplotype. The transfused lymphocytes are recognized as self by the host immune system and are not rejected. The recipient's cells, however, are seen as foreign by the infused lymphocytes, leading to a GVH response. Shared HLA haplotypes are more likely to occur among first-degree family members and in population groups with limited HLA heterogeneity. In the United States, the risk of transfusion of blood from HLA-homozygous donors to unrelated HLA-heterozygous patients is estimated to be approximately 1 in 7174. In Japan, a more genetically homogeneous population, the risk is much greater (1 in 874).[91] The incidence of TA-GVHD in the United States is clearly much lower than would be expected based on HLA considerations alone.[92] Although underreporting may play a role, it is likely that other factors, including the use of blood that is stored for up to 6 weeks (with decreased leukocyte viability) and the rejection of HLA-homozygous cells based on minor transplantation antigens, also are factors.

There is no effective therapy for TA-GVHD. Fortunately, TA-GVHD is effectively prevented by gamma irradiation of blood products before transfusion. One case of TA-GVHD has been documented after irradiation with 1500 rad,[93] and previous studies suggest that irradiation to 2000 rad is required to reduce mitogen-responsive lymphocytes by 5 to 6 logs compared with unirradiated controls.[94] Based on these observations, irradiated blood products are required to receive 2500 rad (25 Gy) to the central part of the container, with 1500 rad (15 Gy) as the minimum dose to any other point.[95] Cellular blood products are required to be irradiated for the following situations: recipients identified to be at risk for TA-GVHD, donations made by blood relatives of the recipient, and donors selected to be HLA-matched with the recipient.[96] At this time, it is recommended that only cellular blood products and fresh plasma be irradiated. TA-GVHD has not been reported to be caused by transfusion of plasma or cryoprecipitate that has been frozen and thawed.

SOLID ORGAN TRANSPLANTATION

Transfusion medicine is integral to the success of any solid organ transplantation program. The role of the transfusion medicine specialist and hematologist focuses on blood group compatibility, histocompatibility, transfusion and coagulation support, and adjunctive treatment of humoral rejection. Improved surgical technique and advances in prevention of allograft rejection have led to tremendous growth in solid organ transplantation during the past decade. During 2002, for example, 25,700 solid organ transplantations were performed, including more than 14,000 kidney, 5000 liver, 2000 heart, and 1000 lung transplantations in the United States. The Annual Report of the United Network for Organ Sharing (UNOS) is available on the Internet (www.optn.org/data/annualReport.asp). The availability of multiple drugs to prevent organ rejection, including prednisone, cyclosporine (Sandimmune, Neoral, SangCya), tacrolimus (Prograf, FK506), mycophenolate mofetil (CellCept), daclizumab (Zenapax), antithymocyte globulins (Atgam, Thymoglobulin, Orthoclone), and rapamycin (Rapamune), has extended graft and patient survival. Designed to suppress T-cell activation and cytokine release, these drugs are not cytotoxic agents and lack direct marrow toxicity.

IMMUNOHEMATOLOGY AND SOLID ORGAN TRANSPLANTATION

Renal Transplantation

Pretransplantation Blood Transfusion

After the initial investigations by Opelz and colleagues,[89] numerous studies documented that pretransplantation blood transfusions promoted prolonged renal allograft survival. As a result, deliberate use of random donor transfusions before cadaver donor renal transplantation and donor-specific transfusions (DSTs) before living-related donor transplants became widespread. A proportion of deliberately transfused patients became HLA alloimmunized, however, and the resulting HLA incompatibility eliminated them as candidates for transplantation. The introduction of cyclosporine in the 1980s led to improved graft survival and the benefit of pretransplantation transfusions became more difficult to document.[90] As a result, the practice of pretransplant transfusion was abandoned.

ABO Compatibility

ABO compatibility between donor antigens and recipient antibodies is critical for successful renal transplantation.[100] ABH antigens are richly expressed on vascular endothelial cells[101] and renal cells[102] and are excreted in the urine.[103] As a result, ABO incompatible grafts are at high risk for humoral rejection, and transplantation against ABO barriers has traditionally been contraindicated.[104,105] Because group O recipients are restricted to group O donors, several experimental protocols have investigated the use of group A_2 donors (who express group A antigens at approximately one-fourth the strength of group A_1 individuals) for group O or group B recipients with low-titer anti-A antibodies.[106,107] Protocols aimed at allowing renal transplantation across the ABO barrier typically involve pretransplant plasmapheresis or immunoadsorption to remove anti-ABO antibodies, in combination with immunosuppressive agents and careful monitoring of antibody titers.[108] Short-term results with such protocols have in some cases been encouraging.[109,110] In some cases, high titers of anti-ABO antibody can continue to circulate in the recipient—but without corresponding damage to the antigen-positive transplanted organ. This phenomenon, termed *accommodation*, is not well understood.[111]

HLA Compatibility

The importance of serologic HLA compatibility between donor antigens and recipient antibodies is well established for renal transplantation. Recipients who express warm-reactive antibodies to HLA class I antigens of the donor are at risk for hyperacute rejection characterized by complement activation, intravascular coagulation in the graft, organ ischemia, and necrosis that may occur within minutes of establishing blood flow to the graft. Several techniques are used for HLA crossmatching, and there is controversy regarding which method has the highest predictive value. Standards of the American Society for Histocompatibility and Immunogenetics (www.ashi-hla.org/) require that the final crossmatch employ a technique with greater sensitivity than the basic microlymphocytotoxicity test. Such techniques may use longer incubation times, more wash steps, an antiglobulin reagent, B-cell targets, dithiothreitol, or flow cytometry.[112,113]

Recognition of the importance of HLA-serologic compatibility led to the practice of monthly HLA antibody screening of serum from HLA-sensitized patients awaiting kidney transplants. Antibody specificities that are identified are recorded and the corresponding antigens avoided when allocating suitable kidney allografts. Some programs also consider compatibility results using archived sera when allocating allografts to recipients who are known to be HLA sensitized. Analysis of recipient HLA specificities has revealed that identification of antibodies directed against common "public antigens" may be more clinically meaningful than antibodies to private HLA antigens.[114–116] Understanding the exact value of HLA matching for long-term graft acceptance is complicated by the power of immunosuppressive medications, the polymorphism of the HLA system, variable response to different loci within the major histocompatibility complex, and the confounding effects from minor histocompatibility antigens. Studies of the precise value of matching have yielded conflicting results; nevertheless, consideration of the extent of match remains a high priority in organ allocation. DNA-based HLA typing continues to advance understanding of the role for HLA matching in renal transplantation.

Routine practice does not require HLA matching of donor and recipient when allocating cadaver kidneys. However, retrospective studies of graft survival have suggested that certain HLA mismatches are associated with a higher incidence of rejection,[117] and large retrospective analyses have provided evidence that greater degrees of HLA matching between the donor and recipient result in longer graft survival.[118,119] For example, Takemoto reported that allograft half-life was 12.5 years among more than 7,600 cadaver-donor transplants without HLA-mismatches compared with 8.6 years among 81,000 HLA-mismatched cadaver-donor transplants.[120] Studies have shown that matching for HLA-DR antigens may be more important than HLA-A,B,C.[96] Although not all have agreed that matching improves outcomes,[121] the potential benefits have prompted organ banks to allocate cadaver organs based on the degree of HLA match rather than simply on the results of HLA compatibility testing. However, matching cadaver organs to distant recipients may carry the disadvantage of prolonged cold-ischemia time. As a result, allocation based on HLA matching combined with limitation of cold-ischemia time is used. Despite the beneficial effects of HLA matching, matched *cadaver* transplants do not survive as well as matched *living-related* transplants. The difference may reflect not only injury to the graft during preservation but also the influence of histocompatibility mismatches not recognized by existing HLA-typing techniques.

Liver Transplantation

ABO Compatibility

Ordinarily, the donor liver must be ABO compatible with the recipient. Transplantation of ABO incompatible livers has occurred by error or under urgent circumstances, with limited success.[122–124] ABO-incompatible liver transplants may occur more frequently in pediatric cases when a compatible donor organ is unavailable and recipient blood group alloantibodies are poorly developed.[125] Data from the UNOS Scientific registry found that ABO mismatch was among the strongest independent predictors of adverse outcome after emergency liver transplantation.[126] In another series, survival of emergently transplanted ABO-incompatible grafts was 30% compared with 76% for emergently transplanted ABO compatible grafts.[127] The immune response to ABO-incompatible grafts is consistent with a pattern of hyperacute rejection.[128] No standards exist regarding transfusion support for ABO-incompatible grafts, but the use of RBCs and FFP compatible with both donor and recipient would seem desirable.

Hemolytic Antibodies of Donor Origin

Passenger lymphocytes that accompany a graft may continue to secrete antibodies directed against blood group antigens during the early postoperative period. If the recipient's native red cells or transfused red cells express the matching antigen, a Coombs-positive hemolytic anemia may appear approximately 1 week after transplant.[129] Although the direct antiglobulin test may only be weakly reactive, rather brisk hemolysis typical of complement fixing ABO antibodies can occur. Acute renal failure from intravascular hemolysis in this setting is rare but has been reported.[130]

Approximately 30% of patients transplanted with ABO-compatible but nonidentical livers have been reported to develop postoperative hemolysis mediated by anti-ABO antibodies produced by passenger lymphocytes.[131] Hemolysis has also been reported to result from non-ABO blood group antigens[128] but is most commonly seen when the donor is group O and the recipient is group A_1. Posttransplant hemolysis has been reported after all types of major solid organ transplants, including liver,[130] kidney,[132] heart–lung,[133] spleen,[134] and pancreas.[135] It is most common after liver transplantation, probably by virtue of the greater number of passenger lymphocytes that accompany this large organ. This phenomenon is uncommon after kidney transplantation because of UNOS policies that reserve group O donors for group O recipients. The diagnosis is confirmed by testing an eluate made from the patient's red cells against non–group O target cells—a test not routinely done by the blood bank in the evaluation of a positive direct antiglobulin test. Treatment consists of transfusion with cells compatible with donor and recipient antibodies. Red cell exchange is usually not required and the condition is generally self-limited because donor lymphocytes are deleted posttransplant.

Alloantibodies to Red Cell Antigens

Patients with clinically significant alloantibodies directed against red cell antigens outside the ABO system pose a unique problem in the setting of the massive transfusion requirements that unpredictably accompany liver transplantation.[136] Depending on the availability of antigen-negative donor units, one strategy is to begin surgery with antigen-negative compatible red cells and then allow transfusion to "wash out" recipient alloantibody before switching to antigen-positive red cells. Approximately 1 blood volume of antigen-negative units can be reserved for the end of the case to reconstitute the patient with compatible blood for the postoperative period. Antibody washout can be roughly predicted from the presurgical antibody titer as measured by twofold serial dilution. Each blood volume of transfusion reduces the titer by one dilution. For example, an antibody that reacts at 1:16 titer requires roughly 4 blood volumes of transfusion to wash out.

Heart and Lung Transplantation

Cardiac transplantation has become an established therapy for life-threatening cardiac dysfunction, including coronary disease, cardiomyopathy, and congenital cardiac defects. One-year patient survival rates of approximately 85% and 5-year survival rates of 70% have been achieved through the use of effective immunosuppressive regimens, improved recipient selection criteria, the use of heart-assist devices to bridge the waiting time between diagnosis and transplantation, the development of percutaneous endomyocardial biopsy for improved detection of early rejection episodes, and more effective management of postoperative infectious complications. As a result of these improvements, research has shifted from short-term problems such as acute rejection to those factors influencing long-term morbidity-free survival.

Cadaver lung transplants and living-related partial lung transplants have been used in the treatment of a variety of end-stage pulmonary diseases, including cystic fibrosis, emphysema, and α_1-antitrypsin deficiency. A variety of techniques have been developed to prevent rejection of the bronchial anastomosis between donor and recipient. Combined heart–lung transplants are infrequent and are used in the treatment of congenital heart disease with Eisenmenger syndrome or primary pulmonary hypertension.

ABO Compatibility

Because ABO antigens are present on cardiac endothelial tissue, ABO compatibility of donor and recipient is a prerequisite for heart transplantation. ABO is a major determinant of waiting time for heart and lung transplant recipients, with group O recipients consistently requiring longer waiting times. As with other solid organ transplants, ABO-compatible but -nonidentical allografts are used. However, ABO-identical transplants may have a better overall survival than ABO-compatible but -nonidentical grafts. ABO-incompatible heart transplants are absolutely contraindicated in adults because of the risk of hyperacute rejection. However, many successful ABO-incompatible heart transplants have been performed in infants.[137] The infant immune system does not produce T cell-independent antibodies, and early ABO-incompatible heart transplantation produces tolerance in the recipient to donor blood group A or B antigens. The primary mechanism underlying this tolerance appears to be specific elimination of donor-reactive B lymphocytes.[138] Thus, a type O infant who receives a type A heart transplant will typically have normal levels of circulating anti-B antibody, but not the usually expected anti-A antibody later in life.

HLA Compatibility

The clinical significance of HLA antibody testing in cardiac and lung transplantation remains controversial and surveyed practices show a lack of consensus.[139,146,147] Recipients with HLA antibodies to donor antigens do not experience hyperacute rejection and some studies have reported no adverse outcomes despite incompatible crossmatches at the time of transplantation.[140] However, most studies have found that patients with HLA antibodies, detected by a pretransplantation HLA crossmatch or by a highly panel-reactive antibody (PRA), have a higher frequency of rejection episodes in the first months after transplantation. Whether this reflects a direct effect of HLA antibodies or represents a marker of recipient cellular immune responsiveness is not resolved. For example, in a review of 500 cardiac transplants at the Cleveland Clinic, sensitized patients (PRA > 10%) had a 1-year graft survival of 76% compared with 89% for nonsensitized patients ($P = 0.02$).[141] As with renal transplants, some studies have suggested that antibodies to class I HLA antigens[142] or antigens specific to the donor[143,144] are more important predictors for early rejection episodes. Other studies have not found HLA antibodies to play a critical role in graft rejection.[145]

Xeno-antibodies

Naturally occurring xeno-antibodies in humans represent a major immunologic barrier to xenotransplants. Similar to ABO antibodies, xeno-antibodies are directed against sugar epitopes, including α-galactose found on the cells of all mammals other than humans and Old World monkeys. Antibodies to α-galactose fix complement avidly and produce a potent hyperacute rejection.[148] As a result, strategies to overcome this immune barrier have been directed against the level of antibody[149] and against prevention of complement activation.[150,151]

TRANSFUSION MEDICINE SUPPORT FOR SOLID ORGAN TRANSPLANTATION

Specialized Blood Components

Cytomegalovirus-Reduced Risk Blood

The implications of CMV infection are different in solid organ transplant recipients compared with bone marrow transplant recipients. After solid organ transplantation, the recipient's immune system is not chimeric, and immunosuppression is less extensive than that required for allogeneic marrow transplantation. As a result, solid organ recipients appear to have better immunity against infections such as CMV, which cause less postoperative morbidity.

Most serious CMV infections result from primary transmission from the donor allograft rather than from blood transfusion.[152,153] CMV-seronegative recipients of CMV-seropositive allografts are therefore at greatest risk for posttransplantation infection regardless of blood transfusion therapies. For example, in a study of liver transplant recipients, it was found that symptomatic CMV disease, CMV hepatitis, invasive fungal disease, and death were each more likely to occur in patients who acquired CMV from the donor organ rather than from transfusion.[154] When the recipient is CMV-seropositive, reactivation infection is more common than transfusion-transmitted disease. Second-strain infection can occur from the allograft, but has not been reported as a result of transfusion. This may result from the fact that the allograft is retained whereas blood donor leukocytes are largely apoptotic and cleared shortly after transfusion. When the organ donor or the recipient is CMV positive, the use of CMV-negative blood components should be considered investigational.

However, when both donor and recipient are CMV-negative, CMV-reduced-risk blood is indicated for lung transplantation.[155] CMV-reduced risk blood is defined as blood from CMV-seronegative donors or leukoreduced blood—either of which can effectively prevent CMV transmission by transfusion. CMV-reduced risk blood is not generally used for adult liver transplant cases because of the large number of products required. CMV-reduced risk blood products are not a strict requirement among most solid organ recipients. For example, Preiksaitis reported the incidence of postoperative CMV among CMV-seronegative recipients who were supported with CMV-untested and nonleukoreduced blood components.[153] Although postoperative CMV was very common (131 [85%] of 154) when the organ allograft was CMV-seropositive, CMV syndromes were at near background levels (3 [2.4%] of 127) when organ donor and recipient were CMV seronegative despite the use of blood components that were not CMV-reduced risk. Among the different categories of transplantation, the incidence of postoperative transfusion-associated CMV was 0 of 57 (0%, renal), 0 of 29 (0%, heart), 2 of 20 (10%, liver), and 1 of 6 (16.7 %, lung).[153] Current interest has centered on the use of PCR for the early detection of CMV infection as a guide to the preemptive use of ganciclovir.[156,157]

γ-Irradiated Blood Components

Patients undergoing solid organ transplantation are not known to be at increased risk for TA-GVHD.[158] As a result, γ-irradiated cellular blood components are not currently required for solid organ transplant recipients preoperatively or postoperatively. Because γ-irradiation results in dramatic elevation of plasma potassium levels in stored red cells, irradiated and stored red cells may increase the risk of hyperkalemic cardiac arrest at the time of massive transfusion.

Massive Transfusion during Liver Transplantation

OLT has become the treatment of choice for life-threatening end-stage hepatic failure.[159] Successful OLT requires a close working relationship between the surgical team, anesthesia services, and blood services because the operation sometimes requires spectacular quantities of blood support. Improved surgical technique, use of venovenous bypass for those cases in which the vena cava is interrupted, argon laser-directed electrocoagulation, and better preservative solutions for storing the donor liver ex vivo have contributed to decreased transfusion requirements during surgery.[160,161] One-year and 5-year patient survival rates are approximately 85% and 75% respectively.

Causes of Bleeding

Intraoperative transfusion requirements for OLT cannot be predicted on the basis of preoperative coagulation screening.[162] Rather, the presence of severe portal hypertension, previous right upper quadrant surgery, vascular abnormalities of the portal vein, poor left ventricular function, pulmonary hypertension, poor nutritional state, or comorbid diseases are the most important predictors of massive transfusion and decreased survival. Prior transjugular intrahepatic portosystemic stent-shunt (TIPSS) does not appear to adversely affect surgical outcomes during OLT.[163]

OLT requires a difficult right upper quadrant dissection of the recipient hepatic bed, which can be complicated by severe portal hypertension, friable collateral vessels, adhesions from prior procedures, or inflammation from the patient's underlying disease. Removal of the liver requires isolating the blood supply of the organ and clamping and cutting the portal vein, hepatic artery, common bile duct, and the hepatic vein or the inferior vena cava above and below the liver. The period after the recipient hepatectomy and before reestablishing blood flow to the new graft is referred to as the anhepatic phase of surgery and is the period of greatest risk.

Patients who require OLT usually have multiple hemostatic abnormalities associated with acute or chronic liver failure. Decreased coagulation factors, splenomegaly with thrombocytopenia, dysfibrinogenemia, and chronic fibrinolysis with elevated fibrin split products may all be present in varying combinations. Some patients develop a profound intraoperative fibrinolysis. Tissue plasminogen activator (tPA)—presumably released from recipient blood vessels or from the vessels of the graft in response to shock, acidosis, pharmacologic pressors, ischemia, or preservation injury—circulates in high concentration. Normally cleared by the liver, tPA released during and immediately after the anhepatic phase of surgery is not cleared from the bloodstream. As a result, tPA activity can reach 10 to 100 times normal levels and a pathologic systemic lytic state ensues.[164,165] A sudden decrease in all coagulation factors occurs with particularly marked declines in fibrinogen and factor VIII.[166] Proteolysis of von Willebrand factor may also occur.[167] Less severe cases may not demonstrate systemic lysis but may lyse clot at sites of previous hemostasis. As the liver allograft begins to function, tPA is rapidly cleared and fibrinolysis decreases.

Transfusion Support During Liver Transplantation Surgery

A rapid transfusion device designed to deliver large volumes of blood components in a rapid fashion is essential for OLT. These devices consist of a sterile holding reservoir, high-capacity blood filter, roller pump, in-line blood warmer and air detection device. Blood is pumped through large-bore catheters placed in the antecubital or central veins. Intraoperative blood recovery devices are a useful adjunct to blood support during OLT, particularly in cases requiring massive transfusion.[168,169] Blood suctioned from the operative field is anticoagulated with citrate and collected in a sterile holding reservoir. The shed blood is then centrifuged, the supernatant discarded, and the residual packed red cells washed with saline. The saline-suspended packed red cells may then be pumped to the rapid transfusion device or transferred to a plastic blood collection bag for later reinfusion.

OLT demands careful but aggressive component therapy guided by the clinical course and the results of intraoperative coagulation monitoring.[170] Serial intraoperative hematocrit and coagulation monitoring using a limited number of tests with rapid turnaround time provides valuable information for rational blood component management. Some OLT centers monitor coagulation using thromboelastography—a method that measures whole blood coagulation by impedance to an oscillating cylinder.[171,172] Other programs use traditional measurements such as the prothrombin time, fibrinogen, and platelet count. Either method of monitoring is valuable, provided that testing is done serially, results are reported rapidly, changes are correlated in the operating room with the clinical picture, and abnormalities are interpreted by someone with experience in the coagulopathy of OLT.

Red cell support must be given in consideration of the competing needs of other patients. Probably as a consequence of postoperative immunosuppression, Rh-negative individuals transfused with Rh-positive blood at the time of transplantation are not likely to make anti-D.[173] Nevertheless, Rh-negative women of childbearing age without anti-D are initially supported in many programs with a reasonable number of D-negative units and then switched to D-positive cells should more blood be needed. In some programs, Rh-negative males and females who are not of childbearing potential are treated from the outset with Rh-positive blood. Because many OLT patients are massively transfused, delayed hemolytic transfusion reactions in the postoperative period if directed against high-frequency antigens can result in dramatic hemolysis.

The use of fresh frozen plasma (FFP), platelet concentrates, and cryoprecipitate is guided by the clinical course and by the results of intraoperative monitoring.[174] Although care must be given to prevent dilutional coagulopathy, it is not necessary to mix equal ratios of red cells and FFP or platelet concentrates. Reasonable goals of component therapy in the absence of fibrinolysis or other complications include an international normalized ratio (INR) of less than 2 or 2.5, a platelet count higher than 50,000 to 100,000/μL, and a fibrinogen concentration more than 100 mg/dL. Antifibrinolytic agents are indicated during or shortly after the anhepatic phase of surgery in those patients who demonstrate a systemic lytic state.[175] A loading dose and continuous infusion of ε-aminocaproic acid,[176] tranexamic acid, or aprotinin[177] has been used with success. Hourly bolus doses have also been used. Tranexamic acid[178,179] or aprotinin[180,181] each reduced operative blood loss during liver transplantation when studied in randomized, prospective, placebo-controlled trials. Because the routine use of antifibrinolytics may result in thrombotic complications in some patients, our program uses antifibrinolytics for those patients who show evidence of fibrinolysis. Recombinant activated factor VII has been used to promote hemostasis during liver transplantation. Although a small pilot study suggested decreased transfusion requirements compared with historical controls,[182] a subsequent controlled trial failed to demonstrate a favorable effect on blood loss. For all patients, local hemostasis provided by meticulous and advanced surgical skill remains critically important.

Metabolic Complications of Massive Transfusion During Liver Transplantation Surgery

Patients undergoing massive transfusion during OLT are susceptible to all the major complications of massive transfusion, including hypothermia, dilutional coagulopathy, electrolyte imbalance, pulmonary dysfunction, and transfusion-transmitted infections. OLT patients are uniquely at risk for life-threatening hypocalcemia as a result of citrate toxicity.[183] Magnesium is also chelated by citrate, and low magnesium concentrations may accompany massive transfusion during OLT surgery.[184] Because the liver is the main organ for citrate metabolism and because OLT patients can receive very rapid infusions of large volumes of FFP that is rich in Na_3-citrate, the quantity of citrate infused per kilogram body weight per minute can quickly exceed the rate of citrate removal.[185] Citrate toxicity is more pronounced if concomitant renal failure is present because the kidney is the major site of citrate excretion. The principal effects of citrate toxicity are cardiovascular. An initial blunted response of cardiac output to left-ventricular volume loading is followed by hypotension resulting from poor cardiac output and decreased systemic vascular resistance. If misinterpreted as hypotension due to hypovolemia, a more rapid transfusion of citrate-rich blood components will worsen cardiac output. Citrate toxicity is aggravated by hypothermia and hyperkalemia. Because a widened QTc interval on the electrocardiogram has low specificity and poor predictive value, intraoperative monitoring of the ionized calcium level is essential during OLT. Untreated severe depression of the ionized calcium or magnesium results in bizarre electrocardiographic disturbances and fatal arrhythmias.

Plasmapheresis and Photopheresis

The indications for plasmapheresis in transplantation patients remain poorly defined and not established by controlled clinical trials. Preoperative plasmapheresis or blood exchange is able to lower titers of ABO antibodies, especially those of the IgM class.[124,149] Plasmapheresis is less effective at reducing titers of HLA antibodies, which are largely IgG in nature. Plasmapheresis has been reported to successfully treat some patients with postoperative HLA-mediated humoral rejection of renal allografts.[187] Photopheresis refers to a treatment in which blood passes along an extracorporeal circuit and is exposed to a photoactive chemical (psoralen) plus ultraviolet light. Used initially in the treatment of Sézary syndrome, photopheresis has been applied to the treatment of solid organ transplant rejection unresponsive to standard therapy. Uncontrolled studies have reported success in cardiac, renal, lung, and liver transplants.[188]

SUGGESTED READINGS

Bensinger WI, Martin PJ, Storer B, et al: Transplantation of bone marrow as compared with peripheral-blood cells from HLA-identical relatives in patients with hematologic cancers. N Engl J Med 344:175, 2001.

Bolan CD, Childs RW, Procter JL, et al: Massive immune haemolysis after allogeneic peripheral blood stem cell transplantation with minor ABO incompatibility. Br J Haematol 112:787, 2001.

Bowden RA, Slichter SJ, Sayers M, et al: A comparison of filtered leukocyte-reduced and cytomegalovirus (CMV)-seronegative blood products for the prevention of transfusion-associated CMV infection after marrow transplant. Blood 86:3598, 1995.

Daly PA, Schiffer CA, Aisner J, et al: Platelet transfusion therapy. One-hour posttransfusion increments are valuable in predicting the need for HLA-matched preparations. JAMA 243:435, 1980

Hanson SR, Slichter SJ: Platelet kinetics in patients with bone marrow hypoplasia: Evidence for a fixed platelet requirement. Blood 66:1105, 1985.

The Trial to Reduce Alloimmunization to Platelets Study Group: Leukocyte reduction and ultraviolet B irradiation of platelets to prevent alloimmunization and refractoriness to platelet transfusions. N Engl J Med 337:1861, 1997

Rebulla P, Finazzi G, Marangoni F, et al, for the Gruppo Italiano Malattie Ematologiche Maligne dell'Adulto: The threshold for prophylactic platelet transfusions in adults with acute myeloid leukemia. N Engl J Med 337:1870, 1997.

Schoemans H, Theunissen K, Maertens J, et al: Adult umbilical cord blood transplantation: A comprehensive review. Bone Marrow Transplant 38:83, 2006.

Takemoto SK, Terasaki PI, Gjertson DW, Cecka JM: Twelve years' experience with national sharing of HLA-matched cadaver kidneys for transplantation. N Engl J Med 343:1078, 2000.

Wandt H, Schaefer-Eckart K, Frank M, et al: A therapeutic platelet transfusion strategy is safe and feasible in patients after autologous peripheral blood stem cell transplantation. Bone Marrow Transplant 37:387, 2006.

West LJ, Pollock-BarZiv, SM, Dipchand AI, et al: ABO-incompatible heart transplantation in infants. N Engl J Med 344:193, 2001.

Worel N, Greinix HT, Schneider B, et al: Regeneration of erythropoiesis after related- and unrelated-donor BMT or peripheral blood HPC transplantation: A major ABO mismatch means problems. Transfusion 40:543, 2000.

REFERENCES

For complete list of references log onto www.expertconsult.com

PART X

CONSULTATIVE HEMATOLOGY

CHAPTER 156

HEMATOLOGIC MANIFESTATIONS OF SYSTEMIC DISEASE: LIVER AND RENAL DISEASE

Peter W. Marks and Rachel Rosovsky

Disorders of the liver and kidney can be associated with very significant hematologic effects. With hepatic dysfunction, effects on red blood cell morphology and coagulation predominate, whereas with renal disease, effects on red blood cell production and platelet function predominate. Understanding the pathogenesis of such disorders facilitates accurate diagnosis and management.

HEMATOLOGIC MANIFESTATIONS OF LIVER DISEASE

Progressive liver disease can eventually result in cirrhosis and is associated with portal hypertension and splenomegaly. Portal hypertension is associated with variceal and gastrointestinal bleeding and resultant anemia. Splenomegaly is associated with any combination of leukopenia, anemia, or thrombocytopenia.[1] Because the liver is integrally involved in the metabolism of lipids, which are major constituents of the red blood cell membrane, abnormalities in erythrocyte size and shape may arise with hepatic dysfunction.[2] The liver is also a vital organ contributing to the blood coagulation process. It is a major site of synthesis for virtually all of the proteins involved in the soluble hemostatic system and is involved in the clearance of products of proteolysis. These features facilitate the delicate balance of the coagulation system. Patients with liver disease, therefore, are at increased risk for developing a variety of hemostatic defects.

This section will discuss several of the hematologic problems commonly encountered in patients with liver disease: red blood cell abnormalities, vitamin K deficiency, bleeding due to hepatic failure, and complications in liver transplantation. It will also touch upon the effects of alcohol on the hematologic system.

RED BLOOD CELL ABNORMALITIES

Morphologic Abnormalities

Abnormalities in lipid metabolism that occur in liver disease can lead to changes in red blood cell size and shape. Macrocytosis may be an initial finding, followed by the development of target cells and acanthocytes (spur cells) (Fig. 156–1A). These changes are associated with abnormal cholesterol loading of the red blood cell membrane. Cholesterol loading of the lipid bilayer acts to restrict the mobility of integral membrane proteins. The erythrocytes are therefore unable to undergo normal deformation as they transit the vasculature.[3] When cholesterol loading is sufficiently severe, passage of such red blood cells through the microcirculation of the spleen leads to cytoskeletal damage and the irreversible deformation of the red blood cell noted morphologically as spur cells.[4]

Spur Cell Anemia

A hemolytic anemia associated with few other hereditary or acquired conditions, spur cell anemia is most commonly observed in chronic or severe liver disease.[5] In contrast to its mild manifestations in individuals with alpha beta-lipoproteinemia (see Chapter 46), in liver disease spur cell anemia may be quite severe and can cause life-threatening declines in hemoglobin concentration. Treatment options for this disorder have been disappointing. Therefore the development of spur cell anemia in a patient with hepatic failure generally is indicative of a very poor prognosis. Depending on the cause, patients may also suffer from disseminated intravascular coagulation, gastrointestinal bleeding, and/or liver failure. There have been a few case reports of clinical improvement using a combination of therapeutic agents such as flunarizine, pentoxifylline, and cholestyramine,[6,7] but for the most part, the only effective treatment has been liver transplantation.[8]

Coagulation Defects and Liver Disease

The clinical manifestations of coagulopathy based on hepatic dysfunction range from asymptomatic laboratory abnormalities to life-threatening hemorrhage. These manifestations of liver disease are the result of a variety of derangements in hemostasis. There is decreased synthesis of clotting factor proteins, which are produced primarily in the liver. In addition, defective forms of fibrinogen may be synthesized in liver disease due to abnormal posttranslational modification of this protein. The defective fibrinogen produced has an inability to polymerize normally into fibrin strands. This defect is manifest in the laboratory with abnormal thrombin and reptilase times (measures of fibrinogen cleavage and polymerization into fibrin), often in the setting of normal immunologic amounts of fibrinogen. Because fibrin is a polymer of many subunits, even small numbers of abnormal fibrin molecules can poison the multimerization process and result in a bleeding diathesis.[9]

Although many assays are available in the coagulation laboratory to elucidate the more precise nature of the factors affected, a carefully performed history and physical examination, in combination with an appropriate initial laboratory evaluation, will often reveal the cause and facilitate the treatment of most hemostatic abnormalities in patients with liver disease.

VITAMIN K DEFICIENCY

Deficiency in vitamin K may occur in a variety of medical and surgical settings. Poor oral intake, broad-spectrum antibiotics, and age are all risk factors for vitamin K deficiency. The uptake of the vitamin is intimately linked to the liver, as biliary salts are required for intestinal absorption.[10] Vitamin K deficiency can therefore be caused by anything that impairs the metabolism of bile acids. This includes intra- or extrahepatic cholestasis, biliary system fistulae or obstruction, primary biliary cirrhosis, or treatment with bile acid binders (ie, cholestyramine).[11] There are also nonhepatic causes of vitamin K deficiency, such as malnutrition or the administration of broad-spectrum antibiotics.[12,13] Finally, the most commonly used oral anticoagulants, coumarin derivatives such as warfarin, act by disrupting the vitamin K cycle.

Vitamin K is fat soluble and is an essential component in the production of several of the coagulation proteins (see Chapter 130).[14] It was initially named "Koagulationsvitamin" in reference to its connection with the coagulation system.[15] Investigation of the underlying cause of the hemorrhagic disease that cattle developed in the early

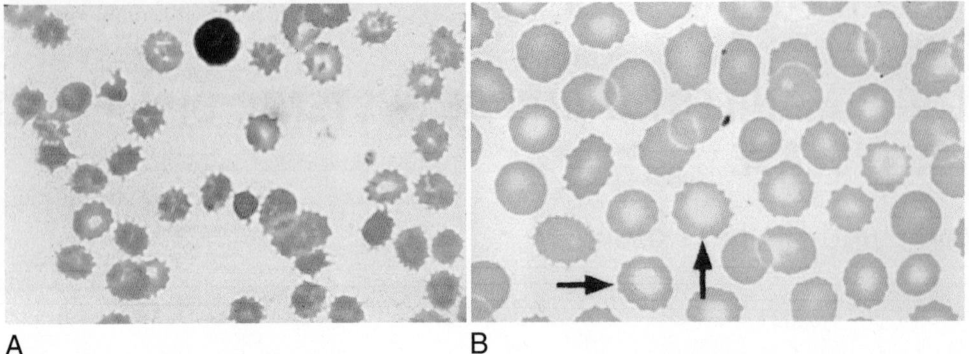

Figure 156–1 Morphology of acanthocytes and echinocytes. **A,** Acanthocytes, or spur cells, are most commonly observed in significant numbers on the peripheral blood smear in cases of liver disease, although they may also be prominent in certain rare disorders (eg, alpha beta-lipoproteinemia). Their characteristic features are spines that seemingly project from the surface of the cell. Such morphologic change represents the result of irreversible cytoskeletal damage due to passage of abnormally stiff cells through the reticuloendothelial system. **B,** Echinocytes, or burr cells, are the hallmark of uremia, although they may be observed as an artifact on less than optimally prepared smears. An undulating or bumpy red blood cell surface characterizes this morphologic change, the cause of which is unknown.

part of the 20th century (eventually found to be due to the ingestion of spoiled sweet clover containing coumarols) helped to elucidate the role and importance of this factor.[16,17] Vitamin K serves as a coenzyme in the posttranslational carboxylation of factors II, VII, IX, and X.[18] This modification creates sites on these proteins for calcium ion coordination and thereby renders them functional.[19,20]

An alteration in the synthesis of vitamin K-dependent coagulation factors is usually reflected by changes in specific laboratory parameters. Initially, there is a prolongation of the prothrombin time (PT) because factor VII, a critical component of the coagulation cascade synthesized in the liver, has a half-life of only 4 to 7 hours. An increase in the activated partial thromboplastin time (PTT) may occur as well when there is a substantial decline in factors II, IX, and X, which have longer half-lives.

Replacement of vitamin K may be warranted when the PT is prolonged by more than 3 seconds or to an International Normalized Ratio (INR) of greater than 1.5. When there is no evidence of active bleeding and the INR is moderately prolonged, vitamin K can be administered orally, subcutaneously, intramuscularly, or intravenously, although the intramuscular route is less preferable in the setting of coagulopathy. Dosing regimens commonly utilized include 5 mg orally or 10 mg subcutaneously once a day for 3 to 5 consecutive days.[21] If there is no improvement in the PT after three doses, however, additional replacement usually provides no further benefit.[22,23] Additionally, in patients with severe liver disease, vitamin K supplementation often has only a modest effect in correcting the prolonged PT.[24] In this setting, inadequate hepatic protein synthetic function is the primary issue.

When the INR is greatly prolonged in the absence of bleeding (INR >9), administration of intravenous vitamin K, either alone or in combination with other agents, may be indicated. In cases of simple vitamin K deficiency, such as that due to dietary deficiency or due to warfarin administration, intravenous administration of doses of between 1 and 2 mg can lead to complete correction of the INR within 4 to 6 hours. In this regard, many clinicians have avoided this route of administration because of reports of fatal allergic reactions in the literature.[25] More recently, the risk of anaphylaxis and the administration of vitamin K has been more thoroughly reviewed. Reports of adverse drug reactions in association with vitamin K were collected and categorized by route of administration, dose, and type of reaction. Although there were more anaphylactic reactions documented with intravenous administration of the drug than any other route of administration, the actual number of reports was relatively small given its widespread use.[26] That being said, it might seem most prudent to administer vitamin K intravenously slowly and only in circumstances when patients are at high risk for hemorrhage or are actively bleeding.

BLEEDING IN FULMINANT COAGULOPATHY

The bleeding patient with liver disease poses many challenges, the most immediate of which is to locate the source of the bleed and then attempt to correct it. Patients with hepatic dysfunction may bleed from varices, ulcers, or disseminated intravascular coagulation, to name a few entities. Such patients generally require some type of plasma component replacement therapy in addition to correction of the underlying anatomic defect.[21,27–30] Patients who are undergoing invasive procedures or who are in imminent danger of bleeding will also need treatment for the purpose of prophylaxis. Each source of therapy must have its particular advantages weighed against its potential detrimental side effects.

Fresh frozen plasma (FFP) has been used as a first-line treatment because it contains all the components of the clotting and fibrinolytic system present in circulating blood, except for platelets. It is currently recommended as an adjunctive hemostatic agent in any patient actively bleeding or for prophylaxis before invasive procedure in patients with coagulopathy due to liver disease.[31–35] Although the recommended dose is weight based (1 mL/kg body weight generally increases clotting factors 1% to 2%), in most clinical situations calculations are not performed. Instead, patients receive on average 4 to 8 units of FFP. Because factor VII has such a short half-life, additional infusions are often required every 6 to 12 hours to maintain a hemostatic effect. This practice of transfusion translates into a fairly large volume load. In some patients with liver disease, who already have an expanded intravascular plasma volume, this therapy is not well tolerated.

Allergic reactions are observed in 1% to 3% of patients treated with FFP and are usually confined to urticaria. Anaphylaxis is rare and can occur in the setting of IgA deficiency. Hemolysis can take place if there is ABO blood group incompatibility, and antibodies against granulocytes present in the donor plasma can cause the very rare complication of transfusion-related acute lung injury.[36] Other potential adverse effects of FFP include the risk of viral transmission. The risk of transmitting human immunodeficiency virus, hepatitis B, or hepatitis C is similar to that of whole blood.[37] Use of solvent/detergent-treated plasma has been explored as a method to lessen the risk of these potential infections.[38] Unfortunately, there appear to be potential hepatic side effects of solvent/detergent-treated plasma in certain populations of patients, and additional development of such products is required.

In severe bleeding episodes, replacement solely with FFP is sometimes insufficient. If the patient is actively bleeding, red blood cell transfusions are required to maintain an adequate hematocrit level and prevent shock. In patients with a platelet count below 50×10^9/L or suspected platelet dysfunction, platelet transfusions may also be

Management of Coagulopathy in Liver Disease

Appropriate management of the patient with liver disease and coagulopathy can prevent complications or minimize bleeding. Because patients with liver disease often have a combination of defects, such as thrombocytopenia from hypersplenism, decreased circulating levels of coagulation factors, and abnormal fibrinogen due to impaired hepatic synthesis, bleeding may be particularly severe and require the administration of multiple different blood products.

A trial of administration of vitamin K 5 to 10 mg a day for 3 to 5 days by the oral (preferred) or subcutaneous route is reasonable in patients with mild to moderately elevated clotting times who are not actively bleeding. In more severe cases of liver disease, the maneuver generally has little or only temporary effect.

In patients who are actively bleeding, fresh frozen plasma (FFP) provides a ready source of all of the coagulation factors. Administration of 15 to 20 mL/kg (equivalent to about 1000 to 1500 mL or four to six bags of FFP) is generally reasonable as a start. Two common mistakes are often made, both related to the relatively short half-life (several hours) of several clotting factors: (a) the units of FFP are given too slowly over a number of hours or (b) after initial administration of FFP and correction of clotting times, additional units are not administered in a timely manner. The solution to the former error is to administer the units over the course of no more than 1 to 2 hours; the solution to the latter is to monitor coagulation parameters and/or empirically give 2 to 4 additional units of FFP approximately every 6 hours.

Dysfibrinogenemia should be suspected when coagulation times fail to correct despite apparently adequate and timely administration of FFP. In this setting, it can be quite difficult to overwhelm the inhibitory effects of abnormal fibrin monomers present in the patient. Administration of cryoprecipitate, 10 to 20 units, in addition to FFP may help in overcoming this barrier. In addition, administration of cryoprecipitate should be considered for rapid replacement of fibrinogen in bleeding patients with fibrinogen levels below 50 to 100 mg/dL.

Moderate to severe thrombocytopenia should also be corrected. In the bleeding patient, platelet transfusion is reasonable if the count falls below 50,000/μL, and certainly if it falls below 20,000/μL. Unfortunately, because of hypersplenism, platelet recovery is often poor. Nonetheless, there is likely some residual hemostatic benefit in the bleeding patient. Additionally, in the rush to transfuse other blood products, an adequate hemoglobin concentration should also be maintained by transfusion of packed red blood cells as necessary.

Recombinant factor VIIa (Novoseven) has been used off-label in the setting of liver disease to try to achieve hemostasis. Doses leading to correction of the prothrombin time in the setting of liver disease are generally only about one-half to one-quarter (25–50 μg/kg) of the doses required for the treatment of hemophilia with inhibitors. The duration of the correction obtained is generally 4 to 8 hours. It should be noted, however, that correction of the prothrombin time does not necessarily correlate with prevention of bleeding. Because of its short half-life, use of recombinant factor VIIa may be most appropriate in certain circumstances, such as when emergency procedures are necessary, or to temporize until more durable measures can be taken. Even in such cases, care should be taken to maintain an adequate fibrinogen level and/or consider the possibility of a dysfibrinogenemia, as much of the action of the clotting cascade ultimately rests on the successful production of fibrin polymers.

helpful.[39] Alternatively, exchange transfusions in combination with platelets and plasma can be effective in controlling bleeding, especially in patients with liver disease who cannot tolerate the volume load associated with FFP.[40]

In cases of advanced liver disease, disseminated intravascular coagulation may be present. Alternatively, in the setting of massive transfusions, hypofibrinogenemia may exist. The use of cryoprecipitate is indicated if the fibrinogen level falls below 100 mg/dL. For every 10 kg of body weight, one unit of cryoprecipitate, which contains factors VIII, XIII, von Willebrand factor, fibronectin, and fibrinogen, will increase the fibrinogen level by approximately 50 mg/dL.

Cryoprecipitate does not contain significant amounts of any of the vitamin K-dependent coagulation factors and therefore, in the setting of vitamin K antagonists or deficiency, prothrombin complex concentrates (PCCs) are sometimes useful. Concomitant administration of antithrombin concentrates or heparin is often given prior to the PCC to decrease the risk of thromboembolic complications, which can occur when using these agents.[41] Two rarer problems associated with the use of PCCs are acute anaphylactic reactions secondary to the presence of foreign proteins and the development of inhibitors. Thus, given the potential hazards of PCCs, they should be used only in emergency situations, such as in the setting of critical bleeding and volume overload in patients with advanced liver disease. When these agents are utilized, laboratory monitoring for disseminated intravascular coagulation is mandatory.[42]

Recombinant factor VIIa (rFVIIa) has shown promising results in the management of patients with coagulopathy due to liver disease.[43,44] It was first approved as an antihemophilic agent, and, since then, it has shown favorable results when used off-label in managing patients with coagulopathies caused by liver disease.[45–47] In nonbleeding cirrhotic patients, for example, rFVIIa transiently reverses prolonged prothrombin times. The duration of this normalization is dose dependent. Transient correction of the PT by rFVIIa was also observed in patients undergoing liver biopsy and in patients experiencing variceal bleeds.[48–50] Finally, as described below, rFVIIa has been used in patients undergoing orthotopic liver transplantation and has possibly resulted in improved hemostasis, less blood loss, reduced blood product requirements, and, in one study, even a slight improvement in survival.[51]

As compared with FFP, rFVIIa has no risk of viral transmission and has the advantage of being administered in a small volume. The observed efficacy with rFVIIa in transiently correcting major laboratory parameters has potentially allowed for safer invasive procedures and decreased use of blood products in patients with liver disease. The optimal dosing schedule and a more complete safety profile of rFVIIa still needs to be determined, however, in large randomized controlled trials. In addition, whether the observed effects translate into improved survival in cirrhotic patients with coagulopathy remains to be seen.

SPECIAL CONSIDERATIONS IN LIVER TRANSPLANTATION

Patients undergoing orthotopic liver transplantation often experience severe hemostatic alterations, of which the most significant is bleeding. The different stages of transplantation, which include the preoperative, anhepatic, reperfusion, and convalescent phases, confer different hemostatic risks.[52] In the preoperative phase, for example, the underlying liver disorder and its subsequent amount of liver parenchymal cell damage is associated with preexisting compromise of the hemostatic system. During the anhepatic phase, a decrease in the hepatic clearance of activated coagulation factors and an absence of clotting factor production causes an increase in tissue plasminogen activator and a decrease in plasminogen activator inhibitor 1, respectively.[53–56] This state of hyperfibrinolysis continues during and after the graft reperfusion phase, where it has been postulated that endothelial cell injury further releases thromboplastic substances, including tissue plasminogen activator.[57] Additional challenges in liver transplantation include the extent of the surgery and the possibility that the transplanted liver may be rejected.

The intense fibrinolytic activity and resultant bleeding problems associated with orthotopic liver transplantation have been controlled in the past with multiple transfusions of packed red blood cells, FFP, and platelet concentrates. In an attempt to reduce the amount of blood loss and resulting transfusion requirement, the use of antifibrinolytic agents has been explored in this setting. Two randomized controlled studies showed that prophylactic therapy with aprotinin significantly decreased hemorrhagic blood loss.[58,59] An additional randomized study compared the antifibrinolytic agent tranexamic acid to aprotinin and found similar safety and efficacy between the two agents.[60] However, there is controversy regarding the overall safety and efficacy of these agents.[61] In any case, reasonable caution should be taken when using antifibrinolytic agents such as aprotinin. The drugs have the potential to disrupt the balance of the coagulation system, and, in the randomized trials, patients at increased risk of thromboembolic complications (ie, with malignancies) were excluded. There have been a few case reports of fatal thromboembolism associated with its use, although it is unclear whether aprotinin was the only cause implicated in these instances.[62] Additionally, allergic reactions and renal dysfunction have occurred.[63–65]

Recombinant factor VIIa (rFVIIa) is another hemostatic agent whose use has been, and continues to be, investigated in the setting of orthotopic liver transplantation. Initial small studies suggested a potential benefit of rFVIIa with a reduction in the number of red blood cell transfusions required.[66,67] However two subsequently conducted randomized controlled trials did not confirm such a benefit.[68,69] Other trials have suggested that use of rFVIIa might be most effective in patients at the highest risk for bleeding.[70] In summary, routine use of rFVIIa in the setting of liver transplantation remains controversial, although there is some evidence to suggest that there may be high-risk situations in which its use is warranted.

EFFECTS OF ALCOHOL

Even in the absence of significant liver disease, chronic alcohol intake frequently leads to a mild to moderate macrocytosis, generally in the 100 to 110 fL range.[71] In addition, the intake of alcohol may be associated with other phenomena such as poor dietary intake and gastrointestinal bleeding, which are associated in turn with megaloblastic anemia due to folate deficiency and with iron deficiency, respectively. If folate and iron deficiencies are simultaneously present, the mean corpuscular volume may actually be normal, but the red blood cell distribution width will be elevated.

Other manifestations of heavy alcohol intake include direct toxic effects on the bone marrow, with reversible suppression of hematopoiesis. Although all lineages can be affected, anemia and thrombocytopenia are most common. Particularly when folate deficiency is present a sideroblastic anemia can occur in which there is defective iron utilization for hemoglobin synthesis.[72] Alcohol also impairs platelet production and function.[73] This is in addition to thrombocytopenia resulting from portal hypertension and splenomegaly. Recovery from significant thrombocytopenia generally occurs rapidly within approximately 1 week of cessation of alcohol intake. The hematologic effects of alcohol are particularly pronounced in patients with hepatic cirrhosis who continue to consume alcohol. These individuals may present with bleeding with moderate to severe pancytopenia and may require significant blood product support.

HEMATOLOGIC MANIFESTATIONS OF RENAL DISEASE

Because the kidney is the locus for the production of the primary driver of red blood cell production, erythropoietin, it should follow that renal injury would be associated with anemia, and this is borne out by fact. Although end-stage renal disease is associated with severe anemia (see later), even modest renal damage, such as that seen in diabetic patients with very modestly elevated serum creatinine levels, can be associated with impaired erythropoietin production.

Renal disease can be associated with subsequent defects in red blood cells, platelets, leukocytes, and coagulation factors. In addition, acquired disorders, such as hemolytic-uremic syndrome, can manifest simultaneously as hematologic and renal disturbances.

Abnormal red blood cell morphology due to uremia is manifest with the presence of echinocytes (burr cells) on the peripheral blood smear (see Fig. 156–1B). The pathogenesis underlying this morphologic change is unknown. Uremic toxins also significantly impair platelet function, leading to an acquired aspirin-like platelet release defect. This finding, in combination with a decreased quantity and/or function of certain clotting proteins, including von Willebrand factor, can lead to significant bleeding complications. Cellular and humoral immunity mediated via lymphocytes are also adversely affected in renal disease, and a wide variety of leukocyte defects have been reported in this setting.[74] In clinical practice, however, hypoproliferative anemia, bleeding complications, and hemolytic-uremic syndrome are the most frequent clinically relevant entities encountered, so they are covered in greater detail here.

MANAGEMENT OF HYPOPROLIFERATIVE ANEMIA

End-stage renal disease is a major health problem in the United States, with incidence increasing every year. The associated anemia is a cause of significant morbidity and mortality. Although the cause of the anemia is multifactorial, reduced erythropoietin production is primarily responsible. Erythropoietin is a glycoprotein hormone synthesized primarily in the kidney.[75,76] This crucial component in the regulation of hematopoiesis is essential for the proliferation, maturation, and differentiation of erythroid precursors (see Chapter 25).[77]

Previously, the great majority of patients on dialysis required chronic blood transfusions. This situation has changed dramatically with the introduction of recombinant human erythropoietin (rHuEPO) into clinical practice. In addition to accelerating erythropoiesis and reducing allogeneic blood transfusions, rHuEPO has been shown to increase exercise capacity and improve quality of life, sleep, cognitive function, and sexual function in anemic patients with chronic renal failure.[78–82] A small number of prospective and retrospective clinical studies have also shown that treatment with rHuEPO decreases the rise in creatinine, slows the decline of glomerular filtration rate, and delays initiation of dialysis in patients with chronic renal failure. The results from these few exploratory clinical trials support the hypothesis that using rHuEPO and correcting anemia may slow the rate of progression of renal failure.[83–85]

Treatment of anemia may also have significant cardiovascular benefits in this population. A few recent studies have shown that left ventricular hypertrophy is directly related to the level of anemia in chronic renal failure patients.[80–82] In addition, left ventricular mass has been shown to be an independent determinant in the survival of patients on dialysis.[86] Thus, treatment with rHuEPO may have benefits in terms of cardiac function, and subsequently, survival for these patients.[87] However, data also suggest that excessive correction of the hemoglobin level to values greater than approximately 12 g/dL may be associated with an increased incidence of cardiovascular and thromboembolic events. Therefore, the use of erythropoiesis-stimulating agents to increase hemoglobin values to greater than 12 g/dL is not routinely recommended.

Although rHuEPO can be administered intravenously or subcutaneously, the subcutaneous route appears to be advantageous. It is easier to administer and can be given less frequently. Hypertension and, to a much lesser degree, thrombosis have been reported in patients on dialysis.[85,88] In addition, a short-lived influenza-like syndrome has been described.[89] Rare side effects include allergic reactions, seizures, hyperkalemia, and thrombocytosis. Pure red blood cell aplasia, thought to be due to the development of antierythropoietin antibodies, is also a rare but serious complication that has primarily been reported with certain preparations of rHuEPO.[86,87,90]

Management of the Anemia of Renal Disease

Recombinant human erythropoietin (rHuEPO) and the longer-acting modified erythropoietin, darbepoetin, have revolutionized treatment of the anemia of renal disease. However, owing to their potential for adverse events, the potential inconvenience of their administration by the parenteral route, and their expense, they should be used thoughtfully and judiciously.

Regardless of the extent of renal insufficiency, patients who are candidates for erythropoietin replacement should have an assessment of their iron stores. Analysis of serum parameters, such as ferritin, iron, and transferrin generally suffice for this purpose. If there is any hint that iron deficiency may be present, it should be addressed prior to, or at least concomitantly with, the administration of rHuEPO. Although oral replacement may be reasonable in a patient with borderline iron stores and renal insufficiency, intravenous replacement with iron dextran, iron gluconate, or iron sucrose should be considered in patients with more severe iron deficiency or renal failure.

In the setting of mild to moderate renal insufficiency, such as that often seen in diabetic patients, it is not unreasonable to initiate therapy on a weekly basis if using rHuEPO or every other week when using darbepoetin when the hemoglobin is less than 9 g/dL. After the hemoglobin concentration increases to greater than 10 g/dL, the frequency of administration or dose can be tapered to maintain a level between 10 and 12 g/dL. In some exceptional circumstances, such as in patients with significant congestive heart failure or pulmonary disease, maintenance of hemoglobin at a higher level may be determined to be beneficial.

If there is no response to erythropoietin after 4 to 8 weeks of weekly therapy with rHuEPO or biweekly therapy with darbepoetin, iron stores should be reevaluated. If adequate, dose escalation of rHuEPO or darbepoetin by 50% and an additional trial for 4 to 8 weeks is reasonable. After that time, however, the drug should be discontinued and consideration be given to the cause for the lack of response, which is otherwise rare in the setting of anemia purely due to renal insufficiency. Usually, a dose of 40,000 U of rHuEPO every 1 to 2 weeks or 200 μg of darbepoetin every 2 to 4 weeks often suffices to maintain a hemoglobin level greater than 10 g/dL.

An increase in the hemoglobin to greater than 10 g/dL after a 4-week course of therapy is frequently the target goal when administering rHuEPO. Some patients may fail to respond or may be resistant to the effects of rHuEPO. The most common cause for a failure in response is iron deficiency anemia.[91] Other contributing factors that may affect the response are cobalamin or folate deficiency, infection, chronic inflammation, secondary hyperparathyroidism, malnutrition, hemoglobinopathies, aluminum toxicity, or bone marrow fibrosis.[89,92–94]

Iron deficiency is almost universal in the dialyzed patient. Gastrointestinal bleeding, blood draws, and hemodialysis all contribute to this iron-deficient state.[95] In addition, by accelerating erythropoiesis, rHuEPO actually can cause functional iron deficiency.[91,92] As a result, iron supplementation in chronic renal failure patients is usually essential. Even with the most rigorous protocols, oral iron preparations have not been as effective as intravenous ones, largely because of poor absorption resulting in failure to maintain adequate hematologic parameters (hemoglobin >11–12 g/dL, transferrin saturation >20%, plasma ferritin concentration >100 ng/mL). Thus, intravenous iron is often administered.[96,97] There are now multiple formulations of intravenous iron available for administration, including iron dextran (InFeD), sodium ferric gluconate complex (Ferrlecit), and iron sucrose (Venofer). The latter two preparations often utilized because they would appear to have more favorable safety profiles.[94,98–100] In particular, anaphylactic reactions appear to be somewhat less common.[101]

A hyperglycosylated rHuEPO, darbepoetin (Aranesp), is available.[102] It has the same mechanism of action as rHuEPO with the advantage of having a two- to threefold longer half-life.[103,104] Consequently, it can be dosed less frequently, allowing for fewer injections.[105,106] Darbepoetin appears to be equivalent to rHuEPO in terms of its clinical outcomes in patients with chronic renal failure, specifically in reaching a target hemoglobin, the time it takes to reach that target, and the percentage of patients who reach that goal.[107,108] It is also a well-tolerated medication and has a safety profile that is similar to that of rHuEPO.[109,110] There have been no antibodies to native or recombinant erythropoietin detected to date in patients treated with darbepoetin.

HEMOSTATIC AGENTS FOR USE IN UREMIA

Bleeding from uremia is one of the major causes of morbidity in patients with end-stage renal disease.[104,105] There are multiple factors contributing to the pathogenesis of this bleeding risk, but recent focus has centered on platelet dysfunction,[107,108,111] abnormal platelet–vessel wall interactions,[109] retention of uremic toxins,[110] presence of anemia, and increased levels of nitrous oxide.[112–114]

The hemorrhagic manifestations commonly seen with uremia include epistaxis, gastrointestinal and genitourinary bleeding, subdural hematomas, hemorrhagic pericarditis, ecchymoses, and prolonged bleeding from skin puncture sites. A number of therapeutic options exist for the treatment of the hemorrhagic diathesis caused by uremia, and these should be considered in any patient who is actively bleeding or about to undergo a surgical procedure.

Correction of anemia with either red blood cell transfusions or recombinant human erythropoietin contributes significantly to reducing the bleeding tendency. Raising the hematocrit to 27% or greater has been shown to decrease the bleeding time and improve platelet function.[115–117] Similarly, hemodialysis has been shown to partially correct the bleeding time and potentially decrease the risk of bleeding.[118]

Perhaps the most convenient and safest treatment for bleeding in the setting of uremia, regardless of whether a patient is being dialyzed, is the use of desmopressin (ddAVP). Possibly through release of von Willebrand factor from endothelial stores and through improved platelet signal transduction, it frequently improves hemostasis. In a randomized placebo-controlled trial, administration of 0.3 μg/kg of ddAVP resulted in a decrease in the bleeding time 1 hour after the infusion. However, the duration of action was relatively short and the improvement lasted only 6 to 12 hours.[119] If a longer duration of action is needed, administration of conjugated estrogens can be considered.[114,120] An intravenous dose of 0.6 mg/kg is given daily for 5 days. Although estrogens are slower in their onset of action, and perhaps somewhat less reproducible in terms of response, their effect can last 7 to 10 days. The mechanism of action of estrogens is not well understood but may be related to their effects on nitrous oxide. Finally, cryoprecipitate, rich in von Willebrand factor and fibrinogen, can also sometimes temporarily correct the bleeding time. It appears to act as quickly and last as long as ddAVP. A commonly used dose is 10 units every 12 to 24 hours.[121]

MANAGEMENT OF HEMOLYTIC-UREMIC SYNDROME AND THROMBOTIC THROMBOCYTOPENIC PURPURA

Hematologic and renal abnormalities can manifest nearly simultaneously and suddenly in two disorders: hemolytic-uremic syndrome (HUS) and thrombotic thrombocytopenic purpura (TTP)(see Chapter 139). Distinguishing between these two entities can be difficult.[122,123] They are both characterized by thrombocytopenia, microangiopathic hemolytic anemia, and platelet aggregation ultimately leading to end organ dysfunction.[124] In HUS, the microvascular thrombi tend to occur within the renal microcirculation, causing acute renal failure. In TTP, the microvascular ischemia occurs in many organs and may affect the cerebral circulation, causing neurologic abnormalities.

Although not infrequently idiopathic, both HUS and TTP have been associated with the administration of various medications such as cyclosporine (HUS) and clopidogrel (TTP). In addition, the occurrence of HUS has been associated with Shiga toxin-producing bacteria (*Escherichia coli* 0157:H7).[119] Interestingly, the clinical course of HUS appears to depend on cause. Children who suffer from postdiarrheal HUS generally improved on their own with supportive care, and they only occasionally require short-term dialysis.[125] Patients with medication-related HUS tend to have poorer prognoses.

Deficiencies in factors of the alternative complement pathway have been associated with HUS, and ADAMTS-13 deficiency has been found in some patients with TTP.[121,126,127] However, rapid determination of the level of these proteins is not yet routinely available, so the distinction between HUS and TTP, when made, generally relies on associated clinical findings.

In adults, HUS and TTP are often managed similarly by clinicians. Plasma-based therapies have been demonstrated to significantly decrease the mortality rates associated with HUS-TTP, and studies have documented the value of plasma exchange over simple plasma infusion.[128,129] The efficacy of plasma exchange possibly comes from its ability to remove the toxic factors implicated in the initiation of these disorders as well as replace a depleted, missing, or inhibited factor such as the ADAMTS-13 protease.[130,131] Some clinicians advocate that plasma exchange should begin promptly in any individual suspected of having HUS or TTP, regardless of whether the former or the latter is more strongly suspected.[132] Daily therapy with total plasma exchange is recommended until remission is evident, as determined by resolution of any renal and/or neurologic failure, normalization of platelet count and lactate dehydrogenase level, and a stable hematocrit level reflecting absence of ongoing hemolysis, or until it is clear that no further clinical benefit is being derived. Further research will hopefully better elucidate the pathogenesis of HUS and TTP and thereby facilitate the development of tailored therapies for each of these entities.

SUMMARY

There are numerous hematologic manifestations of liver and renal disease ranging from morphologic changes of red blood cells to coagulation abnormalities affecting hemostasis. Optimal patient care is facilitated by an understanding of these associated complications and their appropriate management.

SUGGESTED READINGS

Bailie GR, Clark JA, Lane CE, Lane PL: Hypersensitivity reactions and deaths associated with intravenous iron preparations. Nephrol Dial Transplant 20:1443, 2005.

Lodge JPA, Jonas S, Jones RM, et al: Efficacy and safety of repeated perioperative doses of recombinant factor VIIa in liver transplantation. Liver Transpl 11:973, 2005.

Niemann CU, Behrends M, Quan D, et al: Recombinant factor VIIa reduces transfusion requirements in liver transplant patients with high MELD scores. Transfus Med 16:93, 2006.

Planinsic RM, van der Meer J, Testa G, et al: Safety and efficacy of a single bolus administration of recombinant factor VIIa in liver transplantation due to chronic liver disease. Liver Transpl 11:895, 2005.

Xia VW, Steadman RH: Antifibrinolytics in orthotopic liver transplantation: Current status and controversies. 11:10, 2005.

Zipfel PF, Misselwitz J, Licht C, Skerka C: The role of defective complement control in hemolytic uremic syndrome. Semin Thromb Hemost 32:146, 2006.

REFERENCES

For complete list of references log onto www.expertconsult.com

CHAPTER 157

HEMATOLOGIC MANIFESTATIONS OF SYSTEMIC DISEASE: INFECTION, CHRONIC INFLAMMATION, AND CANCER

Peter W. Marks and David S. Rosenthal

Various infections, chronic inflammatory conditions, and malignancies share potential hematologic manifestations. Depending on the nature of the particular condition, such effects may be observed as abnormalities in one or more of the hematopoietic cell lineages or in the function of the blood coagulation cascade. Because hematologic manifestations often are early indicators of systemic disease, familiarity with the disease entities associated with such changes is important knowledge for the practicing clinician.

INFECTIOUS DISEASES

Bacterial, fungal, protozoan, and viral infections may have major hematologic manifestations.[1] In certain cases, such as that of infection with malarial parasites, there is a characteristic finding, such as hemolytic anemia. In other cases, the effects may be more diverse, or an infectious agent may cause different disease manifestations in different individuals. Such is the case for tuberculosis, which can lead to pancytopenia in some individuals and a leukemoid reaction in others. Past medical history may also have an effect on the hematologic manifestation of disease. For example, infection with *Babesia* is often subclinical, yet in the case of individuals who have undergone splenectomy, fulminant manifestations are not uncommon. This section will focus on the etiologic agents and manifestations associated with bacterial, fungal, protozoan, and viral infections, with the exception of human immunodeficiency virus (HIV) infection and infectious mononucleosis associated with Epstein–Barr virus (EBV) infection, which are described in detail in Chapters 158 and 54, respectively.

PANCYTOPENIA

Bacterial, fungal, protozoan, and viral infectious agents are sometimes associated with pancytopenia, which may range from a mild depression in blood counts to severe trilineage aplasia. Pancytopenia may be caused by direct toxic effects leading to bone marrow necrosis, bone marrow replacement (myelophthisis), inhibitory effects of inflammatory mediators, or activation of the reticuloendothelial system leading to hemophagocytic syndrome.[2] Alternatively, it may be the result of persistent congestive splenomegaly resulting from infections such as salmonellosis, tularemia, syphilis, toxoplasmosis, schistosomiasis, malaria, infectious mononucleosis, or hepatitis.[3,4]

Particularly in patients with poor nutritional status, immunocompromise, or previous treatment with chemotherapy, pancytopenia can result from gram-positive, gram-negative, or fungal infections, such as with *Brucella*, *Salmonella typhi*, *Aspergillus*, or *Mucor*. Mycobacterial infections leading to granuloma formation are also associated with pancytopenia,. This feature may be the first symptom of these infections, which tend to manifest less acutely.

Viral infections associated with pancytopenia include those with arboviruses, such as dengue, which cause transient effects, and suspected agents, such as a non-A to -G hepatitis that appears to be associated with more durable aplastic anemia.[5] The latter association with viral infection is suspected, rather than proven, as particularly in young adult males pancytopenia may be preceded clinically by hepatitis. In general, immunosuppressive therapy or allogeneic bone marrow transplantation is the treatment of choice in such cases.

ANEMIA

Infectious agents can cause anemia by a variety of different mechanisms. These broadly fall into the categories of decreased production, increased destruction, or blood loss (Table 157–1). Although the effect of increased destruction by infectious agents is generally confined to the red cell lineage, decreased production is often, but not invariably, associated with general myelosuppression and effects on other cell lineages.

Anemia Caused by Decreased Production

Anemia due to inflammatory changes, frequently described in adults as the anemia of chronic disease or the anemia of chronic inflammation, is one of the most common manifestations of infection. In the pediatric age group, similar, more transient changes are often described as the anemia of acute infection.[6,7]

The anemia of chronic disease can be characterized as a normocytic, normochromic, or mildly microcytic, hypochromic anemia with a low reticulocyte count. Serum iron and transferrin levels are often low in patients with normal to increased body iron stores. The pathophysiology of the anemia of chronic disease has become increasingly defined.[8] The anemia of chronic disease appears to result from a combination of increased levels of hepcidin in combination with the release of several cytokines. In this setting several events occur: (a) Iron becomes trapped in the reticuloendothelial system, (b) erythropoietin levels decrease, and (c) cytokines directly suppress the hematopoiesis in the bone marrow. The iron-regulatory protein hepcidin plays a key role in this process through its eventual effects on diverse aspects of iron metabolism (Fig. 157–1).[9]

Though confined to specific anatomic spaces, several localized infections with bacterial, fungal, or protozoal agents are often associated with the anemia of chronic disease. These include abscesses, cavitary pulmonary disease, chronic infectious arthritis, chronic osteomyelitis, and endocarditis. For example, hypoproliferative anemia may manifest in patients with tuberculosis. In most clinical cases, the degree of anemia tends to correlate with the duration and extent of infection.

Viral infections can also be associated with hypoproliferative anemia. Parvovirus B19 infection is the classic example.[10] This agent infects red blood cell precursors via receptor-mediated entry through the blood group P receptor. It can then replicate in erythroid progenitor cells. Although the transient red aplasia that generally results from parvovirus B19 infection is most often apparent clinically in patients with underlying hematologic conditions, including hemoglobinopathies and in immunodeficiency syndromes, it occasionally manifests in otherwise healthy individuals.[11] A specific example of the manifestation of parvovirus B19 infection in patients with hematologic disorders is the occurrence of aplastic crises in patients with sickle cell disease.[12] Additionally, lack of clearance of the virus in immunocompromised individuals can lead to prolonged periods of anemia. In such cases, treatment with immunoglobulin may prove beneficial.[13]

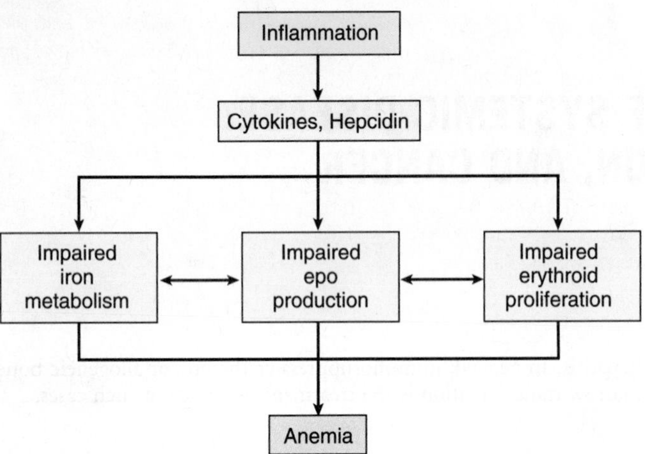

Figure 157–1 Pathophysiology of the anemia of chronic disease. The same potential mechanisms are involved in the hypoproliferative anemia that is frequently seen in infectious diseases, rheumatologic conditions, and malignancy. An inflammatory condition (infection, systemic inflammatory disease, or malignancy) leads to the production of hepcidin and cytokines, which subsequently prevent iron from being released from the reticuloendothelial system, leading to decreased erythropoietin (epo) release and inhibited hematopoiesis.

Table 157–1 Mechanisms of Anemia in Infectious Diseases

Decreased production of red blood cells
Anemia of chronic disease
Anemia of acute infection (pediatrics)
Aplasia
Increased destruction of red blood cells
Parasitization of the erythrocyte
Hemolytic uremic syndrome
Disseminated intravascular coagulation
Effects of enzyme deficiency (G6PD)
Immune-mediated hemolysis
Blood loss
Gastrointestinal (helminthic infections)
Genitourinary (schistosomiasis)
Pulmonary (tuberculosis)

Table 157–2 Causes of Infection-Related Hemolytic Anemia

Erythrocytic parasitization
Malaria
Babesiosis
Bartonellosis
Toxin production
Clostridium perfringens
Immune hemolysis
Cold agglutinin disease
Mycoplasma pneumoniae
EBV
Paroxysmal cold hemoglobinuria (Donath-Landsteiner antibodies)
Secondary and congenital syphilis
Measles
Measles vaccination
Antigen-antibody complex ("innocent bystander")
Haemophilus influenzae
Polyagglutination
Enteric bacteria
Oxidative effects of infection or treatments for infection
G6PD deficiency
Mechanical destruction
DIC
HUS
Endocarditis

DIC, disseminated intravascular coagulation; EBV, Epstein-Barr virus; G6PD, glucose-6-phosphate dehydrogenase; HUS, hemolytic uremic syndrome.

Anemia Caused by Increased Destruction

Hemolytic anemia in the setting of infection can result from various mechanisms, including those related to direct invasion of red blood cells with pathogens, toxin production, resultant immune reactions, inherent increased susceptibility of red cells to hemolysis, and mechanical effects (Table 157–2). Diagnosis of these entities relies on a carefully performed history and physical examination, which in the setting of a heightened index of suspicion should be followed by an appropriate diagnostic evaluation. In some cases, specialized testing, such as serology, molecular diagnostics, or enzymatic assays, is critical to an accurate diagnosis. In other cases, examination of the peripheral blood, through review of thin or thick smears or of special stains, provides the definitive diagnosis. This is the case for infection with intraerythrocytic parasites as in babesiosis or malaria.

Although malaria is perhaps the best-known parasitic infection causing hemolysis, several other agents are capable of producing this effect. Infection may be caused by adherence of agents to the red cell membrane followed by its disruption, or by infestation of the erythrocyte by the parasite, often as an obligatory step in the life cycle of the pathogen. Infection caused by *Bartonella bacilliformis* is an example of the former, whereas infection with tick-borne *Babesia microti* is an example of the latter.[14,15] Bartonellosis (Oroya fever) is like malaria in that it is a vector-borne illness. It is transmitted to humans by the bite of a sand fly found in the high Andes. The disease manifests with fever, chills, and hemolysis within 2 to 3 weeks of infection. Resultant hemolysis can be particularly severe or even fatal if untreated with appropriate antibiotics (eg, tetracycline or chloramphenicol). In the case of malaria, the pathogenesis of erythrocytic infection has been elucidated.[16] In the case of *Plasmodium falciparum*, merozoites, which are abundantly present in the bloodstream, adhere to glycophorin molecules on the surface of red cells. The merozoites are then able to transiently disrupt the membrane and underlying cytoskeletal structure of the erythrocyte in order to gain entry, without causing lysis of the cell. The organisms subsequently feed on hemoglobin, produce various proteins, and eventually undergo destruction in the spleen. Hemolysis can be particularly severe in some cases (Blackwater fever) when acute intravascular hemolysis results from an autoimmune reaction. In this case, the direct antiglobulin (Coombs) test is positive.

The effect of bacterial hemolytic toxins is rarely observed in humans, except in the case of infection by *Clostridium perfringens*.[17] Although clostridial sepsis is rare, it is sometimes seen in the setting of septic abortion, biliary tract disease, traumatic wound infection, or in the setting of severe pancytopenia, such as in individuals undergoing intensive induction or consolidation chemotherapy for hematologic malignancies. The organism produces a lecithinase (α-toxin), which reacts with red cell membrane lipoproteins to release lysolecithin, which is then lytic to the cells.[18] Although the underlying organism is sensitive to antibiotics (eg, metronidazole), fulminant infection in the presence of underlying disease and decreased oxygen-carrying capacity frequently lead to mortality.

Immune mechanisms are ultimately responsible for the hemolytic conditions that result from infection with a variety of pathogens.[19] These can broadly be divided into autoimmune, antigen–antibody complex ("innocent bystander"), and polyagglutination reactions. Certain infectious agents can stimulate antibody production with affinity for red cell surface proteins, thereby causing autoimmune hemolytic anemia. Intravascular and extravascular mechanisms have been defined: the former are generally secondary to immunoglobulin M (IgM) or "cold" antibodies, whereas the latter are generally secondary to IgG or "warm" antibodies. The two most common infections causing cold autoimmune hemolytic anemia are those due to *Mycoplasma pneumoniae* and EBV associated with infectious mononucleosis.[20] Each of these infections results in the production of IgM antibodies to the I system of red cell membrane antigens (I and i are carbohydrate surface antigens). In the case of *M pneumoniae* the target antigen is the I antigen, and in the case of EBV it is the i antigen. These antibodies bind to red cells at temperatures lower than 37°C and fix complement, eventually leading to hemolysis. The incidence of cold autoimmune hemolytic anemia from these infections is relatively low. When it occurs, the mainstay of treatment is supportive care and maintenance of warm body temperature, as low external temperatures can significantly exacerbate hemolysis. Immunosuppressive therapy is not generally indicated. Other bacterial and viral infections such as those with *Legionella*, mumps, rubella, and cytomegalovirus (CMV), as well as vaccination against measles, have also been occasionally associated with cold autoimmune hemolytic anemia. IgG antibodies that react with red cells in the cold cause a rare form of cold autoimmune hemolytic anemia. These Donath–Landsteiner antibodies are responsible for paroxysmal cold hemoglobinuria.[21] Although they may also be idiopathic, in the setting of infection they are associated with syphilis in adults and viral infections, such as varicella, mumps, or measles, in children. Warm autoimmune hemolytic anemia in response to infection is very rare.

Antigen–antibody complexes are a rare cause of hemolysis due to infection through an "innocent bystander" effect. In this case, the infectious agent, or an antibiotic administered for its eradication, leads to antibody formation. These antibody–antigen complexes then attach to the red cell surface and lead to hemolysis. *Haemophilus influenzae* type b meningitis has been associated with this mechanism of hemolysis in children.[22] Polyagglutination is a rare type of hemolysis that results from the exposure of hidden erythrocyte antigens and subsequent reaction with antibodies that would not normally react with intact antigens.[23] For example, neuraminidase, produced by enteric bacteria, can effect such a change, ultimately leading to hemolysis.

An inherent increased susceptibility of red cells to infection occurs in patients with glucose-6-phosphate dehydrogenase (G6PD) deficiency.[24] Although this trait, prevalent in African and Mediterranean populations, is relatively protective against malarial infection, it also makes these individuals susceptible to oxidant stress. G6PD is chiefly responsible for the production of antioxidants in the red cell (reduced glutathione). Decreased production of antioxidants in G6PD deficiency leads to the production of oxidized hemoglobin and oxidized lipids within the red cell. This eventually results in hemolysis within the spleen. Oxidized aggregates of hemoglobin are visible as Heinz bodies on supravital staining of blood smears with methyl or crystal violet (Fig. 157–2). The resultant removal of these Heinz bodies in the process of RBC destruction leads to the characteristic bite cells seen on a peripheral blood smear. Hemolysis in G6PD deficiency may result from infections and from therapeutics used in their management (Table 157–3). Bacterial and viral infections have been implicated, as well as a number of antibiotic and antimalarial agents.

Finally, hemolysis may result from infectious agents. For example, disseminated intravascular coagulation (DIC) caused by bacterial or fungal infection or hemolytic uremic syndrome caused by *Escherichia coli* 0157:H7 infection causes shearing of the erythrocyte within the vasculature, leading to the characteristic microangiopathic changes on the peripheral blood smear. Such mechanical hemolysis may also be seen in severe cases of endocarditis due to turbulent flow through abnormal cardiac valves.

Anemia Caused by Blood Loss

Several infectious agents are associated with disruption of the integrity of the mucosa of the gastrointestinal or genitourinary tracts, and therefore lead to blood loss anemia. Infection with *Helicobacter pylori*, a major causative agent in peptic ulcer disease, is a significant cause of blood loss anemia in developed nations.[25] Worldwide, helminthic infections, such as that of the hookworm, are a major cause of iron deficiency anemia as a result of chronic blood loss through the gastrointestinal tract. Eradication of these infectious agents and iron replacement, if appropriate, lead to resolution of the anemia.

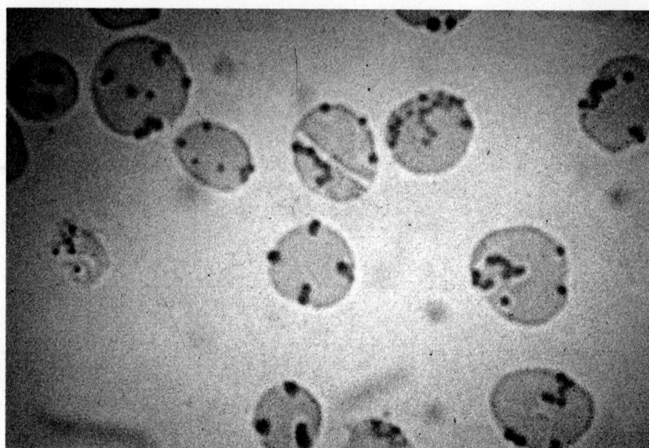

Figure 157–2 Heinz body preparation revealing aggregates of precipitated hemoglobin, such as those that might be present in a G6PD-deficient patient with infection or undergoing treatment with oxidant medications. G6PD, glucose-6-phosphate dehydrogenase.

Table 157–3 Causes of Hemolysis in Patients With G6PD Deficiency

Infectious agents
Salmonella
Escherichia coli
β-Hemolytic streptococci
Rickettsia
Hepatitis viruses
Influenza A
Medications
Antimalarials
Primaquine
Pamaquine
Sulfonamides
Sulfones
Nitrofurans
Sulfapyridine

G6PD, glucose-6-phosphate dehydrogenase.

WHITE BLOOD CELL CHANGES

Changes in leukocyte parameters are often one of the hallmarks of infection. These include changes in number and in cellular morphology. However, the changes encountered may vary significantly, depending on the type of infection and the host affected. For example, certain infections are commonly associated with leukocytosis, whereas others are associated with leukopenia. In addition, the same infectious agent might cause leukocytosis in one individual but leukopenia in another.

Morphologic Abnormalities

Review of the peripheral blood smear can provide significant insight into the possible presence of infection. Early changes in infection may

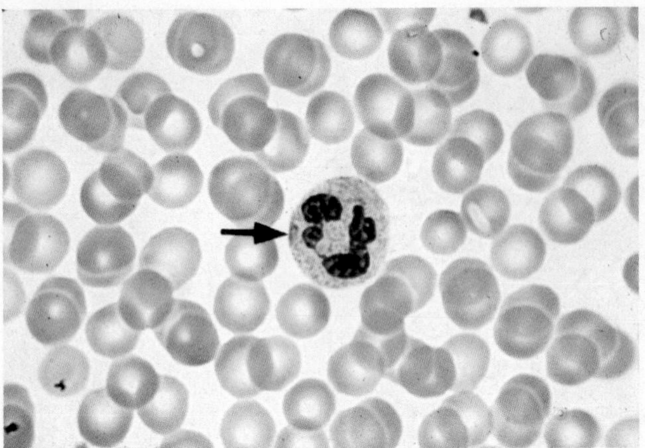

Figure 157–3 Döhle bodies seen on a Wright–Giemsa-stained smear. These *sky blue inclusions* in the cytoplasm of neutrophilic leukocytes represent collapsed stacks of Golgi apparatus. When they are observed, the differential diagnosis is relatively short. When present in the setting of toxic granulations or vacuolization, or both, the likely cause is an infection or significant marrow stimulation, such as that seen with myeloid growth factor administration. When present in nearly all neutrophilic leukocytes, and in the setting of giant platelets, Döhle bodies are indicative of May-Hegglin anomaly, an inherited autosomal dominant disorder.

include an increase in the number of bands, even before the development of overt leukocytosis. A greater shift to immaturity (left shift) may occur when infection is severe, with metamyelocytes or even earlier forms present on the peripheral blood smear. Particularly revealing are the presence of toxic granulations, cytoplasmic vacuolization, and Döhle bodies (Fig. 157–3); their appearance should trigger an assessment for the possibility of infection. Indeed, occasionally, these changes may precede the development of other infectious symptoms and signs. Rarely, in cases of severe systemic infection, organisms may be seen within leukocytes on peripheral blood smear. On Wright–Giemsa-stained smears, both gram-negative and gram-positive organisms stain purple, in contrast to their appearance on traditional gram stains.

Morphologic changes in white blood cells may also be observed on a peripheral blood smear that may underlie a predisposition to infection. For example, pseudo-Pelger–Huët anomaly and hypogranulation of polymorphonuclear leukocytes may indicate an underlying myelodysplastic syndrome.

Leukocytosis

The extent of increase in the white blood cell count may vary depending on the etiologic agent, severity of infection, and host factors. Most limited bacterial infections are associated with a white blood cell count of 12 to 14 × 10^9/L, whereas systemic infections will have a white blood cell count of 15 to 30 × 10^9/L. Massive infections, particularly with certain agents, may produce leukemoid reactions with elevations in the white blood cell count to 150 to 200 × 10^9/L.[26] Such severe elevations in white blood cells often trigger significant concern among clinicians for the possibility of underlying hematologic malignancies. Particularly in the presence of anemia or thrombocytopenia, or both, such elevations in white blood cell can present diagnostic challenges that require resolution through bone marrow examination or other specialized diagnostic testing. Leukemoid reactions are defined as a white blood cell count of greater than 50 × 10^9/L, with or without the presence of immature cells, in the absence of evidence of leukemia.

Various hematologic malignancies may be mimicked by the response to infectious agents (Table 157–4). Among these, a picture that appears like chronic myelogenous leukemia (CML) is probably

Table 157–4 Hematologic Conditions Mimicked by Infections

Condition
CML
Infection in the presence of underlying disorders
Meningitis (*Haemophilus influenzae, Neisseria meningitidis*)
Staphylococcal sepsis
Pneumococcal endocarditis
Salmonellosis
Diphtheria
Bubonic plague
Tuberculosis
AML
Tuberculosis
Recovery from agranulocytosis
CLL
Pertussis
Varicella
Viral exanthems
ALL
Tuberculosis
Infectious mononucleosis
Acute Monocytic Leukemia
Tuberculosis
Myelodysplasia
HIV
Other viral infections

ALL, acute lymphocytic leukemia; AML, acute myeloid leukemia; CLL, chronic lymphocytic leukemia; CML, chronic myeloid leukemia; HIV, human immunodeficiency virus.

the most common. A high white blood cell count with few immature cells may accompany infection when underlying disorders are present, such as malignancy, rheumatologic disease, or glomerulonephritis. A variety of bacterial infections, in the absence of underlying disorders, can also manifest with a similar picture. For example, disseminated tuberculosis may manifest with white blood cell counts of up to 200 × 10^9/L and a moderate left shift.[27] Although bone marrow examination is sometimes necessary to distinguish such conditions, the wide availability of molecular diagnostic testing for the BCR–ABL translocation can help exclude CML from consideration based on a peripheral blood sample.

Laboratory findings suggesting hematologic malignancies other than CML may also be seen. A rebound phenomenon resembling acute myelogenous leukemia (AML) may accompany recovery from antibiotic-induced agranulocytosis and after marrow suppression from severe bacterial and protozoan infections. A mature lymphocytosis, such as that seen in chronic lymphocytic leukemia (CLL), is less likely to be mimicked by infection; although before the introduction of antibiotics, cases of potentially fatal cases of pertussis were reported in the setting of a hematologic picture similar to CLL.[28] More commonly among hematologic conditions mimicked by infection, the presence of immature lymphoid cells resembling lymphoblasts in young adults with infectious mononucleosis occasionally leads to an inappropriate diagnosis of acute lymphocytic leukemia (ALL). Review of a combination of laboratory parameters including heterogeneity of atypical lymphocytes, liver function tests, and serology helps to exclude ALL. Changes indicative of myelodysplasia may also occur with viral infections, and can be difficult to distinguish from an underlying marrow disorder. In addition, certain conditions may be associated with the appearance of nucleated red blood cells in addition to immature myeloid cells (leukoerythroblastic response).[29] These include septicemia, miliary tuberculosis, and histoplasmosis. When concern exists for a potential underlying hematologic disorder in the setting of infection, careful monitoring in the recovery phase from infection is indicated.

Table 157–5 Infections That May Cause Neutropenia in the Normal Host

Bacterial
Salmonellosis
Tularemia
Brucellosis
Rickettsia
Viral
Measles
Varicella (chickenpox)
Rubella
Influenza
Infectious hepatitis
Yellow fever
Sandfly fever
HIV
Colorado tick fever
Dengue fever
Rocky Mountain spotted fever
Protozoan
Malaria
Kala-azar
Relapsing fever
Massive
Miliary tuberculosis

HIV, human immunodeficiency virus.

Neutropenia and Neutrophilia

Although white blood cell counts of less than 1.5 × 10^9/L can occur paradoxically in almost any infection, they are most commonly encountered in patients with compromised bone marrow as a result of chronic debilitation, nutritional deficiency, or chemotherapy. In addition, certain infections characteristically present with neutropenia. These include a few bacterial pathogens, protozoan, and viral infections (Table 157–5). Viral pathogens are notable in this regard, and include infectious hepatitis, influenza, and HIV infection. Neutropenia may also occur late in the course, during the bacteremic phase, of typhoid, paratyphoid, and tularemia. Agranulocytosis, however, is a rare complication of infection. If it occurs after initiation of antibiotic therapy, it is suggestive of an adverse drug reaction. Alternatively, it suggests an underlying primary bone marrow disorder or immunodeficiency syndrome. For example, an aplastic picture may occur in immunosuppressed patients infected with a viral infection such as parvovirus B19.[30]

Neutrophilia usually accompanies the leukocytosis and left shift that occur in infections. More than two-thirds of cases of infection-related neutrophilia are secondary to bacteria.[31] However, neutrophilia is sometimes present in infection in the absence of an increased total white blood cell count. This change may be seen early in the response to infection, as neutrophilic leukocytes are released from the marginated pool in response to inflammatory mediators and catecholamines.

Lymphocytopenia and Lymphocytosis

Lymphocyte counts of less than 1 × 10^9/L are common in acute bacterial, fungal, viral, and protozoan infections, in addition to being quite common in hospitalized patients.[32] Chronic infections with tuberculosis, histoplasmosis, and brucellosis are also associated with lymphocytopenia. Alterations in the numbers of B and T cells may also occur with infection, and changes in T-cell subsets can occur in bacterial, fungal, and viral diseases, in addition to HIV, with which they are classically associated.[33] For example, early in the course of acute bacterial infection, the total number of T cells can decline, whereas the number of B cells increases.

Table 157–6 Infections that May Cause Lymphocytosis

Acute Infection
Pertussis
Infectious mononucleosis
Infectious hepatitis
Acute infectious lymphocytosis
Toxoplasmosis
Cytomegalovirus
Chronic Infection
Tuberculosis
Brucellosis
Syphilis
Congenital
Secondary
Rickettsia

Lymphocytosis is a rare finding in bacterial infections, with the exception of that from *Bordetella pertussis* (Table 157–6). In this case, it is suspected that the toxin produced by the organism inhibits lymphocyte migration out of the bloodstream into tissues. However, rickettsial and viral infections are associated with lymphocytosis (Table 157–6). Acute infectious lymphocytosis, a disorder of unclear etiology suspected to be related to viral infection with an adenovirus or coxsackievirus A, can sometimes be associated with a significant lymphocytosis of 30 to 100 × 10^9/L.

Morphologic abnormalities in lymphocytes, particularly in viral infections such as infectious mononucleosis, can occasionally appear to mimic those of patients with ALL. Although variation in the atypical nature of such lymphocytes is a helpful diagnostic clue on examination of the peripheral blood smear, flow cytometric analysis can help eliminate leukemia from consideration without the need for a bone marrow biopsy.[34]

Other Changes in White Blood Cells

Eosinopenia is generally a correlate of the severity of infection, and its presence may suggest a poor prognosis. Eosinophilia, defined as an absolute count greater than 0.25 × 10^9/L, although rare in typical bacterial, fungal, and viral infections, is common in invasive parasitic disease.[35] Protozoan infection with trichinosis, schistosomiasis, filariasis, and echinococcal disease are frequently accompanied by eosinophilia. Unless invasive, helminthic intestinal infections tend not to cause a change in the eosinophil count. Significant eosinophilia may also be seen in bronchopulmonary aspergillosis, coccidioidomycosis, and *Chlamydia pneumonitis* of infancy. In contrast to eosinophilia, basophilia is rarely seen in response to infection. Its presence suggests an underlying myeloproliferative disorder.

Monocytosis, defined as an absolute count greater than 0.95 × 10^9/L, may be seen in subacute or chronic infections. It may also develop during the recovery phase of any infection. Infections associated with monocytosis include tuberculosis, syphilis, subacute bacterial endocarditis, brucellosis, and many rickettsial and protozoan infections including malaria, trypanosomiasis, and kala-azar. Infection with varicella-zoster can also cause a significant monocytosis. In the case of tuberculosis, the monocyte-to-lymphocyte ratio may reflect the activity of disease. Normally this ratio is about 0.3, and when it exceeds 1 it is associated with active exudates and a poor prognosis.[36] With improvement of disease, this ratio returns toward normal.

PLATELETS AND ABNORMALITIES OF COAGULATION

Thrombocytopenia

Thrombocytopenia in the absence of disseminated intravascular coagulation may be seen in septicemia associated with bacterial, fungal, or viral infections, and can occasionally be quite severe.[37] More than 65% of cases of bacteremia are associated with thrombocytopenia, and about one-third of cases are associated with decreases in platelet counts to below 50 × 10^9/L. The mechanism underlying thrombocytopenia in the absence of DIC may be related to suppression of platelet production, increased platelet utilization, and immune phenomena.

Bacterial and viral infections may also be associated with the development of immune thrombocytopenia. Hepatitis C infection in particular is associated with this complication.[38] Certain antibiotics, such as vancomycin, are also occasionally associated with the development of immune thrombocytopenia.

Thrombocytosis

Infection is one of the more common causes of mild to moderate thrombocytosis to the range of 500 to 700 × 10^9/L, although platelet counts of up to 1000 × 10^9/L may be seen.[39] This is particularly true in chronic infections such as tuberculosis, osteomyelitis, and subacute bacterial endocarditis, as well as during the recovery from infection. In general, elevated platelet counts in the presence of infection are best managed by observation, and there is no role for antiplatelet agents.

Coagulation Abnormalities

Many cases of DIC are associated with an infectious etiology. Possible underlying causes include endothelial surface damage and tissue necrosis. Bacterial, fungal, viral, and protozoan infections have all been implicated (Table 157–7). While treating the underlying infection, supportive care with the transfusion of appropriate blood products is indicated.

Thrombotic complications (aside from DIC) are uncommonly caused by infection, but do occur. These include suppurative thrombophlebitis at intravenous sites in the arms or legs, septic thrombophlebitis of the pelvic veins, and thrombosis caused by aspergillus infection.[40] In such cases, coordinated management is necessary, and may require the administration of antibiotic or antifungal agents along with anticoagulants.

Table 157–7 Infections Frequently Associated With Disseminated Intravascular Coagulation

Bacteria *Neisseria meningitides* *Staphylococcus aureus* *Streptococcus pneumoniae* *Neisseria gonorrhoeae* *Mycobacterium tuberculosis* *Salmonella typhimurium*
Rickettsia
Mycoplasmosis
Histoplasmosis
Aspergillosis
Malaria

CHRONIC INFLAMMATORY DISORDERS

Rheumatoid arthritis is well associated with the anemia of chronic disease. In addition, anemia and other hematologic manifestations may occur in other chronic inflammatory disorders, including systemic lupus erythematosus (SLE), polymyalgia rheumatica, scleroderma, mixed connective tissue disease, and Sjögren syndrome, among others. On some occasions, the hematologic complications may be the dominant symptoms of these conditions.

ANEMIA

Anemia Caused by Decreased Production

The anemia of chronic disease is one of the most common hematologic disorders in chronic inflammatory conditions. The mechanism of pathogenesis is similar to that described for the anemia due to infection (see Fig. 157–1).[41] A combination of inflammatory cytokines, increased hepcidin production leading to the sequestration of iron in the reticuloendothelial system, and decreased erythropoietin production leads to decreased red cell production. Though erythropoietin deficiency does not appear to be the primary event leading to the development of anemia, its therapeutic administration to patients can in many cases overcome other barriers to red cell production, leading to improvement in anemia.[42] In particular, the beneficial effect of erythropoietin has been documented in the management of anemia in rheumatoid arthritis.[43] Recombinant human erythropoietin (rHuEPO) and darbepoetin, a modified erythropoietin with a longer half-life, are available for the treatment of such patients. When using these agents, it is particularly important to assess whether there are adequate iron stores. Iron-deficient individuals will not respond

Treatment of the Anemia of Chronic Disease with Erythropoietin

When administered appropriately, erythropoietin (EPO) can significantly improve the quality of life of patients with anemia of chronic disease. Therapy with either recombinant human erythropoietin (rHuEPO) or with darbepoetin is best considered only for patients with hemoglobin values of less than 10 g/dL, unless specific comorbidities such as significant cardiac or pulmonary disease exist. Though not specifically approved for this indication, a starting dose of 40,000 U rHuEPO weekly or 200 μg darbepoetin every other week is often sufficient to produce a 1 to 2 g/dL improvement in hemoglobin in patients with replete iron stores. After several weeks it may be necessary to decrease the frequency or dose of administration, based on response. If a response is not observed after 4 to 8 weeks of therapy and the patient is iron replete, the dose may be escalated by 50%. Thereafter, a lack of response after 4 to 8 more weeks of therapy should lead to its discontinuation and a search for other potential causes of the anemia. In some cases, bone marrow examination to search for underlying disorders such as myelodysplasia may be indicated.

The single most common reason for a lack of response to erythropoietin in patients with chronic inflammatory disorders, and rheumatoid arthritis in particular, is the concomitant presence of iron deficiency anemia. Given the inconvenience of subcutaneous injections and the cost of erythropoietin, iron stores should routinely be assessed before erythropoietin therapy is initiated. When severe iron deficiency is present, consideration may be given to the administration of intravenous iron. Preparations such as iron dextran, iron sucrose, and iron gluconate are now available for this use. Use of these agents must be tempered somewhat against their side effects, which include a small risk of allergic reactions.

to erythropoietin, and frank iron deficiency may be provoked by the stimulation of erythropoiesis in patients with borderline iron stores.[44]

Chronic inflammatory conditions have also been associated with other causes of hypoproliferative anemia. Acquired pure red cell aplasia has occasionally been associated with both rheumatoid arthritis and SLE.[45,46] The diagnostic distinction between the anemia of chronic disease and acquired pure red cell aplasia is based on the degree of anemia, as well as the finding on bone marrow examination of severe hypoplasia in the setting of relative preservation of other lineages in the latter entity. Unlike the anemia of chronic disease, acquired pure red cell aplasia does not respond to therapy with erythropoietin. Toxic effects of medications should be excluded. Although spontaneous remission sometimes occurs after several weeks, treatment with immunosuppressive or cytotoxic agents is often necessary.[47]

Myelodysplastic syndromes have also been associated with rheumatologic manifestations. Cases have been reported in which arthritis preceded the development of myelodysplasia, as well as cases in which rheumatologic manifestations such as vasculitis occurred subsequent to the diagnosis.[48] Optimal therapy for such patients has yet to be defined, though experimental approaches, such as the administration of antitumor necrosis factor (TNF) therapy, have been investigated.[49]

Anemia Caused by Increased Destruction

Autoimmune hemolytic anemia is associated with several rheumatologic disorders. In particular, in SLE it has also been associated with immune thrombocytopenia (Evans syndrome) and/or with leukopenia. Most typically this is a direct antiglobulin test (Coombs)-positive anemia found in the setting of other indicators of warm autoimmune hemolytic anemia (spherocytes on a peripheral blood smear, increased reticulocyte count, and elevated lactate dehydrogenase [LDH]).

If the anemia is mild and patients are asymptomatic, no specific therapy for autoimmune hemolytic anemia need be administered. Patients with more severe anemia who are symptomatic may be treated for warm autoimmune hemolytic anemia with corticosteroids (prednisone 60–100 mg/day followed by a slow taper). Those who do not respond, or who cannot be weaned off of corticosteroids, are candidates for splenectomy. Therapies used for patients unable to undergo splenectomy or who are refractory to splenectomy include other immunosuppressant and cytotoxic agents, as well as danazol.[50] In addition, responses to anti-CD20 monoclonal antibody have been reported.[51]

Anemia Caused by Blood Loss

Iron deficiency anemia is common in chronic inflammatory disorders, and particularly in patients with rheumatoid arthritis treated with aspirin or other nonsteroidal drugs, which often lead to gastrointestinal blood loss. However, its diagnosis can be particularly challenging, as hallmarks of iron deficiency anemia commonly used in clinical practice may be absent. Surrogate measures of iron stores are affected by the inflammatory response (eg, serum ferritin may be elevated as an acute phase reactant), and patients may be taking medications (eg, methotrexate) that lead to overall elevations in the mean corpuscular volume. The diagnosis is clear when the serum ferritin value is less than 10 μg/L and is highly suggested when the value is less than 30 μg/L, yet iron deficiency may still be present along with much higher ferritin levels.[52] Use of a combination of mean cell volume, transferrin saturation, and ferritin and use of soluble transferrin receptor have been proposed as better noninvasive measures.[53,54] However, the diagnosis of iron deficiency must sometimes rely on bone marrow examination. In such cases, iron staining of a bone marrow aspirate may be preferable to that of a bone marrow biopsy as certain fixatives may leach out iron from the biopsy.

Therapy to remediate iron deficiency in patients with rheumatoid arthritis and other chronic inflammatory conditions may depend on the extent of anemia and on the administration of concomitant medications. In particular, the administration of strong antacid medications, such as proton pump inhibitors, may decrease oral iron absorption. In some cases where administration of such medications is necessary, and the degree of anemia is moderately severe, consideration may be given to the administration of intravenous iron. Rapid repletion of iron by the intravenous route is highly effective, but is occasionally associated with side effects that include allergic reactions.

WHITE BLOOD CELL CHANGES

Two rheumatologic disorders are associated with changes in white blood cell parameters: SLE is often associated with neutropenia, and rheumatoid arthritis is occasionally associated with neutropenia and splenomegaly (Felty syndrome).[55] In SLE, neutropenia is often mild to moderate, is not associated with a significant increased risk for infection, and does not require specific therapy.

Felty syndrome is a more problematic issue in patients with a history of rheumatoid arthritis. It tends to manifest years after the initial diagnosis of rheumatoid arthritis, often when the arthritis is not very active.[56] Various pathophysiologic mechanisms have been proposed, including antineutrophil antibodies and T cell-mediated suppression of neutrophil production.[57] Because hairy cell leukemia and T-γ lymphoproliferative disorder may manifest similarly, they must be considered in the differential diagnosis.

The neutropenia in Felty syndrome may be severe and can be associated with recurrent infections, as well as with leg ulceration. Particularly in infection requiring treatment, use of hematopoietic growth factors, such as granulocyte colony-stimulating factor (G-CSF) or granulocyte–macrophage colony-stimulating factor (GM-CSF), may be beneficial, and prolonged hematologic responses are sometimes observed. However, complications with the use of G-CSF may occasionally include the reactivation of arthritis and the development of vasculitis; these may be minimized by using the lowest possible dose of G-CSF necessary to maintain a white blood cell count higher than 1000 μL.[58] Alternatively, treatment with corticosteroids or cytotoxic agents can lead to improvement of the neutropenia, although no single therapy has a high response rate. The role of splenectomy remains controversial.

An increased incidence of lymphoproliferative disorders, such as lymphoma, has been noted in patients with rheumatologic disorders. This appears to be particularly true for Sjögren syndrome, in which the incidence of non-Hodgkin lymphoma is significantly higher than that of the general population.[59]

PLATELETS AND ABNORMALITIES OF COAGULATION

Thrombocytopenia and Thrombocytosis

Immune-mediated thrombocytopenia is not uncommon in patients with SLE and other rheumatologic disorders; however, in rheumatoid arthritis, this finding is rare. The signs and symptoms, as well as diagnosis and management, are largely similar to that of idiopathic cases of immune-mediated thrombocytopenia.[60] An area of some controversy is the use of splenectomy for patients who have failed first-line therapy with corticosteroids. Although it has been suggested in the past that splenectomy was relatively ineffective treatment for patients with SLE, more recent literature suggests that it may be beneficial.[61,62] Aside from splenectomy, other therapies may be considered. Administration of immunoglobulin may serve as a temporizing measure, whereas other drugs that take longer to act, such as immunosuppressants, cytotoxic agents, or danazol, are tried. The anti-CD20 monoclonal antibody rituximab has been used effectively, without formal regulatory approval, for the management of immune-mediated thrombocytopenia and may be considered as a therapeutic

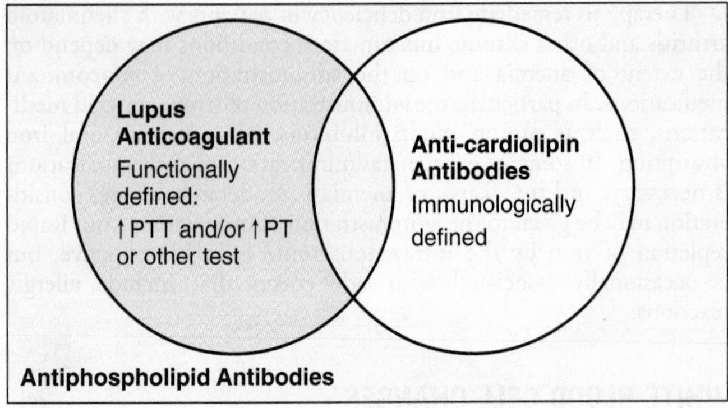

Figure 157–4 Overlap between the detection of lupus anticoagulants and anticardiolipin antibodies. Lupus anticoagulants are defined by their effects on coagulation-based assays, whereas anticardiolipin antibodies are immunologically detected. PTT, partial prothrombin time; PT, prothrombin time.

option.[63] No single therapy has a particularly high response rate, and sometimes it is necessary to move from trials of one therapeutic agent to another.

As opposed to thrombocytopenia, thrombocytosis is relatively common in rheumatoid arthritis as an acute phase reactant. Generally, the platelet count is moderately elevated, although platelet counts of up to 1,000,000/μL may occasionally be seen. Thrombocytosis correlates with elevation in the sedimentation rate and may serve as a marker of disease activity.[64] Complications from such elevated platelet counts, such as thrombosis, are rare. Rebound thrombocytosis may be seen in SLE and other rheumatologic disorders after splenectomy or withdrawal of offending cytotoxic agents. No therapy is generally indicated.

Abnormalities of Coagulation

Lupus anticoagulants and anticardiolipin antibodies are common in patients with SLE and other rheumatologic disorders.[65] Other antibodies potentially affecting coagulation, such as those to β_2-GPI, may also be present.[66] Particularly when present in high titer, anticardiolipin antibodies may be associated with lupus anticoagulant activity and with thrombosis (Fig. 157–4). Despite their name, however, lupus anticoagulants are not specifically associated with lupus and are anticoagulants in vivo only occasionally. In the absence of complications, treatment is not indicated.

Of note, in contrast to many other causes of thromboembolic disease, lupus anticoagulants are associated with both arterial and venous disease. *Antiphospholipid antibody syndrome* is the term that has been used to describe the presence of thromboembolic disease, recurrent fetal loss, and thrombocytopenia in the setting of the presence of a persistent lupus anticoagulant.[67] Once a diagnosis of antiphospholipid antibody syndrome has been made in the setting of thromboembolic disease, long-term anticoagulation is indicated, because of the high risk of recurrent events. Although it was previously thought that increased intensity anticoagulation with warfarin (to an international normalized ratio [INR] of 2.5 to 3.0) was appropriate, standard intensity anticoagulation (to an INR of 2.0 to 2.5) is now considered sufficient.[68,69] However, for specific patients with recurrent events while on warfarin, consideration needs to be given to higher-intensity anticoagulation with warfarin or in some cases to anticoagulation with agents such as low-molecular-weight heparin.

CANCER

Hematologic abnormalities are common in patients with cancer, both as a result of the underlying disease and as a consequence of therapy.[70]

Table 157–8 Mechanisms of Anemia in Cancer

Decreased production of red blood cells
Anemia of chronic disease
Marrow replacement by tumor (myelophthisis)
Nutritional deficiency
Pure red cell aplasia
Effect of cancer chemotherapy
Increased destruction of red blood cells
AIHA
Warm AIHA
Cold AIHA
Drug-induced hemolytic-uremic syndrome
DIC
Effects of enzyme deficiency (G6PD)
Hemophagocytic syndrome
Blood loss
Gastrointestinal blood loss
Colorectal cancer
Genitourinary cancer

AIHA, autoimmune hemolytic anemia; DIC, disseminated intravascular coagulation; G6PD, glucose-6-phosphate dehydrogenase.

In addition, patients with certain hematologic malignancies may be predisposed to infection, which can lead to complications such as DIC.

ANEMIA

Anemia is the most common hematologic abnormality in patients with cancer.[71] It may be observed in about 50% of patients at some time during their course of presentation or treatment. Although there is significant overlap with infection and chronic inflammation in the underlying mechanisms leading to anemia, certain unique causes exist in patients with malignancy, particularly those related to the side effects of therapy (Table 157–8).

Anemia Caused by Decreased Production

Anemia occurs frequently in patients with hematologic or nonhematologic malignancies. Independent of bone marrow invasion, the anemia of chronic disease is common in nonhematologic cancers and may represent the initial finding. The extent of anemia is often, but not invariably, proportional to the stage of disease. The underlying pathophysiology of the anemia of chronic disease is similar to that observed in infection and chronic inflammation (see Fig. 157–1).[72] In addition, this anemia is often responsive to the administration of erythropoietin, and the same caveats hold (see box on Treatment of the Anemia of Chronic Disease with Erythropoietin). Patients will not respond to therapy if they are iron deficient.

Replacement of the marrow space with leukemia may lead to anemia, often in the setting of pancytopenia. Solid tumors can also invade the marrow space causing myelophthisis, manifesting with anemia or pancytopenia if involvement is more extensive. In such cases, a leukoerythroblastic peripheral blood smear may be seen with teardrop forms of erythrocytes, nucleated red cells, and immature white blood cells. The solid tumors most commonly associated with marrow invasion include breast cancer, prostate cancer, small-cell lung cancer, and lymphoma. Treatment of the underlying malignancy is the therapy of choice, although administration of erythropoietin sometimes leads to improvement of the anemia.[73]

Aside from treatment-related anemia, other causes of anemia are less common that those previously noted. Nutritional deficiencies sometimes are found, such as folate deficiency in anorexic patients and vitamin B_{12} deficiency in patients who have undergone gastric or colonic resection (vitamin B_{12} deficiency taking several years to manifest itself). Pure red cell aplasia has a significant association with thymoma; 10% to 15% of patients may present with this complication.[74] Pure red cell aplasia has also been reported in non-Hodgkin lymphomas, non–small-cell lung cancer, breast cancer, and gastric cancer. The mechanism underlying the development of pure red cell aplasia may involve a combination of humoral and cellular events leading to a suppression of erythropoiesis.[75] Although treatment of the underlying disease sometimes leads to improvement in pure red cell aplasia, therapy is frequently required. Corticosteroids, antithymocyte globulin, danazol, and cytotoxic agents have been used.

Anemia has increasingly been recognized as a complication of cancer chemotherapy. Various cytotoxic agents are associated with bone marrow suppression. Although associated effects of the myeloid and megakaryocytic lineages tend to resolve within 1 to 2 weeks with most agents, anemia tends to be long lasting. Cumulative effects of multiple cycles of chemotherapy lead to more pronounced decreases in the number of RBCs. Administration of rHuEPO has been demonstrated in several clinical trials to improve anemia and quality of life in patients receiving cancer chemotherapy.[76,77] Both rHuEPO and darbepoetin have been approved for the treatment of anemia related to cancer chemotherapy, and guidelines for their use in appropriate patient populations are available.[78]

Anemia Caused by Increased Destruction

Several mechanisms may lead to red cell destruction in cancer. These include autoimmune hemolytic anemia and microangiopathic hemolytic anemia, either related to DIC or to drug-induced hemolytic uremic syndrome. Autoimmune hemolytic anemia is most commonly associated with lymphoproliferative disorders. Warm autoimmune hemolytic anemia affects about 25% of patients with CLL. It also occurs in roughly 50% of patients with angioimmunoblastic lymphadenopathy, although it is less frequent in other lymphomas (non-Hodgkin and Hodgkin) and myeloma.[79] Autoimmune hemolytic anemia is a well-described complication of the treatment of CLL with fludarabine, possibly related to induction of immune dysregulation.[80] Use of this agent should be avoided in patients with preexisting autoimmune hemolytic anemia. Warm autoimmune hemolytic anemia is also occasionally associated with solid tumors, including adenocarcinomas and squamous cell carcinomas. Although treatment of the underlying malignancy may lead to resolution of autoimmune hemolytic anemia, therapy directed at management of the anemia is often required. Similar therapies, including immunosuppressants, cytotoxic agents, or splenectomy may be required.

Cold autoimmune hemolytic anemia is also observed in association with lymphoproliferative disorders. Although it is less common than warm autoimmune hemolytic anemia, it is estimated that about 50% of patients who present with apparently idiopathic cold autoimmune hemolytic anemia (unrelated to bacterial or viral infection) have an underlying hematologic malignancy. Keeping patients warm is a mainstay of therapy for patients with cold autoimmune hemolytic anemia. Corticosteroids and splenectomy are generally ineffective. More recently, several case reports have appeared of effective therapy using anti-CD20 monoclonal antibody for patients with cold autoimmune hemolytic anemia. In some instances therapy with this agent addresses both the underlying disorder and the anemia.[81]

Anemia may be seen as one component of microangiopathic change. Moderate- to high-grade DIC is a common complication of certain hematologic malignancies (M3 and M5 AML) and certain advanced solid tumors, particularly mucin-secreting metastatic adenocarcinomas. In such cases, laboratory parameters often reflect a classic DIC pattern, and fragmented erythrocytes are observed on peripheral blood smear. Low-grade DIC leading to anemia and occasional schistocytes on smears of less pronounced or atypical coagulation abnormalities may also be observed, sometimes in patients with metastatic prostate cancer. Therapy with blood products is a temporizing measure. Resolution of the anemia relies on effective treatment of the underlying malignancy.

Hemolytic anemia may also follow the administration of cancer chemotherapy. Microangiopathic change may occur as a component of therapy-induced hemolytic uremic syndrome. Mitomycin C is an agent well known to cause this complication; however, others may do so as well.[82] For example, gemcitabine has also been associated with hemolytic uremic syndrome.[83] Discontinuation of the potentially offending agent is indicated.

Another cause of chemotherapy-induced hemolysis is the administration of doxorubicin, a strong oxidant, to patients with G6PD deficiency. Although hemolysis may be self-limited in patients with the A– genotype, it may be more pronounced in those with the Mediterranean genotype, and require cessation of doxorubicin therapy.

Hemolysis may be seen in conjunction with hemophagocytic syndrome, which may be observed in association with malignancies, as well as with infectious diseases.[84] In particular, hemophagocytic syndrome has been reported is association with non-Hodgkin lymphomas and leukemias. Although therapy for the underlying malignancy may sometimes lead to amelioration of disease, this syndrome often has a fatal outcome.

Anemia Caused by Blood Loss

Iron deficiency anemia often manifests in malignancies of the gastrointestinal tract, particularly colorectal cancers. Genitourinary cancers, such as renal cell carcinoma and bladder cancer, can also lead to iron deficiency, but this occurrence is less common. Although therapy with iron preparations can lead to improvement in anemia, absent a clear understanding of the source of blood loss, the empiric administration of iron should be reserved for those who are too infirm to undergo a diagnostic evaluation. Failure to undertake such an evaluation can lead to serious consequences, such as missing the early detection of a localized colon cancer that later goes on to manifest in metastatic disease.

WHITE BLOOD CELL CHANGES

Leukocytosis

Leukemia often, though not invariably, manifests with an elevated white blood cell count. In addition, several solid tumors are associated with leukocytosis or even leukemoid reactions.[85] The latter may occur in response to a high degree of necrosis with the tumor mass. Malignancies associated with leukocytosis include non–small-cell lung cancer (bronchogenic type), renal cell carcinoma, and gastric carcinoma. Therapy is such cases should be directed at the underlying disease.

Neutropenia

Neutropenia may be the sign of a hematologic malignancy. It also may reflect significant marrow invasion by solid tumors, leading to myelophthisis and a leukoerythroblastic peripheral blood smear.

With solid tumors, neutropenia is most commonly seen as a side effect of chemotherapy. Many cytotoxic chemotherapy agents cause significant myelosuppression, with nadirs in the WBC count that occur days to a few weeks after administration, depending on the specific agent. In certain circumstances when the likelihood of prolonged neutropenia is high, such as with high-dose-intensity chemotherapy for solid tumors, administration of G-CSF or GM-CSF may be indicated. Guidelines have been developed to help clinicians determine when use of such agents is indicated.[86]

Lymphopenias

Treatment with several chemotherapeutic agents can produce deficits in total lymphocyte count or in lymphocyte subsets. Fludarabine and cladribine (2-chlorodeoxyadenosine) are two examples. The deficit in T-cell function following a single 5- to 7-day course of cladribine can last for numerous months, leading to an increased risk for opportunistic infections, such as *Pneumocystis carinii* pneumonia.[87] Strong consideration should be given to the administration of *Pneumocystis carinii* pneumonia prophylaxis, and potentially to antifungal prophylaxis in individuals treated with these agents.

PLATELETS AND ABNORMALITIES OF COAGULATION

Thrombocytopenia and Thrombocytosis

Several hematologic malignancies may manifest with prominent thrombocytopenia. Although this often reflects underlying marrow replacement, in certain instances, such as lymphoproliferative disorders, it may be reflective of an autoimmune disorder. For example, immune-mediated thrombocytopenia may represent an early finding in CLL.

Marrow replacement with solid tumors may also lead to thrombocytopenia. However, the most common circumstance in which thrombocytopenia is encountered in cancer patients is after chemotherapy with cytotoxic agents. Different agents are associated with transient thrombocytopenia, although several drugs, such as mitomycin C and carboplatin, are associated with longer-lasting effects, particularly after several cycles of chemotherapy are administered.

Thrombocytosis may be a prominent presenting feature of the myeloproliferative disorders, as well as myelodysplastic syndrome with the 5q− chromosomal abnormality.[88] A mild to moderate reactive thrombocytosis also frequently occurs in the setting of solid tumors. Whether this contributes to the hypercoagulable state of malignancy is unclear.

Abnormalities of Coagulation

Coagulation abnormalities are frequent in patients with cancer. Bleeding complications resulting from DIC represent one end of the spectrum, and thromboembolic complications resulting from a confluence of factors represent the other end.

DIC has been associated with AML, particularly the M3 and M5 subtypes. It also has been reported in association with other malignancies, particularly mucin-secreting adenocarcinomas such as gastric cancer. In such cases, blood product support is a temporizing measure while therapy for the underlying disease is administered. Chronic low-grade DIC has been associated with metastatic prostate cancer and can manifest atypically. Thrombocytopenia and low fibrinogen levels may be the primary manifestations, rather than abnormalities in coagulation times. Low-dose heparin may be beneficial for some patients, although it must be used cautiously.[89]

A few chemotherapy agents have clinically significant effects on coagulation aside from causing thrombocytopenia. The most notable of these is L-asparaginase, which is associated with the production of abnormal fibrinogen, which can lead to hemorrhagic or thrombotic complications.[90]

Although Trousseau syndrome was long ago identified as a potential complication of malignancy, thromboembolic complications have increasingly been identified as a cause of morbidity and mortality in cancer patients.[91] A variety of factors place patients at increased risk for thrombosis (Table 157–9). In some cases, such as in patients with malignant brain tumors, the risk for thrombosis during the course of illness exceeds 25%. The use of anticoagulants for the prevention of thrombosis in patients with malignancies must be tempered against the potential bleeding complications and the poten-

Table 157–9 Risk Factors for Thrombosis in Cancer

Procoagulants produced by tumors
Tissue factor
Cysteine protease activity
Vascular invasion
(Often observed in renal, gastric, germ cell, lung, adrenocortical tumors)
Host response to tumors
Elevated levels of factors V, VIII, IX, and XI
Decreased levels of protein C, antithrombin
Physical Inactivity
Surgical procedures
Decreased performance status
Depression
Limb immobility
Pathologic fractures
Paresis
Inherited or acquired thrombotic tendencies
Factor V Leiden, prothrombin gene mutation
Lupus anticoagulants
Indwelling venous devices
Central venous catheters
Other intravascular devices (filters, stents)
Chemotherapy-induced changes

Management of Thrombotic Complications in Cancer Patients

Tumor-related effects, host response, and therapeutic interventions combined lead to the high rate of venous thromboembolic disease that is observed in cancer patients. Though the risks of anticoagulation for a given patient should always be carefully considered, the potential benefit of prophylactic or therapeutic anticoagulation should not be underestimated for cancer patients in particular.

Use of low-dose prophylactic anticoagulation for patients with indwelling central venous catheters does not appear to be supported by well-controlled randomized trials.[92,93] Given these data, it would seem most appropriate to initiate therapy with full-intensity anticoagulation with either warfarin or low-molecular-weight heparin whenever a patient is judged to be at sufficiently high risk for catheter-related thrombosis, so long as this risk is felt to outweigh the potential for bleeding complications.

Using warfarin in particular to treat cancer patients with thrombotic complications can be challenging, especially in individuals with poor oral intake or diarrhea. With these individuals, unfractionated heparin or low-molecular-weight heparin may be administered at therapeutic doses. This is preferable to the insertion of mechanical devices. Except in circumstances such as that of recent intracranial surgery, use of vena-caval filters should be avoided because as clots form around the devices, they can impede blood flow and exacerbate swelling of the lower extremities.

If a patient experiences recurrent thrombotic events while receiving standard-dose anticoagulation therapy with warfarin, the intensity of anticoagulation may be increased to a higher target INR. However, it may be preferable to switch to therapeutic doses of low-molecular-weight heparin rather than to increase the intensity of anticoagulation, as in clinical practice this appears to have similar or greater efficacy and is simpler from the standpoint of patient monitoring and compliance. Care should be taken, however, when using low-molecular-weight heparin in patients with evidence of renal impairment, as low-molecular-weight heparin is cleared via a renal mechanism.

Regardless of whether warfarin or low-molecular-weight heparin is used for treatment, long-term anticoagulation should be administered to cancer patients who have experienced a thrombotic event so long as the malignancy is active. In patients with metastatic disease, this often translates into lifetime anticoagulation.

tial difficulty in using anticoagulants with patients receiving chemotherapy.

The high incidence of thrombotic complications in patients with malignancy has led to trials of prophylactic administration of anticoagulants, particularly in the setting of long-term indwelling central venous catheters. Although the use of very low dose anticoagulation (1 mg warfarin daily) or prophylactic dose low-molecular-weight heparin (enoxaparin 40 mg daily) does not appear to be effective in preventing thrombotic complications, the safety and efficacy of prophylaxis with standard treatment doses of anticoagulants remains open.[92,93]

Thromboembolic events in patients with metastatic cancer may best be managed with long-term anticoagulation, if the risk-to-benefit ratio is acceptable (see box on Management of Thrombotic Complications in Cancer Patients). Although use of warfarin is often reasonable as an initial therapy, regulation of the international normalized ratio can be difficult in cancer patients. There is also a significant failure rate. This has led to trials of low-molecular-weight heparin in this setting, as their administration is somewhat easier to regulate. Low-molecular-weight heparin is effective in the treatment and prophylaxis of thromboembolic events in cancer patients.[94]

SUMMARY

Infection, chronic inflammation, and cancer all share in common the potential ability to have profound effects on the blood. In some cases, such as for the anemia of chronic disease, the likely pathogenesis is also shared. Knowledge of the hematologic manifestations of these disorders facilitates their accurate diagnosis and management.

SUGGESTED READINGS

Baillie FJ, Morrison AE, Fergus I: Soluble transferrin receptor: A discriminating assay for iron deficiency. Clin Lab Haematol 25:353, 2003.

Couban S, Goodyear M, Burnell M, et al: Randomized placebo-controlled study of low-dose warfarin for the prevention of central venous catheter-associated thrombosis in patients with cancer. J Clin Oncol 23:4063, 2005.

Galli M, Luciani D, Bertolini G, Barbui T: Anti-beta 2-glycoprotein I, antiprothrombin antibodies, and the risk of thrombosis in the antiphospholipid syndrome. Blood 102:2717, 2003.

Lee AY, Levine MN, Baker RI: Low-molecular-weight heparin versus a coumarin for the prevention of recurrent venous thromboembolism in patients with cancer. N Engl J Med 349:146, 2003.

Rastetter W, Molina A, White CA: Rituximab: Expanding role in therapy for lymphomas and autoimmune diseases. Annu Rev Med 55:477, 2004.

Ridker PM, Goldhaber SZ, Danielson E: Long-term, low-intensity warfarin therapy for the prevention of recurrent venous thromboembolism. N Engl J Med 348:1425, 2003.

Roy CN, Andrews NC: Anemia of inflammation: The hepcidin link. Curr Opin Hematol 12:107, 2005.

Roy CN, Weinstein DA, Andrews NC: 2002 E. Mead Johnson Award for Research in Pediatrics Lecture: The molecular biology of chronic disease: A hypothesis. Pediatr Res 53:507, 2003.

Silverman GJ, Weisman S: Rituximab therapy and autoimmune disorders: Prospects for anti-B cell therapy. Arthritis Rheum 48:1484, 2003.

Young NS, Brown KE: Parvovirus B19. N Engl J Med 350:586, 2004.

REFERENCES

For complete list of references log onto www.expertconsult.com

CHAPTER 158

HEMATOLOGIC MANIFESTATIONS OF AIDS

Alexandra M. Levine

DEFINITION OF AIDS

The definition of acquired immunodeficiency syndrome (AIDS) was initially based exclusively upon clinical symptoms and signs.[1] As knowledge of the viral etiology evolved, the case definition of AIDS underwent multiple revisions by the Centers for Disease Control and Prevention (CDC). Inclusion of specific clinical illnesses in a patient with serologic evidence of infection with the human immunodeficiency virus (HIV) was classified as clinical AIDS, whereas an HIV-infected patient with a CD4 count of less than 200 cells/mL (0.2×10^9/L) was considered to have immunologic AIDS.[2–4] The specific AIDS-defining clinical illnesses employed in the United States are depicted in Table 158–1.

Although this expanded definition is employed in industrialized nations, the World Health Organization (WHO) adopted alternative case-definition systems for the diagnosis of AIDS in resource-poor countries where serologic and immunologic testing are not readily available.[5]

Two major subtypes of HIV have been associated with AIDS.[6] In most areas of the world, HIV-1 is the predominant type, associated with immunodeficiency and clinical AIDS. However, a second type, termed HIV-2, has been isolated from AIDS patients from West Africa, where this retrovirus is endemic.[7] Infection with HIV-2 leads to a more prolonged asymptomatic duration of disease, with less immunodeficiency and a decreased risk of developing full-blown clinical AIDS over time.[7]

EPIDEMIOLOGY OF AIDS

Origin of Human Immunodeficiency Virus-1

HIV-1 is a member of the primate Lentivirinae subfamily of retroviruses,[6,8] RNA viruses that induce a chronic cellular infection by converting their RNA genome into a DNA provirus that is integrated into the genome of the infected cell. Infection by these lentiviruses is characterized by long periods of clinical latency followed by a gradual onset of disease-related symptoms.[6,9–11]

At approximately the same time that AIDS was first recognized in 1981, reports of a similar immunodeficiency syndrome, characterized by wasting and opportunistic infections, was described in several colonies of macaques housed at primate centers in the United States.[10,12,13] The illness, known as simian immunodeficiency syndrome, was associated with infection by a retrovirus, termed simian immunodeficiency virus (SIV).[14] Subsequent testing revealed that over 20% of all symptomatic African green monkeys or African mangabeys tested from the wild had serologic evidence of SIV infection.[15–17] The SIV viral strain infecting these monkeys was subsequently found to be related to HIV-2, a less virulent strain of human immunodeficiency virus, found primarily in West Africa.[7,18] An immunodeficiency virus related to HIV-1 and infecting African chimpanzees was also identified.[19] Recent evidence suggests that the subspecies of chimpanzee *Pan troglodytes* may have been the original reservoir of HIV-1, whereas the Sooty mangabey may have been the original reservoir for HIV-2.[17,20,21] Thus, human AIDS is actually a zoonotic infection, presumably first acquired in hunters who were exposed to the infected blood of their simian prey.

Factors Leading to Current Pandemic of HIV

Although initial transmission of HIV-1 from chimp to man is thought to have occurred several hundred years ago, social circumstances at that time did not promulgate widespread transmission to others. However, by the mid- to late 1960s, political and societal circumstances were beginning to change dramatically in ways that were conducive to the rapid spread of this infection in humans. The movement of previously isolated African peoples from rural villages to large urban centers; a change in sexual habits, resulting in widespread exposure to increasing numbers of sexual partners; the worldwide epidemic of illicit parenteral drug abuse; and the advent of commercial air travel all contributed to the current pandemic of HIV infection.

The WHO has recently estimated that more than 40 million people had been infected by HIV worldwide by 2003,[5] with approximately 28 million of these living in sub-Saharan Africa. The cumulative number of deaths due to HIV/AIDS has surpassed 25 million, with 75% in Africa. Approximately 15,000 new infections occur each day, and HIV/AIDS has now become the fourth most common cause of death, worldwide.

Methods of HIV-1 Transmission

HIV may be transmitted by sexual contact with an infected partner, by parenteral drug use with a contaminated needle, by exposure to infected blood or blood products, and by perinatal exposure from an infected mother to her infant.

Sexual Transmission

HIV-1 has been isolated from the semen of HIV-infected men as well as from cell-free seminal fluid and may be detected during the first 2 to 4 weeks after primary infection.[22,23] Factors associated with increased viral burden in semen include more advanced, clinically symptomatic HIV disease, higher levels of HIV-RNA in blood, CD4 cell counts of less than 200/mL, and presence of seminal fluid leukocytosis. HIV infection has been reported after exposure to infected semen during artificial insemination.[22–24]

HIV has been recovered from cervical and vaginal secretions of HIV-infected women,[25,26] and HIV-infected endothelial cells and macrophages have been detected in cervical biopsies.[27] Factors that influence the levels of HIV-1 in female genital tract secretions include the stage of HIV disease, menstruation status, hormonal parameters, concomitant vaginal infection, age, HIV-1 RNA level in plasma, and antiviral therapy.[28] Although female-to-female transmission of HIV has been reported,[29,30] this appears to be relatively unusual.

HIV transmission may be facilitated by the presence of other ulcerative or nonulcerative sexually transmitted diseases,[31] and HIV has been isolated directly from genital ulcers.[32] Prevention or treat-

Table 158–1 Definitions of AIDS in the United States

A) Clinical AIDS defining conditions in persons infected with HIV
Opportunistic infections
Lymphomas
Kaposi sarcoma
Cervical cancer
Wasting syndrome
AIDS dementia syndrome
Recurrent bacterial pneumonia (≥2 episodes/year)
Mycobacterium tuberculosis
B) Immunologic AIDS
CD4 cell counts <200/μL

ment of sexually transmitted disease has been associated with a decrease in HIV-1 transmission.[33]

Transmission Through Injection Drug Use

Sharing needles and syringes is an important mode of transmission among injection drug users.[34] The use of cocaine or other such non-injection drugs has also been associated with an increased risk of HIV infection,[35] by providing the opportunity for engagement in high-risk sexual behaviors.

Transmission Through Infected Blood Products

The risk of infection with HIV after receiving a single unit of infected blood is approximately 90%.[36] Transfusion of blood products derived from multiple units of pooled blood can also transmit HIV and clearly accounted for the initially high prevalence of HIV infection among patients with hemophilia. Screening of all donated blood for HIV-1 in the United States began in March 1985, and, together with the subsequent routine heat or solvent detergent treatment of clotting factor concentrates, has resulted in a marked decrease in new transfusion-associated HIV infections. Guidelines for proper inactivation of HIV in clotting factor concentrates have been developed.[37,38] Currently, the risk of acquiring HIV through receipt of a unit of blood that tests negative for antibodies to HIV-1 is approximately 1 in 493,000.[39]

Mother-to-Child Transmission

The risk of infection from mother to infant differs in various parts of the world, ranging from approximately 15% in Europe to 15% to 30% in the United States and 40% to 50% in Africa.[40–42] HIV-1 may be transmitted in utero,[43,44] at the time of delivery (intrapartum)[45,46]; or postpartum, through breast-feeding of HIV-1 infected mother's milk.[47,48] Several factors have been shown to predict an increased risk of perinatal transmission. In terms of the mother, more advanced HIV disease,[49,50] higher HIV-1 viral load in the plasma,[51,52] cigarette smoking,[53] and active injection drug use[54] have all been associated with increased risk of transmission. In terms of the details of delivery, premature rupture of the amniotic membranes (>4 hours),[55,56] presence of chorioamnionitis,[54] and vaginal delivery, as opposed to elective cesarean section,[56,57] have each been associated with increased rates of vertical transmission. In terms of the infant, breast-feeding, prematurity, and low gestational age are reported as risk factors for HIV transmission.[55–58] The CDC has made formal recommendations regarding the optimal care for HIV-1-infected pregnant women.[59] These recommendations differ for resource-rich and resource-poor settings. In the United States, the use of antiretroviral agents in pregnancy and delivery, with subsequent administration to the infant for the first 6 weeks of life, has resulted in a dramatic reduction in the rate of transmission, from approximately 25% to 8% with use of zidovudine alone, and even lower with use of combination antiretroviral therapy, termed *highly active antiretroviral therapy* (HAART).[60] With the further use of elective cesarean section and avoidance of breast-feeding, transmission rates have dropped to approximately 2% or less.[56–59] The efficacy of shorter courses of zidovudine or nevirapine (a nonnucleoside reverse transcriptase inhibitor) have been demonstrated and may be more practically feasible in resource-poor regions of the world, although significant hepatic toxicity and development of drug resistance have been reported after use of single-dose nevirapine in this setting.[61–64] The long-term toxicities of in utero exposure to antiretroviral agents are unknown. To date, however, with the exception of efavirenz,[65] there have been no clinical data to indicate any excess in congenital birth defects after use of these antiretroviral agents,[66] nor has there been evidence of an increase in malignant disease among those children exposed in utero.[67] Furthermore, the use of antiretroviral agents during pregnancy has resulted in a 43% decrease in the number of children with perinatally acquired HIV infection in the United States when comparing data from 1992 and 1996.[68]

Transmission to Health Care Workers

HIV may be transmitted from infected patients to health care workers, primarily through accidental needle stick exposures. Risk factors for greater likelihood of infection include presence of more advanced HIV disease in the source patient, occurrence of a deep needle stick injury, presence of visible blood on the needle or device, and prior insertion of the needle directly into a vein or artery.[69] The risk of such iatrogenic infection, from a source patient with full-blown clinical AIDS is approximately 0.3% per exposure. Iatrogenic infection after mucocutaneous exposure to infected fluids is approximately 0.1%, whereas transmission through intact skin, though reported, is exceedingly rare.[69,70] The use of short-course antiretroviral therapy (postexposure prophylaxis) has been associated with significant decreases in the risk of infection, and guidelines have been recommended for use of such prophylaxis.[69,70] Briefly, antiretroviral therapy should be initiated as quickly as possible after exposure, and certainly within 72 hours. Therapy is continued for 4 weeks. The specific regimen to be employed is based on the infection status of the source person, and the degree of risk posed by the exposure.[69]

PATHOGENESIS OF HIV/AIDS

HIV-1 Structure and Gene Products

HIV-1 has three structural genes necessary for replication: *gag, pol,* and *env*.[6] These viral genes encode proteins that are required for binding to the host cell, intracellular synthesis of provirus by reverse transcription, proviral integration into the host-cell genome, and viral assembly and release. The 9-kb genome of HIV-1 also contains at least six additional genes involved in the regulation of viral gene expression and cellular latency: *vif, vpu, vpr, tat, rev,* and *nef* (Fig. 158–1).[6,71]

env

HIV-1 is an icosahedral virion with a protein-rich envelope in a membrane derived from the host cell (see Fig. 158–2).[72] The surface of the virus particle contains a 120-Da glycoprotein (gp120) that is linked noncovalently to a 41-kd transmembrane protein (gp41). Both proteins are derived from a 160-kd precursor protein that is encoded by the *env* gene. The intracellular processing of gp160 involves the assembly of oligomeric trimer complexes, which are glycosylated and subsequently cleaved into the respective gp120 and gp41 components in the Golgi apparatus of the host cell.[73] HIV gp120 serves as a virion receptor for noninfected cells,[74] with virus

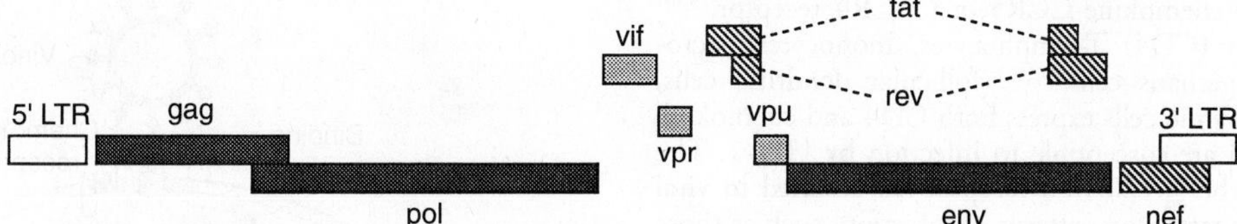

Figure 158–1 Genetic organization of HIV-1. The nine genes of HIV-1 are shown. Structural proteins of the virion and enzymes required for replication are encoded by *gag, pol,* and *env* (*darkly shaded regions*); regulatory proteins (*crosshatched areas*) are encoded by *tat* and *rev*, arising from doubly spliced messages, and *nef.* The *vif, vpr,* and *vpu* genes perform specialized functions relevant to cellular interactions. Two identical long terminal repeats (LTRs) are present at the 5′ and 3′ end of the genome and contain sequences critical for viral transcription and activation by cellular and viral factors.

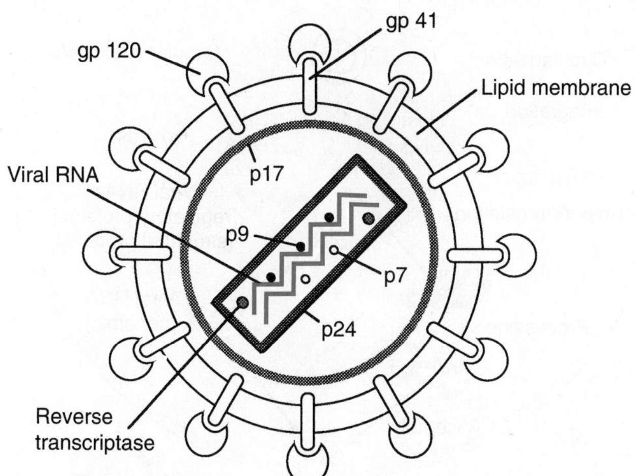

Figure 158–2 Structure of the HIV virion. Two coding strands of genomic RNA are packaged in a nucleoid core with the p7, p9, and p24 proteins and reverse transcriptase. The core is surrounded by the p17 matrix protein lining the inner surface of the envelope. The envelope consists of a lipid bilayer derived from the infected cell and glycoprotein spikes that consist of the outer gp120 molecule, which contains the binding site for CD4, and gp41, which anchors the glycoprotein complex to the envelope and mediates fusion of the viral membrane with the cell membrane during viral penetration.

initially binding to the CD4 antigen on uninfected cells, and then to one of two chemokine coreceptors, CCR5 or CXCR4.[75–77] The CD4-binding domain of gp120 is located on the carboxyl terminal region of the molecule.[78] Within the CD4-binding site of gp120 are a number of regions that display significant genetic variation between different viral isolates without compromising viral binding.[78,79] The binding of CD4 results in a conformational transition in the V3 variable loop of gp120, exposing the chemokine receptor-binding site of the viral particle and increasing the affinity of gp120 binding to CCR5 by 10- to 100-fold.[73,80] The complexing of gp120 with CD4, with subsequent conformational change, also exposes the HIV-1 transmembrane-anchoring protein, gp41, which is necessary for fusion of the viral membrane with the membrane of the newly infected cell.[80] These viral proteins are immunogenic. Consequently, antibodies against both gp120 and gp41 can be detected in the serum of all individuals infected with HIV-1.[81] However, antibodies capable of neutralizing HIV and preventing cellular infection appear to develop only after infection is well established. Furthermore, these antibodies are not capable of efficiently controlling ongoing infection.[73] The envelope genes of HIV-1 demonstrate the greatest genomic diversity when compared to all other genetic components of the virus.[82]

gag

The *gag* gene encodes a 54-kd precursor protein that is cleaved by a viral protease to form four viral core proteins: p24, p17, p9, and p7 (see Fig. 158–2).[6,83] The 24-kd protein (p24) forms the shell of the nucleocapsid. The 17-kd myristoylated matrix protein (p17) is located between the viral envelope and the nucleocapsid and functions to stabilize the virion and, as part of the p54 *gag*-precursor protein, to assist in targeting viral assembly at the cell surface. The 7-kd protein (p7) and the 9-kd protein (p9) are tightly associated with the viral RNA, stabilizing it in the viral ribonucleoprotein core.[83]

pol

The *pol* gene encodes three critical viral proteins. The first, reverse transcriptase, is a 66-kd protein that generates a complementary copy of DNA (cDNA) from the viral RNA genome. The cDNA is then used as a template, generating a double-stranded DNA provirus, which then integrates into the host cellular genome.[84] The *pol* gene also encodes a 31-kd integrase protein that is required for stable integration of proviral double-stranded DNA into host cellular DNA.[85] Additionally, the 5′ region of the *pol* gene encodes a viral protease that cleaves the p54 *gag* precursor protein.[86,87] A defective protease leads to the production of noninfectious virions.[86]

Regulatory and Accessory Genes

After integration of proviral DNA into the host genome, HIV-1 proviral transcription leads to the expression of regulatory proteins designated *tat, rev,* and *nef.*[88] *Tat* is a small nuclear protein that is essential for HIV replication and, in conjunction with other cellular proteins, TAK (Tat-associated kinase) and CycT (cyclin T), assists in viral RNA elongation, resulting in a 1000-fold increase in HIV-1 expression by the infected cells.[89–91]

Rev results in the production of a viral protein that regulates nuclear export of unspliced viral RNA.[92] Like *tat, rev* is essential for viral replication and must bind to a *rev*-responsive element located in the *env* gene.

The *nef* gene product has a role in the modulation and downregulation of the cellular receptor, CD4, as well as HLA class I molecules on the cell surface, and may also play a role in increasing viral infectivity, as well as facilitating the recruitment of uninfected CD4+ lymphocytes.[88,93–96]

The product of the *vpu* accessory gene appears necessary for viral maturation and budding from the host cell, assisting in the membrane transport of *env* gene products,[97] whereas viral infectivity appears to require the protein product of the *vif* gene.[98] Of interest, *vif* also interacts with a cellular RNA editing enzyme, APOBEC3G, which, in the absence of *vif,* induces hypermutation and frequent inactivation of viral proteins.[99] The *vpr* gene product is incorporated into the nascent viral particle, where it helps in the targeting of viral RNA and DNA complexes to the nucleus, and induces cell cycle arrest in infected cells.[88,100]

Life Cycle of HIV-1

After initial infection, HIV-1 gp120 binds to the CD4 surface membrane protein on susceptible target cells, resulting in a further high-affinity binding to the chemokine CCR5 or CXCR4 receptor.[73,101] Human helper-inducer (CD4) T-lymphocytes, monocytes-macrophages, epithelial Langerhans cells,[102,103] follicular dendritic cells, megakaryocytes, and thymic cells express both CD4 and chemokine receptor molecules and are susceptible to infection by HIV-1. The structural diversity of the gp120 viral receptor has resulted in viral strains with selective or restricted patterns of infection, such as those that readily infect monocytes, whereas others are tropic for CD4 lymphocytes.[79,82,104] Macrophage-tropic (M-tropic) strains of HIV use the CCR5 chemokine receptor to infect both macrophages and memory CD4+ lymphocytes, whereas T-tropic strains primarily use the CXC4 chemokine receptor, but may also use CCR5.[101] Additional chemokine receptors CCR2 and CCR3 have also been implicated as coreceptors for HIV infection of certain cell types.[101] In general, upon initial establishment of HIV infection, CCR5 coreceptors are used, allowing infection of macrophages and memory CD4+ T lymphocytes.[105] Over time, HIV variants usually evolve to use the CXCR4 receptor, a change that is associated with more rapid CD4+ cell decline, and clinical progression to AIDS.[106] The importance of chemokine coreceptors in the transmission of HIV has been demonstrated by various experiments in nature; individuals who are homozygous for a deletion allele (32 deletion) of CCR5 are apparently resistant to acquiring HIV-1 infection if exposed, whereas heterozygous, though infectable, do relatively well and are likely to become long-term nonprogressors.[107,108] Aside from the importance of chemokine coreceptors, viral transmission is also markedly enhanced by the presence of dendritic cells which express DC-SIGN, a C-type lectin. These dendritic cells bind to gp 120 and facilitate transfer of cell-associated virus to CD4+ T cells; they are thought to be operative in the transmission of HIV across mucosal barriers.[109,110]

After binding to the CD4 and chemokine receptors on the host cell, the virus envelope fuses with the host cell membrane (Fig. 158–3).[104] This fusion is mediated by a hydrophobic domain on the amino terminal portion of gp41.[80] The internalized nucleocapsid is then destabilized, and it dissociates after binding to the cellular protein cyclophilin A,[111] exposing the viral RNA genome associated with reverse transcriptase. Reverse transcription then proceeds by the synthesis of a single cDNA strand, followed by degradation of the viral RNA by the ribonuclease H activity of viral p66.[112,113] Subsequently, reverse transcriptase then acts as a DNA polymerase, forming a second DNA strand. This synthesis of the double-stranded DNA provirus must proceed rapidly to prevent the degradation of viral RNA by intracellular enzymes.[114] The estimated rate of base substitution errors for HIV reverse transcriptase may be as high as 1 in 1700 to 1 in 2000.[82,113] This results in 5 to 10 nucleoside mutations per virus for each replication cycle and explains the high degree of genomic diversity observed between viral isolates of HIV.[82]

The integration of the proviral material is now necessary for stable infection of the cell. In this regard, viral integrase is capable of both cleaving host DNA and integrating a linear form of the provirus into transcriptionally active regions of host chromosomes.[85,115] Kinetic studies of HIV-1 infection have detected viral DNA present in the cytoplasm within 2 to 3 hours of infection, whereas nuclear viral DNA has been detected by 24 hours.[116]

After successful integration of the viral genome, the HIV-1-infected cell may then develop either a latent or a persistent form of infection. Subsequent HIV-1 transcription and replication can be upregulated via multiple factors, including activation of the infected cell, because HIV-1 does not replicate efficiently in resting lymphocytes or macrophages.[117,118] Cytokines, transactivating factors of other viruses, or cellular transactivating proteins, such as NF-κB, may also enhance HIV proviral transcription.[118,119]

After appropriate activating signals, transcription of the provirus occurs via cellular RNA polymerase, leading to the production of genomic RNA, which is then transported to the cytoplasm. Structural proteins of the *gag*, *pol*, and *env* genes are then synthesized; these are expressed as precursor proteins, which are then cleaved by viral protease to yield mature viral proteins. Proteolysis of proteins by the viral protease is essential for viral maturation and infectivity.[86] The products of the *env* gene, gp120 and gp41, are then transported to the

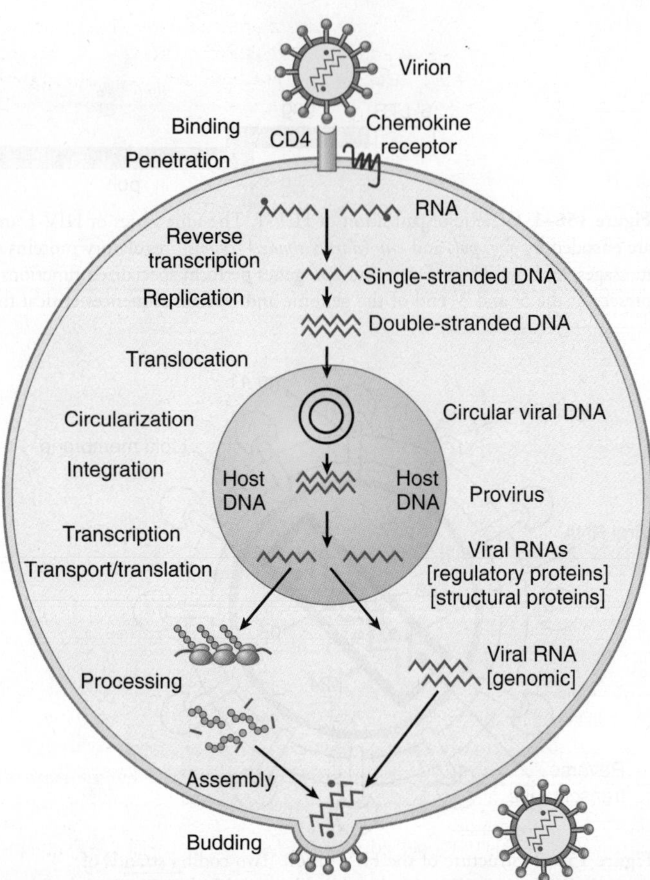

Figure 158–3 HIV life cycle. Binding of the virion to the cell surface is mediated by a specific interaction of the gp120 envelope glycoprotein with the cellular CD4 molecule and members of the chemokine receptor family of proteins (usually CCR5 or CXCR4). Penetration occurs as the viral membrane fuses with the cellular membrane in a process that requires the gp41 envelope molecule. The viral capsid is uncoated and viral genomic RNA is reverse transcribed and duplicated by the viral reverse transcriptase to produce a double-stranded copy of viral DNA. The DNA duplex is transported to the nucleus, where it integrates into host chromosomes. After appropriate activating signals, the provirus is transcribed by cellular RNA polymerase and transported to the cytoplasm. Proteins are translated and processed through biochemical steps that depending on the protein, involve glycosylation (envelope), cleavage (envelope, Gag, Pol), myristoylation (p17), and phosphorylation (Rev, Nef). Packaging of genomic RNA with viral proteins occurs as envelope glycoproteins are inserted into the cell membrane, and a new virion subsequently buds outward from the plasma membrane.

cell membrane. The ribonucleoprotein core assembles in the cytoplasm of the host cell and subsequently moves to the membrane surface for budding. The efficient packaging of the viral RNA with viral proteins is dependent upon packaging signals present in the *Gag* region of the viral RNA, whereas the budding of virus from the cell surface appears to be dependent upon the product of the *vpu* gene, which assists in membrane transport of *env* gene products.[97,120]

An interesting aspect of HIV-1 is its ability to replicate in an ongoing manner, over years, at an exceptionally rapid pace. Thus, approximately 10^9 to 10^{10} new virions are produced every day.[121] With this rapid rate of production and exceptionally high rate of base substitution errors for the HIV reverse transcriptase,[112–114] a high degree of genomic diversity results,[82] with the potential for rapid emergence of new, resistant isolates after exposure to antiretroviral agents.

Although most virally infected, activated CD4+ cells are rapidly destroyed (see below), other cell populations, such as memory CD4+ cells, macrophages, and dendritic cells live for prolonged periods and serve as a reservoir for long-term infection.[122] The latent, proviral infection of long-lived memory CD4+ cells serves as a source for potential reactivation of viral replication throughout the lifetime of the infected individual, despite the use of effective antiretroviral therapy.[121,123]

Mechanisms of Immune Dysfunction

HIV infection results in both aberrant immune regulation as well as immunodeficiency. The numerous defects in cellular immune response observed with HIV infection include decreased lymphocyte proliferation to soluble antigens, decreased helper response in immunoglobulin (Ig) synthesis,[124] impaired delayed hypersensitivity,[1,2] decreased interferon-γ production,[125] and decreased T cell-mediated cytotoxicity of virally infected cells.[126] Defects in B-lymphoid function[127–129] as well as in innate immune function have also been described.[130]

CD4+ Lymphocyte Depletion

Infection with HIV-1 results in a progressive loss of CD4-positive (CD4+) T lymphocytes, resulting from the direct cytopathic effect of HIV on these cells.[131,132] Additionally, the formation of syncytial multinucleated giant cells by a mechanism involving fusion of infected cells expressing viral gp120 with noninfected CD4+ T lymphocytes is another mechanism of CD4 depletion.[133] The propensity of certain viral stains to form syncytia appears to be associated with an aggressive clinical course.[133,134] More recent experimental data suggest that an HIV-1 phenotypic switch from an M-tropic (nonsyncytial) to a T-tropic (syncytial) virus may be the central event in the development of HIV-induced immunodepletion.[134]

The host immunologic response against HIV-infected lymphocytes may also contribute to the progressive loss of CD4+ lymphocytes by antibody-mediated and cytotoxic T cell-mediated mechanisms.[135] Noninfected lymphocytes may also become "innocent bystander" targets for immunologic destruction by binding free gp120 to their surface CD4 protein, which may also lead to apoptosis of these uninfected cells.[136,137] Additionally, the high production of TNF-related apoptosis-inducing ligand (TRAIL) by monocytes in HIV-infected individuals may also contribute to the death of CD4+ T lymphocytes.[138]

Defective production of immunostimulatory cytokines, such as interleukin-2 (IL-2),[139–141] or exaggerated expression of inhibitors of T-lymphocyte proliferation, such as transforming growth factor-β (TGF-β),[142] can contribute to the progressive decline in CD4 lymphocytes. HIV-1 tat protein has also been shown to downregulate IL-7 receptor expression on CD8 T cells; because optimal proliferation and function of these cells requires IL-7 signaling, it is possible that the loss of effective cytotoxic CD8+ cell function may also be involved in HIV-related immune dysfunction.[143] High-level replication and budding of virus, resulting in membrane injury, has also been proposed as a mechanism for lymphocyte cytotoxicity as well. Lastly, thymic dysfunction due to HIV may lead to defective maturation and release of CD4+ lymphocytes into the periphery.[144]

Of interest, although significant CD4+ depletion occurs over time with resultant clinical deterioration, immune defects are present even prior to such profound cellular loss. These defects may relate to the fact that initially HIV-1 selectively infects memory, as opposed to naive CD4+ cells,[145,146] which preferentially express the CCR5 chemokine receptor, more likely to be utilized in the early stages of infection by HIV.[147,148] Furthermore, specific depletion of CD4+ helper cells that specifically stimulate the Th1 immune responses involved in cell-mediated immunity has also been demonstrated in the early phases of HIV infection, again leading to immune defects prior to actual CD4+ depletion in later stages of infection.[149,150]

Recent advances in combination antiretroviral therapy have resulted in marked suppression of viral replication, with resulting reductions of blood and tissue viral reservoirs.[151,152] Efficient viral suppression has resulted in significant and prolonged immunologic reconstitution characterized by increased CD4+ lymphocyte numbers, reduced opportunistic infections, and prolonged survival.[153,154] However, significant deficits in the immunologic repertoire persist, and complete immunologic reconstitution has not yet been attained.[155,156]

Defects in B-Cell Immunity

A number of defects in humoral immunity have been associated with HIV infection. Pronounced polyclonal activation of B lymphocytes is common, resulting in polyclonal hypergammaglobulinemia.[127,128] Spontaneous proliferation of B cells is observed in patients with advanced HIV infection.[128,129] In contrast, antigen-specific B-cell proliferation and antibody production are decreased in patients with AIDS, which may also result from the loss of helper T-lymphocyte activity.[157,158]

The aberrant B-lymphocyte regulation in HIV infection is associated with a pronounced increase in autoimmune phenomena.[159] In addition to an increased frequency of positive antiglobulin test results, antibodies against neutrophils,[160,161] lymphocytes,[162] and platelets[161,163] have also been reported.

Aberrant B lymphoid regulation and function are also operative in the development of aggressive, B-cell lymphomas in HIV-infected patients; in this regard, lymphoma became an AIDS-defining illness in 1992.[4] Of note, the B lymphoma cells are not infected by HIV, but result from the chronic B-cell stimulation and proliferation induced by HIV, with eventual development of genetic errors leading to clonal selection and malignancy.[164] Approximately half of these lymphomas are also associated with Epstein–Barr infection (EBV), which has been shown to be monoclonal, and present within the nucleus of the lymphoma cells.[165,166] These aggressive B-cell lymphomas are most likely to occur during the later stages of HIV infection, with significant CD4+ cell depletion; their incidence has significantly decreased with the widespread use of highly active antiretroviral therapy (HAART).[167] Hodgkin lymphoma (HL), another B lymphocytic malignancy, is also statistically increased in the setting of HIV.[168] Of interest, however, the incidence of HL appears to be increasing in the era of HAART, perhaps reflecting the importance of the cellular milieu of the Reed–Sternberg (RS) cell, which is rich in CD4+ lymphocytes, with paucity of infiltrating CD8+ or natural killer cells.[169–171] As CD4 cells rise with effective use of antiretroviral therapy, the cellular milieu within nodal tissue may become more supportive of further growth and inhibition of apoptosis of the malignant RS cells. Further discussion of these B-cell lymphomas associated with HIV may be found in Chapter 86.

Defects in Immune Accessory Cells and Natural Killer Cells

Monocytes, macrophages, and follicular dendritic cells of the lymph nodes express CD4 antigen and can be infected by HIV.[172,173] Monocytes and macrophages are resistant to HIV-induced cytotoxicity and serve as a chronic reservoir of HIV expression.[172,173] Although functional defects in the chemotaxis of HIV-infected monocytes have been reported,[174] most studies have failed to demonstrate consistent defects.[175,176] Nonetheless, HIV nef protein interferes with the macrophage colony-stimulating factor (M-CSF) receptor signaling pathway, inhibiting the functions of M-CSF in monocytes and macrophages, which suggests that modulation of monocytes and macrophages may be involved in HIV-1 disease progression.[177] The follicular dendritic cells appear to play an important role in HIV clearance in early asymptomatic HIV disease. However, a progressive depletion of these cells is observed over time, resulting in increasing plasma viremia. The loss of follicular dendritic cells results in defective antigen processing in patients with advanced HIV disease.

Natural killer (NK) cell activity is decreased in the blood of HIV-infected individuals.[178,179] In combination with CD4+ helper lymphocyte depletion, decreased NK activity results in defective clearance of virally infected cells. Although the number of NK cells is reported to be normal,[178,179] the defect in NK activity appears to result from a deficiency in the signals for cell activation. These aberrations in innate immunity have been shown to correlate with development of various opportunistic infections in HIV-infected persons.[130] The addition of exogenous IL-2 can improve NK lymphocyte function.[180]

DIAGNOSIS OF HIV INFECTION

The primary diagnostic screening tool for HIV infection is detection of antibody via the enzyme-linked immunoassay (ELISA). However, because a positive ELISA result may not be specific for HIV-1 infection, all positive ELISA screening test results should be verified by immunoblot, using HIV-1-specific antigens.

Employing recent ELISA and immunoblot techniques, the median time from initial infection to first detection of HIV antibody has been estimated to be approximately 2 to 4 weeks, whereas 95% of cases are expected to seroconvert within 5.8 months.[181] Presence of HIV infection for longer than 6 months without detectable antibody is extremely uncommon.[182–184]

The presence of the p24 antigen or HIV RNA in serum or plasma may precede seroconversion by several weeks.[185] This initial rise in p24 antigen correlates with the burst of viremia that occurs shortly after primary HIV infection.[186] Despite these observations, p24 antigen screening of donated units of blood appears to provide no benefit over conventional ELISA and immunoblot techniques.[187]

Testing by polymerase chain reaction (PCR) may detect presence of HIV within days or a week of initial infection. However, PCR is not used as a screening tool, as false-positive results have been detected in as many as 9% of individuals.[184]

MONITORING THE COURSE OF HIV INFECTION OVER TIME

HIV infection results in a progressive process characterized by gradual depletion of immune function and eventual development of rather nonspecific symptoms, followed by specific infections and/or neoplastic disease. Patients who develop full-blown AIDS generally experience relentless deterioration in physical health, ultimately succumbing to one or more complications secondary to acquired immunodeficiency, organ dysfunction, and/or malignancy associated with HIV infection.

The course of HIV infection can be monitored by serial determination of CD4+ cell counts, as well as serial assessment of the quantity of HIV-1 RNA in the plasma; these studies have allowed a more rational basis on which to predict the course of disease in individual patients. In a pivotal study performed by the Multicenter AIDS Cohort (MACS), a longitudinal cohort study of HIV disease in homosexual and bisexual men, the earliest, baseline level of HIV RNA in plasma was found to correlate significantly with prognosis over time.[188] In a subsequent study, use of both viral load and CD4+ cells was found to more accurately predict the prognosis of HIV-infected men.[189] Current guidelines from the US Public Health Department suggest institution of HAART in all patients with symptomatic HIV or AIDS, and in asymptomatic HIV-infected individuals when the CD4 count falls below 350 cells/mL (0.35×10^9/L) or when the HIV viral load reaches 100,000 copies/cc or more, in patients with CD4 cells >350/mL.[190]

HIGHLY ACTIVE ANTIRETROVIRAL THERAPY

In addition to the use of viral load monitoring, the development of potent new antiretroviral agents, including the protease inhibitors,[153] has recently led to a remarkable improvement in the natural history of HIV infection.[154] The use of HAART usually consists of three or four different antiretroviral medications, typically from two or three classes of agents, including the nucleoside (or nucleotide) reverse transcriptase inhibitors (NRTIs), nonnucleoside RT inhibitors (NNRTIs), protease inhibitors (PIs), and fusion inhibitors (Table 158–2).[190] Although a detailed discussion of these agents is outside the scope of this chapter, use of HAART has resulted in stunning clinical improvements, associated with a 73% decrease in the incidence of new opportunistic infections and a 49% decrease in death due to AIDS when data from 1994 were compared to data from 1997–1998.[154] Remarkable decreases in the incidence of cytomegalovirus disease, atypical *Mycobacterium intracellularis* infections, and other serious opportunistic infections have occurred as a consequence of HAART therapy,[191] and improvement in immune function has also been documented.[192] It may now be possible to discontinue the routine use of prophylaxis against *Pneumocystis carinii* or other opportunistic infections in patients who have been successfully treated with HAART.[193] These remarkable improvements in disease outcome have been maintained over time.[194]

Table 158–2 Antiretroviral Therapy

	Trade Name
Reverse transcriptase inhibitors (nucleosides)	
• Zidovudine (ZDV; AZT)	• Retrovir
• Didanosine (ddI)	• Videx
• Zalcitabine (ddC)	• HIVid
• Lamivudine (3TC)	• Epivir
• Abacavir (ABC)	• Ziagen
• Emtricitabine (FTC)	• Emtriva
Reverse transcriptase inhibitors (nonnucleosides)	
• Efavirenz	• Sustiva
• Nevirapine	• Viramune
• Delavirdine	• Rescriptor
RT inhibitors (nucleotides)	
• Tenofovir	• Viread
Protease inhibitors	
• Saquinavir	• Invirase
• Saquinavir	• Fortovase
• Indinavir	• Crixivan
• Nelfinavir	• Viracept
• Ritonavir	• Norvir
• Amprenavir	• Agenerase
• Lopinavir + Ritonavir	• Kaletra
• Atazanavir	• Reyataz
• Fosamprenavir	• Lexiva
• Tipranavir	• Aptivus
• Darunavir	• Prezista
Fusion inhibitor	
• Pentafuside (T20)	• Fuseon
Integrase inhibitor	
• Raltegravir	• Isentress
CCR5 antagonists	
• Maraviroc	• Selzentry
Fixed dose combinations	
• AZT + 3TC	• Combivir
• AZT + 3TC + ABC	• Trizivir
• 3TC + ABC	• Epzicom
• Tenofovir + Emtriva	• Truvada
• Tenofovir + Emtriva + efavirenz	• Atripla

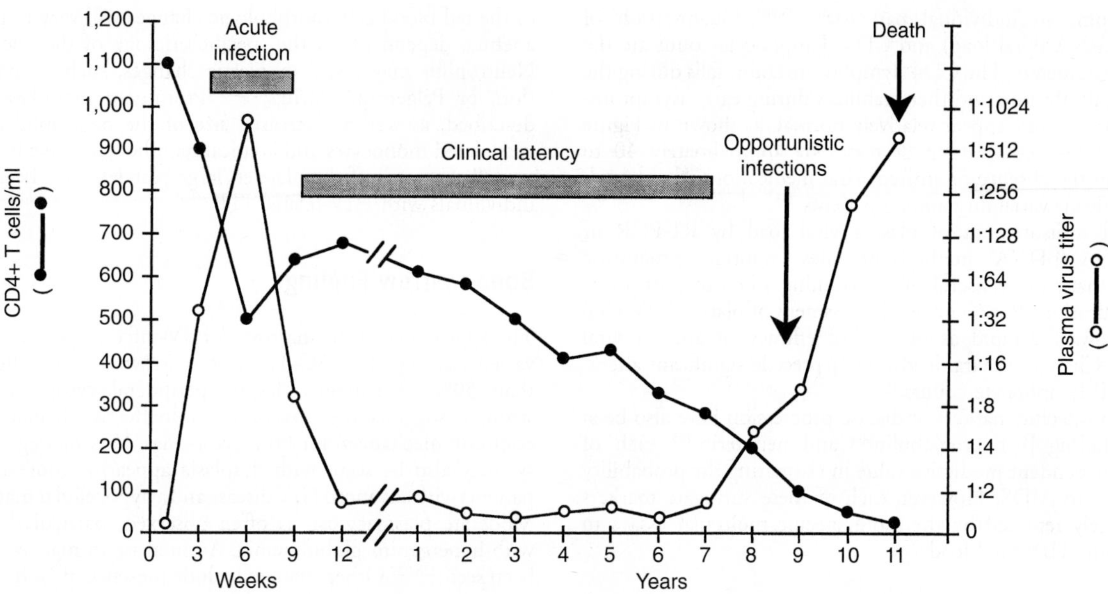

Figure 158–4 Natural history of HIV infection in an infected individual. A typical course of HIV infection is shown. During primary infection, there is active viral replication with viremia and widespread dissemination of virus to lymphoid tissues, during which time a sharp decline in the number of CD4$^+$ lymphocytes occurs. This is followed by a prolonged period of clinical latency, characterized by a slow but progressive decline in CD4$^+$ lymphocytes. When the CD4$^+$ cell number falls to less than 200/μL, the clinical course is generally complicated by opportunistic infections. A quantitative increase in viremia occurs during this time, reflecting increased viral replication.

CLINICAL STAGES OF HIV INFECTION

Acute Retroviral Syndrome

An acute clinical illness is often associated with initial HIV infection, occurring in approximately 50% to 90% of individuals.[186,195,196] This syndrome begins approximately 1 to 3 weeks (range 5 days to 3 months) after primary infection and usually lasts for 1 to 2 weeks. Prominent symptoms include significant fatigue and malaise; fever, which may be as high as 40°C (104°F); headache; photophobia; myalgias; and a morbilliform rash, seen in approximately 40% to 50% of patients. Generalized lymphadenopathy may occur toward the end of the acute illness. The symptoms are quite nonspecific and may be similar to those of other viral illnesses, such as infectious mononucleosis. All symptoms of this acute retroviral syndrome subside within several weeks, coincident with the initial host immune response to HIV, as shown in Fig. 158–4. However, headache may persist as an intermittent complaint, as may generalized lymphadenopathy, termed persistent, generalized lymphadenopathy (PGL), which occurs in approximately 75% of patients.[186,196] Initial attempts to employ HAART therapy in patients with the acute retroviral syndrome, in the hope of preventing or delaying the progression of HIV disease have not yet shown success.

Asymptomatic HIV disease (CDC Category A)

After resolution of the acute retroviral syndrome, the patient usually returns to a state of normal vigor and well-being. During this period, the patient harbors HIV in blood and in genital secretions and may transmit the virus to others. This phase of asymptomatic infection persists for approximately a decade in the absence of therapy and appears similar in all racial and ethnic groups, all geographic areas, both genders, and all risk groups for HIV infection.[197–199] Certain genetic polymorphisms have been described in the chemokine receptor genes that serve as coreceptors for HIV (eg, 32 deletion of CCR5), which predict for better prognosis and longer periods of AIDS-free survival.[107,108]

Symptomatic HIV Disease (CDC Category B)

With time, more significant manifestations of disease occur, with development of fatigue, fevers, weight loss, and/or night sweats. Unusual infections can occur, such as oral candidiasis, herpes zoster, and/or molluscum contagiosus, which, although not serious enough to be considered AIDS-defining, do serve to alert the clinician that underlying immune deficiency may be present.[200] Recurrent episodes of vaginal candidiasis or other gynecologic infections may be the first symptom of Category B disease in women. Immune thrombocytopenic purpura (ITP) may also occur during the course of symptomatic HIV infection. Presence of symptomatic, Category B disease would be an indication for initiation of antiretroviral therapy, even in the absence of surrogate markers of disease progression, such as CD4 cell depletion or elevated HIV-1 viral load in plasma.

AIDS (CDC Category C)

Over time, progression of HIV-induced immunodeficiency is expected, especially in the absence of effective antiretroviral therapy, leading to the development of opportunistic infections, specific neurologic symptoms, wasting syndrome, or malignant disease (Kaposi sarcoma, B-cell lymphoma, invasive cervical cancer).[200] These clinical illnesses are indicative of full-blown clinical AIDS, as depicted in Table 158–1.

The term *immunologic AIDS* is employed in individuals who have not yet developed an AIDS-defining clinical illness but in whom significant CD4$^+$ depletion has occurred, defined as a CD4 cell count lower than 200/μL, or less than 14% CD4$^+$ cells.[4] These individuals are at high risk for rapid development of clinical AIDS, and should clearly be treated with HAART, in an attempt to prevent these illnesses and their resultant morbidity and mortality.

LABORATORY CORRELATES OF DISEASE PROGRESSION

With progression from the initial acute retroviral syndrome to more advanced disease, various laboratory parameters may be used to predict outcome in individual patients.[188,189,201] Quantitation of plasma HIV RNA (viral load) and $CD4^+$ lymphocyte count are the most useful parameters. The $CD4^+$ lymphocyte count falls during the acute retroviral infection and then stabilizes during early asymptomatic infection and may appear relatively normal, as shown in Figure 158–4. The $CD4^+$ count then decreases by approximately 40 to 80 mL/year in the absence of antiretroviral medications,[202] although there is significant variability among patients.[203]

An initial measurement of plasma viral load by RT-PCR or branched-DNA (bDNA) methods provides important prognostic information that can be useful in determining when to start antiretroviral medications.[188,189] The serial assessment of plasma HIV viral load also allows for rapid assessment of efficacy of antiretroviral medications. Changes in viral load usually precede significant alterations in $CD4^+$ lymphocyte counts.[153,189]

Several nonspecific markers of disease progression have also been defined, including β_2-microglobulin[204] and neopterin,[205] each of which has independent predictive value in estimating the probability of progression to AIDS. However, each of these surrogate markers has been largely replaced by the more specific molecular assays to quantify plasma HIV viral load.

ABNORMALITIES OF HEMATOPOIESIS INDUCED BY HIV

Hematopoietic Progenitor Cells (CFU-GEMM)

Early in the AIDS epidemic, the potential for direct infection of the $CD34^+$ hematopoietic progenitor cell was considered, as these cells have been shown to express both the CD4 receptor and the CXCR4 coreceptor necessary for HIV-1 viral entry.[206,207] Furthermore, early experiments indicated that these progenitors were, indeed, infectable by HIV-1.[208,209] However, more recent evidence has indicated that the hematopoietic progenitor cell is not infected by HIV-1.[210–213]

Abnormalities in More Committed Myeloid Progenitors and Marrow Stroma

Although the $CD34^+CFU^-GEMM$ is not infected by HIV per se, the more committed myeloid progenitor cells can be infected and are clearly functionally abnormal, with markedly decreased colony growth.[214] Thus, as a result of cell surface interactions with HIV gp 120/160, decreased colony growth of BFU-E; CFU-GM, CFU-G and CFU-M have all been reported.[214] Likewise, the microenvironment of the marrow, necessary for normal blood cell growth and development, is also abnormal. The multiple cells, such as T cells and macrophages, that comprise this microenvironment (stroma) are infectable by HIV, resulting in decreased production of various hematopoietic growth factors, and further abnormalities of progenitor cell growth.[215–217] Additionally, cytokine dysregulation may lead to decreased growth of hematopoietic colonies, because of excessive production of TNF-α and interferon-γ by HIV-infected stromal cells in the marrow.[214,218,219] All of these factors, along with numerous additional abnormalities, eventually lead to the frequent development of cytopenias, including anemia, neutropenia, and/or thrombocytopenia.

MORPHOLOGIC CHANGES OF HEMATOPOIETIC CELLS IN HIV-1 INFECTION

Peripheral Blood Smears

The peripheral blood smear may be quite variable in patients with underlying HIV infection, dependent on other underlying conditions or infections (see Fig. 158–5A,B).[220] Numerous morphologic changes in red cells, white cells, and platelets have been described. In terms of the red blood cell, morphologic changes will vary in patients with anemia, dependent on the specific etiology of the anemic process. Neutrophils may reveal dysplastic changes, such as hyposegmentation, or PelgerHuët forms.[220,221] Prominent granulation has been described, as well as increased size of the neutrophils.[220,221] Large, vacuolated monocytes and atypical lymphocytes have been described as well. In terms of the platelet, large platelets may be seen in those individuals with HIV-related ITP.

Bone Marrow Findings

The appearance of the marrow in HIV-infected persons can be quite varied (see Fig. 158–5C–H). The marrow is hypercellular in more than 50% of patients, despite peripheral cytopenias.[221–226] This strongly suggests the possibility of ineffective hematopoiesis as a common mechanism for HIV cytopenias. Varying degrees of dysplasia may also be seen, with dysplasia appearing more frequently in patients with advanced HIV disease and a hypocellular marrow.[221,226,227] Moderate plasmacytosis is often observed, particularly in patients with hypergammaglobulinemia. An increase in marrow reticulin has been seen.[226,227] Other changes include presence of "soft" granulomas,

Thrombocytopenia in the HIV-Infected Patient

Thrombocytopenia is relatively common among HIV-infected persons, and may be caused by various medications, by malignant disease within the marrow, or most commonly by immune mechanisms. Immune thrombocytopenic purpura (ITP) is thought to be secondary to molecular mimicry between gp IIb/IIIa on the platelet surface and the outer membrane gp 120/160 of HIV. In addition to immune destruction of antibody-coated platelets through the Fc receptor on macrophages in the spleen, complement-mediated platelet destruction has also been described. The rate and level of platelet production in HIV-infected persons may also be perturbed, due to the direct infection of megakaryocytes. Patients with HIV-related ITP usually do have excessive bleeding, which has been reported in less than 10%. Nonetheless, bleeding may occur and therapy may also be indicated prior to the performance of invasive procedures. The initial therapy of choice for patients with HIV-ITP is effective antiretroviral therapy (HAART). Although many regimens have been shown effective in this regard, zidovudine appears particularly useful, with response rates in the range of approximately 70%. Responses to HAART are relatively rapid, occurring within 1 or 2 weeks, and may be durable. In the patient who does not respond to HAART, or in those with clinical bleeding or requirement for an invasive procedure, high dose intravenous gammaglobulin (IVIg) at a dose of 1000 to 2000 mg/kg may be used effectively, as in HIV-negative patients. Nonetheless, only 25% of patients will sustain prolonged elevation of platelet counts after IVIg. Use of anti-Rh (D) antibody is associated with increase of platelet counts to more than 50,000/dL in approximately 60% of patients, when given intravenously at a dose of 25 µg/kg. Higher doses (75 µg/kg) may also be used, as in patients with HIV-negative ITP. Anti-Rh (D) therapy may only be useful in those Rh-D-positive patients who have a spleen and whose hemoglobin level is high enough to allow the predicted hemolysis, occurring as a consequence of the Anti-Rh (D) therapy; a loss of 1 to 2 g of hemoglobin is expected. Corticosteroids may also be effective in HIV-infected patients with ITP, although this drug may be more problematic in the setting of HIV-induced immunosuppression. Splenectomy may be efficacious, and is not associated with progression of the underlying HIV disease. In patients with platelet counts greater than 20,000/dL, who do not respond to these various therapies, consideration can be given to simply watching without specific further treatment for the ITP.

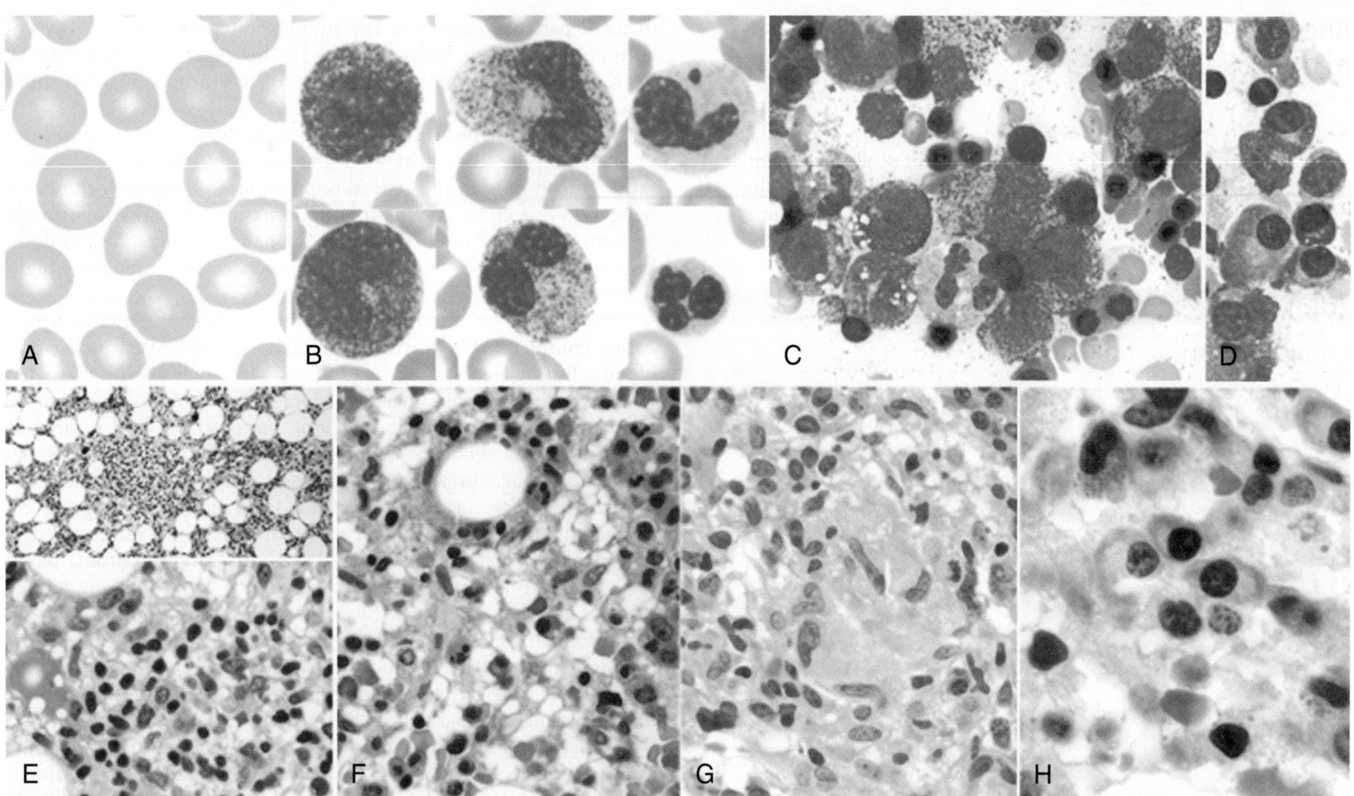

Figure 158–5 Typical peripheral blood and bone marrow findings in HIV (**A–H**). The peripheral smear not uncommonly shows anemia, which is sometimes macrocytic (**A**). There frequently is a neutrophilia with left shift, toxic granulation, and some mild dysplastic change is present in the granulocytes (**B**). In some patients, particularly those with severe disease, some of the segmented neutrophils show cytoplasmic inclusions similar to the Howell–Jolly bodies seen in red cells (**B**, *top, right cell*). These are nuclear in origin and are not microorganisms. The bone marrow is normo- or hypercellular and frequently shows granulocytic hyperplasia with left shift, and megaloblastoid change in the myeloid and erythroid cells lines (**C**). Typically there is also a reactive plasmacytosis (**D**). The biopsy commonly shows atypical reactive lymphoid infiltrates (**E**), poorly formed (**F**) or well-formed granuloma (**G**), and increased plasma cells (**H**).

even in the absence of specific infection other than HIV-1. Additionally, the pathologist should be alert to the possibility of marrow infiltration by lymphoma, Kaposi sarcoma, Hodgkin lymphoma, and/or various fungal and acid-fast organisms. In this regard, bone marrow examination is often requested for the purpose of obtaining a diagnosis in HIV-infected patients with fever of unknown origin. The diagnostic yield from the procedure is rather low, at approximately 20%, with infection due to mycobacterial or fungal infections seen most commonly.[228]

ANEMIA IN HIV INFECTION

Incidence and Risk Factors for Anemia

Anemia is very common in HIV-infected individuals, diagnosed in approximately 10% to 20% at initial presentation and developing in approximately 70% to 80% of patients over the course of disease.[226,227,229] In an attempt to ascertain the precise incidence of anemia in the setting of HIV infection, Sullivan and colleagues evaluated data derived from the case records of 32,867 HIV-infected persons followed from 1990 through 1996.[229] This cohort, termed the Multistate Adult and Adolescent Spectrum of HIV Disease Surveillance Project, is composed of individuals who receive HIV care in hospitals and HIV clinics in nine US cities. Using a hemoglobin level of less than 10 g/dL to define anemia, the 1-year incidence of anemia was 37% among patients with clinical AIDS; 12% among patients with immunologic AIDS; and 3% among HIV-infected individuals with neither clinical nor immunologic AIDS. Using a hemoglobin cutoff value of 12 g/dL as criteria for anemia in a large group of participants from the Women's Interagency HIV Study (WIHS), Levine and colleagues found a higher prevalence of anemia in HIV-infected women compared to HIV-uninfected controls.[230] Thus, 37% of the 2056 HIV infected women were anemic at baseline, compared to 17% of the 569 HIV-negative controls ($P < 0.001$). In the HAART era, an observational cohort study of 6725 HIV-infected patients from across Europe also documented a high prevalence of anemia,[231] with 58% diagnosed with mild anemia, defined as hemoglobin level of 8 to 14 g/dL in males or 8 to 12 g/dL in females, whereas 1.4% had severe anemia, defined as a hemoglobin level of <8 g/dL.[231] These data thus confirm the high incidence of anemia among HIV-infected patients in both the pre-HAART and HAART eras. Further, the frequency and severity of anemia in HIV-infected patients appear to correlate with HIV-related factors, such as CD4 cell counts less than 200 cells/mL (0.2×10^9/L), higher plasma HIV-1 RNA levels and a history of having been diagnosed with a clinical AIDS-defining condition.[229–231]

Etiology of Anemia

The etiology of anemia in the setting of HIV infection is often multifactorial, with numerous different causes having been described, as depicted in Table 158–3.

Anemia Due To Decreased Production of Red Blood Cells

A decrease in production of red blood cells may result from factors suppressing the CD34+ CFU-GEMM progenitor cell, such as inflammatory cytokines or the HIV virus itself.[226] In addition, a blunted production of erythropoietin has been documented in anemic HIV-infected patients, similar to the suppression seen in other states of chronic infection or inflammation. In this regard, a specific defect in the posttranscriptional synthesis of erythropoietin has been described.[232]

Table 158–3 Causes and Mechanisms of Anemia in HIV Infection

Mechanisms of Anemia	Cause of Anemia
Decreased red cell production	Neoplasm infiltrating the marrow Lymphoma Kaposi sarcoma Others Infection Atypical tuberculosis (*Mycobacterium avium intracellularis* or *Mycobacterium avium complex*) *Mycobacterium tuberculosis* Cytomegalovirus B19 parvovirus Fungal infection Medications HIV infection • Abnormal growth of burst-forming units–erythroid • Anemia of chronic disease • Blunted erythropoietin production and response Iron deficiency anemia secondary to chronic blood loss
Ineffective production	Folic acid deficiency Dietary Jejunal pathology: malabsorption B_{12} Deficiency Malabsorption in ileum Gastric pathology
Increased red cell destruction	Coombs-positive hemolytic anemia Hemophagocytic syndrome Thrombotic thrombocytopenic purpura Disseminated intravascular coagulation Medications Sulfonamides, dapsone Oxidant drugs in glucose-6-phosphate dehydrogenase deficiency

Infiltration of the marrow by tumor, such as non-Hodgkin lymphoma, may be associated with anemia.[233] Furthermore, although rather uncommon in the general population, in patients with underlying HIV infection, Hodgkin lymphoma involves bone marrow in 50% to 60%, and often presents with pancytopenia, commonly in association with systemic B symptoms, such as fever, drenching night sweats, and/or weight loss.[234,235]

Involvement of marrow by infection, such as *Mycobacterium avium* complex (MAC), may also lead to the decreased production of red cells (see Fig. 158–6). In addition, MAC may also be associated with cytokine-induced marrow suppression. Other opportunistic infections that may involve the bone marrow and lead to anemia include *M Tuberculosis*, cytomegalovirus, herpes simplex virus, as well as multiple fungal organisms, including histoplasmosis, coccidioidomycosis, and Cryptococcus.[228,236] Aside from inducing hypoproliferative anemia due to involvement of the marrow, these infections may also involve the gastrointestinal (GI) tract, leading to chronic blood loss and eventual iron deficiency anemia.

Infection of the marrow by parvovirus B19 is another cause of hypoproliferative anemia in HIV-infected patients, resulting in specific infection of the pronormoblast (see Fig. 158–7).[237,238] Thus, although marrow failure affecting all three lines has been described in association with parvovirus B19 infection, a pure red cell aplasia is the usual consequence. Parvovirus infection is usually acquired during childhood, leading to "fifth disease," one of the common childhood exanthems. Exposure to the virus leads to an antibody response, with subsequent resistance to further infection. Approximately 85% of adults have serologic evidence of prior parvovirus infection. However, the seroprevalence of such antibodies among HIV-infected patients is only 64%. This would suggest that these individuals may have an ineffective immune response against newly acquired infection, or may have lost prior seropositivity. The diagnosis of parvovirus B19 can be made on marrow examination, revealing giant pronormoblasts with clumped basophilic chromatin and clear cytoplasmic vacuoles; diagnosis can be confirmed by in situ hybridization using sequence-specific DNA probes for parvovirus B19.[239] Therapy for parvovirus-induced red cell aplasia consists of infusions of intravenous (IV) gamma globulin that contain antibodies from plasma donors, most of whom have previously been exposed to parvovirus. Doses of 400 mg/kg/day for 5 to 10 days or 1 g/kg/day for 3 days have been used successfully.[240] Relapse of parvovirus B19-induced red cell aplasia may occur, necessitating retreatment in these individuals.[238]

Hypoproliferative anemia in HIV-infected patients may also commonly occur as a consequence of the use of multiple medications, many of which may cause marrow and/or red cell suppression. Zid-

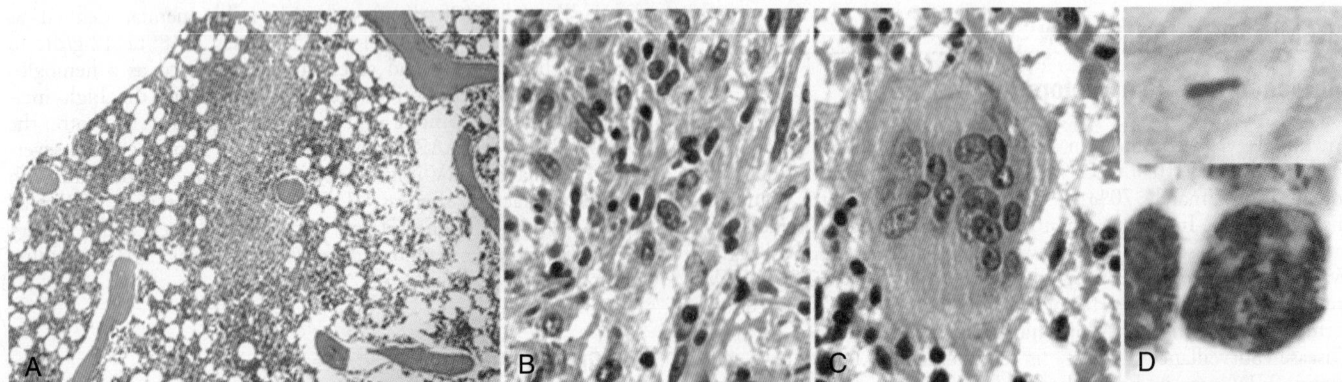

Figure 158–6 Acid-fast organisms in granuloma (**A–D**). Large poorly formed granuloma in the bone marrow (**A**) is composed of loosely aggregated histiocytes, lymphocytes, and plasma cells (**B**), with occasional giant cells (**C**). The acid-fast stain shows rare elongated slightly beaded organisms, typical of *Mycobacterium tuberculosis* (**D**, *top*). In *Mycobacterium avium* complex, the organisms frequently stuff histiocytes (**D**, *bottom*).

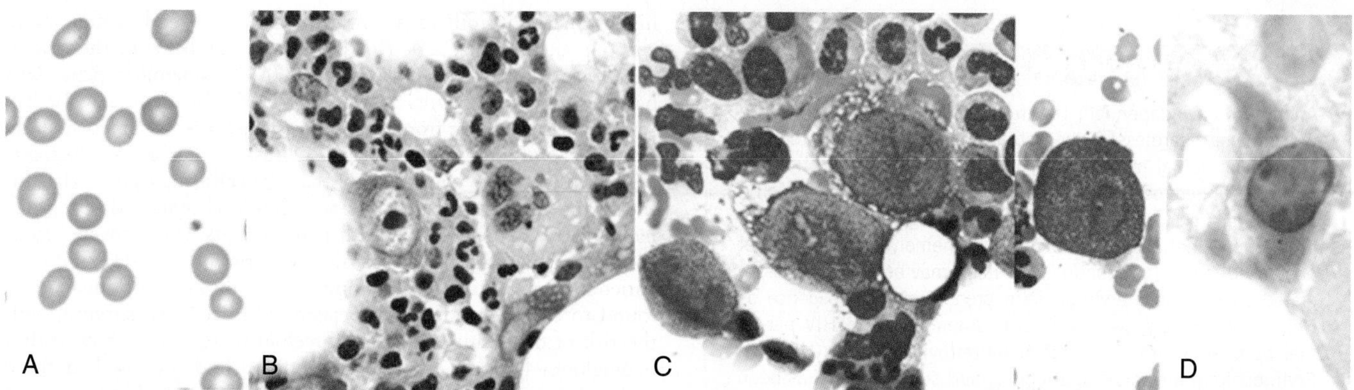

Figure 158–7 Human Parvovirus infection in HIV (**A-D**). The peripheral blood smear shows anemia with no polychromasia (**A**). The marrow biopsy shows mostly granulocytic and megakaryocytic elements with a lack of erythroid forms (**B**), except for rare large pronormoblasts with nuclear inclusions (**B**, *center*). On the aspirate, the large degenerating pronormoblasts have nuclear inclusions that resemble large nucleoli (**C**). These are viral inclusions. Sometimes the pronormoblasts are totally degenerated, and present as only bare nuclei, with the viral inclusion still obvious (**C**, *right*). An immunostain for parvovirus in a degenerated pronormoblasts is illustrated (**D**).

ovudine (AZT), the first licensed antiretroviral agent, is uniformly associated with macrocytosis [mean cell volume (MCV >100 fm)], which can be used as an objective indication that the patient has been compliant with this medication.[241] It is noteworthy that transfusion-dependent anemia (hemoglobin <8.5 g/dL) has been reported in approximately 30% of patients with full-blown AIDS, receiving zidovudine at doses of 600 mg/day. However, the incidence of severe anemia is only 1% when the same dose of zidovudine is used in patients with asymptomatic HIV disease.[242] Azidothymidine has also been associated with bone marrow failure, and should not be used together with myelosuppressive chemotherapy in HIV-infected patients with malignancy.[243] Although other reverse-transcriptase inhibitors, such as lamivudine, didanosine, or stavudine may cause anemia, this outcome is rather unusual. Other commonly used medications that can cause anemia in HIV-infected patients include trimethoprim-sulfamethoxazole, ganciclovir, sulfadiazine, pentamidine, rifabutin, flucytosine, amphotericin, foscarnet, and cidofovir.

Anemia Due To Increased Red Cell Destruction

Increased red cell destruction may be seen in HIV-infected patients with G-6-PD deficiency who are exposed to oxidant drugs, such as dapsone or sulfa-containing therapy, frequently employed for therapy or prophylaxis of *Pneumocystis carinii* infection.[244] Hemolytic anemia may also occur in HIV-infected patients with disseminated intravascular coagulation (DIC) or thrombotic thrombocytopenic purpura (TTP)[245]; presence of fragmented red cells and thrombocytopenia on blood smear will be seen in the latter two conditions, and Heinz bodies will be seen in association with G-6-PD deficiency. Hemophagocytic syndrome (hemophagocytic lymphohistiocytosis), with abnormal activation and proliferation of mature macrophages/histiocytes with increased phagocytic activity has also been described in association with HIV, and may occur as a consequence of acute HIV infection.[246–249] This disorder has recently been shown to result from severe imbalance of IL-18 and IL-18 binding protein, resulting in activation of Th-1 lymphocytes and macrophages, which then escape control by NK-cell cytotoxicity.[250]

An additional cause of red cell destruction in HIV-infected patients is the development of autoantibodies, with resultant positive Coombs test and shortened red cell survival. It is interesting to note that a positive direct Coombs test result has been reported in as many as 18% to 77% of HIV-infected patients, although the incidence of actual hemolysis is quite low.[251] When present, anti-I antibody and antibody against auto-U antigens have been described, occurring in 64% and 32% of HIV-infected patients, respectively.[252–254] A high incidence of positive direct Coombs test results has also been detected in patients with other hypergammaglobulinemic states, indicating that the positive Coombs test seen in HIV-infected patients may simply be secondary to the polyclonal hypergammaglobulinemia that is known to occur in the setting of HIV infection.[254]

Anemia Due To Ineffective Production of Red Cells (B_{12} or Folic Acid Deficiency)

Folic acid is absorbed in the jejunum and is responsible for the one-carbon transfer required in the synthesis of DNA. A deficiency of folic acid leads to a megaloblastic anemia, with large ovalocytes in the blood, hypersegmented neutrophils, and a decrease in all three lines, with resultant anemia, neutropenia, and thrombocytopenia. Because tissue stores of folate are relatively small, a deficiency of folate in the diet lasting as little as 3 to 6 months may lead to anemia. It is thus apparent that HIV-infected patients who are ill and not eating properly, as well as those with underlying disease of the jejunum, may be unable to absorb sufficient folic acid. The classic changes of megaloblastic anemia will be detected upon examination of the bone marrow, whereas serum and red cell folate levels will be low.

Ineffective production of red cells, with peripheral pancytopenia, elevated indirect bilirubin level, and low reticulocyte count may also be seen in vitamin B_{12} deficiency. The absorption of B_{12} requires initial production of intrinsic factor by parietal cells in the stomach, with subsequent absorption of the complex of B_{12} and intrinsic factor within the ileum. Thus, malabsorption of B_{12} can occur in various disorders of the stomach, by production of antibodies to the H^+/K^+ ATP pump or to intrinsic factor (pernicious anemia), or by various disorders of the small bowel and ileum (infection or Crohn disease). Although B_{12} deficiency is unlikely on a dietary basis alone, patients with HIV infection appear to be prone to B_{12} malabsorption, presumably because of the myriad of infections and other disorders that may occur in the small intestine. Negative vitamin B_{12} balance has been documented in approximately one-third of patients with AIDS, the majority demonstrating defective absorption of the vitamin.[255] Diagnosis of B_{12} deficiency can be made by documenting low serum B_{12} levels, along with elevated levels of folic acid, homocysteine, and methylmalonic acid in the serum , whereas the earliest indication of negative B_{12} balance is the finding of low B_{12} levels in blood in patients taking transcobalamin II.[256] Monthly administration of parenteral B_{12} will correct the deficiency and the resultant anemia and pancytopenia in the peripheral blood. Because B_{12} deficiency may also cause neurologic dysfunction (subacute combined degeneration of the cord), with motor, sensory, and higher cortical dysfunction, the possibility of vitamin B_{12} deficiency should also be considered in HIV-infected patients with these neurologic symptoms and signs.

Anemia in the HIV-Infected Patient

Anemia is an independent risk factor for death in HIV-infected individuals, regardless of the actual etiology of the low red cell count. The actual mechanisms or cause of this association are not well understood. There are multiple reasons for an HIV-infected person to become anemic, including decreased red cell production, ineffective production, or hemolysis. In terms of decreased red cell production, HIV itself may be operative, associated with blunted erythropoietin production and response as well as abnormal growth of BFU-E. Anemia due to HIV per se may be treated with highly active antiretroviral therapy (HAART). Erythropoietin may also be effective, and such therapy has been associated with improvements in both hemoglobin levels and in quality-of-life parameters. Multiple medications may cause hypoproliferative anemia, with low reticulocyte count and normal indirect bilirubin levels in the setting of HIV, including zidovudine (AZT), the first of the antiretroviral drugs to be licensed in the United States, as well as lamivudine, didanosine, and stavudine. Prophylactic antiinfective agents such as sulfonamides, trimethoprim, and pyrimethamine and pentamidine may cause anemia and should be considered in the evaluation of these individuals. Other antiinfectives, including antiviral agents such as ganciclovir, foscarnet and cidofovir; and antifungal agents such as flucytosine or amphotericin are relatively common causes of anemia in the HIV-infected patient. In addition, various infections may themselves cause hypoproliferative anemia, as described with atypical TB (MAI/MAC), *Mycobacterium tuberculosis*, cytomegalovirus, B19 parvovirus, and various fungal infections. Development of malignancy, with marrow involvement, may also cause a hypoproliferative anemia, occurring predominantly in patients with Hodgkin Disease and/or non-Hodgkin lymphoma. Furthermore, more "usual" causes of hypoproliferative anemia, such as iron deficiency due to chronic blood loss, should also be considered in HIV-infected patients with low reticulocyte counts, normal indirect bilirubin levels, and hypochromic, microcytic anemia. Multiple causes of ineffective red cell production have also been described in HIV-infected patients, who present with anemia, low reticulocyte levels, and elevation of indirect bilirubin. These include folic acid deficiency, due to inadequate diet or to jejunal pathology; or B_{12} deficiency due to malabsorption in the ileum, or gastric pathology with decreased production or production of antibody to intrinsic factor. Lastly, numerous causes of hemolytic anemia have been described in HIV-infected patients. These individuals present with an elevated reticulocyte count, and elevated indirect bilirubin levels. Coombs positive hemolytic anemia has been described, and is relatively common in patients with HIV-related Castleman disease. Hemophagocytic syndrome has been described, as has thrombotic thrombocytopenic purpura (TTP). Multiple drugs may also be associated with hemolysis in this setting, including sulfonamides, dapsone, and oxidant drugs in the patient with underlying G6PD deficiency.

Consequences of Anemia in HIV Infection

Decreased Survival

Several large cohort studies have shown that anemia is an independent risk factor for shorter survival in HIV-infected patients.[229,231,257,258] In the Multistate Adult and Adolescent Spectrum of HIV Disease Surveillance Project, anemia, defined as a hemoglobin level lower than 10 g/dL or a physician's diagnosis of anemia, was found to be associated with an increased risk of death for all CD4 ranges in this cohort.[229] However, the greatest risk of death was noted in patients with baseline CD4 cell counts greater than 200 cells/mL (0.2×10^9/L), with a relative risk of death 150% higher than for individuals in the same CD4 cell count strata without anemia (RR 2.3, $P < 0.001$). In comparison, the risk of death was increased by approximately 60% for anemic patients with baseline CD4 cell counts lower than 200 cells/mL (0.2×10^9/L). Importantly, recovery from anemia was shown to be independently associated with improved survival. Thus, among anemic patients with baseline CD4 counts lower than 50 cells/mL (0.05×10^9/L), those who remained anemic (hemoglobin level remained <10 g/dL) had a 160% higher risk of death than patients who recovered from anemia following treatment. In another series of 2348 HIV-infected patients from Baltimore, development of any grade of anemia was found to be independently associated with decreased survival, with the risk of death approximately threefold increased in those with a hemoglobin level of 7 to 8 g/dL and fourfold increased in those with a hemoglobin level below 6.5 g/dL.[257] Of significance, use of erythropoietin was associated with a decreased risk of death, as was use of antiretroviral therapy. Similarly, an additional study performed among 6725 European HIV-infected patients demonstrated that hemoglobin level at baseline, together with CD4 count and viral load, were independent prognostic factors for survival.[194,231] For each 1-g/dL decrease in hemoglobin level, the relative hazard of death was 1.39 (95% CI, 1.34–1.43; $P < 0.0001$). Finally, in the large multicenter prospective study of 2056 HIV-infected women, Levine and colleagues confirmed the independent association between anemia and decreased survival.[258] Anemia has also been confirmed as an independent predictor of mortality among HIV-infected persons in resource-poor regions of the world[259] and use of total lymphocyte count and hemoglobin concentration has been suggested as a more cost-effective way to monitor HIV progression in these settings.[260] Further work is required to elucidate the precise mechanisms underlying this strong prognostic association, and it is conceivable that anemia may simply serve as a surrogate marker for more advanced systemic illness.

Disease Progression

Anemia has also been shown to be independently associated with more rapid clinical progression of HIV infection. In one large European study aimed at identifying predictive factors for disease progression among HIV-infected patients receiving HAART, the most recent measured hemoglobin level, CD4 cell count, and HIV-1 viral load, as well as a history of clinical AIDS before initiation of HAART were all independently related to the risk of disease progression.[261] Thus, with mild anemia (hemoglobin of 8–14 g/dL for men and 8–12 g/dL for women), the relative hazard of disease progression or death was 2.2 (95% CI 1.6–2.9, $P < 0.0001$), whereas for severe anemia (hemoglobin <8 g/dL), the relative hazard was 7.1 (95% CI 2.5–20.1, $P = 0.0002$).

Effects on Quality of Life

Presence of anemia has consistently been associated with decreases in quality of life, as measured by the Linear Analogue Scale (LASA), and other such instruments.[262,263]

Effect of Highly Active Antiretroviral Therapy on Anemia

Recent studies have confirmed the ability of HAART to correct or improve the anemia of HIV infection. In a study of 6725 HIV-infected patients from across Europe,[231] use of HAART was statistically associated with improvement in hemoglobin levels. In addition, prolonged HAART use was associated with a greater likelihood of correcting anemia. Thus, 65.5% of the cohort was anemic before the use of HAART, 53% were anemic after 6 months of HAART, and 46% were anemic after 12 months of HAART. In a study of

905 HIV-infected patients from Baltimore, use of HAART was associated with an increase in hemoglobin levels after 1 year of follow-up.[264] Among the patients with a baseline hemoglobin level less than 14 g/dL, 21% of patients receiving HAART recovered from anemia (hemoglobin >14 g/dL) compared to only 8% in those not receiving HAART ($P = 0.0006$).[264] In multivariate analysis, use of HAART was strongly associated with freedom from anemia, after adjusting for CD4 cell count, HIV-1 RNA level, sex, race, history of injection-drug use, and use of various therapies for anemia. More recently, data from the Women's Interagency HIV Study (WIHS) demonstrated that use of HAART for as little as 6 months was independently associated with a higher likelihood of resolution of anemia, and longer use was associated with more profound improvements.[258] In addition, use of HAART for at least 12 months was significantly associated with a reduced risk of developing anemia.[258]

The mechanisms whereby HAART may protect against development of anemia or correct preexisting anemia are not yet fully understood. Nonetheless, because HIV infection directly contributes to the development of anemia, it is conceivable that HAART may protect against or correct anemia simply by decreasing the level of HIV-1 viral burden and/or by overcoming the factors responsible for the anemia of chronic disease. Additionally, use of HAART has been associated with an increase in hematopoietic progenitor cell growth,[265] whereas ritonavir, a protease inhibitor, has also been shown to directly stimulate progenitor cell growth and to inhibit apoptosis of hematopoietic progenitors in vitro.[266]

Use of Erythropoietin in HIV-Infected Patients With Anemia

A blunted response to erythropoietin is extremely common in the setting of HIV infection.[232] The mechanism of this decreased production is likely a posttranscriptional defect, as levels of messenger RNA for erythropoietin are normal although erythropoietin protein levels are decreased.[232] In addition, development of autoantibodies to erythropoietin has been described in HIV-infected patients.[267] Multiple studies have now confirmed the beneficial effect of erythropoietin in HIV-infected patients with anemia, in whom marrow function has been suppressed as a result of HIV or other chronic infectious or inflammatory diseases.[268,269] Erythropoietin is also effective in treating the anemia due to zidovudine or other medications, including cancer chemotherapy, that suppress the marrow.[260,270]

The baseline level of endogenous serum erythropoietin can predict which patients are likely to respond to the therapeutic use of erythropoietin. Thus, patients with a baseline endogenous erythropoietin level of 500 IU/L or less are expected to respond to such therapy, whereas those with endogenous levels greater than 500 IU/L are not. Erythropoietin is administered subcutaneously at a dose of 100 to 200 U/kg body weight, three times weekly until normalization of the red blood cell and then given approximately once every week or every other week to maintain a hemoglobin concentration of approximately 12 g/dL. Recent trials have demonstrated the equivalent efficacy of 40,000 units of erythropoietin given weekly as compared with the original thrice-weekly schedule in anemic HIV-infected patients.[263]

Data from recent studies have indicated that correction of anemia by erythropoietin is associated with improvement in quality of life (QOL) measures,[262,263,271] with the mean Linear Analogue Scale (LASA) QOL score increasing by 41% and the Medical Outcomes Study–HIV (MOS-HIV) overall QOL score increasing by as much as 37% in one study.[262]

Toxicity of erythropoietin is uncommon, consisting primarily of local pain at the site of injection, mild fever, or rash. However, the prevalence of these side effects has been similar to those seen with placebo-treated patients. Development of pure red cell aplasia has been described in HIV-negative patients receiving the Eprex product (epoetin alfa) from Europe, although this complication is uncommon and has not been reported in the setting of HIV.[272]

Currently, several prospective trials have also evaluated the efficacy and toxicity of darbepoetin alfa, a novel erythropoiesis-stimulating protein (NESP), in anemic HIV-infected patients. Compared with conventional erythropoietin, darbepoetin alfa has a longer terminal half-life, owing to the presence of additional sialic acid residues, and thus offers the advantage of a less frequent dosing schedule.[273,274] Preliminary data from one recent study suggested that darbepoetin-alfa given at a dose of 3.0 mg/kg once every 2 weeks is effective in improving the hemoglobin level in the majority of HIV-infected patients as well as in maintaining hemoglobin levels and improving quality-of-life measures.[275]

NEUTROPENIA

Incidence and Etiology of Neutropenia in HIV

Neutropenia is reported in approximately 5% to 10% of patients with early, asymptomatic HIV infection and in more than 50% of those individuals with more advanced HIV-related immunodeficiency.[226,269] In a study of 1729 HIV-infected women, evaluated as part of the Women's Interagency HIV Study, the prevalence of neutropenia (<2000/μL) at baseline was 44%, whereas 7% had less than 1000 neutrophils/μL. Over 7.5 years of follow-up, neutrophil counts lower than 2000/μL occurred on at least one occasion in 79%, whereas absolute neutrophil count (ANC) lower than 1000/μL was documented in 31%.[276] Factors associated with more severe underlying HIV disease, such as lower $CD4^+$ cell counts and higher HIV-1 RNA levels correlated statistically with development of neutropenia on multivariate analysis in this study, whereas prevention of neutropenia was seen in those patients receiving combination antiretroviral therapy without inclusion of zidovudine.[276]

As with other peripheral blood cytopenias in the setting of HIV infection, multiple etiologies may be present, either singly or in combination (Table 158–3).[277] Thus, decreased colony growth of the progenitor cell CFU-GM[278,279] may lead to decreased production of both granulocytes and monocytes. Soluble inhibitory substances produced by HIV-infected cells have been noted to suppress neutrophil production in vitro, suggesting that autoimmunity may play a part in the development of neutropenia in HIV infection.[160,280] However, more recent studies have now shown that the presence of neutrophil-bound immunoglobulin (Ig) correlates best with stage of disease rather than with neutropenia per se.[281] Decreased serum levels of G-CSF have been described in HIV-seropositive subjects with afebrile neutropenia (<1000 neutrophils/mL), indicating that a relative deficiency of this specific hematopoietic growth factor may also contribute to persistent neutropenia.[282] Suppression of myelopoiesis may also occur as a consequence of the inflammatory cytokines induced by HIV infection, such as transforming growth factor-β and tumor necrosis factor-α.[283,284] In a more direct manner, certain HIV-1 proteins, such as tat protein and protein 24 (p24) have also been implicated in suppression of myelopoiesis.[284,285] Other causes of neutropenia in HIV infection include the presence of opportunistic infections, and/or malignancies involving the bone marrow. Finally, myelosuppression and neutropenia may also result from any one of several medications that are commonly prescribed for HIV-infected patients. In a recent study of 87 consecutive HIV-infected patients with ANC levels lower than 2000/μL, only 3 individuals were not receiving drugs associated with neutropenia, and 66% were receiving three or more potentially myelosuppressive medications.[286] The medications most frequently associated with neutropenia in this setting include trimethoprim-sulfamethoxazole, pentamidine, pyrimethamine-sulfadiazine, flucytosine, amphotericin, foscarnet, cidofovir, and ganciclovir, used to treat or prevent various opportunistic infections. In addition, certain antiretroviral agents, such as zidovudine, lamivudine, didanosine, stavudine, abacavir, and indinavir have also been associated with neutropenia.[243,287–289] Chemotherapeutic agents are also commonly associated with neutropenia, as is interferon-alpha.

Abnormalities of Granulocyte and Monocyte Function in HIV

Aside from absolute neutropenia, patients with HIV infection may also experience decreased function of granulocytes and monocytes. Thus, impaired chemotaxis and reduced expression of adhesion molecules on neutrophils has been described. Additionally, abnormal Fc processing by macrophages has been documented, whereas decreased opsonization, decreased production of superoxide with diminished intracellular killing of bacterial or fungal organisms by granulocytes has also been noted.[290–293]

Risk Factors for Infection in Neutropenic HIV-Infected Patients

In patients with cancer who receive chemotherapy, multiple studies have shown that the risk of bacterial infection rises when the ANC falls below 1000 cells/mL and increases further when the ANC falls below 500 cells/mL.[294] Several studies have confirmed the same relationship in patients with HIV infection. Thus, Moore and colleagues found that the risk of bacterial infection increased 2.3-fold for HIV-infected individuals with ANC less than 1000 cells/mL and rose by 7.9-fold in those with ANC levels less than 500 cells/mL.[295] Lower ANC counts have been associated with increased risk of hospitalization for serious infection, as shown in a review of 2047 HIV-positive patients.[296] On multivariate analysis, the severity and duration of neutropenia were found to be significant predictors of the incidence of hospitalization for serious bacterial infections.[296]

In a recent study of 62 HIV-infected patients with ANCs of 1000 cells/mL or less, 24% developed infectious complications, most commonly within 24 hours after the onset of neutropenia.[297] On multivariate analysis, the three factors independently associated with infectious complications included presence of a central venous catheter, neutropenia in the previous 3 months, and a lower nadir of granulocyte count (250 cells/mL in those with infections vs 622 cells/mL in those without). Among patients with medication-associated neutropenia, the most common cause was zidovudine, followed by trimethoprim-sulfamethoxazole, and ganciclovir; neutropenia was less likely to be associated with infection in these patients than in individuals who were neutropenic owing to the use of cancer chemotherapy.[297]

Another more recent study, however, has suggested that the risk of serious infectious complications in neutropenic HIV-infected patients is quite low.[286] In this prospective study of neutropenia (defined as an ANC of 1000 cells/mL or less) in 87 consecutive HIV-infected patients, all except three episodes of neutropenia were associated with known myelosuppressive medications. The majority of patients had received cotrimoxazole (62%), lamivudine (56%), and/or zidovudine (40%).[286] The mean ANC of these individuals was 660 cells/mL (range 100–900 cells/mL) and the median duration of neutropenia was 13 days. Severe neutropenia was, however, uncommon; only three patients had ANC nadirs lower than 200 cells/mL. Of importance, serious neutropenia-related sepsis in this setting was uncommon, with culture-proven infection occurring in only 8% and presumed infection in a further 8% of patients. No patient died of infection. As expected, patients with infections had significantly lower ANC nadirs (mean, 460 vs 710 cells/mL) and significantly lower CD4 cell counts (mean, 64 vs 126/mL), but did not have a longer duration of neutropenia than those patients who did not develop infection.

The state of underlying HIV-1 infection may also influence the risk of febrile neutropenia in HIV-infected patients. Thus, a recent prospective observational cohort study indicated that low $CD4^+$ lymphocyte counts were associated with an increased risk of bacterial infection in HIV-infected neutropenic patients.[286] A similar relationship has also been reported in HIV-negative patients undergoing chemotherapy; in this setting a low pretreatment CD4 count (<450/mm^3) was an independent risk factor for febrile neutropenia and early death.[298]

Of interest, the occurrence of neutropenia (ANC <2000/μL) per se was not associated with decreased survival among a group of 1729 HIV-infected women.[276]

Impact of Highly Active Antiretroviral Therapy on Neutropenia

Recent evidence indicates that use of HAART may be associated with an improvement in leukopenia and neutropenia in treated patients.[266] Thus, in a group of 66 HIV-infected patients treated with HAART, significant increases in total leukocyte counts and absolute granulocyte counts were seen after 6 months of treatment.[266] Of interest, Sloan and colleagues have recently demonstrated a direct stimulatory effect of protease inhibitors on human hematopoiesis.[299] In a prospective study of 1729 HIV-infected women, Levine and colleagues demonstrated that combination antiretroviral or HAART therapy, without zidovudine, were associated with protection against development of neutropenia over time, whereas this protection was lost when zidovudine was part of the antiretroviral regimen.[276] Furthermore, HAART therapy, even when zidovudine was included, was statistically associated with resolution of preexisting neutropenia among these women. These data would indicate that mild to moderate levels of neutropenia may be managed by use of HAART alone, although several months of therapy are required to achieve the desired effect.[276]

Use of Granulocyte–Macrophage Colony-Stimulating Factor or Granulocyte Colony-Stimulating Factor in Neutropenic, HIV-Infected Patients

Granulocyte–Macrophage Colony Stimulatory Factor

When administered subcutaneously to HIV-infected patients with neutropenia, GM-CSF results in dose-dependent increases in granulocytes, monocytes, and eosinophils.[300,301] Therapy with GM-CSF may also improve neutrophil function by enhancing phagocytosis, degranulation, leukotriene B_4 synthesis, release of arachidonic acid, superoxide anion generation, and antibody-dependent cellular cytotoxicity.[302,303] Although there were initial concerns that GM-CSF may increase HIV replication,[304] subsequent in vitro studies have indicated that GM-CSF, in fact, inhibits HIV-1 replication in monocytes and macrophages.[305]

In one study comparing 123 HIV-positive leukopenic patients (defined as a white blood cell count <3 × 10^9/L) treated with subcutaneous GM-CSF versus 121 nontreated leukopenic HIV-positive controls, administration of GM-CSF for 12 weeks was found to significantly increase the total leukocyte count of treated patients.[306] In patients receiving GM-SCF, the total leukocyte count increased by 22% at week 1 and by 65% at week 12, when compared to baseline values ($P < 0.001$), whereas the circulating monocyte levels increased by two- to threefold at week 12 ($P < 0.001$). In contrast, the total leukocyte count decreased by 24% below baseline values at week 12 ($P < 0.001$) in the control group. Of importance, no statistically significant change occurred in HIV p24 antigen levels in patients treated with GM-CSF, even among those who were not receiving antiretroviral therapy.[306]

The safety and efficacy of GM-CSF in HIV-infected patients receiving antiretroviral therapy has also been confirmed in another randomized placebo-controlled trial involving a group of 105 HIV-infected patients.[307] GM-CSF was given at a dose of 125 μg/m^2 twice weekly for 6 months. Patients randomized to antiretroviral therapy plus GM-CSF achieved a greater reduction in plasma viral load, they were more likely to achieve HIV-1 RNA levels below the limit of detection, and they also demonstrated a lower frequency of zidovudine resistance mutations than those who received antiretroviral agents plus placebo. Side effects of GM-CSF include primarily an influenza-like syndrome, with fever, bone pain, myalgia, fatigue, malaise, and headache.

Granulocyte Colony-Stimulating Factor

G-CSF has also been shown to be effective at preventing severe neutropenia and reducing the incidence of bacterial infections and the number of days of hospitalization in neutropenic HIV-infected patients.[308] Kuritzkes and colleagues randomized 258 such patients with CD4 counts below 200 cells/mm^3 and moderate neutropenia (defined as an ANC of 750–1000/mL) to receive G-CSF (1 μg/kg/day or 300 μg three times per week) versus no treatment for 24 weeks.[308] Patients in the control group who developed severe neutropenia (ANC less than 500/mL) were rerandomized to receive G-CSF according to one of the two treatment groups. Treatment with G-CSF was effective at preventing the development of severe neutropenia and in reducing the incidence of bacterial infections, independent of CD4 count, number of prior opportunistic infections, or baseline use of zidovudine. Thus, in an intention-to-treat analysis, the incidence of severe neutropenia was 1.7% in the treated group versus 22% in the control group, whereas the incidence of bacterial infections was 31% lower in the treated group (2.93 vs 4.25/1000 patient days). Furthermore, patients treated with G-CSF had 54% fewer severe bacterial infections and 45% fewer hospital days for bacterial infections. Of importance, there was no difference between the groups in terms of toxicity or HIV RNA levels in plasma. The most frequently reported adverse events were fever, diarrhea, fatigue, nausea, headache, anemia, abdominal pain, vomiting, and myalgia. Thus, it would appear that administration of G-CSF when patients are mildly neutropenic may be superior to waiting for patients to become severely neutropenic. However, as discussed, effective use of HAART may also be equally efficacious in resolving mild to moderate neutropenia.

The early recommendations for dosing of G-CSF included use of 5 mg/kg/day given subcutaneously. Recent evidence suggests, however, that much lower doses of G-CSF may be effective in HIV-infected persons. Thus, an initial dose of 1 mg/kg/day is often initiated and used until the neutrophil count rises to acceptable levels (>1000 cells/mL). This is followed by a titration of dosing, often requiring therapy only once or twice per week, as necessary to maintain the desired response.[309,310]

Thus, use of G-CSF or GM-CSF to improve neutropenia in HIV-infected patients has been shown to be both safe and effective. Although patient survival has not increased as a consequence of G-CSF or GM-CSF,[311] these drugs will allow safer administration of other necessary medications, and will also potentially reduce both the incidence of bacterial infections and number of hospital days.[301,308,311]

THROMBOCYTOPENIA

Thrombocytopenia is relatively common during the course of HIV infection, occurring in approximately 40% of patients and serving as the first symptom or sign of HIV infection in approximately 10%.[312,313] Sullivan and colleagues[313] evaluated the 1-year incidence of thrombocytopenia (<50,000/mL) in a group of 30,214 HIV-infected patients as part of the retrospective Adult and Adolescent Spectrum of Disease Project. The incidence of thrombocytopenia over 1 year was 8.7% in patients with clinical AIDS, 3.1% in patients with immunologic AIDS (CD4 <200 cells/mL), and 1.7% in patients with neither. Development of thrombocytopenia was associated with history of clinical or immunologic AIDS, injection drug use, history of anemia or lymphoma, and African American race. After controlling for multiple factors (AIDS, CD4 count, anemia, neutropenia, antiviral therapy, and receipt of prophylaxis against *P carinii*), thrombocytopenia was significantly associated with shorter survival (risk ratio = 1.7, 95% confidence interval = 1.6–1.8).[313]

More recently, Pearce and colleagues evaluated the incidence of thrombocytopenia, defined as a platelet count lower than 150,000/mL, among 1990 HIV-infected and 553 HIV-negative women who were part of the Women's Interagency HIV Study. At baseline, 15% of HIV-positive women were thrombocytopenic, compared to 1.6% of HIV-negative women ($P < 0.001$).[314] Factors associated with increased risk of thrombocytopenia included HIV infection, low CD4 levels, increasing viral load, smoking, and Caucasian race/ethnicity. Of importance, the study also found thrombocytopenia to be a significant predictor of both all-cause and AIDS-related mortality among women infected with HIV. Thus, HIV-infected women with a platelet count lower than 50,000/mL had a fivefold increased risk of death from any cause compared to women with normal platelet counts (HR = 5.10, 95% confidence interval = 2.71–9.58) and an approximate threefold increased risk of death from AIDS (HR = 3.36, 95% confidence interval = 1.44–7.83). The statistically significant increase in mortality due to thrombocytopenia was maintained even after exclusion of those patients who died of bleeding events.

Mechanisms of Thrombocytopenia in HIV-Related Immune Thrombocytopenic Purpura

Increased Platelet Destruction

As in "de novo" immune thrombocytopenic purpura (ITP), HIV-infected patients with ITP also demonstrate increased platelet destruction via Fcγ-mediated phagocytosis by macrophages in the spleen.[315] In HIV-related ITP, however, multiple mechanisms for development of platelet-associated antibody have been described, often occurring simultaneously in a given patient. Thus, presence of platelet-specific antibodies, immunochemically characterized as antiglycoprotein (GP)IIb and/or GPIIIa, have been detected in HIV-infected patients with ITP, indicating a mechanism similar to that described in de novo disease.[316] However, cross-reactive antibody between HIV gp160/120 and platelet GPIIb/IIIa has also been demonstrated.[317] Thus, Bettaieb and colleagues found that serum antibodies against HIV gp160/120 could be eluted from platelets of patients with HIV-related ITP and that these HIV-specific antibodies shared a common epitope with antibodies against platelet GPIIb/IIIa on the platelet surface. The specific immunodominant epitope against which the antibody is directed in HIV-ITP is the β_3 GPIIIa integrin, GPIIIa49–66, which shares a known epitope region with HIV-1 protein nef.[318–320] Of interest, purified anti-GP IIIa49–66 antibody from patients with HIV-ITP can induce platelet fragmentation by catalyzing hydrogen peroxide generation in a complement-independent manner, serving as yet another mechanism of platelet destruction in this setting.[321] A binding partner of β_3 GPIIIa integrin is talin-H, a cytoskeletal platelet protein that plays a key role in the regulation of integrin activation and can be cleaved during platelet activation and also by HIV-1 protease.[322,323] Following platelet fragmentation by complement independent generation of hydrogen peroxide, talin-H may be exposed, leading to antibody production. In this regard, the talin head has been shown to serve as yet another immunodominant epitope of the antibody response in patients with HIV-ITP.[324] It is thus apparent that molecular mimicry between various HIV-associated and platelet-associated proteins may be operative in the immune destruction of platelets in some cases of HIV-related ITP. A further mechanism of antibody-induced destruction of platelets arises from the nonspecific absorption of immune complexes against HIV onto the platelet Fc receptor, thus providing a "free" Fc portion for subsequent macrophage binding and phagocytosis.[316]

Decreased Platelet Production

Kinetic studies of platelet production and destruction have been performed in patients with HIV-related ITP, with results compared to a group of normal control subjects and to a group of patients with de novo ITP.[315] Mean platelet survival was found to be significantly decreased in patients with HIV-ITP, occurring to the same extent in patients receiving zidovudine and in those who were untreated. It is interesting to note that the mean platelet survival was also significantly decreased in HIV-infected patients with normal platelet counts. In addition to this increased destruction of platelets, mean platelet production was also found to be significantly decreased in patients with untreated HIV-ITP, although those patients receiving zidovudine demonstrated a subsequent increase in platelet production, occurring even in zidovudine-treated HIV-infected individuals without thrombocytopenia. Kinetic studies performed by Cole and colleagues confirmed the decrease in platelet production seen in patients with HIV-ITP, despite a sixfold elevation in thrombopoietin levels and a threefold expansion of megakaryocyte mass when compared to normal controls.[325] This finding suggested the possibility of HIV-induced apoptosis of megakaryocytes.[326] Thus, it is apparent that patients with HIV-ITP, though experiencing a moderate increase in platelet destruction, are also faced with significant decreases in platelet production, which occur even in those individuals with normal platelet counts.[315]

Infection of the Megakaryocyte by HIV

The cause for the reduced production of platelets in the setting of HIV infection may be direct infection of the megakaryocyte by HIV. Thus, Kouri and colleagues first demonstrated that human megakaryocytes bear a $CD4^+$ receptor capable of binding HIV-1,[327] whereas Zucker-Franklin et al showed that HIV-1 could be internalized by human megakaryocytes.[328] The presence of the HIV-1 coreceptor, CXCR4, on megakaryocytic progenitors, megakaryocytes, and platelets was subsequently demonstrated as well.[329] Furthermore, employing in situ hybridization techniques and a ^{35}S HIV riboprobe (antisense to an HIV *env* sequence), HIV transcripts have been detected in megakaryocytes of 5 of 10 patients with HIV-ITP, indicating that the megakaryocyte had been infected by HIV in these cases.[330] Expression of viral RNA was also detected in all 10 patients, using in situ hybridization techniques. Specific ultrastructural damage in the HIV-infected megakaryocytes has been noted, consisting of blebbing and vacuolization of the surface membrane.[331] The documentation of significant increases in platelet production after receipt of zidovudine[332] would be consistent with the hypothesis that a major mechanism of this disorder is the direct infection of the megakaryocyte by HIV.

Recently, Harker and colleagues described three chimpanzees infected with HIV-1 who developed ITP associated with elevated levels of antibody against platelet GPIIIa. Use of recombinant pegylated human megakaryocyte growth and development factor (MGDF) was associated with a decline in antiplatelet antibodies in serum, an increase in peripheral blood platelet counts, and an increase in the number of megakaryocytes and megakaryocyte progenitors in the marrow.[333] These changes would imply that the mechanism of ITP in HIV-infected chimps includes insufficient compensatory increases in platelet production, similar to that decreased in humans.

Therapy for HIV-Related Immune Thrombocytopenic Purpura

The Need for Therapy

HIV-ITP may undergo spontaneous remission in approximately 18% of patients.[163] Furthermore, most patients with HIV-ITP do not experience bleeding, with hemorrhagic events described in only 8% of such individuals.[334] Nonetheless, treatment is indicated when bleeding occurs, in preparation for an invasive procedure, in patients with platelet counts lower than 30,000/μL, or lower than 50,000//μL in those with underlying coagulopathies. As detailed below, antiretroviral therapy is quite effective in patients with HIV-ITP and may serve as the initial reason for starting such antiviral treatment.

Zidovudine

The Swiss Group for HIV Studies was the first to demonstrate the efficacy of zidovudine therapy in patients with HIV-ITP.[332] Ten seropositive patients, with platelet counts ranging from 20,000 to 100,000/mL, received zidovudine at a dose of 2 g/day for 2 weeks, followed by 1 g/day for 6 weeks. This was followed by 8 weeks of placebo. All 10 patients experienced an increase in platelet counts while on zidovudine, with a mean increase of 54,600/mL range (53,200–107,800/mL). In contrast, no patient experienced an increase in platelet count while on placebo. The time to onset of response was approximately 8 days, with full response achieved by day 30. These results were subsequently confirmed by others.[335]

The optimal dose of zidovudine in HIV-ITP was studied by Landonio et al, who compared a dose of 500 mg/day in 35 patients with 1000 mg/day in another group of 36 individuals.[336] The majority of patients in both groups were injection drug users, with similar mean platelet counts (approximately 23,000/mL) and mean $CD4^+$ counts (approximately 400 cells/mL). A response rate of 57% was achieved in the low-dose group, with 11% experiencing complete response. In contrast, a response rate of 72% was achieved in those receiving 1000 mg zidovudine per day, with complete response in 39%. At month 6, a significant difference remained between the groups, with a mean platelet count of 56,000/mL in the low-dose group versus 98,200/mL in those receiving high-dose zidovudine. It is apparent from this study that high-dose zidovudine is advantageous in patients with HIV-ITP.[336]

Highly Active Antiretroviral Therapy in Immune Thrombocytopenic Purpura

Recently, HAART has been shown to be effective in the treatment of HIV-related ITP. In a report of 37 such patients, use of HAART was associated with a significant increase in platelet count, documented after 3 months of treatment, independent of baseline platelet count or the concomitant use of zidovudine.[337] Similarly, in a retrospective study involving 15 patients with HIV-related ITP treated with HAART, 11 (73%) had an increase in platelet count to values of 50,000/mL whereas eight (53%) had an increase in platelet count to values of 100,000/mL after 6 months of HAART therapy.[338] Consistent with these findings, data from the Women Interagency HIV Study demonstrated a strong association between the use of HAART and resolution of thrombocytopenia (defined as a platelet count >150,000/mL).[314] Thus, compared to thrombocytopenic women not receiving antiretroviral therapy, women in a non–AZT-containing HAART regimen were nearly 2 times more likely to improve their thrombocytopenia (OR = 1.84, 95% confidence interval = 1.31–2.59, $P < 0.001$), whereas women in an AZT-containing HAART regimen were even more likely to resolve their thrombocytopenia (OR = 2.85, 95% confidence interval = 1.96–4.15, $P < 0.0001$).[314] Thus, HAART is an important treatment modality in patients with HIV-related ITP and should be the initial treatment of choice in these patients. It is likely that effective use of HAART significantly decreases HIV viral load, and in so doing ameliorates many of the effects of HIV on megakaryocytes and on platelet production as well as platelet destruction.

Interferon-Alpha

A prospective, randomized, double-blind, placebo-controlled trial of Interferon (IFN)-α at a dose of 3 million units thrice weekly given subcutaneously was conducted in 15 patients with HIV-related

ITP.[339] A platelet response was documented in 66%, with a mean increase of 60,000/mL. The average time to response was 3 weeks. When interferon therapy was discontinued, platelet counts returned to baseline values within 3 months, indicating the necessity to maintain IFN-α therapy over time. In an attempt to ascertain the mechanisms by which IFN-α exerts its effects, Vianelli et al demonstrated a prolongation in platelet survival, whereas no significant increase in platelet production was noted.[340]

High-Dose Intravenous Gamma Globulin

Intravenous gamma globulin (IVIG), at a dose of 1000 to 2000 mg/kg, has been used effectively in pediatric and adult patients with de novo ITP, resulting in a significant rise in platelet counts within 24 to 72 hours in the majority of individuals.[341] Bussel and Haimi treated 22 patients with HIV-related ITP employing 1 to 2 g/kg during a 2- to 5-day period, depending upon the platelet response.[342] The average platelet count prior to therapy was 22,000/mL, rising to a mean of 182,000/mL (range 10,000–404,000/mL) within 2 to 5 days. Only two patients did not respond, whereas 77% experienced an increase to more than 100,000/mL, and 86% had an increase to more than 50,000/mL. However, when IVIG was discontinued, only 25% of patients maintained the increased platelet count, whereas the remainder required repeat infusions approximately every 21 days. The major problem with IVIG appears to be cost, which is quite significant. For this reason, IVIG is often reserved for use in patients who are acutely bleeding or require an immediate increase in platelet count, for example, prior to an invasive procedure.

Anti-Rh Immunoglobulin

The use of anti-Rh Ig in nonsplenectomized Rh-positive patients with HIV-related ITP represents another potential mode of therapy.[203] Requirements for effective therapy with anti-Rh (D) include a baseline hemoglobin level adequate to permit a 1- to 2-g decrease due to therapy-related hemolysis, presence of Rh positivity in the patient, and presence of a spleen, the site at which red cells would preferentially be phagocytized. Oksenhendler et al treated 14 Rh-positive patients with HIV-ITP employing 12 to 25 μg/kg of anti-Rh Ig given intravenously over 30 min on two consecutive days.[343] Nine (64%) Rh-positive patients responded with a platelet count above 50,000/mL, with response first noted at a median of 4 days (range 3–12 days), and median response duration of 13 days (range 0–37 days). Maintenance therapy was administered at a dose of 13 to 25 μg/kg IV every 2 to 4 weeks, resulting in a long-term response (>6 months) in five of six such patients. Subclinical hemolysis occurred in all, with a drop of hemoglobin of 0.4 to 2.2 g. Gringeri et al subsequently confirmed these results and also studied the use of intramuscular (IM) anti-D Ig for maintenance treatment after successful induction therapy by the intravenous route.[344] Patients self-administered the IM anti-Rh at a dose of 6 to 13 μg/kg/week. After induction, 83% of patients had achieved a platelet count above 50,000/mL, a response that was maintained in 85% over time. It is thus apparent that anti-Rh Ig may be used safely and effectively in patients with HIV-related ITP, providing an alternative that in some institutions may be as little as one-half the cost of high-dose IVIG.[343,344] Although not yet published in HIV-infected patients, higher dosing schedules of anti-D Ig, using 75 μg/kg/day have been associated with more rapid and durable increases in platelet count when studied in HIV-negative individuals with ITP.[345]

Splenectomy

Splenectomy has been used effectively in patients with de novo ITP who are refractory to corticosteroids, resulting in return to a normal platelet count in approximately two-thirds.[346] At the onset of the AIDS epidemic, several anecdotal case reports described a rapid progression to AIDS postsplenectomy, and the procedure was largely abandoned. More recently, Oksenhendler et al reported long-term experience in a cohort of 185 patients with HIV-ITP.[347] Splenectomy was eventually performed in 68 of these patients, at an average of 13 months from initial diagnosis of HIV-ITP. The mean platelet count presplenectomy was 18,000/mL, rising to 223,000/mL postoperatively. A response was seen in 92% of patients, with complete response (platelet count >100,000/mL) in 85%. Maintenance of the elevated platelet count for longer than 6 months was documented in 82%. In comparing the survival or rate of progression to AIDS in the 68 splenectomized patients versus the 117 who did not undergo the procedure, no difference was found, indicating that splenectomy was not associated with more rapid progression of HIV disease. Similar conclusions were made by Kemeny et al.[348] It is important to note, however, that 5.8% of patients undergoing splenectomy in Oksenhendler series experienced fulminant infection, consisting of *Streptococcus pneumoniae* meningitis in two and *Haemophilus influenzae* sepsis in one. It is thus apparent that patients should undergo prophylactic vaccination prior to splenectomy and that such surgery may ultimately be safer in those HIV-infected patients who can still achieve an appropriate antibody response to vaccination against *S pneumoniae* or *H influenzae.*

Corticosteroids

Corticosteroids remain the initial therapy of choice in patients with de novo ITP and at a dose of 1 mg/kg/day are associated with an 80% to 90% response rate.[349] Similar results have been documented in patients with HIV-related disease.[350] However, the immunosuppressive effects of high-dose corticosteroids have made such therapy far from optimal in HIV-infected patients. Furthermore, because corticosteroids are associated with increased growth of Kaposi sarcoma (KS),[351] the potential development of fulminant KS in HIV-infected patients who are coinfected by Human Herpes Virus 8 (HHV-8) has further dampened the enthusiasm for this therapeutic modality.

Other Causes of Thrombocytopenia in HIV-Infected Patients

Although HIV-ITP is the most common cause of low platelet counts in the setting of HIV, other etiologies may also occur, such as infiltration of bone marrow by malignancy or opportunistic infection. Thrombotic microangiopathy due to TTP or HUS may also occur in the setting of HIV, resulting in characteristic thrombocytopenia. Additionally, multiple drugs used commonly in HIV may also be associated with thrombocytopenia.

THROMBOTIC MICROANGIOPATHY

Prior to the availability of HAART, TMA was well described in HIV-infected patients, seen in approximately 1% to 2%.[244,352–355] Both hemolytic uremic syndrome (HUS) and thrombotic thrombocytopenic purpura (TTP) have been described,[352,354,356,357] with the former more likely to be diagnosed in later stages of HIV infection. HIV-infected patients with TTP tend to present similarly to those without underlying HIV infection, with fragmented schistocytes and thrombocytopenia on peripheral blood smears, as well as fever, subtle abnormalities of renal function, and a variety of neurologic abnormalities, including altered mental status, seizures, transient focal neurologic deficits.[244,352–355]

The actual mechanism of TMA in patients with HIV is unclear, and may involve endothelial cell damage or perturbation, perhaps by HIV, or by CMV, inflammatory cytokines, or toxins produced by *Shigella dysenteriae* and *Escherichia coli* 0157:H7.[358] Nonetheless, similar to de novo TTP,[359] persistence of high-molecular-weight von Willebrand factor (vWF) multimers, with complete deficiency of the vWF-cleaving protease, ADAMTS-13, has been described,[360,361] with demonstration of an IgG1 antibody to ADAMTS-13 in one case.[360]

In terms of therapy for HIV-TTP, several case reports have noted a response to antiretroviral therapy.[361,362] In general, however, treatment is similar to that used for de novo TTP, consisting of plasma exchange, in which plasmapheresis is performed, removing unusually large vWF multimers and antibodies against ADAMTS-13, along with infusion of fresh-frozen plasma or cryosupernatant.[359] Response to such therapy as been reported in more than 50% of HIV infected cases.[244,353–355,357]

VENOUS THROMBOTIC DISEASE

Although numerous case reports of venous thrombosis occurring in HIV-infected patients have been published, an increased incidence of venous thromboembolic disease has only recently been described in the setting of underlying HIV infection.[363–370] In the Multistate Adult and Adolescent Spectrum of HIV Disease Surveillance Project sponsored by the CDC, the incidence of thrombosis among 42,935 HIV-infected individuals was found to be 2.6 per 1000 person-years.[212] The incidence was lower for individuals with immunologic AIDS (1.8 per 1000 person-years) or asymptomatic HIV infection (1.3 per 1000 person-years) than for persons with clinical AIDS (6.2 per 1000 person-years). Factors significantly associated with the risk of thrombosis included an age of 45 years or more, CMV retinitis, other AIDS-defining opportunistic infections, hospitalization, use of megestrol acetate, and use of indinavir.[369] Use of other antiretroviral agents, sex, race, and a history of injection drug use were not associated with an increased risk for thrombosis.

However, in another study that directly compared the risk of venous thromboembolism in HIV-infected patients and HIV-negative controls, no statistically significant difference in the rate of thrombotic disease was reported between the groups, when studied overall (HIV-infected, 2.8%, vs HIV-negative controls, 1.8%).[368] Nonetheless, when considering only those patients under the age of 50 years, the frequencies were significantly different (HIV-infected, 3.31% vs HIV-negative controls, 0.53%, $P < 0.0001$).

In an attempt to determine the incidence of venous thrombosis in HIV-infected patients compared to individuals without HIV infection, and to determine whether the introduction of combination antiretroviral therapy altered the rates of thrombotic disease, Fultz and colleagues retrospectively reviewed the medical charts of 37,535 HIV-infected veterans and 37,535 age-, race-, and site-matched controls.[370] Compared to HIV-negative controls, HIV infection was associated with a 39% increased incidence of thromboembolism in the pre-HAART era (standardized incidence ratio [SIR] = 1.39; 95% confidence interval = 1.26–1.52) and a 33% increased incidence in the post-1996 era (SIR = 1.33; 95% confidence interval = 1.24–1.43). This increased risk of thrombosis was independent of a diagnosis of malignancy, HIV-related opportunistic infection, or use of central venous catheters. Furthermore, thrombosis was significantly associated with increased mortality in all groups. It is thus apparent that venous thrombotic disease is increased in the setting of HIV infection, independent of many of the more commonly known risk factors.

HIV infection is known to result in increased levels of proinflammatory cytokines, such as TNF-α, IL-1, and IL-6, which can contribute to the development of a procoagulant state by upregulation of factor VIII and downregulation of protein S.[371–373] These same cytokines have also been shown to downregulate the expression of numerous proteins necessary for fibrinolysis.[374] Elevated factor VIII levels per se are a component of the inflammatory state,[375] and elevated factor VIII activity has been independently associated with an increased prevalence of deep vein thrombosis in HIV-negative individuals.[376]

Several studies have suggested that progressive HIV infection may be associated with the development of a hypercoagulable state. In one recent study comparing 94 HIV-infected women and 50 HIV-negative controls, Levine and colleagues documented a clear relationship between progressive stages of HIV disease and stepwise increases in factor VIII activity along with decreases in levels of functional protein S, both of which have been associated with increased risk of thromboembolism in HIV-infected individuals.[377] Thus, functional protein S activity progressively decreased from 76% in HIV-negative women, to 67% in those with asymptomatic HIV, 62% in those with immunologic AIDS, and 46% in those with clinical AIDS ($P < 0.0001$), whereas factor VIII activity statistically increased in a stepwise manner, from 116% in HIV negatives, to 149% in asymptomatic HIV, 196% in immunologic AIDS and 211% in patients with clinical AIDS ($P < 0.0001$). Of interest, no patient demonstrated presence of a lupus anticoagulant.[377] Other studies have also reported abnormalities of coagulation proteins in HIV-infected patients, such as acquired deficiencies in protein S,[378–383] protein C,[383,384] and heparin cofactor II.[385] Thus, although the precise mechanisms leading to thromboembolism in HIV are not yet elucidated, it is possible that the progressive proinflammatory milieu of HIV infection may be operative.

The presence of anticardiolipin antibodies has been described in as many as 80% of HIV-infected patients, and their prevalence may be higher in patients with clinical AIDS.[386–388] Patients with antiphospholipid syndrome are at risk for clinical thrombosis, in addition to persistent laboratory abnormalities, including presence of lupus anticoagulant (LA), ACAs, or other antiphospholipid antibodies. Although ACAs may be associated with a hypercoagulable state,[389] most studies have found no correlation between high levels of ACAs and clinical thrombosis in the setting of HIV infection[386–388]; nevertheless, isolated case reports of patients with ACAs and unusual sites of venous thrombosis have been described.[390–392] Furthermore, LA is a stronger predictor of thrombosis than ACAs in patients with antiphospholipid syndrome.[393] Of interest, no case of LA was found among the 92 HIV-infected patients studied by Levine and colleagues.[377]

Although the incidence of venous thrombotic events (VTE) is clearly not as common as the other hematologic disorders described in HIV, an increase in VTE is clearly expected in the setting of HIV infection, possibly as a consequence of cytokine activation in an underlying inflammatory state, or other factors. Clinicians should be alert to the possibility of VTE, and to development of VTE in unusual sites, in the setting of underlying HIV infection.

SUGGESTED READINGS

Biggar RJ, Jaffe ES, Goedert JJ, Chaturvedi A, Pfeiffer R, Engels EA: Hodgkin lymphoma and immunodeficiency in persons with HIV/AIDS. Blood, 108:3786–3791, 2006.

Canon J-L, Vansteenkiste J, Bodoky G, et al: Randomized, double blind, active controlled trial of every 3 week darbepoetin alfa for the treatment of chemotherapy induced anemia. J Natl Cancer Inst 98:273, 2006.

Faller EM, McVey MJ, Kakal JA, MacPherson PA: Interleukin-7 receptor expression on CD8 T-cells is downregulated by the HIV Tat protein. J Acquir Immune Defic Syndr 43:257, 2006.

Hammer SM, Saag MS, Schechter M, et al: Treatment for adult HIV infection: 2006 recommendations of the International AIDS Society—USA panel. JAMA 296:827, 2006.

Herbeuval J-P, Boasso A, Grivel J-C, et al: TNF-related apoptosis-inducing ligand (TRAIL) in HIV-1 infected patients and its in vitro production by antigen-presenting cells. Blood 105:2458, 2005.

Lau B, Gange SJ, Phair JP, Riddler SA, Detels R, Margolick JB: Use of total lymphocyte count and hemoglobin concentration for monitoring progression of HIV infection. J Acquir Immune Defic Syndr 39:620, 2005.

Levine AM, Karim R, Mack W, et al: Neutropenia in human immunodeficiency virus infection: Data from the Women's Interagency HIV Study. Arch Intern Med 166:405, 2006.

Levine AM, Vigen C, Gravink J, Mack W, Watts CH, Liebman HA: Progressive prothrombotic state in women with advancing HIV disease. J Acquir Immune Defic Syndr 42:572, 2006.

Li Z, Nardi MA, Karpatkin S: Role of molecular mimicry to HIV-1 peptides in HIV-1 related immunologic thrombocytopenia. Blood 106:572, 2005.

Mazodier K, Marin V, Novick D, et al: Severe imbalance of IL-18/IL-18BP in patients with secondary hemophagocytic syndrome. Blood 106:3483, 2005.

O'Brien ME, Kupka R, Msamanga GI, Saathoff E, Hunter DJ, Fawzi WW: Anemia is an independent predictor of mortality and immunologic progression of disease among women with HIV in Tanzania. J Acquir Immune Defic Syndr 40:219, 2005

Suzu S, Harada H, Matsumoto T, Okada S: HIV-1 nef interferes with M-CSF receptor signaling through Hck activation and inhibits M-CSF bioactivities. Blood 105:3230, 2005.

Townsend CL, Tookey PA, Cortina-Borja M, Peckham CS: Antiretroviral therapy and congenital abnormalities in infants born to HIV-1-infected women in the United Kingdom and Ireland, 1990 to 2003. J Acquir Immune Defic Syndr 42:91, 2006.

REFERENCES

For complete list of references log onto www.expertconsult.com

CHAPTER 159

HEMATOLOGIC ASPECTS OF PARASITIC DISEASES

David J. Roberts

INTRODUCTION

Parasitic diseases are not common in medical, let alone hematologic, practice in North America or Europe. However, much of the world's population are infected and become symptomatic from a plethora of parasites, and many of these infections represent global public health problems.

Although some significant parasitic diseases are transmitted in temperate climates, the majority of parasites of significance to human health are endemic in the tropical world. This reflects not only socioeconomic circumstances but also the origin of our species in tropical Africa, where the human host, parasites, and also vectors have established complex relationships over evolutionary timescales.[1] Notwithstanding such geographical variation in the incidence of parasitic disease, both travelers and recent migrants now present to hematology clinics and laboratories all over the world with increasing frequency. Even here, there are marked variations in practice in North America and Europe; where the United Kingdom reports more cases of imported malaria than the United States of America and indeed has a 10-fold greater incidence of malaria per capita, reflecting the increased frequency of travel to and from endemic areas compared to North American populations.

Malaria, leishmaniasis, malaria, trypanosomiasis, and babesiosis may present directly or indirectly to hematologists. This account will concentrate on the biological, clinical, and hematologic features of these infections and the hematologic aspects or complications of their treatment. Comprehensive accounts of the general medical aspects of these diseases are provided in many recent textbooks.[2–4]

MALARIA

Malaria is a major public health problem in tropical areas, and it is estimated that it is responsible for 1 to 3 million deaths annually and 300 to 500 million infections.[5] The vast majority of morbidity and mortality from malaria is caused by infection with *Plasmodium falciparum*, although *P vivax*, *P ovale*, and *P malariae* also are responsible for human infections. In endemic areas, a significant proportion of the mortality and morbidity is due to anemia. In Europe and North America, malaria is not infrequently a clinical problem in travelers or recent arrivals from malaria-endemic areas and hematologists may be involved in the diagnosis and management of the disease. Moreover, in nonendemic areas, malaria may cause a fatal transfusion-transmitted infections and detection of blood donors who may be carrying the disease represents a major challenge for blood services.

Epidemiology

Approximately 1000 million people live in areas of endemic or epidemic malaria. The global mortality and morbidity have been recently revised to 350 million cases and 1 million deaths per year following an evaluation of the prevalence of infection in Southeast Asia (Fig. 159–1). There is increasing anecdotal evidence that the incidence of severe disease is now falling, sometimes spectacularly, in many parts of Africa following the widespread introduction of artemisinin combination treatment, impregnated bednets, and residual spraying under the local campaigns.[6] Evidence of more general effectiveness of WHO's "Roll Back Malaria" is yet to appear (rbm.who.int/).

The distribution of malaria is determined by features of host, vector, and parasite. In summary, the global distribution of autochthonous or endogenous malaria is limited by the lower temperature limits for development of the parasite in the mosquito (sporogony) of 20°C for *P falciparum* and 15°C for other human malarias. Within these limits transmission does not occur above 1500 m in arid regions or in the Central and South Pacific (due to the absence of suitable vectors). In addition, *P vivax* malaria is rare in Africa where the population frequency of the blood group Duffy negative (Fya^-Fyb^-) is high. *P ovale* requires a lengthy period of sporogony and is confined to areas of Africa and Southeast Asia with a high density of susceptible *Anopheles* spp.

In some malarious areas the seasonal pattern of clinical malaria is determined by the increase in vector density after rainfall, leading to an increase in new infections as transmission increases. In naïve individuals, parasites can cause chronic infection lasting many months.

The intensity of transmission determines the distribution of clinical symptoms in different age groups. In general, in areas of high transmission younger children suffer from severe disease. Where transmission is less intense, older children suffer from severe disease. Finally, if the rate of transmission is very low, few cases of malaria are seen in any age group and such populations would have little natural immunity. In such areas, a sudden increase in vectorial capacity (through the accidental introduction of efficient vectors or higher density, biting, or survival of the resident vectors), more rapid parasite sporogony, or migration of infected or nonimmune populations can result in epidemics where large numbers fall ill in all age groups. The transition from high to low transmission has been classified by holo-, hyper-, meso-, and hypoendemicity. These categories can be related epidemiologically to age-specific rates of parasite prevalence or splenomegaly and theoretically to the reproductive ratio of malarial infection.[7,8]

Malaria exerts a substantial selection for human traits that protect from infection. Sickle cell trait and thalassemia traits protect from infection and are truly polymorphic characteristics in many parts of the world. Understanding the genetic epidemiology has provided the foundation of population genetics and has provided classic examples of principle of genetic selection in vivo—for example, balancing selection for sickle cell trait and negative epistasis for sickle cell trait and alpha thalassemia. The homozygous forms of these characteristics cause significant clinical disease, for example, sickle cell disease, beta-thalassemia, and G6PDH deficiency. In endemic areas, these genetic diseases represent major public health problems. For a review, see references 9 and 10.

Parasitology

In *P falciparum* (see later for a discussion of the other human parasites) the infective sporozoite forms are inoculated into the bloodstream from the salivary glands of a female *Anopheles* mosquito (Fig. 159–2). These thin, needle-shaped cells, 10 to 12 μm in length circulate briefly with a half-life of approximately 30 minutes, before traversing macrophages and several hepatocytes before residing in a

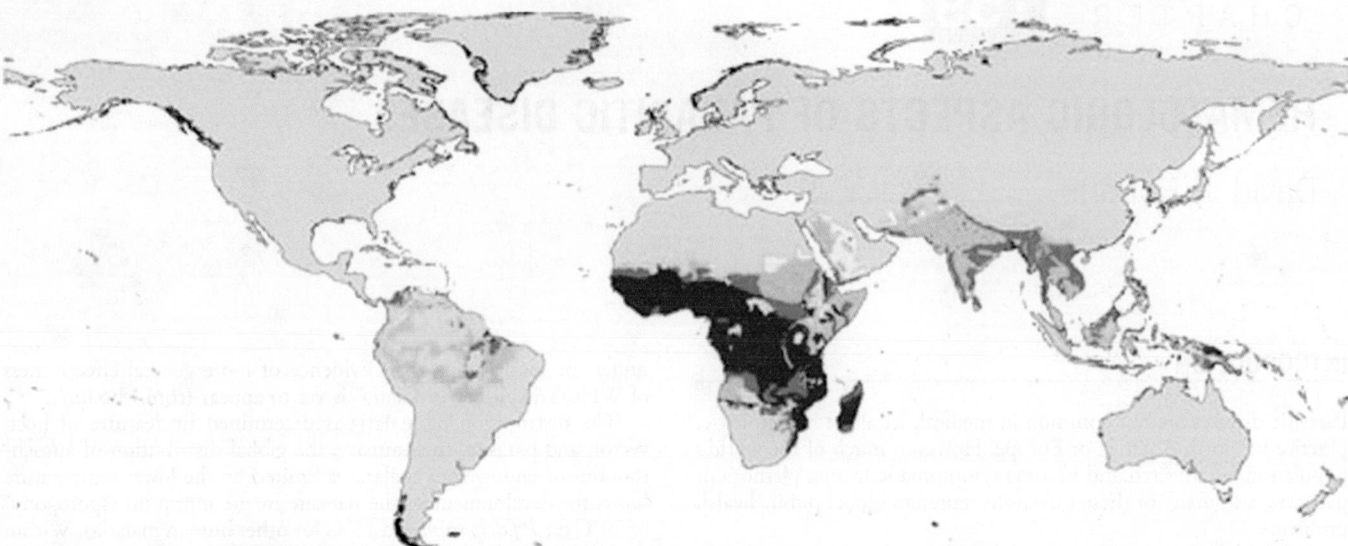

Figure 159–1 Global malaria endemicity. Areas are coloured according to malaria endemicity (prevalence): *light green*, hypoendemic (areas in which childhood infection prevalence is less than 10%); *medium green*, mesoendemic (areas with infection prevalence between 11% and 50%); *dark green*, hyperendemic and holoendemic (areas with an infection prevalence of 50% or more); unclassified areas (*yellow*) represent only 6% of the global population at risk and are due to discrepancies in recent data. Grey areas are a combined mask of areas outside of the transmission limits and areas of population density less than 1 person/km^2 *(Data from Snow RW, Guerra CA, Noor AM, Myint HY, Hay SI. The global distribution of clinical episodes of* Plasmodium falciparum *malaria. Nature 434:214, 2005.)*

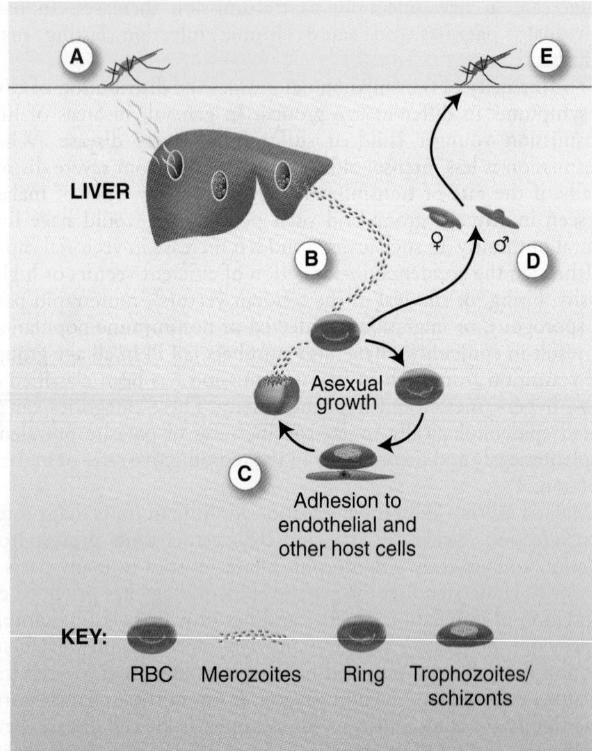

Figure 159–2 *Plasmodia* life cycle. **A,** The asexual life cycle begins when sporozoites from a female mosquito taking a blood meal enter the circulation and invade hepatocytes. **B,** Up to 10, 000 merozoites are formed. Following rupture of the hepatocyte, infective merozoites are released and invade erythrocytes (RBC). **C,** Within RBC, the parasite develops through the stages of rings, trophozoites, and schizonts. Mature schizonts burst to release erythrocytic merozoites that invade new RBC. **D,** A small proportion of merozoites in RBC transform into male and female gametocytes that are ingested by the mosquito. **E,** The male and female gametes fuse and transform into an oocyst, which divides asexually into many sporozoites that migrate to the salivary gland from where they are released during the next blood meal.

single hepatocyte.[11,12] Here rapid multiplication takes place over 5 to 8 days to produce a liver schizont, 80 μm in diameter and containing 30,000 ± 10,000 merozoites that are released into the bloodstream, where they infect erythrocytes.[13] When ready to leave hepatocytes, the parasite induces cell death in the hepatocytes and causes the release of merozoites in membrane-enclosed structures or merosomes that are extruded from the infected cell, so avoiding host cell defense mechanisms.[14]

The merozoites bind and then invade red blood cells (for review of red cell and merozoite interactions see reference 15). The host plasma membrane is invaginated to form the parasitophorous vacuole. For the first 10 hours, the developing parasites appear as fine "ring forms." Between 10 and 15 hours, the cytoplasm thickens and 16 hours after invasion granules of the black pigment hematin, the end-product of hemoglobin digestion, begin to appear. Ligands are expressed at the surface of the infected red blood cell that mediate adhesion to host receptors on venular endothelium. These trophozoites no longer circulate throughout the body but are sequestered in the peripheral circulation. Nuclear division begins, at approximately 30 hours, to form schizonts, containing up to 32 merozoites. At 48 hours, the red blood cell is ruptured to release the merozoites into the circulation to continue further cycles of asexual multiplication.

The erythrocytic cycle of schizogony may achieve a 10-fold increase in parasitemia in vivo and a patent or microscopically detectable infection 6 days after the liver stage is completed. After two or more cycles, the infection becomes clinically apparent by the paroxysms of fever that accompany the release of merozoites. Cycles of schizogony continue until the rate of parasite multiplication is reduced by chemotherapy, specific or nonspecific defense mechanisms, or occasionally, the demise of the host.

Some merozoites do not multiply but become committed during the previous erythrocytic cycle to form male or female gametocytes.[16] Gametocytes are distinguished by dispersed pigment in a single nucleus, in a fully grown parasite, and are sequestered for the first 5 days of their development in the peripheral circulation. Thus 8 to 10 days after the start of clinical infection, mature, crescent-shaped gametocytes appear in the blood.

The sexual phase (or sporogony) of the parasite life cycle begins after a male and female gametocyte are ingested by a feeding female *Anopheles* mosquito. In the midgut of the mosquito the gametocytes shed the red blood cell membrane. This change is apparently precipi-

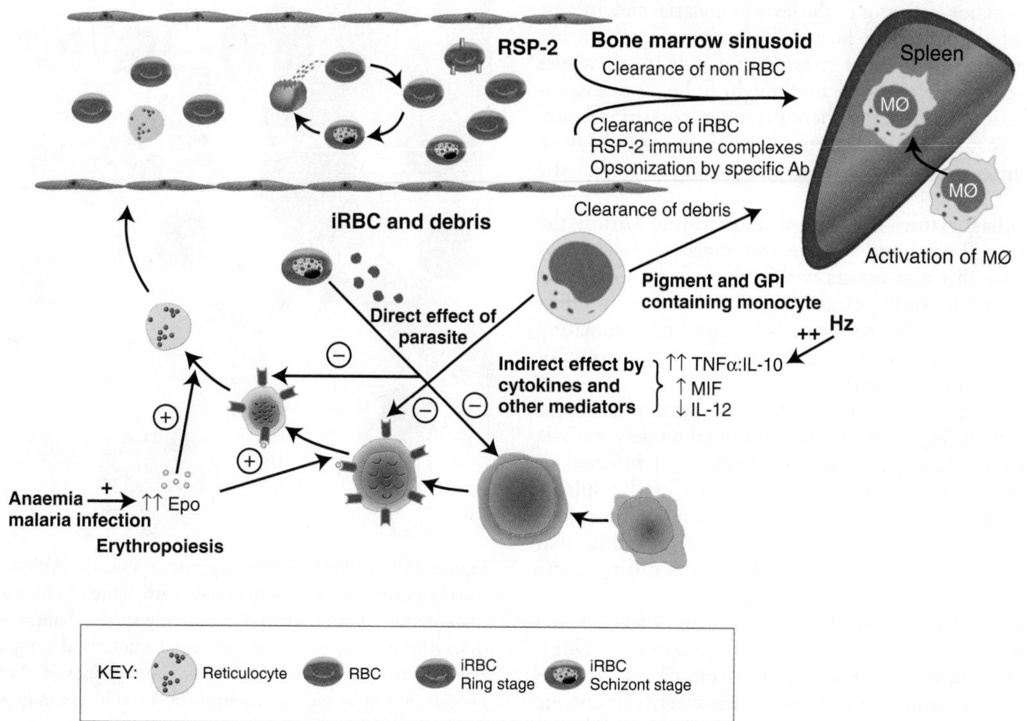

Figure 159–3 Pathogenesis of malarial anemia. Severe malarial anemia is characterized by destruction of infected red blood cell (iRBC) following schizogony and clearance of both iRBC and uninfected RBC. During malarial infection, changes in membrane protein composition occur and the resultant immune complexes of RBC, Ag, and immunoglobulin (Ig) (eg, RBC–RSP2–Ig) are cleared by macrophages to the spleen where they become activated. Pigment-containing macrophages may release inflammatory cytokines and other biologically active mediators such as 4-hydroxy-nonenal (HNE). Macrophage inhibitory factor may be released by macrophages or a *Plasmodial* homolog may suppress erythropoiesis. Malarial pigment or other parasite products may have a direct inhibitory effect on erythropoiesis. Inhibition of erythropoiesis may be at one or more sites in the growth and differentiation of hematopoietic progenitors. Both indirect and direct effects may cause suppression of the bone marrow and spleen resulting in inadequate reticulocyte counts for the degree of anemia. Hz, hemozoin; GPI, glycophosphatidylinositol anchors of merozoite proteins; Epo, erythropoietin; MΦ, macrophage; RSP-2, ring surface protein-2; Ig, immunoglobulin.

tated by the drop in temperature. A female gametocyte forms a single macrogamete, but male gametocytes undergo several rounds of nuclear division to produce flagellated microgametes. These microgametes are motile and migrate to fertilize a macrogamete. The resulting zygote enlarges to form a mobile oökinete and migrates through the epithelial wall of the mosquito midgut to rest finally on the external surface. The oöcyst divides repeatedly to form up to 10,000 sporozoites, which travel up through the hematocelomic fluid to enter the acinar cells of the salivary glands. Once here they are infective when injected into the host.

Major differences exist in the life cycles of other human *Plasmodium* spp. First, in *P vivax* and *P ovale* infections, some sporozoites entering the liver form dormant hypnozoites that only begin to divide after a variable period of some months to cause further blood-stage infections or relapses. Second, the cycle of erythrocytic development in *P malariae* takes 72 hours and thus causes quartan fever (ie, on days 1 and 4).

The Pathophysiology of Malarial Anemia

Malaria gives ample reasons for both increased red cell destruction and reduced red cell production (see Fig. 159–3 for overview).

Loss of Infected Erythrocytes

Destruction of red blood cells is inevitable as parasites complete their 48-hour growth cycle and lyse their temporary host cell. Some parasites may be removed from erythrocytes as immature ring forms by phagocytized cells, leaving the red blood cells with residual parasite antigens to continue to circulate, albeit with reduced survival.[17] Infected erythrocytes may also be phagocytosed by macrophages following opsonization by immunoglobulins and/or complement components.[18,19] Other signals for recognition of infected erythrocytes by macrophages include abnormally rigid membranes and exposure of phosphatidylserine and other altered host antigens.[20–23]

Loss of Uninfected Erythrocytes

The activity and the number of macrophages are increased in malarial infection, and increased removal of uninfected cells may occur. Moreover, the signals for recognition of uninfected erythrocytes for removal by macrophages are enhanced. Uninfected erythrocytes bind increased amounts of immunoglobulin and/or complement as detected in the direct antiglobulin test (DAT or Coombs Test).[24–26] These antibodies do not have a particular specificity but are more likely to represent immune complexes absorbed onto the surface of red blood cells. However, an association between a positive DAT and severe anemia has not been established. More recent studies have shown that red cells from malaria patients were not only more susceptible to phagocytosis but also showed increased surface IgG and deficiencies in CR1 and CD55 compared with controls.[22,23]

Role of the Spleen

Some degree of splenomegaly is a normal feature of malarial infection, and the prevalence of splenomegaly in regions of malarial transmission is used as a major indicator of the level of malarial endemicity. The importance of the spleen in host defence against malaria has been demonstrated in experimental systems, and individuals whose spleens have been surgically removed are thought to be more susceptible to severe infection. Indeed, the phenomenon of parasitic sequestration is thought to have evolved primarily as an immune evasion strategy so the mature parasite can avoid passing through the spleen.[27]

Active erythrophagocytosis is a conspicuous feature within the bone marrow during *P vivax* and *P falciparum* malaria,[28,29] and it is highly probable that this also occurs within the spleen. Cytokines may be responsible for activating macrophages during malaria infection. Children with acute *P falciparum* malaria have high circulating levels of interferon-γ and TNF-α,[30] a synergistic combination of cytokines that activate macrophages.

Several studies have attempted to define the pathophysiologic changes in the spleen during acute malaria. In animal models, malaria is accompanied by increased intravascular clearance of infected or rigid, heat-treated cells by the spleen,[31] alterations in the splenic microcirculation,[32] and myelomonocytic recruitment to the spleen and liver.[33] In studies of human malaria it has been found that increased splenic clearance of heated red cells occurs during acute attacks.[34]

Changes to the uninfected red blood cells during infection also contribute to their own enhanced clearance by phagocytes. Uninfected red cells in children and adults with severe disease are less deformable and this is a significant predictor of the severity of anemia and indeed outcome, consistent with the notion that these cells are being removed by the spleen.[20] It has also been found that immunoglobulin (Ig) G-sensitized red cells are rapidly removed from the circulation by the spleen and that unusually rapid clearance persists well into the convalescent phase.[35]

Thus, all the available evidence points to increased reticuloendothelial clearance in *P falciparum* malaria, persisting long after recovery. These changes are presumably a host defence mechanism, maximizing the clearance of parasitized erythrocytes.

The Role of Ineffective Erythropoiesis in Severe Malarial Anemia

Reticulocytopenia has been confirmed in numerous clinical studies of malarial anemia.[36,37,38] The histopathologic study of the bone marrow of children with malarial anemia shows erythroid hyperplasia with increased numbers of erythroid precursors (Fig. 159–4). However, the maturation is abnormal by light and electron microscopy. Abdalla and Weatherall described the hallmark characteristics of such abnormal maturation, namely cytoplasmic and nuclear bridging and irregular nuclear outline.[39,40] They later confirmed that the distribution of the erythroid progenitors through the cell cycle is abnormal in malarial anemia, with an increased proportion of cells in the G2 phase compared with normal controls.[41] Horstmann and colleagues confirmed these findings using the same criteria as Abdalla, they studied six patients with falciparum malaria before and after treatment.[38]

Ineffective erythropoiesis also contributes to anemia in animal models of malaria. A recent study has shown that vaccinated *Aotus* monkeys, after a challenge infection, may develop moderate to severe anemia following rapid clearance of uninfected erythrocytes but with low reticulocyte counts, indicating bone marrow dysfunction.[42] Erythropoiesis is disrupted in mice during malaria infection. Mice infected with *P berghei* show reduced bone marrow cellularity, erythroblasts, BFU-E, and CFU-E as early as 24 hours postinfection.[43] The cellularity and CFU-S content of the femoral marrow of BALB/c mice infected with *P chabaudi adami* decreases as the parasitemia increases.[44]

Schofield and colleagues have outlined the transcriptional profile of genes in the brain and spleen of mice infected with *P berghei* ANKA. In murine splenocytes, enzymes of the glycolytic pathway and interferon-inducible genes were upregulated whereas genes associated with erythropoiesis were suppressed.[45]

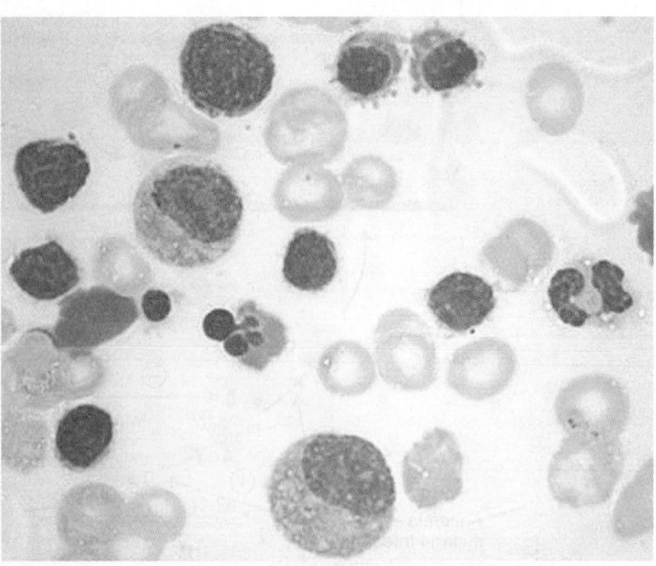

Figure 159–4 Bone marrow aspirate in malaria. Although erythropoiesis is usually normoblastic in individuals with acute or chronic malaria, the examination of bone marrow frequently shows changes reflecting dyserythropoiesis, such as the irregular nuclei and cytoplasmic bridges in erythroblasts seen in this figure. Two young rings of *Plasmodium falciparum* can be seen in an erythrocyte. (*Giemsa stain* × *900*). (*Courtesy of Dr Saad H. Abdalla.*)

Modulation of Erythropoiesis by Cytokines

Given the importance of erythropoietin (Epo) to erythropoiesis, attention has been focused on the levels of this crucial cytokine in malarial infection. Serum Epo was appropriately raised in a single study of African children suffering from malarial anemia.[46,47] However, other studies in adults from Thailand and Sudan have suggested that the Epo concentration, although raised, was inappropriate for the degree of anemia.[48,49] The most recent studies of the level of Epo in African children have shown a supraphysiologic rise in Epo levels compared to age-matched community controls with nonmalarial anemia.[50] These data would support a hypothesis that high levels of Epo in malaria anemia may exert a cytoprotective effect and improve the outcome in severe malaria.

The prime candidates for the host factors mediating dyserythropoiesis are imbalances of the tumor necrosis factor-α (TNF-α), interferon-γ (IFN-γ), and interleukin-10 (IL-10). The concentrations of TNF-α and IFN-γ have been correlated with the severity of the disease.[51–53] Whereas low concentrations of TNF-α (<1 ng/mL) stimulate erythropoiesis, higher levels of TNF-α have been shown to suppress erythropoiesis.[53] Furthermore, it is possible that high levels of these inflammatory cytokines may contribute to reduced and abnormal production of erythrocytes, and also to increased erythrophagocytosis.

Recent evidence has suggested that the release of macrophage inhibitory factor (MIF) inhibits the growth of early erythroid and myeloid progenitors during murine malaria infection[54] and $MIF^{-/-}$ mice are protected from anemia during experimental malaria infection.[55] However, the role of MIF in human malaria infection has not been established.

High levels of the Th2-type cytokine, IL-10, might prevent the development of severe malarial anemia. Low levels of IL-10 have been described in African children with severe malarial anemia.[51] Similarly, defective IL-12 production has been shown experimentally to be associated with increased severity of malaria in a rodent model and low IL-12 levels have been associated with severe malaria in African children.[56–59]

Modulation of Erythropoiesis by Infected Erythrocytes

There is also substantial evidence that lysate of infected erythrocytes may directly modulate the function of host cells. During its blood stage, the malaria parasite proteolyses host hemoglobin in an acidic vacuole to obtain amino acids, releasing heme as a by-product, which is autooxidized to potentially toxic hematin (aquaferriprotoporphyrin IX, H_2O–Fe(III)PPIX). β-Hematin forms as a crystalline cyclic dimer of Fe(III)PPIX and is complexed with protein and lipid products as malarial pigment or hemozoin. Arese and colleagues showed that the function of monocytes and of monocyte-derived macrophages is severely inhibited after ingestion of malaria pigment or hemozoin. These cells were unable to repeat phagocytosis and to generate oxidative burst when appropriately stimulated.[60–62] Furthermore, after phagocytosis of hemozoin human and murine myeloid cells were unable to kill ingested fungi, bacteria, and tumor cells[63] and to respond to IFN-γ stimulation, but instead responded by increased release of interleukin-1β (IL-1β) and TNF-α,[64] macrophage inflammatory protein-1α (MIP-1α) and MIP-1β.[65]

The hemozoin polymer of heme moieties may be complexed with biologically active compounds. The oxidation of membrane lipids catalyzed by the ferric heme produces the lipoperoxides.[62,66] There is accumulating evidence that HNE and other lipoperoxides including 15-hydroxy-arachidonic acid (15-(*R,S*)-HETE) may play a role in the pathophysiology of malaria. Arese and colleagues showed that HNE and HETE are generated in parasitized erythrocytes and that the toxicity of hemozoin was reduced after removal of lipids. HNE also inhibits the upregulation of surface expression of ICAM-1, VCAM-1, and E-selectin following TNF-stimulation.[67] Moreover, endoperoxides produced in pigment-containing monocytes or macrophages may impair erythroid growth.[68] Hemozoin may also directly inhibit erythroid development in vitro and increased levels of plasma hemozoin and pigment in monocytes have been associated with anemia.[50]

Modulation of Erythropoiesis by Infection

In children presenting with acute malaria, bacteremia is associated not only with anemia but also with excess mortality.[69] Parvovirus B19 may cause a transient reticulocytopenia and thus severe and sudden anemia in those suffering from a hemolytic anemia or fetal anemia and intrauterine death.[70] Most children in Africa have serologic evidence of infection early in life. However, acute infection with this virus is uncommon in those presenting with severe malarial anemia.[47,71]

Prevalence and Etiology of Anemia in the Developing World

In endemic areas the etiology of anemia is complex. Acute or chronic malaria infection is a major precipitating factor in children with severe anemia causing admission to hospital.[47]

Longitudinal studies from the Gambia have shown that whereas the mean hemoglobin levels in children varies significantly through the year, anemia is much more common in the rainy season when malaria transmission is its highest.[72] However, the rains are also associated with an increase in water-borne diarrheal disease and poor food supplies. So the seasonal increase in anemia in malaria endemic areas arises on a background of low or frankly deficient stores of hematinics and/or other micronutrients. Iron deficiency, which affects at least 20% of the world's population, is a major factor in the seasonal surge of anemia in the tropical rainy season. Low iron stores at birth and dietary iron deficiency may be exacerbated by hookworm or schistosomal infection. Folate deficiencies and/or increased requirements may occur in many populations, although frank folate deficiency is uncommon. Recent studies have shown that a low baseline hemoglobin level at the start of the season for malaria transmission is a major risk factor for developing severe malarial anemia.[73]

Quantifying the contribution of these individual factors to anemia reliably requires intervention studies. In Tanzania, Menendez and Alonso and their colleagues have shown that iron supplementation and antimalarial prophylaxis prevented 30% and 60%, respectively, of all cases of moderate anemia presenting during the malaria transmission season.[74] The same group preformed another trial, giving sulphadoxine-pyrimethamine or placebo at the same time as routine vaccinations delivered through the WHO Expanded Program on Immunisation (EPI). All children received iron supplementation between 2 and 6 months of age. This simple intervention reduced severe anemia by 50% compared to the placebo group, whereas serologic responses to EPI vaccines were not affected by the intervention.[75]

There is now widespread interest in repeating these trials elsewhere to define strategies to prevent anemia in children living in areas with different patterns of malaria endemicity.[76]

Features of Malarial Anemia

The Spectrum of Disease Caused by Malarial Infection

The signs and symptoms of malarial infection in humans are caused by the asexual blood stage of the parasite. Infection with blood-stage parasites may result in a wide range of outcomes and pathologies. Indeed, the spectrum of severity ranges from asymptomatic infection to rapidly progressive, fatal illness. The clinical presentation of malarial infection is also wide and influenced by age, immune status, and pregnancy and by the species, genotype, and perhaps the geographic origin of the parasite. In endemic areas, many infections present as an uncomplicated febrile illness. In more severe forms of the disease, children may present with prostration or inability to take oral fluids or in younger children and inability to suckle. Alternatively, they may exhibit a number of syndrome(s) of severe disease, including anemia, coma, respiratory distress, and hypoglycemia and may also have a high rate of bacteremia.[69,77]

In most age groups, anemia is frequently accompanied by more than one syndrome of severe disease, and the already substantial case fatality rate of 15% to 20% for severe malaria in African children rises significantly when multiple syndromes of severe disease are present.[77]

The age distribution of anemia and other syndromes of severe disease are a consistent but puzzling feature of the epidemiology of clinical malaria. Children born in endemic areas are protected from severe malaria in the first 6 months of life by the passive transfer of maternal immunoglobulins and by fetal hemoglobin. Beyond infancy, the most common form of presentation of severe disease changes from anemia in children aged 1 to 3 years old, in areas of high transmission, to cerebral malaria in older children, in areas of lower transmission.[78] As transmission intensity declines further, severe malaria is most frequently found in older age groups.

The Clinical Features of Malarial Anemia

The blood stage of falciparum malaria may cause life-threatening anemia; a hemoglobin level of less than 5 g/dL is considered to represent severe disease. Children with anemia may present with malaise, fatigue, and dyspnea or respiratory distress, which usually represents metabolic acidosis, but in an ill child acute respiratory infection must be carefully excluded.[77,79,80]

Acidosis is largely due to excessive lactic acid and other anions. Salicylate toxicity and dehydration may also play a role. However, the majority of children presenting with respiratory distress are severely anemic, have a metabolic acidosis secondary to reduced oxygen-carrying capacity and respond to rapid transfusion of fresh blood (for a review, see reference 81). A minority of those with respiratory distress do not respond to appropriate resuscitation. They probably represent a heterogeneous clinical group and may have renal failure, systemic bacterial infection, or a more profound syndrome of systemic disturbance due to malarial parasites.

Hemolytic Syndromes Including Blackwater Fever

The sudden appearance of hemoglobin in the urine indicating severe intravascular hemolysis leading to hemoglobinemia and hemoglobinuria or blackwater fever received particular attention in early studies of anemia in expatriates living in endemic areas.[82] There was an association between blackwater fever and the irregular use of quinine for chemoprophylaxis. This drug can act as a hapten and stimulate production of a drug-dependent complement-fixing antibody. Recent studies of sudden intravascular hemolysis have shown it is rare in Africa, but more common in Southeast Asia and Papua New Guinea, where some cases are associated with G6PD deficiency and treatment with variety of drugs including quinine, mefloquine, and artesunate.[83] However, in the majority of cases, the cause of sudden hemolysis cannot be accounted for and it seems likely unidentified hemolytic mechanism(s) may operate.

The Hematologic Features of Malarial Infection

The anemia of falciparum malaria is typically normocytic and normochromic, with a notable absence of reticulocytes, although microcytosis and hypochromia may be present because of the very high frequency of alpha and beta thalassaemia traits and/or iron deficiency in many endemic areas.[47,71]

The anemia of malaria may be accompanied by changes in the white cell and platelet counts and in clotting parameters, but these changes are neither in themselves diagnostic nor guide management. Malaria is accompanied by a modest leucocytosis, although leucopenia may also occur. Occasionally, leukemoid reactions have been observed. Leucocytosis has been associated with severe disease.[84,85] A high neutrophil count may also suggest intercurrent bacterial infection. Monocytosis and increased numbers of circulating lymphocytes are also seen in acute infection although the significance of these changes is not established.[86] However, malarial pigment is often seen in neutrophils and in monocytes and has been associated with severe disease and unfavorable outcome.[87,88]

Thrombocytopenia is almost invariable in malaria and so may be helpful as a sensitive, but nonspecific marker, of active infection. However, severe thrombocytopenia ($<50 \times 10^9$/L is rare. Increased removal of platelets may follow absorption of immune complexes, but there is no evidence for platelet-specific alloantibodies.[89] By analogy with erythropoiesis, there may be a defect in thrombopoiesis but this has not been established. Thrombocytopenia is not associated with disease severity, although somewhat paradoxically platelets have been shown to contribute to disease pathology in animal and in human malaria.[90,91] Moreover, in human infections, platelets may form clumps with infected erythrocytes.[92] One explanation of this paradox could be that low levels of platelets might not only be a marker of parasite burden but also be protective from severe disease and/or be associated with antiinflammatory cytokine responses.[93]

Disordered coagulation and clinical evidence of bleeding are not infrequent in nonimmune adults contracting malaria and presenting with severe disease. Patients may present with bleeding at injection sites, gums, or epistaxis. Abnormalities of laboratory tests of hemostasis, suggesting activation of the coagulation cascades, occur in acute infection. However, histologic evidence of intravascular fibrin deposition is notably absent in those dying from severe malaria in adults.[94] Factor XIII, normally responsible for cross-linking fibrin, is inactivated during malaria infection, and these data may explain low levels of fibrin deposition in the face of increased procoagulant activity.[95]

The bone marrow is typically hypercellular. The most striking findings are of grossly abnormal development of erythroid precursors or dyserythropoiesis. The developing erythroid cells typically demonstrate cytoplasmic and nuclear bridging and irregular nuclear outline.[39,40] These changes are probably central to the pathophysiology of malarial anemia and are discussed in detail below. The proportion of abnormal erythroid precursors and the degree of dyserythropoiesis are markedly greater in chronic compared to acute infection, suggesting that the inhibition and abnormal maturation of erythroid precursors may have somewhat differing etiologies in acute and chronic infection.[39]

The role of hematinic deficiency in children presenting with malaria and anemia may be difficult to assess. The relative importance of absolute and functional iron deficiency have not been defined. Nevertheless, many hospitals give a course of iron supplementation after an episode of acute malaria, although no general guidelines have been established. Chronic hemolysis may increase folate requirements, but frank deficiency is uncommon in children presenting with acute malaria, at least in East Africa.[47] Folate deficiency may be more common in West Africa and protocols for folate supplementation after malaria must reflect local experience.

Malarial Anemia in Pregnancy

Pregnancy is accompanied by a series of physiological changes that predispose not only to anemia but also to malaria. Hemodilution causes a physiological decrease in hemoglobin. Moreover, the demand for both iron and folate increases as the fetus grows and often precipitates frank folate or iron deficiency, particularly in multigravid women.

Occult malaria infection, often without fever, may cause anemia and placental dysfunction. This effect is greatest in primigravidae and has been attributed to the adhesion of parasitized erythrocytes to chondroitin sulfate A and hyaluronic acid in the placenta (for reviews, see references 98 and 99).[96,97] Fetal growth is impaired and babies born to women with placental malaria are on average 100 g lighter than controls born to women without malaria. The subsequent contribution of malaria to infant mortality is substantial.[100] Furthermore, the increase in hematopoiesis demanded by hemolysis during malaria infection may precipitate frank folate deficiency. Finally, women who are not immune to malaria are more likely to develop hypoglycemia and pulmonary edema during pregnancy.

The increase in maternal and fetal morbidity and mortality secondary to malaria may be prevented by routine hematinic supplementation and by intermittent treatment with antimalarials during the second and third trimesters with sulphadoxine-pyrimethamine (Fansidar).[101]

Hyperreactive Malarial Splenomegaly

Although splenomegaly, secondary to malarial infection, usually regresses as immunity is acquired, some people living in endemic areas develop progressive, massive splenomegaly.[102] The pathophysiology of such hyperreactive malarial splenomegaly (HMS) is poorly understood but certainly results in B-cell hyperplasia with high levels of polyclonal IgM, reaching a level greater than 2 SD above the local reference mean. The specific antimalarial antibody titer is high, although only a small proportion of the polyclonal IgM response is directed at malarial antigens. B-cell hyperplasia may provoke proliferation of both T cells and macrophages and IgM levels may cause cryoglobinemia and stimulate erythrophagocytosis.

Patients may present typically between 20 and 40 years old, with massive splenomegaly without lymphadenopathy, anemia that may be severe, neutropenia, and thrombocytopenia. The anemia may cause life-threatening hemolytic crises and/or neutropenia associated with severe bacterial infection. Thrombocytopenia is rarely symptomatic. The bone marrow shows hypercellularity, with a lymphocytosis in marrow and peripheral blood. The high IgM levels distinguish HMS from CLL or other lymphoproliferative disorders. However, the polyclonal proliferation of B cells may transform to a true clonal lymphoproliferative disorder. This appears to be derived from a naïve B cell, although the exact classification of such lymphoproliferative disorders is poorly defined,[103] although there is a single report of a high incidence of B prolymphocytic leukemia in one population.[104]

Treatment for HMS is life-long antimalarial prophylaxis. Regression of signs and symptoms returns over 1 to 2 years but may relapse if antimalarial therapy ceases. Splenectomy is contraindicated as it is technically difficult, with considerable interoperative mortality and may predispose to severe infection.

Anemia and *P vivax*, *P ovale*, and *P malariae* Infection

In *P vivax* and *P ovale* malaria, high parasitemias are rare as invasion of erythrocytes is limited to reticulocytes. The parasites do not appear to sequester in the peripheral circulation or to cause organ-specific syndromes. Mortality is limited to occasional deaths from splenic rupture and from intercurrent illnesses in already weakened individuals.

Nevertheless, *P vivax* malaria has been clearly associated with anemia during pregnancy and with low birth weight of children of affected mothers. Here cytokines or other inflammatory mediators appear to cause placental dysfunction.[105] *P malariae* infection is also rarely fatal but is distinguished by the persistence of blood-stage parasites for up to 40 years. It can however cause a progressive and fatal nephrotic syndrome.[106]

Malaria Diagnosis

The diagnosis of malaria is based on the identification of circulating blood-stage parasites. The standard methods of preparing thick and thin films are straightforward and allow a simple method to diagnose infection (Table 159–1).[107–109] However, malaria diagnosis poses particular problems for inexperienced staff. The main biological problem is that the level of circulating parasites is only weakly associated with the overall parasite burden as falciparum-infected erythrocytes are sequestered in capillary venules; thus the parasitemia is not a reliable guide to the severity of disease. Second, missing or delaying the diagnosis of falciparum malaria may result in serious morbidity and mortality. Finally, the most sensitive methods for diagnosis of infection, namely microscopy, require both skill and time.

In endemic areas, laboratory staff are skilled at the examination of thick films and routinely are able to detect 1 parasite in 100 HPFs of a thick film, which corresponds to a sensitivity of approximately 5 to 50 parasites/μL.[107,110] Thin films are used for speciating parasites and the circulating asexual forms of the four main malaria species can be readily identified, whereas the sexual forms (gametocytes) of the species require some skill and regular practice (Figs. 159–5 and 159–6).

Nevertheless, diagnosis of malaria by microscopy in nonendemic countries has proven problematic. Routine laboratories may only achieve sensitivities of the order of 500 parasites/μL using thick films.[110,111] Quality assurance schemes show that performance of routine hematology laboratories in the recognition of and speciation of malaria parasites is poor.[109,111]

There has therefore been a strong drive to use nonmicroscopy methods for malaria diagnosis. It is now apparent that these methods are not sufficiently sensitive for clinical diagnosis, although they may have a role in detecting parasites of more than 500 parasites/μL when experienced staff are not available and/or as part of an out-of-hours service. However, it must be emphasized that these tests are no substitute for careful microscopy. Operationally this means that hematology labs need to make the diagnosis of malaria and must maintain the skills needed for reliable examination of thick films.

A number of methods based on the fluorescent staining of parasite DNA and/or RNA and the concentration of parasites have been devised.[112–114] However attractive these methods may appear, their sensitivity is limited by background staining of cellular debris and the limit of their sensitivity is approximately 100 parasites/μL. The time taken in preparing samples and the specialized equipment and skills needed to use these methods limits their effectiveness in routine practice.

Detection of circulating malarial antigens is another potentially attractive, but ultimately limited, alternative to the laborious method of screening blood films. The widely available tests detect Plasmodium histidine rich protein-2 (Binax test, Launch Diagnostics Ltd), and Plasmodium-specific lactate dehydrogenase (OptiMal-IT test, TCS Biologicals, UK) by immunochromatography.[115] The formulation of the tests using dipstick antigens allows rapid testing to be performed by laboratory staff. However, the sensitivity is 100 to 1000 parasites/μL and this is comparable to the sensitivity achieved by inexperienced but not experienced microscopists. The current recommendations for malaria diagnosis in the United Kingdom emphasize clearly that these tests only have a place when experienced staff are not available.

Amplification of circulating parasite DNA using the repeated rRNA genes is an extremely sensitive method of malaria diagnosis.[116] The sensitivity may be as low as 0.005 parasites/μL or 5 parasites/mL.[117,118] Undoubtedly, this is a useful tool for reference laboratories but is not yet in routine diagnostic use.

Table 159–1 Malaria Diagnosis

Thick and thin films should be prepared for cases of suspected malaria.
Immunochromographic tests lack sensitivity to detect low levels of parasites that may be highly clinically significant.
Routine Giemsa or May–Grünwald–Giemsa stains are unlikely to give satisfactory results as the pH is too low.
Films can be stained with Giemsa or Leishman stain (thin films) or Field stain (thick films). (For details see *Guideline: The Clinical Diagnosis of Malaria*, www.bcshguidelines.org).
200 high-power fields (×100 objectives) should be examined in a thick film.
Asexual parasitemia should be reported after counting 1000 RBCs in a thin film. A graticule or grid may help counting.
If parasitemia is less than 1:1000 RBCs, parasitemia may be counted in a thick film in relation to the number of WBCs.
During active infection, daily parasite count should be obtained.
Counting and speciation of malaria parasites should be verified by a second observer.
Reports on negative films despite a strong clinical suspicion of malaria should be qualified that negative films do not exclude a diagnosis of malaria. Repeat films should be requested if clinically appropriate. Thrombocytopenia may heighten suspicion of malaria.

Treatment

Malaria requires urgent effective chemotherapy to prevent progression of disease and may be the most crucial public health intervention to reduce global mortality from malaria. The drug treatment of malaria must take account of the expected pattern of drug resistance in the area where infection was contracted, the severity of clinical disease, and the species of parasite. The spread of drug-resistant parasites and the optimal use of affordable, effective drugs are of continual concern and these have recently been reviewed (Table 159–2).[119–121] Artemisinin-based combination treatments have been the mainstay of treatment for falciparum malaria in Southeast Asia for more than

Text continued on p. 2353.

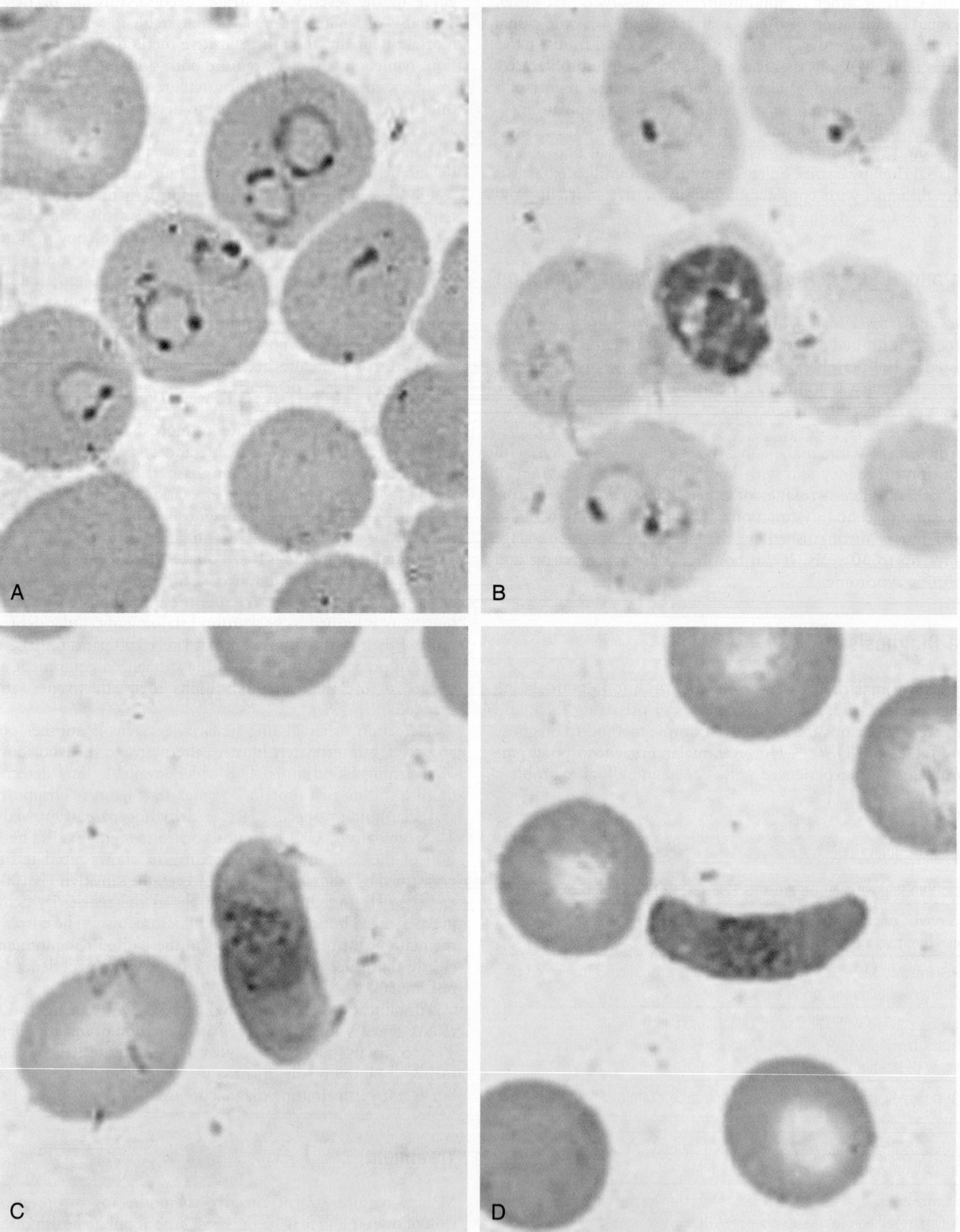

Figure 159–5 Blood stage malaria (thin blood films). *Plasmodium falciparum*: Fine rings (**a**) predominate, with mature trophozoites and schizonts (**b**) appearing uncommonly in the peripheral circulation because infected cells adhere to postcapillary venules. Host cells are not enlarged. Basophilic clefts and spots of irregular shape and size (Maurer clefts and dots) may be seen in erythrocytes containing more mature parasites. They are thought to be aggregates of parasite proteins that are being exported from the parasite to the surface of the red cell. Crescent-shaped male (**c**) and female gametocytes (**d**) are diagnostic. (*Giemsa* × *1500*). *Plasmodium vivax*: All stages of asexual parasites—from young trophozoites

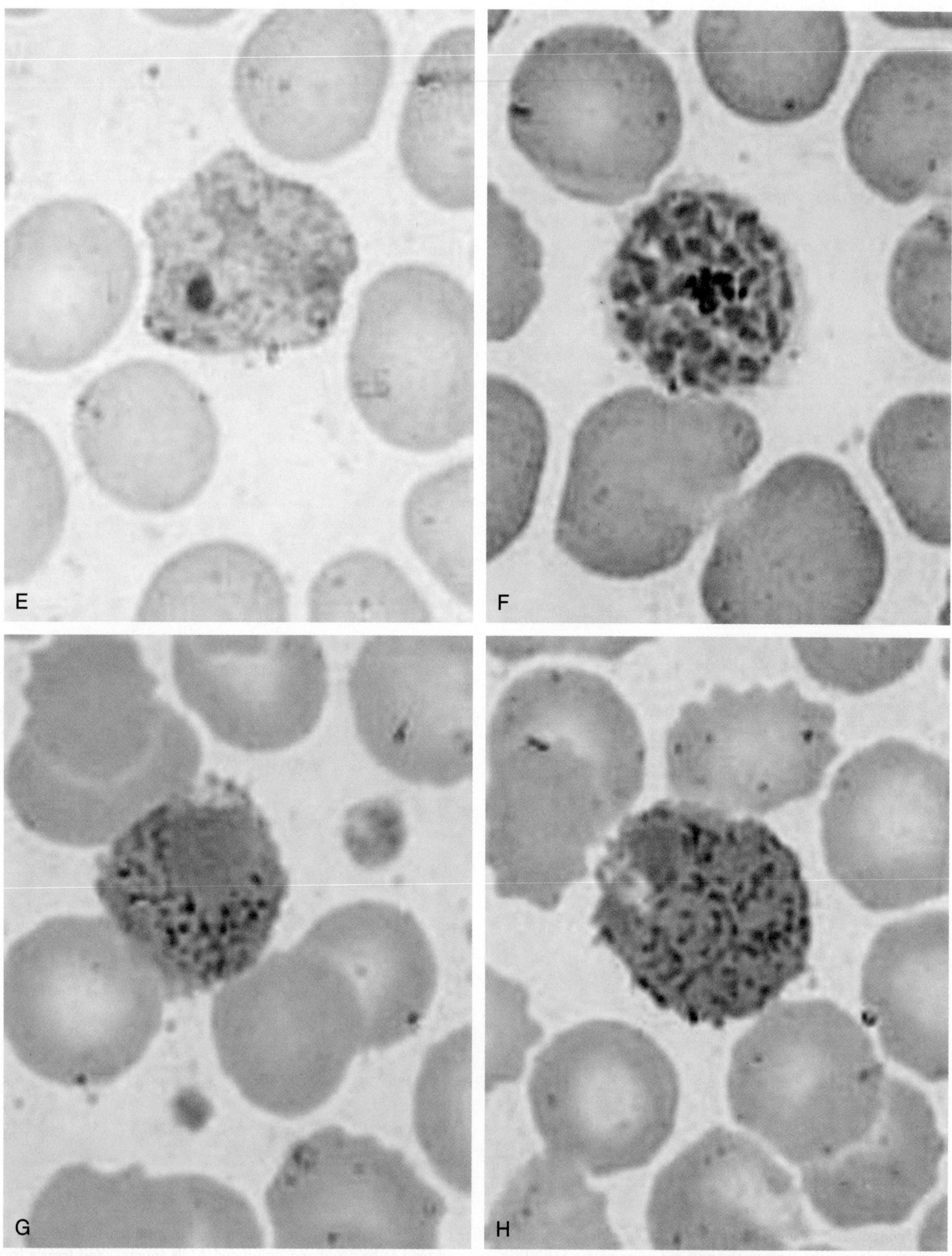

Figure 159–5, cont'd (**e**) to schizonts—appear in the peripheral circulation in vivax malaria together with gametocytes. The parasites are large and ameboid, and produce schizonts with approximately 16 daughter cells (merozoites) (**f**). Pigment is well developed. Host red cells are enlarged and uniformly covered with fine eosinophilic stippling (Schüffner dots). Gametocytes are round, with the male (microgametocytes; (**g**) being approximately 7 μm, and the female (macrogametocytes; (**h**) being 10 μm or more in diameter. (*Giemsa* × *1500*). *Plasmodium ovale*: Intraerythrocytic ring forms

(Continued)

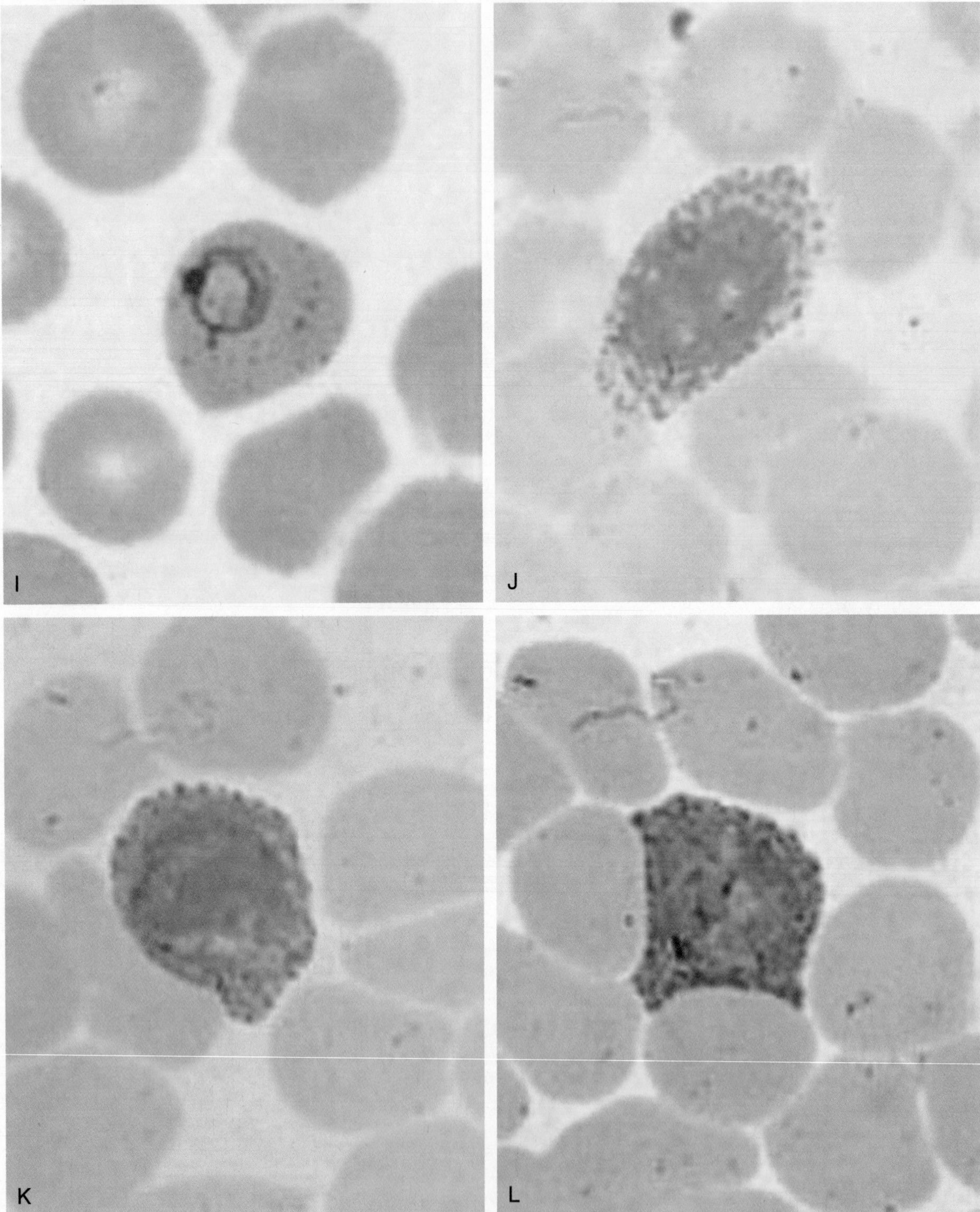

Figure 159–5, cont'd (i) have a prominent nucleus. The older parasites (j) differ from *P vivax* in being more compact and producing about eight merozoites at schizogony. Like *P vivax*, the host red cells contain Schüffner dots and tend to be ovoid and fimbriated. Male (micro-) and female (macro-) gametocytes (**k** and **l**) are smaller than those of *P vivax*. (*Leishman × 1500*). *P malariae*: All intraerythrocytic stages may appear in the peripheral circulation, from young trophozoites

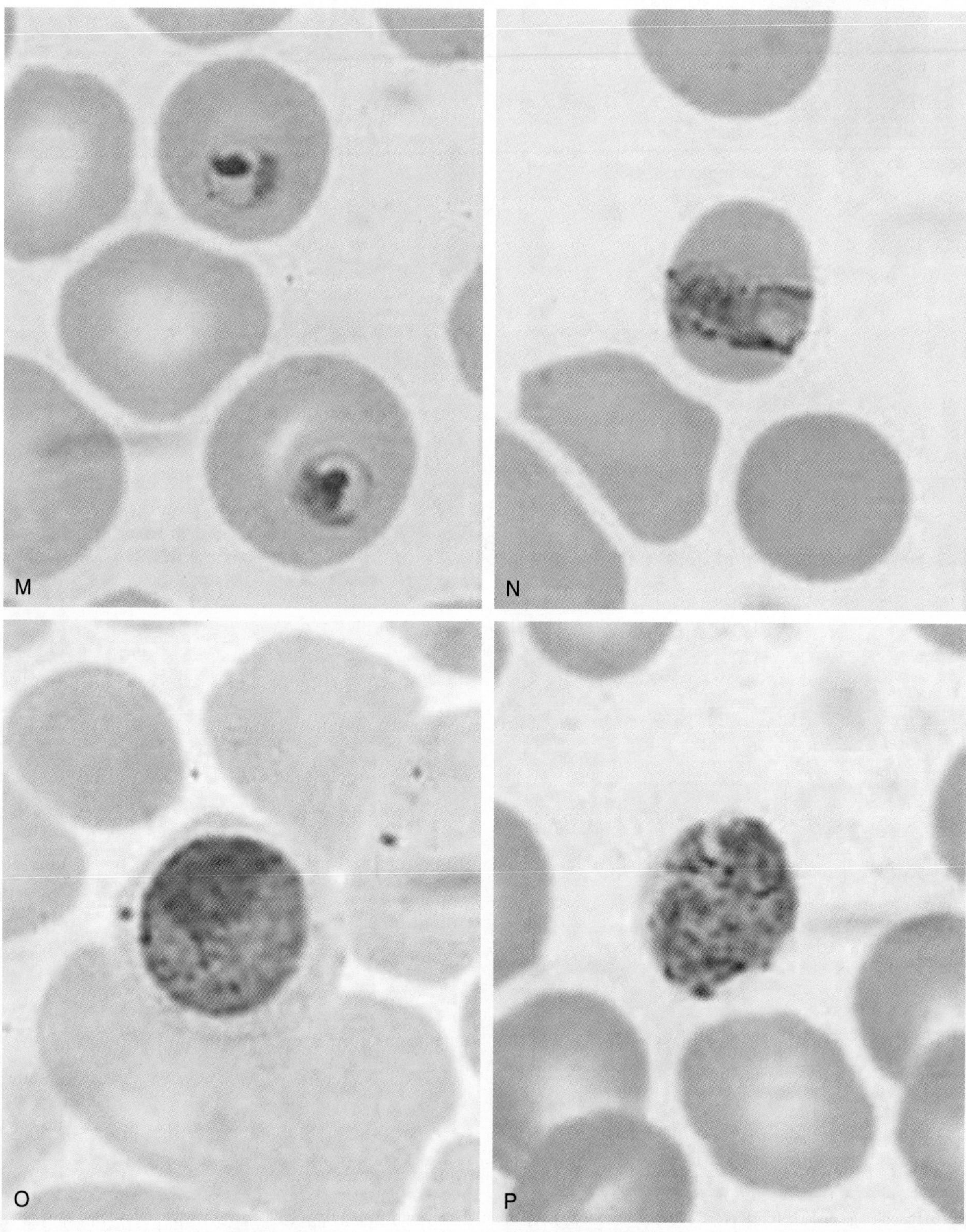

Figure 159–5, cont'd (**m**) to compact schizonts with eight merozoites. Band forms (**n**) stretching across the red cell are common. With special staining, a very fine stippling (Ziemann dots) is sometimes seen. Host red cells are not enlarged. Gametocytes, no larger than their host cells, are round and compact with distinct blackish pigment, being finer in the males (**o**), in which the nucleus is more diffuse and the cytoplasm somewhat mauvish, whereas the granules are fewer and larger in the female (**p**), which stains a bluer color. (*Leishman* × *1500*)

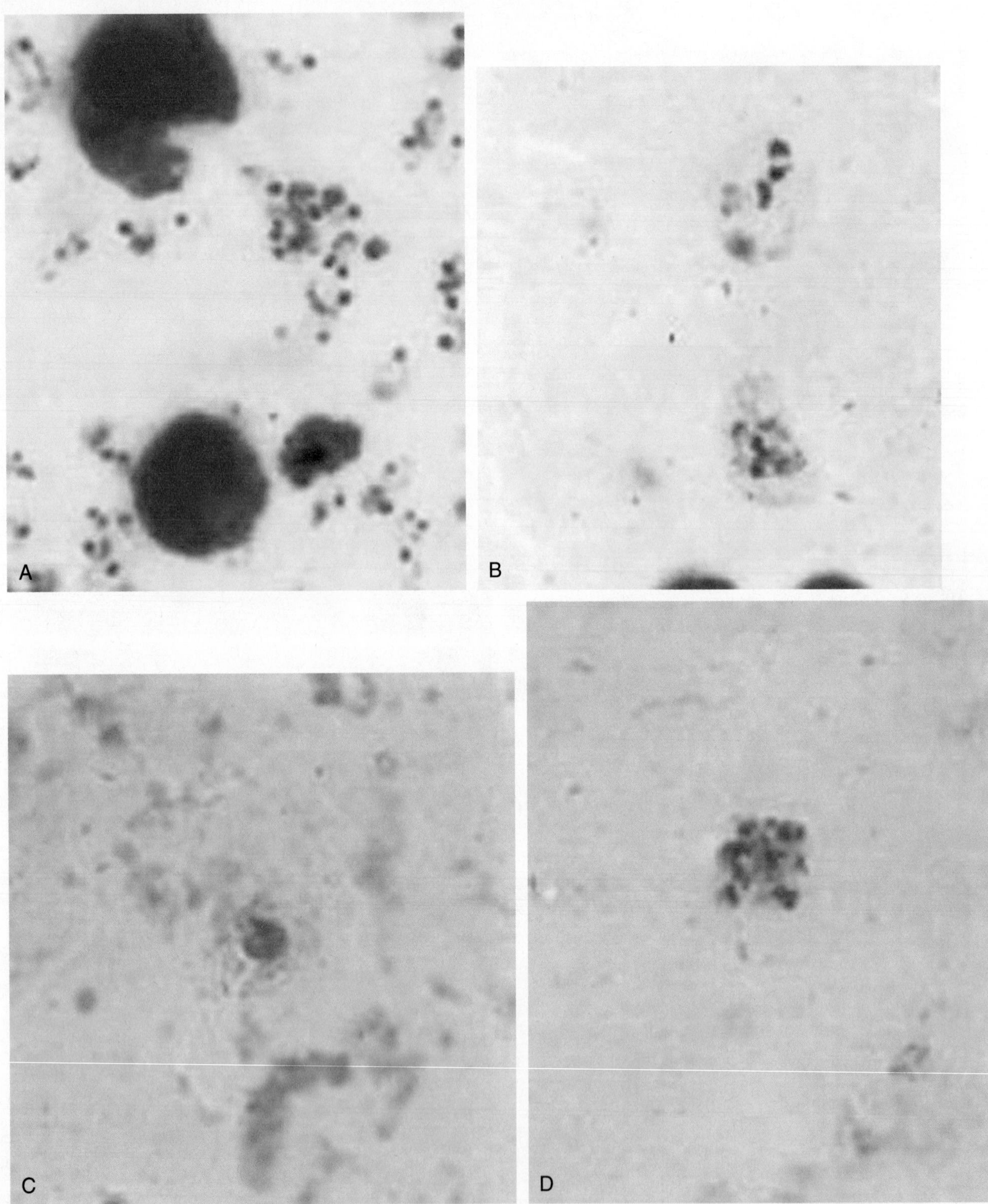

Figure 159–6 Blood-stage malaria (thick blood films). *Plasmodium falciparum*: Usually only young rings (**a**) are seen in acute infections, although sometimes in very large numbers. *Plasmodium vivax*: All stages may be present; here two young trophozoites are seen (**b**), with Schüffner dots seen as "ghost cells" in the thinner parts of the film where the host cell has been hemolyzed. *Plasmodium ovale*: The Schüffner dots of *P ovale* also may show up in a thick film as a ghost cell, but the parasite can be distinguished from *P vivax* by the solid appearance and heavy pigment even of young trophozoites (**c**). *Plasmodium malariae*: Younger parasites can be recognized by their heavy pigment, but this may be so heavy that it obscures the other inner structures. Schizonts containing up to eight merozoites with a central mass of pigment (**d**) are characteristic. *P malariae* is difficult to differentiate from *P ovale* in thick films, in which the parasites are easily confused. However, unlike *P malariae*, *P ovale* may be seen in ghost cells (**c**). (*Field* × *1500*)

Table 159–2 Commonly Used Antimalarial Drugs and Their Side Effects

	Oral Dose	Parenteral Dose	Side Effects
Sulphadoxine-Pyrimethamine	Sulphadoxine 25 mg/kg Pyrimethamine 1.25 mg/kg as a single dose (max 1500 mg Sulphadoxine and 75 mg pyrimethamine)	For IM injection, doses as for oral	Use with caution in first trimester Causes kernicterus in neonates Skin rashes, fatal Stevens–Johnson syndrome
Amodiaquine	10 mg/kg for 3 days	Not used	Hepatitis Fatal agranulocytosis when used for prophylaxis
Artemether	3.2 mg/kg day 1 1.6 mg/kg days 2–7	3.2 mg/kg IM day 1, then 1.6 mg/kg for 3 days, then oral	Reticuolcytopenia
Artesunate	4 mg/kg OD for 7 days	2.4 mg/kg IM day 1, then 1.2 mg/kg for 3 days, then oral	Reticulocytopenia
Artemether/lumofantrine	Fixed dose combination: artemether (20 mg) with lumofantrine (120 mg), twice daily for 3 days if <15 kg then 1 tablet, 15–25 kg 2 tablets, 25–35 kg 3 tablets, >45 kg 4 tablets		
Quinine	10 mg/kg of salt (max 600 mg) 8 hourly for 7 days	20 mg/kg in 10 mL/kg isotonic fluid over 4 hours, then 10 mg/kg over 2 hours given 12 hourly in children and 8 hourly in adults	Thrombocytopenia, intravascular hemolysis (Blackwater fever) when used prophylactically, nausea, tinnitus, deafness
Mefloquine	15 mg/kg base day 1, 10 mg/kg base day 2	Not given	Psychosis, fits
Halofantrine	6 mg/kg base 6 hourly for 3 doses and repeat after 1 week.	Not given	Delay in AV conduction so prolonged QT interval

10 years and are now increasingly recommended as first-line treatment throughout the rest of the world.[122] The hematologic side effects of antimalarial drugs in use today are few. Amodiaquine is associated with neutropenia and agranulocytosis. Artemisinin-based treatments may cause reticulocytopenia but this is not clinically significant.

In severely ill patients, good nursing care is vital. Monitoring and treatment of fits and hypoglycemia is essential and antipyretics should be given.[123]

Certainly, blood transfusion is in principle a straightforward solution to the treatment of severe malarial anemia, although controversy exists over the trigger for transfusion and the rate of administration of blood. The standard regimes of cautious and slow delivery of blood have been challenged by the demonstration that rapid initial flow rates may correct lactic acidosis and hypovolemia. However, in nonimmunes and in pregnant women, blood transfusion must be accompanied by careful hemodynamic monitoring to avoid precipitating or exacerbating pulmonary edema.

No formal controlled trials for the transfusion of patients with malaria have been performed. Whatever clinical guidelines emerge, in reality blood transfusion in the heartland of malaria-endemic areas is beset by many practical and theoretical problems. First, the absence of well-characterized donor panels (and thus systematic blood collection) frequently jeopardizes the supply of blood. Second, even when standard screening for HIV is in place, the residual risk of HIV transmission in the serologic window of infectivity remains at 1 in 2000.[124] At a practical level, positive indirect antiglobulin tests in acute infection may make the exclusion of alloantibodies difficult. Depending on the clinical urgency and transfusion history, the least serologically incompatible blood may have to be given.

One therapeutic option available in North America and in Europe for the urgent treatment of nonimmune patients with severe disease would be an exchange blood transfusion. This procedure removes nonsequestered, infected erythrocytes and possibly circulating toxins. In the absence of evidence from trials for the use of exchange transfusion in malaria, some have suggested that this treatment could be given for hyperparasitemia (>20%) in severely ill nonimmune patients.[125,126]

The salient features that make this clinical problem a major public health concern are the very large numbers of children affected and the difficulty of satisfactory treatment by blood transfusion outside specialist centers.

Malaria as a Transfusion-Transmitted Infection

Malaria is undoubtedly the most common transfusion-transmitted infection in the world. In endemic areas a large proportion of adult donors will be parasitemic, perhaps 20% to 80% depending on the rate of transmission. Here the donor deferral is impractical and treatment of recipients with a course of effective antimalarials is the most practical alternative.

In nonendemic areas, transmission of malaria is an occasional but potentially devastating complication of blood transfusion, and considerable thought and resources are required to combat the problem effectively.

The first case of transfusion-transmitted malaria (TTM) was in 1911.[127,128] Between 1911 and the mid-1970s the incidence of TTM rose to more than 140 cases per year, with *P vivax* the most common species causing infection, although the proportion of cases due to *P falciparum* has steadily increased, perhaps reflecting the speed and destination of international travel. It is striking that the background problem, namely in malaria in returned travelers, is much more common in the United Kingdom than the United States, with the per capita incidence differing by nearly a factor of 10 and a higher proportion of cases due to *P falciparum* in Europe and the United Kingdom compared with the United States.[129]

Recent experience in the United Kingdom and United States has emphasized the seriousness of transfusion-transmitted malaria. Two of the last five cases of malaria due to blood transfusion in the United

Table 159–3 UK Donor Selection Guidelines for Donors "At-Risk" of Transmitting Malaria

Donor "Risk" Category	Guidelines
Resident	Defined as having lived in Sub-Saharan Africa (except South Africa) or Papua New Guinea for a continuous period of 6 months at any time of life. Permanent deferral unless malaria antibody negative at least 6 months after returning from a malarious area. Any subsequent visits to any malarious area each require a 6-month deferral period and a negative antibody test prior to reinstatement.
History of malaria	Permanent deferral unless malaria antibody negative at least 3 years after cessation of treatment or last negative
Undiagnosed febrile illness	While abroad or within 4 weeks of return Deferral for 12 months or 6 months if malarial antibody negative
All other risks	Deferral for 12 months or 6 months if malarial antibody negative

Kingdom were fatal.[130–132] Whereas in the United States, 14 cases of transfusion-transmitted malaria were reported between 1990 and 1999, but only 2 cases between 2000 and 2005.[133]

Detecting these cases after transfusion is frequently delayed as malaria infection acquired in nonendemic countries rarely figures in immediate differential diagnosis and requires careful examination of the blood film.

The mainstay of preventing TTM in the United Kingdom is donor deferral backed up by detection of circulating antibodies to malaria antigens. The guidelines for donor deferral were carefully revised after analysis of circumstances of recent TTM (Table 159–3).[134] These criteria recognize that malaria in the nonimmune is likely to present within 6 months of return from an endemic area and that significant immunity to falciparum malaria may be acquired by residence after 6 months in a malarious area.

The criteria also required that residents, those having had malaria or an undiagnosed febrile illness, may be reinstated if antimalarial antibodies cannot be detected. The importance of antimalarial antibody testing rests on the fact that it is a very sensitive method to detect chronic infection whereas the identification of circulating malarial antigens or nucleic acids or microscopy would fail to detect a level of 1 parasite/mL, which would still give a highly infectious dose in a unit of blood.

The assays for antimalarial antibodies previously used indirect immunofluorescence antibody tests (IFAT) to detect reactivity to a crude parasite lysate as a target antigen. However, an enzyme-linked immunosorbent serologic assay (ELISA) using recombinant malarial antigens have proved to be a more practical if slightly less sensitive alternative to IFAT.[131,134,135] These tests detect antimalarial antibodies in less than 2% of donors who have visited endemic areas. It has been calculated that the return of 90% of malarial antibody-positive visitors to the donor pool releases an extra 50,000 units a year in the United Kingdom, and this is a highly cost-effective process to reduce the attrition of eligible blood donors.

Donor deferral is based on the potential of a donor to carry malaria and is therefore based on the area of travel, length of stay of residence, elapsed time since leaving the endemic area and history of malaria. It has been repeatedly shown that application of even the most thorough donor questionnaires allows some of those carrying malaria to give blood as guidelines are frequently incorrectly applied or questions answered inaccurately in routine practice.[133,136]

In Canada donors reporting diagnosis or treatment of malaria defer permanently[12] and in the United States donors are deferred 3 years after treatment.[133] The criteria will inevitably cause unnecessary deferral of those who never actually had malaria but also permits some individuals with low-level chronic infection to donate as malaria not infrequently presents more than 3 years after returning from endemic areas.[133,132] The last case of malaria transmitted in the United Kingdom was by someone who left a malarious area 8 years previously and the longest recorded case of recrudescence of malaria infection is 44 years for *P malariae.*

In conclusion, permanent deferral of all those visiting malaria-endemic areas is unlikely to be a viable strategy to prevent TTM as donor bases are declining. Preventing malaria transmission through blood transfusion requires comprehensive, regularly reviewed and effectively implemented guidelines for donor deferral and laboratory testing. Even the best strategy is a compromise and medical laboratory staff should be aware of the rarely, but potentially serious, possibility of fever after transfusion that could be caused by malaria.

VISCERAL LEISHMANIASIS

Leishmaniasis is a generic term of infection by 30 or so species of the obligate intracellular parasites from the genus *Leishmania.* Visceral leishmaniasis or Kala-azar presents with a wide spectrum of systemic and hematologic features.

Epidemiology

Visceral leishmaniasis (VL) occurs in all countries bordering the Mediterranean and across the Middle East, including Saudi Arabia and Yemen. Indian VL occurs in the eastern regions (particularly Assam, Bengal, Bihar, Uttar Pradesh, Madras, and Sikkim) and in Nepal and Bangladesh. African Kala-azar is endemic in Kenya, Ethiopia, and the Sudan and sporadic elsewhere in tropical Africa. In the Americas, VL occurs in foci across Mexico, Central America, Colombia, Venezuela, Guyana, Brazil, Bolivia, and northern Argentina (Fig. 159–7).

The total burden of disease is difficult to estimate but significant. Leishmaniasis burden is endemic in 88 countries, with 500,000 new cases of VL per year, with the vast majority occurring in India, Bangladesh, Nepal, Northern Sudan, and northeastern Brazil.[137] VL is associated with poverty and undernutrition in endemic areas, particularly in the hyperendemic foci of southern Sudan and the Ganges river basin. In the Mediterranean area, it is increasingly seen in association with HIV infection, where infection rates in HIV-infected people may be as high as 10%.

Visceral Leishmaniasis (VL) is caused by a number of species of the *Leishmania donovani* complex.[138,139] In the Mediterranean and areas in the Middle East and Central Asia through to China, *Leishmania infantum* predominates whereas *L donovani* is more prevalent in India and Africa. *Leishmania tropica* is a less common cause of VL in these areas. Throughout their range in the Old World, parasites are transmitted by the female sandfly of the *Phlebotomus* genera.

Leishmaniasis is caused by different parasites and vectors in the New World, where *L chagasi* and *L amazonensis* are transmitted by the *Lutzomyia* genera of sandfly.

Leishmania organisms are present in blood and so the disease can be transmitted by blood transfusion, as a sexually transmitted disease, as a congenital infection, by needle sharing for intravenous drug abuse, or within a laboratory by intradermal inoculation of *L donovani* promastigotes.[140,141] Very few cases of *Leishmania* have occurred as transfusion-transmitted infections in Europe or North America, with under 10 cases in infants or immunocompromised patients over the last fifty years. In endemic areas, this problem represents a much greater but unquantified risk.

Parasitology

Leishmania amastigotes live and multiply within macrophages by binary fission. They are round or ovoid bodies, approximately 2 to

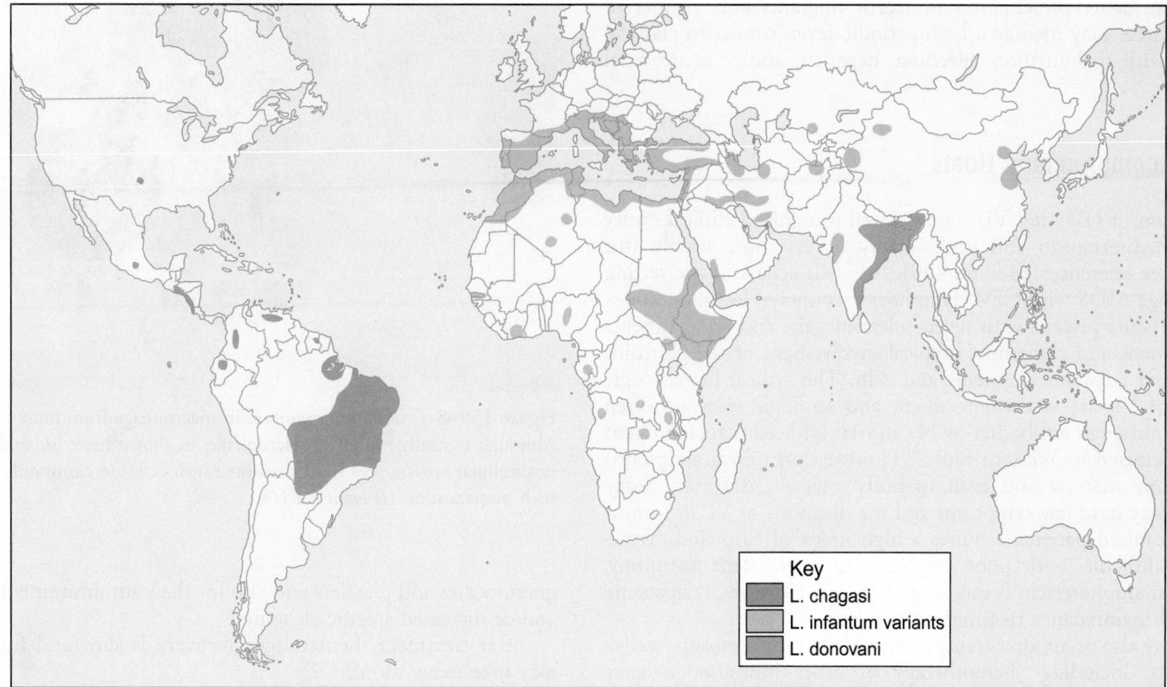

Figure 159–7 Epidemiology of visceral leishmaniasis (VL). VL caused by parasites of the *Leishmania donovani–Leishmania infantum* complex occurs in the Mediterranean littorals, the Middle East, and adjacent parts of the former Soviet Union, the Sudan, east Africa, the Indian subcontinent and China, and South America (*Leishmania chagasi*). An arid, warm environment provides ideal ecologic conditions for the breeding of many species of sandfly. Zoonotic kala-azar due to *L infantum* and *L chagasi* is commonly associated with dry, rocky, hill country where cases are typically scattered. In India, *L donovani* is essentially an anthroponosis. This type of kala-azar may occur in severe epidemic fashion, as can kala-azar in the Sudan.

3 μm in diameter. Occasional rupture of cells allows invasion of uninfected monocytes and macrophages by free forms. Sandflices ingest amastigotes within macrophages from blood or skin. In the insect's stomach, free amastigotes multiply and divide asexually, becoming elongated and developing flagella as metacyclic promastigotes. Within 2 weeks, such infective forms migrate through the lining of the stomach and enter the proboscis of the sandfly, allowing them to be inoculated in the human host while the sandfly takes a blood meal. Promastigotes are taken up by macrophages, where they become amastigotes by simple fission.

The large elongated fusiform promastigote measures 15 to 20 μm in length and 0.5 to 3.5 μm in width. Cultured promastigotes may also demonstrate rounded forms 4 to 5 μm in diameter. In Giemsa or other Romanovsky stains, a large nucleus and smaller distinct rod-like kinetoplast are obvious. The organisms must be distinguished from *Histoplasma capsulatum*.

Pathology

Parasites spread within macrophages to local lymph nodes and then to the liver, spleen, and bone marrow. They are also present more widely, in particular in the gastrointestinal tract and epidermis. In the subclinical cases, a cellular mediated immune response causes a granulomatous lesion and resolution of the infection. However, in clinical VL little if any inflammatory response to the rapidly extensive and expanding parasite-laden parasite macrophages is seen. Where it shows, a granuloma develops at the site of the initial inoculation but may not be apparent at the time of presentation.

Clinical Features of Visceral Leishmaniasis

The spectrum of clinical disease is wide, from asymptomatic infection to acute or chronic illness. Perhaps only 1% to 3% of all infections are symptomatic, with an incubation period of 10 days to 10 years, but it is typically between 3 and 6 months.

The high number of seropositive individuals in relation to clinical cases suggests that spontaneous cure without symptoms or with mild systemic symptoms and hepatosplenomegaly occur in the majority of individuals. In endemic areas, a significant number of seropositive children, who do not develop classical VL, suffer a subclinical form of disease with malaise, fever, poor weight gain, intermittent cough, diarrhea, hepatomegaly, and variable splenomegaly. In these cases, Leishmania were neither cultured nor seen in bone marrow aspirates.[142] There are also reports of VL presenting as mild nonspecific illness with fever, fatigue, cough, and abdominal pain in returning army personnel from the Middle East. In these cases, *L tropica* was isolated from bone marrow or lymph nodes.[143]

Patients with typical, chronic VL often present with malaise and considerable fatigue and the slow onset of low grade fever, anorexia, and weight loss. They usually have anemia, progressive and occasionally massive splenomegaly, hepatomegaly, lymphadenopathy, and hypergammaglobulinemia, with increasing skin pigmentation (hence the name kala-azar from the Hindi for black sickness). Patients may have jaundice, petechia, or purpura, heart murmurs, and edema. The size of the spleen is related to the length of infection and severity of the pancytopenia. In Africa, patients may have diffuse polymorphic papular lesions at presentation. Oral, nasal, nasopharyngeal, and laryngeal ulcers may occur during active disease or after treatment. The large spleen, often extending to the right iliac fossa, may be painful. Other features of acute disease include cough, epistaxis, and in some severe cases concurrent infection of the respiratory or gastrointestinal tracts and/or tuberculosis.

The typical features of VL may be preceded by bacteremia, bacterial infection, acute hepatitis or Guillain–Barré syndrome. VL may be associated with hepatic necrosis, cholecystitis, or neuropathy. Occasionally, lymphadenopathy may occur without systemic features of the disease. Here, histology shows noncaseating granulomas and amastigotes within macrophages.

A more acute presentation in recent migrants and visitors to endemic areas may include a high periodic fever, similar to classical malaria, with malnutrition, bleeding, hepatitis, and/or acute renal failure.

Immunocompromised Hosts

Coinfection of HIV and VL is now a well-recognized clinical entity in the Mediterranean and undoubtedly occurs more widely (for reviews, see references 148 and 149).[144–147] VL occurs in the setting of late-stage AIDS with CD4+ lymphocyte counts of less than 200 × 10^6/L. Patients present with fever, splenomegaly, and pancytopenia with frequent and sometimes atypical involvement of the gastrointestinal and respiratory systems and skin. The typical hematologic features of VL are sometimes absent and serologic tests are often negative, although antibodies to 14- and 16-kd Leishmania antigens may be detected by Western Blot.[150] However, organisms are plentiful in bone marrow and even in buffy coat preparations. Some patients may have few symptoms and the diagnosis of VL in immunocompromised patients requires a high index of suspicion. Treatment is difficult, with poor responses to pentavalent antimony. Liposomal amphotericin is the drug of choice. However, relapses are usual and maintenance treatment is required.

VL may also occur after transplantation, after immunosuppressive treatments, including chemotherapy or other immunodeficiency states.[151,152] Although patients present with a typical combination of fever, pancytopenia, and splenomegaly, the diagnosis may be missed if not considered.

Hematologic Features

VL causes a moderate normocytic, normochromic anemia.[153] The pathogenesis of anemia is multifactorial and includes hemodilution, shortened red cell survival, and reduced erythropoiesis.[154] The plasma is low, with plentiful stored iron typical of the anemia of chronic disease.[155] One report has suggested that that Epo levels are reduced compared to what would be expected for the degree of anemia.[156] Occasionally, folate deficiency secondary to malabsorption and/or increased cell turnover or coexistent iron deficiency are associated with macrocytic or microcytic anemia, respectively.[157]

The direct Coombs test is usually positive for C3 components and IgG and anti-I agglutinins may be present, but the presence and strength of the test is not correlated with the severity of the anemia. The positive DCT appears to be due to absorbed immune complexes onto erythrocytes.[158] The neutrophil survival is reduced and the differential white count shows neutropenia, relative lymphocytosis, and low eosinophil levels, with a white cell count typically in the range 2 to 4 × 10^9 L.

Neutrophil function may be impaired.[159] Pancytopenia is more severe in those with concurrent HIV infection. A leukemoid reaction to infection has been reported.

Typically the platelet count is reduced to 50 to 200 10^9 L as platelet survival is reduced. Mucosal bleeding may occur but extensive purpura is uncommon.

The prothrombin time is usually mildly prolonged to 2 to 4 seconds longer than control, secondary to impaired liver function. Fibrinolytic activity is increased and in advanced cases fibrinogen levels may be reduced. Disseminated intravascular coagulation or vasculitis may occur.[153,160] Full coagulation screening is advisable if a splenic aspirate or bone marrow biopsy is planned.

The bone marrow is usually hypercellular, with increased erythroid, myeloid, and platelet precursors. Lymphocytes may be increased and macrophages contain Leishman–Donovan bodies (Fig. 159–8). If weight loss and malabsorption are extensive, the marrow may undergo gelatinous transformation.[161]

The mechanism of leucopenia and thrombocytopenia is multifactorial. There is evidence for reduced bone marrow production of granulocytes and platelets and also for their autoimmune destruction and/or increased splenic clearance.

After treatment, hematologic recovery is slow and full recovery may take many months.[155]

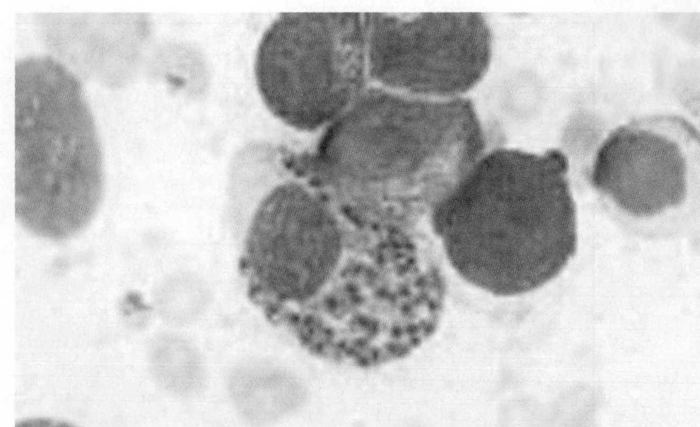

Figure 159–8 *Leishmania infantum* in macrophage from bone marrow. Although typically found in macrophages as shown here, isolated extracellular amastigotes from disrupted host cells are commonly seen in such preparations. (*Giemsa* × *810*)

Laboratory Features

The epidemiologic context and clinical features can suggest a diagnosis of Leishmaniasis. Hematologic and biochemical tests are nonspecific; biochemical tests may show mild elevation of bilirubin and transaminases and more commonly raised alkaline phosphatase. Previously, the nonspecific formol gel test was used to indicate hypergammaglobulinemia. Diagnosis is confirmed by direct examination of parasites by microscopy, culture, or polymerase chain reaction (PCR) (for a detailed review, see reference 162).

Morphology

The pathognomic amastigotes of *Leishmania* spp. can be found in a variety of sources. The diagnosis is often made by splenic puncture or by bone marrow aspiration where large numbers of amastigotes may be seen within macrophages. Amastigotes are stained using Giemsa or other Romanovsky stains and demonstrate a purple nucleus and the large anterior kinetoplast (Fig. 159–8).

In nonimmunocompromised patients, splenic aspirates are positive in more than 95% and bone marrow aspirates positive in more than 85%, buffy coat macrophages positive in more than 70%, and lymph nodes positive in more than 60% of patients with VL. In practice, samples are taken from the least invasive sites first, although lymphadenopathy is not invariable.

Where coinfection of HIV and Leishmania occurs, amastigotes are more reliably found in bone marrow than in peripheral blood and may also be demonstrated in biopsies from a wide variety of sites. Biopsy material can be stained with polyclonal anti-Leishmania serum and indirect immunofluorescence. However, direct demonstration of parasites is less sensitive than culture or PCR.

Splenic Aspiration

Splenic aspiration is rarely performed in North America and Europe but is a common diagnostic procedure in endemic areas. Aspiration is contraindicated in the presence of a bleeding tendency, portal hypertension, or a splenic hydatid cyst. Splenic aspirates are obtained from the middle of the long axis of the spleen. After cleaning the skin, a 21-gauge needle attached to a 5-mL syringe is inserted subcutaneously in line with the long axis of the spleen. The needle should be swiftly inserted to a depth of approximately 2 or 3 cm at an angle of roughly 45° to the skin, applying negative pressure. The needle should be withdrawn immediately while maintaining negative pressure and only taking a few seconds for the entire procedure. The splenic tissue may be expelled from the needle using a small amount of air and by fixing the stain using standard procedures.

Culture

Amastigotes may be grown as motile promastigotes from aspirates on the classical Novy, MacNeal, and Nicolle medium (NNN) or other suitable media, at 22 to 24 °C and populations double only every 2 to 3 days.[163,164] Inoculation of material into the susceptible golden hamster is no longer used to grow parasites.

Molecular Methods

The PCR may detect low levels of infection, and has been used for diagnosis and monitoring of treatment and to genotype the parasites.[165–167] Blood from filter paper can be used to prepare DNA, but as for direct morphology, PCR from bone marrow samples is a more sensitive method to demonstrate parasites.[168] It may be particularly useful for monitoring treatment and relapse in HIV- and *Leishmania*-infected patients.[169]

Serologic Tests

Serologic tests have to be interpreted in the light of the clinical findings. The tests are useful to screen suspected cases or populations for VL. However, they are unreliable in immunocompromised patients, who frequently are seronegative in spite of patient inflection. Conversely, those harboring a subclinical infection may be seropositive but samples may fail to yield evidence of parasites. Finally, serology is positive many years after treatment or self-cure.

An indirect IFAT or ELISA using freeze-dried Leishmania antigen have sensitivity and specificity greater than 95%. A direct agglutination test (DAT) is also available with purified freeze-dried antigen and is a highly sensitive and specific test.[170] The freeze-dried antigen is very stable even when stored in extreme conditions.

The ELISA and immunochromatographic tests using recombinant Leishmania K39 antigen are 100% sensitive and more than 98% specific in Asia.[171,172] The sensitivity and specificity of the DAT and K39 ICT are broadly similar, although the K39 test was less sensitive in the Sudan than in Asia.[173]

Treatment in patients without HIV coinfection may be monitored using urine antigen tests using detection of the K39 and K26 Leishmania antigens. These tests become negative 3 weeks after commencing treatment.

Management

General supportive care is important and includes correction of nutritional and hematinic deficiencies, blood transfusion in severe anemia, and antibiotics for secondary infections.

Specific chemotherapy for VL uses a number of potentially toxic drugs. Intercurrent infections must be identified and treated, and general measures include improvement of nutritional status (for review of treatment, see references 174 and 175). Use of pentavalent antimonials including sodium stibogluconate (Pentostam) and meglutamine antimonate (Glucantime) are now limited, especially in South Asia, by increasing drug resistance.

Amphotericin B is effective against Leishmania and is used in endemic areas where high levels of resistance to pentavalent antimonials are present. It may be given as a slow intravenous infusion in 5% dextrose over 4 to 6 hours, beginning at 0.1 mg/kg a day, increasing to 1 mg/kg until a total dose of 20 mg/kg has been given. Side effects include anaphylaxis, anemia, fever, bone chills, bone pain, and thrombophlebitis. Hypokalemia and hypomagnesemia are significant problems, and potassium loss and supplementation may be reduced by the concurrent use of amiloride to prevent renal tubular potassium leakage.[176]

Reduced toxicity from amphotericin is achieved using liposomal amphotericin preparations (AmiBisome). It is an effective and safe treatment and is used when affordable. The recommended dose is 3 mg/kg/day on days 1 to 5, 14, and 21. Studies have shown a short course of treatment of the single infusion at 5 mg/kg or 5 daily infusions of 1 mg/kg have cure rates of over 90%. In patients with HIV, a dose of liposomal amphotericin at 4 mg/kg/day on days 1 to 5 followed by 4 mg/kg/day on days 10, 17, 24, 31, and 38. The relapse rate is high and close monitoring of patients is required.

Miltefosine is a new drug and effective orally against visceral leishmaniasis in India and Africa.[177,178] The current regimes are 100 mg/day or 2 mg/kg/day in children for 4 weeks. Higher than 95% cure rates have been achieved. Gastrointestinal upset occurs frequently. Miltefosine is teratogenic and may reduce fertility. It has a long half-life and has a low therapeutic index, which may contribute to the development of resistance and so combination chemotherapy is being investigated to combat development of resistance.

Intramuscular paromomycin has been used at a dose of 15 mg/kg/day for 21 days. It has recently been shown to be equivalent to amphotericin B for the treatment of visceral leishmaniasis in India.[179] Moreover, patients treated for VL in Africa with sodium stibogluconate and paromomycin have an improved outcome compared with therapy with sodium stibogluconate alone.[180]

Post-kala-azar dermal Leishmaniasis may occur in up to 10% of patients after treatment for VL. It occurs mainly in India and is common in Africa. It occurs after treatment of visceral Leishmaniasis and may occur up to 10 years after treatment. It presents as a maculopapular rash spreading around the mouth, trunk, and limbs. These nodules and papules contain amastigotes. Prolonged treatment may be required to eliminate infection.

Leishmaniasis as a Transfusion-Transmitted Infection

Leishmaniasis poses problem as a potential transfusion-transmitted infection in endemic areas. The disease can be transmitted by blood and platelet concentrates, although leukodepletion by filtration reduces organisms by many orders of magnitude and so probably also the risk of transmission. In Europe, given the low absolute risk of transmission, donor deferral is used to reduce the risk of donation by anyone who is parasitemic.[181] It is has been noted that service personnel returning from the Middle East represent a group of potential donors who may have been exposed to infection.[182]

AFRICAN TRYPANOSOMIASIS

African Trypanosomiasis is caused by the flagellate protozoa *Trypanosoma brucei* spp, named after David Bruce, a Scottish parasitologist who first demonstrated the parasite in the blood of cattle affected by "nagana." In man, Aldo Castellani demonstrated Trypanosomes in the cerebrospinal fluid of patients with sleeping sickness. Bruce was able to show the protozoa in blood and showed that they were transmitted from antelopes to cattle by the tsetse fly and blood of patients suffering from sleeping sickness.

Epidemiology

Trypanosomes are transmitted by some species of the large and distinctive tsetse flies (*Glossina* spp.) in a sporadic distribution south of the Sahara and north of the Zambezi river. Of the three species, *Trypanosoma brucei brucei* infects animals whereas *T brucei gambiense* causes infection and sleeping sickness in Central and West Africa and

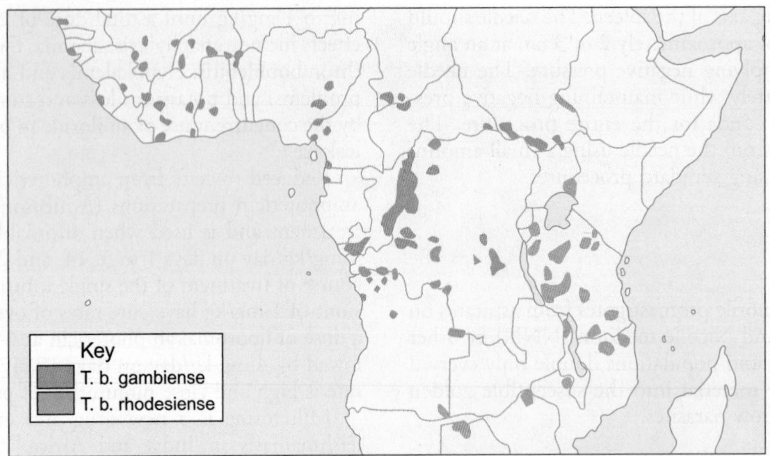

Figure 159–9 Distribution of *Trypanosoma brucei* infection in humans. African trypanosomiasis is confined to equatorial Africa, with a patchy distribution depending on detailed topographical conditions. It is caused by two subspecies of *T brucei*: *T b gambiense* infection is widespread in West and Central Africa, mainly by riverine species of tsetse fly (*Glossina*), but *T b rhodesiense*, transmitted mostly by savannah species, is restricted to the east and east-central areas, with some overlaps between the two. Although domestic pigs form an important reservoir for *T b gambiense* infection, various wild ruminants are the major sources for *T b rhodesiense*. The epidemic reemergence of African trypanosomiasis in recent years is exemplified by the death of at least 96 people in Angola in 2003, when 3,115 cases were confirmed among a suspected 270,000 new cases in that country. In the same year it was estimated that some 500,000 people across Africa were suffering from trypanosomiasis, which was likely to have a mortality rate of approximately 80%. Recent reports indicate a spread of transmission from the northern towards the southern parts of Angola. *(Adapted from WHO Map No. 98005)*

T brucei rhodesiense causes disease in East and Central Africa. *T b gambiense* is transmitted mainly between humans by the *G palpalis* group in foci along watercourses in West and Central Africa. *T b rhodesiense* is transmitted by the *G morsitans* groups widely distributed in the East African Savannah. Here, the disease is clearly a zoonosis, with antelopes and domestic cattle as reservoir hosts and afflicting mainly hunters, guides, and game wardens and may occasionally occur in tourists on safari in the game parks of East Africa (Fig. 159–9).

Historically, the disease has caused major epidemics, causing hundreds of thousands of deaths and has prevented human settlement in large areas of Africa. Over 50 million people are now at risk of trypanosomiasis and it has been estimated that the disease causes over 50,000 deaths each year. Most cases are reported in Zaire and northwestern Uganda, with a few hundred or fewer each year in neighboring East African countries.

Case finding and control measures have substantially reduced the risk of epidemics. Epidemics of disease have been associated with a breakdown in health services, for example, in villages in the areas of Lake Victoria in Uganda and more recently in Zaire, Angola, and southern Sudan.

Parasitology

The small mobile trypomastigotes circulate and may be seen in peripheral blood. These flattened, fusiform organisms are pleomorphic, but typically of a similar size to a red blood cell, approximately 20 μm long and have an undulating membrane, attached to the protruding flagellum, extending from the anterior pole of the elongated body (Fig. 159–10).

Parasites multiply by binary fission and may cause chronic parasitemia and evade humoral immune responses by clonal antigenic variations of the major surface glycoprotein.[183]

When trypomastigotes are taken up in a blood meal, by the tsetse fly, they multiply in the mid gut by simple fission. Later, they penetrate the wall of the gut and migrate to the salivary glands. There, as morphologically distinct epimastigotes, they become infective (or metacyclic) trypomastigotes 15 to 30 days after first infecting the fly. In endemic areas, up to 1% to 5% of flies may be infected. Flies remain infective until they die, several months later.

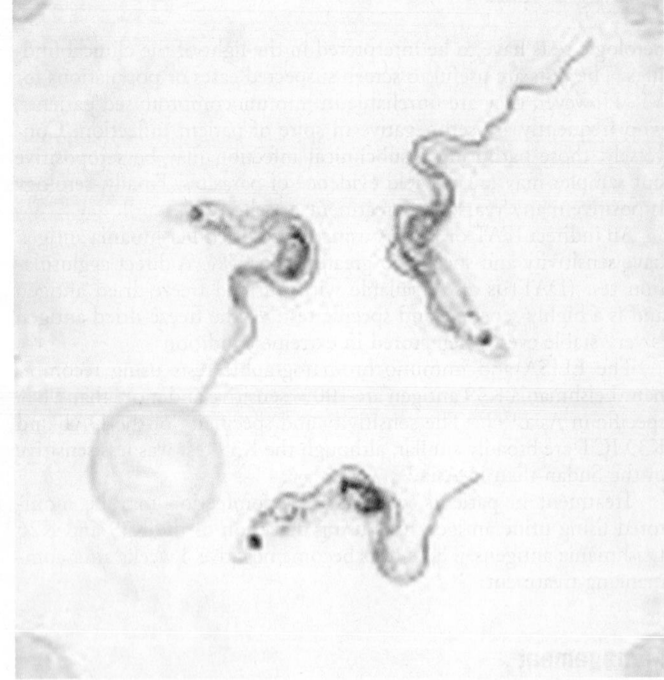

Figure 159–10 Original illustration of *Trypanosoma* (*Trypanozoon*) *brucei gambiense* in human blood by J. Everett Dutton. Polymorphic trypanosomes were first discovered a century ago, in 1895, by Bruce in the blood of domestic cattle suffering from the wasting disease nagana in South Africa. The first observation of these protozoa in humans was by R. M. Forde, who noted, in 1902, "small worm-like, extremely active bodies" in the blood of a sick European seaman in the Gambia. The parasites seen here in a Romanowsky-stained, thin blood film, which were described and named by Dutton in the same year, are responsible for sleeping sickness in west Africa. *(Reproduced by kind permission of the Director, Liverpool School of Tropical Medicine.)*

Pathology

The lymphatic, cardiac, and central nervous systems are involved by the disease. Initially, proliferation of trypanosomes within lymph nodes and the spleen is accompanied by expansion of the lymphocytes, macrophages, and erythrophagocytosis. Polyclonal activation of lymphocytes results in high production of IgM and rheumatoid factor, and anti-DNA antibodies may appear. Later fibrosis and endarteritis supervenes with proliferation of endothelial cells and perivascular infiltration of plasma cells and lymphocytes. The liver shows infiltration of the portal tracts and fatty degeneration.

In *T b rhodesiense*, cardiac involvement may be extensive, with endocarditis, myocarditis, and pericarditis leading to extensive damage and death.

In the second stage of the disease, trypanosomes multiply within the CNS and cause a chronic meningoencephalitis. Edema, hemorrhages, granulomatous lesions, and thrombosis contribute to cerebral degeneration. Lymphocytosis and plasma cells with large eosinophilic inclusions (Mott cells) may be found in the CNS.

Intriguingly, nonpathogenic species of African trypanosomes may be killed by the human high-density lipoprotein (HDL) particles. Haptoglobin-related protein (Hpr), apolipoprotein L-I (apoL-I), and apolipoprotein A-I (apoA-I) act to kill parasites and appear to require assembly for significant biological activity.[184,185] *T brucei rhodesiense* is resistant to killing by human sera as it appears HDL complexes, although internalized, are not targeted to the lysosomes.[186]

Clinical Features

T brucei gambiense

Local inflammation at the site of inoculation causes a distinctive chancre or painful, indurated ulcer appearing 2 to 3 days after an infective bite and lasting for up to a month.

Trypanosomes multiply in the lymphatic system for 6 to 14 days before causing patent infection in the blood, characterized by waves of parasitemia and fever. Later, invasion of the central nervous system may occur by transit of organisms through the choroid plexus and/or endothelial cells.

In the blood stage of infection, fever, headache, and arthralgia are prominent. Lymphadenopathy is common, particularly in the posterior triangle of the neck (Winterbottom sign). There may be intermittent rashes (often circinate erythema), pruritus, or edema. Moderate splenomegaly occurs in 10% to 20% of patients. A few infected patients are asymptomatic.

This early stage of infection may last for up to 2 years or more before CNS involvement, although rapidly progressive disease may occur. The CNS phase of disease is marked by the progressive onset of headache, disinhibited behavioral changes, mood, thought, and sleep disturbance. Wasting is prominent. Signs of diffuse CNS damage in the last phases of the disease include dementia, extrapyramidal and cerebellar dysfunction, and hyperesthesia. Tendon reflexes are increased and signs of UMN lesions widespread. Death usually occurs by intercurrent infection.

T brucei rhodesiense

T brucei rhodesiense is more virulent, causing a more serious acute disease, with systemic features including serous effusions, hepatocellular jaundice, and a mild normocytic, normochromic anemia. Hepatosplenomegaly and lymphadenopathy are common but involvement of cervical lymph nodes is less typical. Myocarditis is rare but may cause death before CNS involvement. Here CNS disease occurs sooner and is more rapidly progressive than *T brucei gambiense* infection and is fatal within 1 to 3 months.

Infection with *T brucei gambiense* may resolve in the vast majority of cases. Where infection persists there is typically a long asymptomatic phase. Numerous lymph nodes are enlarged to 1 to 2 cm in diameter and are soft, mobile, and painless.

The differential diagnosis of trypanosomiasis includes malaria, typhoid, fever, and viral hepatitis in the acute phase, whereas lymphadenopathy may suggest infectious mononucleosis or TB. In the cerebral phase of the disease, syphilis, TB, HIV-associated cryptococcal meningitis, or chronic viral encephalitis must be considered.

Children

Those affected in utero may be born with CNS abnormalities. In children, the disease is more rapidly progressive, and epileptic seizures and psychomotor retardation are the principal features of the disease.

HIV

The frequency of HIV seropositivity has been reported to show no significant differences between those presenting with trypanosomiasis and age-matched controls.[187,188] These results do not exclude that coinfections may modulate the course of the disease or the effectiveness of treatment.

Hematologic and Laboratory Features

The main hematologic features are a normocytic, normochromic anemia and moderate thrombocytopenia.[189] The anemia of trypanosomiasis is multifactorial. Hemodilution, hemolysis, and dyserythropoiesis or ineffective erythropoiesis all contribute to the pathogenesis. Hemolysis may be caused directly by lytic factors released by trypanosomes or indirectly by deposition of immune complexes and subsequent clearance of coated erythrocytes. In vitro studies have suggested that the variant surface glycoprotein from trypanosomes may be shed and taken up onto the erythrocyte membrane, where antibody and complement deposition could contribute to hemolysis. Bone marrow response is inadequate and although the nature of the defect is unclear, there is failure in incorporation of iron into erythroid precursors as is seen in many forms of the anemia of chronic disease. In mice infected with human trypanosomiasis, TNF-α contributes to bone marrow suppression, but detailed studies of the pathogenesis of anemia in human infections have not been reported. Serum IgM levels may be elevated to 4 times normal and with raised IgG levels cause an increased erythrocyte sedimentation rate.

The white cell count may be elevated with monocytosis, lymphocytosis, and circulating plasma cells, but eosinophilia is absent. Plasma cells with eosinophilic inclusion or Mott morular cells may occasionally be seen.

Petechia and purpura may be secondary to vascular injury, thrombocytopenia, and a complex but poorly defined coagulopathy. Abnormal liver function may cause prolonged clotting times. Functionally, both thrombosis and fibrinolysis are increased, and fibrin degradation products (D-dimers) have been are raised in acute disease and in *T b rhodesiense* a frank disseminated intravascular coagulation may become evident.[190]

Examination of the bone marrow shows hypercellularity. Gelatinous degeneration may be seen in wasted patients.

Mononuclear cells are present late in the disease and the cell count corresponds to the degree of neurologic involvement and may reach more than 300/μL in severely ill patients. The CSF protein levels are elevated (0.4 to 1.0 g/L).

As disease progresses, the circulating parasites become scarce. However, anemia and endocrine dysfunction, including amenorrhea, reduced libido, and impotence become apparent.

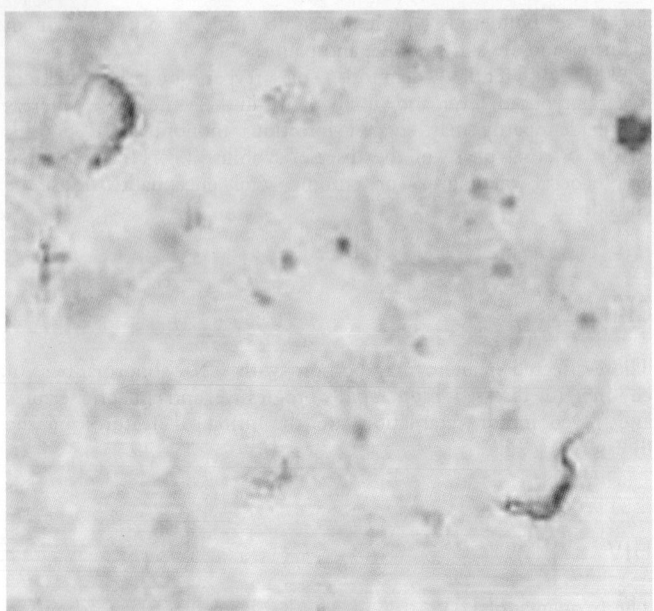

Figure 159–11 *Trypanosoma brucei rhodesiense* in human blood. *T b brucei* parasitizes wild and domestic animals but does not infect humans. The different subspecies can be distinguished with certainty only by biochemical techniques, such as electrophoretic typing of their isoenzymes or by the use of DNA probes. *T b gambiense* and *T b rhodesiense* (and *T b brucei* of animals) are virtually indistinguishable in blood films. Note the small kinetoplast and free flagellum. Both subspecies from humans will infect guinea pigs, but only *T b rhodesiense* is infective to rats, in which the parasites are polymorphic, that is, long, thin, intermediate and short, stumpy forms of trypomastigotes may coincide. (*Giemsa × 900*)

Parasitologic Assays

Direct detection of the parasite is particularly important in the light of the toxicity of the treatment.

Trypanosomes may be detected in lymph node aspirates and in wet and thick blood smears (Fig. 159–11). An aspirate may be taken from enlarged nodes. Aspirated fluid can be examined under a coverslip and motile trypanosomes are typically seen at the edges of the coverslip.

Trypanosomes can be seen in wet smears, where a drop of blood is placed on a slide and examined under a coverslip. Alternatively, thick or thin Giemsa-stained blood films are made as for malaria diagnosis. The sensitivity may be increased by microcentrifugation.[191]

More recent methods to detect the low levels of parasitemia seen in *T b gambiense* include quantitative examination of the buffy coat using acridine orange[192] and small-scale ion-anion exchange chromatography.[193] Here, erythrocytes are retained in the column whereas trypanosomes are eluted and are visible after concentration by centrifugation. The sensitivity of detection with these methods ranges from 10^4 mL for wet smears to 10^2 mL for ion-exchange columns and centrifugation.

In *T b rhodesiense*, examination of the blood is more likely to yield a positive result than aspiration of lymph nodes.

Inoculation of the aspirate or samples into susceptible animals or in vitro culture has been used to detect low level parasitemia. Mice and rats were used to detect *T b rhodesiense*, whereas the multimammate rat (*Mastomys natalensis*) and guinea pigs were used for *T b gambiense.*

Cerebrospinal Fluid

Trypanosomes may be found in the CSF as disease progresses, although a double centrifugation technique may be required to demonstrate organisms. Here, 5 to 10 mL of CSF are centrifuged and the sediment taken up into a capillary tube and recentrifuged before examining the capillary tube under a coverslip (Fig. 159–12).[194]

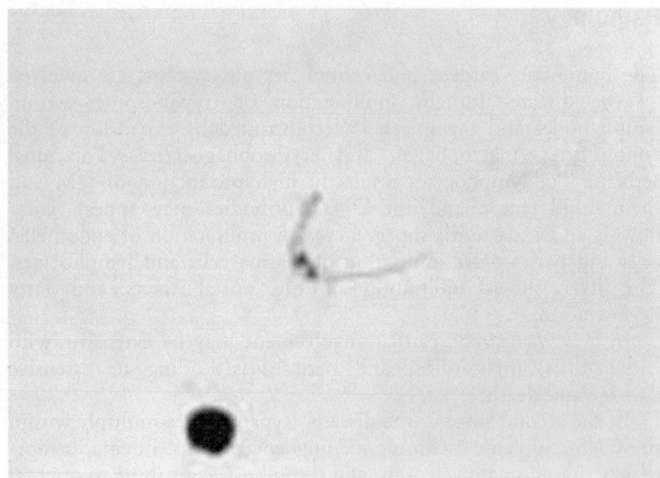

Figure 159–12 Trypomastigote of *Trypanosoma brucei brucei* in cerebrospinal fluid. A single organism is seen in this sample taken from cerebrospinal fluid filtered in a "minicolumn." (*Giemsa × 1200*)

Serology

Serologic tests are use for passive population screening in control programs (for a review, see reference 195). A Card Agglutination Test for Trypanosomiasis (CATT) is robust and can be used without extensive laboratory facilities.[196,197] The test contains freeze-dried trypanosomes with the LiTat 1.3 variant antigens. And can be obtained from the Institute of Tropical Medicine, Antwerp (www.itg.be/itg/). It is quite sensitive (>95%) but lacks specificity due to cross-reactivities with animal *Trypanosoma* spp. Although useful as a patient screening test in hospital for suspected cases of Trypanosomiasis, the predictive value for a positive test falls when screening populations for active cases. It has nevertheless been reported to double the number of active cases found. Some patients may be false-negative using this test if they are infected by parasites that do not express this variant antigen. Further versions of this assay have been developed to use dried blood on filter paper, namely the micro-CATT and macro-CATT, but these are less sensitive than the whole blood assay.

In *T brucei gambiense* serologic tests are not widely available and direct examination of blood and CSF for parasites is the first line of investigation.

The card indirect agglutination trypanosomiasis test (TrypTect CIATT) can detect circulating antigens in *T b gambiense* and *T b rhodesiense* infection by latex agglutination. The sensitivity of the test is 95.8% for *T b gambiense* and 97.7% for *T b rhodesiense* and so significantly higher than that of lymph node puncture, microhematocrit centrifugation, and CSF examination after single and double centrifugation.[198]

A rapid latex agglutination test (LATEX/*T b gambiense*) contains a mixture of three variable surface antigens of the bloodstream form of trypanosomes and has been used to detect antibodies in patients infected with *T b gambiense.* At 1 : 16 serum dilution, test specificity was 99%, whereas sensitivity ranged from 83.8% to 100% depending on the geographic origin of the samples. The test sensitivity falls to 66% for 66 CSF samples from second-stage patients.[199] A rapid latex agglutination test, LATEX/IgM, for the semiquantitative detection of IgM in CSF is available.[200]

Finally, immunofluorescence assays and ELISA tests for antibodies using whole parasites are highly sensitive and specific, although less practical for mass screening.[201]

Treatment

Treatment of Trypanosomiasis depends on the subspecies of trypanosome present. The drugs may be difficult to source and are toxic, so treatment requires expert help.

Early stage *T b gambiense* may be treated with pentamidine for 7 days (IV or more usually IM; 4 mg/kg/day). Hematologic side effects include neutropenia and more general side effects include hypotension, hypercalcemia, hyperkalemia, renal failure, and hyperglycemia. Pentamidine will not cure CNS disease and so examination of the CSF is required after initial treatment of the blood-stage diseases.

Eflornithine (α-difluoromethylornithine) for 14 days (IV; 100 mg/kg, 6-hourly) is effective for CNS treatment for *T b gambiense*.[202] It is a toxic drug suppressing DNA replication by inhibition of ornithine decarboxylase and thus polyamine synthesis and DNA replication. It causes dose-dependent bone marrow suppression with anemia, neutropenia, and thrombocytopenia in the majority of patients. The effects are reversible and are rarely dose-limiting. It is effective neither in children nor in coinfection with HIV, where metarsoprol is required.

Metarsoprol is a trivalent organic arsenical compound and is more toxic but cheaper than eflornithine. It is used in Africa for the treatment of late-stage CNS trypanosomiasis. It is given as three daily IV injections, at a dose of 3.6 mg/kg up to 180 mg, on two occasions a week apart. If the CNS leukocyte count is greater than 20/mm^3, a further three injections are given a week later.

Metarsoprol causes a secondary encephalopathy in 5% to 10% of treated cases and is fatal in half of these.[203] The incidence and severity of encephalopathy may be reduced by concurrent administration of prednisolone (1 mg/kg/day up to 40 mg) started 1 to 2 days before metarsoprol treatment.[204] When steroids are used is necessary to give patients antimalarial and antihelminthic therapy, especially if *Strongyloides stercoralis* is present.

Prior treatment of blood-stage disease with pentamidine may reduce antigen levels and possibly adverse events. Promethazine, anticonvulsants, and antiemetics are important adjunctive treatments prior to commencing CNS therapy.

Polyneuropathy occurs in 10% of cases treated with metarsoprol and may be severe, causing quadriplegia. If neuropathy is suspected, metarsoprol should be stopped immediately and thiamine (100 mg, three times a day) given until symptoms subside.

Patients require prolonged specialist follow-up over 2 years, including blood and CSF examination for parasites. A rising CSF leukocyte count is a good guide to CSF relapse even in the absence of a demonstration of parasites.[205]

In treatment for early-stage *T b rhodesiense*, suramin is given as five IV injections (20 mg/kg, up to 1.5 g) on days 1, 3, 6, 14, and 21. Adverse effects include fever, proteinuria, paresthesia, pruritus, and urticaria. Hemolytic anemia, agranulocytosis, and thrombocytopenia have been reported as side effects.

Combination therapy of antitrypanosomal drugs has now been used to increase the efficacy of treatment and to overcome increasing drug resistance.

It may be possible to use the antitrypanolytic factors in serum to kill pathogenic parasites. The major trypanocidal factor in human serum is apolipoprotein L-1 (apoL-1)[206]; apoL-1 is taken up in the parasite but neutralized in the lysosome by serum resistance-associated protein (SRA), which binds to a specific apoL-1 domain. Truncated apoL-1, which lacks this SRA-binding domain, may kill pathogenic trypanosomes and represents a new avenue for therapy that can be applied to human disease.[207]

Trypanosomiasis as a Transfusion-Transmitted Infection

Trypanosomiasis is a transfusion-transmitted infection. Asymptomatic or early-stage patients with trypanosomiasis are clearly a threat to the blood supply. Patients are excluded in the United Kingdom, Europe, and North America by the general donor queries relating to fever and constitutional symptoms.

In endemic areas, exclusion of infected donors is particularly with early-stage *T b gambiense* is clearly a more complex problem as patients may be asymptomatic for long periods of time if the degree of risk is unknown and no specific screening procedures are in place.

In summary, hematologic involvement in trypanosomiasis is peripheral to the main two features of the disease, but examination of lymph node aspirates, blood, and CSF is essential for diagnosis and management of the disease. Occasional patients may become severely ill and have complex hematologic abnormalities. In endemic areas, trypanosomiasis may pose a risk to the blood supply.

AMERICAN TRYPANOSOMIASIS

American trypanosomiasis (or Chagas disease, named after the Brazilian parasitologist Carlos Chagas), is caused by infection with *T cruzi*. This flagellated protozoon is transmitted by the triatomine insects, the reduviid bugs. The acute phase of infection is characterized by fever and high parasitemia, followed by a chronic phase with positive serology and low parasitemia but with end-organ damage to the heart, peripheral nervous system, and gastrointestinal tract, causing a chronic cardiomyopathy, neuropathy, and megaesophagus and megacolon.

Epidemiology

Chagas disease may occur in the Americas from the southern United States to Chile, but the highest prevalence is in Bolivia and Brazil (Fig. 159–13). There are 10 to 20 million seropositive people in Latin America, although the incidence of new infection is falling rapidly.[208] Infections are found not only in rural areas but also in recent migrants to urban areas in North and South America. It is estimated that approximately 100,000 seropositive individuals are living in the United States. True, endogenous (autochthonous) infection in the United States is vanishingly rare. Visitors to endemic areas are only rarely infected, with only a handful of cases being recorded in intrepid travelers spending time in traditional housing in rural areas. The range of reservoir hosts and species of triatomine bugs transmitting infection is wide.

Parasites may be also transmitted by blood transfusion (see below), vertically from mother to child by breast feeding, organ transplantation, and rarely by sexual transmission. Several outbreaks in Brazil have been reported after contamination of food by triatomine bugs and their feces. Laboratory infection by accidental ingestion or inoculation of parasites is well recorded.

Parasitology

T cruzi parasites are from the order Kinetoplastids and family Trypanosomidae, existing as infective trypomastigotes in the bloodstream of vertebrate hosts. These organisms are fusiform cells, 10 to 20 μm in length, with a distinctive large posterior kinetoplast, containing mitochondrial DNA. They can enter phagocytes, muscle and nerve cells, and a wide variety of other cell types and here transform to oval amastigotes 2 to 5 μm in diameter. They multiply by fission, and amastigotes develop into mature trypomastigotes released on rupture of the cell to begin a new cycle of invasion and multiplication.

Slender, highly motile and broader, less motile trypomastigotes have been distinguished, which may be relatively more infective for host cells and insects, respectively.

The species of triatomine bugs that commonly transmit disease are able to cause extensive infestation of simple mud-and-wattle thatched houses in rural Latin America.[209] Here, Chagas disease is a disease of poverty associated with poor housing. These bugs are infected by circulating trypomastigotes after taking a blood meal on

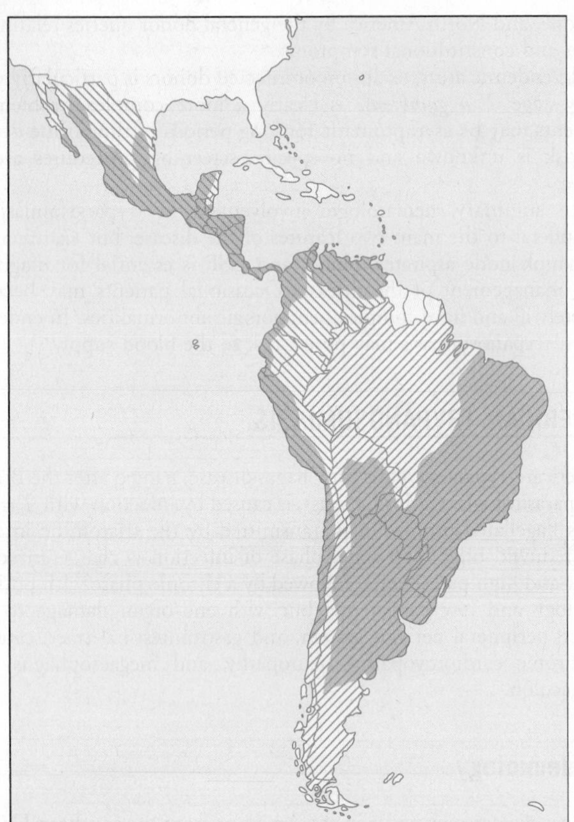

Figure 159–13 Distribution of Chagas disease. Human infection is endemic in parts of Central and South America from the Andes to the Atlantic coast and as far south as the latitude of the River Plate (Río de la Plata) shown here in green. Two major intergovernmental programmes were started in 1991 to eliminate domestic vectors by a combination of spraying residual insecticides in houses, the use of insecticidal paints, and the deployment of fumigant canisters. The countries covered in the two initiatives, the second of which started in 1997, are shown in the figure. The latter program instituted universal blood screening to avoid transmission from infected blood donors. In less than a decade, remarkable progress has been made. Transmission (by the major vector, *T infestans*) was eliminated in Uruguay by 1997 and in Chile by 1999. Major reductions in transmission have also been reported from other endemic countries but, to date, not complete control. *(Southern Cone Initiative; Andean and American Initiative areas.)*

sleeping victims. In the mid gut, trypomastigotes transform into epimastigotes and multiply by fission, before migrating to the hind gut where they develop into metacyclic trypomastigotes, adherent to the epithelium of the rectum. These infective forms are excreted into the feces and people are infected by rubbing this infected material from the bug into the skin or conjunctival membranes. In the human host, multiplication into macrophages is followed by rapid dissemination of trypomastigotes into the blood and hence to tissues.

The genome sequence of *T cruzi* has stimulated a plethora of comparative and genomic approaches to the study of the parasite.[210,211]

Trypanosoma rangeli Infections

The nonpathogenic trypanosomes can be transmitted directly to people by the bite of the triatomine bugs and they exist only as circulating trypomastigotes. No tissue amastigotes exist. Circulating organisms are sparse, but sometimes diagnosis can be made by careful microscopic examination of the distinctive morphology of these organisms in blood smears. The anterior position of the nucleus and small kinetoplast distinguish it from *T cruzi* (Fig. 159–14). The

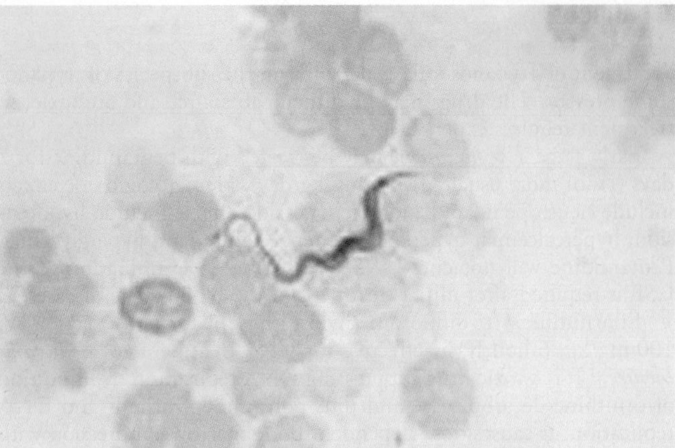

Figure 159–14 *Trypanosoma rangeli. T rangeli* is a long, slender trypanosome also transmitted by reduviid bugs from wild animals to humans. It is readily distinguished by its shape from *T cruzi* in blood films, and appears to be nonpathogenic to humans. (*Giemsa* × *1200*)

antibodies produced to *T rangeli* cross-react with those from *T cruzi* and hence cause false-positive serologic tests for *T cruzi*. However, the species may be differentiated by xenodiagnosis or molecular genetics in specialized laboratories.[212] The importance of recognizing this nonpathogenic infection is to avoid unnecessary treatment for *T cruzi*.

Pathology

There is a wide variation in the pathogenicity of isolates and some regional variation in the clinical spectrum of acute and chronic illness. Molecular typing has demonstrated considerable heterogeneity of *T cruzi* isolates, although the association between strains of parasite and the outcome of infection are unclear. Clearly, the organism must have many mechanisms of the immune evasion to cause chronic infections in a high proportion of individuals. Some of these have been elegantly defined, including resistance to activation of the alternate pathway of complement, specific mechanisms of entering the host cells and evasion of intracellular killing by the oxidative burst and lysozymes. Both $CD4^+$ and $CD8^+$ T cells are important for killing *T cruzi*-infected cells, and interferon-γ has shown to be important to control disease, whereas TGF-β and IL-10 enhance parasite replication.

End-organ damage occurs after tissues have been infected by *T cruzi* amastigotes, but the mechanisms leading to extensive cell damage are not clear. After multiplication, tissue amastigotes form pseudocysts in the heart with little or no inflammatory reaction, although occasionally acute myocarditis with focal hemorrhage and inflammation may lead to heart failure. As the disease progresses, the inflammatory response is increased and is associated with increased tissue damage. There may be an autoimmune component to this inflammatory response but the precise pathogenesis is poorly understood.[213] In the heart, chronic myocarditis leads to a decline in cardiac function. In late-stage disease, amastigotes can be found in almost all organs. Acute myocarditis with focal hemorrhage and inflammation may also lead to heart failure. Involvement of the brain, meninges, liver, lymph nodes, and spleen are common. Damage to the muscle walls and intramural nerve plexus in the esophagus and colon leads to dilation of these structures in the later phases of the disease.

Clinical Features

In about half the patients, a granuloma (or chagoma) occurs where parasites have been inoculated. The tender erythematous papule becomes keratotic and later heals, forming a hyperpigmented scar. When the conjunctiva are inoculated, the extensive unilateral periorbital edema may be prolonged (Romana's sign).

The severity of the acute illness is variable and ranges from asymptomatic infection or a mild febrile illness to a severe, potentially fatal illness with cardiac failure and meningoencephalitis in a minority of cases. Myalgia, generalized lymphadenopathy, hepatosplenomegaly, headaches, facial or generalized edema, vomiting, diarrhea, and anorexia are common features of the acute disease. The disease may be worse in children. The acute illness typically resolves in 4 to 8 weeks.

Chagas disease must be distinguished from typhoid fever, visceral leishmaniasis, brucellosis, toxoplasmosis, and malaria in cases of chronic, febrile illness in endemic areas.

Chronic Disease

The acute phase of *T cruzi* infection is followed by a variable latent or indeterminate phase with no clinical symptoms. Indeed, patients may never present with signs of end-organ damage. However, up to a third of clinically infected patients may develop cardiac involvement and show right-bundle branch block, AV conduction abnormalities, and/or abnormal T and Q waves. The patient may experience palpitations, chest pain, edema, and dizziness or syncope or dyspnea. The heart is enlarged and intramural thrombus may cause sudden death.

In a further minority of chronically infected patients, the gastrointestinal tract is infected with abnormal motility of the esophagus and colon, leading to dysphagia and/or severe constipation. Occasionally other hollow organ systems may be affected.

Pregnancy and Congenital Infection

In pregnant women, Chagas disease can cause spontaneous abortion, premature birth, intrauterine growth retardation, and stillbirth. Congenital infection occurs in 1% to 2% of women with chronic infection. Prompt diagnosis of circulating parasites in neonates at risk of congenital Chagas disease is essential to begin early treatment. It is recognized that infection can also be transmitted by breast feeding. Most children are asymptomatic but 10% to 20% of children have a mild systemic illness with hepatosplenomegaly. More severely affected newborn children have pneumonitis, meningoencephalitis, and diffuse dermal granulomas. Petechiae, purpura, and a generalized bleeding tendency may occur.[214]

Immunocompromised Patients

The disease may recrudesce after chemotherapy for malignant disease, immunosuppressive therapy, or after organ transplantation. The clinical disease may be fulminating with obvious parasitemia. Irregular erythematous indurated lesions have been described during *T cruzi* recrudescence after solid organ transplantation. Here, tissue amastigotes can be demonstrated by fine-needle aspiration.

HIV

Coinfection with *T cruzi* and HIV has been reported from urban centers in Brazil. *T cruzi* develops in end-stage disease with $CD4^+$ T-cell counts of less than 400/μL. Patients may be severely ill, the majority with meningoencephalitis and often with a space-occupying lesion. Typically, the CSF shows a mild lymphocytosis (<100 cells/μL). Parasites may be seen in the blood and occasionally the CSF. Cardiac involvement and heart failure is common.

Hematologic and Laboratory Features

A mild normocytic, normochromic anemia is typical of acute illness. The pathogenesis of the anemia and contributions of hemolysis and bone marrow depression has not been studied in humans, but in experimental infections in mice, uncontrolled infection and TNF-α can be shown to contribute to depressed hematopoiesis. A modest lymphocytosis and increases in liver and muscle enzymes may be present. Nonspecific ECG changes, first-degree heart block, and cardiomegaly suggest early myocardial involvement.

Hematologic abnormalities are not usually found in the late stage of disease where cardiomyopathy with cardiac failure, rhythm disturbance, and angina and systemic emboli from intramural thrombus may occur. Trials of systemic anticoagulation have not been conducted.

Diagnosis

Microscopy

During the acute phase of the disease, motile trypanosomes can be identified in wet preparations or buffy coat preparations using concentration methods and detailed morphology, including Giemsa-stained gently prepared thick and thin films to avoid damage to parasites (Fig. 159–15). Trypanosomes can be aspirated from the chagoma in the acute phase of disease and visualized in a wet preparation of needle aspirates. Parasites may occasionally be found in lachrymal fluid.

Sensitivity is increased by the concentration methods described for *T brucei* above. Organisms may also be sought in centrifuged serum after blood has clotted or by centrifugation after lysis of red blood cells with 0.8% ammonium chloride. Trypomastigotes can also be detected in other specimens including CSF, bone marrow, pericardiac fluid and tissue biopsies. Organisms must be distinguished from the morphologically similar nonpathogenic *T rangeli* (Fig. 159–14 and see above).

After the acute phase, circulating parasites are not visible although inoculation of blood into the susceptible animals (xenodiagnosis), in vitro culture, or molecular methods may demonstrate patent infection. Parasitemia may be obvious in immunocompromised patients in the chronic phase of disease.

Xenodiagnosis

Infection of laboratory triatomine bugs by a seropositive patient is more sensitive than morphology in chronically infected patients. It

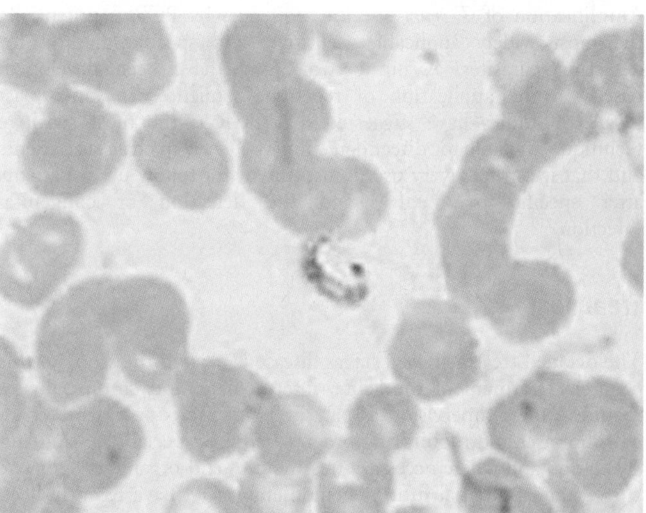

Figure 159–15 *T cruzi* in human blood film. The causative agent occurs in blood films characteristically as short C-shaped or S-shaped trypomastigotes with a prominent kinetoplast. It is otherwise monomorphic. (*Giemsa × 950*)

is also possible to infect susceptible laboratory animals. However, these techniques are only available in specialized centers in Latin America.

In Vitro Culture

Epimastigotes can be cultured using blood agar (Novy Nichol MacNeal [NNN]) medium or other media such Schiender insect medium. After 4 weeks' or more culture at 26°C, epimastigotes may be detected.[215,216]

Serology

Serology is a sensitive method of detecting infection after the acute phase. In Latin America, a number of commercial assays are available using crude epimastigote lysates in a variety of different formats. Serologic tests have used IFAT and ELISA using crude antigen prepared from in vitro cultures of epimastigotes. These tests must be carefully controlled with appropriate positive or negative sera. Chronically infected patients usually give a positive test if titers are greater than 1:80.[217] These have a sensitivity and specificity of more than 95%. These antibodies may cross-react with antibodies to malaria, leishmaniasis, syphilis, and some autoimmune conditions. ELISAs should be used in conjunction with a confirmatory test such as Western blotting.

In South and North America, a number of companies market ELISA-based assays using recombinant antigens, synthetic peptides, or a concentrated extract of excretory-secretory antigens from either Brazil or Tulahuen strain *T cruzi* trypomastigotes (total trypomastigote excretory-secretory antigens [TESAs]). These assays may provide more rapidly available and cheaper tests without loss of sensitivity and specificity (see section Chagas Disease as a Transfusion-Transmitted Infection below for further discussion).

Serologic testing may be useful in the evaluation of people who may have been exposed to Chagas disease, pregnant women, patients about to undergo immunosuppressive treatment or to receive chemotherapy or who have been diagnosed with HIV or other immunosuppressive illness. Children born to seropositive women will have maternally derived IgG anti–*T cruzi* antibodies, but demonstrate IgM anti–*T cruzi* antibodies if congenitally infected.

Molecular Diagnosis

Amplification of *T cruzi*–specific sequences by PCR is potentially the most widely applicable, sensitive, and specific method for detecting parasites. A number of assays have been developed, based on the application of repetitive sequences in kinetoplast DNA.[218] Studies have suggested that PCR is the most sensitive technique available for direct detection of *T cruzi* in chagasic patients and that it can be a very useful instrument for follow-up of patients after specific treatment[218] and the detection of congenital infection.[219]

Treatment

The detailed treatment of Chagas disease is beyond the scope of this chapter. Treatment of the acute, intermediate, and chronic phases requires expert supervision as parasitologic cure is only achieved in half the cases and monitoring progress requires specialist testing and evaluation and where necessary treatment of end-organ damage. The current and potential future chemotherapy[220,221] have recently been reviewed.

Nifurtimox is a synthetic nitrofuran that inhibits pyruvic acid synthesis by inhibition of lactic dehydrogenase. It is given for 30 to 120 days at 3 to 5 mg/kg three times a day. The most serious side effects are peripheral neuropathy, mental disturbance (including psychosis) and hemolytic anemia associated with glucose-6-phosphate dehydrogenase deficiency.

Benznidazole is widely available in Latin America and is given at 2.5 to 5 mg/kg twice a day for 30 to 60 days. Severe hematologic complications are common and bone marrow depression is a serious side effect. Thrombocytopenia may be severe and neutropenia may progress to agranulocytosis. Other serious complications include photosensitivity, neuropathy, and weight loss.[222]

Supportive therapy is required for heart failure and acute meningoencephalitis. Surgery may be required for alleviation of esophageal and chronic dysfunction. In the absence of effective or simple therapy, control of triatomine bugs and an improvement in the housing stock are essential to prevent and control disease.

Trypanosomiasis as a Transfusion-Transmitted Infection

Chagas disease may occur as a TTI and represents a real threat to the safety of the blood supply in endemic areas. It is estimated that 1.5% to 50% of contaminated units cause infection in recipients, a wide range that may reflect the stage of infection in the donor, the type and processing of the component, and the immune status of the recipient.[223]

In endemic areas, seropositivity is high, reaching 50% in some areas of Bolivia and 1% to 2% in major areas in Brazil. Control of blood transfusion–transmitted infection is part of the WHO strategy for control of Chagas disease.[224–226] Serologic screening, tests using synthetic peptide antigens, or a mixture of recombinant antigens to detect anti–*T cruzi* antibodies in chronically infected blood donors, are more than 95% sensitive[227,228] and these serologic tests, replacing those based on crude antigens, have allowed improved coverage of screening of blood donors throughout Latin America.[229]

It is also possible to treat blood with gentian violet (0.25 g/L for 24 hours at 4°C) or with methylene blue to kill circulating organisms. It has also been shown that amotosalen plus UVA photochemical inactivation technology is effective in inactivating *T cruzi*, in platelet concentrates and plasma.[230] In addition, prophylactic benznidazole can be given to immunosuppressed patients receiving blood products in endemic areas.

Outside Latin America, Chagas disease is an occasional cause of TTI, mainly in immunosuppressed patients. It is possible that minor infections are not recognized in healthy individuals. Clearly the high rates of seropositivity in individuals from endemic areas suggest that recent migrants may easily transmit the disease.

In the United Sates, the overall seropositive rate among blood donors is 1:250,000, with local incidence rates reaching 1:7500 or greater in Los Angeles and Miami.[223] These rates are probably underestimates as migration from endemic areas has recently increased. *T cruzi* can be detected by PCR in about half the seropositive donors and remain viable for at least 20 days surviving cryopreservation and thawing.[223] *T cruzi* has been reported to be transmitted after organ transplantation[231,232] and after blood transfusion in seven patients who were immunosuppressed.[233–237]

Donors can be excluded a medical questionnaire eliciting obvious symptoms of acute or chronic disease. Prospective studies have shown these questionnaires would miss many infected donors,[238,239] including those infected congenitally.[240]

In the United States, new tests have been requested by the Food and Drug Administration to combat this threat. A radioimmune precipitation assay (RIPA) is the most sensitive method to detect anti–*T cruzi* antibodies,[241] although RIPA cross-reactivity has been reported in patients with visceral leishmaniasis.[242] It is, however, unsuitable for mass screening. An ELISA based in a concentrated extract of excretory-secretory antigens from either Brazil or Tulahuen strain *T cruzi* trypomastigotes (TESAs)[243,244] had an overall sensitivity of 100% and specificity of more than 94%, and a prototype *T cruzi* lysate-based ELISA has been developed and appears to be 97.7% sensitive and 100% specific.[241]

It is only to be hoped that sensitive screening tests are consistently applied to reduce transmission of Chagas disease by blood products in endemic and nonendemic countries. On a more general note, it is encouraging that the initiatives to control *T cruzi* infection across Latin America are showing real evidence of success.[208,245]

BABESIOSIS

Babesiosis is an intraerythrocytic infection caused by parasites from the order Piroplasmida and the genera Babesiidae. The infection is zoonosis transmitted by hard-bodied ticks and causes fever and hemolytic anemia.[246] Several distinct *Babesia* spp. cause disease in different geographical areas.[247,248]

There are two well-defined *Babesia* species that cause human infection. *Babesia microti* is a parasite of small rodents in northeastern United States and is spread by nymphs, larvae, and adult forms of the hard-bodied ixodid ticks (*Ixodes dammini*). Infection of the white-tailed deer by ticks allows multiplication and spread of the infected ticks. Infections can be transferred to humans by all forms of the tick after prolonged feeding. The infection is therefore most common in people holidaying or working in forested areas of northeastern United States. The offshore islands of Nantucket, Martha's Vineyard, Block Island, and Shelter Island are foci of disease, but it also occurs inland in Connecticut and New York State. Hundreds of cases have been recorded since the first identified case in 1969. Visitors and workers in endemic areas should avoid tick bites using appropriate clothing and repellents.

In Europe, *B divergens* and the morphologically indistinguishable parasite *B bovis* are transmitted to humans by ticks (*Ixodes ricinus*) from cattle. Less than 50 cases have been recorded. European cases of *B microti* and *B canis* infection have also been reported.[247]

A handful of cases of infections with poorly defined *Babesia* spp. have been reported from the western United States. These organisms are morphologically indistinguishable from *B microti* but are distinguished by molecular methods. The MO1-type piroplasm has caused illness in an index case in Missouri in 1992 and the WA1-type and CA1–4 piroplasms caused disease in five cases reported from Washington State and California respectively in 1994.[249,250] A further *B microti*–like organism has been isolated from an asymptomatic woman in Taiwan.[251]

B microti and the WA1-type piroplasms have been transmitted by blood and platelet transfusions. Transplacental infection by *B microti* has been reported.

Parasitology

Parasites appear to be introduced into the bloodstream, where they invade erythrocytes. There they multiply by asexual fission to produce 2 to 4 merozoites. These infective forms are released after lysis of the erythrocyte and begin another cycle of invasion multiplication. Parasites are cleared by macrophages. The contribution of antibodies and cell-mediated immune response has not been defined, although *Babesia bovis* expresses clonally variant antigens on the surface of infected erythrocytes.[27]

Clinical Features

The North American *B microti* infections have an incubation period of several weeks and after infection by blood transfusion clinical symptoms have taken from 17 days to many months to become manifest.[252–255]

The spectrum of clinical disease is wide. *B microti* may cause asymptomatic infection or present with a mild flu-like illness in most cases in people with normal immune and splenic function.[256] The cardinal manifestations are fever and hemolytic anemia. Splenectomy, old age, and immunosuppression, including HIV, may increase the risk of more severe clinical disease.[257–259] The disease may progress to ARDS, disseminated intravascular coagulation, or renal failure.[252] Patients who have had a splenectomy should avoid exposure to ticks in forested areas where the disease is transmitted.

B divergens in Europe predominantly causes symptomatic infection in people who have had a splenectomy.[260,261] Here, the case fatality rate is of the order of 50%.

Patients present with high fever, often with chills and sweats, jaundice, fatigue, malaise, headache, arthralgia, and myalgia. Gastrointestinal disturbances are common and people may complain of dark urine secondary to hemoglobinuria. In some cases, the disease progresses with respiratory failure secondary to ARDS, disseminated in intravascular coagulation and renal failure requiring the appropriate supportive care.[262] Such severe cases resemble severe malaria in nonimmunes and it has been suggested that the pathophysiology-like malaria includes adhesion and sequestration of infected erythrocytes and the release of proinflammatory cytokines. These diseases may be confused with *falciparum* malaria, leptospirosis, or viral hepatitis.

Hematologic and Laboratory Features

The hematologic features of the disease are dominated by substantial intravascular hemolysis.[262,263] Physical examination shows pallor, jaundice, and mild hepatosplenomegaly.

The laboratory findings are those of a compensated intravascular hemolytic anemia and thus feature low hemoglobin and haptoglobin and increased reticulocyte count, serum lactate dehydrogenase, and hemoglobinuria and proteinuria. Moderate thrombocytopenia is common.[255,264] Electron microscopy suggests uninfected erythrocytes are damaged during infection and so likely to be cleared more rapidly than normally.[265] The white cell count is usually decreased with atypical lymphocytosis and occasional evidence of hemophagocytosis. However, leucocytosis may occur, particularly in *B divergens* infections.

The Direct Coombs test is frequently positive for both C3 components and IgG. Polyclonal hypergammaglobulinemia is seen and levels of C3 and C4 are reduced in acute infection.[266] Liver function tests show raised indirect bilirubin and mildly raised transaminase levels.

Diagnosis

The blood films stained with Giemsa or Romanovsky stains show ring-like intraerythrocytic parasites. Morphology is variable and ring, rod, and ameboid forms of babesia parasites may be seen (Fig. 159–16).[246] Occasionally, multiple intraerythrocytic forms can be seen, linked to form a tetrad or colloquially "Maltese Cross." However, at low parasitemia, babesia parasites may easily be mistaken for ring-stage forms of *P falciparum*. Moreover, false-positive sightings *of Babesia* spp. may be due to platelets, nonspecific stain deposit overlying erythrocytes, or indeed other intraerythrocytic inclusions.

Parasitemias are variable and in *B microti* infections may be low or transient.[256] In symptomatic infection, parasitemias typically range from less than 1% to 10% and rarely much higher, more than 70%, in severe infections.

Low-level parasitemias may be detected by inoculation of the blood into susceptible animals, including the golden hamster (*Mesocricetus auratus*), but is not routinely available.

An indirect fluorescent antibody test using crude antigen is available in the United States through the Division of Parasitic Diseases at CDC.[267] Titers greater than 1 : 64 are regarded as positive and has been reported to be 88% to 96% sensitive and 90% to 100% specific.

PCR analysis is the most useful method of detecting or confirming low levels of parasitemia, when serologic tests are positive and can also be used to monitor treatment.[268] Species-specific PCR primers are available to provide precise identification of infected parasites. Nevertheless, some rare forms of piroplasma parasites cannot be classified.

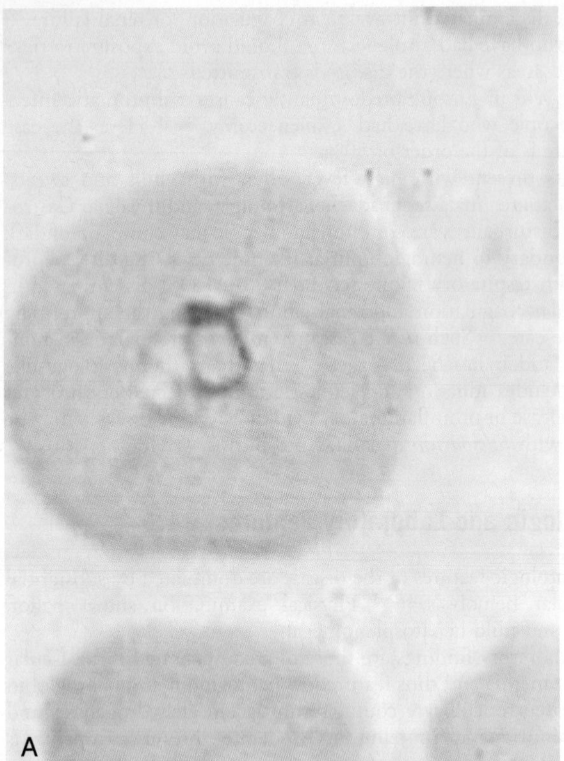

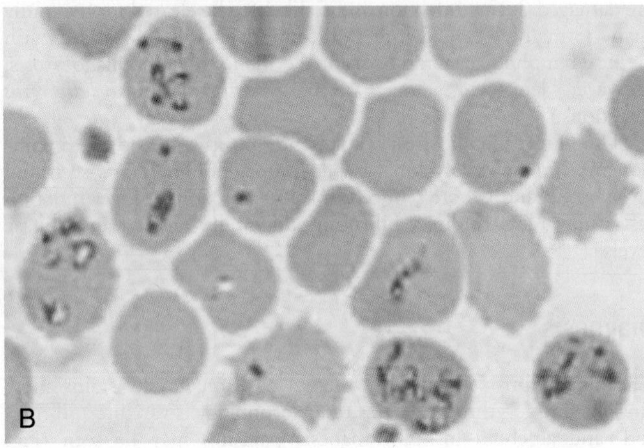

Figure 159–16 Babesia parasites. Human infection with species of piroplasm transmitted by the bite of the tick *Ixodes ricinus* infected from cattle is a rare occurrence. Infection in normal people with this piroplasm may give rise to a self-limiting fever and parasitemia, as in the case of infection with the rodent parasite *Babesia microti* on the northeastern seaboard of the United States via the tick *Ixodes scapularis* (**a**). Heavy red-cell infection may develop, however, in splenectomized patients, leading to fatal hemolytic anemia. This patient died from an infection acquired from the cattle parasite *B divergens* in Scotland (**b**). Other species of *Babesia* that occasionally infect humans, for example, the WA1, CA1, and MO1 isolates from the United States are distinguished by molecular means. (*Giemsa × 700*)

Treatment

Many *B microti* infections are self-limiting, and therapy is used for moderate or severe disease.[269,270] The usual treatment is a 7- to 10-day course of clindamycin (up to 1.2 g twice a day; children 20 to 40 mg/kg/day) and quinine (650 mg three times a day; children 25 mg/kg/day). These two drugs may be given parentally in severe disease.

B divergens infections are often fatal in splenectomized patients and therapy is based on somewhat limited experience. Pentamidine with co-trimoxazole has been used successfully, whereas individual patients treated with pentamidine and co-trimoxazole or quinine, chloroquine, and pyrimethamine have been unsuccessful. Three cases have been treated successfully with large volume exchange transfusions (2–3 blood volumes) and intravenous clindamycin and oral quinine.[271] This regime of clindamycin and intravenous and oral quinine gives the best chance of success in the absence of randomized control RCT evidence.

Atovaquone and azithromycin have also been used successfully and may represent alternative regimes to clindamycin and quinine.

Exchange transfusion has been suggested as a useful adjunctive treatment if the parasitemia rises to greater than 10% and/or in severely ill patients. *B divergens* infections can run a rapidly progressive course and early exchange transfusion should be considered.

The parasite and hemoglobin levels should be regularly monitored during treatment.

Serology and PCR testing of seropositive cases may be helpful in making a diagnosis. An indirect IFAT is available for *B divergens* and *B microti*. The IFAT titer is usually greater than 1:64 in acute infection. The reported sensitivity of the *B microti* IFAT is 88% to 96% and specificity 90% to 100%.[23] Antimalarial antibodies may cross-react in this test.

Babesia and Transfusion-Transmitted Infection

Prevention of babesia as a transfusion-transmitted infection in the United States requires screening donors about a previous history of babesiosis and excluding patients with fever and a low hematocrit level. In the United Kingdom, a conservative approach has been taken and all donors who have visited northeastern United States between May and October are excluded, in addition to the standard criteria of screening out febrile and/or anemic donors.

EOSINOPHILIA

Eosinophilia may be caused by a wide variety of systemic diseases and parasitic infections. The association with parasitic disease is through part of the Th2 T-cell response stimulated by helminths (worms), filaria, and cestodes. In general, protozoan infections, such as malaria, amebiasis, giardiasis, are not associated with eosinophilia. However, case reports do exist suggesting isosporosis, toxoplasmosis, and infection with *Dientamoeba fragilis* can cause eosinophilia.

The rise in absolute eosinophil count depends on the degree of tissue invasion and is therefore modest with tapeworms and adult roundworms resident in the bowel but much higher where invasion occurs, for example, *Toxocara canis* or filaria. Some parasites have migratory larval stages, for example, ascariasis (roundworms) and clonorchiasis.

The differential diagnosis of eosinophilia in those who have lived in tropical areas is therefore wide. Evaluating the patients must begin by establishing the degree of eosinophilia (minimal, $<1 \times 10^9$/L; moderate, 1 to 3×10^9/L; high $>3 \times 10^9$/L), the relation to travel (where necessary), and the presence of symptoms. A wide range of systemic diseases are associated with eosinophilia, and the eosinophil count may be high in drug allergy, pulmonary infiltrate with eosinophilia, and vasculitides.

Eosinophilia in Travelers

Evaluating the cause of eosinophilia in travelers to tropical areas where many parasitic diseases are endemic requires a systematic approach to narrow down likely possibilities by considering existing systemic diseases that may cause eosinophilia (particularly allergy, drug ingestion and autoimmune disease, vasculitis, or arthritis), the areas visited, duration of stay and history of exposure to soil-transmitted nematodes, freshwater potentially infected with schistosomiasis, and rural areas where loiasis, onchocerciasis, and hydatid disease may be contracted.

Physical examination may show subcutaneous swellings associated with filaria or hepatosplenomegaly consistent with schistosomiasis, hydatid disease, or toxocara.

Laboratory examination requires a stepwise approach given the breadth of the differential diagnosis (Table 159–4). The details of specific parasitologic tests are beyond the scope of this chapter, and detailed investigation would certainly require consultation with colleagues in infectious diseases.

Some parasitic causes of eosinophilia may not be diagnosed during the incubation period as larval stages of nematode worms may cause eosinophilic drug migration, but eggs will not be excreted in stools for many months. Moreover, filarial infections do not produce detectable parasites in blood or skin for many months after exposure.

In immunocompromised patients or those about to receive diagnosis, eosinophilia may be crucial, given the risks of giving immunosuppressive therapy such as chemotherapy or hematopoietic stem cell or solid organ transplantation to a patient with a chronic parasitologic infection. Patients with undiagnosed eosinophilia and possible exposure to *Strongyloides* should be given empirical course of treatment.

Table 159–4 Approach to Investigation of Eosinophilia in a Returning Traveler

History	Allergy Drugs and vitamins (L-tryptophan) Regions, localities, and duration of exposure
Physical examination	Skin, subcutaneous tissues Liver/spleen Signs of other systemic disease
Initial investigations	Full blood count and differential white blood cell count Stool examination for ova and parasites (×3) Urine analysis Examination of midday urine for ova and parasites (×3) (in those who have traveled to Africa or the Middle East)
Further investigations as suggested by travel and exposure from history	As suggested by travel and exposure from history *Strongyloides* culture and serology Duodenal aspirate (strongyloidiasis, hookworm) Serology (schistosomiasis, filariasis) Day/night blood films (filariasis)
Further studies if suggested by history and physical examination	Skin snips (onchocerciasis) Chest x-ray (hydatid cyst, tropical pulmonary eosinophilia, paragonimiasis) Soft tissue x-ray (cysticercosis) Sputum examination for ova and parasites (paragonimiasis) Abdominal ultrasound (hydatid cyst) Cystoscopy with or without biopsy (schistosomiasis) Rectal snips (schistosomiasis)

OTHER PARASITIC DISEASES

Many parasitic diseases cause some minor hematologic disturbance. A few may present with distinct hematologic features or indeed syndromes.

Filariasis

Lymphatic filariasis is caused by *Wuchereria bancrofti* and *Brugia malayi*. Infection with *W bancrofti* occurs throughout the tropics but by far the majority of cases are in Asia. The distribution of *B malayi* is more restricted to China, Southeast Asia, and southern India. The male and female adult worms live in the lymphatics and the female worm releases vast number of microfilariae, each 250 to 300 μm in length. Microfilariae develop but do not appear to multiply in the mosquito.

Infection may present with lymphangitis; often recurrent and unlike bacterial infections, the inflammatory features may spread distally. Over time, lymphatic obstruction may cause hydrocele, lymphedema (if severe elephantiasis), chyluria, and tropical pulmonary eosinophilia. *B malayi* causes neither hydrocele nor chyluria.

Filariasis is most easily diagnosed by finding microfilariae in peripheral blood in a wet preparation. Motile microfilariae can be seen under low power and may be concentrated by centrifugation or filtration using a 3-μm filter. They are speciated in thin or thick films by their nuclear distribution and sheath characteristics (Fig. 159–17) and the two pathogenic species must be distinguished from the nonpathogenic species *Mansonella perstans* and *M ozzardi*, which do not have sheaths. Circulating *W bancrofti* antigens can also be detected in the circulation by ELISA or immunochromatographic methods. Adult worms can sometimes be imaged by ultrasound. Filarial DNA from all species can be detected by PCR. Serology is unhelpful as many people become exposed without developing clinical symptoms.

The worms cause marked or severe eosinophilia (see below) with counts greater than 10^9/L. Migration of worms through the lungs may exacerbate the eosinophil count and cause minor respiratory symptoms and fluctuating radiologic signs. Other causes of tropical pulmonary eosinophilia are the worms (helminths) Ascaris, Strongyloides, Schistosoma, and Toxocara. Of these organisms causing pulmonary symptoms and signs, filariasis alone is responsive to diethyl carbamazine. Albendazole and ivermectin may also be used against filarial infection.

Toxoplasmosis

Toxoplasmosis may cause a mild illness or a more prolonged course with constitutional symptoms, atypical lymphocytes and thrombocytopenia. Congenital toxoplasmosis as a result of infection acquired during pregnancy is a cause of neonatal thrombocytopenia, where it may be accompanied by cerebral calcification, hepatitis, and pneumonitis. In immunocompromised patients, new or reactivated toxoplasmosis may cause severe disease, including encephalitis, pneumonitis, and hepatitis. Thrombocytopenia is frequently accompanied by anemia and leucopenia.

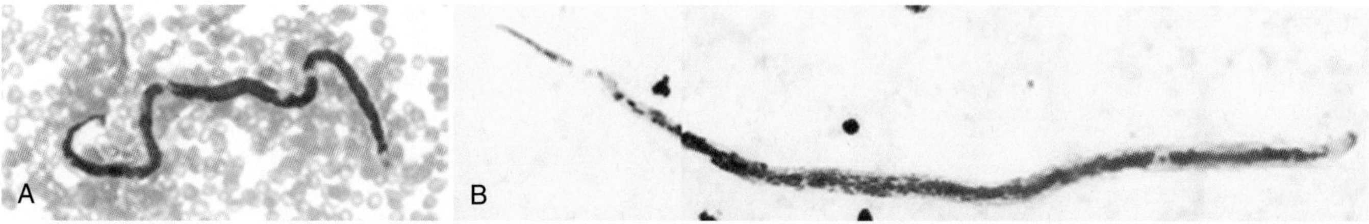

Figure 159–17 Microfilaria (*Brugia malayi*) on thick (**A**) and thin prep (**B**). Speciation is determined by the nuclear distribution and sheath characteristics.

Amebiasis

Amebiasis causes hypochromic, microcytic anemia both as a result of chronic blood loss and as an anemia of chronic disease where disease progresses to formation of a liver abscess. Neutrophilia accompanies severe tissue damage caused by perforation of the bowel or a liver abscess or may be present in a secondary bacterial infection. Sometimes a leukemoid reaction with high white cell count and extreme left-shifted myeloid cells can be seen. Prolonged and/or extensive liver damage may cause prolongation of the prothrombin time.

Giardiasis

Acute giardiasis causes folate deficiency through malabsorption of folate in the small intestine. Chronic infection can cause vitamin B_{12} deficiency as ileal absorption of the vitamin is impaired.

Hookworm Infection

Adult hookworms attach themselves to the lining of the small bowel and take blood meals. The accumulated blood loss may be extensive as worms consume 2.0 mL (*Neomercator americanus*) or 0.5 mL of blood (*Ancylostoma duodenale*) each day. These infections are a common contributing factor to iron deficiency anemia in children where infection is acquired by eating or walking barefoot on larva-infected soil. The disease is usually diagnosed by finding excreted eggs in stool samples, and treatment is with albendazole.

Tapeworm Infection

The fish tapeworm (*Diphyllobothrium latum*) is a rare cause of vitamin B_{12} deficiency. This tapeworm is transmitted in the Far East by eating raw or partially cooked fish. Infection has to be extensive and causes vitamin B_{12} deficiency; however, such cases are rare, even in endemic areas.

Schistosomiasis

Schistosoma hematobium causes blood loss in urine. Infection is acquired by swimming in fresh water, where cercariae from the infected snail host enter the skin and migrate to the blood vessels of the bladder. Chronic blood loss is a cause of iron deficiency anemia in children in endemic areas, but infection is likely to be diagnosed at an early stage in travelers because of the striking symptoms of painless hematuria. Treatment is with praziquantel.

SUMMARY

Parasitic diseases present many problems for global heath. They cause a wide spectrum of hematologic abnormalities, and in endemic areas, a broad knowledge of the parasitic disease is vital for everyday practice. In nonendemic areas, there are a few situations where the diagnosis or management of these diseases may fall within the remit of hematologists and hematology laboratories, particularly malaria and the diagnosis of anemia, cytopenias, eosinophilia, and hepatosplenomegaly. Here, a high index of suspicion is often needed for the diagnosis to be made. A good travel history is crucial to establish exposure to parasitic disease and to prompt the search for the appropriate organisms. Several parasitic diseases pose a threat for the safe supply of blood, and the problems of screening of these infections are far from solved. Beyond everyday practice the pathophysiology and prevention of these diseases pose major challenges for biomedical research and public health.

SUGGESTED READINGS

Antinori S, Calattini S, Longhi E, et al: Clinical use of polymerase chain reaction performed on peripheral blood and bone marrow samples for the diagnosis and monitoring of visceral leishmaniasis in HIV-infected and HIV-uninfected patients: A single-center, 8-year experience in Italy and review of the literature. Clin Infect Dis 44:1602, 2007.

Bailey JW, Williams JE, Bain BJ, Parker-Williams J, Chiodini P: Guideline: The laboratory diagnosis of malaria. wwwbcshguidelinescom. 2007.

Marin-Neto JA, Cunha-Neto E, Maciel BC, Simoes MV: Pathogenesis of chronic Chagas heart disease. Circulation 115:1109, 2007.

Melaku Y, Collin SM, Keus K, Gatluak F, Ritmeijer K, Davidson RN: Treatment of kala-azar in southern Sudan using a 17-day regimen of sodium stibogluconate combined with paromomycin: A retrospective comparison with 30-day sodium stibogluconate monotherapy. Am J Trop Med Hyg 77:89, 2007.

Reithinger R, Dujardin JC: Molecular diagnosis of leishmaniasis: Current status and future applications. J Clin Microbiol 45:21, 2007.

Smith DL, McKenzie FE, Snow RW, Hay SI: Revisiting the basic reproductive number for malaria and its implications for malaria control. PLoS Biol 5:e42, 2007.

Sundar S, Jha TK, Thakur CP, Sinha PK, Bhattacharya SK: Injectable paromomycin for visceral leishmaniasis in India. N Engl J Med 356:2571, 2007.

ter Kuile FO, van Eijk AM, Filler SJ: Effect of sulfadoxine-pyrimethamine resistance on the efficacy of intermittent preventive therapy for malaria control during pregnancy: A systematic review. JAMA 297:2603, 2007.

Tobler LH, Contestable P, Pitina L, et al: Evaluation of a new enzyme-linked immunosorbent assay for detection of Chagas antibody in US blood donors. Transfusion 47:90, 2007.

REFERENCES

For complete list of references log onto www.expertconsult.com

CHAPTER 160

HEMATOLOGIC PROBLEMS IN THE SURGICAL PATIENT: BLEEDING AND THROMBOSIS

Mark T. Reding and Nigel S. Key

INTRODUCTION

Surgical patients often present unique challenges to the consulting hematologist. They may develop hemostatic disorders ranging from unexpected bleeding to pathologic thrombosis, both of which can be potentially life-threatening. Consultation may be sought to assess preoperative bleeding risk and/or to recommend strategies to prevent postoperative thrombosis. The hematologist may be called upon to assist in the management of patients with a previous history of bleeding or thrombosis, and in those with unexplained bleeding or thrombosis in the postoperative period. This chapter will review the preoperative evaluation of bleeding risk, the management of patients with hemostatic abnormalities, perioperative management of patients on long-term oral anticoagulation, and strategies to prevent surgery-induced venous thromboembolism (VTE).

PREOPERATIVE EVALUATION OF HEMOSTATIC RISK

Preoperative evaluation of hemostatic risk begins with a carefully taken history. Particular attention should be directed at specific bleeding symptoms, and any history of bleeding associated with surgical procedures, including circumcision, tonsillectomy, and dental extractions. A detailed family history and record of medication use, including nonprescription medications, should be obtained. In adults, an interview to assess for the presence or absence of bleeding symptoms has a high discriminating power when used in a screening situation, where no bleeding disorder is suspected, but may be less discriminatory for those referred for specialty evaluation.[1] In the pediatric population, the medical history may be less reliable as a screening method because of fewer previous hemostatic challenges.[2]

Obtaining an adequate bleeding history may be complicated by the fact that many hemostatically normal people consider their bleeding to be excessive. Surveys of healthy individuals frequently report excessive nosebleeds (5%–39%), gingival bleeding (7%–51%), easy bruising (12%–24%), menorrhagia (23%–44%), postpartum bleeding (6%–23%), and bleeding following dental extraction (up to 13%) and tonsillectomy (up to 11%).[1,3–5] Thus, a thorough search for objective confirmation of reported symptoms is essential. Also, a constellation of bleeding symptoms, rather than any single symptom, is most helpful in suggesting the presence and etiology of an underlying bleeding disorder.

The need for routine preoperative laboratory testing is controversial. Those in favor of testing point to the asymptomatic nature of some hemostatic abnormalities that may cause surgical bleeding and the occasional failure to obtain a detailed history.[6–8] A prospective study of preoperative screening in children before tonsillectomy found both history and laboratory screening to have high specificity but a low positive predictive value for perioperative bleeding.[7] Another study found that perioperative blood loss in adult cardiothoracic surgery patients could be predicted with a model, which included the bleeding time, prothrombin time (PT), and platelet count.[9] Given the variety of potential hemostatic defects, however, no simple screening system will identify all patients at increased risk of bleeding. Those against routine laboratory testing[10] point to retrospective studies indicating that they rarely detect unexpected bleeding disorders,[11,12] and also emphasize the problems in evaluating false-positive abnormalities. A recent literature review found insufficient evidence to conclude that an abnormal prothrombin time/international normalized ratio (PT/INR) predicts bleeding during invasive procedures.[13] A retrospective review[14] of the value of preoperative platelet count, PT, and activated partial thromboplastin time (aPTT) in 828 patients undergoing major noncardiac surgery found that only 2% had abnormal results, and most were expected on the basis of history and physical examination. Furthermore, no relation between abnormal laboratory tests and intraoperative blood loss or postoperative bleeding complications was found.[14] This is not surprising, given the lack of studies using an evidence-based approach to determine the degree of abnormality in the PT/INR or aPTT at which an invasive procedure may be unsafe.[15] A number of prospective studies have also concluded that routine screening laboratory tests in asymptomatic patients are not predictive of peri- or postoperative bleeding.[16–20] Thus, for an unselected population, in the absence of historical risk factors or physical examination findings suggestive of an underlying bleeding tendency, the likelihood of an unsuspected, clinically significant congenital or acquired coagulopathy is low enough that routine laboratory screening is not warranted,[21] particularly for those undergoing low risk procedures. However, it has been suggested that Ashkenazi Jews should receive special consideration, because of the relatively high prevalence of factor XI deficiency. In this population, screening aPTT might be reasonable to consider.[21]

The bleeding time has long been used to assess primary hemostasis and to predict the risk of hemorrhage associated with invasive procedures. However, there is now general consensus that in the absence of a history of a bleeding disorder, the bleeding time is not useful in this setting.[22] More recently, a platelet function analyzer (PFA-100) has been developed for rapid, quantitative, in vitro global testing of platelet function.[23–27] The clinical sensitivity (94%–95%) and specificity (88%–89%) of this instrument are virtually identical to platelet aggregometery,[27] and it is clearly superior to the bleeding time.[24,28] It has been suggested that the PFA-100 could be used in screening for primary hemostatic defects in routine clinical practice,[29] but such testing has limitations. The PFA-100 has high sensitivity for moderate to severe von Willebrand Disease and severe platelet defects, such as Glanzmann thrombasthenia and Bernard–Soulier syndrome, but it has poor sensitivity for milder intrinsic platelet disorders like storage pool disease, Hermansky–Pudlak syndrome, and primary secretion defects.[28] Although the PFA-100 is most useful when a hemostatic defect is clinically likely, in such cases additional testing is usually necessary to establish a specific diagnosis.[28,30,31] If clinical suspicion is high, further testing is indicated even with normal PFA-100 results.[28] Thus, the PFA-100 should not be used for general unselected screening[31] and adequately designed clinical trials are needed to clarify the role of this device in predicting surgical bleeding risk.[30]

Notwithstanding the ongoing controversy regarding the value of preoperative laboratory screening, it seems reasonable to adopt an approach that it is a compromise, in which the level of hemostatic risk for the proposed surgery or invasive procedure (Table 160–1) forms the basis for an approach to preoperative evaluation (Table 160–2). A hemostatic history should be obtained in all patients, and in those about to undergo a low-risk procedure no laboratory tests are required. For moderate-to-high risk procedures, additional screen-

Table 160–1 Risk of Bleeding With Surgical or Invasive Procedures

Risk	Type of Procedure	Examples
Low	Nonvital organs involved, exposed surgical site, limited dissection	Lymph node biopsy, dental extraction, cataract extraction, most cutaneous surgery, laparoscopic procedures, coronary angiography
Moderate	Vital organs involved, deep or extensive dissection	Laparotomy, thoracotomy, mastectomy, major orthopedic surgery, pacemaker insertion
High	Bleeding likely to compromise surgical result, bleeding complications frequent	Neurosurgery, ophthalmic surgery, cardiopulmonary bypass, prostatectomy or bladder surgery, major vascular surgery, renal biopsy, bowel polypectomy

Table 160–2 Preoperative Hemostatic Evaluation

Routine Screening	
Surgical Risk	**Approach**
Low	History only
Moderate or high	History, PT, aPTT, platelet count
Consultation History	**Approach**
Negative or minimal for bleeding	PT, aPTT, platelet count, biochemical profile, complete blood count with differential, review of peripheral smear
Suggestive of bleeding disorder	Add to above as indicated: platelet function tests, von Willebrand antigen, ristocetin cofactor, factor VIII, factor IX, factor XI, factor XIII assays

ing could include a PT/INR, aPTT, and assessment of the platelet count.

In practice, a hematologist is rarely consulted for routine screening because surgeons have adopted approaches based on their own training and local practice patterns. Rather, consultation is sought because of a history suggesting a bleeding disorder or an abnormal test that is found on screening. The approach of the consultant cannot be one of "routine screening" because the judgment of the referring physician that a bleeding disorder may be present indicates an increased probability of finding an abnormality. If a referral is obtained as a result of an abnormal screening test result, this finding must be pursued and the abnormality fully explained. However, for all referrals the history is still of central importance and must include a thorough review of any bleeding episodes, including hospital records and results of prior hemostatic testing, as well as careful attention to the family history. The physical examination should focus on evidence of bleeding and on identifying systemic disorders such as hepatic or renal disease. If the history of bleeding is negative or minimal, appropriate laboratory testing would include a PT/INR, aPTT and a biochemical profile to evaluate hepatic and renal function. A complete blood count and examination of the peripheral blood smear are useful to identify myeloproliferative disorders, gray platelet syndrome, or thrombocytopenia. If the history is suggestive of a hemostatic abnormality, a full evaluation is indicated and additional specific testing is usually required because von Willebrand disease, mild deficiencies of factors VIII, IX, and XI, severe factor XIII deficiency, platelet function defects, and fibrinolytic abnormalities may not be identified by global screening tests (Table 160–2).

HEMOSTATIC AGENTS

A variety of hemostatic agents are available and may be useful for the prevention or treatment of bleeding in the surgical patient. These agents work through a variety of mechanisms to facilitate hemostasis, including enhancement of primary hemostasis, stimulation of thrombin generation and fibrin formation, and inhibition of fibrinolysis.[32] However, it is important to note that there are a paucity of safety data involving hemostatic agents, as most trials have been designed to assess therapeutic efficacy rather than potential complications including thrombosis.[32,33] The use of desmopressin, fibrin sealants, topical thrombin, antifibrinolytics, and recombinant factor VIIa will be discussed here. Blood products (platelets, fresh frozen plasma, cryoprecipitate) and clotting factor VIII and IX concentrates are discussed elsewhere (Chapters 125 and 151).

Desmopressin

Desmopressin (1-deamino-8-D-arginine vasopressin, or DDAVP) is a synthetic analog of the antidiuretic hormone arginine vasopressin. Intravenous, subcutaneous, or intranasal administration of DDAVP results in transient increases in plasma concentrations of factor VIII and von Willebrand factor as a result of their release from vascular endothelium.[34] Peak levels (typically 2–4 times basal) are achieved 30 to 60 minutes after intravenous and 60 to 90 minutes after subcutaneous or intranasal administration.[35] Doses may be repeated at intervals of 12 to 24 hours, but tachyphylaxis may occur after 3 or 4 doses,[36] limiting further usefulness of DDAVP. Expression of GPIb and GPIIb/IIIa on platelet membranes is also enhanced following administration of DDAVP.[37]

DDAVP is the treatment of choice for patients with mild hemophilia A or type I von Willebrand disease who require low-risk surgical procedures. Moderate- or high-risk procedures usually require administration of clotting factor concentrates.[35] DDAVP may also be useful for patients with congenital or acquired platelet function disorders.[35,37,38] Although initially felt to be promising,[39] the efficacy of DDAVP in reducing blood loss and transfusion requirements associated with cardiopulmonary bypass has not been supported by subsequent clinical trials,[40–43] an impression that has been confirmed by large meta-analyses.[44,45] Worrisome also is the fact that meta-analysis has shown a 2.4-fold increase in perioperative myocardial infarction in cardiac surgery patients treated with DDAVP.[45] Thus, the routine use of DDAVP in cardiac, orthopedic, or other elective surgical procedures is not recommended,[33,46] although certain subgroups of patients, such as those with platelet dysfunction, may benefit.[33,37,46–48] Because of the small but important risk of myocardial infarction,[49] DDAVP should be used with caution in any surgical patient with a history of, or risk factors for, coronary artery disease.[37,46]

Fibrin Sealants

Fibrin sealants (also referred to as "fibrin glue" or "fibrin tissue adhesive") are hemostatic agents composed of purified, virally inactivated human fibrinogen, human thrombin, and sometimes added components such as human factor XIII and bovine aprotinin.[50] These agents reproduce the final steps of the coagulation cascade, resulting in formation of a stable fibrin clot.[51] Commercially available in Europe and Japan for more than 25 years, concern about viral transmission halted development and limited the use of fibrin sealants in the United States until 1998, when licensing was approved by the Food and Drug Administration. Fibrin sealants may be a useful adjunct in achieving surgical hemostasis, reducing the need for postoperative transfusion, and possibly decreasing postoperative wound complications. A relative disadvantage of these agents is that to be effective, they need to be applied to a tissue surface that is dry (and therefore not actively bleeding).

Fibrin sealants are used in cardiovascular surgery to seal suture lines and anastomoses, and are helpful in reducing air leakage in thoracic surgery.[50,52] They may also be used in plastic and reconstructive surgery, hepatic surgery, orthopedic surgery, dental surgery, in the treatment of upper gastrointestinal hemorrhage, to prevent and treat CSF leakage in neurosurgery, and in urologic procedures.[50,52,53] Fibrin sealants may be particularly useful in laparoscopic and bariatric surgery.[52] The use of fibrin sealants has been shown to reduce perioperative blood loss in patients with a variety of congenital bleeding disorders.[54]

In spite of their increasing use across a wide range of surgical specialties over the last several years, recent studies continue to paint a conflicting picture regarding the benefits of fibrin sealants. In a study of 85 patients and 80 controls undergoing unilateral total knee arthroplasty, the use of fibrin sealant (along with autologous platelet gel) resulted in significantly higher postoperative hemoglobin levels, decreased transfusion requirements, and lower incidences of wound leakage and poor healing.[55] In contrast, a meta-analysis of 11 trials investigating the use of fibrin sealant in breast cancer surgery found no benefit in reducing postoperative wound drainage or seroma formation.[56] Some argue that discrepant results between studies may be due to differences in the fibrin sealant preparations used, application techniques, and outcome measures.[52] Regardless, there are few randomized controlled trials in the literature to guide clinical practice, and the methodological quality of the available studies has been criticized.[33,57]

Topical Thrombin

Thrombin derived from bovine plasma has been used for more than 30 years as a topical hemostatic agent in surgical patients. However, plasma-derived bovine thrombin has been associated with the development of antibodies that may cross-react with human blood proteins, leading to hemorrhagic complications.[58–60] Recombinant human thrombin is now being developed as an alternative agent.[61–63] A phase III clinical trial was completed in the fall of 2006 but has not yet been published.

Antifibrinolytics

Antifibrinolytic agents include the synthetic lysine analogs 6-aminohexanoic acid (aminocaproic acid) and 4-(aminomethyl)cyclohexane carboxylic acid (tranexamic acid), and the serine protease inhibitor aprotinin. Although both types of antifibrinolytic agents are used in managing surgical bleeding, the fact that the lysine analogs are orally available facilitates their use in other clinical situations as well.

Aminocaproic acid and tranexamic acid

Both aminocaproic acid and tranexamic acid bind reversibly to the lysine binding site on plasminogen, thereby interfering with fibrin binding, which is required for activation by plasminogen activators.[35] Although tranexamic acid is approximately 10 times more potent than aminocaproic acid and has a longer half-life, both drugs have similar hemostatic effects even in the absence of laboratory signs of excessive fibrinolysis.[64] Extravascular tissue accumulation with inhibition of tissue fibrinolysis and subsequent clot stabilization is thought to explain the efficacy of these drugs.[35]

Because the oral form of tranexamic acid is no longer commercially available in the United States, aminocaproic acid has become the lysine derivative of choice. It is commonly used to treat mucosal hemorrhage (menorrhagia, epistaxis, dental bleeding) in patients with congenital coagulopathies, and is also effective for prevention of oral bleeding in those who require dental work while receiving long-term oral anticoagulant therapy. Although aminocaproic acid is sometimes used to treat bleeding in patients with thrombocytopenia, there is a lack of randomized controlled trials in the literature to guide clinical practice.[38] The use of antifibrinolytic drugs in patients with gastrointestinal bleeding would seem rational given the high concentration of fibrinolytic enzymes in the digestive tract, and a meta-analysis of more than 1200 such patients found reductions in recurrent bleeding, need for surgery, and mortality.[65] However, improvements in the efficacy of other medical and endoscopic treatments have limited the use of these drugs in this setting, although they are still useful for some patients with underlying bleeding disorders.[35] The urinary tract is also rich in plasminogen activators and some clinical trials comparing tranexamic acid or aminocaproic acid with placebo in patients undergoing prostatectomy have shown reduced blood loss, but not a reduced need for transfusion or decreased mortality.[35] Additional data from appropriately designed clinical trials are needed before the routine use of antifibrinolytic agents in urologic surgery can be recommended.[47]

The largest experience with the use of aminocaproic acid in surgical patients exists in those undergoing cardiac surgery. Older meta-analyses have consistently shown that prophylactic treatment of cardiac surgery patients with aminocaproic acid results in a 30% to 40% reduction in postoperative bleeding, without an increase in thromboembolic complications.[45,66–68] Similar results have been shown with tranexamic acid.[37] Other meta-analyses have shown that aminocaproic acid and tranexamic acid are effective in reducing surgical blood loss, but have yielded inconsistent results in reducing transfusion requirements.[46,69] A wide variety of dosing schedules may partly explain these heterogeneous results.[46] A recent meta-analysis showed that both agents were effective in reducing blood loss and transfusion requirements in those undergoing cardiac surgery.[70]

Two randomized controlled trials[71,72] have shown that high-dose tranexamic acid significantly reduces surgical blood loss and transfusion requirements in liver transplant recipients. A recent meta-analysis identified 23 studies with a total of 1407 liver transplant patients who received aminocaproic acid, tranexamic acid, or aprotinin compared with each other or with controls/placebo. This review found that tranexamic acid and aprotinin reduced transfusion requirements without any increased risk for hepatic artery thrombosis, VTE, or perioperative mortality.[73] Additional studies comparing the efficacy of tranexamic acid with aminocaproic acid and/or aprotinin are needed.[37]

A number of studies have demonstrated that antifibrinolytic agents reduce blood loss in orthopedic surgery. A recent meta-analysis[74] identified 43 randomized controlled trials in total hip and knee arthroplasty, spine fusion, musculoskeletal infection, or tumor surgery. Aprotinin and tranexamic acid significantly reduced the number of patients requiring transfusion, with a dose–effect relationship suggested for tranexamic acid. Aminocaproic acid was not found to be effective, although the data were sparse. Similarly, data were too limited to make any definitive conclusions about the safety of these agents in orthopedic surgery patients.

There are case reports of thrombosis associated with both aminocaproic acid and tranexamic acid. However, no significant increase in thrombotic complications has been observed when these drugs have been used in patients undergoing cardiac, liver transplant, or orthopedic surgery, although those studies were not specifically powered to evaluate for thrombotic complications.[35,37,70,73]

Aprotinin

Aprotinin is a polypeptide extracted from bovine lung that inhibits the action of serine proteases including plasmin and kallikrein.[35] In addition to its antifibrinolytic activity, aprotinin is also thought to preserve platelet function and have antiinflammatory effects, both of which may be mediated by inhibition of protease-activated receptors expressed on platelets, vascular endothelium, and neutrophils.[75] The pharmacokinetics of aprotinin are complex and there is wide interindividual patient variability.[46] Renal failure results in reduced clearance and prolonged half-life of this drug. As neither the optimal dose nor the appropriate therapeutic concentration required for effective hemostasis has been definitively established, many different dosing regimens have been used.[46]

A large number of clinical trials have consistently shown that prophylactic administration of aprotinin can improve hemostasis and reduce requirements for transfusion of red blood cells, platelets, and fresh frozen plasma in a majority of patients undergoing cardiopulmonary bypass.[33,37,46] A large meta-analysis of randomized controlled trials using aprotinin in cardiac surgery has also demonstrated decreased mortality and a reduced incidence of repeat thoracotomy, without any increased risk of perioperative myocardial infarction.[45] Furthermore, another meta-analysis of randomized controlled trials showed a lower incidence of stroke in cardiac surgery patients treated with high-dose aprotinin.[76]

Although there is abundant solid evidence that aprotinin effectively reduces blood loss and transfusion requirements in cardiac surgery patients, recent literature highlights the risk of serious adverse events associated with this drug and has fueled much debate. A nonrandomized observational study involving 4374 patients who received elective coronary revascularization compared aprotinin, aminocaproic acid, and tranexamic acid with no treatment.[77] This study found that use of aprotinin was associated with a doubling of the risk of renal failure requiring dialysis, a 55% increase in the risk of myocardial infarction or heart failure, and a nearly doubled increase in the risk of stroke or encephalopathy. Aminocaproic acid and tranexamic acid reduced blood loss to a similar degree, but without any increased risk of adverse renal, cardiac, or cerebrovascular events. The same investigators also recently reported that aprotinin use is associated with an increased risk of long-term (5 years) mortality following coronary artery bypass graft surgery.[78] Another recent cohort evaluation of 3348 patients who underwent cardiothoracic surgery in a single center that reserves aprotinin use for complex surgeries and for those patients whose religious beliefs forbid blood transfusion confirmed an increased risk of postoperative renal dysfunction, but found no increased risk of myocardial or cerebrovascular events.[79] Although aminocaproic acid and tranexamic acid appear to be relatively safe, it is important to note that the numbers of trials and study participants are much smaller for these drugs than for aprotinin. Moreover, trials comparing aprotinin with aminocaproic acid and tranexamic acid have been too few and too small.[33] The Blood Conservation Using Antifibrinolytics: A Randomized Trial in a Cardiac Surgery Population (BART) study plans to enroll 2970 patients undergoing high-risk cardiac surgery to determine whether aprotinin is superior to aminocaproic acid or tranexamic acid in reducing the risk of postoperative bleeding, adverse cardiovascular events, renal failure, and mortality. Although the safety debate remains, and until the results of the BART study are available, aprotinin is still the hemostatic agent of choice but should be limited to use in complex cardiac surgeries or in situations when excessive blood loss is anticipated, such as when antiplatelet agents have already been used.[33]

Although the use of aprotinin in orthotopic liver transplantation was first reported more than 15 years ago, its routine use in this setting has long been debated. Two randomized controlled trials have shown a 30% to 40% reduction in transfusion requirements in liver transplant recipients.[80,81] Aprotinin may also have favorable hemodynamic effects following graft reperfusion,[82] possibly because of inhibition of the release of bradykinin and other vasodilating substances. Prophylactic administration of aprotinin has also been shown to significantly reduce perioperative bleeding in patients undergoing noncardiac thoracic surgery and orthopedic surgery, although the extent of the clinical trial data is more limited.[37]

Because of its bovine origin, aprotinin may cause hypersensitivity reactions. The incidence is less than 1%, increasing to approximately 3% upon reexposure to the drug. Thus, retreatment within 6 months is not recommended.[48,83] In addition to the recent safety concerns noted above, the similar beneficial effects, yet significantly greater cost, of aprotinin compared with aminocaproic acid or tranexamic acid have led some to question the routine use of aprotinin in surgical patients.[48]

Recombinant Factor VIIa

Recombinant factor VIIa (rfVIIa) is a hemostatic agent that is currently licensed in the United States only for the management of bleeding in hemophilia patients with factor VIII or factor IX inhibitors and in those with congenital fVII deficiency. This drug is believed to induce hemostasis at local sites of tissue injury through enhancement of thrombin generation on the surface of thrombin-activated platelets.[84] Recombinant fVIIa also activates thrombin activatable fibrinolysis inhibitor (TAFI), which in turn stabilizes the clot by inhibiting fibrinolysis.[85] The use of rfVIIa in the management of hemophilia and factor VII deficiency is reviewed in Chapters 126 and 127. Accumulating anecdotal experience and case series have generated interest in the use of rfVIIa in other settings, and it is increasingly being used for off-license indications, such as to control refractory bleeding after surgery or major trauma, and to prevent bleeding in surgeries where blood loss is expected to be excessive.

Difficult to control "coagulopathic" hemorrhage commonly occurs without preexisting coagulation deficits in those who suffer major trauma and roughly half of all early trauma deaths are due to hemorrhage. Such bleeding is typically multifactorial, with contributions from the dilution of platelets and clotting factors secondary to large-volume transfusions, excessive transfusion of citrate anticoagulant, hyperfibrinolysis, hypothermia with subsequent slowing of the enzymatic coagulation reactions, and acidosis. In 1999, a report of the successful treatment of a bleeding soldier with rfVIIa[86] generated widespread interest in the use of rfVIIa outside of hemophilia. A number of case reports and series followed, describing favorable results with the use of rfVIIa in trauma patients. A randomized, controlled trial published in 2005[87] that included 143 blunt and 134 penetrating trauma patients currently provides the best evidence regarding the efficacy of rfVIIa in this setting. In a post hoc analysis of the group with blunt trauma, three successive doses of rfVIIa significantly decreased red blood cell transfusion (mean reduction of 2.6 units) and decreased by approximately half the number of patients requiring massive transfusion (more than 20 units of red blood cells). Similar trends were observed in the patients with penetrating trauma but were not statistically significant. Although this study supports the use of rfVIIa in blunt trauma, particularly in coagulopathic patients,[88] many issues require further investigation, including dosing and timing of administration.[89]

Significant hemostatic alterations may result from cardiopulmonary bypass, leading to excessive postoperative bleeding. Hypothermia, hemodilution, and activation of the coagulation, fibrinolytic, and inflammatory pathways all contribute to the complex hemostatic defect associated with cardiopulmonary bypass. In addition, use of newer anticoagulant drugs including direct thrombin inhibitors, low-molecular-weight heparins, pentasaccharides, and platelet inhibitors may also contribute to hemorrhagic risk in cardiac surgery patients.[90] Perioperative bleeding is a major cause of morbidity and mortality and thus the current widespread interest and increasing off-label use of rfVIIa in this patient population.[89] A number of case reports and uncontrolled case series in both adult and pediatric populations have suggested that rfVIIa is effective in decreasing blood loss and transfusion requirements in many patients with intractable bleeding following cardiopulmonary bypass. Although well-designed, randomized, placebo-controlled trials are lacking, considering the current published experience and the pathophysiology of perioperative bleeding in this setting, there appears to be a role for rfVIIa in the treatment of life-threatening, refractory hemorrhage associated with cardiac surgery. There is little evidence to justify the prophylactic use of rfVIIa in these patients. Additional study is urgently needed to address questions regarding optimal dosing, safety, and cost-effectiveness.[89–91]

Elective surgical procedures may potentially be amenable to the possible blood-sparing effects of rfVIIa. A randomized double-blind placebo-controlled trial of 36 patients undergoing retropubic prostatectomy demonstrated greater than 50% reduction in surgical blood loss in patients treated with a single intraoperative dose of rfVIIa.[92] Conversely, however, in a similarly designed trial in 204 noncirrhotic patients undergoing partial hepatectomy, treatment with rfVIIa resulted in a much less dramatic reduction in blood loss.[93] In addition, because the amount of bleeding reported in the control group of the former study has been perceived as excessively high, rfVIIa is not routinely or commonly recommended for elective prostate or other urologic surgery.[89] The published experience in orthopedic, vascular, and obstetric/gynecologic surgery is still too limited and subject to publication bias to draw meaningful conclusions.[89]

Neurosurgical patients are distinct from other groups in that rather than treating massive hemorrhages, the goal is to treat relatively small bleeds within a closed space where even mild or modest benefit may result in significantly better clinical outcomes.[89] A recent, randomized, placebo-controlled study of intracerebral hemorrhage showed that treatment with rfVIIa within 4 hours after the onset of symptoms limits growth of the hematoma, reduces mortality, and improves functional outcomes at 90 days, albeit with a small increase in the frequency of thromboembolic events.[94] Solid evidence supporting the use of rfVIIa for other neurosurgical indications is still limited, but this study has had a major impact on the management of hemorrhagic stroke in North America, and has promoted the implementation of additional ongoing clinical trials.[89]

The primary safety concern with the use of rfVIIa is thrombosis. Most of the initially reported thrombotic events were associated with other risk factors such as preexisting atherosclerotic vascular disease or advanced age.[95] In hemophilia, the risk of thrombosis is estimated to be less than 1%.[96,97] However, with the increasing use of rfVIIa in patients without hemophilia, concerns about the thrombogenic potential of this drug remain. Much of the published literature describing off-label use of rfVIIa reports a very low incidence of thrombotic complications, but it is important to recognize that most of these studies involved patients with already impaired coagulation and were not specifically designed to assess for thrombotic risk. A review based on the FDA MedWatch database[98] has heightened awareness about the thrombogenic potential of rfVIIa. Both arterial and venous thromboembolic events have been reported, and the vast majority have occurred with off-label use of rfVIIa. The thromboembolic event was felt to be the probable cause of death in 72% of the reported fatalities. Half of the thromboembolic events occurred within 24 hours of the last dose of rfVIIa, and many occurred within 2 hours.[98] Similar concerns have been raised by a recent report describing a 9.4% incidence of thromboembolic complications after administration of rfVIIa to trauma patients, with 10 of 14 deaths attributed at least in part to the thromboembolic event.[99] Further studies are clearly needed to better define the efficacy and safety of rfVIIa in surgical and trauma patients.

MANAGEMENT OF PATIENTS WITH HEMOSTATIC ABNORMALITIES

Patients with known hemostatic abnormalities are often referred prior to surgery for assessment of bleeding risk and recommendations regarding perioperative management. The approach to these patients should be according to the following considerations: (a) the risk of bleeding associated with the specific surgery or procedure must be evaluated (Table 160–1); (b) the need for surgery and its urgency must be carefully considered; greater risks are more warranted for correction of life-threatening conditions than for purely elective procedures; (c) the nature and severity of the patient's hemostatic abnormality and the ability to correct it must be recognized; and (d) consideration must also be given to the duration of replacement that will be required, with appreciation of potential bleeding that may be associated with events in the postoperative period such as removal of sutures and deep drains and the need for physical therapy, especially after orthopedic surgery. The following sections discuss perioperative management of some common coagulation abnormalities; the management of congenital factor deficiencies and von Willebrand disease are discussed elsewhere in this text (Chapters 125, 127 and 129).

Thrombocytopenia

Thrombocytopenia is one of the most common acquired hemostatic abnormalities, and the availability of platelet transfusion makes consideration of both emergency and elective surgery reasonable even in severely thrombocytopenic patients. The best index of bleeding risk in thrombocytopenic patients is the platelet count. In nonsurgical patients a threshold platelet count of 10,000/μL is widely used for prophylactic transfusions, yet there is inadequate scientific evidence to determine the platelet count below which the risk of surgical bleeding is increased.[100,101] The American Society of Anesthesiologists Task Force on Blood Component Therapy concluded that prophylactic platelet transfusion in surgical patients is usually indicated when the count is below 50,000/μL and is rarely indicated when the count is above 100,000/μL.[100] Clinical trials addressing this issue are still lacking.[102,103] For low-risk surgery, a single transfusion to increase the platelet count to more than 50,000/μL followed by close observation may suffice, whereas transfusion to maintain the platelet count at greater than 50,000/μL for moderate-risk surgery and greater than 100,000/μL for high-risk surgery is usually appropriate. The optimal duration of postoperative platelet support has not been carefully studied, but even for moderate- or high-risk surgery, platelets may be needed for less than 1 week as they are principally required for primary hemostasis. The platelet count should be monitored closely during the postoperative period, with the expectation that platelet survival will be shortened by infection, fever, or bleeding. In addition, platelet transfusion may be indicated for surgical patients despite an apparently adequate count in the presence of known or suspected platelet dysfunction and microvascular bleeding.

When thrombocytopenia is due to increased platelet destruction (eg, immune thrombocytopenic purpura), prophylactic platelet transfusion is largely ineffective and is indicated only for active, serious bleeding. In preparation for surgery, therapy with steroids and/or intravenous gamma-globulin often will increase the platelet count to a satisfactory level so that transfusion is not needed. Rh_o(D) immune globulin (WinRho) may also be useful in this setting.

Platelet Dysfunction

Patients with platelet dysfunction represent a large group in whom preoperative consultation is sought, typically because of an abnormal bleeding history or the discovery of a prolonged bleeding time or other laboratory assessment of platelet function with a normal platelet count. Drugs are the most common cause of acquired platelet dysfunction. Many commonly used types of medications including aspirin and other nonsteroidal antiinflammatory drugs, antibiotics, antidepressants (SSRIs), cardiovascular drugs, and newer antiplatelet agents, including ADP receptor and GPIIb/IIIa antagonists, can cause platelet dysfunction. Ethanol as well as certain foods and herbal supplements can also inhibit platelets: a careful history is therefore essential. Any drugs that interfere with platelet function should be discontinued before surgery and avoided in the perioperative period if possible.

A number of medical conditions can also cause acquired platelet dysfunction. The etiology may be fairly obvious in cases of renal or liver disease, myeloproliferative disorders, leukemias, myelodysplastic syndromes, or dysproteinemias, but consideration of undiagnosed intrinsic platelet defects (storage pool disease or platelet release defects) or von Willebrand disease may be necessary. Treatment of the underlying disease is the most effective approach, if possible. If not, platelet transfusion may be indicated, but the dose required to achieve hemostasis is difficult to predict and depends in part on the severity of the underlying platelet abnormality. As discussed above, treatment with DDAVP may be appropriate in selected patients. The exact mechanism of action of DDAVP in acquired platelet dysfunction is not well understood, but one study suggests that DDAVP interacts directly with platelets and exerts a priming effect on platelet aggregation stimulated by ADP or collagen.[104] Expression of GPIb and GPIIb/IIIa on platelet membranes is also enhanced following administration of DDAVP.[37]

Renal Disease

Impaired hemostasis has long been recognized in patients with chronic renal failure and is discussed in greater detail in Chapter 156.

The pathogenesis is multifactorial, but is due in large part to alterations in platelet function.[105] Anemia also contributes to platelet dysfunction in chronic renal failure. Red blood cells release ADP, which in turn inactivates vascular prostacyclin (PGI_2), an inhibitor of platelet function.[106] Correction of anemia, now routinely accomplished through the use of recombinant erythropoietin, also improves the rheologic factors that facilitate platelet interaction with the vessel wall. Increase in hematocrit, whether by the use of erythropoietin or transfusions, is accompanied by significant shortening of the bleeding time and improvement of platelet adhesion.[107] In addition to platelet dysfunction and altered balance between mediators of normal endothelial function, the pathophysiology of uremic bleeding is complicated by the comorbidities in this patient population, such as vascular disease and hypertension, and the medical treatment of those conditions.[108]

Owing to the success of erythropoietin, other hemostatic agents now play a smaller, yet still important, role in the management of bleeding in patients with renal insufficiency, particularly those with acute or subacute renal failure. DDAVP was shown in a randomized placebo-controlled trail to normalize bleeding times within 1 hour in uremic patients.[109] DDAVP may be useful for treating acute bleeding, and for prophylaxis prior to biopsy or urgent surgery. Conjugated estrogens also improve bleeding times and reduce or stop bleeding in uremic patients through unknown mechanisms.[110,111] Unlike DDAVP, the clinical effect of conjugated estrogens is delayed for several hours, but they have a much longer duration of action (10–15 days).[35] Thus, conjugated estrogens are more useful for management of chronic recurrent bleeding and perhaps prior to elective surgery. DDAVP and conjugated estrogens may be given concurrently, thereby taking advantage of the different timing of their hemostatic effects.[35] Conjugated estrogens may be given orally or intravenously, usually as five to seven daily doses, and are usually well tolerated, with negligible side effects. Cryoprecipitate can also shorten the bleeding time in patients with renal failure, but concerns about viral transmission and the effectiveness of other hemostatic agents have limited its routine use in this setting.

Liver Disease

Hemostatic alterations in patients with acute or chronic liver disease (Chapter 156) are complex and involve both procoagulant and anticoagulant pathways.[112,113] Although patients with liver disease are typically felt to have deficient hemostasis, this concept has been challenged in recent literature.[113] In fact, patients with liver disease may develop portal vein or hepatic artery thrombosis, which are partly due to a hypercoagulable state.[113]

The coagulopathy of liver disease is usually the result of a combination of several deficits,[114,115] including (a) reduced synthesis of pro- and anticoagulant clotting factors, which is proportional to the extent of hepatocyte damage.[114] Slight prolongation of the PT/INR occurs in mild to moderate liver disease, primarily because of decreased factor VII synthesis. More advanced liver disease is accompanied by additional clotting factor decrements, including factors II, IX, and X, followed by fibrinogen and factor V. Factor VIII levels are typically preserved (and often elevated) even in severe liver disease. (b) Vitamin K deficiency due to impaired enterohepatic recirculation of bile salts and subsequent malabsorption may compound the reduction in clotting factor synthesis. (c) Dysfibrinogenemia due to synthesis of abnormally glycosylated fibrinogen occurs in 60% to 70% of patients with liver disease.[116] This results in a disproportionate prolongation of the thrombin time relative to a mildly prolonged PT/INR and aPTT. (d) Thrombocytopenia is common in advanced chronic liver disease, and occurs in up to 65% of those with cirrhosis.[117,118] Platelet counts rarely drop below 30,000–40,000/μL and spontaneous bleeding on this basis alone is uncommon. Thrombocytopenia results from both hypersplenism and reduced hepatic synthesis of thrombopoietin.[119] Direct ethanol toxicity and folate deficiency may also impair megakaryocyte production. (e) Platelet dysfunction through a variety of mechanisms is also seen in liver disease,[115] although this may be offset by elevated von Willebrand factor levels.[120] (f) Hyperfibrinolysis due to impaired hepatic clearance of plasminogen activators and/or reduced synthesis of endogenous inhibitors of fibrinolysis (α_2-antiplasmin, TAFI) is also common with advanced liver disease.[114,115]

Patients with severe decompensated liver disease and markedly abnormal coagulation tests are at increased risk of bleeding, and surgery should be avoided except as a lifesaving measure. In evaluating hemostasis in patients with less severe disease, the PT/INR and aPTT may be good indicators of decreased synthesis of clotting factors and vitamin K deficiency, but they are poor predictors of bleeding risk. Several published studies have shown the failure of the PT/INR and aPTT to predict bleeding following liver biopsy.[13,121–125] Similarly, preoperative hemostatic testing has generally not been shown to be clinically useful in predicting bleeding during liver transplantation.[126] A study in patients with liver disease found that INRs in the range of 1.3 to 2.0 generally correspond to levels of factors II, V, and VII that are adequate for hemostasis.[127] A preoperative platelet count is needed to identify thrombocytopenia and some assessment of platelet function may be useful to determine whether platelet function is abnormal in the setting of a normal or near-normal platelet count. A thrombin time should also be performed, to evaluate for dysfibrinogenemia. Tests for fibrinogen/fibrin degradation products, D dimer, and euglobulin clot lysis time may be useful in evaluating disseminated intravascular coagulation or accelerated fibrinolysis.

In patients with mild liver disease and mild-moderate PT/INR prolongation (<2.0), serious surgical bleeding is unlikely in the absence of other hemostatic abnormalities, and prophylactic intervention is not necessary for low- or moderate-risk surgery. For high-risk surgery or greater degrees of hemostatic abnormality, transfusion of fresh frozen plasma is the most commonly used approach for correcting the coagulation abnormality, although there are no good prospective studies to guide the use of fresh frozen plasma in this situation. It should be noted that the PT of fresh frozen plasma is approximately 15 seconds, so complete correction of the patient's PT/INR cannot usually be achieved.[128] Administration of platelets should be considered for more severe degrees of thrombocytopenia, although recovery will be decreased in the presence of splenomegaly. Administration of DDAVP may be useful in correcting abnormal platelet function in some cases.[129] Administration of 5 to 10 mg vitamin K will usually shorten the PT/INR if vitamin K deficiency is a contributory factor. As discussed above, antifibrinolytic agents may also be useful in the reduction of perioperative hemorrhage in patients with liver disease.

INTRAOPERATIVE AND POSTOPERATIVE BLEEDING

Excessive bleeding during or after surgery is a serious and potentially life-threatening complication that requires immediate evaluation and a rapid approach to diagnosis and institution of treatment. The first consideration should be to differentiate between "surgical" and "coagulopathic" causes of bleeding. Failure to surgically control bleeding vessels at the operative site is the most frequent cause of postoperative bleeding, and is suggested by evidence of hemorrhage only at the operative site and seen as expanding hematoma, excessive blood in surgical drains, or saturated wound dressings. Conversely, coagulopathic bleeding is suggested by slower "oozing" at the operative site in addition to evidence of bleeding outside the operative field that may be seen as petechiae, purpura, or bleeding at sites of venipuncture, urinary or vascular catheters, or nasogastric and endotracheal tubes.[130] In addition to careful physical examination, laboratory tests including PT/INR, aPTT, and platelet count are an essential part of the evaluation. Other useful tests may include fibrinogen activity, a test for fibrin degradation products or D dimer, and euglobulin lysis time to search for evidence of DIC or fibrinolysis. The peripheral blood smear should also be reviewed to examine platelet morphology and number and to identify possible red blood cell fragmentation that may occur in DIC. The possibility of a preexisting hemostatic abnormality that may have been undetected before surgery should also be considered. Revisiting the patient's family and past medical history, along with a thorough review of preoperative medication use may yield important diagnostic clues.

When evaluating hemostatic tests in surgical patients, changes that normally occur in response to surgery must be considered. These vary depending on the extent of tissue dissection and duration of the procedure. Consumption as well as hemodilution from crystalloid and blood product infusion both lead to acute reductions of coagulation factors and platelets during surgery and in the initial postoperative period. This is typically followed by changes resulting from the acute phase response, including increases in fibrinogen, platelet count, factor VIII, and plasminogen activator inhibitor-1 during the first postoperative week.[131]

Alterations in coagulation factor levels that occur during surgery and in the initial postoperative period can limit the reliability of the PT/INR and aPTT in evaluating the bleeding surgical patient. Clinical practice guidelines have consistently recommended transfusion of fresh frozen plasma when PT/INR and aPTT results exceed the mean reference range by 1.5 times.[100,132–137] However, a prospective study of 16 patients with bleeding caused by dilutional coagulopathy following spinal surgery found significant variability in the PT/INR and aPTT, and suggested that depending on which test system was used, clinical decisions regarding coagulation factor replacement therapy might differ.[138] Conversely, another and larger retrospective study in a similar patient population found that the PT/INR and aPTT had sufficient sensitivity and specificity to be helpful in guiding transfusion therapy,[139] and some consensus panel guidelines do recommend that transfusion of fresh frozen plasma and cryoprecipitate in the bleeding surgical patient be guided by coagulation studies.[140] Additional prospective studies of patients undergoing other types of surgery are needed to more clearly define the role of coagulation testing in the management of surgical bleeding.

Coagulopathy Associated With Massive Blood Loss/Transfusion

Massive bleeding (loss of one or more blood volumes in a 24-hour period) may occur in the setting of severe trauma or major surgery, and requires aggressive transfusion of blood products and other fluids. In addition to a dilutional coagulopathy, other complications including consumptive coagulopathy, hypothermia, electrolyte abnormalities (due to citrate intoxication) and acid–base disturbances may also develop.[141] In patients without a preexisting coagulopathy, replacement of approximately 1.5 blood volumes is the threshold for the development of dilutional coagulopathy.[142] At that point, PT/INR, aPTT, fibrinogen level, and platelet count should be determined. If the PT/INR or aPTT is prolonged greater than 1.5 times control, the fibrinogen level is below 100 mg/dL, or the platelet count is reduced to 50,000 to 70,000/μL, clinical coagulopathy is suspected and appropriate blood product administration is indicated, particularly if additional blood loss is expected. The same coagulation parameters should be measured again with the replacement of each additional half blood volume (ie, 5–6 units of red blood cells).[143] With prolonged hypotension, acidosis, or extensive tissue trauma and ischemia, tissue factor and tissue plasminogen activator may be released into the bloodstream, initiating DIC. Obstetric catastrophes also commonly result in DIC. Consumptive coagulopathy results in hemostatic failure at lower volumes of blood loss or replacement and simple administration of blood components may not correct the coagulopathy. In these circumstances, restoration of systemic and hepatic perfusion (the liver is an important site of clearance of fibrin degradation products and activated coagulation factors) is essential for regaining control of hemostasis.

Cardiopulmonary Bypass

Cardiopulmonary bypass is associated with unique hemostatic changes. Perfusion through the extracorporeal membrane oxygenator has profound effects on platelets and clotting factors: platelet count, hematocrit, and levels of coagulation and fibrinolytic factors are reduced to approximately 50% of baseline after starting bypass, and remain reduced throughout the procedure, with the exception of factor V, which may be further reduced to less than 20%.[144–147] These changes may be caused in part by exposure to artificial surfaces and also by a tissue factor-dependent pathway related to surgical trauma.[148] Cardiopulmonary bypass results in significant platelet dysfunction reflected by release of α-granule contents, the generation of platelet microparticles, abnormal in vitro aggregation tests, and a prolonged bleeding time that usually corrects within 1 hour postoperatively.[144–149] In addition to quantitative and qualitative defects, cardiopulmonary bypass also results in platelet activation, which may contribute to thrombotic and inflammatory complications.[150] Patients with acute ischemic coronary syndromes—who may be candidates for urgent cardiac surgery—are routinely treated with drugs such as GPIIb/IIIa inhibitors that further impair platelet function, which may already be associated with cardiopulmonary bypass. If surgery cannot be delayed, consideration of prophylactic platelet transfusions may be required.[151] Inadequate neutralization of heparin by protamine sulfate given after completion of cardiopulmonary bypass may result in a prolonged aPTT and thrombin time with a normal reptilase time and is an indication for additional protamine sulfate. The use of DDAVP, antifibrinolytic drugs, and rfVIIa to reduce the hemorrhagic complications of cardiac surgery is discussed above.

Orthotopic Liver Transplantation

In addition to the complex coagulopathy of end-stage liver disease, orthotopic liver transplantation is accompanied by major alterations in hemostasis. The surgical procedure itself can be divided into three stages, each with its own profile of coagulation abnormalities.[152] Bleeding during the preanhepatic stage, while the host liver is surgically isolated, is due primarily to the patient's preexisting coagulopathy and is determined by the severity of the underlying liver disease. Excessive fibrinolysis may be encountered during this stage in 10% to 20% of those with cirrhosis. The anhepatic stage begins with surgical removal of the liver. Bleeding during this stage is primarily hemostatic because of DIC and excessive fibrinolysis.[152,153] As the donor liver is reperfused, the postanhepatic stage begins, and serious bleeding is often encountered as a result of a combination of hyperfibrinolysis, metabolic acidosis, hypothermia, electrolyte abnormalities, and sometimes impaired cardiac function.[152,154] The multifactorial nature of the coagulopathy associated with orthotopic liver transplantation requires a combination of therapeutic interventions. In addition to transfusion of blood products, other hemostatic agents such as DDAVP and antifibrinolytics may be useful and are discussed above. There has also been much interest in the use of rfVIIa, and two large randomized, placebo-controlled trials have recently been completed. In one study, a single dose of rfVIIa prior to surgery failed to reduce the number of red blood cell transfusions required.[155] The other study used repeated doses of rfVIIa during surgery, which also failed to reduce the number of red blood cell units transfused or intraoperative blood loss. However, a small but significant increase in the number of patients who avoided red blood cell transfusion entirely was observed in the treatment group.[156] As for other types of surgery, questions about optimal dosing, cost-effectiveness, and safety remain to be answered, and it is still questionable whether rfVIIa should be used as prophylaxis in liver transplant patients outside of a prospective clinical trial.[157]

Perioperative Anticoagulation Management

Hematologists are frequently consulted for advice on the perioperative management of patients on long-term oral anticoagulation. Important considerations to be taken into account include (a) the underlying indication for anticoagulant therapy; (b) in the case of secondary antithrombotic prophylaxis, the remoteness of the most

Table 160–3 Perioperative Management Strategies for Patients on Chronic Oral Anticoagulant Therapy

Clinical Situation	Suggested Anticoagulation Management
Low bleeding risk surgery (dental, cataract, skin)	Reduce dose of OAT to achieve INR ≈ 2
Low thrombotic risk Aortic valve prosthesis without Other thrombotic risk factors* or AF with low stroke risk or VTE > 3 months previously	Stop OAT 4 nights before surgery Safe to operate when INR ≤ 1.4 Restart OAT on evening of surgery Use prophylactic perioperative UFH/LMWH if indicated (depends on type of surgery)
Moderate thrombotic risk Mitral or multiple prostheses or Aortic prosthesis with risk factors for thrombosis or AF at high stroke risk or VTE within past 3 months	Stop OAT 4 days prior to surgery Begin IV UFH† when INR < 2.0 (target APTT = 2–3 × control) Stop heparin 5 hours presurgery Begin UFH prophylaxis and OAT as soon as possible postoperatively; continue heparin until INR has been therapeutic for >48 hours

AF, atrial fibrillation; OAT, oral anticoagulant therapy; UFH, unfractionated heparin; VTE, venous thromboembolism.

*Risk factors include caged-ball or single tilting disc valve, AF, history of stroke/TIA/other embolic event, left ventricular failure, underlying hypercoagulable state, including cancer.

†LMWH at full-treatment doses may also be used for bridging, although an FDA warning about their use in patients with mechanical valve prostheses was issued in 2002 (discussed in text).

Adapted from Dorman BH et al: Identification of patients at risk for excessive blood loss during coronary artery bypass surgery: Thromboelastography versus coagulation screen. Anesth Analg 76(4):694, 1993.

recent thrombotic event; (c) other comorbid conditions that may increase the risk of thrombosis, and/or the potential consequences of thrombosis, while oral anticoagulation is temporarily interrupted; and (d) the risk of bleeding, and/or the potential consequences of bleeding, associated with the procedure. Suggested management strategies are summarized in Table 160–3.

Traditionally, patients on chronic oral anticoagulation were admitted to hospital several days prior to surgery for "bridging" anticoagulation, at which time warfarin was discontinued, and dose-adjusted unfractionated heparin (UFH) was administered by continuous infusion. The short half-life of UFH allows it to be safely discontinued approximately 4 to 6 hours ahead of the procedure. In recent years, there has been a trend toward the use of low-molecular-weight heparins (LMWH) in place of UFH.[158–160] LMWHs have the advantage that in most patients with normal renal function, no monitoring is required, so that therapy can be administered in the outpatient setting. In addition, the risk of heparin-induced thrombocytopenia is less with LMWHs.[161] However, the longer half-life (generally in the range of 4–6 hours) necessitates withdrawal of these agents 12 hours or more preoperatively, although even then, significant circulating anticoagulant activity may remain in the plasma.[162] Bridging with UFH may still be appropriate for some patients, for example those with an estimated creatinine clearance less than 30 mL/min in whom the half-life of LMWHs may be prolonged, in some patients with mechanical prosthetic heart valves (see below), or in those at increased risk of bleeding if treated on an outpatient basis. To date, there are no published randomized control trials data on which to base decisions regarding the relative efficacy and bleeding risks of perioperative anticoagulation management; thus, all recommendations are at best grade 1C+. One concern with the lack of randomized studies is the fact that it has been assumed that heparins are equally efficacious as warfarin in reducing the risk of arterial thromboembolism in patients with atrial fibrillation or mechanical heart valves, whereas in fact there are few data to support this assumption.[163]

In general, as long as it is known to be in the therapeutic range, oral anticoagulation therapy can be continued without any significant increased risk of bleeding in patients undergoing single or multiple dental extractions (see section on management of anticoagulation in patients undergoing dental surgery), joint and soft tissue injections and arthrodesis, cataract surgery, dermal surgery, and upper or lower endoscopy or colonoscopy with or without biopsy.[164,165] For other surgeries, temporary interruption of oral anticoagulation is usually required. Even with a normal diet, 4 to 5 days should be allowed for full or near full reversal of oral anticoagulation targeted to an INR of 2.0 to 3.0. A more rapid reversal over 24 to 36 hours can be achieved if necessary by administration of a small oral dose of vitamin K_1 (1.0–2.5 mg).[166] Large doses of vitamin K_1 (>10 mg) are generally unnecessary for this purpose, and will lead to prolonged refractoriness to warfarin after it is reinitiated. Although frequently used, subcutaneous administration of vitamin K_1 is associated with highly variable absorption, and should be avoided. Intravenous vitamin K_1 has the advantage of more rapid INR reversal compared to the oral route,[167] but it should be administered slowly to avoid anaphylactoid reactions. Urgent reversal of oral anticoagulation prior to surgery may call for the administration of fresh frozen plasma, although large volumes are usually required to reverse the INR, and indeed, complete normalization cannot usually be achieved. Furthermore, the effect is relatively short-lived because of the short half-life (approximately 6 hours) of transfused factor VII. Therefore, concomitant vitamin K_1 administration is also always required to ensure maintenance of adequate hemostasis. Prothrombin complex concentrates (PCCs; 25–50 U/kg) may be used to control hemorrhage in the orally anticoagulated patient who is actively bleeding,[168] and they have been used to expeditiously reverse warfarin therapy prior to emergency surgery.[169] These concentrates are manufactured by fractionation of pooled plasma, and contain all the vitamin K-dependent procoagulant factors (II, VII, IX, and X), with a varying content of heparin and antithrombin, and the vitamin K-dependent anticoagulant proteins C and/or S. They are then subjected to one or more virucidal processes. Concern has been raised that PCCs may be associated with an increased risk of thrombosis.[170] However, the reports of thrombosis with these agents generally preceded the availability of modern day nonactivated concentrates, and occurred in patients with hemophilia who had received >200 U/kg/day for several days. Nonetheless, because the thrombotic risk might be accentuated in the perioperative period, the risk–benefit of these agents to reverse anticoagulation prior to surgery needs to be carefully weighed. Recently, the use of recombinant factor VIIa to reverse anticoagulation prior to emergency surgery has also been reported,[171] but further experience is needed before this approach can be recommended. In either case, the hemostatic agent needs to be supplemented by oral vitamin K_1 therapy to provide sustained correction of the coagulopathy.

Depending on the estimated risk of thrombosis when warfarin is discontinued, bridging with LMWH (or UFH) may be required while the INR is in the subtherapeutic range.[165,172] In this regard, a number of specific issues, which are considered in the next paragraph, surround each of the three most common indications for long-term oral anticoagulation therapy, namely VTE, atrial fibrillation (AF), and mechanical cardiac valve prostheses.[173] Although no LMWH yet has FDA approval for this purpose, large case series support the safety of this approach.[160,174,175] Regardless of whether bridging anticoagulation with UFH or LMWH is employed, the INR should be checked preoperatively to ensure that the pharmacologic effect of warfarin has been adequately reversed. Most surgeries can be safely carried out when the INR is less than 1.5.

Venous Thromboembolism

Patients are generally anticoagulated with warfarin to a target INR of 2.0 to 3.0 for several months to years after an acute episode of

VTE (here defined as deep vein thrombosis ± pulmonary embolism) (see Chapter 135). Before deciding on a perioperative anticoagulation management strategy in these patients, it is helpful to assess separately the risks of bleeding and recurrent VTE in the pre- and postoperative periods.[158] Although somewhat dependent on the type and magnitude of the intervention and method and duration of anesthesia, the risk of thrombosis is magnified up to 100-fold during the postoperative period.[176] In some individuals, for example those with a critically reduced cardiopulmonary reserve, even a minimal risk of pulmonary embolism may be unacceptable. Conversely, the potential consequences of even a modest amount of bleeding may be unacceptable in certain situations, for example, bleeding into an enclosed space such as the central nervous system in a patient undergoing neurosurgery.

It has been estimated that the risk of recurrent VTE after an acute VTE event without anticoagulant therapy is approximately 40% at 1 month and 10% at 2 months.[158] Even in patients appropriately treated with anticoagulants, the cumulative risk of recurrent VTE at 3 months is in the order of 6% to 8%, with approximately three quarters of events occurring within the first 3 to 4 weeks.[176–178] The risk gradually recedes thereafter, such that it is essentially back to baseline by approximately 3 months. However, the baseline risk may itself vary considerably. For example, in the case of an individual with a history of idiopathic VTE (ie, not associated with surgery or trauma), it may be as high as 10% to 15% per annum, at least during the first 2 to 3 years.[179,180] Especially high rates of recurrence may also be seen with underlying cancer, chronic cardiorespiratory disease, or antiphospholipid syndrome.[177,179,180] Therefore, wherever possible, it is usually preferable to delay elective surgery for a minimum of 2 to 3 months after an acute episode of VTE. In the extreme situation where surgery is unavoidable within the first month after an acute VTE, the risk–benefit ratio usually favors bridging with full-dose UFH or LMWH prior to and resuming again as soon as possible after surgery.[160,165,172] Generally speaking, a delay of 12 hours is sufficient to ensure adequate hemostasis after surgery, before heparin is reinitiated, although of course this will also depend on the type of surgery and its customary bleeding risks. When UFH is used, no bolus dose should be administered to avoid over-anticoagulation and the attendant increased risk of bleeding. In the second or third months after an acute VTE, the heightened risk of VTE after surgery still favors full-intensity heparin therapy initiated as soon as possible in the postoperative period. However, the preoperative risk of recurrence has receded to the point where prophylactic doses of subcutaneous heparin or LMWH are probably sufficient.[158] One of these agents should be initiated when the INR is less than 2.0 and continued until approximately 12 hours preoperatively. In most patients who are 3 or more months remote from their most recent episode of VTE, preoperative bridging anticoagulation is usually unnecessary. Standard postoperative prophylaxis with LMWH/UFH is then administered with simultaneous reinitiation of warfarin.

Atrial Fibrillation

Several large prospective studies have established the major risk factors for and rates of embolic stroke and bleeding for patients with nonvalvular atrial fibillation.[181,182] Low thrombotic risk patients include those who are relatively young (<65 years) with "lone" atrial fibrillation and no additional risk factors for stroke, such as a previous history of stroke or transient ischemic attack (TIA), hypertension, diabetes, or left ventricular dysfunction. Their risk of stroke without anticoagulant therapy is estimated to be less than 1% per annum, although there are limited clinical trials data on this topic.[183] At the opposite end of the spectrum, the estimated risk of stroke may approach 15% per annum in elderly patients (>75 years) with a previous history of stroke and one or more of the above risk factors.

A reasonable approach to perioperative anticoagulation management in patients with AF is to discontinue oral anticoagulation 4 to 5 days ahead of the planned surgery, with no bridging therapy except for those at high risk (stroke or TIA within previous month, rheumatic mitral valvular disease, nonvalvular AF with two or more risk factors). A large single-center series using a standardized LMWH bridging algorithm in patients at risk for arterial thromboembolism reported a thromboembolism rate of 0.4%, and a 0.7% incidence of major bleeding.[184]

Mechanical Prosthetic Heart Valves

The major thrombotic risks associated with mechanical prosthetic heart valves are systemic embolization, and valve thrombosis, which usually presents as acute congestive heart failure. These risks are dependent on the location of the valve (higher in the mitral position than the aortic position), number of valves, and type of valve.[185] The earlier model ball-and-cage valves (eg, Starr-Edwards) are considered to be more thrombogenic than the single leaflet tilting disc models (eg, Bjork-Shiley, Medtronic), which in turn are more thrombogenic than the bileaflet tilting disc models (eg St. Jude). The annual risk of thrombosis in patients with mechanical valves not receiving oral anticoagulation will therefore vary with (a) the type and location of the valve(s) and (b) certain comorbidities that increase the thrombotic risk, such as atrial fibrillation, congestive heart failure, enlarged left atrium, left ventricular aneurysm, and intracardiac thrombus. Estimates of the risk of thrombosis without anticoagulation are generally in the range of 8% to 15% per annum, but these figures may be exaggerated owing to the overrepresentation of older-model valves in these series.[186]

It is generally agreed that bridging with UFH or LMWH is unnecessary for the patient with an isolated prosthetic valve in the aortic position without any other major risk factors who is to undergo elective surgery. Warfarin therapy is merely discontinued 4 to 5 days ahead of the procedure, and is reinitiated as soon as possible after surgery with prophylactic doses of UFH or LMWH.[174,187,188] On the other hand, bridging may be indicated for patients with an aortic valve prosthesis and other risk factors for thrombosis, for mitral valve prosthesis, and for multiple valvular prostheses. In this situation, intravenously administered UFH with a target APTT of at least twice the control level is an accepted option. A growing experience with outpatient LMWH bridging (given at full therapeutic doses) suggests that it may be as effective and safe as UFH, at a lower overall cost. However, in 2002, the manufacturers of Enoxaparin issued a drug label "Warning" indicating that the use of Enoxaparin was not recommended for thromboprophylaxis for patients with prosthetic heart valves.[189] This action was prompted by the deaths of two pregnant patients with prosthetic valves from thrombotic complications while taking Enoxaparin. The warning was subsequently reworded to acknowledge that the standard approach—infusional dose-adjusted UFH—has also been associated with adverse thrombotic outcomes in pregnant women with prosthetic heart valves, and that this topic has not been studied adequately.[187,190,191] It is therefore likely that pregnancy represents a very different situation with respect to the failure rate of all heparins in bridging. The accompanying hypercoagulable state and increased plasma volume and glomerular filtration rate (which can affect the volume of distribution of the drug) contribute to the uniqueness of the pregnant patient with a prosthetic valve.[192,193] In the absence of data from randomized controlled trials, consensus is moving toward recommending the use of LMWH without routine monitoring for bridging anticoagulation in nonpregnant patients, based on an absence of evidence of any lesser efficacy or safety.[184,188,191] LMWH is probably also a reasonable option for longer-term prophylaxis in the pregnant patient who cannot take warfarin, although in this situation, routine periodic monitoring of anti-Xa activity is recommended with appropriate dose adjustments to target a peak anti-Xa activity (4–6 hours postdosing) of 0.7 to 1.2 U/mL.[187,191] The relatively low enrollment of subjects with mechanical heart valves receiving LMWH in registries of bridging anticoagulation suggests that there remains some reluctance to use this approach.[160,194,195] Indeed, recent recommendations from the American College of Cardiology and American Heart Association continue to recommend UFH given by continuous infusion rather than LMWHs for bridging in patients at high risk of thrombosis.[187] This category would include all patients with mitral or tricuspid valve replacements and those with an aortic valve replacement and additional risk factors (atrial fibrillation, previous thromboembolism, a "hypercoagulable condition," older-generation mechanical valves, >1 mechanical valve, or a left ventricular ejection fraction < 0.3). It is clear that there is clinical equipoise in the optimal choice of bridging for higher risk patients, and data from prospective randomized clinical trials are urgently required to resolve the issue.

Management of Anticoagulation in Patients Undergoing Dental Surgery

A common reason for hematologic consultation is to provide recommendations for the patient on long-term oral anticoagulation therapy in whom dental surgery, including dental extraction(s), is scheduled. In a randomized clinical trial, a nonsignificant increase in bleeding complications occurred in patients continued on oral anticoagulation without adjustment (other than ensuring the INR was <4.0), compared to an intervention group in which anticoagulation was discontinued for 2 days to achieve an INR less than 2.0.[196] It is likely that the concurrent use of an antifibrinolytic agent mouthwash—which has independently been shown to reduce blood loss in this situation[197,198]—would further diminish the bleeding risk.

Management of Anticoagulation in Patients Undergoing Gastrointestinal Endoscopic Procedures

In deciding on the most appropriate periprocedural management of oral anticoagulant therapy in patients undergoing GI endoscopy, a working knowledge of the bleeding risk associated with the various interventional procedures is required (Table 160–4). Although simple diagnostic colonoscopy is associated with a very low bleeding risk (approximately 0.1%), colonic polyps will be identified in approximately one-third of patients undergoing routine screening. Endoscopic polypectomy may be associated with a significant bleeding risk. Risk factors for hemorrhage include hypertension, polyp size, sessile morphology, and location in the ascending colon. Bleeding is frequently delayed, with a median onset at approximately 5 days, although it may encountered up to 14 days postprocedure.[199] A consensus statement from the American Society for Gastrointestinal Endoscopy recommends continuing warfarin in the therapeutic range in patients who have a low risk of bleeding (eg, upper- or lower-GI endoscopy ± biopsy). On the other hand, interruption of anticoagulation (either temporary cessation or halving the dose for several days preoperatively in all but the highest thrombotic risk patients[200]) is recommended in those undergoing high-risk procedures (Table 160–4). In those patients with the highest risk of thromboembolism (eg, atrial fibrillation with valvular disease and/or prior history of stroke), bridging anticoagulation with heparin is recommended before and after high-risk procedures.[201]

Management of Anticoagulation in Patients Receiving Neuraxial Anesthesia

A special situation concerns the management of perioperative anticoagulation, particularly LMWHs, in patients receiving neuraxial (spinal and epidural) anesthesia or analgesia for surgery. The advantages of these forms of regional anesthesia compared to systemic anesthesia (superior analgesia, decreased transfusion requirements, and lower incidence of thrombotic complications) must be weighed against the risk of spinal hematoma. This rare but potentially disastrous complication is a result of needle- or catheter-induced vascular trauma during placement into the subarachnoid or epidural space. Bleeding usually occurs into the epidural space, probably because of the prominent epidural venous plexus. It presents more frequently as a delayed but progressive sensory or motor deficit, or bladder or bowel dysfunction, rather than radicular back pain. Attention was drawn to this problem in the mid-1990s when multiple cases of spinal hematoma associated with the use of the LMWH Enoxaparin were reported to the US Food and Drug Administration. Significant risk factors that have been identified include the timing of both needle or catheter placement and removal in relation to the last dose of LMWH, the concurrent use of antiplatelet agents, and trauma during the regional anesthetic procedure.[202] Spinal hematomas have been reported with both single-dose and continuous neuraxial anesthesia, although the risk is considered to be much lower with the former procedure. Recommendations designed to minimize the risk of spinal hematoma include (a) placement of the needle at least 10 to 12 hours after the last prophylactic dose, or longer (eg, 20–24 hours) after the last full therapeutic dose of LMWH; (b) similarly, removal of an indwelling catheter should be delayed for at least 10 to 12 hours after a dose of LMWH, most of which have a half-life in the range of 4 to 6 hours.[202] Once-daily prophylactic LMWH regimens are associated with lower trough anticoagulant levels than twice-daily regimens, and they may be a safer choice in patients in whom indwelling catheters are employed,[203] with removal of the catheter scheduled for 20 or more hours after the last dose of drug. It is generally considered safe to administer the next dose of LMWH 2 hours after catheter removal. The synthetic pentasaccharide, Fondaparinux (Arixtra), also carries a black box warning from the FDA, although in fact very little is known about the associated risk of spinal hematoma formation. The long plasma half-life of the agent (21 hours) should be borne in mind when making treatment decisions about its use when regional anesthesia is being concurrently employed.[202] Avoidance of the simultaneous use of antiplatelet agents, including aspirin and nonsteroidal antiinflammatory agents, is advisable in the case of all these anticoagulants. For further information about this topic, the reader is referred to the American Society of Regional Anesthesia and Pain Medicine (ASRA)

Table 160–4 Risk of Bleeding Associated With Various Endoscopic Procedures

Low-Risk Procedures	High-Risk Procedures (Approximate Bleeding Risk (%))
Diagnostic esophagogastroduodenoscopy	Colonoscopic polypectomy (1%–2.5%)
Flexible sigmoidoscopy and colonoscopy ± biopsy	Gastric polypectomy (4%)
Diagnostic endoscopic retrograde cholangiopancreatography	Laser ablation and coagulation (<6%)
Biliary stent insertion without endoscopic sphincterotomy	Endoscopic sphincterotomy (2.5%–5%)
Endosonography	Dilatation of benign or malignant strictures
Push enteroscopy	Percutaneous endoscopic gastrostomy

EGD, esophagogastroduodenoscopy; ERCP, endoscopic retrograde cholangiopancreatography; EUS, endosonography.

Second Consensus Conference on Neuraxial Anesthesia and Anticoagulation.[202]

Prophylaxis for Venous Thromboembolism After Surgery and Trauma

Epidemiology and Natural History

The overall incidence rate of VTE in the community is approximately 1 in 1000 per annum. It has been estimated that hospitalization for surgery accounts for about one-quarter of cases of VTE, and is associated with an almost 22-fold increased risk. Trauma accounts for about half as many additional cases, with a 13-fold increased risk.[176] Additional identified risk factors (which may coexist in these individuals) include malignancy, central vein catheterization, a history of superficial venous thrombosis, and neurologic disease with extremity paresis. Older age is also a strong independent risk factor, whereas hormonal therapies (oral contraceptives, hormone replacement therapy, tamoxifen, and raloxifene) compound the risk in women.[177] In hospitalized patients, DVT is often clinically silent, and pulmonary embolism may be rapidly fatal. It has been estimated that more than 12 million hospitalized patients per annum are at risk of VTE.[204] Because screening for asymptomatic DVT by ultrasonography is expensive yet relatively insensitive,[205] widespread use of prophylaxis is widely acknowledged to be the most effective strategy to minimize the burden of venous thromboembolic disease. This strategy has also been shown to be a cost-effective approach.

Although patients on the surgical and trauma services represent a significant proportion of VTE disease burden, they also provide an important opportunity for prevention through the appropriate design and utilization of validated VTE prophylaxis regimens. A comprehensive treatise detailing the proceedings of the Seventh ACCP (American College of Chest Physicians) Consensus Conference on Antithrombotic Therapy was published in 2004, and is generally accepted as the reference standard for evidence-based VTE prophylaxis in surgical patients.[206] The reader is referred to these guidelines for details of recommended regimens, including dose, frequency, and duration of therapy. Some general principles from this document will be discussed here, with a focus on more recent developments and ongoing controversies in the field.

Using sensitive techniques such as ascending venography, much has been learned about the frequency and natural history of DVT formation after surgical procedures. In many studies, venography was performed at 7 to 14 days postoperatively, to coincide with the termination of pharmacologic prophylaxis. Recently however, it has become clear that DVT formation may continue for up to several weeks after surgery, and the trend in the last several years in certain situations, such as after hip replacement or abdominal/pelvic cancer surgery, has been toward longer duration of therapy, up to 28 to 35 days (discussed further below). Venographic studies have also shown that many DVTs are asymptomatic, that the process is dynamic—with a minority of thrombi extending whereas most resolve spontaneously, and that distal (infrapopliteal) DVTs are much less important from a clinical standpoint, because they are associated with a much lower risk of embolization. These studies have defined the absolute risks of VTE according to these end points, and allowed a given individual's risk of VTE to be assessed preoperatively (Table 160–5). Low-risk individuals are defined as those aged less than 40 years undergoing minor surgery lasting less than 30 minutes, with no additional risk factors. At the other end of the spectrum, very high-risk individuals are those aged more than 40 undergoing major orthopedic lower extremity or spinal surgery, or who have suffered major trauma. A history of prior VTE, or presence of a thrombophilic disorder or cancer further heighten the risk in this group.[206]

Nonpharmacologic Methods of Venous Thromboembolism Prophylaxis

Early ambulation should be a routine component of postoperative care whenever possible. It has been shown to be associated with a lower risk of postoperative VTE, for example after hip replacement surgery.[207] Properly fitted elastic stockings (ie, those not leading to venous compression above the knee) are a useful adjunct in VTE prophylaxis, but are generally insufficient as the sole prophylactic modality. On the other hand, intermittent pneumatic compression devices, both those that provide intermittent calf ± thigh compression or foot pumping action, may be used as the primary modality in all but the highest risk group of patients undergoing high-risk general surgery, or hip or knee surgery, and some forms of neurosurgery. These devices presumably reduce the risk of VTE by preventing venostasis in the immobilized limb(s). Although it has been postulated that they also enhance fibrinolysis by stimulating endothelial release of plasminogen activators, recent data have failed to support this hypothesis.[208,209] Compliance is a constant concern with these

Table 160–5 Recommendations for Prophylaxis of Deep Vein Thrombosis

Approximate Risk Category*	Patients	Calf DVT	DVT	PE	Recommendation
Low	Surgical patients under 40, surgery lasting <30 minutes, no additional risk factors	1%–2%	0.5%–1%	0%–0.1%	Ambulation, leg exercises
Moderate	Surgical patients older than 40, having abdominal or thoracic surgery lasting >30 minutes	20%–30%	2%–10%	1%–3%	Low-dose heparin
	Neurosurgery or other patients with high bleeding risk				Pneumatic compression
High	Hip fracture Hip replacement Knee replacement Open prostatectomy Gynecologic malignancy	40%–80%	20%–40%	5%–10%	Warfarin,† LMWH Warfarin,† adjusted-dose heparin, LMWH LMWH, external pneumatic compression Pneumatic compression Pneumatic compression

DVT, deep vein thrombosis; LMWH, low-molecular-weight heparin; PE, pulmonary embolism.
*Without prophylaxis.
†Given in low-dose regime.

devices, as is the possibility of reduced efficacy in significantly overweight individuals. Intermittent pneumatic compression is often used as an adjunct to pharmacologic prophylaxis in high-risk individuals.[210]

Inferior vena cava filters are occasionally used to prevent pulmonary embolization in patients with extensive trauma in whom the bleeding risks are (sometimes incorrectly) perceived to be too high for the use of pharmacologic prophylaxis [211–213] There are very few prospective randomized trials to support the use of IVC filters,[214] and in one of the few such trials, filter placement was associated with a significantly greater risk of late-onset DVT.[215] Filter deployment may still be a reasonable approach in a patient with a very recent VTE who requires urgent surgery in whom aggressive anticoagulant prophylaxis is not considered feasible. Recently, temporary (retrievable) IVC filters, which generally require removal within 2 to 3 months, are being increasingly used in this type of situation, despite an absence of data from randomized clinical trials.[216–218] However, accumulating experience generally appears to be favorable; for example, in a large retrospective series of almost 450 trauma victims in whom retrievable IVC filters were placed (76% for prophylactic indications), only 3 cases of migration, 2 breakthrough pulmonary emboli, and 6 symptomatic IVC occlusions were recorded.[219]

Table 160–6 Suggested Dosing Regimens for Prophylactic Low-Molecular-Weight Heparins and Pentasaccharide for Orthopedic or General Surgery

Drug	Orthopaedic Surgery	General Surgery
Enoxaparin	30 mg (3000 IU) every 12 hours Begin 12–24 hours after surgery Continue for 7–10 days Consider extended prophylaxis After THA (40 mg once daily Until 28–35 days postsurgery)	40 mg (4000 IU) once daily Begin 1–2 hours presurgery
Dalteparin	5000 IU once daily	2500 IU once daily Begin 1–2 hours presurgery
Tinzaparin	75 IU/kg once daily Begin 1–2 hours preoperatively	
Fondaparinux	2.5 mg once daily Begin 6 hours postsurgery	

IU, international units

Pharmacologic Methods of Prophylaxis

Although the efficacy of aspirin as a primary and secondary intervention in arterial vascular occlusive disorders is now well established, it is not generally recommended for prophylaxis of perioperative VTE, and certainly not as a sole agent. In reality, the true efficacy of aspirin in this situation is probably an understudied area. Intriguingly, in the very large Pulmonary Embolization Prevention (PEP) trial, 160 mg a day of aspirin initiated preoperatively as an adjunctive therapy to conventional prophylaxis was associated with a reduction in symptomatic pulmonary embolism from 1.2% with placebo to 0.7% ($P <$ 0.001), although there was an increased rate of bleeding requiring transfusion.[220]

Several agents form the mainstay for VTE prophylaxis in surgery in the 7th ACCP Conference recommendations (Table 160–6). These are UFH (given subcutaneously, either 5000 Units 2 to 3 times daily without monitoring, or every 8 hours with dose adjustment to maintain a high normal midinterval APTT), LMWH (enoxaparin, tinzaparin, or dalteparin) given subcutaneously once or twice daily (depending on the agent), and warfarin (given postoperatively and adjusted to a target INR of 2.0–3.0). Fondaparinux, a synthetic pentasaccharide that selectively inhibits factor Xa in an antithrombin-dependent manner, is also licensed for VTE prophylaxis in total hip and knee arthroplasty surgery, and hip fracture surgery.[221] Additional antithrombotic agents are currently under development in phase II or III trials, including orally available factor Xa and thrombin inhibitors,[222,223] and inhibitors of the tissue factor–factor VIIa complex, such as recombinant nematode anticoagulant protein (rNAP-c2).[224] Potential drawbacks of these newer agents include the lack of specific antidotes in the event of bleeding,[225] and the fact that many of these drugs are excreted via the kidney, necessitating caution in patients with renal impairment. An advantage of LMWHs and other structurally unrelated molecules over UFH is (respectively) the reduced risk of heparin-induced thrombocytopenia. For example, clinically apparent HIT was present in 2.7% of patients receiving prophylactic doses of UFH after hip surgery, compared to 0% in this cohort who received LMWH ($P = 0.0018$).[226] However, HIT may occur as a rare complication of LMWHs such as Enoxaparin, Tinzaparin, or Dalteparin.[161] On the other hand, although the anti-PF4–heparin antibodies responsible for HIT may be stimulated during Fondaparinux therapy, they do not react against the PF4–Fondaparinux complex,[227] and the clinical syndrome (thrombocytopenia and thrombosis) has not been described with this agent.

In general, all these forms of thromboprophylaxis are associated with roughly a 70% risk reduction in perioperative VTE, but there are some important differences in efficacy that have been demonstrated in specific types of surgery,[206] which are briefly outlined below. Conversely, the bleeding risks are principally related to dose and host risk factors, and to a lesser extent the choice of agent and timing of administration in relation to surgery. In general surgery, it is usually recommended that either UFH or LMWH be given 1 to 2 hours in advance of surgery.[163] In orthopedic surgery in the United States, LMWH is traditionally initiated 12 hours postoperatively, which may in fact be suboptimal when compared to regimens in which these agents are initiated in close proximity to surgery (between 2 hours preoperatively and 6–8 hours postoperatively).[228] Details of suggested dosing schedules are shown in Table 160–6.

Orthopedic Surgery

Major orthopedic surgery (total hip and knee arthroplasty, hip fracture, and spinal surgery) is among the highest risk forms of surgery, with venographically detected DVT occurring in 40% to 70% of patients not receiving prophylaxis.[229] The corresponding rates of death due to PE is 0.1% to 0.4% of patients undergoing total hip replacement, 0.2% to 0.7% undergoing total knee replacement, and 3.6% to 12.9% following hip fracture surgery.[206] Meta-analysis has demonstrated that the protection against proximal DVT afforded by low-dose UFH may be inferior to LMWH. An acceptable alternative to LMWH is warfarin, which is preferred by many orthopedic surgeons. Most commonly, warfarin is initiated the evening of surgery, although in some protocols it is begun on the evening prior to surgery, without any apparent difference in efficacy. Dose adjustment is performed to achieve a target INR of 2.5 ± 0.5. The efficacy of LMWH is either equivalent or slightly superior to warfarin in total hip arthroplasty, and more definitively superior in total knee arthroplasty, albeit at the expense of a mildly increased risk of bleeding.[206]

Fondaparinux (2.5 mg once daily) was compared with enoxaparin (40 mg once daily or 30 mg twice daily) in hip and knee arthroplasty, and in hip fracture repair.[230–233] In a meta-analysis of the major trials, which included 7344 patients, there was a statistically significant 55% relative risk reduction (6.8% vs 13.7%) in the incidence of venographically detected DVT (and proximal DVT). However, there was no difference in the incidence of symptomatic VTE or fatal PE, and major bleeding was more frequently encountered in the fondaparinux group compared to the enoxaparin group (2.7% vs 1.7%).[232,233] It remains an open question whether the higher efficacy at the expense of greater bleeding risk with fondaparinux is explained by the fact that the first dose was usually administered earlier than enoxaparin (6 hours vs 12 hours postoperatively).

Prolonged prophylaxis beyond the usual 7 to 10 days is a pertinent consideration for total hip arthroplasty patients, where the median time to diagnosis of symptomatic VTE (occurring in 2.8% of patients within 3 months) is 17 days postoperatively. In contrast, VTE after total knee arthroplasty (occurring in 2.1% of patients within 3 months) tends to occur much earlier, after a median of 7 days.[229] By meta-analysis, trials in which LMWH prophylaxis was extended for 30 to 42 days were associated with a significant reduction in the frequency of symptomatic VTE, without any increase in major bleeding.[234,235] This was especially true in total hip arthroplasty, where the absolute risk reduction in symptomatic VTE was approximately 2%.[234] Prolonged therapy with warfarin may be similarly effective, although some studies,[236] but not others,[237] have raised concerns about the bleeding risks. As yet, despite early indications of favorable cost-effectiveness, long-term prophylaxis with LMWH or warfarin is not widely used. As an alternative strategy during this period, aspirin is recommended.[238]

Recently, it has been demonstrated that patients with comparatively minor forms of lower-extremity orthopedic surgery, such as therapeutic arthroscopic knee procedures, are also at increased risk of VTE.[239,240] A recent meta-analysis concluded that the total incidence of asymptomatic DVT after knee arthroscopy was 9.9% (95% confidence interval, 8.1%–11.7%), with a proximal DVT incidence of 2.1% (95% confidence interval, 1.2%–3.0%).[241] Routine use of pharmacologic prophylaxis is probably not warranted, although it would be appropriately considered in a patient with a previous history of VTE, or other risk factors, such as prolonged tourniquet time (>60 min), a known thrombophilic disorder, or on estrogen therapy.

Trauma

Up to 60% of trauma patients suffer venographically demonstrated DVT within 14 days of admission,[242] although the range of reported VTE complication rate in trauma varies enormously in the literature, possibly reflecting not only variable study methodologies but also study subject heterogeneity.[243,244] Factors that appear to be independently associated with a greater risk of thrombosis following trauma include (a) age >40 years, (b) lower-extremity fracture, (c) major head injury, (d) more than 3 ventilator days, (e) venous injury, and (f) major surgical procedure.[245] Although there is general agreement that some form of prophylaxis is routinely warranted, there is confusion (even from prospective randomized clinical trials) whether pharmacologic prophylaxis is superior to nonpharmacologic prophylaxis,[243,246,247] and whether LMWH have a specific advantage over UFH.[248,249] Nonpharmacologic methods of prophylaxis may be difficult to apply in some cases with external fixation devices in the lower extremities, and it is therefore recommended that intermittent pneumatic compression alone be used only when both lower extremities are available. Routine surveillance using duplex ultrasound scans are not recommended unless VTE prophylaxis cannot be employed. An extensive review of the scientific evidence and development of evidence-based practice consensus guidelines in trauma surgery published in 2002 recommended that, where feasible, prophylaxis using LMWH rather than UFH be preferred for patients with pelvic, complex lower-extremity, or spinal fractures,[248,250] especially with partial or complete motor paralysis. However, the EAST guidelines acknowledge a paucity of Level 1 evidence to support the prophylaxis algorithms.[250] A subsequent registry of 743 high-risk trauma patients prescribed once-daily prophylactic dose LMWH, regardless of the need for invasive procedures and including those with stable intracranial injuries, did not document any exacerbations of head injury due to bleeding.[251] Notably in this study, the LMWH was initiated an average of 3.3 days after admission. However, for patients at very high risk for both VTE and bleeding with anticoagulation, IVC filter placement—generally using retrievable devices—may occasionally be justified.

Even without the associated risks of surgery, bony fracture and immobilization may be sufficient stimuli to increase the incidence of VTE. For example, a 19% rate of venographically demonstrated DVT was noted in patients requiring plaster immobilization or bracing after a leg fracture or ruptured Achilles tendon. This was reduced to 9% in a matched group treated with prophylactic LMWH throughout the period of immobilization.[252] Here again, however, the evidence overall does not clearly support the need for routine pharmacologic VTE prophylaxis in all patients treated for lower-extremity fracture.

Neurosurgery

Patients undergoing neurosurgery involving craniotomy, particularly when performed for high-grade glioma,[253,254] are also at high risk with respect to the risk for VTE. Symptomatic events occur in as many as 6% of patients within the first 3 months postoperatively.[253] The need for pharmacologic prophylaxis is tempered by the potentially disastrous consequences of intracranial bleeding as a complication of therapy. This concern has led some to recommend a conservative strategy of nonpharmacologic prophylaxis only. In a landmark randomized, placebo-controlled trial, Agnelli and colleagues demonstrated that Enoxaparin 40 mg daily (initiated within 24 hours postoperatively) was associated with a 49% relative risk reduction in venographically demonstrated DVT compared to placebo in patients undergoing elective cranial or spinal surgery (97% for tumors). The rate of symptomatic VTE was reduced from 6% to 1%, with no increase in bleeding.[255] Multimodal prophylaxis combining LMWH, compression stockings, and intermittent pneumatic compression may be even more effective.[256] Yet concerns remain that pre- or early postoperative administration of LMWH is associated with an increased risk of bleeding.[257] In this more than in other areas of surgery, the timing of initiation of heparin/LMWH, dosing, and duration of therapy are critical factors in determining the risk–benefit ratio. In fact, a recent analysis of the literature applied in a decision analysis model comparing mechanical prophylaxis to mechanical prophylaxis ± UFH or LMWH was marginally in favor of the use of pneumatic compression devices alone.[258]

General and Gynecologic Surgery

Rates of asymptomatic VTE in all comers undergoing general surgery without VTE prophylaxis (approximately 20%–25%) are lower than in major orthopedic surgery, although it should be noted that the rates are substantially lower in certain minor forms of surgery, such as appendectomy or abdominal wall surgery The increasing use of laparoscopic techniques has tended to lower the risks that were previously encountered with the corresponding open procedures. Patient-related risk factors include cancer, advancing age, a history of previous VTE, obesity, varicose veins, and estrogen use.

In several meta-analyses, thrombosis prophylaxis using LMWH is uniformly superior to placebo, and equivalent to subcutaneous UFH.[259–261] UFH is also equivalent to LMWH in high-risk urologic or gynecologic surgery. In moderate-risk gynecologic surgery, nonpharmacologic prophylaxis with intermittent pneumatic compression is as efficacious as LMWH,[262] although patients with a history of cancer or DVT, or age more than 60 years may be more prone to fail intermittent pneumatic compression alone.[263] Although bleeding rates are purportedly higher with LMWH than UFH in general surgery, this may be a function of administered dose. A lower dose of LMWH (<3500 anti-Xa units/day) may be as efficacious as UFH, with a bleeding rate that is actually somewhat lower.[260,261]

Cancer increases the risk of postoperative VTE by a factor of approximately 2,[177,264] and patients undergoing major abdominal or pelvic surgery for neoplastic disorders should be considered to be at high risk. This risk may be related to enhanced activation of coagulation, more prolonged immobilization, and/or greater extent of surgery and duration of anesthesia. Low-dose UFH or LMWH combined with intermittent pneumatic compression appears to be ideal VTE prophylaxis.[261,265] Therapy is typically initiated 2 hours preoperatively. Approximately 40% of VTE occurs following discharge, suggesting a possible need for prolonged therapy. Indeed, recent evidence suggests that prolonged administration of Enoxaparin (40 mg once daily) results in a reduction of venographically demonstrated DVT (from 12.0% in the 1-week treatment group to 4.8% in the 4-week treatment group), without any increased risk of bleeding.[266]

Renal Transplantation

In the United States, approximately 14,000 renal transplants are performed annually. Published estimates of the incidence of postoperative VTE have varied from 0.6% to 25%. A retrospective analysis of more than 2000 renal allograft recipients found a 6.2% incidence of symptomatic DVT in patients undergoing kidney or simultaneous kidney–pancreas transplant without prophylaxis in the period between 1985 and 1995.[267] In this study, the incidence of symptomatic DVT following kidney transplantation (4.5%) did not appear to be significantly higher than the rate in general surgical procedures of a comparable magnitude; however, the rate in patients receiving kidney–pancreas allografts (18.1%) was considered to be excessively high.

A number of special considerations apply to the use of prophylactic anticoagulation in renal transplant recipients. Because renal function may remain impaired for several days or more following the procedure, impaired clearance of LMWHs may increase the risk of bleeding. Therefore, UFH may be a better choice for prophylaxis. Furthermore, prophylactic anticoagulation may be of theoretical benefit in the prevention of other vascular complications of renal transplantation. Specifically, it has been demonstrated that common inherited and acquired thrombophilias (factor V Leiden [FV G1691A], prothrombin G20210A mutation, and antiphospholipid antibodies) are associated with an increased risk of primary renal graft thrombosis, and acute vascular rejection. Primary renal graft thrombosis, defined as thrombosis of the renal graft vasculature in the absence of histopathologic evidence of rejection, usually occurs within 10 days of renal transplant, and virtually always results in loss of the graft. Thrombosis is as likely to be arterial as venous, and occurs in approximately 2% (range 1%–6%) of recipients. The usual presentation is with sudden-onset oliguria or anuria associated with a falloff in graft function. In the case of renal vein thrombosis, there may be pain at the graft site, hematuria, and even graft rupture. A number of retrospective case control studies,[268–270] and a prospective study,[271] have demonstrated that one or more of these thrombophilias are associated with an estimated 3- to 10-fold increased risk of renal graft thrombosis. With respect to acute vascular rejection, it is hypothesized that endothelial damage and microvascular thrombosis caused by the underlying thrombophilia increase the likelihood of graft malfunction or loss if the transplanted organ is challenged by an acute rejection episode. Inherited thrombophilias may increase the relative risk of acute vascular rejection by an estimated 4- to 12-fold.[271]

It has not been established by appropriate prospective randomized study whether antithrombotic prophylaxis can prevent early renal graft thrombosis and/or acute vascular rejection. However, small series have suggested that UFH, LMWH, or aspirin (>75 mg daily) may diminish the rate of early allograft thrombosis, compared with historical controls.[272,273] Prophylaxis may be particularly vital in high-risk patients, for example, those with identified thrombophilia, and/or a previous history of early graft loss or VTE.[274] However, the optimal intensity, duration, and composition of prophylactic regimens has not been determined, and opinions differ considerably, from long-term full-intensity anticoagulation begun in the early postoperative period to short-term lower-intensity heparin followed by longer-term aspirin therapy.[275]

COMPLIANCE WITH VENOUS THROMBOEMBOLISM PROPHYLAXIS

Most studies examining the question of compliance with nationally developed guidelines for VTE prophylaxis have concluded that thromboprophylaxis is underutilized, both in terms of the absolute number of eligible but undertreated patients, and the appropriateness (ranging from total omission to suboptimal choice, dose or duration) of therapy. In general, orthopedic services tend to be more (>85%) compliant with published guidelines, probably reflecting the longer history of utilization and widespread awareness of the benefits and risks of VTE prophylaxis by orthopedic surgeons.[276,277] In general surgery, compliance with grade A recommendations may be much lower, sometimes in the 30%–50% range.[278] This reluctance to utilize prophylaxis may be explained by a tendency to underestimate the thrombotic risk in high-risk patients.[204,276] Conversely, despite uncertainties regarding the optimal approach to prophylaxis in neurosurgical patients, 85% of practitioners in the United Kingdom regularly used some form of prophylaxis.[279] Improvement in compliance is probably best achieved by the application of surgical service-specific guidelines, developed in each institution to mirror its own patient population. Like all guidelines, the recommendations should be flexible enough to allow informed physicians to exercise their clinical judgment when assessing risks and benefits of a specific regimen in the case of an individual patient.

Treatment of Postsurgical Venous Thromboembolism

The principles of treatment of acute VTE occurring in the postoperative period do not differ materially from treatment under other circumstances (Chapter 135), with the exception that the bleeding risks associated with anticoagulation are increased. Although virtually all series agree that recent surgery is a risk factor for bleeding,[280] it is difficult to find relevant literature that quantifies the risk (with respect to the rate of decline in the risk after surgery). It is generally recommended that if surgery has involved a vital organ (eg, brain, eye), it is inappropriate to risk full-intensity anticoagulation for 5 to 7 days[254] (or longer—eg at least 7–10 days—when thrombolytic therapy is to be used). This recommendation is supported by animal data demonstrating that the risk of intracranial hemorrhage with full-intensity heparin anticoagulation in the postoperative period following craniotomy dropped off sharply between the 7th and 10th postoperative day.[281] If anticoagulation is strongly contraindicated, placement of an IVC filter may be the only available option. At the other end of the spectrum, anticoagulation after minor procedures in patients judged to be at low risk of bleeding can probably be initiated after 12 to 24 hours. UFH may have certain advantages over LMWH in these circumstances, most notably its short half-life and susceptibility to more complete reversal with protamine, which dictate that it will be more reversible in the event of bleeding.

SUGGESTED READINGS

Adams GL et al: The balance of thrombosis and hemorrhage in surgery. Hematol Oncol Clin North Am 21(1):13, 2007.

Bergqvist D et al: Duration of prophylaxis against venous thromboembolism with enoxaparin after surgery for cancer. N Engl J Med 346(13):975, 2002.

Bonow RO et al: ACC/AHA 2006 guidelines for the management of patients with valvular heart disease: A report of the American College of Cardiology/American Heart Association Task Force on Practice Guidelines (writing committee to revise the 1998 Guidelines for the Management of Patients With Valvular Heart Disease): Developed in collaboration with the Society of Cardiovascular Anesthesiologists: Endorsed by the Society for Cardiovascular Angiography and Interventions and the Society of Thoracic Surgeons. Circulation 114(5):e84, 2006.

Brown JR, Birkmeyer NJ, O'Connor GT: Meta-analysis comparing the effectiveness and adverse outcomes of antifibrinolytic agents in cardiac surgery. Circulation 115(22):2801, 2007.

Caldwell SH et al: Coagulation disorders and hemostasis in liver disease: Pathophysiology and critical assessment of current management. Hepatology 44(4):1039, 2006.

Carless PA, Henry DA: Systematic review and meta-analysis of the use of fibrin sealant to prevent seroma formation after breast cancer surgery. Br J Surg 93(7):810, 2006.

Clark P, Mintz PD: Transfusion triggers for blood components. Curr Opin Hematol 8(6):387, 2001.

Cothren CC et al: Utility of once-daily dose of low-molecular-weight heparin to prevent venous thromboembolism in multisystem trauma patients. World J Surg 31(1):98, 2007.

Crowther MA et al: Oral vitamin K lowers the international normalized ratio more rapidly than subcutaneous vitamin K in the treatment of warfarin-associated coagulopathy. A randomized controlled trial. Ann Intern Med 137(4):251, 2002.

Danish SF et al: Prophylaxis for deep venous thrombosis in craniotomy patients: A decision analysis. Neurosurgery 56(6):1286, 2005; discussion 1292.

Fremes SE et al: Metaanalysis of prophylactic drug treatment in the prevention of postoperative bleeding. Ann Thorac Surg 58(6):1580, 1994.

Geerts WH et al: Prevention of venous thromboembolism: The Seventh ACCP Conference on Antithrombotic and Thrombolytic Therapy. Chest 126(3 Suppl):338S, 2004.

Goldhaber SZ: "Bridging" and mechanical heart valves: Perils, promises, and predictions. Circulation 113(4):470, 2006.

Hedner U: Recombinant factor VIIa: Its background, development and clinical use. Curr Opin Hematol 14(3):225, 2007.

Hirsh J, O'Donnell M, Weitz JI: New anticoagulants. Blood 105(2):453, 2005.

Key NS, Negrier C: Coagulation factor concentrates: Past, present, and future. Lancet 370(9585):439, 2007.

Laupacis A, Fergusson D: Drugs to minimize perioperative blood loss in cardiac surgery: Meta-analyses using perioperative blood transfusion as the outcome. The International Study of Peri-operative Transfusion (ISPOT) Investigators. Anesth Analg 85(6):1258, 1997.

Levy JH: Massive transfusion coagulopathy. Semin Hematol 43(1 Suppl 1): S59, 2006.

Mangano DT, Tudor IC, Dietzel C: The risk associated with aprotinin in cardiac surgery. N Engl J Med 354(4):353, 2006.

Mannucci PM, Levi M: Prevention and treatment of major blood loss. N Engl J Med 356(22):2301, 2007.

Mayer SA et al: Recombinant activated factor VII for acute intracerebral hemorrhage. N Engl J Med 352(8):777, 2005.

Molenaar IQ et al: Efficacy and safety of antifibrinolytic drugs in liver transplantation: A systematic review and meta-analysis. Am J Transplant 7(1):185, 2007.

Peterson P et al: The preoperative bleeding time test lacks clinical benefit: College of American Pathologists' and American Society of Clinical Pathologists' position article. Arch Surg 133(2):134, 1998.

Practice guidelines for blood component therapy: A report by the American Society of Anesthesiologists Task Force on Blood Component Therapy. Anesthesiology 84(3):732, 1996.

Rogers FB et al: Practice management guidelines for the prevention of venous thromboembolism in trauma patients: The EAST practice management guidelines work group. J Trauma 53(1):142, 2002.

Scarpelini S, Rizoli S: Recombinant factor VIIa and the surgical patient. Curr Opin Crit Care 12(4):351, 2006.

Segal JB, Dzik WH: Paucity of studies to support that abnormal coagulation test results predict bleeding in the setting of invasive procedures: An evidence-based review. Transfusion 45(9):1413, 2005.

Seshadri N et al: The clinical challenge of bridging anticoagulation with low-molecular-weight heparin in patients with mechanical prosthetic heart valves: An evidence-based comparative review focusing on anticoagulation options in pregnant and nonpregnant patients. Am Heart J 150(1):27, 2005.

Streiff MB: Vena caval filters: A comprehensive review. Blood 95(12):3669, 2000.

Velmahos GC: The current status of thromboprophylaxis after trauma: A story of confusion and uncertainty. Am Surg 72(9):757, 2006.

REFERENCES

For complete list of references log onto www.expertconsult.com

CHAPTER 161

HEMATOLOGIC CHANGES OF PREGNANCY

Jacob Laubach and Johanna Bendell

The primary physiological hematologic changes during pregnancy relate to the expansion of plasma volume. The greatest increase in plasma volume occurs between 6 and 24 weeks' gestation. After 24 weeks the plasma volume increases, but at a slower rate. In a normal pregnancy the plasma volume increases 40% to 60%,[1] with the change in plasma volume proportional to fetal weight.[2] Erythropoiesis in the first trimester of pregnancy is similar to erythropoiesis in the nonpregnant woman, but increases in the second and third trimesters.[3] Coincident with changes in plasma volume, there is a simultaneous but less than proportional increase in red blood cell mass of 20% to 50%. As a result, a pregnant woman's hematocrit typically lies in the 30% to 32% range.[1] In addition to these physiologic changes, a prothrombotic state develops as pregnancy advances that is believed to prepare the mother and fetus for placental separation during delivery.[4]

ANEMIA IN PREGNANCY

Because of the physiologic decrease in hemoglobin and hematocrit during pregnancy, the Centers for Disease Control and Prevention (CDC) Pregnancy Nutrition Surveillance System has created new standard definitions for anemia in pregnant women.[5] Anemia during pregnancy is quite common; the World Health Organization (WHO) reports 35% to 75% of women in developing countries and 18% of women in industrialized countries develop anemia in pregnancy.[6] The effects of anemia on both the mother and fetus can range from mild to severe. Common maternal signs and symptoms of anemia include tachycardia, pallor, tachypnea, glossitis, fatigue, paresthesias, and headache. Hemoglobin levels less than 6 g/dL in pregnant women can be associated with significant maternal and fetal complications. At these levels, tissue oxygenation decreases and may lead to a state of high-output congestive heart failure in the mother. Meanwhile, multiple studies have shown a correlation between maternal anemia and increased rates of both preterm (<37 weeks' gestation) and low-birth-weight deliveries.[7–15] These studies indicate that anemia in the first or second trimester of pregnancy conveys an increased risk of preterm delivery, whereas third trimester anemia does not. Interestingly, they also demonstrate an increased risk of preterm delivery and low birth weight in women with a relatively high hematocrit (≥40%) in the second or third trimester. In interpreting results from such studies on anemia in pregnancy, it is important to consider confounding factors such as maternal nutrition and health, socioeconomic conditions, and environmental influences that can independently affect pregnancy outcomes.

IRON DEFICIENCY ANEMIA

Iron deficiency is the most common cause of nonphysiologic anemia in pregnancy, accounting for 75% of cases.[16] In the United States, the estimated prevalence of iron deficiency anemia in pregnancy ranges from 3% to 9% during the first trimester to 16% to 55% in the third trimester.[17,18] The prevalence of iron deficiency anemia increases in the setting of poor appetite and nutrition, nausea, and vomiting; second pregnancy in less than 2 years; and chronic illness. Iron deficiency anemia in pregnancy is also seen more often in African American, low-income, and adolescent women.[19–21] That the incidence of iron deficiency anemia increases as pregnancy progresses reflects heightened iron requirements during pregnancy. Total iron stores increase from 2.2 g in a nonpregnant woman to 3.2 g in a pregnant woman at term, creating a 900- to 1000-mg iron requirement during the course of pregnancy.[22] Between 500 and 600 mg are used to increase erythrocyte mass, whereas 300 mg are required by the fetus and placenta. For a woman with adequate iron stores, the average daily iron requirement increases 2 to 4 mg per day, increasing further in the third trimester to 6 to 8 mg per day.[23,24] In addition, iron absorption from the intestine increases as much as 40% during pregnancy.[25] Although a pregnant woman may have iron deficiency anemia, her fetus typically does not develop iron deficiency as a result of active iron transport across the placenta.[26–28] However, infants of iron-deficient mothers do have a higher risk of developing iron deficiency later in infancy.

Symptoms of iron deficiency anemia in pregnant women are similar to those observed in nonpregnant individuals and include fatigue, lethargy, headache, and pica, a condition defined as the consumption of nonnutritive substances such as ice, baking soda, baking powder, clay, or dirt. Exam findings such as pallor, glossitis, and cheilitis in a pregnant woman should prompt the clinician to further evaluate a woman for iron deficiency. Although uncommon, retinal bleeding, conjunctivitis, tachycardia, and splenomegaly can be seen in instances of severe iron deficiency.[29] Microcytosis distinguishes iron-deficiency anemia from physiologic anemia of pregnancy, which is normochromic and normocytic. In turn, iron deficiency must be differentiated from other causes of microcytic anemia such as chronic inflammatory conditions and hemoglobinopathies. A reduced serum ferritin concentration (normal value in pregnancy 55–70 μg/L) and transferrin saturation (<15% in iron deficiency) are useful indicators of iron deficiency in the pregnant patient as in nonpregnant individuals.[29]

Iron deficiency anemia diagnosed during pregnancy is treated as it would be in the nonpregnant woman. Oral iron therapy with 60 to 120 mg per day of elemental iron is recommended. Intravenous iron is appropriate in certain circumstances; evidence from a recently published randomized trial by Al et al supports the use of intravenous iron therapy to replenish iron stores in appropriately selected patients, including those who have not tolerated a trial of oral iron therapy and those with severe iron deficiency.[30]

Because the typical diet in the United States provides only 50% of daily iron requirements for the pregnant woman and because of the relatively high prevalence of iron deficiency among women of child-bearing age, routine iron supplementation in pregnancy is recommended.[16,25] Currently, the CDC, the American Dietetic Association, and the American College of Obstetrics and Gynecology recommend 15 to 30 mg daily of elemental iron to prevent adverse outcomes due to iron deficiency anemia.[31–35] Based on the results of a study by Casanueva et al, weekly therapy with 120 mg of iron appears to be a safe and effective alternative to daily therapy.[36] The side effects associated with iron therapy—constipation, diarrhea, nausea—are well known.

Multiple studies have shown that routine iron supplementation in pregnancy decreases the incidence of iron deficiency anemia.[37–41] Furthermore, in a recent randomized, double-blinded study in which 275 iron-replete pregnant women received either a daily iron supplement or placebo from time of enrollment (all women were enrolled before week 20) to 28 weeks' gestation, the incidence of both low-birth-weight and preterm low-birth-weight infants was lower among women who received daily iron.[42] Nonetheless, there are limits to the effectiveness of routine iron supplementation. After all, the recommendation by prominent public health organizations for universal iron supplementation has not led to a commensurate decrease in the incidence of iron deficiency anemia in pregnancy[43,44] or an increase in maternal hemoglobin levels.[45,46] Clearly, compliance is an important factor in this discussion. A large, multicenter, randomized controlled trial on the benefits of iron supplementation during pregnancy in the United States is needed to draw more definitive conclusions.

MEGALOBLASTIC ANEMIA

Folate deficiency accounts for 95% of megaloblastic anemias in pregnancy.[47] Folate deficiency complicates between 1% and 4% of pregnancies in the United States and affects approximately one-third of pregnancies worldwide.[48] Like iron deficiency anemia, the incidence of megaloblastic anemia in pregnancy is increased in adolescents, women of low socioeconomic status, and women with multiple closely spaced births.[49] The folic acid requirement for the nonpregnant woman is 50 to 100 μg per day, but this increases to 150 μg during pregnancy as red cell mass in the mother increases and as fetal demands for folate grow with cell proliferation.[50]

Several trials have demonstrated a relationship between folic acid supplementation prior to and during pregnancy and a reduced incidence of neural tube defects.[51–54] These led in the early 1990s to a formal recommendation of this practice among women planning to become pregnant. The CDC currently recommends that a pregnant woman receive 400 μg of folate daily to reduce the risk of a neural tube defect.[55] To reduce elevated homocysteine levels observed in individuals with folate deficiency, 400 μg is thought to be the minimum daily dose required.[56] Moreover, it has been suggested that higher doses of folate—up to 5 mg daily—may provide greater benefit to pregnant women with respect to prevention of neural tube defects.[57] To date, though, this recommendation has not been implemented on a broad scale. Women for whom a previous pregnancy has been complicated by neural tube defects should receive 4 mg of folate daily as prophylactic therapy before and during subsequent pregnancies.

Although the mechanism by which folate exerts its protective effect is not fully understood, work by Rothenberg and colleagues has provided important insight in this area. Autoantibodies against folate receptors were found in 9 of 12 women in whom a current or previous pregnancy had been complicated by neural tube defect, whereas such antibodies were detected in only 2 of 20 control individuals.[58] The autoantibodies blocked binding of folate to receptors in an in vitro experimental model. The authors suggest that folate supplementation in individuals with such autoantibodies may exert its protective effect by overcoming this blockade.

The diagnosis of folate deficiency in pregnancy should not be based on serum folate levels, as they can be affected by acute nutritional deficiency, alcohol intake, or hemolysis. Red blood cell folate is a better marker of folate deficiency if low, but it too may be normal in megaloblastic anemia. Furthermore, it is a more useful determinant of folate levels for the previous 1 to 3 months, because red blood cell survival is 120 days. The combination of an elevated homocysteine level and normal methylmalonic acid level has a 99% sensitivity and specificity for diagnosis of folate deficiency.[59]

Vitamin B_{12} deficiency rarely causes anemia in pregnancy. The daily requirement for vitamin B_{12} is small because of large vitamin B_{12} stores within the body. Vitamin B_{12} also has a significant enterohepatic circulation, such that most vitamin B_{12} in bile is reabsorbed. It typically takes several years to manifest vitamin B_{12} deficiency.[60] Vitamin B_{12} deficiency is caused by poor intake, as seen in strict vegetarians who ingest little or no vitamin B_{12}-rich animal and dairy protein, and by poor absorption. Poor absorption of vitamin B_{12} can occur as a result of malabsorption syndromes such as pernicious anemia or Crohn disease. The requirements of vitamin B_{12} during pregnancy are minimal and do not usually affect overall body stores.[49] If vitamin B_{12} deficiency is suspected, a serum vitamin B_{12} level can be obtained, though these levels may be decreased in pregnancy without true body vitamin B_{12} depletion.[61,62] An elevated level of both homocysteine and methylmalonic accurately confirms the diagnosis of vitamin B_{12} deficiency.[56] A woman with vitamin B_{12} deficiency should receive vitamin B_{12} therapy for the duration of her pregnancy. A common repletion schedule involves intramuscular injections of cyanocobalamin or hydroxocobalamin, 1000 μg once weekly for 8 weeks, then monthly. The Shilling test to assess for intrinsic factor deficiency should be deferred during pregnancy so as to limit radiation exposure.

HEMATOLOGIC MALIGNANCIES

Hematologic malignancies are among the most common malignancies diagnosed during pregnancy.[63] They include Hodgkin and non-Hodgkin lymphoma, acute myelogenous leukemia (AML), acute lymphocytic leukemia, chronic myelogenous leukemia (CML), myelodysplastic syndrome (MDS), and essential thrombocytosis (ET).

Hodgkin and Non-Hodgkin Lymphoma

That hematologic malignancies are among the most commonly diagnosed cancers during pregnancy reflects to a large extent the relatively high incidence of Hodgkin lymphoma in women between the ages of 15 and 24.[64] Based on the results of several retrospective studies, Hodgkin lymphoma diagnosed during pregnancy appears to have no significant effect on pregnancy outcome.[65] A single-institution experience published by Dilek and colleagues, however, highlights complications that may occur in pregnant women with Hodgkin disease, as children born to three of five women with the disease had complications, including death.[66] Remission rates and 20-year overall survival among women diagnosed with Hodgkin disease during pregnancy are reportedly similar to those observed in nonpregnant women with the disease.[67,68] In rare instances, Hodgkin lymphoma metastasizes to the placenta, so the placenta and newborn infant should be examined for evidence of malignancy.[69] Staging during pregnancy can be performed with computed tomography, but magnetic resonance imaging is preferred to reduce to exposure of the fetus to radiation.

Like other malignancies managed during pregnancy, treatment of women with Hodgkin disease is challenging. Generally, chemotherapy at any point in pregnancy increases the risk of an unfavorable outcome.[66] The teratogenic effects of chemotherapy and radiation during pregnancy are a primary concern. However, the standard regimen of adriamycin, bleomycin, vinblastine, and dacarbazine does not appear to increase teratogenic risk when given in the second or third trimesters.

Non-Hodgkin lymphoma rarely occurs during pregnancy. There are case reports and case series of women with non-Hodgkin lymphoma who have been successfully treated with chemotherapy during the second and third trimesters of pregnancy.[70] Alkylating agents given in the first trimester can result in fetal malformations or death,[71] although there are reports of children who received chemotherapy in the first trimester with no subsequent deficits.[72] Based on available data, response and recurrence rates among women treated for non-Hodgkin lymphoma during pregnancy are similar to those seen in the treatment of pregnant women with Hodgkin disease.

Acute and Chronic Leukemia

Pregnant women with acute myelogenous leukemia, acute lymphocytic leukemia, and chronic myelogenous leukemia can be treated successfully with standard therapy; however, treatment carries the risk of teratogenic effects related to chemotherapy, including intrauterine growth retardation, fetal malformation, cardiac toxicity, and death. There appears to be no influence of pregnancy on the course of leukemia.

As might be expected, the teratogenic risk associated with chemotherapy is greatest with treatment during the first trimester.[73] In the largest study of its kind, Aviles and Neri followed 84 children born to mothers with hematologic malignancies, including 29 women with acute leukemia and 38 who received treatment during the first trimester. Assessing growth and development, hematologic parameters, psychological characteristics, and cognitive function over 19 years, the authors found no significant, long-term, deleterious consequences related to treatment.[72] A more recent case report and literature review by Niedermeier analyzed the outcomes of 20 women treated for AML during the second or third trimester of pregnancy.[74] Within this series, 11 pregnancies resulted in infants with no abnormality, 4 involved infants with an abnormality, and 5 resulted in spontaneous abortion or stillbirth.

Among acute leukemias arising within the myeloid lineage, acute promyelocytic leukemia is unique in terms of clinical features—particularly disseminated intravascular coagulation and associated bleeding complications—and therapy, which involves all-*trans* retinoic acid (ATRA) in conjunction with traditional chemotherapy. Concern regarding the teratogenic effects of ATRA is warranted. In the 1980s, Lammer and colleagues noted an increased risk of fetal malformation following in utero exposure to the retinoid isotretinoin.[75] And a recent case report by Carradice et al describes a bleeding complication that occurred even after ATRA initiation in a pregnant woman with acute promyelocytic anemia.[76] However, a review of 13 women treated during pregnancy with ATRA for acute promyelocytic anemia found no evidence that the agent leads to fetal malformation when used in the treatment of pregnant women.[77]

Similar concerns regarding toxicity of therapy arise in managing pregnancies conceived prior to and during treatment of chronic myelogenous leukemia. Imatinib, a small-molecule inhibitor against the BCR/ABL tyrosine kinase, is the standard of care for treatment of chronic myelogenous leukemia. In animal studies, imatinib exhibited teratogenicity in rats and impaired spermatogenesis in dogs, monkeys, and rats.[78] Meanwhile, in a series of 19 pregnancies involving a mother or father undergoing imatinib-based therapy for CML, three pregnancies resulted in a spontaneous abortion whereas 2 others produced children with minor malformation.[79] The remaining 13 pregnancies resulted in the delivery of a healthy child. Among mothers in this study who had previously achieved a complete hematologic remission with imatinib and interrupted therapy during pregnancy, a majority (5 of 9) lost the hematologic remission. These findings highlight the important therapy-related implications for mother and fetus, which must be weighed carefully in determining an appropriate course of management. Currently, it is recommended by specialists in the field that patients undergoing treatment with imatinib for CML utilize proper contraception.[79]

Myeloproliferative Disorders

The non-BCR/ABL myeloproliferative disorders include polycythemia vera (PV), essential thrombocytosis (ET), and idiopathic myelofibrosis (MF). In 2001, the World Health Organization expanded its definition of myeloproliferative disorders to include the less common entities chronic neutrophilic leukemia, eosinophilic leukemia, systemic mastocytosis, and chronic myelomonocytic leukemia. Patients with these disorders may suffer from a variety of complications, including thrombosis and hemorrhage. Although their incidence peaks in the sixth or seventh decade, myeloproliferative disorders do occur sporadically in younger individuals and as such can affect pregnant women.

Most literature pertaining to non-BCR/ABL myeloproliferative diseases and pregnancy applies to essential thrombocytosis as it is most likely among this class of diseases to affect women of childbearing age. Data from pregnant women with polycythemia vera and idiopathic myelofibrosis are scant, making it more difficult to draw firm conclusions on pregnancy outcomes. Spontaneous abortion, intrauterine growth retardation, preterm delivery, and placental abruption all appear to occur more frequently in women with essential thrombocytosis than in the general population.[80] Although the precise mechanism has not been fully elucidated, dysregulated placental blood flow and thrombosis are thought to play a primary role in this pathogenesis.

Among pregnant women with an underlying BCR/ABL-negative myeloproliferative disorder, those whose history includes a previous venous or arterial thrombotic event, a prior hemorrhagic event, or a previous pregnancy-related complication are considered high risk for a subsequent complication related to their disease.[81] It is generally agreed that pregnant women with a myeloproliferative disorder should receive low-dose aspirin during pregnancy and for 6 weeks following delivery.[80] Low-molecular-weight heparin should be considered for individuals at high risk for thrombotic complications, though there have been no randomized trials or even large case–control trials to guide this practice.[80] Compressive stockings can be used in this setting as well. Cytoreductive therapy should be avoided during pregnancy if possible. If such therapy becomes necessary, interferon α represents the agent of choice in pregnancy.

Sickle Cell Disease

Many women with sickle cell disease experience more frequent vasoocclusive crises and other sickle cell-related complications during pregnancy.[82] The increased frequency of vasoocclusive crises, particularly during the latter half of pregnancy, likely results from heightened metabolic requirements in pregnancy, increased venous stasis, and the physiologic prothrombotic state of pregnancy. In addition, pathophysiologic changes in the renal and immune function of patients with sickle cell disease increase their susceptibility to urinary tract infections and pyelonephritis. In a recently published retrospective cohort study, Thurman and colleagues compared rates of asymptomatic bacteriuria and pyelonephritis among women with sickle cell trait with those among a cohort of pregnant control patients.[83] The implications of such a study are noteworthy because in the general population, bacteriuria in pregnant women is associated with increased morbidity and mortality for both mother and fetus.[83] The authors found equivalent rates of asymptomatic bacteriuria in the two groups. On the other hand, they detected a higher prevalence of pyelonephritis among the cohort with sickle cell trait.

Other significant complications occur in pregnant women with sickle cell disease as well. For example, the incidence of preeclampsia, thromboembolic events, placental abruption, intrauterine growth retardation, low birth weight, and postpartum infections is higher among women with hemoglobin SS, SC, and Sβ-thalassemia as compared to women without sickle cell disease. One study noted a higher incidence of stillbirths and perinatal mortality among patients with sickle cell disease,[84] whereas another one revealed an increased risk of preterm labor and premature rupture of membranes in women with hemoglobin SS disease.[85] By causing tissue hypoxia, sickling of red blood cells within the placental vasculature causes deleterious effects upon the fetus.[86]

Because of the increased risk for such complications, women with sickle cell disease should receive close medical attention throughout the prenatal period. This includes counseling about intrauterine diagnosis of sickle cell disease when appropriate. Pregnant women can undergo chorionic villi sampling as early as the 9th week of gestation or amniocentesis in the 15th to 16th weeks. A reticulocyte count along with hemoglobin, iron, and folate levels should be obtained to assess for deficiency states and bone marrow suppression. Urinalysis with urine culture is performed as often as every trimester to monitor for asymptomatic bacteriuria. Finally, beginning around 28 weeks of gestation, patients should make weekly clinic visits and begin serial ultrasonography.

Treatment of sickle cell disease during pregnancy warrants careful consideration. With regard to maintenance therapy, hydroxyurea has been used safely throughout pregnancy in patients with sickle cell anemia, though formal studies of its use in this setting have not been performed to date.[87] Women should receive 5 mg of supplemental folic acid daily. Studies examining the benefit of prophylactic blood transfusions or exchange transfusions have not led to definitive conclusions.[82] Though they may lead to alloimmunization, prophylactic transfusions appear to decrease the incidence of vasoocclusive crises and decrease maternal and fetal morbidity and mortality.[88] A conservative approach reserves transfusions for the patient whose hemoglobin levels fall below 6 g/dL, the patient who develops progressive complications related to sickle cell disease, or the patient with obstetric complications.[89] Following this approach, 60% to 75% of women with sickle cell disease will require transfusion therapy during pregnancy. Patients with sickle cell crisis during pregnancy, meanwhile, should receive aggressive analgesic therapy, hydration, and oxygen while undergoing evaluation of infection or other precipitating influence.

At the time of delivery, the pregnant woman with sickle cell disease is managed in a manner similar to those with high cardiac output anemia. Supplemental oxygen, hydration, and adequate anesthesia should be given to prevent sickling of red blood cells and the associated complications. During the postpartum period, meanwhile, hemoglobin levels are followed closely and prophylaxis for venous thromboembolism is administered unless contraindications preclude it.

THALASSEMIAS

Pregnant women with an underlying thalassemia typically have β-thalassemia minor or α-thalassemia trait—conditions with a relatively benign clinical phenotype—rather than β-thalassemia major or hemoglobin H disease. Because of delayed pubertal growth or hypogonadism with associated anovulation, women with β-thalassemia major and hemoglobin H disease rarely become pregnant. Case reports indicate that when it does occur, pregnancy in women with hemoglobin H disease can be complicated by severe hemolytic anemia and hepatosplenomegaly. Pregnancy outcomes among women with β-thalassemia intermedia, meanwhile, were examined in a recently published study by Nassar et al. Following nine pregnancies in five patients with β-thalassemia intermedia, the authors noted a high incidence of intrauterine growth restriction (IUGR) and frequent requirement for red blood cell transfusion, even among women who had not been transfusion dependent prior to pregnancy.[90] One pregnancy resulted in intrauterine fetal demise at 36 weeks. These findings are consistent with previous observations made in reference to a population of pregnant women with thalassemia; an earlier review of the literature found that 50% of pregnancies in this patient population were complicated by preterm delivery, third-trimester stillbirth, or intrauterine growth retardation.[91]

Pregnancy is a common setting for the diagnosis of β-thalassemia minor or α-thalassemia trait in previously asymptomatic women who are found to be anemic on routine laboratory evaluation during pregnancy. Several studies indicate that the physiologic anemia of pregnancy may be exacerbated in women with thalassemia minor, though findings from at least one study suggest otherwise.[92] β-thalassemia minor and α-thalassemia traits do not have an adverse effect on fetal development, fetal morbidity and mortality, or maternal morbidity and mortality.[93,94]

Like those with sickle cell disease, women with thalassemia require vigilant follow-up throughout their pregnancy. This includes interval monitoring of maternal vital signs and fetal heart rate, maternal hemoglobin levels, and fetal growth as assessed by ultrasound beginning around the 24th week of gestation. Patients are screened for folate and iron deficiency. They should also be assessed for iron overload, which can develop in individuals with thalassemia as a result of increased intestinal iron absorption, frequent blood transfusions, and rapid turnover of plasma iron.[90] Prenatal genetic testing can be performed if desired, with results used to counsel parents of the child and guide optimal care of the fetus. In terms of therapy, there are no specific treatment recommendations for women with thalassemia during pregnancy aside from folate supplementation and supportive care. In pregnant women with evidence of iron overload, chelation therapy using deferoxamine has been safely used, though the potential for teratogenicity associated with the agent must be considered in this setting.[95]

OTHER HEMOLYTIC ANEMIAS

Hereditary Spherocytosis

Hereditary spherocytosis is the most common inherited hemolytic anemia among people of northern European descent.[96] Few cases of pregnancy in individuals with hereditary spherocytosis have been reported. Published reports indicate there may be an increased incidence of first-trimester fetal loss patients with hereditary spherocytosis.[97] Because some patients have only low levels of hemolysis under normal conditions, the disease may not become clinically apparent until pregnancy. Pregnant women with hereditary spherocytosis can exhibit a variety of clinical manifestations. These include folate deficiency related to the increased requirements of pregnancy superimposed on chronic hemolysis, hemolytic crisis, and aplastic crisis.[98,99] The results of two small series suggest that pregnancy outcomes for women with hereditary spherocytosis are generally good, with improvements in outcomes for splenectomized patients.[94,100] Care is primarily supportive.

Pyruvate Kinase Deficiency

Pyruvate kinase deficiency is a rare disorder resulting in impaired glycolysis and adenosine triphosphate (ATP) generation. Clinically, most patients with the disorder exhibit a compensated hemolysis. There are very few reports of pregnancy in women with pyruvate kinase deficiency. Published reports indicate that although such women experience increased levels of hemolysis and thus require transfusions, pregnancy outcomes are favorable for both mother and fetus.[101]

Glucose 6-Phosphate Dehydrogenase Deficiency

Favorable pregnancy outcomes observed in women with hereditary spherocytosis and pyruvate kinase deficiency stand in contrast to those in women with glucose 6-phosphate dehydrogenase (G6PD) deficiency. The deficiency of glucose 6-phosphate dehydrogenase in this disorder leads to hemolytic anemia in the face of oxidative stress. The condition increases the risk of spontaneous abortion, low birth weight, and neonatal jaundice.[102] Women with G6PD deficiency should be instructed to strictly avoid medications with oxidative potential. Complications following the ingestion of oxidative drugs can even occur in a carrier of the G6PD deficiency gene if her male fetus has inherited the disease.[103]

Paroxysmal Nocturnal Hemoglobinuria

Paroxysmal nocturnal hemoglobinuria (PNH) is a rare clonal disorder caused by somatic mutation in the membrane-anchoring protein *PIGA*. *PIGA* mutation leads, in turn, to deficient function of critical membrane proteins that in wild-type individuals are anchored by the gene product of *PIGA*. Features of the clinical phenotype include hemolysis, thrombosis, and bone marrow failure. Hemolysis results from deficiency in the membrane proteins CD55 and CD59, which renders affected individuals susceptible to complement-mediated intravascular hemolysis.

The clinical manifestations of PNH can have a devastating impact on pregnancy. Reported cases highlight the significant pregnancy-associated morbidity and mortality in women with this condition.

Complications include severe anemia, thrombocytopenia, thrombotic events, preterm delivery, low-birth-weight infants, neonatal death, and maternal death.[104,105] A study by Ray and colleagues reviewed pregnancy outcomes in 24 women with PNH and found a 20% maternal mortality rate.[105]

Owing to the high-risk nature of their pregnancies, women with PNH require close medical attention in the antenatal, perinatal, and postnatal periods. Prophylactic anticoagulation is recommended because of the high incidence of thrombotic events during pregnancy.[106] Warfarin is contraindicated because of its teratogenicity. Low-molecular-weight heparin, meanwhile, is favored over unfractionated heparin because it less frequently causes heparin-induced thrombocytopenia. Anticoagulation should be interrupted during the perinatal period but, in the absence of contraindications, reinitiated thereafter and continued for 6 weeks postpartum.[106]

Results of a phase III trial by Hillmen and colleagues demonstrated that eculizumab, a humanized monoclonal antibody against the terminal complement protein C5, can reduce levels of hemolysis, stabilize hemoglobin, minimize transfusion requirement, and improve quality of life in patients with PNH.[107] Although the drug offers promise for pregnant women with PNH, it has not yet been studied in this patient population and thus cannot be recommended for use. Red blood cell transfusions are used in the treatment of anemia. In the setting of thrombocytopenia and bleeding, platelet transfusions may also be necessary.

Autoimmune Hemolytic Anemia

Autoimmune hemolytic anemia can occur during pregnancy and lead to anemia. The relatively small size of IgG immunoglobulin molecules allows them to cross the placenta; thus, the IgG subtype of autoimmune hemolytic anemia can adversely affect the fetus. In contrast, the larger IgM antibodies do not cross the placenta. Patients with autoimmune hemolytic anemia are treated with glucocorticoids and, if necessary, intravenous immunoglobulins. Supportive transfusions are administered when needed.[108] In rare instances, pregnancy appears to precipitate the development of autoimmune hemolytic anemia in a previously unaffected woman. The etiology of this phenomenon is not known.[109] Women in this circumstance have been treated in the standard fashion with favorable results.

THROMBOCYTOPENIA IN PREGNANCY

Thrombocytopenia occurs in approximately 7% to 12% of pregnancies. Most cases are attributed to gestational, or incidental, thrombocytopenia and require only routine monitoring.[110–112] On the other hand, several life-threatening syndromes associated with thrombocytopenia such as HELLP and disseminated intravascular coagulation can occur in pregnancy and require urgent evaluation. The various causes of thrombocytopenia during pregnancy are reviewed here.

Gestational (Incidental) Thrombocytopenia

Studies suggest that in up to 75% of cases, thrombocytopenia in pregnancy can be attributed to gestational thrombocytopenia.[112] Women with gestational thrombocytopenia typically have platelet counts in the 70,000 to 150,000/μL range, are otherwise healthy, and have no prior history of idiopathic thrombocytopenic purpura (ITP). Thrombocytopenia in these women most often develops late in the second trimester or in the third trimester. Although the etiology of gestational thrombocytopenia has not been clearly established, it is thought the condition results from pregnancy-related hemodilution and increased platelet clearance.[112]

Women with this condition can be reassured that gestational thrombocytopenia does not cause adverse effects on either the mother or fetus. Physicians could not always provide such reassurance; for many years, even mild thrombocytopenia in an otherwise healthy pregnant woman led to extensive evaluation and prompted concern about perinatal bleeding and adverse outcomes at the time of delivery. In an important study that changed this approach, Burrows and Kelton prospectively followed more than 2000 women who gave birth during a 1-year period at a single Canadian hospital. Eight percent of patients involved in the study were found to have mild thrombocytopenia that had no effect on the mother or fetus.[113]

Idiopathic (Autoimmune) Thrombocytopenic Purpura

Responsible for pregnancy-associated thrombocytopenia in approximately 3% of cases, idiopathic thrombocytopenic purpura (ITP) represents an important diagnostic consideration in this patient population. It is the most common cause of thrombocytopenia during the first two trimesters of pregnancy.[108,114] ITP can recur in a woman with previously documented disease or develop de novo during pregnancy. Pregnancy itself does not exacerbate the disease.

ITP may be difficult to distinguish from gestational thrombocytopenia, as patients with these conditions can present with similar clinical and laboratory findings. Elevated levels of platelet-associated IgG and antibody titers can be found in both conditions.[115] Furthermore, assays that detect antibodies against the glycoprotein receptors IIb/IIIa and Ib/IX are not specific for ITP.[116] Thrombocytopenia in the first trimester or early portion of the second trimester should raise suspicion for ITP, whereas thrombocytopenia that develops later in pregnancy should raise suspicion for gestational thrombocytopenia.

Women with preexisting ITP should be followed carefully during pregnancy, with monthly monitoring during the first two trimesters, biweekly in the third trimester, and weekly in the final weeks of pregnancy.[117] Management of ITP, meanwhile, depends on the maternal platelet count. Patients with severe thrombocytopenia (platelet count <10,000/μL) require immediate treatment. Options include corticosteroids, typically prednisone, at a dose of 1 mg/kg/day initially; high-dose intravenous immune globulin (IVIG) at an initial dose of 1 mg/kg; anti-D immune globulin in conjunction with steroids; or splenectomy for individuals who do not respond to other interventions. As one might expect, each of these therapies has limitations. IVIG, for example, has a relatively short duration of action (3–4 weeks) and thus may require readministration during the course of pregnancy. Though easily administered and relatively inexpensive, corticosteroids increase the incidence of gestational diabetes, pregnancy-induced hypertension, postpartum psychosis, and osteoporosis. Thus, corticosteroids should be avoided if possible. Anti-D immune globulin has been used in pregnant women with ITP, but large safety trials in pregnancy have not been performed.[110] Finally, splenectomy jeopardizes the life of the fetus, particularly when performed early in pregnancy. If it becomes necessary in the management of a pregnant woman with ITP, the procedure should be deferred until the second or third trimester if possible. Agents such as danazol, cyclophosphamide, and vinca alkaloids—though used in the management of ITP in nonpregnant individuals—are teratogenic and should be avoided during pregnancy.[117] Danazol may cause clitoral enlargement and labial fusion in female fetuses when given in the first trimester.[118]

Patients with mildly reduced platelet counts (60,000–100,000/μL) are followed without intervention. Individuals with slightly lower platelet counts (20,000–60,000/μL) do not require specific intervention either, but are more likely to require therapy as their pregnancy progresses. For these individuals, a single dose of IVIG 2 weeks prior to delivery or daily steroid therapy initiated 3 weeks prior to delivery can be administered to raise the platelet count above 50,000/μL.

As discussed previously, maternal antiplatelet IgG can cross the placenta and cause thrombocytopenia in the fetus.[119] Percutaneous umbilical blood sampling (PUBS) is the most accurate means to obtain the fetal platelet count. However, the procedure is associated with a high complication rate and 1% fetal mortality.[120] Intrapartum fetal scalp sampling represents an alternative, but the accuracy of this technique is only 50% to 70%.[121] Meanwhile, the maternal platelet count and antiplatelet antibody level do not accurately predict the fetal platelet count.[122] Overall, 10% of babies born to mothers with ITP have a platelet count less than 50,000/μL whereas fewer than 5% have a platelet count less than 20,000/μL.[114] Treatment of the pregnant woman with IVIG or steroids does not appear to affect the platelet count of her fetus.[123,124] Thrombocytopenia places neonates at risk for bleeding events, including intracranial hemorrhage, though this complication is rare.[125]

In light of the bleeding risk to both mother and fetus, the method of delivery in women with ITP has been a matter of debate. Some clinicians have advocated fetal platelet count monitoring with Cesarean section in instances where the fetal platelet count lies below 50,000/μL. On the other hand, others have argued for vaginal delivery in all pregnant women with ITP, citing the risks associated with fetal platelet count monitoring and the low incidence of fetal intracranial bleeding even with severe thrombocytopenia. At present, available guidelines on the subject suggest that obstetric factors, rather than hematologic ones, should guide the manner of delivery.[126] Following the delivery of a child, cord blood platelet is checked and the newborn platelet count followed because thrombocytopenia most often peaks 4 to 6 days after delivery and resolves as maternal antiplatelet IgG is cleared.

Preeclampsia and HELLP Syndrome

Thrombocytopenia in pregnant woman also occurs in association with preeclampsia and HELLP syndrome, potentially severe multisystem disorders associated with pregnancy. In previously healthy nulliparous women, the incidence of preeclampsia is between 2% and 7%.[127] Thrombocytopenia is observed in 15% to 50% of patients with this condition.[110,128] Clinical manifestations include a maternal syndrome characterized by hypertension, proteinuria, and systemic abnormalities as well as a fetal syndrome characterized by fetal growth restriction, preterm delivery, and hypoxia-induced neurologic damage.[127,128]

In most instances, preeclampsia occurs during a woman's first pregnancy, though it can recur in a subsequent pregnancy or occur for the first time in a woman with one or more previously unaffected pregnancies. Risk factors for the disorder include, but are not limited to, preeclampsia in a previous pregnancy, a family history of preeclampsia, chronic hypertension, obesity, multifetal gestation, rheumatic disease, and preexisting thrombophilia.[127] With respect to thrombophilia, a case control study by Mello and colleagues suggests that the prevalence of an underlying thrombophilia is significantly higher among women who develop preeclampsia during pregnancy than among those who have uneventful pregnancies.[129]

HELLP syndrome—defined by hemolysis, elevated liver enzymes, and low platelets—represents a severe variant of preeclampsia. In the majority of cases, patients who develop the syndrome are Caucasian and multiparious.[130] The median age of affected patients is 25. Meanwhile, the time of presentation during pregnancy ranges from the midtrimester (15%) to term (18%). Thirty percent of patients develop HELLP within 2 days after delivery.[131] Patients typically exhibit vague symptoms such as malaise, fatigue, epigastric or right upper quadrant pain, nausea, vomiting, and flu-like symptoms. Because of the nonspecific nature of these symptoms, diagnosis is often delayed; one study found an average time to diagnosis of 8 days in women with HELLP syndrome.[132] Clinical findings at the time of diagnosis—weight gain or edema, hypertension, and proteinuria—are similar to those observed in preeclampsia.[131]

Although various criteria have been used in diagnosing HELLP syndrome, they generally share the following features: hemolysis as evidenced by schistocytes on the peripheral blood smear, serum LDH greater than 600 U/L and/or serum total bilirubin greater than 1.2 mg/dL, AST greater than 70 IU/L, and a platelet count lower than 100,000/μL.[133] Martin and colleagues have further defined HELLP syndrome on the basis of platelet count. According to this classification, patients with class 1 HELLP syndrome have a platelet count lower than 50,000/μL, those with class 2 disease have a platelet count between 50,000 and 100,000/μL, and individuals with class 3 HELLP syndrome have a platelet count higher than 100,000/μL.[131] As might be expected, women with Class 1 HELLP syndrome required a recovery period in the aftermath of their illness.

Although the precise mechanism through which preeclampsia develops is uncertain, research in the field continues to advance understanding of the underlying pathophysiology. Endothelial cell dysfunction following placentation appears to play a central role in the pathogenesis of the disease. During development of the placenta, placental trophoblast cells interface with the epithelial layer of the uterus, forming the decidua. Penetration and remodeling of maternal spiral arteries beginning at week 9 during pregnancy increases placental perfusion and improves oxygenation for the developing fetus under normal conditions.[134]

Several studies in the late 1990s demonstrated low levels of vascular growth factor ligands—including vascular endothelial growth factor (VEGF), placenta growth factor (PIGF), and vascular endothelial growth factor receptor (VEGFR)-1—in women with HELLP.[132,135,136] In addition, decreased levels of active matrix metalloproteinase were noted in preeclamptic placentas as compared to normal individuals.[137] More recently, attention has focused on the purported antiangiogenic effects of soluble fms-like tyrosine kinase-1 (sFlt-1), a soluble receptor that binds both VEGF and placenta growth factor (PIGF).[138] Circulating levels of sFlt-1 are elevated in women with preeclampsia whereas levels of both VEGF and PIGF are reduced.

The role of immunologic factors in the pathogenesis of preeclampsia has also received recent attention. For example, the interaction between fetal trophoblasts and maternal T cells—primarily NK cells—appears to play a critical role in normal placental development.[139] Studies indicate that decidual NK cells uniquely recognize the HLA groups of infiltrating trophoblasts and suggest that insufficient activation of maternal NK cells may contribute to the development of preeclampsia.[134]

Cellular abnormalities such as those described impair placental implantation and vasculogenesis, leading to fetal hypoxia and the release of vasoactive compounds such as endothelin, nitric oxide, and prostaglandins. High levels of endothelin, a potent vasoconstrictor, are seen in preeclamptic patients, and injection of endothelin into rabbits produces a syndrome similar to HELLP syndrome.[140,141] The activity of endothelin, nitric oxide, and prostaglandins leads to hypertension and platelet activation. In turn, injury to the vascular endothelium results in fibrin deposition, further platelet activation, and the release of additional vasoactive agents such as serotonin and thromboxane A_2. The etiology of thrombocytopenia in preeclampsia is likely related to increased antiplatelet IgG levels[142] or to activation of the coagulation cascade with subsequent consumption of platelets.[143,144]

These events lead to the multisystem dysfunction seen in patients with HELLP syndrome. Fibrin deposition in the hepatic sinusoids causes hepatocellular injury. Patients can develop right upper quadrant pain if intraparenchymal or subcapsular hemorrhage occurs. Disseminated intravascular coagulation (DIC) was observed in 21% of patients with HELLP in one series, whereas placental abruption was seen in 16% of patients.[145] Other manifestations of HELLP syndrome include acute renal failure, pulmonary edema, shock, cerebrovascular accident (CVA), eclampsia,[146] retinal detachment,[140] diabetes insipidus,[147] and increased incidence of cesarean section.[148]

HELLP syndrome is associated with high maternal and neonatal mortality. Maternal mortality ranges from 1.1% to 24.2%.[149] The immediate cause of death is most often rupture of the liver, DIC, acute renal failure, pulmonary edema/acute respiratory distress syndrome (ARDS), shock, or CVA. Perinatal deaths resulting from placental abruption, asphyxia, or extreme prematurity occur in 10% to 15% of patients.[146] Following delivery, infants born to women with preeclampsia or HELLP can develop a self-limited neonatal thrombocytopenia. Uncertainty exists as to whether infant thrombocytopenia in these instances results from preeclampsia/HELLP itself or from a related complication such as neonatal sepsis.[150–152] HELLP recurs in subsequent pregnancies of affected women in 3% to 27% of cases. There is also an increased risk of preeclampsia, placental abruption, and preterm delivery in these pregnancies.[153,154]

In caring for the patient with preeclampsia or HELLP syndrome, the clinician's primary concerns are the mother's health and safety. The clinician must also consider the stage of pregnancy at time of diagnosis, the condition of the fetus, and desires of the patient in making management decisions. Definitive treatment for preeclampsia and HELLP involves delivery of the fetus; it is indicated for women who present after 34 weeks' gestation and those with evidence of multisystem dysfunction. However, conservative, supportive care without immediate delivery can be pursued for the woman who is relatively asymptomatic, hemodynamically stable, less than 32 to 34 weeks' gestation, and without evidence of abnormal coagulation.[155] Magnesium sulfate, which reduces cerebral vasoconstriction and ischemia, should be administered for seizure prophylaxis.[156] Parenteral labetalol or hydralazine is given for blood pressure control. Meanwhile, systemic corticosteroids appear to lessen the risk of maternal ARDS and reduce neonatal complications when administered to women who present at less than 34 weeks' gestation.[157] In addition to these measures, volume status is closely monitored to prevent overexpansion of plasma volume and ensure adequate urine output.

Persistent right upper quadrant pain—which may herald a liver hematoma or rupture, hemodynamic instability, coagulation profile abnormalities, or a decline in clinical status—should prompt delivery by cesarean section. As mentioned previously, delivery is also indicated if the fetus is at least 32 to 34 weeks of gestation at the time signs and symptoms of preeclampsia/HELLP develop. In a clinically stable woman, vaginal delivery can be attempted.[158] When cesarean section is required, transfusion of red blood cells, platelets, and fresh frozen plasma is performed as necessary prior to and during surgery. Severe hypofibrinogenemia should be treated with cryoprecipitate.

Patients are monitored closely in the postpartum period. Magnesium should be continued for 12 to 48 hours after delivery and blood pressure controlled appropriately. Although hypertension typically resolves within 6 weeks after delivery, some women require long-term antihypertensive therapy.[156] Coagulation and platelet abnormalities tend to resolve within the 24 to 48 hours following delivery. Some patients, however, experience an ongoing decline in the platelet count and should be followed until counts normalize. Postpartum eclampsia can occur for up to 48 hours after delivery; thus, patients and health care providers should remain vigilant in monitoring for suggestive signs and symptoms.[159] Treatment options in the setting of severe postpartum preeclampsia and HELLP include corticosteroids and plasmapheresis.[160,161]

In light of the morbidity and mortality associated with preeclampsia and HELLP, considerable research has focused on prevention of these conditions. The efficacy of various preventive strategies—including magnesium supplementation, low-dose aspirin, zinc supplementation, antihypertensive drugs, and heparin therapy among others—has been the focus of observational studies, systematic reviews, and randomized trials. Initial small studies suggested that low-dose aspirin reduces the risk of preeclampsia, although patients who received aspirin had a higher incidence of placental abruption and bleeding.[162] Larger, randomized trials failed to confirm the benefit of low-dose aspirin.[163,164] Antioxidants vitamin C and vitamin E have shown promise in small trials, but further testing needs to be done.[165] Calcium supplementation appeared to be beneficial based on a study of Ecuadorian pregnant teens,[166] but a subsequent randomized study performed in the United States showed no benefit to this intervention.[167] Some clinicians endorse calcium supplementation in patients with low dietary calcium intake, particularly for those expectant mothers at risk for preeclampsia.[168] Supplemental fish oil may lower the risk of preterm delivery in women with previous preterm delivery, twin pregnancies, intrauterine growth retardation, or preeclampsia, but further studies are needed to confirm this benefit.[169]

Thrombotic Thrombocytopenic Purpura–Hemolytic Uremic Syndrome

Thrombotic thrombocytopenic purpura (TTP) and hemolytic uremic syndrome (HUS) are also important considerations in the evaluation of pregnant women with thrombocytopenia. Like preeclampsia/HELLP, they are multisystem disorders associated with high morbidity and mortality in the absence of appropriate therapy. Microvascular injury and platelet agglutination with resulting thrombocytopenia and microangiopathic hemolytic anemia are pathologic hallmarks of TTP and HUS (Fig. 161–1). They are rare conditions overall, but the incidence of both increases in pregnancy.[170] In the case of TTP, in fact, estimates suggest that approximately 10% of cases occur in pregnant or postpartum women.[171]

Because they share many common clinical features, TTP and HUS are often categorized as a single entity, TTP-HUS. However, the pathophysiology underlying the two conditions appears to be distinctive. TTP is associated with unusually large multimers of circulating von Willebrand factor, which foster platelet aggregation and thrombus formation. Under normal circumstances, a von Willebrand factor-cleaving protease referred to as ADAMTS13 cleaves these multimers into smaller multimers of normal size. In TTP, function of the cleaving protease is impaired. ADAMTS13 deficiency characterizes familial TTP. Meanwhile, inhibition of ADAMTS13 protease activity by an autoantibody characterizes the acquired form of TTP. An inhibitory autoantibody can be found in 70% to 85% of patients with TTP.[172] On the other hand, impaired von Willebrand factor-cleaving protease activity does not appear to play a role in the pathogenesis of HUS.[173]

It can be difficult to distinguish TTP and HUS from HELLP syndrome. From a clinical standpoint, this represents an important distinction because accurate diagnosis dictates appropriate therapy. TTP tends to occur earlier in pregnancy, with a mean onset at 23.5

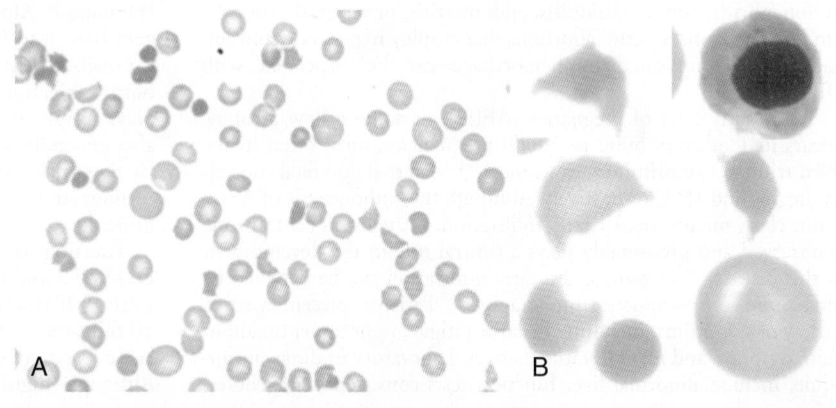

Figure 161–1 Microangiopathic hemolytic anemia, in pregnancy, peripheral blood smear (**A–B**). Evidence of microangiopathy with the formation of schistocytes, fragmented forms and spherocytes, associated with polychromasia and nucleated red blood cells (**A** and **B**, detail).

weeks, although it can occur at any point from the first trimester through the postpartum period.[174] HUS primarily occurs after delivery; 90% of cases occur in the postpartum period, with a mean onset at 26 days after delivery.[175] TTP and HUS do not cause hypertension or liver necrosis. Furthermore, TTP and HUS frequently persist after delivery whereas HELLP typically resolves in the postpartum period.

Early studies of pregnant women with TTP-HUS documented a maternal mortality rate of 44% and a perinatal mortality rate of 80%.[175] Occlusion of vessels within the decidua and resulting placental ischemia primarily account for fetal morbidity and mortality.[176] Treatment of TTP–HUS involves emergent plasmapheresis within 24 to 48 hours of diagnosis. The response rate among pregnant women treated with plasmapheresis for TTP is approximately 75%. By comparison, the overall response rate in patients with TTP is approximately 80% to 90%.[177–179] Long-term sequelae in surviving patients include chronic renal failure, hypertension, and recurrence of TTP–HUS. TTP–HUS recurs in approximately 50% of subsequent pregnancies.[180] Infusion of fresh frozen plasma represents an alternative to plasmapheresis, though plasmapheresis is the preferred treatment modality. The response rate following fresh frozen plasma infusion is 64%.[181] Corticosteroids (prednisolone 200 mg IV per day or prednisone 200 mg PO per day) have also been successfully used in the treatment of pregnancy-associated TTP–HUS, with a response rate of 26%.[179] Conversely, antiplatelet agents such as aspirin do not play a role in the treatment of pregnancy-associated TTP–HUS.[182]

Disseminated Intravascular Coagulation

Disseminated intravascular coagulation (DIC) in the pregnant woman can occur in various clinical settings, including HELLP syndrome, TTP–HUS, placental abruption, amniotic fluid embolism, uterine rupture, intrauterine fetal demise, sepsis, elective abortion, and acute fatty liver of pregnancy.

Severe placental abruption sufficient to cause fetal death occurs in 0.12% of all pregnancies.[183] This condition leads to a consumptive hypofibrinogenemia, and—when fibrinogen levels fall below 100 to 150 mg/dL—bleeding may ensue. Maintenance of adequate urine output and a hematocrit level greater than 30% are important components of care for the woman who has suffered a placental abruption. Either vaginal delivery or cesarean section is appropriate in the context of severe placental abruption. In a woman undergoing cesarean section following abruption, the platelet count should be maintained at 50,000/µL or above through platelet transfusion and fibrinogen replaced with fresh frozen plasma or cryoprecipitate.

Amniotic fluid embolism is a rare but often lethal condition with a mortality rate of approximately 80%.[184] Ten to 15% of these patients develop a coagulopathy. DIC in this setting most likely follows the release of thromboplastin-rich material into the maternal circulation. DIC seen in association with uterine rupture and intrauterine fetal demise presumably occurs through a similar mechanism.[185] On the contrary, bacterial endotoxin or exotoxin mediates sepsis-associated DIC in the pregnant woman with pyelonephritis, chorioamnionitis, endometritis, or septic abortion.[186] On rare occasions, elective abortions that employ hypertonic solution and those complicated by hemorrhage can be associated with DIC.[187]

Acute fatty liver of pregnancy (AFLP), or acute yellow atrophy, occurs in 1 of every 5000 to 10000 pregnancies, most often in the third trimester of primiparous women.[188] Maternal and fetal mortality are 5% and 15%, respectively. Although the pathogenesis of AFLP is not clear, microvesicular fatty infiltration of the liver's central zone is observed and presumably plays a central role in the development of this disease.[189] In some cases, fatty infiltration can be detected by ultrasound or computed tomography.[190] Patients present with a variety of symptoms, including malaise, fatigue, right upper quadrant pain, dyspnea, and mental status changes. Laboratory findings, meanwhile, include abnormal liver function tests consistent with cholestatic disease, elevated ammonia, low fibrinogen and antithrombin levels, and elevated prothrombin time, with evidence of DIC. Hepatic dysfunction can impair gluconeogenesis. Diabetes insipidus may be present. The clinical course of AFLP resembles that of HELLP, TTP, and HUS, although the microangiopathy and thrombocytopenia are not as severe.[191] With supportive care, the condition typically resolves within 10 days after delivery.

BLEEDING DISORDERS

von Willebrand Disease

Affecting approximately 1% of the population, von Willebrand disease (vWD) is the most common inherited disorder of coagulation. By mediating platelet adhesion and functioning as a carrier for circulating factor VIII, von Willebrand factor (vWF) plays a vital role in hemostasis. According to the most widely used classification by Sadler, there are 3 types of vWD: type 1 (partial deficiency of vWF), type 3 (severe deficiency of vWF), and type 2, which includes four subtypes that involve qualitative defects in vWF.[192] Factor VIIIc, vWF antigen (vWF:Ag), and the ristocetin cofactor activity (vWF:RCo) are important components of the laboratory diagnosis. vWD does not impair fertility or increase the likelihood of miscarriage.[193] Thus, the management of pregnancy in patients with the condition is an important feature of the overall care for these individuals.

For the pregnant woman with vWD, bleeding at parturition and in the postpartum period is of primary concern. Related concerns include the administration of anesthesia, perineal hematoma, episiotomy blood loss and healing, and bleeding at surgical sites. Approximately 75% of women with moderate to severe vWD will experience significant peripartum bleeding.[194] And overall, there is a 20% risk of postpartum hemorrhage in women with vWD. In a normal pregnancy, FVIIIc and vWF levels increase, beginning in the second trimester.[195] They peak as the pregnancy nears term. Among many pregnant women with vWD, particularly those with Type 1 disease, a similar increase in FVIII and vWF levels is observed. Factor VIIIc levels in pregnant women with vWD peak at 29 to 32 weeks' gestation whereas vWF:Ag levels peak at approximately 35 weeks' gestation.[196] The risk of peripartum bleeding is related to the level of these factors.[197] In most instances, vWF:Ag, factor VIIIc, and vWF:RCo levels should be assessed during the first and third trimester to determine bleeding risk for individuals with vWD. However, this may be less relevant for patients with Type 3 vWD, wherein levels tend to remain low throughout pregnancy. Patients without a documented bleeding disorder who suffer bleeding complications during pregnancy should be evaluated for vWD because many with the disorder have a mild clinical course and remain undiagnosed for a long period.[198]

As a general rule, therapy can be rendered either in the setting of a spontaneous bleeding event or in a prophylactic context for the high risk individual. Mainstays of therapy for pregnant women with vWD include DDAVP (1-deamino-8-D-arginine-vasopressin), a synthetic analogue of vasopressin, and vWF-FVIII concentrates (Humate-P, Alphanate). Cryoprecipitate can be used on an emergent basis if vWF–FVIII concentrates are unavailable, but is avoided if possible during pregnancy because it poses a small risk of blood-borne infection.[199] Meanwhile, although antifibrinolytic therapy plays a role in the management of individuals with vWD, it is also generally avoided during pregnancy and lactation because of its potential teratogenicity and effects on the newborn. Data concerning the toxicity of antifibrinolytic therapy in pregnancy is limited.

Exerting its effect through the type 2 vasopressin receptors, DDAVP rapidly and transiently increases levels of factor VIII and vWF.[200] It is administered by continuous intravenous infusion over 30 minutes in the setting of an acute bleeding event. On a prophylactic basis, it can be given subcutaneously or inhaled nasally.[200] Although highly effective when used in an appropriate clinical context, DDAVP does have limitations. Patients who have never received DDAVP therapy should be tested for responsiveness to the agent during the second trimester. Because of its potential oxytocic effect, DDAVP is pregnancy risk category B.[196] Owing to its antidiuretic effect, meanwhile, DDAVP can cause fluid retention and hyponatremia. Finally, DDAVP has uncertain utility in the management of women with type 2 and type 3 vWD because of underlying genetic defect in these individuals. VWF–factor VIII concentrate is indicated for these patients.

Multidisciplinary care by an experienced obstetrician and hematologist should be provided for the pregnant woman with vWD. This becomes particularly important as parturition nears. In providing care for this population of patients, clinicians aim to control disease effects in the pregnant and postpartum mother. Factor VIIIc and vWF : RCo levels, PTT, type and cross match, and a complete blood count are obtained at the time of hospital admission. Women with vWD should be monitored for bleeding at the time of delivery, with transfusional products and DDAVP available for use as needed. vWF : RCo and factor VIIIc levels of 50 IU/dL generally serve as a target at parturition and in the postpartum period; expert opinion suggests that women with levels below this should receive replacement products.[201]

In the management of pregnant women with vWD, the provision of regional anesthesia during delivery is an important topic. Some anesthesiologists employ epidural anesthesia in patients with mild disease, with or without the use of DDAVP.[202,203] For patients with moderate to severe disease, an alternative form of analgesia may be considered. If epidural analgesia is utilized in a patient with moderate to severe disease, prophylactic therapy is indicated. The epidural catheter should be removed soon after delivery, as falling factor levels in the postpartum period increase the bleeding risk.[199]

The route of delivery is also an important matter in patients with vWD. To minimize the risk of neonatal hemorrhage, some obstetricians recommend cesarean delivery for patients with type 2, type 3, and clinically moderate type I disease. However, neonatal bleeding occurs in the setting of cesarean delivery as well, and delivery methods have not been rigorously compared.[196,202]

Prenatal testing is a challenge in women with vWD. The specific mutations involved in the pathogenesis of type 1 and type 3 vWD are not known. And multiple mutations are involved in the pathogenesis of type 2 vWD. Fetal blood vWF levels can be obtained in necessary, but there are inherent risks associated with the procedure.[204] Expectant mothers should be informed of these risks in making decisions about prenatal genetic testing (Fig. 161–2).

Hemophilias

The hemophilias (A and B) are X-linked recessive diseases characterized by hemarthrosis and subcutaneous and intramuscular bleeding.[205] Hemophilia A results from deficient production of factor VIII, and hemophilia B, from deficient production of factor IX. As X-linked disorders, hemophilia A and B occur most often in men, but they can occur in women under several circumstances, including X-chromosome inactivation (lyonization), X hemizygosity, and double heterozygosity as can occur in the female offspring of an affected father and carrier mother.[206] In the United States, women account for 1.7% of patients with hemophilia A and 3.2% of patients with hemophilia B.[207] Fifty percent of male offspring from a female carrier inherit the disorder, whereas 100% of male offspring from an affected mother inherit the disease. Female carriers in both disorders can be detected through laboratory screening and pedigree analysis.[208] Women with hemophilia and pregnant women with an affected fetus must be monitored closely during pregnancy for bleeding events that compromise the well-being of either the mother or fetus. Fetal umbilical blood sampling can be used to check factor VIII and factor IX levels. Chorionic villus sampling may also be used.[209]

At parturition, women with hemophilia A whose factor VIIIc level lies below 50% of the normal range should receive purified factor VIII. Levels should be greater than 80% for surgery and maintained at 30% to 40% for 3 to 4 days postoperatively. Rarely, thrombosis can occur in the aftermath of factor VIII replacement therapy.[210] Six to 10% of neonates with hemophilia have hemorrhagic complications in the perinatal period, including intracranial hemorrhage. Vacuum extractors, forceps delivery, and scalp electrodes should be avoided. To date, no studies have rigorously compared vaginal and cesarean delivery in this patient population. Neonatal blood should be assayed for factor VIIIc levels and PTT immediately after birth.[203] Neonates with low factor VIIIc levels may require serial cranial ultrasounds to rule out bleeding.[211]

Hemophilia B is treated in a similar fashion. However, it should be noted that cryoprecipitate contains low levels of factor IX and should not be used as replacement therapy in the management of this condition. Purified factor IX is the agent of choice for patients with hemophilia B. Meanwhile, individuals with other clotting factor deficiencies should receive fresh frozen plasma or specific clotting factor products to maintain factor levels at greater than 25%.[212] One exception to this pertains to the management of patients with factor XIII deficiency; the occurrence of spontaneous recurrent abortions and uterine bleeding in these individuals necessitates regular infusions of

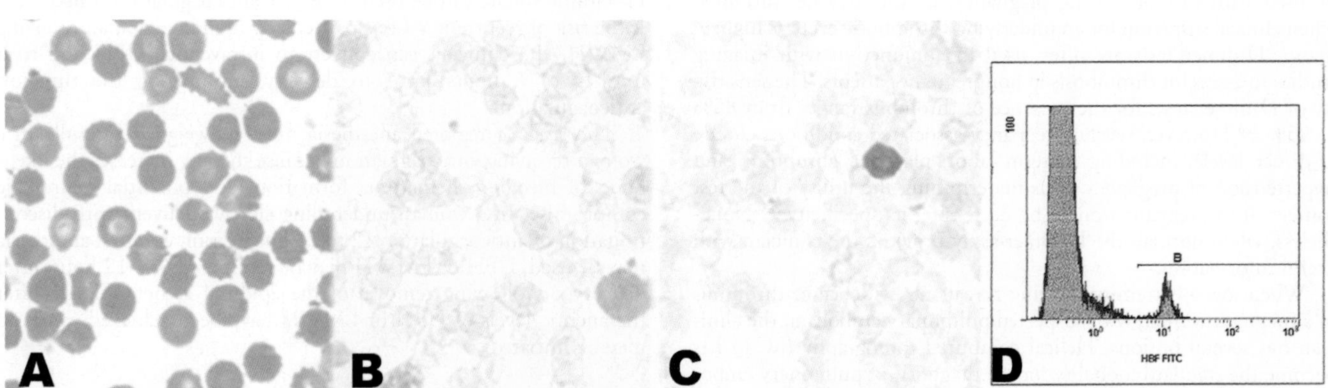

Figure 161–2 Evaluation of fetal–maternal bleed: Kleihauer–Betke test and flow cytometric analysis of Hgb F in red blood cells (**A–D**). The principle behind the Kleihauer–Betke test is that fetal cells are resistant to acid elution. In **A**, a fetal control specimen, none of the cells are eluted of their hemoglobin, whereas in a normal adult control, **B**, essentially all cells are lysed and negative. The rare weakly positive cells (see single cell, right side) are adult cells that contain increased Hgb F, but not at the level of a fetal cell. In the test case (**C**), rare fetal cells in the maternal blood can be detected and enumerated. Note the bight staining in the single positive cell. An alternative to this acid elution test is the direct measure Hgb F in red blood cells with an anti-HgbF antibody and flow cytometric analysis. The histogram shows a large negative peak (left) corresponding to adult cells containing only HgbA. There is an intermediate shoulder to the right corresponding to adult cells containing increased HgbF (**F** cells), and there are fetal cells in a distinct small positive peak, corresponding to cells from the fetal–maternal bleed.

fresh frozen plasma or factor XIII concentrate to maintain pregnancy.[213]

VENOUS THROMBOEMBOLIC DISEASE AND PREGNANCY

VTE disease is a leading cause of maternal morbidity and mortality.[214] The risk of venous thromboembolism increases two- to fourfold during pregnancy and the early postpartum period.[215] In women who have had a previous VTE event, pregnancy appears to increase the risk of a recurrent thromboembolic event.[216] Various factors account for the prothrombotic state associated with pregnancy. Increased estrogen levels early in pregnancy increase venous distention and contribute to venous stasis.[217] Increased plasma volume and compression of the inferior vena cava by the gravid uterus contributes to venous stasis as well.[218] In addition, studies have demonstrated decreased blood flow velocity in pregnant women, particularly in the left leg when pregnant women lie in a supine position. This phenomenon likely explains the increased risk of left leg thrombosis among pregnant women.[219] Furthermore, the concentration of coagulation factors changes during pregnancy. The concentration of vWF, fibrinogen, and prothrombin, along with factors V, VII, VIII, IX, X, and XII increases, whereas the concentration of factor XI and protein S decreases.[220–222] Finally, fibrinolytic activity decreases during pregnancy as the level of plasminogen activator inhibitors 1 and 2 increases.[223] Other factors—including high body mass index, smoking, immobilization, and age more than 35 years—should also be considered when assessing the thrombotic risk of a pregnant woman.

Because of the prothrombotic physiology associated with pregnancy, a clinician's concern for venous thromboembolism in a pregnant woman should prompt immediate evaluation. To assess for lower-extremity thrombosis, venous compression ultrasound remains the initial test of choice. Ultrasound poses no threat to the fetus and can detect thrombosis of the proximal common femoral and popliteal veins with a sensitivity of 95% and specificity of 96%. Despite the efficacy of ultrasound, limitations to its use do exist. The test is less effective for the diagnosis of calf vein thrombosis, with a sensitivity and specificity in the 60% to 70% range.[224] For this reason, a woman with suspected lower-extremity DVT should undergo serial ultrasounds if the initial evaluation is nondiagnostic.[225] Similarly, thrombus in the common iliac vein can evade diagnosis by venous compression ultrasound.

In such cases, other modalities such as contrast venography and magnetic resonance venography (MRV) can be considered. Although contrast venography exposes the fetus to radiation and should thus be used with caution during pregnancy, its use may be warranted when clinical suspicion for an underlying thrombotic event is high.[224] Serum D-dimer tests are often used in conjunction with imaging studies to assess for thrombosis in nonpregnant patients. The sensitivity of D-dimer tests for the presence of thrombus ranges from 85% to 95%.[226] However, several pregnancy-associated conditions elevate D-dimer levels, including preterm labor, placental abruption, and hypertension of pregnancy, thus undermining the utility of the test somewhat in pregnant women by decreasing its specificity.[223] Nonetheless, when normal, the D-dimer assay provides the clinician with useful information.

When lower-extremity imaging reveals no evidence of thrombus in a pregnant woman with suspected pulmonary embolism, the clinician has several options. Helical computed tomography (hCT) has become the standard modality for the diagnosis of pulmonary embolism in nonpregnant individuals at many centers. However, even with abdominal shielding, the procedure results in fetal radiation exposure (approximately 16 mrad) due to internal scatter.[227] Although this low level of radiation exposure probably does not cause harm to the fetus, repeated imaging during the course of pregnancy is to be avoided.[225] Ventilation-perfusion (VQ) scanning is frequently employed in the evaluation of pregnant women with suspected pulmonary embolism, but has limitations as well. Results of a prospective study indicate that when used in this patient population, VQ scanning infrequently yields a conclusively positive result (1.8% of cases) and is often nondiagnostic (24.8% of cases).[228] Finally, pulmonary angiography can be utilized in the evaluation of pulmonary embolism in rare instances when the previously described diagnostic tests yield nondiagnostic results in the face of a high clinical suspicion.

VTE in pregnancy is treated with heparin. Until low-molecular-weight heparin (LMWH) was introduced in the late 1980s, unfractionated heparin (UF) was the anticoagulant of choice for treatment of pregnant women with VTE. Because it does not cross the placenta, UF is nonteratogenic. However, drawbacks to UF therapy—including heparin-associated osteoporosis, heparin-induced thrombocytopenia (HIT), and the drug's unpredictable pharmacokinetics—are well documented.[214] Heparin-associated osteoporosis can develop in women who receive at least 1 month of therapy; it is likely related to a toxic effect of heparin on osteoblasts.[229] Because of its more favorable side-effect profile, reliable pharmacokinetics, and equal efficacy in treating VTE, LMWH now represents the most commonly used anticoagulant for treatment of VTE in pregnancy.[230] The risk of osteoporosis and HIT appears to be less with LMWH-based anticoagulation than with UF-based anticoagulation.[231,232] Though practice patterns vary, it is reasonable to base the initial dose of LMWH on early-pregnancy—rather than current—weight.[233] Because clearance of LMWH increases during pregnancy, twice-daily dosing regimens are preferred to once-daily regimens.[234] In terms of duration of therapeutic anticoagulation, many clinicians continue therapy at full dose through the entire pregnancy and puerperium based on the rationale that pregnancy itself represents a risk factor for recurrent VTE.[230] In contrast, other clinicians advocate initial anticoagulation with full-dose LMWH for a designated period followed by conversion to an intermediate dose. This approach may be beneficial for individuals susceptible to side effects of anticoagulation such as bleeding or osteoporosis.[214]

Warfarin is contraindicated in pregnant women. It crosses the placenta and can cause both fetal hemorrhage and nervous system abnormalities and other teratogenic effects.[235] Warfarin can be used in the postpartum period after initiating therapy with concurrent heparin, and in this setting does not appear to increase the risk of bleeding in children of lactating mothers.[224] Danaparoid, a heparinoid, is recommended for the treatment of HIT in the pregnant woman.[214] This agent does not cross the placenta and has little cross-reactivity with UF and LMWH.

Anticoagulation should be discontinued at the time of parturition. UFH and LMWH should, in most circumstances, be stopped 12 to 24 hours prior to delivery. If delivery is imminent, and there is question as to the level of anticoagulation, activated partial thromboplastin time (aPTT) or activated Factor Xa levels should be checked. Protamine sulfate can be used to reverse anticoagulation if necessary. If the risk of recurrent VTE is particularly high in a woman receiving LMWH, the clinician can convert to intravenous UFH and treat until 4 to 6 hours prior to delivery, minimizing the time off anticoagulation.

The risks of regional anesthesia must be weighed carefully in a woman receiving anticoagulation because therapy increases the likelihood of bleeding, hematoma formation, and potential neurologic compromise. In a woman undergoing elective delivery with discontinuation of anticoagulation 12 to 24 hours prior, epidural anesthesia may be used. UFH or LMWH may be reinitiated 6 to 12 hours after delivery or following removal of the epidural catheter. Then, after therapeutic levels of UFH or LMWH have been achieved, warfarin may be initiated.

PROPHYLACTIC ANTICOAGULATION DURING PREGNANCY

Given the prothrombotic state associated with pregnancy itself, prophylactic anticoagulation should be considered in pregnant women with a prior history of VTE. Recurrence rates for VTE during pregnancy may be as high as 12% based on the results of retrospective studies.[236] Conversely, Brill-Edwards and colleagues prospectively studied 125 pregnant women with prior VTE in a study that excluded women with known thrombophilia.[237] Study subjects did not receive prophylactic anticoagulation during the antenatal period, but did receive anticoagulation therapy for 4 to 6 weeks postpartum. The authors documented a VTE recurrence rate of 2.4%. Women who had a temporary risk factor at the time of their initial VTE event and lacked laboratory evidence of an underlying hypercoagulable disorder at the time of study enrollment experienced no recurrences during pregnancy. Based on the results of this study, routine prophylactic anticoagulation for women with a single previous VTE event is not recommended. However, patients with a known hypercoagulable state, those with multiple previous VTE events, and those considered high risk for recurrent VTE should receive prophylactic anticoagulation during pregnancy and for 4 to 6 weeks postpartum. As previously discussed, prophylactic anticoagulation can be discontinued at parturition and reinitiated 6 to 12 hours postpartum.

The management of pregnant women with prosthetic heart valves is controversial and deserves special attention, though a full review of the topic is beyond the scope of this review. Coupled with the prothrombotic physiology of pregnancy, the presence of a prosthetic valve places such women in an ultra-high risk category. Prior to the introduction of LMWH, options for anticoagulation in this patient population included (a) warfarin throughout pregnancy, (b) warfarin, with UFH during weeks 6 to 12, the period of major organogenesis, and (c) UFH throughout pregnancy.[214] More recently, LMWH has been utilized in this setting, though its safety and efficacy have been questioned on the basis of several studies. Overall, a lack of rigorous, comparative studies hinders evidence-based management of women with prosthetic heart valves. Current recommendations allow for one of three therapeutic strategies, initiated after a thorough discussion of risks and benefits with the patient: (a) warfarin, with LMWH or UF substituted during weeks 6 to 12, (b) dose-adjusted UFH throughout pregnancy, or (c) dose-adjusted LMWH throughout pregnancy.[214]

THROMBOPHILIA AND PREGNANCY

Thrombophilias, inherited and acquired, increase the risk of VTE in pregnant women and adversely affect pregnancy outcomes. Included within this category of diseases are factor V Leiden, prothrombin gene polymorphisms, antiphospholipid antibody syndrome, antithrombin deficiency, along with protein S and C deficiency.

Factor V Leiden Gene Polymorphism

The factor V Leiden gene polymorphism is the most common inherited genetic disorder among pregnant women with a history of VTE, occurring in approximately 44% of cases.[238] It is characterized by a guanine-to-adenine point mutation at position 1691.[239] The mutation, which occurs in 3% of low-risk obstetric patients, impairs cleavage of procoagulant factor Va by activated protein C.[240] The risk of thrombosis is 5- to 10-fold higher in factor V Leiden heterozygotes than in normal individuals and 50- to 100-fold higher in homozygotes than in normal individuals.[241] The incidence of thrombosis in pregnancy among patients with the factor V Leiden gene polymorphism is approximately 17%.[242] A progressive decrease in activated protein C during pregnancy compounds the prothrombotic effect of the factor V Leiden mutation.[243] Besides VTE, women with the Factor V Leiden mutation can develop placental thrombosis and, in turn, complications associated with placental hypoxia such as preeclampsia and HELLP, placental abruption, intrauterine growth restriction, stillbirth, and—likely—first trimester miscarriage.[243]

Women with a documented factor V Leiden polymorphism should receive anticoagulation during pregnancy. An individual with the disorder who has never experienced thrombotic complications receives prophylactic doses of UFH or LMWH. On the other hand, a woman who has experienced a serious thrombotic complication receives therapeutic anticoagulation throughout pregnancy and for 6 to 12 weeks postpartum. Given the frequency of this mutation, a pregnant woman who presents with either a family or personal history of VTE should undergo testing for the factor V Leiden polymorphism to ensure proper risk stratification and therapeutic management.

Antiphospholipid Antibody Syndrome

The antiphospholipid antibody syndrome is the most common form of acquired thrombophilia.[244] Antiphospholipid antibodies include lupus anticoagulant antibodies and anticardiolipin antibodies. They can occur as a manifestation of various conditions, such as systemic lupus erythematosus (SLE) and other rheumatic diseases, infection, and drug reactions. Antiphospholipid antibodies exert their prothrombotic effect through several mechanisms. For example, they inhibit the activity of anticoagulants thrombomodulin, protein S, protein C, β2-glycoprotein I, and prostacyclin.[245–247] They interact with phospholipids on the surface of platelets, increasing platelet adhesiveness and production of von Willebrand mulitmers.[248,249] And in the pregnant patient, antiphospholipid antibodies decrease levels of annexin V, a potent vascular endothelial anticoagulant produced by placental trophoblasts.[250] Nonpregnant individuals with antiphospholipid antibody syndrome can develop arterial and venous thromboses. In the pregnant woman, antiphospholipid antibody syndrome can manifest as thrombotic events, spontaneous abortion, preeclampsia and HELLP syndrome, and intrauterine fetal growth restriction.[251–254]

Antiphospholipid antibodies can be detected in 5% of healthy pregnant women and 37% of pregnant women with SLE.[255] Meanwhile, thrombotic events occur in approximately 5% of pregnant women with antiphospholipid antibodies.[254] All pregnant women with SLE should undergo testing for antiphospholipid antibodies. Women who sustain recurrent spontaneous abortions or a thromboembolic event during pregnancy should also undergo evaluation for the disorder. A history of either vascular thrombosis or fetal loss coupled with the presence of either lupus anticoagulant antibodies or anticardiolipin antibodies establishes the diagnosis of antiphospholipid antibody syndrome.[256] False-negative laboratory results do occur, and do so more frequently in pregnant than in nonpregnant women. This may be due to the increased concentration of clotting factors observed in pregnancy.[257] Women with antiphospholipid antibody syndrome who have sustained prior thrombotic events receive therapeutic anticoagulation during pregnancy. Those with antiphospholipid antibodies but no manifestations of the clinical syndrome should receive prophylactic anticoagulation.

Hyperhomocysteinemia

Homocysteine is a thiol-containing amino acid that plays an important role in several metabolic pathways, including pathways that involve cobalamin (vitamin B_{12}) and folate. In a normal pregnancy, the concentration of homocysteine decreases, presumably as a result of increased glomerular filtration, increased plasma volume and hemodilution, and perhaps uptake by the developing fetus.[258] Individuals who are homozygous for the thermolabile variant of methylenetetrahydrofolate reductase (MTHFR) can develop hyperhomocysteinemia, a condition associated with a number of pregnancy-related complications, including thrombosis, preeclampsia, spontaneous abortion, placental abruption, intrauterine fetal growth restriction, fetal neural tube defects, and stillbirth.[259,260] Although folate supplementation decreases the risk of fetal neural tube defects, it does not appear to decrease the incidence of thrombotic complications.

Prothrombin Gene Mutation

A polymorphism in the prothrombin gene (20210A) occurs in approximately 1% of pregnant women.[241] Among those who harbor the polymorphism, 3% to 10% will develop thrombotic complications during pregnancy. Studies demonstrate an increased risk of preeclampsia and HELLP syndrome,[261] spontaneous abortion,[262] and intrauterine growth retardation[263] in women with the prothrombin gene mutation. Such women are treated like those with the factor V Leiden polymorphism.

SUGGESTED READINGS

Al RA, Unlubilgin E, Kandamir O, et al: Intravenous verses oral iron for treatment of anemia in pregnancy: A randomized trial. Obstet Gynecol 106:1335, 2005.

Ali R, Ozkalemkas F, Ozcelik T, Ozkocaman V, et al: Imatinib and pregnancy. J Clin Oncol 24:3812, 2006.

Ault P, Kantarjian H, O'Brien S, et al: Pregnancy among patients with chronic myeloid leukemia treated with imatinib. J Clin Oncol 24:1204, 2006.

Casanueva E, Viteri FE, Mares-Galindo M, et al: Weekly iron as a safe alternative to daily supplementation for nonanemic pregnant women. Arch Med Res 12:674, 2006.

Clines DB, McMillan R: Management of adult idiopathic thrombocytopenia purpura. Annu Rev Med 56:425, 2005.

Dilek I, Topcu N, Demir C, et al: Hematologic malignancy and pregnancy: A single-institution experience of 21 cases. Clin Lab Haem 28:170, 2006.

Diop S, Sarr P, toure-Fall AO, et al: Normal delivery is still a challenge during pregnancy in sickle cell disease patients. Ann Hematol 84:194, 2005.

Franchini M, Veneri D: The antiphospholipid syndrome. Hematology 10:265, 2005.

Greer IA, Nelson-Piercy C: Low-molecular-weight heparins for thromboprophylaxis and treatment of venous thromboembolism in pregnancy: A systematic review of safety and efficacy. Blood 106:401, 2005.

Harrison, C: Pregnancy and its management in the Philadelphia negative myeloproliferative diseases. Br J Haematol 129; 293, 2005.

Hillmen P, Young NS, Shubert J, et al: The complement inhibitor eculizimab in paroxysmal nocturnal hemoglobinuria. N Engl J Med 355:1233, 2006.

James AH: von Willebrand disease. Obstet Gyncecol Surv 61:136, 2006.

Kujovich JL: von Willebrand disease and pregnancy. J Thromb Haemost 3:246, 2005.

Lam C, Lim K, Karumanchi SA: Circulating angiogenic factors in the pathogenesis and prediction of preeclampsia. Hypertension 46:1077, 2005.

McMullin MF, Bareford D, Campbell P, et al: Guidelines for the diagnosis, investigation and management of polycythaemia/erythrocytosis. Br J Haematol 130:174, 2005.

Mello G, Parretti E, Marozio L, et al: Thrombophilia is significantly associated with severe preeclampsia: Results of a large-scale, case-controlled study. Hypertension 46:1270, 2005.

Nassar AH, Usta IM, Rechdan JB, et al: Pregnancy in patients with beta-thalassemia intermedia: Outcome of mothers and newborns. Am J Hematol 81:499, 2006.

Niedermeier DM, Frei-Lahr DA, Hall PD: Treatment of acute myeloid leukemia during the second and third trimesters of pregnancy. Pharmacotherapy 25:1134, 2005.

Parker C, Omine M, Richards S, et al: Diagnosis and management of paroxysmal nocturnal hemoglobinuria. Blood 106:3699, 2005.

Redman CW, Sargent IL: Latest advances in understanding preeclampsia. Science 308:1592, 2005.

Robertson L, Wu O, Langhorne P: Thrombophilia in pregnancy. Br J Haematol 132:171, 2005.

Sibai B, Dekker G, Kupferminc M: Pre-eclampsia. Lancet 365:785, 2005.

Thrombosis in a pregnant hemophilia A carrier after intrapartum recombinant factor VIII. Obstet Gynecol 105:875, 2005.

Thurman AR, Steed LL, Hulsey T, et al: Bacteriuria in pregnant women with sickle cell trait. Am J Obstet Gynecol 194:1366, 2006.

REFERENCES

For complete list of references log onto www.expertconsult.com

CHAPTER 162

HEMATOLOGIC MANIFESTATIONS OF CHILDHOOD ILLNESS

A. Kim Ritchey, Frank G. Keller, and Sarah H. O'Brien

The hematologic response to systemic illness in children is similar to that in adults. A number of disorders occur more frequently in children, however, and some are unique to the pediatric population. In addition, interpretation of the hematologic response is predicated on knowledge of the normal developmental changes that occur within the hematopoietic system throughout childhood (Table 162–1).

This chapter focuses on the hematologic manifestations of common or unique systemic diseases that occur in the neonate, child, or adolescent. Illnesses that often require hematologic consultation are emphasized. Systemic diseases that produce hematologic abnormalities that are similar in adults and children are discussed in other chapters (see Chapters 156–160). For a comprehensive review of the subject, the reader is referred to a published textbook.[1]

INFECTIOUS DISEASE

Infection, especially viral infection, is the most common problem encountered by the pediatrician. Although most infections do not produce significant hematologic sequelae, all classes of microorganisms have been implicated in the pathogenesis of hematologic abnormalities that range from mild and clinically irrelevant to severe and life-threatening. This section describes the changes seen in red blood cells (RBCs), white blood cells (WBCs), platelets, and the coagulation system that are routinely encountered, are associated with a specific infection, or have a potentially serious clinical impact.

CHANGES IN RED BLOOD CELLS

The anemia of chronic inflammation or infection in children is similar to that seen in adults in terms of both clinical and hematologic findings and pathogenesis.[2] However, anemia with acute infections occurs more commonly in children than in adults.

Anemia of Acute Infections

A mild to moderate anemia of uncertain etiology may occur in the setting of both acute viral infections and more serious bacterial infections. In a study of children with mild viral or bacterial infections in the outpatient setting, anemia was documented in 5% of children 4 to 12 years of age, 17% of children 6 months to 4 years of age, and 33% of infants 6 to 11 months of age.[3] In 14 of 15 young children, the anemia resolved within 3 to 4 weeks. However, multiple mild infections may predispose the infant to the development of a more chronic, mild anemia or low-normal hemoglobin that may be due to iron deficiency, thus warranting a trial of iron supplementation. Among children hospitalized with moderately severe inflammatory processes, the incidence of mild anemia (hemoglobin 10.1 to 11.0 g/dL) is as high as 78%.[4] Specific acute bacterial infections associated with a high incidence of anemia (44%–74%) include bone and joint infections, typhoid fever, brucellosis, and invasive *Haemophilus influenzae* infections.

The anemia associated with *H influenzae* meningitis has been the most thoroughly studied of the anemias of acute infection. A majority of children with *H influenzae* meningitis have mild anemia on admission, with hemoglobin in the 9 to 11 g/dL range, and up to 90% become anemic during the course of the illness.[5] This is in contrast with meningitis secondary to *Streptococcus pneumoniae* or *Neisseria meningitidis,* in which anemia is uncommon. The pathophysiology of the anemia of *H influenzae* disease appears to be multifactorial. Shurin and associates[6] have shown that *H influenzae* capsular polysaccharide, polyribosyl ribitol phosphate, binds to erythrocytes, which, in the presence of antibody and complement, can result in intravascular and extravascular hemolysis. They further hypothesize that polyribosyl ribitol phosphate alone may induce more rapid clearance of RBCs, perhaps on the basis of decreased RBC deformability. In addition, hypoferremia may limit bone marrow response to hemolysis.

Acute Hemolytic Anemia

Acute hemolysis has been observed with infections from all classes of microorganisms but is relatively uncommon. The anemia may be mild to severe, and the condition is manifested in children in either of two ways: (a) clinical presentation with symptoms and signs of infection predominating in a child subsequently found to have anemia or (b) clinical presentation with the manifestations of acute hemolytic anemia.

The mechanism of hemolysis in patients presenting with an infectious disorder depends on the infecting organism, but in most cases hemolysis is extravascular.[7] Reported mechanisms include the following:

- Release of hemolysins (*Clostridium perfringens* sepsis)
- Invasion of the RBC (malaria)
- Alteration of RBC surface:
  - Direct adherence by the organism (*Bartonella*)
  - Alterations of antigenic phenotype by neuraminidase (influenza virus)
  - Cold agglutinins (*Mycoplasma, Listeria,* Epstein-Barr virus [EBV], *Leptospira, Rubella*[8])
  - Absorption of capsular polysaccharide (*H influenzae*)
- Mechanical mechanisms (microangiopathy associated with disseminated intravascular coagulation [DIC] or hemolytic uremic syndrome)
- Oxidative damage in persons with congenital enzyme deficiencies (eg, hepatitis with glucose-6-phosphate dehydrogenase [G6PD] deficiency, *Campylobacter jejuni* infection in the neonate).

Acute, infection-associated hemolytic anemia in one study lagged behind the clinical infection by 3 to 7 days.[9] Most children were shown to have adsorption of microbial antigens to the RBC surface, suggesting an "innocent bystander" mechanism of erythrocyte sensitization, ultimately leading to hemolysis. A minority of patients in this series had classic autoantibody-mediated hemolytic anemia.

Autoimmune hemolytic anemia in children usually is transient, is not associated with underlying systemic disease, and carries a low mortality rate. Children frequently have a history of concurrent or recently resolved infection, especially viral upper respiratory tract infection. Anticytomegalovirus (CMV) immunoglobulin G (IgG) has

Table 162–1 Normal Hematologic Values in Childhood

	Hb (g/dL)		Red Cells Hct (%)		MCV (fL)		White Cells Total (×10³/μL)		White Cells Neutrophils (%)	White Cells Lymphocytes (%)	Coagulation PT (sec)*		Coagulation APTT (sec)*	
AGE	*Mean*	*(Range)*	*Mean*	*(Range)*	*Mean*	*(Range)*	*Mean*	*(Range)*	*Mean*	*Mean*	*Mean*	*(Range)*	*Mean*	*(Range)*
Birth (term)	18.5	(14.5–22.5)	56	(45–69)	108	(95–121)	18.1	(9.3–30.0)	61	31	16	(13–20)	55	(45–65)
2 months	11.2	(9.4–14.0)	35	(28–42)	96	(77–115)								
6 months–2 years	12.5	(11.0–14.0)	37	(33–41)	77	(70–84)	11.3	(6.0–17.5)	32	61				
2–6 years	12.5	(11.5–13.5)	37	(34–40)	81	(75–87)	8.5	(5.0–15.5)	42	50				
6–12 years	13.5	(11.5–15.5)	40	(35–45)	86	(77–95)	8.1	(4.5–13.5)	53	39				
12–18 years							7.8	(4.5–13.5)	57	35				
Male	14.5	(13.0–16.0)	43	(37–49)	88	(78–98)								
Female	14.0	(12.0–16.0)	41	(36–46)	90	(78–102)								

Hb, hemoglobin; Hct, hematocrit; MCV, mean corpuscular volume; PT, prothrombin time; APTT, activated partial thromboplastin time.

*The normal range for the PT and APTT varies between laboratories. The time at which normal adult values are attained is 1 week for the PT and 2 to 9 months for the APTT. The platelet count is within the adult range from birth.

Data from Rudolph AM, Hoffman JIE (eds.): Pediatrics, 17th ed. East Norwalk, Conn, Appleton-Century-Crofts, 1982, p 1036, and from Nathan DG, Oski FA (eds.): Hematology of Infancy and Childhood, 3rd ed. Philadelphia, WB Saunders, 1987, p 1679.

been implicated as the cause of acute autoimmune hemolytic anemia in an infant with CMV disease. In the typical acute, transient cases, 59% to 68% of children have a history of recent infection, whereas 0% to 20% of those with the less common chronic course have such a history of infection.

Aplastic Crisis

Temporary arrest of RBC production has been observed in children with infections, but anemia is uncommon because of the long RBC life span. In two situations, however, severe anemia has been linked with infection and cessation of erythropoiesis: (a) B19 parvovirus infection in patients with an underlying hemolytic anemia and (b) transient erythroblastopenia of childhood.

The B19 parvovirus has been a known pathogen in animals for years but has only recently been linked with human disease.[10] It is the etiologic agent of fifth disease (erythema infectiosum), a mild illness with a characteristic "slapped cheek" facial erythema and a generalized reticular rash. In normal volunteers infected with B19 parvovirus, a mild, transient, and clinically irrelevant drop in the hemoglobin and reticulocyte count was observed.[11] In normal children, this infection usually is not associated with hematologic abnormalities, although reports of both hematologic and nonhematologic effects are increasing.[12] In children with sickle cell disease, spherocytosis, and other hemolytic anemias, B19 parvovirus infection can produce a severe anemia associated with peripheral reticulocytopenia and marrow erythroblastopenia—the "aplastic crisis." Recovery within 1 to 2 weeks is the rule, but transfusion may be necessary.

B19 parvovirus infection also has been associated with prolonged anemia and reticulocytopenia in children with acute lymphoblastic leukemia in remission, those with solid tumors receiving chemotherapy, those with immunodeficiency, those who have undergone renal transplantation, and those with autoimmune hemolytic anemia, and as the initial manifestation of human immunodeficiency virus infection. Human parvovirus also has been identified as a cause of nonimmune hydrops fetalis.[13]

Transient erythroblastopenia in childhood (TEC) is a syndrome characterized by temporary arrest of RBC production with moderate to severe anemia in previously normal infants and toddlers. Although no specific infectious agent has been proved to cause TEC, the frequency of a history of infection within 1 to 3 months, the seasonal clustering, and the similarity to childhood idiopathic thrombocytopenic purpura (ITP) all suggest a possible viral etiology. B19 parvovirus has not been definitively associated with TEC.[14]

CHANGES IN WHITE BLOOD CELLLS

Children, as a rule, have the expected leukocyte response to infection. Infants and young children normally have a lymphocyte predominance (see Table 162–1), however, and any leukocyte response to infection must be judged on the basis of age-related normal values.

The predictive value of the peripheral WBC and differential counts in suspected bacterial infections has been extensively evaluated in infants and children. Todd has shown that in hospitalized children, a neutrophil count greater than 10,000/μL or band count greater than 500/μL is associated with an 80% chance of having a bacterial infection.[15] In children undergoing evaluation for possible meningitis, Lembo and colleagues[16] found that a ratio of immature to total neutrophils greater than 0.12 was more strongly associated with, and more sensitive for, bacterial meningitis than was the total WBC count or the total band count. Febrile children between the ages of 3 and 48 months are at increased risk for bacteremia, especially with *S pneumoniae*. McCarthy and associates[17] demonstrated a threefold increase in risk of bacteremia in febrile (with temperatures greater than 40°C) children, younger than 2 years of age, who had a WBC count of 15,000/μL or greater. In this setting, the WBC count was a more sensitive indicator of the presence of pneumonia or bacteremia than was the absolute neutrophil or band count. The degree of leukocytosis (ie, >25,000/mm² vs >15,000/mm²) probably has no further discriminating ability.[18] Other studies have found both WBC count and absolute neutrophil count to be of value in differentiating bacterial from nonbacterial infection, whereas band count was not helpful.

There are recognized exceptions to the anticipated leukocyte response to infection that may serve as a clue to the diagnosis. In typhoid fever and brucellosis, leukopenia and neutropenia are prominent early in the illness. Shigellosis is associated with a variable leukocyte count, but the count often is normal, with a greater percentage of bands than neutrophils. Illnesses associated with lymphocytosis include pertussis (whooping cough), infectious lymphocytosis, infectious mononucleosis, and other viral infections. Neutropenia can be seen in bacterial sepsis from meningococci, pneumococci, staphylococci, and other bacteria and is associated with a poor prognosis. Black children (and adults) normally have lower WBC and neutrophil counts than those seen in whites; leukocyte and neutrophil response to serious infection may be decreased.[19]

NEUTROPENIA

The most common cause of neutropenia (neutrophil count less than 1500/μL) in children is viral infection. A number of specific viruses are associated with neutropenia, including hepatitis, roseola, rubella, and mumps viruses and adenovirus, coxsackievirus A21, EBV, human herpesvirus-6 (HHV-6), and influenza virus.[20] The most common clinical setting, however, is the incidental discovery of neutropenia in the child with a nonspecific viral syndrome. Usually the neutropenia in this situation continues for less than 30 days and is rarely associated with infectious complications. Neutropenia also has been associated with a number of bacterial, rickettsial, and fungal infections.[21]

EOSINOPHILIA

The most common cause of eosinophilia worldwide is parasitic infection. In the United States, visceral larva migrans (*Toxocara* infestation) is the most common cause of exaggerated eosinophilia (WBC count 30,000–100,000/μL, with 50%–90% mature eosinophils) in children.[22] Mild to moderate eosinophilia (600/μL or greater) is most often seen in allergic children but also is characteristic of *Chlamydia* pneumonitis in infants.

CHANGES IN PLATELETS/COAGULATION

Thrombocytosis

Thrombocytosis (platelet count >500,000/μL) is known as an acute-phase reaction to infection, but it has been infrequently identified in children in the past. There is a particularly high incidence of thrombocytosis in patients with bacterial infections, especially pneumonia with emphysema, and *H influenzae* meningitis. Inflammatory cytokines, such as interleukin (IL)-1, IL-6, and thrombopoietin, may play an etiologic role in the reactive thrombocytosis of infection.[23] Thrombocytosis may be more common in simple acute infections than was previously recognized. Heath and Pearson documented a 13% incidence of thrombocytosis in ambulatory patients; children with an increased platelet count were more likely to have a diagnosis of infection.[24] In a Japanese study of greater than 15,000 platelet counts in more than 7500 hospitalized patients, 6% of patients had thrombocytosis with an age-dependent incidence: 12.5% in neonates, 35.8% in 1-month-old babies, 12.9% in 6- to 12-month-old infants, then decreasing to 0.6% in 11- to 15-year-old children. Infection was the cause of the thrombocytosis in 67.5% of the cases.[25] There were no apparent sequelae to the thrombocytosis, and antiplatelet therapy is not indicated. Although the most common cause of thrombocytosis in children is infection, the list of considerations in the differential diagnosis of an elevated platelet count is extensive[26] and rarely includes underlying childhood malignancy.

Thrombocytopenia

Thrombocytopenia can be seen in patients suffering from infections with all types of organisms. Common viral agents include varicella virus, EBV, rubella virus, mumps virus, measles virus (wild or vaccine strains), HHV-6, hepatitis A virus, and CMV. The primary mechanism of the thrombocytopenia is immune destruction, although a direct viral effect on the platelet, megakaryocyte, or hematopoietic stem cell has been demonstrated. Because childhood ITP is thought to be secondary to infection in most instances, the definitions of "thrombocytopenia with infection" and "childhood ITP" tend to merge. Thrombocytopenia from infection usually is transient, although instances of chronic thrombocytopenia from specific viral infections (eg, varicella) have been documented.[27]

Thrombocytopenia also is associated with bacterial sepsis. The low platelet count may be an isolated finding or associated with DIC. Corrigan documented a 61% incidence of thrombocytopenia in 45 children with sepsis.[28] The degree of thrombocytopenia was mild to moderate (64% had platelet counts greater than 50,000/μL), but platelet counts ranged as low as 8000/μL. There was no evidence of DIC in 39% of those with low platelet counts. Thrombocytopenia in the setting of bacterial sepsis probably is also mediated by an immune mechanism with elevated platelet-associated IgG.

Petechial bleeding without thrombocytopenia can be seen in both bacterial and viral disease, especially that due to meningococci, streptococci, and echoviruses. The explanation for the petechial rash in these infections is either vasculitis or platelet dysfunction.

Disseminated Intravascular Coagulation/Purpura Fulminans

DIC is uncommon after childhood infections and, if present, usually is accompanied by shock, with at least a 50% mortality rate. The most common organisms producing DIC are bacterial, especially the gram-negative bacteria (meningococci, *H influenzae*, *Aerobacter*, and others) but also gram-positive organisms (*Staphylococcus aureus*, group B streptococci, *S pneumoniae*, particularly in the asplenic host, and *Bacillus anthracis*). DIC also is associated with disseminated viral (varicella, measles, rubella), rickettsial (Rocky Mountain spotted fever), fungal, mycoplasmal, and parasitic infections.

Purpura fulminans is a rare syndrome, seen in extremely ill children with DIC. Purpura fulminans is characterized by the rapid progression of ecchymotic skin lesions, especially of the extremities, that may progress to gangrene, ultimately resulting in amputation.[29] This syndrome has been described as a postinfectious purpura, with scarlet fever, upper respiratory tract infection, and varicella as the most common preceding illnesses and a latent period of 0 to 90 days following infection. A similar clinical picture can be seen in children with DIC and acute bacterial sepsis, especially meningococcemia.

There is increasing evidence that DIC with purpura fulminans is associated with deficiency of the naturally occurring anticoagulants. Children with postvaricella purpura fulminans have been shown to have acquired protein S deficiency, anti–protein S antibody, or the presence of a lupus anticoagulant.[30] In children with infectious purpura, protein C activation is impaired as reflected in low levels of protein C, protein S, and antithrombin. These findings are consistent with downregulation of the endothelial thrombomodulin–protein C receptor pathway.[31] The severity of protein C deficiency has been associated with increased morbidity and mortality.[32] There are minimal data on the frequency of inherited thrombophilia in children who develop purpura fulminans. In one report, the frequency of factor V Leiden was not different from that in healthy children; presence of factor V Leiden was not associated with an increased mortality rate, although complications were increased.[33] In another study of 16 children with purpura fulminans 6 of 16 (37%) patients studied had the Factor V Leiden mutation. All of the children in this study survived, but 10 (63%) required amputation.[34]

Treatment of purpura fulminans consists of antibiotics for suspected bacterial infection, volume replacement for shock, and heparin. Although there is controversy regarding the routine use of heparin in DIC, its use in purpura fulminans has been associated with an improved outcome when it is started early in the course of the disease and continued for 2 to 3 weeks.[35] Theoretically to improve the efficacy of heparin, it is reasonable to infuse fresh frozen plasma or antithrombin III (AT III) concentrates[36] if the AT III level is low. There is anecdotal evidence that infusion of AT III concentrates or protein C concentrates partially corrects or normalizes the hemostatic abnormalities.[37,38] However, the KyberSept trial, a double-blind placebo-controlled trial of the use of ATIII concentrates in 2300 adults with sepsis, found no difference in mortality at day 28 after diagnosis.[39] In a phase II trial of protein C concentrate in the treatment of sepsis and purpura fulminans in children, there was dose-dependent activation of protein C and normalization of coagulation imbalances. Although there was no improvement in mortality, the study was not powered to detect these changes.[40]

Recombinant human activated protein C (drotrecogin alfa activated) has been shown to reduce the mortality rate in adults with severe sepsis.[41] In pediatric trials of activated protein C for treatment of sepsis, there was no noticeable improvement in mortality (children have a lower mortality rate than adults) and there were significant bleeding risks.[42,43] Although activated protein C has been used in patients with purpura fulminans, the data do not suggest a beneficial effect on mortality.[44,45] It should be noted, however, that these studies did not address a potential benefit on amputation risk or cosmetic outcome. Recombinant tissue plasminogen activator has been used in an attempt to restore organ perfusion by dissolution of diffuse microvascular thromboses[46]; however, in a retrospective multicenter study of 62 patients with meningococcal purpura fulminans treated with systemic tPA, there was a high incidence of intracerebral hemorrhage without proven efficacy in reduction of mortality or incidence of amputation.[47] Other treatments, such as regional sympathetic blockade, topical nitroglycerin, and local infusion of tissue plasminogen activator, have been used to improve regional blood flow to the affected part. The mortality rate for postinfectious purpura fulminans has declined from 90% in the past to 18%.[29] The outcome for patients with acute bacterial sepsis and purpura fulminans has also improved, but mortality as high as 50% continues to be reported.

Coagulation Inhibitors

Acquired inhibitors of coagulation in children with infection are usually transient and mild, but may be associated with severe bleeding.[48] They are often detected after a viral illness, during antibiotic therapy, or incidentally (frequently prior to tonsillectomy/adenoidectomy). Both specific inhibitors of coagulation factors (especially factors VIII and IX) and lupus anticoagulants have been demonstrated. Although previously thought to be uncommon, studies have found 50% to 90% of children with infection have at least one positive test for an antiphospholipid antibody.[49,50] Significant bleeding is usually seen only in those children with specific factor inhibitors, although hemorrhage also has been described with lupus anticoagulants.[51] In symptomatic patients, treatment with prednisone has been associated with remission of bleeding manifestations. Complete resolution without recurrence is the most common event.

PANCYTOPENIA

Pancytopenia in a child should alert the clinician to the possibility of disorders such as leukemia, aplastic anemia, or disseminated neuroblastoma. Infectious causes of pancytopenia are uncommon, and disseminated disease is most often present. Organisms implicated in patients with pancytopenia include *Mycobacterium tuberculosis*, atypical mycobacteria, *Histoplasma capsulatum*, *Leishmania*, *Salmonella typhi*, *Mucor* species, *Brucella* species, *Fusobacterium necrophorum*, and *Ehrlichia canis*.[21] Virus-associated or reactive hemophagocytic syndrome is an additional, although rare, cause of pancytopenia. Children with human immunodeficiency virus (HIV) infection and concomitant infection with *Mycobacterium avium-intracellulare* or parvovirus B19 have been reported to have pancytopenia.

HUMAN IMMUNODEFICIENCY VIRUS INFECTION IN CHILDREN AND ADOLESCENTS

Infection with HIV is more common in adults but is now recognized as a leading cause of immunodeficiency in infants and children.[52] Acquisition of HIV in a majority of infected children (most of whom are younger than 2 years of age) is by vertical transmission from an infected mother to her infant. Of children younger than 13 years with acquired immunodeficiency syndrome (AIDS), 80% have a parent with AIDS or AIDS-related complex (ARC), 13% have a history of blood transfusion, and 5% have hemophilia or another coagulation disorder.[53] With improvement in screening blood and blood donors for HIV, it is expected that vertical transmission from mother to infant will remain the primary method of transmission. Other "adult" routes of infection (homosexuality, intravenous needle use) are possible, especially in the adolescent and the sexually abused child.

Clinical manifestations of AIDS in children include oral thrush, chronic interstitial pneumonitis, hepatosplenomegaly, lymphadenopathy, and failure to thrive. Other clinical characteristics distinguishing pediatric from adult HIV infection include a shorter incubation period, more pronounced hypergammaglobulinemia, more serious bacterial and CMV disease, and the rare occurrence of Kaposi sarcoma or other malignancies. Multiple, serious bacterial infections and lymphocytic interstitial pneumonitis/pulmonary lymphoid hyperplasia are accepted as indicative of AIDS among children and adults. However, as in adults, there is a broad spectrum of disease manifestations, with all organ systems potentially affected and progressive immune and clinical deterioration.

The diagnosis of HIV infection is now possible in early infancy with the advent of assays to detect HIV DNA and RNA. Other advances in monitoring immune status and new therapies for HIV disease and opportunistic infections have resulted in a decrease in the number of children in the United States with AIDS. The focus of medical management of children with HIV is early aggressive therapy to prevent immunologic deterioration and the clinical manifestations of AIDS.[54] Guidelines for current antiretroviral therapy in children are available on the AIDSinfo Web site (www.aidsinfo.nih.gov).

The hematologic manifestations of AIDS in children are similar to those in adults (see Chapter 158) and depend on the stage of the HIV infection and the presence of coexistent disease.[54,55] Anemia is by far the most common finding (seen in 70%–90% of the cases), although the incidence has decreased with effective antiviral therapy.[56] Severe anemia (hematocrit less than 25%) in one study correlated with development of an opportunistic infection and death within 7 months.[57] Severe autoimmune hemolytic anemia has been described infrequently, but in one case was the presenting manifestation of HIV in a 5-month-old infant.[58] Leukopenia and neutropenia are commonly seen in HIV-infected children (occurring in 47% and 41%, respectively), with severe neutropenia associated with opportunistic infections. Immune neutropenia and also circulating anticoagulants have been described. Lymphopenia is progressive but less prominent in children than in adults until late in the course. Thrombocytopenia is present in 13% to 30% of pediatric AIDS patients and can be associated with clinically significant and even fatal hemorrhage. The mechanism of the thrombocytopenia in most cases is immune destruction, with a high percentage of patients having antiplatelet antibodies or immune complexes,[59] although amegakaryocytic thrombocytopenia has been reported.[60] Variable therapeutic responses to both corticosteroids and intravenous IgG have been demonstrated; some children will have spontaneous remissions.[59,61] Thrombosis has also been described and is associated with severe disease.[62] The evaluation and treatment of hematologic abnormalities in HIV-infected children have been reviewed by Laufer and Scott.[54]

Isolated thrombocytopenia as a presenting manifestation of HIV infection has been reported in a number of children, usually infants and even in a neonate.[63] There have been no associated clinical stigmata of AIDS or ARC, and patients have been responsive to standard treatment (intravenous IgG or prednisone), often with sustained remissions. In a few patients with prolonged follow-up, no further manifestations of HIV infection were seen. Although it has been suggested that HIV testing may be indicated in all children with ITP, it seems most reasonable to check the HIV status of those with risk factors for AIDS and those outside the typical age group for ITP, especially infants.

COLLAGEN VASCULAR DISEASE/ACUTE VASCULITIS

Juvenile Rheumatoid Arthritis

Juvenile rheumatoid arthritis (JRA) includes a group of disorders with varied clinical presentation, course, and outcome. Systemic JRA, which occurs in 30% of patients, is a multisystem disease characterized by fever, rash, polyarticular (often destructive) arthritis, hepatosplenomegaly, and lymphadenopathy. Patients with JRA commonly demonstrate hematologic abnormalities that are proportional to disease activity. In the polyarticular presentation, more than four joints are involved but the systemic findings are absent. This group, which accounts for 25% of patients, also may exhibit hematologic abnormalities. Pauciarticular JRA is characterized by involvement of fewer than four joints and is rarely associated with hematologic abnormalities.

The incidence of anemia is 50% to 60% in patients with systemic or polyarticular JRA and 10% in those with pauciarticular arthritis. The anemia usually correlates with disease activity, worsening during acute flare-ups; however, there is no relationship to the duration of illness. RBCs may be normochromic/normocytic or microcytic/hypochromic. The reticulocyte count usually is low. Iron studies often show low serum iron, increased free erythrocyte protoporphyrin, low-normal or elevated total iron-binding capacity, and normal or low serum ferritin. Serum erythropoietin levels usually are mildly elevated (but not as high as in iron deficiency). The bone marrow does not show erythroid hyperplasia in response to the anemia and has diminished (but not absent) iron stores. The etiology of the anemia may be chronic disease, iron deficiency, or both.

Although it is difficult to differentiate anemia of chronic disease from iron deficiency anemia, studies in patients with systemic-onset chronic JRA suggest defective iron supply as the primary cause.[64] Transferrin receptor levels are inversely related to hemoglobin levels in this population. Determination of serum transferrin receptor levels may be a discriminating assay for diagnosis of iron deficiency in JRA.[65] Oral iron has been effective in raising the hemoglobin in iron-deficient anemic patients with JRA, and intravenous iron has been effective in raising the hemoglobin level in children unresponsive to oral iron.[64] Excessive production of IL-6, as well as of other inflammatory cytokines, has been documented in patients with JRA and may provide an explanation for the abnormalities in iron metabolism. IL-6 may enhance ferritin synthesis and increase hepatic uptake of serum iron. Increased ferritin results in reticuloendothelial iron blockage and diminished iron absorption.[64]

Less common causes of anemia in JRA include erythroid aplasia, suppression of erythropoiesis by circulating inhibitors, hemolysis, and a macrocytic anemia probably related to increased folate clearance and low plasma and RBC folate levels.

In systemic JRA, leukocytosis with mean WBC counts up to 30,000/μL and neutrophilia with a left shift occur in 90% of patients, especially those with active disease. Leukocytosis is less common in polyarticular arthritis and usually absent in pauciarticular disease. Leukocytosis is so prevalent in systemic JRA that the presence of neutropenia should alert the clinician to question the diagnosis and ensure that other possibilities such as systemic lupus erythematosus (SLE) and acute lymphocytic leukemia (ALL) are not overlooked. ALL in children may manifest with fever, joint pain, hepatosplenomegaly, and isolated cytopenias. Because about 4% of children with ALL are misdiagnosed as having JRA, it is important to perform bone marrow aspiration to rule out leukemia in any patient thought to have systemic JRA before initiation of corticosteroid therapy.

Nonetheless, neutropenia has been reported in several patients with JRA.[66] Other causes of neutropenia are bone marrow suppression due to therapy with gold or nonsteroidal antiinflammatory drugs[67] and, in adults, Felty's syndrome, the triad of rheumatoid arthritis, splenomegaly, and neutropenia. Studies of neutrophil function have demonstrated mild defects in chemotaxis and phagocytosis.[68] About 50% of patients with systemic JRA have less than 5% eosinophils on the peripheral smear.[69] Basophilia and plasmacytoid lymphocytes also have been reported. Studies of cellular immunity are conflicting, demonstrating normal or increased T and B lymphocyte number, increased immunoglobulin synthesis and secretion, and either impaired or normal delayed hypersensitivity and lymphoproliferative response to mitogens.[70,71] Monocyte dysfunction with decreased Fc receptor expression, decreased superoxide production, and decreased complement-mediated phagocytosis has been described.[72]

The platelet count is elevated in about half of the patients with systemic JRA. IL-6, a cytokine that stimulates thrombopoiesis, is elevated in patients with active systemic JRA, and increased levels of IL-6 are correlated with elevated platelet counts.[73] Persistent thrombocytosis may serve as an adverse prognostic marker for long-term outcome in JRA.

Thrombocytopenia may result from bone marrow suppression by gold therapy, the rare consumptive coagulopathy, or platelet trapping in Felty's syndrome. Thrombocytopenia is also seen in the potentially life-threatening complication of macrophage activation syndrome (see macrophage activation syndrome below). Because thrombocytopenia is uncommon in JRA, however, an unexplained low platelet count should lead the clinician to consider alternative diagnoses, such as SLE or ALL. On the other hand, isolated thrombocytopenia may be the only presenting sign in a child who later develops JRA or another collagen vascular disease. Therefore, JRA and SLE should be considered in the differential diagnosis of ITP in the child who is older than 9 years and female. Appropriate screening tests for autoantibodies (eg, antinuclear antibody assay, direct Coombs test) should be performed at diagnosis and periodically if new symptoms develop.

DIC may occur in children with systemic JRA after hepatic damage, as part of the macrophage activation syndrome, from aspirin or gold therapy, or during disease flare-ups treated with nonsteroidal antiinflammatory drugs when serum albumin is low.[74] These patients often are very ill and may require early and aggressive medical therapy as well as platelet and coagulation factor replacement to control the coagulopathy. The incidence of coagulation abnormalities in nonbleeding patients with systemic JRA is controversial. One study demonstrated prolonged prothrombin time (PT) and activated partial thromboplastin time (APTT) and elevated fibrinogen, factor VIII, and fibrinopeptide A levels in up to 50% of these patients[75]; other reports have not confirmed such findings. Another study found elevation of D-dimer levels in 96% of systemic-onset JRA patients; serial measurements of D-dimer levels appeared to parallel response to treatment.[76] In apparent distinction, decreased fibrinolytic activity and increased plasminogen activator inhibitor have been found in patients with active JRA, especially those with the systemic form. Antibodies against factor VIII and the lupus anticoagulant are occasionally seen in children with JRA.

Macrophage Activation Syndrome

Macrophage activation syndrome (MAS) is a life-threatening multisystem disorder most closely resembling hemophagocytic lymphohistiocytosis (HLH) that occurs primarily in patients with systemic onset juvenile rheumatoid arthritis (sJRA). This syndrome usually occurs early in the course of active sJRA and can even be a presenting feature,[77] although it has been reported to occur later and during a quiescent phase.[78] It is estimated that approximately 7% of patients with sJRA develop MAS and mortality is between 10% and 20%.[79] MAS has also been reported in other systemic inflammatory disorders including systemic lupus erythematosus and Kawasaki disease.[77]

The main clinical features of MAS include high unremitting fever, hepatosplenomegaly, lymphadenopathy, bleeding, rash, and central nervous system manifestations. Neurologic symptoms include lethargy, irritability, disorientation, headache, seizures, and coma. Children with MAS are acutely ill and almost 50% require ICU care.[80] The diagnosis may be delayed because the presentation mimics an acute exacerbation of sJRA or severe infection. Of interest, some patients have shown a paradoxical improvement in the underlying inflammatory disease at the onset of MAS. Precipitating factors that have been implicated include a flare-up of the underlying disease, aspirin or other nonsteroidal antiinflammatory drug toxicity, viral infections, a second injection of gold salts, methotrexate, and sulfasalazine therapy.[80]

Typical laboratory features include pancytopenia, hypofibrinogenemia (<250 mg/dL), elevated liver enzymes (>40 IU/mL), hypertriglyceridemia (>160 mg/dL), and marked elevation of ferritin (>10,000 ng/mL). Other laboratory findings with less sensitivity and specificity include coagulopathy, hyponatremia, and hypoalbuminemia. The hallmark of this disorder is the presence of hemophagocytic histiocytes usually seen in the bone marrow, although they can be found in the liver and other organs. These characteristic macrophages are regarded as confirmatory evidence rather than a requirement for a diagnosis, because they have not been documented in as many as 20% of patients with the classical clinical and laboratory findings of MAS.[80,81]

There are no accepted diagnostic criteria for MAS in sJRA. Preliminary diagnostic guidelines have been proposed (Table 162–2), although they have not been validated in prospective studies.[81] These guidelines are similar to criteria for the diagnosis of HLH,[82] although there are a number of differences that should be emphasized. Although the diagnostic criteria for HLH include documentation of hemophagocytic histiocytes in bone marrow or other tissue, this is not the case for the MAS guidelines. In MAS, clinical features are less strong discriminators than laboratory features. Although the presence of fever was universal in patients with MAS, it had a low specificity rate because of the high incidence of fever in patients with sJRA without MAS. The pattern of fever may be of more importance because patients with MAS tend to have nonremitting fever as opposed to the high spiking fevers seen in sJRA. The other clinical criteria may occur late in the course of MAS, resulting in abnormal laboratory findings being more helpful in making a diagnosis early in the course of the illness. Because blood counts are usually elevated in patients with sJRA, the decrease in counts seen with MAS may actually result in a "normal" blood count, although in patients with HLH cytopenias are usually well below the normal levels.

The pathogenesis of MAS is similar to that proposed for HLH.[82,83] Indeed it has been proposed that MAS be considered one of the subtypes of acquired HLH.[79] The presentation of MAS is a result of an ineffective immune response to an endogenous or exogenous stimulus leading to an exaggerated inflammatory state produced by a release of high levels of cytokines. These proinflammatory cytokines include tumor necrosis factor alpha (TNF-α), interleukin (IL) 6, IL-8, IL-12, IL-18, macrophage inflammatory protein (MIP 1- a), and interferon gamma (INF-γ) released by stimulated lymphocytes and histiocytes. Defective NK cell function and cytotoxic T-cell activity has been documented in patients with MAS as well as HLH and may be the common pathway leading to the clinical presentation.[84] NK function in patients with active sJRA but without MAS has also been found to be abnormal.[85] This may explain why MAS is almost exclusively seen in the systemic form of JRA and not the other subtypes of the disease. Mutations in the perforin gene have been described in some patients with HLH. The cytotoxic function of NK cells is mediated by the release of perforin and other cytolytic granules into the target cell leading to cell death. Abnormalities of perforin expression have been found in patients with MAS although no mutations have been identified in the few patients studied.[84]

Table 162–2 Preliminary Diagnostic Guidelines for Macrophage Activation Syndrome in Systemic Juvenile Rheumatoid Arthritis[81]*

Laboratory Criteria

1. Decreased platelet count (≤262 × 10⁹/L)
2. Elevated levels of aspartate aminotransferase (>59 U/L)
3. Decreased white blood cell count (≤4.0 × 10⁹/l)
4. Hypofibrinogenemia (≤250 mg/dL)

Clinical Criteria

1. Central nervous system dysfunction (irritability, disorientation, lethargy, headache, seizures, coma)
2. Hemorrhages (purpura, easy bruising, mucosal bleeding)
3. Hepatomegaly (≥3 cm below the costal margin)

Histopathological Criterion

Evidence of macrophage hemophagocytosis in the bone marrow aspirate

Diagnostic rule

The diagnosis of MAS requires the presence of any two or more laboratory criteria or of ≥2 clinical and/or laboratory criteria. A bone marrow aspirate for the demonstration of hemophagocytosis may be required only in doubtful cases.

*The suggested criteria are useful only in patients with active sJRA. The laboratory thresholds are examples only and are not specific for the diagnosis. (See text)

Treatment of MAS should be started promptly and not delayed for lack of hemophagocytosis if the clinical and laboratory features are consistent with the diagnosis. Initial treatment should be high-dose corticosteroid therapy followed by cyclosporine A if there is not a rapid response. Intravenous methylprednisolone with doses from 2 to 30 mg/kg/day have been the most common corticosteroid reported in the literature and is usually effective in controlling hyperinflammation.[80] The corticosteroid of choice used in the treatment of HLH is dexamethasone, but the use of this corticosteroid has not been reported in MAS. Cyclosporine A has been very effective in inducing remissions either when used as initial treatment or in cases of corticosteroid failure.[78,80,86] In addition to immunosuppression, there should be withdrawal of any suspected triggering medications and treatment of infection. Intravenous immunoglobulin therapy has usually been ineffective, although it has been reported to induce a full recovery in one case of a child who failed high-dose corticosteroids.[87] Etanercept has also been reported to induce clinical responses in patients with MAS.[88,89] Etanercept is a recombinant-soluble TNF-α receptor fusion protein that binds to TNF-α, blocking its effect. Although use of this agent to reduce the elevated levels of TNF-α found in this disorder is attractive, it should be used with caution, because there are case reports of MAS developing after the initiation of etanercept.[90]

KAWASAKI SYNDROME

Kawasaki syndrome is an acute multisystem disorder characterized by abrupt onset of fever unresponsive to antibiotics; bilateral conjunctival injection; reddening of the lips, tongue, or oral mucosa; reddening, induration, or peeling of the skin on the hands or feet; polymorphous truncal rash; and cervical lymphadenopathy. This disorder occurs most commonly in children younger than 2 years and has many features of a severe vasculitis. The most serious complication is development of coronary artery aneurysms, which occurs in 20% of children and is responsible for the 3% mortality rate; death often is due to coronary artery thrombosis or rupture. The etiology of Kawasaki disease is unknown. The immunologic and clinical characteristics of this disorder are similar to those of diseases associated with superantigen production, of which toxic shock syndrome is a classic example.[91]

Children with Kawasaki syndrome may have a mild normochromic, normocytic anemia with reticulocytopenia. Rare patients with autoimmune hemolytic anemia have been reported. Leukocytosis is almost universal, with mean neutrophil counts of 21,000/μL. Ninety-five percent of patients have neutrophilia, with a left shift persisting up to 3 weeks. The finding of vacuoles and toxic granulation in neutrophils is a helpful adjunct in the diagnosis of Kawasaki disease. Activated neutrophils and monocytes may play a role in aneurysm development through the production of elastase. Granulocyte colony-stimulating factor levels have been correlated with coronary artery dilatation during the acute phase of Kawasaki syndrome.[92]

Studies of cellular immunity show normal total T-cell numbers but decreased suppressor T cells, causing relatively elevated T helper-cell levels during the first 4 weeks of disease.[93] The change of T-cell subsets plus B lymphocyte stimulation may contribute to the exaggerated production of all major immunoglobulin classes during the first 8 weeks of the disease.[94] An unusual infiltration of IgA-producing plasma cells within vascular tissue in Kawasaki syndrome, with an oligoclonal IgA response, suggests that the immune stimulation is antigen driven.[95] Circulating immune complexes and high C3 (but not C4) levels are found during weeks 1 and 3. During the acute phase, increased levels of the cytokines IL-1, IL-6, IL-8, interferon-γ, and tumor necrosis factor are noted in the circulation, and IL-1, IL-2, interferon-γ, and tumor necrosis factor in blood vessels and skin biopsies.[91] Declining serum IL-6 levels appear to correlate with clinical response after treatment with intravenous immunoglobulin (IVIG).[96]

Impressive thrombocytosis occurs in 85% of patients by the second week, peaking during the third. Platelet counts of up to 2 million are not uncommon, and the mean platelet count is 700,000/μL. Thrombocytosis may serve as a marker of possible atypical Kawasaki disease in infants less than 1 year of age. In a study of more than 25,000 infants with unexplained fever, 8.8% with a platelet count greater than 800,000/uL were found to have Kawasaki disease as opposed to 0.4% of those with a platelet count less than 800,000/uL.[97] Thrombocytosis is preceded by elevated thrombopoietin levels.[98] However, 2% of patients may have thrombocytopenia caused by a consumptive coagulopathy. Platelets demonstrate hyperaggregation on exposure to adenosine diphosphate, epinephrine, and collagen in vitro. These abnormalities may persist for as long as 9 months after diagnosis.[99] During the first month, levels of factor VIII, fibrinogen, thromboxane B_2, and thromboglobulin are increased. AT III and fibrinolysis activity are decreased. The PT, APTT, and thrombin time usually are normal.[100]

Prevention and treatment of existing coronary aneurysms constitute the primary therapeutic goal. Aspirin suppresses platelet aggregation but does not affect aneurysm formation. Combining aspirin with high-dose IVIG infusions reduces aneurysm formation, decreases fever, and normalizes laboratory signs of inflammation.[101] The use of corticosteroids is controversial, with conflicting data regarding increased aneurysm formation after steroid usage.[102–104] However, in a randomized double-blind, placebo-controlled trial a single pulsed dose of intravenous methylprednisolone, in addition to conventional therapy, did not improve coronary artery outcomes.[105] In subgroup analysis of children with persistent fever, coronary outcomes were better in the corticosteroid group. If children at highest risk of primary treatment failure could be identified initially, corticosteroid use may be of benefit in this group. Guidelines for the diagnosis, treatment, and long-term management of Kawasaki syndrome have been published.[106]

HENOCH–SCHÖNLEIN PURPURA

Henoch–Schönlein purpura (HSP) (anaphylactoid purpura) is a systemic vasculitis characterized by unique purpuric skin lesions, transient arthralgias or arthritis (especially affecting the knees and ankles), colicky abdominal pain, and nephritis. Recognition of HSP is important, not so much for its hematologic abnormalities (which are rare) as for the unusual nonthrombocytopenic purpuric lesions, which are frequently confused with the hemorrhagic rash of ITP.

This vasculitis occurs most commonly in children 3 to 7 years old, often 1 to 3 weeks after an upper respiratory tract illness. The presenting sign in 50% of children is a characteristic rash, which may begin as urticaria. As these eruptions fade, they are replaced by brownish-red maculopapular lesions and petechiae. The petechiae coalesce, forming areas of raised or "palpable" purpura on the buttocks, legs, and extensor surfaces of the arms, with a symmetrical distribution. The rash may fade but can recur for months, especially with increased activity. Children younger than 3 years of age often have painful soft tissue swellings of the scalp and face (especially periorbital areas) and on the dorsa of the hands and feet. Infantile acute hemorrhagic edema is an acute vasculitis affecting infants younger than 2 years, which may be a benign form of HSP.

Sixty-seven percent of patients experience colicky abdominal pain, often associated with vomiting, hematemesis, or melena from submucosal hemorrhage and edema of the small bowel wall. With severe edema, the bowel wall may become a leading point for intussusception.[107]

Renal involvement occurs in 50% of patients, especially boys and older children, and may present after initial systemic symptoms. Hematuria, either microscopic or gross, may occur with proteinuria during the first 3 weeks of the illness, but rarely after 6 months. With progressive involvement, hypertension, impaired renal function, and renal failure can occur in up to 15% of children, with an associated mortality rate of 3%.

In occasional patients, an acute scrotum that mimics testicular torsion may develop; however, surgical exploration may not be necessary if appropriate clinical and radiographic features are present. Other rare manifestations of HSP include neurologic, cardiac, and pulmonary events.

Anemia occasionally develops as a result of gastrointestinal tract blood loss or decreased RBC production caused by renal failure. The leukocyte count is normal. Despite the impressive purpura, the platelet count is normal or increased with normal platelet function. Coagulation factor levels usually are normal, although transient decreases in factor XIII activity and vitamin K deficiency from severe vasculitis-induced intestinal malabsorption have been reported. Signs of increased fibrinolysis, as evidenced by elevation of D-dimer and other markers, have been described.[108] Bleeding in the gastrointestinal tract, the lungs, or, rarely, the central nervous system is due to a necrotizing vasculitis and not a hemostatic defect.[107] Hypercoagulability does not play a role with normal frequency of MTHFR, prothrombin, and Factor V Leiden gene mutations.[109]

Henoch–Schönlein purpura is considered an IgA-mediated inflammation of small vessels. Biopsy of skin or other involved tissue reveals a leukocytoclastic vasculitis. Immune complexes of IgA with complement, IgG, or IgM have been found circulating in the serum[110] and deposited in blood vessel walls of kidney, and in intestinal and skin lesions.[111] The mechanism of production, accumulation, and deposition of IgA immune complexes in the blood vessel is unclear. It has been suggested that HSP may be a systemic form of IgA nephropathy.[112] Both disorders have identical features on renal biopsy and are characterized by mesangial proliferation, occasional focal sclerosis, and crescent formation.[113]

Treatment is mainly supportive, although corticosteroids have been found to provide symptomatic relief with severe joint, scrotal, or abdominal pain.[114,115] They do not alter skin involvement or prevent renal involvement. Recent studies have suggested that corticosteroids plus azathioprine, cyclosporin A, or cyclophosphamide may have a role in the management of severe renal involvement.[116–120] The prognosis is good for full recovery, except in the children with renal failure.

CARDIOPULMONARY DISEASE

Congenital Heart Disease

Congenital heart disease occurs in about 1% of live births. Structural heart malformation usually follows predictable patterns such that six defects account for 70% of all cardiac disorders: ventricular septal defect, atrial septal defect, tetralogy of Fallot, patent ductus arteriosus, pulmonary stenosis, and aortic stenosis. Children with cardiac abnormalities may be acyanotic or cyanotic, depending on the underlying lesion. Hematologic abnormalities occur most often in children with cyanotic congenital heart disease (CCHD).

Polycythemia is the bone marrow response to chronic hypoxemia in patients with CCHD. The decreased arterial oxygen content stimulates erythropoietin production, which in turn increases erythropoiesis. The resultant increased RBC mass increases the oxygen-carrying capacity of the blood, resulting in improved tissue oxygenation. With adequate compensation, erythropoietin levels fall to normal, while higher RBC production is maintained. A second compensatory mechanism is an increase in 2,3-diphosphoglycerate (2,3-DPG) levels in the RBC when the arterial oxygen tension is less than 70 mm Hg. The higher 2,3-DPG level causes a right shift of the oxyhemoglobin curve, resulting in greater oxygen release to the tissues.

Polycythemia in the cyanotic child is beneficial up to a point. Because the relationship between the hematocrit and blood viscosity is hyperbolic, minor increases in the hematocrit above 70% cause marked increases in blood viscosity. This higher viscosity results in impaired perfusion within the microvasculature, with ultimately less tissue oxygen delivery. The impairment is magnified in severe polycythemia (hematocrit level greater than 75%) such that headache, irritability, dyspnea, and even formation of pulmonary, renal, or central nervous system thrombi may result.[121] To prevent these complications, the hematocrit level should be maintained around 60% through the use of exchange transfusions. Small aliquots of the patient's blood are slowly removed and replaced by equal volumes of plasma or 5% albumin. Care should be taken to remove blood slowly, because vascular collapse, cyanosis, stroke, and seizures have been reported with too rapid an exchange. Apheresis (erythrocytapheresis) also has been shown to be an effective means of decreasing viscosity in polycythemic patients.

Infants with CCHD are at risk of developing iron deficiency anemia. The deficiency may result from the combination of poor iron stores at birth (especially in premature infants), increased iron needed for enhanced erythropoiesis, poor iron intake due to poor feeding, and ongoing iron losses as a consequence of phlebotomy or exchange transfusion. These children may exhibit symptoms of iron deficiency (irritability, anorexia, poor weight gain) or worsening cyanosis. The hemoglobin may be normal for age but inappropriately low for the degree of hypoxemia. Low RBC indices and hypochromic, microcytic RBCs are the best indices of iron deficiency in this setting.[122] Polycythemic children with iron deficiency anemia are at increased risk for cerebral vein thrombosis because of the poor deformability of the iron-deficient RBC, which further increases blood viscosity.[123] To prevent this complication and to allow for maximal tissue oxygenation, all infants should be fed iron-rich infant formula and receive iron replacement therapy as needed to normalize RBC indices.

Hemolytic anemia, characterized by mechanical destruction of red blood cells and manifested by the presence of schistocytes in the peripheral blood smear, is occasionally seen after the placement of prosthetic heart valves.

Routine screening of patients with congenital heart disease has demonstrated coagulation abnormalities in 20% to 59% of children with acyanotic defects and in 40% to 50% of those with cyanotic heart disease (Table 162–3).[124] Only 11% of children with CCHD have any clinical evidence of bleeding preoperatively. However, children with underlying hemostatic defects have a greater frequency and severity of postoperative bleeding.[124,125] Presurgical screening tests should include at least a platelet count, platelet function assay (eg, closure time), PT, and APTT. Further investigations may be indicated if there is a history of bleeding or abnormal results on screening tests. Children with polycythemia have contracted plasma volumes; therefore, when blood samples are collected, extra care should be taken to ensure the proper 1 : 9 ratio of 3.8% sodium citrate to blood, to prevent artificial abnormalities in coagulation test results.

The etiology of the coagulation abnormalities in CCHD is unclear. Earlier reports suggesting a role for consumptive coagulopathy have not been confirmed. Protein C levels in 8 of 29 term infants with CCHD were significantly lower than in controls with no evidence of familial deficiency. Of these infants, two had thrombotic complications and four had consumptive coagulopathy.[126] Platelets have shortened survival times (even with normal counts), and normal to increased numbers of megakaryocytes in the bone marrow are reported.[127] This increased platelet destruction does not appear to be due to DIC. Both the platelet and coagulation abnormalities are directly proportional to the degree of hypoxemia and polycythemia. For example, children with oxygen saturation greater than 60% have a mean platelet count of 315,000/μL, whereas those with saturation less than 60% have a mean count of 185,000/μL.[127] The mild platelet and coagulation abnormalities usually are decreased or corrected after surgical repair of the heart defect.[124,128] With bleeding, or if surgery is not possible, the coagulopathy may be treated by correction of polycythemia to a hematocrit level of 60% by using slow plasma-exchange transfusion.[129]

Table 162–3 Coagulation Abnormalities in Congenital Heart Disease

Incidence (%)		
Abnormality	***Acyanotic CHD***	***Cyanotic CHD***
Prolonged bleeding time	11	28
Prolonged PT		20
Prolonged APTT		19
Thrombocytopenia	12–40	0–36
Abnormal platelet aggregation	14	38–70
Increased fibrinolysis	12	0–10
Abnormal clot retraction	10	
Low fibrinogen	16	12
Increased fibrin split products		Occasionally
Decreased factors II, V, VII, VIII, IX, X, XI, XII		Occasionally
Decreased protein C		25%*
Decreased large multimers of von Willebrand factor	100†	

CHD, congenital heart disease.

*Data from MacDonald PD, Gibson BE, Braunlie J, et al: Protein C activity in severely ill newborns with congenital heart disease. J Perinatal Med 20:421, 1992.

†Twelve patients studied; true prevalence unknown.

Adapted from Lascari AD: Hematologic Manifestations of Childhood Diseases. New York, Thieme-Stratton, 1984, with permission.

CYSTIC FIBROSIS

Cystic fibrosis (CF) is a multisystem disorder of exocrine gland dysfunction characterized by chronic pulmonary disease, pancreatic exocrine insufficiency, hepatic dysfunction, abnormal reproductive organ function, and intestinal obstruction associated with abnormally high sweat electrolyte levels. It is an autosomal recessive disease with an incidence of 1/2000 live births.

Severe hemolytic anemia due to vitamin E deficiency may be the presenting manifestation of CF. Dolan initially linked deficiency of vitamin E with severe hemolytic anemia in infants who presented with pallor, edema, hypoproteinemia, and thrombocytosis.[130] This complication can be seen as early as 6 weeks of age.

Many children with CF are chronically hypoxic, yet they do not have the expected augmented erythroid response. In a study by Vichinsky and colleagues,[131] none of 42 children with CF had polycythemia, and 30% (especially the boys and the older children) had a normochromic, normocytic or hypochromic, microcytic anemia with reticulocytopenia. In contrast with children with CCHD, there was no appropriate increase in RBC 2,3-DPG levels, no right shift of the oxyhemoglobin curve, and either a low or a normal erythropoietin level. In vitro assays showed normal erythroid progenitor cell numbers and no serum inhibitor of erythropoiesis. Up to 66% of the children studied had abnormalities consistent with iron deficiency, and all responded to oral or parenteral iron therapy.

It appears that the etiology of anemia in CF is multifactorial. A blunted erythropoietic response to hypoxia plus iron deficiency secondary to iron malabsorption or poor dietary iron intake may each be partially responsible for the development of anemia. If iron deficiency persists despite adequate oral supplementation, the possibility of ongoing blood loss, or of iron malabsorption that may necessitate parenteral iron replacement, should be considered. Soluble transferrin receptor levels may be helpful in distinguishing iron deficiency from anemia of chronic inflammation in CF.[132]

Findings of studies of neutrophil function in children with CF are conflicting. Some reports indicate impaired chemotaxis, chemiluminescence, granule release, and superoxide production,[133–135] whereas others have demonstrated factors in patient sputum that actually enhance neutrophil and monocyte responses to stimulants.[136] Although these sputum factors may improve neutrophil killing ability, they also may worsen neutrophil-mediated lung damage through increased release of neutrophil elastase.[137] Evaluation of immune function has revealed impaired lymphoproliferative responses to *Pseudomonas* and other gram-negative bacterial antigens, defective opsonization, increased levels of circulating immune complexes, and decreased numbers of T helper cells in 30% of patients.[138] The contribution of these findings to frequent pulmonary infection is still under investigation.

Children with CF usually do not experience clinically significant bleeding owing to impaired hemostasis, despite the risk of liver disease and vitamin K deficiency from malabsorption. An exception may be infants under 1 year of age, in whom rare case reports of vitamin K-deficient hemorrhage have been reported in association with cystic fibrosis.[139–141] Routine coagulation tests usually yield normal results, with an occasional prolonged APTT reported. A study by Corrigan and colleagues[142] revealed that 60% of 24 patients had a more subtle deficiency of prothrombin activity, thought to be due to vitamin K deficiency. Other investigators, using direct measurement of vitamin K and PIVKA-II (protein induced by vitamin K absence-II), have reported conflicting percentages of patients to be vitamin K deficient.[143,144] Routine vitamin K supplementation is not recommended, although it may be indicated in persons with severe liver disease or confirmed coagulation abnormalities.

Children with CF may have a particularly high predisposition to recurrent venous thrombosis. In a study of 19 patients with recurrent venous thrombosis, 6 had CF, whereas none of 101 thrombosis patients without recurrence had CF. A striking association with respiratory tract colonization with *Burkholderia cepacia* was noted, as was the frequent presence of a central venous catheter. Several of the recurrences occurred while on therapeutic anticoagulation.[145]

GASTROINTESTINAL DISEASE

Milk Protein-Induced Enteropathy and Heiner Syndrome

The association of iron deficiency with dietary intake of cow's milk in young infants is established. A major contributing factor is the relatively poor bioavailability of iron in cow's milk as compared with breast milk. In addition, the rapid growth of infants and corresponding rapid increase in red cell mass necessitates an increased requirement for dietary iron. The role of cow's milk in inducing occult gastrointestinal blood loss in infants was carefully documented more than three decades ago in a sentinel paper that also demonstrated a correlation between the amount of milk ingested and the amount of fecal blood lost.[146] Gastrointestinal blood loss in response to cow's milk ingestion appears to be most prevalent in infants less than 6 months of age, and occurs with diminishing frequency in older infants.[147] The majority of affected infants will outgrow their milk protein sensitivity by 3 years of age. The gastrointestinal blood loss may be ameliorated by heat denaturing of the milk proteins. Occasionally toddlers and older children have been documented to have milk-induced gastrointestinal bleeding with associated iron deficiency anemia.[148,149] Substantially limiting cow's milk consumption and prescribing iron supplementation is sufficient to correct the iron deficiency and associated hypoproteinemia in most children.

A variety of gastrointestinal syndromes associated with cow's milk sensitivity, with varying manifestations and severity, have been described. Associated findings may include vomiting, diarrhea, poor growth, and hypoproteinemia; however, some patients may have occult blood loss and anemia without associated complaints. At the severe end of the spectrum a cow's milk protein-induced enterocolitis may occur.[150] Such patients may present with acute, severe bloody diarrhea, vomiting, abdominal distention, methemoglobinemia and shock, even in the absence of anemia.[150] Even minute amounts of cow's milk protein in human breast milk may be sufficient to precipitate a severe event.[151] In patients with chronic occult gastrointestinal blood loss esophagogastroduodenoscopy may reveal gastritis or gastroduodenitis, and colonoscopy may demonstrate modest histological abnormalities in the proximal colon.[149,152] The immunopathobiology of cow's milk protein allergy syndromes has not been fully elucidated. Most of these syndromes affecting the intestinal tract only are non-IgE mediated.[153,154] Wilson et al reported the frequent presence of precipitating antibodies to milk proteins in the study population as a whole.[155] However, the presence of such antibodies did not appear to predict milk-induced gastrointestinal bleeding. The roles that genetic predisposition, intestinal and immunologic immaturity in young infants, exposure to cow's milk protein in breast milk, gastrointestinal infections, or other factors may play in the development of milk protein enteropathy are not fully understood.

In 1962 Heiner et al described a syndrome in infants and young children that included chronic cough, recurrent lung infiltrates, poor growth, gastrointestinal symptoms and blood loss, iron deficiency anemia, and pulmonary hemosiderosis associated with multiple serum precipitins to cow's milk proteins.[156] Others have confirmed and further detailed this rare syndrome.[157,158] Additional manifestations may include intermittent wheezing, hilar lymphadenopathy, eosinophilia, elevated levels of serum IgE, IgM, or IgA, chronic rhinitis, adenoidal hypertrophy, hypercapnia, and cor pulmonale. A feature of this syndrome is rapid improvement of the pulmonary manifestations after eliminating cow's milk from the diet.

CELIAC DISEASE

Celiac disease, or gluten-sensitive enteropathy, is an inflammatory and malabsorptive process resulting from an aberrant intestinal T-cell immune response to ingested dietary gluten, leading to injury of the mucosa of the small intestine.[159] Classical celiac disease has been characterized as frequently affecting infants and young children, leading to steatorrhea, failure to thrive, weight loss, and nutritional deficiency. With the advent of improved screening techniques, the prevalence is recognized to be greater than previous estimates. Celiac disease broadly affects both children and adults, many of whom may have minimal classical symptoms of the disorder. Treatment is usually institution of a gluten-free diet, with resolution of the process in the majority of cases.

Iron deficiency is frequently present in celiac disease in children and adults and may be the sole recognized manifestation of the disorder.[160] Dietary iron absorption primarily occurs within the proximal small intestine, the same region most affected by celiac disease. As a result iron deficiency in celiac disease appears to be primarily due to impaired absorption of dietary iron, although a component of chronic gastrointestinal blood loss may also apply in a minority of patients.[160,161] Iron deficiency in celiac disease may be refractory to iron supplementation, and a significant percentage of children and adults with iron deficiency anemia that does not respond to therapeutic oral iron replacement have celiac disease.

Folic acid and to a lesser frequency vitamin B_{12} deficiency may also result from the malabsorptive process in celiac disease. Manifestations may include macrocytic anemia, leukocytopenia, and pancytopenia. Neurologic findings may be present with vitamin B_{12} deficiency. Other vitamin and micronutrient deficiencies, including copper and vitamin K deficiency, have been observed in celiac disease. Splenic hypofunction may occur with some frequency in adults with celiac disease, but appears to be less common in children. A number of case reports have suggested an association of pulmonary hemosiderosis with celiac disease.[162,163] The pathophysiology of this association in not known, but the pulmonary process may improve with initiation of a gluten-free diet.

A high index of suspicion is important for diagnosing celiac disease in children, particularly those who are minimally symptomatic. In addition to correcting the nutritional deficiencies and growth failure in children with celiac disease, recognition of the disease and institution of a gluten-free diet may minimize the risk of some of the associated conditions of celiac disease, including the development of non-Hodgkin lymphoma involving the intestinal tract.

INFLAMMATORY BOWEL DISEASE

Anemia is a very common extraintestinal manifestation of inflammatory bowel disease (IBD), particularly in children with Crohn disease, in whom the historical prevalence of anemia approaches 70% to 80%.[164,165] A more recent series suggest that the prevalence of anemia may be declining in Crohn disease, perhaps due to more effective therapy.[166] The etiology of anemia in IBD appears to be multifactorial, but the most common contributing factors are iron deficiency related to chronic gastrointestinal blood loss or iron malabsorption due to intestinal mucosal injury, and decreased absorption and sequestration of iron stores as is seen in the anemia of chronic inflammation. These broad mechanisms for anemia may coexist, and it is sometimes difficult to determine the predominant mechanism. Measurement of serum transferrin receptor can be helpful in this setting to distinguish the contribution of iron deficiency anemia versus anemia of chronic inflammation.[167] Other contributing factors to anemia in IBD may also be present in individual patients, including immune-mediated hemolytic anemia, hemophagocytosis, malnutrition, folate and vitamin B_{12} deficiency, and the suppressive effects of medications on hematopoiesis.[168]

Specific treatment of anemia in IBD may be difficult. Oral iron supplementation is not always effective. Comparative studies of oral versus intravenous iron supplementation suggest the intravenous route may result in better short-term improvement in anemia; however long-term outcome data are lacking.[169,170] Some patients may respond to supplemental erythropoietin administration as well.[171] Patients with IBD may have impaired enterocyte-mediated intestinal absorption of iron, the degree of which appears to correlate with disease activity.[172] The role that induction of hepcidin expression by mediators of inflammation, particularly IL-6, plays in the anemia of IBD is an intriguing area of ongoing investigation.[172]

Other hematologic manifestations of IBD include leukocytosis and thrombocytosis, hyposplenism, an increased propensity toward thrombosis, and therapy-related leukopenia and thrombocytopenia. There may be an increased incidence of immune-mediated thrombocytopenia associated with IBD.[173] The recently described potential association between infliximab, an anti–tumor necrosis factor antibody, and hepatosplenic T-cell lymphoma, bears close observation, and suggests that biologic agents such as infliximab should be used only after careful consideration of the potential benefits and risks of the agent in the individual patient.[174]

ANOREXIA NERVOSA

Anorexia nervosa is a psychiatric disorder occurring in about 1/800 adolescent girls; it is characterized by an inability to maintain a minimal normal body weight, intense fear of being fat, body image distortion, and amenorrhea. The profound weight loss is accompanied by hypothermia, hypotension, edema, lanugo, and metabolic changes and is associated with a mortality rate of 5% to 18%. A mild, normochromic, normocytic anemia with reticulocytopenia occurs in 30% of patients.[175] Acanthocytes or spur cells have been reported and may be due to low serum β-lipoprotein levels. The causes of the anemia probably are decreased RBC production and a relative increase in plasma volume. A few patients have had slightly decreased RBC survival. Serum B_{12} and folate levels usually are normal. Despite low serum iron and decreased marrow iron stores in 80% of patients, iron deficiency anemia is uncommon except during recovery, when iron supplementation is necessary. The severe hypophosphatemia seen during refeeding of severely malnourished patients has been associated with hemolytic anemia.

Fifty percent of patients have leukopenia, with an absolute decrease in numbers of neutrophils, lymphocytes, and monocytes.[176,177] The neutropenia may be quite severe. An increased incidence of infection is not usual, although with increasing use of central venous catheters, more serious bacterial infections are being reported.[177] Bone marrow reserves are normal despite marrow hypoplasia and a normal to slightly decreased size of the marginal pool. Impaired neutrophil chemotaxis, intracellular killing of staphylococci, and decreased complement levels have been demonstrated in patients with anorexia. These findings are associated with occasional skin abscess formation.

Patients with anorexia nervosa have no apparent bleeding diathesis. The platelet count is normal to slightly decreased,[175,178] and in vitro platelet aggregation response to epinephrine, adenosine diphosphate, and collagen is exaggerated. Coagulation defects are uncommon, except for that related to vitamin K deficiency reported in bulimia.

The hematologic changes in anorexia nervosa are directly correlated with total body fat mass depletion.[179] A bone marrow pattern on magnetic resonance imaging suggestive of gelatinous transformation of bone marrow (serous atrophy) is seen in patients with the lowest hematologic parameters. Direct examination of the bone marrow reveals hypoplasia with loss of fat stores and replacement by a gelatinous acid mucopolysaccharide ground substance. Focal or extensive necrosis may be present.[180] Bone marrow histiocytes are relatively increased in number and have prominent blue-green granules. With nutritional supplementation, bone marrow hypoplasia reverses, the gelatinous material disappears, and the hematologic abnormalities, including neutrophil defects and low complement levels, resolve by 8 weeks.

THROMBOEMBOLIC COMPLICATIONS IN CHILDHOOD ILLNESS

Improvements in medical and surgical care, in particular advances in critical and supportive care, have led to increased survival among children with malignancy and chronic illnesses. However, the extended survival of these children has led to new comorbidities in the field of pediatrics, including thromboembolic complications. The increased risk of thromboembolism in children with chronic illnesses is multifactorial and may include the illness itself, medical and surgical interventions, or the central venous line used to administer therapy.

Unlike adults, in whom idiopathic thromboembolism occurs regularly, the majority of thromboembolic events in children are secondary to serious underlying conditions such as cancer, trauma, or surgery.[181] The Canadian Childhood Thrombophilia Registry contains more than 400 children.[182] In this population, over 50% had an underlying systemic illness, with malignancy (25%) and cardiac illness (20%) as the most common entities. This review will focus on four childhood illnesses commonly associated with thromboembolism: malignancy, congenital heart disease, nephrotic syndrome, and systemic lupus erythematosus. In addition to the diseases discussed in this review, other chronic illnesses of childhood have been associated with thromboembolism, including sickle cell anemia (see Chapter 43), juvenile rheumatoid arthritis, inflammatory bowel disease, and cystic fibrosis.

THROMBOEMBOLISM IN PEDIATRIC CANCER

Although thrombosis is a well-known complication of pediatric malignancy, the overall incidence is infrequent compared to adults with cancer. Surprisingly, there have been no large cohort studies to assess the prevalence of thrombosis among all childhood cancer types. Small studies report an incidence of 7% to 14% based on clinical symptoms, which increases to 44% to 50% when children undergo routine radiographic screening.[183–189] Of note, all of these studies were focused on catheter-related thrombosis. As a result, the majority of thrombosis described in the literature is located in the upper venous system. Right atrial thrombi are also frequently seen, with a reported incidence of 9% to 14% in children with indwelling catheters.[185,188] Typically asymptomatic, these thrombi are often found incidentally on routine surveillance echocardiograms for children receiving anthracycline chemotherapy. Although the presence of a central venous line is the most important risk factor in the development of pediatric thrombosis, children with cancer are also at risk for thrombosis at sites other than their catheter.[188,191]

There are several mechanisms by which malignancy alone increases the risk of thromboembolism.[192] These include direct activation of the coagulation system, inhibition of fibrinolysis through secretion of plasminogen activator inhibitor-1, and the release of cytokines, which themselves induce procoagulant and antifibrinolytic activity. Malignant cells can also adhere to platelets, leukocytes, and the endothelium through adhesion molecules present on their surface. Finally, as tumors increase in size, they may compress or occlude blood vessels, leading to reduced blood flow and stasis.

In adults, solid tumors are associated with a higher risk of thromboembolism than hematologic malignancies.[193] In contrast, acute lymphoblastic leukemia (ALL) is the most common malignancy reported in association with thrombosis in children, with a reported incidence rate of 5.2% in a recent meta-analysis.[194] This may simply be due to the fact that ALL is the most common cancer seen in pediatrics. However, brain tumors, the most common solid tumor in children, do appear to have a relatively lower risk of thrombosis. Two large studies reported incidences of 0.6% and 2.8%, as opposed to the 18% to 28% incidence of thrombosis in adults with brain tumors.[195–197] Large cohort studies containing children with all types of malignancies are needed to better understand the true incidence of thromboembolism in pediatric malignancy.

As stated above, the majority of literature on thromboembolism in pediatric cancer focuses on children with acute lymphoblastic leukemia (ALL). As opposed to other types of cancer, cerebral venous thrombosis and stroke are frequently seen, particularly in the setting of asparaginase therapy. Asparaginase, an essential component of induction chemotherapy, reduces the synthesis of both coagulation factors and inhibitors as a consequence of asparagine depletion.[198] Higher incidences of thrombosis appear to be associated with lower doses of asparaginase given for long periods, as well as prednisone (when given instead of dexamethasone).[194]

When treating a thromboembolism in a patient with cancer, low-molecular-weight heparin (LMWH) is likely the best choice. Warfarin, although it is less expensive and can be given orally, is too difficult to regulate in the setting of multiple chemotherapy agents, changing vitamin K stores due to antibiotics and illness, and the frequency of invasive procedures.[189,199,200] A randomized clinical trial in adult cancer patients demonstrated that LMWH was more efficacious and as safe as warfarin in preventing recurrent thromboembolism.[201] There are no specific recommendations for duration of anticoagulation in pediatric cancer patients. However, it seems reasonable to continue or resume some type of anticoagulation in the setting of ongoing risk factors, such as a repeat course of asparaginase in ALL, or anticipated postoperative immobilization in an osteosarcoma patient undergoing resection. LMWH should always be held 24 hours prior to a lumbar puncture or other invasive procedure. However, there is no evidence regarding how to best adjust LMWH in the setting of chemotherapy-induced thrombocytopenia.

Because central venous lines are the most important risk factor in the development of pediatric thrombosis, investigators have sought to determine if thromboprophylaxis is effective in preventing this complication. Earlier studies did show that thromboprophylaxis is tolerable in children with cancer.[189] However, a recent randomized trial demonstrated no difference in the incidence of line-related thrombosis between pediatric cancer patients receiving low-dose warfarin (goal INR 1.3–1.9) and those in the control group.[183] Therefore, routine prophylaxis cannot be recommended at this time.

THROMBOEMBOLISM IN CONGENITAL HEART DISEASE

Although congenital heart disease (CHD) affects only 1% of live births, almost 50% of infants less than 6 months of age and 30% of older children who develop venous thromboembolism have underlying cardiac disorders.[202] Also, the majority of children receiving prophylactic anticoagulation are being treated for complex CHD or severe acquired cardiac diseases such as cardiomyopathy. Children with CHD are at risk for venous, arterial, and intracardiac thromboembolism, as well as embolism to the central nervous system. CHD is the most common associated diagnosis among children hospitalized with arterial ischemic stroke in the United States.[203]

Cardiac catheterization is the most common procedure performed in children with CHD, and is used for both diagnostic and therapeutic purposes. Access is typically obtained through the femoral artery. Historically, thromboembolism of the femoral artery was a common complication of this procedure, particularly in younger patients. In the 1970s, a randomized clinical trial demonstrated that the use of unfractionated heparin prophylaxis reduced the incidence of femoral artery thrombosis from 40% to 8% in children less than 10 years of age.[204] The current recommendation from the American College of Chest Physicians (ACCP) is that all children should undergo prophylaxis with unfractionated heparin prior to cardiac catheterization, using a bolus of 100 to 150 U/kg.[181] Additional doses may be required for prolonged catheterizations.

The Fontan procedure, which diverts systemic venous return directly to the pulmonary arteries, is the definitive palliative surgical treatment for most congenital univentricular heart lesions.[202] Unfortunately, thromboembolic events continue to be a major cause of morbidity and mortality in this procedure. The reported incidence of these complications in cohort studies ranges from 1% to 19%, and include venous thrombosis of the Fontan circuit, right atrial thrombosis, and stroke.[202] Thromboembolic events may occur anytime after the procedure but often present months to years later.[205]

There is no consensus as to the optimal type or duration of anticoagulation that Fontan patients should receive, nor are there any data that any one prophylactic regimen is effective in reducing thromboembolic complications. Institutional protocols, if they exist, range from no anticoagulation to aspirin to warfarin. The ACCP guidelines suggest either therapy with aspirin (5 mg/kg/day) or therapeutic heparin followed by warfarin to achieve a target INR of 2.5, but state that the optimal duration of therapy is unknown.[181] An ongoing multicenter study in Australia and Canada is comparing these two therapies in a randomized clinical trial.[202]

There is even less data on the role of anticoagulation or antiplatelet therapy in other cardiac procedures with the potential risk of thromboembolism. These include the placement of endovascular stents and Blalock–Taussig shunts, as well as Norwood and Glenn procedures, which are typically performed prior to the definitive Fontan procedure. The ACCP recommends perioperative heparin therapy for these procedures.[181] However, the need for ongoing aspirin therapy is not known.

In contrast, long-term anticoagulation therapy is clearly indicated for children with prosthetic heart valves. This population is treated according to adult recommendations. Children with biologic valves should receive 3 months of warfarin, followed by long-term aspirin therapy. Those with mechanical valves must remain on long-term warfarin, with target INRs of 2.5 or 3.0 depending on the specific type of valve.[206]

THROMBOEMBOLISM IN NEPHROTIC SYNDROME

The increased risk of thromboembolism in pediatric nephrotic syndrome is multifactorial.[207] The same urinary losses that lead to profound hypoalbuminemia in these patients also cause acquired deficiencies of anticoagulants such as antithrombin and free Protein S. Most recently, acquired Protein Z deficiency has been reported, with correlation between Protein Z and albumin levels.[208] Increased levels of procoagulants, including fibrinogen, Factor V, and Factor VIII, as well as hypercholesterolemia and increased platelet aggregation, have all been described in nephrotic syndrome. Finally, the therapeutic interventions themselves can increase the risk of thromboembolism. Diuretics cause reduced intravascular volume leading to hemoconcentration, whereas steroids and cyclosporine increase procoagulant activities.

The incidence of thromboembolism in pediatric nephrotic syndrome ranges from 1.8% to 5.4% in published series.[207,209,210] This contrasts with adult nephrotic syndrome, in which incidence rates as high as 44% have been reported.[209] The most common locations in children are the deep veins of the lower extremities and renal veins. Pulmonary embolism, one of the most feared complications of nephrotic syndrome, was traditionally thought to be a rare event. Although clinically diagnosed in less than 1% of children, a frequency of 27% (7/26) was found in a series of nephrotic children who underwent screening with ventilation-perfusion scans.[211] These data suggests that pulmonary symptoms may not always be due to fluid overload in this population, and that pulmonary embolism should at least be considered in any nephrotic patient with a significant change in respiratory status.

Prophylactic anticoagulation is recommended for adult nephrotic syndrome as long as the patient has nephrotic proteinuria and/or severe hypoalbuminemia. The question of prophylactic anticoagulation with LMWH or low-dose aspirin has been raised for nephrotic children with similar features, and/or those with steroid-resistant disease.[212] However, no studies have been performed to evaluate the efficacy or safety of this practice. Therefore, prophylactic anticoagulation remains controversial in pediatric nephrotic syndrome and is generally not used in children without a prior history of thrombosis.[213] One reason for the controversy is that predictors of thrombosis have not been established in this population. Even decreased plasma concentrations of antithrombin, the most recognized risk factor, is not a constant finding in nephrotic children who develop thromboembolism.[212] The most consistent biological risk factor to date is the presence of severe hypoalbuminemia.[207]

For those patients who develop a thrombosis, the ACCP recommends unfractionated heparin or LMWH for 5 to 7 days, followed by LMWH or warfarin for 3 to 6 months.[181] Some form of anticoagulation, however, should be continued or resumed in the setting of active disease. To avoid hemoconcentration, diuretics must be avoided or used judiciously in patients who have experienced a thromboembolic event. Finally, it is important to remember that the efficacy of heparin, especially unfractionated heparin, can be impaired in the setting of decreased antithrombin levels.

THROMBOEMBOLISM IN SYSTEMIC LUPUS ERYTHEMATOSUS

The reported incidence of thromboembolism in pediatric systemic lupus erythematosus (SLE) ranges from 9% to 17%, similar to rates reported in adult SLE patients.[215,216] Compared with malignancy, congenital heart disease, and nephrotic syndrome, thromboembolism in SLE is more likely to be arterial and involve the central nervous system. These events can occur early in the disease process, often at the time of the SLE diagnosis.

The significant association between the presence of antiphospholipid antibodies and thromboembolism is well described in patients with SLE.[217] Antiphospholipid antibodies (APLA) are a heterogenous group of antibodies directed against plasma proteins and phospholipid complexes. They most frequently occur in the setting of SLE, but are also associated with juvenile rheumatoid arthritis, epilepsy, and other diseases.[218] There are multiple subtypes of APLA, including lupus anticoagulants, anticardiolipin antibodies, anti-B2-glycoprotein, and antiprothrombin antibodies. The exact mechanism of APLA-associated thromboembolism has not been elucidated, but recent data suggest that lupus anticoagulant antibodies interfere with the function of the protein C pathway, leading to an acquired activated protein C resistance.[219]

APLA are quite common in the pediatric SLE population. An analysis of 12 reported series of children with SLE reported a global prevalence of 48% for anticardiolipin antibodies, and 23% for lupus anticoagulants.[218] Recent work has focused on the predictive value of APLA subtypes for the risk of thromboembolic events. In a cohort of 58 children with SLE, 7 of whom had 10 thrombotic events, the presence of lupus anticoagulants had the highest predictive power for thromboembolism, with a sensitivity of 100% and a negative predictive value of 100%.[220] The presence of anticardiolipin antibody was also predictive, but only if the antibody was persistent (positive on at least two occasions 3 months apart). Other studies have confirmed the strong predictive power of APLA, in particular lupus anticoagulants, for the risk of thromboembolism.[215,221,222] The association appears to be even stronger than that reported for adult SLE patients, likely because of the lack of other confounders such as older age, pregnancy, and malignancy.[223] In fact, pediatric SLE patients who are negative for antiphospholipid antibodies rarely develop thrombotic events.

On the basis of the above data, it is recommended that children with SLE be routinely screened for lupus anticoagulants, and if antibodies are present on more than one occasion they should be counseled on the presenting symptoms of stroke and other thrombotic events.[222] Prophylaxis with low-dose aspirin may be reasonable, especially in the setting of other thrombotic risk factors. However, there is not yet data to support prophylactic anticoagulation in SLE patients with lupus anticoagulants in the absence of a history of thromboembolism.[215]

It is important to note that transient lupus anticoagulants, perhaps the result of infections or immunizations, have been well described in healthy children. These lupus anticoagulants are often found incidentally in the preoperative evaluation of an elevated APTT in a child undergoing tonsillectomy. These incidentally found antibodies have not been associated with an increased risk of thrombosis.

The management of thromboembolism in SLE patients and APLA is different from most other pediatric thromboembolisms. APLA syndrome, defined by the association of a persistent APLA with symptomatic thromboembolism, has a very high risk of thrombus recurrence off therapy, and most affected children are treated indefinitely.[224] However, the appropriate intensity of this prolonged therapy is not known. Children with systemic inflammatory disorders such as SLE, rheumatoid arthritis, and inflammatory bowel disease are also at risk for thrombus recurrence when their inflammatory process is exacerbated. Children with systemic inflammation and a history of thrombosis should receive prophylactic anticoagulation until the inflammation is well controlled.[181,224]

Hematologic Complications of Solid Organ Transplantation in Children

The frequency and the success of solid organ transplantation in children have been increasing over the last decade. In 2004 there were 1816 transplants in children representing 7% of all recipients.[228,229] This is an increase of 13% over the last decade. Of the transplants in 2004, the majority were renal transplants (765) followed by liver (529) then heart (250–290). The success rate has been also improving impressively, with 5-year survival after kidney transplant at 83% to 90%, liver transplant 79% to 83%, and cardiac transplant 70% to 75%.

Hematologic complications after solid organ transplantation are a common problem. Although most of the evidence regarding type, frequency, and etiology of these complications has been studied in adults, there are increasing reports in children. Following renal transplantation 60% of children are reported to be anemic. After liver transplant, 36% of children will have a hematologic problem and of these 54% are anemic events, 19% anemia and neutropenia, 12% thrombocytopenia, 8% neutropenia, and 2% pancytopenia.[230] After

Thrombophilia Screening in Children with Systemic Disease

In a child with an underlying systemic disease, the importance of prothrombotic traits in the pathogenesis of thromboembolism is unknown. Even the prevalence of thrombophilia among these patient populations is unclear. There does not appear to be an increased incidence of inherited thrombophilia in pediatric SLE patients with thrombophilia.[213] Nephrotic children have a prevalence of Factor V Leiden similar to the normal population.[223] In two studies describing the prevalence of thrombophilia in children with acute lymphoblastic leukemia, one reported 0% prevalence, compared with 84% in the other.[185,187,224] In the setting of leukemia, thrombophilia evaluation is further complicated because the anticoagulants Protein C and Protein S can be reduced by chemotherapy. Lipoprotein (a), another marker of thrombophilia, has been shown to vary depending on stage of disease and response to treatment.[227]

At this time, even screening for inherited prothrombotic traits in children with thromboembolism is of unproven benefit.[179] Therefore, any recommendations for universal thrombophilia screening in children with malignancy or other illness, and using the results to guide clinical management, are premature. It is hoped that future studies will investigate the usefulness of thrombophilia screening in selected populations, such as children with steroid-resistant nephrotic syndrome, or SLE and a positive lupus anticoagulant.

heart, heart–lung, or double lung transplant, 51% of patients have been reported to have hematologic problems: 49% anemia, 14% neutropenia, 14% thrombocytopenia, and 23% anemia plus neutropenia with or without thrombocytopenia.[231] The etiology of these hematologic problems is most commonly a result of infection followed by medication effect. Miscellaneous causes include blood loss, microangiopathic hemolytic anemia, autoimmune cytopenias, posttransplant lymphoproliferative disease (PTLD), and multifactorial.

In the next section, discussion of the hematologic complications of solid organ transplantation is divided into cell type and by organ type when feasible. Incidence, etiology, and natural history of the problem are addressed. Much of the data are derived from adult studies, but information from pediatric studies are emphasized.

RED CELLS

Anemia is a common problem after transplantation. The incidence is reported as follows:

Kidney
- –at time of transplant: 66% [232]
- –after transplant: 60% to 84% [233]

Liver 20% to 35% [230,234,235]

Heart/heart–lung/double lung 30% to 70% [231,236]

There are distinct patterns of presentation of the problems associated with red cells, including early posttransplant anemia, hemolytic uremic syndrome (HUS)/microangiopathic hemolytic anemia (MAHA), late anemia from immunosuppressant drugs, late anemia from other causes, and pure red cell aplasia.

Early Posttransplant Anemia

Early post-transplant anemia is defined as anemia that occurs within 6 months from the time of transplant. The etiologies include:

1) Post-operative hemorrhage
2) Hemolytic anemia secondary to
   a. Passenger lymphocyte syndrome
   b. HUS/MAHA
3) Infection
   a. Sepsis
   b. Viral, esp. CMV, EBV, parvovirus
4) Medication
   a. Immunosuppressive drugs
   b. Nonimmunosuppressive drugs
5) After renal transplantation:
   a. Iron deficiency
   b. Prior uremia/bone disease

Passenger Lymphocyte Syndrome

Passenger lymphocyte syndrome is a graft-versus-host reaction.[237,238] Antibodies made by donor B cells ("passengers") transplanted with the organ are made against host red blood cells. This direct antiglobulin-positive immune hemolytic anemia occurs within 3 to 24 days posttransplant. Rh antibodies, especially anti-D, are the most common type of antibody. The anemia can be mild to severe, but is self-limited lasting about a month. The incidence of this complication increases as the size of the transplanted organ increases:

	Antibody + (%)	Hemolysis (%)
Kidney	17	9
Liver	40	29
Heart/lung	70	70

The incidence also varies depending on blood type of donor and recipient:

–61% with O donor and A recipient

–22% with O donor and B recipient

–17% with AB donor and non-AB recipient

Pediatric cases have been reported following all types of solid organ transplant and the incidence appears to be the same in children and adults, at least following liver transplantation.

Treatment consists of observation alone if mild and transfusion if severe.[237] When transfusing red cells, the ABO type of the transfused product should be identical to or compatible with the recipient serum, regardless of donor type. When transfusing platelets or fresh frozen plasma, the product should be compatible with both recipient and donor. Empiric therapy employed in management of severe cases includes corticosteroids, plasma exchange, and red cell exchange.

Hemolytic Uremic Syndrome/Microangiopathic Hemolytic Anemia

HUS/MAHA following solid organ transplant has been described most often in adults who have the typical clinical presentation for this disorder.[239–241] The majority of cases have been described in renal transplant recipients (90% of cases reported), but it has been seen with all transplant types. The median time of onset is 30 day posttransplant ranging from 8 days to 9 months,[239] and 80% of cases are within 90 days and 96% within a year.[241]

Following renal transplant for HUS, 23% of patients will have a recurrence, but the incidence varies depending on the original type of HUS. When transplant is for diarrhea-associated HUS, the recurrence rate is less than 10%. The incidence increases when the original diagnosis is atypical adult HUS and increases even more with familial HUS (60% recurrence rate), especially if there is factor H deficiency. In children transplanted for HUS there was an 8.8% recurrence rate,[242] although it was 80% for those transplanted for atypical HUS.

The calcineurin inhibitors cyclosporine (CsA) and tacrolimus (TAC) have triggered the HUS in all of the nonrenal transplant cases and half of the renal transplant cases. The possibility of an infectious trigger has been suggested for the development of MAHA.

Treatment consists of discontinuing or decreasing the dose, or switching the calcineurin inhibitor. Plasma exchange is an unproven therapy. The outcome for graft survival is 60% for de novo HUS, but only about 33% for recurrent HUS. In children transplanted for atypical HUS, almost all lost their grafts if they develop recurrent HUS.

Late Posttransplant Anemia

Anemia occurring greater than 6 months after transplant is termed late posttransplant anemia. Causes of late anemia that are common to all solid organ transplants include[230–232,234,236]:

1. Infection
   a. EBV
   b. Parvo
   c. Rarely, CMV
2. Drug effect
   a. Myelosuppression
   b. Hemolytic anemia
   c. Other drug effects (trimethoprim-sulfamethoxazole, dapsone, etc)
3. Rejection/PTLD
4. Anemia of chronic disease
5. Iron deficiency
6. Acute renal failure
7. Uncommon/multifactorial

Etiologies of late anemia in the renal transplant setting include:

1. End stage renal disease
2. Low erythropoietin levels (68% of patients will have levels <2 SD below norm)[232]

Young children postrenal transplant have less anemia than older children and young adults. This may be due to the large donor kidney with higher erythropoietin levels and creatinine clearance relative to the size of the patient.

Immunosuppressant Drugs

There is a wide variation in the reported incidence of anemia secondary to immunosuppressant drugs: 1% to 53%. This variation may be a result of the lack of a specific test for drug-associated anemia and the lack of prospective studies. Indirect evidence for the association, however, is quite strong, that is, the ISD is stopped or changed and the anemia improves. There is a clear association of HUS/MAHA with the immunosuppressant drugs CsA and TAC in the early post-transplant period, but there are a number of studies documenting the association of late anemia with these agents as well.

In a study of children after liver transplant, half of the cases of anemia were attributed to ISD.[230] The diagnosis was usually made by excluding other causes of anemia plus evidence of resolution of the anemia after change in the ISD dose or switch to an alternative drug (median time for resolution—4 months).

In a study of children and young adults following cardiothoracic transplantation, approximately a quarter of the cases of anemia was attributed to tacrolimus, primarily because no other etiology was found.[231] The nadir hemoglobin in these patients was 7.3 to 8.8 g/dL, with reticulocytes from 1.5% to 6.7%. Only one patient had a direct antiglobulin study performed and it was negative. Four of five patients with simultaneous anemia and neutropenia recovered counts within 5 weeks of switching to CsA.

In a study of 50 pediatric renal transplant patients, the prevalence of anemia was 60%, with 30% having hemoglobin levels below 10 g/dL. TAC dose was found to be significantly associated with the presence of anemia.[243]

The association of pure red cell aplasia (PRCA) and TAC was first reported in adults. Two children were reported to develop PRCA while on TAC 8 and 47 months after liver transplantation.[244] Neither had evidence of parvovirus B19 infection. When there was no evidence of spontaneous recovery after 2 to 3 months of observation, they were switched from TAC to CsA and both recovered within 3 weeks.

There are a number of case reports of autoimmune hemolytic anemia associated with the use of TAC in both children and adults. A child with a cold antibody-positive hemolytic anemia 1 year after kidney transplant did not improve when TAC was switched to CsA, but the anemia resolved after switching to sirolimus.[245] A 9-year-old girl with severe anemia related to cold agglutinin production after liver transplantation improved when TAC was stopped.[246] When TAC was subsequently restarted, the anemia worsened, but it resolved without recurrence after switching to CsA. Four children receiving TAC developed either autoimmune hemolytic anemia alone or with thrombocytopenia following liver or intestinal transplantation.[247] TAC was not stopped because of concern for rejection. These patients were treated with corticosteroids and rituximab with a good response, but relapses were seen in two and all required continuous corticosteroid administration. Finally, an 8-year-old developed a warm antibody autoimmune hemolytic anemia 7 years after cardiac transplant while on TAC.[248] The patient was treated with steroids, intravenous immunoglobulin, and rituximab. Although responsive, he had a chronic relapsing course.

Nonimmune hemolysis has also been documented in adults. In a retrospective study of 81 patients (median age 39 years; range 12–66) after lung transplantation, 20% developed hemolytic anemia in the first year after transplant.[249] All were on CsA and none received TAC. The anemia was mild to moderate and there was no evidence of autoantibody formation or MAHA and other causes of anemia were excluded. The authors postulate an auto- or alloimmune mechanism to explain this phenomenon.

Anemia has been reported to be associated with all of the currently used immunosuppressants, including mycophenolate mofetil and sirolimus. Although direct comparison of all of the drugs has not been performed, it appears that TAC and CsA have a similar incidence,[250] with anemia occurring less commonly with the others. One possible mechanism of the development of autoimmune antibodies posttransplant is the chronic T-cell suppression resulting for the use of these agents followed by release of B-cell control. As noted above, treatment has been empiric and has included the standard treatments for autoimmune hemolytic anemia, including rituximab. Reduction in dose or switching the type of the immunosuppressant drug appears to be an effective therapy.

Pure Red Cell Aplasia Associated With Parvovirus B19

PRCA was initially reported in adults in 1986 with multiple reports since that time. Review of the literature in 2006 revealed 91 cases of parvovirus B19 infection posttransplant reported in adults.[249] Seventy-four were in solid organ recipients, with the majority following kidney transplant (71%), followed by heart/lung transplant (16%), then liver transplant (12%). Ninety-nine percent were anemic, with a third also having leukopenia and 18% thrombocytopenia. The average time to onset was 1.75 months posttransplant with a range of 1 week to 96 months. The most reliable test to diagnose infection was the parvovirus B19 PCR, positive in 85% of cases; IgM was positive in 78% and IgG 39%. Treatment with intravenous immunoglobulin was used in 84% of patients and there was a recurrence in 28%. The three deaths were only seen in patients after liver transplant who developed myocarditis and cardiogenic shock. Of interest, in a prospective study of 47 solid organ transplant recipients, none were found to have molecular evidence of parvovirus B19 in the first year posttransplant.[251]

In a review of parvovirus B19 infection in children after transplantation, there were 16 case reports: 5 after liver, heart, and renal transplant each and 1 after bone marrow transplantation.[252] Onset was at a median of 8 months with a range of 1 to 24 months. Although only 3 of 14 tested with IgM positive, all were PCR positive. There were no associated symptoms in 7 of 14, but other reported symptoms include cytopenias, rash, myocarditis, and pneumonia. All 10 patients who received intravenous immunoglobulin treatment were cured.

PLATELETS

Problems with platelets including thrombocytopenia and thrombocytopathy have been reported posttransplant primarily in adults. Following liver transplantation, almost all patients will develop a transient thrombocytopenia. Delayed thrombocytopenia is much less frequent. It has been reported in 12% of children after liver transplant,[230] 8% after cardiothoracic transplant,[229] and outside of the setting of HUS/MAHA very infrequently after kidney transplantation. Causes of platelet problems posttransplant include medication effect, immune etiology, HUS/MAHA, infection, and other miscellaneous causes.

Immediate Thrombocytopenia After Liver Transplantation

More than 90% of adults have been reported to have thrombocytopenia within the first week after liver transplantation.[253–257] Nadir counts usually occur between days 4 and 6 posttransplant, with an average count of 58,000 cu mm (range 19–330). An increase in thrombopoietin is seen on day 4 to 6 and increased reticulated platelets are noted on day 7 to 8. There are few reported clinical sequelae from the mild thrombocytopenia, although the lowest platelet counts have been associated with the most severe and complicated posttransplant course. Resolution is usually seen in 2 weeks. Lack of resolution is associated with poor prognosis for graft and overall survival.

There is controversy regarding the etiology of this transient thrombocytopenia. One theory is that it is a nonimmune consumptive process reflected by increased markers of thrombin generation.[255] The liver may be the site of platelet sequestration. A second theory is that it is unlikely to be a consumptive process because of the lack of platelet activation after day 1. The thrombocytopenia is more likely a result of low levels of thrombopoietin seen pretransplant. With new production and rising levels of thrombopoietin from the new liver, there is a subsequent increase in platelet production resulting in normalization of the platelet count soon after transplantation. Although the specific etiology has not been clarified, there is general consensus that it is not immune mediated.

Lymphocyte-depleting antibodies such as rabbit antithymocyte globulin (rATG) are being used with increasing frequency as induction type therapy in pediatric liver and intestine transplantation. rATG does exacerbate the transient thrombocytopenia seen immediately following solid organ transplant, but resolves in a similar 1- to 2-week period.

Treatment of this transient thrombocytopenia is supportive. Platelet transfusions are of uncertain benefit. Although originally azathioprine was felt to be a cause of this thrombocytopenia, there is no evidence that alteration of azathioprine dose is necessary.

Delayed Posttransplantation Thrombocytopenia

Delayed thrombocytopenia is not a major problem after solid organ transplantation and most of the data are published in adult series. In one retrospective study of 36 adult liver transplant recipients, mild thrombocytopenia (<140,000 cu mm) was seen in 54% of patients at 1 year and 25% at 3 years posttransplant.[258] However, severe thrombocytopenia (<50,000 cu mm) was only seen in 9% of patients at 1 year and in no patients at 3 years posttransplant. The thrombocytopenia was associated with splenomegaly in some patients. No clinical bleeding problems were noted after 1 year from transplant.

In one report, 3 of 25 (12%) pediatric liver transplant recipients were found to have isolated thrombocytopenia.[230] The etiology of the thrombocytopenia in these children was cavernous transformation of the portal vein, autoimmune, and unknown. In two other children in this series, thrombocytopenia was associated with additional cytopenias and the cause was possibly related to TAC.

In a study of 126 children who underwent cardiothoracic transplantation, 9 (8%) were noted to have isolated thrombocytopenia. Infection was the most common etiology.[231] In patients with combined cytopenias including thrombocytopenia, two-thirds were related to either infection or PTLD and 20% possibly secondary to TAC.

Sirolimus has been associated with mild thrombocytopenia in adults although the reported frequency has varied. In a study of renal transplant recipients, 23% were reported to have mild thrombocytopenia,[259] whereas no liver transplant patients on the drug were found to be thrombocytopenic.[260] In 66 pediatric kidney transplant recipients on sirolimus, there were no reported cases of thrombocytopenia.[261] Low platelet counts are usually seen within the first 4 weeks of treatment and are associated with higher sirolimus blood levels.[262,263] Like TAC and CsA, sirolimus has been shown to potentiate agonist-induced platelet aggregation, although this is not the proven explanation for the thrombocytopenia.[264] Twenty-five percent to 50% dose reduction is often effective in resolving sirolimus-mediated thrombocytopenia.

Immune-Mediated Thrombocytopenia Posttransplantation

There are many case reports of immune-mediated thrombocytopenia after all types of solid organ transplantation, in children and adults, and either alone or in combination with other cytopenias.

Eight adults post–liver transplant were reported to have immune thrombocytopenia—incidence of 0.7%.[265] The low platelets were seen on average 53 months after transplantation with a range of 1.9 to 173 months. Three patients had demonstrable antiplatelet antibodies. Steroids provided effective therapy in 4 and rituximab in 4, although splenectomy was ultimately necessary in three. Seven of the eight survive with normal platelet counts. Five children were reported to have severe thrombocytopenia (<10,000 cu mm) within 2 to 4 months after starting TAC.[247,266] All were documented to have antiplatelet antibodies. Responses were seen to steroids, rituximab, or anti-D.

Following heart and/or lung transplantation, two cases in adults[267] have been reported. These cases occurred 60 to 460 days after transplant and responded to prednisone and intravenous immunoglobulin. Acquired Glanzmann thromboasthenia has been reported in two children post–cardiac transplantation.[268,248] Both were receiving TAC and had demonstrable antibodies against GPIIb/IIIa. One patient had multiple autoantibodies and the other subsequently developed additional antiplatelet antibodies. One child responded to prednisone therapy and switching from TAC to CsA. The other responded to rituximab after failing prednisone and intravenous immunoglobulin.

Alloimmune thrombocytopenia was reported in three recipients of organs from the same donor (two kidneys and a liver).[269] Development of HPA-1a (PL^{A1}) antibodies from donor B cells were

Treatment of Immune-Mediated Thrombocytopenia after Solid Organ Transplantation in Children

There is no standard approach to the treatment of immune-mediated thrombocytopenia that occurs after solid organ transplantation. First, all other causes of thrombocytopenia should be ruled out before beginning therapy for what is often a presumptive diagnosis of immune-mediated thrombocytopenia. If the thrombocytopenia is mild to moderate (>20,000–30,000/uL) with no associated bleeding symptoms, we usually observe without intervention and monitor the platelet count on at least a weekly basis. If the platelet count is lower than 10,000 to 15,000/uL or if there is bleeding, immediate treatment is initiated with high-dose corticosteroids: 4 mg/kg/day of prednisone (or IV equivalent) divided in 3 to 4 doses and continued for 4 days. If there is a response (ie, platelet count >20,000/uL), the corticosteroid is dropped to 2 mg/kg/day divided in 2 to 3 doses and then slowly tapered to zero over the subsequent 2 to 3 weeks. Intravenous gammaglobulin or anti-D in standard doses used for childhood ITP can be used if there is no response to high-dose corticosteroids.

For patients who have recurrent or chronic thrombocytopenia requiring multiple courses of treatment to maintain platelet counts greater than 10,000 to 15,000/uL, we have utilized vincristine (1.5 mg/M^2 [max. dose 2 mg] IV weekly ×6) with success. Rituximab (375 mg/M^2 IV weekly ×4) has infrequently been used in this situation. For patients on tacrolimus with refractory thrombocytopenia, serious consideration should be given to switching to an alternative immunosuppressant, since this may be necessary for resolution of the thrombocytopenia. Involvement of both the transplant team and the hematology team is necessary for ideal management of these complex patients.

documented in an example of passenger lymphocyte syndrome. The thrombocytopenia in these cases was particularly refractory to standard treatment except transfusion of HPA-1a-negative platelets. One patient died, another required splenectomy, and one patient's thrombocytopenia resolved after an episode of severe graft rejection.

Infection-Associated Thrombocytopenia Posttransplantation

Although there are few published reports, one would expect the same hematologic problems, including thrombocytopenia, associated with bacterial sepsis or other serious infections as seen in nontransplant patients. Infection with HHV6 and the herpesvirus group has been studied closely.

HHV6 is commonly seen posttransplant, mostly in stem cell transplant recipients. In adults after liver transplant, there are case reports of a syndrome of HHV6 infection with thrombocytopenia, fever, and encephalopathy.[270] This syndrome has not been reported in children with HHV6 infection.[271,272]

Herpesvirus infection after kidney transplantation in children is seen in about a third of patients, with CMV being the most common infection.[273] The hematologic abnormalities associated with herpesvirus infection include thrombocytopenia and leukopenia, with an incidence of 31% and 24% respectively. These and other symptoms of herpesvirus infection occur at the same frequency as nontransplant patients.

There is a case report of a child post–liver transplant who developed measles complicated by autoimmune thrombocytopenia and neutropenia.[274]

WHITE BLOOD CELLS

Leukopenia and neutropenia are uncommonly reported in the literature after solid organ transplantation, although this may not reflect the true incidence seen in practice.[275] In two reviews of hematologic complications in children after transplantation, isolated neutropenia was seen in 2/70 (3%) patients after liver transplant[230] and 9/106 (8%) patients after cardiothoracic transplant.[231] Neutropenia was also seen in combination with other cytopenias. Although there are predominantly case reports in the pediatric literature, in one review of neutropenia after 400 renal transplants in adults, 35 cases (9%) were reported.[276] The etiology of leukopenia or neutropenia is similar in children and adults: immunosuppressive agents, other myelosuppressive drugs (eg ganciclovir), infection (CMV, sepsis, etc), and less frequently interferon, PTLD, hypersplenism, interferon, and idiopathic. Use of TAC is often implicated as a possible contributing factor.

Both filgrastim (G-CSF) and sargramostim (GM-CSF) have been used to treat neutropenia in adults and children. In adults it has resulted in improvement of the white count in more than 90% of patients after three to four doses.[276,277] There was no evidence of precipitation of rejection. In the case reports in children, both agents have been found to be effective in most patients, but there is a suggestion that efficacy may be affected by continuation of TAC.[275,278,279]

Azathioprine is well known to cause myelosuppression and has been associated with moderate to severe neutropenia. Azathioprine is catabolized in vivo by xanthine oxidase and thiopurine methyltransferase (TPMT). TPMT activity can vary considerably depending on a genetic polymorphism. Approximately 0.3% of Caucasians are homozygous and 11% heterozygous for deficiency of TPMT. Severe myelosuppression, including fatal neutropenia, has been documented in transplant patients who are homozygous for TMPT deficiency and receiving azathioprine.[280] There are some data that suggest that monitoring 6-thioguanine nucleotides (the metabolites of azathioprine) may allow for individualized management of azathioprine dosing with fewer side effects, although this has not become common practice.[281,282]

Neutropenia has also been associated with the use of mycophenolate mofetil (MMF) and sirolimus. Neutropenia and thrombocytopenia have been noted as a side effect of MMF since 1998.[283] Leukopenia may affect 5% to 11% of patients on the drug [284] and pseudo-Pelger–Huet anomaly has also been noted.[285] The leukopenia is often seen within 2 to 8 months after starting the drug. Filgrastim has been effective in reversing the neutropenia although some cases required decreasing the dose or stopping the drug. Ganciclovir or valacyclovir are commonly utilized simultaneously with MMF to treat or prevent CMV disease. These drugs are also known to also be associated with neutropenia. There may be an interaction between these drugs that increase the risk for neutropenia.[286] It may be necessary to stop ganciclovir as well as MMF for the neutropenia to improve.[285] Of note, serious infections are infrequently encountered.

In two reports of the use of sirolimus in children, neutropenia was the most common toxicity along with hepatitis, hyperlipidemia, and mouth ulcers.[287,288] It is not clear whether the neutropenia is directly related to serum level of the drug. Most counts will improve with a decrease in the drug dose, although few patients need to have the drug discontinued.

Pancytopenia

Pancytopenia is seen in two settings after solid organ transplantation. The first is early after liver transplant for acute liver failure from acute infectious hepatitis.[289,290] This represents the known aplastic anemia that can be seen in as many as a third of patients after non-A–E hepatitis. Treatment and outcome are similar to patients with posthepatitic aplastic anemia who do not require liver transplantation. The second setting is delayed pancytopenia, which may be secondary to infection with or without PTLD.[230] A number of cases have been associated with the use of TAC.[230,291]

HEMATOLOGIC ASPECTS OF POISONING

It has been estimated that about 6 million children, most younger than 5 years, ingest some toxin each year. The effects of toxins on the blood are diverse, usually nonspecific, and in most situations overshadowed by the nonhematologic manifestations of the exposure.[292] With certain toxins, however, bleeding, anemia, or change in the appearance (color) of the blood may be an important component of the clinical sequelae of an acute exposure.

The abnormalities of hemostasis after poisoning are numerous, and the mechanisms vary. Bleeding may be the only manifestation of warfarin toxicity secondary to an overdose of the drug or ingestion of a rodenticide-containing warfarin. Any hepatotoxic substance (eg, iron, acetaminophen) may lead to decreased synthesis of clotting factors and resultant coagulopathy. Bleeding in these circumstances is delayed for at least 24 hours, although there appears to be an early coagulopathy in iron poisoning that may be due to a direct effect on clotting protein function and not hepatotoxicity.[293] DIC has been seen after ingestion of mushrooms of the *Amanita* genus, or following a bite from the brown recluse spider (*Loxosceles reclusa*). Poisonous snake bites can result in coagulation abnormalities characterized by hypofibrinogenemia with or without thrombocytopenia or a DIC-like syndrome.[292] Severe thrombocytopenia has been described with elemental mercury poisoning.

Acute hemolytic anemia may be the presenting manifestation after exposure to drugs and toxins in children with G6PD deficiency or hemoglobin Zürich or (rarely) in normal children. Severe hemolytic anemia has been seen after the bite of the brown recluse spider and of a rattlesnake, and after a wasp sting.

Exposure to certain toxins may result in characteristic color changes of the blood, which in turn may be reflected clinically in abnormal skin color. The child with methemoglobinemia (see next paragraph) presents with a slate-gray cyanosis unresponsive to 100% oxygen administration. On exposure to air, the blood retains a distinct brown color. Patients with toxic exposure to carbon monoxide or cyanide have increased levels of carboxyhemoglobin or cyanhemoglobin, respectively, resulting in a cherry-red color of the blood and skin, but only with high concentrations of the offending hemoglobin.

Infants (up to 4 months of age) are at particular risk for developing methemoglobinemia because of a reduced amount (approximately 60% of normal) of cytochrome b_5 reductase present in neonatal RBCs. Methemoglobinemia has been described in infants with diarrheal illness and in infants exposed to exogenous agents.[294]

Yano and colleagues[295] described 11 patients with transient methemoglobinemia, all infants younger than 1 month of age, who presented with vomiting, diarrhea, and acidosis. In prospective studies of infants younger than 6 months of age with diarrheal disease, 64% had elevated levels of methemoglobin (with a mean ± SD of 10.5 ± 12.3%), 31% were cyanotic, most infants were small and/or failing to thrive, there was no association of methemoglobinemia and acidosis, and all children recovered from their illness.[296,297] Although most infants with endogenous methemoglobinemia can be managed with support and hydration, treatment with methylene blue (1 mg/kg) is indicated in the symptomatic or more severely affected child (ie, with methemoglobin greater than 20% to 30%).

Nursery epidemics of methemoglobinemia have been reported in normal newborns exposed to disinfectants or aniline dyes used to mark diapers. Infants fed formulas made with well water containing a high concentration of nitrates have developed methemoglobinemia. EMLA cream, a eutectic mixture of the local anesthetics lidocaine and prilocaine, has been effective in decreasing pain in infants undergoing circumcision. Methemoglobinemia has been reported with EMLA use in this situation, but only in overdose.[298] Other ingestions associated with methemoglobinemia include phenazopyridine (Pyridium), dapsone, metoclopramide, and nitroethane (an artificial fingernail remover). Although the list of oxidants reported to cause methemoglobinemia is long,[299] methemoglobinemia due to exogenous agents is uncommonly seen in infants and children.

LEAD POISONING

Lead poisoning in children has been a serious public health problem for decades. However, the most serious toxic effects of lead (eg, encephalopathy) commonly seen in the past are rarely encountered today, primarily because of measures instituted to decrease lead exposure (no-lead paint, no-lead gasoline) and screening programs in high-risk areas. Mean blood lead levels in the United States have declined, from 15 μg/dL between 1976 and 1982 to 3.6 μg/dL between 1988 and 1991.[300] Nonetheless, lead toxicity remains a problem, especially in high-risk children. There is increasing evidence that even low levels of lead exposure are associated with a significant decline in neurodevelopmental outcome,[301] and in 1991 the Centers for Disease Control and Prevention (CDC) lowered the intervention level of lead in the blood from 25 to 10 μg/dL. Reviews of the public health issues relating to lead poisoning in children have been published.[302]

The primary hematologic effect of lead is interference at multiple points along the heme synthetic pathway. The two most important effects are inhibition of δ-aminolevulinic acid (ALA) dehydratase and ferrochelatase, resulting in the accumulation of heme intermediates such as protoporphyrin. A shortened RBC survival time accompanies lead poisoning and probably is due to decreased activity of pyrimidine 5-nucleotidase (also resulting in basophilic stippling of the RBC) and possibly inhibition of G6PD and the pentose shunt.[303]

The anemia of lead poisoning has classically been described as a hypochromic, microcytic anemia, as might be expected from the effects of lead on heme synthesis. Although anemia has been said to be a common finding in lead intoxication, in reality, anemia is uncommon unless the lead poisoning is severe or there is associated iron deficiency.

A strong association exists between lead poisoning and iron deficiency in children. Both tend to occur in the same population of predominantly lower socioeconomic status. Experimentally, iron deficiency has been shown to increase lead absorption, retention in tissues, and toxicity. Iron deficiency also decreases lead excretion during chelation.[304] Lead may impede iron absorption and metabolism, leading to a vicious circle of increasing lead toxicity and worsening iron deficiency. In a study of children with lead poisoning (blood lead of 30 μg/dL or higher), 86% were found to have iron deficiency, and 100% of those with more severe lead poisoning (CDC risk classification III) were iron deficient.[305]

A number of reports in children with lead toxicity have documented the infrequent occurrence of anemia without concomitant iron deficiency. Cohen and colleagues[303] found anemia in 12% and microcytosis in 21% of iron-sufficient children with severe lead poisoning (CDC classes III and IV). The combination of anemia plus microcytosis, however, was found in only 1 of the 58 children in their series. In less severely affected children (CDC classes I to III), Yip and associates[306] found a 30% incidence of anemia, but of those with either mild or no iron deficiency, only 6% were anemic. Clark and coworkers,[307] using multiple linear regression analysis, found transferrin saturation to be the most important predictor of mean corpuscular volume, hemoglobin, and zinc protoporphyrin levels in children with lead poisoning.

Two important points emerge from the foregoing information: (a) children with significant lead poisoning may have neither anemia nor microcytosis and (b) children with documented lead poisoning should be screened for underlying iron deficiency. The immediate treatment and long-term management of lead poisoning can be found in a recent review.[308]

HEMATOLOGIC ASPECTS OF METABOLIC DISEASES

A number of congenital disorders of metabolism may manifest hematologic abnormalities as part of the clinical presentation. Such global metabolic defects have diverse manifestations; especially prominent are neurologic abnormalities, failure to thrive, and unexplained metabolic acidosis. Although the hematologic findings may be overshadowed by the systemic illness, the recognition of a characteristic pattern of signs and symptoms may lead expeditiously to the correct diagnosis. Table 162–4 is a compilation of inborn disorders of metabolism that may manifest in infancy or childhood with hematologic cytopenias.[309] Additional information regarding metabolic disorders is available through OMIM (Online Mendelian Inheritance in Man): www.ncib.nlm.nih.gov/omim/.

SPLENOMEGALY IN CHILDREN

Splenomegaly is a problem frequently encountered by both the pediatrician and the pediatric hematologist. Although the spleen is rarely a site of primary disease, it may reflect systemic involvement in a variety of disorders. The spleen is the largest collection of lymphoid tissue in the body, with a unique association between the bloodstream and the reticuloendothelial compartment of the spleen. Splenomegaly may result when there is antigenic stimulation of the lymphoid system (eg, infection), obstruction of blood flow within or distal to the spleen (eg, portal vein obstruction), exaggeration of one of the normal functions of the spleen because of an underlying abnormality (eg, hemolytic anemia, splenic sequestration), or infiltration of the spleen by a foreign cell (eg, leukemia, storage diseases).

The spleen tip normally is palpable in preterm infants; up to 30% of full-term neonates have a palpable spleen. A spleen can be felt in up to 5% to 10% of normal children, but most of these are in the infant or toddler age group. As a general rule, a spleen easily palpable below the costal margin in any child over the age of 3 to 4 years must be considered abnormal until proven otherwise. That some palpable spleens may indeed be normal is attested to by the study of McIntyre and Ebaugh, who found that 3% of healthy college freshmen have palpable spleens, of which about one-third persist.[310] "Pretenders" of splenomegaly include the left lobe of the liver, a left upper quadrant tumor such as Wilms tumor or neuroblastoma, the "wandering spleen," and the proptotic spleen (seen in children with a depressed diaphragm from obstructive pulmonary disease, such as asthma or bronchiolitis).

The most common cause of acute splenomegaly in children, especially young children, is a viral infection. Splenic enlargement in this setting is mild to moderate and usually transient. When the history and physical findings suggest a viral etiology, a complete blood count with differential, platelet count, and reticulocyte count should be performed to rule out unsuspected leukemia or hemolytic anemia and to determine whether there is an atypical lymphocytosis. The child should be reevaluated in approximately 4 weeks (or sooner if symp-

Table 162–4 Hematologic Manifestations of Metabolic Disease With Onset in Infancy and Childhood

Category	Disease	Defect	Hematologic Finding(s)	Associated Findings
Lysosomal enzyme defects	Gaucher disease, Type 1	Glucocerebrosidase deficiency	Anemia, thrombocytopenia	Splenomegaly, bone abnormalities, delayed puberty, lipid engorged macrophages (Gaucher cell) in bone marrow
	Niemann–Pick disease, Type A	Acid sphingomyelinase deficiency	Anemia	Feeding difficulties, hepatosplenomegaly developmental delay, neurodegenerative course, cherry-red macula, lipid-laden macrophages (foam cells) in bone marrow
	Wolman disease	Acid lipase deficiency	Anemia, thrombocytopenia	Emesis, diarrhea, hepatosplenomegaly, vacuolization of lymphocytes, lipid-laden macrophages in bone marrow, adrenal calcification
	Aspartylglucosaminuria	Aspartylglucosaminidase deficiency	Neutropenia	Recurrent infections, diarrhea, hemias, lens opacities, neurologic abnormalities, vacuolated lymphocytes
Defects of heme synthesis	Congenital erythropoietic porphyria	Uroporphyrinogen III cosynthase deficiency	Anemia, thrombocytopenia	Hemolysis, staining of diapers, photosensitivity, developmental delay, splenomegaly, erythrodontia
	Erythropoietic protoporphyria	Ferrochelatase deficiency	Anemia, thrombocytopenia	Hemolysis, photosensitivity, neurologic abnormalities, hepatobiliary dysfunction
Defects of amino acid metabolism	Tyrosinemia, Type 1	Fumarylacetoacetate hydrolase deficiency	Anemia, thrombocytopenia	Failure to thrive, emesis, hepatopathy, neurologic abnormalities, bleeding, "cabbage-like" odor, renal tubular dysfunction
Defects of organic acid metabolism	Isovaleric acidemia	Isovaleryl-CoA dehydrogenase deficiency	Anemia, thrombocytopenia, neutropenia, pancytopenia	Acidosis, emesis, neurologic abnormalities, odor of "sweaty feet"
	Methylmalonic acidemia	Methylmalonyl-CoA mutase deficiency	Anemia, thrombocytopenia, leukopenia, pancytopenia	Acidosis, neurologic abnormalities, failure to thrive, emesis
	Mevalonic aciduria	Mevalonate kinase deficiency	Anemia, thrombocytopenia	Acidosis, cataracts, neurologic abnormalities, hepatosplenomegaly
Defects of organic acid metabolism	Propionic acidemia	Propionyl CoA carboxylase deficiency	Anemia, thrombocytopenia neutropenia, pancytopenia	Ketotic hyperglycinemia, acidosis, neurologic abnormalities
	Pyroglutamic aciduria	Glutathione synthetase deficiency	Anemia, neutropenia	Hemolysis, neurologic abnormalities, metabolic acidosis

Table 162–4 Hematologic Manifestations of Metabolic Disease With Onset in Infancy and Childhood—cont'd

Category	Disease	Defect	Hematologic Finding(s)	Associated Findings
Membrane transport defects	Lysinuric protein intolerance	*SLC7A7* gene mutations	Anemia, thrombocytopenia, leukopenia, pancytopenia	Malabsorption, protein intolerance, hyperammonemia, neurologic abnormalities, glomerulonephritis, pulmonary hemorrhage, hemophagocytosis
Glycolytic pathway defects	Triosephosphate isomerase deficiency	Triosephosphate isomerase deficiency	Anemia	Hemolysis, neurologic abnormalities, myopathy
	Phosphoglycerate kinase deficiency	Phosphoglycerate kinase deficiency	Anemia	Hemolysis, neurologic abnormalities
Defects of vitamin metabolism	Cobalamin metabolic defects	Cobalamin transport and utilization defects	Anemia, thrombocytopenia, neutropenia, pancytopenia	Megaloblastosis, failure to thrive, neurologic abnormalities
	Folate metabolic defects	Folate transport and utilization defects	Anemia, thrombocytopenia	Megaloblastosis, ringed sideroblasts, diarrhea, failure to thrive, neurologic abnormalities
	Holocarboxylase synthetase deficiency	Holocarboxylase synthetase deficiency	Thrombocytopenia	Acidosis, hyperammonemia, respiratory distress, neurologic abnormalities, skin rash
Defects in metal metabolism	Wilson disease	*ATP7B* gene mutation	Anemia	Hemolysis, liver dysfunction, neurologic abnormalities, Kayser-Fleischer rings, arthropathy
Defects of purine and pyrimidine metabolism	Hereditary orotic aciduria	Uridine-5′-monophosphate synthase deficiency	Anemia, leukopenia	Megaloblastosis, orotic acid crystalluria, immunodeficiency
	Lesch–Nyhan syndrome	Hypoxanthine-guanine phosphoribosyltransferase deficiency	Anemia	Megaloblastosis, hyperuricemia, nephrolithiasis, neurologic abnormalities, self-mutilation
Defects of carbohydrate metabolism	Galactosemia	Galactose-1-phosphate uridyltransferase deficiency	Anemia	Hemolysis, failure to thrive, neurologic findings, jaundice, emesis, diarrhea, hepatic dysfunction, cataracts, gram-negative sepsis
	Glycogen storage disease Type 1b	Deficient hepatic transport of glucose—phosphate	Anemia, neutropenia	Hypoglycemia, acidosis, hepatomegaly, xanthomas, inflammatory bowel disease
	Hereditary fructose intolerance	Aldolase B deficiency	Anemia, thrombocytopenia	Poor feeding, emesis, failure to thrive, neurologic findings, hypoglycemia, liver dysfunction, ringed sideroblasts, coagulopathy, hemophagocytosis, shock
Mitochondrial disorders	DIDMOAD syndrome (Wolfram syndrome)	Mitochondrial DNA deletions	Anemia, thrombocytopenia, neutropenia, pancytopenia	Megaloblastosis, ringed sideroblasts, diabetes insipidus, diabetes mellitus, optic atrophy, deafness
	Pearson syndrome	Mitochondrial DNA deletions	Anemia, thrombocytopenia, neutropenia, pancytopenia	Ringed sideroblasts, vacuolization of marrow precursors, exocrine pancreatic dysfunction, metabolic acidosis
Lipoprotein disorders	Abetalipoproteinemia	Microsomal triglyceride transfer protein defects	Anemia	Hemolysis, acanthocytosis, bleeding, emesis, diarrhea, failure to thrive, neurologic findings
Miscellaneous disorders	Barth syndrome (endocardial fibroelastosis-2)	Tafazzin gene mutations	Neutropenia	Cardiomyopathy, endocardial fibroelastosis, skeletal myopathy, short stature, 3-methylglutaconicaciduria, abnormal mitochondria
	Cyclic hematopoiesis	Neutrophil elastase gene mutation	Neutropenia	Recurrent oral ulcers, poor dentition, recurrent fever, malaise
	Severe congenital neutropenia (Kostmann syndrome)	Neutrophil elastase gene mutation	Neutropenia	Severe invasive infections, acute leukemia
	Wiscott–Aldrich syndrome	*WAS* gene mutations	Thrombocytopenia	Eczema, infections, small platelets

CoA, coenzyme A; DIDMOAD, diabetes insipidus, diabetes mellitus, optic atrophy, deafness.

Table 162–5 Causes of Splenomegaly in Children

Disorders of the Blood
Hemolytic anemia: congenital/acquired
Thalassemia
Sickle cell disease
Leukemia
Osteopetrosis
Myelofibrosis/myeloid metaplasia/thrombocythemia
Infections: Acute and Chronic
Viral
Congenital (eg, TORCH association)
Mononucleosis (eg, EBV, CMV infection)
Virus associated hemophagocytic syndrome
Human immunodeficiency virus
Bacterial
Sepsis/abscess
Brucellosis
Salmonellosis
Tularemia
Tuberculosis
Subacute bacterial endocarditis
Syphilis
Lyme disease
Fungal
Histoplasmosis (disseminated)
Rickettsial
Rocky Mountain spotted fever
Cat scratch disease
Parasitic
Toxoplasmosis
Malaria
Leishmaniasis (kala-azar)
Schistosomiasis
Echinococcosis
Hepatic/Portal System Disorders
Acute/chronic active hepatitis
Cirrhosis/hepatic fibrosis/biliary atresia
Portal or splenic venous obstruction (Banti syndrome)
Autoimmune Disease
Juvenile rheumatoid arthritis
Systemic lupus erythematosus
Autoimmune lymphoproliferative syndrome (Canale–Smith syndrome)
Neoplasms/Cysts
Lymphomas (Hodgkin and non-Hodgkin)
Hemangiomas/lymphangiomas
Hamartomas
Congenital or acquired (posttraumatic) cysts
Storage Diseases/Inborn Errors of Metabolism
Lipidoses: Gaucher disease, Niemann–Pick disease, others
Mucopolysaccharidoses
Defects in carbohydrate metabolism: galactosemia, fructose intolerance
Sea-blue histiocyte syndrome
Miscellaneous Disorders
Histiocytoses
Reactive
Langerhans cell
Malignant
Sarcoidosis
Congestive heart failure
Familial Mediterranean fever

CMV, cytomegalovirus; EBV, Epstein-Barr virus; TORCH, toxoplasmosis, other infections, rubella, cytomegalovirus infection, herpes simplex.

Evaluation and Management of the Child With Splenomegaly

When evaluating the child with chronic splenomegaly, the clinician must consider all of the possibilities noted in Table 162–5. Clues from the history and physical examination may suggest a specific etiology and direct a tailored approach to the diagnostic laboratory evaluation. If, on the other hand, there is no apparent cause of the enlarged spleen, a number of screening laboratory tests should be performed, including a complete blood count with differential, platelet count, and reticulocyte count; evaluation of the peripheral smear; determination of sedimentation rate; liver function tests; determination of antibody titers to Epstein–Barr virus (EBV), cytomegalovirus (CMV), and *Toxoplasma*; antinuclear antibody assay; and ultrasound evaluation of the liver, spleen, and portal system (the last with Doppler flow technique). Further evaluation, including bone marrow examination, may be necessary if the screening tests do not reveal the cause of the splenic enlargement.

Management of splenomegaly usually is that of the underlying disease, when such treatment exists. Splenectomy may be indicated in selected conditions, but the potential benefits from splenectomy must be weighed against the risk of postsplenectomy sepsis, a rapidly progressive bacteremia, most commonly from *S pneumoniae*, with a mortality rate of approximately 50%. The risk of postsplenectomy sepsis depends on the age of the patient and the nature of the underlying disorder. Patients younger than 3 years of age and those with a compromised immune or reticuloendothelial system are most susceptible. When elective splenectomy is indicated, it is advisable (a) to postpone surgery until the patient is at least 5 to 6 years of age; (b) to administer pneumococcal, meningococcal, and *H influenzae* vaccines (if the patient was not previously immunized) at least 1 to 2 weeks before splenectomy; (c) to consider use of prophylactic penicillin for at least 4 years; and (d) to manage significant febrile illnesses as possible postsplenectomy sepsis at all times. In addition to the risk of postsplenectomy sepsis, the rare complication of postsplenectomy portal or splenic vein thrombosis must also be considered.

For children younger than 5 years of age with severe symptoms from hemolytic anemia, hemoglobinopathy, or hypersplenism, partial splenectomy should be considered. In a number of studies, up to 90% of the spleen has been removed safely, with a high rate of success and preservation of splenic function.[311,312] Regrowth of the spleen to variable degrees has been noted, with occasional need for reoperation.

toms persist). If splenomegaly persists beyond 4 to 6 weeks, the splenic enlargement may be considered chronic.

A list of causes of splenomegaly in children is presented in Table 162–5.[313] Symptoms from splenic enlargement are uncommon, although massive splenomegaly may cause abdominal discomfort and early satiety. If the spleen is sufficiently large, there may be increased destruction or sequestration of one or more of the formed elements of the blood (hypersplenism). Cytopenias tend to be mild to moderate, with the platelet count affected the most.

An approach to the pediatric patient with splenic enlargement is outlined in the box on Evaluation and Management of the Child with Splenomegaly.

SUGGESTED READINGS

General

Lascari AD: Hematologic Manifestations of Childhood Diseases. New York, Thieme-Stratton, 1984.

Infectious Disease

Abshire TC: The anemia of inflammation. A common cause of childhood anemia. Pediatr Clin North Am 43:623, 1996.

Ellaurie M, Burns ER, Rubenstein A: Hematologic manifestations in pediatric HIV infection: Severe anemia as a prognostic factor. Am J Pediatr Hematol Oncol 12:449, 1990.

Buranski B, Young N: Hematologic consequences of viral infections. Hematol Oncol Clin North Am 1:167, 1987.

Strausbaugh LJ: Hematologic manifestations of bacterial and fungal infections. Hematol Oncol Clin North Am 1:185, 1987.

Collagen Vascular Disease/Acute Vasculitis

Cazzola M, Panchio L, deBenedetti F, et al: Defective iron supply for erythropoiesis and adequate endogenous erythropoietin production in the anemia associated with systemic-onset juvenile chronic arthritis. Blood 87:4824, 1996.

Newburger JW, Takahashi M, Gerbe MA, et al: Diagnosis, treatment and long-term management of Kawasaki disease: A statement for health professionals from the Committee on Rheumatic Fever, Endocarditis, and Kawasaki Disease, Council on Cardiovascular Disease in the Young, American Heart Association. Pediatrics 114:1708, 2004.

Ravelli R: Macrophage activation syndrome. Curr Opin Rheumatol 14:548, 2002.

Cardiopulmonary Disease

Keevil B, Rowlands D, Burton I, Webb AK: Assessment of iron status in cystic fibrosis patients. Ann Clin Biochem 37:662, 2000.

West D, Scheel J, Stoverk, et al: Iron deficiency in children with cyanotic congenital heart disease. J Pediatr 17:266, 1990.

Gastrointestinal Disease

Halfdanarson T, Litzow MR, Murray JA: Hematologic Manifestations of Celiac Disease. Blood 109:412, 2007.

Semrin G, Fishman D, Gousvaros A, et al: Impaired intestinal iron absorption in Crohn's disease correlates with disease activity and markers of inflammation. Inflamm Bowel Dis 12:1101, 2006.

Tunnessen WW, Oski FA: Consequences of starting whole cow milk at 6 months of age. J Pediatr 111:813, 1987.

Thromboembolic Complications in Childhood Illness

Monagle P, Chan A, Massicotte P, et al: Antithrombotic therapy in children: The Seventh ACCP Conference on Antithrombotic and Thrombolytic Therapy. Chest 126(3 Suppl):645S, 2004.

Schlegel N: Thromboembolic risks and complications in nephrotic children. Semin Thromb Hemost 23(3):271, 1997.

Wiernikowski JT, Athale UH: Thromboembolic complications in children with cancer. Thromb Res 118(1):137, 2006.

Hematologic Complications of Solid Organ Transplantation in Children

Dobrolet NC, Webber SA, Blatt J, et al: Hematologic abnormalities in children and young adults receiving tacrolimus-based immunosuppression following cardiothoracic transplantation. Pediatr Transplant 5:125, 2001.

Iglesias-Berengue J, Lopez-Espinosa JA, Ortega-Lopez J, et al: Hematologic abnormalities in liver-transplanted children during medium- to long-term follow-up. Transplant Proc 35:1904, 2003.

Taylor RM, Bockenstedt P, Su GL, et al: Immune thrombocytopenic purpura following liver transplantation: A case series and review of the literature. Liver Transplant 12:781, 2006.

Hematologic Aspects of Poisoning

Sauter D, Goldfrank L: Hematologic aspects of toxicology. Hematol Oncol Clin North Am 1:335, 1987.

REFERENCES

For complete list of references log onto www.expertconsult.com

CHAPTER 163

THE SPLEEN AND ITS DISORDERS

Susan B. Shurin

Galen described the spleen as the "organ of mystery," with functions related to mood and good or ill humors. It was not until the 18th century that the spleen's relationship to the immune and hematologic systems was appreciated. The complexities of splenic function continue to be the focus of research and observation. The spleen is not necessary to life because its many functions are redundant, overlap with the functions of other organs, and can be assumed by other organs. The spleen, however, is an important part of many disease processes as well as normal function of the immune and hematologic systems. The spleen efficiently phagocytoses erythrocytes, recycles iron, recognizes and destroys pathogens, and induces adaptive immune responses. An appreciation for the subtleties of its anatomy and function is important for the physician evaluating patients with many hematologic, immunologic, and hepatic diseases.

NORMAL SPLENIC ANATOMY AND FUNCTION

Embryology

The spleen arises from the mesoderm. By the ninth week of gestation, layers of the left dorsal mesogastrium condense, and blood vessels appear. Sheaths are formed around arterioles by reticular cells and fibers. Macrophages are present and are phagocytic by the end of the first trimester. Lymphocytes appear during the fourth month. Red and white pulp can be identified by the sixth month. Germinal centers do not develop during fetal life, but primitive inactive follicles are evident at birth.[1] In mice, a homeobox gene, *Hox11* (now known as *Tlx1*), which controls the genesis of the splanchnic mesodermal plate, is essential for development of the spleen.[2] Both the basic helix–loop–helix transcription factor capsulin,[3] and the Wilms tumor suppressor 1 gene (WT1) are indispensable for formation of the spleen.[4] The genetic basis for development of the human spleen is less well understood. The spleen is capable of supporting hematopoiesis during fetal life and, in a variety of pathologic states, postnatally. The circulation of primitive hematopoietic stem cells in peripheral blood during prenatal life through birth makes it difficult to distinguish hematopoiesis dependent on tissues in the organs and the incidental presence of hematopoietic cells within the circulation of those organs.[5,6]

Anatomy

The spleen is the body's largest filter of the blood.[7,8] Located directly below the diaphragm and adjacent to the stomach, it is covered by a fibrous capsule with blood vessels, lymphatics, and nerves coated by peritoneal mesothelium (Figs. 163–1 and 163–2). The splenic artery comes from the celiac axis, enters the capsule at the hilum, and branches into trabecular arteries. The trabecular arteries then branch into central arteries and enter the white pulp. The periarterial lymphoid sheath consists of a cuff of T lymphocytes, plasma cells, and macrophages around the central arteries. As the arteries branch, the sheath narrows. B-lymphocyte clusters appear in follicles along the periarterial lymphoid sheath at arterial branch points.

The components of the white pulp are connected by a reticular network and supporting stromal cells. On the cut surface of the normal spleen, white pulp is visible as white nodules 1 to 2 mm in diameter. Their size varies with age and antigenic stimulation. The nodules are fully developed at birth, increase in size in childhood (especially with immunizations and infections), peak at puberty, and involute in adulthood. Immunologically normal, uninfected adults normally have no evident germinal centers. A mantle zone of B lymphocytes surrounds the follicle, or secondary germinal center. Antigen trapping and processing take place in the marginal zone of the white pulp.[9,10]

The red pulp of the spleen consists of vascular sinuses, the cords of Billroth, and the terminal branches of the penicilliary arteries.[11,12] Vascular sinuses are lined with endothelial cells with long processes and a basement membrane with ring fibers that attach to macrophage dendritic processes. No tight junctions or interdigitations connect the cytoplasmic processes. Intact leukocytes, erythrocytes, and platelets are able to squeeze through the potential spaces between these cells and between the ring fibers. Processes of the reticular cells of the cords of Billroth are outside the sinus walls. Endothelial cells line the sinuses and pulp veins but not the cords. Circulation of blood through red pulp lined with endothelium, or closed circulation, is rapid. Circulation into the cords, or open circulation, is slower and permits the macrophages lining the cord to remove damaged or aged cells.

Functions

The functions of the spleen are summarized in Table 163–1.

The Red Pulp

The function of the red pulp is dominated by splenic macrophages, which are responsible for filtering of the blood, removal of bacteria, and iron recycling.

Removal of Damaged and Aged Formed Elements

The venous system of the red pulp enables it to filter whole blood, removing senescent erythrocytes and other blood cells. Arterial blood is delivered to the cords of the red pulp. The cords have an open system of reticular fibers, fibroblasts, and macrophages without an endothelial lining. Blood passes from the cords into the efferent venous sinuses, which are lined with endothelium with a discontinuous structure. Stress fibers extend beneath the basal plasma membrane and run parallel to the axis of the endothelial cells. These cords direct the blood into sinuses through slits formed by the stress fibers. In many animals, these stress fibers are contractile, and enable the spleen to serve as a reservoir of red cells and reduce blood viscosity when the animal is at rest. There is no evidence that the spleen serves such a function, or is capable of significant changes in volume with rest and exercise, in humans.

As erythrocytes and platelets age, they tolerate the hostile splenic environment less well than when they are healthy with metabolic reserve.[13] The spleen is acidotic (pH 6.8 to 7.2), hypoxic (Po_2 54 mm Hg), and hypoglycemic (glucose concentration approximately 60% of that in venous blood). Damage to aged anucleate cells includes changes in their membrane complex carbohydrates, which facilitate recognition by splenic macrophages and removal from the circulation.[14,15] *Culling* describes the destruction of erythrocytes: the normal removal of aging cells or the removal of damaged cells in pathologic states. Most platelets and leukocytes are not removed by the spleen as they age but adhere to vessel walls and migrate into tissues, where they die. *Pitting* refers to the removal of inclusions from within erythrocytes, which are then released back into the circulation. The erythrocyte membrane is in close apposition to the macrophage membrane, so that aged or damaged glycoproteins, antibody, or complement on the surface of the cell are easily recognized and activate phagocytosis. Particulate matter—Howell–Jolly bodies, Heinz bodies, Pappenheimer bodies, and malarial and other parasites—can be removed and the cell returned to the bloodstream. Membrane-containing adsorbed antibody can be removed and the remainder of the cell released with changes in shape and volume. Internal vesicles near the erythrocyte membrane appear as if they were on the surface of the cell, and are termed *pits* or *pocks*.[16–19] The spleen also normally removes these, with the polished erythrocyte returned to the circulation. The lack of this polishing function can be used to assess splenic dysfunction, as the number of pits or pocks per erythrocyte is increased when the spleen fails to remove them.

Recycling of Iron

Both hepatic and splenic macrophages are important for recycling of iron as erythrocytes are phagocytized and hydrolyzed in the phagolysosome. Degradation of hemoglobin releases heme, which is catabolized into biliverdin, carbon monoxide, and ferrous iron (Fe^{2+}).

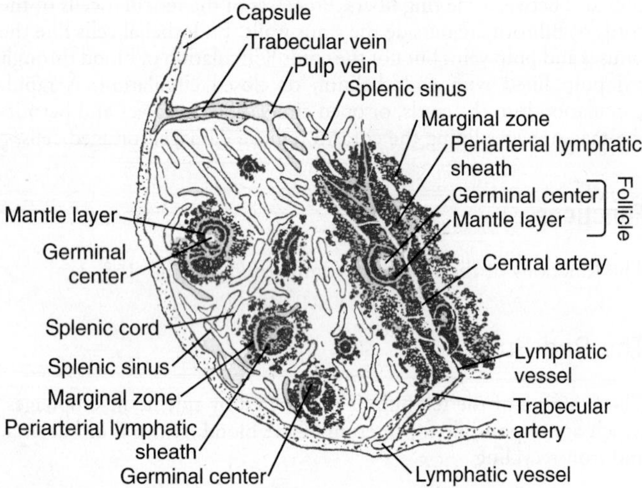

Figure 163–1 Anatomy of the spleen. (From Weiss L, Tavassoli M: Anatomic hazards to the passage of erythrocytes through the spleen. Semin Hematol 7:372, 1970, with permission.)

Iron is then either released as a low-molecular-weight species for rapid reuse or stored as ferritin. As ferritin accumulates, it aggregates into hemosiderin. Iron-laden macrophages are a feature of iron overload states in both the liver and spleen. Erythrocytes that are destroyed intravascularly release hemoglobin that binds to haptoglobin. CD163 on the surface of splenic macrophages mediates endocytosis of circulating hemoglobin and haptoglobin-bound hemoglobin.[20]

Iron is released from stores in splenic macrophages in response to the erythropoietic drive expressed by the bone marrow. The precise mechanisms are not well understood. Uptake of iron is mediated in most cells by a divalent cation transporter, natural-resistance-associated macrophage protein 2 (NRAMP2),[21] in recycling endosomes that express the transferrin receptor. NRAMP2 transports ferritin into the cytoplasm across the endosomal membrane. In addition to the more widely expressed NRAMP2, macrophages and monocytes express NRAMP1, which was initially described as an iron-transporting protein impacting resistance to intracellular pathogens.[22,23] A third molecule involved in iron metabolism in the spleen is lipocalin-2, which is secreted by macrophages and other myeloid cells when activated by exposure to bacterial metabolites. Lipocalin-2 binds to bacterial siderophores and sequesters iron from microorganisms.[24] These and related molecules tightly link the iron-recycling and host resistance functions of the red pulp of the spleen.

Antibody Production

After stimulation and differentiating into antigen-specific plasmablasts in the follicles of the white pulp, plasmablasts and plasma cells lodge in the red pulp, where they are closer to macrophages. A similar translocation occurs in lymph nodes where plasmablasts migrate to the medullary cords. This translocation occurs after upregulation of expression of CXC-chemokine receptor 4 (CXCR4), which binds CXC-chemokine ligand 12 (CXCL12) expressed in red pulp.[25,26]

The White Pulp

The lymphoid region of the spleen incorporates multiple components of the immune system that are organized to enhance recognition and/or response to pathogens. The white pulp contains lymphoid sheaths around branching arterial vessels, similar to the structure of lymph nodes. Specific chemokines attract B and T cells to their appropriate domains. The periarteriolar lymphoid sheath, or PALS, contains T cells that interact with dendritic cells and circulating B cells. T cells and dendritic cells are attracted to PALS through CC-chemokine ligands 19 and 21.[27] Follicles contain B cells where clonal expansion of activated B cells occurs. B-cell migration to follicles requires CSCL13.[28] Expression of all these homeostatic chemokines is reduced when signaling through the lymphotoxin receptor or tumor necrosis alpha receptor 1 is absent, which results in disorganization of the domains of the white pulp.[29–31]

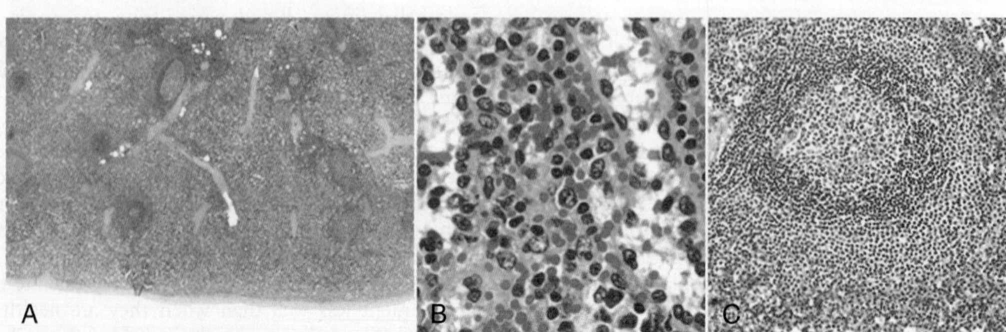

Figure 163–2 Spleen (**A–C**). Low power of spleen (**A**) removed from a patient with ITP. Note capsule (*bottom*), white pulp, and red pulp. High power of red pulp (**B**) showing splenic sinuses (*left* and *right*), and cords (*central*). Detail of white pulp (**C**) illustrating germinal center (*center*) surrounded immediately by mantle zone and then by marginal zone.

Marginal Zone

Leukocytes leave the bloodstream and enter the white pulp in the marginal zone of the spleen via G-protein-coupled receptor functions, similar to migration of leukocytes across endothelial barriers in inflammation. The marginal zone is both a transit area and contains resident cells with complex interactions. Marginal zone metallophilic macrophages form an inner ring close to the white pulp, marginal zone macrophages form an outer ring, and dendritic cells and B cells are located between the two sets of macrophages.[32,33] Both trafficking and retention of dendritic cells and B cells involve complex interactions with integrins and other adhesion molecules.[34,35]

Innate Immunity

The spleen is important in the recognition of antigens, especially when administered intravenously, in the production of antibody, and in the clearance of opsonized and unopsonized particles from the bloodstream (see Table 163–1).[36–38] The spleen is structured to facilitate monitoring of the contents of the blood, with blood flowing through the marginal zone directly along the white pulp. The white pulp is involved in adaptive immunity, whereas the marginal zone is involved in both innate and adaptive immunity (Table 163–2).

Trapping and processing of antigens is a major function of the marginal zone with its abundant blood supply (2 L/minute) and large number of macrophages. Antigens penetrate the germinal center where T lymphocytes predominate. Processing of carbohydrate antigens is a special function of splenic marginal zone lymphocytes.[39] Marginal zone macrophages express lectin receptors and scavenger receptors that efficiently bind polysaccharide antigens. These enable them to bind and clear pathogens—mycobacteria, bacteria, and viruses—without surface opsonins.[40–43] Toll-like receptors important for pattern recognition are expressed on splenic, as on all, macro-

Table 163–1 Functions of the Spleen

Category	Function	Effector Cells/Areas
Clearance/filtration	Antibody-mediated clearance Culling and pitting	Macrophages Reticular meshwork
Immune response		
Marginal zone	Interaction of antigens with effector cells Antigen processing Immune recognition	Monocytes, lymphocytes Macrophages T cells (periarteriolar sheath)
White pulp	Immunoregulation, antibody production Antigen processing, preservation	B cells (lymphoid follicles) Macrophages
Red pulp	Phagocytosis	Macrophages, monocytes, neutrophils
Hematologic	Hematopoiesis Storage of erythrocytes, platelets, leukocytes Finishing/polishing of erythrocytes	Cords and sinuses Reticular meshwork, red pulp Reticular meshwork, macrophages
Hemostasis	Production of factor VIII, von Willebrand factor	Endothelial cells

Table 163–2 Innate Immune Pattern Recognition Receptors That Are Highly Expressed on Splenic Phagocytic Cells*

Name	Abbreviation	Function	Splenic Cells Expressing	Recognizes or Affects	Pathogens Recognized
Toll-like receptor networks	TLR	Pattern recognition of pathogen-associated molecular patterns	Marginal zone macrophages Dendritic cells	Lipopolysaccharide Flagellin Double-stranded RNA	Multiple bacteria, especially gram negative
Natural-resistance-associated macrophage protein-1	NRAMP-1	Solute carrier family 11 (proton-coupled divalent metal ion transporters); phagolysosomal function	Macrophages	Lysosomal targeting	*Mycobacterium tuberculosis* *M avium* *M leprae*
Natural-resistance-associated macrophage protein-2	NRAMP-2	Proton-dependent cation transporter; iron absorption	Macrophages (apical duodenal cells, erythroid cells)	Impairs bacterial gene expression, protein synthesis	*Brucella* spp
Sialic acid binding Ig-like lectin-1; sialoadhesin	SIGLEC1, CD 169	Immunoglobulin superfamily	Splenic and peritoneal macrophages Many hematopoietic cells	Mannose	*Streptococcus pneumoniae*
Specific intercellular adhesion molecule-3 grabbing nonintegrin related 1	SIGNR1, CD 209b	ICAM-3 binding nonintegrin homolog, mannose receptor	Dendritic cells	Polysaccharide antigens, mannosylated lipoarabinomannan (ManLAM)	Fungi, other pathogens
Macrophage receptor with collagenous structure	MARCO	Type 1 scavenger	Marginal zone macrophages	Lipopolysaccharide	*Staphylococcus aureus* *Escherichia coli*

*These receptors contribute to resistance to infection with pathogens in the absence of prior exposure, specific immune responses, or surface opsonic immunoglobulin or complement.

phages; the expression of receptors that bind directly to components of unopsonized pathogens is a feature of splenic macrophages.

Splenic macrophages are more sensitive to small amounts of opsonic antibody or complement on the surface of particles than are macrophages in the liver, lung, or bone marrow.[44] In the absence of a spleen, nonimmune individuals may fail to remove bacteria with little opsonic coating.[45,46] The production of antigen-specific IgM is impaired in the absence of a spleen.[39,47] An asplenic individual has defective recognition of carbohydrate antigens, defective production of IgM early in infection, and defective removal of lightly opsonized particles—all crucial components of response to invasive infection with encapsulated organisms.

Marginal zone B cells are sensitive to detection of blood-borne pathogens. They rapidly differentiate into either antigen-presenting cells or IgM-producing plasma cells. After activation in the marginal zone, some B cells migrate into the white pulp, where they function to activate naïve CD4-positive T cells.[48] Similarly, blood-borne dendritic cells activated in the marginal zone migrate into the white pulp. This process appears to be important in control of certain parasitic infections. In *Leishmania donovani* infection, the spread of infection is inversely proportional to the up- or downregulation of CCR7 expression on activated dendritic cells and migration of APCs into the white pulp.[49]

Adaptive Immunity

The white pulp is both anatomically and functionally similar to lymph nodes.[50] However, all splenic cells enter the white pulp via the marginal zone, as opposed to through high endothelial venules and afferent lymphatic vessels. This exposes incident cells to an environment highly sensitive to detection of blood-borne pathogens. Circulating dendritic cells capture bacteria from the blood and transport them to the spleen, where they mediate the initial differentiation of B cells to plasmablasts or APCs. Activated APCs entering the white pulp activate T cells, resulting in changes in receptor expression that enables them to migrate to the edge of B-cell follicles. Contact between activated T cells induces an isotype switch in follicular B cells, which then migrate to the red pulp and marginal zones, or remain in splenic germinal centers.[51] The white pulp of the spleen is the largest mass of lymphoid tissue in the body. The B lymphocytes, which ultimately produce antibodies, predominate in the nearby germinal centers and mantle zones. These areas all increase in size and activity with immunization or infection. The complex interaction between the cells in close apposition, autocrine and paracrine signaling, and migration of cells into, between compartments of, and ultimately out of the spleen contribute to the extraordinary repertoire of innate and adaptive immunity within the organ.[52] Changes in splenic architecture are quite dramatic with septicemia; the most marked depletion of splenic B areas is seen in overwhelming enterococcemia. Bacterial virulence factors appear to contribute to depletion of B- and T-cell areas.[53]

Hematopoiesis

Active hematopoiesis can be seen in the fetal spleen throughout the second trimester, decreasing in the third trimester.[54] Erythropoiesis and megakaryocytopoiesis predominate, with myelopoiesis present to a lesser extent. As hematopoiesis moves from the hepatic phase into the bone marrow, it becomes less evident within the fetal spleen. The spleen is not normally a site of hematopoiesis in postnatal life in humans, but it is a rich source of hematopoietic stems cells and can support hematopoiesis in a number of pathologic states.[5,6] Extramedullary hematopoiesis is a significant cause of splenomegaly in bone marrow diseases (eg, myelofibrosis or osteopetrosis) and chronic hemolytic anemias (eg, thalassemia). The stromal cells of the spleen appear to be capable of supporting hematopoiesis and may produce the c-*kit* ligand,[55,56] as do marrow stromal cells. When splenic hematopoiesis occurs, the erythrocytes and platelets that circulate tend to be less mature than when hematopoiesis occurs in the bone marrow, which suggests that egress from the spleen is easier than from the marrow.

In rodents, the spleen continues to function as a hematopoietic organ during adult life. In higher mammals, including primates, the resident stem cells are capable of restoring hematopoietic and immunologic function after lethal irradiation.[57]

Storage of Cells

The normal adult spleen contains 20 to 40 mL of blood, and does not serve as a reservoir for blood volume or erythrocytes. This changes in many conditions associated with splenomegaly, especially if portal hypertension is also present. The widening of the pulp cords creates an organ with more storage volume. Vascular pooling of blood and formed elements occurs, regardless of the underlying cause of the splenomegaly.[58] Platelets and granulocytes, however, are normally stored in the red pulp of the spleen. As much as one-third of the total platelet mass may be stored in the spleen and released when cytokines affecting platelet adhesiveness are released.[59,60] The lack of musculature in the human splenic capsule prevents the distention and contraction that occur in many animals, such as dogs, although the spleen appears to contract in divers during periods of breath-hold apnea, with a rapid 20% decrease in volume observed in divers without decrease in splenic arterial blood flow.[61] After splenectomy, platelet counts and granulocyte counts rise significantly, then fall.[62] The circulating masses of these cell pools are chronically increased postsplenectomy, which may contribute to an increased incidence of atherosclerosis years after splenectomy.[63,64]

EXAMINATION OF THE SPLEEN

For adequate examination of the spleen, the patient must be fully supine, relaxed, with arms adjacent to the trunk, and the examiner must be on the patient's right side.[65] Beginning in the right iliac fossa, the examiner's hand gently advances toward the left upper quadrant. This minimizes the likelihood that a grossly enlarged spleen will be unappreciated, and the lower pole and medial border should be easily appreciated. If the spleen cannot be felt with this approach, the left hand of the examiner is placed on the left flank, lifting the lower part of the rib cage to displace the spleen medially toward the examiner's right hand. The splenic notch should be felt in the inferior medial border. Rotating the patient into the right lateral position while still recumbent may make it easier to palpate the spleen. The spleen should move with deep inspiration. It is dull to percussion. The degree of enlargement is usually measured in centimeters below the costal margin. It may be difficult to appreciate even significantly enlarged spleens, depending on the position of the spleen within the abdomen. Normal splenic size in an adult is up to 250 g, and up to 13 centimeters in its long axis. Up to half of spleens weighing 600 to 750 g are not palpable.[66] Greater degrees of splenomegaly are less difficult to appreciate on physical examination.

Up to 15% of normal children and 3% of young adults have palpable spleens, up to 2 cm below the left costal margin, without evidence of illness.[67] The spleen involutes with age, and a spleen that is palpable in an older person is less likely to be a normal variant and more likely to be associated with clinical disease.

IMAGING OF THE SPLEEN

Radionuclide scintigraphy assesses anatomic and functional aspects of the spleen.[68] The most common procedure is a liver–spleen scan in which ^{99m}Tc sulfur colloid is injected intravenously and taken up by hepatic and splenic macrophages. It is the phagocytic activity of macrophages—rather than the presence of the spleen itself or any aspects of lymphoid function—that is assessed. A dynamic ^{99m}Tc scan can also assess the distribution of blood within the portal system and suggest the presence of portal hypertension. Infusion of ^{99m}Tc-labeled

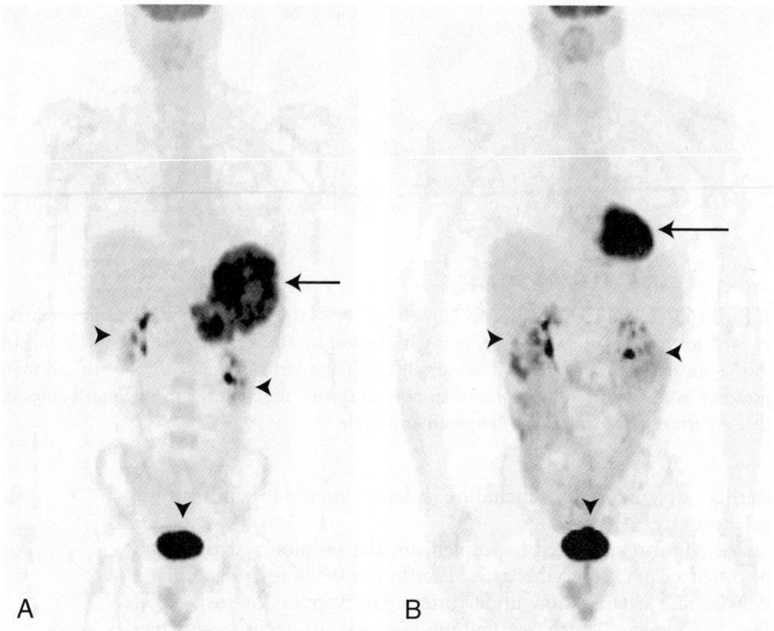

Figure 163–3 PET scanning to image areas of involvement in Hodgkin disease.[89] Panel A shows pretreatment and Panel B shows the same patient after 3 cycles of chemotherapy. The spleen is particularly well imaged on PET scan. *(From Friedberg JW, Chengagi V: PET scans in the staging of lymphoma: Current status. Oncologist 8:438, 2003)*[89]

or ^{111}In-labeled platelets with scintigraphy to determine their relative distribution in the liver and spleen has been used with considerable, but not absolute, success to predict the clinical efficacy of splenectomy in immune thrombocytopenic purpura.[69]

Ultrasonography readily shows the size, shape, and several aspects of splenic anatomy, including the presence of cysts and abscesses.[70] The procedure is noninvasive, painless, of low cost, avoids radiation exposure for patients, and is a good screening study when the spleen is thought to be enlarged. Accessory spleens tend not to be well visualized on routine ultrasonography. Endoscopic ultrasound-guided biopsy in the hands of a skilled operator permits accurate diagnosis of lesions as small as a centimeter or less, which compares well with results obtained using computed tomography (CT).[71–73] High frequency sonography has significantly better resolution, and can visualize both nodularity within the spleen, which occurs in childhood as immunity is acquired, and accessory spleens and splenosis after splenic rupture or trauma.[74]

CT imaging has the advantage of showing the anatomy and some aspects of splenic function.[75] Contrast material in the stomach, small bowel, and colon, given enterally, helps delineate splenic tissue when it impinges on these organs. Intravenous contrast material is required to delineate splenic lesions whose density is the same as normal splenic tissue. Abscesses have a rim of contrast agent enhancement.[76]

CT can be used to estimate the volume of the spleen. Accessory spleens have the same attenuation as a normal spleen, which is somewhat less than that of liver.[77] Accessory spleens are usually located in the gastrosplenic ligament near the hilum. Subcapsular and intrasplenic hematomas and splenic lacerations are clearly seen on CT. Leukemias and many inflammatory diseases produce diffuse splenomegaly. Granulomas and infarcted areas eventually calcify. Cysts, abscesses, and some malignancies have inhomogeneous patterns on CT scan.[78–80] Although not replacing other methods of staging, splenic enlargement on CT may direct follow-up studies and indicate prognosis.[81]

In addition to imaging the spleen, CT can be used to direct therapeutic interventions. Abscesses, hematomas, and cysts can be drained. As long as portal hypertension is not present and vascular lesions have been excluded, thin-needle aspiration under CT guidance is generally a safe intervention.

As with head injury, emergency room CT scanning of patients with abdominal trauma may avoid hospital admission and avoid laparotomy. With mild splenic injury, a single scan may be sufficient to direct management.[82]

Magnetic resonance imaging (MRI) is useful for identifying vascular lesions, which would otherwise require angiography, and splenic infections. It is more difficult to image the contents of the upper abdomen with MRI than with CT because of respiratory motion. With more rapid imaging technology, MRI has gained considerable utility for imaging infectious and vascular lesions of the spleen. Hepatosplenic candidiasis and other infections to which immunocompromised patients are susceptible can be identified noninvasively with modern MRI technology.[83–85]

Perhaps the most valuable use of MRI imaging of the spleen is to obtain a quantitative measurement of iron burden in organs that accumulate iron in iron overload.[86]

Positron-emission tomography (PET) scanning using ^{18}F2-deoxyglucose (FDG) has an increasing role in the diagnosis, staging, and monitoring of lymphoma, both non-Hodgkin and Hodgkin disease. It is more sensitive than CT scanning at identifying nodal disease, and superior to both lymphangiography and CT scanning at imaging the spleen. The availability of more sensitive, specific and less toxic approaches to imaging permits more precise staging of Hodgkin lymphoma without the complications of splenectomy (see Fig. 163–3).[87–89]

The place of PET scanning is expanding in other disorders as whole-body PET scanners and appropriate small-molecule markers for individual diseases are more widely available. Imaging studies in small-animal models are very promising; splenic involvement can be identified with high sensitivity in mice.[90]

TESTS OF SPLENIC FUNCTION

The peripheral blood smear may be the most sensitive tool for identification of functional or anatomic hyposplenia. The presence of Howell–Jolly bodies, which are nuclear remnants normally removed by the spleen, is an excellent indicator of hyposplenism (see Fig. 163–4).[17,18,91] These are rarely seen until the spleen is largely nonfunctional or overwhelmed by other phagocytic functions, such as extravascular hemolysis. Newborn infants commonly have visible Howell–Jolly bodies, and splenic function appears to be at least somewhat impaired in the first week of life.[92] Pappenheimer bodies (siderotic granules normally removed by the spleen) are often seen in hyposplenic states, particularly when a component of hemolysis exists.[93] Erythrocyte morphology reflects the lack of membrane polishing by the spleen, with the presence of acanthocytes and target cells.[14,16,61] Granulocyte and platelet numbers are increased

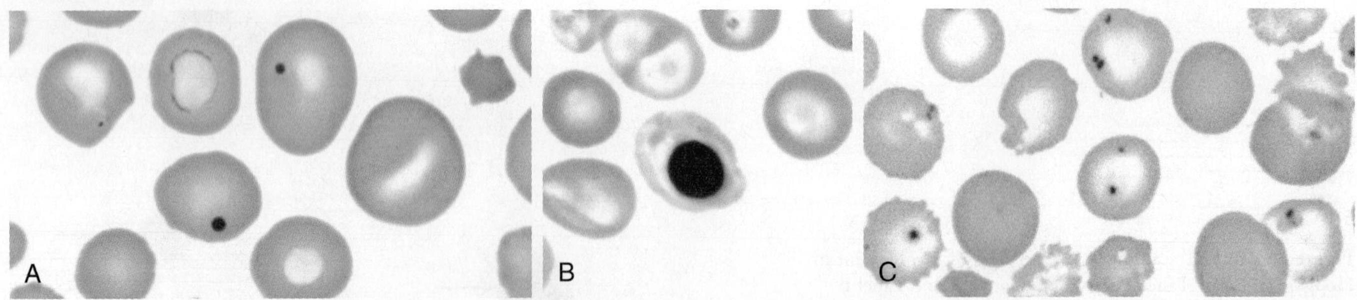

Figure 163–4 Red blood cells with Howell-Jolly bodies (**A**), Nucleated red blood cell (**B**), and cells with Pappenheimer bodies (**C**). Red blood cells with Howell-Jolly bodies are seen in patients with hyposplenism. The cytoplasmic inclusions (**A**) are nuclear remnants which are usually round and stain similar to the nucleus of a nucleated red blood cell (**B**). They occur normally during red cell maturation, but are typically removed by a normal spleen. Their presence in the blood indicates less than normal splenic function. Pappenheimer bodies (**C**), which can also be seen in hyposplenism, are siderotic granules that are irregular in shape, and frequently multiple.

during asplenic states, including splenic infarction and surgical splenectomy.[59,62]

To confirm suspected hyposplenism, the simplest test is a count of pitted or pocked erythrocytes. Fixation in 0.5% to 1.0% glutaraldehyde and examination under interference optics for surface pits reveals endocytic vesicles containing hemoglobin, ferritin, and remnants of mitochondria.[14] These form in mature erythrocytes and are normally removed by the functioning spleen. The number of pitted cells (not the number of pits per cell) is inversely proportional to splenic function, with normal persons having less than 2% pitted cells.

ASPLENIA AND HYPOSPLENIA

Congenital asplenia may be an isolated lesion or associated with severe cyanotic congenital heart disease and bilateral right-sidedness.[94] Life-threatening cardiac lesions, including transposition of the great vessels, pulmonary artery atresia or stenosis, septal defects, anomalous venous drainage, and single atrioventricular valve, are components of this condition. The liver is central, and both lungs have three lobes. The peripheral blood smear shows Howell–Jolly bodies and other signs of hyposplenism. There is considerable variation in the anatomic and functional findings, and it is difficult to predict with accuracy the degree of splenic dysfunction on the basis of the anatomy alone.[95] Children who survive the cardiac difficulties in the neonatal period have a significant incidence of sepsis secondary to a variety of organisms.[96]

Polysplenia is associated with bilateral left-sidedness. Dextrocardia, bilateral superior venae cavae, septal defects, and anomalous pulmonary venous return are associated cardiac lesions. Both lungs have two lobes, the liver is midline, and bowel malrotation is common. The splenic tissue is divided into two to nine masses.[197] The peripheral blood smear usually does not suggest hyposplenism, and no clear association with an increased risk of infection has been documented.

Asplenia occurring without heart disease is less likely to be detected before an infection develops than when associated cardiac lesions bring the patient to medical attention.[98,99] Some of these patients also have situs inversus. Isolated cases of asplenia discovered after death of an otherwise healthy adult or child from overwhelming sepsis with encapsulated organisms have been reported.[100] Familial instances of congenital asplenia are likely to be instances of genetic abnormalities (eg, Hox11/Tlx1), but these are not yet characterized. Examination of a blood smear for Howell Jolly bodies is a simple procedure and may be lifesaving in the rare patients affected with these disorders.[100]

Imaging to determine whether a spleen is present should follow identification of Howell–Jolly bodies on the blood smear of an otherwise healthy person. Immunization with polysaccharide vaccines and early intervention with antibiotics for apparent infection may prove lifesaving for these individuals.[94] Because approximately 20%

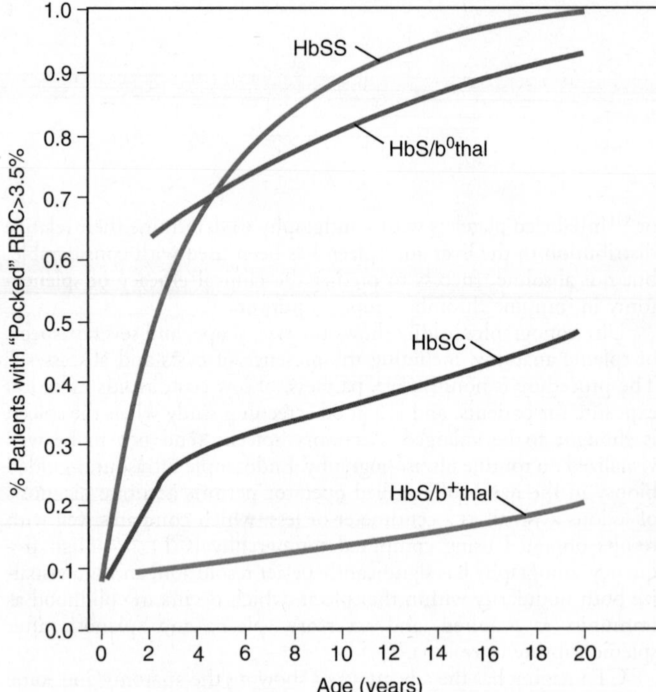

Figure 163–5 Development of functional asplenia in sickle cell disorders. (Pearson HA, Gallagher D, Chilcote R, et al: Developmental patterns of splenic dysfunction in sickle cell disorders. Pediatrics 76:392, 1985. Reproduced by permission of *Pediatrics in Review.*)

of invasive pneumococcal infections in these patients are nonvaccine strains, a high degree of vigilance remains essential, even with more widespread immunization of healthy children.[101]

ACQUIRED HYPOSPLENISM

Infarction in Sickle Cell Disease

The course of sickle cell disease is marked by progressive dysfunction of multiple organs over many years.[102] One of the earliest organs to be affected is the spleen. Serial measurement of pitted erythrocytes in sickle syndromes demonstrates that splenic dysfunction develops progressively over the first few years of life in the major sickle syndromes (Figs. 163–5 and 163–6).[103] The hypoxic, acidotic, hypoglycemic environment of the spleen creates optimal conditions for tactoid formation and for sickling of the poorly deformable erythrocytes, which then block splenic blood vessels and infarct the tissues. Splenic environmental conditions that enhance acidosis or hypoxia, or additional erythrocyte membrane or enzyme abnormalities that promote irre-

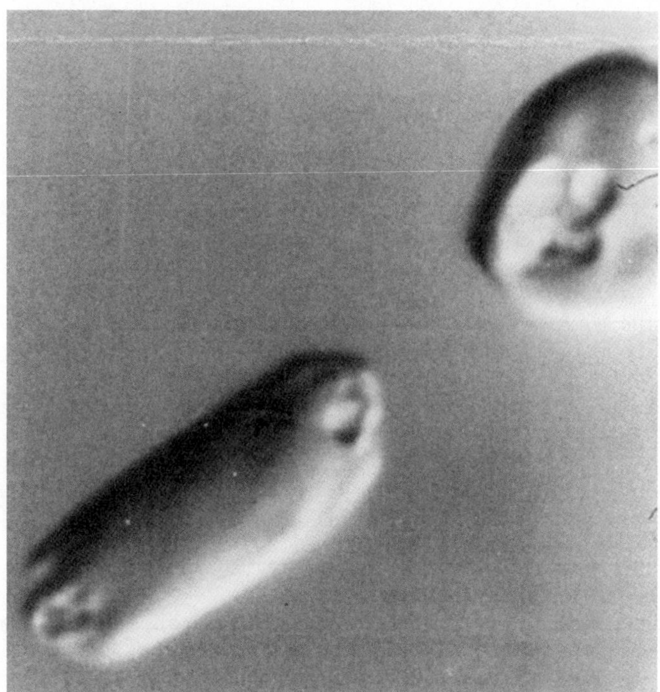

Figure 163–6 Pocked erythrocytes in the sickle hemoglobinopathies. (From Sills R, Oski FA: RBC surface pits in the sickle hemoglobinopathies. Am J Dis Child 133:526, 1979, with permission. Copyright 1979, American Medical Association.)

versible sickling, enhance splenic infarction.[104] The hyposplenism is reversible with transfusion for at least the first few years of life, but becomes irreversible with progressive damage to blood vessels by 6 years of age in patients with sickle cell disease.[105–107]

Splenic sequestration is a manifestation of the infarctive process of sickling in the spleen that extends to involve larger veins.[108,109] The unimpeded flow of well-oxygenated blood in the splenic arterioles into the distensible splenic tissues results in pooling of a large amount of blood, whereas the venous drainage is occluded by sickled hypoxic erythrocytes. Unlike the chronic process of smaller-vessel infarction, the acute splenic sequestration crisis can be life threatening because a large amount of blood can collect in the highly distensible spleen. The tendency to recurrence and the potential for fatal outcome lead to the common recommendation for splenectomy in a patient who has had one severe splenic sequestration crisis, or more than one less severe crisis. Occlusion of venous drainage also occurs in the liver, but the less distensible capsule of the liver and the options for venous drainage through the portal system make this less likely to threaten life.

Immunologic and Autoimmune Diseases

Poor phagocytic function of the spleen is associated with impaired function of the Fc receptors on splenic macrophages in a variety of immunologic, rheumatic, and inflammatory disorders. Among those disorders in which hyposplenism has been clearly defined and associated with a risk of infection are systemic lupus erythematosus, rheumatoid arthritis, sarcoidosis,[110] systemic vasculitis, ulcerative colitis, celiac disease,[111] amyloidosis,[112] chronic graft-versus-host disease,[113] mastocytosis,[114] and congenital[115] and acquired immunodeficiency.[116] The diseases themselves and the immunosuppressive therapies that are used in their management may contribute to the risk of infection in these conditions. Immunization to polysaccharide antigens and recognition of the risk of bacterial infection are important to minimizing the risks of splenic hypofunction.[117]

Splenomegaly and the production of autoantibodies (such as to platelets in idiopathic thrombocytopenic purpura) are features of acquired immunodeficiency syndrome (AIDS). In the late stages of AIDS, atrophy of lymphoid follicles and depletion of T cell-dependent areas are common. It is not clear that impairment of phagocytic function is a component of this splenic atrophy in AIDS.

Therapy-Induced Splenic Hypofunction

Radiation therapy affects splenic function, depending on the dose administered.[118] In general, phagocytic cells are not affected by irradiation, but lymphoid cells are extremely sensitive. B-cell function is nearly ablated with as little as 500 cGy. T-cell lymphoblastogenesis is eliminated by administration of 3000 cGy. With doses of 2000 cGy, splenic hypofunction is usually transient because the macrophages and splenic stroma are not affected, and circulating B and T lymphocytes can repopulate the splenic follicles. Patients receiving irradiation to the bed of a left Wilms tumor are not hyposplenic. However, permanent splenic hypofunction develops with doses of greater than or equal to 4000 cGy, which is standard dosing for Hodgkin disease. The risk of infection is significant after such therapy.

Corticosteroid therapy impairs the affinity of the Fc receptors of splenic macrophages for opsonic immune globulin G (IgG), and decreases the adhesiveness of granulocytes and monocytes.[119,120] This creates a pharmacologic splenectomy acutely with administration of corticosteroids at common therapeutic dosages. The function of the Fc receptors on hepatic, pulmonary, and bone marrow macrophages is far less affected than that of splenic macrophages. The acute rise in platelet count or hemoglobin values seen with corticosteroid therapy in idiopathic thrombocytopenic purpura or autoimmune hemolytic anemia is due to decreased clearance of sensitized cells. With longer therapy, the production of antibodies by splenic lymphocytes is also affected, and splenic function continues to be impaired.

Intravenous IgG appears to decrease the phagocytic function of the spleen by binding to Fc receptors and impeding their recognition of opsonized particles.[121] This is a transient effect because the Fc receptors are internalized and recycled, and opsonic function returns to normal within 2 to 3 weeks.[122] Occupancy and impairment of function of Fc receptors is also seen with administration of anti-D immunoglobulin to Rh-positive patients, which induces a transient hemolytic anemia. Reticuloendothelial blockade, or occupancy of these receptors, refers to the impaired ability of the spleen to recognize and remove other IgG-coated particles, including bacteria, in the presence of these agents.[123]

SPLENOMEGALY AND HYPERSPLENISM

An enlarged spleen is not a disease state in itself but usually indicates some underlying pathology. The processes run the gamut from minor to life threatening, from congenital disorders to those at the end of life, and few organ systems are not represented in the underlying conditions. It is useful to approach splenomegaly by considering the processes that may cause splenic enlargement and then to focus on the specific diagnoses within those categories.

The spleen may be enlarged as a result of infiltration, hypertrophy of normal elements (macrophages and lymphoid components), extramedullary hematopoiesis, inflammatory or immunologic processes, and systemic or portal congestion. The degree of splenomegaly correlates well with involvement of the spleen in many malignant disorders, such as Hodgkin disease.[124] Rarely, anatomic abnormalities will cause splenomegaly. Splenomegaly is important to investigate because it is frequently the presenting finding of a serious disorder whose earlier recognition and treatment may prevent significant long-term morbidity and mortality. The diseases associated with splenomegaly are detailed in Table 163–3.

Hypersplenism refers to nonimmune, indiscriminate destruction of the formed elements of the blood by a spleen that is enlarged, affected by portal hypertension, or both. The bone marrow is hyper-

Table 163–3 Causes of Splenomegaly

Primary Process	Pathogenesis	Examples
Anatomic	Developmental anomalies	Cysts, pseudocysts, hamartomas, peliosis, hemangiomas
Hematologic	Hemolysis	Intrinsic (membrane, enzyme, hemoglobin disorders); extrinsic (immune)
	Extramedullary hematopoiesis	Myeloproliferative diseases/myelodysplasias, myelofibrosis, osteopetrosis
Infectious	Bacteria	Acute and chronic systemic infection, abscesses, SBE
	Mycobacteria	Miliary tuberculosis
	Spirochetes	Syphilis, Lyme disease, leptospirosis
	Viruses	EBV, CMV, HIV, hepatitis A, B, C
	Rickettsia	Rocky Mountain spotted fever, Q fever, typhus disseminated candidiasis,
	Fungi	histoplasmosis, South American blastomycosis
	Parasites	Malaria, babesiosis, toxoplasmosis, *Toxocara canis/cati*, leishmaniasis, schistosomiasis, trypanosomiasis
Immunologic	Collagen vascular diseases	Felty syndrome, SLE, mixed connective tissue disorder, systemic vasculitis, Sjögren syndrome, systemic mastocytosis
	Immunodeficiency	Common variable immunodeficiency
	Immune/inflammatory	Graft-versus-host disease, serum sickness, LGL lymphocytosis, Weber Christian histiocytoses
Neoplastic	Primary malignancies	Lymphomas, leukemias
	Metastatic malignancies	Breast, lung, skin, colon
Infiltrative	Storage diseases	Gaucher disease, Niemann–Pick disease, GM-1 gangliosidosis, glycogen storage disease type IV, Tangier disease, Wolman disease, mucopolysaccharidoses, hyperchylomicronemia types I and IV
Congestive	Portal hypertension	Intrahepatic cirrhosis, extrahepatic cirrhosis (Budd–Chiari syndrome)
	Systemic	Congestive heart failure

CMV, cytomegalovirus; EBV, Epstein–Barr virus; HIV, human immunodeficiency virus; LGL, large granular lymphocyte; SBE, subacute bacterial endocarditis; SLE, systemic lupus erythematosus.

plastic, and the peripheral blood cell counts are decreased as a consequence of destruction of mature formed elements. Splenectomy corrects the cytopenia. Any of the formed elements of the blood—erythrocytes, neutrophils, or platelets—can be affected, alone or in combination. Splenic hypertrophy results in pooling of formed elements and premature destruction of cells by splenic macrophages. Because a normal function of splenic macrophages is to remove senescent cells, this is an exaggeration of a process that is physiologic for splenic macrophages.

Hypersplenism develops in patients who receive chronic transfusion. There are several components to the development of hypersplenism. The antigenic load of allogeneic transfused cells stimulates the immune system. Transfused cells have shorter survival than normal red cells (mean of 60 instead of 120 days, unless specially prepared neocytes are used), which increases the work of splenic macrophages. Finally, iron overload causes hemosiderosis of both the spleen and the liver, so that portal hypertension may develop and further increase splenic pathology. Hypersplenism increases the transfusion requirement in patients who are transfusion-dependent.

SPLENECTOMY

Indications and Timing

Splenectomy should be performed for clinical indications rather than for specific diagnoses. In many instances, removal of the spleen will improve the condition of patients with hemolytic anemia due to intrinsic disorders of erythrocyte membranes and enzyme disorders, and of those with chronic conditions, such as storage diseases and portal hypertension. Specific clinical indices that require intervention should be identified, and parameters that can be used to identify clinical improvement (usually an increase in peripheral blood cell counts, growth, or energy level) should be determined before the procedure is performed. For patients with inherited erythrocyte membrane or enzyme disorders, such as hereditary spherocytosis or pyruvate kinase deficiency, marked reticulocytosis indicating significant metabolic energy required for erythropoiesis, somatic growth failure, or lack of exercise tolerance would be potential indications for splenectomy. Avoidance of formation of gallstones, formerly often considered an indication for splenectomy when a diagnosis of hereditary spherocytosis was made, is less important today because minimally invasive surgical procedures have improved the management of cholelithiasis. Patients with storage disorders such as Gaucher disease develop splenomegaly and hypersplenism. Cytopenias requiring intervention should be present before splenectomy is performed. The clinical benefit to be obtained from splenectomy should at least balance, and preferably outweigh, the potential long-term risks of postsplenectomy septicemia,[125–135] the increased incidence of arteriosclerotic cardiovascular disease,[63] and the shift of storage cells from the spleen to other organs, such as bone marrow, where they may do more harm in the absence of the spleen.[136–140] Not all patients with hemolytic anemias, such as hereditary spherocytosis, need splenectomy. If they develop an aplastic crisis, as with parvovirus B-19 infection, while their spleens are intact, they may need transfusion. Many patients with mild chronic hemolysis and well-compensated anemia may be better off with their spleens remaining intact. Patients with immune thrombocytopenic purpura should undergo surgical splenectomy when the risks of bleeding or of medical therapies (such as long-term corticosteroids) are such that the benefits of splenectomy exceed the risks. These indications for splenectomy are different in adults and in children and are affected by the presence of underlying disorders, such as systemic lupus erythematosus and HIV infection.

Splenectomy for sickle cell disease is usually performed for splenic sequestration that is severe, persistent, or recurrent. In some sickle syndromes, the spleen does not autoinfarct in childhood, and persistent splenomegaly may increase the degree of anemia. The risk of subsequent development of gallstones should be considered in patients with hemoglobinopathies and other hemolytic anemias so that cholecystectomy can be performed simultaneously, if deemed indicated.[141]

The timing of splenectomy—when it is to be performed—should again be chosen to minimize risks and maximize benefits. Immunity to carbohydrate antigens, such as those in the cell walls of encapsulated organisms, such as *Streptococcus pneumoniae*, *Neisseria*, and *Haemophilus influenzae* type b, develops over the first 2 to 3 years of life. When splenectomy can be delayed until the patient is at least 2 and preferably more than 5 years of age, specific immunity and response to administered polysaccharide vaccines will improve host defenses and lessen the risk of postsplenectomy sepsis. When patients have storage diseases, such as Gaucher disease, or hemolytic anemia predisposing to iron overload, such as thalassemia, the presence of the spleen as a preferential site for storage of harmful cellular breakdown products may protect other organs from damage. Delaying splenectomy until a clear clinical indication is present will balance risks optimally.

Relative Contraindications

Extramedullary hematopoiesis is a relative contraindication to splenectomy. In some conditions, splenomegaly reflects the fact that the bone marrow is not the primary site of hematopoiesis. Intrinsic bone marrow pathology, such as myelofibrosis, renders the marrow cavity incapable of supporting hematopoiesis. Myeloid metaplasia may reflect the fact that the spleen has become a predominant site of hematopoiesis. Splenectomy under these circumstances may render the patient pancytopenic and produce massive hepatomegaly. The major conditions leading to this circumstance are malignant osteopetrosis in young children and myelofibrosis in adults. It is important to determine before splenectomy that the patient is not dependent on splenic hematopoiesis for survival.

Portal hypertension is not a contraindication to splenectomy, but it affects the surgical approach. It is helpful to determine before surgery whether the patient is likely to need a shunt to reduce portal hypertension and manage esophageal varices.

Surgical Options

When splenectomy is clearly indicated, acute complications are rarely a consideration in the decision to perform surgery. Nevertheless, advances in surgical procedures have minimized the short-term risks of the procedure itself and of postoperative complications, such as intestinal obstruction from adhesions. Subtotal splenectomy can be performed when total splenectomy is not desirable, such as for the removal of a cyst, a pseudocyst, or tumors; after trauma; or for Gaucher disease.[136,137] Wedge resection with mattress sutures and cyanoacrylate adhesions and microfibrillar collagen omental packs have greatly improved partial splenectomy procedures in the past decade. Laparotomy is required, when extensive peritoneal adhesions are present; for the staging of Hodgkin disease[142,143]; and for removal of most massively enlarged spleens.[144,145] A sufficiently large incision to permit full visualization and mobilization is essential when the spleen is very large or when inspection is a major part of the surgical procedure. A retroperitoneal approach is useful when the spleen is not massively enlarged but needs to be fully removed, such as when cytopenias are the indication for the procedure. This approach shortens the postoperative recovery time and avoids induction of peritoneal adhesions.

Minimally invasive procedures have become standard for most splenectomies. Laparoscopy is now the procedure of choice for splenectomy. Although the operative time is significantly greater than for laparotomy, the postoperative recovery time, the risk of damage to the pancreas, the likelihood of development of subphrenic abscess and peritoneal adhesions postoperatively, and the nutritional and metabolic challenges to the patient are considerably reduced. Laparoscopic splenectomy can be performed even in thrombocytopenic patients. The outcome of laparoscopic splenectomy in ITP is affected by the experience and skill of the surgeon and by obesity of the patient. Extensive presurgical use of corticosteroids may induce obesity and impair tissue healing, resulting in a higher risk of complications of laparoscopic splenectomy than in patients whose splenectomy is performed before these drug effects develop.[146]

Appreciation of the risk of postsplenectomy septicemia[147,148] and refinements in noninvasive, accurate radiologic monitoring techniques have led to more conservative approaches to splenic injury.[128,149] Nonoperative management has increased over time, and has acceptable mortality and complication rates in selected patients, although early discharge may put patients at risk of later complications.[150] Noninvasive imaging and minimally invasive surgical procedures have impacted heavily upon these trends. After traumatic rupture, splenic tissue may regenerate minisplenules in the peritoneal cavity, a process termed *splenosis*.[147,151] Although splenosis is partially protective against postsplenectomy infection in animals,[151,152] its protective value in humans is not known and depends on the adequacy of perfusion of splenic tissue (Fig. 163–7).[153] It is generally valuable to attempt preservation of splenic function when possible after traumatic rupture. Some surgeons are attempting to induce splenosis when traumatic splenectomy is unavoidable, in the hope of minimizing late complications.

As the late complications of splenectomy are better appreciated, surgeons have become increasingly creative at performing procedures that preserve or restore splenic function. Even large cysts that were indications for splenectomy until recently have been managed with spleen-conserving procedures, such as partial or total cystectomy, and can often be performed laparascopically.[154] Pancreatic surgery often requires sacrifice of the spleen; increasing numbers of procedures are being performed with salvage of the spleen.[155,156]

Splenic transplantation is being used as a means of developing immune tolerance, as well as to reduce the risk of infection, in organ transplantation. Allograft spleen has been transplanted within multivisceral grafts with only minimal graft-versus-host disease. To date, there are more animal than human data, and it is unclear how large an impact this approach may have on visceral, especially small bowel and pancreatic, allotransplantation.[157–160]

Complications After Splenectomy

Acute complications in the perioperative period include rupture of the spleen, the development of subphrenic abscess, and injury to the pancreas with the operative procedure. In a healthy patient, the acute risk of splenectomy is low. The degree of splenomegaly greatly affects the risk of rupture and pancreatic injury. The technical difficulty of splenectomy is much greater when the spleen is massively enlarged than when the spleen is small. Rupture of the spleen once the arterial supply has been ligated is rarely a problem. The splenic hilum is retroperitoneal, so that when the spleen is very large, mobilization to access the splenic artery and vein can be difficult. After recovery from surgery, intestinal obstruction due to formation of peritoneal adhesions is a complication that, if it is to occur at all, usually occurs within the first few months.

Two late complications of splenectomy give the greatest concern: overwhelming postsplenectomy septicemia and atherosclerotic heart disease. Both of these complications may develop many years after the splenectomy. The precise risk is not known, and preventive interventions are probably underutilized because patients may not be aware of the risks of splenectomy performed early in life.[161]

Postsplenectomy septicemia is rare but may be rapidly lethal. It is due to the inability of hepatic and pulmonary macrophages to effectively clear organisms from the bloodstream in the absence of protective levels of opsonic IgG antibody. Organisms that enter the bloodstream and would ordinarily be removed by splenic macrophages are able to evade recognition by macrophages whose Fc and C3b receptors appear to be less avid than those of splenic macrophages. Circulation of the blood through the liver and lung is more rapid than through the spleen, and there is little opportunity for macrophages to recognize organisms whose surfaces contain no IgG

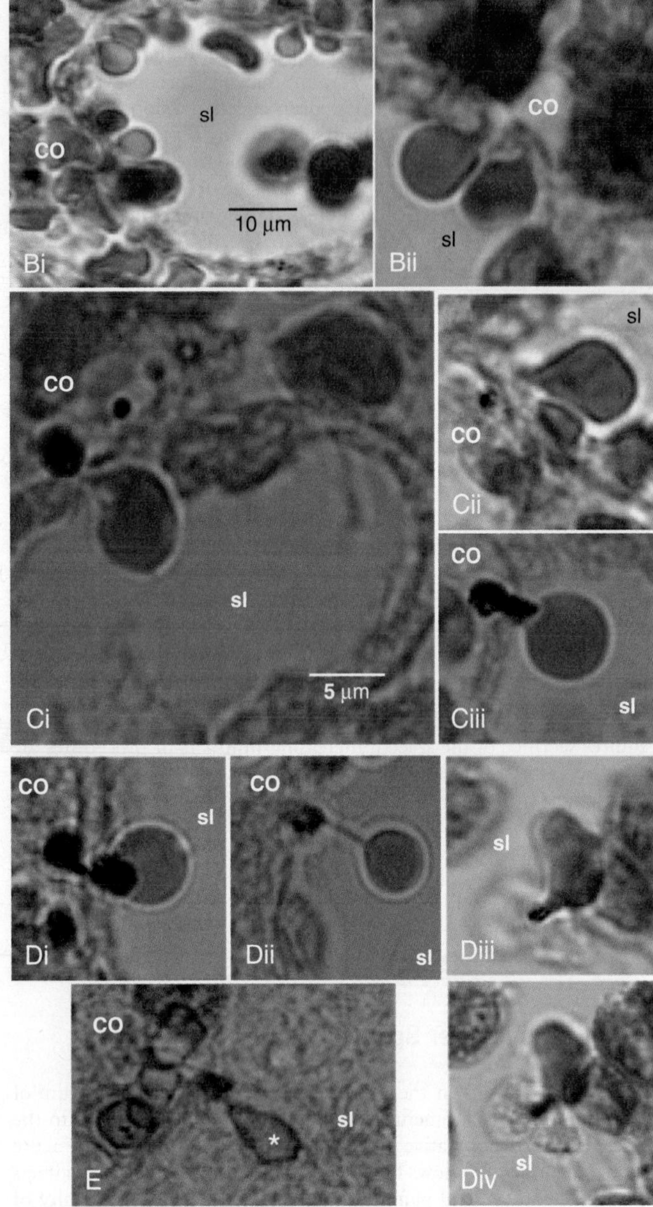

Figure 163–7 Removal of intraerythrocyte dead malarial parasites by isolated perfused human splenic tissue.[153]

and only small amounts of C3bi. Generation of cytokines, including tumor necrosis factor-α, and bacterial endotoxins lead to cardiovascular collapse and shock. It is rare to revive an asplenic patient once the patient is in shock, even with effective antibiotic therapy. The risk that this will happen varies with the indication for splenectomy (Table 163–4) and the patient's medical condition. Factors that impair host defenses significantly increase the risk of infection. These include deficient opsonins (hypogammaglobulinemia and specific antibody production deficiency), reticuloendothelial blockade related to increased phagocytic activity of macrophages in other organs, impaired antigen processing or recognition (AIDS, lymphoma, other malignancies, and some collagen vascular diseases), neutropenia, and high iron load (thalassemia). Patients at the lowest risk are those in whom splenectomy cures the underlying problem, such as isolated ITP, hereditary spherocytosis, and trauma. Patients undergoing splenectomy for trauma have a 50-fold greater risk of septic death than trauma patients with spleens intact. The risk in patients with sickle cell disease is increased 350-fold over that of the general population.

Table 163–4 Incidence of Postsplenectomy Sepsis

Indication for Splenectomy	Cumulative Incidence of Bacterial Sepsis (%)
Trauma	1.5
Hematologic disorders	3.4
Portal hypertension	8.2
Hodgkin disease	10
Sickle cell disease	15
Thalassemia	25

Data from Gorse GJ: The relationship of the spleen to infection. In Bowlder AJ (ed.): The Spleen: Structure, Function, and Clinical Significance. New York, Van Nostrand Reinhold, 1990, p 269, with permission.

Atherosclerosis developing many years after splenectomy may be related to the thrombocytosis that occurs, with enhancement of plaque formation. Statistically, the increased risk of atherosclerosis is not great,[63] but for individuals with other risk factors, such as hypertension, diabetes, high levels of cholesterol or homocysteine, heterozygous protein C or S deficiency, or factor V Leiden, splenectomy may pose a more significant risk. No data are currently available in this area.

Prevention of Complications

Postsplenectomy Septicemia

The major risk of postsplenectomy sepsis is infection with encapsulated organisms such as *Staphylococcus pneumoniae*, *Haemophilus influenzae* type b, and *Neisseria meningitidis*, which require opsonization for effective phagocytosis. Polysaccharide vaccines are available for all three groups (Table 163–4).[162–166] The highest risk period for children is in the first 2 years of life, when their ability to mount an antibody response to purified polysaccharides has not developed completely, so protein-conjugated vaccines are now in widespread use. This has significant potential benefit for patients whose asplenia is not recognized, as they may be immunized as part of their routine care. The antibody responses to vaccines, especially the conjugated vaccines, differ in IgG subclasses from those produced in natural infection. Overwhelming postsplenectomy sepsis, and death from sepsis in functionally hyposplenic patients, should be preventable.[167] It is recommended that immunization be done 3 weeks before the anticipated splenectomy to optimize antigen recognition and processing, and induce more effective immunity.[168] Adults are presumed to be immune to *H influenzae* type b, and may receive the pneumococcal and meningococcal vaccines alone. Reimmunization for children is recommended 2 to 5 years after initial immunization. Repeat administration of pneumococcal vaccine is recommended every 10 years.[169] Because these recommendations change with experience and vaccine usage, it is wise to consult current guidelines for individual patients.[170–172]

There are fewer data on the efficacy of prophylactic antibiotics for asplenic patients, except for young children with sickle cell disease, in whom antibiotics should be initiated as soon as the diagnosis is established. Present recommendations are that twice-daily oral penicillin or amoxicillin be continued in sickle cell patients until 6 years of age. High-risk patients with surgical or functional asplenia, including those with diagnoses of thalassemia, Hodgkin disease, other malignancies, immunodeficiency disease, or chronic graft-versus-host disease, should receive prophylactic antibiotics unless specific contraindications exist. Whether or not such patients receive prophylactic antibiotics, and regardless of their immunization status, they may develop overwhelming infections with other organisms, including gram-negative organisms and *Staphylococcus aureus*. Updated recommendations should be consulted for specific circumstances.

The single most important measure to prevent postsplenectomy septicemia is education of patient, family, and physician. Recognition of the risk, the institution of appropriate preventive measures, and the rapid administration of antibiotics to a patient who is showing signs of infection (fever and chills) can be lifesaving.

Atherosclerosis

The magnitude of the risk of development of atherosclerosis is not clear.[173] Appropriate preventive measures include identifying and minimizing concurrent risk factors, such as obesity, dietary patterns, a sedentary lifestyle, and the presence of other hereditary factors that would predispose to thrombosis. Low-dose aspirin could be considered, but no data exist regarding its efficacy in this situation.

CONCLUSION

Although very little novel information has emerged about clinical aspects of splenic function in recent years, advances in supportive care in several fields have had significant impacts on the management of disorders of the spleen. Better and more effective immunizations, administered widely for indications unrelated to splenic dysfunction, have improved prevention of serious complications of these disorders. Advances in imaging and surgery have transformed the management of splenic trauma and other anatomic disorders, as well as splenic surgery for diagnosis and staging of malignancies.

In contrast to the modest clinical gains, enhanced understanding of the complexity of cross-talk between the cells of the immune and hematopoietic system has transformed our appreciation of the molecular, cellular, system and network basis for long-standing clinical observations about splenic function. The ability of splenic macrophages, in concert with dendritic cells and B cells, to recognize and ingest a variety of microorganisms without specific immunity or previous exposure provides great insight into the reasons that the spleen protects against a variety of very specific infections. More detailed understanding of the impact of the microenvironment on cellular functions, the role of stromal infrastructure on the ability of cells to interact with and respond to invading pathogens, and the sensitive cellular cross-talk among components of the immune system has contributed to an appreciation of clinical observations about the role the spleen plays in normal biology. The sensitive interactions between hematopoiesis, recycling of aging cells, and iron metabolism is most clearly demonstrated in the spleen.

Although not necessary to life under baseline circumstances, the contribution of the spleen to homeostasis under stress is considerable. Ongoing efforts to preserve and manage splenic function will benefit from enhanced appreciation of the underlying biology.

SUGGESTED READINGS

Brendolan A, Orsado MM, Carsetti R, et al: Development and function of the mammalian spleen. Bioessays 29:166, 2007.

Cai W, Olafsen T, Zhang X, et al: PET imaging of colorectal cancer in xenograft-bearing mice by use of an 18F-labeled T84.66 anti-carcinoembryonic antigen diabody. J Nucl Med 48:170, 2007.

Crawford RS, Tabbara M, Sheridan R, et al: Early discharge after nonoperative management of splenic injuries: Increased patient risk caused by late failure? Surgery 142:337, 2007.

Grijalva CG, Nuorti JP, Arbogast PG, et al: Decline in pneumonia admissions after routine childhood immunisation with pneumococcal conjugate vaccine in the USA: A time-series analysis. Lancet 369:1179, 2007.

Haan JM, Boswell S, Stein D, et al: Follow-up abdominal CT is not necessary in low-grade splenic injury. Am Surg 73(1):13, 2007.

Hackett S, Chua-Ausom W, Pootraku P, et al: The magnetic susceptibilities of iron deposits in thalassaemic spleen tissue. Biochim Biophys Acta 1772:330, 2007.

Juweid ME, Stroobants S, Hoekstra OS, et al: Use of positron emission tomography for response assessment of lymphoma: Consensus of the Imaging Subcommittee of International Harmonization Project in Lymphoma. J Clin Oncol 25:571, 2007.

Kato T, Tzakis AG, Selvaggi G, et al: Transplantation of the spleen: Effect of splenic allograft in human multivisceral transplantation. Ann Surg 246:436, 2007.

Matsumoto CS, Fishbein TM: Modified multivisceral transplantation with splenopancreatic preservation. Transplantation 83:234, 2007.

Mattioli G, Pini Prato A, Cheli M, et al: Italian multicentric survey on laparoscopic spleen surgery in the pediatric population. Surg Endosc 21:527, 2007.

Price VE, Blanchette VS, Ford-Jones EL: The prevention and management of infections in children with asplenia or hyposplenia. Infect Dis Clin North Am 21:697, 2007.

Salvia R, Bassi C, Festa L, et al: Clinical and biological behavior of pancreatic solid pseudopapillary tumors: Report on 31 consecutive patients. J Surg Oncol 95:304, 2007.

Stephens DS: Conquering the meningococcus. FEMS Microbiol Rev 31:3, 2007.

Troendle SB, Adix L, Crary SE, Buchanan GR: Laboratory markers of thrombosis risk in children with hereditary spherocytosis. Pediatr Blood Cancer 49:781, 2007.

Valette F, Querellou S, Oudoux A, et al: Comparison of positron emission tomography and lymphangiography in the diagnosis of infradiaphragmatic Hodgkin's disease. Acta Radiol 48(1):59, 2007.

REFERENCES

For complete list of references log onto www.expertconsult.com

CHAPTER 164

APPENDIX: NORMAL BLOOD VALUES: SELECTED REFERENCE VALUES FOR NEONATAL, PEDIATRIC, AND ADULT POPULATIONS

Donald L. Yee, Catherine M. Bollard, and Sharon M. Geaghan

Table 1 Reference Ranges for Leukocyte Counts in Children and Adults*

	Total Leukocytes		Neutrophils**			Lymphocytes			Monocytes		Eosinophils	
Age	**Mean**	**Range**	**Mean**	**Range**	**%**	**Mean**	**Range**	**%**	**Mean**	**%**	**Mean**	**%**
Birth	18.1	9.0–30.0	11.0	6.0–26.0	61	5.5	2.0–11.0	31	1.1	6	0.4	2
12 hours	22.8	13.0–38.0	15.5	6.0–28.0	68	5.5	2.0–11.0	24	1.2	5	0.5	2
24 hours	18.9	9.4–34.0	11.5	5.0–21.0	61	5.8	2.0–11.5	31	1.1	6	0.5	2
1 week	12.2	5.0–21.0	5.5	1.5–10.0	45	5.0	2.0–17.0	41	1.1	9	0.5	4
2 weeks	11.4	5.0–20.0	4.5	1.0–9.5	40	5.5	2.0–17.0	48	1.0	9	0.4	3
1 month	10.8	5.0–19.5	3.8	1.0–9.0	35	6.0	2.5–16.5	56	0.7	7	0.3	3
6 months	11.9	6.0–17.5	3.8	1.0–8.5	32	7.3	4.0–13.5	61	0.6	5	0.3	3
1 year	11.4	6.0–17.5	3.5	1.5–8.5	31	7.0	4.0–10.5	61	0.6	5	0.3	3
2 years	10.6	6.0–17.0	3.5	1.5–8.5	33	6.3	3.0–9.5	59	0.5	5	0.3	3
4 years	9.1	5.5–15.5	3.8	1.5–8.5	42	4.5	2.0–8.0	50	0.5	5	0.3	3
6 years	8.5	5.0–14.5	4.3	1.5–8.0	51	3.5	1.5–7.0	42	0.4	5	0.2	3
8 years	8.3	4.5–13.5	4.4	1.5–8.0	53	3.3	1.5–6.8	39	0.4	4	0.2	2
10 years	8.1	4.5–13.5	4.4	1.8–8.0	54	3.1	1.5–6.5	38	0.4	4	0.2	2
16 years	7.8	4.5–13.0	4.4	1.8–8.0	57	2.8	1.2–5.2	35	0.4	5	0.2	3
21 years	7.4	4.5–11.0	4.4	1.8–7.7	59	2.5	1.0–4.8	34	0.3	4	0.2	3

*Numbers of leukocytes are in thousands per mm^3, ranges are estimates of 95% confidence limits, and percentages refer to differential counts. Neutrophils include band cells at all ages and a small number of metamyelocytes and myelocytes in the first few days of life.

**Normal ranges vary slightly depending on automated analyzer used. The total leukocyte count is used to convert percentage values to absolute counts. Some automated hematology analyzers provide a full or limited differential.

Data from Dallman PR: Blood-forming tissues. In Rudolph AM (ed.): Pediatrics, 16th ed. New York, Appleton-Century-Crofts, 1977, p 1178.

Table 2 Reference Hematologic Values in Children and Adults*

	Hemoglobin (g/dL)		Hematocrit (%)		Red Blood Cell Count (10^{12}/L)		MCV (fL)		MCH (pg)		MCHC (g/dL)	
Age	**Mean**	**−2 SD**	**Mean**	**−2 SD**	**Mean**	**−2 SD**	**Mean**	**−2 SD**	**Mean**	**−2 SD**	**Mean**	**−2 SD**
Birth (cord blood)	16.5	13.5	51	42	4.7	3.9	108	98	34	31	33	30
1–3 days (capillary)	18.5	14.5	56	45	5.3	4.0	108	95	34	31	33	29
1 week	17.5	13.5	54	42	5.1	3.9	107	88	34	28	33	28
2 weeks	16.5	12.5	51	39	4.9	3.6	105	86	34	28	33	28
1 month	14.0	10.0	43	31	4.2	3.0	104	85	34	28	33	29
2 months	11.5	9.0	35	28	3.8	2.7	96	77	30	26	33	29
3–6 months	11.5	9.5	35	29	3.8	3.1	91	74	30	25	33	30
0.5–2 years	12.0	10.5	36	33	4.5	3.7	78	70	27	23	33	30
2–6 years	12.5	11.5	37	34	4.6	3.9	81	75	27	24	34	31
6–12 years	13.5	11.5	40	35	4.6	4.0	86	77	29	25	34	31
12–18 years												
Female	14.0	12.0	41	36	4.6	4.1	90	78	30	25	34	31
Male	14.5	13.0	43	37	4.9	4.5	88	78	30	25	34	31
18–49 years												
Female	14.0	12.0	41	36	4.6	4.0	90	80	30	26	34	31
Male	15.5	13.5	47	41	5.2	4.5	90	80	30	26	34	31

*These data have been compiled from several sources. Emphasis is given to studies employing electronic counters and to the selection of populations that are likely to exclude individuals with iron deficiency. The mean ±2 SD can be expected to include 95% of the observations in a normal population.
Data from Dallman PR: Blood-forming tissues. In Rudolph A (ed.): Pediatrics, 16th ed. New York, Appleton-Century-Crofts, 1977, p 1111.

Table 3 Reticulocyte Counts in Infants and Children by Flow Cytometry

Age	Number	Percentage	Absolute Count (10^9/L)
0–14 days*	21	5.33 + 1.99 (1.61/8.28)	318.44 + 50.04 (238.9/404.1)
14 days–1 years*	32	2.03 + 0.52 (1.09/3.00)	89.00 + 22.94 (45.8/137.8)
1–3 years*	63	2.01 + 0.72 (1.11/5.00)	88.38 + 20.49 (50.2/141.0)
3–8 years*	60	2.19 + 0.66 (0.95/4.03)	98.83 + 27.97 (45.4/163.1)
8–12 years*	18	2.07 + 0.78 (1.18/3.78)	90.20 + 27.16 (54.8/154.4)
12–adult*	14	2.25 + 0.99 (1.32/4.91)	91.62 + 24.80 (58.6/146.2)
Age	**Number**	**Percentage**	**Absolute Count (10^4/μL)**
Term newborns†	150	2.44 + 1.15 (1.1/5.5)	7.42 + 2.50 (4.9/15.0)
Preterm newborns†	30	2.55 + 1.01 (0.9/6.5)	7.18 + 2.88 (4.0/17.1)
1 week–16 years†	750	1.16 + 0.39 (0.6/1.9)	5.87 + 1.23 (5.0/6.5)

*Data from 188 pediatric outpatients (0–18 years of age) for whom all hematologic parameters are within age-appropriate reference ranges. Unpublished data from Lucile Packard Children's Hospital at Stanford. Analysis was performed on Beckton Dickenson FACSCAlibur flow cytometer. Results are expressed as mean +1 SD (min/max).

†Data from Herkner KR, Bock A, et al: Reticulocyte counting and maturity grading in pediatrics using the Sysmex R-1000 automated reticulocyte analyzer. Sysmex J Int 2:4, 1992.

Note: Flow cytometry may yield results 0.5% to 1.0% higher than microscopy following supravital staining.

Table 4 Estimated Blood Volumes

Age	Plasma Volume (PV) (mL/kg)	Red Blood Cell Mass* (RCM) (mL/kg)	Total Blood Volume (mL/kg) From PV	Total Blood Volume (mL/kg) From RCM
Newborn	41.3 46.0	43.1	82.1 78.0	86.1 84.7
1–7 days	51–54	37.9	82–86	77.8
1–12 months	46.1	25.5	78.1	72.8
1–3 years	44.4 47.2	24.9	73.8 81.8	69.1
4–6 years	48.5 49.6	25.5	80.0 85.6	67.5
7–9 years	52.2 49.0	24.3	87.6 86.1	67.5
10–12 years	51.9 46.2	26.3	87.6 83.2	67.4
13–15 years	51.2		88.3	
16–18 years	50.1		90.2	
Adults	39–50	20–35	68–88	55–75

The red cell volume, plasma volume, and total blood volume are calculated from hematocrit (packed cell volume) and isotope dilution after reinjection of red cells labeled with a radioactive isotope.

*Red cell volume is approximately 5 mL/kg less in females compared to males. Performance of a red cell mass is only occasionally indicated in the investigation of polycythemia to differentiate primary of secondary polycythemia (elevated red cell mass) from relative polycythemia (normal red cell mass). Data from Price DC, Ries C: Appendix. In Handmaker H, Lowenstein JM (eds.): Nuclear Medicine in Clinical Pediatrics. New York, Society of Nuclear Medicine, 1975, p 279. Red cell volume reference from ICSH. J Nuclear Med 21:793, 1980.

Table 5 Red Blood Cell Enzyme Activity in Adults and Term Infants*

Enzyme	Adults (*n* = 20)	Infants (*n* = 10)
Hexokinase	12.9 ± 2.1	34.0 ± 6.0
Phosphoglucose isomerase	406 ± 37	560 ± 112
Phosphofructokinase	148 ± 24.5	84.5 ± 24
Aldolase	24.5 ± 3.7	42.0 ± 10.0
Glyceraldehyde-3-phosphate dehydrogenase	885 ± 127	884 ± 245
Triosephosphate isomerase	26,323 ± 3240	29,111 ± 4100
Phosphoglycerate kinase	2795 ± 144	3926 ± 528
Phosphoglycerate mutase	751 ± 99	1049 ± 160
Enolase	252 ± 54	517 ± 121
Pyruvate kinase	179 ± 16	256 ± 50
Lactic dehydrogenase	2033 ± 287	2756 ± 425
Glucose-6-phosphate dehydrogenase	215 ± 18	328 ± 40

*Infant samples were obtained from newborns weighing more than 2800 g whose gestational age was 39 weeks or greater. Blood was drawn within 24 hours of birth. All the newborns were clinically healthy. Adult samples were obtained from healthy, normal volunteers. Units per 100 mL of red blood cells. Data from Oski FA: Red cell metabolism in the newborn infant, V: Glycolytic intermediates and glycolytic enzymes. Pediatrics 44:84, 1969.

Table 6 Red Cell Glycolytic Intermediate Metabolites in Normal Adults, Term Infants, and Premature Infants*

Metabolite	Normal Adults (n = *10)*	Term Infants (n = *10)*	Premature Infants (n = *11)*
Glucose-6-phosphate	24.8 ± 9.8	45.2 ± 8.7	66.8 ± 34.8
Fructose-6-phosphate	5.4 ± 1.0	9.9 ± 2.3	20.5 ± 8.9
Fructose-1,6-diphosphate	4.6 ± 1.0	3.8 ± 0.7	3.6 ± 0.8
Dihydroxyacetone phosphate	4.9 ± 3.5	11.9 ± 5.0	18.6 ± 10.7
Glyceraldehyde-3-phosphate	2.6 ± 0.7	1.9 ± 1.6	6.5 ± 3.2
3-Phosphoglycerate	61.6 ± 12.4	58.2 ± 14.4	47.5 ± 14.2
2-Phosphoglycerate	4.3 ± 1.8	4.9 ± 1.6	4.4 ± 2.5
Phosphoenolpyruvate	8.8 ± 2.6	7.6 ± 2.9	7.4 ± 3.0
Pyruvate	73.5 ± 33.1	70.4 ± 32.3	78.4 ± 4.15
2,3-Diphosphoglycerate	4423 ± 1907	3609 ± 800	3152 ± 2133

*Premature infants had birth weight below 2200 g and gestational age of <37 weeks and were clinically healthy at the time of investigation.
Data from Oski FA: Red cell metabolism in the newborn infant, V: Glycolytic intermediates and glycolytic enzymes. G6PD deficiency. Pediatrics 44:84, 1969; and Beutler E. Blood 84(11):3613, 1994. Units per 100 mL of red blood

Table 7 Reference Values for Hemoglobin F and Hemoglobin A_2 in the First 2 Years of Life*

	Hemoglobin F (%)*		Hemoglobin A_2 (%)[†]	
Age	*Mean*	*±2 SD*	*Mean*	*±2 SD*
1–7 days	75	61–80		
2 weeks	75	66–81		
1 month	60	46–67	0.8	0.4–1.3
2 months	46	29–61	1.3	0.4–1.9
3 months	27	15–56	2.2	1.0–3.0
4 months	18	9.4–29	2.4	2.0–2.8
5 months	10	2.3–22	2.5	2.1–3.1
6 months	7	2.7–13	2.5	2.1–3.1
8 months	5	2.3–12	2.7	1.9–3.5
10 months	2.1	1.5–3.5	2.7	2.0–3.3
12 months	2.0	1.3–5.0	2.7	2.0–3.3
13–16 months	0.6	0.2–1.0	2.6	1.6–3.3
17–20 months	0.6	0.2–1.0	2.9	2.1–3.5
21–24 months	0.6	0.2–1.0	2.8	2.1–3.5

*Data from Schroter W, Nafz C: Diagnostic significance of hemoglobin F and A_2 levels in homo- and heterozygous β-thalassemia during infancy. Helv Paediatr Acta 36:519, 1981.

[†]Data from Metaxotou-Mavromati AD, Antonopoulou HK, Laskari SS, et al: Developmental changes in hemoglobin F levels during the first 2 years of life in normal and heterozygous β-thalassemia infants. Pediatrics 69:738, 1982.

Note: Hemoglobin F increases with beta-thalassemias, hereditary persistence of fetal hemoglobin and bone marrow failure syndromes. Hemoglobin A_2 increases with beta-thalassemias, megaloblastic anemias, and thyrotoxicosis; it may be reduced with iron deficiency, lead poisoning, anemia of chronic disease, sideroblastic anemia, and hypothyroidism.

Table 8 Hemoglobin A Levels (%) in Normal and Heterozygous β-Thalassemia Infants During the First 2 Years of Life

Age (month)	Normal Mean ± SD	Heterozygotes Mean ± SD
1	0.8 ± 0.4	. . .
2	1.3 ± 0.5	1.8 ± 0.3
3	2.2 ± 0.6	3.8 ± 0.9
4	2.4 ± 0.4	4.0
5–6	2.5 ± 0.3	5.2 ± 0.7
7–9	2.7 ± 0.4	5.3 ± 0.7
10–12	2.7 ± 0.4	5.0 ± 0.6
13–16	2.6 ± 0.5	5.4 ± 0.8
17–20	2.9 ± 0.4	5.5 ± 0.6
21–24	2.8 ± 0.4	5.6 ± 0.9

HbA_2 is usually elevated in the β-thalassaemias, and in unstable B-chain hemoglobinopathies. Data from Metaxotou-Mavromati AD, Antonopoulou HK, Laskari SS, et al: Developmental changes in hemoglobin F levels during the first two years of life in normal and heterozygous β-thalassemia infants. Hemoglobin A2: origin, evolution, and after math. Pediatrics 69:736, 1982; and Steinberg MH, Adams JG: Blood 78:2165, 1991.

Table 9 Serum, Ferritin, Iron, Total Iron-Binding Capacity, and Transferrin Saturation in Children and Adults*

Age	Male Subjects		Female Subjects**	
Ferritin	***ng/mL***	***μg/L***	***ng/mL***	***μg/L***
1–30 days***	6–400	6–400	6–515	6–515
1–6 months***	6–410	6–410	6–340	6–340
7–12 months***	6–80	6–80	6–45	6–45
1–5 years[†,‡]	6–24	6–60	6–24	6–60
6–9 years[†,‡]	10–55	10–55	10–55	10–55
10–14 years[†]	23–70	23–70	6–40	6–40
14–19 years[†]	23–70	23–70	6–40	6–40
Iron[§]	***μg/dL***	***μmol/L***	***μg/dL***	***μmol/L***
1–30 days	32–112	5.7–20.0	29–127	5.2–22.7
31–365 days	27–109	4.8–19.5	25–126	4.5–22.6
1–3 years	29–91	5.2–16.3	25–101	4.5–18.1
4–6 years	25–115	4.5–20.6	28–93	5.0–16.7
7–9 years	27–96	4.8–17.2	30–104	5.4–18.6
10–12 years	28–112	5.0–20.0	32–104	5.7–18.6
13–15 years	26–110	4.7–19.7	30–109	5.4–19.5
16–18 years	27–138	4.8–24.7	33–102	5.9–18.3
Iron-Binding Capacity[§]	***μg/dL***	***μmol/L***	***μg/dL***	***μmol/L***
1–30 days	94–232	16.8–41.5	94–236	16.8–42.2
31–182 days	116–322	20.8–57.6	89–311	15.9–55.7
182–365 days	176–384	31.5–68.7	138–365	24.7–65.3
1–3 years	204–382	36.5–68.3	184–377	32.9–67.5
4–6 years	180–390	32.2–69.8	162–352	29.0–63.0
7–9 years	183–369	32.8–66.1	167–336	29.9–60.1
10–12 years	173–356	31.0–63.7	198–383	35.4–68.6
13–15 years	193–377	34.5–67.5	169–358	30.3–64.1
16–18 years	174–351	31.1–62.8	194–372	34.7–66.6

Table 9 Serum, Ferritin, Iron, Total Iron-Binding Capacity, and Transferrin Saturation in Children and Adults*—cont'd

Age	Male Subjects		Female Subjects**	
Ferritin	*ng/mL*	*µg/L*	*ng/mL*	*µg/L*
Transferrin Saturation†,‡,¶	***Male Subjects***		***Female Subjects***	
1–5 years	0.07–0.44		0.07–0.44	
6–9 years	0.17–0.42		0.17–0.42	
10–14 years	0.11–0.36		0.02–0.40	
14–19 years	0.06–0.33		0.06–0.33	
Transferrin§	***g/L***		***g/L***	
1–30 days	0.97–2.05		0.92–2.08	
31–182 days	1.06–3.25		1.28–3.09	
182–365 days	1.78–3.57		1.46–3.64	
1–3 years	1.96–3.65		1.49–3.82	
4–6 years	2.02–3.50		1.74–3.99	
7–9 years	1.49–3.53		1.86–3.68	
10–12 years	1.73–3.80		1.85–3.77	
13–15 years	1.71–3.74		1.93–3.91	
16–18 years	1.94–3.48		1.81–4.16	

*Assessment of iron status may be complicated by the presence of an acute phase reactants and/or liver disease. Serum ferritin is generally the preferred test for assessing iron deficiency. Ferritin levels reflect bone marrow iron stores and are decreased in iron deficiency. Higher ferritin levels (up to 100 µg/L) may be found in patients with iron deficiency and inflammatory disease/malignancy (acute phase response). Soluble transferrin receptor levels are not affected in an acute phase response and therefore may be more useful in selected patient since levels are normal in anemia of chronic disease uncomplicated by iron deficiency.

**Using immunoassay techniques, Ferritin levels in adult women and men may range from 15–200 µg/L to 30–300 µg/L, respectively. Ferritin levels in women following menopause progressively approach those for adult males. Brugnara C: Iron deficiency and erythropoiesis: new diagnostic approaches. Clin Chem 2003 Oct; 49(10):1573--8. Clin Chem 49(10):1573, 2003; and Cook JD: The measurement of serum Narsferrin receptor. Am J. Med Sci. 1999 Oct; 318(4):269--76. Am J Med Sci 318:269, 1999.

***From Soldin SJ, Morales A, et al: Pediatric reference ranges on the Abbott Imx for FSH, LH, prolactin, TSH, T4, T3, free T4, free T3, T-uptake, IgE, and ferritin. Clin Biochem 28:603, 1995. Study was based on hospitalized patients. Values represent 2.5th and 97.5th percentiles.

†From Lockitch G, Halstead AC, et al: Age- and sex-specific pediatric reference intervals for zinc, copper, selenium, iron, vitamins A and E, and related proteins. Clin Chem 34:1625, 1988. Study was based on healthy children; children with anemia, microcytosis, and thalassemia syndromes were excluded. Values represent the 0.025 and 0.975 fractiles.

‡No significant differences between males and females; range derived from combined data.

§From Soldin SJ, Brugnara C, et al: Pediatric Reference Ranges, 2nd ed. Washington, DC, AACC Press, 1997, pp 100, 101, 143.

¶Transferrin saturation calculated from iron (µmol/L)/total iron binding capacity. Transferrin, transferrin saturation and total iron binding capacity results are misleading in patients receiving iron therapy. Note that the lower reference limits for serum iron and transferrin saturation in this study are below the limits used to define acceptable levels for nutritional health for these two analytes (see O'Neal RM, Johnson OC, Schaefer AE: Guidelines for the classification and interpretation of group blood and urine data collected as part of the National Nutritional Survey. Pediatr Res 4:103, 1970).

Table 10 Reference Ranges for Serum Haptoglobin by Age

	Hemoglobin-Binding Capacity (mg/dL)	
Age	***Mean***	***Range (95%)***
Cord blood	0	0
1–7 days	10	0–41
1–4 weeks	28	0–45
1–3 months	59	41–95
3–6 months	91	64–134
6–12 months	115	43–160
1–5 years	109	51–160
5–10 years	107	62–186
>10 years	110	41–165

Data from Kalil M, Badr-El-Din MK, Kassem AS: Haptoglobin level in normal infants and children. Alex Med J 13:1, 1967.

Note: Serum haptoglobin is often used to evaluate hemolysis (especially intravascular) but reduced levels can also result from hepatocellular disease, massive tissue hemorrhage and congenital deficiency states. High levels can be seen with pregnancy and in acute phase responses which may confound assessment for hemolysis.

Table 11 Plasma Levels of Folic Acid and Vitamin B_{12} in Children

Age	Males	Females
Folic Acid	***nmol/L***	***nmol/L***
0–1 years	16.3–50.8	14.3–51.5
2–3 years	5.7–34.0	3.9–35.6
4–6 years	1.1–29.4	6.1–31.9
7–9 years	5.2–27.0	5.4–30.4
10–12 years	3.4–24.5	2.3–23.1
13–18 years	2.7–19.9	2.7–16.3
Vitamin B_{12}	***pmol/L***	***pmol/L***
0–1 years	216–891	168–1117
2–3 years	195–897	307–892
4–6 years	181–795	231–1038
7–9 years	200–863	182–866
10–12 years	135–803	145–752
13–18 years	158–638	134–605

Data were collected from hospitalized patients; 2.5th to 97.5th percentile values adapted from the Hoffman technique. Specimens from >100 patients in each age group were analyzed by radioimmunoassay.

Data from Hicks JM, Cook J, et al: Vitamin B_{12} and folate: pediatric reference ranges. Arch Pathol Lab Med 117:704, 1993.

Note: Serum folate may be decreased despite normal red blood cell folate during periods of systemic illness and decreased short-term folate intake.

Table 12 Serum Erythropoietin Levels in Term Infants During the First Year of Life*

Days After Birth	Erythropoietin (mU/mL)	Hemoglobin (g/dL)	RBC (μ10⁶/μL)
0–6	33.0 ± 31.4 (11)	15.6 ± 2.2 (11)	4.51 ± 0.74 (11)
7–50	11.7 ± 3.6 (7)	12.8 ± 1.1 (5)	3.92 ± 0.35 (5)
51–100	21.1 ± 5.5 (13)	11.4 ± 1.0 (10)	4.09 ± 0.51 (10)
101–150	15.1 ± 3.9 (5)	11.2 ± 1.1 (3)	4.21 ± 0.31 (3)
151–200	17.8 ± 6.3 (6)	—	—
>201	23.1 ± 9.7 (10)	11.8 ± 0.8 (9)	4.57 ± 0.24 (9)

*Values are expressed as means ± SD; parentheses enclose number of specimens. Patients were not transfused and weighed ≥2500 g.
Data from Yamashita H, Kukita J, et al: Serum erythropoietin levels in term and preterm infants during the first year of life. Am J Pediatr Hematol Oncol 16:213, 1994.

Table 13 Plasma Erythropoietin Reference Ranges in Children*

Age (year)	Number	Male Subjects	Number	Female Subjects
1–3	122	1.7–17.9	97	2.1–15.9
4–6	89	3.5–21.9	76	2.9–8.5
7–9	79	1.0–13.5	80	2.1–8.2
10–12	98	1.0–14.0	90	1.1–9.1
13–15	100	2.2–14.4	148	3.8–20.5
16–18	66	1.5–15.2	77	2.0–14.2

*Values are expressed in mIU/mL. Data were obtained from a total of 1122 hospitalized and outpatient children ages 1 to 18 years, using a commercially available enzyme-linked immunosorbent assay methodology. Values are 2.5th to 97.5th percentiles.

Data from Krafte-Jacobs B, Williams J, Soldin SJ: Plasma erythropoietin reference ranges in children. J Pediatr 126:601, 1995.

The measurement of erythropoietin is occasionally indicated in the differentiation of polycythemia vera (decreased) and secondary erythrocytosis (elevated) but in practice the test is unreliable with a broad overlap between the two groups. Erythropoietin levels are usually increased in anemia except in chronic renal failure patients with anemia. Erythropoietin levels may be used to monitor erythropoietin therapy in patients with chronic renal failure. The reference range is method dependent. Adult values are approximately 3 to 16 mIU/mL. Coles PM et al: N Engl J Med 315:283, 1986.

Table 14 Comparison of Selected Coagulation Factor Values in Newborns*

Study	Fibrinogen (mg/dL)	Factor II (U/mL)	Factor VIII (U/mL)	Factor IX (U/mL)	Factor XII (U/mL)	Antithrombin (U/mL)	Protein C (U/mL)
Term							
Hathaway and Bonnar (1987) and Manco-Johnson et al (1988)†	240 (150)	0.52 (0.25)	1.5 (0.55)	0.35 (0.15)	0.44 (0.16)	0.56 (0.32)	0.32 (0.16)
Andrews et al (1987, 1988)‡	283 (177)	0.48 (0.26)	1.0 (0.50)	0.53 (0.25)	0.53 (0.20)	0.63 (0.25)	0.35 (0.17)
Corrigan (1992)§	246 (150)	0.45 (0.22)	1.68 (0.50)	0.40 (0.20)	0.44 (0.16)	0.52 (0.20)	0.31 (0.17)
Preterm							
Hathaway and Bonnar (1987) and Manco-Johnson et al (1988)†	300 (120)	0.45 (0.26)	0.93 (0.54)	0.41 (0.20)	0.33 (0.23)	0.40 (0.25)	0.24 (0.18)
Andrews et al (1987, 1988)‡	243 (150)	0.45 (0.20)	1.1 (0.50)	0.35 (0.19)	0.38 (0.10)	0.38 (0.14)	0.28 (0.12)
Corrigan (1992)§	240 (150)	0.35 (0.21)	1.36 (0.21)	0.35 (0.10)	0.22 (0.09)	0.35 (0.10)	0.28 (0.12)

*Data are expressed as mean and lower limits of normal (in parentheses). Preterm, 30 to 36 weeks' gestational age.

†From Hathaway W, Bonnar J: Hemostatic Disorders of the Pregnant Woman and the Newborn Infant. New York, Elsevier Science, 1987; Manco-Johnson M, Marlar R, et al: Severe protein C deficiency in newborn infants. J Pediatr 113:359, 1988.

‡From Andrews M, Paes B, et al: Development of the human coagulation system in the full-term infant. Blood 70:165, 1987; Andrews M, Paes B, et al: Development of the human coagulation system in the healthy premature infant. Blood 72:1651, 1988.

§From Corrigan JJ Jr: Normal hemostasis in fetus and newborn: coagulation. In Polin RA, Fox WW (eds.): Fetal and Neonatal Physiology. Philadelphia, WB Saunders, 1992, p 1368; From Hathaway W, Corrigan J: Report of scientific and standardization subcommittee on neonatal hemostasis. Thromb Haemost 65:323, 1991.

Note: In summary, plasma levels of the vitamin K-dependent factors (including proteins C and S), contact factors and antithrombin are decreased at birth.

Table 15 Changes in Prothrombin Time (PT), Activated Partial Thromboplastin Time (aPTT), and Thrombin Time (TT) in Term and Premature Infants

	PT	aPTT	TT
Normal control	1	1	1
Term infants (ratio)	1.15–1.3	1.2–1.5	1.16–1.4
(increase in seconds)	(3–4 seconds)		
Small preterm (ratio)	1.30	1.4–2.4	1.31–1.50
(increase in seconds)	(4–5 seconds)		

Owing to the variability of normal values for these tests, the results are expressed as a ratio of the newborn clotting times to the mean value for adult controls. Small preterm: less than 32 weeks of gestational age; data from Hathaway W, Corrigan J: Report of scientific and standardization subcommittee on neonatal hemostasis. Thromb Haemost 65:323, 1991.

Table 16 Reference Values for Coagulation Tests in Healthy Children Aged 1–16 Years Compared With Normal Adults*

Age	1–5 years	6–10 years	11–16 years	Adult
Coagulation Tests	***Mean (Boundary)***	***Mean (Boundary)***	***Mean (Boundary)***	***Mean (Boundary)***
PT (s)	11 (10.6–11.4)	11.1 (10.1–12.1)	11.2 (10.2–12.0)	12 (11.0–14.0)
INR	1.0 (0.96–1.04)	1.01 (0.91–1.11)	1.02 (0.93–1.10)	1.10 (1.0–1.3)
APTT (s)	30 (24–36)	31 (26–36)	32 (26–37)	33 (27–40)
Fibrinogen (g/L)	2.76 (1.70–4.05)	2.79 (1.57–4.0)	3.0 (1.54–4.48)	2.78 (1.56–4.0)
Bleeding time (min)**	6 (2.5–10)†	7 (2.5–13)†	5 (3–8)†	4 (1–7)
II (U/mL)	0.94 (0.71–1.16)†	0.88 (0.67–1.07)†	0.83 (0.61–1.04)†	1.08 (0.70–1.46)
V (U/mL)	1.03 (0.79–1.27)	0.90 (0.63–1.16)†	0.77 (0.55–0.99)†	1.06 (0.62–1.50)
VII (U/mL)	0.82 (0.55–1.16)†	0.85 (0.52–1.20)†	0.83 (0.58–1.15)†	1.05 (0.67–1.43)
VIII (U/mL)	0.90 (0.59–1.42)	0.95 (0.58–1.32)	0.92 (0.53–1.31)	0.99 (0.50–1.49)
vWF (U/mL)	0.82 (0.60–1.20)	0.95 (0.44–1.44)	1.00 (0.46–1.53)	0.92 (0.50–1.58)
IX (U/mL)	0.73 (0.47–1.04)†	0.75 (0.63–0.89)†	0.82 (0.59–1.22)†	1.09 (0.5–1.63)
X (U/mL)	0.88 (0.58–1.16)†	0.75 (0.55–1.01)†	0.79 (0.50–1.17)†	1.06 (0.70–1.52)
XI (U/mL)	0.97 (0.56–1.50)	0.86 (0.52–1.20)	0.74 (0.50–0.97)†	0.97 (0.67–1.27)
XII (U/mL)	0.93 (0.64–1.29)	0.92 (0.60–1.40)	0.81 (0.34–1.37)†	1.08 (0.52–1.64)
PK (U/mL)	0.95 (0.65–1.30)	0.99 (0.66–1.31)	0.99 (0.53–1.45)	1.12 (0.62–1.62)
HMWK (U/mL)	0.98 (0.64–1.32)	0.93 (0.60–1.30)	0.91 (0.63–1.19)	0.92 (0.50–1.36)
XIIIa (U/mL)	1.08 (0.72–1.43)†	1.09 (0.65–1.51)†	0.99 (0.57–1.40)	1.05 (0.55–1.55)
XIIIs (U/mL)	1.13 (0.69–1.56)†	1.16 (0.77–1.54)†	1.02 (0.60–1.43)	0.97 (0.57–1.37)

*All factors except fibrinogen are expressed as units per milliliter, where pooled plasma contains 1.0 U/mL. All data are expressed as the mean, followed by the upper and lower boundaries encompassing 95% of the population. Between 20 and 50 samples were assayed for each value for each age group. Some measurements were skewed due to disproportionate number of high values. The lower limit, which excludes the lower 2.5% of the population, is given.

APTT, activated partial thromboplastin time; HMWK, high molecular weight kininogen; PK, prekallikrein; PT, prothrombin time; VII, factor VII procoagulant; vWF, von Willebrand factor.

†Values that are significantly different from values in adults.

Data from Andrew M, Vegh P, Johnston M, Bowker J, Ofosu F, Mitchell L: Maturation of the hemostatic system during childhood. Blood 80:1998, 1992.

Consult this reference for additional reference range data for the anticoagulant and fibrinolytic systems in these age groups.

**Note: Owing to concerns regarding its reproducibility, sensitivity and specificity, the bleeding time is considered obsolete at many centers, and has often been replaced by tests such as the PFA-100® (see table 18).

Table 17 Reference Values for the Inhibitors of Coagulation in Fetuses, Full-Term Infants, and Adults*

	Fetuses (Weeks Gestation)				
Parameter	*19–23* (n = *20)*	*24–29* (n = *22)*	*30–38* (n = *22)*	*Newborns* (n = *60)*	*Adults* (n = *40)*
ATII (%)	20.2 (12–31)‡	30.0 (20–39)	37.1 (24–55)§	59.4 (42–80)§	99.8 (65–130)
HCII (%)	10.3 (6–16)	12.9 (5.5–20)	21.1 (11–33)§	52.1 (19–99)§	101.4 (70–128)
TFPI (ng/mL)†	21.0 (16.0–29.2)	20.6 (13.4–33.2)	20.7 (10.4–31.5)§	38.1 (22.7–55.8)§	73.0 (50.9–90.1)
PC Ag (%)	9.5 (6–14)	12.1 (8–16)	15.9 (8–30)§	32.5 (21–47)§	100.8 (68–125)
PC Act (%)	9.6 (7–13)	10.4 (8–13)	14.1 (8–18)‡	28.2 (14–42)§	98.8 (68–129)
Total PS (%)	15.1 (11–21)	17.4 (14–25)	21.0 (15–30)§	38.5 (22–55)§	99.6 (72–118)
Free PS (%)	21.7 (13–32)	27.9 (19–40)	27.1 (18–40)§	49.3 (33–67)§	98.7 (72–128)
Ratio of free PS to total PS	0.82 (0.75–0.92)	0.83 (0.76–0.95)	0.79 (0.70–0.89)§	0.64 (0.59–0.98)§	0.41 (0.38–0.43)
C4b-BP (%)	1.8 (0.6)	6.1 (0–12.5)	9.3 (5–14)	18.6 (3–40)§	100.3 (70–124)

*Values are the mean, followed in parentheses by the lower and upper boundaries including 95% of the population. Ag, antigen; Act, activity.
†Twenty samples were assayed for each group, but only 10 for 19- to 23-week-old fetuses.
‡$P < 0.05$.
§$P < 0.01$.
Data from Reverdiau-Moalic P, Delahousse B, et al: Evolution of blood coagulation activators and inhibitors in the healthy human fetus. Blood 88:900, 1996.

Table 18 PFA-100® Closure Times in Healthy Neonates, Children and Adults

	Collagen/Epinephrine (seconds)	Collagen/ADP (seconds)
Term neonates (*n* = 17)	81 (61–108)	56 (48–65)
Children (*n* = 57)	117 (83–163)	91 (72–111)
Adults (*n* = 31)	106 (82–142)	85 (67–111)

Data from Carcao MD, Blanchette VS, Dean JA, et al: Br J Haematol 101(1):70, 1998. Mean and ranges given as 5th to 95th percentiles. Determination of site-specific reference ranges is recommended as longer reference closure times have also been reported. The assay assesses platelet and von Willebrand factor function under shear conditions but abnormal closure times may also occur with anemia, thrombocytopenia, and/or antiplatelet therapy.

Table 19 Complement Fractions C3 and C4 in Males and Females, by Age*

Study	Age	g/L
C3		
Zillow et al (1993)†	Healthy neonates	0.30–0.98
Lockitch et al (1988)†	0–5 days	0.26–1.04
	1–19 years	0.51–0.95
	Adult	0.45–1.8
C4		
Lockitch et al (1988)‡	0–5 days	0.06–0.37
	1–19 years	0.08–0.44
	Adult	0.11–0.5

*Interpretation: Reduced C4 with or without reduced C3 implies classical pathway activation as seen in SLE , immune complex disease and hereditary angioedema due to C1 inhibitor deficiency. Reduced C3 with normal C4 implies activation by the alternative pathway (eg, sepsis). Elevated C3 and/or C4 implies an acute phase response. Primary deficiency is rare and requires functional assay. Wen L, et al: J Allergy Clin Immunol 113:585, 2004.
†From Zilow G, Zilow EP, Burger R, Linderkamp O: Complement activation in newborn infants with early onset infection. Pediatr Res 1993 Aug;34(2):199–203. Results are 0th to 100th percentiles. Thirty-two healthy full-term newborns, birth weights between 2500 and 4020 g, were tested. All mothers (vagina, rectum) and infants (ear, gastric) were culture negative.
‡Lockitch G, Halstead AC, Quigley G, et al: Age- and sex-specific pediatric reference intervals: Study design and methods by measurement of serum proteins with the Behring LN nephelometer. Clin Chem 1988 Aug 34(8):1618–21. Results are 0.025 to 0.975 fractiles.

Table 20 Plasma Levels of Immunoglobulin A in Males and Females, by Age

	Male			Female		
Age	*Number*	*mg/dL*	*g/L*	*Number*	*mg/dL*	*g/L*
Soldin et al (1996)*						
1–30 days	61	1–20	0.01–0.20	56	1–19	0.01–0.19
31–182 days	52	7–56	0.07–0.56	60	1–59	0.01–0.59
183–365 days	37	9–107	0.09–1.07	23	15–90	0.15–0.90
1–3 years	105	18–171	0.18–1.71	127	25–141	0.25–1.41
4–6 years	138	60–231	0.60–2.31	135	47–206	0.47–2.06
7–9 years	111	77–252	0.77–2.52	105	41–218	0.41–2.18
10–12 years	104	61–269	0.61–2.69	115	73–239	0.73–2.39
13–15 years	104	42–304	0.42–3.04	118	82–296	0.82–2.96
16–18 years	112	89–314	0.89–3.14	100	90–322	0.90–3.22
Lockitch et al (1988)†						
0–12 months			0.00–1.00		0–100	
1–3 years			0.24–1.21		24–121	
4–6 years			0.33–2.35		33–235	
7–9 years			0.41–3.68		41–368	
10–11 years			0.64–2.46		64–246	
12–13 years			0.70–4.32		70–432	
14–15 years			0.57–3.00		57–300	
16–19 years			0.74–4.19		74–419	

*Data from Soldin SJ, Bailey J, Beatey J, et al: Pediatric reference ranges for immunoglobulins G, A and M on the Behring nephelometer. Clin Chem 42: S308, 1996.
†Data from Lockitch G, Halstead AC, et al: Age- and sex-specific pediatric reference intervals: Study design and methods illustrated by measurement of serum proteins with the Behring LN nephelometer. Clin Chem 34:1618, 1988. Results are 0.025 to 0.975 fractiles.

IgA levels and immunoglobulin levels in general are used for the assessment of patients with recurrent sinopulmonary infection, sepsis, gastrointestinal infection or other clinical presentations suggestive of immunoglobulin deficiency. If concern regarding presence of a paraprotein electrophoresis ± immunofixation is required. Reference intervals may vary with methodology and with the racial composition of the population.

Table 21 Immunoglobulin E in Males and Females, by Age

Age	Females (KIU/L)	Males (KIU/L)	Age	Females (KIU/L)	Males (KIU/L)
Soldin, Lenherr et al (1995)*					
0–12 months	<8	<12			
1–3 years	<28	<90			
4–10 years	<137	<163			
11–18 years	<398	<179			
Soldin, Morales et al (1995)†					
0–12 months	0–20	2–24			
1–3 years	2–55	2–149			
4–10 years	8–279	4–249			
11–15 years	5–295	7–280			
16–18 years	7–698	5–268			
Cord blood‡		0.02–2.08 IU/mL			
Lindberg and Arroyave (1986)§					
<1 years		0–6.6			
1–2 years		0–20.0			
2–3 years		0.1–15.8			
3–4 years		0–29.2			
4–5 years		0.3–25.0			
5–6 years		0.2–17.6			
6–7 years		0.2–13.1			
7–8 years		0.3–46.1			
8–9 years		1.8–60.1			
9–10 years		3.6–81.0			
10–11 years		8.0–95.0			
11–12 years		1.5–99.7			
12–13 years		3.9–83.5			
13–16 years		3.3–188.0			

*Data from Soldin SJ, Lenherr S, Kumar A: Pediatric reference ranges for IgE. Clin Chem 41:S92, 1995.

†Data from Soldin SJ, Morales A, et al: Pediatric reference ranges on the Abbott Imx for FSH, LH, prolactin, TSH, T4, T3, free T3, T-uptake, IgE, and ferritin. Clin Biochem 28:603, 1995. Study was based on hospitalized patients. Values represent 2.5 and 97.5th percentiles.

‡Data from Ownby DR, Johnson CC, Peterson EL: Maternal smoking does not influence cord serum IgE or IgD concentrations. J Allergy Clin Immunol 88:555, 1991. Values constitute 95% of the measured samples.

§Data from Lindberg RE, Arroyave C: Levels of IgE in serum from normal children and allergic children as measured by an enzyme immunoassay. J Allergy Clin Immunol 78:614, 1986. Three hundred forty-six nonatopic children were selected for study by enzyme-linked immunosorbent assay methodology.

The measurement of IgE levels has limited value in the identification of atopy since there is a large overlap in the expected values between atopic and nonatopic individuals. The use of this test however aids in the monitoring of allergic bronchopulmonary aspergillosis. Hamilton RG: J Allergy Clin Immunol 111:2:687, 2003.

Table 22 Immunoglobulin M in Males and Females, by Age

	Male			Female		
Age	*Number*	*mg/dL*	*g/L*	*Number*	*mg/dL*	*g/L*
Soldin et al (1997)*						
1–30 days	61	12–117	0.12–1.17	56	19–104	0.19–1.04
31–182 days	52	27–147	0.27–1.47	60	9–212	0.09–2.12
183–365 days	37	41–197	0.41–1.97	23	4–216	0.04–2.16
1–3 years	105	63–240	0.63–2.40	127	70–298	0.70–2.98
4–6 years	138	64–248	0.64–2.48	135	81–298	0.81–2.98
7–9 years	111	49–231	0.49–2.31	105	62–270	0.62–2.70
10–12 years	104	58–249	0.58–2.49	115	81–340	0.81–3.40
13–15 years	104	57–298	0.57–2.98	118	69–361	0.69–3.61
16–18 years	112	59–291	0.59–2.91	100	86–360	0.86–3.60
Lockitch et al (1988)†						
0–12 months			0.0–2.16		0–216	
1–3 years			0.28–2.18		28–218	
4–6 years			0.36–3.14		36–314	
7–9 years			0.47–3.11		47–311	
10–11 years			0.46–2.68		46–268	
12–13 years			0.52–3.57		52–357	
14–15 years			0.23–2.81		23–281	
16–19 years			0.35–3.87		35–387	

*Data from Soldin SJ, Bailey J, Beatey J, et al: Pediatric reference ranges for immunoglobulins G, A, and M on the Behring nephelometer. Clin Chem 42:S308, 1996. Plasma or serum.

†Data from Lockitch G, Halstead AC, et al: Age- and sex-specific pediatric reference intervals: Study design and methods illustrated by measurement of serum proteins with the Behring LN nephelometer. Clin Chem 34:1618, 1988. Results are 0.025 to 0.975 fractiles. Plasma or serum.

Reference intervals may vary with methodology and with the racial composition of the population.

Table 23 Plasma Levels of Immunoglobulin G in Males and Females, by Age

	Male			Female		
Age	*Number*	*mg/dL*	*g/L*	*Number*	*mg/dL*	*g/L*
Soldin et al (1997)*						
1–30 days	61	260–986	2.60–9.86	56	221–1031	2.21–10.31
31–182 days	52	195–643	1.95–6.43	60	390–794	3.90–7.94
183–365 days	37	184–974	1.84–9.74	23	407–774	4.07–7.74
1–3 years	105	507–1305	5.07–13.05	127	550–1407	5.50–14.07
4–6 years	138	571–1550	5.71–15.50	135	675–1540	6.75–15.40
7–9 years	111	700–1680	7.00–16.80	105	589–1717	5.89–17.17
10–12 years	104	818–1885	8.18–18.85	115	705–1871	7.05–18.71
13–15 years	104	709–1861	7.09–18.61	118	891–1907	8.91–19.07
16–18 years	112	632–1979	6.32–19.79	100	953–2108	9.53–21.08
Lockitch et al (1988)†						
0–12 months			2.73–16.60		273–1660	
1–3 years			5.33–10.78		533–1078	
4–6 years			5.93–17.23		593–1723	
7–9 years			6.73–17.34		673–1734	
10–11 years			8.21–18.35		821–1835	
12–13 years			8.93–18.23		893–1823	
14–15 years			8.42–20.13		842–2013	
16–19 years			6.46–18.64		646–1864	

*Soldin SJ, Bailey J, Beatey J, et al: Pediatric reference ranges for immunoglobulins G, A, and M on the Behring nephelometer. Clin Chem 42:S308, 1996.

†Lockitch G, Halstead AC, et al: Age- and sex-specific pediatric reference intervals: Study design and methods illustrated by measurement of serum proteins with the Behring LN nephelometer. Clin Chem 34:1618, 1988. Results are 0.025 to 0.975 fractiles.

Normal IgG levels do not exclude humoral immunodeficiency and further functional studies (eg, the assessment of antibody responses post vaccine administration) and/or IgG subclasses (Table 24), may be required if there is a high degree of clinical suspicion.

Reference intervals may vary with methodology and with the racial composition of the population

Table 24 Immunoglobulin G Subclasses*

Age	IgG1	IgG2	IgG3	IgG4
Cord blood, preterm	3.4–9.7	0.7–1.7	0.2–0.5	0.2–0.7
Cord blood, term	5.8–13.7	0.6–5.2	0.2–1.2	0.2–1.0
5 years	5.6–12.7	0.4–4.4	0.3–1.0	0.1–0.8
6 years	6.2–11.3	0.5–4.0	0.3–0.8	0.2–0.9
7 years	5.4–10.5	0.9–3.5	0.3–1.1	0.2–1.1
8 years	5.6–10.5	0.7–4.5	0.2–1.1	0.1–0.8
9 years	3.9–11.4	0.7–4.7	0.4–1.2	0.2–1.0
10 years	4.4–10.8	0.6–4.0	0.3–1.2	0.1–0.9
11 years	6.4–10.9	0.9–4.3	0.3–0.9	0.2–1.0
12 years	6.0–11.5	0.9–4.8	0.4–1.0	0.2–0.9
13 years	6.1–11.5	0.9–7.9	0.2–1.1	0.1–0.8
Adults	4.8–9.5	1.1–6.9	0.3–0.8	0.2–1.1

*Values for males and females, expressed in g/L. Twenty schoolchildren from each age group were tested. Only samples with C-reactive protein within the reference range were included. Enzyme-linked immunosorbent assay methodology was used on serum.

From Miles J, Riches P: The determination of IgG subclass concentrations in serum by enzyme-linked immunosorbent assay: Establishment of age-related reference ranges for cord blood samples, children aged 5 to 13 years and adults. Ann Clin Biochem 31:245, 1994.

Performing IgG subclasses has a limited role for the assessment of antibody-mediated immune function in patients with recurrent sinusitis and respiratory infections. IgG subclass deficiency may be associated with recurrent bacterial infection. Seventy percent of serum IgG is IgG1—selective IgG1 deficiency is rare. The most frequent abnormality is IgG2 deficiency, or a combined IgG2-IgG4, deficiency. IgG2 deficiency may be associated with IgA deficiency in patients with chronic respiratory infection. Decreased IgG3 levels may be seen in primary immunodeficiencies (eg Wiskott–Aldrich syndrome) and in type I diabetes mellitus. The significance of decreased IgG4 in absence of IgG2 deficiency is uncertain. Maguire G. Ann Clin Biochem 39:4:374, 2002.

Table 25 Serum Levels of Immunoglobulin Light Chains in Males and Females*

Age	Kappa (g/L)	Lambda (g/L)	Kappa/Lambda Ratio
Newborn	8.10 (7.7–8.7)	4.70 (4.5–5.0)	1.74 (1.7–1.9)
Premature	4.29 (3.1–4.9)	2.91 (2.6–3.1)	1.70 (1.6–1.9)
1 month	4.46 (3.6–4.8)	2.32 (1.9–3.5)	1.80 (1.6–2.0)
2 months	2.58 (2.4–2.7)	1.88 (1.8–2.0)	1.66 (1.6–1.7)
3 months	2.07 (1.7–2.5)	2.25 (2.0–2.3)	1.09 (1.0–1.3)
4 months	2.09 (1.9–2.4)	2.40 (1.6–2.6)	0.98 (0.8–1.0)
5 months	2.36 (2.0–3.2)	2.54 (2.4–2.9)	1.02 (1.0–1.1)
1 year	4.46 (3.0–5.3)	3.91 (2.7–4.8)	0.99 (0.9–1.2)
2 years	5.32 (3.6–6.4)	3.82 (2.8–4.0)	1.42 (1.3–1.5)
3 years	4.98 (4.1–5.4)	3.67 (3.1–4.8)	1.31 (1.1–1.4)
4 years	6.78 (4.8–8.3)	4.87 (4.0–5.5)	1.51 (1.2–1.7)
5 years	6.58 (5.4–7.1)	4.01 (3.8–4.7)	1.55 (1.3–1.7)
6 years	8.02 (6.0–8.5)	4.01 (3.0–6.0)	1.61 (1.6–1.7)
7 years	5.90 (4.6–7.5)	4.08 (3.9–4.5)	1.64 (1.4–1.8)
8 years	8.34 (7.3–9.1)	4.64 (5.1–6.4)	1.50 (1.4–1.7)
9 years	8.26 (7.1–9.6)	4.95 (3.3–5.5)	1.69 (1.5–1.8)
10 years	9.03 (8.2–9.6)	5.32 (4.9–5.7)	1.80 (1.3–1.9)
11 years	7.18 (6.0–8.3)	4.10 (3.8–4.8)	1.67 (1.4–1.8)
12 years	9.17 (8.2–9.6)	4.90 (4.1–6.0)	1.82 (1.7–2.0)
13 years	9.59 (8.2–10.5)	5.86 (5.3–6.1)	1.64 (1.4–1.7)
14 years	9.45 (8.0–10.8)	5.50 (4.9–5.8)	2.09 (1.9–2.2)
15 years	10.18 (7.2–11.0)	4.75 (4.1–5.0)	2.25 (1.7–2.3)
16 years	9.37 (7.0–11.2)	5.09 (4.6–5.6)	1.89 (1.5–2.2)

*Median and ranges given as 10th to 90th percentiles.

Data from Herkner KR, Salzer H, et al: Pediatric and perinatal reference intervals for immunoglobin light chains kappa and lambda. Clin Chem 38:548, 1992.

The measurement of free light chains is predominantly performed for the diagnosis and monitoring of amyloid, non-secretory myeloma and light chain myeloma. The kappa/lambda ratio is critical since an excess of kappa versus lambda or excess lambda versus kappa light chains is consistent with a plasma cell dyscrasia. Bradwell D. et al: Lancet 36(4);89, 2003.

Table 26 Reference Ranges for Pediatric Lymphocyte Subsets at Different Ages*

Age		Total Lymphocytes	CD4	CD8	CD2	CD3	CD19	Helper/Suppressor Ratio
0–6 months	%	0.62–0.72	0.50–0.57	0.08–0.31	0.55–0.88	0.55–0.82	0.11–0.45	—
(*n* = 10)	A	5.4–7.2	2.8–3.9	0.35–2.5	3.9–5.3	3.5–5.0	0.43–3.3	6.22
6–12 months	%	0.60–0.69	0.49–0.55	0.08–0.31	0.55–0.88	0.55–0.82	0.11–0.45	—
(*n* = 9)	A	5.3–6.7	2.6–3.5	0.35–2.5	3.8–4.9	3.4–4.6	0.43–3.3	6.22
12–18 months	%	0.56–0.63	0.46–0.51	0.08–0.31	0.55–0.88	0.55–0.82	0.11–0.45	—
(*n* = 9)	A	4.9–5.9	2.3–2.9	0.35–2.5	3.5–4.2	3.2–3.9	0.43–3.3	6.22
18–24 months	%	0.52–0.59	0.42–0.48	0.08–0.31	0.55–0.88	0.55–0.82	0.11–0.45	—
(*n* = 10)	A	4.4–5.5	1.9–2.5	0.35–2.5	3.1–3.9	2.8–3.5	0.43–3.3	6.22
24–30 months	%	0.45–0.57	0.38–0.46	0.08–0.31	0.55–0.88	0.55–0.82	0.11–0.45	—
(*n* = 9)	A	3.9–5.2	1.5–2.2	0.35–2.5	2.6–3.6	2.3–3.3	0.43–3.3	6.22
30–36 months	%	0.39–0.53	0.33–0.44	0.08–0.31	0.55–0.88	0.55–0.82	0.11–0.45	—
(*n* = 10)	A	3.3–5.1	1.2–2.0	0.35–2.5	2.2–3.5	1.9–3.1	0.43–3.3	6.22
3 years	%	0.22–0.69	0.27–0.57	0.14–0.34	0.65–0.84	0.55–0.82	0.09–0.29	—
(*n* = 73)	A	1.6–5.4	0.56–2.7	0.33–1.4	1.2–4.1	1.0–3.9	0.20–1.3	3.24

*Values are expressed as 95th percentile reference range.

%, relative percentage; A, absolute cell count $\times 10^9$/L.

Samples analyzed by Epics Profile (Coulter) flow cytometer following whole blood lysis.

Data from Kotylo PK, Fineberg NS, et al: Reference ranges for lymphocyte subsets in pediatric patients. Am J Clin Pathol 100:111, 1993. See also Denny T, Yogev R, et al: Lymphocyte subsets in healthy children during the first 5 years of life. JAMA 267:1484, 1992. Copyright 1992, American Medical Association.

Note: Values may also vary with gender, diurnal rhythm, and other physiological variables.

Table 27 Total Bilirubin in Premature and Full-Term Infants

	Premature	Full-Term
	mg/dL	*mg/dL*
Cord blood*	<2.0	<2.0
0–1 days*	<8.0	<6.0
1–2 days*	<12.0	<8.0
2–5 days*	<16.0	<12.0
>5 days*	<2.0	0.2–1.0
	μmol/L	*mg/dL*
Bottle-fed infants†	<212	<12.4
Breast-fed infants†	<253	<14.8

*Data from Behrman RE (ed.): Nelson Textbook of Pediatrics, 14th ed. Philadelphia, WB Saunders, 1992, p 1803.

†Data from Maisels MJ, Gifford K: Normal serum bilirubin levels in the newborn and the effect of breast feeding. Pediatrics 78:837, 1986. Represents 97th percentile rank for white neonates of >2500 g birth weight.

Note: A clinical practice guideline pertinent to the management of neonatal hyperbilirubinemia is available from the American Academy of Pediatrics: Pediatrics 114(1):297, 2004.

INDEX

Note: Page numbers followed by f refer to figures; page numbers followed by t refer to tables; page numbers followed by b refer to boxed material.

A

D

E

F

G

H

I

J

K

M

O

T

U

V

W

X